Holland–Frei

Cancer Medicine

8

Editors

Waun Ki Hong, MD, DMSc (Hon)
Head and Professor, Division of Cancer Medicine
American Cancer Society Professer
Samsung Distinguished University Chair in Cancer Medicine
The University of Texas M. D. Anderson Cancer Center
Houston, Texas

Robert C. Bast Jr., MD
President for Translational Research
Harry Carrothers Wiess Distinguished University Chair for Cancer Research
Professor of Medicine, Department of Experimental Therapeutics
The University of Texas M. D. Anderson Cancer Center
Houston, Texas

William N. Hait, MD, PhD
Senior Vice-President and Global Head, Oncology Therapeutic Area
Ortho Biotech Oncology Research and Development
Raritan, New Jersey

Donald W. Kufe, MD
Professor of Medicine
Harvard Medical School
Department of Medicine Oncology
Dana-Farber Cancer Institute
Boston, Massachusetts

Raphael E. Pollock, MD, PhD
Head, Division of Surgery
Professor and Chairman, Department of Surgical Oncology
Senator A.M. Alken, Jr. Distinguished Chair
The University of Texas MD Anderson Cancer Center
Houston, Texas

Ralph R. Weichselbaum, MD
Daniel K. Ludwig Professor and Chairman of the Department of Radiation and Cellular Oncology
Director of the Center for Metastasis Research
University of Chicago
Chicago, Illinois

James F. Holland, MD, ScD (hc)
Distinguished Professor of Neoplastic Diseases
Professor, Medicine, Hematology and Medical Oncology
Professor, Oncological Sciences
Mount Sinai Medical Center
New York, New York

Emil Frei III, MD
Director and Physician-in-Chief Emeritus
Richard and Susan Smith Distinguished Professor of Medicine
Harvard Medical School
Dana-Farber Cancer Institute
Boston, Massachusetts

Holland-Frei
Cancer Medicine
8

An approved publication of the

American Association for Cancer Research

2010
PEOPLE'S MEDICAL PUBLISHING HOUSE–USA
SHELTON, CONNECTICUT

People's Medical Publishing House-USA
2 Enterprise Drive, Suite 509
Shelton, CT 06484
Tel: 203-402-0646
Fax: 203-402-0854
E-mail: info@pmph-usa.com

09 10 11 12/PMPH/9 8 7 6 5 4 3 2

ISBN 978–1–60795–014–1
Printed in China by People's Medical Publishing House
Copyeditor/Typesetter: Newgen; Cover designer: Mary McKeon

Library of Congress Cataloging-in-Publication Data

Holland Frei cancer medicine 8. -- 8th ed. / editors, Waun Ki Hong … [et al.].
p.; cm.
Rev. ed. of: Holland Frei cancer medicine 7 / editors, Donald
W. Kufe … [et al.]. 7th ed. 2006.
Includes bibliographical references and index.

ISBN-13: 978-1-60795-014-1
ISBN-10: 1-60795-014-6

1. Cancer. I. Hong, Waun Ki. II. American Association for Cancer Research.
III. Holland Frei cancer medicine 7. IV. Title: Holland Frei cancer medicine eight.
V. Title: Cancer medicine 8.
[DNLM: 1. Neoplasms. QZ 200 H7343 2009]
RC261.C2735 2009
616.99'4—dc22

2009039147

Sales and Distribution

Canada
McGraw-Hill Ryerson Education
Customer Care
300Water St
Whitby, Ontario L1N 9B6
Canada
Tel: 1-800-565-5758
Fax: 1-800-463-5885
www.mcgrawhill.ca

Foreign Rights
John Scott & Company
International Publisher's Agency
P.O. Box 878
Kimberton, PA 19442
USA
Tel: 610-827-1640
Fax: 610-827-1671
Japan
United Publishers Services
Limited
1-32-5 Higashi-Shinagawa
Shinagawa-ku, Tokyo 140-0002

Japan
Tel: 03-5479-7251
Fax: 03-5479-7307
Email: kakimoto@ups.co.jp
United Kingdom, Europe, Middle
East, Africa
McGraw Hill Education
Shoppenhangers Road
Maidenhead
Berkshire, SL6 2QL

England
Tel: 44-0-1628-502500
Fax: 44-0-1628-635895
www.mcgraw-hill.co.uk

Singapore, Thailand, Philippines, Indonesia, Vietnam, Pacific Rim, Korea
McGraw-Hill Education
60 Tuas Basin Link
Singapore 638775
Tel: 65-6863-1580
Fax: 65-6862-3354
www.mcgraw-hill.com.sg

Australia, New Zealand
Elsevier Australia
Tower 1, 475 Victoria Avenue
Chatswood NSW 2067
Australia
Tel: 0-9422-8553
Fax: 0-9422-8562
www.elsevier.com.au

Brazil
Tecmedd Importadora e
Distribuidora
de Livros Ltda.
Avenida Maurilio Biagi 2850
City Ribeirao, Rebeirao, Preto SP
Brazil
CEP: 14021-000
Tel: 0800-992236
Fax: 16-3993-9000
Email: tecmedd@tecmedd.com.br

India, Bangladesh, Pakistan, Sri Lanka, Malaysia
CBS Publishers
4819/X1 Prahlad Street 24
Ansari Road, Darya, New Delhi-
110002
India
Tel: 91-11-23266861/67
Fax: 91-11-23266818
Email:cbspubs@vsnl.com

People's Republic of China
PMPH
Bldg 3, 3rd District
Fangqunyuan, Fangzhuang
Beijing 100078
P.R. China
Tel: 8610-67653342
Fax: 8610-67691034
www.pmph.com

Preface

This 8th edition of *Cancer Medicine* integrates better than ever the new understanding of cancer science and cancer medicine. The explosion of knowledge about genes and cancer, receptors, and signal transduction has led to therapeutics based on this knowledge. Oncologists must now all be familiar with pathways and processes that explain the pathogenesis of neoplasms as well as the new molecules that target these steps. Hundreds of potential drugs are under study, some of which will prove to be of clinical importance. Most of them were selected and developed because of their relationship to the new knowledge, rather than the random screening of chemical compounds, soil samples, and exotic plants that characterized a former era. The early chapters of this book prepare the reader to comprehend the evolving information about the molecular events that lead to cancer and the therapeutics that address them. Concurrent advances in the conduct of surgery and of radiation therapy have improved targeting and decreased collateral damage. Appreciation of the clinical characteristics of the many diseases that comprise the rubric of cancer is essential if we are to realize the full benefits of the new knowledge. These many diseases are covered in later chapters.

The editors have chosen experts who have written authoritatively about the disciplines and diseases covered in their respective chapters. As the world of science and medicine chip away the unknowns of the cancer process and its prevention and therapy, we believe the contents of this work will provide a platform for understanding the current state of accomplishment and for preparing the reader for a critical evaluation of discoveries still to come.

The Editors
2010

Contributors

Stuart A. Aaronson, MD
Professor and Chairman
Department of Oncological Sciences
Mount Sinai School of Medicine
New York, New York

David H. Abramson, MD
Chief, Ophthalmic Oncology Service
Department of Surgery
Memorial Sloan-Kettering Cancer Center
New York, New York

Jeremy S. Abramson, MD
Instructor in Medicine
Department of Medicine
Division of Hematology and Oncology
Massachusetts General Hospital
Boston, Massachusetts

Vandana Gupta Abramson, MD
Assistant Professor of Medicine
Division of Hematology and Oncology
Vanderbilt University School of Medicine
Nashville, Tennessee

Roberto Adachi, MD
Assistant Professor
Department of Pulmonary Medicine
The University of Texas
M. D. Anderson Cancer Center
Houston, Texas

Ranjana Advani, MD
Department of Radiation Oncology
Kovler Viral Oncology Laboratory
University of Chicago
Chicago, Illinois

Sunil J. Advani, MD
Post Doctorate
Department of Radiation Oncology
University of Chicago
Chicago, Illinois

Jaffer A. Ajani, MD
Professor
Department of Gastrointestinal Medical Oncology
The University of Texas
M. D. Anderson Cancer Center
Houston, Texas

James P. Allison, PhD
Chairman, Immunology Program
Department of Immunology
Memorial Sloan-Kettering Cancer Center
New York, New York

Edward P. Ambinder, MD
Department of Medicine
Mount Sinai School of Medicine
New York, New York

Kenneth C. Anderson, MD
Chief
Division of Hematologic Neoplasia
Dana-Farber Cancer Institute
Boston, Massachusetts

Michael Andreeff, MD, PhD
Professor of Medicine
Department of Stem Cell Transplantation
The University of Texas
M. D. Anderson Cancer Center
Houston, Texas

Ana Aparicio, MD
Assistant Professor
Department of Genitourinary (GU) Medical Oncology
Division of Cancer Medicine
The University of Texas
M. D. Anderson Cancer Center
Houston, Texas

Narin Apisarnthanarax, MD
Clinical Research Fellow
Department of Dermatology
University Hospital-Case Western Reserve University
Cleveland, Ohio

Philip M. Arlen, MD
Senior Clinician
Laboratory of Tumor Immunology and Biology
Center for Cancer Research
National Cancer Institute
Bethesda, Maryland

James O. Armitage, MD
Dean, College of Medicine
University of Nebraska Medical Center
Omaha, Nebraska

Rony Avritscher, MD
Assistant Professor
Department of Diagnostic Radiology
The University of Texas
M. D. Anderson Cancer Center
Houston, Texas

Diwakar D. Balachandran, MD
Assistant Professor
Department of Pulmonary Medicine
The University of Texas
M. D. Anderson Cancer Center
Houston, Texas

Aditya Bardia, MBBS, MPH
Fellow, Medical Oncology
Department of Oncology
Johns Hopkins University
Baltimore, Maryland

Lara Bashoura, MD
Assistant Professor
Department of Pulmonary Medicine
The University of Texas
M. D. Anderson Cancer Center
Houston, Texas

Robert C. Bast Jr., MD
President for Translational Research
Harry Carrothers Wiess Distinguished University Chair for Cancer Research
Professor of Medicine
Department of Experimental Therapeutics
The University of Texas
M. D. Anderson Cancer Center
Houston, Texas

Stephen B. Baylin, MD
Professor of Oncology
The Sidney Kimmel Comprehensive Cancer Center at Johns Hopkins
Baltimore, Maryland

Georgia M. Beasley, MD
Resident in Surgery
Department of Surgery
Duke University
Durham, North Carolina

Jonathan S. Berek, MD, MMS
Chairman
Department of Obstetrics and Gynecology
Stanford University Medical School
Palo Alto, California

Ross S. Berkowitz, MD
William H. Baker Professor of Gynecology
Division of Gynecologic Oncology
Department of Obstetrics and Gynecology
Harvard Medical School
Boston, Massachusetts

Leslie Bernstein, PhD
Professor and Director
Department of Cancer Etiology
City of Hope Comprehensive Cancer Center
Duarte, California

Donald A. Berry, PhD
Professor and Head
Division of Quantitative Sciences
The University of Texas M. D. Anderson Cancer Center
Houston, Texas

Cindy Berthelot, MD
Resident
Department of Dermatology
The University of Texas M. D. Anderson Cancer Center
Houston, Texas

Joseph R. Bertino, MD
University Professor of Medicine and Pharmacology
The Cancer Institute of New Jersey
New Brunswick, New Jersey

Gerald P. Bodey, MD
Professor Emeritus
Department of Infectious Diseases
Infection Control and Employee Health
The University of Texas M. D. Anderson Cancer Center
Houston, Texas

Ernest C. Borden, MD
Deputy Director
Taussig Cancer Institute
The Cleveland Clinic
Cleveland, Ohio

Otis W. Brawley, MD
Chief Medical Officer
American Cancer Society
Professor of Hematology, Oncology and Epidemiology
Emory University
Atlanta, Georgia

Robert S. Bresalier, MD
Professor of Medicine
Department of Gastroenterology, Hepatology and Nutrition
The University of Texas M. D. Anderson Cancer Center
Houston, Texas

Marcia S. Brose, MD, PhD
Assistant Professor
Department of Otorhinolaryngology: Head and Neck Surgery
University of Pennsylvania Health System
Philadelphia, Pennsylvania

Kevin M. Brown, PhD
Investigator
Integrative Cancer Genomics Division
Translational Genomics Research Institute (TGen)
Phoenix, Arizona

Thomas A. Buchholz, MD
Professor and Chair
Department of Radiation Oncology Treatment
The University of Texas M. D. Anderson Cancer Center
Houston, Texas

Aman U. Buzdar, MD
Professor
Department of Breast Medical Oncology
The University of Texas M. D. Anderson Cancer Center
Houston, Texas

Michele Carbone, MD, PhD
Professor and Chairman
Department of Pathology
John A. Burns School of Medicine
University of Hawaii
Honolulu, Hawaii

Alan C. Carver, MD
Assistant Professor
Department of Neurology
Mount Sinai School of Medicine
New York, New York

A. Philippe Chahinian, MD
Professor
Department of Medicine
Mount Sinai School of Medicine
New York, New York

Richard Champlin, MD
Professor of Medicine, Chair
Department of Stem Cell Transplantation
The University of Texas M. D. Anderson Cancer Center
Houston, Texas

Joe Y. Chang, MD, PhD
Associate Professor of Radiation Oncology
Department of Radiation Oncology
The University of Texas M. D. Anderson Cancer Center
Houston, Texas

Martin C. Chang, MD, PhD
Department of Pathology
Brigham & Women's Hospital
Boston, Massachusetts

Iona Cheng, PhD
Assistant Professor
Epidemiology Program
University of Hawaii
Cancer Research Center of Hawaii
Honolulu, Hawaii

Yung-Chi Cheng, PhD
Department of Pharmacology
Yale University School of Medicine
New Haven, Connecticut

Michael A. Choti, MD, MBA
Jacob C. Handelsman Professor of Surgery
Department of Surgery
Johns Hopkins University School of Medicine
Baltimore, Maryland

James E. Cleaver, PhD
Professor
Department of Dermatology, School of Medicine
University of California at San Francisco
San Francisco, California

Steven K. Clinton, MD, PhD
Professor of Internal Medicine
Division of Hematology and Oncology
The Ohio State University Medical Center
Columbus, Ohio

Carmel J. Cohen, MD
Professor
Division of Obstetrics and Gynecology
Mount Sinai School of Medicine
New York, New York

Harvey J. Cohen, MD
Professor and Chairman
Department of Medicine
Duke University Medical Center
Durham, North Carolina

Jeffrey I. Cohen, MD
Head, Medical Virology Section
National Institute of Allergy and Infectious Diseases
National Institutes of Health
Bethesda, Maryland

Lorenzo Cohen, PhD
Professor and Program Director
Integrative Medicine Program, Department of Behavioral Science
The University of Texas M. D. Anderson Cancer Center
Houston, Texas

Peter D. Cole, MD
Associate Professor of Pediatrics
Albert Einstein College of Medicine
The Children's Hospital at Montefiore
Bronx, New York

Eric A. Collisson, MD
Helen Diller Family Comprehensive Cancer Center
University of California at San Francisco
San Francisco, California

Michael Colvin, MD
Professor and Director
Duke University, Comprehensive Cancer Center
Durham, North Carolina

James L. Connolly, MD
Professor
Department of Pathology
Harvard Medical School
Boston, Massachusetts

Christopher L. Corless, MD, PhD
Associate Professor of Pathology
Department of Pathology
Oregon Health and Science University
Portland, Oregon

Jorge Cortes, MD
Professor and Deputy Chairman
Leukemia Department
The University of Texas
M. D. Anderson Cancer Center
Houston, Texas

David Cosgrove, MD
Professor
Department of Hematology and Medical Oncology
Johns Hopkins University
Baltimore, Maryland

Richard Cote, MD, FRCPath
Professor and Chairman
Department of Pathology
Miller School of Medicine
University of Miami Health System
Miami, Florida

Kenneth H. Cowan, MD, PhD
Director
Eppley Institute for Cancer Research
University of Nebraska Medical Center
Omaha, Nebraska

Christopher H. Crane, MD
Professor of Radiation Oncology
Department of Radiation Oncology Treatment
The University of Texas
M. D. Anderson Cancer Center
Houston, Texas

Carlo M. Croce, MD
Professor, Director, and John W. Wolfe Chair in Human Cancer Genetics
Department of Molecular Virology, Immunology, and Medical Genetics
Ohio State University
Columbus, Ohio

Chistopher P. Crum, MD
Director, Women's and Perinatal Pathology
Department of Pathology
Brigham & Women's Hospital
Boston, Massachusetts

Steven A. Curley, MD, FACS
Professor of Surgical Oncology
Department of Surgical Oncology
The University of Texas
M. D. Anderson Cancer Center
Houston, Texas

Timothy A. Damron, MD, FACS
David G. Murray Professor of Orthopedic Surgery
Department of Orthopedic Surgery
State University of New York, Upstate Medical University
Syracuse, New York

Siamak Daneshmand, MD
Associate Professor
Surgery for Urology and Oncology
Oregon Health and Science University
Portland, Oregon

Michael D'Angelica, MD
Surgical Oncologist
Hepatopancreatobiliary Service
Memorial Sloan-Kettering Cancer Center
New York, New York

Marta L. Davila, MD
Associate Professor
Deputy Chair Ad Interim
Department of Gastroenterology, Hepatology and Nutrition
The University of Texas
M. D. Anderson Cancer Center
Houston, Texas

John Davis, MD
Assistant Professor
Department of Urology
Division of Surgery
The University of Texas
M. D. Anderson Cancer Center
Houston, Texas

Shaheenah Dawood, MBB.Ch, MRCP (UK)MPH
Medical Oncology Department
Dubai Hospital
Dubai, United Arab Emirates

Lisa M. DeAngelis, MD
Chair
Department of Neurology
Memorial Sloan-Kettering Cancer Center
New York, New York

Katherine DeLellis Henderson, PhD
Assistant Research Scientist
Department of Cancer Etiology
City of Hope Comprehensive Cancer Center
Duarte, California

Samuel R. Denmeade, MD
Assistant Professor of Oncology
Oncology, Division of Experimental Therapeutics
The Sidney Kimmel Comprehensive Cancer Center at Johns Hopkins
Baltimore, Maryland

Maria T. DeSancho, MD
Assistant Professor of Medicine
Department of Medicine
Weill-Cornell Medical College
New York, New York

Mark W. Dewhirst, DVM, PhD
Gustavo S. Montana Professor of Radiation Oncology
Professor of Pathology and Biomedical Engineering
Duke University Medical Center
Durham, North Carolina

Burton F. Dickey, MD
Professor and Chair
Department of Pulmonary Medicine
The University of Texas
M. D. Anderson Cancer Center
Houston, Texas

Nicolas C. Dracopoli, PhD
Vice President
Biomarkers
Ortho Biotech Oncology Research and Development
Radnor, Pennsylvania

Stephen W. Duffy, MsC
Professor of Cancer Screening
Cancer Research UK Centre for Epidemiology, Mathematics and Statistics
Wolfson Institute of Preventive Medicine
London, England

Ira J. Dunkel, MD
Pediatric Oncologist
Department of Pediatrics
Memorial Sloan-Kettering Cancer Center
New York, New York

Madeline M. Duvic, MD
Professor
Department of Dermatology
The University of Texas M. D. Anderson Cancer Center
Houston, Texas

Ann M. Dvorak, MD
Professor
Beth Israel Deaconess Medical Center
Boston, Massachusetts

Harold F. Dvorak, MD
Professor
Beth Israel Deaconess Medical Center
Boston, Massachusetts

George A. Eapen, MD
Associate Professor
Department of Pulmonary Medicine
The University of Texas M. D. Anderson Cancer Center
Houston, Texas

Joseph P. Eder, MD
Associate Professor of Medicine
Department of Medicine
Division of Medical Oncology
Dana-Farber Cancer Institute
Harvard Medical School
Boston, Massachusetts

Suhendan Ekmekcioglu, PhD
Assistant Professor
Department of Experimental Therapeutics
The University of Texas M. D. Anderson Cancer Center
Houston, Texas

Carmen P. Escalante, MD
Professor and Chairman
Department of General Internal Medicine, Ambulatory Treatment and Emergency Care
The University of Texas M. D. Anderson Cancer Center
Houston, Texas

Laura Esserman, MD
Professor, Surgery and Radiology, and Affiliate Faculty, Institute for Health Policy Studies
Department of Surgery
University of California San Francisco Helen Diller Family Comprehensive Cancer Center
San Francisco, California

David S. Ettinger, MD
Alex Grass Professor of Oncology
Department of Oncology
The Sidney Kimmel Comprehensive Cancer Center at Johns Hopkins
Baltimore, Maryland

Douglas B. Evans, MD
Professor and Chairman
Department of Surgery
Donald C. Ausman Family Foundation
Department of Surgery
The Medical College of Wisconsin
Milwaukee, Wisconsin

Scott E. Evans, MD
Assistant Professor
Department of Pulmonary Medicine
The University of Texas M. D. Anderson Cancer Center
Houston, Texas

Michael S. Ewer, MD, MPH, JD
Professor and Special Assistant to the Vice President
Office of Vice President, Medical Affairs
The University of Texas M. D. Anderson Cancer Center
Houston, Texas

Steven M. Ewer, MD
Assistant Professor
Department of Medicine
University of Wisconsin
Madison, Wisconsin

Stefan Faderl, MD
Associate Professor
Department of Leukemia
The University of Texas M. D. Anderson Cancer Center
Houston, Texas

Saadia A. Faiz, MD
Assistant Professor
Department of Pulmonary Medicine
The University of Texas M. D. Anderson Cancer Center
Houston, Texas

Mark K. Ferguson, MD
Professor of Surgery
Section of Cardiac and Thoracic Surgery
The University of Chicago
Chicago, Illinois

Mauro Ferrari, PhD
Professor
Department of Experimental Therapeutics
The University of Texas M. D. Anderson Cancer Center
Houston, Texas

Kathleen M. Foley, MD
Neurologist
Pain and Palliative Care Service
Memorial Sloan-Kettering Cancer Center
New York, New York

Arthur E. Frankel, MD
Professor of Cancer Biology and Medicine
Scott & White Healthcare
Wake Forest University School of Medicine
Winston-Salem, North Carolina

Milo Frattini, PhD
Professor
Laboratory of Molecular Diagnostic
Institute of Pathology
Locarno, Switzerland

Arnold S. Freedman, MD
Associate Professor of Medicine
Department of Medical Oncology
Dana-Farber Cancer Institute
Boston, Massachusetts

Emil Frei III, MD
Director and Physician-in-Chief Emeritus
Richard and Susan Smith Distinguished Professor of Medicine
Harvard Medical School
Dana-Farber Cancer Institute
Boston, Massachusetts

Moshe Frenkel, MD
Associate Professor
Department of General Oncology
The University of Texas M. D. Anderson Cancer Center
Houston, Texas

Michael L. Friedlander, MD, PhD
Professor (Conjoint)
Department of Medicine
Prince of Wales Hospital
Community of Health Services
Sydney, Australia

Valentin Fuster, MD, PhD
Professor
Cardiovascular Institute-Cardiology
Mount Sinai School of Medicine
New York, New York

Robert F. Gagel, MD
Professor and Division Head
Division of Internal Medicine
The University of Texas M. D. Anderson Cancer Center
Houston, Texas

Robert C. Gallo, MD
Director and Professor
Department of Viral Carcinogenesis
Institute of Human Virology of the University of Maryland School of Medicine
Baltimore, Maryland

Chirag D. Gandhi, MD
Assistant Professor of Neurosurgery
Department of Neurological Surgery
UMDNJ-New Jersey Medical School
Newark, New Jersey

M. Kay Garcia, DRN, LAC, DrPH
Advanced Practice Nurse
Clinical Nurse Specialist and Acupuncturist
Integrative Medicine Program
Department of Behavioral Science
The University of Texas M. D. Anderson Cancer Center
Houston, Texas

Adam S. Garden, MD
Professor
Department of Radiation Oncology
The University of Texas M. D. Anderson Cancer Center
Houston, Texas

Juri G. Gelovani, MD, PhD
Professor and Chairman
Department of Experimental Diagnostic Imaging
The University of Texas M. D. Anderson Cancer Center
Houston, Texas

Jeffrey E. Gershenwald, MD
Professor of Surgery and Cancer Biology
Departments of Surgical Oncology and Cancer Biology
The University of Texas M. D. Anderson Cancer Center
Houston, Texas

Teresa Ann Gilewski, MD
Attending Physician
Department of Clinical Oncology
Memorial Sloan-Kettering Cancer Center
New York, New York

Inderbir S. Gill, MD, MCh
Vice Chairman
Glickman Urological and Kidney Institute
Cleveland Clinic Taussig Cancer Institute
Cleveland, Ohio

Edward L. Giovannuci, MD, ScD
Professor of Nutrition and Epidemiology
Department of Nutrition and Department of Epidemiology
Harvard School of Public Health
Boston, Massachusetts

Bonnie S. Glisson, MD
Professor of Medicine
Department of Thoracic, Head and Neck Medical Oncology
The University of Texas M. D. Anderson Cancer Center
Houston, Texas

Gabrielle R. Goldberg, MD
Assistant Professor
Department of Geriatrics and Adult Development
Mount Sinai Medical Center
New York, New York

Jeffrey D. Goldsmith, MD
Department of Anatomic Pathology
Beth Israel Deaconess Medical Center
Boston, Massachusetts

Donald P. Goldstein, MD
Clinical Professor of Obstetrics
Department of Gynecologic Oncology
Brigham & Women's Hospital
Boston, Massachusetts

Ali-Reza Golshayan, MD
Assistant Professor
Department of Medicine
MUSC Hollings Cancer Center
Medical University of South Carolina
Charleston, South Carolina

David W. Goodrich, PhD
Assistant Professor
Department of Pharmacology and Therapeutics
Roswell Park Cancer Institute
Buffalo, New York

Elizabeth M. Grainger, PhD, RD
Senior Research Associate
Comprehensive Cancer Center
The Ohio State University
Columbus, Ohio

Joe W. Gray, PhD
Associate Laboratory Director for Life & Environmental Sciences
Life Sciences Division
Lawrence Berkeley National Laboratory
Berkeley, California

David J. Grdina, PhD
Professor of Radiation and Cellular Oncology
Department of Radiation and Cellular Oncology
The University of Chicago
Chicago, Illinois

F. Anthony Greco, MD
Director of Sarah Cannon Cancer Center
Sarah Cannon Research Institute
Nashville, Tennessee

Elizabeth A. Grimm, PhD
Deputy Division Head of Research Affairs
Division of Cancer Medicine
Professor, Department of Experimental Therapeutics
The University of Texas M. D. Anderson Cancer Center
Houston, Texas

Louise B. Grochow, MD
Associate Professor
Department of Oncology
Johns Hopkins University School of Medicine
Baltimore, Maryland

Luca Grumolato, PhD
Post-Doctoral Fellow
Department of Oncological Sciences
Mount Sinai School of Medicine
New York, New York

José G. Guillem, MD, FACS, FACRS
Director of the Hereditary Colorectal Cancer Family Registry
Colorectal Service, Department of Surgery
Memorial Sloan-Kettering Cancer Center
New York, New York

James L. Gulley, MD, PhD, FACP
Senior Clinician
Laboratory of Tumor Immunology and Biology
Center for Cancer Research
National Cancer Institute
Bethesda, Maryland

William C. Hahn, MD, PhD
Associate Professor of Medicine
Department of Medical Oncology/ Molecular and Cellular
Dana-Farber Cancer Institute
Harvard Medical School
Boston, Massachusetts

John D. Hainsworth, MD
Chief Scientific Officer
Sarah Cannon Research Institute
Nashville, Tennessee

William N. Hait, MD, PhD
Senior Vice-President and Global Head, Oncology Therapeutic Area
Ortho Biotech Oncology Research and Development
Raritan, New Jersey

Stanley R. Hamilton, MD
Professor and Division Head
Department of Pharmacology and Therapeutics
The University of Texas M. D. Anderson Cancer Center
Houston, Texas

Axel R. Hanauske, MD, PhD, MBA
Professor of Medicine
Department of Hematology and Medical Oncology, Palliative Care
Eli Lilly & Co.
Indianapolis, Indiana

Eric K. Hansen, MD
Radiation Oncologist
Department of Radiation Oncology
Providence St. Vincent Medical Center
Portland, Oregon

Curtis C. Harris, MD
Chief, Laboratory of Human Carcinogenesis
National Cancer Institute
Bethesda, Maryland

Harold A. Harvey, MD
Professor, Hematology Oncology
Division of Hematology and Oncology
Milton S. Hershey Medical Center
Hershey, Pennsylvania

Dorothy K. Hatsukami, PhD
Associate Director, Cancer Prevention and Control
Department of Psychiatry
The Cancer Center
University of Minnesota
Minneapolis, Minnesota

Stephen S. Hecht, PhD
Masonic Cancer Center
University of Minnesota
Minneapolis, Minnesota

Steven J. Heller, MD
Johnson & Johnson
Raritan, New Jersey

Daniel Y.C. Heng, MD
Assistant Professor of Medicine
Department of Medical Oncology
Tom Baker Cancer Center
University of Calgary
Calgary, Alberta

Bryan T. Hennessy, MD
Assistant Professor
Department of Gynecologic Medical Oncology
The University of Texas M. D. Anderson Cancer Center
Houston, Texas

Roy S. Herbst, MD, PhD
Professor
Department of Thoracic, Head and Neck Medical Oncology
The University of Texas M. D. Anderson Cancer Center
Houston, Texas

James G. Herman, MD
Associate Professor of Oncology
Department of Oncology
The Sidney Kimmel Comprehensive Cancer Center at Johns Hopkins
Baltimore, Maryland

Diana M. Hey Cauley, PharmD
Clinical Pharmacy Specialist
Genitourinary Medical Oncology
Division of Pharmacy
The University of Texas M. D. Anderson Cancer Center
Houston, Texas

John V. Heymach, MD, PhD
Assistant Professor
Department of Thoracic, Head and Neck Medical Oncology
The University of Texas M. D. Anderson Cancer Center
Houston, Texas

Teru Hideshima, MD, PhD
Principal Associate in Medicine
Department of Medicine
Dana-Farber Cancer Institute
Boston, Massachusetts

James W. Hodge, PhD, MBA
Senior Scientist
Laboratory of Tumor Immunology and Biology
Center for Cancer Research
National Cancer Institute
Bethesda, Maryland

James F. Holland, MD, ScD (hc)
Distinguished Professor of Neoplastic Diseases
Professor, Medicine, Hematology and Medical Oncology
Professor, Oncological Sciences
Mount Sinai Medical Center
New York, New York

Jimmie C. Holland, MD
Chair Emerita
Department of Psychiatry and Behavioral Sciences
Memorial Sloan-Kettering Cancer Center
New York, New York

Waun Ki Hong, MD, DMSc (Hon)
Head and Professor, Division of Cancer Medicine
American Cancer Society Professor
Samsung Distinguished University Chair in Cancer Medicine
The University of Texas M.D. Anderson Cancer Center
Houston, Texas

Richard T. Hoppe, MD
Chairman, Radiation Oncology
Department of Radiation Oncology
Stanford University Medical Center
Stanford, California

Gabriel N. Hortobagyi, MD
Professor and Chairman
Department of Breast Medical Oncology
The University of Texas M. D. Anderson Cancer Center
Houston, Texas

Robert A. Hromas, MD
Deputy Director, Clinical Affairs and Translational Research
University of New Mexico Cancer Center
Professor and Chief, Division of Hematology-Oncology
University of New Mexico Hospital
Albuquerque, New Mexico

Arti Hurria, MD
Director, Cancer and Aging Research Program
Division of Medical Oncology and Therapeutic Research
City of Hope Medical Center
Duarte, California

Patrick Hwu, MD
Professor and Chairman
Department of Melanoma Medical Oncology
The University of Texas M. D. Anderson Cancer Center
Houston, Texas

Rakesh K. Jain, PhD
A. Werk Cook Professor of Radiation Oncology (Tumor Biology)
Department of Radiation Oncology
Harvard Medical School and Massachusetts General Hospital
Boston, Massachusetts

Ahmedin Jemal, DVM, PhD
Program Director, Cancer Occurrence
Department of Epidemiology and Surveillance Research
American Cancer Society
Atlanta, Georgia

Anuja Jhingran, MD
Associate Professor
Department of Radiation Oncology Treatment
The University of Texas M. D. Anderson Cancer Center
Houston, Texas

Carlos A. Jimenez, MD
Associate Professor
Department of Pulmonary Medicine
The University of Texas M. D. Anderson Cancer Center
Houston, Texas

Ellen Jones, MD
Professor
Department of Radiation Oncology
University of North Carolina
Chapel Hill, North Carolina

J. Stephen Jones, MD, FACS
Associate Professor of Surgery and Chairman
Department of Regional Urology
Glickman Urological and Kidney Institute
Cleveland Clinic Taussig Cancer Institute
Cleveland, Ohio

Roy Jones, MD, PhD
Professor
Department of Stem Cell Transplantation
The University of Texas M. D. Anderson Cancer Center
Houston, Texas

V. Craig Jordan, OBE, PhD, DSc
Adjunct Professor
Department of Molecular Pharmacology and Biological Chemistry
Feinberg School of Medicine
Philadelphia, Pennsylvania

Peter Kabos, MD
Clinical Fellow
Horowitz Lab
University of Colorado at Denver
Aurora, Colorado

Barton A. Kamen, MD
Chief Medical Officer
The Leukemia & Lymphoma Society
Mamaroneck, New York

Hagop M. Kantarjian, MD
Professor and Chairman
Department of Leukemia
The University of Texas M. D. Anderson Cancer Center
Houston, Texas

Ahmed O. Kaseb, MD
Assistant Professor
Department of Gastrointestinal Medical Oncology
The University of Texas M. D. Anderson Cancer Center
Houston, Texas

Matthew Kaufman, MD
Attending Physician
CLL Research and Treatment Program
Long Island Jewish Medical Center
New Hyde Park, New York

Richard M. Kaufman, MD
Instructor in Pathology
Department of Pathology
Brigham & Women's Hospital
Boston, Massachusetts

Jonathan J. Keats, PhD
Research Fellow
Department of Hematology and Oncology
Comprehensive Cancer Center
Scottsdale, Arizona

Nancy E. Kemeny, MD
Professor of Medicine
Department of Medicine
Memorial Sloan-Kettering Cancer Center
New York, New York

Samuel Kenan, MD
Professor
Department of Orthopedic Surgery
New York University Medical Center
New York, New York

Merrill S. Kies, MD
Professor
Department of Thoracic, Head and Neck Medical Oncology
The University of Texas M. D. Anderson Cancer Center
Houston, Texas

Jeri Kim, MD
Associate Professor
Department of Genitourinary (GU) Medical Oncology, Division of Cancer Medicine
The University of Texas M. D. Anderson Cancer Center
Houston, Texas

Youn H. Kim, MD
Professor of Dermatology
Department of Dermatology
Stanford University Medical Center
Redwood City, California

Hedy Lee Kindler, MD
Associate Professor of Medicine
Department of Medicine
Section of Hematology and Oncology
The University of Chicago
Chicago, Illinois

Catherine E. Klein, MD
Professor of Medicine
Department of Veterans Affairs
Eastern Colorado Health Care System
Denver, Colorado

H. Phillip Koeffler, MD
Director
Division of Hematology and Oncology
Cedars-Sinai Medical Center
Los Angeles, California

Elise C. Kohn, MD
Head, Molecular Signaling Section
National Cancer Institute
Bethesda, Maryland

Christian Kollmannsberger, MD
Clinical Associate Professor of Medicine
Division of Medical Oncology
University of British Columbia
BC Cancer Agency - Vancouver Cancer Centre
Vancouver, British Columbia

Ritsuko K. Komaki, MD
Professor
Department of Radiation Oncology
The University of Texas M. D. Anderson Cancer Center
Houston, Texas

Robert J. Kreitman, MD
Chief, Clinical Immunotherapy Section
Laboratory of Molecular Biology
National Cancer Institute
National Institutes of Health
Bethesda, Maryland

Deborah Kuban, MD
Professor
Department of Radiation Oncology
Division of Radiation Oncology
The University of Texas M. D. Anderson Cancer Center
Houston, Texas

Donald W. Kufe, MD
Professor of Medicine
Harvard Medical School
Department of Medical Oncology
Dana-Farber Cancer Institute
Boston, Massachusetts

Joy H. Kunishige, MD
The University of Texas
M. D. Anderson Cancer Center
Houston, Texas

Michael E. Kupferman, MD
Assistant Professor
Department of Head and Neck Surgery
The University of Texas
M. D. Anderson Cancer Center
Houston, Texas

Razelle Kurzrock, MD
Professor and Chairman
Department of Investigational Cancer Therapeutics
The University of Texas
M. D. Anderson Cancer Center
Houston, Texas

Raymond S. Lance, MD
Associate Professor
Department of Urology
Eastern Virginia School of Medicine
Norfolk, Virginia

Debra L. Laskin, PhD
Professor and Chair
Department of Pharmacology and Toxicology
Rutgers University, School of Pharmacy
Piscataway, New Jersey

Jeffrey D. Laskin, PhD
Professor
Department of Environmental and Occupational Medicine
University of Medicine and Dentistry of New Jersey
Robert Wood Johnson Medical School
Piscataway, New Jersey

Donghui Li, PhD
Professor of Medicine
Department of Gastrointestinal Medical Oncology Research
The University of Texas
M. D. Anderson Cancer Center
Houston, Texas

Scott M. Lippman, MD
Professor of Medicine and Chairman
Department of Thoracic, Head and Neck Medical Oncology
The University of Texas
M. D. Anderson Cancer Center
Houston, Texas

Jennifer K. Litton, MD
Assistant Professor
Department of Breast Medical Oncology
The University of Texas
M. D. Anderson Cancer Center
Houston, Texas

Christopher J. Logothetis, MD
Professor and Chairman
Department of Genitourinary Medical Oncology
The University of Texas
M. D. Anderson Cancer Center
Houston, Texas

Janina A. Longtine, MD
Associate Professor
Department of Pathology
Harvard Medical School
Boston, Massachusetts

Charles Lu, MD
Associate Professor
Department of Thoracic, Head and Neck Medical Oncology
The University of Texas
M. D. Anderson Cancer Center
Houston, Texas

Kirk A. Ludwig, MD
Associate Professor of Surgery
Chief of Colorectal Surgery
Department of Surgery
Medical College of Wisconsin
Milwaukee, Wisconsin

Donald F. Lynch Jr., MD
Professor and Chairman
Department of Urology
Eastern Virginia School of Medicine
Norfolk, Virginia

Henry T. Lynch, MD
Professor and Chairman
Department of Preventive Medicine
Creighton University Medical Center
Omaha, Nebraska

Cristina Magi-Galluzzi, MD, PhD
Director of Genitourinary Pathology
Department of Pathology at Cleveland Clinic
Assistant Professor of Pathology
Lerner College of Medicine at Case Western Reserve University
Cleveland, Ohio

Robert G. Maki, MD, PhD
Associate Professor
Department of Medicine
Weill Cornell University Medical College
New York, New York

Paul F. Mansfield, MD
Professor of Surgery
Department of Surgical Oncology
The University of Texas
M. D. Anderson Cancer Center
Houston, Texas

Alberto M. Marchevsky, MD
Head, Pulmonary Pathology
Cedars-Sinai Medical Center
Clinical Professor of Pathology
School of Medicine
University of Southern California
Los Angeles, California

Paul Mathew, MD
Assistant Professor
Department of Genitourinary Medical Oncology
The University of Texas
M. D. Anderson Cancer Center
Houston, Texas

Peter M. Mauch, MD
Associate Chief of Academic Operations
Department of Radiation Therapy
Brigham & Women's Hospital
Boston, Massachusetts

Beryl McCormick, MD
Clinical Director
Department of Radiation Oncology
Memorial Sloan-Kettering Cancer Center
New York, New York

Nicole S. McMahon, BS
Graduate Student
Department of Surgical Oncology
Duke University Medical Center
Durham, North Carolina

Anna T. Meadows, MD
Professor
Department of Pediatrics
The Cancer Center at The Children's Hospital of Philadelphia
Philadelphia, Pennsylvania

Jeffrey I. Mechanick, MD
Associate Clinical Professor
Department of Medicine
Mount Sinai School of Medicine
New York, New York

Diane E. Meier, MD
Professor
Department of Geriatrics and Adult Development
Mount Sinai Medical Center
New York, New York

Matthew Meyerson, MD, PhD
Assistant Professor of Pathology
Department of Medical Oncology/Molecular and Cellular
Dana-Farber Cancer Institute
Harvard Medical School
Boston, Massachusetts

Gordon B. Mills, MD, PhD
Professor and Chairman
Department of Systems Biology
The University of Texas M. D. Anderson Cancer Center
Houston, Texas

Bruce D. Minsky, MD
Associate Dean and Professor of Radiation and Cellular Oncology
Department of Radiation and Cellular Oncology
University of Chicago Medical Center
Chicago, Illinois

David L. Mitchell, PhD
Professor of Carcinogensis
Department of Carcinogenesis
The University of Texas M. D. Anderson Cancer Center
Houston, Texas

Rodolfo C. Morice, MD
Professor
Department of Pulmonary Medicine
The University of Texas M. D. Anderson Cancer Center
Houston, Texas

Charles S. Morrow, MD, PhD
Associate Professor
Department of Biochemistry
Wake Forest University School of Medicine
Winston-Salem, North Carolina

Donald L. Morton, MD
Chief, Melanoma Program
Director, Surgical Oncology Fellowship Program
John Wayne Cancer Institute at Saint John's Health Center
Santa Monica, California

Natalie Moryl, MD
Internist
Pain and Palliative Care Service Department of Medicine
Memorial Sloan-Kettering Cancer Center
New York, New York

Jeffrey A. Moscow, MD
Chief, Division of Pediatric Hematology-Oncology
University of Kentucky, College of Medicine
Lexington, Kentucky

David G. Murry, MD
Emeritus Chair, Orthopedic Surgery
Deparment of Orthopedic Surgery
State University of New York, Upstate Medical University
Syracuse, New York

Hyman B. Muss, MD
Professor of Medicine
Lineburger Cancer Center
University of North Carolina at Chapel Hill
Chapel Hill, North Carolina

Piero Mustacchi, MD, ScD [Hon]
Clinical Professor of Medicine and Epidemiology
Department of Medicine and Epidemiology
University of California at San Francisco
San Francisco, California

Joseph L. Nates, MD, MBA, HCA, FCCM
Professor of Critical Care Medicine
Deputy Chair, ICU Medical Director
Department of Critical Care
The University of Texas M. D. Anderson Cancer Center
Houston, Texas

Victor A. Neel, MD, PhD
Director
Division of Dermatological Surgery
Massachusetts General Hospital
Boston, Massachusetts

Alfred I. Neugut, MD, PhD
Myrone M. Studner Professor of Cancer Research
Department of Epidemiology
Columbia University, Mailman School of Public Health
New York, New York

Craig R. Nichols, MD
Professor of Medicine
Department of Medicine
Division of Hematology and Oncology
Oregon Health and Science University
Portland, Oregon

Craig Nolan, MD
Neuro-oncologist
Department of Neurology
Memorial Sloan-Kettering Cancer Center
New York, New York

Larry Norton, MD
Norna S. Sarofin Chair of Clinical Oncology
Department of Clinical Oncology
Memorial Sloan-Kettering Cancer Center
New York, New York

Andrew Novick, MD†
Chair of the Glickman Urological and Kidney Institute
Cleveland Clinic Taussig Cancer Institute
Cleveland, Ohio

Brian O'Sullivan, MD, FRCPI
Professor of Radiation Oncology
Department of Radiation Oncology
Princess Margaret Hospital
Toronto, Ontario

Susan O'Brien, MD
Professor
Department of Leukemia
The University of Texas M. D. Anderson Cancer Center
Houston, Texas

Takao Ohnuma, MD, PhD
Professor of Medicine
Division of Hematology and Oncology
Department of Medicine
Mount Sinai School of Medicine
New York, New York

Maura O'Leary, MD
Administrative Officer
Children's Oncology Group
Bethesda, Maryland

Amir Onn, MD
Adjunct Assistant Professor
Department of Pulmonary Medicine
The University of Texas M. D. Anderson Cancer Center
Kfar Vitkin, Israel

James C. Padussis, MD
Professor of Surgery
Department of Surgery
Duke University Medical Center
Durham, North Carolina

Ben-Ho Park, MD, PhD
Associate Professor of Oncology
Department of Hematology and Medical Oncology
The Sidney Kimmel Comprehensive Cancer Center at Johns Hopkins
Baltimore, Maryland

†Deceased.

Harvey I. Pass, MD
Professor of Cardiothoracic Surgery and Surgery
Department of Cardiothoracic Surgery
New York University School of Medicine and Clinical Cancer Center
New York, New York

Edward F. Patz Jr., MD
James and Alice Chen Professor of Radiology
Department of Radiology
Duke University Medical Center
Durham, North Carolina

C. Leigh Pearce, PhD
Assistant Professor
Department of Preventive Medicine
Keck School of Medicine
University of Southern California
Los Angeles, California

Karl S. Peggs, MA, MB, BCh, MRCP, FRC Path
Investigator
Department of Hematology
UCL Cancer Institute
London, England

Marco A. Pierotti, PhD
Scientific Director
Scientific Management
Fondazione IRCCS Istituto Nazionale dei Tumori
Milan, Italy

Peter W.T. Pisters, MD, FACS
Professor of Surgery
Department of Surgical Oncology
The University of Texas M. D. Anderson Cancer Center
Houston, Texas

Giuseppe Pizzorno, PhD, PharmD
Vice President of Operations
Associate Director for Translational Research
Division Head of Drug Development
Nevada Cancer Institute
Las Vegas, Nevada

William K. Plunkett Jr, PhD
Professor
Department of Experimental Therapeutics
The University of Texas M. D. Anderson Cancer Center
Houston, Texas

Raphael E. Pollock, MD, PhD
Head, Division of Surgery
Professor and Chairman, Department of Surgical Oncology
Senator A.M. Aiken, Jr. Distinguished Chair
The University of Texas M. D. Anderson Cancer Center
Houston, Texas

Kornelia Polyak, MD, PhD
Assistant Professor of Medicine
Department of Medical Oncology/ Molecular and Cellular
Dana-Farber Cancer Institute
Harvard Medical School
Boston, Massachusetts

Kalman D. Post, MD
Chairman Emeritus
Leonard I. Malis, MD / Corinne and Joseph Graber Professor
Department of Neurosurgery
Mount Sinai School of Medicine
New York, New York

S. Egbert Pravinkumar, MD, FRCP
Assistant Professor of Medicine
Department of Critical Care
The University of Texas M. D. Anderson Cancer Center
Houston, Texas

Ching-Hon Pui, MD
Chair and American Society Professor
Department of Oncology
St. Jude Children's Research Hospital
Memphis, Tennessee

Sergio A. Quezada, PhD
Research Fellow
Department of Immunology
Memorial Sloan-Kettering Cancer Center
New York, New York

Derek Raghavan, MD, PhD
M. Frank and Margaret Domiter Rudy Institute (Distinguished) Chair in Translational Cancer Research
Institute Chairman
Cleveland Clinic Taussig Cancer Institute
Cleveland, Ohio

Kristjan T. Ragnarsson, MD
Professor and Chair
Department of Rehabilitation
Mount Sinai School of Medicine
New York, New York

Jamal Rahaman, MD
Fellowship Director
Division of Gynecologic Oncology
Mount Sinai School of Medicine
New York, New York

Kanti R. Rai, MD
Joel Finkelstein Cancer Foundation Professor of Medicine
Division of Hematology and Oncology
Albert Einstein College of Medicine
New Hyde Park, New York

Noopur Raje, MD
Assistant Professor of Medicine
Director, Multiple Myeloma Program
Harvard Medical School
Boston, Massachusetts

Jacob H. Rand, MD
Director
Hematology Laboratories, Pathology Department
Montefiore Medical Center
Bronx, New York

Mark J. Ratain, MD
Leon O. Jacobson Professor of Medicine
University of Chicago Pritzger School of Medicine
Chairman, Committee on Clinical Pharmacology and Pharmacogenomics
Associate Director for Clinical Sciences, Cancer Research Center
University of Chicago Medical Center
Chicago, Illinois

Gregory H. Reaman, MD
Professor of Pediatrics
School of Medicine and Health Sciences
The George Washington University
Bethesda, Maryland

John C. Reed, MD, PhD
President and CEO, Professor and Donald Bren Presidential Chair
The Burnham Institute
La Jolla, California

Marvin S. Reitz, PhD
Professor and Associate Director
Basic Science Division
Institute of Human Virology
University of Maryland School of Medicine
Baltimore, Maryland

Elizabeth Repasky, PhD
Professor of Oncology
Department of Immunology
Roswell Park Cancer Institute
Buffalo, New York

Susan R. Rheingold, MD
Assistant Professor
Division of Oncology
The Children's Hospital of Philadelphia
Philadelphia, Pennsylvania

David C. Rice, MD
Associate Professor
Department of Thoracic and Cardiovascular Surgery
The University of Texas M. D. Anderson Cancer Center
Houston, Texas

Brian I. Rini, MD
Associate Professor of Medicine and Associate Director for Clinical Research
Department of Solid Tumor Oncology
Cleveland Clinic
Cleveland, Ohio

Kenneth V.I. Rolston, MD, FACP
Professor of Medicine
Department of Infectious Diseases/ Infection Control and Employee Health
The University of Texas M. D. Anderson Cancer Center
Houston, Texas

Bruce J. Roth, MD
Professor of Medicine and Urologic Oncology
Department of Hematology and Oncology
Vanderbilt University Medical Center
Nashville, Tennessee

Jack A. Roth, MD
Professor of Surgery
Department of Thoracic and Cardiovascular Surgery
The University of Texas M. D. Anderson Cancer Center
Houston, Texas

Jacob H. Rotmensch, MD
Professor and Chief Gynecologic Oncology
Department of Gynecologic Oncology
University of Chicago Medical Center
Chicago, Illinois

Eric K. Rowinsky, MD
Institute for Drug Development
Cancer Therapy and Research Center
San Antonio, Texas

Eric H. Rubin, MD
Vice President
Oncology Clinical Research
Merck Research Laboratories
North Wales, Pennsylvania

Raymond W. Ruddon, MD, PhD
Professor Emeritus
Department of Pharmacology
University of Michigan Medical School
Ann Arbor, Michigan

Nancy Russell, PhD
Integrative Medicine Program
Department of Behavioral Science
The University of Texas M. D. Anderson Cancer Center
Houston, Texas

Anguraj Sadanandam, PhD
Life Sciences Division
Lawrence Berkeley National Laboratory
Lausanne, Switzerland

Amar Safdar, MD, FACP
Associate Professor
Department of Infectious Diseases
The University of Texas M. D. Anderson Cancer Center
Houston, Texas

Joseph K. Salama, MD
Assistant Professor
Department of Radiation and Cellular Oncology
University of Chicago
Chicago, Illinois

Takeshi Sano, MD
Professor and Chairman
Gastric Surgery Division
Gastroenterological Surgery Cancer Institute Hospital
Tokyo, Japan

David T. Scadden, MD
Director, Center for Regenerative Medicine
Department of Medicine Hematology/Oncology
Massachusetts General Hospital and Harvard Medical School
Boston, Massachusetts

Amy C. Schefler, MD
Vitreoretinal Fellow
Bascom Palmer Eye Institute
University of Miami
Miami, Florida

Charles A. Schiffer, MD
Professor of Medicine and Oncology
Division of Hematology and Oncology
Karmanos Cancer Institute
Wayne State University
Detroit, Michigan

Jeffrey Schlom, PhD
Chief
Laboratory of Tumor Immunology and Biology
Center for Cancer Research
National Cancer Institute
Bethesda, Maryland

Erasmus Schneider, PhD
Director, Division of Translational Medicine, Wadsworth Center
Assistant Director for Oncology, Clinical Laboratory Evaluation Program, New York State Department of Health
Associate Professor, Department of Biomedical Sciences, School of Public Health
Wadsworth Center
New York State Department of Health
SUNY Albany
Albany, New York

David E. Schteingart, MD
Professor, Department of Internal Medicine
Division of Endocrinology and Metabolism
University of Michigan
Ann Arbor, Michigan

David L. Schwartz, MD
Assistant Professor
Department of Radiation Oncology
The University of Texas M. D. Anderson Cancer Center
Houston, Texas

Aleksandar Sekulic, MD, PhD
Assistant Professor
Department of Dermatology
College of Medicine
Mayo Clinic
Scottsdale, Arizona

Vickie R. Shannon, MD
Professor
Department of Pulmonary Medicine
The University of Texas M. D. Anderson Cancer Center
Houston, Texas

Padmanee Sharma, MD, PhD
Assistant Professor
Department of Genitourinary Medical Oncology
The University of Texas M. D. Anderson Cancer Center
Houston, Texas

Sunil Sharma, MD
Chief of the Sections of Phase I and Gastrointestinal Oncology Programs
Nevada Cancer Institute
Las Vegas, Nevada

Steven I. Sherman, MD
Professor and Chairman
Department of Endocrine Neoplasia and Hormonal Disorders
The University of Texas M. D. Anderson Cancer Center
Houston, Texas

Elizabeth Shpall, MD
Professor of Medicine
Department of Stem Cell Transplantation
The University of Texas M. D. Anderson Cancer Center
Houston, Texas

Branimir Sikic, MD
Professor
Department of Medicine-Oncology
Stanford University School of Medicine
Stanford, California

Richard T. Silver, MD
Professor of Medicine
Division of Hematology-Oncology
Department of Medicine
Weill Cornell Medical College
New York, New York

Lewis R. Silverman, MD
Associate Professor
Department of Medicine
Mount Sinai School of Medicine
New York, New York

George W. Sledge Jr., MD
Professor of Medicine and Pathology
Melvin and Bren Simon Cancer Center
Indiana University School of Medicine
Indianapolis, Indiana

Cardinale B. Smith, MD
Fellow
Department of Geriatric and Palliative Care
Mount Sinai Medical Center
New York, New York

Robert A. Smith, PhD
Director of Cancer Screening
Cancer Control Science Department
American Cancer Society
Atlanta, Georgia

Arthur J. Sober, MD
Associate Chief
Department of Dermatology
Massachusetts General Hospital
Boston, Massachusetts

Stephen T. Sonis, DMD, DMSc
Senior Surgeon
Division of Oral and Maxillofacial Surgery
Brigham & Women's Hospital
Boston, Massachusetts

Gabriella Sozzi, PhD
Chief
Cytogenetic and Molecular Cytogenetic Department
Fondazione IRCCS Istituto Nazionale Tumori
Milan, Italy

Paul T. Spellman, PhD
Staff Scientist
Life Sciences Division
Lawrence Berkeley National Laboratory
Berkeley, California

Paul Stauffer, MS, CCE
Professor and Director Hyperthermia Physics
Department of Radiation Oncology
Duke University Medical Center
Durham, North Carolina

John P. Stein, MD (deceased)
Professor of Urology
Keck School of Medicine, USC
Departments of Urology and Preventive Medicine
Norris Comprehensive Cancer Center
University of Southern California
Los Angeles, California

Richard M. Stone, MD
Associate Professor of Medicine
Department of Leukemia
Brigham & Women's Hospital, Dana-Farber Cancer Institute
Boston, Massachusetts

Erich M. Sturgis, MD, MPH
Assistant Professor and Surgeon
Department of Head and Neck Surgery
The University of Texas M. D. Anderson Cancer Center
Houston, Texas

Max W. Sung, MD
Clinical Assistant Professor
Division of Hematology and Oncology
Mount Sinai School of Medicine
New York, New York

Thomas Suter, MD
Professor
Swiss Cardiovascular Center
Bern University Hospital
Bern, Germany

Stephen G. Swisher, MD
Professor and Chairman
Department of Thoracic and Cardiovascular Surgery
The University of Texas M. D. Anderson Cancer Center
Houston, Texas

Chris H. Takimoto, MD, PhD
Senior Director
Department of Translational Medicine
Ortho Biotech Oncology Research and Development
Radnor, Pennsylvania

James A. Talcott, MD, SM
Associate Professor of Medicine
Harvard Medical School
Director, Center for Outcomes Research
Massachusetts General Hospital
Boston, Massachusetts

Ayalew Tefferi, MD
Professor of Medicine
Department of Hematology
Mayo Clinic
Rochester, Minnesota

Richard L. Theriault, DO, MBA, FACP
Professor
Department of Breast Medical Oncology
The University of Texas M. D. Anderson Cancer Center
Houston, Texas

David C. Thomas, MD
Director of Ambulatory Services and Ambulatory Training
Department of Medicine and Department of Rehabilitation Medicine
Mount Sinai School of Medicine
New York, New York

Melanie B. Thomas, MD, MS
Assistant Professor of Medicine
Department of Gastrointestinal Medical Oncology
The University of Texas M. D. Anderson Cancer Center
Houston, Texas

Michael J. Thun, MD, MS
Vice President Emeritus
Epidemiology and Surveillance Research
American Cancer Society
Atlanta, Georgia

Swan N. Thung, MD
Professor
Pathology, Division of Hepatopathology
Mount Sinai School of Medicine
New York, New York

Elizabeth L. Travis, MD
Professor and Associate Vice President of Women Faculty Programs
Department of Experimental Radiation Oncology
The University of Texas M. D. Anderson Cancer Center
Houston, Texas

Jeffrey M. Trent, PhD
President and Research Director
Translational Genomics Research Institute and Van Andel Research Institute
Phoenix, Arizona

David A. Tuveson, MD, PhD
Group Leader
Department of Oncology
Cambridge University
Cambridge, England

Douglas S. Tyler, MD
Vice Chair, Veterans Affairs
Department of Surgery
Duke University Medical Center
Durham, North Carolina

Thomas Uldrick, MD, MS
Staff Clinician
Department of Health and Human Services
National Cancer Institute
Bethesda, Maryland

Sarina van der Zee, MD
Fellow
The Zena and Michael A. Wiener Cardiovascular Institute
The Mount Sinai Medical Center
New York, New York

Ara A. Vaporciyan, MD
Associate Professor
Department of Thoracic and Cardiovascular Surgery
The University of Texas M. D. Anderson Cancer Center
Houston, Texas

Michael A. Via, MD
Clinical Fellow
Department of Medicine
Mount Sinai School of Medicine
New York, New York

Benjamin L. Viglianti, PhD
Research Associate
Department of Radiation Oncology
Duke University Medical Center
Durham, North Carolina

Bert Vogelstein, MD
Investigator
Professor of Oncology
Sidney Kimmell Comprehensive Center at Johns Hopkins University
Baltimore, Maryland

Daniel D. Von Hoff, MD
Physician-in-Chief and Senior Investigator
Director of Translational Research
Translational Genomics Research Institute
Phoenix, Arizona

Evan Vosburgh, MD
Clinical Associate Professor of Medicine
Department of Medicine
Yale University
New Haven, Connecticut

Zeljko Vujaskovic, MD, PhD
Associate Professor of Radiation Oncology, Pathology, and Medical Physics
Department of Radiation Oncology
Duke University Medical Center
Durham, North Carolina

Michael J. Wallace, MD
Associate Professor
Section Chief of Interventional Radiology
Department of Diagnostic Radiology
The University of Texas M. D. Anderson Cancer Center
Houston, Texas

Helen H. Wang, DrPH, MD
Associate Professor
Department of Pathology
Beth Israel Deaconess Medical Center
Boston, Massachusetts

Ralph R. Weichselbaum, MD
Daniel K. Ludwig Professor and Chairman of the Department of Radiation and Cellular Oncology
Director of the Center for Metastasis Research
University of Chicago
Chicago, Illinois

Lawrence Weiss, MD
Director, Pathology Core
Department of Pathology
City of Hope Medical Center
Duarte, California

Talia R. Weiss, BA
Department of Psychiatry and Behavioral Sciences
Memorial Sloan-Kettering Cancer Center
New York, New York

Ainsley Weston, PhD
Associate Director for Science
Office of the Director
National Institute for Occupational Safety and Health
Morgantown, West Virginia

Cheryl L. Willman, MD
Professor
School of Medicine Pathology
University of New Mexico Cancer Center
Albuquerque, New Mexico

Ignacio I. Wistuba, MD
Professor
Department of Pathology Research
The University of Texas M. D. Anderson Cancer Center
Houston, Texas

Robert A. Wolff, MD
Professor of Medicine
Department of Gastrointestinal Medical Oncology
The University of Texas M. D. Anderson Cancer Center
Houston, Texas

James C. Yao, MD
Associate Professor
Department of Gastrointestinal Medical Oncology
The University of Texas M. D. Anderson Cancer Center
Houston, Texas

Sai-Ching Jim Yeung, MD, PhD
Associate Professor
Department of General Internal Medicine, Ambulatory Treatment and Emergency Care and Department of Endocrine Neoplasia and Hormonal Disorders
The University of Texas M. D. Anderson Cancer Center
Houston, Texas

Michael R. Zalutsky, PhD
Professor
Department of Radiology
Medical Physics Program and Biomedical Engineering
Pratt School of Engineering
Duke University
Durham, North Carolina

Ming Zhou, MD, PhD
Assistant Professor
Department of Anatomic Pathology
Cleveland Clinic Lerner College of Medicine of the Case Western Reserve University
Cleveland, Ohio

Contents

Preface . . . . *v*

Part ONE: CARDINAL MANIFESTATIONS OF CANCER

1 **Cardinal Manifestations of Cancer** *1*
James F. Holland, MD, ScD (hc), Emil Frei III, MD, Waun Ki Hong, MD, DMSc (Hon), Donald W. Kufe, MD, Robert C. Bast, Jr., MD, William N. Hait, MD, PhD, Raphael E. Pollock, MD, PhD, Ralph R. Weichselbaum, MD

Part TWO: SCIENTIFIC FOUNDATIONS OF CANCER

Section 1: CANCER BIOLOGY

2 **Molecular Biology, Genomics, Proteomics, and Mouse Models of Human Cancer** *5*
Kornelia Polyak, MD, PhD, Matthew Meyerson, MD, PhD, William C. Hahn, MD, PhD, David A. Tuveson, MD, PhD

3 **Cell Proliferation and Differentiation** *26*
Michael Andreeff, MD, PhD, David W. Goodrich, PhD, H. Phillip Koeffler, MD

4 **Apoptosis and Cancer** *40*
John C. Reed, MD, PhD

5 **Growth Factors and Signal Transduction in Cancer** *51*
Luca Grumolato, PhD, Stuart A. Aaronson, MD

6 **Oncogenes** *68*
Marco A. Pierotti, PhD, Milo Frattini, PhD, Gabriella Sozzi, PhD, Carlo M. Croce, MD

7 **Tumor Supressor Genes** *86*
David Cosgrove, MB, BCh, Ben Ho Park, MD, PhD, Bert Vogelstein, MD

8 **Genomic Alterations and Chromosomal Aberrations in Human Cancer** *102*
Kevin M. Brown, PhD, Jonathan J. Keats, PhD, Aleksandar Sekulic, MD, PhD, Cheryl L. Willman, MD, Jeffrey M. Trent, PhD, Robert A. Hromas, MD

9 **Biochemistry of Cancer** *125*
Raymond W. Ruddon, MD, PhD, Donald W. Kufe, MD

10 **Invasion and Metastases** *141*
Elise C. Kohn, MD

11 **Tumor Angiogenesis** *149*
John V. Heymach, MD, PhD, George W. Sledge Jr., MD, Rakesh K. Jain, PhD

12 **Epigenetic Contributions to Human Cancer** *170*
James G. Herman, MD, Stephen B. Baylin, MD

Section 2: CANCER IMMUNOLOGY

13 **Cancer Immunotherapy** *175*
Karl S. Peggs, MA, MB, BCh, MRCP, FRC Path, Sergio A. Quezada, PhD, Padmanee Sharma, MD, PhD, James P. Allison, PhD

Section 3: CANCER ETIOLOGY

14 **Genetic Predisposition to Cancer** *190*
Henry T. Lynch, MD, Vandana Gupta Abramson, MD, Marcia S. Brose, MD, PhD

15 **Chemical Carcinogenesis** *225*
Ainsley Weston, PhD, Curtis C. Harris, MD

16 **Hormones and the Etiology of Cancer** *237*
Leslie Bernstein, PhD, C. Leigh Pearce, PhD, Iona Cheng, PhD, Katherine DeLellis Henderson, PhD

17 **Ionizing Radiation** *248*
David J. Grdina, PhD

18 **Ultraviolet Radiation Carcinogenesis** *262*
James E. Cleaver, PhD, David L. Mitchell, PhD

19 **Inflammation and Cancer** *270*
Debra L. Laskin, PhD, Jeffrey D. Laskin, PhD

20 **RNA Tumor Viruses** *279*
Robert C. Gallo, MD, Marvin S. Reitz, PhD

21 **Herpesviruses** *291*
Jeffrey I. Cohen, MD

22 **Papillomaviruses and Cervical Neoplasia** *298*
Christopher P. Crum, MD, Martin C. Chang, MD, PhD

23 **Hepatitis Viruses** *302*
Max W. Sung, MD, Swan N. Thung, MD

24 **Parasites** *311*
Piero Mustacchi, MD, ScD [Hon]

Section 4: TRANSLATIONAL CANCER MEDICINE

25 **Molecular Imaging in Clinical Oncology** *318*
Juri G. Gelovani, MD, PhD

26 **Molecular Diagnostics in Cancer** *335*
Bryan T. Hennessy, MD, Robert C. Bast Jr., MD, Gordon B. Mills, MD, PhD

27 **Personalized Medicine in Oncology Drug Development** *347*
William N. Hait, MD, PhD, Nicolas, C. Dracopoli, PhD, Steven J. Heller, MD, Chris H. Takimoto, MD, PhD

28 **Cancer Genome Aberrations: Measures, Causes, and Consequences** 359
Eric A. Collisson, MD, Anguraj Sadanandam, MD, Paul T. Spellman, MD, Joe W. Gray, PhD

29 **Cancer Nanotechnology** *364*
Mauro Ferrari, PhD

Section 5: CANCER EPIDEMIOLOGY, PREVENTION, AND SCREENING

30 **Cancer Epidemiology** ... 371
Michael J. Thun, MD, MS, Ahmedin Jemal, DVM, PhD

31 **Tobacco-Induced Cancers and Their Prevention** ... 386
Stephen S. Hecht, PhD, Dorothy K. Hatsukami, PhD

32 **Nutrition in the Etiology and Prevention of Cancer** ... 398
Elizabeth M. Grainger, PhD, RD, Edward L. Giovannucci, MD, ScD, Steven K. Clinton, MD, PhD

33 **Chemoprevention of Cancer** ... 411
Scott M. Lippman, MD, Waun Ki Hong, MD, DMSc (Hon)

34 **Cancer Screening and Early Detection** ... 419
Robert A. Smith, PhD, Stephen W. Duffy, MSc, Otis W. Brawley, MD

Section 6: CLINICAL TRIALS AND OUTCOMES ASSESSMENT

35 **Statistical Innovations in Cancer Research** ... 446
Donald A. Berry, PhD

36 **Outcomes Research in Oncology** ... 464
James A. Talcott, MD, SM

PART THREE: PRINCIPLES OF CANCER DIAGNOSIS

Section 7: CANCER PATHOLOGY

37 **Principles of Cancer Pathology** ... 473
James L. Connolly, MD, Jeffrey D. Goldsmith, MD, Helen H. Wang, MD, Janina A. Longtine, MD, Ann M. Dvorak, MD, Harold F. Dvorak, MD, Stanley R. Hamilton, MD

Section 8: IMAGING

38 **Principles of Imaging** ... 489
Edward F. Patz Jr., MD

39 **Interventional Radiology for the Cancer Patient** ... 490
Rony Avritscher, MD, Michael J. Wallace, MD

PART FOUR: PRINCIPLES OF THERAPEUTIC MODALITIES

Section 9: SURGICAL ONCOLOGY

40 **Principles of Surgical Oncology** ... 499
Raphael E. Pollock, MD, PhD, FACS, Michael A. Choti, MD, MBA, FACS, Donald L. Morton, MD, FACS

Section 10: RADIATION ONCOLOGY

41 **Principles of Radiation Oncology** ... 510
Joseph K. Salama, MD, Mark W. Dewhirst, DVM, PhD, Ralph R. Weichselbaum, MD

42 **Hyperthermia** ... 528
Benjamin L. Viglianti, MD, PhD, Paul Stauffer, MS, CCE, Elizabeth Repasky, PhD, Ellen Jones, MD, Zeljko Vujaskovic, MD, PhD, Mark W. Dewhirst, DVM, PhD

Section 11: MEDICAL ONCOLOGY

43 **Principles of Medical Oncology** ... 541
William N. Hait, MD, PhD, James F. Holland, MD, ScD (hc), Emil Frei III, MD, Donald W. Kufe, MD Robert C. Bast Jr., MD, Waun Ki Hong, MD, DMSc (Hon)

Section 12: CHEMOTHERAPY

44 **Cytokinetics** ... 550
Larry Norton, MD, Theresa Ann Gilewski, MD

45 **Principles of Dose, Schedule, and Combination Chemotherapy** ... 558
Joseph P. Eder, MD, William N. Hait, MD, PhD, Emil Frei III, MD, Louise B. Grochow, MD

46 **Preclinical and Early Clinical Development of New Anticancer Agents** ... 568
Daniel D. Von Hoff, MD, Axel-R. Hanauske, MD, PhD, MBA

47 **Pharmacology** ... 587
William K. Plunkett Jr., PhD, Mark J. Ratain, MD

48 **Drug Resistance and Its Clinical Circumvention** ... 597
Jeffrey A. Moscow, MD, Erasmus Schneider, PhD, Branimir I. Sikic, MD, Charles S. Morrow, MD, PhD, Kenneth H. Cowan, MD, PhD

Section 13: CHEMOTHERAPEUTIC AGENTS

49 **Folate Antagonists** ... 611
Peter D. Cole, MD, Barton A. Kamen, MD, Joseph R. Bertino, MD

50 **Pyrimidine and Purine Antimetabolites** ... 621
Giuseppe Pizzorno, PhD, PharmD, Sunil Sharma, MD, Yung-Chi Cheng, PhD

51 **Alkylating Agents and Platinum Antitumor Compounds** ... 633
Michael Colvin, MD, William N. Hait MD, PhD

52 **Drugs That Target DNA Topoisomerases** ... 645
Eric H. Rubin, MD, William N. Hait, MD, PhD

53 **Microtubule-Targeting Natural Products** ... 655
Eric K. Rowinsky, MD

Section 14: BIOTHERAPEUTICS

54 **Interferons** ... 679
Ernest C. Borden, MD

55 **Cytokines and Hematopoietic Growth Factors** ... 686
Suhendan Ekmekcioglu, PhD, Razelle Kurzrock, MD, Elizabeth A. Grimm, PhD

56 **Monoclonal Serotherapy** ... 710
Robert C. Bast Jr., MD, Michael R. Zalutsky, PhD, Robert J. Kreitman, MD, Arthur E. Frankel, MD

57 **Vaccines and Immunostimulants** ... 725
James L. Gulley, MD, PhD, FACP, Philip M. Arlen, MD, James W. Hodge, PhD, MBA, Jeffrey Schlom, PhD

Section 15: ENDOCRINE THERAPY

58 **Antiestrogens, Progestins, and Aromatase Inhibitors** *737*
Aman U. Buzdar, MD, Shaheenah Dawood, MBB.Ch, MRCP (UK)MPH, Harold A. Harvey, MD, V. Craig Jordan, OBE, PhD, DSc

59 **Androgen Deprivation Strategies in the Treatment of Advanced Prostate Cancer** *750*
Samuel R. Denmeade, MD

Section 16: GENE THERAPY

60 **Cancer Gene Therapy** *759*
Sunil J. Advani, MD, Ralph R. Weichselbaum, MD, Donald W. Kufe, MD

Section 17: BONE MARROW TRANSPLANTATION

61 **Hematopoietic Cell Transplantation** *776*
Roy Jones, PhD, MD, Elizabeth Shpall, MD, Richard Champlin, MD

PART FIVE: PRINCIPLES OF MULTIDISCIPLINARY MANAGEMENT

Section 18: PSYCHO-ONCOLOGY

62 **Principles of Psycho-Oncology** *793*
Jimmie C. Holland, MD, Talia R. Weiss, BA

Section 19: CANCER REHABILITATION MEDICINE

63 **Principles of Cancer Rehabilitation Medicine** ... *810*
David C. Thomas, MD, Kristjan T. Ragnarsson, MD

Section 20: MULTIDISCIPLINARY MANAGEMENT

64 **Multidisciplinary Management** *823*
James F. Holland, MD, ScD (hc), Emil Frei III, MD, Waun Ki Hong, MD, DMSc (Hon), Donald W. Kufe, MD, Robert C. Bast Jr., MD, Raphael E. Pollock, MD, PhD, Ralph R. Weichselbaum, MD, William N. Hait, MD, PhD,

65 **Cancer and Pregnancy** *830*
Jennifer K. Litton, MD, Richard L. Theriault, DO, MBA, FACP

66 **Cancer and Aging** *838*
Arti Hurria, MD, Hyman B. Muss, MD, Harvey J. Cohen, MD

67 **The Role of Integrative Oncology in Cancer Care** *846*
Lorenzo Cohen, PhD, Nancy Russell, PhD, M. Kay Garcia, DRN, LAC, DrPH, Moshe Frenkel, MD

Section 21: PAIN AND PALLIATION

68 **Palliative Care** *854*
Cardinale B. Smith, MD, Gabrielle R. Goldberg, MD, Diane E. Meier, MD

69 **Management of Cancer Pain** *863*
Natalie Moryl, MD, Alan C. Carver, MD, Kathleen M. Foley, MD

Section 22: CENTRAL NERVOUS SYSTEM

70 **Primary Neoplasms of the Central Nervous System in Adults** *881*
Craig Nolan, MD, Lisa M. DeAngelis, MD

71 **Brain Metastases** *899*
Lisa M. DeAngelis, MD

Section 23: THE EYE

72 **Neoplasms of the Eye** *904*
Amy C. Schefler, MD, David H. Abramson, MD, Ira J. Dunkel, MD, Beryl McCormick, MD

Section 24: ENDOCRINE GLANDS

73 **Neoplasms of the Endocrine Glands: Pituitary Neoplasms** *915*
Chirag D. Gandhi, MD, Kalmon D. Post, MD

74 **Neoplasms of the Thyroid** *923*
Steven I. Sherman, MD

75 **Neoplasms of the Adrenal Cortex** *933*
David E. Schteingart, MD

76 **Tumors of the Diffuse Neuroendocrine and Gastroenteropancreatic Endocrine System** *940*
Evan Vosburgh, MD

Section 25: HEAD AND NECK

77 **Neoplasms of the Head and Neck** *959*
Michael E. Kupferman, MD, Erich M. Sturgis, MD, MPH, David L. Schwartz, MD, Adam Garden, MD, Merrill S. Kies, MD

Section 26: CANCER OF THE THORAX

78 **Cancer of the Lung** *999*
Charles Lu, MD, Amir Onn, MD, Ara A. Vaporciyan, MD, Joe Y. Chang, MD, PhD, Bonnie S. Glisson, MD, Ritsuko Komaki, MD, Ignacio I. Wistuba, MD, Jack A. Roth, MD, Roy S. Herbst, MD, PhD

79 **Malignant Mesothelioma** *1044*
Harvey I. Pass, MD, Michele Carbone, MD, PhD, Hedy Lee Kindler, MD

80 **Thymomas and Thymic Tumors** *1053*
A. Philippe Chahinian, MD, Alberto M. Marchevsky, MD

81 **Tumors of the Heart and Great Vessels** *1062*
Sai-Ching Jim Yeung, MD, PhD, Carmen Escalante, MD, Sarina van der Zee, MD, A. Philippe Chahinian, MD, Valentin Fuster, MD, PhD

82 **Primary Germ Cell Tumors of the Thorax** *1067*
John D. Hainsworth, MD, F. Anthony Greco, MD

Section 27: GASTROINTESTINAL TRACT

83 **Neoplasms of the Esophagus** *1074*
Stephen G. Swisher, MD, David C. Rice, MD, Jaffer A. Ajani, MD, Ritsuko K. Komaki, MD, Mark K. Ferguson, MD

84 **Carcinoma of the Stomach** *1086*
James C. Yao, MD, Christopher H. Crane, MD, Takeshi Sano, MD, Paul F. Mansfield, MD

85 **Treatment of Liver Metastases** *1109*
Nancy E. Kemeny, MD, Michael D'Angelica, MD

86 **Primary Neoplasms of the Liver** *1124*
Max W. Sung, MD, Swan N. Thung, MD

87 **Gallbladder and Bile Duct Cancer** *1132*
Ahmed O. Kaseb, MD, Melanie B. Thomas, MD, MS, Steven A. Curley, MD, FACS

88 **Neoplasms of the Exocrine Pancreas** *1144*
Robert A. Wolff, MD, Christopher H. Crane, MD, Donghui Li, PhD, Douglas B. Evans, MD

89 **Neoplasms of the Small Intestine, Vermiform Appendix, and Peritoneum, and Carcinoma of the Colon and Rectum** *1172*
James C. Padussis, MD, Georgia M. Beasley, MD, Nicole S. McMahon, BS, Douglas S. Tyler, MD, Kirk A. Ludwig, MD

90 **Neoplasms of the Anus** *1194*
Bruce D. Minsky, MD, José G. Guillem, MD

Section 28: GENITOURINARY TRACT

91 **Renal Cell Carcinoma** *1204*
Brian I. Rini, MD, Daniel Y.C. Heng, MD, Ming Zhou, MD, PhD, Andrew Novick, MD, Derek Raghavan, MD, PhD, FACP, FRACP

92 **Tumors of the Renal Pelvis and Ureter** *1212*
Ali-Reza Golshayan, MD, Inderbir S. Gill, MD, MCh, Cristina Magi-Galluzzi, MD, PhD, Derek Raghavan, MD, PhD, FACP, FRACP

93 **Bladder Cancer** *1219*
Derek Raghavan, MD, PhD, FACP, FRACP, John P. Stein, MD, Richard Cote, MD, FRCPath, J. Stephen Jones, MD, FACS

94 **Neoplasms of the Prostate** *1228*
Christopher J. Logothetis, MD, Jeri Kim, MD, John Davis, MD, Deborah Kuban, MD, Paul Mathew, MD, Ana Aparicio, MD

95 **Tumors of the Penis and Urethra** *1255*
Raymond S. Lance, MD, Donald F. Lynch Jr, MD

96 **Testis Cancer** *1263*
Christian Kollmansberger, MD, Siamak Daneshmand, MD, Eric K. Hansen, MD, Christopher L. Corless, MD, PhD, Bruce J. Roth, MD, Craig R. Nichols, MD

Section 29: FEMALE REPRODUCTIVE ORGANS

97 **Neoplasms of the Vulva and Vagina** *1289*
Jacob H. Rotmensch, MD

98 **Neoplasms of the Cervix** *1299*
Anuja Jhingran, MD

99 **Endometrial Cancer** *1325*
Jamal Rahaman, MD, Carmel J. Cohen, MD

100 **Neoplasms of the Fallopian Tube** *1338*
Jamal Rahaman, MD, Carmel J. Cohen, MD

101 **Ovarian Cancer** *1344*
Jonathan S. Berek, MD, MMS, Michael L. Friedlander, MD, PhD, Robert C. Bast Jr., MD

102 **Molar Pregnancy and Gestational Trophoblastic Neoplasia** *1376*
Donald P. Goldstein, MD, Ross S. Berkowitz, MD

103 **Gynecologic Sarcomas** *1384*
Jamal Rahaman, MD, Carmel J. Cohen, MD

Section 30: THE BREAST

104 **Neoplasms of the Breast** *1393*
Gabriel N. Hortobagyi, MD, FACP, Laura Esserman, MD, Thomas A. Buchholz, MD, FACP

Section 31: THE SKIN

105 **Melanoma** *1459*
Jeffrey E. Gershenwald, MD, Patrick Hwu, MD

106 **Other Skin Cancers** *1487*
Victor A. Neel, MD, PhD, Arthur J. Sober, MD

Section 32: BONE AND SOFT TISSUE

107 **Bone Tumors** *1497*
Timothy A. Damron, MD, FACS, David G. Murray, MD

108 **Soft Tissue Sarcomas** *1517*
Peter W.T. Pisters, MD, FACS, Brian O'Sullivan, MD, FRCPI, Robert G. Maki, MD, PhD

Section 33: HEMATOPOIETIC SYSTEM

109 **The Myelodysplastic Syndrome** *1544*
Lewis R. Silverman, MD

110 **Acute Myeloid Leukemia in Adults: Mast Cell Leukemia and Other Mast Cell Neoplasms** *1559*
Charles A. Schiffer, MD, Richard M. Stone, MD

111 **Chronic Myeloid Leukemia** *1582*
Jorge Cortes, MD, Richard T. Silver, MD, Hagop M. Kantarjian, MD

112 **Acute Lymphoblastic Leukemia** *1591*
Stefan Faderl, MD, Ching-Hon Pui, MD, Susan O'Brien, MD, Hagop M. Kantarjian, MD

113 **Chronic Lymphocytic Leukemia** *1604*
Kanti R. Rai, MD, Matthew Kaufman, MD

114 **Hodgkin Lymphoma** *1622*
Peter M. Mauch, MD, Lawrence Weiss, MD, James O. Armitage, MD

115 **Non-Hodgkin Lymphoma** *1645*
Arnold S. Freedman, MD

116 **Mycosis Fungoides and Sézary Syndrome** *1659*
Richard T. Hoppe, MD, Youn H. Kim, MD, Ranjana Advani, MD

117 **Plasma Cell Tumors** *1668*
Noopur Raje, MD, Teru Hideshima, MD, PhD, Kenneth C. Anderson, MD

118 **Myeloproliferative Neoplasms: Essential Thrombocythemia, Primary Myelofibrosis, and Polycythemia Vera** *1686*
Ayalew Tefferi, MD

Section 34: NEOPLASMS IN AIDS

119 **Neoplasms in Acquired Immunodeficiency Syndrome** *1696*
Jeremy S. Abramson, MD, David T. Scadden, MD

Section 35: UNKNOWN PRIMARY SITE

120 **Neoplasms of Unknown Primary Site** *1713*
John D. Hainsworth, MD, F. Anthony Greco, MD

Section 36: PEDIATRIC ONCOLOGY

121 Principles of Pediatric Oncology *1723*
Maura O'Leary, MD, Gregory H. Reaman, MD

Section 37: COMPLICATIONS OF CANCERS AND THEIR TREATMENT

122 Anorexia and Cachexia *1740*
Takao Ohnuma, MD, PhD

123 Antiemetic Therapy *1757*
Aditya Bardia, MBBS, MPH, David S. Ettinger, MD

124 Neurologic Complications *1763*
Lisa M. DeAngelis, MD

125 Dermatologic Complications of Cancer Chemotherapy *1779*
Cindy Berthelot, MD, Joy H. Kunishige, MD, Narin Apisarnthanarax, MD, Madeleine M. Duvic, MD

126 Skeletal Complications *1788*
Samuel Kenan, MD, Jeffrey I. Mechanick, MD, Michael A. Via, MD

127 Hematologic Complications and Blood Bank Support *1797*
Richard M. Kaufman, MD, Kenneth C. Anderson, MD

128 Coagulopathic Complications of Cancer Patients *1813*
Maria T. DeSancho, MD, Jacob H. Rand, MD

129 Urologic Complications *1823*
Christopher J. Logothetis, MD, Diana M. Hey Cauley, PharmD

130 Cardiac Complications *1832*
Michael S. Ewer, MD, MPH, JD, Steven M. Ewer, MD, Thomas Suter, MD

131 Respiratory Complications *1849*
Vickie R. Shannon, MD, George A. Eapen, MD, Carlos A. Jimenez, MD, Rodolfo C. Morice, MD, Elizabeth L. Travis, PhD, Lara Bashoura, MD, Amar Safdar, MD, FACP, Scott E. Evans, MD, Roberto Adachi, MD, Saadia A. Faiz, MD, Diwakar D. Balachandran, MD, Joseph L. Nates, MD, MBA, FCCM S. Egbert Pravinkumar, MD, FRCP, Burton F. Dickey, MD

132 Gastrointestinal and Hepatic Complications in Cancer Patients *1871*
Marta L. Davila, MD, Robert S. Bresalier, MD

133 Oral Complications of Cancer and Their Treatment *1880*
Stephen T. Sonis, DMD, DMSc

134 Gonadal Complications *1891*
Peter Kabos, MD, Catherine E. Klein, MD

135 Endocrine Complications and Paraneoplastic Syndromes *1901*
Sai-Ching Jim Yeung, MD, PhD, Robert F. Gagel, MD

136 Treatment-Related Secondary Cancers *1915*
Susan R. Rheingold, MD, Alfred I. Neugut, MD, PhD, Thomas Uldrick, MD, MS, Anna T. Meadows, MD

Section 38: INFECTION IN THE CANCER PATIENT

137 Infections in Patients With Cancer *1921*
Kenneth V.I. Rolston, MD, FACP, Gerald P. Bodey, MD

Section 39: ONCOLOGIC EMERGENCIES

138 Oncologic Emergencies *1941*
Sai-Ching Jim Yeung, MD, PhD, Carmen Escalante, MD

Section 40: ONCOLOGY AND INFORMATICS

139 Oncology Informatics *1961*
Edward P. Ambinder, MD

Index *1981*

1 Cardinal Manifestations of Cancer

James F. Holland, MD, ScD (hc) ■ Emil Frei III, MD ■ Waun Ki Hong, MD, DMSc (Hon) ■ Donald W. Kufe, MD ■ Robert C. Bast Jr., MD ■ William N. Hait, MD, PhD ■ Raphael E. Pollock, MD, PhD ■ Ralph R. Weichselbaum, MD

Cancer is a singular word that embraces a vast diversity of diseases that can occur in any organ system throughout the animal kingdom. The unique characteristic of cancer is the proliferation of cells of a type different from, if ever so slightly, the normal complement of the organism. The proliferation may be rapid or slow, the accumulation of cells may be massive or miniscule. The essence of the matter, however, is that aberrant cells, distinct from the ordinary evolution of cell types, appear and accumulate. Thus, a cancer differs from hypertrophy and hyperplasia, which involve normal cells.

A cancer cell does not obey the complex rules of architecture and function that govern the usual placement and behavior of cells within a tissue. The wondrous coexistence of cells and tissues of multiple types that make up the eye, the finger, or the kidney, for example, each with appropriate anatomic location with all connections intact to fulfill their appointed tasks, is part of the miracle we call life. The explanation for this marvelous organization is the field of continuing exploration seeking the messages and exquisite controls that exist in multicellular organisms.

Cancer is distinguished from other abnormal cellular growths that lead to benign tumors in its characteristic independence from the restrictions present in normal tissues. Benign tumors expand and compress, but do not attack or invade adjacent tissues. Accumulated cancer cells make a tissue that ignores the anatomic barriers of adjacent cell membranes and basement membranes. Through chemical and mechanical means, the cancer cell insinuates itself between and into the space of the normal cells, killing them by chemical and physical means, the grand usurper. Even though the placenta in mammals shows this behavior, there is self-limitation in location and in survival of the placental invasion. Although leukocytes normally extravasate and permeate tissues, they do not share the other characteristics of cancer. The cancer cell is partially or absolutely insensitive to such normal constraints, and may continue its invasiveness indefinitely.

Upon reaching a circulatory conduit, either a lymphatic or capillary vessel, a process that may not be entirely haphazard, cancer cells often penetrate the wall as part of their invasive behavior. They then may be carried by the lymphatic or venous circulation to remote sites where the possibility of adherence, extravasation, and colonization can occur, establishing metastases. In the absence of an intervening event, and given enough time, with few exceptions, the cancer process, as described, can lead to such anatomic or functional distortions that death ensues.

The cancer process does not start with a fully invasive cancer cell. A disorder in molecular instructions for protein synthesis is the common precursor lesion, nearly always because of qualitatively or quantitatively aberrant ribonucleic acid (RNA) messages transcribed from nuclear deoxyribonucleic acid (DNA). This occurs because of a mutation of the DNA, or because of overexpression of particular genes that encode proteins important as catalysts in pathways for stimulating growth, or because of underexpression of genes whose coded proteins control and inhibit growth. Portions of genes may be lost, translocated, or amplified. Indeed, entire chromosomes may be deleted, replicated, or fused in abnormal ways. All such distortions of DNA can give rise to abnormal or unbalanced RNA messages, leading to qualitative or quantitative differences in proteins that result in disordered cellular function. Sometimes the functional abnormality is so extreme as to be lethal to the cell, initiating the suicidal mechanism of apoptosis. In other instances, the functional abnormality results in disease. Some of these diseases display the characteristics of cancer. Mutation, overexpression, and underexpression of genes can result from a wide spectrum of intrinsic and extrinsic causes, with various pathways that lead not to one final common pathway, but by several converging routes to cells with the phenotypic characteristics of cancer. When these cells are limited to an epithelial layer above the basement membrane, they are called *carcinoma-in-situ* or *intraepithelial neoplasia*. Similar changes probably occur, but are more difficult to recognize, in the mesenchymal tissues. Even cancer cells that do not penetrate the basement membrane, and thus lack one of the cardinal features of true cancer, represent a long series of antecedent molecular abnormalities that eventually lead to this optically recognizable cellular change. Furthermore, these evolving cancer cells are the common, if not the exclusive, precursor of invasive cancer.

In their earliest stages, as proliferating cells accumulate, cancers are almost always asymptomatic. Cancers cause symptoms as they advance as a consequence of their mass, because they ulcerate on an epithelial surface, or because of change in function of the affected structure or organ. Nearly all the symptoms that can be caused by cancer can also be caused more commonly by noncancerous diseases. The astute clinician must include cancer in the differential diagnosis of virtually every symptom, albeit a benign disease may usually explain it. Doctors never diagnose diseases they don't think of. Cancers occur at any age. A longer life span provides greater opportunity for intrinsic organic events or an encounter with environmental carcinogens, however, and greater opportunity for initial DNA mutations to be fully realized as invasive cancers. Thus age is the principal risk factor for most, but not all, cancers.

Such common symptoms as sore throat, runny nose, or a chest cold can sometimes be a result of cancers of pharynx, sinuses, or bronchi, respectively. Indeed, patients with these cancer diagnoses usually have been treated, often repeatedly and for extended periods, for the benign disease because cancer was not considered in the differential diagnosis, and appropriate observations were not made. Cancer symptoms such as diarrhea, constipation, or mild pain often seem commonplace. Cancer symptoms may be intermittent, with spontaneous temporary improvement, a phenomenon that is usually misinterpreted by patients and often by physicians as evidence against the diagnosis of cancer. In fact, recurrent appearance or chronicity of a symptom which in short duration is characteristic of a common benign disease markedly heightens the possibility of an underlying dysfunction caused by cancer.

Cancers cause their symptoms by a few readily understandable mechanisms.

Occlusion of an essential conduit, partial or complete, can be caused by tumor. A tumor mass grows to such size that it partially or completely occludes an essential conduit. Classic presentations are cancer of the bronchus where partial bronchial occlusion causes cough, diminishes ciliary clearance of secretion, and sometimes leads to bronchopneumonia. Complete bronchial occlusion leads to atelectasis and chronic pneumonia. Compromise of the esophageal lumen by tumor mass or muscular dysfunction resulting from infiltration causes dysphagia, which, in its early presentation, is far too often attributed to benign cause. Gastric tumors rarely cause complete obstruction, but often impair normal gastric motility. This defect may lead to easy satiety, anorexia, indigestion, and nausea. Decrease in caliber of the transverse and descending colon, sigmoid or rectum by tumor mass can lead to change in bowel habit, including diminished caliber of stools, constipation and bouts of cramps and/or diarrhea from peristaltic efforts of the proximal gut. Compromise of the lumen of the common bile duct by carcinoma of the head of the pancreas or of the bile duct itself produces obstructive jaundice, not infrequently after minor antecedent digestive complaints or unexplained pruritus ascribed to accumulated bile salts.

Ureteral obstruction by compression from retroperitoneal masses or bladder tumor leads to hydroureter and hydronephrosis, often asymptomatic or revealed by vague discomfort in flank or loin, or by urinary tract infection. Bilateral obstruction leads to uremia with its protean symptomatology. Compromise of the urethra as it courses through the prostate causes diminished urinary stream, inadequate bladder emptying, frequency, urgency, nocturia, and when severe, obstructive uropathy and uremia.

Tumors in the cecum and ascending colon and in the urinary bladder, because their content is not solid and because of greater luminal diameter, uncommonly cause obstruction, but may distort normal function enough to alter bowel or urinary habits.

A mass discovered by palpation or x-ray may be a presenting finding, as in breast carcinoma. Dysfunction from replacement of the substance of a parenchymatous organ by tumor is a subset of mass presentation. The classic example is primary or, more commonly, metastatic brain tumor, which becomes identified by abnormal brain function. Seizure or paralysis, sensory or coordination abnormality, memory defect, and personality change may all be consequences of space occupation. These changes may occur not only because a specific area of the brain is affected, but since the calvarium is not distensible, because of increased intracranial pressure. In other patients, headache may be the only symptom of increased intracranial pressure. Similar dysfunction of the spinal cord with distal motor and sensory phenomena can reflect space occupation by a mass within or impinging on the cord or cauda equina. Hepatic dysfunction from space occupation by primary or metastatic tumor, often with related intrahepatic bile duct compression, can present as jaundice. Sometimes the liver enlarges to enormous size, causing digestive disorders, pain, and a visible and palpable mass in the upper abdomen. Thyroid cancer usually presents as a mass, and uncommonly this results in hypothyroid laboratory values, but rarely in clinical hypothyroidism.

A sarcoma of the soft tissues usually presents as a palpable mass. Testicular cancer ordinarily presents as a mass: the testicle may only be slightly larger than its fellow, but harder and heavier in the examiner's hand. Ovarian cancer may be detected as an adnexal mass.

A new lump or mass, or a changing one, requires exclusion of cancer based on clinical examination, imaging studies, or a biopsy. Most lipomas, and self-discovery of the xiphoid, are two types of lumps that can usually be dismissed on clinical grounds. A dominant breast mass or even a questionable one, requires assessment by appropriate imaging, and often by cytologic or histologic means. A thyroid nodule, an enlarged lymph node that is hard, a node that remains enlarged without infectious explanation for 2 weeks, a skin mass with the characteristics of melanoma or carcinoma, especially if ulcerated, a new subcutaneous or abdominal or scrotal mass all require consideration of cancer and appropriate diagnostic study.

Ulceration on the skin or on an epithelial surface, can lead to blood loss and occasionally can serve as a portal of infection. Skin ulcerations are commonly ignored for weeks or months and are often interpreted as a common injury of unremembered origin that did not heal. Bronchial ulceration results in hemoptysis, usually blood-tinged sputum, and only rarely massive bleeding. Any of the upper alimentary canal cancers can ulcerate and bleed. Usually the bleeding is slow, intermittent, and silent, leading to iron-deficiency anemia. Hematemesis or massive melena is uncommon. Carcinomas of the cecum and ascending colon often present with the symptoms of anemia because of ulceration and bleeding.

Carcinoma of the bladder and carcinoma of the kidney commonly manifest hematuria. Sometimes this is fortuitously discovered as a microscopic or chemical abnormality on routine urinalysis. Clots from renal bleeding can lead to ureteral colic. Hematuria less often heralds prostate cancer, but hematospermia implies prostate disease, benign or malignant, because carcinoma of the seminal vesicle is exceedingly rare.

Endometrial carcinoma most often presents as postmenopausal vaginal bleeding, although any vaginal bleeding outside the normal menstrual cycle is worthy of suspicion. Contact bleeding during intercourse is suggestive of cervical ulceration, most commonly a result of cancer.

Pain is commonly thought of as a surrogate for early cancer, although this is mistaken. Most cancers are initially painless. Pain occurs when a tumor invades, presses on, or stretches a nerve, or when proximal smooth muscle contracts in an attempt to bypass an obstructed or dysfunctional distal segment of a conduit. Most pains of short duration that disappear are not caused by cancer. Cancer must enter the differential diagnosis, however, when pain is recurrent or persistent without ready explanation, or atypical, or present when there is no other recognizable cause. New pain, not necessarily severe, must be carefully interpreted. Abdominal pain and skeletal pain distinct from joint symptomatology deserve particular attention, and early rather than late studies to establish a cause. Pain in a breast mass does not exclude its being cancer.

Weight loss may first indicate an unsuspected cancer, and when combined with grumbling low grade discomforts, malaise, and fatigue, is a cause for particular scrutiny. A wide variety of other diseases can also cause these common symptoms, but cancer should not be at the bottom of the list. If a diagnosis is not established after initial studies a second complete history and physical examination after a short interval is imperative.

Effusion caused by cancer in the pleural, pericardial, or peritoneal cavities can lead to dyspnea and discomfort. Increasing abdominal girth, often with malaise, oliguria, constipation, and weight gain, is a cardinal symptom of ascites. In the thorax, bronchogenic carcinoma, mesothelioma, metastatic breast or ovarian cancer, and primary carcinoma of serous membranes are the frequent causes of malignant effusion. Ascites as a presenting symptom is characteristic of ovarian cancer and cancer of the serous membranes. Pancreatic cancer, mesothelioma, metastatic carcinoma on the peritoneum and in the liver and several non-neoplastic diseases also enter the differential diagnosis.

Perforation caused by invasion of the wall of a hollow viscus causes pain, usually sudden. Cancer is not suspected in most cases when this rare event occurs. Pneumothorax from perforation of the pleura by a primary or metastatic pulmonary tumor is an uncommon emergency. Fistulization of gastric cancer into the transverse colon leads to vague abdominal discomfort, which is misinterpreted or neglected, and then sudden onset of diarrhea with prominent gastrocolic reflex. Appendiceal cancer, albeit a rare tumor, frequently presents as acute appendicitis with peritonitis because of rupture. Perforation of the colon is more frequently caused by diverticulitis than by colon cancer. Ruptured ectopic pregnancy due to choriocarcinoma has been reported. Tracheoesophageal fistulization in the course of esophageal or bronchogenic carcinomas occurs late.

Fever of unknown origin that persists for more than one week must include cancer among its possible causes. Hodgkin disease, other lymphomas, acute leukemia, cancer of the kidney, and cancers of the liver are high on the list of neoplasms that can cause fever. Certain cancers predispose to infections because of ulceration, obstruction, or disordered leukopoiesis.

Endocrine hyperactivity syndromes may occasionally turn out to be caused by cancer. Hyperadrenalism, sometimes first manifest as hirsutism, can indicate adrenal cancer. Cushing syndrome can also result from small cell carcinoma of the lung. Hyperparathyroidism rarely comes from parathyroid cancer but can be mimicked by ovarian cancer and squamous carcinomas. Tumors that secrete thyroid hormone, estrogens, insulin, glucagon, aldosterone, epinephrine, or norepinephrine are often benign tumors of the parent endocrine organ, but cancer must always be considered. Functional neuroendocrine tumors may secrete serotonin and other vasoactive principles that cause the carcinoid syndrome.

Paraneoplastic syndromes may be early symptoms of cancer. Myasthenia gravis, Raynaud syndrome, hypertrophic osteoarthropathy and clubbing, and refractory anemia may herald thymoma, myeloma, lung cancer, and hematologic dyscrasia (and thymoma) respectively. A diligent search must be made for these and other causes.

Absence of cardinal manifestations is usual for cancers detected by screening by Papanicolaou smears, mammography, prostate-specific antigen determinations, colonoscopy, computed tomography, lung scanning, and total skin examination. Asymptomatic cancers discovered by these methods are generally far less advanced than those that cause symptoms. Occasionally, routine chemical or hematologic laboratory data in asymptomatic patients suggest cancer or leukemia. Such incidental discovery reinforces the proposition that early in their pathogenesis, cancers are almost always asymptomatic.

Predispostion to cancer characterizes a broad spectrum of diseases, exposures, and lifestyle behaviors. Patients who have had inflammatory bowel disease, human papilloma virus infection of the cervix, hepatitis B or C infection, those with prior radiation exposure, earlier treatment with alkylating agents, anthracyclines, or podophyllotoxin derivatives, or specific environmental exposures such as asbestos, those who have smoked, heavily imbibed alcohol, or sun worshipped, and those with a strong family history of cancer, particularly those neoplasms known in part to be heredofamilial all are in groups that deserve special consideration for the particular cancers that occur in them at a higher frequency than normal.

Cancerophobia does not predispose to cancer. Depression occurs more frequently with carcinoma of the pancreas than with gastric carcinoma, however, and may be an early symptom of pancreatic neoplasia.

The Present

By the time cancer is diagnosed, it is often past the stage of easy curability. Frequently the earliest symptoms were ignored or rationalized. Mammography, early surgery, and hormonal, chemotherapeutic and immunologic treatment have decreased mortality from breast cancer; cytology and early treatment have diminished cervical cancer mortality; and colonoscopy and polypectomy have decreased colon cancer mortality. Other screening programs portend similar promise by diagnosing cancers before they become symptomatic. Cancer has replaced syphilis as the great imitator. Many symptomatic patients with cancer are still curable with today's therapies. Delay cannot possibly help, however, once an early symptom occurs that eventually proves to be caused by cancer. Inclusion of cancer as a possibility in every differential diagnosis can save lives.

The Future

The expansion of diagnostic techniques based on genomics and proteomics augurs well for earlier identification of cancers. Not only is it reasonable to believe that clinical diagnosis will be accelerated by laboratory methods, but these two disciplines are likely to alter our understanding of the cancer process as it occurs in humans. It is hoped that the consequent impact of this knowledge on cancer prevention and on cancer therapy will be revolutionary. The cardinal manifestations of cancer may then become principally of historical interest while laboratory abnormalities are instrumentally detectable well before clinical presentation. Indeed departure from a population norm may be less significant than departure from one's prior proteomic profile taken as a baseline during health. If such a blue-sky future ever unfolds, public understanding and compliance will still be critical determinants of cancer prevention and early diagnosis.

2 Molecular Biology, Genomics, Proteomics, and Mouse Models of Human Cancer

Kornelia Polyak, MD, PhD ■ Matthew Meyerson, MD, PhD ■ William C. Hahn, MD, PhD ■ David A. Tuveson, MD, PhD

Cancer is a genetic disease. Abnormalities in genes that control cellular proliferation lead to the unrestrained growth that characterizes the malignant cell. Thus, to gain the initiative in cancer detection and treatment, oncologists must begin to understand the molecular roots of the disease: genes, their messenger ribonucleic acids (mRNAs), and the proteins they produce. In short, oncologists should be conversant with the tools of molecular biology.

This chapter is a basic survey of molecular biology and is directed toward the clinician or trainee who wants a fundamental understanding of this discipline. It is "methods-oriented" and will serve as a frame of reference for other chapters in this book. It describes the principles that underlie the procedures used most commonly by molecular biologists and provides examples of clinically relevant situations that draw on particular techniques. It will become apparent that molecular biology already plays an important role in clinical cancer medicine, from the analysis of tumors for prognostic or pathogenetic information to the production of pharmacologic agents, such as colony stimulating factors, interleukins, and erythropoietin.

We will begin with an overview of genes, gene expression, and gene cloning. Our discussion of techniques will follow the flow of genetic information as we explain the procedures used to analyze gene expression at the levels of DNA, RNA, and protein. Good general overviews can be found in several books.[1]

Overview: Gene Structure

Genes and Gene Expression

The gene is the fundamental unit of inheritance and the ultimate determinant of all phenotypes. The DNA of a normal human cell contains an estimated 30,000-120,000 genes, but only a fraction of these are used (or expressed) in any particular cell at any given time. For example, genes specific for erythroid cells, such as the hemoglobin genes, are not expressed in brain cells. The identity of each gene expressed in a particular cell at a given time and its level of expression are defined as the "transcriptome."

According to the central dogma of molecular biology, a gene exerts its effects by having its DNA transcribed into an mRNA, which, in turn, is translated into a protein, the final effector of the gene's action. Thus, molecular biologists often investigate gene expression or activation, by which is meant the process of transcribing DNA into RNA or translating RNA into protein. The process of transcription involves creating a perfect RNA copy of the gene using the DNA of the gene as a template. Translation of mRNA into protein is a somewhat more complex process because the structure of the gene's protein is encoded in the mRNA and that structural message must be decoded during translation.

Functional Components of the Gene

Every gene consists of several functional components, each involved in a different facet of the process of gene expression (Fig. 2-1). Broadly speaking, however, there are two main functional units: the promoter region and the coding region.

The promoter region controls when and in what tissue a gene is expressed. For example, the promoter of the hemoglobin gene is responsible for its expression in erythroid cells and not in brain cells. How is this tissue-specific expression achieved? In the DNA of the gene's promoter region, there are specific structural elements, nucleotide sequences (see Structural Considerations below) that permit the gene to be expressed only in an appropriate cell. These are the elements in the hemoglobin gene that instruct an erythroid cell to transcribe hemoglobin mRNA from that gene. These structures are referred to as *"cis"*-acting elements because they reside on the same molecule of DNA as the gene. In some cases, other tissue type–specific *cis*-acting elements, called *enhancers*, reside on the same DNA molecule but at great distances from the coding region of the gene.[2] In the appropriate cell, the *cis*-acting elements bind protein factors that are physically responsible for transcribing the gene. These proteins are called *trans*-acting factors because they reside in the cell's nucleus separate from the DNA molecule bearing the gene. For example, brain cells would not have the right *trans*-acting factors that bind to the hemoglobin promoter; therefore, brain cells would not express hemoglobin. They would, however, have *trans*-acting factors that bind to neuron-specific gene promoters.

The structure of a gene's protein is specified by the gene's coding region. The coding region contains the information that directs an erythroid cell to assemble amino acids in the proper order to make the hemoglobin protein. How is this order of amino acids specified? As described in detail later, DNA is a linear polymer consisting of four distinguishable subunits called *nucleotides*. In the coding region of a gene, the linear sequence of nucleotides encodes the amino acid sequence of the protein. This genetic code is in triplet form so that every group of three nucleotides encodes a single amino acid. The 64 triplets that can be formed by four nucleotides exceed the 20 distinct amino acids used to make proteins. This makes the code degenerate and allows some amino acids to be encoded by several different triplets.[3] The nucleotide sequence of any gene can now be determined (see below). By translating the code, one can derive a predicted amino acid sequence for the protein encoded by a gene.

Structural Considerations

Fine Structure ■ The basic repeating units of the DNA polymer are nucleotides (Fig. 2-2). Nucleotides consist of an invariant portion, a five-carbon deoxyribose sugar with a phosphate group, and a variable portion, the base. Of the four bases that appear in the nucleotides of DNA, two are purines, adenine (A) and guanine (G), and two are pyrimidines, cytosine (C) and thymine (T). Nucleotides are connected to each other in the polymer through their phosphate

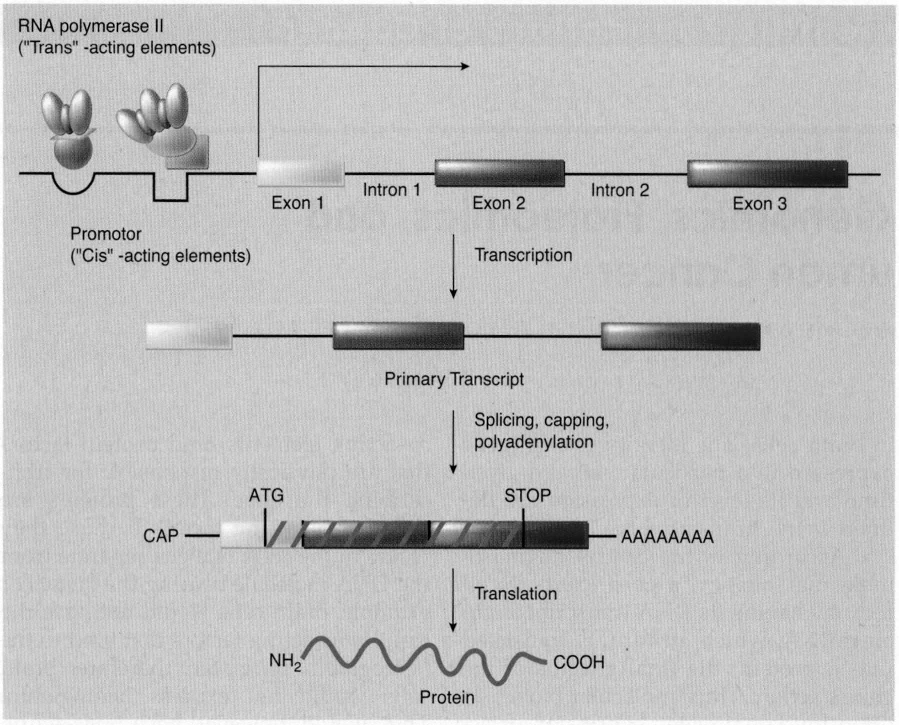

Figure 2-1 Gene expression. A gene's DNA is transcribed into messenger ribonucleic acid (mRNA), which, in turn, is translated into protein. The functional components of a gene are schematically diagrammed here. Areas of the gene destined to be represented in mature mRNA are called *exons*, and intervening areas of DNA between exons are called *introns*. The portion of the gene that controls transcription, and therefore expression, is the promoter. This control is exerted by specific nucleotide sequences in the promoter region (so-called *"cis"*-acting factors) and by proteins (so-called *"trans"*-acting factors) that must interact with promoter DNA and/or ribonucleic acid (RNA) polymerase II for transcription to occur. The primary transcript is the RNA molecule made by RNA polymerase II that is complementary to the entire stretch of DNA containing the gene. Before leaving the nucleus, the primary transcript is modified by splicing together exons (thus removing intron sequences), adding a cap to the 5′ end and adding a poly-A tail to the 3′ end. Once in the cytoplasm, mature mRNA undergoes translation to yield a protein.

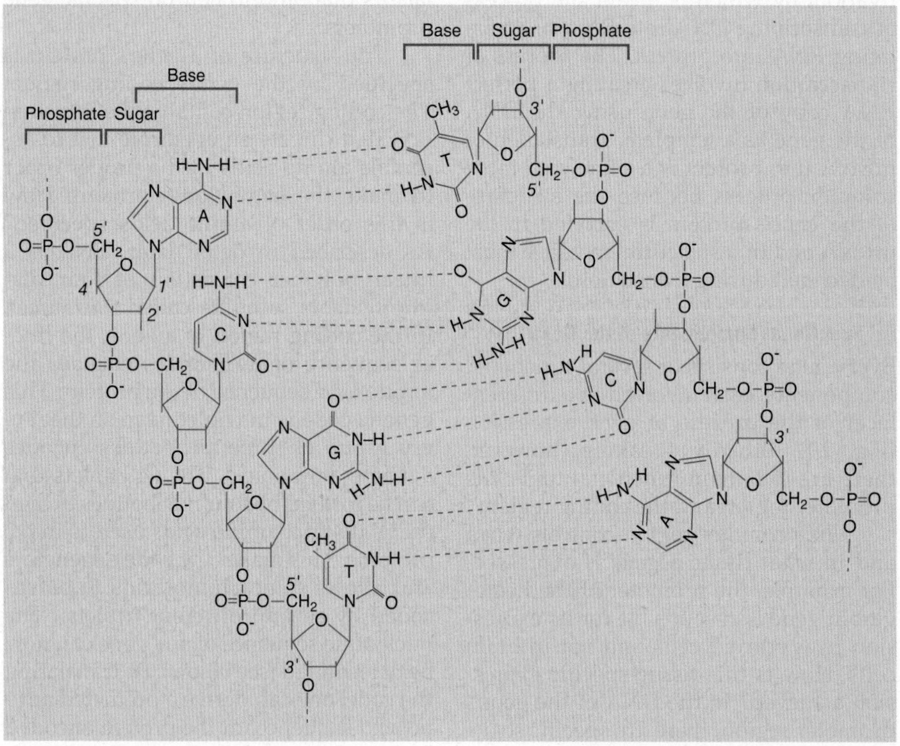

Figure 2-2 Structure of base-paired, double-stranded DNA. Each strand of DNA consists of a backbone of five-carbon deoxyribose sugars connected to each other through phosphate bonds. Note that as one follows the sequence down the left-hand strand (A to C to G to T), one is also following the carbons of the deoxyribose ring, going from the 5′ carbon to the 3′ carbon. This is the basis for the 5′ to 3′ directionality of DNA. The 1′ carbon of each deoxyribose is substituted with a purine or pyrimidine base. In double-stranded DNA, bases face each other in the center of the molecule and base pair via hydrogen bonds (*dotted lines*). Base-pairing is specific so that adenine pairs with thymine and guanine pairs with cytosine.

groups, leaving the bases free to interact with each other through hydrogen bonding. This base-pairing is specific, so that A interacts with T and C interacts with G. DNA is ordinarily double-stranded, ie, two linear polymers of DNA are aligned so that the bases of the two strands face each other. Base-pairing makes this alignment specific, so that one DNA strand is a perfectly complementary copy of the other. This complementarity means that each DNA strand carries the information needed to make an exact replica of itself.

In every strand of a DNA polymer, the phosphate substitutions alternate between the 5′ and 3′ carbons of the deoxyribose molecules. Thus, there is directionality to DNA: the genetic code reads in the 5′-3′ direction. In double-stranded DNA, the strand that carries the translatable code in the 5′-3′ direction is called the *sense strand*, whereas its complementary partner is the *antisense strand*.

Gross Structure In eukaryotes, the coding regions of most genes are not continuous. Rather, they consist of areas that are transcribed into mRNA, the exons, which are interrupted by stretches of DNA that do not appear in mature mRNA, the introns (see Fig. 2-1). The functions of introns are not known with certainty. A purpose of some sort is implied by their conservation in evolution. However, their overall physical structure might be more important than their specific nucleotide sequences because the nucleotide sequences of introns diverge more rapidly in evolution than do the sequences of exons. Overall, DNA that contains genes comprises a minority of total

DNA. Between genes, vast stretches of untranscribed DNA are assumed to play an important structural role.

In the nucleus, DNA is not present as naked nucleic acid. Rather, DNA is found in close association with a number of accessory proteins, such as the histones, and in this form is called *chromatin*.[4] Although many of DNA's accessory proteins have no known specific function, they generally appear to be involved in the correct packaging of DNA. For example, DNA's double helix is ordinarily twisted on itself to form a supercoiled structure.[5] This structure must unwind partially during DNA replication and transcription.[6] Some of the accessory proteins, eg, topoisomerases and histone acetylases, are involved in regulating this process.

Summary

Genes specify the structure of proteins that are responsible for the phenotype associated with a particular gene. Although the nucleus of every human cell contains 30,000-120,000 genes, only a fraction of them are expressed in any given cell at any given time. The promoter (with or without an enhancer) is the part of the gene that determines when and where it will be expressed. The coding region is the part of the gene that dictates the amino acid sequence of the protein encoded by the gene. DNA is a linear polymer of nucleotides. Ordinarily, the nucleotide bases of one strand of DNA interact with those of another strand (A with T, C with G) to make double-stranded DNA. In the cell's nucleus, DNA is associated with accessory proteins to make the structure called *chromatin*.

General Techniques

Restriction Endonucleases and Recombinant DNA

In eukaryotic chromosomes, individual molecules of DNA are several million base pairs long. Because these molecules are far too large to analyze directly, scientists are usually interested in cutting DNA into fragments of manageable size. Fortunately, for molecular biologists, bacteria have evolved a highly diverse set of enzymes, the restriction endonucleases, which cleave DNA internally within the polymer.[7]

In nature, these enzymes have evolved to protect the bacteria from invasion by foreign DNA molecules, such as phage. To discriminate between "domestic" and "foreign" DNA, these enzymes recognize specific nucleotide sequences. DNA without such specific sequences is left undisturbed by the enzymes. However, when a restriction endonuclease spots a recognition site, it binds to the site and cleaves both strands of the DNA to which it has bound. Individual restriction endonucleases recognize specific sequences, usually in the order of four to six bases in length, and these sequences are often palindromes, ie, the 5′-3′ sequence in the upper strand is identical to the 5′-3′ sequence in the lower strand (Fig. 2-3).[8]

Although restriction endonucleases cut DNA into smaller fragments, there is a lower limit to the size of useful fragments. One would not want to cut DNA into such small pieces that the informational content of each piece is negligible. Statistically, the longer a restriction endonuclease's recognition sequence, the less frequently this sequence will occur in a stretch of DNA. Therefore, the enzymes most commonly used to cut DNA into usefully large fragments are those that recognize a 6-nt recognition site (so-called "six-base cutters"). For example, an endonuclease isolated from *Escherichia coli*, called *Eco*RI, recognizes the sequence GAATTC, and wherever this occurs in double-stranded DNA, it will cleave between the G and A (see Fig. 2-3). (Note that the antisense strand, which reads CTTAAG in the 3′-5′ direction, will also read GAATTC in the 5′-3′ direction. This is what is meant by a palindromic sequence.)

Gene Cloning

Mechanics ■ The most powerful technique available for gene analysis, the one technique that is the cornerstone for all others, is gene cloning (see Fig. 2-3). In the gene cloning process, a discrete piece of DNA is faithfully replicated in the laboratory. Cloning provides quantities of specific DNA sufficient for biochemical analysis or for any other manipulation, including joining to a foreign piece of DNA. In the early 1970s, Cohen and colleagues drew on two fundamental properties of bacteria and their viruses (phages) that made this innovation possible: plasmids and DNA ligases.[9]

Plasmids are circular molecules of DNA that replicate in the cytoplasm of bacterial cells, separate from the bacteria's own DNA. In nature, plasmids often carry genetic information useful to the host bacterium, such as genes that confer resistance to antibiotics. For the purposes of gene cloning, plasmids are important because they contain all of the information necessary for directing bacterial enzymes to replicate the plasmid DNA, in some cases, to many thousands of copies per bacterium.

DNA ligases are enzymes produced by bacteria (and some phages when they infect bacteria) that can link or ligate together separate pieces of DNA. The nucleotide sequence in a piece of DNA does not influence the activity of a DNA ligase so that a DNA ligase can join two pieces of DNA that are not ordinarily connected to each other in nature.

In gene cloning, one uses a restriction endonuclease to cut open the circular plasmid DNA in a region of the plasmid not necessary for replication (see Fig. 2-3). Suppose, eg, that the enzyme *Eco*RI cuts open the plasmid in such a nonessential area. *Eco*RI recognizes the sequence GAATTC and cuts both DNA strands between the G and the A nucleotides. Protruding from the cut ends will be single-stranded DNA "tails" with the sequence AATT. (Note that the tail's sequence in the sense strand is the same as the sequence in the antisense strand when the nucleotides are read in the 5′-3′ direction.) Any other piece of DNA that has been cut with *Eco*RI will also have single-stranded AATT tails, and the AATT tails on this foreign piece of DNA can base-pair with the complementary TTAA tails (reading 3′-5′) on the cut plasmid. When this happens, the foreign DNA piece physically closes the gap in the plasmid, forming a closed circular plasmid again (which is necessary for plasmid propagation).

Although the nucleotides at the ends of the plasmid and foreign DNA now abut each other, they are not covalently connected. This is an unstable situation that the DNA ligase rectifies. The DNA ligase covalently joins the plasmid and foreign DNA to create a recombinant plasmid, which still has all of the information needed to be replicated in a bacterium but which also contains a foreign DNA insert. Obviously, the *Eco*RI-cut ends of the plasmid can also base-pair with themselves again to reform the native plasmid, but molecular biologists have developed a number of tricks to suppress this phenomenon. It should be pointed out that single-stranded tails are not always necessary for making recombinant DNA. Under certain conditions, the DNA ligase can join together two fragments of blunt-ended DNA without these tails.

When a recombinant plasmid is reintroduced into a host bacterium (by a process called *transformation*), the plasmid will replicate normally. Now, however, its foreign DNA insert is replicated along with the plasmid into which it was inserted. The transformed bacteria can then be grown to large numbers in liquid culture. With each bacterial cell division, the progeny bacteria contain plasmid molecules that continue to replicate. When the bacterial culture contains the desired quantity of this plasmid (this may be milligrams of plasmid DNA in a 1 L culture), it can be reisolated as pure DNA. The cloned foreign piece of DNA can then be

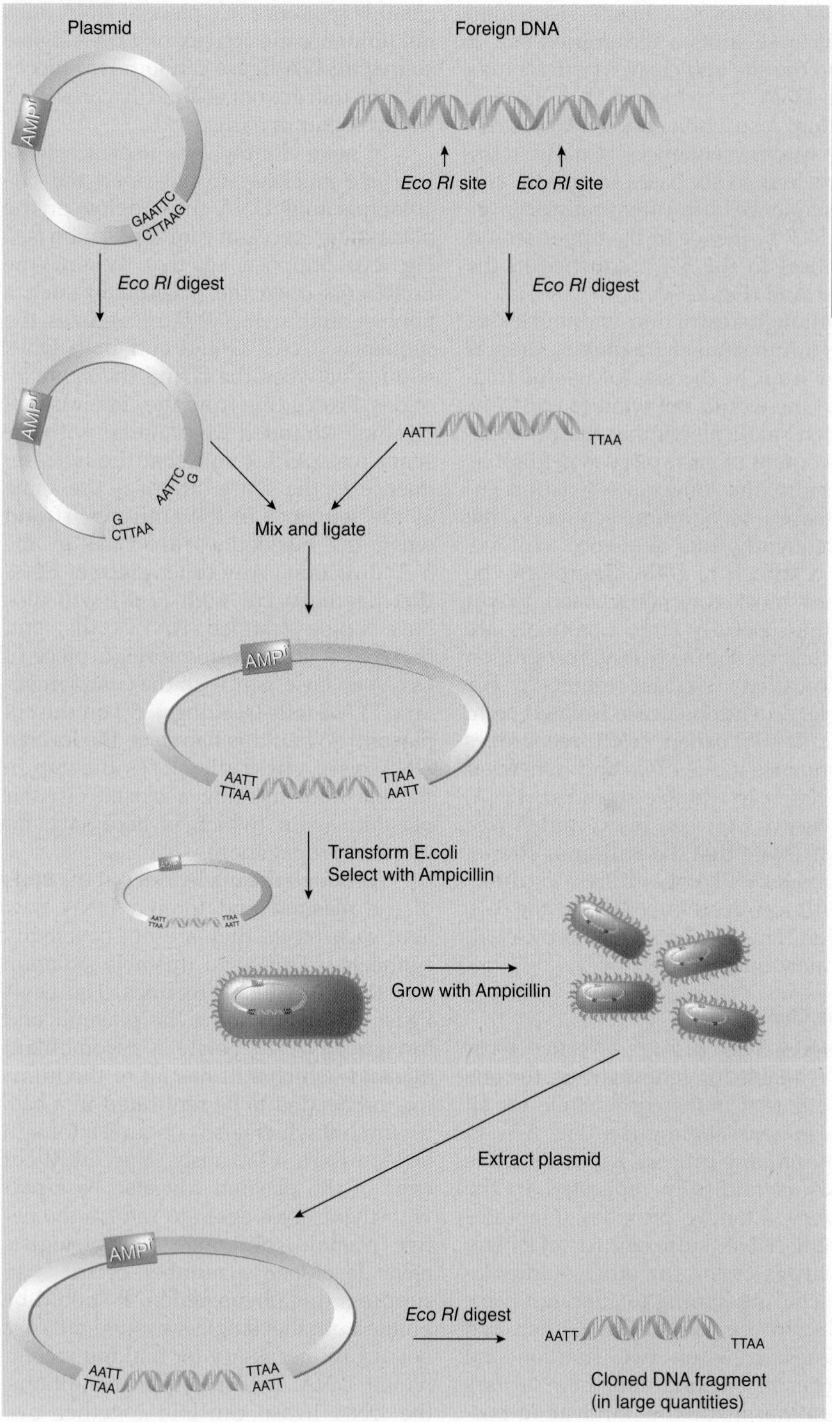

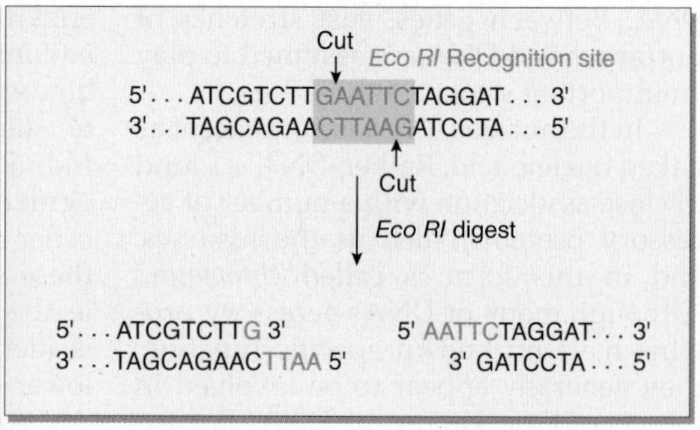

Figure 2-3 ■ Digestion of DNA with the restriction endonuclease *Eco*RI and gene cloning. In this example, a small amount of foreign DNA (a few nanograms) is digested with *Eco*RI. The nucleotide sequence of this stretch of DNA contains the recognition sequence for *Eco*RI, GAATTC (*boxed*). *Eco*RI cuts the DNA in both strands between the indicated nucleotides, resulting in fragments with 5′ single-stranded tails. This foreign DNA can come from any source, the only requirement being that it contains the same restriction endonuclease recognition sites as the vector. Plasmid vector is also digested with *Eco*RI to create a linear DNA molecule. The "sticky" single-stranded ends of the foreign DNA can align and base-pair with the complementary "sticky ends" of the plasmid, after which DNA ligase covalently bonds foreign DNA to plasmid DNA. This recombinant DNA is introduced into *E. coli* by a process called transformation. Because the bacteria themselves are not resistant to ampicillin, growth in ampicillin will select only those bacteria that have taken up the plasmid DNA (which carries an ampicillin resistance gene). The plasmid contains a bacterial origin of replication so that as the bacterial culture grows, plasmids replicate, resulting in several copies in each bacterium. When the culture has grown to sufficient size, plasmid DNA can be isolated biochemically, foreign DNA can be cut from the plasmid using *Eco*RI, and the resulting yield will often be milligrams of DNA, ie, greater than a 10^6-fold amplification.

cut out (with *Eco*RI, in our example) for further analysis or manipulation. One can also use bacterial viruses (or phages) in the same manner by infecting host bacteria with recombinant phage-bearing foreign DNA sequences. In all of these experiments, the plasmid or phage that houses the foreign DNA is called a *vector* because it is the vehicle that directs the foreign DNA into the host bacterium.

These extraordinarily powerful tools, which are now part of the standard armamentarium of all molecular biology laboratories, have been responsible for the development of nearly all of the analytic techniques described later. Several excellent manuals have been published that describe these techniques in detail.[10]

Gene Probes and Hybridization

We shall see in the following sections that what lies at the heart of gene analysis is the ability to identify a specific gene (or mRNA) in a complex mixture of all of the DNA (or RNA) in a cell or tissue. This can be done only when one already has a cloned fragment of DNA from the gene of interest. Such fragments are usually obtained from gene libraries constructed from genomic DNA or complementary deoxyribonucleic acid (cDNA) or generated using polymerase chain reaction (PCR, to be described below). These DNA fragments can be almost any size, from a fraction of the size of the gene (a few hundred or even fewer nucleotides) to the size of an entire gene (several thousand nucleotides). These cloned gene fragments are called *probes* because they are used to probe native DNA or RNA for the gene of interest.

To be useful, a gene probe must contain a sufficient number of nucleotides so that it will recognize the sequences of its corresponding gene. Recognition occurs by a process called *nucleic acid hybridization*, in which two pieces of DNA can align themselves (or anneal) by copies of the specific gene present in the target DNA, this technique can be used quantitatively. For example, in an analysis of primary breast cancer tissue, Southern blotting was used to determine that 30% of these samples contained multiple copies of c-*neu* oncogene DNA, eg, the gene was amplified.[12]

Nucleotide Sequencing

The nucleotide sequence of a gene's coding region encodes the amino acid sequence of its protein. This means that even in the absence of any knowledge about a gene's protein, we can predict the structure of that protein given the nucleotide sequence of the gene. How can the nucleotide sequence of a gene be determined? The major method used for sequencing DNA is the "enzymatic chain termination" method devised by Sanger and colleagues.[13]

The chain termination method relies on properties of enzymes called *DNA polymerases* (Fig. 2-5). These are enzymes that create new DNA polymers starting from individual nucleotides. However, for a DNA polymerase to work, it needs a template of single-stranded DNA on which to create the new polymer. DNA polymerase adds a new nucleotide to the 3′ end of a growing DNA chain, but the base of the new nucleotide must be able to base-pair (ie, be complementary) to the base on the template over which the polymerase is positioned. After the addition of that nucleotide, the polymerase moves to the next nucleotide on the template and adds a new nucleotide to the 3′ end of the growing chain. Again, the new nucleotide must be complementary to the next base in the template. When the process is completed, the DNA polymerase will have made a new DNA chain whose nucleotide sequence is completely complementary to the template DNA.

Nucleotide sequencing is based on the observation that when DNA polymerase adds a synthetic abnormal nucleotide to a growing chain, the polymerization stops. The synthetic terminating nucleotides used most commonly are dideoxynucleotides that have no alcohol substitutions on the 3′ carbon of their deoxyribose groups and thus cannot be joined by a phosphate bridge to the next nucleotide (see Fig. 2-2). For example, in the presence of dideoxyadenosine triphosphate (ATP), chain termination will occur wherever an A appears in the new DNA sequence (a T in the template) (Fig. 2-6). These reactions are performed in vitro in a test tube, where millions of new DNA molecules are being made at once. If normal deoxy-ATP is mixed with dideoxy-ATP in the proper proportion, only a few of these molecules will terminate at each T in the template. This will generate a series of new DNA polymers, each one stretching from the beginning of the chain to the position of an A (ie, a T in the template). If the newly formed DNA is fluorescently labeled, the products can be separated electrophoretically in a polyacrylamide gel or capillary gel (see below). Each step of the ladder is a fragment of DNA that stretches from the start of the new polymer to the position of an A. Four separate reactions are performed using each of the four dideoxynucleotides, each coded with a distinct fluorescent color. The four reactions are run together in a capillary gel, and the order of nucleotides is read by the order of the different colors.

Following the completion of the human genome sequence, genome researchers shifted their efforts from de novo to comparative sequencing. Large-scale sequencing projects have been initiated aimed at comparing groups of healthy and diseased individuals with the goal of understanding genetic variation associated with a particular disorder. The successful completion of these projects requires new sequencing technologies that allow fast, affordable, and accurate

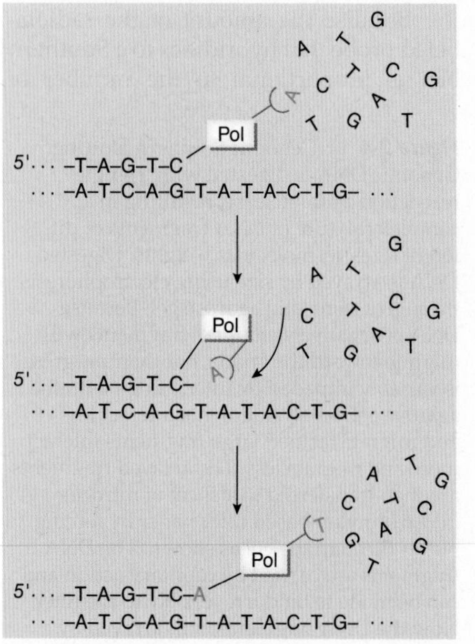

Figure 2-5 DNA polymerase. In this schematic, the enzyme DNA polymerase is creating a new DNA chain (*upper strand*) using a template (*lower strand*). Specific nucleotides are added from the 5′ to the 3′ direction as determined by the next nucleotide in the template.

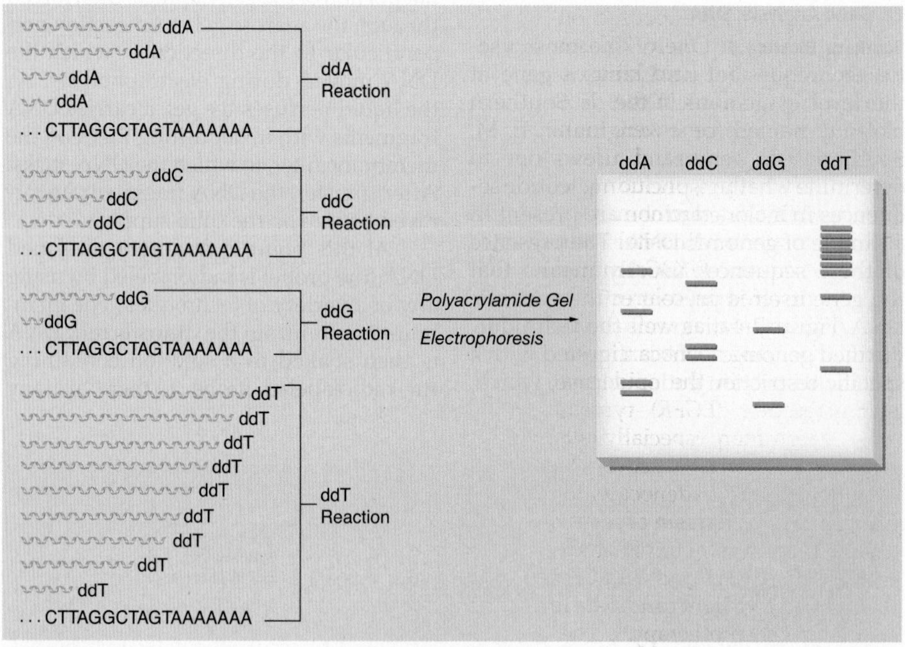

Figure 2-6 DNA sequencing using the chain termination method. In this example, DNA ending with the sequence {156}CTTAGGCTAGTAAAAAAA is being analyzed. Four reactions are performed, each using this DNA as a template for a DNA polymerase reaction and each containing one of the four dideoxynucleotides (dideoxyadenosine triphosphate [ddA], dideoxycytidine triphosphate [ddC], dideoxyguanosine triphosphate [ddG], and dideoxythymidine triphosphate [ddT]). In each reaction, chain elongation will terminate when the dideoxynucleotide is incorporated at the position of its complementary nucleotide in the template. This will result in a family of chains of differing lengths that correspond to the position at which polymerization terminated. In this example, these chains can be resolved by electrophoresis through a urea-containing polyacrylamide gel, in which longer chains run near the top of the gel and shorter chains near the bottom. Each new chain is radioactively labeled, and after autoradiography, the pattern of bands can be read from x-ray film. By noting the order in which bands appear, starting at the bottom of the gel, one can read the sequence of the template by substituting the complement of each dideoxynucleotide at every position. Reading from the bottom yields GAATCCGATCATTTTTTT, and substituting the complementary base at each position yields CTTAGGCTAGTAAAAAAA, the sequence of the template. The use of fluorescent labels in capillary gel electrophoresis is conceptually similar.

sequencing. A variety of array-oriented methods, including oligonucleotide array hybridization, fluorescent detection of the sequencing extension of arrayed PCR products, and chemiluminescent detection of the sequence extension of arrayed PCR products, now offer the potential of increased sequencing throughput and decreased cost.

The applications of DNA sequencing for cancer diagnosis and treatment selection are increasing as our knowledge of cancer-causing mutations continues to grow. In general, tumor suppressor genes are inactivated by loss-of-function mutations in cancer, whereas oncogenes are activated by amplification, translocation, or gain-of-function mutations. A specific example with clinical relevance is the discovery of mutations in the c-kit protein tyrosine kinase gene by DNA sequencing of gastrointestinal stromal tumors (GISTs).[14] This has led to the successful treatment of GIST with the c-kit inhibitor STI-571 or Gleevec.[15]

With the completion of the human genome sequence, targeted sequencing studies of particular gene families have now led to the identification of common cancer-associated mutations. To date, these systematic studies have focused on enzyme families such as protein kinases, protein phosphatases, and lipid kinases. Of note, activating mutations in the *BRAF* serine-threonine kinase gene were found in over half of all melanomas and subsequently in other cancer types, including colorectal, lung, and thyroid carcinomas.[16] Mutations in the phosphatidylinositol 3-kinase catalytic subunit gene *PIK3CA* mutations have been discovered in colorectal carcinoma and glioblastoma, as well as breast carcinomas.[17] In lung adenocarcinoma, activating mutations in the epidermal growth factor receptor (*EGFR*) tyrosine kinase gene are common, especially in East Asian populations.[18] The discovery of *EGFR* mutations in lung adenocarcinoma sheds light on the mechanism of response to the kinase inhibitors gefitinib and erlotinib, whereas the *BRAF* and *PIK3CA* mutation discoveries highlight candidate targets for anticancer chemotherapy.[18] The analysis of *EGFR* mutation is now a useful diagnostic tool for lung carcinoma patients. In myeloproliferative diseases such as polycythemia vera, the *JAK2* V617F activating mutation is a pathognomonic finding.[19] One can anticipate that many different DNA sequencing tests will become part of cancer diagnostics in the setting of treatment with targeted therapies.

The advent of single-template sequencing technologies promises a vast expansion of our abilities to discover cancer-causing mutations and to diagnose them. These array-based DNA sequencing technologies have the capacity to generate millions of DNA sequences in a single experiment and have the promise of complete sequencing of all coding regions in a single analysis.[20] Single-template sequencing methods are able to detect mutations effectively in heterogeneous cancer samples, overcoming one of the major limitations of current sequence detection approaches.[21] During the next several years, it is likely that next-generation DNA sequencing methods will become the technology of choice for cancer mutation detection expanding the clinical research of genome-based diagnosis.

Polymerase Chain Reaction (PCR)

To detect gene sequences by Southern blotting, at least 1-2 mg of genomic DNA is required. This translates into milligram quantities of tissue that must be used fresh or freshly frozen. By amplifying specific fragments of DNA, the PCR lowers the theoretic limit of detectable DNA sequences in a sample to a single molecule of DNA. With some advance knowledge of the nucleotide sequences in the DNA to be detected, microscopically small amounts of tissue, even a single cell, contain enough DNA to be amplified, and the amplified DNA can be easily analyzed. Even fixed tissue in paraffin blocks or on slides can yield sufficient DNA for analysis using PCR.[22] The concepts underlying PCR are diagrammed in Figure 2-7. Two short single-stranded DNA fragments, called primers, have

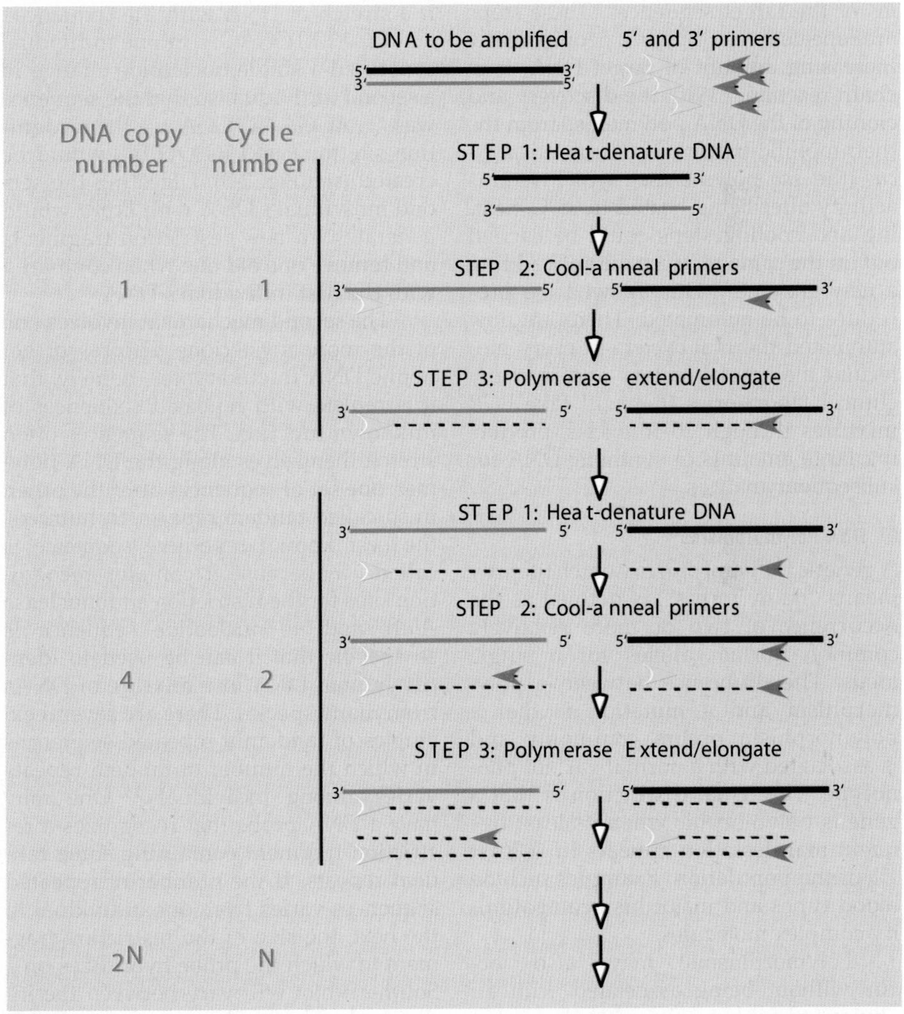

Figure 2-7 Polymerase chain reaction. DNA is mixed with short (10-20 base) single-stranded oligonucleotide primers that are complementary to the 5′ and 3′ ends of the sequence to be amplified. The mixture is heated to denature or "melt" all double-stranded DNA and then cooled to permit the primers to anneal to their complementary sequences on the DNA to be amplified. Note that the 5′ primer will anneal to the lower strand and the 3′ primer will anneal to the upper strand. A heat-resistant (thermostable) DNA polymerase (*Taq* polymerase; see text) was present in the original mixture, and it now synthesizes DNA by starting at the primers and using the strands to which the primers are annealed as a template. This results in the formation of two double-stranded DNA copies for every molecule of double-stranded DNA in the original mixture. The reaction is then heated to melt double-stranded DNA and cooled to allow reannealing, and the polymerase makes new double-stranded DNA again. There are now four double-stranded DNA copies for each original DNA molecule. This process can be repeated *n* times (usually 20-50) to result in 2n copies of double-stranded DNA.

sequences complementary to those that flank the stretch of DNA to be amplified. They are added to the target DNA, the mixture is heated to dissociate the paired double strands of target DNA, and then the temperature is lowered to permit hybridization, or annealing, of the primers to their complementary sequences on the target DNA. A DNA polymerase enzyme is added to the mixture, which will add nucleotides to the 3′ end of the primers using the target DNA as a sequence template. This step generates one copy of each of the strands of one target DNA molecule. The mixture is heated again to dissociate the strands and then cooled to allow more primers to anneal to the target sequences on both the original and new pieces of DNA. DNA polymerase is added again and now generates four copies of the target sequences. These steps are repeated, resulting in a geometrically increasing amount of target DNA, ie, a chain reaction.[23] With the discovery and cloning of the DNA polymerase from the thermophilic bacterium *Thermus aquaticus* (the *Taq* polymerase), which retains activity after being heated to 95°C, heating and cooling steps could be carried out on the same mixture without adding a new enzyme.[24] This allowed the procedure to be automated. There are now automated thermal cyclers in every molecular biology laboratory and in many clinical laboratories that will take PCR mixtures through 20-50 cycles, producing large amounts of synthetic DNA for subsequent analysis.

DNA Polymorphisms

A genetic polymorphism (which literally means "many forms") is defined as the occurrence of two or more relatively common normal alleles for a single locus. The difference between a polymorphism and a mutation is that a polymorphism occurs commonly and is associated with a normal variant phenotype. The usual distinction is that a gene is polymorphic when its least frequent manifestation appears in at least 1% of the population. Examples include blood types and major histocompatibility complex molecules.

Polymorphisms may also occur without being associated with an obvious phenotype. For example, changes in nucleotide sequence within introns or in regions between genes would not necessarily result in altered proteins and would therefore be "silent." However, if these changes are polymorphic, ie, frequent, then there is a high probability that an individual might be heterozygous for the polymorphism. In other words, it would be likely that the two chromosomes of a diploid pair would carry different versions of the polymorphism. Then, if the chromosomal position of the polymorphic change were known, it could be used as a marker for mapping other genes. There are several varieties of DNA polymorphisms, and they provide the basis for gene mapping techniques that have identified several important cancer genes.

RFLPs appear as differences among individuals in the pattern of bands on a Southern blot probed with a single-cloned DNA. There are two mechanisms whereby DNA polymorphisms are detectable by Southern blotting. First, a single nucleotide change might either create or destroy the recognition site for a restriction endonuclease. This would cause an alteration in the Southern blot pattern of that gene when the DNA is digested with a particular restriction endonuclease. For example, if a stretch of DNA with the sequence . . . AGGATTTCGA . . . in one individual contained a single nucleotide change in a second individual so that the sequence was . . . AGGAATTCGA . . ., the recognition site for *Eco*RI (GAATTC) would be created (see Fig. 2-3). Digesting the second individual's DNA with *Eco*RI would generate two new restriction fragments and remove one old one when compared with the first individual's DNA.

The second mechanism involves one of the more mysterious features of genomic DNA in eukaryotes, namely, that it is replete with repeated sequences of unknown function. The sequences often stretch themselves along the DNA polymer, one set of sequences after the other, in so-called tandem repeats. In humans, the best known repetitive sequence is called *alu* (because it contains recognition sites for the restriction endonuclease *Alu*I), and its nucleotide sequence is so specific that it can be used to identify human DNA in a mixture of DNAs from many species. There are several examples of tandemly repeated sequences in which the number of tandem repeats varies among individuals.[25] One may have a DNA probe that recognizes a restriction fragment containing some tandem repeats. If the number of repeated sequences varies from one individual to the next, the size of the restriction fragment to which the probe hybridizes on a Southern blot will vary between the individuals. This will appear as an RFLP. These polymorphisms are called *variable number of tandem repeats* (VNTRs). In other cases, the repeat unit can be as small as two or three nucleotides (ie, di- or trinucleotide repeats), and polymorphisms can be recognized by changes in the size of PCR products containing these repeats (see below).

By either mechanism, these RFLPs are stably inherited in a mendelian fashion, which permits them to be used in gene mapping. RFLPs occur at specific positions (loci) in genomic DNA. If all of the affected individuals in a family with a particular genetic disease inherit the same RFLP, ie, presumptive evidence that the gene for the disease is close (or linked) to the RFLP locus. Linking a disease locus to an RFLP maps the gene for that disease and is the first step toward cloning the gene responsible for the disease. These are the tools of reverse genetics, which have also led to the identification of some of the genes associated with malignant transformation, such as the *BRCA1* gene on chromosome 17, whose mutations are responsible for a relatively significant fraction of heritable breast cancer.[26]

RFLPs have also been used to demonstrate gene loss in cancer (Fig. 2-8A). This approach relies on an individual being heterozygous for an RFLP, ie, having one polymorphism on one chromosome and another polymorphism on the other. If an individual with cancer is heterozygous for a particular RFLP (termed an *informative individual*), his or her tumor can be analyzed by Southern blotting, using the probe that recognizes the polymorphism, and compared with normal tissue analyzed the same way. If one of the RFLPs present in the heterozygous individual's normal DNA is missing from the tumor cell DNA, the tumor is said to have undergone a reduction to homozygosity or a loss of heterozygosity (LOH). This implies a loss of genetic material from the tumor, specifically the DNA that includes the missing RFLP. This is the hallmark of a tumor suppressor gene.[27] It was in this way that the involvement of the suppressor gene *TP53* was found in human colon cancers.[28]

A particularly interesting polymorphism is known as a microsatellite. For unknown reasons, about 50,000 copies of the repetitive sequence dC-dA (tandemly repeated 10-60 times) are dispersed throughout the human genome.[29] Because the longer tandem repeats (VNTRs, as mentioned earlier) have been called minisatellite DNA, the shorter dC-dA repeats are called microsatellite DNA. (The term *satellite* refers to the fact that the buoyant density of repetitive DNA is different from the majority of genomic DNA. This leads to the appearance of small satellite bands distinct from the main DNA band when genomic DNA is purified by density gradient centrifugation.) The number of repeats at a particular locus varies in a polymorphic way among individuals, and because these sequences are stably inherited, they can serve as polymorphic markers. The difference in the number of repeat units between two polymorphic microsatellites can be as small as a few nucleotides. These differences cannot be detected by Southern blotting, which has a resolution of 100 nt.

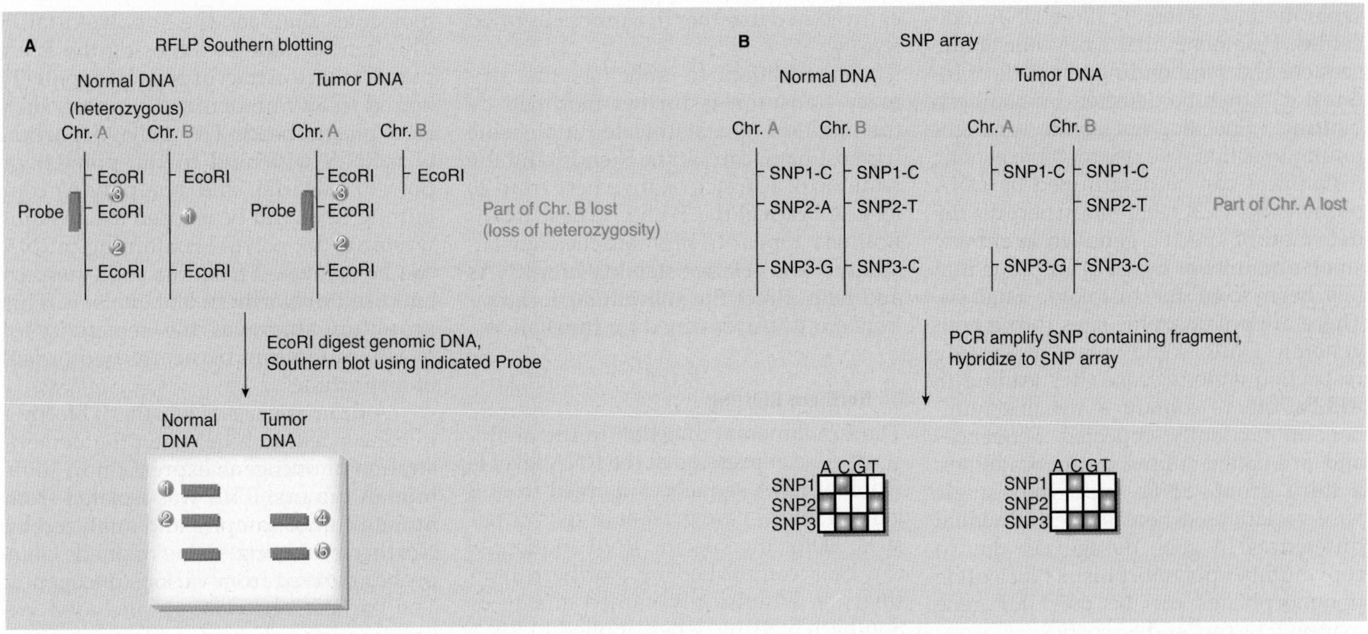

Figure 2-8 Methods to detect loss of heterozygosity in tumor tissue. (**A**) Restriction fragment length polymorphism (RFLP) and Southern blotting. In this example, an individual is heterozygous for an *Eco*RI recognition site: the second *Eco*RI site on chromosome A is absent on its diploid partner, chromosome B. The individual's tumor is assumed to be clonal and to have arisen from a cell that lost the region of chromosome B displayed in the figure. Southern blotting can then be performed using genomic DNA from the individual's normal DNA and tumor DNA in separate lanes of the agarose gel. Probing the DNA with the probe (indicated on the figure) reveals a heterozygous banding pattern in normal DNA (reflecting the presence of both polymorphisms, one on each chromosome pair) and a loss of that pattern in the tumor DNA. This is one of the hallmarks of a tumor suppressor gene. (**B**) Single nucleotide polymorphism (SNP) array. In this example, an individual is heterozygous for SNPs 2 and 3 and homozygous for SNP 1. Following the polymerase chain reaction (PCR) amplification of genomic fragments containing each SNP individually, these fragments are hybridized to an array composed of oligonucleotides complementary to the ones amplified. The loss of a heterozygous SNP signal on the array indicates loss of the chromosomal region containing this SNP.

However, these differences can easily be resolved using PCR. Primers that flank the repeat region are used in a PCR in the presence of radiolabeled deoxynucleotides, and the products are separated on a DNA sequencing-style polyacrylamide gel. Mini- and microsatellite polymorphic markers are much more useful in gene mapping than RFLPs because, unlike RFLPs, which usually have only two alleles, the variable number of repeats creates multiple alleles for each locus, significantly raising the likelihood that an individual will be heterozygous for the marker.

Although the number of repeats in a microsatellite marker is usually stable, in some cancers, most notably colorectal cancer, the number of microsatellite repeats in the tumors differs from that in normal colorectal tissue from the same patient. Because the variability in repeat number occurs at all positions throughout the genome of the tumor, this suggests that the tumors experience overall genetic instability.[30] The basis of this instability is believed to be a mutation in the human homologs of DNA "proofreading" genes that, when mutated in yeast, lead to the appearance of unstable numbers of dC-dA repeats. One of these human genes, *MSH2*, which maps to chromosome 2, is responsible for hereditary nonpolyposis colorectal cancer.[31]

Single nucleotide polymorphisms (SNPs) are one of the most common polymorphism within the human genome.[32] SNPs are single base variations within a coding or noncoding DNA sequence; they occur approximately once every 1350 base pairs in the average individual.[33] Analysis of SNPs has several uses in human cancer genetics. SNP analysis can be used to localize genes causing familiar cancers by linkage analysis.

SNP analysis is a powerful method to determine LOH in human cancers. The major approach for LOH is the use of microarrays (see below) that contain large numbers of human SNPs. PCR amplification of genomic DNA and hybridization to arrays permits the detection of chromosomal regions of LOH (Fig. 2-8B). This provides a high-throughput and automatable method for large-scale LOH analysis.[34] Furthermore, SNP analysis of LOH can be performed on laser-capture microdissected cells from paraffin-embedded tissue specimens, thereby allowing genomic studies on standard pathologic specimens.[35]

In addition to predicting LOH, SNP arrays can also be used for assaying overall genome-wide copy number changes and for identifying amplified chromosomal areas that frequently harbor oncogenes.[36] For example, *ERBB2*, *EGFR1*, *MYC*, and *CCND1* are oncogenes that are commonly overactivated owing to a significant increase in their copy number. In addition, recent studies revealed a high degree of copy number polymorphism among individuals that may be responsible for a larger fraction of interpersonal genetic variations than SNPs are.[37]

Comparative genomic hybridization, employed using whole-chromosome spreads or array-based platforms, is another method used for the detection of chromosomal copy number changes based on the comparison of the hybridization intensity of tumor and normal control DNA samples.[38] The resolution of the best available array comparative genomic hybridization is comparable to that of currently used SNP arrays (5 kb average across the genome). However, SNP arrays can more accurately predict LOH, thus allowing the quantitative determination of both chromosomal losses and gains and allelic changes in a single experiment.

Summary

Genomic DNA is too large to be analyzed easily in the laboratory, but it can be cut into manageable fragments using restriction endonucleases isolated from bacteria. Electrophoresis through an agarose gel can separate these fragments by size. Pulsed-field gel electrophoresis is a variation of this technique that allows the separation of extremely large DNA molecules. Fragments that carry nucleotide sequences corresponding to a gene of interest can then be detected by Southern blotting. Specific nucleotide changes (mutations) that give rise to stable genetic differences can be determined by DNA sequencing. PCR technology permits the detection of specific genes in extremely small amounts of tissue or in tissue that has been fixed for histologic analysis. There are polymorphic sites throughout genomic DNA; some create or destroy restriction endonuclease sites leading to RFLPs; others contain a variable number of tandemly repeated sequences and are called mini- or microsatellites; a third group, SNPs, represents single base variations; whereas interindividual differences in gene dosage are due to copy number polymorphism. Nucleotide polymorphisms can be used for gene mapping or cancer diagnostics.

Gene Expression: mRNA Transcript Analysis

Structural Considerations

The first step in gene expression is transcription of the genetic information in DNA into RNA. The individual building blocks of RNA, ribonucleotides, have the same structure as the deoxyribonucleotides in DNA, except that (1) the 2′ carbon of the ribose sugar is substituted with an OH group instead of H and (2) there are no thymine bases in RNA, only uracil (demethylated thymine), which also pairs with adenine by hydrogen bonding. Just like the DNA polymerases described earlier, the enzyme RNA polymerase II uses the nucleotide sequence of the gene's DNA as a template to form a polymer of ribonucleotides with a sequence complementary to the DNA template.

For transcription to be "correct," RNA polymerase II must (1) use the antisense strand of DNA as a template, (2) begin transcription at the start of the gene, and (3) end transcription at the end of the gene. The signals that ensure correct transcription are provided to the RNA polymerase II by DNA in the form of specific nucleotide sequences in the promoter of the gene. After reading and interpreting these signals, the RNA polymerase generates a primary RNA transcript that extends from the initiation site to the termination site in a perfect complementary match to the DNA sequence used as a template. However, not all transcribed RNA is destined to arrive in the cytoplasm as mRNA. Rather, by an incompletely understood process, sequences complementary to introns (see above) are excised from the primary transcript, and the ends of exon sequences are joined together in a process termed *splicing*.[39]

In addition to splicing, the primary transcript is further modified by the addition of a methylated guanosine triphosphate "cap" at the 5′ end[40] and the addition of a stretch of anywhere from 20 to 40 A bases at the 3′ end.[41] These modifications appear to promote the translatability[42] and relative stability of mRNAs and help direct the subcellular localization of mRNAs destined for translation.

Northern Blotting

The fundamental question in the analysis of gene expression at the RNA level is whether RNA sequences derived from a gene of interest are present in cells or tissues. Detecting specific RNA sequences can be accomplished by Northern blotting, the whimsically named analog of Southern blotting, when applied to RNA analysis. RNA can be isolated from cells in its intact form, free from significant amounts of DNA.[43] Messenger RNA is much smaller than genomic DNA, so it can be analyzed by agarose gel electrophoresis without the enzymatic digestion steps that are necessary for the analysis of high-molecular-weight DNA.

RNA is single-stranded and has a tendency to fold back on itself. This allows complementary bases on the same stretch of RNA to base-pair with each other and to form what is termed *secondary structure*. Because secondary structure can lead to aberrant electrophoretic behavior, RNA is electrophoretically separated by size in the presence of a denaturing agent, such as formaldehyde or glyoxal/dimethyl sulfoxide. After electrophoresis through a denaturing agarose gel, the RNA is transferred to a nitrocellulose or nylon-based membrane in the same manner as DNA for Southern blotting (see Fig. 2-4). Hybridization schemes and blot washing are essentially the same for Northern blotting as for Southern blotting. In this manner, specific RNA sequences corresponding to those in cloned DNA probes can easily be identified.

There is a lower limit to the sensitivity of Northern blotting so that only moderately abundant mRNAs can be detected using this technique. One way to increase the sensitivity of Northern blotting is to enrich the RNA preparation for mRNA. Ordinarily, mRNA makes up <10% of the total RNA content of a cell or tissue. When RNA is isolated from these sources, all RNA species are being isolated, ie, ribosomal and transfer RNA as well as mRNA. As noted earlier, most mRNAs destined for the cytoplasm and translation are modified by the addition of a 3′ poly(A) tract. An RNA preparation can, therefore, be greatly enriched for mRNA species by removing all RNA molecules that lack the 3′ poly(A) tail.[44] This can be done by exposing the RNA preparation to a tract of poly(U) or poly(T) bound to an immobilized support, such as a plastic bead. The poly(A) portion of mRNA will bind to the poly(U) or poly(T) material, and non-poly(A)-containing RNA can be washed away. After washing, the poly(A)-containing mRNA can be recovered from the solid support and used in Northern blot analysis. This procedure improves the sensitivity of Northern blotting by nearly two orders of magnitude.

A dramatic use of Northern blotting in cancer research has been the demonstration of oncogene expression in some human tumors. RNA was isolated from human tumor samples and analyzed by Northern blotting using cloned DNA probes derived from various oncogenes. The earliest observations included expression of c-*abl* and c-*myc* in human tumor cell lines and leukemic blasts.[45] Since then, however, a large number of proto-oncogenes have been shown to be transcribed in primary human tumor tissue.

Complementary DNA ■ The flow of genetic information usually runs from DNA to RNA to protein, according to the so-called central dogma of molecular biology. There are, however, exceptions to this rule, the most prominent of which involves the life cycle of retroviruses. These viruses encode their genetic information in RNA rather than DNA. When they invade a susceptible host cell, they direct the synthesis of a DNA intermediate that is a complementary copy of their genomic RNA. The enzyme that accomplishes this task, reverse transcriptase, is a DNA polymerase (see above) that uses RNA, rather than DNA, as a template to form a cDNA copy of the RNA.[46] This enzyme can be used in vitro to make cDNA copies of any available RNA.

One important application of cDNA synthesis has been the construction of cDNA libraries, which are basically gene libraries consisting only of the genes that are expressed in a cell or tissue of interest.[47] Most of the time, one is not really concerned with all of the DNA in the genome, eg, intron sequences, promoters, and vast regions of "uninformative" DNA that lie between genes. Furthermore, if one were interested in analyzing the genes expressed in a brain cell, why bother making a library that contained sequences for the hemoglobin gene? One way to construct a library comprising only tissue-specific expressed genes would be to clone all of the mRNA in a specific cell or tissue of interest. Unfortunately, there is no way to ligate single-stranded RNA to a double-stranded DNA cloning vector. However, one can use all of the mRNA in a cell as a template for making double-stranded cDNA, which can then be inserted into a cloning vector.

To make a cDNA library, one isolates all of the mRNA from a cell or tissue. Then, using this mRNA as a template, reverse transcriptase makes cDNA copies of each mRNA molecule in the mixture. The cDNA is ligated into a plasmid or phage vector as described earlier (see Fig. 2-3), and the recombinant vectors are introduced into bacteria. After growth on agar plates, each bacterial colony or phage plaque of a cDNA library houses a unique recombinant vector containing the cDNA copy of a single mRNA. Desired clones can be detected by nucleic acid hybridization to the plaques or colonies using a radiolabeled gene probe.[48] Alternatively, if the vector containing the cDNA molecules can direct transcription of mRNA by host bacterial cells, mRNA will be synthesized, and that mRNA will be translated. In this case, each bacterial colony or plaque will produce a different protein, and each protein will have been encoded by an mRNA from the original cell or tissue being investigated. If an antibody directed against a protein of interest is available, the cDNA clone corresponding to the mRNA that encodes that protein can be identified by binding the antibody to the colonies or plaques of the cDNA library.[49] This technique, called *expression cloning*, often employs the bacteriophage λgt11 as the cloning vector.

cDNA libraries can be used to clone cDNA for a known gene to discover the sequence of the mRNA it encodes. One application of this is the generation of expressed sequence tag databases by sequencing clones of various cDNA libraries. Alternatively, cDNA libraries can also be used to identify previously unknown genes. In a process called *differential screening*, cDNAs can be discovered that owe their existence to a particular differentiation or activation state in the cell of origin. For example, this technique has been used to identify genes whose expression is turned on by hormones or by growth factors.[50]

Sequence-Based Gene Expression Profiling

The most comprehensive way to display a unique pattern of gene expression that determines the identity of a cell or tissue would be to construct a cDNA library from it and sequence every clone. This was thought to be an impossible task and rather, a technique called *serial analysis of gene expression* (SAGE) was developed that achieved the same end in a practical manner. In SAGE, the investigator sequences a small and unique fragment of each expressed gene (called a SAGE tag) and quantifies the number of times it appears (called the SAGE tag number). The SAGE tag numbers, therefore, directly reflect the abundance of the corresponding transcript.

The sensitivity and the quantitative accuracy of SAGE are theoretically unlimited. The generation of a SAGE library does not require any prior knowledge of what genes are expressed in the cell of interest. Therefore, SAGE is able to detect and quantify the expression of previously uncharacterized genes.

The generation of a SAGE library used to be a technically challenging multistep procedure that has been described in detail.[51] However, the application of single-molecule sequencing platforms[20] changed this and now SAGE and other sequence-tag-based methodologies are fairly easy to perform. Figure 2-9 outlines the essence of the method.

SAGE has been used for the comparison of gene expression profiles of different cell types from normal and tumor tissue.[52] SAGE is one of the techniques used by the National Cancer Institute–funded Cancer Gene Anatomy Project (CGAP).[53] A goal of this project is to create a catalog of genes expressed in various normal and cancerous tissue types. To date, more than 120 different SAGE libraries have been deposited on the National Center for Biotechnology Education/CGAP SAGEmap Web site (http://cgap.nci.nih.gov/SAGE), which is now the largest source of public SAGE data.[53,54]

DNA Microarray Analysis

Another approach to comparative gene expression profiling employs the use of DNA microarrays, often referred to as DNA chips. Two basic types of DNA microarrays are currently available: oligonucleotide arrays[55] and cDNA arrays.[56] Both approaches involve the immobilization of DNA sequences in a gridded array on the surface of a solid support, such as a glass microscope slide or silicon wafer. In the case of oligonucleotide arrays, 25-nt long fragments of known DNA sequence are synthesized in situ on the surface of the chip using a series of light-directed coupling reactions similar to photolithography. Using this method, as many as 400,000 distinct sequences representing over 18,000 genes can be synthesized on a single 1.3 × 1.3 cm microarray. In the case of cDNA microarrays, cDNA fragments are deposited onto the surface of a glass slide using a robotic spotting device. For both microarray approaches, the next step involves the purification of RNA from the source of interest (eg, from a tumor), enzymatic fluorescent labeling of the RNA, and hybridization of the fluorescently labeled material to the microarray. Hybridization events are then captured by scanning the surface of the microarray with a laser-scanning device and measuring the fluorescence intensity at each position in the microarray. The fluorescence intensity of each spot on the array is proportional to the level of expression of the gene represented by that spot. This process is illustrated in Figure 2-10.

Microarray analysis has proven to be a powerful method for the analysis of gene expression patterns in human cancer and for cancer classification. Gene expression profiles have been used for class prediction, for determining which samples belong to which tumor class, and for class discovery of new tumor types. The first proof of principle for gene expression analysis in cancer was the demonstration that acute myeloid leukemias and acute lymphoid leukemias could be accurately distinguished.[57] Since then, new cancer classes have been discovered in leukemias,[58] lymphomas,[59] brain cancer,[60] breast cancer,[61,62] prostate cancer,[63] and lung cancer[64] among others.

The challenge now is not so much how to generate complex gene expression data but rather how to interpret it. The key is to develop methods for recognizing meaningful gene expression patterns and distinguishing those patterns from noise. Such noise (random gene expression levels) can be generated by (1) variability among microarrays, (2) variability in RNA labeling and hybridization methods, and, perhaps most importantly (3) biologic variability among samples. It is likely that all of the above sources of variability are significant. It has become clear that the successful elucidation of genetic networks through expression profiling requires the expertise of a new generation of scientists, namely, computational biologists. Improvements in DNA microarray fabrication will become valuable only if pattern recognition algorithms are similarly developed. Many of the problems associated with array-based technologies are eliminated with the use of sequence-based methods described earlier. Thus, as sequencing technologies improve and become more and more affordable, sequence-based approaches are likely to decrease or even eliminate the use of arrays for most experiments. It is also likely that the analysis of gene expression profiles that guides treatment planning of individual patients will be increasingly used in the clinical management of cancer patients.

Polymerase Chain Reaction

Another important use of cDNA technology has allowed PCR to be applied

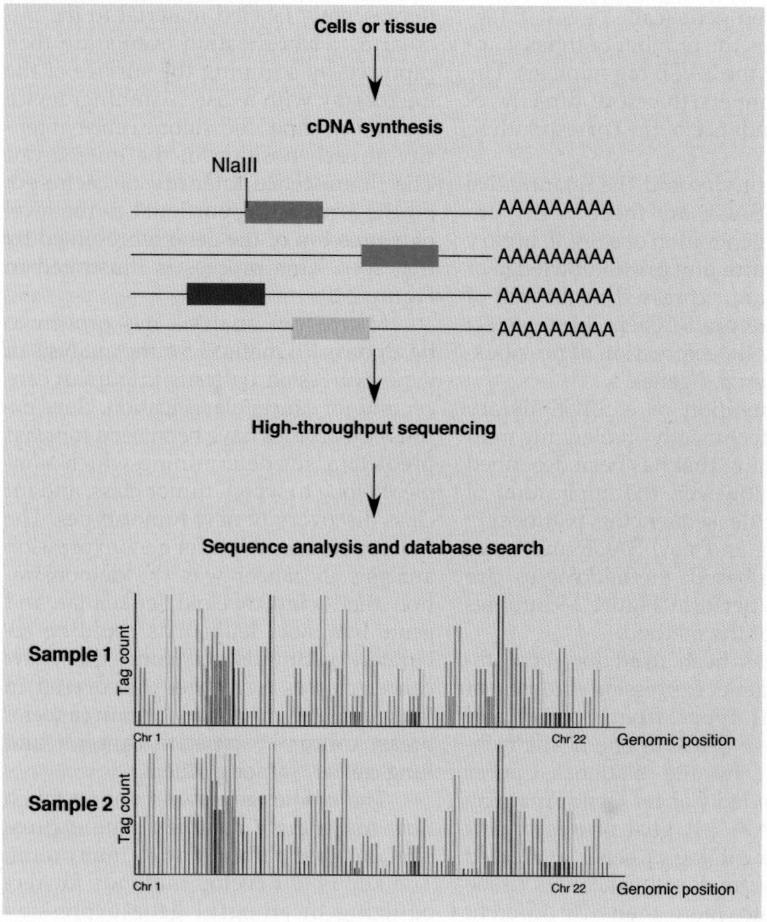

Figure 2-9 Construction and analysis of serial analysis of gene expression (SAGE) libraries. In step 1, a complementary deoxyribonucleic acid (cDNA) library is constructed from the cells or tissue of interest, and the cDNAs are immobilized on magnetic beads at their 3′ ends. In step 2, the cDNAs are subjected to restriction enzyme digestion with a so-called anchoring enzyme. This anchoring enzyme is a frequent cutter restriction endonuclease (usually *Nla*III) that ensures that all of the cDNAs are cut at least once. Subsequently another linker is ligated to the cDNA ends that contains a recognition site for a tagging enzyme. This tagging enzyme is a type two restriction endonuclease (usually *Mme*I) that cuts at some distance to the 3′ side of the actual recognition site. These tags are then directly processed for single-molecule DNA sequencing platform. Data are analyzed by using software that reads the sequence obtained, derives the tags, matches them to their cognate cDNA, and gives the gene expression profile in a numeric format.

to RNA. Because the *Taq* polymerase is a DNA polymerase (see above), it cannot use RNA as a template. Simply adding primers and *Taq* polymerase to an RNA preparation will not result in amplification. However, if an RNA of interest could be made into DNA, then PCR would proceed as usual.

The first step in this analysis is generating a cDNA copy of the mRNA of interest using reverse transcriptase. This can be done using a primer consisting of Ts [complementary to the poly(A) tail] or of a sequence complementary to some portion of the 3′ region of the mRNA. The 5′ primer can then be added along with *Taq* polymerase, and the single-stranded cDNA made in the first step will be amplified as described earlier (see Fig. 2-7). In one of the first applications of this technique, Philadelphia chromosome–positive leukemias were diagnosed by identifying chimeric *bcr-abl* mRNA species in clinical material using PCR. Since then, so-called reverse transcriptase PCR has come into widespread use.[65]

One inherent problem in using PCR to monitor mRNA expression is quantitation of the amplified PCR products. In Northern blotting or nuclease protection analysis, the intensity of the hybridization signal is directly proportional to the amount of target RNA in the sample. Thus, one can compare the number of RNA molecules in one sample with another. With PCR, a slight change in the efficiency of polymerization in an early cycle in one sample will lead to a geometrically increasing discrepancy between the amount of amplified product in that sample compared with another sample, and the amounts of PCR product when the reaction reaches saturation can also differ significantly. Fortunately, a number of techniques have been described for normalizing the products of PCRs to allow quantitative comparisons. Most notably, quantitative real-time PCR[66] is a method for continuous monitoring of amplification. This method makes quantitative comparisons of amplifications during the unbiased linear range in which each cycle gives a constant increase in amplification. In brief, quantitative real-time PCR takes advantage of a fluorogenic probe within the amplified region containing a fluorescent tag on one end and a quencher on the other end. Amplification also leads to digestion of the probe, now liberating a free fluorescent molecule; the increase in fluorescence is proportional to the amplification.

Clinical Application of Gene Expression Profiling

Recently three gene expression profiling-based diagnostic tests have been approved by the Federal Drug Administration (FDA) and introduced into the clinical management of patients diagnosed with early-stage breast cancer: OncotypeDX (Genomic Health, Redwood City, California), MammaPrint (Agendia BV, Amsterdam, the Netherlands), and H/I (AvariaDX, Carlsbad, California).[67] Oncotype DX was developed based on the testing of the expression of a candidate gene set (250 cancer-related genes) by quantitative real-time PCR in a large clinical trial with long-term follow-up (NSABP B14), and identifying a gene signature that predicted clinical outcome.[68] A gene signature composed of 21 genes predicted 10-year breast cancer recurrence. The expression levels of these 21 genes measured by quantitative RT-PCR combined with a quantitative algorithm are used to produce a number between 0 and 100, which is the recurrence score. The recurrence score is categorized into low (score <18), intermediate (score >18 but <30), and high (score ≥30). After the initial publication several follow-up studies have been performed in various cohorts and the Oncotype Dx recurrence score was found to have predictive power beyond that of conventional risk predictors (St. Gallen or National Comprehensive Cancer Network risk stratification guidelines). Mammaprint is evaluating the expression of a 70-gene

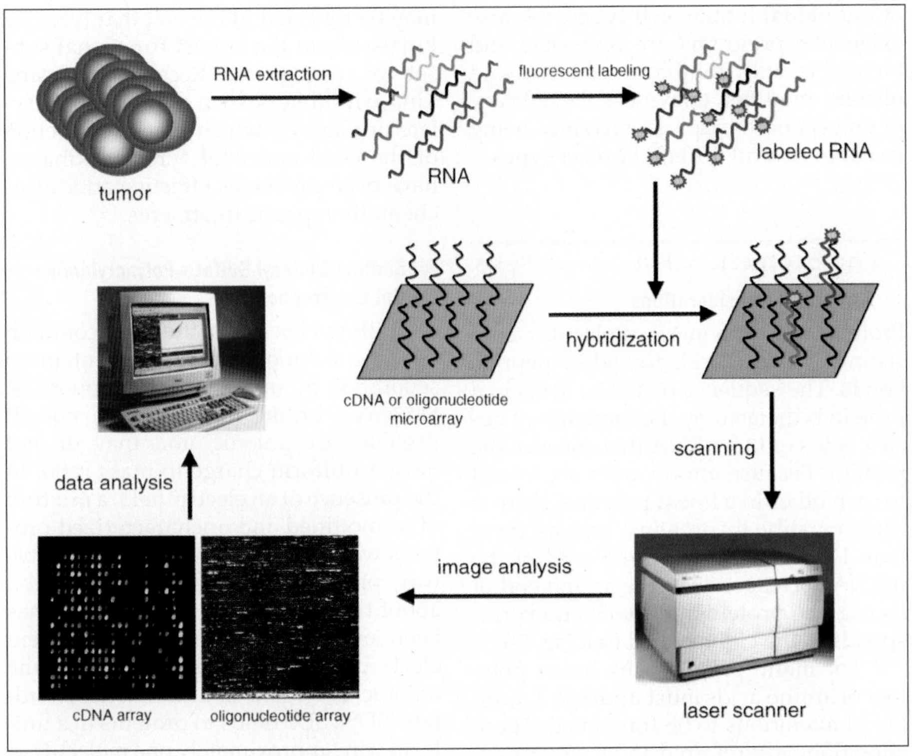

Figure 2-10 DNA microarray analysis. In this example, RNA extracted from a tumor is end-labeled with a fluorescent marker and then allowed to hybridize to a chip derivatized with complementary DNA (cDNAs) or oligonucleotides, as described in the text. The precise location of RNA hybridization to the chip can be determined using a laser scanner. Because the position of each unique cDNA or oligonucleotide is known, the presence of a cognate RNA for any given unique sequence can be determined.

signature derived from 25,000 candidate genes present on a cDNA array used for the initial study.[62] The test was developed at the Netherlands Cancer Institute by using 78 lymph node–negative patients younger than age 55 years who did not carry a *BRCA* gene mutation and who had tumors that were <5 cm in diameter. The end point in the initial study was 5-year distant metastasis recurrence. Patients are classified by calculating the correlation coefficient between a patient's expression levels of the 70 genes and an average good-prognosis expression profile. If the correlation coefficient exceeds 0.4, the patient is classified as having a good prognosis; if less, they are classified as having a poor prognosis. The H/I test is still in the developmental and validation phase, and based on a comparative study it was less accurate predicting outcome than other gene signatures.[69]

Ribozymes and RNA Interference

Some RNA molecules, in addition to proteins, have enzymatic activity. These RNAs, called ribozymes, can cleave RNA at sequence-specific sites.[70] They were originally discovered in *Tetrahymena* when it appeared that some of the primary RNA molecules in that species were capable of splicing out their introns without the aid of any protein enzymes. Ribozymes have also recently been described in higher organisms, and it is likely that they will be found to play a universal and important role in RNA processing. Sequence-specific ribozymes that will destroy specific mRNAs can be synthesized. One application of this technology is the introduction into malignant cells of ribozymes directed against activated oncogenes.

A different method to disrupt cellular RNA molecules is RNA interference (RNAi). RNAi is an evolutionarily conserved mechanism of gene regulation involving the production of short (18-21 nt) double-stranded that RNA results in gene silencing by inducing mRNA degradation. This phenomenon was first described in *Caenorhabditis elegans*[71] and plants[72] and later in *Drosophila melanogaster*.[73] In these model organisms, the introduction of long double-stranded RNA molecules results in potent suppression of the target gene expression in a sequence-specific manner. Subsequently, short RNA duplexes (19-29 nt), known as small interfering RNAs (siRNAs), were shown to induce silencing of genes in mammalian cells.[74] Although the full implications of RNAi on mammalian biology remains incompletely understood, RNAi has been widely adopted in research laboratories, for applications ranging from inhibiting the function of single genes in cell culture to developing gene therapy techniques in vivo to specifically target disease-associated alleles.[75]

Summary

The genetic information in DNA is copied, or transcribed, into mRNA by the enzyme RNA polymerase II. Before being transported to the cytoplasm, primary transcripts in the nucleus are modified by splicing out introns, adding a 5′ cap and adding a 3′ poly(A) tract. Cytoplasmic mRNA can be detected by Northern blotting, nuclease protection assays, or modified PCR. Although nuclease protection assays are technically somewhat more demanding than Northern blotting, they are more sensitive and can provide structural information about mRNA transcripts. A retroviral enzyme called reverse transcriptase can make cDNA copies of mRNA transcripts. These cDNAs can be cloned into cDNA libraries, which are useful for isolating and analyzing expressed genes. In the future, ribozymes and/or RNAi may be useful for the selective elimination of specific mRNA species.

Epigenetic Regulation

In recent decades the search for genes implicated in tumorigenesis focused on genes that are genetically altered in the tumors. However, recent progress in understanding the role of epigenetic regulation of tumor suppressor genes and oncogenes suggests that epigenetic modifications are also likely to play a role in tumorigenesis. Epigenetic regulatory programs depend on DNA methylation, chromatin (histone) modification, and noncoding RNAs. Each of these mechanisms has been shown to play a role in regulating cellular differentiation and tumorigenesis. For example, DNA methylation has been demonstrated to play an important role in silencing gene expression, imprinting, and X-chromosome inactivation.[76] Inherited defects in DNA methylation and imprinting result in developmental defects and increase the risk of tumorigenesis.[76] Recent data also implicate DNA methylation and chromatin changes as initiating events in neoplasia preceding the occurrence of genetic alterations.[77] This was experimentally proven in mice by introducing into the germline a hypomorphic allele of the DNA methyltransferase gene *DNMT1*, which led to 90% decrease in DNA methylation and subsequently to cancer development.[78]

The increased interest in analyzing epigenetic modifications led to the development of novel technologies that allow the analysis of these changes in a comprehensive manner and at genome-wide scale. Methylation-sensitive arbitrarily primed PCR (MS-AP-PCR),[79] methylated CpG island amplification followed by restriction difference analysis (MCA-RDA),[80] CpG island arrays coupled with differential methylation hybridization (DMH),[81] restriction length genome scanning (RLGS) using methylation sensitive enzymes,[82] methyl-CpG binding domain affinity chromatography,[83] and gene expression profiling following demethylation/deacetylation treatment[84] all have been successfully used for the identification of novel methylated loci in different cancer types.[85] Methylation-specific digital karyotyping (MSDK) is a sequence-based technology that enables comprehensive and unbiased genome-wide DNA methylation analysis.[86] Using a combination of a methylation-sensitive mapping enzyme (eg, *Eag*I) and a fragmenting enzyme (eg, *Nla*III), short sequence tags can be obtained and uniquely mapped to genome location. The number of MSDK tags obtained from a sample reflects the methylation status of the mapping enzyme sites.

DNA methylation and chromatin modification are interrelated processes and noncoding RNAs may link the two processes together.[85,87] In the past few years the number and type of known histone modifications increased dramatically, and a large set of enzymes has been identified that play a role in mediating these processes.[87] Thus, the four core histones (H2A, H2B, H3, and H4) have been found to subject to various posttranslational modifications, including acetylation, methylation, phosphorylation, ubiquitination, sumoylation, ADP ribosylation, deimination, and proline isomerization. Most of these modifications regulate transcription by influencing the recruitment of other proteins, and a few of them are also involved in DNA repair and chromatin condensation. Using antibodies specifically recognizing methylated histone H3-lys9 and the recently developed ChIP-on-chip,[88] GMAT (genome-wide mapping technique),[89] and ChIP-Seq[90] technologies, it is possible to analyze heterochromatin changes at a genome-wide scale.

Summary

The role of epigenetic programs in tumor initiation and progression is becoming increasingly clear. In fact, it is hypothesized that epigenetic alterations may precede genetic events and promote the acquisition of these changes. Due to the interest in the field and the development of new technologies, a human epigenome project is planned that will determine the comprehensive epigenetic profiles of individual human cell types. Because epigenetic programs are reversible and targetable with inhibitors of DNA and histone modifier enzymes, the efficacy of epigenetic therapy is currently being tested in several different cancer types.

Gene Expression: Protein Analysis

Structural Considerations

Proteins are polymeric molecules consisting of amino acids linked by peptide bonds. The sequence of amino acids in a protein is dictated by the sequence of nucleic acids in the mRNA that encodes the protein. Because amino acids are joined to each other in a linear polymer, there is directionality to proteins, just as there is to DNA and RNA. The 5′ end of the mRNA corresponds to the amino end of its cognate protein and the 3′ end corresponds to the carboxy end (see Fig. 2-1).

For many proteins, the linear polymer of amino acids must undergo a number of alterations to be functional. These alterations are referred to as *posttranslational modifications*. For example, proteins destined to be secreted from a cell initially exist as propeptides with a 20- to 30-amino acid sequence at their amino ends. This highly hydrophobic tail, called a *leader sequence*, remains embedded in the membranes of the endoplasmic reticulum and secretory granule until the protein is to be secreted, at which point, the leader sequence is cleaved. There are many examples of propeptides that undergo cleavage of specific amino acids before they become mature, functional proteins.

Other posttranslational modifications include the addition of various nonpeptide substituents to the side chains of amino acids. These include simple and complex carbohydrate chains, sulfate groups, and phosphate groups. Phosphorylation of intracellular proteins, usually on serine, threonine, or tyrosine residues, plays an important regulatory role in protein function. For example, many of the cell surface receptors for growth factors, such as the platelet-derived growth factor (PDGF) receptor[91] and the receptor for macrophage colony-stimulating factor (M-CSF),[92] are themselves protein tyrosine kinases. When this type of receptor binds its ligand, the receptor undergoes a conformational change that activates its kinase activity. The activated receptor then adds phosphate groups to some of its own tyrosine residues and to tyrosines in other proteins. These phosphorylations are part of the signal transduction process, whereby a message is sent from the cell surface receptor to the nucleus. The importance of tyrosine phosphorylation in cell growth may be reflected in the fact that tyrosine kinases form the largest functional subset of oncogenes. Recently, tyrosine kinase inhibitors, such as imatinib mesylate or Gleevec, which blocks the action of the c-abl and c-kit tyrosine kinases, have been proven as effective anticancer chemotherapeutic treatments.[15,93]

Sodium Dodecyl Sulfate-Polyacrylamide Gel Electrophoresis

As with nucleic acids, the most common analytic technique applied to proteins is separation by size using electrophoresis. However, unlike nucleic acids, not all proteins are anionic, and they do not have a uniform charge-to-mass ratio. In the presence of an electric field, a mixture of unmodified and uncharacterized proteins would migrate in an unpredictable way, providing little or no information about their structures. This problem has been overcome by performing protein electrophoresis in the presence of the anionic detergent sodium dodecyl sulfate (SDS). SDS binds to proteins in a uniform way, approximately one molecule of SDS for every two amino acids. Thus, all proteins become polyanions in the presence of SDS, and the number of negative charges (supplied by the sulfate group in SDS) is directly proportional to the size, or molecular weight, of the protein.

Because proteins are generally smaller than the most commonly analyzed nucleic acids, electrophoresis is performed through a solid support made of polyacrylamide, which resolves low-molecular-weight molecules better than agarose. In the presence of an electric field, proteins in SDS will migrate toward the anode at a rate inversely proportional to the log of their molecular weights.[94] {Weber, 1969 #1393} Proteins can be analyzed by sodium dodecyl sulfate-polyacrylamide gel electrophoresis (SDS-PAGE) in the presence or absence of β-mercaptoethanol (β-ME), which reduces sulfhydryl groups on the side chains of cysteines that can bind two separate protein chains together. Electrophoresis in the presence of β-ME permits the analysis of protein subunits whereas electrophoresis in the absence of β-ME can reveal multimeric protein associations. SDS-PAGE is routinely employed to test the purity of a protein preparation. It is also an integral component of the techniques of immune precipitation and Western blotting.

Immunoblotting

One of the most valuable immunologic identification techniques is immunoblotting (Fig. 2-11A).[95] A mixture of proteins can be electrophoretically separated by SDS-PAGE, and the separated proteins can be transferred to a nitrocellulose or nylon-based filter by electrophoresis in a direction perpendicular to that of the first electrophoresis. The proteins will remain bound to the membrane support. By analogy to Southern blotting for DNA and Northern blotting for RNA, this technique for protein transfer has been called Western blotting. The protein blot can be soaked in a solution that contains a specific antibody that binds to the protein of interest. The presence of the bound antibody on the blot can then be detected if the antibody is labeled. The label can be an enzyme that reveals its presence by catalyzing a color or light-emitting reaction, or it can be a radionuclide, such as ^{125}I, that can be detected by autoradiography. Alternatively, an unlabeled antibody can be detected by washing the blot in a solution that contains a labeled anti-immunoglobulin antibody. This technique has been used to demonstrate overexpression of the HER2/*neu* protein in some breast cancers in which Southern blotting revealed no gene amplification.[96] Because the protein is the effector of gene function and the determinant of phenotype, overexpression of the protein can be highly significant and is often considered to be the "gold standard" of overexpression.

Immune Precipitation

A primary goal of molecular biology is to use gene probes to detect the presence of a particular gene in a complex mixture of DNAs or RNAs. In a similar way, a specific antibody can be used as a probe to detect the presence of a particular protein in a complex mixture of proteins. An antibody directed against a protein of interest can be added to a mixture of proteins under conditions that allow the antibody to bind to its target protein (Fig. 2-11B). One can then collect all of the immunoglobulins in that mixture by adding a protein that binds to immunoglobulins, such as anti-immunoglobulin antibodies or staphylococcal protein A. These proteins are often bound to a solid support, such as polystyrene beads, which can be removed from the solution by gentle centrifugation. As the beads collect at the bottom of the centrifuge tube, their attached immunoglobulin and target proteins collect there as well. When boiled in SDS and β-ME, the protein complexes dissociate, and they can be electrophoretically separated by SDS-PAGE. This process is called immune precipitation. To document the specificity of the antibody, a second immune precipitation is usually performed with a control antibody that does not bind the protein of interest. The two precipitations can be run side by side on SDS-PAGE, and the protein of interest can be identified by its presence in the experimental lane and its absence from the control lane. The proteins can be identified by staining reactions or, if the protein preparation is radiolabeled, by autoradiography.

An important application of this technique was the demonstration that the protein product of the retinoblastoma susceptibility gene (*Rb*) binds to proteins encoded by DNA tumor viruses. Antibodies directed against adenovirus proteins were used in an immune precipitation of proteins from cells transformed or infected by adenovirus. In addition to the adenovirus proteins, the precipitated proteins contained another protein that was proven to be the protein encoded by the retinoblastoma susceptibility gene.[97] Similar experiments using antibodies directed against the large T antigen of SV40 revealed an interaction between the T antigen protein and the RB protein.[98] In both cases, these interactions appear to be central to the mechanisms whereby these viruses oncogenically transform susceptible host cells.

Enzyme-Linked Immunosorbent Assay

Measurement of serum protein levels can be a valuable tool in cancer screening, cancer diagnosis, and monitoring the results of therapy. One of the most important applications of this approach is the measurement of prostate-specific antigen (PSA) levels for the detection and follow-up of prostate cancer.[99] The method used to measure PSA and other serum protein levels is ELISA.[100] This method is diagrammed in Figure 2-11C. The principle is essentially the same as immune precipitation, except that instead of binding the antibody to protein A beads, the specific antibody is immobilized onto the surface of a transparent plastic plate. The specific test protein then binds to the antibody (ie, the immunosorbent part of the assay), and other proteins are washed away. A second antibody, which recognizes a distinct epitope or antigenic region of the same antigenic protein, is then added. This antibody is covalently coupled to an enzyme (hence the enzyme-linked part). Specific binding of the second antibody leads to an enzyme concentration proportional to the amount of protein. The addition of a substrate for a fluorescent, chemiluminescent, or colorimetric reaction then gives a signal proportional to the amount of enzyme and hence the amount of antigenic protein. Small molecule concentrations (eg, drug levels) can be measured in the same way if there are two independent antibodies, both of which can bind to the molecule at the same time.

Protein Sequencing

The ultimate in protein identification is direct determination of amino acid sequence. Automated sequenators are now available that have considerably simplified this technically demanding analysis. In addition, recent advances in protein chemistry have permitted sequencing to be performed on mere picomoles of protein. In fact, Western blotting can be used to purify small amounts of protein, and the fragment of the blot containing the stained protein of interest can be used directly in an automated sequenator.[101]

Direct protein sequencing was responsible for ushering in the modern era of molecular oncology. The protein encoded by the oncogene v-*sis*, the transforming gene of the simian sarcoma virus, was found to be nearly identical to the empirically determined amino acid sequence of the B chain of human PDGF.[102] This was the first demonstration of a connection between oncogenes and the components involved in normal cellular proliferation.

Mass Spectrometry

Dramatic advances in mass spectrometric methods in recent years have made mass spectrometry a preferred method for protein analysis and offer promise for use in diagnostic analysis as well. Mass spectrometry is a technique to convert molecules into ions and then to measure their mass. The distinct mass of a given protein is a method to identify that protein in a mixture. Furthermore, proteins can be identified unambiguously by tandem mass spectrometry, in which the proteins are first fragmented into peptides and separated, and then the peptides are fragmented further for sequencing.[103] Mass spectrometry is summarized briefly in Figure 2-12. An excellent review article is available.[104]

Engineered Protein Expression

The final goal of many experiments in molecular biology is the use of biologic systems to synthesize the protein encoded by the gene being studied. This process, called engineered protein expression, can be an experimental end in itself. When the expressed protein synthesized by recombinant DNA methods can be shown to have all of the properties of the natural protein, this is considered to be proof that the proper gene has been cloned. Alternatively, expression can be an end in itself when one wants to produce large amounts of a particular protein that might be difficult to obtain from natural sources.

In Vitro Translation ■ One very simple expression method is in vitro translation, in which translation occurs entirely in a test tube. All of the components necessary for translating mRNA can be obtained from cells that are highly efficient in protein synthesis, such as reticulocytes (usually

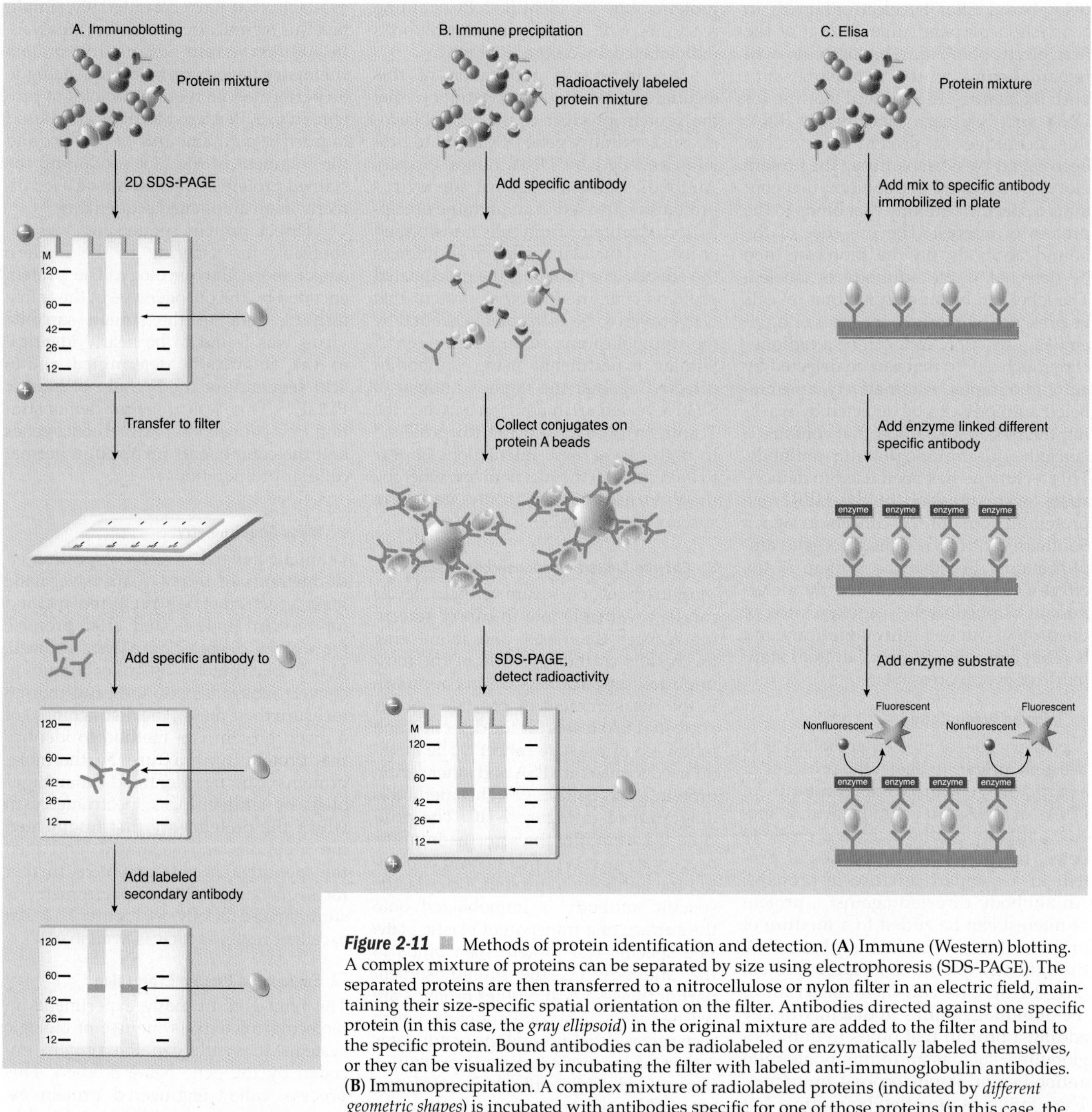

Figure 2-11 ■ Methods of protein identification and detection. (**A**) Immune (Western) blotting. A complex mixture of proteins can be separated by size using electrophoresis (SDS-PAGE). The separated proteins are then transferred to a nitrocellulose or nylon filter in an electric field, maintaining their size-specific spatial orientation on the filter. Antibodies directed against one specific protein (in this case, the *gray ellipsoid*) in the original mixture are added to the filter and bind to the specific protein. Bound antibodies can be radiolabeled or enzymatically labeled themselves, or they can be visualized by incubating the filter with labeled anti-immunoglobulin antibodies. (**B**) Immunoprecipitation. A complex mixture of radiolabeled proteins (indicated by *different geometric shapes*) is incubated with antibodies specific for one of those proteins (in this case, the *gray ellipsoid*). After the antibodies have bound to their protein, small polystyrene or agarose beads containing staphylococcal protein A are added to the mixture. Protein A binds to the antibodies, and when centrifuged, the beads to which the protein A is bound will sediment to the bottom of the centrifuge tube, taking along the antibodies and the specific protein to which they have bound. The unbound proteins remain in the supernatant and can be removed. After boiling to dissociate the protein A/antibody/protein complex, specifically precipitated radiolabeled protein can be visualized by electrophoresis (SDS-PAGE) and autoradiography. (**C**) Enzyme-linked immunosorbent assay (ELISA). To perform ELISA, one needs to develop two independent antibodies that bind to the protein to be detected (*gray ellipsoid* in this example) with high specificity and affinity. One of these antibodies is then coupled to a plate, which is then incubated with the protein mix to be analyzed (this can be tissue, blood, or another body fluid). The specifically bound protein is retained on the plate and is detected with the second antibody generated against it that is coupled to an enzyme or isotope, allowing quantitation of the bound protein. ELISAs are usually very sensitive and can detect picomolar amounts of proteins.

from rabbits) or wheat germ. Under the appropriate conditions, and in the presence of all 20 amino acids, a synthetic or purified RNA added to such a system will be efficiently translated into protein. If a radioactive amino acid, such as [^{35}S]methionine, is included in the mix, the reaction products can be analyzed by SDS-PAGE and autoradiography. Demonstrating an appropriately sized protein or one that is recognized by a specific antibody constitutes good evidence that the mRNA in hand is the one the investigator desires.

Large-Scale Production of Recombinant Proteins ■ In vitro translation can be applied only at a small-scale analytic level. To produce large amounts of protein, one must turn to in vivo expression systems. One of the simplest involves cloning the cDNA for the desired protein into a bacterial plasmid or phage that contains a transcriptional promoter active in bacteria. When introduced into the appropriate bacterial host, large amounts of mRNA will be transcribed, which, in turn, will be translated into protein. The recombinant protein can then be purified away from all of the bacterial proteins. This is the way in which some clinically available interferons[105] have been produced.

As noted earlier, many eukaryotic proteins require posttranslational modifications for maximal activity. Bacteria do not have the machinery required to accomplish complex modifications, such as the addition of specific carbohydrate groups. Moreover, the interior milieu of a bacterial cell is a reducing environment so that disulfide bonds essential to the structure and function of many eukaryotic proteins cannot form. When these modifications are required, mammalian cells can be used for expression. The basic concept is the same as in bacterial systems: a cDNA is cloned into a vector with a eukaryotic transcriptional promoter, and the resulting recombinant DNA is introduced into mammalian cells.[106] However, there are still significant disadvantages in the use of mammalian cells for large-scale recombinant protein production. Mammalian cells are expensive to grow in vitro because they require a medium rich in nutrients and growth factors. Yeast cells, insect cells, and even plant cells are being exploited as an attractive compromise between mammalian cell culture and bacterial culture for protein expression. These eukaryotic cells can execute most of the posttranslational modifications required by mammalian proteins, including disulfide bonding. At the same time, these cells are easier and more economical to grow in vitro. A number of expression vectors analogous to those described here for bacteria and animal cells have been developed for these alternative eukaryotic hosts. Interested readers are referred to other sources for in-depth descriptions.[107]

Methods for Analyzing Protein–Protein Interactions ■ An important and challenging task in postgenomic biology is to understand the function of proteins encoded by the genome and to determine their involvement in signaling pathways and

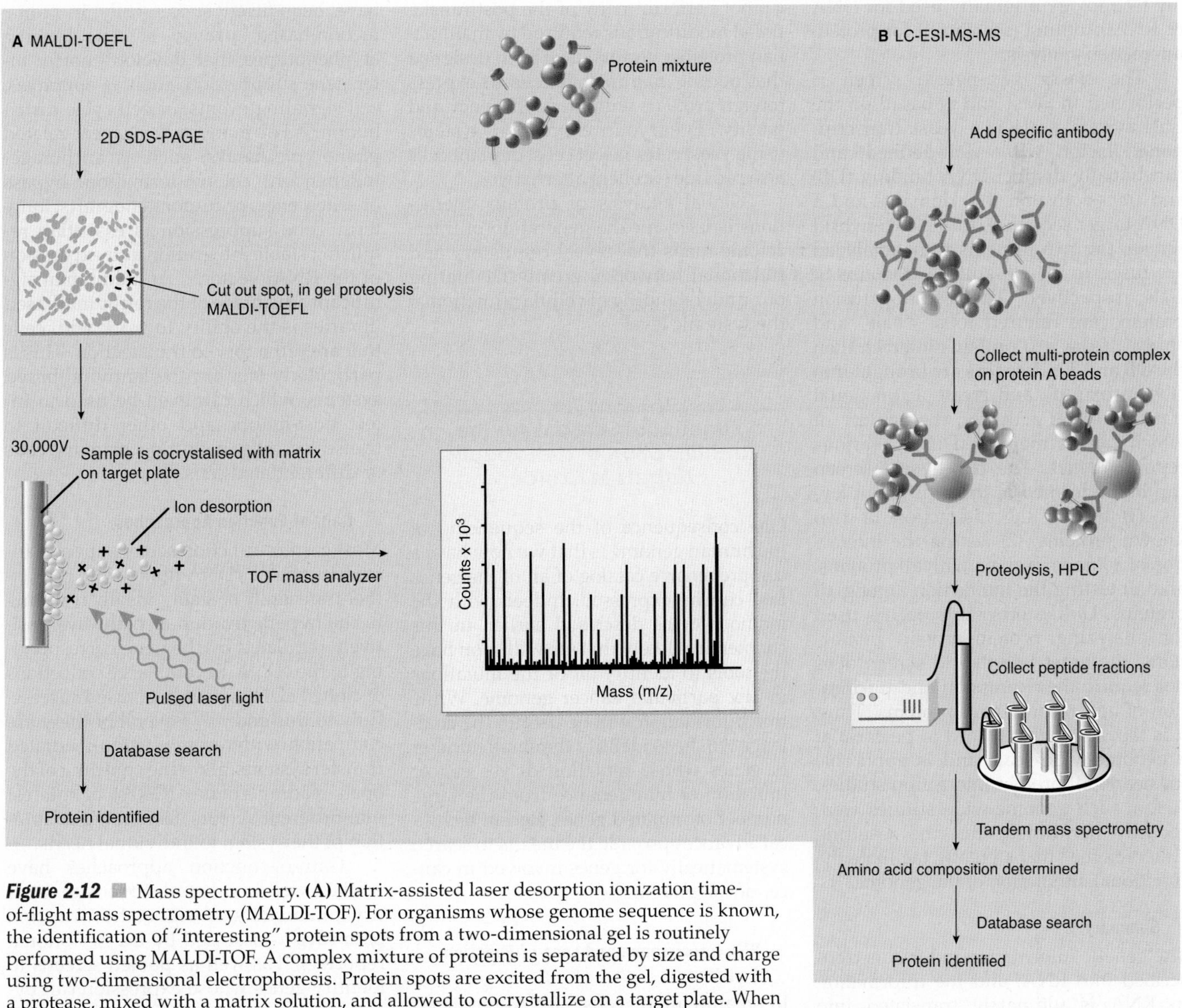

Figure 2-12 ■ Mass spectrometry. **(A)** Matrix-assisted laser desorption ionization time-of-flight mass spectrometry (MALDI-TOF). For organisms whose genome sequence is known, the identification of "interesting" protein spots from a two-dimensional gel is routinely performed using MALDI-TOF. A complex mixture of proteins is separated by size and charge using two-dimensional electrophoresis. Protein spots are excited from the gel, digested with a protease, mixed with a matrix solution, and allowed to cocrystallize on a target plate. When a laser is fired at the target plate, the matrix absorbs the laser light's energy and vaporizes, carrying some of the sample with it into a vacuum space. At the time the laser is fired, a high voltage is applied to the target plate to accelerate the ionized sample's movement toward the time-of-flight (TOF) mass analyzer. The resulting peptide fingerprint can then be used to search databases to determine the identity of the protein. **(B)** The liquid chromatography electrospray ionization tandem mass spectrometry (LC-ESI-MS-MS) can be used to obtain amino acid sequence information, allowing highly refined database searches. The approach employs capillary high-performance liquid chromatography (HPLC), which allows very slow (submicroliter/min) flow rates that are essential for obtaining high-sensitivity ESI-MS-MS of peptides. Following the liquid chromatography and electrospray ionization, the ions are analyzed by linearly linked tandem mass spectrometers that yield amino acid composition information.

cellular networks. One approach to understanding protein function is to investigate its interaction with other proteins of known function. By performing such analysis at a genome-wide level, one can create protein–protein physical interaction networks.[108] These networks can be combined with gene expression or other genomic data to generate regulatory and signaling networks at the cellular level. Several methods allow the characterization of protein–protein interactions at a genome-wide scale.[108] These include comprehensive protein pull-down assays, protein chips, and two-hybrid screens. Comprehensive protein pull-down assays use the combination of immunoprecipitation and mass spectrometric methods discussed earlier, whereas protein chips are the application of the microarray technology originally used for DNA or RNA profiling (see above) for protein interaction analysis.

The classic two-hybrid screen is performed in yeast and is based on the Gal4 system. Gal4 is a yeast transcriptional factor with well-defined and functionally distinct DNA binding (DB) and *trans*-activator (TA) domains and a DNA target sequence. In the two-hybrid screen, the two proteins to be analyzed are fused to the DB and TA domains of Gal4, respectively. The resulting fusion proteins are referred to as "bait" and "prey." If the two proteins interact, then the DB and TA domains are brought into close proximity and create a functional transcriptional activator, the activity of which can be monitored using various reporter genes. The two-hybrid screen can be performed at three different levels: (1) testing the interaction of two known proteins, (2) testing the interaction of a known protein with all proteins, and (3) testing the interaction among all proteins. Unlike other approaches used for analyzing protein–protein interactions, the yeast two-hybrid screen does not require the expression and purification of any recombinant proteins. Thus, it is fairly straightforward to perform at a genome-wide scale and is applicable for nearly all protein interaction studies. A few such genome-wide studies were recently performed, and the resulting "interactome" maps greatly facilitate the functional annotation of the genome.[109]

Summary

The genetic information in DNA is transcribed into RNA, and the information in RNA is ultimately translated into protein. Like DNA and RNA, proteins are also directional. The amino and carboxy termini of proteins are specified by the 5′ and 3′ ends, respectively, of their cognate mRNAs. After translation, proteins may require further modification to be fully functional.

Proteins can be fractionated by size using electrophoresis through polyacrylamide gels in the presence of the anionic detergent SDS (SDS-PAGE). SDS-PAGE is an integral component of the analytic techniques of immune precipitation and Western blotting. Automated analyzers are now available that can directly determine the amino acid sequence of a protein using vanishingly small amounts of material.

The mRNA that encodes a protein can be translated in vitro using cellular extracts of rabbit reticulocytes or wheat germ. The DNA that encodes a protein can be transcribed and the RNA translated in vivo by using appropriate vector and host cell combinations in culture. Bacterial cells are simple and economical vehicles for expressing foreign genes, but they cannot perform many of the posttranslational modifications required by mammalian proteins. Vectors have been designed that permit mammalian cells to express foreign proteins with great efficiency and fidelity. Eukaryotic expression systems using yeast cells, insect cells, or plant cells also provide excellent alternatives.

Global analysis of protein interactions is used for the generation of interactome maps that reveal regulatory and functional networks, greatly facilitating our understanding of cellular function at the systemic level.

Functional Screens for the Identification of Therapeutic Targets in Cancer

One consequence of the sequencing of the human genome is that we now have a comprehensive catalog of all of the genes that can be expressed. Indeed with the methodologies described earlier, in this chapter. it is likely that we will soon have the tools to identify all of the mutations in any particular cancer genome. While this information will be useful, the challenge will be to identify the small number of genes whose mutation drives cancer initiation or maintenance from the large number of mutated genes. Recent technical advances provide the means to search systematically for genes involved in cancer development.

RNA Interference and Loss-of-Function Genetics

In mammalian cells, RNAi-mediated gene suppression can be induced by the introduction of chemically synthesized siRNAs, or plasmids expressing short hairpin RNA, known as shRNAs, which get processed to siRNAs by Dicer.[110] In either case, the siRNA becomes incorporated into the RNA-induced silencing complex (RISC) and directs sequence-specific-mediated degradation or translational suppression of the target mRNA, resulting in decreased protein expression.[111] Although siRNAs are easily synthesized and highly effective in inducing gene knockdown, such oligonucleotide reagents are relatively expensive and can only be used for transient loss-of-function experiments. Vector-based systems offer the possibility of adding selectable markers, such as drug resistance, stable expression of the RNAi construct, as well as being a renewable resource through propagation in bacteria. More recently, inducible RNAi vectors have also been developed, allowing fine temporal and spatial regulation of RNAi-induced gene knockdown.[112]

Both siRNA and shRNA libraries have been used successfully in transfection-based arrayed screens looking at phenotypes that develop shortly after gene suppression, such as apoptosis, cell signaling events, or cell cycle distribution.[113] For many other cancer-related phenotypic assays, such as anchorage-independent colony formation, bypass of senescence, or tumor xenografts, long-term gene suppression is essential, requiring stable integration and expression of the RNAi vector.[114] An additional significant advantage of the retroviral-based libraries is the ability to work with cells that are refractory to transfection. This is particularly true for the lentiviral-based systems, which can even be used to infect post-mitotic and other difficult to transduce cells, including primary cells or differentiated cells.[115]

Gain-of-Function Approaches

Most gain-of-function screens involve introduction of a cDNA library into cells either transiently or stably, ideally resulting in the hyperactivation of pathways positively regulated by the gene corresponding to the cDNA. Several large collections of cloned cDNAs have been used successfully to this end.[116,117] Several of these are compatible with recombination-mediated transfer systems, allowing shuttling of the open reading frames (ORFs) of interest into different vectors, facilitating adaptation of the system to individual needs.

Gain-of-function approaches have worked well in arrayed screens to identify modulators of signal transduction pathways as assessed by transcriptional reporters,[118] as well as pooled screens to identify genes whose expression can bypass senescence or anti-estrogen treatment.[117] Most of these arrayed screens have employed transient expression by transfection, an approach that works well with transcriptional reporter-driven systems focused on short-term events. In contrast, for many screens relevant to oncogenic transformation require long-term expression and selection, necessitating stable integration of cDNA expression vectors.

Another type of gain-of-function approach utilizes microRNA (miRNA) expression libraries to screen using phenotypic assays. miRNAs are endogenous small RNAs that function by downregulating expression of their target genes, either through induction of transcript degradation or translational inhibition. Nearly 500 annotated human miRNAs have been described, most of which do not have identified targets or functions.[119] miRNAs implicated in cancer include let-7, a negative regulator of RAS found upregulated in lung cancers[120]; the miR-17-92 cluster, which is upregulated in lymphomas and can promote lymphomagenesis[121]; and miR-15 and miR-16, negative regulators of BCL2, that are downregulated in chronic lymphocytic leukemia.[122] These examples suggest that true extent of the contribution of miRNAs to tumorigenesis is not yet known. Thus, further functional studies are necessary. For example, recent work using a retroviral expression library of miRNAs identified miR-372 and miR-373 in a Ras-induced senescence bypass screen, suggesting possible oncogenic function for these miRNAs.[123] Future applications of this approach will likely yield many more cancer-relevant miRNAs and the identification of their respective targets are also likely to provide further insight into the oncogenic process.

Summary

Increasingly, unbiased genome-wide functional screens have been used for the identification and validation of novel therapeutic targets in cancer. Although most of these screens are performed in cell culture models, in combination with the analysis of primary human tumor samples several of them resulted in the discovery of genes with key roles in tumorigenesis. Improvements in culture models and the application of these technologies in animal models increase the likelihood that the findings are validated in human cancer patients.

Mouse Models of Human Cancer

Despite advances in our understanding of the biology of cancer at the molecular level, the application of this knowledge to the clinical management of cancer patients has been lagging behind. One of the factors limiting the translation of discoveries made in the laboratory to the clinic has been the availability of in vivo animal models of cancer that faithfully reproduce the human disease. Animals, particularly rodents, have been used in cancer research for decades to explore fundamental biological properties of tumors and to evaluate anti-neoplastic therapies.[124] Initially, such rodent models were largely limited to spontaneous or carcinogen-induced neoplasms, or more commonly the ectopic or orthotopic transplantation of murine or human tumor cells into syngeneic or immunodeficient mice. Although none of these approaches accurately represents the complexity of human cancer, preclinical studies with these models are nonetheless traditionally required as efficacy data during the regulatory approval of investigational new anti-neoplastic agents. Improved animal cancer models became available with the advent of genetically engineered mouse models (GEMM) of cancer following advances in molecular biology and embryology in the early 1980s. GEMM's enabled the direct investigation of potential tumorigenic genes in vivo, and today models that accurately represent nearly every major human cancer exist.[125] The first generation of GEMMs was transgenic tumor-prone mice produced through the ectopic introduction of activated oncogenes. Indeed, such "oncomice" confirmed the tumorigenic properties of c-Myc, Ras, and several viral oncoproteins through the development of lymphoma, breast cancer, and pancreatic cancer.[126] Although many early oncomouse models were informative, most human cancers could not be accurately modeled using this approach, likely due to the nonphysiological properties inherent in ectopic expression cassettes and tissue mosaicism. An alternative early approach to model human cancer was through the disruption or "knockout" of endogenous putative tumor suppressor alleles that were identified in cancer prone kindreds. Indeed, knockout mice confirmed Knudsen's hypothesis of tumor suppressor gene function, although the tumor spectrum in such KO mice oftentimes was quite distinct from the cognate human condition. A detailed description of the basic methodologies required for the generation of transgenic and knockout mice can be found in an excellent manual on the manipulation of the mouse embryo.[127] These early mouse models were very powerful in validating the cancer-relevant role of particular genes or their combination in tumorigenesis and allowed the identification of cooperating genetic alterations by insertional mutagenesis. However, a major drawback of these early mouse models is that genetically engineered mutations are present in every cell of the mouse. This is problematic for multiple reasons. First, it can lead to embryonic lethality or abnormalities if the affected oncogene or tumor suppressor gene is required for normal development. Second, with the exception of hereditary cancer predisposition syndromes, the modus operandi of these mutational events does not reproduce the human disease because the majority of human tumors evolve owing to acquired somatic genetic changes. Third, it did not allow the interrogation of the role of cancer-relevant genes in a particular organ type or stage of tumorigenesis. Recognizing these deficiencies, investigators have been developing ever more sophisticated mouse models that more faithfully reflect the human disease.

Currently used mouse models are very different from those first-generation ones.[128] Constitutive and generalized expression systems have been replaced with inducible and cell type–specific platforms, and conditional gene targeting strategies are usually favored over germline loss-of-function mutations. At present, tetracycline (TET), tamoxifen (TAM), and Cre/loxP and their various combinations are the most popular choices for conditional gene expression and targeting. The TET system allows both temporally and cell type–specific gene expression. It has two different variations, TET-OFF and TET-ON, depending on whether the expression of the targeted gene (regulated by a TET-responsive transactivator) is expressed in the presence (TET-ON) or absence (TET-OFF) of TET.[129] The Cre/loxP system is used for the conditional inactivation (tumor suppressor genes) or activation (oncogenes) of endogenous genes.[130] This approach is based on the use of a bacterial enzyme (Cre recombinase) that specifically catalyzes the recombination of loci flanked by its recognition sites (loxP). For example, when a tumor suppressor gene of interest is flanked by two loxP sites, expression of the Cre recombinase will lead to the deletion of that gene.[130] Because the Cre expression can be regulated, eg, by the TET system, spatially and temporally, inactivation of such a tumor suppressor can now be achieved at will, in a specific cell compartment and at specific times during development or tumorigenesis. Using these state-of-the-art strategies, GEMM's have now been developed that faithfully model the development of preinvasive and invasive carcinomas of the lung, pancreas, prostate, ovary, and breast.[125] Such models oftentimes demonstrate additional pathophysiological sequelae, including cachexia and metastasis, and somatic biochemical and genomic alterations that are common in the cognate human malignancy. A major advance using these GEMM's is the identification of new pathways in human cancers by cross-species comparisons.[131]

Investigations are now underway to determine the role of GEMMs of cancer in diagnostic and therapeutic development. Unanswered questions about GEMMs include the absence of evidence demonstrating a superior predictive therapeutic utility of GEMMs to xenografted tumor models, and whether species-specific differences in drug metabolism, the tumor microenvironment, and cell intrinsic pathways will preclude the translation of information in GEMMs to the clinical setting. Nonetheless, several recent publications suggest that these models will be informative in the preclinical assessment of anti-neoplastic agents.[132]

Summary

Animal rodent models are required components in anticancer drug development. Therefore, the recent generation of GEMMs that faithfully recapitulate the human disease is a major accomplishment in cancer research. Current efforts will determine the opportunities and limitations that these models will afford in the area of basic cancer biology and preclinical applications.

Selected References

The complete reference list can be found at www.CANCERMEDICINE8.com

1. Alberts B, Johnson A, Lewis J, et al. *Molecular Biology of the Cell*. 4th ed. Garland Press; 2002; Lewin B. *Genes VII*. 7th ed. Oxford: Oxford University Press; 1999; Watson JD, Gilman M, Witkowski J. *Recombinant DNA*. 2nd ed. New York: W. H. Freeman; 1992.
2. Atchison ML. Enhancers: mechanisms of action and cell specificity. *Annu Rev Cell Biol*. 1988;4:127; McKnight S, Tjian R. Transcriptional selectivity of viral genes in mammalian cells. *Cell*. 1986;46(6):795.
3. Nirenberg MW, Leder P. RNA codewords and protein synthesis. *Science*. 1964;145:1399.
4. Laskey RA, Earnshaw WC. Nucleosome assembly. *Nature*. 1980;286(5775):763.
5. Bauer WR, Crick FHC, White JH. Supercoiled DNA. *Sci Am*. 1980;243:100.
6. Wang JC. DNA topoisomerases. *Annu Rev Biochem*. 1985;54:665.
7. Smith HO. Nucleotide sequence specificity of restriction endonucleases. *Science*. 1979;205(4405):455.
8. Roberts RJ. Restriction and modification enzymes and their recognition sequences. *Nucleic Acids Res*. 1982;10(5):r117.
9. Cohen SN, Chang AC, Boyer HW, et al. Construction of biologically functional bacterial plasmids in vitro. *Proc Natl Acad Sci USA*. 1973;70(11):3240.
10. Ausubel FM, Brent R, Kingston RE, et al. *Current Protocols in Molecular Biology*. New York: John Wiley & Sons; 1998; Sambrook J, Russell D. *Molecular Cloning: A Laboratory Manual*. 3rd ed. Cold Spring Harbor, NY: Cold Spring Harbor Laboratory Press; 2001.
11. Southern EM. Detection of specific sequences among DNA fragments separated by gel electrophoresis. *J Mol Biol*. 1975;98(3):503.
12. Slamon DJ, Clark GM, Wong SG, et al. Human breast cancer: correlation of relapse and survival with amplification of the HER-2/neu oncogene. *Science*. 1987;235(4785):177.
13. Sanger F, Nicklen S, Coulson AR. DNA sequencing with chain-terminating inhibitors. *Proc Natl Acad Sci USA*. 1977; 74(12):5463.
14. Nakahara M, Isozaki K, Hirota S, et al. A novel gain-of-function mutation of *c-kit* gene in gastrointestinal stromal tumors. *Gastroenterology*. 1998;115(5):1090.
15. Joensuu H, Roberts PJ, Sarlomo-Rikala M, et al. Effect of the tyrosine kinase inhibitor STI571 in a patient with a metastatic gastrointestinal stromal tumor. *N Engl J Med*. 2001;344(14):1052.
16. Davies H, Bignell GR, Cox C, et al. Mutations of the *BRAF* gene in human cancer. *Nature*. 2002;417(6892):949.
17. Samuels Y, Wang Z, Bardelli A, et al. High frequency of mutations of the *PIK3CA* gene in human cancers. *Science*. 2004;304(5670):554.
18. Lynch TJ, Bell DW, Sordella R, et al. Activating mutations in the epidermal growth factor receptor underlying responsiveness of non-small-cell lung cancer to gefitinib. *N Engl J Med*. 2004;350(21):2129; Pao W, Miller V, Zakowski M, et al. EGF receptor gene mutations are common in lung cancers from "never smokers" and are associated with sensitivity of tumors to gefitinib and erlotinib. *Proc Natl Acad Sci USA*. 2004;101(36):13306; Paez JG, Janne PA, Lee JC, et al. EGFR mutations in lung cancer: correlation with clinical response to gefitinib therapy. *Science*. 2004;304(5676):1497.
19. James C, Ugo V, Le Couedic JP, et al. A unique clonal JAK2 mutation leading to constitutive signalling causes polycythaemia vera. *Nature*. 2005;434(7037):1144; Kralovics R, Passamonti F, Buser AS, et al. A gain-of-function mutation of JAK2 in myeloproliferative disorders. *N Engl J Med*. 2005;352(17):1779; Levine RL, Wadleigh M, Cools J, et al. Activating mutation in the tyrosine kinase JAK2 in polycythemia vera, essential thrombocythemia, and myeloid metaplasia with myelofibrosis. *Cancer Cell*. 2005;7(4):387.
20. Hodges E, Xuan Z, Balija V, et al. Genome-wide in situ exon capture for selective resequencing. *Nat Genet*. 2007;39(12):1522; Margulies M, Egholm M, Altman WE, et al. Genome sequencing in microfabricated high-density picolitre reactors. *Nature*. 2005;437(7057):376; Shendure J, Porreca GJ, Reppas NB, et al. Accurate multiplex polony sequencing of an evolved bacterial genome. *Science*. 2005;309(5741):1728.
21. Thomas RK, Nickerson E, Simons JF, et al. Sensitive mutation detection in heterogeneous cancer specimens by massively parallel picoliter reactor sequencing. *Nat Med*. 2006;12(7):852.
23. Mullis KB, Faloona FA. Specific synthesis of DNA in vitro via a polymerase-catalyzed chain reaction. *Methods Enzymol*. 1987;155:335; Saiki RK, Gelfand DH, Stoffel S, et al. Primer-directed enzymatic amplification of DNA with a thermostable DNA polymerase. *Science*. 1988;239(4839):487.
25. Nakamura Y, Leppert M, O'Connell P, et al. Variable number of tandem repeat (VNTR) markers for human gene mapping. *Science*. 1987;235(4796):1616.
30. Aaltonen LA, Peltomaki P, Leach FS, et al. Clues to the pathogenesis of familial colorectal cancer. *Science*. 1993;260(5109):812; Thibodeau SN, Bren G, Schaid D. Microsatellite instability in cancer of the proximal colon. *Science*. 1993;260(5109):816.
32. Wang DG, Fan JB, Siao CJ, et al. Large-scale identification, mapping, and genotyping of single-nucleotide polymorphisms in the human genome. *Science*. 1998;280(5366): 1077.
42. Filipowicz W. Functions of the 5,-terminal m7G cap in eukaryotic mRNA. *FEBS Lett*. 1978;96(1):1; Shatkin AJ. mRNA cap binding proteins: essential factors for initiating translation. *Cell*. 1985;40(2):223.
45. Westin EH, Wong-Staal F, Gelmann EP, et al. Expression of cellular homologues of retroviral onc genes in human hematopoietic cells. *Proc Natl Acad Sci USA*. 1982;79(8):2490; Eva A, Robbins KC, Andersen PR, et al. Cellular genes analogous to retroviral onc genes are transcribed in human tumour cells. *Nature*. 1982;295(5845):116.
46. Baltimore D. RNA-dependent DNA polymerase in virions of RNA tumour viruses. *Nature*. 1970;226(252):1209; Temin HM, Mizutani S. RNA-dependent DNA polymerase in virions of Rous sarcoma virus. *Nature*. 1970;226(252):1211.
47. Efstratiadis A, Kafatos FC, Maniatis T. The primary structure of rabbit beta-globin mRNA as determined from cloned DNA. *Cell*. 1977;10(4):571; Rougeon F, Mach B. Stepwise biosynthesis in vitro of globin genes from globin mRNA by DNA polymerase of avian myeloblastosis virus. *Proc Natl Acad Sci USA*. 1976;73(10):3418.
48. Grunstein M, Hogness DS. Colony hybridization: a method for the isolation of cloned DNAs that contain a specific gene. *Proc Natl Acad Sci USA*. 1975;72(10):3961; Benton WD, Davis RW. Screening lambdagt recombinant clones by hybridization to single plaques in situ. *Science*. 1977; 196(4286):180.
51. Velculescu VE, Zhang L, Vogelstein B, et al. Serial analysis of gene expression. *Science*. 1995;270(5235):484.
55. Chee M, Yang R, Hubbell E, et al. Accessing genetic information with high-density DNA arrays. *Science*. 1996;274(5287):610; Lockhart DJ, Dong H, Byrne MC, et al. Expression monitoring by hybridization to high-density oligonucleotide arrays. *Nat Biotechnol*. 1996;14(13):1675.
57. Golub TR, Slonim DK, Tamayo P, et al. Molecular classification of cancer: class discovery and class prediction by gene expression monitoring. *Science*. 1999;286(5439):531.
61. Perou CM, Sorlie T, Eisen MB, et al. Molecular portraits of human breast tumours. *Nature*. 2000;406(6797):747.
62. van de Vijver MJ, He YD, van't Veer LJ, et al. A gene-expression signature as a predictor of survival in breast cancer. *N Engl J Med*. 2002;347(25):1999.
70. Zaug AJ, Been MD, Cech TR. The *Tetrahymena* ribozyme acts like an RNA

base-pairing. Hybridization occurs by the specific pairing of A to T bases and of G to C bases (see Fig. 2-2). Perfectly matched sequences pair more tightly than sequences containing mismatches, and long-matched sequences pair more tightly than shorter-matched sequences. Hybridization is the concept that underlies molecular biology methods, such as Southern blotting, microarray analysis, and PCR (see below).

Summary

Genes can be cut from total genomic DNA using restriction endonucleases that recognize specific nucleotide sequences. Individual genes can be captured and replicated in bulk for detailed analysis. This process is called *cloning* and employs bacterial plasmids and viruses (phage) as carriers for the cloned genes. Enzymes called DNA ligases join foreign DNA to plasmid or phage vectors, which can then replicate within bacterial cells to create gene libraries. Using nucleic acid hybridization, cloned genes act as probes to detect the presence of their native counterparts in complex mixtures of DNA or RNA.

Gene Analysis: DNA

Southern Blotting ■ One of the most useful techniques for analyzing a gene at the level of genomic DNA is Southern blotting, named for its originator, E. M. Southern.[11] In general, it allows one to determine whether specific nucleotide sequences in a cloned probe are present in a sample of genomic DNA. The presence of these sequences usually means that the gene itself is present in the genomic DNA. Figure 2-4 diagrams the technique. Purified genomic DNA is digested with a specific restriction endonuclease, which, as described earlier, will produce an array of differently sized DNA fragments. Electrophoresis through an agarose gel then separates these fragments according to size. (Because the phosphate groups in DNA make the molecules negatively charged, they will migrate toward the anode in an electric field. The semiporous agarose will allow molecules of DNA to pass with varying degrees of ease, at a rate inversely proportional to their size. At any time after electrophoresis begins, small molecules will be closer to the anode than large molecules.) The agarose gel is usually cast in the form of a flat rectangle a few millimeters thick.

The final goal of Southern blotting is to identify specific fragments of cut DNA using nucleic acid hybridization. Because the agarose gel used in electrophoresis is thick and the DNA fragments can move within it, DNA in the gel is not in a suitable form for further analysis. The DNA fragments must be transferred to a solid support to which they are irreversibly bound to carry out nucleic acid hybridization studies. Thus, after electrophoresis, a paper-thin membrane microfilter (made of nitrocellulose or nylon) is placed over the flat portion of the gel. Liquid is then forced through the agarose gel in a direction perpendicular to the direction in which the DNA moved during electrophoresis. As the liquid perfuses the gel, it carries DNA fragments with it, depositing them on the membrane filter, to which the DNA sticks. After transfer, the DNA fragments are arrayed by size on the solid support.

At this point, a fragment of cloned DNA (the probe) is radiolabeled by using any of a variety of techniques. The membrane containing the transferred DNA is then soaked in a solution containing the radiolabeled probe. If there are any sequences in the genomic DNA that are complementary to those in the probe, the probe will hybridize to those sequences on the filter. The unbound probe can be washed away, and the remaining specifically hybridized probe can be visualized by exposing the filter to x-ray film.

What results from these studies is a pattern of one or more bands on x-ray film. Each band corresponds to a restriction endonuclease–generated DNA fragment containing nucleotide sequences complementary to those in the radioactive probe. For any particular gene probe, the size (ie, length) of the band it identifies will be the same from individual to individual (although see below for a discussion of restriction fragment length polymorphisms [RFLPs], an important exception). Therefore, if a gene has undergone a structural rearrangement, as, eg, when the c-*abl* oncogene is translocated from chromosome 9-22, the pattern may change. Suppose, eg, that the c-*abl* probe ordinarily recognizes a 2000-base *Eco*RI fragment in normal genomic DNA. If the translocation break point in a chronic myelogenous leukemia (CML) patient occurs within that fragment, part of the c-*abl* gene and one of its *Eco*RI sites will move to chromosome 22. Southern blot analysis of the patient's DNA may now detect either (1) a larger fragment than normal if the recipient chromosome has an *Eco*RI site farther away than the old *Eco*RI site or (2) a smaller fragment if it has an *Eco*RI site closer than the old one. Southern blotting is thus a sensitive technique for detecting large structural rearrangements in the genome, such as those that are occasionally associated with malignancy.

Because the amount of the radiolabeled probe that hybridizes to a Southern blot is proportional to the number of

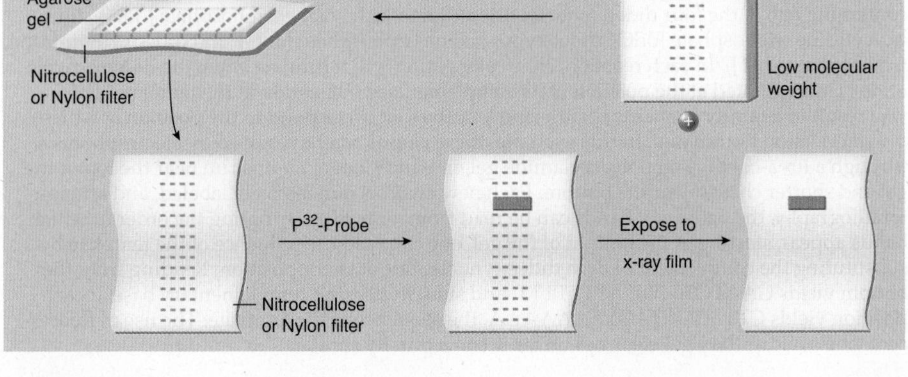

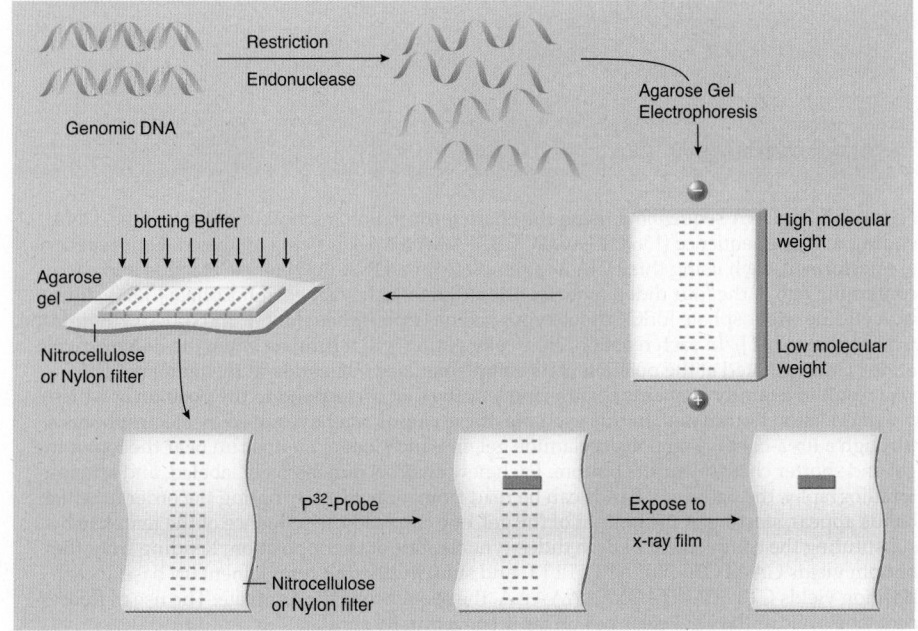

Figure 2-4 ■ Genomic Southern blotting. Genomic DNA is digested with a single restriction endonuclease, resulting in a complex mixture of DNA fragments of different sizes, ie, molecular weights. Digested DNA is arrayed by size using electrophoresis through a semisolid agarose gel. Because DNA is negatively charged, fragments will migrate toward the anode, but their progress is variably impeded by interactions with the agarose gel. Small fragments interact less and migrate farther; large fragments interact more and migrate less. The arrayed fragments are then transferred to a sheet of nitrocellulose or nylon-based filter paper by forcing buffer through the gel as shown. The DNA fragments are carried by capillary action and can be made to bind irreversibly to the filter. Now the DNA fragments, still arrayed by size on the filter, can be probed for specific nucleotide sequences using a ^{32}P-radiolabeled nucleic acid probe. The probe will hybridize to complementary sequences in the DNA, and the position of the fragment that contains these sequences can be revealed by exposing the filter to x-ray film.

restriction endonuclease. *Nature.* 1986;324 (6096):429.
71. Fire A, Xu S, Montgomery MK, et al. Potent and specific genetic interference by double-stranded RNA in *Caenorhabditis elegans. Nature.* 1998;391(6669):806.
76. Jones PA, Takai D. The role of DNA methylation in mammalian epigenetics. *Science.* 2001;293(5532):1068; Feinberg AP, Tycko B. The history of cancer epigenetics. *Nat Rev Cancer.* 2004;4(2):143; Herman JG, Baylin SB. Gene silencing in cancer in association with promoter hypermethylation. *N Engl J Med.* 2003;349(21):2042.
77. Feinberg AP, Ohlsson R, Henikoff S. The epigenetic progenitor origin of human cancer. *Nat Rev Genet.* 2006;7(1):21; Baylin SB, Ohm JE. Epigenetic gene silencing in cancer-mechanims for early oncogenic pathway addiction? *Nat Rev Cancer.* 2006;6:107; Holm TM, Jackson-Grusby L, Brambrink T, et al. Global loss of imprinting leads to widespread tumorigenesis in adult mice. *Cancer Cell.* 2005;8(4):275.
78. Gaudet F, Hodgson JG, Eden A, et al. Induction of tumors in mice by genomic hypomethylation. *Science.* 2003;300(5618):489.
82. Costello JF, Fruhwald MC, Smiraglia DJ, et al. Aberrant CpG-island methylation has non-random and tumour-type-specific patterns. *Nat Genet.* 2000;24(2):132.
87. Kouzarides T. Chromatin modifications and their function. *Cell.* 2007;128(4):693.
90. Mikkelsen TS, Ku M, Jaffe DB, et al. Genome-wide maps of chromatin state in pluripotent and lineage-committed cells. *Nature.* 2007.
93. Druker BJ, Sawyers CL, Kantarjian H, et al. Activity of a specific inhibitor of the BCR-ABL tyrosine kinase in the blast crisis of chronic myeloid leukemia and acute lymphoblastic leukemia with the Philadelphia chromosome. *N Engl J Med.* 2001;344(14):1038.
103. Wilm M, Shevchenko A, Houthaeve T, et al. Femtomole sequencing of proteins from polyacrylamide gels by nano-electrospray mass spectrometry. *Nature.* 1996;379(6564):466; Shevchenko A, Chernushevich I, Wilm M, et al. De Novo peptide sequencing by nanoelectrospray tandem mass spectrometry using triple quadrupole and quadrupole/time-of-flight instruments. *Methods Mol Biol.* 2000;146:1.
105. Goeddel DV, Yelverton E, Ullrich A, et al. Human leukocyte interferon produced by *E. coli* is biologically active. *Nature.* 1980;287(5781):411; Derynck R, Remaut E, Saman E, et al. Expression of human fibroblast interferon gene in *Escherichia coli. Nature.* 1980;287(5779):193; Nagata S, Taira H, Hall A, et al. Synthesis in *E. coli* of a polypeptide with human leukocyte interferon activity. *Nature.* 1980;284(5754):316.
109. Ito T, Chiba T, Yoshida M. Exploring the protein interactome using comprehensive two-hybrid projects. *Trends Biotechnol.* 2001;19(10 Suppl):S23; Uetz P, Giot L, Cagney G, et al. A comprehensive analysis of protein-protein interactions in *Saccharomyces cerevisiae. Nature.* 2000;403(6770):623; Fromont-Racine M, Rain JC, Legrain P. Toward a functional analysis of the yeast genome through exhaustive two-hybrid screens. *Nat Genet.* 1997;16(3):277.
115. Moffat J, Grueneberg DA, Yang X, et al. A lentiviral RNAi library for human and mouse genes applied to an arrayed viral high-content screen. *Cell.* 2006;124(6):1283.
125. Frese KK, Tuveson DA. Maximizing mouse cancer models. *Nat Rev Cancer.* 2007;7(9):645.
126. Hanahan D, Wagner EF, Palmiter RD. The origins of oncomice: a history of the first transgenic mice genetically engineered to develop cancer. *Genes Dev.* 2007;21(18):2258.

3 Cell Proliferation and Differentiation

Michael Andreeff, MD, PhD ■ David W. Goodrich, PhD ■ H. Phillip Koeffler, MD

The biology of cell division, differentiation, and apoptosis is exceedingly similar in both normal and cancer cells. The cancer cell differs from its normal counterpart in that it is aberrantly regulated. Cancer cells generally contain the full complement of biomolecules that are necessary for survival, proliferation, differentiation, cell death, and expression of many cell type–specific functions. Failure to regulate these functions properly, however, results in an altered phenotype and cancer.

Four cellular functions tend to be inappropriately regulated in a neoplasm. First, the normal constraints on cellular proliferation are ineffective. Second, the differentiation program can be distorted. The tumor cells may be blocked at a particular stage of differentiation, or they may differentiate into an inappropriate or abnormal cell type. Third, chromosomal and genetic organization may be destabilized such that variant cells arise with high frequency. Some variants may have increased motility or enzyme production that permits invasion and metastases. Finally, the tightly regulated cell death program (apoptosis) may be dysregulated.[1]

To comprehend the biology of cancer, it is necessary to understand how these functions are controlled in normal cells and how they become uncontrolled in cancer cells. This chapter focuses on the biology of cell proliferation and differentiation, and how these functions are linked in the development of neoplasia. Pathways describing the regulation of apoptosis are discussed in Chapter 4.

Proliferation

Tumor Growth and Cell Proliferation In Vivo

Fundamentally, cancer is a disease of abnormally excessive cell proliferation. It is the increase in tumor cell number, and thus tumor burden, that ultimately accounts for the adverse effects on the host. Indeed, the goal of most current cancer therapy is to reduce the number of tumor cells and to prevent their further accumulation. To better accomplish this goal, a more complete description of the unique characteristics of tumor cell proliferation is required. This task is made difficult by the fact that the mechanisms that underlie tumor and normal cell proliferation are very similar. In this section, we will review current understanding of the complex molecular mechanisms involved in the regulation of cell proliferation with particular emphasis on the aberrations in this system that occur in malignant cells.

One hallmark feature of cancer is that most are genetically clonal suggesting they arise by expansion of a single cell. In cancers where preneoplastic lesions can be identified, however, the preneoplastic cells are likely to be genetically distinct from the overtly neoplastic cells. These observations suggest a model for the genesis of cancer through continual genetic evolution of mutant cells by a process of natural selection. Genetically abnormal cells are generated as a result of environmental insult or normal errors in replication. Some small fraction of these cells escape normal controls on cell proliferation and increase their number. As this pool of mutant cells proliferate, additional mutant variants are continuously generated. If the result of these additional mutations provides a selective growth advantage, then the mutant variant will increase its relative number. Through multiple rounds of proliferation, mutation, and selection, a neoplastic variant evolves to cause cancer (Fig. 3-1). The model predicts that two parameters will critically affect the rate of this clonal evolution, the mutation rate and the rate of proliferation. It follows that mutations that increase the rates of proliferation or mutation rate will increase the rate of neoplastic transformation. Such mutations are, therefore, more likely to be detected in cancer cells than other types of mutations. Further, if such a mutation is inherited, the incidence of cancer within such a family is expected to be significantly higher than normal. As we shall discuss below, both of these predictions are generally confirmed by available observations.

A key assumption of this model is that the genetic potential to form cancer cells exists within the DNA of normal cells. This assumption has been validated upon the discovery that the cancer genes of acutely transforming retroviruses are captured from the genomes of their hosts.

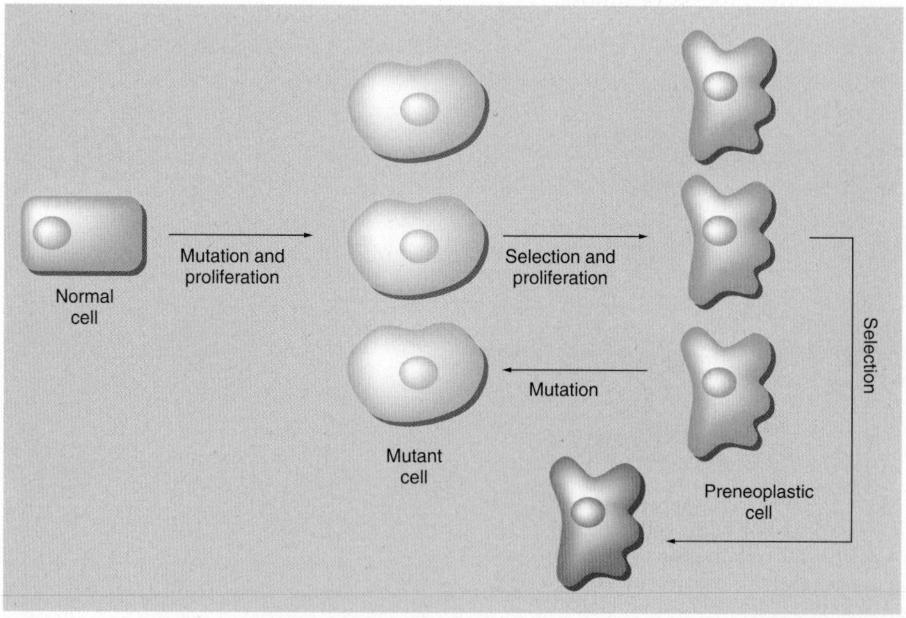

Figure 3-1 ■ Evolution of neoplastic cells. Genetic analysis of cancer suggests that neoplastic cells arise through an accumulation of mutations. The genetic clonality observed in most cancers suggests they arise from a single neoplastic cell that has undergone multiple rounds of mutation, proliferation, and selection. This hypothesis is summarized in the diagram. Normal cells undergo random mutagenesis generating several distinct variants. Variants that survive undergo additional rounds of mutation and selection. Subvariants escaping normal growth controls can expand to form preneoplastic lesions. Additional mutations within the population of preneoplastic cells gives rise to clonal variants that proliferate into cancer.

Previously, it had been assumed that cancer genes evolved de novo in viruses. In retrospect, that normal cells have the genetic potential to evolve into cancer cells is logical based on biological arguments. For example, it is clear that human cells possess an intrinsic proliferative capacity that is in vast excess of that required to meet the needs of normal growth and development. Normal human cells can divide as often as once or twice a day in vivo. A cell dividing at this rate would generate a cell number equal to the total number of cells in an adult human in <2 months. We have evolved highly regulated mechanisms to restrain this proliferative capacity to appropriate times and places. It is this excess proliferative capacity that provides the genetic foundation upon which a cancer cell is built. The key in understanding tumor cell proliferation, then, is to characterize the mechanisms that are normally utilized to restrain the proliferation of normal cells and to understand how they fail during cancer.

Cell Cycle Control

The cell division cycle can be divided into two functional phases, S and M phases, and two preparatory phases, G1 and G2 (Fig. 3-2). S phase is defined as the phase in which the DNA is replicated. The time it takes a typical human cell to complete S phase is about 8 h and is invariant under normal circumstances. Fully replicated chromosomes are segregated to each of the two daughter nuclei by the process of mitosis during M phase. The length of M phase is about 1 h and is also normally invariant. G1 phase precedes S phase, whereas G2 phase precedes M phase. G1 and G2 phases are required for the synthesis of cellular constituents needed to support the following phase and ultimately to complete cell division. In mammalian cells, the length of G2 phase is about 2 h. The length of G1 phase is highly variable and can range from about 6 h to several days or longer. In human cells, the varying length of G1 phase accounts for most of the differences in the time it takes to execute a cell division cycle between different cell types or between cells growing under different conditions. Cells that persist in G1 phase for extended periods of time enter a distinct state called G0. Although such cells are metabolically active, they are not actively proliferating. Cells in G0 can reenter the cell cycle or they can remain in G0 indefinitely.[2]

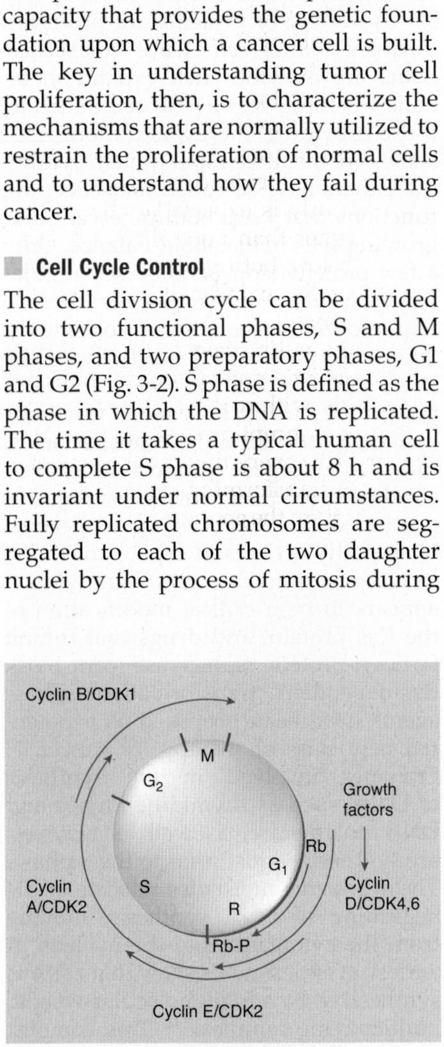

Figure 3-2 Cyclin-dependent kinase (CDK) regulation of the cell cycle. The phases of the cell division cycle are shown. Transition from one phase to the next requires transit of a checkpoint like the restriction point (R) during the G0/G1 to S phase transition. Transit of the checkpoint is mediated by activation of cyclin-dependent kinases. The timing of activation of individual CDKs during the cell cycle is shown by the respective arrows. Activation of cyclin D/CDK4,6 is coincident with phosphorylation of the retinoblastoma tumor-suppressor protein (Rb) and transit of the R checkpoint.

A successful cell division cycle requires the orderly and unidirectional transition from one cell cycle phase to the next. Certain events must be completed before others are begun. For example, beginning mitosis before the completion of DNA replication would obviously be deleterious to the cell. In theory, the ordering of cell cycle events may be accomplished in a manner analogous to the substrate-product relationship of a metabolic pathway. The product of one reaction serves as the substrate for the next. The rate of the first reaction, therefore, limits that of the next. Hence, regulation of the system is inherent in the biochemical events of the process itself. The prevailing view, however, is that the timing and ordering of cell cycle transitions is dependent on separate positive and negative regulatory circuits.[3] The regulatory circuits enforce a series of checkpoints, allowing passage only after completion of critical cell cycle events. Two classes of regulatory circuits exist, intrinsic and extrinsic. Intrinsic regulatory pathways are responsible for the precise ordering of cell cycle events. Since the length of S, G2, and M phases in mammalian cells is normally invariant, the transitions between these phases are controlled predominantly by intrinsic regulatory pathways. Extrinsic regulatory pathways function in response to environmental conditions or in response to detected cell cycle defects. Both types of regulatory circuits can use the same checkpoints. Deregulation of intrinsic regulatory pathways can contribute to cancer. For example errors in the spindle-assembly checkpoint can lead to chromosomal imbalance and aneuploidy, a feature characteristic of virtually all cancers. Dysregulation of proteins that control this checkpoint have been detected in human cancer.[4,5] However, we will focus our attention on the extrinsic regulatory circuits where differences between normal and neoplastic cells are most commonly observed.

Passage of the cell cycle checkpoints ultimately requires the activation of intracellular enzymes known as cyclin-dependent kinases (CDKs). CDKs are extremely well conserved through evolution. CDKs exist in all eukaryotic cells from fungi to plants to mammals. In fact, CDKs from human cells can functionally substitute for the enzymes in yeast. The structural and functional conservation of these enzymes through evolution suggests that they are centrally important for the cell cycle in all eukaryotic cells. The requirement for these enzymes for cell cycle transitions has been amply documented, particularly in organisms like yeast that are amenable to genetic manipulation. Since activation of CDKs is the central event in cell cycle transitions, it is not surprising that their activity is exquisitely regulated at several levels (Fig. 3-3).[6,7] The active CDK holoenzyme is composed of a catalytic subunit and the cyclin regulatory subunit. Each cyclin is synthesized at a particular stage of the cell cycle. For example, cyclin E is synthesized in late G1 and early S phase; cyclin A is synthesized during S and G2 phases; and cyclin B is synthesized in G2 and M phases. Therefore, a given catalytic subunit cannot become active until an

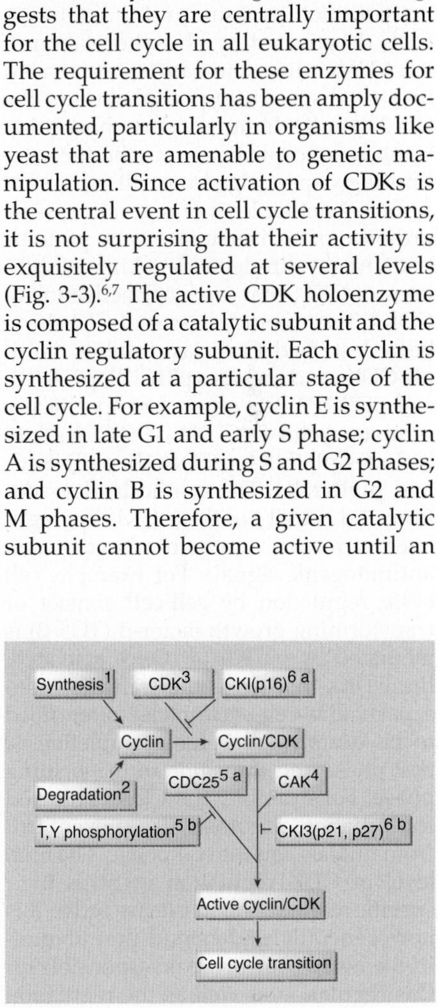

Figure 3-3 Regulation of cyclin-dependent kinases (CDKs). The activity of CDKs is controlled at several levels. (1) Synthesis of cyclins occurs at specific times during the cell cycle or in response to certain growth factors (see Fig. 3-2). (2) Degradation of cyclins occurs at specific times during the cell cycle and is mediated by ubiquitin-dependent proteolysis. (3) The cyclin subunit must complex with the catalytic CDK subunit. (4) The assembled complex requires phosphorylation by CAK to reach maximum specific activity. (5) The assembled complex is inactivated by phosphorylation on specific residues in the ATP-binding site of the enzyme (5 b) and can be reactivated by dephosphorylation of these residues by cdc25 (5 a). (6) CKIs can inhibit assembly of the cyclin/CDK complex (6 a) or the activation of the assembled complex (6 b).

appropriate cyclin is synthesized. Upon synthesis, a cyclin can assemble with an appropriate catalytic subunit. However, this complex requires phosphorylation on threonine by another regulated kinase, the CDK-activating kinase or CAK. CAK is itself a CDK composed of cyclin H and CDK7 proteins. Hence the levels of CAK influence the activity of assembled CDKs. Another level of regulation is deactivation of the CDK by phosphorylation of its ATP-binding site by yet another regulated kinase activity. This kinase activity is unusual in that it has dual specificity for both tyrosine and threonine. A CDK deactivated by phosphorylation of its ATP-binding site can be reactivated by a dual specificity phosphatase of the Cdc25 family. In fact, dephosphorylation by these phosphatases may be the rate-limiting step in triggering cell cycle transitions. Another level of regulation is the presence of a diverse family of proteins known as cyclin-dependent kinase inhibitors, or CKIs, that can block activation of CDKs. Two distinct classes of CKIs have been described. One class inhibits multiple CDKs and includes p21CIP1, p27KIP1, and p57KIP2. The other class specifically inhibits cyclin D/CDK4 or 6 CDKs and includes p16INK4, p15INK4B, p18INK4C, and p19INK4D. The synthesis, degradation, and activity of these CKIs are regulated in response to both mitogenic and antimitogenic signals. For example, cell cycle regulation by cell-cell contact or transforming growth factor-β (TGF-β) is mediated by p27KIP1.[8,9] Once activated, the CDKs that drive the transition into a particular cell cycle phase often need to be deactivated before completion of that phase and transition to the ensuing phase. For example, the CDKs required for initiation of mitosis also prevent exit from mitosis and into G1 phase. The final level of CDK regulation involves their specific degradation in precise order. It is now generally understood that ubiquitin-mediated proteolysis is responsible for this regulation as well as the regulation of a host of other cell cycle regulators.[10,11] Hence, synthesis, posttranslational modification, and programmed degradation all contribute to the regulation of CDKs.

The G0 to S Checkpoints

As discussed earlier, the time it takes to progress through the S, G2, and M phases of the cell cycle is relatively invariant. The length of G1 phase on the other hand is variable. In addition, cells can exit the cell cycle for extended periods of time and mammalian cells do so during the G1 phase of the cell cycle. Cells that have exited the cell cycle are said to be in a G0 state, or "quiescent." Most cells in adults are in G0. This absence from the cell division cycle can be temporary or permanent as in terminally differentiated cells, for example. Cells in G0 can be very active functionally and metabolically, and proliferation of G0 cells can be initiated by changes in cell density, the presence of mitogens or growth factors, or the supply of nutrients. These cells then reenter the cell cycle, beginning a sequence of events that culminates in cell division. Hence, the G0/G1 to S phase transition is highly regulated, and the result of this regulation, by and large, determines the growth fraction of a population of cells.

The transition from G0/G1 to S phase is regulated by two major checkpoints called competence and the restriction point (R). These checkpoints are located ~12 and 2 h before the start of the S phase, respectively. At least three growth factors, provided in serum, are required sequentially to transit these checkpoints following resumption of proliferation of fibroblasts in vitro: platelet-derived growth factor (PDGF), epidermal growth factor (EGF), and insulin-like growth factor (IGF-1). As mentioned earlier, extracellular TGF-β has the opposite effect. It inhibits the growth of various epithelial cells by modulating expression of CKIs. Paracrine production of TGF-β could limit growth of both normal and cancer cells, and experimental models suggest that it may play a role in the regression of breast cancers in response to hormonal or drug therapies.[12,13] Once the R point has been passed, the cell is committed to a round of cell division. The cell now completes S, G2, and M phases without the need for additional growth factors or even additional protein synthesis. Once initiated, the cell cycle is not free running; the competence and restriction checkpoints must be passed in each subsequent G1 phase, thus requiring the continued presence of growth factors. The switching of cells back and forth between quiescence and cycling depends on extracellular conditions and is regulated differently in normal and tumor cells.

Growth factor receptors are complex, large proteins that span the plasma membrane. They have a specific domain that recognizes the growth factor on the outside of the cell, and their cytoplasmic portion may have an enzymatic function, such as a protein tyrosine kinase. Binding of a growth factor or ligand to its receptor can induce transmission of a signal to the cytoplasm through activation of the kinase.[14,15] The next step is a transduction of the cytoplasmic signal to the cell nucleus. This is accomplished by a heterogeneous group of molecules known as second messengers and includes various proteins that are phosphorylated by kinases, small molecules such as inositol phosphates and cyclic AMP, and ions, including Ca^{2+}, H^{+}, and Zn^{2+}. Within the nucleus, genes are then activated in response to these second messengers. As an illustration of this general scheme, upon binding of EGF to the extracellular domains of its receptor, autophosphorylation occurs in the intracellular domain of the protein. This phosphorylated domain facilitates the formation of a protein complex containing Grb2 and Sos. This complex activates the Ras protein by catalyzing exchange of Ras-bound GDP for GTP. The GTP-bound form of Ras activates the c-Raf kinase. This kinase then triggers a phosphorylation cascade ultimately activating mitogen-activated protein kinase. This kinase may phosphorylate and regulate transcription factors such as Jun, Fos, and Myc.

A variety of proteins are produced during G1 after cells leave quiescence. Some are enzymes that expand metabolic functions lost by G0 cells, such as those providing energy, and more ribosomes are made for rapid protein synthesis. Others have so-called housekeeping functions that keep both quiescent and growing cells in metabolic balance. Only a few proteins appear to be key regulatory molecules. For example, enzymes are required for the synthesis of isoprenoids, which are necessary for activity of the Ras oncogene, and for the synthesis of polyamines, which have many functions including ionic binding to nucleic acids. The Ras oncogene product is synthesized as a precursor protein that requires posttranslational processing to become biologically active and capable of transforming mammalian cells. Farnesylation appears to be a critical modification of the Ras protein, and drugs that inhibit farnesyl-protein transferase can block Ras-dependent transformation. These agents have been proposed as a potential new class of therapy for cancer.[16,17] Enzymes involved in the synthesis of DNA, such as thymidine kinase and DNA polymerase, as well as histones, are synthesized just prior to the S phase. These enzyme molecules relocate at the beginning of DNA synthesis, moving from the cytoplasm into the nucleus. A variety of experiments show that DNA is synthesized by a high-molecular-weight, multienzyme complex.[18-20] This complex contains many enzymes known to be involved in the process of DNA replication, but its size and other features are still a matter of debate. After DNA synthesis has commenced, cell growth becomes relatively independent of external controls. The daughter cells, now in the G1 phase, will then either pass through another cycle or arrest in a quiescent G0 state, depending, once more, on external conditions. If these conditions are not adequate, the cell will become arrested before it reinitiates DNA synthesis.

How is reentry into the cell cycle from G0 ultimately controlled? Like other cell cycle transitions, activation of CDKs is required. G0 cells are devoid of significant CDK activity. In the presence of mitogenic growth factors, expression of D-type cyclins (cyclins D1, D2, and D3) is stimulated and continues throughout G1 phase as long as the growth factors are present.[21] D-type cyclins complex with either CDK4 or CDK6 catalytic subunits to form a holoenzyme modified by CAK. All of the relevant substrates for cyclin D/CDK4 or 6 have probably not been enumerated. However, one important substrate is likely the retinoblastoma tumor-suppressor protein (Rb) and the other members of its gene family p107 and p130. Rb is constitutively expressed and constrains cells from progressing through the G1 phase of the cell cycle (Fig. 3-4).[22] Rb complexes with many cellular proteins including the E2F transcription factors. When in complex with E2F, Rb represses transcription from E2F-dependent promoters. Upon phosphorylation by cyclin D/CDK4 or 6,[23] Rb loses its ability to restrain the cell cycle.[24] This response is presumably because it can no longer complex with E2F and/or repress E2F-dependent transcription.[25] The E2F family contains at least eight members (E2F-1 through E2F-8) that encode nine protein species.[26,27] Most E2F proteins function as transcriptional activators when in heterodimeric complex with one of the E2F-related proteins DP-1, 2, or 3. The heterodimeric complex binds a specific DNA sequence and activates transcription from the promoters of many genes important for S phase including dihydrofolate reductase, DNA polymerase α, and thymidine kinase.[28] Perhaps most importantly, E2F influences the expression of cyclin E.[29] In fact, of many E2F-dependent genes, cyclin E is the only one deregulated upon loss of Rb in normal cells.[30] Cyclin E expression begins in late G1 phase and complexes with CDK2. Cyclin E/CDK2 activity is necessary and sufficient for the start of S phase.[31] Forced expression of cyclin E/CDK2 activity can trigger the start of S phase in the absence of Rb phosphorylation and derepression of other E2F-dependent genes, suggesting that cyclin E is a primary target for regulation by cyclin D/CDK4 or 6, Rb, and E2F.[32,33] E2F proteins can also function as transcriptional repressors when in complex with members of the retinoblastoma protein family. Some E2F proteins appear to function as constitutive transcriptional repressors and do not bind retinoblastoma protein family members.

DNA Damage-Induced Checkpoints

Upon nuclear DNA damage, normal cells initiate a response that includes cell cycle checkpoint activation, apoptotic cell death, and transcriptional induction of genes involved in DNA repair. Induction of apoptosis is an important response to DNA damage and is discussed in detail in a separate chapter. Normal cells in G1 phase prior to the R point will arrest in G1 phase upon sensing DNA damage. This arrest is presumably induced to prevent the replication of damaged DNA. Replication of damaged DNA can result in the incorporation of heritable genetic mutations. If cells are past the R point or within S phase, DNA replication is slowed, again to allow time for DNA repair. If cells sense DNA damage while in G2 phase, a G2 cell cycle arrest will occur. Different types of DNA damage can interfere with normal mitosis, resulting in heritable genetic mutations or cell death.

The tumor-suppressor genes ATM and p53 play an important part in responses to damaged DNA.[34,35] For example, cells containing mutations in p53 fail to arrest in G1 or undergo apoptosis efficiently upon irradiation. Cells containing mutations in ATM are also deficient for cell cycle arrest as well as some forms of DNA repair. The p53 protein functions as a transcription factor by binding specific DNA sequences and regulating transcription from promoters containing those sequences. In normal cells, DNA damage induces an increase in p53 levels by inhibiting the normal rapid turnover of the protein. The p53 protein is normally targeted for ubiquitin-dependent proteolysis by association with the Mdm2 protein. This association is inhibited by phosphorylation of p53 on specific amino-terminal residues that is triggered by DNA damage.[36] Phosphorylation on these amino-terminal residues also facilitates dephosphorylation or acetylation of p53 carboxy-terminal residues. These modifications increase the affinity of p53 for its DNA-binding site by distinct mechanisms[37,38] and hence increase its ability to activate transcription. The transcription of a number of genes can be affected by activation of p53. However, the ability of p53 to directly increase expression of p21CIP1 is probably important for p53-dependent G1 cell cycle arrest observed upon DNA damage. As discussed earlier, p21CIP1 is a CKI that can inhibit the activity of multiple CDKs, including cyclin D/CDK4 or 6 as well as cyclin E/CDK2. In summary, DNA damage generates a signal that can activate p53 by posttranslational modification. Increased p53 activity upregulates p21CIP1, which prevents activation of CDKs, required for the G1 to S transition (Fig. 3-4).

ATM is the gene whose mutation is responsible for ataxia telangiectasia. Immunodeficiency, progressive cerebellar ataxia, radiosensitivity, cell cycle checkpoint defects, and cancer predisposition characterize this disease. ATM encodes a protein containing a phosphatidyl-inositol 3-kinase-like domain, implicating it in signal transduction. Like p53 mutant cells, mutant ATM cells are defective in the G1/S checkpoint activated after radiation-induced DNA damage. This defect is attributable to the lack of p53 activation that normally occurs, suggesting that ATM may participate in

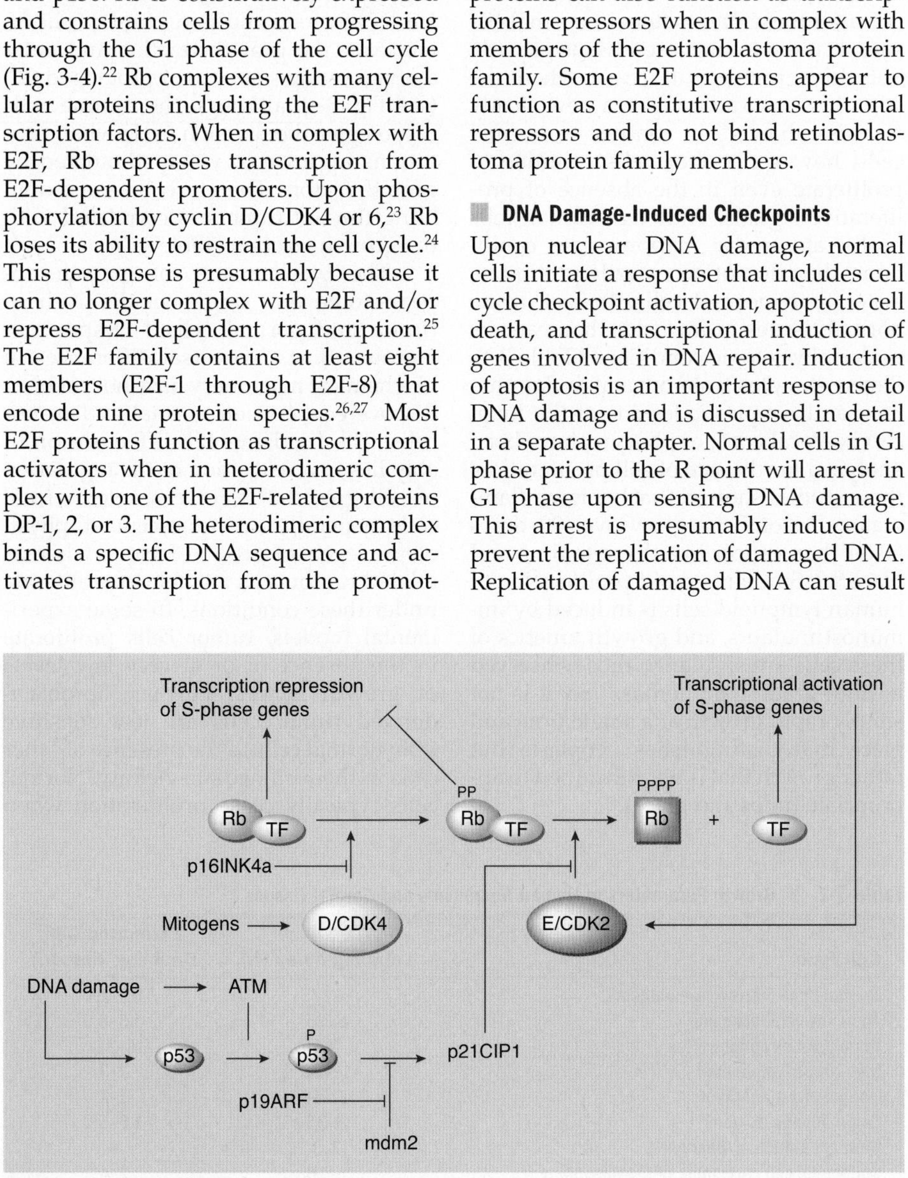

Figure 3-4 G1 phase checkpoints mediated by p53 and Rb. The figure depicts how Rb can enforce a G1 checkpoint by association with transcription factors (TF) and repression of genes containing the relevant TF DNA-binding site. The genes regulated by Rb/TF complexes include cyclin-dependent kinases (CDKs) thereby comprising a positive feedback loop. This feedback is damped by the presence of CKIs like p16INK4a and p21CIP1. CKI expression can be modulated by the p53 DNA damage response pathway as indicated. Phosphorylation status of proteins is indicated by "P" where relevant.

the same pathway as p53. ATM protein, and the related ATR protein, can, in fact, associate with and phosphorylate p53 at its amino-terminal sites.[39,40] The p53-directed kinase activity of the ATM protein is itself activated by DNA damage. ATM protein, therefore, contributes to the activation and stabilization of p53 by phosphorylating amino-terminal sites during the radiation-induced DNA damage response. ATM protein may play a role in sensing DNA damage and generating the DNA damage signal.

Environmental agents like radiation or DNA-damaging chemicals most commonly induce DNA damage. Rarely, DNA damage can be generated by mistakes in the normal execution of the cell cycle or as a consequence of normal metabolic activity through the generation of reactive oxygen species. However, a form of DNA damage eventually occurs in all normal cells as they suffer replicative senescence. Normal cells have a limited replicative lifespan both in vivo and in vitro; a cell can undergo only a finite number of cell divisions. This limit is thought to be imposed, at least in part, by levels of telomerase activity.[41,42] Telomerase is an enzymatic activity within cells that is required to maintain the integrity of DNA ends.[43] DNA polymerases involved in DNA replication synthesize DNA in the 5′-3′ direction and require a primer and template. The requirement for a primer ensures that some genetic information will be lost from the 5′ end of DNA during each round of DNA replication. Telomerase adds DNA of a particular sequence to the ends of DNA without the need for a separate primer or template, thus protecting cells from loss of genetic information. Telomeric DNA also protects chromosomes from degradation or recombination. Without telomeric DNA, chromosomes become unstable. As normal cells become senescent, they lose telomerase activity and their cell division cycle is arrested. This cell cycle arrest may be mediated by the DNA damage checkpoint since shortened telomeric DNA is associated with DNA strand breaks that may be sensed as damaged DNA. Consistent with this hypothesis, shortening of telomeric DNA triggers a p53-dependent cell cycle arrest by accumulation of single-stranded DNA.[44] However, there is some controversy as to whether telomere shortening itself is a trigger for replicative senescence.[45]

Replicative senescence is defined as a state of permanent exit from the cell division cycle, typically in the G1 phase. Like quiescent cells, senescent cells are metabolically active and resistant to apoptosis. However, senescent cells exhibit characteristics that distinguish them from quiescent cells, in particular the expression of a unique form of beta-galactosidase activity.[46] While first discovered as a response of cells cultured in vitro to lack of telomerase activity and a limited replicative life span, senescence is now recognized to be triggered in response to a variety of stresses including DNA damage, oncogene activation, constitutive growth factor stimulation, and oxidative stress among others. This more general cellular senescence may provide a barrier to tumorigenesis in vivo in response to such stresses, as preneoplastic lesions often exhibit markers of senescence.[47]

Checkpoint Defects in Tumor Cells

To maintain tissue homeostasis and to support normal development, each organ maintains tight controls over Tc, growth fraction, and cell loss. Physiologic stimuli can alter these parameters in normal tissues, leading to increased tissue growth, but this growth will cease when the stimulus is withdrawn or a new steady state is achieved. In contrast to normal cells, however, tumor cells continue to proliferate even in the absence of proliferative signals. Although tumor cells proliferate under inappropriate conditions, they do not necessarily proliferate faster than normal cells. In fact, some normal tissues grow faster than cancers under physiologic conditions (Table 3-1). Biopsy samples from normal, inflammatory, and neoplastic lesions of the lung, cervix, vocal cord, or pharynx have been analyzed for the rate of cell proliferation; these studies showed that benign inflammatory lesions can grow over 20 times faster than cancer in a discrete time and place.[48-50] Similarly, rapid proliferation of human lymphoid cells is induced by immunostimulants, and growth kinetics of these cells are similar to those observed in high-grade lymphomas.[51] So, it is not simply rapid growth at a single time and place that distinguishes neoplasia but rather growth that is not restrained to appropriate times and places.

It generally is believed that neoplastic cells multiply exponentially during the early phases of tumor cell growth. As the tumor mass increases, however, the rate of growth declines. Measuring tumor growth over time describes a curve with an exponential increase in the early period, then a flattening out of the growth rate over time (ie, Gompertzian curve).[52] Several mechanisms have been invoked to explain this change in growth rate with larger tumors: (a) decrease in the growth fraction, (b) increase in cell loss (ie, exfoliation, necrosis), (c) nutritional depletion of tumor cells resulting from outgrowth of available blood supply, or (d) lengthening of Tc. Experimental tumor models suggest that cell cycle time changes only slightly when tumor growth decreases.[53] Under adverse conditions, tumor cells often leave the growth fraction and enter a nongrowing state (G0 or prolonged G1) (see Fig. 3-1), although these same cells can reenter the division cycle when conditions improve or when stimulated by growth factors. Therefore, the mass doubling time of tumors is correlated with the growth fraction (Table 3-2).

The biochemistry of growth appears to be very similar qualitatively in tumor and normal cells.[54] Despite numerous efforts, universal differences in biochemical machinery have not yet been discovered between normal and tumor cells. The fundamental difference probably lies in a relaxation of the regulation of cell growth.[53,55] For example, normal cells generally are quiescent at physiologic levels of growth factors, whereas related tumor cells are able to proliferate under these conditions. In some experimental models, tumor cells proliferate in the absence of or at very low levels of growth factors. Further, fibroblast-derived tumor cells are less sensitive than normal cells to the presence of other cells in their immediate vicinity. Normal cells typically cease proliferation when

Table 3-1 Growth Parameters of Human Neoplasms and Normal Tissues

Cell Type	Labeling Index (%)	Estimated Cell Doubling Time (d)
Normal bone marrow myeloblasts	32-75	0.7-1.1
Acute myeloid leukemia	8-25	0.5-8.0
Normal B-cell lymphocytes	0-1	14-21+
High-grade lymphoma	19-29	2-3
Normal intestinal crypts	12-18	1-2
Colon adenocarcinoma	3-35	1.6-5.0
Normal epithelium/pharynx	2-3	–
Squamous cell carcinoma of the nasopharynx	5-16	2-4
Normal epithelium/bronchus	–	9-10
Epidermoid carcinoma of the lung	5-8	8-10
Normal epithelium/cervix	4-8	–
Squamous cell carcinoma of the cervix	13-40	–
Ovarian carcinoma	3-20	5-6
Benign mole of skin	0.3	–
Malignant melanoma of skin	12.8	–

Table 3-2 **Correlation Between Mass Doubling Time and Growth Fraction**

Cell Type	Growth Fraction (%)	Estimated Cell Doubling Time (d)
Experimental tumors		
NL1210 (mouse)	86	0.5
B 16 (mouse)	55	1.9
LL (mouse)	38	2.9
DMBA (rat)	10	7.4
Human tumors		
Embryonal carcinoma	90	27
Lymphoma (high grade)	90	29
Squamous cell carcinoma	25	58
Adenocarcinoma	6	83

the in vitro culture becomes confluent, but tumor cells can reach several fold higher densities in culture. Also, cells of normal solid tissue lie on a secreted extracellular matrix (ECM) that is composed of various proteins that stimulate cell growth.[56] Tumor cells often are partly or completely independent of ECM for optimal growth, and they may secrete little matrix material.[57]

What molecular defects bring about the relaxed growth requirements in neoplastic cells? Defects can occur at several levels. For example, limiting growth factors may not be needed because tumor cells inappropriately produce their own (ie, an autocrine mechanism). Alternatively, receptors may be produced in excess, as is the case for EGF receptors in numerous clinical tumors, leading to adequate stimulation at the low growth factor concentrations found in vivo. Moreover, mutations that alter intracellular signaling mechanisms may bypass growth factor dependence. Mutated forms of proto-oncogenes and inactivated tumor-suppressor genes can activate growth in these ways. We will focus here on defects that occur in cell cycle regulatory proteins that enforce the checkpoints discussed earlier.

Like normal cells, the transit of cell cycle checkpoints in cancer cells ultimately requires the activation of CDKs. Due to the complexity of CDK regulation, defects leading to inappropriate activation of CDKs can occur at several levels. The overexpression of cyclin D1 has been detected in many human cancers due to gene amplification or translocation of the cyclin D1 gene.[58] The cyclin D1 gene is located on chromosome 11q13. This chromosomal region is amplified in a wide variety of human cancers including small cell lung tumors (10%), primary breast cancers (13%), bladder cancer (15%), esophageal carcinoma (34%), and squamous cell carcinoma of the head and neck (43%) among others.[59] Of course, other potential oncogenes could be contained within the amplified region. However, cyclin D1 is likely important since its expression is consistently elevated in these tumors. Cyclin D1 overexpression can also be observed in tumors, such as sarcomas, colorectal tumors, and melanomas, without amplification of the gene. In some cases, cyclin D1 expression is activated by chromosomal translocation. In parathyroid adenoma, Motokura and colleagues[60] have identified cyclin D1 as being translocated to the parathyroid hormone gene, thereby deregulating cyclin D1 expression. Translocation of the cyclin D1 gene with immunoglobulin heavy chain gene transcriptional control elements has also been observed in B-cell lineage mantle cell lymphomas. Cyclin D1 is a growth factor–responsive cyclin that plays an important role in regulating the G0/S checkpoint. Deregulated expression of cyclin D1 could inappropriately increase cyclin D1/CDK4 activity and drive transit of the checkpoint even in the absence of appropriate growth factors. Direct evidence that forced expression of cyclin D1 can facilitate tumorigenesis has been obtained from transgenic mice in which overexpression of cyclin D1 has been targeted to the mammary epithelium. These mice develop ductal hyperproliferation and eventual mammary tumor formation.[61]

CDK activation can also be accomplished by inactivation of CKIs. Genetic mutation of CKI genes has also been observed frequently in human cancer. In this scenario, loss of a CKI relieves one constraint on the activation of CDKs and provides a proliferation stimulus. In particular, the INK4 locus within chromosomal region 9p21 is one of the most frequently mutated areas in human cancers.[62] This locus is also frequently methylated in some tumor types including bladder cancer and leukemia. Extensive methylation of DNA prevents efficient transcription of genes within the methylated region, thus silencing gene expression. Three proteins are encoded by the INK4 locus including the CKIs p16INK4a and p15INK4b as well as p19ARF (see below). It is likely that p16INK4a is a bona fide tumor-suppressor gene, since many of the mutations detected in tumors specifically target expression of this protein, and because germ line mutations that specifically map to p16INK4a have been detected in kindreds with familial melanoma and pancreatic adenocarcinoma. In addition, mutations in CDK4 that prevent binding with p16INK4a, thus relieving it of p16-mediated inhibition, have also been found in melanoma-prone families. Loss of p16INK4a may facilitate activation of cyclin D1/CDK4 or 6, which is likely to affect regulation of the G0/S checkpoint. Mutation of other CKIs in human cancer is rare, suggesting that they may be required for execution of the cell cycle. However, expression of p27KIP1 is inversely correlated with clinical outcome in a limited number of cancers, including melanoma and carcinoma of the oral cavity.

CDK activation also requires dephosphorylation of inhibitory threonine/tyrosine phosphorylation sites by the Cdc25 family of dual specificity phosphatases. In vitro evidence exists that the Cdc25 family members are potential oncogenes.[63] Forced expression of Cdc25 can cooperate with Ha-Ras or loss of Rb to induce oncogenic transformation of primary cells. Overexpression of Cdc25 has also been detected in some primary human tumors. Cdc25A may be a direct transcriptional target for the myc oncogenes.[64] Inappropriately high Cdc25 levels may provide an oncogenic stimulus by inappropriately activating CDK activity.

One of the most important genes involved in human cancer is the Rb tumor-suppressor gene. An interesting feature of retinoblastoma is that close to 40% of cases are hereditary, and susceptibility to retinoblastoma is inherited as a simple autosomal dominant trait with high (90%) penetrance. The simple genetics of retinoblastoma has provided the means to molecularly clone the gene responsible; mutational inactivation of both alleles of Rb is necessary and sufficient for retinoblastoma.[65] Mutation of Rb is observed at high frequency in osteosarcoma and soft-tissue sarcoma as well. Rb mutations can also be detected in a wide variety of clinically important cancers including carcinoma of the breast, prostate, bladder, kidney, liver, pancreas, cervix, and lung, as well as leukemia. Further, expression of wild-type Rb cDNA in cancer cells can inhibit their tumorigenicity.[66] As mentioned earlier, cyclin D/CDK4 or 6 phosphorylation, which, in turn, is regulated by p16INK4a, inhibits Rb function. This finding suggests that these three proteins function in the same biochemical pathway (Fig. 3-4). Support for this functional interrelation comes from the observation that deregulation of any one of these proteins greatly decreases the likelihood of detecting defects in the other proteins. For example, tumor cells that lose p16INK4a or overexpress cyclin D1 generally retain wild-type Rb. Cells lacking wild-type Rb typically express normal levels of cyclin D1 and p16INK4a. In addition, induction of cell cycle arrest by forced expression of p16INK4a only occurs in cells that contain functional Rb. If mutations in any of the members of this pathway are considered, disruption of this p16INK4a/cyclin D1/CDK4 or 6/Rb pathway may occur in most human cancers (Fig. 3-5).[2] Since this pathway is important for regulation of the G0 to S phase transition, it has a major influence on the growth fraction of normal tissues.

The p53 gene is the most frequently mutated gene in human cancer.[67] Germ line p53 mutation is involved in the cancer-prone Li-Fraumeni syndrome.[68] Mice lacking p53 due to genetically engineered disruption are also cancer prone. Wild-type p53 is critically important for operation of the DNA damage-induced checkpoint (see above). Upon sensing DNA damage, p53 is activated, resulting in either G1 cell cycle arrest or apoptosis. These responses either allow time for the cell to repair the damage or to rid the body of cells with damaged DNA. Loss of p53 function, therefore, decreases genomic stability. Loss of genomic stability can increase the accumulation of additional genetic mutations required for neoplastic transformation. The *Mdm2* gene encodes a protein that binds p53 and targets its destruction by the ubiquitin-proteosome pathway. Too much Mdm2 protein may be analogous to p53 inactivation since any p53 synthesized would be rapidly degraded. Mdm2 was originally identified as an oncogene amplified in a spontaneously transformed mouse cell line. Overexpression of Mdm2 mediated by gene amplification can also be detected in many human cancers, particularly sarcoma.[69] The protein-protein interaction between Mdm2 and p53 has recently become a therapeutic target: disruption would abolish p53 degradation, result in increased p53 levels and apoptosis. Indeed, several inhibitors of this interaction have been described[70] and have shown to induce apoptosis in p53 wild-type malignancies.[71] Interestingly, the p19ARF protein encoded by the INK4a locus also regulates p53 function.[72] The p19ARF protein can bind Mdm2 and prevent Mdm2 from targeting p53 for degradation. Consistent with the ability of p19ARF to activate p53, forced expression of p19ARF can cause a p53-dependent cell cycle arrest. As discussed previously, mutations of the INK4 locus that inactivate p19ARF, as well as p16INK4a, are commonly observed in human cancer. Inactivation of p19ARF may contribute to tumorigenesis since Mdm2-mediated degradation of p53 would be unimpeded. The functional interrelation between p19ARF, Mdm2, and p53 defines another cell cycle checkpoint control pathway (Fig. 3-5). Deficiencies in this pathway also play a vital role in neoplastic transformation.

Although cancer cells use the same cell cycle machinery as normal cells, the cell cycle checkpoints in tumor cells are relaxed. Of the scores of proto-oncogenes and tumor-suppressor genes that have been identified to date, most function in signal transduction pathways that mediate mitogenic stimulation. These signal transduction pathways eventually converge on the cell cycle checkpoint that control the G0/G1 to S phase transition and activate appropriate CDKs. Influencing the transit of this checkpoint has a major influence on the proliferation of normal and tumor cells by affecting both Tc and growth fraction. Increased proliferation, in turn, increases the rate of evolution toward neoplasia (see above). Despite the number and variety of genes involved in signal transduction, relaxation of the G1/G0 to S checkpoint controls in tumor cells is mediated by disruption of a relatively small number of pathways. The Rb and TP53 growth control pathways figure prominently among them. These two pathways are the most frequently mutated in human cancer cells. Disruption of the Rb or p53 pathways probably occurs in virtually every human cancer.

Aurora kinases are a recently discovered family of kinases (A, B, and C) consisting of highly conserved serine/threonine protein kinases found to be involved in multiple mitotic events: regulation of spindle-assembly checkpoint pathway, function of centrosomes and cytoskeleton, and cytokinesis. Aberrant expression of Aurora kinases may lead to cancer. For this reason the Aurora

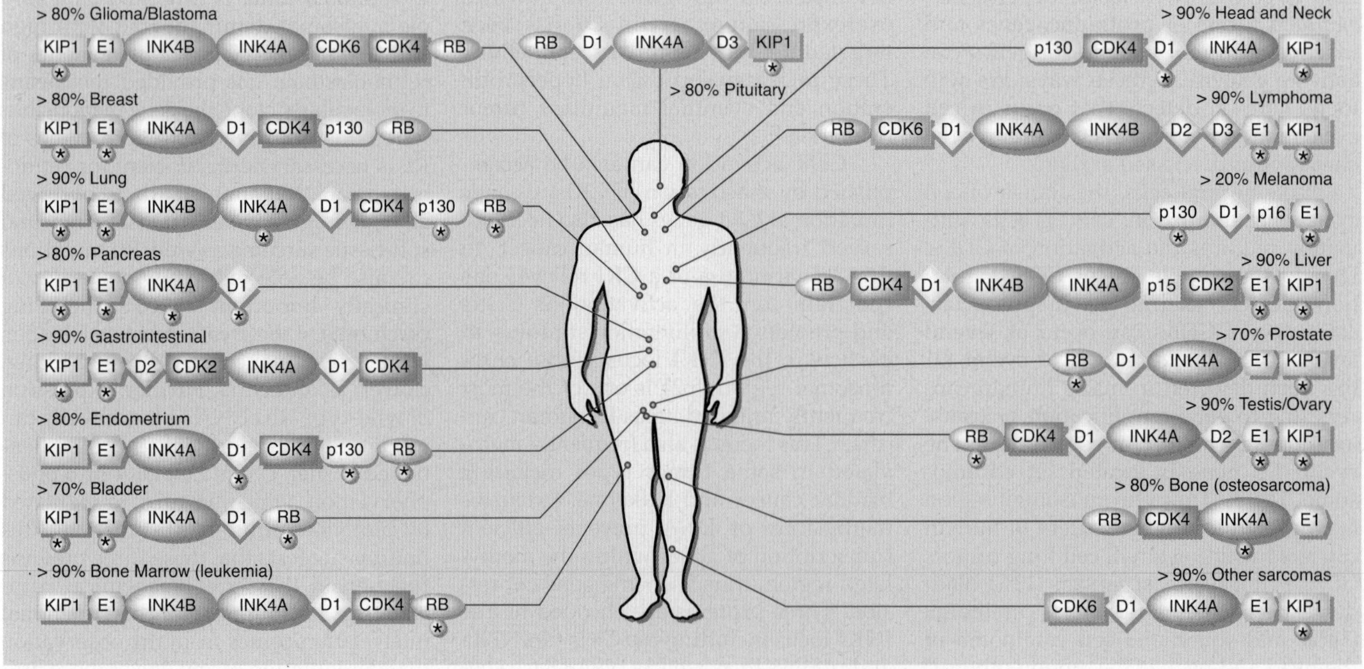

Figure 3-5 Deregulation of the Rb growth control pathway in human cancer. The figure depicts several clinically important human cancers and the genetic or epigenetic alterations of the Rb growth control pathway that have been identified in such cancers. Members of this pathway include CKIs, cyclins, cyclin-dependent kinases (CDKs), and the Rb family of proteins. The percentages given indicate fraction of cases where alteration in any of the indicated pathway components has been detected. Alterations with a demonstrated correlation with prognosis are indicated with an asterisk. *Source:* Adapted from Ref. 2.

kinases are potential targets in the treatment of cancer. Some Aurora kinase inhibitors have shown clinical activity in a wide range of tumor types.[73,74]

Over the last several years, studies have shown that genes involved in the circadian rhythm can be dysregulated in cancer.[75-78] The *Per1* and *Per2* genes normally are transcriptionally activated by the Clock and Bmal genes in the morning. As they accumulate, they relocalize from the cytoplasm to the nucleus and downregulate the Clock and Bmal genes by late afternoon. Furthermore, the Clock and Bmal complex can activate other genes with E-boxes, often these target genes are associated with enhanced proliferation. In addition, *Per* proteins can bind to the CHK2 and ATM genes to enhance the inabilities to mediate apoptosis after exposure to DNA-damaging agent. Decrease expression of the *Per* genes has been detected in a variety of leukemias and cancers including acute lymphocytic and myelocytic leukemia, B-cell lymphomas, breast, lung, and colon cancers. Inactivating the *Per* genes provides a growth advantage to the cancer cell by allowing the Clock/Bmal complex to turn on genes associated with proliferation.

Insights into the mechanisms of cell cycle control have provided entirely new approaches to cancer therapy. Kinase inhibitors such as flavopiridol, UCN-01, proteosome inhibitors (eg, bortezomib), and Aurora kinase inhibitors are being tested in clinical trials and are quickly becoming part of the therapeutic armamentarium.

Apoptosis and Proliferation

There are at least two interesting connections between regulators of cell proliferation and apoptosis. One is based on the observation that many slowly proliferating tumors such as chronic lymphocytic leukemias,[79] low-grade non-Hodkin lymphomas,[80] multiple myelomas,[81] colon,[82] and breast cancers[83] overexpress the anti-apoptotic proteins Bcl-2 and Bcl-XL. The interaction between Bcl-2 and calcineurin may be relevant to the inhibition by Bcl-2 of cell proliferation as NF-AT-inducible genes are important for proliferation in some types of cells. There is emerging evidence that Bcl-2 and its close relatives exert at least two distinct functions: they not only inhibit apoptosis but also restrain cell cycle entry.[84-86] These two functions can be genetically separated as mutation of a conserved tyrosine residue (Y28) at the C-terminal end of the BH4 region of Bcl-2 does not affect its anti-apoptotic activity, but markedly reduces its ability to restrain reentry of quiescent cells into the cell cycle.[86] The inhibitory effect of Bcl-2 on entry into the cell cycle may contribute to the better prognosis of patients whose breast cancer tissue shows abnormally high levels of Bcl-2.[87] Delayed cell cycle entry could result in longer time to relapse. Quiescent leukemic progenitor cells also overexpressed Bcl-XL and Bcl-2, as compared to their proliferating counterparts.[88] When Bcl-2 antisense oligonucleotides were used in vitro in primary AML samples, recruitment of leukemic cells into the cell cycle was observed.[89] The precise mechanism by which Bcl-2 affects cell cycle progression remains to be determined. Disruption of the interactions of Bcl-2 proteins with their pro-apoptotic counterparts results in apoptosis induction, and several small molecule inhibitors are now in early clinical trials[90-92] Mcl-1, another Bcl-2 family member, was recently found to be essential for the survival of hematopoietic stem cells[93] and of acute and chronic leukemias and can be targeted by MAPK signaling inhibition.[90]

Downstream of Bcl-2, a member of caspase inhibitors termed "inhibitors-of-apoptosis" (IAP) proteins, may also affect cell cycle regulation: survivin itself is expressed in a cell cycle–dependent manner and is regulated by the MAPK and PI3K signaling pathways.[94] Maximal expression is in G2/M and recent studies suggest that survivin plays a role in cell cytokinesis. Its downregulation can cause G2 block and polyploidization. For details of survivin's anti-apoptotic function, see Chapter 4. Downregulation of survivin expression with antisense oligonucleotides or MAPK and PI3K inhibitors[94] has resulted in cell cycle arrest, and to a lesser degree, in apoptosis, confirming its dual function.

Differentiation

All tumors show abnormalities in differentiation (ie, anaplasia). The presence of immature and the lack of mature, terminally differentiated cells is a hallmark of cancer, with rare exceptions: in chronic myelogenous leukemias (CML), the number of mature granulocytes is actually increased, at least at early stages of the disease, and it takes several years and additional genetic alterations of immature blast cells until they predominate. Similarly, in myelodysplastic syndromes, mature appearing granulocytes can be clonal.[95] Hence, the differentiation block characteristic for most cancers is not absolute. The anaplasia of tumors can provide insights into their etiology, degree of malignancy, prognosis, and sensitivity to therapeutic intervention by differentiation- or maturation-inducing agents. These differences in phenotype arise from differences in gene expression, not in gene content. The genes expressed by a particular cell only comprise ~10-20% of the coding capacity of the genome. In humans, there are over 30,000 genes that code for proteins; however, an individual cell generally expresses only 10,000-20,000 genes. Genes expressed by a particular cell depend on its embryonic lineage, developmental stage of the organism, tissue and cellular environment, and functions that the cell must fulfill. The mechanisms that regulate gene expression are incompletely understood; however, they most certainly entail the sequential action of cell-type-specific or cell-lineage-specific transcription factors that repress or activate the differentiation-specific genes. The transcription of genes itself is regulated by a complex enzymatic machinery. Histone acetylation/deacetylation and methylation/demethylation of target genes have recently been the focus of detailed studies and provide the basis for "transcription therapy."[96] Programs of gene expression generally are instituted early in embryogenesis and sequentially altered as development proceeds.[97,98] Posttranscriptional modifications, such as phosphorylation and ubiquination of many genes, add further complexity to the regulation of gene expression. Messenger RNA transcripts can be silenced by short "interference" RNAs (siRNA),[99] short hairpin RNAs (shRNA), or cDNA/RNAi hybrid molecules.[100-103]

Some genes are expressed by many, if not all, cell types. These "housekeeping" genes generally encode proteins that participate in basic or universal cellular functions. Other genes that are expressed only in specific cell types and/or stages of development are said to be cell-type or differentiation-specific genes. Thus, the expression of specific gene products marks both the cell lineage and the stage of differentiation.

Differentiation and Cell Proliferation

Differentiation begins shortly after the first few cell divisions that follow fertilization. Throughout development, and in adult organisms, the ability of a cell to proliferate is intimately connected to its state of differentiation. Adult tissues generally express a variety of factors that act to maintain both the proliferation and the differentiation status of the cells. These include secreted molecules, transmembrane receptors, intracellular signaling molecules, and transcription factors. For example, myoD[104] and C/EBP-α[105] are nuclear factors that activate the transcription of muscle- and adipocyte-specific genes, respectively; in addition, both proteins are potent inhibitors of cell proliferation.

Transcription factors are the engines that drive proliferation and differentiation of cells. Their disruption is associated with cancer.[106,107] One of the earliest revelations of this fact was the identification of retroviral oncogenes that were associated with the development of cancer. For example, the avian myeloblastosis virus causes myeloblastic leukemia in chickens. The virus overexpresses the transcription factor *myb*. Likewise, avian myelocytomatosis virus produces a variety of cancers in chickens. This virus has a dysregulated *myc* oncogene. Both *myc* and *myb* have subsequently been identified as dysregulated in a variety of human cancers. A second manner, in which cancer-related dysregulated transcription factors were discovered, was by analysis of chromosomal translocations. One of the genes at the chromosomal rearrangement is often a transcription factor that becomes dysregulated, such as the fusion of the *PML* and *RAR* (retinoic acid receptor) genes in acute promyelocytic leukemia. *RAR* is a transcription factor often involved in differentiation; however, when fused to *PML*, the fusion product behaves as a repressor of differentiation-related target genes.

Some transcription factors are necessary for differentiation of stem cells to their mature progeny. Dysfunction of these transcription factors can be associated with a block in differentiation, resulting in the cell remaining in the proliferative pool. This provides them with a growth advantage compared to their normal counterpart, thus setting the stage for the development or progression of cancer. For example, the CCAAT/enhancer-binding protein-alpha (C/EBPα) is a transcription factor mutated in ~7-15% of AMLs.[108,109] Also, members of a family with an increased proclivity to develop AML were found to have a germ line mutation of one allele of C/EBPα.[110] Another leukemia-prone syndrome has a germ line mutation of one allele of the transcription factor RUNX1. These individuals with the germ line C/EBPα and RUNX1 mutation have a long latency period (10-30 years) before developing leukemia, suggesting additional mutations are necessary for progression to leukemia.[111] In addition, these families suggest that haploinsufficiency of either of these transcription factors increases the risk of development of AML. Besides mutations, expression and/or activity of C/EBPα can be disrupted in a variety of cancers. For example, the AML-1/ETO and the PML/RARα leukemia-associated fusion proteins can inappropriately sequester C/EBPα in the cytoplasm, as well as blunt its transcription.[112] The BCR-ABL fusion product, found in chronic myelogenous leukemia, inhibits the efficient translation of C/EBPα. Also, tumors derived from the lung, liver, and breast have a low expression of C/EBPα compared to surrounding normal tissues. The mechanism of gene silencing in these cancers is not clear.

Besides acting as a transcription factor, C/EBPα can bind and block the activity of E2F and the cyclin-dependent kinase-2 (CDK2) and CDK4, and it can increase levels of $p21^{WAF1}$, a cyclin-dependent kinase inhibitor. Thus C/EBPα can directly slow proliferation, independent of its transcriptional activity. These antigrowth effects are lost with dysregulation of C/EBPα. Taken together, an altered C/EBPα can foster aberrant cell growth at the same time as it loses its capacity to induce differentiation. Experimental forced expression of C/EBPα in leukemia cells induces their terminal differentiation, suggesting that induction of expression of C/EBPα may be a worthwhile therapeutic target in selected cancers and leukemias.

In early embryos, cell proliferation is the primary means by which the cell mass increases. As the organism develops, however, proliferation becomes restricted. Some differentiated cells continue to proliferate, but others irreversibly lose this ability. Embryonic cells often display traits that confer on them a selective growth advantage over that of an adult cell. They proliferate vigorously,[113] are capable of extensive migration, secrete factors that increase the local supply of blood, and produce enzymes capable of degrading basement membranes.[114] These traits also are characteristic of tumor cells, including the ability to increase local blood supply (ie, angiogenesis).[115] Recent data suggest that tumor angiogenesis is an important, negative prognostic indicator for carcinomas and leukemias.[116,117] Angiogenesis is now being extensively investigated as a potential target for cancer therapy.[118] Thus, in adult organisms, mutations or conditions that activate portions of embryonic programs for gene expression or inactivate portions of the adult program can produce cells with many properties of malignant tumor cells.[119]

Stem Cells

Stem cells have the capacity for both self-renewal (ie, proliferation without a change in phenotype) and differentiation (ie, changing into a new phenotype). Some stem cells have already undergone considerable differentiation, so further differentiation is restricted to a single cell type or lineage. Other stem cells are multipotent and differentiate into a variety of cell types (ie, hematopoietic stem cells). It has been difficult to demonstrate cells in adults that are totipotent (ie, capable of differentiating into most or all of the cell types that comprise the organism), but the recent cloning of animals from mature cells demonstrates the persistence of stem cell characteristics even in fully differential cells.[120] Recently, neuronal stem cells were shown to produce a variety of blood cell types[121] and adult human mesenchymal stem cells that are present in adult marrow were shown to have the potential to differentiate to lineages of mesenchymal tissues, including bone, cartilage, fat, tendon, muscle, marrow stroma, neuronal cells, and myocytes.[122-125] Conversely, primitive hematopoietic stem cells were reported to give rise to muscle,[126] liver,[127,128] intestinal,[128,129] pulmonary epithelial,[130,131] and neuronal cells.[132,133] Engraftment and differentiation by a single, bone marrow-derived stem cell in liver, lungs, GI tract, and skin were reported.[130] Some of these data were obtained from experiments where hematopoietic cells or whole bone marrow cell populations including stromal cells being transplanted into sex mismatched hosts, and sex-chromosome differences were used to determine the origin of immune histochemically identified organ cells.[134-136] However, colocalization of markers is technically challenging and recent reports have explained some of the published data as results of cell fusions rather than of "transdifferentiation"[137,138] or have failed to confirm previous reports. Weissman's group, transplanting single green fluorescent protein-marked hematopoietic stem cells into lethally irradiated nontransgenic mice, did not find convincing evidence of bone marrow–derived neuronal cells, liver, kidney, gut, skeletal muscle, cardiac muscle, or lung cells.[139] Another recent report was unable to confirm the ability of bone marrow cells to differentiate into neuronal cells.[140]

While dedifferentiation or "transdifferentiation" of adult stem cells remain uncertain or very rare, embryonic stem (ES) cells have great value for the study of differentiation, for the elucidation of organ-specific coordinated gene expression programs, and for the development of regenerative medicine applications.[141] These studies have now been extended to cells of human origin.[142,143] ES cells are pluripotent cell lines derived from the inner cell mass (ICM) of blastocyst stage embryos[113] and have been successfully gene-marked.[144] They have the ability to differentiate into myocytes with structural and functional properties of cardiomyocytes[145] and into many other cell types.[146-151] Their therapeutic utility for cancer and degenerative disease is presently under investigation in preclinical model systems.

Mesenchymal stem cells (MSC) can be isolated from bone marrow samples and subsequently expanded over a million-fold in culture. MSC differentiate into adipocytes, osteocytes, chondrocytes, tenocytes, marrow stromal cells, muscle and perhaps neuronal cells[125,152] and are being used in early clinical trials to enhance bone marrow grafting and to suppress graft vs host disease in allogeneic bone marrow transplants.[153] An intriguing finding is the observation that MSC can contribute to the formation of stroma in solid tumors and tumor metastases and that they can deliver therapeutic genes such as interferon-beta and induce tumor regressions.[154-156]

In general, stem cell differentiation results in two types of changes: the expression of specialized, differentiation-specific gene products and a partial or complete restriction of the cell's capacity for further proliferation. It then follows that another mechanism by which tumor cells might arise is through mutations that render a stem cell partly or wholly unable to differentiate.

Some cells, particularly in adults, are terminally differentiated. These cells were believed to be irreversibly blocked in their ability to proliferate, although they may perform specialized functions for a long period of time. Perhaps with the exception of CML, tumors of terminally differentiated cells are not found. Thus, tumors of mature muscle or nerve cells do not occur, although tumors of less differentiated myoblastic or neuronal stem cells do. Cell proliferation appears to be incompatible with the expression of a terminally differentiated program of gene expression. Thus, irreversible arrest of cell division and expression of the terminally differentiated phenotype are interdependent. This concept, however, has recently been called into question by the discovery that fully differentiated cells can develop features of stem cells, including cells that underwent epithelial-mesenchymal transition.[157]

In many tissues, continuous proliferation is restricted to a subpopulation of cells, the stem cells, which undergo self-renewal, as well as differentiation, into cell types with a more restrictive proliferative potential. It then follows that mutations or conditions that interfere with the differentiation of stem cells will result in unbalanced proliferation and, thus, uncontrolled growth of the tissue. Mutations that drive proliferation are associated with an accumulation and overgrowth of less-differentiated cells in the tissue. A common feature of tumor cells is their failure to differentiate terminally under appropriate conditions either in vivo or in culture.[158-160]

Extracellular Factors That Control Differentiation

During embryogenesis and in a number of adult tissues, differentiation depends on external factors. These include insoluble factors such as ECM and both the proximity and type of neighboring cells, as well as a growing list of soluble factors. In model systems, differentiation can be induced by a variety of biologic agents and drugs (Table 3-3). Both the ECM and differentiation-promoting soluble factors may be produced in an autocrine or paracrine fashion.

Cell-cell and cell-ECM interactions are important for both the induction and maintenance of differentiation in several cell lineages. Although our understanding at a molecular level of insoluble factors is still incomplete, progress has been made in identifying key molecules and pathways through which these factors act. In the case of the ECM, specific cell surface receptors bind to particular components of the ECM.[161] It now appears that the binding of an ECM component to its cellular receptor activates an intracellular signal transduction pathway that is analogous to the signaling pathways that have been identified for polypeptide GFs and growth inhibitors. Tumor cells often lose their ability to sense the ECM or neighboring cells.[162]

The soluble factors that regulate differentiation can be broadly classified into those that bind to cell surface receptors and those that freely cross the plasma membrane and bind to cytoplasmic or nuclear receptors. The first class includes molecules such as the fibroblast growth factors (FGFs) (TGF-β, IGF-1, and b-FGF) and hematopoietic factors such as colony-stimulating factor-1 (CSF-1), granulocyte colony-stimulating factor (G-CSF), granulocyte-macrophage colony-stimulating factor (GM-CSF), stem cell factor (SCF), Flt-3 Ligand, and the interleukins. These are all polypeptides, and many were first identified as GFs or growth inhibitors. It is now clear, however, that these factors have a multitude of effects depending on the target cells and the cellular microenvironment.[163]

For example, basic FGF was identified as a fibroblast mitogen in brain and pituitary extracts, but recent data suggest that FGF induces mesodermal differentiation in early embryos, is angiogenic, and is a survival factor for endothelial cells.[164,165] FGF also inhibits the differentiation of some cells. Terminal differentiation into mature myotubes cannot occur unless it is withdrawn from proliferating myoblasts. Similarly, TGF-β was first identified as a stimulator of anchorage-independent growth in mesenchymal cells and later as an inhibitor of epithelial cell proliferation.[166,167] Like FGF, TGF-β stimulates the differentiation of some cells (ie, keratinocytes or intestinal epithelial cells) but inhibits differentiation in others (ie, myoblasts or preadipocytes). In some human tumor cells cultured in vitro or in athymic mice, TGF-β both inhibits tumor growth and promotes a more differentiated phenotype in the remaining cells. Other studies suggest that TGF-β induces the expression of one or more inhibitors of cyclin-dependent protein kinases (eg, p21, p27, p16); inhibition of these kinases, in turn, prevents the phosphorylation and, thus, inactivation of the RB protein, thereby inhibiting cell proliferation.[168-171]

Table 3-3 **Induction of Differentiation in Culture**

Stem Cell	Differentiation Markers	Inducers
Preadipocyte	Adipocyte	Insulin, cort, cell density
Basal keratinocyte	Cornified envelope	RA deficiency, cell density
Myoblast	Myotube	GF deficiency, cell density
Squamous cell carcinoma	Cornified envelope	GF deficiency, cort
Embryonal carcinoma	Endoderm, mesoderm, ectoderm	RA, ara-C, mito, HMBA, coculture with blastocyst
Neuroblastoma	Neuron, neurotransmitter, action potential	PI, 6TG, ara-C, MTX, dox, bleo, RA, GF deficiency
Melanoma	Dendrite, melanin, tyrosinase	PI, dox, DMSO, TPA, RA, MSH
Colon adenocarcinoma	Mucus, dome formation, CEA, columnar cell	NMF, DMSO, butyrate, low glucose, IFN, HMBA, cell density
Breast adenocarcinoma	Casein, dome formation	RA, PGE, DMSO
Bladder transitional cell carcinoma	Keratin filament, loss of surface antigen	HMBA
Erythroleukemia	Mature erythroid cell, hemoglobin	Dox, ara-C, 6TG, mito, dact, aza, hemin, DMSO, HMBA, CSF, RA, IFN
Promyelocytic	Granulocyte, macrophage	IFN, CSF, vitD, TPA, DMSO, NMF, dact, HMBA, aza, ara-C, RA
Myelocytic leukemia	Granulocyte, macrophage	CSF, RA, vitD, ara-C, dact, DMSO, TPA, cort, dox

Abbrevations: ara-C, Cytarabine; aza, 5-azacytidine; bleo, bleomycin; CEA, carcinoembryonic antigen; cort, glucocorticoids; CSF, colony stimulating factor; dact, dactnomycin; DMSO, dimethylsulfoxide; dox, doxorubicin; GF, growth factor; HMBA, hexamethylbisacetamide; IFN, alpha- or gamma-interferon; mito, mitomycin C; MSH, melanocyte-stimulating hormone; MTX, methotrexate; NMF, *N,N*-dimethylformamide; PGE, prostaglandin E; PI, phosphodiesterase inhibitor; RA, retinoic acid; TPA, 12-*O*-tetradecanoylphorbol-13-acetate; vitD, 1,25-dihydroxy vitamin D; 6TG, 6-thioguanine.
Source: Data from Ref. 211, 212, and 219.

Another family of extracellular proteins is the CCN protein family, which is composed of six members: Cyr61, CTGF, NOV, WISP-1, WISP-2, and WISP-3 (officially known as CCN1-6, respectively).[172] The CCN gene contains four conserved modular domains that share sequence similarity with other protein families: IGF-binding protein (IGFBP), von Willebrand type C (VWC), thrombospondin type 1 (TSP1), and a C-terminal domain (CT). Cyr61 (CCN1) is a secreted, cysteine-rich, heparin-binding protein that associates with the extracellular matrix and the cell surface. Integrins, including $\alpha v\beta 3$, $\alpha v\beta 5$, $\alpha 6\beta 1$, and $\alpha IIb\beta 3$, have been identified as receptors of Cyr61. Through these receptors, Cyr61 probably exerts its effects on cellular activity in a variety of tissue types. It is highly expressed in many breast, brain, and esophageal cancers and melanomas, and high expressions have been associated with a worse prognosis.[173-176] Furthermore, forced expression of Cyr61 in "normal" cell lines from these same tissues allows them to form tumors in immunodeficient mice. Dysregulation of various cellular signaling pathways, such as the receptor tyrosine kinases (eg, epidermal growth factor receptor), can cause a cascade of signaling that induces expression and secretion of CCN1 (Cyr61), which, in a paracrine and autocrine fashion, stimulates integrins to provide growth signals for the cancer and precancer cells.

The membrane-permeable regulators of differentiation include retinoic acid (ie, vitamin A) and its derivatives (RA).[177] There is strong evidence that concentration gradients of RA are critical for the morphogenesis of some tissues in the early embryo.[120] RA can stimulate or inhibit growth and differentiation depending on the cell type. In general, RA is required for the differentiation of many epithelial cells. It diffuses freely into cells, whereupon it binds to specific nuclear protein receptors (ie, the retinoic acid receptors [RARs]). In addition, other nuclear proteins, called RAR coregulators, have been found that interact with RARs and modulate their actions in various cell types.[178] These differences may explain why specific cells and tissues differ in their responses to RA. Some differentiation-specific genes that are regulated by RA contain sequences specific to the initiation of transcription,[179] to which RA-RAR complexes bind and thereby activate transcription.[120,180] In acute promyelocytic leukemia (APL), RAR fuses with the PML gene in the reciprocal translocation t(15;17) and with PLZF in t(11;17).[181] The ensuing fusion proteins PML/RARα and PLZF/RARα inhibit transcription by inducing the N-Cor/sin3A/HDAC1 corepressor complex (Fig. 3-6). This transcriptional silencing in APL is mediated through deacetylation of the core proteins of nucleosomes, histones H2A, H2B, H3, and H4 (Fig. 3-7). Lysines (k) in the amino-terminal tails of H2A, H2B, H3, and H4 are acetylation/deacetylation sites for histone acetylatransferases (HATs) and histone deacetylases (HDACs).[182-184] With inhibition of HDACs by HDAC inhibitors such as suberoylanilide hydroxamic acid (SAHA),[182] histones are acetylated, and the DNA that is tightly wrapped around a deacetylated histone core relaxes (Fig. 3-8). Other HDAC inhibitors include trichostatin A and depsipeptide; SAHA and depsipeptide are in clinical trials. In RA-resistant PLZF-RARα leukemias, the combined exposure to ATRA and SAHA resulted in therapeutic effects. This therapeutic concept has been termed "transcription therapy."[96,185-187]

The sex steroids, estrogen and testosterone, may regulate differentiation by similar mechanisms. Another nuclear receptor, the peroxisome proliferator-activated receptor-γ (PPARγ), has recently been identified as a potential target for cancer therapy. In addition, PPARγ ligand has been used in a clinical trial for prostate cancer,[188] resulting in stabilization of the disease. It is highly expressed in normal adipose tissues, monocytes, leukemias, and epithelial malignancies. PPARγ ligands signal differentiation, growth arrest, and apoptosis. PPARγ must form a heterodimer with RXR to bind DNA and activate transcription. In the absence of ligand, the heterodimer associates with a complex of corepressor proteins that silence target promoters by deacetylating histones in the adjacent chromatin. Ligand binding induces a conformational change in the receptor, which dissociates the corepressor complex, and permits the heterodimer to interact with coactivator complexes (p160/CBP and DRIP). The complexes acetylate histones and allow transcription (reviewed in Ref. 190). Somatic loss-of-function PPARγ mutations were found in colon cancers and a PAX8-PPARγ fusion was recently identified in human thyroid follicular carcinomas carrying the translocation t(2;3)(q13;p25). PPARγ ligation may affect tumor growth indirectly through regulation of the tumor-suppressor gene PTEN.[189,190] In a clinical trial, PPARγ ligation resulted in the induction of differentiation in liposarcomas.[191]

Tumor cells often produce factors that affect both growth and differentiation. Basic FGF can confer neoplastic properties when expressed in an inappropriate cell type (eg, a fibroblast). In addition, inappropriate expression of FGF by one cell may stimulate the growth and affect the differentiation of neighboring cell types.[165]

Intracellular Regulators

External factors and intrinsic programs of gene expression control cellular differentiation. In either case, the expression of differentiation-specific genes generally is under the control of a small number of master regulatory genes. Genes recently have been identified that are potential "master regulators" of developmental stages and differentiation-specific gene expression. The most globally acting master regulatory genes are known as homeotic genes, which were first identified as genetic loci that determined the

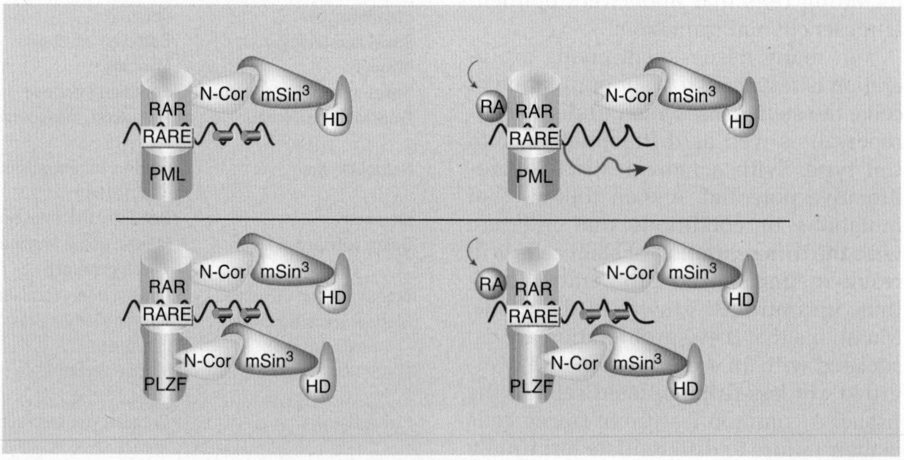

Figure 3-6 RARα fusion proteins induce N-CoR/Sin3A/HDAC1, corepressor complex and inhibit transcription. A model for the interactions of APL fusion proteins with the N-CoR-mSin3-histone deacetylase complex. PML-RARα interacts with N-CoR (or SMRT) and recruits the mSin3-HD complex, decreasing histone acetylation and producing repressive chromatin organization and transcriptional repression. RA induces dissociation of the N-CoR-mSin3-HD complex, recruitment of coactivators with histone acetyltransferase activity (not shown), increased levels of histone acetylation, chromatin remodeling and transcriptional activation. PLZF-RARα has two N-CoR-binding sites that, even in the presence of RA, recruit the N-CoR-mSin3-HD complex and maintain transcription repression. *Source:* Redrawn from Ref. 182.

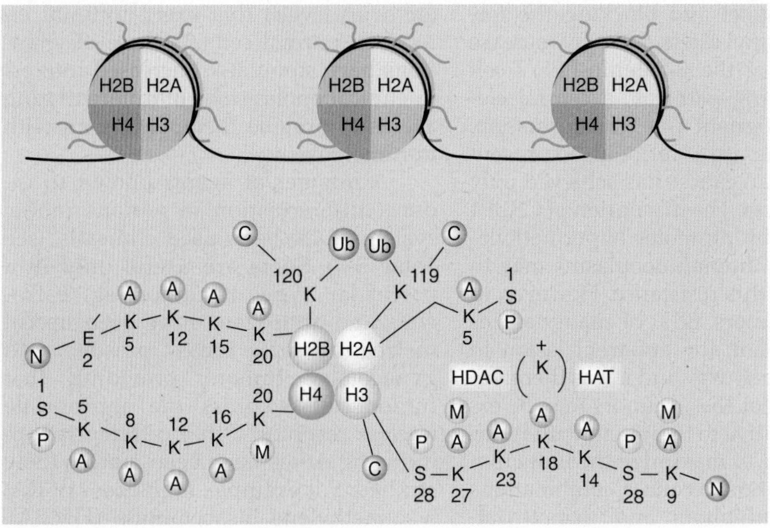

Figure 3-7 Schematic of the structure of histones in nucleosomes. (**A**) The core proteins of nucleosomes are designated H2A (histone 2A), H2B (histone 2B), H3 (histone 3), and H4 (histone 4). Each histone is present in two copies, so the DNA (black) wraps around an octomer of histones—the core nucleosome. (**B**) The amino-terminal tails of core histones. Lysines (K) in the amino-terminal tails of histones H2A, H2B, H3, and H4 are potential acetylation/deacetylation sites for histone acetyltransferases (HATs) and histone deacetylases (HDACs). Acetylation neutralizes the charge on lysines. A, acetyl; C, carboxyl terminus; E, glutamic acid; M, methyl; N, amino terminus; P, phosphate; S, serine; Ub, ubiquitin. *Source:* Reprinted by permission from Macmillian Publishers Ltd: Nat Rev Cancer, Marks P, Rifkind RA, Richon VM, et al. Histone deacetylases and cancer:causes and therapies, 1:194–202, copyright 2001.

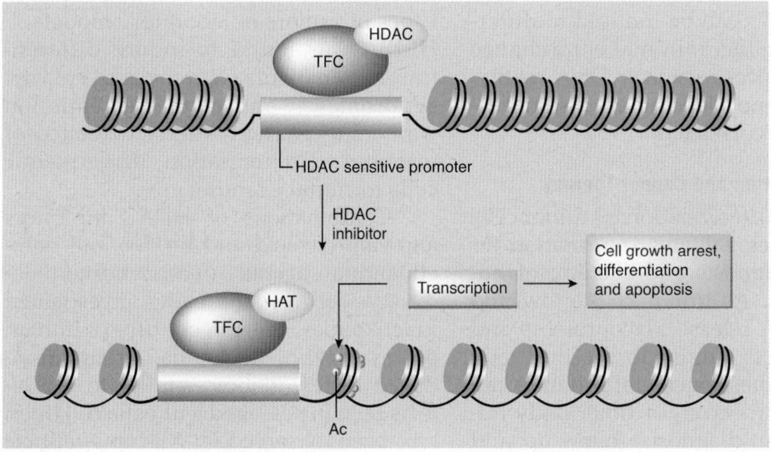

Figure 3-8 Proposed mechanism of action of histone deacetylase inhibitors. With inhibition of histone deacetylases (HDACs) by HDAC inhibitors such as suberoylanilide hydroxamic acid, histones are acetylated, and the DNA that is tightly wrapped around a deacetylated histone core relaxes. It has been proposed that there are specific sites in the promoter region of a subset of genes (eg, SP1 sites) that recruit the transcription factor complex (TFC) with HDAC and that the accumulation of acetylated histones in nucleosomes leads to increased transcription of this subset of genes (eg, *CDKN1A*, which encodes WAF1), which, in turn, leads to downstream effects that result in cell-growth arrest, differentiation and/or apoptotic cell death acetyltranferase. *Source:* Reprinted by permission from Macmillian Publishers Ltd: Nat Rev Cancer, Marks P, Rifkind RA, Richon VM, et al. Histone deacetylases and cancer:causes and therapies, 1:194–202, copyright 2001.

developmental and spatial fates of cells in embryos of the fruit fly *Drosophila*. Similar genes have been identified in the genomes of higher organisms, including humans. Individual homeotic genes are expressed at different times during development and also are expressed in different adult tissues. Some homeotic genes code for extracellular factors, whereas others code for nuclear proteins that are probably transcriptional regulatory factors. Homeotic genes regulate programs of differentiation as opposed to individual differentiation-specific genes. They appear to act by initiating cascades of gene expression that involve regulatory genes having a more restricted range of actions.[192,193] Some homeotic genes may function as tumor suppressors in normal tissues; others may promote tumorigenesis when mutated or deregulated. Mutations in homeotic genes may reactivate portions of an embryonic program of gene expression or suppress portions of an adult program of gene expression.[194-196]

DNA Methylation

In many cases, cells must go through one or more rounds of DNA replication before they can differentiate. This requirement may be because there often is a need to modify the pattern of DNA methylation before differentiation begins. DNA methylation in eukaryotes involves addition of a methyl group to the carbon/5 position of the cytosine ring.[197] Changes in DNA methylation commonly are introduced during DNA replication. DNA methylation is essential for development in the mouse and plays an important role in inactivation of the X-chromosome and genomic imprinting.[198] It may also contribute to the control of tissue-specific gene expression. The most direct mechanism by which DNA methylation can interfere with transcription is to prevent the binding of basal transcriptional machinery or ubiquitous transcription factors that require contact with cytosine in the major groove of the double helix. Most mammalian transcription factors have GC-rich-binding sites and many have CpGs in their DNA recognition elements. Binding by several of these factors is indeed impeded or abolished by methylation of CpG, though some factors, notably Sp1, are indifferent to methylation status. The highest density of nonmethylated CpGs in the vertebrate genome are found in CpG islands, which usually contain promoter or other regulatory DNA that is required for active transcription of a gene. CpG island chromatin is enriched in hyperacetylated histones and deficient in linker histones. These are essential features of transcriptionally competent chromatin templates. In contrast, chromatin assembled on artificially methylated DNA becomes associated with hypoacetylated histones, refractory to nuclease or restriction endonuclease digestion and transcriptionally silent. Many tumor-suppressor and other cancer-related genes have been found to be hypermethylated in human cancer cells and primary tumors (Table 3-4).[199] The different classes of genes that are silenced by DNA methylation include tumor-suppressor genes, genes that suppress tumor invasion, and metastasis; DNA repair genes; genes for hormone receptors; and genes that inhibit angiogenesis. The methylation of DNA on specific cytosine residues is believed to contribute to the changes in gene expression that occur during development. Presumably, DNA methylation affects gene expres-

Table 3-4 **Genes Silenced by Aberrant DNA Methylation**

Tumor suppressor
p15 INK4B (cyclin kinase inhibitor)
p16 INK4A (cyclin kinase inhibitor)
p73 (p53 homology)
ARF/INK4A (regulate level p53)
Wilms tumor
von Hippel-Lindau (VHL)
Retinoic acid receptor-β (RARβ)
Estrogen receptor
Androgen receptor
Mammary-derived growth inhibitor
Hypermethylated in cancer (HIC1)
Retinoblastoma (Rb)
Invasion/metastasis inhibitor
E-cadherin
Tissue inhibitor metalloproteinases-3 (TIMP-3)
mts-1
CD-44
DNA repair/detoxify carcinogens
Methylguanine methyltransferase
HMLH1 (mismatch DNA repair)
Glutathione S-transferase
BRCA-1
Angiogenesis inhibitor
Thrombospondin-1 (TSP-1)
TIMP-3
Tumor antigen
MAGE-1

Source: Data from Ref. 200.

sion because the transcriptional regulatory proteins that bind to methylated DNA differ from those that bind to unmethylated DNA. Many neoplastic tissues have hypermethylated genes relative to their normal counterparts[200-204] and, indeed, pharmacologic agents that alter the pattern of DNA methylation induce differentiation in a number of cultured cell lines: 5-azacytidine and recently deoxyazacytidine (DAC) have shown promise in vitro and in clinical trials in leukemias.[198,199] Gene silencing by hypermethylation of promoter genes has been recognized as an important mechanism of carcinogenesis that has great promise for cancer prevention and therapy ("epigenetic therapy"). In breast cancer, demethylating agents have been proposed to reactivate silenced genes, including the estrogen receptor and RARβ genes. As discussed earlier, the first described alteration in the retinoid pathway was the leukemogenic role of the PML-RAR fusion protein. Later, evidence supported the role of RARβ2 as a tumor-suppressor gene: the induction of RARβ2 related to the chemopreventive effects of retinoids, the loss of RARβ2 expression in human neoplasms, frequent chromosomal losses at 3p21-3p24 where RARβ2 is located, and the methylation-mediated silencing of RARβ2.[205] Subsequently, the epigenetic silencing of the cellular retinol-binding protein-1 gene (CRBP1) was reported as a common alteration in human cancer.[206] The loss of CRBP1 may compromise retinoic acid metabolism by diminishing retinol transport and blocking the formation of retinyl esters and may increase the activity of the β-catenin-LEF/T-cell factor signaling pathway, a central element in malignant cell transformation. Until now, the use of retinoids to prevent or treat human cancer has achieved only modest success. The disruption of CRBP1 and RARβ2 by promoter hypermethylation in many human neoplasms may in part explain this resistance. However, in colorectal tumors, 30% of malignancies did not present any apparent lesion in the retinoid pathway and it was therefore postulated that these tumors may be extremely sensitive to treatment with retinoids. In order to maximize the induction of differentiation in cancer, combinations of HDAC inhibitors and demethylating agents have been proposed.[198] DNA methylation is probably not a universal mechanism for differentiation, however, and some cells can be induced to differentiate with either minimal or no change in cell cycle progression.[207] DNA methylation and gene silencing are also not always strictly correlated.

Differentiation and Cancer Therapy

Analysis of differentiation by tumor cells often provides valuable information for both the diagnosis and therapy of human cancers. As tumor cells grow and die, they can release glycoproteins and other products similar to those of fetal tissues, and these oncofetal products can be detected in serum or other body fluids to assist in diagnosis, follow-up, and selection of therapies. Examples include estrogen receptors and α-lactalbumin in breast cancer, prostate-specific antigen and prostatic acid phosphatase in prostate cancers, and myoglobin and desmin in sarcomas.[208]

Elevations of these markers in the serum often predict relapse of the neoplasm before any sign by routine examination or radiographic tests. In general, the specificity of such markers for a given neoplasm is poor because minor elevations also occur with inflammatory and other benign conditions or with several types of neoplasms. In carcinoma of unknown primary site, tissue markers for neuroendocrine differentiation select for a subgroup of patients with improved response to chemotherapy.[209]

Some tumor cells can be induced to differentiate terminally. This has been shown most extensively in cultured cell lines (see Table 3-3) but also in experimental animals.[171,210,211] After tumor cells have been induced to undergo terminal differentiation, their ability to grow as a tumor often is stably suppressed. In contrast to most anticancer drugs, which have nonspecific toxicity to both normal and cancer cells, drug-induced differentiation can be demonstrated with agents (or drug levels) that exert minimal effects on normal cells.[210] These observations have stimulated increased interest in clinical applications of differentiating agents to provide therapeutic gain with minimal toxicity.[212]

A number of agents known to induce differentiation in various model systems have been used clinically (see Table 3-3). Some are useful only in a particular type of tumor; eg, estrogens and androgens have been useful in treating some breast, prostate, and gynecologic tumors, providing that tumor cells express the appropriate nuclear receptor. Other differentiation-inducing drugs have been more widely studied. For example, high doses of RA, hexamethylene bisacetamide (HMBA), or 5-azacytidine, an inhibitor of DNA methylation, can induce differentiation and inhibit the growth of several types of tumors in laboratory models.[211] HMBA was found to induce differentiation in patients with myelodysplastic syndromes,[213] and complete remission was achieved with direct evidence of terminal differentiation of leukemic cells to clonal granulocytes.

Combinations of HDAC inhibitors (eg, valproic acid and SAHA) and demethylating agents (5-azacytidine, deoxyazacytidine) are being investigated in leukemias. In fresh cultures of human promyelocytic leukemia, retinoid-induced differentiation, similar to the effects seen in passaged leukemia cell lines, has been observed.[214] All-trans-retinoic acid has been used in clinical therapy of promyelocytic leukemia with promising results,[215,216] and retinoids have been used in combination with interferon-α to produce responses in patients with squamous cell cancer of the skin or cervix.[217] Because differentiating agents may inhibit tumor cell growth by multiple mechanisms, it is difficult to prove specific differentiating actions of these agents when used in patients.[216,218] For example, retinoids not only induce differentiation in leukemia but also downregulate anti-apoptotic genes.[219] An exception are studies in leukemias where sequential samples are readily available, differentiation markers are well established, and the clonality of differentiated cells can be ascertained by methods such as molecular cytogenetics (FISH).[213]

Retinoids and other differentiating agents are also used in clinical trials to prevent cancer in patients with premalignant lesions or a high risk for developing cancer of the breast, cervix, colon, skin, lung, or oral cavity. Early results are encouraging, including the reversal of oral leukoplakia and prevention of second neoplasms in patients with treated squamous cell carcinoma of the head and neck.[218,220] Greater knowledge about the molecular basis for the control of differentiation should lead to more accurate predictions, however, as well as rational design of therapies for controlling tumor growth by manipulating the state of differentiation.[211,221,222]

Selected References

The complete reference list can be found at www.CANCERMEDICINE8.com

1. Evan GI, Vousden KH. Proliferation, cell cycle and apoptosis in cancer. *Nature.* 2001;411:342–348.
8. Polyak K, Lee M-H, Erdjument-Bromage H, et al. Cloning of p27Kip1, a cyclin-dependent kinase inhibitor and a potential mediator of extracellular antimitogenic signals. *Cell.* 1994;78:59–66.
11. Koepp DM, Harper JW, Elledge SJ. How the cyclin became a cyclin: regulated proteolysis in the cell cycle. *Cell.* 1999;97:431–434.
15. Druker BJ, Mamon HJ, Roberts TM. Oncogenes, growth factors, and signal transduction. *N Engl J Med.* 1989;321:1383–1391.
22. Goodrich DW, Wang NP, Qian YW, Lee EY, Lee WH. The retinoblastoma gene product regulates progression through the G1 phase of the cell cycle. *Cell.* 1991;67:293–302.
26. Trimarchi JM, Lees JA. Sibling rivalry in the E2F family. *Nat Rev Mol Cell Biol.* 2002;3:11–20.
27. Iaquinta PJ, Lees JA. Life and death decisions by the E2F transcription factors. *Curr Opin Cell Biol.* 2007;19:649–657.
38. Waterman MJ, Stavridi ES, Waterman JL, Halazonetis TD. ATM-dependent activation of p53 involves dephosphorylation and association with 14-3-3 proteins. *Nat Genet.* 1998;19:175–178.
40. Khanna KK, Keating KE, Kozlov S, et al. ATM associates with and phosphorylates p53: mapping the region of interaction. *Nat Genet.* 1998;20:398–400.
45. Stewart SA, Weinberg RA. Senescence: does it all happen at the ends? *Oncogene.* 2002;21:627–630.
46. Prieur A, Peeper DS. Cellular senescence in vivo: a barrier to tumorigenesis. *Curr Opin Cell Biol.* 2008;20:150–155.
51. Tannock I. Cell kinetics and chemotherapy: a critical review. *Cancer Treat Rep.* 1978;62:1117–1133.
59. Sherr CJ. Cancer cell cycles. *Science.* 1996;274:1672–1677.
67. Prives C, Hall PA. The p53 pathway. *J Pathol.* 1999;187:112–126.
68. Akashi M, Koeffler HP. Li-Fraumeni syndrome and the role of the p53 tumor suppressor gene in cancer susceptibility. *Clin Obstet Gynecol.* 1998;41:172–199.
70. Vassilev LT, Vu BT, Graves B, et al. In vivo activation of the p53 pathway by small-molecule antagonists of MDM2. *Science.* 2004;303:844–848.
71. Kojima K, Konopleva M, Samudio IJ, et al. MDM2 antagonists induce p53-dependent apoptosis in AML: implications for leukemia therapy. *Blood.* 2005;106:3150–3159.
75. Gery S, Koeffler HP. The role of circadian regulation in cancer. *Cold Spring Harb Symp Quant Biol.* 2007;72:459–464.
77. Gery S, Gombart AF, Yi WS, et al. Transcription profiling of C/EBP targets identifies *Per2* as a gene implicated in myeloid leukemia. *Blood.* 2005;106:2827–2836.
79. Robertson LE, Plunkett W, McConnell K, Keating MJ, McDonnell TJ. Bcl-2 expression in chronic lymphocytic leukemia and its correlation with the induction of apoptosis and clinical outcome. *Leukemia.* 1996;10:456–459.
84. Mazel S, Burtrum D, Petrie HT. Regulation of cell division cycle progression by bcl-2 expression: a potential mechanism for inhibition of programmed cell death. *J Exp Med.* 1996;183:2219–2226.
85. O'Reilly LA, Huang DC, Strasser A. The cell death inhibitor Bcl-2 and its homologues influence control of cell cycle entry. *EMBO J.* 1996;15:6979–6990.
88. Konopleva M, Zhao S, Hu W, et al. The anti-apoptotic genes Bcl-XL and Bcl-2 are over-expressed and contribute to chemoresistance of non-proliferating leukaemic CD34+ cells. *Br J Haematol.* 2002;118:521–534.
90. Konopleva M, Contractor R, Tsao T, et al. Mechanisms of apoptosis sensitivity and resistance to the BH3 mimetic ABT-737 in acute myeloid leukemia. *Cancer Cell.* 2006;10:375–388.
91. Schimmer AD, Kantarjian H, O'Brien S, et al. A phase I study of the pan Bcl-2 family inhibitor obatoclax mesylate in patients with refractory hematologic maligancies. *Clin Cancer Res.* 2008;In Press.
92. Konopleva M, Watt J, Contractor R, et al. Mechanisms of antileukemic activity of the novel Bcl-2 homology domain-3 mimetic GX15-070 obatoclax. *Cancer Res.* 2008;68:3413–3420.
93. Opferman JT, Iwasaki H, Ong CC, et al. Obligate role of anti-apoptotic MCL-1 in the survival of hematopoietic stem cells. *Science.* 2005;307:1101–1104.
94. Carter BZ, Milella M, Altieri DC, Andreeff M. Cytokine-regulated expression of *survivin* in myeloid leukemia. *Blood.* 2001;97:2784–2790.
95. Andreeff M, Stone R, Michaeli J, et al. Hexamethylene bisacetamide in myelodysplastic syndrome and acute myelogenous leukemia: a phase II clinical trial with a differentiation-inducing agent. *Blood.* 1992;80:2604–2609.
96. Pandolfi PP. Histone deacetylases and transcriptional therapy with their inhibitors. *Cancer Chemother Pharmacol.* 2001;48 (Suppl 1):S17–S19.
100. Paddison PJ, Caudy AA, Bernstein E, Hannon GJ, Conklin DS. Short hairpin RNAs shRNAs) induce sequence-specific silencing in mammalian cells. *Genes Dev.* 2002;16:948–958.
106. Tenen DG. Disruption of differentiation in human cancer: AML shows the way. *Nat Rev Cancer.* 2003;3:89–101.
107. Kelly LM, Gilliland DG. Genetics of myeloid leukemias. *Annu Rev Genomics Hum Genet.* 2002;3:179–198.
108. Nerlov C. C/EBPalpha mutations in acute myeloid leukaemias. *Nat Rev Cancer.* 2004;4:394–400.
110. Smith ML, Cavenagh JD, Lister TA, Fitzgibbon J. Mutation of CEBPA in familial acute myeloid leukemia. *N Engl J Med.* 2004;351:2403–2407.
117. Weidner N, Semple JP, Welch WR, Folkman J. Tumor angiogenesis and metastasis—correlation in invasive breast carcinoma. *N Engl J Med.* 1991;324:1–8.
121. Bjornson CR, Rietze RL, Reynolds BA, Magli MC, Vescovi AL. Turning brain into blood: a hematopoietic fate adopted by adult neural stem cells in vivo [see comments]. *Science.* 1999;283:534–537.
125. Pittenger MF, Mackay AM, Beck SC, et al. Multilineage potential of adult human mesenchymal stem cells. *Science.* 1999;284:143–147.
132. Mezey E, Chandross KJ, Harta G, Maki RA, McKercher SR. Turning blood into brain: cells bearing neuronal antigens generated in vivo from bone marrow. *Science.* 2000;290:1779–1782.
139. Wagers AJ, Sherwood RI, Christensen JL, Weissman IL. Little evidence for developmental plasticity of adult hematopoietic stem cells. *Science.* 2002;297:2256–2259.
140. Castro RF, Jackson KA, Goodell MA, et al. Failure of bone marrow cells to transdifferentiate into neural cells in vivo. *Science.* 2002;297:1299.
149. Kaufman DS, Hanson ET, Lewis RL, Auerbach R, Thomson JA. Hematopoietic colony-forming cells derived from human embryonic stem cells. *Proc Natl Acad Sci USA.* 2001;98:10716–10721.
155. Studeny M, Marini FC, Dembinski J, et al. Mesenchymal stem cells: potential precursors for tumor stroma and targeted-delivery vehicles for anti-cancer agents. *J Natl Cancer Inst.* 2004;96:1593–1603.
156. Vermeulen K, Van Bockstaele DR, Berneman ZN. The cell cycle: a review of regulation, deregulation and therapeutic targets in cancer. *Cell Prolif.* 2003;36:131–149.
157. Mani SA, Guo W, Liao MJ, et al. The epithelial-mesenchymal transition generates cells with properties of stem cells. *Cell.* 2008;133:704–715.
175. Xie D, Yin D, Tong X, et al. Cyr61 is overexpressed in gliomas and involved in integrin-linked kinase-mediated Akt and beta-catenin-TCF/Lef signaling pathways. *Cancer Res.* 2004;64:1987–1996.
181. Grignani F, De Matteis S, Nervi C, et al. Fusion proteins of the retinoic acid receptor-alpha recruit histone deacetylase in promyelocytic leukaemia. *Nature.* 1998;391:815–818.
182. Marks P, Rifkind RA, Richon VM, et al. Histone deacetylases and cancer: causes and therapies. *Nat Rev Cancer.* 2001;1:194–202.
187. Konopleva M, Andreeff M. Role of peroxisome proliferator-activated receptor-gamma in hematologic malignancies. *Curr Opin Hematol.* 2002;9:294–302.
200. Jones PA, Baylin SB. The fundamental role of epigenetic events in cancer. *Nat Rev Genet.* 2002;3:415–428.

4 Apoptosis and Cancer

John C. Reed, MD, PhD

Programmed cell death plays critical roles in a wide variety of physiologic processes during fetal development and in adult tissues. In most cases, physiologic cell death occurs by a process known as "apoptosis." Defects in apoptotic cell death contribute to neoplastic diseases, by preventing or delaying normal cell turnover, thus promoting cell accumulation. Defects in apoptosis also facilitate tumor progression, by rendering cancer cells resistant to death mechanisms relevant to metastasis, hypoxia, growth factor deprivation, chemotherapy, and irradiation. Knowledge of the molecular mechanisms responsible for the regulation and execution of apoptosis has provided insights into the pathobiology of cancer and has suggested a variety of novel therapeutic strategies that may eventually improve the efficacy of cancer treatment.

It is now well established that defects in the normal mechanisms that control programmed cell death (PCD) occur commonly in cancers. Cell numbers in the body are governed not only by cell division, which determines the rate of cell production, but also by cell death, which sets the rate of cell loss. In the course of a typical day, an average adult produces, and in parallel eradicates ~50-70 billion cells, representing approximately 1 million cells per second. Normally, these two processes of cell division and cell death are tightly coupled so that no net increase in cell numbers occurs, or so that such increases represent only temporary responses to environmental stimuli. However, alternations in the expression or function of the genes that control PCD can upset this delicate balance, contributing to the expansion of neoplastic cells.[1,2]

Defects in normal programmed cell death mechanisms play a major role in the pathogenesis of tumors (Table 4-1), allowing neoplastic cells to survive beyond their normally intended lifespan, subverting the need for exogenous survival factors, providing protection from hypoxia and oxidative stress as tumor mass expands, and allowing time for accumulative genetic alterations that deregulate cell proliferation, interfere with differentiation, promote angiogenesis, and increase cell motility and invasiveness during tumor progression. In fact, apoptosis defects are recognized as an important complement to proto-oncogene activation, as many deregulated oncoproteins that drive cell division also trigger apoptosis (eg, Myc; E1a; cyclinD1).[3] Defects in apoptosis facilitate metastasis by allowing epithelial cells to survive in a suspended state, without attachment to extracellular matrix.[4] They also promote resistance to the immune system, in as much as many of the weapons cytolytic T cells (CTL) and natural killer (NK) cells use for attacking tumors depend on integrity of the apoptosis machinery.[5] Finally, cancer-associated defects in apoptosis play a role in chemoresistance and radioresistance, increasing the threshold for cell death, and thereby requiring higher doses for tumor killing.[6,7] Thus, defective apoptosis regulation is a fundamental aspect of the biology of cancer.

Table 4-1 ■ Cancer and Apoptosis: Pathogenesis, Progression, Therapy Resistance

Cell accumulation (cell death < cell division)
Longevity (accumulation of genetic lesions)
Proto-oncogene tolerance (nullify pro-apoptotic effects)
Genomic instability (tolerate DNA mistakes)
Immune surveillance (resistance to immune attack)
Growth facor/hormone-independence (survival without paracrine/endocrine growth factors)
Angiogenesis (resistance to hypoxia; hypoglycemia)
Metastasis (survival without attachment)
Chemoresistance/radioresistance (increased threshold for cell death)

Apoptosis is defined by its morphologic features. As viewed with the assistance of the light- (or preferably electron-) microscope, the characteristics of the apoptotic cell include chromatin condensation and nuclear fragmentation (pyknosis), plasma membrane blebbing, and cell shrinkage. Eventually, the cell breaks into small membrane-surrounded fragments (apoptotic bodies), which are cleared by phagocytosis, without inciting an inflammatory response. The release of apoptotic bodies is what inspired the term "apoptosis" from the Greek, meaning "to fall away from" and conjuring notions of the falling of leaves in the autumn from deciduous trees.[8]

In recent years, the molecular machinery responsible for apoptosis has been elucidated, revealing a family of intracellular proteases—Caspases—which are responsible directly or indirectly for the morphologic and biochemical changes that characterize the phenomenon of apoptosis.[9,10] Diverse regulators of the Caspases have also been discovered, including activators and inhibitors of these cell death proteases. Inputs from signal transduction pathways into the core of the cell death machinery have also been identified, demonstrating ways of linking environmental stimuli to cell death responses or cell survival maintenance. Knowledge of the molecular mechanisms of apoptosis is providing insights into the pathogenesis and progression of cancer, and is beginning to suggest new approaches to the treatment of neoplastic diseases.

In this chapter, some of the genes involved in apoptosis regulation are described, and examples of cancer-associated defects in the expression or regulation of those genes or their encoded proteins are provided. In addition, some of the emerging strategies for restoring apoptosis sensitivity to tumors based on pharmacologic manipulation of cell death proteins are explained.

Apoptosis Caused by Caspases

What causes the morphologic changes that we recognize as "apoptosis" and the biochemical changes often associated with this phenomenon? The answer is proteases. Specifically, activation of a family of intracellular cysteine proteases that cleave their substrates at aspartic acid residues, known as "Caspases" for Cysteine Aspartyl-specific Proteases.[11] These proteases are present as inactive zymogens in essentially all animal cells, but can be triggered to assume active states, generally involving their proteolytic processing at conserved aspartic acid (Asp) residues. During activation, the zymogen pro-proteins are cleaved to generate the large (~20 kDa) and small (~10 kDa) subunits of the active enzymes, typically liberating an N-terminal prodomain from the processed polypeptide chain. The active enzymes consist of heterotetramers comprising two large and two small subunits, with two active sites per molecule.[9,10]

The observation that Caspases cleave their substrates at Asp residues and that they are also activated by proteolytic processing at Asp residues makes evident that these proteases collaborate in proteolytic cascades, where Caspases activate themselves and each other. Humans contain 10 Caspases. They can be subgrouped according to either their amino-acid sequence similarities or their protease specificities. From a functional perceptive, it is useful to view the Caspases as either upstream "initiator" Caspases or downstream "effector" Caspases.[12] The zymogen forms of upstream initiator Caspases possess large N-terminal prodomains, which function as protein interaction modules, allowing them to interact with various proteins that trigger Caspase activation. In contrast, the proforms of downstream effector Caspases contain only short N-terminal prodomains, serving no apparent function. Downstream Caspases are largely dependent on upstream Caspases for their proteolytic processing and activation. The substrates of effector Caspases include protein kinases (often separating the autorepressing regulatory domains from catalytic domains) and other signal transduction proteins, cytoskeletal and nuclear matrix proteins, chromatin-modifying (eg, poly-ADP-ribose polymerase) and DNA repair proteins, and inhibitory subunits of endonucleases (CIDE-family proteins).[9,10,12]

Inactivating mutations in genes encoding Caspases in human malignancies have been reported. For example, homozygous deletions of the *CASPASE-3* gene were identified in MCF7 cells, a breast cancer cell line commonly employed as an experimental model.[13] Similarly, missense mutations in the *CASPASE-8* gene have been documented as well as gene silencing in association with hypermethylation of CpG islands, in neuroblastomas and some other types of solid tumors.[14,15] Frame-shift mutations that disrupt the reading-frame of the *Caspase-5* gene have been cited in colon cancers that have microsatellite instability (MSI), a DNA mismatch repair enzyme defect associated with mutations in homopolymeric stretches of nucleotides throughout the genome.[16] Thus, precedence exists for cancer-associated mutations in Caspase-encoding genes, presumably contributing to apoptosis-resistance states. However, because of redundancy among Caspases, these defects do not prevent apoptosis altogether, leaving alternative routes of apoptosis intact.

Caspase Activation Pathways: An Overview

Several pathways for activating Caspases exist, although details remain sketchy for some of them (Fig. 4-1). The simplest is exploited by CTL cells and natural killer (NK) cells, which introduce apoptosis-inducing proteases, particularly granzyme B, into effective intracellular compartments of target cells via perforin-dependent mechanisms.[17] Unlike the Caspases, granzyme B is a serine protease. However, similar to the Caspases, granzyme B specifically cleaves its substrates at Asp residues. Granzyme B is capable of cleaving and activating multiple Caspases and some Caspase substrates.[18] Endogenous and viral inhibitors of granzyme B have been identified, accounting for resistance to this apoptosis inducer.[19-21]

Another Caspase-activation pathway is represented by tumor necrosis factor (TNF)-family receptors. Eight of the ~30 known members of the TNF family in humans contain a so-called Death Domain (DD) in their cytosolic tails.[22] Several of these DD-containing TNF-family receptors use Caspase activation as a signaling mechanism, including TNFR1/CD120a; Fas/APO1/CD95; DR3/Apo2/Weasle; DR4/TrailR1; DR5/TrailR2; and DR6. Ligation of these receptors at the cell surface results in receptor clustering and recruitment of several intracellular proteins, including certain pro-Caspases, to the cytosolic domains of these receptors, forming a "death-inducing signaling complex" (DISC) that triggers Caspase activation and leads to apoptosis.[23,24] The specific Caspases summoned to the DISC are Caspase 8 and, in some cases, Caspase 10. These Caspases contain so-called death effector domains (DEDs) in their N-terminal prodomains that bind to a corresponding DED in FADD, a bipartite adapter protein containing a DD and a DED. FADD functions as a molecular bridge between the DD and DED domain families, and is in fact the only protein in the human genome with this dual domain structure.[25] Consequently, cells from mice in which the *FADD* gene has been knocked out are resistant to apoptosis induction by TNF-family cytokines and their receptors.[26] Cells derived from *Caspase 8* knock-out mice also fail to undergo apoptosis in response to ligands or antibodies that activate TNF-family death receptors, demonstrating an essential role for this Caspase in this pathway.[27] However, mice lack the highly homologous protease, Caspase 10, which is found in humans, having arisen from an apparent gene duplication on chromosome.[2,25] Thus, it is presently unclear to what extent Caspases 8 and 10 display redundancy in human cells.

Mitochondria also play important roles in apoptosis, releasing cytochrome *c* (cyt *c*) into the cytosol, which then causes assembly of a multiprotein Caspase-activating complex, referred to as the "apoptosome."[28,29] The central compo-

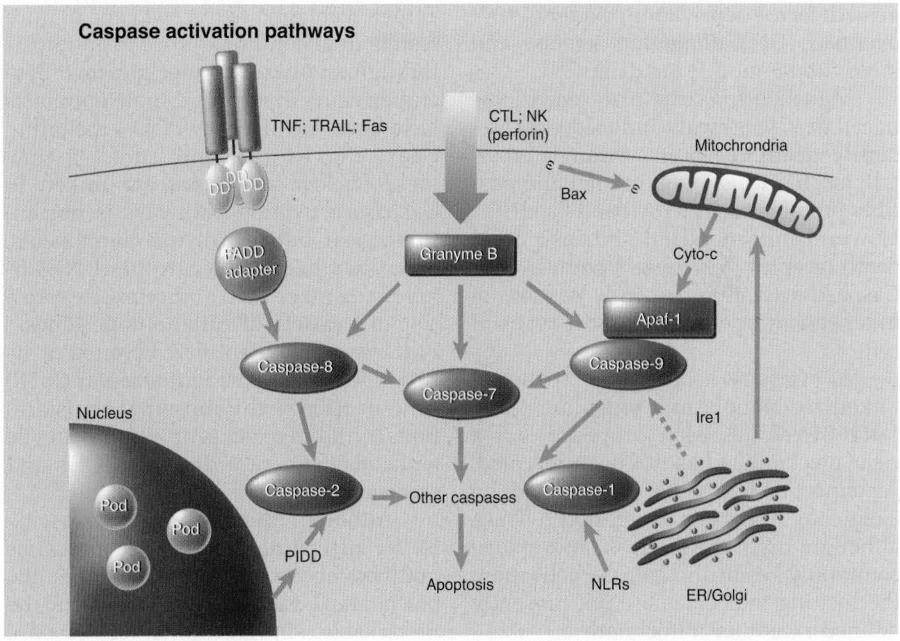

Figure 4-1 The major pathways for Caspase activation in mammalian cells are presented. The extrinsic (*left*) is induced by members of the TNF family of cytokine receptors such as TNFR1, Fas, and the TRAIL Receptors. These proteins recruit adapter proteins to their cytosolic Death Domains (DDs), including FADD, which then bind DED-containing pro-Caspases, particularly pro-Caspase 8, inducing their activation. CTLs and NK cells introduce the protease granzyme B into target cells (*middle*). This protease cleaves and activates multiple members of the Caspase family. The intrinsic pathway (*right*) is initiated by release of cytochrome *c* from mitochondria, induced by various stimuli, including elevations in the levels of pore-forming pro-apoptotic Bcl-2 family proteins such as Bax. In the cytosol, cytochrome *c* binds and activates APAF-1, allowing it to be associated with and activate pro-Caspase 9. Active Caspase 9 (intrinsic) and Caspase 8 (extrinsic) have been shown to directly cleave and activate the effector protease, Caspase 3. Other Caspases also become involved in these pathways (not shown), thus the schematic represents an over simplification of the events that occur in vivo. Poorly defined pathways linking nuclear structures called PML oncogenic domains (PODs) (*lower left*) and stress in the Golgi and endoplasmic reticulum (ER) (*lower right*) to Caspase activation have also been described.

nent of the apoptosome is APAF1, a Caspase-activating protein that oligomerizes upon binding cyt *c* and specifically binds pro-Caspase 9. APAF1 and pro-Caspase 9 interact with each other via their caspase recruitment domains (CARDs). Such CARD–CARD interactions play important roles in many steps in apoptosis pathways. In addition to cyt *c*, mitochondria also release several other proteins of relevance to apoptosis, including Endonuclease G, AIF (anactivator of nuclear endonucleases), Smac (Diablo), Omi (HtrA2) and ARTS—antagonists of a family of Caspase-inhibitory proteins known as the IAPs (see below). However, the central importance of the cyt *c*–dependent pathway for apoptosis is underscored by the observation that cells derived from mice in which either the *apaf1* or *pro-Caspase 9* genes have been ablated are incapable of undergoing apoptosis in response to agents that trigger cyt *c* release from mitochondria.[30] Nevertheless, such cells can die by nonapoptotic routes, demonstrating that mitochondria control both Caspase-dependent and Caspase-independent cell death pathways.[31] The mitochondrial pathway for apoptosis is activated by myriad stimuli, including growth factor deprivation, oxidants, Ca^{2+} overload, DNA-damaging agents, and microtubule-modifying drugs.[29,32]

Mitochondria can also participate in cell death pathways induced via TNF-family death receptors, through cross-talk mechanisms involving Bid and possibly proteins such as BAR and Bap31.[33-36] However, mitochondrial ("intrinsic") and death receptor ("extrinsic") pathways for Caspase activation are fully capable of independent operation in most types of cells.[37]

A Caspase activation pathway linked to endoplasmic reticulum (ER)/Golgi stress has been proposed, but a clear mechanism has not been revealed. A connection between Caspase 2 and the Golgi has also been suggested.[38] Thus, although organellar stress and injury commonly result in Caspase activation, the inciting molecules are not presently defined except for mitochondria.

The tumor suppressor p53 induces apoptosis via several mechanisms. One of these involves p53-mediated induction of the gene encoding PIDD, a DD-containing protein that binds the bipartite adapter protein RAIDD, containing DD and CARD domains, which in turn binds the CARD of pro-Caspase 2 to form the "PIDDosome."[39]

Caspase 1 and its close relatives Caspases 4 and 5 are primarily responsible for proteolytic cleavage and activation proinflammatory cytokines pro-IL 1β, pro-IL 18, and pro-IL 33. However, when excessive, these caspases induce apoptosis. Among the proteins that activate inflammatory Caspases are the NLR-family members. The NLRs include 22 members in humans. All NLRs contain a nucleotide-binding oligomerization domain called NACHT and sensory domains consisting of Leucine-Rich Repeats (LLRs). The LLRs are thought to directly or indirectly bind pathogen-derived molecules and mediators elaborated by tissue injury, thus inducing NLR oligomerization. Several NLRs directly bind pro-Caspase 1 via CARD domains or indirectly via PYRIN domains (PYD) that associate with the bipartite adapter protein ASC, which contains PYD and CARD domains, the latter binding the CARD of pro-Caspase 1. The Caspase-activating complexes involving NLRs have been termed "inflammasomes."[40] Another version of Caspase-1 activator is found in AIM2. The AIM2 protein contains an ASC-binding PYD and a DNA-binding Hin200 domain. Certain classes of DNA molecules induce Caspase-1 activation and cell death via AIM2.[41-43]

Finally, a nuclear pathway for apoptosis regulation centers on discrete nuclear organelles, called PML oncogenic domains (PODs) or nuclear bodies (NBs). Targeted ablation of the *pml* gene in mice results in general resistance to apoptosis through an unknown mechanism.[44] Several proteins that can promote apoptosis have been localized to PODs, including Daax, Zip Kinase, and Par4.[45-49] How these nuclear structures are linked to Caspase activation pathways is not entirely clear but one of the components, Daxx, has been shown to bind NF-κB-family member RelB and repress expression of a variety of antiapoptotic genes.[50] PML was first identified because of its fusion to the retinoic acid receptor (*RAR*) gene in t(15;17) chromosomal translocations found in acute promyelomonocytic leukemias, where it disrupts PODs and creates an apoptosis-resistant state.[51]

Although diverse mechanisms exist for activating initiator Caspases, as outlined above, in most instances the biochemical mechanisms appear to be remarkably similar. Much of Caspase activation can be explained by the "induced proximity model," where adapter proteins bring Caspases into close opposition, causing their dimizeration and stabilizing the active conformation.[52]

Protein Domains Involved in Apoptosis Regulation

The proteins that directly control the intrinsic, extrinsic, and other less understood Caspase-activation pathways often exist as families that can be recognized based on their amino-acid sequences and/or structural similarity. Moreover, interactions among these proteins are commonly mediated by domains that are intimately associated with apoptosis regulation, including Caspase recruitment domains (CARDs), Death Domains (DDs), Death Effector Domains (DEDs), Bcl-2 Homology (BH) domains of Bcl-2 family proteins, and Baculovirus IAP Repeat (BIR) domains of IAP-family proteins. A summary is provided below of some of the proteins that constitute these families of apoptosis regulators follows, along with information about their mechanisms; examples of alterations in cancer, and strategies for exploiting the information for devising new cancer therapies.

Death Domain Proteins

The death domain (DD) is a protein interaction module consisting of a compact bundle of six helices.[53] Death domains bind each other, probably forming oligomers of unknown stoichiometry. Specificity for partner selection among DDs is dictated by differences in surface residues. DDs appear to be capable of undergoing a conformational change to an open extended structure upon dimerization in some cases.[54]

Several of the members of the TNF-family of cytokine receptors contain DDs in their cytosolic regions, including TNFR1, Fas [Apo1], DR3 [Apo2], DR4 [Trail-R1], DR5 [Trail-R2], DR6 in humans, mice, and probably other mammals. The p75 Nerve Growth Factor receptor (p75-NGFR) also contains a modified ("type II") DD[55] and has been reported to induce apoptosis under some circumstances.[56] The TNF-family receptors, TNFR1, DR3, and DR6 are known to bind an adapter protein TRADD, via its homologous DD.[57-60] The DD of TRADD is capable of binding certain other DD-containing proteins, including the adapter protein FADD. The FADD (Mort1) protein contains two protein interaction modules, a DD and a DED. FADD links TNF-family death receptors to Caspases, using its DD to bind TRADD or to interact directly with the cytosolic DD of the TNFR-family member Fas, and employing its DED to bind DED-containing Caspases. Experimental evidence has demonstrated the presence of FADD within the receptor complexes of all known DD-containing members of the TNF-family except p75-NGFr. Thus, this protein plays a central role in linking Caspases to TNF-family death receptors, a notion borne out by gene ablation studies in mice, which have demonstrated an inability of TNFR1, Fas, and other death receptors tested thus far to induce apoptosis in the absence of FADD.[26,61-63]

The TNF family receptors member, Fas (Apol; CD95) is a potent inducer of apoptosis. Fas plays a critical role in immune system homeostasis, eradicating potentially autoreactive lymphocytes and downregulating immune responses after elimination of foreign antigen by reducing the numbers of expanded clones of antigen-specific T cells and B cells in peripheral lymphoid organs.[22,64,65] Germ line mutations in Fas and Fas-Ligand (FasL) have been discovered as the underlying basis for the lymphoproliferative autoimmune phenotype of *lpr/lpr* and *gdl/gdl* strain mice, respectively.[66,67] Similarly, causative mutations have been identified in the *FAS* gene of humans in patients with Autoimmune Lymphoproliferative Syndrome (ALPS). Thus, the Fas/FasL system plays a critical role in lymphocyte homeostasis in vivo. FasL is also a principal weapon used by cytolytic T cells for inducing apoptosis of virus-infected, tumorigenic, and allogenic cells.[65] Unfortunately, preclinical liver toxicity has precluded attempts to apply FasL or agonistic anti-Fas antibodies for the treatment of cancer.[68]

At least some of the mutant Fas proteins found in humans with ALPS have been shown to operate as trans-dominant inhibitors of wild-type Fas, probably explaining the dominant inheritance pattern of this disorder. In contrast, mutations in the *fas* gene of *lpr*-strain mice produce a similar autoimmune lymphoproliferative disorder with a recessive inheritance pattern.[66] FasL, like most TNF family members, is a trimer, and the receptor probably also forms trimers and perhaps higher-order oligomers, thus explaining why some Fas mutants display dominant-negative effects on wild-type Fas, whereas others do not. Indeed, mutant versions of Fas from some patients with hereditary ALPS have been demonstrated to antagonize wild-type Fas, probably forming mixed oligomers of wild-type and mutant molecules.[69]

Somatic mutations in the *FAS* gene have been found in multiple myelomas and non-Hodgkin lymphomas (NHLs). In a study of 150 cases of NHLs, where the coding regions of the gene were systematically sequenced, *FAS* gene mutations were found in 16 (11%) of the tumors.[70] Missense mutations within the DD of the receptor were associated with retention of the wild-type allele, suggesting a dominant-negative mechanism, whereas missense mutations outside the death domain were associated with allelic loss.[70]

Fas expression confers important prognostic information for some patients with leukemia. The *FAS* gene encodes two protein isoforms through alternative mRNA splicing: full-length Fas that has a transmembrane domain and a soluble form of Fas that lacks this transmembrane domain.[71] Soluble Fas is secreted into the extracellular environment where it acts as a decoy and binds FasL. As such, soluble Fas is an inhibitor of apoptosis. In a study of 59 patients with adult T-cell leukemia, increased serum levels of soluble Fas were associated with reduced survival and remained an important predictor in multivariate analysis even after accounting for other clinical risk factors.[72] Higher levels of soluble Fas in serum have also been correlated with disease progression and advanced clinical stage in B-CLL.[73,74] In addition to squelching Fas-induced apoptosis through secretion of soluble Fas, another suppressor of Fas, called DcR3, has been identified that is overexpressed in some tumors. DcR3 represents a member of the TNF-family that competes with Fas for binding to Fas L but lacks a DD and does not transduce apoptotic signals, functioning as a "decoy" receptor.[75]

TRAIL is a TNF-family ligand that has shown promise for the treatment of cancer. Unlike many other TNF-family cytokines, TRAIL does not induce inflammatory reactions and appears to be well tolerated in preclinical animal models, provided the recombinant protein is prepared in a careful manner.[76] The version of TRAIL currently being used in humans clinical trials is a soluble trimer, representing the extracellular domain of TRAIL. TRAIL induces apoptosis via two DD-containing receptors, TRAIL-R1 (DR4) and TRAIL-R2 (DR5). In addition to these death receptors, however, at least three TNF-family proteins have been identified that compete for binding to TRAIL but do not deliver death signals into cells. These "decoy" receptors, include DcR1, DcR2, and Osteoprogenerin (OPG) (Fig. 4-2).[75] It has been speculated that differences in the ratios of death and decoy receptors explain the selective toxicity of TRAIL to tumor cells versus normal cells, although this is probably not always true, representing an oversimplification of the mechanisms that account for the observed differential sensitivity to TRAIL. Agonistic antibodies to the TRAIL receptors, DR4 and DR5 that trigger tumor cell apoptosis are currently in clinical development.[77] The observation that tumor suppressor p53 can induce transcription of the death receptors Fas and DR5 in some types of tumor cells[78,79] may explain in part the synergistic antitumor activity in mouse models reported when combining cytotoxic anticancer drugs with TNF-family death ligands or agonistic antibodies that bind TNF-family death receptors.[80]

Besides the DD-containing TNF-family receptors, additional DD-containing proteins have been implicated in apoptosis, such as the DAP kinase-1, which modulates apoptosis induction by TNF-family death receptors through unclear mechanisms.[81] This kinase has

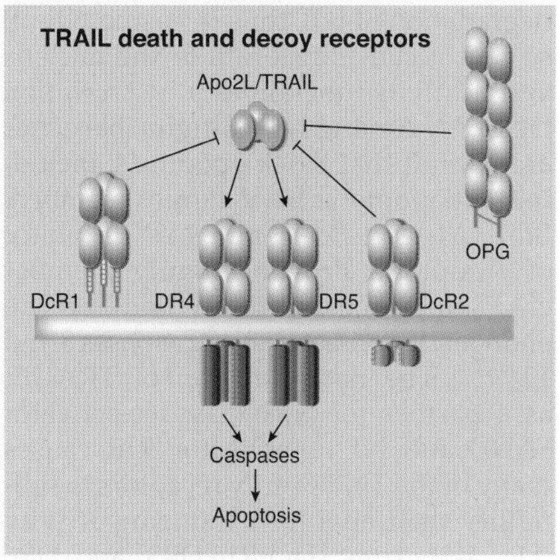

Figure 4-2 In humans, five receptors have been identified for TRAIL. Two of these, DR4 (TRAIL-R1) and DR5 (TRAIL-R2), are transmembrane proteins containing cytosolic DDs that engage the Caspase activation machinery. The others function as "decoys," competing for binding to TRAIL but lacking the capacity to signal into the cell death pathway. DcR1 is a GPI-linked protein, attached to the membrane via lipid modification. DcR2 is a transmembrane protein containing a nonfunction, truncated DD. OPG is a secreted protein. Differences in the ratios of TRAIL-binding death and decoy receptors may account in some cases for differential sensitivity of normal and tumor cells to this death-ligand.

been implicated in suppression of metastasis. In a recent study, DAPK1 has been implicated in autophagy, where it phosphorylates the BH3 domain of autophagy protein Beclin and frees it from Bcl-2 (see below for more on BH3 protein and Bcl-2 family).[82] Several cytoskeleton-associated ankyrin-family proteins contain DDs, but their relevance to apoptosis remains uncertain. Given evidence however that Caspase-8 activation is triggered by suspension of adherent epithelial cells,[83,84] an event that disturbs the cytoskeleton, it is intriguing to speculate a possible role in the phenomenon of "anoikis" (ie, apoptosis induced by depriving cells of integrin-mediated attachments to extracellular matrix). Avoidance of anoikis represents an important aspect of tumor invasion, metastasis, and angiogenesis.[85] It is also fundamental to correct positioning of cells during development, possibly accounting for the embryonic lethality of *fadd* and *Caspase-8* gene ablation in mice. The DD-containing, p53-induced protein PIDD and its role in Caspase 2 activation has been described above.[39]

The DDs, however, are not always involved in Caspase activation. In fact, some of the signal transduction pathways in which non–Caspase activating DD-proteins are involved indirectly regulate apoptosis through effects on NF-κB, suppressing rather than inducing apoptosis. For example, the RIP protein, binds TRADD and activates kinases that induce degradation of IκB, thus releasing NF-κB so that it can translocate to the nucleus and fulfill its function as a transcription factor.[86-88] Among NF-κB-inducible genes are several that block apoptosis, including antiapoptotic Bcl-2 family members Bfl-1 (A1) and Bcl-X, and IAP (Inhibitor of Apoptosis Proteins)-family member cIAP2 and probably cIAP1, and FLIP, an endogenous antagonist of Caspases 8 and 10.[49,89-93] The dual function of TRADD, as a partner for both Caspase-activator FADD and NF-κB-activator RIP, causes many of the TNF-family receptors to self-nullify their apoptosis-inducing activity (Fig. 4-3). Thus, TNFR1, DR3, and DR6 are uncertain apoptosis inducers, unless NF-κB induction is inhibited, in which case they typically elicit robust apoptotic responses.[94,95] In contrast, Fas and the Trail-receptors DR4 and DR5 only rarely activate NF-κB, probably because these receptors complexes contain FADD but not TRADD.[55,56,96,97] In fact, it is because TRAIL receptors (DR4; DR5) do not induce NF-κB-mediated pro-inflammatory responses in vivo that TRAIL is under incistigation for use in the treatment of cancer, whereas NF-κB-inducing TNF proved to be unacceptable

Death Effector Domain (DED) Proteins

The structure of the DED is similar to the DD, comprising 6 helices.[98] DEDs are found in Caspases 8 and 10 in humans. The prodomain regions of pro-Caspases 8 and 10 contain two tandem DEDs, which are responsible for their interactions with the DED of FADD, thus mediating their recruitment to death receptor complexes. Multiple DED-containing modulators of apoptosis have been identified, some of which enhance and others that inhibit Caspase-activation by TNF-family death receptors.[99] Among these, the DED-containing protein FLIP (also known as Flame, CASH, Clarp, MRIT, Casper, I-Flice, Usurpin) has emerged as an important suppressor of apoptosis in cancer (Fig. 4-4). FLIP shares extensive amino-acid sequence similarity with pro-Caspases 8 and 10, containing two N-terminal DEDs followed by a pseudo-Caspase domain that lacks critical residues required for protease activity, including the catalytic cysteine.[100,101] FLIP associates with pro-Caspase 8 and also competes with pro-Caspases 8 and 10 for binding to FADD, thus squelching death receptor signaling. An interesting finding is that some tumors have been reported to contain inappropriately elevated levels of FLIP, rendering them resistant to apoptosis induction by Fas-expressing cytolytic T cells.[102] FLIP-mediated resistance to Fas may even allow tumor cells to tolerate expressing FasL, using this death ligand as a weapon against neighboring normal cells and triggering apoptosis of immune cells.[103-105] Downregulation of FLIP using antisense oligonucleotides or drugs that reduce FLIP protein levels can restore sensitivity of tumor cell lines to apoptosis induced by TRAIL or FasL,[106,107] suggesting opportunities for improved cancer therapy. The mechanisms responsible for increased expression of FLIP in tumors are unknown. Because FLIP is an NF-κB-inducible gene,[108] tumor-associated increases in NF-κB activity may play a role.

CARD-Family Proteins ■ Several pro-Caspases contain N-terminal CARDs in their prodomains, including Caspases 1, 2, 4, 5, and 9 in humans. The overall structure of the CARD is similar to DDs and DEDs, comprising 6 helices.[109-112] Homotypic interactions among CARD-carrying proteins play important roles in Caspase activation throughout animal evolution. One of the paradigms used for Caspase activation is embodied in CED-4/Apaf-1 family proteins. These proteins contain a CARD domain in combination with a nucleotide-binding oligomerization domain, known as a NBARC[113] domain (Nucleotide-Binding domain homologous to Apaf-1, CED-4 and plant R gene products).[114] The N-terminal CARDs of Apaf-1 in humans and CED-4 in the nematode *Caenorhabditis elegans* mediate interactions with the CARDs of specific initiator Caspases, pro-Caspase 9 and pro-CED 3, respectively.[115-117] Oligomerized APAF-1 and CED-4 activate Caspases by the induced proximity mechanism.[118-120]

With the CED-4 protein of *C. elegans*, binding and activation of the Caspase pro-CED 3 is spontaneous. In contrast, the human APAF-1 protein contains, in addition, regulatory domain comprising several WD repeat domains, which renders it dependent on cyt *c*.[28,121] Biochemical analysis of human Apaf 1 using in vitro reconstituted systems with purified components indicates that cyt *c*, in combination with dATP, induces oligomerization of APAF-1 molecules, followed by binding to and activation of pro-Caspase 9.[119,120] Several mechanisms for suppressing Caspase activation by APAF 1 have been identified in tumors, including: (1) expression of a splice variant that produces a shorter, noncatalytic isoform of pro-Caspase 9 that can compete with full-length pro-Caspase 9 for binding APAF 1; (2) phosphorylation of human Caspase 9 by the kinases Akt or Erk1/2; (3) overexpression of heat shock proteins, that bind either APAF 1 or pro-Caspase 9; (4) overexpression of TUCAN/Cardinal (CARDS), a CARD-containing antagonist of Caspase 9 that prevents its association with APAF 1; (5) Caspase-9-binding IAP-family proteins; (6) silencing of the *APAF1* gene by methylation; and (7) alkalinization of the cytosol, induced probably by the Na^+–H^+ exchanger in response to Protein Kinases activated by growth factors.[122-128]

Besides regulating Caspase activation, several CARD-family proteins have been reported to induce or inhibit NF-κB activation. For example, *BCL-10*

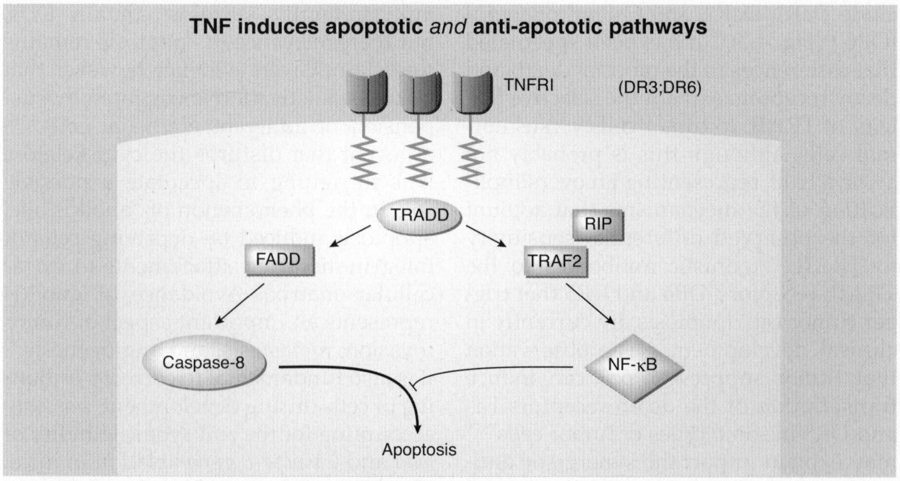

Figure 4-3 ■ Opposing pathways for cell death and cell survival are induced by TNF-family receptors. Several TNF-family receptors simultaneously engage parallel pathways for apoptosis and apoptosis suppression, including TNFR1, DR3, and DR6. The DD-containing adapter protein TRADD binds DDs in the cytosolic domains of TNF-family receptors. TRADD can associate with FADD, which in turn binds Caspases 8 and 10, triggering their activation. However, TRADD can also bind RIP and TRAFs, inducing activation of protein kinases that lead to NFxB activation. NFxBiifamily transcription factors induce expression of several antiapoptotic genes. Some TNF-family receptors activate only one of these two pathways. For example, Fas and TRAIL receptors induce Caspase activation but fail to interact with the proteins required for NFxB responses. Conversely, multiple TNF-family receptors, including TNFR2, CD30, and CD40 activate the NFxB pathway but do not recruit TRADD or FADD to their cytosolic domains (not shown).

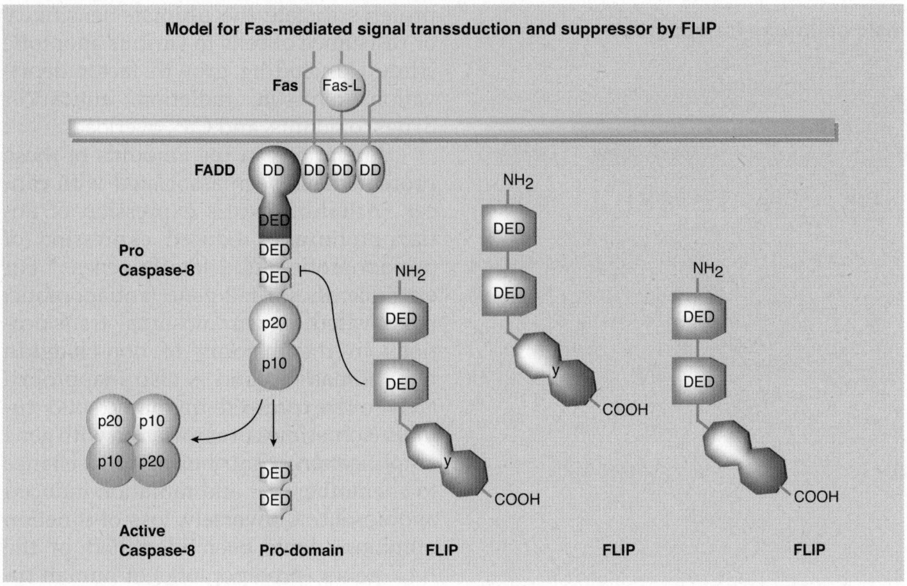

Figure 4-4 The TNF-family receptor Fas contains a cytosolic DD that binds the bipartite adapter protein, FADD. The DD of FADD interacts with Fas, and its DED binds the DEDs in pro-Caspase 8. Recruitment of pro-Caspase 8 to clustered receptors on the plasma membrane induces proteolytic processing and activation of pro-Caspase 8, releasing the active protease into the cytosol. FLIP contains DED domains that compete for binding to pro-Caspase 8 and FADD, squelching signaling by Fas. Overexpression of FLIP occurs in many cancers.

(also known as huE10 and CIPER) is a gene initially identified because of its involvement in chromosomal translocations found in lymphomas that arise in mucosal areas (MALTomas).[129] Bcl 10 induces NF-κB activation, and ablation of the *bcl-10* gene in mice precludes NF-κB activation via antigen receptors in T and B lymphocytes.[130] Mutant versions of Bcl-10 have been reported in cancers, although the frequency of such gene mutations is debated.[129,131,132] These truncated forms of Bcl-10 display NFxB-inducing activity and manifest transforming activity in classical rodent cell-based assays in vitro.[129]

IAP Family Proteins The IAPs (Inhibitor of Apoptosis Proteins) represent a family of evolutionarily conserved apoptosis suppressors.[133-135] Although these proteins can interact with a variety of biochemical pathways in cells, the fundamental mechanisms of action of most if not all IAP-family proteins involve direct binding to Caspases—acting as endogenous inhibitors of the cell death proteases.[133]

IAPs are found in the genomes of mammals, insects, and certain animal viruses. All members of this family, by definition, contain at least one copy of a so-called BIR (*baculovirus iap repeat*) domain, a zinc-binding fold,[136-138] which is important for their antiapoptotic activity. In addition to 1-3 copies of a BIR domain, many IAP family proteins also contain other domains, including RING zinc-fingers, CARDs, Ubiquitin-conjugating enzyme (E2s) domains, or putative nucleotide-binding domains. An interesting finding is that the RINGs of IAPs have recently been implicated in interactions with the cellular components of the ubiquitination machinery,[139] thus controlling turnover of these proteins and other proteins with which they associate. Also, the BIR-containing protein, Apollon (Bruce), contains a domain with ubiquitin-conjugating enzyme (E2) activity, further suggesting links of BIR-family proteins to the cellular ubiquitination machinery.[140] Although IAP-family proteins all contain BIR domains, the mere presence of a BIR domain does not necessarily indicate antiapoptotic activity. For example, BIR-containing proteins that regulate mitosis and meiosis but have no apparent effect on cell death regulation have been described in yeast and *C. elegans*.[141,142]

Several IAPs have been shown to bind and potently inhibit activated Caspases. Among the Caspases bound by human IAP family members XIAP, cIAP1, and cIAP2 are the effector Caspases 3 and 7 as well as the initiator Caspase 9.[143-145] (Fig. 4-5). In the case of XIAP, it was shown that the second BIR domain and the linker region between BIR1 and BIR2 are required for binding and suppressing Caspases 3 and 7, whereas the third BIR domain binds Caspase 9.[136,146-148] Thus, different domains in the multi-BIR containing IAPs are responsible for finding to different Caspases. IAP family member, Livin (ML-IAP), contains a single BIR and finds Caspase 9 but not Caspases 3 and 7.[149] Surviving also contains a single BIR and reportedly associates with Caspase 9, although its mechanism of Caspase suppression is poorly defined and may require partner proteins or interactions with other IAP family members.[150-152] IAPs lack activity against many members of the Caspase family of cell death proteases. Thus, overexpression of IAPs may block some apoptosis pathways but not others. This stands in marked contrast to the baculovirus p35 protein, an apoptosis suppressor that displays broad activity against Caspases but for which no cellular homolog has been identified.[19] Nevertheless, human IAPs such as XIAP can arrest apoptosis induced via either the intrinsic (mitochondrial) or extrinsic (death receptor) pathways, probably because they target effector caspases which are common to both pathways (Fig. 4-5).[148]

Overexpression of IAP-family gene has been documented in cancers. For example, overexpression of the IAP member *Survivin* has been observed in many common types of cancer.[153] Survivin is highly expressed in the developing fetus but largely absent from normal adult tissues.[154] Through unclear mechanisms, Survivin becomes overexpressed in cancers. Indeed, genome-wide transcription profiling suggests that *Survivin* is among the most tumor-specific genes thus far identified.[155] The promoter of the *Survivin* gene is normally cell cycle regulated, becoming activated specifically in late G2/M-phase.[156] Moreover, the Survivin protein is associated with the chromosomes during mitosis and the mitotic spindle apparatus, where it plays a critical role in ensuring proper control chromosome segregation during anaphase and in the final execution of cytokinesis. Suppression of *Survivin* expression using antisense methods or dominant-inhibitory mutants results in polyploidy, aneuploidy, and apoptosis.[157] Apparent Survivin orthologs in yeast and *C. elegans* also participate in cell cycle regulation but lack effects on cell life/death,[142,158] suggesting that *Survivin* evolved this function later as a possible way of creating a cell cycle checkpoint that ensures apoptotic elimination of cells, that fail to properly sort their genetic material during cell division.

Elevated expression of other IAP-family members in cancer also occurs.[159] For example, Livin (ML-IAP; KIAP; Ts-IAP; ILP2) is scarcely expressed in normal tissues but reportedly found at high levels in melanomas or renal cancers.[149,160,161] Examples of overexpression of XIAP, cIAP1, and cIAP2 in cancers have also been reported, sometimes in association with adverse clinical outcome.[133,134] Antisense-mediated reductions on XIAP or cIAP1 can induce apoptosis of tumor cell lines in culture or sensitize cells to cytotoxic anticancer drugs. Although its overall relevance to apoptosis re-

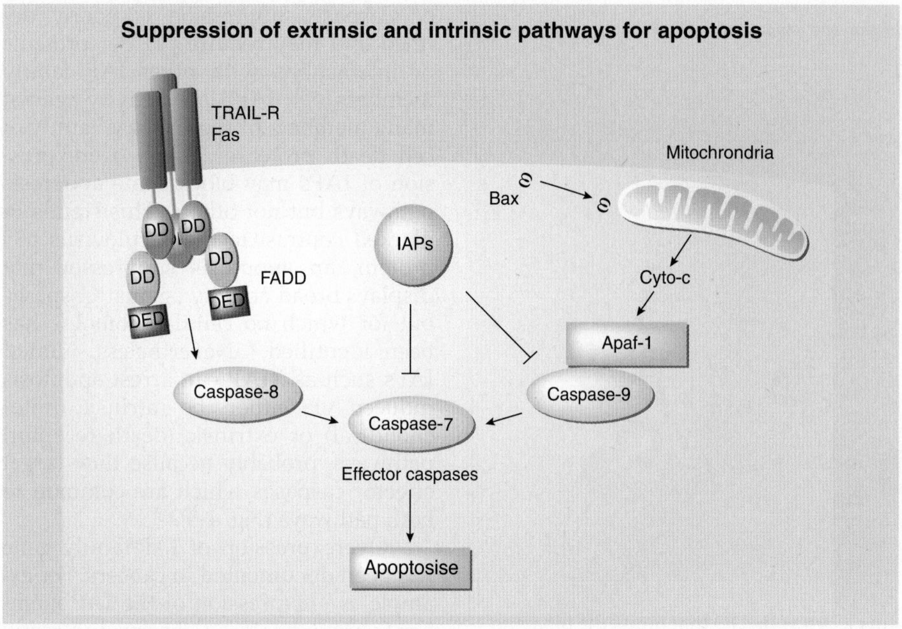

Figure 4-5 ■ Several IAP-family proteins in humans have been shown to directly bind Caspases. XIAP, cIAP1, and cIAP2, eg, can find active Caspases 3 and 7, representing downstream effector Caspases that function at the convergence of apoptosis pathways. XIAPs, cIAP1, cIAP2, and Livin also find active Caspase 9, the apical protease in the mitochondrial pathway for apoptosis.

mains uncertain, antisense-mediated downregulation of IAP-family member Apollon can sensitize tumor cell lines to apoptosis induced by anticancer drugs.[162] These types of antisense experiments provide proof of concept evidence that the pathological elevations of IAPs found in cancers are important for maintaining tumor cell survival and resistance to chemotherapy.

Endogenous antagonists of the IAPs help to keep these apoptosis suppressors in check, promoting apoptosis. Three of these naturally occurring IAP antagonists, SMAC (Diablo), HtrA2 (Omi), and ARTS are sequestered inside mitochondria, becoming released into the cytosol during apoptosis.[163,164] SMAC and HtrA2 have N-terminal leader sequences that are removed by proteolysis upon import into mitochondria, exposing a novel tetra-peptide motif that binds the BIR domains of IAPs. These IAP antagonists compete with Caspases for binding to IAPs, thus freeing Caspases from the grip of the IAPs and promoting apoptosis. Synthetic peptides that mimic SMAC and HtrA2 induce apoptosis or sensitize tumor cell lines to apoptosis induced by cytotoxic anticancer drugs.[165-167] Structural information derived from high-field NMR and x-ray crystallography indicate that a tetra-peptide motif is sufficient to bind the BIRs of IAPs, suggesting a path to drug discovery where small-molecule chemical compounds that occupy the same tetra-peptide–binding motif on BIRs can be envisioned as new apoptosis-sensitizing agents for cancer. At present, compounds based on this SMAC-mimicking mechanism are in clinical testing as well as antisense-based DNA drugs that target mRNAs encoding IAP family members. It remains to be determined whether tumors downregulate expression of their endogenous IAP antagonists such as SMAC and HtrA2 as a strategy for achieving apoptosis resistance.

BCL-2 Family Proteins ■ The mitochondria-dependent pathway for apoptosis is governed by Bcl-2-family proteins. Bcl-2, Bcl-X^L, Bak, and many other members of the Bcl-2 family have a hydrophobic stretch of amino acids near their carboxyl terminus that anchors them in the outer mitochondrial membrane.[29] In contrast, other Bcl-2 family members such as Bid, Bim, and Bad lack these membrane-anchoring domains but target mitochondria in response to specific stimuli. Still others have the membrane-anchoring domain but keep it latched against the body of the protein, until stimulated to expose it (eg, Bax).[168]

Bcl-2 family proteins are conserved throughout metazoan evolution, with homologs found in vertebrate and invertebrate animal species. Several types of animal viruses also harbor Bcl-2 family genes within their genomes, including herpes simplex viruses implicated in cancer such as the Epstein-Barr Virus (EBV) and Kaposi sarcoma herpes virus (KSHV). Both pro-apoptotic and antiapoptotic Bcl-2 family proteins have been delineated.[169-173] The relative ratios of anti- and pro-apoptotic Bcl-2 family proteins dictate the ultimate sensitivity or resistance of cells to various apoptotic stimuli, including growth factor deprivation, hypoxia, radiation, anticancer drugs, oxidants, and Ca^{2+} overload.

Alterations in the amounts of these proteins have been associated with cancer, including excess expression of antiapoptotic and reduced expression of pro-apoptotic *BCL-2* family genes.[174] For example, the *BCL-2* gene (antiapoptotic) is activated by chromosomal translocations in the majority of non-Hodgkin lymphomas[175,176] and is also inappropriately overexpressed in many solid tumors (sometimes in association with gene amplification), contributing to resistance to chemotherapy- and radiation-induced apoptosis.[177] Conversely, loss-of-function mutations have been identified in the *BAX* genes (pro-apoptotic) of human tumors[178] and analysis of *bax* -/- knockout mice indicates that *bax* is a tumor suppressor in vivo.[179] Transcription of the human *BAX* gene is also directly regulated by p53, thus providing another connection of this important tumor suppressor to apoptosis pathways.[180]

In humans, at least 26 members of the Bcl-2 family gene family have been identified. These genes encode the antiapoptotic proteins, Bcl-2, Bcl-X^L, Mcl-1, Bfl-1 (A1), Bcl-W, and Bcl-B (Boo;Diva) as well as the proapoptotic proteins Bax, Bak, Bok (Mtd), Bad, Bid, Bim, Bik, Hrk, Bcl-X^S, APR (Noxa), PUMA, p193, Bcl-Gs, Bcl-rambo (Mil), Nip3, and Nix (BNIP). Some of the Bcl-2 family genes produce two or more proteins through alternative mRNA splicing, sometimes exerting opposing effects on cell death regulation (eg, Bcl-X$_L$ vs Bcl-X$_S$). Gene ablation studies in mice suggest that each of the Bcl-2 family members plays unique roles in controlling cell survival in vivo, reflecting their tissue-specific patterns of expression or cell-context-dependent requirements for these proteins.

Based on their predicted (or experimentally determined) 3-dimensional structures, Bcl-2 family proteins can be broadly divided into two groups. One subset of these proteins is similar in structure to the pore-forming domains of bacterial toxins, such as the colicins and diphtheria toxin.[181-184] These helical pore-like proteins include both antiapoptotic proteins (Bcl-2, Bcl-X^L, Mcl-1, Bfl-1, Bcl-W, and probably Bcl-B) as well as pro-apoptotic proteins (Bax, Bak, Bok, and Bid). Most of the proteins in this subcategory can be recognized by conserved stretches of amino-acid sequence homology, including the presence of Bcl-2 Homology (BH) domains, BH1, BH2, BH3, and sometimes BH4. However, this is not uniformly the case, as the Bid protein contains only a BH3 domain but has been determined to share the same overall protein-fold with Bcl-X^L, Bcl-2, and Bax.[182,183] Where tested to date, these proteins have all been shown to form ion-conducting channels in synthetic membranes in vitro, including Bcl-2, Bcl-X^L, Bax, and Bid, but the relevance of this in vitro activity to their in vivo functions is uncertain.[185-189]

The other subset of Bcl-2 family proteins appears to have in common only the presence of the BH3 domain, including Bad, Bik, Bim, Hrk, Bcl-GS, p193, APR (Noxa), and PUMA. These "BH3-only" proteins are uniformly pro-apoptotic. Their cell death–inducing activity depends, in most cases, on their ability to dimerize with antiapoptotic Bcl-2 family members, functioning as trans-dominant inhibitors of proteins such as Bcl-2 and Bcl-X^L.[173,190] However, some of these proteins (eg, Bid, Bim) can also dimerize with pro-apoptotic proteins (eg, Bax; Bak), functioning as agonists of the killers, in addition to dimerizing with antiapoptotic proteins (eg, Bcl-2; Bcl-X^L), functioning as antagonists (Fig. 4-6).[191,192] Binding of Bid to Bax or Bak promotes their insertion into and oligomerization in membranes, causing permeabilization of the outer mitochondrial membrane and release of molecules such as cyt *c*, SMAC, and Omi into the cytosol.[193,194]

The BH3 domain has been shown to mediate dimerization among Bcl-2 family proteins. This domain consists of an amphipathic a-helix of ~16 amino-acid length that inserts into a hydrophobic crevice on the surface of antiapoptotic proteins such as Bcl-X^L.[195] Thus, mutations in the BH3 domain of proteins such as Bad, Bik, Bim, Bcl-GS, and Hrk that abolish their ability to bind other Bcl-2 family member also abrogate their capacity to induce apoptosis. Proof-of-concept experiments performed with synthetic peptides representing the BH3 domain have suggested a path forward in terms of drug discovery. For example, BH3 peptides directed against antiapoptotic proteins overexpressed in cancers (eg, Bcl-2; Bcl-X^L) can restore sensitivity to apoptosis, at least in vitro.[196] Accordingly, small-molecule chemical compounds have been delineated that interact with the same BH3-binding pocket on Bcl-2 and Bcl-X^L, nullifying their cytoprotective actions, and promoting tumor cell apoptosis.[197-199] At present, several BH3 mimicking compounds are in clinical development.

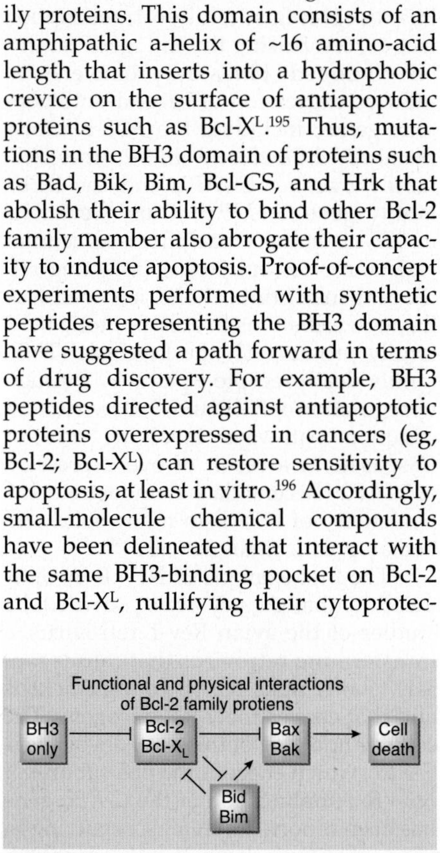

Figure 4-6 ■ Network of interactions among Bcl-2-family proteins. The functional and physical interactions among Bcl-2-family proteins are depicted.

The BH3-only proteins link a wide variety of environmental stimuli to the mitochondrial pathway for apoptosis (Fig. 4-7). For example, the transcription factor p53 directly induces expression of BH3-only proteins Noxa (APR) and PUMA,[200-202] thus linking p53 to the death machinery. The BH3-only protein BFM is associated with the actin cytoskeleton.[203] Circumstances that perturb the cytoskeleton, such as cell detachment from extracellular matrix, release BFM, allowing it to dimerize with antiapoptotic proteins on the surface of mitochondria and induce apoptosis. Thus, BFM may represent an important defense mechanism against metastasis. Bid is cleared by Caspase 8 in the context of signaling by apoptosis-inducing TNF-family receptors, removing the N-terminal 52 amino acids and exposing both the BH3 dimerization domain as well as generating a novel N-terminus that becomes myristoylated, facilitating targeting of the Bid protein into membranes.[34,189,204,205]

This Caspase-8-mediated activation of Bid represents an important mechanism accounting for cross-talk between the death receptor (extrinsic) and mitochondrial (intrinsic) pathways. Isoforms of the BH3-only protein, Bim, associate with microtubules via direct binding to microtubule-associated dynein light chain (DLC).[206] Disruption of these protein interactions frees microtubule-associated isoforms of Bim, allowing them to dimerize via the BH3 domain with antiapoptotic Bcl-2 family proteins on the surface of mitochondria. The BH3-only protein Bad translocates between the cytosol and mitochondria, depending on whether it is phosphorylated. Several protein kinases, including Akt (PKB), PKA, Raf1, Rsk1, and Pak1 have been reported to phosphorylate BAD, thus inactivating the protein such that it cannot dimerize with and antagonize Bcl-2 or Bcl-X^L.[207,208] Evidence has been presented that BAD is inactivated by this phosphorylation mechanism in many cancers. Finally, expression of some pro-apoptotic Bcl-2 family proteins is controlled at the level of mRNA splicing, with specific signals switching mRNA splicing patterns to produce versions of the proteins with pro-apoptotic activity (eg, Bcl-X^S; Bcl-Gs).[209,210]

In addition to their well-known roles in controlling outer mitochondrial membrane permeability, Bcl-2 family proteins also have important functions in ER membranes.[211] Although details are still being actively investigated, an interesting observation is that pro-apoptotic proteins Bax and Bak interact with and stimulate

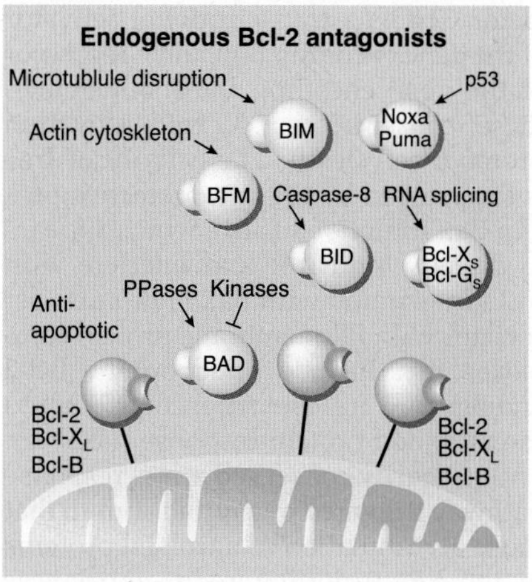

Figure 4-7 ■ BH3-only proteins link cell-death stimuli to the mitochondrial pathway for apoptosis. Multiple proapoptotic BH3-only proteins have been identified that dimerize with and antagonize antiapoptotic Bcl-2 family proteins such as Bcl-2 and Bcl-X^L on the surface of mitochondria. BFM associates with the actin cytoskeleton but is released when the cytoskeleton is disrupted, translocating to mitochondria. BFM may be important therefore for apoptosis that results when cells detach from extracellular matrix. This cause of apoptosis has been termed "anoikis." Longer isoforms of BIM associate with proteins that bind microtubules. Disruption of microtubules therefore may release BIM. The BAD protein is regulated by phosphorylation. Several kinases, including Akt, have been reported to phosphorylate and thereby inhibit dimerization of BAD with Bcl-X^L. Phosphatases counteract this effect, and activate BAD, allowing it to induce apoptosis. BID is cleaved by Caspase 8 in the context of apoptosis induction by TNF-family death receptors. The uncleaved BID protein is inactive in the cytosol, whereas cleavage produces a truncated protein that targets mitochondrial membranes and dimerizes with other Bcl-2 family proteins. NOXA and PUMA are proteins whose expression is induced by p53. The activation of p53 is induced by DNA damage, thus linking DNA-damage (caused, for example, by anticancer drugs or x-irradiation) to apoptotic responses. Bcl-Gs and Bcl-X^S are apoptosis-inducing apoptosis proteins produced as a result of alternative mRNA splicing. Longer forms of these proteins lack pro-apoptotic activity. Switching to production of the short forms promotes apoptosis.

the ER membrane signaling protein Ire1. Ire1 is a transmembrane protein of the ER, which contains a cytosolic protein kinase domain and a endoribonuclease domain, conferring dual catalytic activities. The kinase activity results in initiation of a kinase casade that includes Apoptotic Signaling Kinase-1 (Ask1), an upstream activator of kinases that activate JNK and p38 MAPK. JNK phosphorylates and inhibits antiapoptotic protein Bcl-2 while also phosphorylating and stimulating pro-apoptotic protein Bim. In addition, p38 MAPK stimulates the transcription factor CHOP, a transcriptional activator of the gene encoding Bim and a repressor of the gene encoding Bcl-2. Altogether, these consequences of Ire1 activation promote cell death. The activity of Ire1 is suppressed by the cytoprotective protein Bax Inhibitor-1 (BI-1), which appears to directly bind Ire1 and interfere with Ire1's interaction with Bax.[212] BI-1 also associates with ER membrane protein complexes that include antiapoptotic Bcl-2 and Bcl-X_L.[213] Ire1 is a major contributor to the unfolded protein response (URP), an evolutionarily conserved stress response pathway triggered by myriad stimuli that cause accumulation of unfolded proteins in the ER, including redox-imbalances (including ischemia-reperfusion injury), ER Ca^{2+} dysregulation, protein glycosylation disturbances, and proteasome inhibitors. Thus, Bcl-2 family proteins play important roles as modulators of the UPR and ER stress signaling.

An additional ER-related function of Bcl-2 family proteins concerns Ca^{2+} homeostasis. Antiapoptotic proteins Bcl-2 and Bcl-X_L reportedly interact with inositol triphosphate receptors (IP3Rs) and cause passive leakage of Ca^{2+} from ER, resulting in lower resting levels of this divalent cation within the lumen of the ER. The consequence is that stimuli that cause Ca^{2+} discharge from ER produce less of a corresponding rise in cytosolic free Ca^{2+}, having a wide variety of consequences that can be important for cell death regulation.[211] Bax and Bak have opposing effect on ER Ca^{2+}, whereas the aforementioned BI-1 protein phenocopies Bcl-2 and Bcl-X_L with regard to Ca^{2+} and seems to be required for Bcl-X_L to regulate ER Ca^{2+}.[214] More work is required to reveal the full implications of these ER-associated activities of Bcl-2 family proteins and their interaction partners in ER membranes.

Alternative Forms of Cell Death

Apoptosis represents only one cell death mechanism. Necrosis is a Caspase-independent route of cell death, typically characterized by loss of osmotic stability of cells, with organellar swelling and plasma membrane rupture. The release of intracellular components to the extracellular milieu generally triggers an inflammatory response, unlike apoptosis. Many cell death stimuli that operate through the mitochondrial or ER pathways for apoptosis trigger parallel Caspase-dependent and Caspase-independent cell death mechanisms. In general, Caspase-dependent kills faster than the Caspase-independent mechanisms, but Caspase suppressors (either pharmacological or endogenous) can unmask the latter and thus result in nonapoptotic cell death. Caspase-independent mediators of nonapoptotic cell death that are released by mitochondria include the endonuclease Endo-G, the flavoprotein Apoptosis Inducing factor (AIF), a modulator of transcription factors called Bit, and other proteins.[215] How the ER induces Caspase-independent cell death is uncertain, but liberation of Ca^{2+} from the lumen of this organelle is likely to be involved, which can have several downstream consequences, including activation of calpain-family cysteine proteases and induction of Ca^{2+}-dependent swelling and rupture of mitochondria.[211,216]

Besides apoptosis and necrosis, autophagic cell death has recently been recognized as a route of cellular demise with relevance to cancer. Autophagy is an evolutionarily conserved process whereby intracellular macromolecules and organelles are encased in a membranous vesicle (the autophagosome) for delivery to lysosomes, where the sequester cargo undergoes degradation and recycling into anabolic pathways. At least in yeast for which the genetics of this pathway have been worked out in some detail, autophagy is induced under times of nutrient deprivation, allowing cells to generate ATP through catabolism of organelles and other cellular structures. Although autophagy evolved in eukaryotes as a survival mechanism, excessive autophagy leads to nonapoptotic cell death.[217] It is controversial whether the presence of autophagic morphological features concomitant with cell death is causal versus merely coincidental. Nevertheless, under some conditions, specific components of the autophagy machinery appear to promote cell death.[218]

Malignant cells often display abnormally low levels of autophagy.[219,220] The connection between cancer and decreased autophagy was solidified with the discovery that the BECLIN1 gene locus, which is mutated in 40-75% of prostate, breast, and ovarian cancers,[219,220] encodes an evolutionarily conserved component of the autophagic machinery.[221,222] Unlike many tumor suppressors, biallelic inactivation of the BECLIN1 locus has not been observed, suggesting that partial loss (ie, haploinsufficiency) of the Beclin-1 protein is positively selected during tumorigenesis but that complete loss of Beclin-1 function is not compatible with tumor progression. An interesting observation is that, Beclin binds Bcl-2,[223] and several other proteins via a BH3-like domain and this interaction is controlled by protein phosphorylation.[224,225]. In this regard, recent data suggest that autophagy and apoptosis may be antagonistic processes because caspases have been reported to suppress the autophagic program in tumor cells.[226] In addition, antiapoptotic Bcl-2 family proteins (eg, Bcl-2; Bcl-X_L) bind and suppress autophagy protein Beclin.[227,228] If apoptosis and autophagy are mutually exclusive, then it may be important to understand how cancer therapies predicated on induction of apoptosis interact with the autophagy machinery of cells.

Signal Transduction and Apoptosis Dysregulation in Cancer

In addition to genes that encode "core" components of the apoptosis machinery, tumor-associated alterations have been identified in genes that provide important regulatory inputs into the expression of apoptosis genes or the regulation of their encoded proteins. This includes many transcription factors and growth factor receptors. However, ultimately, many of these signaling molecules funnel into common pathways linked to the apoptosis machinery. Two prominent examples are described here, namely, NF-κB and Akt. For more comprehensive summaries of signal transduction inputs into the core apoptosis machinery, the reader is referred to other works.[190,229-232]

NF-κB

NF-κB represents a family of transcription factors, comprising the REL gene family. NF-κB directly binds the promoters and induces expression of several antiapoptotic genes, including the *BCL-2* family members *BCL-X* and *BFL-1*, the IAP-family member *C-IAP2*, and the DED-family gene *C-FLIP*.[233] Thus, elevations in NF-κB activity can increase cellular resistance to apoptosis, affecting (1) the Intrinsic (mitochondrial) pathway through elevations in antiapoptotic Bcl-2 family proteins, (2) the Extrinsic (TNF-family death receptor) pathway through upregulation of FLIP, and (3) downstream common pathways involving effector Caspases, as a result of overexpression of cIAP2. Recent data demonstrate hyperactivity of NF-κB in many solid and hematopoietic malignancies.[234]

The first example of NF-κB involvement in malignancy was provided by studies of the avian Rev-T retrovirus, a transforming retrovirus that causes rapidly fatal lymphomas in young chickens and that carries the v-Rel oncogene. The cellular homolog of this viral oncogene is *C-REL*, which encodes the p65 subunit of NF-κB. Amplification of the *C-REL* gene has been reported in NHLs, occurring in ~23% of diffuse large B-cell lymphoma and commonly associated with extranodal presentation.[235] Other genetic alterations associated with dysregulation of NF-κB include chromosomal translocations involving the IκB family member *BCL-3* in B-CLL.[236] IκB family proteins bind and sequester NF-κB complexes, preventing the transcription factor from entering the nucleus. Typically, IκB is regulated by ubiquitin-mediated turnover by the 26s proteasome. Mutations in IκB thus may enhance NF-κB activity, either by producing unstable proteins or by reducing the affinity of IκB for NF-κB. The anticancer activity of drugs that inhibit the proteasome may be attributable in part to suppression of IκB degradation, thereby inhibiting NF-κB induction, although it is clear that other mechanisms such as ER stress induced by accumulation of unfolded proteins also contribute significantly.[211,237] Kinases that induce phosphorylation of IκB, a prerequisite for Ubiquitination and subsequent degradation, also have emerged as attractive drug-discovery targets (Fig. 4-8).

AKT

The protein kinase Akt (PKB) plays important roles in linking growth factor receptors and oncoproteins to apoptosis pathways (Fig. 4-9). The murine gene encoding Akt was first discovered by virtue of its similarity to the *v-akt* oncogene found in some murine leukemia viruses and through its activation in thymomas caused by retrovirus insertions near the *c-akt* gene.[238] Humans contain three *AKT* genes. Akt can phosphorylate multiple proteins within the core apoptosis machinery, some of which have been mentioned above. For example, the pro-apoptotic Bcl-2 family member BAD is a target of Akt, where phosphorylation of BAD inhibits its ability to heterodimerize with Bcl-X_L.[208] Akt also can phosphorylate human Caspase 9, blocking apoptosis downstream of mitochondria.[123] Another substrate of Akt that is relevant to apoptosis is Forkhead Transcription Factors (FKHD). Some FKHD family members appear to control apoptosis, perhaps by affecting transcription of the gene encoding FasL.[239] Phosphorylation of FKHD by Akt prevents its entry into the nucleus. Akt may also play a role in NF-κB activation.[240] Moreover, Akt has been implicated in suppression of Nur77 (TR3), an orphan member of the retinoid/steroid family of transcription factors implicated in apoptosis induction.[241] Akt also opposes apoptosis induced by the kinase Ask1[242] and promotes p53 degradation through effects on Mdm2.[243]

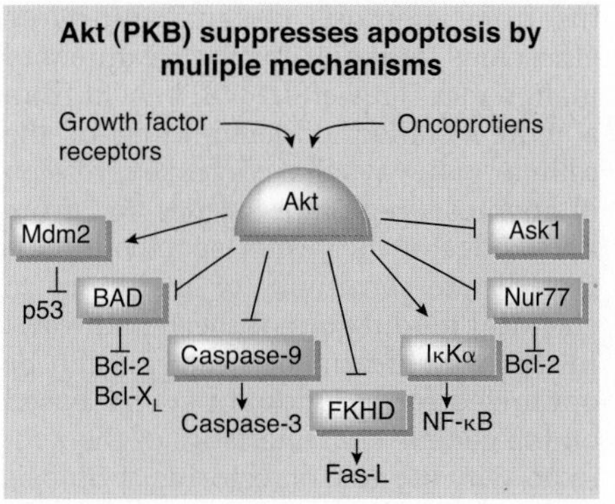

Figure 4-9 ■ The protein kinase Akt (PKB) is activated in response to second-messagers produced by PI3K, a lipid kinase that is activated by many growth factor receptors and oncoproteins. PTEN is a lipid phosphatase that prevents accumulation of these second messagers, the expression of which is lost in many tumors through gene deletions, gene mutations, and other mechanisms.[227] Akt can phosphorylate and either activate (*arrows*) or inactivate (⊥) multiple proteins directly or indirectly relevant to apoptosis.[226] Phosphorylation of BAD prevents dimerization with Bcl-X^L. Phosphorylation of human pro–Caspase-9 suppresses its activation, as well as reducing cellular activity of processed (active) Caspase-9. Phosphorylation of ForkHead family transcription factors by Akt results in their sequestration in the cytosol, preventing their transcriptional induction of pro-apoptotic gene such as *FasL*. Akt may also phosphorylate and suppress Nur77 (TR3), an orphan member of the retinoid/steroid family of transcription factors implicated in apoptosis induction. Akt may also enhance NFκB activity, through poorly understood mechanisms, in some types of cells. Akt opposes activation of Ask1, a protein kinase implicated in apoptosis. Finally, phosphorylation of Mdm2 by Akt promotes its entry into the nucleus, where it binds and induces Ubiquitination and proteasome-dependent degradation of p53.

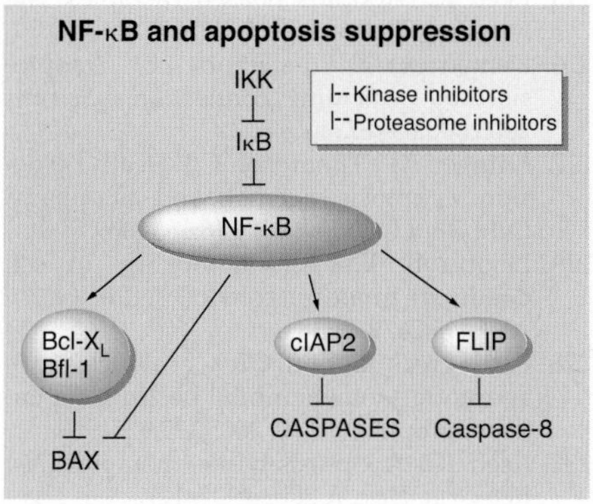

Figure 4-8 ■ NF-κB-family transcription factors induce the expression of multiple anti-apoptotic genes, including *BCL-2* family members *BCL-X and BFL1 (A1),* IAP family member *C-IAP2,* and Caspase-8 antagonist, *FLIP.* NF-κB can also suppress expression of pro-apoptotic gene *BAX,* in some tumor cells. NF-κB activation can be induced by at least two pathways. The "classical" pathway is presented, showing NF-κB under suppression by IxB-family proteins. IxBs are targeted for Ubiquitination and proteasome-dependent degradation when phosphorylated by IκB Kinases (IKKs). Several types of upstream kinases can activate the IKKs. Drugs that inhibit IKKs, as well as proteasome inhibitory drugs, represent novel approaches for interfering with NF-κB activation in tumor cells.

In recent years, evidence of hyperactivity of kinase Akt has been found for many types of human cancers.[208,244] The Akt protein contains a PH domain which binds phospholipid second-messengers produced by Phosphatidyl-Inositol 3′ Kinase (PI3K). Elevations in the levels of these lipid second-messengers result in recruitment of Akt to the plasma membrane, where it becomes activated by phosphorylation.[244] These phospholipid second-messengers are destroyed by PTEN, a lipid phosphatase and important tumor suppressor. Deletions and somatic point mutations that inactivate PTEN occur commonly in cancers.[245] Other mechanisms for deregulating Akt activity have also been described in cancers, including amplification of the *AKT2* gene in breast and ovarian cancers, and overproduction of an Akt-binding protein called Tcl1, as a result of chromosomal translocations in T-cell pro-lymphocytic leukemia (T-PLL). Consequently, Akt has emerged as an attractive candidate for drug discovery, using small-molecule compounds to target the ATP-binding site of the kinase, thereby inhibiting its catalytic activity.

Therapeutic Opportunities from Apoptosis Research

Emerging knowledge about the proteins that constitute the apoptosis core machinery and their upstream inputs has revealed multiple new opportunities for therapeutic intervention, some of which are already under investigation in clinical trials. These opportunities include both discovery and development of new agents (many of which were mentioned above) as well as the potential for more effective exploitation of existing anticancer agents through a deeper understanding of their effects on apoptosis pathways. With respect to new agents in clinical trials, a prominent example of a new strategy for attacking apoptosis resistance mechanisms in cancer is found in nuclease-resistant (phosphorothioate) antisense oligonucleotides directed against *BCL-2* mRNA, currently in Phase III trials for patients with melanoma and CLL. Antisense-based inhibitors of XIAP and Survivin are also in clinical testing. Recombinant TRAIL and agonistic antibodies directed against the TRAIL receptors, TRAIL-R1 (DR4) are also in clinical trials, and may one day provide new arrows for the quivers of medical oncologists. Chemical mimics of SMAC are being evaluated now, a class of agents that often demonstrates striking synergy with TRAIL.

A wide variety of existing and emerging anticancer agents that alter transcriptional mechanisms also indirectly regulate the expression of apoptosis genes and provide opportunities for modulating apoptosis resistance. Prominent among these are members of the retinoid/steroid family of transcription factors that require small ligands for their transcriptional activation. For example, it has been shown that expression of *BCL-2* in mammary epithelium is estrogen-dependent. By negating the transcriptional activity of the Estrogen Receptor (ER), antiestrogens such as Tamoxifen reduce *BCL-2* expression and promote apoptosis of breast cancer cells,[245] probably explaining in part the beneficial effects of antihormonal agents in the treatment of ER-positive breast cancers. Similarly, vitamin D (1,25 (OH)2-cholcalcitriol) and more potent synthetic analogs lacking hypercalcemic effects, activate the vitamin D Receptor (VDR) and suppress expression of several antiapoptotic *BCL-2* family genes, including *BCL-2*, *BCL-XL*, and *MCL-1*, restoring apoptosis sensitivity.[246,247] The retinoid, *all-trans* retinoic-acid (ATRA), and newer Retinoic Acid Receptor-X (RXR)-selective compounds (eg, Bexaretinone) also suppress expression of antiapoptotic *BCL-2* family genes (*BCL-2*; *BCL-XL*) in leukemias and some types of solid tumors. Thiazoladine-dione drugs (currently in use for treatment of Type II diabetes) that bind PPARγ, another member of the steroid/retinoid family of transcription factors, also reduce expression of *BCL-2* or other antiapoptotic *BCL-2* family proteins in some breast, prostate, or colon cancer cell lines.[248] Some PPARγ modulatory drugs also seem to reduce levels of FLIP, the Caspase-8 antagonist, thereby sensitizing tumor cells to the TNF-family death ligands.[106]

Many additional agents can indirectly modulate apoptosis pathways. Histone deacetylase (HDAC) inhibitors, eg, can reduce transcription of antiapoptotic Bcl-2 family genes and c-FLIP in cancers.[219] Upstream of Akt, compounds that inhibit PI3Ks are also in clinical testing. Similarly, small-molecule drugs and monoclonal antibodies directed against various cell-surface growth factors receptors that possess protein tyrosine kinase activity (eg, HER 2; EGFR; IGFR) are expected to shut down the Akt pathway and thus render tumor cells more sensitive to apoptosis.

Altogether therefore, prospects are bright for translation of concepts emerging from apoptosis research into more efficacious therapies for the treatment of malignancy. This effort will benefit from a more detailed understanding of the cellular pathways that control expression of apoptosis-regulatory genes and from knowledge of the tumor-specific lesions that dictate sensitivity or resistance to chemical modulators of these pathways. In this way, treatment strategies can be optimized for individual patients based on the genetic characteristics of their tumors, with the goal of restoring apoptosis sensitivity and encouraging cancer cells to commit suicide by activating their endogenous pathways for programmed cell death.

Acknowledgments

The author thanks M. Hanaii and T. Siegfried for manuscript preparation, and gratefully acknowledges the generous support of the National Institutes of Health (NIH).

Selected References

The complete reference list can be found at www.CANCERMEDICINE8.com

10. Cryns V, Yuan Y. Proteases to die for. *Genes Dev.* 1999;12:1551–1570.
24. Yuan J. Transducing signals of life and death. *Curr Opin Cell Biol.* 1997;9:247–251.
25. Reed JC, Doctor K, Rojas A, et al. Comparative analysis of apoptosis and inflammation genes of mice and humans. 2002. [In press]
28. Reed JC. Cytochrome C: can't live with it; can't live with-out it. *Cell.* 1997;91:559–562.
29. Green DR, Reed JC. Mitochondria and apoptosis. *Science.* 1998;281:1309–1312.
32. Kroemer G, Reed JC. Mitochondrial control of cell death. *Nat Med.* 2000;6:513–519.
37. Vaux DL, Strasser A. The molecular biology of apoptosis. *Proc Natl Acad Sci USA.* 1996;93:2239–2244.
65. Krammer PH. CD95's deadly mission in the immune system. *Nature.* 2000;407:789–795.
75. Ashkenazi A, Dixit VM. Apoptosis control by death and decoy receptors. *Curr Opin Cell Biol.* 1999;11:255–260.
85. Frisch SM, Ruoslahti E. Integrins and anoikis. *Curr Opin Cell Biol.* 1997;9:701–706.
100. Wallach D. Placing death under control. *Nature.* 1997;388:123–126.
101. Tschopp J, Irmler M, Thome M. Inhibition of Fas death signals by FLIPs. *Curr Opin Immunol.* 1998;10:552–558.
121. Abrams JM. An emerging blueprint for apoptosis in drosophila. *Trends Cell Biol.* 1999;9:435–440.
133. Deveraux QL, Reed JC. IAP family proteins: suppressors of apoptosis. *Genes Dev.* 1999;13:239–252.
134. La Casse EC, Baird S, Korneluk RG, MacKenzie AE. The inhibitors of apoptosis (IAPs) and their emerging role in cancer. *Oncogene.* 1998;17:3247–3259.
135. Miller L. An exegesis of IAPs: salvation and surprises from BIR motifs. *Trends Cell Biol.* 1999;9:323–328.
153. Ambrosini G, Adida C, Altieri DC. A novel anti-apoptosis gene, Survivin, expressed in cancer and lymphoma. *Nat Med.* 1997;3:917–921.
167. Herr I, Debatin K-M. Cellular stress response and apoptosis in cancer therapy. *Blood.* 2001;98:2603–2614.
170. Adams J, Cory S. The Bcl-2 protein family: arbiters of cell survival. *Science.* 1998;281:1322–1326.
171. Reed JC. Bcl-2 family proteins. *Oncogene.* 1998;17:3225–3236.
184. Schendel S, Montal M, Reed JC. Bcl-2 family proteins as ion-channels. *Cell Death Differ.* 1998;5:372–380.
190. Huang DC, Strasser A. BH3-only proteins-essential initiators of apoptotic cell death. *Cell.* 2000;103:839–842.
194. Korsmeyer SJ, Wei MC, Saito M, et al. Pro-apoptotic cascade activates BID, which oligomerizes BAK or BAX into pores that result in the release of cytochrome *c*. *Cell Death Differ.* 2000;7:1166–1173.
207. Franke TF, Cantley LC. A bad kinase makes good. *Nature.* 1997;390:116–117.
208. Datta S, Brunet A, Greenberg M. Cellular survival: a play in three Akts. *Genes Dev.* 1999;13:2905–2927.
211. Kim I, Xu W, Reed JC. Cell death and endoplasmic reticulum stress: disease relevance and therapeutic opportunities. *Nat Rev Drug Discov.* 2008;7:1013–1030.
215. Reed JC. Apoptosis-based therapies. *Nat Rev Drug Discov.* 2002;1:111–121.
216. Demaurex N, distelhorst C. Apoptosis—the calcium connection. *Science.* 2003;300:65–67.
217. Edinger AL, Thompson CB. Death by design: apoptosis, necrosis and autophagy. *Curr Opin Cell Biol.* 2004;16:663–669.
218. Levine B, Yuan J. Autophagy in cell death: an innocent convict? *J Clin Invest.* 2005;115:2679–2688.
228. Pattingre S, Tassa A, Qu X, et al. Bcl-2 antiapoptotic proteins inhibit beclin 1-dependent autophagy. *Cell.* 2005;122:927–939.
232. Reed JC. Apoptosis-based therapies. *Nat Rev Drug Discov.* 2002;1:111–121.
233. Karin M, Lin A. NFkappaB at the crossroads of life and death. *Nat Immunol.* 2002;3:221–227.
248. Elstner E, Linker-Israeli M, Umiel T, et al. Combination of a potent 20-epi-vitamin D3 analogue (KH 1060) with 9-cis-retinoic acid irreversibly inhibits clonal growth, decreases bcl-2 expression, and induces apoptosis in HL-60 leukemic cells. *Can Res.* 1996;56:3570–3576.

5 Growth Factors and Signal Transduction in Cancer

Luca Grumolato, PhD ■ Stuart A. Aaronson, MD

The evolution of multicellular organisms has involved the development of intercellular communication required for processes such as embryonic development, tissue differentiation, and systemic responses to wounds and infections. These complex signaling networks are in large part mediated by growth factors, cytokines and hormones. Such factors can influence cell proliferation in positive or negative ways, as well as induce a series of differentiated responses in appropriate target cells. The interaction of a growth factor with its receptor by specific binding in turn activates a cascade of intracellular biochemical events that is ultimately responsible for the biologic responses observed. Cytoplasmic molecules that mediate these responses have been termed second messengers. The eventual transmission of biochemical signals to the nucleus leads to effects on the expression of cassettes of genes involved in mitogenic and differentiation responses.

The pathogenic expression of critical genes in growth factor signaling pathways can also contribute to altered cell growth associated with malignancy. The v-*sis* oncogene of simian sarcoma virus, which encodes a growth factor homologous to the B chain of human platelet-derived growth factor (PDGF-B), is the paradigm for such genes.[1] The normal counterparts of other oncogenes have been shown to encode membrane-spanning growth factor receptors.[2,3] Other genes that act early in intracellular pathways of growth factor signal transduction have been implicated as oncogenes as well. Present knowledge indicates that the constitutive activation of growth factor signaling pathways through genetic alterations affecting these genes contributes to the development and progression of most if not all human cancers.

This chapter focuses on normal aspects of growth factor signaling, particularly those mediated by growth factor receptors possessing intrinsic protein tyrosine kinase activity. In addition, examples are provided where abnormalities in early steps in these pathways involving alterations in growth factor expression and/or receptor signaling have been implicated in the etiology of human malignancies. Finally, we will discuss how this knowledge may be useful in efforts to design new approaches toward therapeutic intervention with the malignant process. The limits of space preclude a discussion of several important families of ligands and their receptors. These include the cytokines and their receptors, which lack intrinsic tyrosine kinase activity but associate with cytoplasmic tyrosine kinases. Other ligand/receptor families will not be discussed.

Background

Hormones that act at great distances from the cells producing them have been known for many years. Hormones as signaling molecules were isolated from tissue fluids and readily characterized by their in vivo effects. In contrast, knowledge of growth factors is relatively recent. Growth factor activity capable of stimulating the growth of chicken embryonic nerve cells was found to be released by mouse sarcoma cells.[4] During purification of this nerve growth factor (NGF), a second activity that promoted eyelid opening and incisor eruption in newborn mice and rats was discovered. Because of recognition of its effects on epithelial cells, this factor was designated epidermal growth factor (EGF).[5]

An important discovery concerning growth factors came from the demonstration of a unique enzymologic activity associated with binding of EGF to its receptor.[5] Studies of the product of the viral oncogene, v-src, had led to the demonstration of its ability to act as a protein kinase.[6,7] Many protein kinases had been previously identified, but these had the capacity to phosphorylate serine and/or threonine residues. Moreover, it was well established that phosphorylations and dephosphorylations affected the activities of a variety of proteins. However, the src product was subsequently shown to have a unique specificity as a protein kinase in that it was capable of phosphorylating tyrosine residues.[8] Cohen then showed that addition of EGF led to phosphorylation of its purified receptor on tyrosine residues.[5] Subsequent studies have demonstrated that tyrosine kinase activity is central to the functions of a large number of mitogenic signaling molecules.

Several major modes of action for growth factors have been described. Sporn and Todaro[9] defined autocrine and paracrine as major modes of action for growth factors in addition to the classical means by which hormones travel great distances from their sites of production (Fig. 5-1). The autocrine mode refers to the ability of growth factor to act on the same cell releasing it. In the paracrine mode, the released growth factor from one cell acts on a nearby or adjacent cell. Certain growth factors also exist as membrane-anchored forms, which can bind and activate membrane receptors only on adjacent cells. This process, considered a variant of the paracrine mode, has been termed juxtacrine[10] and is capable of delivering spatially localized intercellular stimuli. A number of researchers have observed that factors that are produced in cells but are not detectably secreted nevertheless can induce observable phenotypic changes in those cells. The suggestion has been made that this represents an "intracrine" mode of action, whereby the factor interacts with its receptor for example, within the Golgi apparatus.[11,12] A sixth mode of action, in which the growth factor is bound to and stored within the extracellular matrix before presentation to the receptor on the cell surface, has also been demonstrated.[13]

Growth Factor Receptors with Tyrosine Kinase Activity

Growth factors mediate their diverse biologic responses by binding to and activating cell-surface receptors with intrinsic protein kinase activity.[14] To date, more than 50 receptor tyrosine kinases (RTKs),

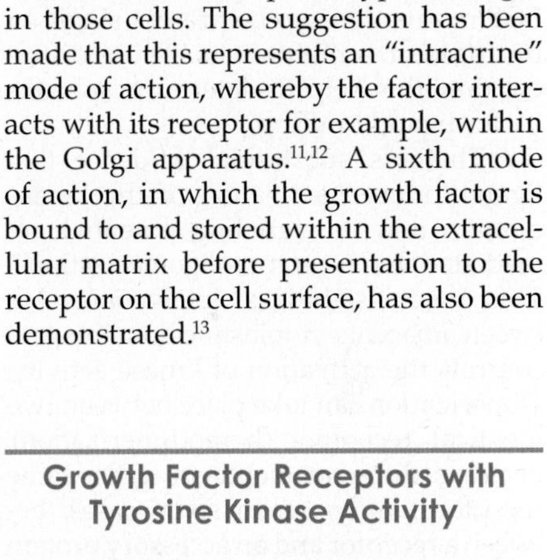

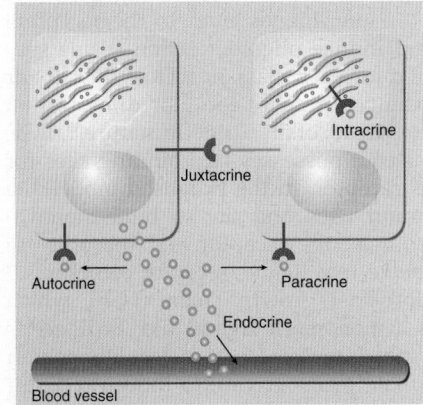

Figure 5-1 ■ Modes of action for growth factors.

which belong to at least 18 different receptor families, have been identified. All RTKs contain a large, glycosylated, extracellular ligand-binding domain, a single transmembrane region, and a cytoplasmic portion with a conserved protein tyrosine kinase domain. In addition to the catalytic domain, a juxtamembrane region and a C-terminal tail can be identified in the cytoplasmic portion. Because of their structure, RTKs can be visualized as membrane-associated allosteric enzymes with the ligand-binding and protein tyrosine kinase domains separated by the plasma membrane. Their role is to catalyze the transfer of the γ-phosphate of adenosine triphosphate (ATP) to tyrosine residues of exogenous substrates as well as within their own polypeptide chain. Tyrosine phosphorylation represents the language that these receptors use to transduce the information carried by the growth factor.

On the basis of sequence similarity, it is possible to classify these receptors into related groups.[15] Characteristic structural features of their extracellular domains include cysteine-rich motifs, immunoglobulin-like repeats (Ig-like), fibronectin type III repeats (FNIII), and EGF motifs that can be present singly or in different combinations. These different domains help to determine specificity for ligand binding.

There is substantial evidence that ligand-induced activation of the kinase domain and its signaling potential are mediated by receptor oligomerization.[16] This event stabilizes interactions between adjacent cytoplasmic domains and controls the activation of kinase activity. Dimerization can take place between two identical receptors (homodimerization), between different members of the same receptor family, or, in some cases, between a receptor and an accessory protein (heterodimerization).[16] Heterodimerization of RTKs has been shown, on the one hand, to increase the repertoire of ligands that can be recognized by each receptor alone and, on the other hand, to expand the diversity of signaling pathways that can be recruited by a given receptor.

How ligands bind to the receptors and induce oligomerization seems specific for each class of RTKs.[17] PDGF, for example, induces receptor dimerization by virtue of its dimeric nature.[18] EGF, instead, possesses two binding sites for its receptor. In the proposed model, the ligand uses one site to bind monovalently to the receptor and the other to bridge two ligand/receptor complexes.[19] Fibroblast growth factor (FGF), which is a monomeric ligand like EGF, needs instead an accessory molecule, heparan sulfate proteoglycan, to induce receptor dimerization.[20,21] Interestingly, the insulin receptor (IR) family exists as disulfide-bonded homo- or heterodimers of receptor subunits.[22] Thus, ligand binding does not induce receptor dimerization but presumably causes a conformational change in the preformed dimeric receptor, which leads to receptor activation.

The activation of intrinsic protein kinase activity results in autophosphorylation of specific tyrosine residues in the cytoplasmic portion of the RTK. Moreover, tyrosine phosphorylation in the kinase domain stimulates the intrinsic catalytic activity of the receptor. Recently, biochemical and structural studies have revealed some of the molecular mechanisms that mediate such activation. There is substantial evidence that autophosphorylation occurs in *trans* by a second RTK after dimerization induced by ligand binding. In the unphosphorylated state, the receptor possesses a low catalytic activity due to the particular conformation of a specific domain in the kinase region, which interferes with the phosphotransfer event. Phosphorylation of the kinase domain removes this inhibition, and the catalytic activity is enhanced and persists for some time independently of the presence of the ligand. Although kinase activity is at a low basal level in the monomeric state, this activity is sufficient to induce trans-autophosphorylation once the dimer forms. Autophosphorylation also occurs outside the kinase domain and serves the important function of creating docking sites for downstream signal transduction molecules (see below). The main function of the transmembrane domain is to anchor the receptor in the plane of the plasma membrane, thereby connecting the extracellular environment with internal compartments of the cell. It was initially thought that this domain represented a passive anchor of the receptor to the membrane.[16] However, point mutations in the transmembrane domain of one receptor, the neu/erbB-2, enhance its transforming properties. This transmembrane mutation may have a stabilizing effect on conformation, which results in dimerization and constitutive activation of receptor signaling.[23] Genetic alterations in this domain have, in fact, demonstrated an active role of this region in RTK dimerization and demonstrated that dimerization is not sufficient, but proper alignment must also occur for activation and signaling.[24]

The juxtamembrane sequence that separates the transmembrane and cytoplasmic domains is not well conserved between different families of receptors. However, juxtamembrane sequences are highly similar among members of the same receptor family. Studies indicate that this domain plays a role in modulation of receptor functions by heterologous stimuli, a process termed receptor transmodulation.[16] For example, addition of PDGF to many types of cells causes a rapid decrease in high-affinity binding of EGF to its receptor. This has been shown to be a downstream effect of PDGF receptor activation in which protein kinase C, itself a serine protein kinase, is activated and, in turn, phosphorylates a site in the juxtamembrane domain of the EGF receptor.[16] This region may also play a role in signaling, as has been suggested by the capacity to bind specific substrates in a ligand-dependent manner. For example, it has been shown that *eps8* directly binds to the juxtamembrane domain of the EGFR in a phosphotyrosine- and SH2-independent manner.[25]

The tyrosine kinase domain is the most conserved among tyrosine kinase receptors, and an intact protein tyrosine kinase domain is absolutely required for receptor signaling. For example, mutation of a single lysine in the ATP-binding site, which blocks the ability of the receptor to phosphorylate tyrosine residues, completely inactivates receptor biologic function. The kinase domain of some RTKs (eg, PDGF and FGF receptors) is split by insertions of up to 100 mostly hydrophilic amino acid residues. Kinase insertion sequences are highly conserved between species, suggesting an important role of this domain in receptor function. In fact, this region contains important autophosphorylation sites that have the function of coupling with signal-transducing molecules. Thus, it appears that the role of the kinase insert region is to mediate receptor interactions with second messengers.[16]

The C-terminal tail sequences are among the most divergent between known RTKs.[14] The C-terminal domain of the receptor is thought to play an important role in regulating kinase activity. This region typically contains several tyrosine residues, which are phosphorylated by the activated kinase. In fact, the receptor, itself, is often the major tyrosine phosphorylated species observed following ligand stimulation. Specific amino acid sequences in this domain play an important role in determining activation of specific signal-transducing molecules by RTKs as described in the Growth Factor Receptor Signaling section of this chapter. The ability to molecularly clone related genes based upon the conserved nature of their kinase domains has led to the identification of a number of structurally related members of several receptor families as listed below.

Classification of Growth Factors and Their Receptors

Platelet-Derived Growth Factor Family

PDGF is the major protein growth factor in human serum and is a markedly heat-stable, cationic protein that consists of four related but nonidentical polypeptide chains. While PDGF-A and PDGF-B have been extensively studied since the 1970s, PDGF-C and PDGF-D were only identified in 2000[26-28] and 2001,[29-31] respectively, using bioinformatics approaches. The PDGF ligands contain a characteristic motif named cystine knot and formed of regularly spaced cysteine residues that allow intra- and intermolecular bonds.[32] All PDGF molecules form disulfide-linked homodimers, but PDGF-A and PDGF-B can also exist as heterodimers. Unlike PDGF-A and PDGF-B, which are secreted as active ligands, PDGF-C and PDGF-D become active following cleavage of their N-terminal domain.[33] PDGF-AB is the major PDGF form found in platelets and is released into serum upon blood clotting. However, there is evidence for the natural occurrence of each of the other forms. Connective tissue and glial cells in culture are highly sensitive to the mitogenic effects of PDGF,[18] and these cells express PDGF receptors. As shown in Figure 5-2, receptors of the PDGF family exhibit several distinctive features. Their extracellular regions show primary sequence characteristics and the same spacing of cysteine residues, consistent with the organization of five immunoglobulin-like domains.[34] Another feature of the PDGF receptor family is the presence of a large kinase insert within the tyrosine kinase domain. These 80 to 100 amino acid stretches are highly divergent among different family members. There are reports that the kinase insert is required for interaction with certain substrates,[35] and deletions in this domain impair receptor mitogenic signaling.[36] As the four PDGF ligands, the two PDGF-Rs are encoded by distinct genes[32,37] and form homo- or heterodimers.[38] Ligands have different affinity for the different receptor combinations: AA binds αα, CC and AB bind αα and αβ, BB binds all the three receptor dimers, and DD binds αβ and ββ.[33] This is an example of the fine degree of regulation that can evolve in the interactions of ligands with their receptors. Presumably, in the case of PDGF, this relates to quantitative regulation of responses based upon differential availability in tissues of ligands and receptors, since there is evidence that the two PDGF receptors themselves are each capable of mediating the major known PDGF responses, including mitogenic signaling and chemotaxis.[34] Gene inactivation of the PDGF receptors and ligands has demonstrated that this signaling is essential during embryonic development. In particular, these studies have shown that PDGF-B and PDGF-Rβ are crucially involved in vessel formation, while PDGF-A/C and PDGF-Rα play a broader role in different processes, such as central nervous system, neural crest, and organ development.[32,39] More specific strategies, including conditional knockout and knockin approaches, have been used to address the primary functions of PDGF signaling during development.[39,40]

The transforming protein expressed by SSV shares close structural similarities with PDGF-B chain homodimers.[41] PDGF-B has been detected in human tumor cells[42] that also possess PDGF receptors. These findings, taken together with the demonstration that the normal PDGF-B gene can act as an oncogene when expressed at high levels,[43] suggest that PDGF-B plays a role in the development of certain human cancers. The PDGF-A chain is frequently expressed by human tumor cells, and AA homodimers are produced by osteosarcoma,[44] melanoma,[45] and glioblastoma cells,[46] which can display autocrine activation of PDGF signaling.[47] Of note, a translocation between chromosomes 17 and 22 in dermatofibrosarcoma protuberans has been shown to bring the PDGF-B gene under the control of the widely expressed collagen type 1 alpha 1 promoter, leading to an autocrine loop.[48] The more recently discovered PDGF-C and -D ligands have been reported to possess transforming capacity in some glioblastomas[49] and may be involved in different types of cancers, including Ewing sarcoma, medulloblastoma, and prostate cancer.[32] Aberrant stimulation of PDGF signaling in cancer can also be caused by ligand-independent activation of PDGF-Rs. For example, mutations in the catalytic and juxtamembrane domains of PDGF-Rα have been identified in gastrointestinal stromal tumor (GIST), a rare malignancy of mesenchymal origin.[50] Of note, PDGF-Rα and c-kit (discussed later) mutations in GIST are mutually exclusive, indicating that these RTKs activate common oncogenic downstream pathways in this type of cancer.[50,51] Another mechanism of ligand-independent activation of PDGF-Rs has been described in hematological malignancies, where gene translocations can provoke the fusion of PDGF-Rα or PDGF-Rβ catalytic domain with different partner proteins.[50]

Colony-stimulating factor 1 (CSF-1) or macrophage-colony-stimulating factor (M-CSF) also belongs to this family.[52] This molecule promotes the growth and maturation of monocytes and macrophage precursors. It also enhances the phagocytic and tumoricidal activity of human macrophage/monocytes and induces them to secrete a variety of different cytokines. Two active forms, one of which is secreted and the other cell associated, arise from differential splicing. The *c-fms* proto-oncogene encodes the CSF-1 receptor,[3] another member of the PDGF receptor family. The CSF-1 receptor is expressed in cells of the monocyte/macrophage lineage, as well as in the CNS and placental trophoblasts.[53] Several studies have reported elevated CSF-1 serum concentration in patients affected with different types of cancer,[54] and it has been proposed that CSF-1 can stimulate tumor growth and progression to metastasis.[55] For example, one study showed that the invasiveness of breast carcinoma is promoted through a paracrine positive loop between cancer cells secreting CSF-1 and macrophages producing EGF.[56]

Stem cell factor (SCF),[57] also designated kit ligand, mast cell growth factor, or steel factor (SLF), is a hematopoietic and tissue growth factor that binds to the receptor encoded by the c-kit proto-oncogene.[53] The naturally occurring form of this secreted molecule is a 165 amino acid polypeptide, which is heavily N- and O-glycosylated and exists as a dimer. Alternative splicing of the gene results in secreted and membrane-bound forms. The SCF/kit ligand is present at relatively high levels in human plasma relative to most other cytokines. This growth factor does not stimulate hematopoietic colony formation itself but has been shown to augment the in vitro proliferation of both myeloid and lymphoid hematopoietic progenitor cells in the presence of other cytokines.[57] It has been proposed that SCF, produced locally at high concentrations by bone marrow stromal cells, acts as an "anchor" factor and permits stem cells to respond to physiologic concentrations of cytokines. It also promotes the activation of skin mast cells and basophils. SCF receptor, encoded by the *c-kit* proto-oncogene, contains in its extracellular portion five immunoglobulin-like domains, which determine the binding specificity and facilitate dimerization. An intracellular juxtamembrane domain separates the transmembrane region and the kinase domain. It has been shown that *c-kit* is frequently mutated in GIST. Activating mutations in *c-kit* gene have been reported isn exon 9, 11, and 13, encoding the extracellular dimerization domain, the juxtamembrane domain, and the kinase domain, respectively.[58] Other malignancies showing activation of SCF-c-kit signaling through an autocrine or paracrine mechanism include small cell lung cancer (SCLC) and testicular germ cell tumor.[58]

The Flt3 receptor was cloned by low-stringency hybridization with a *c-fms* probe and is expressed in pre-B, monocytic and myeloid cell lines.[53] It contains, as the other members of this family of RTKs, an extracellular domain with five immunoglobulin-like domains, a transmembrane region, a cytoplasmic juxtamembrane domain, and two kinase domains linked by a kinase insert domain.[59]

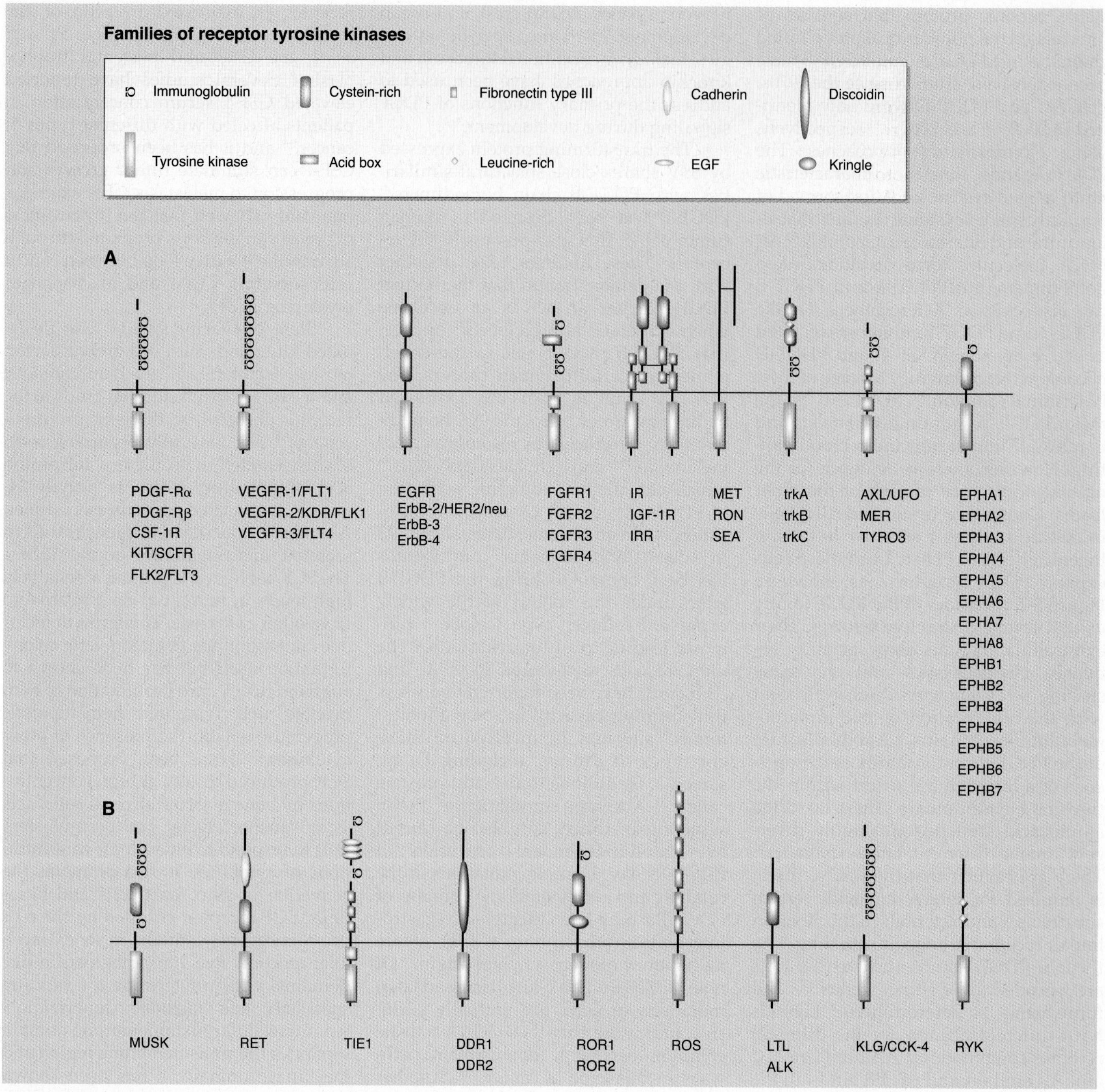

Figure 5-2 ■ Families of receptor tyrosine kinases.

The Flt3 ligand is a transmembrane protein that undergoes proteolytic cleavage to generate a soluble factor with a certain similarity in the conserved cysteine residues with the kit ligand.[53] Flt3 is expressed at high levels in CD34+ "short-term" hematopoietic stem cells, and the Flt3 ligand exerts a proliferative effect on both the myeloid and lymphoid lineages, usually in combination with other cytokines.[59] Activating mutations of Flt3 are the most frequent genetic abnormality in acute myeloid leukemia (AML) and include in-frame tandem duplications in the juxtamembrane domain or missense point mutations in the kinase domain.[59]

Vascular Endothelial Growth Factor Family

Efforts to identify factors that control angiogenesis led to the identification of a potent mitogen for vascular endothelial cells of small and large vessels.[60] Vascular endothelial growth factor (VEGF), also designated vascular permeability factor (VPF), is a glycosylated, dimeric heparin-binding protein (mol. wt. 45,000 Da) able to stimulate angiogenesis and to increase the permeability of capillary vessels to different macromolecules. The potent mitogenic effects of VEGF are restricted to cells of vascular endothelial origin. Similarly to PDGF, VEGF contains a cystine-knot domain, and the two growth factors are thought to derive from a common ancestor polypeptide.[61] The most abundant and active member of the family, VEGF-A, is a glycosylated, dimeric heparin-binding protein able to stimulate angiogenesis and to increase the permeability of capillary vessels to different macromolecules. Alternative splicing originates several isoforms of VEGF-A. The predominant human isoforms, VEGF-A-121 and 165, are secreted from producing cells, whereas VEGF-A-189 and 206 are not efficiently secreted and seem to bind tightly to cell-surface heparin-like molecules.[62] Substantial evidence indicates that the binding of the best-studied form VEGF-A-165 to its receptor is dependent on cell-surface-associated heparin-like molecules. Four additional endothelial growth factors, which are structurally related to VEGF, have been reported.[63-65] VEGF-B and its alternatively spliced isoform, described as VEGF-related factor (VRF),[66] are predominantly expressed in embryonal and adult myocardial and skeletal muscle tissues. VEGF-B isoforms can bind VEGFR-1 but not VEGFR-2 or VEGFR-3.[64] Inactivation of the gene encoding VEGF-B suggested an involvement of this growth factor in heart development and inflammatory angiogenesis.[64] VEGF-C is a ligand for VEGFR-2 and VEGFR-3 receptors, and it is expressed in different organs including the heart, small intestine, placenta, ovary, and the thyroid gland.[64] Mice lacking both VEGF-C alleles die of edema due to incomplete development of lymphatic vessels, while the loss of one VEGF-C allele provokes less severe defects in lymphatic vasculature.[65] VEGF-D binds VEGFR-2 and VEGFR-3 and has both angiogenic and lymphangiogenic properties. VEGF-D is present in most human tissues, with highest expression levels in the lung and skin during development.[65] It has been shown that both VEGF-C and VEGF-D play important roles in promoting tumor-induced lymphangiogenesis.[67,68] Another member of the VEGF family of growth factors, VEGF-E, was discovered in the genome of a parapoxvirus, which provokes skin lesions with extensive capillary proliferation.[69] VEGF-E is a potent angiogenic factor that binds with high affinity to the VEGFR-2 receptor.[65] Recently a new VEGF was identified in snake venom and called VEGF-F.[65]

Three high-affinity receptors for VEGF have been identified.[62,65] These receptors, termed VEGFR-1/Flt-1 (fms-like tyrosine kinase-1),[70] VEGFR-2/KDR/Flk-1 (kinase insert domain containing receptor/fetal liver kinase-1),[71] and VEGFR-3/Flt-4 (fms-like tyrosine kinase-4)[72] are characterized by an extracellular region containing seven (VEGFR-1 and 2) or six (VEGFR-3) Ig-like domains and a tyrosine kinase interrupted by a large kinase insert. VEGFRs are expressed by vascular endothelial cells although expression has also been detected in certain hematopoietic cells, such as monocytes, and in melanoma cell lines. VEGFR-1 was initially considered a "decoy receptor" reducing the levels of circulating VEGF, but more recent studies have shown that VEGFR-1 can mediate mitotic signals and be involved in the recruitment of endothelial progenitor cells.[73] VEGFR-2 is reported as a major regulator of vasculogenesis and angiogenesis. Its biologic role has been clarified by disruption of this gene in mouse embryos, which failed to develop both endothelial and hematopoietic cells.[74] Heparan sulfate proteoglycan and neurophilin can act as co-receptors by enhancing binding of several VEGF isoforms to VEGFR-2.[62] VEGFR-3 expression pattern and knockout studies suggest that this receptor is essential during embryogenesis for the development of blood vessels, but it becomes redundant in mature vessels.[64] A recent study revealed that VEGF-A can promote cell migration and proliferation through direct activation of PDGF-Rα and PDGF-Rβ in human mesenchymal stem cells, providing evidence of cross-talk between VEGF and PDGF signaling pathways.[75]

Placenta-derived growth factor (PlGF) is another member of this family originally discovered in the placenta[76] and also expressed in the heart and lungs. PlGF forms homodimers or heterodimers with VEGF and binds to VEGFR-1.[65] PlGF inactivation revealed that this growth factor is not involved in embryonic angiogenesis but it is required in angiogenesis, plasma extravasation, and collateral growth in response to ischemia and inflammation or during wound healing.[77] PlGF has been implicated in colorectal cancer, acute lymphoblastic leukemia (ALL), and Ewing sarcoma.[65]

Epidermal Growth Factor Family

EGF consists of 53 amino acids constrained by three internal disulfide bonds and is generated from a 1200 residue precursor that contains eight units similar to EGF and is detected as a glycosylated membrane protein.[78,79] Other members of this widely expressed EGF family include TGF-α (transforming growth factor-α),[80] amphiregulin (AR), or schwannoma-derived growth factor (rat homolog of AR), heparin-binding EGF (HB-EGF), betacellulin, the poxvirus mitogens (vaccinia, Shope, and myxoma growth factors), epiregulin, and the neuregulin family. All of these molecules share sequence similarity, at least 28% sequence identity, and 100% conservation of the six cysteine residues present within the mature sequence of EGF. With the exception of the neuregulins, all of these proteins are able to bind to the EGF receptor and show mitogenic effects on EGF-responsive cells.[81]

It has been shown for EGF and TGF-α that the membrane-bound forms may interact with receptors on the surface of adjacent cells, thereby potentially contributing to cell–cell adhesion and to cell–cell stimulation.[80] Since many of these molecules bind and activate the same receptor, there appears to be substantial functional redundancy within this family. Nonetheless, quantitative differences in their biologic activities have been demonstrated. The findings that TGF-α is found in culture fluids from various oncogenically transformed cells[82] gave rise to its designation as a "transforming growth factor." TGF-α and EGF are almost indistinguishable in their ability to bind, activate, and down-modulate the EGF receptor in mammalian cells.[82]

AR was initially purified from conditioned medium of a human breast adenocarcinoma, MCF-7, treated with phorbol 12-myristate 13-acetate.[83] AR is a potent stimulator of normal keratinocytes and mammary epithelial cells. Relative to EGF, AR contains a very basic 40 amino acid stretch at its N terminus, which is also rich in potential N- and O-linked glycosylation sites. Within this region, there are also two putative nuclear localization signals. In fact, AR has been detected in the nucleus and in the cytoplasm of treated cells. The biologic importance of its nuclear localization is not yet understood. AR is a heparin-binding growth factor, whose bioactivity can be inhibited by heparan sulfate.[83] It has also been shown that extracellular heparan sulfate proteoglycans are essential for mediation of its mitogenic signal by EGFR.[84] AR participates in the development of kidney and postnatal mammary gland[85,86] and it plays a role in liver regeneration.[87]

HB-EGF is a more potent mitogen for smooth-muscle cells than either EGF or TGF-α.[88] It is also active on fibroblasts but not endothelial cells. Like TGF-α and AR, HB-EGF is secreted by means of proteolytic processing of a transmembrane precursor. At least five different forms with N-terminal heterogeneity have been identified.[89] It has also been demonstrated that the membrane-anchored form of HB-EGF acts as the diphtheria toxin receptor.[90] Betacellulin is a potent mitogen for retinal pigment epithelial cells and vascular smooth-muscle cells.[91] Epiregulin was identified as a novel EGFR ligand, which stimulates the proliferation of fibroblasts, hepatocytes, and smooth-muscle cells.[92]

Purification of rat and human stimulatory proteins for the second member of the EGF receptor family (see below) led to the isolation of cDNAs encoding novel EGF-related proteins. The 44 kDa rat factor, termed Neu differentiation factor (NDF), stimulates p185neu tyrosine phosphorylation and induces the production of milk components in certain breast carcinoma cell lines. The homologous human factors, termed heregulins (HRGs) or neuregulins (NRGs), were found to be mitogenic for certain mammary tumor cells.[93] At least 26 different NRG-1 isoforms have been described, including the acetylcholine receptor inducing activity (ARIA) and glial growth factors (GGF). NRG isoforms are encoded by the same gene through alternative splicing and are classified into three groups based on their N-terminal domain: HRG (type I), GGF (type II), and sensory and motor neuron-derived factor (SMDF, type III).[94] Another characteristic used to classify NRG-1 isoforms is the presence of exon α or β, which encode the which encode part of the EGF motif. It has been shown that β isoforms have higher receptor affinity and are generally more potent than α isoforms.[94] Like TGF-α, NRGs display a wide distribution in many tissues and organs. Moreover, the expression patterns of some isoforms are tissue-specific. For example, the α2 isoform is the predominant form in mesenchymal tissues, whereas the β1 isoform is enriched in brain tissue and spinal cord.[94,95] Three other genes with a high degree of homology to NRG-1 and displaying different affinities for EGFRs have been identified. NRG-2 and -3 are expressed predominantly in neural tissues both in embryos and adults. NRG-4 was instead detected in adult pancreas and weakly in muscle.[81,94]

EGF family ligands have been classified based on their affinity for one of four members of the EGF/ErbB receptor family,[81] which includes the EGFR, ErbB-2 (also known as HER-2, for homolog of the human EGF receptor, or *c-neu* for homolog of the rat proto-oncogene *neu*), ErbB-3, and ErbB-4. The first group of ligands binds to the EGFR and includes EGF, TGF-α, AR, HB-EGF, betacellulin, and epiregulin. The second group, represented by betacellulin, HB-EGF, and epiregulin, binds the EGFR and ErbB-4. All NRGs bind to ErbB-3 and ErbB-4. Although no direct ligand for ErbB-2 has been identified, it has been shown that this receptor is the preferred heterodimerization partner of the other ErbB receptors. In the case of ErbB-3, heterodimerization is essential for NRG signaling since this unique receptor possesses an impaired kinase activity.[96] ErbB receptor heterodimerization allows the receptors to work synergistically by expanding the array of signaling events that can be activated by a single molecule.[81]

The EGFR was identified and isolated by biochemical techniques and shown to be the cellular homolog of the *v-erbB*, a retroviral oncogene.[2] The other members were isolated from genomic DNAs and cDNA libraries by low-stringency hybridization techniques using conserved tyrosine kinase domain probes. The extracellular domains of each of these molecules contain cysteine-rich motifs in two distinct regions and an uninterrupted tyrosine kinase domain. Whereas the EGFR and ErbB-2 are expressed in a wide variety of cell types, the expression of ErbB-3 is restricted to cells of epithelial or neuroectodermal origin.[81]

Fibroblast Growth Factor Family

FGFs comprise a 22 member family that exhibits mitogenic activity upon a wide variety of cells of mesenchymal, neuronal, and epithelial origin.[97,21] These proteins can bind to and have their biologic activities modulated by heparin. The family includes acidic FGF (aFGF, FGF-1), basic FGF (bFGF, FGF-2), int-2 (FGF-3), hst/KS3 (FGF-4), FGF-5, FGF-6, keratinocyte growth factor (FGF-7), androgen-induced growth factor (AIGF or FGF-8), and glia-activating factor (GAF or FGF-9).

The first to be isolated, bFGF, was recognized in certain hormone preparations by its mitogenicity for fibroblasts and chondrocytes and was later purified from bovine pituitary. aFGF was purified independently from acidic extracts of bovine brain.[97] Both acidic and basic FGF are angiogenic in vivo and are involved in various processes, including neuronal regeneration and bone development.[98] Both are single-chain polypeptides of about 17,000 Da with 55% amino acid sequence identity. A striking feature of their structures, in contrast to those of many other family members, is the lack of a consensus secretory signal peptide. This has generated a great deal of speculation regarding their mode of release from cells. It has been argued that they are liberated by lysis or escorted out of intact cells by other proteins. The presence of a nuclear translocation signal and detection of aFGF and bFGF in the nuclei of endothelial and mesenchymal cells, respectively,[99,100] have suggested that these growth factors may also act internally without requiring a secretory signal sequence.[98]

Analysis of DNA of mammary tumors induced by mouse mammary tumor virus (MMTV) revealed that the viral genome frequently integrates within a genetic locus termed *int-2* and thereby activates expression of this gene by insertional mutagenesis. The protein encoded by int-2, renamed FGF-3, is predicted to be 245 amino acids long and highly similar to aFGF and bFGF. Transgenic mouse experiments have shown that FGF-3 expression leads to mammary gland hyperplasia in female mice and benign epithelial hyperplasia in the prostate of males.[101] The normal expression of *int-2* is apparently limited to embryonic tissues.[97] A recent study revealed that individuals affected with a particular form of deafness presented a missense mutation in the FGF-3 gene, indicating an important role of this growth factor in the development of the inner ear.[102]

FGF-4 and FGF-5 were uncovered during searches for oncogenes in human tumor cells.[21,97] FGF-4 was isolated independently from a human stomach tumor (hst) and a Kaposi sarcoma (KS3). It is mitogenic for vascular endothelial cells, human melanocytes, and mouse NIH/3T3 fibroblasts. The FGF-5 gene was also isolated by DNA transfection but by use of a selection system in which cell proliferation was dependent on abrogation of growth factor requirements. FGF-5 was found to be mitogenic for mouse fibroblasts and bovine heart endothelial cells.[103] Knockout studies have demonstrated that FGF-4 is required at a very early stage of development involving implantation of the embryo.[104] The inactivation of the FGF-5 gene is associated with a very different phenotype, in which affected mice develop apparently normally and show only increased hair length following birth.[105]

FGF-6 was isolated by low-stringency hybridization and was shown to act as a transforming gene for NIH/3T3 cells by transfection analysis.[21] KGF (FGF-7) was isolated from media conditioned by a human embryonic lung fibroblast cell line and was found to be a potent mitogen for epithelial cells but to lack activity on fibroblasts or endothelial cells.[106] Thus, KGF was distinct in its target cell specificity not only from other members of the FGF family but also from other known polypeptide growth factors as well. KGF is expressed by stromal, but not epithelial, cells of most major epithelial tissues.[107] There is evidence that KGF plays a role in epithelial renewal during wound repair[108] and as a stromal mediator of epithelial cell proliferation/differentiation in sex hormone-responsive tissues.[109] All of these findings support the concept that this factor is important in the normal mesenchymal stimulation of epithelial cell growth.

AIGF (FGF-8) was isolated from media conditioned by a cell line derived from a testosterone-dependent mouse mammary tumor cell line.[97] Target cells include epithelial and fibroblast cells and its expression appears to be restricted to the testes in the adult, and during the period of embryonic reproductive tract development.[21]

Little information is as yet available concerning most of the more recently identified FGF family members. GAF (FGF-9)[97] was purified from supernatants of a human glioma cell line. FGF-10 was identified by homologous-based PCR and has target cell specificity most similar to FGF-7. Other FGF family members have been recently identified by degenerate PCR or by homology searches of genome databases. Several lack secretory signal peptides and/or possess nuclear localization signals, and their functions remain to be defined.[97]

The prototype FGF receptor closely resembles the PDGF receptor family but instead contains extracellular domain variants with two or three immunoglobulin-like motifs instead of five. Moreover, the kinase insert within the tyrosine kinase domain of this receptor family is shorter (14 amino acids) than in members of the PDGF receptor (Fig. 5-2). Four distinct but related genes, FGFR1, FGFR2, FGFR3, and FGFR4, have been identified.[21] Adding to this complexity are findings of alternatively spliced forms of FGF receptors expressed in different cell types. In the case of the FGFR1 and FGFR2 genes, multiple forms of the FGF receptor are generated via alternative splicing. The second half of Ig domain III represents one site of alternative splicing in both FGFR1 and -2. Binding studies have shown that alternative splicing in this domain is important in determining ligand-binding specificities.[110]

Tissue-specific alternative splicing in the third Ig domain and tissue-specific differential gene expression occur in vivo and regulate responsiveness to different FGF ligands. The complexity of heterodimeric interactions among different FGFRs remains to be elucidated.[21,97,111]

The Insulin Family

The diversity of metabolic effects of insulin has been studied intensively for decades.[112] Its primary in vivo functions involve the regulation of rapid anabolic responses such as glucose uptake, lipogenesis, and amino acid and ion transport. In addition to its effects on metabolism, insulin stimulates DNA synthesis and cell growth. The insulin-like growth factors, IGF-I and IGF-II, were first recognized as serum factors, antigenically distinct from insulin. These molecules are induced by growth hormone and serve as its effectors in stimulating growth of skeletal tissues.[113]

IGF-I, insulin, and IGF-II share around 50% amino acid sequence similarity.[113] Insulin is synthesized as a 109 amino acid precursor (preproinsulin), which is processed to a 6 kDa protein consisting of two chains (A and B) linked by two disulfide bonds. The structures of IGF-I and IGF-II are analogous to proinsulin in that they consist of a single polypeptide chain. In vivo studies indicate that IGF-I acts in an autocrine or paracrine mode since infusion of IGF-I does not give rise to its growth-promoting actions.[113] Although it is not known whether overexpression of insulin family members can lead to transformation, addition of exogenous IGF-I or supraphysiologic levels of insulin to mouse NIH/3T3 cells overexpressing IGF-I receptors induced morphologic transformation and enabled the cells to grow in soft agar and form tumors in nude mice.[114]

IGFs are bound to carrier proteins and are maintained at steady concentrations in the blood stream. The carrier proteins belong to a class of proteins that have high affinity and specificity for the IGFs and are designated as insulin-like growth factor-binding proteins (IGFBP). Six different IGFBPs have been identified in humans, and it seems that they are well conserved among mammals. The IGFBPs are involved in modulation of the proliferative and mitogenic effects of the IGFs at endocrine, paracrine, and autocrine levels.[115-117]

The IR is the prototype for a family of RTKs, which function as a heterotetrameric aggregation of two α and two β subunits (Fig. 5-2). The extracellular ligand-binding subunit, which contains a single cysteine-rich cluster, is disulfide-linked to the transmembrane β subunit, which contains the cytoplasmic tyrosine kinase domain.[118] The IR binds insulin with ~100-fold greater affinity than it does IGF-I or IGF-II (100 pM versus 10 nM). The IGF-I receptor is closely related to the IR in sequence and structure but binds IGF-I with highest affinity (100 pM), followed by IGF-II and insulin.[118] IGF-II is also bound by another receptor, which has been shown to be identical to the cation-independent mannose-6-phosphate receptor. The IGF-II receptor binds IGF-II and IGF-I with high affinity but does not bind insulin, and it appears to have a role in limiting IGF-II bioavailability.[119] A third member of the IR family, the insulin receptor-related receptor (IRR), shares their structural features. However, the ligand for IRR has not been identified,[120] and it is possible that this receptor may form heterodimers with the IR or IGF-R, in a way analogous to the ligandless ErbB-2 in the EGF signaling.

Increased expression of IGF-I, IGF-II, IGF-IR, or combinations thereof has been observed in different types of cancer, including glioblastoma, medulloblastoma, breast, colorectal, and pancreas carcinomas, and ovarian cancer.[119] These data, together with studies using cellular and animal models, suggest a role of this signaling in cancer growth and metastasis and support the idea of the IGF system as a potential target for cancer therapy.[117,119,121]

Hepatocyte Growth Factor

Hepatocyte growth factor (HGF) was isolated from plasma[122] or platelets.[123] HGF levels were found to increase dramatically following acute liver injury; thus, HGF was reasoned to play an important role in liver regeneration. The biochemical and biologic properties of HGF were found to differ from those of other known growth factors. The molecular weight of native HGF is around 90,000 Da and consists of two polypeptide chains of about 70,000 and 34,000 Da linked by disulfide bonds. HGF cDNA is encoded as a single 728 amino acid protein that is processed by proteolytic cleavage into heavy and light chains.[124] HGF is structurally related to plasminogen, containing serine-protease domains and disulfide bond-linked intrachain structures known as "kringles." Neither plasminogen nor plasmin have HGF-like activity, and HGF is not likely to be a protease since the histidine and serine residues in the region corresponding to the catalytic site are replaced by other amino acids.[124] HGF is mitogenic for a variety of epithelial cells, as well as endothelial cells and melanocytes, and is also capable of inducing certain cell types to undergo morphogenesis when suspended in a semisolid matrix. Thus, HGF/scatter factor is a mitogen, motogen, and a morphogen.[125] The HGF gene knockout is an embryonic lethal, leading to obvious abnormalities in liver and placenta development, as well as in the migration of myoblasts from the somites to the limbs and in motoneuron axon guidance.[126,127] The increase of HGF/SCF levels following liver, kidney, or heart injury and the expression of HGF/SCF and its receptor in mesenchymal stem cells strongly suggest the involvement of this growth factor in wound healing and tissue repair.[128,129]

A ligand related to HGF, termed "HGF-like" or macrophage-stimulating protein (MSP),[130] is a heterodimer of a heavy chain of 53 kDa (α) and a light chain of 25 kDa (β). MSP shares with HGF the overall four kringle/protease domain-like structure. Liver appears to be the main source of MSP, and its major activity to date is stimulating macrophage migration.

c-met was initially identified as a rearranged oncogene in a human osteogenic sarcoma cell line transformed in vitro with a chemical carcinogen.[131] This proto-oncogene encodes a 190 kDa glycoprotein that is processed to form a heterodimer comprised of a 50 kDa β-chain and 145 kDa α-chain. The extracellular, membrane-spanning, and tyrosine kinase domains are located on the β-chain (Fig. 5-2). The juxtamembrane domain contains serine and tyrosine residues that, upon phosphorylation, are involved in the degradation of the receptor, while the C-terminal tail is a unique docking site for the recruitment of several downstream signaling molecules.[132] MET is expressed in a variety of tissues, but the highest levels are found in epithelial cells. The expression of HGF is detected in mesenchymal cells of various organs and in particular in stromal and non-parenchymal cells neighboring epithelia.[131] The MET receptor initiates all of the known responses to HGF/SF mitogenesis, including motility and morphogenesis.[133,125]

Ron/Stk was isolated as a *c-met*-related gene by means of degenerate oligonucleotides.[134] *Ron* cDNA encodes a glycosylated protein, which shares overall similar topology with the HGF receptor, displays 63% sequence identity in its catalytic domain, and has a similar tissue distribution. The ligand for RON is MSP.[135]

Neurotrophin Family

In addition to NGF,[4] which was discovered several decades ago, the neurotrophin family includes brain-derived neurotrophic factor (BDNF), neurotrophin-3 (NT-3), neurotrophin-4 (NT-4), neurotrophin-5 (NT-5), and neurotrophin-6 (NT-6). These factors mediate cell interactions regulating neuron survival during development and function in the adult nervous system as well.[136,137]

Neurotrophins are 12-13 kDa proteins derived from 30-35 kDa precursors, proneurotrophins, by proteolytic cleavage. Both neurotrophins and proneurotrophins are secreted and can have opposite effects on target cells, such as survival versus apoptosis or synaptic long-term potentiation versus depression.[138] NGF is a basic 118 amino acid protein that acts on sensory and sympathetic neurons in the peripheral nervous system.[4] NGF is also present in the brain, where it serves a trophic function in the development and maintenance of cholinergic neurons of the basal forebrain.[137] BDNF supports the survival of neural crest-derived embryonic sensory neurons in vitro, and is expressed mainly in the CNS. NT-3 shows a strong sequence similarity to both NGF and BDNF and displays a high degree of regional specificity. Gene inactivation studies have shown that NT-3 participates in the development of the central and peripheral nervous system, in particular for sensory neurons and the enteric nervous system.[137,139] NT-4 was isolated from *Xenopus* as a molecule with the capacity to stimulate sensory neurons in culture. Another growth factor was almost simultaneously isolated from human and rat and termed NT-5, but was later shown to reflect the same gene. NT-4/5 is the least conserved factor among the family, and the inactivation of its gene provoked a mild phenotype, with reduced visceral afferent fibers in the small intestine and defects in nutrient feedback from the gastrointestinal tract.[140,141] While members of the NGF family share considerable sequence similarity, they have unique biologic activities and cooperate to support the development and maintenance of the vertebrate nervous system.

The neurotrophins interact with two distinct classes of receptors.[136,142] One is the p75/p80 low-affinity NGF receptor (p75NTR) protein. This receptor is a glycoprotein that is highly conserved across species and is broadly expressed in neuronal and non-neuronal tissues. Its extracellular region contains a cysteine-rich domain, whereas the intracellular domain is not related to any known protein and has no known enzymatic function. Low-affinity binding (Kd of 10^{-9} M) of all tested neurotrophins is mediated via this p75NTR, although its physiologic functions are not yet well understood.[142] p75NTR was recently found to function as a co-receptor for other ligands. Hempstead and colleagues showed that the NGF precursor binds with high-affinity p75NTR and its co-receptor sortilin, but not Trks, and induces apoptosis in neuronal and glial cells.[143,144] Finally, p75NTR can form a complex with the co-receptors NogoR and LINGO-1 to mediate the effects of the myelin-based growth inhibitors, Nogo, myelin-associated glycoprotein, and oligodendrocyte myelin glycoprotein.[145]

The *trk* genes encode the second class of neurotrophin receptors (Fig. 5-2). *Trk or trkA* was discovered in efforts to isolate oncogenes from human tumor cells.[146] The other two members of the family, *trkB and trkC*, were isolated by screening mammalian cDNA libraries with the *trkA* proto-oncogene as probe.[142] In contrast to p75NTR, the cytoplasmic regions of p140 trkA, p140 trkB, and p145 trkC contain tyrosine kinase catalytic domains. Their extracellular regions contain Ig-like and FNIII domains, in addition to cysteine clusters alternated with leucine motif repeats. Structural studies have shown that NGF binds the membrane-proximal Ig-C2-like domain of trkA, which induces receptor dimerization, phosphorylation of cytoplasmic tyrosine, and recruitment of adaptor proteins that mediate the signaling cascades.[147,148]

Each member of the trk family can bind at least one member of the neurotrophin family.[136,149] Although there are obvious preferences for binding of a particular neurotrophin to one of the trk family members, there is some promiscuity. In particular, the presence or absence of short sequences of amino acids in the juxtamembrane region of each trk, determined by alternative splicing, has profound effects on the specificity of the receptors for different neurotrophins. In summary, trkA binds and becomes activated by NGF, and NT-3 in the presence of the insert region. TrkB binds and is activated by BDNF, while the splice variant containing the insert in the juxtamembrane region also binds NT-3 and NT-4. *The trkC* product is activated by NT-3 but not NGF or BDNF.[147] Thus, at least three high-affinity receptors confer different but not absolute specificities for these related ligands.

Ligands for the Axl/SKY/MER Family

Protein S acts by indirectly inhibiting proteases involved in the coagulation cascade, although the precise mechanism remains unclear. Other functions, not directly involving coagulation, had been proposed for protein S.[150] This 70 kDa protein contains several modules, including an N-terminal region containing vitamin K-dependent α-carboxylation sites, a thrombin-sensitive module, a series of EGF-like repeats that undergo hydroxylation modification, and a module with homology to steroid-binding globulin. *Gas6* was cloned as a growth arrest-specific gene[151] and shares all but the thrombin-sensitive module with protein S. Coagulation factors such as thrombin are able to activate intracellular signaling via G protein-coupled cell-surface receptors. Thus some proteases and protease regulators may serve to integrate coagulation with associated cellular responses required for tissue repair and growth. Protein S and Gas6 serve as ligands for a subfamily of RTKs comprising Sky/Tyro3, Axl/Ufo, and Mer (Fig. 5-2). *Axl* (from the Greek word *anexelekto* or uncontrolled) was identified as a transforming gene from patients with chronic myelogenous leukemia and myeloproliferative disorders, respectively, by DNA transfection-tumorigenicity analysis.[152] The murine homolog, adhesion-related kinase (*Ark*), was cloned on the basis of relatedness to the tyrosine kinase domain of one of the FGF receptors. The encoded Axl/Ark proteins define a family of RTKs, which feature a new sequence in their cytoplasmic tyrosine kinase domains and an extracellular domain that juxtaposes two Ig-like domains and two FN type III repeats. A similar external domain topology has been observed among several neural cell adhesion molecules and a receptor tyrosine phosphatase.[153] Axl expression has been detected in the majority of cell types examined, with the exception of lymphocytes and granulocytes. Another member of this family is Sky (Tyro3), showing around 64% amino acid identity with axl. Sky is expressed predominantly in the brain, kidney, testis, and ovary and it has been proposed that it may be involved in cell adhesion and/or survival, particularly in the CNS.[152,154,155]

A third family member, *c-mer,* was isolated from a human B-lymphoblastoid cDNA expression library.[152] Sequence comparisons showed that this gene is the human homolog of the chicken retroviral oncogene, *v-nyk* (renamed *v-eyk*), a truncated tyrosine kinase whose expression by retroviral infection produced sarcomas in chickens. The designation *c-mer* was based on its expression pattern in monocytes and tissues of epithelial and reproductive origin. Gas6 activates all three receptors, while Protein S is specific for Sky.[154] The crystal structure of a minimal Gas6–Axl complex has been recently published[156]: the two Ig-like domains of an Axl monomer are linked to the steroid-binding globulin domain of a Gas6 molecule. Lateral diffusion of these 1:1 complexes induces the formation of a circular 2:2 assembly.[155,156] Of note, it has been shown that Axl constitutively interacts with interleukin (IL) 15 receptor a, and that both receptors can be triggered by IL-15 in mouse fibroblasts.[157] There is evidence that this family of receptors plays a role in regulation of macrophage activation and that compromised signaling results in a hyperactive immune system and may contribute to autoimmune diseases.[152] Their expression in neural tissues argues for neurotrophic roles as well.[154]

The Ephrin Family

Ligands, named ephrins, do not function as typical soluble ligands but as membrane-bound molecules. The ephrins are divided into two groups: ephrin-A subclass, which is anchored to the membrane by a glycosyl phosphatidylinositol (GPI) linkage, and ephrin-B, which possesses a transmembrane domain.[158] The EPH receptors are the largest subfamily of RTKs (Fig. 5-2). These genes encode proteins of ~130 to 135 kDa, classified into two groups (A and B) based on relatedness of their extracellular domain sequences. With few exceptions, ephrin-A binds to EPHA receptors, whereas ephrin-B binds to EPHB receptors.[158] Ephrins bind EPH on juxtaposed cell surfaces with nanomolar affinity, which then leads to the formation of a tetramer comprising two receptors and two ligands. These complexes can aggregate in larger clusters according to the density of Ephrin and EPH on the cell surfaces.[159] Activation by Ephrin induces EPH phosphorylation by the receptors themselves (transphosphorylation) or by other kinases such as those belonging to the SRC family.[159] It has been shown that the transmembrane ephrin-B molecules can signal bidirectionally following binding and activation of receptors in a neighboring cell.[160]

Although the EPH receptors and their ligands are differentially expressed, all members are expressed with a specific distribution in both the developing and adult nervous system, implicating a possible role in a variety of developmental processes. It is now clear that these receptors and their ligands mediate contact-dependent cell interactions. In particular, it has been shown that they play a role in the repulsion mechanisms that guide migrating cells and neuronal growth cones to their specific targets. This ligand–receptor system plays an important role in patterning of embryonic structure of the brain and somites. Repulsive interactions and complementary expression patterns have also been shown in the vasculature systems where EPH receptors are implicated in a demarcation between arterial and venous systems and vasculature remodeling.[158] Of note, it has been shown that ephrins can also modulate the balance between self-renewal and differentiation in different types of precursor and stem cells.[159]

Agrin Family

Agrin, named from the Greek word *agrein* (to aggregate), is a heparin sepharose proteoglycan that is capable of inducing aggregation of acetylcholine receptors (AchRs) in myotubes at the postsynaptic membrane.[161] Agrin is a component of the extracellular matrix that is also capable of inducing aggregation of several other synaptic proteins. MuSK (muscle-specific kinase) is a novel RTK characterized by an extracellular portion containing four immunoglobulin-like domains (Fig. 5-2). MuSK knockout mice have established its central role in AchR clustering. MuSK is crucial for Agrin signaling at the neuromuscular junction, but evidence indicates that Agrin does not directly bind MuSK. Indeed, a recent study showed that the LDL receptor-related protein 4 may be the long-sought and elusive receptor for Agrin, required for Agrin-induced phosphorylation of MuSK in the formation of neuromuscular synapses.[162]

GDNF Family

Glial cell line-derived neurotrophic factor (GDNF), neurturin (NRTN), artemin (ART), and persephin (PSP) are members of the GDNF family of neurotrophic factors that, based on their cysteine knot structure, represent a subgroup of the TGF-β protein superfamily.[163] GDNF was initially identified as a trophic factor for midbrain dopaminergic neurons. GDNF is the most potent survival factor for motor neurons yet identified and has received attention as a potential therapeutic agent for the treatment of neurodegenerative diseases.[164] GDNF also acts as a morphogen in kidney development. NRTN and ART have similar biologic properties to GDNF, whereas PSP is expressed at low levels in most tissues and is not a trophic factor for peripheral neurons.[163] GDNF acts through a receptor complex that consists of the *c-ret* proto-oncogene,[165] encoded RTK (Fig. 5-2) and a ligand-binding component, the GDNF family receptor α (GFRα). GFRα was identified by expression cloning as a novel GPI-linked protein.[166] The four GRFα receptors provide specificity for the ligand, with GDNF preferentially binding GRFα1, NRTN to GRFα2, ARTN to GRFα3, and PSPN to GRFα4. A dimeric GDNF family member first binds to GFRα, and this complex then interacts with RET to induce its dimerization and activation.[167,168]

The RET extracellular domain shows a unique feature, the presence of sequences similar to cadherin repeats. This motif is known to play an important role in Ca^{2+}-dependent homophilic binding in other proteins.[169] So far, only RET, among all RTKs, is known to contain this sequence (Fig. 5-2). RET is essential for the development of the sympathetic, parasympathetic, enteric nervous systems and the kidney.[169]

Angiopoietins

The TIE (tyrosine kinase with immunoglobulin and epidermal growth factor homology domains) family of RTKs includes two receptors that are exclusively expressed in endothelial cells[170] (Fig. 5-2). The angiopoietins were originally identified as ligands for Tie2: Ang1 and Ang2 are the best characterized, while Ang4 and its mouse ortholog Ang3 were identified later.[171] No specific ligand has been identified for Tie1, but it has been shown that at high concentrations Ang1 binds to Tie1 through integrins.[172] While Ang1 and Ang2 bind to the same region in the extracellular portion of Tie2, only Ang1 is capable of promoting Tie2 autophosphorylation. Tie2 activation by Ang1 is required to maintain the resting state of the endothelium, whereas Ang2 destabilizes the quiescent endothelium and primes the response to exogenous stimuli.[171] Ang1 or Tie2 knockout mice are embryonic lethal and show a similar phenotype, with severe vascular remodeling defects. Interestingly, Ang2 transgenics phenocopy Ang1- or Tie2-deficient mice, while inactivation of the Ang2 gene only induces a very mild phenotype.[172]

DDR Ligands

Discoidin domain receptors (DDRs) are now referred to as DDR1 and DDR2.[173] As shown in Figure 5-2, these receptors possess several features that are shared with the TRK family in their kinase domains. However, the extracellular domains contain a motif with homology to discoidin-1, a lectin found in *Dictyostelium discoideum*, where it is involved in cell aggregation.[174] These receptors are widely and differentially expressed during development and in adulthood.[173] A unique feature of DDR1 and DDR2 is the fact that both receptors have collagens as ligands. Whereas DDR1 activation is achieved by type I to type VI and type VIII collagens, DDR2 is only activated by fibrillar collagens.[173] Stimulation of DDR kinase activity requires the native triple-helical structure of collagen and occurs over an extended period of time. DDR1 null mice are viable but small and have mammary gland and kidney defects,[175,176] while the knockout of DDR2 leads to dwarfism and shortening of long bones.[177]

Other RTKs

The identification of new RTKs implies the existence of new growth factors as well. Several RTKs await the assignment of ligands. ROR1 and ROR2[178] were originally identified based on the similarity of their TK domains to the *trk* family of neurotrophin receptors (Fig. 5-2). Both are widely expressed and at high levels during early embryonic development. Dror, the corresponding gene in *Drosophila*,[179] is expressed specifically in the developing nervous system.[178] The ROR extracellular domains also show sequence similarity with the cysteine-rich domain of frizzled proteins, which act as Wnt receptors, and there is evidence that ROR2 is involved in non-canonical Wnt signaling.[180,181]

Ros is the cellular counterpart of *v-ros*, originally identified in the avian sarcoma virus UR2.[182] This RTK has an unusually large extracellular domain of nearly 2,000 amino acids, and is closely related to the product of the sevenless gene from *Drosophila*. Ros is expressed during mammalian embryonic development and persists in the male reproductive tract. Male mice homozygous for deletion of this gene are sterile.[183]

Leukocyte tyrosine kinase (LTK) is expressed in B-lymphocyte precursors, forebrain neurons in the mouse, as well as in placenta and hematopoietic cells in human.[184] A related gene identified as rearranged with the NPM nucleolar phosphoprotein gene in most anaplastic large cell non-Hodgkin lymphomas[185] is termed anaplastic lymphoma kinase (*ALK*). *Alk* is normally expressed in the small intestine, testis, and brain but not in normal lymphoid cells.[186] The *Drosophila* homolog of *Alk* is the receptor for the secreted molecule Jelly belly.[187] It has been suggested that ALK is the receptor for pleiotrophin family members,[188] but this idea is still controversial.

KLG (for kinase like gene) was isolated from a cDNA library prepared from embryonic chicken tissues using as a probe the *v-sea* oncogene.[189] KLG is a member of the immunoglobulin gene superfamily, with seven Ig-like loops in its extracellular domain (Fig. 5-2). Its human homolog, CCK-4/PTK7, was isolated from a colon carcinoma.[190] Recent studies indicate that this receptor is a regulator of planar cell polarity in vertebrates.[191] *RYK* (for related to tyrosine kinase)[192] is ubiquitously expressed and encodes a protein consisting of a WIF (Wnt inhibitory factor) containing extracellular domain.[193] The functional significance of KLG and Ryk is not known because efforts to demonstrate their tyrosine kinase activity have not as yet been successful. Both proteins contain several sequence substitutions in the conserved TK catalytic domain, similar to those present in the tyrosine kinase defective ErbB-3. Ryk has recently been implicated in Wnt signaling.[194,195]

Abnormalities Associated with Growth Factors in Cancer Cells

The role of growth factors in transformation was demonstrated by findings that the *v-sis* oncogene encoded a protein closely related to human PDGF-B.[1] MMTV induction of mammary carcinoma in mice correlated with integration of the provirus in the region of the *int-2* (FGF-3) gene. Moreover, the FGF-4 and FGF-5 genes were isolated by their ability to cause transformation of mouse fibroblasts in vitro.[21,97] The expression of any growth factor and its specific receptor by the same cell might establish an autocrine loop that contributes to tumor progression. Autocrine-transforming interactions have been identified in a number of human malignancies. At least one PDGF chain and one of its receptors have been detected in a high fraction of sarcomas and in glial-derived neoplasms.[196-198] In tissue culture, such tumor cells exhibit evidence of a functional autocrine loop, in which chronic PDGF receptor activation can be demonstrated by the detection of tyrosine phosphorylated receptors and/or down-regulation of the receptor protein. TGF-α is often detected in carcinomas that express high levels of EGF receptors.[199] Since many more ligands for tyrosine kinase receptors have recently been identified, the contribution of autocrine loops to human malignancies is probably much more extensive than is presently documented.

Growth factors also contribute to tumor progression by a paracrine mode. For example, continuous stimulation by growth factors in paracrine as well as autocrine modes during chronic tissue damage and repair associated with cirrhosis and inflammatory bowel disease may predispose to tumors.[200] Some tumor cells produce paracrine-acting angiogenic growth factors such as the VEGFs. Such growth factors cause the paracrine stimulation of endothelial cells inducing neoangiogenesis and lymphangiogenesis, which contribute to tumor progression.[201]

Aberrations Affecting Growth Factor Receptors in Tumor Cells

Although growth factor receptors can be constitutively activated by autocrine loops, a number of other mechanisms have been identified by which growth factor receptors can become transforming. The paradigm for such alterations is *v-erbB*, the oncogenic counterpart of the EGFR receptor, transduced as the viral oncogene of avian erythroblastosis virus.[2] The mechanism of *v-erbB* activation involved deletion of its ligand-binding domain, resulting in a truncated EGFR. More subtle mutational changes are responsible for oncogenic activation of *v-fms*, whose normal homolog is the CSF-1 receptor.[3] Here, a small genetic alteration affecting the external domain of the molecule was responsible for constitutive activation of this receptor as an oncogene.[202] *V-ros* and *V-kit* (see sections above) represent other examples.[53] Neu was initially identified as an oncogene by NIH/3T3 transfection analysis[203] of cDNA from ethylnitrosourea-induced rat neuroblastomas. The transforming gene was identified as having a specific mutation in its transmembrane domain responsible for oncogenic activation.[204]

Alterations affecting a large number of RTKs have been implicated in human malignancies as summarized in Table 5-1. One mechanism involves the amplification or overexpression of a normal receptor. As shown in Table 5-1 examples include the *EGFR*, *ErbB-2*, and *c-met* (see reviews[205,131]). *ErbB-2* was initially identified as an amplified gene in a primary human breast carcinoma and a salivary gland tumor. Moreover, ErbB-2 overexpression beyond some critical threshold level in NIH/3T3 fibroblasts was shown to be sufficient to induce the malignant phenotype. Clinical studies have indicated that the normal *ErbB-2* gene is frequently amplified and/or overexpressed in human breast carcinomas and in ovarian carcinomas, and detection in breast carcinomas of high ErbB-2 levels is a prognostic indicator of poor survival.[81,205]

Whereas ErbB-2 overexpression has been observed primarily in adenocarcinomas, overexpression of an apparently normal EGFR has been reported frequently in squamous cell carcinomas

Table 5-1 **Genetic Alterations of Growth Factor Signaling in Cancer**

Growth Factor Receptor	Oncogenic Activation Mechanism	Cancer
PDGFR (and)	Autocrine activation	Osteosarcoma, melanoma, glioblastoma
	Tel-PDGFR- t(5;12) translocation	Chronic myelomonocytic leukemia (CMML)
CSF-1R/fms	Extracellular domain mutations	AML, myelodysplastic syndrome (MDS)
CSFR/kit	Point mutations and deletions	AML, mastocytomas, gastrointestinal stromal tumors
Flk2/Flt3	Internal tandem duplication (juxtamembrane domain)	AML, MDS, PML
VEGFR1, -2, -3	Paracrine activation	Tumor angiogenesis and lymphangiogenesis
EGFR	Autocrine activation, amplification/overexpression (amplification)	Squamous cell carcinoma, glioblastoma, other cancers
	Extracellular domain deletions	Glioblastoma
ErbB-2	Amplification/overexpression, amplification	Breast and ovarian carcinoma
FGFR1	Chromosomal translocations (ZNF198-FGFR1, FOP-FGFR1, CEP110-FGFR1,BCR-FGFR1)	Myeloid malignancies
FGFR3	IGH/MMSET t(4;14)-FGFR3 translocation	Multiple myelomas
c-met	Gene rearrangement: Tpr-met t(1;7)	Gastric carcinomas
	Amplification/overexpression	Thyroid, ovarian and colorectal cancers
	Point mutations	Hereditary and sporadic papillary renal carcinoma
TrkA	Gene rearrangement: Tpm-TrkA t(1;1)	Papillary thyroid carcinoma
TrkC	Gene rearrangement: Tel-TRKC t(12;15)	Congenital fibrosarcoma, acute myeloid leukemia, human breast carcinoma
Ret	Gene rearrangements: Ret/PTC (at least 10 PTC loci)	Papillary thyroid carcinomas
	Germline point mutations	Men2A, Men2B, FMTC
Tie1, Tie2	Paracrine activation	Tumor angiogenesis and lymphangiogenesis
Alk	Gene rearrangement: NPM-Alk t(2;5)	Anaplastic large-cell lymphomas

Abbreviations: AML, acute myeloid leukemia; PML, promyelocytic leukemia; tpr, translocated promoter region.

and glioblastomas. In many cases, the EGFR appears to be activated by autocrine stimulation by one of its ligands, most commonly TGF-α. Genomic alterations such as mutation or rearrangement have also been shown to activate the transforming capacity of RTKs in human malignancies (Table 5-1). In some human tumors, deletions within the external domain of the EGFR receptor or mutations in its tyrosine kinase domain[206,207] are associated with its constitutive activation.[81] The *ret* gene is activated by rearrangement, as a somatic event, in about one-third of papillary thyroid carcinomas. Germ-line mutations affecting the cysteine residues in the extracellular region are responsible for multiple endocrine neoplasia (MEN) 2A and for the familial medullary thyroid (FMTC) carcinoma syndrome. In contrast, a substitution of methionine by threonine at codon 918 in the catalytic region of the tyrosine kinase has been reported in MEN 2B.[208] These mutations have been shown to up-regulate RET catalytic function, resulting in its genetic transmission as an oncogene.

MET is overexpressed and/or mutationally activated in a variety of human tumors. A direct role of MET in hereditary papillary renal carcinoma (HPRC) has also been established.[131] This hereditary disease is characterized by multiple, bilateral renal papillary tumors, in which mutations activate constitutive kinase activity and transforming properties. Somatic mutations in MET have also been detected in some sporadic renal papillary tumors.[131] Several other receptors including the PDGF-β, trkA, trkC, and Alk, have been shown to be oncogenically activated in human malignancies by gene rearrangements that lead to fusion products containing the activated TK domain.[53,209-211]

Signaling Pathways of Tyrosine Kinase Receptors

Molecules, known as adaptor and scaffolding proteins,[212] play an integral role in intracellular signaling both by recruiting various proteins to specific locations, and by assembling networks of proteins particular to RTK cascades. One such adaptor, Grb2, is important in the activation of the small G-protein Ras (Fig. 5-3). These adaptor proteins often contain a variety of motifs that mediate protein–protein interactions. Src homology 2 (SH2) domains are protein motifs that bind to specific phosphorylated tyrosine containing sequences, dictating particular binding partners. SH3 domains recognize and bind to proline-rich sequences in target proteins.[213] Thus, in the case of an adaptor protein such as Grb2, which contains both SH2 and SH3 sequences, an adaptor protein can bring a cytoplasmic protein via its SH3 domain to an activated RTK via an SH2 domain binding to phosphorylated tyrosine residues of the receptor.

Another form of adapter, a docking protein, provides multiple binding sites on which effector molecules can attach, thereby expanding the magnitude of

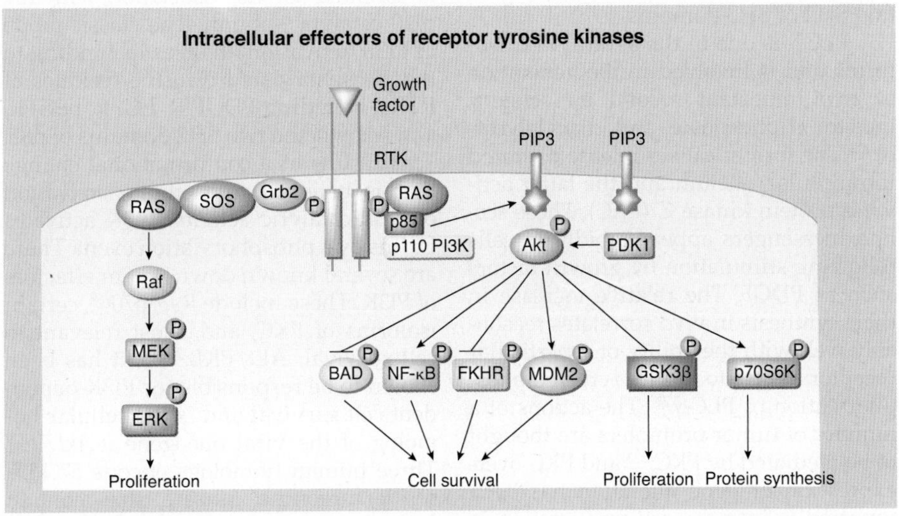

Figure 5-3 Intracellular effectors of receptor tyrosine kinases.

responses from an activated RTK. One such docking protein, IRS-1, is a substrate of the IR.[214] It contains tyrosine phosphorylation sites and two other important domains: a pleckstrin homology domain (PH) that binds to specific phosphoinositides and a phosphotyrosine-binding (PTB) domain that, like the SH2 domains, binds to phosphorylated tyrosine containing sequences. These two domains are believed to properly position IRS-1 adjacent to the receptor. Proteins that attach to the phosphorylated tyrosine residues phosphorylated in response to IR activation include PI3K, Shp-2, Nck, and Grb2.

Another concept that has surfaced in mammalian signaling is the importance of so-called scaffolding proteins in signaling cascades. Scaffolding proteins allow the formation of multienzyme complexes. The activation of a signaling cascade by a growth factor is an extremely rapid process and is not likely to occur as a result of two proteins randomly floating in the intracellular milieu. Scaffolding proteins ensure the close proximity of the necessary components. Moreover several enzymatic components of a particular signaling cascade may be shared, although the substrates of each may differ. Thus, scaffolding proteins ensure the proper routing of signals by preventing unwanted cross-talk between pathways.[212]

The PDGF system has served as the prototype for identification of the components of signaling cascades. Certain molecules become physically associated and/or phosphorylated by the activated PDGF receptor kinase. Those identified to date include phospholipase C (PLC)-γ,[215] phosphatidylinositol-3'-kinase (PI3K) regulatory subunit (p85),[216] NCK,[217] the phosphatase SHP-2,[218] Grb2,[219] CRK,[220] *RAS* p21 GTPase-activating protein (GAP),[221] *SRC*, and *SRC*-like tyrosine kinases.[222] Many of these molecules contain SH2 or SH3 domains.

PLC-γ is one of the several PLC isoforms and is involved in the generation of two important second messengers, inositol triphosphate and diacylglycerol.[223] The former causes release of stored intracellular calcium and the latter activates protein kinase C (PKC). These second messengers appear rapidly in cells following stimulation by growth factors such as PDGF. The relative increase in their synthesis in vivo correlates reasonably well with the ability of a particular receptor kinase to induce tyrosine phosphorylation of PLC-γ.[215] The actions of a number of tumor promoters are thought to be mediated by PKC,[223] and PKC overexpression or gene alteration has been reported to increase cell proliferation in culture.[224]

PI-3-Kinase and Survival Signaling

The regulation of cell survival and cell death is of extreme importance. During development, certain cells are eliminated by apoptosis (programmed cell death) and others permitted to survive. This is essential for organs and systems to form correctly. The deregulation of these processes can lead to a variety of malformations resulting in deformities or, in extreme cases, incapability with life. In adulthood, regulation of cell survival is equally important for proper homeostasis. Damaged cells must be removed and terminally differentiated cells must be sustained. A failure for this to occur may result in either the accumulation of mutations leading to cancer or, alternatively, to degenerative diseases.

PI3K is a lipid kinase that catalyzes the transfer of the γ-phosphate from ATP to the D3 position of the phosphoinositide (PtdIns) generating PtdIns3P, 4P2, and PtdIns3, 4, 5P3. These lipids can act in a variety of cascades, promoting the activation of several proteins[225] (Fig. 5-3). PI3K activation has been demonstrated to play an important role in cell survival signaling in a number of cell types.[226] There are three classes of PI3Ks, which exhibit variability with respect to their method of activation or their preferred lipid substrate.

The prototypical class 1 PI3K consists of two subunits encoded by two distinct loci: a regulatory and a catalytic subunit. The regulatory subunit is a 50-85 kDa protein that is tightly associated with the p110 catalytic subunit. The most well-studied regulatory subunit is p85. p85 has several characteristic protein domains, including two SH2 domains, which can bind to the phosphorylated tyrosines of several RTKs, thereby facilitating its activation,[226] an SH3 domain that binds to proline-rich regions of several proteins, and an inter-SH2 region that is essential for its association with the p110 catalytic subunit. The classic mode of PI3K activation involves its binding to the phosphorylated tyrosine residues of RTKs, including PDGF-R, EGFR, bFGFR, and trka via the two SH2 domains of p85. This results in a conformational change that is believed to facilitate activation of p110 catalytic activity. PI3K activates PtdIns by a phosphorylation event. There are several known downstream effectors of PI3K. These include Rac, $p70^{s6k}$, certain isoforms of PKC, and, most relevant to cell survival, Akt/PKB.[226] Akt has been shown to be responsible for PI3K-dependent cell survival and is the cellular homolog of the viral oncogene *v-Akt*.[226,227] Three human homologs encode 57 kDa serine/threonine kinases that contain an N-terminal PH domain, which binds to the activated PtdIns products of PI3K. These lipids are believed to mediate the localization of this cytoplasmic protein to the plasma membrane. In addition, phosphorylation of two residues, a serine and a threonine, is required for full activation. These phosphorylation events are catalyzed by two different kinases: one of which, PDK1 (PtdIns(3,4,5)P3 dependent kinase), specifically phosphorylates Thr308 and the other, PDK2, phosphorylates Ser473. The identity of PDK2 has been elusive for years, but recent studies have suggested that a complex of the mTOR (mammalian target of rapamycin) kinase and the adaptor rictor may be responsible for this critical phosphorylation of Akt.[226-229]

Akt promotes survival and prevents apoptosis in various cell types including cerebellar granule neurons, superior cervical neurons, myeloid cells, and myc-overexpressing fibroblasts. The mechanism of Akt-induced survival has begun to be understood. Akt phosphorylates the pro-apoptotic Bcl-2 (B-cell CLL/lymphoma 2) family member, BAD (Bcl2-associated agonist of cell death). When BAD is phosphorylated, it gains affinity for the cytosolic protein 14-3-3 and forms a complex with this protein. Nonphosphorylated BAD can heterodimerize with the antiapoptotic Bcl-2 family member $Bcl\text{-}X_L$. Upon phosphorylation of BAD, its binding to 14-3-3 decreases formation of the $BAD\text{-}Bcl\text{-}X_L$ heterodimer, thus permitting free $Bcl\text{-}X_L$ to protect the cell from apoptosis[226,227] (Fig. 5-3). However, the expression of BAD is not ubiquitous, and in certain cell types in which PI3K/Akt prevents apoptosis, BAD is not expressed. Akt also phosphorylates the Forkhead-related transcription factor (FKHR) creating a binding site for 14-3-3, which retains FKHR in the cytoplasm and inhibits its transcriptional gene targets including pro-apoptotic proteins such as BIM and FAS ligands. There is also evidence that Akt can indirectly increase the function of the NFkB transcription factor complex, which has pro-survival functions. Akt has been reported to activate IkB kinase (IKK), which induces degradation of the NFkB inhibitor, IkB. Studies indicate that Akt may increase p53 degradation through phosphorylation of MDM2.[226,227] Thus, Akt has multiple pro-survival functions. There is also evidence that activated Akt and/or PDK1 exert positive effects on cell growth through phosphorylation of proteins such as p70S6K, involved in protein synthesis, and inhibitory phosphorylation of GSK3, which normally targets cyclin D1 for degradation. Thus, the functions of PI-3-kinase are complex and extend beyond pro-survival functions in the coördinated responses of a cell to growth factor signaling (Fig. 5-3).[226,227]

PI-3-Kinase Signaling in Cancer

PIK3CA, which encodes the p110α catalytic subunit, was found to be amplified in a high percentage of ovarian tumors and ovarian tumor cell lines.[230] Recent studies have identified frequent mutations in the kinase and helical domains of PIK3CA, in particular in colon, breast, endometrial, brain, and gastric tumors.[231,232] There is also evidence of Akt involvement in human malignancies. Akt1 was found to be amplified 20-fold in a primary gastric adenocarcinoma.[233] Additional studies have shown genomic amplification and overexpression of Akt2 in pancreatic and ovarian carcinoma cell lines, as well as in some ovarian and breast carcinomas.[227] (Table 5-1). Overexpression of Akt2 occurs more frequently in undifferentiated and, thus, more aggressive tumors. Recently, a missense mutation in the PH domain of Akt1 was identified in breast, colon, and ovarian cancers, which results in prolonged Akt activation due to its pathological localization to the plasma membrane.[234]

Further evidence of the involvement of the PI3K/Akt pathway in cancer stems from the discovery of the PTEN (phosphatase and tensin homolog) tumor suppressor, a gene inactivated by mutation in a high fraction of glial and endometrial tumors as well as in melanoma, prostate, renal, and small cell lung carcinomas.[235] (Table 5-1). PTEN has high sequence homology to dual specificity phosphatases but its activity on artificial substrates is significantly weaker than other dual specificity phosphatases. However, PTEN was shown to dephosphorylate the third position of phosphatidylinositol both in vitro and in vivo. Thus, PTEN directly opposes PI3K activity by dephosphorylating its activated lipid products. Therefore, the tumor suppressor activity of PTEN is mediated via its ability to oppose both PI3K and Akt; both of which have been shown to be themselves oncogenic.[235]

Ras

Ras proteins are a major point of convergence in RTK signaling and are an important component of the cellular machinery necessary to transduce extracellular signals.[236] (Fig. 5-3). Ras small GTP-binding proteins are membrane-bound intracellular signaling molecules that mediate a wide variety of cellular functions including proliferation, differentiation, and survival. This family consists of ten highly conserved proteins including H-, N-, and K-Ras, R-Ras, Rap1(A and B), TC21 (R-Ras2), and R-RAS3.[236,237] Ras proteins are synthesized in the cytosol and become associated with the inner leaflet of the plasma membrane via posttranslational modifications, including a form of fatty acid lipidation, isoprenylation, on Cys-186. The C-terminal CAAX box (Cys, two aliphatic amino acids, followed by any residue) is an essential motif required for Ras function as it targets the unprocessed protein for this essential modification.[238] Ras acts as a molecular switch alternating from an inactive GDP-bound state to an active GTP-bound state. The paradigm for Ras activation involves the recruitment of a guanine nucleotide exchange factor (GNEF) to the membrane in response to growth factor binding and subsequent activation of a RTK.[236] GNEFs promote the release of GDP from the catalytic pocket of Ras, and the relative abundance of intracellular GTP as compared to GDP ensures preferential binding of GTP. The best example of a Ras GNEF is SOS (son of sevenless), which is brought to the membrane by its stable association with the adaptor protein Grb2.[239] Additional Ras GNEFs have been cloned and include GRF1 and 2 and Ras GRP. The exact specificity of their interactions with different Ras family members and the nature of the stimuli that activate these various exchange factors is presently under investigation.[240]

Although Ras is a GTPase, its intrinsic GTPase activity is actually quite low and requires additional proteins known as GTPase-activating proteins (GAPs) to promote GTP hydrolysis. GAPs can accelerate GTP hydrolysis by several orders of magnitude and are, thus, negative regulators of Ras functions.[241] The mechanism by which GAP accelerates the GTPase reaction is complex and not completely understood. Currently, several GAPs for Ras have been identified including p120 GAP, NF1-GAP/neurofibromin, and GAP1^m, as well as GAPs with preferential activity on related proteins such as R-Ras.[241] Of particular interest is NF1 as it is found to be frequently inactivated by mutation in patients with the familial tumor syndrome, neurofibromatosis type I.

Ras Function

Ras mediates important cellular processes such as proliferation, survival, and differentiation. The exact contribution of H-, N-, and K-Ras isoforms is not clear, as targeted knockouts to *H- and N-Ras* genes resulted in mice that did not exhibit an abnormal phenotype, whereas a *K-Ras* knockout is an embryonic lethal and exhibits liver and hematopoietic defects.[238] Therefore, there may be a certain degree of redundancy between these three Ras proteins.

Ras and Cancer

Ras is involved in a high fraction of human cancers (Table 5-1). Ras has been shown to be oncogenically activated by mutations in over 15% of all human tumors, and in some cancers such as pancreatic carcinoma the frequency is as high as 90%.[242] The initial evidence for Ras involvement in cancer came from the discovery of transforming retroviruses, Harvey and Kirsten sarcoma viruses, which contained *H- and K-ras* cellular-derived oncogenes. The first human oncogenes were identified by transfecting genomic DNA from human tumor cell lines into NIH3T3 mouse fibroblasts and isolating the DNA fragments from the transformed foci. These were shown to be the human homologs of the viral *ras* genes.[243]

The major hotspots for activating Ras mutations are all located near the bound nucleotide, particularly in proximity to the nucleotide phosphate groups. Naturally occurring mutations in human tumors have been found at residues 12, 13, 59, and 61, with positions 12 and 61 being the most common.[238,242] Most of these mutations decrease the intrinsic rate of GTP hydrolysis by Ras and make the molecule significantly less sensitive to GAP-stimulated GTP hydrolysis. Thus, the outcome is a predominantly GTP-bound form that is constitutively active and essentially independent of growth factor stimulation. Ras-transformed cells appear refractile and spindle-shaped, have disorganized actin filaments, and have a decreased affinity for the substratum. They can proliferate in the absence of adhesion (anchorage independence) or in the presence of low serum concentration. Of note, Ras alone is unable to transform primary mouse or human fibroblasts.[243] When oncogenic Ras is introduced into such cells by retroviral-mediated gene transfer, the cells undergo permanent growth arrest, also termed senescence, characteristic of primary cells passed for multiple generations in culture.[244] This senescence response appears to be dependent on the function of certain genes such as *p16*^{INK4a} and *p53*, which act as tumor suppressor genes. The inactivation of these tumor suppressor genes plays a critical role in cancer development. In fact, inactivation of *p53* or *p16*^{INK4a} allows Ras to transform cells, which may help to explain the selective pressure for loss of these tumor suppressor genes in tumors containing Ras oncogenic mutations.[244]

Additional members of the Ras family of GTP-binding proteins can cause cellular transformation when overexpressed in rodent fibroblasts. These include R-Ras,[245] TC21/R-Ras2,[246] and R-Ras3.[247] In fact, TC21 is mutated infrequently in cancers. The other transforming members have not been shown to be oncogenically activated in human tumors.

Signaling Downstream of Ras

Ras mediates its multitude of biologic effects via several downstream effectors. Several proteins have been shown to directly bind to Ras either in vivo or in vitro in a GTP-dependent manner by such methods as yeast two-hybrid or co-immunoprecipitation. These include A, B, and C-Raf, Ral GDS, RGL II, the PI3K, MEKK1, AF6, and PKCζ.[236] Whether they are all true physiologic effectors of Ras remains uncertain. It has been demonstrated that PI3K can be activated independently of RTKs by Ras, providing a direct connection between Ras and PI3K pro-survival signaling.[248]

Ras→Raf→MAPKinase Cascade

The most well-studied effector of Ras is the serine/threonine kinase Raf. Raf has been shown to bind to Ras and in many cases it has been demonstrated to be indispensable for Ras functions such as cellular transformation.[249] In fact, activated Raf or v-Raf, a truncated form of Raf, was initially isolated as a retroviral oncogene. There are three known mammalian Raf isoforms, designated A-, B-, and C-Raf (also known as Raf-1). C-Raf is ubiquitous in its tissue expression, whereas A-Raf and B-Raf expressions are more restricted. A-Raf is expressed mainly in steroid-responsive tissues, particularly in urogenital tissues, whereas B-Raf is restricted to neural-derived tissues.[250] The N terminus of the protein has a negative regulatory role in Raf activation while the C terminus contains the kinase domain. Ras-mediated activation of Raf requires its binding to the N terminus.

It is believed that interaction of Ras with Raf allows translocation of Raf to the membrane (Fig. 5-3), where additional steps leading to its full activation can occur.[236] Several phosphorylation events on both serine/threonine and tyrosine residues are believed to have a role in the full activation of Raf, and major differences in certain phosphorylation sites between B-Raf and C-Raf indicate that regulation of these two isoforms may differ significantly.[250]

Once activated, Raf can phosphorylate MEK (mitogen/extracellular-signal-regulated kinase kinase), also known as Map kinase kinase (MKK), a dual specificity kinase, on Ser_{218} and Ser_{222} leading to its activation[251] (Fig. 5-3). There are two isoforms of MEK, designated MEK1 and 2, both of which are expressed ubiquitously with an approximate sequence identity of 80%. MEK, once activated, can, in turn, activate MAP Kinase or extracellular signal-regulated kinase (ERK).[251] Activation occurs via tandem phosphorylations on both threonine and tyrosine (Thr_{183}-Glu-Tyr_{185}) with the phosphorylation on tyrosine occurring first. There are two ERK isoforms (1 and 2), ubiquitously expressed and with very similar sequence (90%). These proteins, 44 and 42 kDa, respectively, translocate to the nucleus where they can activate a variety of proteins through phosphorylation on serine or threonine. ERK can phosphorylate several of the members of the ETS family of transcription factors, explaining its ability to activate transcription of certain genes.[251] The ETS transcription factors are helix-turn-helix proteins. A member of this family, $p62^{TCF}$/Elk-1, in complex with the serum response factor (SRF), transactivates the serum response element (SRE), which can be found in several promoters, including that of *c-fos*. Phosphorylation of ElK-1 by ERK dramatically increases *c-fos* transcription. ERK can also activate a variety of protein kinases via phosphorylation. For example, p90 RSK is a serine/threonine kinase that has a role in protein translation and is a substrate for the ERKs.[251]

In addition to positive regulation of the MAP kinase pathway by phosphorylation, there are negative regulatory mechanisms that serve to attenuate activation of this cascade. A principal mode of this negative regulation is through a variety of phosphatases, a majority of which have a dual specificity, meaning that they can dephosphorylate both serine/threonine and tyrosine residues.[251] This is consistent with the knowledge that ERK must be phosphorylated on both threonine and tyrosine to achieve maximal activation. There are several known MAP kinase phosphatases that differ in terms of substrate specificity.

ERK activation can lead to increased DNA synthesis and cell proliferation. In fact, *cyclin D1* expression is induced by activated forms of Ras, Raf, and MEK.[252] Dominant negative mutants of members of this cascade can also block this induction in response to growth factor stimulation. Of particular interest is the fact that *cyclin D1* can be rearranged or amplified in human tumors and tumor cell lines (Table 5-1), thus implicating this G1 cyclin in human cancer.[253]

Raf and Cancer

Knowledge of the importance of RTK signal transduction in cancer has recently led to screening of tumor cell lines for mutations in these pathways. Davies et al.[254] identified B-raf mutations in around 66% of human melanoma cell lines and primary tumors (Table 5-1). Of note, the nucleotide changes observed were not consistent with mutations typically induced by UV. Lower frequencies of analogous mutations were observed in colon carcinoma and SCLC[254] (Table 5-1). These mutations were further shown to oncogenically activate B-raf as determined by NIH3T3 transfection analysis, although the transforming efficiency was significantly lower than observed with Ras. These findings increase the number of human tumors, which exhibit mutational activation of growth factor signal transduction pathways.[254]

Other MAP Kinases

In addition to the ERKs, there are other MAP kinases belonging to distinct MAPK cascades with both different upstream activators and downstream effectors. The c-Jun N-terminal kinase (JNK)/stress-activated protein kinase (SAPK) and p38 MAP kinase have been demonstrated to modulate cellular responses to a wide variety of extracellular stimuli including mitogens, inflammatory cytokines, and UV irradiation.[255] In contrast to its ability to activate the MAPK/ERK cascade, H-Ras only minimally perturbs JNK/SAPK. However, overexpression of the constitutively activated mutants of the small G-proteins, Rac and Cdc42, leads to the robust stimulation of JNK/SAPK activity.[255] The pathways leading to JNK activation mirror those seen for ERK. Thus, a variety of MKKs have been discovered that can phosphorylate the various JNK isoforms.[255]

As with the ERKs, the end result of JNK activation is the phosphorylation of certain transcription factors within their activation domains, increasing the transcriptional activity of promoters containing response elements for these factors. JNK can phosphorylate ATF2, ATFa, c-Jun, and Jun-d, as well as ElK-1 and SAP1.[255] Phosphorylation of c-Jun by JNK increases its half-life, preventing ubiquitin-mediated degradation of this shortly lived protein.[256] Evidence from experiments performed using knockout cells of an upstream activator of JNK (MKK4) have demonstrated that JNK plays a role in AP-1 transcription-dependent events in response to stress.[257]

MAP kinase cascades also activate transcription factors such as *c-fos* and *c-jun*. Of note, these genes were initially discovered as retroviral oncogenes in mice and chickens, respectively. The FBJ and FBR murine viruses contain the *fos* sequence under the viral LTR promoter and exhibit changes in regulatory phosphorylation sites that make them more active than the proto-oncogene.[258] ASV17 is a chicken retrovirus containing a Jun oncogene fused to the viral Gag sequence and has lost regulatory phosphorylation sites.[259] Overexpression of *c-fos* can cause cell transformation[260] as well. Fos and Jun together comprise the AP-1 transcription factor. This dimer, in response to UV irradiation, environmental stresses, and PKC activation, binds to AP-1 target sequences such as 12-*O*-tetradecanoylphorbol-13-acetate (TPA) responsive elements.[261]

Growth Factor Signaling and Cancer Therapy

Since many of the signaling pathways involved in cellular transformation by oncogenes have been elucidated, efforts are underway to develop treatment strategies that target these specific signaling molecules or their downstream effectors. One of the important advantages of rationally based targets is that reagents are generally available with which to monitor in vivo inhibition of the target molecule. This makes correlation of clinical response with pharmacodynamic analyses of target suppression feasible and should speed the process of clinical testing. Another advantage is that some of these agents appear to have less inherent toxicities than standard chemotherapeutic regimens. Such approaches rely on the concept of "oncogene addiction," which implies that tumor cells, despite their complex pattern of mutational events, can become particularly dependent on one or a few signaling pathways for their growth and/or survival. These pathways are thought to counterbalance other pro-apoptotic signals also triggered by the oncogenic alterations in the tumor (eg, c-myc overexpression is known to stimulate both proliferation and apoptosis): once the pro-survival signal is blocked, the tumor cell undergoes what has been defined as "oncogenic shock" and dies.[262,263] This idea is supported by studies with tumor cell lines[264] as well as in genetically modified mice, in which complete regression of tumors induced by oncogenes, such as *H-Ras, K-Ras, and c-myc*, was achieved by switching off the expression of that particular oncogene.[265] In some tumors, growth factor signaling may contribute to the progression to a more aggressive disease. In both cases, treatments targeting the aberrantly activated signaling pathway, either alone or in combination with traditional chemo- or radiation therapy, have yielded extraordinary results for certain types of malignancies. In many cases, however, additional genetic lesions, often activating the same signaling pathway, were shown to bypass the targeted oncogene, with important consequences for clinical treatment (see below).

Monoclonal Antibodies

One possible target for therapeutic intervention is the initial triggering of growth factor signaling at the surface of tumor cells. Monoclonal antibodies can be generated to specifically neutralize the activities of growth factors or interfere with ligand–receptor interactions. Monoclonal antibodies have also been applied to interfere with receptors overexpressed in certain types of cancer.[266] For example, administration of monoclonal ErbB-2 or EGFR receptor antibodies were shown to inhibit tumor cell growth.[267,268] Trastuzumab (herceptin, Genentech), a humanized monoclonal antibody against ErbB-2, became the first clinically approved drug targeting an oncogene product. Experimental evidence further indicated that trastuzumab enhances the responsiveness of ErbB-2 overexpressing breast cancer cells to taxanes, anthracyclines, and platinum compounds.[269] Moreover, a phase III trial indicating that trastuzumab added to first-line therapy for metastatic breast cancer provided a significant benefit with respect to survival[270] led to regulatory approval for its use with paclitaxel in first-line therapy. Trastuzumab clinical trials were the first to include patients with a genetic abnormality in their tumor cells (*ErbB-2* gene amplification) and to show that a targeted therapy might be effective as a single agent. A chimeric monoclonal (IMC-C225; cetuximab; erbitux, ImClone Systems) against the EGFR[271] has been approved for the treatment of colorectal and head and neck cancers in combination with chemotherapy and radiotherapy, respectively.[269,270,272] Of note, a recent study reported that cetuximab significantly increased the survival of colorectal cancer patients with wild-type K-Ras, but it had no effects in the presence of K-Ras mutations, accounting for 40% of the tumors.[273] This stresses the need to identify the particular genetic context of a given tumor for a successful therapeutic intervention, as is further discussed below for tyrosine kinase inhibitors.

Neoangiogenesis, which can be a limiting factor in tumor growth and, thus, play an important role in tumor progression, is another example of a tumor-related process successfully targeted by monoclonal antibodies. In fact, bevacizumab (avastin), developed by Genentech, is a humanized monoclonal antibody directed against VEGF approved for treatment of advanced colon carcinoma and NSCLC. Whether this monoclonal antibody acts by inhibiting tumor angiogenesis or by normalizing such vessels and actually improving access of traditional agents to the tumor is being evaluated, but there is little question that this approach can have therapeutic effects.[266] Targeting neoangiogenesis has the advantage that drug resistance is less likely to develop in normal endothelial cells than in the genetically unstable tumor cells. Moreover, the new therapy might be applicable to a wide range of tumors as well as complement-existing therapies. Other agents are under investigation with several directed against VEGF or its major receptor, VEGFR2.

Another strategy based on monoclonal antibodies or modified growth factors involves the delivery of cytotoxic agents, such as toxins or radioisotopes, to tumor cells that overexpress a particular RTK.[274] In addition to targeting an overexpressed receptor on which tumor proliferation is dependent, this approach could provide a means of targeting chemotherapeutic agents internalized by the receptor to sites within the tumor cell. As with other receptor targeting strategies, the efficacy of this approach would be expected to depend upon the differential magnitude of receptor expression by the tumor as opposed to normal cells, as well as accessibility of tumor cells to the systematic administration of such agents.[275]

Tyrosine Kinase Inhibitors

Increased understanding of the important role of growth factor signal transduction in cancer has also led to intensive efforts focused on the development of small molecule inhibitors of specific target molecules, including RTKs (Table 5-2). The most exciting progress to date has come from investigations of imatinib (Glivec, STI-571, Gleevec), a low-molecular-weight inhibitor of the non-RTK Abl, developed by Novartis. *Abl* is translocated in chronic myelogenous leukemia (CML) as part of the Philadelphia chromosome to create the *Bcr-Abl* oncogene.[276] Imatinib interacts with the ATP-binding pocket of the Abl kinase domain and stabilizes a catalytically inactive conformation of this oncogene product.[277,263,266] Clinical trials rapidly confirmed the efficacy of this compound in CML and, therefore, Bcr-Abl as a target in this disease. Remarkable responses were observed in the chronic phase of the disease with complete clearing of Ph+ cells from the circulation in 95% of patients, who had failed standard therapy. Only 9% of patients relapsed over a median follow-up of 18 months,[277] leading to regulatory approval. Imatinib is most effective in the chronic phase with fewer responses and more relapses with patients in myeloid blast crisis. Unfortunately, during the progression of the disease, cancer cells often develop resistance, either through mutations that interfere with the binding of imatinib to Abl or through amplification of the *Bcr-Abl* gene.[263,277] Imatinib was shown to inhibit other related tyrosine kinases, in particular Kit and PDGF-R, for which activating mutations have been identified in GIST. Remarkable clinical activity was observed in this chemotherapy-refractory tumor, leading to approval for use of imatinib in such patients.[278] The effectiveness of this drug in GIST depends on the location of the Kit and PDGF-R mutations. In particular, imatinib is efficacious against tumors harboring mutations in the juxtamembrane domain, but it is generally inactive when the mutations occur in the tyrosine kinase domain.[279] In fact, de novo mutations in the tyrosine kinase domain of Kit and PDGF-R are commonly found in GIST patients that have acquired resistance to imatinib treatment.[279] Other tumors with c-kit or PDGF-R activating mutations are currently being evaluated for treatment efficacy by imatinib.[277,266,279]

Another tyrosine kinase receptor successfully targeted by small molecule inhibitors is the EGFR. Gefitinib (Iressa) and erlotinib (Tarceva), developed by AstraZeneca and OSI/Genentech, are reversible competitive inhibitors of ATP binding by the EGFR kinase and have been approved for patients with advanced NSCLC having failed conventional chemotherapy. The first clinical trials showed that only a relatively small fraction of NSCLC patients responded to these drugs. Later studies revealed that sensitivity to these inhibitors correlates with activating mutations in the EGFR kinase domain, present in ~10% of NSCLC patients, usually non-smokers, and more frequent in women and in individuals of Asian descent.[280] Despite the initial remission, NSCLCs responsive to gefitinib or erlotinib invariably develop resistance. In 50% of the cases, an additional mutation in EGFR (T790M) causes a weaker interaction of the inhibitors with the kinase.[280] Of note, mutations in analogous positions of Abl, Kit, and PDGF-R confer resistance to imatinib: these events affecting the conserved threonine residue near the catalytic site are referred to as gatekeeper mutations, because they cause a steric hindrance that interferes with the binding of the inhibitor.[281] Second generation tyrosine kinase inhibitors that irreversibly compete for the ATP binding to EGFR and whose activity is not affected by the T790M mutation[281,282] are being preclinically and clinically tested. Another mechanism of resistance to gefitinib and erlotinib has recently been identified and involves amplification of the MET receptor, resulting in the activation of ErbB-3 and bypass of the EGFR.[283] These results underline the potential interest of a therapeutic strategy that simultaneously targets different components of a signaling pathway. In this respect, lapatinib (Tykerb), developed by GlaxoSmithKline, is the first dual inhibitor of EGFR and ErbB-2, approved in 2007 for use in combination with capecitabine for advanced and metastatic breast cancer.[284] Other more promiscuous small molecule inhibitors that target different tyrosine kinases involved in both tumorigenesis and angiogenesis, such as sorafenib (Nexavar, Bayer) and sunitinib (Sutent, Pfizer), have been recently approved for the treatment of certain cancers, including advanced renal cell carcinoma, hepatocellular carcinoma, and imatinib-refractory GIST.[279,285] The promising results obtained with the aforementioned tyrosine kinase inhibitors are stimulating the development of new small molecule inhibitors, targeting either specific growth factor receptors, such as EGFR, MET, and IGF-R, as well as multiple kinases.[117,282,283,286,287]

Inhibition of Growth Factor Downstream Signaling

Downstream components of growth factor signaling pathways activated in cancer cells are also potential therapeutic targets. There has been extensive preclinical and clinical evaluation of inhibitors of activated Ras. Most approaches have focused on efforts to inhibit Ras membrane localization required for its function by interfering with the farnesylation or geranylation steps. To date, clinical trials have involved farynesyl transferase inhibitors. Unfortunately, most of these agents have shown unacceptable toxicities, limiting enthusiasm for this class of agents. However, most of these agents are not specific for Ras farnesylation, and the prenylation pathway through geranylgeranyl transferase is a known alternative pathway for K- and N-Ras membrane targeting. Thus, whether agents, which target Ras through this alternative pathway, will lead to new anticancer agents remains to be resolved.[288,289]

Raf and MEK have also emerged as key targets for anticancer drug design based on the fact that a broad array of solid tumors utilize this important pathway. The development of agents has largely focused on the design of small molecule inhibitors of enzyme function. The multi-kinase inhibitor sorafenib, which also targets Raf ATP-binding sites, was shown to have antitumor activity in xenograft models of colon, pancreatic, and ovarian cancers[290] and was approved in 2005 for treatment of advanced renal carcinoma.[289] This is an area of increased emphasis with the recent discovery that B-Raf oncogenic mutations commonly occur in melanoma, colon, and NSLCs.[290] Since the Ras/Raf/MAPK pathway has pleiotropic effects on proliferation, motility, and cell survival, inhibitors of this pathway might be expected to exert multiple adverse effects on tumor cells. An orally active MEK inhibitor, PD184352, has been reported to be active in preclinical *in vivo* tumor growth models,[291] but it failed phase II trials in patients with breast, colorectal, and pancreatic cancers.[289] A derivative of PD184352 developed by Pfizer, PD0325901, has shown better results and it is currently being tested in clinical trials.[232,289] Other MEK inhibitors, such as AZD6244 (Array BioPharma), XL518 (Exelixis), and RDEA119 (Ardea Biosciences), are also being evaluated for their potential use in the treatment of malignancies with activation of this pathway.[232] Another obvious candidate as a therapeutic target is the PI3K-Akt pathway, in efforts to inhibit its antiapoptotic functions. Several small molecules targeting PI3K have been developed, including isoform-specific or pan-PI3K inhibitors. All of these compounds compete for the ATP binding in the catalytic pocket of PI3K, and some have moved from the preclinical phase to phase I trials in patients.[232] Of note, a recent study in a mouse model of K-Ras-induced lung cancer has shown that the PI3K-mTOR and MEK inhibitors NVP-BEZ235 and ARRY-142886 were ineffective when used alone, but they synergized to significantly reduce the size of tumors,[292] indicating that combinations of drugs targeting different downstream branches of a pathway may increase their therapeutic potential.

Growth Factors to Alleviate the Secondary Effects of Cancer Therapy

While attacking growth factor signal transduction is becoming an increasing focus of cancer drug development, growth factors, themselves, have also been applied clinically in efforts to ameliorate the toxicities of conventional therapies to rapidly proliferating normal tissues. For example, Amgen has successfully developed erythropoietin and G-CSF, which specifically stimulate erythrocyte and granulocyte production, as the drugs, Epogen and Neupogen, respectively. Moreover, second generation versions of each that require less frequent administration have been developed and approved for clinical use. Toxicity to the normal gastrointestinal tract is a complication of a number of cancer therapies. Oral mucositis associated with increased need for pain medication and parenteral nutrition can be debilitating to patients as can bowel irritation associated with bleeding or diarrhea. As discussed earlier, FGF-7 (KGF) is a growth factor that acts specifically on epithelial cells. Amgen has developed KGF as a drug, Kepivance/Palifermin, approved for clinical use in ameliorating oral mucositis associated with bone marrow transplantation for hematopoietic tumors.[293] Conceivably, the ability to protect normal rapidly proliferating cells of the bone marrow and gastrointestinal tract from the toxicities of certain cancer therapies may allow the use of more intensive treatment with greater likelihood of cure.

The recent advances in targeting specific growth factor signaling aberrations in human cancer cells argue strongly that the knowledge that has been gained concerning the important role of growth factor signal transduction in cancer is leading to a promising new era in cancer therapeutics. Increasing understanding of the molecular basis for the selectivity of the successful targeted drugs, as well as the mechanisms of acquired resistance to these therapies, strongly suggests that, in the future, treatments will likely involve a combination of targeted agents tailored to the specific genetic alterations of a given tumor. In this respect, recent and astonishing technical advances, potentially allowing a better genetic classification of tumors, such as the isolation of single circulating cancer cells for the analysis of mutations in a particular gene,[294] or, longer term, the whole genome sequencing of a tumor,[295] open new perspectives that were unimaginable until now.

Selected References

The complete reference list can be found at www.CANCERMEDICINE8.com

1. Doolittle RF, Hunkapiller MW, Hood LE, et al. Simian sarcoma virus onc gene, v-sis, is derived from the gene (or genes) encoding a platelet-derived growth factor. *Science.* 1983;221:275–277.
2. Downward J, Yarden Y, Mayes E, et al. Close similarity of epidermal growth factor receptor and v-erb-B oncogene protein sequences. *Nature.* 1984;307:521–527.
3. Sherr CJ, Rettenmier CW, Sacca R, Roussel MF, Look AT, Stanley ER. The c-fms proto-oncogene product is related to the receptor for the mononuclear phagocyte growth factor, CSF-1. *Cell.* 1985;41:665–676.
4. Levi-Montalcini R. The nerve growth factor 35 years later. *Science.* 1987;237:1154–1162.
5. Cohen S. Nobel lecture. Epidermal growth factor. *Biosci Rep.* 1986;6:1017–1028.
6. Brugge JS, Erikson RL. Identification of a transformation-specific antigen induced by an avian sarcoma virus. *Nature.* 1977;269:346–348.
7. Levinson AD, Oppermann H, Levintow L, Varmus HE, Bishop JM. Evidence that the transforming gene of avian sarcoma virus encodes a protein kinase associated with a phosphoprotein. *Cell.* 1978;15:561–572.
14. Aaronson SA. Growth factors and cancer. *Science.* 1991;254:1146–1153.
15. Blume-Jensen P, Hunter T. Oncogenic kinase signalling. *Nature.* 2001;411, 355–365.
16. Schlessinger J. Cell signaling by receptor tyrosine kinases. *Cell.* 2000;103:211–225.
21. Wilkie AO, Patey SJ, Kan SH, van den Ouweland AM, Hamel BC. FGFs, their receptors, and human limb malformations: clinical and molecular correlations. *Am J Med Genet.* 2002;112:266–278.
39. Hoch RV, Soriano P. Roles of PDGF in animal development. *Development.* 2003;130:4769–4784.
50. Heinrich MC, Corless CL, Duensing A, et al. PDGFRA activating mutations in gastrointestinal stromal tumors. *Science.* 2003;299:708–710.
53. Scheijen B, Griffin JD. Tyrosine kinase oncogenes in normal hematopoiesis and hematological disease. *Oncogene.* 2002;21:3314–3333.
61. Holmes DI, Zachary I. The vascular endothelial growth factor (VEGF) family: angiogenic factors in health and disease. *Genome Biol.* 2005;6:209.
65. Otrock ZK, Makarem JA, Shamseddine AI. Vascular endothelial growth factor family of ligands and receptors: review. *Blood Cells Mol Dis.* 2007;38:258–268.
81. Yarden Y. The EGFR family and its ligands in human cancer. signalling mechanisms and therapeutic opportunities. *Eur J Cancer.* 2001;37(suppl 4), S3–8.
94. Stove C, Bracke M. Roles for neuregulins in human cancer. *Clin Exp Metastasis.* 2004;21:665–684.
97. Powers CJ, McLeskey SW, Wellstein A. Fibroblast growth factors, their receptors and signaling. *Endocr Relat Cancer.* 2000;7:165–197.
110. Thisse B, Thisse C. Functions and regulations of fibroblast growth factor signaling during embryonic development. *Dev Biol.* 2005;287:390–402.
117. Pollak M. Insulin and insulin-like growth factor signalling in neoplasia. *Nat Rev Cancer.* 2008;8:915–928.
124. Nakamura T, Nishizawa T, Hagiya M, et al. Molecular cloning and expression of human hepatocyte growth factor. *Nature.* 1989;342:440–443.
127. Boccaccio C, Comoglio PM. Invasive growth: a MET-driven genetic programme for cancer and stem cells. *Nat Rev Cancer.* 2006;6:637–645.
137. Snider WD. Functions of the neurotrophins during nervous system development: what the knockouts are teaching us. *Cell.* 1994;77:627–638.
138. Lu B, Pang PT, Woo NH. The yin and yang of neurotrophin action. *Nat Rev Neurosci.* 2005;6:603–614.
146. Klein R, Jing SQ, Nanduri V, O'Rourke E, Barbacid M. The trk proto-oncogene encodes a receptor for nerve growth factor. *Cell.* 1991;65:189–197.
147. Huang EJ, Reichardt LF. Trk receptors: roles in neuronal signal transduction. *Annu Rev Biochem.* 2003;72:609–642.
152. Lemke G, Lu Q. Macrophage regulation by Tyro 3 family receptors. *Curr Opin Immunol.* 2003;15:31–36.
159. Pasquale EB. Eph receptor signalling casts a wide net on cell behaviour. *Nat Rev Mol Cell Biol.* 2005;6:462–475.
161. Bezakova G, Ruegg MA. New insights into the roles of agrin. *Nat Rev Mol Cell Biol.* 2003;4:295–308.
163. Airaksinen MS, Saarma M. The GDNF family: signalling, biological functions and therapeutic value. *Nat Rev Neurosci.* 2002;3:383–394.
172. Fiedler U, Augustin HG. Angiopoietins: a link between angiogenesis and inflammation. *Trends Immunol.* 2006;27:552–558.
173. Vogel W. Discoidin domain receptors: structural relations and functional implications. *FASEB J.* 1999;13(suppl):S77–82.
181. Green JL, Kuntz SG, Sternberg PW. Ror receptor tyrosine kinases: orphans no more. *Trends Cell Biol.* 2008;18:536–544.
205. Roskoski R, Jr. The ErbB/HER receptor protein-tyrosine kinases and cancer. *Biochem Biophys Res Commun.* 2004;319:1–11.
212. Pawson T, Scott JD. Signaling through scaffold, anchoring, and adaptor proteins. *Science.* 1997;278:2075–2080.
223. Berridge MJ, Irvine RF. Inositol phosphates and cell signalling. *Nature.* 1989;341:197–205.
226. Cantley LC. The phosphoinositide 3-kinase pathway. *Science.* 2002;296:1655–1657.
232. Yuan TL, Cantley LC. PI3K pathway alterations in cancer: variations on a theme. *Oncogene.* 2008;27:5497–5510.
238. Santos E, Nebreda AR. Structural and functional properties of ras proteins. *FASEB J.* 1989;3:2151–2163.
243. Barbacid M. ras genes. *Annu Rev Biochem.* 1987;56:779–827.
250. Wellbrock C, Karasarides M, Marais R. The RAF proteins take centre stage. *Nat Rev Mol Cell Biol.* 2004;5:875–885.
251. Lewis TS, Shapiro PS, Ahn NG. Signal transduction through MAP kinase cascades. *Adv Cancer Res.* 1998;74:49–139.
255. Davis RJ. Signal transduction by the JNK group of MAP kinases. *Cell.* 2000;103:239–252.
263. Weinberg RA. The biology of cancer. *Garland Science.* 2006. "the rational treatment of cancer', p725-796
270. Slamon DJ, Leyland-Jones B, Shak S, et al. Use of chemotherapy plus a monoclonal antibody against HER2 for metastatic breast cancer that overexpresses HER2. *N Engl J Med.* 2001;344:783–792.
277. Druker BJ. Perspectives on the development of a molecularly targeted agent. *Cancer Cell.* 2002;1:31–36.
280. Sharma SV, Bell DW, Settleman J, Haber DA. Epidermal growth factor receptor mutations in lung cancer. *Nat Rev Cancer.* 2007;7:169–181.
283. Engelman JA, Zejnullahu K, Mitsudomi T, et al. MET amplification leads to gefitinib resistance in lung cancer by activating ERBB3 signaling. *Science.* 2007;316:1039–1043.
291. Sebolt-Leopold JS, Herrera R. Targeting the mitogen-activated protein kinase cascade to treat cancer. *Nat Rev Cancer.* 2004;4:937–947.

6 Oncogenes

Marco A. Pierotti, PhD ■ Milo Frattini, PhD ■ Gabriella Sozzi, PhD ■ Carlo M. Croce, MD

Since the early proposals of Boveri more than a century ago, multiple experimental evidences have confirmed that at the molecular level, cancer is due to lesions in the cellular DNA. First, it has been observed that a cancer cell transmits to its daughter cells the phenotypic features characterizing the "cancerous" state. Second, most of the recognized mutagenic compounds are also carcinogenic, having as a target cellular DNA. Finally, the karyotyping of several types of human tumors, particularly those belonging to the hematopoietic system, led to the identification of recurrent qualitative and numerical chromosomal aberrations, reflecting pathologic rearrangements of the cellular genome. Taken together, these observations suggest that the molecular pathogenesis of human cancer is due to structural and/or functional alterations of specific genes whose normal function is to control cellular growth and differentiation or, in different terms, cell birth and cell death.[1,2]

The identification and characterization of the genetic elements playing a role in the scenario of human cancer pathogenesis have been made possible by the development of DNA recombinant techniques during the last two decades. One milestone was the use of the DNA transfection technique that helped clarify the cellular origin of the "viral oncogenes." The latter were previously characterized as the specific genetic elements capable of conferring the tumorigenic properties to the RNA tumor viruses also known as retroviruses.[3,4] Further, the transfection technique led to the identification of cellular transforming genes that do not have a viral counterpart. Besides the source of their original identification, viral or cellular genome, these transforming genetic elements have been designated as proto-oncogene in their normal physiologic version and oncogene when altered in cancer.[5,6] A second relevant experimental approach has regarded the identification and characterization of clonal and recurrent cytogenetic abnormalities in cancer cells, especially those derived from the hematopoietic system. Several oncogenes have been thus defined by molecular cloning of the chromosomal breakpoints including translocations, inversions, etc. Additional oncogenes have been identified through the analysis of chromosomal regions anomalously stained (homogeneously staining regions [HSR]), representing gene amplification. Finally, the detection of chromosome deletions has been instrumental in the process of identification and cloning of a second class of cancer-associated genes, the tumor suppressors. Contrary to the oncogenes that are activated by dominant mutations and whose activity is to promote cell growth, tumor suppressors act in the normal cell as negative controllers of cell growth and are inactive in tumor cells. In general, therefore, the mutations inactivating tumor suppressor genes are of the recessive type. More recently, using the high-throughput technologies, several genes have been demonstrated to be altered (mainly due to hyperactivating mutations) in human cancers. One of these, *BRAF*, represents the most relevant gene in melanoma development.[7] In the last subgroup, we can also number those obtained by the analysis of the protein kinases (kinome)[8] or phosphatases (phosphatome)[9] of the human genome or of several isoforms of a relevant protein involved in cancer development such as PI3K.[10]

Furthermore, a third class of cancer-associated genes has been defined thanks to the analysis of tumors of a particular type, that is, tumors in which an inherited mutated predisposing gene plays a significant role. These tumors include cancers in patients suffering from hereditary nonpolyposis colorectal cancer (HNPCC) syndromes.[11]

The genes implicated in these tumors have been defined as mutator genes or genes involved in the DNA-mismatch repair process. Although not directly involved in the carcinogenesis process, these genes, when inactivated, expose the cells to a very high mutagenic load that eventually may involve the activation of oncogenes and the inactivation of tumor suppressors.[12]

In this chapter, the methods by which oncogenes were discovered will be first described. The various functions of cellular proto-oncogenes will then be presented, and the genetic mechanisms of proto-oncogene activation will be summarized. Then, the role of specific oncogenes in the initiation and progression of human tumors will be discussed. Finally, the discovery that oncogenes may represent relevant target for new drugs will be described.

Discovery and Identification of Oncogenes

The first oncogenes were discovered through the study of *retroviruses*, RNA tumor viruses whose genomes are reverse-transcribed into DNA in infected animal cells.[13] During the course of infection, retroviral DNA is inserted into the chromosomes of host cells. The integrated retroviral DNA, called the provirus, replicates along with the cellular DNA of the host.[14] Transcription of the DNA provirus leads to the production of viral progeny that bud through the host cell membrane to infect other cells. Two categories of retroviruses are classified by their time course of tumor formation in experimental animals. Acutely transforming retroviruses can rapidly cause tumors within days after injection. These retroviruses can also transform cell cultures to the neoplastic phenotype. Chronic or weakly oncogenic retroviruses can cause tissue-specific tumors in susceptible strains of experimental animals after a latency period of many months. Although weakly oncogenic retroviruses can replicate in vitro, these viruses do not transform cells in culture.

Retroviral oncogenes are altered versions of host cellular proto-oncogenes that have been incorporated into the retroviral genome by recombination with host DNA, a process known as retroviral *transduction*.[15] This surprising discovery was made through study of the Rous sarcoma virus (RSV) (Fig. 6-1). RSV is an acutely transforming retrovirus first isolated from a chicken sarcoma over 80 years ago by Payton Rous.[16] Studies of RSV mutants in the early 1970s revealed that the transforming gene of RSV was not required for viral replication.[17-19] Molecular hybridization studies then showed that the RSV transforming gene (designated v-*src*) was homologous to a host cellular gene (c-*src*) that was widely conserved in eukaryotic species.[20] Studies of many other acutely transforming retroviruses from fowl, rodent, feline, and nonhuman primate species have led to the discovery of dozens of different retroviral oncogenes (see the discussions below and also Table 6-1). In every case, these retroviral oncogenes are derived from normal cellular genes captured from the genome of the host. Viral oncogenes

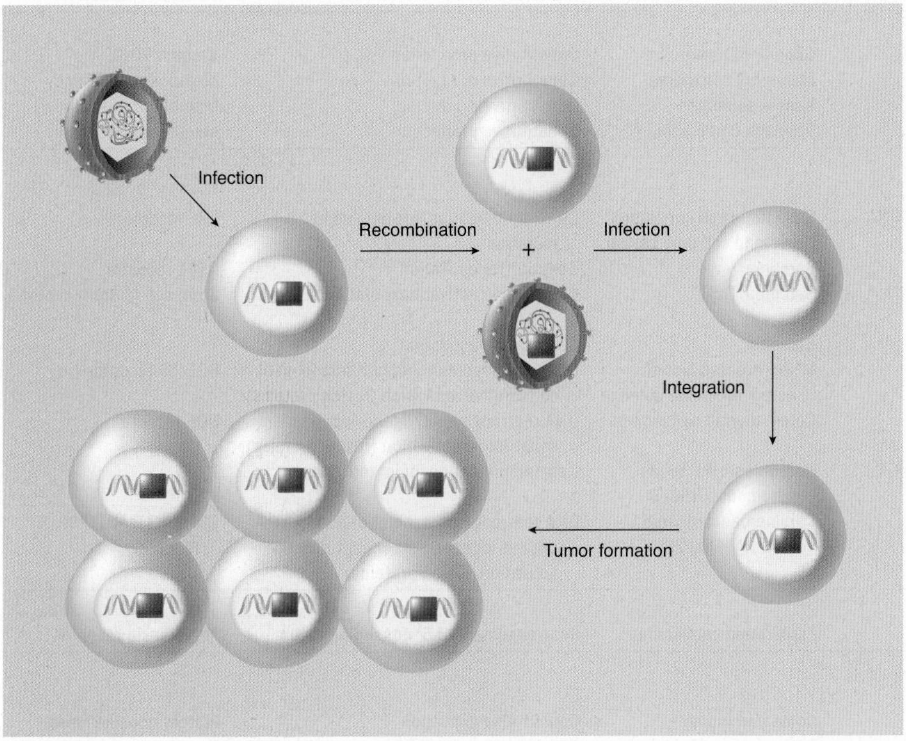

Figure 6-1 ■ Retroviral transduction. An RNA tumor virus infects a human cell carrying an activated *src* gene (red box). After the process of recombination between retroviral genome and host DNA, the oncogene *c-src** is incorporated into the retroviral genome and is re-named *v-src*. When the retrovirus carrying *v-src* infects a human cell, the viral oncogeneis rapidly transcribes and is responsible for the rapid tumor formation.

are responsible for the rapid tumor formation and efficient in vitro transformation activity characteristic of acutely transforming retroviruses.

In contrast to acutely transforming retroviruses, weakly oncogenic retroviruses do not carry viral oncogenes. These retroviruses, which include mouse mammary tumor virus (MMTV) and various animal leukemia viruses, induce tumors by a process called *insertional mutagenesis* (Fig. 6-2).[12] This process results from integration of the DNA provirus into the host genome in infected cells. In rare cells, the provirus inserts near a proto-oncogene. Expression of the proto-oncogene is then abnormally driven by the transcriptional regulatory elements contained within the long terminal repeats of the provirus.[21,22] In these cases, proviral integration represents a mutagenic event that activates a proto-oncogene. Activation of the proto-oncogene then results in transformation of the cell, which can grow clonally into a tumor. The long latent period of tumor formation of weakly oncogenic retroviruses is therefore due to the rarity of the provirus insertional event that leads to tumor development from a single transformed cell. Insertional mutagenesis by weakly oncogenic retroviruses, first demonstrated in bursal lymphomas of chickens, frequently involves the same oncogenes (such as *myc*, *myb*, and *erb B*) that are carried by acutely transforming retroviruses.[23-25] In many cases, however, insertional mutagenesis has been used as a tool to identify new oncogenes, including *int-1*, *int-2*, *pim-1*, and *lck*.[26]

The demonstration of activated proto-oncogenes in human tumors was first shown by the DNA mediated transformation technique.[27,28] This technique, also called *gene-transfer* or *transfection* assay, verifies the ability of donor DNA from a tumor to transform a recipient strain of rodent cells called NIH 3T3, an immortalized mouse cell line 29 (Fig. 6-3).[30] This sensitive assay, which can detect the presence of single-copy oncogenes in a tumor sample, also enables the isolation of the transforming oncogene by molecular cloning techniques. After serial growth of the transformed NIH 3T3 cells, the human tumor oncogene can be cloned by its association with human repetitive DNA sequences. The first human oncogene isolated by the gene-transfer technique was derived from a bladder carcinoma.[31,32] Overall, approximately 20% of individual human tumors have been shown to induce transformation of NIH 3T3 cells in gene-transfer assays. The value of transfection assay was recently reinforced by the laboratory of Robert Weinberg, which showed that the ectopic expression of the telomerase catalytic subunit (hTERT), in combination with the simian virus 40 large T product and a mutated oncogenic H-ras protein, resulted in the direct tumorigenic conversion of normal human epithelial and fibroblast cells.[33] Many of the oncogenes identified by gene- transfer studies are identical or closely related to those oncogenes transduced by retroviruses. Most prominent among these are members of the ras family that have been repeatedly isolated from various human tumors by gene transfer.[34,35] A number of new oncogenes (such as *neu*, *met*, and *trk*) have also been identified by the gene-transfer technique.[36,37] In many cases, however, oncogenes identified by gene transfer were shown to be activated by rearrangement during the experimental procedure and are not activated in the human tumors that served as the source of the donor DNA,[38] as in the case of *ret* that was subsequently found genuinely rearranged and activated in papillary thyroid carcinomas.[39,40]

Chromosomal translocations have served as guideposts for the discovery of many new oncogenes.[41,42] Consistently recurring karyotypic abnormalities are found in many hematological and solid tumors. These abnormalities include chromosomal rearrangements as well as the gain or loss of whole chromosomes or chromosome segments. The first consistent karyotypic abnormality identified in a human neoplasm was a characteristic small chromosome in the cells of patients with chronic myelogenous leukemia (CML).[43] Later identified as a derivative of chromosome 22, this abnormality was designated the Philadelphia chromosome, after its city of discovery. The application of chromosome banding techniques in the early 1970s enabled the precise cytogenetic characterization of many chromosomal translocations in human leukemia, lymphoma, and solid tumors.[44] The subsequent development of molecular cloning techniques then enabled the identification of proto-oncogenes at or near chromosomal breakpoints in various neoplasms. Some of these proto-oncogenes, such as *myc* and *abl*, had been previously identified as retroviral oncogenes. In general, however, the cloning of chromosomal breakpoints has served as a rich source of discovery of new oncogenes involved in human cancer. More recently, the use of high-throughput sequencing technologies and bioinformatics from the Human Genome Project led to the discovery of new genes involved in cancer development, such as *BRAF* and *PI3K*.[7,10]

Oncogenes, Proto-oncogenes, and Their Functions

Proto-oncogenes encode proteins that are involved in the control of cell growth. Alteration of the structure and/or ex-

Table 6-1 ■ **Oncogenes**

Oncogene	Chromosome	Identification Method	Neoplasm	Mechanism of Activation	Protein Function
Growth factors					
v-sis	22q12.3-13.1	Sequence homology	Glioma/fibrosarcoma	Constitutive production	B-chain PDGF
int2	11q13	Proviral insertion	Mammary carcinoma	Constitutive production	Member of FGF family
KS3	11q13.3	DNA transfection	Kaposi sarcoma	Constitutive production	Member of FGF family
HST	11q13.3	DNA transfection	Stomach carcinoma	Constitutive production	Member of FGF family
Growth factor receptors					
Tyrosine kinases: integral membrane proteins					
EGFR	7p1.1-1.3	DNA amplification/DNA sequencing	Squamous cell carcinoma Non-small cell lung cancer	Gene amplification/protein/point mutation	EGF receptor
v-fms	5q33-34 (FMS)	Viral homologue	Sarcoma	Constitutive activation	CSF1 receptor
v-kit	4q11-21 (KIT)	Viral homologue/DNA sequencing	Sarcoma/GIST	Constitutive activation/point mutation	Stem cell factor receptor
v-ros	6q22(ROS)	Viral homologue	Sarcoma	Constitutive activation	?
MET	7p31	DNA transfection	MNNG-treated human osteocarcinoma cell line	DNA rearrangement/ligand-independent constitutive activation (fusion proteins)	HGF/SF receptor
TRK	1q32-41	DNA transfection	Colon/thyroid carcinomas	DNA rearrangement/ligand-independent constitutive activation (fusion proteins)	NGF receptor
NEU	17q11.2-12	Point mutation/DNA amplification	Neuroblastoma/breast carcinoma/NSCLC	Gene amplification/point mutation	?
RET	10q11.2	DNA transfection	Carcinomas of thyroid Men 2A/Men 2B	DNA rearrangement/point mutation (ligand-independent constitutive activation/fusion proteins)	GDNF/NTT/ART/PSP receptor
Receptors lacking protein kinase activity					
mas	6q24-27	DNA transfection	Epidermoid carcinoma	Rearrangement of 5' noncoding region	Angiotensin receptor
Signal transducers					
Cytoplasmic tyrosine kinases					
SRC	20p12-13	Viral homologue	Colon carcinoma	Constitutive activation	Protein tyrosine kinase
v-yes	18q21-3 (YES)	Viral homologue	Sarcoma	Constitutive activation	Protein tyrosine kinase
v-fgr	1p36.1-36.2 (FGR)	Viral homologue	Sarcoma	Constitutive activation	Protein tyrosine kinase
v-fes	15q25-26 (FES)	Viral homologue	Sarcoma	Constitutive activation	Protein tyrosine kinase
ABL	9q34.1	Chromosome translocation	CML	DNA rearrangement (constitutive activation/fusion proteins)	Protein tyrosine kinase
Membrane-associated G proteins					
H-RAS	11p15.5	Viral homologue/DNA transfection	Colon, lung, pancreas carcinomas	Point mutation	GTPase
K-RAS	12p11.1-12.1	Viral homologue/DNA transfection	AML, thyroid carcinoma, melanoma/colon/lung	Point mutation	GTPase
N-RAS	1p11-13	DNA transfection	Carcinoma, melanoma	Point mutation	GTPase
BRAF	6	DNA sequencing	Melanoma, thyroid, colon, ovary	Point mutation	Ser/Thr kinase
gsp	20	DNA sequencing	Adenomas of thyroid	Point mutation	Gs alpha
gip	3	DNA sequencing	Ovary, adrenal carcinoma	Point mutation	Gi alpha
GTPase exchange factor (GEF)					
Dbl	Xq27	DNA transfection	Diffuse B-cell lymphoma	DNA rearrangement	GEF for Rho and Cdc42Hs
Vav	19p13.2	DNA transfection	Hematopoietic cells	DNA rearrangement	GEF for Ras?
Serine/threonine kinases: cytoplasmic					
v-mos	8q11 (MOS)	Viral homologue	Sarcoma	Constitutive activation	Protein kinase (ser/thr)
v-raf	3p25 (RAF-1)	Viral homologue	Sarcoma	Constitutive activation	Protein kinase (ser/thr)
pim-1	6p21 (PIM-)	Insertional mutagenesis	T-cell lymphoma	Constitutive activation	Protein kinase (ser/thr)
Cytoplasmic regulators					
v-crk	17p13 (CRK)	Viral homologue		Constitutive tyrosine phosphorylation of cellular substrates (eg, paxillin)	SH-2/SH-3 adaptor
Transcription factors					
v-myc	8q24.1 (MYC)	Viral homologue	Carcinoma myelocytomatosis	Deregulated activity	Transcription factor
N-MYC	2p24	DNA amplification	Neuroblastoma: lung	Deregulated activity	Transcription factor
L-MYC	1p32	DNA amplification	Carcinoma of lung	Deregulated activity	Transcription factor
v-myb	6q22-24	Viral homologue	Myeloblastosis	Deregulated activity	Transcription factor
v-fos	14q21-22	Viral homologue	Osteosarcoma	Deregulated activity	Transcription factor API
v-jun	p31-32	Viral homologue	Sarcoma	Deregulated activity	Transcription factor API
v-ski	1q22-24	Viral homologue	Carcinoma	Deregulated activity	Transcription factor
v-rel	2p12-14	Viral homologue	Lymphatic leukemia	Deregulated activity	Mutant NF-kappa B
v-ets-1	11p23-q24	Viral homologue	Erythroblastosis	Deregulated activity	Transcription factor
v-ets-2	21q24.3	Viral homologue	Erythroblastosis	Deregulated activity	Transcription factor
v-erbA1	17p11-21	Viral homologue	Erythroblastosis	Deregulated activity	T3 Transcription factor
v-erbA2	3p22-24.1	Viral homologue	Erythroblastosis	Deregulated activity	T3 Transcription factor
Others					
BCL2	18q21.3	Chromosomal translocation	B-cell lymphomas	Constitutive activity	Antiapoptotic protein
MDM2	12q14	DNA amplification	Sarcomas	Gene amplification/increased protein	Complexes with p53

Abbreviations: AML, acute myeloid leukemia; CML, chronic myelogenous leukemia; GTPase, guanosine triphosphatase; PDGF, platelet-derived growth factor.

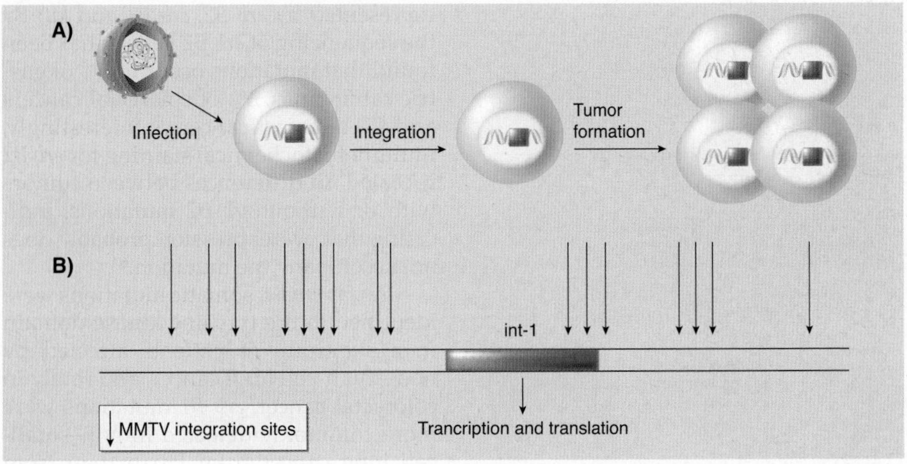

Figure 6-2 Insertional mutagenesis. (**A**) The process is independent from genes carried by the retrovirus. Retrovirus, eg, MMTV, infects a human cell. The proviral DNA is integrated into the host genome in infected cells. Rarely, the provirus inserts near a proto-oncogene (eg, *int-1*) and activates the proto-oncogene. Activated proto-oncogene results in cell transformation and in tumor formation. (**B**) Sites of integration of MMTV retrovirus near the proto-oncogene *int-1*. All sites determine *int-1* activation.

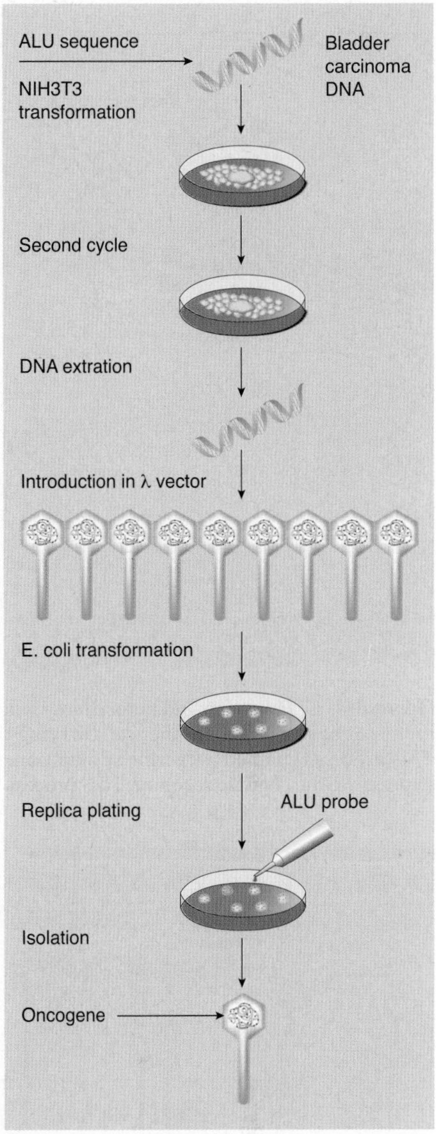

Figure 6-3 Transfection assay. DNA from a tumor (eg, bladder carcinoma) is used to transform a rodent immortalized cell line (NIH3T3). After serial cycles, DNA from transformed cells was extracted and then insertedinto β vector, that was subsequently used to transform anappropriate *Escherichia coli* strain. Using a specific probe (Alu in the figure) it was possible to isolate and then char-acterize the involved human oncogene.

pression of proto-oncogenes can activate them to become oncogenes capable of inducing in susceptible cells the neoplastic phenotype. Oncogenes can be classified into five groups based on the functional and biochemical properties of protein products of their normal counterparts (proto-oncogenes). These groups are (1) growth factors, (2) growth factor receptors, (3) signal transducers, (4) transcription factors, and (5) others, including programmed cell death regulators. Table 6-1 lists examples of oncogenes according to their functional categories.

Growth Factors

Growth factors are secreted polypeptides that function as extracellular signals to stimulate the proliferation of target cells.[45,46] Appropriate target cells must possess a specific receptor in order to respond to a specific type of growth factor. A well-characterized example is platelet-derived growth factor (PDGF), an approximately 30-kd protein consisting of two polypeptide chains.[47] PDGF is released from platelets during the process of blood coagulation. PDGF stimulates the proliferation of fibroblasts, a cell growth process that plays an important role in wound healing. Other well-characterized examples of growth factors include nerve growth factor (NGF), epidermal growth factor, and fibroblast growth factor.

The link between growth factors and retroviral oncogenes was revealed by study of the *sis* oncogene of simian sarcoma virus, a retrovirus first isolated from a monkey fibrosarcoma. Sequence analysis showed that *sis* encodes the beta chain of PDGF.[48] This discovery established the principle that inappropriately expressed growth factors could function as oncogenes. Experiments demonstrated that the constitutive expression of the sis gene product (PDGF*b*) was sufficient to cause neoplastic transformation of fibroblasts but not of cells that lacked the receptor for PDGF.[49] Thus, transformation by sis requires interaction of the sis gene product with the PDGF receptor (PDGFR). The mechanism by which a growth factor affects the same cell that produces it is called *autocrine stimulation*[50] (Fig. 6-4). The constitutive expression of the *sis* gene product appears to cause neoplastic transformation by the mechanism of autocrine stimulation, resulting in self-sustained aberrant cell proliferation. This model, derived from experimental animal systems, has been recently demonstrated in a human tumor. Dermatofibrosarcoma protuberans (DP) is an infiltrative skin tumor that was demonstrated to present specific cytogenetic features: reciprocal translocation and supernumerary ring chromosomes, involving chromosomes 17 and 22.[51,52] Molecular cloning of the breakpoints revealed a fusion between the collagen type Ia1 (COL1A1) gene and PDGF-β gene. The fusion gene resulted in a deletion of PDGF-β exon 1 and a constitutive release of this growth factor. Subsequent experiments of gene transfer of DP's genomic DNA into NIH 3T3 cells directly demonstrated the occurrence of an autocrine mechanism by the human rearranged PDGF-β gene involving the activation of the endogenous PDGF receptor.[53,54] Another example of a growth factor that can function as an oncogene is *int-2*, a member of the fibroblast growth factor family. *Int-2* is sometimes activated in mouse mammary carcinomas by MMTV insertional mutagenesis.[55]

Growth Factor Receptors

Some viral oncogenes are altered versions of normal growth factor receptors that possess intrinsic tyrosine kinase activity.[56] Receptor tyrosine kinases, as these growth factor receptors are collectively known, have a characteristic protein structure consisting of three principal domains: (1) the extracellular ligand-binding domain, (2) the transmembrane domain, and (3) the intracellular tyrosine kinase catalytic domain (Fig. 6-5). Growth factor receptors are molecular machines that transmit information in a unidirectional fashion across the cell membrane. The binding

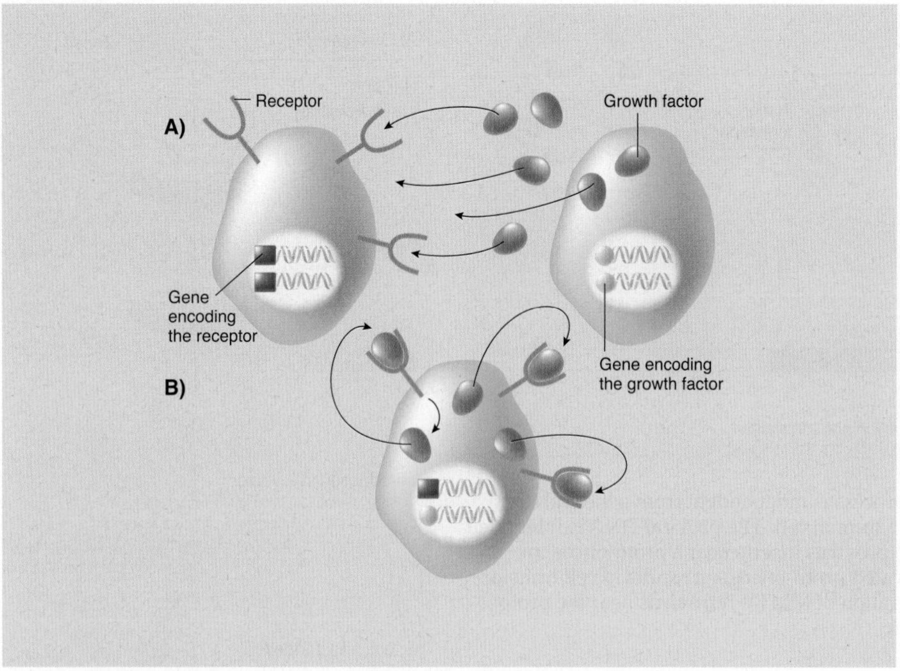

Figure 6-4 ■ Paracrine and autocrine stimulation. (**A**) A growth factor produced by the cell on the right stimulates another cell carrying the appropriate receptor (*left*) on cell membrane. This process is named paracrine stimulation. (**B**) A growth factor is produced by the same cell expressing the cognate receptor. This process is designated autocrine stimulation.

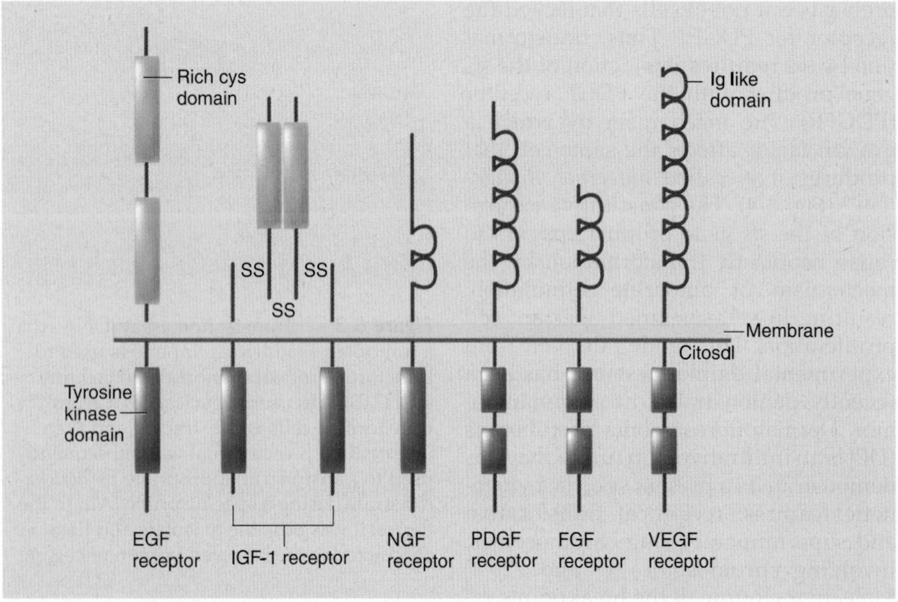

Figure 6-5 ■ Representative examples of tyrosine kinase receptor families.

of a growth factor to the extracellular ligand-binding domain of the receptor results in the activation of the intracellular tyrosine kinase catalytic domain. The recruitment and phosphorylation of specific cytoplasmic proteins by the activated receptor then trigger a series of biochemical events generally leading to cell division.

Because of the role of growth factor receptors in the regulation of normal cell growth, it is not surprising that these receptors constitute an important class of proto-oncogenes. Examples include *erb B1*, *erb B2*, *fms*, *kit*, *met*, *ret*, *ros*, and *trk*. Mutation or abnormal expression of growth factor receptors can convert themv into oncogenes.[57] For example, deletion of the ligand-binding domain of *erb B* (the epidermal growth factor receptor) is thought to result in constitutive activation of the receptor in the absence of ligand binding.[58] Point mutation in the tyrosine kinase domain or of the extracellular domain and deletion of intracellular regulatory domains can also result in the constitutive activation of receptor tyrosine kinases. Relevant examples are represented by *erb B2*, *erb B1* and *kit*. By the sequencing of *erb B2* gene, it has been found that mutations occur in 5% of gastric carcinomas, 3% of colorectal cancers and 4% of breast cancers.[59] Interestingly, immunohistochemical staining for *erb B2* revealed no differences between tumors with or without *erb B2* mutations, indicating that overexpression probably does not accompany the mutation.[60]

As far *erb B1*, somatic mutations were identified in the tyrosine kinase domain in a subgroup of patients affected by non–small-cell lung cancer, and rarely in colorectal cancer. *erb B1* mutations were more commonly detected in non–small-cell lung cancer from Japan than from United States, thus suggesting that ethnic differences may exist in *erb B1* mutation occurrence. In addition, it seems that *erb B1* mutations occur more frequently in never smokers female patients, generally affected by an adenocarcinoma.[61] Germ-line mutations occurring in epidermal growth factor receptor (EGFR) exon 21 are reported in patients showing multiple lung adenocarcinomas.[62]

The proto-oncogene *kit* encodes a transmembrane tyrosine kinase glycoprotein. Binding of its cognate ligand stem cell factor (SCF) to *kit* results in receptor homodimerization, activation of *kit* tyrosine kinase activity and resultant phosphorylation of a variety of substrates, including Akt and STAT3. Three general mechanisms of kit activation in tumor cells have been described: (1) autocrine and/or paracrine stimulation of the receptor by its ligand, SCF; (2) cross-activation by other kinases and/or loss of regulatory phosphatase activity; and (3) acquisition of activating mutations of several different exons of the kit gene. *Kit* mutations (typically in exon 17) are most commonly found in mastocytosis/mast cell leukemia, acute myelogenous leukemia (AML), seminoma/dysgerminoma, and sinosal natural killer/T-cell lymphoma. In gastrointestinal stromal tumors (GISTs), more heterogeneous mutations are described: mutations most commonly occur in the juxtamembrane exon 11 of the gene (in about 65% of all GISTs) whereas about 10% of GISTs have kit exon 9 mutations and 2% exon 13 or exon 17 mutations. In GIST showing any alterations in the kit gene, point mutations may occur in pdgfra, a gene belonging to the same family as kit. Approximately 5% of GIST have a constitutively activating mutations in pdgfra, mostly (80%) found in exon 18 and the rest either in exon 12 (10-15%) or 14 (1-5%).[63] *kit* and *pdgfra* mutations are mutually exclusive. Patients with kit or pdgfra mutations show worse prognosis with respect to patients with wild-type sequences of both genes. Gastric GISTs with exon 11 deletions are more aggressive than those with substitutions. The less common *kit* exon 9 codons 502-503 duplication occurs predominantly in small intestinal GISTs. pdgfra mutations are associated with gastric GISTs, epithelioid morphology and a less malignant course of disease.[64] Germ-line mutations in kit gene have been found in patients manifesting multiple GIST arising at earlier age, urticaria pigmentosa, melanocytic nevi, melanomas, achalasia or neuronal hyperplasia of the mesentheric plexus.[65]

Increased expression through gene amplification and abnormal expression in the wrong cell type are additional mechanisms through which growth factor receptors may be involved in neoplasia. The identification and study of altered growth factor receptors in experimental models of neoplasia have contributed much to our understanding of the normal regulation of cell proliferation.

Signal Transducers

Mitogenic signals are transmitted from growth factor receptors on the cell surface to the cell nucleus through a series of complex interlocking pathways collectively referred to as the signal transduction cascade.[66] This relay of information is accomplished in part by the stepwise phosphorylation of interacting proteins in the cytosol. Signal transduction also involves guanine nucleotide-binding proteins and second messengers such as the adenylate cyclase system.[67] The first retroviral oncogene discovered, *src*, was subsequently shown to be involved in signal transduction.

Many proto-oncogenes are members of signal transduction pathways.[68,69] These consist of two main groups: nonreceptor protein kinases and guanosine triphosphate (GTP)-binding proteins. The nonreceptor protein kinases are subclassified into tyrosine kinases (eg, *abl*, *lck*, and *src*) and serine/threonine kinases (eg, *raf-1*, *mos*, and *pim-1*). GTP-binding proteins with intrinsic guanosine triphosphatase (GTPase) activity are subdivided into monomeric and heterotrimeric groups.[70] Monomeric GTP-binding proteins are members of the important *ras* family of proto-oncogenes that includes H-*ras*, K-*ras*, and N-*ras*.[71] Heterotrimeric GTP-binding proteins (G proteins) implicated as proto-oncogenes currently include *gsp* and *gip*. Signal transducers are often converted to oncogenes by mutations that lead to their unregulated activity, which in turn leads to uncontrolled cellular proliferation.[72]

Transcription Factors

Transcription factors are nuclear proteins that regulate the expression of target genes or gene families.[73] Transcriptional regulation is mediated by protein-binding to specific DNA sequences or DNA structural motifs, usually located upstream of the target gene. Transcription factors often belong to multigene families that share common DNA-binding domains such as zinc fingers. The mechanism of action of transcription factors also involves binding to other proteins, sometimes in heterodimeric complexes with specific partners. Transcription factors are the final link in the signal transduction pathway that converts extracellular signals into modulated changes in gene expression.

Many proto-oncogenes are transcription factors that were discovered through their retroviral homologues.[74] Examples include *erb A*, *ets*, *fos*, *jun*, *myb*, and *c-myc*. Together, fos and jun form the AP-1 transcription factor, which positively regulates a number of target genes whose expression leads to cell division.[75,76] *Erb A* is the receptor for the T3 thyroid hormone, triiodothyronine.[77] Proto-oncogenes that function as transcription factors are often activated by chromosomal translocations in hematologic and solid neoplasms.[78] In certain types of sarcomas, chromosomal translocations cause the formation of fusion proteins involving the association of *EWS* gene with various partners and resulting in an aberrant tumor-associated transcriptional activity. Interestingly, a role of the adenovirus *E1A* gene in promoting the formation of fusion transcript fli1/ews in normal human fibroblasts was recently reported.[79] An important example of a proto-oncogene with a transcriptional activity in human hematologic tumors is the c-*myc* gene, which helps to control the expression of genes leading to cell proliferation.[80] As will be discussed later in this chapter, the c-*myc* gene (which is encoded for a nuclear DNA-binding protein belonging to the helix-loop-helix/leucine zipper superfamily, involved in transcriptional regulation) is frequently activated by chromosomal translocations in human leukemia and lymphoma.

Programed Cell Death Regulation

Normal tissues exhibit a regulated balance between cell proliferation and cell death. Programmed cell death is an important component in the processes of normal embryogenesis and organ development. A distinctive type of programmed cell death, called apoptosis, has been described for mature tissues.[81] This process is characterized morphologically by blebbing of the plasma membrane, volume contraction, condensation of the cell nucleus, and cleavage of genomic DNA by endogenous nucleases into nucleosome-sized fragments. Apoptosis can be triggered in mature cells by external stimuli such as steroids and radiation exposure. Studies of cancer cells have shown that both uncontrolled cell proliferation and failure to undergo programmed cell death can contribute to neoplasia and insensitivity to anticancer treatments.

The first proto-oncogene shown to regulate programmed cell death is *bcl-2*. It was the study of chromosomal translocations in human lymphoma that lead to the discovery of *bcl-2*. Experimental studies show that *bcl-2* activation inhibits programmed cell death in lymphoid cell populations. The dominant mode of action of activated *bcl-2* led to classify it as an oncogene. The *bcl-2* gene encodes a protein localized to the inner mitochondrial membrane, endoplasmic reticulum, and nuclear membrane. The mechanism of action of the bcl-2 protein has not been fully elucidated, but studies indicate that it functions in part as an antioxidant that inhibits lipid peroxidation of cell membranes.[82] Moreover, bcl-2 homologues, some of which bind to bcl-2, have been identified, suggesting that bcl-2 functions at least in part through protein-protein interaction. Site-directed mutagenesis of bcl-2 protein BH1 and BH2 domains showed that these two regions are important for binding of bcl-2 to bax, a member of the bcl-2-family that promotes cell death and whose interaction with bcl-2 is necessary to regulate the apoptotic pathway[11] (Fig. 6-6). Although translocation is the main mechanism of *bcl-2* gene activation, *bcl-2* point mutations and amplification also have been reported. Mutations clustering in the *bcl-2* open-reading frame occur in high-grade B-cell lymphomas transformed from low grade follicular lymphomas carrying *bcl-2* gene rearrangement.[82] The amplification of the *bcl-2* gene, which leads to increased protein production, has been detected

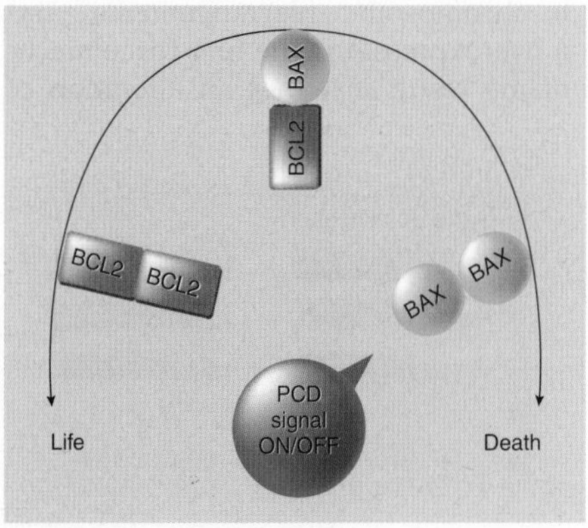

Figure 6-6 ■ Effect of bcl-2 activity on the control of the cell life. In the presence of BAX only, the cell goes to apoptosis. bcl-2 regulates the cycle of the cell by the interaction with BAX. When bcl-2 is overexpressed, the cell cycle is deregulated and the apoptosis is prevented, eventually leading to tumor formation. This is an important cause for tumor formation. *Abbreviations*: PCD, program cell death or apoptosis.

in about 30% of high-grade diffuse large cell lymphomas (DLCL) lacking bcl-2 translocation.[83] Clinical relevance of bcl-2 expression has been shown in solid tumors, such as breast, prostate, thyroid, and lung.[84-87]

The second oncogene more recently shown to be involved in apoptosis is caspase-9, which is activated by the following intrinsic pathway. Release of cytochrome c into the cytosol results in activation of the caspase adaptor Apaf-1 and procaspase-9, which form a holoenzyme complex named apoptosome. Caspase-9, in turn, activates downstream caspases, most importantly caspase-3 and also caspase-6, 7, and 8, which results in DNA fragmentation and apoptosis.[11,88] It has been demonstrated that Akt may regulate apoptosome function by phosphorylation of caspase-9 at the Ser-196 level.[89] This phosphorylation event has relevant functional consequences, leading to the suppression of apoptosis caspase-9-mediated. The Akt suppression is specific for caspase-9 and probably is due to the inactivation of the intrinsic catalytic activity. More recently it has been demonstrated that bax is also involved, leading to caspase-9 stimulation (through Apaf-1) in response to mitochondrial membrane damage.[90]

Mechanisms of Oncogene Activation

The activation of oncogenes involves genetic changes to cellular proto-oncogenes. The consequence of these genetic alterations is to confer a growth advantage to the cell. Four genetic mechanisms activate oncogenes in human neoplasms: (1) mutation, (2) gene amplification, (3) chromosome rearrangements, and (4) overexpression. The first three mechanisms result in either an alteration of proto-oncogene structure or an increase in proto-oncogene expression (Fig. 6-7). Because neoplasia is a multistep process, more than one of these mechanisms often contribute to the genesis of human tumors by altering a number of cancer-associated genes. Full expression of the neoplastic phenotype, including the capacity for metastasis, usually involves a combination of proto-oncogene activation and tumor suppressor gene loss or inactivation.

Mutation

Mutations activate proto-oncogenes through structural alterations in their encoded proteins. These alterations, which usually involve critical protein regulatory regions or directly the catalytic domain, often lead to the uncontrolled, continuous activity of the mutated protein. Various types of mutations, such as base substitutions, deletions, and insertions, are capable of activating proto-oncogenes.[91] Retroviral oncogenes, for example, often have deletions that contribute to their activation. Examples include deletions in the amino-terminal ligand-binding domains of the erb B, kit, ros, met, and trk oncogenes.[6] In human tumors, however, most characterized oncogene mutations are base substitutions (point mutations) that change a single amino acid within the protein.

Point mutations are frequently detected in the ras family of proto-oncogenes (K-*ras*, H-*ras*, and *Nras*). The human *ras* genes encode for similar membrane-bound 21 kd proteins (189 amino acids) involved in signal transduction, with a guanine nucleotide-binding activity as well as an intrinsic GTPase activity. When activated, ras proteins transduce the signal by linking tyrosine kinases to downstream serine/threonine kinases, such as raf, and mitogen-activated protein kinases (MAPKs)[92] (Fig. 6-8). Stabilization of ras proteins in their active state causes a continuous flow of signal transduction, which results in malignant transformation. This status can be achieved after point mutation, mainly at codon 12 level, with a smaller number involving other regions such as codons 13 or 61. In addition, it has been recently shown that K-*ras* mutation may also occur at a certain frequency at codon 146 in several neoplastic diseases.[93] Mutations of ras in human tumors have been linked to carcinogen exposure: for example, the occurrence of K-*ras* mutations in non-small-cell lung cancer seems to be due to smoking exposure, in particular to benzoapyrene.[94] It has been estimated that as many as 15% to 20% of unselected human tumors may contain a ras mutation. Mutations in K-ras predominate in tumors derived from endodermal tumors, including carcinomas of pancreas (90%), colorectal (40%) and lung.[71,92] This finding is due to the fact that K-*ras*, but not H-*ras* or N-*ras*, promotes the expansion of an endodermal stem/progenitor cell and blocks its differentiation.[95] N-*ras* mutations are preferentially found in hematologic malignancies, with up to a 25% incidence in AMLs and myelodysplastic syndromes. The majority of thyroid carcinomas have been found to have ras mutations distributed among K-*ras*, H-*ras*, and N-*ras*, without preference for a single *ras* family member, but showing an association with the follicular type of differentiated thyroid carcinomas. As a prognostic tool, a link between poor outcome and specific types of K-*ras* mutations has been hypothesized. Demonstration of such a prognostic effect, not yet firmly established, otherwise may allow appropriate targeting of intensive follow-up and adjuvant therapy.[96] Moreover, again in colorectal cancer, the identification of K-ras mutations in stool samples may be used in early diagnosis,[97] and in plasma samples for monitoring patients' follow-up:[98]

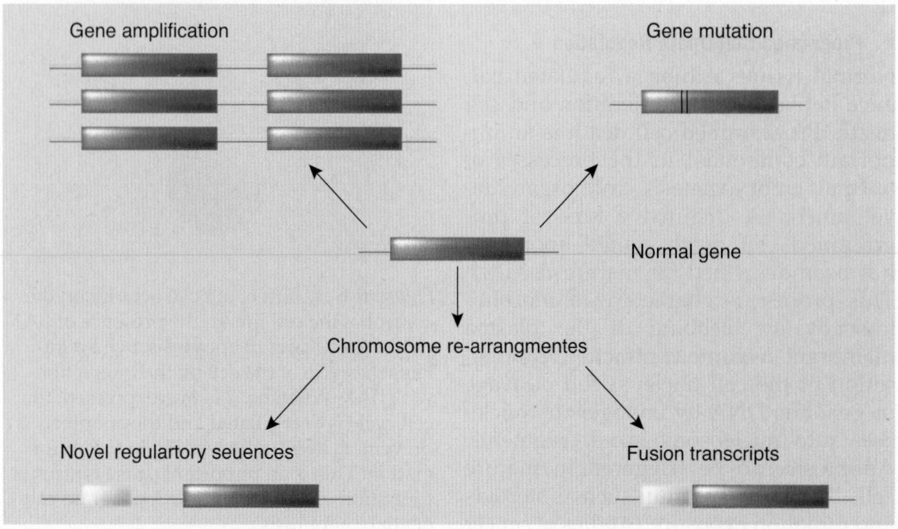

Figure 6-7 Schematic representation of the main mechanisms of oncogene activation (from proto-oncogenes to oncogenes). The normal gene (proto-oncogene) is depicted with its transcribed portion (*rectangle*). In the case of gene amplification, the latter can be duplicated 100-fold, resulting in an excess of normal protein. A similar situation can occur when following chromosome rearrangements such as translocation, the transcription of the gene is now regulated by novel regulatory sequences belonging to another gene. In the case of point mutation, single amino acid substitutions can alter the biochemical properties of the gene product, causing, in the example, its constitutive enzymatic activation. Chromosome rearrangements, such as translocation and inversion, can then generate fusion transcripts resulting in chimericoncogenic proteins.

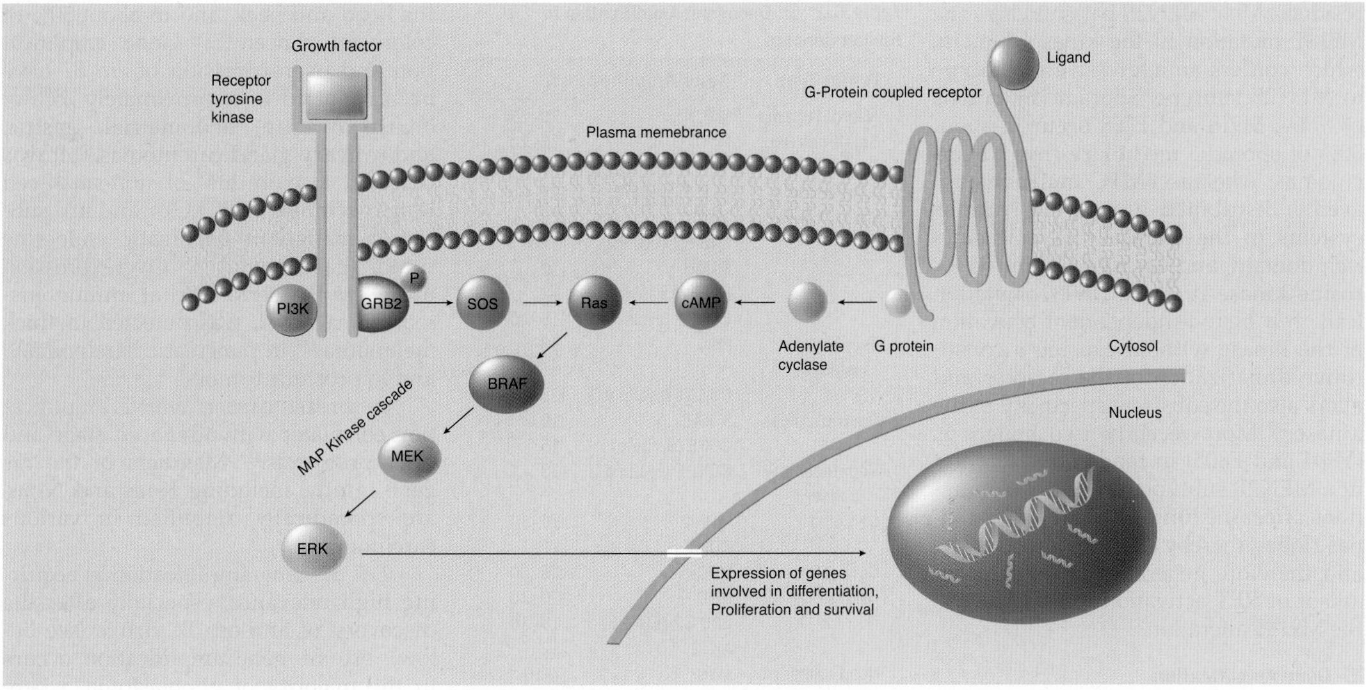

Figure 6-8 The ras-raf-MAPK signaling pathway.

In addition to cancer, *ras* mutations are involved in other diseases. Specifically, N-*ras* mutations cause a human autoimmune lymphoproliferative syndrome,[99] while H-*ras* and K-*ras* germ-line mutations underlie disorders of the Noonan syndrome spectrum.[92] The last data, coupled with the evidence that cancers rarely occur in these individuals, is leading to a re-evaluation of the effective role played by *ras* genes in carcinogenesis.

Another example of activating point mutations is represented by those occurring in *BRAF* gene, the first result of the human genome project in the screening of cancer genes using high-throughput genomic technologies.[7] The *BRAF* sequence contains the three conserved regions CR1, which encodes for the putative zinc finger domain, CR2, where several serine/threonine-rich regions are located, and CR3, which corresponds to the kinase domain. BRAF is recruited to the plasma membrane upon binding to ras-GTP and represents a key point in the signal transduction through the mitogen-activated protein (MAP) kinase pathway (see Fig. 6-8). The most common oncogenic mutation of BRAF, occurring in more than 90% of cases, changes the valine residue at position 600 within the BRAF kinase domain to glutamic acid (600), thus mimicking the phosphorylation of threonine 599 and serine 602, two major points of BRAF regulation which lead to a protein with high activity, able to constitutively activate ERK protein.[11] In tissue specimens, BRAF mutations were found in melanomas (75%), thyroid (45%), colorectal (12%), and ovarian cancer (14%).[7,100] BRAF mutations may also occur in acute lymphoblastic leukemia (ALL).[101] Furthermore, it has been shown that *BRAF* mutations occur in colorectal cancer only when tumors do not carry mutations in the K-*ras* gene, and in papillary thyroid carcinoma when *RET* or *TRK* rearrangements are absent. These mutual exclusions have led to the assumption that *BRAF* and K-*ras* alterations, or *BRAF, RET* and *TRK* alterations, could have the same functional effect in colorectal or in thyroid carcinogenesis, respectively.[11,100,102] As regards colorectal cancer, *BRAF* mutations are frequently present in sporadic cases with methylated hMLH1, but not in HNPCC-related cancers, thus representing a possible strategy for exclusion criteria for HNPCC.[103] Moreover *BRAF* mutations are frequently found in hyperplastic polyps and in serrated adenomas,[104] suggesting that they represent an early and critical event in these types of lesions. *BRAF* mutations may have an influence on patients' prognosis depending on the tumor type where they occur: in ovarian cancer *BRAF* mutations are associated with type I tumors, that are slow growing and generally confined to the ovary at diagnosis.[105] and with the aggressive tall-cell variant in papillary thyoid carcinomas.[100] *BRAF* mutations, especially the V600E change, that is very easy to investigate, are now acquiring a role in early diagnosis or disease monitoring in patients' follow-up: indeed, they are investigated to improve the diagnosis in fine-needle aspiration biopsy with cytological findings suspicious for papillary thyroid carcinomas.[106] On the contrary, in melanoma BRAF mutations could be only used to monitor in serum the follow-up of patients receiving biochemotherapy[107] and not for early diagnosis because they even precede the neoplastic transformation, since all types of nevi besides Spitz and Blue nevi show *BRAF* alterations at a high frequency.[108] However, the real role of BRAF mutations in cancerogenesis is brought into question by a recent discovery: surprisingly, it has been demonstrated that the typical BRAF V600E mutation leads to synthesis and secretion of the IGFBP7 protein, which acts through autocrine/paracrine pathways to inhibit the MAPK signaling and induce senescence and apoptosis.[109] A deepen analysis of the interplay between BRAF V600E change and IGFBP7 is therefore urgently required.

Another significant example of activating point mutations is represented by those affecting the ret proto-oncogene in multiple endocrine neoplasia (MEN) type 2 (2A and 2B) syndrome and familial medullary thyroid carcinomas (FMTC). MEN 2A is associated most frequently with mutations of codon 634 (85%), particularly C634R. This germline point mutation affecting one of the cysteine residues located in the juxtamembrane domain of the ret receptor has been found to confer an oncogenic potential to the latter as a consequence of the ligand-independent activation of the tyrosine kinase activity of the receptor. Experimental evidence has pointed out that these cysteine residues-involving mutations promote ret homodimerization via the formation of intermolecular disulfide bonding, most likely as a result of an unpaired number of cysteine residues. Most MEN2B patients carry the M918T mutation in the kinase domain, which confers an aggressive phenotype to MEN2B subtype. Sporadic mutations of V804, M918 and E768 occur in about 50% of sporadic medullary thyroid carcinomas, whereas FMTC mutations are evenly distributed among the various cysteins in the extracellulary cysteine-rich domain, and occasionally in the tyrosine kinase domain. M918T mutation lead to a ligand-independent activation of the kinase without causing a constitutive dimerization of the receptor and alters also the substrate specificity of the kinase.[110] More recently, two mutations (V804 and E805) in tandem were found in a MEN2B subtype. These novel mutations affect the hinging motion of the kinase lobes, thereby altering the active site and, therefore, generate a different mechanism of RET activation with respect to the M918T alteration.[111]

Gene Amplification

Gene amplification refers to the expansion in copy number of a gene within the genome of a cell. Gene amplification was first discovered as a mechanism by which some tumor cell lines can acquire resistance to growth-inhibiting drugs.[112] The process of gene amplification occurs through redundant replication of genomic DNA, often giving rise to karyotypic abnormalities called double-minute chromosomes (DMs) and HSRs.[113] DMs are characteristic minichromosome structures without centromeres. HSRs are segments of chromosomes that lack the normal alternating pattern of light and dark staining bands. Both DMs and HSRs represent large regions of amplified genomic DNA, containing up to several hundred copies of a gene. Amplification leads to the increased expression of genes, which in turn can confer a selective advantage for cell growth.

The frequent observation of DMs and HSRs in human tumors suggested that the amplification of specific proto-oncogenes may be a common occurrence in neoplasia.[114] Studies then demonstrated that three proto-oncogene families—*myc*, *erb B*, and *ras*—are amplified in a significant number of human tumors (Table 6-2). About 20% to 30% of breast and ovarian cancers show c-myc amplification, and an approximately equal frequency of c-myc amplification is found in some types of squamous cell carcinomas.[115] N-*myc* was discovered as a new member of the *myc* proto-oncogene family through its amplification in neuroblastomas.[116] Amplification of N-*myc* correlates strongly with advanced tumor stage in neuroblastoma[117] (Table 6-3), suggesting a role for this gene in tumor progression.[118] L-*myc* was discovered through its amplification in small-cell

Table 6-2 ■ Oncogene Amplification in Human Cancers

Tumor Type	Gene Amplified	%
Neuroblastoma	MYCN	20-25
Small-cell lung cancer	MYC	15-20
Glioblastoma	ERB B1 (EGFR)	33-50
Breast cancer	MYC	20
	ERB B2 (EGFR2)	~20
	FGFR1	12
	FGFR2	12
	CCND1 (cyclin d1)	15-20
Esophageal cancer	MYC	38
	CCND1 (cyclin d1)	25
Gastric cancer	K-RAS	10
	CCNE (cyclin e)	15
Hepatocellular cancer	CCND1 (cyclin d1)	13
Sarcoma	MDM2	10-30
	CDK4	11
Cervical cancer	MYC	25-50
Ovarian cancer	MYC	20-30
	ERB B2 (EGFR2)	15-30
	AKT2	12
Head and neck cancer	MYC	7-10
	ERB B1(EGFR)	10
	CCND1(cyclin d1)	~50
Colorectal cancer	MYB	15-20
	H-RAS	29
	K-RAS	22

carcinoma of the lung, a neuroendocrine-derived tumor, and in bladder neoplasia.[119] Furthermore, c-*myc* activation may be mediated by APC and/or β-catenin alterations in several tumors, leading to an increase of c-myc transcription through an accumulation of β-catenin into the cytoplasm and the nucleus.[120] A nuclear accumulation of c-myc may identify high-risk subsets of patients with synovial sarcoma of the extremities.[121] Amplification and overexpression of c-*myc*, in combination with *erb B2* alterations, have been reported to be associated with tumor progression from noninvasive to invasive[122] and with poor prognosis[123] in patients with breast carcinoma. In melanoma[124] and in medulloblastoma,[125,126] c-myc expression seems to be a useful prognostic marker able to identify high-risk patients. Amplification of *erb B*, the epidermal growth factor receptor, is found in up to 50% of glioblastomas, in 10% to 20% of squamous carcinomas of

Table 6-3 ■ Correlation of N-myc Copy Number with Stage and Survival in Neuroblastoma

Tumor Type	No. of Cases	%
Benign ganglioneuromas	0/64	(0%)
Low stages	31/772	(4%)
Stage 4-S	15/190	(8%)
Advanced stages	612/1.974	(31%)
Total	658/3000	(22%)

the head and neck, and in about 50% of colorectal cancer.[127,128] Gene amplification and overexpression of *erb B2* have been reported in approximately 25% of breast, ovarian, endometrial, gastric, and salivary gland carcinomas.[129] It was detected also in 16% of non-small-cell lung carcinoma (NSCLC)[130] and in a subset of malignant pancreatic endocrine tumor (gastrinoma).[11,131] Overexpression of the *erb B2*, performed at immunohistochemical level, was detected in thick melanoma,[132] in pancreatic carcinoma,[133] and in prostatic tumors.[134]

In breast cancer, *erbB-2* amplification correlates with advanced stage and poor prognosis.[135] Members of the ras gene family, including K-*ras* and N-*ras*, are sporadically amplified in various carcinomas.

Erb B1 gene amplification is acquiring high relevance, especially after the discovery of anti-erb B1 drugs (see below). erb B1 gene amplification occurs in the majority of glioblastoma, where it represents an independent factor of worse prognosis, and in up to 30% of colorectal, non-small-cell lung and breast cancer (where it is mutual exclusive with respect to *erb B2* gene amplification). In glioblastoma, *erb B1* gene amplification is accompanied in >50% of cases by gene rearrangement, the most common of which is the loss of the 2-7 exons of the extracellular *erb B1* domain, leading to the so-called *erb B1* variant III, which is constitutively activated.[136]

Chromosomal Rearrangements

Recurring chromosomal rearrangements are often detected in hematological malignancies as well as in some solid tumors.[41,137,138] These rearrangements consist mainly of chromosomal translocations and, less frequently, chromosomal inversions. Chromosomal rearrangements can lead to hematological malignancy by two different mechanisms: (1) the transcriptional activation of proto-oncogenes or (2) the creation of fusion genes. Transcriptional activation, sometimes referred to as gene activation, results from chromosomal rearrangements that move a proto-oncogene close to an immunoglobulin or T-cell receptor gene (see Fig. 6-7). Transcription of the proto-oncogene then falls under the control of regulatory elements from the immunoglobulin or T-cell receptor locus. This circumstance causes deregulation of proto-oncogene expression, which can then lead to neoplastic transformation of the cell.

Fusion genes can be created by chromosomal rearrangements when the chromosomal breakpoints fall within the loci of two different genes. The resultant juxtaposition of segments from two different genes gives rise to a composite structure consisting of the head of one gene and the tail of another gene. Fusion genes encode chimeric proteins with transforming activity. In general, both genes involved in the fusion contribute to the transforming potential of the chimeric oncoprotein. Mistakes in the physiologic rearrangement of immunoglobulin or T-cell receptor genes are thought to give rise to many of the recurring chromosomal rearrangements found in hematologic malignancy.[139] Examples of molecularly characterized chromosomal rearrangements in hematologic and solid malignancies are given in Table 6-4. In

Table 6-4 ■ **Molecularly Characterized Chromosome Rearrangements in Tumors**

Affected Gene	Rearrangements	Disease	Protein Type
Hematopoietic tumor			
Gene fusion			
c-ABL (9q34)	t(9:22) (q34:q11)	Chronic myelogenous leukemia and acute leukemia	Tyrosine kinase activated by BCR
BCR (22q11)			
PBX1(1q23)	t(1:19)(q23:p13.3)	Acute pre-B-cell leukemia	Homeodomain
E2A(19p13.3)			HLH
PML(15q21)	t(15:17) (q21:q11-22)	Acute myeloid leukemia	Zn finger
RAR(17q21)			
CAN(6p23)	t(6:9) (p23:q34)	Acute myeloid leukemia	No homology
DEK(9q34)			
REL	ins(2:12) (p13:p11.2-14)	Non-Hodgkin's lymphoma	NF-κB family
NRG		No homology	
Oncogenes juxtaposed with IG loci			
c-MYC	t(8:14) (q24:q32) t(2:8) (p12:q24) t(8:22) (q24:q11)	Burkitt's lymphoma. BL-ALL	HLH domain
BCL-1 (PRADI?)	t(11:14) (q13:q32)	B-cell chronic lymphocyte leukemia	PRADI-GI cyclin
BCL-2	t(14:18) (q32:21)	Follicular lymphoma	Inner mitochondrial membrane
BCL-3	t(14:19) (q32:q13.1)	Chronic B-cell leukemia	CDC10 motif
IL-3	t(5:14) (q31:q32)	Acute pre-B-cell leukemia	Growth factor
Oncogenes juxtaposed with TCR loci			
c-MYC	t(8:14) (q24:q11)	Acute T-cell leukemia	HLH domain
LYLA	t(7:19) (q35:p13)	Acute T-cell leukemia	HLH domain
TALA/SCL/TCL-5	t(1:14) (q32:q11)	Acute T-cell leukemia	HLH domain
TAL-2	t(7:9) (q35:q34)	Acute T-cell leukemia	HLH domain
Rhombotin 1/Ttg-1	t(11:14) (p15:q11)	Acute T-cell leukemia	LIM domain
Rhombotin 2/Ttg-2	t(11:14) (p13:q11) t(7:11) (q35:p13)	Acute T-cell leukemia	LIM domain
HOX 11	t(10:14) (q24:q11) t(7:10) (q35:q24)	Acute T-cell leukemia	Homeodomain
TAN-1	t(7:9) (q34:q34.3)	Acute T-cell leukemia	Notch homologue
TCL-1	t(7q35-14q32.1) or inv t(14q11-14q32.1) or inv	B-cell chronic lymphocyte leukemia	
Solid tumors			
Gene fusions in sarcomas			
FLI1,EWS	t(11:22) (q24:q12)	Ewing's sarcoma	Ets transcription factor family
ERG,EWS	t(21:22) (q22:q12)	Ewing's sarcoma	Ets transcription factor family
ATV1,EWS	t(7:21) (q22:q12)	Ewing's sarcoma	Ets transcription factor family
ATF1,EWS	t(12:22) (q13:q12)	Soft-tissue clear cell sarcoma	Transcription factor
CHN,EWS	t(9:22) (q22 31:q12)	Myxoid chondrosarcoma	Steroid receptor family
WT1,EWS	t(11:22) (p13:q12)	Desmoplastic small round cell tumor	Wilms' tumor gene
SSX1,SSX2,SYT	t(X:18) (p11.2:q11.2)	Synovial sarcoma	HLH domain
PAX3,FKHR	t(2:13) (q37:q14)	Alveolar	Homeobox homologue
PAX7,FKHR	t(1:13) (q36:q14)	Rhabdomyosarcoma	Homeobox homologue
CHOP,TLS	t(12:16) (q13:p11)	Myxoid liposarcoma	Transcription factor
var,HMG1-C	t(var:12) (var:q13-15)	Lipomas	HMG DNA-binding protein
HMG1-C?	t(12:14) (q13-15)	Leiomyomas	HMG DNA-binding protein
Gene fusions in thyroid carcinomas			
RET/ptc1	inv(10) (q11.2:q2.1)	Papillary thyroid carcinomas	Tyrosine kinase activated by H4
RET/ptc2	t(10:17) (q11.2:q23)	Papillary thyroid carcinomas	Tyrosine kinase activated by Rla(PKA)
RET/ptc3	inv(10) (q11.2)	Papillary thyroid carcinomas	Tyrosine kinase activated by ELE1
TRK	inv(1) (q31:q22-23)	Papillary thyroid carcinomas	Tyrosine kinase activated by TPM3
TRK – T1(T2)	inv(1) (q31:q25)	Papillary thyroid carcinomas	Tyrosine kinase activated by TPR
TRK – T3	t(1q31:3)	Papillary thyroid carcinomas	Tyrosine kinase activated by TFG
Hematopoietic and solid tumors			
Oncogenes juxtaposed with other loci			
PTH deregulates PRAD1	inv(11)(p15:q13)	Parathyroid adenoma	PRADI-GI cyclin
BTG1 deregulates MYC	t(8:12)(q24:q22)	B-cell chronic lymphocytic	MYC-HLH domain

Abbreviations: IG, immunoglobulin; TCR, T-cell receptor; HLH, helix-loop-helix structural domain; zn, zinc; HMG, high mobility group; H4; ELE1; TPR and 1TFG, partially uncharacterized genes with a dimerizing coiled-coil domain; RIa, regulatory subunit of PKA enzyme; TPM3, isoform of nonmuscle tropomyosin.

some cases, the same proto-oncogene is involved in several different translocations (ie, c-*myc*, *ews*, and *ret*).

Gene Activation ■ The t(8;14)(q24;q32) translocation, found in about 85% of cases of Burkitt's lymphoma, is a well-characterized example of the transcriptional activation of a proto-oncogene. This chromosomal rearrangement places the c-*myc* gene, located at chromosome band 8q24, under control of regulatory elements from the immunoglobulin heavy-chain locus located at 14q32.[140] The resulting transcriptional activation of c-*myc*, which encodes a nuclear protein involved in the regulation of cell proliferation, plays a critical role in the development of Burkitt's lymphoma.[141] The c-*myc* gene is also activated in some cases of Burkitt's lymphoma by translocations involving immunoglobulin light-chain genes.[142,143] These are t(2;8)(p12;q24), involving the κ locus located at 2p12, and t(8;22)(q24;q11), involving the λ locus at 22q11 (Fig. 6-9). Although the position of the chromosomal breakpoints relative to the c-*myc* gene may vary considerably in individual cases of Burkitt's lymphoma, the consequence of the translocations is the same—deregulation of c-*myc* expression, leading to uncontrolled cellular proliferation. Moreover, again in lymphoma, c-*myc* gene mutations can occur in the gene transactivation domain and in the coding region after translocation into the *Ig* gene.[144] Mutations can occur in the noncoding gene exon 1 and at the exon 1/intron 1 boundary with or without c-*myc* gene translocation.[144] This region is considered the c-*myc* regulatory region and is responsible for its mRNA stability. In Burkitt's lymphoma, mutations frequently occur at sites of phosphorylation, a finding that suggests that they may have a pathogenetic role.

In some cases of T-cell ALL (T-ALL), the c-*myc* gene is activated by the t(8;14)(q24;q11) translocation. In these cases, transcription of c-*myc* is placed under the control of regulatory elements within the T-cell receptor a locus located at 14q11.[145] In addition to c-*myc*, several proto-oncogenes that encode nuclear proteins are activated by various chromosomal translocations in T-ALL involving the T-cell receptor a or β locus. These include *HOX11*, *TAL1*, *TAL2*, and *RBTN1/Tgt1*.[146-148] The proteins encoded by these genes are thought to function as transcription factors through DNA-binding and protein-protein interactions. Overexpression or inappropriate expression of these proteins in T-cells is thought to inhibit T-cell differentiation and lead to uncontrolled cellular proliferation.

A number of other proto-oncogenes are also activated by chromosomal translocations in leukemia and lymphoma. In most follicular lymphomas and some large cell lymphomas, the *bcl-2* gene (located at 18q21) is activated as a consequence of t(14;18)(q32;q21) translocations.[149,150] Overexpression of the bcl-2 protein inhibits apoptosis, leading to an imbalance between lymphocyte proliferation and programmed cell death.[151] Mantle cell lymphomas are characterized by the t(11;14)(q13;q32) translocation, which activates the cyclin D1 (*bcl-1*) gene located at 11q13.[152,153] cyclin D1 is a G1 cyclin involved in the normal regulation of the cell-cycle. In some cases of T-cell chronic lymphocytic leukemia and prolymphocytic leukemia, the *tcl-1* gene at 14q32.1 is activated by inversion or translocation involving chromosome 14.[154] The *tcl-1* gene product is a small cytoplasmic protein whose function is not yet known.

Gene Fusion ■ The first example of gene fusion was discovered through the cloning of the breakpoint of the Philadelphia chromosome in CML.[155] The t(9;22)(q34;q11) translocation in CML fuses the c-abl gene, normally located at 9q34, with the *bcr* gene at 22q11 (Fig. 6-10).[156] The *bcr/abl* fusion, created on the der(22) chromosome, encodes a chimeric protein of 210 kD with increased tyrosine kinase activity and abnormal cellular localization.[157] The precise mechanism by which the *bcr/abl* fusion protein contributes to the expansion of the neoplastic myeloid clone is not yet known. The t(9;22) translocation is also found in up to 20% of cases of ALL. In these cases, the breakpoint in the *bcr* gene differs somewhat from that found in CML, resulting in a 185-kD bcr/abl fusion protein.[158] It is unclear at this time why the slightly smaller bcr/abl fusion protein leads to such a large difference in neoplastic phenotype. Inhibition of bcr/abl tyrosine kinase activity has been introduced as a chemotherapeutic approach in patients with CML. Administration of imatinib resulted in an antileukemic effect in CML patients in whom treatment with standard chemotherapy had failed.[159] However, cases of imatinib-resistance have also been recently documented.[160] Cause of such a failure is due to either bcr/abl gene amplification or single amino acid substitutions affecting residues that are in

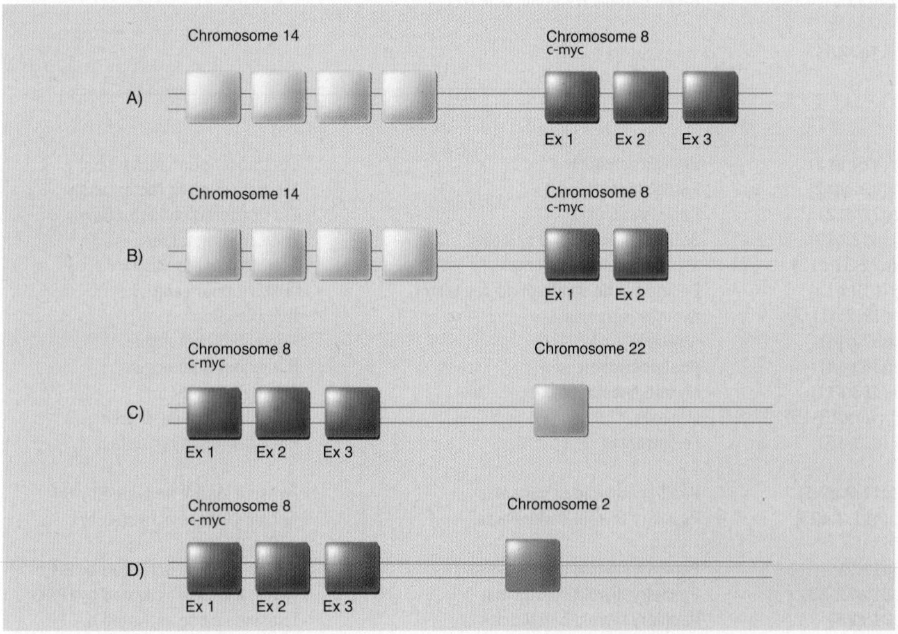

Figure 6-9 ■ c-*myc* translocations found in Burkitt lymphoma. (**A**) t(8;14)(q24;q32) Translocation involving the locus of immunoglobulin heavy chain gene located at 14q32. (**B**) t(8;14)(q24;q32) translocation where only 2 exons of c-myc are translocated under regulatory elements from the immunoglobulin heavy chain locus located at 14q32. (**C**) t(8;22)(q24;q11) translocation involving the *l* locus of immunoglobulin light chain gene at 22q11. (**D**) t(2;8)(p12;q24) translocation involving the *k* locus of immunoglobulin light chain gene located at 2p12.

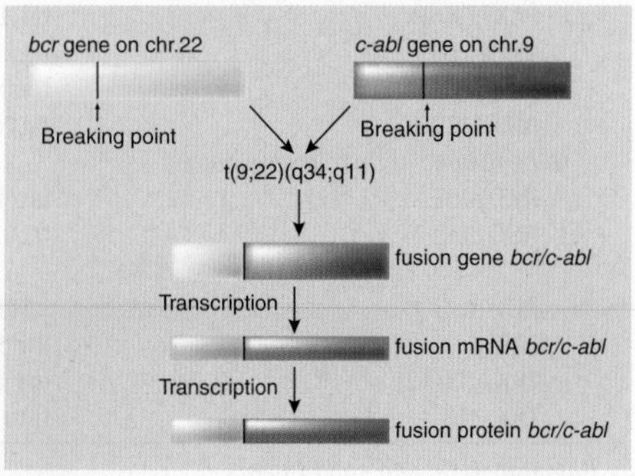

Figure 6-10 ■ Gene fusion. The t(9;22)(q34;q11) translocation in CML determines the fusion of the c-*abl* gene with the *bcr* gene. Such a gene fusion encodes an oncogenic chimeric protein of 210 KD.

direct contact with ATP or are within the ATP pocket of the kinase domain of abl, resulting in structural changes that could influence inhibition sensitivity. Strategies for overcoming resistance have been suggested, exploiting dependence of bcr/abl protein on the molecular chaperone heat shock protein 90.[161]

In addition to *c-abl*, two other genes encoding tyrosine kinases are involved in distinct gene fusion events in hematologic malignancy. The t(2;5)(p23;q35) translocation in anaplastic large cell lymphomas fuses the *NPM* gene (5q35) with the *ALK* gene (2p23).[162] *ALK* encodes a membrane spanning tyrosine kinase similar to members of the insulin growth factor receptor family. The NPM protein is a nucleolar phosphoprotein involved in ribosome assembly. The *NPM/ALK* fusion creates a chimeric oncoprotein in which the ALK tyrosine kinase activity may be constitutively activated. The t(5;12)(q33;p13) translocation, characterized in a case of chronic myelomonocytic leukemia (CMML), fuses the tel gene (12p13) with the tyrosine kinase domain of the platelet-derived growth factor receptor *b* gene (PDGFR-b at 5q33).[163] The tel gene is thought to encode a nuclear DNA-binding protein similar to those of the ets family of proto-oncogenes.

Gene fusions sometimes lead to the formation of chimeric transcription factors.[78,137] The t(1;19)(q23;p13) translocation, found in childhood pre-B-cell ALL, fuses the *E2A* transcription factor gene (19p13) with the *PBX1* homeodomain gene (1q23).[164] The E2A/PBX1 fusion protein consists of the amino-terminal transactivation domain of the E2A protein and the DNA-binding homeodomain of the PBX1 protein. The t(15;17)(q22;q21) translocation in acute promyelocytic leukemia fuses the *PML* gene (15q22) with the *RARA* gene at 17q21.[165] The PML protein contains a zinc-binding domain called a RING finger that may be involved in protein-protein interactions. *RARA* encodes the retinoic acid alpha-receptor protein, a member of the nuclear steroid/thyroid hormone receptor superfamily. Although retinoic acid binding is retained in the fusion protein, the *PML/RARA* fusion protein may confer altered DNA-binding specificity to the RARA ligand complex.[166] Leukemia patients with the *PML/RARA* gene fusion respond well to retinoid treatment. In these cases, treatment with all-trans retinoic acid induces differentiation of promyelocytic leukemia cells.

The *ALL1* gene, located at chromosome band 11q23, is involved in approximately 5% to 10% of acute leukemia cases overall in children and adults.[167,168] These include cases of ALL, AML, and leukemias of mixed cell lineage. Among leukemia genes, *ALL1* (also called *MLL* and *HRX*) is unique because it participates in fusions with a large number of different partner genes on the various chromosomes. Over 20 different reciprocal translocations involving the *ALL1* gene at 11q23 have been reported, the most common of which are those involving chromosomes 4, 6, 9, and 19.[169] In approximately 5% of cases of acute leukemia in adults, the *ALL1* gene is fused with a portion of itself.[170] This special type of gene fusion is called self-fusion.[171] Self-fusion of the *ALL1* gene, which is thought to occur through a somatic recombination mechanism, is found in high incidence in acute leukemias with trisomy 11 as a sole cytogenetic abnormality. The *ALL1* gene encodes a large protein with DNA-binding motifs, a transactivation domain, and a region with homology to the *Drosophila trithorax* protein (a regulator of homeotic gene expression).[172,173] The various partners in *ALL1* fusions encode a diverse group of proteins, some of which appear to be nuclear proteins with DNA-binding motifs.[174,175] The ALL1 fusion protein consists of the amino terminus of ALL1 and the carboxyl terminus of one of a variety of fusion partners. It appears that the critical feature in all ALL1 fusions, including self-fusion, is the uncoupling of the ALL1 amino-terminal domains from the remainder of the ALL1 protein.

Solid tumors, especially sarcomas, sometimes have consistent chromosomal translocations that correlate with specific histological types of tumors.[176] In general, translocations in solid tumors result in gene fusions that encode chimeric oncoproteins. Studies thus far indicate that in sarcomas, the majority of genes fused by translocations encode transcription factors.[177] In myxoid liposarcomas, the t(12;16)(q13;p11) fuses the *FUS* (*TLS*) gene at 16p11 with the *CHOP* gene at 12q13.[178] The FUS protein contains a transactivation domain that is contributed to the FUS/CHOP fusion protein. The CHOP protein, which is a dominant inhibitor of transcription, contributes a protein-binding domain and a presumptive DNA-binding domain to the fusion. Despite knowledge of these structural features, the mechanism of action of the FUS/CHOP oncoprotein is not yet known. A variant transcript, consisting of exons 1 to10 of EWS and exons 2 to 4 of *CHOP*, was recently described.[179] In Ewing's sarcoma, the t(11;22)(q24;q12), fuses the *EWS* gene at 22q12 with the *FLI1* gene at 11q24.[180] Like FUS, the EWS protein contains three glycine-rich segments and an RNA-binding domain. The FLI1 protein contains an ets-like DNA-binding domain. The EWS/FLI1 fusion protein combines a transactivation domain from EWS with the DNA-binding domain of FLI1. In alveolar rhabdomyosarcoma, the t(2;13)(q35;q14) fuses the *PAX3* gene at 2q35 with the *FKHR* gene at 13q14.[181] The PAX3 protein, a transcription factor that activates genes involved in development, is a paired-box homeodomain protein with two distinct DNA-binding domains. The FKHR protein encodes a conserved DNA-binding motif (the fork head domain) similar to that first identified in the *Drosophila* fork head homeotic gene. The PAX3/FKHR fusion protein is a chimeric transcription factor containing the PAX3 DNA-binding domains, a truncated fork head domain, and the carboxy-terminal FKHR regions.

In DP, an infiltrating skin tumor, both a reciprocal translocation t(17;22)(q22;q13) and supernumerary ring chromosomes derived from the t(17;22), have been described.

Although early successful studies in this field have been performed with lymphomas and leukemia, as we have discussed before, the first chromosomal abnormality in solid tumors to be characterized at the molecular level as a fusion protein was an inversion of chromosome 10 found in papillary thyroid carcinomas.[182] In this tumor, two main recurrent structural changes have been described, including inv(10) (q112.2; q21.2), as the more frequent alteration, and a t(10;17)(q11.2; q23). These two abnormalities represent the cytogenetic mechanisms which activate the proto-oncogene *ret* on chromosome 10, forming the oncogenes ret/ptc1 and RET/ptc2, respectively. Moreover, other chromosomal rearrangements leading to ret activation were recently described. The *ret/ptc3* and *ret/ptc4* oncogenes are generated by the fusion of the tyrosine kinase domain of ret and a gene named *ELE1a-ARA70* (or *RFG*), located in the same region 10q11.2.[183,184] In this case a paracentric inversion of the long arm of chromosome 10 occurs. Translocations of *ret/ptc4* are very frequent events in thyroid cancerogenesis of children of the Chernobyl-contaminated areas. That accident led to the occurrence of new forms of ret rearrangements in papillary thyroid cancers, named *ret/ptc5-9*, *ret/PCM1*, and *ELKS/ret*. For instance, ret/ptc5 fusion partner protein is a coiled-coil protein expressed on the Golgi surface. The fusion partner proteins *ret/ptc6* and 7 display rearrangements with the transcriptional intermediary factor 1-alpha and gamma, respectively. RET/ptc8 fusion partner protein is kinectin, whereas in *ret/ptc9* ret rearranges with a putative cytoplasmic protein possibly involved in intracellular-transport processes. *ret/PCM1* lead to a centrosomal protein production, displaying distinct cell-cycle distribution. The *ELKS/ret* oncogene is retrotranscribed into an ubiquitously expressed mRNA with unknown function.[185-190] Virtually all breakpoints in the *RET* gene occur within intron 11, leading intact the tyrosine kinase domain of the receptor and enabling the *RET/PTC* oncoprotein to bind to SHC via Y1062 and activate the downstream cascade 191. Somatic chromosomal rearrangements involving the *RET* gene represent the most frequent genetic alteration in PTC, although wide variations in frequency ranging from 5% to 70% have been observed in different geographic areas.[192] Recent results suggest that a broad variability in the reported prevalence of RET/PTC rearrangements is at least in part a result of the use of different detection methods and tumor genetic heterogeneity.[193] Alterations of chromosome 1 in the same tumor type have then been associated to the activation of NTRK1 (chromosome 1), an NGF receptor, which, like *RET*, forms chimeric fusion oncogenic proteins in papillary thyroid carcinomas.[194] A comparative analysis of the oncogenes originated from the activation of these two tyrosine kinase receptors has allowed the identification and characterization of common cytogenetic and molecular mechanisms of their activation. In all cases, chromosomal rearrangements fuse the tk portion of the two receptors to the 5′ end of different genes that, because of their general effect, have been designated as "activating genes." In the majority of cases, the latter belong to the same chromosome where the related receptor is located, 10 for RET and 1 for NTRK1.

Furthermore, although functionally different, the various activating genes share the following three properties:

1. They are ubiquitously expressed.
2. They display domains demonstrated or predicted to be able to form dimers or multimers.
3. They translocate the tk-receptor-associated enzymatic activity from the membrane to the cytoplasm.

These characteristics can explain the mechanism(s) of oncogenic activation of *ret* and *NTRK1* proto-oncogenes. In fact, following the fusion of their tk domain to the activating gene (1) *ret* and *NTRK1*, whose tissue-specific expression is restricted to subsets of neural cells, become expressed in the epithelial thyroid cells; (2) their dimerization triggers a constitutive, ligand-independent trans-autophosphorylation of the cytoplasmic domains and, as a consequence, the latter can recruit SH2- and SH3-containing cytoplasmic effector proteins, such as Shc and Grb2 or phospholipase C gamma (PLC.), thus inducing a constitutive mitogenic pathway; and (3) the relocalization in the cytoplasm of *ret* and *NTRK1* enzymatic activity could allow their interaction with unusual substrates, perhaps modifying their functional properties.

In conclusion, in PTCs, the oncogenic activation of ret and NTRK1 proto-oncogenes following chromosomal rearrangements occurring in breakpoint cluster regions of both proto-oncogenes could be defined as an ectopic, constitutive, and topologically abnormal expression of their associated enzymatic (tk) activity.[195] RET rearrangements are mutually exclusive with NTRK1 rearrangements and BRAF mutations and show similar but distinct gene expression patterns in papillary thyroid carcinomas.[100] Overall, papillary carcinomas with RET/PTC rearrangements typically present at younger age and have a high rate if lymph-node metastases, clinical papillary histology, and possibly more favourable prognosis.[191]

Protein Overexpression and Constitutive Phosphorylation

Protein overexpression refers to a general deregulation driven by a mechanism not understood or not investigated. An example is Akt, three serine-threonine kinases that represent major effectors-mediating survival signal. Generally, Akt proteins possess six sites of phosphorylation: Ser124 and Thr450 are basally phosphorylated, Tyr315 and Tyr316 depend on Src, Thr308 represents the major site of regulation and is phosphorylated by 3-phosphoinositides-dependent protein kinase 1 (PDK1), Ser473 is only required for maximal Akt activity but the mechanism by which it is phosphorylated remains controversial. Akt is phosphorylated and therefore activated after cell stimulation from different growth factors and from a series of interleukins, while its action is inhibited by PTEN, which dephosphorylates PIP3 and PIP2. Once activated, Akt dissociates from the plasma membrane and translocates to both the cytoplasm and the nucleus. Akt inhibits directly, through phosphorylation of Bad and caspase-9, indirectly, by inducing de novo gene expression of IKK protein kinase and transcription factors. Akt determines cell survival also by virtue of its involvement in cell-cycle progression.[196] Analyses of tissue specimens pointed out that the protein encoded by Akt3 is overexpressed in poorly differentiated breast and prostate cancers and may contribute to the progression of sporadic melanoma.[197] Akt1 is especially involved in the pathogenesis of sporadic thyroid cancer, whereas Akt2 seems to be the isoform which plays a pivotal role in several human tumors such as ovarian, pancreatic, thyroid and colorectal cancer.[197,196] A specific role for Akt3 in the genesis of ovarian cancer has been recently proposed, focused on the modulation of G2-M phase transition.[198] Akt activation is related to worse prognosis in several tumors, including oral squamous cell carcinoma, non-small-cell lung cancers, colorectal, ovarian, breast, follicular thyroid, endometrial, prostate and pancreatic cancers.[199-201] Mutations in Akt genes are rare. In a screening of 294 cancer tissues, only Akt2 was detected with point mutations in 2% of gastric carcinomas and in 2.5% of lung cancers.[202] Recently a novel E17K mutation occurring in the Akt1 has been found at low frequency in breast, colorectal and ovarian cancers.[203]

New Markers from Large-Scale Genomic Analysis

Kinases

A recent analysis organized the protein kinase complement of the human genome (the so-called "kinome") into a dendrogram containing nine broad groups of genes.[204] Using high-throughput sequencing technologies and bioinformatics from the human genome project, one major branch of the histogram, containing three of the nine major groups, was selected for mutational analysis. The selected groups included the 90 tyrosine kinase genes (TK group), the 43 tyrosine kinase-like genes (TKL group), and the 5 receptor guanylate cyclase genes (RGC group). The analysis took into consideration all exons encoding their predicted kinase domains in 35 colorectal cancer cell lines and in 147 colorectal specimens.[205] Thirty-five different types of somatic mutations were identified in 7 genes (*NTRK3, FES, KDR, EPHA3, NTRK2* belonging to the TK group, *MLK4* to *TKL* and *GUCY2F* to *RGC*) and the data suggest that a minimum of 30% of colorectal cancers contain at least one mutation in the tyrosine kinome, whose members represent an attractive target for chemotherapeutic intervention.[205]

Phosphatases

The protein tyrosine phosphatases (PTPs), gene superfamily (the so-called "phosphatome") is composed of three main families: (1) the classic PTPs, including the receptor PTPs (RPTPs) and the nonreceptor PTPs (NRPTPs); (2) the dual specificity phosphatases (DSPs), which can dephosphorylate serine and threonine in addition to tyrosine residues; and (3) the low molecular weight phosphatases (LMPs).[206] Using high-throughput technologies, a mutational analysis of all the coding exons of 53 classic PTPs (21 RPTPs and 32 NRPTPs), 32 DSPs and 1 LMP was performed in 175 colorectal cancers.[9] Six genes containing somatic mutations were identified, including three members of the RPTP subfamily (*PTPRF, PTPRG,* and *PTPRT*), and three members of the NRPTP subfamily

(*PTPN3*, *PTPN13*, and *PTPN14*). Overall, 77 mutations were identified, in aggregate, affecting 26% of colorectal tumors analyzed. The great majority of the mutations would result in proteins devoid of phosphatase catalytic activity.[9] The identification of protein phosphatases mutated could lead to reactivation of their activity through new targeted pharmacologic treatments or, better, inactivate the corresponding kinases that phosphorylate substrates normally regulated by the mutant phosphatases.

PI3K Isoforms

Phosphatidylinositol 3-kinases (PI3K) belong to the lipid kinase family that regulate signal transduction.[207] Hidden Markov models identified eight *PI3K* and *PI3K*like genes, including two uncharacterized genes, in the human genome. By the analysis of the predicted kinase domains of these genes in 234 colorectal cancers, it has been found that *PIK3CA* was the only gene with somatic mutations,[10] which affect 32% of colorectal cancers. A *PIK3CA* mutation was also observed in a very advanced tubulovillous adenoma greater than 5 cm in diameter, suggesting that *PIK3CA* mutations arise late in colorectal tumorigenesis. Hyperactivating *PIK3CA* mutations were also identified in several cancers from colon, lung, ovaries, liver, brain, stomach and breast.[208] In breast carcinomas, *PIK3CA* mutations, especially those at exon 9, occur in about half of lobular carcinomas.[209] In colorectal cancers, *PIK3CA* mutations display a gender bias occurring at higher frequencies in women. This is specifically observed in colorectal cancer, because in breast cancers male display *PIK3CA* mutations at an overall frequency similar to that observed in female. Therefore it seems that *PIK3CA* mutations display gender- and tissue-specific patterns.[210] The analysis of *PIK3CA* mutations in patients affected by hereditary colorectal cancers revealed alteration in 21% of FAP invasive carcinomas, in 21% of HNPCC invasive carcinomas and in 15% of sporadic invasive carcinomas, thus demonstrating that *PIK3CA* mutations are involved in both type of familial colorectal carcinogenesis (FAP and HNPCC) without an evident segregation (at odds with BRAF), and with a similar extent that seen in sporadic patients.[211] Moreover, the clustering of mutations in exon 9 (regulatory region) and 20 (catalytic domain) in the *PIK3CA* gene makes the gene an excellent marker for early detection of cancer or for monitoring tumor progression. In addition to point mutations, PIK3CA may be altered through gene amplification. For example, this type of PIK3CA activation is observed in ovarian cancer, where it is associated with early tumor-associated death.[212] Finally, in addition to their role in cancer, oncogenic *PIK3CA* mutations contribute to the pathogenesis of skin tumors lacking malignant potential, including epidermal nevi and seborrheic keratoses.[213]

Oncogenes in the Initiation and Progression of Neoplasia

Human neoplasia is a complex multistep process involving sequential alterations in proto-oncogenes (activation) and in tumor suppressor genes (inactivation). Statistical analysis of the age incidence of human solid tumors indicates that five or six independent mutational events may contribute to tumor formation.[214] In human leukemias, only three or four mutational events may be necessary, presumably involving different genes.

The study of chemical carcinogenesis in animals provides a foundation for our understanding of the multistep nature of cancer.[215] In the mouse model of skin carcinogenesis, tumor formation involves three phases, termed *initiation*, *promotion*, and *progression*. Initiation of skin tumors can be induced by chemical mutagens such as 7,12-dimethyl-benzanthracene (DMBA) (Fig. 6-11). After application of DMBA, the mouse skin appears normal. If the skin is then continuously treated with a promoter, such as the phorbol ester TPA, precancerous papillomas will form. Chemical promoters such as TPA stimulate growth but are not mutagenic substances. Over a period of months of continuous application of the promoting agent, some of the papillomas will progress to skin carcinomas. Treatment with DMBA or TPA alone does not cause skin cancer. Mouse papillomas initiated with DMBA usually have H-*ras* oncogenes with a specific mutation in codon 61 of the H-*ras* gene. The mouse skin tumor model indicates that initiation of papillomas is the result of mutation of the H-*ras* gene in individual skin cells by the chemical mutagen DMBA. For papillomas to appear on the skin, however, growth of mutated cells must be continuously stimulated by a promoting agent. Additional unidentified genetic changes must then occur for papillomas to progress to carcinoma.

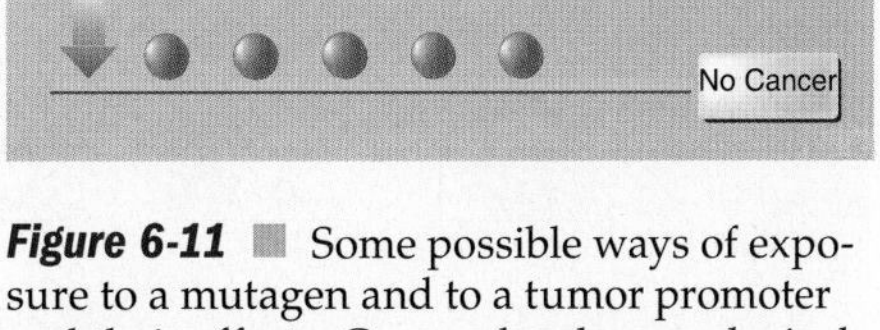

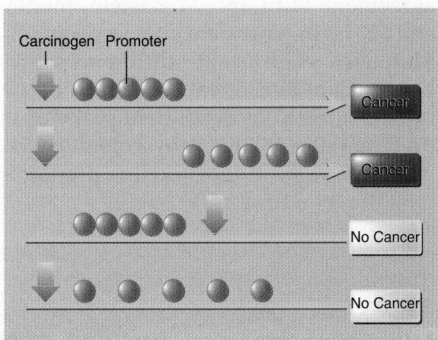

Figure 6-11 Some possible ways of exposure to a mutagen and to a tumor promoter and their effects. Cancer develops exclusively when the exposure to promoter follows the exposure to carcinogen (mutagen, eg, 7,12-dimethyl-benzanthracene) and only when the intensity of the exposure to promoter is higher than a threshold.

Although a single oncogene is sufficient to cause tumor formation by some rapidly transforming retroviruses such as RSV, transformation by a single oncogene is not usually seen in experimental models of cancer. Other rapidly transforming retroviruses carry two different oncogenes that cooperate in producing the neoplastic phenotype. One well-characterized example of this type of cooperation is the avian erythroblastosis virus, which carries the *erb A* and *erb B* oncogenes.[216] Cooperation between oncogenes can also be demonstrated by in vitro transformation studies using nonimmortalized cell lines. For example, studies have shown cooperation between the nuclear myc protein and the cytoplasmic-membrane-associated ras protein in the transformation of rat embryo fibroblasts.[217] As previously reported, a cooperation between SV40 large T product and mutated H-*ras* gene also has been found necessary to transform normal human epithelial and fibroblast cells, provided that they constitutively expressed the catalytic subunit of telomerase enzyme, indicating a more complex pattern in the neoplastic conversion of human cells.

Collaboration between two different general categories of oncogenes (eg, nuclear and cytoplasmic) can often be demonstrated but is not strictly required for transformation.[218] These transgenic mice strains, in fact, generally show an increased incidence of neoplasia and the tumors that result frequently are clonal, implying that other events are necessary. The production of transgenic mice expressing a single oncogene such as myc has also demonstrated that multiple genetic changes are necessary for tumor formation.[219] (For a review on the mouse model of cancer, see *Oncogene*, Vol. 18, issue 2, N. 38, September 1999.)

Cytogenetic studies of the clonal evolution of human hematologic malignancies have provided much insight into the multiple steps involved in the initiation and progression of human tumors.[220] The evolution of CML from chronic phase to acute leukemia is characterized by an accumulation of genetic changes seen in the karyotypes of the evolving malignant clones. The early chronic phase of CML is defined by the presence of a single Philadelphia chromosome. The formation of the *bcr/abl* gene fusion as a consequence of the t(9;22) translocation is thought to be the initiating event in CML.[156] The biologic progression of CML to a more malignant phenotype corresponds with the appearance of additional cytogenetic abnormalities such as a second Philadelphia chromosome, isochromosome 17, or trisomy 8.[221] These karyotypic changes are thought to reflect additional genetic changes involving an increase in oncogene dosage and loss or inactivation of tumor suppressor genes. Although the karyotypic changes in evolving CML are somewhat variable from patient to patient, the accumulation of genetic changes always correlates with progression from differentiated cells of low malignancy to undifferentiated cells of high malignancy.

The initiation and progression of human neoplasia involve the activation of oncogenes and the inactivation or loss of tumor suppressor genes. The mechanisms of oncogene activation and the time course of events, however, vary among different types of tumors. In hematologic malignancies, soft-tissue sarcomas, and the papillary type of thyroid carcinomas, initiation of the malignant process predominantly involves chromosomal rearrangements that activate various oncogenes.[137] Many of the chromosomal rearrangements in leukemia and lymphoma are thought to result from errors in the physiologic process of immunoglobulin or T-cell receptor gene rearrangement during normal B-cell and T-cell development. Late events in the progression of hematologic malignancies involve oncogene mutation, mainly of the *ras* family, inactivation of tumor suppressor genes such as *TP53*, and sometimes additional chromosomal translocations.[222]

In lung cancers, the initiation of neoplasia has been shown to involve oncogene and tumor suppressor gene mutations. These mutations are generally thought to result from chemical carcinogenesis, especially in the case of tobacco-related lung cancer, where a novel tumor suppressor gene (designated *FHIT*) has been found to be inactivated in the majority of cancers, particularly in those from smokers.[223,224] Later, K-*ras* (especially in the adenocarcinoma subtype) and *TP53* alterations drive the malignant transformation of lung cancer.[225]

As far as colorectal cancer is concerned, intensive screening for genetic alteration led to the identification of two major types of colorectal cancer that are distinct by their carcinogenic process. One is characterized by normal karyotype, normal DNA index,[226] and genetic instability at microsatellite loci (MSI) and was called RER-positive tumor for replicative error-positive phenotype and now is called MSI-positive cancer.[227] The second one is represented by alterations of *APC*, K-*ras* and *TP53* genes and genetic losses at microsatellite loci.[228] The second type led to the association between the stepwise progression from normal to dysplastic epithelium to carcinoma and the accumulation of multiple clonally selected genetic alterations. This model, first proposed by Vogelstein in 1990,[229] suggests that APC (or, better, the APC-β-catenin pathway) represents the initial mutational event that determines hyperplastic proliferation and then early adenoma formation. The stage of late adenoma is achieved with K-ras protein stabilization. Loss of tumor suppressor genes at chromosome 18q (such as *DCC*) and mutations in the *TP53* gene lead to carcinoma in situ formation (Fig. 6-12). However, this stepwise model of colorectal tumorigenesis has been mainly validated conceptually, and there is mounting evidence that alternative genetic events may occur during colorectal carcinogenesis, sometimes preferentially, sometimes randomly, sometimes with an overlap.[227] An extensive analysis of the four molecular markers showed a wide spectrum of combination of mutations with a prevalence of two pathways, which cumulatively encompass about 40% of analyzed cases: the *APCK-Ras-TP53-DCC* and the *APC-TP53-DCC* pathway. These results strongly support the existence of two preferential pathways followed by sporadic colorectal cancer with microsatellite stability: a K-*ras* dependent, in agreement with the Vogelstein model, and a K-*ras* independent one, respectively. Moreover, significant differences between colon and rectal tumors could be outlined: the K-*ras* dependent pathway is preferentially followed by colon cancer, while the K-*ras* independent is predominant in rectal tumors.[230]

In melanoma, *BRAF* mutations occur in the vast majority of cases and represent a very early event, since they were also detected in prenoeplastic lesions such as nevi besides Spitz and Blue nevi.[7,108]

Gene amplification is often seen in the progression of some carcinomas and other types of tumors. Amplification of the *erb B2* oncogene may be a late event in the progression of breast cancer.[135] Members of the *myc* oncogene family are frequently amplified in small-cell carcinoma of the lung.[119] As mentioned previously, amplification of N-*myc* strongly correlates with the progression and clinical stage of neuroblastoma.[118] Although there is variability in the pathways of human tumor initiation and progression, studies of various types of malignancy have clearly confirmed the multistep nature of human cancer.

Oncogenes as Target of New Drugs

Several oncogenes act in key points of cell life. Most of them, in fact, codify for growth factor receptor, or are involved in the signal transduction. Therefore, they represent a natural target for the development of new drugs, that are able to block selectively the cells carrying a deregulation in the drug target. Here are summarized the new insights in targeted therapies.

ERB B2

ERB B2 gene amplification occur in a consistent fraction of breast cancers. An antibody (trastuzumab) against erb B2 receptor has entered clinical practice, with evident benefit for patients. Trastuzumab is indicated for patients affected by a metastatic breast cancer, but it is now under evaluation the possibility to administer the drug also in adjuvant therapy. Unfortunately, not all patients showing *erb B2* gene amplification may benefit from trastuzumab administration. This is probably due to the deregulation of *erb B2* downstream members. Indeed, at preclinical level, it has been demonstrated that activating point mutations in the *PIK3CA* gene as well as the

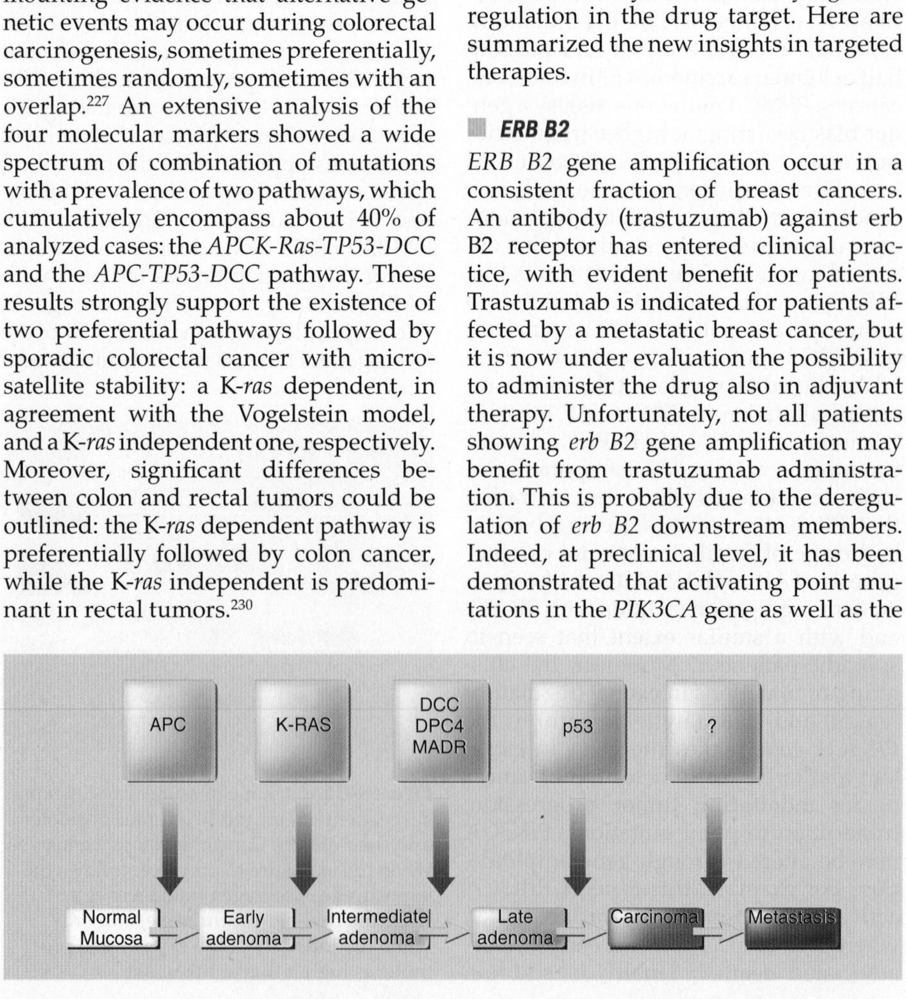

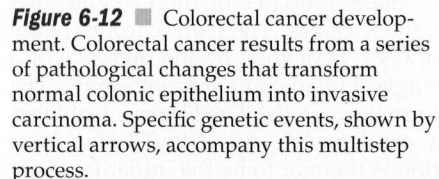

Figure 6-12 Colorectal cancer development. Colorectal cancer results from a series of pathological changes that transform normal colonic epithelium into invasive carcinoma. Specific genetic events, shown by vertical arrows, accompany this multistep process.

loss of expression of PTEN protein lead to trastuzumab resistance.[248]

ERB B1

ERB B1 codify for a receptor tyrosine kinase playing an important role in cancer cell proliferation, angiogenesis and metastasis. Therefore, targeting erb B1 is a valuable molecular approach in cancer therapy. Two classes of erb B1 antagonists have been successfully tested in phase III trials and are now in clinical use: monoclonal antibodies and small-molecule tyrosine kinase inhibitors. Monoclonal antibodies, represented by cetuximab and panitumumab, are able to bind to the extracellular domain of the receptor when it is in the inactive configuration, compete for receptor binding by occluding the ligand-ligand region, and thereby block ligand-induced tyrosine kinase of the receptor. Small-molecule tyrosine kinase inhibitors, represented by gefitinib and erlotinib, compete reversibly with ATP to bind to the intracellular catalytic domain of the receptor and, therefore, inhibit receptor autophosphorylation and downstream signaling.[136]

In non-small-cell lung cancer, only 10 to 20% of patients have a partial response to gefitinib/erlotinib. Several retrospective and prospective studies confirmed that patients carrying an *EGFR* mutation were particularly sensitive to gefitinib/erlotinib, with a response rate up to 80% of mutated patients. Many types of mutations in the erb B1 have been reported, but so far only four drug-sensitive mutations have been validated, including exon 19 deletion, exon 21 L858R substitution, exon 18 (G719A/C) and exon 21 L861Q) substitutions. In addition, erb B1 gene copy number gain (chromosome 7 high polysomy or gene amplification) is emerging as another relevant method for patient selection.[231] Patients characteristics associated with increased responsiveness to gefitinib/erlotinib are never smoking history, Asian ethnicity, female gender, and adenocarcinoma histology. Intrinsic resistance to these drugs is due to the presence of alterations occurring at downstream members of *erb B1* receptor, typically represented by point mutations of K-*ras* gene. Acquisition of drug resistance in patients initially responsive to gefitinib/erlotinib has been linked to a specific secondary somatic mutation *T790M* occurring in the *erb B1* gene.[231] Novel inhibitors are currently under evaluation to specifically act against the *T790M* mutation.[232]

Clinical management of advanced colorectal cancer by the class of monoclonal antibodies represents very promising targeted compounds. Cetuximab or panitumumab monotherapy are associated with response rates of 9-12%, that increase to 20% when the drugs are used in combination with irinotecan in patients who had not had a response to previous therapy with irinotecan. A patient with advanced colorectal cancer must show EGFR overexpression in the primary tumor, as detected by immunohistochemistry, to be eligible for the treatment. Such a methodology, however, does not seem to represent the gold standard to evaluate *erb B1* alterations. On the contrary, recent data indicate that the assessment of *erb B1* gene copy number could be a promising approach to predict the efficacy of monoclonal antibodies against *erb B1*. In addition, the detection of gene or protein alterations of *erb B1* downstream members, such as K-*ras* or *BRAF* point mutations, and the loss of expression of PTEN protein, clearly predict the resistance to cetuximab/panitumumab.[233]

Cetuximab and panitumumab are effective also in 10-13% of patients affected by head and neck squamous cell carcinoma, but in this case the analysis of erb B1 and its downstream members has not been accomplished yet.[234]

KIT-pdgfra

Of great relevance, it has been recently demonstrated that imatinib, an inhibitor of tyrosine kinase activity in bcr-abl-positive leukemia was effective in treating GIST (Fig. 6-13). In this pathology, kit and pdgfra mutational status predicts for the likelihood of achieving response to targeted drug. Patients with an exon 11 kit mutation have a partial response rate up to 85-90%, while those with an exon 9 kit mutation have a partial response rate of around 50%. Patients who have GIST with kit exon 11 mutation also have longer median time to treatment failure as compared to those with GIST harboring other types of mutations. Patients who have no detectable mutation of kit or pdgfra respond less frequently to imatinib than those with exon 11 mutants, but still up to 39% do respond. The rare patients who have GIST with kit exon 13 or 17 mutation of pdgfra mutation may also respond to imatinib. Taken together, these results suggest that treatment with imatinib should be considered for virtually all patients who present with metastatic GIST regardless of the mutational status of the tumour. The rare patients who have GIST with a mutation known to be resistant to imatinib, such as pdgfra exon 18 mutation D842V, may be the only exception to this rule. Interestingly, the pdgfra exon 18 D842V mutation is functionally equivalent to the kit exon 17 D816V mutation, that has never been found in GIST.[63] On the contrary, the kit exon 17 D816V mutation is observed in leukemia, where it confers resistance to imatinib treatment. A majority of patients with a GIST metastatic disease ultimately cease to respond to imatinib. The reasons for failure usually include secondary mutations at the ATP/imatinib binding pocket (exon 13 or exon 14) or in the activation loop (exon 17) of the kit protein kinase that prohibit imatinib binding. Patients who progress despite imatinib dose escalation are candidates for a trial with other tyrosine kinase inhibitors. Sunitinib (SU11248) is an inhibitor of kit, pdgfra, fms-like tyrosine kinase-3 and vascular epidermal growth factor receptor-2, and has been approved by the Food and Drug Administration for the treatment of GIST patients whose disease has progressed on imatinib or are unable to tolerate treatment with imatinib.

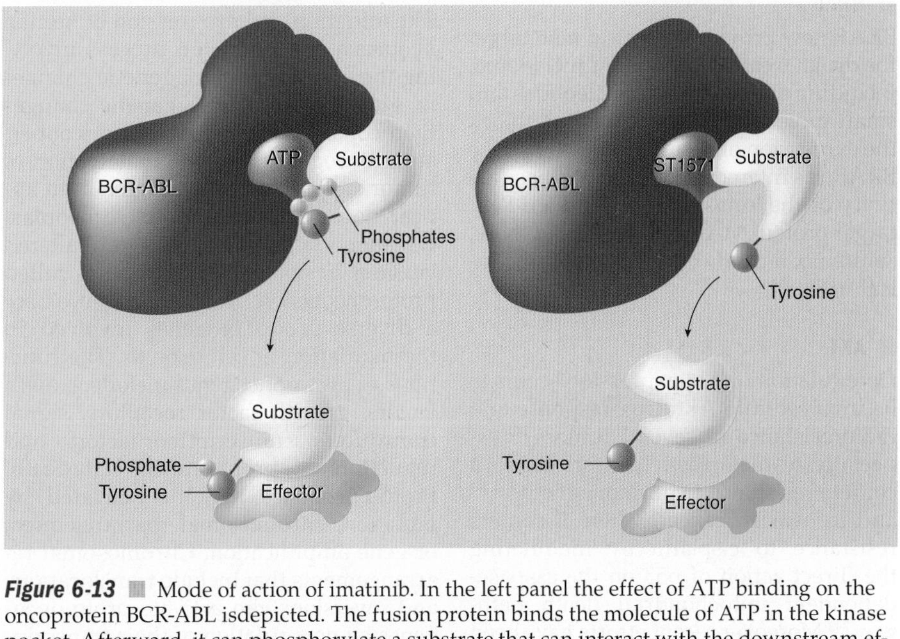

Figure 6-13 Mode of action of imatinib. In the left panel the effect of ATP binding on the oncoprotein BCR-ABL isdepicted. The fusion protein binds the molecule of ATP in the kinase pocket. Afterward, it can phosphorylate a substrate,that can interact with the downstream effector molecules. When imatinib is present (*right panel*), the oncoprotein bindsimatinib in the kinase pocket (competing with ATP) and then the substrate cannot be phosphorylated.

RET

Recently, various kinds of therapeutic approaches, including tyrosine kinase inhibition, gene therapy with dominant negative RET mutants, monoclonal antibodies against oncogenes products, and nuclease-resistant aptamers that recognize and inhibit RET, have been developed. The use of these strategies in preclinical models has provided evidence that RET is indeed a potential target for selective cancer therapy. However, a clinically useful therapeutic option for treating patients with RET-associated cancer is still not available.[235] An anilinoquinazoline, ZD6474, that also possesses an anti-angiogenic effect through VEGFR inhibition, seems to be promising.[191]

RAS

A number of different approaches aimed at abrogating K-*ras* activity have been explored in clinical trials. Usually, the inhibitors directly addressed to K-ras are too toxic for human cells. Currently, the most promising agents are represented by aminobiphosphonates, that have entered clinical practice in the treatment of bone metastases from several neoplasms, including breast and prostate adenocarcinomas.[236]

K-*ras* mutations play also a role in the efficacy of treatment targeted to receptor tyrosine kinase upstream activated, such as EGFR. Indeed, K-*ras* mutations are associated with resistance to EGFR inhibitors gefitinib and erlotinib in non-small-cell lung cancer[237] and represent an independent predictive and prognostic factor in cetuximab or panitumumab-treated advanced colorectal cancer patients.[233,238]

BRAF

BRAF now provides a critical new target for drugs treating malignant melanoma, including antisense oligonucleotides and small molecules. These inhibitors block the expression of BRAF protein, block the BRAF/ras interaction, block its kinase activity or the kinase activity of the *BRAF* target protein MAP kinase. One of these, sorafenib, recently entered phase III clinical trials.[239]

AKT

Deregulation of Akt expression seems to be involved into Akt drug response and radioresistance in several tumors,[240] especially in metaplastic cancer, where it confers resistance to hormone therapy,[241] and in ovarian cancer, where it confers resistance to cisplatin by modulating the direct action of p53 on the caspase-dependent mitochondrial death pathway.[242] Moreover recent efforts have been made in the development of small-molecule inhibitors that directly bind to Akt, such as triciribine and pyridine derivatives. However several drawbacks have been found because of issues toxicity due to the involvement of Akt in insulin signaling.[197]

PIK3CA

Due to the relevance in carcinogenesis, PIK3CA represents a natural target with specific drugs. Most of these have been developed, but many of these showed high toxicity for human cells. Some of these entered clinical trials.[243] *PIK3CA* mutations are linked, at least at preclinical level, to resistance against cetuximab and trastuzumab in metastatic colorectal and breast cancers, respectively.[244]

BCL-2

Many groups have been working to develop anticancer drugs that block the function of antiapoptotic bcl-2 members, thus favoring cell death. Methods include the downregulation of bcl-2 expression through antisense oligonucleotides, or the use of peptides or small organic molecules to the bcl-2 binding pocket, preventing its sequestration of proapoptotic proteins. One of the most promising aspects of these small-molecule inhibitors in treating cancer is that their targets and mechanisms of action are different from those of cytotoxic drugs and radiation. This makes it feasible to combine small-molecule inhibitors with other treatments, creating a synergistic therapy, without likely development of cross-resistance or increased toxicity.

Summary and Conclusions

The initiation and progression of human neoplasia is a multistep process involving the accumulation of genetic changes in somatic cells. These genetic changes then consist of the activation of cooperating oncogenes and the inactivation of tumor suppressor genes, which both appear necessary for a complete neoplastic phenotype. Oncogenes are altered versions of normal cellular genes called proto-oncogenes. Proto-oncogenes are a diverse group of genes involved in the regulation of cell growth. The functions of proto-oncogenes include growth factors, growth factor receptors, signal transducers, transcription factors, and regulators of programmed cell death. Proto-oncogenes may be activated by mutation, chromosomal rearrangement, or gene amplification. Chromosomal rearrangements that include translocations and inversions can activate proto-oncogenes by deregulation of their transcription (eg, transcriptional activation) or by gene fusion. Tumor suppressor genes, which also participate in the regulation of normal cell growth, are usually inactivated by point mutations or truncation of their protein sequence coupled with the loss of the normal allele.

The discovery of oncogenes represented a breakthrough for our understanding of the molecular and genetic basis of cancer. Oncogenes have also provided important knowledge concerning the regulation of normal cell proliferation, differentiation, and programmed cell death. The identification of oncogene abnormalities has provided tools for the molecular diagnosis and monitoring of cancer. Most important, oncogenes represent potential targets for new types of cancer therapies. The goal of these new drugs will be to kill cancer cells selectively while sparing normal cells. One promising approach entails using specific oncogene targets to trigger programmed cell death. The first example of the accomplishment of such a goal is represented by the inhibition of the tumor specific tyrosine kinase bcr/abl in CML, by imatinib.[245] The same compound has been proven active also in a different tumor type, GIST where it inhibits the tyrosine kinase receptor c-kit[246] and in chordomas, where it switches off the PDGFR.[247] Another example is represented by gefitinib and C-225, which inhibit the intracellular tyrosine kinase and the extracellular domain, respectively, of erb B. Thereafter, a plethora of new targeted drugs has entered clinical trials, with evident benefit for the treatment of several neoplastic disease that were, before targeted therapies development, very hard to be treated and cured. The use of high-throughput technologies for the identification of new oncogenes and the rapidly expanding knowledge of the molecular mechanisms of cancer hold great promise for the development of better combined methods of cancer therapy in the near future.

Selected References

The complete reference list can be found at www.CANCERMEDICINE8.com

2. Bernards R, Weinberg RA. A progression puzzle. *Nature.* 2002;418(6900):823.
5. Butel JS. Viral carcinogenesis: revelation of molecular mechanisms and etiology of human disease. *Carcinogenesis.* 2000;21(3):405–426.
7. Davies H, Bignell GR, Cox C, et al. Mutations of the BRAF gene in human cancer. *Nature.* 2002;417(6892):949–954.
8. Bardelli A, Parsons DW, Silliman N, et al. Mutational analysis of the tyrosine kinome in colorectal cancers. *Science.* 2003;300(5621):949.
9. Wang Z, Shen D, Parsons DW, et al. Mutational analysis of the tyrosine phosphatome in colorectal cancers. *Science.* 2004;304(5674):1164–1166.

11. Vogelstein B, Kinzler KW. Cancer genes and the pathways they control. *Nat Med.* 2004;10(8):789–799.
15. Varmus HE. Form and function of retroviral proviruses. *Science.* 1982;216(4548):812–820.
18. Martin GS. Rous sarcoma virus: a function required for the maintenance of the transformed state. *Nature.* 1970;227(262):1021–1023.
28. Krontiris TG, Cooper GM. Transforming activity of human tumor DNAs. *Proc Natl Acad Sci USA.* 1981;78(2):1181–1184.
30. Perucho M, Goldfarb M, Shimizu K, et al. Human-tumorderived cell lines contain common and different transforming genes. *Cell.* 1981;27(3 Pt 2):467–476.
45. Hanahan D, Weinberg RA. The hallmarks of cancer. *Cell.* 2000;100:57–70.
50. Sporn MB, Roberts AB. Autocrine growth factors and cancer. *Nature.* 1985; 313(6005):745–747.
51. Minoletti F, Miozzo M, Pedeutour F, et al. Involvement of chromosomes 17 and 22 in dermatofibrosarcoma protuberans. *Genes Chrom Cancer.* 1995;13:62–65.
61. Paez JG, Janne PA, Lee JC, et al. EGFR mutations in lung cancer: correlation with clinical response to gefitinib therapy. *Science.* 2004;304(5676):1497–1500.
63. Joensuu H. Gastrointestinal stromal tumor (GIST). *Ann Oncol.* 2006 Sep;17(suppl 10):x280–286.
71. Malumbres M, Barbacid M. RAS oncogenes: the first 30 years. *Nat Rev Cancer.* 2003 Jun;3(6):459–465.
82. Danial NN. BCL-2 family proteins: critical checkpoints of apoptotic cell death. *Clin Cancer Res.* 2007 Dec 15;13(24):7254–7263.
102. Rajagopalan H, Bardelli A, Lengauer C, et al. Tumorigenesis: RAF/RAS oncogenes and mismatch-repair status. *Nature.* 2002;418(6901):934.
110. Santoro M, Melillo RM, Carlomagno F, et al. Minireview: RET: normal and abnormal functions. *Endocrinology.* 2004 Dec;145(12):5448–5451.
111. Cranston AN, Carniti C, Oakhill K, et al. RET is constitutively activated by novel tandem mutations that alter the active site resulting in multiple endocrine neoplasia type 2B. *Cancer Res.* 2006 Oct 15;66(20):10179–10187.
113. Cowell JK. Double minutes and homogeneously staining regions: gene amplification in mammalian cells. *Annu Rev Genet.* 1982;16:21–59.
115. Brison O. Gene amplification and tumor progression. *Biochim Biophys Acta.* 1993;1155(1):25–41.
129. Press MF, Bernstein L, Thomas PA, et al. HER-2/neu gene amplification characterized by fluorescence in situ hybridization: poor prognosis in node-negative breast carcinomas. *J Clin Oncol.* 1997; 15(8):2894–2904.
136. Ciardiello F, Tortora G. EGFR antagonists in cancer treatment. *N Engl J Med.* 2008 Mar 13;358(11):1160–1174.
140. Siebert R, Matthiesen P, Harder S, et al. Application of interphase fluorescence in situ hybridization for the detection of the Burkitt translocation t(8;14)(q24;q32) in B-cell lymphomas. *Blood.* 1998;91(3):984–990.
154. Pekarsky Y, Hallas C, Croce CM. Molecular basis of mature T-cell leukemia. *JAMA.* 2001;286(18):2308–2314.
156. Shtivelman E, Lifshitz B, Gale RP, Canaani E. Fused transcript of abl and bcr genes in chronic myelogenous leukaemia. *Nature.* 1985;315(6020):550–554.
158. Ottmann OG, Druker BJ, Sawyers CL, et al. A phase 2 study of imatinib in patients with relapsed or refractory Philadelphia chromosome-positive acute lymphoid leukemias. *Blood.* 2002;100(6):1965–1971.
162. Duyster J, Bai RY, Morris SW. Translocations involving anaplastic lymphoma kinase (ALK). *Oncogene.* 2001;20(40):5623–5637.
165. Salomoni P, Pandolfi PP. The role of PML in tumor suppression. *Cell.* 2002; 108(2):165–170.
171. Schichman SA, Canaani E, Croce CM. Self-fusion of the ALL1 gene. A new genetic mechanism for acute leukemia. *JAMA.* 1995;273(7):571–576.
177. Barr FG. Gene fusions involving PAX and FOX family members in alveolar rhabdomyosarcoma. *Oncogene.* 2001;20(40):5736–5746.
191. Ciampi R, Nikiforov YE. RET/PTC rearrangements and BRAF mutations in thyroid tumorigenesis. *Endocrinology.* 2007 Mar;148(3):936–941. Epub 2006 Aug 31.
196. Shinohara M, Chung YJ, Saji M, Ringel MD. AKT in thyroid tumorigenesis and progression. *Endocrinology.* 2007 Mar;148(3):942–947. Epub 2006 Aug 31.
197. Amaravadi R, Thompson CB. The survival kinases Akt and Pim as potential pharmacological targets. *J Clin Invest.* 2005 Oct;115(10):2618–2624.
204. Manning G, Whyte DB, Martinez R, et al. The protein kinase complement of the human genome. *Science.* 2002;298(5600):1912–1934.
207. Vivanco I, Sawyers CL. The phosphatidylinositol 3-Kinase AKT pathway in human cancer. *Nat Rev Cancer.* 2002;2(7):489–501.
215. Weinberg RA. Oncogenes and multistep carcinogenesis. In: Weinberg RA, ed. *Oncogenes and the Molecular Origins of Cancer.* New York, NY: Cold Spring Harbor; 1989:307–326.
219. Pelengaris S, Khan M, Evan G. c-MYC: more than just a matter of life and death. *Nat Rev Cancer.* 2002;2(10):764–776.
221. Rowley JD. Chromosome abnormalities in human cancer. In: De Vita VT, Hellman S, Rosenberg SA, eds. *Principles and Practice of Oncology.* Philadelphia: Lippincott; 1989:81–87.
223. Sozzi G, Veronese ML, Negrini M, et al. The FHIT gene at 3p14.2 is abnormal in lung cancer. *Cell.* 1996;85:17–26.
229. Fearon ER, Vogelstein B. A genetic model for colorectal tumorigenesis. *Cell.* 1990;61:759–767.
233. Frattini M, Saletti P, Romagnani E, et al. PTEN loss of expression predicts cetuximab efficacy in metastatic colorectal cancer patients. *Br J Cancer.* 2007 Oct 22;97(8):1139–1145.
240. Bussink J, van der Kogel AJ, Kaanders JH. Activation of the PI3-K/AKT pathway and implications for radioresistance mechanisms in head and neck cancer. *Lancet Oncol.* 2008 Mar;9(3):288–296.
244. Jhawer M, Goel S, Wilson AJ, et al. PIK3CA Mutation/PTEN expression status predicts response of colon cancer cells to the epidermal growth factor receptor inhibitor cetuximab. *Cancer Res.* 2008;68(6):1953–1961.
245. Goldman JM, Melo JV. Targeting the BCR-ABL tyrosine kinase in chronic myeloid leukemia. *N Engl J Med.* 2001; 344(14):1084–1086.
246. Heinrich MC, Blanke CD, Druker BJ, Corless CL. Inhibition of KIT tyrosine kinase activity: a novel molecular approach to the treatment of KIT-positive malignancies. *J Clin Oncol.* 2002;20(6):1692–1703.
247. Casali PG, Messina A, Stacchiotti S, et al. Imatinib mesylate in chordoma. *Cancer.* 2004;101(9):2086–2097.

7 Tumor Suppressor Genes

David Cosgrove, MB, BCh ■ Ben Ho Park, MD, PhD ■ Bert Vogelstein, MD

A genetic basis for the development of cancer has been hypothesized for over a century, supported by familial, epidemiologic, and cytogenetic studies. However, only in the past 35 years has definitive evidence emerged that cancer is a genetic disease. It is now known that cancers arise through a multistage process in which inherited and somatic mutations of cellular genes lead to repeated waves of clonal selection in which cells with the most robust and aggressive growth properties prevail. Two classes of genes, proto-oncogenes and tumor suppressor genes, are primary targets for the mutations, because these genes control the ratio of cell birth and cell death. In all normal tissues of the adult, this ratio is exactly 1.0; mutations increase the ratio. A third class of genes, called genomic stability genes, do not alter the ratio when mutated, but can indirectly contribute to tumorigenesis through an acceleration of mutations in proto-oncogenes and tumor suppressor genes.

The vast majority of the mutations that contribute to the development and behavior of cancer cells are somatic (ie, arising during tumor development) and are present only in the neoplastic cells of the patient. A small fraction of mutations in cancer cells are constitutional and thus present in all somatic cells of affected individuals. Such mutations not only predispose to cancer, but can also be passed on to progeny.

The identification and function of proto-oncogenes and their oncogenic variants are reviewed in other chapters of this book. We provide a brief summary of their general properties as a comparison to tumor suppressor genes. More than 100 different proto-oncogenes have been identified through various experimental strategies. In general, proto-oncogenes have critical roles in a variety of growth regulatory pathways, and their protein products are distributed throughout many subcellular compartments. The mutant alleles present in cancers have sustained gain-of-function alterations resulting from point mutations, chromosomal rearrangements, or gene amplifications of the proto-oncogene sequences. In the overwhelming majority of cancers, mutations in proto-oncogenes arise somatically in the tumor cells, although germline mutations activating the function of the rearranged during transfection (*RET*) gene have been identified in patients with multiple endocrine neoplasia type 2 and in familial medullary thyroid cancer, and germline mutations in the metastasis (*MET*) gene have been identified in hereditary papillary renal cell carcinoma.

Whereas oncogenic alleles harbor activating mutations, tumor suppressor genes are defined by their inactivation in human cancer. As reviewed below, the existence of many tumor suppressor genes has been hypothesized and, thus far, approximately 30 tumor suppressor genes have been described and definitively implicated in cancer development. As in the case of proto-oncogenes, the cellular functions of tumor suppressor genes appear to be diverse.

Defects in genomic stability genes have also been implicated in a broad spectrum of human cancers. Like tumor suppressor genes, the genomic stability genes are inactivated in human cancers. However, unlike the mutations in tumor suppressor genes, mutations in genomic stability genes are much more often inherited in mutant form. For example, inherited mutations in the breast cancer 1 early onset (*BRCA1*) or breast cancer 2 early-onset (*BRCA2*) genes play a key role in hereditary breast and ovarian cancers, but these genes are rarely mutated somatically in nonfamilial forms of breast cancers. Similarly, inherited mutations of nucleotide excision repair (*NER*) genes give rise to xeroderma pigmentosa, but somatic mutations of these genes have only rarely been reported in nonfamilial forms of cancer.

Enormous progress has been made in the identification of inherited and somatic mutations in proto-oncogenes, tumor suppressor genes, and genomic stability genes in human cancers. The function of these genes has been elucidated, in part, through the analysis of a variety of model systems employing mice, flies, worms, and other organisms, and through the investigation of human cancer cell lines. The principal aims of this chapter are to review the somatic cell genetic and epidemiologic studies that established the existence of tumor suppressor genes; to describe the identification and cloning of representative tumor suppressor genes, such as the retinoblastoma and *TP53* genes; to highlight selected studies of the function of tumor suppressor genes in the regulation of cell birth and cell death; and to illustrate an example of a genomic stability gene that plays a causal role in common human cancers.

Genetic Basis for Tumor Development

The inherited basis of human cancer has been appreciated for almost 150 years. In 1866, Broca described a family in which many members developed breast or liver cancer, and he proposed that an inherited abnormality within the affected tissue allowed for tumor development.[1] Following the rediscovery of Mendel's work, studies of the rates of spontaneous mammary tumor formation in various inbred strains of mice led Haaland to argue that tumorigenesis could behave in a formal sense as a Mendelian genetic trait.[2] Similarly, Warthin's analysis of the pedigrees of cancer patients at the University of Michigan Hospital between 1895 and 1913 identified four multigenerational families with susceptibilities to specific cancer types that appeared to be transmitted as autosomal dominant Mendelian traits (Fig. 7-1).[3] Although these and other studies suggested the existence of an inherited genetic basis for some cancers, other explanations for familial clustering were certainly possible (eg, shared exposure to a carcinogenic agent in the environment

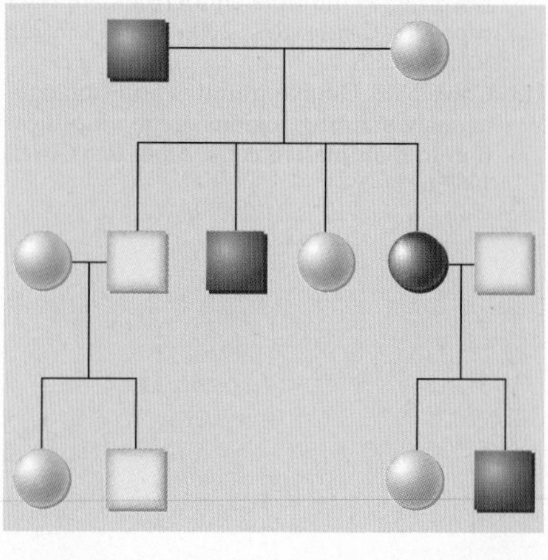

Figure 7-1 ■ The inheritance of cancer in a family. The affected members with cancer are indicated by shaded squares (males) or circles (females). This family demonstrates a dominant pattern of inheritance, meaning that each offspring has a 50% chance of inheriting a germline mutation that predisposes to a high probability of developing cancer.

or diet). Furthermore, it was highlighted that most cancers in humans appeared to arise as sporadic, isolated cases.

A role for somatic mutations in the development of cancer was first proposed by Boveri, who noted that, in sea urchin eggs fertilized by two sperm, abnormal mitotic divisions leading to the loss of chromosomes occurred in daughter cells, and atypical tissue masses could be seen in the resulting gastrula.[4] He believed that these abnormal tissues appeared physically similar to the poorly differentiated tissue masses seen in tumors and hypothesized that cancer arose from a cellular aberration producing abnormal mitotic figures. Boveri's hypothesis apparently did not gain favor at the time, initially because of the lack of direct experimental support from studies of the karyotypes of animal and human tumors. Such karyotypes were impossible to obtain with the available technology. Once the karyotypic studies were performed decades later, and appeared to support his hypothesis, Boveri was still doubted because of uncertainty about whether the changes in chromosome number in tumors were a cause or an effect of the neoplastic process.

A landmark observation in the search to identify a genetic basis for cancer was reported by Rous in 1911, when he showed that sarcomas could be reproducibly induced in chickens by cell-free filtrates of a sarcoma that had previously arisen in another chicken.[5] Although this observation provided strong evidence that neoplasms could be virally induced, the observation also provided support for the view that cancer could be attributed to discrete genetic elements. Sixty years after Rous's initial report, the oncogenic region of the Rous sarcoma virus was identified. Further characterization and cloning of the transforming sequences demonstrated that the oncogenicity of the virus depended on *vsrc*, a transduced and mutated copy of the *csrc* cellular proto-oncogene. Subsequently, all oncogenes of acutely transforming ribonucleic acid (RNA) tumor viruses have been found to be transduced cellular genes. (In fact, they were defined as proto-oncogenes). The viral oncogenes cause transformation because they are mutated versions of cellular proto-oncogenes or are expressed at abnormally high levels. In human cancers, somatic mutations generate oncogenic alleles from proto-oncogenes.

Oncogenes play a role in most forms of human cancer, but are particularly prominent in "liquid" tumors, such as leukemias and lymphomas, as well as in sarcomas. Such cancers often have characteristic chromosomal translocations that alter proto-oncogenes at the breakpoints, fusing them with unrelated genes and endowing the fusion product with new properties that increase cell birth or decrease cell death.

Somatic Cell Genetic Studies of Tumorigenesis

The studies of Ephrussi et al.[6] and Harris[7] provided compelling evidence that the ability of cells to form a tumor behaves as a recessive trait at the cellular level. They observed that the growth of murine tumor cells in syngeneic animals could be suppressed when the malignant cells were fused to nonmalignant cells, although reversion to tumorigenicity often occurred when the hybrids were propagated for extended periods in culture. The reappearance of malignancy was found to be associated with specific chromosome losses. The interpretation of those authors, that malignancy can be suppressed in somatic cell hybrids, was subsequently supported by additional studies of mouse, rat, and hamster intraspecies somatic cell hybrids, as well as by interspecies hybrids between rodent tumor cells and normal human cells.[8,9] The karyotypic instability of the rodent–human hybrids, however, complicated the analysis of the human chromosomes involved in the suppression process. Stanbridge and his colleagues overcame this problem by studying hybrids made by fusing human tumor cell lines to normal, diploid human fibroblasts.[10,11] Their analysis confirmed that hybrids retaining both sets of parental chromosomes were suppressed, with tumorigenic variants arising only rarely after chromosome losses in the hybrids. Moreover, it was demonstrated that the loss of specific chromosomes, and not simply chromosome loss in general, correlated with the reversion to tumorigenicity. Tumorigenicity could be suppressed even if activated oncogenes, such as mutant *ras* genes, were expressed in the hybrids.[11,12]

The observation that the loss of specific chromosomes was associated with the reversion to malignancy suggested that a single chromosome (and perhaps even a single gene) might be sufficient to suppress tumorigenicity. To directly test that hypothesis, the technique of microcell-mediated chromosome transfer was used to transfer single chromosomes from normal cells to tumor cells. It was found that the transfer of a single chromosome 11 into the HeLa cervical carcinoma cell line suppressed the tumorigenic phenotype of the cells.[13] Similarly, transfer of chromosome 11 into a Wilms tumor cell line was found to suppress tumorigenicity, whereas the transfer of several other chromosomes had no effect.[14] Many studies have demonstrated that transfer of even very small chromosome fragments will specifically suppress the tumorigenic properties of certain cancer cell lines.

Although tumorigenic growth in immunocompromised animals can often be suppressed in hybrids resulting from fusion between malignant and normal cells or by transfer of unique chromosome fragments, other traits characteristic of the parental tumor cells, such as immortality and anchorage-independent growth in vitro, may be retained. This observation is consistent with the notion that most malignant tumors arise as a result of multiple genetic alterations. Suppression of tumorigenicity following cell fusion or microcell chromosome transfer might thus represent correction of only one of many alterations.

In summary, somatic cell genetic approaches provided early and persuasive evidence for the existence of critical growth-regulating genes in normal cells that can suppress phenotypic traits of immortal or even fully cancerous cells.

Retinoblastoma: A Paradigm for Tumor Suppressor Gene Function

Essentially concurrent with the initial cell fusion experiments of Harris and colleagues, Knudson's analysis of the age-specific incidence of retinoblastoma led him to propose that two "hits" or mutagenic events were necessary for retinoblastoma development.[15] Retinoblastoma occurs sporadically in most cases, but, in some families, it displays an autosomal dominant inheritance. In an individual with the inherited form of the disease, Knudson proposed that the first hit is present in the germline, and thus in all cells of the body. However, the presence of a mutation at the susceptibility locus was argued to be insufficient for tumor formation, and a second somatic mutation was hypothesized to be necessary for promoting tumor formation. Given the high likelihood of a somatic mutation occurring in at least one retinal cell during development, the dominant inheritance pattern of retinoblastoma in some families could be explained. In the nonhereditary form of retinoblastoma, both mutations were proposed to arise somatically within the same cell. Although each of the two hits could theoretically have been in different genes, subsequent studies (see below) led to the conclusion that both hits were at the same genetic locus, ultimately inactivating both alleles of the retinoblastoma 1 (*RB1*) susceptibility gene. Knudson's hypothesis served not only to illustrate mechanisms through which inherited and somatic genetic changes might collaborate in tumorigenesis, but also to link the notion of recessive genetic determinants for human cancer to somatic cell genetic findings on the recessive nature of tumorigenesis.

The first clue to the location of a putative gene responsible for inherited retinoblastoma was obtained from karyotypic analyses of patients with retinoblastoma. Constitutional deletions of chromosome 13 were observed in some cases.[16] Subsequent cytogenetic studies of patients with retinoblastoma identified detectable germline deletions of chromosome 13 in only about 5% of all patients. However, in cases where deletions were observed, the common region of deletion was centered around chromosome band 13q14.[17] When compared with karyotypically normal family members, patients with deletions of 13q14 were found to have reduced levels of esterase D, an enzyme of unknown physiologic function.[18] This finding implied that the esterase D gene might be contained within chromosome band 13q14. Indeed, analysis of the segregation patterns of esterase D isozymes and retinoblastoma development in families with inherited retinoblastoma established that the esterase D and *RB1* loci were genetically linked.[19]

Subsequently, a child with inherited retinoblastoma was found to have esterase D levels approximately one-half of normal, although no deletion of chromosome 13 was seen in karyotype studies of his blood cells and skin fibroblasts.[20] Interestingly, tumor cells from this patient had a complete absence of esterase D activity, despite harboring one apparently intact copy of chromosome 13. Based on these findings, it was proposed that the copy of chromosome 13 retained in the tumor cells had a submicroscopic deletion of both the esterase D and *RB1* loci. Moreover, it was concluded that the initial *RB1* mutation in the child was recessive at the cellular level (ie, cells with inactivation of one *RB1* allele had a normal phenotype). However, the effect of the predisposing mutation could be unmasked in the tumor cells by a second event, such as the loss of the chromosome 13 carrying the wild-type *RB1* allele. This proposal was entirely consistent with Knudson's two-hit hypothesis.[15,21]

To establish the generality of these observations, Cavenee and colleagues undertook studies of retinoblastomas, both inherited and sporadic, by using deoxyribonucleic acid (DNA) probes from chromosome 13. Probes detecting DNA polymorphisms were used, so that the two parental copies of chromosome 13 in the cells of the patient's normal and tumor tissues could be distinguished from one another. By using such markers to compare paired normal and tumor samples from each patient, the Cavenee group was able to demonstrate that loss of heterozygosity (LOH—ie, the loss of one parental set of markers) for chromosome 13 alleles had occurred during tumorigenesis in more than 60% of the cases studied.[22] LOH for chromosome 13, and specifically for the region of chromosome 13 containing the *RB1* gene, occurred via a number of different mechanisms (Fig. 7-2). In addition, through study of inherited cases, it was shown that the copy of chromosome 13 retained in the tumor cells was derived from the affected parent and that the chromosome carrying the wild-type *RB1* allele had been lost.[22,23] These data established that the unmasking of a predisposing mutation at the *RB1* gene, whether the initial mutation had been inherited or had arisen somatically in a single developing retinoblast, occurred by the same chromosomal mechanisms.

Patients with the inherited form of retinoblastoma were known to be at an increased risk for the development of a few other cancer types, particularly osteosarcomas. LOH for the chromosome 13q region containing the *RB1* locus was seen in osteosarcomas arising in patients with the inherited form of retinoblastoma,

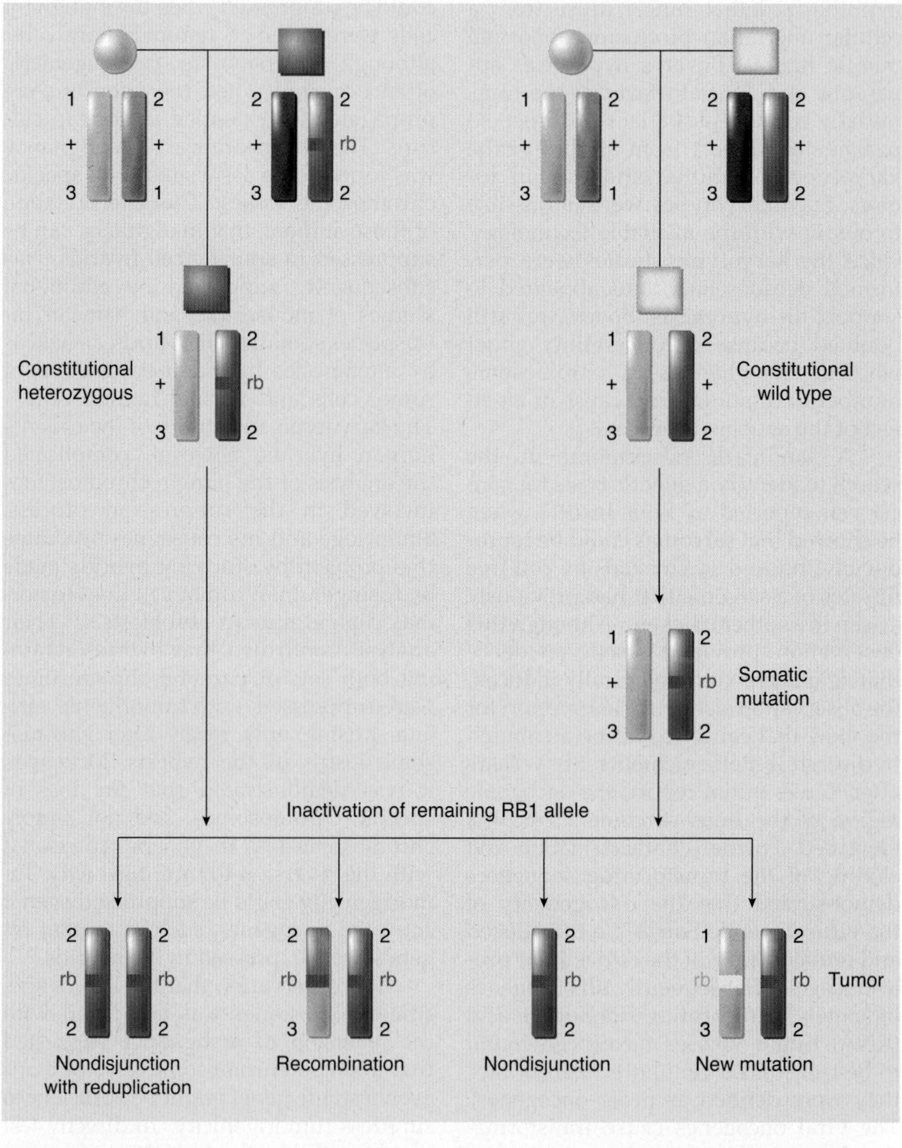

Figure 7-2 Chromosomal mechanisms that result in loss of heterozygosity for alleles at the retinoblastoma predisposition (*RB1*) locus at chromosomal band 13q14. In the inherited form of the disease (*top left*), the affected son inherits a mutant *RB1* allele (*rb*) from his affected father and a normal *RB1*allele (+) from his mother. Thus, he has one wild-type and one mutant *RB1* allele in all his cells (ie, constitutional genotype for *RB1* is *rb* /+). The two copies of chromosome 13 in his normal cells (one from each parent) can be distinguished using polymorphic DNA markers flanking the *RB1* locus (the polymorphic alleles are designated by number). A retinoblastoma can arise after inactivation of the remaining wild-type *RB1* allele. Among the genetic mechanisms found to inactivate the remaining wild-type *RB1* allele during tumor development are chromosome nondisjunction and reduplication of the remaining copy of chromosome 13, mitotic recombination, nondisjunction, and new RB mutations that inactivate the remaining *RB1* allele. Shown at the *top right* is the situation in the non-inherited (sporadic) form of the disease. A somatic mutation arises in a developing retinal cell and inactivates one of the *RB1* alleles. A retinoblastoma will develop if the remaining *RB1* allele is inactivated by one of the mechanisms shown.

suggesting that inactivation of both *RB1* alleles was critical to the development of osteosarcomas in those with inherited retinoblastoma.[24,25] Chromosome 13q LOH was also frequently observed in sporadic osteosarcomas. These molecular studies of retinoblastomas and osteosarcomas provided strong support for Knudson's two-hit hypothesis and suggested that a variety of tumors might arise through the inactivation of various tumor suppressor loci.[11,21,23] In addition, the studies demonstrated that the inherited and sporadic forms of a specific tumor type both appeared to arise as a result of genetic alterations in the same gene.

Cloning and Analysis of the RB1 Gene

The molecular cloning of the *RB1* gene was facilitated by the identification in the chromosome 13q14 region of an anonymous DNA marker that detected DNA rearrangements in retinoblastomas.[26] Analysis of the DNA sequences flanking this DNA marker revealed a gene with the properties expected of *RB1*.[27-29] The *RB1* gene has a complex organization, with 27 exons spanning more than 200 kb of DNA, and an RNA transcript of about 4.7 kb. The *RB1* gene appears to be expressed ubiquitously rather than to be restricted to retinoblasts and osteoblasts.

Cloning of *RB1* allowed study of mutations that inactivate the gene. Although gross deletions of *RB1* sequences have been observed in a small subset of retinoblastoma and osteosarcoma cases, most tumors appear to express full-length *RB1* transcripts and lack detectable gene rearrangements when analyzed by Southern blotting.[30-33] Hence, the detection of inherited and somatic mutations in the *RB1* gene in most cases has required detailed characterization of its sequence. Extensive analysis of mutant *RB1* alleles has provided definitive molecular evidence supporting Knudson's two-hit model. As predicted, patients with inherited retinoblastoma have been found to have one mutated and one normal allele in their constitutional (blood) cells. In retinoblastomas of such individuals, the remaining *RB1* allele has been found to be inactivated by somatic mutation, usually by loss of the normal allele through a gross chromosomal event (Fig. 7-2), but in some cases by point mutation. Multiple tumors arising in an individual patient with inherited retinoblastoma were all found to contain the same germline mutation, but different somatic mutations affected the remaining *RB1* allele. The vast majority of patients with a single retinoblastoma and no family history of the disease have two somatic mutations in their tumors and two normal alleles in their constitutional cells.

The observation that *RB1* is ubiquitously expressed is rather puzzling, given the restricted spectrum of tumors that develop in patients with germline *RB1* mutations. Patients with germline mutations of *RB1* are at elevated risk only for the development of a rather limited number of tumor types, including retinoblastomas in childhood, osteosarcomas, soft-tissue sarcomas, and melanomas later in life. *RB1* germline mutations fail to predispose to most common cancers, despite the fact that somatic *RB1* mutations have been observed in a wide variety of cancer types, including breast, small cell lung, bladder, pancreas, and prostate cancers.[34] It is possible that retinoblastoma protein functions differently in retinal epithelial cells than in other cell types, so that the *RB1* gene acts as a "gatekeeper" in retinal cells but not in other cell types.

Function of Retinoblastoma Protein P105-RB

The protein product of the *RB1* gene is a nuclear phosphoprotein known as p105-Rb or, more commonly, pRB. Its molecular weight is about 105,000 Da. Studies by Whyte and colleagues provided critical insights into pRB function, connecting human tumorigenesis with experimental tumors caused by DNA tumor viruses. They demonstrated that pRB formed a complex with the E1A oncoprotein encoded by the murine DNA tumor virus adenovirus type 5.[35] Prior studies of E1A had established that it had many effects on cell growth, including cell immortalization and cooperation with other oncogenes (eg, mutated ras oncogene alleles) in neoplastic transformation. It was thus hypothesized that functional inactivation of pRB through its interaction with E1A might contribute to some of E1A's transforming functions. Additional support for that proposal was provided by data establishing that mutations inactivating the ability of E1A to bind to pRB also inactivated E1A's transforming function.[36,37]

The significance of physical interaction between pRB and a DNA tumor virus oncoprotein was further supported by the subsequent demonstration that other DNA tumor virus oncoproteins also formed complexes with pRB, including SV40 T antigen and the E7 proteins of human papillomavirus (HPV) types 16 and 18 (Fig. 7-3).[38,39] Many of the mutations that inactivated the transforming activities of these oncoproteins also inactivated their ability to interact with pRB. Furthermore, E7 proteins from "high-risk" HPVs (ie, those linked to cancer development), such as HPV 16 and 18, formed complexes more tightly with pRB than did E7 proteins of "low-risk" viruses (eg, HPV types 6 and 11). These studies of pRB provided compelling evidence that DNA tumor viruses might transform cells at least in part by inactivating tumor suppressor gene products. In addition, given the critical dependence of DNA tumor viruses on harnessing the cell's machinery for replication of the viral genome, the studies also provided support for the hypothesis that pRB might control normal cell growth by interacting with cellular proteins that regulate the cell's decision to enter into the DNA synthesis (S) phase of the cell cycle.

The functional activity of pRB is regulated by phosphorylation during nor-

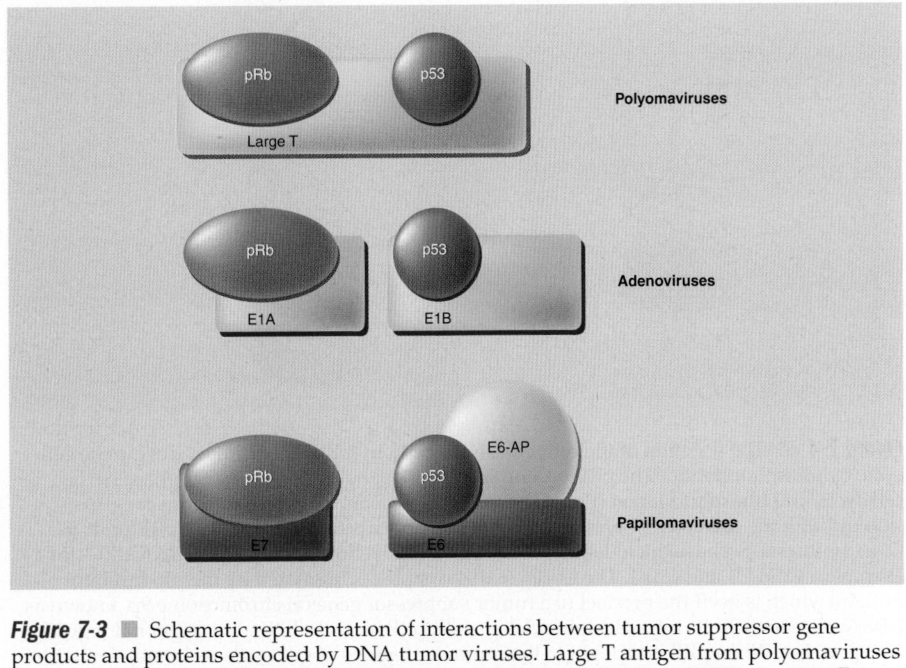

Figure 7-3 ■ Schematic representation of interactions between tumor suppressor gene products and proteins encoded by DNA tumor viruses. Large T antigen from polyomaviruses (such as simian virus 40 [SV40]) bind both the retinoblastoma (pRB) and TP53 proteins. For the adenoviruses and the high-risk human papillomaviruses (HPV types 16 and 18), various viral protein products complex with pRB and TP53. A cellular protein known as E6-associated protein (E6-AP) cooperates with the HPV E6 protein to complex and degrade TP53.

mal progression through the cell cycle. Accordingly, pRB appears to be predominantly unphosphorylated or hypophosphorylated in the G1 phase of the cell cycle and maximally phosphorylated in G2 (Fig. 7-4). The critical phosphorylation events regulating the function of pRB are likely to be mediated at the boundary between the G1 and S phases of the cell cycle by cyclin and cyclin-dependent kinase (Cdk) protein complexes.[34,40] When it is not phosphorylated, pRB forms complexes with proteins in the E2F family and inhibits transcription by recruiting proteins involved in transcriptional repression.[40] When phosphorylated, pRB can no longer efficiently form complexes with E2Fs (Fig. 7-4). The E2F proteins, when dimerized with their differentiation-regulated transcription factor partner(DP) proteins, are then capable of activating the expression of a number of genes that are likely to regulate or promote entry into S-phase, including DNA polymerase α, thymidylate synthase, ribonucleotide reductase, cyclin E, and dihydrofolate reductase.[40] That E2F family members directly affect cellular proliferation was recently shown in conditional mouse knockout models.[41] Several other cellular proteins that bind to pRB have been identified, but their functions and the significance of their interactions with pRB remain less-well characterized than the interactions of pRB with E2Fs. Future studies will undoubtedly shed further light on the means by which loss of pRB function, and that of pRB homologs p107 and p130,[42] contribute to cancer development.

TP53 Gene

Studies in the late 1970s revealed that a cellular phosphoprotein with a relative molecular mass of about 53,000 Da formed a tight complex with SV40 T antigen; hence, the name of the TP53 protein.[43-45] Further work established that TP53 also formed a complex with other viral oncogene products, including the adenovirus E1B protein, and that TP53 was present at low levels in normal cells and high levels in many tumors and tumor cell lines.[43,46-48] These initial findings suggested that increased levels of TP53 might contribute to cancer. Consistent with that notion, gene transfer studies provided data demonstrating that *TP53* functioned as an oncogene in in vitro experiments.[47,49-51] However, subsequent studies in human tumors showed that *TP53* was in reality a tumor suppressor gene.[52]

The rationale for the human cancer studies was the observation that chromosome 17p LOH was common in a number of tumor types, including colorectal, bladder, breast, and lung cancer.[53,54] Detailed mapping showed that region 17p, which was lost in colorectal cancers, included the *TP53* gene.[52] Analysis of the sequence of the *TP53* alleles retained in those cancers with 17p LOH demonstrated that the remaining *TP53* allele was mutated,[52] in perfect accord with Knudson's hypothesis for the alterations expected in tumor suppressor genes. These observations were soon extended to other cancer types, and they explained many previous observations concerning TP53 that had been confusing when *TP53* was believed to be an oncogene.[55-59] Additional evidence that *TP53* functions as a tumor suppressor gene in human cancer is provided by gene transfer studies, but such overexpression studies cannot be easily interpreted, as many genes with no role in neoplasia can inhibit the growth of transfected cells.[60-63] Based on the types of tumors in which *TP53* mutations have been found, and the prevalence of *TP53* mutations in those tumor types, *TP53* is believed to be the most frequently mutated gene in human cancer.[64]

Detailed characterization of the particular base substitutions in the *TP53* gene revealed distinctly different spectra of *TP53* mutations in various types of cancer. For example, most *TP53* mutations in colorectal cancers appear to have arisen spontaneously as a result of deamination of methylated cytosine bases, leading to C > T transition mutations. By contrast, many of the *TP53* mutations seen in lung cancers are transversion mutations (eg, G > T) that may have arisen as result of direct interactions of *TP53* gene sequences with carcinogens present in tobacco smoke. Furthermore, some of the most compelling data to link mutagenic and carcinogenic agents with cancer induction come from study of the *TP53* mutations seen in squamous cell cancers of the skin or in hepatocellular cancers. In squamous cell cancers arising in ultraviolet light–exposed skin, a sizable fraction of the *TP53* mutations appear to have arisen from the generation of pyrimidine dimer premutagenic lesions. Similar studies of the *TP53* gene in hepatocellular cancers arising in individuals from geographic areas with very high exposures to aflatoxin identified mutations that are similar to those generated by aflatoxin in in vitro studies.[64]

Germline mutations in the *TP53* gene have been seen in those affected by Li–Fraumeni syndrome (LFS) and in a small subset of pediatric patients with sarcomas or osteosarcomas that do not meet the more strict criteria for diagnosis of LFS.[65-67] Those with LFS are at risk for

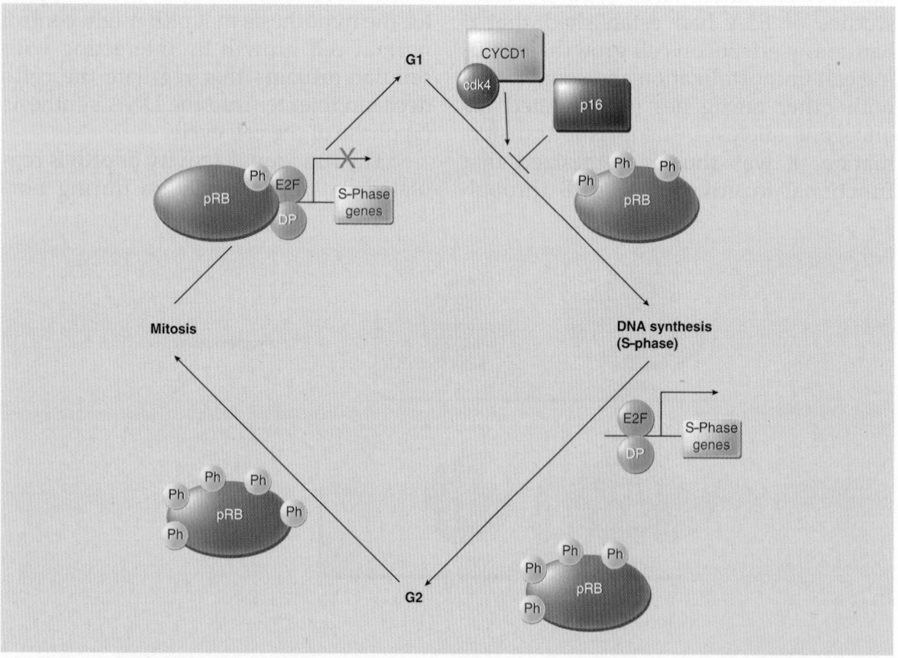

Figure 7-4 The function of the retinoblastoma protein (pRB) is regulated during the cell cycle by phosphorylation. The pRB protein is hypophosphorylated in the G1 phase of the cell cycle, and phosphorylation (Ph) of specific sites appears to increase during progression through the cell cycle. A protein complex that appears to phosphorylate pRB prior to DNA synthesis (S-phase) includes a cyclin (Cyc) and a cyclin-dependent kinase (Cdk)—for example, cyclin D1 and Cdk4. The CycD1/Cdk4 complex is regulated by the p16 inhibitor protein, which is itself the product of a tumor suppressor gene on chromosome 9p, known as *CDKN2* (see text). In its hypophosphorylated state, pRB binds to E2F transcriptional regulatory proteins. When pRB is brought to the promoter regions of genes via its interaction with E2F proteins, pRB represses the expression of the E2F/DP target genes. Phosphorylation of pRB releases it from the E2F/DP protein complex and results in gene activation, including those genes involved in DNA synthesis. The figure also indicates that pRB phosphorylation increases in G2 with pRB dephosphorylated at or near anaphase.

developing a number of tumors, including soft-tissue sarcomas, osteosarcomas, brain tumors, breast cancers, and leukemias. Between one-half and two-thirds of patients with LFS have germline mutations in the central core domain of the *TP53* coding sequences that resemble the somatic mutations frequently seen in sporadic cancers.[68] Some LFS patients and families with phenotypic features of LFS have germline mutations in a gene termed *hCHK2* that phosphorylates *TP53* and controls the cell's response to DNA-damaging events.[69]

In addition to somatic and inherited mutations in the gene, *TP53* function can be inactivated by other mechanisms. As noted above, most cervical cancers contain high-risk or cancer-associated HPV genomes (ie, HPV type 16 or 18). The *E6* gene product of high-risk, but not low-risk, HPV types binds to a cellular protein known as E6-AP (for E6-associated protein) and stimulates TP53 degradation.[70-74] A cellular TP53-binding protein known as mouse double minute 2 (MDM2) is overexpressed in a subset of soft-tissue sarcomas as a result of gene amplification involving chromosome 12q sequences.[75] More recent studies have identified another TP53-binding protein, MDM4, which is overexpressed in a variety of cancers as a result of gene amplification of chromosome 1q sequences.[76] DNA transfection studies have shown that both the *MDM2* and *MDM4* genes can function as oncogenes when overexpressed. The oncogenic function is presumably mediated through their binding to and inactivation of TP53. Both proteins mask TP53's transcriptional activation domain and promote TP53's ubiquitination and subsequent degradation by the proteasome.[77-79] Consistent with the notion that MDM2 is a critical inhibitor of TP53 function, sarcomas with *MDM2* amplification and overexpression rarely harbor somatic mutations in *TP53*.[80] Disruption of the *MDM2* and *MDM4* genes in the germline of mice is lethal, probably because such disruption allows unregulated activity of *TP53*. Accordingly, disruption of the murine *TP53* gene rescues MDM2-deficient and MDM4-deficient mice from embryonic lethality.[81,82] Other mechanisms of regulating TP53 function have also been described, including mutation of a nuclear-cytoplasmic shuttle protein called nucleophosmin in almost 100% of adult acute myelogenous leukemias that demonstrate cytoplasmic localization of this protein, with the notable exception of acute promyelocytic leukemia.[83]

TP53 Function ■ The TP53 protein has been shown to function as a transcriptional regulatory protein.[84,85] In its wild-type state, the TP53 protein is capable of binding to specific DNA sequences with its central core domain (Fig. 7-5). The amino terminal sequences of TP53 function as a transcriptional activation domain, and the carboxyl terminal sequences appear to be required for TP53 to form dimers and tetramers with itself. TP53 activates transcription of a number of genes with roles in the control of the cell cycle, including *WAF1/CIP1/p21* (which encodes a regulator of Cdk activity),[86] *MDM2* (as noted above, encoding a protein that is a known negative regulator of *TP53*), and 14-3-3σ (a regulator of G2/M progression),[87] and various genes that likely function in apoptosis, including *PUMA* and *NOXA*. Experimental disruption of these genes by targeted homologous recombination can recreate some of the phenotypes associated with *TP53* inactivation.[88,89]

The vast majority of the somatic mutations in TP53 are missense mutations leading to amino acid substitutions in the central portion of the protein (exons 5-9).[64] Consistent with the structure of the TP53 protein, these missense mutations have marked effects on the TP53 protein's ability to bind to its cognate DNA recognition sequence through either of two mechanisms.[90] Some mutations (eg, mutations at codons 248 or 273) alter *TP53* sequences that are directly responsible for sequence-specific DNA binding. Other mutations (eg, codon 175) appear to affect the folding of *TP53* and thus indirectly affect its ability to bind to DNA. Recently, evidence that these missense mutations can confer "gain of function" rather than a dominant negative effect was demonstrated via "knock in" mouse models, whereby precise missense mutations were introduced into the endogenous *TP53* gene.[91-95]

Under some circumstances, TP53 acts at the G1/S checkpoint to regulate the cell's decision to synthesize DNA, although TP53 also appears to have a critical function at G2/M.[96,97] In other settings, TP53 appears to exert control over the cell's decision to undergo apoptosis or programmed cell death.[85] Of particular interest with regard to cancer treatment are data suggesting that some tumor cells lacking TP53 function are less sensitive to irradiation and chemotherapeutic agents such as cisplatin.[91,98,99] However, studies of other tumor cells suggest that *TP53* status shows a very different relationship to chemotherapeutic response, with cells that lack functional TP53 being markedly sensitive to DNA-damaging agents but resistant to 5-fluorouracil.[100] Thus far, studies of primary human cancers have emphasized that a rather complex relationship is likely to exist between *TP53* mutational status and the responsiveness of cancer cells to chemotherapy or radiation therapy, or both. In particular, it is difficult to distinguish the effects of *TP53* mutation on the natural progression of disease from its effects on responses to treatment and other cellular stresses.[101,102] Hopefully, further research

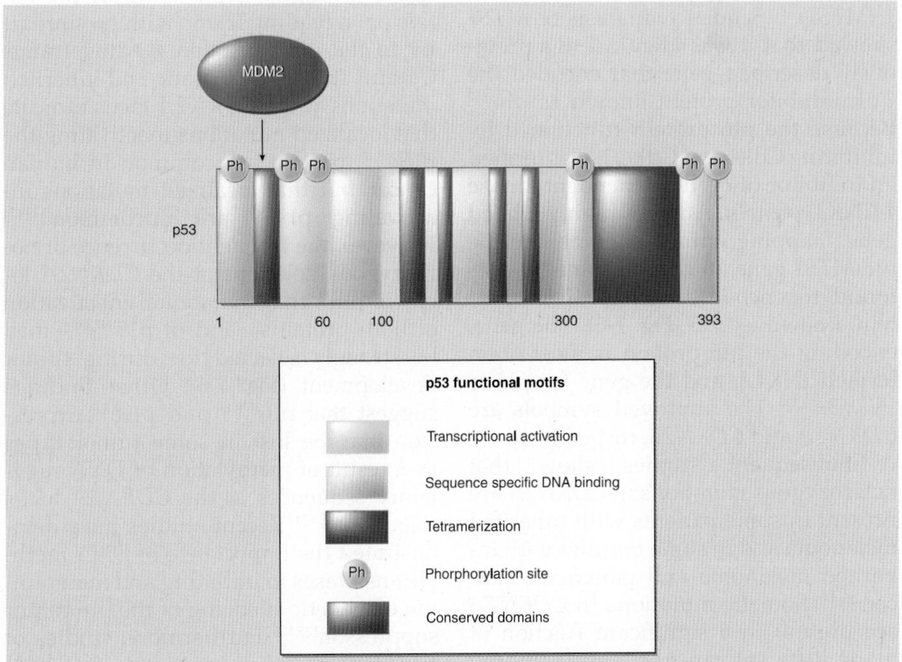

Figure 7-5 ■ TP53 functional motifs. Sequences of TP53 involved in transcriptional activation, sequence-specific DNA binding, tetramerization, and binding by the MDM2 protein are indicated. The five distinct regions of TP53 sequence that are highly conserved between TP53 proteins of diverse species are indicated. In addition, the locations of several sites in the protein that are phosphorylated (Ph) and that regulate TP53 function are indicated.

on *TP53* will clarify our understanding of its normal functions, the basis for its frequent inactivation in many different cancers, and the consequences of its inactivation on tumor growth and response to therapy.

Cyclin-Dependent Kinase Inhibitor 2A Locus

Studies of the cyclin-dependent kinase inhibitor 2A (CDKN2A) locus on chromosome 9p illustrate well how observations from initially disparate lines of investigation often converge to implicate a particular locus as a critical factor in cancer development. The LOH of chromosome 9p was frequently found in many different tumor types, including melanomas, gliomas, nonsmall cell lung, bladder, head and neck cancers and leukemias.[103-106] Of considerable interest were observations establishing that a subset of such tumors had homozygous (complete) deletions affecting the 9p21 region,[107-109] strongly supporting the existence of a tumor suppressor gene in the region. In addition to the frequent somatic alterations of chromosome 9p sequences in cancers, linkage studies of some families with inherited melanoma indicated a melanoma predisposition gene mapped to essentially the same region of 9p.[110] These observations stimulated great interest in the chromosome 9p region presumed to contain the tumor suppressor gene or genes. One of the genes identified in the region as a result of positional cloning efforts was initially termed multiple tumor suppressor 1 (*MTS1*).[111] Sequence analysis of *MTS1* showed that it was identical to a previously described gene that encoded the Cdk inhibitor protein known as p16.[112] Because the p16 protein functioned by inhibiting Cdk4 and Cdk6, it was termed an inhibitor of cyclin-dependent kinase 4 (INK4) protein. Another highly related gene, mapping immediately next to the *p16/MTS1* gene on chromosome 9p, was found to encode a second INK4 protein, known as p15 (Fig. 7-6). The gene, encoding the p16 protein is most often termed *INK4A*, and the gene for p15 is *INK4B*.[113,114] The approved symbols are *CDKN2A* and *CDKN2B*, respectively.

Subsequent studies show that heterozygous mutations in *CDKN2A* are present in some patients with inherited melanoma and in some families with inherited melanoma and pancreatic cancer.[115-118] Somatic mutations in *CDKN2A* are present in a significant fraction of many different cancer types, including but not limited to melanomas, gliomas, pancreatic and bladder cancers, and leukemias. In some tumors, deletions affecting the *CDKN2A* gene also involve the *CDKN2B* gene. In rare tumors, deletions inactivate *CDKN2B* but not *CDKN2A*.[119] The prevalence and specific nature of *CDKN2A* mutations vary markedly from one tumor type to another. In contrast to other tumor suppressor genes, such as *RB1* and *TP53*, homozygous deletion is a fairly common mechanism of *CDKN2A* inactivation in cancer.[120]

Detailed studies of the *CDKN2A* locus led to the identification of a novel alternative transcript containing nucleotide sequences identical to those in transcripts for the $p16^{INK4A}$ protein, but with unique 5′ sequences (Fig. 7-6).[113,114,121] The alternative CDKN2A locus transcript encodes a protein known as p19 alternative reading frame ($p19^{ARF}$), with p19 denoting its apparent weight. The human version of the mouse $p19^{ARF}$ protein is sometimes called $p14^{ARF}$ because of its smaller apparent molecular weight in gel electrophoresis studies. However, both proteins appear to have identical functions, and the discussion below uses the $p19^{ARF}$ terminology because that is the term found more frequently in the literature.

The $p19^{ARF}$ protein contains sequences from a distinct first exon (exon 1β). Exon 1β is located upstream of exon 1α, the first exon present in transcripts for p16 (Fig. 7-6). Exon 1β is spliced to exon 2, which, along with exon 3, is present in the transcripts for both the $p19^{ARF}$ and $p16^{INK4A}$ proteins. However, the $p19^{ARF}$ protein shares no sequence similarity with the $p16^{INK4A}$ protein because $p19^{ARF}$ synthesis initiates at a unique methionine codon in exon 1β and continues through exon 2, using an alternative open reading frame with no similarity to the $p16^{INK4A}$ open reading frame. Careful studies of somatic and inherited mutations at the *CDKN2A* locus indicate that localized mutations inactivating the $p16^{INK4A}$ protein are common in human cancer, but that localized mutations inactivating $p19^{ARF}$ are uncommon.[113,114] However, the frequent occurrence of homozygous deletions at the *CDKN2A* locus implies that mutational inactivation of both proteins—and of $p15^{INK4B}$—may be strongly selected for during tumor development (Fig. 7-6). Other findings suggest that $p16^{INK4A}$ and $p19^{ARF}$ expression may be lost in some tumor types as a result of methylation of DNA regulatory sequences at the *CDKN2A* locus (Fig. 7-6).[122-124] Recent studies have demonstrated the importance of DNA methyltransferases in initiating and maintaining epigenetic silencing of the p16 tumor suppressor.[125,126] Furthermore, studies of mice with germline inactivation of $p19^{ARF}$ and $p16^{INK4A}$ indicate that these proteins function as tumor suppressor genes in vivo.[127-129]

The mechanism through which the $p16^{INK4A}$ protein controls tumorigenic growth is apparently through its inhibition of Cdk4 activity. As indicated above, phosphorylation of pRB impedes its ability to transcriptionally regulate E2F-target genes (Fig. 7-4). The cyclin D1/Cdk4 complex has a critical role in regulating pRB phosphorylation and function.[123] Hence, the $p16^{INK4A}$ protein, by virtue of its regulation of Cdk4 activity, is, in turn, a critical factor in regulating pRB phosphorylation. Presumably, inactivation of $p16^{INK4A}$ results in inappropriate phosphorylation of pRB and a subsequent inability of hyperphosphorylated pRB to bind E2Fs and appropriately regulate gene expression at the G1–S transition.

Initially, insights into the means by which p19ARF functioned as a growth regulator and tumor suppressor in vitro and in vivo were lacking, in part because the p19ARF protein lacks significant similarity to proteins with well established function. It is now clear that p19ARF binds directly to the MDM2 protein, and its binding blocks both MDM2-induced degradation of TP53 and the effects of MDM2 on TP53-mediated transcriptional activation of genes.[114] Hence, p19ARF function may be important for maintaining the appropriate function of TP53 in cells, much as p16INK4A function is critical for appropriate pRB function.

Contrary to this, however, is the fact that alterations of p19ARF and TP53 often coexist in cancer cells, suggesting that they do not alter the same pathway, whereas Rb and p16INK4A alterations are mutually exclusive, supportive of the fact that they affect the same pathway.[130] Nevertheless, these findings emphasize the concept that oncogenes and tumor suppressor genes do not function in isolation. Rather, they function in intricately linked cascades or networks that have important consequences for both tumorigenesis and therapy (Fig. 7-7).[85,131]

Adenomatosis Polyposis Coli Gene

Identification and Germline Mutations Hereditary colorectal cancer syndromes are usually subdivided into polyposis and nonpolyposis types. The polyposis types are those in which up to thousands of benign tumors (polyps) can be seen prior to cancer development. In the nonpolyposis types, few, if any, polyps are noted prior to cancer diagnosis, despite the elevated risk of cancer and the fact that most colorectal cancers are believed to arise from adenomatous precursor lesions.

One of the polyposis syndromes is known as familial adenomatous polyposis (FAP) or adenomatosis polyposis coli (APC). FAP is an autosomal dominant disorder affecting about 1 in 8000 individuals in the United States. The syndrome is characterized by the development of hundreds of adenomatous polyps in the colon and rectum of affected individuals by early adulthood. The lifetime risk of

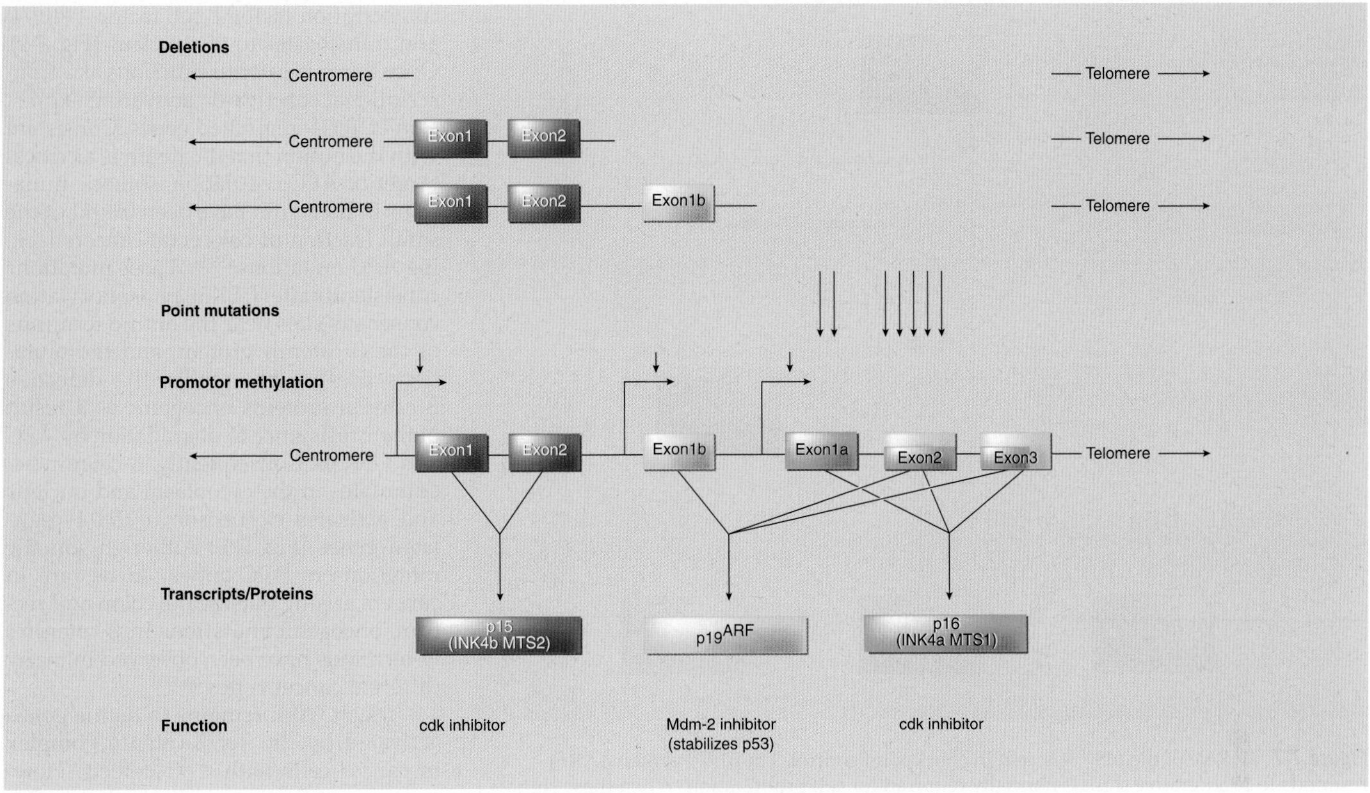

Figure 7-6 ■ Genomic structure, mutations, and transcripts of the *CDKN2B* (p15) and *CDKN2A* (p16/p19 ^{ARF}) locus. The origins of the p15, p16, and p19^{ARF} transcripts are shown schematically, along with a representative depiction of genomic deletions, point mutations (*arrows*), and promoter methylation (*arrowheads*) noted in human cancers. The exons of the *CDKN2B* and *CDKN2A* loci are shown as *rectangles*. The transcripts/proteins and presumed functions of the transcripts/proteins are indicated. The *red rectangles* indicate the open reading frame in transcripts encoding p15; the *yellow rectangles* indicate the open reading frame present in transcripts encoding p19ARF; and the *lavender rectangles* indicate the open reading frame present in transcripts encoding p16. The size of the locus, exons, and transcripts are not shown to scale.

colorectal cancer in those with the classic form of FAP is extremely high, approaching 100% by age 60 years.

An observation that greatly aided localization of the *APC* gene was the demonstration by Herrera and Sandberg, in 1986, of an interstitial deletion of chromosome 5q in a patient with features of FAP, but without any family history of the syndrome.[132] Subsequent DNA linkage studies confirmed that, in multiple kindreds with FAP, or the related condition known as Gardner syndrome, the polyposis phenotype segregated with DNA markers near 5q21.[133,134] In 1991, positional cloning efforts identified the *APC* gene as the specific gene responsible for FAP.[135-138] The *APC* gene is large, with more than 15 exons, and alternative splicing affects the 5′ untranslated portion of transcripts. The predominant *APC* transcript encodes a 2843–amino acid protein expressed in many adult tissues.

In the great majority of individuals with FAP, heterozygous germline mutations can be identified in the *APC* gene.[139-141] All of the germline *APC* mutations in those with FAP appear to inactivate APC protein function. The overwhelming majority of these germline mutations are localized nonsense or frameshift mutations in the 5′ half of the coding region of *APC* (Fig. 7-8). Consistent with Knudson's two-hit hypothesis, inactivation of the remaining wild-type APC allele by somatic mutation in those carrying a germline *APC* mutation is observed in the cancers that arise.[142,143] Correlations between the location of a particular germline *APC* mutation and clinical features have been found,[144] although clear insights into the molecular basis for the predisposition to extracolonic tumors (eg, jaw osteomas and desmoid tumors) in FAP patients with variant phenotypes are lacking. However, some light has been shed on the variability in polyp number seen in families with polyposis.[142,145] Mutations in the 5′ region of the *APC* gene appear to be correlated with an attenuated phenotype attributable to reentry of the ribosome on the APC transcript downstream of the premature stop codon, resulting in an APC protein that retains some of its normal activity.[145] Mutations in 3′ third of the *APC* gene are also associated with a milder polyposis phenotype than are mutations in the central third of the gene, perhaps because the mutated APC proteins similarly retain some tumor suppressor activity. Unexpectedly, extracolonic features such as desmoid tumors appear to be more common in patients with 3′ mutations.[142] Finally, a missense mutation in the middle of the *APC* gene has been found to predispose to colorectal cancers in Ashkenazi Jewish families.[146] This mutation does not alter the function of the gene product, but creates a "hot-spot" that appears to be highly mutable, resulting in somatic deletions or insertions of surrounding nucleotides that produce truncations.

Somatic Mutations in Sporadic Colon Tumors ■ Whereas germline *APC* mutations are an uncommon cause of colorectal cancer in the general population and are present in only about 0.5% of all colon cancers, somatic *APC* mutations are present in the vast majority of sporadic colorectal adenomas and carcinomas.[147] The initial observation suggesting that *APC* inactivation might be common in colon tumors was the observation that the chromosome 5q region containing the *APC* gene was affected by LOH in many sporadic colorectal adenomas and carcinomas.[54,148] Since the identification of the *APC* gene, detailed analyses of the somatic mutations inactivating the *APC* gene in colorectal tumors have been carried out. The somatic *APC* mutations in sporadic tumors are similar in nature and location to the germline *APC* mutations found in those with FAP (Fig. 7-8). Present findings suggest that up to 90% of colorectal tumors, regardless of their size or partic-

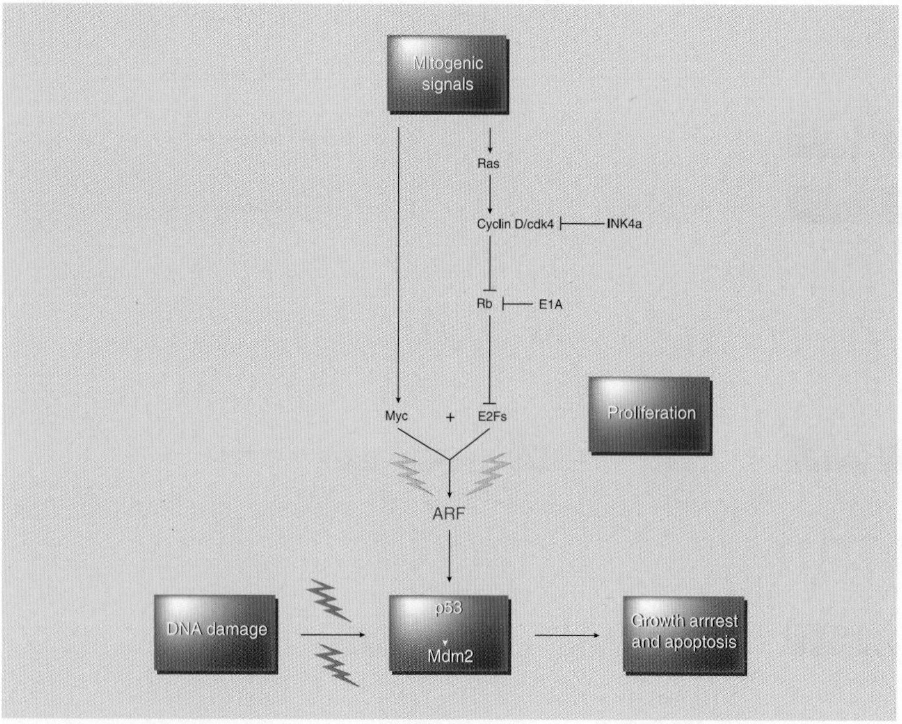

Figure 7-7 ■ Role of the p19ARF protein in checkpoint control. The p19ARF protein (ARF) responds to proliferative signals normally required for cell proliferation. When these signals exceed a critical threshold, the ARF-dependent checkpoint (*yellow lightning bolts*) is activated, and ARF triggers a TP53-dependent response that induces growth arrest or apoptosis, or both. Signals now known to induce signaling via the ARF-TP53 pathway include Myc, E1A, and E2F-1. In principle, "upstream" oncoproteins, such as products of mutated *ras* alleles, constitutively activated receptors, or cytoplasmic signal transducing oncoproteins, might also trigger ARF activity via the cyclin D-Cdk4-RBE2F or Myc-dependent pathways, both of which are normally necessary for S-phase entry. In inhibiting cyclin Ddependent kinases, p16INK4A can dampen the activity of mitogenic signals. In the figure, E1A is shown to work, at least in part, by opposing RB function. For simplicity, Myc and E2F-1 are shown to activate only TP53 via the effects on ARF, though highly overexpressed levels of these proteins can activate TP53 in ARF-negative cells, albeit with an attenuated efficiency. ARF activation of TP53 likely depends on inactivation of Mdm2-specific function(s). DNA damage signals (eg, ionizing and ultraviolet radiation, hypoxic stress) activate (*blue lightning bolts*) TP53 through multiple signaling pathways.

ular histopathologic features, harbor somatic mutations that inactivate *APC*.[142,149]

Function ■ The *APC* gene encodes a large protein of roughly 300 kDa that is hypothesized to regulate cell adhesion, cell migration, or apoptosis in the colonic crypt. The localization of the APC protein in the basolateral membrane of colonic epithelial cells, with an apparent increase in APC expression in cells near the top of the crypt implies that APC may regulate shedding or apoptosis of cells as they reach the crypt apex.[150] Perhaps consistent with this view, restoration of APC protein expression in colorectal cancer cells lacking endogenous APC expression has been reported to promote apoptosis.[151,152]

The APC protein binds to a number of proteins, including β-catenin, γ-catenin (also known as plakoglobin), glycogen synthase kinase 3β (GSK3β), end-binding protein 1 (EB1), human Drosophila large discs (hDLG), microtubules, and the related proteins axin and conductin.[153] With the exception of β-catenin, GSK3β, and the conductin and axin proteins, the significance and role of APC's interactions with its various binding partners is not well understood. Several lines of evidence imply that APC has a critical function in regulating β-catenin.[153,154] β-Catenin is an abundant cellular protein, first identified because of its role in linking the cytoplasmic domain of the E-cadherin cell–cell adhesion molecule to the cortical actin cytoskeleton, via β-catenin's binding to α-catenin. The truncated (mutant) APC proteins present in many colorectal cancers lack some or all of the repeat motifs crucial for binding to β-catenin. APC not only binds to β-catenin, but, in collaboration with the GSK3β enzyme and other proteins, such as axin and conductin, it appears to regulate the abundance of β-catenin in the cytosol via phosphorylation. In colorectal cancers in which *APC* is mutated and unable to bind or effectively coordinate the regulation of β-catenin, β-catenin accumulates in the cell, complexes with the transcription factor T cell factor-4 (Tcf-4) and translocates to the nucleus (Fig. 7-9). Once there, β-catenin functions as a transcriptional coactivator, activating expression of Tcf-4–regulated genes. Consistent with the notion that β-catenin is a critical target of *APC* regulation, somatic mutations in β-catenin have been found in the small fraction of colorectal cancers lacking *APC* mutations.[155-157] These mutations consistently alter GSK3β phosphorylation consensus sites near the amino terminus of the β-catenin protein, and the mutations presumably render the defective β-catenin proteins oncogenic as a result of their resistance to degradation by APC and GSK3β. Consequently, β-catenin accumulates in the cytoplasm and nucleus and activates expression of Tcf-4–regulated genes (Fig. 7-9). Although somatic mutations in *APC* appear to be rare in cancers arising outside the colon and rectum, oncogenic mutations in β-catenin's N-terminus have been observed in many different cancer types.[158,159]

Much work remains to define genes activated by the Tcf/β-catenin complex in cancer cells with *APC* defects. However, recent findings indicate that proto-oncogenes such as *c-myc* and cyclin D1 (*CCND1*), extracellular proteases such as matrix metalloproteinase 7 (MMP-7), growth inhibitory cytokines such as bone morphogenetic protein 4 (BMP-4), and nuclear receptor factors such as the peroxisome proliferator–activator receptor δ (PPARδ) may be critical targets.[160-166] Like *c-myc* and *CCND1*, other Tcf/β-catenin targets with increased expression as a result of *APC* or β-catenin mutations presumably promote cell growth or inhibit cell death, or both. Further work on APC function should offer crucial insights into the carcinogenesis of colon and other cancers, thus providing novel strategies and targets for therapy and chemoprevention.[167]

Wilms Tumor Gene

Wilms tumors are the most common renal neoplasm in children, accounting for approximately 6% of all pediatric cancers.[168] Wilms tumors are similar to retinoblastomas in a number of ways: both can occur bilaterally or unilaterally, with single or multiple foci, and in a sporadic or inherited fashion. The two-mutation model originally proposed for retinoblastoma was also proposed to explain Wilms tumor.[169] However, hereditary cases are not as common among Wilms tumor patients as they are in retinoblastoma patients. Almost all patients inheriting a mutation at the *RB1* locus develop a retinoblastoma, but only approximately 50% of individuals carrying a germline mutation predisposing to Wilms tumor develop the disease (ie, lower penetrance).[168]

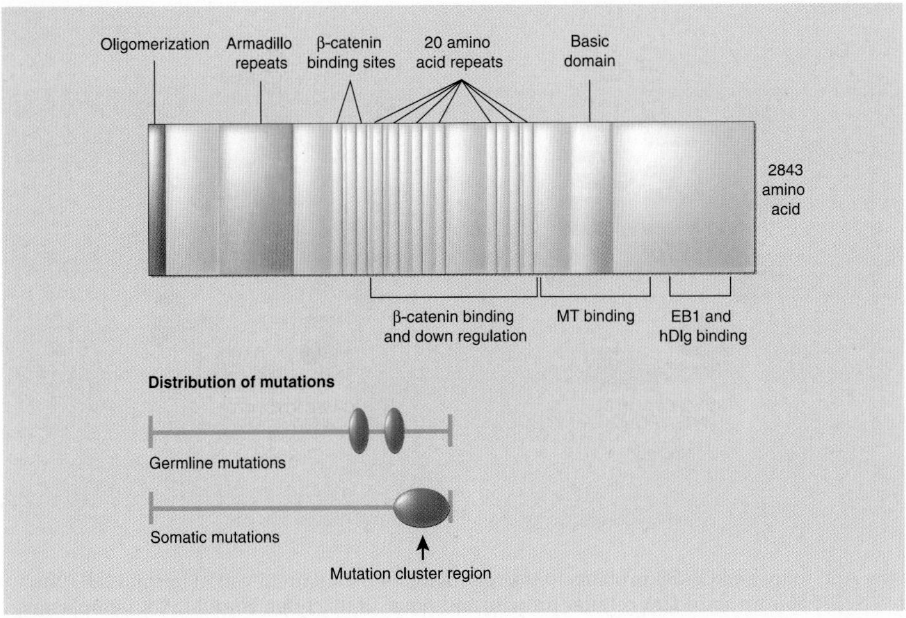

Figure 7-8 Schematic representation of Apc protein domains with respect to mutational analysis results. The relative positions of various Apc domains. A putative domain involved in homo-oligomerization of Apc is located at the aminoterminus. Also noted are a series of repeats of unknown function with similarity to the *Drosophila* armadillo protein, sequences known to mediate binding to β-catenin and its downregulation, a basic domain in the carboxy-terminal third of the protein that appears to facilitate complexing with microtubules (MT), and sequences near the carboxy-terminus of Apc that are known to interact with the EB1 and human homolog of the *Drosophila* disc large (hDlg) protein. Germline mutations in the *APC* gene (predominantly chain terminating) are dispersed throughout the 5′ half of the sequence, with two apparent "hot spots" at codons 1061 and 1309. Somatic mutations in the *APC* gene in colorectal cancer appear to cluster in a region termed the "mutation cluster region," and mutations at codons 1309 and 1450 are most common.

Perhaps the first finding to offer insight into an inherited genetic basis for Wilms tumor was a report in 1964 describing six patients with Wilms tumor and sporadic aniridia (ie, congenital absence of the iris).[170] It was proposed that the simultaneous occurrence of these two very rare conditions might result from chromosomal aberrations affecting two or more loci, a situation now often called a contiguous gene syndrome—mutation of one locus presumably leading to aniridia and mutation of another leading to Wilms tumor. This hypothesis was subsequently supported by the discovery of interstitial deletions of chromosome 11p13 in peripheral blood samples from children with the WAGR syndrome (Wilms tumor with aniridia, genitourinary abnormalities, and mental retardation) of Wilms tumor.[171] Cytogenetic studies of tumor tissues in a few cases of sporadic-type Wilms tumors revealed deletions or translocations of chromosome band 11p13.[172,173] Subsequent studies of paired samples of Wilms tumor and normal cells from patients, using probes that detect restriction fragment length polymorphisms (RFLPs) on chromosome 11p, revealed that LOH of 11p occurred frequently in Wilms tumors of both the inherited and sporadic types.[174-177]

The Wilms tumor 1 (*WT1*) gene was identified in 1990 by virtue of mutations inactivating the gene in patients with the WAGR syndrome and by analysis of somatic mutations in the gene in tumors from a minority of patients with unilateral Wilms tumor and no associated congenital malformation.[178] *WT1* is encoded by 10 exons and its transcripts are subject to alternative splicing.[179,180] In contrast to the rather ubiquitous expression of the *RB1*, *TP53*, and *APC* genes, expression of the *WT1* gene appears to be restricted to embryonic kidney and a small subset of other tissues.[181,182] *WT1* messenger ribonucleic acids (mRNAs) encode proteins with molecular masses of 45,000-49,000 Da and 4 zinc-finger motifs. Based on their predicted amino acid sequences the WT1 proteins were suspected from the outset to function in transcriptional regulation.[181] Several studies provide evidence to support that notion, although some WT1 isoforms may have a role in RNA processing, rather than in transcription regulation.[180,181] WT1 proteins suppress the transcriptional activity of promoter elements from a number of growth-inducing genes, including the genes for early growth response (EGR1), insulin-like growth factor-2 (IGF-2), and platelet-derived growth factor A chain (PDGFA), suggesting that WT1 may function in gene repression.[183] Other studies suggest that WT1 can activate or repress gene expression, depending on the cell type and promoter context.[184] Consistent with the notion that WT1 may have a physiologic function in transcriptional activation, recent work indicates that WT1 activates expression of amphiregulin, a member of the epidermal growth factor family.[185] Loss of amphiregulin expression may contribute to loss of appropriate differentiation during Wilms tumor development. Adding to the complex nature of WT1's role as a transcriptional regulator, recent studies suggest that certain *WT1* splice variants have dramatically different effects in their ability to regulate gene expression.[186,187]

WT1 inactivation clearly contributes to Wilms tumor development in those with the WAGR syndrome. Moreover, approximately 10% of apparently sporadic Wilms tumors harbor detectable somatic mutations in the *WT1* gene.[188] Nevertheless, much evidence indicates that Wilms tumors arise through mutations in genes other than *WT1*. First, the chromosome 11p allelic losses seen in Wilms tumor frequently involve band 11p15, but not band 11p13, where the *WT1* gene resides.[188-190] Second, the 11p15 region harbors a gene responsible for Beckwith-Wiedemann syndrome (BWS), a congenital disorder in which affected individuals manifest hyperplasia of the kidneys, endocrine pancreas, and other internal organs; macroglossia; and hemihypertrophy.[191,192] Those affected by BWS are also at increased risk of developing embryonic tumors, such as hepatoblastoma and Wilms tumor. Finally, linkage studies of three families with dominant inheritance of Wilms tumor exclude linkage of the susceptibility locus in those families to any part of chromosome 11p.[193,194] These data suggest that germline mutations in any one of at least three different genes (ie, *WT1*, the *BWS* gene, and at least one gene not on chromosome 11p) predispose to Wilms tumor. Whether a combination of inherited and somatic mutations in more than one of those genes is ultimately required for the transformation of a developing kidney cell into a Wilms tumor, or whether alternative genetic pathways for the development of Wilms tumors exist, remains to be established. The genetic heterogeneity observed among Wilms tumors provides an important contrast to the apparently less complex genetic pathway of retinoblastoma.

Neurofibromatosis 1 and 2 Genes

Neurofibromatosis 1 Gene Von Recklinghausen's disease, also called neurofibromatosis 1 (NF1), is a dominantly inherited syndrome with variable disease manifestations. The consistent feature is that tissues derived from the neural crest are commonly affected. In addition to the nearly uniform development of neurofibromas, NF1 patients are at elevated risk for developing pheochromocytomas,

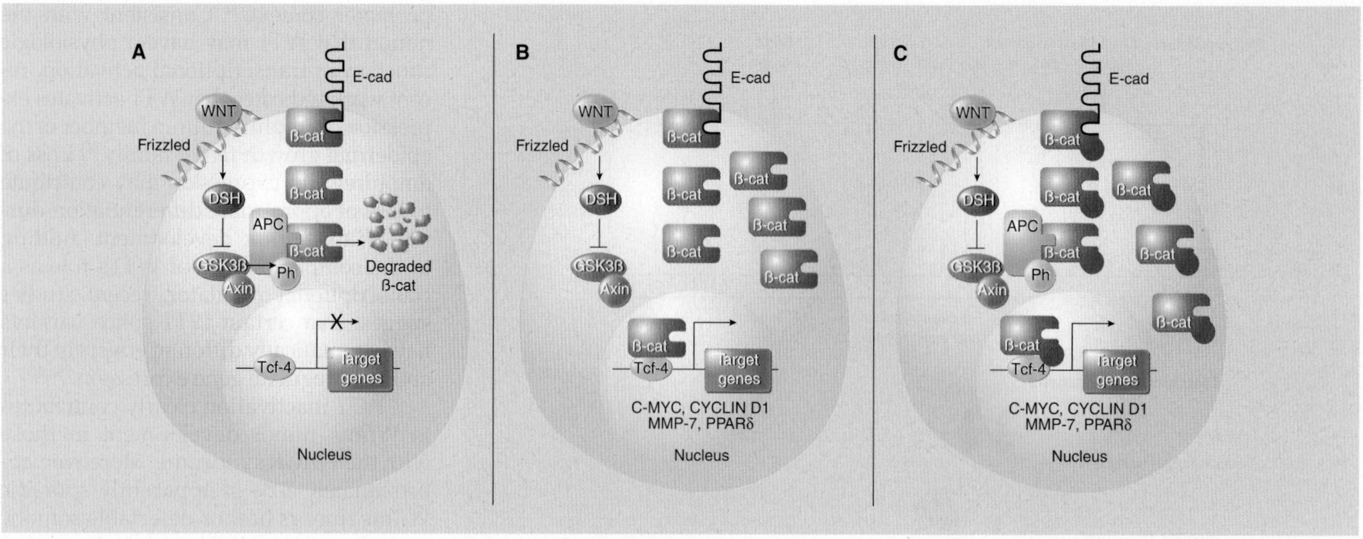

Figure 7-9 ■ A model indicating the function of the Apc, axin, and Gsk3β proteins in the regulation of β-catenin (β-cat) in normal cells, and the consequence of Apc or β-cat defects in cancer cells. β-Cat is an abundant cellular protein, and much of it is often bound to the cytoplasmic domain of the E-cadherin (E-cad) cell–cell adhesion protein. **(A)** In normal cells, the proteins glycogen synthase kinase 3β (Gsk3β), Apc, and axin function to promote degradation of free cytosolic β-cat, probably as a result of phosphorylation of the N-terminal sequences of β-cat by Gsk3β. Gsk3β activity and β-cat degradation are inhibited by activation of the wingless (Wnt) pathway, as a result of the action of the Frizzled receptor and disheveled (Dsh) signaling protein. **(B)** Mutation of Apc in colorectal and other cancer cells results in accumulation of β-cat, binding to Tcf-4, and transcriptional activation of Tcf-4 target genes, such as *c-myc*, cyclin D1, *MMP-7,* and *PPARδ* (see text). **(C)** Point mutations and small deletions in β-cat in cancer cells inhibit phosphorylation and degradation of β-cat by Gsk3β and Apc, with resultant activation of *c-myc* and other Tcf-4 target genes.

schwannomas, neurofibrosarcomas, and primary brain tumors.[195-197] The *NF1* gene was initially localized to the pericentromeric region of chromosome 17q by linkage analyses.[198,199] Subsequently, karyotype studies of two NF1 patients identified germline chromosomal rearrangements involving band 17q11.[200,201] In further work, both patients were found to have genetic alterations of a localized region of band 17q11. Intensive positional cloning efforts in this chromosome region led to the identification of the *NF1* gene in 1991.[202-204] The *NF1* gene is large, spanning roughly 350 kb of DNA, and it encodes a protein product with a molecular mass of about 300 kDa.[195,197,205] Although germline mutations in the *NF1* gene are believed to underlie the development of the associated disease features in all or nearly all NF1 patients, specific germline *NF1* mutations have been identified in approximately one-half to two-thirds of NF1 patients.[195,197,205,206] Difficulties in identifying germline mutations in the *NF1* gene in the remaining NF1 patients may be a result of the inherent inefficiencies and insensitivity associated with mutation detection strategies in such a large gene.

In addition to germline *NF1* mutations in those patients with NF1, the *NF1* gene is affected by somatic mutations in a fraction of colon cancers, melanomas, neuroblastomas, and bone marrow cells from patients with the myelodysplastic syndrome.[195,205,207-209] Consistent with its presumed tumor suppressor role, the mutations inactivate *NF1.* Studies of leukemias arising in pediatric neurofibromatosis patients provide the clearest evidence that both copies of the *NF1* gene are inactivated during tumorigenesis,[210] as predicted by the Knudson model. Like the *RB1, TP53,* and *APC* genes, the *NF1* gene is expressed ubiquitously. Thus, as for other inherited cancer syndromes, the basis for the tissue specificity of the malignant tumors observed in neurofibromatosis patients is puzzling. The NF1 protein product, termed neurofibromin, is a member of the guanosine triphosphate (GTPase)–activating protein family (GAPs).[195, 211-213] Perhaps the best studied GAP is Ras-GAP, which markedly enhances the GTPase activity of the wild-type K-Ras, H-Ras, and N-Ras proteins. Although the means through which *NF1* defects alter cell growth is not well understood, it is likely that inactivation of neurofibromin function leads to alterations in signaling pathways regulated by small Ras-like GTPase proteins.[214]

Neurofibromatosis 2 Gene ■ Neurofibromatosis 2 (NF2—also known as central neurofibromatosis) is an autosomal dominant disorder that is distinct from NF1 in both genetic and clinical features.[195,215,216] A hallmark of NF2 is the occurrence of bilateral schwannomas that affect the vestibular branch of the eighth cranial nerve (acoustic neuromas). NF2 patients are also at elevated risk for meningiomas, spinal schwannomas, and ependymomas. The neurofibromatosis 2 (*NF2*) gene was mapped to chromosome 22q by a combination of linkage analyses and LOH studies[217-219] and was cloned in 1993 using positional cloning approaches.[220,221] Germline mutations inactivating the *NF2* gene were observed in those patients with NF2, and somatic *NF2* mutations were also observed in a subset of sporadic schwannomas and meningiomas. Somatic *NF2* mutations in most other tumor types appear to be infrequent. However, preliminary studies indicate that the *NF2* gene may be frequently affected by somatic mutations in malignant mesotheliomas[222,223] despite this tumor type not being seen at increased frequency in patients with NF2.[216] The *NF2* gene encodes a protein with strong similarity to a cytoskeletal protein family thought to act as linker proteins between integral membrane proteins and scaffolding proteins of the filamentous submembrane lattice.[221] Consequently, *NF2* gene alterations might contribute to tumor development, at least in part, by effects on cell shape, cell–cell interactions, or cell movement (or a combination). Mouse studies confirm the importance of *NF2* in tumor development. Although *NF2* null mice typically develop osteosarcomas and not schwannomas, recent studies that used a conditional NF2 inactivation system in mouse Schwann cells appear to recapitulate the disease phenotype observed in humans.[224]

von Hippel-Lindau Gene

von Hippel-Lindau (VHL) syndrome is a rare dominant disorder predisposing affected individuals to the development of hemangioblastomas of the central nervous system and retina, renal carcinomas of clear cell type, and pheochromocytomas.[225-227] The *VHL* gene was mapped to chromosome 3p by linkage analysis. As with many other inherited cancer genes, LOH studies established that the *VHL* gene behaves as a typical tumor suppressor gene, with both alleles inactivated during tumorigenesis.[226,228] Positional cloning efforts identified the *VHL* gene in 1993.[229] Germline mutations inactivating one *VHL* allele are seen in the majority of individuals in families displaying features of the VHL syndrome.[225-227] As with some other inherited cancer syndromes, preliminary genotype–phenotype relationships have been observed. Specifically, a certain class of *VHL* germline mutations is associated with the development of renal cancer only, a second class is linked to predisposition to both renal cancer and pheochromocytoma, and yet a third mutation class is associated only with pheochromocytoma.[226] Somatic mutations in the *VHL* gene are also seen in more than 80% of sporadic renal cell carcinomas of the clear cell type, but not in renal cell carcinomas of other histopathologic types (eg, papillary type).[226,227] Approximately 20% of sporadic clear cell renal cancers do not carry a detectable mutation in the *VHL* gene. However, in many of these cases, the *VHL* gene may be inactivated by epigenetic silencing,[230] a mechanism noted earlier in this chapter in connection with inactivation of the *CDKN2A* locus. In tumor types other than clear cell renal cancer, inactivation of the *VHL* gene appears to be uncommon.[226]

The *VHL* gene encodes a 213–amino acid protein whose major function appears to be in the regulation of angiogenesis through protein degradation. The protein encoded by *VHL* is part of a ubiquitin ligase complex that degrades hypoxia-induced factor 1α (HIF-1α) in the presence of oxygen. In the absence of oxygen in normal cells, or when *VHL* is mutated in tumor cells, the HIF-1α transcription factor is stabilized, leading to the expression of cytokines such as vascular endothelial growth factor and the stimulation of angiogenesis. Further biochemical and cell biology studies on *VHL* and renal cell carcinomas are likely to offer definitive insights into angiogenesis, one of the most important stromal processes associated with neoplasia.[231,232]

Genomic Stability Genes

Several recessive cancer predisposition syndromes resulting from inactivation of genes that function in DNA damage recognition and repair have been described, including ataxia-telangiectasia (AT), Bloom syndrome, xeroderma pigmentosum, and Fanconi anemia. In each case, the specific cancer type and the DNA-damaging agents that increase cancer risk are distinct. Although AT heterozygotes may subtly increase the risk of breast cancer,[233] in other recessive cancer syndromes, only homozygotes appear to clearly increase cancer risk. That observation contrasts sharply with the picture in the dominant cancer predisposition syndromes discussed earlier (eg, inherited retinoblastoma, familial adenomatous polyposis, NF1, and NF2), where heterozygotes have a clearly elevated cancer risk. Homozygotes for tumor suppressor gene mutations rarely if ever exist, probably because the condition is lethal during embryogenesis. It is important to remember that the tumor suppressor genes do not only function as guardians against cancer; their main function is the control of normal cell balance, and their inactivation is expected to be incompatible with normal embryonic development.

Because recessive cancer syndromes are quite rare, this discussion of the role of genomic stability genes in cancer will focus on syndromes that are inherited in an autosomal dominant fashion. These syndromes include the most common types of familial cancers, predisposing to tumors of the colon, breast, and other organs.

DNA Mismatch Repair Gene Defects and Hereditary Nonpolyposis Colorectal Cancer Familial clustering of colon cancer has long been recognized, with approximately 5% of all colon cancers attributable to inheritance of a gene defect with a strong effect on cancer risk and another 10-15% with a moderate effect on risk. Germline *APC* mutations are responsible for 0.5-1% of colorectal cancer cases in the Western world, and hereditary nonpolyposis colorectal cancer (HNPCC) is responsible for 2-4%.[234-236]

Diagnostic criteria for identifying those individuals and families most likely to be affected by HNPCC have been determined,[234-237] despite the absence of overt clinical findings prior to cancer diagnosis, and the potential for chance clustering of colon cancer within a family. Representative diagnostic criteria include (1) exclusion of familial polyposis; (2) colorectal cancer in at least three relatives, one of them being a first-degree relative of the others; (3) two or more successive generations affected; and (4) at least one of the affected individuals being younger than 50 years of age at the time of diagnosis. Although not all individuals affected by HNPCC meet these criteria, familial aggregations of colorectal cancer that are likely to have a genetic basis distinct from that underlying the majority of HNPCC cases can be excluded.[234,236]

Several genes responsible for HNPCC have been identified, including two on chromosome 2p (mutS homologs 2 and 6 [*MSH2, MSH6*]) and another on chromosome 3p (mutS homolog 1 [*MLH1*]). Together, germline mutations in these three genes account for virtually all classic HNPCC cases.[234,236-239] The protein products of the *MSH2* and *MLH1* genes appear to have critical roles in the recognition and repair of DNA mismatches (Fig. 7-10). A number of other gene-encoding proteins that function in

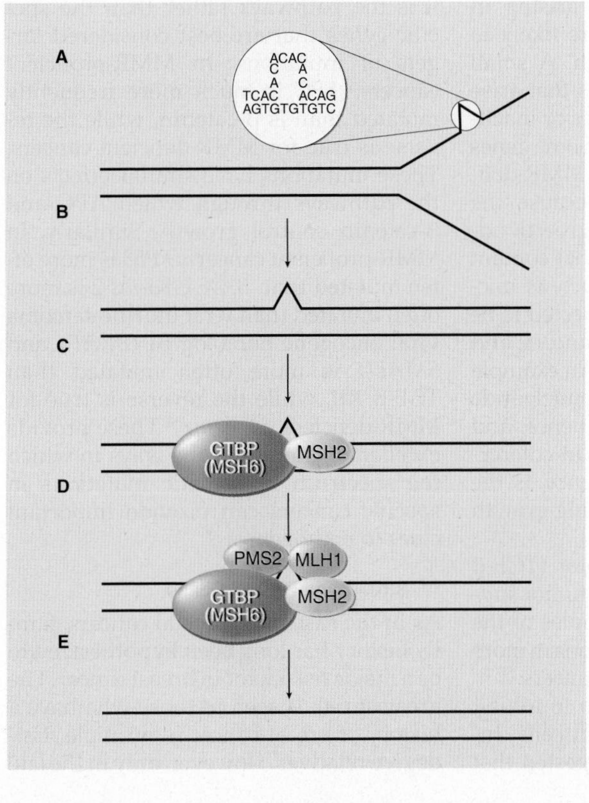

Figure 7-10 Mismatch repair pathway in human cells. **(A, B)** During DNA replication, DNA mismatches may arise, such as from strand slippage (shown) or misincorporation of bases (not shown). **(C)** The mismatch is recognized by MutS homologs, perhaps most often Msh2 and GTBP/Msh6, although another MutS homolog, Msh3, may substitute for GTBP/Msh6 in some cases. **(D, E)** MutL homologs, such as Mlh1 and Pms2, are recruited to the complex and the mismatch is repaired through the action of a number of proteins, including an exonuclease, helicase, DNA polymerase, and ligase.

mismatch repair have been identified, and mutations inactivating the postmeiotic segregation 2 (*PMS2*) genes have been seen in a small fraction of those with HNPCC-like disease.[234,236-240]

In cells with one normal and one mutant allele of a DNA mismatch repair gene, DNA repair is minimally impaired, if at all. However, inactivation of the remaining allele can occur as a result of somatic mutation in a normal epithelial cell. This "second hit" abrogates mismatch repair function, and hundreds to thousands of mutations may thereby occur during each subsequent cell-division cycle. Because these mutations preferentially arise in mononucleotide, dinucleotide, and trinucleotide repeat tracts (ie, microsatellite sequence tracts), the phenotype is often called the microsatellite instability (MSI) phenotype.

Germline mutations in the known mismatch repair (MMR) genes have been detected in only 2-4% of colorectal cancer patients, although approximately 10-15% of all colon cancers display the MSI phenotype.[234,237-239,241-243] Clearly, only a small fraction of the sporadic colorectal cancers with the MSI phenotype develop as the result of a germline mutation in a known mismatch repair gene. Somatic mutations in mismatch repair genes have been found in some sporadic colorectal cancers with the MSI phenotype.[244] In most sporadic cases, however, inactivation of the *MLH1* gene occurs as a result of epigenetic inactivation.[245,246] The basis for this inactivation and the molecular mechanism or mechanisms underlying the accompanying methylation of the *MLH1* gene promoter are unknown.

Many of the mutations arising in cells with MMR-deficiency are likely to be detrimental to cell growth. A small fraction of the total mutations that arise presumably activate oncogenes or inactivate tumor suppressor genes. Some genes are preferentially mutated in MMR-deficient cancers, presumably because the mutations confer a selective growth advantage. For instance, genes that contain repetitive DNA sequences, such as microsatellite tracts, might be expected to be targets of mutation in these cancers, and data support this prediction. An example of a gene that contains a mononucleotide repeat tract in its coding sequence, and that is frequently inactivated in colorectal cancers with MMR-deficiency, is the type II receptor for transforming growth factor-β (TGF-β).

The TGF-β type II receptor (TGF-β RII) is a compelling candidate tumor suppressor gene, because both copies of the gene are inactivated by mutations in more than 90% of MSI colorectal cancers.[247,248] The TGF-β cytokine is known to inhibit the growth of many epithelial cells. Intriguingly, one study has suggested that germline mutations in the cytoplasmic domain of the TGF-β type II receptor is associated with HNPCC,[249] although this observation has not been confirmed in additional HNPCC kindreds. A downstream effector of the TGF-β pathway, small mothers against decapentaplegic 4 (*SMAD4*), also called deleted in pancreatic cancer 4 (*DPC4*), has been identified as a tumor suppressor gene. *SMAD4* is somatically mutated in 45-50% of pancreatic cancers, in 10-20% of colorectal cancers, and in a very small fraction of other cancers.[250-252] Germline inactivating mutations in *SMAD4* are found in a major fraction of patients with juvenile polyposis syndrome (JPS).[253] Patients with JPS develop benign (hamartomatous, not adenomatous) polyps of the intestinal tract and are at increased risk of colorectal and gastric cancer. Germline mutations of a receptor for bone morphogenetic protein (BMP), a TGF-β family member, have also been described to lead to JPS.[254] Taken together, the TGF-β signaling pathway has been shown to play a central role in both predisposition and progression of colorectal cancers.[255]

Another recently suggested candidate for somatic inactivation in MMR-deficient colorectal cancers is the B cell lymphoma 2 (BCL-2)–associated X protein (*BAX*) gene,[256] which is a potential TP53-regulated gene, encoding a BCL-2–related proapoptotic protein. Finally, there are data suggesting that gain-of-function mutations in β-catenin arise preferentially in MSI colon cancers,[156,157,257] although the β-catenin mutations are not present in a microsatellite tract. These mutation comparisons emphasize that it is the pathways rather than the specific genes that are best considered targets of mutations. In MMR-proficient cancers, *APC* is much more frequently mutated than is β-catenin, while the reverse is true for MMR-deficient cancers. These mutations have similar effects on the pathways through which APC and β-catenin control growth. Similarly, in MMR-proficient cancers, *TP53* is more often mutated than *BAX*, c-Ki-*ras*-2 is more often mutated than v-raf murine sarcoma viral oncogene homolog B1 (*BRAF*), and *SMAD4* is more often mutated than TGF-β RII, while the reverse is true for MMR-deficient cancers.[258] These provide excellent examples of the ways in which the spectrum of somatic mutations in specific cancers can provide important clues to pathogenesis.

BRCA1 and BRCA2 Genes

As in the case of colorectal cancers, family history has long been hypothesized to be a major risk factor in breast cancer. The greatest risk is seen in those who have a history of breast cancer in multiple first-degree relatives. However, only in the late 1980s was evidence obtained that predisposition to breast cancer in some families could be attributed to a highly penetrant autosomal dominant allele. In 1990, Hall and colleagues reported the localization of one such breast cancer predisposition gene, *BRCA1*, on chromosome 17q21.[259] Others found that germline *BRCA1* mutations substantially increase the risk not only of breast cancer but also of ovarian cancer.[260,261] Intensive research efforts were focused on the region of chromosome 17q harboring *BRCA1*, and the gene was ultimately identified by positional cloning approaches in 1994.[262,263]

Studies of germline *BRCA1* mutations in breast cancer patients have yielded important results. In studies of families with four or more cases of breast or ovarian cancer (or both) diagnosed before age 60 years, germline *BRCA1* mutations were identified in nearly 50% of families studied.[264-266] In fact, germline *BRCA1* mutations may account for cancer predisposition in roughly 75% of families who manifest both breast and ovarian cancer.[264,265] Many distinct germline *BRCA1* mutations have been identified, although most of the mutations result in the synthesis of a truncated BRCA1 protein.[264,265] Whereas most germline *BRCA1* mutations have been identified in only one or a few families, some mutations have been found recurrently. The 11 most common mutations account for about 45% of the total BRCA1 mutations observed.[265,266] In fact, the two most common mutations in *BRCA1* (185delAG and 5382insC) account for approximately 10% of the total. Of note, the 185delAG frameshift mutation at codon 185 of *BRCA1*, involving a deletion of two bases (adenine and guanine), has been identified in more than 20 Jewish families with familial breast or ovarian cancer. Moreover, population surveys of Ashkenazi Jews, chosen without regard to a family history of cancer, indicate that approximately 1% carry the 185delAG mutation.[265-267] Based on studies of families with germline *BRCA1* mutations, the lifetime risks of breast cancer and ovarian cancer in those carrying an inactivating mutation are estimated to be 85% and 50%, respectively.[264,265,268] Whether specific germline *BRCA1* mutations confer a greater risk of breast and ovarian cancer than do other mutations remains uncertain.

As with most tumor suppressor genes and their associated familial cancer syndromes, germline mutations of *BRCA1* lead to the presence of a mutant allele in every cell of the body. Cancers then arise through inactivation of the second wild-type allele by the mechanisms outlined in Figure 7-2. In the case of *BRCA1* (and *BRCA2*), LOH of the remaining wild-type allele is usually responsible for the second "hit" leading to inactivation of the *BRCA1* gene. In addition, LOH of the *BRCA1* locus was found in approximately 50% of unselected breast cancers and 65-80% of unselected ovarian cancers.[265,269] Because most breast and ovarian cancers are not associated with a hereditary predisposition (ie, they are sporadic), these studies of unselected cancers led investigators to hypothesize that BRCA1 would play an important role in the development of sporadic breast and ovarian cancers. However, despite these LOH data, sporadic breast and ovarian cancers rarely harbor mutations in the *BRCA1* gene, demonstrating that at least one-wild type allele is still present in most of these sporadic cancers.[265,269] Somewhat surprisingly, this finding would suggest that BRCA1 does not have a role in the genesis of the more common, nonfamilial forms of breast and ovarian cancers. However, it is still possible that downstream effectors of the BRCA1 protein are altered in sporadic breast and ovarian cancers, suggesting that the pathway, rather than the gene, is an important contributor to the carcinogenic process of these cancers.[270]

Although germline mutations in the *BRCA1* gene underlie cancer predisposition in roughly 40-50% of families with multiple breast cancer cases, another highly penetrant autosomal dominant susceptibility gene termed *BRCA2* plays a critical role in a significant fraction of the families with multiple breast cancer cases lacking *BRCA1* mutations. The *BRCA2* gene was mapped to chromosome 13q12-13 in 1994,[271] and identified by positional cloning strategies in 1995.[272] Although germline mutations in *BRCA1* and *BRCA2* appear to confer essentially similar lifetime risks of female breast cancer (ie, approximately 80%), the risk of ovarian cancer is reduced to approximately 10% in those with *BRCA2* mutations as compared with approximately 40-50% in those with *BRCA1* mutations. The risk of male breast cancer is markedly elevated in *BRCA2* mutation carriers, with a lifetime risk of approximately 7%, as opposed to a 1% lifetime risk of in *BRCA1* mutation carriers.[273] There also appears to be an elevated risk of pancreatic and perhaps several other cancers in both male and female *BRCA2* mutation carriers.[265] As is the case for *BRCA1*, LOH of the *BRCA2* locus at 13q12, but not at the *RB1* locus at 13q14, has been observed in some sporadic breast, pancreatic, head and neck, and other cancers, suggesting that *BRCA2* may be a target for somatic mutations in cancer. However, as with *BRCA1*, detections of somatic *BRCA2* mutations in sporadic cancers have been few,[265] once again suggesting that perhaps the pathway, rather than the gene, is the target of genetic alteration in sporadic forms of these cancers.

The *BRCA1* and *BRCA2* genes each encode a large nuclear protein. The amino acid sequences of the two proteins have only short regions of similarity with one another or other well-characterized proteins. Although their lack of obvious functional motifs stymied initial attempts to define the cellular functions of BRCA1 and BRCA2, several lines of evidence indicate that both proteins interact directly or indirectly with homologs of yeast Rad51, a protein that functions in the repair of double-stranded DNA breaks.[274-281] Moreover, the BRCA1, BRCA2, and Rad51 proteins all appear to be present in a stable multiprotein complex in the cell's nucleus. Consequently, it has been suggested that BRCA1 and BRCA2 may function in the response to or repair of DNA damage, particularly double-strand DNA breaks.[282] Other findings imply that BRCA1 and perhaps BRCA2 may have a role in regulating transcription.[283] Although the DNA repair and transcription regulation functions may be distinct, it is entirely possible that the two functions are linked in a process sometimes called transcription-coupled DNA repair.[276] There is precedent for this idea, in that some nucleotide excision repair genes causing xeroderma pigmentosum can also function in transcription,[284] and repair of certain types of DNA damage is known to be coupled to transcription.[285]

As with other genes that confer site-specific predisposition to cancer yet are ubiquitously expressed in adult tissues, it is not clear why germline mutations in *BRCA1* and *BRCA2* markedly increase the risk of only selected cancer types (eg, breast and ovarian). One suggestion is that breast and certain other epithelial cells may be particularly susceptible to the type of DNA damage that arises in cells with *BRCA1* or *BRCA2* defects. Loss of BRCA1 or BRCA2 function would then lead to markedly increased rates of mutation acquisition only in certain cell types. Alternatively, the processes in which BRCA1 and BRCA2 function may have many backup systems or fail-safe mechanisms in most normal cell types, but not in breast and other selected epithelial cell types. A third possible explanation for the tissue specificity of the cancers seen in *BRCA1* and *BRCA2* mutation carriers is that inactivation of either BRCA1 or BRCA2 is most often associated with a detrimental or even a lethal effect in stem cells other than those of the breast or ovary. Finally, although the observations thus far have implicated BRCA1 and BRCA2 predominantly in maintenance of genome integrity, other functions for the proteins are possible, with evidence of a link between the estrogen receptor and BRCA1 function, and of BRCA1 interaction with inactivated X chromosomes, found only in female cells, thus providing another potential explanation for this tumor suppressor's tissue and gender specificity.[286,287]

Candidate Tumor Suppressor Genes

The tumor suppressor genes discussed above and others summarized in Table 7-1 are distinguished by the fact that germline-inactivating mutations in the genes are associated with inherited cancer predisposition. The link between germline mutation and elevated cancer risk provides incontrovertible evidence of the gene's role in tumorigenesis. Other findings, such as the demonstration in sporadic cancers of LOH of one tumor suppressor gene allele accompanied by somatic mutation of the remaining allele, offer evidence for a more widespread role for many of the inherited cancer genes. Although the tumor suppressor genes in Table 7-1 are definitively linked to inherited cancer syndromes, it is possible that germline mutations in other bona fide tumor suppressor genes may be associated with a more modest cancer risk, as has already been demonstrated for the I1307K mutation in *APC*.

Tumor suppressor genes that are not found to be mutated in the germline may still frequently be inactivated by somatic mutations in sporadic forms of cancer. In these cases, their principal role may relate to tumor progression rather than tumor initiation. Because the evidence in favor of involvement of these genes does not include predisposition by inheritance in mutant form, confidence in the role of these genes in human tumorigenesis is not as high as for those listed in Table 7-1. Nevertheless, when such a gene can be shown to be mutated in a large number of cases of a given tumor type, and when the mutations are clearly inactivating (eg, truncating mutations), the likelihood that they play a role in tumorigenesis is high. A complete accounting of such genes can be found in Vogelstein and Kinzler[130] and Futreal and colleagues.[288]

An increasing number of genes with decreased or absent expression in cancers are being discovered through microarrays, serial analysis of gene expression, and other global gene expression techniques.[130] These genes are sometimes termed tumor suppressors solely on the basis of their reduced expression. A small subset of these genes may, indeed, have critical roles in growth regulation, but expression data provide insufficient evidence to invoke causality. The altered expression of genes in cancers more often reflects the effect rather than the cause of the neoplastic process (ie, the altered growth and differentiation properties of cancer cells and their abnormal microen-

Table 7-1 Tumor Suppressor and Stability Genes Associated with Inherited Cancer Predisposition Syndromes

Gene[a]	Syndrome	Hereditary Pattern	Second Hit	Pathway[b]	Major Hereditary Tumor Types[c]
Tumor Suppressor Genes					
APC	FAP	Dominant	Inactivation of wt allele	APC	Colon, thyroid, stomach, intestine
AXIN2	Attenuated polyposis	Dominant	Inactivation of wt allele	APC	Colon
CDH1 (E-cadherin)	Familial gastric carcinoma	Dominant	Inactivation of wt allele	APC	Stomach
GPC3	Simpson-Golabi-Behmel syndrome	X-linked	?	APC	Embryonal
CYLD	Familial cylindromatosis	Dominant	Inactivation of wt allele	APOP	Pilotrichomas
EXT1, EXT2	Hereditary multiple exostoses	Dominant	Inactivation of wt allele	GLI	Bone
PTCH	Gorlin	Dominant	Inactivation of wt allele	GLI	Skin, medulloblastoma
SUFU	Medulloblastoma predisposition	Dominant	Inactivation of wt allele	GLI	Skin, medulloblastoma
FH	Hereditary leiomyomatosis	Dominant	Inactivation of wt allele	HIF1	Leiomyomas
SDHB, SDHC, SDHD	Familial paraganglioma	Dominant	Inactivation of wt allele	HIF1	Paragangliomas, pheochromocytomas
VHL	von Hippel-Lindau	Dominant	Inactivation of wt allele	HIF1	Kidney
TP53 (p53)	Li-Fraumeni	Dominant	Inactivation of wt allele	TP53	Breast, sarcoma, adrenal, brain, ...
WT1	Familial Wilms tumor	Dominant	Inactivation of wt allele	TP53	Wilms
STK11 (LKB1)	Peutz-Jeghers	Dominant	Inactivation of wt allele	PI3K	Intestinal, ovarian, pancreatic
PTEN	Cowden	Dominant	Inactivation of wt allele	PI3K	Hamartoma, glioma, uterus
TSC1, TSC2	Tuberous sclerosis	Dominant	Inactivation of wt allele	PI3K	Hamartoma, kidney
CDKN2A (p16INK4A, p14ARF)	Familial malignant melanoma	Dominant	Inactivation of wt allele	RB	Melanoma, pancreas
CDK4	Familial malignant melanoma	Dominant	?	RB	Melanoma
RB1	Hereditary retinoblastoma	Dominant	Inactivation of wt allele	RB	Eye
NF1	Neurofibromatosis	Dominant	Inactivation of wt allele	RTK	Neurofibroma
BMPR1A	Juvenile polyposis	Dominant	Inactivation of wt allele	SMAD	Gastrointestinal
MEN1	Multiple endocrine neoplasia type I	Dominant	Inactivation of wt allele	SMAD	Parathyroid, pituitary, islet cell, carcinoid
SMAD4 (DPC4)	Juvenile polyposis	Dominant	Inactivation of wt allele	SMAD	Gastrointestinal
BHD	Birt-Hogg-Dube	Dominant	Inactivation of wt allele	?	Renal, hair follicle
HRPT2	Hyperparathyroidism jaw-tumor	Dominant	Inactivation of wt allele	?	Parathyroid, jaw fibroma
NF2	Neurofibromatosis	Dominant	Inactivation of wt allele	?	Meningioma, acoustic neuromas
Stability Genes					
MUTYH	Attenuated polyposis	Recessive	None required	BER	Colon
ATM	Ataxia-telangiectasia	Recessive	None required	CIN	Leukemias, lymphomas, brain
BLM	Bloom	Recessive	None required	CIN	Leukemias, lymphomas, skin
BRCA1, BRCA2	Hereditary breast cancer	Dominant	Inactivation of wt allele	CIN	Breast, ovary
FANCA, FANCC, FANCD2, FANCE, FANCF, FANCG	Fanconi anemia A, C, D2, E, F, and G	Recessive	None required	CIN	Leukemias
NBS1	Nijmegen breakage	Recessive	None required	CIN	Lymphomas, brain
RECQL4	Rothmund-Thomson	Recessive	None required	CIN	Bone and skin
WRN	Werner	Recessive	None required	CIN	Bone and brain
MSH2, MLH1, MSH6, PMS2	HNPCC	Dominant	Inactivation of wt allele	MMR	Colon, uterus
XPA, XPC; ERCC2, ERCC3, ERCC4, ERCC5; DDB2	Xeroderma pigmentosum	Recessive	None required	NER	Skin

[a]Representative genes of all major pathways and hereditary cancer predisposition types are listed. Approved gene symbols are provided for each entry; alternative names are in parentheses.
[b]In many cases, the gene has been implicated in several pathways. The single pathway that is listed for each gene represents a "best guess" (when one can be made) and should not be regarded as conclusive.
[c]In most cases, the nonfamilial tumor spectrum caused by somatic mutations of the gene includes those occurring in familial cases but also additional tumor types. For example, mutations of *TP53* and *CDKN2A* are found in many more tumor types than those to which Li-Fraumeni and familial malignant melanoma patients, respectively, are predisposed.
Abbreviations: APC, adenomatous polyposis coli; APOP, apoptotic pathway; BER, base excision repair; CIN, chromosomal instability; FAP, familial adenomatous polyposis; GLI, glioma associated oncogene; HIF1, hypoxia inducing factor 1; MMR, mismatch repair; NER, nucleotide excision repair; PI3K, phosphatidylinositol 3-kinase; RB, retinoblastoma; RTK, receptor tyrosine kinase pathway; SMAD, SMA and MAD related protein 4; wt, wild type.
Source: Adapted from Ref. 130.

vironment as compared with normal cells in the tissue or organ from which the cancer arose). Moreover, many genes that play no role in cancer can dramatically alter cell growth when expressed exogenously at a high, unphysiologic level, rendering functional analyses of such candidates problematic. In the end, the mutational and functional evidence should be carefully weighed before a conclusion can be drawn that a gene has a causal role in tumorigenesis and that it should appropriately be designated a tumor suppressor gene.

Summary

There is now overwhelming evidence that mutations in tumor suppressor genes are major molecular determinants for most common human cancers. Thus far, more than 30 tumor suppressor genes have been identified by molecular cloning techniques. In some cases, these genes are inactivated in the germline, and their inactivation predisposes to cancer. Far more frequently, these same tumor suppressor genes are inactivated by somatic mutations during tumor development. Although much has been learned about tumor suppressor genes, a great deal of work remains. Advancements in our understanding of tumorigenesis will continue with the identification of additional tumor suppressor genes, the detailed characterization of their normal cellular functions, and the elucidation of the frequency and spectrum of mutations and other mechanisms that inactivate both the genes and their protein products in human tumors. These findings will not only provide new insights into cancer pathogenesis, but should also prove beneficial in the diagnosis and appropriate management of patients with cancer.

Selected References

The complete reference list can be found at www.CANCERMEDICINE8.com

1. Broca P. Etiologie des productions accidentelles. *Traite des Tumerus.* 1866;147–157.
4. Boveri T. *The Origin of Malignant Tumors.* Baltimore, MD: Williams and Wilkins; 1929.
10. Stanbridge EJ, Der CJ, Doersen CJ, et al. Human cell hybrids: analysis of transformation and tumorigenicity. *Science.* 1982;215(4530):252–259.
15. Knudson AGJ. Mutation and cancer: statistical study of retinoblastoma. *Proc Natl Acad Sci U S A.* 1971;68(4):820–823.
19. Sparkes RS, Murphree AL, Lingua RW, et al. Gene for hereditary retinoblastoma assigned to human chromosome 13 by linkag to esterase D. *Science.* 1983;219 (4587):971–973.
21. Knudson AG Jr. Hereditary cancer, oncogenes, and antioncogenes. *Cancer Res.* 1985;45(4):1437–1443.
22. Cavenee WK, Dryja TP, Phillips RA, et al. Expression of recessive alleles by chromosomal mechanisms in retinoblastoma. *Nature.* 1983;305(5937):779–784.
26. Dryja TP, Rapaport JM, Joyce JM, Petersen RA. Molecular detection of deletions involving band q14 of chromosome 13 in retinoblastomas. *Proc Natl Acad Sci U S A.* 1986;83(19):7391–7394.
35. Whyte P, Buchkovich KJ, Horowitz JM, et al. Association between an oncogene and an anti-oncogene: the adenovirus E1A proteins bind to the retinoblastoma gene product. *Nature.* 1988;334(6178):124–129.
43. DeLeo AB, Jay G, Appella E, Dubois GC, Law LW, Old LJ. Detection of a transformation-related antigen in chemically induced sarcomas and other transformed cells of the mouse. *Proc Natl Acad Sci U S A.* 1979;76(5):2420–2424.
52. Baker SJ, Fearon ER, Nigro JM, et al. Chromosome 17 deletions and p53 gene mutations in colorectal carcinomas. *Science.* 1989;244(4901):217–221.
54. Vogelstein B, Fearon ER, Hamilton SR, et al. Genetic alterations during colorectal-tumor development. *N Engl J Med.* 1988;319(9):525–532.
64. Hollstein M, Hergenhahn M, Yang Q, Bartsch H, Wang ZQ, Hainaut P. New approaches to understanding p53 gene tumor mutation spectra. *Mutat Res.* 1999;431(2):199–209.
69. Bartek J, Falck J, Lukas J. CHK2 kinase—a busy messenger. *Nat Rev Mol Cell Biol.* 2001;2(12):877–886.
75. Oliner JD, Kinzler KW, Meltzer PS, George DL, Vogelstein B. Amplification of a gene encoding a p53-associated protein in human sarcomas. *Nature.* 1992;358(6381):80–83.
76. Marine JC, Jochemsen AG. Mdmx and Mdm2: brothers in arms? *Cell Cycle.* 2004;3(7):900–904.
85. Vogelstein B, Lane D, Levine AJ. Surfing the p53 network. *Nature.* 2000;408(6810): 307–310.
86. el-Deiry WS, Tokino T, Velculescu VE et al. WAF1, a potential mediator of p53 tumor suppression. *Cell.* 1993;75(4):817–825.
88. Waldman T, Kinzler KW, Vogelstein B. p21 is necessary for the p53-mediated G1 arrest in human cancer cells. *Cancer Res.* 1995;55(22):5187–5190.
89. Yu J, Wang Z, Kinzler KW, Vogelstein B, Zhang L. PUMA mediates the apoptotic response to p53 in colorectal cancer cells. *Proc Natl Acad Sci U S A.* 2003;100(4):1931–1936.
91. Jeffers JR, Parganas E, Lee Y, et al. Puma is an essential mediator of p53-dependent and -independent apoptotic pathways. *Cancer Cell.* 2003;4(4):321–328.
100. Bunz F, Hwang PM, Torrance C, et al. Disruption of p53 in human cancer cells alters the responses to therapeutic agents. *J Clin Invest.* 1999;104(3):263–269.
111. Kamb A, Gruis NA, Weaver-Feldhaus J, et al. A cell cycle regulator potentially involved in genesis of many tumor types. *Science.* 1994;264(5157):436–440.
120. Cairns P, Polascik TJ, Eby Y, et al. Frequency of homozygous deletion at p16/ CDKN2 in primary human tumours. *Nat Genet.* 1995;11(2):210–212.
123. Jacobs JJ, Kieboom K, Marino S, DePinho RA, van Lohuizen M. The oncogene and Polycomb-group gene bmi-1 regulates cell proliferation and senescence through the ink4a locus. *Nature.* 1999;397(6715):164–168.
125. Bachman KE, Park BH, Rhee I, et al. Histone modifications and silencing prior to DNA methylation of a tumor suppressor gene. *Cancer Cell.* 2003;3(1):89–95.
130. Vogelstein B, Kinzler KW. Cancer genes and the pathways they control. *Nat Med.* 2004;10(8):789–799.
131. Schmitt CA, Fridman JS, Yang M, et al. A senescence program controlled by p53 and p16INK4a contributes to the outcome of cancer therapy. *Cell.* 2002;109(3):335–346.
135. Groden J, Thliveris A, Samowitz W, et al. Identification and characterization of the familial adenomatous polyposis coli gene. *Cell.* 1991;66(3):589–600.
142. Kinzler KW, Vogelstein B. Lessons from hereditary colorectal cancer. *Cell.* 1996;87(2):159–170.
144. Nieuwenhuis MH, Vasen HF. Correlations between mutation site in APC and phenotype of familial adenomatous polyposis (FAP): a review of the literature. *Crit Rev Oncol Hematol.* 2007;61(2):153–161.
151. Morin PJ, Vogelstein B, Kinzler KW. Apoptosis and APC in colorectal tumorigenesis. *Proc Natl Acad Sci USA.* 1996;93(15):7950–7954.
163. Park BH, Vogelstein B, Kinzler KW. Genetic disruption of PPARdelta decreases the tumorigenicity of human colon cancer cells. *Proc Natl Acad Sci USA.* 2001;98(5):2598–2603.
167. Gerner EW, Ignatenko NA, Lance P, Hurley LH. A comprehensive strategy to combat colon cancer targeting the adenomatous polyposis coli tumor suppressor gene. *Ann N Y Acad Sci.* 2005;1059:97–105.
169. Knudson AG Jr, Strong LC. Mutation and cancer: a model for Wilms' tumor of the kidney. *J Natl Cancer Inst.* 1972;48(2):313–324.
174. Fearon ER, Vogelstein B, Feinberg AP. Somatic deletion and duplication of genes on chromosome 11 in Wilms' tumours. *Nature.* 1984;309(5964):176–178.
178. Call KM, Glaser T, Ito CY, et al. Isolation and characterization of a zinc finger polypeptide gene at the human chromosome 11 Wilms' tumor locus. *Cell.* 1990;60(3):509–520.
188. Haber DA, Housman DE. The genetics of Wilms' tumor. *Adv Cancer Res.* 1992;59:41–68.
195. Gutman D. Neurofibromatosis type 1. In: Kinzler KW, ed. *The Genetic Basis of Human Cancer.* New York: McGraw-Hill; 1998:423–442.
210. Shannon KM, O'Connell P, Martin GA, et al. Loss of the normal NF1 allele from the bone marrow of children with type 1 neurofibromatosis and malignant myeloid disorders. *N Engl J Med.* 1994;330(9): 597–601.
214. Patrakitkomjorn S, Kobayashi D, Morikawa T, et al. NF1 tumor suppressor, neurofibromin, regulates the neuronal differentiation of PC12 cells via its associating protein, collapsin response mediator protein-2. *J Biol Chem.* 2008;283(14):9399–9413.
224. Giovannini M, Robanus-Maandag E, van der Valk M, et al. Conditional biallelic Nf2 mutation in the mouse promotes manifestations of human neurofibromatosis type 2. *Genes Dev.* 2000;14(13):1617–1630.
226. Linehan WM. Renal carcinoma. In: Kinzler KW, ed. *The Genetic Basis of Human Cancer.* New York: McGraw-Hill; 1998:455–474.
234. Boland CR. Hereditary nonpolyposis colorectal cancer. In: Kinzler KW, ed. *The Genetic Basis of Human Cancer.* New York: McGraw-Hill; 1998:333–346.
237. Lynch HT, de la Chapelle A. Genetic susceptibility to non-polyposis colorectal cancer. *J Med Genet.* 1999;36(11):801–818.
245. Herman JG, Umar A, Polyak K, et al. Incidence and functional consequences of hMLH1 promoter hypermethylation in colorectal carcinoma. *Proc Natl Acad Sci U S A.* 1998;95(12):6870–6875.
255. Xu Y, Pasche B. TGF-beta signaling alterations and susceptibility to colorectal cancer. *Hum Mol Genet.* 2007;16(Spec No 1): R14–20.
259. Hall JM, Gryfe R, Kim H, et al. Linkage of early-onset familial breast cancer to chromosome 17q21. *Science.* 1990;250(4988): 1684–1689.
264. Collins FS. BRCA1—lots of mutations, lots of dilemmas. *N Engl J Med.* 1996;334(3):186–188.
288. Futreal PA, Coin L, Marshall M, et al. A census of human cancer genes. *Nat Rev Cancer.* 2004;4(3):177–183.

8 Genomic Alterations and Chromosomal Aberrations in Human Cancer

Kevin M. Brown, PhD ▪ Jonathan J. Keats, PhD ▪ Aleksandar Sekulic, MD, PhD ▪
Cheryl L. Willman, MD ▪ Jeffrey M. Trent, PhD, Robert A. Hromas, MD

Introduction

Increasingly, cancer is recognized as a heterogeneous collection of diseases whose initiation and progression are promoted by the aberrant function of genes that regulate DNA repair, genome stability, cell proliferation, cell death, adhesion, angiogenesis, invasion, and metastasis in complex cell and tissue microenvironments.[1,2] Variant or aberrant function of these so-called cancer genes may result from naturally occurring DNA polymorphisms, changes in genome copy number (through amplification, deletion, chromosome loss, or duplication), changes in gene and chromosome structure (through chromosomal translocation, inversion, or other rearrangement that leads to chimeric transcripts or deregulated gene expression), and point mutations (including base substitutions, deletions, or insertions in coding regions and splice sites). Beyond perturbations of the DNA sequence itself, heritable epigenetic modifications of the genome, including DNA methylation, genomic imprinting, and histone modification by acetylation, methylation, or phosphorylation, have also been shown to play a critical role in tumorigenesis.[3,4] Inactivation of genes that normally suppress the cancer phenotype (tumor suppressor genes) have been shown to occur through mutation, deletion, and epigenetic modifications, whereas activation of genes that promote the cancer phenotype (oncogenes) may occur through mutation, amplification, epigenetic modifications, and structural chromosomal rearrangements.[1,2] Strikingly, the function of the same cancer-promoting gene may be disrupted through different molecular mechanisms in tumors of different lineages. Although the vast majority (90%) of cancer genes identified to date are mutated or altered through chromosomal aberrations in somatic tissues, 10% are altered in the germline, thereby transmitting heritable cancer susceptibility through successive generations.[5]

Overwhelming evidence supports the hypothesis that cancer is caused by the stepwise accumulation of numerous genetic and epigenetic aberrations.[1] Since the initial discovery of a recurring chromosomal abnormality in a human cancer in 1960 by Nowell—the "Philadelphia chromosome" fragment associated with chronic myelogenous leukemia (CML)[6]—and the determination by Rowley in 1973, using newly developed chromosomal banding techniques, that the Philadelphia chromosome was actually a balanced reciprocal translocation between chromosomes 9 and 22 (Fig. 8-1),[7,8] it has become clear that many aberrations are shared both within and across cancer types. The discovery of such commonalities has served to greatly increase our understanding of the development; progression; and in many cases, clinical behavior of human neoplasms.

Importantly, such discoveries have directly led to the development and clinical application of effective "targeted" therapies, resulting in improved treatment of cancer. It is particularly fitting that one of the first successful targeted cancer therapies was developed to the first reported chromosomal abnormality in human cancer. The seminal discovery of the t(9;22) Philadelphia chromosome translocation[6-8] laid the foundation for the subsequent cloning and characterization of the *BCR-ABL* chimeric fusion gene arising from the t(9;22), the determination that *BCR-ABL* encoded a constitutively active tyrosine kinase, and the ultimate development of one of the first successful targeted cancer therapies by Drucker and colleagues—the selective tyrosine kinase inhibitor imatinib, or Gleevec, for the treatment of CML.[9-11] This paradigm has been repeated with dramatic success. Several newly introduced cancer drugs targeted to specific genomic lesions have shown clinical efficacy: imatinib/Gleevec, not only for the selective inhibition of the ABL kinase in CML but also the PDGFR and KIT tyrosine kinases altered by genomic changes in gastrointestinal stromal tumors and hypereosinophilic syndromes;[12-14] trastuzumab/Herceptin, the neutralizing antibody targeted to the Her2/ErbB2 tyrosine kinase receptor whose encoding gene *ERBB2* is amplified and overexpressed in 25-30% of breast carcinomas;[15,16] and gefitinib/Iressa or erlotinib/Tarceva, shown to have striking effectiveness in 5-10% of lung adenocarcinoma patients with European ancestry and 25-30% of Japanese patients who harbor activating mutations in the *EGFR* gene.[17,18] Clinical trials are ongoing for numerous novel therapeutic agents directed against genomic targets in cancer.

These successes in leveraging genomic discovery as the basis to develop clinically useful disease subclassifications and targeted therapies have served as much of the impetus behind continued

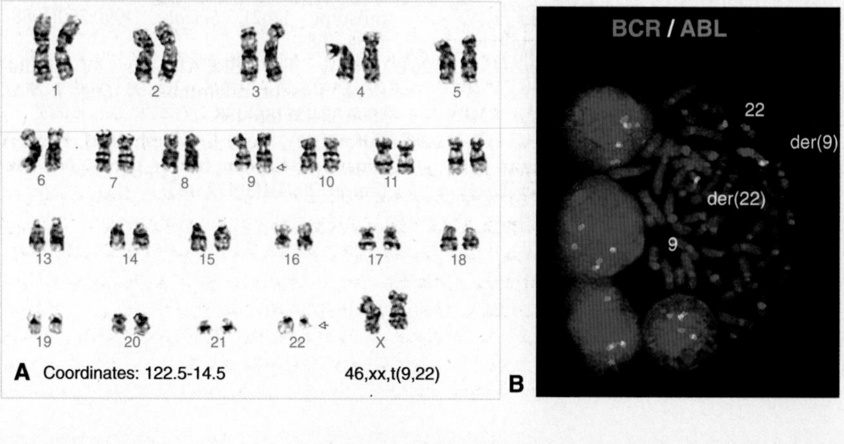

Figure 8-1 ▪ **(A)** Chromosome G-banded karyotype of metaphase chromosomes from a case of chronic myelogenous leukemia (CML): 46,XX, t(9;22). **(B)** Interphase and metaphase FISH detection of the t(9;22) *BCR-ABL* gene fusion using fluorescently labeled genomic probes for *BCR* (green) and *ABL* (red). Note that the fusion of *BCR* and *ABL* probes results in a yellow signal indicating colocalization of the red and green probes as a result of the t(9;22). (Courtesy of Dr. Susana Raimondi of St. Jude's Children Research Hospital.)

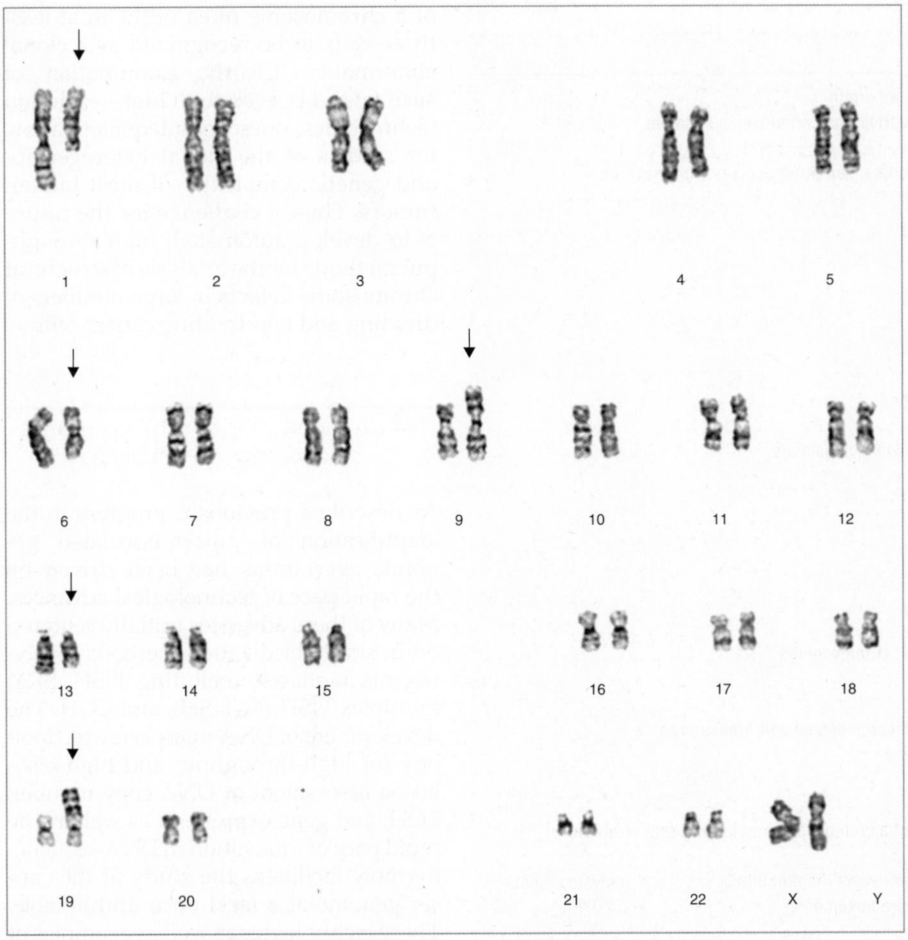

Figure 8-2 Chromosome G-banded karyotype of metaphase chromosomes from a case of pediatric B precursor acute lymphocytic leukemia (ALL) with the recurrent t(1;19)46,XX,t(1;19)(q23;p13.3),del(6)(q21q25),i(9)(q10),del(13)(q22q32). (Courtesy of Dr. Andrew Carroll, University of Alabama at Birmingham).

rent translocation, whereas others have numerous aberrations and very complex karyotypes. In solid epithelial-derived tumors, cytogenetic analyses have identified many structural chromosomal aberrations, but in contrast to hematopoietic and mesenchymal tumors, very few are recurrent.[1,43] The sheer number and variety of chromosome aberrations in many tumors have led some to assert that many aberrations are "noise," but the majority of the evidence support the view that the seemingly random aberrations generated by failures in the maintenance of genomic integrity are the result of selection in the evolution of a tumor.[1,2] In contrast, recurrent structural aberrations are frequent transforming events in sarcomas, leukemias, and lymphomas. Indeed, the majority of cancer genes identified to date reside at the break point of recurrent cytogenetic abnormalities in hematopoietic neoplasms despite the fact that hematopoietic tumors constitute only 10% of human cancers.[4,5,45] Although there is wide agreement that recurrent aberrations are particularly important for cancer development,[1,2] identifying the important cancer-related genes in many recurrent cytogenetic abnormalities is not always straightforward because aberrations may contain multiple genes, and more than one may be involved in different structural aberrations that contribute to the cancer phenotype.

One of the simplest and most common abnormalities in cancer cells is a gain or a loss of a whole chromosome resulting from defective chromosome segregation during telophase in mitosis or defective cytokinesis. Gains or losses of whole chromosomes or individual chromosome arms are displayed in written karyotypes as a plus sign (+) or a minus sign (–) before the designated number of the chromosome gained or lost (see Table 8-1). The functional consequence of these chromosome aberrations, which occur particularly frequently in solid tumors, may be hard to establish because the aberrations may extend over tens of thousands of megabases and may affect hundreds to thousands of genes. It has been easier to establish the cancer relevance of more limited regions of chromosomal gain and loss, created by amplification or deletion, as these smaller aberrations have been shown to alter the dosage of known oncogenes or tumor suppressor genes. Deletions are indicated by the abbreviation "del" and insertions by "ins" (see Table 8-1), with each abbreviation coming before the number of the chromosome involved. Restricted regions of the genome may also be amplified and the amplified fragments may be present in small extrachromosomal acentric fragments (so-called double minutes or dmin), integrated into chromosomes in homogeneous staining regions (HSRs), or dispersed throughout the genome (see Table 8-1). Adding to the complexity, amplified DNA fragments may contain DNA from different chromosomal regions.[2] Classic examples of oncogene activation in solid tumors include *ERBB2* in breast cancers and *MYC* in a variety of tumor types. The amplification of several cancer genes has been associated with therapeutic resistance, such as amplification of the *BCR-ABL* gene in CML patients resistant to imatinib/ Gleevec,[9,46] amplification of *DHFR* in patients resistant to methotrexate,[47] and amplification of the androgen receptor AR in prostate cancers resistant to endocrine therapy.[48] Loss of specific regions of the genome is often associated with loss of tumor suppressor genes, such as *TP53, RB1, PTEN,* and *CDKN4.* Inactivation of the remaining normal allele of carriers with inherited mutations of *RB1, BRCA1, BRCA2, TP53,* and *PTPRJ,* or in somatic cancer cells that have acquired mutations in one allele of these genes, is critical for the promotion of tumorigenesis. Based on these data, it is reasonable to expect that many more critical "cancer genes" will soon be identified in other less well-studied regions

Table 8-1 ■ ISCN Abbreviated Terms and Symbols

Term (Symbol)	Description
add	Additional material of unknown origin
approximate sign (~)	Denotes intervals and boundaries of a chromosome segment
C	Constitutional anomaly
comma (,)	Separates chromosome numbers, sex chromosomes, chromosome abnormalities
Cp	Composite karyotype
Del	Deletion
Der	Derivative chromosome
Dic	Dicentric
Dmin	Double minute
Dup	Duplication
Fis	Fission, at the centromere
Hsr	Homogeneously staining region
I	Isochromosome
Idem	Denotes the stemline karyotype in subclones
Ider	ISO derivative chromosome
Idic	ISO dicentric chromosome
Inc	Incomplete karyotype
Ins	Insertion
Inv	Inversion
Mar	Marker chromosome
minus sign (−)	Loss
multiplication sign (×)	Multiple copies of rearranged chromosomes
Or	Alternative interpretation
P	Short arm of chromosome
parentheses ()	Surround structurally altered chromosome and breakpoints
plus sign (+)	Gain
Q	Long arm of chromosome
Qpd	Quadruplication
question mark (?)	Questionable identification of a chromosome or chromosome structure
R	Ring chromosome
semicolon (;)	Separates altered chromosomes and breakpoints in structural rearrangements involving more than one chromosome
Slant line (/)	Separates clones
T	Translocation
Tas	Telomeric association
Trc	Tricentric chromosome
Trp	Triplication

of chromosome gain and loss in human cancers.

As previously described, recurrent structural chromosomal rearrangements occur frequently in hematopoietic neoplasms, sarcomas, and in some epithelial solid tumors. These structural changes may involve equal exchange of material between two chromosomes (referred to as "balanced") or may be nonreciprocal, in which portions of the genome are gained or lost as a consequence of the genomic alteration. One of the most common cytogenetic alterations in cancer is "translocation," where material between two or more chromosomes is exchanged (see Table 8-2; Fig. 8-3). Translocations are identified by the abbreviation t, with the chromosomes involved noted in the first set of parentheses and the break points in the second set of parentheses (see Table 8-2). Translocations may occur as a consequence of abnormal double-strand break (DSB) repair or through other means of intra- or interchromosomal recombination.[2] Translocations may result if DSBs occur in two distinct chromosomes simultaneously and the DSBs are aberrantly repaired; if the free end of one chromosome is ligated to another chromosome rather than its cognate free chromosome fragment, a translocation may result. In balanced reciprocal translocations (see Fig. 8-3), both chromosomes ligate each other's free ends, resulting in two abnormal chromosomes that are reciprocal products of each other. In an unbalanced translocation, only one set of DSBs is ligated, resulting in one abnormal chromosome; the unligated free chromosome fragments are often unstable and lost in the next mitosis. Another structural cytogenetic defect seen in cancer is an inversion (inv) (see Tables 8-1 and 8-2 and Fig. 8-3). Chromosome inversions may occur if two DSBs occur simultaneously in the same chromosome; instead of repairing the proper free ends to each other, the middle fragment of the chromosome inverts and is ligated to the opposite free ends.

In traditional cytogenetic analysis using chromosome banding techniques, structural abnormalities such as a translocation are required to be seen in at least 2 of 20 metaphase chromosome spreads using light microscopy to be recognized as "clonal" for that tumor.[43,44] Gain or loss of a chromosome must occur in at least three cells to be recognized as a clonal abnormality. Clearly, examination of such few cells, even with high-resolution technologies, does not adequately allow for studies of the clonal heterogeneity and genetic complexity of most human tumors. Thus, a challenge for the future is to develop automated, high throughput methods for the analysis of structural chromosome defects in large numbers of dividing and nondividing cancer cells.

Newer Methods of Chromosome and Genome Analysis

As described previously, progress in the identification of cancer-associated genomic aberrations has been driven by the rapid pace of technological advances. Many of these advances initially centered on in situ hybridization methods involving me taphases, including FISH, SKY, multiplex FISH (M-FISH), and CGH. The development of DNA microarray technology for high-throughput and high-resolution assessment of DNA-copy number, LOH, and gene expression as well as the rapid pace of innovation in DNA sequencing now facilitates the study of the cancer genome at a level once unthinkable. These technologies as well as examples of integrative analysis of genomic data are briefly described below.

Fluorescence In Situ Hybridization

FISH[19-22,49] is a technique in which DNA probes are labeled with various fluorochromes (eg, rhodamine), followed by hybridization to either metaphase spreads or interphase cells and are detected using fluorescence microscopy (see Figs. 8-1B and 8-4). FISH has had a dramatic impact on the sensitivity, detection, and analysis of chromosome aberrations in cancer cells and has been rapidly adapted to the clinical diagnostic setting. The ability to detect chromosomal aberrations in interphase cells has been a particularly dramatic advance and has facilitated the analysis of genomic aberrations in all cancers but particularly in solid tumors that have been less adaptable to in vitro culture and metaphase analysis. A large number of commercially available probes are now available for FISH analysis of chromosome aberrations in metaphase spreads and interphase nuclei. These probes include chromosome-specific centromere probes that unequivocally detect the number of copies of a specific chromosome presents in interphase and metaphase; whole chromosome paints that color an entire chromosome; large DNA probes (derived from YAC or BAC clones, see Table 8-2) from specific regions of the genome that efforts to comprehensively discover and catalog genomic alterations in human cancer. Discovery over the past decades has been steadily driven by a rapid pace of technological advance. Today, in addition to high-resolution chromosome banding and advanced chromosomal imaging technologies, chromosome aberrations in cancer cells can be analyzed with an increasing number of large-scale, comprehensive genomic and molecular genetic technologies discussed and illustrated throughout this chapter. These techniques include fluorescence in situ hybridization (FISH),[19-22] spectral karyotyping (SKY),[19] chromosome microdissection FISH (micro-FISH),[23-27] comparative genomic hybridization (CGH)[28-32] as well as microarray-based methods to detect fine-scale changes in chromosomal copy number, identify regions of loss of heterozygosity (LOH),[2,31,33] catalog epigenetic changes, and characterize patterns of gene expression. Advances in sequencing technology have further pushed the envelope of cancer gene discovery. Improvements in high-throughput Sanger sequencing have made possible multiple ambitious mutation screens on the level of entire gene families[34-37] and even the near complete protein-coding genome,[38-41] whereas the recent development of massively parallel sequencing methodologies has at last made the possibility of sequencing and assembling entire cancer genomes a reality.[42]

Extensive catalogs of these genome-level data are maintained and made available to the research community; notably, cytogenetic aberrations observed in more than 48,000 human tumors have been compiled and are now maintained and regularly updated online (see The Mitelman Database of Chromosome Aberrations in Cancer at the US National Cancer Institute [NCI] Cancer Genome Anatomy Project [CGAP] Web site: <http://cgap.nci.nih.gov>).[43] Data from countless microarray studies are warehoused by multiple entities, including the US National Center for Biotechnology Information (NCBI Gene Expression Omnibus;http://www.ncbi.nlm.nih.gov/geo/) and the European Bioinformatics Institute (EBI Array Express; <http://www.ebi.ac.uk/microarray-as/ae/>). On the DNA sequence level, the Wellcome Trust Sanger Institute Cancer Genome Project maintains a highly useful database of somatic mutations identified in human cancer (Catalogue of Somatic Mutations in Cancer [COSMIC] database; <http://www.sanger.ac.uk/genetics/CGP/cosmic>) as well as a detailed census of all human genes that have been causally linked to tumorigenesis (Cancer Gene Census; <http://www.sanger.ac.uk/genetics/CGP/Census>).[4,5]

Despite the commonalities observed within and between individual types of cancer, the genetic heterogeneity of human cancer is striking and appears to parallel the wide range of patient responses to many anticancer therapies in use today. Comprehensive discovery and the functional analysis of the full spectrum of genomic changes in each human cancer are widely considered to be essential for continued advances in cancer diagnosis, treatment, and the development of new and more effective therapies with curative intent. A detailed understanding of the genomic lesions underlying cancer will facilitate the identification of the cellular pathways and networks perturbed by genomic mutations, improve cancer diagnosis through molecular classification, enhance the selection of therapeutic targets for drug development, promote the development of faster and more efficient clinical trials using agents targeted to specific genomic abnormalities, and create markers for early detection and recurrence surveillance. To meet these challenges, the US National Cancer Institute (NCI) and National Human Genome Research Institute (NHGRI) launched a large collaborative project in 2006, the Cancer Genome Atlas (TCGA; see <http://cancergenome.nih.gov/>). Using multiple state-of-the-art genomic technologies to comprehensively identify all genomic alterations associated with multiple cancer types, the TCGA effort began with large pilot studies of glioblastoma multiforme,[39] ovarian cancer, and lung cancer. Similarly ambitious studies are beginning to be nucleated by members of the International Cancer Genome Consortium (ICGC; <http://icgc.org>), with a goal of comprehensively cataloging all genomic aberrations associated with at least 50 different cancers. The ultimate success of these as well as other comprehensive, large-scale projects will continue to rapidly advance our understanding of cancer genetics and genomics and will potentially revolutionize our approach to the diagnosis and treatment of cancer.

Chromosome Nomenclature and Cancer Cytogenetic Aberrations

Normal human diploid cells have 22 pairs of autosomes (nonsex chromosomes), numbered from chromosome 1 (the longest human chromosome) to 22 (the smallest double-stranded DNA fragment), and two sex chromosomes (X or Y) (Fig. 8-2). Traditional cytogenetic analyses are performed on metaphase chromosomes spreads (karyotypes) and, hence, can be obtained only from actively dividing cells. This essential characteristic has complicated the cytogenetic analysis of many tumors, particularly solid tumors, which may be difficult to adapt to short-term in vitro cultures to derive metaphases. Cells under analysis must be suspended and exposed to a hypotonic solution, fixed, and stained according to a variety of protocols. Brief exposure of metaphase chromosomes to mitotic inhibitors, DNA-binding agents to elongate chromosomes, or amethopterin or fluorodeoxyuridine to synchronize cells has resulted in longer, more distinct chromosomes. To enhance the likelihood of obtaining acceptable metaphases from hematopoietic as well as solid tumors, phytohemagglutinin-stimulated conditioned medium, recombinant colony-stimulating factors, and other lineage-specific growth factors are frequently added to the culture medium.

Banding of human chromosomes is essential for traditional cytogenetic investigations because it allows the identification of individual chromosomes and creates regional markers for physical mapping and topography. A band is defined as a chromosome area that is distinguished from adjacent segments by appearing darker or lighter through one or more banding techniques, including quinacrine–mustard (Q bands) and trypsin–Giemsa (G bands) staining (see Fig. 8-2). Typically, approximately 600 bands can be discerned under high-power microscopy in a metaphase spread using standard chromosome banding techniques. Each chromosome band and sub-band is numbered from the centromere to the telomere of each arm, allowing investigators to consistently refer to specific chromosomal bands and regions. International standards have been developed and are applied to the descriptive nomenclature that defines chromosome topography and karyotypic aberrations (insertions, deletions, translocations, amplifications) in cancer cells (see Table 8-1).[44] This cytogenetic nomenclature is under constant refinement with the use of state-of-the-art means of chromosome analysis, including SKY, CGH, and FISH (see <http://cgap.nci.nih.gov>). The long arm from the centromere of each chromosome is termed the "q" arm, and the short arm is termed the "p" arm. Visual karyotypes, derived from chromosome metaphases of actively dividing cells, are usually displayed with the long arm of each chromosome on the bottom (see Fig. 8-2). When a karyotype is displayed in written form, the total number of chromosomes (the modal number) is followed by the sex chromosomes.

There is considerable variability in the degree to which cancer genomes are aberrant at the chromosomal level in different human tumors. Some cancers are characterized by a single signature chromosomal abnormality, such as a recur-

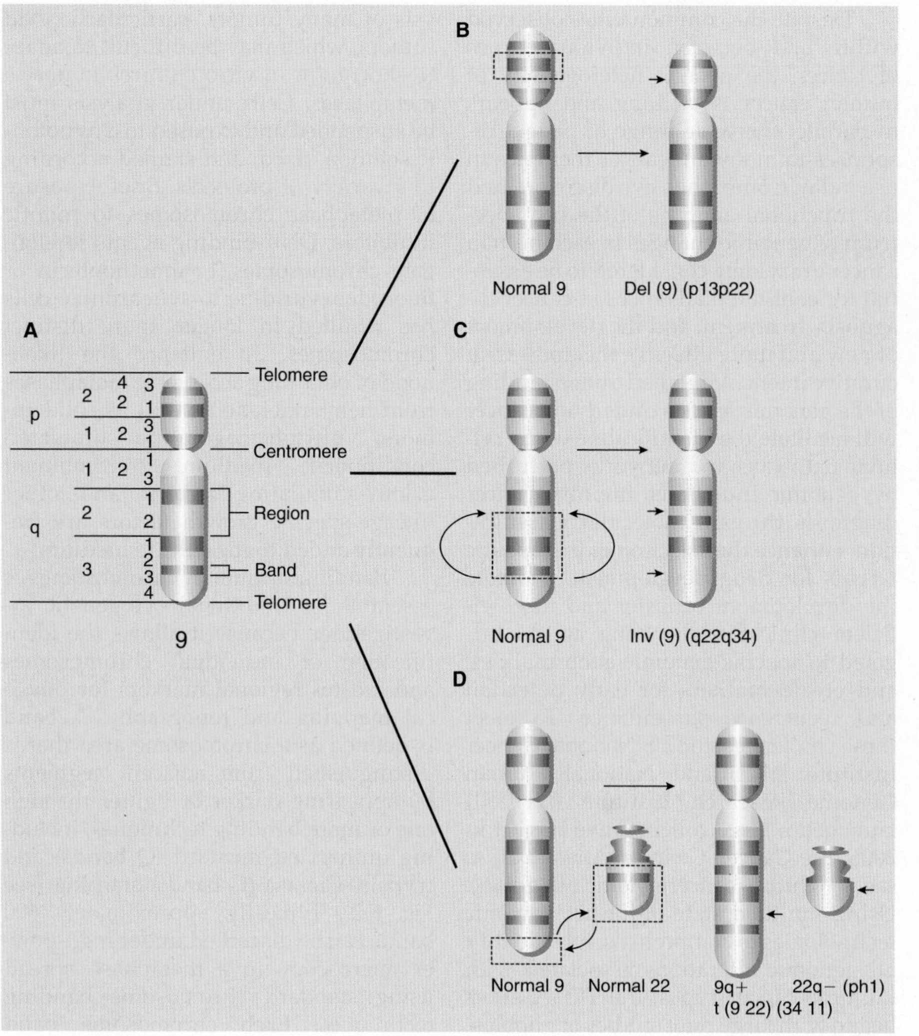

Figure 8-3 Schematic diagram illustrating a normal chromosome and three chromosomal abnormalities observed in human neoplasms. **(A)** Diagram of the banding pattern of a normal chromosome 9. The chromosome arms (p, short arm; q, long arm), regions, and band numbers are indicated on the left of the chromosome; specific chromosome structures are indicated on the right of the chromosome. **(B)** Diagram of the mechanism of an interstitial deletion of the short arm of chromosome 9, a common abnormality in acute lymphoblastic leukemia. Chromosome breaks occur in bands 9p13 and 9p22, and the intervening chromosomal segment (band 9p21 and parts of bands 9p13 and 9p22) is lost [del(9)(p13p22)]. **(C)** Diagram of the mechanism of a paracentric inversion. Chromosome breaks occur in two bands within a single chromosome arm, in this case, within 9p22 and 9q34; the intervening segment is inverted and the chromosome breaks are repaired [inv(9)(q22q34)]. **(D)** Diagram of the mechanism of the reciprocal translocation involving chromosomes 9 and 22, t(9;22)(q34;q11), which gives rise to the Philadelphia (Ph1) chromosome in the malignant cells of patients with chronic myelogenous leukemia. Breaks occur in bands q34 and q11 of chromosomes 9 and 22, respectively, followed by a reciprocal exchange of chromosomal material. This rearrangement results in the translocation of the ABL oncogene, normally located at 9q34, adjacent to the BCR gene on chromosome 22, giving rise to a chimeric BCR-ABL gene, whose protein product plays a role in the transformation of myeloid cells.

can be used to screen for regional aberrations such as amplifications, or structural chromosomal aberrations including recurring translocations; and genomic DNA probes for specific human genes. Particularly useful for the detection of structural rearrangements are new "break-apart" and "dual-fusion" probes for the specific chromosomal aberrations seen in hematopoietic malignancies and sarcomas.[50-52] Break-apart FISH probes are derived from two adjacent regions of the genome and are differentially labeled; these two probes move apart only in the event of a structural chromosomal rearrangement in the interval normally flanked by the probes. Such probes are independent of the partner gene and are particularly useful in detecting structural rearrangements in "promiscuous" cancer genes that may be translocated to many different partner genes on different chromosomes (eg, *ALK, BCL6, ETV6 [TEL], EVI1, EWSR1, IGH, MLL, MYC, NUP98, PDGFR, RARA, RET,* and *RUNX1 [AML1]*). Highly recurrent translocations, such as t(9;22) in CML, can be identified using "dual-fusion" assays with FISH probes derived from two independent regions of the genome that are differentially labeled; these probes fuse only when the specific translocation is present. FISH technologies are also very useful for the detection of specific gene amplifications, such as *ERBB2* in breast cancer, in both interphase cells and metaphase chromosomes. Another highly interesting application of FISH techniques is the integration of FISH and immunophenotyping (called FICTION).[52] FICTION is useful for mapping the actual cells that carry specific chromosomal abnormalities. A particularly striking recent discovery with this technique was that lymphoma-associated endothelial cells contain the same specific translocation as the surrounding tumor cells,[53] suggesting that lymphoma may arise in a multipotent progenitor cell capable of both lymphoid and endothelial differentiation. Although other explanations include cell fusion or the uptake of apoptotic material, this observation is very intriguing.

Given suitable probes, interphase FISH enhances cytogenetic analysis in specimens with a low mitotic index, such as in myeloma or chronic lymphocytic leukemia (CLL), and in specimens that tend to have poor chromosome morphology in metaphase spreads, such as in ALL. Interphase FISH can be scaled up to analyze hundreds of cells and thereby increase the sensitivity of analysis and the detection of clonal chromosomal abnormalities in far greater numbers of cells than traditional chromosome banding techniques and metaphase analysis. FISH also increases the sensitivity of detecting cytogenetic abnormalities—particularly cryptic translocations or smaller structural rearrangements—and is useful for monitoring the response to treatment and as a sensitive minimal residual disease detection assay. The current sensitivity of interphase FISH is approximately 5% abnormal cells. FISH analysis of metaphase chromosomes is particularly useful for detection of cryptic translocations (such as the *BCR-ABL* translocation in CML or the recently discovered inv(7)(p15q34) cryptic translocation in T-ALL resulting in aberrant *HOX* gene expression[54]), resolving complex chromosomal rearrangements, and identifying the origin of "marker" chromosomes, which are unknown chromosome fragments in metaphase spreads.

Table 8-2 ■ Glossary

Amplification:	An increase in the number of copies of a DNA segment.
Alu element:	Alu sequences are a family of short interspersed repeats and are the most abundant repeat sequences in the human genome, comprising 5-10% of the total human genome sequence. Alu sequences can be found at sites of chromosome aberrations in human cancer and may foster chromosomal rearrangements.
BAC:	Bacterial artificial chromosome; a cloning vector that contains very large (45-70 kb) human genomic DNA fragments; BAC clones covering >98% of the human genome are now available for FISH chromosomal studies.
Centromere:	The constriction along the length of the chromosome that is the site of the spindle fiber attachment. The position of the centromere determines whether chromosomes are metacentric (X-shaped, such as chromosomes 1, 3, 16, 19, 20) or acrocentric (inverted V-shaped, such as chromosomes 13-15, 21, 22, Y).
CGH:	Comparative genomic hybridization. CGH is a fluorescent molecular cytogenetic technique for determining copy number gains and losses and amplifications between two samples of DNA, by competitively hybridizing differentially labeled DNA from these samples to normal metaphase chromosomes (Fig. 8-8).
Clone:	In traditional chromosomal banding studies and analysis of metaphase chromosome spreads, a "clone" is defined as two cells with the same additional or structurally rearranged chromosome or three cells with loss of the same chromosome.
Deletion:	A segment of a chromosome is missing as the result of two breaks and loss of the intervening piece (Fig. 8-3)
Diploid:	Normal chromosome number and composition of chromosomes.
Epigenetic:	Epigenetics is the study of the heritable changes in gene function that result from modifications to the genome (such as methylation or chromatin remodeling) rather than changes in the primary DNA sequence itself.
FISH:	FISH is a technique in which DNA probes are labeled with various fluorochromes (eg, rhodamine), followed by hybridization to either metaphase spreads or interphase cells and detected using fluorescence microscopy (Figs. 8-1B and 8-4).
Fosmid:	A cloning vector used for large segments of genomic DNA. Often used when constructing stable genomic libraries.
Hyperploid:	Additional chromosomes, therefore the modal number is 47 or greater.
Hypoploid:	Loss of chromosomes, eg, modal number 45 or less.
Haploid:	Only one-half the normal complement, ie, 23 chromosomes.
Inversion:	Two breaks occur in the same chromosome with rotation of the intervening segment. If both the breaks are on the same side of the centromere, it is called a paracentric inversion. If they are on opposite sides, it is called a pericentric inversion (Fig. 8-3).
Isochromosome:	A chromosome that consists of identical copies of one chromosome with loss of the other arm. Thus, an isochromosome for the long arm of No. 17 [i(17q)] contains two copies of the long arm (separated by the centromere) with the loss of the short arm of the chromosome.
Karyotype:	Arrangement of chromosomes from a particular cell according to a well-established system such that the largest chromosomes are first and the smallest ones are last. Normal female karyotype is 46, XX; normal male karyotype is 46, XY.
DNA polymorphism:	One of two or more alternate forms (alleles) of a chromosomal locus that differ in nucleotide sequence or have variable numbers of repeated nucleotide units.
Single nucleotide polymorphism (SNP):	SNPs (pronounced "snips") are heritable DNA sequence variations that occur when a single nucleotide (A, T, C, or G) in the genome sequence is changed. Most SNPs involve the replacement of cytosine (C) with thymine (T). Occurring every 100-300 bases along the human genome, SNPs are the most frequent type of human DNA polymorphism. They are heritable and stable from generation to generation.
SKY:	SKY (Fig. 8-5) and M-FISH (Fig. 8-6) are molecular cytogenetic techniques that permit the simultaneous visualization of all human chromosomes in different colors, facilitating karyotype analysis. For these techniques, chromosome-specific probe pools (referred to as "chromosome painting" probes) generated from flow cytometric-sorted chromosomes are amplified and then fluorescently labeled and hybridized to metaphasic chromosomes.
Translocation:	A break in at least two chromosomes with exchange of material; in a reciprocal translocation, such that there is no obvious loss of chromosomal material (Fig. 8-3).
UPD:	Uniparental disomy; the presence of two copies of a chromosome or chromosomal segment originating from one parent, with no copies contributed by the other.
YAC:	Yeast artificial chromosome; a yeast cloning vector that contains large human genomic DNA fragments.

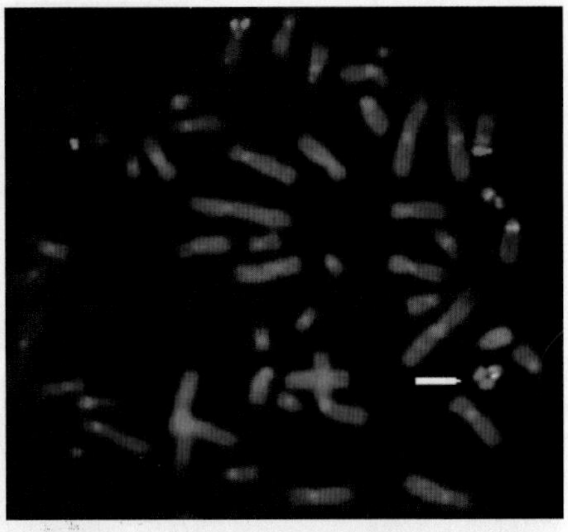

Figure 8-4 ■ FISH analysis of gene amplification in acute myeloid leukemia using BAC probes to *TEL* and *RUNX1*. The green fluorescence shows the *TEL* gene located on chromosome 12 and the red fluorescence shows the *RUNX1* gene on chromosome 21. Note the amplification of RUNX1 on chromosome 21 indicated by the arrow. (Courtesy of Dr. Kathy Richkind, Genzyme Genetics.)

Spectral Karyotyping and Multiplex Fluorescence In Situ Hybridization

SKY (Fig. 8-5) and M-FISH (Fig. 8-6) are molecular cytogenetic techniques that permit the simultaneous visualization of all human chromosomes in different colors, facilitating karyotype analysis. For these techniques, chromosome-specific probe pools (referred to as "chromosome painting" probes) generated from flow cytometric-sorted chromosomes are amplified and then fluorescently labeled using degenerate oligonucleotide-primed polymerase chain reaction. Both SKY and M-FISH use a combinatorial labeling scheme with different fluorochromes that can be spectrally distinguished but use different fluorescence detection methods. In SKY, image acquisition is performed using epifluorescence microscopy, CCD imaging, and Fourier transform spectroscopy.[19] With this approach, the entire fluorescence emission spectrum can be analyzed with a single exposure. In M-FISH, separate images are captured for each of the five fluorochromes using filters, and then computer software is used to combine the images. In both M-FISH and SKY, unique pseudocolors are ultimately assigned to each individual chromosome based on their overall specific fluorescence signature (see Figs. 8-5 and 8-6).

SKY and M-FISH are useful in detecting and mapping structural chromosomal rearrangements, detecting unknown "marker" chromosomes, identifying cryptic translocations, and in characterizing complex chromosomal rearrangements. With the advent of M-FISH and SKY, it is clear that many malignancies have a far greater fraction of cytogenetic abnormalities than was previously thought. For example, previously, only 50% of AML could be found to have cytogenetic abnormalities by careful conventional cytogenetics. Using M-FISH and SKY, the percentage of AML that have cytogenetic abnormalities is 80% (see Fig. 8-5).[55] However, SKY and M-FISH may not have high enough resolution to identify the exact chromosomal region involved in abnormalities.

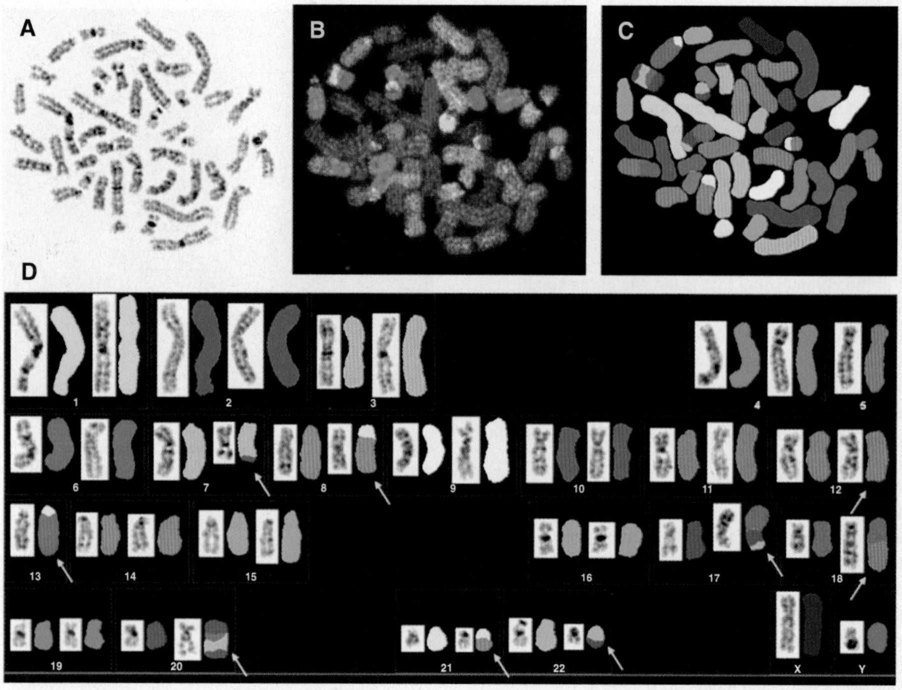

Figure 8-5 Complex karyotype detected in a patient with acute myeloid leukemia, analyzed using spectral karyotyping (SKY). **(A)** Inverted and contrast-enhanced DAPI image of the metaphase cell. (**B** and **C**) The same metaphase cell with chromosomes shown in SKY display colors (B) and SKY classification colors (C). **(D)** Karyotype of the same cell with each chromosome represented twice by its inverted DAPI-stained image on the left and SKY image shown in classification colors on the right. Arrows denote structurally rearranged chromosomes. The karyotype interpretation is as follows: 44,XY,-5,der(7)t(7;17)(q22;?),der(8)(8qter→8q21?.2::8p21→cen→8q21?.2::21q21→21q21::21q21→21qter),der(12)ins(12;5)(p12;?q31?q22),-13, der(13)ins(13;21)(q11;q?q?),der(17)(13qter→13q14::17p11→cen→17q21::17?→17?::22q?→22q?), der(18)(18pter→cen→18q21.322::5?q22→5?q11. 2),der(20)(20pter→cen→20q11::13q12→13q14 or 13q14→13q12::22q11→22q13 or 22q13→22q11::17q2?3→17qter), der(21)t(8;21)(?p21;q11),der(22)t(20;22)(q1?;q11). (Courtesy of Dr. Krzysztof Mrózek, The Ohio State University.)

Chromosome Microdissection FISH

One additional tool that is increasingly being used to investigate the origins of complex chromosome alterations is the combination of chromosome microdissection and FISH (micro-FISH). This approach, initially developed in the laboratory of the authors,[27] essentially involves the dissection of one to five copies of target chromosomal material using micromanipulator-controlled glass microneedles on an inverted microscope; targeted material may include chromosomal breakpoint regions (for a translocation), HSRs (for an amplified intrachromosomal segment), dmin or rings (for extrachromosomal material), or essentially any recognizable chromosomal material. Dissected chromosome fragments are subsequently transferred to a "collection drop" (containing buffers, reagents, and a "universal primer") to facilitate amplification of a general representation of the dissected chromosomal fragment. The amplified material is then labeled with a fluorochrome in a secondary PCR and hybridized to normal metaphases (micro-FISH), revealing the chromosomal constitution of the dissected fragments (such as those from complex chromosomal rearrangements, see Fig. 8-7).[23-27] A specific example of the recent use of micro-FISH from the laboratory of the authors combined chromosomal microdissection with G-banding and FISH to map a recurrent melanoma breakpoint on chromosome band 6q14.3, thereby identifying a novel association between the mitotic checkpoint protein TTK and chromosomal instability. *TTK* is commonly lost through unbalanced nonreciprocal translocation of t(4;6)(q33;q14.3). Loss of *TTK* alleles results in loss of heterozygosity (LOH) and amplification of the remaining allele via whole chromosome duplication.[56]

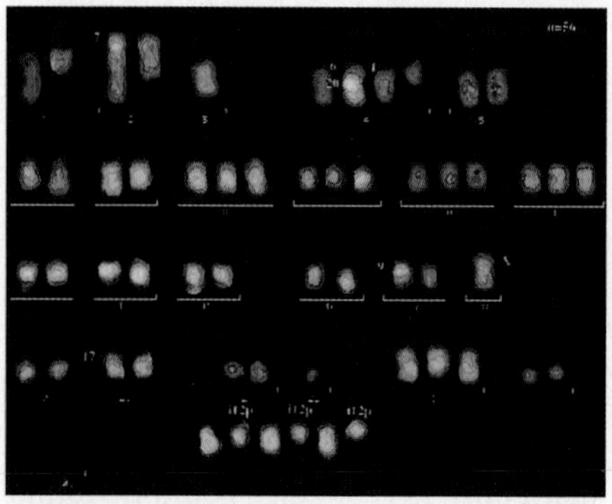

Figure 8-6 M-FISH studies performed on a germ cell tumor, demonstrating the isochromosome 12p and also the general amplification of 12p material that is very common in all germ cell tumors. The amplified oncogene on 12p has not yet been identified. (Courtesy of Dr. Octavian Henegariu.)

Largely because of the tedious, time-consuming, and highly complex protocols for capturing, amplifying, labeling, and then analyzing results from metaphase spreads, micro-FISH has had limited application. However, conceptually, this approach has continued utility in several ways for cases of importance in both medical genetics and malignancy. This method is clearly useful in characterizing cases with copy number "neutral" changes, including balanced reciprocal translocations and inversions. In addition, micro-FISH can be of value in cases for which there is clinically useful diagnostic cytogenetic material available but no remaining sample for more "advanced" molecular studies (eg, diagnostic samples from 5q deletions patients with MDS). Finally, although still largely confined to the research laboratory, micro-FISH is once again becoming of interest as microdissected, amplified labeled material that can now be hybridized to DNA microarrays (essentially using a modification of the approach described below for array-based CGH) to closely pinpoint the aforementioned breakpoints of reciprocal translocations.

Comparative Genomic Hybridization

CGH is a fluorescent molecular cytogenetic technique for determining copy number gains and losses between two samples of DNA by competitively hybridizing differentially labeled DNA from these samples to normal metaphase chromosomes (Fig. 8-8). It is a powerful tool for screening chromosomal copy number changes in tumor genomes and has the advantage of analyzing entire genomes in a single experiment. As it is dependent on DNA for analysis, it is particularly applicable to the study of tumors that do not yield sufficient metaphases for chromosome analysis, and it can be applied to small numbers of microdissected cells, fixed or frozen samples as well as paraffin-embedded tissues. CGH is based on quantitative two-color FISH; equal amounts of tumor DNA and normal reference DNA that are labeled with distinct fluorochromes are mixed together and competitively hybridized to normal metaphase spreads (see Fig. 8-8A). The fluorescence intensity ratio between labeled tumor DNA and normal chro-

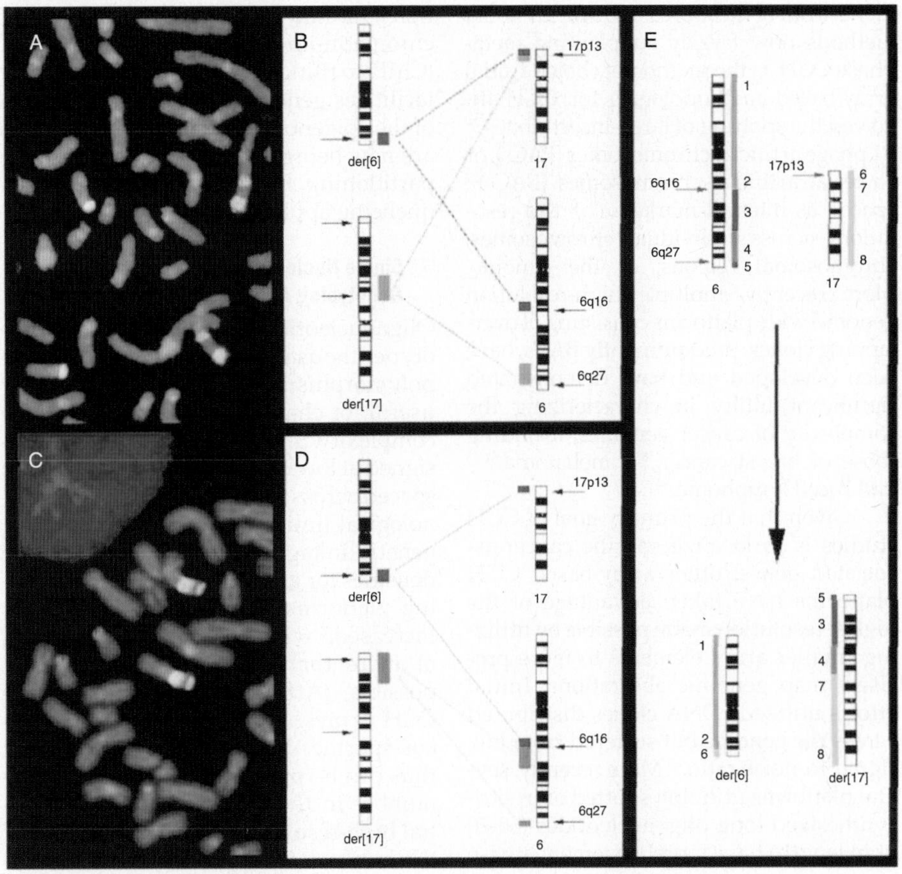

Figure 8-7 Characterization of a complex chromosome rearrangement involving 6q and 17p by microfluorescence in situ hybridization (micro-FISH) in the UACC-930 melanoma cell line. **(A)** Microdissected probes from the breakpoint of der(6) (red) and the proximal breakpoint of der(17) (green) were hybridized back to normal metaphase chromosomes. Microdissected DNA from the proximal breakpoint of der(17) mapped to the proximal region of the 17p13 breakpoint and the distal region of the 6q27 breakpoint; DNA from the breakpoint of der(6) mapped to the distal region of the 17p13 breakpoint and the proximal region of 6q16 breakpoint. **(B)** The micro-FISH results detected in panel A are illustrated. **(C)** Microdissected probes from the breakpoint of der(6) (red) and the distal breakpoint of der(17) (green) were hybridized to a normal metaphase. The probe from the distal breakpoint of der(17) was localized to the distal region of the 6q16 breakpoint and the distal region of the 6q27 breakpoint. **(D)** The micro-FISH result detected in panel C is illustrated. **(E)** A summary of micro-FISH results; the complex chromosomal rearrangement includes an inversion involving 6q, inv(6)(q16q27), and a translocation involving the inverted 6q and 17p13. (Reproduced with permission from Guan XY, et al.[25])

mosome DNA is measured by scanning along each chromosomal region in the metaphase spread. This provides information about the relative copy number of tumor versus normal DNA by chromosomal region. Thus, gains and losses can be digitally visualized (see Fig. 8-8B). CGH is limited by the fact that it will only detect gains or losses present in a large fraction of the tumor cells and cannot detect balanced chromosomal translocations or other aberrations. This limits its effectiveness, especially in hematologic malignancies, where most translocations are balanced. The use of CGH is still mostly investigational, and it is rarely used in the clinical diagnostic setting. However, this technique is powerful because it does not require advance knowledge of cytogenetic abnormalities. It also precludes the selection of a subpopulation of the tumor under analysis during the short-term in vitro culture necessary to obtain metaphases. CGH has been applied to many tumor types and revealed novel regions of chromosome gain and loss in cancers of the colon, breast, prostate, cervix, glioblastomas, and lymphomas.[57]

Microarray-Based CGH

Conventional metaphase CGH suffers from significant limitations in resolution and sensitivity, as well as in accuracy of mapping genomic aberrations back to genomic reference sequence. The rapid development of microarray-based methods and their application to assaying DNA copy number have led to tremendous improve-

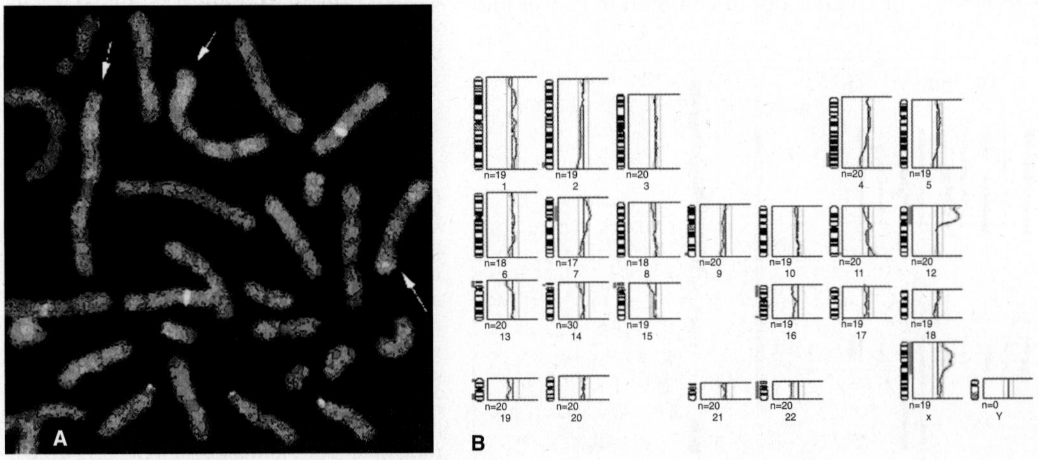

Figure 8-8 CGH on a germ cell tumor sample. The arrows indicate the amplification of 12p material common in these tumors. **(A)** This photomicrograph demonstrates the annealing of fluorescently labeled normal chromosomes to a tumor specimen. **(B)** The diagram demonstrates the computer analysis of gains or losses of tumor DNA compared to normal DNA. Right of the line indicates gain, and left of the line indicates loss of chromosomal material relative to normal. Note the marked gain of material on chromosome 12. (Courtesy of Dr. Octavian Henegariu.)

ments in all of these areas, with array-CGH methods now largely supplanting metaphase CGH as the method of choice. Initial array-based methodologies for CGH involved the spotting of large-insert clones,[30] P1 phage artificial chromosomes (PACs), or bacterial artificial chromosomes (BACs)[29] spaced as interval markers (1-3 Mb resolution) across individual chromosomes, chromosomal regions, or the genome. More recently, multiple high-resolution genome-wide platforms consisting of overlapping clones, predominantly BACs, have been developed and have demonstrated significant utility in characterizing the complexity of cancer genomes, including those of breast cancer,[58-60] melanoma,[61-63] and B-cell lymphoma.[64]

Given that the primary goal of CGH studies is to localize specific cancer-associated genes, other array-based CGH platforms have taken advantage of the higher resolution made possible by utilizing smaller array elements to more precisely map genomic aberrations. Initial efforts utilized cDNA clones distributed across the genome but suffered from low signal-to-noise ratio.[65] More recently, several platforms utilizing spotted or in situ-synthesized long oligonucleotides (60-70 nt in length) have largely overcome these sensitivity issues. Importantly, given that probes for these platforms are designed *in silico* and synthesized on the array, the resolution of these arrays is flexible, allowing for exon- and even tiling-level analysis capable of detecting microdeletions (Fig. 8-9).[66,67] In a manner similar to BAC CGH arrays, oligonucleotide CGH arrays have now been widely applied toward cataloging DNA copy number aberrations in cancer genomes.

Oligoarrays designed for DNA copy number analysis are now being adapted for applications beyond copy number analysis. Although CGH arrays are of limited utility in mapping balanced chromosomal translocations from whole genomes, such mapping may be performed by hybridizing individual chromosomes or chromosomal segments isolated via chromosome microdissection[68] or flow-sorting. Hybridization of chromatin-immunoprecipitated DNA (ChIP) to tiling- or CpG island arrays now facilitates genome-wide characterization of the epigenome.[69,70] Finally, CGH arrays are now being used as a tool for genome partitioning to facilitate targeted resequencing applications.[71,72]

Single Nucleotide Polymorphism Genotyping Arrays

Oligonucleotide arrays designed to genotype thousands of single nucleotide polymorphisms (SNPs) are similarly useful for characterizing tumor genome complexity. SNP arrays were initially designed at low density (6000-10,000 probes spaced across the genome) owing to technological limitations, largely facilitating genetic linkage analysis. Oligonucleotide densities for genome-wide SNP genotyping platforms have since progressively increased, with the rapid genotyping of more than one million SNPs now possible (Affymetrix, Illumina). Like CGH arrays, SNP arrays quantitate locus-specific hybridization signal and thus can be used to estimate DNA copy number in the genome. One of the initial high-resolution SNP array studies of the human cancer genome involved the genotyping of the NCI-60 cell line panel using 100K-element SNP arrays, leading to the discovery of high-level, focal amplifications of the microphthalmia-associated transcription factor *MITF* in 10-20% of melanoma tumors.[73] SNP arrays have since been applied to a wide range of cancers, including lung cancer,[74] melanoma,[73,75,76] breast cancer,[38] colorectal cancer,[38] glioblastoma,[39,40] and pancreatic cancer.[41]

Given that these arrays have been designed to provide genotype data on dense panels of informative polymorphic markers, they provide the added benefit of simultaneously allowing for assessment of LOH in addition to DNA copy number. Importantly, LOH in the absence of copy number aberration (eg, copy neutral LOH; uniparental disomy, or UPD) is not uncommon in cancer and may also provide evidence for the presence of mutated tumor suppressors.[77-79] Although SNP-based LOH is ideally assessed via genotyping patient-matched pairs of tumor and normal tissue, LOH may also be inferred from extended regions of homozygosity, albeit with some loss of power.[80,81] Genome-wide SNP studies of multiple cancers, including AML,[79,82] neuroblastoma,[83] colorectal cancer,[84,85] melanoma,[75] basal cell carcinoma,[78] and lung cancer,[74] have revealed genomic regions subject to copy neutral LOH.

Gene Expression Profiling

The development of cDNA and oligonucleotide microarrays for simultaneous quantitation of thousands of mRNA transcripts has had a dramatic impact on our understanding of human cancer. Although various microarray platforms utilize diverse manufacturing, labeling, and analysis methods, the general principle of a microarray analysis remains the same. RNA isolated from an individual sample is typically enzymatically copied, labeled, and hybridized to the surface of a microarray, which contains thousands of immobilized cDNA or oligonucleotide probes. Each probe on the array is derived from the coding sequence of an individual gene and located at a unique location on the array surface. The signal at each microarray spot is quantitated, and the signal for each gene can thus be compared to those from other samples (single-color arrays) or alternatively to that from a competitively cohybridized reference sample (two-color arrays). Although originally designed to assay the expression of individual genes, array-based methods have more recently been adapted to profile and map global transcription on the exon- and genome-levels[86] as well as to profile the expression of mature human micro-RNAs (miRNAs).[87]

Gene expression profiling (GEP) via microarrays continues to play a significant role in the identification of prognostic and diagnostic genetic markers that may also serve as targets for novel therapies. Gene

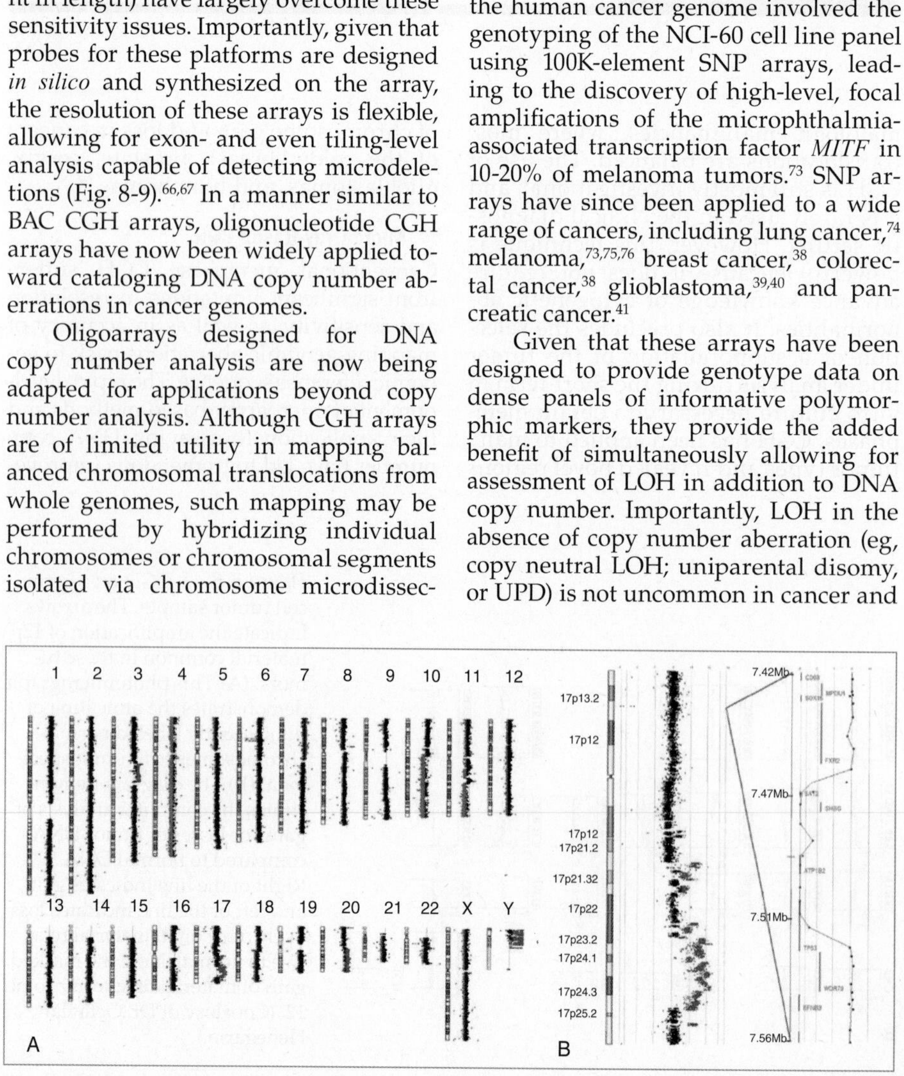

Figure 8-9 High-resolution array-based CGH analysis of a melanoma cell line. **(A)** CGH log2 ratio data for the cell line are plotted for the genome. **(B)** CGH log2 ratio data are plotted for chromosome 17 (left) as well as a focal region of homozygous deletion with a breakpoint within the *TP53* tumor suppressor (right). Regions of DNA copy loss plotted to the left of the axis and regions of gain are plotted to the right. Individual log2 ratio data (dots) and log2 ratio moving average (line) are shown.

expression patterns have been widely used to subclassify cancers into homogeneous entities not easily discernable using traditional histopathologic or cytogenetic techniques, for instance, in diffuse large B-cell lymphoma (DLBCL),[88,89] lung cancer,[90] and breast cancer.[91,92] In some instances, specific subgroups have been shown to represent distinct disease states that respond differently to standard therapies. Gene expression profiles have also been widely mined to specifically identify sets of genes predictive of disease progression, response to therapy, or metastasis[93-95] as well as the presence of specific recurrent cytogenetic abnormalities[96-98] or gene mutations.[99-102] Data from such microarray experiments can aid in the search for new therapeutic targets and in the identification of novel diagnostic markers.

Intriguingly, expression profiles have also been used to identify novel recurrent chromosomal aberrations in human cancer. Outlier analysis methods such as Cancer Outlier Profile Analysis (COPA) have been applied to identify genes that are dramatically over- or underexpressed in a subset of samples within a specific tumor type. Such "outlier" expression patterns may be indicative of recurrent underlying chromosomal aberrations or mutations resulting in altered gene expression. Importantly, COPA was successfully used to identify strong outlier profiles for two ETS-family transcription factor genes (*ERG* and *ETV1*) across several prostate cancer data sets; subsequent investigation revealed the presence of recurrent fusions of *TMPRSS2* and these two ETS-related genes in prostate cancer (Fig. 8-10).[103,104] Based on these data, *TMPRSS2* fusions with an additional ETS-family transcription factor (*ETV4*) have since been identified[105] as well as additional fusions between ETS-family genes and a prostate-specific androgen-induced gene (*SLC45A3*), a prostate-specific androgen-repressed gene (*C15orf21*), an endogenous retroviral element, and a highly expressed housekeeping gene (*HNRPA2B1*).[106] These ETS-family gene aberrations represent the first high-frequency gene fusion event associated with a carcinoma, challenging the long-held notion that gene fusions or balanced chromosomal aberrations play only a minor role in the pathogenesis of epithelial tumors.

DNA Sequencing Approaches

Until recently, widespread sequencing of DNA has largely centered around improvements to the Sanger method originally developed in the 1970s.[107] Progressive advances in this methodology, including fluorescent-labeled nucleotides, capillary electrophoresis, and improved laboratory automation have allowed for scaling of this method to enable the sequencing of simple as well as complex genomes. Nonetheless, genome-scale sequencing projects using this methodology continue to be expensive, logistically challenging efforts. Despite these challenges, several large-scale efforts aimed at identifying novel mutations associated with specific cancers have recently been launched utilizing Sanger-based methods. These studies include a screen of 518 protein kinases across several hundred human cancer samples of various types,[34-37] approximately 1300 genes in glioblastomas multiforme,[39] more than 18,000 genes across a small set of breast and colorectal tumors,[38] and more than 20,000 genes in glioblastoma multiforme[39,40] and pancreatic cancer.[41] Notably, such screens have led to the identification of activating BRAF mutations in a large percentage of human melanomas[108] and nevi,[109] as well as ERBB2 mutations in human breast cancer.[110]

Paired-end sequencing, in which both ends of thousands of individual DNA clones (or alternatively DNA fragments) are sequenced, has clear application to the characterization of genomic

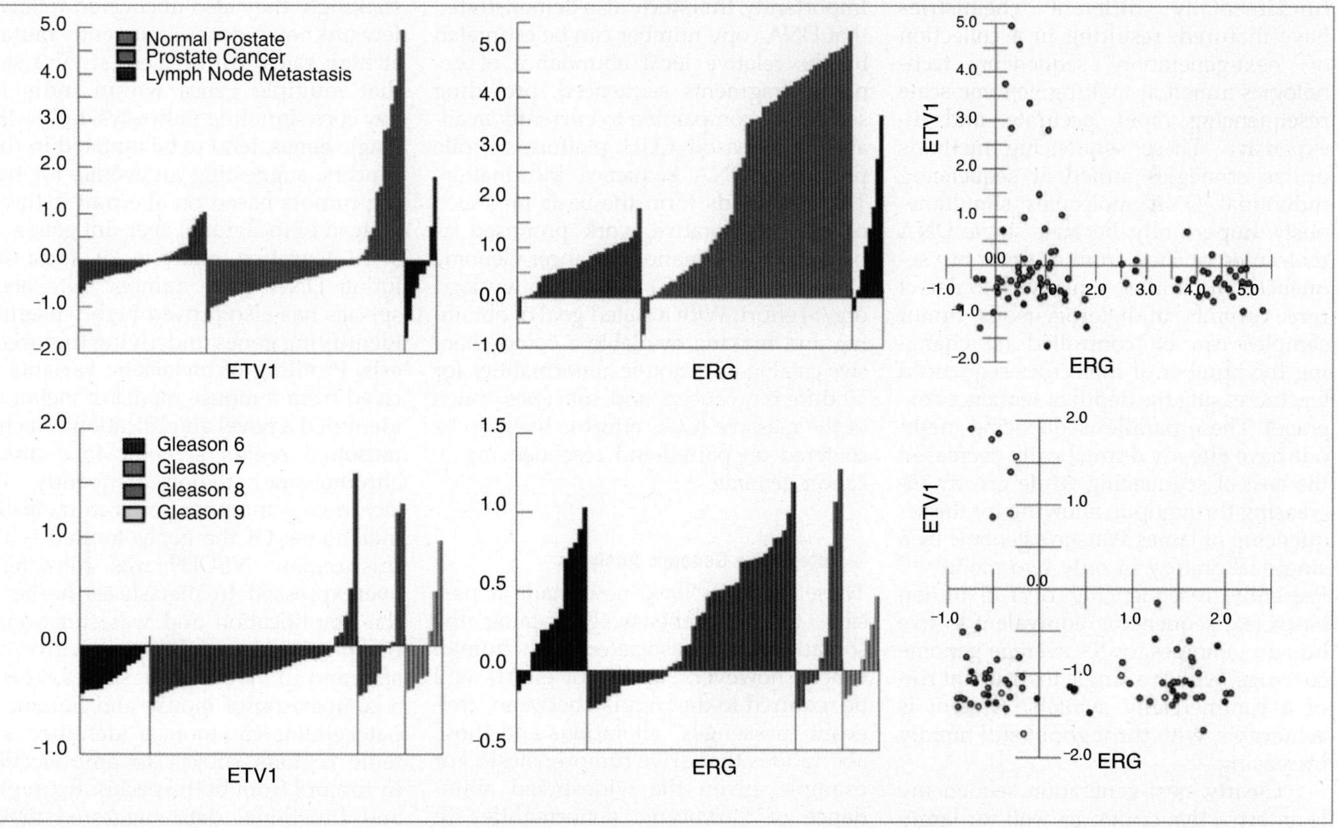

Figure 8-10 COPA analysis identifies ETS-family gene fusions in prostate cancer. Tomlins and colleagues analyzed two sets of prostate cancer expression array data 179,180 using cancer outlier profile analysis (COPA) to identify "outlier" genes dramatically overexpressed in subsets of samples. COPA of these data revealed *ETV1* and *ERG* as outlier genes across both prostate cancer gene expression data sets, with overexpression in prostate cancer being driven by recurrent gene fusion events to TMPRSS2. *ETV1* and *ERG* expression (normalized expression units) are shown from all profiled samples both gene expression studies. Sample classes are indicated according to the color scale. In one data set,[179] prostate cancer samples were classified based on the Gleason grade. Scatter plots of *ERG* and *ETV1* expression across all of the profiled samples are shown (right). (From Tomlins SA, Rhodes DR, Perner S, et al. Recurrent fusion of TMPRSS2 and ETStranscription factor genes in prostate cancer. Science. 2005;310:644–648. Reprinted with permission from AAAS.)[104]

aberrations in human cancer. The paired-end sequencing approach was initially utilized in the sequencing of the human HPRT locus;[111] given that data related to the orientation and spacing of two ends of clones of known size is of significant utility in genome assembly, this method was subsequently widely applied toward the shotgun sequencing and assembly of numerous genomes. This same orientation and spacing data are also of considerable use for comparing cancer genomes to a reference genome sequence; instances where the orientation and or distance of end-pairs are inconsistent with a reference genome are suggestive of genomic rearrangements. This approach was initially applied to a BAC library from the MCF-7 breast cancer cell line genome,[112] and has since been applied toward characterizing the structural variation across the germline human genome[113] as well as the identification of fusion transcripts[114-116] via paired-end sequencing of transcripts. Despite these advances, the relatively high cost associated with Sanger-based sequencing of the large number of inserts necessary for full genome coverage has limited the application of this approach toward large-scale characterization of cancer genomes.

Over the past several years, efforts to develop sequencing platforms with fundamentally different chemistries have matured, resulting in a collection of "next-generation" sequencing technologies aimed at making genome-scale resequencing rapid, accurate, and inexpensive. These sequencing methods utilize strategies aimed at sequencing individual DNA molecules simultaneously. Importantly, because single DNA molecules isolated from a tumor are sequenced in parallel, sensitivity to detect rare variants in heterogeneous tumor samples can be controlled by changing the number of molecules sequenced (eg, increasing the depth of sequence coverage). These parallel sequencing methods have already dramatically decreased the cost of sequencing while greatly increasing throughput, allowing for the sequencing of James Watson's genome by a single laboratory in only two months.[117] Presently, resequencing of 1-15 billion bases (eg, sequencing equivalent to five human genomes, or 5X average genome coverage) within a single instrument run of a commercially available system is achievable, with throughput still rapidly increasing.

Clearly, next-generation sequencing is an attractive option as well for large-scale candidate gene sequencing studies. Such studies require an additional means to partition or enrich samples for the desired genomic regions prior to sequencing; several approaches for genome partitioning aimed toward targeted and exon resequencing have recently been reported, including solid-phase BAC[72] or oligonucleotide[71] array-based DNA capture as well as multiplex amplification using inversion probes.[118] An alternative strategy also applied toward gene resequencing is the mass sequencing of gene transcripts. Transcriptome sequencing methods are attractive in that they simultaneously quantitate relative expression levels and identify sequence variants, fusion transcripts, and alternative splice events; such methods have already been applied using Sanger-based approach (serial analysis of gene expression [SAGE],[119] di-Tags[115,116]). Nonetheless, this method may miss sequence variants that are expressed at low to zero levels in the tissue analyzed as well as fail to detect nonsense sequence variants owing to nonsense-mediated transcript decay.

To date, sufficient progress has been made in parallel-sequencing methodologies to make the sequencing of complete cancer genomes achievable, as evidenced by the recent report of the application of this methodology to characterize genomic aberrations in two lung cancer genomes.[42] This study utilized a paired-end approach, demonstrating strikingly complex genomic rearrangements (Fig. 8-11) including those resulting in previously unreported fusion transcripts. Importantly, this study also demonstrated that DNA copy number can be estimated by the relative local abundance of genomic fragments sequenced, providing sensitivity comparable to currently available array-based CGH platforms while providing DNA sequence information. These methods form the basis for much of the collaborative work proposed as part of the International Cancer Genome Consortium (ICGC) (<http://www.icgc.org/>) effort. With a stated goal of obtaining and making available a comprehensive catalog of genomic abnormalities for 50 different cancers and subtypes, much of the massive ICGC effort is likely to be centered on paired-end resequencing of cancer genome.

Integrative Genomic Analyses

These methods have now made it possible to comprehensively catalog the somatic events associated with human cancer; however, significant efforts will be required to distinguish between irrelevant "passenger" alterations and those aberrations that drive tumorigenesis. For example, given the widespread abundance of karyotypic abnormalities in many cancers, array-based CGH or LOH profiling of even a small number of samples often implicates numerous chromosomal regions harboring large numbers of genes, most of which are unlikely to play a significant functional role in cancer. Methods aimed at prioritizing chromosomal loci based on the observation of recurrent changes have proven useful;[120] these methods, however, may require large sample sets and are less effective in identifying genes that are more frequently activated or inactivated via mutation, methylation, transcriptional repression, or other means, rather than larger-scale genomic aberration. Furthermore, genomic alterations of multiple genes within an individual pathway may be functionally equivalent (and mutually exclusive); thus, specific pathways may collectively be subject to genomic aberrations at a frequency far higher than any of its individual gene components. Thus, the integration of multiple types of genomic data will clearly be necessary to unravel the complexity of somatic cancer genetics.

Three recent high-profile studies have integrated high-resolution DNA copy number, gene expression data, and large-scale sequencing data to provide a clearer picture of the mutational complexity and underlying core pathways in human glioblastoma[39,40] and pancreatic cancer.[41] Although these studies did indeed identify countless novel genes mutated in individual cancers (on average 63 and 47 mutations per pancreatic tumor and glioblastoma, respectively), more strikingly they also uncovered relatively few unknown genes recurrently mutated at high rates. All of these studies show that multiple genes within individual key core signaling pathways, rather than single genes, tend to be mutated in these cancers, suggesting an avenue for treating tumors based on aberrant pathways instead of individual aberrant genes.

Integrative analysis of high-resolution DNA copy number data across species has also proved highly useful in identifying genes underlying tumorigenesis. Profiling of metastatic variants derived from a mouse model of melanoma identified a novel amplification of a chromosomal region syntenic to a human chromosomal region frequently subject to copy number gains in metastatic melanoma. Of the genes located within this region, NEDD9 was consistently overexpressed in metastases harboring the amplification and was functionally demonstrated to enhance in vitro invasion and in vivo metastasis.[121] Likewise, a comparison of mouse and human hepatocellular carcinomas identified syntenic regions subject to amplifications in tumors from both species. Expression and functional data suggested that of the genes located within the common amplicon, only *cIAP1* and *Yap* were consistently overexpressed in samples with the amplification and accelerated tumorigenesis.[122]

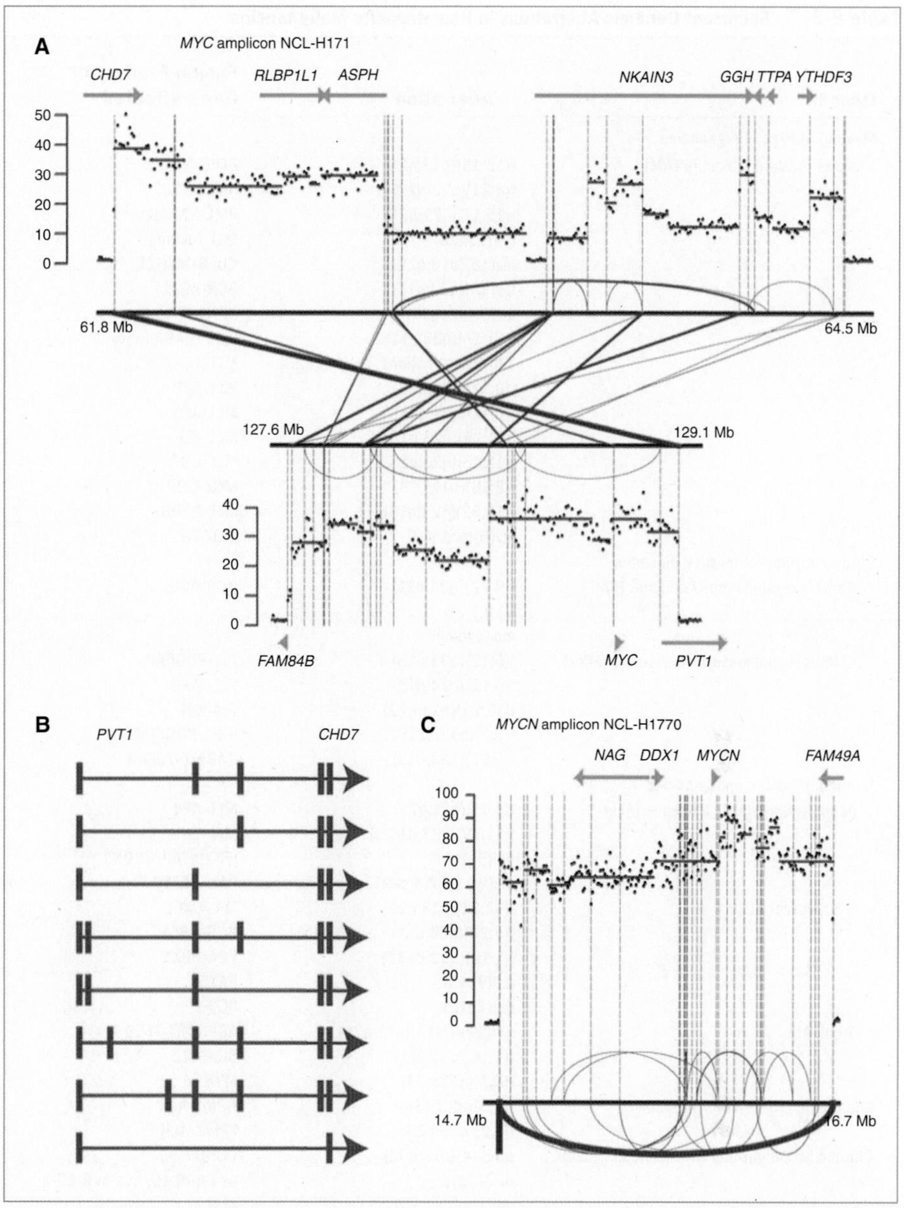

Figure 8-11 Complex amplicons observed in the lung cancer cell lines NCI-H2171 and NCI-H1770 via massively parallel paired-end sequencing. **(A)** The *MYC* amplicon of NCI-H2171 involves two regions of chromosome 8q, both of which show extensive variation in copy number. Breakpoints between and within the two regions are shown in blue lines, with the thickness of the line proportional to the number of paired-end reads spanning the same breakpoint. The locations of the breakpoints frequently correspond to changes in copy number. **(B)** A *PVT1-CHD7* fusion gene is created by the most commonly seen breakpoint in the MYC amplicon. Extensive splicing of the PVT1 moiety was seen on RT-PCR, but the three most common transcripts accounted for 23 of 30 of colonies sequenced. **(C)** The *NMYC* amplicon of NCI-H1770 showed up to 85-fold amplification of a 2-Mb region. The most common breakpoint observed demarcated the 5→ and 3→ borders of the amplicon and suggested tandem insertion of the 2-Mb region, but several other rearrangements were seen within the amplicon, both inverted (arcs above the line) and noninverted (arcs below the line). (Reprinted by permission from Macmillan Publishers Ltd: *Nat Genet* 40, 722-729, copyright 2008.[42])

Ultimately, functional studies are needed to clearly validate the role of any candidate gene identified via genomic methods in tumorigenesis. Although such validation is commonplace on a gene-by-gene basis, recent studies have demonstrated the power of integrating genomic data with data from high-throughput functional genomics tools for activating and inactivating specific genes. Boehm and colleagues utilized a library of activated kinases to screen for those that could replace signaling through the phosphatidylinositol-3-kinase (PI3K) pathway to transform human embryonic kidney (HEK) cells.[123] Of the six kinases identified, I kappa-B kinase epsilon (*IKBKE*) was shown to be amplified and overexpressed in human breast cancer cell lines and tumors, whereas suppression of IKBKE expression in cells harboring these amplifications induced cell death. Ebert and colleagues conversely used high-throughput RNA interference to screen for those genes on chromosome band 5q for which loss of function in hematopoietic progenitor cells phenocopy 5q⁻ myelodysplastic syndrome,[124] implicating the ribosomal subunit protein RPS14 in 5q⁻ disease etiology.

Cancer Genome Analysis: From Application to Discovery

A comprehensive and detailed review of all of the recurrent genomic and chromosomal aberrations in human cancer, the structure and function of the genes that are altered or disrupted by each of these aberrations, the functional consequences of these aberrations on cellular networks and pathways and their mechanisms of transformation, their various means of detection, and their use in cancer diagnosis and therapy would necessitate an entire textbook. Progress in this field is so rapid and evolves in such constantly surprising directions that remaining up to date is a true challenge. Thus, in addition to the tables of recurrent genomic aberrations in hematopoietic cancers (Table 8-3) and solid tumors (Table 8-4) provided in this chapter, the reader is directed to the many online repositories, catalogs, and resources mentioned throughout this chapter as well as to the disease-oriented chapters in this book for a more thorough discussion and review of the various cancer-associated genomic and chromosomal abnormalities and their clinical significance. We present here a detailed discussion of multiple myeloma and malignant melanoma as illustrative examples of the impact of improved genome technology on our understanding of human cancer.

Table 8-3 **Recurrent Genomic Aberrations in Hematopoeitc Malignancies**

Cancer	Aberration	Fusion Product or Gene Affected
Myeloid lineage malignancies		
Acute myeloid leukemia (AML)	t(12;15)(p13;q25)	ETV6-NTRK3
	t(8;21)(q22;q22)	AML1-ETO
	t(15;17)(q22;q21)	PML-RAR(alpha)
	der(11q23)	MLL fusions
	inv(16)(p13;q22)	CBFB-MYH11
	t(9;22)(q34;q11)	BCR-ABL1
	inv(3)(q21q26)	RPN1-EVL1
	t(11;17)(q23;q11)	PLZF-RAR(alpha)
	11q translocations, del(11)(q23)	MLL
	t(9;11)(q22;q23)	MLL-AF9
	t(6;11)(q27;q23)	MLL-AF6
	t(11;19)(q23;p13.1)	MLL-ELL
	t(11;16)(q23;p13.3)	MLL-CBP
	t(8;16)(p11;p13)	MOZ-CBP
	t(11;22)(q23;q13)	MLL-P300
	inv(8)(p11q13)	MOZ-TIF2
Chronic myeloproliferative diseases		
Chronic myelogenous leukemia (CML)	t(9;22)(q34;q11)	BCR-ABL1
	i(17q)	
	monosomy 7	
Chronic myelomonocytic leukemia (CMML)	t(5;12)(q33;p13)	TEL-PDGFRB
	t(9;12)(p24;p13)	TEL-JAK2
	t(12;21)(p13;q22)	TEL-ABL
	t(5;7)(q33;q11)	HIP1-PDGFRB
	t(5;17)(q33;p13)	RAB5-PDGFRB
Lymphoid lineage malignancies		
Acute lymphoblastic leukemia (ALL)	t(4;11)(q21;q23)	MLL-AF4
	t(11;19)(q23;p13.3)	MLL-ENL
	del(9p)	IFN/MTAP/CKDN2
	dic(9;12)(p13;p13)	PAX5/ETV6
B-precursor ALL	t(12;21)(p13;q22)	TEL-AML1
	t(9;22)(q34;q11)	BCR-ABL1
	t(1;19)(9q23;q32)	E2A-PBX1
	del(9p13)	PAX5
	del(7p12)	IKZF1
T-cell ALL	der(17)t(X;17)(p11;q25)	ASPSCR1-TFE3
	t(1;14)(q32;q11)	SIL-SCL
	t(6;7)(q23;q34)	MYB
Anaplastic large T-cell lymphoma	t(2;5)(p23;q35)	NPM1-ALK
	t(1;2)(q25;p23)	TPM3-ALK
Chronic lymphoproliferative leukemia (CLL)	t(11;14)(q13;q32)	CCND1
	del(13q)	hsa-miR-15, hsa-miR-16-1
	del(11q)	ATM
	trisomy 12	
	del(17p)	TP53
	del(6q)	
	trisomy 19	
B-cell lymphoma	t(11;14)(q13;32)	CCND1
	t(14;18)	BCL2
		MYC
		BCL6
MALT lymphoma	t(11:18)(q21;q21)	AIP2-MALT1
	t(14;18)(q32;q21)	MALT1
	t(1;14)(p22;q32)	BCL10
	t(3;14)(p14;q32)	FOXP1
Lymphoplasmacytoid lymphoma	t(9;14)(p13;q32)	PAX5
Mantle cell lymphoma	t(11;14)(q13;32)	CCND1
Follicular lymphoma	t(14;18)(q32;q21)	BCL2
	del(6q)	
	+7	
	der(18)t(14;18)	
	del(17p)	
	+12	
Burkitt lymphoma	t(8;14)(q24;q32)	MYC
	t(2;8)(p11;q24)	MYC
	t(8;22)(q24;q11)	MYC
Multiple Myeloma	t(11;14)(q13;32)	CCND1
	t(6;14)(p21;q32)	CCND3
	t(4;14)(p16;q32)	FGFR3, MMSET
	t(14;16)(q32;q23)	MAF
	t(14;20)(q32;q12	MAFB

Multiple Myeloma

Multiple myeloma is a hematological malignancy that affects approximately 20,000 individuals each year in the United States.[125] This neoplasia is characterized by an accumulation of plasma cells in the bone marrow, resulting in anemia and chronic infections as the expanding tumor suppresses normal hematopoiesis. Although we have recently seen significant improvements in patient outcome, myeloma still accounts for a disproportionate number of deaths, with roughly 11,000 people dying each year of this malignancy.[125] Given the relatively low incidence of this disease, it is surprising that many of the initial applications of new technologies have occurred in this field. The early adoption of new technologies has been driven by several characteristics of the disease. First, a better understanding of this cancer is desperately needed as the median survival for patients with this terminal malignancy has only recently improved beyond 3 years. In addition, unlike other cancers with an equally dismal prognosis, the tumor cells can easily be isolated from patients by a bone marrow biopsy and purified by anti-CD138 sorting. Much of the recent progress made in understanding the pathogenesis of multiple myeloma was dependent on the application of these new technologies.

The foundation that underpins much of our current understanding of myeloma genetics is based on the use of G-banding techniques on metaphase chromosome spreads (ie, conventional cytogenetics) in the 1970s and 1980s. In 1984, Lewis and McKenzie published a meta-analysis of the first 27 published myeloma karyotypes and in the process, correctly identified the majority of the chromosome abnormalities identified to date.[126] Their observations provided the basis for the dichotomy that divides myeloma into two broad categories of hyperdiploid myeloma (48-74 chromosomes) and nonhyperdiploid myeloma (patients with hypodiploid, pseudodiploid, and tetraploid genomes). In the case of hyperdiploid patients, the chromosomes that account for the increased chromosome count are not random but typically represent trisomies of chromosomes 3, 5, 7, 9, 11, 15, 19, and 21.[127] Beyond this broad generic classification, the whole genome scan provided by conventional cytogenetics identified frequent deletions of chromosome 13, rearrangements at 14q32, and amplifications of 1q. Unfortunately, even though conventional cytogenetics laid a solid foundation for the field, it is not broadly applicable as metaphase chromosomes are only generated from one-third of patients due to the low proliferative index of this tumor.

Table 8-4 Recurrent Chromosomal Abnormalities in Malignant Solid Tumors

Tumor Type	Chromosome Abnormality	Fusion Product or Gene Affected
	del(14q32)	TRAF3
Epithelial Tumors		
Bladder cancer, squamous cell	monosomy 9 trisomy 7	CDKN2/P16
Bladder cancer, transitional cell	monosomy 9, del9p	CDKN2A
	trisomy 7	EGFR
	del(13q)	RB
	del(1p)	
	monosomy 11, del(11p)	HRAS1
	del(17p13)	P53
	add(1q32)	MDM4
Breast	i(1q)	
	t(1;16)	
	+7p11.2	EGFR
	add(8q)	MYC
	add(11q)	CCND1
	del(16q)	E-cadherin
	add(17q11-12)	ERBB2
	add(20q12)	AIB1
	add(17q)	TBX2/RPS6KB1
	add(6p21)	CCND3, P21/WAF1
	t(12;15)(p13;q25)	ETV6-NTRK3
Cervical	add(4p16)	FGF4
	add(8q24.21)	MYC
	del(18q21)	SMAD4
Colon	del(17p)	TP53
	del(18q)	DCC/DPC4
	del(5q)	APC
	del/mut(2q)	MSH2
	del/mut(3q)	MLH1
	del/mut(7p)	PMS1/2
Endometrial-endometrioid type	add(1q25-q42) add(9pter-13.1)	
Endometrial-serous type	add(3q26.1)	
	add(8q)	?MYC
Esophagus	del(8q22)	FEZ1
	del(13q)	ING1/WWOX
	del(13q)	RB
	del(17p)	P53
	del(3p21)	DLC1
Head/neck	add(11q13)	CCND1/PRAD1
	del(18q)	
	del(13q)	ING1
	del/mut(10q23)	PTEN
Lung carcinoma, small cell	del(3p14-23)	FHIT
Lung cancer, nonsmall cell	del (3p)	VHL/FHIT/PTPRG
	del (9p21)	CDKN2A
	del(13q14) del(17p13)	RB P53
	del(5p15.33)	TERT
	add(7p)	EGRFR
Prostate	del(10q24-25)	MXI1
	del(10q23)	PTEN
	del(17q21)	BRCA1
	loss of Y	

(Continued)

Although conventional cytogenetics methods are not informative in all myeloma patients, they are still applied as a common clinical test with a significant bearing on prognosis. First, patients with nonhyperdiploid karyotypes do poorly compared with their hyperdiploid counterparts.[128] Second, the presence of monosomy 13 is associated with a poor prognosis, and although controversial, monosomy 13 appears to be a poor prognosis marker irrespective of ploidy status.[128-130] Finally, the suppression of detectable chromosome abnormalities by conventional cytogenetics is a strong predictor of a long-term and durable remission irrespective of the level of remission achieved by therapy.[131]

Although conventional cytogenetics only provides a low-resolution view of the genome, some of the observed abnormalities have provided the basis for fundamental observations regarding the origin of myeloma. For example, Bergsagel and colleagues developed the seminal hypothesis that myeloma is characterized by illegitimate IgH rearrangements based on the frequent rearrangements of 14q32 detected by metaphase cytogenetics and the ubiquitous presence of similar rearrangements in mouse plasmacytomas.[132] The work of this group using a directed Southern blot assay identified the majority of the known IgH translocations, many of which are essential to the current prognostic models that exist in the field.[133]

The limited applicability of Southern blots to patient studies and the low proliferative index of the tumor, which compromises both conventional cytogenetic and spectral karyotype studies, resulted in the rapid adoption of interphase FISH in the myeloma field. The application of interphase FISH in myeloma differs from its application in many hematological malignancies where FISH results are diagnostic [ie, t(9;22) in CML and t(11;14) in mantle cell lymphoma]. In myeloma, most of the tests used in clinical labs are prognostic tests, designed to identify deletions of 13q14 and 17p13; the presence of an IgH translocation (breakapart FISH probes); a variety of specific IgH translocations including t(4;14), t(11;14), t(14;16), and t(14;20) (fusion FISH strategies); and hyperdiploid karyotypes based on trisomies of chromosomes 3, 9, 11, 15 and 19. The introduction of these tests has resulted in a variety of prognostic systems based on single events such as 13q14 deletions or t(4;14).[134,135] However, these single parameter models have been replaced by the multiple parameter models developed by the groups of Rafael Fonseca and Herve Avet-Loiseau that combine multiple interphase FISH results or a clinical feature with interphase FISH results, respective-

Table 8-4 ■ **Recurrent Chromosomal Abnormalities in Malignant Solid Tumors *(Continued)***

Tumor Type	Chromosome Abnormality	Fusion Product or Gene Affected
	del(8p), add8q	
	del(11p)	KAI1
	del(1q)	HPC1/PCAP/PRCA1
	add(8q22-q24)	MYC
	del(8p11-p23)	NKX3-1
	del(12p13)	CDKN1B
	del(13q14)	RB1
	t(21q22)	TMPRSS2-ERG
	t(21q22)(7p21)	TMPRSS2-ETV1
	t(21q22)(17q21)	TMPRSS2-ETV4
	t(6;16)(p21;q22)	RPS10-HPR
Renal cell carcinoma, papillary	t(X;1)(p11.2;q21.2)	PRCC-TFE3
	t(X;17)(p11.2;q25)	
	+7	MET
	Del(7q)	HPRC
Renal carcinoma, clear cell	del(3p25)	VHL
	t(3;8)(p21;q24)	HRCA1
	t(6;11)	Alpha/TFE3
	t(3;8)	FHIT/TCR8
	t(2;3)	DIRC2
Thyroid carcinoma	inv10(q11.2;q21.2)	RET-H4(PTC1)
	t(10;12)	RET-ELK4
	t(10;17)	RET-ELK5
	inv(1q22)	NTRK1-TPM3
	inv(7q21–22q34)	AKAP9–BRAF
	t(2;3)(q13;p25)	PAX8–PPARG
	t(1;3)	NTRK1-TPR/TFG
Mucoid carcinoma (salivary gland)	t(11;19)(q21;p13)	MECT1-MAML2
Mesenchymal Tumors		
Lipoma	add(12q)	MDM2
	t(12;16)	CHOP-FUS
Chondrosarcoma	trisomy 7	
	add(20p)	
	add(20q)	
Synovial sarcoma	t(X;18)(p11.2;q11.2)	SYT-SSX1/SSX2
Rhabdomyosarcoma (alveolar type)	t(2;13)(q35;q14)	PAX3-FKHR
	t(1;13)(p36;q14)	PAX7-FKHR
Extraskeletal myxoid chondrosarcoma	t(9;22)(q22;q12)	EWS-CHN/TEC
Fibrosarcoma	add(12q)	MDM2
	add(14q21-24)	
	add(7q31)	
	add(8q)	?MYC
Congenital fibrosarcoma	t(12;15)(p13;q25)	ETV6-NTRK3
Fibromyxoid sarcoma	t(7;16)	FUS-CREB3L2
Central Nervous System Tumors		
Anaplastic astrocytoma	del(9p)	CDKN2A
	del(13q)	RB
Glioblastoma	+7	
	del(10q)	PTEN/MXI1
	del(9p)	CDKN2A
	del(22q)	NF2

(Continued)

ly (Fig. 8-12A and B).[136,137] Although the methodology and stratification are different in these two studies, both conclude that t(4;14), t(14;16), t(14;20), and deletions of 17p13 are markers of poor prognosis. The true culmination of these findings is best highlighted by the Mayo Clinic mSMART protocol that directs patients into specific therapeutic regiments based on the genetic abnormalities identified by conventional cytogenetics and interphase FISH.[138]

The use of global GEP has built on the fundamental genetic classes identified by cytogenetics and FISH. The first significant applications of GEP in the field of myeloma provided class identifiers that divide myeloma into seven or eight groups, depending on the application of an unsupervised or a supervised analysis.[139,140] In a supervised approach, Bergsagel and colleagues defined eight distinct groups, in what are termed the TC groups, based on the overexpression of target genes associated with IgH translocations and the expression of the D-type cyclins (Fig. 8-13). Moreover, even the seven unsupervised groupings defined by Shaughnessy and colleagues are largely defined by the known IgH translocations and the associated overexpressed target gene signatures.[140] Although myeloma is a relatively rare disease, the strong correlation between specific translocations and overexpressed target genes helped provide the basis for the development of the COPA algorithm developed by Arul Chinnaiyan's group at the University of Michigan that resulted in the identification of *TMPRSS2-ETS* gene fusions in prostate cancer.[104]

Beyond simple classification strategies, the true power of GEP in myeloma appears to be the development of a robust prognostic model. Although the current prognostic models that include FISH assays have a much greater predictive value than those based on clinical features alone, many of the patients in the good prognosis subgroups still do poorly clinically. Using GEP, Shaugnessy and colleagues identified a 70- or a 17-gene signature that could identify the patients with a poor prognosis irrespective of their FISH-based classification (Fig. 8-13).[141] Unfortunately, this GEP-based prognostic model is limited in its application to all MM patients, as it requires large amounts of tumor cells and specialized facilities; however, with the advent of new technologies we may see this model replace the FISH-based models in the coming years.

The use of conventional cytogenetics, SKY, FISH, and GEP has been invaluable in defining molecular subgroups and prognostic models in myeloma. However, less the contribution of conven-

Table 8-4 **Recurrent Chromosomal Abnormalities in Malignant Solid Tumors *(Continued)***

Tumor Type	Chromosome Abnormality	Fusion Product or Gene Affected
Schwannoma	del(22q)	NF2
Embryonic Tumors		
Ewing tumors	t(11;22)(q24;q12)	EWSR1-FLI1
	t(21;22)(q12;q12)	EWSR1-ERG
Medulloblastoma	i(17q)	
	del(17p)	REN
Neuroblastoma	del(1p32 to p36)	
	add(2p24)	MYCN
Wilms' tumor	del(11p13)	WT1
Mesoblastic nephroma	t(12;15)(p13;q25)	ETV6-NTRK3
Retinoblastoma	del(13q14)	RB
Clear cell sarcoma of soft parts	t(12;22)(q13;q12)	EWSR1-ATF1
Malignant melanoma	del(1p11-22)	
	del(6q11-q27)	
	del(9p)	CDKN2A
	add(4q11-q12)	KIT
	add(12q14)	CDK4
	add(11q13)	CCND1
	add(3p14)	MITF
Germ cell tumors		
Testicular tumors	i(12p), add(12p)	?CyclinD2
Other tumors		
Dermatofibrosarcoma protuberans	+ring chromosome	
	t(17;22)(q2;q13)	COL1A1-PDGFB

tional cytogenetics to the identification of IgH translocations, none of the aforementioned technologies has identified an underlying genetic cause of myeloma. One of the first technologies that promised to identify previously unknown abnormalities was CGH. The initial application of CGH in myeloma using metaphase CGH provided the first unbiased glimpse of the myeloma genome, as it could be performed on all patients. However, these studies only refined most of the previous findings from conventional cytogenetics and SKY studies.[142] The promise of CGH as a discovery platform was only recently met with the development of array-based copy number analysis platforms that interrogate 22,000-500,000 regions of the genome simultaneously and thus are capable of identifying single gene abnormalities. Several groups have now screened the myeloma genome using the various platforms with variable success in identifying novel events.[127,143-145] Most groups have still focused on whole genome analyses, but finally these studies have resolved the standard hyperdiploid and nonhyperdiploid categories into additional subgroups, largely based on deletions of chromosomes 13, 1p, 8, and amplifications of 1q (Fig. 8-14).[127] A good example of using CGH to identify novel events in myeloma was recently published by Keats et al. using an array-based CGH platform with 44,000 probes.[145] In this study, they elected to study only regions of the genome with homozygous deletions, as these inherently small regions of the genome contain a limited number of genes that are predicted to be tumor suppressor genes. Using this strategy they identified 46 candidate genes, of which 5 were involved in the regulation of the NF-kB pathway. Ultimately, the integration of CGH and GEP data sets resulted in the identification of nine deregulated genes in the NF-kB pathway. One of these genes, TRAF3, was inactivated in 13% of patients making it the most frequently inactivated tumor suppressor identified in myeloma to date.

The development of RNAi has revolutionized the biological sciences; in most situations, RNAi is used as a methodology to address a specific problem in a hypothesis driven project. Recently, however, genome-scale RNAi screening has been used to discover genes that are required for malignant proliferation and mammary cell survival.[146-148] Using an RNAi screen of 2500 genes in three myeloma cell lines Staudt and colleagues identified IRF4 as an essential gene in myeloma.[148] An interesting finding is that this gene is not mutated and is only very rarely overexpressed in myeloma by an IgH translocation. Yet the expression of this gene is required for the survival of both normal and myeloma plasma cells. This "nononcogene addiction" of myeloma cells to IRF4 represents a novel concept in the pathogenesis of any malignancy that will need to be investigated in other diseases in the future.

The genetic underpinnings of myeloma have slowly been elucidated with the application of each new technology. In the last 10 years in particular, the field has changed drastically from a disease characterized by two broad cytogenetic groups to one with well-accepted subentities with defined prognostic outcomes. Although most of the discoveries made to date have affected only prognosis, we are finally seeing the development of novel targeted therapies for the specific IgH translocations and inhibitors of the NF-kB pathway.

Malignant Melanoma

Malignant melanoma continues to pose a substantial clinical challenge. The American Cancer Society estimates that in 2008 there will be 62,480 new cases of melanoma in the United States and that about 8420 people will die of this disease.[149] Melanoma continues to rank as the sixth most common cancer in men and seventh most common cancer in women. As it affects disproportionately high numbers of younger individuals, melanoma represents one of the leading cancers in terms of average years of life lost per person.[150] Current diagnostic and prognostic methods for early disease detection, which rely primarily on classic microscopic tissue morphology and the thickness of the primary tumor measured in millimeters, fall short of providing a fully accurate, individualized assessment of risk of disease progression. Similarly, the lack of adequate approaches to properly define disease subgroups on a molecular level has historically precluded rational treatment design and selection. However, rapid advances in genomic strategies in recent years have facilitated an exponential increase in our understanding of the molecular underpinnings of melanoma. These insights are likely to markedly affect the diagnosis, prognosis, classification, and treatment of melanoma.

Early cytogenetic studies of cutaneous melanoma provided an important initial outline of the dynamic genomic landscape in this disease. The most common recurring cytogenetic abnormalities involved rearrangements of chromosome 1p, multiple abnormalities of chromosome 6, and extra copies of chromosome 7.[151,152] Iso(1q) or del(1p) appears to occur in approximately 60% of all melanomas, whereas chromosome 6 rearrangements were reported in more than 80% of cases. However, the only karyotypic abnormality seen in both dysplastic nevi and melanoma were deletions of chromosome 9, especially 9pter-p22 (now known to harbor the tumor suppressor *CDKN2A*). In addition, translocations involving the terminal region of chromosome 10q24-26 were reported in both early and late melanomas suggesting it might represent an early event in oncogenesis of melanoma.[153] Although these reports identified only broad genomic regions of involvement and not individual genes, early functional studies by Trent and colleagues provided an initial validation of these cytogenetic findings by demonstrating that insertion of a normal chromosome 6 into melanoma cells harboring chromosome 6 aberrations could revert some features of the malignant phenotype.[154]

The convergence of melanoma cytogenetics and the study of familial melanoma cases, which account for approximately 10% of all melanomas,[155] served to elucidate some of the primary mechanisms underlying the etiology of both familial and sporadic melanoma as well as other cancers. Study of such families provided evidence linking heritable susceptibility to melanoma to an interval centered on chromosome band 9p21,[155,156] a region previously shown to be subject to deletion in both melanoma and dysplastic nevi. Subsequently, the *CDKN2A* locus located in this area was identified as a potential tumor suppressor in cancer cell lines from various tissue types[157] including melanoma,[158] and mutations cosegregating with melanoma susceptibility have since been identified in 10-40% of melanoma families.[159-162] Consistent with cytogenetic data implicating the *CDNK2A* locus in sporadic disease, *CDKN2A* has been demonstrated to be frequently subject to genomic aberration in sporadic melanoma; the gene is deleted in approximately 50% of melanomas, inactivated by point mutations in approximately 9% of tumors,[163] and epigenetically silenced in 20-75% of melanomas.[163,164] These data firmly estab-

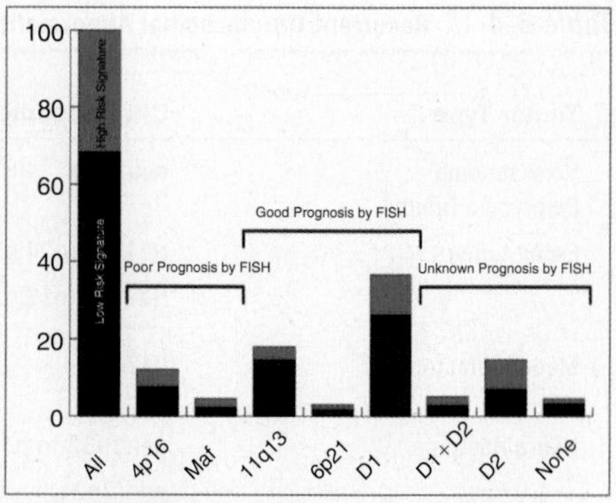

Figure 8-13 ■ Gene expression models of myeloma. Patients' samples from the Multiple Myeloma Research Consortium Genomics Initiative were classified according to the TC Classification scheme proposed by Bergsagel et al. that uses gene expression results to stratify patients into interphase FISH-related prognostic groups. To identify the patients with a predicted poor prognosis irrespective of TC group the 17-gene model proposed by Shaugnessy et al.[141] was applied and samples with an index associated with poor prognosis are highlighted in red.

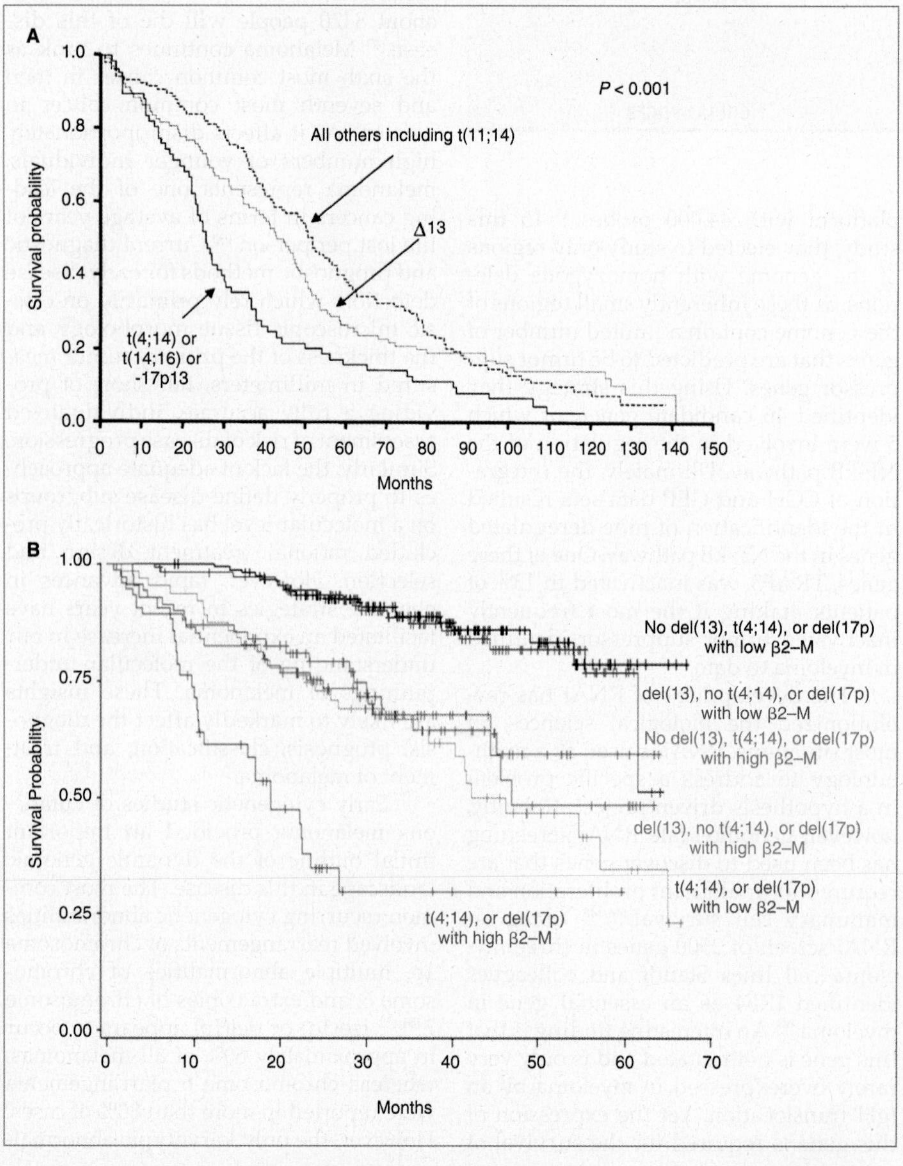

Figure 8-12 ■ **(A)** Interphase FISH-based model proposed by the Mayo Clinic based on the detection of del(13), del(17p), t(4;14), t(11;14), and t(14;16). This research was originally published in Blood. Fonseca R, et al. Clinical and biologic implications of recurrent genomic aberrations in myeloma. *Blood.* 2003;101:4569-4575. © The American Society of Hematology. **(B)** Combined interphase FISH and clinical feature model proposed by the Intergroupe Francophone du Myelome based on the detection of del(13), del(17p), t(4;14), and the level of beta-2-microglobulin in the serum. This research was originally published by Avet-Loiseau H, et al. Genetic abnormalities and survival in multiple myeloma: the experience of the Intergroupe Francophone du Myelome. *Blood.* 2007;109:3489-3495. © The American Society of Hematology.

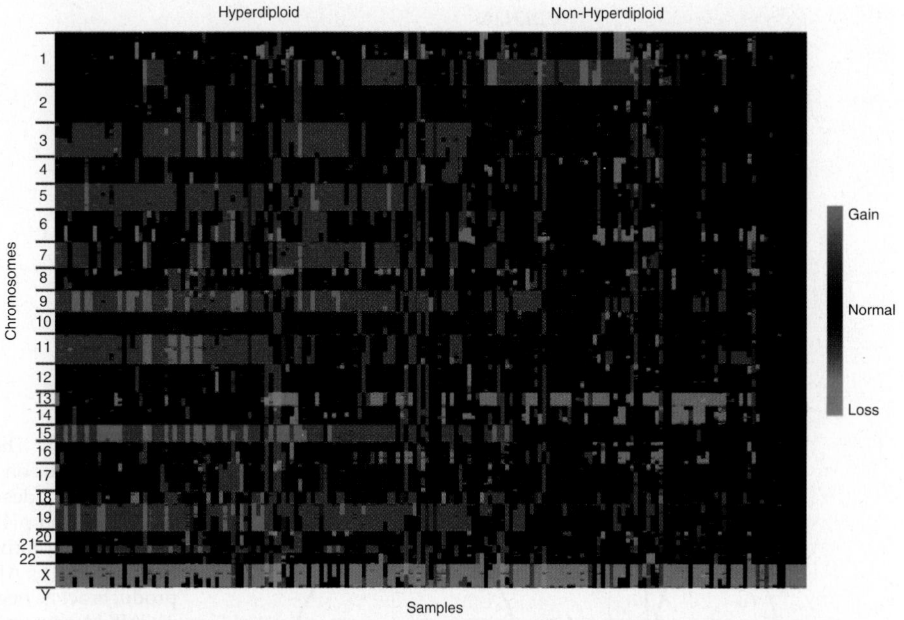

Figure 8-14 Hierarchal clustering of aCGH data from myeloma patients shows the hyperdiploid and nonhyperdiploid dichotomy. A total of 102 myeloma patients were assayed on the Agilent 44B array CGH platform and the detected regions of gain or loss are summarized. On the left the characteristic whole chromosome gains of the odd number chromosomes in hyperdiploid myeloma are clearly seen. On the left relatively few gains are seen with gains of 1q and deletions of chromosome 13 being the most common abnormalities seen in nonhyperdiploid patients.

lished *CDKN2A* as a critical player in both familial and sporadic disease.

The gene structure of the *CDKN2A* locus is unique in the genome, encoding for two overlapping but very disparate proteins, $p16^{INK4A}$ and $p14^{ARF}$ (Fig. 8-15). Although structurally unique, the protein products of both genes act as tumor suppressors by negatively regulating cell cycle progression. The $p16^{INK4A}$ protein regulates the RB1 (retinoblastoma gene) pathway, whereas $p14^{ARF}$ regulates the TP53 (tumor protein 53) pathway, with both pathways acting as key negative regulators of cell cycle progression. Therefore, genetic or epigenetic changes resulting in a functional loss of $p16^{INK4A}$ and $p14^{ARF}$ ultimately lead to uninhibited cellular growth and proliferation.

Importantly, the identification of *CDKN2A* as a major melanoma tumor suppressor locus has highlighted these two critical pathways as recurrent targets of genomic aberration in melanoma. In the RB1 pathway, cyclin-dependent kinase 4 (*CDK4*), cyclin D1 (CCND1), and RB1 itself are all occasionally targeted. A small fraction of melanoma-prone families have been shown to carry germline *CDK4* mutations,[165-168] with most of these rare mutations changing the arginine at position 24 to cysteine (R24C). This substitution blocks the binding of CDK4 to $p16^{INK4A}$ but preserves the CDK4-CCND1 interaction, resulting in a constitutively active CDK4/CCND1complex. In sporadic disease, this same *CDK4* mutation has been reported;[167] however, focal amplifications of CDK4 appear more common.[62,161] Aberrations of *CCND1* in melanoma are relatively rare, occurring mainly as amplifications in approximately 4% of tumors,[62,63,76] whereas direct inactivating mutations in the *RB1* gene occur in approximately 6% of sporadic melanoma tumors.[163] Consistent with the notion that such aberrations in the same pathway may be functionally similar, familial melanoma patients tend to have either $p16^{INK4A}$ mutations or $CDK4^{R24C}$ mutations but not both. In sporadic disease, amplifications of *CDK4* likewise tend to occur in tumors without $p16^{INK4A}$ deletions.[62]

In contrast to many cancers, melanomas display a surprisingly low frequency of *TP53* mutations (9%).[169] Although most other tumors inactivate this pathway directly at the level of *TP53*, melanoma appears to largely rely on inactivation of the pathway at the level of *CDKN2A* and its product, $p14^{ARF}$. Most *CDKN2A* mutations affect $p16^{INK4A}$, either alone or in combination with $p14^{ARF}$, suggesting that $p16^{INK4A}$ is the principal susceptibility gene at this locus. However, reports of families with mutations in $p14^{ARF}$ alone raise the possibility that loss of $p14^{ARF}$ could be sufficient to lead to a melanoma phenotype.[170-172] Although conclusive evidence of independent roles for $p16^{INK4A}$ and $p14^{ARF}$ loss in development of melanoma in humans is still pending, genetic studies in mouse suggest that both genes are essential for melanoma suppression. Disruption of either gene in mouse germline DNA leads to increased melanoma susceptibility;[173,174] however, tumors arising in mice with germline deletion of $p19^{ARF}$ (a mouse ortholog of human $p14^{ARF}$) appear to acquire somatic mutations in the $p16^{INK4A}$/RB1 pathway. In contrast, tumors arising in mice with disrupted $p16^{INK4A}$ tend to develop mutations in the $p19^{ARF}$/p53 pathway. This complex interplay of genetic alterations provides further support for the essential tumor suppressor role of both genes, at least in mouse models of melanoma.

More recently, newer genomic approaches have had a similarly dramatic impact on our understanding of the basic underpinnings of melanoma development as well as potential therapeutic avenues for more effective treatment. Perhaps most notably, one of the initial findings reported from a large DNA sequencing-based mutation screen of 518 protein kinases conducted as a part of the Wellcome Trust Sanger Institute Cancer Genome Project was the presence of recurrent activating point mutations in BRAF kinase in numerous cancers. The cancer with the highest mutation rate was melanoma (59% for cell lines, 67% in melanoma tumors, and 80% in short term cultures);[108] subsequently, activating BRAF mutations were also detected in most of common benign nevi, suggesting a possible critical early role in development of melanoma. Importantly, the vast majority of BRAF mutations target a single residue, changing the valine at position 600 to glutamic acid (V600E), thus potentially providing a uniform therapeutic target. Several inhibitors of BRAF have thus far been developed and extensively tested in clinical trials, with no significant benefit observed in these studies to date. These first generation BRAF inhibitors had a relatively low specificity; newer drugs that are expected to provide more specific inhibition of BRAF are presently under development. With the recent emergence of next-generation sequencing platforms that can facilitate even more ambitions mutation screens, it is likely that sequencing will continue to contribute to the identification of numerous additional potential therapeutic targets.

The application of array-based, genome-wide analytical approaches has similarly accelerated the study of melanoma, suggesting new avenues for the

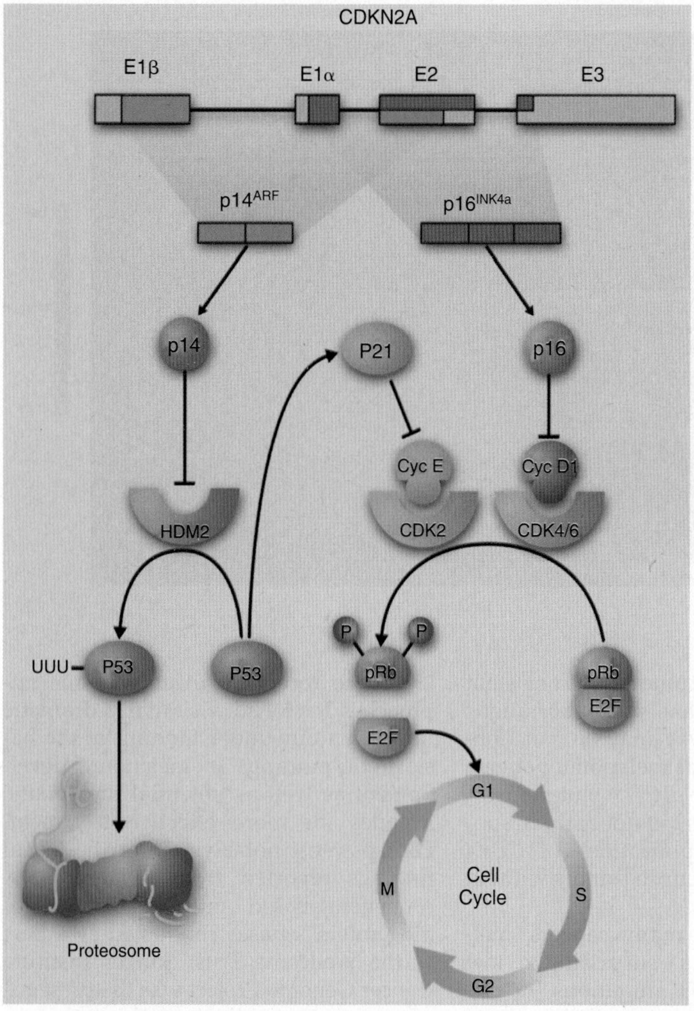

Figure 8-15 ■ The *CDKN2A* locus and cell cycle control. The *CDKN2A* locus on chromosome 9p21 has an unusual structure because it encodes for two overlapping but very distinct proteins: p16INK4A and p14ARF. This is accomplished through selective use of an alternative first exon (exon E1a in p16INK4A and exon E1b in p14ARF). Although structurally very different, both protein products act as negative regulators of cell cycle progression. The p16INK4A protein inhibits the activation of CDK4 and CDK6 by cyclin D1 (CCND1), thereby preventing the subsequent phosphorylation of RB1. Underphosphorylated RB1 sequesters the transcription factor E2F and prevents it from inducing the progression from G1 to S phase of the cell cycle. The absence of functional p16INK4A, therefore, leads to hyperphosphorylation of RB1 with resulting release of E2F and uninhibited cell cycle progression. In contrast, p14ARF regulates tumor protein 53 (p53) activity by inhibiting MDM2, a ubiquitin ligase that otherwise targets p53 for degradation by proteasome. High levels of p14ARF stabilize p53, permitting it to induce p21WAF1/CIP1, a cell cycle inhibitor that blocks CDK2/cyclin E (CCNE1)–mediated phosphorylation of RB1. In the absence of functional p14ARF, uncontrolled ubiquitination and degradation of p53 removes this important cell cycle brake, leading ultimately to hyperphosphorylation of RB1 and cell cycle progression. *Source:* From Ref. 181.

diagnosis of histologically challenging cases, highlighting new melanoma oncogenes underpinning disease etiology and even fundamentally altering our understanding of melanoma as a collection of molecularly distinct diseases. Toward improved diagnosis, the identification of melanoma-specific genomic alterations may provide a basis for distinguishing melanomas from benign nevi in cases with challenging histology. An examination of gene copy number changes in 132 primary melanomas and 54 benign nevi demonstrated significant copy number alterations in 127 (96.2%) melanomas and in only seven (13%) nevi. All seven nevi with copy number changes were Spitz nevi, and six of them harbored an isolated gain involving 11p that was not observed in any of the melanoma samples, suggesting a potential clinical utility of this finding in differentiation of Spitz nevi from melanoma.[175]

Garraway and colleagues used SNP array-based gene copy number interrogation across a panel of human cancer cell lines, identifying the microphthalmia-associated transcription factor (*MITF*) as a novel lineage-specific survival oncogene in melanoma.[73] SNP profiling of the NCI-60 cell line panel identified recurrent amplifications of a small region of chromosome arm 3p only in melanoma samples. Subsequent interrogation of expression microarray data from these cell lines for genes differentially expressed between samples with and without 3p amplification identified *MITF* as the only such gene located within the affected 3p region. Overall, amplifications of *MITF*, in some cases strikingly focal,[76] appear to occur in 10-15% of human melanomas and are more frequently found in metastases. Consistent with this difference, high MITF protein expression levels in tumors were also subsequently linked to poor prognosis. In vitro, coexpression of MITF with active BRAF (V600E) was oncogenic, whereas reduction of MITF activity leads to an increased sensitivity of melanoma cells to chemotherapeutic agents.

A recent landmark study of gene copy number alterations in a large set of primary melanomas via array-based CGH identified numerous large as well as focal chromosomal aberrations, including those to *CDKN2A*, *CCND1*, and *CDK4* previously described. More important, however, the integrative analysis of these CGH data, sequencing data (eg, *NRAS* and *BRAF* mutation status), and data on anatomic site and associated sun exposure of the primary tumor lend strong support to the hypothesis that melanoma consists of several genetically distinct entities, fundamentally altering our understanding of this disease (Fig 8-16).[62] The vast majority of melanomas arising on skin with evidence of chronic sun-induced damage were observed to have mutations in either BRAF or NRAS but not both, whereas most melanomas in other groupings (eg, acral melanomas, mucosal melanomas, melanomas arising on nonchronically sun-damaged skin) had mutations in neither. Instead, melanomas from these other groups frequently had DNA copy number increases in *CDK4* and *CCND1*. Further supporting this notion that these subgroups represent molecularly distinct entities, these groupings can be largely distinguished from each other based on overall pattern of genomic alteration and *BRAF* mutational status.[62]

Patterns of co-occurrence observed in melanoma CGH and mutation data highlight two key pathways that appear to be aberrant in the majority of melanomas. Curtin and colleagues noted a clear mutual exclusivity of alterations involving the members of a single signal-

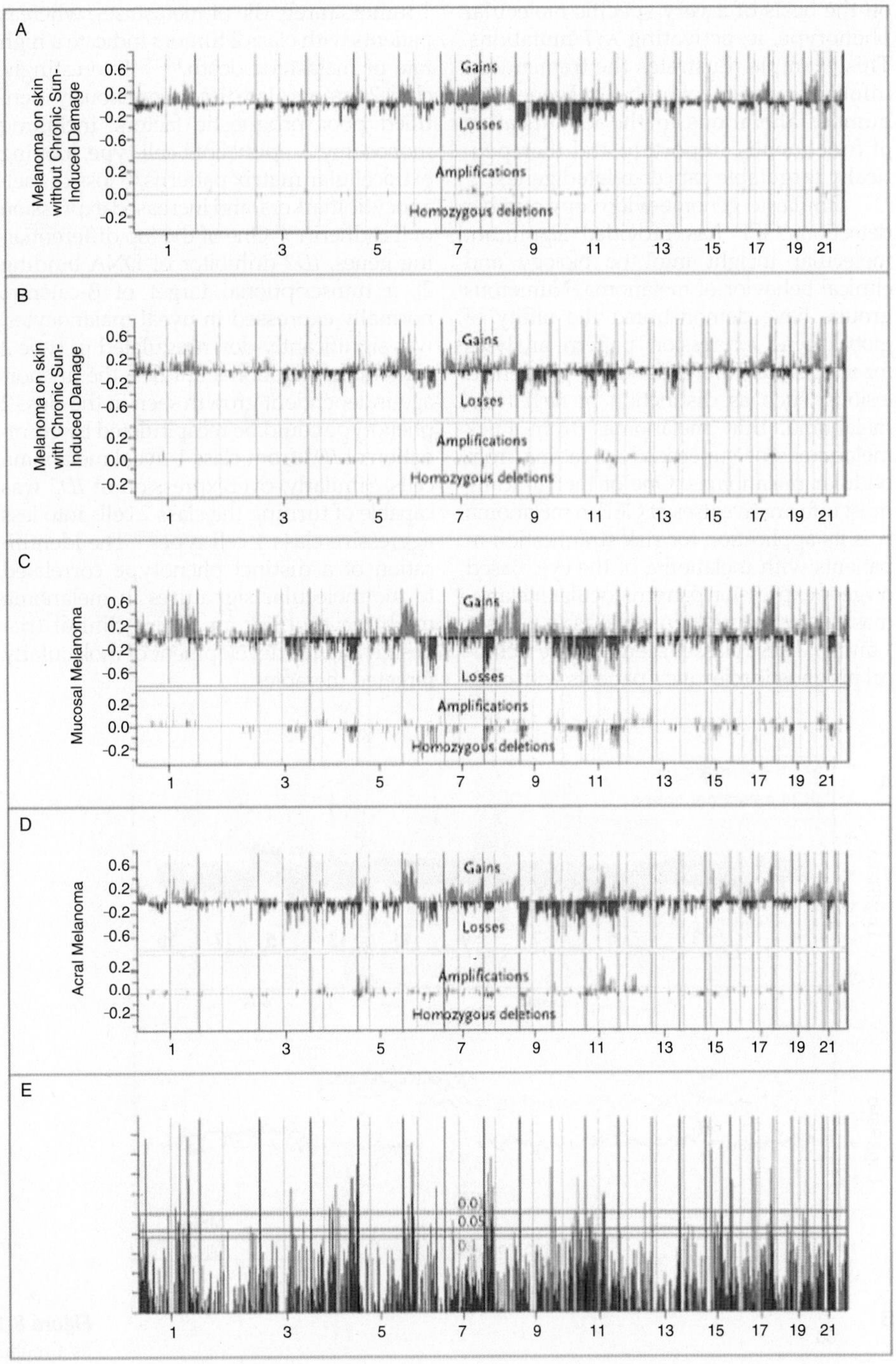

Figure 8-16 Changes in the number of copies of DNA in subgroups of melanoma. CGH analysis was performed on four subgroups of melanoma according to the anatomic location and the level of sun exposure. This included melanomas arising in the skin without chronic sun damage **(A)**, melanomas arising in the skin with chronic sun damage **(B)**, mucosal melanomas **(C)**, and acral melanomas **(D)**. Two histograms are shown for each group of melanoma (Panels A, B, C, and D) and for the four groups combined (Panel E). In each panel, the upper plots show low-level gains (green) and losses (red), and the lower plots show amplifications (green) and homozygous deletions (red) for each type. Vertical dashed lines represent the location of the centromere. The x axis represents genomic position, with the bacterial artificial chromosomes ordered according to position in the genome beginning at 1p and ending at 22. The y axis represents the fraction of the samples with a given clone altered. Panel E shows the statistical differences between the changes in the number of copies in the four groups. The magnitude of the F statistic is shown as the height of the vertical bars, and their global significance is indicated with horizontal dashed lines that show the max T-adjusted p-value cutoffs (red, $p = 0.01$; blue, $P = 0.05$; and green, $P = 0.1$).
Source: From Ref. 62.

ing pathway, NRAS-BRAF-MAPK pathway.[62] Similar to the mutual exclusivity of *BRAF* and *NRAS* mutations that had been previously described, tumors with activating mutations in *NRAS* or *BRAF* also do not contain amplifications of downstream MAPK target genes, such as *CDK4* or *CCND1*, suggesting that aberration at any of several levels is sufficient to activate the pathway and drive tumor progression.[62,63] Likewise, an observation of frequent co-occurrence of *BRAF* activation and *PTEN* inactivation or deletion indicates that, in addition to *BRAF* activation, melanomas likely require PI3K pathway activation.[63] However, *NRAS*-activating mutations do not co-occur with *PTEN* mutations, consistent with the notion that unlike BRAF, which cannot induce PI3K activation, NRAS alone stimulates both BRAF/MAPK and PI3K pathways.[63] Effective antimelanoma therapy will likely require simultaneous inhibition of both MAPK and PI3K pathways.

Given the multiple types of aberrations that may either activate or inactivate a cancer gene, individual genomic methods often identify only a small fraction of samples with alterations in a given gene. This "tip of the iceberg" phenomenon is illustrated by the identification of *KIT* aberrations in melanoma. An investigation of a cohort of 102 melanoma tumors identified *KIT* gene amplification in seven samples.[61] However, subsequent targeted sequencing of the *KIT* gene in all 102 samples identified activating mutations and/or copy number increases of *KIT* in 39% of mucosal and 36% of acral melanomas as well as in 28% of melanomas from chronically sun-damaged skin but none in melanomas from skin without chronic sun damage.[61] As a protein kinase, KIT represents an ideal "druggable" therapeutic target that is already being explored in other malignancies. Indeed, identification of *KIT* mutations in melanoma has spurred several ongoing clinical trials evaluating the utility of KIT inhibitors for the treatment of melanoma. Importantly, many of these trials have adopted a new paradigm in clinical cancer research—selection of patients on the basis of a very specific molecular phenotype, ie, activating *KIT* mutations. This example illustrates the tremendous informative value of high-level gene copy number alterations in the identification of functionally important and therapeutically targetable cancer-related genes.

Similar to genome-wide copy number detection, GEP has provided significant molecular insight into the biology and clinical behavior of melanoma. Numerous groups have demonstrated the utility of global gene expression pattern analyses for successful differentiation of pigmented lesions, such as distinction of nevi from melanoma, thin melanomas from thick melanomas or superficial spreading from nodular melanomas. One of the clinically most informative uses of GEP in melanoma was its application for risk stratification in patients with melanoma of the eye. Based on gene expression patterns, ocular melanomas cluster naturally in two classes (classes 1 and 2). These classes seem to have a clinical prognostic relevance; patients with class 1 tumors rarely die of metastases, whereas patients with class 2 tumors indicate a high rate of metastatic death.[176,177] Interestingly, class 2 tumors also display previously identified poor prognostic factors, including monosomy 3, epithelioid cell type, looping extracellular matrix patterns,[176] loss of melanocytic markers, and increased expression of E cadherin.[178] One of the top differentiating genes, *ID2* (inhibitor of DNA binding 2), a transcriptional target of β-catenin, normally expressed in uveal melanocytes, was significantly downregulated in type 2 tumors. In functional studies, the anchorage-independent growth seen in the class 2 phenotype could be recapitulated by elimination of *ID2* from class 1 uveal melanoma cells. Similarly, overexpression of *ID2* was capable of turning the class 2 cells into less aggressive class 1 cell type.[178] The identification of a distinct phenotype correlated to the molecular signatures in melanoma might have utility for future clinical trial design and for development of molecularly targeted therapies.

Although the majority of genomic advances in melanoma have been achieved through examinations of human specimens, comparative genomics has provided invaluable insights that would likely not have been reached by single-species studies. A recent study took advantage of a mouse melanoma model, combined with high-resolution genomic analysis of mouse and human melanoma tissues, to identify genes contributing to the process of melanoma metastasis.[121] In this study, focal genomic amplification in mouse tumors that have acquired metastatic potential corresponded to a much larger recurrent amplification detected in human melanomas. Integration of the copy number and gene expression data in the mouse model pointed to *NEDD9* as the single gene implicated in the amplified region (Fig. 8-17). Subsequent analysis of human melanoma tissues confirmed significantly higher expression levels of NEDD9 in metastatic compared with primary melanomas. However, forced overexpression

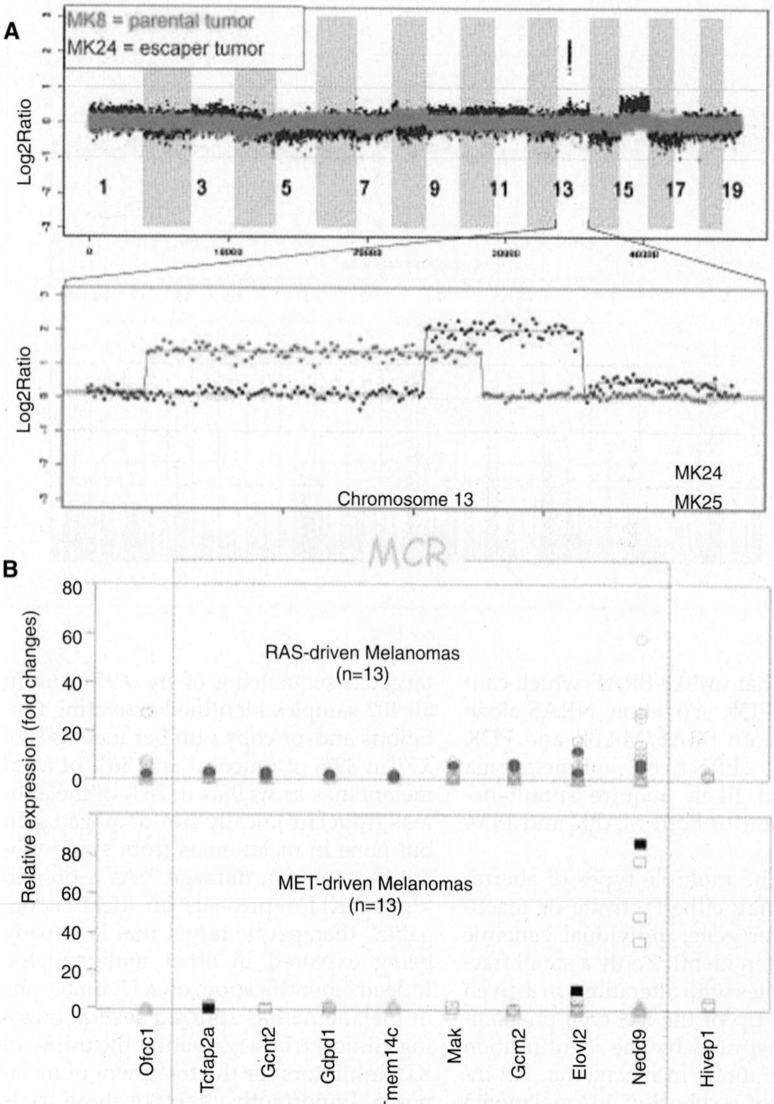

Figure 8-17 Comparative genomics identifies *NEDD9* as a melanoma metastasis gene. **(A)** A metastatic mouse melanoma cell line (M24) was compared to its parental, nonmetastatic line (M8) by high-density array CGH profiling. The numbers in the white and gray bars represent individual mouse chromosomes. The upward deflection of signal (blue) indicates gains and downward deflection (blue) indicates losses of genetic material. Note a high-amplitude focal amplicon on chromosome 13 and a gain of whole chromosome 15 in the metastatic MK24 but not in parental MK8 cell line. Bottom panel shows the expanded view of the bracketed region on chromosome 13 in M24 and in another metastatic mouse melanoma line MK65. Note an overlap of the two amplicons that outlines a common amplified region. **(B)** This common amplified region on chromosome 13 contains 8 genes. Gene expression analyses of the resident genes by real-time qPCR was carried out on independent set comprising 13 Ras-driven melanomas and 4 MET-driven melanomas along with 4 normal melanocyte cultures. Of the eight genes, only *NEDD9* exhibited consistent overexpression in samples with and without genomic amplification when compared to nontransformed primary melanocyte cultures. *Source:* From Ref. 121.

of NEDD9 conferred metastatic potential on primary melanocytes and inhibition of NEDD9 in mouse melanoma tumors by siRNA significantly reduced their metastatic potential. These data suggest that NEDD9 might represent a viable therapeutic target for treatment of melanoma and illustrate the power of cross-species approaches for identification of cancer-related genes in melanoma.

Summary

It is commonly accepted that cancer is a genetic disease caused by the acquisition of a number of genetic abnormalities resulting in the development of a malignant phenotype. The analysis of metaphase karyotypes provided our first broad glimpse into the anatomy of a malignant cell and identified many of the basic abnormalities that characterize cancer (ie, amplifications, deletions, and translocations). In contrast, many of the specific abnormalities that are common to most cancers were identified through the analysis of cancer causing viruses or linkage studies in families with hereditary cancers. Unlike most of the metaphase studies, these detailed studies identified many human genes with small, often single nucleotide, abnormalities (ie, HRAS/KRAS and TP53). The development of microarray-based technologies has drastically improved our understanding of cancer and facilitated the identification of numerous novel oncogenes and tumor suppressor genes in a variety of cancers (ie, TMPRSS-ETS fusions, BRAF activation, WTX and TRAF3 inactivation). This progress has not only improved our understanding of cancer but also facilitated the development of improved diagnostic tests and new-targeted therapies such as Gleevec and Herceptin. Recent technological innovations have made possible even more ambitious efforts to comprehensively catalog all genomic aberrations associated with human cancer. Although significant challenges will remain, including integration and analysis of these massive data sets, functional characterization of novel cancer genes, and development of novel therapeutics, these data should rapidly advance our understanding of cancer genetics and potentially revolutionize our approach to the diagnosis and treatment of cancer.

Selected References

The complete reference list can be found at www.CANCERMEDICINE8.com

1. Hanahan D, Weinberg RA. The hallmarks of cancer. *Cell*. 2000;100:57–70.
2. Albertson DG, Collins C, McCormick F, Gray JW. Chromosome aberrations in solid tumors. *Nat Genet*. 2003;34:369–376.
3. Feinberg AP, Tycko B. The history of cancer epigenetics. *Nat Rev Cancer*. 2004;4:143–153.
4. Ushijima T. Detection and interpretation of altered methylation patterns in cancer cells. *Nat Rev Cancer*. 2005;5:223–231.
5. Futreal PA, Coin L, Marshall M, et al. A census of human cancer genes. *Nat Rev Cancer*. 2004;4:177–183.
6. Nowell P. A minute chromosome in human granulocytic leukemia. *Science*. 1960;132:1497.
7. Caspersson T, Farber S, Foley GE, et al. Chemical differentiation along metaphase chromosomes. *Exp Cell Res*. 1968;49:219–222.
8. Rowley JD. Letter: A new consistent chromosomal abnormality in chronic myelogenous leukaemia identified by quinacrine fluorescence and Giemsa staining. *Nature*. 1973;243:290–293.
9. Ren R. Mechanisms of BCR-ABL in the pathogenesis of chronic myelogenous leukaemia. *Nat Rev Cancer*. 2005;5:172–183.
10. Druker BJ, Talpaz M, Resta DJ, et al. Efficacy and safety of a specific inhibitor of the BCR-ABL tyrosine kinase in chronic myeloid leukemia. *N Engl J Med*. 2001;344:1031–1037.
11. Deininger M, Buchdunger E, Druker BJ. The development of imatinib as a therapeutic agent for chronic myeloid leukemia. *Blood*. 2005;105:2640–2653.
12. Clark MA, Fisher C, Judson I, Thomas JM. Soft-tissue sarcomas in adults. *N Engl J Med*. 2005;353:701–711.
13. van der Zwan SM, DeMatteo RP. Gastrointestinal stromal tumor: 5 years later. *Cancer*. 2005;104:1781–1788.
14. Muller AM, Martens UM, Hofmann SC, et al. Imatinib mesylate as a novel treatment option for hypereosinophilic syndrome: two case reports and a comprehensive review of the literature. *Ann Hematol*. 2006;85:1–16.
15. Marty M, Cognetti F, Maraninchi D, et al. Randomized phase II trial of the efficacy and safety of trastuzumab combined with docetaxel in patients with human epidermal growth factor receptor 2-positive metastatic breast cancer administered as first-line treatment: the M77001 study group. *J Clin Oncol*. 2005;23:4265–4274.
16. Buzdar AU, Ibrahim NK, Francis D, et al. Significantly higher pathologic complete remission rate after neoadjuvant therapy with trastuzumab, paclitaxel, and epirubicin chemotherapy: results of a randomized trial in human epidermal growth factor receptor 2-positive operable breast cancer. *J Clin Oncol*. 2005;23:3676–3685.
17. Paez JG, Janne PA, Lee JC, et al. EGFR mutations in lung cancer: correlation with clinical response to gefitinib therapy. *Science*. 2004;304:1497–1500.
18. Lynch TJ, Bell DW, Sordella R, et al. Activating mutations in the epidermal growth factor receptor underlying responsiveness of non-small-cell lung cancer to gefitinib. *N Engl J Med*. 2004;350:2129–2139.
19. Schrock E, du Manoir S, Veldman T, et al. Multicolor spectral karyotyping of human chromosomes. *Science*. 1996;273:494–497.
20. Speicher MR, Gwyn Ballard S, Ward DC. Karyotyping human chromosomes by combinatorial multi-fluor FISH. *Nat Genet*. 1996;12:368–375.
21. Fauth C, Speicher MR. Classifying by colors: FISH-based genome analysis. *Cytogenet Cell Genet*. 2001;93:1–10.
22. Lichter P. Multicolor FISHing: what's the catch? *Trends Genet*. 1997;13:475–479.
23. Gracia E, Ray ME, Polymeropoulos MH, et al. Isolation of chromosome-specific ESTs by microdissection-mediated cDNA capture. *Genome Res*. 1997;7:100–107.
24. Guan XY, Trent JM, Meltzer PS. Generation of band-specific painting probes from a single microdissected chromosome. *Hum Mol Genet*. 1993;2:1117–1121.
25. Guan XY, Zhang HE, Zhou H, et al. Characterization of a complex chromosome rearrangement involving 6q in a melanoma cell line by chromosome microdissection. *Cancer Genet Cytogenet*. 2002;134:65–70.
26. Meloni-Ehrig AM, Chen Z, Guan XY, et al. Identification of a ring chromosome in a myxoid malignant fibrous histiocytoma with chromosome microdissection and fluorescence in situ hybridization. *Cancer Genet Cytogenet*. 1999;109:81–85.
27. Meltzer PS, Guan XY, Trent JM. Telomere capture stabilizes chromosome breakage. *Nat Genet*. 1993;4:252–255.
28. Kallioniemi A, Kallioniemi OP, Sudar D, et al. Comparative genomic hybridization for molecular cytogenetic analysis of solid tumors. *Science*. 1992;258:818–821.
29. Pinkel D, Segraves R, Sudar D, et al. High resolution analysis of DNA copy number variation using comparative genomic hybridization to microarrays. *Nat Genet*. 1998;20:207–211.
30. Solinas-Toldo S, Lampel S, Stilgenbauer S, et al. Matrix-based comparative genomic hybridization: biochips to screen for genomic imbalances. *Genes Chromosomes Cancer*. 1997;20:399–407.
31. Knuutila S, Autio K, Aalto Y. Online access to CGH data of DNA sequence copy number changes. *Am J Pathol*. 2000;157:689.
32. Menten B, Pattyn F, De Preter K, et al. arrayCGHbase: an analysis platform for comparative genomic hybridization microarrays. *BMC Bioinformatics*. 2005;6:124.
33. Hampton GM, Larson AA, Baergen RN, et al. Simultaneous assessment of loss of heterozygosity at multiple microsatellite loci using semi-automated fluorescence-based detection: subregional mapping of chromosome 4 in cervical carcinoma. *Proc Natl Acad Sci USA*. 1996;93:6704–6709.
34. Bignell G, Smith R, Hunter C, et al. Sequence analysis of the protein kinase gene family in human testicular germ-cell tumors of adolescents and adults. *Genes Chromosomes Cancer*. 2006;45:42–46.
35. Davies H, Hunter C, Smith R, et al. Somatic mutations of the protein kinase gene family in human lung cancer. *Cancer Res*. 2005;65:7591–7595.
36. Greenman C, Stephens P, Smith R, et al. Patterns of somatic mutation in human cancer genomes. *Nature*. 2007;446:153–158.
37. Stephens P, Edkins S, Davies H, et al. A screen of the complete protein kinase gene family identifies diverse patterns of somatic mutations in human breast cancer. *Nat Genet*. 2005;37:590–592.
38. Wood LD, Parsons DW, Jones S, et al. The genomic landscapes of human

breast and colorectal cancers. *Science*. 2007;318:1108–1113.
39. McLendon R, Friedman A, Bigner D, et al. Comprehensive genomic characterization defines human glioblastoma genes and core pathways. *Nature*. 2008.
40. Parsons DW, Jones S, Zhang X, et al. An Integrated Genomic Analysis of Human Glioblastoma Multiforme. *Science*. 2008.
41. Jones S, Zhang X, Parsons DW, et al. Core Signaling Pathways in Human Pancreatic Cancers Revealed by Global Genomic Analyses. *Science*. 2008.
42. Campbell PJ, Stephens PJ, Pleasance ED, et al. Identification of somatically acquired rearrangements in cancer using genome-wide massively parallel paired-end sequencing. *Nat Genet*. 2008;40:722–729.
43. Mitelman F, Johansson B, Mertens F. Mitelman database of chromosome aberrations in cancer. 2005 http://cgap.nci.nih.gov/chromosomes/mitelman.
44. Mitelman F. ISCN 1995: an international system for human cytogenetic nomenclature. Basel: Switzerland, 1995.
45. Mitelman F, Johansson B, Mertens F. Fusion genes and rearranged genes as a linear function of chromosome aberrations in cancer. *Nat Genet*. 2004;36:331–334.
46. Gorre ME, Mohammed M, Ellwood K, et al. Clinical resistance to STI-571 cancer therapy caused by BCR-ABL gene mutation or amplification. *Science*. 2001;293:876–880.
47. Banerjee D, Mayer-Kuckuk P, Capiaux G, et al. Novel aspects of resistance to drugs targeted to dihydrofolate reductase and thymidylate synthase. *Biochim Biophys Acta*. 2002;1587:164–173.
48. Koivisto P, Kononen J, Palmberg C, et al. Androgen receptor gene amplification: a possible molecular mechanism for androgen deprivation therapy failure in prostate cancer. *Cancer Res*. 1997;57:314–319.
49. Jain KK. Current status of fluorescent in-situ hybridisation. *Med Device Technol*. 2004;15:14–17.
50. van der Burg M, Poulsen TS, Hunger SP, et al. Split-signal FISH for detection of chromosome aberrations in acute lymphoblastic leukemia. *Leukemia*. 2004;18:895–908.
51. van Zutven LJ, Velthuizen SC, Wolvers-Tettero IL, et al. Two dual-color split signal fluorescence in situ hybridization assays to detect t(5;14) involving HOX11L2 or CSX in T-cell acute lymphoblastic leukemia. *Haematologica*. 2004;89:671–678.
52. Kearney L, Horsley SW. Molecular cytogenetics in haematological malignancy: current technology and future prospects. *Chromosoma*. 2005;114:286–294.
53. Streubel B, Chott A, Huber D, et al. Lymphoma-specific genetic aberrations in microvascular endothelial cells in B-cell lymphomas. *N Engl J Med*. 2004;351:250–259.
54. Speleman F, Cauwelier B, Dastugue N, et al. A new recurrent inversion, inv(7)(p15q34), leads to transcriptional activation of HOXA10 and HOXA11 in a subset of T-cell acute lymphoblastic leukemias. *Leukemia*. 2005;19:358–366.
55. Rowley JD. The role of chromosome translocations in leukemogenesis. *Semin Hematol*. 1999;36:59–72.
56. Dennis TR, Cunliffe HE, Wattendorf DJ, et al. TTK (hMps1) kinase mitotic checkpoint gene: relationship to chromosome 6q14.3 rearrangements and centrosome amplification in melanoma. *Mol Cancer Res*. 2008. In press.
57. Lichter P, Joos S, Bentz M, Lampel S. Comparative genomic hybridization: uses and limitations. *Semin Hematol*. 2000;37:348–357.
58. Chin K, DeVries S, Fridlyand J, et al. Genomic and transcriptional aberrations linked to breast cancer pathophysiologies. *Cancer Cell*. 2006;10:529–541.
59. Neve RM, Chin K, Fridlyand J, et al. A collection of breast cancer cell lines for the study of functionally distinct cancer subtypes. *Cancer Cell*. 2006;10:515–527.
60. Jonsson G, Staaf J, Olsson E, et al. High-resolution genomic profiles of breast cancer cell lines assessed by tiling BAC array comparative genomic hybridization. *Genes Chromosomes Cancer*. 2007;46:543–558.
61. Curtin JA, Busam K, Pinkel D, Bastian BC. Somatic activation of KIT in distinct subtypes of melanoma. *J Clin Oncol*. 2006;24:4340–4346.
62. Curtin JA, Fridlyand J, Kageshita T, et al. Distinct sets of genetic alterations in melanoma. *N Engl J Med*. 2005;353:2135–2147.
63. Jonsson G, Dahl C, Staaf J, et al. Genomic profiling of malignant melanoma using tiling-resolution arrayCGH. *Oncogene*. 2007;26:4738–4748.
64. Mestre-Escorihuela C, Rubio-Moscardo F, Richter JA, et al. Homozygous deletions localize novel tumor suppressor genes in B-cell lymphomas. *Blood*. 2007;109:271–280.

9 Biochemistry of Cancer

Raymond W. Ruddon, MD, PhD ▪ Donald W. Kufe, MD

Biochemistry of Cancer in Context

The field of cancer biochemistry evolved from a number of disciplines, through information developed down parallel timelines, in some cases based on work initiated a century or more ago. In others, knowledge evolved over a much shorter and more recent time span. Eventually, this information converged into a matrix supporting our current understanding of cancer.

The biochemical differences between normal and malignant cells were originally discovered through studying patterns of enzymatic activity. In the 1920s, Warburg studied glycolysis in a wide variety of human and animal tumors and found a general trend toward increased glycolysis over oxidative phosphorylation in tumor cells.[1] He noted that when normal tissue slices were incubated in a nutrient medium containing glucose, but without oxygen, there was a high rate of lactic acid production (anaerobic glycolysis); however, if the normal tissue slices were incubated with oxygen, lactic acid production stopped. In tumor tissue slices, the rate of lactic acid production was higher in the absence of oxygen than in normal tissues, and the presence of oxygen slowed but did not eliminate lactic acid formation in the tumor slices. Warburg concluded that cancer cells have an irreversible injury to their respiratory mechanism, which increases the rate of lactic acid production even in the presence of oxygen. He regarded the persistence of glycolysis as the crucial biochemical lesion in neoplastic transformation.

This old idea still has some credence in that there are hypoxic areas in the core of tumors, where the glycolytic pathway predominates, and glucose transporters are increased.[2] This has clinical implications because hypoxic cells do not respond as well to certain anticancer drugs or radiation therapy. The ability of lactate and pyruvate—endpoints of glycolysis—to enhance tumor progression appears to be mediated by the activation of hypoxia inducible factor-1 (HIF-1).[3] In addition to increased activity of enzymes of the glycolytic pathway, such as hexokinase, phosphofructokinase, and pyruvate kinase in cultured cancer cells, hypoxia is also a common feature of many human solid cancers. These effects have been linked to tumor progression, metastasis, and multidrug resistance.[4] Oncogenes such as *ras*, *src*, and *myc* enhance aerobic glycolysis by increasing the expression of glucose transporters and glycolytic enzymes (reviewed in Ref.3).

Cancer cells react to hypoxic conditions by upregulating the expression of HIF-1, which is a transcription factor that in turn upregulates the expression of genes involved in glycolysis, glucose transport (GLUT-1), angiogenesis (VEGF), cell survival, and erythropoiesis. HIF-1 expression has been observed in cancers of the brain, breast, colon, lung, ovary, and prostate and their metastases but not in the corresponding normal tissues. Its expression in tumors correlates with poor prognosis.

Interest in tumor metabolism has been stimulated once again by modern techniques such as positron emission tomography (PET), sensitive mass spectrometry (MS), and high-resolution nuclear magnetic resonance spectroscopy (NMR). PET uses fluorine-18 labeled fluorodeoxyglucose (FdG) to detect tissue regions of high glucose uptake, which is indicative of upregulated glycolysis and increased metabolic rate. FdG PET imaging has shown that most primary and metastatic human cancers have increased glucose uptake.[4] This is indicative of a "glycolytic switch" in cancer cells and may be a precursor of tumor angiogenesis and metastasis.[4]

NMR and MS can now be used to measure metastatic profiles of cancer cells and the metabolic phenotype of tissues and organs. This science of "metabolomics" (see below) can provide metabolic biomarkers of tumors such as production of the end products of glycolysis, lipid levels indicative of cell membrane turnover, and alterations in amino acid and nucleotide levels.[5]

It remains unexplained why cancer cells prefer glycolysis, which generates only 2 mols of ATP per molecule of glucose, over oxidative phosphorylation, which when coupled to glycolysis produces 30 mols of ATP per molecule of glucose. Thompson's group has demonstrated that cancer cells increase the ability to transport glucose through upregulation of glucose transporters.[2] This allows cancer cells to spare pyruvate, which during oxidative phosphorylation is converted to lactate. This excess pyruvate is then available for fatty acid synthesis for new membrane production. Recent advances in clinical oncology take advantage of the Warburg principle. That tumor cells have a greater avidity for glucose than normal cells forms the basis for PET, whereby radiolabeled glucose accumulates to a greater extent in cancer than in normal tissues, thus allowing sensitive nuclear imaging.

Because mitochondria contain the enzymatic cascades for oxidative phosphorylation, it has been suggested that damage to mitochondria may be involved in the disruptions of oxidative metabolism seen in malignant tumors. Mutations of mitochondrial DNA (mtDNA) have recently been observed in a variety of human cancers, including bladder, head and neck, lung,[6] and ovarian[7] cancers. An interesting finding was that in the bladder cancers, the mutation hot spots were primarily in a nicotinamide adenine dinucleotide dehydrogenase (NADH) subunit,[6] a key component of the electron transfer machinery, supporting a mechanism for the alterations in oxidative metabolism seen in malignant cells. Because mitochondrial DNA is exposed to high levels of reactive oxygen species generated during oxidative phosphorylation, it is not surprising that mtDNA is highly susceptible to mutational events. The mutational rate of mtDNA is estimated to be 10 times higher than that of nuclear DNA.[7] Mitochondria also play a key role in apoptosis, and alterations in those mitochondria-mediated events are seen in cancer cells.

Based on the work done approximately 50 years ago on the production of hepatic cancer by feeding aminoazo dyes, the Millers advanced the "deletion hypothesis" of cancer.[8] This hypothesis was based on the observation that a carcinogenic aminoazo dye covalently bound liver proteins in animals undergoing carcinogenesis, whereas little or no dye binding occurred with the protein of tumors induced by the dye. They suggested that carcinogenesis resulted from "a permanent alteration or loss of protein essential for the control of growth."

Approximately 10 years later, Potter suggested that the proteins lost during carcinogenesis may be involved in the feedback control of enzyme systems required for cell division,[9] and he proposed the "feedback deletion hypothesis."[10] Potter postulated that "repressors" crucial to the regulation of genes involved in cell proliferation are lost or inactivated by the action of oncogenic agents, either by interacting with DNA to block repressor-gene transcription or by reacting directly with repressor proteins and inactivating them. This prediction anticipated the discovery of tumor-suppressor proteins, such as p53 and RB, by about 25 years.

Biochemical studies of cancer were also aided by the "minimal-deviation" hepatomas developed by Morris.[11] These tumors were induced in rats by feeding them the carcinogens such as fluorenylphthalamic acid, fluorenylacetamide, or trimethylaniline. These hepatocellular carcinomas are transplantable in an inbred host strain of rats and have a variety of growth rates and degrees of differentiation. The term *minimal deviation* was coined by Potter[10] to convey the idea that some of these neoplasms differ only slightly from normal hepatic parenchymal cells. He reasoned that if the biochemical lesions present in the most minimally deviated neoplasm could be identified, the crucial changes defining the malignant phenotype could be determined. As Weinhouse[12] has indicated, studies of these tumors greatly advanced our knowledge of the biochemical characteristics of the malignant phenotype, and they have ruled out many secondary or nonspecific changes that relate more to tissue growth rate than to malignancy.

The extensive biochemical analyses of the Morris minimal-deviation hepatomas led Weber to formulate the "molecular correlation concept" of cancer that states that "the biochemical strategy of the genome in neoplasia could be identified by elucidation of the pattern of gene expression as revealed in the activity, concentration, and isozymic pattern of key enzymes and their linking with neoplastic transformation and progression."[13] Weber proposed three general types of biochemical alterations associated with malignancy: (1) transformation-linked alterations that correlate with the events of malignant transformation and that are probably altered in the same direction in all malignant cells; (2) progression-linked alterations that correlate with tumor growth rate, invasiveness, and metastatic potential; and (3) coincidental alterations that are secondary events and do not correlate strictly with transformation or progression. He maintained that enzymes involved in the regulation of rate and direction of flux of competing synthetic and catabolic pathways would be the enzymes most likely to be altered in the malignant process (see "Metabolomics"). In contrast, enzymes that are not rate limiting and that do not regulate reversible equilibrium reactions would be of lesser importance. As one would expect, a number of enzyme activities that Weber and others have found to be altered in malignant cells are those involved in nucleic acid synthesis and catabolism. In general, the key enzymes in the de novo and salvage pathways of purine and pyrimidine biosynthesis are increased and the opposing catabolic enzymes are decreased during malignant transformation and tumor progression. Weber noted that the degree of neoplasia was related to the concentrations of certain regulators of key metabolic pathways. The question of why anaplastic, rapidly growing tumors tend to be biochemically alike, whereas more well-differentiated tumors display a vast array of phenotypic characteristics was approached by Knox.[14] He thought that the majority of biochemical components in tumor tissues are "normal," in the sense that they are produced by certain specialized adult normal cells or by normal cells at some stage of their differentiation. In cancer cells, it is the combination and proportions of these normal components that are abnormal. The biochemical diversity of cancer cells, then, would depend on the cell of origin of the neoplasm and its degree of neoplasticity.[14] All too frequently, in the histopathologic or biochemical characterization of cancer, a biochemical component that is present or absent, or increased or decreased, is not considered in relation to the particular cell of origin of a tumor, its differentiation state, or its degree of neoplasticity.

The data on enzyme patterns of cancer cells indicate that undifferentiated, highly malignant cells tend to resemble one another and fetal tissues more than their adult normal counterparts, whereas well-differentiated tumors tend to resemble their cell of origin more than other tumors. Between these two extremes lie several levels of neoplastic gradation leading to the vast biochemical heterogeneity of tumors. This heterogeneity also exists for tumors of the same tissue type arising in different patients or even in the same patient at different stages of the disease. The advent of global transcriptional profiling using microarray technologies confirms these observations and has had major impact on our thinking about diagnosis, prognosis, and treatment.

Undifferentiated tumors tend to converge to a more fetal-like state as demonstrated by the frequent production of oncodevelopmental gene products. A number of cancer-cell characteristics, such as invasiveness and metastasis, are also seen in embryonic tissues. For example, the developing trophoblast invades the uterine wall during the implantation step of embryonic development. During organogenesis, embryonic cells dissociate themselves from the surrounding cells and migrate to new locations, a process not unlike metastasis. Thus, it is not surprising that fetal-like stem cells may exist in cancer and that these "cancer stem cells" may be the ultimate progenitor of the entire malignancy.

Many malignant neoplasms produce polypeptides, oligosaccharides, and lipids that are more fetal like and inappropriate for the cell types of their tissue of origin, indicating a derangement in the flow of genetic information in the transformed malignant cell. This derangement could occur by means of an alteration of gene expression, resulting from gene amplification, rearrangement, translocation, or point mutations. Any of these mechanisms could result in the so-called derepression of genes normally present in tissue stem cells but not at all or only minimally expressed in normal adult cells. The inappropriate production by cancer cells of certain proteins and other cellular products has been called *ectopic production*, and it has been observed that the pattern of ectopically produced proteins and hormones often resembles more closely that of the embryonic or fetal state than of the adult state of differentiation. This observation has led to the concept that the expression of these genes in cancer cells results from the derepression of "oncodevelopmental genes," ie, genes expressed normally during embryonic development that are usually shut off or only minimally transcribed by differentiated adult cells. Examples of these ectopic proteins are alphafetoprotein (AFP), human chorionic gonadotropin (hCG), and carcinoembryonic antigen (CEA), which are used as diagnostic tumor markers.

Biochemical Basis of Malignant Transformation

Treatment of animals or cells in culture with carcinogenic agents is a means of studying discrete biochemical events that lead to malignant transformation. Studies of cell transformation in vitro, however, have many pitfalls. For example, "tissue culture artifacts" include overgrowth of cells not characteristic of the original population of cultured cells (eg, overgrowth of fibroblasts in cultures that were originally primarily epithelial cells), selection for a small population of variant cells with continued passage in vitro, or appearance of cells with an abnormal chromosomal number or structure (karyotype). Changes in the characteristics of cultured cell populations can lead to "spontaneous" transformation that mimics some of the changes seen in populations of cultured cells treated with oncogenic agents. Thus, it is often difficult to distinguish the critical malignant events from the noncritical ones.

Malignant transformation can also be induced by treatment of susceptible experimental animals with carcinogenic chemicals, oncogenic viruses, or irradiation. Identification of critical biochemical changes in vivo is even more complex because it is difficult to discriminate toxic from malignant events and to determine what role myriad factors, such as the nutritional state of the animal, hormone levels, or endogenous infections with microorganisms or parasites, might play. Moreover, tissues are a mixture of cell types, and it is difficult to determine in which cells the critical transformation events are occurring and what role the microenvironment of the tissue plays.

Most studies that are designed to identify discrete biochemical events occurring in cells during malignant transformation have therefore been done with cultured cells because clones of relatively homogeneous cell populations can be studied and the cellular environment defined and manipulated. Recent evidence suggests the existence of cancer stem cells, ie, cancer cells of tissue stem cell origin that generate progeny that can populate the entire malignant cell population.

It is likely that tissue stem cells are the targets of malignant transformation in vivo because they are the cells with proliferative capacity. It also appears that the cancer stem cells maintain the proliferative capacity of the tumor. There is good evidence to support this concept. For example, when mouse myeloma cells were placed in an in vitro colony-forming assay, only one in several thousand cells was able to form colonies, and when transplanted in vivo only 1-4% formed spleen colonies.[15] For solid cancers, similar data have been obtained: only 1 in 1000 to 1 in 5000 lung cancer, ovarian cancer, or neuroblastoma cells were able to form colonies in soft agar,[16] again suggesting that there is a subpopulation of cancer cells that proliferate to maintain progressive tumor growth. It has now been possible to distinguish the genetic and phenotypic characteristics of the subset of cells that are the more aggressive, self-renewing cells in a cancer. Al-Hajj et al.[17] found that when human breast cancer cells derived from breast cancer patients were grown in immunocompromised (SCID) mice, only a minority of breast cancer cells were able to form tumors. As few as 100 out of tens of thousands of cells were able to do this. The tumorigenic subpopulation was identified by their cell surface markers and identified as having a $CD44^+/CD24^-$ phenotype. When these cells were passaged into additional mice, tumors were generated that contained both $CD44^+/CD24^-$ cells and nontumorigenic cells. These data demonstrate that only a few cells from human breast cancers have the ability to proliferate extensively, whereas the majority of cells from these tumors have only limited proliferative capacity in vivo. Similarly, a cancer stem cell population has now been identified in other human cancers. These data are consistent with the concept that it is a cancer stem population lurking within a human cancer that are the cells responsible for the aggressive growth of cancers. It further suggests that this is the cell population for which biochemical markers need to be developed and implemented clinically to discern which neoplasms are the ones to treat aggressively and which ones may be more indolent and less dangerous. This would be a big help, eg, in discriminating which breast ductal carcinomas in situ (DCIS tumors) should undergo more extensive surgery and chemotherapy or hormonal therapy and which may be managed less aggressively. Similarly, such markers could be used to know which prostate cancers should be excised, irradiated, or left for "watchful waiting."

In addition, it is the cancer stem cell population for which therapies should be targeted and developed. Currently available chemotherapeutic drugs were developed largely on the basis of their ability to shrink a tumor mass in an experimental model and in a human clinical trial. Because most cells in a cancerous tissue have limited proliferative potential, the ability of a drug to decrease a tumor mass largely reflects the ability of the drug to kill this less aggressive, potentially less dangerous type of cell, leaving behind the more proliferative clones. Thus, drugs more specifically targeted to the cancer stem cell population should result in more effective and durable responses.

The ultimate criterion that establishes whether cells have been transformed is their ability to form a tumor in an appropriate host animal. The ability to generate immortalized "normal" cell lines of a given differentiated phenotype from human embryonic stem cells has enhanced the ability to study cells of a normal genotype from a single source.[18]

Over the past 60 years, scientists focused on identifying the phenotypic characteristics of in vitro–transformed cells that correlate with the growth of a cancer in vivo. This approach has tremendously increased our knowledge of the biochemistry of cancer cells. However, many of the biochemical characteristics initially thought to be closely associated with the malignant phenotype of cells in culture were subsequently found to be dissociable from the ability of those cells to produce tumors in animals. Furthermore, individual cells of malignant tumors growing in animals or in humans exhibit marked biochemical heterogeneity, as reflected in their cell surface composition, enzyme levels, immunogenicity, response to anticancer drugs, and so on. This has made it extremely difficult to identify the essential changes that produce the malignant phenotype. However, Hahn and colleagues[19] showed that ectopic expression of the human telomerase catalytic subunit (human telomerase reverse transcriptase [hTERT]) in combination with the oncogenes *H-ras* and SV40 virus large-T antigen can induce tumorigenic conversion in normal human epithelial and fibroblast cells, suggesting that disruption of the intracellular pathways regulated by these gene products is sufficient to produce a malignant cell. Additional work indicates the importance of the stroma to this process because cancer cells of epithelial origin require specific interactions with blood vessels (angiogenesis) and matrix proteins.[20]

Table 9-1 lists the properties of transformed malignant cells growing in cell culture or in vivo.[21] Some of these characteristics may be seen both in transformed cells in culture and in tumors growing in experimental animals or patients. In addition, hyperproliferative conditions in patients, such as inflammatory bowel disease or psoriasis, may display some of these characteristics. Thus, for diagnostic purposes, it is important to use a number of characteristics that define the malignant state.

Immortality of Transformed Cells in Culture

Normal diploid mammalian cells have a limited life expectancy in culture. For example, normal human fibroblast lines may live for 50-60 population doublings[22] (the "Hayflick index"), but then viability begins to decrease rapidly unless they transform spontaneously or are transformed by oncogenic agents. However, malignant cells, once they become established in culture, will generally live for an indefinite number of population doublings, provided the right nutrients and growth factors are present. This fundamental difference may be related to the continual shortening of chromosomal telomeres each time cells divide. In human cells, telomeres are made up of an average of 5000-15,000 base-pair repeats containing the sequence (TTAGGG)n together with telomere-binding proteins.[23] Younger cells have longer telomeres. Every time a cell divides, 50-100 base pairs are lost, and a cellular signal is eventually triggered to stop cell division. Cells of higher eukaryotic organisms maintain telomere length by the activity of telomerase.

This is a ribonucleoprotein complex that contains several proteins and ribonucleic acid (RNA). The catalytic component of this complex is a reverse transcriptase,

Table 9-1 ■ Properties of Transformed Malignant Cells

A. In vitro alterations

1. Cytological changes resembling those of cancer cells in vivo, including increased cytoplasmic basophilia, increased number and size of nuclei, increased nucleus:cytoplasmic ratio, and formation of clusters and cords of cells.
2. Alteration in growth characteristics:
   "Immortality" of transformed cells in culture. Transformed malignant cells become "immortal" in that they can be passaged indefinitely.
   Decreased density-dependent inhibition of growth or loss of "contact inhibition." Transformed cells frequently grow to a higher density than their normal counterparts, and they may "pile up" in culture rather than stop growing when they make contact.
   Decreased serum requirement. Transformed cells usually require lower concentrations of serum or growth factors to replicate in culture than nontransformed cells require.
   Loss of anchorage dependence and acquisition of ability to grow in soft agar. Transformed cells may lose their requirement to grow attached to surfaces and can grow as free colonies in a semisolid medium.
   Loss of cell cycle control. Transformed cells fail to stop at cell cycle checkpoints when they are subject to metabolic restriction of growth.
   Resistance to cell death.
3. Changes in cell membrane structure and function, including increased agglutinability by plant lectins; alteration in composition of cell surface glycoproteins, proteoglycans, glycolipids, and mucins; appearance of tumor-associated antigens; and increased uptake of amino acids, hexoses, and nucleosides.
4. Loss of cell-cell and cell-extracellular matrix interactions that foster cell differentiation.
5. Loss of response to differentiation-inducing agents and altered cellular receptors for these agents.
6. Altered signal-transduction mechanisms, including constitutive rather than regulated function of growth factor receptors, phosphorylation cascades, and dephosphorylation mechanisms.
7. Ability to produce tumors in experimental animals. This is the sine qua non that defines malignant transformation in vitro. If the cells believed to be transformed do not produce tumors in appropriate animal hosts, they cannot be defined as "malignant." However, failure to grow in an animal model does not rule out that they may be tumorigenic in a different type of animal (eg, syngeneic vs allogeneic).

B. In vivo alterations

1. Increased expression of oncogene proteins as a consequence of chromosomal translocation, amplification, or mutation.
2. Loss of tumor suppressor gene protein products because of deletion, mutation, or silencing.
3. Activation of telomerase
4. Alterations in DNA methylation patterns.
5. Genetic imprinting errors that lead to overproduction of growth-processing substances (eg, IGF-2).
6. Increased or unregulated production of growth factors (eg, TGF-α), tumor angiogenesis factors, PDGF, hematopoietic growth factors (eg, CSFs, interleukins).
7. Genetic instability leading to progressive loss of regulated cell proliferation, increased invasiveness, and increased metastatic potential. "Mutator" genes may be involved in this effect.
8. Alteration in enzyme patterns. Malignant cells have increased levels of enzymes involved in nucleic acid synthesis and produce higher levels of lytic enzymes (eg, proteases, collagenases, glycosidases).
   Production of oncodevelopmental gene products. Many cancers produce increased amounts of oncofetal antigens (eg, carcinoembryonic antigen), placental hormones (eg, human chorionic gonadotropin), or placental-fetal type isoenzymes (eg, placental alkaline phosphatase).
9. Ability to avoid the host's antitumor immune response.

hTERT, that uses the RNA contained in the complex as a template for reverse transcription to replicate the DNA sequences in the telomere. Germ cells and pluripotent tissue stem cells have telomerase activity; however, telomerase is turned off in cells from most tissues as they differentiate. Most human cancers appear to be able to reactivate telomerase activity, thus rejuvenating their proliferative capacity;[24] however, 10-15% of human cancers do not express telomerase and apparently maintain telomere length by a different mechanism.[25] Telomerase has been a target of interest for both diagnostic and therapeutic approaches to cancer. A potential problem with the use of telomerase inhibitors for cancer therapy is their slow onset of action because tumor cells can continue to proliferate until telomere length reduces to a critical length. Moreover, normal stem cells, such as those involved in hematopoiesis and wound healing, are negatively affected by telomerase inhibition.[25] There are also data indicating that restoring telomerase in human cells extends their life span,[26] suggesting that senescence can be overcome and perhaps providing a way to maintain human stem cells for replacement of aging or damaged tissues.

Transformed cells that become established in culture also frequently undergo karyotypic changes, usually marked by an increase in chromosomes (polyploidy). This suggests that cells with increased amounts of certain growth-promoting genes are generated and/or selected during passage in culture. The more undifferentiated cells from cancers of animals or patients also often have an atypical karyotype, suggesting that the same selection process may occur in vivo with progression over time of malignancy from a lower to a higher grade. In fact, it is highly unusual for a metastatic deposit from a recurrent cancer to be more differentiated than the primary tumor.

Decreased Requirement for Growth Factors

Other properties that distinguish transformed cells from their nontransformed counterparts are decreased density-dependent ("contact") inhibition of proliferation[27] and the requirement for growth factors for replication in culture. Cells transformed by oncogenic viruses require lower concentrations of serum for growth than do normal cells.[28] For example, 3T3 fibroblasts transformed by SV40,[29] polyoma,[30] murine sarcoma virus,[31] or Rous sarcoma virus[32] are all able to grow in a culture medium that lacks certain serum growth factors, whereas uninfected cells are not able to grow. Cancer cells can produce their own growth factors that may be secreted and activate proliferation in neighboring cells (paracrine effect), or, if the same malignant cell type has both the receptor for a growth factor and the means to produce the factor, self-stimulation of cell proliferation (autocrine effect) may occur.[33]

Loss of Anchorage Dependence

Most freshly isolated normal animal cells and cells from cultures of normal diploid cells do not grow well when they are suspended in fluid or a semisolid agar gel. If these cells make contact with a suitable surface, however, they attach, spread, and proliferate, a process termed *anchorage-dependent growth*. When removed from this attachment the cells rapidly undergo a form of programmed cell death termed "anoikis" (*gr.* homeless). In contrast, many cell lines derived from tumors and cells transformed by oncogenic agents exhibit *anchorage-independent growth* and proliferate without attachment to a surface. This property of transformed cells has been used to develop clones of malignant cells.[33] The ability to grow cancer cells derived from human tumors in soft agar allowed investigators to test their sensitivity to chemotherapeutic agents and to screen for potential new anticancer drugs.[34] However, because a very low percentage of cells in a human cancer are clonogenic, the usefulness of these assays has been limited.

Loss of Cell Cycle Control and Resistance to Cell Death

Normal cells respond to a variety of suboptimal growth conditions by entering a quiescent (G0) phase of the cell cycle. There appears to be a decision point in the G1 phase of the cell cycle, at which time the cell must make a commitment to continue into the S phase, the DNA synthesis step, or to stop in G1 and wait until conditions are more optimal for cell replication to occur. If this waiting period is prolonged, the cells are said to be in a G0 phase. Once cells make a commitment to divide, they must continue through S, G2, and M to return to G1. If normal cells are blocked in S, G2, or M for any length of time, they die. The events that regulate the cell cycle are referred to as *cell cycle checkpoints*. This loss of cell cycle checkpoint control by cancer cells may contribute to their increased susceptibility to anticancer drugs. Normal cells use these checkpoints to protect themselves from exposure to growth-limiting conditions or toxic agents. In contrast, cancer cells can continue through these checkpoints into cell cycle phases that make them more susceptible to the cytotoxic effects of certain drugs that require movement through the cell cycle. For example, if the DNA of normal cells is damaged, they arrest in G1 so that the DNA can be repaired prior to replication. If irreparable damage occurs, normal cells will activate cell death pathways mediated by p53 or Rb. Another checkpoint in the G2 phase allows repair of chromosome breaks before chromosomes are segregated at mitosis. A postmitotic checkpoint prevents endoreduplication, ie, cytokinesis without adequate segregation of duplicated chromosomes to daughter cells. Cancer cells exhibiting poor or absent checkpoint controls replicate the damaged DNA, thus accounting for persisting and accumulating mutations.

Protein Synthesis, Bioenergetics, and Cell Survival

Abnormal regulation of protein synthesis can transform cells through changes in the expression and activity of translation factors such as elongation initiation factor-2 alpha (eIF2 alpha) and its specific protein kinase, PKR.[35,36] There is also abundant evidence suggesting that the effect of growth factors requires transient inhibition of protein synthesis.[37] In fact, a variety of processes important to cell proliferation are stimulated by inhibitors of protein synthesis including RNA synthesis,[38] polyamine transport,[39] ATP turnover,[40] expression of early growth response genes such as *c-fos* and *cjun*,[40,41] activation of ribosomal protein S6 kinase,[42] MAP kinases,[43] and JNK/SAPK kinases.[44] In addition, exposure of 3T3 cells to cycloheximide or puromycin results in induction of DNA synthesis and cell division.[45] These effects are linked to signal-transduction pathways through the activation of phospholipase C, an enzyme that mediates the release of intracellular calcium from the endoplasmic reticulum by generating inositol tris phosphates. Intracellular calcium activates a series of calmodulin-dependent enzymes, including elongation factor-2 kinase, a ubiquitous enzyme frequently activated in transformed cells[46] that regulates protein elongation.[47]

Protein synthesis accounts for a major percentage of energy consumption. In the presence of adequate nutrients, protein synthesis is stimulated and cell death pathways such as autophagy (see below) are inhibited (Fig. 9-1). The mammalian target of rapamycin (mTOR) pathway integrates the cellular response to growth factors and nutrients through regulation of protein synthesis.[48] In yeast, TOR provides a link between cellular growth and the availability of extracellular nutrients.

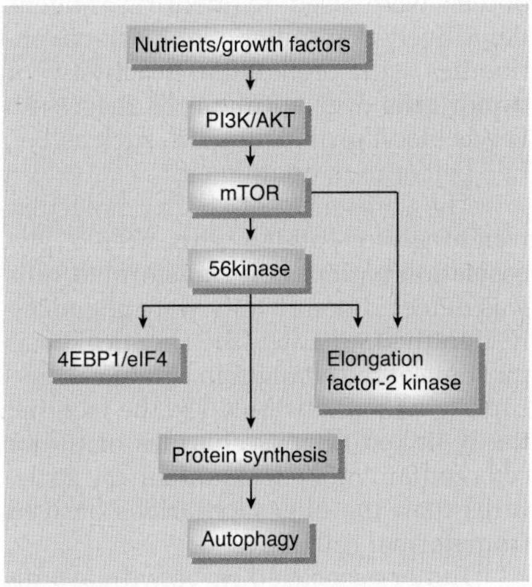

Figure 9-1 In the presence of nutrients (glucose, amino acids, growth factors) protein synthesis is stimulated and autophagy is inhibited. This is mediated through activation of mTOR (via activation of PI3 kinase and AKT and inactivation of the tuberous sclerosis complex [TSC1 and 2]). mTOR phosphorylates S6 kinase and increases the translation of mRNAs that encode ribosomal and other proteins involved in translation. This initiates translation by phosphorylating 4EBP1, an inhibitor of initiation, causing its disassociation from eIF4E. Active eIF4 promotes cell proliferation by increasing translation of cyclin D1, c-Myc, and VEGF. mTOR and S6 kinase also release the cellular check on peptide elongation by phosphorylating and inactivating eEF-2 kinase. eEF2-kinase phosphorylates eEF-2, a 100kDa protein that mediates the translocation step in peptide-chain elongation by inducing the transfer of peptidyl-tRNA from the ribosomal A to P site. Phosphorylation of eEF-2 at Thr56 by eEF-2 kinase decreases the affinity of the elongation factor for ribosomes and terminates elongation. Activation of TOR in yeast inhibits induction of autophagy via phosphorylation of the APG1- APG-13 complex a process inhibited by rapamycin in both yeast and mammalian cells.

In mammals, TOR is also regulated by growth factors through the PI3K/Akt pathway.[49] Substantial cross talk exists between the PI3K/AKT pathway and the Ras/Raf/ERK1/2 pathways. For example, EGF activation of both ERK1/2 and Akt blocked the induction of autophagy, whereas PTEN, a negative regulator of Akt, stimulated autophagy in HT-29 colon cancer.[50] Activating Ras mutations also induced autophagy in colon cancer cells, and this was blocked by feeding amino acids.[51,52] The importance of this pathway to sustaining cancer viability makes the individual components attractive for drug development.

In the absence of nutrients, protein synthesis is inhibited and autophagy is activated. Nutrient/growth factor deprivation and ATP depletion activate autophagy by inhibiting mTOR (via activation of TSC2 by 5 AMP kinase) and decreasing phosphorylation of S6 kinase and 4EBP1.[53,54] Under these conditions, initiation of translation is repressed by the reformation of the 4EBP4/eIF4E inhibitory complex, and elongation is inhibited through activation of eEF-2 kinase. Thus, eukaryotic cells have evolved a mechanism to withstand starvation by decreasing energy use through inhibiting protein synthesis and increasing energy production through autophagic recycling of amino acids produced from digestion of cellular organelles and proteins.

Alterations in biochemical balance ("bioenergetics") can ultimately lead to cell death. Cells die through several mechanisms including apoptosis, necrosis, or autophagy. Necrosis and autophagy are tightly linked to the state of nutrient-dependent cellular bioenergetics. For example, autophagy is a mechanism by which cells respond to nutrient deprivation and is known to occur in yeast, plants, worms, flies, mice, and humans.[55] In yeast, nutrient deprivation activates a programmed genetic response that results in two outcomes: (1) self-digestion of cytoplasm and organelles and the recycling of amino acids for energy use and (2) the budding of an immortal spore. This form of self-digestion in unicellular organisms leads to self-preservation in times of famine. Autophagy finds its counterpart in multicellular organisms, as high up the animal kingdom as *Homo sapiens*. At the cellular level, nutrient deprivation prompts cells to exit the cell cycle, shrink, autodigest long-lived proteins and damaged organelles, and recycle the components for synthesis of macromolecules or oxidation in mitochondria to maintain cellular ATP. Autophagy may thus result in cellular destruction or alternatively cellular "hibernation" until the supply of nutrients is restored.

Three recent papers highlight aspects of autophagy relevant to cancer biology. For example, Kuma and colleagues[56] asked, "How do newborns survive after being cut off from the maternal blood supply and before adequate nutrients are available through suckling?" In this remarkable set of experiments, it was shown that at birth there is upregulation of autophagy in several organs most notably heart, diaphragm, alveolar cells, and skin. Mice lacking *Atg5*, a gene whose product is critical for the formation of autophagosomes, appear normal at birth but die within 24 h of delivery. The animals have reduced circulating amino acids and die secondary to energy depletion. Electrocardiograms performed on the newborns pups revealed cardiac ischemia. Thompson's laboratory[57] looked at the role of autophagy in the survival of immortalized hematopoietic precursors and primary bone marrow cultures deprived of an obligate growth factor (IL-3). They found that cells in which apoptosis was inactivated by deleting *Bax* and *bak* survived for >6 weeks in the absence of IL-3 by using autophagy to supply precursors for ATP. Upon re-addition of IL-3, cells increased glucose transport and recovered size and ability to proliferate. Finally, Boya and colleagues[58] found that nutrient-deprived HeLa cells underwent autophagy and prevented apoptosis (believed to occur through sequestration of damaged mitochondria). However, blocking the autophagic pathway with either small interfering RNAs against key autophagy genes (*beclin1*, *Atg10*, or *Atg12*) or with drugs (3-methyladenine, hydroxychloroquine, bafilomycin A1, or monensin) triggered apoptosis.

Eventually, cells deprived of nutrients will deplete ATP below a critical concentration compatible with life. When this occurs, cellular transporters will no longer function, electrochemical gradients will collapse, and cells ultimately undergo necrosis.[59] Thompson's group has suggested that necrotic cell death can be programmatically activated in response to overwhelming DNA damage. In this model, DNA damage activates poly-ADP ribose polymerase (PARP), which in turn ADP-ribosylates nucleosomal proteins to allow more efficient DNA repair. This reaction depletes NAD and inhibits glycolysis. Because cancer cells are reliant on glycolysis for ATP generation, PARP activation will ultimately initiate necrotic cell death.

Changes in Cell Membrane Structure and Function

The plasma membrane plays an important role in the "social" behavior of cells, including communication with other cells, cell movement and migration, adherence to other cells or structures, access to nutrients in the microenvironment, and recognition by the body's immune system. Alterations of the plasma membrane in malignant cells may be inferred from a variety of properties that characterize their growth and behavior, eg, the loss of density-dependent inhibition of growth, decreased adhesiveness, loss of anchorage dependence, and invasiveness through normal tissue barriers. In addition, a number of changes in the biochemical characteristics of the surfaces of malignant cells have been observed. These include appearance of new surface antigens, proteoglycans, glycolipids, and mucins, and altered cell–cell and cell–extracellular matrix communication.

Alterations in Cell Surface Glycolipids, Glycoproteins, Proteoglycans, and Mucins

Aberrant glycosylation was first suggested as the basis for the tumor-associated determinants of glycolipids by the finding of a remarkable accumulation of fucose-containing glycolipids in human adenocarcinomas.[60] These identifications were confirmed once monoclonal antibodies were used to identify antigens definitively. A number of monoclonal antibodies with preferential reactivity for tumor cells over normal cells react with Lewis blood group antigens, such as Le_x, Le_a, Le_b, or their analogues.[60]

The presence of high molecular weight glycopeptides with altered glycosylation patterns on transformed cells was detected before they were chemically identified.[61,62] Later, the chemical basis for some of the changes in tumor cell glycoproteins was attributed to the fact that the N-linked oligosaccharides of tumor cells contain more multiantennary structures than the oligosaccharides derived from normal cells.[63]

Tumor-associated carbohydrate antigens can be classified into three groups[60]: (1) epitopes expressed on both glycolipids and glycoproteins, (2) epitopes expressed only on glycolipids, and (3) epitopes expressed only on glycoproteins. To the first group belongs the lacto series structure that is found in the most common human cancers, such as lung, breast, colorectal, liver, and pancreatic cancers. The common backbone structure for these epitopes is Ga1β1→3G1cNacβ1→3Ga1 (type 1 blood group) or Galβ1→4G1cNacβ1→3Ga1 (type 2 blood group). The second group of epitopes, expressed exclusively on glycolipids, is mostly on the ganglio or globo series structures. This series of epitopes is expressed abundantly only on certain types of human cancers, such as melanoma, neuroblastoma, small-cell lung carcinoma, and Burkitt lymphoma. The third group of epitopes, seen only on glycoproteins, is the multiantennary branches of N-linked carbohydrates and the alterations of O-linked carbohydrate chains seen in some mucins.

Tumor-associated carbohydrate antigens can also be classified by the cell types expressing them as those (1) expressed on only certain types of normal cells (often only in certain developmental stages) and greatly accumulated in tumor cells, (2) expressed only on tumor cells, eg, altered blood group antigens or mucins, and (3) expressed commonly on normal cells but present in much higher concentrations on tumor cells, eg, the GM3 ganglioside in melanoma and L_{ex} in gastrointestinal cancer.[60]

A variety of chemical changes in tumor cells has been identified that can explain altered glycosylation patterns. These result from three kinds of altered processes: (1) incomplete synthesis and/or processing of normally existing carbohydrate chains and accumulation of the resulting precursor form, (2) activation of glycosyltransferases that are absent or have low activity in normal cells, and (3) organizational rearrangement of tumor cell membrane glycolipids.[64]

Moreover, the glycosyl epitopes found in glycolipids and glycoproteins make up microdomains that are involved in cell adhesion and signal-transduction events. They function as a "glycosynapse" in mediating these events.[65] The cell motility, altered adhesive properties, and invasiveness observed in cancer cells are regulated by these glycosynapse complexes.[66]

Interest in the carbohydrate components of the cell surface has been heightened by the fact that many monoclonal antibodies developed to tumor-associated antigens recognize these carbohydrate moieties or peptide epitopes exposed by altered glycosylation. Moreover, many of these blood group–specific antigens are seen at certain stages of embryonic development and thus fit the definition of oncodevelopmental antigens. Thus, the field of "chemical glycobiology" is making significant contributions to our understanding of the cell surface biochemistry of normal and malignant cells.[67]

Role of Glycosyl Transferases and Oligosaccharide-Processing Enzymes

The substitution of additional carbohydrate moieties on blood group-related structures is not the only aberrant modification of glycoproteins or glycolipids observed in cancer cells. Increased branching of asparagine-linked oligosaccharides and incomplete processing of these oligosaccharides have also been noted in certain cell surface as well as secretory glycoproteins.[68,69] The increased activity of specific *N*-acetylglucosaminyl transferases in tumor cells appears to be responsible for the appearance of tri- and tetra-antennary structures, whereas the analogous glycoprotein in normal cells is often a biantennary structure. Unusually high expression of *N*-acetylglucosaminyltransferase IVa has been observed in human choriocarcinoma cell lines and may be the enzymatic basis for the formation of abnormal biantennary sugar chains on hCG.[70] Similarly, the extra fucosylations that appear on membrane glycoproteins and glycolipids are associated with the induction of an unusual α-fucosyltransferase in chemical carcinogen-induced precancerous rat liver and in the resulting hepatomas.[71] These investigations strongly suggest that the regulation of glycosyltransferase genes is important in malignant transformation.[72]

The use of inhibitors of glycosylation and oligosaccharide-processing supports the importance of glycosylation patterns of cell surface glycoproteins and glycolipids in the malignant phenotype. For example, tunicamycin, an inhibitor of addition of N-linked glycans to nascent polypeptide chains, castanospermine, an inhibitor of glucosidase, and KI-8110, an inhibitor of sialyltransferase activity, all reduce the number of lung metastases in murine experimental tumor models.[73-75] In addition, swainsonine (an inhibitor of glucosidase) was shown to reduce the rate of growth of human melanoma xenografts in athymic nude mice,[76] and castanospermine was observed to inhibit the growth of v-*fms* oncogene-transformed rat cells in vivo.[77] These results support the hypothesis that the synthesis of highly branched complex type oligosaccharides is associated with the malignant phenotype and may provide tumor cells with a growth advantage.

Mucins ■ Mucins are a type of highly glycosylated proteins that contain more than 50% of their molecular mass as *O*-linked oligosaccharides. A feature common to the mucins is a domain with tandem repeats that are rich in serines, threonines, and prolines. The serine and threonine residues function as sites for the extensive *O*-glycosylation. Twenty mucins have been identified to date. There are two classes of mucins: the secreted mucins and the membrane-bound (transmembrane) mucins. The secreted mucins contribute to the formation of a physical barrier that affords protection to epithelia in the respiratory system, gastrointestinal tract, and other specialized organs with secretory functions. The membrane-bound mucins also contribute to this protective mucous gel through glycosylated ectodomains that are tethered to transmembrane subunits at the apical cell surface. The mucous gel protects the epithelia from diverse forms of stress that include low pH (gastric mucosa), toxins, proteases, microorganisms, and reactive oxygen species. The membrane-bound mucins also signal the presence of external stress to the interior of epithelial cells to activate a repair and survival response.

The membrane-bound mucins MUC1 (CA15-3), MUC4, and MUC16 (CA125) are aberrantly overexpressed in diverse human tumors. For example, with transformation and loss of polarity, carcinoma cells express MUC1 at high levels over the entire cell surface and in the cytoplasm.[78] At the cell membrane, MUC1 associates with members of the ErbB family of receptor tyrosine kinases and integrates ErbB receptor signaling with the Wnt pathway.[79,80] MUC1 is overexpressed in most carcinomas of the breast, prostate, lung, pancreas, ovary, and other transformed epithelia. Multiple myeloma cells, lymphomas, and certain leukemias also express MUC1 at high levels. Estimates indicate that of the 1.4 million tumors diagnosed annually in the United States, greater than 900,000 exhibit MUC1 overexpression. Notably, overexpression of MUC1 is sufficient to induce anchorage-independent growth and tumorigenicity.[81,82]

Overexpression of MUC1 is also sufficient to confer resistance to induction of cell death by genotoxic anticancer agents.[83,84] How MUC1 contributes to these characteristics of the transformed phenotype is not precisely known. However, the MUC1 transmembrane subunit is targeted to the nucleus where it contributes to the regulation of gene expression.[81,85-87] MUC1 is also targeted to mitochondria where it attenuates the activation of the intrinsic apoptotic pathway.[83,88] The MUC1 cytoplasmic domain interacts directly with-β catenin,[89] p53,[85] estrogen receptor α,[86] and IκB kinases.[90] These findings have indicated that the MUC1 transmembrane subunit has a chaperone-like function with diverse client proteins.

MUC4 is a transmembrane mucin that is overexpressed by pancreatic and certain other cancers. Like MUC1, MUC4 consists of a heavily *O*-glycosylated ectodomain with tandem repeats that is noncovalently tethered to a transmembrane subunit.[91] However, unlike MUC1, the extracellular region of the MUC4 transmembrane subunit contains EGF-like domains that can function as intramembrane ligands for ErbB2.[92] MUC4 sequesters ErbB2 at the apical membrane of normal epithelial cells and thereby prevents the formation of activated ErbB2-ErbB3 heterodimers.[93] However, MUC4-mediated sequestration of ErbB2 is abrogated by loss of polarity associated with stress or transformation.[93,94]

Overexpression of MUC4 has been correlated with pancreatic tumor progression.[95] Moreover, silencing MUC4 has been associated with decreased pancreatic tumor cell growth and metastasis.[96] MUC4 expression is upregulated in pancreatic cancer cells by diverse signals induced by TGF-β, TGF-β, interferon-γ, TNF-α, and retinoic acid.[97] Like MUC1 and MUC4,[98] MUC16 is overexpressed in ovarian cancer. Also known as CA125, MUC16 was first identified as a serum marker used to monitor the clinical course of women with ovarian cancer.[99] Cloning of the gene encoding CA125 demonstrated that this glycoprotein is a mucin family member and was designated MUC16.[100] The functional role of MUC16 in ovarian cancer remains unclear, although like MUC1 and MUC4, MUC16 has a transmembrane subunit that may contribute to the malignant phenotype.

The overexpression of MUC1, MUC4, and MUC16 in human cancers has generated interest in these mucins as attractive targets for antibody serotherapy and for anticancer vaccines. These topics are covered in other chapters in this text.

Proteoglycans ■ The proteoglycans are high molecular weight glycoproteins that have a protein core to which are covalently attached large numbers of side chains of sulfated glycosaminoglycans as well as *N*-linked and/or *O*-linked oligosaccharides. They are categorized on the basis of their glycosaminoglycans into several types, including heparan sulfate, chondroitin sulfate, dermatan sulfate, and keratan sulfate.[101] The glycosaminoglycans have different repetitive disaccharide units bound to the core protein through a common glycosaminoglycan linkage region: G1cNacβ1→3Ga1β1→3Ga1β1→4Xylβ→1OSer. The structure of the sulfated glycopeptides from the carbohydrate–protein linkage region of some of the proteoglycans has been determined.[102]

Proteoglycans interact via their multiple binding domains with many other structural macromolecules, giving them the capacity "to function as a multipurpose 'glue' in cellular interactions."[103] They bind together extracellular matrix (ECM) components, such as hyaluronic acid, collagen, laminin, and fibronectin; mediate binding of cells to the ECM; act as a reservoir for growth factors; and "present" growth factors to growth factor receptors on cells. The proteoglycans also act as cell adhesion factors by promoting organization of actin filaments in the cell's cytoskeleton. Proteoglycans have been shown to undergo both quantitative and qualitative changes during malignant transformation, and alterations have been reported in breast, colon, and liver carcinomas, in glioma cells, and in transformed murine mammary cells and 3T3 fibroblasts.

Two putative tumor-suppressor genes are glycosyl transferases required for the biosynthesis of the proteoglycan heparan sulfate.[104] Mutations of these genes, called *ext1* and *ext2*, have been associated with the development of skeletal dysplasias, and these findings suggest that alterations in the synthesis of heparan sulfate precursor polysaccharide are involved in dysregulation of heparan sulfate production and function in tumor formation.

Modification of Extracellular Matrix

The ECM plays a key role in regulating cellular proliferation and differentiation. In the case of tumors, it is now clear that development of a blood supply and interaction with the mesenchymal stroma on which tumor cells grow are involved in their growth, invasive properties, and metastatic potential. This topic is covered in detail in Chapter 10, "Invasion and Metastases." Here, we focus only on some of the key biochemical features.

The ECM components include collagen, proteoglycans, and glycoproteins, such as fibronectin, laminin, and entactin. Basement membranes are a specialized type of ECM. These membranes serve as a support structure for cells, act as a "sieving" mechanism for transport of nutrients, cellular metabolic products, and migratory cells (eg, lymphocytes) and play a regulatory role in cell proliferation and differentiation.[105] Basement membranes also prevent the free passage of cells across them, but there are mechanisms that permit the passage of inflammatory cells. It is also clear that basement membranes act as regulators of cell attachment, through cellular receptors called integrins (see below). There is also "cross talk" between epithelial cells and their ECM to create a microenvironment for accurate signal transduction for growth factors and other regulatory molecules. It has been shown, eg, that exogenous reconstituted basement membranes stimulate specific differentiation of a variety of cell types, including mammary cells, hepatocytes, endothelial cells, lung alveolar cells, uterine epithelial cells, Sertoli cells, and Schwann cells.[106]

Cell-Extracellular Matrix and Cell-Cell Adhesion

Cells in tissues are attached to one another and to the ECM. Disruption of these adhesion events leads to increased cell motility and potential invasiveness of cells through the ECM. In addition, most cell types require attachment to the ECM for normal growth, differentiation, and function. This attachment is responsible for what was termed "anchorage dependence." Normal cells that are detached from their binding to the ECM undergo apoptosis, whereas tumor cells that are less dependent on this attachment are free to proliferate and invade tissues.

Cell adhesion to the ECM is mediated by cell surface receptors called *integrins*. Integrins are a family of proteins consisting of heterodimers that are integral membrane proteins with a specific arginine, glycine, aspartic acid (RGD) amino acid sequence involved in binding to the ECM.[107] Integrins also link the external ECM cytoskeleton to the intracellular actin cytoskeleton, and via this connection a linkage to control of gene expression in the cell nucleus is established. In this way, cell–ECM interactions can control gene readout involved in cell differentiation and function. Cell–ECM interactions occur via focal adhesions that consist of clusters of ECM-bound integrins, and these, in turn, connect to actin fibrils and the signal-transduction machinery inside the cell. These signaling pathways include the focal adhesion kinase (FAK) pathway that participates in the control of anchorage dependence and growth factor signaling pathways, such as the *ras-raf*–mitogen-activated kinase, protein kinase C, and phosphatidylinositol 3-kinase pathways.[108] Thus, integrins cooperate with growth factors to enhance mitogenic signaling. Alterations in integrin receptor expression observed in cell–cell interactions are also important for the normal regulation of cell proliferation and differentiation. These interactions are mediated by a family of cell adhesion molecules (CAMs), which act as both receptors (on one cell) and ligands (for another cell). The expression of CAMs is programmed during development to provide positional and migratory information for cells. A large family of CAMs has been identified. One group of these, called cadherins, comprise a superfamily of Ca^{2+}-dependent transmembrane glycoproteins that play an essential role in the initiation and stabilization of cell–cell contacts. Regulation of cadherin-mediated cell–cell adhesion is important in embryonic development and maintenance of normal tissue differentiation.[109,110]

The extracellular domain of various cadherins is responsible for cell–cell homotypic binding (a given cadherin domain for a given cell type), and the conserved cytoplasmic domains interact with cytoplasmic proteins called *catenins.* Each cadherin molecule can bind to either β-catenin or γ-catenin, which in turn bind α-catenin. α-Catenin links the cadherin complex to the actin cytoskeleton. Cell lines that lack α-catenin lose normal cell–cell adhesiveness and have increased invasiveness.[111]

E-cadherin is the predominant type of cadherin expressed in epithelial tissue. Alterations of E-cadherin expression and function have been observed in human cancers.[112] In addition, downregulation of E-cadherin correlates with increased invasiveness, metastasis, and poor prognosis in cancer patients. Suppression of this invasive phenotype can be achieved by transfection of E-cadherin cDNA (complementary deoxyribonucleic acid) into carcinoma cells, and contrarily, invasiveness of E-cadherin gene-transfected cells can be restored by exposure of the cells to E-cadherin antibodies or an E-cadherin antisense RNA.[112] Germline mutations of the E-cadherin gene (*cdh1*) have been found in New Zealand Maori families with a dominantly inherited susceptibility to gastric cancer.[113]

The cellular binding protein for E-cadherin is β-catenin, the intracellular location of which can be cell membrane associated, cytoplasmic, or nuclear. Early mutations in the human colon cancer progression pathway affect the cellular distribution of β-catenin. In patients with colon cancer, the normal colonic epithelial cells adjacent to neoplastic lesions had mostly cell surface membrane–associated expression of β-catenin, whereas cytoplasmic expression of β-catenin was observed in aberrant crypt foci.[114] Nuclear expression was observed in more advanced dysplasias and increased as adenomas progressed to carcinomas. These latter changes are also observed in less- differentiated areas of tumors and are accompanied by loss of E-cadherin expression at the invasive front of breast carcinomas, possibly as a consequence of hypermethylation of the E-cadherin promoter.[115]

Production of Lytic Enzymes

Transformed malignant cells in culture and human cancer cells in vivo produce a variety of lytic enzymes that degrade the ECM and allow cancer cells to invade tissues, lymphatic channels, and the vasculature. These proteases include plasminogen activator, cathepsins, adamalysin-related membrane proteases, and a number of matrix metalloproteases (MMPs).[116] The MMPs are a large family of proteases that includes collagenases (MMPs 1, 2, and 9) and stromelysins (MMPs 3 and 11). Collagenases have been found at elevated levels in melanoma and in cancers of the colon, breast, lung, prostate, and bladder. Usually, these elevated levels correlate with higher tumor grade and invasiveness. MMP-2 and MMP-9 levels are significantly elevated in the serum of patients with metastatic lung cancer, and in those patients with high levels, response to chemotherapy is diminished.[117] The production of MMPs by tumor cells appears to be mediated, at least in part by "extracellular matrix metalloproteinase inducer," (EMMPRIN; CD147), a member of the immunoglobulin superfamily that is enriched on the surface of cancer cells.[118,119] Overexpression of EMMPRIN can promote anchorage-independent cell growth and render cells less sensitive to chemotherapy.[118]

Biochemical Basis of Cancer Epigenetics

Cancer cells have altered gene expression that includes chromosomal translocations and inversions, gene deletions, gene amplifications, point mutations, and duplications or losses of whole chromosomes. However, much of the malignant phenotype is produced by epigenetic changes, whose biochemical basis we discuss herein.

Alterations in Chromatin Structure and Function

Chromatin in higher organisms is organized into nucleosomes that are tuna fish can–shaped structures made up of two molecules each of the core histones H2A, H2B, H3, and H4, forming an octamer core around which approximately two turns of DNA are wrapped. In a tightly wrapped conformation, DNA transcription into messenger ribonucleic acid (mRNA) is inhibited. The initiation of gene transcription requires a partial unwrapping of this octamer core, which is regulated by biochemical alteration of the core histones. This involves chemical modifications that regulate the acetylation, methylation, phosphorylation, and ubiquitination of histones. Combinations of these covalent histone modifications have been called the "histone code," by which is meant that specific alterations of histones at specific times in the cell cycle "mark" histone tails by these chemical modifications in a way that enables them to recruit or "derecruit" other chromatin modifying proteins such as transcriptional coactivators or repressors to promoter regions.[120] Some of the histone modifications appear to involve reciprocal alterations that affect DNA transcription. For example, Nakayama and colleagues[121] have shown in fission yeast that histone H3 methylation on lysine-9 is linked to H3 deacetylation on lysine-14, both of which events are necessary for formation of heterochromatin, the form that is inactive in transcription. In contrast, the "on" state of chromatin active in gene transcription is related to acetylation of lysine-14 and phosphorylation of serine-10.[121]

Other similar reciprocal chromatin activating and deactivating events have been observed in mammalian (HeLa) cells, in which methylation of arginine-3 of histone H4 facilitates subsequent acetylation of H4 amino acid "tails," leading to transcriptional activation of nuclear hormone receptor.[122]

Some gene-silencing events require both histone deacetylation and DNA methylation. Methylation of DNA by DNA methyltransferase recruits methyl-binding proteins and histone deacetylases. This coupling of DNA methylation and histone deacetylation correlates with silent transcriptional regions in chromatin.[123] These processes of controlling chromatin structure and function are key to understanding cell differentiation and the altered gene expression that occurs in malignant transformation.

Some of the genes involved in the acetylation and deacetylation of histones have been identified.[124] There are two categories of acetylation genes: *hat1* and *hat2*. Acetylation of histone H4, eg, reduces the affinity of the histone amino terminal tail for DNA and allows a reduction of DNA wrapping around the histone octamer and a subsequent decrease in the tightness of nucleosome packaging. This makes more DNA sequences available for transcription. Deacetylation of histone H4 by deacetylases (HDAC1 and HDAC2), on the other hand, increases affinity of H4 for DNA and results in tighter packing of nucleosomes and less transcription. Mutations in yeast deacetylases have been identified that allow H3 and H4 acetylation to be maintained. This would be expected to result in constitutively unfolded regions of chromatin and increased gene transcription. Disruption of deacetylase activity that alters expression of many genes in yeast, as well as in mammalian cells, has been observed. Mutations in histone acetylases, deacetylases, and components of these complexes have significant effects in yeast, and similar mutations may have implications for human disease, including cancer. Recent data have shown that members of the HDAC1 and HDAC2 family of genes belong to a network of genes coordinately regulated and involved in chromatin remodeling during cell differentiation.[125]

In addition to acetylation, phosphorylation of histones is also important for chromatin structure and function.[126] A fifth histone, H1, interacts with DNA, links adjacent nucleosome cores, and further condenses chromatin structure. Phosphorylation of H1 is thought to play a role in increased gene transcription. Phosphorylation of histone H3, on the other hand, is required for proper chromosome condensation and segregation during mitosis.[126] In addition, during the immediate–early response of mammalian cells to mitogens, histone H3 is rapidly and transiently phosphorylated by a kinase called Rsk-2.[127] This suggests that chromatin remodeling is part of the cascade involved in mitogen-activated protein kinase-regulated gene expression.

A "cancer-chromatin connection" is implicated by the observations relating to the role of the tumor-suppressor gene *rb* in the regulation of the histone deacetylase HDAC1.[128] RB acts as a strong transcriptional repressor by forming a complex with the transcriptional activating factor E2F and HDAC1, tethering these activities to E2F-responsive promoters, including the cyclin E promoter region. Repression of E2F-bound promoters by RB is released by mitogenic signals that activate cyclin-dependent kinase phosphorylation of RB, thereby releasing RB from the complex and allowing histone acetylation to occur. This increases accessibility of gene promoter sequences to transcriptional activators. Point mutations of the *rb* gene observed in some tumors abolish RB-induced repression and RB-associated deacetylase activity, allowing increased E2F-mediated gene expression. Viral oncoproteins can disrupt the interaction between RB and HDAC1. In addition, unoccupied retinoic acid receptors (RARs) have been shown to repress transcription of target genes by recruiting the histone deacetylase complex to these genes.[129] Mutant forms of RAR-α result from chromosomal translocations seen in human acute promyelocytic leukemia (APL). These mutant forms prevent appropriate deacetylase activity and result in gene activation. This deregulation can be diminished by all-*trans* retinoic acid, at doses that induce APL cell differentiation suggesting that oncogenic alterations in RARs mediate leukemogenesis via aberrant regulation of histone acetylation.

DNA Methylation

Methylation of DNA on cytosine in CpG islands is another mechanism for regulating gene expression. Hypermethylated DNA sequences are usually less expressed, and hypomethylated sequences are more expressed. CpG islands are short sequences rich in CpG dinucleotides found in the 5'-regulatory regions of about half of all human genes. Alterations in DNA methylation patterns have been observed in tumor cell lines, animal tumor models, and primary human cancers. Feinberg and colleagues[130] observed an average of 8-10% reduction in genomic 5-methylcytosine content in colon adenomas and adenocarcinomas. Interestingly, three patients with the highest 5-methylcytosine content in their normal colon appeared to have a germline predisposition to cancer (Lynch syndrome). Hypermethylation of DNA is postulated to be involved in the loss of tumor-suppressor gene function. Hypermethylation of the regulatory sequences of some of those genes, including *TP53*, *p15*, *p16*, E-cadherin, *vhl*, and *hmlh1*, has been observed, but whether this is a cause of tumor-suppressor gene silencing is still unclear. Aberrantly methylated CpG sequences have been detected in serum and tissue of patients with colorectal,[131] non–small-cell lung,[132] liver,[133] and prostate[134] cancers.

DNA methyltransferase activity has been reported to be overexpressed in a number of human cancer cell lines and tissues, although the incidence and extent of this is still being debated.[135] So far, three DNA methyltransferases have been detected in mammalian cells, and the activity of one of these, DNMT1, is threefold higher in *fos* oncogene-transformed fibroblasts than in normal fibroblasts, and the transformed cells contain more 5-methylcytosine than normal fibroblasts.[136] Transfection of the *dnmt1* gene into fibroblasts induces transformation, whereas inhibition of *dnmt1* expression by an antisense oligonucleotide reverses *fos*-induced transformation. These results suggest that oncogene-induced malignant transformation is mediated through alterations in DNA methylation.

Genomic imprinting is an epigenetic modification of the genome that allows only the maternal or paternal allele of a gene to be expressed. Approximately 30 mammalian genes are known to be imprinted.[137] In a number of human cancers, loss of imprinting (LOI) occurs, allowing both the maternal and paternal alleles to be expressed. If this affects a growth factor, such as insulin-like growth factor-2 (IGF-2), cells obtain a double dose of a growth stimulatory signal. LOI of IGF-2 has been observed in approximately 45% of patients with colorectal cancer.[138] Notably, this LOI could also be detected in the circulating leukocytes of affected patients, suggesting that this is an alteration that precedes the onset of neoplasia and could be used as a screening test for cancer susceptibility. Somewhat paradoxically, LOI can be reversed by drugs that are DNA methyltransferase inhibitors, such as 5-aza-2-deoxycytidine, suggesting that an aberrant DNA methylation event induces LOI.[139] LOI of the *igf2* gene appears to be involved in tumor progression, leading to a more invasive phenotype.[140]

DNA Repair

DNA repair mechanisms are covered extensively in Chapter 2, "Molecular Biology, Genomics, and Proteomics" and Chapter 5, "Signal Transduction." It is sufficient to note here that a number of biochemical mechanisms are invoked by human cells when their DNA is damaged by internal metabolic events (eg, oxidative stress, cytosine deamination) or exogenous factors (eg, chemical carcinogens, irradiation). These repair mechanisms include (1) photoactivation repair for removal of UV-induced pyrimidine dimers, (2) strand break repair for excision and repair of a length of DNA sequence, (3) base excision repair producing apurinic or apyrimidinic sites in DNA, (4) nucleotide excision repair, and (5) O6-alkylguanine-DNA alkyltransferase that recognizes and removes small alkyl adducts from DNA.

DNA repair is usually very accurate, but if repair cannot occur prior to or during DNA replication, it may be error prone, potentially leading to a mutagenic and carcinogenic event. A number of inherited defects in DNA repair systems predispose individuals to getting cancer. These syndromes include xeroderma pigmentosum, ataxia telangiectasia, Fanconi anemia, Bloom syndrome, and Cockayne syndrome.

Biochemistry of Cellular Differentiation

All tissues in the body contain cells that can divide and renew themselves. A subset of the cell population in any tissue can differentiate into the functional cells of that tissue. The normal process of cellular differentiation ultimately leads to an adult, "terminally" differentiated cell that cannot, under ordinary circumstances, divide again. These fully differentiated cells carry out the recognizable functions of most tissues in the body. Carcinogenesis alters cells to produce a state of increased proliferation and decreased differentiation; the genes controlling cell proliferation are inappropriately expressed and the genes controlling differentiation are repressed.

As tissues develop, some cells retain the capacity to divide, whereas others divide and then differentiate into cells with a more restricted phenotype.[141] These latter cells are then said to be pluripotent rather than totipotent, ie, they are now committed to develop into one of the cell types peculiar to their tissue of origin. Embryologists have traditionally defined the commitment of a cell to one general pathway of differentiation rather than another as *determination*. They reserve the term *differentiation* for the final events in which a terminally differentiated cell arises from a pluripotent one. However, biochemically, this is probably an artificial distinction because the total process most likely represents a continuum of biochemical and molecular events leading from a totipotential cell to a terminally differentiated one. The final characterization of differentiation requires the identification of the particular biochemical events that led to the uniquely specialized adult cell.

By definition, the process of differentiation requires a heritable alteration in the pattern of gene readout in one of the two progeny cells arising from the same parent cell. Because all the cells in the body are derived from a single cell, the fertilized ovum, this process must entail the expression of characteristics in one progeny cell that are not expressed in the other progeny cell from the same parent cell. This process must continue to occur throughout embryonic development to generate the wonderful diversity of cell types present in the adult organism.

The discovery of human embryonic stem cells and embryonic germ cells,[142] and recent data showing that even adult tissues such as brain, liver, and muscle contain stem cells that can be induced to differentiate into a variety of cell types,[143] have drastically altered the question: What is a stem cell? These findings indicate that the plasticity of certain cells in adult tissues is far beyond what was imagined a few years ago. It also raises the question of what is the target cell for the malignant transformation process. If these pluripotent stem cells are present in all tissues in the body, why are not all tissues equally susceptible to carcinogenesis? Yet we know that brain tumors and sarcomas, although not rare, occur much less often than epithelial cell tumors (carcinomas) and that cancers of heart muscle are very rare. One explanation is that muscle cells and brain cells are less exposed to environmental agents and hormonal influences that can activate the carcinogenic process. There are data, however, that damage to these tissues can activate endogenous stem cells to proliferate and move to areas of the lesion.[144] These data imply that these same cells would also be susceptible to carcinogenic damage because they are the cells that have the proliferative capacity to undergo mutagenic damage as they replicate their DNA. This also raises the question of the ability of cells in adult tissues to de-differentiate in response to tissue damage and the question of whether stem cells in adult tissues are really de-differentiated adult cells. The answer to these questions will affect how one approaches the field of cancer prevention, initiation, progression, and treatment because it depends on the cell type being targeted. If we learn that the origin of cancer is a stem cell, then this cell must be isolated, studied, and characterized for treatments to be effective.

Induction of Differentiation in Cancer Cells

There are a number of examples of animal malignant tumors or human cancer cells in culture that can be induced to lose their malignant phenotype by treatment with certain differentiation-inducing agents. These include induction of differentiation of the Friend virus–induced murine erythroleukemia by dimethyl sulfoxide (DMSO); differentiation of murine embryonal carcinoma cells by exposure to retinoic acid, cAMP analogues, hexamethylene bisacetamide, or sodium butyrate; and differentiation of human acute promyelocytic (HL-60) cells in culture by a number of anticancer drugs, sodium butyrate, DMSO, vitamin D3, phorbol esters, or retinoic acid analogues.[145]

Being able to treat cancer through induction of cellular differentiation is an attractive idea because the therapy could be target-cell specific and most likely be much less toxic than standard chemotherapeutic agents. The best example of this is the treatment of APL in patients with all-*trans* retinoic acid. A more recent example is induction of solid tumor differentiation by the peroxisome proliferators-activated receptor γ (PPAR γ) ligand troglitazone in patients with liposarcoma.[146] PPAR γ is a nuclear receptor that forms a heterodimeric complex with the retinoid X receptor (RXR). This complex binds to specific recognition sequences on DNA and, after binding ligands for either receptor, enhances transcription of differentiation-inducing genes, including those for the adipocyte-specific pathway. PPAR γ appears to act as a tumor suppressor in the prostate and thyroid gland, but not in the colon, where its actions are more complex.[147] Nevertheless, agents that can exploit the proliferation-inhibiting effects of PPAR γ in cancer tissue and have minimal metabolic side effects may be good targets for drug discovery.

Biochemistry of Signal Transduction

This topic is covered in further detail in Chapter 5. A large number of growth factors, cytokines, hormones, and exogenous chemicals can trigger cellular responses via receptor-mediated events that foster cellular proliferation and/or differentiation. Sometimes these factors do both. The intracellular signaling pathways that accomplish this are varied and complex. Frequently, these pathways are inappropriately activated in cancer cells by either inappropriate expression of an oncogene coding for a growth factor, a growth factor receptor, or components of intracellular signaling pathways. There is significant cross talk between these signaling pathways such that up- or downregulation of one of them may trigger responses in another one. Thus, inhibition of one component of a signal-transduction pathway may be compensated by upregulation of another. This has important therapeutic implications because a drug that blocks an early or upstream component of a given pathway may be circumvented by activation of another parallel pathway. A goal, then, is to try to target the downstream events where transduction pathways converge in their ability to stimulate gene activation events. Alternatively, if a cancer is driven by a single or limited alteration in signal transduction (eg, bcr-abl kinase in chronic phase CML), targeting an upstream signaling mechanism can be effective.

An example of the cross talk among ligand-receptor triggered events is the binding of platelet-derived growth factor (PDGF) to its receptor R-PDGFR.[148] This induces dimerization of the receptor, which in turn triggers signal-transduction pathways. The PDGF receptor becomes autophosphorylated on multiple tyrosines by activation of its receptor tyrosine kinase. This fosters binding to specific Src homology 2 domain (SH2)-containing proteins that are part of the Grb2-Sos-Ras-Raf-Mek-Erk pathway. In addition, there is cross talk with the phosphatidyl inositol kinase (PI3K) pathway. PI3K can also stimulate Rac guanosine triphosphatase (GTPase), which can activate JAK/STAT signaling events. Activation of the SH2 domain protein PLC-γ1 can also potentially stimulate protein kinase C (PKC) signaling pathways. Thus, cytoplasmic signaling proteins form networks of interactions rather than simple linear pathways.[148] These diverse signaling pathways, in turn, induce broadly overlapping sets of genes.[149]

The redundancy and interactions of signal-transduction pathways is only one example of the complexity of protein–protein and cell component interactions in cells, both normal and malignant. These findings have led to a new field of study, called "systems biology." The science of systems biology is revealing that the interactions among DNA, RNA, proteins, carbohydrates, lipids, and indeed all the components of cells and tissues, are extremely more complex than had been realized previously.

The goal of systems biology is to integrate biological information across several hierarchical levels, including DNA, RNA, protein, protein–protein interactions, gene regulatory networks, cellular communication systems, tissue and organ interactions (eg, hormonal signaling), and ecological systems.

A clue as to how complex this will be can be seen from the incredibly complex genetic and protein–protein interaction networks in lower organisms. For example, global mapping of a yeast genetic interaction network containing 1000 genes revealed more than 4000 interactions.[150] A single large network of 1548 proteins in yeast showed 2538 interactions.[151] Seventy-two percent of 1393 characterized proteins with at least one partner of known function predicted 364 previously uncharacterized functions. In *C. elegans*, more than 4000 protein–protein interactions were identified in a subset and the current version of the "Worm Interactions" contains more than 5500 interactions.[152]

In *Drosophila*, a total of 10,623 predicted gene transcripts that were isolated and screened against DNA libraries produced a map of 7048 proteins and 20,405 interactions.[153] Statistical modeling of the networks showed two levels of organization: short-range organization, most likely corresponding to more localized pathways, and a global organization, presumably corresponding to broader, more complex connecting pathways. Analysis of these interactions found known pathways, extended pathways, and previously unknown pathway components.

These data provide some insights into how complex a problem it will be to define the systems biology of human beings. Nevertheless, recent technological advances allow some approaches to this issue. It will require interactions among biologists, chemists, physicists, engineers, computer scientists, and mathematicians to figure all this out. The technologies of gene expression arrays, proteomics, molecular imaging, electrical engineering, nanotechnology, and microfluidics will all be involved in developing the "lab-on-a-chip" or the "nanolab" of the future.[154]

One of the neat new technologies involves the use of nanowire sensors, of nanometer (10^{-9} m) or less diameter (see "Nanotechnology"), coated with a probe molecule to sense a particular signature of gene or protein expression. These nanowires can also have built-in mechanisms that produce an electrochemical signal that can detect, with great sensitivity, molecular interactions. A visionary's view of this is that this scale of instrumentation can lead to hand-held, microfluidics-based systems to detect single cell genomic or proteomic expression enabling a physician to analyze a patient's blood sample of a few microliters (obtained by a finger prick) to assess up to 10,000 functions. The impact of this sort of technology on the future of medicine is mind boggling indeed.

Guanosine triphosphate (GTP)-binding protein (G-protein) signaling events are another ubiquitous pathway for gene activation, some of which are mediated by cAMP and have protean effects on cellular processes.[155] Mutations in components of G-protein coupled pathways have been observed, some of which appear to be involved in a number of human diseases, including tumor formation.[155,156]

Alterations of other signal-transduction pathways also correlate with malignant transformation. For example, cellular transforming events induced by the viral oncogene v-*fps* correlate with activation of the endogenous STAT3 signal-transduction pathway.[157] TGF-β signaling is mediated via the SMAD family of transducer proteins, and somatic mutations of one of these, SMAD4, are frequently observed in pancreatic cancers and, less frequently, in colon, breast, and lung cancers.[158] Functionally disruptive mutations of SMAD2 have been observed in colorectal and lung cancers.

These observations increase the long list of signal-transduction components that are known to be altered in cancer, such as Ras, Myc, Src, and Erb B. Thus, it is clear that disruption of signal-transduction pathways is a commonly observed event in human cancer and provides a target for therapeutic intervention.

Many signal-transduction events involve phosphorylation steps including (1) receptors coupled to tyrosine kinase activity; (2) receptors coupled to guanine nucleotide-binding proteins, which in turn may activate or inhibit adenylate cyclase, activate phosphoinositide hydrolysis leading to protein kinase C activation and intracellular Ca^{2+} release, or modulate cell membrane ion channels; and (3) intracellular receptors, such as those for steroid hormones, thyroid hormone, and retinoic acid, all of which have DNA-binding domains as well as ligand-binding domains and can interact directly with DNA to modulate gene transcription. All of these receptor-mediated signal-transduction mechanisms are potential sites for upregulation or deregulation in cancer cells, eg, by oncogene activation or overexpression or by tumor-suppressor gene inactivation.

Protein Kinases

Both tyrosine- and serine/threonine-protein kinases play critical roles in cancer. Prototypes include the mitogen-activated protein kinases (serine/threonine) and receptor-coupled/oncogene kinases (tyrosine). Many growth factor receptors mediate their cellular effects by intrinsic tyrosine kinase activity, which in turn may phosphorylate other substrates involved in mitogenesis. A number of transforming oncogene products have growth factor or growth factor receptor–like activities that work via a tyrosine kinase–activating mechanism. For example, the *v-src* gene product is itself a cell membrane–associated tyrosine kinase. The *v-sis* oncogene product is virtually homologous to the β chain of PDGF. The *v-erb* product is a truncated form of the epidermal growth factor (EGF) receptor. The *fms* gene product is analogous to the receptor for CSF-1. The *met* and *trk* proto-oncogene products are receptors for hepatocyte growth factor (HGF) and nerve growth factor (NGF), respectively. In chronic myelogenous leukemia (CML), the BCR-ABL translocation that causes activation of this RTK in CML can be inhibited by imatinib (Gleevec).[159] Because this agent has relatively specific activity vs BCR-ABL and *c-kit*, this has led to the development of other specific, targeted agents that promise to improve the therapeutic index of anticancer chemotherapy.

Some of the key substrates for receptor–tyrosine kinase-coupled activity are (1) phospholipase Cγ (PLCγ), which activates phosphatidyl inositol hydrolysis, releasing the second messengers diacylglycerol (DAG) and inositol triphosphate (INSP3) that activate PKC and mobilize intracellular calcium release, respectively (a number of tumor promoters also activate PKC); (2) the GTPase-activating protein (GAP) that modulates *ras* proto-oncogene protein function; (3) *src*-like tyrosine kinases; (4) PI3K that associates with and may modulate the transforming activity of polyoma middle T antigen and the *v-src and v-abl* gene products; and (5) the *raf* proto-oncogene product that is itself a serine/threonine protein kinase.

Thus, activation of protein kinases is a key mechanism in regulating signals for cell proliferation. The substrates of these kinases include transcription regulatory factors, such as those linked to mitogenic signaling pathways, eg, proteins encoded by the *jun, fos, myc, myb, rel,* and *ets* proto-oncogenes.

The ErbB (HER) family of receptor tyrosine kinases (RTKs) are important therapeutic targets.[160-162] Four members of this family of RTKs have been identified: epidermal growth factor receptor (EGFR, or ErbB1, HER1), ErbB2 (HER2, Neu), ErbB3 (HER3), and ErbB4 (HER4). These receptors share an amino acid homology of 40-50% and have common functional characteristics, yet differences in expression in various tissues and different phenotypes observed in knockout mice indicate that they have nonredundant functions. At least 25 ligands, with different binding affinities, are known for various members of this family. However, no endogenous high-affinity ligand specific for ErbB2 is known. When these RTKs are activated, they, in turn, activate a number of downstream signaling partners (eg, the MAP kinases ERK1/2) that induce a variety of cellular events that regulate cell proliferation and differentiation.

Dysregulated function and/or overexpression of the ErbB family are observed in a wide variety of human cancers, including breast, prostate, lung, ovarian, and renal cancers as well as glioblastomas. Therapeutic modalities aimed at blocking the dysregulated activities of these receptors include small molecules such as erlotinib (Tarceva) and gefitinib (Iressa)[160,161] and antibodies such as trastuzumab (Herceptin) and cetuximab (Eribtiux), targeted at ErbB2 in breast cancer and EGFR in colon cancer, respectively.[163]

A recent observation links various levels of activation of EGFR to different cellular functions. It was observed that the EGFR-mediated effects on DNA synthesis, cell adhesion, and cell motility differ depending on levels of saturation of the receptor.[162] For example, even though exogenously added EGF has no additional effects on DNA synthesis that is already maximally stimulated by subsaturating levels of EGFR occupation by endogenous ligand, added EGF can still induce integrin expression, integrin-mediated adhesion, and motility in cultured human colon cancer cells. These data suggest that these activities may be additional targets for EGFR-modulating agents.

Lipid Kinases

PI3-kinase catalyzes the conversion of phosphatidylinositol 4-phosphate and phosphatidylinositol (4,5)-bisphosphate to phosphatidylinositol (3,4)-bisphosphate and phosphatidylinositol (3,4,5)-trisphosphate, respectively, thereby generating phosphoinosides that can signal and/or attract enzymes such as Akt to the plasma membrane. The activation of PI3-kinase in normal cells is dependent on the control of growth factor–receptor interactions but can be autonomous in cancers. The phosphorylation of Akt by PI3-kinase can activate pathways that promote cell growth and inhibit cell death. The activity of PI3-kinase and Akt are normally balanced by the opposing effects of protein phosphatases.

Protein Phosphatases

Protein phosphatases (PTPases) play a regulatory role in certain cellular metabolic functions such as the activation–inactivation steps for glycogen synthase and phosphorylase. PTPases also play a role in the activity of various receptors and in the function of certain cell cycle regulating genes. For example, expression of a truncated, abnormal protein tyrosine phosphatase in BHK cells produces multinucleated cells, possibly by dephosphorylating the cyclin-dependent kinase p34cdc2. Activation of p34cdc2 requires dephosphorylation of a tyrosine residue, and this activation drives the cell from the G2 into the M phase. The truncated phosphatase apparently interferes with the normal synchrony between nuclear formation and cell division.

PTPases are a diverse family of enzymes that exist in cell membranes and in intracellular locations. Some are associated with receptors that have tyrosine kinase activity. The aberrant phosphorylation state of tyrosine in certain key proteins, such as c-Src or c-Raf, that can lead to cellular transformation could theoretically come about as a result of deregulation of a protein kinase or underexpression of a protein phosphatase. For example, cells treated with vanadate, a PTPase inhibitor, have increased protein phosphotyrosine levels and a transformed phenotype.[164] Further evidence that PTPases are involved in cancer is the observation that a receptor-linked PTPase located on chromosome 3, which has a deletion in renal cell and lung carcinomas, suggesting that this PTPase gene may act as a tumor-suppressor gene. Thus, one could predict that a high level of expression of specific PTPases may be able to reverse the malignant phenotype, and one can think of strategies, then, to transfect these genes into tumor cells or deliver inducers of the enzymes to tumor cells.

The PTPase PTEN is mutated in human brain, breast, and prostate cancers.[165] This was discovered by mapping homozygous deletions on human chromosome 10q23 that occur at high frequency in human cancers. Mutations of the *pten* gene were detected in 17% of primary glioblastomas as well as in human-derived cancer cell lines and xenografts of glioblastoma (31%), prostate cancer (100%), and breast cancer (6%). PTEN is a protein tyrosine phosphatase that dephosphorylates PIP3 in the phosphatidyl inositol pathway (AKT/PI3 kinase). Loss of PTEN activity increases PIP3 phosphorylation and leads to cellular transformation. Thus, PTEN is considered to have tumor suppressor function, and this protein and its substrates are potential targets for new therapeutic agents.

An effect of PTPases opposite to that of PTEN has been observed in metastatic human colon cancer. Saha and colleagues[166] have observed that the PRL-3 protein tyrosine phosphatase gene was overexpressed in each of 18 colon cancer metastases, as compared to nonmetastatic tumors and normal colorectal epithelium. This somewhat counterintuitive observation reminds us that the dysregulated state of phosphorylation events can have inhibitory or stimulatory effects on the cancer process depending on the cell type and the microenvironment. Nevertheless, it does suggest that enzymes such as that encoded by PRL-3 can be targets for another approach to anticancer drug discovery.

Biochemistry of the Cell Cycle

Cell cycle checkpoints provide "go/no-go" decision points that determine whether a cell progresses to the next cell cycle phase. Many of the biochemical mechanisms involved in these checkpoint controls have been identified. Most of what we know about cell cycle regulation originally came from lower organisms, including yeast.[167] One of the first genes identified as an important cell cycle regulator in yeast was *cdc2/cdc28*. Activation of this kinase requires association with a regulatory subunit called cyclin A. It is now known that sequential activation and inactivation of cyclin-dependent kinases (cdks) is the primary means of cell cycle regulation.

The role of various cdks, cyclins, and other gene products in regulating checkpoints at G1 to S, G2 to M, and mitotic spindle segregation have been described in detail elsewhere[167-169] and in Chapter 3, "Cell Proliferation and Differentiation." Alterations of one or more of these checkpoint controls occur in most, if not all, human cancers at some stage in their progression to invasive cancer.

Alteration of the G1/S checkpoint occurs in many human cancers. Cyclin D1 gene amplification occurs in a subset of breast, esophageal, bladder, lung, squamous cell carcinomas, and certain lymphomas. Cyclins D2 and D3 are over-expressed in some colorectal carcinomas. In addition, the cyclin D–associated kinases cdk4 and cdk6 are over-expressed or mutated in some cancers. Mutations or deletions in the cdk4 and cdk6 inhibitor INK4 have been observed in familial melanomas, and in biliary tract, esophageal, pancreatic, head and neck, non–small-cell lung, and ovarian carcinomas. Inactivating mutations of cdk4 inhibitory modulators p15, p16, and p18have been observed in a wide variety of human cancers. Cyclin E is also amplified and overexpressed in some breast and colon carcinomas and leukemias.

The retinoblastoma gene is an important regulator of the G1/S checkpoint. Phosphorylation of RB by cyclin D–dependent kinase releases RB from the transcriptional regulator E2F and activates E2F function. Inactivation of *rb* by genetic alterations occurs in retinoblastoma and is also observed in other human cancers, eg, small-cell lung carcinomas and osteogenic sarcomas. Mutations in the *rb* gene increase the expression of enzymes involved in DNA synthesis (dihydrofolate reductase, thymidylate synthase, ribonucleotide reductase) and in experimental systems affect sensitivity to antimetabolite chemotherapeutic drugs.[170]

The *TP53* gene product is an important cell cycle checkpoint regulator at both the G1/S and G2/M checkpoints but does not appear to be important at the mitotic spindle checkpoint because gene knockout of *TP53* does not alter mitosis. The *TP53* tumor-suppressor gene is the most frequently mutated gene in human cancer, indicating its important role in conservation of normal cell cycle progression.[171] One of the essential roles of p53 is to arrest cells in G1 or G2 after genotoxic damage, to allow for DNA repair prior to DNA replication and cell division. In response to massive DNA damage, p53 triggers apoptosis. Preclinical evidence also suggests that p53 status can affect the sensitivity to drugs and radiation. In most cases, cell lines with wild-type p53 are more sensitive to DNA-damaging drugs.[172] Using homologous recombination to delete p53, it was shown that p53 affected sensitivity to fluoropyrimidines.[173] Because p53 transcriptionally regulates numerous genes through activation or repression, the status of p53 can also have effects on antimicrotubule drugs and irradiation.[174]

The spindle assembly checkpoint machinery involves genes called *bub* (budding uninhibited by benomyl) and *mad* (mitotic arrest-deficient).[169] There are three *bub* genes and three *mad* genes involved in the formation of this checkpoint complex. A protein kinase called Mps1 also functions in this checkpoint function. The chromosomal instability, leading to aneuploidy in many human cancers, appears to be caused by defective control of the spindle assembly checkpoint. Mutant alleles of the human *bub1* gene have been observed in colorectal tumors displaying aneuploidy. Mutations in these spindle checkpoint genes may also result in increased sensitivity to drugs that affect microtubule function because drug-treated cancer cells do not undergo mitotic arrest and go on to die.

Future Directions of Cancer Biochemistry

The ability to generate robust data from cells, tissues, and whole organisms will inevitably lead to further integration of biochemistry with other areas of science. Efforts are underway to understand the entire spectrum of enzyme reactions through identifying and characterizing all protein kinases at the genetic, biochemical, and structural levels. Understanding how the cell integrates these reactions to convert substrate to product and how the steady state is disrupted in disease will be the challenge of the future. The direction that biochemistry is moving is exemplified by the new area of metabolomics.

Metabolomics

Genomics is the global study of gene expression, transcriptomics, the genome-wide study of mRNA, and proteomics the study of protein expression. Metabolomics is the study of the metabolome, the repertoire of biochemicals or small molecules that are produced by cells and tissues. The metabolome represents the final products of interactions among gene expression, protein expression, and the environment. Estimates indicate that there may be as few as 2500 small molecules in the human metabolome. Metabolite profiles are often generated by high throughput NMR and mass spectroscopy. Stable isotope-based dynamic metabolic profiling is also used to study metabolic fluxes (fluxomics). Metabolomics is being applied to tumor cells and to biofluids (blood and urine) from patients with cancer with a goal of attempting to link genetic alterations associated with transformation to downstream metabolic changes. For example, recent studies have demonstrated that K-Ras mutations at codon 12 are associated with increased glycolysis, whereas codon 13 mutants increase oxidative pentose phosphate pathway activity and pyruvate dehydrogenase flux.[175] In other studies, functional genomics has been combined with metabolomics to identify features of neuroendocrine cancers that have a poor outcome.[176] Metabolomics is also being used to study the effects of anticancer agents. In this context, treatment of myeloid leukemia cells with imatinib is associated with increased glucose carbon flow toward nucleic acid and fatty acid synthesis.[177] Although still at an early stage, metabolomics has the potential to provide new biomarkers for the diagnosis and monitoring of cancer, and to identify new therapeutic targets for anticancer drug discovery.

Nanotechnology

Nanotechnology is another field of research that will have a great impact on how we approach the science of cancer biochemistry. In one sense, nanotechnology is nothing more than a new name for things that exist on a small scale, the things that are on the size of groups of atoms, in other words, "chemistry." The term, however, has taken on the meaning for things manufactured by human ingenuity to be on the scale of molecules that nature-invented. The term derives from the Greek word "nanos" for dwarf. In its technical usage, nano- is a prefix for something that is a one billionth part (10^{-9}) of a specified unit, eg, nanometer, nanosecond. In the fields of chemistry and physics, the term is usually used to define particles of 1-100 nm in diameter. This is equivalent to about the size of 200 gold atoms assembled together.

The field of nanotechnology now encompasses several fields including physics, chemistry, engineering (eg, nanomaterials, nanoelectronics, microfluidics), computer science, biology, and medicine. In the field of medicine, all of these disciplines will need to work together to harness the new breakthroughs in diagnostic techniques and therapeutics that will drive the future of medical practice.

Carbon nanotubes and nanowires are being used to detect specific DNA sequences and proteins.[154] Up to 1000 nanowire detectors (about 8 nm in diameter) can be condensed into an area about the size of a single cell. Potentially, each nanowire could contain a different antibody or oligonucleotide to detect a protein or mRNA sequence.[154] On one chip, it would be possible to carry out 1000 single cell experiments (the "lab-on-a-chip"). As an example, single strand DNA can be bound to a nanowire, and the binding of complementary mRNA will cause a signal to be generated, indicating a specific hybridization has occurred. Thus, this can be used to detect gene expression patterns in a few cells and potentially in a single cell when coupled to microfluidic techniques that can separate and detect single cells in a fluid sample.[154,178] Another method for this is the so-called nanocantilever array. Here, the biomarker proteins bind to antibodies attached to cantilevers and this binding causes the cantilevers to deflect, producing a signal that can be detected by laser beam or electronically.

One can envision using similar nanodevices for molecular detection in vivo. For example, implantable sensors could be designed to emit a signal that could be detected outside the body. A big challenge for this is the potential for nonspecific binding of tissue and serum proteins on the sensing surfaces; however, methods to circumvent such "biofouling" can be developed. One nifty futuristic concept is the coupling of nanosensing devices with a drug delivery system that could be implanted on the same minichip into a tumor vascular bed. For example, a sensor that detects the presence of a tumor biomarker or tumor physiological parameter such as low pH or low oxygen tension could produce a signal that would trigger the connected drug delivery platforms. One can also envision a multifunctional nanoparticle, which would have on its surface multiple tumor targeting moieties such as antibodies to cell surface markers such as EGFRs and other upregulated GFRs.[178]

Various "nanovectors" can be designed to deliver drugs to targeted tissues. These include liposomes with surface complexed antibodies to tumor antigens, "nanoshells" composed of gold over a silica core, and various polymer-coated particles such as dendritic polymers (see below). Several types of nanoparticles can also be used for in vivo molecular imaging by, eg, enhancing MRI contrast or ultrasound imaging. Not only can multiple targeting modalities be put on the surface of nanovectors, but they could also be loaded with multiple drugs each with a different time-release "minipump" such as an ultrasound or electronically signaled release mechanism. An example of this is the design of nanoparticle-RNA aptamer bioconjugates that target prostate-specific membrane antigen on the surface of prostate cancer cells and that are composed of a controlled release polymer that releases an RNA aptamer targeted to block a tumor growth factor or other tumor-related process.[179]

Baker and colleagues have designed dendritic polymers that function as multifunctional delivery devices.[180] The dendritic polymer–nanoparticle targets intracellular folate and selectively delivers methotrexate intracellularly. It also emits an optical imaging signal through attachment of flourescein to the nanovector. In cell culture systems, the nanovector-delivered methotrexate killed a 100-fold more cancer cells than free methotrexate added to the culture medium.

Micro RNA

Another "hot topic" in cancer biochemistry is the discovery of micro RNAs and their role in cell regulatory pathways. Micro RNAs (miRNAs) are small RNAs that have gene-silencing activity. Unlike siRNAs that are derived from dsRNAs, which are produced from aberrant gene expression such as genes from viruses that have infected cells, miRNAs are transcribed from noncoding genes in the genome (what used to be called "junk-DNA"). Some estimates are that introns and other noncoding RNAs make up 98% of the transcriptional output of the human genome. There is speculation that this large amount of miRNAs provides the functional regulator that makes humans so different from mice, with which we share about 95% of the same genes. Like siRNA, miRNA is also processed by Dicer into about 22 nt long sequences.[181]

The expression of miRNAs correlates to a cell's developmental lineage and stage of differentiation and also reflects the differentiation state of tumors.[182] In general, a downregulation of miRNAs in cancers compared with normal tissues has been observed. However, of the 200 plus miRNAs described in humans, some clusters are overexpressed in some cancers. For example, a cluster of miRNAs derived from the *mir*-17-92 miRNA gene locus is overexpressed in human B cell lymphomas.[183] Similarly, in breast cancer two miRNAs, *mir*-21 and *mir*-155 are upregulated.[184] Three miR-

NAs are downregulated in breast cancer: *mir*-10b, *mir*-125b, and *mir*-145. Thus, it appears that miRNAs can act either as oncogenes or tumor suppressor genes. There is evidence of interaction between miRNA expression and the *ras* and *myc* oncogenes.[181,185] c-Myc has been shown to activate expression of a cluster of six miRNAs on human chromosome 13, and two of these miRNAs, *mir*-17-5p and *mir*-20a negatively regulate E2F1, which is one of the promitogenic genes turned on by c-Myc.[185]

Cancer Prevention

A discussion of future directions of cancer biochemistry should include the topic of cancer prevention. One of the clues about how body metabolism can affect cancer risk is the role of caloric restriction. It has been known for over 70 years that limiting food consumption in rodents increased their life span (reviewed in Ref. [186]). This is also true for yeast, round worms (*C. elegans*), fruit flies (*Drosophila*), and most likely primates. Since nature has a way of creating an evolutionary continuum, it is probably also true for humans. This observation related to the number of calories in the diet; hence the term "caloric restriction" (CR) is used to define the phenomenon. In general, calorie restricted diets contain 60-70% of what animals would eat ad libitum. The phenotype that a CR diet produces includes lower body temperature, blood glucose, and insulin levels, reduced body fat, and lower total body weight.[186] Although the size of organs in such CR fed animals is lower, brain size is not reduced. CR animals are also more resistant to temperature and oxidative stress. Evolutionarily, this makes sense because an organism that could survive in times of food scarcity would have a reproductive advantage.

CR diets not only slow the aging process but prevent the commencement of late-onset diseases including cancer. An example from animal studies is that CR extends the life span of tumor suppressor–deficient mice (eg, $p53^{-/-}$) that have a high frequency of cancers and die early (reviewed in Ref. 186).

The genes that play a role in regulating the CR response include the *sir*2 (silent information regulator 2) family of genes. The *sir*2 was first found in yeast where it mediates gene-silencing events. The *sir*2 ortholog in mammals is called *sirt*1, and it appears to mediate physiological events that result from a CR diet (reviewed in Ref. 186). *sir*2 also has an ortholog in *C. elegans*, and its expression is a determinant of life span in that organism. Since yeast and *C. elegans* diverged about 1 billion years ago, this suggests the evolutionary conservation of this process.

The *sir*2 gene product (called sirtuin) is an NAD-dependent histone deacetylase and the *sirt*1 product in mammalian cells deacetylates histones and nonhistone substrates. Because histone deacetylation is a mechanism to shut down expression of some genes (see above), this suggests a way that the "metabolic thermostat" could be turned down, allowing cells to survive longer. Support for the role of the *sir*2-related genes in CR comes from experiments in which the *sir*2 gene was deleted in yeast (CR did not extend life span in this case) and CR was shown to increase the silencing activity of *sir*2.[187] Moreover, a group of compounds known as STACs (sirtuin activating compounds) extend the replicative life span of yeast, *C. elegans*, and *Drosphila* as well as of human cells in culture.[188] Resveratrol, one of the STACs , responsible for this mechanism, is a naturally occurring polyphenol antioxidant found in raspberries, blueberries, peanuts, grapes, grape skins, and red wine. There is anecdotal epidemiological data that indicate that one or more glasses of wine a week may lower the risk of upper digestive tract cancers and cardiovascular disease. Since dark chocolate also contains similar antioxidants, this suggests an attractive dietary regimen for wine and chocolate lovers.[189,190]

Another mechanistic link of *sirt*1 activity to cancer prevention comes from studies showing that *sirt*1 is a negative regulator of PPARγ activity. PPARγ overexpression is associated with aging changes and cancer progression in colon, bladder, breast, and prostate (reviewed in Ref. 186). Thus, inhibition of PPARγ activity may be another mechanism of cancer prevention by *sirt*1 activation.

Acknowledgment

The authors thank Eileen Ferguson, Department of Pharmacology, University of Michigan Medical School, for her careful preparation of the manuscript.

Selected References

The complete reference list can be found at www.CANCERMEDICINE8.com

1. Warburg O. *The Metabolism of Tumors.* London: Arnold Constable; 1930.
2. Edinger AL, Thompson CB. Akt maintains cell size and survival by increasing mTOR-dependent nutrient uptake. *Mol Biol Cell.* 2002;13:2276–2288.
3. Lu H, Forbes RA, Verma A. Hypoxia-inducible factor 1 activation by aerobic glycolysis implicates the Warburg effect in carcinogenesis. *J Biol Chem.* 2002;277:23111–23115.
5. Griffin JL, Shockcor JP. Metabolic profiles of cancer cells. *Nat Rev Cancer.* 2004;4:551–561.
6. Fliss MS, Henning U, Caballero OL, et al. Facile detection of mitochondrial DNA mutations in tumors and bodily fluids. *Science.* 2000;287:2017–2019.
10. Potter VR. Biochemical perspectives in cancer research. *Cancer Res.* 1964;24:1085–1098.
13. Weber G. Enzymology of cancer cells (part one). *N Engl J Med.* 1977;296:486–493.
17. Al-Hajj M, Wicha MS, Benito-Hernandez A, Morrison SJ, Clarke MF. Prospective identification of tumorigenic breast cancer cells. *Proc Natl Acad Sci USA.* 2003;100:3983–3988.
23. Blackburn EH. Switching and signaling at the telomere. *Cell.* 2001;106:661–673.
32. Graeber TG, Eisenberg D. Bioinformatic identification of potential autocrine signaling loops in cancers from geneexpression profiles. *Nat Genet.* 2001;29:295–300.
37. Herschman HR. Primary response genes induced by growth factors and tumor promoters. *Annu Rev Biochem.* 1991;60:281–319.
51. Furuta S, Hidaka E, Ogata A, et al. Ras is involved in the negative control of autophagy through the class I PI3- kinase. *Oncogene.* 2004;23:3898–3904.
55. Shintani T, Klionsky DJ. Autophagy in health and disease: a double-edged sword. *Science.* 2004;306:990–995.
59. Edinger AL, Thompson CB. Death by design: apoptosis, necrosis, and autophagy. *Curr Opin Cell Biol.* 2004;16:663–669.
64. Hakomori S-I. Aberrant glycosylation in cancer cell membranes as focused on glycolipids: overview and perspectives. *Cancer Res.* 1985;45:2405–2417.
65. Hakomori S-I. The glycosynapse. *Proc Natl Acad Sci USA.* 2002;99:225–232.
66. Ruddon RW. *Cancer Biology.* 4th Ed. New York: Oxford University Press; 2007:123–126.
67. Bertozzi CR, Kressling LL. Chemical glycobiology. *Science.* 2001;291:2357–2364.
81. Li Y, Liu D, Chen D, et al. Human DF3/MUC1 carcinoma-associated protein functions as an oncogene. *Oncogene.* 2003;22:6107–6110.
89. Huang L, Chen D, Liu D, et al. MUC1 oncoprotein blocks GSK3β-mediated phosphorylation and degradation of β-catenin. *Cancer Res.* 2005;65:10413–10422.
90. Ahmad R, Raina D, Trivedi V, et al. MUC1 oncoprotein activates the IκB kinase β complex and constitutive NF-κB signaling. *Nat Cell Biol.* 2007;9:1419–1427.
96. Singh AP, Moniaux N, Chauhan SC, et al. Inhibition of MUC4 expression suppresses pancreatic tumor cell growth and metastasis. *Cancer Res.* 2004;64:622–630.
99. Bast RC Jr, Feeney M, Lazarus H, et al. Reactivity of a monoclonal antibody with human ovarian carcinoma. *J Clin Invest.* 1981;68:1331–1337.
103. Ruoslahti E. Proteoglycans in cell regulation. *J Biol Chem.* 1989;264:13369–13372.
106. Streuli CH, Bissell MJ. Expression of extracellular matrix components is regulated by substratum. *J Cell Biol.* 1990;110:1405–1415.
108. Giancotti FG, Ruoslahti E. Integrin signaling. *Science.* 1999;285:1028–1032.
110. Uemura T. The cadherin superfamily at the synapse: more members, more missions. *Cell.* 1998;93:1095–1098.
112. Guilford P. E-cadherin downregulation in cancer: fuel on the fire? *Mol Med Today.* 1999;5:172–177.

116. Liotta LA, Kohn EC. The microenvironment of the tumourhost interface. *Nature.* 2001;411:375–379.
120. Berger SL. The histone modification circus. *Science.* 2001;292:64–65.
123. Rice JC, Allis CD. Gene regulation: code of silence. *Nature.* 2001;414:258–259.
130. Feinberg AP, Gehrke CW, Kuo KC, Ehrlich M. Reduced genomic 5-methylcytosine content in human colonic neoplasia. *Cancer Res.* 1988;48:1159–1161.
131. Toyota M, Ho C, Ahuja N, et al. Identification of differentially methylated sequences in colorectal cancer by methylated CpG island amplification. *Cancer Res.* 1999;59:2307–2312.
137. Tilghman SM. The sins of the fathers and mothers: genomic imprinting in mammalian development. *Cell.* 1999;96:185–193.
140. Christofori G, Naik P, Hanahan D. Deregulation of both imprinted and expressed alleles of the insulin-like growth factor 2 gene during beta-cell tumorigenesis. *Nat Genet.* 1995;10:196–201.
143. Blau HM, Brazelton TR, Weimann JM. The evolving concept of a stem cell: entity or function? *Cell.* 2001;105:829–841.
148. Pawson T, Saxton TM. Signaling networks—do all roads lead to the same genes? *Cell.* 1999;97:675–678.
153. Giot L, Bader JS, Brouwer C, et al. A protein interaction map of *Drosophila melanogaster. Science.* 2003;302:1727–1736.
154. Heath JR, Phelps ME, Hood L. Nanosystems biology. *Mol Imaging Biol.* 2003;5:312–325.
159. Druker BJ, Sawyers CL, Kantarjian H, et al. Activity of a specific inhibitor of the BCR-ABL tyrosine kinase in the blast crisis of chronic myeloid leukemia and acute lymphoblastic leukemia with the Philadelphia chromosome. *N Engl J Med.* 2001;344:1038–1163.
160. Moasser MM, Basso A, Averbuch SD, Rosen N. The tyrosine kinase inhibitor ZD1839 ("Iressa") inhibits HER2-driven signaling and suppresses the growth of HER2-overexpressing tumor cells. *Cancer Res.* 2001;61:7184–7188.
165. Li J, Yen C, Liaw D, et al. *PTEN*, a putative protein tyrosine phosphatase gene mutated in human brain, breast, and prostate cancer. *Science.* 1997;275:1943–1947.
167. Johnson DG, Walker CL. Cyclins and cell cycle checkpoints. *Ann Rev Pharmacol Toxicol.* 1999;39:295–312.
169. Orr-Weaver TL, Weinberg RA. A checkpoint on the road to cancer. *Nature.* 1998;392:223–224.
171. Levine AJ. p53, the cellular gatekeeper for growth and division. *Cell.* 1997;88:323–331.
178. Ferrari M. Cancer nanotechnology opportunities and challenges. *Nat Rev Cancer.* 2005;5:161–171.
180. Quintana A, Raczka E, Piebler L, et al. Design and function of a dendrimer-based therapeutic nanodevice targeted to tumor cells through the folate receptor. *Pharm Res.* 2002;19:1310–1916.
181. Meltzer PS. Small RNAs with big impacts. *Nature.* 2005;435:745–746.
186. Guarente L, Picard F. Calorie restriction-The SIR2 connection. *Cell.* 2005;120:473–482.

10 Invasion and Metastases

Elise C. Kohn, MD

Invasion and metastasis are the most insidious and life-threatening aspects of cancer.[1-3] The capacity for invasion may not be expressed initially or in all tumors. Those tumors with minimal or no invasion may be extirpated successfully leading to cure in some patients, but this occurs only in tumors with minimal or no invasion. Most cancers, however, gradually unmask their invasive potential, progressing over time to frank malignancy from preexisting carcinoma in situ, adenomas, or disorders of epithelial proliferation. Once the neoplasm becomes invasive, it can disseminate through shedding and through lymphatics and/or vascular channels that it has induced through tumor-stimulated lymphangiogenesis, angiogenesis, and other perturbations of the local microenvironment.[4] Invasion and metastases kill hosts through two processes: local invasion and distant organ colonization and injury. Local invasion can compromise the function of involved tissues by local compression, local destruction, or prevention of normal organ function. The most significant turning point in cancer, however, is the establishment of distant organ colonization. The patient can no longer be cured by local therapy at this point.

Our understanding of invasion and metastasis continues to advance and is now driving development of a large number of new therapeutic agents. However, our ability to detect occult metastatic disease or metastatic potential prior to development of occult disease still lags. Commensurate with this is some improvement in overall survival of advanced solid tumor patients. Some patients with cancer have benefited from improved screening techniques that detect early stage cancer. Examples are Papanicolaou (Pap) screening for cervical cancer and magnetic resonance scanning and mammography for breast cancer. Still, approximately 30% of patients will have clinically detectable metastases at the time of initial diagnosis, and a further 30% of patients will harbor occult metastases, relative proportions that have not changed for decades. The relapse rate for stage I disease in breast cancer and most other early stage solid tumors patients who have less than 1 cm tumors remains approximately 20%, indicating that the development of metastatic potential is an early event. Improved classification of tumors has led to more targeted and logical application of therapy in many diseases, bringing much of the scientific progress to the patient. We now recognize premalignant risk lesions with high propensity for progression, allowing therapeutic and preventive intervention in some tumors. However, for most solid tumors, once metastatic, there is limited potential for cure or prolonged tumor-free time (Fig. 10-1).

Tumors of comparable size and histology can have widely divergent metastatic potential, depending on their genotype and local environmental influences. Cancer is a disease of signaling caused by expression of genetic changes. Aberrant signaling is driven through genetic changes of germ line and somatic mutation leading to changes in the pattern of intrinsic cellular and microenvironment signaling. Metastatic potential is influenced by all components of the local microenvironment, including sister tumor cells, local stroma, inflammation, and local vascular activity. These dynamic interactions result in elaboration of cytokines driving changes in the local immune response, and stromal–tumor interactions. This complexity underscores the importance of understanding the molecular events of the metastatic process and using that understanding to develop biomarker panels, through which to predict presence and location of active metastatic disease and occult metastases, and to identify and develop therapeutic targets. The malignant phenotype is thus the culmination of a series of genetic changes in the primary tumor and its metastases through which investigation of the activation, regulation, and manipulation of regulatory elements can be exploited as a new frontier for metastases research.

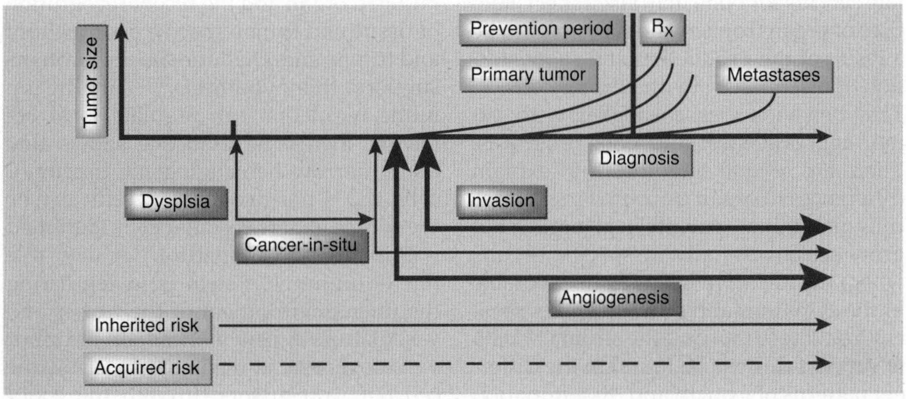

Figure 10-1 Temporal progression of cancer. Diagnosis and treatment of cancer occurs generally late in the course of disease. At this time, a high proportion of patients have obvious or occult metastases. Acquisition of the invasive and angiogenic phenotypes occur very early, in some cancers, perhaps more than 5 to 10 years prior to presentation. This demonstrates a window of opportunity to intervene with anti-invasive and antimetastasis therapies.

Molecular Events Underlying the Metastatic Phenotype

Tumor-induced neovascularization and invasion are obligate early events.[1] The angiogenic switch has been shown to precede actual malignant transformation in some cancers.[5] Local microinvasion can occur early, even though distant dissemination may not be evident or may not yet have begun. Invasion is a more efficient process than metastasis, where microinvasion may be ongoing without subsequent entry into the vascular portals of dissemination. Millions of cells are shed into the circulation daily from locally invasive cancer, but only a small fraction (0.01%) is successful at initiating colonies.[1,6] Thus, further understanding and molecular dissection of the processes of invasion and metastasis are needed (Table 10-1). A number of studies have sought to identify the molecular events underlying development of the metastatic phenotype. Golub and others postulated that the metastatic phenotype was preexistent in a tumor. Several groups have now reported different gene cassettes as predictive of metastasis (and survival) in different cancers—obtained using gene expression arrays.[7-10] Whether there are different cassettes from different cancers, different cancer microenvironments such as metastatic sites vs primary sites, or the different cassettes are a result of statistical overfitting where the number of potential genetic events is far in excess of the number of cases tested may be less important than the finding that the genes validate their potential. Results from these studies are being advanced translationally into the clinical arena and may prove to be an important mechanism for subsetting disease and triaging patients into a more individual or fitted therapeutic plan.

Tumor–Host and Tumor–Stromal Interactions

Cancer is a derangement in the proper sorting of cell populations causing a violation of normal tissue boundaries. Tissue architecture, normally maintained by basement membrane delineation of tissue boundaries and cell–cell communication, suppresses inappropriate intermixing of cells from different tissue types. Normal cells remain confined to their home territory because they are held in check by intercommunication with neighboring cells and the surrounding extracellular matrix. Appropriate sorting of parenchymal tissue cells during morphogenesis and wound healing is tightly regulated by soluble and solid phase stimuli. In contrast, successful malignant tumor cells are resistant to the regulatory signals because they appropriate, misinterpret, or disregard these signals.[4] The process of metastasis is a cascade of linked sequential steps involving multiple host–tumor interactions (Table 10-2). Metastasis is a highly selective competition, favoring the survival of minor subpopulation(s) of tumor cells that preexist within the primary tumor.

The distribution of metastases varies widely depending on the histologic type and anatomic location of the primary tumor and the characteristics of the local microenvironment.[1,6] On one hand, the most frequent organ location of distant metastases in many types of cancers still appears to be the first capillary bed or lymphatic tree encountered by the circulating cells. This may explain why lung and liver metastases are the first parenchymal metastases seen from most systemic cancers. On the other hand, there are many metastatic sites that cannot be predicted on the basis of anatomic considerations alone and might be considered examples of organ tropism. The mechanisms for this homing are becoming understood as we learn more about the local microenvironment of the tumor and secondary sites. The predilection of breast and prostate cancers for bone may also reflect a degree of organ tropism and may, in part, be a result of the production and sequestration of osteopontin by the tumor cells.[11,12] This behavior was correlated with tumor aggressiveness and poor prognosis. There are several hypotheses to explain differences in organ tropism. First, tumor cells disseminate equally in all organs but grow selectively only in specific organs where the microenvironment is favorable in the cytokines and growth factors present from the tumor and the stroma.[1,4] Data to support this can be found in the different patterns of growth and dissemination that are observed when subcutaneously implanted xenografts are compared to orthotopic implants.[6] Preferential growth and homing may be induced by the local microenvironment. Second, circulating tumor cells may adhere specifically to the endothelial luminal surface only in the targeted organ and the recent recognition of tissue and tumor-specific endothelium and tumor-endothelium-specific proteins supports this hypothesis.[13-15] Finally, immune regulation can regulate local behavior. Increasing evidence shows that bone marrow hemangiogenic precursor cells, CD34 positive marrow cells, can be the source of new vascular cells identified within tumor vasculature.[16] A new role for the immune system is in regulating the microenvironment of the tumor and vasculature. A new mechanism of tumor vasculogenesis is mediated by dendritic cell (DC) precursors through the cooperation of beta-defensins and vascular endothelial growth factor-A (VEGF-A).[17] This finding identified a subset of DC precursors having both leukocyte and endothelial cell markers. Furthermore, this

Table 10-1 ■ Metastasis Facts

- Up to 60% of patients with invasive cancer have overt or occult metastases at diagnosis.
- Acquisition of the invasive phenotype is an early event in cancer progression.
- Millions of tumor cells are shed daily into the circulation.
- Less than 0.01% of circulating tumor cells successfully initiate a metastatic focus.
- Angiogenesis is a ubiquitous and early event that is necessary for and promotes metastatic dissemination.
- Invasion and angiogenesis use the same signal transduction programs and gene expression cassettes.
- Circulating tumor cells can be detected in patients who do not develop overt metastatic disease.
- Metastases may be as susceptible to anticancer therapy as their primary tumors.
- Therapeutic intervention against targets of invasion and metastasis may alter both the metastatic process and angiogenesis.

Table 10-2 ■ Tumor–Host Interactions During the Metastatic Cascade

1. Tumor initiation	Carcinogenic insult, oncogene activation or derepression, genomic instability, germ line mutations, stem cell activation
2. Promotion and progression	Genetic, and epigenetic instability, promotion-associated genes and growth factors, mutation or loss of suppressor gene products, changes in the local microenvironment owing to stromal or inflammatory response to the aberrant premalignant state, carcinogen exposure, organ stress
3. Uncontrolled proliferation	Autocrine growth factors or their receptors, receptors for most hormones such as estrogen, activated stroma, paracrine stimulation through elaboration of cytokines and growth factors, increased vascularity
4. Angiogenesis	Multiple angiogenesis factors including known growth factors, elaborated from tumor, stroma, vasculature, and inflammatory cells
5. Invasion of local tissues, blood, and lymphatic vessels	Serum chemoattractants, autocrine motility factors, attachment receptors, degradative enzymes, loss of expression of proteinase inhibitors, leaky vessels, heterotypic cell-cell adhesion
6. Circulating tumor cell arrest and extravasation	Homotypic and heterotypic aggregation of tumor and other cells
a. Adherence to endothelium	Tumor cell interaction with fibrin, platelets, clotting factors
b. Retraction of endothelium	Adhesion of tumor, endothelial cells, and stromal cells to
c. Adhesion to basement membrane	integrins and other receptors for matrix proteins
d. Dissolution of basement membrane	Metalloproteinases, serine proteinases, heparinase, cathepsins
e. Migration	Autocrine motility factors, chemotaxis factors
7. Colony formation at secondary site	Co-optation of receptors normally used for homeostatic control
	Response to local (normal) tissue growth factors, angiogenesis factors
	Mutation, overexpression and/or loss of metastasis suppressor and promoting genes
8. Evasion of host defenses and resistance to therapy	Resistance to killing by host immune cells; failure to express or blocking of tumor-specific antigens; promoting immune infiltration, amplification of drug-resistant genes; immune tolerance to tumor antigens

cell subset had a plasticity—the ability to form vascular precursors—for which outcome was microenvironment specific. This transition into vascular cells and structures was dependent on CCR6 stimulation followed by VEGF action through vascular endothelial growth factor receptor-2 (VEGFR-2), a receptor for which therapeutic interventions have been developed successfully. Accumulating evidence also indicates a more complex role of the immune system in regulating the development of local tumor vasculature.[18] The role of the microenvironment for both stromal cells and tumor cells is increasingly complex and important and will have an important role in how we rethink therapeutic intervention for invasive and metastatic disease.

The microenvironment is a network of scaffolding made out of collagens, glycoproteins, growth factors, and glycans coupled with the cellular component comprising the normal stromal elements, fibroblasts, endothelial cells, and immune cells into which the tumor cells invade and grow.[1] The scaffolding materials form structures, such as the basement membrane surrounding epithelial and endothelial structures, that separate tissue compartments. Tumor cells penetrate the basement membrane to enter the underlying interstitial stroma during a transition from in situ to invasive carcinoma.[2,19] This process of invasive behavior and the phenotypic and genotypic changes associated with it is often called epithelial–mesenchymal transition, one with involvement of the transforming growth factor-β/SMAD family of cytokines.[20,21] The basement membrane is a dense meshwork of type IV collagen, glycoproteins, such as laminin, fibronectin, proteoglycans, and embedded growth factors. Loss of continuity of the basement membrane is the distinguishing feature for malignancy. Benign proliferative disorders may have disorganized epithelial–stromal architecture without clear disruption. Extreme forms can mimic the appearance of invasive carcinoma. Thus, the sine qua non of cancer is its capacity for invasion, not unchecked proliferation (Fig. 10-2).

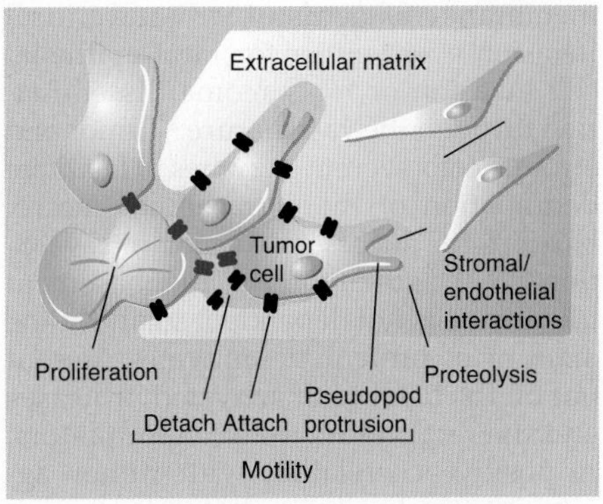

Figure 10-2 Cell invasion of the extracellular matrix. Physiologic or malignant invasion is motility coupled to adhesion and proteolysis. The advancing pseudopod, extended through calcium-regulated actin polymerization, may focus the action of cell surface proteinases, receptors, and activators. Matrix degradation is balanced by endogenous inhibitors of proteolysis to provide adhesive traction and to contain the event to the local microenvironment. Signal-transduction pathways cycle the individual invading cell through pseudopod protrusion, proteolysis, antiproteolysis, adhesion, and detachment.

Adhesion

Both cell–cell interactions and cell–stroma interactions play an important role during invasion. Connections through cell-adhesion molecules stabilize tissue integrity, whereas loss or alteration of these cell surface proteins is associated with increased metastatic potential. Cell polarity and organization during spreading and migration is regulated by cell interaction with extracellular matrix proteins, through the integrin family, and with other cells, through the transmembrane glycoprotein cadherins. Activation of these cell surface receptors transmits external signals into the cell and thus directs cell behavior.

Homotypic Cell–Cell Interactions

The cadherins are transmembrane glycoproteins that mediate extracellular calcium-dependent homotypic cell–cell interactions.[22,23] E-(epithelial) cadherin, the most extensively studied, is involved in epithelial cell–cell communication. It is found at the cell membrane in adherens junctions in complex with a family of distinct but related cytoplasmic proteins, α and β catenins, and plakoglobin and armadillo.[24,25] Cadherin–catenin complexes are linked to the cytoskeleton through direct interactions between α-catenin and α-actinin.[26,27] E-cadherin functions as a metastasis suppressor molecule in several cell lines and cancer types.[28,29] In these studies, loss of gene expression was correlated with increased invasiveness and metastatic potential, and replacement or augmentation of gene expression resulted in suppression of the invasive phenotype. Loss of E-cadherin in ovarian surface epithelial cells is associated with loss of cell–cell contact and increase in motile and metastatic potential during progression of the transformation of ovarian surface epithelium to ovarian carcinoma.[30] Human breast adenocarcinoma cells (MCF-7), but not normal mammary epithelial cells, induced endothelial cell dissociation, which correlated with the loss of E-cadherin expression at the site of tumor cell–endothelial cell contact.[31]

There are situations in which E-cadherin is normal but other members of the complex are not. For example, when E-cadherin was expressed in invasive breast cancer MCF-7-10A cells, they exhibited the ability to aggregate, but their morphology was unaltered and the cells remain invasive. These cells had reduced expression of plakoglobin and reduced phosphorylation of β-catenin as compared with the less invasive MCF-7 human breast cancer cells.[32] β-Catenin, under normal conditions, binds to the tumor-suppressor gene product, adenomatous polyposis coli (APC).[33] APC–β-catenin interactions promote APC hyperphosphorylation, resulting in targeted degradation of β-catenin. Alternatively, β catenin, if not degraded and when not involved in the APC cell adhesion complex, can move into the nucleus where it interacts with T Cell Factor (TCF) family members, stimulating gene transcription and promoting cell proliferation. This complex process also involves the WNT/frizzled pathway.[24,34,35] Thus, intercellular adhesion mediated by cadherin–catenin complexes or the release of the catenins plays a role in both structural morphology and functional differentiation. Any loss of this control mechanism may facilitate the invasive process.

Furthermore, cadherins cross talk with the receptor tyrosine kinases and other signaling proteins. Interaction with the epidermal growth factor receptor (EGFR) induces tyrosine phosphorylation of β-catenin and leads to disassembly of the cadherin–catenin complex.[36] This leads to either degradation of β-catenin or its translocation to the nucleus and interaction with the transcriptional apparatus. Bidirectional regulation is seen in which E-cadherin interacts with EGFR to decrease its mobility and ligand affinity.[37] These behaviors have a net function to increase the invasive and metastatic potential.

Heterotypic Cell–Cell Interactions

The selectins are a family of calcium-dependent adhesion proteins that mediate heterotypic interaction.[38] The importance of heterotypic interaction is more prominent now that the interaction of tumor cells with stromal components, such as inflammatory and endothelial cells, is recognized not just biologically but also as points for therapeutic targeting. First recognized for their involvement in leukocyte rolling, the selectins were identified as involved in endothelial cell–leukocyte interactions. The rolling process involves dynamic tethering and release of the leukocytes on the endothelium, with rapid cycling of selectin–selectin ligand binding.[39] Similar interactions have now been demonstrated for the interaction of tumor cells and endothelium. The target binding sites for the selectins are structures containing sialyl-Lewis[a] and sialyl-Lewis[x], are expressed on tumor cells.[40] Sialyl-Lewis[a] is also useful as a biomarker, as it is recognized by the CA19-9 antibody. Selectins function in heterotypic binding of tumor cells to endothelium.[41] P(platelet)-selectin has been shown to be involved in tumor cell–platelet interactions to facilitate metastasis.[42]

Heterotypic Cell–Matrix Interactions

The integrins are a family of transmembrane glycoproteins that are expressed by the cell as alpha–beta heterodimers.[43] Although originally identified as cell adhesion molecules, integrins are major signaling molecules for inhibition of apoptosis, induction of gene expression, and stimulation of cell proliferation, invasion and metastasis,[37,39] and angiogenesis.[43-47] Integrin ligands include a variety of extracellular molecules, such as collagens, laminin, tenascin, fibronectin, vitronectin, von Willebrand factor, and thrombospondin.[26] Integrin signaling depends on the dynamic formation of cellular focal adhesions, specialized sites at which cells form outside–in signaling complexes. These signaling complexes regulate cell shape, migration, and proliferation, and create a framework for the association of important signaling molecules. Protein phosphorylation, mobilization of calcium, and guanosine triphosphate (GTP) exchange are common signals involved in propagation of integrin-mediated information. Integrins also have extensive cross talk with different classes of transmembrane receptors, such as the receptor tyrosine kinases, allowing propagation of proliferation and invasion messages through multiple mechanisms.[45,48-51] Furthermore, these proteins have been targeted successfully for therapeutic manipulation. The integrin $\alpha v\beta 3$ plays a fundamental role in angiogenesis and invasion.[51] It mediates cellular adhesion to extracellular matrix proteins and cross talks with receptor tyrosine kinases, such as the VEGFR-2 and Ephrin A2.[52-54] Integrin $\alpha v\beta 3$ is expressed minimally in normal or resting blood vessels but is upregulated significantly on the endothelium of neovessels.[55] It has been targeted for the development of molecular therapeutics.

Proteolysis

The process of invasion is dynamic. It requires ongoing protein synthesis and degradation. Degradation of basement membrane collagen is an early and critical invasion event either for local epithelial cell invasion or for sarcoma dissemination through the vasculature.[2] Tumor and stromal cells secrete enzymes to facilitate degradation of the extracellular matrix barriers for successful tumor intravasation.[56-59] Degradation of the basement membrane is not dependent solely on the amount of proteolytic enzymes present but on the balance of activated proteases and their naturally occurring inhibitors. A positive correlation with tumor aggressiveness has been shown for a variety of degradative enzymes, including heparinases, seryl-, thiol- (cathepsins), and metal-dependent enzymes.

Matrix metalloproteinases (MMPs) are a family of more than 25 neutral metalloenzymes secreted as latent proenzymes. They require activation through proteolytic cleavage of the amino terminal domain, and their activity depends on the presence of Zn^{2+} or Ca^{2+}. Five MMP subclasses have been defined and grouped according to substrate specificity: interstitial collagenases, gelatinases, stromelysins, membrane-type MMPs (MT-MMPs), and elastases.[57-61] Increased MMP activity has been detected and shown to correlate with invasion and metastatic potential in a wide range of cancers, including ovary, lung, prostate, breast, and pancreas cancers.[62] Type IV collagen is a critical component of the basement membrane architectural scaffolding, on which laminin, heparan sulfate, proteoglycan, and minor components of the basement membrane are assembled. It is classically degraded by MMP-2 (gelatinases) and this was the logic behind using these MMPs as the first therapeutic protease targets.[63,64]

These enzymes are inhibited by members of the endogenous tissue inhibitor of metalloproteinase (TIMP) family.[65,66] The relationship between the levels of activated MT-MMPs, MMPs, and free TIMPs is a major determinant of the balance between matrix degradation and matrix formation or stabilization in the tumor microenvironment.[67] Selectivity can be shown by the example of the action of TIMP-2 but not TIMP-1 on basic fibroblastic growth factor (bFGF)-induced stimulation of endothelial cell proliferation that is independent of its ability to inhibit MMP. The TIMPs have now been shown to have multiple MMP-independent activities.[68,69] These proteins may also act as cytokines and recognize specific receptors. TIMP-1 inhibited angiogenesis in vivo and both capillary endothelial cell proliferation and migration in vitro and it functions as an anti-apoptotic factor in lymphoma cells. Furthermore, TIMP-1 has been shown to be a molecular marker for breast cancer.[70]

Plasminogen activators—tissue-type plasminogen activator (tPA) and urokinase plasminogen activator (uPA)—are serine-specific proteases that convert inactive plasminogen to active plasmin, a trypsin-like enzyme that degrades a variety of proteins, including fibrin, fibronectin, type IV collagen, vitronectin, and laminin.[71] uPA is involved primarily in cell-mediated proteolysis during macrophage invasion, wound healing, embryogenesis, invasiveness, and metastasis, where it has the ability to activate latent collagenases and proplasminogen activators, and to degrade TIMPs. uPA directly activates latent growth factors, such as the precursor form of hepatocyte growth factor/scatter factor (pro-HGF/SF) and indirectly latent transforming growth factor (TGF)-β through activation of plasminogen.[72] The interaction of uPA and its receptor plays an important role in direct and indirect extracellular matrix degradation, thus potentiating invasive and angiogenic events.

uPA binds to specific cell surface receptors (uPAR).[73] Both uPA and its inactive zymogen (pro-uPA) bind with high affinity to uPAR. High levels of uPA have been observed in human tumors and a multitude of carcinoma cell lines. Elevated expression of uPA and plasminogen activator inhibitor-1 (PAI-1) in tumor extracts has been shown to correlate with increased invasion, increased incidence of relapse, and shorter overall survival. The action of uPA can be counteracted by naturally occurring inhibitors including members of the SERPIN (serine protease inhibitor) family, PAI-1, PAI-2, and protease nexin-1.[74,75] Receptor-bound active uPA is inhibited by PAI-1, PAI-2, and PN-1. Unlike the uPAR–uPA complex that remains stable at the cell surface, the uPAR–uPA-inhibitor complex is internalized quickly by the cell and degraded.[76-78] The PAI-1 is produced primarily by endothelial cells and also by a number of other cell types.

Tumor Cell Migration

Migration is necessary early in invasion, whether physiologic or malignant.[1] Immune cells must exit the vasculature and migrate to the site of infection or inflammation; similarly, endothelial cells must migrate from their quiescent home for vascular budding and neoangiogenesis, and tumor cells must migrate from their primary site. The invading cell couples local proteolysis with coordinated and temporally limited attachment and detachment to achieve forward locomotion. Tumor cells have a motile response to many agents, including host-derived motility and growth factors and cytokines,

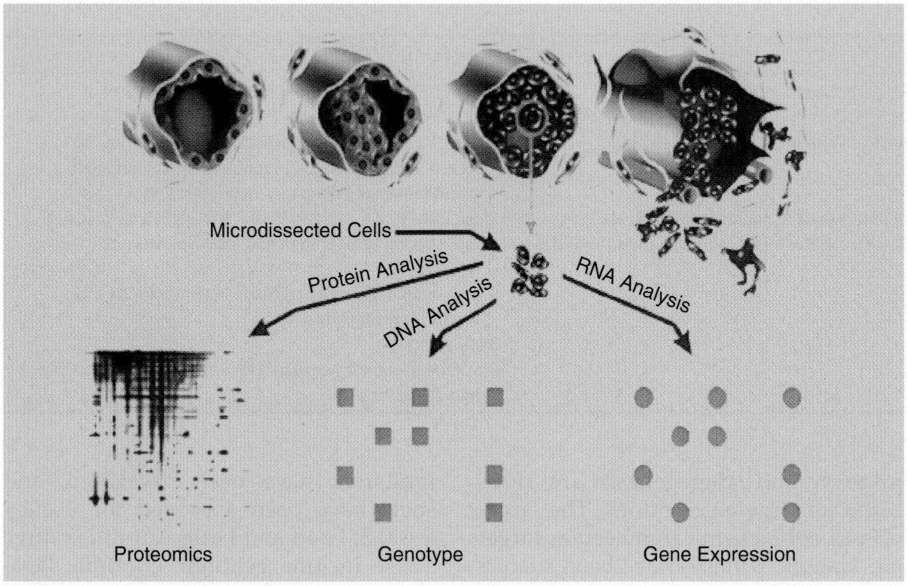

Figure 10-3 ■ Application of microdissection to the study of invasion and metastases. Isolation of involved and stromal cells independently can allow for dissection of the genotypic, gene expression, and proteomic events underlying acquisition of invasive behavior and its use for metastatic dissemination. DNA, RNA, and protein can be retrieved from selectively microdissected cells and applied to two-dimensional electrophoresis, oligonucleotide arrays for genomic analysis, and for cDNA microarrays and establishment of cDNA libraries. Differential analysis of these tools using invasive and metastatic versus noninvasive or nonmetastatic cell materials has already yielded new information in the regulation of cancer dissemination.

extracellular matrix components, and tumor-secreted factors.[79] Pseudopodia protruding in response to chemoattractants may serve multiple functions, including acting as sense organs for the migrating cell to locate directional clues, secrete motility-stimulating factors, provide propulsive traction for locomotion, and induce matrix proteolysis to assist in the penetration of the matrix.[80,81] Tumor cell migration is dynamic and complex allowing the responding cell(s) to respond to multiple stimuli in additive or synergistic fashions to dictate the direction, location, and magnitude of the migratory response.

Tumor cells secrete factors that function as autocrine motility factors. The first described autocrine motility factor, autotaxin, or lysophospholipase D.[82-84] Autotaxin stimulates tumor cell motility and also was found to induce angiogenesis in xenograft systems. LPA is produced, in part, by autotaxin cleavage of lysophosphatidic acid. LPA is therefore a mechanism through which the pro-invasive and proangiogenic activity of autotaxin is propagated. LPA is a potent growth, motility, and angiogenic factor and its pathway, the target of many molecular therapeutics.[85,86] The requirement for autotaxin in angiogenesis is further stressed by the embryonic lethality of its knockout in mice demonstrated by profound vascular defects.

A wide variety of growth factors and cytokines stimulate tumor cell and endothelial cell motility, including the insulin-like growth factors (IGF), hepatocyte growth factor (HGF), FGF, TGF-β, and cytokines of the CCR and CXC family.[87,88] Many of these are felt to be part of the controversial process of epithelial–mesenchymal transition, a process that occurs in the acquisition of the metastatic phenotype.[89] HGF is a paracrine motility factor that stimulates motility of epithelial and endothelial cells. HGF, the preferred ligand for the *c-met* protooncogene product, induces the scatter or chemokinetic locomotion of epithelial colonies, resulting in an invasive phenotype in vivo. HGF /scatter factor (HGF/SF) and its receptor *c-met* can play an important role during tumor progression and has been shown to be mutated.[90,91] These factors primarily stimulate chemotactic, or directed, or chemokinetic, random, motility and may thus play a role in the tumor cell homing to secondary sites. Therefore, the response of the tumor cell to motility stimulation by autocrine factors, matrix components, and host-derived growth factors is important in the initiation of tumor cell locomotion, its directedness, and the determination of the metastatic focus and are thus a potentially important target for molecular therapeutic intervention.

Angiogenesis

Neovascularization, or angiogenesis, covered in more detail elsewhere in this compendium, is a prerequisite for the local expansion of tumor colonies beyond the size restricted by oxygen and nutrient diffusion. Tumor vascularization is, thus, one of the rate-limiting steps for tumor metastasis and growth.[92,93] New capillaries provide cancer cells with conduits for entry into the circulation, nutrition, and exposure to stimulants and modifiers. Angiogenesis is necessary at the beginning and end of the metastatic cascade. The process of blood vessel formation is functionally similar to tumor cell invasion and can be considered as a form of regulated invasion,[1,3] using the same software and hardware as invading tumor cells. Many autocrine and paracrine cytokines and growth factors discussed above for tumors are also important in the local microenvironment as angiogenic factors causing a pleiotropic response of enzyme production, migration, and/or proliferation in endothelial cells. It has been argued that nonvascularized primary tumors may be maintained as dormant, small tumor nodules, kept constant by a balance of cell proliferation and apoptosis,[94] a concept not yet proven clinically. A tumor mass larger than 0.125 mm^3 has outgrown its capacity to acquire nutrients by simple diffusion and must initiate angiogenesis through host vessel initiation of capillary sprouts in the direction of the tumor.[95] Neovascularization is thus a permissive event that allows metastatic dissemination of invasion-competent cells. The parallel between the cellular and molecular biology of angiogenic physiologic invasion and malignant invasion stresses how therapeutics targeted at invasion may have benefits as antiangiogenic agents. The cassette of events necessary for neovascularization and vascular extension is similar to those required by tumor cells in local extension and dissemination. Thus, genetic and molecular regulation of components of invasion and metastases may be expected to cross over to angiogenic events, such that agents targeted to the biochemical and signaling events in invasion and metastasis should have biological activity in the local microenvironment.[4]

Invasion as a Therapeutic Molecular Target

Invasion and subsequent metastasis are very complicated multistep processes and are not monogenic in molecular origin. Loss of function/loss of suppressor and gain of function/oncogenic overexpression or overactivation of physiologically important signals combine to regulate invasion and metastasis. The metastatic phenotype requires gain of function pro-invasive and proangiogenic events for success and inhibition of regulatory events guarding density independence, cell–cell

Table 10-3 ■ **Metastasis Targets and Agents**

Targeted Therapies	Example Agents	Effects
Growth factors	cetiximab (anti-EGFR), pertuzumab, erlotinib and gefitinib bevacizumab VEGFR2-selective kinase inhibitors, eg, cefiranib, sorafenib, sunitinib, axitinib Multi target kinase inhibitors such as imatinib (PDGFR, abl, kit), sorafenib (VEGFR2, raf), dasatinib (src, abl), sunitinib (PDGFR, VEGFR, FGFR)	Block EGFR signaling, proliferation invasive behavior Neutralizes VEGF Inhibits VEGFR2 signaling signaling by complexing the ligand, reduced vascular proliferation, and remodeling in endothelium and lymphangioendothelium Block PDGFR, kit, abl, raf, VEGFR RTK signaling, vascular and stromal proliferation and invasive behavior
Cell adhesion	FAK and Src inhibitors	Blocks endothelial cell and tumor cell interaction with matrix, may regulate MMP activation
Signaling	[See text below]	Blockade of signals necessary for angiogenesis, invasion, and metastasis

adhesion, and cell–matrix attachment. Two classes of invasion and metastasis-associated gene products can be identified: (1) those that regulate outside–in events and (2) those that provide intracellular regulation. Acquisition of invasive potential is an early event in the malignant process, occurring in both the host and malignant components of the tumor and is often preceded by local angiogenesis at the in situ cancer.[4] The biochemical events underlying invasion are shared in the different proinvasive cells and thus are logical molecular targets for therapeutic application (Table 10-3 and Fig. 10-4).[1,4,96]

Receptor Tyrosine Kinase Metastasis Targets and Other Kinase Targets

Kinases that lie at nodal intersection points in signaling pathways regulating invasion and angiogenesis are recognized as targetable entities. The largest classes of biochemical molecular targets are kinases. Kinases have been successfully inhibited most commonly with small molecules that mimic ATP and compete for binding in the ATP binding pocket, thus reducing or blocking kinase function. Receptor tyrosine kinases targeted to date are broad in number and selectivity.[99] Kinase inhibitors approved for use in the United States include those targeting EGFR and members of the HER family of receptors, VEGF receptor 2, the type III receptor tyrosine kinases (c-kit, abl) and platelet-derived growth factor receptors, src, focal adhesion kinase (FAK) and others.[99,100] Several small molecule EGF receptor (HER1) and EGF receptor family (HER2, 3, and 4) kinase inhibitors have been developed, and some have been approved for use by the U.S. Food and Drug Administration. These include gefitinib, erlotinib, lapatinib, cetuximab, and trastuzumab.[101-104] Imatinib mesylate has been shown to be remarkably successful in its inhibition of the bcr–abl fusion kinase in chronic myelogenous leukemia as well as inhibition of c-kit in gastrointestinal stromal tumors and dermatofibrosarcoma protuberans.[105-107] A key finding in the studies of imatinib was the rapid reduction in vascular circulation in the tumor bed as imaged using positron emission tomography and dynamic contrast enhanced magnetic resonance imaging. Another approach to block ligands and receptors has been high affinity neutralizing monoclonal antibodies. VEGF ligand binding with bevacizumab, and receptor kinase inhibition with sorafenib and other investigational agents has yielded success in several difficult cancers, such as the very vascular clear cell carcinoma of the kidney.[108-110]

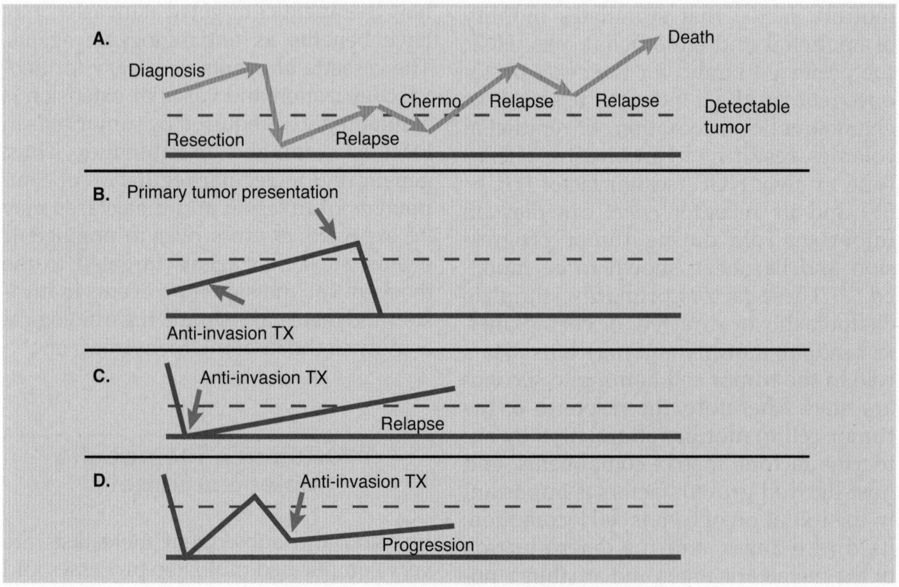

Figure 10-4 ■ Therapeutic uses of anti-invasion therapies. **(A)** Time course of solid tumor presentation, response, and progression. **(B)** Prevention. Invasion and angiogenesis, which use the same molecular and biochemical processes as malignant invasion, occur early. As such, a preventative intervention can be approached in high-risk individuals. **(C)** Adjuvant therapy. At the completion of diagnosis, optimal cytoreduction by surgery and therapies, and anti-invasive therapy may be applied as adjuvant treatment to slow the time to relapse or prevent relapse entirely. **(D)** Maintenance. Invasion and angiogenesis are dynamic processes, ongoing throughout the cancer process. Thus, intervention with anti-invasive therapy after optimal treatment or after treatment for relapse may prolong the time to the next relapse and maintain the tumor in a more dormant or slowly progressing state.

Antiadhesive Agents

A limited number of agents that affect tumor or endothelial cell adhesion have entered clinical trials, but several are under development. These include peptidomimetics and monoclonal antibodies that target integrins and downstream cytoplasmic kinases. In recent times, the role of src and FAK in aspects of vascular development and extension, invasion, and metastasis has been applied to therapeutic development. Application of agents, such as dasatinib, a multifunctional src/abl inhibitor, to solid tumors has been advanced and surrogate markers of target inhibition are under development.[111-114] Similarly, biochemical targeting of FAK has had preliminary success with low toxicity.[115,116] Maturation of preclinical and clinical studies is necessary to show whether this targeting of src and/or FAK is modulating adhesion, invasion, and angiogenesis as predicted or if other downstream functions are modulated.

Antiangiogenesis Therapies

Activated endothelial cells utilize similar mechanisms for neovascularization of cancers and for vascular remodeling during wound healing but each process has selective components as well. These have been targeted with success, and some antiangiogenic agents are now FDA-approved for use in selected cancers. Thalidomide, a cause of profound birth defects when used as a sedative, has shown promise for the treatment of both prostate cancer and multiple myeloma.[117,118] Although described as an antiangiogenic agent, its actual mechanism of action in patients in these settings is still unclear. Imatinib mesylate, described above as an inhibitor of receptor tyrosine kinases, has clinically evident antiangiogenic activity. Fluoro-deoxyglucose positron emission tomography (FDG-PET) and dynamic contrast-enhanced magnetic resonance imaging (DCE-MRI) are two techniques that are used to monitor and quantitate vascular flow.[119] Endothelial cell-specific reagents include those targeted at VEGF, including monoclonal anti-VEGF antibody (bevacizumab) and the small molecules directed against the VEGF receptor(s).[108-110,120,121] Bevacizumab has been approved for use in second line therapy in colon cancer. This drug and other agents, alone and in combination with chemotherapies, are in advanced phase clinical trials against cancers at several sites, including lung, renal cell and ovarian carcinomas. Highly selective inhibitors of VEGF receptors have been studied clinically for some time, but the response has been disappointing. However, a newer series of inhibitors that are more promiscuous in their activity, inhibiting several targets, are more promising.[99] Sorafenib (BAY 43-9006) touted initially as an raf kinase inhibitor has similar activity against VEGFR2.[122] Clinical responses and disease stabilization have been observed in multiple cancer types, especially renal cell carcinoma and hepatocellular carcinoma, previously considered generally therapy resistant.[122,123] Enthusiasm has been renewed with the advent of these newer agents for targeting the vasculature along with improved clinical assessment tools such as FDG-PET and DCE-MRI.[119] These new results have proven that components of the activated local microenvironment within cancers provide druggable targets.

Therapeutic Disruption of the Tumor Microenviroment

Therapeutic efforts in cancer prevention and treatment are being focused at the level of signaling pathways or selective modulatory proteins. Many or most of the signaling events important in transformation and survival are also active in the angiogenic and metastatic processes.[4] Two types of proteins have proven druggable: kinases and G-protein coupled receptors. Successful targeting of the tumor microenvironment has included selective targeting to the stromal components through direct angiogenesis inhibition such as through bevacizumab, neutralizing antibody against VEGF[110] and also against the interactive tumor microenvironment.[110,112,116,124,128] Agents such as the approved kinase inhibitors sunitinib and sorafenib are multipotent, targeting a variety of serine/threonine and tyrosine kinases involved both in activation and proliferation of stromal components and tumor cells. Targets such as Raf-1 kinase, abl, kit, PDGFR, and others are found on solid tumor cells and on endothelial cells, pericytes, and/or fibroblasts, all involved in making the local environment conducive to vascular advancement and tumor metastasis. Controversy exists as to whether agents should be selective only against invasion or against metastasis or pluripotence also.[99] Agents such as lapatinib, selective to the HER family of receptor tyrosine kinases have activity in tumors and support structures overexpressing the HER2 oncogene, whereas use of imatinib, sorafenib, and sunitinib may target more broadly.

Key questions that need to be considered in targeting the tumor and its microenvironment are as follows:

1. Is/are the target(s) present on the target cells (tumor, vascular, stromal)?
2. Did the agent dysregulate/inhibit its target in the expressing cell?
3. What other putative (off-target) targets were modified by the agent?
4. Is the modified target necessary and/or sufficient for clinical activity?

These questions are important to address as most solid tumors are driven by broad genomic disruption and therefore rarely dependent on a single translocation, such as Philadelphia chromosome, or mutation KIT in gastrointestinal stromal tumor. Thus, inhibition of a target that may be present, involved biologically, but insufficient by itself may be interpreted as a negative clinical study if translational endpoints addressing biochemical or genetic effects are not addressed. Furthermore, as there are many deregulated pathways in solid tumors, and many of those pathways may be upregulated in activated stroma, it is important to consider that "off-target" effects may in fact be therapeutically valuable.

Rational combination therapy incorporating agents that target selectively, such as bevacizumab, and those that are more promiscuous, such as sorafenib, take advantage of the concept that modulation of multiple key signaling nodes may result in more than additive effects.[4,128-131] Mathematically, effective disruption of a key pathway at one node requires at least 90% inhibition. However, in most situations, there are alternative pathways downstream that may overcome that inhibition. Alternatively, a combination targeting unique but interactive signaling events may require less inhibition, thus potentially resulting in the same or greater activity with lower doses of each drug. This was applied to target the tumor microenvironment using bevacizumab to neutralize VEGF and disrupt angiogenesis and vascular remodeling, in combination with sorafenib. Sorafenib, originally developed as a raf-1 kinase inhibitor, is also a potent inhibitor of the VEGFR2 receptor tyrosine kinase. A phase I trial to test the combination concept demonstrated an interactive effect on toxicity, but a surprising activity with prolonged disease stabilization and unexpected number of partial responses in ovarian cancer (43%).[129,130] Tumor vascular flow was reduced during combinatorial therapy as measured by dynamic contrast enhanced magnetic resonance imaging (Azad, Kohn et al., in preparation). Proof of mechanism studies will help interpretation of the value of this combination.

Chronic Low-Dose Chemotherapy

Another approach to targeting the tumor and microenvironment is the application of low dose chemotherapy applied more frequently, with or without inclusion of antiangiogenic therapy. It was initially tested in a model using continuous low-dose vinblastine with a neutralizing VEGFR2 antibody, leading to the tag term: Less is more. The concept proposed was that this approach made the chemotherapeutic agent a more selective antivascular therapy, so stated because there was little or no effect on proliferation of the tumor.[132-135] This apparent advance could also be reasoned to be one of addressing pharmacokinetics determining the effect of continuous low dose, raising and stabilizing a C_{min} rather than testing the effect of C_{max}, where the target is the largest net exposure attainable, especially over a threshold. The total drug exposure with metronomic therapy may be similar or greater to that with pulse therapy. Newer data suggest that the low-dose chemotherapy may improve susceptibility to antiangiogenic agents. Further laboratory and clinical trials are required to test this hypothesis.

Summary

The study of molecular mechanisms underlying invasion and its subsequent association with angiogenesis and metastasis has led to dramatic advances in our understanding of cancer and has identified multiple therapeutic targets. Neovascularization, eg, uses the same cassettes of genes and proteins in vascular sprout formation that cancer cells utilize for invasion consistent with the observation that anti-invasive drugs can also be antiangiogenic. The dissection of the invasive and metastatic processes has created new directions for cancer marker development and application. Importantly, molecular advances have allowed confirmation that invasion and acquisition of the metastatic phenotype are early events in cancer progression. Further application of this critical knowledge will advance our ability to identify patients who are at the highest risk for disseminated disease, to better develop therapeutics for those key patients, and, perhaps, to prevent many patients from receiving treatment that they might not have needed.

Selected References

The complete reference list can be found at www.CANCERMEDICINE8.com

1. Liotta LA, Kohn EC. The microenvironment of the tumor-host invasion field. *Nature*. 2001;411:375–379.
5. Hanahan D, Folkman J. Patterns and emerging mechanisms of the angiogenic switch during tumorigenesis. *Cell*. 1996;86:353–364.
6. Fidler IJ, Hart IR. Biologic diversity in metastatic neoplasms: origins and implications. *Science*. 1982;217:998.
8. Ramaswamy S, Ross KN, Lander ES, Golub TR. A molecular signature of metastasis in primary solid tumors. *Nat Genet*. 2003;33:49–54.
9. Wang Y, Klijn JG, Zhang Y, et al. Gene-expression profiles to predict distant metastasis of lymph-node-negative primary breast cancer. *Lancet*. 2005;365:671–679.
13. Hardwick JS, Yang Y, Zhang C, et al. Identification of biomarkers for tumor endothelial cell proliferation through gene expression profiling. *Mol Cancer Ther*. 2005;4:413–425.
16. Peters BA, Diaz LA, Polyak K, et al. Contribution of bone marrow-derived endothelial cells to human tumor vasculature. *Nat Med*. 2005;11:261–262.
17. Conejo-Garcia JR, Benencia F, Courreges MC, et al. Tumor-infiltrating dendritic cell precursors recruited by a beta-defensin contribute to vasculogenesis under the influence of VEGF-A. *Nat Med*. 2004;10:950–958.
20. Valcourt U, Kowanetz M, Niimi H, Heldin CH, Moustakas A. TGF-beta and the Smad signaling pathway support transcriptomic reprogramming during epithelial–mesenchymal cell transition. *Mol Biol Cell*. 2005;16:1987–2002.
23. Jou TS, Stewart DB, Stappert J, et al. Genetic and biochemical dissection of protein linkages in the cadherin–catenin complex. *Proc Natl Acad Sci USA*. 1995;92:5067–5071.
24. Agnieszka Kobielak A, Fuchs E. α-catenin: at the junction of intercellular adhesion and actin dynamics. *Nat Rev Mol Cell Biol*. 2004;5:614–625.
30. Hoffman AG, Burghardt RC, Tilley R, Auersperg N. An in vitro model of ovarian epithelial carcinogenesis: changes in cell–cell communication and adhesion occurring during neoplastic progression. *Int J Cancer*. 1993;54:828–838.
39. BarthelSR,GavinoJD,DeschenyL,Dimitroff CJ. Targeting selectins and selectin ligands in inflammation and cancer. *Expert Opin Ther Targets*. 2007;11(11):1473–1491.
42. Borsig L, Wong R, Feramisco J, et al. Heparin and cancer revisited: mechanistic connections involving platelets, P-selectin, carcinoma mucins, and tumor metastasis. *Proc Natl Acad Sci USA*. 2001;98:3352–3357.
46. Chicurel ME, Singer RH, Meyer CJ, Ingber DE. Integrin binding and mechanical tension induce movement of mRNA and ribosomes to focal adhesions. *Nature*. 1998;392:730–733.
48. Raghavan S, Vaezi A, Fuchs E. A role for αβ1 integrins in focal adhesion function and polarized cytoskeletal dynamics. *Dev Cell*. 2003;5:415–427.
51. Guo W, Giancotti FG. Integrin signalling during tumour progression. *Nat Rev Mol Cell Biol*. 2004;5:816–826.
56. Liotta LA, Tryggvason K, Garbisa S, et al. Metastatic potential correlates with enzymatic degradation of basement membrane collagen. *Nature*. 1980;248:67–68.
59. Davis GE, Senger DR. Extracellular matrix mediatesamolecularbalancebetweenvascular morphogenesis and regression. *Curr Opin Hematol*. 2008 May;15(3):197–203[Review].
62. Decock J, Paridaens R, Ye S. Genetic polymorphisms of matrix metalloproteinases in lung, breast and colorectal cancer. *Clin Genet*. 2008;73:197–211.
63. Overall CM, Kleifeld O. Tumour microenvironment—opinion: validating matrix metalloproteinases as drug targets and anti-targets for cancer therapy. *Nat Rev Cancer*. 2006;6:227–239.
71. Dass K, Ahmad A, Azmi AS, Sarkar SH, Sarkar FH. Evolving role of uPA/uPAR system in human cancers. *Cancer Treat Rev*. 2008;34:122–136.
74. Potempa J, Korzus E, Travis J. The serpin superfamily of proteinase inhibitors: structure, function, and regulation. *J Biol Chem*. 1994;269:15957–15960.
84. Mills GB, Moolenaar WH. The emerging role of lysophosphatidic acid in cancer. *Nat Rev Cancer*. 2003;3:582–591.
87. Cardones AR, Murakami T, Hwang ST. CXCR4 enhances adhesion of B16 tumor cells to endothelial cells in vitro and in vivo via beta(1) integrin. *Cancer Res*. 2003;63:6751–6757.
89. Yang J, Weinberg RA. Epithelial-mesenchymal transition: at the crossroads of development and tumor metastasis. *Dev Cell*. 2008;14:818–829.
90. Bellon SF, Kaplan-Lefko P, Yang Y, et al. c-Met inhibitors with novel binding mode show activity against several hereditary papillary renal cell carcinoma-related mutations. *J Biol Chem*. 2008;283:2675–2683.
93. Liotta LA, Kleinerman J, Saidel G. Quantitativerelation-shipsofintravascular tumor cells: tumor vessels and pulmonary metastases following tumor implantation. *Cancer Res*. 1974;34:997–1003.
95. Folkman J. Tumor angiogenesis: therapeutic implications. *N Engl J Med*. 1971;285:1182.
97. Eccles S, Welch DR. Metastasis: recent discoveries and novel treatment strategies. *Lancet*. 2007;369:1742–1757.
98. Bidard F-C, Pierga J-Y, Vincent-Salomon A, Poupon M-F. A "class action" against the microenvironment: do cancer cells cooperate in metastasis? *Cancer Metastasis Rev*. 2008;27:5–10.
108. Rini BI, Small EJ. Biology and clinical development of vascular endothelial growth factor-targeted therapy in renal cell carcinoma. *J Clin Oncol*. 2005;23:1028–1043.
112. Park SI, Zhang J, Phillips KA, et al. Targeting SRC family kinases inhibits growth and lymph node metastases of prostate cancer in an orthotopic nude mouse model. *Cancer Res*. 2008 May 1;68(9):3323–3333.
113. Serrels A, Macpherson IR, Evans TR, et al. Identification of potential biomarkers for measuring inhibition of Src kinase activity in colon cancer cells following treatment with dasatinib. *Mol Cancer Ther*. 2006;5:3014–3022.
115. Roberts WG, Ung E, Whalen P, et al. Antitumor activity and pharmacology of a selective focal adhesion kinase inhibitor, PF-562,271. *Cancer Res*. 2008;68:1935–1944.
116. Halder J, Lin YG, Merritt WM, et al. Therapeutic efficacy of a novel focal adhesion kinase inhibitor TAE226 in ovarian carcinoma. *Cancer Res*. 2007;67:10976–10983.
119. Rajendran JG, Krohn KA. Imaging hypoxia and angiogenesis in tumors. *Radiol Clin North Am*. 2005 Jan;43(1):169–187.
121. Ellis LM. Bevacizumab. *Nat Rev Drug Discov*. 2005;Suppl:S8–S9.
124. Alessandro R, Spoonster J, Wersto RP, Kohn EC. Signal transduction as a therapeutic target. *Curr Topic Microbiol Immunol*. 1996;213:167–188.
125. Adachi Y, Yoshio-Hoshino N, Nishimoto N. The blockade of IL-6 signaling in rational drug design. *Curr Pharm Des*. 2008;14:1217–1224.
127. Ramachandran R, Hollenberg MD. Proteinases and signalling: pathophysiological and therapeutic implications via PARs and more. *Br J Pharmacol*. 2008; 153:S263–S282.
128. Coleman RL, Kohn EC. Rationale for combination use of targeted agents in ovarian cancer: Do we have one? *Cancer*. 2008;113(4):665–667.
129. Azad NS, Posadas EM, Kwitkowski V, et al. Combination targeted therapy with sorafenib and bevacizumab results in enhanced toxicity and antitumor activity. *J Clin Oncol*. 2008:26:3709–3714.
130. Cannistra SA. Challenges and pitfalls of combining targeted agents in phase I studies. *J Clin Oncol*. 2008;26:3665–3667.
131. Royal RE, Libutti SK. Combining agents that target the tumor microenvironment improves the efficacy of anticancer therapy. *Clin Cancer Res*. 2008;14:270–280.
132. Kerbel R, Folkman J. Clinical translation of angiogenesis inhibitors. *Nat Rev Cancer*. 2002;2(10):727–739.
134. Hanahan D, Bergers G, Bergsland E. Less is more, regularly: metronomic dosing of cytotoxic drugs can target tumor angiogenesis in mice. *J Clin Invest*. 2000;105:1045–1047.

11 Tumor Angiogenesis

John V. Heymach, MD, PhD ■ George W. Sledge Jr., MD ■ Rakesh K. Jain, PhD

Angiogenesis, the growth of new capillary blood vessels, is central to the growth and metastatic spread of cancer. Nearly four decades ago, it was recognized to be a potential therapeutic target for the treatment of cancer.[1] Since that seminal observation, the field has undergone explosive growth that has taken it from theory to clinical validation of angiogenesis as a therapeutic target, and antiangiogic therapy is now in routine clinical use. Bevacizumab, a monoclonal antibody targeting vascular endothelial growth factor (VEGF), has undergone the most extensive clinical evaluation to date and is now a standard agent for the treatment of colorectal, lung, renal cell, and breast cancer as well other malignancies. Several other antiangiogenic agents are in routine use for renal cell cancer.

While the progress of the field is encouraging, the clinical benefits of antiangiogenic agents have been relatively modest thus far, and key questions remain unanswered: How should antiangiogenic therapy be combined with other therapeutic regimens and treatment modalities? In what tumor types, and at what stage(s), should these agents be used? Can markers be developed to identify patients most likely to benefit, or experience toxicities, from treatment? The ultimate impact of antiangiogenic therapy in the treatment of cancer will be determined at least in part by the ability of basic researchers and clinicians to address these questions.

An understanding of the cellular and molecular basis of tumor angiogenesis is therefore important for clinicians who diagnose and treat cancer by various modalities. This chapter is focused on certain general principles of tumor angiogenesis that are intrinsic to the behavior of human cancer, and lessons that can be gleaned from the clinical testing and use of angiogenesis inhibitors to date.

Rationale for Targeting Tumor Vasculature

The enormous progress that has been made in understanding molecular and genetic events that underlie the transformation of a normal cell to a cancer cell is reflected in many chapters in this book. Not surprisingly, most therapeutic approaches that have arisen from this research are targeted at the cancer cell, with a number of notable successes, such as therapies targeting BCR-ABL oncogene in CML or mutated c-KIT in gastrointestinal stromal tumors. In these cases, it appears that cell survival and other key processes are highly dependent on a single activated pathway. For the vast majority of solid tumors, targeting a single molecular pathway in the cancer cell has produced much more modest benefits. Experimental and clinical evidence reviewed in this chapter indicates that it is prudent to develop cancer therapies against another target, the microvascular endothelial cell, with the understanding that the 2 targets are not mutually exclusive.

Consider a cancer cell that has progressed through a series of mutations so that by activation of certain oncogenes and by loss of specific suppressor genes, it has become self-sufficient in growth signals, insensitive to antigrowth signals, unresponsive to apoptotic signals, capable of limitless replicative potential, and tumorigenic.[2] Current evidence argues that these neoplastic properties may be necessary but not sufficient for a cancer cell to expand into a population that is symptomatic, clinically detectable, metastatic, and lethal. For a tumor to develop a metastatic and/or a lethal phenotype, it must first recruit and sustain its own private blood supply, a process called tumor angiogenesis.[2]

A tumor can recruit vessels through at least 4 mechanisms: (1) co-option of existing vessels; (2) sprouting from existing vessels (angiogenesis); (3) formation of new vessels de novo, typically from bone-marrow derived cells in the adult (vasculogenesis); and (4) intussusception, the insertion of interstitial tissue columns into the lumen of preexisting vessels (reviewed in Ref. 3).

Nonangiogenic Tumors Are Harmless

There is an early stage of neoplastic development when tumors are not yet able to recruit new microvascular endothelial cells and cannot induce angiogenesis. As a result, most human tumors remain in situ and dormant at a microscopic size and are harmless to the host.[4] Nonangiogenic human tumors in mice are not only harmless throughout the normal life span of a mouse but usually cannot expand beyond a volume of approximately 1-2 mm^3.

Cancer Without Disease: Prolonged Survival With Nonangiogenic, Dormant Tumors ■ Nonangiogenic tumors in humans also stop expanding at a microscopic size of approximately 1 mm or less. For over 100 years, pathologists performing autopsies on individuals who died of automobile accidents or other trauma have documented the presence of in situ carcinomas. These findings, summarized by Black and Welch in 1993,[5] reveal that for a given age group, a large number of individuals harbor in situ carcinomas but a very small percentage in that age group are diagnosed with cancer during life. For example, carcinoma in situ is found in the breasts of 39% of women age 40-50 years who died of trauma, but only 1% are ever diagnosed with cancer in this age range. Carcinoma in situ of the prostate is diagnosed in 46% of men age 60-70 years who died of trauma, but only 1% are diagnosed during life. Carcinoma in situ is found in more than 98% of individuals age 50-70 years who died of trauma but is diagnosed in only 0.1% during life. What keeps these in situ carcinomas in check? One explanation is the potential contribution of host-derived factors that prevent in situ carcinomas from switching to the angiogenic phenotype. Among factors that could offer such protection, the role of physiologic levels of endogenous angiogenesis inhibitors is intriguing (see the sections on endogenous angiogenesis inhibitors).[6]

Disease of Cancer Requires Expansion of Tumor Mass ■ The disease brought about by cancer is not manifest until after continuous expansion of a tumor mass takes place, beyond the microscopic size of the restricted nonangiogenic tumor in situ cancer. However, expansion of the tumor mass beyond the initial microscopic size of a nonangiogenic tumor is dependent on recruitment of endothelial cells. Such endothelial cell recruitment begins when tumor cells undergo a switch to the angiogenic phenotype.[7-9] The angiogenic phenotype is driven by a number of changes which may include (1) increased expression by tumor cells of angiogenic proteins such as VEGF and basic fibroblast growth factor (bFGF); (2) increased expression of angiogenic proteins from stromal cells (ie, stromal fibroblasts), a process induced by the tumor itself; (3) decreased expression of endogenous angiogenesis inhibitors (ie, thrombospondin [TSP]-1) by the tumor and by stromal fibroblasts; and (4) recruitment of bone marrow–derived endothelial cell precursors (see below for a detailed discussion of the switch to the angiogenic phenotype). Other mechanisms will unquestionably be uncovered.

Expansion of the tumor mass can produce symptomatic, detectable, and potentially lethal cancer either from a local mass that mechanically interferes with function (ie, a brain tumor or an intestinal obstruction from ovarian cancer), from a dispersed mass (ie, multiple metastases), from release of cytokines that interfere with hemostasis and result in abnormal clotting or bleeding (the 2 most common causes of death in cancer patients), or from cytokines that produce cachexia (ie, tumor necrosis factor [TNF]-α) or interfere with other functions (ie, inappropriate hormone release). In summary, in its simplest terms, absence of tumor angiogenesis prevents expansion of the tumor mass beyond a microscopic size, thereby avoiding metastatic spread and tumor-related symptoms, and hence, "cancer without disease."[6] Recruitment of microvascular endothelial cells is also necessary for expansion of a normal tissue mass and for expansion of an organ mass, eg, after partial hepatectomy.[10] In fact, angiogenesis is fundamental to reproduction, development, and repair, but such physiologic angiogenesis occurs mainly as short-lived capillary blood vessel growth that usually lasts only days (ovulation angiogenesis), weeks (wound healing angiogenesis), or months (fetal and placental angiogenesis but then it is always down-regulated spontaneously and on a predictable timetable.[11,12]

Historical Background

More than 100 years ago, it was observed that tumors were often more vascular than corresponding normal tissues.[13] This tumor hyperemia observed during surgery was generally explained by simple dilation of existing host blood vessels.[14] Vasodilation was thought to be a side effect of metabolites or of necrotic tumor products escaping from the tumor. Three reports, although largely overlooked, suggested that tumor hyperemia could be related to new blood vessel growth, ie, to neovascularization and not solely to vasodilation. A 1939 article showed that whereas neovascularization of a wound in a transparent chamber in a rabbit ear regressed completely after the wound healed,[15] a tumor implant in the chamber was associated with accelerated growth of new capillary blood vessels. The other 2 reports, in 1945 and 1947, demonstrated that new vessels in the neighborhood of a tumor implant arose from host vessels and not from the tumor itself.[16] These articles notwithstanding, debate continued in the literature for two more decades about whether a tumor could expand to a large size (centimeters) by simply living on preexisting vasculature (vessel co-option).[17] Even among the few investigators who accepted the concept of tumor-induced neovascularization, it was generally assumed that this vascular response was an inflammatory reaction, a side effect of tumor growth, not a requirement for tumor growth.[18] It is now recognized that the 2 processes are often linked and that the recruitment of inflammatory cells plays a key role in initiating and promoting tumor angiogenesis.

Beginning of Angiogenesis Research

Hypothesis: Tumor Growth Depends on Angiogenesis

In 1971, Folkman proposed a new view of the role of blood vessels in tumor growth. He hypothesized that tumor growth is angiogenesis-dependent.[1] This hypothesis suggested that tumor cells and vascular endothelial cells within a neoplasm may constitute a highly integrated ecosystem and that endothelial cells may be switched from a resting state to a rapid growth phase by a "diffusible" chemical signal from tumor cells. An additional speculation was that angiogenesis could be a relevant target for tumor therapy (ie, antiangiogenic therapy). Folkman proposed these ideas from experiments he performed with Frederick Becker in the early 1960s, which revealed that tumor growth in isolated perfused organs was severely restricted in the absence of vascularization of the tumors (Fig. 11-1).[19-23]

These concepts were not accepted at the time. Although a few investigators in the early 1970s perceived that tumors could actually induce neovascularization, the belief persisted that such neovascularization was an inflammatory host response to necrotic tumor cells or possibly a host defense detrimental to the tumor. Another obstacle to research on tumor angiogenesis was the conventional wisdom at that time that any new vessels induced by a tumor, like new vessels in a wound, would become established and thus could not be made to involute. From this assumption, scientists concluded that antiangiogenic therapy could never regress a tumor; therefore, it would be fruitless to try to discover angiogenesis inhibitors. In this pessimistic atmosphere, it took many years for compelling evidence to be generated that would convince scientists that tumor growth depended on neovascularization. Eventual acceptance of Folkman's 1971 hypothesis was slow because it would be two more years before the first vascular endothelial cells were successfully cultured in vitro, 8 years before it was possible to grow capillary endothelial cells in vitro, 11 years before the discovery of the first angiogenesis inhibitor, and 13 years before the purification of the first angiogenic protein.[24-28]

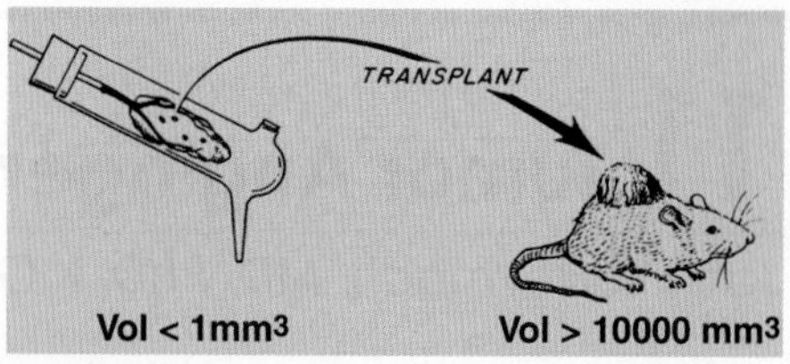

Figure 11-1 ■ Tumors remain avascular in isolated perfused organs.[20] Whole organs, supported by perfusion, allow growth of tumors in isolation from a host. The tumor remains very small, less than 1 mm^3 in an avascular environment compared to growth in mice, which can exceed 10,000 mm^3.

Throughout the 1970s, laboratory studies were devoted to demonstrating that tumor vessels were new proliferating capillaries; the sequential steps of the angiogenic process could be identified; qualitative and quantitative bioassays for angiogenesis could be developed; viable tumor cells released diffusible angiogenic factors that stimulated new capillary growth and endothelial mitosis in vivo, despite the arrest of tumor cell proliferation by irradiation; necrotic tumor products were not angiogenic per se; and angiogenesis itself could be inhibited.[29-32] Because of these efforts to provide supporting evidence that tumor growth was angiogenesis dependent, the field of angiogenesis research began. Today the field has broadened to include a wide spectrum of basic science disciplines, from developmental biology to molecular genetics, as well as a variety of clinical specialties, which include, in addition to oncology, cardiology, dermatology, gynecology, ophthalmology, and rheumatology.

Experimental Evidence ■ By the mid-1980s, considerable experimental evidence had been assembled to support the hypothesis that tumor growth is angiogenesis dependent. The idea could now be stated in its simplest terms: "Once tumor take has occurred, every further increase in tumor cell population must be preceded by an increase in new capillaries that converge upon the tumor."[33] The hypothesis predicted that if angiogenesis could be completely inhibited, tumors would become dormant at a small, possibly microscopic, size.[22] It forecasted that whereas the presence of neovascularization would be necessary but not sufficient for expansion of a tumor, the absence of neovascularization would prevent expansion of a primary tumor mass beyond 1-2 mm^3 and restrict a metastasis to a microscopic dormant lesion (Fig. 11-1).

The hypothesis that tumors are angiogenesis dependent is now supported by a large body of preclinical evidence[34] including pharmacological and genetic studies, as well as clinical studies discussed in a later section. Some of the observations supporting the angiogenic hypothesis included:

1. Tumors implanted into subcutaneous transparent chambers grow slowly before vascularization, and tumor volume increases linearly. After vascularization, tumor growth is rapid and tumor volume may increase exponentially.[35,36]
2. Tumors grown in the vitreous of the rabbit eye remain viable but are restricted to diameters of less than 0.50 mm for as long as 100 days. Once such a tumor reaches the retinal surface, it becomes neovascularized and within 2 weeks can undergo a 19,000-fold increase in volume over the avascular tumor.[37]
3. The limit of oxygen diffusion is approximately 100-200 µm. Tumor cells that exceed these distances from a capillary vessel become necrotic, as determined by intravital microscopy of tumors in transparent skin chambers in mice (Fig. 11-2).[38]
4. In transgenic mice that develop carcinomas of the beta cells in the pancreatic islets, large tumors arise from a subset of preneoplastic hyperplastic islets but only after they have become vascularized.[8]
5. In colon carcinomas arising in rats after carcinogen exposure, there is an early phase (tumor diameter < 3.5 mm) during which the tumor is temporarily supplied by preexisting host microvessels that are dilated and widened.[39] This stage is similar to "co-option" of blood vessels.[40] Subsequently, new capillary vessels sprout and proliferate (angiogenesis), which leads to increasing microvessel density and is accompanied by rapid tumor growth.
6. A neutralizing antibody to VEGF was administered to mice bearing tumors that induced angiogenesis solely by VEGF.[41] Tumor growth was inhibited by more than 90%. The antibody had no effect on the tumor cells in vitro.[42] This observation has been replicated using a variety of methods to block VEGF, including a fusion protein engineerd from VEGF receptors (VEGF trap).[43] Similar results were seen with an antibody directed against another angiogenic factor, bFGF.[44]
7. Specific immunologic inhibition of the $a_v b_3$-integrin on capillary endothelial cells resulted in apoptosis of proliferating endothelial cells, blocked neovascularization, and induced tumor regression.[45]
8. An angiogenesis inhibitor, TNP-470 (AGM- 1470), a synthetic analog of fumagillin, selectively inhibited proliferating endothelial cells in vitro and in vivo.[46] It potently inhibited tumor growth in vivo but did not inhibit tumor cells in vitro. In preclinical studies, it has a broad spectrum of antitumor activity, with complete regressions observed in 7 tumor types in mice, including neurofibrosarcoma, neurofibroma, breast cancer, gastric cancer, and choriocarcinoma, as well as mouse reticulum sarcoma and gastric carcinoma.[47]
9. Endogenous specific inhibitors of endothelial proliferation and of angiogenesis inhibit tumor growth in a variety of murine cancer models. These inhibitors include angiostatin, a 38 kDa internal fragment of plasminogen (generated by Lewis lung carcinoma); endostatin, a 20 kDa internal fragment of collagen XVIII (generated from a murine hemangioendothelioma); a 53 kDa conformationally changed fragment of antithrombin III (generated from human small cell lung cancer); and tumstatin, a 28 kDa internal fragment of collagen IV (a 3 noncollagenous 1 [NC1] domain) (Table 11-1).[48-55]
10. Id1 and Id3 are helix-loop-helix proteins that may control differentiation by interfering with deoxyribonucleic acid (DNA) binding of transcription factors. After targeted disruption of 1 allele of Id1 and 2 alleles of Id3, 3 different types of implanted tumors failed to induce angiogenesis, their growth was severely restricted, and they did not metastasize.[56,57] However, when these mice were injected with bone marrow from wild-type

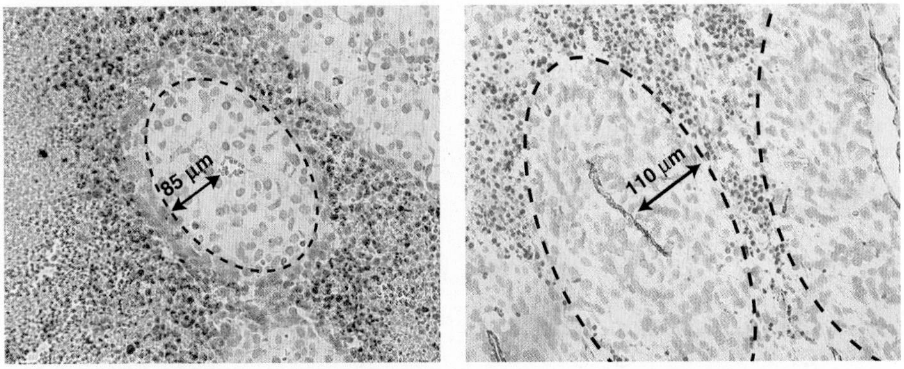

Figure 11-2 (**A**) A cuff of live tumor cells around a microvessel in a human melanoma growing in a SCID mouse has an average radius of 85 microns. The appearance of an ellipsoid is due to the way the section is cut. (**B**) A cuff of rat prostate cancer cells around a microvessel has an average radius of 110 microns.[558]

Table 11-1 **Examples of Regulators of Angiogenesis**

Proangiogenic Molecules	Antiangiogenic Molecules	Transcription Factors, Oncogenes, and Other Regulators
Vascular endothelial growth factor (VEGF)	Interferon-α,β,γ	Hypoxia inducible factor (HIF)-1α, 2α
	Thrombospondin-1,2	Nuclear Factor-κB (NF-κB)
Basic fibroblast growth factor (bFGF)	Angiopoietin 2	Epidermal growth factor receptor (EGFR)
Transforming growth factor-α (TFG-α)	Tissue Inhibitors of MMPs (TIMPs)	
Platelet-derived growth factor (PDGF)		Ras
Epidermal growth factor (EGF)	Endostatin	p53
Angiopoietins	Angiostatin	Von Hippel-Lindau
Interleukin-6	Interleukin-12	Cadherin
Interleukin-8	Endostatin	Integrin
Matrix metalloproteinases (MMPs)	Thrombospondin-1	Semaphorin
Hepatocyte growth factor (HGF)		Id1, Id2
Stromal cell-derived Factor-1α (SDF-1α)		Prolyl hydroxylases
Delta-like ligand 4 (DLL4)		myc
Ephrins		
Monocyte chemoattractant protein-1 and other chemokines		

mice containing normal Id1 and Id3 markers, progenitor endothelial cells expressing Id1 and Id3 circulated from the bone marrow to the tumor vascular bed. The increase in progenitor endothelial cells correlated with and permitted the tumors to undergo increased tumor neovascularization and tumor growth.[57]

Biology of Tumor Angiogenesis

The Role of Angiogenesis in Preneoplasia and Early Tumorigenesis

In the experiments with isolated perfused organs by Folkman and colleagues more than three decades ago, it was observed that the growth of tumors was severely restricted in diameter in the absence of angiogenesis.[20,58] This and other studies led to the proposal that the growth of solid tumors is dependent on new capillary sprouts (termed angiogenesis), and that without angiogenesis solid tumors might become completely dormant.[1] This raised the possibility that angiogenesis might be a therapeutic target not only for the treatment of advanced cancers, but potentially for chemoprevention as well. In recent years, angiogenesis has been validated as a therapeutic target for advanced cancers though a growing body of preclinical and clinical studies. The study of angiogenesis inhibitors for blocking the earliest steps in the development of cancer (chemoprevention) has lagged behind, despite the strong support for the concept provided by preclinical studies (reviewed in Refs. 59, 60).

Preclinical Studies Demonstrating a Role for Angiogenesis in Early Tumorigenesis

In the 1970s, it was shown by Gullino et al. that pre-cancerous tissues demonstrate signs of early angiogenesis, and it was suggested that blocking this process may be used to prevent cancer.[61] Later, using transgenic mouse models of tumorigenesis, Hanahan and colleagues demonstrated that some pre-malignant lesions undergo "angiogenic switch" early in carcinogenesis reflecting a change in the net balance between angiogenic stimulators and inhibitors.[8,9] VEGF and matrix metalloproteinase-9 were shown to play important roles in the angiogenic switch in these models.[62-64] In a murine model of pancreatic islet carcinoma, 4 different antiangiogenic agents were tested (TNP-470, endostatin, angiostatin, or the matrix metalloproteinase inhibitor BB-94) and had distinct activity profiles in terms of their ability to prevent tumor formation (chemoprevention), slow the growth of small tumors (early intervention), and regress established tumors.[8,65,66] In another study, established mammary cancer cells (ie, previously transformed cells but not primary tumors) were implanted in a dorsal skinfold window chamber in rats, and were found to induce angiogenesis long before the tumor population would have reached the limiting size of a non-neovascularized tumor, ie, 0.2-2 mm. Concomitant implantation of the cancer cells with a truncated soluble receptor for VEGF led to tumor cell apoptosis, tumor regression, and suppression of tumor growth before the appearance of neovascular sprouts. This receptor, however, had no effect on tumor cells in vitro, while it had a potent antiproliferative effect on endothelial cells.[67] These and other preclinical studies suggest that angiogenesis is an early and critical step in tumorigenesis, and that antiangiogenic agents may inhibit the tumor progression and growth.

Recent studies have further elucidated the properties of angiogenic vessels occurring during preneoplasia. Using a spontaneous carcinogenesis model in the skin of mice, it was observed that even during the hyperplastic/dysplastic stage, a rise in interstitial fluid pressure (IFP) could be detected.[68] Furthermore, nascent vessels demonstrated altered permeability, vessel compression, and decreased perivascular coverage. Lymphatic vessels were observed to be partly compressed and nonfunctional at this stage. This suggests that many of the changes typically associated with vasculature in established tumors actually occur during the preneoplastic stage.

Preneoplasia Is Associated with Increased Angiogenesis in Human Tumors

Studies from human clinical specimens provide further support for the hypothesis that angiogenesis occurs early in tumor progression, typically during the preneoplastic stage. In cervix cancer, eg, an initial mild increase in vessel density has been detected in the early dysplastic (cervical intraepithelial neoplasia [CIN] I) stage. Mid–late dysplasias (CIN II–III) exhibited a readily apparent angiogenic switch, wherein new vessels became densely apposed along the basement membrane underlying the dysplastic epithelium.[69,70] Biopsies from lung cancer patients and high-risk individuals have shown that preneoplastic lesions ranging from hyperplasia and metaplasia to carcinoma in situ are associated with increased microvessel density in the surrounding mucosa.[71-73] A distinctive pattern known as angiogenic squamous dysplasia[72] has also been identified. The specific angiogenic stimulators in bronchial preneoplastic lesions have not been established, but elevated levels of VEGF,[71] EGFR,[74] and COX-2[75] have been observed.

Role of Angiogenesis in the Metastatic Spread of Cancer

In addition to its role in enabling the growth of small pre-malignant or malignant lesions, angiogenesis contributes to the hematogenous metastatic spread of tumors. This metastatic spread may be facilitated by the presence of "mosaic" blood vessels in tumors, in which both endothelial and tumor cells form the luminal blood surface, facilitating the shedding of tumor cells into the circulation. In one study, approximately 15% of vessels in a colon cancer xenograft model were mosaic vessels in which tumor cells appeared to directly contact the luminal vessel surface without endothelial cells acting as a barrier.[76] Similar numbers of mosaic tumor vessels were detected in human tumor biopsies. These observations suggest that the irregular architecture and function of tumor vessels may facilitate tumor cell shedding into the circulation and metastatic spread.

Micrometastases also appear to be dependent on angiogenesis in order to progress into clinically evident tumors. They may remain dormant in distant sites for an extended period of time but a small fraction of these acquire an adequate blood supply to permit the development of tumors; angiogenesis inhibitors can inhibit this process in a variety of murine models.[77-82] The continued growth of both the primary tumor and metastases thereafter depend on the maintenance of an adequate blood supply. In theory, angiogenesis inhibitors may therefore offer benefit when used for chemoprevention as well as in treatment of early stage, occult metastatic, or advanced disease.[59,83,84]

Taken together, these preclinical and clinical studies provide evidence that the induction of angiogenesis is an early and important step in tumor progression, likely occurring in precancerous lesions, and is involved in metastatic spread. For these reasons, angiogenesis is a rational target for chemoprevention. Additional studies will be needed to elucidate the key regulators of early angiogenesis, and to identify the different types of antiangiogenic agents that may be optimal for chemoprevention, advanced disease, and other applications.

Regulators of Angiogenesis

The Discovery of Diffusible Factors Stimulating Tumor Angiogenesis

The observation in the 1970s that tumors implanted into the avascular cornea or onto the vascularized chick chorioallantoic membrane induced an ingrowth of new capillaries indicated that tumors released diffusible angiogenic factors.[9]

This result motivated the development of in vitro and in vivo bioassays to guide the search for tumor-derived angiogenic factors.[85]

Fibroblast Growth Factors ■ bFGF or FGF-2 was the first angiogenic protein to be isolated and purified from a tumor (1982), followed shortly by acidic FGF (aFGF or FGF-1).[28,86,87] Acidic and bFGFs stimulate endothelial cell mitosis and migration in vitro and are among the most potent angiogenic proteins in vivo. They have high affinity for heparin and heparan sulfate, are stored in extracellular matrix, but lack a signal sequence for secretion.[88] The expression of bFGF receptors is very low. Although many different cells synthesize bFGF, including tumor cells of the central nervous system, sarcomas, genitourinary tumors, and even endothelial cells in the tumor vasculature, it is not clear how bFGFs, in the absence of a signal sequence, are exported from tumors, unless proteinases or heparanases mediate release of FGF from extracellular matrix.[88-92] Identification of an FGF-binding protein secreted by tumors into the extracellular matrix may illuminate a mechanism of tumor mobilization of stored FGFs.[93-95] Furthermore, some tumors recruit macrophages[96] and activate them to secrete bFGF,[89] whereas others attract mast cells, which, because of their high content of heparin, could sequester bFGF. In spontaneous tumors that arise in transgenic mice, aFGF and bFGF are exported into conditioned medium by angiogenic tumor cells but not by pre-angiogenic cells in earlier stages of tumor progression.[38,97] bFGF is not a specific endothelial mitogen, but has several cell targets including fibroblasts, smooth muscle cells, and neurons. Therefore, it is puzzling why experimental tumors transfected with bFGF containing an engineered signal sequence stimulate mainly endothelial proliferation almost to the exclusion of smooth muscle and fibroblast proliferation.[44,98] However, the ability of endothelial-derived angiopoietin-2 to repel smooth muscle or to prevent smooth muscle or pericytes from intimate contact with endothelial cells may explain this phenomenon in part (see Angiopoietins below).[99-101] bFGF interferes with adhesion of leukocytes to endothelium, and it has been suggested that tumors that elaborate bFGF may produce a form of local immunologic tolerance.[102-104]

Abnormally elevated levels of bFGF are found in the serum and urine of cancer patients and in the cerebrospinal fluid of patients with different types of brain tumors.[105,106] High bFGF levels in renal carcinoma correlate with a poor outcome.[107] Also, bFGF levels in the urine of children with Wilms' tumor correlate with stage of disease and tumor grade.[108]

VEGF Family ■ Dvorak first proposed that tumor angiogenesis is associated with increased microvascular permeability.[109] This led to the identification of vascular permeability factor (VPF).[110-112] VPF was subsequently sequenced by Ferrara and in 1989 was reported to be a specific inducer of angiogenesis called VEGF.[111-113] At the same time, a novel angiogenic protein was first isolated and purified from a tumor (sarcoma 180) in the Folkman lab, and in a collaboration with Ferrara was shown to be VEGF.[113] Since then, more than 40 angiogenic inducers have been identified, most of them as tumor products (Table 11-1).[3,114] VEGF is an endothelial cell mitogen and motogen that is angiogenic in vivo.[115-117] Its expression correlates with blood vessel growth during embryogenesis and is essential for development of the embryonic vascular system.[118,119] VEGF expression also correlates with angiogenesis in the female reproductive tract, and in tumors.[62,120-122] VEGF is a 40-45 kDa homodimeric protein with a signal sequence secreted by a wide variety of cells and the majority of tumor cells. VEGF exists as 5 different isoforms of 121, 145, 165, 189, and 206 amino acids, of which $VEGF_{165}$ is the predominant molecular species produced by a variety of normal and neoplastic cells. Two receptors for VEGF are found mainly on vascular endothelial cells, the 180 kDa fms-like tyrosine kinase (Flt-1)[123] and the 200 kDa human kinase insert domain-containing receptor (KDR) and its mouse homolog, Flk-1.[124] VEGF binds to both receptors, but KDR/Flk-1 transduces the signals for endothelial proliferation and chemotaxis.[125-128] Other structural homolog of the VEGF family include VEGF-B, VEGF-C, VEGF-D, and VEGF-E.[129,130] VEGF-C and -D bind to Flt-4, which is preferentially expressed on lymphatic endothelium.[131,132]

Klagsbrun et al. discovered that neuropilin-1, a neuronal guidance molecule, is a co-receptor for $VEGF_{165}$, but not for VEGF.[133,134] This finding provides a molecular mediator that coordinates growth in the vascular system with the nervous system. Other neuronal guidance proteins and/or their receptors are also angiogenesis regulators. For example, neuropilin is a receptor for VEGF and for semaphorin. Semaphorin repels neurite outgrowth and is also an angiogenesis inhibitor. Ephrins are neural guidance molecules, but also genetically determined arteries and veins during embryogenesis. EphrinB2 is expressed by tumor vascular endothelium. Perhaps in part because of the overlap between regulators of the nervous and vascular systems, angiogenesis in brain tumors has distinctive characteristics such as high IFP and low oxygen tension that contribute to the malignant behavior of these tumor.[135]

Neuropilin is not a tyrosine kinase receptor and is expressed on nonendothelial cells, including tumor cells. This allows VEGF that is synthesized by tumor cells to bind to their surface. Surface-bound VEGF could make endothelial cells chemotactic to tumor cells, or it could act in a juxtacrine manner to mediate co-option of microvessels by tumor cells. Neuropilin also binds placenta growth factor-2 (PlGF-2) and heparin is essential for the binding of $VEGF_{165}$ and PlGF-2 to neuropilin-1.[40,136] The natural cell surface polysaccharide in vivo is heparan sulfate, not heparin. Heparan sulfate may act as a template to accelerate the interaction of VEGF or PLGF-2 with VEGF. VEGF expression by tumors is up regulated by hypoxia and is often elevated near areas of tumor necrosis.[137-140] Hypoxia activates hypoxia inducible factor-1 (HIF-1), which binds to the Hypoxia Response Element (HRE sequence) in the VEGF promoter, which leads to VEGF mRNA transcription.[125,139] Independent of this, hypoxia stabilizes the VEGF mRNA.

VEGF Signal Transduction ■ While VEGF-A binds VEGFR1 with a higher affinity than VEGFR-2, the majority of biological effects of VEGF-A on tumor endothelium are thought to be mediated through VEGFR-2. On ligand binding, VEGFR-2 dimerizes, resulting in activation of the tyrosine kinase and autophosphorylation of residues including Tyr^{951}, Tyr^{996}, Tyr^{1054}, Tyr^{1175}, and Tyr^{1214}.[141] Phosphorylation of these residues induces the activation of signal transduction molecules including PI3K, phospholipase C-g (PLC-g), Akt, Src, Ras, and mitogen-activated protein kinase (MAPK) (Fig. 11-3). Phosphorylation of Tyr^{1175} results in the binding and phosphorylation of PLC-g, which subsequently promotes the release of Ca^{2+} from internal stores and activation of protein kinase C (PKC). PKC activation and Ca^{2+} mobilization are considered critical for VEGF-A induced cell proliferation and nitric oxide production respectively.[142]

The PI3K pathway is paramount in the regulation of cell proliferation, survival, and migration. VEGF-A has been shown to promote phosphorylation of p85 subunit of PI3K and enhance PI3K enzymatic activity. The mechanism by which VEGF-A results in activation of PI3K remains unclear, although studies have implicated a role for Src kinases, b-catenin, and VE-cadherin.[143,144] VEGFR-2 induced activation of PI3K results in accumulation of phosphatidylinositol-3, 4,5-triphosphate (PIP_3), which induces phosphorylation of Akt/PKB. Once activated, Akt/PKB phosphorylates and thus inhibits proapoptotic proteins BAD, and caspase-9.

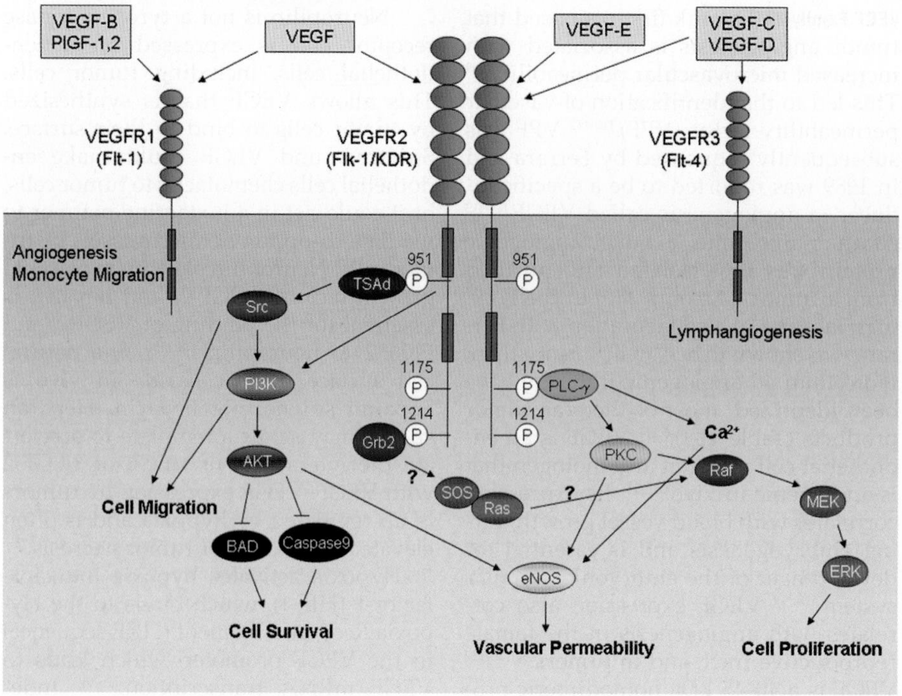

Figure 11-3 ■ VEGFR signal transduction. VEGF family members, VEGF, VEGF-B, VEGF-C, VEGF-D, VEGF-E, and PlGF bind 3 VEGFR tyrosine kinases, resulting in dimerization, receptor autophosphorylation, and activation of downstream pathways. Signal transduction via VEGFR2 is shown. Ligand binding to VEGFR2 activates signal-transduction molecules phospholipase C-γ (PLC-g), PI3K, Akt, Ras, Src, and MAPK and regulates cell proliferation, migration, survival, and vascular permeability.

Members of the Src family kinases, Src, Fyn, and Yes, are expressed in endothelial cells. Following VEGFR-2 autophosphorylation, T cell specific adapter (TSAd) binds Tyr[951] and then associates with Src. Src kinases control actin stress fiber organization and may mediate VEGF-A induced PI3K activation. Ligand binding to VEGFR-2 also initiates activation of the Ras pathway, triggering signaling through the Raf-1-MEK-ERK signal cascade[141] known to be important in growth factor-induced cell proliferation. This activation may occur through multiple routes.[141,145]

Biological Function of VEGF ■ In its initial discovery, VEGF was identified as a mediator of vessel permeability.[129,146] This capacity to render small veins and venules hyperpermeable is a critical function of VEGF. VEGF is indeed one of the most potent regulators of vascular permeability, and the observation that tumor-associated blood vessels are hyperpermeable is attributed to tumor-secreted VEGF. While the mechanisms by which VEGF increases microvascular permeability are incompletely understood, it may be at least in part due to VEGF-induced endothelial fenestrations,[119] opening of junctions between adjacent endothelial cells,[147] and through a calcium-dependent pathway involving nitric oxide (NO) production.[148-150]

In addition to its effect on vascular permeability, VEGF is a survival factor for endothelial cells, inhibiting endothelial cell apoptosis through activation of the PI3K-Akt pathway[151] and increasing in the anti-apoptotic protein bcl-2.[152] In vivo, VEGF blockade has been demonstrated to cause increases in apoptosis of immature, non-pericyte covered vessels.[153] VEGF is an endothelial cell mitogen though VEGFR-2-mediated signal transduction through Erk1/2 and JNK/SAPK as well as possibly protein kinase C.[152,154] While VEGF is not as potent an endothelial cell mitogen as other factors such as bFGF, VEGF has a broader range of activity for processes critical for angiogensis. VEGF induces expression of matrix-metalloproteinases and serine proteinases involved in degradation of the basement membrane, which is necessary for endothelial cell sprouting and invasion.[152] In addition, VEGF facilitates endothelial cell migration through FAK and p38 MAPK-induced actin reorganization.[3,147,152,155]

Circulating VEGF may be one of the angiogenic signals by which tumors recruit bone marrow derived cells, including endothelial progenitors and myeloid cells whose recruitment is thought to be mediated by VEGFR-2 and VEGFR-1, respectively.[156-160] A growing body of evidence suggests that VEGF-receptor bearing bone-marrow derived cells contribute to initiating tumor formation, by creating a "metastatic niche," and/or help promote tumor angiogenesis[56,57,161-163] although there appear to be VEGFR-1 independent mechanisms as well.[164] Circulating endothelial and myeloid cells are also being studied as potential biomarkers, as noted later in the chapter, and may contribute to resistance to VEGF pathway inhibitors.[165,166] It is worth noting that VEGF in the circulation may not all be tumor derived. VEGF serum concentrations closely correlate with platelet counts in cancer patients. VEGF is stored in platelets, transported, and released from them.[167] Furthermore, Pinedo and colleagues report that platelet counts have prognostic significance for cancer patients: higher platelet counts correlate with a worse prognosis.[168,169] Therefore, it is possible that for those types of tumors that recruit bone marrow-derived endothelial cells, communication from tumor to bone marrow may be mediated in part by the VEGF in circulating platelets.

Angiopoietins ■ Angiopoietin-1 is a 70 kDa ligand that binds to a specific tyrosine kinase expressed only on endothelial cells, called Tie2 (also called Tek). A ligand for Tie1 has not been elucidated.[133,170-173] Like VEGF, angiopoietin-1 is an endothelial cell specific growth factor. Angiopoietin-1, however, is not a direct endothelial mitogen in vitro. Rather, it induces endothelial cells to recruit pericytes and smooth muscle cells to become incorporated in the vessel wall. Pericyte and smooth muscle recruitment are mediated by endothelial production of PDGF-BB (and probably other factors) when Tie2 is activated by angiopoietin-1.[174] There is increased vascularization in mice that overexpress angiopoietin-1 in the skin.[173] The vessels are significantly larger than normal and the skin is reddened. The vessels are not leaky and there is no skin edema, in contrast to dermal vessels of mice overexpressing VEGF. In double transgenic mice expressing both angiopoietin-1 and VEGF in the skin, dermal angiogenesis is increased in an additive manner, but the vessels do not leak.[175] This model closely approximates angiogenesis in healing wounds (ie, relatively nonleaky vessels with pericytes and some perivascular smooth muscle cells contained in the vascular wall). In contrast, tumor vessels are leaky and thin-walled with a paucity of pericytes. Angiopoietin-2, produced by vascular endothelium in a tumor bed, blocks the Tie2 receptor and acts to repel pericytes and smooth muscle.[170] Nevertheless, tumor vessels remain thin "endothelium-lined tubes" even though some of these microvessels reach the diameter of venules. A key point is that angiopoietins and VEGF together play a role in angiogenesis, and the activity of both is context-dependent with different activities observed in angiogenic versus mature vessels. As an example, for rapidly proliferating endothelium, VEGF antagonism or withdrawal may result in apoptosis and microvessels regression; mature vessels appear to be much less dependent on this pathway.[175]

Other Soluble Factors Regulating Angiogenesis ■ Interleukin-8 (IL-8) is a proinflammatory chemotactic cytokine produced by monocytes, macrophages, and tumor cells.[176] IL-8 induces endothelial cell proliferation and chemotaxis as well as promotes endothelial cell survival.[176,177] The effects of IL-8 are mediated through interactions with 2 cell-surface G protein-coupled receptors, CXCR1 and CXCR2 and activation of subsequent downstream signaling molecules including PI3K and MAPK.[178] Hepatocyte growth factor/scatter factor (HGF/SF) is the ligand for c-Met.[179] Originally identified as a mitogen for primary cultured hepatocytes, HGF has since been shown to facilitate tumor angiogenesis. c-Met is expressed on endothelial cells, and activation by tumor-secreted HGF/SF augments matrix degradation and endothelial cell invasion.

Endogenous Inhibitors of Angiogenesis

Endogenous angiogenesis inhibitors block vascular endothelial cells from proliferating, migrating, or increasing their survival in response to a spectrum of proangiogenic proteins, including VEGF, bFGF, IL-8, PDGF, and PD-ECGF. Natural angiogenesis inhibitors include interferon-alfa (IFN-α), interleukin-12 (IL-12), platelet factor 4, TSP-1, angiostatin, endostatin, arrestin, canstatin, tumstatin, PEX (matrix metalloproteinase 2), pigment epithelium–derived factor, and antiangiogenic antithrombin III (an internal fragment of antithrombin III, named aaAT).[27,45,46 48,50,53,180,181]

The first clue to the existence of endogenous angiogenesis inhibitors came from the discovery that IFN-α inhibited endothelial cell migration and that platelet factor 4 inhibited endothelial proliferation.[182-184] Both were subsequently shown to inhibit angiogenesis.[182-186] However, Bouck was the first to show that a tumor could generate an angiogenesis inhibitor. Bouck and her colleagues subsequently proposed that the angiogenic phenotype was the result of a net balance of endogenous inhibitors and stimulators of angiogenesis.[187] A nontumorigenic hamster cell line became tumorigenic in association with the loss of a suppressor gene and concomitant with the onset of angiogenic activity. The nontumorigenic line secreted high levels of an angiogenesis inhibitor, a truncated form of TSP-1, that decreased by about 96% in the tumorigenic cells.[188] TSP-1 was shown to be regulated by the wild-type tumor suppressor *p53* in fibroblasts and in mammary epithelial cells.[189,190] Loss of p53 function in the transformed derivatives of these cells dramatically decreased the level of the angiogenesis inhibitor. Restoration of p53 upregulated TSP-1 and raised the antiangiogenic activity of the tumor cells. Deletion of TSP-1 led to accelerated growth of breast cancers that arise spontaneously in neu-transgenic mice.[191] The demonstration by Rastinejad and colleagues that the switch to an angiogenic phenotype involved a negative regulator of angiogenesis generated by the tumor per se suggested to Folkman a unifying angiogenic mechanism to explain a well-recognized but previously unsolved clinical and experimental phenomenon: the inhibition of tumor growth by the tumor mass. In this phenomenon, "the removal of certain tumors, eg, breast carcinomas, colon carcinomas, and osteogenic sarcomas can be followed by rapid growth of distant metastases."[192,193] Postoperative chemotherapy was introduced mainly to prevent or delay the growth of secondary metastases. Several studies in terminally ill patients demonstrated the suppression of a secondary tumor by a primary tumor.[194] A primary tumor can suppress metastases originating from a different type of tumor (eg, a breast cancer can inhibit melanoma metastases). In melanoma, partial spontaneous regression of the primary tumor may be followed by rapid growth of metastases, and when ionizing radiation is employed to regress a small cell lung cancer, distant metastases may undergo rapid growth.[53,195] Once it was demonstrated that a tumor could generate a negative regulator of angiogenesis, then it became clear that a primary tumor, while stimulating angiogenesis in its own vascular bed, could possibly inhibit angiogenesis in the vascular bed of a distant metastasis.[188] However, at least two conditions would be necessary: first, the primary tumor (ie, the first tumor to grow) would need to generate an angiogenic promoter in excess of an inhibitor in its own vascular bed, and, second, the putative inhibitor would need to have a longer half-life in the circulation than the angiogenic promoter. After arriving in the Folkman laboratory in 1991, O'Reilly and his colleagues validated this hypothesis by discovering angiostatin, endostatin, and antiangiogenic antithrombin over the next 8 years.[48-50,52,53]

Angiostatin ■ Angiostatin is a 38 kDa internal fragment of plasminogen that was purified from the serum and urine of mice bearing a subcutaneous Lewis lung carcinoma that suppressed growth of its lung metastases by inhibiting their angiogenesis (Fig. 11-4).[48] Angiostatin is not secreted by tumor cells but is generated through proteolytic cleavage of circulating plasminogen by a series of enzymes released from the tumor cells. At least one of these tumor-derived enzymes, urokinase plasminogen activator (uPA), converts plasminogen to plasmin, whereas a phosphoglycerate kinase from hypoxic tumor cells then reduces the plasmin so that it can be converted to angiostatin by one of several different metalloproteinases.[196] Other types of tumors have since been reported to generate angiostatin (eg, human prostate cancer).[197,198]

Angiostatin and its isoforms induce cell arrest and apoptosis of endothelial cells and inhibit endothelial migration, angiogenesis in vitro, and angiogenesis in the quail chorioallantoic membrane.[199-201] Angiostatin can also be generated by different enzymes and by other cell types; can inhibit other tumor types by its antiangiogenic action; can decrease activity of the MAPKs, ERK-1 and ERK-2 in endothelial cells; can upregulate E-selectin in proliferating endothelial cells; and can be delivered in vivo by gene therapy.[196,197,202-204] Angiostatin also binds specifically to adenosine triphosphate (ATP) synthase, a transmembrane protein expressed by vascular endothelial cells, and to a fragment of vitronectin. It can potentiate radiation therapy of experimental tumors.[205-208] It also appears to inhibit proliferation of circulating precursor endothelial cells derived from bone marrow.[209] Angiostatin effectively blocks endothelial cell migration induced by plasmin binding to a_vb_3-integrin.[210,211] Angiostatin may act at least in part by transiently increasing ceramide, a sphingolipid second messenger implicated in a proapoptotic pathway, and by increasing RhoA, an effector of cytoskeletal structure.[212] Other mechanisms of angiostatin have been reported. Angiostatin, but not plasminogen, specifically binds to tyrosine kinase substrate annexin II through the lysine-binding domain in endothelial cells.[213] Angiostatin inhibits signaling of HGF in endothelial cells (and smooth muscle cells) by blocking HGF-induced signaling of c-MET, Akt, and ERK-1/2,[214] and down-regulates expression of VEGF expression in tumor cells.[215] This implies that angiostatin may act as a direct and an indirect inhibitor of angiogenesis.

When angiostatin was delivered to mice bearing a variety of tumors, it showed significant efficacy either alone or in combination with endostatin, as a fusion protein of angiostatin and endostatin, or in combination with IL-12.[215-218] When 3 different types of murine tumors were engineered to produce granulocytemacrophage colony-stimulating factor (GM-CSF), the level of angiostatin in the serum increased 4-fold above

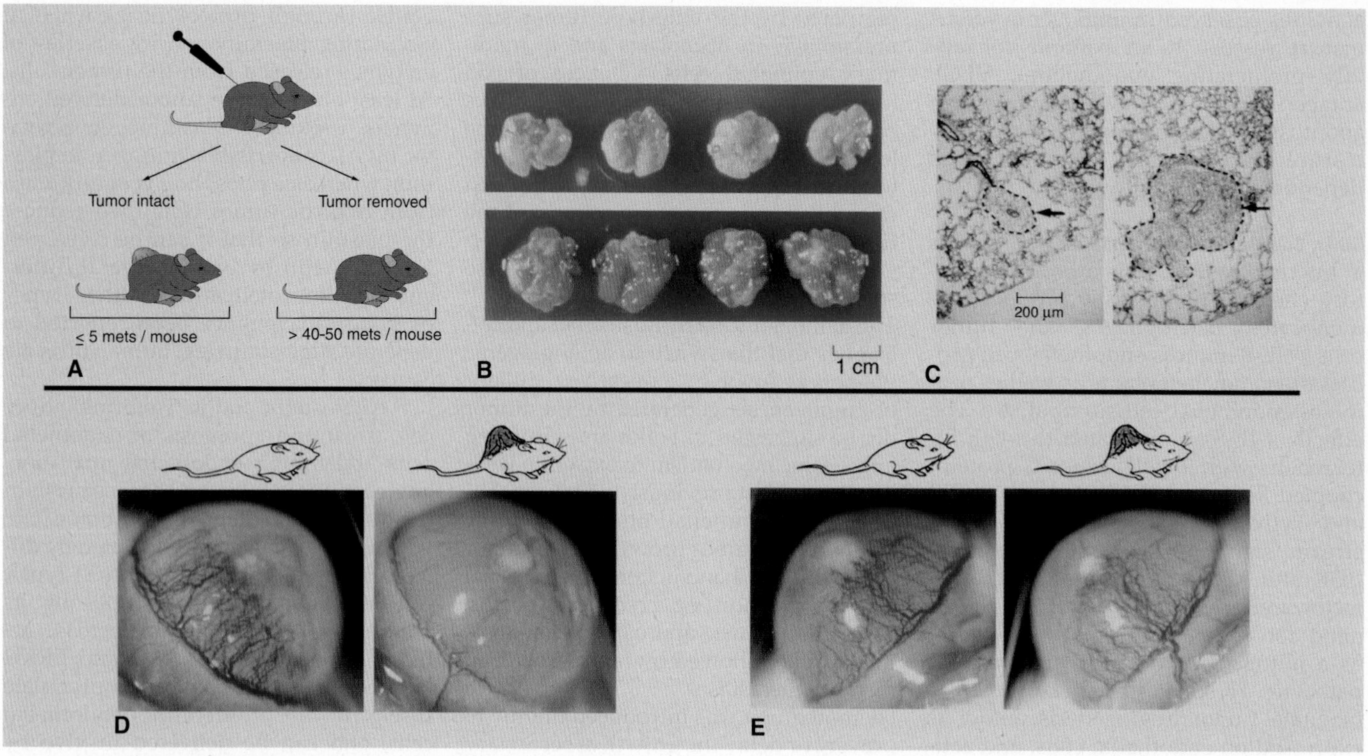

Figure 11-4 ■ (**A**) Mice bearing Lewis lung carcinoma.[448] Tumors were resected when tumor size reached 1.5-2 cm^2 and the animals were killed after 5 or 15 days. (**B**) *Upper panel*: lungs from animals still bearing the primary tumor. Lower panel: lungs removed at the same time from animals in which the tumor had been resected and the animals killed 15 days later. (**C**) *Left panel*: microscopic pulmonary metastasis in an animal in which a primary tumor is in place at the same time as the right panel. There is no evidence of angiogenesis as only a single central microvessel stained with antibody to von Willebrand factor. This dormant metastasis is approximately 200 microns in its longest diameter. Right panel: lung metastasis from an animal euthanized 5 days after the primary tumor was removed, showing 8 or 9 new vessels in an enlarging metastasis.[42] (**D**) A human prostate carcinoma (LNCaP) growing on the dorsum of a SCID mouse inhibits cornea neovascularization induced by an implanted sustained release pellet of bFGF (80 ng) (right panel). Left panel depicts bFGF-induced corneal neovascularization at 5 days in the absence of a primary tumor. LNCaP prostate cancer generates angiostatin. (**E**) A human colon cancer that does not produce an angiogenesis inhibitor, growing in a SCID mouse as a control for **D**.

controls and directly correlated with GM-CSF production.[219] Angiostatin levels directly correlated with macrophage metalloelastase production, which appeared to mediate cleavage of angiostatin from plasminogen. Metastases were suppressed in all 3 tumor systems.

Endostatin ■ A strategy similar to the one that uncovered angiostatin (eg, suppression of tumor growth by tumor mass) was employed by O'Reilly and colleagues with murine hemangioendothelioma and human small cell lung cancer to discover endostatin and aaAT.[50,52,53] Both endostatin and aaAT are generated from larger parent proteins by enzymes released by the tumor cells. Endostatin is a 20-22 kDa internal fragment of collagen XVIII.[50,52,220,221] It is the first of a group of endogenous angiogenesis inhibitors that are predominantly extracellular proteins, which generally require proteolytic processing to become active.[3,222] Like angiostatin, endostatin is a specific inhibitor of endothelial cell proliferation and migration.[223,224] At least two enzymes produced by tumor cells are necessary to cleave endostatin from collagen XVIII: an elastase and a cathepsin.[225,226] Endostatin is present in basement membranes and vessel walls and is especially rich in elastic fibers of the aorta and sparse elastic fibers of veins.[227]

Novel mechanisms have recently been reported for the antiangiogenic action of endostatin, although we are a long way from a complete picture. Endostatin blocks the binding of $VEGF_{121}$ and $VEGF_{165}$ to the KDR/Flk-1 receptor, blocks tyrosine phosphorylation of this receptor, and blocks activation of its intracellular signaling events, ERK, p38 MAPK, and p125FAK.[228] This receptor mediates endothelial cell motility and proliferation. Endostatin also blocks VEGF. Although endostatin does not bind to VEGF,[228] it does down-regulate VEGF expression in tumor cells (similar to the effect of angiostatin).[215] Endostatin can therefore be considered to act as both a direct and an indirect angiogenesis inhibitor. In bFGF-treated endothelial cells, endostatin induces endothelial cell apoptosis, in part by activating tyrosine kinase signaling of the Shb adaptor protein.[229] However, endostatin does not compete with binding of bFGF to tissues and does not affect bFGF receptor signaling.[230] Endothelial cell migration, which is critical for new sprout formation during angiogenesis, requires continuous turnover of cell–cell interactions and of cell–matrix interactions.[231] Endostatin prevents bFGF-induced or VEGF-induced loss of endothelial cell-cell adhesions or endothelial cell adhesion to basement membrane. Another antiangiogenic mechanism of endostatin in addition to its antiproliferative and antimotility effect on angiogenic endothelial cells is the stabilization of newly formed endothelial tubes. Endostatin decreases formation of VEGF-induced microvessels sprouting from aortic rings in vitro.[232] Endostatin also binds and inhibits the catalytic activity of MMP-2.[233,234] As a result, endothelial cell invasion is inhibited and tumor cell invasion may also be decreased. Endostatin also inhibits integrin-dependent endothelial cell migration because it binds to α_5- and α_v-integrins on the endothelial cell surface, in particular $\alpha_5\beta_1$.[235] It has been proposed that $\alpha_5\beta_1$-integrin may be a functional receptor for endostatin.[34]

A wide variety of tumors in many different laboratories have been inhibited by endostatin in mice and rats without evidence of toxicity or drug resistance.[236] These include lung adenocarcinoma, thyroid carcinoma, colon carcinoma, leukemia, human non-small cell lung cancer, human pancreatic cancer, human neuroblastoma, mammary cancer (soluble endostatin from *E. coli*), colon cancer metastases to the liver, spontaneous mouse mammary carcinoma (delayed onset, decreased tumor burden, and prolonged survival), and spontaneous pancreatic islet carcinomas.[237-244] Several interesting characteristics of endostatin make it advantageous for clinical use in cancer patients. First, it is not toxic.[245] At this time, endostatin is in phase 1 and 2 clinical trials, and, to date, it has been used in not more than approximately 120 patients. However, all centers report that there are virtually no side effects, even in patients who have been on endostatin injected daily subcutaneously without interruption for up to 3.5 years.

Tumstatin ■ Tumstatin (28 kDa) is the NC1 domain fragment of the α_3 collagen molecule and exhibits antiangiogenic activity in both the in vitro and in vivo assays.[54,246-249] Tumstatin (α_3(IV)NC1) binds to endothelial cells via $\alpha_v\beta_3$-integrin and $\alpha_6\beta_1$-integrin [54,246,248,249] and induces apoptosis of proliferating endothelial cells.[247] Cell biologic experiments demonstrated that the antiangiogenic activity of tumstatin is dependent on $\alpha_v\beta_3$-integrin binding on proliferating endothelial cells.[54,249] These experiments support the notion that through the action of endogenous inhibitors such as tumstatin, $\alpha_v\beta_3$-integrin could also function as a negative regulator of angiogenesis.[54,250-252]

Antiangiogenic Conformation of Antithrombin III ■ A human small cell lung carcinoma suppressed angiogenesis and tumor growth at remote sites in immunodeficient mice. These cells generated an enzyme in vitro that converted the 58 kDa conformation of circulating antithrombin III to a 53 kDa form of the protein in which the externally configured stressed loop of antithrombin was retracted into the body of the molecule.70 The 53 kDa "cleaved" form is a specific endothelial inhibitor and a potent angiogenesis inhibitor and has no thrombin binding activity. Antithrombin III has no anti-endothelial or antiangiogenic activity. The enzymes that induce this conformational change have not yet been elucidated. Human pancreatic cancer also generates the 53 kDa cleaved antiangiogenic antithrombin.[237]

Other Pathways Regulating Angiogenesis

Hypoxia Inducible Factor-1 ■ Expression of angiogenic factors including VEGF is positively regulated by hypoxia through the stabilization of the transcription factor HIF-1.[253,254] HIF-1 is a transcription factor comprised of 2 subunits, HIF-1α and HIF-1β. While HIF-1β is expressed constitutively, expression of HIF-1α is tightly regulated. The stability of HIF-1α is primarily controlled by hypoxia. When oxygen is abundantly present, prolyl hydroxylases modify proline residues 402 and 564 on HIF-1a allowing it to bind the VHL tumor suppressor gene, which targets it for degradation.[254] Following binding of the HIF-1α and -β subunits, HIF-1 transverses to the nucleus and modulates the expression of numerous genes involved in angiogenesis, cell survival, invasion, and glucose metabolism.[254] Indeed, HIF-1α is thought to be the key regulator of potent proangiogenic factors including VEGF.

Although initially thought to be primarily regulated by hypoxia, recent studies have revealed a number of non-hypoxic regulators including receptor tyrosine kinases such as EGFR,[255] the PI3K/AKT/mTOR pathway; and metabolic pathways including the tricarboxylic acid (Krebs) cycle (reviewed in Refs. [256, 257]). Alterations in these pathways have been shown to contribute to inherited cancer syndromes, highlighting their role in carcinogenesis. For example, germline mutations in the VHL gene underlying Von-Hippel Lindau disease, leads to a markedly elevated risk of developing renal cell carcinoma (RCC), hemangioblastomas of the CNS, and other tumor types. The VHL protein encoded by this gene is part of protein complex that targets HIFs for degradation.[256] Sporadic mutations in the VHL gene also occur in sporadic clear-cell RCC. A second syndrome, hereditary leiomyomatosis and RCC, results from mutations in the fumarate hydratase (FH) gene.[258] FH is a mitochondrial protein involved in the TCA cycle. Although the mechanism(s) by which FH mutations promote tumorigenesis are still under investigation, it appears that loss of FH function results in an increase in HIFs by causing a buildup of intracellular fumarate, which inhibits the enzymes (HIF hydroxylases, also known as EGLNs) that hydroxylate HIFs and target them for VHL-mediated degradation. A third hereditary syndrome, tuberous sclerosis complex, is caused by mutations in the tuberous sclerosis complex, resulting in elevated HIFs via the mTOR pathway.[259,260] Several other syndromes have also been identified that resulted in elevated levels of HIFs and downstream HIF-regulated gene products, causing a "pseudohypoxic" state.[257,259] The observations that multiple inherited cancer syndromes involve pathways that converge on HIFs support the hypothesis that dysregulation of the pathways regulating angiogenesis are likely to play a role in driving early tumorigenesis. Several drugs targeting HIFs are currently in clinical development.

Oncogenes as Regulators of Angiogenesis

It is widely established that activation of proto-oncogenes can induce tumorigenesis. In tissue culture, expression of activated oncogenes increases cell proliferation and decreases apoptosis.[261] While these changes contribute to tumorigenesis by altering the equilibrium between cell proliferation and apoptosis, there is considerable evidence that this alone is not sufficient to produce expansive tumor growth.[262,263] Rather, tumors must also acquire an adequate vascular supply to grow beyond 1-2 mm in diameter. In support of this concept, published reports have demonstrated that transfection of tumor cells with oncogenes results in enhanced production of proangiogenic molecules,[264] and the in vivo growth of oncogene-driven tumors can be restricted with angiogenesis inhibitors.[265] In lung cancer patients, eg, mutations in K-Ras, p53, and epidermal growth factor receptor (EGFR) are among the oncogenes that have been linked to angiogenesis. Oncogenes shown to play a role in regulating angiogenic factors include Ras, p53, Myc, and EGFR.

Ras ■ Ras is one of the most commonly activated oncogenes, occurring in 17-25% of all human tumors.[266] In tissue culture studies, transfection of transformed murine endothelial cells with the Ras oncogene results in elevated production of VEGF, and treatment of these cells with the PI3K inhibitor, wortmannin, abrogates VEGF expression, indicating that mutated Ras regulates VEGF expression in a PI3K dependent manner.[267] K-Ras gene mutations were positively associated with high VEGF expression in human non-small cell lung cancer (NSCLC) specimens[268] and other disease types. More direct evidence for the involvement of Ras in regulation of angiogenesis comes from a transgenic model of melanoma, in which down-regulation of the Ras oncogene in a melanoma driven by doxycycline-inducible Ras led to massive apoptosis of microvascular endothelium in the tumor bed starting within 6 hours. Tumor cells began to die days later, and large tumors had completely disappeared by 12 days.[269]

p53 ■ In addition to its role in the regulation of cell cycle and apoptosis, emerging data indicates that p53 indirectly promotes tumor vascularization by altering the expression of proangiogenic and antiangiogenic molecules. In tissue culture studies, fibroblasts expressing wild-type p53 secrete high levels of the antiangiogenic glycoprotein, TSP-1. However, loss of wild-type p53 and expression of the mutant form results in diminished TSP-1 mRNA and protein.[189] Furthermore, in fibroblasts transfected with a temperature sensitive form of p53 display a mutant phenotype at 37°C and a wild-type phenotype at 32.5°C, while VEGF expression is elevated in mutant but not wild-type p53 expressing cells.[270] In support of the hypothesis that wild-type p53 regulates angiogenesis in human cancers, immunohistochemical evaluation of 73 NSCLC clinical specimens revealed a strong statistical association between p53 nuclear localization and microvessel count.[271] Additionally, in an analysis of 107 NSCLC patients, p53 was determined to be significantly associated with VEGF expression and microvessel count.[272] It is likely that loss of wild-type p53 elaborates tumor cell expression of additional proangiogenic factors in NSCLC. Wild-type p53 has been demonstrated to promote Mdm2-mediated ubiquitination and degradation of HIF-1α.[273] The loss of wild-type p53 is associated with elevated levels of HIF-1α in tissue culture and augments hypoxia-induced VEGF expression.[273]

Myc ■ Myc is a pleiotropic transcription factor overexpressed in many cancer types that plays a role in regulating angiogenesis, inflammation, and many other processes. Myc activity has been shown to be regulated by Ras pathway activation[264] that in turn regulates angiogenesis at least in part through effects on TSP-1. Myc has also been shown to interact with the HIF-1α pathway to induce angiogenesis by an hypoxia- independent mechanism[274] and regulate the recruitment of mast cells required for myc-driven tumorigenesis in a transgenic mouse model.[275]

EGFR Family ■ EGFR is a member of the erbB family of receptor tyrosine kinases, which also includes HER2/Neu, HER3 (ErbB3), and HER4 (ErbB4). An expanding body of evidence indicates that activation of EGFR leads to enhanced production of proangiogenic molecules. Initial experiments using prostate cancer cell lines demonstrated that stimulation of tumor cells with EGF elevated HIF-1a expression.[276] EGF has been shown to increase VEGF production in some tumor cell lines[277,278] and, conversely, treatment of tumor cells with EGFR inhibitors can decrease VEGF expression in various tumor types.[255,278-280] In NSCLC cell lines, EGF activates HIF-1α and induces expression of the chemokine receptor CXCR4 in tissue culture.[245] Moreover, in an immunohistochemical study of 172 NSCLC patients, expression of EGFR was associated with HIF-1α positivity.[281]

Like EGFR, HER2/Neu has also been shown to play a role in regulating angiogenesis. Blockade of HER2 using the monoclonal antibody trastuzumab (Herceptin) has been shown to block the production of multiple angiogenic factors and induce vessel normalization and regression in an murine model of human breast cancer, and enhance the effects of VEGF pathway blockade.[282,283]

Therapeutic Approaches to Targeting Tumor Vasculature

Angiogenesis Inhibitors versus Vascular Targeting Agents

Angiogenesis is the formation of new vessels from preexisting vasculature. Angiogenesis inhibitors are therefore typically targeted at the early stages in this process, including endothelial sprouting and survival mechanisms, which are often VEGF-dependent. Vascular targeting agents (VTAs), also known as vascular disrupting agents (VDAs), differ from angiogenesis inhibitors in that they target established abnormal tumor vasculature.[284] VTAs can induce rapid collapse of tumor vasculature, and their effects on normal vasculature can cause a host of side effects including acute coronary syndromes, thrombophlebitis, and tumor pain. None of these agents is currently in routine clinical use for cancer but several are currently in advanced clinical testing including AS1404, which is currently in phase 3 trials for NSCLC.

Antiangiogenic Effects of Chemotherapy and Other Therapeutic Agents

Multiple preclinical studies have suggested that several "classical" chemotherapeutic agents may also have potent antiangiogenic or vascular-targeting effects. Preclinical studies suggest that low dose, frequent dosing schedules ("metronomic dosing") may enhance the antiangiogenic effects of chemotherapy.[285-287] Several of these regimens are undergoing clinical evaluation. It also appears that among chemotherapy drugs, certain agents—particularly taxanes and vinca alkaloids—may have relatively more potent antiangiogenic effects than other drugs[287] that may help explain why there are differences in the degree of enhancement observed when antiangiogenic agents such as bevacizumab are added to chemotherapy. This prompted further examination of a wide variety of drugs, which were initially thought to target primarily tumor cells. Many of these were subsequently found to have antiangiogenic effects, prompting the term "accidental antiangiogenics."[288]

Targeting VEGF Pathway

VEGF is the prototypic member of a family of structurally related, homodimeric growth factors that includes placental growth factor (PlGF), VEGF-B, VEGF-C, VEGF-D, and VEGF-E. As described earlier, VEGF family members bind to a family of transmembrane receptor tyrosine kinases that include VEGFR-1 (Flt-1), VEGFR-2 (KDR, Flk-1), and VEGFR-3 (Flt-4) (Fig. 11-3). The effects of VEGF or VEGFR on vascular permeability and endothelial proliferation, migration, and survival are thought to be primarily mediated by VEGFR-2 while VEGFR-3 is primarily expressed on lymphatic endothelium (reviewed in Refs. [141,148]). Agents targeting the VEGF pathway include monoclonal antibodies that bind the ligand (ie, bevacizumab) or block the receptor (IMC-1121b), as well as small molecule receptor tyrosine kinase inhibitors (RTKIs) such as PTK787, ZD6474, and SU11248. Because of the structural similarity of the different receptor tyrosine kinase domains, RTKIs typically inhibit multiple receptors. These profiles of receptor specificity for each inhibitor, as well as their pharmacokinetics and potency for receptor inhibition, are likely to be the key determinants of their clinical activity. Representative agents targeting the VEGF pathway that are currently in clinical testing are listed in Table 11-2.

Combinations of Antiangiogenics with Chemotherapy: Mechanisms for Enhanced Antitumor Activity

Preclinical and clinical studies have demonstrated that antiangiogenic therapy improves the outcome of cytotoxic therapies.[289,290] This finding is paradoxical. It was initially expected that targeting the tumor vasculature would drastically diminish the delivery of oxygen and therapeutics to the solid tumor, producing hypoxia that would cause many chemotherapeutics, as well as radiation, to be less effective.[289,290] Tumor vasculature is known to be structurally and functionally abnormal, with tortuous, highly permeable vessels. Blood flow within these intra-tumoral vessels is nonuniform. Proliferating tumor cells compress blood and lymphatic vessels resulting in a microenvironment typified by interstitial hypertension (elevated hydrostatic pressure outside the blood vessels), acidosis, and hypoxia.[291,292] This deficient vascular network and interstitial hypertension impairs drug delivery to tumor cells. Moreover, hypoxia renders tumor cells resistant to radiation and several cytotoxic agents, and increases genetic instability selecting tumor cells that have a greater metastatic potential. In addition to the direct effects on tumor cells, hypoxia leads to vascular abnormalization by signaling via PHD2 in tumor endothelial cells[293] and, along with the low pH within the tumor microenvironment, weakens the cytotoxic functions of tumor infiltrating immune cells. Collectively, the abnormal vasculature within solid tumors creates

Table 11-2 VEGF Pathway Inhibitors in Clinical Development

Type	Agent	Target	Phase of Development
Monoclonal antibody	Bevacizumab (Avastin)	VEGF-A	Phase 3-4; FDA approved for CRC, breast cancer, and NSCLC
	IMC-1121B	VEGFR-2 extracellular domain	Phase 3
Soluble decoy receptor	VEGF Trap	VEGF-A, VEGF-B and PIGF	Phase 3
Antisense Oligonucleotide	VEGF-AS (Veglin)	VEGF, VEGF-C, VEGF-D	Phase 1
Peptide	Dehydrodidemnin B (Aplidin)	VEGF	FDA approved for MM
Adnectin	CT-332	VEGFR-2	Phase 2
RTKIs	Vandetanib	VEGFR-2, EGFR, and RET	Phase 3
	Sorafenib	VEGFR-2 and 3, PDGFR-β, Flt-3, c-Kit, and B-Raf	Phase 3; FDA approved for renal cell and hepatocellular cancers
	AZD2171 (cediranib)	VEGFR-1,2,3 and c-Kit	Phase 3
	Sunitinib	VEGFR-1, 2, PDGFR, c-Kit, RET, and Flt-3	Phase 2/3; FDA approved for renal cell carcinoma and gastrointestinal stromal tumors
	AG-013736 (axitinib)	VEGFR-1,2,3, and PDGFR	Phase 3
	AMG 706	VEGFR-1,2,3, PDGFR, and c-Kit	Phase 2
	Vatalanib	VEGFR-1,2,3, PDGFR, c-Kit	Phase 3
	BIBF 1120	VEGFR-1,2,3, PDGFR, FGFR-1/3	Phase 3
	CEP-7055	VEGFR1,2,3	Phase 1
	CHIR258	VEGFR1,2 and FGFR1,3	Phase 1
	GW786034 (pazopanib)	VEGFR2	Phase 3
	OSI-930	VEGFR, c-Kit	Phase 1 solid tumors
	BMS-582664	VEGFR2, FGFR	Phase 1
	XL184	VEGFR-2, MET, RET	Phase 3

Abbreviations: AML, acute myelogenous leukemia; CRC, colorectal cancer; EGFR, Epidermal growth factor receptor; FDA, Food and Drug Administration; GBM, glioblastoma multiforme; MM, multiple myeloma; NSCLC, non-small cell lung cancer; PIGF, placental growth factor; PDGFR, platelet-derived growth factor receptor; RCC, renal cell carcinoma; RTKI, small molecule receptor tyrosine kinase inhibitor; VEGF, vascular endothelial growth factor; VEGFR, vascular endothelial growth factor receptor.

a significant barrier to delivery and efficacy of cancer therapeutics.

One proposed mechanism to explain the enhancement in efficacy of chemotherapy by antiangiogenic therapy is that these agents have the potential to "normalize" tumor vessels. In animal models of cancer, inhibition of VEGF signaling results in a vasculature network that more closely resembles vessels within normal tissue. This "normalized" vasculature is less leaky, less dilated, and has less tortuous vessels with a more normal basement membrane and increased pericyte coverage. Concurrent with these changes in vascular morphology, within the tumor there is a decrease in IFP, increased oxygenation, and improved delivery of concurrently administered chemotherapeutics (Fig. 11-5).[294-302] Evidence from a phase 1/2 clinical trial in locally advanced rectal carcinoma patients receiving bevacizumab and chemotherapy (with radiation) corroborate with preclinical findings. Bevacizumab treatment was associated with a decrease in tumor IFP and an increase in mature, pericyte-covered vessels.[303,304]

Antiangiogenic Agents in Combination With Radiotherapy

A growing body of evidence suggests that antiangiogenic therapy may enhance the efficacy of radiotherapy for solid tumors. There are several proposed mechanisms through which this enhancement may occur. First, radiotherapy may act by "normalizing" the disorganized and hyperpermeable vasculature in tumors.[289,305] Vessel normalization would permit a more effective delivery of oxygen to tumor tissue, resulting in a reduction in tumor hypoxia and augmenting radiation-induced cytotoxicity in part by increasing the formation of oxygen free radicals. This reduction in hypoxia may be transient, however, as prolonged use of antiangiogenic agents may eventually also reduce the "normalized" vessels within tumors resulting in an inadequate intra-tumoral vascular supply, such that the tumor would again be hypoxic with reduced radiosensitivity. This concept is supported by mouse xenografts showing the existence of a period of time ("normalization window") during which radiation therapy used in conjunction with an antiangiogenic agent is most effective.[301,306]

Antiangiogenic therapy may act to enhance the anti-endothelial effects of radiotherapy. While it was initially assumed that the antitumor effect of radiotherapy was due to direct action on tumor cells, more recent evidence has demonstrated that radiotherapy also induces endothelial cell apoptosis.[306-308] Other studies have confirmed these results.[309] Thus, the exact mechanism(s) of interaction between antiangiogenic agens and radiation remains unclear.

Nevertheless, several preclinical studies demonstrating that antiangiogenic agents can synergize with or potentiate the effects of radiotherapy.[205,206,310-312] There are several credible explanations for the effect. As aforementioned, VEGF is a survival factor for endothelial cells. Thus, blockade of VEGF signaling on endothelial cells renders the tumor-associated vasculature more sensitive to radiotherapy. In addition, radiation induces VEGF expression which then contributes to radioresistance by blocking radiation-induced endothelial cell apoptosis.[313,314]

One possible cause for concern in testing combinations of antiangiogenic therapy and radiotherapy is the observation from preclinical studies that at least some of the toxicities of radiotherapy such as intestinal radiation damage may also be due to endothelial apoptosis.[315] In lung cancer patients treated with the combination of bevacizumab, chemotherapy, and radiotherapy, trachea-esophageal fistulas have been observed.[316] Clearly additional studies will be needed to assess the feasibility and efficacy of these combinations.

Clinical Advances in the Use of Antiangiogenic Therapy

The hypothesis that tumor angiogenesis could serve as a target for cancer therapy is now strongly supported by results of a number of randomized phase 3 clinical trials across multiple, different tumor types (Table 11-3). As discussed below, bevacizumab, a monoclonal antibody targeting VEGF, is now a standard therapy for metastatic colorectal, non-small cell lung, breast, and other tumor types,[317,318] VEGFR tyrosine kinase inhibitors (TKIs) such as sunitinib and sorafenib are now approved for RCC and other diseases.[319,320] These coupled with our increased understanding of the biological pathways underlying tumor angiogenesis and the development of improved agents for targeting these pathways, have led to a dramatic increase in the number of clinical trials employing antiangiogenic therapy either alone or in combination with other therapeutic modalities. Currently, the majority of these agents target the VEGF

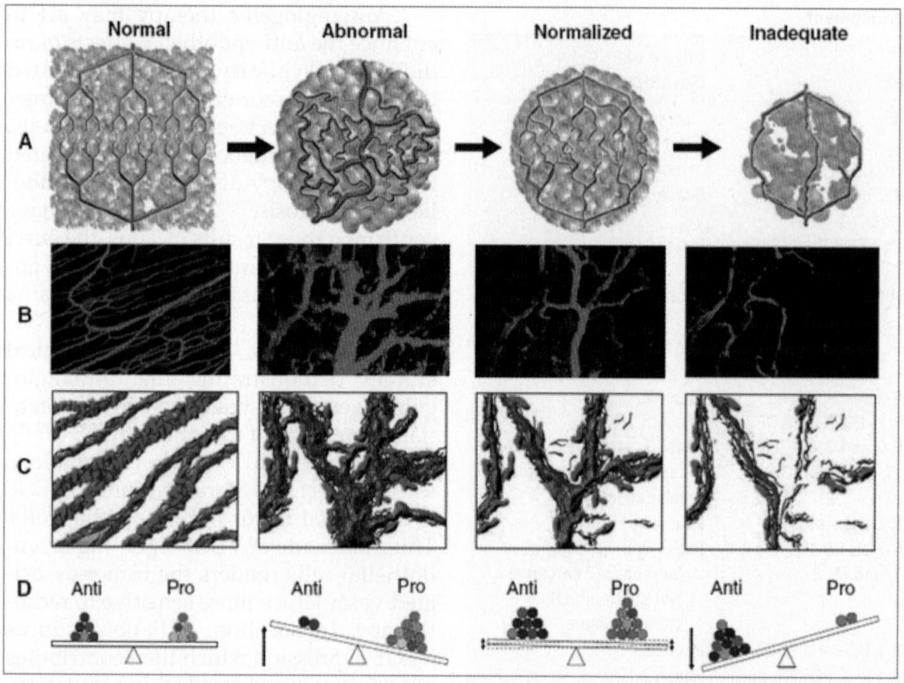

Figure 11-5 Changes in tumor vasculature during treatment with antiangiogenic agents.[289] (**A**) The tumor vascular network is structurally and functionally abnormal. Antiangiogenic therapies might initially improve both the structure and the function of tumor vessels. Continued or aggressive antiangiogenic regimens may eventually result in a vascular supply that is inadequate to support tumor growth. (**B**) Vascular normalization due to inhibition of VEGFR2. On the left is a two-photon image depicting normal blood vessels in skeletal muscle; subsequent representative images show human colon carcinoma vasculature in mice C at day 0, 3, and 5 after treatment with a VEGR2-specific antibody. (**C**) Diagram illustrating the concomitant changes in basement membrane (blue) and pericyte (red) coverage during vessel normalization. (**D**) These changes in the vasculature may reflect changes in the balance of proangiogenic and antiangiogenic factors in the microenvironment.

pathway because of its role as a key regulator of tumor angiogenesis.

VEGF Pathway Inhibitors as Anticancer Therapy: Clinical Experience

Clinical trials of one of the earliest VEGF pathway inhibitors, bevacizumab, began in 1997. When used as monotherapy for the treatment of advanced solid tumors, the clinical activity of these agents, as judged by objective tumor responses, has generally been low with the exception of RCC. For example, no partial or complete remissions were observed in 25 patients treated in a phase 1 trial of bevacizumab.[321] Furthermore, in 243 previously treated patients with colorectal cancer, there was a 3% objective response rate for bevacizumab monotherapy, compared to 9.2% for FOLFOX4 chemotherapy and 21.8% for the combination. Low response rates have also been reported for VEGFR TKIs when used as single agents as discussed below. For this reason, VEGF pathway inhibitors have often been developed as part of combination regimen with chemotherapy or other targeted therapeutics. Major findings in the clinical development of VEGF pathway inhibitors for several common tumor types are reviewed below.

Renal Cell Cancer

One tumor type for which VEGF pathway inhibitors appear to be particularly promising, even when used as monotherapy, is metastatic RCC. These tumors are often marked by inactivation of the von Hippel-Lindau gene leading to VEGF overexpression (reviewed in Ref. [322]). In randomized studies, both bevacizumab and sorafenib have been shown to significantly prolong time to progression compared to placebo controls.[323,324] Sunitinib also demonstrated substantial antitumor activity in metastatic RCC, with a 40% objective response rate in phase 2 testing.[325]

After initial phase 2 trials suggested the potential for therapeutic activity in renal cell cancers, phase 3 trials evaluated anti-VEGF therapies either alone or in combination with other targeted or biological agents. Cytokine therapies (IFN-α- and IL-2-based therapies) have long been the mainstay of therapy for renal cell cancers, so it was rational to evaluate anti-VEGF therapy in the context of such agents. Phase 3 trials examining 2 small molecule RTKIs of VEGF receptors (sorafenib and sunitinib) as well as monoclonal anti-VEGF therapy (bevacizumab) have now been reported, and consistently favor the addition of (or replacement with) anti-VEGF therapy to standard cytokine therapy, or the addition of anti-VEGF therapy following cytokine therapy.

Trials of Anti-VEGF Therapy versus Cytokine Therapy ■ Motzer and colleagues compared the use of sunitinib (at a dose of 50 mg orally daily for 4 weeks, followed by 2 weeks without treatment) or IFN-α (9 MU subcutaneously 3 times weekly) in patients with previously untreated, metastatic RCC.[320] The primary endpoint of progression-free survival (PFS) was significantly improved in patients receiving sunitinib (11 vs 5 months, $p < 0.001$). Patients receiving sunitinib also experienced higher response rates and improved quality of life.

Trials of Cytokine Therapy With or Without Anti-VEGF Therapy ■ Escudier et al.[326] performed a placebo-controlled phase 3 trial comparing the use of IFN-α-2a to IFN-α-2a plus bevacizumab in patients with previously untreated metastatic renal cell cancer. PFS was significantly longer (10.2 vs 5.4 months, $p = 0.0001$) in patients receiving the combined biologic approach. At the time of publication, survival analysis was immature but trended in favor of the bevacizumab-containing arm.

Trials of Anti-VEGF Therapy Following Cytokine Therapy ■ Escudier et al.[319] performed a phase 3 trial of sorafenib (400 mg twice daily) versus a placebo in patients who had progressed following first-line cytokine therapy for advanced renal cell cancer. Median PFS was 5.5 months in the sorafenib group and 2.8 months in the placebo group ($p < 0.01$). An initial analysis of overall survival showed that sorafenib reduced the risk of death (hazard ratio, 0.72; 95% CI, 0.54-0.94; $p = 0.02$), although this benefit was not statistically significant using the O'Brien–Fleming method.

Therapy Following Initial Anti-VEGF Treatment ■ The demonstration of a beneficial effect for anti-VEGF therapy in renal cell cancer has fundamentally altered the treatment landscape for this disease. Nevertheless, anti-VEGF therapy is not curative and only modestly prolongs survival, leaving room for substantial therapeutic improvement. A recent evaluation by Tamaskar et al.[327] suggests that patients progressing on one VEGF-targeting agent may still respond to another. Whether this cross-sensitivity is a function of the promiscuity of RTKIs such as sunitinib and sorafenib, or of differential pharmacokinetics, or of varying affinities for VEGF receptors, is unknown.

Table 11-3 **Selective Phase 3 Studies of Approved Antiangiogenic Agents**

Tumor Type	Regimen	n	Primary Endpoint	HR (Primary Endpoint)	Median OS (m)	Median PFS (m)	ORR, %	References
Colorectal (previously untreated)	IFL + placebo	411	OS		15.6	6.2	34.8	317
	IFL + BV	402		0.66	20.3**	10.6**	44.8*	
Colorectal (previously treated)	FOLFOX4	286	OS		10.8	4.7	8.6	331
	FOLFOX4 + BV	291		0.75	12.9*	7.3**	22.7**	
	BV	243			10.2	2.7	3.3	
NSCLC (previously untreated, non-squamous)	PC	444	OS		10.3	4.5	15	318
	PC+BV	434		0.79	12.3	6.2	35	
Breast cancer (previously treated)	PCI	241	PFS			8.0	44	365
	PC + BV 7.5	248		0.79	NR	8.7*	55	
	PC + BV 15	247		0.72	NR	8.8*	63	
Breast cancer (previously untreated)	Paclitaxel	354	PFS		25.2	5.9	21.2	363
	Paclitaxel + BV	368		0.60	26.7	11.8**	36.9**	
RCC (previously untreated)	IFN	363	OS		NR	5.2	13.1	436
	IFN + BV	369		NR	NR	8.5**	25.5**	
RCC (previously untreated)	IFN-α	375	PFS		NR	11	6	320
	Sunitinib	375		0.42	NR	5	31**	
RCC (previously treated)	Placebo	452	OS		15.9	2.8	2	319
	Sorafenib	451		0.72	19.3	5.5	10	
Hepatocellular Carcinoma (previously untreated)	Placebo		OS, SFP		7.9	4.1†	1	367
	Sorafenib			0.69	10.7**	4.9†	2	

*$p < 0.05$, **$p < 0.001$, †Results for symptomatic free progression.

Abbreviations: BV, bevacizumab, IFL, irinotecan, bolus fluorouracil, and leucovorin, FOLFOX 4, fluorouracil, oxaliplatin, leucovorin, HR =Hazard Ratio, IFN, interferon, NR, not reported, NSCLC, non-small cell lung carcinoma, PC, paclitaxel and carboplatin, PFS, progression-free survival, OS, overall survival, ORR, objective response rate, RCC, renal cell carcinoma, SFP, symptomatic free progression.

mTOR Inhibition in Renal Cell Cancer ■ Two recent trials[328,329] have recently examined the role of mTOR inhibition in patients with advanced renal cell cancer. While mTOR has several biologic roles, one is as a downstream effector of VEGF signaling. In a trial comparing the mTOR inhibitor temsirolimus versus IFN-α versus the combination of temsirolimus plus IFN-a as front-line therapy, Hudes et al.[330] demonstrated the superiority of temsirolimus to IFN-α, with a significant improvement in overall survival (10.9 vs 7.3 months, p = 0.008); the combination arm was not superior to IFN monotherapy. In addition, the temsirolimus group had fewer serious adverse events than the IFN-α group. In a placebo-controlled randomized phase 3 trial in the post-VEGF tyrosine kinase inhibition setting, the mTOR inhibitor everolimus significantly prolonged PFS when compared to placebo (4 vs 1.9 months, $p < 0.001$).[331] Overall survival was not significantly different, perhaps due to the fact that crossover was allowed for patients progressing on placebo. Though toxicities were generally mild, significant increases in severe (grade 3 or 4) toxicities were seen for stomatitis, $p = 0.03$; infections, $p = 0.03$; hypercholesterolaemia, $p = 0.03$; hyperglycaemia, $p < 0.0001$; lymphopenia, $p = 0.002$; and hypophosphataemia, $p = 0.01$.

Antiangiogenic Therapy as Adjuvant Therapy in Renal Cell Cancer ■ The advent of multiple active antiangiogenic agents in an amazingly brief period has led to the development of several adjuvant trials in renal cell cancer. These include: E2805, a double-blind placebo-controlled trial comparing sunitinib, sorafenib, and no active therapy; the SORCE trial, which compares sorafenib with a placebo for 1, 2, or 3 years of therapy; and the STAR trial, which compares sunitinib to placebo as adjuvant therapy in high-risk renal cancer. These trials, if positive, will mark a turning point in the history of this disease.

Prediction of Therapeutic Benefit in Renal Cell Cancer ■ Currently there is no reproducible means of predicting response to therapy for anti-VEGF agents in renal cell cancer. Curiously, and perhaps surprisingly, a recent analysis of patients treated with anti-VEGF therapy for metastatic renal cell cancer failed to demonstrate a statistically significant increase in response in patients with *VHL* inactivation.[330]

Future Directions in Renal Cell Cancer ■ The existence of multiple agents targeting the same general pathways raises the question of whether such agents could be useful combined in a "horizontal" approach to the VEGF pathway. While several ongoing trials are examining this approach, an instructive example of this general approach is the ongoing E2804 trial, a randomized phase 2 comparison of bevacizumab versus temsirolimus plus bevacizumab versus bevacizumab plus sorafenib versus sorafenib plus temsirolimus. This trial will examine both toxicity and efficacy issues for the "horizontal" combinations.

Colorectal Cancer

Advanced colorectal cancer represented the first human cancer in which a phase 3 trial demonstrated clinical benefit, and to this day represents among the best studied of human solid tumors with regard to antiangiogenic therapy. In 2004, results of a phase 3, randomized, placebo-controlled study were reported comparing standard IFL chemotherapy (irinotecan, fluorouracil, and leucovorin) with or without bevacizumab in patients with previously untreated metastatic colorectal cancer.[317] Patients treated with IFL plus bevacizumab had a significantly longer overall survival and PFS as well a higher overall response rate (Table 11-3). This trial provided definitive evidence that the addition of an angiogenesis inhibitor to chemotherapy could prolong survival and, based on the results of this trial, bevacizumab received approval from the U.S. Food and Drug Administration for use in combination with fluorouracil-containing chemotherapy as first-line treatment for metastatic colorectal cancer.

Subsequent studies have built upon this original finding. In a trial of previously treated patients with colorectal cancer, patients treated with bevacizumab combined with FOLFOX4 chemotherapy (fluorouracil, oxaliplatin, leucovorin) had a prolonged survival compared to those treated with FOLFOX4 alone[331] although the magnitude of this benefit (2.1 months) appeared to be smaller than that observed in the first-line trial (4.7 months), presumably related to the more advanced nature of the disease.

The first adjuvant trial of anti-VEGF therapy to be reported, the NSABP C-08 trial, randomized patients with colorectal cancer to receive either a standard chemotherapy regimen, or to receive chemotherapy plus bevacizumab, with the latter being administered for a total of one year. As recently reported at the 2009 American Society of Clinical Oncology meetings, the addition of bevacizumab to chemotherapy did not result in a statistically significant improvement in the primary study endpoint of disease-free survival. The reasons for this failure are uncertain, but suggest that much is yet to be learned regarding the role of anti-VEGF therapy as adjuvant therapy. N. Wolmark, G. Yothers, M. J. O'Connell, S. Sharif, J. N. Atkins, T. E. Seay, L. Feherenbacher, S. O'Reilly, C. J. Allegra A phase III trial comparing mFOLFOX6 to mFOLFOX6 plus bevacizumab in stage II or III carcinoma of the colon: Results of NSABP Protocol C-08 ASCO Meeting Abstracts Jun 20 2009: LBA4

Preclinical data had previously suggested that the combination of EGFR-targeted therapy plus anti-VEGF therapy might result in superior antitumor activity. This hypothesis was directly examined in two phase 3 trials. In the first of these, the PACCE trial, previously untreated metastatic colorectal cancer patients were randomized to receive fluorouracil, leucovorin, bevacizumab and irinotecan or oxaliplatin, with or without the pan-HER inhibitor panitumumab. This trial was prematurely halted due to decreased PFS and increased toxicity in panitumumab-treated patients in the oxliplatin portion of the trial.[332] A second phase 3 trial (the CAIRO2 trial) evaluated the addition of cetuximab to bevacizumab in the context of capecitabine and oxaliplatin chemotherapy for previously untreated metastatic colorectal cancer. Regrettably, this trial similarly demonstrated both inferior PFS and quality of life for patients receiving combined biologic therapy. Response rate and overall survival were not significantly altered by the addition of anti-EGFR therapy.[333] A biologic explanation for these results is currently awaited.

Biomarker analyses of colorectal cancer trials have been largely unavailing. Expression levels of VEGF-A, TSP, and microvessel density performed in a subset analysis of the original Hurwitz trial were not associated with clinical outcome.[334] Similarly, analysis of oncogenes known to play a role in colorectal cancer (eg, K-Ras, b-raf, and p53) failed to demonstrate an association with clinical outcome.[335] As in metastatic breast cancer, the presence of clinically significant hypertension has been associated with clinical outcome in a phase 2 trial analysis.[336]

The status of anti-VEGF therapy in advanced colorectal cancer is complicated by the rapid changes occurring in this disease in recent years, where the addition of novel chemotherapeutic and biologic agents has altered overall survival to a significant degree. Though bevacizumab is the best-studied antiangiogenic agent in advanced colorectal cancer, other agents have now been examined in phase 3 trials. An interim analysis from a randomized phase 3 trial comparing FOLFOX4 chemotherapy alone or in combination with the oral small molecule receptor TKI vatalanib (PTK787) as first-line therapy for metastatic colorectal cancer showed a nonstatistically significant trend toward improved PFS in the combination arm as judged by central review.[337] Complete results, including overall survival, are not yet available.

Non-Small Cell Lung Cancer

Angiogenesis Inhibitors as Single Agents for Advanced NSCLC ■ When tested as monotherapy for advanced NSCLC, inhibitors directed at VEGF have generally led to low rates of objective tumor responses. In the phase 2 trial of chemotherapy with or without bevacizumab, 19 patients in the control arm received high-dose, single-agent bevacizumab on progression, and although 5 had disease stabilization, there were no objective responses.[338]

VEGFR TKIs have demonstrated clear evidence of antitumor activity as single agents in NSCLC, although to date there are no studies demonstrating that they prolong overall survival compared to chemotherapy or other targeted agents. Vandetanib (ZD6474), a dual VEGFR/EGFR inhibitor, has been one of the most extensively tested thus far. In a randomized phase 2 trial involving 168 patients with locally advanced or metastatic, platinum-refractory NSCLC, a statistically significant but modest improvement in median PFS was observed in patients receiving vandetanib compared to gefitinib (11.0 vs 8.1 weeks, $p = 0.011$).[339] Vandetanib was also directly compared to chemotherapy (carboplatin and paclitaxel), or the combination of vandetanib with chemotherapy, in a phase 2 study in 181 previously untreated NSCLC patients.[340] A trend toward inferior PFS was observed in the vandetanib arm compared to chemotherapy alone (11.5 vs 23.1 weeks, p = NS). Phase 3 trials of vandetanib in NSCLC patients are ongoing, both as monotherapy and in combination with chemotherapy.

Sorafenib has also shown evidence of single-agent activity in advanced, recurrent NSCLC. In a randomized discontinuation phase 2 clinical trial (ECOG2501), NSCLC patients with stable disease during treatment with sorafenib (N = 97) were randomized to either continue sorafenib or receive placebo.[341] Patients on the sorafenib arm had a significantly longer PFS compared to those receiving placebo (3.6 vs 1.9 months, $p = 0.01$). Interestingly, despite this PFS improvement, although only a single patient had an objective response, illustrating that for NSCLC, as in RCC,[319] objective tumor response rates may not be the most appropriate metric for benefit in early testing.

Sunitinib has also demonstrated encouraging single-agent activity in patients with recurrent NSCLC.[342] Objective tumor responses were observed in 7 of 63 patients (ORR 11.1%), and 70% of patients demonstrated at least some degree of tumor shrinkage. The safety profile was considered acceptable overall, but 2 patients, both with squamous cell histology, died of treatment-related pulmonary hemorrhage. This toxicity has been seen with other angiogenesis inhibitors, as described below, and has led to the exclusion of patients with squamous histology from treatment with bevacizumab and several other agents.

Other VEGFR TKIs that have demonstrated single-agent activity in advanced NSCLC include vatalanib (PTK787) , axitinib (AG-013736),[343] and XL647,[344] and TKI blocking EGFR, Her2, and VEGFR2.

Bevacizumab With Chemotherapy for Advanced NSCLC ■ Given their modest single agent activity, angiogenesis inhibitors have most commonly been tested in combination with chemotherapy for NSCLC. Bevacizumab has been the most extensively tested agent in NSCLC to date. Initial phase 2 testing in chemonaive, advanced NSCLC patients suggested that bevacizumab improved objective response rates and time to progression when added to the standard doublet chemotherapy regimen of carboplatin and paclitaxel.[338] This study also revealed an unanticipated and concerning side effect: severe pulmonary hemorrhage, which occurred in 6 out of 67 patients who had received bevacizumab, and was fatal in 4 cases. Tumor characteristics associated with significant hemoptysis were central location, proximity to major blood vessels, necrosis and cavitation before or during therapy, and squamous histology. Since squamous cell tumors are more commonly located centrally and have a greater tendency to cavitate than adenocarcinomas, it is unclear whether histology alone is the primary risk factor for hemoptysis, or simply a surrogate for other risk factors.

Based on the promising outcomes with bevacizumab in this phase 2 trial, a randomized phase 2/3 trial was conducted by the Eastern Cooperative Oncology Group (ECOG), E4599, comparing standard carboplatin and paclitaxel (CP) for 6 cycles with or without bevacizumab in 878 patients with previously untreated, advanced (Stage IIIB or IV) non-squamous NSCLC.[318] Patients receiving CP with bevacizumab had a significantly improved median overall survival (12.3 vs 10.3 months, hazard ratio 0.77, $p = 0.003$), PFS (6.2 vs 4.5 months, $p < 0.0001$), and response rate (35% vs 15%, $p < 0.001$) compared to CP alone (Table 11-3). The main grade 3 or higher toxicities associated with bevacizumab were clinically significant bleeding (4.4% vs 0.7% in the standard chemotherapy arm), febrile neutropenia, and hypertension. The overall rate of fatal hemoptysis with bevacizumab when squamous histology was excluded was approximately 1%. This may be considered an acceptable risk in light of the absolute improvements in survival of 7% and 8% at 1 and 2 years, respectively.

Interestingly, unplanned subset analyses of E4599 found that the survival benefit was confined primarily to male participants, although females did benefit in terms of response and PFS.[345] The reason for this apparent gender-based difference in benefit is unclear. In elderly patients, defined as greater than 70 years old, there also appeared to be an increase in toxicity but no obvious improvements in overall survival.[346]

This was the first randomized phase 3 study in advanced NSCLC that demonstrated superior overall survival when targeted therapy is combined with standard chemotherapy. A similar randomized phase 3 trial testing bevacizumab in combination with another standard doublet of cisplatin and gemcitabine (GC) has recently been reported (AVAIL).[347] In this study, a total of 1,043 patients were randomized to either low- (7.5 mg/kg) or high- (15 mg/kg) dose bevacizumab once every 3 weeks with GC, compared to GC alone. In this study PFS and objective response rates were significantly improved in the bevacizumab containing arms compared to GC but overall survival was not improved. There were no significant differences in efficacy or toxicity between the low and high doses of bevacizumab. This clinical result is consistent with the vascular normalization hypothesis.[348]

Based on these results, some oncologists regard bevacizumab in combination with CP as a new standard of care for patients with non-squamous NSCLC. Given the results of the AVAIL trial, however, it remains an open question as to whether a similar degree of benefit can be expected when bevacizumab is combined with any platinum-containing doublet for untreated NSCLC patients, and whether additional clinical criteria such as sex or age should be used in selecting patients for treatment.

VEGFR TKIs With Chemotherapy as First-Line NSCLC Therapy ■ VEGFR TKI/chemotherapy combinations are also being evaluated in randomized trials for first-line treatment of advanced NSCLC treatment. In a preliminary analysis, the ESCAPE (Evaluation of *Sorafenib*, Carboplatin and Paclitaxel Efficacy in NSCLC) trial comparing CP chemotherapy with or without sorafenib in 926 patients showed no overall or PFS benefit for the sorafenib-containing arm.[349] Another TKI, AZD2171 (cediranib) was recently tested with CP in a planned phase 2/3 trial by the National Cancer Institute of Canada (NCIC trial BR24)[350] in 296 patients. Although evidence of improved PFS and objective response rates was observed in the cediranib arm, the trial was discontinued at a pre-planned analysis at the end of the phase 2 component of the trial because of an excess of dose-related adverse effects including dehydration, diarrhea, and fatigue. A similar trial is currently being planned at a lower dose of cediranib. As noted previously, vandetanib with CP (VCP) was recently compared to CP or vandetanib alone in 181 patients.[340] VPC could be safely administered, even in patients with squamous cell histology and treated brain metastases. Patients receiving VPC had a trend toward improved objective response rate (32 vs 25%) and longer PFS (24 vs 23 weeks; hazard ratio = 0.76, one-sided P = 0.098) compared to CP. Taken together, trials of VEGFR TKIs with chemotherapy for first-line NSCLC treatment have been somewhat disappointing thus far, with modest gains, at most, in efficacy and significant toxicities in some cases.

VEGFR TKIs With Chemotherapy for Recurrent NSCLC ■ Vandetanib has also been evaluated in combination with docetaxel for patients previously treated with platinum-containing chemotherapy.[351] A total of 127 patients were randomized to receive docetaxel with either low dose (100 mg once daily) or high dose (300 mg once daily) vandetanib. This study met its primary endpoint of prolonged median PFS in the vandetanib arm, although, interestingly, a trend toward greater benefit was observed in the low-dose arm (19, 17, and 12 weeks in low dose, high dose, and control arms, respectively). There was no significant difference in survival between the treatment arms. Based on these results, a randomized, phase 3 trial of vandetanib 100 mg daily with docetaxel versus docetaxel was conducted. Preliminary results from this study suggest a significantly improved PFS in the vandetanib arm although full results of this trial have not yet been reported.

Antiangiogenic Agents in Combination With Other Targeted Therapies for NSCLC ■ The molecular pathways regulating tumor angiogenesis, as well as tumor cell survival, are complex and in at least some cases redundant.[263,352] It is not surprising, therefore, that therapeutic approaches targeting a single pathway do not typically provide long-term disease control and tumor resistance inevitably develops. Combinations of targeted agents may therefore provide improved clinical outcomes while avoiding the toxicities associated with chemotherapy. In NSCLC, and several other diseases, dual blockade of the EGFR and VEGF pathways is being studied clinically because both are validated therapeutic targets that are known to be interrelated. VEGF is downregulated by EGFR inhibition, likely through both HIF-α dependent and independent mechanisms,[255,280,281,353-355] and EGFR, like VEGFR-2, may be expressed on tumor-associated endothelium.[356-358] Acquired resistance to the EGFR inhibitor was found to be associated with increased VEGF levels and increased tumor angiogenesis in preclinical studies.[359]

Clinically, inhibition of both VEGF and EGFR has been investigated using combinations of individual drugs, or single multitargeted TKIs such as vandetanib as discussed above. In a randomized phase 2 trial, bevacizumab and erlotinib (BE) was compared to chemotherapy alone (docetaxel or pemetrexed) or chemotherapy with bevacizumab (Table 11-3) in patients with refractory or recurrent NSCLC.[360] A trend toward improved PFS, and improved tolerability, was observed in the BE arm compared to chemotherapy. A randomized phase 3 trial of BE compared to erlotinib was subsequently conducted in 636 second-line patients (BETA trial, for BEvacacizumab/TArceva). Preliminary reports from this study indicate that patients in the BE arm did have improved PFS (3.4 vs 1.7 months) and objective response rate compared to the erlotinib arm, but overall survival was not improved (9.3 vs 9.2 months). Combinations of VEGFR TKIs, including sorafenib, sunitinib, and cediranib, with EGFR inhibitors are also under investigation.[361]

Antiangiogenic Therapy for Operable NSCLC ■ The use of angiogenesis inhibitors in the neoadjuvant or adjuvant setting is also being investigated in NSCLC patients with operable disease. In one preoperative trial, the VEGFR TKI pazopanib was found to have significant antitumor activity, with 87% of patients demonstrating a reduction in tumor volume.[362] A phase 3 randomized trial testing is also underway testing whether the addition of bevacizumab to 4 cycles of standard chemotherapy improves outcomes compared to chemotherapy alone for fully resected Stage IB-IIIA NSCLC (ECOG1505).

Breast Cancer

Anti-VEGF therapy has been studied extensively in patients with advanced breast cancer, in both the front-line and refractory metastatic disease settings, and is now being explored in the adjuvant disease setting. Multiple agents have been examined in the phase 2 and phase 3 settings, as well as combinatorial therapies involving HER2-targeted therapy, hormonal therapy, and chemotherapy.

After initial phase 2 trial results suggested modest but real biologic activity for the anti-VEGF monoclonal antibody bevacizumab in heavily pretreated metastatic breast cancer, several large phase 3 trials were initiated combining bevacizumab with chemotherapy in both front-line and more refractory metastatic breast cancer. The first of these trials compared capecitabine alone or in combination with bevacizumab in the setting of anthracycline- and taxane-treated advanced breast cancer. This trial failed to achieve a statistically significant improvement in either progression-free or overall survival, though a significant improvement in response rate was reported.

Subsequently investigators examined the combination of paclitaxel and bevacizumab in the context of front-line therapy for metastatic breast cancer.[363] This trial was based on prior preclinical studies demonstrating synergistic activity for the combination of bevacizumab and taxane-based chemotherapy against endothelial cells.[364] Patients enrolled in this trial (E2100) had either hormone-sensitive or estrogen receptor, progesterone receptor, and HER2 negative breast cancer; or, if HER2-positive, must have received prior HER2-targeted therapy (but not chemotherapy) in the metastatic setting. Patients could have received hormonal therapy in either the adjuvant or metastatic setting, and could have received adjuvant chemotherapy, including taxane-based chemotherapy if more than a year prior to study entry.

The result of this trial represented the basis for the subsequent regulatory approval of bevacizumab in metastatic breast cancer. PFS, the primary trial endpoint, was doubled (11.8 months for paclitaxel plus bevacizumab vs 5.9 months for paclitaxel alone), and a statistically significant improvement in response rate was observed. Overall survival was not significantly improved, though this trial was relatively underpowered for a survival endpoint. Of note, an analysis of the PFS endpoint suggested that no particular breast cancer subgroup gained preferential benefit with the addition of bevacizumab. Toxicities were consistent with the known patterns observed in other bevacizumab trials.

After initial reporting of the E2100 trial, other phase 3 trials examined the combination of bevacizumab with chemotherapy in the front-line metastatic breast cancer setting. The AVADO trial was a front-line metastatic chemotherapy trial comparing docetaxel with docetaxel plus bevacizumab (in 1 of 2 doses).[365] This trial demonstrated a statistically significant improvement in PFS for both bevacizumab-containing arms when compared with the chemotherapy-alone arm. As in E2100, no overall survival advantage was observed, though an improvement in response rate was noted. Neither dose of bevacizumab was obviously superior. The RIBBON-1 trial compared the addition of bevacizumab to a variety of front-line chemotherapy agents (with the exception of the weekly paclitaxel schedule examined in E2100). This trial has been reported as positive for its primary endpoint of PFS.

Numerous other therapeutic strategies are being examined with anti-VEGF therapy in the metastatic breast cancer setting. These include the combination of anti-VEGF therapy with both front-line hormonal therapy and with anti-HER2 therapy, with promising initial phase 2 results. These in turn have led to the development of ongoing phase 3 trials comparing hormonal therapy ± bevacizumab or HER2-targeted therapy. The combination of HER2-targeted therapy with anti-VEGF therapy is of particular interest, given preclinical data suggesting that HER2 is an upstream regulator of VEGF expression in HER2-positive breast cancer, and that the combination of HER2-targeted therapy with anti-VEGF therapy results in synergistic antitumor activity.

The addition of anti-VEGF therapy to standard hormonal therapy is also being examined in the setting of front-line hormone-sensitive (ER- and/or PR-positive) metastatic breast cancer. Based on preclinical data suggesting synergistic antitumor activity between hormonal therapy and anti-VEGF therapy, as well as promising phase 2 data from the metastatic disease setting, C40503 will randomize patients receiving front-line hormonal therapy (either tamoxifen or an aromatase inhibitor) to receive bevacizumab or a placebo.

Promising results in the front-line metastatic breast cancer have also led to the development of ant-VEGF therapies in the adjuvant (microscopic metastatic disease) setting. The E5103 trial, ongoing in the Breast Cancer Intergroup of North America, randomizes women with lymph node-positive and high-risk lymph node-negative hormone-sensitive HER2-negative and triple-negative breast cancers to receive either a standard chemotherapy (doxorubicin plus cyclophosphamide followed by weekly paclitaxel) or to chemotherapy plus bevacizumab (either for the course of chemotherapy or to a total of a year's worth of anti-VEGF therapy). Disease-free survival is the primary endpoint in this ongoing trial. Similarly, the ongoing BETH trial examines the role of anti-VEGF therapy for HER2-positive tumors in the adjuvant setting. Between them, these trials should provide useful proof-of-concept data for the role of bevacizumab in the adjuvant setting. Both E5103 and BETH include important correlative analyses.

In addition to monoclonal anti-VEGF therapy with bevacizumab, numerous other anti-VEGF agents are being explored in the setting of metastatic breast cancer. Several oral small molecule RTKIs of the VEGF receptors (eg, sorafenib, sunitinib, and axitinib) have been examined in the phase 2 disease setting, both as monotherapy and in combination with chemotherapy, with initial promising results. These results, in turn, have led to ongoing phase 3 trials in the metastatic disease setting. Similarly, phase 1 and 2 trials are exploring the combination of small molecule RTKIs of the VEGF receptors.

Multiple phase 3 trials demonstrate the benefit of anti-VEGF therapy in the front-line metastatic disease setting. Nevertheless, the lack of an overall survival advantage in these trials, the real toxicity of anti-VEGF therapy, and the price of these novel agents have limited the regular use of these agents in the metastatic setting. Concerns regarding the therapeutic index for such agents are perhaps best answered by turning anti-VEGF therapy into true "targeted" therapy, targeted in the clinical sense of being able to correlate a biomarker with outcome for either progression-free or overall survival. Ongoing analyses are attempting this difficult goal. Examination of the phase 3 E2100 trial, as mentioned above, offered no ready surrogate marker of benefit related to breast cancer biology. In contrast, examinations of host biology appear to provide potential clues to therapeutic individualization. Analysis of the E2100 proof-of-concept trial suggests that patients experiencing Common Toxicity Criteria Grade 3 or 4 hypertension had a greater than 1 year improvement in overall survival than patients not experiencing clinically significant hypertension.[366] An analysis of single nucleotide polymorphisms for VEGF and VEGFr-2 demonstrated statistically significant improvements in overall survival for patients with the VEGF-2578 AA and -1154 AA SNPs. While these studies clearly require confirmation, they suggest the possibility that the host is "wired" for response to anti-VEGF therapy, and that VEGF SNPs and their physiologic effects are "imprinted" on the patient's cancer.

Hepatoma

Hepatoma (hepatocellular carcinoma) is an important cancer on a global basis, and has been characterized by remarkably poor prognosis and few active agents for decades. The advent of antiangiogenic therapy has reinvigorated therapeutic attacks on hepatoma.

In a randomized placebo-controlled phase 3 trial, sorafenib prolonged overall survival (5.5 m vs 2.5 m for control[367] (Table 11-3). Multiple antiangiogenic agents are currently under investigation.

Other Malignancies

Antiangiogenic therapies (particularly anti-VEGF therapies) have been examined in numerous other human malignancies, with initial positive results (and a few signal failures) in several cancers. Many of these approaches are discussed elsewhere in this book, and will be summarized only briefly here, as they have not yet passed the test of a positive phase 3 randomized controlled trial.

Pancreatic cancer: A large phase 3 trial comparing gemcitabine plus bevacizumab versus gemcitabine plus placebo has been reported as a negative trial. Pancreatic cancer continues to elude our best therapeutic efforts.

Ovarian cancer: Early results from phase 2 trials of anti-VEGF agents in ovarian cancer have demonstrated antitumor activity as well as significant reductions in ascites. These in turn have led to the development of ongoing phase 2 trials.

Glioma: Several phase 2 trials of anti-VEGF therapy as monotherapy have suggested that bevacizumab has therapeutic activity in advanced gliomas. These promising results have led to a submission to the Food and Drug Administration for accelerated approval, as well as to the development of a proof-of-concept phase 3 trial.

Non-Hodgkin's lymphoma: Positive early results for anti-VEGF therapy have been reported from several phase 2 trials, and have led to the development of phase 3 trials, which are ongoing.

Toxicities of Antiangiogenic Therapy

Angiogenesis inhibitors have been developed with the hope that they would provide a relatively nontoxic means to slow or prevent tumor growth that could be used over long periods of time, toward the goal of converting cancer into a manageable, chronic condition. Based on the clinical experience to date, it appears that they do in fact have a generally favorable side effect profile that is nonoverlapping with chemotherapy. Certain toxicities have emerged, however, that appear to be specific to entire classes of agents and, in some cases, potentially life-threatening.

Pure VEGF antagonists (eg bevacizumab) offer an important window into the physiologic and pathophysiologic effects of VEGF blockade; agents that combine VEGF blockade with blockade of other kinases (eg, sorafenib and sunitinib) add side effects specific to the kinases blocked. Additional drug-specific idiosyncratic side effects may also occur. In addition, as antiangiogenic agents are regularly combined with chemotherapeutic agents across a broad array of diseases, and frequently prolong PFS, chemotherapy-related side effects may be increased related to increased duration of their use. For instance, in the E2100 phase 3 breast cancer trial patients receiving bevacizumab in addition to paclitaxel-based chemotherapy suffered statistically significant increases in grade 3 and 4 toxicities for infection, fatigue, and sensory neuropathy, in addition to VEGF-related side effects such as hypertension, cerebrovascular ischemia, headache, and proteinuria.[363] It seems likely that the increased rates of infection, fatigue, and sensory neuropathy seen in E2100 were a function of prolonged exposure to chemotherapy, as patients receiving bevacizumab not only had prolonged PFS, but also received increased duration of taxane-based chemotherapy.

The availability of multiple phase 3 trials allows us to gauge these toxicities across large populations, while smaller studies have focused on individual toxic effects. In this section, we will focus on toxicities that are VEGF-related and mechanistic in nature (ie, were a function of a ligand-receptor interaction in a normal tissue organ). These side effects include toxicities that are seen across most disease treated with anti-VEGF therapy, as well as side effects that—while mechanistic—are seen more commonly with specific diseases (eg, bowel perforation and pulmonary hemorrhage). Side effects unrelated to VEGF inhibition observed with nonspecific RTKIs will not be discussed here.

Hypertension ■ The most commonly reported toxicity in patients receiving anti-VEGF therapies is hypertension. It is generally mild-to-moderate in nature, though very rarely severe hypertension (malignant hypertension) has been reported. Hypertension is thought to be related to alterations in endothelial function related to blockade of the nitric oxide pathway downstream from the VEGF receptor.[368] In contrast to anti-VEGF therapy, VEGF infusions are associated with decreases in blood pressure. Management of anti-VEGF-related hypertension has not been carefully studied in the clinic, though it appears responsive to standard antihypertensive agents, and is reversible on discontinuation of anti-VEGF therapy. For patients experiencing mild-to-moderate degrees of hypertension, anti-VEGF therapy may be continued in the presence of appropriate antihypertensive therapy. Recent data suggests that the presence of hypertension may be associated with improved outcome, and as such hypertension may represent a type of pharmacokinetic or pharmacodynamic surrogate biomarker of response.[369] Analysis of the E2100 phase 3 breast cancer trial demonstrated a relationship between hypertension and particular single nucleotide polymorphisms for VEGF, though this finding awaits and requires confirmation.[366]

Arterial Thromboembolic Events ■ An increased incidence of thromboembolic and cardiovascular events has been observed in some but not all clinical trials of VEGF inhibitors. These events, while uncommon, may be serious and life threatening. Data pooled from five phase 3 trials with bevacizumab (all of which excluded patients with a recent history of stroke or heart attack) demonstrated a hazard rate of 2.0 for such events, with an increase in absolute risk from 1.7% in control patients to 3.8% in bevacizumab-treated patients. There was no associated increase in venous thromboembolic events. Cerebrovascular ischemia reported with bevacizumab may involve either transient ischemic attacks or stroke; myocardial infarction and angina have also been reported to occur with increased frequency.[370] These toxicities are more common in the elderly (age >65) and in patients with a prior history of arterial thromboembolic events. Management of these complications is similar to those in patients not receiving anti-VEGF therapy. In contrast to hypertension, which is generally readily managed with antihypertensive therapy, discontinuation of VEGF-targeted therapy in the presence of arterial thromboembolic events seems appropriate.

Patients receiving VEGF-targeted therapy frequently experience headaches, and occasionally these headaches may prove severe, with severe headaches occurring approximately 3% of the time in phase 3 trials. These headaches are traditionally migraine-like in nature, and anecdotally respond to anti-migraine agents such as serotonin receptor-active agents. Headaches may recur, and patients experiencing headaches may require chronic anti-migraine medications such as beta-blocker therapy if the patient's cancer continues to respond to anti-VEGF therapy. The relationship of such headaches to more severe central nervous system ischemic events is unknown.

Reversible Posterior Leukoencephalopathy Syndrome ■ RPLS is a rare central nervous system complication of anti-VEGF therapy. RPLS is a subacute neurologic syndrome typically consisting of headache, cortical blindness, and seizures, and has been reported anecdotally in patients receiving VEGF-targeting therapy. The etiology of RPLS is not well understood at present, nor is its relationship to VEGF inhibition, though it has been suggested that vasospasm of the posterior cerebral arteries may be important. Immediate cessation of anti-VEGF therapy, and appropriate anti-hypertensive management (a potential predisposing factor) are indicated.[371,372]

Nephrotoxicity ■ Nephrotoxicity, in the form of proteinuria, is common in patients receiving prolonged anti-VEGF therapy with as many as 40% of patients having at least some degree of proteinuria. More severe protein loss (eg, nephrotic syndrome) is rare, occurring in approximately 1-2% of patients. While not well studied, proteinuria is reversible when anti-VEGF therapy is provided, and patients may be re-challenged. A standard approach has been to discontinue bevacizumab temporarily if urine protein excretion is 2 g/24 h or greater and then resumed when protein excretion is less than 2 g/24 h. Bevacizumab treatment should be discontinued if nephrotic-range proteinuria develops. From a mechanistic standpoint, VEGF is important in renal glomerular homeostasis, so the renal effects of anti-VEGF therapy are perhaps unsurprising.[373] A recent investigation has associated bevacizumab-induced proteinuria with renal thrombotic microangiopathy, suggesting that VEGF plays a critical role in protection against this condition.[374]

Pulmonary Hemorrhage ■ Hemorrhage was reported in the initial phase 2 trial of lung cancer patients, where fatal hemorrhagic events were observed.[338] This trial suggested that patients with squamous cell cancer histology were at increased risk for this complication, and along with patients with gross hemoptysis (1/2 tsp or more per event) and those being treated with anticoagulant therapy or nonsteroidal anti-inflammatory agents, were excluded from the proof-of-concept phase 3 NSCLC trial conducted by the ECOG (E4599). Despite these exclusions, the rate of life-threatening pulmonary hemorrhage was 1.9% (with 1.2% fatal events), suggesting that we remain imperfect at predicting which patients will experience this complication.[318] The discussion of pulmonary hemorrhagic events should be part of the informed consent discussion for all lung cancer patients receiving bevacizumab or other VEGF-targeting agents. The mechanism of this side effect is unknown as is its dose-response relationship. The relationship with squamous cell lung carcinoma may be related to the tendency of these cancers to undergo central necrosis; central cavitation is common in lung cancers treated with anti-VEGF therapy.

Bowel Perforation ■ Bowel perforation has been seen predominantly in patients with advanced colorectal cancer and ovarian cancer, though it has been reported to occur in virtually every cancer treated with bevacizumab, albeit less commonly in cancers not involving the abdomen or pelvis. One recent analysis has suggested a 30-day mortality of 12.5% for patients undergoing this complication, suggesting its seriousness.[375] A recent review of the experience of bowel perforation in patients with advanced colorectal cancer has suggested that the incidence of bowel perforation seems to be higher in patients with an intact primary tumor, recent history of sigmoidoscopy or colonoscopy, or previous abdominal or pelvic radiotherapy. Interestingly, a prior history of peptic ulcer disease, diverticulosis, or use of nonsteroidal anti-inflammatory drugs was not obviously associated with an increased risk of bowel perforation.[376] At present we lack any useful exclusion factors that might prevent patients from developing this complication. The etiology of this side effect is uncertain, though preclinical evidence suggests that anti-VEGF therapy may greatly reduce the vascular density of normal intestinal villi.[377] This may be exacerbated when anti-VEGF therapy is combined with radiation.[310]

The management of bowel perforation involves awareness and recognition of symptoms and emergent surgical intervention. Surgical intervention in the face of anti-VEGF therapy may itself be associated with an increased risk of postsurgical complications such as further bowel perforation and abdominal fistulae. These, however, should not prevent a life-saving surgical intervention.[52,378]

Lessons from Clinical Studies of Antiangiogenic Therapy and Future Directions

Mechanisms of Resistance to VEGF Pathway Inhibitors

The therapeutic efficacy of conventional chemotherapy for most solid tumors is limited in part by the emergence of drug resistance by rapidly mutating tumor cells. Because antiangiogenic agents are directed against tumor endothelium, which was presumed to be diploid and genetically stable, it was initially thought that tumors will not develop resistance to antiangiogenic therapy[52,378] as they do to cytotoxic chemotherapy. Clinical experience thus far, however, suggests that virtually all tumors do eventually progress despite treatment with a VEGF inhibitor. Recent studies have suggested several potential mechanisms by which tumors may initially have or acquire resistance, or at least decreased sensitivity, to VEGF pathway inhibitors.[166,379]

Incomplete Target Inhibition ■ Drugs may not be present at sufficiently high concentrations at their targets for a sufficiently long time to cause a sustained inhibition of VEGF receptor signaling and tumor angiogenesis. In trials of VEGFR inhibitors SU5416 and SU6668, tumor biopsies taken prior to and during treatment revealed that VEGFR phosphorylation was inhibited by less than 50% in all cases, providing a potential explanation for the lack of significant clinical activity observed in these trials.[380,381] This incomplete target inhibition may be because drugs are not present within the tumor at sufficiently high concentrations, or for prolonged enough periods of time, to effectively inhibit angiogenesis. For other TKIs such as gefitinib and imatinib, incomplete target inhibition has been shown to result from genetic changes, eg, secondary mutations in EGFR or BCR-ABL, or epigenetic changes reducing the intracellular concentrations of the inhibitor.[382-384] It is not yet known whether mutations may be present within VEGFR in tumor endothelium.

Bypass of the VEGF Pathway Through Expression of Additional Angiogenic Factors ■ Genetic mutations or the activation of pathways such as hypoxia-inducible factor-1 may lead to the expression of additional angiogenic factors (or the loss of angiogenic inhibitors) by malignant cells in the tumor.[254,385] In turn, these changes may promote the proliferation and survival of tumor endothelial cells even in the presence of VEGF blockade. It has been observed, eg, that advanced stage breast cancers express a greater number of proangiogenic factors than early stage cancers, [386] which may help explain why previously untreated patients with metastatic breast cancer appeared to have a greater benefit from the addition of bevacizumab to standard chemotherapy than previously treated patients.[387,388]

Altered Threshold for Hypoxia-Induced Apoptosis ■ Certain changes within a tumor cell may make it less sensitive to the diminished vascular supply and resulting hypoxia induced by antiangiogenic therapy. For instance, it has been demonstrated in murine xenograft models that tumor cells bearing mutated p53 are less sensitive to hypoxic conditions in vitro and respond somewhat less well to a VEGF receptor-2 inhibitor.[389]

Genetic Alterations Within Tumor Endothelium ■ The assumption that tumor endothelium are normal diploid cells and therefore presumably genetically stable has been challenged by the recent observations from murine studies[390] and biopsies from patients with lymphoma[391] that tumor endothelial cells may harbor cytogenetic abnormalities. The functional significance and relevance of this finding to other tumor types is not yet known, but it supports the mounting evidence that tumor endothelial cells, like tumor cells, are likely to be a complex therapeutic target.

Genetic Variability in Host ■ Recent studies have suggested that polymorphisms in the VEGF gene are associated with the risk of developing cancer[392-394] and may also influence the response to bevacizumab when given with chemotherapy to breast cancer patients.[366] Polymorphisms in other genes regulating angiogenesis, such as IL-8 and the HIF family, have been described as well. The availability of high throughput methods for analyzing polymorphisms on a genome-wide basis should facilitate the analysis of genetic differences in the host and their impact on response to angiogenesis inhibitors.

Potential Biomarkers for VEGF Pathway Inhibitors

The Critical Need for Biomarkers for VEGF Pathway Inhibitors ■ In recent years, there has been significant progress in the clinical development of antiangiogenic therapy, particularly inhibitors of the VEGF pathway. Despite this progress, benefits to date have been modest, are seen only in subsets of patients, and inevitably yield to therapeutic resistance. The mechanisms by which tumors develop resistance to VEGF inhibition are not fully understood, and understanding them is critical for identifying patients with resistance and building combination regimens to overcome it. Furthermore, the biological activity of these agents remains difficult to assess because they do not typically lead to objective responses as judged by tumor shrinkage when used as monotherapy. As an illustration of this point, in a phase 1 trial of bevacizumab, no objective responses were observed out of 25 patients.[395] Thus, there is an urgent need for biomarkers for identifying which patients are most likely to respond to treatment or develop therapeutic resistance, selecting the optimal drug dosage, and determining whether the intended molecular target has been effectively inhibited.[396-398] Ideally such methods should be noninvasive and practical for routine clinical care. There are currently no validated biomarkers for in routine clinical use. There are, however, a number of different biomarkers under investigation in clinical and preclinical studies (Table 11-4). These can be divided into invasive markers that assess changes in tissue or vasculature directly; circulating markers detectable in blood or urine, and radiographic markers. Several of these are discussed below.

***Invasive Markers* ■** Serial biopsies taken prior to and during treatment have the potential to directly demonstrate drug effects on tumors and other tissues at the cellular and molecular level but are typically not practical to obtain outside the setting of a clinical trial. This approach has been used to demonstrate that bevacizumab induces changes in microvessel density, tumor-cell apoptosis, and proliferation in rectal cancer patients.[303,304,399] Changes in tumor IFP, a key parameter impacting vascular function, have also been demonstrated.[304,305] This approach may also provide insights into the lack of significant clinical activity seen for some agents. For example, in clinical trials of SU5416 and SU6668, 2 of the earliest VEGFR TKIs in clinical development, it was observed that VEGFR and other key targets were incompletely inhibited in post-treatment tumor biopsies[380,381] suggesting that higher drug concentrations, or more potent inhibitors, may be required. In addition, studies of changes in gene expression in cancer cells and tumor-associated macrophages (TAMs) after VEGF blockade with bevacizumab have shown upregulation of the SDF1a-CXCR4 pathway and of the VEGF receptor NRP1 in rectal cancer patients.[400]

***Table 11-4* ■ Surrogate Markers under Investigation for the Evaluation of Efficacy of Antiangiogenic Agents**

Marker	Parameter Evaluated	Comments/ Limitations	References
Tumor-based			
Tissue biopsy	Immunohistochemistry: Protein expression as a marker Microvascular density Perivascular cell coverage of tumor vessels Cell proliferation/apoptosis Genomic analyses	Not easily available in some tumors	303, 304, 334, 335, 343, 380
Interstitial fluid pressure measurement	Tumor interstitial fluid pressure	Limited accessibility in some tumors	303, 304, 437, 438
Measurements of tissue oxygenation	Tumor oxygen tension	Difficult accessibility in some tumors	439
Skin wound healing	Wound healing time	Investigated as biomarker of efficacy and indicator of side effects	440
Circulating markers in blood or urine			
Blood CECs, CPCs, or CEPs	Concentration of viable CEC/ CPCs/CEPs	Unclear origin, viability and surface phenotype of the circulating cells	303-306, 410, 415, 420, 421, 425, 441
Circulating proteins (cytokines, angiogenic factors, etc)	Concentration of levels of cytokines, angiogenic factors, markers of hypoxia, endothelial damage, and other factors in the blood	Can be done using commercially available multiplexed assays, ELISAs.	306, 405, 410-412, 414, 442, 443
Protein level in urine	Urine MMPs, VEGF, etc.	Limited to excreted proteins, depends on factors that might be altered by treatment such as renal function (eg proteinuria)	444
Radiographic			
CT imaging	Blood flow and volume, permeability-surface area product, mean transit time	Resolution, measurement of composite parameters	303, 304, 445
PET imaging	Tracer uptake	Resolution, measurement of composite parameters	303-305, 445
MRI	Blood flow, permeability	Resolution, measurement of composite parameters	306, 431, 446, 44790

Abbreviations: CAF, circulating angiogenic factor; CECs, circulating endothelial cells; CEPs circulating endothelial progenitors; CT, computer tomography; MMPs, matrix metalloproteinases; MRI, magnetic resonance imaging; PET, positron emission tomography; VEGF, vascular endothelial growth factor.

Circulating Protein Markers in Blood and Urine ■ Tumor angiogenesis is regulated by a balance between pro angiogenic and antiangiogenic factors and cytokines released by tumor cells, stroma, and by inflammatory cells. Many of these factors can be detected in circulation and other biologic fluids and serve as biomarkers for monitoring anti-VEGF therapies.[379,396-398]

Plasma and serum levels of VEGF and soluble VEGFR-2 have been investigated as pharmacodynamic biomarkers of activity of VEGF inhibitors, prognostic markers, and predictive markers of clinical benefit. In preclinical models, rapid increases of plasma VEGF, and decreases in soluble VEGFR-2, have been observed in both non-tumor bearing and tumor-bearing mice.[401-403] These increases were induced in a dose-dependent manner, and correlated with the treatment efficacy, suggesting that they may be useful for selecting the appropriate drug dosage.

These markers have also been evaluated in clinical trials. Bevacizumab (alone and with cytotoxics) has been shown to increase both serum and plasma total VEGF levels.[303,305,321,323] Interestingly, free serum VEGF concentrations decreased to undetectable levels even with low doses of bevacizumab in one of the studies.[321] Most VEGFR TKIs have been shown to induce similar changes. The most widely studied is sunitinib maleate (SU11248, Sutent®, Pfizer), which along with other TKIs has been shown to consistently induce on-therapy increases in VEGF plasma levels, and decreases in soluble (s)VEGFR-2, that are rapidly reversible when the therapy is stopped.[306,404-409] In 1 study, changes in sVEGFR-2 correlated with plasma levels of the drug.[410] Collectively, these findings suggest that VEGF and sVEGFR-2 may be useful pharmacodynamic markers.

Baseline levels of VEGF may also be predictive of benefit for some drugs although this has not been consistently observed in all studies. NSCLC patients with high VEGF were more likely to respond to the combination of bevacizumab with chemotherapy compared to chemotherapy alone.[411] Interestingly, a trend in the opposite direction was observed for the TKI vandetanib, as patients with low VEGF appeared to derive a greater clinical benefit from the vandetanib containing arm compared to the control arm in 3 randomized phase 2 studies.[412] It appears that the predictive value of markers such as VEGF will depend on the specific drug and disease setting.

Recent technological advances such as multiplex bead assays have permitted investigators to assess a much wider variety of factors. A signature derived from a profile of 35 cytokines and angiogenic factors was shown to be predictive of vandetanib benefit in a randomized phase 2 study.[413] Among these circulating biomarkers, PlGF has been shown to be consistently increased by anti-VEGF therapy in cancer patients regardless of the tumor type or agent used, suggesting that it might be an additional pharmacodynamic biomarker for antiangiogenic therapy.[303,305,306,405,414,415] Future studies will establish if PlGF levels have any predictive value for this therapy. Finally, this approach may also prove to be useful for identifying potential mechanisms of therapeutic resistance. Several candidates are SDF1α-CXCR4 pathways, bFGF, IL-6, HGF, and IL-8.[305,306,413,415,416]

Circulating Endothelial Cells (CECs) and Progenitors (CEPs) ■ Mature CECs (derived from existing vessels) and bone marrow-derived circulating precursor cells (CPCs) or endothelial precursors (CEPs), which can differentiate into mature endothelial cells and contribute to neovascularization, have been investigated as biomarkers for antiangiogenic therapy.[57,158,159,306,410,417-420] Consistent with preclinical models,[421,422] increases in mature CECs during treatment—which have a large percentage of apoptotic cells and are thought to represent cells shed from tumor endothelium—may be associated with benefit in patients treated with antiangiogenic or vascular targeting agents.[410,423-425] CPCs, by contrast, appear to decrease with bevacizumab[303-305] or sunitinib treatment.[415] Despite these encouraging results, the clinical application of circulating cells as biomarkers will require standardization and further phenotypic definition of cell populations.[426-428]

Imaging ■ A number of different techniques are under investigation for assessing parameters related to tumor vasculature such as perfusion, permeability, hypoxia, and metabolic activity. These include dynamic contrast-enhanced MRI (DCE-MRI), CT, and positron emission tomography (reviewed in Refs. 397, 398, 429–435). These methods have the important advantage of permitting longitudinal assessments noninvasively. There are a number of limitations for each of these methods, however. There is significant heterogeneity in blood flow and permeability within tumors, and the currently available methods generally lack the spatial resolution to assess this. Furthermore, most assess composite parameters, which depend on both tumor blood flow and permeability.[379] The cost of these studies may also limit their use, particularly for large randomized clinical trials needed to validate their utility.

Concluding Remarks

Nearly four decades ago, tumor angiogenesis was recognized as a potential therapeutic target for the treatment of cancer.[1] Since that seminal observation, the field has moved from conception to the clinical testing of dozens of new agents. Angiogenesis inhibitors are now part of the standard treatment regimens for lung, colorectal, renal, breast, and several other types of cancers. While these recent advances have validated antiangiogenic therapy as treatment modality, and provided benefit to countless patients, it is also true that the clinical gains thus far have been been modest. As the field moves from infancy into adolescence, a number of key issues will need to be addressed in order for the antiangiogenic therapy to realize its therapeutic potential for cancer patients. Among these issues are understanding the mechanism(s) by which antiangiogenic therapy enhances the efficacy of chemotherapy and radiotherapy, and designing combinations appropriately; identifying critical pathways driving angiogenesis other than VEGF, and developing drugs to inhibit them; creating biomarkers for identifying which patients will benefit (or experience toxicity) from a given agent; and exploring the application of angiogenesis inhibitors to earlier stages of cancer, with the goal of rendering microscopic tumors dormant.

Acknowledgments

This chapter is dedicated to Judah Folkman, MD, for his pioneering work in tumor angiogenesis and for his generous mentorship.

The authors thank Monique Nilsson, PhD, Terry Shackleford, PhD, and Dan Duda, DMD , PhD for editorial assistance and critically reviewing the manuscript.

Selected References

The complete reference list can be found at www.CANCERMEDICINE8.com

1. Folkman J. Tumor angiogenesis: therapeutic implications. *N Engl J Med.* 1971;285:1182–1186.
3. Carmeliet P, Jain RK. Angiogenesis in cancer and other diseases. *Nature.* 2000;407:249–257.
6. Folkman J, Kalluri R. Cancer without disease. *Nature.* 2004;427:787.
7. Gimbrone MA, Jr., Leapman SB, Cotran RS, et al. Tumor dormancy in vivo by prevention of neovascularization. *J Exp Med.* 1972;136:261–276.
8. Folkman J, Watson K, Ingber D, et al. Induction of angiogenesis during the transition from hyperplasia to neoplasia. *Nature.* 1989;339:58–61.
28. Shing Y, Folkman J, Sullivan R, et al. Heparin affinity: purification of a tumor-derived capillary endothelial cell growth factor. *Science.* 1984;223:1296–1299.
40. Holash J, Maisonpierre PC, Compton D, et al. Vessel cooption, regression, and growth in tumors mediated by angiopoietins and VEGF. *Science.* 1999;284:1994–1998.

41. Kim KJ, Li B, Winer J, et al. Inhibition of vascular endothelial growth factor-induced angiogenesis suppresses tumour growth in vivo. *Nature.* 1993;362:841–844.
48. O'Reilly MS, Holmgren L, Shing Y, et al. Angiostatin: a novel angiogenesis inhibitor that mediates the suppression of metastases by a Lewis lung carcinoma. *Cell.* 1994;79:315–328.
50. O'Reilly MS, Boehm T, Shing Y, et al. Endostatin: an endogenous inhibitor of angiogenesis and tumor growth. *Cell.* 1997;88:277–285.
58. Folkman J, Long DM, Becker FF. Tumor behavior in isolated perfused organs: in vitro growth and metastases of biopsy material in rabbit thyroid and canine interstitinal segment. *Ann Surg.* 1963;164:491–502.
61. Gullino PM. Angiogenesis and oncogenesis. *J Natl Cancer Inst.* 1978;61:639–643.
65. Bergers G, Javaherian K, Lo KM, et al. Effects of angiogenesis inhibitors on multistage carcinogenesis in mice. *Science.* 1999;284:808–812.
68. Hagendoorn J, Tong R, Fukumura D, et al. Onset of abnormal blood and lymphatic vessel function and interstitial hypertension in early stages of carcinogenesis. *Cancer Res.* 2006;66:3360–3364.
110. Senger DR, Galli SJ, Dvorak AM, et al. Tumor cells secrete a vascular permeability factor that promotes accumulation of ascites fluid. *Science.* 1983;219:983–985.
111. Ferrara N, Henzel WJ. Pituitary follicular cells secrete a novel heparin-binding growth factor specific for vascular endothelial cells. *Biochem Biophys Res Commun.* 1989;161:851–858.
123. de Vries C, Escobedo JA, Ueno H, et al. The fms-like tyrosine kinase, a receptor for vascular endothelial growth factor. *Science.* 1992;255:989–991.
131. Kaipainen A, Korhonen J, Mustonen T, et al. Expression of the fms-like tyrosine kinase 4 gene becomes restricted to lymphatic endothelium during development. *Proc Natl Acad Sci U S A.* 1995;92:3566–3570.
135. Jain RK, di Tomaso E, Duda DG, et al. Angiogenesis in brain tumours. *Nat Rev Neurosci.* 2007;8:610–622.
148. Ellis LM, Hicklin DJ. VEGF-targeted therapy: mechanisms of anti-tumour activity. *Nat Rev Cancer.* 2008;8:579–591.
149. Weis SM, Cheresh DA. Pathophysiological consequences of VEGF-induced vascular permeability. *Nature.* 2005;437:497–504.
157. Rafii S, Lyden D, Benezra R, et al. Vascular and haematopoietic stem cells: novel targets for anti-angiogenesis therapy? *Nat Rev Cancer.* 2002;2:826–835.
158. Asahara T, Murohara T, Sullivan A, et al. Isolation of putative progenitor endothelial cells for angiogenesis. *Science.* 1997;275:964–967.
247. Maeshima Y, Sudhakar A, Lively JC, et al. Tumstatin, an endothelial cell-specific inhibitor of protein synthesis. *Science.* 2002;295:140–143.
254. Semenza GL. Targeting HIF-1 for cancer therapy. *Nat Rev Cancer.* 2003;3:721–732.
283. Izumi Y, Xu L, di Tomaso E, et al. Tumour biology: herceptin acts as an anti-angiogenic cocktail. *Nature.* 2002;416:279–280.
285. Browder T, Butterfield CE, Kraling BM, et al. Antiangiogenic scheduling of chemotherapy improves efficacy against experimental drug-resistant cancer. *Cancer Res.* 2000;60:1878–1886.
288. Miller KD, Sweeney CJ, Sledge GW, Jr. Redefining the target: chemotherapeutics as antiangiogenics. *J Clin Oncol.* 2001;19:1195–1206.
289. Jain RK. Normalization of tumor vasculature: an emerging concept in antiangiogenic therapy. *Science.* 2005;307:58–62.
291. Jain RK. Normalizing tumor vasculature with anti-angiogenic therapy: a new paradigm for combination therapy. *Nat Med.* 2001;7:987–989.
293. Mazzone M, Dettori D, de Oliveira RL, et al. Heterozygous deficiency of PHD2 restores tumor oxygenation and inhibits metastasis via endothelial normalization. *Cancer Cell.* Cell. 2009; 136:839-851.
301. Winkler F, Kozin SV, Tong RT, et al. Kinetics of vascular normalization by VEGFR2 blockade governs brain tumor response to radiation: role of oxygenation, angiopoietin-1, and matrix metalloproteinases. *Cancer Cell.* 2004;6:553–563.
304. Willett CG, Boucher Y, di Tomaso E, et al. Direct evidence that the VEGF-specific antibody bevacizumab has antivascular effects in human rectal cancer. *Nat Med.* 2004;10:145–147.
306. Batchelor TT, Sorensen AG, di Tomaso E, et al. AZD2171, a pan-VEGF receptor tyrosine kinase inhibitor, normalizes tumor vasculature and alleviates edema in glioblastoma patients. *Cancer Cell.* 2007;11:83–95.
307. Garcia-Barros M, Paris F, Cordon-Cardo C, et al. Tumor response to radiotherapy regulated by endothelial cell apoptosis. *Science.* 2003;300:1155–1159.
310. Kozin SV, Boucher Y, Hicklin DJ, et al. Vascular endothelial growth factor receptor-2-blocking antibody potentiates radiation-induced long-term control of human tumor xenografts. *Cancer Res.* 2001;61:39–44.
317. Hurwitz H, Fehrenbacher L, Novotny W, et al. Bevacizumab plus irinotecan, fluorouracil, and leucovorin for metastatic colorectal cancer. *N Engl J Med.* 2004;350:2335–2342.
318. Sandler A, Gray R, Perry MC, et al. Paclitaxel-carboplatin alone or with bevacizumab for non-small-cell lung cancer. *N Engl J Med.* 2006;355:2542–2550.
319. Escudier B, Eisen T, Stadler WM, et al. Sorafenib in advanced clear-cell renal-cell carcinoma. *N Engl J Med.* 2007;356:125–134.
320. Motzer RJ, Hutson TE, Tomczak P, et al. Sunitinib versus interferon alfa in metastatic renal-cell carcinoma. *N Engl J Med.* 2007;356:115–124.
347. Manegold C, von Pawel J, Zatloukal P, et al. Randomised, double-blind multicentre phase III study of bevacizumab in combination with cisplatin and gemcitabine in chemotherapy-naïve patients with advanced or recurrent non-squamous non-small cell lung cancer (NSCLC): BO17704 J Clin Oncol, 2007 *ASCO Annual Meeting Proocedings.* 2007;25:LBA7514.
361. Adjei A, Mandrekar S, Marks R, et al. A Phase I study of BAY 43–9006 and gefitinib in patients with refractory or recurrent non-small-cell lung cancer (NSCLC). J Clin Oncol, 2005 *ASCO Annual Meeting Proocedings.* 2005;23:3067.
364. Sweeney CJ, Miller KD, Sissons SE, et al. The antiangiogenic property of docetaxel is synergistic with a recombinant humanized monoclonal antibody against vascular endothelial growth factor or 2-methoxyestradiol but antagonized by endothelial growth factors. *Cancer Res.* 2001;61:3369–3372.
365. Miles D, Chan A, Romieu G, et al. Randomized, double-blind, placebo-controlled, phase III study of bevacizumab with docetaxel or docetaxel with placebo as first-line therapy for patients with locally recurrent or metastatic breast cancer (mBC): AVADO. ; 2008;26:LBA1011-.
377. Kamba T, McDonald DM. Mechanisms of adverse effects of anti-VEGF therapy for cancer. *Br J Cancer.* 2007;96:1788–1795.
400. Xu L, Duda DG, di Tomaso E, et al. bevacizumab, an anti-VEGF antibody, upregulates SDF1alpha; CSCR4, CSCL6 and neuropilin 1 in tumors in rectal cancer patients. Cancer Res. 2009: In press.
408. Rosen L, Mulay M, Long J, et al. Phase I trial of SU011248, a novel tyrosine kinase inhibitor in advanced solid tumors. *Proc Am Soc Clin Oncol.* 2003;22:191 (Abstract 765).
424. Heymach J, Kulke M, Fuchs C, et al. Circulating endothelial cells as a surrogate marker of antiangiogenic activity in patients treated with endostatin. *Proc Am Soc Clin Oncol.* 2003;22:979.
427. Duda DG, Cohen KS, Scadden DT, et al. A protocol for phenotypic detection and enumeration of circulating endothelial cells and circulating progenitor cells in human blood. *Nat Protoc.* 2007;2:805–810.
430. Cheng HL. Dynamic contrast-enhanced MRI in oncology drug development. *Curr Clin Pharmacol.* 2007;2:111–122.
433. Miller JC, Pien HH, Sahani D, et al. Imaging angiogenesis: applications and potential for drug development. *J Natl Cancer Inst.* 2005;97:172–187.
436. Rini BI, Halabi S, Rosenberg JE, et al. Bevacizumab plus interferon alfa compared with interferon alfa monotherapy in patients with metastatic renal cell carcinoma: CALGB 90206. *J Clin Oncol.* 2008;26:5422–5428.
439. Dunst J, Hansgen G, Krause U, et al. A 2-week pretreatment with 13-cis-retinoic acid + interferon-alpha-2a prior to definitive radiation improves tumor tissue oxygenation in cervical cancers. *Strahlenther Onkol.* 1998;174:571–574.
442. Hanrahan EO, Lin HY, Du DZ, et al. Correlative analyses of plasma cytokine/angiogenic factor (C/AF) profile, gender and outcome in a randomized, three-arm, phase II trial of 1st-line vandetanib (VAN) and / or carboplatin plus paclitaxel (CP) for advanced non small cell lung cancer (NSCLC). *Proc ASCO.* 2007.
445. Jennens RR, Rosenthal MA, Lindeman GJ, et al. Complete radiological and metabolic response of metastatic renal cell carcinoma to SU5416 (semaxanib) in a patient with probable von Hippel-Lindau syndrome. *Urol Oncol.* 2004;22:193–196.
447. Sorensen AG, Batchelor TT, Zhang W-T, et al. "A Vascular normalization index" as a mechanistic biomarker to predict survival after a single dose of cediranib in recurrent glioblastoma patients . *J Clin Oncol.* Cancer Res. 2009;69:5296-5300.
448. Holmgren L, O'Reilly MS, Folkman J. Dormancy of micrometastases: balanced proliferation and apoptosis in the presence of angiogenesis suppression. *Nat Med.* 1995;1:149–153.

12 Epigenetic Contributions to Human Cancer

James G. Herman, M.D. ■ Stephen B. Baylin, M.D.

Over the past 15 years, an exciting advance in our understanding of the mechanisms underlying cancer development has been our growing appreciation that these diseases are not driven solely by genetic changes, but also by epigenetic changes. Strictly speaking, the term epigenetic refers to heritable changes in gene expression, in dividing somatic cells, which are mediated by alterations other than changes in the primary base sequence of DNA.[1,2] This definition the two critical characteristics encompasses of epigenetic alterations in cancer in terms of their clinical importance. First, that the genes affected by epigenetic changes in cancer remain wild type for DNA sequence rather than harboring irreversible mutations. Second, and closely related, the changes are, then, potentially reversible if gene repression is altered such that the wild type gene function can be restored.[3,4-6]

This recognition of epigenetic changes, which are fundamental to cancer initiation and progression, is occurring in the midst of a dynamic explosion of knowledge as to how the human genome is normally controlled, via chromatin packaging of DNA, to regulate gene expression in different tissues and during devlopment.[1,2] For example, epigenetic processes play a fundamental role during normal embryonic development and adult cell renewal. As such, these processes control the emergence of different cellular phenotypes, all with the exact underlying DNA sequence, which occur during development and differentiation. While this knowledge of gene regulation continues to grow rapidly, our understanding of the complete spectrum of epigenetic changes that are key to cancer development is likely to be still in its early stages. However, there is much that has already been learned, and this knowledge in the understanding of basic cancer biology and carcinogenesis already has palpable translational implications, which are discussed in this chapter.

Mechanisms Involved in Epigenetic Regulation of Gene Expression

Formation of Chromatin

While all of the fundamental information for gene expression lies in the primary base sequence of DNA, which can be viewed as a "hard drive" for storage of this essential coding, the patterns of gene expression in cells is determined by how this DNA is modified following synthesis and how it is packaged into the nucleus by the proteins, or chromatin, by which it is arranged.[1,2] The latter processes of packaging might, then, are viewed as the "software," which provides the readout of the hard drive information contained in the DNA sequence. The primary role of the DNA modification and chromatin packaging is to balance the genome such that the majority of DNA is encompassed in a silent or low transcription state to guard against unwanted expression of repeat sequences, potential transposable elements, and viral insertions accrued over evolution.[1,2,7] The first element of DNA packaging is its interactions with proteins forming chromatin. The fundamental scaffolding proteins for chromatin are the histone proteins, and their assembly with DNA, in turn, forms the key element, or nucleosomes (Fig. 12-1), which are essential for arranging DNA in the nucleus.[8] Nucleosomes consist of ~146 bp of DNA wrapped twice around an octamer of the core histone proteins, H2A, H2B, H3, and H4.[8] For functional mediation of gene expression profiles from DNA, nucleosomes must not only be properly distributed linearly along DNA, but must also be arranged into higher order, multinucleosome structures[1,9] (Fig. 12-2). These dynamics are mediated by chromatin remodeling proteins, and the more widely and irregularly spaced the nucleosomes are in their linear placement along DNA, and the less compacted the higher order structures, the more "open" the chromatin is and the more available is the DNA for active gene transcription (Fig. 12-2). This is often the case in areas in and around active gene promoters. Conversely, the more regular and evenly the nucleosomes are spaced, and the more compacted their higher order structures (Fig. 12-2), the more "closed" is the chromatin and the more repressive for gene transcription. This latter configuration dominates most of the human genome, as noted earlier, to prevent unwanted gene expression and to facilitate chromosome structure.

Integrally involved with this dynamic chromatin structure is a dependency of nucleosome function on states of chromatin, which are determined by differing ratios of active and repressive histone "modifications."[2,9] These consist of additions or modifications to key amino acids, primarily located in the tails of the histones that stick out from the nucelosome assembly,[8] in the form of lysine acetylation, lysine and arginine methylation, serine and threonine phosphorylation, glutamic acid ADP-ribosylation, and lysine ubiquitination and sumoylation.[9]

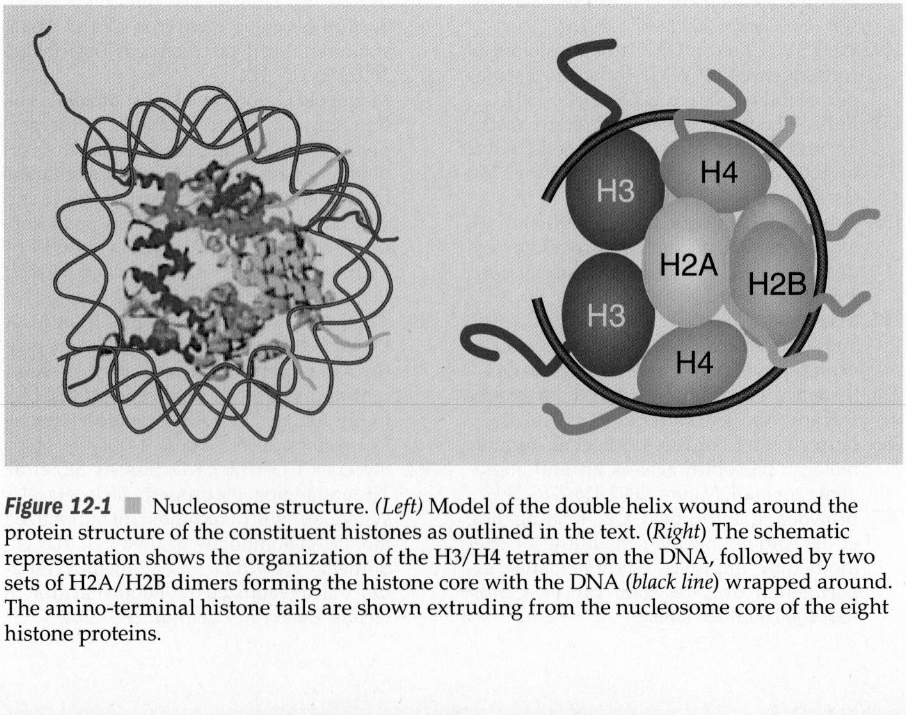

Figure 12-1 ■ Nucleosome structure. *(Left)* Model of the double helix wound around the protein structure of the constituent histones as outlined in the text. *(Right)* The schematic representation shows the organization of the H3/H4 tetramer on the DNA, followed by two sets of H2A/H2B dimers forming the histone core with the DNA (*black line*) wrapped around. The amino-terminal histone tails are shown extruding from the nucleosome core of the eight histone proteins.

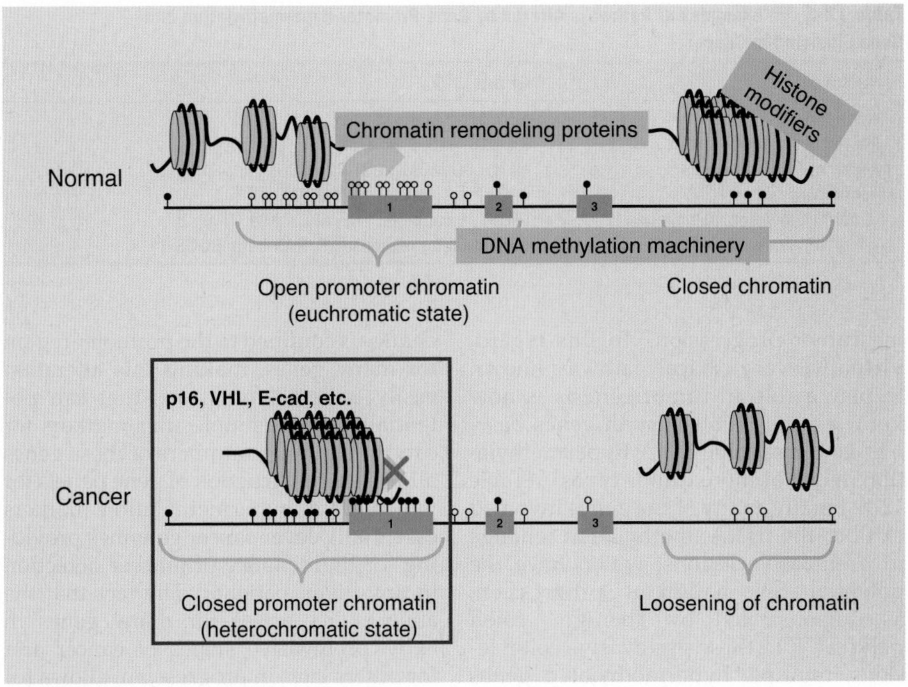

Figure 12-2 Depiction of the packaging arrangement of human DNA (straight black line). Top panel shows that for normal cells a more linear arrangement of nucleosomes (yellow circles with DNA wrapped around as outlined in Fig. 12-1) depicting the "open" arrangement of chromatin around most gene promoters containing CpG islands (unmethylated CpG sites shown as white lollipops), which are being actively transcribed or can be induced to transcribe (large light blue arrow). Exons 1 through 3 of the model gene are depicted by the numbered light blue boxes. Regions of DNA within the body of the gene and extending beyond the third exon are depicted as being in the closed, transcriptionally repressed, conformation typical of the majority of the normal human genome. This closed structure is represented by the more packed, three dimensional organization of the nucleosomes and the CpG sites in the closed regions are depicted as being methylated (black lollipops). The text in yellow squares depicts the chromatin remodeling protein complexes, histone modifying enzymes, and enzymes performing DNA methylation (DNA methylation machinery), which are responsible for DNA packaging as discussed in the text. The bottom panel depicts the altered chromatin patterns present in a typical cancer cell with a switch in positions of the normal closed and open chromatin regions in the genome. Many closed regions now have an open chromatin with loss of DNA methylation, while a large group of gene promoters have assumed a closed chromatin with abnormal, CpG island DNA methylation and repressed transcription (large red X over the transcription start site depicted by the light blue arrow.

The balance of these marks form a very complex "histone code" that participates, along with nucleosome positioning, in packaging the genome such that both constitutive and cell type dependent chromatin patterns of open and/or closed configurations are maintained from cell division to cell division and ensuring that these patterns remain stable in non-dividing cells.[9] It is in this way that cells maintain a "memory" for patterns of gene expression and chromosome structure that facilitate normal patterns of development and the maintenance of mature cell renewal and differentiation states.[9]

The best characterized of the histone modifications, mentioned earlier, are lysine methylation and acetylation, which are most closely associated with either high or low states of gene transcription. These marks in turn are established by families of enzymes consisting of histone methyltransferases (HMTs) that catalyze the methylation,[9] histone demethylases that remove these methyl additions,[9,10] and histone acetylases or (HATs) and histone deactylases (HDACs), which place and remove the acetyl groups, respectively.[9,11] For these dynamic events, examples of key methylation marks associated with gene states are methylation of lysine 4 of histone 3 (H3K4me3), which is associated with open chromatin typical of active transcription, and methylation of lysine 9 or lysine 27 (H3K9me3, H3K27me3), which is characteristic of repressed gene expression.[9,12] Adding to the information contained in this histone code is the fact that lysine methylation may be present in either monomeric, dimeric, or trimeric, states.[2,9] There is also a regulated balance for histone acetylation in which enzymatic activity of the HAT's and HDAC's determine states of histone lysine acetylation that are typical of open, transcriptionally active chromatin, and deactylation, more associated with closed chromatin and repressed transcription.[9] Key examples of such active marks at gene promoters are H3K9- and H4K16acetyl.[9]

DNA Methylation

While not present in all multicellular organisms, humans, other mammals, and other higher organisms add an additional layer of epigenetic regulation. Working in close concert with chromatin states to package the human genome is a key modification consisting of methylation added directly to postreplicated DNA.[11,13] This step consists of attachment of a methyl moiety to the C5 position of the base, cytosine, only when it is located preceding a guanine or in a "CpG" dinucleotides context. The methyl group is transferred from S-adenosyl methionine to DNA through catalysis by a family of DNA methyltransferase (DNMT) enzymes.[11,13] The role of this DNA methylation is closely tied to the distribution of the CpG dinucleotide in human and other genomes. This is a nonrandom and uneven distribution in which there has been a global and progressive depletion of CpGs over evolution because of deamination of methylated CpGs to change the cytosines (Cs) to thymidines (Ts).[11,13] Failure to repair these thymidines then results in transition of the Cs to T's. However, there remains interspersed conservation of nondepleted, CpG rich stretches (~0.4 to several thousand kb) or so called "CpG islands", which are particularly important to the DNA methylation patterns.[11,13] These islands, especially when found in the 5' end of about 50% of human genes,[11,13] remain non-DNA methylated while the majority of the CpG' sites in the remainder of DNA are methylated[11,13] (Fig. 12-2).

This pattern of DNA methylation, depicted in Figure 12-2, works in tight concert with the nucleosome positioning and histone modifications previously discussed to determine the epigenetic regulation of the genome. Thus, methylated DNA associates with, and helps maintain in a tight heritable state, the relatively transcriptionally inert status of the majority of the genome, which is most apparent in the closed chromatin or "heterochromatic regions" concentrated in pericentromeric parts of chromosomes. In contrast, the non-DNA methylated CpG islands associated with gene start sites appear to reflect and facilitate a transcriptional ready and/or active transcription state.[11,14] This tight interaction between histone modifications and DNA methylation is reflected in the fact that transcriptional repression is associated with DNA methylation is required to maintain the repression of the most closed chromatin states. Thus, deactylated histone lysines, such as for H3K9, and repressive methylation marks, such as H3K9me3, associate with methylated DNA.[11,13] In turn, such marks, and particularly H3K9me, appear important for targeting of DNA methylation.[11,13]

Altered Chromatin in Cancer or the "Cancer Epigenome"

Loss of DNA Methylation

Virtually all cancer types harbor what appears to be a marked shift in the chromatin packaging patterns, described in the previous sections, for normal cells[3] (Fig. 12-2). This has been best studied to date for DNA methylation, where there are at least two major changes that are now well appreciated. First, there are global losses of this modification from the widespread regions of the genome, which harbor DNA methylation in normal cells[3,4] (Fig. 12-2). Indeed, this was the first chromatin abnormality well cataloged for cancer,[15] although much remains to be learned about the ramifications of this change. Since these are generally areas of closed chromatin where the DNA methylation helps to maintain transcriptionally repressed DNA, such losses could associate with abnormal transcription.[4] Indeed, a number of genes with oncogenic potential, and which normally have low expression in normal cells, have now been reported to be upregulated in association with cancer specific decreases in promoter DNA methylation.[4] Also, pericentromeric regions are a target for DNA methylation losses in multiple cancer types and this may play a role in the genesis of chromosomal instability in neoplasia.[4,15]

Gene Promoter DNA Hypermethylation

The best studied chromatin change, which is associated with epigenetic abnormalities in cancer, and the one with the most recognized ramifications, to date, entails localized increases in DNA methylation in gene promoter CpG islands, which are protected from this change, as discussed earlier, in normal cells (Fig. 12-2).[3-5] This change is associated with tight transcriptional repression of genes and can, thus, serve as an alternative to gene mutations for loss of function of a number of well-characterized tumor-suppressor genes.[3-5] In addition to these classic-suppressor genes, data derived from random screens of cancer cell DNA for DNA hypermethylated genes, indicate that hundreds of such genes appear to exist, for several cancer types analyzed, in a given patient's tumor.[3-5,16] While all of these gene changes may not be pivotal for driving the initiation or progression of the particular cancers that harbor them, many, including the classic-suppressor genes, do encode for genes for which loss of function would be important for tumor development.[3-5] Many genes, which are seldom or never mutated in cancers, may still have important roles in tumorigenesis, since they undergo promoter DNA hypermethylation and silencing during tumor progression.[3] In this regard, virtually every critical pathway known to play a role in tumorigenesis is now known to be involved with genes bearing cancer specific DNA hypermethylation in one or more tumor types[3-5] (Table 12-1). Finally, many of the genes involved exhibit the DNA methylation change in preinvasive lesions, which have the potential for malignant progression, as demonstrated by "benign" colon polyps.[3-5,17] In these preinvasive colon lesions, multiple hypermethylated genes are already present and encode for key genes that, when inactivated, would deregulate key pathways, such as the Wnt pathway, which are well known to drive the initiation and progression of all colon cancers.[3-5,17] These findings have led to the hypothesis that epigenetic changes may be in many cases important for tumor initiation and for the appearance of abnormally expanding cells, which arise in cancer risk states, such as chronic inflammation.[17-19]

Table 12-1 ■ **Examples of Pathways Altered by Gene-Promoter Hypermethylation and Gene Silencing in Cancer**

Pathway	Genes 3-5
Wnt pathway	APC, SFRP family, SOX17
Altered cell-cycle control	Rb, p16, p15, p14, p73
Repair of DNA damage	MLH1, O6-MGMT, GST-Pi, BRCA1
Apoptosis	DAP kinase, caspase 8, TMS-1
Tumor-cell invasion, angiogenesis,	THBS1, E-cadherin, VHL, APC, LKB1, TIMP- 3,
Tumor architecture	Growth-factor response ER, RAR-beta, SOCS-1*

Clinical Implications of Altered DNA Methylation in Cancer

Although, the full impact of understanding chromatin alterations in cancer are just beginning to emerge, important progress is being made in at least two broad categories of translational application. First, is the use of DNA hypermethylated gene promoter sequences as tumor biomarkers, and second is the use of epigenetic therapies, which may be efficacious because they target reversal of abnormal gene silencing.[4-6,20]

Cancer DNA Methylation Biomarkers

There are some simple advantages that the detection of DNA methylation changes in cancer allow over other molecular approaches. First, the overall frequencies of methylation changes appear to be greater in many instances than mutational changes.[16] This appears to be true for all major solid and liquid cancer types examined thus far, although the specific genes altered are different among tumor types. A second advantage of the detection of DNA methylation changes associated with gene silencing is that this change is confined to the promoter region for many genes, making this alteration easily targeted for assays that can potentially serve as molecular markers for cancer. The large numbers of these genes allows for construction of gene panels for which DNA hypermethylation markers essentially cover cancer genomes providing for high chance of marker detection in any given patient.[21] The fact that the abnormality arises for many genes in early, preinvasive stages of cancer and for others later in progression, allows for potential uses of such markers in cancer risk assessment, early diagnosis, molecular restaging of tumors, and prediction of tumor behavior. Thus, the high frequency, early occurrence of such changes, and the ability to assay methylation of each gene with a single assay, facilitate the use of such approaches for the early detection of cancer. Examples of each of the marker possibilities mentioned earlier include those listed in Table 12-2. Thus, for cancer risk assessment, detection of DNA hypermethylated gene sequences in sputum DNA now holds considerable promise for predicting which individu-

Table 12-2 ■ **Examples of Using Gene Promoter DNA Hypermethylated Sequences as Cancer Biomarkers: Nearing Clinical Use**

Early diagnosis and/or detection of high risk states:
Detection of CpG-island DNA hypermethylation of gene panels in sputum from individuals at high risk for lung cancer[5,22]
Detection of *GSTP1* DNA hypermethylation in prostate biopsies and urine specimens prostate cancer[27,28]
Prognosis:
Detection of DNA hypermethylation in gene panels in tumor, and lymph node DNA, to restage stage 1 nonsmall cell lung carcinoma and predict early recurrences[31]
Detection of DNA hypermethylation to predict sensitivity of glioblastomas to Temazolamide[32-34]
Hypermethylation of specific genes
Whole DNA-methylome profiles
Histone-modification maps
Prediction:
CpG-island hypermethylation as a marker of response to chemotherapy, hormone therapy and targeted-therapy e.g., MGMT in patients with glioma and temozolomide treatment

als at high risk for developing lung cancer will actually manifest this disease within a defined period after initiation of marker monitoring.[5,22] Detection of colon cancer has been explored by detection of altered DNA methylation in either the blood or stool.[23-26] Detection of such genes in urine can potentially stratify the risk for, or provide for early diagnosis of, bladder cancer[27] and in prostate biopsies for improvement in the diagnosis of prostate cancer.[28]

A second area in which the changes of DNA methylation may be used in the management of cancer follows the observation that these genes are part of key pathways in the development of cancer. This allows the use of DNA methylation in these genes to potentially be used as prognostic or predictive biomarkers (Table 12-2). In general, the presence of DNA methylation for most genes has been associated with adverse outcome, thus providing a prognostic biomarker. This is consistent with the role that silencing of key tumor suppressor genes can play in altering key signaling pathways. Thus, tumors with alterations of single genes, or multiple genes, are more aggressive or molecularly advanced, and thus lead to worse outcomes.[29,30] Recently, detection of a small panel of DNA hypermethylated genes simultaneously in tumor and mediastinal lymph node DNA provides an extremely promising approach to restaging of stage 1 lung cancer patients to stage 3, thus predicting which of these individuals has a high risk of rapid recurrence.[31]

Another useful tool for the management of patients by medical oncologists is the possibility that DNA methylation in specific genes may affect the cancer cell sensitivity to different therapies. For example, silencing of a DNA repair gene may increase likelihood of tumor response to DNA damaging agents that would be repaired by this protein. The most clear example of this has been demonstrated for patients with the virulent brain tumor, glioblastoma, where detection of tumor DNA hypermethylation for the DNA damage repair gene, *O6-MGMT*, predicts for higher likelihood of response and post-treatment period of freedom from disease recurrence, for patients treated with the DNA alkylating agent, Temazolamide.[32-34] Other studies have suggested that sensitivity to cisplatin may be mediated by silencing of *FANCF* in ovarian cancer[35,36] and sensitivity of colon cancer to topoisomerase inhibitors may be mediated by silencing of the Werner syndrome gene (*WRN*).[37] Before clinical use, these studies need to be confirmed in additional populations and ideally in prospectively evaluated patients. However, such developments might greatly aid in optimizing the therapeutic choices offered to patients, who only have one opportunity for first line therapy. An ever-increasing number of larger and larger clinical trials seeking to validate the marker approaches and push their incorporation into standard oncology practice. Finally, other DNA methylation changes, such as losses of normal DNA methylation in tumor DNA, and changes in chromatin marks for active or repressed gene function, will almost certainly appear as promising molecular cancer markers.

"Epigenetic" Cancer Therapy

This type of therapy refers to cancer treatments based on the concept of reverting abnormal gene expression patterns toward normal as a means of cancer treatment. To date, two classes of drugs, which may achieve this goal, those which can experimentally induce DNA demethylation (5-aza-cytidine, azacytidine and 5-aza-2'-deoxycytidine, or decitabine) and those which inhibit histone deactylases (SAHA), have been approved by the FDA for treatment of the preleukemic state, myelodysplasia (MDS), and cutaneous T-cell lymphoma, respectively. Both azacitidine[38] and decitabine[39,40] have shown clinical benefit, and most recently, in a randomized phase III trial, azacitidine has shown a survival benefit.[41] Although, in both instances, these drugs achieve impressive response rates, and durable responses, in previously refractory diseases, it must be cautioned that their exact mode of efficacy remains to be proven—ie, they may not work clinically, solely, or partially—through the epigenetic effects, they mediate experimentally.[40,42,43] Thus use of the these drugs in other hematologic malignancies is the focus of many ongoing trials and potentially promising results are being seen especially for the DNA demethylating agents in acute myelogenous (AML) and chronic myelogenous (CML) leukemias.[39,44] Also, there is experimental evidence for synergy of DNA demthylating, and histone deactylase inhibition, for re-expression of DNA hypermethylated cancer genes.[45] Thus, multiple trials are exploring the clinical potential of using combination therapies with these agents. Most of these trials are joined with studies trying to examine whether DNA demethylation and re-expression of abnormally silenced genes corresponds with, or predicts, therapeutic response. Probably, over the next few years, all of these clinical studies will establish the true position of these drugs, and their mechanism of clinical efficacy, in the clinical arena.

The use of these therapies in solid tumors is less well explored, but has been examined in a few trials with less success than in studies of AML and MDS.[46,47] However, the universal presence of the therapeutic targets, as discussed in multiples sections of this chapter, makes the potential for such approaches as compelling in these cancers as in the hematologic malignancies. It is certain that, over the next few years, many trials will appear for epigenetic therapy approaches in solid tumors and, as in the leukemias, these will include studies to elucidate the precise mechanisms underlying clinical efficacy. All of these investigations, plus those in the hematologic malignancies, will not only guide the use of currently existing agents, but foster the development of newer and possibly more potent and specific drugs, as well. As we learn more about what precisely mediates abnormal DNA methylation and the components of chromatin which collaborate to initiate and maintain such changes, new molecular targets will almost surely emerge. Combination therapies exploiting these targets will likely follow.

Summary

Work over the past decade, especially for DNA methylation changes, has amply established that, from initiation through progression to advanced stages, cancer is a disease of epigenetic as well as genetic alterations. These studies, closely entwined with an explosion of basic knowledge about how chromatin constituents package the human genome to regulate gene expression patterns, are providing a rich substrate for new cancer biomarker and therapy strategies. There is enormous potential for these strategies to enter usage in the cancer clinical arena over the next decade.

References

1. Allis CD, Jenuwein T, Reinberg D, eds. *Epigenetics*. Cold Spring Harbor, New York: Cold Spring Harbor Laboratory Press; 2006.
2. Jenuwein T. The epigenetic magic of histone lysine methylation. *Febs J*. 2006;273:3121–3135.
3. Jones PA, Baylin SB. The epigenomics of cancer. *Cell*. 2007;128:683–692.
4. Esteller M. Epigenetics in cancer. *N Engl J Med*. 2008;358:1148–1159.
5. Herman JG, Baylin SB. Gene silencing in cancer in association with promoter hypermethylation. *N Engl J Med*. 2003;349:2042–2054.
6. Egger G, Liang G, Aparicio A, Jones PA. Epigenetics in human disease and prospects for epigenetic therapy. *Nature*. 2004;429:457–463.

7. Bestor TH. The host defence function of genomic methylation patterns. *Novartis Found Symp.* 1998;214:187–195; discussion 195–199, 228–232.
8. Kornberg RD, Lorch Y. Twenty-five years of the nucleosome, fundamental particle of the eukaryote chromosome. *Cell.* 1999;98:285–294.
9. Allis CD, Jenuwein T, Reinberg D. Overview and concepts. In: CD Allis TJ, Reinberg D, eds. *Epigenetics.* Cold Spring Harbor, NY: Cold Spring HarborLaboratory Press; 2007.
10. Agger K, Christensen J, Cloos PA, Helin K. The emerging functions of histone demethylases. *Curr Opin Genet Dev.* 2008;18:159–168.
11. Bird A. DNA methylation patterns and epigenetic memory. *Genes Dev.* 2002;16:6–21.
12. Ringrose L. Polycomb, trithorax and the decision to differentiate. *Bioessays.* 2006;28:330–334.
13. Li E, Bird, A. DNA methylation in mammals. In: CD Allis TJ, D Reinberg, eds. *Epigenetics.* Cold Spring harbor, NY: Cold Spring Harbor laboratory Press; 2007.
14. Robertson KD. DNA methylation and human disease. *Nat Rev Genet.* 2005;6:597–610.
15. Feinberg AP, Tycko B. The history of cancer epigenetics. *Nat Rev Cancer.* 2004;4:143–153.
16. Schuebel KE, Chen W, Cope L, et al. Comparing the DNA hypermethylome with gene mutations in human colorectal cancer. *PLoS Genet.* 2007;3:1709–1723.
17. Baylin SB, Ohm JE. Epigenetic gene silencing in cancer—a mechanism for early oncogenic pathway addiction? *Nat Rev Cancer.* 2006;6:107–116.
18. Ohm JE, McGarvey KM, Yu X, et al. A stem cell-like chromatin pattern may predispose tumor suppressor genes to DNA hypermethylation and heritable silencing. *Nat Genet.* 2007;39:237–242.
19. Feinberg AP, Ohlsson R, Henikoff S. The epigenetic progenitor origin of human cancer. *Nat Rev Genet.* 2006;7:21–33.
20. Laird PW. The power and the promise of DNA methylation markers. *Nat Rev Cancer.* 2003;3:253–266.
21. Esteller M, Corn PG, Baylin SB, Herman JG. A gene hypermethylation profile of human cancer. *Cancer Res.* 2001;61:3225–3229.
22. Belinsky SA. Gene-promoter hypermethylation as a biomarker in lung cancer. *Nat Rev Cancer.* 2004;4:707–717.
23. Grady WM, Rajput A, Lutterbaugh JD, Markowitz SD. Detection of aberrantly methylated hMLH1 promoter DNA in the serum of patients with microsatellite unstable colon cancer. *Cancer Res.* 2001;61:900–902.
24. Lenhard K, Bommer GT, Asutay S, et al. Analysis of promoter methylation in stool: a novel method for the detection of colorectal cancer. *Clin Gastroenterol Hepatol.* 2005;3:142–149.
25. Chen WD, Han ZJ, Skoletsky J, et al. Detection in fecal DNA of colon cancer-specific methylation of the nonexpressed vimentin gene. *J Natl Cancer Inst.* 2005;97:1124–1132.
26. Petko Z, Ghiassi M, Shuber A, et al. Aberrantly methylated CDKN2A, MGMT, and MLH1 in colon polyps and in fecal DNA from patients with colorectal polyps. *Clin Cancer Res.* 2005;11:1203–1209.
27. Chan MW, Chan LW, Tang NL, et al. Hypermethylation of multiple genes in tumor tissues and voided urine in urinary bladder cancer patients. *Clin Cancer Res.* 2002;8:464–470.
28. Tokumaru Y, Harden SV, Sun DI, Yamashita K, Epstein JI, Sidransky D. Optimal use of a panel of methylation markers with GSTP1 hypermethylation in the diagnosis of prostate adenocarcinoma. *Clin Cancer Res.* 2004;10:5518–5522.
29. Brock MV, Gou M, Akiyama Y, et al. Prognostic importance of promoter hypermethylation of multiple genes in esophageal adenocarcinoma. *Clin Cancer Res.* 2003;9:2912–2919.
30. Kawakami K, Brabender J, Lord RV, et al. Hypermethylated APC DNA in plasma and prognosis of patients with esophageal adenocarcinoma. *J Natl Cancer Inst.* 2001;92:1805–1811.
31. Brock MV, Hooker CM, Ota-Machida E, et al. DNA methylation markers and early recurrence in stage I lung cancer. *N Engl J Med.* 2008;358:1118–1128.
32. Esteller M, Garcia-Foncillas J, Andion E, et al. Inactivation of the DNA-repair gene MGMT and the clinical response of gliomas to alkylating agents. *N Engl J Med.* 2000;343:1350–1354.
33. Hegi ME, Diserens AC, Gorlia T, et al. MGMT gene silencing and benefit from temozolomide in glioblastoma. *N Engl J Med.* 2005;352:997–1003.
34. Stupp R, Hegi ME, Mason WP, et al. Effects of radiotherapy with concomitant and adjuvant temozolomide versus radiotherapy alone on survival in glioblastoma in a randomised phase III study: 5-year analysis of the EORTC-NCIC trial. *Lancet Oncol.* 2009.
35. Olopade OI, Wei M. FANCF methylation contributes to chemoselectivity in ovarian cancer. *Cancer Cell.* 2003;3:417–420.
36. Taniguchi T, Tischkowitz M, Ameziane N, et al. Disruption of the Fanconi anemia-BRCA pathway in cisplatin-sensitive ovarian tumors. *Nat Med.* 2003;9:568–574.
37. Agrelo R, Cheng WH, Setien F, et al. Epigenetic inactivation of the premature aging Werner syndrome gene in human cancer. *Proc Natl Acad Sci USA.* 2006;103:8822–8827.
38. Silverman LR, Demakos EP, Peterson BL, et al. Randomized controlled trial of azacitidine in patients with the myelodysplastic syndrome: a study of the cancer and leukemia group B. *J Clin Oncol.* 2002;20:2429–2440.
39. Wijermans P, Lbbert M. Epigenetic therapy with decitabine for myelodysplasia and leukemia. *Fut Oncol.* 2005;1:585–591.
40. Daskalakis M, Nguyen TT, Nguyen C, et al. Demethylation of a hypermethylated P15/INK4B gene in patients with myelodysplastic syndrome by 5-Aza-2′-deoxycytidine (decitabine) treatment. *Blood.* 2002;100:2957–2964.
41. Fenaux P, Mufti GJ, Hellstrom-Lindberg E, et al. Efficacy of azacitidine compared with that of conventional care regimens in the treatment of higher-risk myelodysplastic syndromes: a randomised, open-label, phase III study. *Lancet Oncol.* 2009;10:223–232.
42. Sigalotti L, Altomonte M, Colizzi F, et al. 5-Aza-2′-deoxycytidine (decitabine) treatment of hematopoietic malignancies: a multimechanism therapeutic approach? *Blood.* 2003;101:4644–4646; discussion 4645–4646.
43. Gore SD, Baylin S, Sugar E, et al. Combined DNA methyltransferase and histone deacetylase inhibition in the treatment of myeloid neoplasms. *Cancer Res.* 2006;66:6361–6369.
44. Issa JP, Gharibyan V, Cortes J, et al. Phase II study of low-dose decitabine in patients with chronic myelogenous leukemia resistant to imatinib mesylate. *J Clin Oncol.* 2005;23:3948–3956.
45. Cameron EE, Bachman KE, Myohanen S, Herman JG, Baylin SB. Synergy of demethylation and histone deacetylase inhibition in the re- expression of genes silenced in cancer. *Nat Genet.* 1999;21:103–107.
46. Schrump DS, Fischette MR, Nguyen DM, et al. Phase I study of decitabine-mediated gene expression in patients with cancers involving the lungs, esophagus, or pleura. *Clin Cancer Res.* 2006;12:5777–5785.
47. Momparler RL, Cote S, Eliopoulos N. Pharmacological approach for optimization of the dose schedule of 5-Aza-2′-deoxycytidine (Decitabine) for the therapy of leukemia. *Leukemia.* 1997;11(Suppl):S1–S6.

13 Cancer Immunotherapy

Karl S. Peggs, MA, MB, BCh, MRCP, FRC Path ■ Sergio A. Quezada, PhD ■ Padmanee Sharma, MD, PhD ■ James P. Allison, PhD

Cancer and the Immune System: A Brief History

Immunosurveillance

The idea that the immune system is capable of recognizing and responding to cancer is not novel. Paul Ehrlich (1854-1915) was perhaps first among the early visionaries to speculate that the immune system played a key role in suppressing tumors and that the incidence of cancer would be much greater were it not for the ability of the immune system to identify and eliminate nascent tumor cells, a concept that would later become known as the immune surveillance hypothesis when revisited over 50 years later by F. Macfarlane Burnet and Lewis Thomas.[1-3] However, proof of concept remained elusive. While it was established that chemically-induced tumors were immunogenic in murine models, spontaneously arising tumors behaved differently and were not rejected in similar experimental systems.[4] These data informed a growing consensus that naturally arising tumors were non-immunogenic and that the antigens targeted by the immune system in chemically-induced tumors were perhaps unique to this setting. The scientific basis supporting immunosurveillance was further undermined by experiments showing that athymic mice do not have an increased frequency of tumors induced by a chemical carcinogen.[5] Thus even though a notable excess of a variety of cancers occurring in immunosuppressed organ transplant recipients was recognized as inferential that immune surveillance occurred in humans, it remained frustratingly apparent by the early 1980s that definitive support from murine models was still lacking.[3] Furthermore, while certain tumors were many 100-fold more common in immune suppressed individuals (eg, some skin cancers, Kaposi sarcoma, and lymphomas), the frequency of noncutaneous, nonvirally-induced cancers was generally not increased, suggesting a potentially unique role for immune surveillance in malignancies associated with oncogenic viruses.[6,7] It was at this time that further inferential evidence in humans was beginning to emerge from the demonstration of increased rates of malignancies in patients with the newly defined acquired immunodeficiency syndrome.[8,9] However, the marked association with virally-induced cancers was similarly striking.

Multiple strands of evidence would need to coalesce to rekindle enthusiasm for the therapeutic potential of immune-based strategies. A critical cornerstone was provided by the works of Aline van Pel, Thierry Boon, and Pierre van der Bruggen, demonstrating firstly that specific immunity to spontaneous tumors could be induced by vaccinating mice with mutagenized tumor cells,[10] and subsequently in identifying a tumor-specific antigen that could be recognized by human cytolytic T cells.[11] These studies showed that spontaneous tumors were not inherently deficient in tumor antigens, but instead failed to stimulate an effective immune response. Critically, this failure could be overcome by vaccination in mouse models. The molecular definition of tumor antigens revolutionized the field of tumor immunology by legitimizing the mechanism by which the adaptive immune system discriminates between normal and neoplastic cells. The detection of tumor-specific responses in humans fueled speculation that these responses could be similarly manipulated to induce tumor erradication.[12] Simultaneously, it engendered rapid development of a new field within tumor immunology searching for tumor-associated antigens. Many tumor antigens have since been cloned. They can be broadly segregated into five major categories: (a) differentiation antigens, eg, melanocyte differentiation antigens, tyrosinase, gp-100, and Melan-A/MART-1; (b) mutational antigens, eg, abnormal forms of the tumor suppressor p53; (c) over-expressed normal antigens, eg, HER-2/neu, galectin-9; (d) cancer-testis antigens (CTAs), eg, MAGE, LAGE and NY-ESO-1; and (e) viral antigens, eg, EBV, HERV.[13,14]

Immunoediting

The demonstration of tumor-specific antigens in spontaneously arising tumors that could be recognized by the immune system gave further credence to the theory of immune surveillance, but fell short of providing definitive proof. Indeed, antigenicity is necessary but not sufficient for immunogenicity. The idea remained controversial until 2001, when an landmark paper by Robert Schreiber in collaboration with Lloyd Old demonstrated that lymphocytes and the immune stimulator IFN-γ cooperate to inhibit the development of spontaneous and carcinogen-induced tumors in mice genetically engineered to lack a functional immune system (RAG-2$^{-/-}$).[15] Moreover, they also recognized that some tumor cells escape detection and eventually cause cancer. They posited that the cellular composition of these tumors, driven by the selective pressure exerted by immune system, becomes serially less immunogenic, having undergone a process at the cellular level ghosting Darwinian environmental selection. They suggested a model in which immune surveillance exerts a selective pressure such that any cells that eventually escape and outgrow are inherently less immunogenic than the starting population (immunoediting), perhaps as a consequence of downregulation of the molecules that are required for immune recognition. Experimental support for this idea was provided by data demonstrating that tumor cells from immunodeficient mice were more immunogenic than those from immunocompetent mice. Although sustaining the concept of immune surveillance, these data raised a potentially formidable obstacle to the delivery of clinically useful immunotherapies, suggesting that by the time a cancer becomes detectable it is already beyond the capabilities of the host immune system to eradicate it. Critically, from the therapeutic standpoint, however, they showed that it was possible to make these cells visible to the immune system by increasing their antigen expression. Similar findings were obtained in RAG-1$^{-/-}$ mice,[16] and additional studies in mice specifically deficient in αβ or γδ T cells demonstrated that both cell types play critical and distinct roles in immune surveillance.[17-19] NK and NKT cells were also implicated as mediators of protection in experiments in which they were depleted with either anti-NK1.1 monoclonal antibody or anti-asialo-GM1 prior to challenge with a chemical carcinogen.[16] Further dissection of the critical effector mechanisms underlying host resistance to both chemically induced and spontaneous tumors has emerged from studies on IFN-γ and perforin demonstrating that deficiencies in either of these key immunologic molecules manifests with increased susceptibility to tumor growth.[15,20-26]

The central tenets of immunoediting have evolved slightly since inception, but may be considered to consist of three processes occurring either independently or sequentially.[27-30] First, "elimination" in which immunity functions as an extrinsic tumor suppressor (equivalent to the original concept of immunosurveillance); second, "equilibrium" in which cancerous cells survive but are held in check by the immune system; and third "escape" in which tumor cell variants with either reduced immunogenicity or the capacity to attenuate or subvert immune responses grow into clinically apparent cancers. Data supporting the equilibrium process have remained relatively elusive, and largely inferred from clinical observation. For example, the development of melanoma of donor origin in two recipients of renal allografts from the same donor who had been considered cured of melanoma treated 16 years previously.[31] More recently Schreiber's group has shown clearer evidence to support the existence of such a state in a mouse model of primary chemical carcinogenesis, demonstrating it to be mechanistically distinguishable from elimination and escape.[32] Following exposure to the carcinogen approximately 20% of animals developed fatal tumors, but some survived with no overt evidence of tumor growth (apparent elimination). Immune suppression in these mice, however, resulted in the unmasking of dormant tumors which then spread, ultimately killing the host. This effect was observed either following T cell depletion or following neutralization of IFN-γ or IL-12, but not following depletion of natural killer cells suggesting a specific role for adaptive immunity in the maintenance of equilibrium. Furthermore, examination of stable dormant lesions revealed cancerous cells with similar morphological features to those in progressive lesions but with a lower proliferative index and increased apoptosis. The lesions were infiltrated with T cells suggesting a possible ongoing interaction with the host immune system. Engraftment of these cancerous cells into immunodeficient mice following a short period of ex vivo culture resulted in tumor growth. In contrast, transfer into immunocompetent recipients failed to induce tumor growth. Finally, tumor outgrowth occasionally occurred following a period of dormancy in immunocompetent animals, and in these cases tumor cells were able to grow following transfer to immunocompetent mice, suggesting they had become less immunogenic. These data supported the idea that tumor cells are unedited in equilibrium but become edited when they spontaneously escape immune control.

Immune Tolerance

The overall debate over the significance of immune surveillance in human cancers had one further concept to fully embrace, fostering the incorporation of significant advances in our understanding of the mechanisms controlling immunological tolerance. In 2005, Gerald Willimsky and Thomas Blankenstein suggested that sporadic tumors in mice do not lose immunogenicity as would be predicted by models invoking immunoediting as the major reason for tumor escape, but rather induce tolerance to evade immune detection.[33] The idea itself was not new and indeed had been part of the original immunoediting model. The message was simple and had major implications for the successful application of immune-based therapies. Progression of cancer may not depend solely on intrinsic adaptions of the tumor cells to evade detection, but rather on changes exerted on host immunity to induce a state of functional inertia. These mechanisms are neither mutually exclusive nor entirely separable, as upregulation of the surface expression of immuno-inhibitory ligands by tumor cells can potentially abrogate immune responses just as efficiently as downregulation of immunostimulatory elements. Their studies involved the use of mouse model in which a viral cancer-promoting gene (SV40 large T) was controlled to activate rarely in random tissues. Although immune responses to the SV40 large T protein were initially detected in the mice, they subsequently developed immune tolerance, while the tumors remained capable of eliciting vigorous immunity when transferred into identical but tumor-free mice (with no clear evidence for immunoediting).

The apparent contradictions between this study and those supporting a more central importance for tumor-intrinsic editing may reflect differences in inherent tumor immunogenicity. More immunogenic tumors will, by definition, generate a more robust immune response. This likely relates partly to the ability of dendritic cells (DCs) to present tumor debris in an "immunogenic" fashion, which in itself may reflect activation by secondary danger signals. In this setting evolutionary pressures may be higher and immunoediting may be critical to immune evasion. For less immunogenic tumors that do not efficiently activate cellular antigen-presenting machinery, arousal of the immune system is minimal and escape variants are therefore less likely to be sculpted by immunoediting. In these cases tolerance or immunological ignorance may play variable roles.

Early Failures—Lessons Learned

The apparent confirmation of the validity of the immune surveillance hypothesis led to great enthusiasm for the development of immune-based anticancer therapies. However, attempts to target human cancers by immunotherapy have been significantly less successful than initially envisaged possible, leading to the marginalization of immunotherapies from mainstream oncology practice. In patients presenting with cancer, endogenous antitumor immunity has been insufficient to eliminate the tumor. Immunological ignorance may contribute to tumor outgrowth, but antitumor responses are detectable in many of these patients. Indeed, it is clear from the detailed studies of immunoediting in mouse models that even when immunosurveillance fails, the relationship between immunity and cancer is far from over. It is therefore likely that failure to eradicate tumors relates to limitations of effector function of the tumor-specific T cells. For maximal antitumor responses it is necessary for appropriately targeted and activated effectors expressing T cell receptors (TCRs) of sufficient avidity to migrate into tumor sites and maintain effector function within immunologically hostile tumor microenvironments. The presence of even large numbers of T cells capable of recognizing tumors is not singularly sufficient to mediate tumor regression, as evidenced by unrestricted tumor growth in TCR transgenic mice in which all of the T cells are capable of recognizing the tumor antigen.[34] Clinical studies of active immunization have shown that despite expansion of tumor-reactive T cells to levels of up to 40% of the circulating $CD8^+$ T cell repertoire tumor growth may continue apparently unimpeded.[35] There is now ample experimental evidence that functional systemic antitumor activity may not translate into tumor rejection, either because of lack of infiltration of T cells into the tumor[36] or because of local suppression of function within the tumor microenvironment. Although tumor-specific immunity is compromised in tumor-bearing mice, there is often no generalized immune deficiency,[37] indicating that tumors can specifically suppress the induction of effective antitumor immunity. This concept is perhaps best highlighted by concomitant immunity, wherein a mouse injected with a tumor will reject a subsequent challenge with the same tumor at a distant site, despite continued growth at the site of initial challenge.[38-40] Intriguingly, however, it has been known for some time that the initial generation of concomitant immunity is eventually subverted during primary tumor progression by the establishment of $CD4^+$ T cell-mediated immune suppression.[41,42] Despite these findings the majority of approaches to tumor immunotherapy have until recently remained grounded in infectious disease principles. It had been established in the 1980s that antigen-specific $CD8^+$ cytotoxic T cells (CTLs) were able to induce fully protective immunity against the influenza virus, leading to the development of effective vaccines.[43] The critical role of DCs in mediating these immune responses was recognized soon thereafter in the work of Ralph Steinman and others.[44] On the basis of growing evidence that tumors express antigens that can be presented by professional APCs to induce the generation of tumor-specific CTLs, tumor immunotherapists aimed to parallel the successes achieved in developing vaccines for infectious diseases. Strategies have included vaccination with peptide, DNA or antigen-pulsed DCs. Alternate approaches have been pursued based on directly enhancing effector number or function by adoptive transfer of T cells expanded from tumor-infiltrating lymphocytes (TILs), T cells activated ex vivo with cytokines, T cells together with cytokines, and more recently T cells engineered to express receptors specific for tumor-associated antigens (either TCRs or chimeric antigen receptors (CAR).[45-49] While these approaches have resulted in some impressive responses (reviewed later), they all potentially remain limited by the locally immunosuppressive microenvironment within the tumor, as evidenced by the evolution of such strategies to incorporate lymphodepleting or non-myeloablative conditioning to enhance responses. Since tumors can be viewed as taking advantage of immunological ignorance, anergy and suppression, effectively subjugating host responses to create isolated nodes of immune privilege within an otherwise immunologically intact host, they share many similarities with chronic pathogens such as *Mycobacteria tuberculosis, Listeria monocytogenes* and *Leishmania major.* In this context the challenges of delivering effective vaccines or immunotherapies are much more closely aligned with those associated with therapy of these established chronic infections than with acute infectious pathogens, in which the majority of the successes have come with prophylactic vaccination strategies. Further consideration of the mechanisms underlying the tumor escape phase of the immunoediting model may enlighten strategies to enhance the effectiveness of immunotherapies.

Mediators of Immune Escape

As previously discussed, the significant changes occurring in the escape phase may be broadly considered as those intrinsic to the tumor cells themselves and those involving the local tumor microenvironment, although the two overlap. Classic examples of the former include downregulation of costimulatory molecules (eg, B7 molecules) by the tumor leading to activation of tumor-reactive T cells in the absence of appropriate costimulation and induction of anergy,[50] or tumor antigen loss or downregulation of major histocompatibility complex (MHC) molecules which can render the tumor cells essentially invisible to the immune system.[51] Further examples include mutations conferring increased resistance to apoptosis induction or cell-mediated cytotoxicty, such as overexpression of anti-apoptotic molecules (eg, FLIP and BCL-XL),[52,53] and mutations in FAS or the TRAIL receptor death receptor 5 (DR5).[54-56] Increased expression of T-cell inhibitory molecules such as programmed cell death ligand 1 (PD-L1), B7-H3, B7x, HLA-G, and HLA-E by the tumor cells themselves or surrounding parenchyma (stromal or antigen presenting cells [APCs]) can directly inhibit effector T cell function, and in many cases expression levels by the tumor or its microenvironment have been found to correlate inversely with tumor outcomes.[57-65] Further proposed mediators of local immune suppression include soluble suppressive factors elaborated by the tumor or parenchyma such as interleukin (IL)-10, transforming growth factor-β (TGF-β), VEGF, or gangliosides.[66-72] Indoleamine 2,3-dioxygenase (IDO) expression by tumor cells or IDO-competent APCs, such as some plasmacytoid DCs (pDCs), can also contribute to acquired tolerance, both by direct suppression of T cells and by enhancement of local regulatory T cell (Treg) mediated suppression.[73,74] IDO catalyzes the rate-limiting step in tryptophan degradation, and the combination of local reduction in tryptophan levels (possibly via the intermediacy of causing cellular stress responses in effector T cells) and the production of immunomodulatory tryptophan metabolites appears to exert tolerogenic activity. Furthermore, IDO-expressing pDCs resident within tumor-draining lymph nodes appear to directly activate mature Treg, which can subsequently cause upregulation of PD-L1 by other DCs which in turn inhibits effector T cell proliferation.[75] It has become clear that these regulatory networks are therefore extremely complex.[76] The presence of an array of other cell types capable of actively suppressing immune reactions such as $CD4^+CD25^+$ Treg, IL-10-secreting Treg, CD1d-restricted (NKT) T cells, immature and plasmacytoid DCs (iDCs and pDCs) and myeloid-derived suppressor cells (MDSCs) (noncell-autonomous suppression) within the tumor or tumor draining lymph nodes is clearly critical to induction and/or maintenance of local immune privilege in a number of systems.[74,77] Such cells may be preferentially recruited to these sites, or expanded or induced therein.

Non Cell-Autonomous Suppression

A number of $CD4^+$ T cell subtypes with regulatory or suppressive activity are now recognized. They fall broadly into one of two categories: Those produced by the thymus, express CD4, CD25, GITR, OX40 and cytotoxic T-lymphocyte-associated-antigen 4 (CTLA-4), and appear crucially dependent on the expression of the X-linked forkhead/winged helix transcription factor, Foxp3, for their development (so-called "naturally occurring" Treg);[78-84] and those which arise from naïve $CD4^+$ T cells as a result of "tolerogenic" encounters in the periphery. The latter "inducible" or "adaptive" Treg include interleukin (IL)-10-producing, Foxp3-negative Tr1 cells,[85-87] TGF-β-producing Th3 cells,[88,89] and extra-thymically generated $CD4^+CD25^+Foxp3^+$ iTreg cells.[90-95] In addition, $CD4^+CD25^-Foxp3^+$ T cells with regulatory capabilities have been recognized.[96] The acquisition of regulatory phenotype and suppressive functions by conventional nonregulatory $CD4^+$ T cells following exposure to antigens under certain conditions is now recognized as a major contributor to the maintenance of T cell homeostasis and control of inflammation. Of particular note, since thymic involution occurs relatively early in humans compared to mice, and telomere length in human Treg is considerably shorter, it is conceivable that peripheral conversion plays a far more important role in the maintenance of tolerance (and perhaps in immune subversion by tumors) in humans than in mice.[97-99] Furthermore, if antigen encounter is required for conversion, it seems plausible that the regulatory pool expands at the expense of potential effector T cells, since precursors recognizing tumor antigens will be redirected into a suppressor rather than effector phenotype.[100,101] Characterization of the conditions that drive such peripheral conversion is ongoing, but factors such as suboptimal antigen stimulation in combination with TGF-β appear to be important, both of which are likely to be relevant within the tumor microenvironment.[93,102] IDO produced by either tumor cells or parenchyma (eg, pDCs) also favors conversion,[75,103,104] and retinoic acid appears to be a key mediator in establishing intestinal tolerance.[105-108] Regulatory T cells require TCR triggering to become functional, and at least some tumor-associated Treg are specific for tumor antigens,[109] but once activated they suppress in an antigen-independent manner. While adaptive Tr1 and Th3 cells exert suppression mostly through soluble factors (IL-10 and/or TGF-β), their $Foxp3^+$ counterparts suppress via a variety of mechanisms, the relative importance of which remain to be fully elucidated in any given situation. Possible mechanisms include those involving CTLA-4, membrane-bound TGF-β, and pericellular generation of adenosine.[110-116] Their expansive capacity to suppress multiple immune effector populations, including $CD4^+$ and $CD8^+$ T cells, B cells and NK cells,[117] makes them potentially attractive "nodal" targets for therapeutic intervention within immunosuppressive networks. To add further to this complexity, $CD8^+$ T cells with suppressor activity have also been described.[118-121] The dominant inhibitory potential of Treg populations in murine models of malignancy is well established,[122] and more recently their potential role in human malignancies has been demonstrated.[123] The mechanisms driving Treg expansion and accumulation in patients with cancer are not fully understood, but both proliferation of pre-existing Treg and conversion from naïve precursors are likely to be involved.[101,124,125] Their relative abundance predicts for tumor outcomes in murine models,[126,127] and correlates inversely with outcomes in several epithelial carcinomas, including ovarian,[123,128] breast,[129] and hepatocellular carcinoma.[130] Intriguingly, in hematological malignancies this association is reversed and high levels of Treg appear to confer improved prognoses (eg, cutaneous T cell, follicular and Hodgkin lymphoma[131-133]). The level of infiltration of a tumor by Treg alone may not be the best predictor of outcome. Hodgkin lymphoma tumors contain significant populations of both IL-10-secreting Tr1 and $CD4^+CD25^+$ Treg which induce a profoundly immunosuppressive environment.[134] Combined assessment both of cells expressing Foxp3 and of cells expressing TIA-1 (cytotoxic granule-associated RNA binding protein) offers a better predictor of response,[133] highlighting the potential importance of assessing the relative prevalence of multiple infiltrating cellular populations. Indeed, identification of specific immunological signatures (based on flow cytometry, PCR or microarray analyses[135]) that predict outcomes, or guide the institution or monitoring of therapies would be useful adjuncts to modern clinical practice. For example, it is plausible that tumors that contain few TILs, including Treg, will respond well to treatments that aim to enhance CTL numbers, function or migration, While those that contain significant numbers of Treg would benefit from therapies aimed at reducing Treg number or function. In addition, Treg represent another regulatory mechanism that may be enhanced in response to, and hence limit the efficacy of, current immunotherapeutic interventions. For example, IL-2 has entered clinical trials for a number of human cancers such as melanoma, renal cell carcinoma, rhabdomyosarcoma and ovarian cancer. Its initial use was based on the idea that it may directly enhance effector function of both innate and adaptive immune systems. However, IL-2 is recognized as crucial for the homeostasis and function of $CD4^+CD25^+$ Treg in vivo,[136-138] and administration to patients with cancer results in increases in the numbers of peripheral Treg cells and stimulation of expression of CXC-chemokine receptor 4 (CXCR4) and CCR4 on Treg promoting their migration toward CXCL12 and CCL2 within the tumor microenvironment.[139-141] Since the targets of many cancer vaccination strategies are self antigens, it is perhaps no surprise that "therapeutic" cancer vaccines can induce amplification of tumor-specific Treg.[142,143] The "immunogenicity" or "tolerogenicity" of DCs thus becomes an increasingly important consideration in vaccination programs since even conventionally "mature" DCs can activate and expand autoantigen-specific Treg cells.[144,145]

Multiple suppressive APC populations have been described, and postulated to play a part in the generation of local immune privilege within tumors. Developing tumors may selectively recruit suppressive APCs or convert stimulatory APCs into suppressors, mirroring the situation with suppressive T cell populations. The molecular mechanisms underpinning active immune suppression by DC and myeloid populations have not been fully elucidated, but include secretion of IL-10 and TGF-β, expression of FAS ligand, PD-L1, and elaboration of intracellular IDO.[146-150] IDO-competent DCs can induce apoptosis of activated T cells, or either T cell anergy or conversion of effectors into Treg as previously outlined.[75,103,151,152] The local balance of stimulatory vs suppressive APCs is probably critical in determining the eventual outcome of T cell encounter with antigen in these sites. It has also become clear that the interaction between DCs and Treg is likely a two-way process.[153-155] MDSCs are a heterogeneous group of cellular precursors of macrophages, granulocytes, DCs and myeloid cells at earlier stages of differentiation, which express both the myeloid differentiation antigen Gr-1 (Ly6G and Ly6C) and CD11b in mice, and are generally defined as $CD14^-CD11b^+$ cells in humans (expressing CD33 but lacking expression of mature myeloid or lymphoid markers).[156-158] Specific phenotypic markers that are reflective of suppressor function remain relatively poorly defined.[159] They consist of two major subsets of $Ly6G^+Ly6C^{low}$ granulocytic and $Ly6G^-Ly6C^{high}$ monocytic cells in mice. Numbers may correlate with clinical outcomes in human cancer.[160] Several tumor-derived cytokines have been implicated in the expansion of MDSC, including VEGF, IL-1β, and GM-CSF.[161-163] The mechanism of MDSC-mediated suppression is complex, involving contributions from either iNOS or arginase 1,[147,164-167] which enable MDSCs to inhibit T cell responses in various ways, including induction of apoptosis, inhibition of proliferation, or induction of a regulatory phenotype. Nitration of tyrosines in the TCR-CD8 complex appears to render CD8-expressing T cells unable to bind peptide-MHC complexes and to respond to the specific peptide, although they retain their ability to respond to nonspecific stimulation.[168] Type 2 macrophages found at tumor sites have also been implicated in suppression of tumor immunity and seem to share some functional properties with immature myeloid cells.[169,170]

It is perhaps unsurprising given the multitude of potential local immunosuppressive mechansims engaged within an actively growing tumor, that even in those cancer immunotherapies that succeed in inducing systemic immunity, translation into clinically significant effects are rare. It is likely that these mechanisms will need to be addressed in order to improve outcomes. What remains wholly unclear is how effectively this aim can be met, and how many of the disparate targets will need to be tackled at any one time in order to generate locally curative immunity.

Moving Toward Clinically Effective Immunotherapies

Just as the basic idea of immune surveillance is not new, attempts to exploit the immune system to combat cancer have a similarly long history. In 1891 William Coley (1862-1936), a bone surgeon at New York Cancer Hospital which later became part of the Memorial Sloan-Kettering Cancer Center, learned from hospital notes of a patient who had been seen 7 years earlier with an inoperable malignant tumor in his neck, which had disappeared following a bacterial skin infection. The infection was erysipelas caused by *Streptococcus pyogenes*. After a considerable search (detailed eloquently by Stephen Hall in his book *A Commotion in the Blood*[171]) Coley was able to track him down and found him to remain free from any evidence of cancer. He reasoned that somehow the infection had been the precipitant of the remarkable recovery. Indeed, there was already clear precedent in the published literature of the time. Almost 25 years earlier in 1867 a German professor named Busch had intentionally infected a female patient with erysipelas in order to cure a large tumor.

An impressive though short-lived partial response was documented. Coley found more than 20 published accounts before 1890 linking infection with erysipelas and antitumor responses. On this background, and somewhat less encumbered by current regulatory issues, he pursued his own clinical trial using live bacteria, evolving to the use of heat-killed bacteria following some infection-related deaths.[172,173] It is remarkable to consider that even a minority of these patients were cured. The first patient he infected with erysipelas was apparently cured, dying 10 years later of unknown causes, as was the first patient treated with his mixed Coley toxins, dying 25 years later of a heart attack. Ultimately the antitumor effects were probably attributable to the production of tumor necrosis factor (TNF) in response to bacterial endotoxins.[174,175] While TNF itself has proven too toxic for reliable clinical usage, it is perhaps fitting that members of the TNF superfamily and their receptors remain important targets for current approaches to immunotherapy. The rest of the chapter will discuss the strategies which have arisen from the studies already mentioned, briefly exploring recent approaches to promote DC function but concentrating largely on adoptive cellular therapies and immunostimulatory monoclonal antibodies.

Adoptive Cell Therapy and Development of Personalized Immunotherapies

The growing appreciation that tumor-bearing hosts often do mount antitumor responses, and that the greatest concentration of accessible tumor-specific cells may reside within the tumor itself (albeit held in check by local immunoparetic factors) has informed the development of the field of adoptive cellular therapy (ACT). Furthermore, the failure of active immunization to effect major clinical responses has clearly not always reflected a lack of systemic antitumor immunity, although it has been argued that at least part of this failure relates to stimulation mainly of low-avidity effector T cells, itself reflecting the impact of central deletional tolerance on the anti-self T cell repertoire. These cells may be detectable by conventional immune monitoring techniques, but have little chance of rejecting established tumors, particularly as access to and function within the tumor microenvironment are also likely to be limiting factors. Adoptive immunotherapy allows the identification of rare cells with relatively high affinity for tumor antigen that can be selected in vitro and expanded before transfer to the host. These cells can be activated ex vivo and directly administered, in the hope of avoiding the tolerizing factors present at the tumor site. Initially based on the idea that significantly increasing the number of tumor-reactive T cells will bypass all peripheral and local regulatory mechanisms, flooding the tumor and leading to prompt tumor rejection, modern approaches now recognize the importance of further manipulation of the host to optimize the chances of therapeutic success. These approaches have been developed in parallel with, and in many cases informed, studies advancing our knowledge of the factors limiting antitumor immunity, establishing that the administration of large numbers of activated high affinity "tumor-specific" T cells to a lymphodepleted host can overcome inhibitory factors and mediate effective cancer immunotherapy in some cases of human malignancy, particularly melanoma. Approaches to date have been largely based on the in vitro expansion of T cells obtained from tumor infiltrates, and to a lesser degree from peripheral blood or lymph nodes biopsies. Transfers are often combined with administration of the T cell growth factor IL-2. It is likely that such strategies will continue to evolve, incorporating advances in immunostimulatory antibody research (see below).

Much of the pioneering work that laid the foundations for subsequent investigation of passive anticancer immunotherapy through ACT was performed by Nicholas Mitchison in the early 1950s,[176,177] and it is perhaps germane to reflect that the enhancing activity of host irradiation and well as the significance of antigen dose in determining immune response was already established in these seminal works.[178-180] The further development of ACT owes much to work of the groups of Alexander Fefer, Martin Cheever and Philip Greenberg at University of Washington, as well as those of Steven Rosenberg and Nicholas Restifo at National Cancer Institute. Fefer advanced the concept of "chemoimmunotherapy" in the late 1960s, demonstrating that an established syngeneic lymphoma (FBL-3 or Friend virus-induced lymphoma) could be eradicated after therapeutic combination of high doses of the alkylating agent cyclophosphamide and the transfer of immune cells from a mouse previously sensitized (or challenged) with the same tumor.[181-183] Further studies helped to define some of the mechanisms underpinning this antitumor activity, demonstrating that it was either directed against tumor or virus antigens,[182,183] that T cells were the major mediators,[184] and that this activity could also be isolated from nonsensitized mice, although with a much diminished potency.[185] This last point is significant since it suggests that a population of tumor-reactive T cells may be present in naive animals. The work was extended to show that antitumor activity was enhanced in cells that had been re-sensitized and expanded with irradiated tumor in vitro,[186-188] or even with cells that had been only primarily sensitized in vitro.[189] An important advance during this work was the introduction of IL-2 in the in vitro system which allowed further expansion of tumor-reactive T cells.[189] Finally, it was demonstrated that tumoreactive T cells could be cultured in vitro for long periods of time and that after adoptive transfer they would proliferate and mediate specific tumor rejection which could be significantly augmented by the in vivo administration of IL-2.[190-192] These studies were amongst the first to highlight the potential benefits of the use of IL-2 both in vitro and in vivo in mediating efficient expansion and enhancing tumor rejection.

Contemporaneously, Rosenberg also demonstrated the benefits of IL-2 in cancer immunotherapy. In what would become one of the cornerstones of ACT, a series of studies were published on the use of "T cell growth factor" (TCGF or IL-2) to clone and expand T cells,[45,193,194] including its use for the isolation and expansion of T cells infiltrating solid tumors.[195] Importantly, human lymphocytes grown in TCGF where capable of killing autologous tumor cells in vitro.[196] This initial observation led to a series of publications documenting the role of IL-2 in the "lymphokine-activated killer" cell phenomena (LAK)[197] and the capacity of these cells to kill fresh tumor cells in vitro as well as to induce regression of established disseminated lymphoma after adoptive transfer in animal models.[198] These studies were not limited to lymphoma and follow-up studies rapidly transitioned to treatment of established murine melanoma.[199] One notable feature of Rosenberg's approach to immunotherapy was its fast translation into clinical trials. In early 1984 the first phase I study on the use of LAK cells in humans was published.[200] This trial demonstrated proof of concept, showing that large numbers of cells could be obtained by in vitro expansion of lymphocytes derived from peripheral blood, which could then be safely transferred back into patients with cancer. The study also documented evidence of migration of these cells into several organs and tissues including tumor. Two additional studies would be instrumental in the advancement of ACT into the clinical setting, both relating to the in vivo administration of IL-2 in murine models.[201,202] Following phase I assessment of the safety of systemic administration of IL-2 in humans, [203] a much larger study combining LAK and IL-2 administration was performed[204,205] in which more than 100 patients were treated with several courses of IL-2 and very high numbers of autologous LAK cells (up to 18.4×10^{10} cells). Complete or partial responses were seen in 21% of patients.[205] Despite the favorable results obtained in these early clinical trials, data from murine models would redirect research away from LAK cells and toward the transfer of highly specific tumor-reactive T cells. The new approach was based in the isolation and in vitro expansion of TILs with IL-2.[195] These expanded TILs were 50-100 times more efficient than LAK cells in the treatment of various types of tumors, and their potency was significantly enhanced when their transfer was combined with in vivo administration of cyclophosphamide and IL-2.[45] Clinical trials mirroring the murine experience and combining cyclophosphamide, TILs and IL-2 have yielded complete and partial responses in up to 31% of patients with metastatic melanoma.[206]

These early studies have helped to inform the evolution of ACT as a form of personalized immunotherapy.[207-209] The transition of ACT into the clinical setting has, however, not been without difficulties. These can be considered in two groups: factors relating to difficulties in generating appropriate products for adoptive transfer, and factors relating to host or tumor resistance to transferred populations.

Generation of Cellular Therapy Products

One major limitation has been the difficulty in accessing tumor samples containing sufficient numbers of viable TILs for successful isolation and expansion, which remains a limiting step in 60-70% of cases.[210] Alternative strategies for isolation of tumor-reactive lymphocytes (TRLs) would facilitate more widespread application. Such approaches include the use of T cells from peripheral blood or lymph node biopsies.[211-214] Stimulation with antibodies directed against CD3 and the co-stimulatory receptor CD28 expressed on T cells are now widely used for the ex vivo expansion of large numbers of TRLs, while 4-1BB (see below) has recently attracted more attention both for activation and selection protocols.[215-218] The identification and cloning of T cells with specificity to antigens that either are more abundant on or, less commonly, specific to tumor cells (NY-ESO-1, MART-1, tyrosinase, gp-100, p53) has also contributed greatly to the development of alternatives to isolation of TILs. In vitro enrichment of such TRLs from peripheral blood by stimulation with their cognate antigen can be followed by expansion protocols as previously outlined. Much has been learned about the optimal characteristics of the transferred cells, in terms of maximizing persistence and antitumor activity. Long term in vitro culture has been demonstrated to be detrimental and the level of differentiation of T cells to be critical.[219] IL-2 drives differentiation of T cells to intermediate and late effector stages of differentiation. Furthermore, IL-2 may not be the optimal cytokine to use to enhance activity in vivo since it also expands Treg and is associated with significant toxicity. The first issue may be addressed by the use of IL-7, IL-15 and IL-21 which seem to more specifically target effector T cells when applied either alone or in combination,[220] rescuing tolerant $CD8^+$ T cells,[221] and generating less differentiated cells which appear to mediate greater antitumor immunity.[222-224] IL-2 seems to be required not only for the expansion but also for the long-term persistence of the adoptively transferred T cells. More recent work in murine models suggests that co-transfer of $CD4^+$ T cells can supply IL-2 and sustain TRLs for long periods of time therefore increasing the antitumor effect of ACT.[225-227] Numerous studies have demonstrated the requirement for $CD4^+$ T cell help in the generation and/or maintenance of $CD8^+$ T cell memory. In addition to provision of cytokine support, they have roles in DC conditioning and in recruitment and activation of macrophages and eosinophils which can mediate antitumor effects.[224,228,229]

More recent efforts have focused on genetic modification of T cells to engineer improved antitumor effects. Such approaches include the transfer of CAR that have antibody-based external receptor structures and cytosolic domains that encode signal transduction modules of the TCR.[230] These allow redirection of T cell specificity in an MHC unrestricted manner, while delivering the equivalent intracellular signaling of TCR ligation. Furthermore, the impact of triggering can be enhanced by engineering the cytolsolic domain for additional provision of counterfeit co-stimulatory signaling following ligation (mimicking CD28, 4-1BB or OX40 ligation). Although incorporation of a CD28 component results in IL-2 release and limited proliferation (plus enhanced resistance to the suppressive effects of Treg[231]), T cell activation remains incomplete and can be further enhanced by inclusion of the 4-1BB or OX40 signaling domains within the construct.[232,233] A number of early trials have suggested that persistence of transgene-expressing cells may be limited to periods of days to weeks following transfer.[49,234-237] This may relate in part to the potential immunogenicity of the CAR. However, lessons learnt from earlier ACT studies may also be pertinent, and current approaches are focusing on the use of central rather than effector memory populations,[238,239] and on the use of T cells specific for herpes viruses which are maintained at relatively high levels in humans due to persistent stimulation via their native TCR by the "latent" viral reservoir.[49] Central memory cells represent the least differentiated end of the spectrum of antigen-experienced T cells and retain the developmental options of naive T cells including the capacity for marked clonal expansion. An alternative strategy to redirect T cell specificity relies on transduction of TCR genes from tumor-reactive clones, although this has the relative disadvantage of conferring MHC-restricted targeting.[48,240-242] In the first clinical trial using this approach a MART-1-reactive TCR was transduced into human lymphocytes, inducing the capacity to secrete effector cytokines and display lytic activity when co-incubated with $MART\text{-}1^+$ tumor cells. Following recipient lymphodepletion, these cells were infused into patients with melanoma who subsequently received infusions of IL-2 with the suggestion that the T cells may have effected clinical responses in 2 of 17 patients.[48] Potential factors limiting efficacy in this study include variable persistence of gene-modified cells, and relatively low levels of surface expression of the introduced TCR. The latter relates to competition of exogenous TCR chains with endogenous TCR chains for assembly with CD3 components and also to the formation of mixed dimers of exogenous and endogenous TCR chains, restricting avidity.[243] Indeed, gene optimization that elicits only modest increases in TCR expression may result in marked enhancement of antitumor activity.[244] An alternate and perhaps complementary approach is to engineer cells in ways to enhance survival, eg, by transducing cells with chimeric GM-CSF-IL-2 receptors (designed to deliver an IL-2 signal when binding GM-CSF in an autocrine loop[245]), CD28,[246] or the catalytic subunit of telomerase.[247] The ability to further modify these lymphocytes, to make them less subject to the suppressive influences present in the tumor microenvironment such as the introduction of genes encoding dominant-negative TGF-β, or inhibitory RNAs to prevent the expression of inhibitory molecules such as CTLA-4 and PD-1, could potentially further enhance the activity of the transferred cells.[248] Alternatively, overexpression of selected co-stimulatory ligands may induce auto- and transcostimulation, resulting in potent antitumor activity.[249]

Role of Lymphodepletion

Transfer of tumor-specific T cells into unmanipulated hosts is often accompanied by a failure to demonstrate engraftment or persistence of transferred cells, or only modest antitumor effects on bulky tumors,[250-252] and it is likely that further attention to both intrinsic and extrinsic inhibitory factors will be critical to successful clinical application. Profound lymphodepletion of the host substantially increases the effectiveness of cell transfer therapy, likely by a number of mechanisms including elimination of cytokine sinks (lymphocytes competing with transferred cells for homeostatic cytokines such as IL-7 and IL-15), elimination of Treg and myeloid suppressor cells, and provision of an environment driving homeostatic proliferation.[225,253-255] The Treg content of the adoptively transferred population may also be important.[225] In addition to effects on immune cells, host irradiation can sensitize the stromal cells surrounding the tumor[256] and induce upregulation of adhesion molecules on tumor vasculature.[257,258] Finally, host irradiation releases LPS from commensal gut microflora which further matures DCs to activate tumor-reactive T cells,[259] and escalation to ablative conditioning with hematopoietic stem cell rescue may further promote the expansion and function of adoptively transferred CD8$^+$ T cells.[260]

Current Position of Adoptive T-Cell Transfer

Experience with ACT is therefore generally encouraging, but it is important to recognize that use of TILs may favor inclusion of those with an immune system inherently more capable of mediating antitumor activity. Since the level of tumor infiltration with TILs has been shown to correlate with outcome in a number of studies of human malignancy, the ability to generate a therapeutic product from TILs could be a predictive biomarker for outcome. The achievement of higher response rates in the significantly less selected groups receiving CAR- or TCR-transduced ACT will be an important step forward in this regard, but current results have demonstrated results more typical of other single-agent immunotherapeutic approaches. In the absence of large randomized studies it is impossible to assess the relative contributions of lympho-depleting chemo-radiotherapy, IL-2 and ACT to overall results. The number of randomized studies performed in the field remains limited (reviewed in Ref. 212) and only one of these had a positive outcome. Intriguingly, this was in patients with hepatocellular carcinoma rather than the more commonly treated melanoma or renal cancer. Patients received peripheral blood T cells activated in vitro with anti-CD3 and IL-2 in the adjuvant setting following surgical resection of the primary tumor (n = 150). Tumor recurrence was reduced 41% in those receiving ACT with longer progression free survival (p = 0.01), and a trend toward longer overall survival (p = 0.09).[261] There was no such benefit in a more recent trial of patients with stage III melanoma randomized to receive TIL plus IL-2 or IL-2 alone.[262,263] One further major problem with the application of ACT is that it is a highly personalized treatment and does not easily fit into current modes of oncological practice. Generation of appropriate cellular products is labor-intensive and requires significant laboratory expertise. Furthermore, each patient essentially requires the generation of new reagent limiting the opportunities for easy commercialization, and suggesting that delivery may be considered more service-oriented rather than product-related (as in the case of most drugs). This aspect, combined with increasing awareness that minimizing ex vivo T cell manipulation may be advantageous in terms of clinical outcomes, is driving the current evolution of clinical strategies. The issue is also informed by topical debate concerning the nature of the best targets for immunotherapy in terms of public vs private antigens. While we have historically focused on "public" or shared tumor antigens such as MART-1 and gp-100, accepting that antitumor efficacy may then be inextricably linked to tissue-specific toxicity, "private" or patient-specific antigens generated as a consequence of the evolution of the malignant phenotype and inherent genetic instability within these lesions have a number of attractive advantages,[264,265] an idea we shall return to later.[266] The acceptance of tissue-specific toxicity leads to the concept of "dispensible tissues,"[267] which may be acceptable in the case of vitiligo with therapies targeting melanoma or B cell deficiency following anti-CD20 therapy, but will be more of an issue if the target is shared by a vital organ.[235] The parallel development of "off the shelf" reagents for enhancing immunity offers a number of interesting approaches to further enhance the efficacy of ACT. However, it remains unclear what overall contribution ACT will continue to provide if these strategies can be optimized in a way that targets private antigens by enhancing in vivo immunogenicity, effectively tailoring personalized therapy with the use of less "patient-centric" reagents.

Promoting DC Function

Detailed discussion of the newer approaches aimed at enhancing antigen presentation in efforts to improve antitumor immunity is beyond the scope of this chapter. However, a few deserve brief mention. DCs are uniquely specialized to present processed antigens to stimulate antigen-specific effector responses. Progress in our understanding of factors associated with DC-induced immunogenicity rather than tolerogenicity have informed the development of clinical therapeutics, yet it remains apparent that even conventionally "mature" DCs (with high levels of expression of co-stimulatory molecules) can mediate immune suppressive activity.[142,268-270] Cytokines known to enhance DC immunogenicity (eg, IFNs, IL-15, TNF, and IL-1) are generally insufficient to induce robust adaptive immunity when given in isolation.[271] By contrast, Toll-like receptor (TLR) agonists are showing some early promise in clinical studies, particularly in combination with other therapeutic modalities. Unmethylated CpG-oligodeoxynucleotides (ODNs) bind TLR9 on pDCs and B cells, inducing Th1 polarized immune responses and regression of established tumors in mice, as well as activity in phase I and II clinical trials.[272-279] TLR9-activated APCs activate NK cells, enhance expression of Fc receptors on polymorphonuclear leukocytes, and promote CTL activation. However, it is important to remain aware that in some settings TLR ligands provoke immunosuppressive or tolerogenic responses.[280,281] The context of TLR signaling may well be important and much remains to be learned about how the immune system discriminates between pathogenic inflammatory insults and the "beneficial" inflammation associated with commensal organisms or wound healing in order to iterate either immune activation or suppression in the light of apparently similar inflammatory signaling. The imidazoquinolone Imiquimod ligates TLR7 (and to a lesser degree TLR8) and when applied topically stimulates recruitment of pDCs and myeloid-derived DCs into tumors, both of which are implicated in subsequent antitumor activity.[282] It may also directly induce upregulation of vascular E-selectin and inhibit Treg function (including both Treg and novel $\gamma\delta$ suppressor populations),[283-285] and has been demonstrated to exhibit exciting clinical activity in vulval intraepithelial neoplasias.[286,287] Activation of invariant NKT cells by the CD1d-reactive glycolipids α-galactosylceramide (a-GalCer) or its analog a-C-galactosylceramide (a-C-GalCer) provides an alterative route to DC maturation, enhancing antitumor activity in a number of murine models.[288-290]

Another attractive target for enhancing APC performance is CD40. This molecule belongs to the TNF receptor (TNFR) superfamily (see below), and ligation is crucial for development of competent cellular immune responses, at least in part through the induction of IL-12 secretion by DCs. It is also critical for affinity maturation and heavy chain class switching during humoral responses.[228,291] It is constitutively expressed by B cells and DCs, and is also expressed by macrophages, T cells and nonhematopoietic cells such as vascular endothelium.[292] Its ligand CD40L is principally expressed by activated

CD4+ T-helper cells, although it is also expressed by pDCs, activated NK cells and platelets. CD40 ligation is critical for licensing of DCs, providing the temporal bridge between CD4+ T cell help and effective generation of CD8+ CTL responses by "conditioning" DCs (enhancing activation and costimulatory capacity). This activity may be reliant on CD27:CD70 interactions, as blocking CD70 during anti-CD40 treatment abrogates protection in a murine lymphoma model.[293] CD40 stimulation can potentially effect antitumor responses in a number of ways.[294,295] First, the expression of CD40 by a number of lymphoma and carcinoma tumor cells suggests that monoclonal antibodies to CD40 could elicit complement- or antibody-dependent cellular cytotoxicity (CDC or ADCC). Second, CD40 signaling has been reported to directly induce apoptosis in some tumor cells, notably in high grade B-cell non-Hodgkin lymphomas (NHLs) and epithelial carcinomas.[296-298] Finally, by enhancing antigen-presenting capacity CD40 ligation may directly, particularly in the case of B-cell lymphomas, or indirectly enhance presentation of tumor antigens to the immune system, at least partially overcoming the requirement for CD4+ T cells help in the generation of effective and durable antitumor CTL responses.[299-301] CD40 ligation by either CD40L or stimulatory anti-CD40 monoclonal antibodies in vitro or in vivo enhances antitumor vaccine efficiency in a number of murine models of malignancy.[294,302] By extension, forced expression of CD40L by either DC vaccines or B-cell tumors such as chronic lymphocytic leukemia using recombinant adenoviral vectors can enhance antitumor T cell responses and induce some level of clinical response.[303,304] Of note, however: These responses may be transient and associated with rapid engagement of host immune inhibitory circuits (eg, Treg), suggesting that combinatorial approaches might be more effective.[143] Clinical trials with recombinant CD40L trimer or anti-CD40 antibodies have suggested that in vivo triggering of CD40 on tumors and/or APCs can induce responses in a minority of patients, particularly in B-cell lymphomas or melanoma, although toxicities including systemic inflammatory syndromes and venous thromboses have been documented.[305-307] Nevertheless, these agents may prove to be valuable components of future therapeutic combinatorial strategies.[308]

Directly Promoting T-Cell Function

Immune activation is critically regulated by two major families of co-receptors expressed by T cells: the immunoglobulin-like (Ig) superfamily and the TNFR superfamily.[309,310] Costimulatory members of the former include CD28 and inducible T-cell co-stimulator (ICOS), while OX40, CD27, 4-1BB, CD30, GITR (glucocorticoid-induced TNFR family related gene), and HVEM (herpes-virus entry mediator) are members of the latter. The most well-established inhibitory members of the immunoglobulin "co-stimulatory" family include CTLA-4 and programmed cell death 1 (PD-1). B and T lymphocyte attenuator (BTLA) is the most recently described member of the family and also appears to mediate inhibitory effects on T cell activation.[311] The identities of the receptors for the newer members of the B7 ligand family (B7-H3 and B7x/B7-H4) remain elusive, but these receptors may also mediate significant inhibitory activity, perhaps more so in the periphery given the tissue distribution of these more recently identified ligands. Stimulatory or blocking monoclonal antibodies (Fig. 13-1) are being extensively investigated for their abilities to enhance T cell numbers, function, and maintenance of immunological memory.[312,313]

Stimulatory Antibodies to 4-1BB (CD137), OX40 (CD134), and GITR—Accentuating the Positive?

A number of the members of the TNFR family are appealing candidates for the development of targeted therapeutics. To date there have been relatively few data regarding agonistic anti-CD27 antibodies in murine tumor models, although it does appear to be a potentially interesting target for boosting antitumor immunity.[293] Greater attention has been focused on 4-1BB and OX40. 4-1BB is expressed on activated T cells (including Treg and NKT cells), activated NK and DCs, eosinophils, mast cells and endothelial cells in some metastatic tumors.[310,314-316] Its ligand 4-1BBL is expressed on activated DCs, B cells and macrophages. Ligation on T cells results in upregulation of anti-apoptotic genes and protection from activation-induced cell death (AICD),[317] enhancing establishment of durable memory CTLs.[318] The upregulation of 4-1BB on antigen-experienced T cells suggests that anti-4-1BB may differentially target these primed T cells, preferentially influencing those T cells with highest avidity receptors and partially explaining why 4-1BB costimulation may be superior to CD28 costimulation for the generation of antigen-specific cells for adoptive therapies.[219] While it is assumed that co-stimulation of CD8+ T cells is the principal mechanism of action of anti-4-1BB, various other immunomodulatory activities may contribute. In this respect, a common theme developing in our understanding of the function of immunostimulatory antibodies is their possible mutliplicity of function, reflecting the cellular distribution of the receptors. Thus (a) activation of APCs,[316] (b) reduction in Treg suppressive capacity[319] or enhancement of effector resistance to suppression,[320] and (c) co-stimulation of CD4+ and CD8+ T cells are all supported by experimental data. Furthermore, activated NK cells (possibly equivalent to IFN-producing killer DCs, IKDC[321-323]) and NKT cells may be relevant targets for antitumor activity.[315,324-326] Reverse signaling into cells expressing the ligands for a number of Ig or TNFR superfamily members (see also GITR:GITRL, CTLA-4:B7 and PD-1:PD-L1 below) is another recurring theme of recent investigations into immune modulating functions of these molecules. In the case of 4-1BBL this may result in enhanced production of inflammatory mediators or enhanced cell adhesion, facilitating egress of immune effectors into sites of inflammation.[327,328] There are conflicting data as to whether 4-1BB ligation on Treg results in enhanced or reduced suppressive capacity,[319,329,330] and synergy of antitumor activity with approaches that are thought to target Treg number or function has been taken as evidence that any 4-1BB-mediated inhibitory effects on Treg function may be relatively modest.[331-333] Forced expression of 4-1BBL in murine tumors enhances immunogenicity, reducing engraftment rates in immune competent recipients, although growth of untransfected cells is only modestly affected in relatively poorly immunogenic tumors.[334] Agonistic anti-4-1BB monoclonal antibodies enhance antitumor CTL responses, enabling rejection of established syngeneic tumor cell lines.[335-337] Activity appears critically dependent on CD8+ T cells and (in most studies) NK cells, with the role of CD4+ T cells varying in different tumor models.[315,336-339] Just as with other immunostimulatory antibodies, combination with vaccination strategies enhances activity in poorly immunogenic tumor models.[340,341] Co-administration with transgenic tumor-specific CTL enhances antitumor activity, apparently via a reduction in AICD rather than enhanced proliferation.[342] These data demonstrate the activity of anti-4-1BB antibodies in the absence of CD4+ T cell help, albeit in immunodeficient hosts (RAG2$^{-/-}$) lacking normal regulatory mechanisms. Early experience with a humanized clinical grade antibody (BMS-663513) has targeted mainly patients with melanoma and renal cell carcinoma.[343] The antibody was well tolerated with some evidence of activity (6% partial responses in melanoma patients), once again demonstrating the probable need to evaluate combinatorial approaches (and also define the optimal dosing strategy).[331,344,345] Two particularly

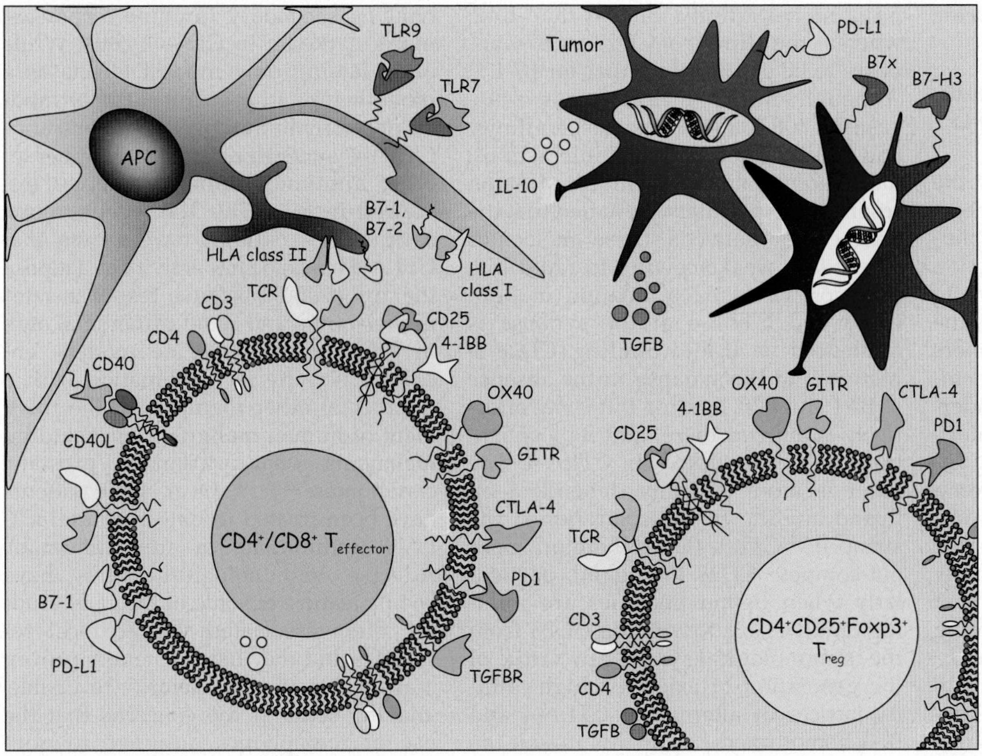

Figure 13-1 Potential targets for immunostimulatory therapies. The majority of T cell co-receptors that are upregulated upon activation of effector cells are also expressed by regulatory T cell populations and both cell types may be important targets for therapeutic interventions.

intriguing and seemingly paradoxical features of anti-4-1BB monoclonal antibodies are their ability to ameliorate autoimmunity[346-348] and to suppress humoral immunity in mice.[349] Although the precise mechanism(s) remain obscure, possibilities include effects on Treg function, interference with CD4+ T cell activation (possibly via the intermediacy of expansion of IFNγ-secreting CD11c+CD8+ T cells[350]), or IFNγ-dependent induction of IDO.[347,348] This highlights the potential importance of the timing of immunomodulatory interventions, as CD4 downregulation may be induced by AICD, which can also occur in CD8+ T cells if exposure to anti-4-1BB occurs immediately after antigen encounter.[351,352] While this suppressive activity has been proposed to be advantageous in terms of limiting possible antibody-mediated toxicities, it is recognized that it might also be deleterious to the development of optimal anticancer immunity.

OX40 is expressed transiently on activated CD4+ and CD8+ T cells, functioning as a late co-stimulatory receptor.[310,353] It is also expressed by NKT cells, where triggering may be required for optimal activation by a-GalCer,[354] and Treg. Its ligand OX40L is expressed in a similar distribution to 4-1BBL, on activated DCs, B cells and macrophages, as well as activated T cells and endothelial cells.[310] OX40 ligation regulates CD4+ and CD8+ T cell survival and memory generation, preventing T cell tolerance.[355-358] It also impairs the suppressor functions of Treg,[359,360] allowing tumor-resident DCs to traffic to draining lymph nodes to prime tumor-specific CD8+ CTL.[81] Furthermore, OX40 triggering appears to be antagonistic for Foxp3 induction in antigen-responding naïve CD4+ T cells, effectively suppressing the generation of iTreg,[361,362] and blocks the generation of IL-10-producing Tr1 cells,[363] suggesting that OX40 may antagonize the generation of a number of different inducible Treg populations. 4-1BB and OX40 act independently to facilitate robust CD8 and CD4 recall responses, overlapping in their intracellular signaling pathways,[364] yet neither 4-1BB nor GITR signaling seem to block the generation of Tr1,[363] and there are currently no reports illustrating whether they influence Foxp3+ iTreg induction. As with 4-1BBL, forced expression of OX40L by tumor cells increases immunogenicity, with tumor rejection dependent on both CD4+ and CD8+ T cells.[365] Furthermore, intratumoral injection of DCs modified to have enhanced expression of OX40L can effect tumor rejection in murine models that is dependent on CD8+ CTL responses, themselves dependent on CD4+ T cells and NKT cells.[354] Agonistic anti-OX40 antibodies also increase antitumor activity in a number of transplantable tumor models.[366] Concomitant activity on both effector and regulatory compartments may be a prerequisite of effective rejection of established tumors.[81] In preclinical models OX40 ligation enhances several other immunostimulatory approaches.[367-371]

In common with both 4-1BB and OX40, GITR is transiently expressed on activated T cells.[372,373] It is also constitutively expressed at high levels on Treg with further induction following activation.[374,375] Its ligand GITR-L is expressed at low levels on B cells, macrophages and some DCs, transiently increasing following activation. GITR ligation stimulates both proliferation and function of CD4+ and CD8+ T cells.[376] Its activity on Treg has remained more contentious.[80,377,378] Anti-GITR antibodies reduce suppression in co-cultures of CD4+CD25− effectors and CD4+CD25+ Treg, but whether this relates to reduced Treg suppressor function, increased resistance of effectors to the preserved suppressor function of Treg, or a combination of both, has yet to be definitively demonstrated. Experiments using mixtures of GITR+/+ and GITR−/− effector and regulatory cells suggest that ligation of GITR on the effector population rather than the regulatory population is critical for abrogating suppression,[378] suggesting that enhanced effector resistance to suppression may be key in in vitro assays. Injection of adenovirus expressing recombinant GITR-L into B16 melanoma promotes T-cell infiltration and reduced tumor volumes,[379] while agonistic anti-GITR antibodies have been shown to enhance both rejection of established methylcholanthrene-induced fibrosarcomas, and to enhance systemic antitumor responses and concomitant immunity when given following B16 melanoma challenge.[380,381] Furthermore, the same antibody also enhances the impact of DNA-vaccination in terms of generation of systemic immunity and enhancing resistance to challenge with murine melanoma.[382]

Stimulation Through Checkpoint Blockade of CTLA-4 (CD152), PD-1 (CD279), PD-L1 (CD274)—Eliminating the Negative

In contrast to the TNFR superfamily, the existence of co-inhibitory receptors mediating direct downregulation of lymphocyte activation and/or effector function has been a recognized feature of the Ig superfamily for some time. Indeed, the co-inhibitory receptor-ligand members outnumber the co-stimulatory members within this superfamily, engendering the idea of regulatory or inhibitory checkpoint blockade as a therapeutic anticancer strategy by James Allison over a decade ago.[383] Blockade of inhibitory immune checkpoints for therapeutic benefit offers considerable promise, particularly as combination with other treatment modalities that promote cross-priming of antitumor immunity may yield additive or synergistic activity. The strategy that is the most advanced in clinical development involves antibodies which block CTLA-4.[313]

CTLA-4 is expressed by activated $CD4^+$ and $CD8^+$ T cells, though its surface expression is tightly regulated with a short half-life. While expression is difficult to detect on resting T cells, it influences some the earliest events in T cell activation,[384,385] being rapidly mobilized from intracellular vesicles in the proximity to the MTOC to the immune synapse after TCR engagement.[386] In the unphosphorylated state, an intracellular localization motif mediates rapid binding to AP-2, endocytosis and lysosomal targeting.[387] It is constitutively expressed by natural and inducible $Foxp3^+$ Treg, although the majority of CTLA-4 is again found intracellularly, even following activation. CTLA-4 shares the B7-1 (CD80) and B7-2 (CD86) ligands with CD28, a critical co-stimulatory molecule. Ligation of CD28 in concert with TCR stimulation enhances T-cell proliferation by inducing production of IL-2 and anti-apoptotic factors, decreasing the number of ligated TCRs that are required for a given biological response.[388] CTLA-4 engagement selectively blocks augmentation of gene regulations by CD28-mediated co-stimulation, but does not ablate gene regulation induced by TCR triggering alone.[389] The function of CTLA-4 as a negative regulator of CD28-dependent T cell responses is most strikingly demonstrated by the phenotype of CTLA-4 knock-out mice, which succumb to a rapidly lethal polyclonal CD4-dependent lymphoproliferation within 3 to 4 weeks of birth.[390,391] CTLA-4 has significantly higher affinities for both B7 ligands than does CD28, and has a higher affinity for B7-1 than B7-2, whereas the affinity of CD28 for B7-2 appears to be greater than that for B7-1.[392] Although initial measurements suggested a 100-1000 fold increased affinity and avidity for CTLA-4:B7 interactions, more recent data using surface plasmon resonance experiments revealed that the interactions between these molecules are 10-fold weaker owing to rapid dissociation rates. Accumulation of both CD28 and CTLA-4 at the synapse is influenced by ligand binding. CD28 is recruited to the synapse in the absence of B7-1 and B7-2 binding but is not effectively stabilized there, and its localization can be disrupted by CTLA-4. The latter is more critically dependent on ligand binding for concentration at the synapse.[393] CTLA-4 may, therefore, both out-compete CD28 for ligand, particularly when ligand densities are limiting, and be able to exclude CD28 from the immunological synapse by virtue of the generation of extended high affinity lattices of alternating CTLA-4 and B7-1 homodimers.[394] For this reason the tight spatial and temporal regulation of CTLA-4 expression is likely to be critical for determining the outcome of CD28-mediated signaling. Furthermore, CTLA-4 ligation induces decreased production of cytokines (particularly IL-2 and its receptor) and cell cycle arrest in G1, suggesting that both ligation-dependent and ligation-independent mechanisms contribute to its negative regulatory function. Finally, CTLA-4 has an important role in Treg-mediated suppression, as evidenced by the recent demonstration that Treg-specific CTLA-4 deficiency in conditional knock-out (CKO) mice is associated with a profound reduction in their suppressive capacity.[112] CKO mice developed a lethal autoimmune lymphoproliferative syndrome with a slightly slower tempo than CTLA-$4^{-/-}$ mice. The mechanism(s) by which CTLA-4 mediates these Treg-associated effects remain(s) unclear, but may be dependent on reverse signaling into B7-expressing cells.[110,111] Certain subsets of DCs are induced to express IDO subsequent to CTLA-4 binding to DC-associated B7,[110,395] and induction of constitutive expression of inducible cAMP early repressor/cAMP response element modulator (ICER/CREM) attenuates IL-2 production in activated $CD25^+Foxp3^-$ T-cell effectors following similar B7-mediated "signaling."[111] Furthermore, Treg-mediated suppression during in vitro suppressor assays is associated with reduced activation of APCs (evidenced by reduced surface expression of B7 molecules[112]).

Antibody-mediated blockade of CTLA-4 is particularly effective at enhancing secondary immune responses, more markedly in $CD4^+$ T cells. While often having only modest effects as a monotherapy in preclinical tumor models of poorly immunogenic tumors, anti-CTLA-4 synergizes with a number of other antitumor immunotherapies (reviewed in Refs. 310, 314). Furthermore, early clinical studies have shown that CTLA-4 blockade has activity as a monotherapy (5-15% objective response rates in melanoma and renal carcinoma) and, in keeping with murine models, enhanced activity in combination with a number of other therapies in the treatment of human malignancies including melanoma, renal, ovarian and prostatic carcinomas.[309,396-400] Over 4000 patients have been treated to date with anti-CTLA-4 (ipilimumab or tremelimumab). Adverse immunological events have been a feature of some of the early studies, often associated with clinical responses, but they have generally proven manageable and the majority reversible, allaying some of the concerns that the use of therapeutics designed to nonspecifically enhance immune reactivity and to interfere with tumor-induced tolerance might uncouple mechanisms of self-tolerance systemically resulting in uncontrolled autoimmunity. This is a theoretical concern for agents inducing immunostimulation either by agonism of co-stimulatory pathways, antagonism of co-inhibitory pathways, or subversion of Treg-mediated suppression. The severe toxicity experienced by normal volunteers receiving a "super-agonistic" co-stimulatory antibody directed toward CD28 (TGN1412) highlights the need for careful evaluation of these new therapeutics,[401,402] although other targets which do not obviate the requirement for TCR signaling in inducing T cell activation (a feature of super-agonists) will likely have more favorable toxicity profiles, as is the case with CTLA-4 blockade. The association between adverse immune events and responses with anti-CTLA-4 is apparent across tumor types. For example, in patients with enterocolitis, response rates of 45% and 46% have been reported for metastatic melanoma and renal cell cancer, respectively.[403] What remains less clear is whether this association is an inevitable outcome of the mechanism of action of this new class of immunotherapeutics, or whether a narrow therapeutic window exists in which beneficial antitumor activity can be dissociated from adverse immune events, as has been hinted in some studies.

PD-1 is more broadly expressed than CD28 or CTLA-4. It can be detected on activated $CD4^+$ and $CD8^+$ T cells, as well as B cells, monocytes and at lower levels on NKT cells. It binds to 2 separate ligands, PD-L1 and PD-L2, which exhibit distinct expression profiles (reviewed in Ref. 151). PD-L1 is broadly expressed, and can be detected on resting and activated T cells (including $CD4^+CD25^+Foxp3^+$ Treg), B cells, macrophages, DCs, and mast cells. In addition, its expression on nonhematopoietic cells (including cornea, lung, pancreatic islets, placental syncytiotrophoblast, keratinocytes, and vascular endothelium) may have relevance to the function of this receptor-ligand pair. This broad nonhematopoietic expression pattern suggests that inhibition through the PD-L1/PD-1 axis may not be restricted solely to the interaction of T cells and professional APCs, but that it may also be relevant during the effector phase of the immune response in peripheral tissues, perhaps helping to prevent immune mediated tissue damage directly at the tissue interface. By comparison, PD-L2 has a much more limited expression profile. It is not expressed on naïve nor activated T cells, but is instead restricted to activated macrophages, myeloid DCs and mast cells, suggesting that it fulfills a role that differs from that of PD-L1. The phenotype of $PD\text{-}1^{-/-}$ mice provides perhaps the most direct evidence for an inhibitory role of this receptor.[404,405] These mice can develop an array of autoimmune pathologies characterized by high titers of autoantibodies, in keeping with a negative regulatory effect on T and/or B cells. PD-L1 and PD-L2 may also regulate T cell responses through reverse signaling. Cross-linking antibodies against PD-L2 directly induce DCs to produce immunomodulatory cytokines such as IL-6 and TNF-a,[406,407] at the same time as protecting them from cell death.[408] In addition, PD-1-Ig inhibits DC activation and increases IL-10 production independently of any influence on IDO.[409]

PD-L1 was recently demonstrated to bind B7-1 with an affinity intermediate between those of CTLA-4 and CD28 for B7-1.[410] This interaction was specific and bidirectional, allowing suppression of T cell proliferation and cytokine production either through B7-1 or PD-L1. T cell activation signals delivered through the TCR and CD28 will thus be integrated with cell intrinsic co-inhibitory signals delivered through CTLA-4 and PD-L1 (via B7-1 on the APC, and potentially also via B7-1 and PD-1 on other T cells), and PD-1 and B7-1 (via PD-L1 on the APC, and potentially via CTLA-4, PD-1 and PD-L1 on other T cells). Finally, inhibitory signaling through PD-1 and B7-1 (via PD-L1 on nonhematopoietic tissues) may influence the final outcome of antigen encounter in the periphery. This leads to an almost bewildering complexity of possible cell intrinsic inhibitory signals that is almost certainly further complicated by the influence of the temporal expression profiles of the various "receptors" and "ligands." The hierarchy of the relative importance of individual elements remains unclear, and is likely to differ between T cell subsets. It is also likely that there is some redundancy within such complex and apparently overlapping systems. The physiological relevance of some of these findings also remains uncertain, but members of the PD-1:PD-L1/PD-L2 grouping clearly make attractive therapeutic targets for attempts to enhance antitumor immunity. Combinatorial blockade of CTLA-4 and PD-L1 might concomitantly eliminate cell intrinsic negative signaling through CTLA-4, B7-1, PD-L1, and PD-1 while favoring positive signaling through CD28. Recent data highlight the relevance of this pathway to chronic T cell responses to pathogens.[411-414] During chronic LCMV infection, antigen-specific $CD8^+$ T cells are impaired. These "exhausted" T cells demonstrate a selective upregulation of PD-1, and in vivo administration of anti-PD-L1 antibodies restores their activity as indicated by increased proliferation and cytokine production, and by a significant reduction in viral load.[411] Similarly, upregulation of PD-1 on HIV-specific $CD8^+$ T cells has been associated with T cell exhaustion and disease progression in humans.[412] Finally, a recent report shows that in HIV patients with progressive disease both PD-1 and CTLA-4 are up-regulated on virus-specific $CD4^+$ T cells, and that their expression directly correlates with disease progression and inability to produce IL-2 upon re-stimulation.[415] Together these data suggest that blockade of PD-1 and/or PD-L1 can restore functionality of the T cell compartment and could be applied, not only to reinvigorate responses to chronic infections, but also to enhance T cell activity toward other chronic pathologies such as cancer.

PD-L1 is expressed by a variety of human and murine tumors, and PD-1 is also expressed by TIL, leading to the hypothesis that this molecule may be important in restricting intratumor effector T cell responses. In humans, myeloid DCs isolated from tumor or lymph nodes from ovarian carcinoma patients express high levels of PD-L1, and are capable of enhancing T cell activity only following PD-L1 blockade.[416] Likewise, pDCs in tumor draining lymph nodes produce high levels of IDO which results in Treg activation, upregulation of PD-L1 on the DCs and negative regulation of T cell responses.[75] PD-L1 is expressed on several human carcinomas (mammary, cervical, lung, ovarian, colonic, renal), as well as melanoma, glioblastoma and some hematopoietic malignancies.[57,417-421] Its expression has been directly correlated with poor prognosis in bladder, breast, kidney, gastric and pancreatic cancer.[59,419,422] Forced expression of PD-L1 on murine tumor lines diminished T cell activation and tumor killing in vitro, and markedly enhanced tumor growth in vivo, While anti-PD-L1 antibodies blocked these effects.[423,424] In the 4T1 mammary carcinoma model, PD-L1 is upregulated in vivo by the tumor, making it refractory to immunotherapy with the anti-4-1BB antibody. Co-administration with anti-PD-L1 resulted in dramatic tumor rejection.[425] Likewise, anti-PD-L1 antibody delayed in vivo growth of PD-L1-expressing murine myeloma cell lines. PD-L1 blockade has also been shown to synergize with ACT to induce rejection of squamous cell carcinoma.[424] Furthermore, adoptive transfer of $PD1^{-/-}$ tumor-reactive $CD8^+$ T cells caused rejection of B16 melanoma while neither wild type nor $CTLA\text{-}4^{-/-}$ tumor-reactive $CD8^+$ T cells were capable of inducing rejection.[417] In this study, blockade of PD-L1 in the effector phase but not during T cell priming also mimicked the results obtained with $CD8^+$ $PD\text{-}1^{-/-}$ T cells. This is in keeping with a model wherein CTLA-4 may play a more vital role in the control of $CD4^+$ T cell responses,[426] whereas PD-1 is essential in the regulation of $CD8^+$ effector T cell responses within the tumor.

While PD-L1 blockade has been proven effective at enhancing antitumor T cell responses, very few studies have examined the ability of PD-1 blockade to directly promote antitumor T cell responses in vivo. Among these, anti-PD-1 antibodies (as well as genetic ablation) were shown to reduce dissemination of B16 melanoma to the liver following injection into the spleen. In the same study, CT26 colon carcinoma injected intravenously was prevented from disseminating to the lungs by anti-PD-1 therapy.[427] A more recent study also demonstrated that PD-1 (as well as PD-L1) blockade resulted in a small but significant decrease in growth of murine pancreatic carcinoma.[428] A fully human anti-PD-1 monoclonal antibody has recently been developed and its ability to enhance the function of human tumor-specific T cells has been tested in vitro.[429] Vaccine-induced melanoma-reactive $CD8^+$ T cells showed an increase in number, IFN-γ production and killing of $MART\text{-}1^+/gp100^+$ melanoma targets upon re-stimulation in vitro with the blocking anti-PD-1 antibody. There were no apparent effects on cell death, suggesting that the augmented in vitro responses were mostly due to increased proliferation of tumor-reactive T cells rather than decreased cell death. While these results are promising, a better understanding of the mechanisms underpinning bidirectional regulation through PD-L1 and B7-1 may help to inform future trials and perhaps to help decide which molecule (PD-L1 or PD-1) makes the optimal target for cancer immunotherapy.

Other inhibitory members of the Ig superfamily offer further possible targets for co-inhibitory blockade although the impact such interventions would have on antitumor activity remains more speculative at present. Thus the as yet unidentified receptor for the B7x (B7-H4) ligand,[430-432] offers one such possibility.[433,434] The current literature on B7-H3 and antitumor responses remains somewhat contradictory (reviewed in Ref. 310). BTLA (B- and T-lymphocyte attenuator, CD272) is also a potential target, offering the unique example of an Ig superfamily member whose ligand is a member of the TNFR family (HVEM),[435] establishing a previously unsuspected link between these two important families of co-stimulatory molecules (reviewed in Ref. 437).

Targeting Treg Suppressive Capacity

Approaches aimed at reducing suppressor function or Treg numbers are attractive therapeutic strategies given the apparent importance of Treg populations in mediating local immune privilege within tumor sites. Small-molecule inhibitors of Treg function would be useful additions to our current therapeutic armamentarium. From the preceding discussions it is apparent that therapies directed toward members of both the Ig and TNFR superfamilies potentially act on regulatory as well as effector compartments. This duality of function, simultaneously enhancing effector function and reducing suppressor function (and/or increasing resistance to suppression) may be critical to the early successes these approaches have enjoyed in preclinical and clinical applications. TLR8 triggering also appears to reverse Treg-mediated suppression, and to have additional inhibitory effects on suppressive $\gamma\delta$ populations.[284,285]

An alternative approach to reducing suppressive capacity of Treg is that of depletion. The recognition that subversion of Treg may play a critical role in establishing and maintaining intratumoral tolerance is partly based on observations of tumor outcomes following CD25-directed depletion. Anti-CD25 monoclonal antibodies (eg, PC61) have antitumor activity in a number of murine tumor models.[122,437-440] While effective when given prior to tumor engraftment they have only limited activity in the therapeutic setting once tumor growth is established. Rather than relating to depletion of activated effectors as initially surmized, it is now recognized that failure in the therapeutic setting may relate to lack of effector infiltration and accumulation within established tumors, further illustrating the principle that systemic generation of immune responses may be insufficient to effect antitumor activity.[36] Furthermore, depletion of Treg may be relatively short-lived, both because of rapid proliferation of naturally occurring Treg and peripheral conversion of $CD4^+Foxp3^-$ precursors.[97,100] The duration of depletion likely relates to the functional half-life of the depleting agent. Studies in humans have used either IL-2 or anti-CD25 as a delivery vehicle for a variety of toxins. Denileukin difitox (Ontak) is a fusion protein created by replacing the receptor finding domian of diptheria toxin with IL-2, which directs the cytocidal action of diphtheria toxin to cells that overexpress the IL-2 receptor. Ex vivo studies indicate that it interacts with the high- and intermediate-affinity IL-2 receptor on the cell surface and undergoes internalization. Subsequent cleavage in the endosome releases the diphtheria toxin into the cytosol, which then inhibits cellular protein synthesis, resulting in rapid cell death. It is characterized by a relatively short half-life (60 minutes) compared with monoclonal antibodies. Preliminary studies in ovarian and renal cell carcinoma demonstrate an early reduction in circulating Treg cells following denileukin diftitox therapy with preservation of the $CD4^+CD25^{int}$ memory T cell pool,[441] but possible depletion of $CD25^+$ effector cells with prolonged/repeated administration.[442] Administration prior to tumor RNA-transfected DC vaccines enhanced tumor immunity as measured by subsequent in vitro analyses of cytokine production in recall responses to the DC vaccine. The in vivo antitumor efficacy is still under preclinical evaluation. However, the data from murine models suggest that the demonstration of antitumor activity may be more difficult than enhancement of systemic immunity, and the issue of the duration of depletion that can be achieved remains perhaps critical.[443,444] The same issues may pertain to other depletion strategies, such as those that use a fusion of anti-CD25 monoclonal antibody to a truncated form of the bacterial *Pseudomonas* exotoxin A,[445] or those to ricin.[446] For these reasons, approaches that target Treg function rather than number have potential advantages. Furthermore, if such approaches could be targeted to the tumor microenvironment, systemic toxicities and particularly the risk of harmful autoimmunity, might be restricted. Our knowledge of the pathways involved in Treg generation and accumulation within the tumor now allows consideration of a number of novel therapeutic strategies. Thus, inhibition of the IDO pathway or TGF-β might reduce the rate of peripheral conversion and influence immune privilege status within the tumor.[125,447-450]

Cytokines—Intercellular Mediators of Immunity

Some of the possible uses of cytokines have been described in the section on ACT. Few have shown evidence of a potent ability to enhance antitumor activity in vivo, partially because of their pleiotropic effects and adverse side effect profiles at high doses (eg, IL-2 and type I IFN). IL-15 and IL-21, both members of the common γ-chain group, have attracted more attention recently. IL-15 is likely to have differing roles in mouse and human $CD4^+$ memory T cell homeostasis, since human $CD4^+$ memory cells constitutively produce and proliferate in response to it while it is not produced by mouse T cells.[451,452] Other sources of physiologically active IL-15 include monocytes, macrophages, DCs and stromal cells. It is recognized to activate NK cells, be critically involved in the maintenance of durable high avidity $CD8^+$ memory T cell responses, and to promote MHC class I expression by DCs. [453,454] IL-15 is capable of enhancing $CD8^+$ T cell responses to vaccines and to enhance antitumor activity when either supplied exogenously or engineered to be secreted by tumor vaccines.[220,223,455] Clinical application is keenly awaited. IL-21 is produced by NKT and $CD4^+$ T cells and enhances the proliferation and function of $CD8^+$ T cells, NK and NKT cells, as well as influencing B-cell differentiation.[456] Furthermore, it appears to reduce the suppressive capacity of Treg.[457] It has been demonstrated to enhance antitumor activity in a number of preclinical murine models either as a monotherapy or in combinatorial approaches with other cytokines (IL-15, IL-2), apoptosis-inducing antibodies (anti-DR5), CD1d reactive glycolipids (aGalCer), or co-stimulatory agonists.[458-461] Early phase clinical studies of recombinant human IL-21 suggest that it is relatively well tolerated and mediates biological activity in terms of activation of NK and $CD8^+$ T cells, although it is too early to assess possible antitumor efficacy.[462,463]

Not all cytokines are immunostimulatory. Tumor cells can produce immunosuppressive cytokines or induce their production by regulatory infiltrates or stromal cells. Both IL-10 and TGF-β provide possible targets for therapeutic intervention. Targeting TGF-β has shown efficacy in murine tumor models[67,69] and clinical grade antibodies (used in systemic sclerosis) are available, as are those for IL-10.

Combinatorial Immunotherapeutics

It is clear from preclinical models and early clinical experience that multimodal approaches may be required to successfully eradicate poorly immunogenic tumors. The recent literature demonstrates the potential for many combinations to give synergistic or additive effects. Attempting to choose rationally those approaches which are likely to be best is very challenging, but considering approaches under a number of basic headings allows the identification of potentially attractive combinations. We can perhaps simplistically think of modern strategies as (a) improving antigen presentation or immunogenicity (eg, vaccines, CpG), (b) improving T-effector function, numbers or persistence directly (eg, agonistic anti-TNFR antibodies, cytokines), (c) removing or disabling immunological checkpoints, either cell intrinsic or cell extrinsic (eg, CTLA-4 or PD-1 blockade, Treg depletion, and possibly agonistic anti-INPR antibodies), (d) "resetting" the system and taking advantage of proliferative advantages in a lymphopenic environment (eg, ACT), and (e) improving antigen specificity or TCR avidity for tumor antigens (eg, CAR and TCR gene therapies). It has also become apparent that some agents bridge these categories, so the duality of enhancing effector function and reducing suppression afforded by, eg, CTLA-4 blockade, or OX40 stimulation, may be achieved with one agent. Since recent data highlight the ability of regulatory checkpoints to limit the efficacy of any directly stimulatory strategy, the inclusion of at least one therapy aimed at disabling immune checkpoints is theoretically attractive. So, eg, combination of anti-CTLA-4 with vaccines,[464-466] CpG,[467] Treg depletion[468] or anti-4-1BB[469] markedly enhances activity. Similarly diverse synergy is seen when combining anti-4-1BB antibodies with other modalities.[344,345,367] One example of combining three of these strategies is provided in a preclinical model using antibodies directed toward the death-inducing TNF-related apoptosis-inducing ligand receptor (TRAIL-R), CD40 and 4-1BB which has been shown to augment antitumor activity in TRAIL-sensitive murine tumor models.[308] Induction of tumor apoptosis and antigen release from tumor cells and recruitment of innate immune cells into the tumor site by anti-DR5 (anti-TRAIL-R), coupled with augmentation of DC function induced by anti-CD40, and improved induction, activation and survival of tumor-specific CTL facilitated by anti-4-1BB (possibly with further effects on Treg), are all likely to be important contributors to the favorable antitumor activity.[470,471] Furthermore, anti-CD40 can be substituted by CpG, utilizing NKT activation to amplify DC function, with similar results.[325] One potential advantage of approaches relying on the synergy of multiple components is that they might reduce the toxicity induced by higher doses of each agent administered as monotherapy (eg, immune responses may be constrained toward tumor-related antigens rather than ubiquitous self antigens). Appropriate timing of sequential therapies is likely to become an important factor in such combinatorial approaches.

New Mechanisms of Antitumor Activity Demand New Response Criteria

The mechanisms underlying the antitumor activity of immunostimulatory therapies are indirect, relying on the activation of tumor-reactive immune effector cells, and contrasting with the direct activity of most conventional chemotherapeutics. The kinetics of clinical responses may therefore differ significantly, potentially taking longer to become manifest. This issue is well illustrated by early experience with CTLA-4 blockade. Over 4000 patients have been treated to date with either anti-CTLA-4 (Ipilimumab or Tremelimumab) or anti-PD-1 antibody. The majority of the clinical experience has been with anti-CTLA-4 (Ipilimumab) antibody in the setting of metastatic melanoma,[396-399] although patients with prostate cancer,[400] renal cell carcinoma,[474] ovarian cancer,[397] and urothelial carcinoma of the bladder[473,474] have also shown similar clinical responses, immune responses, or immune-related adverse events as a result of therapy.

The tempo and patterns of clinical responses for anti-CTLA-4 have been striking, but do not always fit with conventional cancer therapies such as cytotoxic chemotherapy or currently approved monoclonal antibodies.[475-477] Cytotoxic chemotherapies act directly on tumor cells to elicit cell death. Similarly, rituximab and cetuximab, monoclonal antibodies currently approved as cancer therapeutics, both lead to tumor cell destruction as a result of Fc receptor activity and antibody-dependent cell-mediated cytotoxcity.[478-481] In contrast, anti-CTLA-4 antibody generates antitumor responses not because of a direct action on tumor cells but rather due to the activation of tumor-specific T cells which must expand and differentiate in order to become effector cells that can elicit tumor cell death. This indirect method of generating cancer cell death means that antitumor responses take longer to become detectable by radiographic images or changes in blood-based tumor markers, thus making it difficult to predict or categorize these responses by standard methods, including the Response Evaluation Criteria in Solid Tumors (RECIST)[482] that are used to objectively evaluate therapeutic efficacy of anticancer agents.

While response to chemotherapy is usually apparent after 1 or 2 cycles of treatment, clinical responses with anti-CTLA-4 therapy can range from detectable antitumor responses within a few weeks to months after starting treatment to a prolonged period of stable disease followed by detectable tumor regression or even a period of progressive disease followed by tumor regression at a later time. This variation in clinical responses with anti-CTLA-4 therapy is best illustrated by the pooled results from 6 studies that enrolled 356 patients with metastatic melanoma to receive single or multiple ipilimumab doses ranging from doses of 0.1 mg/kg to 20 mg/kg administered as monotherapy (n = 209), combination with dacarbazine (n = 35), or combination with IL-2 (n = 26) or combination with melanoma peptide vaccine (n = 76) to yield clinical responses in 46 of 356 patients with an overall objective response (OR) rate of 12.9%.[475] Many responses occurred later than is typical with cytotoxic agents. Complete responses (CR) occurred in 11 patients from 10-106 weeks, and partial responses (PR) in 35 patients from 5-62 weeks following therapy. Clinical responses were documented in 28/46 patients at time points beyond 12 weeks from initiation of treatment. From this group of 28 patients, 18 patients were found to have an OR after having a short period of stable disease lasting for only 2 months or a prolonged period of stable disease lasting as much as 16 months before tumor regression was appreciated. Strikingly, 4 patients had progressive disease as determined by standard RECIST criteria prior to documented clinical responses. Objective clinical responses seen in this cohort of patients are durable and still ongoing in 25/46 patients for 5+ years in some patients. Therefore, antitumor responses induced as a result of anti-CTLA-4 therapy may not fit with standard RECIST criteria thus prompting the need for novel efficacy criteria to evaluate this class of immunotherapeutic agents.[483] Consequently, although conventional chemotherapy treatment strategies would consist of changing to a different chemotherapy regimen in a patient who has nonresponding (ie, stable) or progressive disease, it is clear that in the setting of anti-CTLA-4 therapy careful consideration must be given to the fact that patients may benefit at a later time from continued therapy or without additional therapies. Clinical trial design must take this unique feature of anti-CTLA-4 therapy into account in order to establish endpoints that can accurately reflect the efficacy of this and other agents in this class of drugs.

As is the case for clinical responses, adverse events associated with anti-CTLA-4 therapy are different than those seen with conventional chemotherapeutic agents and appear to be related to the systemic activation of the immune system and development of inflammatory-like conditions such as colitis, uveitis, hypohysitis, and dermatitis.[398,401,474,484-486] These adverse events have been termed immune related adverse events or irAEs. Most irAEs have been manageable and reverse either spontaneously or with corticosteroids. Unlike previously approved cytokine therapies such as high-dose IL-2, which requires a medical setting comparable to an intensive care unit for administration due to its potential serious toxicities related to capillary leak syndrome,[487] anti-CTLA-4 therapy is administered in clinical trials as a single intravenous infusion per dose in an outpatient setting. Most irAEs that occur as a result of treatment can be managed in the outpatient setting. The use of corticosteroids to treat irAEs does not appear to affect the antitumor action of anti-CTLA-4 antibody.[488] Although some studies suggest a correlation between irAEs and antitumor responses, there have been patients who respond to anti-CTLA-4 therapy without experiencing an irAE. Further investigation is ongoing to understand the relationship between anti-CTLA-4 antibody treatment, antitumor responses and irAEs.[472-474,489] Most clinical trials to date using this new class of immunotherapeutic agents have been conducted in the metastatic disease setting; however, the first clinical trial in the pre-surgical setting is ongoing with anti-CTLA-4 antibody and provides the opportunity to conduct detailed analyses on tumor tissues, which are limited in the metastatic setting, in order to correlate immunologic changes within the tumor microenvironment with those that occur within the systemic circulation, thereby identifying potentially relevant biomarkers that can be used to monitor patients with metastatic disease who receive anti-CTLA-4 therapy.[473,489] In addition, the acceptable safety profile to-date observed with anti-CTLA-4 in patients with localized disease participating in the pre-surgical clinical trial suggests that investigation of this therapy in the neoadjuvant and adjuvant settings may be feasible. Additional clinical trials with appropriate endpoints and the identification of biomarkers that will predict for or allow for the selection of patients for treatment will ensure that this class of cancer therapeutics results in clinical benefit in a greater proportion of patients.

Paradigm Shift—From Immune Adjuvants to Immunosupportive Therapies?

Recent attention has also focused on the potential for immunotherapies to augment conventional chemotherapy or radiotherapy,[345,490,491] and on trying to optimize the immunogenicity of cell death. While apoptosis has long been considered as non-immunogenic or even tolerizing, more recent data suggest that not all forms of apoptosis are necessarily immunologically equivalent. Massive apoptosis may change a normally tolerogenic cross-presentation of antigen[492] into an effective cross-priming event,[493] and stressed apoptotic tumor cells have an enhanced capacity to activate DCs and induce specific CTLs, possibly via the intermediary of heat shock protein induction.[494] Uric acid release by injured cells is a key endogenous danger signal improving cross-priming,[495] HMGB1 (high mobility group box 1) released during late apoptosis initiates an inflammatory response through binding TLR4 on DC,[496,497] and calreticulin exposure on the cell surface may also be important in distinguishing between immunogenic and non-immunogenic cell death by targeting cells for phagocytosis by DCs.[498,499] Furthermore, apoptotic cells express phosphatidylserine residues on their plasma membrane, which can bind with MFGP-E8 (milk fat globule protein E8) released in response to GM-CSF, enhancing phagocytic uptake by APCs. This helps to explain the mechanism of GM-CSF-induced potentiation of antitumor immunity, but MFGP-E8-mediated uptake of apoptotic cells is a key determinant of GM-CSF-triggered tolerance and MFG-E8 attenuates the vaccination activity of GM-CSF-secreting tumor cells through Treg induction, providing a further potential target for enhancing vaccine efficacy.[500] As it has become apparent that several classes of anticancer drugs have extrinsic activities that favor immunogenic cell death (eg, anthracyclines increase calreticulin exposure and HMGB1 release, gemcitabine both enhances antigen cross-presentation by DC and eliminates $CD11b^+$/$Gr\text{-}1^+$ MDSC), and that others may favor generation of immunity through suppression of inhibitory populations (eg, gemcitabine as described, and cyclophosphamide, which may preferentially impair Treg proliferation at lower doses[501]), it has become clear that such considerations may favor future choices for combination with immunotherapies. These approaches have shown promise in preclinical models despite concerns that cytotoxic drugs might be detrimental to immunotherapies. Cytotoxic chemotherapies appear capable of inducing an appropriate milieu for presentation of tumor antigens.[502] Further beneficial effects likely include increased antigen cross-presentation,[503] partial activation of DCs,[504] and partial sensitization of tumor cells for CTL mediated lysis.[505] While there is currently scant evidence from studies in humans to define the relative importance of these considerations to therapeutic outcomes, the attraction of enhancing the immunogenicity of cell death in vivo, and one shared by agents such as CpG, is that the tumor might be turned into its own polyvalent cellular vaccine, allowing presentation of private tumor epitopes and favoring tumor-specific immunity. This would obviate the requirement for an absolute knowledge of the relevant target antigens. We are beginning to appreciate the impact of genetic instability within tumors on the generation of potentially immunogenic neo-antigens,[264-266] and it is possible that we will shift to a position wherein conventional anticancer therapies become viewed as immunosupportive, rather than one in which cancer immunotherapies are viewed as adjuvants.

Major challenges will need to be faced in the coming years. Identification of the best combinatorial strategies will continue to be informed by careful mechanistic studies in mouse models. The identification of robust predictors of response will perhaps parallel attempts to tailor chemotherapeutics according to the genetic profile of the tumor or of tumor infiltrates. Finally, attempts to manipulate the host in order to achieve such favorable immunological profiles will be required to prove the therapeutic worth of cancer immunotherapies in comparative studies, confirming them to be much more than modern biomarkers for disease outcome.

Acknowledgments

Our research was funded in part by Leukaemia Research Fund, UK, Irvington Institute Fellowship Program of the Cancer Research Institute, USA, UTMDACC Physician Scientist Award, a Bladder Cancer SPORE Career Development Award 5P50 CA091846 04 (PP-CDP4), American Society of Clinical Oncology Career Development Award, a Prostate Cancer Foundation Award, and Doris Duke Clinical Scientist Development Award.

Disclosure

James P. Allison is coinventor of intellectual property concerning CTLA-4 that is held by University of California, Berkeley and is a consultant for Medarex and Bristol Squibb, who are involved in the clinical development of anti-CTLA-4.

Selected References

The complete reference list can be found at www.CANCERMEDICINE8.com

11. van der BP, Traversari C, Chomez P, et al. A gene encoding an antigen recognized by cytolytic T lymphocytes on a human melanoma. *Science.* 1991;254(5038):1643–1647.
15. Shankaran V, Ikeda H, Bruce AT, et al. IFNgamma and lymphocytes prevent primary tumour development and shape tumour immunogenicity. *Nature.* 2001; 410(6832):1107–1111.
32. Koebel CM, Vermi W, Swann JB, et al. Adaptive immunity maintains occult cancer in an equilibrium state. *Nature.* 2007.
46. Rosenberg SA, Packard BS, Aebersold PM, et al. Use of tumor-infiltrating lymphocytes and interleukin-2 in the immunotherapy of patients with metastatic melanoma. A preliminary report. *N Engl J Med.* 1988;319(25):1676–1680.
48. Morgan RA, Dudley ME, Wunderlich JR, et al. Cancer regression in patients after transfer of genetically engineered lymphocytes. *Science.* 2006;314(5796):126–129.
73. Munn DH, Mellor AL. Indoleamine 2,3-dioxygenase and tumor-induced tolerance. *J Clin Invest.* 2007;117(5):1147–1154.
78. Takahashi T, Kuniyasu Y, Toda M, et al. Immunologic self-tolerance maintained by CD25+CD4+ naturally anergic and suppressive T cells: induction of autoimmune disease by breaking their anergic/suppressive state. *Int Immunol.* 1998; 10(12):1969–1980.
81. Piconese S, Valzasina B, Colombo MP. OX40 triggering blocks suppression by regulatory T cells and facilitates tumor rejection. *J Exp Med.* 2008;205(4):825–839.
82. Fontenot JD, Gavin MA, Rudensky AY. Foxp3 programs the development and function of CD4+CD25+ regulatory T cells. *Nat Immunol.* 2003;4(4):330–336.
90. Walker MR, Kasprowicz DJ, Gersuk VH, et al. Induction of FoxP3 and acquisition of T regulatory activity by stimulated human CD4+. *J Clin Invest.* 2003;112(9):1437–1443.
92. Apostolou I, von Boehmer H. In vivo instruction of suppressor commitment in naive T cells. *J Exp Med.* 2004;199(10):1401–1408.
109. Wang HY, Lee DA, Peng G, et al. Tumor-specific human CD4+ regulatory T cells and their ligands: implications for immunotherapy. *Immunity.* 2004;20(1):107–118.
110. Fallarino F, Grohmann U, Hwang KW, et al. Modulation of tryptophan catabolism by regulatory T cells. *Nat Immunol.* 2003;4(12):1206–1212.
112. Wing K, Onishi Y, Prieto-Martin P, et al. CTLA-4 control over Foxp3+ regulatory T cell function. *Science.* 2008;322(5899): 271–275.
123. Curiel TJ, Coukos G, Zou L, et al. Specific recruitment of regulatory T cells in ovarian carcinoma fosters immune privilege and predicts reduced survival. *Nat Med.* 2004;10(9):942–949.
125. Ghiringhelli F, Puig PE, Roux S, et al. Tumor cells convert immature myeloid dendritic cells into TGF-{beta}-secreting cells inducing CD4+CD25+ regulatory T cell proliferation. *J Exp Med.* 2005;202(7):919–929.
126. Quezada SA, Peggs KS, Curran MA, Allison JP. CTLA4 blockade and GM-CSF combination immunotherapy alters the intratumor balance of effector and regulatory T cells. *J Clin Invest.* 2006;116(7):1935–1945.
176. Mitchison NA. Passive transfer of transplantation immunity. *Nature.* 1953;171 (4345):267–268.
190. Cheever MA, Greenberg PD, Fefer A, Gillis S. Augmentation of the anti-tumor therapeutic efficacy of long-term cultured T lymphocytes by in vivo administration of purified interleukin 2. *J Exp Med.* 1982;155(4):968–980.
198. Eberlein TJ, Rosenstein M, Rosenberg SA. Regression of a disseminated syngeneic solid tumor by systemic transfer of lymphoid cells expanded in interleukin 2. *J Exp Med.* 1982;156(2):385–397.
205. Rosenberg SA, Lotze MT, Muul LM, et al. A progress report on the treatment of 157 patients with advanced cancer using lymphokine-activated killer cells and interleukin-2 or high-dose interleukin-2 alone. *N Engl J Med.* 1987;316(15):889–897.
208. Dudley ME, Wunderlich JR, Robbins PF, et al. Cancer regression and autoimmunity in patients after clonal repopulation with antitumor lymphocytes. *Science.* 2002;298(5594):850–854.
221. Teague RM, Sather BD, Sacks JA, et al. Interleukin-15 rescues tolerant CD8+ T cells for use in adoptive immunotherapy of established tumors. *Nat Med.* 2006;12(3):335–341.
222. Gattinoni L, Klebanoff CA, Palmer DC, et al. Acquisition of full effector function in vitro paradoxically impairs the in vivo antitumor efficacy of adoptively transferred CD8+ T cells. *J Clin Invest.* 2005;115(6):1616–1626.
228. Schoenberger SP, Toes RE, van der Voort EI, Offringa R, Melief CJ. T-cell help for cytotoxic T lymphocytes is mediated by CD40-CD40L interactions. *Nature.* 1998;393(6684):480–483.
239. Berger C, Jensen MC, Lansdorp PM, Gough M, Elliott C, Riddell SR. Adoptive transfer of effector CD8+ T cells derived from central memory cells establishes persistent T cell memory in primates. *J Clin Invest.* 2008;118(1):294–305.
240. Stanislawski T, Voss RH, Lotz C, et al. Circumventing tolerance to a human MDM2-derived tumor antigen by TCR gene transfer. *Nat Immunol.* 2001;2(10):962–970.
241. Kessels HW, Wolkers MC, van den Boom MD, van der Valk MA, Schumacher TN. Immunotherapy through TCR gene transfer. *Nat Immunol.* 2001;2(10):957–961.
264. Sjoblom T, Jones S, Wood LD, et al. The consensus coding sequences of human breast and colorectal cancers. *Science.* 2006;314(5797):268–274.
285. Peng G, Wang HY, Peng W, Kiniwa Y, Seo KH, Wang RF. Tumor-infiltrating gammadelta T cells suppress T and dendritic cell function via mechanisms controlled by a unique toll-like receptor signaling pathway. *Immunity.* 2007;27(2):334–348.
286. van Seters M, van Beurden M, ten Kate FJ, et al. Treatment of vulvar intraepithelial neoplasia with topical imiquimod. *N Engl J Med.* 2008;358(14):1465–1473.
289. Fujii S, Shimizu K, Smith C, Bonifaz L, Steinman RM. Activation of natural killer T cells by alpha-galactosylceramide rapidly induces the full maturation of dendritic cells in vivo and thereby acts as an adjuvant for combined CD4 and CD8 T cell immunity to a coadministered protein. *J Exp Med.* 2003;198(2):267–279.
291. Ridge JP, Di Rosa F, Matzinger P. A conditioned dendritic cell can be a temporal bridge between a CD4+ T-helper and a T-killer cell. *Nature.* 1998;393(6684):474–478.
299. French RR, Chan HT, Tutt AL, Glennie MJ. CD40 antibody evokes a cytotoxic T-cell response that eradicates lymphoma and bypasses T-cell help. *Nat Med.* 1999;5(5):548–553.
306. Vonderheide RH, Flaherty KT, Khalil M, et al. Clinical activity and immune modulation in cancer patients treated with CP-870,893, a novel CD40 agonist monoclonal antibody. J Clin Oncol. 2007;25(7): 876–883.
335. Shuford WW, Klussman K, Tritchler DD, et al. 4-1BB costimulatory signals preferentially induce CD8+ T cell proliferation and lead to the amplification in vivo of cytotoxic T cell responses. *J Exp Med.* 1997;186(1):47–55.
340. Wilcox RA, Flies DB, Zhu G, et al. Provision of antigen and CD137 signaling breaks immunological ignorance, promoting regression of poorly immunogenic tumors. *J Clin Invest.* 2002;109(5):651–659.
355. Bansal-Pakala P, Jember AG, Croft M. Signaling through OX40 (CD134) breaks peripheral T-cell tolerance. *Nat Med.* 2001;7(8):907–912.
380. Ko K, Yamazaki S, Nakamura K, et al. Treatment of advanced tumors with agonistic anti-GITR mAb and its effects on tumor-infiltrating Foxp3+CD25+CD4+ regulatory T cells. *J Exp Med.* 2005; 202(7):885–891.
383. Leach DR, Krummel MF, Allison JP. Enhancement of antitumor immunity by CTLA-4 blockade. *Science.* 1996;271(5256): 1734–1736.
397. Hodi FS, Mihm MC, Soiffer RJ, et al. Biologic activity of cytotoxic T lymphocyte-associated antigen 4 antibody blockade in previously vaccinated metastatic melanoma and ovarian carcinoma patients. *Proc Natl Acad Sci USA.* 2003;100(8): 4712–4717.
410. Butte MJ, Keir ME, Phamduy TB, Sharpe AH, Freeman GJ. Programmed death-1 ligand 1 interacts specifically with the B7-1 costimulatory molecule to inhibit T cell responses. *Immunity.* 2007;27(1): 111–122.
411. Barber DL, Wherry EJ, Masopust D, et al. Restoring function in exhausted CD8 T cells during chronic viral infection. *Nature.* 2006;439(7077):682–687.

14 Genetic Predisposition to Cancer

Henry T. Lynch, MD ■ Vandana Gupta Abramson, MD ■ Marcia S. Brose, MD, PhD

The way we think about heredity and cancer underwent a sea change during the twentieth century. When familial adenomatous polyposis (FAP) was described over 100 years ago,[1,2] hereditary cancer syndromes were thought to be very rare. Seventy years ago, a case-control study showed that a positive family history for cancer of the stomach or colon meant a threefold increased risk for those cancers in family members.[3] In the 1960s, family studies suggested an autosomal dominant mode of genetic transmission for certain clusters of carcinoma of breast, ovary, and colon,[4] a notion that was seriously questioned by many and categorically rejected by some. In the 1980s, the gene for FAP was linked to 5q,[5] then mapped to 5q21,[6,7] ushering in the molecular era in cancer research. The transformation was completed during the 1990s as molecular geneticists made links between mutations and cancers of diverse anatomic sites. There are now more than 70 germline mutations known to be responsible for cancer susceptibility, and it seems that the genetic basis for yet another cancer syndrome is revealed monthly.

The human genome has been mapped, making it almost certain that more cancer susceptibility genes will be found.[8] But the brave new world of molecular biology still must have clinicians in it. Cancer geneticists will not be able to match a subset of our 30,000-40,000 genes to hereditary disorders without good, descriptive family studies. Unfortunately, it is rare to pick up a medical chart and find useful information about the family history of cancer.[9,10] A clinician armed with knowledge about the general features of inherited cancer syndromes (Table 14-1) and a willingness to ask about family history constitutes a tremendously effective screen for hereditary cancer.

Table 14-1 ■ **General Features of Hereditary Cancer Syndromes**

Same or linked forms of cancer in two or more close relatives
Earlier than usual cancer onset in one or more relatives
Bilateral cancer in paired organs
Multiple primary tumors in the same individual
Specific constellation of tumors are part of known cancer syndrome
Evidence of autosomal dominant transmission of cancer susceptibility

The estimated number of new cases of cancer diagnosed in the United States during 2008 is 1,437,180 and the estimated mortality is 565,650.[11] If 5-10% of those cases have a primary hereditary etiology (a conservative estimate), then approximately 100,000 cancers each year will be attributable to genetic factors. Molecular genetics promises unprecedented power to control or prevent those cancers by testing unaffected members of families whose histories suggest a hereditary syndrome. An individual carrying a cancer-causing germline mutation can be enrolled in surveillance and management programs tailored to the natural history of a particular hereditary disorder, whereas those lacking the mutation can be managed according to the general population cancer screening guidelines.

This rough magic is not without difficulties and drawbacks. Genetic counseling is mandatory, both before and after testing is undertaken. Almost none of the screening and surveillance measures counseled in this chapter has been evaluated in controlled studies; such studies will need to be undertaken where feasible. Ethical and medicolegal dilemmas will certainly arise as patients and their physicians confront privacy and insurability issues. Nevertheless, the translation of genetic knowledge to clinical practice should yield a significant reduction in cancer morbidity and mortality.

Importance of Family History

The concept of family history-based "targeted cancer surveillance" for cancer control was proposed a quarter-century ago.[12] In 2004, Guttmacher and colleagues[13] commented that a clinician's ignorance with regard to a patient's family history of cancer can easily result in a failure to offer potentially lifesaving early surveillance. The U.S. Surgeon General, in conjunction with other government health agencies, including the NIH, was concerned enough about this matter to launch a campaign to promote the awareness of the medical value of family history and to facilitate data collection and analysis.[13,14]

A careful assessment of cancer of all anatomic sites is mandatory in compiling a cancer family history, because the diagnosis of a hereditary cancer syndrome may often be established through recognition of the pattern of multiple primary cancers. This, of course, is most evident in the hereditary breast-ovarian cancer (HBOC) syndrome. Other examples include colorectal cancer (CRC) and carcinoma of the endometrium and ovary among other cancer types in the Lynch syndrome (LS); sarcoma, breast cancer, brain tumors, leukemia, lymphoma, laryngeal carcinoma, lung cancer, and adrenal cortical carcinoma in the SBLA (Li-Fraumeni) syndrome; medullary thyroid carcinoma (MTC) and pheochromocytoma (PTC) in MEN2a and MEN2b; melanoma and pancreatic cancer in the *CDKN2A* (*p16*) mutation in the familial atypical multiple mole melanoma (FAMMM) syndrome; diffuse gastric cancer and lobular breast cancer with *CDH1* mutation in hereditary diffuse gastric cancer (HDGC); and the list goes on. Knowledge of the integral tumors in the differing hereditary cancer syndromes provides important clues in concert with the natural history of the tumors' cancer complement; therein, screening and management may differ strikingly based on the differences in the tumors, age of onset (frequently earlier than their sporadic counterparts), pathology, accelerated carcinogenesis that impacts on the frequency of screening, bilaterality in paired organs that can provide the need for prophylactic surgery as in the contralateral breast in the case of ipsilateral breast cancer, and the location of the cancer may also be important, as in the case of CRC and its proximal proclivity in the LS. All of this information must be embraced in the genetic counseling program. This way, in identifying individuals at high risk, we can then ensure the search for the identification of pathogenic mutations either in the family or for the particular syndrome, such as *BRCA1* and *BRCA2* in HBOC. Clearly, DNA may be of extraordinary value in mutation identification through testing of the most informative family member.

Unfortunately, family history is still notoriously neglected by physicians as well as their patients. However, genetic counselors have been contributing immensely to rectifying this problem and are making a difference. It is important to realize that genetic counseling must be considered to be mandatory before DNA testing. However, this dictum has not been routinely followed by commercial testing laboratories wherein they may send a blood collection kit to the physician or, in some cases, directly to the patient and therein do not demand genetic counseling before the DNA collection.

Genetic Basis of Cancer Syndromes

Breast-Ovarian Cancer Syndrome

Overview ■ In the United States, one in seven women will develop breast cancer in her lifetime. Some women, however, are at an even greater risk of developing the disease. The HBOC syndrome is characterized by the clustering of breast cancer alone, or breast and ovarian cancer, in a single family. The HBOC syndrome was first described in the 1970s with an autosomal dominant mode of genetic transmission.[15,16]

Familial breast cancer accounts for 5-10% of all breast cancer, and a substantial number of these cases can be linked to mutations in the genes *BRCA1* or *BRCA2*.[17,18] Familial cases of ovarian cancer comprise up to 8% of all ovarian cancer, and recent reports suggest that most of these may be accounted for by mutations in *BRCA1* or *BRCA2*,[19] and less frequently by mismatch repair (MMR) mutations as part of the LS.[20,21]

BRCA1 was first linked to chromosome 17q21[22,23] and subsequently isolated in 1994.[24] The existence of breast cancer families without associated mutations in *BRCA1* led to the discovery of a second breast cancer susceptibility gene, *BRCA2*, on chromosome 13q12.[25,26] The scientific and clinical impact of the discovery of these two genes will be discussed below.

***BRCA1* and *BRCA2*: Gene Structure and Function** ■ *BRCA1* and *BRCA2* encode large proteins of 1863 and 3350 amino acids, respectively. Both are complex genes made up of more than 20 exons. Neither gene bears significant homology with other known genes, with the exception of the BRCT domain in the C-terminus of *BRCA1*, a domain found in more than 40 other genes associated with response to DNA damage.[27] It is clear that both *BRCA1* and *BRCA2* are important components of the pathway that protects cells from the effects of DNA damage (reviewed by Venkitaraman[28]). The majority of mutations identified thus far lead to protein truncation, and it is believed that cancer develops when the second copy is lost. Therefore, it is thought that *BRCA1* and *BRCA2* behave like classic tumor suppressor genes, with the loss of one copy predisposing the carrier to the development of the characteristic cancers of this classic cancer syndrome.

Several lines of investigation have implicated *BRCA1* and *BRCA2* in DNA damage response pathways. An association between *BRCA1* and p53 and the subsequent enhancement of p53 activity incriminates *BRCA1* in p21-mediated cell cycle arrest following DNA damage.[29] In addition, *BRCA1* has been shown to form complexes with both *BRCA2*[30] and *Rad51*,[31] the human homologue of the *Escherichia coli* gene *RecA*, which is essential to normal recombination and genome stability. Colocalization of *BRCA1*, *BRCA2*, and *Rad51* in "nuclear dot" structures is seen to disappear following the treatment of cells with DNA-damaging agents that cause double-stranded chromosome breaks.[32] In addition, mouse embryonic stem cells that are homozygous for *BRCA1* null and *BRCA2* truncations are hypersensitive to ionizing radiation and other forms of oxidative damage.[33] The complex network of interactions connecting *BRCA1* and *BRCA2* to cell cycle checkpoints and homologous DNA damage repair has been reviewed recently.[34]

BRCA1 may also play a role in transcription regulation, cell cycle control, and development.[35] Both BRCA1 and BRCA2 are nuclear proteins.[36-39] BRCA1 has been shown to associate with the RNA polymerase holoenzyme[40] and bind CREB,[41] implicating it in transcriptional regulation. BRCA1 protein levels also have been shown to be altered by variations in hormone levels.[42] During the cell cycle, BRCA1 and BRCA2 mRNA levels have been found to increase from low levels at the start of G1 to maximum levels at the G1/S transition in parallel to cyclin A levels. Phosphorylation of BRCA1 also occurs in a cell cycle-dependent manner, suggesting that it may play a role in the G1/S checkpoint control.[43] Mice with homozygous deletion of *BRCA1* or *BRCA2* die as embryos, revealing a key role for *BRCA1* and *BRCA2* in development.[44-46] However, mice homozygous for a partial deletion of *BRCA2* are viable but show growth retardation and the development of thymic lymphomas.[47,48] Homozygous deletion of *BRCA1* in mouse mammary tissue has been found to lead to the development of tumors.[49]

***RAD51* 135G→C Modifies Breast Cancer Risk Among *BRCA2* Mutation Carriers** ■ Breast cancer risk in mutation carriers is modified by variable genetic or environmental factors that cluster in families. *BRCA1* and *BRCA2* interact with *RAD51*, which has a single-nucleotide polymorphism (SNP) that has been suggested as a possible modifier of breast cancer risk in *BRCA1* and *BRCA2* mutation carriers.[50] Findings disclosed a statistically significant increased risk among *BRCA2* mutation carriers through 135G→C, which may modify the risk of breast cancer in *BRCA2* mutation carriers by altering the expression of *RAD51*, which is the first gene to be reliably identified as a modifier of risk among *BRCA* mutation carriers.[50]

***PTEN* and Breast Cancers with *BRCA1* Mutation** ■ Saal et al.[51] note that Pten contributes to the formation of basal-like mammary tumors in mice. In humans, loss of PTEN expression is significantly associated with the basal-like breast cancer (BBC) subtype of breast cancer with poor prognosis. Importantly, *BRCA1* is a cancer-susceptibility gene involved in double-strand DNA break (DSB) repair, which leads to breast cancers that are nearly always of the BBC type.

BBC comprises 10-20% of all breast cancer and is one of the subtypes with the worst prognosis. BBCs are highly proliferative, poorly differentiated, and genomically unstable. They are ER-, PR-, and Her2-neu-; these are initiated by a *BRCA1* mutation.

PTEN is a tumor suppressor that inhibits downstream signaling. The model developed by Saal et al. implies that BBCs may be strongly associated with aberrant *PTEN-PI3K* pathway signaling. Importantly, therapy targeted to this pathway may be an effective way to treat and possibly even prevent some sporadic and hereditary BBCs.

The DSB repair in breast cancer may make it possible that other grossly rearranged genes also contribute to tumor suppression, observations that are analogous to those in LS, where lack of MMR leads to microsatellite instability (MSI), which, in turn, leads to the mutation of *TGFBR2* and other genes that drive tumor progression.

Clinical Aspects of *BRCA1* and *BRCA2* ■ It is estimated that a family history of breast cancer in the general population confers a 1.7 relative risk (RR) of developing the disease.[52-54] The majority of these families will not have a mutation in *BRCA1* or *BRCA2*. However, in a woman who develops breast cancer before the age of 40, the chance that she carries a mutation in *BRCA1* may be as high as 10%, or even 20% if she is Ashkenazi Jewish.[18,55-57] This may not be true for *BRCA2*, which may be associated with a slightly older age of diagnosis.[58]

The transmission of the heritable susceptibility to these cancers follows an autosomal dominant pattern. It is estimated that carriers have a 50-85% chance of developing breast cancer by the age of 70 and a 16-60% risk of developing ovarian cancer.[59,60] Initial reports of a higher than background incidence of prostate cancer have not been confirmed, but there is evidence from several studies of *BRCA1* mutation carriers for an increased risk of colon cancer (RR 2), pancreatic cancer (RR 2-3), gastric cancer (RR 3-7), and fallopian tube cancer (RR 50-100).[61,62] *BRCA2* mutations are associated with an increased incidence of male breast cancer (RR 50-100),[63] as well as an increased risk of prostate cancer (RR 5), pancreatic cancer (RR 4), gall bladder and bile duct cancer (RR 5), stomach cancer (RR 3), and malignant melanoma (RR 3).[64]

Of the women seen in American cancer risk evaluation clinics, *BRCA1* accounts for up to 20-30% of breast-ovarian cancer families, whereas *BRCA2* accounts for 10-20%. Multiple less penetrant cancer genes that may occur at a higher frequency most probably account for the rest of inherited breast cancer risk in families with multiple cases of breast cancer not attributable to *BRCA1* or *BRCA2*.[65,66]

Together, *BRCA1* and *BRCA2* account for most cases of familial ovarian cancer.[19]

The prevalence of certain *BRCA1* and *BRCA2* mutations is occasionally higher than expected due to the increased transmission of a few mutations ("founder effect") in several subpopulations. Characteristic founder mutations for *BRCA1* and *BRCA2* have been identified in families of Ashkenazi Jewish descent and in Iceland, Finland, Hungary, Russia, France, Holland/Belgium, Sweden/Denmark, and Norway. Most of what we know about *BRCA1* and *BRCA2* has come from the studies of Caucasians in the United States and Europe. Significantly less is known about the rates of *BRCA1* and *BRCA2* mutations in families from other ethnic or racial backgrounds.

BRCA1-associated tumors are more likely to be aneuploid, have a high S-phase component,[67] be high grade,[68,69] and be estrogen receptor and progesterone receptor negative.[70] Whether these characteristics result in poorer survival has been difficult to study due to multiple confounding variables, although some studies suggest that this may be the case.[71,72] Evidence from the Breast Cancer Linkage Consortium revealed that unlike *BRCA1*, *BRCA2* tumors are largely indistinguishable from sporadic tumors in their mitotic rate or degree of polymorphism.[67]

BRCA1 Mutation and Early Age Predict Rapid Breast Cancer Growth ■ Tilanus-Linthorst and colleagues assessed tumor volume doubling time through MRI and/or mammography in 100 breast cancer cases. Forty-three women with *BRCA1* mutations, 16 with *BRCA2* mutations, and 41 high-risk women without an identified mutation were studied. Tumor growth rate was inversely proportional to increased age ($P = 0.004$) and was twice as fast in *BRCA1* ($P = 0.003$) or *BRCA2* ($P = 0.03$) mutation carriers as in other high-risk patients of the same age.[73]

Pathologic tumor size decreased with increasing age ($P = 0.001$). Specifically, median size was 15 mm for patients less than 40 years old compared with 9 mm in older patients ($P = 0.003$); tumors were largest in young women with *BRCA1* mutations. The authors concluded that tumors grow more quickly in *BRCA1* mutation carriers and in young women. A patient's age and risk group should therefore be taken into account in screening protocols.[73] Because *BRCA1/2* mutation carriers develop breast carcinoma at an early age, we recommend the initiation of screening at age 40 or 10 years earlier than the development of disease in other family members. For screening, we recommend alternating MRI and mammography every 6 months since the tumor can exhibit rapid growth.

Breast-Cancer Stromal Cells with *TP53* Mutations ■ Patocs and colleagues[74] discuss the phenomenon of "cross-talk" between a cancer and its microenvironment, the importance of which is being increasingly recognized. They hypothesize that "mutational inactivation of the tumor-suppressor gene *TP53* and genomic alterations in stromal cells of a tumor's microenvironment contribute to the clinical outcome." Noteworthy is the finding that only a single microsatellite locus (2p25.1) in stromal cells from hereditary breast cancer was associated with mutated *TP53*. However, 66 such loci were found in cells from sporadic breast cancer. A specific set of five loci were linked to an increased loss of heterozygosity and allelic imbalance in the stroma of specific tumors associated with nodal metastases in the absence of *TP53* mutations. Somatic *TP53* mutations in stroma, but not epithelium, of sporadic breast cancers were associated with regional nodal metastases ($P = 0.003$). Stroma-specific loss of heterozygosity or allelic imbalance was concluded to be associated with somatic *TP53* mutations and regional lymph node metastases in sporadic breast cancer but not in hereditary breast cancer. These observations, therefore, suggest that *TP53*-mutated stroma, or loss of heterozygosity or allelic imbalance at five specific stromal markers accelerates tumor progression.

Pathology Differences Between BRCA1 and BRCA2 ■ Compared with *BRCA2* tumors, *BRCA1* tumors are more proliferative, are more likely to be aneuploid, have increased numbers of tumor infiltrating lymphocytes, and are more likely to be "triple negatives" (ER-, PR-, Her-2-). *BRCA1* tumors are also more likely to be medullary cancers and less likely to be tubular-lobular group cancers or carcinomas in situ.

Genome-Wide High-Density SNP Linkage Analysis of Non-*BRCA1/2* Breast Cancer Families ■ Gonzales-Neira and colleagues[75] estimate that approximately 30% of hereditary breast cancer cases involve *BRCA1/2* mutations. The search for additional high-risk breast cancer predisposition genes, to date, has been unsuccessful. However, Gonzales-Neira et al.[75] used SNP markers for whole-genome screening of 19 non-*BRCA1/2* breast cancer families using 4720 genome-wide SNPs. They identified five regions on chromosomes 2, 4, 7, 11, and 14, as candidate breast cancer susceptibility genes.

Risk Evaluation and Screening ■ The first and most important step in any cancer risk evaluation program is the recording of an accurate medical history and cancer pedigree. Where possible, it is recommended that all reported cancers be confirmed by documentation from a hospital record. This is especially true in the case of ovarian cancer, which may be mistaken for stomach, colon, endometrial, or liver cancer as the information is passed through the family. The pedigree helps in identifying the type of cancers and the transmission pattern. Once an accurate pedigree is attained and a diagnosis of hereditary cancer is suspected, recommendations can be made regarding the advisability of increased cancer surveillance and DNA testing. However, it is extremely important that the clinician and genetic counselor be aware of the enormous genotypic and phenotypic heterogeneity in hereditary breast cancer, as shown in Figure 14-1.

There are several useful models that assist the provider in the evaluation of a patient's risk for the development of breast cancer.[76] These models are based on documented breast cancer risk factors. Other models are available that estimate the probability that the pattern of cancers in a family may be the result of a mutation in *BRCA1* or *BRCA2*. These models take into account, to varying degrees, the number of cancers, age at diagnosis, location in the pedigree, and relationship of others in the family who have had breast or ovarian cancer. Although every model has its strengths and weaknesses, knowledge of the appropriate use of different models can help give a range of probabilities that the patient may carry a mutation in one of the two most common susceptibility genes.[76]

Owing to the expense and difficulty in testing for mutations in *BRCA1* and *BRCA2*, an effort is made to target the testing to the mutations that are felt to be likely in that individual. For example, families of Ashkenazi Jewish descent can be screened relatively quickly and inexpensively first for the three founder mutations, 185delAG, 5382insC in *BRCA1*, and 6174delT in *BRCA2*. These three mutations are thought to account for more than 90% of mutations in this population.[60,77]

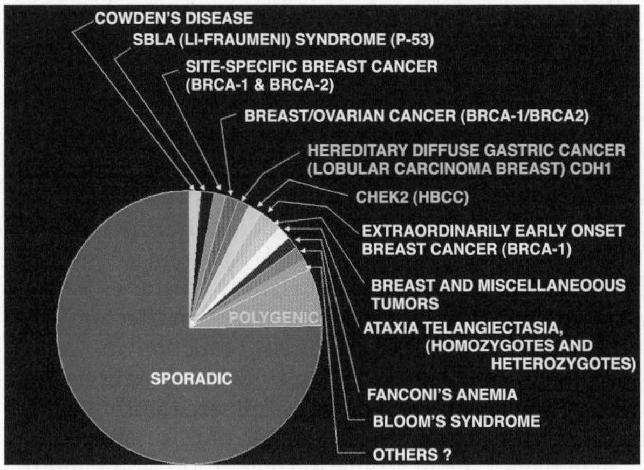

Figure 14-1 ■ Schematic diagram depicting heterogeneity in breast cancer. Note especially the two most recently described types of hereditary breast cancer, shown in yellow text: lobular carcinoma of the breast due to mutation of *CDH1* in the hereditary diffuse gastric cancer syndrome, and hereditary breast and colorectal cancer (HBCC) due to mutation of *CHEK2*. *Source*: Adapted from Lynch HT, et al. Surg Clin North Am 70:753, 1990.

Where possible, testing is performed on an individual who has been affected with breast or ovarian cancer, thereby increasing the chance that if a genetic alteration exists, it will be identified. Once a mutation is identified in a family, testing of that one mutation can be carried out in the other high-risk individuals. The exception to this approach is in the Ashkenazi Jewish population, where the risk of having more than one founder mutation is sufficient to always warrant screening for all three. In a family where no mutation has been identified, a negative result on testing is uninformative, whereas a negative test on an individual from a family with a known mutation defines the woman's chance of acquiring breast or ovarian cancer similar to that of the general population.

For those who desire genetic testing, adequate genetic counseling is required before and after the acquisition of any testing results. Once testing has been obtained, those with positive test results have many treatment options available to them including various screening methods, chemoprevention, and prophylactic surgery. Ideally, screening by frequent clinical breast exams, yearly mammography, ultrasound, and MRI will identify most but, unfortunately, not all, breast cancer at stage I or II disease. New evidence that MRI is a more sensitive tool than breast exams, mammography, or ultrasound for the screening of *BRCA1* mutation carriers, particularly in young women with dense breasts, has been reported recently,[78] although the impact on mortality is unknown. Chemoprevention with tamoxifen has been shown to reduce the risk of breast cancer in *BRCA1/2* mutation carriers by 50%,[79] although at the price of increased risk of cardiovascular effects and endometrial cancer. Whether newer anti-estrogens, such as raloxifene and anastrazole, will be more successful chemopreventive agents remains to be determined (see recent review by Cuzick and colleagues[80]).

Prophylactic Surgery and HBOC ■ Prophylactic mastectomy and prophylactic oophorectomy among patients at an inordinately high risk for HBOC were initially discussed by Lynch and colleagues in the early 1970s.[15,16,81-85] Prophylactic contralateral mastectomy in high-risk women with ipsilateral breast cancer was also considered a logical option, given the enormous risk of bilaterality in hereditary cases.[86]

Hartmann and colleagues[87] initially used "high-risk" criteria such as the number of a patient's breast cancer-affected first- and second-degree relatives for consideration of prophylactic mastectomy. They found that in these high-risk women, prophylactic mastectomy produced a 90% reduction in the risk of breast cancer, with a significant reduction in mortality. Seven breast cancers occurred in their study after subcutaneous bilateral mastectomy; there were none after total mastectomy.[87] Subsequently,[88] they employed genetic testing to distinguish the *BRCA1/2* mutation carriers in this cohort and showed that prophylactic mastectomy is a viable option in *BRCA1/2* mutation carriers; breast cancer did not develop in any of the women with a confirmed *BRCA1* or *BRCA2* mutation after a median follow-up of 16 years.

A prospective study by Meijers-Heijboer and colleagues[89] also showed significant benefit of prophylactic mastectomy among *BRCA1/2* mutation carriers. These investigators studied 76 women, who eventually underwent prophylactic mastectomy, and 63 women, who declined the surgery and chose regular surveillance. Findings disclosed an absence of breast cancer among those undergoing prophylactic mastectomy during a follow-up of 2.9 (±1.4) years. In comparison, eight breast cancers developed in those women who elected regular surveillance after a mean follow-up of 3.0 (±1.5) years ($P = 0.003$; hazard ratio [HR], 0; 95% confidence interval [CI], 0-0.36). The authors concluded that, "in women with a *BRCA1* or *BRCA2* mutation, prophylactic bilateral total mastectomy reduces the incidence of breast cancer at three years of follow-up." A significantly greater number of women in the prophylactic mastectomy group, as opposed to those in the surveillance group, had undergone a premenopausal oophorectomy (44 vs 24 [58% vs 38%], $P = 0.03$), implying a possible protective effect from prophylactic oophorectomy. Recent studies[90,91] have, in fact, found risk-reducing effects of prophylactic salpingo-oophorectomy on both breast and ovarian cancer in patients who carry a *BRCA1* or *BRCA2* mutation.

Rebbeck and colleagues[92] showed a statistically significant reduction in breast cancer risk following bilateral prophylactic oophorectomy among *BRCA1* mutation carriers, which was greater in women who were followed for 5 or more years after surgery. In addition, prophylactic salpingo-oophorectomy also showed a potential for the reduction of risk for ovarian cancer. Hormone replacement therapy did not negate this reduction in breast cancer risk after bilateral prophylactic oophorectomy. The authors stated that the most probable mechanism for the decreased risk was the reduction of ovarian hormone exposure.[92]

Rebbeck and colleagues[91] prospectively studied 551 women with *BRCA1* or *BRCA2* germline mutations identified from registries; 259 had undergone bilateral prophylactic oophorectomy and 292 matched controls had not undergone the procedure. Study subjects were followed for a minimum of 8 years. Findings disclosed that "Six women who underwent prophylactic oophorectomy (2.3 percent) received a diagnosis of stage I ovarian cancer at the time of the procedure; two women (0.8 percent) received a diagnosis of papillary serous peritoneal carcinoma, 3.8 and 8.6 years after bilateral prophylactic oophorectomy. Among the controls, 58 women (19.9 percent) received a diagnosis of ovarian cancer, after a mean follow-up of 8.8 years. With the exclusion of the six women whose cancer was diagnosed at surgery, prophylactic oophorectomy significantly reduced the risk of coelomic epithelial cancer (hazard ratio, 0.04; 95 percent confidence interval, 0.01 to 0.16)...." In addition, a subgroup analysis of 241 women without a history of breast carcinoma and/or prophylactic mastectomy was performed to determine the effect of bilateral prophylactic oophorectomy on breast cancer risk. The finding revealed that "Of 99 women who underwent bilateral prophylactic oophorectomy and who were studied to determine the risk of breast cancer, breast cancer developed in 21 (21.2 percent), as compared with 60 (42.3 percent) in the control group (hazard ratio, 0.47; 95 percent confidence interval, 0.29 to 0.77)." The authors concluded that bilateral prophylactic oophorectomy reduced the risk of ovarian cancer and breast cancer in those women who were harbingers of *BRCA1* or *BRCA2* germline mutations.

Kauff and colleagues[90] compared the effect of prophylactic salpingo-oophorectomy to that of surveillance on the incidence of breast cancer and ovarian cancer in harbingers of *BRCA* mutations. They studied 170 women (35 years of age or older) who had declined bilateral oophorectomy and chose surveillance for ovarian cancer. They found that "The time to breast cancer or *BRCA*-related gynecologic cancer was longer in the salpingo-oophorectomy group, with a hazard ratio for subsequent breast cancer or *BRCA*-related gynecologic cancer of 0.25 (95 percent confidence interval, 0.08 to 0.72)."

A more recent study by Kauff and colleagues[93] notes that prophylactic salpingo-oophorectomy now provides an option for the reduction of *both* breast and ovarian cancers for women with *BRCA1* and *BRCA2* mutations. These authors studied 1079 women (30 years of age and older) with *BRCA1* or *BRCA2* mutations. Women self-selected prophylactic salpingo-oophorectomy or observation and answered a questionnaire, followed by a medical record review. During a 3-year follow-up, prophylactic salpingo-oophorectomy was associated with "an 85% reduction in *BRCA1*-associated gynecologic cancer risk (hazard ratio [HR] = 0.15; 95% CI 0.04-0.56) and a 72% reduction in *BRCA2*-associated breast cancer risk (HR = 0.28; 95% CI 0.08-0.92)." The authors noted that, "While protection against *BRCA1*-associated breast cancer (HR = 0.61; 95% CI 0.30-1.22) and *BRCA2*-associated gynecologic cancer (HR = 0.00; 95% CI, not estimable) was suggested, neither effect reached statistical significance." The authors concluded that the protection conferred by prophylactic salpingo-oophorectomy against breast and gynecologic cancers may differ between carriers of *BRCA1* and *BRCA2* mutations, and that studies evaluating the efficacy of risk-reduction strategies in *BRCA* mutation carriers should be stratified by the specific gene mutated.

BRCA1/2 Concerns About Prophylactic Surgery ■ We have identified the *BRCA1/BRCA2* germline mutation status of 1252 individuals from 95 families with HBOC (H.T.L., unpublished data). To date, we have counseled 687 women from 83 of these families. Pertinent insights about their interest in surgical prophylaxis have emerged. For example, before receiving their DNA results, 362 of these women were asked if they would consider a prophylactic mastectomy. A total of 138 out of 362 (38%) women said they would consider prophylactic mastectomy if they were positive for the mutation. Interestingly, 5 out of 307 (2%) women said they would consider prophylactic mastectomy even if negative for the mutation. This reflects, in part, the anxiety of many women about the 1:7 lifetime general-population breast cancer risk and a general conception, based on the experiences of friends or family, that the disease is uniformly terminal. It may also reflect a lack of belief that a negative mutation finding would remove them from the greater HBOC lifetime breast cancer risk, since many have been labeled "high risk" for years based on family history, and/or many of their relatives may have been affected with breast cancer.

If positive for the mutation, 172 (51%) out of the 336 women who answered the question said that they would consider bilateral prophylactic oophorectomy and, if negative, 14 (5%) out of 289 women would still consider this surgery. Following disclosure of mutation status, we found that 27 out of 142 (19%) mutation-positive women had undergone prophylactic mastectomy, and 46 out of 131 (35%) had undergone a bilateral prophylactic oophorectomy.

Metcalfe and colleagues[94] evaluated the rate of prophylactic contralateral mastectomy in an international cohort of women with HBOC. This study included 927 *BRCA1* or *BRCA2* mutation positive women with unilateral breast cancer. Subjects were followed prospectively for a minimum of 1.5 years, after which time information was obtained on prophylactic surgery, tamoxifen use, as well as the occurrence of contralateral breast cancer. Two hundred fifty-three women (27.3%) underwent contralateral prophylactic mastectomy following the diagnosis of breast cancer. This international study involved 43 centers in 8 countries (Austria, Canada, France, Israel, Italy, Norway, Poland, and the United States). Large differences in contralateral prophylactic mastectomy rates were noted by country, ranging from 0% in Norway to 49.3% in the United States. In addition, "Among women from North America, those who had a prophylactic contralateral mastectomy were significantly younger at breast cancer diagnosis (mean age, 39 years) than were those without preventive surgery (mean age, 43 years). Women who initially underwent breast-conserving surgery were less likely to undergo contralateral prophylactic mastectomy than were women who underwent a mastectomy (12% *v* 40%; $P < 10^{-4}$)...." Prophylactic contralateral mastectomy was more frequently chosen by women who had elected to undergo prophylactic bilateral oophorectomy (33%) than by those with intact ovaries (18%; $P < 10^{-4}$). The authors concluded that patients' age, type of initial cancer surgery, as well as prophylactic oophorectomy were all predictive of prophylactic contralateral mastectomy in breast cancer-affected women with a *BRCA* mutation. Acceptance of contralateral prophylactic mastectomy appeared to be significantly higher in North America than in Europe.

Rebbeck and colleagues,[95] in their update of their study of the efficacy of bilateral prophylactic mastectomy for breast cancer risk reduction in women with *BRCA1* and *BRCA2* mutations, note that research in this area is limited despite the clinical use of this risk-management strategy. Their study estimated the degree of breast cancer risk reduction after surgery in women who carry these mutations. Their results showed that breast cancer was diagnosed in 2 (1.9%) out of 105 women who had bilateral prophylactic mastectomy and in 184 (48.7%) out of 378 matched controls who did not have the procedure. Mean follow-up was 6.4 years. The authors note, "Bilateral prophylactic mastectomy reduced the risk of breast cancer by approximately 95% in women with prior or concurrent bilateral prophylactic oophorectomy and by approximately 90% in women with intact ovaries." They concluded that, overall, bilateral prophylactic mastectomy reduced the risk of breast cancer in women with *BRCA1/2* mutations by approximately 90%.

Despite the decrease in risk, the role of lumpectomy in the presence of a BRCA mutation remains unclear. In the setting of a *BRCA1* or *BRCA2* mutation, Robson and colleagues[96] suggest that the significant risks of contralateral breast cancer and late metachronous ipsilateral breast cancer, "may prompt the serious consideration of bilateral mastectomy as a preventive measure." However, limited data are available on whether this decrease in breast cancer risk translates into increased survival when compared with multimodality surveillance of mutation carriers.

Breast Cancer Susceptibility Genes Other Than _BRCA1/BRCA2_ ■ de Jong and colleagues[97] have provided an extensive review focusing on genes other than the high-penetrance *BRCA1/BRCA2* mutations that are involved in breast cancer susceptibility, including the discovery of 13 polymorphisms in 10 genes that are either associated with breast cancer susceptibility or that are in strong linkage disequilibrium with breast cancer-causing variants. They discuss recent data that assume that hypermethylation of the promotor region of a gene can also be one of the "hits" acquired in malignant neoplastic development due to silencing of the gene. Germline mutations in other genes of interest found to predispose to breast cancer include the *TP53* gene in the Li-Fraumeni syndrome (LFS), the *ATM* gene in ataxia telangiectasia, the *PTEN* gene in Cowden syndrome (CS), and the *LKB1* gene in Peutz-Jeghers syndrome (PJS). Polymorphisms in *HRAS1, GSTM1, GSTP1, CYP1B1* (codon 119), *CYP2D6, CYP19*, and *VDR* (*Apa*I and poly-A) are also implicated. The group also found a decreased risk of breast cancer in women homozygous for the variant allele for the intron 3, exon 4, and intron 6 polymorphisms in the *Tp53* gene, the *Xba*I polymorphism in the *ER* gene, and the PROGINS polymorphism in the *PR* gene. The authors suggest that carriers of these polymorphisms may represent a subpopulation in whom prevention strategies in the future may be applied less intensively than for the general population. Little is known of how the combinations of such polymorphisms might affect breast cancer risk.

The *CHEK2**1100delC variant is an example of a novel lower penetrance allele associated with increased breast cancer risk. The *CHEK2**1100delC variant predisposes to breast cancer in multiple-case families in whom *BRCA1* and *BRCA2* mutations have been excluded. In a large case-control study, de Bock and colleagues[98] found that harboring the *CHEK2**1100delC mutation increases breast cancer risk, albeit to a lesser degree than *BRCA1* or *BRCA2* mutations. How this information should be incorporated into clinical practice is not yet clear, but the authors suggest that "intensive surveillance, and possibly preventive measures should be considered for newly diagnosed breast cancer cases carrying the *CHEK2**1100delC variant."

Cybulski and colleagues[99] have also recently examined the *CHEK2* gene, which has been associated with a predisposition to breast and PC in North America and Europe. It is noteworthy that this CHEK2 protein participates in the DNA damage response involving multiple cell types and thereby becomes a good candidate for a multisite cancer susceptibility gene. These investigators identified three founder alleles to be present in Poland; two resulted in truncated CHEK2 protein, and the third led to a missense substitution of an isoleucine for a threonine. The majority of common cancer anatomic sites associated with protein-truncating alleles included cancers of the thyroid (odds ratio [OR] 4.9; $P = 0.0006$), breast (OR 2.2; $P = 0.02$), and prostate (OR 2.2; $P = 0.04$). In addition, the missense variant I157T was associated with an increased risk of breast cancer (OR 1.4; $P = 0.02$), colon cancer (OR 2.0; $P = 0.001$), kidney cancer (OR 2.1; $P = 0.0006$), PC (OR 1.7; $P = 0.002$), and thyroid cancer (OR 1.9; $P = 0.04$). Thus, the range of cancers associated with mutations of the *CHEK2* gene may far exceed breast cancer alone.

Summary ■ With the identification of *BRCA1* and *BRCA2*, we have been able to directly impact the care of people who come from families with mutations in these genes. With further characterization of additional cancer-prone genes, we hope to gain further insights into the mechanisms that underlie the development of these cancers and their potential for cancer prevention and cure. The cloning of the human genome and the identification of additional risk-associated genes continues to expand the clinical management of individuals with a strong family history of breast and ovarian cancers.[100] Thus, the role of genetic counseling by individuals who specialize in cancer risk assessment will continue to grow in importance. Similarly, an increased understanding of the function of these genes may have significant implications for the treatment of these tumors in the future.[101]

Colorectal Carcinoma

Overview ■ Colorectal cancer (CRC), while highly prevalent worldwide, is nevertheless one of the most preventable cancers. Its etiology is the product of both genetic and environmental factors and their interaction.

Approximately 148,810 new cases of CRC were diagnosed in the United States during 2008, and the estimated mortality of the disorder for that year was approximately 49,960.[11] Known hereditary syndromes will account for at least 10% of those, and it is likely that more subtle susceptibility factors contribute to the pathogenesis of many more. A large prospective study[102] recently confirmed what more than a dozen retrospective studies had asserted, that a family history of CRC confers increased risk of the disease.

In 1985, analysis of a large colon cancer-prone Utah kindred pointed to the existence of a partially penetrant gene, inherited in an autosomal dominant manner.[103] The missense mutation in the *APC* gene described by Laken and colleagues (I1307K)[104,105] is an example of such a mutation. Other low-penetrance mutations may prove to be important contributors to colon cancer risk and are discussed elsewhere in this chapter. This section will review four inherited syndromes featuring increased risk for colon cancer: FAP, hereditary nonpolyposis colorectal cancer (LS), familial juvenile polyposis (FJP), and PJS.

CRC's familial component is extremely high, with estimates ranging to about one-fourth of the total CRC burden; at least 10% of CRC is hereditary. Remarkable advances in molecular genetics during the past two decades have led to the discovery of a molecular basis for several highly penetrant CRC-prone disorders, the most noteworthy of which are FAP, linked to the *APC* tumor suppressor gene; LS, attributable to several MMR genes, including *MLH1, MSH2*, and *MSH6*; autosomal dominantly inherited hamartomatous polyposis syndromes responsible for CRC that include PJS due to *STK11/LKB*, and juvenile polyposis (JP) linked to mutations in *SMAD4* and *BMPR1A*. Autosomal recessive mutations in the *MYH* MMR gene in its biallelic presence gives rise to a phenotype comparable in many ways to attenuated FAP. These syndromes and their recognition through molecular genetic testing provide unique opportunities for clinicians to identify their distinguishing multiple colonic polyp phenotypes; occasional extracolonic polyp stigmata such as perioral pigmentations in PJS, and sebaceous cysts and congenital hypertrophy of the retinal pigmentation in FAP. Clearly, these pre-morbid stigmata can expedite the identification of candidates for molecular genetic testing, so that significant clues of who needs testing can be more readily discerned. There is a need for the molecular geneticist to obtain help in terms of an accurate diagnosis in order to determine where to look in the genome based on the hereditary cancer syndrome of concern.[106] Family history will be important and its full interpretation may be dependent on the physician's knowledge of these syndromes. Their respective natural histories, differing tumor complements, and pathology features will be important for structuring a lifetime screening and management program.[107]

Familial Adenomatous Polyposis ■ The historical concept of the hereditary basis for CRC has been aided significantly by the detailed description provided by Bussey.[108] Specifically, this history begins with observations by Menzelio[109] who, in 1721, may have reported the first example of a patient with a large number of polyps in the gastrointestinal (GI) tract. This multiple polyp phenotype provided powerful evidence of this physical "anchoring point," thereby fueling in a tangible way that subsequently served as a basis for both its cancer association and its significant presence in close family members through transmission from one generation to the next, as described subsequently. This concrete phenomenon, inherent in the polyp, provides sharp contrast to the struggle for legitimizing a genetic basis for the LS, which albeit manifesting occasional colonic adenomas had lacked multiple adenomas as a physical guide to CRC and ultimately its genetic transmission.

Many decades later, more definition of histology, number and location of polyps and associated lesions, and possible familial incidence, began being identified. The science of histopathology, initiated in the early 1860s, recognized the importance of intestinal polyps. In 1881, Woodword[110] divided polyposis into "primary" (no apparent antecedent disease), and "secondary" (when polyps followed previous inflammation and ulcers of the colon).

In 1882, Cripps[1] reported polyposis coli in two members of the same family (brother and sister). This was likely the first indication that it was familial and possibly of genetic origin. Bussey[108] believes that this important observation dates the point at which the history of FAP started. In 1890, Bickersteth[111] reported a family with affected members in two generations (mother and son), which strengthened the issue of FAP's inheritance. In 1887, Smith[2] mentioned the presence of "adenocarcinoma" of the colon when describing three members of a family with multiple polyps.

At the end of the nineteenth century, three of the four most prominent features of FAP had been recognized: (1) there was a large number of polyps; (2) histologically, they were adenomatous; and (3) they were inherited. The fourth feature, the association with CRC, is mentioned in 1887 by Smith.[2]

St. Mark's Hospital and Cancer Registry ■ The first register of polyposis families contributed significantly to the number of patients available for clinical and pathology investigation. Therein, Cuthbert Dukes, consultant pathologist at St. Mark's Hospital, London, pioneered family studies, and the importance of the family pedigree. This FAP registry at St. Mark's Hospital was established in 1925. As of 1990, there were over 510 families, 63 of whom showed the adenomatous type; 1238 members of these families were seen to have polyposis. Other families in this polyposis registry include 37 with PJS, 64 with JP, and 46 with miscellaneous types.

New technology with the sigmoidoscope with self-contained illumination was introduced at the beginning of the twentieth century. Barium enema was improved by double-contrast technique.

It is noteworthy that before World War II about 65% of FAP patients had CRC on first examination; this has fallen to about 5%. However, Arvenitis et al.[112] at the Cleveland Clinic showed 59% of patients with FAP in 1990 dying of metastatic CRC.

By World War II, Dukes decided puberty was the right time to commence regular annual sigmoidoscopic examination of the children of a polyposis patient. Hill et al.[113] and Morson et al.[114] subsequently described the natural history of FAP (number of adenomas, age range of onset, adenoma-carcinoma sequence)

Prophylactic Colectomy in FAP ■ Bussey[108] notes that through the advent of safe surgical treatment, patients in the benign stage of FAP could benefit from cancer prevention by total removal of the colon and rectum. Two views emerged: one view advocating total proctocolectomy and ileostomy whereas the second view argued that an ileostomy posed a severe handicap to an individual. It was reasoned that the risk of rectal cancer following colectomy and ileorectal anastomosis would be minimal when rectal examinations were carried out every 6 months. It then became a policy at St. Mark's Hospital to retain the rectum. Therein, the first ileorectal anastomosis was conducted in 1948. Many surgical innovations have been adopted since, including abdominal perineal resection, mucosectomy, and ileal pouch reservoir to protect against rectal carcinoma.

Associated Extracolonic Lesions ■ In 1953, Gardner and Richards[115] published on a polyposis family wherein affected members also exhibited (a) multiple osteomas of the cranium and mandibles; (b) multiple epidermoid cysts; and (c) fibromas of the skin. This was subsequently called Gardner syndrome. Further study of this large Utah family added dental abnormalities (supranumerary teeth) and desmoid tumors of the abdominal wall and extension of adenomas to any part of the skeletal system.[116]

In 1975, Utsunomiya and Nakamura[117] found that x-rays of the mandibles among more than 90% of all Japanese polyposis patients they examined had occult osteomas in this area, a finding that was subsequently confirmed at other centers. Lewis et al.,[118] in 1984, added congenital hypertrophy of the retinal pigment epithelium (CHRPE). In 1985, Bulow et al.[119] showed that about one-third of FAP patients also had gastric polyps mainly of two types: adenomas and fundic gland polyps.

Bulow[120] cites an 1861 clinical patient report by Luschka[121] that may have been FAP. The first definitive report of a patient with multiple colonic polyposis was published in 1881 by Sklifasowski.[122] The first familial example was that of a brother and sister with FAP reported by Cripps[1] in 1882. Additional cases of CRC in patients with FAP were reported by Smith in 1887.[2] The histologic changes from adenoma to adenocarcinoma were first described by Handford.[123] Lockhart-Mummery[124] was the first to report that the relevant hereditary factor in this disease is not the cancer per se, but rather the presence of multiple adenomas, which have a tendency to undergo malignant transformation. This sentinel report, emanating from the histories of three FAP families, formed the basis for the now renowned St. Mark's Hospital Polyposis Registry in London, England. Herrera et al.[5] in 1986 examined a patient with multiple developmental abnormalities as well as multiple colonic polyps. Interstitial deletion of chromosome 5 was observed. In 1987, Bodmer et al.[125] provided evidence that the FAP gene, now known as *APC*, was on chromosome 5. Since then, there have been abundant advances in the understanding of the genotypic and phenotypic heterogeneity of this *APC* mutation.

FAP is inherited in an autosomal dominant pattern. The incidence is 1 in 6,000 to 1 in 13,000; Powell and colleagues estimated that more than 50,000 families in the United States could benefit from genetic counseling for this disorder.[126] Affected individuals carry germline mutations of the *APC* gene on chromosome 5q21-q22.[6,7,125,127,128] About one-third of FAP patients have no family history and probably represent new mutations. Many mutations of *APC* have been described; 80% of them are truncating. There is some correlation between the position of the truncating mutation and phenotype (discussed below).

APC is a large gene, with 15 exons encoding a 2,843 residue protein. The gene product participates in several functions, including differentiation, proliferation, apoptosis, adhesion, migration, and chromosomal segregation.[129] First, APC may negatively regulate the Wnt-1 signaling pathway by binding to β-catenin.[130,131] Mutated APC product, unable to bind, allows cytoplasmic and nuclear accumulation of β-catenin, with persistent activation of downstream transcription and growth factors. APC protein also colocalizes with the microtubule cytoskeleton, leading to the speculation that APC is involved in cell migration and cell adhesion.[132] Finally, APC might be involved in cell cycle regulation.[133]

Affected individuals have multiple colonic adenomas and, if untreated, will inevitably develop CRC. Adenomas arise in the mid to late teens; 95% of mutation carriers have adenomas by age 35. More than 90% of FAP patients develop duodenal adenomas, but carcinoma supervenes in only about 5%. Gastric polyposis is seen in at least 50% of affected patients; most of the polyps are fundic gland polyps, but gastric adenomas do occur. Although fundic gland polyps are considered to be benign, there are reports of dysplasia in fundic gland polyps and reports of carcinoma arising adjacent to, or in continuity with, fundic gland polyps.[134] Abraham and colleagues[135] have shown that FAP-associated fundic gland polyps often have sporadic *APC* alterations that sporadic fundic gland polyps lack, suggesting that the polyps arising in the hereditary setting are neoplastic. Gastric carcinoma risk, however, is not appreciably elevated in Western FAP patients. In contrast, Japanese and Korean families with FAP have a threefold to fourfold excess risk for gastric carcinoma.[136]

Extraintestinal manifestations of FAP include desmoid tumor, hepatoblastoma, thyroid carcinoma, medulloblastoma, and a litany of benign lesions: sebaceous or epidermoid cysts, lipomas, osteomas, supernumerary teeth, congenital hypertrophy of retinal pigment epithelium, and juvenile nasopharyngeal angiofibromas. Brain tumors, particularly medulloblastomas, are a feature of the Turcot's variant of FAP.[137]

The attenuated variant of FAP (AFAP) presents a particularly difficult diagnostic challenge.[138-140] Adenomas can be sparse (one or two in some patients, dozens in others) and are often right-sided. The adenomas appear at a later age (35-40 years) than in classic FAP, as do colon carcinomas (55 years). Upper GI manifestations (fundic gland polyps and duodenal adenomas) are seen with the same, or possibly a greater, frequency as in classic FAP. The first AFAP families to be described had mutations near the proximal end of the *APC* gene; the phenotype has since been seen in families with mutations at the extreme distal end as well.

Genetic testing is available for FAP. If a mutation is found in an affected family member, then other at-risk family members can easily be tested for the mutations. Genetic testing is not recommended for children less than 10 years old. If no mutation is found in an affected family member, the test is considered uninformative; a negative result in that setting does not rule out FAP.

Two recent studies compared the phenotype of FAP families with and without documented mutations. Moisio and colleagues[141] identified 38 different germline mutations in *APC* in 47 out of 65 (72%) Finnish FAP kindreds. Families without detectable *APC* mutations differed from mutation positive families by having an older mean age of polyposis diagnosis (38.6 years [48 individuals] vs 30.0 years [140 individuals]; $P = 0.001$) and a lower proportion of kindreds with extracolonic disease (6/18 vs 5/47; $P = 0.04$). Heinimann and colleagues[142] studied 36 FAP families, 72% of which were positive for the *APC* germline mutation. The mean age at diagnosis of colonic adenomas was 35.2 years in *APC*-positive families vs 45.3 years in *APC*-negative families. Gastric polyps were found in 14 patients, all of whom were *APC* positive. Finally, patients who were *APC* negative showed a lower number of colonic adenomas at diagnosis and fewer extracolonic manifestations. These authors concluded that patients from FAP families who lacked *APC* germline mutations presented with a notably milder disease phenotype when compared with the *APC*-positive families.

Randomized, controlled trials demonstrating the efficacy of screening and management regimens have not been performed and are not likely to be. Nevertheless, the following recommendations are generally agreed upon: affected or at-risk individuals should have annual flexible sigmoidoscopy beginning by age 12. If the family history suggests AFAP, then colonoscopy is required (because the adenomas are more proximal), but can begin later (age 20). Prophylactic colectomy should be considered once multiple adenomas have appeared. However, it may be that prophylactic colectomy can be temporarily postponed in AFAP when management by polypectomy is possible; we are following several mutation carriers who develop one or two new adenomas every year but who have not developed carcinoma. Endoscopic surveillance of the rectum and anus should be continued after prophylactic colectomy. A baseline upper endoscopy is advisable by age 20, with follow-up examinations every 2 to 3 years unless symptoms occur. Annual thyroid palpation is suggested, and children at risk for FAP should have serum α-fetoprotein testing every 6 months until 6 years of age in the interest of early detection of hepatoblastoma.

When duodenal adenomas are discovered, they should be removed endoscopically if feasible. Often, however, the adenomas are too numerous to remove; in that case, annual surveillance with biopsy of grossly suspicious lesions is a prudent course. It is hoped that chemoprevention will help control duodenal adenomas, but results thus far have not been encouraging (reviewed by Hawk and colleagues[143]).

Desmoid tumors can be a difficult management problem. These locally aggressive soft-tissue tumors typically arise in the abdominal wall or bowel mesentery. Relentless recurrences are the rule.[144,145] The difficulty of surgical cure, complete with the fact that surgery may initiate the pathogenesis of desmoids, has led to the recommendation that only symptomatic desmoid tumors should be surgically resected.[146] Desmoid tumors may occur in excess in certain FAP families.[145,147,148]

I1307K Ashkenazi Mutation ■ First described by Laken and colleagues,[104] the I1307K mutation/polymorphism is carried by approximately 6% of Ashkenazi Jews and a lower proportion of other Jews; it has not been seen in non-Jews.[104,149,150] Carriers have an approximately twofold risk of CRC compared with non-carriers.[104] Rozen and colleagues[151] studied the I1307K *APC* gene variant in 718 Israeli Jews wherein "I1307K occurred in 6.2% Ashkenazi participants, in 1.5% of non-Ashkenazi control participants (p= 0.02) and in 10% of Ashkenazim with *familial* neoplasia (relative risk 1.73 [not significant when compared with controls]; 95% confidence interval, 0.7-3.2). Colorectal neoplasia was detected in carriers at a younger age ($p<0.05$) without excess risk for multiple colorectal neoplasia or non-colorectal neoplasia. I1307K attributable risk for colorectal neoplasia was 0.5-0.6%. Compared with non-carriers, both Ashkenazi and non-Ashkenazi I1307K carriers had similar flanking polymorphic markers ($p<0.01$)."

The conclusion from this study was that this low penetrant genetic variant poses an approximate 1.7 RR for neoplasia in mutation carriers who have familial CRC and that it appears to be clinically equivalent to "obtaining a family history of sporadic colorectal neoplasia and promoting early screening. I1307K is a founder genetic variant in Jews of different ethnic origin, mainly Ashkenazim, but it explains only partially their higher instance of colorectal carcinoma."[105]

Locker and colleagues[151] studied 215 Ashkenazi Jews with a personal history of CRC. Clinical and family history, pathology reports, and slides were obtained, and blood was drawn for I1307K determination. The presence of the mutation was determined by PCR from white blood cell DNA. CRC pathology slides were read in a blinded manner. Of the 215 enrolled patients, 26 (12.1%) tested positive for I1307K. There was no difference in the pathologic features between CRC in Ashkenazi I1307K mutation carriers compared with noncarriers. There was no difference in the age at diagnosis or history of a second or other primary cancers. Carriers had an increased likelihood of having a first-degree relative with CRC (50%) compared with noncarriers (28%, $P < 0.04$). There was no distinguishing feature found other than family history that characterizes I1307K-positive CRC. The investigators found no group of Ashkenazi Jews with CRC for whom screening for I1307K would be clinically useful.

***MYH (MUTYH)* Mutations and CRC** ■ *MYH* is a DNA-base-excision-repair gene located on chromosome 1p. Mutations in this gene predispose to an autosomal recessively inherited colonic polyposis that shows an average of 55 adenomas in an affected individual.[152] This disorder is rare, accounting for approximately 1 out of 10,000 in the general population and accounting for about 5% of persons with a FAP-type phenotype.[152] This represents a high risk for colorectal neoplasia.

Nielsen and colleagues[153] provided a recent characterization of *MUTYH*-

associated polyposis (MAP) as an autosomal recessively inherited disorder wherein carriers of biallelic *MUTYH* germline mutations harbor an approximately 60% risk for development of CRC. It is estimated that in the general population approximately 1.5% of individuals are heterozygous carriers of the *MUTYH* mutation and therein progeny of MAP patients are at an increased risk of inheriting two *MUTYH* mutations and in this biallelic state they show an enormously increased risk for manifesting CRC. These authors combined data from the literature as well as 40 Dutch MAP patients in order to construct a Markov model for developing a societal cost-utility analysis of genetic screening of MAP families, which involved testing the spouse when heterozygous and testing the progeny of that spouse. Results showed that the cost of genetic screening families of MAP patients when compared to the absence of screening was estimated at €25,000 per quality-adjusted life year (QALY). Findings showed that "For a *MUTYH* heterozygote index-patient, the ratio was €51,500 per QALY...." These results were shown to be sensitive to several of the parameters in the model, including the cost for molecular genetic testing. It was concluded that genetic screening in families of MAP patients was found to be acceptable in concert with international standards. Recommendations were, therefore, posed that genetic testing of spouses and/or children should be discussed with an offer to counselees.

Nielsen and colleagues,[153] in their review of MAP, note that Al-Tassan and colleagues[154] reported that *MYH* is the first autosomal recessive inherited disorder demonstrating an increased risk for developing colorectal adenomas and carcinomas. In the majority of MAP patients, colonic polyposis and subsequent CRC occur in the majority of patients. Interestingly, biallelic *MUTYH* mutations are found in 10-25% of patients with "between 10 and a few hundred adenomas and in 1% of patients with a colorectal carcinoma. Patients with more than 10 adenomas are currently being offered MUTYH mutation analysis. Siblings of a MAP patient have a 25% risk of having inherited biallelic mutations and are eligible for genetic testing."[153]

Sensitivity with the penetrance of CRC in MAP patients ranges between 40% and 70%. The percentage of MAP patients reported to develop CRC lies between 50% and 70%. MAP patients have between 10 and about 100 adenomas at a mean age of 50; they are advised to have colonoscopic screening from age 25.

Lefevre and colleagues[155] found that there were 9 women and 22 men with a mean age of 54 years (range 22-68 years) at the time of diagnosis. The mean number of polyps was 63. Eighteen patients (58%) had a CRC. Biallelic *MYH* mutations were found in six patients (19.3). It was concluded that *MYH* is responsible for about 1.4% of all adenomatous polyposis and about 20% of adenomatous polyposis without an identified *APC* mutation.

Familial Juvenile Polyposis ■ Sporadic juvenile polyps are relatively common (one autopsy study of patients under 21 years reported a prevalence of 1%).[156] Usually solitary, the polyps are innocuous and do not confer increased risk for cancer of the colon.[157] The discovery of multiple juvenile polyps in a patient without a family history of polyposis can create a diagnostic dilemma. The clinical diagnosis of JP requires histologic confirmation of a juvenile polyp, plus the presence of any of the following: more than five juvenile polyps in the colorectum, juvenile polyps elsewhere in the GI tract, or a family history of polyposis. Even when there are multiple juvenile polyps and a family history of polyposis, the diagnosis of JP must be made with care, because CS and Bannayan-Riley-Ruvalcaba (BRR) syndrome have similar polyps but a very different spectrum of associated lesions.[158]

Three variants of JP have been described: a rare, usually fatal JP of infancy with diarrhea, protein-losing enteropathy, and alopecia; juvenile polyps of the colorectum; and generalized JP. (The division between the latter two may be an artifact of variable penetrance, as both the colorectal and generalized forms have been described in one kindred. Extraintestinal anomalies, while not common, have been reported in association with juvenile polyps; these include hydrocephalus, thyroglossal duct cyst, tetralogy of Fallot, coarctation of the aorta, idiopathic hypertrophic subaortic stenosis, and malrotation of the gut.)

The inheritance pattern is autosomal dominant. A gene for FJP has been mapped on to a locus on chromosome 18q21.[159] The gene encodes a component of the TGFβ signaling pathway *MAD4*.[160,161] Mutations in *MADH4* account for about 20% of FJP cases. A second gene, bone morphogenetic protein receptor 1A (*BMPR1A*), has been implicated in another 20% of FJP.[162] *BMPR1A* is a member of the TGFβ superfamily, and is part of the pathway mediated by *MADH4* signaling.

Juvenile polyps may be found in the colorectum (98%), stomach (14%), duodenum (2%), and small bowel (7%).[163,164] Although the polyps are considered benign, FJP patients are at increased risk for CRC. The cumulative lifetime risk was estimated by Järvinen to be 50%,[165] an estimate that compares remarkably well to a report from the University of Iowa describing a large FJP kindred in which 16 out of 29 (55%) affected individuals developed GI cancer.[166] Eleven members of the Iowa kindred had colon cancer and six had gastric cancer.

Affected individuals need regular endoscopic surveillance. Scott-Conner and colleagues[164] recommend upper and lower GI endoscopy beginning at age 15 and continuing every 3 years as long as no lesions are detected. If a family carries a *MADH4* or *BMPR1A* mutation, at-risk individuals can be tested to determine whether surveillance is needed. Small number of polyps can be managed by polypectomy; in these cases, endoscopy should be repeated yearly until the patient is free of polyps. If there are multiple polyps in the colon, subtotal colectomy is recommended if the rectum can be cleared endoscopically; otherwise, total colectomy is a consideration. For young children with large numbers of polyps, regular colonoscopy with removal of the largest polyps is an option as a temporizing measure until puberty has been attained. Multiple gastric polyps, particularly if dysplasia is present, should prompt consideration of gastrectomy.

Children with large numbers of polyps present a difficult management problem. Colectomy is the prudent choice, but we believe regular colonoscopy with removal of the largest polyps until the patient attains puberty is also an option.[166]

Peutz-Jeghers Syndrome ■ Peutz-Jeghers syndrome (PJS) is inherited in an autosomal dominant pattern and has been mapped on to a locus on chromosome 19p13.3.[167,168] The gene responsible for the syndrome encodes a serine threonine kinase, STK11 (also known as LKB1).[167] Abnormal (ie, inactive) forms of this kinase may lead to defective control of cellular growth and differentiation. Not all PJS families can be linked to 19p13.3, leading to speculation that there is a second locus for the syndrome.[169,170] The incidence of PJS is unknown; it is thought to be about one-tenth as common as FAP.[103]

The diagnosis of PJS requires histologic confirmation of a hamartomatous, Peutz-Jeghers-type polyp. Because such polyps can be seen in individuals who do not have PJS, clinical diagnosis also requires at least two of the following: small bowel polyposis, family history of PJS; or pigmented macules of buccal mucosa, lips, fingers, and toes.[171] Genetic testing for the syndrome is being developed.[172]

Peutz-Jeghers polyps have been found in the entire GI tract. The small bowel is the site affected most often, but stomach and colon are involved as well; esophageal polyps are rare. The polyps are almost always multiple but tend to number in the dozens rather than the hundreds. Peutz-Jeghers polyps have also been described in respiratory mucosa and the urinary tract. One member of the Dutch family originally studied by Peutz suffered from severe nasal polyposis and eventually developed a nasal carcinoma.[173]

PJS carries an increased risk for malignancy. Giardiello and colleagues[171] found a RR for cancer 18 times that of the general population in 31 PJS patients. Malignancies involved pancreas (4), breast (2), stomach (2), colon (2), lung (2), and endometrium (1). Spigelman and colleagues[174] reported that 72 retrospectively studied PJS patients were 13 times more likely than the general population to develop a malignancy. The tumors involved colon, stomach, small intestine, ovary, fallopian tube, thyroid, and lung. Investigators from the Mayo Clinic[175] found a RR for cancer of 9.9 in 34 PJS patients, with cancers of the colon (7), breast (6), lung (3), and cervix (2) predominating. The Mayo Clinic group found a particularly high incidence of breast and gynecologic cancers, contributing to a relative cancer risk of 18.5 in women, compared with 6.2 in men.

The Dutch family originally described by Peutz has been updated, and the findings further demonstrate that PJS is a cancer-prone condition.[173] Of the 22 affected individuals, 7 developed carcinoma (3 colon, 1 stomach, 1 GI not otherwise specified, 1 breast, and 1 nasal cavity). All patients with malignancy were dead of their disease before the age of 50 years.

Nearly every female PJS patient will have ovarian involvement by sex cord tumor with annular tubules (SCTAT). The tumors are bilateral in at least two thirds of the cases (in contrast to SCTAT in the sporadic setting, which is almost always unilateral). An unusual form of cervical cancer, minimal deviation adenocarcinoma (adenoma malignum), is also characteristic of PJS. This rare tumor accounts for 1-3% of all cervical adenocarcinoma but, in one series, affected 4 out of 27 women with PJS.[176]

The surveillance protocol advocated by the St. Mark's Polyposis Registry[177] includes yearly hemoglobin and yearly ultrasound of the pelvis in females and of the pancreas in all patients. Testicular ultrasound should also be carried out in males with feminizing features. Biannual upper and lower endoscopy with small-bowel X-ray are recommended. Regular mammography and cervical smear are critical surveillance measures. Tomlinson and Houlston[178] suggest that upper endoscopy, colonoscopy, and small-bowel x-ray begin in the second decade and that mammography begin at age 25.

The GI polyps may be associated with bleeding, obstruction, or intussusception. Conservative removal (snare polypectomy) is favored over segmental resection of bowel to avoid the development of a short bowel syndrome.

Differentiating among juvenile polyposis syndrome (JPS), CS, BRR syndrome, and PJS can be difficult.[158] Table 14-2 outlines the genetic and clinical features of the hamartomatous polyposes.

Familial Nonsyndromic CRC and Colonic Adenomas ■ Colons with dysplastic susceptibility genes appear as probable candidates for an as yet unknown subset of "sporadic" colon neoplasia (adenomas and CRC) in so-called average-risk older adults. It has been estimated that 35% of CRC risk may be heritable.[179] With respect to non-syndromic CRC, it is estimated that about 20% of individuals report CRC in a first-degree relative and therein it is hypothesized that the so-called familial cancer clusters may have a genetic basis.[180] This subject has been given appropriate emphasis by Cannon-Albright and colleagues,[181] who suggested that colonic adenomas were autosomal dominantly inherited with the estimated penetrance in the range of 40% by age 60 with an increase to about 60% by age 80. These findings were given further support by Winawer and colleagues,[182] who identified an approximately 2.5-fold increase for CRC among first-degree relatives of adenoma probands when compared with spouse controls. Furthermore, advanced adenomas and familial risk for CRC indicate that probands with this pathology pose a higher predisposition to advanced adenomas in CRC. These are certainly areas of keen interest for genetic and biomedical investigation in the search for CRC susceptibility loci and, eventually, identification of pathogenic CRC germline mutations.

Chan and colleagues[183] evaluated the association of family history of CRC in concert with cancer recurrence and survival in CRC-affected individuals. Among the 1087 eligible patients, 195 (17.9%) had a family history of CRC in a first-degree relative. Furthermore, cancer recurrence or death "occurred in 57 of 195 patients (29%; 95% confidence interval [CI], 23%-36%) with a family history of colorectal cancer and 343 of 892 patients (38%; 95 CI 35-42%) without a family history. Compared with patients without a family history, the adjusted hazard ratios (HRs) among those with 1 or more affected first-degree relatives were 0.72 (95% CI 0.54-0.96) for disease-free survival, 0.74 (95% CI 0.55-0.99) for recurrence-free survival, and 0.75 (95% CI 0.54-1.05) for overall survival...." Of further interest was the fact that the reduction in CRC recurrence or death, in combination with a family history, became stronger with an increased number of CRC-affected first-degree relatives. In addition, the improved disease-free survival associated with a family history was independent of tumoral MSI or MMR status. These authors appropriately concluded that, "among patients with stage III colon cancer receiving adjuvant chemotherapy, a family history of colorectal cancer is associated with a significant reduction in cancer recurrent and death." Similar findings have been identified in the LS.[184]

Lynch Syndrome and Other Forms of Hereditary Nonpolyposis Colorectal Cancer (HNPCC) ■ ***History of Lynch Syndrome*** ■ The history of LS dates to an observation of Aldred Warthin, pathologist at the University of Michigan School of Medicine.[185] He became deeply moved when his seamstress, in 1895, told him that she would most probably die of cancer of the colon, stomach, or her female organs, because of the enormous proclivity to these cancers in her family. Unfortunately, just as she had told Warthin, she died at a young

Table 14-2 ■ **Hamartomatous Polyposis Syndromes**

Syndrome	Phenotype	Mutations
Peutz-Jeghers	Perioral pigmentations, pigmentations of fingers, upper and lower GI hamartomatous lesions, small bowel and pancreas cancer, colorectal cancer, and sexcord tumors with annular tubules (SCTAT) of the ovary	*LKBI/STK11* gene[543]
Familial juvenile	GI hamartomatous polyps, increased polyposis risk of GI malignancy (stomach, colorectum), diagnosis made only when features classic for other syndromes are not present	*SMAD4/DPC4* gene[161] *BMPRIA* gene[162] *PTEN* gene[544]
Cowden syndrome	Colonic hamartomatous polyps but firm association with colorectal cancer yet to be identified, benign and malignant neoplasms of the thyroid, breast, uterus, and skin (multiple trichilemmomas)	*PTEN/MMAC1/DEP1*[367,377] (Finding a germline *PTEN* mutation is molecular evidence for the Cowden syndrome, but absence of an identifiable *PTEN* mutation is nondiagnostic)
Bannayan-Ruvalcaba-Riley	Microcephaly, fibromatosis, hamartomatous polyposis, hemangiomas, speckled penis; colorectal cancer has not been identified	*PTEN*

age of metastatic endometrial carcinoma. Warthin listened intently, developed her pedigree, and along with other similar cancer prone families published this work in 1913.[186] He updated the family in 1925.[187] The seamstress's family has since been known as Family G.

Lynch and colleagues[4] described the natural history and genetics of two large Midwestern kindreds (Families N and M) in 1966. The clinical genetic features in these families were similar to those of Family G.[4] Dr. A. James French, Warthin's successor as chairman of pathology at the University of Michigan, heard about Lynch's research on Families N and M,[4] and recalled that Warthin, his predecessor, had discovered a similar family (Family G) in 1895. Lynch was then invited by French to take custody of all the detailed documents and pathology specimens which the meticulous Warthin had investigated, catalogued, and published over a span of more than 30 years.[186,187] Family G was then updated and published in 1971.[188] This material is discussed in a more detailed review of the history of LS.[189] Through the use of conversion technology,[190] an *MSH2* mutation was identified in Family G in the year 2000. The family was most recently updated in 2005.[191]

Mismatch Repair Mutations ■ LS is inherited in an autosomal dominant pattern. A germline mutation in one of the genes responsible for DNA MMR can be demonstrated in approximately 40-60% of families meeting clinical criteria for LS (Table 14-3). The incidence has not been definitely established, but a large-scale molecular screening study from Finland indicates that the disorder accounts for about 2% of the CRC burden in that country.[192] Other estimates of its frequency range much higher.[20,21]

Mutations in six different MMR genes have been identified in LS patients[193,194]: *MLH1*,[195] located on chromosome 3p21.3; *MSH2*[196,197] and *MSH6*,[198] both located on 2p21; *PMS2*,[199] located on 7p22; *MLH3*,[200,201] located on 14q24.3; and possibly *PMS1*,[199] located on 2q31-q33. Approximately 90% of the identified LS mutations involve *MLH1* or *MSH2*, while mutations in the *MSH6* gene account for approximately 10%. *MSH6* mutations appear to predispose to an atypical form of LS characterized by an excess of endometrial cancer and a deficit of CRC [202].

Microsatellite Instability ■ All cells of individuals affected with LS carry a nonfunctioning allele of a DNA MMR gene; if the wild-type allele is lost or inactivated, the cell can no longer repair DNA mismatches that inevitably arise during DNA replication. Cells with defective DNA MMR accumulate mutations at a very high rate (as much as 1000 times to that of the normal cells). Because DNA mismatches are more likely to occur in DNA microsatellites (areas with multiple repeats of one nucleotide or one pair of nucleotides), defective DNA MMR leads to the phenomenon of MSI, in which the progeny of the defective cells have varying lengths of a given microsatellite.

Table 14-3 ■ Cardinal Features of Lynch Syndrome

- Autosomal dominant inheritance pattern seen for syndrome cancers in the family pedigree.
- Earlier average age of CRC onset than in the general population: average age of 45 years in Lynch syndrome vs 63 years in the general population
- Proximal (right-sided) colonic cancer predilection: 70-85% of Lynch syndrome CRCs are proximal to the splenic flexure
- Accelerated carcinogenesis (tiny adenomas can develop into carcinomas more quickly): within 2-3 years in Lynch syndrome vs 8-10 years in the general population
- High risk of additional CRCs: 25-30% of patients having surgery for a Lynch syndrome-associated CRC will have a second primary CRC within 10 years of surgical resection if the surgery was less than a subtotal colectomy
- Increased risk for malignancy at certain extracolonic sites:
  - Endometrium (40-60% lifetime risk for female mutation carriers)
  - Ovary (12-15% lifetime risk for female mutation carriers)
  - Stomach (higher risk in families indigenous to the Orient, reason unknown at this time)
  - Small bowel
  - Hepatobiliary tract
  - Pancreas
  - Upper uro-epithelial tract (transitional cell carcinoma of the ureter and renal pelvis)
  - Brain (in the Turcot's syndrome variant of the Lynch syndrome)
- Sebaceous adenomas, sebaceous carcinomas, and multiple keratoacanthomas in the Muir-Torre syndrome variant of Lynch syndrome
- Pathology of CRCs is more often poorly differentiated, with an excess of mucoid and signet-cell features, a Crohn-like reaction, and a significant excess of infiltrating lymphocytes within the tumor
- Increased survival from CRC
- The sine qua non for diagnosis is the identification of a germline mutation in a mismatch repair gene (most commonly *MLH1*, *MSH2*, or *MSH6*) that segregates in the family: ie, members who carry the mutation show a much higher rate of syndrome-related cancers than those who do not carry the mutation

The predilection of DNA mismatches for mono- and dinucleotide repeats plays a deciding role in the genetic mutations contributing to carcinogenesis. Nearly all colon cancers with MSI have mutations in the transforming growth factor β type II receptor (*TGFβIIR*) and *BAX* genes, and those mutations are located in repeating sequences. Mutation of *TGFβIIR* leads to escape from the growth inhibitory effects of TGFβ, whereas mutation of *BAX* interferes with its pro-apoptotic effect. Thus, carcinogenesis in colon cancers with MSI may involve mutations in critical genes different from those involved in other colon cancers (such as *APC*, *K-ras*, *TP53*).

Individuals carrying germline mutations of *MLH1* or *MSH2* have a lifetime risk for CRC on the order of 80%.[203] The cancers tend to arise proximal to the splenic flexure (70%). The average age at diagnosis is 45 years. Multiple synchronous and metachronous colon cancers are a feature of the syndrome, with 30% of patients developing a second colon cancer within 10 years if a limited operation (right hemicolectomy or segmental resection) is carried out for the initial cancer. Even when total abdominal colectomy is performed, the rectum is still at risk; Rodriguez-Bigas and colleagues[204] reported that 12% of LS patients had rectal cancer within 12 years after colectomy.

The colon cancers arising via the MSI pathway, whether hereditary or sporadic, often have clinicopathologic clues to their molecular pathogenesis. Such tumors are usually located proximal to the splenic flexure, and may have mucinous or signet ring cell morphology.[205] Medullary carcinoma, a subtype recently recognized in the World Health Organization classification, is found almost exclusively in tumors with high levels of MSI (MSI-H).[206] There is commonly a host lymphoid response, either in the form of lymphoid aggregates at the edge of the tumor or lymphocytes infiltrating the tumor. The latter have been found to be the single best marker of MSI status.[207] Jass has developed an algorithm for identifying MSI-H colon cancer.[205]

When one suspects that a tumor is MSI positive, immunohistochemical stains for the protein product of the DNA MMR genes *MLH1* and *MSH2* can be a useful confirmatory tool. For example, Marcus and colleagues found that 37 out of 38 neoplasms known to be MSI-H (by PCR analysis) demonstrated the absence of MLH1 or MSH2 expression, and 34 out of 34 microsatellite stable (MSS) tumors had intact staining.[208] There are, however, important differences between hereditary and sporadic MSI-H cancers that must be understood. Essentially, all sporadic MSI-H colon cancers are the result of hypermethylation of the *MLH1* promoter site. In this situation, no protein is produced and immunohistochemical stains are negative. In the hereditary setting, one allele carries a germline mutation; when the second allele is lost or inactivated, it is possible that the mutant allele will produce a truncated or otherwise altered protein that stains normally but functions abnormally, thus resulting in a falsely normal immunohistochemical stain. Salahshor and colleagues,[209] for example, described intact staining for MLH1 in 2 out of 15 MSI-H cancers from patients with known mutations of *MLH1*. In a large series of unselected cases, Lindor and colleagues[210] found that 27 out of 818 tumors with intact staining of MLH1 and MSH2 were MSI-H. The authors concluded that immunohistochemistry (IHC) is a specific (100%) and sensitive (92.3%) screening tool, but that some MSI-H tumors will be missed if only IHC is performed. We believe the same general rule applies to testing in the hereditary setting, but would emphasize the possibility of falsely normal staining; if clinical features suggest LS, negative IHC should not be taken as definitively ruling out the syndrome.

MSI, IHC, and MMR Mutations ■ Lagerstedt-Robinson and colleagues[211] provided elucidation of the molecular genetic status of LS based on the large Swedish HNPCC Registry where they employed current diagnostic strategies for efficiently detecting MMR mutations, and where they noted the range of challenges encountered in such detection. Their study involved 285 families that had been accumulated on the basis of referral for family history for early-onset CRC, arising from careful collection and verification of reported family history with families classified as meeting the Amsterdam criteria, as showing a specified lesser strength of family history, or as a singleton patient with CRC onset before the age of 50 years. Tumor tissue from the youngest available family member was subjected to MSI analysis. IHC was also performed, but only on MSI-positive tumors. Mutational testing of the four most commonly mutated MMR genes (*MSH2*, *MLH1*, *MSH6*, and *PMS2*), including rearrangement studies for detection of large deletions, was conducted on the youngest member of families fulfilling the Amsterdam criteria I (AC-I) and non-AC-I families with a patient younger than age 50, and on all patients with tumors showing MSI. Pathologic mutations were found in 88% of AC-I, 59% of non-AC-I families, and 80% of the early-onset MSI-positive singleton patients. In families meeting Amsterdam features but without demonstrated MSI, 29% were found to have pathologic germline mutations. In a few instances, loss of staining with IHC was found in tumors that were MSI negative. MMR mutations were found in many tumors, with some but not all interpreted as likely being pathologic according to the accepted criteria, mainly cosegregation with disease in multiple similarly affected families.

The authors concluded that MSI alone could not be used as a basis for selecting patients for mutational testing, given the modest but real fraction of patients with MSI-negative tumors in which mutations were found. In addition, since IHC predicted mutations in a few MSS tumors, but missed other MSI-positive tumors, neither MSI nor IHC was felt to serve as a stand-alone screen.[211,212]

Lagerstedt Robinson and colleagues[211] developed a clinical algorithm for testing, which was initiated by a positive family history or early cancer onset where MSI testing was performed and positive tumors were then subjected to IHC followed by mutational testing. When a mutation was not identified, the tumors were then tested for the presence of a *BRAF* mutation, which is a good surrogate for methylation testing to identify non-LS epigenetic silencing of MLH1. Nevertheless, those patients who were mutation negative received clinically oriented recommendations for empiric screening which, nevertheless, was only slightly less aggressive than that for mutation positive patients.[20,21,213]

Lynch and colleagues[212] concluded that a significant contribution of the study by Lagerstedt Robinson and colleagues[211] dealt with a further demonstration of a central role for MSI combined with IHC in selecting subjects for MMR mutation testing, a finding consistent with the work of Hampel and colleagues[214] who identified an even tighter correlation between MSI and IHC, which often accounted for discrepant findings on the basis of technical limitations in the handling of tissues. Hampel and colleagues[214] and Lagerstedt Robinson and colleagues[211] have reminded us that, at least in sufficiently compelling clinical findings, in concert with Amsterdam criteria, that mutational testing may be warranted even when neither MSI nor IHC is informative. Unfortunately, however, they were unable to provide data on mutation yield in MSS/IHC-negative patients whose clinical picture was less striking because these patients were not tested for MMR mutations. Genetic counseling will help frame the issue for the patient.[213] An Amsterdam criteria-positive patient may have such a high probability of a mutation that MSI and IHC can be dispensed with altogether and models purporting to provide a priori probabilities without and with these screens can be used, much as they are in *BRCA* testing strategies."[212]

A major question relates to how the clinician should interpret these various strategies (family history, Amsterdam criteria, molecular features) for arriving at a LS diagnosis. Lynch and colleagues[212] have suggested that the clinical presentation of LS becomes less obvious than their family history of early CRC onset alone, and therein the greater becomes the role for MSI and IHC. For example, "MSI-negative/IHC-negative tumors perhaps warrant no further molecular genetic evaluation. In clinically marginal cases, if MSI is present and accompanied by loss of MLH1 protein, an argument can be made for proceeding next with *BRAF* mutation testing for methylation assay, rather than expensive *MLH1* mutation testing, because the presence of a *BRAF* mutation quite conclusively rules out Lynch syndrome."[215,216] Finally, when a decision is made to perform MSI, we at Creighton University, as well as other groups dealing with LS, routinely do IHC staining at the same time and proceed with mutational testing if either test is informative. The performance of both tests will then serve in a quality assurance role when discrepancies between MSI and IHC occur, as they do in up to 10% of cases, because further assessment of technical issues involved in the discrepancy can lead to performance improvement.[210] When the tumor is MSI-positive, IHC will then direct mutational testing to a specific MMR gene, which MSI alone is not capable of doing.[217] Finally, of further assistance to clinicians, a number of practice guidelines have been developed by various professional organizations and agencies,[218-221] which may prove useful for diagnosis, surveillance, and management of patients with consideration of LS. Therein, the findings and conclusions of the research by Lagerstedt Robinson and colleagues[211] are consistent with these guidelines.

Effect of TP53 Polymorphism ■ Jones and colleagues[222] note that a common G-to-C polymorphism at codon 72 in the *TP53* gene has been found to be associated with an increased risk for carcinoma of the lung, nasopharynx, oral cavity, prostate, and breast cancer. These authors suggested that this mutation may also be a marker for genetic susceptibility in CRC and therein they investigated this *TP53* polymorphism and age of onset in LS. Their findings disclosed that LS patients who were heterozygous for this polymorphism developed their CRC 13 years earlier than LS patients who were homozygous for the wild-type allele. They, therefore, concluded that adding an individual's *TP53* status to other genetic and environmental risk factors may improve risk estimates and help to identify those who are genetically susceptible to earlier onset of LS-associated cancers.

Methylation and Transcriptional Silencing of the MLH1 Gene ■ Hitchins and colleagues[223] note that biallelic promoter methylation and transcriptional silencing of the *MLH1* gene "occurs in the majority of sporadic colorectal cancers exhibiting microsatellite instability due to defective DNA mismatch repair. Long-range epigenetic silencing of contiguous genes has been found on chromosome 2q14 in colorectal cancer...." These investigators hypothesized that epigenetic silencing of *MLH1* could occur on a regional scale affecting additional genes within 3p22, as opposed to a focal event. They noted that the cluster of genes flanking *MLH1* is specifically methylated in the microsatellite-unstable group of cancers extended across 1.1 Mb. They concluded that their results showed that "coordinate epigenetic silencing extends across a large chromosomal region encompassing *MLH1* in microsatellite-unstable colorectal cancers. Simultaneous epigenetic silencing of this cluster of 3p22 genes may contribute to the development or progression of this type of cancer."

***BRAF* Mutation** ■ Recently, Domingo and colleagues[216] note that the oncogenic V600E hotspot mutation within *BRAF*, a kinase-encoding gene from the RAS/RAF/MAPK pathway, was found to be associated with sporadic MSI-H CRC. These authors analyzed the *BRAF*-V600E hotspot mutation and identified same "in 40% (82/206) of the sporadic MSI-H tumours analyzed but in none of the 111 tested HNPCC tumours or in the 45 cases showing abnormal MSH2 immunostaining." They concluded that detection of the V600E mutation in an MSI-H CRC tumor is used against the presence of a germline mutation in either *MLH1* or *MSH2*. Hence, screening for MMR genes will not be necessary in those patients who are positive for the V600E when there is no other significant evidence suggesting an MMR-associated LS mutation. Therefore, the testing of the *BRAF* hotspot, "is a reliable, fast, and low cost strategy which simplifies genetic testing for HNPCC."

Bessa and colleagues[224] note that MMR deficiencies are the hallmark of LS tumors, but in approximately 15% of CRC these deficiencies are frequently associated with somatic methylation of the MMR gene *MLH1*. However, the oncogenic mutation in the *BRAF* gene "has been involved in sporadic CRC showing MMR deficiencies as a result of MLH1 promoter methylation ... BRAF V600E mutation was analyzed in CRC patients with MMR deficiencies (microsatellite instability and/or lack of MLH1/MLH2 protein expression) in the EPICOLON population-based study." These investigators then found deficiencies in 119 out of the 1222 CRC patients who harbored tumors showing either MSI (n = 111) or loss of protein expression (n = 81). BRAF mutation was identified in 22 (18.5%) of the patients, none of whom had an unambiguous germline mutation. It was concluded that detection of the BRAF V600E mutation not only simplified but also, moreover, improved the cost effectiveness of genetic testing for LS, particularly in patients with an incomplete or unknown family history.

Prevalence of a Large Genomic Deletion Encompassing Exons 1-6 of the *MSH2* Gene ■ More than 400 different pathogenic mutations have been registered in the International Database of Mutations in HNPCC Kindreds (available at http://www.insight-group.org/). Although detection of mutations is usually performed by sequencing, we have reported that one class of mutations, namely, large structural rearrangements such as large deletions, is difficult to detect by that method. They can be readily identified by Southern hybridization,[225] multiplex ligation-dependent probe amplification,[226] after conversion to haploidy,[190,227] and by PCR, as reviewed by Lynch and colleagues.[228]

Wagner and colleagues[229] identified a large genomic deletion encompassing exons 1-6 of the *MSH2* gene, referred to as the American Founder Mutation (AFM), in several of the Creighton University LS families, and considered it to be the most common mutation responsible for the syndrome in the United States. Lynch and colleagues[228] updated these findings based on the study of 566 family members of 9 probands, whom have been identified to be at risk and counseled; 137 of these family members have been tested, with 61 showing carriage of the founder mutation. Three families were tentatively linked genealogically to a German immigrant couple that arrived in the United States and settled in Pennsylvania in the early 1700s. On the basis of this understanding, it was calculated that 18,981 Americans (95% CI 6,038-34,466) would carry the AFM mutation.[230] More recently, Clendenning and co-workers at The Ohio State University[231] have investigated these families and 32 additional families that had been found to have the mutation. Although haplotype analysis gave evidence for a common ancestor among all of the families, the Clendenning group traced extended families back to the eighteenth century without any evidence of further convergence among them. Characterization of the genomic sequence "flanking the deletion and the identification of a common disease haplotype of between 0.6 and 2.3 Mb in all probands provides evidence for a common ancestor between these extended families. The DMLE+2.2 software predicts an age of ~500 years (95% CI, 425-625) for this mutation. Taken together, these data are suggestive of an earlier founding event than was first thought, which likely occurred in a European or a Native American population. The consequences of this finding would be that the AFM is significantly more frequent in the United States than was previously predicted." The Creighton group has tracked movements of branches of the family from Pennsylvania, through North Carolina, Alabama, Kentucky, Missouri, Iowa, Nebraska, Utah, Texas, and California, and documented carriers of the mutation who have been diagnosed in 14 states. Furthermore, the deletion was not found among 417 European and Australian families with LS. This study is being expanded, wherein current estimates indicate that as many as 16,000 descendants from this original cohort are at increased risk for carriage of this *MSH2*del1-6 mutation.[230]

Extracolonic Cancers ■ Extracolonic cancers are common in LS.[232] Endometrial carcinoma heads the list; women with LS have a 20-60% lifetime risk for endometrial cancer.[203,233] There is also an increased risk for carcinoma of the stomach, ovary, renal pelvis and ureter, small bowel, hepatobiliary tract, and pancreas. Glioblastoma multiforme is seen in some LS families. (Families with colon cancer and brain tumors described under the eponym "Turcot syndrome" have included FAP families with medulloblastoma and LS families with glioblastoma.[137]) Muir-Torre syndrome (MTS) (benign and malignant sebaceous skin tumors in combination with colon cancer and other internal malignancies) has been shown by mutational analysis to be a variant of LS.[234] Although the RR for breast cancer is not increased in LS, breast cancers arising in LS demonstrate MSI,[235] suggesting that breast cancer is a tumor integral to LS in some families, albeit with lower penetrance (see Table 14-3).

Finally, Watson and colleagues have provided further information on the subject of extracolonic and extraendometrial cancer in LS based on pooled data from four LS research centers (the Danish hereditary colon cancer registry in Copenhagen, Denmark; the Foundation for the Detection of Hereditary Tumours in Leiden, Holland; the LS registry in Helsinki, Finland; and the Hereditary Cancer Center at Creighton University in Omaha, Nebraska) in a retrospective cohort study, which was able to produce absolute incidence estimates for these cancer types and to evaluate several potential risk modifiers. The cohort included 6041 members of 261 families with LS-associated *MLH1* or *MSH2* mutations. All were mutation carriers by test, probable mutation carriers (CRC or endometrial cancer affected), or first-degree relatives of these. It was found that: "Among mutation carriers and probable carriers, urologic tract cancer ($N = 98$) had an overall lifetime risk (to age 70) of 8.4% (95% CI: 6.6-10.8); risks were higher in males ($p < 0.02$) and members of *MSH2* families ($p < 0.0001$). Ovarian cancer ($N = 72$) had an lifetime risk of 6.7% (95% CI: 5.3-9.1); risks were higher in women born after the median year of birth ($p < 0.008$) and in members of *MSH2* families ($p < 0.006$). Brain tumors and cancers of the small bowel, stomach, breast and biliary tract were less common. Urologic tract cancer and ovarian cancer occur frequently enough in some LS subgroups to justify trials to evaluate promising prevention interventions. Other cancer types studied occur too infrequently to justify strenuous cancer control interventions."

Genotype-Phenotype Heterogeneity ■ LS, not unlike other autosomal dominantly inherited disorders, is noteworthy for genotypic and phenotypic heterogeneity.[21,202,236] *MSH2* mutations may predispose to the more severe phenotypic cancer phenomenon in LS, inclusive of an excess of extracolonic cancer compared to its *MSH1* counterpart. This was investigated by Vasen and colleagues[237] in a study that included 138 families with LS wherein mutations were identified in 79 families (34 with *MLH1*, 40 with *MSH2*, 5 with *MSH6*). These investigators found that the lifetime risk for developing cancer at any anatomic site was significantly higher for *MSH2* mutation carriers as opposed to *MLH1* mutation carriers ($P < 0.01$). With respect to specific anatomic sites, findings disclosed that, "The risk of developing colorectal or endometrial cancer was higher in *MSH2* mutation carriers than in *MLH1* mutation carriers, but the difference was not significant ($p = .13$ and $p = .057$, respectively). *MSH2* mutation carriers were found to have a significantly higher risk of developing cancer of the urinary tract ($p < .05$). The risk of developing cancer of the ovaries, stomach and brain was also higher in the *MSH2* mutation carriers than in the *MLH1* mutation carriers, but the difference was not statistically significant." Of equal interest is the observation of a significantly higher risk of developing cancer of the urinary tract in those who were carriers of the *MSH2* mutation.

Hendriks and colleagues[238] performed mutation analysis on 20 families with a germline mutation in *MSH6* wherein they compared the cancer risks between *MSH6* and *MLH1/MSH2* mutation carriers. They identified a total of 146 *MSH6* mutation carriers, among whom the cumulative risk for CRC was 69% and only 30% for women. Endometrial carcinoma was present in 71% of the women by age 70. Considering all LS-related tumors, they were significantly lower in *MSH6* mutation carriers compared with *MLH1* or *MSH2* mutation carriers ($P = 0.002$). Among females with *MSH6* mutations, the risk of CRC was significantly lower ($P = 0.0049$) and the risk for endometrial cancer significantly higher ($P = 0.02$) than in *MLH1* and *MSH2* mutation carriers.

Childhood Cancer and MMR ■ Bandipalliam,[239] de Vos and colleagues,[240] and Scott and colleagues[241] have described lymphomas as integral to the LS tumor spectrum in patients showing biallelic germline mutations in MMR genes. This syndrome is characterized by a constitutional biallelic inactivation of the MMR genes, which contribute to a recessive disorder in accordance with an MMR-deficiency syndrome which predisposes to "childhood malignancies such as lymphoma, leukemia, brain and gastrointestinal tumors and features of neurofibromatosis type 1."[242] To date, however, lymphomas have only been considered to be an integral component of LS's tumor spectrum in patients with biallelic MMR germline mutations. However, Pineta and colleagues[242] discuss several cases of lymphomas that were not related to an MMR deficiency syndrome in LS kindreds. Herein, they note that, "Only two cases have been studied in depth: an HNPCC patient with a MSI+ T-cell non-Hodgkin lymphoma with no detected germline mutation; and a *MLH1*-mutation carrier with a MSI- follicular lymphoma and normal MLH1 expression (Rosty et al., 2000[243]; Herano et al., 2002[244])."[242] Pineta and colleagues[242] describe a patient with an *MSH2* germline mutation who manifested three metachronous CRCs and subsequently developed a B-cell non-Hodgkin lymphoma (NHL). The lymphoma showed loss of expression of the MSH2 protein, accompanying MSI and loss of the wild-type MSH2 allele. These authors suggested that the inactivation of both alleles of *MSH2* played an etiologic role in the lymphomagenesis. They believe that this is the first report of a MSI+ lymphoma with "concomitant loss of the MSH2 protein, linked to a heterozygous germline mutation of the *MSH2* gene...." These investigators suggest that the loss of both copies of an MMR gene may provide a crucial etiologic event in lymphomagenesis. In this family, the findings of Pineta and colleagues suggest that lymphomagenesis "may be caused by the inactivation of both *MSH2* alleles in individuals with heterozygous mutations." Furthermore, their results reveal that the "lymphoma carried a biallelic deletion of exons 9 and 10, while a diploid dose was maintained in the rest of the MSH2 exons ... demonstrating that the wild-type allele was inactivated in the lymphoma. Similar results were obtained in the colorectal cancer sample taken from the proband."[242]

Menko and colleagues[245] note that *PMS1*, *PMS2*, *MLH3*, and *EXO1* mutations, while not fully clarified as high-penetrance LS genes, may, nevertheless, apparently play a very small role.[246-248] (cited by Menko and colleagues) Although childhood and hematological cancers are not generally considered as part of the LS tumor spectrum, Menko and colleagues note that there has been recent evidence of homozygous mutations in the MMR genes, *MLH1*, *MSH2*, and *PMS2*, in children with hematological malignancies, solid tumors, and, surprisingly, clinical signs (multiple *café-au-lait spots*) of neurofibromatosis type 1.[249-256] (cited by Menko and colleagues) Given this background, Menko and colleagues described a child with multiple café-au-lait spots in association with an oligodendroglioma at age 10, followed by rectal carcinoma at age 12. These lesions were ascribed to a homozygous *MSH6* mutation with predicted pathogenic effects. This child was the youngest of a sibship of four, involving consanguineous, healthy parents. He died at age 12 of complications of the oligodendroglioma. Importantly, he lacked axillary freckling, neurofibromas, or Lisch noduli. His siblings, two sisters and a brother, were normal. There was an unconfirmed history of CRC in the proband's maternal grandfather, which was diagnosed at age 47.

MSI testing showed the rectal cancer to be MSI-H phenotype (BAT25, BAT26, and D5S346), while the brain tumor was MSI-stable. Immunohistochemical staining for MLH1 and MSH2 expression was normal in the rectal cancer, while MSH6 expression was absent. However, in the brain tumor, MSH6-positive cells were identified. A screening test for Fanconi anemia (FA) was negative and no germline *NF1* gene defect was present.

Given that the patient reported by Menko and colleagues[245] was homozygous for an *MSH6* mutation, it is, therefore, noteworthy that heterozygous carriers of the *MSH6* germline mutation show a characteristic phenotype of adult-onset CRC and endometrial cancer.[202] However, Menko and colleagues note that homozygosity for the *MSH6* defect, "Apparently leads to the clinical picture of café-au-lait spots and childhood malignancies...."

Menko and colleagues conclude that, next to *MLH1*, *MSH2*, and *PMS2*, *MSH6* is also involved in the clinical syndrome of childhood tumors and café-au-lait spots, a fact that has been confirmed by a recent report of this syndrome in siblings with homozygous *MSH6* frameshift mutation,[257] which appears to confirm this association. Menko and colleagues also note that the finding in the brain vs the rectal tumor may indicate that biallelic MMR gene defects are associated with various pathways of carcinogenesis.

In their literature review, Menko and colleagues note that Trimbath and colleagues[253] have also reviewed the subject of café-au-lait spots, childhood colorectal neoplasia, and recessive inheritance in past reports of neurofibromatosis and Turcot syndrome.[253]

Nakagawa and colleagues[258] note that mutations in the *PMS2* gene are rare in the etiology of LS. They provide evidence from five published cases which suggested that, contrary to the Knudson principle, *PMS2* mutations cause LS or Turcot syndrome only when they are biallelic in the germ line or abnormally expressed.

Unusual Tumors ■ Molecular pathogenesis of tumors outside the usual LS spectrum remain controversial. Broaddus and colleagues[259] described two young *MSH2* mutation carriers, one age 34 who developed an adrenal cortical carcinoma, and the second a 39-year-old woman who had a diagnosis of anaplastic carcinoma of the thyroid, tumors that are not usually associated with LS. Both of these patients were members of AC-I^{+} families. The adrenal tumor and the thyroid tumor each showed complete loss of immunohistochemical expression for MSH2 protein. However, neither of these tumors was found to be MSI-H in accordance with the National Cancer Institute's panel of five microsatellite markers.

Other rare tumors in LS include a report[260] of a malignant fibrous histiocytoma arising in a patient with a germline *MSH2* mutation and a positive family history. A male with a germline *MLH1* mutation and a positive family history developed infiltrating ductal carcinoma of the breast 30 years after early-onset CRC. The breast tumor had MSI positivity—BAT-26 and BAT-40. Wild-type *MLH1* allele was lost in the breast tumor tissue compared to normal tissue and was related to the underlying germline mutation of *MLH1*.[261] Berends and colleagues[262] reported a female with an *MSH2* germline mutation, ovarian cancer, and three metachronous CRCs; she was also found to have an adrenal cortical carcinoma. It is of further interest that the original proband in Family N[4] manifested adrenal cortical carcinoma. The dilemma remains as to whether these tumors are related to defects in DNA MMR, or whether they have arisen independently of this MMR defect.

Table 14-4 ■ **Amsterdam I and Amsterdam II Criteria, and Bethesda Guidelines**

Amsterdam I criteria[263]
At least three relatives with histologically verified colorectal cancer:
1. One is a first-degree relative of the other two
2. At least two successive generations affected
3. At least one of the relatives with colorectal cancer diagnosed at <50 yrs of age
4. Familial adenomatous polyposis has been excluded
Amsterdam II criteria[265]
At least three relatives with an hereditary nonpolyposis colorectal cancer-associated cancer (colorectal cancer, endometrial, stomach, ovary, ureter/renal pelvis, brain, small bowel, hepatobiliary tract, and skin [sebaceous tumors]):
1. One is a first-degree relative of the other two
2. At least two successive generations affected
3. At least one of the hereditary nonpolyposis colorectal cancer-associated cancers should be diagnosed at <50 yr of age
4. Familial adenomatous polyposis should be excluded in any colorectal cancer cases
5. Tumors should be verified whenever possible
Bethesda Guidelines for testing of colorectal tumors for microsatellite instability[266]
1. Individuals with cancer in families that meet the Amsterdam criteria
2. Individuals with two HNPCC-related cancers, including synchronous and metachronous colorectal cancers or associated extracolonic cancers[a]
3. Individuals with colorectal cancer and a first-degree relative with colorectal cancer and/or HNPCC-related extracolonic cancer and/or a colorectal adenoma; one of the cancers diagnosed at age <45 yr, and the adenoma diagnosed at age <40 yr
4. Individuals with colorectal cancer or endometrial cancer diagnosed at age <45 yr
5. Individuals with right-sided colorectal cancer with an undifferentiated pattern (solid/cribiform) on histopathology diagnosed at age <45 yr[b]
6. Individuals with signet-ring-cell-type colorectal cancer diagnosed at age <45 yr[c]
7. Individuals with adenomas diagnosed at age <40 yr

[a] Endometrial, ovarian, gastric, hepatobiliary, or small-bowel cancer or transitional cell carcinoma of the renal pelvis or ureter.
[b] Solid/cribiform defined as poorly differentiated or undifferentiated carcinoma composed of irregular, solid sheets of large eosinophilic cells and containing small gland-like spaces.
[c] Composed of >50% signet ring cells.

Pedigree Assessment and Lynch Syndrome ■ The diagnosis of LS is partially based on pedigree assessment. Still widely used are the AC-I, shown in Table 14-4,[263] which helped standardize reporting of LS but had limitations as a case-finding tool, notably the failure to acknowledge any contribution from extracolonic cancer. The importance of extracolonic cancer was demonstrated by Wijnen and colleagues,[264] who found three independent variables predictive of germline mutations in *MSH2* or *MLH1*: fulfillment of the AC-I, the presence of endometrial cancer in the kindred, and early age at diagnosis of CRC. New criteria (Amsterdam II) developed by the International Collaborative Group on HNPCC[265] are listed in Table 14-4, as are the Bethesda Guidelines, which have more recently been shown to be useful.[266,267]

Finally, a more detailed algorithmic approach to diagnosis of LS has recently been advocated by Lipton et al.[268] Chao and colleagues[269] have suggested an algorithm that calls attention to the fact that *MLH1/MSH2* mutations account for approximately 90% of LS families wherein 24% of these mutations are missense. Therein, interpretation of missense variants is dependent on certain associated clinical and molecular characteristics. These authors divided their database into "non-overlapping training and validation sets and tested MAPP-MMR." Results showed that "MAPP-MMR significantly outperformed other missense variant classification algorithms (sensitivity, 94%; specificity, 96%; positive predictive value, 98%; negative predictive value, 89%), such as SIFT and PolyPhen. MAPP-MMR is an effective bioinformatic tool for missense variant interpretation that accurately distinguishes *MLH1/MSH2* deleterious variants from neutral variants."

MAPP is a relatively new algorithm[270] and has been used to predict the clinical consequences of missense variants.[271] MAPP has been customized for specific proteins and therein has been optimized specifically for *MLH1/MSH2* "and developed MAPP-MMR, an application that distinguishes *MLH1/MSH2* deleterious variants from neutral variants more effectively than any other computational approach."[269]

A portion of the variation in clinical phenotypes is attributable to missense mutations.[272] For example, a number of missense variants showed minimal or conflicting supporting evidence that are classified as variants of uncertain significance (VUS). However, only 40-60% of families meeting clinical criteria for LS harbor identifiable MMR germline mutations,[273] suggesting that other genes, including modifier genes, may be of etiologic importance. Medical nomenclature is moving in the direction of using the term Lynch syndrome to designate the specific hereditary cancer syndrome caused by germline mutations in the MMR genes and to use the "older" term hereditary nonpolyposis colorectal cancer (HNPCC) to cover the broader category of hereditary predisposition to CRC lacking an excess of polyps. Familial CRC type X, discussed subsequently, is an example of this phenomenon.

CRC Prevention: Colonoscopy Screening ■ The most important reason for diagnosing LS with a high level of certainty is its highly significant clinical implications. It is noteworthy that surveillance for CRC in those harboring a mutation is highly effective and considerably less costly than a lack of CRC surveillance.[274,275]

Because of the early age of CRC onset in LS and its penchant for the proximal colon, full colonoscopy should be initiated by age 20-25 in germline mutation carriers and those at risk on the basis of pedigree analysis. Colonoscopy should be performed at least every 1 to 2 years, given the problem of accelerated carcinogenesis of CRC in LS.[21,276] We prefer every other year in high-risk patients who have not had DNA testing and annually in patients with LS germline mutations or who are obligate gene mutation carriers by their position in the pedigree.

Järvinen and colleagues[274] showed the benefit of colonoscopic screening in LS through a controlled clinical trial extending over 15 years.[274] The incidence of CRC was compared in two cohorts of at-risk members of 22 LS families. CRC developed in eight screened subjects (6%), compared with 19 controls (16%; P = 0.014). The CRC rate was reduced by 62%. All CRCs in the screened group were local, causing no deaths, compared with nine deaths caused by CRC in the controls. It was concluded that CRC screening at 3-year intervals more than cuts in half the risk of CRC, prevents CRC deaths, and decreases overall mortality by about 65% in LS families. The relatively high incidence of CRC even in the screened subjects (albeit without deaths) argues for shorter screening intervals, eg, 1 year. In addition, Vasen and colleagues[277] discovered five interval cancers in LS patients within 3 years 6 months following a normal colonoscopy.

In reviewing this subject, Church[278] has suggested that interval CRCs develop from normal epithelium within 3 years or from adenomas that were missed. It is important to realize that colonoscopy "miss" rates are as high as 29% for polyps <5 mm in diameter.[279] Patients should be advised that colonoscopy is not a perfect screening procedure, and the option of prophylactic colectomy should be discussed.[280,281]

Surgical Measures ■ Subtotal colectomy as a prophylactic measure among LS patients remains controversial, but patients who carry germline mutations should be offered this option as an alternative to lifetime colonoscopic surveillance. Genetic counseling must be provided so that patients can be in a better position to evaluate the various management strategies. Church[281] and Lynch[280] both suggest that prophylactic surgery should be an option for patients likely to show reduced compliance for colonoscopy.

Syngal and colleagues[282] examined the life expectancy and quality-adjusted life expectancy benefits resulting from endoscopic surveillance and prophylactic colectomy among carriers of germline mutations for LS. Both risk-reduction programs showed large gains in life expectancy for mutation carriers, with benefits of 13.5 years for surveillance and 15.6 years for prophylactic proctocolectomy at 25 years of age, compared with no intervention. The benefits of prophylactic colectomy decreased with increasing age.

Gynecologic Screening and Surgical Management ■ Women who carry a germline mutation for LS should have annual screening for endometrial cancer beginning at age 30-35 years. Endometrial aspiration and transvaginal ultrasound are advised for screening; however, we lack evidence-based data showing survival benefit from such screening. Prophylactic hysterectomy and oophorectomy can be considered when childbearing is completed. Schmeler and colleagues[283] have shown a significant reduction in endometrial and ovarian cancer among those patients with LS who underwent prophylactic surgery vs those who did not have surgical prophylaxis.

Those with a family history of kidney cancer and/or hematuria should have annual ultrasound and urinalysis with cytologic examination. This screening should begin at age 30, or at first evidence of hematuria. Evidence-based data showing survival advantage for urologic, gastric, and small bowel screening were not available. Periodic upper endoscopy should be performed in families with gastric or small bowel cancer, and those of oriental origin.

Tobacco Use in Lynch Syndrome ■ To our knowledge, the first study documenting the role of an environmental factor modulating the phenotype of LS was reported by Watson and colleagues,[284] who analyzed smoking history among germline mutation carriers from the Creighton University LS database. Findings disclosed that tobacco users had a higher incidence of CRC than non-users, reflected in a HR of 1.43 ($P < 0.04$). *MLH1* carriers (vs *MSH2* carriers) and males (vs females) were at statistically significant increased risk of tobacco-associated CRC. However, Cox proportional hazards modeling failed to demonstrate a significant correlation between CRC risk and increased pack-years of use. Cox proportional hazards modeling also failed to show a significant association between alcohol use and CRC risk ($P > 0.40$), and there was no significant association between alcohol's interaction with cigarette smoking and CRC risk. It was, therefore, concluded that tobacco use, *MLH1* mutation carriers (as opposed to *MSH2*) and a male sex were significantly associated with an increased risk of CRC (HRs 1.43, 2.07, and 1.58, respectively). Alcohol use did not alter CRC risk. These findings support the need for smoking cessation as an integral part of LS management.

Familial Colorectal Cancer Type X ■ As mentioned earlier, approximately 60% of families fulfilling AC-I for LS harbor a hereditary abnormality in a DNA MMR germline mutation. The remainder (40%) do not have an MMR mutation. Lindor and colleagues[285] studied 161 AC-I$^+$ pedigrees from families divided into those with (group A) vs those without (group B) MMR deficiency through tumor testing. This involved 3422 relatives for the analysis. Findings disclosed that group A families showed an increased incidence of LS-related cancers, while group B families showed an increased incidence that was restricted to CRC (SIR, 2.3; 95% CI, 1.7-3.0), and was to a lesser extent than group A (SIR, 6.1; 95% CI 5.2-7.2) (P < 0.001). These authors concluded that families that were AC-I$^+$ but lacked evidence of DNA MMR defect do not share the same cancer incidence as families with LS with hereditary MMR deficiency. Members of such families have a lower incidence of CRC than those in LS families, and incidence may not be increased for other LS-associated cancers. Furthermore, they indicated that such families should not be described or counseled as LS; therein, they suggested a designation of "familial colorectal cancer type X."[285]

In a somewhat similar study, Llor and colleagues[286] assessed the relevance of clinically defined LS patients without characteristic mutator pathway alterations and identified their phenotypic cancer features in a prospective population-based cohort that included 1309 newly diagnosed CRC patients. All patients with evidence of MMR aberrations were analyzed for MSI; IHC for MLH1, MSH2, and MSH6; germline mutations in *MLH1* and *MSH2*.

Results disclosed that 25 patients (1.9%) fulfilled AC-I for LS, but 15 (60%) patients of that group did not have MSI and had normal expression of MMR proteins. Compared with LS patients with MSI, these patients showed mostly left-sided tumors without lymphocytic infiltrate; were older; had fewer family members affected with CRC or endometrial cancer; more often fulfilled AC-II.

In addition, they showed that "Like unstable HNPCC patients, this group without mutator pathway alterations had a significant percentage of synchronous and metachronous adenomatous polyps and cancers."[286] Putative LS families with an autosomal dominant inheritance pattern but without evidence of MMR deficiency showed a lesser penetrance than LS kindreds with molecular deficiency.

In summary, there are certain distinctive clinical/pathologic features of the AC-I+ families lacking MSI/MMR mutations, which include the following: they are *older* than those with MSI; tumors are less commonly *proximal*, less often clearly differentiated and *mucinous*, and more often show DNA *aneuploidy*. There is also a higher proportion of polyps in families lacking MSI/MMR, but differences do not reach statistical significance.[285,287] They do not present with *multiple cancers*; there is lesser *penetrance* than AC-I+ families with MSI/MMR deficiency, and a lower incidence of CRC and endometrial cancer; more than half of the families showed only CRCs in their pedigrees.[285,288]

No genes have been identified as altered in AC-I+ families with MSS; MSS tumors develop at a later age (53 years vs 41 years for MSI tumors).[289]

Inflammatory Bowel Disease ■ Van Limbergen and colleagues[290] discuss progress that has been made during the past decade in the understanding of the molecular genetics of inflammatory bowel disease (IBD). Concordance data in twin/family studies of IBD have proven to be of great value for genome-wide linkage analysis involving multiple IBD families; this research has led to the identification of IBD susceptibility loci. Specifically, the IBD1 locus on chromosome 16 has led to the discovery "of the NOD2/CARD15 gene as the first susceptibility gene in Crohn's disease ... This landmark finding has led to the redirection of basic research in IBD with interest focused principally on regulation of the innate immune response and mucosal barrier function...."[290] More currently, new insights into primary pathogenic mechanisms have been reached through the use of genome-wide association studies, which has led to several newly discovered genes "such as the Interleukin-23 receptor (IL23R) and ATG16L1 (autophagy-related 16-like 1) genes are strongly implicated...." Collectively, this research has helped to change some of the fundamental understanding of IBD pathophysiology and will have important implications for clinical practice.

Li-Fraumeni Syndrome

Li-Fraumeni syndrome (LFS) is inherited as an autosomal dominant.[291,292] Its incidence is unknown. Mutations in the *p53* gene on chromosome 17p31 are found in about 70% of classical LFS families,[293,294] but *p53* has been ruled out in some classic families,[295] suggesting that this syndrome is genetically heterogeneous. Genetic testing for *p53* mutations is available.

The tumor spectrum in LFS was characterized by Lynch and colleagues[296] with the acronym SBLA (*s*arcoma, *b*reast cancer, brain tumors, *l*eukemia, lymphoma, laryngeal carcinoma, lung cancer, and *a*drenal cortical carcinoma). Melanoma, germ cell tumor, pancreatic, gastric, and prostatic carcinomas have also been described in LFS. The clinical diagnosis requires one patient with sarcoma under age 45, a first-degree relative with any type of cancer under age 45, and a third affected family member with sarcoma (any age) or other cancer (less than 45 years old). However, its extensive genotypic and phenotypic heterogeneity must be considered when evaluating suspect families.[297]

The risk of developing noncutaneous malignancy is 50% by age 30 and 90% by age 70. Hisada and colleagues[298] studied the incidence of second and third primary cancers in members of 24 LFS kindreds. The cumulative probability of a second primary cancer was 57% at 30 years after the first cancer diagnosis. Sarcomas and carcinoma of the breast accounted for 46 out of the 72 cancers identified.[297] Brain tumors may show an extraordinarily high frequency in certain families.[297]

Annual physical examinations with blood cell counts are advised for LFS patients. Careful attention should be given to sites known to be at risk in LFS. Annual mammography, clinical breast examination, and frequent breast self-examination starting at age 25 are particularly important. Recent interest has focused on the role of MRI, particularly in young patients with dense breasts.

Malignant Melanoma

Inherited risk factors are thought to account for approximately 5-10% of melanoma, but gene and mutation frequencies are unknown. Melanoma syndromes have been described as dysplastic nevus syndrome,[299] also known as the FAMMM,[300] occasionally, pancreatic carcinoma, and melanoma-astrocytoma syndrome.[301] Three putative melanoma-susceptibility genes have been nominated. The first was *CMM1*, which was mapped on to chromosome 1p36. However, no candidate gene at this locus has been identified. A second susceptibility locus was mapped on to 9p21; the culprit gene is *CDKN2* (*p16*).[302-304] Finally, germline mutations in the *CDK4* gene on chromosome 12q14 have been documented in rare melanoma-prone families.

Hereditary predisposition to melanoma should be suspected in a patient with findings of invasive melanoma in at least two first-degree relatives and/or multiple atypical nevi in the patient.[300] Early age at melanoma diagnosis and multiple primary melanomas are typical of melanoma-prone families. Although not all melanoma kindreds have dysplastic nevi, 10-100 nevi on the upper trunk and limbs, with variability in mole size, shape, and color, are characteristic of many *CDKN2* mutation carriers. Histologically, such nevi show the architectural and cytologic atypia of a dysplastic nevus.

The FAMMM syndrome, as mentioned, is associated with pancreatic cancer.[304] Bergman and colleagues[305] found that the risk for pancreatic cancer in these families is elevated by a factor of 13.4. Astrocytomas and sarcomas occur to excess in some melanoma families.[304] Lynch and colleagues,[304] in a study of Creighton University's familial pancreatic cancer resource composed of 159 families, identified 19 (12%) which showed the FAMMM cutaneous phenotypes. In eight of these families with FAMMM-pancreatic carcinoma (FAMMM-PC), the *CDKN2A* germline mutation was identified. One of the patients with the *CDKN2A* mutation had a sarcoma at age 23 and expired from this disease. Her father had classical FAMMM phenotypic features and manifested a sarcoma, esophageal carcinoma, two malignant melanoma primaries, and died of metastatic cancer. Findings from this study support the existence of the FAMMM-pancreatic cancer (FAMMM-PC) syndrome due to the *CDKN2A* germline mutation.[304]

Various mutations of *CDKN2* have been described. In Dutch melanoma kindreds, a 19-bp deletion has been implicated.[306] Whelan and colleagues[307] linked melanoma/pancreatic cancer predisposition to a missense mutation (Gly93Trp).

Genetic testing for mutations in *CDKN2* is available clinically, but its use is limited by debate over how to use the results.[304,308,309] Four healthy carriers of *CDKN2* mutations, all children of parents who died of pancreatic carcinoma, are being followed (H.T.L., unpublished data, 2004). Regular endoscopic ultrasound (EUS) of the pancreas is ongoing. However, the risks and benefits of EUS have not been established. Study of pancreatic juice for biomarker association is underway in families from the Creighton University resource that show the FAMMM in association with pancreatic cancer and the *CDKN2A* mutation.

Individuals in melanoma-prone kindreds should perform monthly skin self-examination, possibly with the assistance of a spouse or significant other. Comprehensive dermatologic evaluation by a knowledgeable dermatologist should be done semi-annually. Any suspicious lesions should be excised. Sunburn should be avoided, and use of ultraviolet A/B-blocking sunscreens is encouraged.

Multiple Endocrine Neoplasia

Multiple Endocrine Neoplasia Type 1 Multiple endocrine neoplasia type 1 (MEN1) is a rare autosomal dominant disorder associated with several endocrine tumors that cause as much harm by the hormones they oversecrete as by their malignant potential. The prevalence of MEN1 is around 2 per 100,000, and the tumors most commonly seen include parathyroid adenomas (90%), gastrinomas (40%), insulinomas (10%), and other GI endocrine tumors, as well as prolactinomas (20%) and other tumors in the anterior pituitary.[310] Gastrinomas are commonly found in the duodenum, and carcinoid tumors, thyroid adenomas, adrenal adenomas, angiofibromas, and lipomas are also seen more commonly than in the general population.[310]A diagnosis of MEN1 is made in an individual with two of the three primary classes of MEN1 tumors (parathyroid, entero-pancreatic endocrine, and pituitary tumors). Familial MEN1 is diagnosed with one case and at least one first-degree relative with one of the three component tumor types (reviewed by Brandi and colleagues[310]). MEN1 was first recognized as a familial disorder by Wermer[311] (for a review see Marx[312]).

MEN1 often presents as primary hyperparathyroidism (HPT) and less commonly as Zollinger-Ellison syndrome (ZES), insulinoma, or a pituitary tumor. The majority of those affected will have HPT, with 50% experiencing symptoms by the age of 25 and almost 100% by age 50 years.[313] As is the case with other familial cancer syndromes, the presentation may be multifocal, as opposed to the solitary tumors found in most sporadic cases. Management of these tumors can be difficult due to the nature of the hormones they secrete. In addition, these tumors are often small, multiple, and difficult to remove surgically.

The *MEN1* gene was discovered by positional cloning following its localization on chromosome 11q13.[314,315] *MEN1* encodes menin, a protein that has been shown to inhibit growth of ras-transformed fibroblasts.[316] More recently, it has been shown that inactivation of menin by antisense RNA antagonizes TGFβ-mediated cell growth inhibition, implicating this pathway in menin-related tumor suppression.[317] The majority of mutations documented at this time led to early termination of the protein product, suggesting that it is a classic tumor suppressor gene.[315] Recent evidence now suggests that menin binds DNA, regulates cell proliferation,[318] and induces apoptosis,[319] while additional cellular functions continue to be elucidated. Mutations in the *MEN1* gene occur throughout the gene and no strong genotype/phenotype associations have been identified. Furthermore, some sporadic parathyroid adenomas, gastrinomas, and insulinomas, along with other sporadic endocrine tumors, have been found to be associated with somatic mutations in the *MEN1* gene.[320-323]

It is now expected that most, if not all, families with MEN1 will carry mutations in this gene. Clinical DNA testing exists and can save an individual from a MEN1 family from periodic biochemical testing of serum calcium, parathyroid hormone, and prolactin, which otherwise is begun as an adolescent. However, genetic testing of individuals at this young age is controversial as it is not clear that parathyroidectomy in childhood is indicated, since it may not decrease disease-related morbidity or mortality. The fact that biochemical testing is readily available and often less expensive than mutational analysis of *MEN1* makes the role of clinical DNA testing uncertain at present. However, patients with a possible family history and symptoms that do not meet the criteria for MEN1, such as an isolated primary hyperthyroidism, may benefit from genetic testing. As we learn more about the *MEN1* gene, and can develop effective treatment strategies based on the knowledge of carrier status, DNA testing may take on a more important role.

Multiple Endocrine Neoplasia Type 2 MEN2 families are predisposed to develop the triad of MTC, PTC, and parathyroid hyperplasia with HPT (for a review, see Machens[324]). MEN2A, which encompasses the majority of the cases, usually presents with MTC, which has been documented in infancy and is the major source of mortality in MEN2. MEN2B families have very early onset, aggressive MTC, as well as HPT and characteristic developmental abnormalities involving hyperplasia of the autonomic nerves of the intestines and characteristic facies due to the disorganized growth of axons on the lips, oral mucosa, and conjunctiva.

Familial MTC (FMTC), the third manifestation of MEN2, consists of families in which only MTC is present. The MTC in FMTC is often later in onset and has a better prognosis than in MEN2A and MEN2B.

MEN2 is caused by mutations in *RET*.[325,326] *RET* is located on chromosome 10q11.2, has 21 exons, and encodes a transmembrane receptor tyrosine kinase. Unlike all other known familial cancer syndrome genes, *RET* is a proto-oncogene. Mutations that increase RET activity lead to the subsequent development of cancer and somatic overgrowth and those that inactivate RET cause Hirschsprung disease (HD), a congenital absence of sympathetic neurons in the distal colon and rectum resulting in severe bowel dysfunction.[327] Unlike most other familial cancer syndromes, MEN2 has a very strong genotype-phenotype association. Ninety-eight percent of MEN2A and 85% of FMTC families have missense mutations altering a cysteine residue in the extracellular juxtamembrane cysteine-rich region (exons 10 and 11), while a few FMTC families have missense mutations in the intracellular tyrosine kinase domain encoded by exon 13. The outcomes of these FMTC patients also vary by genotype; in one study, of all carriers of the *RET* oncogene who had thyroidectomy, the 11 with mutations in codons 790, 791, 804, or 891 were cured, but the 5 with mutations in codons 618, 620, 630, or 634, which are associated with aggressive disease, had recurrence of disease.[328] Ninety-five percent of MEN2B families have a single mutation, M918T (exon 16), also in the intracellular tyrosine kinase domain (reviewed by Eng[329]).

Prior to the availability of clinical DNA testing for *RET* mutations, biochemical screening and imaging of individuals at risk for this syndrome began at the age of 4 or 5 and continued into early adulthood. However, as it is now known that 95% of MEN2A and MEN2B, and 85% of FMTC families had documented mutations in *RET*,[330,331] genetic testing is more accurate and has replaced biochemical screening in the diagnosis and management of MEN2. DNA testing for the few common mutations known to be associated with MEN2 can exclude germline *RET* mutations in >99% of those at risk and patients with sporadic MTC.[332] In a family with a known mutation, DNA testing is 100% accurate and can save a non-carrier from unnecessary and uncomfortable biochemical screening. As opposed to MEN1 in which the role of DNA testing remains unclear, early diagnosis with DNA testing in MEN2 is essential. Owing to the high mortality and very early onset of MTC in MEN2, prophylactic thyroidectomy in all mutation carriers should be performed by age 5 years in MEN2A and no later than age 6 months in MEN2B on the basis of positive DNA testing alone.[310,333]

Neurofibromatosis

Neurofibromatosis Type 1 Neurofibromatosis type 1 (NF1) is inherited in an autosomal dominant pattern. The disease incidence is 1 in 3000, with one-third to one half of cases representing new mutations. The implicated gene (*NF1*) is a large gene (59 exons) located on chromosome 17q11.2. Many different mutations of *NF1* have been reported; most (70-80%) are truncating mutations. A protein truncation test is available for clinical genetic testing.

Clinical diagnosis of NF1 requires two or more of the following: (1) café-au-lait spots, (2) two neurofibromas or one plexiform neurofibroma, (3) multiple axillary or inguinal freckles, (4) sphenoid wing dysplasia or congenital bowing or thinning of long bone cortex, (5) bilateral optic nerve gliomas, (6) two or more iris hamartomas, (7) a first-degree relative with NF1 by these criteria.[334] In addition to the lesions listed above, mutation carriers are at risk for neurofibrosarcoma (3-15% of affected individuals), PTC, duodenal carcinoid, neuroblastoma, ependymoma, rhabdomyosarcoma, and Wilms' tumor (WT). Children with NF1 are at increased risk for juvenile myelomonocytic leukemia (juvenile chronic myelogenous leukemia) and the monosomy 7 syndrome, a childhood myelodysplasia.

The *NF1* gene encodes a guanosine triphosphatase-activating protein known as neurofibromin. The gene product negatively regulates signals transduced by ras proteins. Side and colleagues[335] note that NF1 apparently "functions as a tumor-suppressor gene in immature myeloid cells but inactivation of both NF1 alleles has not been demonstrated in leukemic cells from patients with neurofibromatosis type 1."

There are few screening recommendations for patients with NF1. Blood pressure should be monitored twice a year (PTC). Neurologic symptoms (headaches, hearing loss, visual change) should be sought and investigated.

Neurofibromatosis Type 2 ■ NF2 is also autosomal dominant. Disease incidence is 1 in 35,000, with about one-half of cases representing new mutations. The *NF2* gene is on chromosome 22q12.2. Genetic testing is available clinically.

The consensus criteria for NF2 require either (1) bilateral VIII nerve masses or (2) a first-degree relative with NF2 in a patient with one of the following: unilateral VIII nerve mass, a plexiform neurofibroma, two or more neurofibromas, two or more gliomas, two or more meningiomas, posterior subcapsular cataract at a young age, imaging evidence of an intracranial or a spinal cord tumor.[334]

Patients are at risk for central nervous system (CNS) tumors, the most common of which are vestibular schwannomas, schwannomas at other sites, meningiomas, and ependymomas. Although these tumors are often benign and slow growing, their location within the CNS may lead to intracranial and intraspinal involvement with a high rate of morbidity and mortality. Affected individuals also typically develop hearing loss (often bilateral), imbalance, tinnitus, facial weakness and headache, and posterior capsular lens opacities. The average age at onset is in the mid-twenties.[336]

NF2 patients may be clinically subdivided into a severe type and a mild subtype, a classification that is based on the age at onset of symptoms, the number and type of tumors developing, and the duration of disease.[337] The severe type is termed the Wishart form of the disease, which is usually manifested before 25 years of age. These patients rarely survive past 50 years of age. Those with the mild subtype, referred to as Gardner subtype, present with symptoms usually later in life (after 25 years of age), develop a lesser number of more slow-growing tumors, have only bilateral vestibular schwannomas, and generally survive beyond the fifth decade. Ruttledge and colleagues[337] suggest that the majority of familial occurrences of NF2 involve only one form of the disease (ie, Wishart type or Gardner subtype), but they note that Kanter and colleagues[338] have shown that some families will manifest both extremes with intermediate cases occurring within these families.

Baser and colleagues[339] evaluated genotype-phenotype correlations for a variety of non-VIII nerve tumors in 406 patients from the population-based United Kingdom *NF2* registry. Findings disclosed statistically significant genotype-phenotype correlations for intracranial meningiomas, spinal tumors, and peripheral nerve tumors. Individuals with constitutional *NF2* missense mutations, splice-site mutations, large deletions, or somatic mosaicism "had significantly fewer tumors than did people with constitutional nonsense or frameshift *NF2* mutations. In addition, there were significant intrafamilial correlations for intracranial meningiomas and spinal tumors, after adjustment for the type of constitutional *NF2* mutation. The type of constitutional *NF2* mutation is an important determinant of the number of NF2-associated intracranial meningiomas, spinal tumors, and peripheral nerve tumors."

Annual neurologic examination, to include audiologic and ophthalmologic tests, is advised.

Retinoblastoma

Retinoblastoma is the most common intraocular cancer in children. Its incidence is between 1 out of 13,500 and 1 out of 25,000 live births, affecting males and females equally. Most (90%) retinoblastomas are diagnosed before 3 years of age; bilateral tumors tend to be diagnosed at an earlier age than unilateral ones (12 months vs 18 months).

Only 10% of affected patients have a family history of retinoblastoma, but hereditary retinoblastoma is autosomal dominant, with 90% penetrance. Many apparently sporadic cases represent new germline mutations of the gene (*RB*), which is on chromosome 13q14. The gene product is a negative regulator of cell growth. Dephosphorylated RB controls the cell cycle at the restriction point between G1 and S phase, and inhibits a variety of transcription factors. Cells lacking RB function proceed unchecked through the cell cycle. Patients with bilateral retinoblastoma are considered to carry germline mutations of *RB*. Approximately 20% of unilaterally affected individuals also harbor a germline mutation.

Genetic testing is available and is cost effective. Noorani and colleagues[340] compared molecular and conventional screening of retinoblastoma relatives. The cost (in 1994 Canadian dollars) of conventional screening was $31,430 for a prototype family with seven at-risk relatives. This involved three clinic examinations and eight examinations under anesthesia over the first 3 years of life for each relative. The molecular strategy (a search for *RB1* germline mutation in the proband and the testing of relatives for that mutation), coupled with clinical follow-up similar to conventional strategy for relatives with the mutation, gave an expected cost of $8674.

Small retinoblastomas can be treated by cryosurgery, photocoagulation, or radiation therapy. Larger tumors usually require enucleation, emphasizing the importance of early detection.

Second malignant tumors (nonocular) are seen in hereditary retinoblastoma. The incidence has been reported as 4.4% at 10 years, 18.3% at 20 years, and 26.1% at 30 years.[341] Radiation therapy for retinoblastoma contributes to this risk but does not account for all of it. Osteosarcoma and melanoma are the most common second tumors, but brain tumors, sarcomas, leukemias, lymphomas, and pinealoblastoma have been reported.[342] Screening for second tumors is difficult because of the multiple possible sites of involvement.

Nevoid Basal Cell Carcinoma Syndrome (Gorlin Syndrome)

The nevoid basal cell carcinoma syndrome (NBCCS) is a rare disorder featuring the early onset of multiple basal cell carcinomas. An enormous number of additional features comprise the phenotype and have been used to enumerate major and minor diagnostic criteria (see below). There is marked variation in clinical expression within and between families, but Wicking and colleagues[343] find no convincing evidence of nonpenetrance. The inheritance pattern is autosomal dominant. Wicking and colleagues[343] estimate the new mutation rate to be at least 14% when they include those families wherein both parents had been examined clinically and radiologically and where paternity was confirmed. However, these authors call attention to the work of Shanley and colleagues,[344] who indicated that the new mutation rate may be as high as 81% when all patients with unremarkable family histories were defined.

The gene is *PTCH* on chromosome 9q22.3, a human homolog of the *Drosophila* segment polarity gene *patched*.[343,345,346] Genetic testing is available.[343]

The diagnosis of NBCCS can be established on the basis of two major criteria or one major and two minor criteria.[347] Major criteria are (1) multiple (>2) basal cell carcinoma, one basal cell carcinoma diagnosed at <30 years, or >10 basal cell nevi; (2) any odontogenic keratocyst (proven on histology) or polyostotic bone cyst; (3) palmar or plantar pits (≥ 3); (4) ectopic calcification: lamellar or early (<20 years) falx calcification; and (5) family history of NBCCS. Minor criteria are (1) congenital skeletal anomaly: bifid, fused, splayed, or missing rib or bifid, wedged, or fused vertebra; (2) occipitofrontal head circumference >97th percentile, with frontal bossing; (3) cardiac or ovarian fibroma; (4) medulloblastoma; (5) lymphomesenteric cysts; and (6) congenital malformation: cleft lip or palate, polydactyly, eye anomaly (cataract, coloboma, microphthalmia).

Because affected individuals develop multiple basal cell carcinomas by age 40, regular dermatologic screening is advised, with early excision of tumors. Clinicians should be aware that about 5% of patients with NBCCS will develop a medulloblastoma during the first few years of life.[347]

von Hippel-Lindau Disease

von Hippel-Lindau (VHL) disease is inherited as autosomal dominant. Disease incidence is 1 in 36,000. The *VHL* gene is on chromosome 3p25-p26. The gene encodes a protein involved in the transduction of growth signals. Hundreds of different mutations have been described, including missense, non-sense, and deletion mutations. Genetic testing (mutation analysis and linkage analysis) is clinically available.

VHL disease is characterized by multiple cysts in kidney, liver, and pancreas; retinal and cerebellar hemangioblastoma, and increased risk for renal cell carcinoma (RCC) and PTC. Angiomas and cysts of the spleen are occasionally described. Retinal angiomas may also occur, usually in young adulthood, and may produce visual loss. RCC can occur alone or with PTC; occasionally, PTC occurs alone. Because PTC is an integral lesion in other hereditary syndromes (MEN2 and NF1), genetic testing for *VHL* and *RET* mutations has been advocated for patients with familial, multiple, or early-onset PTC.[348] RCC occurs in as many as 75% of affected individuals, with an average age at diagnosis of 40-45 years. Pancreatic neoplasms (cystadenocarcinoma, islet cell tumor) cluster in certain families.

Kaelin discusses the *von Hippel-Lindau* tumor suppressor gene (*VHL*) on chromosome 3p25 and how, in its mutated or silenced form, it contributes to >50% of sporadic clear cell RCCs. The *VHL* germline mutations give risk to VHL. This disease is characterized by "an increased risk of blood vessel tumors (hemangioblastomas) and RCCs. In this setting, *VHL* inactivation gives risk to premalignant renal cysts. Additional genetic alterations are presumably required for conversion of these cysts to renal cell carcinomas."[349]

Affected individuals are advised to have annual neurologic and ophthalmologic examination; annual red blood cell count (renal cysts and cerebellar hemangioblastoma can produce erythropoietin); regular imaging of CNS, kidneys, and pancreas; and annual chemical screening for PTC.[350]

Wilms Tumor

The principal gene for WT (*WT1*) is located at chromosome 11p13. There is a second predisposition locus (WT2) at 11p15.5. A third locus is proposed (WT3) but has not been localized. The *WT1* gene encodes a protein that suppresses transcription downstream from epidermal growth factor receptor 1 and insulin-like growth factor II. Clinical genetic testing is not yet available.

WT affects 1 in 10,000 children. Only 1% of those affected have inherited a germline mutation from a parent. Another 10-30% have new germline mutations of *WT1*. *WT1*-related syndromes may present as unilateral or bilateral WT only, WAGR syndrome (Wilms' tumor-aniridia-genitourinary anomalies-retardation), or Drash syndrome (childhood renal failure secondary to mesangial sclerosis). Hemizygosity for *WT1* is associated with developmental anomalies of the genitourinary tract. Aniridia associates with WT because the gene mutated in aniridia is adjacent to *WT1*; thus, aniridia is rare in the general population (1 in 70,000), but WT occurs in 1 of 70 children with aniridia.

WT is also seen in association with Beckwith-Wiedemann syndrome. The WT2 locus on 11p15 appears to be involved in the genetic events responsible for Beckwith-Wiedemann, but the precise gene has not been identified. The disorder features hemihypertrophy, enlarged organs, prominent eyes, and neonatal hypoglycemia. Affected individuals are at risk for hepatoblastoma, adrenocortical carcinoma, and gonadoblastoma in addition to WT.

Hartley and colleagues[351] note that approximately 20% of second primary tumors that develop in WT survivors are leukemias and that they have an atypical distribution, with myeloid leukemias predominating. The cytotoxic therapy for WT may be responsible for some of the myeloid neoplasms, but some of the cases may represent an underlying predisposition to the development of a second primary cancer. It is noteworthy that both WT and leukemia/lymphoma occur in NF1. WT is also an uncommon component of the LFS.

Although the coexistence of WT and leukemia/lymphoma in families may be uncommon, families of this type may provide important models for elucidating the expression of *WT1* and other genes that may be associated with WT in hematologic forms of cancer. Hartley and colleagues[351] suggest that "Expression and interaction of these genes with other tumor-suppressor genes may have widespread implications for development of second malignancies in certain survivors of WT and of specific tumors in close relatives who may be carriers of germline mutations."[351]

Cancer-Associated Genodermatoses

Rees[352] indicates that humans show a >100-fold variation in their sensitivity to the deleterious effects of ultraviolet radiation, wherein the principal determinants are melanin pigmentation as well as differences in skin inflammation and repair processes. Therein, there is a high heritability for pigmentation. Furthermore, susceptibility to cutaneous cancer, which is a key marker of sun sensitivity, appears to be less heritable. Rees indicates that, despite a large number of murine coat-color mutations, there exists only one gene in humans, namely, the melanocortin 1 receptor (*MC1R*), and therein it is known to account for substantial variation in skin cancer incidence as well as substantial variation in skin cancer incidence as well as in skin and hair color. It is, therefore, of interest that, "Most persons with red hair are homozygous for the alleles of the *MC1R* gene that show varying degrees of diminished function. More than 65 human *MC1R* alleles with nonsynonomous changes have been identified, and current evidence suggests that many of them vary in their physiological activity, such that a graded series of responses can be achieved on the basis of (i) dosage effects (of one or two alleles) and (ii) individual differences in the pharmacological profile in response to ligand." This author concludes that this single locus that has been identified within a Mendelian framework, "can contribute significantly to human pigmentary variation."

Ataxia-Telangiectasia

Ataxia-telangiectasia (A-T) is inherited as an autosomal recessive disorder. The frequency of gene mutations in the general population is around 1.4%,[353] and disease incidence is 1 in 30,000 to 1 in 100,000. Cerebellar ataxia is present in all patients, becoming evident as the child learns to walk. The ataxia is truncal at first but gradually comes to include ataxia of gait, intention tremor, dystonia, slurred speech, and apraxia of eye movements. Oculocutaneous telangiectasia begins in late childhood. Other cutaneous signs are vitiligo, café-au-lait spots, and premature graying of the hair. Cellular and humoral immune deficiency is common, probably accounting for frequent sinopulmonary infections. Endocrine dysfunction (glucose intolerance, hypogonadism) is seen in half of affected individuals. A-T patients are unusually sensitive to ionizing radiation, and conventional radiation therapy regimens can be fatal.

The A-T gene is located on chromosome 11q22-23[354,355] and is designated *ATM*.[356] A-T variants (Nijmegen breakage syndrome and Berlin breakage syndrome) are both linked to 8q21, indicating that they are not allelic with A-T. Most reported A-T mutations result in truncated protein. There are several hundred mutations, with very few spontaneously recurring *ATM* mutations, making population screening difficult.[357] Radioresistant DNA synthesis is the best diagnostic test for A-T. The test is available from a few reference laboratories.

Approximately 15% of A-T patients will die of cancer, with non-Hodgkin's lymphoma, leukemia, and gastric cancer predominating. Medulloblastoma and glioma have also been described in A-T patients. McConville and colleagues[358] describe 14 families with *ATM* mutations and a less severe phenotype and suggest that cancer predisposition may be variable among families. This heterogeneity could result from the position of the *ATM* mutation or the type of mutation involved (eg, missense vs large deletion).

Heterozygotes are at increased risk for breast cancer. Swift and colleagues[359] reported a 6.8-fold increased risk in such patients. Athma and colleagues[353] found increased risk for breast cancer in both younger women (2.9 RR) and in women older than age 60 (6.4 RR). We believe that heterozygous women should begin breast cancer screening at age 30, with regular self-examination and yearly mammograms.

Bloom Syndrome

Bloom syndrome (BS) is a rare (about 170 known cases), autosomal recessive disease that occurs more frequently among Ashkenazi Jews. The *BLM* gene is on chromosome 15q26.1. Multiple mutations are possible; the predominant mutation is referred to as "blm," which is a 6-bp deletion, and 7-bp insertion at nucleotide position 2281 in the *BLM* cDNA.[360] Founder mutations have been described in Ashkenazi Jews.[360] BS somatic cells are hypermutable, with markedly elevated chromosome breakage and sister chromatid exchange.

Affected individuals present with short stature, sun-sensitive facial erythema, malar hypoplasia, nasal prominence, small mandible, and dolichocephalic skull.[361] There is immunodeficiency, manifested by bronchitis and bronchiectasis. The hypermutable DNA is responsible for increased frequency of malignancy, with leukemia and lymphoma predominating in younger patients and carcinomas of larynx, lung, esophagus, colon, breast, and cervix seen in adults. The carcinomas arise about 20 years earlier than expected for the general population.[362]

Gruber and colleagues[363] found that Ashkenazi Jews with CRC were more than twice as likely to be heterozygous for the *BLM* mutation than Ashkenazi Jewish controls without CRC (OR 2.45; 95% CI 1.3-4.8; $P = 0.0065$). In contrast, the Israeli Ashkenazi Jewish population controls showed an absence of *BLM* carriers, thereby decreasing the likelihood that the results could be biased. Their data were supported by findings in a recent mouse model[364] of BS, which tested the effect of Blm haplo-insufficiency and the risk of cancer in mutation carriers. Mice that were heterozygous for *Blm* developed twice the number of intestinal tumors when crossed with mice carrying a mutation of the *Apc* tumor suppressor gene.[364] Gruber and colleagues[363] concluded that, "Our data similarly show that carriers of a *BLM* mutation have an increased risk for CRC. Possible mechanisms of carcinogenesis include (i) haploinsufficiency, in which a half dose of *BLM* gene product is insufficient for full *BLM* function in the maintenance of genomic integrity, giving rise to an increased mutation rate in the heterozygous cell, and (ii) loss of the normal *BLM* allele in a colonic stem cell, giving rise to a cell clone with the same hypermutability as the BS cell. Whichever the mechanism, our data confirm the importance of genomic instability as a critical element in the pathogenesis of cancer."[363]

Cowden Syndrome and Multiple Hamartoma Syndromes

Cowden syndrome (CS) is an autosomal, dominantly inherited, rare disorder that was the first of the multiple hamartoma syndromes to lend itself to genetic characterization. This syndrome has shared overlapping presentations with BRR syndrome and the JPS. Of greatest interest to the practicing oncologist is the fact that CS patients carry a 25-50% lifetime risk of breast cancer and a 3-10% lifetime risk of thyroid cancer (for reviews see Eng[318] and Pilarski[365]). Breast cancer associated with CS often occurs at an earlier age than sporadic breast cancer, with an average age of diagnosis between 38 and 46 years.[366] Unlike CS, BRR does not carry an increased risk of cancer but is now known to be caused by mutations in the same gene, *PTEN*.[367,368]

CS is associated with multiple hamartoma, including GI hamartomatous polyps and benign and malignant neoplasms of the breast, thyroid, endometrium, and skin. It is also associated with facial trichilemmomas, acral keratosis, and verucoid or papillomatous papules in virtually all cases. CS is associated with CNS defects in 40% of cases.[369] Cerebellar dysplastic gangliocytoma, also known as Lhermitte-Duclos disease (LDD), is now established as part of the clinical spectrum of CS.[370] Although 90% of CS patients demonstrate symptoms by the age of 20, only 10% exhibit symptoms before age 10.[371]

In 1996, CS was mapped on to the locus 10q22-23,[371] a region frequently deleted in thyroid tumors.[372] Somatic mutations spanning this region were also commonly found in glioblastoma, breast cancers (in association with CS), and advanced PC.[373] In 1997, *PTEN* was isolated and identified as the gene responsible for CS. *PTEN* consists of 9 exons spanning 100 kb of DNA.[367,373-375] PTEN is a major lipid 3-phosphatase, which signals down the PI3 kinase/AKT pro-apoptotic pathway. Furthermore, PTEN is a protein phosphatase, with the ability to dephosphorylate both serine and threonine residues. The protein-phosphatase activity has also been shown to regulate cell-survival pathways, such as the mitogen-activated kinase (MAPK) pathway. Although it is well established that PTEN's lipid-phosphatase activity, via the PI3K/AKT pathway, mediates growth suppression, there is accumulating evidence that the protein-phosphatase/MAPK pathway is equally important in the mediation of growth arrest and other crucial cellular functions.[376] All genetic and biochemical studies indicate that *PTEN* acts as a classic tumor-suppressor gene.

In 1996, the International Cowden Syndrome Consortium created a set of major and minor criteria to aid in the diagnosis of CS. Using these criteria to identify 37 CS families and 7 BRR families, 81% of patients had a *PTEN* mutation.[377] Mutations were scattered throughout the gene, but a mutation "hotspot" in exon 5 accounted for 43% of the mutations found in the region encoding the protein tyrosine phosphatase. When mutations in exons 7 and 8, which encode potential phosphorylation sites, were included, the mutation rate increased to 77%.[378] Novel mutations have recently been reported involving larger gene deletions and mutations in the promoter region explaining the presence of disease in patients who were mutation negative.[379]

PTEN screening of BRR families revealed that approximately 60% had mutations for this gene.[318] However, only 10% of JPS patients were *PTEN* mutation carriers, and many of those already showed signs of CS or subsequently developed them. Thus, JPS is thought to be a variant of CS with incomplete expressivity.[158] The clinical significance of this association is that patients with JPS and a mutation in *PTEN* may benefit from enhanced screening of the breast, thyroid, skin, and uterus. Finally, when patients with symptoms suggestive of CS but not fulfilling the CS criteria ("CS-like syndromes") were screened for mutations in *PTEN*, only 1 in 64 (2%) of patients carried mutations,[378] supporting the strict use of the International Cowden Consortium criteria for CS.

Attempts to correlate the *PTEN* genotype and phenotype have been limited by small sample size. *PTEN* mutations are associated with LDD in some families,[367,380] but are not clustered in a specific region of the gene. It has been shown recently that as many as 83% of sporadic LDD harbor germline mutations in *PTEN*, supporting a role for *PTEN* testing in these individuals.[381] A trend for greater organ site involvement (5 vs 4 or fewer sites) has been associated with mutations in the protein tyrosine phosphorylase core region; however, larger sample sizes are needed to verify these results.[377] A screen of 177 breast cancer patients with a family history of breast cancer but negative for *BRCA1* and *BRCA2* failed to show *PTEN* coding mutations.[382] Therefore, there appears to be no increased risk of breast cancer in the absence of the other manifestations of CS, and the screening of these patients for *PTEN* in this instance is unwarranted.

Identification of a *PTEN* mutation in a patient is diagnostic for either CS or BRR, but a negative mutation screen is nondiagnostic.[158] *PTEN* carriers should be screened for thyroid and breast cancers starting in their twenties or 5 years earlier than the youngest relative who developed disease. Despite the fact that CS is thought to be inherited in an autosomal dominant pattern, approximately half of individuals with CS do not have a known family history of CS. Although this may imply a problem with identifying affected relatives, this may also indicate variable expression of the phenotype or a de novo mutation in the individual.[383] Future work will likely focus on the variable phenotype of *PTEN* mutations and the altered activity of the P13 kinase/AKT pro-apoptotic pathway; these studies may provide potential targets for novel therapies in the future.

Fanconi Anemia

Fanconi anemia (FA) is inherited as an autosomal recessive disorder. There are five complementation groups: FA-A at 16q24.3, FA-B (unmapped), FA-C at 9q22.3, FA-D at 3p26-p22, and FA-E (unmapped). The carrier frequency is higher in Ashkenazi Jews (1 in 100), and a founder mutation of FA-C has been described in that population.[384] The cells of homozygotes have chromosomal instability that can be demonstrated as enhancement of chromosome breakage in a mitomycin C chromosome stress test.[385]

Progressive pancytopenia is the principal feature of FA, presenting as anemia, bleeding, and easy bruising in children. Multiple congenital abnormalities are seen in roughly two thirds of FA patients; these include hyperpigmentation of the skin, café-au-lait spots, skeletal deformities, renal malformations, microphthalmia, ear anomalies and deafness, congenital heart disease, and hypogonadism.

FA patients are at risk for myelodysplastic syndromes and leukemia, usually acute myelogenous leukemia. Hepatocellular carcinoma has been described in about 5% of patients, possibly secondary to anabolic steroid therapy for anemia. Squamous carcinomas of the upper aerodigestive tract, cervix, vulva, and anus can also complicate the course of FA. The FA-A locus on 16q24.3 is an area that often shows loss of heterozygosity in breast cancer. Cleton-Jansen and colleagues[386] have shown that the *FA-A* gene is not the culprit gene in breast cancer, concluding that "Another tumour suppressor gene in this chromosomal region remains to be identified."

Werner Syndrome

Werner syndrome (WS) is inherited as autosomal recessive. The incidence is estimated at 1 in 50,000 to 1 in 100,000. Its phenotype is characterized by premature aging, with growth arrest at puberty, cataracts occurring in the second and third decades, premature atherosclerosis, and adult-onset diabetes. The average life span is 47 years.

The WS locus, WRN, maps on to chromosomal region 8p12.[387-392] The gene encodes a DNA helicase of 1432 amino acid residues. Bennett and colleagues[387] note that the helicase consensus domain region of WRN has sequence homology with the bacterial RecQ family of helicases, including BLM, the BS gene product.[393] Bennett and colleagues[387] identified MMR in fibroblastoid cells but not in lymphoblastoid cells, a finding that is consistent "with the possibility that WRN protein could have a cell type- and/or tissue-specific role in mismatch repair. Alternatively, a mutation in *WRN* could predispose cells to mutations in other genes required for mismatch repair activity, at least one of which could be an unknown gene."[387]

Malignant neoplasms associated with WS include sarcoma, melanoma, and carcinoma.[394] Organs at risk for carcinoma include thyroid, stomach, liver, breast, and bile duct. Melanomas may arise in unusual locations, such as the nasal cavity.

Risks and benefits of cancer screening in this syndrome have not been established, but regular melanoma surveillance seems reasonable.

Xeroderma Pigmentosum

Xeroderma pigmentosum (XP), mentioned earlier, is inherited as autosomal recessive. The incidence is 1 in 1,000,000 in the United States but 1 in 40,000 in Japan. XP is genetically heterogeneous, with causative loci mapped on to 9q34.1 (XP-A), 2q21 (XP-B), 3p25.1 (XP-C), 19q13.2 (XP-D), 11p12-p11 (XP-E), 16p13.2-p13.1 (XP-F), and 13q32-q33 (XP-G). All of the culprit genes play roles in excision repair of DNA pyrimidine dimers induced by ultraviolet light. Mutation analysis is not available as a clinical test.

Affected individuals show an extraordinary hypersensitivity to sun exposure, manifested by childhood onset of photosensitivity, freckling, and irregular pigmentation. Kraemer and colleagues[395] indicate that the frequencies for malignant melanoma and epithelial cancers (squamous and basal cell carcinoma) are respectively 2000- and 4800-fold higher in XP patients than their occurrence in the general population of the United States. The median age of the initial cancer in XP is about 8 years, which is close to a half-century earlier than its occurrence in the general population of the United States. Lanza and colleagues[396] note that XP lacks the marked spontaneous chromosomal instability that characterizes other hereditary disorders that show hypersensitivity to mutations with the predisposition to neoplasia, inclusive of AT, FA, and BS. Cellular hypersensitivity to ultraviolet radiation is the hallmark of XP. Laboratory testing for XP is available from reference laboratories.

XP patients are at increased risk for noncutaneous malignancies as well. Brain tumors, leukemias, and carcinomas of lung and stomach have been described. Cultured cells from XP patients are hypersensitive to DNA-binding carcinogens in cigarette smoke and charbroiled food. Neurologic abnormalities are described in 20% of XP patients, and genetic evidence suggests overlap between XP and

Cockayne's syndrome (dwarfism with microcephaly, progressive neurologic degeneration, and photosensitivity).[397]

Affected individuals must avoid exposure to carcinogenic effects of sunlight.[398] Assiduous protection from sunlight must begin in infancy, with wide-brimmed hats, long sleeves, and outdoor activities limited to after sunset. Regular examination of skin and eyes, with early excision of lesions, is mandatory. Avoidance of cigarette smoke and grilled food is probably advisable.[399]

Other Cancers with Familial Clusterings

Familial Pancreatic Cancer

Anecdotal case reports and epidemiologic studies have suggested that pancreatic cancer clusters in some families. Although chance aggregations or a common environmental exposure could account for some familial clusters, evidence for a genetic basis continues to accumulate. Ghadirian and colleagues[400] performed a population-based case-control study in Quebec, Canada, and found that 7.8% of pancreatic cancer patients reported a positive family history of pancreatic cancer, compared with 0.6% of controls. Falk and colleagues[401] studied pancreatic cancer in Louisiana and found similar results, as evidenced by an increased risk for pancreatic cancer among persons reporting any cancer in a close relative (OR 1.86; 95% CI 1.42-2.44). The highest risk was seen in those with a history of pancreatic cancer in a close relative (OR 5.25; 95% CI 2.08-13.21).

The National Familial Pancreas Tumor Registry at Johns Hopkins is based on at least two first-degree relatives who have pancreatic cancer.[402] Analysis of these families indicates that even second-degree relatives of affected patients are at increased risk for pancreatic cancer.

When a familial aggregation of pancreatic cancer is recognized, a variety of hereditary cancer disorders needs to be considered. These include HNPCC (*MSH2, MLH1*), PJS, FAMMM, familial breast cancer (*BRCA2*), and hereditary pancreatitis.[304] (All of these conditions are discussed elsewhere in this chapter.)

Hereditary pancreatitis is characterized by recurrent episodes of severe chronic pancreatitis. Affected individuals are at risk for pancreatic pseudocysts, pancreatic exocrine failure, diabetes mellitus, and pancreatic cancer. A gene for hereditary pancreatitis has been mapped to chromosome 7q35.[403] This gene encodes a cationic trypsinogen that, when mutated, fails to inactivate trypsin, resulting in autodigestion of the pancreas. Presumably, chronic epithelial injury and regeneration increase the risk for pancreatic cancer.

Rebours and colleagues[404] evaluated a standardized incidence ratio (SIR) of pancreatic adenocarcinoma (PA) in an exhaustive national (France) series of patients with hereditary pancreatitis with major attention devoted to the search for risk factors. The inclusion criteria involved the study of recurrent, acute, or chronic pancreatitis in two first-degree relatives or three or more second-degree relatives in at least two generations. PC was determined by histological records. The investigation include 200 patients in 78 families. Ten PAs were diagnosed (median age 55 year). In addition, the "SIR of PC for the whole population, men, and women were 87 (95% CI 42-113), 69 (25-150), and 142 (38-225), respectively, with no influence of genetic mutation. At ages 50 and 75 yr, the cumulated risk of PC was 11% and 49% for men and 8% and 55% for women, respectively. Smoking and diabetes mellitus were the main associated risk factors."[404] These authors concluded that patients with hereditary pancreatitis have a marked relative and absolute increased of PC when compared with the general population. The risk appears to be accentuated among cigarette smokers, while there was no correlation with the type of *PRSS1* mutation.

Whitcomb and colleagues identified the first genetic defect of the cationic trypsinogen gene (*PRSS1*), namely, the R122H mutation,[405] which was independently confirmed by Férec and colleagues.[406]

Rebours and colleagues[404] also note that chronic alcoholic pancreatitis, while debated, is nevertheless considered as a risk factor of PA.

Even when known hereditary syndromes are excluded, familial aggregations of PC remain. The inheritance pattern in these families appears to be autosomal dominant.

Surveillance of high-risk patients is evolving. Brentnall and colleagues[407] used EUS, endoscopic retrograde cholangiopancreatography (ERCP), spiral computed tomography, and serum carcinoembryonic antigen and CA19-9 analysis to follow 14 patients from three PC kindreds. Seven patients underwent pancreatectomy on the basis of abnormalities on ultrasonography and ERCP. All seven had histologic dysplasia in the resected specimen; there were no occult carcinomas.

Given the known heterogeneity in PC, it is likely that many differing cancer susceptibility loci will ultimately be identified. For example, Eberle and colleagues[408] have identified a susceptibility locus that maps on to chromosome 4q32-34, in an autosomal dominantly inherited pancreatic cancer family. In the case of *BRCA2*, which predisposes to the HBOC syndrome, Murphy and colleagues[409] found that *BRCA2* mutations significantly increase the risk of PC in individuals with these mutations. Indeed, these investigators indicate that *BRCA2* mutations pose the most common inherited genetic alteration to date that has been identified in familial PC.

van der Heijden and colleagues[410] describe the FA pathway in PC cells wherein biallelic *BRCA2* mutations that can cause FA are present in approximately 7% of PCs. Attention was given to recent findings that several sequence changes in *FANCC* and *FANCG* occur in PC. Therein, they note that functional defects in the Fanconi pathway can give rise to multiple hypersensitivity to interstrand cross-linking agents such as mitomycin C. Importantly, once the functional implications of these mutations in the Fanconi pathway are more fully comprehended, it may then be possible to initiate clinical trials for the treatment of PC with crosslinking pharmaceutical agents of Fanconi-defective cancers. This research is in full accordance with recent developments of targeted chemotherapeutics, wherein the targeting of specific genetic defects in cancer has been taking place. One such example is imatinib, which has been shown to be of significant therapeutic promise in patients with chronic myelogenous leukemia[411,412] and in GI stromal tumor (GIST).[413-416]

van der Heijden and colleagues[410] note that FA-defective cell lines of CAPAN1, PL11, and Hs766T are all hypersensitive to mitomycin C when compared with other PC cell lines. These authors call attention to their previous studies[417] as an explanation of anecdotal observations wherein a subset of PCs were highly sensitive to mitomycin-containing regimens. Therein, they suggest that, "pancreatic cancers might be genetically tested for defects in the pathways that repair interstrand crosslinks, such as the FA pathway. Patients with a defect in one of the repair pathways could then be treated rationally with crosslinking agents, possibly at a much lower dose than is customary."

In dealing with a disease as deadly as PC, one must constantly search for new agents that may hold promise. Clearly, this work of van der Heijden and colleagues[410] must be pursued to the fullest possible extent, given their extremely provocative basic science results. The heterogeneity of hereditary pancreatic cancer is demonstrated in Table 14-5.

A hospital-based case-control study[418] involving 808 patients with pathologically verified PC compared cases with 808 healthy, frequency-matched controls. Significant risk factors for PC were cigarette smoking (approximately 23% of PC cases in the study), diabetes

Table 14-5 Genetic Syndromes with Inherited Predisposition to Pancreatic Cancer

Familial Syndrome[a]	Gene (locus)	Relative Risk	Frequency[b]	References
Peutz-Jeghers syndrome	*STK11* / *LKB1* (19p13.3)	132	4%	167,168,543,545-547
Familial pancreatitis	*Cationic trypsinogen* (7q35)	50-60	Unknown	405,548,549
Familial pancreatic cancer syndrome	unknown (4q32-34)	18-57	Unknown	408,550
FAMMM syndrome	*p16*^{INK4a} / *MTS1* (9p21)	13-22	98%	551-554
Hereditary breast-ovarian cancer syndrome	BRCA2 (13q12)	10	7%	555-557
Familial adenomatous polyposis	*APC* (5q21)	5	40%	7,558-562
HNPCC[c]	*hMSH2* (2p22-21) *hMLH1* (3p21.3)	Unknown	4-11%	563-565
Ataxia telangiectasia	*ATM* (11q22-23)	Unknown	Unknown	566,567

[a] All of the above syndromes are inherited in an autosomal dominant manner, except ataxia telangiectasia, which is an autosomal recessive disorder.
[b] Frequency refers to the frequency of genetic mutation found in sporadically occurring pancreatic carcinomas.
[c] HNPCC: hereditary nonpolyposis colorectal cancer, also known as cancer family syndrome or Lynch syndrome II. HNPCC is typically caused by germline mutations in DNA mismatch repair genes including *hMSH2, hMLH1, hPMS2*, and *hMSH6*. *hMSH2* and *hMLH1* mutations account for half to two thirds of HNPCC. The frequency refers to a defect in any one of the five DNA mismatch repair genes causing HNPCC.
Source: Reproduced by permission from Yee and colleagues *Cancer Biol Ther* 2003;2:1:38-47.

mellitus (approximately 9%), family history of PC (approximately 5%), heavy alcohol consumption (3%), and a history of pancreatitis. Results showed synergistic interactions between cigarette smoking and family history of PC as well as diabetes mellitus in women, in accordance with an additive model. These authors concluded that "The significant synergy between these risk factors suggests a common pathway for carcinogenesis of the pancreas. Determining the underlying mechanisms for such synergies may lead to the development of pancreatic cancer prevention strategies for high-risk individuals."

Familial Gastric Cancer

Gastric cancer has many similarities to esophageal carcinoma in that its incidence shows marked geographic variation. For example, its incidence is exceedingly high in Japan (160/100,000 per year) with high rates also noted in Finland and Chile. In contrast, its incidence is low in the United Kingdom (10/100,000 per year) as well as in the United States, where rates have been declining during the past several decades.

There are two types of gastric adenocarcinoma that can be distinguished histopathologically: (1) intestinal type and (2) diffuse type. Molecular pathology supports the theory that those differences emerge through specific genetic pathways for the two tumor types.[419] The *intestinal* type shows components of glandular or intestinal architecture and tubular structures. The *diffuse* type shows non-coherent, single cells, often with signet-ring cell morphology, and it frequently presents as linitis plastica. Separation of gastric cancer into intestinal and diffuse types is exceedingly useful genetically and epidemiologically.

The intestinal type shows a greater frequency than its diffuse counterpart. In general, the intestinal type is more commonly related to environmental exposures; these include diet (salted fish and meat, and smoked foods), smoking, alcohol, and infection with *Helicobacter pylori*. Indeed, there may be a genetic-environmental interaction in the etiology of gastric carcinoma and *H. pylori* susceptibility.[420-422] El-Omar and colleagues[423] have shown that the eradication of *H. pylori* infection leads to resolution of the gastric inflammation and resolution of hypochlorhydria and atrophy in about half of the patients. Importantly, will eradication of *H. pylori* be effective in hereditary forms of gastric cancer?

In contrast, the diffuse type has a low but relatively stable incidence in most parts of the world. In general, it is related to host factors (discussed subsequently).

Familial Risk Factors ■ We estimate that between 5% and 10% of gastric cancer involves familial clustering. Familial risk for gastric carcinoma was investigated by Hemminki and Jiang[424] employing the nationwide Swedish Family Cancer Database that comprises 10.2 million individuals, with over 34,000 gastric carcinomas. This is the largest study on familial gastric cancer published to date. Standardized incidence rates (SIRs) were 1.31 (95% CI 0.97-1.70) and 1.47 (1.08-1.92) when a parent presented with gastric cancer or gastric adenocarcinoma, respectively. Risk was 1.59 (1.10-2.16) in offspring whose diagnosis was at an age greater than 50 years. Sibling risk for gastric cancer was 3.16 and 5.75 when diagnosed earlier than age 50. Population-attributable proportion of gastric cancer was 0.45%. These authors concluded that environmental factors, possibly *H. pylori* infections, provided the main explanation for familial clustering of gastric cancer. The population-attributable proportion of familial gastric cancer was much lower than that cited in the literature.

Palli and colleagues[425] studied 1016 gastric cancer patients and 1623 population-based controls. Their study was adjusted for potential confounders including diet. Their results showed an increased risk for gastric cancer among those with the following relatives affected: sibling (OR 2.6); parent (OR 1.7) [mother affected, OR 2.3; father affected, OR 1.3]; two or more siblings (OR 8.5); both parents (OR 3.0).

Hereditary Gastric Carcinoma ■ The differential diagnosis of hereditary gastric cancer includes its integral involvement in HNPCC (LS).[426] Following CRC, the second most common cancer in LS in Western countries is endometrial carcinoma; however, gastric cancer is the more prominent extracolonic cancer in Japan and Korea. FAP, LFS, and PJS are other examples of hereditary syndromes showing an increased risk for gastric cancer.

Hereditary Diffuse Gastric Cancer *(HDGC)* ■ Hereditary diffuse gastric cancer (HDGC) is an autosomal dominantly inherited syndrome. Clinical criteria for defining HDGC families include the following: (1) two or more documented cases in first-/second-degree relatives, at least one diagnosed at less than age 50 years; and (2) three or more documented diffuse gastric cancers in first-/second-degree relatives independent of age of onset.

Germline mutations in *CDH1*, which encodes E-cadherin, were first identified in HDGC by Guilford and colleagues, in three Maori HDGC kindreds.[427] Within the past 10 years, *CDH1* mutations have been found in over 50% of families with at least two cases of gastric cancer, with one diagnosed as diffuse gastric cancer before the age of 50 years.[428] The syndrome's penetrance is 70-80%, and the average age of onset of HDGC is about 37 years.

Lobular carcinoma of the breast has been identified as an integral lesion in *CDH1* mutation carriers.[429] Although there are not yet definitive data available on surveillance or risk reduction programs for women with known *CDH1* mutations or untested women from *CDH1*-positive families, these women's lifetime risk of 39-52% for lobular breast cancer[428,430] mandates careful attention. It is suggested that they follow the recommendations for other high-risk women with hereditary breast cancer predisposition.

Screening ■ Screening for diffuse gastric carcinoma includes endoscopy, EUS of the stomach, and multiple gastric biopsies. However, this has been exceedingly unproductive in terms of identifying *early* (and potentially curable) cancer in HDGC in patients with *CDH1* mutations. Early diagnosis is clearly the best chance for curative resection, but it is a formidable task. Initial symptoms may be those of advanced disease and they are often non-specific. When first diagnosed, most cases are locally advanced where over two thirds present with lymph node involvement. Survival is poor when the disease has advanced beyond the mucosa or submucosa. Lesions tend not to form a grossly visible exophytic mass; rather, they spread submucosally. Emerging new screening technologies include color or fluorescent stains to aid in endoscopic detection. EUS is mainly used to stage a previously diagnosed tumor, but it may be useful in identifying early diffuse type gastric cancer.

Prophylactic Surgery ■ Lewis et al[431] reported their findings on prophylactic gastrectomy in six asymptomatic members of two HDGC families (two males and four females), ages 22, 27, 28, 35, 39, and 40, all of whom were positive for *CDH1* mutations. Each of these individuals, when subjected to a research protocol of microscopic sectioning at the time of prophylactic total gastrectomy, had microscopic foci of cancer often at multiple sites, with overlying normal gastric mucosa.

Huntsman and colleagues[432] and Chun and colleagues[433] have discussed the potential efficacy of surgical prophylaxis. They note that the decision for prophylactic gastrectomy must consider the 2-4% risk of mortality and nearly 100% long-term morbidity (chronic diarrhea, dumping syndrome, and weight loss). Ten percent show post-operative complications including infection, myocardial infarction, or leak. Combined results of prophylactic gastrectomy in 10 asymptomatic *CDH1* mutation carriers in three HDGC families showed that despite negative endoscopic examinations and biopsies, all 10 were found to have pathologic evidence for early gastric cancer. Thus, even with intensive endoscopic examinations and random gastric biopsies, this screening approach may be inadequate for early diagnosis and prevention of gastric cancer in HDGC families.

Given the dismal screening results, prophylactic surgery should be presented as a viable option for *CDH1* mutation carriers with positive family histories of diffuse gastric cancer. Although the morbidity of this operation may be higher than that for other genetic diseases, it must be realized that the alternative is a mortality risk of over 80% at a young age.[431] For those not desiring prophylactic gastrectomy, we recommend that there be frequent (q 6-12 months) and highly detailed endoscopic mucosal examination with multiple biopsies of even the most subtle of lesions.

Genetic Counseling and Gastric Cancer ■ Lynch and colleagues[434] performed mutation-based genetic counseling in an HDGC family that harbored the *CDH1* mutation (see Fig. 14-2). A family information service (FIS) was provided,[435] during which 24 family members were thoroughly educated about the clinical and genetic features of HDGC. After giving individual signed consent, they were tested for the *CDH1* mutation, of which 9 were found to be positive and 15 negative. Three of the *CDH1* mutation positives were affected and are deceased due to diffuse gastric carcinoma (Fig. 14-2).

None of the 19 patients counseled wanted their results sent to their physicians once they recognized the potential for insurance discrimination. None had undergone EUS. Three who were positive for the *CDH1* mutation expressed strong interest in prophylactic gastrectomy, and one of these has recently undergone prophylactic total gastrectomy and was found to be negative for meta-

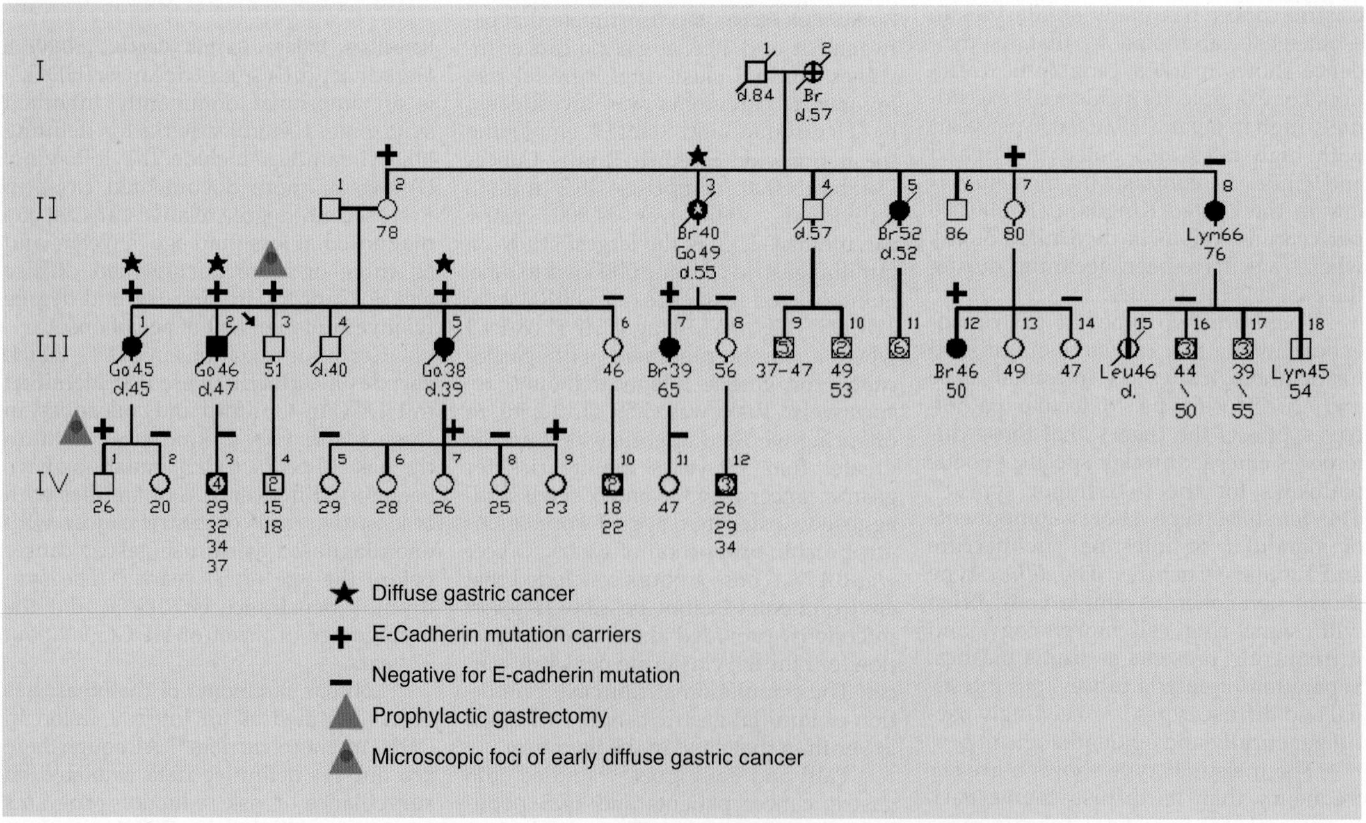

Figure 14-2 ■ Pedigree of family showing *CDH1* (*E-cadherin*) germline mutation.

static disease. This individual (III-3), the proband in this family, during the genetic counseling process, was advised about the importance of undergoing total prophylactic gastrectomy. He realized that he was positive for the *CDH1* germline mutation. He was told about the fact that many patients who had undergone prophylactic total gastrectomy had evidence of microscopic metastatic disease in the surgical specimen. He eventually became resigned to the need for this and underwent the procedure. The examination of the entire stomach revealed three foci of intramucosal signet-cell carcinoma, each <0.5 mm in dimension. There was no evidence of lymph node involvement or distal metastatic spread.[436]

HDGC poses a challenge to genetic counselors as well as clinical geneticists when discussing genetic testing in concert with the decision for and the timing of prophylactic total gastrectomy. Reasons for this include HDGC's 70-80% penetrance, and the wide range in age of onset within and between HDGC families. In our experience, the average age of onset of HDGC has been 38 years, but it may range from 16 to 82 years.[428] Complex medical, ethical, and psychological, as well as medicolegal ramifications (eg, the level of the patient's understanding) may impact heavily on decisions for both testing and surgery.[437]

In conclusion, surveillance, even with intensive endoscopic examinations and random gastric biopsies, may be inadequate for the early diagnosis and prevention of diffuse gastric cancer in HDGC families, hence justifying the consideration of prophylactic surgery, among *CDH1* mutation carriers. The genetic counselor must discuss the option for prophylactic gastrectomy. Clearly, there is a need for a multidisciplinary group of clinicians, geneticists, and genetic counselors to educate and support the family member in order to enable him or her to make decisions about diagnostic and management options for the future.

FAP and Gastric Cancer ■ Gastric cancer occurs in excess in patients with FAP, particularly in Japanese FAP families. However, this was not the case in studies of non-oriental patients with FAP in the Johns Hopkins registry[438] where there was not an increased RR for gastric cancer. Similar results were reported by Jagelman and colleagues,[439] who found gastric cancer in 7 out of 1255 patients with FAP, compared to 10 patients with periampullary carcinoma and 29 with carcinoma elsewhere in the duodenum.

Hyperplastic Polyps ■ A predisposition to gastric cancer may be inherited with a tendency to form hyperplastic polyps. Carneiro and colleagues[440] described a large pedigree characterized by autosomal dominantly inherited predisposition to gastric polyposis coupled with a high incidence of gastric carcinoma. Two of the gastric carcinomas were of the diffuse type and one of these appeared to have originated from hyperplastic polyps. Hyperplastic polyps were found in five of the seven family members without carcinoma of the stomach. The remaining two individuals had marked fobeolar hyperplasia. Chronic atrophic gastritis (CAG) with complete intestinal metaplasia was observed in three of the patients. It was concluded that, "Fobeolar hyperplasia/hyperplastic polyps may play a key role in the development of diffuse carcinomas in this inherited polyposis confined to the stomach with the hyperplastic phenotype."[440]

Gastrointestinal Stromal Tumor (GIST), Imatinib (Glivec) ■ Hirota and colleagues[441] studied a family with multiple GIST tumors, which harbored a new type of germline mutation of the KIT gene observed at Asp-820 in tyrosine kinase (TK) II domain. These authors indicate that mutations in the TK II domain have been identified in mast cell and germ cell tumors, but heretofore had not been found in GIST tumors. Thus, their family represents the first recorded case of GISTs with TK II known mutations. Furthermore, they note that, "Because interleukin 3-dependent Ba/F3 murine lymphoid cells transfected with the mutant KIT complementary DNA grew autonomously without any growth factors and formed tumors in nude mice, the mutation was considered to be gain-of-function type."

Nishida and colleagues[442] note that in the first reported case of familial GISTs there was a germline mutation at the juxtamenbrane domain of the KIT gene. They note, however, that following the original report of Hirota and colleagues,[441] several additional familial GIST cases were described.[443-446] Furthermore, four of these five GIST families manifested the KIT mutation at the juxtamenbrane domain,[442,443,445,446] while the remaining family carried the mutation at the TK I domain.[444]

Until recently, there has not been any effective treatment for unresectable metastatic GIST tumor, a lesion that has been invariably fatal. For example, Joensuu and colleagues[416] described a patient with metastatic GIST treated with intensive doxorubicin-based chemotherapy without response. However, imatinib (Glivec) was started and dramatically reduced metastases. The patient had a complete response within 1 month of the start of ST1571, as evidenced by negative findings on PET and MRI. Toxicity of ST1571 was minimal (mild dyspepsia and slightly increased frequency of bowel movements).

Renal Cell Carcinoma

Approximately 2% of renal cell carcinomas (RCCs) have a familial basis. As with cancers of many other organs, RCC is not a single entity, but rather several histologically distinct patterns, often with a different molecular pathogenesis and different syndromic associations.[447,448] von Hippel-Lindau disease, the most common, is discussed elsewhere in this chapter.

Hereditary papillary RCC (HPRC1) is characterized by multiple, bilateral, low-grade renal carcinomas.[449] The gene (*MET*) is on chromosome 7q33.1-34. It is a proto-oncogene encoding a cell-surface receptor for hepatocyte growth factor (HGF). Normal signaling by the receptor tyrosine kinase requires the presence of the HGF ligand. Activating missense mutations in *MET* lead to constitutive signaling, with activation of downstream pathways.

Extrarenal neoplasms have been described in families with papillary RCC.[450] These include carcinomas of the stomach, rectum, breast, lung, pancreas, and bile duct. It is not clear whether these associations are significant.

Penetrance appears to be low (as low as 30% for some mutations). Subclinical disease is often discovered when gene carriers undergo renal imaging. Annual renal imaging beginning at age 30 years is recommended. Familial papillary RCC has also been described in association with papillary carcinoma of the thyroid.[451] That report, describing one kindred, mapped susceptibility to chromosome 1q21.

Hereditary leiomyomatosis and renal cell cancer (HLRCC) is inherited as an autosomal dominant disorder that involves smooth-muscle tumors of the skin and uterus and/or renal cancer. The disorder has been mapped on to chromosome 1q42.3-43. Toro and colleagues[452] investigated the role of the *fumarate hydratase* (*FH*) gene in HLRCC. They *FH* mutations in 31 families; 20 different mutations were identified, 18 of which were novel. Eighty-one patients (47 women and 34 men) had cutaneous leiomyomas. Ninety-eight percent (46/47) of women with cutaneous leiomyomas also had uterine leiomyomas. The authors identified 13 individuals in 5 families with unilateral and solitary renal tumors, while 7 individuals from 4 families had papillary type II RCC, and an additional individual manifested a collecting duct carcinoma of the kidney.

Tomlinson and colleagues[453] confirmed the association of uterine leiomyomata as being common tumors in this syndrome that also predisposes to multiple fibroids, cutaneous leiomyomata, and RCC.

Chromosome 3 translocations have been associated with risk for clear cell

RCC.[454] Early studies suggested a susceptibility gene at 3p14, possibly involving the *FHIT* tumor suppressor gene. Subsequently, a variety of chromosome 3 breakpoints have been described, all contained within the pericentromeric regions of 3p and 3q. Further, analysis of tumors from affected patients show loss of the derived chromosome and a somatic mutation of the von Hippel-Lindau (*VHL*) gene on the retained chromosome 3.[455] The proposed model for cancer development in this condition is (1) an inherited chromosome 3 translocation; (2) loss of the derivative chromosome (with loss of the VHL locus); and (3) somatic mutation of the VHL allele on the normal chromosome 3. Individuals from kindreds with chromosome 3 translocations and RCC should be offered surveillance recommendations similar to those for von Hippel-Lindau syndrome.

Familial clear cell RCC independent of VHL and chromosome 3 translocations has been described.[456] Because more than half of RCC cases in these families are diagnosed before age 50, annual renal imaging should be offered to at-risk relatives beginning at age 20.

Skates and Iliopoulos[457] discuss the role of molecular markers for RCC in several known hereditary disorders that predispose to this cancer. Therein, they discuss several defined germline mutations in tumor suppressor genes or oncogenes that predispose to the predisposition for RCC. They note, for example, that patients with inactivating mutations in the *Birt-Hogg-Dube* tumor suppressor gene have a risk of developing oncocytic/chromophobe kidney tumors.[458] (cited by Skates and Iliopoulos)

Tuberous sclerosis predisposes to the development of renal tumors. Angiomyolipoma is the most common renal manifestation, but multifocal, bilateral RCC in young patients has been described.[459]

Familial Prostate Cancer

Interest in familial PC risk dates back nearly a half-century to the report by Morganti and colleagues[460] describing an 11-fold increased risk for carcinoma of the prostate in first-degree relatives of index cases compared with age-matched controls. Later, Woolf[461] showed a threefold increased risk for relatives of affected individuals, and in 1982 Cannon and colleagues[462] concluded that PC had a stronger familial aggregation in a Utah Mormon genealogic database than breast or colorectal carcinoma. More recent epidemiologic studies confirm these findings and indicate that risk is related to the number of family members affected and the age of the proband at diagnosis.[463]

Segregation analysis has suggested that a highly penetrant autosomal dominant mutant gene could account for 9% of all PC s and 40% of those diagnosed before age 55.[464] Some candidate genes have been identified, the significance of which is unknown at this time. Risks and benefits of surveillance are unproven, but regular screening by serum prostate-specific antigen and regular digital rectal examination are reasonable. In high-risk families, screening should begin before age 50. The role of transrectal ultrasound and random prostate biopsies is yet to be evaluated.

Prostate Cancer Genetics ■ The search for the role of heredity in PC during the current 5-year period showed an exponential increase and has been addressed in no less than 112 papers in English (Medline search results).[465] Difficulty in identifying genes that predispose to PC is likely due to late age of diagnosis, heterogeneity of the disease, phenocopies (individuals with sporadic forms of the disease interspersed with hereditary cases) in high-risk pedigrees, and genetic complexity.[465,466]

***Identification of Novel Prostate Cancer Susceptibility Loci* ■** Performing a genome-wide linkage scan for PC susceptibility genes in their study of 36 Jewish families, Friedrichsen and colleagues showed significant linkage to peak at 7q11-21,[465] while a genome-wide scan by Tavtigian and colleagues[466] of large, high-risk pedigrees from Utah has provided evidence for linkage to a locus on chromosome 17p. Positional cloning and mutation screening within the defined 17p interval, identified a gene, namely ELAC2, harboring mutations (including a frameshift and a non-conservative missense change) that segregated with PC in two pedigrees.

Xu[467] studied 772 hereditary PC families from the International Consortium for Prostate Cancer Genetics. This author found that the PC-susceptibility gene linked to 1q24-25 was identified in a defined subset of PC families. However, they accounted for only a relatively small proportion of all families, appearing to play a more prominent role in a subset of families wherein several members were affected at an early age and wherein male-to-male disease transmission was present. A candidate gene in the region, *RNASEL*, on chromosome 1q25, was recently identified as a candidate gene for hereditary PC by Wang and colleagues[468] in association with an increased risk of familial, but not sporadic, PC. However, these results were not confirmed in a large case-control study from Sweden arguing against a significant role for *RNASEL*[469] in PC and suggesting that another gene in the region is behind the increased risk. The HPC1 locus on chromosome 1q24-q25 was identified by linkage analysis of 91 families with three or more affected first-degree relatives.[470,471] In contrast, the search for linkage at chromosome 1q42.2-43 was negative in one study.[472] A putative PC susceptibility gene has been mapped on to Xq27-28,[473] a finding that correlates with suggestions of an X-linked mode of inheritance for PC susceptibility.[474]

***Prostate Cancer Risk Associated with Known Cancer Genes* ■** *CHEK2,* the upstream regulator of *p53,* may also contribute to PC risk,[475] implicating the DNA-damage-signaling pathway in the development of PC. This observation was confirmed when two truncating mutations of *CHEK2* were shown to confer moderate risk of PC.[476]

The Breast Cancer Linkage Consortium found that male carriers of *BRCA2* mutations are at increased risk of PC (OR 4.78; 95% CI 1.87-12.25; $P = 0.001$), whereas risk of *BRCA1* mutation carriers was not significantly increased. Thus, HBOC syndrome should be ruled out in families with clusters of prostatic carcinoma. Prostate tumors with frequent genetic aberrations have been observed in the chromosomal region 12p12-13 harboring *CDKN1B.*[477] Segregation in families with PC was primarily contributed by affected offspring whose age at diagnosis was <65 years. *CDH1* has also been associated with prostate carcinogenesis,[478] with the –160 single nucleotide polymorphism acting as a low-penetrant PC susceptibility gene that could explain a proportion of familial PC. Taken together, these findings suggest that germline mutations of *CHEK2, BRCA2, CDKN1B,* and *CDH1* may play a role in PC susceptibility.

Prostate Cancer in Lynch Syndrome ■ Soravia and colleagues[479] suggest that PC may be an integral lesion in the LS. They report a family wherein the proband had three metachronous adenocarcinomas of the colon and rectum at ages 54, 57, and 60, and presented with an adenocarcinoma of the prostate at age 61. These investigators performed immunohistochemical (IHC) staining of colonic, rectal, and prostatic tumor tissues and therein found a lack of expression of MSH2 and MSH6. MSI was evidenced in the rectal, colonic, and prostatic tumors. As the family fit the Amsterdam criteria for the LS, molecular genetic studies were initiated following the proband's son's manifestation of colorectal cancer at age 35. "Southern blotting analysis of genomic DNA led to identification of a novel genomic deletion encompassing exon 5 of the MSH2 gene...." These authors indicate that, to the best of their knowledge, this represents the first report wherein MSI and IHC analysis of the prostate adenocarcinoma clearly linked its cause to the germline MMR mutation. They also note that there have been occasional reports[480,481] of prostate carcinoma in LS kindreds and, therefore, appropriately suggest that PC be included in the LS tumor spectrum.

HNPCC or the LS, as discussed previously, shows a significant increased risk for carcinoma of the ureter and renal pelvis, but to date not the urinary bladder. A statistically significant risk ($P < 0.001$) for these lesions was found in patients with the MTS (a variation of HNPCC manifesting sebaceous adenomas, sebaceous carcinomas, and multiple keratoacanthomas) as opposed to HNPCC patients who lacked MTS cutaneous features.

This demonstrates the importance of inquiring into the presence of cancers of all anatomic sites when investigating any patient's family cancer history. In addition, multicase families, particularly when extended, with pathology verification of cancer, are ideal candidates for formal linkage analysis in the search for genetic susceptibility loci. Such efforts will be of value to molecular geneticists in the search for germline mutations that may predispose to urologic cancer as well as to other cancer types.

Lung Cancer

Although the vast majority of cases of lung cancer are associated with tobacco exposure, only 10-15% of smokers will develop lung cancer.[482] In an effort to determine whether a genetic predisposition to malignancy may exist in smokers who develop lung cancer, Lynch and colleagues[483] evaluated cancer risk in the relatives of 254 consecutively ascertained probands with histologically verified lung cancer and in relatives of 231 probands with other smoking-associated cancers. Although no strong evidence for increased risk of lung cancer in relatives of lung cancer probands was seen, there was a significant increased risk for cancers of all anatomic sites ($P < 0.001$). Conversely, there were no significant excesses of cancer at all anatomic sites in relatives of probands with other smoking-associated carcinomas. The observed increased risk for cancer at all anatomic sites in the relatives of lung cancer probands could result from an underlying hereditary susceptibility to cancer in general in these families.

More recent studies have shown evidence of familial clustering of lung cancer, including an increased risk for first-degree relatives of individuals with cancer.[484,485] The increased risk persists even after adjustment for age, gender, and smoking habits. A recent meta-analysis of 28 case-control and 17 cohort studies showed an approximately twofold increase in the risk of lung cancer in individuals with a family history of lung cancer (RR 1.8; 95% CI 1.6-2.0).[486] The risk was found to be greater in relatives of individuals diagnosed at a young age and in those with multiple affected family members. Eleven studies examined risk of lung cancer among non-smokers who had family members with lung cancer. In these individuals, risk was elevated, although not to the degree of smokers (RR 1.51; 95% CI 1.11-2.06).

Lung cancer presents a model for how the genetics of toxin metabolism may lead to cancer predisposition. Susceptibility to lung cancer in smokers may, in part, be attributable to inter-individual variability in metabolic activation or detoxification of tobacco carcinogens. The glutathione *S*-transferase M1 (GSTM1) genetic polymorphism has been extensively studied in this context. The glutathione *S*-transferase enzyme family is known to play a role in catalyzing the detoxification of tobacco carcinogens. A recent meta-analysis of the results of 98 genetic association studies examining the relationship between the GSTM1 null variant and lung cancer risk included 19,638 lung cancer cases and 25,266 controls.[487] The GSTM1 null variant was associated with a small increase in the risk of lung cancer (OR 1.22; 95% CI 1.14-1.30). Subset analysis revealed that the increased risk of lung cancer associated with GSTM1 null variant was evident in East Asians (OR 1.38; 95% CI 1.24-1.55) but not in Caucasians. Furthermore, evaluation of only the five largest studies revealed no increase in risk of lung cancer in subjects with the GSTM1 null variant. A number of additional studies searching for associations between lung cancer and common genetic polymorphisms have been performed, but no convincing evidence for low penetrance susceptibility genes has emerged from this line of investigation.

Bailey-Wilson and colleagues[488] recently conducted a genome-wide analysis of 52 families of individuals with lung cancer who had several first-degree relatives with lung cancer.[488] Their results localized a region on chromosome 6q23-25 as a major susceptibility locus for lung cancer. When effects of age and personal smoking were incorporated, there was still support for linkage in the region, albeit less strongly. Future cohort studies are needed to identify other genetic determinants of lung cancer and to validate previous retrospective, case-control studies. Such studies cannot only lead to breakthroughs in our understanding of the pathogenesis of lung cancer, but they can help identify a subpopulation of individuals, both smokers and those who are exposed to second-hand tobacco smoke, who would benefit from screening for lung cancer.

Familial Neuroblastoma

Neuroblastoma is a common tumor of childhood, with almost all cases occurring before the age of 10.[489] The tumor has been seen to occur in patients with other neural crest malignancies or disorders, including neurofibromatosis type 1 and congenital central hypoventilation syndrome.[490,491] No genetic links to neurofibromatosis have been found and co-occurrences with neuroblastoma are thought to be related to chance alone.[492] However, constitutional mutations in the PHOX2B gene, which is the major gene affected in the congenital hypoventilation syndrome, are seen in familial neuroblastoma and in 2.3% of cases of neuroblastoma.[493,494]

Several chromosomal regions are potential sites for a neuroblastoma susceptibility gene, including 17q, 1p, 11q, and 14q. Chromosome 1p deletions have been reported in as many as 80% of near-diploid neuroblastomas that have been karyotyped, making this a particularly promising locus.[495] These deletions on chromosome 1 have variable proximal break points, but a region of consistent deletion has been mapped on to sub-bands of 1p36, possibly marking the location of a tumor suppressor gene important in malignant transformation or progression of neuroblastoma. Further support for this locus comes from the study of a sib pair with neuroblastoma. A1p36 deletion was identified in both tumors through use of double-color fluorescence in situ hybridization, and neither tumor showed evidence of *MYCN* amplification, another common genetic alteration in neuroblastoma. Haplotype analysis showed that the siblings inherited the same paternal 1p36→pter chromosome region in both tumors. However, the maternal 1p region was deleted. These data suggest that the siblings inherited a predisposition to neuroblastoma in the paternal 1p36 region and that tumors developed as a consequence of somatic loss of the maternal 1p36 allele. Although these data are promising, consistent evidence of chromosome abnormalities in neuroblastoma has yet to be seen.

A family history of neuroblastoma is present in 1-2% of cases.[496,497] The median age of diagnosis in familial forms of neuroblastoma is 9 months, compared with 2-3 years in sporadic cases. Despite the difficulties in identifying a neuroblastoma susceptibility gene, there is convincing evidence that hereditary predisposition to neuroblastoma segregates as an autosomal dominant Mendelian trait with low penetrance.[498] Thus, efforts to identify a susceptibility locus have continued. Maris and colleagues[499] performed linkage analysis on 10 North American families with multiple neuroblastomas and identified a locus at 16p12-13 consistent with linkage (lod = 3.46). Informative recombinants defined a large (26 cM) interval not yet amenable to gene mutation screening. However, subchromosomal deletions were identified in 5/12 familial (42%) and 55/259 nonfamilial (21%) neuroblastomas at the same locus, narrowing the interval to approximately 13 cM. These data suggest that a gene for hereditary neuroblastoma in some North American families is located at 16p12-p13 and that inactivation of this gene may contribute to the pathogenesis of sporadic neuroblastomas.[500] More recently, Longo and colleagues[498] studied European pedigrees and found a linkage to chromosome 2p and 12p (lod = 3.01, $P < 0.0001$). Their analysis excluded linkage to 16p and confirmed that neuroblastoma is a heterogeneous disease and its genetic determination likely involves multiple loci.

Hematologic Malignancy

Most studies dealing with familial aggregations of hematologic neoplasms have lacked adequately matched controls and have focused on the same hematologic malignancy that was present in the proband. In an attempt to address this issue, Shpilberg and colleagues[501] investigated the familial aggregation of hematologic cancers in 4061 family members of 189 patients with a variety of hematologic neoplasms. They compared their findings with control groups of 955 relatives of 36 patients with non-malignant hematologic disorders and 508 relatives of 33 patients with type 2 diabetes mellitus. They found that the majority of hematologic cancers among family members differed from those of the probands. Specifically, "The odds ratio for haematological neoplasms among relatives of the index cases adjusted for age, sex, ethnicity, number of relatives in the family, and degree of familial linkage in the study group versus the two control groups was 3.62 (95% confidence interval, 1.44-9.07, P < 0.01)." These findings lend support to the idea of a genetic predisposition to cancer in a subset of patients, with diverse familial clustering of the hematologic neoplasms. Therefore, they suggest that the familial aggregation of hematologic cancer is not necessarily disease specific, which is consistent with an abnormality in the pluripotent hematopoietic stem cell.[501] Alternatively, more differentiated hematologic cells of different types may be susceptible to genetic damage in some families.

Families prone to hematologic malignancies have received a paucity of attention when compared to families with solid tumors. Conversely, hematologic malignancies have had more extensive cytogenetic investigation.[502]

Acute Myelogenous Leukemia ■ We have studied a family[503] with acute myelogenous leukemia (Fig. 14-3) wherein many clues were present that appear to link the presumptive genetic susceptibility of solid tumors to hematologic cancer in this family. Review of the pedigree shows several examples of key individuals with solid tumors having progeny with hematologic cancer and, conversely, patients with hematologic cancer having progeny with solid tumors. The pedigree appears to be consistent with an autosomal dominant predisposition to both hematologic and solid tumors. In the absence of a hereditary cancer disorder such as the LFS, these findings appear to be unique, as the hematologic cancers are predominantly AML. There are no premonitory stigmata that may associate this susceptibility to AML.

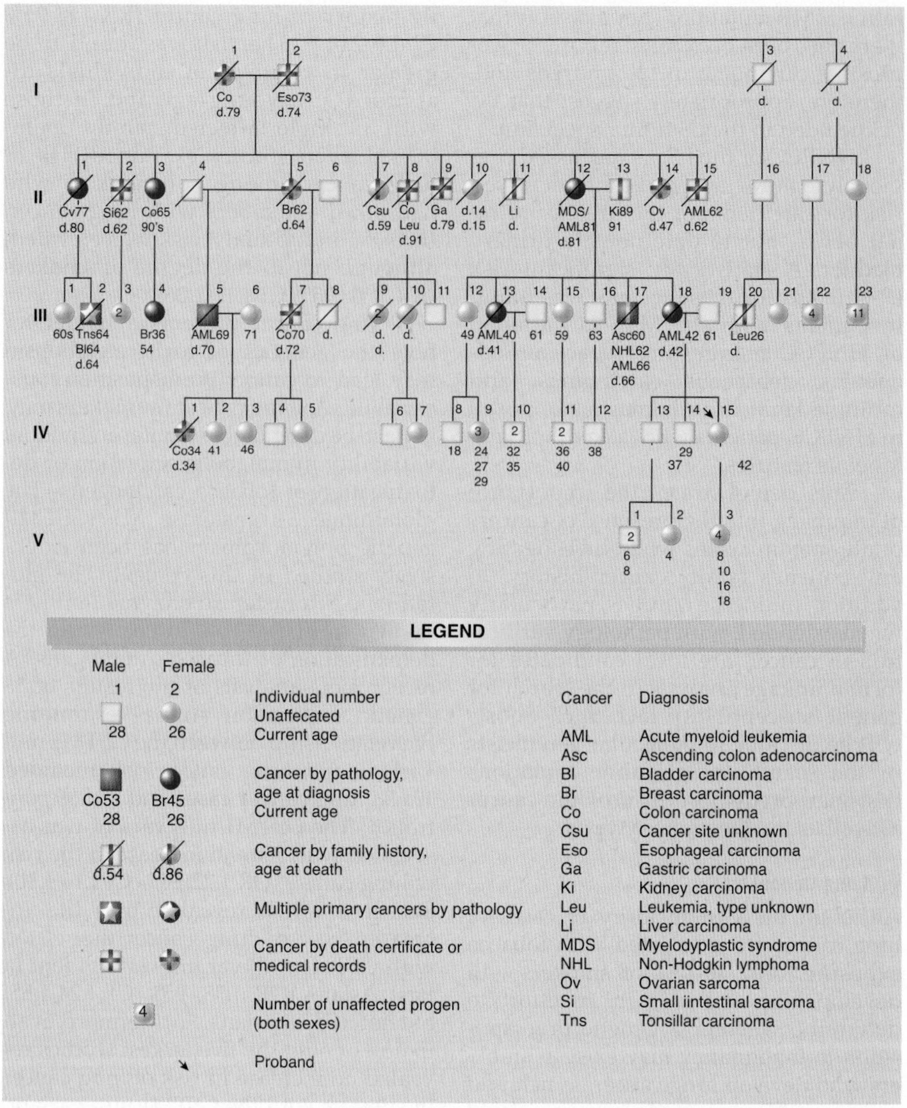

Figure 14-3 ■ Pedigree for hematologic and solid tumor prone family manifesting acute myelogenous leukemia. *Source*: Reprinted from Cancer Genet Cytogenet, 137, Lynch H, et al, Family with Acute Myelogenous Leukemia, Breast, Ovarian,and Gastrointestinal Cancer, 8-14 Copyright 2002, with permission from Elsevier.

Chronic Lymphocytic Leukemia (CLL) ■ Lynch et al[504] described a large multigeneration family with a pedigree (Fig. 14-4) that was consistent with an autosomal dominant mode of genetic transmission for susceptibility to CLL. Because of this family's unique features, it was further investigated by Raval and colleagues[505] in the search for a predisposing mutation. This led to the discovery that loss or reduced expression of death-associated protein kinase 1 (DAPK1) underlies cases of heritable predisposition to CLL and the majority of sporadic CLL, with epigenetic silencing of DAPK1 by promoter methylation occurring in almost all sporadic CLL cases. The research also identified the disease haplotype segregating with the CLL phenotype in this large family. DAPK1 expression of the CLL allele is downregulated by 75% in germline cells due to increased HOXB7 binding, and promoter methylation results in additional loss of DAPK1 expression in affected family members. Thus, reduced expression of DAPK1 can result from a germline mutation as well as from epigenetic or somatic events causing or contributing to the CLL phenotype.[505]

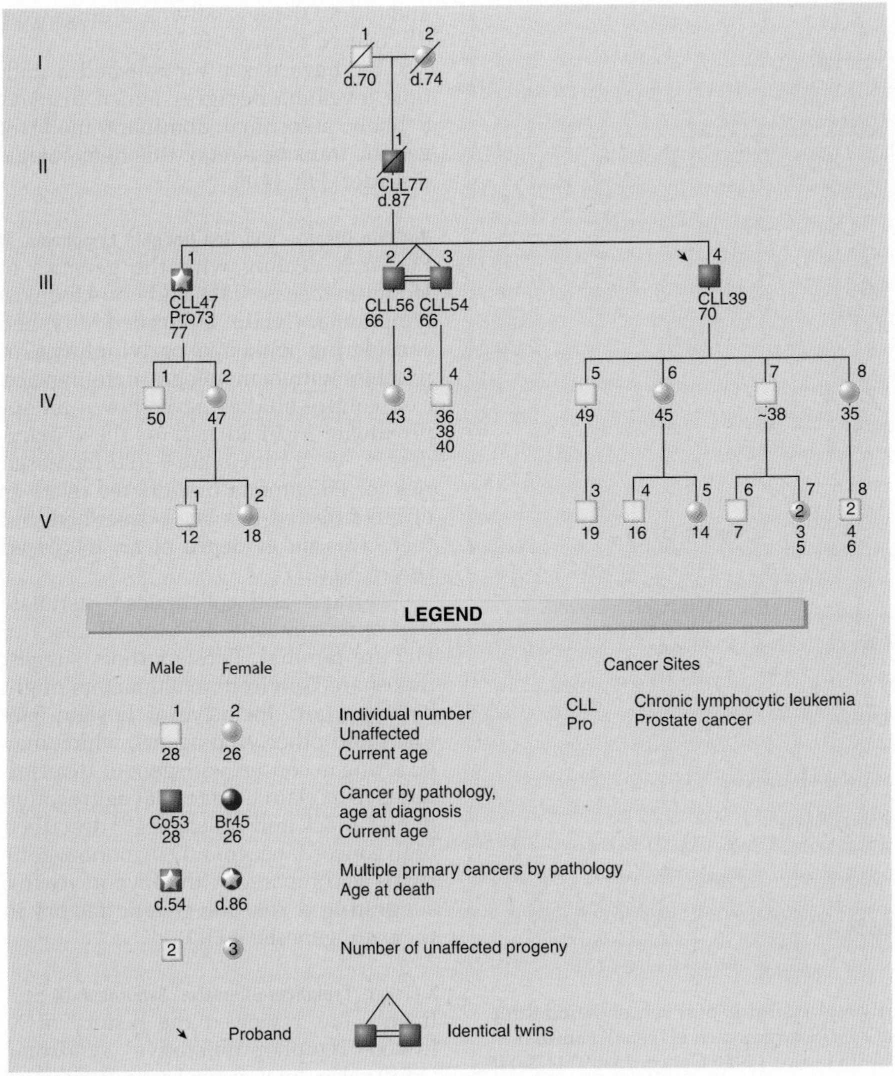

Figure 14-4 Pedigree of a family in which the father and all four children are CLL-affected, findings consistent with an autosomal dominantly inherited predisposition to CLL. *Source*: Lynch HT, et al. Hereditary chronic lymphocytic leukemia: An extended family study and literature review. Am J Med Genet 2002;115:113-117.

Lynch and colleagues had provided FISs to this large family before the *DAPK1* mutation was identified, and followed up with personal genetic counseling result-disclosure settings for those family members who agreed to receive their DNA test results.[506]

Note that the pedigree shows CLL in a father (II-1) and all four of his children (III-1, III-2, III-3, III-4). (Finding a male-to-male transmission excluded X-linked inheritance.) The occurrence of CLL in identical twins in this sibship adds to the likelihood of a primary hereditary etiology. Therefore, hereditary factors appear to be a major contributing causal factor in a subset of CLL cases.[507-509] CLL has also been reported in association with breast cancer.[510]

Yuille and colleagues,[511] employing family history questionnaires on 268 CLL-affected individuals, found that a family history of lymphoproliferative disorder (LPD) in a first-degree relative was present in 33 (12%) of those responding to the survey, while 15 (6%) reported CLL in a first-degree relative. The largest number of CLL affected found in any one of their families was three patients. In their literature survey of CLL families, they identified 81 familial reports of which "64 were two-case families. Thirty-eight contained an affected sibling, and 16 contained an affected parent and affected offspring. Six pairs of monozygotic twins have been reported. In two of these cases, a first-degree relative was also affected. In five of the families with two or more cases of CLL, other relatives were affected ... The largest CLL family reported to date is a six-case family comprising three affected siblings and three affected cousins."[512] Yuille and colleagues[511] suggest that there is an approximate 30-fold increase in risk for CLL in relatives of CLL affecteds.

To date, there has not been any evidence of predisposition genes identified specifically for CLL. However, hematologic cancers inclusive of CLL have been identified in a litany of Mendelian inherited hematologic cancer-prone disorders, particularly such chromosomal breakage syndromes as Bloom syndrome, Fanconi aplastic anemia, and ataxia telangiectasia.[513]

Multiple Myeloma The etiology of multiple myeloma (MM) remains obscure, although there are reports of familial clustering that suggest a host susceptibility factor which may act in concert with environmental effects. Lynch and colleagues[514] reported a family with MM (Fig. 14-5). Their extended MM family comprised a sibship of 7, wherein 3 patients showed histologically verified MM while two had a monoclonal gammopathy of unknown significance (MGUS). Other tumors in the family included acute lymphocytic leukemia, malignant melanoma, and PC. Their review of the literature clearly indicates that a subset of familial MM may also include other hematologic cancers as well as solid tumors. More recently, Lynch and colleagues[515] have emphasized the genotypic/phenotypic heterogeneity of MM by describing 39 MM-prone families, with some of the families showing cases of plasma cell dyscrasias, differing hematological malignancies, and/or solid tumors.

Shoenfeld and colleagues,[516] in their review, identified 36 reports of familial MM and added one family of their own. Interestingly, the patients did not show any significant clinical differences from those with nonfamilial myeloma when considering gender, age, distribution of monoclonal proteins, clinical and laboratory data, and prognosis. They did observe an increased incidence of immunoglobulin abnormalities in healthy relatives of the patients manifesting MM.

Horwitz and colleagues[517] described a family wherein multiple myeloma was present in three siblings, two of whom had a history of a monoclonal gammopathy. Their literature review disclosed 38 pairs of siblings with plasma cell disorders, whereas eight families showed a third affected sibling and four families had a fourth affected relative, thereby suggesting that some cases of multiple myeloma may have an hereditary basis. They suggested that other family members may be at increased risk for developing the disease. These authors also noted in their review of the literature that only two other families had three siblings with MM, but they state that, "five other sibships had combinations of myeloma and monoclonal gammopathy, and two had three siblings with monoclonal gammopathies only. Furthermore, another close relative was affected [with MM] in four of these families. Since approximately 3%

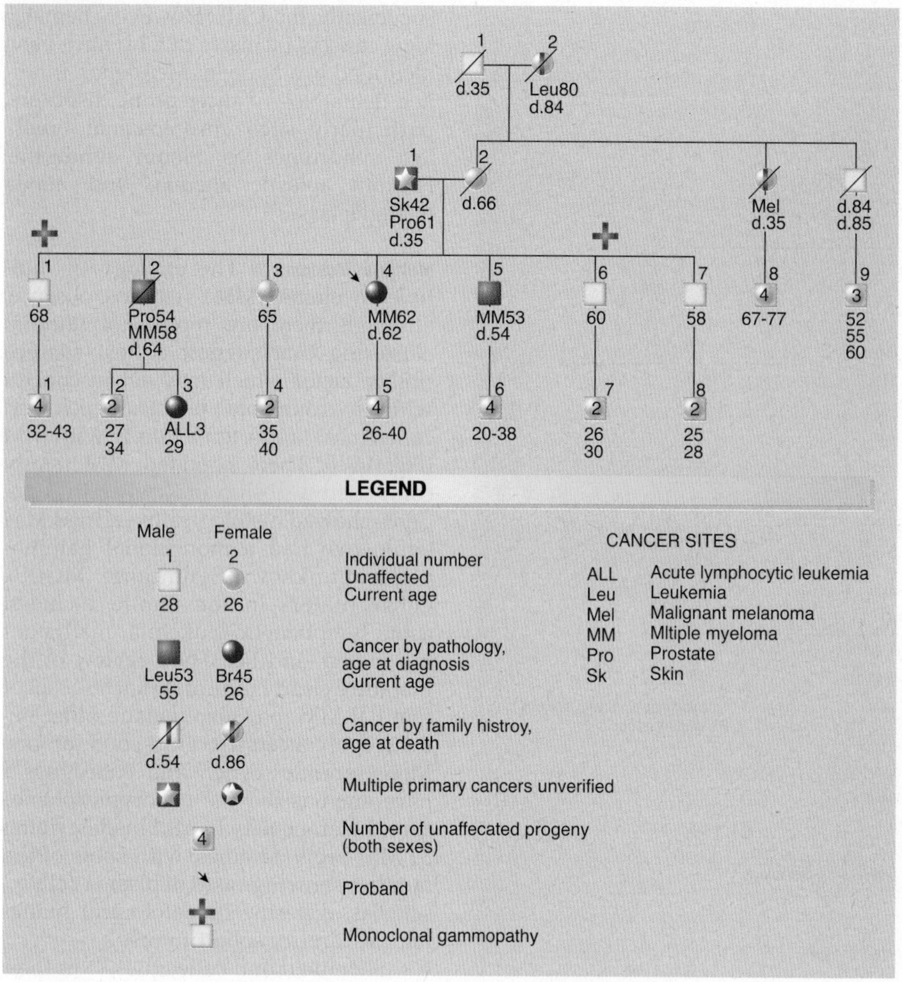

Figure 14-5 ■ Pedigree of multiple myeloma family with a sibship of seven, showing three siblings with verified MM and two siblings with MGUS. (*Source*: Lynch HT, et al. Familial multiple myeloma: A family study and review of the literature. J Natl Cancer Inst 93:1479-1483, 2001.

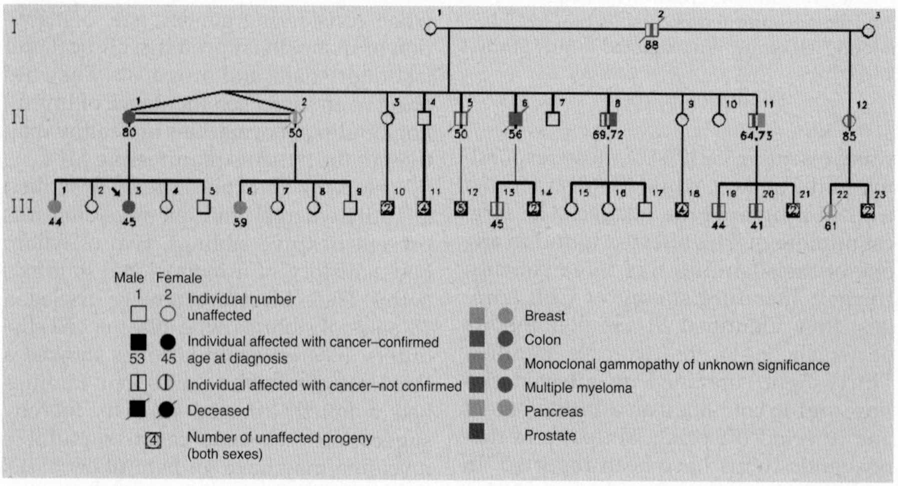

Figure 14-6 ■ Pedigree of a multiple myeloma family displaying a likely autosomal dominant mode of genetic transmission of this hematologic disorder.

of the elderly have benign [monoclonal] gammopathies,[518] the presence of several individuals with such an abnormality in a single family might not be unusual. On the other hand, frank myeloma in three siblings should be very rare."

Bizzaro and Pasini[519] studied a family in which five siblings had a monoclonal gammopathy. MGUS was diagnosed in two of these individuals, following which a family study showed that one sister had died from multiple myeloma, and four of the seven living siblings were discovered to have MGUS.

We have recently published a multiple myeloma pedigree which displays a likely autosomal dominant mode of genetic transmission of this hematologic disorder (Fig. 14-6).[520]

Hodgkin Disease and Non-Hodgkin Lymphoma ■ Research dealing with the genetics of Hodgkin disease (HD) and non-Hodgkin lymphoma (NHL) is limited.[521] When considering leukemia or lymphoma in relatives with hematologic malignancies, case-control studies have shown an approximate 3.62-fold risk for these disorders.[501] An approximate 9-fold increased risk for HD among first-degree relatives of HD affected has been described, but there was no evidence of an increased risk in NHL.[522]

Ferraris and colleagues[523] estimate that approximately 4.5% of all cases of HD are familial. These authors suggest that shared environmental factors might be important, inclusive of Epstein-Barr virus and other viral agents, which may be acting in concert with genetic determinants to explain the familial aggregation of HD. Mack and colleagues[524] described high concordance for HD in monozygotic twins as compared with dizygotic twins, suggesting a role for genetic factors in the pathogenesis of HD.

X-Linked Lymphoproliferative Syndrome ■ Sullivan[525] has reviewed the history of X-linked lymphoproliferative syndrome (XLP), also known as Duncan disease. Purtilo and colleagues, some 30 years ago, performed an autopsy on an 8½-year-old male who died following infectious mononucleosis (IM). This was the third male sibling in the family to have died following a bout of IM. This led to their seminal publication in 1975, which described X-linked recessive combined variable immunodeficiency.[526] More than 80 families have now been reported to the XLP syndrome registry established by Purtilo and colleagues.[527]

XLP is characterized by an enormous sensitivity to EBV. The phenotype features severe or fatal IM, acquired hypogammaglobulinemia, and malignant lymphoma. Sullivan[525] lists the following phenotypic features: (1) life-threatening EBV infection (58% with a mortality of 96%); (2) immunodeficiency in 31% with a mortality of 45%; (3) lymphoma or Hodgkin disease in 30% with a mortality of 69%; and (4) aplastic anemia in 3% with a 50% mortality. Most of the lymphomas are extranodal non-Hodgkin lymphomas, with distal small bowel the site at highest risk.

Genetic linkage studies have localized the XLP locus to the long arm of the X chromosome in Xq24-q25. Coffey and colleagues[528] identified a gene termed *SH2D1A* "that is mutated in XLP patients and encodes a novel protein composed of a single SH2 domain. *SH2D1A* is expressed in many tissues involved in the immune system. The identification of *SH2D1A* will allow the determination of its mechanism of action as a possible regulator of the EBV-induced immune response." EBV infection in susceptible infants is initially asymptomatic, but by adolescence or early adulthood, IM will occur with 100% mortality by the age of 40.

Clinical Translation

Overview

Figure 14-7 shows our recommendations for evaluating and testing individuals suspected of having a hereditary cancer syndrome. Family history and physical examination is used to tentatively classify an index patient as sporadic, familial, or hereditary. Family histories are updated regularly, sometimes resulting in reclassification of risk status. Screening and genetic testing options depend on the specific syndrome under consideration. Worth re-emphasizing here is the potential power of such testing when a cancer susceptibility mutation can be identified and at-risk family members can be tested. Individuals who are positive for the mutation can enter surveillance and management programs tailored to the natural history of the particular syndrome involved. In some circumstances, prophylactic surgery may be an option. Individuals lacking the mutation can follow general population screening guidelines. Whether positive or negative, patients in this situation require compassionate genetic counseling.[82] (For more thoughts on the importance of family history, and information regarding the National Health Institute's family history project, see Guttmacher.[13])

It is important to be aware of factors that might obfuscate pedigree interpretation. These include incomplete gene penetrance in key relatives, early death before phenotype expression, incomplete family history, false paternity, cancer occurrences that may be sporadic, limited patient and/or physician cooperation, records lost or destroyed, and small family size.

We recommend comprehensive education of all at-risk patients as part of genetic counseling. Detailed coverage of the genetics and natural history of the particular hereditary cancer syndrome, as well as the advantages and disadvantages of DNA testing, can be provided in a large group family information session (FIS).[435] Key relatives in the geographic catchment area may attend the FIS at a designated time so that they can be provided with this educational experience. Alternatively, genetic counseling can be offered as a series of appointments with a genetic counselor and medical team. Informed consent for genetic testing is an extremely complex and important issue in genetic testing and must be obtained with care through a detailed discussion with each participant (see Table 14-6 for essential components). Before blood is collected for DNA testing, patients must be advised of the potential for fear, anxiety, apprehension, and intrafamily strife. When a cancer-causing germline mutation is identified, additional genetic counseling on an individual basis at the time of disclosure of these results is required.

Hudson et al.[529] discuss the Genetic Information Nondiscrimination Act (GINA) of 2008, which has been officially signed by President George Bush. It is important to note that GINA addresses only employment and health insurance, excluding life insurance, disability insurance, or long-term-care insurance. Importantly, it prohibits health insurers from using an individual's genetic information for determining eligibility or

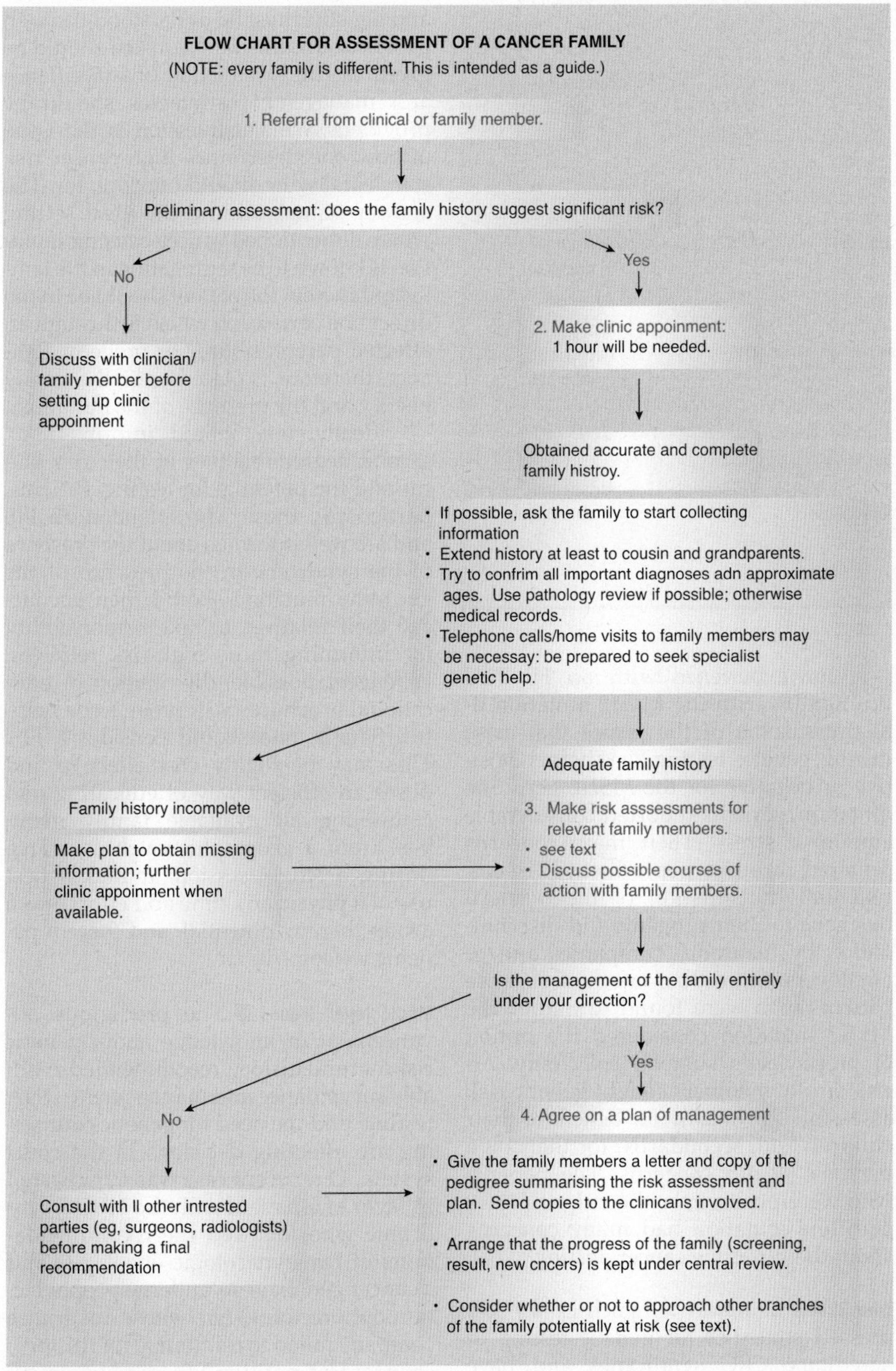
FLOW CHART FOR ASSESSMENT OF A CANCER FAMILY
(NOTE: every family is different. This is intended as a guide.)
1. Referral from clinical or family member.
Preliminary assessment: does the family history suggest significant risk?
No
Yes
Discuss with clinician/ family menber before setting up clinic appoinment
2. Make clinic appoinment: 1 hour will be needed.
Obtained accurate and complete family histroy.
• If possible, ask the family to start collecting information
• Extend history at least to cousin and grandparents.
• Try to confrim all important diagnoses adn approximate ages. Use pathology review if possible; otherwise medical records.
• Telephone calls/home visits to family members may be necessay: be prepared to seek specialist genetic help.
Adequate family history
Family history incomplete
Make plan to obtain missing information; further clinic appoinment when available.
3. Make risk asssessments for relevant family members.
• see text
• Discuss possible courses of action with family members.
Is the management of the family entirely under your direction?
Yes
No
4. Agree on a plan of management
Consult with ll other intrested parties (eg, surgeons, radiologists) before making a final recommendation
• Give the family members a letter and copy of the pedigree summarising the risk assessment and plan. Send copies to the clinicans involved.
• Arrange that the progress of the family (screening, result, new cncers) is kept under central review.
• Consider whether or not to approach other branches of the family potentially at risk (see text).

Figure 14-7 ■ Algorithm depicting the process for the study and genetic counseling of families being observed by the Creighton Cancer Genetic Research Team. *Source:* Reproduced with permission from Lynch HT, et al. Cancer 1999;86:2449-2456. *Abbreviations*: FIS, Family Information Session; ACS, American Cancer Society.

Table 14-6 ■ Content of Informed Consent for Genetic Testing

- Purpose of the test: if testing is part of a research study, the purpose, aims, and design of the research study
- Practical aspects of the testing, including cost, turnaround time, documentation of results
- Predictive value of a positive, negative, or indeterminate result, and corresponding cancer risk information
- Options for cancer risk management in the setting of a positive, negative, or indeterminate result
- Possible psychological implications of testing
- Individualized assessment of insurance and employment discrimination risks
- Alternatives to genetic testing, including the possibility of delaying decision making

Table 14-7 ■ Hereditary Cancer Syndromes for Which Clinical Genetic Testing Is Available

Cancer Syndrome	Associated Cancers and Other Features	Gene(s)	Mode of Inheritance
Breast-ovarian cancer syndrome	Early-onset breast cancer Ovarian cancer Prostate cancer Male breast cancer	*BRCA1* *BRCA2*	Autosomal dominant
Hereditary nonpolyposis colorectal cancer	Early onset colon cancer Endometrial cancer Stomach cancer Ovarian cancer Other genitourinary cancers Absence of polyposis	*MLH1* *MSH2* *MSH6*	Autosomal dominant
Familial adenomatous polyposis	Polyposis (> 100 colon polyps) Early-onset colon cancer Desmoid tumors Epidermoid tumors	*APC*	Autosomal dominant
Li-Fraumeni syndrome	Early-onset breast cancer Childhood sarcoma Brain cancer Leukemia Adrenocortical cancer	*TP53*	Autosomal dominant
von Hippel-Lindau	Renal cell cancer Hemangioblastomas of cerebellum brain stem, spine Retinal angioma Pheochromocytoma	*VHL*	Autosomal dominant

premiums; in addition, an insurer is prohibited from requesting or requiring that a person undergo a genetic test.

GINA is timely, given the fact that genomic information has grown exponentially, wherein it has revolutionized "nearly all areas of biomedical research and, many believe, promising an eventual transformation of health care...." This law, along with the Health Insurance Portability and Accountability Act (HIPAA) should assuage the fears and anxieties of patients contemplating DNA mutation testing or those who have already been tested, and may remain concerned about being discriminated against by health insurers or employers.

We subscribe to the updated guidelines proposed by the American Society of Clinical Oncology,[530] which state that predisposition testing should be offered only when (1) there is a strong family history of cancer, (2) the test can be adequately interpreted, (3) the results will influence medical management of the patient or family members, and (4) laboratories are committed to the validation of testing methodologies. Table 14-7 details hereditary cancer syndromes for which clinical genetic testing is currently available.

Our experience with an HNPCC (LS) family with the *MSH2* mutation illustrates some of the issues that arise during genetic testing.[531] Whether positive or negative for the *MSH2* germline mutation, patients reported considerable emotional stress. Their main concerns centered around reproductive issues, potential transmission of the deleterious gene to their progeny, and discrimination by insurance companies and/or employers. More than one half of those patients who were found to harbor the *MSH2* mutation considered the option of prophylactic subtotal colectomy. At-risk family members sought genetic risk assessment primarily for benefit to their children and, secondarily, for their own personal health concerns. The patients who were positive for the culprit *MSH2* germline mutation had many concerns about their lifetime cancer destiny.

Who Should Be Tested? ■ Lynch et al.[107] expressed strategies for genetic testing in hereditary CRC syndromes and have used this as a model for all forms of hereditary cancer syndromes. With respect to who should have their DNA tested for cancer-causing mutations, it is crucial that the patient receive genetic counseling. Once he/she is thoroughly familiar with the HIPAA[532] consenting process. Needed before testing is a pedigree of the individual's family that is highly consistent with a hereditary breast and/or ovarian cancer syndrome. It would be helpful if the known germline mutation predisposing to cancer is present in the family. Patients at acceptable high cancer risk status, and therefore informative, should be the one(s) offered testing initially, as this will help should there be a distinguishing syndrome stigmata (phenotype) such as multiple trichilemmomas in CS. Risks and benefits must be understood through genetic counseling and consent should be given. A full explanation of surveillance and management strategies should be provided. A major question is the issue of how one determines high cancer risk status and what should one look for. The answer centers around the ideal setting where a mentioned cancer-causing mutation is known to be segregating in the family and therein the patient should be in the direct line of descent, which is through an affected parent, sibling, or progeny. Reliance, therefore, is placed upon the family history and the presence of the mutation.

Ideally, one should inform first-/second-degree relatives of their risk status and the potential for testing. Patients, particularly those who attended an FIS and are well informed about the presence of the syndrome in the presence of the germline mutation should then encourage their relatives to take responsibility for informing these high-risk relatives. Whenever possible, distribution of educational brochures will prove to be helpful. Finally, one should consider a FIS. This may be highly cost effective and poses an efficient way of educating and counseling all available family members from a geographic catchment area during a single session. It makes best use of a physician's time and effort, has a group therapy potential, and therein patients welcome it.

Medicolegal Issues ■ The prodigious advancement in knowledge about genetic risk, natural history, recommended available surveillance and management, DNA testing, and the need for genetic counseling are affecting decisions in the court system. One recent case was adjudicated in favor of a patient with the HBOC syndrome who followed the recommendations of her gynecologic oncologist and a cancer geneticist to undergo prophylactic oophorectomy, but whose insurance company failed to reimburse for this procedure. Her petition for reimbursement was denied at the district court level, but the Nebraska Supreme Court rendered a favorable decision on her part, ordering the insurance company to provide reimbursement for this indicated procedure.[533]

Standard-of-care concerns apply to physicians as well. In the Safer case,[534] a diagnosis of FAP was established in the father of the litigant at age 35. The patient later died. The surviving spouse claimed that although the surgeon discussed her husband's diagnosis, treatment, and cancer management, he failed to disclose the genetic risk for FAP, even though the hereditary nature of FAP was known. The patient's children, then ages 10 and 17, were not advised to seek early colon surveillance. Subsequently, one of the children, at age 36, experienced lower abdominal pain and underwent surgery and extensive chemotherapy for CRC arising in FAP. A claim of negligence was filed against the estate of the surgeon, alleging (1) that he had a duty to warn those known to be at risk of avoidable harm from a genetically transmissible condition existing in his patient, (2) that the physician's duty did extend to members of the immediate family of his patient, and (3) that he had breached these duties.[270] The suit was won by the plaintiff in 1996. Similar cases are likely to become more common as advances in molecular genetics outstrip the ability of physicians to stay current in a very complex field. The physician must not only obtain a sufficiently detailed family history; but also he or she must be able to suggest appropriate surveillance and management for the affected family. Finally, genetic testing is not indicated in all heritable cancer syndromes, and current recommendations will continually change as knowledge in the field advances. For these reasons, updated guidelines[530] have been published and will be periodically updated by the American Society of Clinical Oncology for genetic testing for heritable cancer syndromes, to help educate clinicians in the appropriate use of genetic testing.

Conclusions/Future Directions

The rapid progress in the identification of hereditary cancer syndromes and their molecular genetic etiology during the past decade suggests very strongly that research progress in this new millennium will yield an astounding mass of new clinically translational data, particularly when considering the extant heterogeneity in these disorders.

Here are some predictions for the future:

More High-Prevalence, Low-Penetrance Mutations Will Be Found That Contribute to Familial Clustering of Cancer ■ We predict that more highly penetrant, as well as low-penetrance gene mutations, will be identified and will contribute to what we now construe as familial clustering of cancer. Laken and colleagues,[104] as noted earlier, reported a low-penetrance mutation within the *APC* gene. A T-to-A transversion of nucleotide 3920 was identified, resulting in a substitution of lysine for isoleucine at codon 1307 (I1307K). This mutation was found in 6.1% of the 766 Ashkenazi Jewish patients, but none of the 243 non-Ashkenazim had the mutation.

Laken and colleagues[104] then examined 211 Ashkenazim with CRC and found that 10.4% of them harbored the I1307K mutation. The authors also observed the mutation more commonly (28%) in Ashkenazim with CRC and a first- or second-degree relative with CRC and/or adenomatous polyps than in Ashkenazim with CRC and an unknown or negative family history. They estimated that carrying this mutation resulted in a doubling of CRC risk over the patient's lifetime. The mutation itself is not pathogenic, but the T-to-A transversion creates a poly-A tract at higher risk for subsequent mutations.

Tomlinson and colleagues[535] subsequently identified a novel susceptibility gene mapped on to chromosome 15q14-q22 in an Ashkenazi family with dominantly inherited predisposition to colorectal adenomas and carcinomas. The authors refer to this previously undescribed susceptibility gene on chromosome 15q as *CRAC1* (colorectal adenoma and carcinoma). Interestingly, there were two cases of pancreatic cancer in the family with the suggestion that this could also be part of the phenotype attributable to mutations in the gene. Of further interest is the fact that the family fulfills the Amsterdam criteria for HNPCC but differs in that several of the patients have more colonic adenomas than expected. Genetic linkage analysis excluded germline mutations in *MSH2, MLH1, PSM1, PMS2,* and *MSH6.*

Varley and colleagues[536] suggest that certain *p53* alleles confer low-penetrance predisposition to the development of cancer. They found a narrow spectrum of *p53* mutations in children with adrenocortical tumors; some of the mutations had been inherited and some of the families in question had other cancers. No family met criteria for LFS.

Role of Modifier Genes Will Be More Fully Explored and Clarified ■ Complex genetic and environmental interactions almost certainly influence phenotypic expression in hereditary syndromes. In the Min mouse, inheritance of the Mom1 locus decreases the size and number of intestinal polyps.[537] In human populations, Moisio and colleagues[538] have shown that genetic polymorphisms in carcinogen metabolism might modify phenotype in HNPCC. They found that in patients carrying germline mutations of *MLH1,* a particular N-acetyltransferase 1 allele was associated with younger patient age at diagnosis and tumor location in the distal colon. As mechanisms for genotype-environment interactions are elucidated, there will be more opportunities for therapeutic intervention, which leads to our next suggestion.

Ability to Modulate the Effects of Deleterious Mutations Through Chemoprevention Will Continue to Grow ■ Quite a large body of literature exists on chemoprevention in colon cancer (reviewed by Hawk and colleagues[143]), most of it pertaining to cyclooxygenase inhibitors. Tamoxifen, an anti-estrogen, has been shown to have activity as a chemopreventive agent for breast cancer in patients with DCIS and those with a high risk of breast cancer. Additional indications are currently under study. Many pharmacologic agents under development or currently in trials will undoubtedly aid our ability to inhibit or reverse the process of carcinogenesis.[539]

Microarray Technology Will Make Genetic Testing More Widely Available and Less Expensive ■ The newly developed cDNA microarray analysis provides new methodology for cancer genetic research. Bennicelli and Barr[540] have studied the implications of microarray techniques with respect to the biology of sarcomas. Specifically, these authors have shown how relevant knowledge with respect to a better comprehension of sarcoma biology can be obtained through comparative genomic hybridization and microarray techniques. They showed how these powerful technologies "will facilitate the rapid acquisition of data that provide insight into the molecular genetic and biologic basis of sarcomas."

Finally, these microarray techniques should advance our cause significantly in terms of ferreting out differences between hereditary forms of cancer such as colon, breast, ovary, and endometrium, in the respective hereditary cancer syndromes, and their sporadic counterparts. For example, Kurian and colleagues[541] note that this "mini-revolution is sweeping the world of science and medicine. DNA chip or microarray technology will have a more profound impact than other recent major advances, including DNA sequencing and the polymerase chain reaction (PCR)."

Gene Therapy Will Become a Reality ■ We will have the ability to alter cellular function or structure at the molecular level by replacing lost or defective genes or adding genes known to produce beneficial proteins. Everything from inborn errors of metabolism to atherosclerosis to cancer should be amenable to treatment with molecular techniques. For example, Phase I clinical trials show that *p53* replacement therapy induces tumor regression in lung cancer patients.[542] Patients known to carry mutations in cancer-susceptibility genes should be ideal candidates for molecular intervention.

In the next decade, molecular and genetic approaches will likely take center stage in the prevention, diagnosis, and treatment of cancer. Valuable information on the science and ethics of this expanding field is increasingly available and regularly updated for clinicians, health care providers, and the public by major organizations such as the National Institutes of Health (http://www.genetests.org/). It will be essential that physicians remain well informed so that they may successfully harness the power of these approaches to the benefit of the patients who seek their assistance.

Selected References

The complete reference list can be found at www.CANCERMEDICINE8.com

4. Lynch HT, Shaw MW, Magnuson CW, et al. Hereditary factors in cancer: study of two large Midwestern kindreds. *Arch Intern Med.* 1966;117:206–212.
5. Herrera L, Kakati S, Gibas L, et al. Brief clinical report: Gardner's syndrome in a man with an interstitial deletion of 5q. *Am J Med Genet.* 1986;25:473–476.
7. Kinzler KW, Nilbert MC, Su L-K, et al. Identification of FAP locus genes from chromosome 5q21. *Science.* 1991;253:661–665.
13. Guttmacher AE, Collins FS, Carmona RH. The family history—more important than ever. *N Engl J Med.* 2004;351:2333–2336.
15. Lynch HT, Krush AJ, Lemon HM, et al. Tumor variation in families with breast cancer. *JAMA.* 1972;222:1631–635.
20. Lynch HT, de la Chapelle A. Genomic medicine: hereditary colorectal cancer. *N Engl J Med.* 2003;348:919–932.
22. Hall JM, Lee MK, Newman B, et al. Linkage of early-onset breast cancer to chromosome 17q21. *Science.* 1990;250:1684–1689.
23. Narod SA, Feunteun J, Lynch HT, et al. Familial breast-ovarian cancer locus on chromosome 17q12-q23. *Lancet.* 1991;388:82–83.
61. Brose MS, Rebbeck TR, Calzone KA, et al. Cancer risk estimates for BRCA1 mutation carriers identified in a risk evaluation program. *J Natl Cancer Inst.* 2002;94:1365–1372.
68. Marcus JN, Watson P, Page DL, et al. Hereditary breast cancer: pathobiology, prognosis, and BRCA1 and BRCA2 gene linkage. *Cancer.* 1996;77:697–709.
79. Narod SA, Brunet J-S, Ghadirian P, et al. Tamoxifen and risk of contralateral breast cancer in *BRCA1* and *BRCA2* mutation carriers: a case-control study. *Lancet.* 2000;356:1876–1881.
88. Hartmann LC, Sellers TA, Schaid DJ, et al. Efficacy of bilateral prophylactic mastectomy in BRCA1 and BRCA2 gene mutation carriers. *J Natl Cancer Inst.* 2001;93:1633–1637.
91. Rebbeck TR, Lynch HT, Neuhausen SL, et al. Prophylactic oophorectomy in carriers of *BRCA1* or *BRCA2* mutations. *N Engl J Med.* 2002;346:1616–1622.
95. Rebbeck TR, Friebel T, Lynch HT, et al. Bilateral prophylactic mastectomy reduces breast cancer risk in BRCA1 and BRCA2 mutation carriers: The PROSE Study Group. *J Clin Oncol.* 2004;22:1055–1062.
96. Robson M, Svahn T, McCormick B, et al. Appropriateness of breast-conserving treatment of breast carcinoma in women with germline mutations in *BRCA1* or *BRCA2*: a clinic-based series. *Cancer.* 2005;103:44–51.
104. Laken SJ, Petersen GM, Gruber SB, et al. Familial colorectal cancer in Ashkenazim due to a hypermutable tract in *APC. Nat Genet.* 1997;17:79–83.
105. Locker GY, Kaul K, Weinberg DS, et al. The I1307K APC polymorphism in Ashkenazi Jews with colorectal cancer: clinical and pathological features. *Cancer Genet Cytogenet.* 2006;169:33–38.
107. Lynch HT, Boland CR, Rodriguez-Bigas MA, et al. Who should be sent for genetic testing in hereditary colorectal cancer syndromes? *J Clin Oncol.* 2007;25:3534–3542.
137. Hamilton SR, Liu B, Parsons RE, et al. The molecular basis of Turcot's syndrome. *N Engl J Med.* 1995;332:839–847.
140. Lynch HT, Smyrk T, McGinn T, et al. Attenuated familial adenomatous polyposis (AFAP): a phenotypically and genotypically distinctive variant of FAP. *Cancer.* 1995;76:2427–2433.
166. Howe JR, Mitros FA, Summers RW. The risk of gastrointestinal carcinoma in familial juvenile polyposis. *Ann Surg Oncol.* 1998;5:751–756.
184. Watson P, Lin K, Rodriguez-Bigas MA, et al. Colorectal carcinoma survival among hereditary nonpolyposis colorectal cancer family members. *Cancer.* 1998;83:259–266.
196. Fishel R, Lescoe MK, Rao MRS, et al. The human mutator gene homolog MSH2 and its association with hereditary nonpolyposis colon cancer. *Cell.* 1993;75:1027–1038.
204. Rodriguez-Bigas MA, Vasen HFA, Pekka-Mecklin J, et al. Rectal cancer risk in hereditary nonpolyposis colorectal cancer after abdominal colectomy. *Ann Surg.* 1997;225:202–207.
210. Lindor NM, Burgart LJ, Leontovich O, et al. Immunohistochemistry versus microsatellite instability testing in phenotyping colorectal tumors. *J Clin Oncol.* 2002;20:1043–1048.
213. Lynch HT, Boland CR, Gong G, et al. Phenotypic and genotypic heterogeneity in the Lynch syndrome: diagnostic, surveillance and management implications. *Eur J Hum Genet.* 2006;14:390–402.
214. Hampel H, Frankel WL, Martin E, et al. Screening for Lynch syndrome (hereditary nonpolyposis colorectal cancer). *N Engl J Med.* 2005;352:1851–1860.
221. Lynch P. Standards of care in diagnosis and testing for hereditary colon cancer. *Fam Cancer.* 2008;7:65–72.
229. Wagner A, Barrows A, Wijnen JT, et al. Molecular analysis of hereditary nonpolyposis colorectal cancer in the United States: high mutation detection rate among clinically selected families and characterization of an American founder genomic deletion of the *MSH2* gene. *Am J Hum Genet.* 2003;72:1088–1100.
230. Lynch HT, de la Chapelle A, Hampel H, et al. The American founder mutation for Lynch syndrome: prevalence estimates and implications. *Cancer.* 2006;106:448–452.
256. Gallinger S, Aronson M, Shayan K, et al. Gastrointestinal cancers and neurofibromatosis type 1 features in children with a germline homozygous *MLH1* mutation. *Gastroenterology.* 2004;126:576–585.
267. Umar A, Boland CR, Terdiman JP, et al. Revised Bethesda Guidelines for hereditary nonpolyposis colorectal cancer (Lynch syndrome) and microsatellite instability. *J Natl Cancer Inst.* 2004;96:261–268.
272. Peltomäki P, Vasen H. Mutations associated with HNPCC predisposition—Update of ICG-HNPCC/INSiGHT mutation database. *Dis Markers.* 2004;20:269–276.
283. Schmeler KM, Lynch HT, Chen L-M, et al. Prophylactic surgery to reduce the risk of gynecologic cancers in the Lynch syndrome. *N Engl J Med.* 2006;354:261–269.
284. Watson P, Ashwathnarayan R, Lynch HT, Roy HK. Tobacco use and increased colorectal cancer risk in patients with hereditary nonpolyposis colorectal cancer (Lynch syndrome). *Arch Intern Med.* 2004;164:2429–2431.
285. Lindor NM, Rabe K, Petersen GM, et al. Lower cancer incidence in Amsterdam-I criteria families without mismatch repair deficiency: Familial colorectal cancer type X. *JAMA.* 2005;293:1979–1985.
286. Llor X, Pons E, Xicola RM, et al. Differential features of colorectal cancers fulfilling Amsterdam criteria without involvement of the mutator pathway. *Clin Cancer Res.* 2005;11:7304–7310.
291. Li FP, Fraumeni JF. Soft-tissue sarcomas, breast cancer, and other neoplasms: a familial syndrome? *Ann Intern Med.* 1969;71:747–752.
293. Malkin D, Li FP, Stron LC, et al. Germ line p53 mutations in a familial syndrome of breast cancer, sarcomas and other neoplasms. *Science.* 1990;250:1233–1238.
300. Lynch HT, Fusaro RM, Albano WA, et al. Phenotypic variation in the familial atypical multiple mole- melanoma syndrome (FAMMM). *J Med Genet.* 1983;20:25–29.
304. Lynch HT, Brand RE, Hogg D, et al. Phenotypic variation in eight extended *CDKN2A* germline mutation familial atypical multiple mole melanoma-pancreatic carcinoma-prone families: the familial atypical multiple mole melanoma-pancreatic carcinoma syndrome. *Cancer.* 2002;94:84–96.
318. Eng C. PTEN: one gene, many syndromes. *Hum Mutat.* 2003;22:183–198.
426. Aarnio M, Salovaara R, Aaltonen LA, et al. Features of gastric cancer in hereditary non-polyposis colorectal cancer syndrome. *Int J Cancer (Pred Oncol).* 1997;74:551–555.
431. Lewis FR, Mellinger JD, Hayashi A, et al. Prophylactic total gastrectomy for familial gastric cancer. *Surgery.* 2001;130:612–617.
433. Chun YS, Lindor NM, Smyrk TC, et al. Germline E-cadherin gene mutations: is prophylactic total gastrectomy indicated? *Cancer.* 2001;92:181–187.

15 Chemical Carcinogenesis

Ainsley Weston, PhD ■ Curtis C. Harris, MD

Human chemical carcinogenesis is a multistage process that results from exposures, usually in the form of complex chemical mixtures, often encountered in the environment or through our lifestyle and diet (Table 15-1).[1-4] A prime example is tobacco smoke, which can cause cancers at multiple sites including the lung, the bladder, and the head and neck.[5-7] Although most chemical carcinogens do not react directly with intracellular components, they are activated to carcinogenic and mutagenic electrophiles by metabolic processes evolutionarily designed to rid the body of toxins and to modify endogenous compounds. Electrophilic chemical species are naturally attracted to nucleophiles like deoxyribonucleic acid (DNA) and protein, and through covalent bonding to DNA genetic damage results. Once internalized, carcinogens are subject to competing processes of metabolic activation and detoxification, although some chemical species can act directly. There is considerable variation among the human population in these competing metabolic processes, as well as the capacity for repair of DNA damage and cellular growth control. This is the basis for interindividual variation in cancer risk, and is a reflection of gene-environment interactions, which embodies the concept that heritable traits modify the effects of chemical carcinogen exposure.[8] Such variations in constitutive metabolism and DNA repair contribute to the relative susceptibility of individual members of the population to chemical exposures. For example, only 10% of tobacco smokers develop lung cancer, albeit that tobacco use accounts for other fatal conditions, including chronic obstructive pulmonary disease, stroke, and heart disease. Within the conceptual framework of multistage carcinogenesis, the primary genetic change that results from a chemical-DNA interaction is termed *tumor initiation*.[9,10] Thus, initiated cells are irreversibly altered and are at a greater risk of malignant conversion than are normal cells. The epigenetic effects of tumor promoters facilitate the clonal expansion of the initiated cells.[10] Selective, clonal growth advantage causes a focus of preneoplastic cells to form. These cells are more vulnerable to tumorigenesis because they now present a larger, more rapidly proliferating, target population for the further action of chemical carcinogens, oncogenic viruses, and other cofactors. Additional genetic and epigenetic changes continue to accumulate.[10,11] The activation of oncogenes, and the inactivation of tumor suppressor and DNA-repair genes, leads to genomic instability or the so-called *mutator phenotype* and an acceleration in the genetic changes taking place.[12,13] This scenario is followed by malignant conversion, tumor progression, and metastasis. The underlying molecular mechanisms that govern chemical carcinogenesis are becoming increasingly understood, and the insights generated are assisting in the development of better methods to investigate human cancer risk and susceptibility.[14] The results of such studies are intended to mold strategies for prevention and intervention. Moreover, insights into the normal operations of so-called *gatekeeper* genes,[15] like the tumor suppressor *TP53*, have provided an opportunity to develop new, targeted, therapeutic approaches.[16,17]

Table 15-1 ■ **Selected Examples of Human Chemical Carcinogenesis**

Organ System (Specific Pathology)	Chemical Carcinogen	Cocarcinogen
Lung	Metals: As, Be, Cd, Cr, Ni	–
	BCME	–
(Small cell and squamous cell)	Tobacco smoke	Asbestos
	Diesel exhaust	–
Pleural mesothelium	Asbestos	–
Oral cavity	Smokeless tobacco	–
	Betel quid	Slaked lime [$Ca(OH)_2$]
Esophagus	Tobacco smoke	Alcohol
Nasal sinuses	Snuff	Powdered glass
	Isopropyl alcohol	–
Skin (scrotum)	Cutting oil	–
	Coal soot[a]	–
Liver (angiosarcoma)	Aflatoxin B1	HBV, HCB
	Vinyl chloride	Alcohol
Bladder	Aromatic amines (eg, 4-ABP and benzidine)	–
	Aromatic amines from tobacco smoke[b]	–
ALL	Benzene	–
Lymphatic and hemapoietic malignancies	Ethylene oxide	–

Note: A comprehensive treatise on the evaluation of the carcinogenic risk of chemicals to humans can be found in the ongoing International Agency for Research on Cancer monograph program initiated in 1971.[4]
[a] Early report of occupational chemical carcinogenesis from 225 years ago.[1]
[b] Strong circumstantial evidence.[58]
Abbreviations: 4-ABP, 4-aminobiphenyl; ALL, acute lymphoblastic leukemia; BCME, bischloromethyl ether; HBV, hepatitis B virus; HCV, hepatitis C virus.

Multistage Carcinogenesis

Carcinogenesis can be divided conceptually into four steps: tumor initiation, tumor promotion, malignant conversion, and tumor progression (Fig. 15-1). The distinction between initiation and promotion was recognized through studies involving both viruses and chemical carcinogens.[9,18] This distinction was formally defined in a murine skin carcinogenesis model in which mice were treated topically with a single dose of a polycyclic aromatic hydrocarbon (ie, initiator), followed by repeated topical doses of croton oil (ie, promoter),[9] and this model has been expanded to a range of other rodent tissues, including bladder, colon, esophagus, liver, lung, mammary gland, stomach, and trachea.[19] During the last 50 years, the sequence of events comprising chemical carcinogenesis has been systematically dissected and the paradigm increasingly refined, and both similarities and differences between rodent and human carcinogenesis have been identified.[20,21] Carcinogenesis requires the malignant conversion of benign hyperplastic cells to a malignant state, and invasion and metastasis are manifestations of further genetic and epigenetic changes.[22-24] The study of this process in humans is necessarily indirect and uses

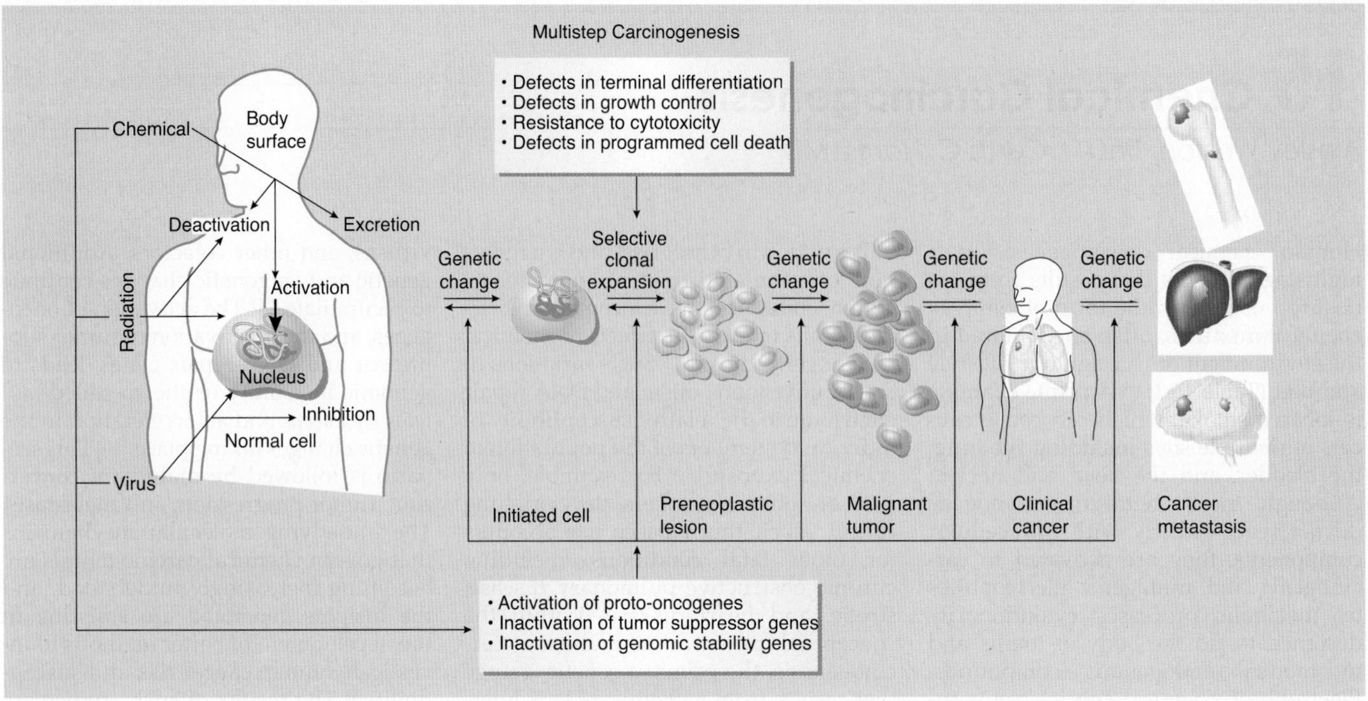

Figure 15-1 Multistage chemical carcinogenesis can be conceptually divided into four stages: tumor initiation, tumor promotion, malignant conversion, and tumor progression. The activation of proto-oncogenes and inactivation of tumor suppressor genes are mutational events that result from covalent damage to DNA caused by chemical exposures. The accumulation of mutations, and not necessarily the order in which they occur, constitutes multistage carcinogenesis. *Source*: From Refs. 26,99.

information from lifestyle or occupational exposures to chemical carcinogens. Measures of age-dependent cancer incidence have shown, however, that the rate of tumor development is proportional to the sixth power of time, suggesting that at least four to six independent steps are necessary.[25] Partial scheduling of specific genetic events in this process has been possible for some cancers. Examples of sequential genetic and epigenetic changes that occur with the highest probability are those found in the development of lung cancer[26,27] and colon cancer.[28,29]

Tumor Initiation

The early concept of tumor initiation indicated that the initial changes in chemical carcinogenesis are irreversible genetic damage. However, recent data from molecular studies of preneoplastic human lung and colon tissues implicate epigenetic changes as an early event in carcinogenesis. DNA methylation of promoter regions of genes can transcriptionally silence tumor suppressor genes.[24] For mutations to accumulate, they must arise in cells that proliferate and survive the lifetime of the organism. A chemical carcinogen causes a genetic error by modifying the molecular structure of DNA that can lead to a mutation during DNA synthesis. Most often, this is brought about by forming an adduct between the chemical carcinogen or one of its functional groups and a nucleotide in DNA[7,19] (the process by which this occurs for the major classes of chemical carcinogens is discussed in detail under "Carcinogen Metabolism"). In general, a positive correlation is found between the amount of carcinogen-DNA adducts that can be detected in animal models and the number of tumors that develop.[30-33] Thus, tumors rarely develop in tissues that do not form carcinogen-DNA adducts. Carcinogen-DNA adduct formation is central to theories of chemical carcinogenesis, and it may be a necessary, but not a sufficient, prerequisite for tumor initiation (the concept of so-called nongenotoxic carcinogens is also explored under "Carcinogen Metabolism"). DNA adduct formation that causes either the activation of a proto-oncogene or the inactivation of a tumor suppressor gene can be categorized as a tumor-initiating event (see "Tumor Progression," "Oncogenes and Tumor Suppressor Genes" in this chapter).

Tumor Promotion

Tumor promotion comprises the selective clonal expansion of initiated cells. Because the accumulation rate of mutations is proportional to the rate of cell division, or at least the rate at which stem cells are replaced, clonal expansion of initiated cells, produces a larger population of cells that are at risk of further genetic changes and malignant conversion.[24,27,28] Tumor promoters are generally nonmutagenic, are not carcinogenic alone, and often (but not always) are able to mediate their biologic effects without metabolic activation. These agents are characterized by their ability to reduce the latency period for tumor formation after exposure of a tissue to a tumor initiator, or to increase the number of tumors formed in that tissue. In addition, they induce tumor formation in conjunction with a dose of an initiator that is too low to be carcinogenic alone. Croton oil (isolated from *Croton tiglium* seeds) is used widely as a tumor promoter in murine skin carcinogenesis, and the mechanism of action for its most potent constituent, 12-*O*-tetradecanoylphorbol-13-acetate, which occurs via protein kinase C activation, is arguably the best understood among tumor promoters.[34] Chemicals or agents capable of both tumor initiation and promotion are known as complete carcinogens, eg, benzo[*a*]pyrene and 4-aminobiphenyl. Identification of new tumor promoters in animal models has accelerated with the sophisticated development of model systems designed to assay for tumor promotion. Furthermore, ligand-binding properties can be determined in recombinant protein kinase C isozymes that are expressed in cell cultures.[35] Chemicals, complex mixtures of chemicals, or other agents that have been shown to have tumor-promoting properties include dioxin, benzoyl peroxide, macrocyclic lactones, bromomethylbenzanthracene, anthralin, phenol, saccharin, tryptophan, dichlorodiphenyltrichloroethane (DDT), phenobarbital, cigarette-smoke condensate, polychlorinated biphenyls (PCBs), teleocidins, cyclamates, estrogens and other hormones, bile acids, ultraviolet light, wounding, abrasion, and other chronic irritation (ie, saline lavage).[19] In addition, protein kinase C is activated and cellular diacylglycerol elevated in laboratory animals maintained on high-fat diets.[36,37]

Malignant Conversion

Malignant conversion is the transformation of a preneoplastic cell into one that expresses the malignant phenotype. This process requires further genetic changes. The total dose of a tumor promoter is less significant than frequently repeated administrations, and if the tumor promoter is discontinued before malignant conversion has occurred, premalignant or benign lesions may regress. Tumor promotion contributes to the process of carcinogenesis by the expansion of a population of initiated cells, with a growth advantage, that will then be at risk for malignant conversion. Conversion of a fraction of these cells to malignancy will be accelerated in proportion to the rate of cell division and the quantity of dividing cells in the benign tumor or preneoplastic lesion. In part, these further genetic changes may result from infidelity of DNA synthesis.[38] The relatively low probability of malignant conversion can be increased substantially by the exposure of preneoplastic cells to DNA damaging agents,[19,39] and this process may be mediated through the activation of proto-oncogenes and inactivation of tumor suppressor genes.

Tumor Progression

Tumor progression comprises the expression of the malignant phenotype and the tendency of malignant cells to acquire more aggressive characteristics over time. Also, metastasis may involve the ability of tumor cells to secrete proteases that allow invasion beyond the immediate primary tumor location. A prominent characteristic of the malignant phenotype is the propensity for genomic instability and uncontrolled growth.[40] During this process, further genetic and epigenetic changes can occur, again including the activation of proto-oncogenes and the functional loss of tumor suppressor genes. Frequently, proto-oncogenes are activated by two major mechanisms: in the case of the *ras* gene family, point mutations are found in highly specific regions of the gene (ie, the 12th, 13th, 59th, or 61st codons), and members of the *myc*, *raf*, *HER2*, and *jun* multigene families can be overexpressed, sometimes involving amplification of chromosomal segments containing these genes. Some genes are overexpressed if they are translocated and become juxtaposed to a powerful promoter, eg, the relationship of *bcl-2* and immunoglobulin heavy chain gene promoter regions in B-cell malignancies. Loss of function of tumor suppressor genes usually occurs in a bimodal fashion, and most frequently involves point mutations in one allele and loss of the second allele by a deletion, recombinational event, or chromosomal nondisjunction. These phenomena confer to the cells a growth advantage as well as the capacity for regional invasion, and ultimately, distant metastatic spread. Despite evidence for an apparent scheduling of certain mutational events, it is the accumulation of these mutations, and not the order or the stage of tumorigenesis in which they occur, that appears to be the determining factor.[26-28] Recent evidence from microarray expression analysis of human cancers supports an alternative, and not mutually exclusive, mode of tumor progression. Gene expression profiles of a primary cancer and its metastases are similar, indicating that the molecular progression of a primary cancer is generally retained in its metastases.[41,42] These results have clinical implications in molecular diagnosis of primary cancers and therapeutic strategies.

Gene-Environment Interactions and Interindividual Variation

A cornerstone of human chemical carcinogenesis is the concept of gene-environment interactions (Fig. 15-2).[8] Potential interindividual susceptibility to chemical carcinogenesis may well be defined by genetic variations in the host elements of this compound system. Functional polymorphisms in human proteins that have, or may have, a role in chemical carcinogenesis include enzymes that metabolize (ie, activate and detoxify) xenobiotic substances, enzymes that repair DNA damage, cell surface receptors that activate the phosphorylation cascade and cell-cycle control genes (ie, oncogenes and tumor suppressor genes that are elements of the signal transduction cascade).

When chemicals or xenobiotics encounter biologic systems, they become altered by metabolic processes. This is an initial facet of gene-environment interaction. The interindividual variation in carcinogen metabolism and macromolecular adduct formation arising from such processes was recognized >25 years ago.[43,44] The cytochrome P450 (CYP) multigene family is largely responsible for the metabolic activation and detoxication of many different chemical carcinogens in the human environment.[45] Cytochrome P450s are Phase I enzymes that act by adding an atom of oxygen onto the substrate; they are induced by polycyclic aromatic hydrocarbons and chlorinated hydrocarbons.[46] Phase II enzymes act on oxidized substrates and also contribute to xenobiotic metabolism. Some Phase II enzymes are methyltransferases, acetyltransferases, glutathione transferases, uridine 5′-diphosphoglucuronosyl transferases, sulfotransferases, nicotinamide adenine dinucleotide (NAD)- and nicotinamide adenine dinucleotide phosphate (NADP)-dependent alcohol dehydrogenases, aldehyde and steroid dehydrogenases, quinone reductases, NADPH diaphorase, azo reductases, aldoketoreductases, transaminases, esterases, and hydrolases. The pathways of activation and detoxification are often competitive, providing yet further potential for individual differences in propensity for

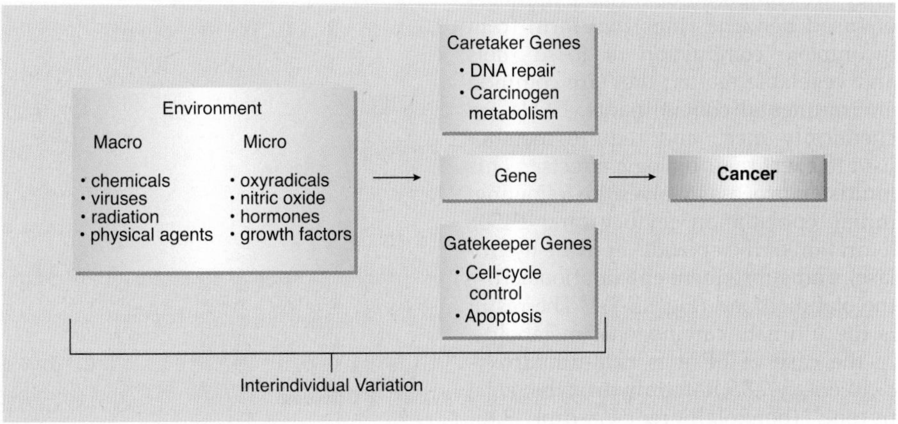

Figure 15-2 The concept of gene–environment interaction is multifaceted: (1) environmental chemicals are altered by the products of metabolic genes; (2) environmental chemicals disrupt the expression (induce or inhibit) of carcinogen metabolizing genes; and (3) environmental exposures cause changes (mutations) in cancer-related genes. The cancer-related genes have been classified as gatekeeper (eg, APC) and caretaker genes (eg, MSH1 and MLH1). The interaction of these genes with external and internal environmental agents can lead to the derangement of regulatory pathways that maintain genetic stability and cellular proliferation.

carcinogen metabolism to DNA damaging species. This scenario is further complicated by a second facet of gene-environment interaction that leads to enzyme induction or inhibition. In this case, environmental exposures alter gene expression, and genes responsible for carcinogen metabolism can be upregulated or repressed by certain chemical exposures.

A third facet of gene-environment interaction occurs when the chemical alters gene structure. Once a procarcinogen is metabolically activated to an ultimate carcinogenic form, it can bind covalently to cellular macromolecules, including DNA. This DNA damage can be repaired by several mechanisms.[47-49] Differences in rates and fidelity of DNA repair potentially influence the extent of carcinogen adduct formation (ie, biologically effective dose) and, consequently, the total amount of genetic damage. The consequences of polymorphisms in genes controlling the cell cycle (serine/threonine kinases, transcription factors, cyclins, cyclin-dependent kinase inhibitors, and cell surface receptors) are much less clear. However, molecular epidemiologic evidence suggests that certain common variants of these types of genes have a role in susceptibility to chemical carcinogenesis.[50,51] The evaluation of polymorphisms as potential biomarkers of susceptibility in the human population is discussed under "Implications for Molecular Epidemiology, Risk Assessment, and Cancer Prevention."

Carcinogen Metabolism

Polycyclic aromatic hydrocarbons (PAHs), eg, benzo[*a*]pyrene (BP), were the first carcinogens to be chemically isolated.[52] They are composed of variable numbers of fused benzene rings that form from incomplete combustion of fossil fuels and vegetable matter; they are common environmental contaminants. PAHs are chemically inert, and require metabolism to exert their biologic effects.[53] This multistep process involves the following: initial epoxidation (cytochrome P450), hydration of the epoxide (epoxide hydrolase), and subsequent epoxidation across the olefinic bond (Fig. 15-3).[45] The result is the ultimate carcinogenic metabolite; in the case of BP it is *r*7,*t*8-dihydroxy-*c*9,10 epoxy-7,8,9,10-tetrahydroxybenzo[*a*]pyrene (benzo[*a*]pyrene-7,8-diol 9,10-epoxide, BPDE).[54] The biology of cytochrome P450 (eg, CYP1A1) metabolism has been elucidated providing a molecular basis for inducibility and interindividual variation and variations in cytochrome levels among humans have been documented.[55] The arene ring of BPDE opens spontaneously at the 10th position, revealing a carbonium ion that can form a covalent addition product (adduct) with cellular macromolecules, including DNA. Several DNA adducts can be formed, the most abundant being at the exocyclic amino group of deoxyguanosine ([7R]-*N*2-[10-{7ß,8a,9a-trihydroxy-7,8,9,10-tetrahydro-benz[*a*]pyrene}yl]-deoxyguanosine; BPdG). One electron oxidation has been suggested as an alternative pathway of PAH activation, here a radical cation forms at the meso position (L-region). The resulting DNA adducts at the C8 of guanine (BP-6-C8Gua and BP-6-C8dGua), the N7 of guanine and adenine (BP-6-*N*7Gua and BP-6-*N*7Ade) likely undergo spontaneous depurination (Fig. 15-4). Firm evidence for the exfoliation of these adducts in urine has been provided.[56,57]

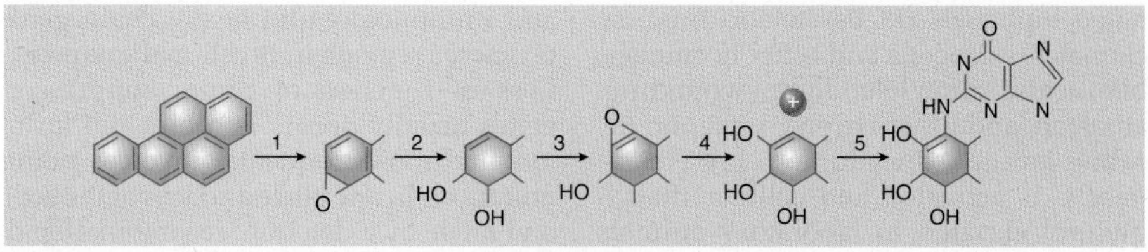

Figure 15-3 Metabolic activation of benzol[*a*]pyrene. (1) Cytochrome P450 (CYP1A1) catalyses initial epoxidation across the 1-2, 2-3, 4-5, 7-8 (shown), 9-10 and 11-12 positions. (2) With the exception of the 1-2 and 2-3 oxides that convert to phenols, epoxide hydrolase may catalyze the formation of dihydrodiols. (3) Benzo[*a*]pyrene-7, 8-dihydrodiol is further metabolized at the olefinic double bond by cytochrome P450 (CYP1B1 and CYP3A4) to form avicinal diol-epoxide (r7, t8-dihydroxy-c9, 10 epoxy-7,8,9,10-tetrahydroxybenz[*a*]pyrene). (4) The highly unstable arene ring opens spontaneously to form a carbocation. (5) This electrophic species forms a covalent bond between the 10 position of the hydrocarbon and the exocyclic amino group of deoxyguanosine.

Aromatic amines are found in cigarette smoke, diesel exhaust, industrial environments and certain cooked foods. The compound, 4-aminobiphenyl, is thought to be responsible for bladder cancer among tobacco smokers and rubber industry workers.[58] In addition, nitrated polycyclic aromatic hydrocarbons are environmental contaminants that are related to aromatic amines by nitroreduction. Aromatic amines can be converted to an aromatic amide that is catalyzed by an acetyl coenzyme A-dependent acetylation.[59] The acetylation phenotype varies among the population. Persons with the rapid acetylator phenotype are at a higher risk of colon cancer, whereas, those who are slow acetylators are at risk of bladder cancer.[60] This latter association may result from the fact that activation of aromatic amines by N-oxidation is a competing pathway for aromatic amine metabolism. The N-hydroxylation products when protonated (eg, in the urinary bladder) are reactive and can cause DNA damage.

An initial activation step for both aromatic amines and amides is N-oxidation by CYP1A2. The reactions

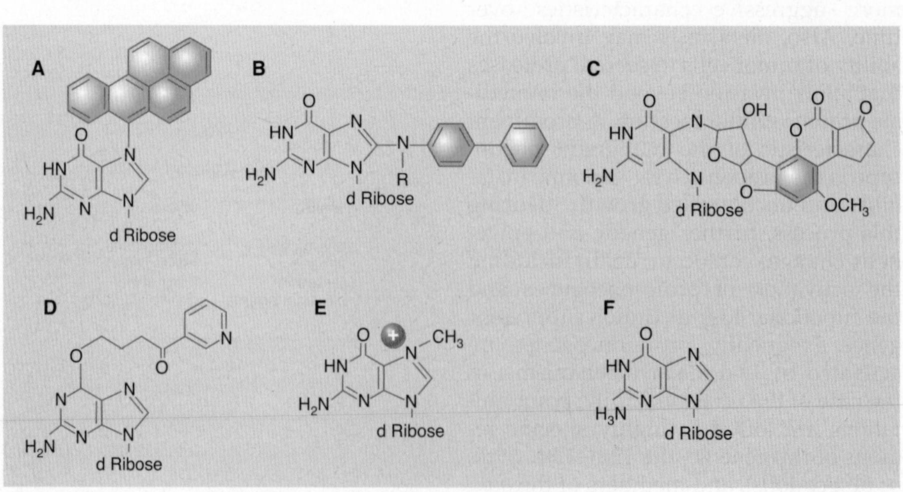

Figure 15-4 Examples of carcinogen–DNA adducts: (**A**) N7(benzo[*a*]pyren-6-yl)guanine; (**B**) *N*-(deoxyguanosin-8-yl)-{acetyl}aminobiphenyl (when R= H the adduct is not acetylated [R can also be an acetyl group]); (**C**) 8,9-dihydro-8-(N5-formyl- 2′, 5′, 6′-triamino-4′-oxo-N5-pyrimidyl)-9-hydroxy-aflatoxin B1; (**D**) O6-[4-Oxo-4(3-pyridyl)butyl]guanine, amutagenic lesion formed by the metabolism of the tobacco-specific nitrosamine, NNK 73,74 ; (**E**) *N*7-methyldeoxygua-nosine; and (**F**) 3-methyladenosine. Adducts **E** and **F** can also result as the small alkyl products of NNK metabolism.[73,74]

Table 15-2 Chronic Inflammation and Infection Can Increase Cancer Risk

Disease	Tumor Site	Risk
Inherited		
Hemochromatosis	Liver	219
Crohn disease	Colon	3
Ulcerative colitis	Colon	6
Acquired		
Viral		
Hepatitis B	Liver	88
Hepatitis C	Liver	30
Bacterial		
Helicobacter pylori	Gastric	11
PID	Ovary	3
Parasitic		
Schistosoma hematobium	Urinary bladder	2-14
Schistosoma japonicum	Colon	2-6
Liver fluke	Liver	14
Chemical/physical/metabolic		
Acid reflux	Esophagus	50-100
Asbestos	Lung pleural	>10
Obesity	Multiple sites	1.3-6.5

"18% of human cancers, ie, 1.6 million per year, are related to infection." B. Stewart and P. Kleihues, World Cancer, Report, IARC Press, Lyon 2003, p. 57.
Rheumatoid arthritis is an example of a chronic inflammatory disease without a marked increased cancer risk, eg, joint sarcoma.
Oncogenic human papilloma viruses are examples of cancer-prone chronic infections without inflammation.

of *N*-hydroxyarylamines with DNA appear to be acid catalyzed, but they can be further activated by either an acetyl coenzyme A-dependent *O*-acetylase or a 3′-phosphoadenosine-5′phosphosulfate-dependent *O*-sulfotransferase. The *N*-arylhydroxamic acids arise from the acetylation of *N*-hydroxyarylamines or N-hydroxylation of aromatic amides; they are not electrophilic and require further activation. The predominant pathway here occurs through acetyltransferase-catalyzed rearrangement to a reactive *N*-acetoxyarylamine. Sulfotransferase catalysis forms *N*-sulphonyloxy arylamides. This complex pathway results in two major adduct types, amides (acetylated) and amines (nonacetylated).

Heterocyclic amines form in food cooking from pyrolysis (>150°C) of amino acids, creatinine, and glucose. They have been recognized as food mutagens, shown to form DNA adducts and cause liver tumors in primates.[61] These compounds are activated by CYP1A2, and their metabolites form DNA adducts in humans. The *N*-hydroxy metabolites of heterocyclic amines like 2-amino-3-methyl-imidazo-[4,5-*f*]quinoline (IQ) can react directly with DNA. Enzymic O-esterification of *N*-hydroxy metabolites plays a key role in activating food mutagens, and because the *N*-hydroxy metabolites are good substrates for transacetylases these chemicals may be implicated in colorectal cancer.

Aflatoxins (B1, B2, G1, and G2), metabolites of *Aspergillus flavus*, contaminate cereals, grain, and nuts. A positive correlation exists between dietary aflatoxin exposure and the incidence of liver cancer in developing countries, where grain spoilage is high. Aflatoxins B1 and G1 have an olefinic double bond at the 8,9-position that can be oxidized by several cytochrome P450.[62] This implies that the olefinic 8,9-bond is the activation site. Further support for this mechanism comes from studies of DNA adducts and the prevalence of *TP53* mutations in liver cancer. In people with liver cancer from parts of China and Africa, where food spoilage caused by molds is high, G:C to T:A transversions in codon 249 are frequent.[63] This phenomenon is consistent with metabolic activation of aflatoxin B1 and the formation of depurinating carcinogen-deoxyguanosine adducts.

Carcinogenic *N*-nitrosamines are ubiquitous environmental contaminants and can be found in food, alcoholic beverages, cosmetics, cutting oils, hydraulic fluid, rubber, and tobacco.[64] Tobacco-specific *N*-nitrosamines (TSNs), eg, 4-(methylnitrosoamino)-1-(3-pyridyl)-1-butanone (NNK), are not formed by pyrolysis, which accounts for the highly carcinogenic nature of snuff and chewing tobacco.[65] TSNs are not symmetric so both small alkyl adducts and large bulky adducts can be formed; eg, NNK metabolism gives rise to either a positively charged pyridyl-oxobutyl ion or a positively charged methyl ion, both of which are able to alkylate DNA.[65] Endogenous nitrosamines form when an amine reacts with nitrate alone or nitrite in the presence of acid. Thus, nitrite (used to cure meats) and l-cysteine, in the presence of acetaldehyde (from alcohol), form *N*-nitrosothiazolidine-4-carboxylic acid. *N*-nitrosodimethylamine undergoes α-hydroxylation, catalyzed primarily by the alcohol inducible CYP2E1, to form an unstable α-hydroxynitrosamine. The breakdown products are formaldehyde and methyl diazohydroxide. Methyl diazohydroxide and related compounds are powerful alkylating agents that can add a small functional group at multiple sites in DNA.

Nongenotoxic carcinogens may function at the level of the microenvironment by dysregulation of hormones and growth factors, or indirectly inducing DNA damage and mutations through the action of free radicals.[66] These chemicals are none or poorly reactive and are resistant to activation through metabolism. They are also characterized by their persistence in biological systems and consequently tend to accumulate in the food chain. However, they can stimulate oxyradical formation by at least three mechanisms: organochlorine species interact with the Ah receptor which can lead to cytochrome P450 induction and associated oxyradical formation; interaction with other receptors, like IFN-γ, can stimulate elements of the primary immune response and again generate oxyradicals; and agents like asbestos can promote oxyradical formation through interaction with ferrous metal. The resulting oxyradicals can then damage DNA. Some of the so-called "nongenotoxic" carcinogens might more appropriately be considered to be "oxyradical triggers." Indeed, chronic inflammatory states, which involve oxyradical formation, can also be cancer risk factors.[66]

Chronic Inflammation and Cancer

More than a century ago, the German pathologist, Virchow proposed that inflammation was associated with cancer.[67] Infection and inflammation significantly contribute to about 25% of cancer cases worldwide (Table 15-3).[68] Free radicals, endogenous chemicals, are released during the inflammatory response. These reactive oxygen species (ROS) and reactive nitrogen species (RNS) are generated as a physiological protective response to pathogenic microorganisms and toxic agents. During chronic inflammation, eg, chronic viral hepatitis, and oxyradical overload conditions, eg, hemochromatosis, these free radicals can induce genetic and epigenetic changes including somatic mutations in cancer-related genes and posttranslational modifications in proteins involved in DNA repair, apoptosis, and arachidonic acid cascade (Fig. 15-5).[68] Epigenetic transcriptional silencing of cancer-related genes including p16, RUNX3, and MLH1, by DNA methylation of their promoter regions has been associated with chronic inflammation in ulcerative colitis and Barretts esophagus.[69,70] MicroRNA expression is also regulated by inflammatory cytokines and free radicals.[71-75] These non-protein coding small RNAs of about 22 base pairs regulate mRNA stability and translation into proteins.[71,76] MicroRNA genes are regulated by transcription factors including the p53 tumor suppressor protein[75] and are involved in carcinogenesis including tumor invasion and metastasis.[77,78] Not surprisingly, microRNAs are also clinical biomarkers associated with diagnosis, prognosis, and therapeutic outcome of cancer.[71,79-83]

DNA Damage and Repair

The DNA damage initials a complex network of signaling cascades.[84,85] The

Table 15-3 Examples of Disease Susceptibility and Disease Syndromes Associated with Mutations in DNA-Repair Genes

Gene	Function	Pathology of Cancer
Cancer susceptibility		
MMR[a]		
MLH1	Damage recognition	HNPCC2[b], glioma
MLH2	DNA binding	HNPCC1, ovarian cancer
MSH3	–	Endometrial cancer
MSH6	Sliding clamp	Endometrial cancer, HNPCC1
PMS1	Damage recognition	HNPCC3
PMS2	Repair initiation	HNPCC4, glioblastoma
NER		
BRCA-1	Directs *p53* transcription toward DNA-repair pathways	Breast cancer, ovarian cancer
RB1	Cell-cycle restriction	Retinoblastoma, breast cancer, and progression osteosarcoma
DSB		
BRCA-2	Regulation of RAD51	Breast cancer, pancreatic cancer
HR		
RAD54	Helicase	Colon cancer, breast cancer, NHL
Other		
TP53 (DSB, NER, HR)	Cell-cycle control; exonuclease; apoptosis; DNA binding	Colon cancer, common somatic defect in human cancer in general; inherited in Li-Fraumeni syndrome and some breast cancers
hOgg1 (Various)	Glycosylase	Cancer susceptibility
Xeroderma pigmentosum (XP)		
NER		
XPD	DNA helicase	Skin and neurologic, but later onset than XPA
XPB	DNA helicase	Skin lesions
XPG	Endonuclease	Acute sun sensitivity, mild symptoms; late skin cancer
XPC (and BER)	Exonuclease	Mental retardation; skin sensitivity; microcephaly
DDB1 and DDB2	Binds specific DNA damage	XPE–Mild skin sensitivity
XPA	Damage sensor	XPA–Skin and neurologic problems: the most severe XP
XPC	Damage sensor	XPC–Skin, tongue, and lip cancer
XPE	Damage sensor	XPE–Neurologically normal
PRR		
POLH	Polymerase	XPV–Mild to severe skin sensitivity; neurologically normal
Other syndromes		
NER		
Cockaynes		
CSB	ATPase	Cutaneous, ocular, neurologic, and somatic abnormalities; short stature, progressive deafness, mental retardation, neurologic degeneration, early death; sometimes presents together with XPB
Juberg-Marsidi		
ATRX	Putative helicase	Thalassemia/mental retardation
SB		
Nijmegen		
NBS1	Nibrin, cell-cycle regulation	Microencephaly; mental retardation; immunodeficiency; growth retardation; radiation sensitivity; predisposition to malignancy
Ataxia-telangiectasia		
ATM	Phosphorylation	Neurologic deficiencies, manifest by inability to coordinate muscle actions; skin and corneal telangiectases. Leukemia, lymphoma, and other malignancies (breast cancer?)
MRE11(Ataxia-like)	Exonuclease	DNA damage sensitivity; genomic instability; telomere shortening; aberrant meiosis; severe combined immunodeficiency
PRKDC	Ser/Thr kinase	SCID
Bloom's		
BLM	DNA helicase	High rate of spontaneous lymphatic and other malignancy; high-rate SCE[c]
Fanconi anemia		
FANCA-G	Protein control	Multiple congenital malformations; chromosome breaks; pancytopenia Telomere shortening
Werner		
WRN	DNA helicase/exonuclease	Premature senility, short stature, exonuclease rapidly progressing cataracts, loss of connective tissue and muscle, premature arteriosclerosis, increase risk of malignancy
RecQ4	DNA helicase	Osteosarcoma; premature aging

[a] **Repair mechanisms**: BER, base excision; DSB, double-strand break; HR, homologous recombination; MMR, mismatch; NER, nucleotide excision; PRR, postreplication; SB, strand break.
[b] **Diseases**: HNPCC, hereditary nonpolyposis colon cancer; NHL, non-Hodgkin lymphoma.
[c] **Other abbreviations**: SCE, sister chromatid exchange; SCID, severe combined immunodeficiency.

chemical structure of DNA can be altered by a carcinogen in several ways: the formation of large bulky aromatic adducts, small alkyl adducts, oxidation, dimerization, and deamination. In addition, double- and single-strand breaks can occur. Chemical carcinogens can cause epigenetic changes, such as altering the DNA methylation status that leads to the silencing of specific gene expression.[86] A complex pattern of carcinogen-DNA adducts likely results from a variety of environmental exposures, because of the mixture of different chemical carcinogens present.

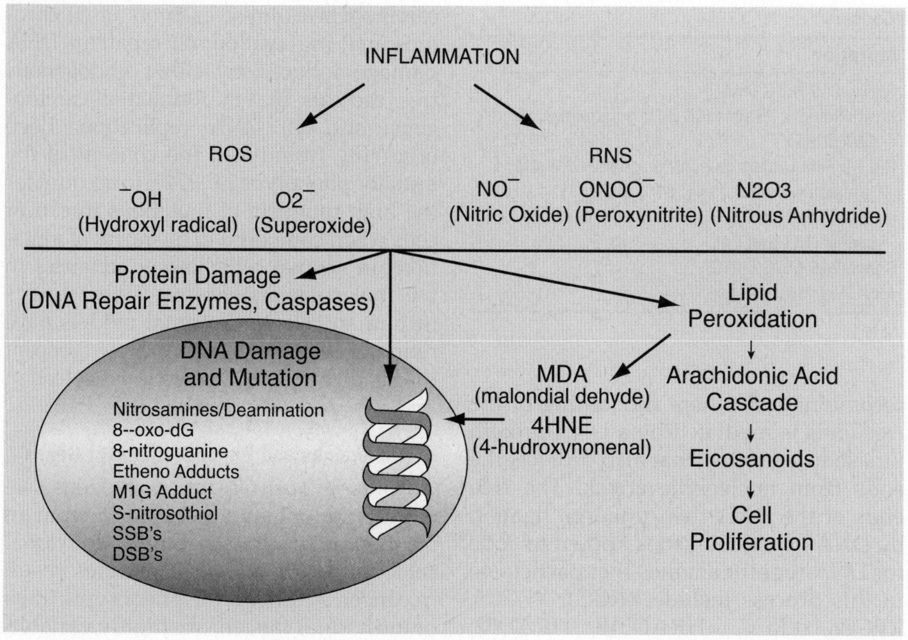

Figure 15-5 Several reactive oxygen (ROS) and reactive nitrogen species (RNS) are generated during chronic inflammation. The reactive species can induce DNA damage, including point mutations in cancer-related genes, and modifications in essential cellular proteins that are involved in DNA repair, apoptosis, and cell cycle, either directly or indirectly through the activation of lipid peroxidation and generation of reactive aldehydes, eg, malondialdehyde (MDA) and 4-hydroxynonenal (4-HNE).[161]

BPDE reacts with the exocyclic (N2) amino group of deoxyguanosine and resides within the minor groove of the double helix; it is typical of polycyclic aromatic hydrocarbons. This adduct, BPdG, is probably the most common, persistent adduct of benzo[*a*]pyrene in mammalian systems, but others are possible. Adducts like BPdG are thought to induce *ras* gene mutations, which are common in tobacco-related lung cancers.[87] Aromatic amine adducts are more complex, because they have both acetylated and nonacetylated metabolic intermediates, and they form covalent bonds at the C8, N2, and sometimes O6 positions of deoxyguanosine as well as deoxyadenosine. The major adducts, however, are C8-deoxyguanosine adducts, which reside predominantly in the major groove of the DNA double helix (see Fig. 15-4).[59]

Aflatoxin B1 and G1 activation through hydroxylation of the olefinic 8,9-position results in adduct formation at the N7-position of deoxyguanosine. These are relatively unstable with a half-life of ~50 h at neutral pH; depurination products have been detected in urine.[88] The aflatoxin B1-*N*7-deoxyguanosine adduct also can undergo ring opening to yield two pyrimidine adducts; alternately, aflatoxin B1-8,9-dihydrodiol could result, restoring the DNA molecular structure if hydrolysis of the original adduct occurs.[89]

DNA alkylation can occur at many sites either following the metabolic activation of certain *N*-nitrosamines, or directly by the action of the *N*-alkylureas (*N*-methyl-*N*-nitrosourea) or the *N*-nitrosoguanidines. The protonated alkyl-functional groups that become available to form lesions in DNA generally attack the following nucleophilic centers: adenine (N1, N3, and N7), cytosine (N3), guanine (N2, O6, and N7), and thymine (O2, N3, and O4). Some of these lesions are known to be repaired (*O*6-methyldeoxyguanosine), while others are not (*N*7-methyldeoxyguanosine), which explains why *O*6-methyldeoxyguanosine is a promutagenic lesion and *N*7-methyldeoxyguanosine is not.[64,90]

Another potentially mutagenic cause of DNA damage is the deamination of DNA-methylated cytosine residues. 5-Methylcytosine comprises ~3% of deoxynucleotides. In this case, deamination at a CpG dinucleotide gives rise to a TpG mismatch. Repair of this lesion most often restores the CpG; however, repair may cause a mutation (TpA).[91] Deamination of cytosine also can generate a C to T transition if uracil glycosylation and G-T mismatch repair are inefficient.

Oxyradical damage can form thymine glycol or 8-hydroxydeoxyguanosine adducts. Exposure to organic peroxides (catechol, hydroquinone, and 4-nitroquinoline-*N*-oxide) leads to oxyradical damage; however, oxyradicals and hydrogen peroxide can be generated in lipid peroxidation and the catalytic cycling of some enzymes, as well as environmental sources (eg, tobacco smoke).[68,92] Certain drugs and plasticizers can stimulate cells to produce peroxisomes, and oxyradical formation is mediated through protein kinase C when inflammatory cells are exposed to tumor promoters like phorbol esters.[93,94] Oxyradicals can contribute to deamination through induction of NO synthetase.[95]

Maintenance of genome integrity requires mitigation of DNA damage. Thus, diminished DNA-repair capacity is associated with carcinogenesis, birth defects, premature aging, and foreshortened life span. DNA-repair enzymes act at DNA damage sites caused by chemical carcinogens, and six major mechanisms are known: direct DNA repair, nucleotide excision repair, base excision repair, nonhomologous end joining (double-strand break repair), mismatch repair, and homologous recombination (postreplication repair).[48,91]

In the presence of nonlethal DNA damage, cell-cycle progression is postponed for repair mechanisms. This highly coordinated process involves multiple genes. A DNA-damage recognition sensor triggers a signal transduction cascade and downstream factors direct G1 and G2 arrest in concert with the proteins operationally responsible for the repair process. Although there are at least six discrete repair mechanisms, within five of them there are numerous multiprotein complexes comprising all the machinery necessary to accomplish the step-by-step repair function.

Generically, DNA repair requires damage recognition, damage removal or excision, resynthesis or patch synthesis, and ligation. Recent advances have led to the cloning of more than 130 human genes involved in five of these DNA-repair pathways. A list of these genes and their specific functions was published elsewhere.[96] These genes are responsible for the fidelity of DNA repair, and when they are defective the mutation rate increases. This is the mutator phenotype.[97] Mutations in at least 30 DNA-repair associated genes have been linked to increased cancer susceptibility or premature aging (Table 15-4).[96] Moreover, the role of common polymorphisms in some of these genes are associated with increased susceptibility in a gene-environment interaction scenario (this is discussed under "Implications for Molecular Epidemiology, Risk Assessment, and Cancer Prevention"). Indeed, molecular epidemiologic evidence suggests that tobacco-smoking-related lung cancer is associated with a polymorphism in the nucleotide excision repair gene, XPC (ERCC2).[98]

Direct DNA repair is effected by DNA alkyltransferases. These enzymes catalyze translocation of the alkyl moiety from an alkylated base (eg, *O*6-methyldeoxyguanosine) to a cysteine residue at their active site in the absence of DNA strand scission. Thus, one molecule of the enzyme is capable of repairing one DNA alkyl lesion, in a suicide

Table 15-4 **Mutational Spectra of TP53 in Human Cancers**[a]

Carcinogen Exposure	Neoplasm	Mutation
Aflatoxin B1	Hepatocellular carcinoma	Codon 249 (AGG 6 AGT)
Sunlight	Skin carcinoma	Dipyrimidine mutations (CC 6 TT) on nontranscribed DNA strand
Tobacco smoke	Lung carcinoma	G:C 6 T:A mutations on nontranscribed DNA strand (frequently codons: 157, 248, and 273)
Tobacco and alcohol	Carcinoma of the head and neck	Increased frequency p53 mutations (especially codons 157 and 248)
Radon	Lung carcinoma	Codon 249 (AGG 6 ATG)
Vinyl chloride	Hepatic angiosarcoma	A:T 6 T:A transversions

[a]For reviews see Refs, 116, 124, 127, 166.

mechanism. The inactivation of this mechanism by promoter hypermethylation is associated with Kras G to A mutations in colon cancer.[99]

In DNA nucleotide excision repair, lesion recognition, preincision, incision, gap-filling, and ligation are required, and the so-called excinuclease complex comprises 16 or more different proteins. Large distortions caused by bulky DNA adducts (eg, BPDE-dG and 4ABP-dC) are recognized (XPA) and removed by endonucleases (XPF, XPG, FEN). A patch is then constructed (pol, pol e) and the free ends are ligated.

Base excision repair also removes a DNA segment containing an adduct; however, small adducts (eg, 3-methyladenine) are generally the target so that there is overlap with direct repair. The adduct is removed by a glycosylase (hOgg1, UDG), an apurinic endonuclease (APE1 or HAP1) degrades a few bases on the damaged strand, and a patch is synthesized (pol ß) and ligated (DNA ligases: I, II, IIIa, IIIß, and IV).

DNA mismatches occasionally occur, because excision repair processes incorporate unmodified or conventional, but noncomplementary, Watson-Crick bases opposite each other in the DNA helix. Transition mispairs (G-T or A-C) are repaired by the mismatch repair process more efficiently than transversion mispairs (G-G, A-A, G-A, C-C, C-T, and T-T). The mechanism for correcting mispairings is similar to that for nucleotide excision repair and resynthesis described earlier, but it generally involves the excision of large pieces of the DNA containing mispairings. Because the mismatch recognition protein is required to bind simultaneously to the mismatch and an unmethylated adenine in a GATC recognition sequence, it removes the whole intervening DNA sequence. The parental template strand is then used by the polymerase to fill the gap.

Double-strand DNA breaks can occur from exposure to ionizing radiation and oxidation. Consequences of double-strand DNA breaks are the inhibition of replication and transcription, and loss of heterozygosity. Double-strand DNA break repair occurs through homologous recombination, where the joining of the free ends is mediated by a DNA-protein kinase in a process that also protects the ends from nucleolytic attack. The free ends of the DNA then undergo ligation by DNA ligase IV. Genes known to code for DNA-repair enzymes that participate in this process include XRCC4, XRCC5, XRCC6, XRCC7, HRAD51B, HRAD52, RPA, and ATM.[95]

Postreplication repair is a damage-tolerance mechanism and it occurs in response to DNA replication on a damaged template. The DNA polymerase stops at the replication fork when DNA damage is detected on the parental strand. Alternately, the polymerase proceeds past the lesion, leaving a gap in the newly synthesized strand. The gap is filled in one of two ways: either by recombination of the homologous parent strand with the daughter strand in a process that is mediated by a helical nucleoprotein (RAD51); or when a single nucleotide gap remains, mammalian DNA polymerases insert an adenine residue. Consequently, this mechanism may lead to recombinational events as well as base-mispairing.

Persistent non-repaired DNA damage blocks the replication machinery. Cells have evolved translesion synthesis (TLS) DNA polymerases to bypass these blocks.[100] Most of these TLS polymerases belong to the recently discovered Y-family, have much lower stringency than replicative polymerases, and thus are error prone. An increased mutation frequency is an evolutionary trade-off for cellular survival.

Mutator Phenotype

Cancer cells contain substantial numbers of genetic abnormalities when compared with normal cells. These abnormalities range from gross changes such as nondiploid number of chromosomes, ie, aneuploidy, and translocations or rearrangements of chromosomes, to much smaller changes in the DNA sequence including deletions, insertions, and single nucleotide substitutions. Therefore, carcinogenesis involves *errors* in (1) chromosomal segregation; (2) repair of DNA damage induced by either endogenous free radicals or environmental carcinogens; and (3) DNA replication. Loeb originally formulated the concept of the mutator phenotype in 1974[101] to account for the high numbers of mutations in cancer cells when compared to the rarity of mutations in normal cells. Recent advances in the molecular analysis of carcinogenesis in human cells and animal models have refined the mutator phenotype[13] concept that is also linked to the clonal selection theory proposed by Nowell (Fig. 15-6).[102]

Oncogenes and Tumor Suppressor Genes

Chronic exposures to carcinogens, accumulation of mutations, development of the mutator phenotype, and clonal selection during several decades result in cancer. Although the phenotypic traits of individual cancers are highly variable, commonly acquired capabilities include limitless replicative potential, self-sufficiency in growth signals, insensitivity to antigrowth signals, evading apoptosis, tissue invasion, sustained angiogenesis, and metastasis.[103,104] These phenotypic traits reflect a complex molecular circuitry of biochemical pathways and protein machines within cancer cells.[21]

The genes encoding the proteins within the cancer-associated molecular circuitry are of many functional classes and, historically, have been conceptually divided into oncogenes and tumor suppressor genes.[21,104] Detailed descriptions of oncogenes and tumor suppressor genes are found in Chapters 4 to 7. The *ras* oncogene and the *TP53* tumor suppressor gene will be used as examples of molecular targets of chemical carcinogens.

Activated *ras* genes predominate as the family of oncogenes to be isolated from solid tumors that are induced by chemicals in laboratory animals. Members of the *ras* gene family code for proteins of molecular weight 21,000 (p21); these proteins are membrane bound, have GTPase activity, and form complexes with other proteins. The *ras* genes code for small G-proteins (guanine nucleotide binding) that exert a powerful proliferative response through the signal transduction cascade. The first direct evidence of proto-oncogene activation by a chemical carcinogen was obtained from in vitro studies.[105] A wild-type recombinant clone of the human *Ha-ras* gene (pEC) was modified with benzo[*a*]pyrene diolepoxide. The treated plasmid was then used to transfect murine NIH-3T3 cells, with the result that the transformed cell foci contained the same point mutations (in either codon 12 or 61) known to exist in activated *ras* genes isolated from human tumors including the bladder (pEJ). In animal models of chemical carcinogen-

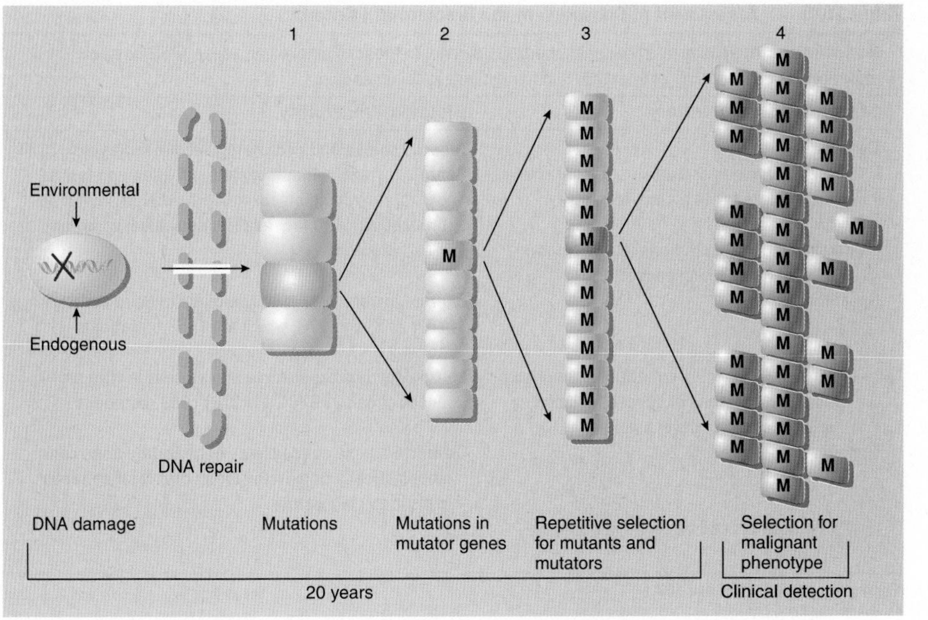

Figure 15-6 Mutation accumulation during tumor progression. (1) Random mutations result when DNA damage exceeds the cell's capacity for error-free DNA repair. (2) These random mutations can result in clonal expansion and mutations in mutator genes (M). (3) Repetitive rounds of selection for mutants yield coselection mutants in mutator genes. (4) From this population of mutant cancer cells, there is selection for cells that escape the host's regulatory mechanisms for the control of cell replication, invasion, and metastasis. *Source*: Modified from Ref. 13.

esis and surveys of different types of human tumors that arise from a variety of environmental exposures, *ras* mutations have been found.[35,106,107] For example, tobacco smoke can mutate *K-ras* during the molecular pathogenesis of human lung adenocarcinoma.[108] In rodents, polycyclic aromatic hydrocarbons (3-methylcholanthrene, 7,12-dimethylbenz[*a*]anthracene, and benzo[*a*]pyrene) have been used repeatedly to produce both benign tumors and malignant carcinomas. A large proportion of these premalignant and malignant lesions have mutations in either the 12th or 61st codons. Similarly, treatment of rats with either 7,12-dimethylbenz[*a*] anthracene or *N*-methyl-*N*-nitrosourea resulted in the development of mammary carcinomas containing *ras* codon 12 or 61 mutations. These types of mutations also have been observed in mouse skin after initiation with 7,12-dimethylbenz[*a*] anthracene and tumor promotion with 12-*O*-tetradecanoylphorbol-13-acetate. Mutations in *ras* have been found in mouse liver after treatment with vinyl carbamate, hydroxydehydroestragole, or *N*-hydroxy-2-acetylaminofluorene. The same point mutations have been found in murine thymic lymphomas after treatment with *N*-methyl-*N*-nitrosourea or γ-radiation, and in other rodent skin models after treatment with methylmethanesulfonate, α-propiolactone, dimethylcarbamyl chloride, or *N*-methyl-*N*9-nitro-*N*-nitrosoguanidine.

These data indicate that chemical carcinogens may produce site-specific mutations based, in part, on nucleoside selectivity of the ultimate carcinogen. Persistence of a specific mutation, however, also depends on the amino acid substitution in that the function of the mutant protein is altered to confer on the cell a selective clonal growth advantage. The types of mutations that are found in chemically activated *ras* genes cause conformational changes that alter protein binding (GTPase-activating protein) in such a way that the *ras*-MAP kinase pathway is permanently activated. Data support the hypothesis that *ras* activation is associated with malignant conversion as well as tumor initiation. Transfection of activated *ras* genes into benign papillomas that did not contain a constitutively activated *ras* gene caused malignant progression.[107] These and other results implicate *ras* mutations in chemical carcinogenesis. Similarly, malignant transformation occurred when immortalized human bronchial epithelial cells were transfected with an activated *ras* gene.[109,110] *Ki-ras* gene mutations are also one of many changes that can arise either early or late in the development of colorectal carcinoma.[111] These findings indicate that the accumulation of mutations, and not necessarily the order in which they occur, contributes to multistage carcinogenesis. Furthermore, the stage of carcinogenesis in which each mutation occurs is not necessarily fixed. In the model for human colorectal carcinoma, *ras* mutations most often occur during malignant conversion, but can be an early event (ie, tumor initiation), but in the rodent skin models, *ras* mutations appear to be primarily a tumor-initiating event. These differences may reflect the type of exposure, both in terms of chemical class and chronic vs acute exposure, or they may be a function of tissue type.

The *TP53* tumor suppressor gene is central in the response pathway to cellular stress.[112] For example, DNA damage caused by chemical carcinogens activates the p53 tumor suppressor protein by posttranslational modification to transduce signals to "guard the genome"[113] by engaging cell-cycle checkpoints and enhancing DNA repair, and as a fail-safe mechanism, to cause replicative senescence or apoptotic death.[114,115] Mutations in the *TP53* gene or inactivation of its encoded protein by viral oncoproteins generally lead to a loss of these cellular defense functions. Not surprisingly, *TP53* mutations are common in human cancer.[116-120]

Molecular analysis of *TP53* can give clues to the environmental etiology of cancer (Table 15-4). It is implicit from the preceding text (see "DNA Damage and Repair") that the covalent binding of activated carcinogens to DNA is not random. Therefore, the formation of a particular DNA lesion to some extent may be deduced from the resulting mutation. A dramatic example of this phenomenon is the previously mentioned *TP53* codon 249 mutation, which is detected in almost all aflatoxin-related hepatocellular carcinomas.[117,121,122] The striking nature of this association could arise by two distinct mechanisms. First, the third base in codon 249 (AGG) may be unusually susceptible to activated aflatoxin B1 mutations. As discussed earlier, aflatoxin B1-8,9-oxide causes a promutagenic lesion by covalently binding to the N7 position of deoxyguanosine. Alternately, cells bearing the codon 249 lesion may have an important selective growth advantage. Evidence that a combination of these factors is responsible has been presented as well.[121] Another prominent example where circumstantial evidence points to specific molecular events is that of *TP53* mutations indicative of pyrimidine dimer formation in ultraviolet light–related skin cancers.[123] In the case of tobacco smoking and lung cancer, G:C to T:A transversions indicate the formation of adducts from activated bulky carcinogens (eg, polycyclic aromatic hydrocarbons).[116,124,125]

Assessment of Causation by the Bradford-Hill Criteria

Results obtained from molecular epidemiologic studies can be used for the assessment of causation. Using the "weight of the evidence" principle, Bradford-Hill proposed criteria in the assessment of cancer causation, including strength of association (consistency, specificity, and temporality) and biologic plausibility.[126] These criteria can be applied for the analysis of data obtained in molecular epidemiologic studies.[127] Cigarette smoking has been established as a major risk factor for the incidence of lung cancer (Table 15-5). Codons 157, 248, and 273 of *TP53* are designated as mutational hotspots in lung cancer. The majority of mutations found at these codons are G to T transversions. Furthermore, besides lung cancer, codon 157 also constitutes one of the hotspots for G to T transversions in breast, and head and neck cancers. In smoking-associated lung cancer, the occurrence of G to T transversions has been linked to the presence of benzo[*a*]pyrene in cigarette smoke. Interestingly, codon 157 (GTC to TTC) mutations are not found in lung cancer from never smokers.[116-118] A dose-dependent increase in *TP53* G to T transversion mutations with cigarette smoking has been reported in lung cancer.[128] Benzo[*a*]pyrene diolepoxide, the metabolically activated form of benzo[*a*]pyrene, has been shown to bind to guanosine residues in codons 157, 248, and 273, which are mutational hotspots in lung cancer.[129] Also, cigarette-smoke condensate or benzo[*a*]pyrene neoplastically transforms in vitro human bronchial epithelial cells.[130] In general, molecular and epidemiologic data provide only circumstantial evidence for causation. Bradford-Hill criteria provide a framework for the logical consideration of converging lines of evidence in cancer etiology.

Table 15-5 **Assessment of Causation by the Bradford-Hill Criteria**[a]

Hypothesis: The chemical carcinogen, benzo[α]pyrene, in tobacco smoke can cause TP53 hotspot mutations at codons 157, 248, and 273 in human lung carcinogenesis

Strength of Association	Biologic Plausibility
Consistency	Tobacco smoke and benzo[*a*]pyrene are mutagens
Cigarette smoking or exposure to coal smoke is associated with a dose-response	Benzo[α]pyrene is metabolically activated and forms benzo[*a*]pyrene diolepoxide-DNA adducts in human bronchus in vitro (75-fold interindividual variation)
Increase in *TP53* mutations (G to T transversions in human lung cancer)	
Specificity	Benzo[α]pyrene diol-exposide binds to Gs in codons 157, 248, and 273, which are *TP53* mutational hotspots
Codon 157 (GTC 6 TTC) mutations are uncommon in other types of cancer, including in lung cancer from never smokers	Benzo[α]pyrene exposure to human cells in vitro produces codon 248 (CGG ≥CTG) *TP53* mutations
Temporality	Cigarette-smoke condensates or benzo[*a*]pyrene can neoplastically transform human bronchial epithelial cells in the laboratory
TP53 mutations can be found in bronchial dysplasia	

[a]For reviews see Refs. 126 and 160.

Implications for Molecular Epidemiology, Risk Assessment, and Cancer Prevention

Molecular epidemiology (use of biochemical and molecular biological methods to buttress epidemiological studies) has resulted from the confluence of several disciplines.[131] It encompasses the detection of carcinogen-macromolecular adducts (DNA as a direct genotoxic measure and protein as a surrogate), normal DNA sequence variants (heritable variations), and mutations in target genes (somatic changes). Therefore, these investigations use epidemiologic methods to investigate all aspects of gene-environment interactions and risk assessment in human populations (Fig. 15-7).

The biologically effective dose of a chemical carcinogen is governed by the amount that reaches a target tissue in a form that becomes activated to a chemical species capable of causing DNA lesions.[132] Humans are most commonly exposed to complex mixtures of chemicals. Human carcinogen dosimetry at the molecular level requires sensitive and specific methods for carcinogen-macromolecular adduct quantitation. The low levels of adducts that are present in human DNA samples challenge the detection limits of conventional assay systems, and complex mixtures of adducted materials confound simple assay systems.

The most commonly used methods for carcinogen-DNA dosimetry in humans are ^{32}P-nucleotide postlabeling, immunoassays, fluorescence spectroscopy, electrochemical conductance, liquid chromatography/electrospray ionization/tandem mass spectrometry (LC/ESI/MS/ MS), and gas chromatography/mass spectroscopy (GC/MS). Each of these techniques currently has its own advantages and limitations, and within the framework of epidemiologic surveys, multiple corroborative end-point analyses seem to provide the most useful information. These methodologies, their application, and their limitations are reviewed extensively elsewhere.[3,32]

For exposure to tobacco smoke, GC/MS has provided a tool to measure aromatic amine protein adducts such as 4-aminobiphenyl hemoglobin. These studies have shown a dose-response relationship between the extent of smoking, type of tobacco used, and the adduct levels.[133] Similarly, tobacco-specific nitrosamine globin adducts have been used to monitor the dose in smokers and snuff dippers. A corroborative approach to the measurement of benzo[*a*]pyrene-DNA adducts has been used in the monitoring of both tobacco and coal smoke exposure. In this study, both GC/MS and fluorescence line-narrowing spectroscopy were used to detect adducts exfoliated in urine.[57,134]

In the case of aflatoxin B1, levels of adducts exfoliated in human urine were measured by GC/MS. 8,9-Dihydro-8-(*N*5-formyl-2′,5′,6′-triamino-4′-oxo-*N*5-pyrimidyl)-9-hydroxy-aflatoxin B1 (aflatoxin-*N7* guanine) adducts correlated with environmental exposure and disease outcome. Similarly, aflatoxin-albumin adducts provided a corroborative surrogate. Both of these markers were also correlated with 6-hydroxycortisol levels, indicating a role for CYP3A4 in aflatoxin B1 activation. Particularly, the presence of aflatoxin-*N7* guanine adducts in urine was associated with liver cancer.[135,136] Based on these findings, a randomized clinical trial of the *interceptor molecule*, chlorophyllin (Derifil), was performed. The test drug or placebo was taken three times daily and urinary AFB1-*N7*-Gua was monitored by GC/MS. After 12 weeks, adduct levels were >100% higher among 90 persons taking the placebo than those (n = 90) taking chlorophyllin.[137]

Interindividual variation in cancer susceptibility, and, consequently, meaningful human cancer risk assessment, involve determination of inherited host factors as well as exposure assessment. Metabolic polymorphisms have been determined by the use of indicator drugs (eg, caffeine, debrisoquine, dextromethorphan, dapsone, and isoniazid); however, these assays are being replaced by direct genetic assays.[138-140] This approach has allowed the investigation of diverse host factors for which indicator drugs were not available, and it has been applied to a wide variety of cancers, including lung, head, and neck.[141-143] Thus, genetic indicators of propensity for carcinogen activation and detoxification, DNA-repair capacity, and cell-cycle control are all features of molecular epidemiologic

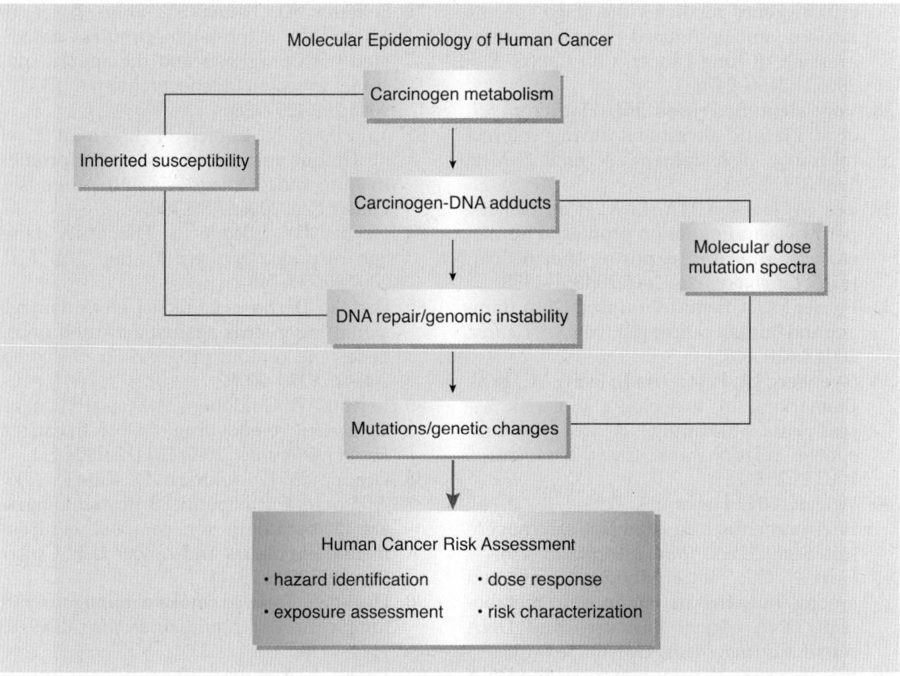

Figure 15-7 Facets of molecular epidemiology that investigate gene–environment interactions. Once internalized, chemical carcinogens are metabolized to reactive species that cause DNA damage (carcinogen DNA adducts). The innate ability to repair DNA damage may reduce or ablate the overall damage burden. Alternately, genetic changes (mutations, clastogenesis) may occur. Carcinogen metabolism and DNA repair are categorizable genetic traits (host factors). DNA adducts (molecular dose) and mutational spectra are measures of exposure. Information from assays designed to investigate host factors and measure exposure can be used for human cancer risk assessment.

studies that are complementary to adduct studies because of the implications for a biologically effective dose after exposure.[3]

Cytochrome P450 polymorphisms, involved in carcinogen activation, and glutathione-*S* transferases, uridine diphosphate (UDP) glucuronosyltransferases, sulfotransferases, and *N*-acyltransferases, involved in both carcinogen activation and detoxification, could explain variations in cancer susceptibility among the human population. Evidence that absent protection of a functionally intact *GSTM1* gene correlates with an increased risk of tobacco-related lung cancer.[144,145] Similarly, UDP glucuronosyltransferases (eg, *UGT1A1*, *UGT1A9*, *UGT2B7*) have been implicated in cancers of the head and neck. Persons inheriting reduced activity variants of *NAT1* and *NAT2* genes, resulting in the slow acetylator phenotype, are at a greater risk of aromatic amine-induced bladder cancer. This may include persons exposed through tobacco smoke inhalation.[60] Even though the inducible form of arylhydrocarbon hydroxylase (AHH) (*CYP1A1* and *CYP1A2*) has long been suspected of increasing cancer susceptibility in PAH-exposed persons, molecular epidemiologic studies remain inconclusive. Studies of *CYP2D6* metabolizer status and tobacco smoke-related lung cancer are similarly confusing.[8] However, analysis of multiple traits, eg, *CYP1A1* and *GSTM1*, in the same population may help to resolve these issues. Currently, there is a need for improved epidemiologic study design that integrates DNA adduct measures with indicators of metabolic capacity.[146-148]

Many DNA-repair genes have been described recently, and a growing number of polymorphisms have been identified for which molecular epidemiologic studies have provided evidence that genetic variation in these attributes can be a human cancer risk factor.[98,149-151] Typically, these types of molecular epidemiological studies initially focus on high exposure groups such as workers, patients taking therapeutic drugs, and tobacco smokers. Several polymorphisms in DNA-repair genes have now been implicated in tobacco-related neoplasams.[152]

Molecular characterization of tumors, ie, molecular profiling, is an important tool that has both etiologic and clinical application. Molecular profiling is a rapidly advancing area that is being propelled by DNA and protein microarray research.[41,42,153-155] During chemical carcinogenesis, the genome becomes altered and mutations accumulate. These mutations become evident in genes responsible for growth control and cellular homeostasis (including protooncogenes, tumor suppressor genes, and some DNA-repair genes), because corruption of these functions is part of carcinogenesis. In respect to chemical carcinogenesis, the most studied genes are Kirsten *ras* (*Kras*) and *TP53*. *Kras* is mutated in ~30% of lung adenocarcinomas, and may prove to be an indicator of prognosis or a guide to treatment.[108] The *TP53* tumor suppressor gene is mutated in most types of human cancers and it is the most commonly mutated gene yet known (eg, mutations in *TP53* are found in ~50% of lung cancers). Unlike *ras* gene mutations that are found in highly specific regions (codons 12, 13, 59, and 61), *TP53* mutations occur more widely. This is presumably because a positive growth advantage is conveyed only with specific *ras* mutations and the loss of *TP53* tumor suppressor function can occur with less specificity. However, for some malignancies, *TP53* mutations have provided clues to cancer etiology (see Table 15-4).[126,156] *TP53* is further distinguished from other genetic lesions in that several possible mutant phenotypes can exist. Mutations may simply lead to the absence of *TP53*, an inactive mutant protein may exist, or the mutant might convey a growth advantage. Several studies have investigated *TP53* expression, and even though its role in prognosis has not been clearly defined, it may be that it will provide a guide to treatment options.[157,158]

The goal of molecular epidemiology is to identify risk factors for disease and outcome. Variations among humans in carcinogen biodistribution, metabolism, DNA adduct formation, DNA repair, and potential responses to tumor promoters have important implications in determining cancer risk. An increased understanding of the molecular basis of these differences and their connection with critical steps in carcinogenesis may assist in future predictions of disease risk before the clinical onset of disease.

The facets of molecular epidemiology of human cancer risk are the assessment of carcinogen exposure and inherited and acquired host cancer-susceptibility factors. The interaction between these facets determines cancer risk. When combined with carcinogen bioassays in laboratory animals and classic epidemiology, molecular epidemiology can contribute to the four critical aspects of cancer risk assessment: (1) hazard identification, (2) dose-response assessment, (3) exposure assessment, and (4) risk characterization. Important bioethical considerations accompany the identification of high-risk individuals; these include autonomy, privacy, justice, and equity. Benefits of the knowledge of risk for an individual may be offset by specific concerns relating to that individual's responsibility to family members and psychosocial anxiety regarding the genetic testing of children.

Therefore, the uncertainty of current individual risk assessments and the limited availability of genetic counseling services dictate caution. In addition, it is widely held that genetic testing should be restricted to those situations that are amenable to preventative or therapeutic intervention.[159]

Acknowledgments

We thank Glory Johnson, Karen MacPherson, and Dorothea Dudek for editorial assistance. We also thank Drs. Mark Toraason and Steven H. Reynolds for thoughtful suggestions. This research was supported [in part] by the Intramural Research Program of the NIH, National Cancer Institute, Center for Cancer Research.

Selected References

The complete reference list can be found at www.CANCERMEDICINE8.com

3. Poirier MC, Santella RM, Weston A. Carcinogen macromolecular adducts and their measurement. *Carcinogenesis.* 2000;21:353–359.
4. International Agency for Research on Cancer. IARC Monographs on the Evaluation of Carcinogenic Risks to Humans. Overall Evaluation of Carcinogenecity. Monographs Volumes 1 to 76. Lyon: IARC; 1971–2000. US Library of Congress call number—RC268 6 I57; 2000.
6. Vineis P, Marinelli D, Autrup H, et al. Current smoking, occupation, *N*-acetyltransferase-2 and bladder cancer: a pooled analysis of genotype-based studies. *Cancer Epidemiol Biomarkers Prev.* 2001;10:1249–1252.
7. Luch A. Nature and nurture—lessons from chemical carcinogenesis. *Nat Rev Cancer.* 2005;5:113–125.
10. Yuspa SH. Overview of carcinogenesis: past, present and future. *Carcinogenesis.* 2000;21:341–344.
13. Loeb LA, Loeb KR, Anderson JP. Multiple mutations and cancer. *Proc Natl Acad Sci USA.* 2003;100:776–781.
14. Hussain SP, Harris CC. Molecular epidemiology and carcinogenesis: endogenous and exogenous carcinogens. *Mutat Res.* 2000;462:311–322.
15. Kinzler KW, Vogelstein B. Gatekeepers and caretakers. *Nature.* 1997;386:761–763.
17. Dey A, Verma CS, Lane DP. Updates on p53: modulation of p53 degradation as a therapeutic approach. *Br J Cancer.* 2008;98:4–8.
19. Yuspa SH, Poirier MC. Chemical carcinogenesis: from animal models to molecular models in one decade. *Adv Cancer Res.* 1988;50:25–70.
26. Russo AL, Thiagalingam A, Pan H, et al. Differential DNA hypermethylation of critical genes mediates the stage-specific tobacco smoke-induced neoplastic progression of lung cancer. *Clin Cancer Res.* 2005;11:2466–2470.
28. Vogelstein B, Fearon ER, Hamilton SR, et al. Genetic alterations during colorectal-tumor development. *N Engl J Med.* 1988;319:525–532.
29. Lea IA, Jackson MA, Li X, et al. Genetic pathways and mutation profiles of human cancers: site- and exposure-specific patterns. *Carcinogenesis.* 2007;28:1851–1858.
32. Poirier MC. Chemical-induced DNA damage and human cancer risk. *Nat Rev Cancer.* 2004;4:630–637.
33. Swenberg JA, Fryar-Tita E, Jeong YC, et al. Biomarkers in toxicology and risk assessment: informing critical dose-response relationships. *Chem Res Toxicol.* 2008;21:253–265.
40. Wogan GN, Hecht SS, Felton JS, et al. Environmental and chemical carcinogenesis. *Semin Cancer Biol.* 2004;14:473–486.
43. Harris CC. Interindividual variation among humans in carcinogen metabolism, DNA adduct formation and DNA repair. *Carcinogenesis.* 1989;10:1563–1566.
49. Friedberg EC. A brief history of the DNA repair field. *Cell Res.* 2008;18:3–7.
52. Phillips DH. Fifty years of benzo(a)pyrene. *Nature.* 1983;303:468–472.
54. Cooper CS, Grover PL, Sims P. The metabolism and activation of benzo[*a*]pyrene. In: Bridges JW, Chasseaud L, eds. England: Wiley and Sons, Ltd.; 1983:295–396.
55. Nebert DW, Dalton TP. The role of cytochrome P450 enzymes in endogenous signalling pathways and environmental carcinogenesis. *Nat Rev Cancer.* 2006;6:947–960.
56. Cavalieri EL, Rogan EG. A unifying mechanism in the initiation of cancer and other diseases by catechol quinones. *Ann N Y Acad Sci.* 2004;1028:247–257.
58. Poirier MC, Beland FA. Aromatic amine DNA adduct formation in chronically-exposed mice: considerations for human comparison. *Mutat Res.* 1997;376:177–184.
59. Beland FA, Poirier MC. DNA adducts and carcinogenesis. In: Sirica AE, ed. New York: Plenum Publishing Corp.; 1989:57–80.
61. Knize MG, Felton JS. Formation and human risk of carcinogenic heterocyclic amines formed from natural precursors in meat. *Nutr Rev.* 2005;63:158–165.
66. Abdollahi M, Ranjbar A, Shadnia S, et al. Pesticides and oxidative stress: a review. *Med Sci Monit.* 2004;10:RA141–RA147.
70. Schulmann K, Sterian A, Berki A, et al. Inactivation of p16, RUNX3, and HPP1 occurs early in Barrett's-associated neoplastic progression and predicts progression risk. *Oncogene.* 2005;24:4138–4148.
73. O'Connell RM, Taganov KD, Boldin MP, et al. MicroRNA-155 is induced during the macrophage inflammatory response. *Proc Natl Acad Sci USA.* 2007;104:1604–1609.
77. Huang Q, Gumireddy K, Schrier M, et al. The microRNAs miR-373 and miR-520c promote tumour invasion and metastasis. *Nat Cell Biol.* 2008;10:202–210.
78. Ma L, Weinberg RA. MicroRNAs in malignant progression. *Cell Cycle.* 2007;7.
79. Schetter AJ, Leung SY, Sohn JJ, et al. MicroRNA expression profiles associated with prognosis and therapeutic outcome in colon adenocarcinoma. *JAMA.* 2008;299:425–436.
81. Yanaihara N, Caplen N, Bowman E, et al. Unique microRNA molecular profiles in lung cancer diagnosis and prognosis. *Cancer Cell.* 2006;9:189–198.
84. Harper JW, Elledge SJ. The DNA damage response: ten years after. *Mol Cell.* 2007;28:739–745.
85. Bartek J, Bartkova J, Lukas J. DNA damage signalling guards against activated oncogenes and tumour progression. *Oncogene.* 2007;26:7773–7779.
86. Lettini AA, Guidoboni M, Fonsatti E, et al. Epigenetic remodelling of DNA in cancer. *Histol Histopathol.* 2007;22:1413–1424.
88. Groopman JD, Johnson D, Kensler TW. Aflatoxin and hepatitis B virus biomarkers: a paradigm for complex environmental exposures and cancer risk. *Cancer Biomark.* 2005;1:5–14.
90. Hecht SS. Tobacco smoke carcinogens and lung cancer. *J Natl Cancer Inst.* 1999;91:1194–1210.
97. Loeb LA. A mutator phenotype in cancer. *Cancer Res.* 2001;61:3230–3239.
98. Zhou W, Liu G, Miller DP, et al. Gene-environment interaction for the ERCC2 polymorphisms and cumulative cigarette smoking exposure in lung cancer. *Cancer Res.* 2002;62:1377–1381.
104. Croce CM. Oncogenes and cancer. *N Engl J Med.* 2008;358:502–511.
112. Vousden KH, Lane DP. p53 in health and disease. *Nat Rev Mol Cell Biol.* 2007;8:275–283.
115. Serrano M, Blasco MA. Cancer and ageing: convergent and divergent mechanisms. *Nat Rev Mol Cell Biol.* 2007;8:715–722.
118. Petitjean A, Mathe E, Kato S, et al. Impact of mutant p53 functional properties on *TP53* mutation patterns and tumor phenotype: lessons from recent developments in the IARC TP53 database. *Hum Mutat.* 2007;28:622–629.
120. Soussi T, Wiman KG. Shaping genetic alterations in human cancer: the p53 mutation paradigm. *Cancer Cell.* 2007;12:303–312.
122. Hussain SP, Schwank J, Staib F, et al. *TP53* mutations and hepatocellular carcinoma: insights into the etiology and pathogenesis of liver cancer. *Oncogene.* 2007;26:2166–2176.
135. Groopman JD, Kensler TW. The light at the end of the tunnel for chemical-specific biomarkers: daylight or headlight? *Carcinogenesis.* 1999;20:1–11.
138. Nebert DW, Russell DW. Clinical importance of the cytochromes P450. *Lancet.* 2002;360:1155–1162.
152. Neumann AS, Sturgis EM, Wei Q. Nucleotide excision repair as a marker for susceptibility to tobacco-related cancers: a review of molecular epidemiological studies. *Mol Carcinog.* 2005;42:65–92.
153. Shih W, Chetty R, Tsao MS. Expression profiling by microarrays in colorectal cancer (Review). *Oncol Rep.* 2005;13:517–524.
161. Hussain SP, Harris CC. Inflammation and cancer: an ancient link with novel potentials. *Int J Cancer.* 2007;121:2373–2380.

16 Hormones and the Etiology of Cancer

Leslie Bernstein, PhD ▪ C. Leigh Pearce, PhD ▪ Iona Cheng, PhD ▪
Katherine DeLellis Henderson, PhD

Substantial and convincing bodies of experimental, clinical, and epidemiologic evidence indicate that hormones play a major role in the etiology of several human cancers. The concept that hormones can increase the incidence of neoplasia was first proposed by Bittner,[1] on the basis of experimental studies of estrogens and mammary cancer in mice. This theory has been refined into epidemiologic hypotheses related to cancers of the breast, endometrium, prostate, ovary, thyroid, bone, and testis.[2,3] The underlying mechanism proposed for these cancers is that neoplasia is the consequence of prolonged hormonal stimulation of the target organ, the normal growth and function of which is controlled by one or more steroid or polypeptide hormones. Evidence is mounting to show that the amount of hormone to which a tissue is effectively exposed is under strong genetic control.[4] Therefore, although external factors such as physical activity or exogenous hormone use may modify hormone profiles, the current evidence supports a multigenic model of cancer susceptibility where sequence variants in genes encoding proteins involved in steroid-hormone biosynthesis, metabolism or intracellular signaling, and transport, and deoxyribonucleic acid (DNA) binding, repair, and transactivation are also important determinants of individual cancer risk.[4,5]

The major carcinogenic consequence of this hormonal exposure at the end organ is cellular proliferation, although direct carcinogenesis resulting from metabolic activation and direct DNA binding is another potential mechanism. The emergence of a malignant phenotype depends on a series of somatic mutations that occur during cell division, but the entire sequence of genes involved in progression from normal cell to a particular malignant phenotype is not known (Fig. 16-1). Candidate genes include those in the endocrine and growth factor pathways,[4-6] as well as DNA repair genes, tumor-suppressor genes, and oncogenes.[7,8] Germ line mutations have been described in two such tumor-suppressor genes, *BRCA1* and *BRCA2*, that are associated with susceptibility to breast and ovarian cancers.[9-12] Germ line mutations in TP53 are also associated in certain kindreds with an increased risk of breast cancer.[13] However, mutations in these genes do not appear to be involved in the majority of sporadic breast cancer. The *HER2/neu* oncogene, which is amplified in some breast cancers, is associated with poor prognosis, and probably represents one critical event in the latter part of breast cancer progression.[14]

Neoplasia of hormone-responsive tissues currently accounts for >30% of all newly diagnosed male cancers and almost 40% of all newly diagnosed female cancers in the United States. Given that endogenous hormones apparently affect the risk of these cancers and their overall frequency, concern exists about the effects on cancer risk if the same or closely related hormones are administered for therapeutic purposes (eg, as contraceptives, as menopausal hormone therapy, or for the prevention of miscarriage).[15] This chapter focuses on breast, endometrial, and ovarian cancers among women and prostate cancer among men and provides a review of the epidemiologic and endocrinologic evidence for the role of hormones in cancer development. It also reviews the current status of the relationship between exogenous hormones and risk of cancers of the breast, endometrium, and ovary. Other less common cancers (eg, cervical cancer, clear cell vaginal adenocarcinoma, thyroid cancer, testicular cancer, and osteosarcoma) appear to have a hormonal basis as well, but are not reviewed here.

Breast Cancer

Breast cancer is the most common cancer in women; the American Cancer Society estimates that approximately 180,000 new cases of invasive breast cancer and 68,000 new cases of breast carcinoma in situ were diagnosed in the United States in 2008. Approximately 40,000 women died due to breast cancer in 2008.[17] A perceptible decline in breast cancer mortality has occurred since 1990,[17,18] resulting from increasing use of mammographic screening and tamoxifen therapy as well as newer forms of chemotherapy including therapy that targets *HER2/neu*.[19,20] Available evidence regarding the hormonal etiology of breast cancer is most consistent with the hypothesis that estrogen is the primary stimulant for breast cell proliferation.[2,3] The simultaneous presence of progesterone further increases the rate of proliferation.[21] This latter conclusion is based largely on the fact that breast mitotic activity peaks during the luteal phase of the menstrual cycle[22] and it is consistent with the increasing number of publications demonstrating that added progestins substantially augment the increased risk of breast cancer from estrogen therapy.[23-27]

The most consistently documented, hormonally related risk factors for breast cancer are early age at menarche, late age at menopause, late age at first full-term pregnancy, and excess weight among postmonstrual women (Table 16-1). The age incidence curve for breast cancer emphasizes the importance of ovulation in determining risk.[15] Cases first occur during early adulthood, and the rate of increase in incidence then rises sharply with age until the time of menopause, when it slows dramatically. The rate of increase in the postmenopausal period is approximately one-sixth the rate of increase in the premenopausal period. This age incidence curve appears, then, to be shaped in a major way by the effects of ovarian activity. Therefore, it is critical to understand the determinants, both genetic and environmental, of the onset, regularity, and cessation of ovulation in order to continue to develop effective prevention modalities for breast cancer.

Reproductive Factors

Early age at menarche is an established risk factor for breast cancer.[3] In general, risk decreases ~5–6% for each year that menarche is delayed and this relationship may be further modified by the age at onset of regular ovulatory menstrual cycles. In a study of young women, Henderson and colleagues[28] reported that women with menarche at age 12 years or younger who experienced rapid onset of regular cycles had nearly a fourfold greater risk of breast cancer than women with later menarche who experienced a long duration of irregular cycles.

These observations suggest that regular ovulatory cycles increase a woman's risk of breast cancer, and they support results from an earlier study that compared circulating hormone levels in daughters of women with breast cancer with those in age-matched daughters of women who do not have breast cancer (controls).[29] Daughters of women with

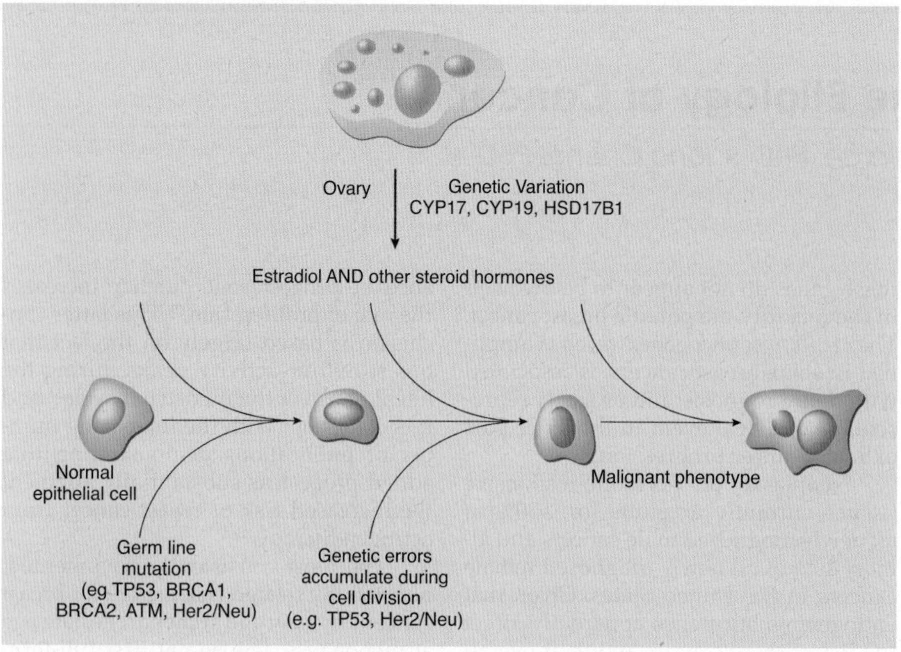

Figure 16-1 Estradiol and, other steroid hormones (eg, progesterone) drive breast cell proliferation, which facilitates the accumulation of random DNA copying errors in critical genes on the pathway to a malignant phenotype. Germ line mutations in relevant tumor-suppressor genes accelerate the transformation to the malignant phenotype.

breast cancer, who as a group have nearly twice the breast cancer risk of the general population, have higher levels of circulating estrogen and progesterone than daughters of controls.

Although menarche and the onset of ovulation are to some extent genetically determined,[30] it is also critical to establish behaviors that may alter the number of ovulatory menstrual cycles a woman experiences during her reproductive years. Strenuous physical activity may delay menarche.[31] For example, in one study, the mean age at menarche of ballet dancers was 15.4 years compared to 12.5 years for reference subjects. Moderate physical activity during adolescence can lead to anovulatory menstrual cycles. Girls who regularly engaged in moderate levels of physical activity (averaging at least 600 kcal of energy expended per week during a 9-month school year) were nearly three times more likely to have anovulatory menstrual cycles than girls who were less physically active.[32] Bernstein and colleagues have reported that lifetime patterns of leisure-time exercise activity significantly impact the risk of breast cancer in young women (<40 years of age),[33] older, postmenopausal women (55-64 years of age),[34] African American women,[35] and Asian American women.[36] Evidence continues to accumulate in support of a protective effect of physical activity on breast cancer risk with risk reductions observed in both case-control and cohort studies, although results vary with respect to the subgroups of women who benefit the most.[37-39]

Table 16-1 **A Summary of Established Hormonal Risk and Protective Factors for Breast Cancer**

Risk factors (increased exposure to estrogen and/or progesterone)
Early menarche
Late menopause
Obesity (postmenopausal women)
Hormone replacement therapy
Protective factors (reduced exposure to estrogen and/or progesterone)
Lactation
Early age at full-term pregnancy
Physical activity (exercise)

In the same way that early onset of menarche and regular onset of ovulation represent greater exposure to estrogen and result in greater risk of breast cancer, late occurrence of menopause and extended exposure to ovulatory cycles at the end of menstrual life also increase risk. The breast cancer risk of women whose natural menopause occurs before age 45 years is approximately one-half that of women whose menopause occurs after age 55 years.[40] Artificial menopause, induced by bilateral oophorectomy or by pelvic irradiation, also markedly reduces breast cancer risk; this reduction is greater than that associated with natural menopause among women who have induced menopause before age 50 years.[40-42] Following natural menopause, endogenous estrogen exposure declines gradually due to the continuing, but declining function of the ovaries and the continuing, persistent ovarian production of a small amount of testosterone, a metabolic precursor of estrogen.

The relationship between weight and breast cancer risk depends on menopausal status. Among postmenopausal women, a 10 kg increment in body weight results in about an 80% increase in breast cancer risk.[43] One explanation for this effect is that heavier postmenopausal women have higher circulating estrogen levels than would be expected because of the conversion of an adrenal androgen, androstenedione, to estrone by the aromatase enzyme present in body fat. In premenopausal women, the relationship between weight and risk is less clearly established, but if anything, the situation is the reverse of that in postmenopausal women; here, high weight is associated with reduced risk.[44] This may result from a reduction in the frequency of ovulatory menstrual cycles associated with high body weight.

Assuming ovarian activity affects breast cancer risk, case-control and cohort studies of breast cancer should find higher levels of circulating estradiol among breast cancer patients than among healthy women. Bernstein and colleagues[45] described the results of two concurrent case-control studies of premenopausal women in the United States (Los Angeles) and China (Shanghai). Overall, breast cancer patients had 14% higher serum estradiol concentrations, with a case-to-control excess of 17% in Chinese women and 11% in white American women, respectively. Los Angeles control women had 21% greater estradiol concentrations than did Shanghai control women, and adjustment for body weight only accounted for 25% of this difference. The results from a pooled analysis of nine prospective studies of endogenous hormones and postmenopausal breast cancer risk provide strong evidence that high estradiol concentrations are predictive of breast cancer risk, with women in the highest quintile of estradiol exposure having a twofold greater risk of breast cancer than those in the lowest exposure quintile.[46] Considering free estradiol, the bioavailable fraction that circulates in blood, women in the highest quintile of exposure have >2.5 times greater breast cancer risk than those in the lowest quintile.

Age at First Birth

Having a first full-term pregnancy at a young age (ie, before age 20 years) lowers a woman's breast cancer risk by about 50% relative to nulliparous women. Full-term pregnancies at later ages provide smaller increments of protection.[47] Women who have a late first full-term pregnancy (ie, after age 30 years) have greater risk of breast cancer than nulliparous women have. This paradoxical cross-over effect of a late first full-term pregnancy has been repeatedly confirmed by epidemiologic studies.

The immediate effect of a full-term pregnancy on breast cancer risk is a short-term increase. Among women who have given birth within the past 3 years, breast cancer risk is nearly three times higher than that of women of the same age, parity, and age at first birth whose most recent birth occurred at least 10 years earlier.[48] On the basis of these results, it appears that a first pregnancy confers two contradictory effects on risk of breast cancer: a short-term increase in risk, followed in the long term by a substantial reduction in risk.[48]

This apparent paradox has a physiologic explanation based on patterns of estrogen as well as prolactin secretion and metabolism during pregnancy. During the first trimester, the level of bioavailable estradiol rapidly rises, an effect that is more apparent during the first than in subsequent pregnancies.[49] Thus, in terms of estrogen exposure to the breast, the net effect during this early part of pregnancy is an increased risk that is equivalent to the exposure from several ovulatory cycles over a relatively short period of time.[50] At a molecular level, it is likely that the hormonal changes during pregnancy induce irreversible differentiation and apoptosis in some cells that have already accumulated one or more of the relevant somatic mutations necessary for breast cancer development. In the long run, however, this negative effect of early pregnancy on risk of breast cancer can be overridden by two beneficial hormonal consequences of completing the pregnancy. It has been reported that prolactin levels are substantially lower in parous compared with nulliparous women.[51-53] Prolactin, a polypeptide hormone, regulates lactation and appears to enhance estrogen effects on breast tissue. In addition, parous women have been reported to have lower levels of bioavailable estradiol than nulliparous women.[50]

Evidence is fairly convincing that lactation reduces the risk of breast cancer among premenopausal women,[54-56] but is less consistent for postmenopausal women.[55,57] In two publications, Enger and colleagues showed substantial breast cancer risk reductions for parous premenopausal and postmenopausal women in the United States who breastfed for >15 months (35% reduction for premenopausal women and 30% reduction for postmenopausal women relative to similar women who never lactated).[54,57] In the United States, rates of breast-feeding have varied over time; some studies may have not observed lower risk of breast cancer among women who have breast fed due to the small proportion of women with a sufficient duration of lactation. Among premenopausal and postmenopausal women in Shanghai, where breast-feeding often extends to >1 year per child, a strong dose-response effect of decreasing breast cancer risk with increasing breast-feeding duration was observed.[58] The time when supplementary feedings are introduced to the infant as well as the frequency and duration of each breast-feeding episode may also contribute to the inconsistent findings. Lactation may reduce breast cancer risk by reducing the total number of ovulatory menstrual cycles a woman experiences during her reproductive years because breast-feeding results in a substantial delay in reestablishing ovulation following a completed pregnancy.

Diet

Much attention has focused on dietary differences between countries, particularly fat consumption patterns, to explain both the international pattern of breast cancer occurrence and changes in rates of breast cancer following migration to high-risk, usually Western nations, from low-risk countries.[59] International breast cancer mortality rates correlate highly with per capita consumption of fat in the diet (correlation coefficient, r = 0.93). When international breast cancer incidence rates rather than mortality rates are considered, the magnitude of the correlation coefficient is still very high (r = 0.84).[59] As implied previously, nutrition may influence breast cancer occurrence by modifying age at menarche and body weight, but the correlation of fat consumption with international breast cancer mortality remains highly significant, even after statistical adjustment for these factors.

It has been theorized that fat intake in the diet may be an important contributor to breast cancer risk. Many case-control studies of fat consumption and breast cancer find only small differences between cases and controls. Similarly, most of the cohort studies that have used food-frequency questionnaires to study the relationship with either total fat, saturated fat, or vegetable fat have found little or no difference in breast cancer risk over a wide range of fat intake. In a meta-analysis of studies of total fat intake and breast cancer risk, the extent of increase in risk comparing women in the highest intake category with the lowest intake category was 14% for case-control studies (summary odds ratio, OR = 1.14; 95% confidence interval (CI) = 0.99-1.32) and 11% for cohort studies (OR = 1.11, 95% CI = 0.99-1.25).[60] The Women's Health Initiative randomized trial of >48,000 women tested the hypothesis that reducing intake of total fat to 20% of energy, increasing consumption of vegetables and fruits to at least five servings daily and grains to at least six servings daily would lower cancer risk, particularly breast cancer risk.[61] Risk of breast cancer, during 8.1 years average follow-up after randomization, produced results that were not quite statistically significant (relative risk, RR = 0.91, 95% CI = 0.83-1.01), but were suggestive of an impact of diet on breast cancer risk, as when women who adhered to the diet were compared to the non-dietary intervention group, the RR was lower.

High-fiber diets may protect against breast cancer, perhaps because fiber reduces the intestinal reabsorption of estrogens excreted via the biliary system.[62] Assessment of fiber intake in epidemiologic studies has been problematic because of a paucity of data on the fiber content of individual foods and disagreement about the most appropriate methods of biochemical analysis to determine the different types of fiber. Case-control, but not cohort studies, have shown a consistent inverse association between dietary fiber intake and breast cancer risk.[63]

Several investigations have been undertaken to demonstrate a reduction in serum estrogen levels following dietary interventions that reduce fat or increase fiber intake.[64,65] A meta-analysis of these studies demonstrated a 7.4% average reduction in estradiol levels of premenopausal women and a 23% reduction in estradiol in postmenopausal women following trials of reduced dietary fat intake.[65] This analysis could not distinguish between a direct dietary effect on hormone levels and an indirect effect that was due to disruption of ovulatory cycles in premenopausal women; nevertheless, whatever the mechanism, such a reduction in estradiol levels is potentially very important.

Exogenous Hormones

Oral contraceptives and menopausal hormone therapy are the exogenous counterparts to endogenous hormonal exposures experienced by women and therefore are of concern as potential contributors to breast cancer risk.

Oral Contraceptives The relationship of oral contraceptive use to breast cancer risk has been the topic of many review articles. A combined analysis of 54 studies that included >150,000 women has provided many important answers about the risk of breast cancer among users of combination oral contraceptives, that is, oral contraceptives that provide an estrogen and progestin in combination in a single pill.[66] This analysis indicates that a modest increased risk of breast cancer is observed among current (RR = 1.24) and recent (RR = 1.16) combination oral contraceptive users. Age at first combination oral contraceptive use modifies the association with recent use. For recent users, the risks are highest for those who began combination oral contraceptive use before the age of 20 years. However, total duration of combination oral contraceptives use was not associated with increased risk of breast cancer, once recency of use was taken into account.

The pooled analysis compiled studies that mainly focused on younger women since most of these studies were conducted at a time when oral contraceptive users had not achieved their perimenopausal and postmenopausal years.[66] The Women's Contraceptive and Reproductive Experiences (Women's CARE) Study, a population-based case-control study conducted in five geographic regions of the United States,[67] involved >4500 newly diagnosed breast cancer patients and >4500 control subjects, who were between the ages of 35 and 64 years. It was specifically designed to assess the impact of oral contraceptives among women who were no longer using oral contraceptives. Relatively few participants in the Women's CARE Study were current oral contraceptive users; many of the women had stopped use at least 20 years earlier. No significant associations were observed between duration of use, estrogen dose of the formulation, age at first use, interval since last use, or use in relation to timing of pregnancy and breast cancer risk. Further, results for younger women (35-44 years) were similar to those for older women (45-64 years) who were more likely to have used earlier formulations, but were less likely to have recently used oral contraceptives.

The International Agency for Research on Cancer has completed a new review (published in 2008) of the existing literature on combination oral contraceptives and breast cancer risk concluding that breast cancer risk is increased in current or recent oral contraceptive users, particularly among women under age 35 years whose first oral contraceptive use was before age 20 years.[68] The increase in risk disappeared as age at current or recent use increased and, following cessation of oral contraceptive use, any increase in risk disappears within 10 years.

Hormone Therapy ■ Hormone therapy has evolved over time. Originally designed to reduce the symptoms of menopause, hormone therapy gained popularity because of its efficacy in reducing the risk of osteoporosis and its purported benefits in reducing the risk of heart disease. Initially formulated as estrogen therapy, the number of women using hormone therapy increased through the mid-1970s, until concerns were raised about the carcinogenic potential of estrogen therapy on the endometrium. In the 1980s cyclic estrogen-progestin regimens became widely recommended and prescribed to eliminate the increase in endometrial cancer associated with estrogen-alone therapy. Initially, these were prescribed as sequential regimens with estrogen given during the first 15-20 days of a 28-day cycle followed by 5-10 days when both estrogen and progestin were given. More recently, continuous-combined regimens have gained favor because they reduce menstrual-like bleeding episodes and because of their ease of administration.

Most studies that have included sufficiently large numbers of women who have used estrogen therapy for extended periods of time (eg, for >10 years) indicate a modest increase in breast cancer risk among exposed women with risk increasing ~3% per year of use.[69] Among studies conducted in the United States, where the use of conjugated equine estrogens is the norm, early estimates were that breast cancer risk increased about 2.2% per year of use of a standard dose regimen (0.625 mg/day).

The Collaborative Group on Hormonal Factors in Breast Cancer pooled data from 51 epidemiologic studies and >160,000 women to assess the impact of hormone therapy on breast cancer risk.[54] Where information was available regarding type of hormone preparation used, 80% of women in these studies had used mostly estrogen-only therapy, and 12% of women had used combination hormone therapy. This study showed that hormone therapy (primarily estrogen therapy) increased breast cancer risk with RRs of 1.09, 1.15, and 1.14 comparing ever users to never users in cohort studies, population-based case-control studies, and hospital-based case-control studies, respectively. Risk was substantially elevated among women who had used hormone therapy for at least 15 years (RR = 1.58). Risk increased by 2.3% ($p = 0.0002$) for each year of use among women who had used hormone therapy within 5 years of diagnosis or an equivalent reference date (Fig. 16-2). However, women who stopped hormone therapy use five or more years earlier had only a modest, nonsignificant increase in risk, regardless of duration of use.

Consistent with these estimates are the results from the Million Women Study, conducted in the United Kingdom, which recruited a cohort of women aged 50-64 years who had undergone routine mammography.[16] In this study, incidence of breast cancer was significantly greater among current users of estrogen therapy than among women who had never used hormones (RR = 1.30, 95% CI = 1.22-1.38). Risk increased with increasing duration of use among these current estrogen therapy users, with 5-9 years of use associated with a RR of 1.32 and 10 or more years of use associated with a RR of 1.37.

The Women's Health Initiative randomized trial compared an estrogen-alone regimen to placebo among women 50-79 years of age who had previously had a hysterectomy and assessed the impact of a combined estrogen plus progestin regimen vs placebo among women 50-79 years of age who had an intact uterus. The estrogen alone regimen consisted of 0.625 mg/day of conjugated equine estrogen,[70] and the combined regimen consisted of 0.625 mg/day of conjugated equine estrogen and 2.5 mg/day of medroxyprogesterone acetate.[26] The results for the estrogen therapy study were somewhat surprising in that, after an average follow-up of 7.1 years, the RR of breast cancer was not elevated (RR = 0.80, 95% CI = 0.62-1.04).[71] In the trial, the reduction in risk was greater and was statistically significant for ductal cancer although even in a trial this large, numbers were too small to demonstrate a difference in risk by tumor histology. In comparison to ductal tumors, risk appeared elevated for lobular cancers and the comparison of ductal to lobular cancer was of borderline statistical significance ($p = 0.054$). A similar, nonstatistically significant difference was observed by stage with risk reduced for localized cancers but not for regional cancers ($p = 0.09$).

For combined hormone therapy, the Women's Health Initiative assessed only the continuous-combined regimen. Three population-based observational studies, published in 1999 and 2000, showed that a combined regimen conferred a greater risk of breast cancer than did an estrogen-alone regimen.[23,24,72] For example, Ross and colleagues found that the increment in risk for each 5 years of use was nearly four times greater for combined hormone therapy users than for estrogen therapy users.[24] Results from the Women's Health Initiative trial arm comparing a continuous CHT to placebo provided a risk estimate that was similar to those from these prior studies (RR = 1.24, 95% CI = 1.01-1.54).[26]

Lee et al.[73] conducted a meta-analysis of the results of studies that have evaluated the impact of combined hormone therapy on breast cancer risk, separating results for use of sequential (cyclic) combined regimens from those for use of continuous-combined regimens and including results from the Collaborative Group on Hormonal Factors in Breast Cancer[66] and the Women's Health Initiative.[26] Overall, users of a combined regimen had substantially elevated risk with risk increasing 7.6% per year of use.[73] Not all studies provided data on progestin schedule. Those that did have shown a small difference in risk between sequential and continuous-combined regimens (increase in breast cancer risk per year of use of 8.9% and 10.3%, respectively). Notably, results from Scandinavian studies have shown that continuous regimens

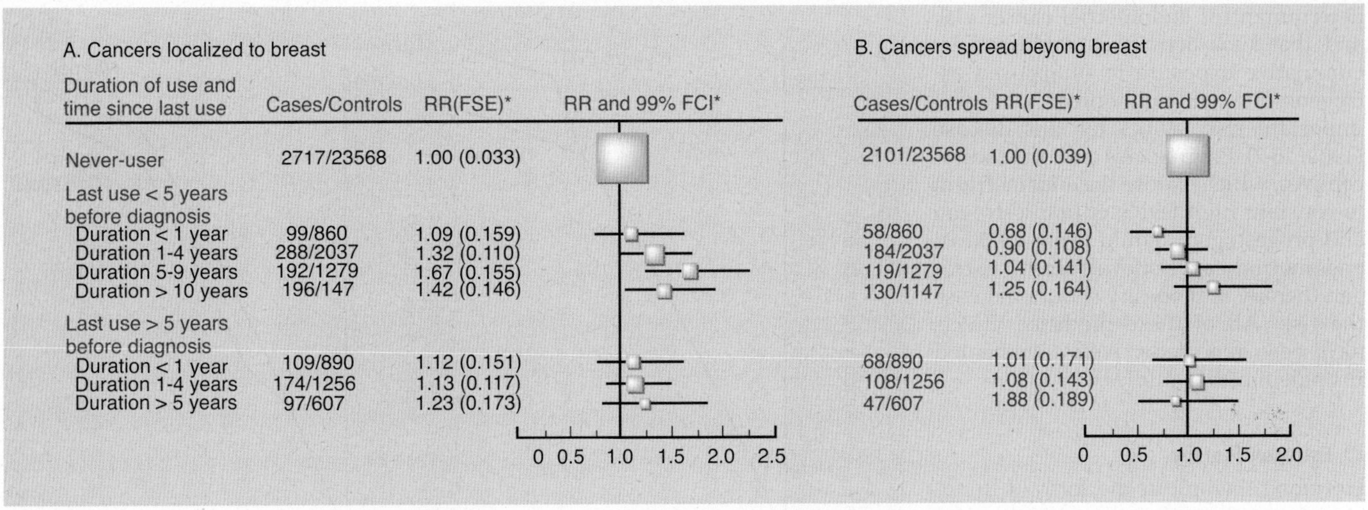

Figure 16-2 Relative risk of breast cancer by duration and time since last use of hormone therapy according to extent of tumor spread relative to never users, stratified by study, age at diagnosis, time since menopause, body mass index, parity, and the age of a woman when her first child was born. "Last use within 5 years before diagnosis" includes current users. *Floated standard errors (FSE) and confidence intervals (FCI) calculated from floated variance for each category.

had a greater impact on risk than sequential regimens. This difference was not as apparent among studies from the United States or the United Kingdom (Million Women Study). In the United States, the total dose of progestin is comparable in continuous-combined compared to sequential regimens, whereas in Scandinavia continuous-combined regimens provide a substantially higher dose of progestin. Thus, evidence is quite strong that the progestin component of combined regimens adds substantially to any increase in breast cancer risk conferred by estrogen alone and that differences in results between the United States and Scandinavia are likely due to differences in the progestin dose administered.

Recently the Women's Health Initiative investigators published an update on health risks and benefits of combined hormone therapy, examining risk following cessation of hormone therapy.[74] Risk for invasive breast cancer remained elevated after an average of 2.4 years of follow-up after use was stopped among women who had been randomized to the estrogen plus progestin arm of the trial evaluating combined therapy (RR = 1.27, 95% CI = 0.91-1.78) although the confidence interval did not exclude 1.0.[74]

Combined hormone therapy preferentially increases risk of lobular and ductal-lobular breast cancers, particularly those judged to have >50% lobular component.[75] Among older women, ages 55-74 years, current users of combined therapy were at 2.7-fold greater risk of lobular carcinoma and 3.3-fold greater risk of ductal-lobular carcinoma compared to women who had not used combined therapy.

Declining use of combined therapy has had a marked impact on breast cancer incidence rates in the United States and Germany.[76-78] It is important to note that rates of breast cancer in the United States began to decline before publication of the Women's Health Initiative result for combined therapy in 2002.[25] An evaluation of data from the Surveillance, Epidemiology, and End Results (SEER) registries for 1975 to 2003 shows a decline in invasive breast cancer from 1999 onward in women 45 years or older, with a sharp decrease in incidence in 2002 and 2003, particularly of estrogen receptor positive tumors, in women 59-69 years of age.[77] Data from a mammography registry in San Francisco indicate that hormone therapy prescribing peaked in 1999; the subsequent decline in prescribing combined therapy was amplified by the publication of the Women's Health Initiative in 2002.[79] Robbins and Clarke confirm this in their analysis of breast cancer incidence across 58 counties in California, clearly demonstrating that breast cancer rates declined between 2001 and 2004, with the rate of decline paralleling the reduction in prescriptions of combined therapy recorded by the California Health Interview Survey.[80] Although some have suggested that part of this decline in breast cancer incidence among older women might be due to decreasing use of mammographic screening, rates of in situ breast cancer, which is diagnosed almost exclusively by mammography, have not decreased in parallel with the decrease in invasive breast cancer,[77] and in California, the California Health Interview Survey has not indicated any significant change in the proportion of women reporting a screening mammogram within the prior 2 years.[80]

Endometrial Cancer

Among the hormone-related cancers, etiologically the best understood is endometrial cancer. All the major demographic characteristics of the disease, as well as the major nondemographic risk factors, are explicable on the basis of cumulative exposure of the endometrium to that fraction of estrogen which is unopposed by the modifying influences of progesterone.[2,3]

Mitotic Activity in the Endometrium

Key and Pike summarized the existing data on endometrial mitotic activity during normal menstrual cycles.[81] Mitotic rates are low during days 1-4 of the cycle, then increase rapidly and remain stable thereafter until day 19, after which rates essentially drop to zero for the remainder of the cycle. There appears to be a lag period of about 4 days before the full stimulatory effects of unopposed estrogen or the modifying influence of progesterone on endometrial mitotic activity are fully apparent.

The cellular basis for the antiestrogenic activity of progestogens on the endometrium is well understood.[2] Progestogens reduce the concentration of estrogen receptors and increase the activity of the 17-β-hydroxysteroid dehydrogenase type II enzyme, which converts estradiol to estrone,[82,83] a biologically less-potent estrogen because of its lower affinity for cellular estrogen receptors. Luteal phase progesterone causes endometrial cells to differentiate to a secretory state and progestogen withdrawal leads to cyclic sloughing of endometrial tissue.

On the basis of the concept that frequency of mitotic activity is the primary determinant of endometrial cancer risk and that such activity is controlled by cumulative exposure to unopposed estrogens, one can readily predict the most important risk factors for this disease (Table 16-2). Pregnancies and oral contraceptives, which expose the endometrium to constant high levels of both estrogen and progestogen, should protect against endometrial cancer development. Estrogen therapy and obesity should increase the risk. All of these predicted effects have been repeatedly well documented in epidemiologic studies.[2]

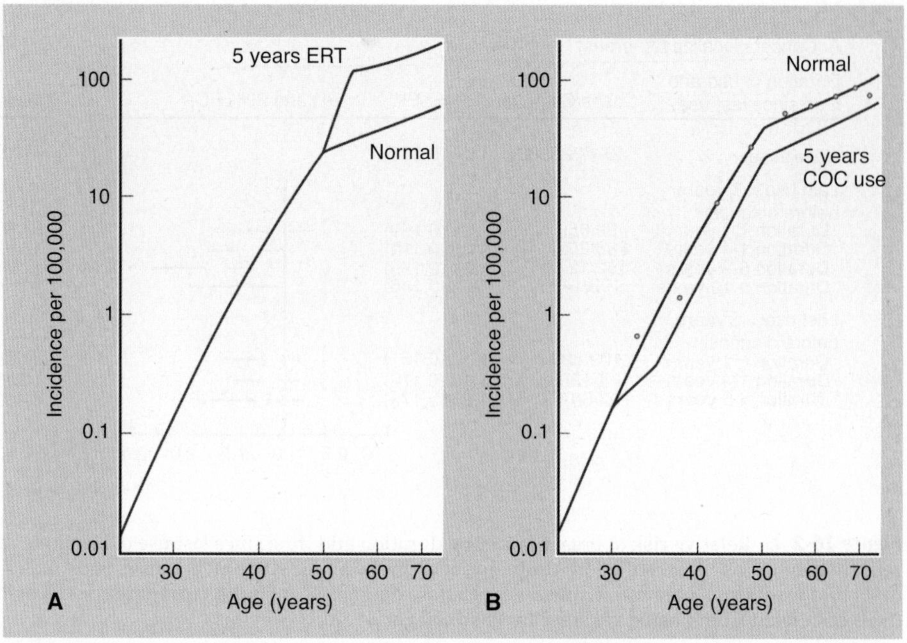

Figure 16-3 ■ Age-specific incidence rates for cancers of the endometrium in women using estrogen therapy (ERT) (**A**) and combination oral contraceptives (COCs) (**B**) for 5 years. Data are from the UK Birmingham Cancer Registry for the years 1968 to 1972. These data largely avoid problems arising from the high hysterectomy and oophorectomy rates in the United States, which artificially distort the age-incidence curves. *Dots,* actual incidence data; *solid lines marked "normal,"* mathematical models predicting these rates from the major known risk factors for these cancers.[15]

Estrogen Therapy

Hormone therapy in the form of unopposed estrogen therapy gained widespread popularity in the United States during the 1960s and 1970s.[84] Concomitant with this increasing usage, incidence rates of endometrial cancer in postmenopausal women also increased rapidly, especially in western US states, where use of estrogen therapy was particularly common.[85] By 1975, the results of epidemiologic case-control studies, demonstrating a strong overall association between estrogen therapy and risk of endometrial cancer, were being published.[86,87] Literally dozens of studies have now documented a high relative increase in the risk of endometrial cancer following estrogen therapy. Risk is strongly related both to dose and duration of use, but high relative increments in risk follow even moderate doses taken for intermediate length periods of time. Women who use estrogen therapy for 5 years or longer have ~3.5-fold increase in risk compared to that of women who have never used such therapy (Fig. 16-3A).[15]

Although use of estrogen clearly increases the incidence of aggressive endometrial cancer, the overall mortality from endometrial cancer among affected users somewhat paradoxically is much lower than among nonusers who develop endometrial cancer.[88] In fact, such women have little reduction in life span when compared to healthy women of the same age. The reasons for this are not completely known, but this phenomenon likely can be explained by the increased medical surveillance among estrogen users. Women who use estrogen therapy tend to be closely monitored because the drug frequently induces vaginal bleeding. Part of the favorable survival experience may also result from patients with estrogen-induced benign hyperplasia being misdiagnosed as having endometrial cancer. Although past users of estrogen therapy have a risk of endometrial cancer that is intermediate between that for current users of comparable duration and lifetime nonusers, risk in such women remains substantially elevated over baseline even after many years without treatment.[89]

Table 16-2 ■ **A Summary of Established Hormonal Risk and Protective Factors for Endometrial Cancer**

Risk factors (increased exposure to "unopposed" estrogen)
• Estrogen replacement therapy
• Obesity
• Sequential oral contraceptives
• Late menopause
Protective factors (decreased exposure to "unopposed" estrogen)
• Pregnancy
• Combination oral contraceptives

As noted earlier, the newer regimens of hormone therapy typically follow one of two patterns. They either provide a sequence of estrogen and estrogen plus progestin like that of sequential oral contraceptives or estrogen and progestin are given together daily throughout the cycle. The sequential regimen attempts to reproduce the hormonal pattern of the normal menstrual cycle, albeit at lower levels of both estrogen and progestogen. One therefore might predict that this method of hormone therapy administration would only partially offset the increased risk of endometrial cancer that is associated with unopposed estrogen therapy. Pike and colleagues showed that if progestins are added for <10 days per month, the risk is only slightly reduced.[90] However, regimens that include progestins for >10 days in a month, or where progestins are given continuously with estrogen, do not increase risk of endometrial cancer.[90]

The Million Women Study conducted in Great Britain, which included 716,738 postmenopausal women without prior cancer or hysterectomy who were recruited between 1996 and 2001, also provides data on this issue.[16] Relative to women who had never used any hormonal therapy, endometrial cancer risk was substantially lower among women who had used continuous-combined therapy as their most recent hormone therapy with a RR of 0.71 (95% CI = 0.56-0.90). For women using cyclic combined hormone therapy, however, risk did not differ from that of nonusers (RR = 1.05, 95% CI = 0.92-1.22). The number of cases among women taking estrogen-alone therapy was small, as this has rarely been given to women with an intact uterus since the mid-to-late 1970s. Among women on estrogen-alone therapy, the RR of endometrial cancer was substantially lower than prior studies had observed (RR = 1.45, 95% CI = 1.02-2.06). As expected, based on the fact that obesity increases endometrial cancer risk through an estrogen pathway causing endometrial proliferation,[81,91] the reduction in risk on combined therapy was greatest among obese women and the increase in risk for estrogen-alone therapy was greatest among nonobese women.

In reporting results of the Million Women Study, the authors also provided an extensive assessment of the literature on the impact of combined hormone therapy on endometrial cancer risk, calculating a summary estimate of RR comparing users to nonusers of continuous-combined therapy and cyclic combined therapy across studies with published data and including their own study.[16] Overall, they estimated that the RR for continuous-combined hormone therapy across all studies was 0.88 (95% CI = 0.75-1.03) compared to never users. This estimate, however, was based on relatively few cases—with only 265 cases identified across six studies, including the Women's Health Initiative.[92] In the meta-analysis included in the Million Women Study publication,[16] the estimated RR of endometrial cancer associated with use of cyclic combined hormone therapy was 1.14 (95% CI = 1.01-1.28). This estimate was based on a total of 456 cases, from six studies, four of which overlap with the studies of continuous-combined therapy. Overall, it appears that regimens in which estrogen and progestin are taken daily together (continuous-combined hormone therapy) provide a slight protection against endometrial cancer relative to the risk among women who had never used any hormonal regimen, whereas cyclic use of progestins results in a risk of endometrial cancer that is slightly higher than that of women who had never used hormone therapy.

Tamoxifen, an antiestrogen to the breast, acts as an estrogen agonist in the endometrium, and the risk of endometrial cancer is elevated by tamoxifen in a fashion analogous to that of estrogen therapy.[93] Furthermore, the increase in risk is greater among women who previously used estrogen therapy and among those with high body mass.[93] The molecular basis of this agonist effect on the endometrium as opposed to the antagonist activity of tamoxifen on the breast, however, is not totally understood.

Body Weight[66]

Unlike breast cancer where high body weight is associated with low risk among young women and high risk among older women, high body weight leads to increased risk of endometrial cancer at all ages.[38] Studies of postmenopausal women show at least a doubling of risk of endometrial cancer between thin and heavy women.[94,95] Adipose tissue is rich in an aromatase enzyme system that converts androstenedione to estrone. In turn, estrone can be converted directly to estradiol. In addition, protein binding of estrogens in blood is lower in obese women, so the amount of bioavailable estradiol in postmenopausal women is higher than would be expected from the peripheral conversion of androstenedione to estrone alone.

The explanation for the substantially increased risk of endometrial cancer with obesity in premenopausal women is less obvious.[95] Although obesity does appear to be associated with slightly increased levels of bioavailable estradiol in premenopausal women, this alone appears to be insufficient to account for such a profound effect. The more likely explanation is that obesity in premenopausal women is associated with amenorrhea and subnormal luteal phase progesterone levels, thus resulting in prolonged exposure of the endometrium to unopposed estrogen derived from peripheral conversion in adipose tissue.[96]

Among postmenopausal women, obesity becomes a more important factor in determining endometrial cancer risk as use of combined hormone therapy has declined since publication of the Women's Health Initiative results. Results from the American Cancer Society Cancer Prevention Study II Nutrition Cohort show that the risk of endometrial cancer associated with obesity is strongly influenced by whether a women has used combined hormone therapy.[97] Increasing body size, measured by body mass index (kg/m^2), is associated with increasing endometrial cancer risk among postmenopausal women with no prior history of hormone therapy use but has no impact on endometrial cancer risk among women who have used combined hormone therapy.[97]

Oral Contraceptives

The role of estrogens as the principal cause of endometrial cancer is further supported by the markedly increased risk after a relatively short duration of use of sequential oral contraceptives, which deliver an unopposed estrogen during most of the monthly cycle.[95,98] As potent as estrogen therapy and sequential oral contraceptives are in modifying the risk of endometrial cancer, these effects can be mitigated by the simultaneous administration of progestogens. A series of case-control and cohort studies has consistently demonstrated that combined oral contraceptives, which deliver estrogen and progestogen simultaneously during each day of use, decrease the risk of endometrial cancer by 11.7% per year of use (Fig. 16-3B).[15] Use of unopposed estrogen therapy for at least 3 years following discontinuation of oral contraceptive use may counter the reduction in risk observed for oral contraceptive use.[99]

Parity

The other major, established risk factor for endometrial cancer, low parity, also is readily explained by the unopposed estrogen hypothesis.[94] The highest risk of endometrial cancer occurs in nulliparous women, and an incremental decrease in risk occurs with each increment in parity. Nulliparous women have a risk of endometrial cancer that is three to five times that of women with parity of greater than three. This effect is expected as no endometrial mitotic activity occurs during pregnancy because of the persistently high progesterone levels.

Ovarian Cancer

Existing epidemiological data on hormonal exposures across the four major histopathological subtypes of epithelial ovarian cancer (serous, endometriod, clear cell and mucinous) suggest that risk factors are consistent across all subtypes except perhaps mucinous tumors. Traditionally, the cell of origin of epithelial ovarian cancer (herein referred to as ovarian cancer) has been described as the single layer of cells lining the surface of the ovary; because these cells replicate during or after each ovulation any respite from ovulation would be protective against ovarian cancer.[100] This hypothesis called "incessant ovulation" is supported by epidemiologic data, which consistently demonstrate that the risk of developing ovarian cancer decreases with increasing parity[101-103] and with combination oral contraceptive use (Table 16-3),[103-108] both of which induce anovulation. However, emerging evidence that serous tumors of the fallopian tube and peritoneum share the same epidemiology as serous ovarian cancers has brought into question the notion that it is the actual act of ovulation and subsequent wound healing that underlies the epidemiology of the disease; instead, it may be the hormonal milieu induced as a result of parity and oral contraceptive use.[109] Further, clear evidence of an association between menopausal hormone therapy exists, suggesting that the hormonal milieu influences risk of ovarian cancer rather than ovulation itself.

As with breast and endometrial cancer, the age-incidence curve for ovarian cancer emphasizes the importance of menopause in determining risk. The age-incidence curve of ovarian cancer can be brought into line with the familiar linear log-log plot of other non-hormone-dependent epithelial tumors, if ovarian age is considered as starting at menarche, but increasing at a reduced rate (~30% of normal) during periods of anovulation, including the postmenopausal years.[15]

Table 16-3 A Summary of Established Hormonal Risk and Protective Factors for Ovarian Cancer

Risk factors (increased number of ovulations)
• Late menopause
Protective factors (decreased number of ovulations)
• Pregnancy
• Oral contraceptives

Parity

Parity has been consistently identified as a protective factor against ovarian cancer.[101-103] After a woman's first birth, risk is reduced ~40% with a 10% reduction in ovarian cancer associated with subsequent births.[102-104,110-112] While part of the greater reduction in risk with the first birth may be an artifact of including infertile women who are at increased risk of ovarian cancer[113] in the nulliparous reference group, this does not fully explain the greater reduction in risk seen with a first birth. An older age (35 years or older) at birth may be more protective than a birth at a young age (under 25 years),[103,104,114] but this result has not been observed in all studies and requires further follow-up.[102,111]

Oral Contraceptives

Epidemiologic studies have consistently demonstrated that oral contraceptive use decreases the risk of ovarian cancer, in a duration-dependent manner analogous to the protective effect observed for endometrial cancer.[103-108] A collaborative analysis of 45 epidemiological studies has shown that any use of oral contraceptives was associated with a 27% reduction in ovarian cancer risk (95% CI = 0.70-0.76), with risk reduced 20% with each 5 years of use.[108] This pooled analysis also showed an attenuation in the risk reduction over time; women whose use ended <10 years previously had a 29% reduction in risk per 5 years of use whereas women who last used oral contraceptives 20-29 years previously had only a 15% reduction per 5 years of use. Clearly though, the reduction in risk persisted for decades. In this study, substantial statistically significant heterogeneity was observed across histopathological subtypes with no statistically significant risk reduction for mucinous tumors.

It has been hypothesized that the blocking of ovulation is the mechanism through which both parity and oral contraceptives protect against ovarian cancer; however, an alternate explanation has arisen. The average daily exposure to progesterone during the normal menstrual cycle is ~3.5 ng/mL compared to 9.2 ng/mL for women taking oral contraceptives.[115,116] Likewise, pregnancy is associated with high progesterone levels. Thus the high levels of progesterone achieved through oral contraceptive use and pregnancy may explain their protective effects. A study of female macaque monkeys has shown that progestins used in oral contraceptives induce apoptosis in the ovarian epithelium which could protect against ovarian cancer.[117] Also, in vitro evidence that estrogen can increase ovarian tumor cell growth exists and this effect can be blocked by progesterone.[118,119]

Hormone Therapy

The epidemiologic evidence regarding hormone therapy and ovarian cancer risk has become much clearer in the recent years. We have conducted a detailed meta-analysis of the published literature through 2007 from population-based case-control studies[104,120-126] and cohort studies[127-131] and have found that use of menopausal estrogen therapy increases ovarian cancer risk by 22% for each 5 years of use ($p < 0.0001$). These results are consistent in all but one of the publications, which showed no association.[120]. Across the 13 publications showing an association, the dose-response relationship is clear.

The results with regard to menopausal estrogen-progestin therapy, while not as consistent, still provide a clear picture. The meta-analysis of population-based case-control studies,[104,120,122-125,128] cohort studies,[129-131] and the Women's Health Initiative[92] show a 10% increase in risk of ovarian cancer per 5 years of combined hormone therapy use ($p = 0.001$). The difference in risk between estrogen only therapy and combined hormone therapy use is statistically significant ($p = 0.004$), suggesting that the addition of a progestin to estrogen therapy ameliorates the effect of the estrogen. These analyses provide further support for a protective effect of progestins on ovarian cancer risk.

It is not clear whether the effect of combined hormone therapy differs depending on whether the sequential or continuous-combined regimen is prescribed. Four studies shed some light on this question. The Million's Women Study[130] did not find a difference in ever use risk estimates associated with combined therapy for these two regimens; however, no duration of use information was provided. The National Institutes of Health American Association for Retired Persons cohort study reports higher risk associated with sequential combined therapy than with continuous-combined therapy, but both regimens were associated with increased risk.[129] A case-control study report shows a reduced risk of ovarian cancer associated with both types of combined therapy regimens,[125] whereas a case-control study from Sweden found that sequential combined therapy increased risk, but continuous-combined therapy did not.[124] The total dose of progestin delivered between sequential and continuous-combined regimens in the United States and the United Kingdom do not differ, but in Sweden the progestin dose in continuous-combined is much higher than that in sequential formulations; this may explain the lack of association with this regimen in the Swedish study.[27] Further follow-up is needed in this area.

Given these findings for menopausal hormone therapy, the interpretation of the observations that parity and oral contraceptive use reduce risk can be viewed in a new light, specifically that the mechanism of action of these two protective factors may act by increasing exposure to progestins. This is more consistent with emerging views that the single layer of cells on the surface of the ovary may not be where ovarian cancer originates.

Prostate Cancer

Prostate cancer is the most frequently diagnosed cancer in American men, with an estimated 186,320 cases diagnosed in 2008.[17] It is also the second leading cause of cancer deaths in males, exceeded only by lung cancer, with ~29,000 deaths from prostate cancer occurring annually.[17] The prostate is an androgen-regulated organ, with androgens considered as the major stimulus for cell division in prostatic epithelium.[5,132] Thus androgens are strong candidates as major contributors to prostatic carcinogenesis. Until recently only indirect evidence supported a causal role for androgens in prostate cancer development. Results from the Prostate Cancer Prevention Trial (PCPT), using an agent that reduces androgen action in the prostate, provided the first direct evidence in support of an important androgen role in this process.[133] Assessing the role of androgens in prostate cancer development has been difficult in part because of a lack of easily measurable hormonal events in men as exist in women (eg, menarche, menopause, reproductive experiences). Furthermore, use of exogenous androgens in men is relatively uncommon.

The epidemiology of prostate cancer is dominated by three observations: (1) the profound international and racial-ethnic variation in incidence and mortality historically reported to be as much as 80-fold between the extremes of high-risk (African Americans) and low-risk (native Japanese and Chinese) populations[134]; (2) the occurrence of occult, subclinical prostate cancer at a relatively comparable prevalence across populations[135]; and (3) the strong relationship between prostate cancer incidence and aging.[5] Prostate cancer is extremely rare before age 50 years, but it is still the most common cancer of American men, in large part because the rate of increase in prostate cancer incidence with aging is greater than for any other cancer.

Some of the indirect evidence for a role of androgens in prostate cancer development has come from comparisons of hormonal profiles of healthy men from racial-ethnic groups at high, intermediate, and low risk of prostate cancer. Although studies have not shown differences in testosterone levels between whites and African Americans,[10,136,137] recent evidence suggests that African Americans have higher estradiol levels than whites and Latinos.[138] Asian men, while showing no evidence of low circulating testosterone levels relative to whites and African Americans at any age, have substantially reduced levels of androstanediol glucuronide.[139,140] This hormone reflects 5α-reductase activity (5α-reductase is the prostatic enzyme that bioactivates testosterone to dihydrotestosterone, the most biologically potent human androgen). Based on these results and the presumptive role of androgens in prostate cell proliferation, Ross and colleagues proposed that a 5α-reductase inhibitor might be an effective chemopreventive agent for prostate cancer.[139]

Several additional indirect lines of evidence point to a role of androgens in prostate cancer pathogenesis. Androgens are required for prostate cancer development or progression in most animal models of prostatic adenocarcinoma.[141] Prostate cancer has never been reported to occur in eunuchs or in men with genetically determined decreased 5α-reductase activity, groups with very low androgen activity and highly underdeveloped prostates.[5] Prostate cancers, at least early in their course, are almost uniformly androgen-dependent, and androgen ablation therapy has been the mainstay for treating early metastatic prostate cancer for many decades.

The role of circulating androgens and prostate cancer risk has been investigated by several studies, yielding inconsistent results. A large pooled analysis of 18 prospective studies from the Endogenous Hormones and Prostate Cancer Collaborative Group found no association between the risk of prostate cancer and circulating levels of testosterone, dihydrotestosterone, dehydroepiandrosterone sulfate, androstenedione, androstanediol glucuronide, estradiol.[142] Circulating sex hormone–binding globulin was associated with a decreased risk of prostate cancer, with a relative risk reduction of 14% when comparing the fifth highest level to the lowest fifth. Sex hormone–binding globulin regulates circulating levels of free testosterone and estradiol and may also play a role in steroid signaling.[143] Although the majority of circulating androgens do not appear to influence prostate cancer risk, an important consideration of these studies is whether a single hormone measurement can accurately reflect the average hormone profile of an individual.

The most convincing evidence for a role of androgens in prostate cancer development comes from the PCPT.[133] In the PCPT, 18,882 healthy men aged 55 years and older, with normal range prostate specific antigen values (PSAs), were randomized to receive 5 mg daily of finasteride, a 5α-reductase inhibitor, or placebo. After 7 years, all men were designated for an end-of-trial prostate biopsy. Prostate cancer incidence in the treatment arm was reduced ~25%. However, paradoxically, there was a statistically significant 25% *increase* in high grade prostate cancer incidence in the therapeutic arm. These disparate findings have created substantial controversy regarding the role of 5α-reductase inhibitors in prostate cancer prevention in healthy men, as well as substantial disagreement regarding the underlying cause of these curious results. It has been argued, for example, that this finding represents an artifact of disruptive morphological changes induced by finasteride in the prostate, or that the increased risk of high grade prostate cancer is the result of detection bias due to finasteride-induced reduction in prostate volume.[144] Others have argued that these results reflect, with a clear biological basis; for example, Ross and colleagues consider that high grade prostate cancer precursor cells, possibly with androgen receptor alterations (amplification, gene mutations) thrive in an androgen-depleted environment, that prostate cancer cells with somatic mutations of the 5α-reductase type II gene respond differently to an inhibitor than those without such changes, and that finasteride, by virtue of increased intraprostatic levels of testosterone, selectively stimulates prostate cancer precursor lesions.[145] Understanding the true nature of these results will have enormous public health implications.

Genetic Determinants

Familial Risk

A family history of breast cancer is associated with an increased risk of the disease.[4] This is particularly apparent when the family history includes a woman who was affected at an early age or had bilateral disease. Whereas a two- to threefold increase in the risk of the disease has been observed in first-degree relatives of women with breast cancer overall, a ninefold increase in risk has been found in the first-degree relatives of premenopausal women with bilateral breast cancer. Very high risks (ie, fivefold or greater) also have been found in women with more than one first-degree relative with breast cancer. Similarly, population-based case-control studies have described a two- to threefold increased risk of ovarian cancer in first-degree relatives of ovarian cancer patients.[146,147] Heritability estimates for both breast and ovarian cancers are ~25%.[148] The impact of family history on endometrial cancer risk is less clear. Some studies have shown an association between family history and risk of this cancer,[149-152] but this finding has not been consistent.[153] Also, unlike breast and ovarian cancers, heritability estimates from twin studies do not suggest a strong genetic component for endometrial cancer.[148]

Prostate cancer is a highly familial disease. Men with a first-degree relative with prostate cancer have approximately a two- to threefold increase in risk compared to men with no such history and this increase is observed across different racial-ethnic groups.[154] As with breast cancer, risk is elevated further when multiple first-degree relatives are affected or when affected relatives are diagnosed at relatively young ages.[155] This strong familial risk has led to the development of several prostate cancer family registries, searching for a single locus, high penetrance gene responsible for this familial risk. Exciting developments from a linkage analysis of prostate cancer in conjunction with follow-up association studies have identified chromosome 8q24 as a susceptibility locus for prostate cancer.[156] Through fine-mapping and genome-wide association studies, multiple independent variants at 8q24 have been discovered that consistently impact prostate cancer risk.[157-159] The population attributable risks associated with these variants range from 8% to 68% depending on the variants and populations considered.[157-159]

Genes

Significant efforts have been directed toward identifying major genes influencing risk of breast and ovarian cancers using high-risk families. Extraordinary success has been achieved using this approach to identify the highly penetrant, major disease-causing genes, *BRCA1* and *BRCA2*. Yet, mutations in *BRCA1* and *BRCA2* explain <10% of the breast[160-162] or ovarian cancer cases.[163] Although *BRCA1* and *BRCA2* are quite important to carriers, a large gap exists in understanding the genetic etiology of breast and ovarian cancers in the general population. All of these observations combined with the epidemiology described earlier are consistent with a multifactorial etiology for each of these cancers, with hormonal, genetic, and environmental factors playing a role. Most likely, the common forms of breast, ovarian, and endometrial cancers are complex genetic diseases with locus and allelic heterogeneity.

Such complex traits are marked by minor susceptibility genes associated with modest increases in risk, but high population attributable risk, because the risk allele may be quite common in the population. These types of genes, such as those involved in reproductive endocrinology, may act alone or in combination with common variants of other genes and environmental factors to increase the risk of breast, ovarian, or endometrial cancer. Ultimately, common variants in several such genes involved in the biology of the breast, ovary, or endometrium could give rise to a "polygenic" etiology of cancer.

Exactly which genes and variants are associated with these cancers is unknown, but candidate genes can be selected based on an understanding of the epidemiology, biology, and etiology of the cancer. Table 16-4 shows one potential list of candidate genes and their related pathways. These genes may harbor risk variants for breast, ovarian, or endometrial cancer. For example, one of the most extensively studied genes in all three of these female hormone-related cancers is the progesterone receptor gene (*PGR*). Two variants have been studied in a number of studies. The first is a nonsynonymous single nucleotide polymorphism (SNP) in exon four of the gene (V660L) and the second is a SNP in the promoter region of the gene (+331G/A). Both SNPs may have functional consequences.[164,165]

A meta-analysis of the association between the V660L variant and breast cancer risk was recently published.[166] Overall, breast cancer risk increased 7% per copy of the L-allele carried (95% CI = 1.02-1.13; $p = 0.01$). However, substantial heterogeneity of risk estimates was observed across the published studies (p for heterogeneity $= 0.01$), suggesting that any association with breast cancer may not be robust. This variant has also been studied extensively in association with ovarian cancer; a large pooling effort, the Ovarian Cancer Association Consortium, reported no overall association with the V660L SNP ($p = 0.38$) after studying >4700 cases.[116] Of note, however, is that this pooled analysis did observe an association between this SNP and risk of the endometrioid subtype of ovarian cancer ($p = 0.04$).

Observing variation in the relationships between genes and histological subtypes of a cancer, such as observed for the PGR V660L SNP and ovarian cancer, has profound implications for study design when attempting to unravel the genetic contributions to disease. If the effects are limited to particular subtypes, as is the case here, then sample sizes needed for these large genotyping efforts are much larger than initially believed. This variant (V660L) has also been explored with regard to endometrial cancer risk and a nonsignificant protective effect has been observed.[165]

The PGR +331G/A variant has also been studied in all three of these hormone-related female cancers. +331G/A has also been reported to have a functional consequence on the transcription of the receptor.[165] Initially, it was reported that the variant allele was associated with an increased risk of breast cancer[167]; however, subsequent studies failed to confirm this association.[166,168-171] One study has shown an association between this variant and an increased endometrial cancer risk,[165] but this finding remains to be confirmed. Similar to the V660L findings with ovarian cancer, the results for the +331G/A variant also illustrate the importance of large studies and collaborative efforts. A collaborative analysis from the Ovarian Cancer Association Consortium showed that the +331G/A PGR promoter polymorphism is associated with a modest decrease in risk of endometrioid and clear cell subtypes of ovarian cancer.[116,172] Without collaborative efforts, these associations would not be detected given the small sample sizes in each study.

The relationship between genetic control of androgen biosynthesis and metabolic pathways and prostate cancer risk remains unclear. A number of years ago, Ross and colleagues published a description of a polygenic model of prostate cancer development related to genetic control of androgen pathways to the prostate.[5] Although both genetic control of androgen biosynthesis outside the prostate and transport of androgens to the prostate are of interest, most research to date has centered around androgen signaling within prostatic epithelial cells, especially in regard to (1) the androgen receptor (AR) gene encoding the androgen receptor, which is responsible both for androgen transport within prostate cells and for transactivation of genes with androgen response elements in their promoter region; (2) the steroid 5α-reductase type II (*SRD5A2*) gene, which encodes the type 2 5α-reductase enzyme responsible for metabolic activation of testosterone to dihydrotestosterone in prostatic cells although other candidate genes in this pathway have also been studied; (3) the cytochrome P450 17α-hydroxylase (*CYP17*) gene, which mediates both 17-α-activity, converting pregnenolone to dehydroepiandrosterone and 17,20-lyase activity, generating androstenedione from progesterone.

The polymorphic CAG repeat in exon 1 of the androgen receptor gene has been proposed to predict androgen receptor transactivation activity and, therefore, prostate cancer risk[173]; support for this hypothesis has been inconsistent,[174-176] with the largest study to date, the Multiethnic Cohort Study, demonstrating no association.[174] A missense substitution polymorphism (A49T) in the *SRD5A2* gene has also been linked to prostate cancer risk, but this result has not been easily reproduced.[177-179] Similarly, the 5′ promoter polymorphism (T27C) in the *CYP17* gene has been associated with prostate cancer in some,[180,181] but not all studies,[182,183] with the Breast and Prostate Cancer Cohort Consortium reporting no association.[184] The lack of consistency in these genetic association studies of androgen genes highlights the need for careful interpretation and replication in multiple well-defined study populations. As with female hormone–related cancers, much work still needs to be done in a more systematic pathway driven approach to fully identify the possible contribution of the candidate androgen genes and prostate cancer risk.

Table 16-4 Candidate Genes and Pathways Relevant to Breast, Ovarian, and Endometrial Cancer Risk

Pathway	Genes
Gonadotropin signaling	*GNRH1, GNRHR, CGA, FSHB, LHB, FSHR, LHCGR, INHA, INHBA, INHBB, ACVR1, ACVR2*
Sex steroid hormone biosynthesis	*CYP11, CYP17, HSD3B1, HSD3B2, CYP19, HSD17B1, HSD17B2, HSD17B3, STAR*
Glucocorticoid synthesis	*CRH, CRHR1/2, POMC (ACTH), MC2R (ACTHR), CYP21, CYP11B*
Endogenous/exogenous hormone metabolism	*AKR1C1, AKR1C2, AKR1C3, AKR1C4, COMT, CYP1A1, CYP1A2, CYP3A4, CYP3A5, CYP1B1, CYP21, HSD3B1, HSD3B2, HSD17B1, HSD17B2, SRD5A1, SRD5A2, SULT1A1, UGT1A*
Hormone transport/action	*ESR1, ESR2, PGR, SHBG*
Growth hormone/insulin-like growth factor signaling axis	*GH1, GHR, GHRH, GHRHR, IGF1, IGF2, IGF1R, IGF2R, IGFALS, IGFBP1, IGFBP2, IGFBP3, IGFBP4, IGFBP5, IGFBP6, POU1F1, SST, SSTR1, SSTR2, SSTR3, SSTR4, SSTR5*

Conclusion

As our understanding of the relationship between epidemiologic risk factors and the circulating levels of the relevant hormones grows, avenues for primary prevention are becoming apparent. The control of obesity has obvious implications for both endometrial cancer and postmenopausal breast cancer. More information on the relationship between childhood diet and physical activity and the onset of puberty, in conjunction with the hormonal physiology of adolescence and young adulthood, may provide increasing avenues for preventing breast, ovarian, and endometrial cancers in women. A large hormonal chemoprevention trial for breast cancer using the antiestrogen drug tamoxifen has already proven successful and an additional national trial using an alternative selective estrogen receptor modulator, raloxifene, without the same estrogen agonist effects on the endometrium, is underway. In the future, aromatase inhibitors, which are effective in breast cancer therapy, may prove to be effective in breast cancer prevention. Hormonal chemoprevention of ovarian and endometrial cancer is already occurring in the population as a whole through the widespread use of combination oral contraceptives, and of endometrial cancer with increasing use of combined hormone therapy. A national trial to prevent prostate cancer through use of finasteride, a 5α-reductase inhibitor, has been completed and provides convincing evidence for the role of androgens in the development of this disease. A growing knowledge of the mutations and polymorphisms in genes causing increased risk of these cancers should lead to better definition of individual susceptibility. It should then be possible to focus intervention strategies on the higher-risk subgroups of the population.

Selected References

The complete reference list can be found at www.CANCERMEDICINE8.com

2. Henderson BE, Ross RK, Bernstein L. Estrogens as a cause of human cancer: the Richard and Hinda Rosenthal Foundation award lecture. *Cancer Res.* 1988;48:246–253.
15. Henderson BE, Ross RK, Pike MC. Hormonal chemoprevention of cancer in women. *Science.* 1993;259:633–638.
20. Berry DA, Cronin KA, Plevritis SK, et al. Effect of screening and adjuvant therapy on mortality from breast cancer. *N Engl J Med.* 2005;353:1784–1792.
21. Key TJ, Pike MC. The role of oestrogens and progestagens in the epidemiology and prevention of breast cancer. *Eur J Cancer Clin Oncol.* 1988;24:29–43.
22. Ferguson DJ, Anderson TJ. Morphological evaluation of cell turnover in relation to the menstrual cycle in the "resting" human breast. *Br J Cancer.* 1981;44:177–181.
25. Writing Group for the Women's Health Initiative Investigators. Risks and benefits of estrogen plus progestin in healthy postmenopausal women: principal results from the Women's Health Initiative randomized trial. *JAMA.* 2002;288:321–333.
26. Chlebowski RT, Hendrix SL, Langer RD, et al. Influence of estrogen plus progestin on breast cancer and mammography in healthy postmenopausal women: the Women's Health Initiative Randomized Trial. *JAMA.* 2003;289:3243–3253.
27. Lee SA, Ross RK, Pike MC. An overview of menopausal oestrogen-progestin hormone therapy and breast cancer risk. *Br J Cancer.* 2005;92:2049–2058.
33. Bernstein L, Henderson BE, Hanisch R, et al. Physical exercise and reduced risk of breast cancer in young women. *J Natl Cancer Inst.* 1994;86:1403–1408.
38. Vainio H, Bianchini F. *IARC Handbooks on Cancer Prevention: Weight Control and Physical Activity.* Lyon, France: International Agency for Research on Cancer; 2002.
46. Key T, Appleby P, Barnes I, et al. Endogenous Hormones and Breast Cancer Collaborative Group. Endogenous sex hormones and breast cancer in postmenopausal women: reanalysis of nine prospective studies. *J Natl Cancer Inst.* 2002;94:606–616.
48. Liu Q, Wuu J, Lambe M, et al. Transient increase in breast cancer risk after giving birth: postpartum period with the highest risk (Sweden). *Cancer Causes Control.* 2002;13:299–305.
59. Armstrong B, Doll R. Environmental factors and cancer incidence and mortality in different countries, with special reference to dietary practices. *Int J Cancer.* 1975;15:617–631.
61. Prentice RL, Caan B, Chlebowski RT, et al. Low-fat dietary pattern and risk of invasive breast cancer: the Women's Health Initiative Randomized Controlled Dietary Modification Trial. *JAMA.* 2006;295:629–642.
63. Key TJ, Allen NE, Spencer EA, et al. Nutrition and breast cancer. *Breast.* 2003;12:412–416.
65. Wu AH, Pike MC, Stram DO. Meta-analysis: dietary fat intake, serum estrogen levels, and the risk of breast cancer. *J Natl Cancer Inst.* 1999;91:529–534.
66. Collaborative Group on Hormonal Factors in Breast Cancer. Breast cancer and hormonal contraceptives: collaborative reanalysis of individual data on 53,297 women with breast cancer and 100,239 women without breast cancer from 54 epidemiological studies. *Lancet.* 1996;347:1713–1727.
68. International Agency for Research on Cancer. *Combined Estrogen-Progestogen Contraceptives and Combined Estrogen-Progestogen Menopausal Therapy.* Volume 91. Lyon, France: International Agency for Research on Cancer; 2008:528.
70. The Women's Health Initiative Steering Committee: effects of conjugated equine estrogen in postmenopausal women with hysterectomy. *JAMA.* 2004;291:1701–1712.
73. Lee SA, Ross RK, Pike MC. An overview of menopausal estrogen-progestin hormone therapy and breast cancer risk. *Br J Cancer.* 2005;92:2049–2058.
76. Radvin PM, Cronin KA, Howlader N, et al. The decrease in breast-cancer incidence in 2003 in the United States. *N Engl J Med.* 2007;356:1670–1674.
81. Key TJ, Pike MC. The dose-effect relationship between "unopposed" oestrogens and endometrial mitotic rate: its central role in explaining and predicting endometrial cancer risk. *Br J Cancer.* 1988;57:205–212.
90. Pike MC, Peters RK, Cozen W, et al. Estrogen-progestin replacement therapy and endometrial cancer. *J Natl Cancer Inst.* 1997;89:1110–1116.
92. Anderson GL, Judd HL, Kaunitz AM, et al. Effect of estrogen plus progestin on gynecologic cancers and associated diagnostic procedures: the Women's Health Initiative randomized trial. *JAMA.* 2003;290:1739–1748.
93. Bernstein L, Deapen D, Cerhan JR, et al. Tamoxifen therapy for breast cancer and endometrial cancer risk. *J Natl Cancer Inst.* 1999;91:1654–1662.
97. McCullough ML, Patel AV, Patel R, et al. Body mass and endometrial cancer risk by hormone replacement therapy and cancer subtype. *Cancer Epidemiol Biomarkers Prev.* 2008;17:73–79.
100. Fathalla MF. Factors in the causation and incidence of ovarian cancer. *Obstet Gynecol Surv.* 1972;27:751–768.
103. Whittemore AS, Harris R, Itnyre J. Characteristics relating to ovarian cancer risk: collaborative analysis of 12 US case-control studies. II. Invasive epithelial ovarian cancers in white women. Collaborative Ovarian Cancer Group. *Am J Epidemiol.* 1992;136:1184–1203.
104. Pike MC, Pearce CL, Peters R, et al. Hormonal factors and the risk of invasive ovarian cancer: a population-based case-control study. *Fertil Steril.* 2004;82:186–195.
108. Collaborative Group on Epidemiological Studies of Ovarian Cancer. Ovarian Cancer and oral contraceptives: collaborative reanalysis of data from 45 epidemiological studies including 23,257 women with ovarian cancer and 87,303 controls. *Lancet.* 2008;371:303–314.
109. Jordan SJ, Green AC, Whiteman DC, et al. Serous ovarian, fallopian tube and primary peritoneal cancers: a comparative epidemiological analysis. *Int J Cancer.* 2008;122:1598–1603.
113. Ness RB, Cramer DW, Goodman MT, et al. Infertility, fertility drugs, and ovarian cancer: a pooled analysis of case-control studies. *Am J Epidemiol.* 2002;155: 217–224.
116. Pearce CL, Wu AH, Gayther SA, et al. Progesterone receptor variation and risk of ovarian cancer is limited to the invasive endometrioid subtype: results from the ovarian cancer association consortium pooled analysis. *Br J Cancer.* 2008;98:282–288.
120. Purdie DM, Bain CJ, Siskind V, et al. Hormone replacement therapy and risk of epithelial ovarian cancer. *Br J Cancer.* 1999;81:559–563.
129. Lacey JV, Jr., Brinton LA, Leitzmann MF, et al. Menopausal hormone therapy and ovarian cancer risk in the National Institutes of Health-AARP Diet and Health Study Cohort. *J Natl Cancer Inst.* 2006;98:1397–1405.
130. Beral V, Bull D, Green J, et al. Ovarian cancer and hormone replacement therapy in the Million Women Study. *Lancet.* 2007;369:1703–1710.
134. Ross RK, Schottenfeld D. Prostate cancer. In: Schottenfeld D, Fraumeni JF, eds. *Cancer Epidemiology and Prevention.* New York: Oxford University Press; 1996:1180–1206.
139. Ross RK, Bernstein L, Lobo RA, et al. 5-alpha-reductase activity and risk of prostate cancer among Japanese and US white and black males. *Lancet.* 1992;339:887–889.
145. Ross RK, Skinner E, Cote RJ. Prevention of prostate cancer with finasteride. *N Engl J Med.* 2003;349:1569–1572.
147. Stratton JF, Pharoah P, Smith SK, et al. A systematic review and meta-analysis of family history and risk of ovarian cancer. *Br J Obstet Gynaecol.* 1998;105:493–499.
148. Lichtenstein P, Holm NV, Verkasalo PK, et al. Environmental and heritable factors in the causation of cancer—analyses of cohorts of twins from Sweden, Denmark, and Finland. *N Engl J Med.* 2000;343:78–85.
153. Olson JE, Sellers TA, Anderson KE, et al. Does a family history of cancer increase the risk for postmenopausal endometrial carcinoma? A prospective cohort study and a nested case-control family study of older women. *Cancer.* 1999;85:2444–2449.

17 Ionizing Radiation

David J. Grdina, PhD

The hazards of exposure to ionizing radiation were recognized shortly after Roentgen's discovery of the X-ray in 1895. Acute skin reactions were observed in many individuals working with early X-ray generators, and by 1902 the first radiation-induced cancer was reported arising in an ulcerated area of the skin. Within a few years, a large number of such skin cancers had been observed, and the first report of leukemia in five radiation workers appeared in 1911.[1] Many experimental and epidemiologic studies have since confirmed the oncogenic effects of radiation.

There are a number of characteristics specific to ionizing radiation that differentiates it from chemical toxic agents or other physical carcinogens. Notable among these is its ability to penetrate cells and to deposit energy within them in a random fashion, unaffected by the usual cellular barriers presented to chemical agents. All cells in the body are thus susceptible to damage by ionizing radiation; the amount of damage incurred will be related to the physical parameters that determine the radiation dose received by the particular cells or tissue.

This chapter reviews briefly the principal cellular effects of radiation, as well as what is known about cellular and molecular mechanisms for radiation carcinogenesis and pharmacologic countermeasures that can mitigate against these processes. The term carcinogenesis is used in its broad sense to include the development of all types of malignant neoplasms. Human risk estimates, derived primarily from epidemiologic studies following relatively high-dose radiation exposures, are also presented. However, few reliable human data are available on its oncogenic effects in the dose range below 10 to 20 cGy.

Development of Radiation Injury

Figure 17-1 is a representation of the interaction of ionizing radiation with biologic tissues and the subsequent development of radiation injury. Such radiation is of two major types, electromagnetic waves or ionizing particles. In either case, interaction with orbital electrons results in ionizations and excitations. The initial deposition of energy in irradiated cells thus occurs in the form of ionized and excited atoms or molecules distributed at random throughout the cells. It is the ionizations that cause most of the chemical changes in the vicinity of the event; this energy may be subsequently transferred through a chain of chemical reactions, finally producing irreversible damage to critical molecules of biologic importance to the cell. It appears that most of the energy that goes into producing excited molecules yields relatively few chemical reactions and is eventually dissipated in the form of heat.

The ionizing event involves the ejection of an orbital electron from a molecule, producing a positively charged or "ionized" molecule. These molecules are highly unstable and rapidly undergo chemical change. This change results in the production of free radicals; these are atoms or molecules containing unpaired electrons. Since the majority of the cell is composed of water, the most common products of this process are the result of the decomposition of water giving rise to both superoxide anion (O_2^-) and hydrogen peroxide (H_2O_2). Also included in this class of radiation-induced reactive oxygen species (ROS) is the highly reactive hydroxyl radical, which has as a result a very short life span and can diffuse only on the average about 4 nm before reacting with other molecules.[2] Paradoxically, the yields of secondary ROS products such as superoxide anion and hydrogen peroxide produced in this manner are significantly lower than that observed following normal metabolism indicating the existence of an amplification mechanism to account for the ultimate magnitude of damage that is observed.[3] One possible mechanism to account for this amplification of ROS production is the inter-mitochondrial communication that results in a subsequent magnification of the ROS damage signal.[4] Following the initiation of oxidative stress as a result of this radiation-induced process, a persistent elevation of oxidative stress can be maintained through the generation of a ROS cascade. One such process has been described in which a ROS cascade can emanate from the mitochondria as a result of O_2^- generation resulting in unstable mitochondrial membrane potentials and redox transitions. This process is referred to as "reactive oxygen species (ROS)-induced ROS release," or RIRR. Under conditions of an excessive oxygen stress burden, the increase in ROS within the mitochondria reaches a threshold that triggers the opening of either the mitochondrial permeability transition (MPT) pore or the inner membrane anion channel (IMAC), which in turn leads to the simultaneous collapse of mitochondrial membrane potential and a transient increase in ROS generation by the electron transfer chain. Release of this ROS burst into the cytosol functions as a second messenger to activate RIRR in neighboring mitochondria.[5,6] In the dose range of 1 to 10 Gy, radiation can produce a transient generation of reactive oxygen or nitrogen within minutes accompanied by a reversible depolarization of mitochondrial membrane potential.[4] In this manner radiation damage in a single mitochondrium could be transmitted via a reversible Ca^{2+}-dependent mitochondrial permeability transition to adjacent mitochondria resulting in the amplification of ROS generation as proposed by the RIRR model. ROS amplification and propagation resulting from such a cascade can then damage important biological targets such as DNA, the nuclear matrix, cytoplasmic transport mechanisms, and both mitochondrial and cellular membranes resulting in cell death. Chemical damage produced from these processes may be repaired before it is irreversible by the recombination of radicals and dissipation of the associated energy. The ROS amplification process may also be interfered with by endogenous antioxidants such as superoxide dismutases (SODs) or exogenously added antioxidants such as the sulfhydryl compounds, a class of

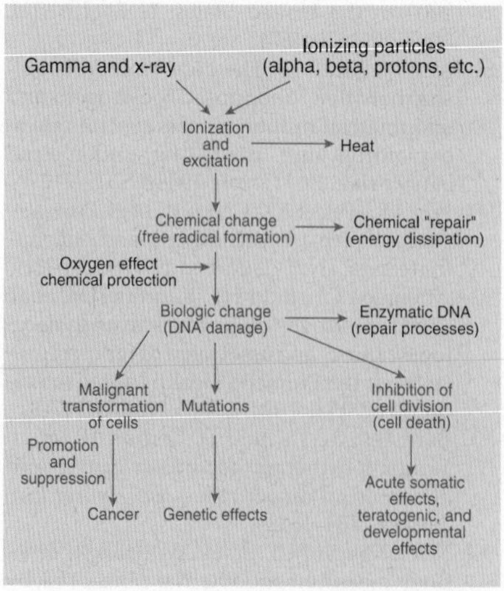

Figure 17-1 Development of radiation injury.

drugs extensively studied for development as radioprotectors.

As the initial ionizing events are similar for all types of radiation, their biologic effects are also qualitatively similar. However, densely ionizing radiations such as alpha particles produce more biologic damage per unit of energy absorbed. The relative biologic effectiveness (RBE) of different types of radiation relative to X-rays is thus related to their linear energy transfer (LET), a measure of the density of the ionizations produced along the radiation track. The initial critical biologic change is thought to be damage to deoxyribonucleic acid (DNA) molecules in the cell. The time required for the entire chain of physical and chemical events as shown in Figure 17-1 from the initial interaction until the production of DNA damage is of the order of a microsecond or less. The subsequent development of biochemical and physiologic changes, however, may take hours to days, whereas the induction of cancer may take many years.

Principal Cellular and Tissue Effects of Radiation

Cell Killing

Radiation can kill cells by two distinct mechanisms. The first is apoptosis, also called programmed cell death or interphase death.[7-9] Cells undergoing apoptosis as an immediate consequence of radiation damage usually die in interphase within a few hours of irradiation, irrespective of and without intervening mitosis. They share distinct morphologic changes, including loss of normal nuclear structure and degradation of DNA that can be demonstrated by a classical pattern of "laddering" on DNA blots. It has long been known that apoptotic cell death can be induced by exposure to relatively low doses of radiation in a few cell types including small lymphocytes, type A spermatogonia, and oocytes.[7] However, apoptosis may also be a significant cause of death in a broader variety of cell types exposed to higher radiation doses, particularly those of hematopoietic or lymphoid origin.

Early investigations have suggested that radiation-induced apoptosis is dependent upon the functional activity of the p53 gene, but it soon became evident that p53-independent pathways may also be involved, such as that mediated by the Bcl-2/BAX family,[10] all of which converge on the activation of proteases called caspases.[11] It has been proposed that p53-dependent apoptosis may involve the transcriptional induction of redox-related genes with the formation of reactive oxygen species, leading to cell death by oxidative stress.[12] DNA damage is thought to be important in triggering the apoptotic response.[13,14] However, there is also evidence for a role of membrane damage and signaling pathways outside the nucleus that involve tyrosine kinases, especially ceramide in the apoptopic process.[15] Apoptosis may serve as a protective mechanism for the elimination of heavily DNA damaged and thus potentially mutated cells from an irradiated population.

Another potential mechanism for removing heavily damaged cells from an irradiated population is the induction of an irreversible G1/S arrest.[16] This is observed, for example, following irradiation of human diploid fibroblasts which are very resistant to apoptosis. The fraction of cells irreversibly blocked in G1/S is reduced if the cells are allowed to repair potentially lethal damage prior to assaying for survival.[16] This arrest is p53- and ATM-dependent[17-19]; no arrest occurs following irradiation of ATM homozygotic cells,[16] nor of $p53^{-/-}$ cells from patients with the Li Fraumeni syndrome.[17] The activation of the p53/p21 pathway by radiation damage in some human tumor cells also suppresses the progression of G1 cells into the DNA synthetic (S) phase of the cell cycle, as well as enhancing apoptotic cell death.[20,21] Interestingly, overexpression of the *C-MYC* oncogene can attenuate this effect in irradiated cells.[22] It has been hypothesized that the absence of a G1 arrest is responsible for the genetic instability that occurs in irradiated cells lacking normal p53 function; cells with extensive genetic damage will progress through the cell cycle and continue proliferation rather than becoming arrested in G1 and undergoing apoptotic cell death or becoming senescent. However, the G1 arrest is only one aspect of a complex cellular response to DNA damage.

The second mechanism for cell killing is radiation-induced reproductive failure. Radiation in sufficient doses can inhibit mitosis, ie, the cell's ability to divide and proliferate indefinitely. The inhibition of cellular proliferation is the mechanism by which radiation kills most mammalian cells. The nature and kinetics of the cytotoxic effects of radiation have been reviewed elsewhere.[7,17] As radiation kills cells by inhibiting their ability to divide, its effects in human beings occur primarily in tissues with high cell turnover or renewal rates characterized by a large amount of proliferative activity. These include tissues such as the bone marrow and the mucosal lining of the stomach and small intestine. Symptoms of acute exposure to whole-body irradiation in human beings are usually observed only following doses of 100 cGy or greater, whereas significant cell killing in vitro can be detected with doses as low as 10 cGy.

Another important somatic effect related to cell killing arises from irradiation of the developing embryo and fetus.[23,24] Whereas irradiation of experimental animals with doses in the order of 200 to 400 cGy during the first trimester of pregnancy has led to a variety of congenital anomalies in the offspring, no such effects were found in large populations of mice exposed to doses below 25 cGy.[23] Moreover, no increase in the frequency of congenital anomalies has been observed in human beings, even following relatively high radiation doses.

Recent epidemiologic studies on the atom bomb survivors of Hiroshima and Nagasaki have focused on mental retardation and other measures of intelligence such as test scores and school performance.[24] These are presumably more sensitive indicators of radiation effects owing to cell depletion amongst the neuroblasts during development. Neuroblasts comprise by far the largest population of cells in the early fetus and continue proliferating until the fifth or sixth month of pregnancy. The number of children with such disorders in the atom bomb survivor study is small, and the mean values for all end points are not significantly different from those in controls for the dose groups below 50 to 100 cGy. The Committee on the Biologic Effects of Ionizing Radiations of the National Research Council (BEIR V Committee)[25] concluded that for mental retardation, the best documented of the developmental abnormalities, the prevalence appeared to increase with dose in a linear manner for individuals irradiated between 8 and 15 weeks, the most sensitive time period after conception. However, the data do not exclude a threshold in the range of 20 to 40 cGy and, indeed, best fit a threshold dose-response relationship with a lower bound of 12 to 20 cGy.[25] On the assumption of a linear, non-threshold relationship, however, the magnitude of the risk would be approximately a 4% chance of occurrence per 10 cGy for exposure at 8 to 15 weeks of gestational age, with less risk occurring for exposure at other ages.

Mutagenesis

The mutagenic effects of ionizing radiation were first described by Herman Muller, in 1927, in his classic experiments with the fruit fly *Drosophila*. Subsequent experiments showed the dose-response relationship for such mutations to be a linear function of exposure over a wide range of radiation doses from as low as 10 to as high as 1000 cGy. Studies of the induction of single-gene mutations in human cells have been limited to several genetic loci. Of particular note is the X-chromosomal gene for hypoxanthine-guanine phosphoribosyltransferase (HPRT), first recognized through its human germinal mutations and then extensively studied as a useful reporter gene for somatic mutations in vitro and in vivo in animals and humans.[26,27] The results of most of these studies also suggest that the induction of mutations in human cells is a linear function of dose with doses as low as 10 cGy, and perhaps as low as 1 cGy, and that the dose-rate effect appears to be relatively small.[28,29] DNA structural analyses show that the majority of radiation-induced mutations in human cells result from large-scale genetic events involving loss of the entire active gene and often extending to other loci on the same chromosome.[30]

The major potential consequence of radiation-induced mutations in human populations is heritable genetic effects resulting from mutations induced in germinal cells. Such effects have been examined in several different animal systems.[25,31] For high dose–rate exposure, the induced mutation rate per gamete generally falls in the range of 10^{-4} to 10^{-5} per cGy. The rates per locus are in the range of 10^{-7} to 10^{-8} per cGy. Protraction of exposure appears to decrease the mutation rate in rodent systems by a factor of 2 or greater. When all of the experimental data for the various genetic end points are considered, the genetic doubling dose (radiation dose necessary to double the spontaneous mutation rate) for low dose–rate exposure appears to be in the range of 100 cGy. Although significant heritable genetic effects of radiation have not yet been demonstrated in human populations, a doubling dose of 100 cGy is not inconsistent with the absence of a statistically significant increase in hereditary disease among the children of atom bomb survivors.[32] Indeed, 100 cGy represents approximately the lower 95% confidence interval (CI) for the human doubling dose calculated from the atom bomb survivor data.[25]

Chromosomal Aberrations

Radiation can induce two types of chromosomal aberrations in mammalian cells. The first have been termed "unstable" aberrations in that they are usually lethal to dividing cells. They include such changes as dicentrics, ring chromosomes, large deletions, and fragments. These types of aberrations do not allow the equal distribution of genetic material into daughter cells; in many cases, the frequency of such aberrations correlates well with the cytotoxic effects of radiation.

The second type has been termed "stable" aberrations. These include changes such as small deletions, reciprocal translocations, and aneuploidy changes that do not preclude the cell from dividing and proliferating. Figure 17-2 shows a karyotype of a human cell showing a stable aberration. Radiation-induced reciprocal translocations such as have occurred in this cell may be passed on through many generations of cell replication and emerge in clonal cell populations.[33,34]

It is well known that such deletions and translocations can result in gene mutations. It is tempting to speculate that they may play a more fundamental role in the process of radiation carcinogenesis. Typically, cancer cells are aneuploid and contain multiple stable chromosomal aberrations. In a number of cases, specific chromosomal abnormalities are associated with specific tumor types. In some instances, such as the chromosome 8:14 translocation in Burkitt lymphoma, the chromosomal change results in the activation of a specific oncogene. In others, such as the chromosome 13q14 deletion found in retinoblastoma (RB), tumor development has been ascribed to loss or inactivation of the RB tumor-suppressor gene. Although radiation-induced cancers show multiple unbalanced chromosomal rearrangements, few show such specific translocations as would be associated with the activation of specific oncogenes or known tumor-suppressor genes.[35]

Neoplastic Transformation In Vitro

An important cellular effect of radiation is neoplastic transformation, or the conversion of a normal cell to one with the phenotype of a cancer cell, including the ability to form an invasive, malignant tumor upon re-injection into syngeneic hosts. Most human cancers have been shown to be clonal in origin. That is, all of the cells within a tumor are descendants of a single cell that has undergone the process of neoplastic transformation. The transformation of one or more normal cells in a tissue in vivo is presumed to represent the earliest step in the overall process of carcinogenesis. Whether or not such a transformed cell can successfully give rise to an invasive, malignant tumor depends upon a number of tissue and systemic factors. Although a number of different in vitro transformation systems involving various species and cell types are under investigation, those that generate reliable quantitative data have been restricted to rodent cells, and in none of these is the entire process of malignant transformation measured.[36,37] Rather, surrogate features of transformation are assayed such as changes in colony morphology, focus formation, or growth under anchorage-independent conditions.

Studies of cellular and animal models for radiation carcinogenesis indicate that it is a progressive, multistep process by which normal cells acquire the various phenotypic characteristics of cancer cells.[38] There appear to be three major independent stages in the malignant transformation of cells in vitro: the development of morphologic changes; cellular immortality; and tumorigenicity.[36] Morphologic changes are many and varied, including the development of abnormalities in cytology, growth pattern, and the control of cell proliferation. Immortalization occurs frequently in rodent cells but extremely rarely in human cells, either spontane-

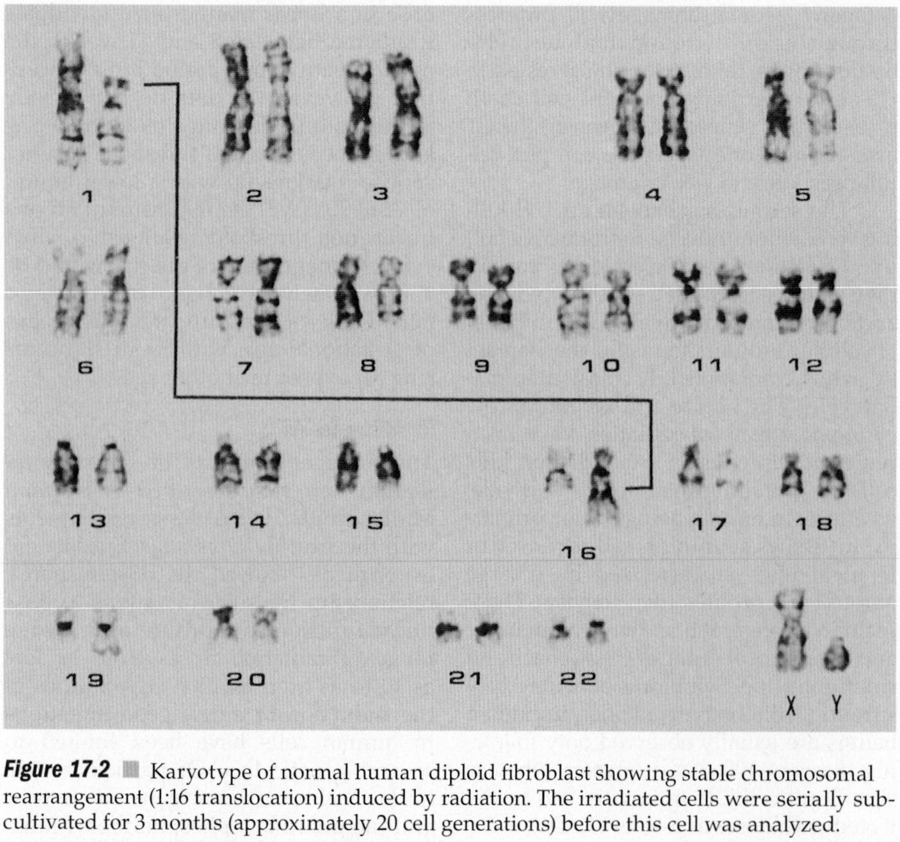

Figure 17-2 Karyotype of normal human diploid fibroblast showing stable chromosomal rearrangement (1:16 translocation) induced by radiation. The irradiated cells were serially subcultivated for 3 months (approximately 20 cell generations) before this cell was analyzed.

ously or as a result of treatment with radiation or chemical carcinogens. It can be induced, however, by transfection of human diploid cells with certain oncogenes and/or genes associated with tumor viruses such as the SV40 T antigen or the E6/E7 genes of human papillomavirus 16, and have been associated with the production of telomerase. Immortalization may thus be an important rate-limiting step in human cell transformation and perhaps in human carcinogenesis in vivo.[36] Tumorigenicity also appears to be an independent phenotype that generally occurs only in previously immortalized cells. A subpopulation of such immortal cells may undergo additional genomic rearrangements that give them a selective growth advantage in vivo perhaps related to factors present in the host animal.[39]

Incubation of cells with various agents either immediately preceding or following exposure or during the 4- to 6-week post-irradiation expression period for transformation can markedly modify the ultimate yield of transformed cells.[40-42] The phosphorothioate drug amifostine as well as its methylated analog were both effective in protecting C3H/10T½ cells against the transforming effects of either low LET gamma rays or fission spectrum neutrons.[40,41] In contrast, the phorbol ester compound 12-*O*-tetradecanoyl-phorbol-13-acetate (TPA) acts as a potent promoter of X-ray transformation, if applied repeatedly beginning either immediately after irradiation or several weeks later. In addition to amifostine, a number of additional drugs have been demonstrated to protect against radiation-induced transformation. These include selenium, retinoids, carotenoids, and ascorbic acid, as well as certain protease inhibitors that have shown promise as chemopreventive agents in vivo.[43-45] Transformation can also be modulated by hormones, growth factors, and anti-inflammatory agents.[43]

It has thus become evident that a number of noncarcinogenic secondary factors can markedly modulate the frequency of radiation-induced transformation. As transformation can be markedly enhanced, suppressed, or completely inhibited by such factors, they may become the controlling ones in the overall process of transformation of cells exposed to radiation. In many cases, the effects of such agents in vitro have been predictive of those observed in experimental animal systems. It therefore seems likely that secondary factors may be of importance in human radiation carcinogenesis, although there are few epidemiologic data to support this contention.

Radiation-induced Genomic Instability

This term refers to a phenomenon observed in a number of different cellular systems whereby radiation exposure appears to induce a type of transmissible genetic instability in individual cells that is transmitted to their progeny, leading to a persistent enhancement in the rate at which genetic changes arise in the descendants of the irradiated cell after many generations of replication. The occurrence of such a process could enhance the probability that a single cell lineage would acquire the multiple sequential and interacting gene mutations necessary to convert a normal cell to a full malignant cell. It would also imply that radiation could act at any point in this carcinogenic process. This phenomenon has been termed a non-targeted effect of radiation, as genetic damage occurs in cells that in themselves received no direct radiation exposure. The end points studied include malignant transformation, specific gene mutations, and chromosomal aberrations. Typically, this phenomenon is studied by examining the occurrence of such genetic effects in clonal populations derived from single cells surviving radiation exposure.[45] Figure 17-3 shows this schematically.

Early evidence for the existence of such a phenomenon was derived from an examination of the kinetics of radiation-induced malignant transformation of cells in vitro.[46,47] These results suggested that transformed foci did not arise from a single, radiation-damaged cell. Rather, radiation appeared to induce a type of instability in 20% to 30% of the irradiated cell population; this instability enhanced the probability of the occurrence of a second, neoplastic transforming event. This finding is in contradistinction to the classic theories of carcinogenesis in which the initiating event is thought to be rare and likely mutagenic in nature. This second event was a rare one, however, occurring with the frequency of ~10^{-6}, and involved in the actual transformation of one or more of the progeny of the original irradiated cells after many rounds of cell division. This second transforming event occurred with the constant frequency per cell per generation, and had the characteristics of a mutagenic event.[48] Thus, neoplastically transformed foci did not appear to arise

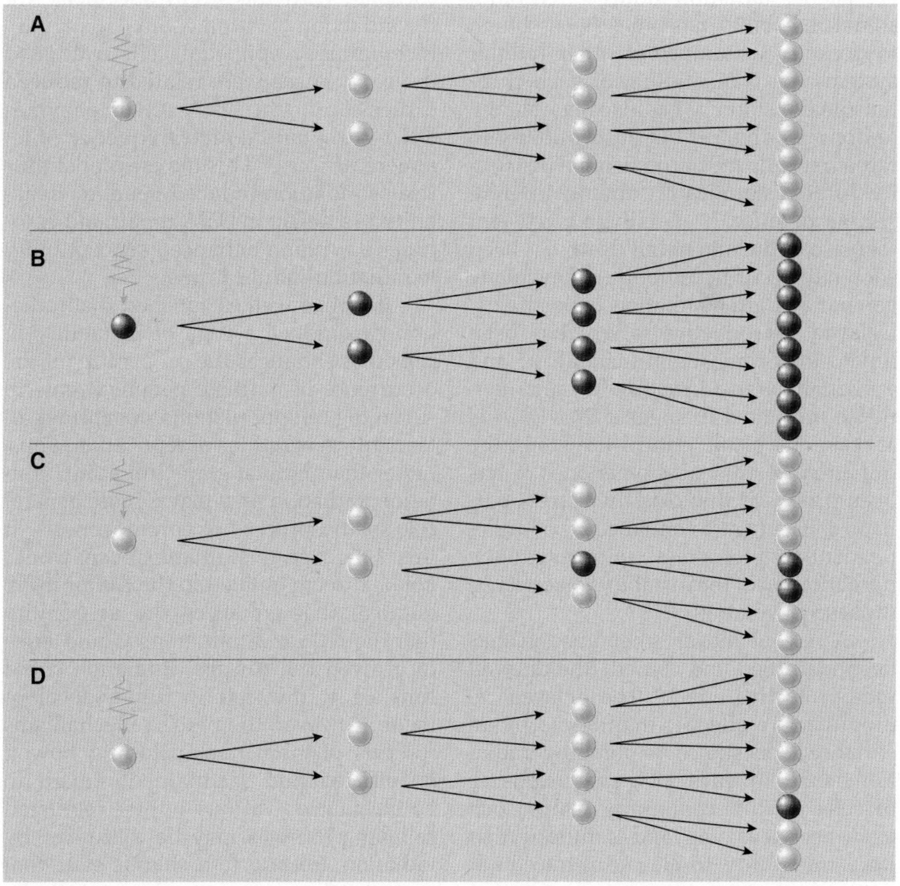

Figure 17-3 Schematic of radiation-induced mutagenesis. *Gray circles* represent normal wild-type cells, while *colored circles* represent mutated cells. **(B)** is an example of a cell directly mutated by radiation exposure; the mutation is transmitted to all of its progeny. However, most of the cells in the irradiated population will retain the wild-type phenotype **(A)**. **(C)** and **(D)** are examples of mutations arising as a result of radiation-induced genomic instability. The irradiated cell and its immediate progeny are wild type, but the frequency with which mutations arise amongst the more distant descendants of the irradiated cell is elevated.

from the original irradiated cell but rather from one or more of its progeny.

This phenomenon was subsequently demonstrated in a number of experiment systems for various genetic end points.[49-52] In terms of mutagenesis, ~10% of clonal populations derived from single cells surviving radiation exposure showed a significant elevation in the frequency of spontaneously arising mutations as compared with clonal populations derived from non-irradiated cells.[53,54] This increased mutation rate persisted for ~30 to 50 generations post-irradiation. The molecular structural spectrum of these late-arising mutants resembles those of spontaneous mutations in that the majority of them are point mutations,[54,55] whereas direct X-ray-induced mutations involve primarily deletions. An enhancement of both minisatellite[56] and microsatellite[57] instability has also been observed in the progeny of irradiated cells selected for mutations at the *thymidine kinase* locus.

An enhanced frequency of nonclonal chromosomal aberrations was first reported in clonal descendants of mouse hematopoietic stem cells 12 to 14 generations after exposure to alpha radiation.[58] Persistent radiation-induced chromosomal instability has since been shown to occur in a number of other cellular systems.[59-62] Transmission of such chromosomal instability has also been shown to occur in vivo,[63,64] but susceptibility to radiation-induced chromosomal instability differed significantly among different strains of mice.[65,66] Finally, a persistent increase in the rate of cell death has been shown to occur in cell populations many generations after radiation exposure.[67-69] Delayed reproductive failure has been linked to chromosomal instability[70] and malignant transformation,[71,72] and evidence presented to suggest that DNA is at least one of the critical targets in the initiation of this phenomenon.[73] It has been proposed that oxidative stress perhaps consequent to enhanced, p53-independent apoptosis may contribute to the perpetuation of the instability phenotype in these populations.[70,72,74]

A recent novel phenomenon has been identified and coined "the delayed radioprotective effect." The delayed radioprotective effect is manifested by an enhanced resistance to ionizing radiation hours to days following exposure of cells to thiol-containing drugs such as *N*-acetylcysteine and captopril that have the ability to elevate intracellular antioxidant enzymes such as manganese superoxide dismutase (MnSOD).[75,76] The underlying mechanism of action responsible for this effect is the activation of the redox-sensitive nuclear transcription factor κB (NFκB) by thiol-reducing agents that subsequently results in the elevated transcription of MnSOD. The resulting 10- to 20-fold elevation of intracellular MnSOD facilitates the prevention and removal of radiation-induced oxidative damage and can enhance survival of cells by 10% to 30%. The ability to elevate and maintain prolonged enhanced intracellular antioxidant levels through this mechanism may therefore facilitate the prevention of the genomic instability phenotype if persistent oxidative stress is indeed a causative factor.

Of importance in terms of radiation carcinogenesis and potential chemoprevention strategies are the emerging observations indicating that persistent oxidative stress and genomic instability occur in vivo and may be related to the induction of cancer. The transmission of radiation-induced chromosomal instability in vivo has been demonstrated in several distinct experimental models,[63,64,77] and evidence presented to suggest that instability induced in X-irradiated mouse hematopoietic stem cells may be related to the occurrence of the nonspecific genetic damage found in radiation-induced leukemias in these mice.[78] Sensitivity to mammary tumor induction was found not only to be strain specific but also to correlate with the strain specificity for the induction of chromosomal instability in mammary epithelial cells irradiated in vivo.[77] These were related to reduced expression of the DNA repair enzymes DNA-PKcs[79] and a high frequency of telomere fusions.[80] This mouse model thus relates radiation-induced genomic instability to a defect in DNA repair and associates it with an enhanced susceptibility to radiation-induced cancer.

It is thus well established that radiation can induce a type of instability in cells that enhances the probability of the occurrence of multiple genetic events in surviving cell populations, sometimes after many generations of replication. Thus, rather than inducing an "initiating" mutation, radiation may play a more general role in the process of carcinogenesis. If this is the case, the initiating event would not be directly related to the tumor itself, but one that enhances the probability that the required mutations would arise in a given cell lineage. Radiation could thus act at any state in tumor development. However, the precise mechanisms for this phenomenon including how it is initiated and maintained remain to be elucidated. Various tightly regulated cellular processes may be disrupted by radiation, leading to a chaotic state that perturbs the normal regulatory and signaling pathways, thus disrupting cellular homeostasis, a state from which the cell never completely recovers.[73] It is tempting to speculate that the various factors known to modulate malignant transformation in vitro may act on this process. Interestingly, this concept is consistent with the emerging findings in human populations, which suggest that some types of radiation-induced cancer may follow a relative risk model (see below); ie, a given dose of radiation increases the rate of occurrence of cancer at all follow-up times rather than inducing a specific cohort of new tumors.

Bystander Effects in Irradiated Cell Populations

It has long been thought that the cell nucleus is the target for the important biologic effects of radiation; these effects occur in the irradiated cell as a direct result of DNA damage that has not been correctly restored by enzymatic repair processes. However, recent evidence shows that targeted cytoplasmic radiation is significantly mutagenic.[81] Moreover, it has become evident that damage signals may be transmitted from irradiated to non-irradiated cells in the population, leading to the occurrence of biologic effects in cells that received no radiation exposure.[82] This phenomenon has been termed the "bystander" effect of radiation; it could be of considerable importance in the carcinogenic effects of very-low doses of densely ionizing radiation such as alpha particles released by radon. Only a small fraction of a person's bronchial epithelial cells, the presumed target for lung cancer, will actually be hit by an alpha particle from residential radon exposure during an exposed person's lifetime.

The experimental model used to study this effect has generally involved the exposure of monolayer cultures of cells to very-low fluences of alpha particles, fluences whereby a very small fraction of the cell population will actually be hit by a particle. In the initial study, an enhanced frequency of sister chromatid exchanges (SCE) was observed in 20% to 40% of cells exposed to fluences by which only 1/1000 to 1/100 cells were traversed by an alpha particle.[83] Evidence has been presented that this effect involves the secretion of cytokines or other factors by irradiated cells that leads to an upregulation of oxidative metabolism in bystander cells.[84,85] There is also evidence that incubation with conditioned medium from irradiated cells has cytotoxic effects on non-irradiated cells, which may be related to the release of a factor(s) into the medium, including reactive oxygen species.[86] These findings are reminiscent of the reports that clastogenic activity can be isolated from the plasma of radiation-exposed people.[87]

Of particular note is the observation that an enhanced frequency of specific gene mutations[88,89] as well as chromosomal aberrations[90,91] occur in bystander cells in populations exposed to very-low fluences of alpha particles. As a result, the induced mutation frequency per alpha particle track increases at low fluences where bystanders as well as directly irradiated cells are at risk for the induction of mutations. This leads to hyperlinearity of the dose-response curve in the low-dose region.

Changes in gene expression also occur in bystander cells in monolayer cultures; the expression levels of p53, p21^{Waf1}, CDC2, cyclin-B1, and rad51 were significantly modulated in non-irradiated cells in confluent human diploid cell populations exposed to very-low fluences of alpha particles.[82] As seen in Figure 17-4, clusters of cells showed enhanced expression of p21^{Waf1} as determined by in situ immunofluorescence staining techniques, although only ~1% to 2% of the cell nuclei were actually traversed by an alpha particle. This phenomenon involved cell-to-cell communication via gap junctions.[92] Evidence that the upregulation of the p53 signaling pathway in bystander cells is a consequence of DNA damage is supported by the observation that p53 was phosphorylated on serine 15.[92] Interestingly, however, DNA damage in bystander cells appears to differ from that occurring in directly irradiated cells; whereas the mutations induced in directly irradiated cells were primarily partial and total gene deletions, >90% of those arising in bystander cells were point mutations.[93] This would be consistent with the evidence that oxidative metabolism is upregulated in bystander cells,[84,85] and has led to the hypothesis that the point mutations are a result of oxidative base damage occurring in bystander cells.[93] The activation of MAP K proteins and their downstream effectors in bystander cells[85] is of particular interest in terms of the preliminary evidence that membrane signaling is involved in the bystander effect in monolayer cultures.[94]

In sum, the results of these studies of bystander effects indicate clearly that damage signals can be transmitted from irradiated to non-irradiated cells. In confluent monolayer cultures, this phenomenon involves gap junction–mediated cell-to-cell communication, and appears to involve both the induction of reactive oxygen species and the activation of extranuclear signal transduction pathways. Some evidence suggests that regulation of the p53 damage-response pathway may be central to this phenomenon. These findings could potentially be of considerable significance in terms of residential radon exposure where the mutagenic and carcinogenic effect could be greater than that predicted on the basis only of those bronchial epithelial cells actually traversed by an alpha particle.

Adaptive Responses ■ The original description of an adaptive response was made by investigators working with human lymphocytes in which they observed that following exposure to a very-low dose of ionizing radiation in the range of 1 to 10 cGy cells acquired an enhanced resistance to a second but much larger dose of 2 Gy or more.[95] The expression of an adaptive response was linked to the requirement of de novo protein synthesis since inhibitors of protein synthesis such as cyclohexamide were found to be inhibitory to this inductive effect.[96] An important candidate in this process has been identified as manganese superoxide dismutase (MnSOD), an antioxidant enzyme localized in the mitochondria of cells. As an example, it has been demonstrated that mouse skin JB6P+ epithelial cells exposed to 10 cGy exhibited an enhanced resistance to a subsequent dose of 2 Gy during which time a number of NFκB-regulated genes including MnSOD, p65, phosphorylated extracellular signal-related kinase, cyclin B1, and 14-3-3ζ were elevated.[97] The importance of elevated MnSOD synthesis in the adaptive response process has been observed in cells following exposure to not only a low dose of ionizing radiation[97] but also the cytokine TNFα[98] and numerous reductive agents such as amifostine and N-acetylcysteine.[76,99] Treatment of cells with NFκB inhibitors and/or antisense MnSOD oligomers or siRNA MnSOD completely inhibited the adaptive response induced by these agents.[97,98] Three generalized examples of adaptive responses are presented in Figure 17-5. Both the radiation- and cytokine-induced adaptive responses are the result of oxidative damage-initiated processes in contrast to the thiol-induced reductive response in which NFκB is activated following the reduction of cysteine residues on its p50 and p65 subunits,[100,101] a process that can be maintained in a persistent manner with chronic thiol exposure.[102]

A genomic approach has been taken to identify genes whose changes in expression could be correlated with the demonstration of a radiation-induced adaptive response. Using cell lines known to be either adaptable or non-adaptable, cells were irradiated initially with 5 cGy followed hours later with a challenge dose of 2 Gy. The adaptable cell lines exhibited an increase in the expression of genes related to DNA repair and stress response with a corresponding decrease in expression of genes related to cell cycle control and apoptosis.[103] One of the difficulties in studying the radiation-induced adaptive response is the lack of a generalized response in all cell systems. However, this response or lack thereof takes on an importance with regard to the potential consequences of low-dose radiation exposures both in the context of the working environment and associated protection standards as well as in the medical use of low-dose diagnostic procedures that many times precede the initiation of radiation-based therapies.

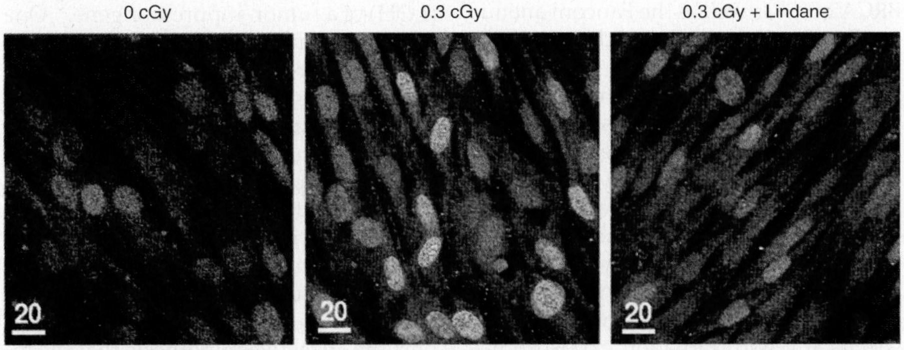

Figure 17-4 ■ Bystander effect of radiation. The expression of p21^{Wafl} was determined in individual cells in monolayer cultures of human diploid fibroblasts by in situ immunofluorescence. In cultures exposed to 0.3 cGy (<1-2% of nuclei traversed by an alpha particle), enhanced expression occurred in many nonirradiated cells occurring in clusters (*center panel*). The effect was suppressed by incubation with lindane, an inhibitor of gap junctionmediated intercellular communication (*right panel*).

Molecular Mechanisms

DNA Damage and Genetic Changes

It is well accepted that DNA damage is central to the biologic effects of ionizing radiation. It is the production of this damage by ionization, resulting specifically in the efficient induction of DNA strand breaks, which differentiates ionizing radiation from most other physical and chemical carcinogens. Although ionizing radiation can produce a broad spectrum of DNA lesions including damage to nucleotide bases, un-repaired or miss-repaired DNA double-strand breaks (DSB) are thought to be the principal lesions responsible for the induction of genetic changes in mammalian cells, including chromosomal abnormalities and gene mutations.[104,105] In contrast, base damage is generally the predominate

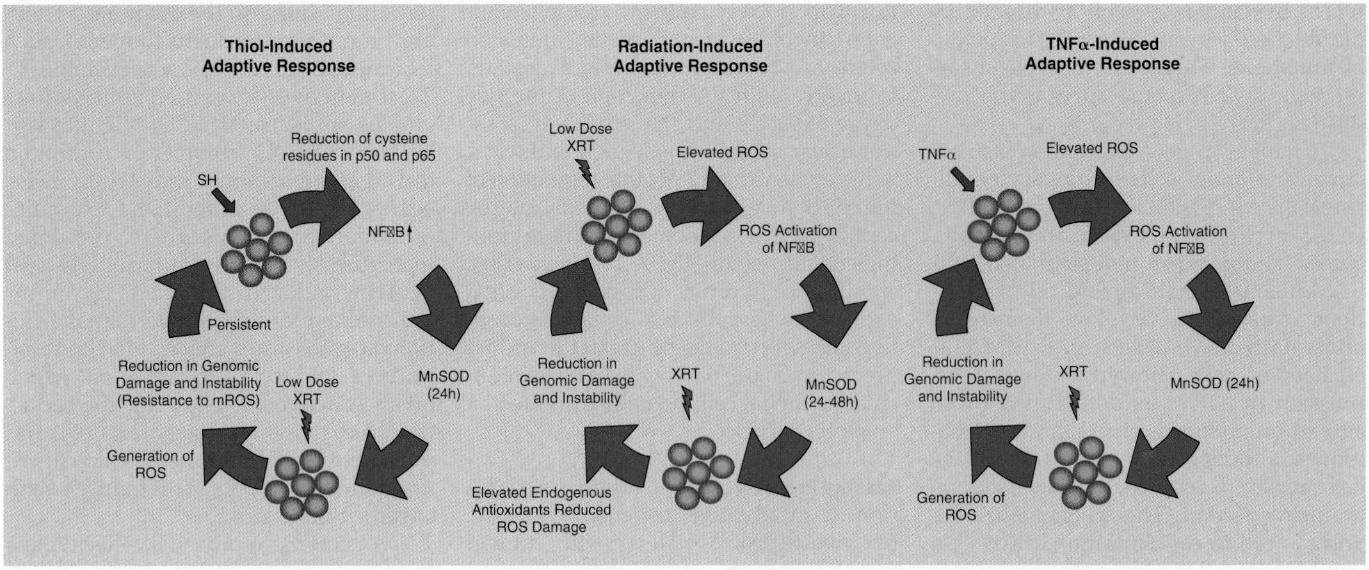

Figure 17-5 Models of adaptive responses: a non-oxidative damage–mediated event induced through the reducing action of free thiols as contrasted to oxidative damage–initiating events induced through the oxidizing action of ionizing radiation and selected cytokines such as tumor necrosis factor α (TNFα). Adaptive responses in general refer to a reduced damaging effect of a relatively high dose of a deleterious agent when induced following exposure to a previous low-dose or nontoxic priming agent.

mechanism for the production of such changes by most chemical carcinogens.

Track analysis studies of x-ray interactions in DNA have provided evidence for clustered damage, which has a high probability of producing complex DSB.[104] This results from the fact that radiation interactions are usually associated with the production of several closely associated ion pairs. Certain types of DNA base damage such as 8-hydroxydeoxyguanosine and thymine glycols have significant potential biologic importance, but the available data suggest that such isolated base damage by itself probably plays a minor role in radiation mutagenesis.[105] However, recent evidence suggests that clustered DNA damage may include abasic sites, oxidized purines, or oxidized pyrimidines.[106] This study, which employed a new method of measuring clustered lesions in genomic DNA, concluded that amongst all complex damage induced by ionizing radiation, the majority represented clustered damage rather than simple DSB. The DNA repair proteins Ku70/80 appear to mediate the repair of such damage.[107] The increased efficiency of DNA breaks induced by high-LET radiation appears to result primarily from their greater complexity.[108] Substantial yields of DSB may also result from secondary electrons with energies well below the ionizing threshold.[109]

Cells possess a complex set of signaling pathways for recognizing such DNA damage and initiating its repair, which are only recently becoming better understood. The ATM gene is one of the prime sensors of DNA damage, which activates by phosphorylation a variety of proteins involved in cell cycle control and DNA repair. Two mechanistically distinct pathways that function in complementary ways are involved in the repair of DSB: non-homologous end joining (NHEJ), which requires little sequence homology between the DNA ends and is thus error prone, and homologous recombination (HR), which uses extensive homology and is generally error-free.[110] NHEJ involves a complex of proteins, including Ku70, Ku80, the DNA-PK catalytic subunit DNA-PKcs, XRCC4, and ligase IV. The NBS1/MRE11/RAD50 complex[111] is also involved in the nucleolytic processing stages of NHEJ; this complex also contributes to HR. HR also involves a complex of proteins, notably RAD51 and other factors in the RAD50 epistasis group.[112] Strong links have been established between recombinational repair and the breast cancer susceptibility proteins BRCA1 and BRCA2,[113-115] as well as the Fanconi anemia family of proteins.[116] Thus, the metabolic repair of radiation-induced DNA strand breaks involves a large complex of proteins, many of which are associated with clinical syndromes of radiosensitivity and cancer susceptibility.

Un-repaired or miss-repaired DSB lead primarily to large-scale genetic changes that are frequently manifested by chromosomal aberrations. However, the search for genetic changes associated specifically with radiation exposure has proven very disappointing. There is no evidence of site specificity for mutations induced by radiation. The spectrum of molecular-structural changes associated with direct radiation-induced mutations involves primarily partial and total gene deletions, thus differing from that for spontaneous mutations where point mutations predominate. However, there appears to be no site specificity for DNA breakpoints that lead to deletions and, similarly, sequence analyses of radiation-induced point mutations have generally shown no site specificity.[117] Furthermore, no genetic alterations unique to radiation have as yet been found in radiation-induced tumors.

Tumor-Suppressor Genes

It is known that unbalanced translocations can lead to deletions. As certain cancers that are known to be induced by radiation (such as some types of leukemia and sarcoma) are specifically those in which deletions occur, it has been proposed that the most likely mutational event in the initiation of radiation carcinogenesis involves loss of heterozygosity (LOH) of a tumor-suppressor gene.[35] One specific example of this phenomenon is the RB tumor-suppressor gene located on chromosome 13q14. The hypersensitivity of retinoblastoma patients to the induction of secondary cancers following radiotherapy, primarily osteosarcomas in the treatment field, is presumably the result of radiation-induced LOH of the *RB* gene.[118] However, RB is a rare disorder and there are few other examples from animal or human carcinogenesis to support the attractive hypothesis that the induction of LOH at tumor-suppressor loci is a general phenomenon in the initiation of radiation carcinogenesis.

Much interest has centered about the p53 gene as it appears to play an important role in cell cycle control, radiosensitivity, the development of genetic instability leading to cell transformation, and perhaps in the response of human tumors to radiation or chemotherapy. p53 mutations have been found in a wide spectrum of human cancers,[119] and in mouse skin tumors induced by ionizing radiation.[120] Mutations of p53 have also been associated with lung cancer induced in underground miners by alpha radiation.[121] Although some strains of knockout mice, either hemizygous and homozygous for the p53 gene, are more susceptible to radiation-induced tumors,[122] LOH at this locus may not be the initiating event.[123] Indeed, there is increasing evidence that p53 mutations may arise late in the development of tumors.[124,125] LOH for p53 mutation in knockout mice may also be a secondary event.[123] It is of interest in this context that the expression of p53 mutations also appears to occur late in the process of radiation-induced malignant transformation, during the growth of the visible-transformed foci,[126] consistent with the findings in some human tumors.[124]

Another area of interest is the role of p53 in the control of cellular radiosensitivity, as it has been proposed that p53 status may be a determinant in the therapeutic responsiveness of certain types of human tumors.[127,128] The absence of normal p53 function is associated with enhanced resistance of human diploid fibroblasts to radiation-induced reproductive failure.[17,129] A similar effect has been described in hematopoietic cell lineages in transgenic mice.[130] For cell types that readily undergo apoptosis, such as those of hematopoietic origin, the lack of an apoptotic response in p53-deficient cells renders them more resistant to radiation. The role of p53 status in the radiosensitivity of cells derived from human solid tumors, however, remains unclear[131-133] and may depend upon tumor type.

Oncogenes

Although the involvement of various oncogenes in experimental and human carcinogenesis is well established, no data have emerged from animal models to suggest a general role for oncogene activation in radiation-induced cancer. Activation of members of the *RAS* family has been reported in a small fraction of certain mouse lymphomas,[134,135] and amplification and rearrangement of *C-MYC* was found in a small percentage of radiation-induced murine osteosarcomas.[136] Radiation-induced skin papillomas in Car-S mice were notable in their lack of *HRAS* mutations, as compared with papillomas induced by a chemical carcinogen or TPA.[137] However, these scattered results have not proven to form a consistent pattern of oncogene activation in radiation carcinogenesis. One special case is the activation of the RET oncogene, which has been associated with susceptibility to the induction of papillary carcinoma by radiation in children.[138]

Experimental Radiation-Induced Carcinogenesis

General Characteristics of Radiation Carcinogenesis

Ionizing radiation has been called a "universal carcinogen" in that it will induce cancer in most tissues of most species at all ages, including the fetus. It is one of the few definitely established carcinogens in human beings, and perhaps the only one for which firm dose-response data in human populations is available. It is, however, a relatively weak carcinogen and mutagen. The cancers induced by radiation are of the same histologic types as occur naturally, but the distribution of types may differ. For example, a higher percentage of small-cell carcinomas of the lung occur as a result of exposure to alpha radiation in uranium miners; radiation generally induces follicular and papillary carcinomas of the thyroid rather than anaplastic and medullary carcinomas; and chronic lymphocytic leukemia is apparently not induced by radiation, whereas other common types of leukemias are. There is a distinct latent period between exposure to radiation and the clinical appearance of a tumor.

Dose-Response Relationships

It has been generally accepted that radiation carcinogenesis is a stochastic process; ie, the probability of the occurrence of the effect increases with dose with no threshold, but the severity of the effect is not influenced by dose. This is in contradistinction to a nonstochastic or deterministic effect for which both the probability and the severity of the effect vary with dose. There is no clear experimental evidence to suggest that the grade of malignancy, including its invasive or metastatic properties, is a function of dose; radiation-induced cancer appears to be an all-or-none effect. Stochastic effects are those that may arise from damage to a few cells or even a single cell. If this is the case, any dose, no matter how small, carries with it the finite probability of producing the effect. Studies of radiation-induced carcinogenesis in experimental animals and human populations have been designed to test this hypothesis, as most environmental exposures are in the low-dose range. Unfortunately, it is very difficult to obtain statistically significant data in either human or animal studies at doses below 10 to 20 cGy of low LET radiation.

Many earlier studies of the effects of radiation in small animals involved its life-shortening properties. Although this effect was originally ascribed to "radiation-induced aging" in which the natural causes of death were accelerated by radiation, a critical examination of this phenomenon by use of techniques such as serial sacrifice experiments and life table analyses has shown that practically all of the life-shortening effect of radiation in experimental animals can be accounted for by the induction of cancer, except perhaps in the high, sublethal dose range.[139,140] Thus, the dose-response relationship for life-shortening in animals should reflect that for cancer deaths from all types of radiation-induced tumors in that species. A generally linear response has been observed for life-shortening in a number of different studies.[141]

The dose-response relationships for the induction of cancers in specific tissues of small animals vary with site, sex, and species.[142-144] For low LET radiation, the frequency of induced cancers generally rises with dose in the range of 0 to 300 cGy. In some cases, tumor incidence levels off at higher doses and may even decline. This phenomenon is thought to reflect cell killing. The carcinogenic effect of low LET radiation in rodents is usually reduced with protraction of exposure. In the dose range up to 200 to 300 cGy, the dose-response curves for individual tumor types vary but generally assume a linear-quadratic to near-linear relationship.

For high LET radiation, the rise in cancer incidence with dose is much steeper. The dose-response curves are approximately linear within the range of 0 to 20 cGy, although in some cases they bend over, reaching a plateau at higher doses.[142,145] In contradistinction to low LET radiation, significant increases in cancer and life-shortening can be observed after doses as low as 10 cGy of neutrons, alpha particles, or heavy ions.[142,145,146] RBE values in the range of 3 to 15 have been estimated for the carcinogenic effects of these radiations at low doses. There is usually no dose-rate effect for high LET radiation exposure. However, an outstanding example is the induction of mouse mammary tumors by low doses of fast neutrons, in which protraction of exposure appears to increase the carcinogenic effect by a factor of 2 to 3 at doses of 2.5 to 10 cGy.[145]

Modifying Factors

As in the case of neoplastic transformation, radiation-induced carcinogenesis in experimental animals can also be modulated by noncarcinogenic secondary factors. Post-irradiation treatment with the tumor-promoter TPA is known to enhance ultraviolet light-induced mouse skin cancer; a similar phenomenon has

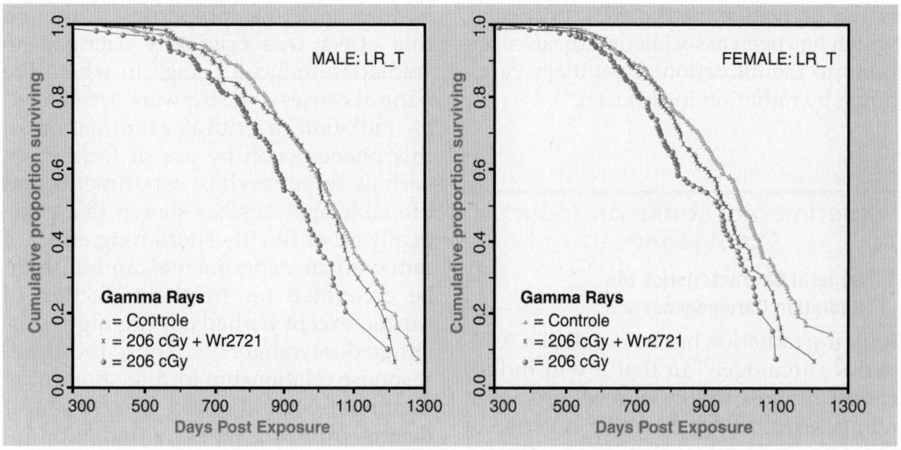

Figure 17-6 Survival curves resulting from lymphoreticular cancers (LR-T), as determined by histopathological analysis of tissues taken from deceased animals that had been irradiated (206 cGy) either with or without amifostine. LR-T includes histiocytic leukemia and lymphoma, lymphocytic-lymphoblastic leukemia and lymphoma, myelogenous leukemia, undifferentiated leukemia and lymphoma, and mixed histiocytic leukemia and lymphoma.

been shown for the induction of malignant squamous cell carcinoma of the skin of mice by ionizing radiation.[147]

The induction of carcinogenesis in experimental animals can also be suppressed by treatment with certain agents that are known to inhibit radiation-induced transformation in vitro. An example of this includes amifostine, which is the only drug currently approved for clinical use as a radioprotector by the FDA.[148] As described by Kaplan-Meyer plots in Figure 17-6, inoculation of B6CF1 hybrid mice with a single dose of 400 mg/kg of amifostine 30 min prior to whole-body irradiation with 2 Gy of low LET radiation significantly protected against carcinogenesis in both male and female animals. As discussed earlier, the reduction in cancer deaths due to lymphoreticular tumors by amifostine is reflected by a shift in the Kaplan-Meyer survival curves for drug-treated irradiated animals to those describing the survival of non-irradiated control animals.[149-151] Causes of death due to lymphoreticular tumors that included leukemias and lymphomas were determined by both gross and microscopic analysis of individual animals by veterinarian pathologists.[149] Likewise, certain protease inhibitors, have also been shown to suppress the induction of cancer in several different tumor systems.[44,152] It is well known that the hormonal environment is important in certain radiation-induced rodent cancers, particularly ovarian and mammary tumors. These and other observations again emphasize the importance of noncarcinogenic secondary factors in experimental radiation carcinogenesis. However, the extent to which such factors are important in radiation-induced cancer in human populations is not clear.

Genetic Susceptibility to Radiation-Induced Cancer

The discovery that mutations in a number of specific genes are associated with an enhanced predisposition to single or multiple cancer types has stimulated renewed interest in the potential role of genetic susceptibility in the carcinogenic effects of radiation.[152,153] However, the known genes are highly penetrant and code for rare hereditary disorders. Should a significant fraction of the population be genetically predisposed to radiation-induced cancer, perhaps from mutations in more common but weakly penetrant genes, this fact could be of considerable importance in the development of protection standards.[154]

Although there is little evidence at present to suggest that such genetic factors are involved in most human cancers, they do appear to play a role in these rare hereditary disorders which may serve as models for radiation-genetic interactions. For example, patients with hereditary retinoblastoma whose somatic cells are heterozygous for the *RB* gene are at markedly increased risk for the development of radiation-induced bone sarcomas,[118] whereas patients with the nevoid basal cell carcinoma syndrome are at high risk for the development of basal cell cancers in irradiated areas. Radiation has also been associated with an enhanced incidence of early onset breast cancer, although the hereditary nature of radiation-induced breast cancer and its relation to the breast cancer susceptibility genes *BRCA1* and *BRCA2* remain to be clarified. Interestingly, transgenic mice heterozygous for either the p53[122] or ATM[155] tumor-suppressor genes also show an increased sensitivity to radiation-induced cancer; ATM and p53 heterozygosity is associated, respectively, with the human cancer-prone disorders ataxia telangiectasia and the Li-Fraumeni syndrome. It is not clear the extent to which more common, low-penetrance susceptibility genes may play a role in genetic predisposition to radiation-induced cancer.[152,154]

Human Epidemiologic Studies

There is now a large body of data on radiation-induced cancer derived from epidemiologic studies in irradiated human populations, and it is primarily on the basis of these data that risk estimates are derived. These data are reviewed and analyzed in detail in the latest reports from the BEIR V Committee[25] and the United Nations Scientific Committee on the Effects of Atomic Radiation (UNSCEAR 2000).[156] They are derived primarily from two sources: (1) the long-term follow-up of survivors of the nuclear bombings of Hiroshima and Nagasaki[157,158] and (2) populations exposed to medical x-rays.[159,160] Information is also available from certain occupational exposures, particularly from individuals with pulmonary and skeletal exposure to alpha radiation. The results of these studies have yielded significant dose-response data for the induction of cancer in at least five tissue sites. Such dose-response data are extremely important in ascribing radiation as the causal agent for the increased incidence of cancer, as well as for estimating the risks associated with a given exposure. Unfortunately, however, the epidemiologic studies yielding useful dose-response data generally involve relatively high-dose exposures (>10 cGy). Thus, risk estimates in the low-dose range must be derived from an extrapolation from the high-dose data. The shape of the dose-response relationship becomes of critical importance in making such extrapolations.

The observed dose-response curves from the human epidemiologic studies appear to be either linear or linear-quadratic in form (ie, a linear component at low doses with a quadratic component at higher doses); although a threshold (dose below which there is no effect) cannot be formally excluded at very low doses.[161,162] A linear curve implies a constant risk per cGy at all doses, whereas the linear-quadratic model implies a smaller risk per cGy in the low-dose range. The assumption of a linear model simplifies the extrapolation from high to low doses and the corresponding estimation of risks. Furthermore, it is a conservative technique; ie, if anything, it would overestimate rather than underestimate the potential risk. There is no evidence for a proportionally greater effect at low doses, except possibly for very low fluences of alpha particles if a bystander effect occurs in vivo.

A final parameter of importance in determining the hazards of a given dose of radiation is the choice of risk models. For many years, risks were estimated on the basis of an absolute risk model. This model assumed that a specific number of excess cancers was induced by a given radiation dose. Radiation-induced cancers occurred in addition to the natural incidence. Thus, the increased risk could be expressed as the number of excess cancer cases (or cancer deaths) per 10^6 exposed people per year per cGy (the rate per year) or as the total number of excess cancers per 10^6 exposed people per cGy (the total risk or lifetime yield of cancers to be expected from a given radiation dose). The absolute risk model generally assumes a linear dose-response relationship, although with certain corrections it can be applied to a linear-quadratic relationship. Because the radiation exposure in Hiroshima included a small fraction of neutrons, the doses in the atom bomb survivor studies are expressed in Sieverts (Sv) rather than Gy, a term that takes into account the RBE of neutrons. For our purposes, however, we can consider that 1 Sv equals ~1 Gy.

An analysis of the recent data from the atom bomb survivors suggests that some types of radiation-induced cancer more likely follow a relative-risk model.[25,157] This is also true for several different tumor types in mice.[139] The relative risk model implies that radiation increases the natural incidence of cancer at all ages by a dose-dependent factor. As the excess cancer risk is proportional to the natural incidence, radiation-induced cancers would occur primarily at the times when natural tumors arose, independent of the age at irradiation. Thus, the largest cohort of radiation-induced cancers would occur in older individuals. The relative risk model appears to fit the epidemiologic data for several solid tumors, although it does not appear to be valid for leukemia or bone and lung cancers. In general, the risk estimates derived from the studies involving medical exposures are similar to those of the atom bomb survivors[160,163,164]; differences in the case of high-dose radiation therapy exposures can be ascribed to cell killing and the effect of dose fractionation.[159] A significantly reduced effect with fractionation for high-dose exposure was observed for lung cancer.[165] This was not the case for breast cancer, although a reduced effect was associated with low dose–rate protracted exposure.[164]

Leukemia

At one time, leukemia was thought to be the major radiation-induced cancer to arise from whole-body exposure. We now know the two reasons for this assumption: (1) the spontaneous occurrence of leukemia is low, and thus radiation-induced cases are more readily recognizable and (2) the latent period in human beings is very short relative to other types of cancer, thus leukemias are recognized earlier. Excess leukemias begin appearing within 2 years after acute radiation exposure, reach a peak incidence within 10 years, and then fall off steadily. This is in contradistinction to other cancers for which the minimum latent period is generally 10 to 15 years, and the appearance of new radiation-induced tumors increases up to 50 years or longer after irradiation. The major sources of data for the induction of leukemia are from the 86,500 members of the life span study of the atom bomb survivors from whom DS86 (1986) dose estimates are available[157] and from a study of ~14,000 patients in the United Kingdom who were treated with radiation for ankylosing spondylitis of the spine.[166]

Figure 17-7A shows the dose-response relationship for the induction of leukemia in the atom bomb survivors, based on the DS86 dosimetry measurements of organ-absorbed dose. A new dosimetry system, DS02, has recently been implemented to replace the DS86. The changes in dose estimates were smaller than what was anticipated, with the primary systematic change being an increase of about 10% in γ-ray estimates for both Hiroshima and Nagasaki. For both solid cancer and leukemia, estimated age-time patterns and sex difference are virtually unchanged by the dosimetry revision.[167] The data are best described by a linear-quadratic dose-response model in the dose range of 0 to 3 Sv. On the basis of these data,[157] the relative risk at 1 Sv (~100 cGy) is 5.62, and the absolute risk is estimated to be 2.61 excess cancer deaths/10^4 persons exposed/year/Sv. This latter figure is approximately fourfold higher than that estimated from the data for the British ankylosing spondylitis patients. This may be ascribed to the younger age of the atom bomb survivors at the time of irradiation and the fact they received a single acute whole-body exposure.[25] Children appear to be twice as sensitive as adults to the leukemogenic effects of radiation. Studies of in utero exposures to medical x-rays suggest that the unborn child may be as much as 10 times more sensitive than adults to the induction of leukemia following in utero irradiation,[168,169] although no difference was found in the leukemia risk between exposure in utero and during the first 5 years of life among the atom bomb survivors.[170]

Radiation-induced leukemia in human populations differs in several characteristics from solid tumors. These include the unusually short latent period, high relative risk (Table 17-1), and the fact that the epidemiologic data best fit a linear-quadratic dose-response relationship. This may be related to the nature of the hematopoietic system, which contains less stroma than do most tissues. Therefore, there may be fewer constraints on cell proliferation, in essence allowing a few transformed cells to grow rapidly and be detected earlier as a clinical cancer.

Other Tumors

Figure 17-7B shows the dose-response relationship for all cancers except leukemia; the data are best described by a linear model in the dose range of 0 to 3 Sv. Table 17-1 shows the various risk estimates for all types of cancer in which mortality was significantly increased among the atom bomb survivors. These data are based upon ~86,500 subjects, of which 50,000 were exposed to >0.005 Sv

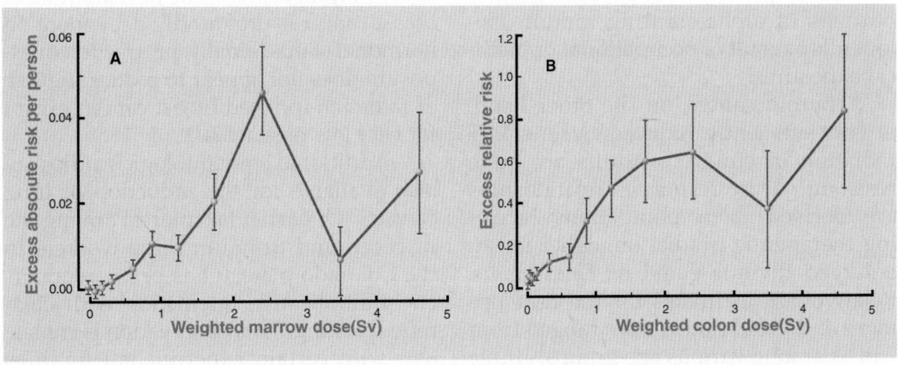

Figure 17-7 Dose-response curves for the induction of cancer in human populations receiving uniform whole-body radiation exposure, derived from epidemiologic data from the atomic bomb survivors of Hiroshima and Nagasaki. **(A)** Leukemia. There is a statistically significant upward curvature in the dose range 0.3 Sv and a statistically significant departure from this in the higher dose range. **(B)** All cancers except leukemia. There is no statistically significant nonlinearity in the range 0.3 Sv, but the leveling off in the higher dose range is marginally significant. *Source:* From Ref. 143.

Table 17-1 Summary Measures of Radiation Dose-Response for Mortality at Statistically Significant Tissue Sites in Atom Bomb Survivors of Hiroshima and Nagasaki[a]

Site of Cancer	Relative Risk per Sv[a]	Excess deaths (No./10⁴/Persons Exposed/Yr/Sv)	Attributable Risk (%)[b]
Leukemia	5.62	2.61	54
All cancers (except leukemia)	1.53	10.6	7.2
Female breast	2.41	1.48	25
Lung	1.53	1.67	10
Esophagus	1.53	0.42	11
Stomach	1.24	2.11	4.6
Colon	1.65	0.73	12
Ovary	1.94	0.61	15
Urinary tract	1.80	0.48	13
Multiple myeloma	2.15	0.17	17

[a] Includes both sexes, all ages at exposure;1950 to 1990 data. Estimates based on weighted organ dose measurements. Data
[b] Percentage of all cancer observed that can be attributed to the radiation exposure.
Source: From Ref. 157.

(0.5 cGy). The most recent estimates indicate that there have thus far been about 100 excess leukemias and 440 other cancer deaths attributable to radiation exposure.[158] There have been a total of about 9300 cancer deaths overall, thus ~6% of all cancer deaths in the population exposed to >0.005 Sv are associated with radiation, although the overall mortality rate is not significantly increased. As can be seen in Table 17-1, the relative risk at 1 Sv is considerably lower for all other cancer types than it is for leukemia. The excess of cancer deaths/10^4 persons exposed/year/Sv is ~13 for all cancers, including leukemia, ranging from 0.17 to 2.11 in individual tissues.

In addition to breast and lung cancers and leukemia, dose-response data from human epidemiologic studies are available for two other sites not shown in the atom bomb survivor data in Table 17-1; these are thyroid and bone cancers. The incidence of bone cancer was not significantly elevated in the atom bomb survivor studies; the relative and absolute risks are low for the induction of this type of cancer by low LET radiation. The dose-response data have come from studies of persons with elevated body burdens of alpha-emitting radium isotopes as a result of occupational or medical exposures.

Thyroid cancer, on the other hand, is very efficiently induced by low LET radiation in children. Adults are quite resistant. Dose-response relationships are derived from populations receiving therapeutic irradiation, either for an enlarged thymus gland or *Tinea capitis*. Relative risk estimates for the development of thyroid cancer have ranged from 7 to 69 among various age groups, ethnic origins, and different studies.[25] However, cancer death rates are not significantly elevated in these populations, since radiation apparently induces only papillary and follicular type tumors, most of which are curable and tend to progress slowly. Studies of populations exposed from the Chernobyl reactor accident also indicate a significant increase in the incidence of thyroid cancers in children, presumably from radioactive iodine released as a consequence of the accident.[156,171] However, there has been no clear evidence of an increase in overall cancer incidence or mortality including leukemia in the exposed population, nor of any other public health impact aside from the psychological one.[156] On the other hand, increased cancer death rates at several different sites are appearing among the workers at the Mayak Nuclear Weapons facility in the former Soviet Union.[172]

In addition to the results from the atom bomb survivors, dose-response data are available for breast cancer from several medically exposed populations.[173,174] The results of these studies are generally consistent in terms of risk estimates. Taken as a whole, however, several other interesting findings have emerged. Radiation-induced breast cancers are similar in histopathologic types and age distribution to those arising spontaneously. Women younger than 20 years of age at exposure are at a higher relative risk than adults, similar to the observations for leukemia. As in the case of thyroid cancer, the development of breast cancer is profoundly dependent on hormonal status. Finally, protraction of exposure does not appear to reduce the risk of radiation-induced breast cancer, except for very low dose rates.[164]

Additional epidemiologic studies are also available for the induction of lung cancer.[25] Of particular interest among the underground uranium mine workers in the Colorado plateau has been an apparent multiplicative interaction with cigarette smoking. This observation is consistent with certain experimental findings on alpha radiation–induced lung cancer. However, statistically significant evidence for a more than additive effect between smoking and low LET radiation on lung cancer has not been observed in other epidemiologic studies. This important question needs further investigation.

Finally, it is of passing note that data are now emerging from the studies of the atomic bomb survivors indicating an increase in noncancer mortality, among the irradiated survivors.[158,173] Increasing trends are observed for disorders of the circulatory, digestive, and respiratory systems with doses >0.5 Sv. The data suggest that 0.8% of noncancer deaths may be associated with the radiation exposure.[158]

Radiation-induced Secondary Tumors

An increase in secondary tumors in the treatment field has now been observed in patients treated for several different types of cancer by radiation therapy, often in conjunction with chemotherapy. In some cases, the incidence of radiation-associated secondary tumors appears to be proportional to dose at the treatment portal, although some epidemiologic data suggest that for leukemia in particular the tumor incidence may decline at high doses, owing to killing of the target cells. The extent to which genetic factors may play a general role in susceptibility to treatment-induced secondary tumors in cancer patients is unclear. Radiation alone used in conventional treatment regimens may not be a very potent inducer of secondary tumors. This prediction arises from the localized nature of the exposure during clinical radiotherapy, in which the dose to normal tissues is minimized, and from the fact that ionizing radiation tends to be cytotoxic rather than mutagenic. The high radiation doses employed may thus kill potentially transformed cells in the treatment field. Exceptions may be the treatment of Hodgkin disease in which lower radiation doses are delivered to a relatively large volume of tissue, and in the use of Intensity Modulated Radiation Therapy (IMRT). IMRT involves the use of more fields with a larger normal tissue volume exposed to lower doses.[174] It has been estimated that IMRT is likely to almost double the incidence of second malignancies compared with conventional radiotherapy from about 1% to 1.75% for patients surviving 10 years.[175] The risk may be even higher for pediatric patients.

Low-Dose Exposures

Sufficient data are now available from the atomic bomb survivors to allow an analysis of those survivors who received <0.5 Sv; these data are providing preliminary estimates of risk for doses as low as 5 to 10 cGy.[162] They indicate a statistically significant risk in this range consistent with a linear dose-response relationship, with an upper confidence limit on any possible threshold of 6 cGy. There have been a number of epidemiologic studies over the past two decades, however, that purport to show a carcinogenic effect of environmental radiation exposures in the dose range well below 10 cGy. The populations involved are varied but include military personnel exposed during nuclear bomb testing, workers in various nuclear and weapons facilities, and members of the general population living near nuclear facilities or exposed to fallout.

There have been several reports analyzing various of these low-dose epidemiologic studies.[176-178] On the basis of the relative and absolute risk estimates shown in Table 17-1, a significant increase in radiation-associated cancer incidence in populations of these sizes exposed to doses in the range of 10 cGy or less would imply a markedly enhanced sensitivity at low doses; ie, the dose-response curve should show marked hyperlinearity with the excess cancer incidence rising rapidly at very low doses. There are no experimental data to support such a phenomenon; indeed, a careful analysis of nearly all of these low-dose studies indicates no significant increase in the incidence of all cancers or of cancers at specific sites. Analyses of a large number of radiation workers from the United Kingdom[179] and Canada[180] indicate that the risk estimates for leukemia and all cancers were consistent with an extrapolation from the atom bomb survivor data, providing no evidence for an unexpected increase in sensitivity at low doses such as to suggest that the current radiation protection standards might be appreciably in error.

There has also been considerable concern about the risk of lung cancer from exposure to naturally occurring radon in the air of homes and the workplaces. The results of several recent epidemiologic studies, however, have been conflicting. For example, a clear association between radon exposure and lung cancer was identified in studies in Sweden and the United Kingdom, whereas equally rigorous investigations in Canada, China, and Missouri found no evidence of excess risk. When a meta-analysis of eight case-control studies was carried out,[181] a positive trend was found consistent with projections of the high-dose data from radon-exposed underground miners. Most radon-induced cancers are expected to occur in cigarette smokers. Overall, however, the carcinogenic risks of residential radon appear to be small,[182] probably of the magnitude of that attributable to passive smoking.[183]

Because the carcinogenic effects of radiation are apparently so small at these low doses, it appears unlikely that they will ever be defined by epidemiologic studies alone. This will likely require a better understanding of the basic mechanisms of radiation carcinogenesis, including the role of factors such as bystander effects, induced genomic instability, and the adaptive response to protracted radiation exposure. In the meantime, risk estimations must be made by extrapolation from the epidemiologic studies at higher doses.

Risk Assessment

Table 17-2 shows the lifetime excess cancer risk estimates following exposure to 1 cGy as determined by the BEIR V Committee.[25] These estimates were derived from a composite of the epidemiologic data from the atom bomb survivors and various medical X-ray exposures. They were derived by use of the relative risk model, on the assumption of a linear-quadratic dose-response relationship for leukemia and a straight linear relationship for other tumors. In addition, characteristics such as the latent period, age at exposure, time after exposure, and interaction effects were taken into consideration.

The risk estimates shown in Table 17-2 are for the mean of all ages at exposure. For children younger than 20 years of age, excess cancer mortality per cGy is about 50% higher than the mean for all tumors, whereas it is much lower at ages >65 years. The leukemia risk, on the other hand, rises quite steeply in middle and old age, where the risk is nearly four times that of young adults and twice that of children.[25] The lifetime excess deaths from all cancers including leukemia for acute radiation exposure as shown in Table 17-2 are ~800 per 10^6 exposed people per cGy. The recent UNSCEAR committee report[156] estimates that the yield may be 20% to 40% higher on an individual basis; this represents approximately a 1:1000 (0.1%) effect per cGy. For example, a person receiving 10 cGy acute whole-body exposure would have a 1% chance of developing a lethal cancer during his or her lifetime as a result of this radiation exposure, whereas the chances of dying of cancer unrelated to radiation exposure are ~18%. This risk would be lower for low dose–rate, protracted exposure (see Table 17-2). It should be emphasized, however, that these risks are for uniform whole-body irradiation. Of concern, however, is the rapidly increasing frequency of pediatric patients undergoing computed tomography (CT) diagnostic procedures. Whole-body CT scans, depending upon the machine used, can deliver doses in excess of 10 cGy.[184] The estimated lifetime cancer mortality risk attributed, for example, to radiation exposure of a small child is an order of magnitude higher than that for an adult.[185] If the current trend continues, pediatric CT will result in a significantly increased lifetime risk over adult CT due to both the increased dose per milliampere-second and the increased lifetime risk per unit dose used.

It is often the perception of risk rather than the actual risk itself, which is particularly important in the promotion and regulation of health and safety.[186] For example, members of the League of Women Voters and a group of college students were asked to order their perception of the risk of fatality for 30 activities and technologies. Both placed nuclear power in first position ahead of smoking, ingestion of alcoholic beverages, and riding in motor vehicles. The risk experts ranked smoking and motor vehicle accidents first (there are about 50,000 motor vehicle deaths in the United States each year, at least 50% of them involving alcohol or drug use), whereas they ranked nuclear power twentieth, in the same range as the ingestion of food coloring and the use of home appliances.

It is of interest to compare the risk of death from various activities associated with everyday living.[187,188] Table 17-3 shows such a comparison. In general, it turns out that the risk from radiation exposure is relatively small when compared with other risks associated with everyday living. Similarly, a comparison of occupational hazards shows that the risks to radiation workers are much lower than those associated with many other occupations. In this context, it is of interest to note the estimation that >430,000 excess deaths each year are associated with cigarette smoking in the United States.[186] On the assumption that 40% of the population smokes, such an excess death rate would be comparable with that resulting from ~350 cGy of uniform whole-body radiation exposure.

Of concern to the clinical oncologist, however, is the increasingly apparent risk of inducing a secondary malignant tumor as a result of the successful treatment of cancer by high doses of radiation, often in conjunction with chemotherapy. This will, of course, depend upon the particu-

Table 17-2 Lifetime Excess Cancer Risk Estimates for Whole-Body Radiation Exposure to 1.0 cGy

	Cancer Deaths per 10^6 Persons Exposed (Excess per cGy)		
Type of cancer	Acute Exposure[a]	Protracted Exposure[b]	Expectation[a]
Leukemias	95	48	6850
Non-leukemias	695	347	176,450
All cancers	790	395	183,300

[a] Estimates from BEIR V Committee report.[25] See text for discussion of these estimates. Normal expectation is the number of cancer deaths (lifetime risk) expected to occur in the general population of 10^6 people.

[b] Derived from acute exposure data by applying a dose-rate effectiveness factor of 2.

Table 17-3 **Risks of Death From Various Activities**[a]

Activity	Risk of Death (Per Million/Yr)
Being a person age 55 years (all causes)	10,000
Smoking a pack of cigarettes daily (all causes)	3500
Rock climbing for 2 h (accident)	500
Canoeing for 20 h (drowning)	200
Motorcycling for 1000 miles (accident)	200
Traveling 1500 miles by car (accident)	40
Being a pedestrian (accident)	40
Working 1 week as a firefighter (accident)	15
Working 1 week in agriculture (accident)	10
Fishing (drowning)	10
Eating (choking on aspirated food)	8
Skiing for 10 h (accident)	8
Working 1 month in a typical factory (accident)	5
Traveling 5000 miles by air (accident)	5
Having a chest radiograph (radiation-induced cancer)	1
Visiting Denver for 2 months (cancer from cosmic rays)	1
Living in the vicinity of a nuclear power plant (radiation-induced cancer)	<0.1

[a] Estimates derived from various sources.

lar tissue sites included in the radiation field. One could then derive rough risk estimates for radiation alone on the basis of the type of information shown in Table 17-1. The information in Table 17-1, however, was derived from presumably normal people in the general population exposed to tens to hundreds rather than thousands of cGy. As discussed earlier, a number of factors might determine susceptibility to secondary tumors in cancer patients treated with high doses of radiation. Cell killing is one of them; patients treated with radiation for carcinoma of the cervix have not shown an increase incidence of leukemia, presumably because the bone marrow cells in the radiation field are killed by the high radiation doses. On the other hand, a risk factor would be the irradiation of large tissue volumes as in the treatment of disorders such as Hodgkin disease; genetic factors would be another. It is well known, for example, that retinoblastoma patients are at very high risk for developing secondary tumors in the irradiated field. The extent to which genetic hypersusceptibility may be important in some of the more common cancers remains to be determined.

In most cases, it would seem that benefit-risk estimation would be positive; ie, the benefit of treatment would outweigh the risk of developing secondary tumors. However, information concerning the relative carcinogenicity of various combinations of radiation and chemotherapeutic agents is now becoming available, and it appears that certain combinations may be more carcinogenic than others. Clearly, additional knowledge is needed to devise effective treatment regimens which might minimize their carcinogenic effects, and thus the risk of developing secondary treatment-induced tumors, while producing an optimal therapeutic gain.

Acknowledgments

I acknowledge the support of Research Grant DE-FG02-05ER64086 from the US Department of Energy (DJG) and National Cancer Institute Grant RO1 CA99005 (DJG).

Selected References

The complete reference list can be found at www.CANCERMEDICINE8.com

1. Upton AC. Historical perspectives on radiation carcinogenesis. In: Upton AC, Albert RE, Burns, FJ, Shore RE, eds. *Radiation Carcinogenesis*. New York: Elsevier; 1986:1–10.
2. Roots R, Okada S. Protection of DNA molecules of cultured mammalian cells from radiation induced single strand scissions by various alcohols and SH compounds. *Int J Radiat Biol*. 1972;21:329–342.
7. Little JB. Cellular effects of ionizing radiation. I & II. *N Engl J Med*. 1968;278:308–315, 369–376.
13. Radford IR. DNA lesion complexity and induction of apoptosis by ionizing radiation. *Int J Radiat Biol*. 2002;78:457–466.
17. Little JB. Failla Memorial Lecture. Changing views of cellular radiosensitivity. *Radiat Res*. 1994;140:299–211.
24. Miller RW. Effects of prenatal exposure to ionizing radiation. *Health Phys*. 1990;59: 57–61.
26. Albertini RJ. Validated biomarker responses influence medical surveillance of individuals exposed to genotoxic agents. *Radiat Prot Dosimetry*. 2001;97:47–54.
37. Little JB. The relevance of cell transformation to carcinogenesis in vivo. In: Baverstock KF, Strather JW, eds. *Low Dose Radiation—Biological Basis of Risk Assessment*. London: Taylor and Francis; 1989:439–445.
38. Cox R. The multi-step nature of carcinogenesis and the implications for risk analysis. *Int J Radiat Biol*. 1998;73:373–376.
40. Hill CK, Nagy B, Peraino, C, Grdina, DJ. 2-[(aminopropyl)amino]ethanethiol (WR1065) is anti-neoplastic and anti-mutagenic when given during ^{60}Co gamma-ray irradiation. *Carcinogenesis*. 1986;7:665–668.
41. Balcer-Kubiczek EK, Harrison GH, Hill CK, Blakely WF. Effects of WR-1065 and WR-151326 on survival and neoplastic transformation in C3H/10T½ cells exposed to TRIGA or JANUS fission neutrons. *Int J Radiat Biol*. 1993;63:37–46.
44. Kennedy AR. Anticarcinogenic activity of protease inhibitors. In: Troll W, Kennedy AR, eds. *Protease Inhibitors as Cancer Chemopreventive Agents*. New York: Plenum Press; 1993:9–91.
45. Little JB. Radiation carcinogenesis. *Carcinogenesis*. 2000;21:397–404.
50. Little JB. Radiation-induced genomic instability. *Int J Radiat Biol*. 1998;74:663–671.
54. Little JB, Nagasawa H, Pfenning T, Vetrovs H. Radiation-induced genomic instability: delayed mutagenic and cytogenetic effects of X rays and alpha particles. *Radiat Res*. 1997;148:299–307.
61. Marder BA, Morgan WF. Delayed chromosomal instability induced by DNA damage. *Mol Cell Biol*. 1993;13:6667–6677.
66. Ponnaiya B, Cornforth MN, Ullrich RL. Radiation-induced chromosomal instability in BALB/c and C57BL/6 mice: the difference is as clear as black and white. *Radiat Res*. 1997;147:121–125.
67. Seymour CB, Mothersill C, Alper T. High yields of lethal mutations in somatic mammalian cells that survive ionizing radiation. *Int J Radiat Biol Relat Stud Phys Chem Med*. 1986;50:167–179.
68. Chang WP, Little JB. Delayed reproductive death in X-irradiated Chinese hamster ovary cells. *Int J Radiat Biol*. 1991;60:483–496.
72. Redpath JL, Gutierrez M. Kinetics of induction of reactive oxygen species during the post-irradiation expression of neoplastic transformation in vitro. *Int J Radiat Biol*. 2001;77:1081–1085.
75. Murley JS, Kataoka Y, Weydert CJ, Oberley LW, Grdina DJ. Delayed cytoprotection after enhancement of *Sod2* (*MnSOD*) gene expression in SA-NH mouse sarcoma cells exposed to WR-1065, the active metabolite of amifostine. *Radiat Res*. 2002;158: 101–109.
76. Murley JS, Kataoka Y, Cao D, Li JJ, Oberley LW, Grdina DJ. Delayed radioprotection by NFκB-mediated induction of Sod2 (MnSOD) in SA-NH tumor cells after exposure to clinically used thiol-containing drugs. *Radiat Res*. 2004;162:536–546.
82. Little JB. Genomic instability and bystander effects: a historical perspective. *Oncogene*. 2003;22:6978–6987.
86. Mothersill C, Seymour CB. Cell–cell contact during gamma irradiation is not required to induce a bystander effect in normal human keratinocytes: evidence for

release during irradiation of a signal controlling survival into the medium. *Radiat Res.* 1998;149:256–262.

90. Little JB, Nagasawa H, Li GC, Chen DJ. Involvement of the nonhomologous end joining DNA repair pathway in the bystander effect for chromosomal aberrations. *Radiat Res.* 2003;59:262–267.
91. Azzam EI, de Toledo SM, Gooding T, Little JB. Intercellular communication is involved in the bystander regulation of gene expression in human cells exposed to very low fluences of alpha particles. *Radiat Res.* 1998;150:497–504.
95. Olivieri G, Bodycote J, Wolff S. Adaptive response of human lymphocytes to low concentrations of radioactive thymidine. *Science.* 1984;223:594–597.
97. Fan M, Ahmed KM, Coleman MC, Spitz DR, Li JJ. Nuclear factor-kB and manganese superoxide dismutase mediate adaptive resistance in low-dose irradiated mouse skin epithelial cells. *Cancer Res.* 2007;67:3220–3228.
98. Murley JS, Kataoka Y, Baker LL, Diamond AL, Morgan WF, Grdina DJ. Manganese superoxide dismutase (SOD2)-mediated delayed radioprotection induced by the free thiol form of amifostine and tumor necrosis factor α. *Radiat Res.* 2007;167:465–474.
99. Murley JS, Kataoka Y, Weydert CJ, Oberley LW, Grdina DJ. Delayed radioprotection by nuclear transcription factor κB-mediated induction of manganese superoxide dismutase in human microvascular endothelial cells after exposure to the free radical scavenger WE1065. *Free Radic Biol Med.* 2006;40:1004–1016.
100. Matthews JR, Wakasugi N, Virelizier, Yodoi Y, Hay RT. Thioredoxin regulates the binding activity of NF-κB by reduction of a disulphide bond involving cysteine 62. *Nucleic Acids Res.* 1992;20:3821–3830.
101. Murley JS, Kataoka Y, Hallahan DE, Roberts JC, Grdina DJ. Activation of NFκB and *MnSOD* gene expression by free radical scavengers in human microvascular endothelial cells. *Free Radic Biol Med.* 2001;30: 1426–1439.
102. Murley JS, Nantajit D, Baker KL, Kataoka Y, Li JJ, Grdina DJ. Maintenance of manganese superoxide dismutase (SOD2)-mediated delayed radioprotection induced by repeated administration of the free thiol form of amifostine. *Radiat Res.* 2008;169:(in press).
104. Goodhead DT. Initial events in the cellular effects of ionizing radiations: clustered damage in DNA. *Int J Radiat Biol.* 1994;65:7–17.
110. Jackson SP. Sensing and repairing DNA double-strand breaks. *Carcinogenesis.* 2002;23:687–696.
117. Grosovsky AJ, de Boer JG, de Jong PJ, et al. Base substitutions, frameshifts, and small deletions constitute ionizing radiation-induced point mutations in mammalian cells. *Proc Natl Acad Sci USA.* 1988;85:185–188.
122. Kemp CJ, Wheldon T, Balmain A. p53-deficient mice are extremely susceptible to radiation-induced tumorigenesis. *Nat Genet.* 1994;8:66–69.
139. Storer JB, Mitchell TJ, Fry RJ. Extrapolation of the relative risk of radiogenic neoplasms across mouse strains and to man. *Radiat Res.* 1988;114:331–353.
140. Thomson JF, Grahn D. Life shortening in mice exposed to fission neutrons and gamma rays. VII. Effects of 60 once-weekly exposures. *Radiat Res.* 1988;115:347–360.
145. Ullrich RL. Tumor induction in BALB/c mice after fractionated or protracted exposures to fission-spectrum neutrons. *Radiat Res.* 1984;97:587–597.
148. Grdina DJ, Murley JS, Kataoka Y. Radioprotectants: current status and new directions. *Oncology.* 2002;63:2–10.
149. Grdina DJ, Carnes BA, Grahn D, Sigdestad CP. Protection against late effects of radiation by *S*-2-(3-aminopropylamino)-ethylphosphorothioic acid. *Cancer Res.* 1991;51:4125–4130.
150. Carnes BA, Grdina DJ. *In vivo* protection by the aminothiol WR-2721 against neutron-induced carcinogenesis. *Int J Radiat Biol.* 1992;61:567–576.
151. Grdina DJ, Carnes BA, Nagy B. Protection by WR-2721 and WR-151327 against late effects of gamma rays and neutrons. *Adv Space Res.* 1992;12:257–263.
154. Baria K, Warren C, Eden OB, et al. Chromosomal radiosensitivity in young cancer patients: possible evidence of genetic predisposition. *Int J Radiat Biol.* 2002;78:341–346.
160. Little MP, Weiss HA, Boice JD Jr, et al. Risks of leukemia in Japanese atomic bomb survivors, in women treated for cervical cancer, and in patients treated for ankylosing spondylitis. *Radiat Res.* 1999;152: 280–292.
174. Goffman TE, Glatstein E. Intensity-modulated radiation therapy. *Radiat Res.* 2002;158:115–117.
185. Brenner DJ, Elliston CD, Hall EJ, Berdon WE. Estimated risks of radiation-induced fatal cancer from pediatric CT. *AJR.* 2001;176:289–296.

18 Ultraviolet Radiation Carcinogenesis

James E. Cleaver, PhD ▪ David L. Mitchell, PhD

Mad dogs and Englishmen go out in the mid-day sun. —Noel Coward

Historical Perspective

Skin tumors in man account for about 30% of all new cancers reported annually.[1,2] Epidemiological and laboratory studies provide evidence for a direct causal role of sunlight exposure in the induction of cancer,[3,4] and the high rate of skin carcinogenesis is a direct result of the high dose rate from the ultraviolet light component. Both basal cell and squamous cell carcinomas are found on sun-exposed parts of the body (eg, the face and trunk in men, face and legs in women) and their incidence is correlated with cumulative sunlight exposure. Tumor incidence and mortality increase with decreasing latitude, corresponding to exposure; skin cancers are less frequent in dark-skinned populations than in lighter-skinned peoples; and tumor incidence increases with occupational exposure, such as in ranchers and fishermen.[5,6]

Exposure to direct sunlight in the mid-United States latitudes results in the accumulation of a mean lethal dose to unprotected human cells within ~30 min.[7] The only other human carcinogen that even approaches these exposure levels would be cigarette smoke in very heavy smokers. Variations in individual susceptibility are also clearly observed in skin carcinogenesis. Human skin can be classified into types I-IV, ranging from individuals who always burn and never tan, to those who tan but never burn; skin cancer susceptibility varies accordingly.[8] But the most dramatic examples of variations in human susceptibility occur in certain human genetic disorders, especially xeroderma pigmentosum (XP), Cockayne syndrome (CS), trichothiodystrophy (TTD), basal cell nevus syndrome (BCNS), the porphyrias, and phenylketonuria.[9] Other disorders associated with acquired sun sensitivity include polymorphous light eruption, actinic reticuloid and prurigo, solar urticaria, lupus erythematosus, and Darier's disease, as well as medication and immunological status. Sunlight exposure also has a major immunosuppressive effect leading to loss of antigen-presenting Langerhans cells and the appearance of dyskeratotic keratinocytes (apoptotic sunburn cells) in the upper epidermis, together with the erythemal sunburn response associated with vasodilation caused by a release of prostaglandin.[10] Immunosuppression in organ transplant and HIV patients also increases skin cancer incidence.[11]

Epidemiology

Skin Cancer Frequency and Age of Onset

The ultraviolet component of sunlight is well-established for squamous and basal cell cancers but still controversial for melanoma.[12-14] Non-melanoma skin cancers are by far the most common cancers that occur in the United States each year,[2,15] comprising 30% to 40% of all cancers and have been increasing steadily for a century.[16,17] Human epidemiological data show that skin cancer risk are associated with geographical locations, skin type, and various photosensitizing, enhancing, and protective applications.[4,5,17-21] There is also a possibility of greater risk when the exposure is received during childhood and adolescence.[4,22] Non-melanoma skin cancer is therefore one of the few malignancies for which there is clear evidence for the identification of the initiating agent. The relationship of melanoma to sun exposure and the possible action spectrum is less clear[12] but may be related to acute burns rather than accumulated dose.[4,23] Neonatal sunburn in mice can induce melanoma, but not exposures later in life.[14]

The importance of DNA as a chromophore for the shorter wavelengths is highlighted by the autosomal recessive disease XP, in which a failure in DNA repair causes a major increase in squamous and basal cell carcinoma and melanoma.[9,12] Median onset for skin cancer in the general United States population occurs at 50-60 years of age; in XP patients, carcinogenesis is accelerated and median onset is within the first decade (Fig. 18-1). This early onset is a direct consequence of sunlight-induced changes in DNA of skin cells.

Sunlight Spectrum and Wavelengths Responsible for Skin Cancer

Ultraviolet radiation (UVR) is divided into three wavelength ranges on the basis of differences in photochemistry and biological importance. UVA (320-400 nm) is photocarcinogenic and involved in photoaging but is weakly absorbed in DNA and protein. The relevant chromophores may therefore involve reactive oxygen species (ROS), which secondarily cause damage to DNA.[24] UVB (290-320 nm) overlaps the upper end of the DNA and protein absorption spectra and is the range mainly responsible for skin cancer through direct photochemical damage to DNA. UVC (240-290 nm) is not present in ambient sunlight but is readily produced by low pressure mercury sterilizing lamps (254 nm) that

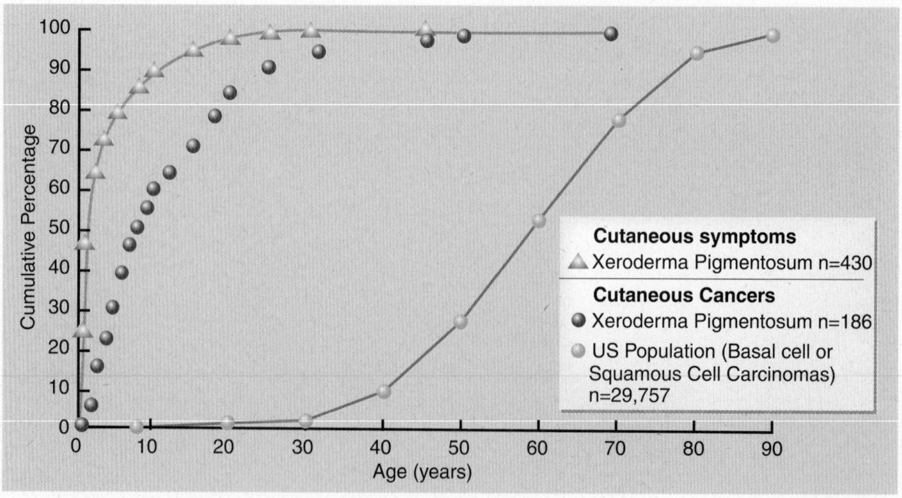

Figure 18-1 ▪ Age at onset of XP symptoms. Age at onset of cutaneous symptoms (generally sun sensitivity or pigmentation) was reported for 430 patients. Age at first skin cancer was reported for 186 patients and is compared with age distribution for 29,757 patients with basal cell carcinoma or squamous cell carcinoma in the United States general population. *Source:* From Ref. 185.

coincides with the peak of DNA absorption (260 nm), and extensively used in experimental studies. Absorption of UVR by stratospheric ozone greatly attenuates these wavelengths, so that negligible radiation shorter than 300 nm reaches the earth's surface. Hence, although UVA and UVB lights constitute a minute portion of the emitted solar wavelengths (10^{-9}), they are primarily responsible for the sun's pathological effects.

Physical shielding of the critical cells of the skin is achieved by melanin pigment and keratin layers; intracellular defenses depend upon repair of DNA damage, antioxidant enzymes (superoxide dismutase, glutathione reductase, etc.), endogenous free radical quenchers, and inducible detoxifying enzymes and biochemical systems.[24] Melanin has multiple functions that can be either harmful or beneficial to the organism.[25] On the one hand, it can be photoprotective, acting as a weak natural sunscreen and scavenger of active chemical species produced by solar UVR. On the other hand, melanin can itself produce active radical species that can damage DNA and has the capacity to bind to drugs in ways that can either benefit or harm the cell.[26] In black skin, melanosomes, the cellular compartments in which melanin is sequestered, are oval, single, and densely packed with melanin and clustered around the nucleus. UVR is blocked from the nucleus and free radicals are absorbed. In contrast, in white skin, melanosomes are round, aggregated, and lightly melanotic. UVR can bypass the clusters to enter the nucleus.

Sunlight-Induced Photoproducts in DNA

The absorption spectrum of DNA correlates well with UV-induced lethality, mutation, and photoproduct formation.[27-31] The energy absorbed by DNA produces molecular changes, some of which involve single bases, others resulting in interactions between adjacent and nonadjacent bases, and still others between DNA and proteins. The relative proportion of DNA photoproducts varies across the UV spectrum.

Dimerizations between adjacent pyrimidines are the most prevalent photoreactions resulting from direct absorption of UVR by DNA. The two major photoproducts are the cyclobutane pyrimidine dimer (CPD) and, at about 25% the frequency, the [6-4] pyrimidine dimer [(6-4)PD] (Fig. 18-2). The distribution of these photoproducts in human chromatin depends on base sequence, secondary DNA structure, and DNA-protein interactions.[31-33] Because cytosine more efficiently absorbs longer wavelengths of UVR than thymine, CPDs containing this base are formed more readily after UVB irradiation.[34] In conjunction with [6-4]PDs, which are preferentially induced at thymine-cytosine dipyrimidines, cytosine CPDs may play a major role in UVB (solar) mutagenesis.[35] Methylation at PyrCG sequences in the p53 gene enhances the formation of CPDs and (6-4)PDs at sites that are hotspots for mutations.[36,37] The [6-4]PD can further undergo a UVB-dependent conversion to its valence photoisomer, the Dewar pyrimidinone (Fig. 18-2).[38] Other less common lesions include purine-purine and purine-pyrimidine photoadducts, photohydrations, and photooxidations.[39] The total yield of these photoproducts is only 3-4% of the yield of CPDs, but a minor biological role as premutagenic lesions in specific sites cannot be excluded.

UVA primarily produces damage indirectly through ROS that in turn react with DNA to form base damage, strand breaks, and DNA-protein cross-links that may be an important pathogenic component of sunlight. Significant levels of cell killing and mutation induction have been observed in human epidermal cells after irradiation with UVA.[27,29] These data are consistent with earlier studies that suggested that the lethal effects of UVA are not mediated by CPD damage[40,41] and that free radical scavengers can mitigate cytotoxicity.[42] The biological importance of UVA is perhaps best illustrated by the demonstration that it causes significant levels of tumorigenesis in hairless mice.[43] Recent evidence suggests that UVA may also induce significant levels of CPDs in human cells by photosensitized triplet energy transfer and that these lesions should be taken into account to fully understand the biological effects of UVA.[44]

Genetic Factors in Skin Carcinogenesis

Excision of UV Photoproducts

The idea that DNA damage is an essential component of photocarcinogenesis arose from the discovery that cells from patients suffering from XP are deficient in DNA nucleotide excision repair (NER) of UV damage.[9,45,46] Two major pathways of NER are known: transcription coupled repair (TCR) and global genome repair (GGR). These pathways remove pyrimidine dimers and large chemical adducts in DNA and replace the damaged site with a newly synthesized polynucleotide patch ~29 bases in length (Fig. 18-3).[47,48] TCR removes damage more rapidly from the transcribed strands of transcriptionally active genes, whereas GGR acts on nontranscribed regions more slowly[49] and is regulated by p53 through control of XPC and XPE(p48) expression.[50]

Excision repair is a heterogeneous process both between species and within the genome. There is considerable difference between CPDs and [6-4]PDs in their rates of excision from the overall genome of rodent and human fibroblasts and skin,[51] even though the basic mechanisms and patch sizes are essentially the same.[52] [6-4]PDs are the more rapidly excised, 50% being removed from human

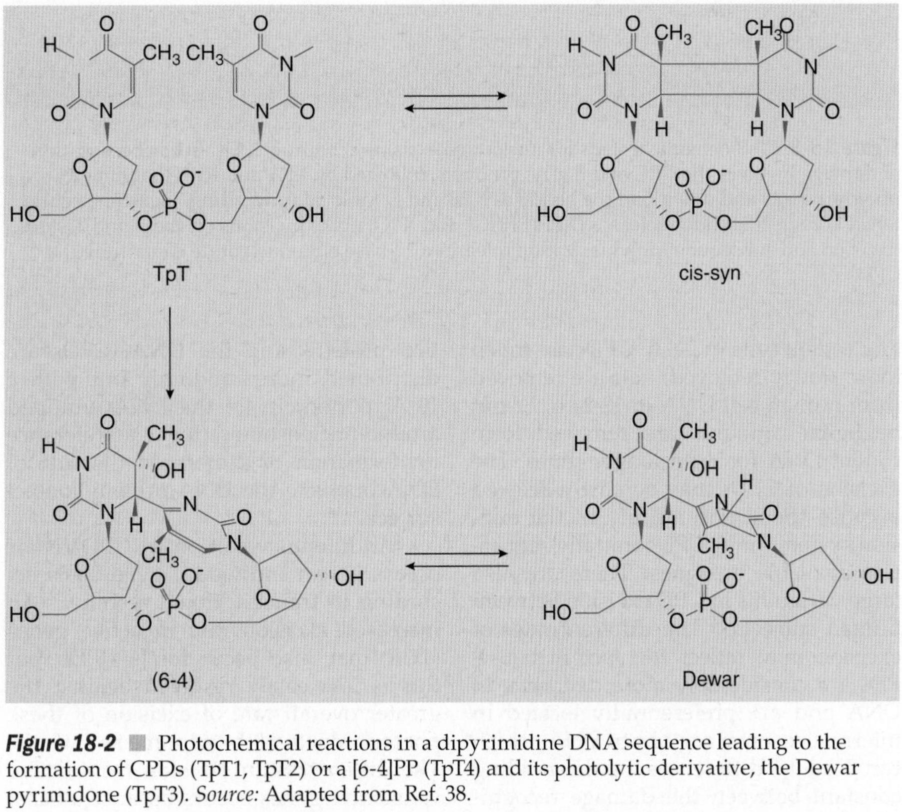

Figure 18-2 Photochemical reactions in a dipyrimidine DNA sequence leading to the formation of CPDs (TpT1, TpT2) or a [6-4]PP (TpT4) and its photolytic derivative, the Dewar pyrimidone (TpT3). *Source:* Adapted from Ref. 38.

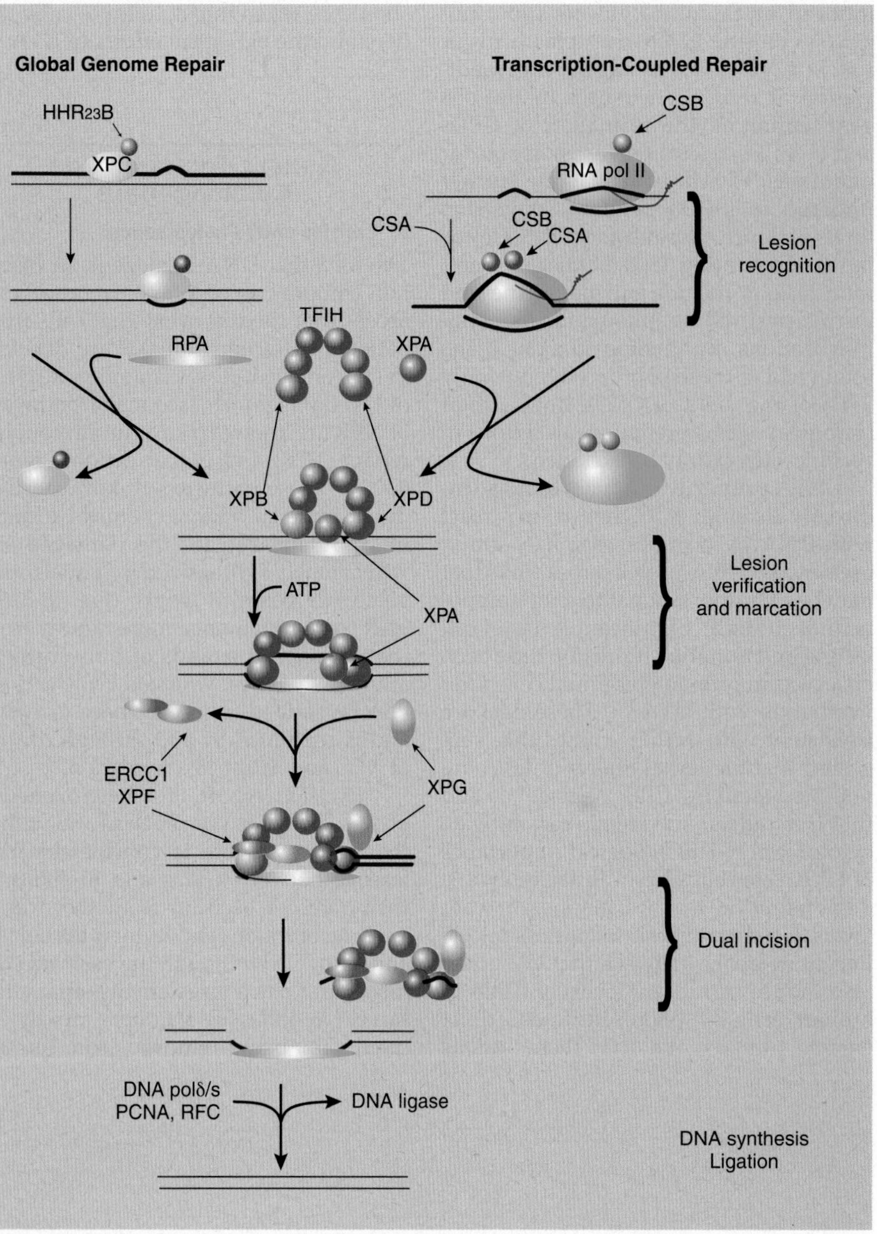

Figure 18-3 Biochemical steps for nucleotide excision repair of CPDs. Initial recognition of damage involves the XPC and E gene products, followed by XPA and RPA that bind to photoproducts and download the helicases XPB and D for local unwinding. Excision occurs when UV-specific endonucleases (XPF/ERCC1 and XPG) make incisions on the 5' and 3' sides. Excision and subsequent polymerization releases a 29-base oligonucleotide containing the CPD.

and rodent cells in 2-6 h. CPDs are much more slowly removed; half are removed from human cell DNA in 12-24 h,[53,54] but negligible amounts are removed from rodent DNA for even longer times. The excision of CPDs may be partly delayed because the strong affinity of the excision system for [6-4]PDs initially sequesters available enzymes. There are also large variations in CPD excision between human subjects.[54] The different rates of excision may reflect the fact that [6-4] PDs are considerably more distortive in DNA and are preferentially located in internucleosomal regions of DNA, which can lead to differences in the binding constant between the damage recognition proteins and the DNA. CPDs are distributed more randomly but with a 10 A° periodicity in the DNA wrapped around nucleosomes, due to a preference for formation of dimers on the side of DNA opposite the DNA-protein contact surface.[55,56]

Additional variation in CPD repair occurs on an individual gene basis according to transcriptional activity.[57] An increased excision rate in active genes (TCR) may also occur for [6-4]PDs, but this is less easily resolved against the greater overall rate of excision of these photoproducts in the genome as a whole. The differences in excision from active vs inactive genes occurs because a basal transcription factor, TFIIH, and two gene products, CSA and CSB, regulate basal transcription and bypass of damage by RNA polymerase II.[58,59] A detailed study of the promoter and first exons of the *PGKI* gene has indicated that excision is slow in regions of promoter binding but increases immediately after the transcription start site.[60] Many of the genes that regulate TCR are associated with the human disorders: XP, CS, TTD, and other disorders. Two of the helicases in TFIIH correspond to the *XPB* and *XPD* genes, and others are known to play a role from their analogs in the yeast transcription factor b.[61]

Mutagenicity of UV Photoproducts and Low-Fidelity DNA Polymerases

Most photoproducts act as blocks to the replicative class B polymerases, Pol A, D, and E. They can, however, depending on their structures, be bypassed during DNA replication to different degrees by damage-specific class Y DNA polymerases.[46,62,63] The class Y polymerases, Pol H, I, and K, have low fidelity due to expanded active sites.[64] Pol H and I are paralogs, both being closely related to the yeast yRad30 gene product. The expanded active sites allow the polymerases to read-through noninformative sequence information. Pol H has the greatest capacity to replicate a large variety of DNA lesions,[65] and preferentially inserts adenine in the nascent strand opposite the lesion (called the "A rule").[66] Hence, Pol H can replicate a thymine-containing CPD with low fidelity,[67,68] and its absence has the most recognizable pathological consequence in the human XP-V complementation group.[69,70] Pol I preferentially inserts guanines and is capable of replicating C-containing photoproducts.[71,72] Pol H or I therefore can insert bases opposite dipyrimidine photoproducts, but the 3' complementary base will be mismatched either by an erroneous insertion or the distortion caused by the photoproduct. Pol K or Z can complete the replicative bypass by extension from the mismatched 3' terminus.[73-75] The absence of Pol H results in increased mutagenesis,[76,77] but the absence of Pol Z has the converse effect of reducing mutation rates.[78]

This mechanism has two important implications regarding the mutagenicity of different photoproducts. First, mutations will most often occur where cytosine is a component of the photoproduct since insertion of adenine opposite thymine is a correct and nonmutagenic event. Hence, most CPDs, because they form between two thymine bases, are not mutagenic. Second, the more distortive a lesion is the more likely it will block DNA synthesis and results in a lethal rather than mutagenic event. Since the [6-4]PD is considerably more distortive than the CPD (ie, it causes a 47° as opposed to a 7° helical bend), it is more likely to be lethal than mutagenic. Because damage bypass and base insertion depend on a variety of conditions, both CPDs and [6-4]PDs contribute to mutagenesis and tumorigenesis in a complex manner.

Sites of mutations have been compared with sites of photoproduct induction in target genes using episomal plasmids and chromosomal genes. Sites and frequencies of mutation hotspots in the *lacI* gene transfected into human cells were identical to those determined in *Escherichia coli.*[79] Sites of transition mutations correlated with sites of increased [6-4]PD induction[80-82] (Table 18-1). In a shuttle vector system in which photoproduct induction and sites of mutation were examined in the *supF* gene, transfection into SV40-transformed human fibroblasts and monkey kidney cells indicated a similar correlation.[83] In the *supF* gene inserted into the mouse L cell chromosome[84] and in the endogenous *APRT* gene of CHO cells,[85] most of the mutations consisted of cytosine-to-thymine transitions occurring at thymine-cytosine and cytosine-cytosine sequences. Due to the strand specificity of repair, there is a bias between mutations in the coding and the noncoding strands of expressed genes that differs according to the NER capacity of the cells.[86,87]

Table 18-1 ■ **UVC-Induced Mutations Observed in Shuttle Vector pZ189 Replicated in XP or Normal Human Cells[a]**

Mutations	Number of Plasmids with Base Changes[b] XP	Normal
Independent plasmids sequenced[c]	61 (100%)	89 (100%)
Point mutations		
• Single base substitution	47[d] (77%)	48 (53%)
• Tandem base substitutions[e]	12 (20%)	16 (18%)
• Multiple base substitutions[f]	1[d] (2%)	24 (28%)
Base insertions and deletions		
• Single base insertion	0	2
• Single or tandem base deletions	1	3
Types of Single or Tandem Base Substitutions and Number of Changes		
Transitions	67[d] (94%)	61 (75%)
• GC to AT	66[d] (93%)	59 (73%)
• AT to GC	1 (1%)	2 (2%)
Transversions	4[d] (6%)	20 (25%)
• GC to TA	0[d]	8 (10%)
• GC to CG	1 (1%)	5 (6%)
• AT to TA	3 (4%)	6 (8%)
• AT to CG	0	1 (1%)

[a]Modified from Ref. 145.
[b]50 to 300 J/m² for XP cells, 100 to 5,000 J/m² for normal cells.
[c]From separate transfections or different mutations in the same transfection including all experiments.
[d]$p < 0.01$ versus normal.
[e]Two base substitutions 0 to 2 bases apart, or 3 adjacent base substitutions.
[f]At least 2 base substitutions more than 3 bases apart.

Because CPDs and [6-4]PDs can both form at sequences shown to be mutation hotspots in shuttle vectors, the identity of the mutagenic lesion has been tested by photoreactivation of the *supF* sequence in plasmids before transfection.[88,89] Enzymatic photoreversal of CPDs reduced the mutation frequency in normal cells by 75% and in XP group A cells by 90%. These results are different from *E. coli* and suggest that [6-4]PDs may be less mutagenic in human cells. A subsequent analysis using photoreactivation suggested that CPDs occurring at dipyrimidine sites containing at least one cytosine base were the predominant mutagenic lesions induced in human cells and that [6-4]PDs at these sites accounted for only about 10% of the mutations.[88] However, this same study indicated that the frequencies of both CPDs and [6-4]PPs at individual dipyrimidine sites did not correlate with mutation frequency, suggesting that, although UV-induced lesions are required for mutagenesis, mutation hotspots are determined by other factors.

A comparison of photoproduct yields, rates of repair, and mutations in the *PGKI* and p53 genes, however, has shown that regions of high UV-induced mutation can be caused by either or both high photoproduct yield and low repair.[60,90-92] DNA repair at individual nucleotides in the p53 tumor suppressor gene, eg, was highly variable and sequence-dependent with slow repair observed at seven of eight of the positions associated with mutations.[90] UV-induced mutations in the p53 gene are a probable step in the formation of squamous cell carcinoma[93,94] and may arise at DNA repair "coldspots" as well as at photoproduct "hotspots."

Mechanism of Nucleotide Excision Repair

Pyrimidine dimers are repaired by a complex multistep process, which involves many interacting gene products that give rise to complex, overlapping symptoms in skin, brain, and other organ systems in patients with mutations in these genes. Several components of NER such as *ERCC1*,[95,96] *XAB2*,[97] and *HR23B*[98] have rarely been found among clinically recognized syndromes. Inactivation of the *ERCC1* gene produces UV-sensitive cells and causes lethal liver failure in mice,[95] and one neonatal lethal mutation in *ERCC1* has been reported in a human patient.[99]

NER involve sequential steps of photoproduct recognition, assembly of the excision complex, displacement of the excised fragment, and polymerization of the replacement patch by assembly of individual factors at sites of DNA damage rather than by preassembly of a complete holocomplex.[100] Photoproduct recognition proceeds through three stages: initial binding by the DDB1/DDB2(XPE) complex,[101] recruitment of XPC/HR23B/centrin via ubiquitylation by the E3 ligase activity of DDB1/DDB2,[98,102-104] and eventual displacement by XPA/RPA that appears to be the final binding complex. XPA/RPA interacts with the unwinding activity of TFIIH and the 3' and 5' nucleases, and binds to the damaged site with a high affinity for the [6-4]PP.[105,106]

The p48 subunit of XPE is inducible by p53 in human cells, but not in rodent cells due to mutation or methylation of the p53 response elements in the promoters.[107] Hence rodent cells fail to repair CPDs in nontranscribed DNA. There is a strong dependence of p48 mRNA levels on basal p53 expression that may provide a link between p53 and NER.[108] The XPC-hHR23B complex initiates NER specifically in nontranscribed DNA.[98,103] The XPC protein binds to the undamaged strand opposite a pyrimidine dimer, inserting a peptide chain within the helix to displace the dimer to an extrahelical position.[109,110] Stable association of TFIIH with DNA lesions is dependent on the integrity of XPA and XPC proteins. TCR is initiated by the arrest of RNA polymerase II at a damaged base, in association with the specific TCR factors CSA, CSB, and XABP, a binding partner of XPA.[111]

Subsequent to or in concert with the binding reactions, DNA is unwound further by the 10 subunit transcription factor TFIIH that contains the 3'-5' (XPB) and 5'-3' (XPD) helicases. The XPG nuclease cuts 3' to the lesion and the ERCC1-XPF nuclease cuts 5' to the CPD. A 27-29 nt oligonucleotide containing the photoproduct is then released.[112] Once this oligonucleotide is removed, the resulting gap is filled in by the combined action of DNA Pol D, proliferating cell nuclear antigen (PCNA), single strand binding protein, and ligase I.[47]

Xeroderma Pigmentosum

XP is a rare autosomal recessive disease that occurs at a frequency of about 1:250,000 in the United States.[9] Affected patients (homozygotes) have sun sensitivity resulting in progressive degenerative changes of sun-exposed portions of the skin and eyes, often leading to neoplasia. Some XP patients have, in addition, progressive neurologic degeneration. Obligate heterozygotes (parents) are generally asymptomatic. The median age of onset is 1-2 years of age, with skin rapidly taking on the appearance of that seen in individuals with many years of sun exposure. Pigmentation is patchy, and skin shows atrophy and telangiectasia with development of basal and squamous cell carcinomas. The frequency of cancers is about 2000 times that seen in the general population under 20 years of age, with an ~30-year reduction in life span.

Cells from patients with XP excise pyrimidine dimers at reduced rates of 0-90% of normal, except for the variant group, which has near-normal rates.[113] The reductions are similar in all tissues thus far investigated, including skin in vivo, peripheral lymphocytes, fibroblasts, liver cell cultures, and tumor cells. There are seven complementation groups among patients who are deficient in excision repair, and an eighth, the XP variant, has a defect in the low-fidelity polymerase Pol H (Table 18-2).

Compared with normal cells, cells from XP groups A and D are very sensitive to the lethal effects of UV light and are unable to excise the CPD and the [6-4] PP. XP group A cells also have a reduced capacity to repair the Dewar pyrimidinone, an important lesion induced with increased efficiency by UVB light.[35,51,114]

Group C is one of the largest groups and is often referred to as the common or classic form of XP. The patients show only skin disorders, which vary considerably in severity, depending on the climate.[115] Tumors of the tongue have been observed in several patients. Cells have low but heterogeneous levels of excision repair (10-20% of normal) and are less sensitive to killing by UV light and chemical carcinogens than cells in groups A, B, D, and G. One characteristic of repair unique to this group is that the reduced repair is confined to nontranscribed regions of the genome.[116] These cells insert repair patches into the transcriptionally active regions of their genome at normal rates, corresponding to [6-4]PP and CPD excision.[116] This raises the dilemma that high rates of cell killing, somatic mutation, and cancer from UV light in XP group C are associated with repair deficiencies in the nontranscribed regions of the genome. This in turn suggests that activating rather than silencing mutations may be important, or that mutations arise from unrepaired lesions in the nontranscribed strand of active genes. Alternatively, global repair deficiencies may cause an overall increase in genomic instability leading to chromosomal aberrations.

Group E is a rare group that exhibits mild symptoms and residual levels of repair that are between 50% and 100% of normal and lack a DNA-binding protein, p48, that is associated with a larger protein, p127.[117] XPE patients carry mutations in the p48 gene,[118] but some apparent XPE patients who had normal p48 were found to be members of other groups who had been misassigned.[119] The role of this protein is still unclear but it is dependent on p53 and involved in repair of nontranscribed regions of DNA.[101,108,118]

XP variant cells have normal excision repair but lack a DNA low-fidelity class Y DNA polymerase, *hRAD30A* (Pol H) that is required for accurate replication of pyrimidine dimers.[69,70] In its absence XP variant cells are very susceptible to UV-induced mutagenesis[76] and exhibit essentially the same symptoms as other XP patients, but lack neurological complications. Carcinogenesis from UV damage in XP patients arises therefore from the loss of either NER capacity or Pol H; both lead to an increase in the amount of persistent DNA damage that becomes the substrate for error generation (mutations, gene rearrangements, deletions, and genomic instability).

Table 18-2 ■ **Complementation Groups in XP and UV-Sensitive Chinese Hamster Ovary (CHO) Cells**

Group	Human Chromosome Location	CNS Repair Disorders	Relative DNA Repair (%)
Xeroderma pigmentosum			
A	9q34.1	Yes	2-5
B (Cockayne, TTD and *ERCC3*)[a,b]	2q21	Yes	3-7
C	3q25	No	5-20
D (Cockayne, TTD and *ERCC2*)[a,b]	19q13.2	Yes	25-50
E	11p11-12	No	50
F	16q13.1	No	18
G (Cockayne)	13q32.3	Yes	<2
Variant *CHO (ERCC)*[c]	6p21	No	100
1	19q13.2	–	Low
2 (XPD)	19q13.2	–	Intermediate
3 (XPB)	2q21	–	Intermediate
4 (XPF)	16q13.1	–	Low
5 (XPG)	13q 32.3	–	Intermediate

[a]Patients also exhibit symptoms commonly associated with Cockayne syndrome: dwarfism, cutaneous features, mental retardation. Group B and ERCC3 represent the same complementation group as Groups D and ERCC2, F and ERCC4, G and ERCC5.
[b]Some patients also have symptoms of trichothiodystrophy.
[c]Genes in the ERCC series are found in human and rodent cells, and were first identified through selection of UV-sensitive hamster cells. ERCC1 does not correspond to any XP group, but the corresponding human genes are identified for others. Relative repair in the ERCC series is classified approximately on the basis of relative sensitivity to DNA damage.
Source: Thanks to L.H. Thompson for providing this summary of gene locations and group assignments. Further details can be found in the websites http://xpmutations.org and http://www.cgal.icnet.uk/DNA_Repair_Genes.html

Cockayne Syndrome

CS is an autosomal recessive disease characterized by cachectic dwarfism, retinal abnormalities, microcephaly, deafness, neural defects, and retardation of growth and development after birth. A major symptom is cerebellar degeneration and Purkinje cell loss causing difficulties in walking and balance.[120] Solar carcinogenesis is not seen in patients with CS, setting this disease apart from XP. CSB knockout mice, however, are sensitive to UVB carcinogenesis.[121]

CS patients are distributed unevenly within the complementation groups with significantly more group A than B patients.[122] Three patients from two families are known from XP complementation group B with additional CS symptoms.[123] as are a few XP-D and XP-G patients. The UV sensitivity of most CS cells lies in a narrow range, with a D37 about half of normal, and in the same range as that of XP-C cells. Characteristic cellular changes in CS include a failure of DNA and RNA synthesis to recover to normal levels after UV irradiation.[124] The excision of DNA photoproducts from total genomic DNA of CS cells is normal, but repair of transcriptionally active genes is reduced.[125] The CS gene products are involved in coupling excision repair to transcription, but their precise function is not yet clear. They may be involved in the ubiquitination and degradation of stalled RNA Pol II at damaged sites.

Cockayne syndrome and XP group C therefore make an interesting contrast. CS cells repair transcriptionally inactive genes, whereas XP-C cells repair only transcriptionally active genes that represent <1-2% of the whole genome. But whereas XP-C shows elevated carcinogenesis, CS does not, indicating that defective global repair is required for carcinogenesis. The defect in CS cells therefore involves too small a total amount of the genome to trigger genomic instability that is carcinogenic. Mice with defects in XP or CS genes, however, both show elevated carcinogenesis,[126] which raises questions of the different roles of NER in humans and mouse strains.

Trichothiodystrophy

TTD is a rare autosomal recessive disorder characterized by sulfur-deficient brittle hair and ichthyosis. Hair shafts split longitudinally into small fibers, and this brittleness is associated with levels of cysteine/cystine in hair proteins that are 15-50% of those in normal individuals. Patients also show physical and mental retardation of varying severity and often have an unusual facial appearance, with protruding ears and a receding chin. Mental abilities range from low normal to severe retardation.[127] Several categories of the disease can be recognized on the basis of UV sensitivity and DNA repair.[128,129] The most severe cases have repair deficiencies and complementation properties that place them in XP groups B and D.[128]

In a detailed analysis of mutations in the *XPD* gene, those that gave rise to XP symptoms corresponded to missense mutations in the DNA helicase motifs of the gene whereas those that gave rise to TTD were mis-sense mutations in the RNA helicase motifs and the C-terminal end of the protein.[130] Some TTD cases do not have mutations in *XPB* or *XPD* and are due to mutations in a small 8-kDa component of TFIIH that appears to regulate the overall level of the transcription factor.[131] Most cases of TTD therefore affect the function of TFIIH in gene transcription and the symptoms of this disease indicate a role for this factor in development and hair growth.

Carcinogenesis

Carcinogenesis often appears to proceed by a multistep process, the first being an initiation event with subsequent promotional events that can often occur much later. One view of carcinogenesis correlates initiation with the induction of a small number of somatic mutations in a few critical genes, and promotion with further alterations in gene expression, copy number, and karyotype. Carcinogenesis appears to involve a process that destabilizes the genome with resulting variations in the activity of a large number of genes that change and develop over time. Genes that are mutated or destabilized include those for cell cycle regulation, checkpoint, and damage response, detoxifying carcinogenic chemicals, DNA repair, and some 50 or more dominantly acting proto-oncogenes activated by mutation, deletion, translocation, or amplification, and tumor suppressor genes whose loss may contribute to the development of cancer.[132,133]

Skin cancers include at least three categories of tumor type: squamous cell carcinoma (SCC), basal cell carcinoma (BCC), and melanoma. SCCs and BCCs appear to originate from different locations in the skin, and melanoma from the pigment cells. The initial damage produced by solar UVB to the skin is eliminated either by repair or by proliferation and exfoliation from the skin's surface. Some cells in the skin also die by apoptosis following exposure ("sunburn cells") resulting in the elimination of damaged cells. Stem cells for the epithelium are thought to reside in the bulge region of the hair follicles,[134] but there are also secondary stem cells at the base of each column of epidermal transit amplifying cells in the epidermal proliferative units.[135] Whether SCCs and BCCs come from different stem cells is currently unknown. A very low frequency of quiescent cells has been observed to retain DNA damage for long periods seemingly without repair or proliferation.[136] The carcinogen-retaining cells may be stem cells, or damaged cells with the potential to become mutants once stimulated to proliferate.

The progression of molecular changes involved in SCC appears to be initiated by inactivating mutations in p53 that result in expanding clones in the sun-exposed areas of the skin that are initially confined within the proliferating units.[137] These clones can be very frequent and can break out of the confines of the columnar structure of the proliferative units after chronic UVB irradiation.[137] Over 90% of SCCs are reported to have p53 mutations that are characteristic of UV exposure, being in dipyrimidine sequences with notable frequencies of CC to TT changes.[93,94,138] Loss of p53 functions can also increase genomic instability during DNA replication when subjected to further UV irradiation.[139-141] Several investigations have also identified activating mutations in the H-*ras* and N-*ras* oncogenes at codon 61, from solar UV exposure.[142-144] However, although over 75% of UV-induced mutations are generally C to T transitions at TC or CC CPD photoproduct sites, the H-*ras* and N-*ras* activation occurred in tumors at a TT site and are transversions not previously identified in model culture systems.[145]

Subsequent to the expansion of p53 mutant clones additional factors come into play with other alterations in gene expression and copy number that have not yet been fully explored. Changes have been observed for example in EGF, *ras*, NFkb, JNK2, presenilin, MMP9, as well as various chromosomal regions identified by allelotyping that control tumor initiation and papilloma to carcinoma conversion.[146-148] There may be an important role for the immune system in SCC formation since immune suppression in organ transplant patients enhances SCC formation, and gamma-delta T cells negatively regulate tumor formation.[149]

BCCs are exemplified by the hereditary disease basal cell nevus syndrome (BCNS). The defect in basal cell nevus syndrome appears to be in the human homolog of the *Drosophila* gene *PATCHED* (*PTC*). The gene is involved in embryonic patterning as well as determining the fate of multiple structures in the developing embryo. Both somatic mutations in sporadic BCCs and single allele mutations in patients with BCNS[150,151] have provided strong evidence that this tumor suppressor is important in BCC tumorigenesis.

The patched protein (PTC) is a transmembrane receptor, and with the coreceptor membrane protein Smoothened (SMO) regulates signal transduction by the extracellular protein Hedgehog (hH) that binds to PTC.[152] PTC represses the pathway by inhibiting signaling by SMO.[153,154] SMO is released from PTC repression if (a) Hh binds to PTC, (b) PTC is mutationally inactivated, or (c) SMO mutation impedes PTC-SMO protein interaction.[155] Once released from PTC repression, SMO signaling activates transcription factor Gli that in turn upregulates expression of *PTC* itself and of a variety of other genes depending on tissue, organism, and stage of development. Mutations in *SMO* have been identified in BCCs and in these tumors, as in BCCs with *PTC* mutations, in situ studies detect increased *PTC* transcript in BCCs as compared to overlying epidermis and stroma.[156,157] Thus, increased *PTC* message levels correlate with decreased PTC protein function. More than 50% of BCCs and 90% of SCCs also contain mutations in p53 with a specific signature induced by ultraviolet light and many other gene amplifications and deletions have been detected.[158]

Melanoma occurs in a hereditary form among ~5% to 12% of all patients.[159] Although this is clinically and histologically indistinguishable from nonfamilial melanoma, there are differences in the age of diagnosis, lesion thickness, and frequency of multiple lesions.[160-162] Significant differences occur in the genetic changes in melanomas according to whether the sites are exposed to chronic (face and hands) or intermittent (trunk and legs) sun damage or are not exposed at all (palms and soles).[163] Melanomas that are not driven by high levels of sun exposure involve a series of mutations, deletions, and amplifications (copy number changes) along the MAP kinase pathway.[159,164-169] This pathway involves N-*ras*, *BRAF*, p16, the pair of *Cyclin D1* and *CDK4*, and *PTEN*. Copy number changes of *Cyclin D1* and *CDK4* are mutually exclusive, as are mutations in *ras* and *BRAF*. *PTEN* being a negative regulator on a parallel *RAS*-activated pathway can occur along with mutations in the *BRAF* arm, but is retained in melanomas on chronically sun-exposed skin.

BRAF, a cytoplasmic serine/threonine kinase regulated by *RAS*, is mutated in a large fraction of melanoma on unexposed skin.[170] BRAF has been successfully targeted by a small molecule inhibitor in clinical trials in combination with chemotherapy, and may become the first line of treatment for certain classes of melanoma.[171] The role of sun damage in chronically exposed regions remains to be fully explored, but melanomas in these regions have fewer mutations and less copy number changes.

Prevention

Nearly all organisms have behaviors or natural features that lower exposure of DNA to solar UVR and reduce the amount of photodamage. Human behaviors include wearing clothes, hats, sunglasses, and sunscreens and general occupational and recreational lifestyles. Other human behaviors can put individuals at greater risk of skin cancer. Over the past few years, the growth in the cosmetic skin-tanning industry has been considered a major contributor to increased skin cancer frequencies, including melanoma.[172] To reduce the risk of skin cancer, the cosmetic tanning industry uses lamps that emit primarily UVA and are thus considered "safe." Recent data showing CPD induction by UVA call this strategy into question.[44] Along similar lines, sunscreen manufacturers have relied primarily on UVB-blocking strategies based on the idea that UVA does not play a significant role in skin cancer. Both of these strategies are questionable because evidence from the Xiphophorus fish melanoma model suggests that UVA may be more effective than UVB in melanoma formation,[173] although this is not supported by recent evidence in mice.[13] The use of UVB sunscreens may even increase melanoma risk by extending exposure to UVA.[174]

In addition to photoprotection, strategies for removing potentially harmful DNA damage within a short time after UV exposure have been researched. One such "morning after" cream contains the bacterial DNA repair enzyme T4 endonuclease V packaged in engineered delivery vehicles that can traverse the stratum corneum, reach cell nuclei in the skin, and repair UV-induced CPDs.[175] This strategy has been shown to enhance DNA repair and reduce cell killing, mutagenesis, and immunosuppression. Similar applications using photolyase are apparently more effective than T4 endonuclease in repairing CPDs from normal human skin cells in vivo.[176] A more controversial therapeutic approach involves the use of thymidine dinucleotides and oligonucleotides that mimic telomeres to stimulate excision repair, decrease UV-induced mutations, and reduce photocarcinogenesis in mice.[177] These and other xenogenic agents delivered to the epidermis in liposomes may have broad applications as active ingredients in modern skin-care products.

Recently, a controversial model has been proposed that questions the net beneficial effects of sunlight on human health. Specifically, the conversion of 7-dehydrocholesterol to cholecalciferol (vitamin D3) and the further production of metabolites 25-hydroxyvitamin D and 1,25-dihydroxyvitamin D (calcitriol) may play a role in reducing various neoplasms in addition to its well-known role in regulating calcium and bone density. Cedric and Frank Garland proposed UVB/vitamin D/cancer theory in 1980 after seeing the map of colon cancer mortality rates in the United States.[178,179] This suggested an inverse correlation between latitude (ie, sunlight exposure) and various solid cancers, including brain, gastric, colon, lung, melanoma, pancreatic, pleural, rectal, and thyroid solid cancers, as well as non-Hodgkin's lymphoma.[180,181] The results are somewhat inconclusive however. Although a significant inverse correlation can be found between vitamin D and colon, esophageal, oral, pancreatic and rectal cancers, and leukemia, no similar correlation was found with bladder, gastric, lung, prostate, and renal cancers.[182] Epidemiological studies can yield variable results and research in the role of vitamin D as a chemopreventive agent needs to enter a more hypothesis-driven phase to explore the mechanisms of this phenomenon.[183] Along these lines, 25-hydroxyvitamin D3, the prohormone of 1,25-dihydroxyvitamin D3 was shown to inhibit the proliferation of primary prostate cancer cells.[184] Should further research support the vitamin D hypothesis, sunlight then becomes a double-edged sword, necessary for the beneficial, chemopreventive effects of vitamin D metabolism yet responsible for inducing most of the skin tumors in the human population. The solution to this problem may require dietary supplementations with vitamin D3 that yield plasma concentrations of 25-hydroxyvitamin D equivalent to those produced by sunlight.

Selected References

The complete reference list can be found at www.CANCERMEDICINE8.com

3. Fitzpatrick TB, Sober AJ. Sunlight and skin cancer. *N Engl J Med.* 1985;313:818–820.
4. Armstrong BK, Kricker A. The epidemiology of UV induced skin cancer. *J Photochem Photobiol B.* 2001;63:8–18.
8. Vitaliano PP, Urbach F. The relative importance of risk factors in nonmelanoma skin cancer. *Arch Dermatol.* 1980;116:454–456.
9. Bootsma D, Kraemer KH, Cleaver JE, Hoeijmakers JHJ. Nucleotide excision repair syndromes: xeroderma pigmentosum, Cockayne syndrome, and trichothiodystrophy. In: Vogelstein B, Kinzler KW, eds. *The Genetic Basis of Human Cancer.* McGraw-Hill; 1998:245–274.
10. Kripke ML. Immunological effects of ultraviolet radiation. *J Dermatol.* 1991;18: 429–433.
12. Kraemer KH, Lee MM, Andrews AD, Lambert WC. The role of sunlight and DNA repair in melanoma and nonmelanoma skin cancer. The xeroderma pigmentosum paradigm. *Arch Dermatol.* 1994;130:1018–1021.
13. De Fabo EC, Noonan FP, Fears T, Merlino G. Ultraviolet B but not ultraviolet A radiation initiates melanoma. *Cancer Res.* 2004; 64:6372–6376.
17. Gallagher RP, Ma D, McLean DI, Yang CP, Ho V, Carruthers JA, et al. Trends in basal cell carcinoma, squamous carcinoma and melanoma of the skin from 1973 through 1987. *J Am Acad Dermatol.* 1990;23:413–421.
23. Armstrong BK. Epidemiology of malignant melanoma: intermittent or total accumulated exposure to the sun? *J Dermatol Surg Oncol.* 1998;14:835–849.
33. Mitchell DL, Jen J, Cleaver JE. Sequence specificity of cyclobutane pyrimidine dimers in DNA treated with solar (ultraviolet B) radiation. *Nucleic Acids Res.* 1992;20:225–229.
44. Courdavault S, Baudouin C, Charveron M, et al. Larger yield of cyclobutane dimers than 8-oxo-7,8-dihydroguanine in the DNA of UVA-irradiated human skin cells. *Mutat Res.* 2004;556(1–2):135–142.
45. Cleaver JE. Defective repair replication in xeroderma pigmentosum. *Nature.* 1968;218: 652–656.
47. Sancar A. Mechanisms of DNA excision repair. *Science.* 1994;266:1954–1956.
48. Sancar A, Sancar GB. DNA repair enzymes. *Annu Rev Biochem.* 1988;57:29–67.
49. Hanawalt PC. Transcription-coupled repair and human disease. *Science.* 1994;266:1957–1958.
51. Mitchell DL, Nairn RS. The biology of the (6-4) photoproduct. *Photochem Photobiol.* 1989;49:805–819.
54. Freeman SE. Variations in excision repair of UVB-induced pyrimidine CPDs in DNA of human skin *in situ*. *J Invest Dermatol.* 1988;90:814–817.
57. Mellon I, Bohr VM, Hanawalt PC. Preferential repair of an active gene in human cells. *Proc Natl Acad Sci USA.* 1986;83:8878–8882.
59. Licht CL, Stevnser T, Bohr VA. Cockayne syndrome group B cellular and biochemical functions. *Am J Hum Genet.* 2003;73:1217–1239.
65. Johnson RE, Washington MT, Prakash S, Prakash L. Fidelity of human DNA polymerase h. *J Biol Chem.* 2000;275:7447–7450.
69. Johnson RE, Kondratick CM, Prakash S, Prakash L. *hRAD30* mutations in the variant form of xeroderma pigmentosum. *Science.* 1999;264:263–265.
70. Masutani C, Kusumoto R, Yamada A, et al. The *XPV* (xeroderma pigmentosum variant) gene encodes human DNA polymerase h. *Nature.* 1999;399:700–704.
77. Wang YC, Maher VM, Mitchell DL, McCormick JJ. Evidence from mutation spec-

tra that the UV hypermutability of xeroderma pigmentosum variant cells reflects abnormal error-prone replication on a template containing photoproducts. *Mol Cell Biol*. 1993;13:4276–4283.

80. Brash DE, Haseltine WA. UV-induced mutation hotspots occur at DNA damage hotspots. *Nature*. 1982;298:189–192.
87. Dumaz N, Drougard C, Sarasin A, Daya-Grosjean L. Specific UV-induced mutation spectrum in the p53 gene of skin tumors from DNA-repair-deficient xeroderma pigmentosum patients. *Proc Natl Acad Sci USA*. 1993;90:10519–10533.
88. Brash DE, Seetharam S, Kraemer KH, et al. Photoproduct frequency is not the major determinant of UV base substitution hot spots or cold spots in human cells. *Proc Natl Acad Sci USA*. 1987;84:3782–3786.
89. Protic-Sabljic M, Tuteja N, Munson PJ, et al. UV light-induced cyclobutane pyrimidine dimers are mutagenic in mammalian cells. *Mol Cell Biol*. 1986;6:3349–3356.
93. Ziegler A, Jonason AS, Leffell DJ, et al. Sunburn and p53 in the onset of skin cancer. *Nature*. 1994;372:773–776.
94. Brash DE, Rudolph JA, Simon JA, et al. A role for sunlight in skin cancer: UV-induced p53 mutations in squamous cell carcinoma. *Proc Natl Acad Sci USA*. 1991;88:10124–10128.
106. Wood RD. DNA damage recognition during nucleotide excision repair in mammalian cells. *Biochimie*. 1999;81:39–44.
111. Lindsey-Boltz LA, Sancar A. RNA polymerase: the most specific damage recognition protein in cellular responses to DNA damage. *Proc Nat Acad Sci USA*. 2007;104:13213–13214.
113. Zelle B, Lohman PH. Repair of UV-endonuclease-susceptible sites in the 7 complementation groups of xeroderma pigmentosum A through G. *Mutat Res*. 1979;62:363–368.
121. Friedberg EC, Meira LB, Cheo DL. Database of mouse strains carrying targeted mutations in genes affecting cellular responses to DNA damage. Version 2. *Mut Res*. 1998; 407:217–226.
126. Berg RJ, Rebel H, van der Horst GT, et al. Impact of global genome repair versus transcription-coupled repair on ultraviolet carcinogenesis in hairless mice. *Cancer Res*. 2000;60:2858–2863.
127. Lehmann AR, Arlett CF, Broughton BC, et al. Trichothiodystrophy, a human DNA repair disorder with heterogeneity in the cellular response to ultraviolet light. *Cancer Res*. 1988;48:6090–6096.
130. Itin PH, Sarasin A, Pittelkow MR. Trichothiodystrophy: update on the sulfur-deficient brittle hair syndromes. *J Am Acad Dermatol*. 2001;44:891–920.
134. Rochat A, Kobayashi K, Barrandon Y. Location of stem cells of human hair follicles by clonal analysis. *Cell*. 1994;76:1063–1073.
137. Zhang W, Remenyik E, Zelterman D, et al. Escaping the stem cell compartment:sustained UVB exposure allows p53-mutant keratinocytes to colonize adjacent epidermal proliferating units without incurring additional mutations. *Proc Natl Acad Sci USA*. 2001;98:13948–13953.
138. Nataraj AJ, Trent JC, Ananthaswamy HN. p53 gene mutations and photocarcinogenesis. *Photochem Photobiol*. 1995;62:165–177.
142. Ananthaswamy HN, Price JE, Goldberg LH, Bales ES. Detection and identification of activated oncogenes in human skin cancers occurring on sun-exposed body sites. *Cancer Res*. 1988;48:3341–3346.
151. Hahn H, Wicking C, Zaphiropoulous PG, et al. Mutations of the human homolog of Drosophila patched in the Nevoid Basal Cell Carcinoma Syndrome. *Cell*. 1996;85:841–851.
152. Toftgard R. Hedgehog signalling in cancer. *Cell Mol Life Sci*. 2000;57:1720–1731.
156. Gailani MR, Bale AE. Developmental genes and cancer: role of patched in basal cell carcinoma of the skin. *J Natl Cancer Inst*. 1997;89:1103–1109.
159. Goldstein AM, Tucker MA. Genetic epidemiology of cutaneous melanoma: a global perspective. *Arch Dermatol*. 2001;137: 1493–1496.
166. Bastian B, LeBoit PE, Hamm H, et al. Chromosomal gains and losses in primary cutaneous melanomas detected by comparative genome hybridization. *Cancer Res*. 1998;58:2170–2175.
169. Pollock PM, Trent JM. The genetics of cutaneous melanoma. *Clin Lab Med*. 2000;20: 667–690.
170. Davies H, Bignell GR, Cox C, et al. Mutations of the *BRAF* gene in human cancer. *Nature*. 2002;417:949–954.
180. Van der Rhee HJ, de Vries E, Coebergh JW. Does sunlight prevent cancer? A systematic review. *Eur J Cancer*. 2006;42:2222–2232.
181. Spina CS, Tangpricha V, Uskokovic M, et al. Vitamin D and cancer. *Anticancer Res*. 2006;26:2515–2524.
185. Kraemer KH, Lee MM, Scotto J. Xeroderma pigmentosum:cutaneous, ocular and neurological abnormalities in 830 published cases. *Arch Dermatol*. 1987;123:241–250.

19 Inflammation and Cancer

Debra L. Laskin, PhD ■ Jeffrey D. Laskin, PhD

An association between inflammation and cancer was first proposed by the German pathologist, Rudolph Virchow in the mid- nineteenth century.[1] He observed leukocytes in neoplastic tissues and suggested that inflammation is one of the predisposing factors in tumorigenesis. Over the past 150 years, evidence has continued to accumulate supporting a strong link between cancer and inflammatory cells, in particular macrophages. These cells release a myriad of inflammatory mediators that have been implicated in the initiation, promotion, and progression phases of cancer development. In the progression phase, it appears that cancer cells usurp or "hijack" normal processes of macrophage-mediated tissue repair and remodeling and use them for their own benefit. This suggests that efficacious therapy against cancer should include combined targeting of tumor cells and the inflammatory microenvironment.

The Inflammatory Response

In response to tissue injury, irritation, or infection, the body mounts an inflammatory response. Characterized by pain, swelling, redness and heat, acute inflammation is an attempt by the immune system to destroy injurious and invading agents, to repair damaged tissue and to restore normal tissue architecture and structure. Major cellular effectors of the inflammatory response are neutrophils and macrophages of the innate immune system. These phagocytic leukocytes emigrate to sites of injury or infection in response to cell and bacterial-derived chemoattractants. Once localized at inflammatory sites, neutrophils and macrophages are activated by products released from damaged tissues and cells and from invading pathogens for cytotoxic and microbicidal activity. This involves phagocytosis and the release of cytotoxic and proinflammatory mediators including reactive oxygen species (ROS), reactive nitrogen species (RNS), eicosanoids and proteolytic enzymes, as well as cytokines such as tumor necrosis factor-alpha (TNFα), interleukin (IL)-1 and IL-6, and chemokines that attract additional inflammatory cells to the site. Under homeostatic conditions, acute inflammation is a rapid and self-limiting process; inflammatory mediators are induced in a tightly regulated sequence, and immune cells move in and out of the affected area, destroying infectious agents, and initiating a late tissue repair and remodeling phase. However, acute inflammation does not always resolve, for example, in the presence of persistent infection or a foreign body (eg, asbestos). This leads to a state of chronic inflammation, characterized by a dense accumulation of activated macrophages and in some cases, lymphocytes in inflamed tissue. Continuous release of cytotoxic and proinflammatory mediators by these cells amplifies and maintains the inflammatory response leading to various chronic diseases and potentially, cancer.

Chronic Inflammation and Cancer

Epidemiologic data have suggested that nearly 25% of cancer deaths are linked to persistent infection and ensuing chronic inflammation.[2] Increased risk of cancer is also associated with chronic inflammation caused by chemical and physical agents.[3,4] The observation that most tumors contain large numbers of inflammatory cells and that the presence of these cells in the tumor correlates with poor clinical prognosis in a number of different types of cancer provides strong support for a role of chronic inflammation in tumorigenesis.[5-7] Additional support comes from findings that cancers frequently arise at sites of chronic inflammation (Table 19-1). The most common example is in patients with inflammatory bowel disease (eg, Crohn disease), who have a strong predisposition for developing intestinal malignancies. Similarly, gastric cancers develop frequently in patients suffering from chronic gastritis associated with *Helicobacter pylori* infection. A high incidence of malignant mesothelioma has also been reported in construction workers with lung scaring and persistent inflammation as a consequence of occupational exposure to asbestos.[8] In a number of these pathologies, long-term use of anti-inflammatory drugs, like aspirin or selective cyclooxygenase-2 (COX-2) inhibitors, is associated with reduced risk of developing malignancies providing further support for a link between cancer and inflammation.[9] It is important to note, however, that in some types of cancer, chronic inflammation is present prior to the malignant change, while in other cancers, an oncogenic change induces a chronic inflammatory microenvironment that promotes the development of a tumor. This suggests that inflammation can contribute to cancer development at multiple stages in the carcinogenic process. For example, at early times, mediators such as ROS and RNS produced by inflammatory macrophages can induce mutations leading to genomic instability, alterations in epigenetic events, and inappropriate gene expression, while mediators released by these cells after the tumor is established enhance proliferation and survival of initiated cells, as well as tumor invasion, metastasis, and angiogenesis.[10-12]

Macrophages

Macrophages are key to both acute and chronic inflammation. These mononuclear phagocytes are derived from

Table 19-1 ■ **Examples of Chronic Inflammatory Conditions Associated With Neoplasia**

Pathologic Condition	Etiologic Agent	Characteristic Neoplasia
Inflammatory bowel disease	Gut pathogens	Colorectal cancer
Gastritis	*H. pylori* infection	Gastric cancer
Asbestosis	Asbestos	Mesothelioma
Silicosis	Silica	Lung cancer
Bronchitis	Tobacco smoke; nitrosamines	Lung cancer
Hepatitis	Hepatitis B and/or C virus	Liver cancer
Cystitis	Gram-negative pathogens; schistosomiasis; carcinogens	Bladder cancer
Pancreatitis	Tobacco, genetic factors	Pancreatic cancer
Skin inflammation	Ultraviolet light	Melanoma
AIDS	HIV	Non-Hodgkin lymphoma; squamous cell carcinomas; Kaposi sarcoma

bone marrow precursors that enter the blood and differentiate into monocytes. The majority of monocytes (>95%) localize in tissues and mature into macrophages where they develop specialized functions depending on the needs of the tissue. Thus in the liver, resident macrophages or Kupffer cells develop a high phagocytic capacity, while in the lung, alveolar macrophages acquire the capacity to release large quantities of highly reactive cytotoxic oxidants. Macrophages contribute to a number of innate immune responses. Through the process of phagocytosis, they function as scavengers, ridding the body of worn-out cells and debris, as well as viruses, bacteria, apoptotic cells, and some tumor cells.[13] Macrophages are also one of the most active secretory cells in the body releasing a vast array of mediators including proteases, complement proteins, cytokines, growth factors, eicosanoids, and oxidants that regulate all aspects of host defense, inflammation, and homeostasis. Additionally, as professional antigen-presenting cells, macrophages are key cells involved in initiating specific immune responses of T lymphocytes.

Accumulating evidence suggests that the diverse biological activities of macrophages are mediated by functionally distinct subpopulations that are phenotypically polarized by inflammatory mediators they encounter in their microenvironment.[3,11,14,15] Polarized macrophages are broadly classified into two major groups: classically activated M1 macrophages and alternatively activated M2 macrophages (Table 19-2). M1 macrophages are activated by type 1 cytokines like interferon-γ (IFNγ) and TNFα, or after recognition of pathogen associated molecular patterns or PAMPs (eg, lipopolysaccharide [LPS], lipoproteins, dsRNA, lipoteichoic acid) and endogenous "danger" signals (eg, heat shock proteins, HMGB1). Alternatively activated M2 macrophages are further subdivided into M2a (activated by IL-4 or IL-13), M2b (activated by immune complexes in combination with IL-1β or LPS), and M2c (activated by IL-10, transforming growth factor–β [TGFβ] or glucocorticoids) subclasses. M1 macrophages release the proinflammatory cytokine, IL-12, promoting strong T-helper cell-1 (Th1) immune responses. In addition, they are powerful effector cells that kill microorganisms and tumor cells and produce cytotoxic mediators (eg, ROS and RNS) and proinflammatory cytokines (eg, TNFα, IL-1, IL-6). In contrast, M2 macrophages support T-helper cell-2 (Th2) associated effector functions. M2 macrophages release the anti-inflammatory cytokine, IL-10, and exert immunosuppressive/anti-inflammatory activity. M2 macrophages also play a role in the resolution of inflammation through phagocytosis of apoptotic neutrophils and increased synthesis of mediators important in wound repair, tissue remodeling, and angiogenesis. Similar functions are exerted by tumor-associated macrophages (TAMs), which display an M2 alternative activation phenotype. It appears that tumors co-opt the normal physiologic actions of macrophages that occur during development and repair in favor of tumor progression.[16,17]

Table 19-2 Activated Macrophage Subpopulations

Macrophage Type		Activating Signals	Phenotype
M_1: Classically activated		IFNγ priming followed by: TNFα GM-CSF LPS Activation of PAMP	–Release proinflammatory cytokines (TNFα IL-1, IL-6, IL-12, IL-23, M1 chemokines) –Express MHC-II –Present antigen to T cells –Promote Th1 responses (cell mediated immunity) –Microbicidal activity –Cytotoxicity –Tissue injury/destruction –Tumor resistance
M_{2a}		IL-4/ IL-13	–Phagocytosis –Stimulate proliferation –Promote tissue repair –Express MHC-II –Present antigen to T cells –Promote Th2 responses –Express scavenger receptors
M_2: Alternatively activated	M_{2b} Type II	Immune complexes + TLR agonists or IL-1β	–Microbicidal activity (release inflammatory mediators) –Phagocytosis –Express MHC-II –Present antigen to T cells –Promote Th2 responses –Express scavenger receptors
	M_{2c} TAM	IL-10 TGFβ Glucocorticoids	–Release IL-10, TGFβ, VEGF, PDGF, fibronectin, MMPs –High levels arginase –Immunosuppressive –Inhibit T cell proliferation –Anti-inflammatory (down regulate M_1 responses) –Release extracellular matrix –proteins (via TGFβ) –Promote wound repair, tissue Remodeling, and angiogenesis –Chronic inflammation

The Tumor Microenvironment

It is now well recognized that a tumor is not simply a mass of transformed cells, but rather a complex unit composed of tumor cells, epithelial cells, stromal fibroblasts, vascular cells (endothelial cells, smooth muscle cells), and infiltrating immune cells (eg, macrophages, neutrophils, dendritic cells, lymphocytes, mast cells) that create a tumor microenvironment.[18-21] Tumor progression involves extensive cross talk between the different cell types in the microenvironment and the surrounding tissue or stroma. This results in suppression of anti-tumor adaptive immune responses, and the release of cytokines and growth factors that support tumorigenesis (Fig. 19-1). Thus, cancer cells alter macrophage and stromal cell functioning such that they provide a permissive and supportive environment for tumor progression. This involves local extracellular matrix remodeling, stimulation of cancer cell proliferation and survival, promotion of cancer cell motility and invasiveness, and induction of angiogenesis.

Tumor-Associated Macrophages

Macrophages represent a major component of the tumor microenvironment and they play a key role in determining outcomes. Initially recruited for tumor destruction, their cytotoxic activity is quickly thwarted by tumor cells, which "re-educate" them to be pro-tumorigenic and release mediators that stimulate tumor cell proliferation, promote angiogenesis, facil-

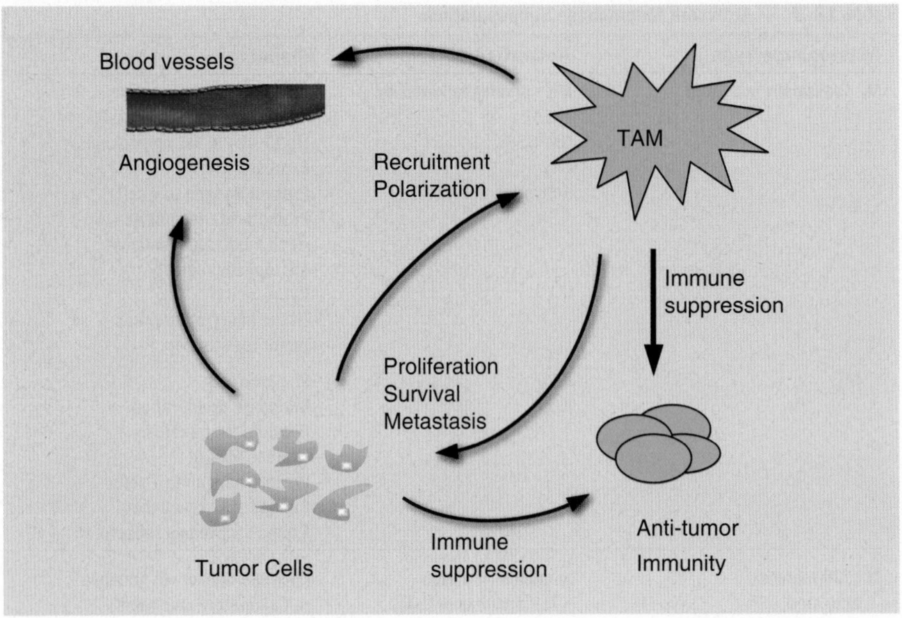

Figure 19-1 ■ Macrophage tumor cell interactions in the tumor microenvironment

itate tumor invasion and metastasis, and suppress anti-tumor immunity.[3,5,7,21-23]

Both clinical and experimental studies support a role of TAMs in tumor progression. Thus, in many human cancers, a high density of TAMs and expression of genes or proteins associated with macrophage infiltration (eg, CD68) or differentiation (eg, colony stimulating factor-1 [CSF-1]) correlates with poor patient prognosis.[5,24-26] Genetic studies have also demonstrated that rates of tumor growth and metastasis are directly correlated with the TAM content of the tumor. For example, in transgenic animals, which are depleted of macrophages due to loss of CSF-1, progression of preinvasive lesions to malignancies is significantly slower, and tumor metastases and angiogenesis are reduced.[27-29] Similarly, in breast cancer cell xenografts, suppression of CSF-1 using siRNA, which reduces the number of TAMs, is accompanied by a marked reduction in tumor growth and angiogenesis.[30] In contrast, the growth of transplanted tumors is significantly increased in mice deficient in SH2-containing inositol-5′-phosphatase (SHIP), which exhibit a spontaneous drift towards M2 macrophage polarization.[31]

TAMs are recruited into the tumor microenvironment by inflammatory mediators released from tumor cells. Most notable are C-C chemokines including CCL2, also known as macrophage chemotactic protein (MCP)-1, as well as CCL3, CCL4, CCL5, and CCL8.[32] Additional tumor-derived mediators that contribute to TAM recruitment include macrophage-colony stimulating factor (M-CSF) or CSF-1, vascular endothelial cell growth factor (VEGF), platelet derived growth factor (PDGF) and TGFβ.[16,33] Recent evidence suggests that TAMs may also be recruited to tumors by HMGB1 released from necrotic tumor cells.[34] In addition to acting as chemoattractants for monocytes/macrophages, CSF-1 and TGFβ promote survival and polarization of infiltrating macrophages into a pro-tumorigenic phenotype. The fact that these polarized cells release high levels of IL-10 and low levels of IL-12 led to their description as M2 macrophages.[35] High IL-10 production by TAMs has been described in numerous experimental models of cancer, and in cancer patients, IL-10 expression is linked to immune suppression.[36,37] One of the main consequences of IL-10 production is autocrine suppression of NF-κB, an important transcription factor regulating proinflammatory cytokine release and cell growth.[23] This leads to decreased production of IL-12 and reduced specific anti-tumor immunity. TAMs are also a source of other potent immunosuppressive molecules including PGE_2 and TGFβ, which contribute to tumor immune evasion.[23,26]

TAMs release many other mediators that contribute to tumor progression and metastasis. These include growth factors that stimulate tumor cell proliferation, like epidermal growth factor (EGF), hepatocyte growth factor (HGF), PDGF, and members of the fibroblast growth factor (FGF) family, as well as IL-6, TNFα and chemokines such as CXCL8 (IL-8) and CXCL12.[26] TAMs also contribute to tumor progression by producing factors that stimulate angiogenesis (eg, VEGF), and the degradation and remodeling of the interstitial matrix (eg, matrix metalloproteinase [MMP]-9, TGFβ). Another pro-tumorigenic mediator released by TAMs is arginase-1, which stimulates production of polyamines, important mediators of cellular proliferation, reduces nitric oxide production and consequent tumor cytotoxicity, and suppresses anti-tumor T-cell activity.[14] TAMs also induce expression of the cell adhesion molecule, VCAM-1 on stromal cells, a step thought to be key for tumor cell dissemination.[38]

Accumulating evidence suggests that TAMs also play a major role in identifying "fertile" sites for productive metastatic tumor growth.[39,40] Thus, TAMs localize at pre-metastatic sites, attracted by chemokines, VEGF-1 receptor, and the presence of endothelial cells capable of expressing high levels of MMP-9. Through the release of VEGF, TGFβ, and TNFα, TAMs "bookmark" these pre-metastatic niches. This involves up regulation of S100 proteins that act as chemoattractants for tumor cells.[33] MMP-9 derived from TAMs has also been implicated in tissue remodeling required for metastatic tumor cell survival at these sites.[41]

Inflammatory Mediators Implicated in Cancer Initiation, Promotion, and Progression

Chronic inflammation is associated with continuous production of proinflammatory cytokines, growth factors, eicosanoids, and proteolytic enzymes that play important roles in tumor initiation, promotion, and progression (Table 19-3). These mediators are generated in large

Table 19-3 ■ **Inflammatory Mediators and Tumorigenesis**

Tumorigenic Process	Inflammatory Mediator	Origin
Initiation	ROS, RNS, COX-2	M1 macrophages, PMN
Promotion	TNFα	M1/M2 macrophages
Proliferation/survival	EGF, HGF, bFGF, PDGF, IL-1, IL-6, CXCL8, TNFα, COX-2, TGFβ	TAM, tumor cells stromal cells
Invasion/metastasis	MMPs, uPA, TGFβ, TNFα, IL-1, IL-6, CSF-1, EGF, VEGF, chemokines	TAM, tumor cells stromal cells
Angiogenesis	VEGF, IL-1, CXCL8, COX-2, NOS-2, chemokines	TAM, tumor cells, stromal cells
Immune suppression	IL-10, IL-17, IL-23, TGFβ, COX-2/PGE2	TAM, Treg, MDSC tumor cells

part by TAMs. The combined activity of mediators released from these cells, as well as tumor cells and stromal cells, is key in determining clinical outcome.[2]

Proinflammatory Cytokines

Cytokines consist of a group of cell-derived proteins that mediate immunity, inflammation and hematopoiesis. They are produced de novo in response to immune or inflammatory stimuli and generally act at very low concentrations over short distances and time spans.. Cytokines act by binding to specific membrane receptors, which then signal the cell via second messengers, often tyrosine kinases, resulting in activation of transcription factors, predominantly NF-κB, AP-1, and STAT, and altered gene expression. Responses to cytokines include increasing or decreasing expression of membrane proteins (including cytokine receptors), proliferation, and secretion of effector molecules. Cytokines may act on the cells that secrete them (autocrine action), on nearby cells (paracrine action), or in some instances, on distant cells (endocrine action). Most notable among the proinflammatory cytokines implicated in the carcinogenic process are TNFα, IL-1 and IL-6, as well as various chemotactic cytokines, referred to as chemokines.

TNFα ■ Considered an early response cytokine produced mainly by macrophages, TNFα appears to orchestrate the inflammatory response.[42] In this capacity, it up regulates cell adhesion molecules on endothelial cells and recruits and activates inflammatory cells. TNFα and its receptors have been detected in many malignancies including those derived from breast, prostate, bladder, and colorectal tissue, and their presence is associated with poor patient prognosis, loss of hormone responsiveness, and cachexia.[43] TNFα is often found in association with IL-1, IL-6, and CSF-1 at relatively low levels, where its pro-tumorigenic actions appear to overwhelm its potential cytotoxic activity.[44]

Experimental evidence for a role of TNFα in tumorigenesis comes from the findings that transgenic mice lacking TNFα or its receptor, TNFR1, are resistant to chemically induced carcinogenesis in the skin, liver, and colon.[45-48] Pharmacologic inhibition of TNFα production has also been reported to reduce the incidence of chemically induced skin tumors.[49] TNFα stimulates the production of ROS and RNS, and it activates NF-κB mediated anti-apoptotic gene expression.[42] It also stimulates tumor cell production of CCL2 (MCP-1), a key cytokine involved in recruitment of macrophages into the tumor microenvironment. These data, together with findings that TNFα is produced by premalignant cells, provides support for the idea that this cytokine plays a role in tumor initiation and may function as an endogenous tumor promoter.[43,50,51] TNFα has also been reported to up regulate MMP-9 and VEGF expression implicating this cytokine in tumor invasion and metastasis.[52] This is consistent with the findings that TNFR1-/- mice are resistant to the development of liver metastasis in experimental colon cancer, while overexpression of the TNFα gene in mice confers a metastatic phenotype on primary tumor cells.[43] The fact that genetic polymorphisms that enhance TNFα production are associated with increased risk of cancer, provides additional support for the idea that TNFα plays a key role in tumorigenesis.[43]

IL-1 ■ The IL-1 family consists of proinflammatory and immunoregulatory cytokines and includes IL-1α, IL-1β, IL-1 receptor antagonist, IL-18, and IL-33.[53] Members of the IL-1 family are important regulators of acute inflammation. They induce expression of numerous proinflammatory genes, including COX-2, inducible nitric oxide synthase (iNOS), MMPs, and various chemokines. IL-1 also stimulates endothelial cells to secrete chemokines such as CCL2 (MCP-1) and CCL8 (IL-8), up regulates expression of cell adhesion molecules (eg, E-selectin, I-CAM-1, and VCAM-1) important in migration of leukocytes and tumor cells, and pro-angiogenic VEGF, and stimulates tumor cell proliferation. These activities are key in promoting inflammatory cell accumulation in the tumor microenvironment, tumor survival and invasiveness, and angiogenesis.

The role of IL-1 family members in tumor growth and progression is well established in several different human cancers.[54,55] In experimental models, genetic ablation of IL-1β prevents tumor metastasis, while high concentrations of IL-1β promote inflammation and tissue damage, as well as tumor invasiveness, metastasis, and angiogenesis. Conversely, delivery of IL-1 receptor antagonists to the tumor site reduces local inflammation, inhibits cancer progression, and decreases metastasis.[56]

IL-6 ■ Another cytokine implicated in carcinogenesis is IL-6.[57,58] This promitogenic cytokine modulates the expression of genes involved in cell cycle progression, apoptosis, and angiogenesis. IL-6 belongs to a larger family of cytokines that signal through a common gp130 receptor expressed on many cell types. Binding of IL-6 to gp130 leads to activation of associated Janus kinases (JAKs). JAKs phosphorylate gp130 resulting in the recruitment and activation of STAT1 and STAT3 transcription factors and stimulation of cellular proliferation.[52] IL-6 has been implicated in the pathogenesis of a number of human cancers including lymphoma, gastric carcinoma, ovarian and prostate cancer, and multiple myeloma.[57-59] High serum IL-6 levels in colon cancer patients are also directly correlated with tumor burden.[60] Experimentally, mice lacking IL-6 are less susceptible to developing tumors when compared to wild type mice, and it has been suggested that IL-6 is essential for ras-driven tumorigenesis.[61,62] Recent studies have also demonstrated that IL-6 and its downstream effector STAT3, are required for the growth of colitis-associated colorectal cancer in mice, and they may also be important in inducing tumor-associated inflammation and promoting cell cycle progression.[63,64]

Chemokines ■ These are cytokines that function to recruit leukocytes to sites of inflammation. Two major groups have been identified based on the positions of the first two cysteine residues in their primary structure, CXC and CC chemokines. Whereas CXC chemokines attract neutrophils and lymphocytes, CC chemokines act on macrophages, eosinophils, dendritic cells, NK cells, and lymphocytes. Receptors for chemokines are transmembrane proteins linked to a Gi protein signaling pathway. The contribution of chemokines and their receptors to tumor progression is well established.[32,33,65] Most tumor cells produce both CXC and CC chemokines. However, clinical and experimental studies indicate that it is the CC chemokines (eg, CCL2, CCL3, CCL4, CCL5, and CCL8) that are mainly involved in recruitment of TAMs into the tumor microenvironment. Most notable among these is CCL2 (MCP-1) which is frequently identified in tumors, and levels of this chemokine correlate with TAM abundance.[26] Interestingly, TAMs have also been reported to generate CCL2, suggesting the existence of an amplification loop within the tumor.[65] Of note, CXC chemokines such as the neutrophil chemoattractant, CXCL8 or IL-8, are also secreted by tumor cells; however these cytokines appear to play a more prominent role in tumor growth, invasion, and angiogenesis.[66,67] This is supported by findings that chronic polymorphonuclear leukocyte (PMN) infiltrates are not commonly detected in tumors. In both mouse and human tumors, expression of CXC chemokines is correlated with increased neovascularization and reduced survival. Moreover, experimental depletion of chemokines results in attenuation of tumor growth and angiogenesis.[68] The metastatic potential of chemokines is attributed to their ability to induce expression of MMPs, which facilitate tumor invasion. Chemokines also direct the migration of metastatic tumor cells to distant organs.[33]

CSF-1

Also known as M-CSF, CSF-1 is a key regulator of proliferation, differentiation and survival of macrophages and monocytes, and their bone marrow precursors. CSF-1 is a dimeric polypeptide growth factor that binds to a cell surface tyrosine kinase receptor on macrophages. It is released by tumor cells and is a major mediator of TAM recruitment to the tumor microenvironment and tumor cell survival. Loss of CSF-1 is associated with decreased macrophage recruitment, stroma formation, and tumor growth.[27] Similarly, macrophage accumulation in the tumor microenvironment is reduced and spontaneous mammary tumor progression is delayed in CSF-1-/- mice, a response restored by overexpression of CSF-1 in transplanted tumor cells.[28] These data provide a causal link between CSF-1-dependent infiltrating macrophages and the malignant potential of epithelial cells. CSF-1 is widely overexpressed in tumors of the breast, uterus, ovary, and prostate, and this is associated with intense macrophage infiltration during the development of tumors and poor clinical prognosis.[19] These findings, together with the observation that blockade of CSF-1 in mice bearing established tumors results in suppression of tumor growth, strongly supports a role of CSF-1 in tumor progression.[30]

TGFb

TGFβ is a multifunctional polypeptide involved in the regulation of cell growth and differentiation, extracellular matrix production and tissue remodeling, and immune suppression. TGFβ appears to play a dual role in carcinogenesis, acting initially as a tumor suppressor and subsequently, as the tumor progresses, as a pro-oncogenic factor, stimulating tumor invasion, angiogenesis, and metastasis, and inhibiting immune surveillance.[69-71] TGFβ is up regulated in a number of human cancers and has been shown to be a predictor of cancer recurrence and mortality. Clinical studies have also documented that elevated levels of TGFβ are prognostic indicators of metastasis to bone and regional lymph nodes in cancer of the breast, prostate, liver, and bladder.[70-72] Experimental studies have confirmed that TGFβ is a key cytokine mediating tumor progression. Inoculation of mice with prostate cancer cells over expressing TGFβ leads to the development of tumors that are 50% larger than controls, and significantly more likely to metastasize.[73] Similarly, pretreatment of mammary adenocarcinoma cells with TGFβ increases their ability to degrade basement membrane and invade local tissue.[70] The pro-tumorigenic activity of TGFβ is due, in large part to its ability to stimulate tumor cells, macrophages and stromal cells to produce MMPs, enzymes that facilitate tumor invasion and metastasis, and up regulate VEGF, as well as connective tissue growth factor, which contribute to angiogenesis.[74] TGFβ is also a potent inducer of epithelial to mesenchymal transition, an important step in tumor invasion and metastasis.[75,76] TGFβ is produced by TAMs, tumor cells, and stromal cells in the tumor microenvironment. TGFβ plays an essential role in suppressing innate and adaptive immune responses in the tumor microenvironment, a process referred to as "immunoediting," and inhibiting TGFβ results in tumor rejection.[52,77,78] Major cellular targets for TGFβ include cytotoxic T lymphocytes, antigen presenting dendritic cells, natural killer (NK) cells, and neutrophils.[71]

Proteases

Proteolytic enzymes released by TAMs and other cells in the tumor microenvironment contribute to the continuous tissue remodeling that characterizes cancer. Prominent among these are MMPs, a class of zinc dependent endopeptidases capable of degrading extracellular matrix. Family members include collagenases, gelatinases, stromelysins, and membrane type MMPs. Other proteases produced by TAMs include plasmin, urokinase-type plasminogen activator (uPA), and the uPA receptor.[79] The activity of extracellular matrix degrading proteases is normally under tight control. Cancer cells disrupt these regulatory mechanisms allowing proteases to act on basement membrane and interstitial matrices, facilitating tumor invasion and metastasis.[80] Proteases also trigger the release of growth factors and angiogenic factors sequestered in neoplastic stroma, promoting cancer cell proliferation and survival, and angiogenesis.[39,81] Of note are MMP-2 and MMP-9, which are key mediators of angiogenesis and tumor growth. Expression of these proteases is increased in several different human tumors and strongly correlates with nodal status and tumor stage, and with more aggressive neoplastic behavior.[82] Findings that tumor xenographs transplanted into mice lacking MMP-9 display reduced vascularity provides direct evidence for a role of this protease in tumor progression.[83,84]

Cyclooxygenase-2 (COX-2)

Another active protein found in inflamed and malignant tissues is COX-2, an inducible enzyme mediating the production of prostaglandins from arachidonic acid. One of the principal metabolic products derived from the action of COX-2 is PGE_2.[85] COX-2 and PGE_2 are highly expressed in colorectal, gastric, esophageal, breast, colon, and prostate cancer, and in non-small cell squamous carcinoma.[86,87] Strong epidemiological and experimental evidence implicates the COX-2/PGE_2 pathway in the pathogenesis of these malignancies. Thus COX-2 expression correlates with poor prognosis, and administration of COX-2 inhibitors reduces the risk of developing some types of cancers and decreases morbidity.[9,88,89] Cancer progression has also been reported to be slow in COX-2 knockout mice and in mice treated with a selective COX-2 inhibitor or other nonsteroidal anti-inflammatory drugs.[9,90] Similarly, functional inactivation of PGE_2 degrading enzymes correlates with increased tumorigenesis in several organs including colon, lung, and bladder, while mice lacking PGE_2 receptors exhibit reduced tumor growth.[91,92] These data, together with findings that mice overexpressing COX-2 are more prone to develop tumors, provide additional evidence for a role of COX-2/PGE_2 in tumorigenesis.[93,94]

Accumulating evidence suggests that COX-2 functions as an interface between inflammation and cancer. It is induced by a multitude of proinflammatory cytokines and growth factors present in the tumor microenvironment via the transcription factor, NF-κB.[95] In various tumor models, COX-2 activation is associated with increased cellular proliferation and invasiveness, and suppression of apoptosis, which is thought to be due to PGE_2-induced production of IL-6, CCL8, VEGF, iNOS, MMP-2, and MMP-9.[96,97]

Reactive Oxygen and Nitrogen Species

ROS and RNS including superoxide anion, hydroxyl radical, nitric oxide and peroxynitrite are produced in significant quantities via enzyme-catalyzed reactions and during mitochondrial respiration. Whereas the generation of low levels of ROS and/or RNS under physiologic conditions functions to regulate cellular signaling pathways including kinases, transcription factors and proteases, production of large quantities of these mediators by inflammatory macrophages during acute inflammatory responses is important in destruction of invading pathogens and foreign materials. Evidence suggests that uncontrolled or excessive production of ROS and/or RNS by inflammatory cells causes oxidative and nitrosative stress and promotes tissue injury. Many biological molecules including lipids, proteins, and DNA are targets for modification by ROS/RNS with diverse pathologic consequences. For instance, peroxidation of membrane lipids by ROS can induce the generation of additional proinflammatory mediators including prostaglandins, thromboxanes, and leukotrienes. ROS and RNS have been implicated in each of the stages of carcinogenesis. Oxidative damage to DNA can lead to mutations, strand breaks, replication errors, and genomic instability, and can inactivate DNA repair enzymes, which can contribute to tumor initiation.[98] ROS and RNS can also activate cell signaling pathways such as the mitogen activated protein (MAP) kinases and transcription factors (eg, AP-1, NF-κB), and alter proteins like p53 that regulate tumor cell proliferation, apoptosis, transformation, survival, and production of pro-tumorigenic inflammatory mediators, suggesting an important role in tumor promotion. This is supported by findings in mouse models, that selective inhibitors of inducible nitric oxide synthase (iNOS or NOS-2), the enzyme mediating nitric oxide production in macrophages, can suppress chemically induced skin papilloma formation, as well as the development of adenocarcinomas in the colon.[99,100]

ROS and RNS released in the tumor microenvironment have also been implicated in tumor migration, invasion, and metastasis.[2,101] One mechanism underlying these actions is activation of transcription factors such as hypoxia inducible factor (HIF)-1α, which leads to induction of VEGF, a key mediator of angiogenesis and tumor progression. Activation of HIF-1α, as well as NF-κB, also leads to up regulation of MMPs and tissue inhibitors of metalloproteinases, which are important in tumor invasion and metastasis.[102,103] Oxidative stress has also been reported to modulate integrin expression and to suppress anoikis, which may also promote metastasis.[104]

ROS and RNS may also contribute to tumor survival and progression by facilitating immunosuppression. Both reactive species up regulate the activity of myeloid-derived suppressor cells (MDSCs), which are abundant in the tumor microenvironment and function to inhibit anti-tumor adaptive immunity.[3,105] In combination with nitric oxide, MDSC-derived ROS contribute to the generation of peroxynitrite, which has been reported to alter T cell antigen recognition and induce T cell tolerance. In addition, nitric oxide up regulates the activity of suppressor T cells (Treg) and this may also contribute to immune suppression.[106]

NF-κB: A Link Between Cancer and Inflammation

NF-κB is a ubiquitous transcription factor that plays a central role in coordinating innate and adaptive immune responses. Recent studies suggest that it is also key in cancer development and progression.[95,107] NF-κB has been described as a potential molecular bridge between inflammation and cancer.[50] Constitutive NF-κB activation is observed in most cancer cells and tissues.[108] This is thought to be due to the presence of inflammatory mediators such as TNFα and IL-1, as well as ROS and RNS, in the tumor microenvironment. A number of inflammatory molecules implicated in carcinogenesis are transcriptionally activated in both TAMs and tumor cells by NF-κB including proinflammatory proteins (eg, iNOS, COX-2, TNFα, IL-6, IL-1), as well as mediators involved in tumor survival (eg, c-FLIP, c-IAP, BCL-2, p53), proliferation (eg, cyclin D1, c-myc), invasion (eg, MMPs, uPA, ICAM-1, VCAM), angiogenesis (eg, VEGF, FGF, HGF, PDGF), and metastasis (eg, VEGF).[108] Tumor-derived cytokines further activate NF-κB in TAMs, thereby creating a sustained chronic inflammatory state within the tumor microenvironment.[109] NF-κB has been reported to play a role in tumor promotion driven by chronic inflammation in several different experimental models. Knockout mice lacking key NF-κB regulatory enzymes exhibit reduced tumorigenesis, a response correlated with decreased TNFα and IL-6 production.[110] The NF-κB pathway also appears to be involved in promoting metastasis by repressing maspin, an inhibitor of tumor metastasis.[110,111]

Recent studies have demonstrated that Toll-like receptors (TLRs) play an important role in activation of NF-κB during carcinogenesis. TLRs such as TLR4 are ubiquitously expressed on TAMs and tumor cells.[112] Ligands for TLR include microbial components such as LPS, as well as endogenous factors released from injured or dying cells including HSP 60, HSP 70, and HMGB1, during which time initiate a process known as the "sterile inflammatory response." Engagement of TLRs on tumor cells up regulates cell-signaling pathways leading to NF-κB activation, promoting an anti-apoptotic, proinflammatory, and promitogenic microenvironment. Thus NF-κB may be a major factor that controls the ability of preneoplastic and malignant cells to survive and avoid or escape apoptosis.[33]

Inflammation and Tumorigenesis

Tumorigenesis involves initiation, promotion, and progression. During the initiation phase, mutations in DNA, activation of oncogenes, or inactivation of tumor suppressor genes, causes a change in the cells such that they become capable of forming tumors. This is followed by a promotion phase when initiated cells proliferate forming a premalignant mass. Subsequently during the tumor progression phase, these cells transform into malignant cells that proliferate and eventually metastasize. Accompanying this process is angiogenesis, the formation of new blood vessels that supply required nutrients to the tumor. Through the release of inflammatory mediators, chronically activated macrophages participate in each of these stages.

Tumor Initiation and Promotion

The process of tumor initiation involves irreversible and persistent DNA damage and the accumulation of mutations in dividing cells. This can lead to activation of proto-oncogenes and/or inactivation of tumor suppressor genes. Evidence suggests that macrophages present at sites of chronic inflammation are directly involved in this process. Macrophages release significant quantities of ROS and RNS that can cause mutations and/or modify proteins that are involved in DNA repair, cell cycle control, and apoptosis.[4,68] Oxidative and nitrosative DNA damage products, such as 8-oxo-deoxyguanosine and 8-nitrodeoxyguanosine, as well as membrane lipid peroxidation products (eg, malondialdehyde, 4-hydroxynonenal), capable of forming DNA adducts, have been identified in human tumors and these are thought to be important in initiation of inflammation driven cancer.[10,113,114] The presence of RNS is also associated with the generation of carcinogenic p53 mutations that occur in approximately 50% of cancers.[4] Inflammation has also been linked to epigenetic alterations that can influence gene expression including DNA methylation and histone modification, and these may also contribute to tumor initiation.

Tumor promotion involves the survival and clonal expansion of initiated cells. Inflammatory macrophages are central to this process through the generation of mediators that promote survival, inhibit apoptosis, and stimulate proliferation. A key signaling molecule in this activity is the transcription factor NF-κB.[50,108] It appears that NF-κB plays a dual role in tumor promotion, regulating anti-apoptotic genes that prevent the death of cells with malignant potential, and stimulating the production of proinflammatory cytokines that are important for tumor cell growth. NF-κB is activated by ROS and RNS, as well as TNFα released from inflammatory macrophages. These mediators also activate AP-1, another transcription factor important in regulating genes involved in neoplastic transformation and proliferation including GM-CSF, MMP-3 and MMP-9.[10,50] Macrophage-derived TNFα has been implicated in the process of tumor promotion in models of chemically induced liver, colon and skin cancer, an activity that is dependent on NF-κB and

AP-1. Experimental findings that selective depletion of TNFα or NF-κB induces apoptosis and reduces the incidence of tumor formation provides additional evidence for a role of these mediators in tumor promotion.[108]

Tumor Progression

Tumor progression involves proliferation of malignant cells, invasion, and metastasis. This is accompanied by angiogenesis and immune suppression. Inflammatory mediators released from TAMs, as well as activated stromal cells and cancer cells in the tumor microenvironment are thought to play a role in each of these stages.

Tumor Cell Proliferation ■ A key step in tumor progression is proliferation of initiated and transformed malignant cells. TAMs release a number of promitogenic factors that stimulate tumor cell proliferation. These include EGF, HGF, FGF, PDGF, and TFGβ, as well as TNFα, IL-1, IL-6, and various chemokines.[5,19,21,115] Many of these mediators are also released by stromal cells within the tumor microenvironment. TAMs also synthesize ornithine and promitogenic polyamines. L-arginine is the substrate for macrophage biosynthesis of nitric oxide via iNOS. Tumor cells markedly inhibit TAM production of nitric oxide by diverting L-arginine metabolism to ornithine biosynthesis, a precursor for polyamine synthesis and a key factor required for tumor cell proliferation. TAM density has been reported to positively correlate with tumor cell proliferation in several different human cancers suggesting that these cells are a major source of mitogenic mediators.[5] This is supported by experimental findings that macrophage depletion results in reduced tumor cell proliferation in animal models.[116-118]

Tumor Invasion and Metastasis ■ The final stage in tumor progression is metastasis, which is thought to be responsible for up to 90% of deaths associated with solid tumors.[71] It is a complex process that involves de-adhesion of metastatic cells from the tumor cell mass, extracellular matrix remodeling, intravasation of tumor cells into the blood, localization in organs, and reestablishment of malignant growths at secondary permissive sites.[80,119] Experimental and clinical data strongly implicate TAMs and inflammatory mediators in each of these processes. Invasion of tumor cells into adjacent tissue involves breakdown of the connective tissue barriers surrounding the tumor. These consist of cell–cell adherent junctions, basement membranes, and interstitial tissue stroma. At the early stages of this process, TAMs have been identified in areas of basement membrane degradation during the transition to malignancy, and at the invasive front of more advanced tumors.[22] Moreover, TAMs localized at these sites express high levels of proteolytic enzymes including MMPs. It has been suggested that tumors exploit the normal matrix remodeling capacities of macrophages enabling them to egress into and through the surrounding stroma.[120,121] Intravasation of tumor cells into blood or lymph vessels often occurs at sites where clusters of macrophages are attached to vessels. It appears that tumor cells and macrophages migrate together in response to EGF and CSF-1, respectively.[122] Findings that inhibition of either of these mediators blocks migration of both cell types in vivo suggests that tumor cells communicate with macrophages and follow them during invasion. One of the key TAM-derived mediators of tumor invasion is TNFα which up regulates expression of MMPs leading to degradation of basement membrane and extracellular matrix.[43] Through the actions of MMPs and other proteases, TAMs are thought to aid tumor progression by creating a path through the extracellular matrix for tumors cells to follow.[123,124] The observation that macrophage localization and expression of proteases correlates closely with the depth of tumor invasion and histological grade in various cancers provides evidence for a role of TAMs in this process.[115] Experimental studies have suggested that macrophages also promote metastasis by the release of the TNFα related cytokine, RANKL, which transcriptionally represses expression of the metastasis tumor suppressor gene maspin.[39] TAMs also produce osteonectin or SPARC, a matricellular glycoprotein that modulates integrin-extracellular matrix interactions, an important step in the metastatic process.[125]

High numbers of TAMs in primary tumors are directly correlated with early metastasis in several different cancer types.[115,126] In mouse models of cancer, depletion of macrophages results in reduced rates of metastases.[28,127] Moreover, exogenous administration of TAM-derived cytokines such as TNFα, IL-1, or IL-6 promotes tumor metastasis, while inhibition of these mediators prevents tumor invasion and localization at distant sites.[12,128] It has been suggested that release of prometastatic cytokines by TAMs occurs in response to tumor cell-derived proteoglycans acting via TLR2.[129]

A question arises about the mechanisms underlying homing of metastatic tumor cells to distal sites. According to Stephen Paget's original 1889 "seed and soil hypothesis," colonization and proliferation of a tumor cells are dependent on a receptive microenvironment within distant target organs.[130] Evidence suggests that TAMs and bone marrow-derived hematopoietic cells precondition these sites for tumor cell implantation, proliferation, and survival.[41,131,132] TAMs accumulate at premetastatic niches in response to chemokines released from localized tumors cells that have broken away from the primary nonmetastic tumor, and identified a receptive site.[80,133] Once localized at these sites, macrophages release mediators such as MMPs which alter the surrounding tissue, making them more receptive for tumor cell implantation and growth.[41] Macrophages also secrete VEGF, TGFβ, and TNFα that induce expression of chemotactic factors such as CXCL12 and S100 proteins stimulating the recruitment of additional macrophages and tumor cells to these premetastatic niches.[19,119] Recent experimental studies have also provided evidence for the preconditioning of local lymph nodes as a common initial metastatic site for many tumor types, which may act as a gateway to distant metastasis.[134]

Immune Suppression

Tumor development is almost always accompanied by recruitment and activation of adaptive and innate immune cells.[135] These include anti-tumor dendritic cells, NK cells, cytotoxic T lynphocytes and B cells, and pro-tumorigenic TAMs, MDSCs, and regulatory T cells (Treg). The outcome of the malignant process appears to depend on the balance in the activity between these different immune cell types. Although initially, anti-tumor immune activity may prevail, as the tumor progresses, selective pressures drive tumor cells to develop strategies to evade immune recognition and destruction. This process termed "immunoediting," involves the redirection of adaptive cytotoxic effector functions away from anti-tumor immunity and towards proinflammatory and proangiogenic effector pathways.[136] Recent evidence suggests that this involves shifting the balance away from production of anti-tumor cytokines such as IL-12 and interferon-γ towards the production of the pro-tumorigenic cytokines, IL-10, IL-17, IL-23, and TGFβ.[136,137]

The immunosuppressive activity of TAMs is mediated by cytokines such as IL-10 and TGFβ. Evidence suggests that tumor cells also release these immunosuppressive mediators, as well as IL-4, IL-6, and PGE2, which inhibit the cytotoxic activity of M1 polarized macrophages, and suppress MHC-II expression and antigen presentation.[138,139] Of particular importance in suppressing adaptive immunity is IL-10, which blocks M1 macrophage activity and, together with TGFβ, induces an M2 phenotype in infiltrating macrophages.[35] These cytokines also inhibit maturation of antigen presenting dendritic cells. The immunosuppressive activity of TAMs is also exerted indirectly through the release of chemokines that preferentially attract T cell subsets (eg, Treg) lacking cytotoxic activity. Treg possess a characteristic anergic phenotype and through the production of TGFβ, IL-10, and IL-23, suppress the activity of cytotoxic T cells, NK cells, dendritic cells, and macrophages. Suppression of T cell mediated anti-tumor activity by Treg is associated with increased tumor growth. Inhibition of anti-tumor T cell-dependent immunity also occurs via production of indoleamine dioxygenase metabolites by TAMs, as well as MDSCs.[126] These consist of a heterogeneous group of immature myeloid cells which inhibit T cell activation and cytotoxic activity. Tumor growth is associated with expansion of the MDSC population, which is thought to be mediated by tumor-derived GM-CSF, CSF-1, IL-13, and VEGF. The immunosuppressive activity of MDSCs is due to production of ROS and RNS and immunosuppressive cytokines.

IL-23 is a key mediator involved in immunoediting.[136] In addition to stimulating IL-10 production and inhibiting the function of cytotoxic T cells, IL-23 acts in concert with TGFβ and IL-6 to promote the development Th17 cells, a memory T cell subset characterized by the production of IL-17. This cytokine acts on stromal cells, epithelial cells, endothelial cells, and macrophages to stimulate the release of mediators that promote a proinflammatory/pro-tumorigenic environment including IL-1, IL-6, TNFα, PGE_2, ICAM, and various chemokines. IL-17 also stimulates angiogenesis and induces expression of MMPs.[140] IL-23 and IL-17 are significantly elevated in most human cancers and this correlates with the presence of macrophages, as well as neutrophils in the tumor microenvironment. The observation that mice lacking IL-23 are resistant to chemically induced tumor formation, and that this is linked to reduced expression of IL-17 and MMPs and attenuated angiogenesis, provides strong support for a role of these cytokines in tumor progression.[136]

Angiogenesis

The growth and survival of solid tumors and their progression to invasive phenotypes depends on angiogenesis; the formation of new blood vessels from pre-existing ones. Angiogenesis promotes not only tumor growth, but also the progression of tumor cells from a pre-malignant to a malignant and invasive phenotype. Angiogenesis also facilitates emigration of inflammatory cells into the tumor microenvironment. The initiation of angiogenesis in developing tumors is referred to as the "angiogeneic switch" and is determined by a balance between the genetic status of the tumor, signals from stromal cells and TAMs in the tumor microenvironment, and the appearance of hypoxia.[141,142] Tumor associated vessels promote tumor growth by providing oxygen and nutrients and favor tumor metastasis by facilitating tumor cell entry into the circulation. A diverse group of inflammatory mediators, generated in large part by TAMs, is involved in angiogenesis. These include VEGF, FGF, IL-1, CCL8, TNFα, COX-2, and nitric oxide, as well as various MMPs and chemokines.[21,26,143] These molecules, which are expressed in a coordinated spatial and temporal fashion, induce proliferation and migration of endothelial cells, matrix remodeling, and the eventual formation of stabilized vessels. It is now well established that TAMs recruited into the tumor microenvironment play a pivotal role in triggering tumor angiogenesis.[144,145] TAMs cluster in "hot spots" in avascular hypoxic areas of tumors along a trail of necrotic debris.[146,147] Hypoxia, or cytokines generated in response to hypoxia such as VEGF, are thought to act as chemoattractants for macrophages.[148] Hypoxia also activates transcription factors such as HIF-1α and HIF-2α in macrophages, as well as tumor cells, triggering a proangiogenic program leading to expression of VEGF, a key mediator of angiogenesis. VEGF is also up regulated in macrophages by tumor cell-derived CSF-1, and knockdown of CSF-1 in experimental models results in reduced VEGF expression and impaired angiogenesis.[149] In addition to hypoxia, VEGF is strongly induced by a number of macrophage and tumor cell-derived mediators (eg, EGF, HGF, IL-1β, IL-6, CCL8, PDGF, TGFβ, and TNFα), and by various oncogenes (eg, *ras,* and erbB-2/Her2, activated EGF receptor and bcr-abl).[20] Additional proangiogenic mediators generated by TAMs in response to local hypoxic conditions include TNFα, FGF, MMPs, and CXCL8, which act in concert with tumor and stromal cell-derived mediators to stimulate endothelial cell proliferation and promote cross talk between tumor cells and endothelial cells.

Strong clinical evidence supports a role of TAMs in angiogenesis. In several human tumors, a correlation between local macrophage density and expression of VEGF and PDGF, and areas of intense angiogenesis, defined by the presence of microvessels, has been described.[26,146] The finding that TAMs are recruited into premalignant lesions immediately before the transition to malignancy and that depletion of macrophages results in a 50% reduction in vascular density and is associated with increased necrosis, provides additional support to this idea.[5]

Therapeutic Implications

A key role of chronic inflammation in tumorigenesis has clearly been established. Thus therapies directed at reducing inflammation or inhibiting the function of inflammatory mediators should reduce cancer risk. Consistent with this idea is the finding that cancer risk among long-term users of aspirin and nonsteroidal anti-inflammatory drugs is reduced by as much as 40–50%.[19] Future, more specific, therapies that target individual mediators or pathways leading to their production may prove more effective in treating cancer. For example, since activation of NF-κB is observed in many human and experimental cancers, inhibitors of this transcription factor may be clinically efficacious and this is under clinical investigation. An alternative approach is to block NF-κB regulated genes such as TNFα, VEGF, or MMP-9. Targeting TAMs or molecules that attract TAM to the tumor microenvironment and mediate their function is another therapeutic strategy. It may also be possible to reorient TAM towards an M1 cytotoxic macrophage phenotype by treating patients with IL-2 or IFNγ, and this has been attempted with limited success.[150,151] Adoptive transfer of ex vivo-generated macrophages in patients with cancer may also be a potential approach.[143] Transfection of these cells with anti-cancer genes or therapeutic genes, or tagging them with chemotherapeutic or angiostatic drugs is another possibility. With all of these approaches, however, it will be important to avoid negative side effects that may be due to compensatory responses of immune cells in the tumor microenvironment. It may be that combined immunotherapy and angiostatic therapy is required for effective anti-tumor responses and better prognosis in cancer patients.

Acknowledgments

Supported by NIH grants GM034310, ES004738, CA132624, ES005022, AR055073 and CA072720.

Selected References

The complete reference list can be found at www.CANCERMEDICINE8.com

1. Balkwill F, Mantovani A. Inflammation and cancer: back to Virchow? *Lancet.* 2001;357:539–545.
2. Hussain SP, Harris CC. Inflammation and cancer: an ancient link with novel potentials. *Int J Cancer.* 2007;121:2373–2380.
3. Mantovani A, Sica A, Allavena P, et al. Tumor-associated macrophages and the related myeloid-derived suppressor cells as

a paradigm of the diversity of macrophage activation. *Human Immunol.* 2009;70: 325-330.
6. Allavena P, Sica A, Garlanda C, Mantovani A. The Yin-Yang of tumor-associated macrophages in neoplastic progression and immune surveillance. *Immunol Rev.* 2008;222:155–161.
10. Kundu JK, Surh YJ. Inflammation: gearing the journey to cancer. *Mutat Res.* 2008;659:15–30.
11. Sica A, Larghi P, Mancino A, et al. Macrophage polarization in tumour progression. *Semin Cancer Biol.* 2008;18:349–355.
12. Mantovani A, Allavena P, Sica A, Balkwill F. Cancer-related inflammation. *Nature.* 2008;454:436–444.
13. Zhang X, Mosser DM. Macrophage activation by endogenous danger signals. *J Pathol.* 2008;214:161–178.
14. Van Ginderachter JA, Movahedi K, Hassanzadeh Ghassabeh G, et al. Classical and alternative activation of mononuclear phagocytes: picking the best of both worlds for tumor promotion. *Immunobiology.* 2006;211:487–501.
15. Martinez FO, Sica A, Mantovani A, Locati M. Macrophage activation and polarization. *Front Biosci.* 2008;13:453–461.
17. de Visser KE. Spontaneous immune responses to sporadic tumors: tumor-promoting, tumor-protective or both? *Cancer Immunol Immunother.* 2008;57:1531–1539.
20. Ariztia EV, Lee CJ, Gogoi R, Fishman DA. The tumor microenvironment: key to early detection. *Crit Rev Clin Lab Sci.* 2006;43:393–425.
26. Allavena P, Sica A, Solinas G, et al. The inflammatory micro-environment in tumor progression: the role of tumor-associated macrophages. *Crit Rev Oncol Hematol.* 2008;66:1–9.
32. Kakinuma T, Hwang ST. Chemokines, chemokine receptors, and cancer metastasis. *J Leukoc Biol.* 2006;79:639–651.
33. Raman D, Baugher PJ, Thu YM, Richmond A. Role of chemokines in tumor growth. *Cancer Lett.* 2007;256:137–165.
39. DeNardo DG, Johansson M, Coussens LM. Immune cells as mediators of solid tumor metastasis. *Cancer Metastasis Rev.* 2008;27:11–18.
40. Le Bitoux MA, Stamenkovic I. Tumor-host interactions: the role of inflammation. *Histochem Cell Biol.* 2008;130:1079–1090.
42. Sethi G, Sung B, Aggarwal BB. TNF: a master switch for inflammation to cancer. *Front Biosci.* 2008;13:5094–5107.
50. Pikarsky E, Porat RM, Stein I, et al. NF-kappaB functions as a tumour promoter in inflammation-associated cancer. *Nature.* 2004;431:461–466.
52. Lin WW, Karin M. A cytokine-mediated link between innate immunity, inflammation, and cancer. *J Clin Invest.* 2007;117:1175–1183.
54. Apte RN, Voronov E. Is interleukin-1 a good or bad "guy" in tumor immunobiology and immunotherapy? *Immunol Rev.* 2008;222:222–241.
55. Voronov E, Carmi Y, Apte RN. Role of IL-1-mediated inflammation in tumor angiogenesis. *Adv Exp Med Biol.* 2007;601:265–270.
57. Naugler WE, Karin M. The wolf in sheep's clothing: the role of interleukin-6 in immunity, inflammation and cancer. *Trends Mol Med.* 2008;14:109–119.
59. Rose-John S, Schooltink H. Cytokines are a therapeutic target for the prevention of inflammation-induced cancers. *Recent Results Cancer Res.* 2007;174:57–66.
65. Balkwill F. Cancer and the chemokine network. *Nat Rev Cancer.* 2004;4:540–550.
68. Allavena P, Garlanda C, Borrello MG, et al. Pathways connecting inflammation and cancer. *Curr Opin Genet Dev.* 2008;18:3–10.
69. Jakowlew SB. Transforming growth factor-beta in cancer and metastasis. *Cancer Metastasis Rev.* 2006;25:435–457.
74. Bierie B, Moses HL. Tumour microenvironment: TGFbeta: the molecular Jekyll and Hyde of cancer. *Nat Rev Cancer.* 2006;6:506–520.
80. Gupta GP, Massague J. Cancer metastasis: building a framework. *Cell.* 2006;127:679–695.
85. Greenhough A, Smartt HJ, Moore AE, et al. The COX-2/PGE2 pathway: key roles in the hallmarks of cancer and adaptation to the tumour microenvironment. *Carcinogenesis.* 2009;30:377-386
95. Karin M. The IkappaB kinase—a bridge between inflammation and cancer. *Cell Res.* 2008;18:334–342.
101. Hussain SP, He P, Subleski J, et al. Nitric oxide is a key component in inflammation-accelerated tumorigenesis. *Cancer Res.* 2008;68:7130–7136.
103. Halliwell B. Oxidative stress and cancer: have we moved forward? *Biochem J.* 2007;401:1–11.
107. Karin M. Nuclear factor-kappaB in cancer development and progression. *Nature.* 2006;441:431–436.
108. Aggarwal BB, Vijayalekshmi RV, Sung B. Targeting inflammatory pathways for prevention and therapy of cancer: short-term friend, long-term foe. *Clin Cancer Res.* 2009;15:425–430.
110. Maeda S, Omata M. Inflammation and cancer: role of nuclear factor-kappaB activation. *Cancer Sci.* 2008;99:836–842.
112. Chen R, Alvero AB, Silasi DA, et al. Cancers take their Toll—the function and regulation of Toll-like receptors in cancer cells. *Oncogene.* 2008;27:225–233.
113. Valko M, Rhodes CJ, Moncol J, et al. Free radicals, metals and antioxidants in oxidative stress-induced cancer. *Chem Biol Interact.* 2006;160:1–40.
115. Guruvayoorappan C. Tumor versus tumor-associated macrophages: how hot is the link? *Integr Cancer Ther.* 2008;7:90–95.
125. Sangaletti S, Di Carlo E, Gariboldi S, et al. Macrophage-derived SPARC bridges tumor cell-extracellular matrix interactions toward metastasis. *Cancer Res.* 2008;68:9050–9059.
126. Talmadge JE, Donkor M, Scholar E. Inflammatory cell infiltration of tumors: Jekyll or Hyde. *Cancer Metastasis Rev.* 2007;26:373–400.
130. Fidler IJ. The pathogenesis of cancer metastasis: the "seed and soil" hypothesis revisited. *Nat Rev Cancer.* 2003;3:453–458.
133. Bidard FC, Pierga JY, Vincent-Salomon A, Poupon MF. A "class action" against the microenvironment: do cancer cells cooperate in metastasis? *Cancer Metastasis Rev.* 2008;27:5–10.
135. de Visser KE, Coussens LM. The inflammatory tumor microenvironment and its impact on cancer development. *Contrib Microbiol.* 2006;13:118–137.
136. Langowski JL, Kastelein RA, Oft M. Swords into plowshares: IL-23 repurposes tumor immune surveillance. *Trends Immunol.* 2007;28:207–212.
137. Mumm JB, Oft M. Cytokine-based transformation of immune surveillance into tumor-promoting inflammation. *Oncogene.* 2008;27:5913–5919.
138. Croci DO, Zacarias Fluck MF, Rico MJ, et al. Dynamic cross-talk between tumor and immune cells in orchestrating the immunosuppressive network at the tumor microenvironment. *Cancer Immunol Immunother.* 2007;56:1687–1700.
139. de Visser KE, Eichten A, Coussens LM. Paradoxical roles of the immune system during cancer development. *Nat Rev Cancer.* 2006;6:24–37.
144. Shojaei F, Zhong C, Wu X, et al. Role of myeloid cells in tumor angiogenesis and growth. *Trends Cell Biol.* 2008;18:372–378.
145. Ruegg C. Leukocytes, inflammation, and angiogenesis in cancer: fatal attractions. *J Leukoc Biol.* 2006;80:682–684.

20 RNA Tumor Viruses

Robert C. Gallo, MD ■ Marvin S. Reitz, PhD

Retroviruses are enveloped viruses that contain a diploid RNA genome and are defined by the presence of reverse transcriptase (RT), a DNA polymerase that transcribes RNA into DNA, which is then inserted into the host cell chromosome. These processes often lead to the capture and/or alteration of genetic material and the transfer of information between cells, with neoplastic transformation of the infected cell being an occasional outcome of infection. Retroviruses are also associated with immunodeficiencies and with neurologic diseases, although infection is often asymptomatic. Retroviruses can also enter the germ line and be present as a part of the genetic complement of all members of a species. These viruses are called endogenous retroviruses.

Retroviruses were discovered early in the twentieth century. Ellerman and Bang showed the transmission of leukemia in chickens by a cell-free filtrate,[1] and Rous was able to transmit sarcomas in chickens by a similar means.[2] These findings were extended to mammals by Bittner in the case of breast tumors in mice[3] and by Gross for murine leukemias.[4] Gross recognized the importance of inoculating newborn mice for development of leukemia and in many respects his work heralded the beginning of modern studies of retroviruses. Jarrett showed that a similar virus was responsible for leukemia in cats, which was the first demonstration of naturally transmitted leukemia in an outbred species.[5,6] Kawakami and Theilen and colleagues first showed that retroviruses could cause leukemia in primates, specifically in gibbon apes and new world monkeys.[7-9]

Biologic assays for these viruses were in use from the 1950s, but a more fundamental understanding of their life cycle was considerably advanced in the early 1970s by the discovery that they contained RT.[10,11] This provided a far simpler and quicker assay for retroviruses, as well as providing a sensitive and relatively simple tool for their general detection. Another important finding in the 1970s was that some retroviruses (eg, Rous sarcoma virus) contained genes for cell transformation and tumorigenesis (called oncogenes) that represented captured cellular genes (proto-oncogenes).[12] This realization led to the identification of dozens of similar genes and to an appreciation of their roles in cell growth and neoplastic transformation.

Despite this work and the interest it engendered, it was widely believed during the 1970s that retroviruses did not play a role in human disease, and that they were likely not even present in the human population. Several discoveries made it clear that this was not the case. First, human T-cell leukemia virus type I (HTLV-I), the first infectious human retrovirus, was discovered by Gallo and his colleagues and shown to be a unique virus.[13-16] HTLV-I was soon established as the etiologic agent of adult T-cell leukemia, a type of leukemia endemic to various locales, including southern Japan and the Caribbean.[17-21] This was quickly followed by the discovery of HTLV-II,[22] a related virus that (although widespread) has not been compellingly associated with any disease.

Several years later, an epidemic of immunodeficiency and malignancies appeared within gay communities, especially in the United States. The first member of another group of human retroviruses was isolated from people with this disease,[23] and when it became possible to culture the virus on a large scale,[24] it was proven to be the etiologic agent of the new disease, called AIDS.[25,26] This virus, now called human immunodeficiency virus type 1 (HIV-1), has become established over much of the world, as has AIDS itself, and HIV-1 represents a current global medical and economic catastrophe. As with HTLV-I, a related virus, HIV-2, was discovered.[27] As with HTLV-II and I, HIV-2 appears to be far less pathogenic than HIV-1.[28]

This chapter summarizes important aspects of the classification and replication cycle of retroviruses and considers some of the pathogenic mechanisms of retroviruses. We also consider endogenous retroviruses and the development of retroviral vectors for gene delivery and therapy.

Classification

The retroviridae are a large family of viruses that are composed of a core structure surrounded by an envelope containing a lipid bilayer. The core or capsid contains proteins specified by the *gag* and *pol* genes (Fig. 20-1). The former are primarily structural and enclose the products of the latter, which are enzymatic and include RT and a viral protease that processes the Gag proteins. The capsid also encloses two copies of the single stranded genomic RNA. The area between the capsid and the lipid envelope bilayer is occupied by another Gag protein called the matrix protein (MA). The lipid membrane contains the viral glycoproteins, including a transmembrane protein (TM) and a large surface protein (SU). The entire virion, or extracellular viral particle, is 100 nm in diameter.

Retroviruses have been classified using a variety of criteria.[29] They were originally categorized according to their biologic effects. The subfamilies included oncoviruses, which cause leukemias or other malignancies in their hosts; lentiviruses, or "slow" viruses, which cause slow degenerative diseases in their hosts; and spumaviruses, or foamy viruses, which produce a "foamy" cytopathic effect in infected cultures. The subfamilies have been divided further based on their genomic structures (Table 20-1). They have been historically classified on the basis of the morphology of budding and mature virions in electron micrographs (Table 20-2). As mentioned earlier, they can also be classified as exogenous or endogenous depending upon whether they are transmitted by infection or genetically within the germ line of a species.

Structure

The simplest retroviruses contain three major genes (*gag*, *pol*, and *env*), all of which are contained in the virion. The genomic RNA, which is generally about 8 to 9500 nucleotides long, contains repeat regions at both ends, called the R region. The DNA form of the genome integrated in the host cell genome contains the R region and other regulatory sequences in structures called the large terminal repeat (LTR) (Fig. 20-1). Retroviruses often become replication-defective by loss of large regions of their genomes, which are sometimes replaced by oncogenes derived from the host cell. We now describe the genome and proteins of replication competent retroviruses.

Long Terminal Repeat (LTR)

The viral LTR provides important functions in the viral replication cycle. The

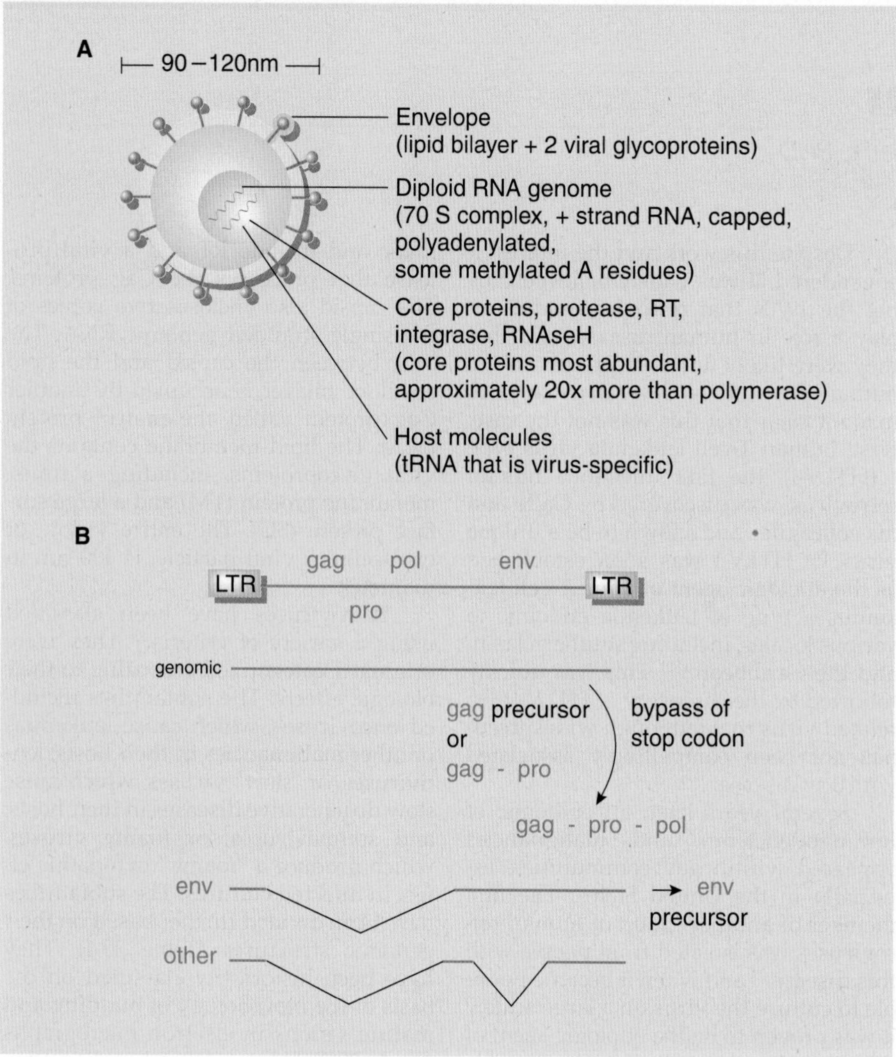

Figure 20-1 (**A**) Structure of typical retrovirus virion. (**B**) Structure of typical retroviral genome. All replication-competent retroviruses generate a full-length genomic ribonucleic acid (RNA) that encodes the gag and pol products and a singly spliced RNA that encodes the env product. Some retroviruses also generate smaller multiply spliced messages. *Abbreviations*: env, envelope; gag, core proteins; pol, polymerase; pro, protease.

Table 20-2 **Retrovirus Morphology**

A-type particles
Intracellular core formation and budding
Intracisternal A-type particles (IAP) are products of endogenous proviruses
Noninfectious
B-type particles (MMTV)
Core formation occurs in the cytoplasm
After budding at the plasma membrane, maturation to an eccentric core occurs
Prominent surface spikes
C-type particles
Most oncornaviruses
Initially form electron-dense patches at the plasma membrane
Budding at plasma membrane
Maturation of core to yield centrally located cores
Spikes may or may not be prominent
D-type particles
Mason-Pfizer monkey virus, simian AIDS virus
Intracellular nucleocapsid formation, budding at plasma membrane
Eccentric core
Less prominent spikes
Lentiviruses
Visna-maedi, EIAV, CAEV, SIV, HIV, FIV, BIV
Core formation and budding as for C-type particles
Condensed mature core forms pyramidal shape
Spumaviruses
IAP-like cores

LTR is required for integration of the genome into host cell DNA and DNA elements within the LTR regulate viral RNA expression. The LTR consists of three areas, the U3, R, and U5 regions (Fig. 20-2). The U5 region is adjacent to the binding site of the primer for DNA synthesis, which is a cellular transfer RNA (tRNA).[30,31] The U5 is the first region to be reverse-transcribed as synthesis proceeds left to right. The R region is synthesized next, at which point the RT must jump to the 3' R region, where the newly synthesized R cDNA hydrogen bonds (hybridizes). Synthesis proceeds through U3 right to left (see Fig. 20-2). Reverse transcription results in synthesis of a double-stranded DNA with U3, R, and U5 regions at both ends. This DNA is integrated into host cell DNA. After integration, RNA transcription initiates in the 5' LTR and terminates in the 3' LTR, and results in a full-length RNA with R regions at both ends.

Table 20-1 **Retrovirus Groups**

Oncornaviruses
Avian leukosis-sarcoma viruses (ALSV)
Avian reticuloendotheliosis virus
Mammalian leukemia and sarcoma viruses (mouse/cat type C viruses)
Mouse mammary tumor virus
Primate type D viruses (Mason-Pfizer monkey virus/simian AIDS virus)
Human T-cell leukemia virus/bovine leukemia virus/simian T-cell leukemia virus
Lentiviruses (including immunodeficiency viruses)
Spumaviruses

The U3 region contains promoter regions for the cellular RNA polymerase II, and includes canonical CCAT and TATAA boxes (Fig. 20-2).[32,33] These drive RNA transcription, which initiates at the CAP site[34] at the junction of U3 and R. Upstream from the promoter region, the U3 contains sequences called enhancers that respond to host cell transcriptional regulatory factors and help to regulate levels of viral RNA expression. Examples include NFkB binding sites in the HIV LTR,[35,36] cAMP-responsive element (CRE) binding sites in the HTLV-I U3,[37] and glucocorticoid receptor binding sites in the U3 of the murine mammary tumor virus (MMTV).[38] The types of enhancers that are contained in a viral LTR help to determine in what kind of cell the virus can replicate. The R region has a transcriptional termination-RNA polyadenylation signal (AATAAA) that functions in the 3' LTR. The promoter in the 3' LTR does not function in the presence of the 5' LTR, but can become active if the upstream LTR is deleted.

Leader Sequence

The leader sequence is the RNA sequence located between the 3' end of the 5' LTR and the initiation codon of the *gag* gene. This stretch of RNA contains three important regions. One is the primer binding site (PBS), to which (as mentioned earlier) a cellular tRNA hydrogen bonds and serves as the primer for first strand cDNA (-strand cDNA) synthesis. A second feature of the leader sequence is a splice donor that is

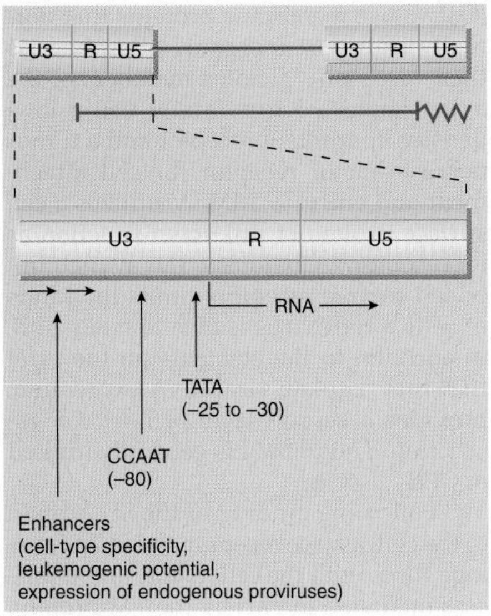

Figure 20-2 Long terminal repeat (LTR) structure. Replication-competent retroviruses contain identical LTRs at the 5' and 3' ends. The U3 portion of the 5' LTR contains all of the enhancer and promoter elements necessary for efficient initiation of transcription of either retroviral or cellular genes. *Abbreviation*: CA, capsid; FeLV, feline leukemia virus; IN, integrase; MA, matrix protein; MMTV, Maloney mammary tumor virus; MuLV, murine leukemia virus; NC, nuclear capsid; PR, protease; RT, reverse transcriptase.

used for generating all spliced subgenomic messenger RNAs (mRNA). These spliced mRNAs code for all viral proteins except those from *gag* and *pol*. The third feature of the leader sequence is a packaging signal by which genomic RNA is recognized by Gag proteins and incorporated into functional virion cores.[39]

Gag

The *gag* gene is always at the 5' end of the central unique (non-LTR) region of the retroviral genome. The Gag proteins are translated from a full-length (unspliced) mRNA as a polyprotein precursor that is processed into three to five mature Gag proteins by the viral protease (one of the proteins encoded by the *pol* gene). The protease (Pro) is translated along with the other *pol* products as extensions of the Gag polyprotein from the same unspliced mRNA by mechanisms that differ from one retroviral group to another.[40-42] The Pol precursor protein is also processed by the viral Pro.

There are three major Gag proteins. These include a nucleic acid binding protein (NC), a small basic protein that is located within the virion capsid and is bound to the genomic RNA. Its positive charge neutralizes the negative charge of the RNA and facilitates RNA packaging and dimerization. The NC also has a zinc finger motif, which is important in RNA binding.[43,44] The motif consists of an arrangement of cysteine and histidine residues present in a specific pattern that facilitates high affinity binding to RNA, and is required for RNA packaging into the virion. The capsid protein (CA) is the major structural protein of the capsid; it forms the shell on the surface of the capsid. The matrix protein (MA) is located between the capsid surface and the envelope bilayer. It interacts with the cytoplasmic tail of the TM envelope protein and CA on the capsid surface. Its interaction with the lipid bilayer requires that MA be myristoylated[45,46]; a lack of myristoylation prevents functional capsid formation.[47]

Pol

The *pol* gene as mentioned earlier is synthesized as an extension of the *gag* gene and encodes enzymatic activities. These include Pro and the viral enzymes required for reverse transcription and integration of viral DNA into the host chromosome. Because viruses require far greater amounts of structural proteins than enzymes, they have had to evolve mechanisms that make synthesis of the *pol* products relatively inefficient. The mechanisms that have been evolved vary among the viruses, as summarized in Figure 20-3. Murine leukemia virus (MuLV) has a stop codon that generally terminates Gag translation. At a low frequency, however, read-through occurs because of suppressor tRNA activity, resulting in a full-length Gag-Pol precursor.[47,48] Other viruses have semi-overlapping reading frames for Pol or Pro and Pol and synthesis of the extended translational products occurs because slippage at short A-rich regions and downstream secondary structure of the RNA result in a shift in mid-translation to alternate reading frames.[49-51]

The function of Pro is to cleave the Gag and Gag-Pol polyprotein precursors into the proper mature proteins. As Pro becomes concentrated in nascent virions, it dimerizes and becomes more active. There are three different enzymatic activities encoded by *pol* that play a role in viral DNA synthesis. These include a DNA polymerase (RT), a ribonuclease H (RNaseH) (which removes the template RNA after strand cDNA synthesis), and an integrase (IN), which catalyzes the integration of viral DNA into host cell DNA. The RT and RNaseH are generally contained in a single mature peptide. The three-dimensional structures of the HIV-1 Pro and RT have been solved[52] and have provided a basis for rational design of anti-HIV drugs. HIV IN has an additional function beyond catalysis of integration; it contains a nuclear localization signal, which facilitates transport of the preintegration complex of viral DNA and several viral proteins

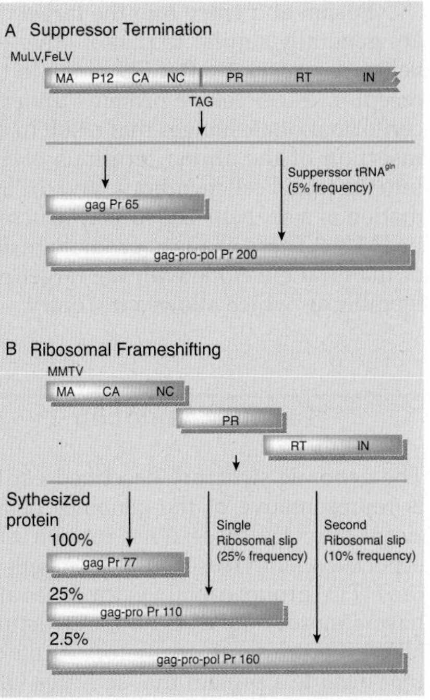

Figure 20-3 Alternative methods different retroviruses use to bypass the gag stop codon to generate the pro-pol products from the full-length genomic transcripts.

to the nucleus and helps in infection of nondividing cells.[53]

Envelope

The *env* gene encodes a precursor polypeptide containing the signal peptide, which guides the insertion of Env proteins into the cell membrane, the transmembrane protein (TM), and the outer large surface protein (SU). The precursor polypeptide, like those for the Gag and Pol proteins, is proteolytically processed, but in this case, cleavage involves cellular proteases. The Env proteins are translated from a spliced mRNA that utilizes the cellular splicing machinery, the splice donor upstream of *gag*, and a splice donor upstream from the initiation codon of *env*.[54,55] The TM and SU proteins are organized into a trimer structure on the virion surface that can be visualized by electron microscopy.

The TM protein is generally the smaller of the two, and penetrates the viral envelope bilayer. The cytoplasmic domain is in contact with the viral MA protein and the extracellular or ectodomains, binds to the SU protein, and retains it on the virion surface.[56] Besides its function of retaining and distributing SU, TM plays a role in the fusion of the viral envelope with the target cell membrane during infection.[56] The SU protein is generally heavily glycosylated and is the outermost viral protein.[57] Its major function is to bind to a specific cell surface protein that serves as the receptor for the virus. Because it is the outermost viral protein, it is the main target of neutralizing antibodies made by the host.[58]

Fusion and entry into the target cell are generally similar to that of other enveloped viruses.[56] After SU binds to the receptor, the envelope proteins undergo conformational changes that result in the insertion of the amino terminus of TM into the target cell membrane and the formation of a six-helix coiled-coil structure in TM.[59,60] These changes promote fusion of the viral envelope with the target cell membrane, which allows viral entry.

Genomic Variation

The genomic structure described earlier is representative of the genomes of the simplest retroviruses; other retroviruses, especially lentiviruses and members of the HTLV group, contain extra genes and have a more complex genomic structure. HIV-1 encodes six regulatory proteins that include a protein that activates viral RNA expression, another that regulates viral RNA splicing patterns, and proteins that interfere with host immune functions. The extra genes result in a more complicated RNA splicing pattern as well, including multiple splicing for many of the regulatory genes. Similarly, HTLV-I (and the related bovine leukemia virus) encodes extra proteins. HTLV-I encodes at least five additional proteins, including (like HIV) a protein that activates viral RNA expression and another that regulates viral RNA splicing patterns. Recently, evidence has been presented[61] that a protein called HBZ (for HTLV-I bZIP protein) is transcribed from the 3' LTR and translated from minus strand viral RNA, and is expressed in infected T cells and in uncultured ATL cells as a 31-kDa protein. The HBZ protein binds to cellular bZIP transcription factors including members of the CREB and Jun families[61] to repress Tax-mediated viral transcription and support ATL cell proliferation. At present, this appears to represent a novel genetic feature of HTLV-I. MMTV and the spumaviruses also encode additional proteins, including those that activate viral RNA expression. Other retroviruses, especially those that are acutely transforming (such as the avian and mammalian sarcoma viruses), are generally replication-defective and have parts of their genomes deleted and replaced with captured cellular genes that confer transforming capability. These viruses require a replication competent helper virus for transmission and replication.

Replication Cycle

The replication cycle includes a number of stages, including entry and the establishment of infection in the target cell, the insertion of viral DNA into the host cell genome (called the provirus), and the synthesis, assembly, and release of virion particles. This process, called horizontal transmission, is summarized in Figure 20-4. In addition, cell replication of a retrovirally infected cell results in concurrent replication of the provirus. This is called vertical transmission, and is the only means of replication for most endogenous viruses, which are present as germ line infections but are generally replication-defective.

The first step in infection is the engagement of a specific cell surface protein by SU on the virion surface. A number of retroviral cell surface receptors have been identified to date. The first receptor to be identified was the HIV receptor CD4, which is present on the surface of helper T cells.[62] It has subsequently been shown that the HIV SU requires a second receptor for functional binding and entry.[63] Following CD4 binding, SU must bind to one of several chemokine receptors, which are in the protein superfamily of G protein-coupled seven transmembrane serpentine receptors.[63-68] The receptor for one type of MuLV is a multiple membrane-spanning cell surface protein that normally serves as a transporter protein for cationic amino acids.[69] Another type of MuLV and gibbon ape leukemia virus (GaLV) use membrane proteins that normally transport inorganic phosphate as their receptors.[70,71] Some members of the avian leukosis virus family use a low-density lipoprotein receptor and a tumor necrosis factor receptor for cell attachment and entry.[72,73] MMTV utilizes a cell surface protein of unknown function as its receptor.[74] Obviously, the availability of cell surface receptors limits the kinds of cells a retrovirus is able to enter, and, in addition to the elements on the viral LTR that regulate viral RNA expression, provides a second level of host cell restriction. Thus, HIV-1 is generally limited to CD4+ T cells.

Following binding of the SU protein to the cell surface receptor, the viral envelope fuses with the cell membrane, a process mediated in part by the TM protein. This causes internalization of the naked core of the virion, which begins to disassemble in the cytoplasm. This makes the RT-RNA complex accessible to DNA precursors, and reverse transcription takes place (Fig. 20-5). The tRNA hybridized to the PBS serves as the initiation point for the synthesis of the first strand (-strand) of cDNA,[30,31] which is synthesized in a leftward direction. This results in a single strand of cDNA that is known as strong stop DNA and contains U5 and R sequences.[75] The strong stop cDNA and RT then jump to the other end of the tem-

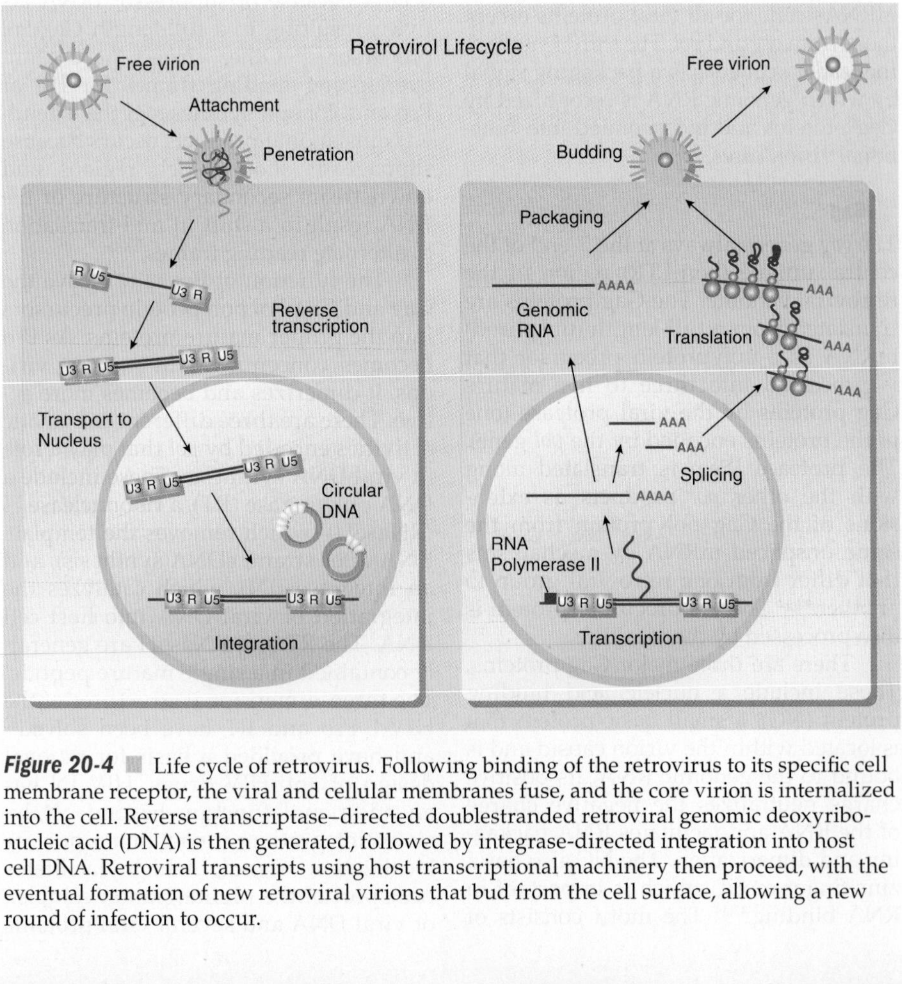

Figure 20-4 Life cycle of retrovirus. Following binding of the retrovirus to its specific cell membrane receptor, the viral and cellular membranes fuse, and the core virion is internalized into the cell. Reverse transcriptase–directed doublestranded retroviral genomic deoxyribonucleic acid (DNA) is then generated, followed by integrase-directed integration into host cell DNA. Retroviral transcripts using host transcriptional machinery then proceed, with the eventual formation of new retroviral virions that bud from the cell surface, allowing a new round of infection to occur.

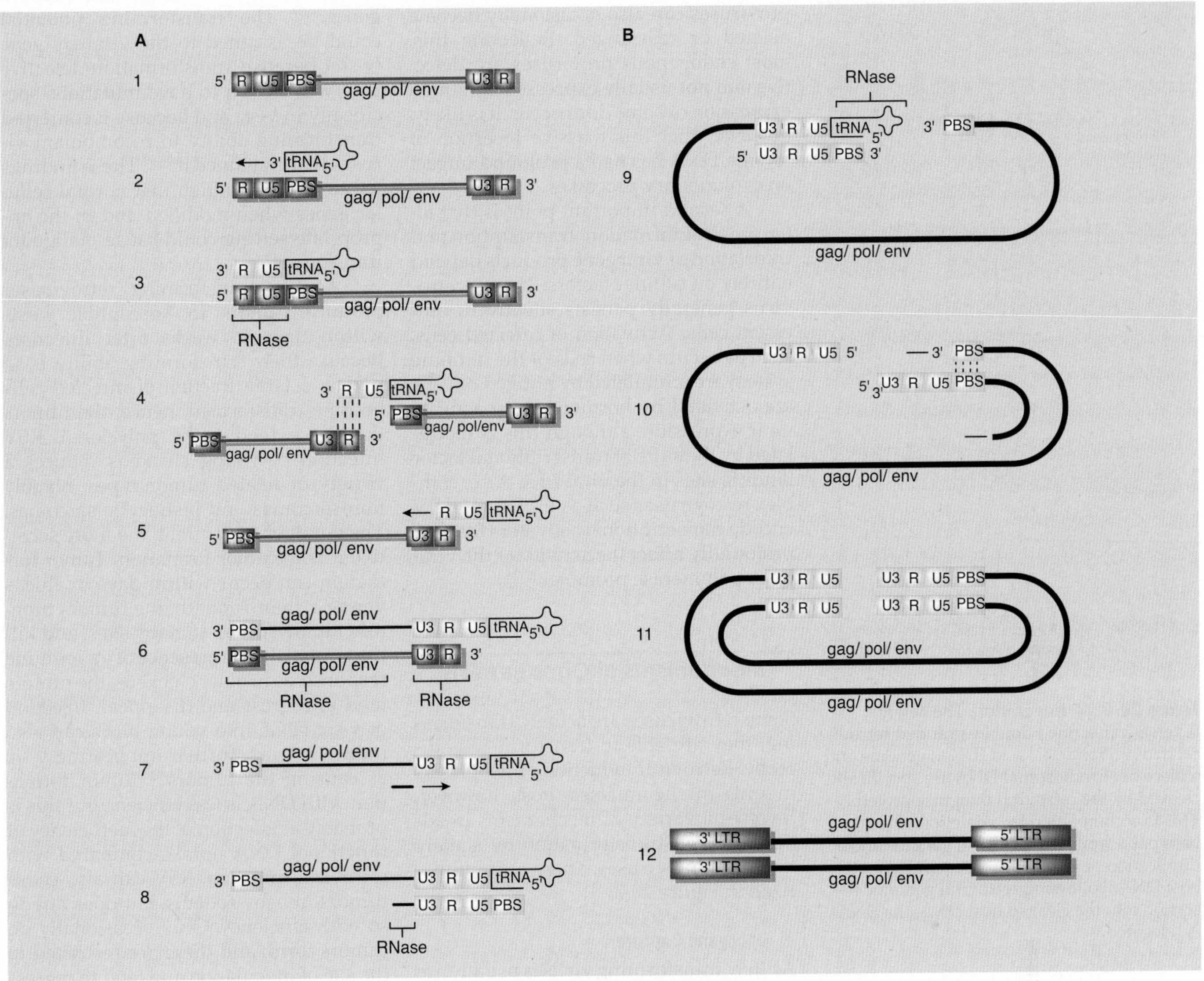

Figure 20-5 Reverse transcription. From a single-stranded ribonucleic acid genomic precursor (**A**), reverse transcriptase synthesizes a double-stranded deoxyribonucleic acid (DNA) provirus ready for integration into host cell DNA (**B**).

plate RNA, where the R -strand cDNA hybridizes to the 3' R region and serves as the primer for the continuation of -strand cDNA synthesis through the U3, *env*, *pol*, and *gag*. The RNaseH removes the template RNA except for a nuclease-resistant polypurine tract immediately upstream from the downstream LTR. The residual polypurine tract RNA residue serves as the primer for second strand (+strand) U3-R-U5 DNA synthesis before it is degraded. RNaseH degrades the tRNA primer and the RT jumps again, this time to the other end of the complete –strand cDNA. The U3-R-U5 +strand cDNA then serves as the primer for the completion of the +strand, resulting in a double-stranded RNA with complete LTRs at both ends.

After DNA synthesis is completed, it is inserted into the host cell genome by the activity of the viral IN protein, as shown in Figure 20-6. The IN catalyzes cleavage of both viral and host cell DNA. The cleavage of viral DNA eliminates several base pairs from each end of the viral DNA and creates staggered single-stranded ends. The cleavage of host cell DNA also creates staggered ends. These are repaired, resulting in the duplication of four to six base pairs of the host cell DNA at the insertion junctions. The viral DNA is inserted into the cleaved host DNA. The integrated viral DNA is called the provirus. Purified IN has been shown to perform all of these functions in vitro, indicating that no additional cellular proteins are required for integration.[76,77]

The integrated provirus serves as a template for the transcription of viral RNA. Cellular RNA polymerase II, which also transcribes cellular mRNA, is used along with other cellular factors for transcription of viral RNA. The full-length transcript can either serve as viral genomic RNA and become packaged into virions or used for translation of the Gag and Pol proteins, although the factors that determine this are not clear. RNA splicing, which generates mRNA for all the other viral proteins, and RNA export from the nucleus to the cytoplasm, also relies for the most part on host cellular factors. As mentioned earlier, however, some viruses that have a complex genome and mRNA splicing pattern, such as HTLV and HIV, encode proteins that regulate splicing and actively facilitate nuclear export.[78-80] The Gag and Pol proteins are translated on free ribosomes.[81] The protein at the amino terminus, MA, is myristoylated co-translationally,[45,46] which directs the Gag and Gag-Pol precursor polypeptides to the inner face of the cell membrane. Here the precursor Gag protein interacts with the packaging signal on the viral RNA to initiate the formation of nascent cores. Cleavage of the Gag and Gag-Pol precursors by the viral protease takes place soon after the virion buds off from the cell surface.[82]

In contrast to Gag and Gag-Pol, Env proteins are synthesized on ribosomes associated with the endoplasmic reticulum.[81] They are glycosylated extensively

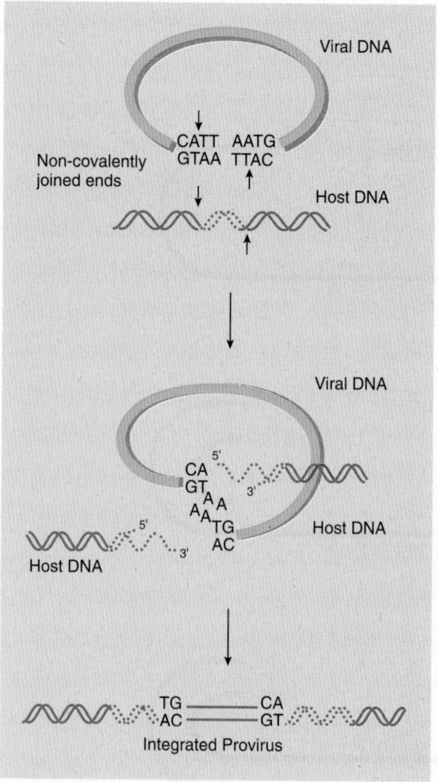

Figure 20-6 Integration. The newly reverse-transcribed double-stranded retroviral deoxyribonucleic acid (DNA) genome and a piece of chromosomal DNA are specifically cleaved by the retroviral integrase protein. This is accompanied by a deletion of two base pairs from the retroviral genome and a duplication of four to six base pairs from the host DNA. Following retroviral genomic insertion into the cleaved host DNA, the DNA is relegated.

here and within the Golgi apparatus and transported to the cell surface, where the signal peptide is removed and cleavage to the mature TM and SU proteins occurs by the action of cellular proteases. The MA protein recognizes the cytoplasmic tail of the TM protein by mechanisms that are not clear, and thereby facilitates the assembly of the core with the envelope to form a complete virion.

A few important points with regard to the retroviral replication cycle should be kept in mind. First of all, proviral formation, which is the product of the integration reaction, results in a stable genetic copy of the virus. This copy is stable; it cannot be removed from the infected cell, and infected cells can and do persist for the life of the host. Furthermore, whenever the cell divides, the provirus is passed on to both daughter cells. As a further consequence, when germ line cells are infected, they become part of the genome of subsequent offspring. As a result, 5% or more of the human genome consists of proviruses from past retroviral infections. Integration, however, is not always accurate, and deletions and rearrangements can occur. Integrated proviruses can also occasionally become deleted or rearranged. Reflecting this, most endogenous proviruses are defective and not usually expressed, although expression of some does occur. It is likely, however, that this massive insertion of foreign DNA has had a profound impact on evolutionary processes.

A second important point is that after proviral formation, transcription and translation of viral gene products depend entirely on cellular factors. Thus, a retrovirus generally persists silently in quiescent cells. Activation of infected cells, such as occurs when cells of the immune system are stimulated by antigen or cells are activated by hormones, can activate viral expression, although this is modulated by the suite of transcriptional factor binding sites in the viral LTR. Also, complex retroviruses such as HTLV and HIV encode transcriptional activators that can profoundly affect the activity of the viral RNA polymerase promoter.[83-88]

Mechanisms of Oncogenesis

Some retroviruses are acutely transforming; they are able to transform cells directly. Retroviral induction of neoplasias in vivo in the infected host, however, involves a variety of mechanisms in addition to cell transformation by acutely transforming viruses. These are summarized in Figure 20-7.

Oncogene Capture

Acutely transforming viruses usually are generated when a cellular proto-oncogene is captured by insertion into the viral genome during viral replication. This process usually causes genetic changes in the proto-oncogene, resulting in an oncogene, or dominant transforming gene. The same process usually also results in a replication-defective virus that requires a helper virus for its replication. The helper virus provides viral proteins to form the virion in which the RNA of the defective virus is packaged. These mixed particles are called pseudotypes.

The first discovered oncogenic virus was Rous sarcoma virus (RSV), which was shown to be a transmissible agent causing sarcomas in chickens.[2] This was one of the first identified retroviruses. RSV was the first acutely transforming virus of many that was shown to have acquired its oncogenicity by the capture of a cellular gene, in this case one called *src*.[12] This was perhaps made possible in part because RSV, unlike most acutely transforming viruses, is replication competent and does not require a helper virus, thus making it simpler to study. The *src* gene in RSV is inserted as a separate gene immediately 3' of the other viral genes.[34,89] The transforming potential could be assigned to the viral *src* gene (v-*src*) because transformation-defective RSV was shown to have mutations specifically in v-*src* and because it conferred transforming ability to recombinant viruses that contained it.[90-92] These findings led to the recognition that normal cellular genes when modified and in the appropriate setting could cause malignant transformation.

Acutely transforming retroviruses produce tumors in susceptible hosts within days to weeks after infection. Because their transforming ability is so potent, a large fraction of infected cells become transformed; hence, the tumors that arise tend to be polyclonal. RSV infection of young chickens induces a variety of related tumor types, notably fibrosarcomas and histiocytic sarcomas. The younger the animal, the more sensitive it is to tumor formation. Tumor formation can occur within days in chicks younger than 1 month, the tumors progress rapidly, occur at many sites, and kill the animal. In the presence of an immune response, as in older chickens, the tumors tend to regress and disappear. Injection of v-*src* DNA into young birds can also induce tumors, further implicating v-*src* as causing the tumors.[93] Tumor formation with DNA is less efficient, but this is probably a reflection of the inefficiency of functional DNA uptake compared with retroviral infection. RSV can also cause tumors in baby rodents, but does not do so with efficiency. Only occasionally do tumors form, and these are restricted to the site of inoculation and tend to regress as the animal becomes older and presumably more immunocompetent. The lower tumorigenic potential probably reflects the reduced replication rate of RSV on rodent cells.[94,95]

A more typical acutely transforming oncogene-containing retrovirus is typified by Abelson murine leukemia virus (A-MuLV). Infection of a nude mouse with a replication competent MuLV[96,97] resulted in the replacement of most of the MuLV genes with a modified copy of the proto-oncogene c-*abl*,[98] a tyrosine kinase that has recently become well known because it is the target of the anticancer drug Gleevec. Like most viral oncogenes and their cellular counterparts (summarized in Table 20-3), the *abl* portion of v-*abl* differs genetically from c-*abl*. The resultant recombinant virus, A-MuLV, is unable to synthesis any of the viral genes, and only codes for a fusion protein containing part of Gag and Abl (v-Abl). The presence of the amino-terminal portion of Gag on v-Abl causes it to be myristoylated and transported to the cell membrane, and this is critical for transformation by A-MuLV. The result of the lack of functional viral genes is that A-MuLV

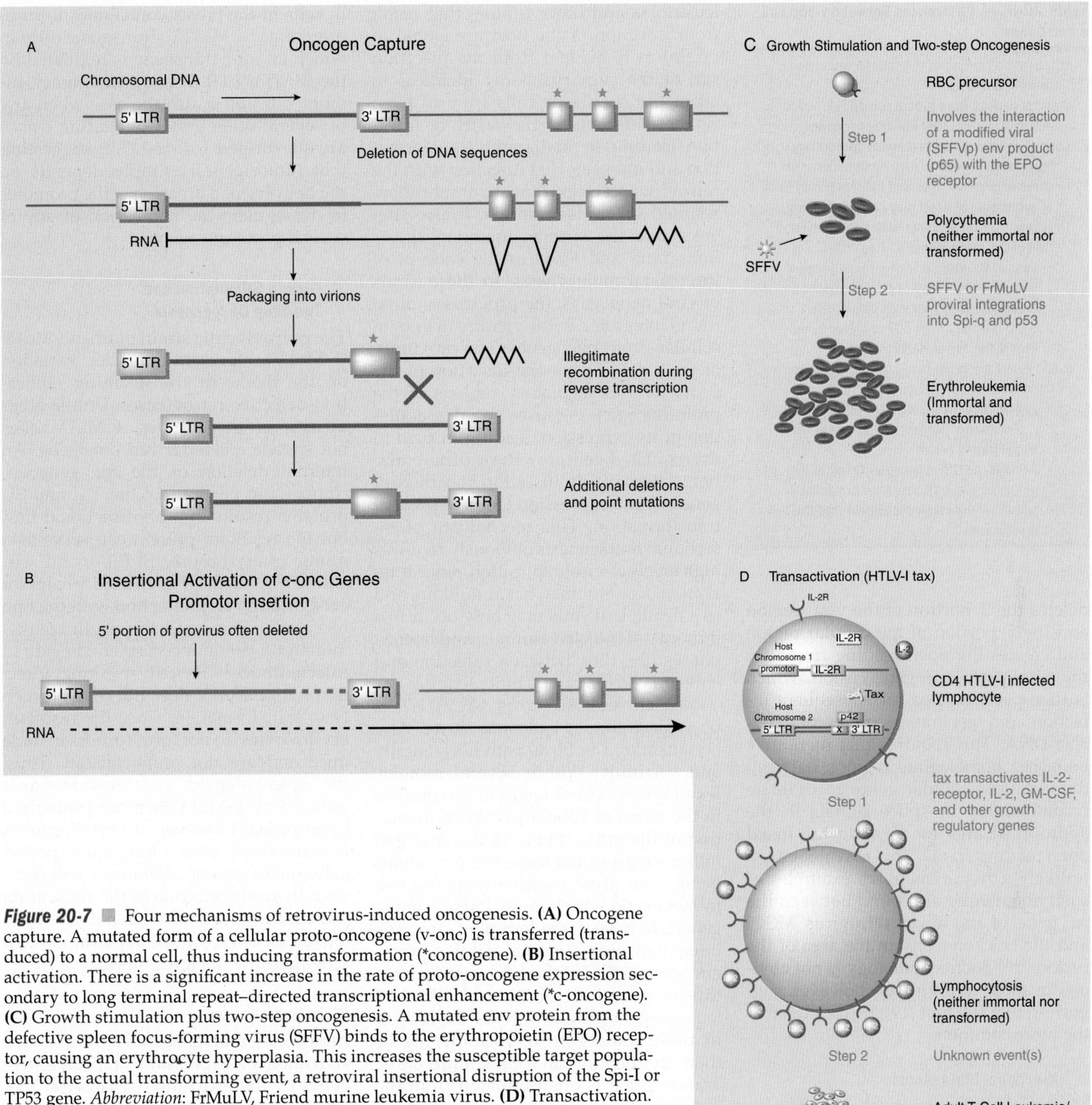

Figure 20-7 Four mechanisms of retrovirus-induced oncogenesis. **(A)** Oncogene capture. A mutated form of a cellular proto-oncogene (v-onc) is transferred (transduced) to a normal cell, thus inducing transformation (*concogene). **(B)** Insertional activation. There is a significant increase in the rate of proto-oncogene expression secondary to long terminal repeat–directed transcriptional enhancement (*c-oncogene). **(C)** Growth stimulation plus two-step oncogenesis. A mutated env protein from the defective spleen focus-forming virus (SFFV) binds to the erythropoietin (EPO) receptor, causing an erythrocyte hyperplasia. This increases the susceptible target population to the actual transforming event, a retroviral insertional disruption of the Spi-I or TP53 gene. *Abbreviation*: FrMuLV, Friend murine leukemia virus. **(D)** Transactivation. The viral transactivating protein (tax in the case of human T-cell leukemia virus type I) causes expansion of the potential target population through transactivation of growth regulatory genes. Some unknown second event then induces the actual transformation of a clone of these cells.

is replication-defective. It is able to infect and transform target cells only with the assistance of a helper virus. A-MuLV induces B-cell lymphomas in young mice, but adult animals are generally resistant to A-MuLV lymphomagenesis.[99]

Several models have been put forth for how cellular sequences are acquired by retroviral genomes, summarized in Figure 18-7A. In one scenario, a retrovirus integrates into the host cell genome just upstream from a proto-oncogene.[100] A subsequent deletion removes the 3' portion of the provirus and the 5' portion of the proto-oncogene, fusing the viral genome with cellular sequences and resulting in a reading frame for a fusion protein, generally including part of the *gag* gene. This gene is transcribed under the regulation of the viral LTR, processed, and co-packaged into a pseudotype retroviral particle with the helper virus genome. When the pseudotype infects a target cell, RT mediates recombination between the 3' ends of the two viral RNAs, which places a 3' LTR on the end of the transduced cellular gene, which allows the resultant double-stranded DNA to be integrated into the host cell DNA.

The second model for the formation of acutely transforming viruses is shown in Figure 18-7B. In this model, a replication competent virus again integrates upstream from a proto-oncogene. On rare occasions the termination signal in the 3' LTR is not recognized and transcription proceeds through the downstream gene. The large combined transcript then undergoes splicing or recombination that

Table 20-3 ■ Differences Between v-onc and c-onc Genes

Often only a portion of the cellular oncogene is present in v-onc.

v-onc is derived from processed mRNA, which is devoid of introns and flanking sequences.

Loss of cellular control elements (promoters/repressors as well as RNA destabilizers) for some oncogenes (myc and mos) elevated level of expression in itself may be transforming.

Deletions/rearrangements may affect the structure of the protein itself:

- Loss of C-terminal Tyr-containing region of *c-src* causes loss of phosphorylation-mediated control by host cell kinases.
- *v-erb* B differs from EGF receptor by deletion of the extracellular domain.

v-onc genes are often fused to viral sequences important for transforming function:

- *gag-abl* acquires a myristoylation signal □ membrane localization important for transforming activity.
- *v-fms* is the CSF-1 receptor fused to the gag gene product, the latter providing a signal sequence for placement into the cell membrane.

deletes the 3' portion of the viral region and the 5' portion of the cellular region and creates the open reading frame for the viral-proto-oncogene fusion, which is then pseudotyped for subsequent infection and generation of an integratable DNA. This requires that there may be either homologous regions between the viral and cellular genes to facilitate recombination or splice signals in the appropriate area for forming the fused open reading frame. This may not be too unlikely a requirement, as examples of such homologies are found between the *pol* gene of the avian retrovirus MC29 and the chicken c-*myc* in the area of the fusion.[100,101] Such a homology is not obvious in most retroviruses, however, suggesting that the first scenario is probably the more common.

Insertional Mutagenesis

Most of the retroviruses that cause neoplasms in their hosts are not acutely transforming viruses, contain the minimum complement of *gag*, *pol*, and *env* genes, and are replication competent. Because many of these viruses induce leukemias and are genetically somewhat related, they are collectively referred to as leukemia viruses. Representatives include avian, murine, feline, and gibbon ape leukemia viruses. The kinds of leukemias induced vary with the viral strain; thus, some strains of gibbon ape leukemia virus are associated with lymphocytic leukemia,[7,102] whereas another strain is associated with myeloid leukemia.[103] Their lack of acutely transforming oncogenes means that they are not competent for direct transformation, and do not transform target cells in vitro. The leukemias and other tumors that result from infection of the host are clonal in origin, as is evident from the insertion site of the provirus being identical in all of the neoplastic cells from a given tumor. This reflects the rarity of infection leading to malignant transformation and indicates that infection with the retrovirus preceded (and, by implication, resulted in) transformation. It also suggests that the specific insertion site is important, and leads to the concept of insertional mutagenesis. In these kinds of viral neoplasias, the provirus is often found integrated in the vicinity of known cellular proto-oncogenes. The proximity of the viral LTR (or the insertion of the provirus into regulatory regions of the proto-oncogene) causes a dysregulation of its expression, leading in turn to dysregulated cell growth or differentiation. Alternatively, insertion may disrupt genes whose expression tends to prevent transformation. This mechanism of insertional mutagenesis obviously requires high levels of viral replication, since integration occurs somewhat at random, and as a result, leukemia may only occur in a minority of infected animals, and latency phases (the time between infection and leukemia onset) can be quite lengthy.

Avian leukosis virus (ALV) is the protypical simple leukemia virus. ALV is transmitted in birds both horizontally and vertically. Within several months, B-cell lymphoblasts begin to accumulate in the bursa of Fabricius.[104] With involution of the bursa, many of the enlarged follicles regress, but some tumor nodules persist and grow, eventually giving rise to metastatic lymphomas. These tumors generally have a predominant provirus integrated near c-*myc*, a cellular proto-oncogene.[105-107] Further suggesting that this is a critical mechanism for ALV leukemogenesis, c-myc RNA expression in these tumors is significantly higher than in the normal cell counterparts. Transcription is often initiated from the 3' LTR,[108] resulting in a chimeric viral-cellular transcript, but continued expression of viral genes and viral replication is no longer needed.

Another well-studied system in which insertional mutagenesis appears to play a critical role is MMTV and murine mammary tumors. As with ALV, MMTV can be transmitted either horizontally or vertically. As with ALV, there is generally a predominant provirus in the mammary tumor cells, with implications similar to those in the case of ALV. Integration was found to occur around but not within a 30 kbp sequence containing the *int*-1 proto-oncogene.[109-111] *Int*-1 expression generally only occurs in the neural tube of mid-gestational embryos and in testicular post-meiotic cells, suggesting that inappropriate expression in cells in the breast contributes to tumorigenesis by MMTV. Transgenic mice in which an int-1 transgene is regulated by the MMTV LTR develop mammary tumors, but this is also the case when any of several other genes (including c-*myc*) are substituted for *int*-1,[112-115] suggesting that tumorigenesis simply depends on the delivery of a breast-specific promoter to dysregulate the expression of any of several proto-oncogenes.

Growth Stimulation and Two-Step Oncogenesis

The polycythemic strain of Friend MuLV (F-MuLV) represents another variation on the theme of transforming replication-defective retroviruses. Unlike other viruses of these types, F-MuLV does not encode a cell-derived oncogene. An internal deletion of the *env* gene encompassing portions of the TM and SU proteins results in a nonfunctional Env, but the resultant protein can serve as a mimic of erythropoietin (Epo) and activate the growth of erythroid precursor cells through an interaction with the Epo receptor.[116] This results in erythroleukemia and a pronounced splenomegaly in infected mice.[117] Strictly speaking, infection with F-MuLV does not result directly in transformation, since the resultant erythrocytes do not form tumors in nude mice and are not immortalized. Thus, the splenomegaly and erythrocytosis induced by F-MuLV is more properly a hyperplasia. However, if erythrocytosis is maintained, after a long latent period subsequent genetic alterations will occasionally transform one of the replicating cells, leading to a monoclonal erythroid leukemia. These events are summarized schematically in Figure 18-7C.

Transactivation

Insertional mutagenesis leading to the activation of expression of proto-oncogenes by the proximity of the viral LTR or the interruption of negative regulatory sequences by the integration event is referred to as *cis* activation. The genomes of some leukemia viruses are more complex than the simple leukemia viruses described earlier such as ALV and MuLV and contain extra genes that perform regulatory functions. The two prototypical examples are HTLV and bovine leukemia virus (BLV). These viruses (like the simple leukemia viruses) are replication competent, do not contain transduced proto-oncogenes in their genomes, and induce monoclonal hematopoietic malignancies only in the minority of infected hosts. However, they are like the acutely transforming viruses in that they transform cells in culture and do not appear to require a specific integration site for oncogenesis (Fig. 18-7D). HTLV is the causative agent for adult T-cell leukemia (ATL), a monoclonal T-cell lymphoma/leukemia with frequent cutaneous manifestations that is endemic to several areas including southern Japan and the Caribbean,[17-19,21,118] and is also the cause of a neurologic disease resembling multiple sclerosis, called tropical spastic paraparesis or HTLV-associated myelopathy.[119]

HTLV and BLV code for proteins, respectively, called Tax[84-86] and p34 Tax,[120] that activate expression by binding to the viral LTR in cooperation with transcription factors. This type of activation by a protein product rather than a DNA regulatory region is called *trans* activation, and these viral proteins are called transactivators. HTLV-I codes for several other proteins as well, including Rex, a protein that regulates the complex pattern of splicing the mRNAs of HTLV-I.[79,80] Three proteins of unknown function are encoded by HTLV-I: p30(II), which is another transactivator that bind to CREB binding protein/p300 (CBP/p300),[121] a transcriptional factor; p12(I), which activates the transcriptional factor NFAT and binds to the cytoplasmic domain of the IL-2 receptor[122,123]; and p13(II), which localizes to mitochondria and interacts with farnesyl pryrophosphate synthetase, an enzyme involved in activation of the proto-oncogene *ras*.[124,125] Most interest has focused on Tax, however, since it is clearly critical to the viral replication cycle through transactivation of the viral LTR, and because its transactivation extends to cellular genes, including those for the IL-2 receptor, lymphotoxin, and granulocyte-macrophage stimulating factor.[126-129] The cross-transactivation of cellular genes leads to the idea that dysregulation of growth regulatory genes by Tax may play an important role in its pathogenesis.

There is a body of experimental evidence suggesting that Tax could indeed play a role in leukemogenesis. The HTLV-I provirus in T cells transformed by HTLV-I infection or in leukemic ATL cells often has extensive deletions, but the Tax open reading frame is always preserved. Mice that are transgenic for Tax develop fibrosarcomas or lymphocytic leukemia when the transgene is regulated by the viral LTR or a T-cell-specific promoter, respectively.[130,131] Tax directly transforms a rat fibroblast cell line and transforms primary rat embryo cells in cooperation with *ras* in vitro,[132,133] showing that Tax indeed has oncogenic properties. Interestingly, when Tax was inserted into the genome of a replication competent but transformation-defective mutant of herpesvirus saimiri, human hematopoietic cells infected in vitro by the chimeric virus were transformed, and the transformed cells resembled ATL cells in morphology and cell surface phenotype,[134] suggesting that Tax is indeed important in ATL pathogenesis. It is likely that, as with F-MuLV leukemogenesis, a second step is required for ATL to occur. For one thing, the rarity of ATL as an outcome of HTLV-I infection indicates that a simple infection is not sufficient, and the lack of a common set of integration sites supports the idea that insertional mutagenesis does not play a role. Most tellingly, the leukemic cells do not express viral RNA until after they are put into culture,[135] indicating that by the time the cells are leukemic, they no longer require viral expression, and suggesting there must be subsequent genetic steps in ATL leukemogenesis.

Recently a better understanding has begun to emerge about the signaling pathways used by Tax for transactivation and transformation. Tax associates with members of the ATF/CREB family of transcriptional factors,[136-140] and the HTLV-I LTR has three ATF/CREB binding sites. Several cellular genes, such as serum responsive factor (SRF) and NFkB/Rel, are transactivated by Tax through the same pathway. Tax also transactivates its LTR, as well as some cellular gene promoters such as those for IL-2 and the IL-2 receptor, directly through NFkB.[141-143] This depends on an interaction of Tax and MEKK1, which leads to phosphorylation of the NFkB inhibitor IkB. Phosphorylation of IkB targets its removal by ubiquitination and degradation in the proteasome, which unmasks the nuclear localization signal of NFkB. This allows it to be transported to the nucleus, where it activates gene expression by binding to NFkB enhancer elements, which are present in the viral LTR. In addition to contributions to cell transformation from the activation of signaling pathways, Tax also appears to directly affect the cell cycle. Tax can bind to the cell cycle inhibitor p16/INK4a and interfere with its ability to inhibit the activity of CDK4, a cyclin kinase important for G1-S progression.[144,145] Tax also mediates the phosphorylation of cyclin D3[146] and upregulates the expression of E2F[145,147] through ATF/CREB signaling, and both of these likely contribute to dysregulation of the cell cycle. Dysregulation of the cell cycle often leads to p53-mediated apoptosis.[148] It appears that Tax also dysregulates activities of p53 required for cell cycle arrest and apoptosis,[149-151] which allows unregulated hyperproliferation and immortalization of cells expressing Tax. Tax appears to inhibit p53 functions in part by an NFkB-dependent mechanism and in part by competing with p53 for binding to CBP/p300. Tax also has been reported to inhibit MAD1, a protein involved in another stage of the cell cycle, the G2/M transition.[152] It is interesting that Tax interferes with the p16/INK4a and p53 pathways, as alteration of these genes or their activities are quite common in naturally occurring cancers.

The protein called HBZ, mentioned earlier and translated from the minus strand of viral RNA, could also be a determinant of HTLV-I leukemogenesis. HBZ appears to be the only viral gene product expressed in ATL cells. HBZ heterodimerizes with members of the CREB and Jun families[61] and supports proliferation of ATL cells.

Retroviruses are also associated with immunodeficiency in infected animals, as in the case of FeLV.[153] The best known example of an immunopathogenic virus is, of course, HIV-1, which is the cause of AIDS. Infection with HIV-1 also leads to an increased incidence in several kinds of tumors, most of which are linked to viruses coinfecting HIV-infected individuals. The clearest example is that of human herpesvirus 8 (HHV-8) (also known as Kaposi sarcoma herpesvirus [KSHV]).[154] HHV-8 is clearly the cause of Kaposi's sarcoma (KS) and a B-cell lymphoma called peripheral effusion lymphoma (PEL).[155] In the absence of HIV-1 or other immunosuppressive conditions, HHV-8 appears to cause these diseases only rarely. HIV-1 infection raises the risk of these diseases by many orders of magnitude.[156] A greatly elevated incidence of non-Hodgkin lymphoma (NHL) is also seen in a setting of HIV infection,[156] and at least a substantial portion of these AIDS-NHL cases is associated with Epstein-Barr virus (EBV) infection. Infection with HIV-1 also appears to increase the risk of childhood leiomyosarcomas (associated with EBV) and of cervical cancer and hepatocarcinoma. The two latter cancers are associated with human papilloma virus and hepatitis B and C virus infections, respectively. Infection with these viruses tends to be higher in HIV-infected people, but there also appears to be a higher risk of cancer in people who are coinfected with HIV and one of these viruses.

It is also possible that HIV may play a more direct role in tumorigenesis. Mice that are transgenic for Tat, the HIV transactivator protein that is functionally homologous to HTLV-I Tax, develop KS-like lesions.[157] A subset of AIDS-NHL is not associated with EBV, and the reasons for its increased incidence are not clear. Conversely, HTLV-I infection can lead to a loss of function of immune cells in vitro, and immunodeficiency occurs in HTLV-I infected people, although this may be an epiphenomenon of the associated leukemogenesis.

Endogenous Retroviruses

Endogenous retroviruses are part of the normal genetic complement of species and make up an extremely large fraction (up to 5%) of various mammalian genomes. Many of these appear to have emerged after speciation, based on differences in their type and number among species. Since retroviruses insert at random, and since there are so many of them present, it is clear that they have played a profound if unclear role in evolution. It is less clear whether any of them play a role in human cancer or other diseases. First, they are for the most part defective because of large deletions, although some only have a few point mutations and a very few may be replication competent. A second property of this type of retrovirus is that they are generally not expressed even at the RNA level. This may be because of mutations in the regulatory regions of their LTRs, because of their location in transcriptionally inactive areas of the chromatin, or because of methylation of promoter sequences in the LTR. When endogenous viruses are expressed as RNA, protein, or virions, it is usually in normal placentas or in teratomas, which may reflect the presence of hormone-responsive elements in the LTRs of many endogenous retroviruses. It is possible that integration of endogenous retroviruses may result in recessive mutations. The Hr (hairless) and D (dilute brown) recessive phenotypes in mice are associated with the presence of endogenous retroviruses at the affected loci,[158-160] and reversion of the mutation is associated with proviral deletion, raising the possibility that there may be analogous situations in humans. Indeed, insertion of a GaLV-related provirus upstream from a duplicated pancreatic amylase gene appears to have allowed its expression in saliva,[161-163] and may have led to the prevalence of starch-rich foods in the human diet.

One specific endogenous retroviral RNA is highly expressed in placenta. Its protein product, syncytin, may be important in human placental morphogenesis, and dysregulation of its expression is associated with pre-eclampsia.[164,165] In general, expression or the lack of expression of endogenous retroviral genes has not been associated with human diseases, although the AKR strain of mice develops leukemia by a complex process that involves expression and recombination of endogenous MuLVs.[166-168] However, a recent report has suggested an association between expression of an endogenous retrovirus related to MuLV and a subset of prostate cancers.[169]

The integration pattern and the content of endogenous retroviruses can differ among members of the same species, suggesting that they are not entirely stable and that many of them are not currently essential to their hosts. Their existence as fixed genetic elements, however, suggests that they were important at one time. Retroviruses that use the same receptor exhibit interference with each other. This is because infection either blocks or downregulates the cell surface expression of the receptor, rendering the cell refractory to superinfection. It may be that endogenous retroviruses provided protection by interference against pathogenic retroviruses that no longer exist, and are therefore no longer important.

Retroviral Vectors and Gene Therapy

As the understanding of the roles of specific genes in different diseases has evolved, treatment of diseases by gene therapy, or the delivery of desired genes, has become more of a possibility. One of the main obstacles has been efficient and specific delivery of a gene to the appropriate tissue and cell type. Delivery by transfection of DNA, or introduction into cells in which the membrane has been partially permeabilized by chemicals or an electrical charge, is relatively inefficient, not very specific, and not generally suitable for delivery in vivo. Delivery by gene gun, which shoots DNA on the surface of gold microparticles into skin and muscle, and direct injection of DNA result in expression of proteins in vivo, but they are not very specific and may be best suited for the delivery of DNA vaccines.

An alternative is to use a recombinant virus to deliver the gene of interest into the appropriate tissue. This method of gene delivery is called transduction. Viruses can be highly tissue-specific, and in principle transduction appears to represent the best approach to gene delivery. Different viruses have been used for gene delivery, including adenovirus, which has disadvantages of a lack of persistence and the likelihood of immune responses against viral proteins upon repeated administration. Retroviral vectors are perhaps the best studied and most promising transducing vectors.[170-173] They integrate, so they theoretically only need to be administered once. In addition, as seen with the acutely transforming replication-defective retroviruses, the vector genome does not need to be able to code for any viral proteins to be integrated. Their tissue and cell tropisms can be altered by pseudotyping them with different envelope proteins.[174] The only requirements for transduction of the gene of interest are that the vector RNA contains the proper packaging signal and has LTRs at both its ends. The proteins required to form virions are provided by cell lines that express all the viral proteins from genes that cannot themselves be packaged. When the vector RNA containing the gene of interest is transfected into a packaging cell line, only the vector RNA is packaged into the virion. Since the pseudotyped RNA does not code for viral proteins, the virions are only capable of a single round of infection and integration. This allows the stable expression of the gene of interest in the absence of any of the retroviral proteins, which would be likely to elicit an immune response that would eliminate the genetically altered cells. The majority of retroviral vectors to date have been based on the Moloney strain of MuLV (Mo-MuLV).[170-173] Mo-MuLV vectors efficiently infect a wide variety of cell types, including those of human origin. More recently, retroviral vectors based on lentiviruses have shown promise. These have the advantage of being able to transduce nondividing cells by the same mechanisms that allow natural lentiviruses to infect resting cells.[175,176]

There are several potential problems with retroviral vectors. One is the possible generation of replication competent helper viruses during the packaging of the vector, which can occur by homologous recombination. Two approaches have been used to minimize this possibility. One is to place the viral structural genes on different genetic units, so that multiple recombination events must occur before a replication competent helper virus is generated. A second approach, not mutually exclusive with the first, is to minimize areas of homology among the units expressing the helper virus proteins and the vector by, for example, using heterologous promoters for helper virus RNA transcription. Another potential problem derives from one of the advantages of retroviral vectors, namely, integration. As mentioned earlier, insertion in the vicinity of a proto-oncogene could lead to tumorigenesis. Although the risk appears small, it is not zero. This was the apparent reason for three of seven monkeys developing lymphomas in one gene therapy study.[177] Mo-MuLV does not replicate well in human cells, but this is not the case for other potential retroviral vectors. Minimizing integration events by, for example, rigorously excluding the presence of replication competent helper viruses helps to avoid this problem, but does not completely eliminate it. Indeed, treatment of young severe combined immunotherapy X1 patients with a lentiviral vector devoid of replicating helper virus appears to have resulted in insertion near the LMO2 proto-oncogene promoter followed by a leukemia-like clonal T-cell outgrowth in several of the patients.[178] Another problem is that expression is not maintained indefinitely; retroviral promoters have a tendency to become inactivated over time. A further limitation is that the genetic capacity of retroviruses is only about 8 to 9 kb, which restricts their ability to deliver genes to a single gene or two.

Conclusions

The study of retroviruses has led to much of today's techniques and understanding of molecular biology. This is obviously especially true in the case of cell transformation and tumorigenesis, since many retroviruses either cause cancers or (in the case of acutely transforming viruses) capture cellular genes that have the potential to contribute to neoplastic transformation. Retroviruses were the first example of a reversal of the normal order of the flow of genetic information, ie, from RNA to DNA. The identification and elucidation of reverse transcription provided the means for cloning and characterizing mRNA, which greatly facilitated understanding gene expression and function. Studies of the regulation of viral transcription, including transactivation of transcription by viral proteins such as Tat and Tax, have increased knowledge about transcriptional regulation. Much has been learned about RNA splicing from studies of retroviral RNA processing, especially studies of mechanisms of viral proteins that specifically regulate this process (Rex and Rev). Studies of ribosomal slippage and termination suppression, mechanisms used by retroviruses to translate reading frames in transcripts downstream from the first reading frame, have helped to elucidate aspects of regulation of translation. We have gained valuable insight on the biochemistry of membranes and membrane fusion from work done on viral entry, and gaining knowledge of the forces involved in viral protein processing and virion assembly has contributed to a better understanding of protein processing and protein-protein interactions. An understanding of how retroviruses package and deliver genetic material holds promise that these viruses will be successfully used to deliver therapeutic genes to appropriate cells and tissues in human diseases. This has been achieved in vitro and to some extent in animals in the laboratory, but clinical success in humans has proven more elusive. However, new generations of vectors currently being studied and developed are bringing us closer to realizing this goal, and it is likely only a matter of time before retroviral viral vectors are used successfully in a clinical setting.

Perhaps among the most important contributions of retroviral research to human health were the discovery of HTLV-I and HIV-1, two pathogenic human retroviruses. During the 1970s, much of the research carried out with retroviruses came under the aegis of the Virus Cancer Program (VCP) as part of President Nixon's War on Cancer. The VCP was ended because of a lack of discovery of human cancer viruses and the growing feeling that human retroviruses did not exist. Shortly thereafter, however, HTLV-I was discovered and linked to ATL. Although this discovery has not led to better treatment for ATL, it has led to better prevention of infection by, for example, screening blood samples and by avoiding transmission by breast-feeding, a common route of infection of babies. Ironically, the most important consequence of the VCP and retroviral research was the relatively rapid discovery and characterization of a virus not directly linked with cancer, but with immunodeficiency. HIV-1 was discovered and shown to be the cause of AIDS and a blood test was developed in a relatively short span of time, and therapies based on structural determinations of its reverse transcriptase and protease were developed and are being successfully used. This rapid progress would have been far slower had the means for isolating, culturing, and characterizing retroviruses not already been in place.

Selected References

The complete reference list can be found at www.CANCERMEDICINE8.com

13. Kalyanaraman VS, Sarngadharan MG, Poiesz B, Ruscetti FW, Gallo RC. Immunological properties of a type C retrovirus isolated from cultured human T-lymphoma cells and comparison to other mammalian retroviruses. *J Virol.* 1981;38(3):906–915.
14. Poiesz BJ, Ruscetti FW, Gazdar AF, Bunn PA, Minna JD, Gallo RC. Detection and isolation of type C retrovirus particles from fresh and cultured lymphocytes of a patient with cutaneous T-cell lymphoma. *Proc Natl Acad Sci USA.* 1980;77(12):7415–7419.
15. Poiesz BJ, Ruscetti FW, Reitz MS, Kalyanaraman VS, Gallo RC. Isolation of a new type C retrovirus (HTLV) in primary uncultured cells of a patient with Sezary T-cell leukaemia. *Nature.* 1981;294(5838):268–271.
16. Reitz MS, Poiesz BJ, Ruscetti FW, Gallo RC. Characterization and distribution of nucleic acid sequences of a novel type C retrovirus isolated from neoplastic human T lymphocytes. *Proc Natl Acad Sci USA.* 1981;78(3):1887–1891.
17. Catovsky D, Greaves MF, Rose M, et al. Adult T-cell lymphoma-leukaemia in Blacks from the West Indies. *Lancet.* 1982;1(8273):639–643.
18. Hinuma Y, Nagata K, Hanaoka M, et al. Adult T-cell leukemia: antigen in an ATL cell line and detection of antibodies to the antigen in human sera. *Proc Natl Acad Sci USA.* 1981;78(10):6476–6480.
19. Kalyanaraman VS, Sarngadharan MG, Nakao Y, Ito Y, Aoki T, Gallo RC. Natural antibodies to the structural core protein (p24) of the human T-cell leukemia (lymphoma) retrovirus found in sera of leukemia patients in Japan. *Proc Natl Acad Sci USA.* 1982;79(5):1653–1657.
20. Robert-Guroff M, Ruscetti FW, Posner LE, Poiesz BJ, Gallo RC. Detection of the human T cell lymphoma virus p19 in cells of some patients with cutaneous T cell lymphoma and leukemia using a monoclonal antibody. *J Exp Med.* 1981;154(6):1957–1964.
21. Yoshida M, Miyoshi I, Hinuma Y. Isolation and characterization of retrovirus from cell lines of human adult T-cell leukemia and its implication in the disease. *Proc Natl Acad Sci USA.* 1982;79(6):2031–2035.
22. Kalyanaraman VS, Sarngadharan MG, Robert-Guroff M, Miyoshi I, Golde D, Gallo RC. A new subtype of human T-cell leukemia virus (HTLV-II) associated with a T-cell variant of hairy cell leukemia. *Science.* 1982;218(4572):571–573.
23. Barre-Sinoussi F, Chermann JC, Rey F, et al. Isolation of a T-lymphotropic retrovirus from a patient at risk for acquired immune deficiency syndrome (AIDS). *Science.* 1983;220(4599):868–871.
24. Popovic M, Sarngadharan MG, Read E, Gallo RC. Detection, isolation, and continuous production of cytopathic retroviruses (HTLV-III) from patients with AIDS and pre-AIDS. *Science.* 1984;224(4648):497–500.
25. Gallo RC, Salahuddin SZ, Popovic M, et al. Frequent detection and isolation of cytopathic retroviruses (HTLV-III) from patients with AIDS and at risk for AIDS. *Science.* 1984;224:500–503.
26. Sarngadharan MG, Popovic M, Bruch L, Schupbach J, Gallo RC. Antibodies reactive with human T-lymphotropic retroviruses (HTLV-III) in the serum of patients with AIDS. *Science.* 1984;224(4648):506–508.
55. Weiss SR, Varmus HE, Bishop JM. The size and genetic composition of virus-specific RNAs in the cytoplasm of cells producing avian sarcoma-leukosis viruses. *Cell.* 1977;12(4):983–992.
61. Mesnard JM, Barbeau B, Devaux C. HBZ, a new important player in the mystery of adult T-cell leukemia. *Blood.* 2006;108(13):3979–3982.
75. Haseltine WA, Kleid DG, Panet A, Rothenberg E, Baltimore D. Ordered transcription of RNA tumor virus genomes. *J Mol Biol.* 1976;106(1):109–131.
79. Ohta M, Nyunoya H, Tanaka H, Okamoto T, Akagi T, Shimotohno K. Identification of a cis-regulatory element involved in accumulation of human T-cell leukemia virus type II genomic mRNA. *J Virol.* 1988;62(12):4445–4451.
80. Seiki M, Inoue J, Hidaka M, Yoshida M. Two cis-acting elements responsible for posttranscriptional trans-regulation of gene expression of human T-cell leukemia virus type I. *Proc Natl Acad Sci USA.* 1988;85(19):7124–7128.
84. Felber BK, Paskalis H, Kleinman-Ewing C, Wong-Staal F, Pavlakis GN. The pX protein of HTLV-I is a transcriptional activator of its long terminal repeats. *Science.* 1985;229(4714):675–679.
85. Fujisawa J, Seiki M, Kiyokawa T, Yoshida M. Functional activation of the long terminal repeat of human T-cell leukemia virus type I by a trans-acting factor. *Proc Natl Acad Sci USA.* 1985;82(8):2277–2281.
87. Sodroski J, Rosen C, Goh WC, Haseltine W. A transcriptional activator protein encoded by the x-lor region of the human T-cell leukemia virus. *Science.* 1985;228(4706):1430–1434.

98. Reddy EP, Smith MJ, Srinivasan A. Nucleotide sequence of Abelson murine leukemia virus genome: structural similarity of its transforming gene product to other *onc* gene products with tyrosine-specific kinase activity. *Proc Natl Acad Sci USA*. 1983;80(12):3623–3627.
100. Varmus HE. Form and function of retroviral proviruses. *Science*. 1982;216(4548):812–820.
101. Walther N, Lurz R, Patschinsky T, Jansen HW, Bister K. Molecular cloning of proviral DNA and structural analysis of the transduced *myc* oncogene of avian oncovirus CMII. *J Virol*. 1985;54(2):576–585.
105. Fung YK, Fadly AM, Crittenden LB, Kung HJ. On the mechanism of retrovirus-induced avian lymphoid leukosis: deletion and integration of the proviruses. *Proc Natl Acad Sci USA*. 1981;78(6):3418–3422.
106. Hayward WS, Neel BG, Astrin SM. Activation of a cellular *onc* gene by promoter insertion in ALV-induced lymphoid leukosis. *Nature*. 1981;290(5806):475–480.
107. Neel BG, Hayward WS, Robinson HL, Fang J, Astrin SM. Avian leukosis virus-induced tumors have common proviral integration sites and synthesize discrete new RNAs: oncogenesis by promoter insertion. *Cell*. 1981;23(2):323–334.
108. Payne GS, Bishop JM, Varmus HE. Multiple arrangements of viral DNA and an activated host oncogene in bursal lymphomas. *Nature*. 1982;295(5846):209–214.
109. Nusse R, Varmus HE. Many tumors induced by the mouse mammary tumor virus contain a provirus integrated in the same region of the host genome. *Cell*. 1982;31(1):99–109.
111. van Ooyen A, Nusse R. Structure and nucleotide sequence of the putative mammary oncogene int-1; proviral insertions leave the protein-encoding domain intact. *Cell*. 1984;39(1):233–240.
114. Sinn E, Muller W, Pattengale P, Tepler I, Wallace R, Leder P. Coexpression of MMTV/v-Ha-ras and MMTV/c-myc genes in transgenic mice: synergistic action of oncogenes in vivo. *Cell*. 1987;49(4):465–475.
116. Li JP, D'Andrea AD, Lodish HF, Baltimore D. Activation of cell growth by binding of Friend spleen focus-forming virus gp55 glycoprotein to the erythropoietin receptor. *Nature*. 1990;343(6260):762–764.
117. Ruscetti SK, Janesch NJ, Chakraborti A, Sawyer ST, Hankins WD. Friend spleen focus-forming virus induces factor independence in an erythropoietin-dependent erythroleukemia cell line. *J Virol*. 1990;64(3):1057–1062.
119. Gessain A, Barin F, Vernant JC, Gout O, Maurs L, Calender A, de TG. Antibodies to human T-lymphotropic virus type-I in patients with tropical spastic paraparesis. *Lancet*. 1985;2(8452):407–410.
121. Zhang W, Nisbet JW, Bartoe JT, Ding W, Lairmore MD. Human T-lymphotropic virus type 1 p30(II) functions as a transcription factor and differentially modulates CREB-responsive promoters. *J Virol*. 2000;74(23):11270–11277.
122. Albrecht B, D'Souza CD, Ding W, Tridandapani S, Coggeshall KM, Lairmore MD. Activation of nuclear factor of activated T cells by human T-lymphotropic virus type 1 accessory protein p12(I). *J Virol*. 2002;76(7):3493–3501.
126. Fujii M, Sassone-Corsi P, Verma IM. c-fos promoter trans-activation by the tax1 protein of human T-cell leukemia virus type I. *Proc Natl Acad Sci USA*. 1988;85(22):8526–8530.
127. Inoue J, Seiki M, Taniguchi T, Tsuru S, Yoshida M. Induction of interleukin 2 receptor gene expression by p40x encoded by human T-cell leukemia virus type 1. *EMBO J*. 1986;5(11):2883–2888.
133. Tanaka A, Takahashi C, Yamaoka S, Nosaka T, Maki M, Hatanaka M. Oncogenic transformation by the *tax* gene of human T-cell leukemia virus type I in vitro. *Proc Natl Acad Sci USA*. 1990;87(3):1071–1075.
134. Grassmann R, Dengler C, Muller-Fleckenstein I, et al. Transformation to continuous growth of primary human T lymphocytes by human T-cell leukemia virus type I X-region genes transduced by a herpesvirus saimiri vector. *Proc Natl Acad Sci USA*. 1989;86(9):3351–3355.
136. Adya N, Giam CZ. Distinct regions in human T-cell lymphotropic virus type I tax mediate interactions with activator protein CREB and basal transcription factors. *J Virol*. 1995;69(3),1834–1841.
138. Suzuki T, Fujisawa JI, Toita M, Yoshida M. The trans-activator tax of human T-cell leukemia virus type 1 (HTLV-1) interacts with cAMP-responsive element (CRE) binding and CRE modulator proteins that bind to the 21-base-pair enhancer of HTLV-1. *Proc Natl Acad Sci USA*. 1993;90(2):610–614.
141. Ballard DW, Bohnlein E, Lowenthal JW, Wano Y, Franza BR, Greene WC. HTLV-I tax induces cellular proteins that activate the kappa B element in the IL-2 receptor alpha gene. *Science*. 1988;241(4873):1652–1655.
142. Leung K, Nabel GJ. HTLV-1 transactivator induces interleukin-2 receptor expression through an NF-kappa B-like factor. *Nature*. 1988;333(6175):776–778.
144. Low KG, Dorner LF, Fernando DB, Grossman J, Jeang KT, Comb MJ. Human T-cell leukemia virus type 1 Tax releases cell cycle arrest induced by p16INK4a. *J Virol*. 1997;71(3):1956–1962.
145. Suzuki T, Kitao S, Matsushime H, Yoshida M. HTLV-1 Tax protein interacts with cyclin-dependent kinase inhibitor p16INK4A and counteracts its inhibitory activity towards CDK4. *EMBO J*. 1996;15(7):1607–1614.
149. Akagi T, Ono H, Tsuchida N, Shimotohno K. Aberrant expression and function of p53 in T-cells immortalized by HTLV-I Tax1. *FEBS Lett*. 1997;406(3):263–266.
151. Pise-Masison CA, Radonovich M, Sakaguchi K, Appella E, Brady JN. Phosphorylation of p53: a novel pathway for p53 inactivation in human T-cell lymphotropic virus type 1-transformed cells. *J Virol*. 1998;72(8):6348–6355.
152. Jin DY, Spencer F, Jeang KT. Human T cell leukemia virus type 1 oncoprotein Tax targets the human mitotic checkpoint protein MAD1. *Cell*. 1998;93(1):81–91.

21 Herpesviruses

Jeffrey I. Cohen, MD

Eight herpesviruses have been isolated from humans: herpes simplex viruses 1 and 2, varicella-zoster virus, cytomegalovirus, human herpesviruses 6 and 7, Epstein-Barr virus (EBV), and Kaposi sarcoma–associated herpesvirus (KSHV). Two of these herpesviruses are associated with human tumors. EBV has been detected in lesions from patients with nasopharyngeal carcinoma, Burkitt lymphoma, Hodgkin disease, and certain other lymphoid tumors. KSHV is associated with Kaposi sarcoma, primary effusion lymphoma, and Castleman disease.

Properties of Herpesviruses

Herpesviruses are enveloped virions containing a deoxyribonucleic acid (DNA) core surrounded by a nucleocapsid and tegument. Infection of cells with herpesviruses begins with fusion of the virion envelope with the cell membrane or endocytosis of the virion. The viral capsid is released into the cytoplasm and is transported to the nucleus where the linear viral DNA circularizes. In infections that result in production of progeny viruses and lysis of the host cell, viral genes are transcribed in the nucleus and their proteins are synthesized in the cytoplasm. Early lytic replication is associated with inhibition of host DNA, RNA, and protein synthesis. Virion DNA is replicated and assembled into nucleocapsids in the nucleus, which subsequently are enveloped and virions are released from the cell. All herpesviruses have the capacity to establish latent infection as well as to undergo lytic infection. The capacity to establish latent infection in vivo and to reactivate from latency ensures a source of virus to infect previously uninfected individuals. Most adults latently harbor herpes simplex 1, varicella-zoster virus, human herpesvirus 6 and 7, and EBV.

Oncogenic Features of Herpesviruses

Several features of herpesvirus replication are important for the maintenance of latency and for oncogenicity. Herpesviruses must maintain their viral genome in the cell, avoid killing the cell, avoid destruction of the cell by the immune system, and activate appropriate cellular growth control regulatory pathways. Because EBV is the best-studied of the oncogenic human herpesviruses, it will be used to illustrate the principles of herpesvirus infection relevant to oncogenicity.

First, viral DNA must be maintained in the cell. EBV establishes latent infection in B lymphocytes. The EBV genome is usually maintained in B cells either as a multicopy circular episome in the host cell, or rarely by integrating the viral DNA into the host genome. Episomes are formed by fusion of direct repeat sequences present at both termini of the linear genome present in virions.

Second, a cell transformed by a virus must avoid immune clearance. Replication of EBV may require 100 viral proteins; however, latent infection of B cells with EBV results in expression of 12 or fewer genes.[1,2] This limited repertoire of gene products prevents frequent viral replication, with death of the infected cell, and restricts the ability of the immune system to recognize and destroy a cell latently infected with the virus.

Third, specific viral proteins interact with other cell proteins or directly transactivate other cell genes to provide additional functions necessary for immortalization. Several EBV proteins interact with cellular proteins to activate transcription of viral and cellular genes or to engage signal transduction pathways in the cell (see below).

EBV: An Oncogenic Human Herpesvirus

Effect on B-Cell Growth In Vitro

Infection of primary B cells with EBV in vitro results in transformation of the cells, which can then proliferate indefinitely. B-cell activation antigens, including CD23, are expressed on the surface of the EBV-transformed B cells and a soluble form of CD23 is secreted from the cells. CD23 may be a growth factor for B cells. EBV infection of Burkitt lymphoma cells in vitro results in upregulation of a number of cellular proteins, including CD44, and two G protein–coupled peptide receptors.[3]

EBV Gene Expression in Transformed Lymphocytes

Eight EBV proteins and several nontranslated RNAs are expressed in latently infected B lymphocytes that have been growth transformed by EBV in vitro (Table 21-1). The EBV nuclear proteins EBNA-1, EBNA-2, EBNA-LP, EBNA-3A, EBNA-3B, and EBNA-3C comprise the EBV nuclear antigen complex. EBNA-1 binds to the oriP sequence (origin of viral DNA replication) on EBV DNA and allows the virus genome to be maintained as an episome in transformed B cells.[4] EBNA-1 also transactivates its own expression. EBNA-1 transcripts are initiated from one of four different promoters. The Cp and Wp promoters are used to express EBNA-1 in lymphoblastoid cell

Table 21-1 **Selected EBV Genes and Their Cellular Homologs and Activities**

Gene	Expression Class	Cellular Homolog	Activity
EBNA-1	Latent, lytic	None	Episome maintenance, transactivates viral genes, inhibits apoptosis
EBNA-2	Latent	Notch	Transactivates viral and cellular genes, inhibits apoptosis
EBNA-3A,B,C	Latent	None	Regulates EBNA-2 activity, transactivates cellular genes
EBNA-LP	Latent	None	Increases EBNA-2 activity
LMP1	Latent, lytic	CD40	Transactivates cellular genes, inhibits apoptosis
LMP2	Latent	None	Prevents EBV reactivation, transactivates Akt
EBERs	Latent	None	Upregulates cellular genes
BARF-1	Lytic	CSF-1R	Inhibits interferon-α
BCFR1	Lytic	IL-10	Inhibits interferon-γ and IL-12
BNLF2a	Lytic	None	Blocks antigen-specific CD8 T-cell recognition
BHRF1	Lytic	Bcl-2	Inhibits apoptosis
BALF1	Lytic	Bcl-2	Regulates BHRF1 activity
BZLF1	Lytic	None	Inhibits interferon-γ effects, inhibits function of p53, inhibits TNF-α, initiates lytic infection

lines in vitro; the Qp promoter is used in tissues from Burkitt lymphoma, nasopharyngeal carcinoma, and Hodgkin disease; and the Fp promoter is used during lytic replication.[5] Transgenic mice expressing EBNA-1 develop B-cell lymphomas.[6] EBNA-1 inhibits its own protein degradation by proteosomes[7] and limits its own translation,[8] both of which may reduce its presentation to CD8+ cytotoxic T cells; however, EBNA-1 remains a target for CD4+ cells.[9-11] EBNA-1 inhibits apoptosis induced by expression of p53.[12]

EBNA-2 transactivates expression of the EBV genes LMP1[13] and LMP2,[14] and the cellular genes CD23, CD21, *c-myc*, and *c-fgr*,[15,16] which encodes a protein tyrosine kinase and is a member of the *src* gene family. EBNA-2 is targeted to the LMP1, LMP2, Cp EBNA, and CD23 promoters by the GTGGGAA-binding protein Jκ, and thereby activates these promoters.[17] EBNA-2 is a functional homolog of the Notch receptor, which uses Jκ to regulate gene expression during development.[18] EBNA-2 also interacts with the DNA-binding protein PU-1 to transactivate the LMP1 promoter[19] and with AUF to transactivate the EBNA Cp promoter.[20] The transactivation domain of EBNA-2 is essential for B-lymphocyte transformation.[21] This domain interacts with transcription factors TFIIB and the TATA-binding protein-associated factor TAF40.[22] EBNA-2 inhibits apoptosis mediated by Nur77.[23]

EBNA-LP interacts with and enhances the ability of EBNA-2 to transactivate LMP1 and LMP2.[24] Although EBNA-LP binds to the retinoblastoma protein and p53 in vitro,[25] the significance of these interactions is uncertain. Deletion of the carboxy terminus of EBNA-LP markedly reduces the ability of the virus to transform B lymphocytes.[26]

EBNA-3A, EBNA-3B, and EBNA-3C are distantly related to each other. The EBNA-3 proteins bind to Jκ preventing it from binding DNA, thereby inhibiting transactivation by EBNA-2.[27] EBNA-3C upregulates expression of LMP1 and CD21. EBNA-3C binds to Nm23-HI, a human metastasis suppressor protein, and inhibits the protein's ability to suppress migration of Burkitt lymphoma cells.[28] EBNA-3C degrades the retinoblastoma protein and enhances kinase activity by disrupting p27.[29,30] EBNA-3A and EBNA-3C are essential for B-lymphocyte transformation in vitro, while EBNA-3B is dispensable.[31,32]

LMP1 functions as a transforming oncogene in nude mice.[33] Expression of LMP1 in EBV-negative Burkitt lymphoma cells results in B-cell clumping and increased villous projections. Upregulation of bcl-2, bfl-1, and A20, and inhibition of Bax, by LMP1 in B cells protects the cells from apoptosis.[34,35] Expression of LMP1 in epithelial cells inhibits differentiation of the cells.[36]

LMP1 is a functional homolog of CD40, a member of the tumor necrosis factor receptor (TNFR) family. The carboxy terminus of LMP1 interacts with the TNFR-associated factors (TRAFs) 1, 2, 3, and 5, TRADD, RIP, and Janus-activated kinase-3 (JAK3) in vitro.[37-39] LMP1 functions as a constitutively active form of CD40 resulting in activation of NF-κB, stress-activated protein kinases, signal transducers and activators of transcription (STATs), adhesion molecules, the B7 co-stimulatory molecule, *c-jun* N-terminal kinase, and B-cell proliferation. LMP1 can functionally substitute for CD40 in transgenic mice.[40] LMP1 upregulates expression of intracellular adhesion molecules, Fas, CD40, and matrix metalloproteinase-9[41] in B cells and epidermal growth factor in epithelial cells.[42] LMP1 induces expression of a cellular microRNA which modulates interferon responsive genes.[43] LMP1 inhibits phosphorylation of Tyk2 resulting in inhibition of interferon-alpha signaling.[44]

LMP1 is essential for transformation of B lymphocytes by EBV.[45] Expression of LMP1 in the skin of transgenic mice induces epithelial hyperplasia with increased expression of keratin 6.[46] Expression of LMP1 in lymphocytes of transgenic mice results in the development of B-cell lymphomas; these tumors contain elevated levels of the anti-apoptotic proteins Bcl-2 and A20, and show activation of Akt, NF-κB, and Stat3.[47,48] Analysis of EBV-containing human lymphomas shows that LMP1 localizes with TRAF-1, TRAF-3, and that activated NF-κB is present.[49]

LMP2 is dispensable for transformation of B cells,[50] but induces a transforming phenotype in epithelial cells and promotes their motility.[51,52] LMP2 prevents lytic reactivation of EBV-infected primary B cells in response to activation of the B-cell receptor complex by cross-linking of surface immunoglobulin. LMP2 associates with the *src* family and *syk* protein-tyrosine kinases that are coupled to the B-cell receptor complex.[53] Binding of LMP2 to these proteins results in their constitutive phosphorylation, which inhibits their ability to mediate signaling for virus reactivation.[53,54] B cells from transgenic mice expressing LMP2 survive even without normal B-cell receptor signaling activity.[55] LMP2 activates beta-catenin and Ras/phosphatidylinositol 3-kinase/Akt signaling pathways in epithelial cells resulting in transformation of the cells.[56,57] LMP2 also activates mTOR and increases c-myc expression.[58]

The two EBV-encoded RNAs, EBER-1 and EBER-2, are the most abundant EBV RNAs in latently infected B cells; however, they are not required for latent or lytic EBV infection, but may contribute to B-cell transformation.[59,60] The EBERs upregulate expression of bcl-2 and IL-10[61] and interact with the double-stranded RNA-activated protein kinase, and interferon-inducible oligoadenylate synthetase.[62,63] The EBV-encoded BART RNAs are expressed during latency and encode microRNAs that regulate LMP1 expression.[64]

EBV Genes Expressed During Productive Infection

Infection of epithelial cells with EBV results in productive infection, with replication of virus and lysis of infected cells. Immediate-early genes encode regulators of virus gene expression, including the BZLF1 and BRLF1 proteins, which act as switches to initiate lytic infection. The BZLF1 protein inhibits TNF-α signaling by reducing expression of the TNF receptor.[65] BZLF1 protein also inhibits the expression of the interferon-γ receptor and the activity of interferon-γ,[66] and inhibits the function of p53.[67] Early genes encode proteins involved in viral DNA synthesis, such as the viral DNA polymerase and thymidine kinase. Late genes encode structural proteins of the virus, including the viral capsid antigen and the major envelope glycoprotein gp350.

Three viral genes expressed during productive infection are functional homologs of cellular genes and are important for the survival of EBV-infected B cells. The EBV BCRF-1 protein is homologous to interleukin-10 and has interleukin-10 activity.[68] BCRF-1 is a B-cell growth factor and inhibits interferon-γ release from activated human peripheral blood mononuclear cells and secretion of interleukin-12 from macrophages. Because interferon-γ is important for the activity of T cells, expression of BCRF-1 during lytic infection may inhibit the ability of cytotoxic T cells to destroy EBV-infected cells.

The EBV BARF-1 protein acts as a soluble receptor for colony stimulating factor 1.[69] BARF-1 inhibits interferon-α secretion by human monocytes. Because interferon-α inhibits outgrowth of EBV-infected B cells in vitro, BARF-1 may act in concert with BCRF-1 to inhibit interferon and promote increased survival of EBV-infected cells. The EBV BNLF2a protein interacts with the TAP complex to block antigen-specific CD8 T-cell recognition.[70] The EBV BHRF1 protein is homologous to bcl-2 and protects Burkitt lymphoma cells from apoptosis.[71] EBV BALF1 is also homologous to bcl-2 and antagonizes the anti-apoptotic effect of BHRF1.[72]

Animal Models

EBV-infected cell lines produce B-cell tumors when inoculated intracerebrally into nude mice. Inoculation of peripheral blood leukocytes from EBV-seropositive humans into mice with severe combined immunodeficiency (SCID) results in development of human B-cell lymphomas in the animals. Inoculation of these mice with peripheral blood leukocytes from EBV-seronegative humans results in engraftment of a human immune system, and if these latter mice are subsequently injected with cell-free EBV, the animals develop immunoblastic lymphomas. These B-cell tumors express the full complement of EBNA and LMP genes characteristic of latently infected, growth-transformed cell lines.[73] Cotton-top tamarins inoculated with a large dose of cell-free EBV develop multifocal large cell lymphomas over the ensuing few weeks. These tumors express EBNA-1, EBNA-2, EBNA-LP, and LMP1[74] and are monoclonal or oligoclonal in origin. Inoculation of Rag2 knockout mice with CD34+ human cord blood cells followed by injection with EBV results in EBV+ B-cell proliferative lesions in the liver and spleen,[75] while inoculation of NOD/SCID mice with human CD34+ cells followed by injection with EBV results in lymphomas that express the EBV latency genes.[76] Inoculation of NOD/SCID mice with human fetal thymus and liver followed by CD34+ cells results in MHC class I and II T-cell responses to EBV.[77]

Clinical Aspects

EBV infection is usually spread by saliva. The virus infects B cells directly, or oropharyngeal epithelial cells and then spreads to subepithelial B cells.[78] During primary infection, up to a few percent of the peripheral blood B lymphocytes are infected with EBV and have the capacity to proliferate indefinitely in vitro. Natural killer (NK) cells, suppressor T cells, and HLA- and EBNA- or LMP-restricted cytotoxic T cells control the latently infected B lymphocytes. T- and B-cell interactions release lymphokines and cytokines, giving rise to many of the clinical manifestations of acute infectious mononucleosis. After recovery, the fraction of B cells latently infected with EBV in the peripheral blood remains at 1 in 10^5 to 1 in 10^6. These lymphocytes are the primary site of EBV persistence and a source of virus for persistent infection of epithelial surfaces.

The B-cell tumors that occur early after EBV infection are usually lymphoproliferative processes, in which latent virus infection in B cells is the principal cause of proliferation. Oral hairy leukoplakia may be the epithelial counterpart. In contrast, Burkitt lymphoma and nasopharyngeal carcinoma occur long after primary EBV infection and viral gene expression is less important to the growth of the malignant cells.

Lymphoproliferative Disease ■ EBV is associated with B-cell lymphoproliferative disease in patients with congenital or acquired immunodeficiency. X-linked lymphoproliferative syndrome is an inherited immunodeficiency of males who have apparently normal cellular and humoral immune responses before infection with EBV. With EBV infection, most of the patients die of a fatal lymphoproliferative disorder or fulminant hepatitis, but some survive with hypogammaglobulinemia. The gene mutated in X-linked lymphoproliferative syndrome has been identified as SAP,[79] which encodes an SH2-containing protein that interacts with the signaling lymphocyte-activation molecule (SLAM) on B and T cells, and with 2B4 on NK and T cells. Anti-CD20 antibody (rituximab) has been effective in treating some patients with X-linked lymphoproliferative disease and acute EBV infection.[80]

EBV is also associated with fatal infectious mononucleosis in persons with no known underlying genetic predisposition or in patients with congenital immunodeficiencies. EBV lymphoproliferative disease occurs in patients who are immunosuppressed as a result of transplantation or acquired immunodeficiency syndrome (AIDS).[81,82] Risk factors for development of lymphoproliferative disease include EBV-seronegativity prior to transplant and receipt of T-cell-depleted bone marrow or anti-lymphocyte antibody. Lymphoproliferative lesions are most commonly seen in the lymph nodes, liver, lungs, kidney, bone marrow, or small intestine. Tumors in transplant patients are usually classified as lymphomas or immunoblastic sarcomas; some patients have hyperplastic lesions. The proliferating lymphocytes in these tumors generally do not have chromosomal translocations.

AIDS-related lymphomas may be systemic (nodal or extranodal) lymphomas, primary central nervous system lymphomas, or primary effusion lymphomas. Primary effusion lymphomas often contain EBV in addition to KSHV. While most B-cell tumors in transplant recipients and central nervous system lymphomas in AIDS patients contain EBV, about 50% of other lymphomas in AIDS patients contain EBV. Tumors in patients with AIDS are usually either immunoblastic lymphomas or Burkitt lymphomas; most of the latter have c-*myc* translocations.

Tissues from transplant recipients or AIDS patients with EBV lymphoproliferative disease show expression of EBERs, EBNA-1, EBNA-2, and LMP1 (Table 21-2). The EBV viral load in the peripheral blood has been used to predict development of disease and to follow patients after therapy. The expression of these EBV genes, which are targets for cytotoxic T cells, has important implications for therapy. Infusion of EBV-specific cytotoxic T cells, non-irradiated donor leukocytes, or HLA-matched allogeneic cytotoxic T cells have been effective in some cases for treatment of EBV lymphoproliferative disease.[83-87] Anti-CD20 antibody (rituximab) has induced remissions in some patients, and has been used in some studies as pre-emptive therapy when EBV viral DNA in the blood is rising in transplant recipients at risk of lymphoproliferative disease,[88] although other studies suggest that preemptive therapy may be unnecessary.[89]

Burkitt Lymphoma ■ Seroepidemiologic studies show a strong association between Burkitt lymphoma and EBV in Africa. More than 90% of African Burkitt lymphomas are associated with EBV, whereas only ~20% of Burkitt lymphomas in the United States are associated with the virus. African patients with Burkitt lymphoma often have high levels of antibody to EBV antigens, and the virus can be recovered from the tissue.

Burkitt lymphomas contain chromosomal translocations that result in c-*myc* dysregulation. The most common chromosomal translocation, t(8;14), places a portion of the c-*myc* oncogene adjacent to an immunoglobulin heavy chain gene. Less common translocations involve the c-*myc* oncogene and the κ or λ immunoglobulin light chain genes t(2;8) and t(8;22), respectively. These translocations result in high constitutive expression of c-*myc*. Dysregulated expression of c-*myc* in EBV-immortalized lymphoblastoid cell lines results in highly transformed

Table 21-2 **■ Diseases Associated with EBV Latent Gene Expression**

Disease	EBERs	EBNA-1	EBNA-2	LMP1	LMP2
Burkitt lymphoma	+	+	–	–	–
Nasopharyngeal carcinoma	+	+	–	+	+
Hodgkin disease	+	+	–	+	+
Peripheral T-cell lymphoma	+	+	–	+	+
Lymphoproliferative disease	+	+	+	+	+

cells that form tumors when injected into immunodeficient mice.[90] Transgenic mice that express a mutated human c-*myc* that is fused to the Igλ, locus, develop tumors that have histologic and phenotypic features of Burkitt lymphomas.[91]

EBV-associated endemic Burkitt lymphoma is thought to develop in steps. First, EBV infection may expand the pool of differentiating and proliferating B cells. Second, chronic endemic malaria may cause T-cell suppression and B-cell proliferation. Third, enhanced proliferation of differentiating B cells may favor the chance occurrence of a reciprocal c-*myc* (t[8;14] or t[8;22]) translocation placing c-*myc* partially under the control of immunoglobulin-related transcriptional enhancers, with development of a monoclonal tumor.

Nasopharyngeal Carcinoma ■ The nonkeratinizing nasopharyngeal carcinomas are uniformly associated with EBV. Patients with nasopharyngeal carcinoma have high levels of antibodies to EBV antigens. A prospective study of Taiwanese men showed that those with IgA antibodies to viral capsid antigen (VCA) and anti-EBV deoxyribonuclease antibodies had an increased risk for developing nasopharyngeal carcinoma when compared to those men without these antibodies.[92] These antibodies are useful in screening patients for early detection of nasopharyngeal carcinoma and are prognostic for patients after treatment. Another study showed that quantifying the level of EBV DNA in plasma of patients with advanced nasopharyngeal carcinoma was useful for monitoring patients and predicting outcomes.[93] Nasopharyngeal carcinoma tissue contains EBV genomes in every cell. These tumors are monoclonal with regard to EBV infection, indicating that EBV infection precedes malignant cell outgrowth at the cellular level. Unlike Burkitt lymphoma, the association of EBV with nasopharyngeal carcinoma is uniform and universal. Infusions of EBV-specific cytotoxic T cells resulted in remissions in some patients with refractory nasopharyngeal carcinoma.[94]

Hodgkin Disease ■ Persons with a history of infectious mononucleosis are at a greater risk of developing Hodgkin disease.[95] Patients with Hodgkin disease generally have higher titers of antibody to EBV VCA than does the general population. Tissues from ~40-60% of patients with Hodgkin disease contain EBV genomes. Cases of Hodgkin disease in patients with human immunodeficiency virus (HIV) or from developing countries are more likely to contain EBV genomes than persons without HIV or from developed countries.[96] The EBV genome is present in Reed-Sternberg cells and the viral genome is monoclonal. EBV is more often associated with aggressive subtypes (especially mixed cellularity) of Hodgkin disease. Tumors from patients with EBV+ Hodgkin disease and some from patients with lymphoproliferative disease arise from post-germinal center cells.[2,97] Infusion of cytotoxic T cells generated from 11 patients with relapsed Hodgkin disease and measurable disease resulted in complete remissions in two patients, partial remission in one patient, stable disease in five patients, and no response in three patients.[98] Infusion of arginine butyrate and ganciclovir to induce EBV thymidine kinase expression with phosphorylation of ganciclovir and induction of apoptosis resulted in antitumor responses in some patients with EBV B-cell malignancies.[99]

Other Tumors Associated with EBV ■ EBV has also been detected in non-Hodgkin's lymphomas. EBV-positive diffuse large B-cell lymphoma has a poorer prognosis than EBV-negative lymphoma.[100] Treatment of patients with EBV+ non-Hodgkin's lymphoma in remission with autologous antigen-presenting cells transduced with LMP2 resulted in increased frequencies of LMP2-specific cytotoxic T cells and tumor responses in several patients with relapsed disease.[101] EBV DNA and latency proteins have been detected in tissues from patients with peripheral T-cell lymphomas.[102] EBV DNA has also been detected in central nervous system lymphomas from patients with no underlying immunodeficiency, T cells in patients with virus-associated hemophagocytic syndrome, nasal T-cell lymphoma, carcinoma of the palatine tonsil, laryngeal carcinoma, and angioimmunoblastic lymphadenopathy. EBV DNA and nuclear antigens have been detected in to thymic carcinomas and in B cell lesions from patients with lymphomatoid granulomatosis.

EBV DNA has been found in leiomyosarcomas in AIDS patients,[103] and viral RNA and EBNA-2 have been detected in smooth muscle tumors in organ transplant recipients.[104] About 7% of primary gastric carcinomas are EBV+, especially in undifferentiated lymphoepithelioma-like carcinomas.

Although some reports suggested that EBV is associated with breast carcinomas, in most of these studies EBV was detected by PCR and viral proteins were found in only a fraction of the tumor cells.[105,106] More recent studies using in situ hybridization and immunohistochemistry have generally not supported an association of EBV and breast carcinoma.[107,108]

KSHV and Malignancies

In 1994, Chang et al. detected sequences of a new human herpesvirus (KSHV) in Kaposi sarcoma tissues from patients with AIDS.[109] Sequence analysis indicates that KSHV, like EBV, is a member of the gamma-herpesvirus subfamily. KSHV is present in B cells in asymptomatic persons. B-cell lines derived from primary effusion lymphomas maintain KSHV in a latent state and can be induced to undergo lytic virus replication by the addition of phorbol ester or butyrate. Foscarnet, ganciclovir, and cidofovir, but not acyclovir, inhibit virus production when these cells are induced to replicate virus.[110]

Infection of dermal microvascular endothelial cells in vitro with KSHV results in transformation of the cells with maintenance of long-term infection. The cells become spindle-shaped and show loss of contact inhibition with anchorage-independent growth.[111] KSHV also transforms bone marrow-derived endothelial cells; however, the virus is present in only a small fraction of the cells.[112] Cystine transporter xCT and integrin α3β1 are cellular receptors for HHV8.[113,114]

Viral Proteins

KSHV encodes a large number of cellular homologs (Table 21-3) that have been grouped into different classes, depending on when they are expressed in primary effusion lymphoma cell lines.[115] Expression of the KSHV K1 gene in rodent fibroblasts results in transformation of the cells.[116] The K1 protein induces tyrosine phosphorylation in cells[117] and activates the Akt signaling pathway.[118] The K1 protein inhibits apoptosis[119] and results in constitutive calcium-dependent signal activation in B cells in the absence of exogenous stimuli.[120]

The KSHV K2 gene encodes an interleukin (IL)-6 homolog (vIL-6). IL-6 is a B-cell growth factor and acts as an autocrine growth factor for lymphoid tumors resulting in proliferation.[121] vIL-6 prevents death of IL-6-dependent B9 cells in vitro,[122] promotes hematopoiesis, and induces vascular endothelial growth factor (VEGF) to promote angiogenesis.[123] The K3 (modulator of immune recognition 1 [MIR1]) and K5 (MIR2) proteins induce rapid endocytosis of MHC class I molecules and interferon-gamma receptor 1 from the surface of cells by ubiquitination of these proteins.[124-126] The K5 protein also downregulates ICAM-1 and B7.2, which results in inhibition of NK cell-mediated cytotoxicity,[127] and removes CD31 from the surface of endothelial cells.[128]

Table 21-3 Selected KSHV Genes and Their Cellular Homologs and Activities

Gene	Expression Class	Cellular Homolog	Activity
K1	II	ITAM motif	Transformation, activates signaling pathways
K2	II	IL-6	B-cell growth factor, angiogenesis, hematopoiesis
K3	III	None	Reduces surface MHC class I
K4	II	MIP-1α	Chemokine receptor antagonist; angiogenesis; chemotaxis
K4.1	II	MIP-1α	Chemokine receptor agonist; angiogenesis; chemotaxis
K5	II	None	Inhibits NK-cell activity; reduces surface MHC class I
K6	II	MIP-1α	Chemokine receptor agonist; angiogenesis; chemotaxis
K8	III	None	Inhibits p53
K9	II	IRF	Represses interferon activity, transformation, inhibits p53
K10.5 (LANA-2)	II	IRF	Represses interferon activity; inhibits apoptosis; inhibits p53
K11.1	I	IRF	Represses interferon activity
K12 (Kaposin A)	II	None	Transformation
K12 (Kaposin B)	II	None	Increases cytokine mRNA stability
K14	II	OX-2	Induces proinflammatory cytokines
K15 (LAMP)	III	None	Binds TRAFs, inhibits B-cell receptor signaling
ORF4	II	CR2	Complement-binding protein
ORF16	II/III	Bcl-2	Inhibits apoptosis
ORF50	III	None	Increases CD21 and CD23 expression
ORF71	I	FLIP	Inhibits apoptosis; activates NF-κB
ORF72	I	Cyclin D	Cell-cycle progression, inhibits Rb
ORF73 (LANA-1)	I	None	Episome maintenance, inhibits p53 and Rb
ORF74	II	GPCR	Angiogenesis, transformation, and proliferation

Expression class I = latent gene, expressed in uninduced primary effusion lymphoma cells, not induced by phorbol ester; class II = expressed in uninduced cells, induced by TPA; class III = lytic gene, expressed only after induction by TPA (includes many structural proteins and DNA replication enzymes).
FLIP = FLICE inhibitory protein; GPCR = G protein–coupled receptor; IRF = interferon regulatory factor; ITAM = immunoreceptor tyrosine-based activation motif; MHC = major histocompatibility complex; MIP = macrophage inflammatory protein; NK = natural killer; Rb = retinoblastoma protein; TRAFs = TNFR-associated factors.

The KSHV K4, K4.1, and K6 genes encode three chemokines: the viral macrophage inflammatory proteins (MIP)-II, -III, and -I, respectively. vMIP-I inhibits replication of HIV strains dependent on CCR5.[122] Each of the viral chemokines partially block HIV infection of peripheral blood mononuclear cells and induce angiogenesis. vMIP-I and vMIP-III are chemokine receptor agonists for CCR8[129] and CCR4,[130] respectively, while vMIP-II is a broad-spectrum chemokine receptor antagonist. vMIP-II is a chemoattractant for eosinophils,[131] binds to both CC and CXC chemokines, and blocks calcium mobilization induced by chemokines.[132]

The KSHV K8 and ORF50 proteins transactivate expression of other KSHV genes during lytic viral replication. K8 and ORF50 inhibit the activity of p53.[133,134] ORF50 (RTA) activates CD21 and CD23.[135] The KSHV K9, K11.1, and K10.5 proteins are referred to as viral interferon regulatory factor (vIRF)-1, -2, and -3, respectively. Each of these proteins inhibits virus-mediated activation of the interferon-α promoter.[136] vIRF1 inhibits MHC-1 transcription and surface expression.[137] vIRF1 and vIRF3 inhibit p53-mediated apoptosis[138,139] and transform NIH 3T3 cells, which can then induce tumors in nude mice.[140] vIRF3 (also called LANA2) protects cells from p53-induced apoptosis.[141,142] KSHV ORF45 blocks the activity of IRF7 and inhibits the activation of interferon-α and -β.[143]

The KSHV K12 locus encodes several proteins termed kaposins. Kaposin A induces transformation of cells; injection of these transformed cells into nude mice results in highly vascularized sarcomas.[144] Kaposin B increases expression of cytokines by activating MAP kinase-associated protein kinase 2 and inhibiting the degradation of cytokine mRNA.[145] The KSHV K14 protein, a homolog of the cellular OX2 protein, stimulates monocytes to produce proinflammatory cytokines such as TNF-α, IL-1β, and IL-6.[146] KSHV ORF4 protein inhibits the complement system.[147] KSHV ORF16 encodes a homolog of bcl-2 and inhibits bax-induced apoptosis.[148] The ORF71 gene encodes a homolog of cellular FLIP (FLICE inhibitory protein) that blocks apoptosis. KSHV ORF71 activates NF-κB, promotes tumor growth, and is required for survival of KSHV-infected lymphoma cells.[149-153] KSHV ORF72 encodes a cyclin D homolog that binds to and activates cdk6 and phosphorylates p27, and stimulates cell-cycle progression in normally quiescent fibroblasts.[154,155] The viral cyclin protein phosphorylates and thereby inactivates the retinoblastoma tumor-suppressor protein[156] and impairs lymphatic function in transgenic mice.[157]

KSHV ORF73 encodes LANA1 that localizes with viral DNA episomes and tethers them to chromosomes during cell division.[158] KSHV LANA1 is required for persistence of the episome in dividing cells and transactivates its own promoter. In addition, LANA1 inhibits the activity of both p53 and the retinoblastoma protein,[159,160] upregulates expression and stabilizes β-catenin,[161] induces nuclear accumulation of hypoxia-inducible factor,[162] and activates c-myc.[163] Expression of LANA in transgenic mice results in follicular hyperplasia and development of lymphomas.[164] LANA inhibits TGF-β signaling.[165] KSHV ORF74 encodes a G protein–coupled receptor that is homologous to the cellular IL-8 receptor; unlike the latter protein, however, the KSHV receptor is constitutively active and induces cellular proliferation.[166] ORF74 protein induces angiogenesis,[167] activates the Akt signaling pathway,[168] and induces proliferation of endothelial cells with lesions that resemble Kaposi sarcoma in transgenic mice.[169,170] ORF74 activates NF-κB and c-*jun*-N-terminal kinase, and upregulates IL-1, IL-8, tumor necrosis factor (TNF), fibroblast growth factor (FGF), and inhibits viral lytic gene expression.[171]

KSHV K15 encodes the latency-associated membrane protein (LAMP) and interacts with TRAFs 1, 2, and 3.[172] K15 suppresses tyrosine phosphorylation and intracellular calcium mobilization, inhibiting B-cell receptor signaling.[173] KSHV encodes multiple microRNAs that target thrombospondin 1 and inhibit TGF-β activity.[174]

Clinical Aspects

Seroprevalence rates for KSHV vary from <5% in normal blood donors in the United States or United Kingdom to 30-35% in HIV-positive homosexual men.[175] Antibody to KSHV is more common in African and Mediterranean populations. At least 85% of patients with Kaposi sarcoma have antibodies to KSHV.[176] The prevalence of Kaposi sarcoma is lower in women than in men, and HIV-seropositive women have a much lower incidence of antibody to KSHV than do seropositive men. KSHV seropositivity in HIV-positive homosexual men is predictive of subsequent development of Kaposi sarcoma.[177] Levels of KSHV DNA are higher in patients with active Kaposi sarcoma or multicentric Castleman disease, than in those in re-

Table 21-4 ■ **Diseases Associated with KSHV Gene Expression**

Gene	Kaposi Sarcoma	Primary effusion Lymphoma	Castleman's Disease
LANA	+	+	+
K12 (Kaposin)	+	+	–
ORF72 (v-cyclin)	+	+	–
ORF71 (v-FLIP)	+	+	+
ORF74 (GPCR)	+	–	–
K10.5 (vIRF3)	–	+	+
K9 (vIRF1)	–	–	+
K2 (vIL-6)	–	±	+

mission, and are also elevated in patients with primary effusion lymphoma.[178] The virus is not thought to be pathogenic in most healthy individuals and can persist in a latent phase for life; however, in immunocompromised persons, it is strongly associated with Kaposi sarcoma. Thus, while infection with KSHV appears to be required for development of Kaposi sarcoma, it is probably not sufficient by itself and other cofactors, such as HIV and impaired cellular immunity, are important. KSHV is thought to be sexually transmitted in homosexual men,[175] and has been associated with sexual transmission and intravenous drug use in women.[179] In endemic populations (eg, Africa), KSHV may be transmitted vertically from mother to child and between siblings and has been transmitted by renal allografts.[180,181]

Kaposi Sarcoma

KSHV has been found in nearly all biopsies of classic Kaposi sarcoma, African endemic Kaposi sarcoma, Kaposi sarcoma in HIV-seronegative transplant recipients and homosexual men, and Kaposi sarcoma in patients with AIDS.[182] KSHV is present in the endothelial and spindle cells of the tumor, but not in normal endothelium.[183] Most of the tumor cells are latently infected with the virus, but 1-5% of the spindle cells in HIV-positive Kaposi sarcoma show lytic KSHV infection. Kaposi sarcoma can be polyclonal, oligoclonal, or monoclonal. KSHV is also present in the peripheral blood mononuclear cells of ~50% of patients with Kaposi sarcoma, and its presence is predictive of development of the malignancy.[175] KSHV has also been detected in the saliva of patients with Kaposi sarcoma, and, infrequently, in semen. Several KSHV proteins are expressed in Kaposi's tissues (Table 21-4). Foscarnet and ganciclovir reportedly reduce the frequency of new Kaposi sarcoma lesions in some, but not all, studies.[184,185] Cidofovir had no effect on treatment of established lesions.[186] In contrast, HIV protease inhibitors have been reported to induce regression of Kaposi sarcoma lesions.[187] IL-12, in combination with liposomal doxorubicin, resulted in tumor responses in AIDS patients with Kaposi sarcoma receiving HAART; responses were maintained with IL-12 therapy.[188] Sirolimus inhibited progression of Kaposi's lesions in kidney transplant patient after cyclosporine was discontinued.[189]

Primary Effusion Lymphoma

KSHV has also been found in primary effusion lymphomas in patients with AIDS.[183,190] These body cavity-based lymphomas of B-cell lineage are located in the pleural, peritoneal, or pericardial space and usually contain EBV as well as KHSV genomes. Some KSHV-positive lymphomas have been found in patients without AIDS.

Multicentric Castleman Disease

KSHV has also been detected in biopsies from some patients with multicentric Castleman disease, especially in the variant known as the plasma cell type.[183,191,192] This disease is usually polyclonal and presents as generalized lymphadenopathy, fever, and hypergammaglobulinemia. KSHV is detected more frequently in biopsies from HIV-positive patients than in biopsies from those patients without HIV. KSHV is present in the immunoblastic B cells of the mantle zone of the lesions.

Other Diseases

KSHV is associated with fever, plasmacytosis, and bone marrow failure after kidney and stem-cell transplantation[193] and has been reported to cause a relapsing inflammatory syndrome.[194] While initial reports detected KSHV sequences in cells from multiple myeloma, prostatic carcinoma, angioimmunoblastic lymphadenopathy with dysproteinemia, angiosarcoma, and pulmonary hypertension, other studies have not confirmed these findings.

Suggested Reading

Bajaj BG, Murakami M, Robertson ES. Molecular biology of EBV in relationship to AIDS-associated oncogenesis. Cancer Treat Res. 2007;133:141-62.

Bashoff C, Endo Y, Collins PD, et al. Angiogenic and HIV-inhibitory functions of KSHV-encoded chemokines. *Science.* 1997;278:290–294.

Bollard CM, Aguilar L, Straathof KC, et al. Cytotoxic T lymphocyte therapy for Epstein-Barr Virus+ Hodgkin's disease. *J Exp Med.* 2004;200:1623–1633.

Brady G, MacArthur GJ, Farrell PJ. Epstein-Barr virus and Burkitt lymphoma.

Carbone A, Cesarman E, Spina M, Gloghini A, Schulz TF. HIV-associated lymphomas and gamma-herpesviruses. Blood. 2009;113:1213-24.

Carbone A. Emerging pathways in the development of AIDS-related lymphomas. *Lancet Oncol.* 2003;4:22–29.

Cohen JI, Bollard CM, Khanna R, Pittaluga S. Current understanding of the role of Epstein-Barr virus in lymphomagenesis and therapeutic approaches to EBV-associated lymphomas. Leuk Lymphoma. 2008;49 Suppl 1:27

Cohen JI. Epstein-Barr virus infection. *N Engl J Med.* 2000;343:481–492.

Coscoy L. Immune evasion by Kaposi's sarcoma-associated herpesvirus. *Nat Rev Immunol.* May 2007;7(5):391–401.

Cosmopoulos K, Pegtel M, Hawkins J, Moffett H, Novina C, Middeldorp J, Thorley-Lawson DA. Comprehensive profiling of Epstein-Barr virus microRNAs in nasopharyngeal carcinoma. J Virol. 2009;83:2357-67.

Delecluse HJ, Feederle R, O'Sullivan B, Taniere P. Epstein Barr virus-associated tumours: an update for the attention of the working pathologist. J Clin Pathol. 2007;60:1358-64.

Di Lorenzo G, Konstantinopoulos PA, Pantanowitz L, Di Trolio R, De Placido S, Dezube BJ. Management of AIDS-related Kaposi's sarcoma. Lancet Oncol. 2007;8:167-76.

Dittmer DP, Krown SE. Targeted therapy for Kaposi's sarcoma and Kaposi's sarcoma-associated herpesvirus. Curr Opin Oncol. 2007;19:452-7.

Dupin N, Fisher C, Kellam P, et al. Distribution of human herpesvirus-8 latently infected cells in Kaposi's sarcoma, multicentric Castleman's disease, and primary effusion lymphoma. *Proc Natl Acad Sci USA.* 1999;96:4546–4551.

Ganem D. KSHV infection and the pathogenesis of Kaposi's sarcoma. *Annu Rev Pathol.* 2006;1:273–296.

Gasperini P, Sakakibara S, Tosato G. Contribution of viral and cellular cytokines to Kaposi's sarcoma-associated herpesvirus pathogenesis. J Leukoc Biol. 2008 ;84:994-1000

Haque T, Wilkie GM, Jones MM, et al. Allogeneic cytotoxic T-cell therapy for EBV-positive posttransplantation lymphoproliferative disease: results of a phase 2 multicenter clinical trial. *Blood.* 2007;110:1123–1131.

Hislop AD, Taylor GS, Sauce D, Rickinson AB. Cellular responses to viral infection in humans: lessons from Epstein-Barr virus. *Annu Rev Immunol.* 2007;25:587–617.

Hum Pathol. 2007;38:1293-304.

J Clin Pathol. 2007;60:1397-402.

Kapatai G, Murray P. Contribution of the Epstein Barr virus to the molecular pathogenesis of Hodgkin lymphoma. J Clin Pathol. 2007;60:1342-9.

Kennedy G, Komano J, Sugden B. Epstein-Barr virus provides a survival factor to Burkitt's lymphomas. *Proc Natl Acad Sci USA*. 2003;100:14269–14274.

Kieff E, Rickinson AB. Epstein-Barr virus and its replication. In: Knipe DM, Howley PM, eds. *Fields Virology*. Philadelphia: Lippincott Williams & Wilkins; 2007:2603–2654.

Kimura H, Ito Y, Suzuki R, Nishiyama Y. Measuring Epstein-Barr virus (EBV) load: the significance and application for each EBV-associated disease. Rev Med Virol. 2008;18:305-19.

Klein E, Kis LL, Klein G. Epstein-Barr virus infection in humans: from harmless to life endangering virus-lymphocyte interactions. Oncogene. 2007;26:1297-305

Küppers R. The biology of Hodgkin's lymphoma. Nat Rev Cancer. 2009 Jan;9(1):15-27.

Kutok JL, Wang F. Spectrum of Epstein-Barr virus-associated diseases. *Annu Rev Pathol*. 2006;1:375–404.

Laurent C, Meggetto F, Brousset P. Human herpesvirus 8 infections in patients with immunodeficiencies. Hum Pathol. 20081;39:983-93.

Leen AM, Heslop HE. Cytotoxic T lymphocytes as immune-therapy in haematological practice. Br J Haematol. 2008;143:169-79.

Liebowitz D. Epstein-Barr virus and a cellular signaling pathway in lymphomas from immunosuppressed patients. *N Engl J Med*. 1998;338:1413–1421.

Lo AK, To KF, Lo KW, et al. Modulation of LMP1 protein expression by EBV-encoded microRNAs. *Proc Natl Acad Sci USA*. 2007;104:16164–16169.

Martin JN, Ganem DE, Osmond DH, et al. Sexual transmission and the natural history of human herpesvirus 8 infection. *N Engl J Med*. 1998;338:948–954.

Milone MC, Tsai DE, Hodinka RL. Treatment of primary Epstein-Barr virus infection in patients with X-linked lymphoproliferative disease using B-cell-directed therapy. *Blood*. 2005;105:994–996.

Moore PS, Bashoff C, Weiss RA, Chang Y. Molecular mimicry of human cytokine and cytokine response path-way genes by KSHV. *Science*. 1996;274:1739–1744.

Park S, Lee J, Ko YH, et al. The impact of Epstein-Barr virus status on clinical outcome in diffuse large B-cell lymphoma. *Blood*. 2007;110:972–978.

Paya CV, Fung JI, Nalesnik MA, et al. Epstein-Barr virus induced posttransplant lymphoproliferative disorders. *Transplantation*. 1999;68:1517–1525.

Ressing ME, Horst D, Griffin BD, Tellam J, Zuo J, Khanna R, Rowe M, Wiertz EJ. Epstein-Barr virus evasion of CD8(+) and CD4(+) T cell immunity via concerted actions of multiple gene products. Semin Cancer Biol. 2008;18:397-408.

Rezk SA, Weiss LM. Epstein-Barr virus-associated lymphoproliferative disorders.

Samols, MA, Skalsky RL, Maldonado AM, et al. Identification of cellular genes targeted by KSHV-encoded microRNAs. *Plos Pathogens*. 2007;35:e65.

Savoldo B, Goss JA, Hammer MM, et al. Treatment of solid organ transplant recipients with autologous Epstein Barr virus-specific cytotoxic T lymphocytes (CTLs). *Blood*. 2006;108:2942–2949.

Shair KH, Bendt KM, Edwards RH, et al. EBV latent membrane protein 1 activates Akt, NFkappaB, and Stat3 in B cell lymphomas. *PLoS Pathogens*. 2007;3:e166.

Soni V, Cahir-McFarland E, Kieff E. LMP1 TRAFficking activates growth and survival pathways. Adv Exp Med Biol. 2007;597:173-87.

Straathof KC, Bollard CM, Popat U, et al. Treatment of nasopharyngeal carcinoma with Epstein-Barr virus—specific T lymphocytes. *Blood*. 2005;105:1898–1904.

Thorley-Lawson DA, Allday MJ. The curious case of the tumour virus: 50 years of Burkitt's lymphoma. Nat Rev Microbiol. 2008;6:913-24

Thorley-Lawson DA, Gross A. Persistence of the Epstein-Barr virus and the origins of associated lymphomas. *N Engl J Med*. 2004;350:1328–1337.

Timms JM, Bell A, Flavell JR, et al. Target cells of Epstein-Barr-virus (EBV)-positive post-transplant lymphoproliferative disease: similarities to EBV-positive Hodgkin's lymphoma. *Lancet*. 2003;361:217–223.

Uchida J, Yasui T, Takaoka-Shichijo Y, et al. Mimicry of CD40 signals by Epstein-Barr virus LMP-1 in B lymphocyte responses. *Science*. 1999;286:300–303.

van Esser JW, Niesters HG, van der Holt B, et al. Prevention of Epstein-Barr virus-lymphoproliferative disease by molecular monitoring and preemptive rituximab in high-risk patients after allogeneic stem cell transplantation. *Blood*. 2002;99:4364–4369.

Wagner HJ, Cheng YC, Huls MH, et al. Prompt versus preemptive intervention for EBV lymphoproliferative disease. *Blood*. 2004;103:3979–3981.

Williams H, Crawford DH. Epstein-Barr virus: the impact of scientific advances on clinical practice. *Blood*. 2006;107:862–869.

Selected References

The complete reference list can be found at www.CANCERMEDICINE8.com

75. Traggiai E, Chicha L, Mazzucchelli L, et al. Development of a human adaptive immune system in cord blood cell-transplanted mice. *Science*. 2004;304:104–107.

83. O'Reilly RJ, Small TN, Papadopoulos E, et al. Biology and adoptive cell therapy of Epstein-Barr virus-associated lymphoproliferative disorders in recipients of marrow allografts. *Immunol Rev*. 1997;157:195–216.

84. Rooney CM, Smith CA, Ng YC, et al. Infusion of cytotoxic T cells for the prevention and treatment of Epstein-Barr virus-induced lymphomas in allogeneic transplant recipients. *Blood*. 1998;5:1549–1555.

85. Haque T, Wilkie GM, Taylor C, et al. Treatment of Epstein-Barr-virus-positive post-transplantation lymphoproliferative disease with partly HLA-matched allogeneic cytotoxic T cells. *Lancet*. 2002;360:436–442.

92. Chien Y-C, Chen J-Y, Liu M-Y, et al. Serological markers of Epstein-Barr virus infection and nasopharyngeal carcinoma in Taiwanese men. *N Engl J Med*. 2001;345:1877–1882.

93. Lin JC, Wang WY, Chen KY, et al. Quantification of plasma Epstein-Barr virus DNA in patients with advanced nasopharyngeal carcinoma. *N Engl J Med*. 2004;350:2461–2470.

99. Perrine SP, Hermine O, Small T, et al. A phase 1/2 trial of arginine butyrate and ganciclovir in patients with Epstein-Barr virus-associated lymphoid malignancies. *Blood*. 2007;109:2571–2578.

101. Bollard CM, Gottschalk S, Leen AM, et al. Complete responses of relapsed lymphoma following genetic modification of tumor-antigen presenting cells and T-lymphocyte transfer. *Blood*. 2007;110:2838–2845.

103. McClain KL, Leach CT, Jensen HB, et al. Association of Epstein-Barr virus with leiomyosarcomas in young people with AIDS. *N Engl J Med*. 1995;332:12–18.

104. Lee ES, Locker J, Nalesnik M, et al. The association of Epstein-Barr virus with smooth-muscle tumors occurring after organ transplantation. *N Engl J Med*. 1995;332:19–25.

107. Chu PG, Chang KL, Chen Y-Y, et al. No significant association of Epstein-Barr virus infection with invasive breast carcinoma. *Am J Pathol*. 2001;159:571–578.

108. Deshpande CG, Badve S, Kidwai N, et al. Lack of expression of the Epstein-Barr virus (EBV) gene products, EBER, EBNA1, LMP1, and LMP2A, in breast cancer cells. *Lab Invest*. 2002;82:1993–1999.

176 Simpson GR, Schulz TF, Whitby D, et al. Prevalence of Kaposi's sarcoma-associated herpesvirus infection measured by antibodies to recombinant capsid protein and latent immunofluorescence antigen. *Lancet*. 1996;348:1133–1138.

179. Cannon MJ, Dollard SC, Smith DK, et al. Blood-borne and sexual transmission of human herpesvirus 8 in women with or at risk for human immunodeficiency virus infection. *N Engl J Med*. 2001;344:637–743.

180. Regamey N, Tamm M, Wernli M, et al. Transmission of human herpesvirus 8 infection from renal-transplant donors to recipients. *N Engl J Med*. 1998;339: 1358–1363.

185. Martin DF, Kuppermann BD, Wolitz RA, et al. Oral ganciclovir for patients with cytomegalovirus retinitis treated with ganciclovir implant. Roche Ganciclovir Study Group. *N Engl J Med*. 1999;340:1063–1070.

188. Little RF, Aleman K, Kumar P. Phase 2 study of pegylated liposomal doxorubicin in combination with interleukin-12 for AIDS-related Kaposi sarcoma. *Blood*. 2007;110:4165–4171.

189. Stallone G, Schena A, Infante B, et al. Sirolimus for Kaposi's sarcoma in renal-t transplant recipients. *N Engl J Med*. 2005;352:1317–1323.

191. Soulier J, Grollety L, Oksenhendler E, et al. Kaposi's sarcoma-associated herpesvirus-like DNA sequences in multicentric Castleman's disease. *Blood*. 1995;86:1276–1280.

193. Luppi M, Barozzi P, Schultz TF, et al. Bone marrow failure associated with human herpesvirus 8 infection after transplantation. *N Engl J Med*. 2000;323:1378–1385.

22 Papillomaviruses and Cervical Neoplasia

Christopher P. Crum, MD ■ Martin C. Chang, MD, PhD

The causal relationship between human papillomaviruses (HPVs) and cervical neoplasia is an accepted fact, and this virus has been the focus of strategies designed to elucidate mechanisms of virus-induced tumorigenesis, to improve the diagnosis and screening of uterine cervical neoplasms, and to exploit the host immune response to prevent these diseases. Technological advances have dictated both the tempo and the direction of this research, which began with descriptive and experimental pathology, progressed to molecular biology, and finally involved molecular immunology in efforts to both implicate the virus directly in producing neoplasia and to unravel the mechanisms of host response and prevention with vaccines.

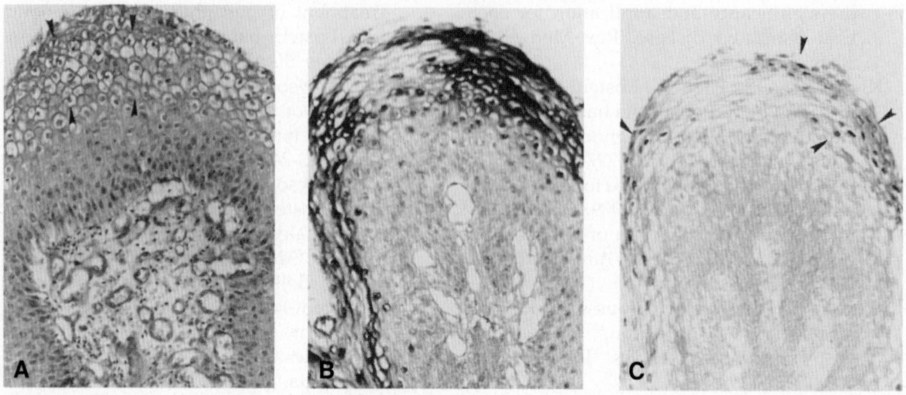

Figure 22-1 ■ Histopathology of a classic human papillomavirus (HPV) infection (condyloma) of the cervix associated with low-risk HPV types (HPV type 6 or 11). (**A**) Morphologic features of HPV infection include nuclear atypia in the superficial epithelial cells with prominent cytoplasmic halos (*arrowheads*). The lower cell layers contain minimal cytologic atypia. (**B**) Appearance following in situ hybridization with a biotin-labeled mixed deoxyribonucleic acid (DNA) probe containing HPV types 6 and 11 (VIRATYPE, Life Technologies, Gaithersburg, MD). The dark staining in the superficial cell nuclei and cytoplasm represents viral DNA and ribonucleic acid produced during viral replication. (**C**) An immunoperoxidase stain for HPV capsid proteins, highlighting several dark-staining nuclei in the superficial epithelium (*arrowheads*).

Definitions, Tissue Specificity, and Mechanisms of Infection and Transformation

Definitions

Genital "infections" are best defined by the presence of clinically or colposcopically identifiable flat or raised lesions that contain papillomaviral deoxyribonucleic acid (DNA), the prototype of which is genital warts. In this instance, infectious virus is likely to be identified within the epithelium (Fig. 22-1). More recently, the term infection has been expanded to include HPV-related precancerous lesions, or even cancers—the term being used loosely to denote the presence of viral DNA. However, integrated viral DNA rather than virions is more likely to be identified in advanced lesions (Fig. 22-2).[1] As is detailed subsequently (see "Risk Factors"), HPV DNA may be associated with no visible abnormality; active, clinically, or morphologically conspicuous infection; and advanced neoplasia (Tables 22-1 and 22-2). The hallmark of significant HPV infection is a morphologic transformation of the target tissue. This is not synonymous with the term transformation as classically applied to changes in cultured cells produced after introduction of HPV nucleic acids. Rather, it defines the morphologic alterations that can be most consistently associated with the presence of HPV nucleic acids. Depending on host factors and HPV type involved in the infection, it may be defined as a low- or high-grade genital precancer, either of which is distinct from the normal epithelium (Figs. 22-1 and 22-2).

Specificity

The squamous epithelium is most susceptible to HPV infections. In particular, squamocolumnar junctions, where basal or reserve cells are undergoing expansion in the form of squamous or columnar cell differentiation (transformation zones), are most vulnerable to the genital papillomaviruses.[2,3] These transformation zones contain multipotent cells that by virtue of their biology or location render them uniquely vulnerable and may be found in the larynx, oropharyngeal mucosa, anus, esophagus, subungual mucosa (nail bed), and conjunctiva. Kreider and colleagues demonstrated that some of these sites are particularly vulnerable to experimental infection with genital viruses.[4] This indicates that the genital HPV types require specific conditions provided by certain locales for infection to occur or characteristics facilitating morphologic transformation once infection has taken place. One component of this equation is the infection of cells that are either undergoing shifts in differentiation or are capable of doing so once infected.[5-7]

Mechanism of Infection

Papillomaviruses are epitheliotropic, circular, double-stranded DNA viruses that infect the squamous epithelium. The interval from exposure to the development of a lesion varies from a few

Table 22-1 ■ **Definitions**

HPV = Human papillomavirus.

CIN = Cervical intraepithelial neoplasia, synonymous with papillomavirus-related squamous intraepithelial lesions. Low-grade CIN (CIN I) is synonymous with flat or exophytic condyloma and exhibits nuclear atypia, principally in the upper epithelial layers. High-grade CIN (CIN II or III) is characterized by atypia in all epithelial layers. HPV-related lesion = Includes HPV infections such as condylomata, but also includes any lesion associated with papillomaviruses, including high-grade CIN and various invasive carcinomas.

Occult or latent HPV = Defined as the presence of HPV DNA in the absence of morphologic evidence of HPV infection (ie, no lesion is present).

High-risk HPV = HPV with documented association with cancer (this is not an assessment of cancer risk and will vary between high-risk HPVs).

Low-risk HPV = HPV with no association with cancer.

VLP = Viral-like particle; pertains to papillomavirion-like particles generated in vitro.

Table 22-2 Genital HPVs and Relationship to Disease

HPV(s)	Associated Diseases
16	More than 50% of high-grade CIN and carcinomas (both squamous and adenocarcinoma)
18	10% of squamous carcinomas, 50% of adenocarcinomas and adenocarcinomas in situ, and 90% of neuroendocrine carcinomas
31, 45	5% to 10% of CIN, squamous carcinomas
33, 39, 51, 52, 55, 56, 58, 59, 68	Less than 3% (each) of CIN, squamous carcinomas
6, 11, 40, 42, 53, 54, 57, 66, 84	Low-risk HPVs, essentially never detected in carcinoma
61, 62, 64, 67, 69-72, 81, cp6108, iso39	Insufficient data to ascertain risk

Source: Adapted from Refs. 14, 28, 55.

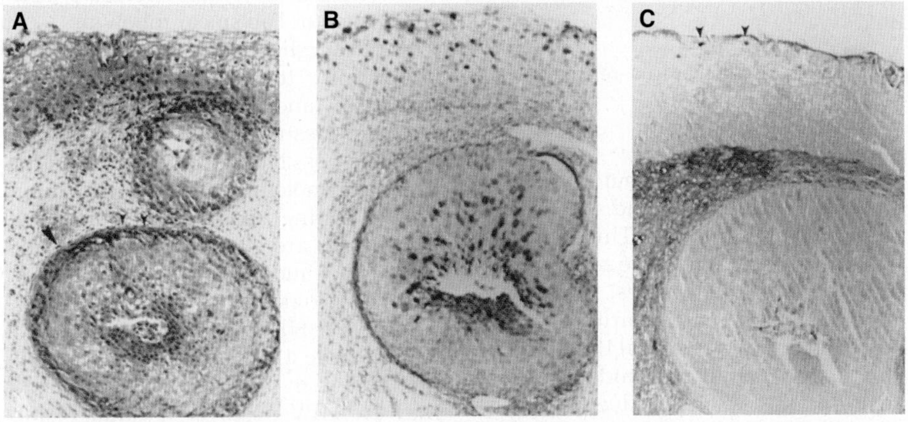

Figure 22-2 Histopathology of cervical intraepithelial neoplasm associated with high-risk human papillomavirus (HPV) types (ie, 16, 31, 33, 35, and so on). (**A**) Lesion involving the superficial and crypt (gland) epithelium (*large arrowhead*). Koilocytotic atypia is present (upper right), but, in addition, nuclear atypia is conspicuous in the lower cell layers (*small arrows*). (**B**) Appearance following in situ hybridization with a mixed probe containing HPV types 31, 33, and 35. Note the similar distribution of staining as in Fig. 22-1B. In contrast to Fig. 22-1C, capsid proteins are infrequently identified by immunostaining, with rare positive nuclei observed (*arrowheads*).

weeks to several months and perhaps longer.[8] It is presumed that the virus gains access to the cervix or lower female genital tract through defects in the epithelium that expose the basal epithelial cells to virion particles.[3] In support of this hypothesis is the demonstration of papillomavirus DNA and ribonucleic acids in basal cells and the observation that experimental infection of the squamous mucosa by HPV is enhanced by disturbing the epithelial surface (and hence exposing the basal cells) prior to exposure.[5] As the cells containing the viral DNA approach the upper layers of the epithelium, the virus replicates and assembles into virions, which can be detected by electron microscopy or immunohistochemistry (Fig. 22-1).[9] Some of the superficial cells in the infected epithelium characteristically display enlarged, hyperchromatic nuclei, with or without cytoplasmic halos (koilocytotic atypia), and the mature virus usually concentrates in this cell population (Fig. 22-1)[9,10] Uncoupling of cell-cycle control also occurs in these cells, the nuclei of which may express cell-cycle proteins (Ki-67, cyclin E, p16ink4).[11,12] The genital squamous epithelium is the principal site for HPV infection, but infection may occur in other sites, as discussed above. Moreover, HPV nucleic acids have been isolated from neoplasms not clearly derived from squamouscommitted epithelial cells, most notably adenocarcinomas and undifferentiated carcinomas (small cell carcinoma).[13,14]

Mechanisms of Neoplastic Transformation

The mechanism by which HPV infection produces neoplastic transformation has been progressively elucidated and consists of at least four components (Fig. 22-3).[3] The first is the direct effects of the viral oncoproteins on the cell-cycle, mediated via interactions between E6 and E7 oncoproteins of cancer-associated (high-risk) HPVs and the tp53 and Rb proteins, respectively (Fig. 22-3). A direct influence of these oncoproteins on other cell-cycle regulators, such as cyclin E, has also been demonstrated.[4] Compensatory elevation in expression of the cyclin-dependent kinase inhibitor p16 results from the above disturbances.[11,12] The second effect is also mediated via viral oncoproteins and consists of abnormalities in centrosome duplication, leading to genomic instability, subsequently reflected in progressive allelic imbalance.[15,16] The latter include alterations in 3p and specific amplifications at 3q25-27.[17,18] The third component is mediated via E6 and consists of telomerase upregulation and a disruption of normal replicative senescence.[19] These events occur ultimately as a function of expression of viral oncoproteins (E6 and E7). A fourth mechanism is the inactivation of tumor suppressor genes by methylation.[20]

HPV and Human Genital Neoplasia

Risk Factors

HPV infection is ubiquitous in the young, sexually active population, peaks in the early reproductive years, is often transient, and becomes increasingly less prevalent with increasing age.[21,22] However, persistent infection by the same HPV type is strongly associated with the risk of a current or subsequent cervical neoplasm.[23] At least 30 HPV types are associated with cervical neoplasia, with a broad gradient of risk imposed by these HPV types. Types 6 and 11 are prototypical "low-risk" HPVs associated with genital warts (condylomata).[24,25] In contrast, type 16 is the prototypical "high-risk" HPV, present in more than 50% of cervical carcinomas.[26] HPV 18 predominates in glandular and neuroendocrine carcinomas.[13,14,27] However, all of these HPVs may be found in women with normal cytology. A variety of other HPVs are associated with cancer at a lower frequency. Currently, these "intermediate-risk" and the high-risk types are combined into a single category. The presence of any HPV, high- or low-risk, does not exclude the subsequent emergence of another HPV infection of different risk, meaning that infection with one virus may serve as a surrogate marker for subsequent infection by a high-risk HPV.[8] Predictably, most HPVs detected in women with normal Pap smears have some association with cancer risk, albeit low.[28]

If a woman is found to harbor a high-risk HPV in her genital tract, what is her risk of developing a high-grade squamous intraepithelial lesion (HSIL)? In general, approximately 15% of reproductive-age women will score positive for high-risk HPVs. The risk of HSIL ranges from less than 5% to over 80%, depending on whether the Pap smear is normal, contains a minor or nondiagnostic atypia (atypical squamous cells of undetermined significance [ASCUS]), or is HSIL.

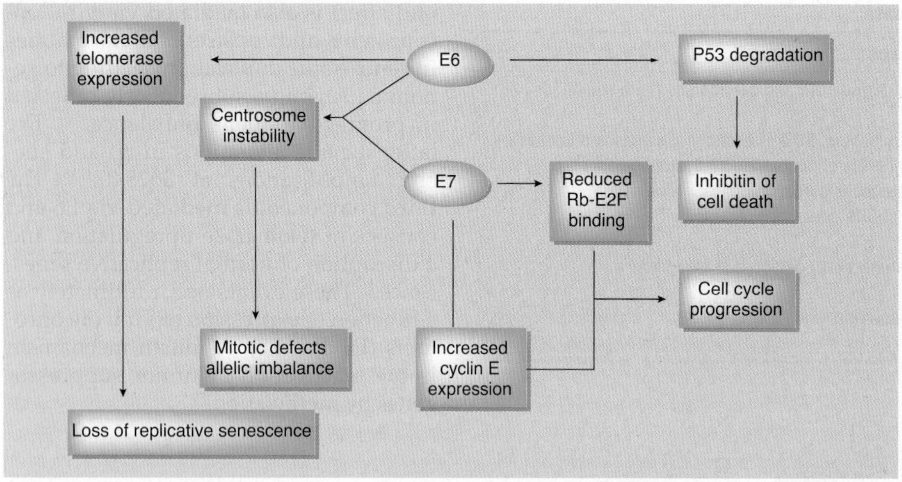

Figure 22-3 Schematic of potential mechanisms of human papillomavirus–related neoplastic transformation.

Repeated detection of the same HPV type—even in the presence of a normal Pap smear—increases the risk to nearly 20%.[23] There is a strong theoretic basis for assuming that intratypical sequence variants influence outcome following infections by HPV 16.[29] However, the use of this information in patient management awaits greater consistency in study design and outcome and a clearer understanding of the mechanisms influencing the relationship between intratypical variants and the risk of developing high-grade cervical intraepithelial neoplasia (CIN) or cancer.

Young, sexually active women are at greatest risk of HPV infection and preinvasive cervical neoplasia, and this risk drops significantly with increasing age. As many as 39% of adolescents may score positive at a single visit.[21] The index of HPV detection drops further with the approach of menopause, presumably signifying a longstanding and effective immune response to the virus that follows the onset of sexual activity and exposure to HPVs in early life.[23,24]

The risk of anogenital neoplasia or HPV infection in immunosuppressed individuals is well documented, particularly in transplantation patients.[30] Human immune deficiency virus (HIV) infection has been the most intensively studied. The risk of HPV positivity and persistent positivity is increased in women who are HIV positive.[31] Furthermore, persistence was 1.9 (95% confidence interval [CI] 1.5-2.3) times greater if the subject had a CD4 cell count <200 cells/µL (vs >500 cells/µL) in one study.[32] The risk of a subsequent squamous intraepithelial lesion is significantly higher in HIV-infected women.[33] The proportion of advanced precursor lesions is not significantly higher, but the risk of lesion persistence is.[32,33] The risk of invasive carcinoma in HIV-infected women is controversial but may be influenced by the level and duration of immunosuppression.[34,35] This is in contrast to gay men, who have a high risk of anal cancer that is greatest in the HIV-infected group, particularly since the initiation of anti-retroviral therapy.[36]

In summary, a multitude of factors, virus and host related, influence the risk of papillomavirus-related anogenital neoplasia before, during, and following exposure and lesion progression.

Applications to Clinical Medicine Background

The prevention of cervical cancer is based on the Pap smear. Because the majority of cervical cancers are preceded by a cervical precursor (CIN) lesion, often by many years, the detection of these precursors is fundamental to cancer prevention. Precursor lesions are recognized clinically on colposcopy, where precursor lesions can be identified following the application of acetic acid.[37] The use of colposcopy has maximized the targeting of lesions for biopsy, and outpatient removal is the usual approach, including cryotherapy, laser, and, recently, loop electrical excision.[38] The latter procedures target the entire transformation zone, removing the lesion and replacing the process of chronic repair with a brief period of reepithelialization. Recurrence after removal or ablation is linked to either inadequate excision or infection by another HPV following therapy. The former is increased when margins are positive. Infection with new HPV types appears to explain why many "recurrences" following ablation for high-grade precursors are low-grade in nature. Reinfection with the same HPV type is uncommon except in immunosuppressed women.

HPV Testing in Management of the Abnormal Pap Smear

HPV testing has emerged as a viable management tool for a subset of women with abnormal cervical cytology. Because HPV is so strongly linked to cervical neoplasia and because high-risk HPV types predominate in the cervix, a substantial proportion of women with a cytologic diagnosis of low- or high-grade precancerous changes will score positive. For this reason, HPV testing is of limited value in this population. However, women with nondiagnostic squamous atypias (ASCUS) present a management dilemma in which the clinician must decide between colposcopy or Pap smear follow-up.

HPV testing offers the additional opportunity to triage the patient into colposcopy and follow-up groups by immediately testing the cytologic sample, which is possible with the newer liquid-based technologies. Newer generations of HPV testing, such as the Hybrid Capture II test, are extremely sensitive and will detect more than 95% of women with histologically proven preinvasive disease.[39] If HPV negative, women with ASCUS have a less than 1% risk of high-grade CIN, in contrast to a 20% risk if they are HPV positive.[39] Similar results have been seen with the management of abnormal glandular cells on the smear.[40] Recently, the test has been approved as an adjunct to the Pap smear for screening women over age 30. The basis for this approach lies in the high negative predictive value of both a normal smear and negative HPV assay, which may permit a longer cytology screening interval. This concept is currently being introduced into and tested in the practice setting, but long-term studies are needed to ascertain the safety of extending follow-up intervals to 3 years.[41]

Surrogate Markers of HPV Infections for Diagnosis

The laboratory management of early cervical neoplasia is based on criteria derived from prior studies correlating the high-risk prototypes (such as type 16) with high-grade squamous intraepithelial lesions (CIN grades II and III).[42] However, the distinction of a preinvasive lesion from a benign inflammatory process may be difficult and can influence management decisions.

Improving the precision of these diagnoses has been the focus of studies designed to identify biomarkers that may simplify the distinction of HPV-related neoplasia from its mimics. Because HPVs disrupt cell function, it is logical to presume that alterations in host genes may serve as "surrogate markers" for HPV infection. Host genes reported to be upregulated in cervical neoplasia include telomerase, p16ink4, cyclin E, Ki-67, MN, and others.[11] Some of these, such as Ki-67, cyclin E, and p16ink4, have practical value in triaging histologic abnormalities.[11,12] As the identification and screening of new biomarkers evolve, it is possible that screening of Pap smears, or cervical samples for host gene alterations, will become standard practice. However, whether such markers will exceed the sensitivity and specificity of HPV testing remains to be determined.

Clinical Management

Management of HPV-related cervical neoplasms continues to be defined and redefined, in step with the methods used for lesion removal. Most women with low- or high-grade CIN on Pap smear or an atypical smear that is HPV positive will be referred to colposcopic examination. Of those who have a negative examination or a low-grade CIN on biopsy, 10-13% will develop a biopsy-proven high-grade CIN within 2 years. Many practitioners will follow patients with low-grade abnormalities and negative colposcopy by repeat cytology in 6-12 months, with attention to this risk.

Biopsy-proven high-grade CIN is typically managed by the loop electrical excision procedure or cone biopsy. Thus, the outcome of a given case will be dependent on the application of the histologic criteria for distinguishing low- from high-grade squamous intraepithelial lesions.[43] Long-term follow-up of all women with cervical abnormalities, treated or otherwise, customarily includes Pap smear evaluations but may eventually include periodic HPV testing as well.

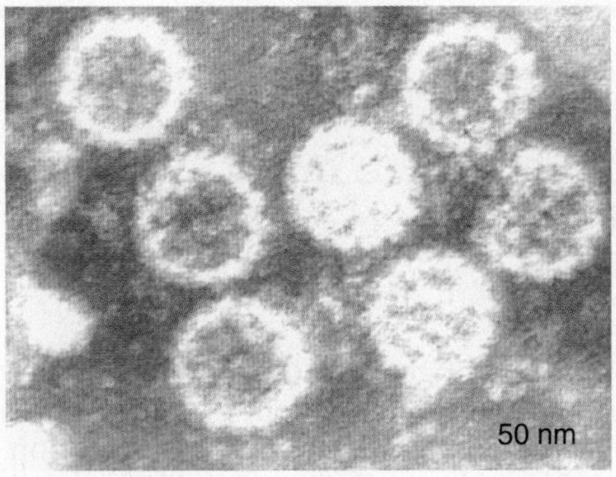

Figure 22-4 ■ Electron micrograph depicting papillomaviruslike particles generated in vitro. *Source*: Courtesy of Ian Frazer, MD, Princess Alexandra Hospital, Queensland, Australia.

Prevention

Efforts to elucidate the immune response to HPV have evolved from studies of fusion proteins and linear epitopes to the production in vitro of virus-like particles (VLPs) (Fig. 22-4).[44-47] VLPs are produced by expressing the entire late region of papillomaviruses in eukaryotic systems, contain the conformational epitopes operative in generating host immunity, and can be used to study (or generate) host immunity.[48,49] This avenue of investigation was the most promising because it offered the advantage of intact particles that were highly immunogenic. Recent large-scale trials have validated the merits of VLP vaccination, demonstrating high efficacy for both preventing infection and lesions attributed to the HPV type(s) targeted in the vaccine.[50,51] Trials are ongoing that test multivalent vaccines containing not only HPV 16 but also HPVs 18, 6, and 11 (the latter two target genital warts). These trials have shown a high efficacy (95% or higher) for preventing both cervical and genital infection by the HPV types targeted in women who have not been exposed.[52] Predictably, efficacies in women who have been exposed are lower, and the overall reduction in HPV-related disease is under 20%.[53] However, vaccine efficacy against non-vaccine types has been recorded to be 27% and cross protection against specific types such as 31, 45 and 52 has been reported. Thus the benefit obtained by the vaccination with HPV 16 and 18 is substantial.[54] Nevertheless, regional variations in HPV types associated with high-grade precursors and invasive carcinomas of the cervix, particularly HIV-infected women, may impose limitations on widespread use of the current vaccine and necessitate expanding the number of HPVs covered.

Selected References

The complete reference list can be found at www.CANCERMEDICINE8.com

10. Purola E, Savia E. Cytology of gynecologic condyloma acuminatum. *Acta Cytol.* 1977;21:26–31.
12. Sano T, Masuda N, Oyama T, Nakajima T. Overexpression of p16 and p14ARF is associated with human papillomavirus infection in cervical squamous cell carcinoma and dysplasia. *Pathol Int.* 2002;52:375–383.
25. Gissmann L, Wolnik L, Ikenberg H, et al. Human papillomavirus types 6 and 11 DNA sequences in genital and laryngeal papillomas and in some cervical cancers. *Proc Natl Acad Sci USA.* 1983;80:560–563.
38. Ferenczy A. Management of the patient with an abnormal Papanicolaou test. Recent developments. *Obstet Gynecol Clin North Am.* 1993;20:189–202.

23 Hepatitis Viruses

Max W. Sung, MD ■ Swan N. Thung, MD

Viruses which selectively infect the liver include the hepatitis A, B, C, D, E viruses, and, more recently, F, GBV-C, TTV, SENV, and NV-F viruses. Hepatitis viruses may cause transient infection which is effectively cleared by host immune responses (A, E), persists with chronic hepatitis, cirrhosis and hepatocellular carcinoma (B, C, D) or persists without associated clinical disease (GBV-C, TTC, SENV, NV-F). Recent studies have indicated that polyviral coinfections may alter the clinical course of these viruses. Table 23-1 summarizes the characteristics of hepatitis viruses.

Hepatitis B Virus

Hepatitis B virus (HBV) is a partially double-stranded DNA virus packaged with a core protein (HBcAg) and DNA polymerase, and enclosed by envelope proteins (HBsAg).[1] Following receptor mediated entry into hepatocytes, the virus enters the nucleus, where the rcDNA is converted to double-stranded circular DNA (cccDNA). cccDNA can remain episomal without integration in host genome; pregenomic RNA is transcribed from cccDNA and in turn converted by reverse transcriptase to HBV rcDNA. Nevertheless, cccDNA is often integrated but in a random fashion in host genome and may play a role in the malignant transformation of infected cells. Protein synthesis proceeds from four open reading frames (ORFs): The envelope proteins (large, middle, and major HBsAg) from the pre-S1, pre-S2, and S gene sequences; the e antigen (HBeAg) and HBcAg from the pre-C and C gene sequences; the DNA polymerase protein from the P gene; and the trans-activator X protein from the X gene. HBeAg contains peptides from the pre-C gene sequence, which permit the protein to be secreted; in contrast, HBcAg lacks these peptides and remains in the cell. HBsAg contains mostly small envelope proteins and is secreted without HBV DNA. DNA replication proceeds via reverse transcription of pregenomic RNA transcribed from cccDNA. It should be noted that HBsAg is secreted at up to 1000 times the rate of infectious virus. The virus itself is not cytopathic; hepatocyte destruction results from immune-mediated responses to viral antigens, leading to hepatic necrosis and inflammation.

In most adult patients, viral infection is cleared by neutralizing antibodies and cytolytic T lymphocytes.[2] Viral infection persists in up to 10% of adults and 90% of neonates following acute infection. The frequency of viral persistence following acute infection is related to age, sex, and immune deficiency. Persistence occurs in 90% of infants under 1 year of age, 30% of children aged 1 through 5 years, and 10% of adults; in men twice as often as in women; and in immune-deficient individuals, such as those with human immunodeficiency virus (HIV) infection, renal insufficiency requiring hemodialysis, or Down syndrome.[3] Patients exposed to large pools of potentially infected plasma, such as those with hemophilia, are also at risk for chronicity.

Chronically infected patients have positive serum HBV DNA and HBsAg. Serum HBeAg may also be present. Clearance of the virus may occur spontaneously, with seroconversion of HBeAg in 10% and of HBsAg in 1-2% of cases per year.[3] Chronically infected patients exhibit a wide range of pathology, from asymptomatic carrier status to mild or severe hepatitis, cirrhosis, or hepatocellular carcinoma (HCC) in various combinations.[4,5] Asymptomatic patients with negative HBsAg, positive anti-HBc and low titers of HBV DNA in the serum may undergo reactivation or exacerbation of HBV infection following chemotherapy or immunosuppressive treatment. It is important to note that in up to 15% of HBsAg carriers, HBeAg seroconversion may be associated with persistent high levels of HBV DNA and with high-grade histologic activity indicative of active viral replication. These patients have been found to acquire a mutation in the pre-C region, which ablates the synthesis of HBeAg.[6]

HBV is transmitted parenterally from infected patients, in whom concentrations in the blood approach 10^{10}/mL (concentrations in body secretions, such as semen and saliva, are only one-thousandth of that in blood).[7] Settings in which HBV may be transmitted include those involving parenteral exposure to infected blood products: transfusions, use of contaminated needles in intravenous drug administrations, sexual intercourse, and perinatal or in utero exposures (mother to infant).[8-11] Infants of HBeAg+ mothers have a 70% chance of infection and a 90% risk of chronic infection.[12] Transmission has also been reported in institutions for the mentally retarded, day care centers, and family environments with close interpersonal contacts.[13,14] The virus has been shown to be quite stable at ambient temperatures, and contamination of surfaces in the homes of chronically infected persons has been documented.[15] The mode of transmission in intrafamilial contacts may be inapparent percutaneous exposure—although oral spread cannot be excluded, because the accidental ingestion of HBsAg+ human serum has been reported to result in HBV infection.

HBV and HCC

Epidemiologic Considerations ■ The evidence for an epidemiologic association between chronic HBV infection and HCC is overwhelming. An estimated 387 million people worldwide are chronic carriers of HBV, and the risk of HCC developing in this population is more than 200 times the risk found in the noninfected population.[16] In low endemic areas, HCC was found in about 0.4% of autopsies; in high endemic areas, where HBV infection is 10 times higher, 20-40% of all cancers are HCCs.

In a prospective study from Taiwan, 22,707 men were tested for HBsAg, with 3454 positive results (15.2%).[17] In the 7-year follow-up, 116 cases of HCC were diagnosed.[18] All of the men with HCC had previously tested positive for HBsAg, except for 3 who had serologic markers of previous HBV infection. None of the HBsAg negative controls developed HCC. HBsAg carriers at especially high risk were those with active infection (HBeAg/HBV DNA+) and those with cirrhosis. In another prospective study of 824 Alaska natives who were HBsAg carriers, the annual incidence for HCC was 3.87 per 100,000 population, accounting for 57% of cancer-related deaths. In the non-carrier Alaska native population, HCC accounted for 2% of all cancer-related deaths.[19] In another prospective study from Taiwan (The REVEAL-HBV Study), 3653 HBsAg carriers were followed for 11.4 years, and HCC was diagnosed in 164 patients. The cumulative incidence rates of HCC were 1.3% for patients with less than 300 copies/ml serum HBV DNA

Table 23-1 ■ **Hepatitis Viruses**

Hepatitis Virus	HAV	HBV	HCV	HDV	HEV
Structure					
Family	Picornaviridae	Hepadnaviridae	Flaviviridae	Deltaviridae	Caliciviridae/togavirus
Size (nm)	28	42	38-50	36	30
Genome	Single-stranded RNA	Partially relaxed double-stranded DNA	Single-stranded RNA	Single-stranded RNA	Single-stranded RNA
	(+) 7.5 kb	3.2 kb	(+) 9.6 kb	(+) 1.7 kb	(+) 7.8 kb
	P1 (structural)	Precore, Pre-S1, Pre-S2	Core, E1, E2, p7 (structural)	HDAg	ORF-1, ORF-2, ORF-3
	P2, P3 (nonstructural)	Envelope, core polymerase, X	NS2, NS3, NS4a, NS4b, NS5a, NS5b (nonstructural)		
Replication	Cytoplasm	Nucleus	Cytoplasm	Nucleus	Not known
	RNA-RNA polymerase	Reverse transcription of pregenomic RNA transcribed from covalently closed circular DNA	RNA-RNA polymerase	RNA-RNA polymerase	Not known
Envelope proteins	None	L, M, S (HNsAg) HBsAg	E1, D2	Yes (major HBsAg from HBV)	None
Capsid proteins	VP1, VP2, VP3	HBcAg	NS2, NS3, NS4	Small and large HDAg (p24, 27)	2
Genomic integration	No	No/Yes	No	No	No
Genotypes	4	8 (A to H)	6 (15 subtypes)	3	3
Serotypes	1	4 (adw, adr, ayw, ayr)	?	?	1
Clinical					
Incubation period	30 days	75 days	50 days	75 days	40 days
Transmission	Fecal–oral	Parenteral	Parenteral	Parenteral	Fecal–oral
Tissues infected	Liver	Liver, blood mononuclear cells	Liver, blood mononuclear cells	Liver	Liver
Virus persistence	No	Yes	Yes	Yes	No
Association with HCC	No	Yes	Yes	No	No
Acute hepatitis	Yes	Yes	Yes	Yes	Yes
Chronic hepatitis	No	Yes	Yes	Yes	No
Progression to chronic hepatitis after acute infection	0%	1-10% adults, 90% neonates	50-80%	2-5% coinfection, 70-90% super infection	0%
Diagnosis					
Acute	IgM anti-HAV	IgM anti-HBc, HBsAg, HBeAg, HBV DNA	HCV RNA, anti-HCV	IgG anti-HDAg (>1:1000), HDV RNA)	IgM anti-HEV, HEV RNA
Chronic	NA	HBsAg, HBeAg,+ HBV DNA	HCV RNA, anti-HCV	IgG anti-HDAg (>1:1000)	NA
Past infection	IgG anti-HAV[a]	Anti-HBs, anti-HBc, anti-HBe	Anti-HCV	IgG anti-HDAg (<1:1000)	IgG anti-HEV
Treatment					
Acute	–	–	–	–	–
Chronic	–	Interferon-α, lamivudine, adefovir, entecavir	Pegylated interferon-α + ribavirin	Interferon-α	–
End stage	Transplantation	Transplantation + HBIg	Transplantation	Transplantation	Transplantation
Prevention					
Pre-exposure	HAV vaccine	HBV vaccine	–	HBV vaccine	Sanitation of water supply
Postexposure	HAV vaccine + Ig	HBV vaccine + HBIg			

Abbreviations: DNA, deoxyribonucleic acid; HAV, hepatitis A virus; HBcAg, hepatitis B core antigen; HBeAg, hepatitis B enzyme antigen; HBIg, hepatitis B immunoglobulin; HBsAg, hepatitis B surface antigen; HBV, hepatitis B virus; HCC, hepatocellular carcinoma; HCV, hepatitis C virus; HDAg, hepatitis D antigen; HDV, hepatitis D virus; HEV, hepatitis E virus; Ig, immunoglobulin; IgG, immunoglobulin G; IgM, immunoglobulin M; RNA, ribonucleic acid.

[a]Also post vaccination.

at baseline, compared to 14.9% for those with serum HBV DNA of 1 million copies/ml or greater.[20]

These two studies not only indicate an association between HBV and HCC, but also strongly suggest a causal relationship (Fig. 23-1). Carcinogenesis is generally accepted to be a multistep process involving initiation, promotion, and progression. The question arises as to whether, despite this overwhelming epidemiologic evidence, HBV infection alone can be responsible for all of those processes.

Mechanisms of Oncogenicity ■ Application of the technology of molecular biology to HBV infection gave several clues regarding the mechanisms by which HBV infection leads to HCC. A uniform mechanism valid for every HCC is still elusive, however. The subsections that follow review the genetic organization of HBV during infection and the possible mechanism or mechanisms by which it can cause HCC.

Integration of HBV DNA ■ The availability of cloned HBV DNA made it possible to detect HBV DNA in HCCs. Epidemiologic studies based on serologic markers were confirmed, because all the HCCs induced by HBV infection contained chromosomally integrated HBV DNA in various forms. The long latency period that elapses between infection

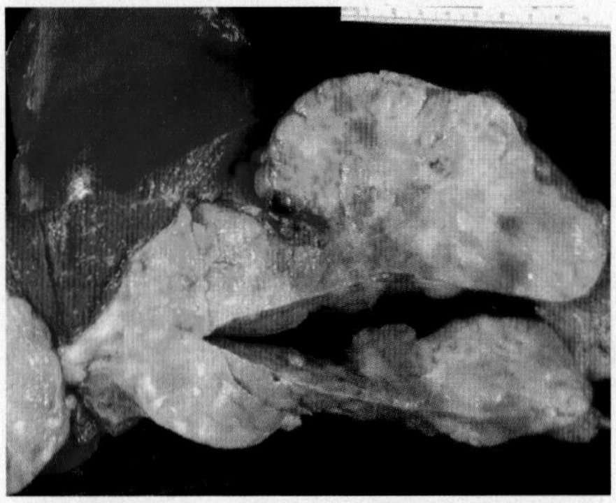

Figure 23-1 ■ Hepatocellular carcinoma in noncirrhotic HBV-infected liver.

and development of HCC makes it very unlikely that the HBV DNA codes for a dominantly acting, classic oncogene. Furthermore, during the latency period, the HBV DNA becomes fragmented and rearranged; thus, neither the inserted HBV DNA sequences nor the chromosomal sites of insertion are uniform in the various HCCs.

Chromosomally integrated HBV DNA may release the growth control of hepatocytes by coding for a factor (similar to the X protein), which activates otherwise dormant genes and protooncogenes, or which silences anti-oncogenes; by inserting HBV DNA sequences that can activate and influence the transcription of cellular genes; by causing chronic inflammation with cell death and hepatocyte regeneration and with fibrosis; and by activating the immune system, thereby liberating cytokines at the wrong time in the wrong place. A comprehensive characterization of gene expression profiles of HBV-related HCC and noncancerous liver samples has been reported using 5′-read expressed sequence tag clusters to a complement DNA (cDNA) microarray system containing 12,393 genes.[21] Altered transcription of multiple genes was noted, including many genes involved in cell cycle regulation and biotransformation, but no overriding trends could be identified.

Activation of Oncogenes, Growth Factors, and Receptors ■ Although the DNA sequences of the woodchuck hepatitis virus are not integrated adjacent to the coding sequences of the *myc* gene, rearrangements of the *myc* gene with a 5 to 50 times higher expression were found in several HCCs. The rearrangements found in woodchuck HCCs are similar to those found in human B- and T-cell leukemias, Burkitt lymphoma, and mouse plasmacytoma.[22]

Mutations and activation of the genes belonging to the *ras* family are associated with a wide variety of human cancers. Mutations in the *ras* genes are not regularly found in human HCCs, but activated H-*ras* and K-*ras* genes have been detected in some HCCs.[23,24] In other tissues, high expression of *ras* genes—as well as mutated sequences—is associated with malignant transformation; the role of the *ras* gene in HCCs therefore cannot be overlooked.

Among the growth factors analyzed in HCCs, insulin-like growth factor 2 (*IGF2*), originally called somatomedin A, seems to be involved in the development of HCCs. The *IGF2* RNAs are differentially spliced: the most abundant species found in fetal woodchuck liver represent the predominant species in both precancerous liver nodules and HCCs in the woodchuck. Furthermore, the pattern of *IGF2* RNAs in precancerous liver nodules is similar to that found in fully malignant HCCs. Thus, the activation of *IGF2* transcripts may contribute to the growth of precancerous nodules.[25]

Because the development of carcinomas can be viewed as a disturbance of the signal transducing system, it is intriguing that HBV DNA is sometimes integrated in a frame next to a liver cell sequence that bears a striking homology not only to the *v-erb-A* oncogene, but also to the DNA-binding domains of the human glucocorticoid receptor, estrogen receptor genes, and the retinoic acid receptor. The inappropriate expression of such genes because of HBV DNA integration might be a contributory factor to the development of HCC.

The HBV DNA integration into chromosomal DNA was found to have a relationship to oncogenes, receptors, growth factors, and (in at least one case) a normal protein, cyclin A.[26] Cyclins A and B are well conserved during evolution and play an important role in mitotic division. HBV DNA is inserted into the intron of cyclin A, and this insertion might influence the progression phase of HCCs.

This brief and by no means complete summation of the insertion sites of HBV DNA leads unequivocally to the conclusion that the integration of HBV DNA can be viewed only as guilt by association; the "smoking gun" has yet to be identified.

Tumor Suppressor Genes ■ Several lines of evidence indicate that HBV DNA insertion into chromosomes may be associated with inactivation of a tumor suppressor gene. First, the long latency period that elapses between infection and development of HCC and the fact that not all infections lead to HCC are compatible with the notion, as seen in retinoblastoma, that one allele is altered genetically, and the other is somatically mutated. Indeed, in children with the Beckwith–Wiedemann congenital malformation syndrome, 10% of the cases are associated with mutations on chromosome 11, leading to tumor formation, including hepatoblastoma, Wilms tumor, rhabdomyosarcoma, and adrenal carcinoma. It has been shown that chromosome 11 codes for a tumor suppressor gene and that the malignant phenotype could be repressed when the normal chromosome 11 was present in somatic hybrids between tumorigenic and nontumorigenic cells.[27] The loss of that normal chromosome led to a reversion to the malignant phenotype. (The suppressor gene in retinoblastoma was mapped to chromosome 13.)

In 45% of HCC cases, alleles from chromosome arm 11p are missing, and in 50% of HCCs, alleles from chromosome arm 13q are missing.[28] In addition, HBV DNA integration was mapped to chromosome 11 in many cases. It has also been shown that the *TP53* gene functions as a tumor suppressor, and in many human cancers, including HCC, mutations occur in that gene, with the mutated gene subsequently acting as an oncogene.[29,30] Furthermore, although evidence—albeit circumstantial—for the role of suppressor genes in HCC is furnished by transgenic mice carrying the *TEAD1* gene (TEA domain family member 1) coding for T-antigen (SV40 transcriptional enhancer factor), the tumorigenic activity of the SV40 T antigen is associated with its ability to bind to the suppressor gene product. In transgenic mice expressing SV40 T antigen, HCC develops after a long period of hyperplasia.[31] Furthermore, mouse hepatocytes immortalized by T antigen were transfected with a selectable gene and HBV DNA. All of the cells in which HBV replicated displayed malignant growth characteristics and were tumorigenic.

It has been well documented that aflatoxin B1 exposure is associated with a specific mutation at codon 249 in the *TP53* tumor suppressor gene in hepatic tumors.[29] Studies of tumor specimens from patients with HCC have also shown a strong association of codon 249 mutations with HBsAg positivity in the serum and HBV DNA in tumor tissue, suggesting an association of HBV with these mutations.

Role of HBx Protein ■ The HBx protein coded by the X gene of HBV has transactivating activity on a number of viral and cellular genes that may be involved in the development of HCC.[32] For instance, the HBx protein has been shown to transactivate c-fos, c-jun, c-myc, EGF and MHC I. It has also been shown to bind and inactivate the *TP53* tumor suppressor protein, and to interact with members of the bZip family and with the P13K p85 subunit of the P13K Akt signaling pathway.[33,34] Its genomic localization is analogous to that of the human T-cell lymphotropic viruses

(HTLV-I and -II, and HIV), that is, it is at the 3′ end of the linearized genome.

Interestingly, other DNA viruses with oncogenic activity also code for transactivating activity. For example, the T antigen of *TEAD1*, the MS-EA protein of Epstein–Barr virus, the IE protein of herpes simplex, and the *tat* protein of HIV (which, despite being an RNA virus, shares some steps in its replicative cycle with HBV). The sequence coding for the HBx protein is well conserved among the various subtypes of HBV and in the woodchuck and ground squirrel hepatitis viruses. Despite the similar genetic organization of the hepadnaviruses, duck hepatitis virus does not contain the sequences coding for the HBx protein, and infection with that virus does not lead to HCC. In many HCCs, viral DNA is inserted near or within the coding sequences of the HBx protein; thus, it is possible that expression of this protein, or of a fusion protein with cellularly coded genes, plays an important role in the development of HCC.[35]

That specific cellular proteins, in concert with virally coded proteins, are involved in HCC is suggested by the finding that chimpanzees infected with HBV display the classic symptoms and signs of hepatitis as judged morphologically in the liver, and by the appearance in those primates of elevated serum enzymes, together with viral antigens and the corresponding antibodies. In contrast to the human disease, however, HBV infection in the chimpanzee does not lead to HCC. Recent studies with HBx-expressing transgenic mice under authentic promoter control showed a high rate of HCC development (86%).[36]

HBV-Induced Hepatocytic Hyperplasia and Necrosis ■ As a consequence of HBV infection leading to HCC: hepatocytic nodules, ground glass–appearing cells (containing HBsAg and displaying hyperplasia), necrotic inflammation, fibrosis, portal inflammation, and, in many cases, cirrhosis, can be detected in the liver. The causal relation between the infection and the liver cell injury has not been elucidated. The evidence that the immune system is involved is only circumstantial.[37]

The availability of vaccines and the production of viral antigens by recombinant DNA technology made it possible to determine that the production of antibodies against HBsAg is T cell-dependent; HBcAg is more immunogenic and elicits antibodies in T cell-dependent and -independent ways.[38,39] HBcAg-specific, functionally competent CD4 helper and CD8 suppressor T cells were detected in chronic infection, but HBsAg-specific T-cells were not found.[40] The T-cell clones that were HBcAg-specific were d-related human leukocyte antigen (HLAdr)-restricted and secreted interleukin-2 (IL-2), interferon-γ, and tumor necrosis factor. For such involvement of the immune system, HBV is obliged to enter the cells of the immune system to present the antigen. There are indications that, albeit rarely, lymphocytes and monocytes are infected with HBV in vivo. Although immune system involvement could adequately explain the cascade of events that lead from infection through inflammation, necrosis, and regeneration, with subsequent genetic changes leading to HCC, the results obtained with transgenic mice indicate that HCC can develop without the contributions of the immune system. Transgenic mice carrying HBV DNA sequences have been produced in several laboratories.[41] The livers of these animals synthesize HBsAg and secrete virus into the serum, but the immune system is tolerant. In one case, a programmed response characterized by inflammation, regenerative hyperplasia, and aneuploidy led to the development of HCC. The incidence of HCC was influenced by sex and age and was directly related to liver cell injury and nonsecreted HBsAg content of the liver cells.

To summarize, several factors, directly or indirectly, alone or in combination, can lead to HCC, but the integration of HBV DNA in one form or another is obligatory in HBV-associated hepatocarcinogenesis.

Primary Prevention

Pre-exposure Prophylaxis ■ Effective vaccines for prophylaxis against HBV infection were first introduced by Krugman in 1981, using inactivated human HBsAg+ serum. The HBsAg particles were subsequently purified from seropositive human sera and used in the plasma-derived vaccine. Advances in genetic engineering enabled the large-scale production of HBsAg protein product by viral expression vectors coding the S gene in bakers' yeast.[42] More than 90% of patients developed adequate levels of anti-HBs (10 mIU/mL) following a series of three injections at 0, 1, and 6 months; in these subjects, protection from subsequent hepatitis B infection was almost complete.[43] Some patients develop "breakthrough" HBV infection despite protective levels of anti-HBs; one of these subjects was shown to have acquired an infection with an HBsAg mutant virus, in which a mutation in the S gene resulting in an amino acid substitution at position 145 rendered the virus insensitive to the neutralizing antibody raised by conventional HBsAg vaccine.[44,45]

Of vaccinated subjects, 90% retain detectable levels and 80% retain protective levels of anti-HBs 5 years after vaccination.[46] The side effects of vaccination include mild pain at the site of injection and mild temperature elevation. No cases of HIV transmission have been reported with either the plasma-derived or recombinant vaccine. However, 5% of vaccinated subjects develop an inadequate response (between 2.1 and 9.9 mIU/mL), and another 5% produce no anti-HBs. Lack of response may be due to immune suppression, such as in subjects with renal failure or HIV infection; to older age (>60 years); or to route of injection (intramuscular is superior to subcutaneous or intradermal administration). In 25% of nonresponders or inadequate responders, an additional dose produced adequate levels of anti-HBs; an additional series of three injections produced adequate anti-HBs in 50-60%. For the remaining 15-25% of nonresponders, other approaches include coadministration of the vaccine with interferon-α or IL-2, and the use of HBsAg vaccines which incorporate pre-S1 and/or pre-S2 antigens.[47]

Despite the development of safe and effective vaccines for HBV infection, the incidence of hepatitis B in the United States has increased. In contrast, a decrease in HBV infection incidence has been demonstrated following vaccination programs in Taiwan and Switzerland. The failure in the United States may be attributable to inadequate vaccination of high risk subjects (only 10% were vaccinated) and the fact that 30-40% of new HBV cases did not fall into the high risk category.[48,49] The current recommendation for a universal hepatitis B vaccination program in childhood should result in the vaccination of all subjects and should effectively reduce the incidence of HBV infection.[50] Such an approach has reduced the prevalence rate of HBsAg+ serum by 99% in Alaska and from 9.8% to 0.7% in children 15 years and younger in Taiwan.[51,52]

The effectiveness of HBV vaccination in the primary prevention of chronic HBV infection and HCC has already been demonstrated in pilot vaccination projects. In Taiwan, universal HBV vaccination was initiated with newborns of HBsAg+ mothers in 1984 and was extended to all children by 1989. The average annual incidence of HCC in children has since decreased to 0.36 from 0.70 per 100,000 children (1981-1986 to 1990-1994).[53]

Postexposure Prophylaxis ■ For prevention after HBV exposure, such as after delivery of a neonate from an infected mother, after needle-stick puncture from an infected patient, or after sexual intercourse with an infected partner, administration of hepatitis B immunoglobulin (HBIg) followed by HBV vaccination has been more than 90% effective.[54] Vaccination without HBIg produced only 70-80% anti-HBs responses.

Blood Donor Screening ■ With the introduction of HBsAg antibody screening in blood donors, the incidence of transfusion-associated hepatitis decreased to 6% from 33% of hepatitis cases over 3 decades. Since the addition of anti-HCV screening, only 0.3% of hepatitis in the United States is transfusion related.[55]

Secondary Prevention

Screening for HCC ■ Locally advanced and metastatic HCC usually responds poorly to anticancer treatments. Early HCC is, however, effectively treated by surgical and nonsurgical modalities, with prolonged survival. It is not clear whether lead-time bias might be responsible, in part, for the survival prolongation.

Because of the high prevalence of HBV infection in certain regions of China, a screening program for HCC was instituted for adults over the age of 35 with chronic HBV infection. The screening tests used were serum α-fetoprotein and liver ultrasonography performed every 6 months. The α-fetoprotein has a sensitivity of 70%, given that up to 30% of HCCs do not secrete it. The specificity of α-fetoprotein depends on the threshold level chosen. For levels of more than 1000 ng/mL, α-fetoprotein is close to 100% specific. For levels of 20-200 ng/mL, false positives outnumber true positives. Liver ultrasonography has up to 70% sensitivity for the detection of HCCs less than 2 cm, but has poor specificity. However, the combination of α-fetoprotein and ultrasonography increases both sensitivity and specificity. Of the 1.3 million people screened in the Chinese program, 500 cases of HCC were detected.[52] A similar screening program was reported from Alaska; it screened 1400 HBsAg carriers and detected 20 cases of HCC.[19,52] A randomized study demonstrating the survival benefit for the screened population as compared with controls has yet to be completed.

Treatment of Chronic HBV Infection ■ For the treatment of chronic HBV infection to be effective, it must eliminate viral replication, resolve hepatic necrotic inflammation, and prevent progression to cirrhosis and HCC. The most effective treatment to date is interferon-α given at a dose of 5 MU daily or 10 MU three times weekly for 12-24 weeks. Meta-analysis of 15 randomized controlled trials showed that interferon-α produced seroconversion of HBeAg in 33% of recipients as compared with 12% of untreated controls.[56] Seroconversion of HBsAg occurred in 10% of treated patients as compared with rare instances in controls. Of patients who clear HBeAg, 65% also clear HBsAg at a mean follow-up of 4.3 years. Of patients who clear both HBeAg and HBsAg, 50-100% also clear serum HBV DNA, with improvement in hepatic necrotic inflammation and normalization of serum alanine aminotransferase (ALT). It should be noted that some patients might clear HBeAg, but still maintain high serum levels of HBV DNA. These patients, who are HBsAg+ and anti-HBe+, may have acquired mutations in the pre-C sequence that ablated synthesis of HBeAg, but that did not affect viral replication.

Factors predicting a favorable response to interferon-α include high serum ALT, low serum HBV DNA, and active hepatic necrotic inflammation.[57] Patients with normal ALT or high serum HBV DNA rarely respond to interferon. It should be noted that Asian patients who demonstrate predictors favorable to interferon, do not respond as well as Caucasian and African American patients.[58] Patients receiving interferon-α treatment, particularly those with more severe hepatitis, may experience a flare-up of hepatic necrotic inflammation, but will not usually require treatment interruption. Prednisone priming before treatment with interferon-α has been reported in pilot studies to be more effective than interferon-α alone. This approach carries the risk of fatal hepatitis exacerbation in cirrhotic patients, and is not recommended as standard treatment.[59,60]

Recently, a number of nucleoside and nucleotide analogs have been shown to be effective and well tolerated in the treatment of chronic HBV infection, with reduction of serum HBV DNA levels and improvement of serum aminotransferase levels. These analogs (lamivudine, adefovir, entecavir), which have been approved by the FDA for the treatment of chronic HBV infection, vary in efficacy, adverse effects and rate of resistance due to the development of resistant mutants. Prolonged administration of lamivudine for 1 year has been shown in a randomized trial to produce sustained suppression of serum HBV DNA (44% vs 16%), HBeAg seroconversion (32% vs 11%), sustained normalization of serum ALT (41% vs 7%), and decreased hepatic fibrosis (5% vs 20%).[61] However, viral resistance in HBV mutants with substitutions in the YMDD motif of the polymerase gene occurred in 38% of patients after 2 years and in 67% of patients after 4 years of lamivudine therapy.[62] Phase III trials of adefovir administered for 48 weeks have shown reduction of HBV DNA levels to undetectable in 39% adefovir-treated subjects compared to 0% controls. ALT normalization was shown in 55% versus 16% and HBeAg seroconversion in 14% versus 6%, adefovir-treated and control subjects, respectively. Lamivudine-resistant HBV infection can be effectively treated by adefovir, although adefovir itself can give rise to resistance at cumulated rates of 0%, 3%, 5% at weeks 48, 96, and 144, respectively.[63] Phase III trials of entecavir compared to lamivudine for 48 weeks have shown higher HBV DNA resolution rates (67% vs 36%), but HBeAg serocoversion rates were similar (21% vs 18%).[64] Entecavir is effective against lamivudine-resistant HBV and suppressed HVA DNA levels to less than 300 copies/mL in 34% by week 96.[65] Other analogs such as emtricitabine and tenofovir have been approved by the FDA for treatment of HIV infection, and has also been shown to be effective against HBV in HIV-infected patients.

HBV reactivation from an inactive HBsAg carrier state, resulting in elevation in serum aminotransferases, increase in serum HBV DNA and reemergence of HBeAg, has been noted in patients receiving chemotherapy, including rituximab, and may persist for up to 1 year following cessation of chemotherapy. Serologic profiles for these patients include positive anti-HBc, positive or negative HBsAg, and low titers of serum HBV DNA. HBV reactivation may result in mild elevations of serum aminotransferases leading to a delay in chemotherapy to acute liver failure. Treatment with lamivudine, starting at least 7 days before initiation of chemotherapy and continued up to 1 year following completion of chemotherapy can be recommended, based on studies that showed efficacy in preventing HBV reactivation with initiation of chemotherapy and at time of lamivudine withdrawal.[66,67]

For patients with liver cirrhosis caused by chronic HBV infection, orthotopic liver transplantation may provide a long-term survival benefit. Recurrence of HBV infection, however, occurs at rates of 40% and 50% at 1 and 3 years following transplantation. Recurrence is particularly high in patients with positive serum HBV DNA at the time of surgery: 83% at 3 years post-transplantation as compared with 58% at 3 years post-transplantation in patients negative for HBeAg and HBV DNA at the time of surgery.[68,69] Long-term therapy with high-dose HBIg post-transplantation reduced HBV recurrence to 35% from 75% and increased survival to 82% from 50% at 3 years post-transplantation.[85] The addition of lamivudine to HBIg has been shown in pilot trials to further reduce HBV recurrence and may improve graft survival. These studies indicate that patients with HBV-related cirrhosis but with negative HBeAg and HBV DNA may benefit from liver transplantation followed by chronic treatment with lamivudine and HBIg.[70]

The effectiveness of interferon-α in the secondary prevention of HCC in patients with chronic HBV infection has been demonstrated. In one study, 101 men with chronic HBV infection were randomized to placebo or interferon-α treatment. Follow-up was between 1.1 and 11.5 years after the end of therapy. HCC was detected in 1 of 67 treated patients as compared with 4 of 34 placebo controls ($p = .013$).[71] In another study, the cumulative occurrence rate of HCC in 313 patients (94 treated with interferon-α, 219 not treated) was assessed at the end of 3, 5, and 10 years. Rates for treated versus untreated patients were 4.5% versus 13.3% at 3 years, 7.0% versus 19.6% at 5 years, and 17.0% versus 30.8% at 10 years ($p = .0124$).[72]

The role of HCV in HCC. HDV ("delta virus") is an RNA virus with envelope proteins that are derived from HBV.[73] HDV infection therefore requires the presence of HBV and can occur concurrently (HDV/HBV coinfection) or in the setting of an established chronic HBV infection (HDV superinfection). Acute HDV/HBV coinfection is self-limiting, with 2-5% persisting as chronic HDV infection. However, acute HDV superinfection can persist in 70-90% of cases, and progression to cirrhosis is more accelerated than with chronic HBV infection alone.[74]

Acute HDV superinfection generally induces an exacerbation of chronic HBV hepatitis, but may induce fulminant hepatitis in 17% of cases.[75] Diagnosis of acute and chronic HDV infection is made by the presence in serum of immunoglobulin G anti-hepatitis D protein (IgG anti-HDAg) at titers of more than 1:1000, or of HDAg, or of HDV RNA.[91] Serum IgG anti-HDAg may persist in low titers (<1:1000) after resolution of HDV infection.[76]

The association of HDV with HCC is not well defined. Patients with HBV-associated cirrhosis and HCC have a prevalence of chronic HDV infection similar to that of patients with HBV-associated cirrhosis without HCC. Chronic HDV infection, however, may accelerate the development of cirrhosis, thereby increasing the risk for HCC.[77]

Prevention is of particular importance for patients with chronic HBV infection because of the aggressive clinical course of HDV superinfection. Treatment of chronic HDV/HBV infection with interferon-α requires higher doses than does HBV infection alone; moreover, the time to response is longer (4-6 months), and the rate of relapse after cessation of treatment (90%) is higher.[78]

Like HBV, HDV is transmitted through parenteral exposure; preventive measures are geared toward safe practices in blood banks, abstinence from intravenous drug use, and vaccination against HBV. No commercial vaccine is currently available for HDV.

Hepatitis C Virus

Hepatitis C virus (HCV) was first isolated from non-A, non-B infectious plasma in 1989.[79] HCV is a member of the family Flaviviridae, which includes yellow fever virus, dengue viruses, and Japanese encephalitis virus. HCV measures 30-60 µm and is an enveloped virus with a single-stranded, linear, positive-sense RNA genome approximately 9.5 kb in length.[80]

The virus contains one large ORF capable of encoding a polyprotein precursor of 3011 amino acids. Structural proteins are encoded at the 5′ end. The 5′ noncoding region precedes the large coding sequence and represents the most highly conserved sequence among the various viral isolates.[81] The 5′ noncoding region contains a series of three short ORFs. The amino terminal of the transcript is cleaved to produce the core protein, an unglycosylated, basic, 19-22 kDa protein (p22). Two putative enveloped glycoproteins of 33-35 kDa and 70-72 kDa are designated E1 and E2, respectively, followed by a small integral protein, p7. The amino terminal of E2 contains a hypervariable region that exhibits significant variation between HCV isolates. Four nonstructural domains follow (NS2 to NS5). The NS2 region is extremely hydrophobic, but its function has not been identified. The NS3 region encodes a 60 kDa protein that contains a viral protease involved in polyprotein processing and a putative helicase enzyme that is probably involved in unwinding the RNA genome for replication. The NS4 region is also extremely hydrophobic and shows 50% sequence homology among the various HCV types. The function of NS4 is not known. The NS5 region encodes a 116 kDa RNA-dependent RNA polymerase that replicates the RNA genome.

Phylogenetic analysis of the NS5 and E1 nucleotide sequences from samples obtained worldwide led to the identification of six major genetic groups and more than 100 subgroups.[82] Genotypes 1 to 3 are distributed worldwide, accounting for 70-80% of HCV infection in Western countries. Genotypes 4 and 5 are distributed primarily in Africa, and genotype 6 in Asia. Response to treatment with interferon-α is poor in patients with genotype 1 HCV infection.[83] Several reports have suggested correlations between these various genotypes and the severity of liver disease, the outcome of interferon treatment, and the development of HCC.[84] In addition, the population of HCV genomes ("quasi-species") shows genetic heterogeneity in infected individuals, which may be the reason that clearing the virus in the host is difficult.

HCV is the most common cause of nonalcoholic liver disease and the leading reason for orthotopic liver transplantation in the United States.[85] Although HCV incidence has declined since 1989 because of blood donor screening, an estimated 38,000 new cases occur annually in the United Sttes.[86] Previously, more than 150,000 individuals were acutely infected with HCV annually.[87] Nearly 4 million people in the United States are currently infected with the virus. The infection is more common in minority populations (3.2% of African Americans and 2.1% of Mexican Americans) than in non-Hispanic white populations (1.5%).

HCV is transmitted through blood and blood products. Risk factors include blood transfusion and intravenous drug use. Sexual and perinatal transmissions are less important routes of transmission. Perinatal transmission occurs more readily when the mother is coinfected with HIV.[88] In approximately 40% of patients with HCV, no recognizable risk factors are present.[85]

The clinical presentation of acute hepatitis C is mild and produces symptoms in only 20% of patients.[89] However, 80% of patients acutely infected with HCV do not clear the virus; they become chronically infected with HCV. Of chronically infected individuals, 20% develop cirrhosis within 20 years, and once the disease is established, they go on to develop HCC at a rate of 1-4% per year.[90] Fulminant hepatitis is rare in hepatitis C.

HCV infection is diagnosed with a third-generation enzyme-linked immunosorbent assay (ELISA) for antibodies to HCV. The test incorporates antigens from the nucleocapsid, NS3, NS4, and NS5 regions.[91] It has a sensitivity of 97%, but false positives require confirmation with a third-generation recombinant immunoblotting assay. In patients with negative anti-HCV because of recent acute infection or immunosuppression, direct detection of HCV RNA with reverse transcriptase PCR is required to assess for active infection.[92] Seroconversion of anti-HCV does not occur until the 9th week following acute HCV infection. It should also be noted that patients who successfully clear the virus may remain positive for anti-HCV for many years.[93,94]

Quantitative methods of HCV RNA, by either PCR or signal amplification, are currently being used to identify candidates for interferon therapy, to monitor viral load during the course of chronic infection and antiviral treatment, and, prior to liver transplantation, to predict recurrent infection in the allografts.[95]

HCV and HCC

A significant proportion of patients with HCC are infected with HCV.[96-98] Patients with well-documented transfusion-related hepatitis C progressed from acute to chronic hepatitis, to cirrhosis, and finally to HCC after 7-23 years (Fig. 23-3). Similar observations were made in chimpanzees years after inoculation with serum from a patient with chronic non-A, non-B hepatitis.

The epidemiologic evidence for an association of HCV with HCC is compelling. Case-control studies from Japan, Italy, Spain, South Africa, and Taiwan have shown that the prevalence of anti-HCV positivity in patients with HCC is substantially higher than in control populations. From 60-70% of Japanese patients with HCC were seropositive for antibodies to HCV. A similar prevalence was reported in Western Europe. HCV RNA and the viral proteins can be detected in both the tumor and the surrounding cirrhotic nodules of the HCC patients. In a prospective study, 246 patients with well-compensated cirrhosis who were positive for anti-HCV by ELISA were followed for 10 years. Of these 246 patients, 56 developed HCC (annual incidence of 2.2%).[99]

The role of HCV in the malignant transformation of hepatocytes is not clear, however. Although 30% of HCCs in HBV carriers developed in the absence of cirrhosis, HCC arising in chronic HCV infection is, with only rare exceptions, associated with cirrhosis.[100-102] Findings suggest an indirect role of HCV in hepatocarcinogenesis, probably through the continuous cell regeneration that results from the chronic micro-inflammatory process, which predisposes hepatocytes to mutations and malignant transformation.[103-105] Case-control studies have suggested a synergism in the development of HCC of chronic HCV infection with HBV markers and a history of alcohol intake.[106] Recent studies in transgenic mice expressing the HCV core protein have suggested that the core protein may have a more direct role in hepatocarcinogenesis by binding to nuclear factors that regulate growth and by accumulating reactive oxygen species.[107]

It should be noted that an increased risk for non-Hodgkin lymphoma and cholangiocarcinoma have been demonstrated in epidemiologic studies of patients with chronic HCV infection.[108-110] Intrahepatic B cells in patients with chronic HCV infection have been shown to be infected with HCV, clonally expanded, and activated to secrete IgM molecules, suggesting a role for HCV-induced B-cell expansion resulting in mixed cryoglobulinemia or non-Hodgkin lymphoma.[111] Several studies have shown an increased risk for cholangiocarcinoma in anti-HCV+ patients.[112,113] The detection of HCV RNA in cholangiocarcinomas further supports the potential role of HCV in the pathogenesis of cholangiocarcinoma.[114,115]

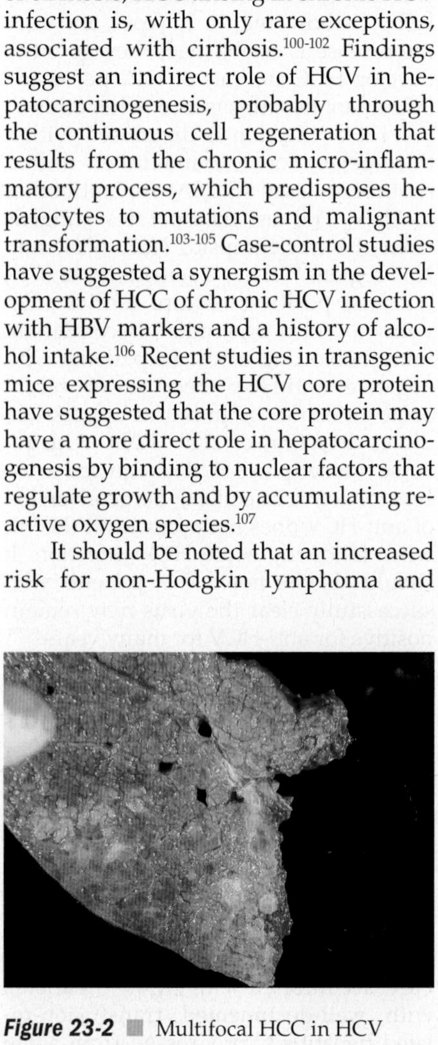

Figure 23-2 ■ Multifocal HCC in HCV cirrhosis.

Prevention and Treatment

Little is known about either passive or active immunity to HCV. Recent studies have shown that reinfection with HCV following a previous infection is quite common.[116,117] That finding suggests that long-lasting immunity to HCV infection is nonexistent. HCV has the ability to mutate rapidly under immune pressure and to exist simultaneously as a series of related but immunologically distinct variants, any one of which can become the predominant strain when a coexistent strain comes under immune pressure.[118] This coexistence of multiple mutants has been termed "quasi-species." Neutralizing antibodies to HCV have been shown to develop, but they are strain-specific and are ineffective against the emerging strains. Major efforts are under way to develop a vaccine that would bypass these obstacles and provide protective immunity.

Before the discovery of HCV, interferon-α was found to be beneficial in patients with chronic non-A, non-B hepatitis.[119] Subsequent randomized controlled trials for chronic hepatitis using HCV RNA and antibody assays have shown that interferon-α administered for 6 months produced disappearance of serum HCV RNA, normalization of serum aminotransferases, and improvement in hepatic inflammation in up to 50% of treated patients.[120] However, relapses following cessation of treatment were common, with increases in serum HCV RNA, elevation of serum aminotransferases, and increased hepatic inflammation. Sustained responses were seen in 6-15% of patients treated with interferon-α. More recently, the combination of interferon-α with ribavirin at a dose of 1000-1200 mg daily has produced sustained responses in 30-40% of patients.[121] Pegylated interferon-α monotherapy, which produces sustained responses in 35-40% of cases, is superior to interferon-α monotherapy.[122] The combination of pegylated interferon-α with ribavirin is currently the standard treatment, with resolution of HCV RNA in 54% 47% of patients treated with pegylated interferon-α monotherapy (p = .01).[123] The duration (6-12 months) and ribavirin dose (800-1400 mg/d) in the combination regimen is modified dependent on genotype and possibly in patients with rapid viral response, who achieve undetectable HCV RNA after 4 weeks of treatment.

For patients with end stage liver cirrhosis from chronic HCV infection, orthotopic liver transplantation may prolong survival. Recurrence of HCV infection is close to 100% post transplantation, but unlike recurrent HBV infection, the clinical course is indolent, and liver cirrhosis may not appear until many years after the surgery.[124] In approximately 10% of cases, however, progression of recurrent hepatitis C to liver failure occurs within a few years because of cirrhosis or massive hepatic necrosis. Fibrosing cholestatic hepatitis post transplantation has also been reported.[125,126] Treatment with interferon-α post-transplantation showed a 28% response in normalization of ALT and a 100% response in reduction of HCV RNA. HCV RNA invariably returned to the pretreatment level after cessation of treatment, however.[127] In studies before 1989, HBIg administration was shown to reduce HCV seroconversion in transplantation patients[128]; however, HBIg is no longer effective because, in 1990, donor screening for anti-HCV eliminated plasma rich in anti-HCV. Based on these data, a monoclonal antibody directed against HCV has been evaluated in an HCV-infected mouse model and is currently in phase I/II clinical trials in patients with chronic HCV infection and post-liver transplantation.[129]

Primary Prevention ■ Prevention of HCV transmission has made great strides since the introduction of HCV screening in 1990 with the first-generation anti-HCV assay. With the refinement of diagnostic assays, the incidence of post-transfusion HCV hepatitis in the United States has been reduced to less than 0.3%. However, post-transfusion HCV hepatitis remains a problem in many parts of the world where donor screening has not been systematic and where contaminated instruments have been used in blood procurement, mass immunization, and surgical or dental procedures. Currently, the major identifiable risk is intravenous drug use with contaminated needles; transmission during sex or birthing is rare. With the lack of an effective HCV vaccine, pre-exposure prophylaxis is not possible. Since the introduction of blood donor screening in 1990, the plasma pools for HBIg and hyperimmunoglobulin are devoid of anti-HCV antibodies and hence not likely to be effective for postexposure prophylaxis.

Secondary Prevention ■ Although interferon-α has been used for the treatment of chronic HCV infection, an international survey also found it to be effective in secondary prevention of HCC. The overall relative HCC risk was 3 times higher in untreated patients than in interferon-treated anti-HCV+ patients and more than 6 times higher in untreated versus treated anti-HCV+/anti-HBc-patients.[130] In a report by the International Interferon-α Hepatocellular Carcinoma Study Group, which involves 21 centers, data on HCC occurrence were collected on 637 patients. Of these 637 patients, 281 received interferon and 356 did not. For anti-HCV+ patients without HBV markers, 29 of 129 untreated patients (20%) and 6 of 116 treated patients (5%) developed HCC.[131] The efficacy of chronic low-dose pegylated interferon-α monotherapy for viral nonresponders is being studied in the Hepatitis C Long-term Treatment Against Cirrhosis (HALT-C) study. Follow-up of 1043 subjects showed no difference between treated vs untreated controls in reduction in liver disease progression (at 3.5 years) or rate of HCC development (at 4.6 years).[132]

Multiple Viral Coinfections ■ The interaction of hepatitis viruses with other viruses in terms of viral replication, chronic liver disease, and development of HCC has generated considerable interest because of the similar mode of transmission of these viruses leading to a substantial group of patients with multiple viral infections.

HIV-HCV ■ Approximately 30% of patients with HIV infection have coinfection with HCV. In high risk groups such as intravenous drug users, the coinfection rate is as high as 73%. Patients with HIV-HCV coinfection have increased HCV viral replication, more rapid progression to cirrhosis and HCC, when compared to patients with HCV infection alone.[133]

HBV-HIV ■ Chronic HBV infection has been reported in 6-14% HIV positive patients. In HIV patients, serum HBV DNA levels and the risk for chronic HBV infection is higher compared to patients with HBV infection alone.[134] There is however no definitive evidence that HBV-HIV coinfection leads to more rapid progression to cirrhosis or HCC, even though the HIV-1 secreted *tat* protein has been shown to enhance malignant transformation of hepatocytes in laboratory studies. HBV, in turn, has not been shown to enhance HIV pathogenesis although the HBV-secreted X protein has also been shown to enhance HIV-1 replication and transcription in preclinical studies.[135]

HBV-HCV ■ Concurrent HBV infection has been reported in 2-10% of patients with HCV infection, and concurrent HCV infection in 5-20% of patients with HBV infection. These doubly infected patients have higher probability of liver cirrhosis and HCC. Although it has been shown in both animal and clinical studies that HCV inhibits HBV replication, the resulting HBV and HCV virological profile can be quite variable.[136]

HBV-HDV ■ Superinfection of HDV in patients with chronic HBV infection has been reported to result in more severe hepatic inflammation, leading to fulminant hepatitis in some cases. However, there is no definitive evidence for increased risk for HCC in doubly infected patients compared to patients with HBV infection alone, although HDV can exacerbate HBV hepatitis and cirrhosis and hence increase the risk of HCC.[137]

HCV-SENV ■ SENV is a single-stranded circular DNA virus-related to TTV, and up to a third of patients with chronic HCV infection have been reported to have positive serum SENV DNA. There is however no evidence that SENV affects HCV replication or the clinical course of chronic HCV infection. SENV also does not affect response of doubly infected patients to treatment with interferon-α and ribavirin.[138]

HCV-NV-F ■ NV-F is a hepatotropic virus-like agent, the DNA of which has been detected in the serum of patients with chronic hepatitis. In a study of 101 HCV-infected patients, 30 had positive serum NV-F DNA and these patients had significantly higher serum aminotransferase levels and higher Knodell histologic activity scores compared to the patients without serum NV-F DNA.[139] It is speculated that NV-F infection in HCV patients may lead to increased hepatic inflammation and may account for the hepatitis "flares" seen in these patients.

Selected References

The complete reference list can be found at www.CANCERMEDICINE8.com

1. Pugh JC, Bassendine MF. Molecular biology of hepadnavirus replication. *Br Med Bull.* 1990;46:329–353.
17. Beasley RP, Hwang LY, Lin CC, Chien CS. Hepatocellular carcinoma and hepatitis B virus. A prospective study of 22,707 men in Taiwan. *Lancet.* 1981;2:1129–1133.
18. Beasley RP. Hepatitis B virus. The major etiology of hepatocellular carcinoma. *Cancer.* 1988;61:1842–1856.
19. McMahon BJ, Alberts SR, Wainwright RB, et al. Hepatitis B sequelae. Prospective study in 1400 hepatitis B surface antigen-positive Alaska native carriers. *Arch Intern Med.* 1990;150:1051–1054.
20. Chen CJ, Yang HI, Su Jun, et al. Risk of hepatocellular carcinoma across a biological gradient of serum hepatitis B virus DNA level. *J Am Med Assoc.* 2006;295:65–73.
21. Xu XR, Huang J, Xu ZG, et al. Insight into hepatocellular carcinogenesis at transcriptome level by comparing gene expression profiles of hepatocellular carcinoma with those of corresponding noncancerous liver. *Proc Natl Acad Sci USA.* 2001;98:150–194.
29. Hsu IC, Metcalf RA, Sun T, et al. Mutational hotspot in the p53 gene in human hepatocellular carcinomas. *Nature.* 1991;350:427–428.
30. Bressac B, Kew M, Wands J, Ozturk M. Selective G to T mutations of p53 gene in hepatocellular carcinoma from southern Africa. *Nature.* 1991;350:429–431.
32. Colgrove R, Simon G, Ganem D. Transcriptional activation of homologous and heterologous genes by the hepatitis B virus X gene product in cells permissive for viral replication. *J Virol.* 1989;63:4019–4026.
34. Andrisani OM, Barnabas S. The transcriptional function of the hepatitis B virus X protein and its role in hepatocarcinogenesis. *Int J Oncol.* 1999;15:373–379.
51. Harpaz R, McMahon BJ, Margolis HS, et al. Elimination of new chronic hepatitis B virus infections: results of the Alaska immunization program. *J Infect Dis.* 2000;181:413–418.
52. Ni YH, Chang MH, Huang LM, et al. Hepatitis B virus infection in children and adolescents in a hyperendemic area. Fifteen years after mass hepatitis B vaccination. *Ann Intern Med.* 2001;135:796–800.
53. Chang MH, Chen CJ, Lai MS, et al. Universal hepatitis B vaccination in Taiwan and the incidence of hepatocellular carcinoma in children. *N Engl J Med.* 1997;336:1855–1859.
55. Alter HJ, Houghton M. Clinical Medical Research Award. Hepatitis C virus and eliminating post-transfusion hepatitis. *Nat Med.* 2000;6:1082–1086.
59. Perrillo RP, Schiff ER, Davis GL, et al. A randomized, controlled trial of interferon alfa-2b alone and after prednisone withdrawal for the treatment of chronic hepatitis B. The Hepatitis Interventional Therapy Group. *N Engl J Med.* 1990;323:295–301.
61. Dienstag JL, Schiff ER, Wright TL, et al. Lamivudine as initial treatment for chronic hepatitis B in the United States. *N Engl J Med.* 1999;341:1256–1263.
62. Liaw RF. Impact of YMDD mutations during lamivudine therapy in patients with chronic hepatitis B. *Antivir Chem Chemother.* 2001;12(suppl 1):67–71.
63. Hadziyannis S, Tassopoulos N, Chang TT, et al. Adefovir dipoxil (ADV) demonstrated sustained efficacy in HBeAg-chronic hepatitis B (CHB) patients [abstract 492]. *J Hepatol.* 2005;42:178.
64. Chang TT, Gish RG, de Man R, et al. A comparison of entecavir and lamivudine for HBeAg-positive chronic hepatitis B. *N Engl J Med.* 2006;354:1001–1010.
65. Sherman M, Yurdaydin C, Sollano J, et al. Entecavir for treatment of lamivudine-refractory, HBeAg-positive chronic hepatitis B. *Gastroenterol.* 2006;130:2039–2049.
66. Jang JW, Choi JY, Bae SH, et al. A randomized controlled study of preemptive lamivudine in patients receiving tran-

sarterial chemo-lipiodolization. *Hepatol.* 2006:43:233–240.
70. Rao W, Wu X, Xiu D. Lamivudine or lamivudine combined with hepatitis B immunoglobulin in prophylaxis of hepatitis B recurrence after liver transplantation: a metaanalysis. *Transpl Int.* 2008 Nov 6.
71. Lin SM, Sheen IS, Chien RN, et al. Long-term beneficial effect of interferon therapy in patients with chronic hepatitis B virus infection. *Hepatology.* 1999;29:971–975.
72. Ikeda K, Saitoh S, Suzuki Y, et al. Interferon decreases hepatocellular carcinogenesis in patients with cirrhosis caused by the hepatitis B virus: a pilot study. *Cancer.* 1998;82:827–835.
77. Benvegnu L, Fattovich G, Noventa F, et al. Concurrent hepatitis B and C virus infection and risk of hepatocellular carcinoma in cirrhosis. A prospective study. *Cancer.* 1994;74:2442–2448.
93. Gretch D, Lee W, Corex L. Use of aminotransferase, hepatitis C antibody, and hepatitis C polymerase chain reaction RNA assays to establish the diagnosis of hepatitis C virus infection in a diagnostic virology laboratory. *J Clin Microbiol.* 1992;30:2145–2149.
94. Takaki A, Wiese M, Maertens G, et al. Cellular immune responses persist and humoral responses decrease two decades after recovery from a single-source outbreak of hepatitis C. *Nat Med.* 2000;6:578–582.
95. Iino S, Komata M, Kumada H, et al. Quantification of HCV RNA by branched DNA probe assay. *J Med Pharm Sci.* 1993;2:327.
97. Saito I, Miyamura T, Ohbayashi A, et al. Hepatitis C virus infection is associated with the development of hepatocellular carcinoma. *Proc Natl Acad Sci USA.* 1990;87:6547–6549.
101. Levrero M, Tagger A, Balsano C, et al. Antibodies to hepatitis C virus in patients with hepatocellular carcinoma. *J Hepatol.* 1991;12:60–63.
103. Theise ND, Lapook JD, Thung SN. A macroregenerative nodule containing multiple foci of hepatocellular carcinoma in a noncirrhotic liver. *Hepatology.* 1993;17:993–996.
104. Theise ND, Schwartz M, Miller C, Thung SN. Macroregenerative nodules and hepatocellular carcinoma in 44 sequential adult liver explants with cirrhosis. *Hepatology.* 1992;16:949–955.
105. Tarao K, Ohkawa S, Shimizu A, et al. Significance of hepatocellular proliferation in the development of hepatocellular carcinoma from anti-hepatitis C virus–positive cirrhotic patients. *Cancer.* 1994;73:1149–1154.
106. Tagger A, Donato F, Ribero ML, et al. Case-control study on hepatitis C virus (HCV) as a risk factor for hepatocellular carcinoma: the role of HCV genotypes and the synergism with hepatitis B virus and alcohol. Brescia HCC Study. *Int J Cancer.* 1999;81:695–699.
107. Koike K, Moriya K, Kimura S. Role of hepatitis C virus in the development of hepatocellular carcinoma: transgenic approach to viral hepatocarcinogenesis. *J Gastroenterol Hepatol.* 2002;17:394–400.
112. Shaib YH, El-Serag HB, Davila JA, et al. Risk factors of intrahepatic cholangiocarcinoma in the United States: a case-control study. *Gastroenterology.* 2005;128:620–626.
118. Ogata NR, Alter HJ, Miller RH, Purcell RH. Nucleotide sequence and mutation rate of the H strain of hepatitis C virus. *Proc Natl Acad Sci USA.* 1991;88: 3392–3396.
119. Hoofnagle JH, Mullen KD, Jones DB, et al. Treatment of chronic non-A non-B hepatitis with recombinant human α interferon. *N Engl J Med.* 1986;315:1575–1578.
120. Davis GL, Balart LA, Schif ER, et al. Treatment of chronic hepatitis C with recombinant interferon alfa. A multicenter randomized, controlled trial. *N Engl J Med.* 1989;321:1501–1506.
128. Feray C, Gigou M, Didier S, et al. Incidence of hepatitis C in patients receiving different preparations of hepatitis B immunoglobulins after liver transplantation. *Ann Intern Med.* 1998;128:810–816.
129. Ilan E, Arazi J, Nussbaum O, et al. The hepatitis C virus (HCV)-Trimera mouse: a model for evaluation of agents against HCV. *J Infect Dis.* 2002;185:153–161.
130. Bonino F, Oliveri F, Colombatto P, Brunetto MR. Impact of interferon-α therapy on the development of hepatocellular carcinoma in patients with liver cirrhosis: results of an international survey. *J Viral Hepat.* 1997;4(suppl 2):79–82.
131. International Interferon-a Hepatocellular Carcinoma Study Group. Effect of interferon-α on progression of cirrhosis to hepatocellular carcinoma: a retrospective cohort study. *Lancet.* 1998;351:1535–1539.
132. Lok AS, Seeff LB, Morgan TR, et al. Incidence of hepatocellular carcinoma and associated risk factors in hepatitis C-related advanced liver disease. *Gastroenterology.* 2009 Jan;136:138–148.
133. Puoti M, Bruno R, Soriano V, et al. Hepatocellular carcinoma in HIV-infected patients with chronic hepatitis C. *Am J Gastroenterol.* 2001;96:179–183.
134. Gilson RJ, Hawkins AE, Beecham MR, et al. Interactions between HIV and hepatitis B virus in homosexual men: effects on the natural history of infection. *AIDS.* 1997;11:597–606.
135. Gomez-Gonzalo M, Carretero M, Rullas J, et al. The hepatitis B virus X protein induces HIV-1 replication and transcription in synergy with T-cell activation signals: functional roles of NF-kappaB/NF-AT and SPI-binding sites in the HIV-1 long terminal repeat promoter. *J Biol Chem.* 2001;276:35435–35443.
136. Chu CM, Yeh CT, Liaw YF. Low-level viremia and intracellular expression of hepatitis B surface antigen (HBsAg) in HBsAg carriers with concurrent hepatitis C virus infection. *J Clin Microbiol.* 1998;36:2084–2086.
137. Fattovich G, Giustina G, Christensen E, et al. Influence of hepatitis delta virus infection on morbidity and mortality in compensated cirrhosis type B. The European Concerted Action on Viral Hepatitis (Eurohep). *Gut.* 2000;46:420–426.
138. Dai CY, Chuang WL, Chang WY, et al. Co-infection of SENV-D among chronic hepatitis C patients treated with combination therapy with high-dose interlferon-alfa and ribavirin. *World J Gastroenterol.* 2005;11:4241–4245.
139. Yeh CT, Hsu CW, Chuang ML, et al. Impact of novel hepatotropic virus-like agent NV-F during chronic hepatitis C virus infection. *J Infect Dis.* 2008; 198:1742–1748.

24 Parasites

Piero Mustacchi, MD, ScD [Hon]

The intensity of parasitic infection frequently correlates with its prevalence.[1] Thus, when relatively uncommon neoplasms are noted with undue frequency in countries with a high prevalence of parasitic diseases, the question of the role of parasites arises. In this respect, the two most intriguing examples are probably the relationships of schistosomiasis to bladder cancer and that of malaria to Burkitt lymphoma. Classic references have been presented before.[2]

Schistosomiasis and Cancer of the Bladder

Epidemiologic Aspects

The data associating schistosorniasis (frequently called bilharzia in Africa) and neoplasia are overwhelming, but explanations for this association remain specuiative.[3,4] Data published so far have been retrospective and, therefore, have yielded only relative frequencies, with their well-known inherent limitations.

Geography

In Africa, squamous cell carcinoma of the bladder is greatly overrepresented among the fellaheen of Egypt and the Africans of Mozambique, Zimbabwe, and Zambia (formerly Rhodesia), all countries where *Schistosoma haematobium* is endemic. An age-standardized mortality rate for bladder cancer of 10.8 per 100,000 males places Egypt at the top of the list of the 54 countries providing data for the 1987 WHO database.[5] Observations made in Ghana and Tanzania[6] suggest an association, however, and none emerges from Tanzania, Uganda, or French-speaking West Africa, where *S. haematobium* is endemic but bladder cancer apparently is rare.

No prospective study measuring the risk of developing bladder cancer in infected and uninfected persons is yet available. Although differences in relative frequencies may reflect differences in risk, the interplay of other factors, such as geopolitical variations in case finding, can result in spurious differences and erroneous associations. If the postulated association is correct, one of several conditions must obtain: the worm (1) produces a carcinogen, (2) carries a virus, or (3) is cocarcinogenic to some other insult. In this case, there are many unanswered questions regarding geographic differences in vesical cancer observed where schistosomiasis is endemic. These range from whether there is geographic uniformity in the host's reaction to infection to whether other environmental variables (such as the bright food coloring used in the candy popular in the Nile delta) interact and are additionally responsible for vesical neoplasia.

Age and Sex

Egyptian data from the Alexandria Cancer Registry disclose a 5-fold sex-linked disparity in the annual age-adjusted incidence rate of bladder cancer: 19.2 per 10^5 males and 3.6 per 10^5 females.[5] Bilharzial (ie, schistosomal) bladder cancer (BBC) attacks men preferentially and seems to be especially common in those with HLA-B16 and Cwt antigens.[7] In Egyptian hospital series, the mean age of patients is 41 years, about 5 years younger than that of patients with non-BBC,[5,8] and the sex ratio ranges from 5:1 to 9:1. Possibly reflecting the lower frequency of schistosomal infestation prevalent in the early 1990s (as compared with the 1960s), mean patient age increased from 47 ± 13.6 to 53 ± 12.2 years.[9] In Ghana, 5 of 13 males with bladder cancer came to autopsy before age 36 years.[10] In Mozambique, too, BBC occurs earlier in life, but the sex ratio (MIF 1.75:1) is not as striking as in Egypt.[11] Whether this difference from Egypt reflects a greater susceptibility of females in Mozambique, a reduced risk in males, or simply a vagary resulting from underreporting remains unresolved.

Urban/Rural Distribution

In Egypt, additional support for an association with bilharzial infection can be found in the relative paucity of bladder cancer cases (10 among 33 cancers) reported from hospitals serving the nonparasitized Italian and Greek residents of metropolitan Cairo, compared with the large number observed in hospitals attending to Egyptian peasants (45 among 74 cancers).[7,9] In Egypt, clinical history of urinary schistosomiasis is associated with increased bladder cancer risk: this explains some 16% of the bladder cancer cases.[12]

Frequency and Severity of Infection

The association of bladder cancer with schistosomal infection seems to become stronger with longer-standing and more severe infection.[8] In the Nile delta, *Schistosoma* ova in the urine correlate with bladder status: cytologically benign epithelium, squamous metaplasia, benign tumors, and, finally, cancer.

The severity of infection tends to rise sharply with opportunities for exposure. In Egypt, it is directly related to the extent of perennial irrigation through canals, which creates a constant risk of reinfection, and inversely related to control measures and availability of safe and effective therapy. In Ghana, where different agricultural conditions prevail, schistosomiasis is essentially a prepubertal disease, and only a small proportion of the population is infested, as compared with the extent in Egypt. Comparative studies in these two countries indicate a rather clear and direct relationship between parasitic infection with *S. haematobium* and frequency of bladder cancer.[10] Thus, the peculiar agricultural setting of the Nile valley singles out this region for a dose–response relationship not encountered in other parts of Africa.

Variability in Diagnostic Criteria of Schistosomiasis

Many reports of schistosomal bladder cancer fail to define the diagnostic criteria for infection. Ruling out a diagnosis of schistosomiasis because of the absence of ova in the centrifuged urine specimen would be unrealistic in many cases of contracted bladder due to bilharzial fibrosis, in which the dense scar tissue precludes shedding of ova from the submucosa. Conversely, sound epidemiologic practices require that when evidence of infestation in ova-negative bilharzial patients is sought by rectal scrapings or radiographic studies, the same diagnostic refinements be used in every member of the group studied.

One study conducted in the Nile delta concluded that only 11% of the men and 3% of the women could be considered infected, on the basis of presence of schistosomal ova in the initial urinalysis. On the basis of this diagnostic criterion, only a suggestive association of infection and cancer of the bladder was demonstrated (p = .04). By expanding the criteria for diagnosis of schistosomiasis to include the presence of ova in any centrifuged urine sample, and other evidence of infection obtained by endoscopic or radiologic procedures, the prevalence of infection was increased 3-fold. After correcting for age, sex, and residence, the relative risk of developing bladder cancer among the bilharzial patients was double that in the comparison population group. By adopting the expanded definition of schistosomiasis, the probability that the association of infection and cancer occurred by chance was much lower ($p = .042$).[10]

Geographic Variability in Schistosomal Virulence

Within East Africa, a coastal strain of *S. haematobium* is more virulent than that at Lake Victoria, where infested bladders do not show severe changes.

When *Schistosoma mansoni* is considered, the Brazilian and Puerto Rican strains are the most virulent, as measured by the production of liver disease in infested mice. Under the same experimental conditions, the Egyptian strain caused the least liver damage and the Tanzanian strain produced the fewest eggs.[13] Variability in *S. mansoni* virulence has been cited to explain the high frequency of liver cancer in Mozambique but not in Egypt, even though schistosomal liver cirrhosis is common in both countries. This type of explanation is, at best, tentative because other, as yet undetected, environmental carcinogenic hazards can be at work.

Progression of Bilharzial Bladder Cancer

Although traditionally considered a disease of slow growth rate with a tendency to recur locally rather than to metastasize, BBC often shows a high proliferative index and a low rate of apoptosis. An over representation of the protein encoded by the *MDM2* gene found in the majority of the studied cases, may account for the frequent inactivation of the *TP53* control pathway observed in BBC, thereby underlining the accumulation of DNA damage and the aggressive clinical course of BBC.[14]

Monosomy 9 may be an early chromosomal change in the urothelium of the bilharzial infected bladder, and a predictor of incipient carcinoma in patients with bilharzial cystitis.[15]

Role of Urinary Infection

Although the causative role of schistosomiasis is now accepted, various associated factors have been proposed in the induction of BBC[16] especially infection with the liberation of N-nitroso compounds.[16] In Egypt, but not in Mozambique, bladder calculi and incrustations of vesical ulcers are frequent complications of schistosomal infection. The experimental work linking some nitroso products of bacterial metabolism to carcinogenesis may perhaps reinvigorate the old carcinogenic hypothesis of the early Egyptian workers who implicated "alkaline urine." In fact, the urinary excretion of nitrite and N-nitroso compounds is increased in patients with *S. haematobium* infection.[17] The prevalence of urinary nitrites found in symptomatic active bilharzial cystitis increases in patients who also have schistosomal bladder cancer.[18,19] In noncancerous bladders, infection with *S. haematobium* increases significantly the ability of the vesical bacterial flora to reduce nitrates to the nitrite precursors of N-nitroso compounds.[20]

Compared to controls, schistosome-infested patients have a 3-fold higher urinary nitrate and the proposition that this is due to the ability of their inflammatory cells to synthesize nitric oxide, seems plausible.[21,22] The endogenous production of nitric oxide and alkylation of DNA by N-nitroso compounds formed by reaction of nitrite with urinary secondary amines, could account for the significant excess of transitions at CpG dinucleotides in the *TP53* gene in BBC as compared with the nonbilharzial counterpart.[23] Moreover, inactivation of *TP53* could be responsible for the conversion of a low-grade tumor to an invasive one.[24,25] The detection of multiple *TP53* mutations in invasive BBC of the squamous cell variety is suggestive of the involvement of a carcinogenic agent with maintenance of preferential activation of the H-*ras* gene.[26] On the other hand, in bladder cancer, the presence or absence of schistosomal ova does not seem to affect the expression of CD44.[27]

Urinary tract infection has been associated with increased chromosomal breakage in the urothelium. The frequency of micronuclei is reduced significantly after antihelminthic treatment.[28] Urothelial carcinogenesis in the presence of schistosomiasis seems to proceed along different pathways from those linked to cigarette smoking, which appears to have a significant impact on mutation of the *TP53* gene with A:T to G:C transitions, that are not observed in BBC.[29] The latter also displays p16^{INK4} alterations more frequently than other bladder tumors.[30]

Carbohydrate antigen 19-9 (CA 19-9) seems to be elevated only in transitional cell carcinoma of the schistosomal bladder, but not in the other histologic varieties.[31]

Apoptosis in Schistosomal Bladder Cancer

Certain genes, such as Bcl-2, contribute to oncogenesis by suppressing apoptosis. In the presence of schistosomiasis Bcl-2 was significantly expressed in squamous cell bladder cancer as compared with the transitional cell cancer[32] but this was not confirmed in another study.[33]

Pathology of Benign and Preneoplastic Schistosomal Bladder Lesions

An intense, delayed-sensitivity reaction is elicited by viable *Schistosoma* eggs plugging the vesical venules leading to tubercules, nodules, or polyps. In bilharzial cystitis, the papilloma, covered as it is by one or two layers of flattened cells, which merge with the transitional epithelium at its base, is essentially a granuloma and not a precancerous lesion. With recurrent inflammation and fibrosis, some transitional epithelial cells become sequestered in the vesical submucosa and acquire a globular arrangement around a central cavity. When they open into the bladder cavity, the cystic formations become pseudoglandular. These structures, as part of cystitis glandularis, are at times precancerous; an adenocarcinoma may arise from the columnar epithelium, into which their lining has differentiated.

In patients with schistosomiasis, squamous metaplasia is frequently encountered because it is a common concomitant of chronic inflammation. This type of metaplasia is a nearly consistent precursor of bladder cancer, and for this reason, leukoplakia acquires clinical importance as a precancerous condition.

Site of Origin

In patients in Western countries, bladder cancer frequently arises in the trigone; in patients in Egypt, it usually develops in areas remote from the ureters, mostly in the anterior and posterior bladder walls. This peculiarity tends to strengthen its association with schistosomal infection because the scanty or altogether absent submucosal tissue of the trigone discourages significant deposition of ova (Table 24-1).

Histologic Classification

Table 24-2 contrasts the overrepresentation of squamous cell carcinoma of the bladder in countries like Egypt, Kuwait, Mozambique, South Africa (Bantu population),[34] and Zimbabwe, where the association with schistosomiasis is considered important, with the Ugandan and white

Table 24-1 ■ Anatomic Distribution of Vesical Cancer in Egypt and the United States

Site	Egypt (%)	United States (%)
Trigone	3	21
Lateral wall	34	47
Anterior wall	22	8
Posterior wall	30	18
Vault	11	6

Table 24-2 ■ **Histologic Distribution of Bladder Cancer in Africa**

Type	Egypt	Kuwait	East Africa	South Africa		Uganda	Zimbabwe
				Bantus	Whites		
Squamous	232	100	58	16	11	26	207
Transitional	134	23	28	2	0	31	63
Anaplastic	2	1	13	4	129	7	7
Adenoearcinoma	20	4	0	1	1	5	20
Total	388	128	99	23	140	69	297

South African experiences where the reverse applies.

Within the same country, squamous cell carcinoma of the bladder is markedly overrepresented only in areas where schistosomiasis is endemic.[35,36] Moreover, the more intense the infection, the greater is the proportion of squamous cell cancers with a reciprocal decrease in the frequency of transitional cell neoplasms (Fig. 24-1).[37] Adenocarcinoma of the bilharzial bladder is particularly aggressive: This may be explained by its proneness to develop gross chromosomal aberrations combined with high cell proliferation.[38]

A rare, though distinct, variant of squamous cell cancer is verrucous carcinoma of the bilharzial bladder (Fig. 24-2). Despite reports to the contrary, a large proportion develop into invasive squamous cell carcinoma, with which they share the same adverse prognosis.[39]

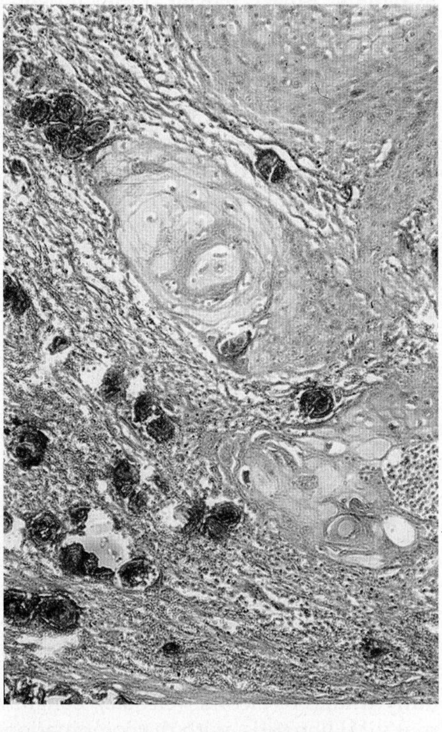

Figure 24-1 ■ Bilharzial bladder cancer. Infiltrating, well-differentiated squamous cell carcinoma with adjacent calcified *S. hematobium* eggs (H&E ×100). *Source*: Courtesy of Drs M.R. Mahran and M. El-Baz, Mansoura University, Egypt.

Experimental Data

Half a century ago, papillomatous hyperplasia of the vesical wall was observed in African sooty monkeys within 3 months of infection with *S. haematobium*. More recently, carcinoma of the bladder was diagnosed in a baboon killed 26 weeks after infection.[40] In a number of nonhuman primates, infection with *S. haematobium* resulted in epithelial proliferation, squamous metaplasia, and transitional cell carcinoma. of the urinary bladder.[41] The American opossum has also been found experimentally suitable for infection with *S. haematobium*.[42] These experimental observations are important because eggs of *S. haematobium*, lyophilized worms, and urine from bilharzia patients have not been found to be carcinogenic to mice.[43,44] Furthermore, *Schistosoma* ova, alone or in the presence of 3-methylcholanthrene, lacked urothelial topical carcinogenicity or cocarcinogenicity in mice.[45] However, 2-acetyl-aminofluorene appears to promote malignant and benign bladder neoplasms of mice infested with schistosomes more often than does either agent alone.[46] Similarly, N-methyl-N-nitrosourea and *S. haematobium* caused bladder tumors in 5 of 16 hamsters, whereas no oncogenic effect was seen with either alone. All 3 *S. haematobium* infected baboons treated with N-butyl-N-butazolnitrosamine developed extensive bladder cancer.[47]

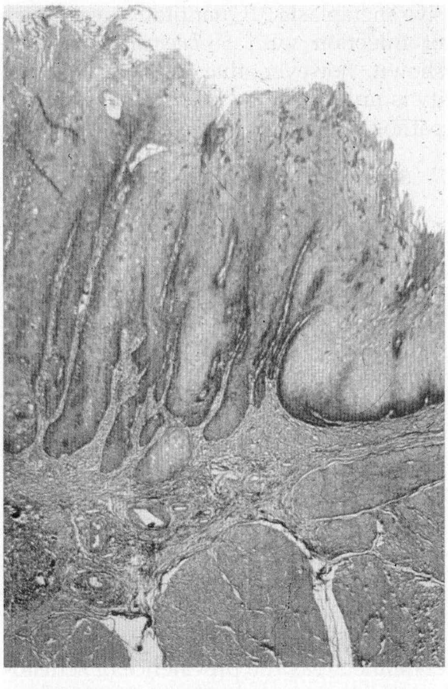

Figure 24-2 ■ Verrucous carcinoma (noninvasive) of bladder with superficial filamentous elongated surface projections (H&E ×40). *Source*: Courtesy of Drs M.R. Mahran and M. El-Baz, Mansoura University, Egypt.

Cancer development was thought to have been accelerated by schistosomal infection, presumably acting as a late-stage cocarcinogen by virtue of its direct proliferative effect on the urothelium.[48] Similarly, an increased incidence of hepatoma has been described after administration of carcinogen to mice infested with *S. mansoni*.[43] This occurs even though the toxic morphologic alterations occurring in the liver are fewer than those observed in noninfected mice exposed to the same hepatocarcinogen.[49]

Helminthic Infestations and Viruses

In one study, human papilloma virus was not detected in 25 cases of BBC.[50] Another study[51] found the virus in 23 of 40 cases. In 1 of 4 capuchin monkeys, C-type virus particles were found in a papillary carcinoma induced by *S. haematobium* that had not been present earlier in the normal bladder tissue. In mice infected with *S. mansoni*, the parasitic disease may enhance the acute effect of hepatitis virus, but no evidence has been found as yet that the chronic cirrhosis-like picture results from this.[52]

Metabolic Observations During Schistosomiasis

Increased urinary excretion of free 3-hydroxykynurenine, 3-hydroxyanthranilic acid, and 2-amino-3-hydroxyacetophenone has been documented in some patients with bladder cancer. These orthoaminophenol derivatives of tryptophan are generally excreted as conjugates of sulfuric acid or glucuronic acid. They are related to the carcinogenic metabolites of β-naphthylamine and are themselves carcinogenic to mice.

The relative resistance of the trigone to schistosomal bladder cancer would make less tenable an etiologic hypothesis predicated on the topical action of an endogenous urinary carcinogen, were it not for the increased activity of urinary β-glucuronidase in vesical infections, including schistosomiasis. Under these circumstances the enzymatic release of the active carcinogen from its glucuronide could well become a significant biologic factor that determines the anatomic localization of the neoplasm. In the study of bilharzial cancer, the metabolism of tryptophan along the formylkynurenine pathway leading to nicotinic acid has elicited considerable interest.[53] The justification for this interest originally stemmed from industrial oncology; however, epidemiologic support is also derived from the high prevalence of classic pellagra that used to be observed in Egypt but not in other parts of Africa where squamous bladder cancer is infrequently reported despite endemic schistosomiasis. In pellagra, exaggeration of the pathway from tryptophan to nicotinic acid occurs, producing larger amounts of tryptophan intermediates along the formylkynurenine pathway.

Our understanding of the role played by *Schistosoma* infection in disturbed tryptophan metabolism is complicated by geographic variations of dietary habits. In fact, serotonin metabolites such as 5-hydroxyindoleacetic acid, which are excreted in large amounts by plantain-eating Africans, are low in Africans on other diets.[54,55] Similar differences attributable to dietary habits have been found between bilharzial patients in Mozambique and in South Africa. Egyptian peasants are not plantain eaters but subsist mostly on beans, lentils, and rice. Those with bilharzial cancer metabolize tryptophan in a manner reminiscent of the pattern seen in many patients with spontaneous bladder cancer, with increased excretion of 3-hydroxyanthranilic acid, anthranilic acid, 5-hydroxyindoleacetic acid, and kynurenine. The excretion of these metabolites is enhanced by a loading dose of tryptophan.

Schistosomiasis should not be considered the only causal factor in the associated excretion of abnormal tryptophan metabolites because, with or without cancer, vesical schistosomiasis is almost universally accompanied by urinary tract infection. The bacterial flora may, thus, contribute to a spurious accumulation of some metabolites of tryptophan. Moreover, untreated pellagra is associated with increased urinary excretion of anthranilic acid, acetylkynurenine, and 5-hydroxyindoleacetic acid.

Potentially carcinogenic metabolites of tryptophan, which may be the true oncogenic agent in the presence of bilharzial bladder inflammation, are principally determined by hepatic metabolic patterns. Factors that bear on this are coincident infestation of the liver by *S. mansoni*, pyridoxine deficiency, and chronic protein starvation. In the presence of advanced abnormalities in any of these factors, lesser amounts of potential carcinogenic metabolites might be formed owing to lack of hepatic enzymes or cofactors. No mutagens were detected by the Ames test in the urine of patients suffering from bilharzial bladder cancer[56] or in soluble extracts of eggs and adult *Schistosoma japonicum* worms.[57] A weak promoting activity was noted for *S. japonicum* soluble egg antigen, which resulted in the recovery of Epstein–Barr virus (EBV) from cultured human lymphoid cells that harbored the viral genome.[57]

The hepatic drug metabolizing capacity of mice infected with *S. mansoni* is markedly reduced.[58] The mutagen inactivating potential of *S. japonicum*-infected mouse liver is similarly reduced.[59] This results in longer persistence of the mutagen in the animal body.[60] It seems likely that the carcinogen dose is a determining factor in the aggressiveness of a bladder tumor, and that a low-grade carcinoma can be converted into a high-grade one if exposed continuously to low doses of N-nitroso compounds.[61] This would explain, at least in part, the overrepresentation of deeply invasive squamous cell cancers in the bilharzial urinary bladder.[61] The significant excess of transitions at CpG dinucleotides in the *TP53* gene in bilharzial bladder cancer has been attributed to the endogenous production of nitric oxide provoked by the inflammatory response to schistosomal ova,[62] while the possible role of human papilloma virus is still uncertain.[63,64]

A study of the frequency of mutant active ras oncogenes in bilharzial bladder cancer concluded that it was not higher than in nonbitharzial cancer.[65] In view of its isolation from direct exposure to putative carcinogens present in the urine, a defunctionalized bilharzial bladder might seem an unlikely site for the development of neoplastic changes. Nonetheless, adenocarcinoma has been reported in a defunctionalized bladder showing extensive metaplasia.[66] Quantitative estimates of infection with *S. haematobium* have shown, however, that its overall severity is unlikely to be the sole factor in the pathogenesis of endemic vesical cancer[67]

Schistosomiasis and Cancer of Other Sites Large Intestine

Although acknowledging the frequency of benign schistosomal polyposis, Egyptian data tend to discount any association of *S. mansoni or S. haematobium* with cancer of the large intestine. On the other hand, in Asia, intestinal infestation with *S. japonicum* is considered a significant contributory factor to the development of cancer of the colon and rectum. *S. japonicum* lays a very large number of eggs (2000 per day per pair of worms) while *S. mansoni's* eggs are considerably less and, thus, cause fewer pathologic problems.[68]

In one report from China, where in endemic areas the prevalence of schistosomiasis may reach 44 per 100,000 persons, 48% of colectomy specimens for colorectal carcinoma obtained from 1951 to 1974 were associated with *S. japonicum* infestation. Associated inflammatory changes, pseudopolyps, and transitional mucosal changes of schistosomal granulomatous disease progressing to mucosal atypia and to carcinoma were reminiscent of bowel carcinoma in patients with ulcerative colitis, save for the ova deposited in all layers of the bowel.[69] Nonetheless, 92% of cancers were well differentiated, compared with 69% in the group without schistosomiasis. An ecologic study of 49 Chinese rural counties indicates that both schistosomal infestation and dietary factors contribute to the remarkable geographic variation of colon cancer in China.[70]

In Shanghai, patients with intestinal schistosomiasis and cancer of the large intestine are, on average, 6 years younger than patients with spontaneous intestinal cancer.[71,72] However, Chinese patients whose history of schistosomiasis entailed an elevated relative risk (RR) of rectal cancer (RR 8.3; CI 3.1 to 22.6) did not show a parallel increase in their RR for cancer of the colon.[73]

Compared to controls, Chinese patients with schistosomal rectal cancer showed a higher proportion of base-pair substitutions at CpG nucleotides and a higher frequency of arginine missense mutations, conceivably the result of genotoxic agents produced endogenously through the course of schistosomiasis japonica.[74]

The Breast

In Egyptian hospital material, the male-to-female breast cancer ratio is substantially greater than in the West. If corroborated by incidence studies, this observation would be a valuable epidemiologic observation worthy of further investigation. Hyperestrogenism secondary to bilharzial liver fibrosis has been invoked as one possible cause.

The Liver

Conflicting observations on the association of schistosomiasis and hepatic cancer are difficult to reconcile without further data. In Egypt[5] and Mozambique, 11 bilharzial liver cirrhosis is very common; carcinoma of the liver, however, is prevalent only in Mozambique, where it is the most common cancer among males. The association of cirrhosis from *S. japonicum* with hepatoma has been reported only infrequently and appears, thus, not to be causal.

In Japan, liver cancer correlated highly with three factors: HBsAg (OR 0.0), history of schistosomiasis (OR 9.5), daily intake of alcohol (OR 3.2), concurrent viral hepatitis, with the combination of hazards acting multiplicatively or at least synergistically.[75-79] In experimental animals, infection with *S. japonicum*, alone[80] or in combination with N-2-fluorenyl acetamide, induced or accelerated the occurrence of liver tumors.[81]

Disturbing are the reports of decreased response to hepatitis B vaccine among children of mothers with schistosomiasis, since the vaccine protects against hepatocellular carcinoma and may diminish the severity of liver disease in patients with schistosomiasis.[82] The relationship between schistosomiasis and hepatocellular carcinoma is confounded by coinfection with hepatitis B virus.[83-85] However, remnants of schistosomal eggs were found in the severe granulomatous reaction present within a well-differentiated hepatocellular carcinoma that had developed in a hepatitis-B and-C, seronegative chimpanzee.[86]

Lymphoma

Eight cases of solitary follicular lymphoma of the spleen were found among 863 spleens removed from patients with hepatosplenic schistosomiasis. The rarity of an isolated tumor at this site and of this type suggests a causal link, possibly mediated by cycles of follicular hyperplasia and involution occurring in the spleen in the course of advanced schistosomiasis.[87] In a Nigerian series, lymphoreticular tumors were overrepresented in infected individuals (16%) as compared with uninfested ones.[88] The occurrence of an isolated, primary T-cell lymphoma of the bladder may represent an unusual immune response to schistosomiasis.[89] In a group of 254 individuals with *S. mansoni*, 6 developed a documented lymphoma.[90]

Other Organs

Immunohistochemically confirmed invasive squamous cell carcinoma of the prostate was diagnosed in three prostatic schistosomiasis patients coming from a population where prostatic cancer is uncommon[91,92] and male breast cancer strikingly high. This suggests that in schistosomiasis, impaired liver detoxication mechanisms may result in increased estrogen and diminished androgen levels. Coexistent schistosomiasis and prostatic carcinoma have been reported in unusually young patients.[93,94] On the other hand, the Egyptian cases indicate no relationship between bilharziasis and cancer of the lungs, pancreas, prostate, seminal vesicles, urethra, vulva, vagina, cervix uteri, body of the uterus, or ovaries.[5] As would be expected, surgical or autopsy material in countries with high schistosomal endemicity from time to time shows the presence of *Schistosoma* ova in various tissues, including cancerous ones. The literature contains a number of isolated reports of such coincidences. Moreover, in areas where infestation is endemic, schistosomal tissue reaction may be so intense and proliferative as to be mistaken clinically for cancer of the large intestine[95] or the cervix.[96]

Evaluation of Carcinogenicity of Schistosomiasis

According to accepted international criteria, infection with *S. haematobium* is carcinogenic to humans (group 1); infection with *S. mansoni* is not classifiable as to its carcinogenicity to humans (group 3); infection with *S. japonicum* is possibly carcinogenic to humans (group 2B).[97]

East Asian Distomiasis

Liver and Pancreas

Clonorchis sinensis is endemic in parts of Japan, Korea, and China; a similar species, *Opisthorchis viverrini*, causes distomiasis in Thailand. Liver fluke infections have been associated with multifocal intrahepatic bile duct adenocarcinoma in those areas of Asia where distomiasis is endemic: Thailand, where 70-90% of the population of the northeast part of the country are infected with *O. viverrini*, has the highest recorded incidence of cholangiocarcinoma in the world. Similarly in Korea, where infestation with *C. sinensis* is widely prevalent, cholangiocarcinoma accounts for more than 20% of liver cancers.[98] In Indonesia, Taipei, and Taiwan, where distomiasis is considered uncommon, cholangiocarcinorna is infrequent. Imported cases of distomiasis are seen in the United States, where up to 26% of Southeast Asian immigrants have active liver fluke infection.[99] Since the parasite can live up to 30 years, it represents a long-term hazard to infected persons.[100]

Human infection results from eating raw or undercooked parasitized freshwater fish. In humans, the ingested parasites excyst in the duodenum and ascend the bile ducts and canaliculi, where they mature, causing biliary epithelial hyperplasia and fibrosis. Similarities between the histopathologic responses in infected humans and experimental animals have been documented, including the development of cholangiocarcinoma in dogs and cats experimentally infected with *Clonorchis*. Hamsters administered dimethylnitrosamine for 10 weeks after infection with *Opisthorchis* developed mucin-secreting cholangiocarcinomas, whereas noninfected animal controls failed to develop tumors. This observation, as well as other observations,[101] are in keeping with experimental evidence pointing to infection as a promoter.[102] In the Far East, nitrosamines are commonly found in such traditional Chinese preserved foods as salted fish, dried shrimp, and sausage.[103] Precursors of nitroso compounds have been identified in the body fluid of men infested with *O. viverrini*.[104] Pancreatic ducts may also be infected with *C. sinensis*; this frequently results in squamous metaplasia and mucous gland hyperplasia. In one instance in the United States, an immigrant with *C. sinensis* in the common bile duct developed a well-differentiated ductal adenocarcinoma of the pancreas.[105]

Evaluation of Carcinogenicity of Distomiasis

Infection with *O. viverrini* is carcinogenic to humans (group 1); infection with *O. felineus* is not classifiable as to its carcinogenicity to humans (group 3); infection with *C. sinensis* is probably carcinogenic to humans (group 2A).[106]

Malaria

The geographic distribution of Burkitt lymphoma in the classic malarial belt initially suggested the possible role of an arthropod vector in oncogenesis. This fits with the notion that the risk for this lymphoma declines with increasing westernization and effective malaria eradication.[107,108] The possibility that drugs taken for malaria prophylaxis could have contributed to the development of Burkitt lymphoma[109,110] was considered unlikely because no increase (and indeed a decrease) in endemic Burkitt lymphoma (eBL) was observed in the Malagasy Republic[111] and in Imesi, West Africa,[112] where intensive antimalarial prophylaxis was practiced; moreover, cases occur[113] among persons not receiving malaria prophylaxis.

More significant are the epidemiologic observations that have linked eBL to the combined effect of malaria and infection with the EBV.[114] Endemic BL is only found in areas where malaria is holoendemic or hyperendemic; within these areas, it is absent in malaria-free pockets, such as urban centers. Within endemic areas, the peak incidence of eBL follows closely the incidence of severe *Plasmodium falciparum* malaria, and malarial prophylaxis reduces the incidence of the lymphorna.[111,112]

Vigorous cellular and serologic responses occur during malarial infection.[115] This renders plausible the argument that persistent reticuloendothelial stimulation experienced among malarial populations conditions the EBV-infected African patient to develop a neoplasm rather than a self-limited disease, such as infectious mononucleosis.[116] This view finds support in the observation that each one of the erythrocytic, exoerythrocytic, and sexual forms of the parasite is structurally differentiated and probably contains a multitude of biologically active antigenic constituents.[117,118] In this respect, it is interesting to note that in endemic malarial areas, the distribution of hyper-reactive malarial splenomegaly parallels the distribution of eBL, and that the peak age incidence of eBL follows closely the peak age incidence of severe *P. falciparum* malaria.[113] In Uganda, odds ratios for Burkitt lymphoma in children increased with increasing antibody levels against EBV ($p < 0.0001$) and malaria ($p = 1.05$).[114]

In situ hybridization for the detection of FBER-I and EBER-2 RNA has demonstrated that acute infection with malaria leads to colonization of lymph nodes by virus-infected lymphoblasts in 60% of the cases.[119,120]

One way of explaining the observation that the malaria patient harboring a multitude of parasite derived antigens becomes a host susceptible to eBL is the suggestion that malaria patients produce so many nonspecific and "useless" antibodies that they are unable to recognize and respond to the threat posed by a small clone of malignant lymphoid cells.[121] This view is supported by experimental data. In mice, antigenic stimulation and immune suppression often result in an increased incidence of lymphomas. Mice repeatedly injected with *Plasmodium berghei* sometimes develop malignant lymphoma that is morphologically similar to Burkitt lymphoma and sometimes develop persistent antigenic stimulation without significant tumorigenesis.[122-124] Lymphomas are frequently induced by Moloney leukemogenic virus in mice infected with *P. berghei* but rarely occur in mice given either plasmodium or virus alone.[125] Acute malaria, which increases B-cell proliferation, also impairs EBV-specific T-cell responses.[126] This results in a larger pool of EBV-infected cells with increased likelihood for chromosomal translocation and lymphomagenesis.[127] In children, the risk of developing Burkitt lymphoma is related to antibody titers against EBV capsid antigens.[128] The clinical manifestations probably are promoted by other environmental factor(s), such as holoendemic malaria[129] and phorbol exposure.[130]

Of considerable interest are studies on the frequency of sickle-cell trait in eBL patients and controls. Persons with sickle trait are not protected from being bitten by mosquitoes or from malarial infection, but they are protected against the lethal effect of overwhelming *P. falciparum* malaria in early childhood and from the intense reticuloendothelial stimulation that sometimes progresses to hyper-reactive malarial splenomegaly.[131] The cystein-rich interdomain region 1 alpha of the *P. falciparum* membrane has been identified as a polyclonal B-cell activator that preferentially activates the memory compartment where EBV is known to persist.[132] Sickle cells exposed to low oxygen tension do not support the growth of parasites in vitro. A similar phenomenon may explain why children with the sickle-cell trait have a lower *P. falciparum* parasitemia. As a result, a lower mortality rate, lower IgM levels, and reduced lymphoproliferation (as measured by spleen size) are found among individuals with hemoglobin AS genotype. However, most studies attempting to relate eBL to AS hemoglobinopathy have failed to reach statistical significance.[126] Other hemoglobinopathies, such as hereditary ovalocytosis, also protect against malaria. If eBL turns out to be underrepresented in populations where both ovalocytosis and malaria are prevalent, as in Papua, New Guinea,[133] such information would provide strong supporting evidence for malaria as a cofactor in the genesis of eBL.[126] In this event, the observation that in Uganda malarial endemicity also correlates with non-Burkitt non-Hodgkin lymphoma, would acquire added significance.[134]

The small differences in titers of malarial antibodies observed in Burkitt lymphoma patients and controls[135] were attributed to the fact that many in the experimental group had received several courses of antimalarial drugs, which may have lowered the level of malaria-specific antibodies.[116] A probable role of malaria emerges also from the following considerations. African children with eBL develop autoantibodies, the elevated titers of which show no linear correlation with EBV titers for viral capsid antigen (VCA) or Epstein–Barr nuclear antigen (EBNA),[136] suggesting that a factor independent of EBV causes an immunologic imbalance and autoantibody production. The notion that this could be due to malaria is supported by the observation that Caucasians suffering from acute *P. falciparum* malaria develop autoantibodies,[137,138] and that experiments in vitro demonstrated that normal human lymphocytes can produce autoantibodies as a response to malarial antigens.[139]

In the genesis of eBL, regardless of whether malaria is considered the initiator and EBV the promoter or vice versa, neither hypothesis accounts for the fact that in vitro infection of B-cells with EBV and stimulation with malaria antigens has yet to produce a cell that carries the chromosomal tumorigenic translocations found in both sporadic and eBL.[128] Overexpression of *c-myc* appears to be central to the pathogenesis of Burkitt and atypical Burkitt lymphomas. Although *c-myc* translocation occurs in all cases of Burkitt lymphoma, differences are seen in the translocation patterns in the endemic and sporadic varieties of the disease. Typically, sporadic Burkitt lymphoma has translocations involving sequences within or immediately 5′ to *myc* on chromosome 8 and sequences within or near the immunoglobulin heavy chain S region on chromosome 14. In contrast, eBL tends to be characterized by a translocation involving sequences on chromosome 8 further upstream from *myc* and sequences within or near the JH region on chromosome 14.[140] Thus, it seems likely that other unidentified factors (genetic, nutritional, or environmental) play a significant role in tumorigenesis.

American Burkitt Lymphoma

By the early 1970s, approximately 100 cases of Burkitt lymphoma had been confirmed by the American Burkitt Lymphoma Registry.[141] Space-time clustering is suggested by the American data.[142,143] Although malaria is associated with Burkitt lymphoma in Africa, the relative rarity of the tumor in relation to the holoendemic nature of malaria indicates that a combination of genetic factors plus specific environmental factors may be operative. Host and environmental factors other than malaria are probably important in North American cases.[141]

Cancer in Animals

Observations made by Fibiger[144] on gastric cancer in rats infested with a nematode are now all but discredited. A question that remains to be evaluated is whether the nematode helped localize some unidentified carcinogens in the diet, similar to the induction of sarcomas at the site of subcutaneous injection of sodium chloride in rats being fed 3-methylcholanthrene.

Sarcoma is an almost inevitable complication of infection of the liver or the subcutaneous tissues of rats with *Cysticercus fasciolaris*, the larval form of the common tapeworm of the cat, *Taenia taeniaformis*. Washed, ground-up *C. fasciolaris* produced peritoneal sarcomas in half the injected rats, the proportion reaching 91% if the animals were genetically related to the parasitized host. The active agent appears to be associated with the calcium carbonate corpuscles of the parasite, but the mechanism is not clear.[145] Although not directly implicated in vesical carcinogenesis, there is suggestive evidence that infestation with another nematode, *Trichosomoides crassicauda*, increases the incidence of tumors in the bladders of rats receiving 2-acetylaminoluorine.[146]

Another nematode, *Spirocerca lupi* has been associated with the development of esophageal sarcoma in dogs. Here the reported association seems to be described only in the southern United States, thereby adding a possible geographic dimension to the problem.

Some neoplastic responses to parasitic infestation are a kind of cecidiosis and may represent the end of a hypothesized evolutionary sequence by which parasite secretions stimulate the host to form protective structures (cecidia) that benefit the parasite.

Selected References

The complete reference list can be found at www.CANCERMEDICINE8.com

3. Mostafa, MH, Sheweita P, O'Connor, PJ. Relationship between schistosomiasis and bladder Cancer. *Clin Microbiol Rev.* 1999;12:97–111.
5. Bedwani R, El-Khwsky F, La Vecchia C, et al. Descriptive epidemiology of bladder cancer in Egypt. *Int J Cancer.* 1993;55:351.
7. Wishahi M, El-Baz HG, Shaker LA. Association between HLA-A, B, C and DR antigens and clinical manifestations of Schistosoma haematobiuin in the bladder. *Eur Urol.* 1989;16:138.
8. Aboul Nasr A, Gazyerli M, Fawn RM, El-Sibal L. Epidemiology and pathology of cancer of the bladder in Egypt. *Acta Unio Int Contra Cancrum.* 1962;18:528.
10. Mustacchi P, Shimkin MB. Cancer of the bladder and infestation with Schistosomiasis haernatobium. *J Natl Cancer Inst.* 1958;20:825.
12. Bedawi R, Renganathan E, El-Khwsky F, et al. Schistosomiasis and the risk of bladder cancer in Alexandria, Egypt. *Br J Cancer.* 1998;77:1186.
15. Ghaleb AH, Pizzolo JG, Melamed MR. Aberrations of chromosomes 9 and 17 in bilharzial bladder cancer as detected by fluorescence in situ hybridization. *Am J Clin Path.* 1996;106:234.
17. Tricker AR, Mostafa HH, Spiegelhalder P, Preussman P. Urinary nitrite and nitroso compounds in bladder cancer patients with schistosomiasis (bilharziasis). *IARC Sci Publ.* 1991;105:178.
18. El-Aaser AA, El-Merzahani MM, El-Bolkain Ibrahim AS. A study on the etiological factors of bilharzial bladder cancer in Egypt. 5-urinary nitrites in a rural population. *Tumori.* 1980;66:400.
19. Tricker AR, Mostafa MH, Spiegelhalder B. Preussman R. Urinary excretion of nitrate, nitrite and N-nitroso compounds in Schistosomiasis and bilharzias bladder cancer patients. *Carcinogenesis.* 1989;10:547–52.
21. Abdel Mohsen MA, Hassan AAM, El-Sewedy SM, et al. Biomonitoring of N-nitroso compounds, nitrite and nitrate in the urine of Egyptian bladder cancer patients with or without Schistosorna haeinatobium infection. *Int J Cancer.* 1999;82:789.
22. Badawi AF. Nitrate, nitrite and N-nitroso compounds in human bladder cancer associated with schistosomiasis. *Int J Cancer.* 2000;85:598.
24. Badawi AA. Molecular and genetic events in schistosomiasis associated human bladder cancer: role of oncogenes and tumor suppressor genes. *Cancer Letters.* 1996;105:123.
27. Gadalla HA, Kamel NA, Badary FA, Elanany FG. Expression of CD44 protein in bilharzial and nonbilharziala bladder cancers. *BJU Int.* 2004;93:151–155.
33. Badr KM, Nolen JD, Derose PB, Cohen C. Muscle invasive schistosomal squamous cell carcinoma of the urinary bladder: frequency and prognostic significance of p53, BCL-2, HER2/neu and proliferation (M1B-1). *Hum Path.* 2004;35:184–189.
35. Kitinya JN, Lauren PA, Eshleman IJ, et al. The incidence of squamous and transitional cell carcinomas of the urinary bladder in northern Tanzania in areas of high and low levels of endemic Schistosoma haematobium infection. *Trans R Soc Trop Med Hyg.* 1986;80:935.
36. Thomas JE, Nassett MT, Sigola LB, Taylor P. Relationship between bladder cancer incidence, Schistosoma haematobiurn infection, and geographical region in Zimbabwe. *Trans R Soc Trop Med Hyg.* 1990;84:551.
38. Shabaan AA, Elbaz AE, Tribukait B. Primary nonurachal adenocarcinoma in the bilharzial urinary bladder: deoxyribonucleic acid flow cytometric and morphologic characterization in 93 cases. *Urology.* 1998;51:469.
41. Kuntz RE, Cheever AW, Myers BJ. Proliferative epithelial lesions of the urinary bladder of nonhuman primates infested with Schistosoma haematobium. *J Natl Cancer Inst.* 1972;48:223.
44. Shimkin MB, Mustacchi PO, Cram EB, Wright WH. Lack of carcinogenicity of lyophilized Schistosoma in mice. *J Natl Cancer Inst.* 1955:16:47.
51. Khaled HM, Raafata A, Mokhtar N, et al. Human papilloma virus infection and overexpression of p53 protein in bilharzial bladder cancer. *Tumori.* 2001;87:256–261.
57. Ishii A, Matsuoka H, Aji T, et al. Evaluation of the mutagenicity and the tumor promoting activity of parasite extract: Schistosoma japonicum infection and Clonorchis sinensis. *Mutat Res.* 1989;224:229.
59. Matsuoka H, Aji T, Ishii A, et al. Reduced levels of mutagen processing potential in the Schistosoma japonicum infected mouse liver. *Mutat Res.* 1989;227:153.
61. Badawi AF, Mostafa MR, O'Connor PJ. Involvement of alkylating agents in schistosome-associated bladder cancer: the possible basic mechanisms of induction. *Cancer Lett.* 1992;63:171.
62. Warren W, Biggs PJ, El-Baz M, et al. Mutations in the p53 gene in schistosomaal bladder cancer: a study of 92 tumors from Egyptian patients and a comparison between mutational spectra from schistosomal. and nonschistosomal urothelial tumors. *Carcinogenesis.* 1995;16: 1181–1189.
65. Fujita J, Nakayama H, Onoue H, et al. Frequency of active ras oncogenes in human bladder cancers associated with schistosomiasis. *Jpn J Cancer Res. (Gann)* 1987;78:915.
68. Ishii A, Matsuoka H, Aji T, et al. Parasite infection and cancer with special emphasis on Schistosoma japonicum infections (Trematoda). A review. *Mutat Res.* 1994;305:273.
70. Guo W, Zheng W, Li JY, et at Correlation of colon cancer mortality with dietary factors, serum markers and schistosomiasis in China. *Nutr Cancer.* 1993;20:13.
73. Xu Z, Su DL. Schistosoma japonicum and colorectal cancer: an epidemiologic study in the People's Republic of China. *Inter J Cancer.* 1984;34:315.
74. Zhang R, Takahashi S, Orita S, et al. p53 gene mutations in rectal cancer associated with schistosomiasis japonica in Chinese patients. *Cancer Letters.* 1998;131:215.
77. Iida F, Iida R, Kamijo H, et al. Chronic Japanese schistosomiasis and hepatocellular carcinoma: ten years of follow-up in Yamanashi prefecture, Japan. *Bull WHO.* 1999;77:573.
79. Badawi AA, Michael MS. Risk factors for hepatocellular carcinoma in Egypt: the role of hepatitis-B viral infection and schistosomiasis. *Anticancer Res.* 1999;19:4563.
85. Hassan MM, Zaghloul AS, El-Serag HB, et al. The role of hepatitis C in hepatocellular carcinoma: a case control study among Egyptian patients. *J Clin Gastroenterol.* 2001;33:123–126.
89. Mourad WA, Khalil S, Radwi A, Peracha A, Ezzat A. Primary T-cell lymphoma of the urinary bladder. *Am J Surg Pathol.* 1998;22:373–377.
90. Ferraz AA, de Sa VC, Lopes EP, et al. Lymphoma in patients harboring hepatosplenic mansonic schistosomiasis. *Arq Gastroenterol.* 2006;43:85–88.
106. IARC Monographs on the evaluation of carcinogenic risks to humans, Vol. 61. Lyon: IARC;1994:162.
108. Ojesina AI, Akang EE, Ojemakinde KO. Decline in the frequency of Burkitt's lymphoma relative to other childhood malignancies in Ibadan, Nigeria. *Ann Trop Paediatr.* 2002;22:159–163.
110. Sadoff L. Antimalarial drugs and Burkitt's lymphoma. *Lancet.* 1973;2:1262.
113. Aghai E, Hulu N, Virag I, et al. Childhood non-Hodgkin's lymphoma–a study of 17 cases in Israel. *Cancer.* 1974;33:1411.
116. Carpenter LM, Newton R, Casabonne D, et al. Antibodies against malaria and Epstein-Barr virus in childhood Burkitt lymphoma: a case-control study in Uganda. *Int J Cancer.* 2008;122:1319–1323.
120. Facer C, Khan G. Detection of EBV RNA (EBER-I and EBER-2) in malaria lymph nodes by in situ hybridization. *Microbiol Immunol.* 1997;41:891–894.
126. Whittle HC, Brown J, Marsh K, et al. T-cell control of Epstein-Barr virus-infected B-cells is lost during P. falciparum malaria. *Nature.* 1984;312:449.
127. Magrath I. The pathogenesis of Burkitt's lymphoma. *Adv Cancer Res.* 1990;55:145.
134. Schmauz R, Mugerwa JW, Wright DH. The distribution of non-Burkitt, non-Hodgkin's lymphoma in Uganda in relation to malarial endemicity. *Int J Cancer.* 1990;46:650.
135. Morrow RH. Epidemiological evidence for role of falciparum malaria. In: Lenoir G, O'Conor G, Olweny C, eds. *Burkitt's Lymphoma: A Human Cancer Model.* Lyon: IARC Science Publication No.60; 1985:177–185.
136. Vainio E, Lenoir GM, Franklin RM. Autoantibodies in three populations of Burkitt's lymphoma patients. *Clin Exp Immunol.* 1983;54:387.
140. Bishop PC, Rao K, Wilson WH. Burkitt's lymphoma: molecular pathogenesis and treatment. *Cancer Invest.* 2000;18:574.

25 Molecular Imaging in Clinical Oncology

Juri G. Gelovani, MD, PhD

Introduction

The discovery of x-rays by Wilhelm Conrad Röntgen in 1895 and radioactivity by Henri Becquerel in 1896[1] revolutionized medical diagnosis and therapeutic interventions. The first radioactive tracer studies in animals were performed using lead-210 and bismuth-210 by George de Hevesy in 1925, and the next year (1926) Herman Blumgart and Otto Yens performed the first diagnostic radiotracer study in humans using bismuth-214.[2] Over the next century, anatomic and functional imaging methods, such as computed tomography (CT), ultrasonography (US), and magnetic resonance imaging (MRI) rapidly developed and became standard in the diagnosis of different diseases, including cancers. While these methods can reveal gross pathomorphological and pathophysiological features of disease, molecular imaging aims to elucidate the genetic, metabolic, and molecular pathophysiological mechanisms and biomarkers of various diseases noninvasively, repetitively, and over the entire body. Molecular imaging can be defined as the in vivo characterization and measurement of biologic processes at a cellular and molecular level.

Historically, radionuclide-imaging approaches are considered the roots of modern molecular imaging. However, the scope of nuclear imaging applications was initially limited to thyroid scintigraphy with I-131, Ga-67 bone scan, and the assessment of renal and hepato-billiary functions. The introduction into clinical practice of more complex radiolabeled agents, including small molecules (^{131}I-metaiodobenzylguanidine, MIBG) and peptides (^{111}In-pentetreotide, octreotide) followed by MRI spectroscopy represents the next stage in the development of molecular imaging.

Currently, the most advanced molecular imaging agents and approaches utilize positron emission tomography (PET) imaging. Significant advances have also been made in magnetic resonance imaging and spectroscopy, (US), and optical (ie, near-infrared, NIR) imaging techniques. Especially promising is the optoacoustic imaging modality.[3-5]

Because of the large number and variety of modern molecular imaging modalities, agents, and applications in oncology, it will not be possible to present an in-depth review of the whole field of molecular imaging in oncology within the current chapter. Therefore, the focus of this chapter will be mostly on nuclear imaging modality of PET and several radiolabeled PET agents (radiotracers) in oncology.

In the current mainstream clinical practice, PET with ^{18}F-labeled glucose analog 2′-fluoro-2′-deoxyglucose (^{18}F-FDG) represents the most widely used molecular imaging radiotracer. However, with the discovery of novel PET radiotracers soon it will be possible to quantitatively assess a variety of other biochemical and signal transduction pathways, including angiogenesis, hypoxia, proliferation, apoptosis, multidrug resistance, and growth factor receptor status. Emergence of hyperpolarized MR spectroscopic imaging opens the possibility for development of novel imaging applications for investigation of the same highly important cancer signaling and biochemical pathways, but without the use of radioactivity. Further, we will review the most widely used clinical molecular imaging applications in different tumor types.

Breast Carcinoma

Breast Carcinoma Diagnostic Imaging

Breast cancer remains the most commonly diagnosed cancer and the second leading cause of cancer death in women.[6] For screening of breast carcinoma, conventional anatomic imaging using mammography remains the standard, which has contributed to increased detection rates, earlier diagnoses, and, therefore, a significant improvement in treatment outcomes. From both the molecular-biological and diagnostic imaging perspectives, breast carcinoma has been investigated extensively. A variety of imaging approaches have been developed to date including digital mammography, MRI, MR spectroscopy (MRS), dynamic contrast-enhanced MRI (DCE-MRI), ^{18}F-FDG PET, ^{18}F-FLT PET, gamma scintigraphy with ^{99m}Tc-Sestamibi, and NIR fluorescence-based optical imaging techniques. Due to variability in the levels of glucose metabolism (utilization) by different types of breast carcinomas, ^{18}F-FDG PET is not currently used for screening. Similarly, gamma scintigraphy with ^{99m}Tc-Sestamibi has been shown to have high sensitivity (Fig. 25-1), but a relatively low specificity for detecting breast carcinomas and has not been approved for screening.[7]

MRI has attained a significant role in diagnosis and monitoring of breast carcinoma.[8] In BRCA1 and BRCA2 mutation carriers, MRI was shown to be more sensitive for detecting breast cancers than mammography, US, or clinical breast examination (CBE) alone.[9] Whether surveillance regimens that include MRI will reduce mortality from breast cancer in women at high genetic risk requires further investigation. Imaging abnormal tumor vasculature with dynamic contrast-enhanced MRI (DCE-MRI) of breast has shown adequate sensitivity and specificity for screening individuals with high risk of breast carcinoma.[10] DCE-MRI is a functional imaging methodology which takes advantage of the hyperpermeable tumor microvasculature due to increased production of pro-angiogenic factors (ie, vascular endothelial growth factor, VEGF) by the tumor cells. Therefore, DCE-MRI is emerging as a powerful high resolution imaging approach for screening high-risk patients and for detecting high-grade ductal carcinoma in situ (Fig. 25-2). However, there are also a number of limitations, including the overlap in enhancement patterns between malignant and benign disease, the failure to resolve microscopic disease particularly in the neoadjuvant setting, and the inconsistent predictive value of the en-

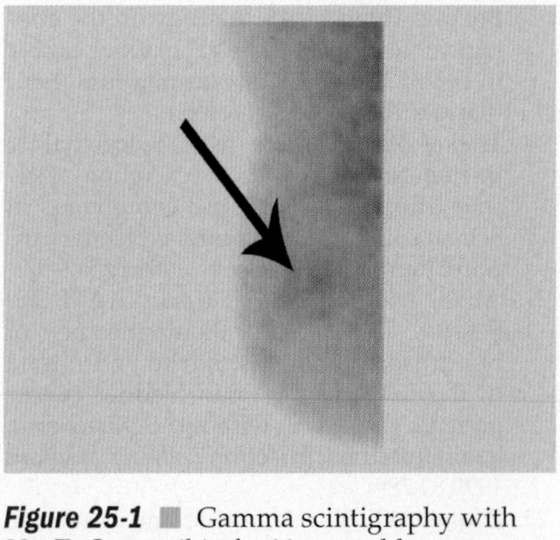

Figure 25-1 Gamma scintigraphy with 99mTc-Sestamibi of a 46-year-old woman shows focal increased radiotracer uptake (arrow) in upper right breast. Pathologic findings showed 0.6-cm infiltrating lobular carcinoma with extensive lobular carcinoma in situ. Source: From Ref. 7.

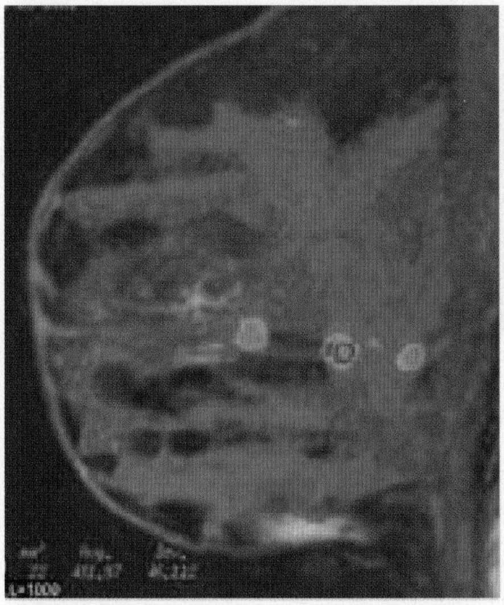

Figure 25-2 Small foci of carcinoma are detectable within an area of DCIS on DCE-MRI examination with multiple islands of increased contrast uptake seen on the positive integral map (in red). *Source*: From Ref. 11.

hancement pattern for clinical outcome. Careful consideration should be given to the technical requirements of individual examinations and the need for automation of post-processing techniques to appropriately handle the growing volume of data acquired.[11] In addition, new large-molecular weight contrast agents, breast carcinoma-targeted gadolinium-labeled agents and ultra-small SPIO conjugates may in the future improve the specificity and accuracy of tumor detection.[12-17] In the context of molecular imaging, MRS has been effective in the differential diagnosis of benign and malignant lesions.[18] Currently, there is evidence of increased choline metabolism in breast cancer cells, as determined by in vivo MRS. In breast malignancies, ^{1}H-MRS achieved a high-overall sensitivity (82%). Most test cases were infiltrating duct carcinoma, but infiltrating lobular, medullary, mucinous and adenoid cystic carcinomas were also positive by ^{1}H-MRS. Large lesional size is a pre-requisite for ^{1}H-MRS testing, and technical problems account for some of the false negative results.[19]

During the past several years, significant advances have been made in optical imaging of breast carcinoma using methods of NIR fluorescence imaging, diffusive optical tomography, and optical coherence tomography. Diffuse optical spectroscopic imaging (DOSI) is a noninvasive imaging modality that uses NIR light to quantitatively characterize the optical properties of thick tissues. Although NIR methods were first applied to breast transillumination (also called diaphanography) nearly 80 years ago, quantitative DOSI methods employing time- or frequency-domain photon migration technologies have only been used for breast imaging during the last decade. DOSI employs broadband technology both in NIR spectral and temporal signal domains in order to separate absorption from scattering and quantify uptake of multiple molecular probes based on fluorescence contrast or absorption (ie, differential absorption of certain spectrum by deoxyhemoglobin and oxyhemoglobin). Additional dimensionality can be generated by co-registering the functional images obtained by DOSI with corresponding x-ray mammograms, breast CT images, or MRI, which provide structural information or vascular flow information, respectively.[20] Fluorescently labeled molecular agents are routinely used in basic biological and preclinical research in oncology, including fluorescent antibodies, peptides, poly-nucleotides, etc. In combination with the rapidly developing imaging methods and instrumentation (ie, DOSI) several fluorescent optical imaging agents based on the FDA-approved breast carcinoma targeting agents (ie, Herceptin) will likely be translated into the clinic in the near future. For example, noninvasive NIR optical imaging with indocyanine green (ICG) has already been used for detection of sentinel lymph nodes in other types of cancer.[21]

Optical coherence tomography (OCT) is an optical imaging modality that performs high-resolution, cross-sectional, subsurface tomographic imaging of the microstructure of tissues. The physical principle of OCT is similar to that of B-mode ultrasound imaging, except that it uses infrared light waves rather than acoustic waves. The in vivo resolution is 10–25 times better than with high-frequency ultrasound imaging (about 10 microns), but the depth of penetration is limited to 1–3 mm, depending on tissue structure, depth of focus of the probe used, and pressure applied to the tissue surface. In the last decade, OCT technology has evolved from an experimental laboratory tool to a new diagnostic imaging modality with a wide spectrum of clinical applications in medical practice of ophthalmology and gastroenterology.[22] OCT functions as a type of "optical biopsy" to provide cross-sectional images of tissue structure on the micron scale. It is a promising imaging technology because it can provide images of tissue in situ and in real time, without the need for excision and processing of specimens. Recently, the diagnostic efficacy of OCT was validated by conventional histopa-

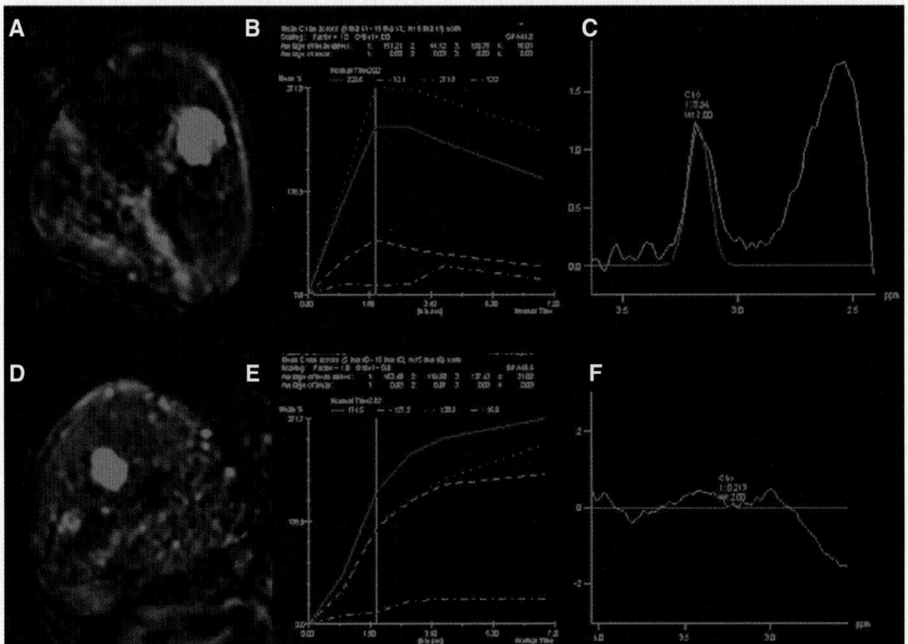

Figure 25-3 Dynamic magnetic resonance imaging (MRI) and proton magnetic resonance spectroscopy (1H-MRS) of the breast. In the same patient, an invasive ductal carcinoma is located in the upper outer quadrant of the left breast (**A–C**) and a fibroadenoma in the upper outer quadrant of the right breast (**D–F**). Both lesions are rounded in shape with inhomogeneous enhancement (**A,S:** subtraction images in the early phase), whereas they are clearly differentiated by the dynamic enhancement/time curves (**B,E:** traced in red and green for the carcinoma and red, yellow and green for the fibroadenoma, relative to intralesional regions of interest [ROIs]) and by the spectrum (**C,F**). Whereas the carcinoma displays a curve with a washout and a gross peak of choline-containing compounds at 3.2 ppm, the fibroadenoma displays a curve with a continuous increase and absence of significant peak at 3.2 ppm. The broad and elevated peak around 2.5 ppm in the spectrum of the cancer is probably due to peritumoural lipids. The curves with slight enhancement (yellow and blue above and blue below) refer to the ROIs positioned in the adipose tissue or in healthy portions of the breast. *Source*: From Ref. 19.

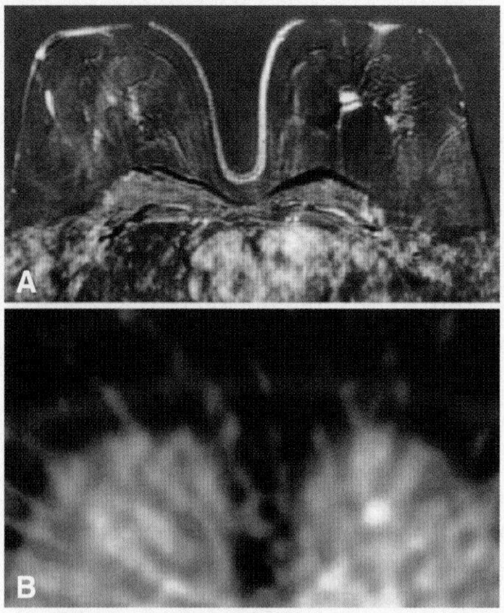

Figure 25-4 Breast carcinoma (histology: pT1N0) of the central part of the left breast in a 77-year-old patient. (**A**) Magnetic resonance mammography: In the subtraction image the tumour can be easily detected. The time–signal intensity curve shows a fast increase of the signal intensity and a washout phase indicating a malignant tumor. (**B**) ^{18}F-FDG PET: in the corresponding image of the same patient the tumor shows strong glucose uptake. In both imaging modalities, tumor location and tumor size were identical. Small foci of glucose uptake are seen in the chest wall on outside the breasts. *Source*: From Ref. 25.

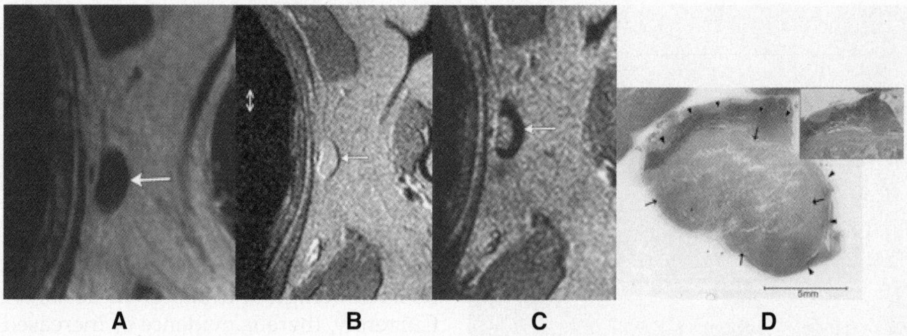

Figure 25-5 Partial SI decrease in 0.7–1.0-cm metastatic lymph node in the left axilla of a 45-year-old woman with primary stage pT2N1 tumor. (**A**) T1-weighted 3D and (**B**) T2*-weighted FFE transverse non-enhanced MR images (24/7) show lymph node (arrow). (**C**) USPIO-enhanced T2*-weighted FFE transverse MR image (683/14) shows same lymph node (arrow) with partial SI decrease, which is indicative of metastatic involvement. (**D**) Photomicrograph of histopathologic specimen of same lymph node confirms presence of metastatic tissue (arrows). Peripheral zone is non-metastatic tissue (arrowheads). (Hematoxylin-eosin stain; original magnification, X5; inset, X25.) *Source*: From Ref. 28.

thology of surgically resected breast tissue specimens containing fibrocystic changes, benign fibroadenomas, and invasive ductal carcinomas.[23] With the development of micro-miniaturized flexible probes, OCT may become potentially useful for invasive visualization of breast lesions at a microscopic resolution that is not achievable by currently available clinical imaging methods.[24]

Breast Carcinoma Staging and Restaging

Both MRI and ^{18}F-FDG PET have demonstrated efficacy in the staging and restaging of breast cancer. MRI is more accurate in comparison with conventional mammography and US in the assessment of the local extent of disease and is superior in sensitivity as compared to PET for diagnosis of the primary lesions.[25-27] MRI using ultrasmall superparamagnetic iron oxide (USPIO) contrast agents had shown promise for evaluation of lymph node involvement. Several studies demonstrated that USPIO-enhanced MRI has a node-by-node sensitivity, specificity, and accuracy reaching 100%, 98%, and 98%, respectively. USPIO-enhanced MRI appears valuable for assessment of axillary lymph node metastases in patients with breast carcinomas and is superior to nonenhanced MRI (Fig. 25-5).[28]

Because of differences in the magnitude of glycolysis among different breast tumors, ^{18}F-FDG PET had historically demonstrated variable sensitivity and specificity for all breast cancers, ranging between 66% and 96% and 83% and 100%, respectively. ^{18}F-FDG PET is the least sensitive for detection, staging, and restaging of tubular, lobular, and in situ carcinoma.[29-32] However, ^{18}F-FDG PET is better than MRI for detection of nodal involvement in the axilla, with a sensitivity ranging from 79% to 100% and a specificity ranging from 50% to 100%. In spite of this, the majority of studies indicate the need for conventional sentinel node mapping in addition to ^{18}F-FDG PET, because of its insensitivity in the detection of micrometastatic desease.[33-36]

In terms of distant staging, PET has been shown to be the most sensitive modality which can detect distant lesions identified by CT or radionuclide bone scanning, and frequently reveals previously unsuspected lesions.[37-39] Also, ^{18}F-FDG PET has become the preferred imaging modality for restaging, because of its higher sensitivity and specificity compared to conventional imaging.[40-42]

Imaging of breast tumor proliferation with ^{18}F-3′-fluorothymidine (^{18}F-FLT) PET is a relatively new and promising imaging application, because of the lower tissue background activity in the mediastinal area and resulting higher target tumor to background contrast ratio, which can facilitate the detection of intrathoracic lymph node metastases.[43,44] ^{18}F-FLT PET is also of value for monitoring of therapy, as will be discussed below.

Monitoring Therapy of Breast Carcinoma

Molecular PET imaging with ^{18}F-FDG and ^{18}F-FLT can predict treatment response early after initiation of therapy long before changes in tumor size will take place, as measured by conventional anatomic imaging. ^{18}F-FDG PET is predictive of which patients will respond to neoadjuvant chemotherapy when baseline PET imaging results are compared with those obtained after the first cycle of chemotherapy.[45-48] Patients with locally advanced breast carcinoma who exhibit limited or no decline in ^{18}F-FDG utilization have higher recurrence and mortality risks. Also, tumor perfusion changes over the course of neoadjuvant chemotherapy as measured directly by ^{15}O-water or indirectly by dynamic ^{18}F-FDG predict disease-free survival and overall survival.[49] However, increase in glucose metabolism, or so-called "metabolic flare" on ^{18}F-FDG PET images induced by 30 mg of estradiol challenge is associated with improved efficacy of hormonal therapy and significantly longer overall survival in patients with estrogen receptor(ER)-positive breast carcinomas.[50]

In molecular pathophysiology of breast carcinoma, ER expression plays an important role in breast carcinoma behavior and is critical for response to endocrine therapies such as tamoxifen and aromatase inhibitors. In routine clinical practice, ER expression is determined in biopsy material. In an advanced disease, tumor tissue biopsies are difficult and are associated with significant sampling error and inconsistencies due to interlesional heterogeneity. This and other considerations motivated the development of PET imaging agents for the assessment of ER status of primary and metastatic tumor lesions, of which the most successful has been ^{18}F-16alpha-17beta-fluoroestradiol (^{18}F-FES). Several PET imaging studies with ^{18}F-FES in breast carcinoma patients demonstrated efficacy for detection of ER-expressing tumors and prediction of responsiveness to endocrine therapy (Fig. 25-6).[51-54]

PET imaging of tumor proliferative activity with 3′-deoxy-3′-[18F]fluorothymidine (^{18}F-FLT) has become a useful tool in clinical research.[55] In a recent clinical study,[56] ^{18}F-FLT PET was performed

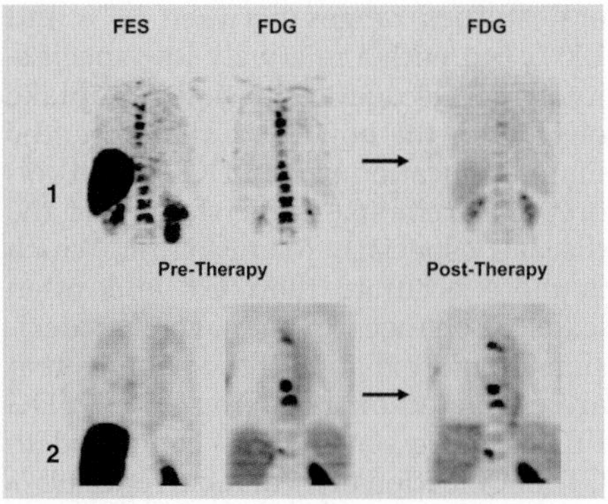

Figure 25-6 ■ Two patients with documented bone metastases from an ER+ primary breast cancer imaged pre-hormonal therapy with FES (first column) and FDG (second column). Patient 1 has high FES uptake at all sites of active disease, indicating preserved ER expression. This patient subsequently responded to hormonal therapy (post-therapy scan in column 3). Patient 2 has no FES uptake at active sites of disease seen by FDG-PET, suggesting loss of ER expression, and had no response to hormonal therapy. *Source*: From Ref. 51.

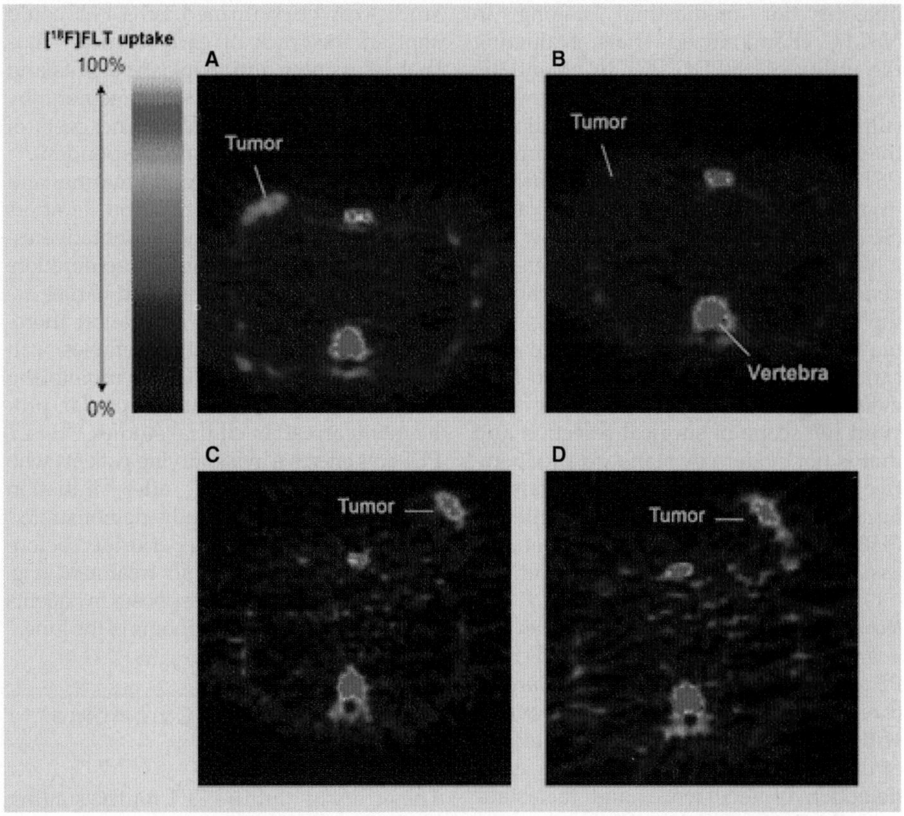

Figure 25-7 ■ ^{18}F-FLT PET images in responding and nonresponding patients 1 week after administration of combination chemotherapy. Pretreatment (**A**) and posttreatment (**B**) transaxial images of patient with grade II lobular breast cancer that responded to treatment. Pretreatment (**C**) and posttreatment (**D**) transaxial images of patient with grade II invasive ductal breast cancer that did not respond to treatment. *Source*: From Ref. 56.

before and 1 week after initiation of combination chemotherapy with 5-fluorouracil, epirubicin and cyclophosphamide (FEC). This study demonstrated that significant decrease in ^{18}F-FLT PET could predict response to therapy or stable disease already after 1 week after initiation of combination chemotherapy (Fig. 25-7). Other studies[57] demonstrated that a decrease in ^{18}F-FLT PET signal in tumors determined at two weeks after the end of the first course of chemotherapy is a useful predictor of long-term efficacy of chemotherapy regimens for women with breast cancer.

DCE MRI has also been shown effective in predicting which patients will respond to preoperative chemotherapy. Changes in the kinetics of Gd-contrast agent extravasation and intratumoral distribution before and early after initiation of chemotherapy predict response to chemotherapy administered in a neoadjuvant setting, and therefore spare patients who do not respond to therapy an unnecessary delay of surgery.[58-60]

Non-Small Cell Lung Carcinoma

Non-Small Cell Lung Carcinoma Diagnosis

Non-small cell lung carcinoma remains the leading cause of death due to cancer in both men and women in the United States.[61] Currently, ^{18}F-FDG PET/CT is the most sensitive noninvasive fusion imaging modality for the evaluation of a solitary pulmonary nodule. One study[62] revealed PET to have a specificity of 77%, sensitivity of 93%, positive predictive value of 72%, and negative predictive value of 94%. However, some reports suggest that in lesions with a high pretest probability, a negative finding on a ^{18}F-FDG PET image would likely not change management and is thus of no added value.[63]

Lung nodule dynamic contrast material–enhanced CT is widely available and has high negative predictive value and lower cost compared with those of FDG PET. However, in an analysis of 42 nodules imaged with both FDG PET and dynamic contrast-enhanced CT, FDG PET was found to be preferable to dynamic contrast-enhanced CT because of much higher specificity and only slightly lower sensitivity.[64] Both dynamic contrast-enhanced CT and FDG PET are suboptimal for evaluating nodules smaller than 8 mm, and, on the basis of Fleischner Society guidelines, these modalities should be followed by conventional CT except for nodules 4 mm or smaller in patients without increased risk for malignancy, in whom such nodules do not warrant follow-up.[65] When tissue diagnosis is indicated, FDG PET can help guide the biopsy location by helping discriminate viable from necrotic tumor. Because of the relatively low specificity of FDG PET, evaluation with the tracer FLT (chemical name, 3′-deoxy-3′-[fluorine 18]fluorothymidine) and PET, which helps assess cellular proliferation, has been suggested as an alternative.

Staging and Restaging of NSCLC ■ PET imaging with ^{18}F-FDG has a significant diagnostic and prognostic value in the initial staging, restaging, and surveillance of non-small cell lung cancer (NSCLC). ^{18}F-FDG PET in combination with conventional radiologic imaging brings significant changes in clinical management of NSCLC. In particular, PET imaging can improve initial staging and guide surgical and radiotherapy planning. After the end of treatment, PET has greater diagnostic accuracy than other imaging modalities for the detection of tumor recurrence. The recent development of fused PET/CT imaging has improved the radiologic evaluation of NSCLC patients by combining metabolic and anatomic imaging; however, this has resulted in more complexity in the image interpretation. It is important for the interpreting physician to understand the role PET/CT plays in the staging, assessment of treatment, and follow-up after therapy in the multidisciplinary management of patients with NSCLC. ^{18}F-FDG PET alone is superior to CT, in terms of sensitivity and specificity for the diagnosis and staging of lung cancer. Several studies[66,67] have demonstrated the benefit of ^{18}F-FDG PET in the management of lung carcinoma patients, primarily due to a more accurate staging. ^{18}F-FDG PET appears superior to CT imaging for mediastinal staging in NSCLC. Randomized trials evaluating the utility of ^{18}F-FDG PET in potentially resectable NSCLC report conflicting results in terms of the relative reduction in the number of noncurative thoracotomies. PET has not been studied as extensively in patients with small cell lung cancer (SCLC), but the available data show that it has good accuracy in staging extensive- versus limited-stage disease. Although the current evidence is conflicting, PET may improve results of early-stage lung cancer by identifying patients who have evidence of metastatic disease that is beyond the scope of surgical resection and that is not evident by standard preoperative staging procedures. Further trials are necessary to establish the clinical utility of PET as part of the standard preoperative assessment of early-stage lung cancer.[68]

Monitoring Therapy of NSCLC ■ For several years, molecular imaging with ^{18}F-FDG PET has become part of the standard of care in presurgical staging of patients with NSCLC, focusing on the detection of malignant lesions at early stages, early detection of recurrence, and metastatic spread. Currently, there is an increasing interest in the role of ^{18}F-FDG-PET beyond staging, such as the evaluation of biological characteristics of the tumor and prediction of prognosis in the context of treatment stratification and the early assessment of tumor response to therapy. Meta-analysis of previously published studies revealed that the degree of FDG uptake is of prognostic value at initial presentation, after induction treatment before resection, and in case of recurrence. At initial presentation, as well as posttreatment, FDG-PET is a better predictor of survival than TNM system staging or CT response.[69] Also, FDG-PET can distinguish patients with a good prognosis from those with a poor outcome, which may help in deciding on the most appropriate treatment and which may be of particular value in stratifying patients for clinical trials. FDG-PET is also of value in predicting outcome of induction therapy and it probably also has a predictive value early in the course of first-line therapy in the case of advanced disease. There are indications that FDG-PET can predict response and patient outcome as early as after one course of (induction) chemotherapy. However, monitoring tumor response with FDG-PET is still in its infancy. The methods of measurement of FDG uptake currently are diverse and timing with respect to anticancer therapy and used thresholds to define response are variable. Therefore, further study is required to deal with these major issues before it is possible to draw definite conclusions on FDG-PET as a tool for therapy response monitoring. If the results of the reviewed studies can be confirmed, FDG-PET could shorten the track of early clinical trials that assess new antineoplastic agents and could improve patient management by reducing morbidity, efforts, and costs of ineffective treatment in nonresponders.[70]

PET imaging using thymidine and analogs labeled with positron emitters provides noninvasive and quantitative estimates of regional cellular proliferation. Therefore, a more accurate and earlier assessment of response to anti-cancer therapies, especially cytostatic therapies, can be done using ^{18}F-FLT PET for monitoring changes in therapy-induced cellular proliferation arrest. In clinical studies, ^{18}F-FLT PET was effective in identifying patients who would respond early after initiation therapy.[71-74] A recent study demonstrated that ^{18}F-FLT PET imaging performed before and 7 days after gefitinib treatment (Fig. 25-8) was able to predict responses in patients with advanced adenocarcinoma of the lung.[75]

Small Cell Lung Carcinoma

Small Cell Lung Cancer

The utility of ^{18}F-FDG PET for the staging and management of patients with small cell lung carcinoma has been demonstrated in several studies.[76-82] Generally, as for other tumor types, high ^{18}F-FDG uptake in SCLC tumors is a predictor of poor outcome.[83] Metabolic response to therapy measured by repetitive ^{18}F-FDG PET (decrease in ^{18}F-FDG uptake) is a predictor of longer median time to progression of the disease.[84]

Colorectal Carcinoma Staging and Restaging

Diagnostic sensitivity of ^{18}F-FDG PET in colon carcinoma as reported by several studies ranges between 95% and 100%, but with a relatively low specificity, which is due to physiologic uptake of FDG in the bowel.[85,86] Therefore, the main application of ^{18}F-FDG PET in colorectal carcinoma is for staging of the disease, especially for restaging, which is more accurate than CT and often leads to changes in management decisions in more than half the patients that are evaluated for restaging.[87-91] ^{18}F-FDG PET is more sensitive as compared to CT for detection of local recurrence (95% and 65%, respectively) and comparably sensitive in detecting metastasis to the liver (98% and 93%, respectively). Combined PET/CT imaging with ^{18}F-FDG improves the accuracy of staging and restaging of colorectal carcinomas from 78% to 89%,[92] although this is not yet adequate. Suboptimal sensitivity and image resolution of ^{18}F-FDG is inadequate to detect lymph node micrometastatic disease. Also, due to a relatively high rate of false-positive results in patients with no clinical risk, patients with colon carcinomas have little additional benefit from ^{18}F-FDG PET compared to conventional imaging.[93]

MRI is the most accurate modality for the initial staging of rectal carcinoma, with similar, if not better sensitivity and specificity of endoluminal US imaging[94-97] and for the assessment of the extent of local invasion and characterization of regional nodal status. The accuracy of MRI ranges between 66% and 92% for Dukes staging of the primary tumor and between 60% and 90% for characterization of pelvic lymph node involvement. MRI, particularly unenhanced single-shot spin-echo echo planar imaging (SS SE-EPI), has good sensitivity and posi-

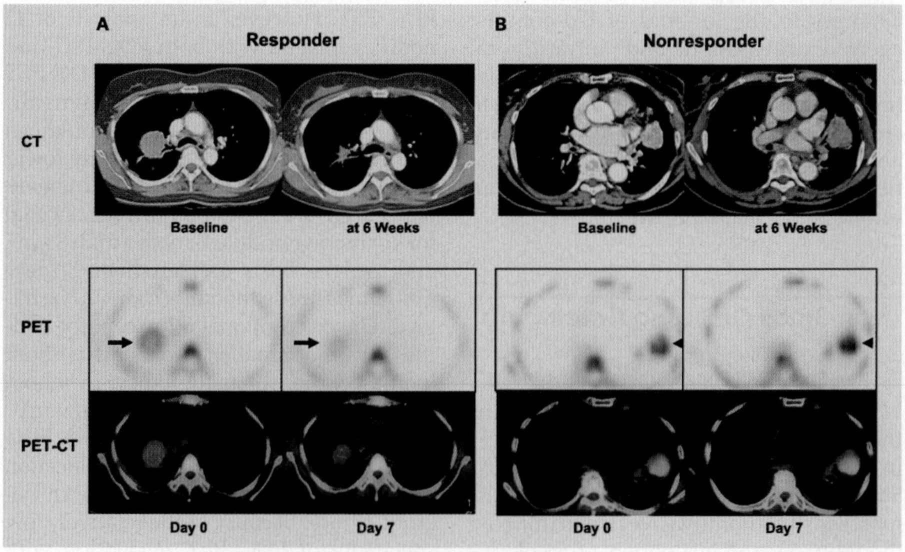

Figure 25-8 ■ PET images of a patient (**A**) show markedly decreased FLT uptake (SUV_{max} = 4.8 → 2.3) at 7 days after gefitinib therapy. The subsequent CT scan at 6 wks reveals tumor shrinkage. PET images of another patient (**B**) show no visible change at 7 days after gefitinib therapy (SUV_{max} = 7.2 → 8.0) and increase in tumor size at 6 weeks. *Source*: From Ref. 75.

tive predictive value for detecting liver metastases from colorectal carcinoma. Its sensitivity is better than that of FDG-PET/CT, especially for small lesions.[98]

The use of intravenous SPIOs has been shown to further improve the detection of lymph node metastases of colorectal carcinoma and other pelvic and abdominal malignancies with sensitivity and specificity of 93% and 100%, respectively.[99-102]

Monitoring Therapy of Colorectal Carcinoma

Among the MRI-based methods, DCE-MRI[103,104] and diffusion-weighted MRI (DW-MRI) for measurement of apparent diffusion coefficient (ADC) of water have shown promise for monitoring therapy of colorectal carcinoma.[105,106] In one of the studies,[107] comparison of mean ADC and cumulative radiation dose showed a significant decrease of mean ADC at the 2nd (P = 0.028), 3rd (P = 0.012), and 4th (P = 0.008) weeks of treatment. Posttreatment edema and fibrosis are considered the reasons for decrease in ADC of tumor lesions. In another more recent study, ADC measurements were performed to assess early response to chemotherapy in patients with colorectal and gastric hepatic metastases.[108] In the latter study, pre-therapy mean ADCs in responding lesions were significantly lower than those of non-responding lesions (P = 0.003). An early increase in ADCs (on day 3 or 7) was observed in responding lesions but not in non-responding lesions (P = 0.002). Weak but significant correlations were found between final tumor size reduction and both pretreatment ADCs (P = 0.006) and early ADC changes (day 3, P = 0.004; day 7, $P < 0.001$).

MRS of ^{19}F has also been used for pharmacokinetic studies with 5-FU and prediction of responses to 5-FU therapy.[109] The maximum level of 5-FU catabolites, as measured by ^{19}F-MRS, is predictive of treatment response in patients with large liver metastases, but not in small metastatic lesions in the liver, which is probably due to low volumetric resolution of MRS.[110]

^{18}F-FDG PET has been shown useful for prediction of therapeutic efficacy and clinical outcome in patients with colorectal carcinomas. ^{18}F-FDG-PET performed early after initiation of chemotherapy mainly depicts chemosensitivity. When performed at later time points or after completion of chemotherapy, chemoresistance of metastases is identified by persistent ^{18}F-FGD uptake.[111] For example, at 4 to 5 weeks after the initiation of therapy with 5-FU with or without interferon-α, the relative ^{18}F-FDG uptake in tumors distinguished responders from non-responders, both by lesion-by-lesion and overall patient response assessment with sensitivity of 100%; specificity of 90% and 75%, respectively.[112] Quantitative, dynamic ^{18}F-FDG PET identified patients who were not responsive to FOLFOX combination therapy or chemo-radiotherapy. Pre-treatment ^{18}F-FDG PET imaging had also been predictive of therapeutic outcome.[113,114] One of the studies,[115] demonstrated that a change in the maximum standardized uptake value of 62.5% or higher and a change in total lesion glycolysis of 69.5% or higher had significantly improved disease-specific (P = 0.08 and 0.03, respectively) and recurrence-free (P = 0.02 and 0.01, respectively) survival.

Also, ^{18}F-FDG PET was shown useful for monitoring of the efficacy of radiofrequency and cryosurgical ablation and chemoembolization of hepatic metastases, and was shown to be more sensitive and accurate in detection of recurrence, as compared to MRI and CT.[116,117]

^{18}F-FLT PET appears to be the most promising candidate for the characterization of tumor proliferation and, therefore, can be used in combination with ^{18}F-FDG for differential diagnosis of cancers (^{18}F-FDG and ^{18}F-FLT positive) and inflammatory lesions (^{18}F-FDG positive and ^{18}F-FLT negative).[118-120] However, ^{18}F-FLT PET is relatively insensitive for detectiing hepatic metastases, which is due to high normal level of ^{18}F-FLT-derived radioactivity in the liver (due to hepatobilliary clearance) and therefore is not suitable for restaging. There are mixed reports regarding the efficacy of ^{18}F-FLT PET for monitoring therapy in rectal carcinomas. For example, in one of the recent studies[121] the degree of change in ^{18}F-FLT uptake 2 weeks after initiation and after completion of neoad-

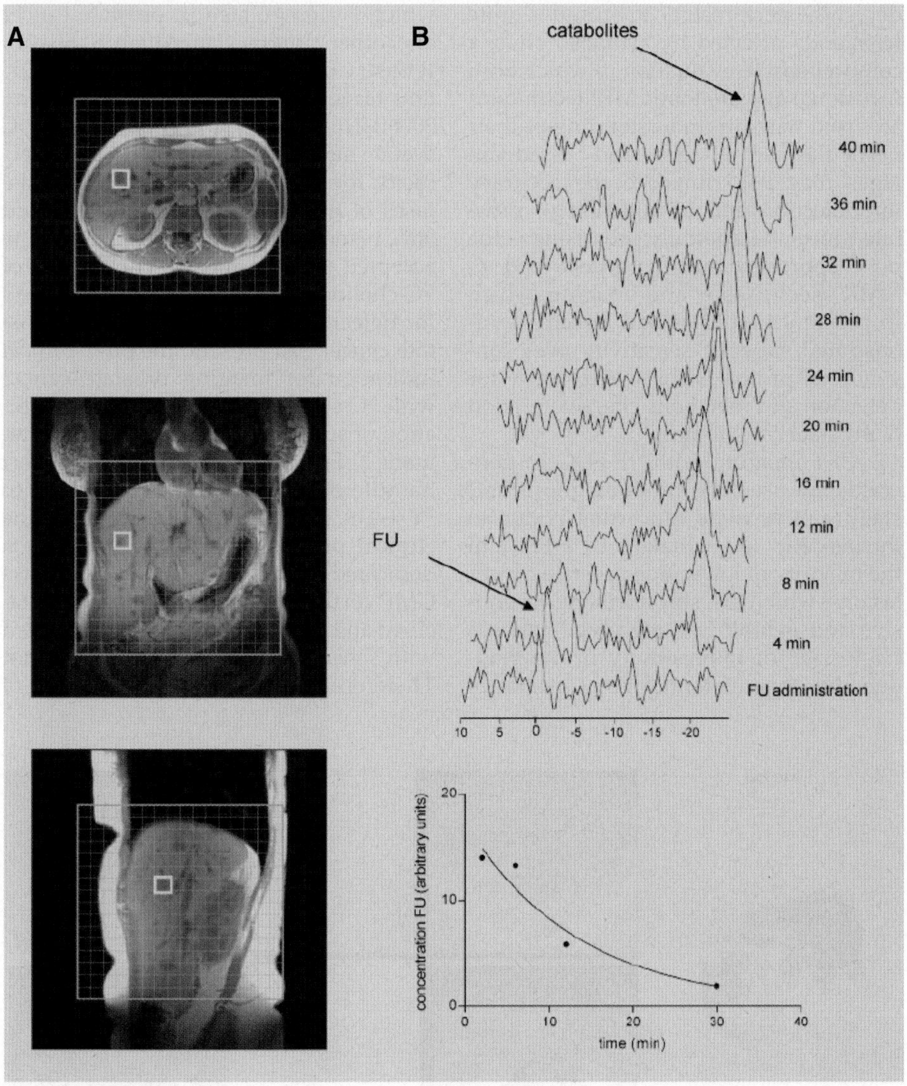

Figure 25-9 ^{19}F MRS of a metastasis in the liver of patient number 30. (**A**) Three orthogonal T1-weighted MR images of slices through the liver are shown with the grid for 3D CSI projected on top of the images. ^{19}F MRS was performed with an optimized CSI (see Patients and Methods). (**B**), ^{19}FMR spectra are shown, selected from the voxel indicated by a white square. They show the changes in signals of FU and catabolites with time after FU administration. The fitted curve FU versus time is shown on the lower right. The half-life of FU in this patient was 9.4 min (R2 of fit¼0.93). Assuming an FU half-life in blood of 5-15 min, this patient is classified as a "non-trapper." *Source*: From Ref. 109.

juvant therapy did not correlate with histopathological tumor regression. Another study[122] demonstrated that the decrease in ^{18}F-FLT uptake along with the decrease in ^{18}F-FDG uptake correlated with the long-term outcome of chemoradiotherapy. Therefore, the role of ^{18}F-FLT in monitoring chemo-radiotherapy of colorectal carcinomas deserves further investigation.

Prostate Carcinoma

Prostate Carcinoma Diagnosis, Staging, and Re-Staging

Prostate cancer is one of the most common cancers in men and the third leading cause of cancer death in men,[123] especially in African-American patients.[124] However, clinical behavior of prostate cancers varies substantially from patient to patient: some cancers are indolent with a relatively favorable prognosis, other cancers are characteristically more aggressive, metastatic, and cause high morbidity and mortality. Recent application of increasingly sophisticated molecular approaches to the study of prostate cancer in this "post-genomic" era has resulted in a rapid increase in the identification of somatic genome alterations and germline heritable risk factors in this disease. These findings are leading to a new understanding of the pathogenesis of prostate cancer and to the generation of new targets for diagnosis, prognosis, and prediction of therapeutic response.[125,126]

Therefore, in addition to more accurate staging of disease, molecular imaging of prostate cancer aims to provide the ability to differentially diagnose indolent versus aggressive cancer types, to permit noninvasive molecular profiling of key biomarker determinants of responsiveness to therapy and overall prognosis. The routine measurement of serum prostate-specific antigen (PSA) has made several anatomical imaging approaches for the initial screening and for therapy monitoring almost obsolete.

Molecular imaging using T2-weighted MRI has been widely used for diagnostic imaging of prostate cancer, but its accuracy for detectiing and localizing prostate cancer is still unsatisfactory. Endorectal coil MRI had improved the accuracy of diagnosis and staging of localized prostate cancer. DCE-MRI can be used to differentiate cancer from normal tissue and further improve the utility of MRI of prostate carcinoma. The advantages of DCE-MRI include the direct depiction of tumor vascularity and, possibly, obviation of an endorectal coil; however, there also are disadvantages, such as limited visibility of cancer in the transitional zone. DCE-MRI was shown to be more sensitive than T2W images for tumor localization (50% vs 21%; $p = 0.006$) and similarly specific (85% vs 81%; $p = 0.593$).[127,128]

Diffusion-weighted imaging (DWI) measures the restriction of diffusion and the reduction of ADC values in cancerous tissue. While this technique allows short acquisition time and provides high contrast resolution between cancer and normal tissue, individual variability in ADC values may erode diagnostic performance.[129,130] For better differentiation of tumor tissue versus normal prostate tissue, selective excitation pulse sequences have also been used to reduce contamination from lipid and water.[131,132]

The application of MRS for characterization of prostate carcinoma lesions is based on the higher ratio of choline and creatine to citrate concentrations in tumor tissue when compared to normal prostate tissue.[133-135] MRS also permits detection of prostate cancer in the transitional zone. However, MRS requires a long acquisition time, does not directly depict the periprostatic area, and is quite frequently affected by artifacts. Thus, a comprehensive evaluation in which both functional and anatomic MRI techniques are used with an understanding of their particular advantages and disadvantages may help improve the accuracy for detection and localization of prostate cancer.[136] Especially promising is the novel approach using hyperpolarized ^{13}C NMR spectroscopy and imaging, which in preclinical studies had already demonstrated superior sensitivity over conventional proton NMR spectroscopy for detection and metabolic characterization of prostate carcinomas.[137]

PET imaging with ^{18}F-FDG in general is not used for initial diagnosis and staging of prostate cancerthat is due to intrinsically low uptake of ^{18}F-FDG in the majority of low-grade prostate cancer lesions, which are still hormone responsive and exhibit low glycolytic activity. High level of radioactivity in the bladder (due to preferential renal clearance of ^{18}F-FDG) often generates image reconstruction artifacts that obscure prostate and confound interpretation of imaging results. This is why several studies have shown ^{18}F-FDG PET to have markedly lower sensitivity for the presence of prostate cancer than conventional anatomical imaging.[138-140] Nevertheless, several studies had demonstrated that decrease in ^{18}F-FDG uptake correlates with response to therapy.[141,142]

Due to inadequacy of ^{18}F-FDG PET for initial detection and staging of prostate cancer, several other PET imaging agents have been investigated, including choline labeled with either ^{11}C[143] or ^{18}F-labeled fluoromethyl and fluoroethyl choline.[144-147] Choline is critical for biosynthesis of cellular membrane and maintenance of its function. The rate limiting stem in choline accumulation is via phosphorylation by the choline kinase, which is upregulated in prostate cancer and other tumors (Janardhan S, Srivani P, Sastry GN. Choline kinase: an important target for cancer. Curr Med Chem. 2006;13(10):1169-86). ^{11}C-choline and ^{11}C acetate have similar sensitivity and specificity for detection lymph node metastases of prostate carcinoma of 80% and 96%, respectively.[148-152] However, it is now accepted that the routine clinical use of ^{11}C-choline PET cannot be recommended for detecting and staging primary prostate cancer . At present, the only clinical indication for imaging prostate cancer with ^{11}C-choline-PET (Fig. 25-10) is evaluation of suspected recurrence after treatment.[153] Furthermore, a relatively short half-life of ^{11}C (~20 min) as compared to ^{18}F (~110 min) limits its use in routine clinical practice due to the need for a dedicated clinical cyclotron, in-house GMP-certified radiotracer production facility, and practical limitations associated with scheduling of imaging procedures. Therefore, several ^{18}F-labeled analogs of

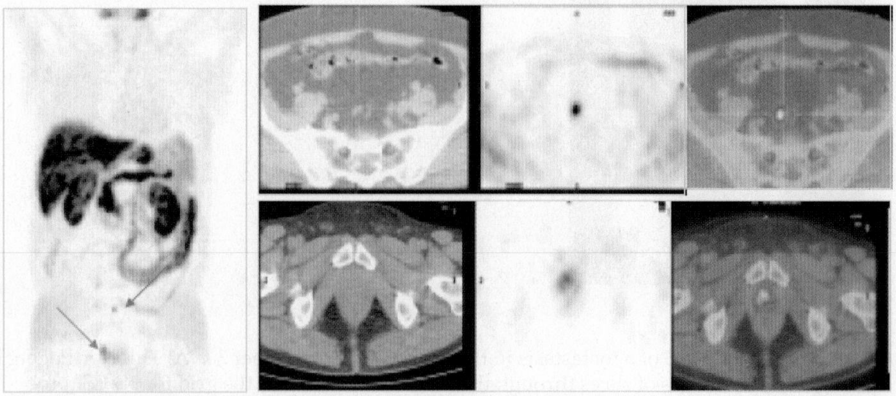

Figure 25-10 A 66-year-old patient with biopsy-proven primary PCa; PSA: 7 ng/mL. ^{11}C-choline PET/CT identified intraprostatic cancer (*lower arrow*) and pre-sacral, lymph-node metastasis (diameter of metastatic deposit: 10 mm, *upper arrow*). Another LNMin the right obturator region (diameter of metastatic deposit: 1.2 mm) was not visualized. Upper images show CT, PET, and PET over CT in two different, transverse, image planes. *Source*: From Ref. 153.

choline have been developed to date and evaluated to certain extent for PET imaging and staging of prostate carcinomas. In general, it has been demonstrated that ^{18}F fluorocholine and ^{18}F fluoroethylcholine exhibit sensitivity and specificity similar to that of ^{11}C choline for detection of primary and metastatic lesions.[154-156]

^{11}C-labeled acetate has also been explored as a potential radiotracer for PET imaging of prostate carcinoma. The rationale for using radiolabeled acetate for imaging of tumors is that it is the precursor to synthesis of acetyl-CoA, which is further utilized in the tricarboxylic acid (TCA) cycle and fatty acid synthesis (FAS). Both TCA and FAS are known to be upregulated, albeit differentially, in the majority of malignancies,[157-159] which has been found to have increased activity in malignant cells of epithelial origin.[90] PET with ^{11}C-acetate has higher sensitivity for detection and staging of primary and metastatic prostate carcinomas, as compared with ^{18}F-FDG, with sensitivities ranging between 59% and 83%. However, the lack of discrimination between prostate carcinoma and benign prostatic hyperplasia has been identified as the major limitation for ^{11}C-acetate PET.[160-163]

PET with ^{11}C-methionine had also shown effectiveness in the evaluation of prostate cancer patients, although its utility or limitations are not sufficiently explored yet. Only a few studies have been reported to date demonstrating that ^{11}C-methionine PET has suitable sensitivity for detection of prostate carcinoma lesions when compared to conventional imaging modalities.[164,165]

Another novel molecular PET imaging agent labeled with ^{18}F, anti-1-amino-3-^{18}F-fluorocyclobutane-1-carboxylic acid (^{18}F-FACBC), has shown promising results in detecting recurrence of prostate carcinoma.[166] Fifteen patients with a recent diagnosis of prostate cancer (n = 9) or suspected recurrence (n = 6) and a mean PSA of 15.0 ng/mL were studied. The ^{18}F-FACBC PET/CT images were compared with clinical, conventional images and pathologic follow-up. In 8 patients with newly diagnosed prostate cancer, ^{18}F-FACBC PET/CT had accurately detected malignancy in 40 of 48 prostate sextants. Pelvic nodal metastases were identified in 7 of 9 patients and were indeterminate in 2 of 9. In all 4 patients who had proven recurrence, ^{18}F-FACBC PET/CT identified malignancies (Fig. 25-11). Larger clinical studies are needed to evaluate ^{18}F-FACBC PET/CT.

Bones and lymph nodes are the most common sites of prostate cancer metastases. Gamma scintigraphy with ^{99m}Tc-methylene diphosphonate (^{99m}Tc-MDP) has been widely used for imaging of bone metastases. Recently, ^{18}F-fluoride had re-emerged as a very effective radiotracer for molecular imaging of bone

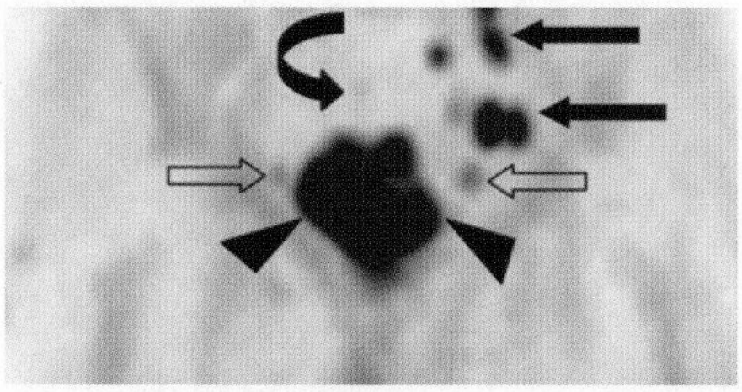

Figure 25-11 ^{18}F-FACBC PET imaging results in a 73-year-old man with extensive invasive prostate carcinoma, with bilateral obturator and left iliac chain lymph nodal involvement. Maximum-intensity-projection image demonstrates extent of large prostate primary (arrowheads) as well as bilateral obturator (open arrows) and left iliac (solid straight arrows) nodes. Bladder activity is not present (curved arrow at bladder location). *Source*: From Ref. 166.

metastatic disease. Increased ^{18}F-fluoride uptake in metastatic bone lesions reflects osteoblastic activity within these lesions. In a thoroughly conducted study, the efficacy of detection of bone metastases by ^{99m}Tc-MDP planar bone scintigraphy, ^{99m}Tc-MDP SPECT, ^{18}F-fluoride PET, and ^{18}F-fluoride PET/CT was compared in 44 patients with high-risk prostate cancer.[167] The sensitivity, specificity, positive predictive value, and negative predictive value were 70%, 57%, 64%, and 55%, respectively, for planar bone scintigraphy, 92%, 82%, 86%, and 90%, for single photon emission computed tomography (SPECT), 100%, 62%, 74%, and 100%, for ^{18}F-fluoride PET, and for ^{18}F-fluoride PET/CT were 100% for all parameters. This particular study demonstrated that ^{18}F-fluoride PET/CT is a highly sensitive and specific imaging modality for the detection of bone metastases in high-risk patients. ^{18}F-fluoroethylcholine PET/CT has also been shown useful for detection of bone metastases.[168,169]

Imaging Andogen Receptor Status

There has been considerable interest in the development of in vivo techniques that would permit noninvasive assessment of androgen receptor status in prostate carcinomas. The 16-[18F]fluoro-5-dihydrotestosterone (FDHT), is an androgen analog, that has been shown to accumulate in AR-expressing tissues.[170] Few clinical studies have been conducted to date using ^{18}F-FDHT PET, but all had demonstrated potential utility for the assessment of AR-expressing hormone-responsive versus AR-mutant hormone non-responsive tumor burden in patients with advanced prostate carcinomas. Results of one such study,[171] conducted in 20 patients with advanced prostate carcinoma, had corroborated the results of conventional diagnostic imaging in 12 of 19 patients (sensitivity of 63%), including the 2 patients with innumerable lesions. ^{18}F-FDHT PET detected 24 of 28 known lesions (86%) in the remaining 10 patients. In addition, ^{18}F-FDHT PET detected 17 unsuspected lesions in 5 of these 10 patients. All 12 patients with positive ^{18}F-FDHT PET underwent a repeat PET study after receiving flutamide for 1 day (250 mg t.i.d.). In all of these patients, there was a statistically significant decrease in tumor uptake of ^{18}F-FDHT after flutamide (p = 0.002). The mean PSA in patients with positive FDHT-PET was significantly higher than that in patients with negative FDHT-PET (p = 0.006). In another study, diagnostic sensitivities of ^{99m}Tc-methylene diphosphonate (bone metastases seeking agent for gamma camera imaging), ^{18}F-FDG and ^{18}F-FDHT have been compared as part of the study carried out in seven patients with advanced prostate carcinoma for the assessment of radiation dosimetry of diagnostic doses of ^{18}F-FDHT.[172] An interesting inverse relationship between the level of ^{18}F-FDG and ^{18}F-FDHT accumulation was observed in individual metastatic lesions in several patients (Fig. 25-12). The latter observation suggests that prostate carcinoma lesions with mutant AR (low ^{18}F-FDHT accumulation) are more metabolically active (high ^{18}F-FDG accumulation) and vice versa and could be differentially diagnosed using this dual-radiotracer PET imaging approach.

Several novel molecular imaging agents are currently in development for diagnosis and monitoring of therapy of prostate carcinoma patients. Among one of the most interesting ones are radiotracers targeting prostate-specific membrane antigen (PSMA), which are currently in preclinical studies.[173-175]

Lymphoma

Diagnosis and Staging

Lymphoma is the most common primary hematopoietic malignancy in the United States.[176] Chemotherapy and radiation therapy for both Hodgkin and non-Hodgkin lymphoma is determined by the stage of the disease. Staging of lymphomas is based on the number of sites involved in the disease, nodal or extranodal involvement, and the localization of the bulk of the disease. Therefore, noninvasive whole body anatomic, functional, and molecular imaging approaches play a significant role in diagnosis and staging of lymphomas. Physical examination and a CT combined with bone marrow and other biopsies in certain situations have been the mainstay of the staging of lymphomas.[177] MRI has not been used extensively, and in comparative studies no great differences in accuracy have been found between CT scans and MRI.[178-180] 67-Gallium scintigraphy was formerly

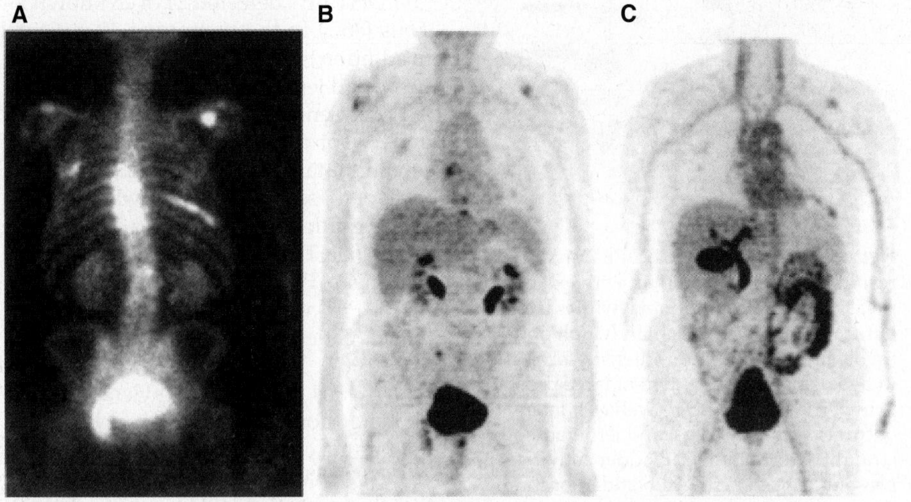

Figure 25-12 ■ Comparative whole-body images of a 75-year-old man with progressive prostate cancer metastatic to bones of the thoracic spine, left rib cage, and scapula: planar λ-camera image of ^{99m}Tc-methylene diphosphonate (**A**); 1-pixel-thick coronal PET image of ^{18}F-FDG (**B**); and 1-pixel-thick coronal PET image of ^{18}F-FDHT (**C**). *Source*: From Ref. 172.

considered valuable for detecting lymphoma involvement, but ^{18}F-FDG-PET has been shown to be significantly more sensitive, and ^{67}Ga scintigraphy has now largely been abandoned.[181-189] However, the standard procedures fail to identify a considerable number of sites, particularly extranodal lesions.

^{18}F-FDG PET has been used as an additional method for staging in several clinical trials, most of which suffer from methodological problems associated with the lack of validation, as it is impossible to biopsy all affected lymph nodes or organs. Therefore, a reference standard based on all available evidence from CT, FDG-PET, and all available clinical information including follow-up must be used instead. Nevertheless, it is currently accepted that ^{18}F-FDG-PET is more accurate than CT for diagnosing both nodal and extranodal disease in Hodgkin lymphoma and aggressive non-Hodgkin lymphoma. ^{18}F-FDG-PET also has had a strong impact on the staging of Hodgkin lymphoma and aggressive non-Hodgkin lymphomas, affecting treatment planning.[190-198] However, ^{18}F-FDG PET does not permit differentiation of lymphomas from inflammatory lymphadenopathy due to other causes. ^{18}F-FDG PET is also relatively insensitive for low-grade lymphomas, and in particular for mucosa-associated lymphoid tissue lymphoma.[199-202] ^{18}F-FDG PET has superior sensitivity and specificity for the staging of lymphomas compared with those of conventional imaging once the diagnosis of lymphoma has already been made. In some cases, in which ^{18}F-FDG PET findings did not match with those observed on CT, the ^{18}F-FDG PET positive lesions have been confirmed by biopsy.[203]

Restaging and Therapy Monitoring in Lymphoma

Molecular imaging with ^{18}F-FDG PET has a sensitivity of 87% and a specificity of 93% for the diagnosis of recurrent disease, compared to that of CT, which is 93% and 90%, respectively. Conventional imaging approaches for restaging of lymphoma have positive and negative predictive values of 72% and 67%, respectively, while ^{18}F-FDG PET has a significantly better positive and negative predictive values of 95% and 83%, respectively.[204] With the introduction of combined PET/CT imaging instrumentation and imaging protocols, ^{18}F-FDG PET/CT is becoming the most prescribed study necessary for follow-up of patients with lymphoma. Despite this, ^{18}F-FDG PET/CT findings do not predict outcome uniformly well. In one study, ^{18}F-FDG PET predicted complete remission more effectively in patients with moderate risk (stage I-III, no relapse, and no more than 2 different prior therapy regimens) than in patients with high-risk disease, with a negative predictive values of 90% versus 50–67% at conventional imaging.[205] In another study, the change in the magnitude of ^{18}F-FDG uptake from baseline to post-therapy PET/CT was on average 72.9% after 2 cycles of chemotherapy and 79.8% after 4 cycles of chemotherapy, with no statistically significant difference (*P* value: 0.24). Therefore, larger, prospective, randomized trials are required to validate ^{18}F-FDG PET/CT as a method for monitoring treatment response in lymphomas.

Although ^{18}F-FDG PET-CT is currently most widely used for treatment response assessment in lymphoma patients, it has its limitations. These limitations are particularly evident in some histological subtypes of lymphomas, which demonstrate variable uptake of ^{18}F-FDG. Follicular lymphoma is often positive at PET, demonstrating 40% more abnormal nodal disease sites than CT alone, but the uptake of ^{18}F-FDG is disease grade-dependent. The sensitivity of ^{18}F-FDG-PET for chronic lymphocytic leukemia is unacceptably low, detecting less than 60% of the abnormal nodes identified by CT.[206] In mucosa-associated lymphoid tissue (MALT) lymphomas, the uptake of ^{18}F-FDG in the organs affected by lymphoma is poor, while the involved lymph nodes are usually well identifiable.[207] Therefore, the use of ^{18}F-FDG PET in response assessment in certain subtypes is prone to significant error unless the patient has pre-treatment functional imaging and, therefore, additional molecular PET imaging agents are needed to address these limitations.

PET with ^{18}F-FLT was shown to be effective in the detection and assessment of lymphoma proliferation, and in differentiating between high- and low-grade lymphomas and tumor grading.[208] In high-grade non-Hodgkin lymphoma patients, chemotherapy is associated with an early decrease ^{18}F-FLT uptake.[209] However, when PET imaging with ^{18}F-FDG and ^{18}F-FLT was compared for functional diagnosis of residual lymphomas after chemoradiotherapy, the overall survival for patients with a negative PET scan was significantly higher than for patients with positive PET, irrespective of the tracer used.[210] ^{18}F-FLT alone was able to distinguish patients with long and short overall survival, although there was no statistically significant difference in survival between cases that were ^{18}F-FDG and ^{18}F-FLT negative compared to those that were ^{18}F-FDG negative alone. Furthermore, ^{18}F-FDG detected more lesions than did ^{18}F-FLT, but the additional biological characterization of tumor tissue with respect to proliferation by ^{18}F-FLT might provide additional valuable information for the detection of recurrence.

MRI can also provide additional valuable information for monitoring treatment response in lymphoma patients, particularly in assessing bone marrow. The signal intensity of active, untreated disease is relatively high on T2 weighted images due to an excess of free water. After successful treatment, the cellular and water content of the tumor decreases, and the residual tissue (collagen and fibrotic components) predominantly contribute to the reduced signal.[211] The sensitivity of MRI for treatment response monitoring varies from 45% to 90%, with a specificity ranging from 80% to 90%.[212,213] The potential role of new contrast agents, such as USPIOs, which are taken up by normal and hypercellular bone marrow, but not by neoplastic lesions, is unclear at present.[214] MR lymphangiography (MRL) using the intravenously administered contrast agent Ferumoxtran-10 with a long plasma circulation time is a novel cellular imaging tool for the evaluation of nodal involvement noninvasively. Ferumoxtran-10 belongs to a class of nanoparticle-based contrast agents known as USPIO. It is commercially known as Sinerem® in Europe,[215] but are not yet FDA-approved.

Phosphorus 31 (^{31}P) MRS has also been studied for monitoring treatment responses in lymphomas by measuring phosphomonoester-to-nucleotide triphosphate ratio, which decreases after treatment in responders but not in nonresponders. Moreover, the phosphomonoester-to-nucleotide triphosphate ratio before therapy was shown to predict the outcome of treatment in non-Hodgkin lymphoma.[216] Certainly, this is an emerging technique that needs larger multicenter trials, but which could have enormous implications for detecting responses to lymphoma therapy in the future.

Melanoma

Diagnosis and Staging of Melanoma

A recent and very thorough review of literature had analyzed 28 ^{18}F-FDG PET imaging studies involving 2,905 patients, who met the inclusion criteria.[217] The pooled estimates of ^{18}F-FDG PET for the detection of metastasis in the initial staging of CMM included a sensitivity of 83% (95% confidence interval [CI]: 81%, 84%); specificity, 85% (95% CI: 83%, 87%); positive likelihood ratio (LR), 4.56 (95% CI: 3.12, 6.64); negative LR, 0.27 (95% CI: 0.18, 0.40); and diagnostic odds ratio, 19.8 (95% CI: 10.8, 36.4). Results from 8 studies suggested that ^{18}F-FDG PET was associated with 33% disease management changes (range, 15–64%). Compared with previous meta-analyses,[218,219] this overall estimate is slightly better for sensitivity (83% vs 79%), but comparable for specificity (85% vs 86%). Therefore, there is a good evidence that ^{18}F-FDG PET is useful for the initial staging of patients with CMM, especially as adjunctive role in Stages III and IV, to help detect deep soft-tissue, lymph node, and visceral metastases. ^{18}F-FDG PET/CT imaging seems to be more accurate than ^{18}F-FDG PET alone, as suggested by 4 eligible studies.

As in many other tumor types, one of the main limitations of ^{18}F-FDG PET is its poor sensitivity to detection of micrometastatic disease sites. For example, one study has demonstrated that the median tumor volume per lymph node was 28.3 mm^3, whereas for ^{18}F-FDG PET to demonstrate disease in regional lymph nodes with 90% sensitivity, the volume of tumor should be 78 mm^3.[220] In another study, ^{18}F-FDG PET demonstrated very low sensitivity (14.3%; 95% CI, 2.5–44%) and positive predictive value (50%; 95% CI, 9–90%) for localizing the subclinical nodal metastases. The specificity, net present value, and diagnostic accuracy were 94.7%, 75%, and 73%, respectively.[221] Also, as for other tumor types, inflammatory lymphadenopathy contributes to false-positive results of ^{18}F-FDG PET.

Therefore, other radiotracers had also been evaluated for initial detection and for monitoring treatment response in melanoma, including ^{11}C-methionine,[222] ^{18}F-FLT,[223] ^{11}C-L-thyrosine,[224] and 6-[^{18}F] fluoro-L-dopa.[225] All these radiotracers demonstrated promise, but the literature describing clinical studies using these alternative radiotracers is rather scarce, and additional clinical studies are needed to assess their diagnostic accuracy in melanoma patients.

MRI was shown to be more sensitive than CT for detection of melanoma metastases that involve the brain, liver, and skeleton.[226] Potential single metastatic deposits demonstrated on MRI usually require biopsy for confirmation. Comparison of the whole-body MRI with whole-body CT in 41 Stage III and IV melanoma patients demonstrated that whole-body MR imaging detected more lesions and led to alteration in treatment plan in 24% of the patients. MRI could be useful for further characterizing individual metastasis, for example, prior to surgery, but it would not be a first-line investigation for staging.

Head and Neck Cancer

Diagnosis and Staging of Head and Neck Carcinoma

^{18}F-FDG PET has become a widely accepted molecular imaging modality for evaluation of head and neck squamous cell carcinomas (HNSCC). ^{18}F-FDG PET may assist in the identification of the primary carcinoma in about 25% of cases, although it is not a substitute for careful endoscopic examination and clinical experience. When used as an initial staging study for patients with advanced HNSCC, PET may identify sites of possible distant metastases or second primary carcinomas in approximately 20% of cases, and over 70% of these are likely to be true positive sites of malignancy.[227] PET has limited value in the setting of the detection of occult nodal metastases and is not recommended for this purpose. One of the most widespread applications of ^{18}F-FDG PET has been for the assessment of recurrent disease following therapy for HNSCC. Studies have generally demonstrated that PET has a high sensitivity for identifying recurrent carcinoma (84–100%) with moderate specificities (61–93%).[228-235] One larger study included 143 patients, in which the ^{18}F-FDG PET was performed after treatment consisting of surgery (64%), radiation (97%), or chemoradiation therapy (65%).[236] The overall sensitivity and specificity of PET was 96% and 72% respectively. When performance was analyzed at local, regional, and distant sites, the specificity of ^{18}F-FDG PET was higher at regional (95%) and distant (95%) sites, but lower (79%) at local sites due to false positive readings. False positive results are typically due to treatment-related effects, inflammation, infection, or recent biopsies. The overall positive predictive value of PET was 69%, while the negative predictive value was 96%. Other studies had demonstrated that PET/CT has been shown to be more accurate than PET alone (96% vs 90%, $P = 0.03$).[237] Also ^{18}F-FDG PET/CT was significantly more accurate than ^{18}F-FDG PET alone or CT alone for detection of malignancy in the head and neck with sensitivity of 98%, specificity of 92%, and an accuracy of 94%.[238]

Monitoring Therapy of Head and Neck Carcinoma

For monitoring treatment response in HNSCC, the optimal timing of ^{18}F-FDG PET following radiation therapy remains unclear, although studies have suggested higher accuracy at intervals of 3 months or greater following completion of radiation. The role of ^{18}F-FDG PET/CT for intensity modulated radiation therapy planning is currently being evaluated and remains controversial. Novel radioactive tracers may enable PET to identify sites of DNA replication (with ^{18}F-FLT), protein metabolism (^{11}C-methionine), hypoxia (with ^{18}F-FMISO or $^{60/61}$Cu-ATSM), and other processes linked to malignancy. For example, hypoxic imaging with PET may be achieved using ^{18}F-misonidazole (^{18}F-FMISO) that accumulates selectively in hypoxic conditions, but shows minimal uptake in tissues with normal oxygenation. Early studies have suggested that FMISO may have value in imaging head and neck cancers, and may have prognostic value for outcomes following radiation therapy.[239] Other studies demonstrated the feasibility of $^{60/61}$Cu-ATSM-guided intensity–modulated radiotherapy (IMRT) approach through co-registering hypoxia $^{(60)}$Cu-ATSM PET to the corresponding CT images for IMRT planning (Fig. 25-13).[240,241] Additional investigation and clinical trials are necessary to validate the utility of these novel radiotracers for molecular imaging of head and neck cancers.

Although melanoma patients with regional nodal metastases are frequently imaged with CT and MRI scans, the efficacy of routine radiologic staging in asymptomatic patients with microscopic nodal involvement has not been well established. Several studies suggest that the vast majority of asymptomatic patients with a new diagnosis of microscopic SLN-positive melanoma do not harbor radiologically detectable SDM and can proceed to complete lymph node dissection without immediate CT or MRI staging.[242] MRI for nodal staging Feasibility studies using SPIO contrast-enhanced demonstrated sensitivity as high as 96% and a specificity as high as 97% according to nodal group.[243-247]

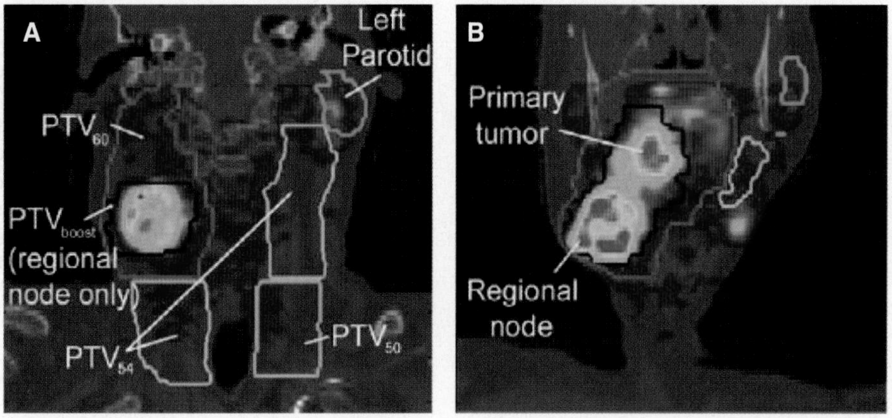

Figure 25-13 ■ Coronal images of the HNSCC patient with overlay of a pre-treatment ^{61}Cu-ATSM PET image. The ^{61}Cu-ATSM retention was the highest in PTVboost, in which (**A**) the regional node and (**B**) the regional node and the primary tumor are shown. The regional node contained a more complex distribution of ^{61}Cu-ATSM retention than the primary tumor. The plane in image (**A**) is inferior to the plane in image (**B**). *Source*: From Ref. 241.

Thyroid Carcinoma

Gamma scintigraphy and SPECT with ^{131}I and ^{123}I radioiodine are the main techniques for staging and leading approaches to treatment of thyroid cancer. However, as thyroid cancer dedifferentiates during progression of the disease, the expression of sodium-iodide symporter (NIS) decreases, and the accumulation of radioiodine decreases. In contrast, the glycolytic activity increases during dedifferentiation, as reflected by increased magnitude of ^{18}F-FDG accumulation in high-grade thyroid carcinoma lesions. In a study involving 108 patients,[248] who were suspected of having recurrence or metastasis and whose ^{131}I whole body scans were negative, ^{18}F-FDG PET revealed recurrence or metastases in 59 patients (sensitivity 93.7%), whereas thyroglobulin (Tg) levels were elevated in 41 (sensitivity 65.1%). In 35 of 45 patients in remission, ^{18}F-FDG PET was negative (specificity 77.8%). Of 40 patients with a negative radioiodine scan showing diffuse hepatic uptake, metastases occurred in 23 patients and remission in 17. ^{18}F-FDG PET showed 100% sensitivity and 76.5% specificity in the detection of recurrence in those 40 patients. In another study, conducted in patients with elevated thyroglobulin levels and a negative finding on a total-body radioiodine scintigraphic scan, ^{18}F-FDG PET was found to be 95% sensitive and 88% accurate for identification of disease sites, and, in 38% of the cases, the discovery of additional sites of disease led to a change in surgical planning.[249] A recent review of the literature[250] provides an overview of the efficacy of ^{18}F-FDG PET in diagnostic imaging of well-differentiated follicular and papillary thyroid cancer. Integration of PET/CT imaging has improved diagnostic accuracy and patient management in differentiated thyroid cancer, which affected patient treatment in 48% of patients when compared with standard ^{18}F-FDG PET and CT performed and analyzed separately.[251]

Gastro-Esophageal Cancer

Accurate staging of esophageal cancer is important when determining which patients will potentially benefit from curative surgery. There is an ongoing debate regarding the impact of ^{18}F-FDG PET and PET/CT imaging on management of patients with gastroesophageal cancers. A recent report based on the literature review concluded that currently ^{18}F-FDG PET has no role in the primary detection of gastric cancer due to its low sensitivity. ^{18}F-FDG PET shows, slightly better results in the evaluation of lymph node metastases in gastric cancer compared to CT and could have therefore a role in the preoperative staging.[252] A recent study, however, reported that the addition of ^{18}F-FDG PET to routine preoperative staging resulted in the exclusion from surgery of 19 (25%) patients who prior to the introduction of ^{18}F-FDG PET would have undergone attempted resection. This study concluded that ^{18}F-FDG PET should be performed in all patients under consideration for esophagogastric resection in order to avoid resection in patients with disseminated disease.[253] The combination of CT and endoscopic US has the highest sensitivity for the detection of small paraesophageal lymph nodes. However, the specificity of ^{18}F-FDG PET (90%) is higher, and ^{18}F-FDG PET has higher accuracy for staging of M1a lymph nodes.[254] In pre-surgical staging for the presence of resectable versus nonresectable disease, ^{18}F-FDG PET is also more accurate than CT (88% vs 65%).[255] ^{18}F-FDG PET appears to be more sensitive, although less specific than CT, for detection of regional recurrence of the disease (92% and 83% vs 83% and 92%, respectively). However, ^{18}F-FDG PET is significantly more sensitive and specific than CT for detection of distant disease sites (95% and 80% vs 79% and 70%, respectively). Also, ^{18}F-FDG PET and PET/CT imaging can accurately stratify patients in terms of responsiveness at an early stage of neoadjuvant chemotherapy.[256-258] According to results of some studies, ^{18}F-FDG PET/CT is as sensitive and specific in detection of recurred gastric cancer except peritoneal seeding.[259] However, additional PET/CT on contrast CT does not seem to increase diagnostic accuracy in detection of recurrent gastric cancer.[260] Further studies are warranted to validate the role of PET/CT in detection of gastric cancer recurrence.

The utility of USPIO contrast-enhanced MRI has been recently evaluated for detection of lymph node metastases in gastric cancer. One of the studies demonstrated that USPIO contrast-enhanced MR had 96.2% sensitivity, 98.3% specificity, 90.1% positive predictive value, 99.0% negative predictive value, and 97.1% accuracy.[261] Therefore, the assessment of lymph node metastases from USPIO-post-contrast MRI is a promising new methodology for diagnosis of regional lymph node metastases in gastric cancer.

Hepatocellular Carcinoma

Accurate diagnosis and staging of hepatocellular carcinoma (HCC) is critical, because aggressive locoregional intervention in advanced HCC is possible in absence of extrahepatic metastases. However, in presence of extrahepatic spread, HCC is categorized as systemic disease and the treatment is limited with poor prognosis. Ttriple-phase CT and contrast-enhanced MRI are widely accepted imaging modalities for staging HCC with accuracies exceeding 80%. Nevertheless, CT and MRI have a limited ability to identify distant metastases. Several studies have demonstrated efficacy of ^{18}F-FDG PET in detecting distant metastases of HCC. The magnitude of ^{18}F-FDG uptake appears to be proportionally related to the expression of molecular markers involved in tumor progression and metastasis. However, the role of ^{18}F-FDG PET remains limited in the screening or diagnosis of primary HCC because of its low sensitivity.[262-264]

PET with another radiotracer, ^{11}C-acetate, is currently undergoing evaluation in HCC patients. Histopathologic validation of PET imaging results suggests that the well-differentiated HCC tumors are detected by ^{11}C-acetate and the poorly differentiated types are detected by ^{18}F-FDG.[265] Addition of ^{11}C-acetate to ^{18}F-FDG PET/CT increases the overall sensitivity for the detection of primary HCC but not for the detection of extrahepatic metastases (Fig. 25-14). ^{18}F-FDG, ^{11}C-acetate, and dual-tracer PET/CT have a low sensitivity for the detection of small primary HCC, but ^{18}F-FDG PET/CT has a relatively high sensitivity for the detection of extrahepatic metastases of HCC.[266] Another group has also reported that ^{11}C-acetate PET/CT was complemen-

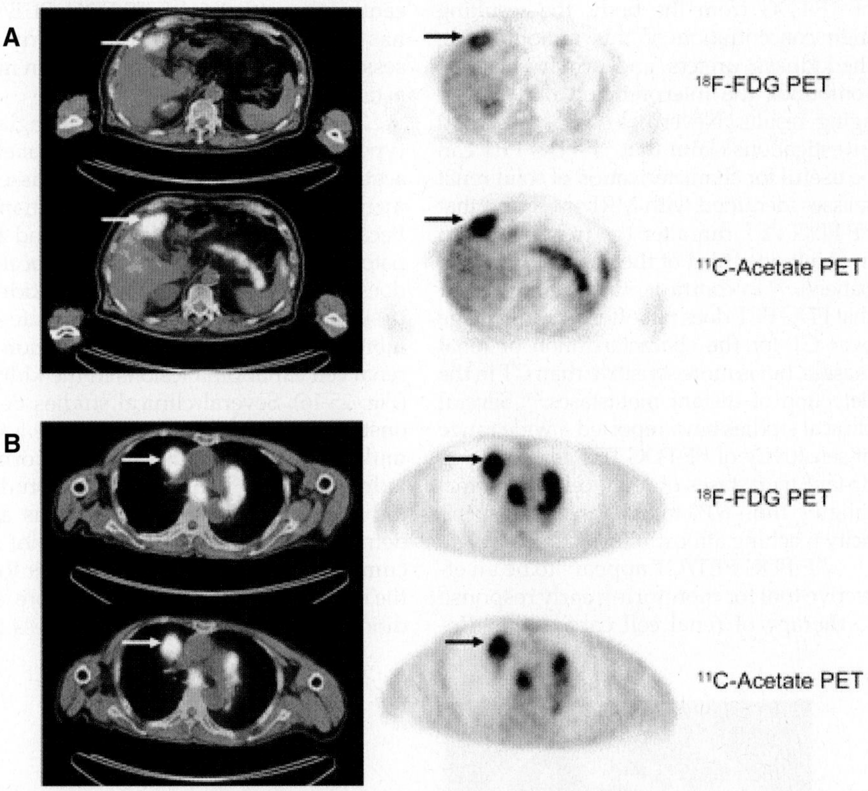

Figure 25-14 Detection of HCC with ^{18}F-FDG PET/CT and ^{11}C-acetate PET/CT on transaxial sections of liver and chest. Panels on left show PET/CT, and panels on right show PET. (**A**) Primary HCC of liver was markedly positive for uptake with both tracers (*arrows*). (**B**) Metastatic HCC of upper lobe of right lung was markedly positive for uptake with both tracers (*arrows*). *Source*: From Ref. 266.

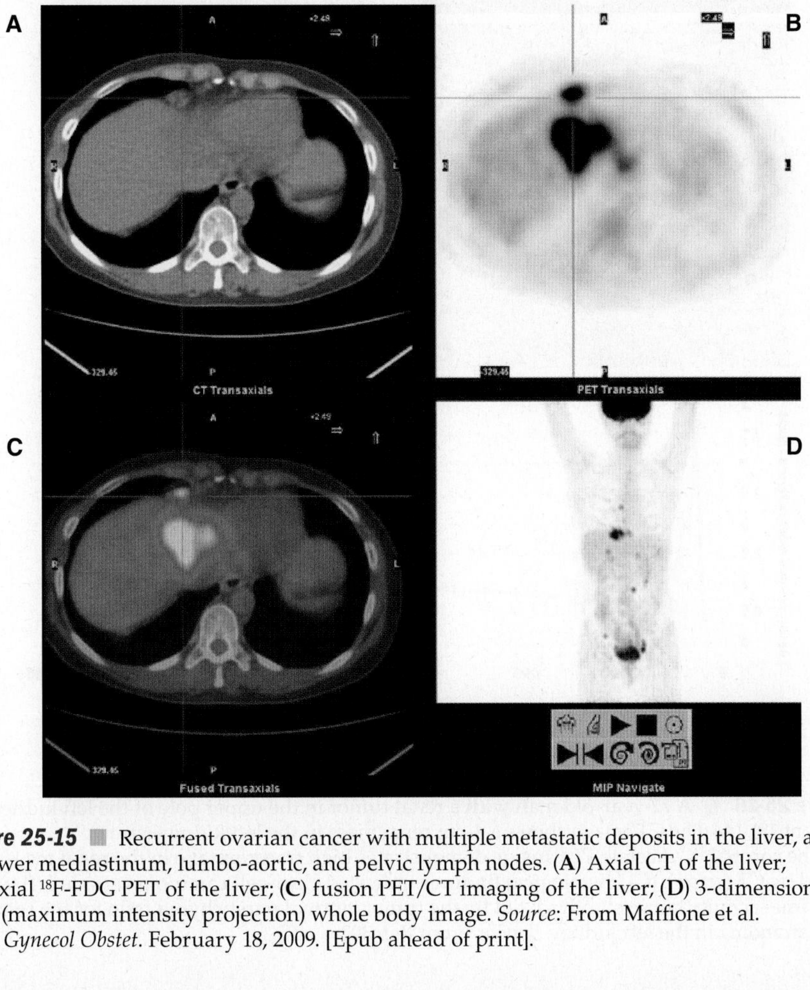

Figure 25-15 Recurrent ovarian cancer with multiple metastatic deposits in the liver, and in lower mediastinum, lumbo-aortic, and pelvic lymph nodes. (**A**) Axial CT of the liver; (**B**) axial ^{18}F-FDG PET of the liver; (**C**) fusion PET/CT imaging of the liver; (**D**) 3-dimensional MIP (maximum intensity projection) whole body image. *Source*: From Maffione et al. *Arch Gynecol Obstet*. February 18, 2009. [Epub ahead of print].

tary to ^{18}F-FDG PET/CT in the evaluation of primary HCC in relation to the degree of tumor cellular differentiation.[267] On an individual patient basis, dual-tracer PET/CT had a sensitivity of 98%, a specificity of 86%, a positive predictive value of 97%, a negative predictive value of 90%, and an accuracy of 96% in the detection of HCC metastasis. The lesion-based and patient-based detection sensitivities were 60% and 64%, respectively, by ^{11}C-acetate PET/CT and 77% and 79%, respectively, by ^{18}F-FDG PET/CT, and they were complementary. Dual-tracer PET/CT was more effective than single-tracer PET/CT in identifying candidates for curative therapy with negative predictive value of dual-tracer, ^{18}F-FDG PET/CT, and ^{11}C-acetate PET/CT: 90%, 49%, and 37%, respectively.[268]

Ovarian Carcinoma

As for all other cancer types, surgical staging is the mainstay for ovarian cancer. ^{18}F-FDG PET imaging (Fig. 25-15) results have a strong correlation with second-look surgery for restaging and prediction of the progression- and disease-free survival.[269] CT with ^{18}F-FDG PET staging can improve with postoperative staging in 87% of patients, as compared with 53% by CT staging alone.[270] For the evaluation of recurrence, ^{18}F-FDG PET has demonstrated sensitivity of 80% and a specificity of 100%, as compared with for conventional imaging that has sensitivity 55% and specificity 100%, respectively, and with 75% and 100%, respectively, of the CA-125 levels in blood.[271] However, the efficacy of ^{18}F-FDG PET for initial diagnosis, staging, and restaging in ovarian carcinomas is still being debated. Meta-analysis of several published studies[272-275] revealed quite variable sensitivity of ^{18}F-FDG PET for staging of ovarian carcinomas, ranging from 58% to 91%, pointing towards inadequacy of ^{18}F-FDG PET for staging and diagnosis of recurrence. Other studies however, have revealed that FDG PET and FDG PET/CT are superior to conventional imaging and therefore are appropriate imaging studies to use, particularly when there is an elevated serum CA-125 level.[276-279] Also, in monitoring response to therapy in advanced-stage ovarian cancer ^{18}F-FDG PET has shown promise.[280] In recurrent disease, ^{18}F-FDG PET/CT altered management in close to 60% of patients, detected more sites of disease than abdominal and pelvic CT, was superior in the detection of nodal, peritoneal, and sub-capsular liver disease and offered the opportunity for technology replacement in this setting.[281] Overall results of clinical studies support an increasing role of ^{18}F-FDG PET/CT for the detection of recurrent ovarian cancer and highlights the potential for ^{18}F-FDG PET/CT to replace the current surveillance techniques in detecting recurrent disease.

Testicular Cancer

Several clinical studies have investigated the clinical role of ^{18}F-FDG PET in the primary tumor staging and in the control of therapy either in seminomatous germ cell tumors (SGCT) or in nonseminomatous germ cell tumors (NSGCT).[282,283] Although molecular imaging with ^{18}F-FDG PET has been reported as a sensitive method for diagnosis and staging of testicular cancer, other studies revealed no additional benefit over CT for the initial staging of testicular carcinomas.[284-286] ^{18}F-FDG PET appears to be superior to conventional imaging for restaging for testicular cancer, by depicting it sooner and being more sensitive for small lesions.[287-289] The specificity and sensitivity, respectively, of ^{18}F-FDG PET were 100% and 80% versus 74% and 70% for CT in an investigation of residual tumor after chemotherapy.[290] Another prospective study designed to investigate whether ^{18}F-FDG PET can help improve the prediction of viable tumor in postchemotherapy seminoma residuals revealed that the specificity of ^{18}F-FDG PET is significantly better than that of using a diameter of 3 cm or greater as a threshold for residual disease at CT.[291] ^{18}F-FDG PET also appears to result in prognostic data in relapse prior to high-dose chemotherapy. In an investigation of relapsed disease, sensitivities and specificities, respectively, for the prediction of failure of high-dose chemotherapy were as follows: ^{18}F-FDG PET, 100% and 78%; radiologic monitoring, 43% and 78%; and serum tumor marker, 15% and 100%.[292] However, a multicenter clinical trial involving 111 high-risk patients with NSGCT, who were studied with ^{18}F-FDG PET scanning within 8 weeks of orchidectomy or marker normalization, demonstrated that out of the 87 ^{18}F-FDG PET-negative patients who proceeded to surveillance, 33 of the 87 patients relapsed within 12 months. As with most other tumor types, inflammatory processes cause false-positive results, especially in sarcoidosis with characteristically high ^{18}F-FDG uptake in the lesions.[293,294] Therefore, ^{18}F-FDG PET is not sufficiently sensitive and specific for the assessment of the risk of relapse and for guidance of management of renal carcinoma patients.

Renal Cell Carcinoma

Renal cell carcinomas exhibited relatively low levels of glycolysis and, thus, low levels of ^{18}F-FDG accumulation, which limits the application of ^{18}F-FDG PET for the evaluation of renal cell carcinomas. Moreover, due to predominantly renal clearance of ^{18}F-FDG from the body, the resulting high concentration of this radiotracer in the kidneys, ureters, and urinary bladder, confounds the interpretation of PET imaging results. Nevertheless, some clinical investigations claim that ^{18}F-FDG PET can be useful for characterization of solid renal masses identified with MRI or CT and that ^{18}F-FDG PET can alter the treatment plan in about one-third of the studied cohort of patients.[295] In contrast, other studies report that FDG PET does not offer any advantage over CT for the characterization of renal masses, but is more sensitive than CT in the detection of distant metastases.[296] Several clinical studies have reported a wide range of sensitivity of ^{18}F-FDG PET for detecting distant metastases of renal cell carcinoma, ranging from 60% to 87%, and with specificity reaching almost 100%.[297-299]

^{18}F-FDG PET/CT appears to be an effective tool for monitoring early response to therapy of renal cell carcinomas. Recently, the efficacy of ^{18}F-FDG PET/CT has been demonstrated for the early assessment of response to sunitinib in metastatic renal carcinoma.[300]

Several other molecular imaging–type PET tracers, such as ^{11}C-labeled acetate, are being studied for the assessment of renal function and malignancy. Because of extensive utilization and hepatobilliary route of clearance, ^{11}C-acetate does not accumulate in normal kidney tissue, urine, and bladder. ^{11}C-acetate exhibits variable levels of accumulation in renal cell carcinoma lesions in the kidney (Fig. 25-16). Several clinical studies demonstrated that renal cell carcinomas accumulate ^{11}C-acetate higher than the normal kidney tissue.[301,302] However, other studies did not support these observations and demonstrated that ^{11}C-acetate did not accumulate in renal carcinomas higher than the normal kidney tissue.[303] Therefore, additional studies are needed to assess the

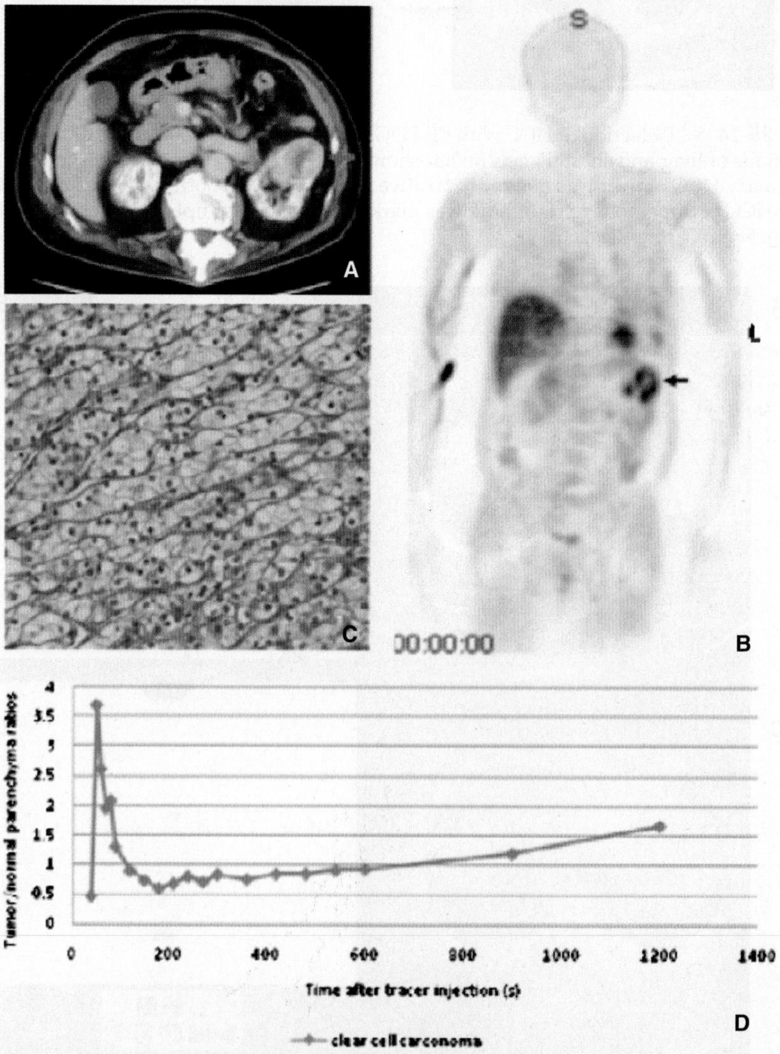

Figure 25-16 A 77-year-old man with a renal tumor in the upper pole of the left kidney (patient 19). **(A)** The CT image shows a 4-cm renal mass in the left kidney (*arrow*). **(B)** The coronal ^{11}C-Acetate PET image demonstrates high tracer uptake in the renal mass detected by CT (*arrow*). **(C)** Histological findings indicated clear-cell carcinoma, grade 1/(H&E). **(D)** Time–activity curve standardized by the tumor/normal parenchyma ratio for the renal cell carcinoma in the left kidney. *Source*: From Ref. 302.

efficacy of ^{11}C-acetate PET/CT for diagnosis, staging, and detection of recurrence of renal carcinomas.

Another recently reported novel molecular PET imaging agent is ^{124}I-labeled G250 chimeric antibody that recognizes carbonic anhydrase-IX, which is overexpressed in clear-cell renal carcinomas. The sensitivity of ^{124}I-cG250 PET for clear-cell kidney carcinoma was 94%; the negative predictive value was 90% and specificity and positive predictive accuracy were both 100%.[304] In this study, ^{124}I-cG250 PET identified accurately clear-cell renal carcinoma; a negative scan was highly predictive of a less aggressive phenotype. Larger clinical studies are warranted.

Bladder Carcinoma

As in case of renal cell carcinoma, renal clearance and urinary excretion of 18F-FDG into the urinary tract complicates the evaluation of pelvic region and urinary bladder, in particular. For this reason, 18F-FDG PET has not been useful in local staging but can be used for the assessment of lymph node involvement and detection of distant metastases.[305-307] Both hydration and furosemide-induced forced dieresis have improved the clearance of ^{18}F-FDG-derived radioactivity from kidneys and bladder, while delayed PET imaging revealed only a background level of radioactivity in the bladder in bladder-preserved patients and affected staging of more than a half of patients involved in the study. Unfortunately, in patients with cystectomy such an improvement in background radioactivity could not be effectively achieved in most cases, because urinary diversion usually results in higher residual activities due to slow washout of pooled urinary ^{18}F-FDG and, therefore, larger residual urinary volumes.[308]

To overcome the problem of renal-urinary clearance of ^{18}F-FDG, other molecular PET imaging agents, such as ^{11}C-choline have been studied in patients with urinary bladder cancer, because there is very little, if any urinary excretion of ^{11}C-choline.[309] Therefore, the sensitivity of ^{11}C-choline PET/CT was assessed for preoperative detection of positive lymph nodes in bladder cancer and shown to range between 60% and 100%, which was only minimally better than that of CT alone.[310,311]

In a recent clinical study, the efficacy of USPIO contrast-enhanced and diffusion-weighted MRI have been compared with conventional MRI techniques, with the aim of improving staging of normal-sized lymph nodes in 21 bladder and/or prostate cancer patients. Patients preoperatively underwent 3-T MRI before and after administration of lymphotropic USPIO using conventional MRI sequences combined with DW-MRI and the results of imaging were validated by histopathologic analysis of lymph nodes obtained by surgery. The USPIO-DW-MRI had detected 92% of metastatic lymph nodes identified by histopathologic examination. The conclusion of this study was that USPIO-DW-MRI is a fast and accurate method for detecting pelvic lymph node metastases, even in normal-sized nodes of bladder or prostate cancer patients.[312]

Cervical Cancer

Cervical cancer is the third most common female cancer in the United States and a leading cause of mortality worldwide.[313] Among the molecular imaging modalities, the highest sensitivity for detection of cancer lesions and recurrent disease, as much as 94–100%, is with ^{18}F-FDG PET.[314-319] However, careful histopathologic validation of results of FDG PET imaging in cervical carcinoma patients are still needed to fully assess the sensitivity and specificity of this molecular imaging modality. This is because, especially in the early stage of the disease the sensitivity of FDG PET for detection of pelvic lymph node metastases was reported to be significantly lower—53%, although the specificity was 90%.[320] For detection of recurrent cervical cancer and restaging, ^{18}F-FDG PET is significantly more accurate than CT or MR imaging.[321] Addition of ^{18}F-FDG PET imaging in patient management plan and decision-making process affects the outcome: a positive finding on a PET scan after treatment correlates with a 32% 5-year survival rate, as compared with 80% for a negative finding.[322] Comparison of ^{18}F-FDG PET with MRI demonstrated that the positive predictive value of ^{18}F-FDG PET in pelvic and paraaortic regions appears to be sufficient and negates the need for lymph node biopsies, while the accuracy of conventional MRI for nodal staging was insufficient and did not affect patient management. On the other hand, other studies[323] reported a staging ^{18}F-FDG PET/CT sensitivity, specificity, positive-predictive value, and negative-predictive value of 72%, 99.7%, 81%, 99.5%, and 99.3%, respectively, for the detection of lymph nodes metastasis in 47 patients affected by clinically early cervical cancer. These values go up to 100%, 99.6%, 81%, 100%, and 99.6% if only lymph nodes larger than 5 mm are considered. However, ^{18}F-FDG PET covers an important and confirmed role in the detection of disease relapse and hence modifying the patients' management. A study conducted in 150 patients with cervical carcinoma[324] determined that in 73.8% of them ^{18}F-FDG PET gave a significant added value over conventional imaging (in particular detecting extra-pelvic metastasis, due to its whole-body field of view). In another single institution prospective study of 92 women after 3 months of therapy, it was found that whole-body ^{18}F-FDG PET was predictive of survival. Therefore, the role of ^{18}F-FDG PET in the staging phase of cervical cancer is not yet fully established, although it appears that the use of hybrid PET/CT scanner, instead of PET alone, greatly improves the method's accuracy especially for early stage disease and larger multi-institutional studies should be conducted to determine the impact of this molecular imaging modality.

Pancreatic Adenocarcinoma

Pancreatic adenocarcinoma is the fourth leading cause of death from cancer in the United States and is increasing in incidence. CT is the most widely available and best-validated modality for imaging patients with pancreatic adenocarcinoma. To maximize the diagnostic efficacy of CT, use of a pancreas protocol is mandatory. The sensitivity of CT for diagnosis of pancreatic adenocarcinoma (89–97%) and its positive predictive value for predicting unresectability (89–100%) are high. The positive predictive value of CT for predicting resectability (45–79%) is low because the diagnostic criteria for diagnosing vascular invasion by tumor favors specificity over sensitivity to avoid denying surgery to patients with potentially resectable tumor. Furthermore, the sensitivity of CT for small hepatic and peritoneal metastases is limited. MRI has not been shown to perform better than CT for the diagnosis and staging of pancreatic adenocarcinoma, but can be helpful as an adjunct to CT, particularly for evaluation of small hepatic lesions that cannot be fully characterized by CT. Ultrasound is often the first study obtained in patients with obstructive jaundice or unexplained abdominal pain, but its utility for diagnosis and staging of patients with pancreatic adenocarcinoma is limited. PET/CT combines the functional information provided by PET with the anatomic information provided by CT and is a promising modality for imaging of patients with pancreatic adenocarcinoma, but its utility has not been established. Endoscopic ultrasound is generally considered superior to CT for the diagnosis and local staging of pancreatic cancer, but is limited by availability and inability to assess for distant metastases.[325] For detection of primary pancreatic adenocarcinoma, the sensitivity of ^{18}F-FDG PET is significantly higher than that of the helical CT, although PET does not have spatial resolution adequate for determination of resectability.[326-328] Nevertheless, a recent study in 56 pancreatic carcinoma patients demonstrated that FDG-PET is useful for the detection of small early pancreatic cancers.[329] Also, ^{18}F-FDG PET showed almost 98% sensitivity in patients with normal serum glucose values[330] and 93% specificity in differentiation of pancreatic adenocarcinoma from chronic pancreatitis.[331,332] ^{18}F-FDG PET/CT had much better sensitivity for detection of distant metastases not identifiable using conventional radiologic imaging, and influenced management decisions in 16% of patients with pancreatic cancer in terms of respectability.[333] Comparison of CT and ^{18}F-FDG PET/CT based planning of radiation therapy in locally advanced pancreatic carcinoma revealed that the co-registration of PET and CT information in unresectable locally advanced pancreatic carcinomas may improve the delineation of gross tumor volume and theoretically reduce the likelihood of topographic misses.[334] In routine clinical practice, ^{18}F-FDG PET is complementary to CT or MRI in detection of recurrent pancreatic cancer and is superior in sensitivity compared to CT or MRI alone for detection of local and extraabdominal recurrences, as well as hepatic metastases.[335]

Neuroendocrine Tumors

Neuroendocrine tumors (NETs), such as carcinoid and pancreatic islet cell tumors were the second major type of tumors after thyroid carcinomas for which molecular imaging had been developed using gamma scintigraphic techniques. NETs express cell membrane neuroamine uptake receptors (ie, somatostatin receptors). Diagnostic assessment of this heterogeneous group of tumors involves blood, urine, and biochemical examination as well as imaging modalities. Once the diagnosis of suspected NET has been ascertained by the identification of typical biochemical markers, different imaging modalities have been used for staging of gastro-entero-pancreatic tumors: CT, MRI, US, angiography, and endoscopy.[336-338] CT, US, and MRI are most frequently employed, however, neither of these technologies is capable of providing information about the functional status of NET. Moreover, CT, US, and MRI are much less precise and much slower in detecting response to therapy of NET when compared with functional imaging. Among the most effective molecular imaging approaches in NETs are ^{123}I-metaiodobenzylguanidine SPECT, somatostatin receptor scintigraphy (SRS), vasoactive intestinal peptide receptor scintigraphy, and ^{18}F-FDG PET, which will be discussed and compared further.

One of the most extensively studied radiotracers for molecular imaging of neuroendocrine carcinomas is the analog of hydroxytryptophan (5-HTP), the ^{11}C-labeled serotonin (^{11}C-5HTP), which has been utilized for staging of carcinoid tumors using PET. In combination with pre-treatment with carbidopa, which is used to inhibit amino acid decarboxylase activity in peripheral tissues and to prevent renal excretion, ^{11}C-5HTP PET can detect very small lesions in the pancreas and thoraxthat are not detectable with ^{111}In-Octreotide scintigraphy, MRI, and CT.[339-341] Other PET tracers, such as ^{11}C-dihydroxyphenylalanine (for carcinoids and endocrine pancreatic tumors), ^{11}C-hydroxyephedrine (for phaeochromocytomas), and ^{11}C-metomidate (for adrenal cortical tumors), have been developed and partly characterized in clinical studies.[342] ^{18}F-FDG PET has also been applied for initial diagnosis and staging of neuroendocrine carcinomas, but its limitations became evident in well-differentiatedNETs, which do not exhibit increased glycolytic activity and do not effectively accumulate ^{18}F-FDG.[343-345]

Because of the short half-life of ^{11}C (20.3 minutes), other ^{18}F-radiolabeled tracers (with almost 2 h half-life of physical decay) have been explored for imaging of neuroendocrine neoplasia. One of the most studied radiotracers is the L-3,4dihydroxy-6-(18)F-fluoro-phenylalanine (^{18}F-FDOPA), an analog of L-3,4 dihydroxyphenylalanine (L-DOPA). ^{18}F-FDOPA is widely used for the assessment of various Parkinsonian syndromes, because it is uptaken by the cells and utilized as a precursor for the neurotransmitter dopamine. NETs exhibit active uptake of amino acids, including ^{18}F-FDOPA, and convert them by means of decarboxylation into biogenic amines, which are stored in cell vesicles. Pretreatment with a decarboxylase inhibitor carbidopa blocks aromatic amino acid decarboxylase enzyme and decreases catabolism of ^{18}F-FDOPA, while increasing its effective uptake and accumulation in NETs.[346,347] One of the studies demonstrated, that for NETs, ^{18}F-FDOPA PET was more accurate (sensitivity, 100%; specificity, 91%) in the detection of skeletal lesions than ^{111}In-Octreotide scintigraphy and CT, but was quite insensitive (sensitivity, 20%; specificity, 94%) in the lung, probably because of the respiratory motion and lesion "smearing" during image acquisition. ^{111}In-Octreotide scintigraphy is best for imaging of tumor lesions in the liver (sensitivity, 75%; specificity, 100%); but is less accurate than ^{18}F-FDOPA PET in other organs.[348] However, ^{18}F-FDOPA PET is less sensitive than ^{18}F-FDG PET and standard imaging procedures for the staging of SCLC .[349]

Most of the NETs over-express somatostatin receptors (SSTRs). Therefore, several radiolabeled somatostatin analogs have been developed for diagnostic imaging and staging of SSTR-positive NETs using a gamma camera and SPECT, as well as PET. SRS using ^{111}In-DTPA- D-Phe1-octreotide (^{111}In-DTPA-OC; Octreoscan) is considered the "gold standard" in the diagnosis, staging and follow-up of patients with NETs. However, the use of more suitable somatostatin analogs {DOTA-TOC (1,4,7,10-tetraazacyclododecane-1-,4,7,10-tetraacetic acid), DOTA-NOC (DOTA-1-Nal3-octreotide), DOTATATE (DOTA-D-Phe1-Tyr3-Thr8-octreotide) DOTA-NOC-ATE((DOTA-1Nal3,Thr8)-octreotide), DOTA-BOC-ATE ((DOTA, BzThi3, Thr8)-octreotide)}(2,14) tagged with positron emitting radionuclides (^{68}Ga, ^{64}Cu) in PET/CT has lead to levels of sensitivity and specificity almost two orders of magnitude higher than those historically achieved by ^{111}In-DTPA-Octreotide SPECT. Baum and colleagues had pioneered the use of ^{68}Ga-DOTA-NOC and ^{68}Ga-DOTA–TATE for routine PET/CT imaging of patients with NETs.[350] In one of their studies comparing the diagnostic efficacy of PET/CT imaging with ^{68}Ga-DOTA-NOC and ^{68}Ga-DOTA–TATE, it has been demonstrated for the first time that ^{68}Ga-DOTA-NOC (Fig. 25-17) is superior to ^{68}Ga-DOTA–TATE in diagnostic sensitivity for NETs.[351]

Many molecular imaging and therapy modalities for NETs are currently under investigation or being developed; nevertheless, no single imaging technique identifies all the metastatic sites of NETs. The best results may be obtained using a combination of functional imaging tests such as PET and and morphologic imaging with CT or MRI. The usefulness of these modalities, however, has to be evaluated by well-designed and multicenter studies.

Conclusion

During the past two decades, several methods in molecular and cellular biology and genetics have been translated from in vitro to the whole body noninvasive in vivo imaging applications, which started the new era in molecular-genetic imaging. Molecular imaging had made a very significant impact in the clinic, both in terms of improving early detection and pre-operative (pre-treatment) staging and early assessment of treatment response and more accurate prognosis. Currently, a large number of novel imaging agents and methods for noninvasive visualization and quantification of a variety of cellular and subcellular targets, signaling, and metabolic processes, are in development. These molecular imaging agents and methods could be applicable to different cancer types that share molecular-pathophysiological mechanisms of cancer development and progression. However, most of the novel molecular imaging agents are still only investigational and have not undergone clinical translation,

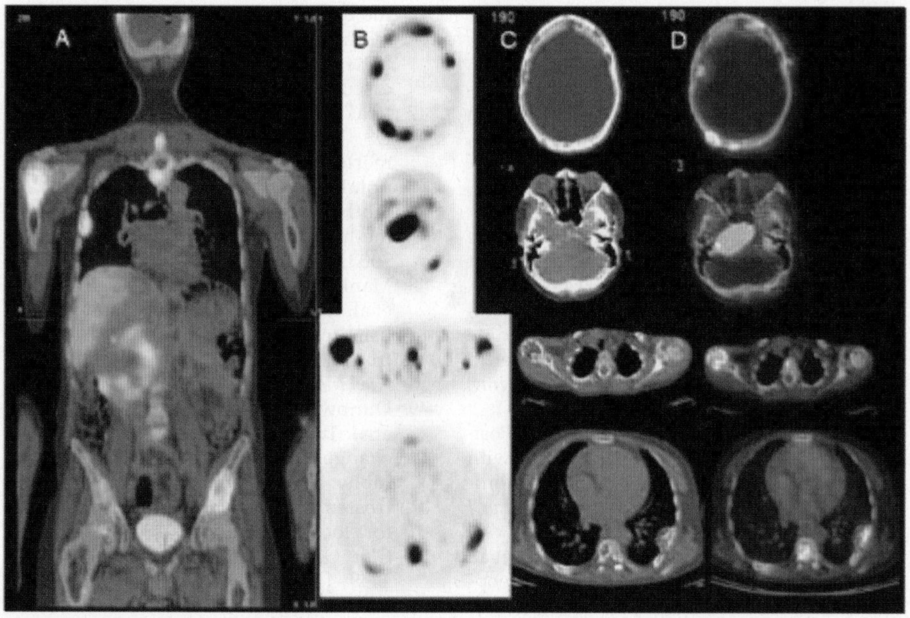

Figure 25-17 (A) ^{68}Ga-DOTA-NOC receptor PET/CT (maximum intensity projection images (MIP) image in a 24-year old paraganglioma patient 7 years after the first PRRT with 90Y DOTA-TOC (1.85 GBq). (B) Transversal PET slices (C), CT scans (D), and fused images show multiple osteolytic lesions in the skull, the humeri, the ribs and the vertebra with intense SMS-receptor expression. *Source*: From Parsad et al, 2007.

rigorous clinical studies, and have not been approved by the FDA yet. Because the majority of novel molecular imaging agents and approaches to date had been developed by the academia, there are both financial and regulatory barriers that hinder their clinical translation, FDA approval, and reimbursement approval. Extension of basic and pre-clinical research into clinical-translational phase (phase 1 and 2 studies), and carefully designed phase 3 and 4 studies are urgently needed to enrich the "toolbox" of molecular imaging agents and approaches in clinical oncology. Further improvements in sensitivity and resolution of diagnostic imaging instrumentation, as well as the development of novel imaging modalities and combined imaging modalities will further increase the role and impact of molecular imaging in oncology.

Selected References

The complete reference list can be found at www.CANCERMEDICINE8.com

2. Patton DD. The birth of nuclear medicine instrumentation. Blumgart and Yens, 1925. *J Nucl Med*. 2003;44:1362.
3. Wang LV. Ultrasound-mediated biophotonic imaging: a review of acousto-optical tomography and photo-acoustic tomography. *Dis Markers*. 2003–2004;19(2–3):123–138.
4. Wang LV. Prospects of photoacoustic tomography. *Med Phys*. December 2008;35(12):5758–5767.
6. Ries L, Eisner M, Kosary C, et al. *SEER Cancer Statistics Review, 1975–2001*. Bethesda, MD: National Cancer Institute; 2004.
7. Brem RF, Floerke AC, Rapelyea JA, Teal C, Kelly T, Mathur V. Breast-specific gamma imaging as an adjunct imaging modality for the diagnosis of breast cancer. *Radiology*. June 2008;247(3):651–657.
9. Warner E, Plewes DB, Hill KA, et al. Surveillance of BRCA1 and BRCA2 mutation carriers with magnetic resonance imaging, ultrasound, mammography, and clinical breast examination. *JAMA*. September 15, 2004;292(11):1317–1325.
10. Kriege M, Brekelmans CT, Boetes C, et al. Efficacy of MRI and mammography for breast-cancer screening in women with a familial or genetic predisposition. *N Engl J Med*. 2004;351:427–437.
11. Turnbull LW. Dynamic contrast-enhanced MRI in the diagnosis and management of breast cancer. *NMR Biomed*. January 2009;22(1):28–39.
12. Daldrup-Link HE, Rydland J, Helbich TH, et al. Quantification of breast tumor microvascular permeability with feruglose-enhanced MR imaging: initial phase II multicenter trial. *Radiology*. 2003;229:885–892.
14. Artemov D, Mori N, Okollie B, Bhujwalla ZM. MR molecular imaging of the Her-2/neu receptor in breast cancer cells using targeted iron oxide nanoparticles. *Magn Reson Med*. 2003;49:403–408.
15. Turetschek K, Floyd E, Helbich T, et al. MRI assessment of microvascular characteristics in experimental breast tumors using a new blood pool contrast agent (MS-325) with correlations to histopathology. *J Magn Reson Imaging*. 2001;14:237–242.
16. Turetschek K, Roberts TP, Floyd E, et al. Tumor microvascular characterization using ultrasmall superparamagnetic iron oxide particles (USPIO) in an experimental breast cancer model. *J Magn Reson Imaging*. 2001;13:882–888.
17. Turetschek K, Floyd E, Shames DM, et al. Assessment of a rapid clearance blood pool MR contrast medium (P792) for assays of microvascular characteristics in experimental breast tumors with correlations to histopathology. *Magn Reson Med*. 2001;45:880–886.
18. Jacobs MA, Barker PB, Bottomley PA, Bhujwalla Z, Bluemke DA. Proton magnetic resonance spectroscopic imaging of human breast cancer: a preliminary study. *J Magn Reson Imaging*. 2004;19:68–75.
20. Tromberg BJ, Pogue BW, Paulsen KD, Yodh AG, Boas DA, Cerussi AE. Assessing the future of diffuse optical imaging technologies for breast cancer management. *Med Phys*. June 2008;35(6):2443–2451.
21. Fujiwara M, Mizukami T, Suzuki A, Fukamizu H. Sentinel lymph node detection in skin cancer patients using real-time fluorescence navigation with indocyanine green: preliminary experience. *J Plast Reconstr Aesthet Surg*. 2008.
22. Fujimoto JG. Optical coherence tomography for ultrahigh resolution in vivo imaging. *Nat Biotechnol*. November 2003;21(11):1361–1367.
23. Hsiung PL, Phatak DR, Chen Y, Aguirre AD, Fujimoto JG, Connolly JL. Benign and malignant lesions in the human breast depicted with ultrahigh resolution and three-dimensional optical coherence tomography. Radiology. September 2007;244(3):865–874.
24. Boppart SA, Luo W, Marks DL, Singletary KW. Optical coherence tomography: feasibility for basic research and image-guided surgery of breast cancer. *Breast Cancer Res Treat*. March 2004;84(2):85–97. Review.
25. Walter C, Scheidhauer K, Scharl A, et al. Clinical and diagnostic value of preoperative MR mammography and FDG-PET in suspicious breast lesions. *Eur Radiol*. 2003;13:1651–1656.
26. Rieber A, Schirrmeister H, Gabelmann A, et al. Pre-operative staging of invasive breast cancer with MR mammography and/or PET: boon or bunk? *Br J Radiol*. 2002;75:789–798.
27. Heinisch M, Gallowitsch HJ, Mikosch P, et al. Comparison of FDG-PET and dynamic contrast-enhanced MRI in the evaluation of suggestive breast lesions. *Breast*. 2003;12:17–22.
28. Memarsadeghi M, Riedl CC, Kaneider A, et al. Axillary lymph node metastases in patients with breast carcinomas: assessment with nonenhanced versus uspio-enhanced MR imaging. *Radiology*. November 2006;241(2):367–377.
29. Walter C, Scheidhauer K, Scharl A, et al. Clinical and diagnostic value of preoperative MR mammography and FDG-PET in suspicious breast lesions. *Eur Radiol*. 2003;13:1651–1656.
30. Wahl RL, Cody RL, Hutchins GD, Mudgett EE. Primary and metastatic breast carcinoma: initial clinical evaluation with PET with the radiolabeled glucose analogue 2-[F-18]-fluoro-2-deoxy-D-glucose. *Radiology*. 1991;179:765–770.
32. Adler LP, Crowe JP, al-Kaisi NK, Sunshine JL. Evaluation of breast masses and axillary lymph nodes with [F-18] 2-deoxy-2-fluoro-D-glucose PET. *Radiology*. 1993;187:743–750.
33. Adler LP, Crowe JP, al-Kaisi NK, Sunshine JL. Evaluation of breast masses and axillary lymph nodes with [F-18] 2-deoxy-2-fluoro-D-glucose PET. *Radiology*. 1993;187:743–750.

34. Wahl RL, Siegel BA, Coleman RE, Gatsonis CG. Prospective multicenter study of axillary nodal staging by positron emission tomography in breast cancer: a report of the staging breast cancer with PET study group. PET Study Group. *J Clin Oncol.* 2004;22(2): 277–285.

36. Utech CI, Young CS, Winter PF. Prospective evaluation of fluorine-18 fluorodeoxyclucose positron emission tomography in breast cancer for staging of the axilla related to surgery and immunocytochemistry. *Eur J Nucl Med.* 1996;23:1588–1593.

37. Avril N, Rose CA, Schelling M, et al. Breast imaging with positron emission tomography and fluorine-18 fluorodeoxyglucose: use and limitations. *J Clin Oncol.* 2000;18:3495–3502.

38. van der Hoeven JJ, Krak NC, Hoekstra OS, et al. 18F-2-fluoro-2-deoxy-d-glucose positron emission tomography in staging of locally advanced breast cancer. *J Clin Oncol.* 2004;22:1253–1259.

39. Yang SN, Liang JA, Lin FJ, Kao CH, Lin CC, Lee CC. Comparing whole body (18) F-2-deoxyglucose positron emission tomography and technetium-99m methylene diphosphonate bone scan to detect bone metastases in patients with breast cancer. *J Cancer Res Clin Oncol.* 2002;128:325–328.

41. Vranjesevic D, Filmont JE, Meta J, et al. Whole-body (18)F-FDG PET and conventional imaging for predicting outcome in previously treated breast cancer patients. *J Nucl Med.* 2002;43:325–329.

42. Moon DH, Maddahi J, Silverman DH, Glaspy JA, Phelps ME, Hoh CK. Accuracy of whole-body fluorine-18-FDG PET for the detection of recurrent or metastatic breast carcinoma. *J Nucl Med.* 1998;39:431–435.

43. Smyczek-Gargya B, Fersis N, Dittmann H, et al. PET with [18F]fluorothymidine for imaging of primary breast cancer: a pilot study. *Eur J Nucl Med Mol Imaging.* 2004;31:720–724.

44. Been LB, Elsinga PH, de Vries J, et al. Positron emission tomography in patients with breast cancer using (18)F-3′-deoxy-3′-fluoro-l-thymidine ((18)F-FLT)-a pilot study. *Eur J Surg Oncol.* February 2006;32(1):39–43.

45. Walter C, Scheidhauer K, Scharl A, et al. Clinical and diagnostic value of preoperative MR mammography and FDG-PET in suspicious breast lesions. *Eur Radiol.* 2003;13:1651–1656.

46. Gennari A, Donati S, Salvadori B, et al. Role of 2-[18F]-fluorodeoxyglucose (FDG) positron emission tomography (PET) in the early assessment of response to chemotherapy in metastatic breast cancer patients. *Clin Breast Cancer.* 2000;1:156–161; discussion 162–163.

47. Krak NC, van der Hoeven JJ, Hoekstra OS, Twisk JW, van der Wall E, Lammertsma AA. Measuring [(18)F]FDG uptake in breast cancer during chemotherapy: comparison of analytical methods. *Eur J Nucl Med Mol Imaging.* 2003;30:674–681.

48. Mankoff DA, Dunnwald LK, Gralow JR, et al. Changes in blood flow and metabolism in locally advanced breast cancer treated with neoadjuvant chemotherapy. *J Nucl Med.* 2003;44:1806–1814.

49. Dunnwald LK, Gralow JR, Ellis GK, et al. Tumor metabolism and blood flow changes by positron emission tomography: relation to survival in patients treated with neoadjuvant chemotherapy for locally advanced breast cancer. *J Clin Oncol.* September 20, 2008;26(27): 4449–4457.

50. Dehdashti F, Mortimer JE, Trinkaus K, et al. PET-based estradiol challenge as a predictive biomarker of response to endocrine therapy in women with estrogen-receptor-positive breast cancer. *Breast Cancer Res Treat.* February 2009;113(3):509–517.

26 Molecular Diagnostics in Cancer

Bryan T. Hennessy, MD ■ Robert C. Bast Jr., MD ■ Gordon B. Mills, MD, PhD

Introduction

Molecular diagnostics involves the use of molecular biomarkers (Box 1) to detect, diagnose, or monitor cancer, as well as to estimate probable patient outcomes or to predict therapeutic interventions that are likely to benefit the patient. Ultimately, the development of molecular diagnostics is expected to facilitate the individualization of cancer treatment. Individualized cancer therapy is regarded as a "holy grail" by cancer researchers, since it is hoped that this approach will maximize treatment benefit for individual cancer patients, while minimizing toxicity. Important progress has already been made in developing and applying molecular diagnostics to clinical management. This chapter provides an overview of the current status of molecular diagnostics for cancer. It will also review potential approaches to the future development of individualized cancer therapies, as well as new techniques and likely problems and hurdles that will need to be addressed and overcome.

Box 1 ■ Cancer Biomarkers

The most general definition of a cancer biomarker includes any characteristic of tumor cells, stroma, normal tissues or body fluids that can aid in detecting, diagnosing, monitoring, defining prognosis, or predicting response or toxicity from treatment. Thus biomarkers can include alterations in DNA, RNA, protein, carbohydrate or lipid as well as biophysical characteristics of tumor cells or tissues. Pathologic examination and imaging techniques have provided conventional tumor histologic and staging information (eg, histotypes, tumor size, lymph node status) that have guided patient management to date, but do not take into account the full heterogeneity of cancers and normal tissues at a molecular level. Individualization of screening, prevention and treatment should be substantially improved by considering the profile of multiple novel molecular biomarkers.

Box 2 ■ An Optimal Screening Test

Four critical terms describe the validity of a screening test: *sensitivity*, *specificity*, and *positive* and *negative predictive values*. Sensitivity, one measure of how good a test is, is the proportion of cases of the disease that are detected by the test (number of true positives/number of true positives plus false negatives). Specificity is the proportion of cases without disease that are detected as negative by the test (number of true negatives/number of true negatives plus false positives). When a test result is a continuous variable, sensitivity and specificity are inversely related and a cutoff for the presence of disease is placed in an arbitrary fashion that indicates the clinical effect of a wrong result. In some cases, the sequencing of two tests for screening (a primary and a secondary test) can allow optimization of sensitivity and/or specificity beyond that achievable with only the primary test prior to definitive treatment (eg, ultrasound-guided breast biopsy following mammography). The prevalence of the disease in a population also affects screening test performance: in low-prevalence settings, even very good tests have poor positive predictive values (the proportion of patients with positive test results who are correctly diagnosed, that is, number of true positives/number of true positives plus false positives). Hence, knowledge of the approximate prevalence of the disease is a critical prerequisite to interpreting screening test results. It is thus easier to effectively screen for common diseases, an inherent problem with devising effective screening strategies for diseases such as ovarian and pancreatic cancers.

Molecular Biomarkers for Screening and Early Detection of Cancer

Early detection implies the diagnosis of cancer at its earliest stage of development, ideally prior to metastasis, when locoregional therapy can achieve cure. Thus early detection is expected to improve patient outcomes using conventional treatment strategies. Early detection and cancer prevention could both be facilitated by the identification of individuals at high risk for developing specific cancers.[1-4] Screening is a term often used for approaches that facilitate early cancer detection. Screening technologies must be capable of detecting small tumors at an early stage. Further, an effective cancer screening approach must be cost effective, acceptable to patients and associated with limited morbidity. Since screening of the entire population is often not practicable, guidelines for patient risk assessment are often necessary to appropriately target approaches to cancer prevention and early cancer diagnosis. As our understanding of the molecular heterogeneity of cancer rapidly advances, novel criteria can be added to these and other conventional criteria (sensitivity, specificity and positive and negative predictive values [Boxes 2 and 3]) that describe an ideal screening biomarker. Thus, as most cancer treatments are effective in only a minority of cancer patients, future useful screening biomarkers will also guide appropriate therapies in individual patients.

Newer radiologic techniques such as ultrasound and magnetic resonance imaging (MRI) afford increasingly more sensitive noninvasive diagnostic procedures for early detection of small tumors. However, while patients with certain tumor types have benefited from such radiologic advances, patients with other cancers such as epithelial ovarian and pancreatic tumors have not. These and other tumor types continue to be commonly diagnosed at an advanced stage and are thus associated with very poor patient outcomes. Novel molecular screening techniques have the potential to address tumor molecular heterogeneity, revolutionize early cancer detection and at the same time facilitate accurate risk assessment and individual treatment planning.

■ Molecular Biomarkers in Current Clinical Practice for Screening and Early Detection

The major factors that are utilized to guide and/or effect cancer screening are risk determination, regular self-assessment and/or physician examination, strategic use of radiologic imaging approaches, and use of a limited number of molecular markers. Risk assessment is initially used to stratify a patient to screening or, if the risk is high enough, prevention. It is currently largely based on patient-specific factors that are determined from a routine history and physical examination, including age, family history, and social factors such as tobacco use. Risk prediction currently involves a limited number of specific molecular biomarkers.

Prostate Cancer ■ Serum prostate specific antigen (PSA) measurement is now routinely recommended in men older than 50 years because of the frequency of prostate cancer in this age group. PSA is normally present in the blood at very low levels; normal PSA levels are between 0 and 4.0 ng/mL. Increased levels of PSA

Box 3 ■ A Suitable Cancer for Screening

There are disease-specific considerations for the successful implementation of screening. Lead time and length time biases are important considerations (Fig. 26-1); these biases can distort the apparent value of screening programs and randomized controlled trials are the only way to avoid them. Further, the presence of a premalignant stage likely facilitates and may be important to the development of an effective screening strategy. Since the inappropriate application or interpretation of screening tests can raise needless anxiety, initiate unnecessary and harmful diagnostic testing, and squander healthcare resources, these concepts are crucial considerations for the implementation of a successful screening strategy.

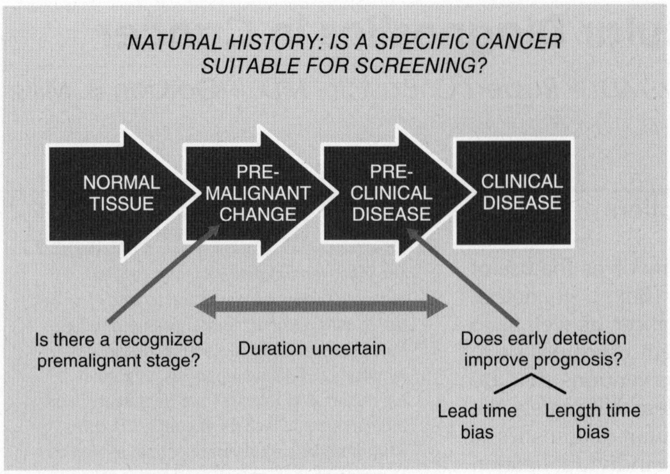

Figure 26-1 ■ Disease-specific considerations for implementation of successful screening. The presence of a recognized premalignant stage facilitates effective screening. Lead time bias occurs when early diagnosis falsely appears to prolong survival. Length time bias occurs when screening over-represents less aggressive disease (eg, with prostate cancer).

may suggest the presence of prostate cancer. As many as 15% of all prostate cancers can occur, however, in the absence of an elevated PSA level. Further, PSA levels can be also elevated due to prostate infection, irritation, benign prostatic hypertrophy or recent ejaculation. Thus, PSA is not an adequately sensitive or specific marker for prostate cancer screening. As a result, PSA screening remains controversial, despite widespread use.[5] Most PSA in the blood is bound to serum proteins. A small amount is not protein bound and is called free PSA. In prostate cancer the ratio of free PSA to total PSA is decreased. The risk of cancer increases if the free to total ratio is less than 25%. Measuring the ratio of free to total PSA may be particularly promising for eliminating unnecessary biopsies in men with PSA levels between 4 and 10 ng/mL.

Breast Cancer ■ In families with a significant history of breast cancer, key cancer risk biomarkers (usually hereditary mutations) can now be identified in a significant minority of cases. Current clinical models can predict an individual woman's probability of having a genetic mutation based on the family history (eg, BRCAPRO model).[6] The incorporation of such models into assessment of a woman with a significant family history of breast cancer can be useful in guiding specific molecular tests that further stratify risk and guide subsequent screening or prevention. *BRCA1* and *BRCA2* are well known hereditary predictive biomarkers of high breast cancer risk,[7] and inherited mutations in these genes account for 5-10% of all breast cancers and for ≥65% of inherited breast cancers.[8,9] *BRCA1*/*BRCA2* mutations are associated with a 55-87% lifetime risk of developing breast cancer, in addition to a mutation type-specific high risk of ovarian cancer.[10] In addition, approximately 12% of high-risk women found to be negative for *BRCA1* and *BRCA2* mutations are estimated to carry another cancer predisposing genomic alteration.[11] This suggests that improved testing approaches and identification of additional biomarkers of risk are needed. Less well-studied breast cancer susceptibility genes include *CHEK2, ATM, NBS1, LKB1, PTEN, p53, XRCC1,* and *STK11,* but these are not commonly sequenced due to the rarity of inherited mutations in breast cancer patients.[12-14]

Colon Cancer ■ Key familial cancer risk biomarkers have also now been identified for colorectal cancer.[15] Familial adenomatous polyposis (FAP) and hereditary nonpolyposis colon cancer (HNPCC) represent predisposing genetic syndromes for early-onset familial/hereditary colon cancer. These syndromes are characterized by germline mutations in the adenomatous polyposis coli (*APC*) and *DNA* mismatch repair genes, respectively. Currently, management guidelines entail cancer prevention with FAP (colectomy) and intensive screening with HNPCC (because of the lower risk of colorectal cancer associated with the latter). In addition, persistent inflammatory bowel disease (chronic ulcerative or Crohnscolitis) place patients at high risk for colorectal cancer.

Regular self-assessment and physician examination are important in screening for early cancer detection. Greater population awareness increases the effectiveness of such strategies. Specific screening recommendations that involve diagnostic procedures are generally only applied to the population when there is conclusive evidence of an associated survival benefit and when the cancer is a common cause of mortality, the latter for reasons that include cost effectiveness. Thus, to facilitate earlier detection of colorectal cancer and with compelling evidence that removal of adenomas can prevent incident cancers, it is now recommended that people be screened beginning at 50 years of age by annual fecal occult blood testing and/or one of the following: flexible sigmoidoscopy or double contrast barium enema every 5 years or colonoscopy every 10 years.[16,17] Increasingly, the ability of colonoscopy to visualize small lesions throughout the entire colon has made this the screening method of choice.

Radiologic Techniques ■ Many efforts to facilitate cancer screening rely on radiology As an example, annual mammography is recommended for women aged 40 years and older.[18] Studies are also presently investigating imaging modalites as initial screening for other forms of cancer. Although routine chest films have not been shown to improve outcomes of lung cancer patients, computed tomography (CT) is much more sensitive and is the subject of current lung cancer screening studies (eg, NELSON trial) in people at increased risk from cigarette smoking.[19] Radiologic imaging is usually also necessary for definitive documentation of early tumors that are detected by other screening approaches prior to biopsy confirmation (eg, ultrasonography with an elevated PSA). Further, investigative molecular approaches to facilitate early diagnosis of cancer are also utilizing novel imaging techniques such as positron emission tomography (PET).[20,21]

More specific guidelines have been developed for high risk patients with strong family histories of cancer, particularly for carriers of genomic biomarkers of high cancer risk. When the cancer risk associated with the specific (usually hereditary) biomarker is high enough, recommendations focus on prevention rather than early detection. Since prevention strategies generally impact quality of life to a greater degree than does screening, the identification of inherited mutations associated with a very high cancer risk necessitates patient education and careful shared decision making. Prophylactic surgery and chemoprevention are particularly effective risk reduction techniques that are reserved for people at highest risk. Celecoxib is an effective agent for the prevention of colorectal adenomas but, because of potential cardiovascular events, cannot currently be routinely recommended for this indication.[22] Some molecular biomarkers not only allow risk assessment, but also facilitate individualized treatment planning. *BRCA2* mutation carriers are at high risk of hormone receptor-positive breast cancer, and treatment with tamoxifen or another antihormonal therapy may result in benefit. However, anti-hormonal therapies have little preventive effect in *BRCA1* mutation carriers since most of these develop hormone receptor-negative tumors. Prophylactic surgery (mastectomy and/or oophorectomy) has been shown to have the greatest protective effect for *BRCA1*/BRCA2 mutation carriers to date, reducing the risk of breast cancer by up to 90%.[7,8,23,24] Currently, there are many factors (eg, ethics, cost) to consider in discussing options for early detection and prevention with very high risk patients and this area of medicine is a rapidly evolving specialty.[25-28]

Ovarian Cancer Screening ■ Early detection of ovarian cancer may significantly improve the survival of women with this disease.[29] Given its prevalence, strategies for early ovarian cancer detection must have relatively high sensitivity (>75%) and an extremely high specificity (99.6%) to attain a positive predictive value of at least 10%. Transvaginal sonography (TVS), serum markers, and a combination of the two modalities have been evaluated for early detection. Serum CA125 has received most attention but lacks the sensitivity or specificity to function alone as a screening test. Greater specificity can be achieved by combining CA125 and TVS and/or by monitoring CA125 over time. Two-stage screening strategies promise to be cost effective, where abnormal serum assays prompt TVS to detect lesions that require laparotomy. Accrual has been completed for a 200,000 woman trial in the United Kingdom that will test the ability of a rising CA125 to trigger TVS and subsequent exploratory surgery. Data from the first 2 years of accrual suggest that this strategy could increase the fraction of disease detected in early stage with adequate sensitivity and specificity. As only 80% of ovarian cancers express CA125, other markers will be required to detect all early stage tumors. The development of technologies that measure multiple serum markers simultaneously, linked to the creation of statistical methods that enhance sensitivity without sacrificing specificity, hold great promise.

Future Approaches to Early Detection and Screening

While current approaches to early detection have impacted mortality from certain forms of cancer, there are many tumor types that have not been detected with these approaches and continue to present with advanced disease. Some such tumors, including pancreatic and ovarian cancers, are associated with production of known serum markers (CA19-9 and CA125, respectively), but these markers generally lack the necessary sensitivity and specificity for effective screening when used alone on a single occasion. However, it can be expected that increasing understanding of the complex molecular basis of cancer and availability of novel molecular technologies will unearth multiple new approaches to facilitate early detection and possibly ultimately prevention of these and other forms of cancer.

Current Molecular Biomarkers for Predicting Outcomes and Therapy Responsiveness

Although molecular biomarkers that facilitate prediction of outcomes in cancer patients are useful, greater clinical utility lies in biomarkers that predict benefit for particular patients from specific cancer therapies. Indeed, there is considerable overlap between both types of biomarkers, since those biomarkers that predict benefit for particular patients from specific cancer therapies will therefore predict improved outcomes.

Breast Cancer

Hormone Receptors ■ Hormone receptor-positive breast cancer comprises approximately 70% of all breast cancers and is marked by the expression of estrogen receptor (ER) alpha and/or progesterone receptor (PR). These two hormone receptors are biomarkers that identify breast tumors that are sensitive to growth inhibition by anti-hormonal treatments, including ER partial agonists/antagonists (eg, tamoxifen), ER downregulators (eg, fulvestrant) and aromatase inhibitors (eg, letrozole).[30,31] In clinical practice, hormone receptor protein expression is therefore routinely assessed in all breast cancers using immunohistochemistry (IHC). Despite at least 5 years of adjuvant anti-hormonal therapy, however, a significant fraction of women with early stage hormone receptor-positive breast cancer relapse, and the majority of women with metastatic hormone receptor-positive breast cancer eventually develop resistance to anti-hormonal manipulation. Thus, over 25,000 women die each year despite having presented with hormone receptor-positive breast tumors, more annual deaths than are caused by all other types of breast cancer combined.

Multiparameter Gene Expression Profiles ■ Our ability to predict the likelihood of cure for patients with hormone receptor-positive breast cancer after treatment with anti-hormonal drugs has improved dramatically. *Oncotype Dx* (Table 26-1), based on the expression of 21 genes, predicts the benefit for individual node-negative hormone receptor-positive breast tumor patients from adjuvant tamoxifen and selects patients for cytotoxic chemotherapy based on features associated with tamoxifen resistance.[32] However, despite the clinical utility of this approach, this and similar assays do not significantly increase our understanding of anti-hormone resistance mechanisms in hormone receptor-positive breast cancer beyond the known roles of tumor grade, HER2, and ER and PR levels.[30,32,33] The mechanisms that account for primary and acquired resistance to anti-

Table 26-1 ■ **The Panel of 21 Genes in *Oncotype Dx* and Their Subdivision Based on Function**

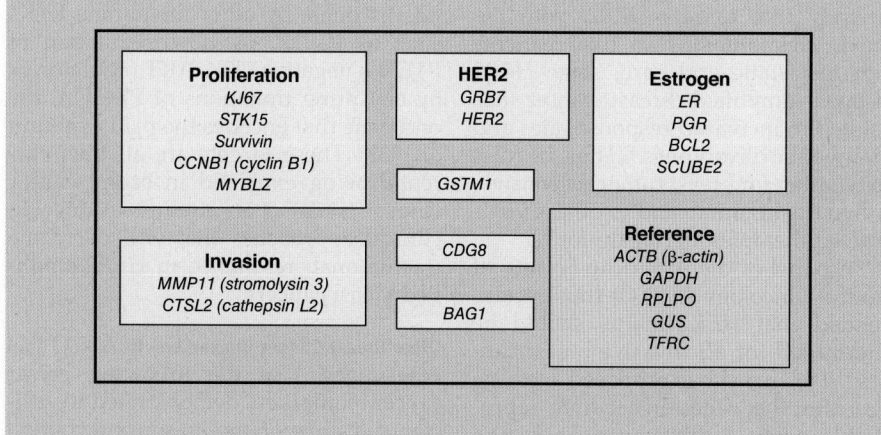

Group	Genes
Proliferation	*KJ67*, *STK15*, *Survivin*, *CCNB1 (cyclin B1)*, *MYBLZ*
HER2	*GRB7*, *HER2*
Estrogen	*ER*, *PGR*, *BCL2*, *SCUBE2*
	GSTM1
	CDG8
	BAG1
Invasion	*MMP11 (stromolysin 3)*, *CTSL2 (cathepsin L2)*
Reference	*ACTB* (β-*actin)*, *GAPDH*, *RPLPO*, *GUS*, *TFRC*

hormonal therapies are not well defined. Although HER2 amplification is uncommon in unselected hormone receptor-positive breast tumors, clinical data and preclinical models utilizing forced overexpression of HER2 implicate a potential role for alterations in signaling pathway(s) downstream from epidermal growth factor receptor (EGFR)/HER2 in anti-hormone therapy resistance.[32,34] The phosphatidylinositol-3-kinase (PI3K)/AKT and mitogen-activated protein kinase (MAPK) pathways are major mediators of the effects of membrane receptor tyrosine kinases (RTKs) such as HER2 and may play a major role in mediating resistance to anti-hormonal therapies.

Several other multiparameter gene expression platforms are under development, but few have been subjected to rigorous assay quality control and clinical validation.[35] In addition to *Oncotype Dx*, other assays include the MammaPrint test, the Rotterdam Signature, and the Breast Cancer HOXB13:IL17BR Gene Expression Ratio.[32,36-40] Only *Oncotype Dx* and the MammaPrint assays are available commercially, and the laboratory that performs the *Oncotype Dx* has been certified by the Clinical Laboratory Improvement Amendments (CLIA) to perform the test for clinical use. The MammaPrint assay has recently received clearance by the US Food and Drug Administration (FDA) as a class 2, 510(k) product, which ensures independent review of data and labeling, conformance of the device sponsor to good manufacturing practices (the so-called quality system regulations), and postmarketing surveillance and reporting to the FDA. The FDA does not evaluate treatment outcomes as a result of use of this prognostic device.

HER2 ■ The oncogene encoding *HER2* is amplified and the protein therefore overexpressed in 15-20% of invasive breast cancers. *HER2* overexpression is associated with an aggressive breast tumor phenotype and reduced survival rates.[41] Combining trastuzumab (Herceptin), a recombinant humanized monoclonal antibody that targets *HER2*, with cytotoxic chemotherapy to treat patients with metastatic and early stage *HER2* oncogene-amplified breast cancer has resulted in increased response rates and improved survival times.[42] Thus, *HER2* is a biomarker for breast tumor responsiveness to trastuzumab and to other *HER2*-targeted therapies (eg, lapatinib).[43]

A panel of the American Society of Clinical Oncology (ASCO) thus recommended that *HER2* status should be determined for all invasive breast cancers.[44] This panel has proposed a testing algorithm that relies on accurate, reproducible assay performance, including newly available types of bright-field in situ hybridization (ISH), and has specified elements to reliably reduce assay variation (eg, specimen handling, assay exclusion, and reporting criteria). A positive HER2 result is IHC staining of 3+ (uniform, intense membrane staining of >30% of invasive tumor cells), a fluorescent in situ hybridization (FISH) result of more than 6 *HER2* gene copies per nucleus, or a FISH ratio (*HER2* gene signals to chromosome 17 signals) of more than 2.2. A negative HER2 result is an IHC staining of 0 or 1+, a FISH result of less than 4.0 *HER2* gene copies per nucleus, or a FISH ratio of less than 1.8. Equivocal results require additional action for final determination. To perform HER2 testing, laboratories should demonstrate 95% concordance with another validated test for positive and negative assay values. The ASCO panel has strongly recommended validation of laboratory assay or modifications, use of standardized operating procedures, and compliance with new testing criteria to be monitored with the use of stringent laboratory accreditation standards, proficiency testing, and competency assessment. The panel also recommended that HER2 testing be done in a College of American Pathologists (CAP)-accredited laboratory.

A significant fraction of patients with *HER2*-amplified breast cancers have tumors that initially do not respond to trastuzumab or that acquire resistance to trastuzumab after an initial period of response.[43] The PI3K/AKT and MAPK pathways are major downstream *HER2* mediators.[45] Trastuzumab decreases AKT activation induced by *HER2* and this downregulation is associated with tumor growth inhibition by trastuzumab. Preclinical evidence has implicated persistent HER2-independent activation of the central critical signaling node AKT despite trastuzumab therapy as a major mechanism that leads to trastuzumab resistance.[46-49] This persistent AKT activation (phosphorylation) despite trastuzumab therapy may be mediated by a cleaved form of *HER2* that does not bind trastuzumab, by other membrane RTKs such as IGF1R, by downregulation of PTEN, a negative PI3K/AKT regulator, or by activating mutations of PIK3CA, the oncogene that encodes the p110α subunit of PI3K. These targets are all thus currently being exploited in breast cancer clinical trials in an attempt to develop clinical approaches that will overcome trastuzumab resistance in *HER2*-amplified breast cancers.

Other Breast Cancer Biomarkers ■ ASCO has determined that the following breast cancer biomarkers demonstrated insufficient current evidence to support routine use in clinical practice[35]: DNA/ploidy by flow cytometry, p53, cathepsin D, cyclin E, proteomics, certain multiparameter assays, bone marrow micrometastases, and circulating tumor cells.

Lung Cancer

EGFR ■ The EGFR tyrosine kinase inhibitors gefitinib and erlotinib are effective therapies for certain non-small cell lung cancer patients, in particular patients whose tumors harbor somatic mutations or amplification of the *EGFR* gene.[50-53] However, the clinical use of *EGFR* inhibitors is not restricted to patients with lung tumors that possess *EGFR* gene abnormalities for two major reasons. The benefit of *EGFR* inhibitors does not seem to be confined to patients with lung tumors that possess *EGFR* gene abnormalities. Further, there are clinical and demographic factors (female sex, a history of never smoking, Asian origin) that predict responsiveness to *EGFR* inhibitors with a similar accuracy to *EGFR* gene anomalies.

As with HER2-targeted therapies, despite initial benefit, all lung cancer patients ultimately develop resistance to *EGFR* inhibitors. Studies over the last few years have identified two different EGFR tyrosine kinase inhibitor resistance mechanisms, a secondary mutation in EGFR (EGFR 790M) and MET amplification.[54] These findings have led to clinical trials using novel therapies that can overcome these resistance mechanisms and that have shown promise in laboratory studies. Ongoing research efforts will likely continue to identify other resistance mechanisms, and these findings will hopefully translate into effective therapies for non-small cell lung cancer patients.

K-*Ras* ■ Emerging data implicate somatic mutations of the K-*ras* oncogene as a mechanism of de-novo resistance to EGFR inhibition in patients with non-small cell lung cancer, and to anti-*EGFR* monoclonal antibodies in patients with metastatic colorectal cancer.[55] However, the low sensitivity of K-*ras* mutations for determining nonresponsiveness to EGFR inhibitors in both tumor types makes it clear that additional mechanisms of resistance to EGFR inhibitors exist.

ERCC1 ■ Adjuvant cisplatin-based chemotherapy improves survival among patients with completely resected non small-cell lung cancer. Patients with excision repair cross-complementation group 1 (ERCC1)-negative tumors appear to benefit from adjuvant cisplatin-based chemotherapy, whereas patients with ERCC1-positive tumors do not.[56] However, this biomarker has not been introduced into routine clinical practice at this time.

Gastrointestinal Stromal Tumors (GIST): KIT and PDGFRA

GIST generally arises from primary activating mutations in the *KIT* or platelet derived growth factor receptor A (*PDGFRA*) genes that result in constitutive activation of RTK activity.[57] Imatinib (Gleevec) provides targeted therapy for GIST by inhibiting the KIT and PDGFRA tyrosine kinases. Clinical benefit is achieved in approximately 85% of patients with unresectable or metastatic disease, with a median progression-free survival of 20-24 months. The mechanisms of acquired resistance to imatinib are heterogeneous, with most involving the emergence of secondary mutations in *KIT* exons 13, 14, or 17. In patients with *GIST* tumors possessing imatinib-resistant mutations, novel kinase inhibitors such as sunitinib can inhibit the function of the mutant protein and restore antitumor activity. Experimental treatment options for imatinib-resistant tumors beyond those currently available consist of other *KIT*-targeting inhibitors (eg, nilotinib and dasatinib) or agents targeting alternative pathways, such as anti-angiogenic agents, mammalian target of rapamycin, *raf* kinase, and chaperone inhibitors.

Chronic Myeloid Leukemia (CML): Bcr-Abl Translocation

The majority of cases of CML arise due to constitutive activation of the Abl kinase as a result of the breakpoint cluster region (Bcr) Abl translocation (Philadelphia chromosome). Targeted therapy with imatinib, which inhibits Abl, has markedly improved the outlook for patients with CML. However, imatinib resistance can emerge despite initial benefit.[58] Bcr-Abl signaling is reactivated at the time of resistance, predominantly due to novel mutations in the kinase domain of Abl that interfere with drug binding. This discovery prompted the development of new Abl kinase inhibitors, among which nilotinib and dasatinib have gained regulatory approval. Despite excellent results in patients with imatinib-resistant or -intolerant CML treated with nilotinib or dasatinib, all available Abl inhibitors exhibit inactivity in the face of certain kinase domain mutations and early indications suggest that the cross-resistant *Bcr-Abl (T315I)* mutant is disproportionately represented among patients who relapse despite these novel therapies. Thus, at present, the development of a T315I inhibitor remains a high priority in CML.

Lymphoma: CD20 and Other Biomarkers

Biomarker-targeted therapeutic approaches have had a significant impact in the treatment of non-Hodgkin lymphoma (NHL).[59,60] The development of the chimeric antibody rituximab as an antibody targeted to the biomarker CD20 heralded a new era in treatment approaches for NHL. While rituximab was first shown to be effective in the treatment of relapsed follicular lymphoma, it is now standard monotherapy for front-line treatment of follicular lymphoma, and is also used in conjunction with chemotherapy for other indolent, intermediate and aggressive CD20-positive B-cell lymphomas. The development of rituximab has led to the subsequent development and approval of the radioimmunoconjugates of rituximab, ^{90}Y-ibritumomab tiuxetan and ^{131}I-tositumomab. Since rituximab is a chimeric antibody, there is also a focus on developing fully humanized antibodies, such as IMMU-106 (hA20), in order to minimise infusion reactions and eliminate the development of human antibodies against the drug.

Further clinical evaluation of antibodies has been based largely on knowledge of antigen expression on the surface of lymphoma cells and has led to the development of antibodies against CD22 (unconjugated epratuzumab and calicheamicin conjugated CMC-544 [inotuzumab ozogamicin]), CD80 (galiximab), CD52 (alemtuzumab), CD2 (MEDI-507 [siplizumab]), CD30 (SGN-30 and MDX-060 [iratumumab]), and CD40 (SGN-40).[60] Furthermore, agonists to TRAIL (tumor necrosis factor-related apoptosis-inducing ligand) are currently being investigated as treatments for NHL as well as of advanced solid tumors. Knowledge of the ability of cancer cells to become resistant to a targeted therapy by activating an alternative pathway has driven studies that combine antibodies such as epratuzumab plus rituximab (ER) or ER plus chemotherapy with CHOP (cyclophosphamide, doxorubicin, vincristine, and prednisone [ER-CHOP]), inotuzumab ozogamicin plus rituximab, alemtuzumab plus CHOP (CHOP-C), and now the combination of TRAIL agonists plus rituximab. Antibody-based therapeutic approaches have had a profound impact on NHL treatment, and it is almost certain that the optimum methods of incorporating these drugs in NHL treatment will continue to be refined.

Molecular Biomarkers for Monitoring of Cancer

A number of circulating biomarkers are used for monitoring of cancer response to therapy and/or for the early detection of recurrent disease in cancer patients.

Alpha-Fetoprotein (AFP) and Human Chorionic Gonadotropin (hCG)

Many germ cell tumors (most male testicular cancers, gestational trophoblastic disease (choriocarcinoma) and rare female ovarian cancers) produce circulating tumor markers (AFP, hCG, lactate dehydrogenase [LDH]).[61] These biomarkers are useful in the diagnosis and staging of germ cell tumors, to monitor therapeutic response and to detect early tumor recurrence. Since recurrent germ cell tumors are curable in many cases with cytotoxic chemotherapy, particularly when the recurrence is detected early, increasing levels of tumor markers during patient follow-up is an indication that salvage therapy should be initiated, even if no evident disease is found. The half-life of the markers must be taken into consideration when evaluating therapeutic responses. Further, marker monitoring has been introduced in the staging of germ cell tumors.

AFP is a glycoprotein normally produced by the fetal yolk sac, the liver and the gastrointestinal tract, but not in adult tissues. It is re-expressed in the germ cell tumors, including yolk sac tumors and embryonal carcinomas. hCG is a glycoprotein produced by syncytiotrophoblastic cells and it consists of two subunits, α and β. The α subunit is common to three pituitary trophic hormones: FSH, LH, and TSH; the β subunit makes hCG enzymatically and immunologically distinct. Assays measure only the β subunit (β-hCG). In males, it is highly specific for testicular cancer and is produced specifically by choriocarcinoma cells and by 5-10% of pure seminomas. LDH reflects "tumor burden," growth rate and cellular proliferation, and is of independent prognostic significance. LDH measurements detect multiple isoenzymes. LDH is increased in about 80% of advanced seminomas and in about 60% of advanced nonseminomatous germ cell tumors. The LDH isoenzyme 1 seems to be more specific and sensitive for germ cell tumors than isoenzymes 2-5.[62]

CA125

CA125, an abbreviation for cancer antigen 125, is a tumor marker that may be elevated in the blood of patients with specific types of cancer. It is a mucinous glycoprotein and a product of the MUC16 gene. As discussed above, CA125 is best known as a marker for ovarian cancer but may also be elevated in endometrial cancer, fallopian tube cancer, lung cancer, breast cancer and gastrointestinal cancers, and also in a number of relatively benign conditions such as endometriosis and ovarian disorders. Thus, CA125, when used alone on a single occasion, is not sensitive or specific enough for ovarian cancer screening.[29] However, serum CA125 level is very useful for following ovarian cancer patient response to treatment, for predicting prognosis in women with ovarian cancer after therapy, and for detecting a recurrence of ovarian cancer. During first-line platinum-based chemotherapy for women with ovarian cancer, CA125 levels should be followed regularly (eg, every 3 weeks) and the CA125 level at nadir, 3-month normalization of CA125 and CA125 half-life are all strong predictors of subsequent progression-free survival and overall survival times.[63-65] The failure of serum CA125 to normalize after initial treatment with surgery and platinum-based chemotherapy is a particularly ominous indication of a poor prognosis in women with ovarian cancer.

In women with previously treated ovarian cancer that is presently in clinical remission, the National Comprehensive Cancer Network (NCCN-www.nccn.org) recommends evaluation of serum CA125 level at each follow-up visit if the CA125 level was elevated at the time of the initial diagnosis. Follow-up visits every 2-4 months are recommended for 2 years after initial definitive therapy, then at 6-month intervals for another 3 years followed by annual follow-up visits. After a documentation of CA125 elevation in such women, the median time to a clinical relapse of ovarian cancer is 2-6 months. However, in the absence of definitive evidence that early therapy improves outcomes, there is a lack of consensus regarding the timing of treatment for recurrent ovarian cancer in women who are found to have an elevation in serum CA125.

CA15-3 and CA27.29

CA15-3 and CA 27.29 are well-characterized assays that allow the detection of circulating MUC1 antigen in peripheral blood.[35] Several studies support the prognostic relevance of this circulating marker in early stage breast cancer but it has yet to be determined if MUC1–based serum markers will have utility in making treatment decisions in this setting.[66,67] ASCO regards available data as insufficient to recommend using CA15-3 or CA 27.29 for breast cancer screening, diagnosis or staging, or for monitoring patients for recurrence after primary therapy, as there is no hard evidence that early detection of recurrence improves survival.[35] In contrast, for monitoring patients with metastatic breast cancer during active therapy, CA27.29 or CA15-3 can be used in conjunction with diagnostic imaging, history, and physical examination. Although present data are insufficient to recommend the use of CA15-3 or CA 27.29 alone for monitoring response to treatment, an increasing CA15-3 or CA27.29 may be used to indicate treatment failure in the absence of readily measurable disease. However, caution should be used when interpreting a rising CA27.29 or CA15-3 level during the first 4-6 weeks of a new therapy, given that spurious early rises may occur.

CA19-9

Carbohydrate antigen 19-9 is elevated primarily in the serum of patients with gastrointestinal tract carcinomas. The greatest utility of serum CA19-9 is in monitoring response to treatment in patients with pancreatic cancer. For patients with locally advanced or metastatic pancreatic cancer undergoing active therapy, ASCO recommends that serum CA19-9 levels be measured every 1-3 months.[68] Elevations in serial CA19-9 determinations suggest progressive disease in the face of treatment but confirmation of this should be sought with other studies such as CT scanning before a therapy change is initiated.

Carcinoembryonic Antigen (CEA)

CEA is a glycoprotein involved in cell adhesion.[69] It is normally produced during fetal development and is not usually present in the blood of healthy adults, although levels are raised in heavy smokers. Serum CEA may be elevated in patients with colorectal carcinoma, gastric carcinoma, pancreatic carcinoma, lung carcinoma, breast carcinoma and medullary thyroid carcinoma. ASCO has set forth clinical practice guidelines for the monitoring of serum CEA levels in patients with colorectal cancer.[68] For colorectal cancer, it is recommended that serum CEA be ordered preoperatively, if it would assist in staging and surgical planning. Postoperative CEA levels should be performed every 3 months for patients with stages II and III colorectal cancer for at least 3 years if the patient is a potential candidate for surgery (eg, liver resection) or chemotherapy for metastatic disease. CEA is also the marker of choice for monitoring the response of metastatic colorectal cancer to systemic therapy.

In terms of other biomarkers, ASCO regards current data as insufficient to recommend the routine use of p53, ras, thymidine synthase, dihydropyrimidine dehydrogenase, thymidine phosphorylase, microsatellite instability, 18q loss of heterozygosity, or deleted in colon cancer (DCC) protein in the management of patients with colorectal cancer.

For monitoring metastatic breast cancer patients during therapy, the ASCO guidelines[35] support the use of CEA in conjunction with diagnostic imaging, history, and physical examination. As with CA15-3 and CA27.29, present data are insufficient to recommend the use of CEA alone for monitoring response to breast cancer treatment. However, in the absence of readily measurable disease, an increasing CEA may be used to indicate treatment failure. Caution should also be used when interpreting a rising CEA level during the first 6 weeks of a new breast cancer therapy as spurious early rises may occur.

PSA

The measurement of serum PSA is important in many respects in men with an established diagnosis of prostate cancer. The rate of rise of PSA has value in predicting prostate cancer prognosis.[5] Men with prostate cancer whose PSA level increased by more than 2.0 ng/mL during the year before the diagnosis of prostate cancer have a higher risk of death from prostate cancer after radical prostatectomy. In addition, the design of an optimal strategy for the treatment of prostate cancer requires assessment of risk. PSA level along with the clinical stage of disease and the Gleason tumor grade are all components of most nomograms and predictive models that are used for such risk assessment.[70] Further, as with CA125, the serum PSA level is monitored regularly during prostate cancer therapy and is a good indicator of disease response to treatment.

For prostate cancer patients who are initially treated with curative intent, a serum PSA level should be checked every 6-12 months for 5 years and annually thereafter (www.nccn.org). A rising PSA level indicates a biochemical failure and often precedes a clinically detectable recurrence by several years. Since a biochemical failure may represent an isolated local recurrence, it is important to identify those patients without identifiable distant metastases, since these patients may be candidates for salvage therapy.

Novel Molecular Biomarkers and Platforms for Their Detection

Malignant tumors are usually characterized by multiple molecular anomalies that are responsible for the specific behavior of each individual tumor, and some of these changes are likely to be detectable from early stages of tumor development. Hence the rationale that novel molecular technologies may allow identification of sensitive and specific biomarkers that will facilitate early cancer detection, personalized therapy planning and monitoring of treatment responses. Novel high-throughput molecular technologies that comprehensively characterize the cancer genome and proteome are presently adding many new possibilities for the identification of biomarkers to the more fully explored potential of more traditional and moderate-throughput investigative approaches. Ideally, with technological advances, one can foresee molecular biomarkers that will perform more than one purpose. For example, screening biomarkers could conceivably be used to facilitate prognostication and individualized treatment planning.

Novel high-throughput and comprehensive genomic and proteomic technologies are being widely developed for early cancer detection as well as prognostication, prediction and target identification. These techniques include gene methylation analysis, gene microarrays and comparative genomic hybridization (CGH, eg, Affymetrix Inc., CA; Agilent Technologies, CA), mass spectrometry/spectroscopy (MS, eg, Ciphergen, CA; Sequenom Inc., CA), and bead-based analysis methods (eg, Illumina Inc., CA; Luminex, TX). Many of these technologies are only beginning to be applied to the discovery of cancer-related molecular marker panels in various clinical settings.[71-75] Gene expression profiles have already been extensively explored in identifying good and poor prognosis subsets of various human tumors.[76] DNA methylation changes are also common molecular alterations in cancer cells and methylation analysis to detect early cancer cell DNA methylation aberrations in, for example, blood, feces and urine is currently being investigated. Together, these genomic and proteomic platforms have the advantage of comprehensively probing the genome and proteome and thus of identifying a large number of potential biomarkers for follow-up studies. Further, the incorporation of information to develop meta-signatures reflecting global DNA, RNA, and protein abnormalities may be capable of outperforming data derived from a single technology that examines only one of these platforms.[77] For example, proteomic studies can augment genomic panels by providing information on posttranslational modifications and on the relative levels and activation of proteins. As such data sets become available, systems for effective data management, integrated analysis of pathways, and "meta-analysis" become critical to the successful development of molecular markers.[78-80]

While most current molecular cancer biomarkers were discovered through the study of limited numbers of genes/proteins, the novel technologies (eg, gene microarrays) introduced in the preceding paragraph have already been used successfully to develop multimarker (eg, multigene) panels for prediction of cancer responses to specific therapies (see above). These multimarker panels may offer a particularly accurate means of early cancer detection, risk prediction and for planning individualized cancer treatment and prevention strategies. A high-throughput proteomic technology allows concurrent analysis of the expression and activation of multiple specific kinases and other proteins.[81-85] This platform (reverse phase protein lysate array [RPPA]) is particularly suited to explore the role of kinase signaling in cancer and the molecular effects of novel agents (eg, tyrosine kinase inhibitors [TKIs]) during treatment and in high risk tissue during chemoprevention (Fig. 26-2).

Novel molecular biomarkers in cancer may be present in the germline genome or may occur in a somatic or acquired fashion in the genome and/or proteome of a particular tissue at high risk of carcinogenesis or possessing malignant transformation. In addition, novel cancer biomarkers are likely to be present in the circulation, either in the form of circulating tumor cells or specific markers or groups ("signatures") of markers.

Novel Germline Biomarkers

Novel biomarkers for high cancer risk and for toxicity and efficacy associated with particular anticancer treatments are likely to be present in the germline genome. Recent studies have begun to identify polymorphisms in the germline genome that are associated with toxicity and efficacy of the *EGFR* inhibitor erlotinib in lung cancer treatment.[86] Recent large scale studies of the germline genome have also begun to uncover novel cancer susceptibility markers.[87,88] Kammerer et al.[87] carried out association studies using 16,000 single nucleotide polymorphisms (SNPs) and identified the intercellular adhesion molecule (*ICAM*) gene region as a novel breast and prostate cancer susceptibility locus. As our ability to predict high cancer risk and likely therapy outcomes utilizing novel germline biomarkers improves further, early detection and prevention strategies must increasingly focus on specific molecular cancer subtypes that will allow us to better define biomarkers of likely benefit from specific therapies.[89]

Tissue-Specific Biomarkers of High Risk and for Early Detection of Cancer

Cellular atypia or early malignant change may be present as an early indicator of high cancer risk in specific tissues. With availability of less invasive ways to obtain cells likely to be at risk of or to harbor early neoplastic change in tissue at risk of cancer (eg, in sputum, bronchial washings, feces, urine or nipple aspirate), the study of tissue markers for screening of carcinogenesis risk and of early malignant transformation becomes more feasible. To date, however, the cost, invasiveness, lack of large prospective outcome validation studies, and absence of standardized guidelines has confined most

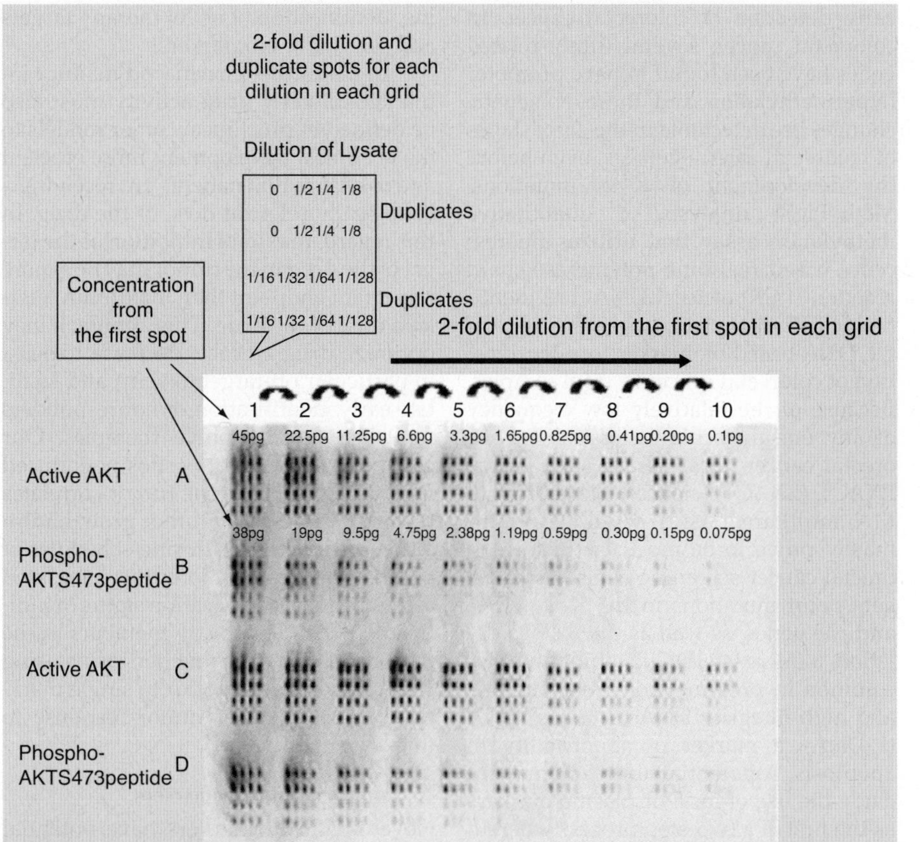

Figure 26-2 Sensitivity and reproducibility of reverse phase protein lysate arrays (RPPA). Here, protein lysates from cell lines have been serially diluted on a nitrocellulose-coated slide followed by probing with monospecific antibodies to total or phosphorylated Akt and signal detection and amplification. Serial dilution curves are used for quantification purposes. *Source:* From Ref. 81.

of these potentially useful approaches to small clinical studies.

Lung Cancer ■ Although screening to detect lung cancer at an early stage using routine cytological examination of sputum did not decrease cancer-specific mortality, the application of molecular detection methods to sputum and bronchial washings is now being studied in an attempt to detect molecular changes associated with premalignant and early malignant bronchial epithelial cells.[90] For example, FISH with locus-specific probes to chromosomal regions 5p15, 7p12 (EGFR), 8q24 (C-Myc), and the centromere of chromosome 6 may significantly improve the sensitivity for detection of malignancy in sputum and bronchial washing specimens.[91]

Colorectal Cancer ■ Malignant cells may be shed into feces during early stages of colorectal cancer development and fecal tests for DNA and other molecular markers are being developed, as are novel endoscopic imaging techniques to detect early colorectal cancer.[92] Several studies have attempted to detect tumor-specific DNA aberrations including APC or *ras* gene mutations or DNA hypermethylation in stool and even plasma to facilitate early detection of colorectal cancer. In colorectal cancer, several tumor-related genes have been found to have promoter hypermethylation and these epigenetic changes are detectable in the early stages of colorectal carcinogenesis, even before the development of K-*ras* mutations. MethyLight analysis, a quantitative methylation assay that utilizes fluorescence-based real-time polymerase chain reaction (PCR) of fecal DNA, has identified SFRP2 methylation as a sensitive single DNA-based biomarker for identification of colorectal cancer in stool samples. Because of the relatively low frequency of any one molecular alteration in colorectal cancer, fecal assays such as the EXACT (EXACT Sciences, Marlborough, MA) multitarget assay panel[93] may ultimately prove to be most useful for colorectal cancer screening. This assay targets point mutations in the K-*ras*, *APC*, and *p53* genes, as well as the *BAT-26* deletion, a microsatellite instability marker common in proximal colorectal tumors, and high-integrity DNA or "long" DNA (L-DNA), a marker of abnormality in apoptosis. A potential approach may include the use of fecal or plasma markers as the first of a two-step process wherein only those found to have a high suspicion of early neoplasia will then undergo colonoscopy.

Breast Cancer ■ Cellular atypia in breast biopsies is associated with a 2- to 10-fold increase in the risk of breast cancer. Atypia can also be detected by a number of other less invasive methods including nipple fluid aspiration, ductal lavage, and periareolar fine needle aspiration.[4] The cellular yield from such methods offers the possibility for detailed molecular study of cellular changes associated with atypia and early carcinogenesis, molecular markers leading to a predisposition to cancer in individual women and of potential prevention and therapeutic targets, particularly with the application of novel high-throughput approaches to the study of DNA, RNA, and protein.[94,95] However, current approaches are most applicable to high content analysis of small numbers of samples.

Cancer-Specific Biomarkers

As discussed in much detail above, progress has already been made in the identification of single biomarkers and multimarker panels (eg, *Oncotype Dx*) in tumor material to facilitate prediction of cancer responses to specific therapies. However, although this is particularly true of breast cancer, progress in this regard is sorely needed in other forms of cancer. Together, the novel genomic and proteomic platforms listed above have the advantage of comprehensively probing the cancer genome and proteome and thus of facilitating identification of novel therapy targets and predictive biomarkers.

In the future, pharmacodynamic biomarkers of early drug activity must also be defined in preclinical tumor models to make clinical development more efficient and to ensure that patients are receiving a biologically relevant dose of the drug. In this regard, maximal inhibition of the target of the drug in the tumor may be a more important endpoint than maximum tolerated dose of the drug. This approach may optimize drug efficacy, decrease toxicity, in particular off-target toxicity, and facilitate early identification of nonresponders for triage to alternative therapies. Our group has shown that perifosine-induced inhibition of AKT in the tumor correlates remarkably well with tumor growth inhibition using multiple dosing schedules of perifosine.[85] Furthermore, the integrated assessment of the activation status of multiple PI3K/AKT pathway members in the tumor soon after starting perifosine using RPPA may prove superior to single markers for prediction of tumor response to this drug.

Serum and Urine Biomarkers

Novel serum biomarkers have potential utility in cancer screening, in prediction of tumor responsiveness to specific therapies and in monitoring tumor responses to therapy. As discussed above, while conventional serum cancer biomarkers are used routinely for cancer monitoring, their application to screening is limited by their lack of adequate sensitivity and specificity.[96-98] Specificity can be improved by monitoring increases in individual marker levels over time, but marker panels will almost certainly be required to increase sensitivity for screening. The conventional concept concerning the screening utility of serum biomarkers is that their detection should trigger clinical assessment by imaging and biopsy, or increased surveillance if appropriate. Alternatively, novel serum markers might be used following screening by other means to increase the specificity of the latter approach. Thus, a novel biomarker may allow definition of an equivocal mammographic lesion as appropriate for serial monitoring or immediate biopsy.

MS-based approaches to identify novel serum biomarkers have been studied for some time based on the hypothesis that proteomic panels could identify tumors from an early stage of development. Ovarian cancer has been the subject of several such studies because of diagnosis in advanced stages, poor patient outcomes and the absence of a well-established screening method. Two general approaches have been utilized: identification of distinctive signatures and discovery of discrete markers that might be assembled into panels. Algorithms for ovarian cancer-specific signatures have evolved over time but none has been prospectively validated with large numbers of early stage or preclinical cases. Three serum biomarker panels have been detected from surface-enhanced laser desorption and ionization time of flight (SELDI-TOF) MS peaks representing 14 differentially expressed serum proteins in ovarian cancer, and the combination of 4 component proteins (transthyretin, beta-hemoglobin, apolipoprotein AI and transferrin) with CA125 has been shown to significantly improve detection of early stage ovarian cancer.[99] However, all such serum biomarker panels require prospective validation.

In the urine, the sensitivity of FISH or of cytokeratin (eg, keratin 19, 20) detection using IHC or reverse transcriptase (RT) PCR may be higher than that of conventional cytology for bladder and urothelial cancer screening.[100] A commercial kit (UroVysion) containing hybridization probes for chromosomes 3, 7, 9p21, and 17 is used for FISH analysis of urine. The sensitivity and specificity associated with this analysis were 60% and 82.6%, respectively, for detection of bladder cancer. In contrast, the sensitivity and specificity associated with urine cytology were 24.1% and 90.5%, respectively. Thus, a FISH assay for chromosomes 3, 7, 9, and 17 may have a higher sensitivity than cytology and a similar specificity for the detection of urothelial cancers. Table 26-2 shows the sensitivity,

Table 26-2 ■ **Sensitivity, Specificity and Positive Predictive Value of Urine Cytology, Bladder Tumor Antigen (BTA) Immunoassay, Nuclear Matrix Protein-22 (NMP22) Detection, ImmunoCyt, and Urine FISH for Early Detection of Bladder Cancer**

	Sensitivity (%)	Specificity (%)	PPV (%)
PSA	72	93	25
Urine cytology	48-73	48-100	48-69
BTA	53	77	63
NMP22	71	66	21
ImmunoCyt	78-81	74-100	26
FISH	69-71	78-95	68

Note: Serum prostate specific antigen (PSA) in prostate cancer screening is shown only as a point of reference. ImmunoCyt is currently approved by the U.S. Food and Drug Administration for the monitoring of recurrent bladder cancer. ImmunoCyt uses a cocktail of three monoclonal antibodies to detect bladder cancer cells in the urine. One antibody is directed against a high molecular-weight form of glycosylated carcinoembryonic antigen, 19A211. The other two antibodies, LDQ10 and M344, are directed against mucins that are specific for bladder cancer and are labeled with fluorescein.
Source: From Ref. 101.

specificity, and positive predictive value of various approaches that have been investigated as potential tools to facilitate bladder cancer screening.[101]

Circulating Tumor and Other Cells

Circulating tumor cells (CTCs) have potential utility in cancer screening, target identification, response prediction and in monitoring response to treatment. Indeed, the predictive and prognostic utility of CTCs have already been demonstrated in metastatic breast cancer.[102] In this study, immunomagnetic enrichment (CellSearch, Veridex, LLC) was used to quantify CTCs. Initial studies of the utility of CTCs in breast cancer screening are proceeding.[103] In ovarian cancer, peripheral blood CTC-specific *p53* sequences are detectable in some FIGO stage III/IV ovarian cancer patients, suggesting that this approach may be useful as a building block toward early detection.[104]

The use of CTCs to study novel molecular biomarkers is limited currently to gene expression signatures because of the need for substrate amplification. However, CTCs have the potential to facilitate early access to the tumor genome and proteome for novel molecular studies of biomarkers and therapy targets in cancer.[105,106] CTCs may ultimately facilitate therapy targeting before definitive treatment and treatment monitoring. A major challenge is the difficulty in harvesting CTCs and of exploring molecular markers in a limited number of cells. Alternative methods of enrichment of CTCs are being explored and include the enhanced density gradient system.[107] We are currently investigating novel methods of DNA and protein extraction to allow detection of mutations and protein expression/activation changes in CTCs, the latter utilizing RPPAs.[108-110] Circulating endothelial cells (CECs) and bone marrow-derived endothelial precursor cells play an important role in tumor neovascularization and growth and, while largely studied thus far for a role in therapy monitoring, also have potential to yield insights into the early origin and pathogenesis of different cancers.[111-113]

Novel Molecular Imaging Approaches

Novel molecular imaging approaches such as PET are making feasible the potential incorporation of important and novel cancer molecular markers and signaling pathways into imaging strategies to enhance early detection, response prediction, and treatment monitoring. It is theoretically possible to image any potential cancer-specific biomarker or target in tumors in vivo by selecting and labeling an appropriate ligand (eg, radiolabeled fluoroestradiol [FES]-PET).[114] Novel CT and MRI-based techniques have refined imaging of other cancer-specific processes such as angiogenesis. Such technologies are new, and the most feasible and appropriate approaches to their application to early cancer detection and in the monitoring of treatment responses remains to be defined.

Challenges in Validation of Novel Molecular Biomarkers

With the use of novel technologies to profile the cancer genome or proteome to define new biomarker panels, limitations in reproducibility occur that are in large part attributable to the simultaneous assay of many gene or protein markers with a limited number of cancer specimens. The resultant large number of potential biomarker combinations introduces a significant likelihood that uncovered associations are simply the result of chance. It is thus critical to adopt a rigorous training, test, and validation approach to novel biomarker studies if they are to meaningfully impact patient management. Most studies that have defined novel biomarker panels have not impacted patient management to date, either because they did not rigorously attempt to deal with this multiple parameter problem or because they did not adopt sufficiently robust statistical approaches to validation. The importance of bioinformatic and biostatistical support for the development of novel molecular diagnostics cannot be overemphasized.

Rigorously validated panels of molecular markers are required before their implementation as routinely used tools in patient management. There are several examples of preliminary panels,[115,116] but their applicability is still being validated. A major hindrance to the design of novel molecular studies for biomarker discovery and validation is the frequent lack of availability of adequately preserved and appropriately annotated samples in large numbers that can be mated to specific technologies. In particular, novel high-throughput approaches are often limited in their utility to fresh frozen specimens (paraffin-embedded samples are much more plentiful). Thus, a popular model for biomarker development has been discovery using novel high-throughput profiling technologies (eg, transcriptional profiling) in frozen tissue, followed by validation using moderate-throughput technologies (eg, RT-PCR) applied to paraffin-embedded tissue. It is critical to define the specific tissue type in which a molecular marker will be validated for clinical use.[117,118] Novel comprehensive approaches to biomarker discovery using proteome- or genome-wide expression profiling have now begun to redefine ways in which tumor banks collect and store tumor samples, with a major emphasis currently placed on fresh frozen specimens.[119,120]

Presently, it is not possible to apply all available investigative technologies to every person, or even every patient at high risk for the development of cancer. Even putting cost issues aside, one challenge is to obtain adequate material from biopsy, cellular or serum specimens. For microarray (transcriptional or CGH) analysis, several hundred nanograms of genomic *DNA* or *RNA* are required, but the amount of DNA and RNA available from a fine needle aspirate (FNA) is in picograms. In the case of 1-5 CTCs in 10 mL of blood, the yield of DNA and RNA is even smaller. Amplification by PCR can increase mRNA yield but PCR-generated mistakes are not uncommon. Further, direct amplification of protein is not possible and, although it is feasible to translate mRNA in vitro, it is doubtful that this will significantly enhance protein yield and it will not allow assessment of post-translational protein modifications. Sensitive methods including MALDI-TOF-MS along with post-hybridization signal amplification in RPPAs do magnify detection limits. However, these major difficulties need to be addressed to facilitate the routine application of novel molecular technologies to cancer diagnostics.

Recommendations

There are a number of important requirements for an effective program that is dedicated to the discover of novel cancer biomarkers. These include collaborative approaches, appropriate human tissue sample sets, an integrated informatics platform, identification and quantitation of candidate biomarkers in tumor tissue, mouse models of disease, standardized reagents for analyzing candidate biomarkers in tissue and fluid along with implementation of automation. As revealed by the Human Genome Project, standards, reagents, tools, and automation are absolutely necessary for advancement in biomarker development. Indeed, the Microarray Gene Expression Data (MGED) Society has established standards for presenting and exchanging gene microarray data (Minimum Information about a Microarray Experiment [MIAME]) and plans to expand these standards to other high-throughput genomic and proteomic technologies in the future. With proteomic biomarkers in particular, technology improvements for better fractionation of the proteome, selection of specific biomarkers from complex mixtures, and multiplexed assay of biomarkers will also greatly enhance progress. A fully integrated biomarker discovery program will center around core resources for technology development and assessment, tissue sample set handling and storage, reagents and bioinformatics.[121] New technologies should be evaluated through pilot projects and "biomarker mines" comprised of individual investigators and smaller research teams. Upon standardization, new technologies can be tested in the clinical setting by cancer site teams dedicated to biomarker discovery at a particular cancer site (Fig. 26-3).

It is necessary to have comprehensive tumor banks with appropriately preserved specimen sets (frozen and paraffin-embedded). As studies characterize tissues using high-throughput genomic, transcriptional and proteomic approaches for biomarker discovery, it is critical that adequate and centralized computational infrastructure be developed to allow storage, utilization, and integration of the vast and heterogeneous data derived from novel "omics" technologies.[122] Such a computational resource should be made available to all investigators in a manner that is easy to use, that protects confidentiality, and avoids duplication of efforts. These resources should facilitate data mining, retrieval, and automated analysis with statistical software packages such as R or Matlab, thus facilitating data integration across genomic, transcriptional, and proteomic platforms and between datasets as well as analysis of the association of specific aberrations and changes with clinical endpoints. Repeated updating should be facilitated as novel "omics" technologies are continually introduced and upgraded. Access would also allow and encourage novel biostatistical approaches that further our ability to work with and integrate large amounts of data across multiple platforms so as to advance understanding of the pathogenesis of and ability to detect early cancer.

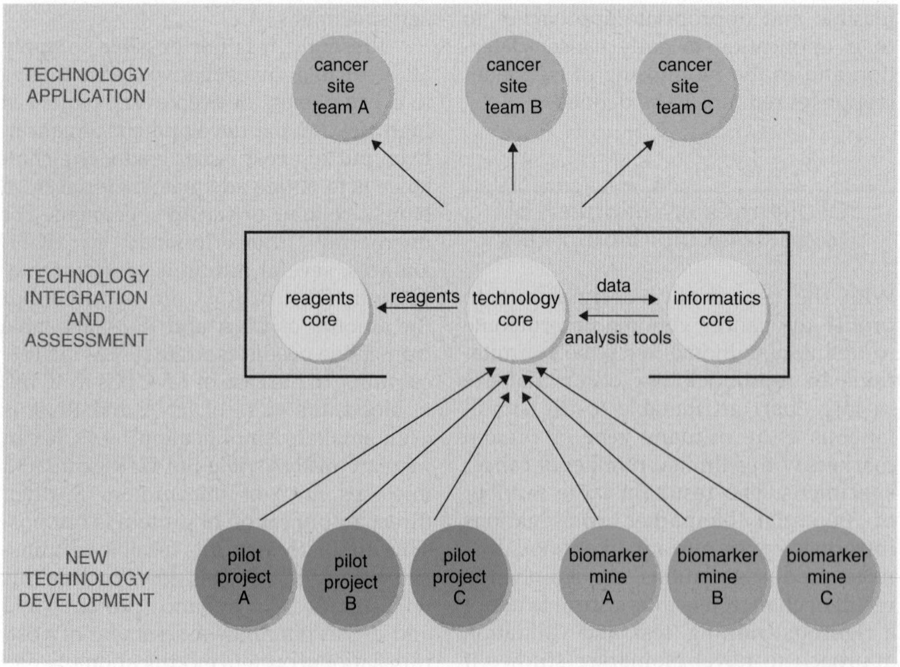

Figure 26-3 ■ A fully integrated clinical biomarker discovery technology program centers around core resources for technology development and assessment, reagents, sample set handling and storage, and informatics. New technologies should be evaluated through pilot projects and "biomarker mines" that are comprised of individual investigators and smaller research teams. Upon standardization by these core teams, new technologies can be tested in the clinical setting by cancer site teams dedicated to biomarker discovery at a particular cancer site. *Source:* From Ref. 121.

The selection of novel biomarkers from data derived using novel high-throughput technologies needs careful consideration. New and increasingly robust approaches to biomarker selection include "extreme" sample training (extreme in terms of the clinical endpoint), dimension reduction-based penalized logistic regression, cancer outlier profile analysis, and multinomial probit regression with Bayesian gene selection.[123-126] New biomarkers should ideally be assessed for potential introduction into clinical management (ie, for validation) by measuring the impact of the biomarker on outcomes and costs in a prospective, randomized experiment.[127] However, study costs and regulatory and healthcare market constraints often make such clinical trials impractical. Researchers and policymakers are thus increasingly using simulation modeling to predict the effects of new biomarkers on outcomes. The latter approach can optimize sensitivity, specificity, and cost in addition to identifying leverage points where more definitive biomarkers may be needed. This approach has already been used to assess the cost effectiveness of flexible sigmoidoscopy for colorectal cancer screening.

Recently, a Committee on Developing Biomarker-Based Tools for Cancer Screening, Diagnosis and Treatment of the Institute of Medicine of the National Academies put together a formal set of recommendations for development of biomarker-based tools for cancer (Box 4).

Conclusion

In summary, significant progress has already been made in the development of molecular diagnostics in certain forms of cancer such as breast cancer. Recent molecular studies have revealed the biologic heterogeneity and complexity of cancer and this necessitates the application of more global studies of the cancer genome and proteome to identify novel biomarkers that facilitate further advances in the understanding, treatment and early detection of cancer. Indeed, the application of high-throughput technologies such as transcriptional profiling is already significantly advancing the ability to

Box 4 Summary of Recommendations to Develop Biomarker-Based Tools for Cancer

Methods, Tools, and Resources Needed to Discover and Develop Biomarkers

1. Federal agencies should develop an organized, comprehensive approach to biomarker discovery, and foster development of novel technologies.
2. Industry and other funders should establish international consortia to generate and share precompetitive biomarker data.
3. Funders should place a major emphasis on developing pathway biomarkers to broaden applicability.
4. Funders should sponsor demonstration projects to develop biomarkers that can predict efficacy and safety in patients for drugs already on the market.
5. Government agencies and other funders should sustain support for high-quality biorepositories of prospectively collected samples.

Guidelines, Standards, Oversight, and Incentives Needed for Biomarker Development

6. Government agencies and other stakeholders should develop a transparent process to create well defined consensus standards and guidelines for biomarker development, qualification, validation and use.
7. The FDA and industry should work together to facilitate the codevelopment and approval of diagnostic-therapeutic combinations.
8. The FDA should clearly delineate and standardize its oversight of biomarker tests used in clinical decision making.
9. The Centers for Medicare and Medicaid Services should develop a specialty area for molecular diagnostics under the CLIA.

Methods and Processes Needed for Clinical Evaluation and Adoption

10. The Centers for Medicare & Medicaid Services should revise and modernize its coding and pricing system for diagnostic tests.
11. The Centers for Medicare and Medicaid Services, as well as other payors, should develop criteria for conditional coverage of new biomarker tests.

As a component of conditional coverage, procedures for high-quality population-based assessments of efficacy and cost effectiveness of biomarker tests should be established.

Source: from the Institute of Medicine of the National Academies.

predict responsiveness to specific cancer treatments. Improving understanding of the molecular heterogeneity of cancer along with rapid improvements in molecular technologies that can profile this heterogeneity have also unearthed further possibilities for the development of molecular diagnostics in cancer. It is expected that these approaches will eventually not only advance our ability to diagnose cancer at an early stage but will also allow simultaneous profiling of molecular targets that will facilitate individualization of patient care to a point where current standard therapies in many cases may become obsolete. The achievement of these goals necessitates overcoming many challenges that lie in the way of the successful implementation of both traditional and novel molecular technologies to cancer diagnostics. As high-throughput technologies acquire an increasing foothold in the development of novel molecular cancer diagnostics, the establishment of robust collaborations and bioinformatics approaches to high-throughput data storage, integration, analysis and validation will be critical.

Selected References

The complete reference list can be found at www.CANCERMEDICINE8.com

1. Fisher B, Costantino JP, Wickerham DL, et al. Tamoxifen for the prevention of breast cancer: current status of the National Surgical Adjuvant Breast and Bowel Project P-1 study. *J Natl Cancer Inst.* 2005;97:1652–1662.
6. Berry DA, Iversen ES Jr, Gudbjartsson DF, et al. BRCAPRO validation, sensitivity of genetic testing of BRCA1/BRCA2, and prevalence of other breast cancer susceptibility genes. *J Clin Oncol.* 2002;20:2701–2712.
11. Walsh T, Casadei S, Coats KH, et al. Spectrum of mutations in BRCA1, BRCA2, CHEK2, and TP53 in families at high risk of breast cancer. *JAMA.* 2006;295:1379–1388.
14. Johnson N, Fletcher O, Naceur-Lombardelli C, et al. Interaction between CHEK2*1100delC and other low-penetrance breast-cancer susceptibility genes: a familial study. *Lancet.* 2005;366:1554–1557.
16. Winawer SJ, Zauber AG, Ho MN, et al. Prevention of colorectal cancer by colonoscopic polypectomy. *N Engl J Med.* 1993;329:1977–1981.
18. Berry DA, Cronin KA, Plevritis SK, et al. Effect of screening and adjuvant therapy on mortality from breast cancer. *N Engl J Med.* 2005;353:1784–1792.
22. Bertagnolli MM, Eagle CJ, Zauber AG, et al. Celecoxib for the prevention of sporadic colorectal adenomas. *N Engl J Med.* 2006;355:873–884.
23. Meijers-Heijboer H, van Geel B, van Putten WL, et al. Breast cancer after prophylactic bilateral mastectomy in women with a BRCA1 or BRCA2 mutation. *N Engl J Med.* 2001;345:159–164.
30. Early Breast Cancer Trialists' Collaborative Group (EBCTCG). Effects of chemotherapy and hormonal therapy for early breast cancer on recurrence and 15-year survival: an overview of the randomised trials. *Lancet.* 2005;365:1687–1717.
31. Goss PE, Ingle JN, Martino S, et al. A randomized trial of letrozole in postmenopausal women after five years of tamoxifen therapy for early-stage breast cancer. *N Engl J Med.* 2003;349:793–802.
32. Paik S, Shak S, Tang G, et al. A multigene assay to predict recurrence of tamoxifen-treated, node-negative breast cancer. *N Engl J Med.* 2004;351:2817–2826.
35. Harris L, Fritsche H, Mennel R, et al. American Society of Clinical Oncology. American Society of Clinical Oncology 2007 update of recommendations for the use of tumor markers in breast cancer. *J Clin Oncol.* 2007;25:5287–5312.
36. van de Vijver MJ, He YD, van't Veer LJ, et al. A gene-expression signature as a predictor of survival in breast cancer. *N Engl J Med.* 2002;347:1999–2009.
38. Wang Y, Klijn JG, Zhang Y, et al. Gene-expression profiles to predict distant metastasis of lymph-node-negative primary breast cancer. *Lancet.* 2005;365:671–659.
40. Ma XJ, Wang Z, Ryan PD, et al. A two-gene expression ratio predicts clinical outcome in breast cancer patients treated with tamoxifen. *Cancer Cell.* 2004;5:607–616.
41. Slamon DJ, Clark GM, Wong SG, et al. Human breast cancer: correlation of relapse and survival with amplification of the HER-2/neu oncogene. *Science.* 1987;235:177–182.
42. Romond EH, Perez EA, Bryant J, et al. Trastuzumab plus adjuvant chemotherapy for operable HER2-positive breast cancer. *N Engl J Med.* 2005;353:1673–1684.
43. Geyer CE, Forster J, Lindquist D, et al. Lapatinib plus capecitabine for HER2-positive advanced breast cancer. *N Engl J Med.* 2006;355:2733–2743.
45. Hennessy BT, Smith DL, Ram PT, Lu Y, Mills GB. Exploiting the PI3K/AKT pathway for cancer drug discovery. *Nat Rev Drug Disc.* 2005;4:988–1004.
46. Nagata Y, Lan KH, Zhou X, et al. PTEN activation contributes to tumor inhibition by trastuzumab, and loss of PTEN predicts trastuzumab resistance in patients. *Cancer Cell.* 2004;6:117–127.
47. Berns K, Horlings HM, Hennessy BT, et al. A functional genetic approach identifies the PI3K pathway as a major determinant of Trastuzumab resistance in breast cancer. *Cancer Cell.* 2007;12:395–402.
49. Lu Y, Zi X, Zhao Y, et al. Insulin-like growth factor-I receptor signaling and resistance to trastuzumab (Herceptin). *J Natl Cancer Inst.* 2001;93:1852–1857.
50. KrisMG, Natale RB, Herbst RS, et al. Efficacy of gefitinib, an inhibitor of the epidermal growth factor receptor tyrosine kinase, in symptomatic patients with non-small cell lung cancer: a randomized trial. *JAMA.* 2003;290:2149–2158.
52. PaezJG, Janne PA, LeeJC, et al. EGFR mutations in lung cancer: correlation with clinical response to gefitinib therapy. *Science.* 2004;304:1497–1500.
53. LynchTJ, Bell DW, Sordella R, et al. Activating mutations in the epidermal growth factor receptor underlying responsiveness of non-small-cell lung cancer to gefitinib. *N Engl J Med.* 2004;350:2129–2139.
54. Engelman JA, Janne PA. Mechanisms of acquired resistance to epidermal growth factor receptor tyrosine kinase inhibitors in non small cell lung cancer. *Clin Cancer Res.* 2008;14:2895–2899.
56. Olaussen KA, Dunant A, Fouret P, et al. DNA repair by ERCC1 in non-small-cell lung cancer and cisplatin-based adjuvant hemotherapy. *N Engl J Med.* 2006;355:983–991.
59. McLaughlin P, Grillo-López AJ, Link BK, et al. Rituximab chimeric anti-CD20 monoclonal antibody therapy for relapsed indolent lymphoma: half of patients re-

spond to a four-dose treatment program. *J Clin Oncol*. 1998;16:2825–2833.

68. Locker GY, Hamilton S, Harris J, et al, for the American Society of Clinical Oncology Tumor Markers Expert Panel. American Society of Clinical Oncology 2006 Update of Recommendations for the Use of Tumor Markers in Gastrointestinal Cancer. *J Clin Oncol*. 2006;24:5313–5327.
72. Rouzier R, Rajan R, Wagner P, et al. Microtubule-associated protein tau: a marker of paclitaxel sensitivity in breast cancer. *Proc Natl Acad Sci USA*. 2005;102:8315–8320.
73. Chang JC, Wooten EC, Tsimelzon A, et al. Gene expression profiling for the prediction of therapeutic response to docetaxel in patients with breast cancer. *Lancet*. 2003;362:362–369.
75. Ayers M, Symmans WF, Stec J, et al. Gene expression profiles predict complete pathologic response to neoadjuvant paclitaxel and fluorouracil, doxorubicin, and cyclophosphamide chemotherapy in breast cancer. *J Clin Oncol*. 2004;22:2284–2293.
76. Bild AH, Yao G, Chang JT, et al. Oncogenic pathway signatures in human cancers as a guide to targeted therapies. *Nature*. 2006;439:353–357.
79. Rhodes DR, Yu J, Shanker K, et al. Large-scale meta-analysis of cancer microarray data identifies common transcriptional profiles of neoplastic transformation and progression. *Proc Natl Acad Sci USA*. 2004;101:9309–9314.
82. Tibes R, Qiu Y, Lu Y, et al. Reverse phase protein array (RPPA): validation of a novel proteomic technology and utility for analysis of primary leukemia specimens and hematopoietic stem cells. *Mol Cancer Ther*. 2006;5:2512–2521.
83. Stemke-Hale K, Gonzalez-Angulo AM, Lluch A, et al. An integrative genomic and proteomic analysis of PIK3CA, PTEN, and AKT mutations in breast cancer. *Cancer Res*. 2008;68:6084–6091.
84. Hu J, He X, Baggerly KA, et al. Non-parametric quantification of protein lysate arrays. *Bioinformatics*. 2007;23:1986–1994.
85. Hennessy BT, Lu Y, Poradosu E, et al. Quantified pathway inhibition as a pharmacodynamic marker facilitating optimal targeted therapy dosing: proof of principle with the AKT inhibitor perifosine. *Clin Cancer Res*. 2007;13:7421–7431.
93. Imperiale TF, Ransohoff DF, Itzkowitz SH, et al. Fecal DNA versus fecal occult blood for colorectal-cancer screening in an average-risk population. *N Engl J Med*. 2004;351:2704–2714.
100. Junker K, Fritsch T, Hartmann A, et al. Multicolor fluorescence in situ hybridization (M-FISH) on cells from urine for the detection of bladder cancer. *Cytogenet Genome Res*. 2006;114:279–283.
102. Cristofanilli M, Budd GT, Ellis MJ, et al. Circulating tumor cells, disease progression, and survival in metastatic breast cancer. *N Engl J Med*. 2004;351:781–791.
108. Becker FF, Wang XB, Huang Y, et al. Separation of human breast cancer cells from blood by differential dielectric affinity. *Proc Natl Acad Sci USA*. 1995;92:860–864.
111. Furstenberger G, von Moos R, Lucas R, et al. Circulating endothelial cells and angiogenic serum factors during neoadjuvant chemotherapy of primary breast cancer. *Br J Cancer*. 2006;94:524–531.
113. Houghton J, Stoicov C, Nomura S, et al. Gastric cancer originating from bone marrow-derived cells. *Science*. 2004;306:1568–1571.
114. Linden HM, Stekhova SA, Link JM, et al. Quantitative fluoroestradiol positron emission tomography imaging predicts response to endocrine treatment in breast cancer. *J Clin Oncol*. 2006;24:2793–2799.
118. Paik S, Kim C-y, Song Y-k, Kim W-s. Technology insight: application of molecular techniques to formalin-fixed paraffin-embedded tissues from breast cancer. *Nat Clin Pract Oncol*. 2005;2:246–254.
119. Segal E, Friedman N, Kaminski N, Regev A, Koller D. From signatures to models: understanding cancer using microarrays. *Nat Genetics*. 2005;37(suppl):S38–45.
121. Aebersold R, Anderson L, Caprioli R, et al. Perspective: a program to improve protein biomarker discovery for cancer. *J Proteome Res*. 2005;4:1104–1109.
122. Almeida JS, C Chen, R Gorlitsky, et al. Data integration gets "Sloppy." *Nature Biotech*. 2006;24:1070–1071.
127. Hartwell L, Mankoff D, Paulovich A, Ramsey S, Swisher E. Cancer biomarkers: a systems approach. *Nat Biotechnol*. 2006;24:905–908.

27 Personalized Medicine in Oncology Drug Development

William N. Hait, MD, PhD ▪ Nicholas C. Dracopoli, PhD ▪ Steve Heller, MD ▪ Chris H. Takimoto, MD, PhD

Introduction

Drugs used to treat patients with cancer are highly effective in a limited number of patients and less effective in most. If it were possible to identify those patients who were most responsive to a drug or a combination of drugs, one could "personalize" treatment. It would then be possible to spare those unresponsive patients the toxicities of cancer chemotherapy. Even drugs that are relatively less toxic, such as hormonal therapies for breast or prostate cancer, or agents that block growth-factor receptors or inhibit their tyrosine kinase domains, can produce side effects that for many other chronic illnesses would not be acceptable.

Therefore, it is anticipated that the tools of modern cancer biology and pharmacology, when properly applied, will be able to identify "responders" and treat these patients while sparing the others. In fact, several well-known examples exist. For example, hormonal therapy for breast cancer such as tamoxifen or aromatase inhibitors are effective in ~60% of patients whose cancer express estrogen and progesterone receptors, but virtually ineffective in those who do not. As breast cancers express hormone receptors in ~50% of patients, treating a non-selected population would lead to an apparent response rate of 30%. In contrast, by treating only ER/PR-positive patients, the apparent response rate would double. A similar analysis carried out for trastuzumab would be as follows: Approximately 30% of patients' breast cancers express HER-2/neu and of those patients who are "Her-2 positive" approximately 30% respond to trastuzumab. Therefore, if trastuzumab were used to treat an unselected population of patients, the apparent response rate would be 9%. In contrast, if only HER-2/neu-positive patients are treated, the observed response rate is three times greater. Unfortunately, for most other patients with solid tumors, and most liquid tumors with the exception of chronic myeloid leukemia (CML), there is no similarly predictive biomarker. For example, the epidermal growth factor receptor (EGFR) is expressed to some degree in most carcinomas, and even the overexpression of the receptor has limited predictive value for drugs that target EGFR including cetuximab, panitumumab, gefitinib, erlotinib and lapatinib. Nonetheless, several important lessons can be learned from the limited examples where predictive biomarkers exist. First, in both cases the ability to predict response relates to the predictive biomarker also being the target for the drug; the same is true for BCR-ABL and imatinib. In contrast, the presence of most targets has little or no predictive utility. For example, our most active chemotherapeutics target DNA or microtubules. These structures are present in every cancer cell and therefore cannot distinguish responders from non-responders. In contrast, drugs that target the enzymes of DNA synthesis such as thymidylate synthase (fluoropyrimidines),[1] and dihydrofolate reductase (methotrexate, pemetrexed)[2,3] have targets whose expression are predictive of response, but are rarely used.

In general, it has been far easier to identify factors that predict non-responsiveness than it is to predict response to therapy. For example, Kirby-Bauer type drug-sensitivity assays, where a patient's cancer cells grown in tissue culture are screened against a panel of drugs, have a far greater ability to identify drug resistance than drug sensitivity, ie, they rarely tell you what drug the patient would respond to.[4] Recent attention has turned to transcriptional profiling using either microarray or quantitative PCR techniques. In the former, a gene expression pattern is identified for responders that are different from the non-responders. This profile is then prospectively applied to a validation set of samples to determine the predictive value, sensitivity, and specificity of the test. Of the profiles in clinical use, such as Oncotype Dx (Genomic Health, Redwood City, California),[5] MammaPrint (Agendia BV, Amsterdam, Netherlands),[6] and H/I (AvariaDX, Carlsbad, California),[7] these tests are better in identifying the patients unlikely to benefit from treatment than the potential responders. Therefore, in the face of limited success to date, it may be valuable to step back and revisit the principles of pharmacology that determine a drug's efficacy. First, the target must be present in the target tissue. Second, the drug must reach the target at sufficient concentration of the active moiety to produce the expected effect. Third, the drug:target interaction must not be short-circuited by drug resistance mechanisms.

It may also be useful to conceptualize the ideal predictive biomarker as we enter into this new frontier. First, the biomarker should predict with high sensitivity (the percentage of true positives of all positive cases in the population) and specificity (the percentage of true negative of all negative cases in the population) for a meaningful response to treatment. In this setting, the test should have high *positive predictive value* (PPV), defined as the percentage of patients

$$\text{PPV} = \frac{\text{Number of true positives (responders)}}{\text{Number of true positives} + \text{Number of false positives}}$$

with a positive test result who respond to the treatment.

For example, the positive predictive value of having a positive test for Her-2/neu overexpression is 9/9 + 21 = 0.30, assuming 30% of patients have a positive test for HER-2/Neu, and 30% of these 30% respond (9% true positives for response) to trastuzumab.

The relationship of predictive to prognostic biomarkers is also of practical importance. Demonstrating the true benefit of a drug may be easier if the predictive biomarker is also an indicator of poor prognosis. For example, overexpression of HER-2/neu not only predicts response to trastuzumab but also is a predictor of a poor prognosis. Thus, in a clinical study where overall survival is the end point, patients in the control arm will have a poor prognosis, shortened survival and this would allow more rapid completion of the clinical trial and higher likelihood that progression-free survival at an early time point would reveal a true difference between treated and control arms. In contrast, problems can arise if the predictive biomarker is an indicator of a good prognosis. For example, activating mutations in the EFGR catalytic domain predict for response to gefitinib [8,9] yet because these mutations unexpectedly turned out to be good prognostic markers,[10] clinical trials enriched for patients whose tumors harbored this biomarker would have to be powered appropriately if overall survival was the agreed upon end point. If PFS was the end point of the trial one might observe no difference between treatment and controls if the analysis was carried out early.

Finally, within our current armamentarium, we may not have drugs or combination of drugs that will be effective even when properly applied to the majority of cancer patients. If this continues to be the case, how will we treat patients who show a predictive profile for nothing? Of course, we would like to offer these individuals clinical trials, but this may be unsatisfying for many individuals. In this case, we would enter into a discussion of risk, ie, if your chances of responding were only 10%, would you want to be treated; what if it were 5% or 1%? Should a drug be offered to a patient whose chance of benefit is this low, ie, treating 95-99% of patients to benefit 1-5%. Furthermore, as most current therapies have significant side effects, are non-curative and often produce remissions lasting a few months, it does not seem like the proper thing to do; even if we could afford to do it.

Additional concerns have been raised over the commercial viability of segmenting the population based on genotypic or phenotypic profiles. It has been argued that the this approach could limit the utility and therefore market value for a drug to so few or so little, that it would not be economically feasible for the medication to be developed. If so, who will develop these medications for this small number of patients with life threatening diseases; all difficult questions for a modern society.

Thus, personalized medicine is a far more complex proposition than merely getting the right drug to the right patient at the right time. In this chapter, we will try to uncover some of the key issues that will help us move toward this idealized state of future medicine.

Biomarkers in Drug Development

A biomarker is a characteristic that is objectively measured and evaluated as an indicator of normal biologic or pathogenic processes or pharmacological responses to a therapeutic intervention. Biomarkers can be classified into several types as shown in Table 27-1. These include predictive, prognostic and surrogate end points. In this section we focus on predictive markers, which are used to identify patients within a population who have a higher probability of responding to treatment than the population in entirety. The development and validation of these markers are constrained by the limited numbers of individuals exposed to effective doses of the experimental compounds and the short timelines required to have an impact on the commercialization of a new product. The symbiotic development of molecular profiling technologies and completion of the human genome sequence and, most recently, the human haplotype map (HapMap), created new opportunities for the comprehensive discovery of markers to help predict drug efficacy or reduce risk of drug toxicity. Although these approaches are beginning to have an impact on drug development, most current examples still date to the pre-genomic era.

Table 27-1 ■ Classification of Biomarkers

Type	Definition	Example
Predictive	Identifies patients most likely to respond or least likely to experience toxicity	Her-2/neu; estrogen receptor
Pharmacodynamic	Determine whether a drug hits the target and has the expected impact on the biological pathway Evaluate mechanism of action	Phosphorylated targets of tyrosine kinases
Prognostic	Predicts course of disease independent of any specific treatment modality	Approved tests (eg, CellSearch, Mammaprints)
Surrogate	Approved registration end point	Commercial diagnostic tests (eg, LDL, HbA1c, viral load, blood pressure)

Novel biomarkers and disease genes share many parallels in their applications in clinical development and target discovery and validation. Both emerged in the pre-genomic era, and began by biological analysis of small numbers of candidate genes that led to the discovery of genes with large effect sizes for monogenic conditions such as cystic fibrosis,[11] and Huntington disease,[12] and drug metabolizing genes such as the cytochrome P450s[13,14] and thiopurine methyl transferase (TPMT).[15] In these studies, variants in individual candidate genes were associated with different drug metabolizing phenotypes, and these associations were subsequently confirmed by exhaustive biological analyses.

Over the past 25 years, increasingly comprehensive tools and genetic maps were developed to discover novel genes for multigenic diseases and other complex conditions. This era began in the early 1980s with the development of restriction fragment length polymorphism (RFLP) maps that covered the entire human genome.[16] Despite their utility, RFLP maps were rapidly replaced by more informative microsatellite maps in the late 1980s,[17,18] which were in turn replaced by comprehensive single nucleotide polymorphism (SNP) maps.[19,20] Genetic maps and tools for linkage analyses were refined again in 2005 with the publication of the first generation HapMap.[21] These tools, while still evolving, now provide clinical investigators a foundation upon which the human genome can be probed for genetic association with various phenotypes of interest, including identification of disease and drug response markers.

Drug development provides some unique challenges for these methods because few patients have are exposed to new drugs in the development process. In phase 1 single and multiple ascending dose studies, many subjects are exposed to a sub-therapeutic dose of the experimental drug or placebo control. Phase 2a studies provide the first opportunity to search for associations in groups of subjects exposed to an effective dose; these associations can subsequently be validated in larger phase 2b and 3 studies. The timing of when patient samples from clinical studies become available for exploratory research further complicate biomarker identification for a new drug. Molecular profiling studies often begin after the clinical trial has been designed and initiated. This temporal misalignment creates a situation in which the marker discovery lags behind the clinical studies, thereby limiting the potential impact of molecular profiling technologies on the overall drug discovery process.

Molecular Profiling

Molecular profiling methods fall into two basic categories: genomic markers and dynamic markers. Genomic markers are stable within a single subject and can be screened in a single sample from a patient enrolled in a clinical study. In contrast, epigenetic changes to DNA, mRNA, and protein levels are dynamic and must be measured multiple times in each patient during a clinical study to determine baseline levels and subsequent changes determined by disease progression, drug response, or other variables.

The Human Genome ■ The completion of the draft human genome in 2001[22,23] was only the first step in developing a comprehensive map of human variation that is necessary to associate individual genetic changes to disease and drug response phenotypes. The subsequent publication of the HapMap[21] was a major step in this direction. The haplotype map was developed by using the genome sequence as a template to discover millions of SNPs and analysis of the distribution of >1 million SNPs in 269 DNA samples from three different human populations (African, Caucasian, East Asian). Analysis of the patterns of SNPs across the genome identified discrete blocks of linkage disequilibrium, the situation in which some genetic markers occur more or less frequently in a population than expected frequencies. That is to say that the genome consists of blocks with little genetic recombination interspersed by regions of higher recombination. The identification of these blocks has a profound impact on strategies for genetic analyses because it is possible to utilize "tagged SNPs" for each of the blocks and identify a SNP or SNPs that represent almost all the genetic variation in a single block. This permits the creation of a comprehensive reference set of "tagged SNPs" that will allow more efficient screening of the human genome. At this time, it appears that sets of 300,000 to 500,000 SNPs[21] will be able to capture almost all the variation in the human genome. Before completion of the haplotype map, the same task required approximately 1,500,000 unselected SNPs.[19] Thus, for the first time, the haplotype map, combined with improved high-throughput methods of SNP genotyping, provide a means of efficiently, if not yet inexpensively, screening the entire human genome.

Although the haplotype map and the concomitant genotyping methodologies are significant advances, will they allow us to identify genes with low biological effect size? To date, we have been disappointed by the promise of genomic technologies to revolutionize the way in which drugs are discovered. With few exceptions, and despite significant effort, we have failed to identify complex disease genes for almost two decades using the successive waves of RFLPs, microsatellite, and SNP maps. In retrospect, we now understand the major limitations of these previous approaches, and can be more confident that the comprehensive haplotype map addresses many of these issues.

However, the haplotype map introduces new uncertainties that will need to be resolved. It will be necessary to answer questions relating to the sample sizes required for association studies to address the large multiple testing issue, especially for developing multiple SNP profiles, and for analytical methods that minimize over fitting of data to limited clinical trial sample sizes. Recent genome-wide association studies found that both novel and known genes (eg, FGFR2) of modest effect size are associated with genetic susceptibility to breast cancer.[24,25] These results demonstrate that large collaborative studies are able to collate samples sets of sufficient size to detect novel genes that may account for a significant portion of common disease predisposition and may underlie differential response to drug treatment.

The development of novel, highly parallel sequencing technology platforms has made it possible to not only screen for previously characterized SNPs, but also to begin to profile human tumors for de novo mutations. Recent sequence profiles of >20,000 transcripts from breast and colorectal cancers[26,27] have provided the first comprehensive view of somatic mutations occurring in human cancer. These studies showed that there were about 10-15 mutations in each tumor responsible for the initiation, progression, or maintenance of each tumor.[27] However, the profile of mutations between tumors varied greatly and only a very few genes (*KRAS, PTEN, PIK3CA*, etc.) were mutated frequently, and a much larger set of genes had less frequent mutations. Consequently, in addition to germline SNP analyses and transcriptional profiling, comprehensive mutation screening in human tumors will be essential to identify "addictive" pathways for the selection of individualized therapies in the future.

The Human Transcriptome ■ Gene expression profiling is the most advanced of the comprehensive molecular profiling technologies. Unlike the haplotype map, it was possible to create growing lists of human genes from large expressed sequence tag (EST) libraries[28] and the partially completed genomic sequence before the completion of the human sequence in 2003. These data were used to develop cDNA arrays and ordered oligonucleotide arrays that can be used to determine relative expression levels of increasingly larger representations of the human transcriptome. For several years, it has been possible to screen almost all known human transcripts using commercially available arrays from several companies. These technologies have been readily available to many investigators. Consequently, expression arrays have been the most widely used tool for scanning dynamic markers because of their comprehensive coverage and relative cost-effectiveness.

Expression profiling has been particularly useful in oncology because it provides a means of visualizing the impact of molecular changes occurring in the tumor, and because of the availability of banked tumor samples for molecular analyses. Although human cancers appear to emerge through events in a small number of key regulatory pathways,[29] it is not possible to detect the underlying genomic (amplifications, deletions, rearrangements and mutations) and epigenomic (methylation, acetylation, etc.) changes occurring in any one tumor with a single technology. Consequently, expression profiling provides a single means of identifying the downstream effect of these molecular events. If changes at any point in any of these key regulatory pathways (eg, apoptosis, cell cycle control) have similar biological effects, then it is likely that global profiling may identify common transcription patterns that could be associated with different disease outcomes and response to therapy.[30,31]

The Human Proteome ■ Biological samples contain complex mixtures of proteins that are more difficult to measure than changes in gene expression. Consequently, protein profiling is less advanced than gene expression profiling for comprehensive analyses of biological samples. Although derived from less than 30,000 genes, alternative splicing and post-translation modifications combine to generate more than 100,000 different proteins.[32] Initially, two-dimensional gel electrophoresis was used to generate profiles of several hundred highly expressed proteins.[33] More recently, combination of a variety chromatographic methods and mass spectrometry has been utilized to generate spectra derived from thousands of proteins from biological samples.[32] Although this is a significant advance, the sensitivity of current proteomic methods is still too low to detect many biologically active proteins such as the cytokines and other signaling proteins.[34]

Plasma protein profiling provides an indirect measure of disease state or drug response through analysis of the plasma proteome. Unlike RNA expression profiling, which requires samples of nucleated cells, protein profiling can be used to screen proteins in plasma[34] as well as enucleated cells such as platelets.[35] The plasma proteome has, consequently, become the object of much interest and provides unique opportunities for biomarker discovery in diseases that, unlike cancer, are not amenable to pretreatment biopsies. The plasma proteome, however, offers some unique challenges because of the vast dynamic range of protein levels (approximately 10^{10} from albumin to the interleukins), the complexity of the sample (several thousand proteins), and the massive dilution of any leaked or secreted protein from a localized disease or inflammatory response into approximately 2.5 L of adult human plasma. Despite these difficulties, the plasma proteome offers a complementary approach to expression profiling and provides a synergistic approach to genetic analyses for the discovery of novel biomarkers.

Proteomic profiling techniques are used to compare plasma from cancer patients and normal controls to search for markers of early stage disease. This could be used to detect lesions before the onset of symptomatic disease and permit excision of the localized tumor before the development of distant metastases. For example, conventional therapy of stage I ovarian cancer (localized within the ovary) has a 95% 5-year survival rate, compared to <40% for more advanced ovarian cancers that have already disseminated at the time of diagnosis.[36] Early experiments using SELDI-TOF mass spectrometry identified patterns of peptides that distinguished between plasma derived from patients with ovarian cancer and normal controls.[36,37] Subsequent validation studies have suggested that these ovarian cancer profiles may have been artifacts,[38] but numerous other proteomic studies have suggested the plasma may contain secreted proteins derived from the tumor or from the host response to the malignancy. These studies include the identification of plasma protein profiles to identify patients with early breast[39] and prostate cancers.[40-42] The development of plasma proteomic profiles for early detection of disease would be of enormous benefit. The profiles could be used to identify patients with otherwise undetectable disease and many more cancer patients could be identified while the disease is amenable to surgical excision.[42] In addition, patients at higher risk could also be identified earlier using proteomic profiling and steered toward adjuvant treatment to increase the chance of a successful clinical outcome.

Applications in Drug Development

There are still few examples of genomics being reduced to clinical practice. The best examples all consist of single genes with relatively large effect sizes that effect drug metabolism or transport and can be used to predict safer or more effective doses of a variety of compounds. In contrast, few definitive pharmacogenomic markers have emerged from the spate of molecular profiling studies over the past few years. This is not unexpected as pharmacogenomic analyses cannot move any faster than the clinical development process, but also reflects some of the difficulties of discovering and validating predictive markers during drug development. However, we are beginning to see the first clinical impact from large retrospective studies using molecular profiling strategies to stratify cancer patients and predict risk of disease recurrence. For example, multiplex-quantitative PCR has been used to stratify risk of recurrence in node-negative[5] and locally advanced[43] breast cancer patients. Microarrays have been widely used to define molecular subtypes of many tumor types, and to stratify risk of disease recurrence[6,44] in breast cancer patients. The success of these approaches suggests that their early implementation in drug development may eventually have a similar impact on predicting response for new therapeutics.

Drug Safety

The three examples below all involve adjusting the dose of a drug to achieve maximum efficacy and minimize the risk of adverse events. The *TPMT* and uridine diphosphate-glucuronosyltransferase (*UGT1A1*) genes are involved in drug transport and metabolism and hence involve pharmacokinetic changes. The vitamin K epoxide reductase complex 1 (*VKORC1*) gene is the target of the drug warfarin, and variants in this gene affect the pharmacodynamic response to therapy with this agent.

TPMT ■ *TPMT* catalyzes thiopurine drugs (azathioprine, 6-mercaptopurine, and thioguanine) used for the treatment of a variety of conditions including acute lymphocytic leukemia[45] and several autoimmune diseases.[35] *TPMT* activity is trimodal, with ~90% of individuals having high activity, ~10% with intermediate activity, and <1% having no detectable activity. Three genetic variants in the *TPMT* gene have been shown to account ~90% of the heterozygous or homozygous mutations, leading to the development of tests to predict the risk of acute myelosuppression resulting from standard doses of thiopurine drugs. The known variants in the *TPMT* gene only account for about two thirds of the phenotypic variability of this enzyme in red blood cells.[46] This shows that other genetic and environmental factors regulating the *TPMT* activity are still to be discovered, and that current *TPMT* tests will still have some false-negative results in which wild-type homozygous or heterozygous patients will have a worse response to therapy than predicted by the TPMT test.

UGT1A1 ■ Uridine diphosphate-glucuronosyltransferase (*UGT1A1*) is an example of an early stage application of pharmacogenetics in the clinic. *UGT1A1* controls glucuronidation of bilirubin[47] and regulates the amount of serum bilirubin. Polymorphisms in this gene have been shown to be responsible for Gilbert and Crigler-Najjar syndromes and to be associated with increased risk of severe adverse events (neutropenia and diarrhea) in patients treated with Irinotecan,[47] a topoisomerase 1 inhibitor widely used in the treatment of colorectal cancer. These *UGT1A1* polymorphisms have also been shown to be associated with reversible hyperbilirubinemia after the treatment of HIV patients with the protease inhibitors atazanavir and indinavir.[48,49] The *UGT1A1*28* allele differs from the wild-type allele by the presence of seven, rather than six, dinucleotide repeats.[47] This dinucleotide repeat variant has been shown to cause reduced enzyme activity and to be associated with higher risk of adverse events in patients treated with Irinotecan, as well as hyperbilirubinemia in patients treated with protease inhibitors.

UGT1A1 polymorphisms could be used to minimize grade 4 adverse events in chemotherapy regimens including Irinotecan. A prospective study showed that grade 4 neutropenia could be reduced by 50% by excluding all patients with *UGT1A1*28* homozygotes, and by 100% by excluding all patients with at least one *UGT1A1*28* allele.[50,51] While eliminating severe neutropenia, this would result in withholding therapy from 10% or >50% of the patients, respectively. Consequently, for genetic testing to be useful for Irinotecan, it will be necessary to define different doses for UGT1A1*28 heterozygotes and homozygotes in order to define a therapeutic window that would allow all colorectal cancer patients to benefit from therapy, rather than just excluding patients at elevated risks of the adverse events from a therapy from which they could otherwise benefit.

VKORC1 ■ Polymorphisms in the VKORC1 have been shown to affect individual response to warfarin.[52] In contrast to the previous two examples that describe pharmacokinetic effects of drug metabolism or transport genes, the *VKORC1* variants result in pharmacodynamic differences in response to warfarin therapy. Analysis of five haplotypes in this gene showed that patients can be separated into high, intermediate, and low responders, and that these groups are, in turn, correlated with *VKORC1* expression levels. The *VKORC1* haplotypes account for ~25% of the variance in warfarin maintenance dose among the three responder groups. In addition, *CYP2C9* polymorphisms account for ~8% of the variance,[52] demonstrating that the pharmacodynamic effect of differential *VKORC1* transcription levels is about three times that of the pharmacokinetic effect of *CYP2C9* polymorphisms. These data suggest that a genetic test could be developed that accounts for approximately one-third of the variability in warfarin maintenance dose, and that this test could be beneficial in reducing initial dose for patients homozygous for the *VKORC1 A/A* haplotype.

Drug Efficacy

Targeted therapies offer some the best examples of how pharmacogenomics is applied to current clinical practice. A targeted therapy is one that is directed at interrupting a known mechanism of action in a specific target. These include therapies that require a clinical test to determine the presence of a specific abnormality in a subset of patients, as well as therapies against abnormalities that occur in almost all cases of the indication and do not require a test after the initial diagnosis.

HER2 ■ The human epidermal growth factor receptor 2 (HER2) is the first and best example of clinical pharmacogenomics. Trastuzumab is a monoclonal antibody against the HER2 antigen expressed in approximately 30% of breast cancers.[53] Trastuzumab was initially developed for advanced breast cancers with either amplified *HER2* gene detected by fluorescent in situ hybridization (FISH) or over expressed HER2 protein detected by immunohistochemistry. Tumors with high expression of HER2 are less differentiated and have increased risk of recurrence and death. Treatment with trastuzumab as a single agent resulted in response rates in HER2-positive patients of ~30%. Recently, three independent clinical studies have shown that the benefits of trastuzumab are applicable to early stage breast cancer patients as well.[54,55] These studies showed that the addition of trastuzumab to standard adjuvant cytotoxic therapy, or use of trastuzumab for 1 year after the completion of adjuvant therapy, showed significantly increased disease-free survival in HER2-positive patients. These studies confirm a new paradigm for oncology drug development and most, if not all, targeted oncology compounds are likely to follow similar developmental pathways.

EGFR ■ The EGFR is a member of the same family of tyrosine kinase inhibitors as HER2[56] and is the target for the monoclonal antibody (cetuximab) and small molecule kinase inhibitors (gefitinib and erlotinib) for use in second line treatment of colorectal and non-small cell lung cancers, respectively.[57] Cetuximab is approved for the treatment of EGFR-positive metastatic colorectal cancer in combination with Irinotecan. Response rates to these therapies are typically between 10% and 15% in Caucasian patients, but response to gefitinib has been shown to be twofold to threefold higher in a select subset of patients with non-small cell lung cancer. Typically, the responsive patients have significant clinical benefit, whereas the majority of patients seem to derive little or no benefit from these therapies. This is almost the perfect case for the development of predictive markers to guide use of agents targeted at EGFR because of this bimodal distribution of response.

The recent discovery of activating mutations in the tyrosine kinase domain of EGFR in non-small cell lung cancer patients[8,9,58] provides a proof of principle for the utility of pharmacogenomic tests. These studies identified mutations or small deletions in the majority of responsive patients, suggesting that these tumors were dependent on constitutive EGFR signaling, and that interruption of this signaling cascade was an effective treatment option for this subset of patients. However, the situation became more complex after the observation that increase in EGFR gene copy number in some non-small cell lung cancers was associated with response to erlotinib.[59] It would not be possible to utilize the activating mutations alone as the predictive marker, since utilization of just the activating mutations as a predictive marker would lead to a number of false negatives.

Surprisingly, the situation in colorectal cancer turned out to be quite different. Relatively large surveys of responding and non-responding tumors did not reveal activating mutations in the tyrosine kinase domain of EGFR.[60] Although the response to cetuximab in some colorectal cancer patients suggests that a subset of these tumors are also dependent on EGFR signaling, this response is evidently not driven by activating mutations in the EGFR kinase domain. More recently, the expression of the EGFR ligands, amphiregulin, and epiregulin, have been shown to be associated with response to cetuximab in colorectal cancer,[61] suggesting that an autocrine stimulation loop may be present in those colorectal cancers that are "addicted" to EGFR signaling.

Tubulin ■ Microtubules are heterodimers consisting of α- and β-tubulins. Agents such as paclitaxel and taxotere are widely used cytotoxic therapies that work by stabilizing tubulin polymerization and inhibiting cell division. Early work revealed that mutations in *p53* could lead to altered sensitivity to antimicrotubule drugs through upregulation of microtubule-associated proteins.[62] Subsequent molecular profiling of breast cancer biopsies revealed expression profiles predictive of response to combination therapies including paclitaxel.[63,64] Later analyses confirmed these data and showed how the levels of another microtubule-binding protein, MAP Tau, are associated with the response to paclitaxel in breast cancer. These observations led to the development of a satisfying model suggesting competition of MAP Tau and paclitaxel during microtubule assembly, and that the tubulin stabilization therapies might be most effective in tumors with low levels of MAP Tau.[65] Subsequent studies of ixabepilone, a newer tubulin polymerizing agent that also binds to β-tubulin, have confirmed these results and shown that MAP-Tau expression is highly correlated with the estrogen receptor (ER) expression and can be used to identify ER and MAP Tau negative subsets of breast cancer patients with a twofold increase in response to single agent ixabepilone in the neoadjuvant setting.[66]

BCR-ABL ■ Chronic myeloid leukemia (CML) arises after the fusion of the BCR and ABL genes to form a constitutively activated tyrosine kinase fusion protein BCR-ABL.[67] Resistance to imatinab, a potent inhibitor of the BCR-ABL tyrosine kinase, is caused by mutations in the ATP-binding site of the ABL kinase. Recently, development of a second generation BCR-ABL kinase inhibitor, dasatanib (or BMS-354825), has shown activity against 14 of 15 imatinab-resistant mutations.[68] Only the T315I mutation was resistant to both imatinab and dasatanib. These data suggest the possibility of developing pharmacogenomic tests for mutations in the BCR-ABL tyrosine kinase to be used in patients developing resistance to imatinab therapy. Consequently, it may be possible to use pharmacogenomic analyses to both select first line therapies (as described for EGFR activating mutations above) as well as selecting second-line therapies for patients developing resistance to an ongoing treatment.

Translational Research and Drug Development

In a recent review, Lawrence Lesko of the U.S. Food and Drug Administration (FDA) highlighted the importance of personalized medicine to the Critical Path Initiative, which is designed to accelerate the development of novel medical therapies.[69] There is little doubt that the future will see the growth of personalized medical therapies in every day medical practice. However, before this approach can gain widespread acceptance, the role of personalized therapy will have to be developed, tested, and validated in clinical trials. Numerous reviews have emphasized how biomarkers, molecular profiling, and individualized therapies are changing the drug development landscape.[70,71] However, there are only a few illustrative examples of well-designed, development plans for molecularly targeted therapies[72-74] In this section, we will highlight how the integration of biomarkers and personalized medical therapy through translational research can optimize the testing of new medical therapies and how these changes are creating new paradigms for cancer drug development.

Translational research in oncology therapeutics can be defined as the integration of predictive, prognostic, and pharmacodynamic biomarkers into the drug development plan using scientific concepts and hypothesis-testing clinical trials to optimize the validation of new therapies. Inherent in this change is the prima facie acknowledgment that developing modestly effective blockbuster drugs for all patients with a common general diagnosis using a "one-drug-fits-all" mentality is not a tenable long-term strategy.[75] Instead, testing individualized, highly effective targeted therapies in well-defined, molecularly characterized subgroups of patients, the so-called niche buster approach,[76] may be a more sustainable model for therapeutic pipelines of the future.

Our classical approach to oncology drug development needs updating. Traditionally, preclinical efficacy and toxicity studies in animal models are followed by a first-in-human phase 1 dose-escalation study designed to define an agent's toxicities, pharmacokinetics, and maximum tolerated dose (MTD).[77] Next, single arm phase 2 studies are performed at the MTD in patients with a uniform disease diagnosis to screen for antitumor activity, typically assessed by tumor shrinkage. Finally, large placebo-controlled, randomized phase 3 studies attempt to quantify the magnitude of benefit of the experimental agent over existing treatment options, and if positive, provide the basis for drug registration. However, this rigid structure may not be well suited to the modern era, and may account, at least in part, for the large number of late failures in phase 3 oncology trials.[78,79]

But what are the alternatives? Workman has proposed a series of conceptual goals, called the pharmacological audit trail, which is designed to guide the development of a new, targeted therapy through the early stages of clinical development.[80] The components of pharmacological audit trail link essential parameters of drug pharmacology to desired clinical effects (Fig. 27-1). It represents a practical effort to define the relationship between molecular target status, pharmacokinetics, pharmacodynamics, subsequent biological changes, and ultimately, clinical outcomes. The pharmacological audit trail begins during preclinical testing immediately after a potential therapeutic agent is discovered and extends to first-in-human trials through to the demonstration of proof-of-concept and clinical activity. These questions are addressed in the clinical development space historically occupied by phase 1 and early phase 2 clinical trials. The overall purpose of the pharmacological audit trail is to improve the quality of decision making at these early stages of the drug development process.

Selecting the Right Drug

Personalized medicine is challenging us to determine "the right drug for the right patient at the right dose and time" for any specific cancer therapeutic target.[75] Selecting the right drug for clinical development requires the identification of a validated therapeutic target and the discovery of an appropriate agent that modulates this target. A detailed description of non-clinical drug development is beyond the scope of this discussion,[81] but one of the key deliverables required early in preclinical testing is the characterization of the mechanistic pharmacology of a novel therapeutic. This includes the demonstration that the drug hits its putative target, thereby modulating downstream biological processes, ultimately resulting in antitumor efficacy in model systems. Typically, oncology efficacy studies are conducted in human tumor cell lines grown in vitro and in human tumor in vivo xenograft models. The expression of the molecular target within and between various tumor types and in normal tissues should be characterized at this stage of testing. This information can guide strategic planning for future clinical studies. Finally, a drug must demonstrate appropriate pharmacological characteristics such as adequate formulation properties and viable animal pharmacokinetics, and it must pass animal safety pharmacology and toxicology studies before advancing into first-in-human trials.

Predictive biomarker discovery is the cornerstone of personalized medicine and optimal success is dependent on the discovery of biomarker assays that are simple, sensitive, and readily applied to clinical specimens. Assays such as analysis of circulating tumor cells, plasma protein profiles, or IHC performed on formalin-fixed, paraffin-embedded tumor tissues are more advantageous than tests that require fresh tumor biopsies. During preclinical development, putative predictive biomarkers can be analyzed in a series of human tumor cell lines, in fresh or in banked human specimens before prospective clinical testing. This early investment in assay method development is essential if a biomarker is to be developed simultaneously with a therapeutic agent entering clinical trials.

Robust pharmacodynamic biomarker assays related to drug mechanisms of action are also important during preclinical development. In vivo efficacy experiments can define how drug-induced biomarker changes relate to antitumor efficacy end points such as growth inhibition, apoptosis, or tumor shrinkage. Technical issues related to biomarker assay implementation, tissue collection, processing, storage, and assay reproducibility should also be characterized to the fullest extent possible. Rigorous evaluation of putative biomarker assays is important for testing clinical hypotheses: does the agent modulate the therapeutic target and does this modulation correlate with desired outcomes? The tools essential for evaluating these key issues in early drug development must be forged at the preclinical stage.

Ultimately, these laboratory tests provide the reference database for the clinical evaluation of a novel targeted agent. Specific critical performance criteria derived from preclinical studies can provide

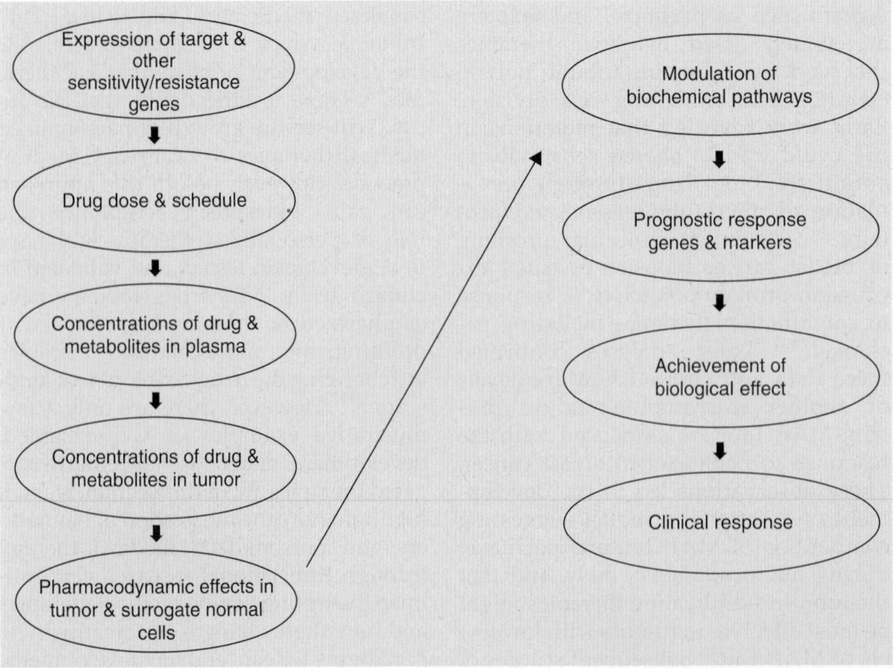

Figure 27-1 The pharmacological audit trail. *Source*: Adapted with permission from the American Association for Cancer Research from Workman, Paul. Auditing the pharmacological accounts for Hsp90 molecular chapterone inhibitors: unfolding the relationship between pharmacokinetics and pharmacodynamics. Mol Cancer Ther. 2003;2(2):131-138, Fig. 1, p. 132.

benchmarks for the evaluation of a drug's pharmacokinetic and pharmacodynamic behavior. Frequently, these benchmarks can be assessed in first-in-human studies. For example, if the minimal threshold plasma drug concentrations or tumor tissue exposures required for drug activity in preclinical animal models are not achieved in clinical studies, then a serious problem is identified. Pharmacodynamic benchmarks can also be evaluated in early clinical trials. If 80% or greater inhibition of a key signaling pathway in human tumor xenografts is required for tumor growth inhibition in nude mice, then this level of targeted inhibition might serve as a critical performance criterion for clinical studies. If maximal pathway inhibition in patient's tumors is 50% or less and there is no other evidence of antitumor efficacy in a clinical trial, then the further development of the targeted agent must be questioned. Alternatively, if this benchmark is achieved or surpassed in the clinical study, the biomarker assay could be used to explore a minimal effective biological dose. For a biomarker end point to be sufficient to guide major drug development decisions, it must be evaluated rigorously before initiating clinical trials.[70,80]

Recently, the FDA has proposed the exploratory IND mechanisms for early clinical testing of novel agents as part of the critical path initiative.[82] These exploratory IND trials, also referred to as phase 0 studies, are of limited duration and, by definition, cannot have therapeutic intent. Specific examples of exploratory IND trials include microdose pharmacokinetic studies, assessments of drug target modulation, or measurement of an agent's pharmacological effect after a single or limited number of repeat doses. In some phase 0 trials, testing of a pharmacodynamic biomarker may be the primary clinical end point. Although a phase 0 trial may move a novel agent into the clinic more rapidly than through a traditional IND mechanism, it does not obviate the need to conduct a traditional phase 1 dose escalation study to determine toxicity. Thus, it may represent more of a drug discovery tool than a development tool by efficiently weeding out undesirable candidates early in the developmental timeline. At present, only a few targeted cancer therapies have been studied in a phase 0 trial,[83] however, the early entry of agents into clinical testing may yield valuable information for some classes of novel agents.

Selecting the Right Dose and Schedule

Once a drug enters first-in-human testing, a careful review of a drug's pharmacokinetic and on-target pharmacodynamic behavior is required (Fig. 27-1). Specific questions to be examined include whether the drug achieves adequate systemic concentrations in the plasma, and at the target site? The systemic delivery question can be addressed by classical pharmacokinetic assessments, although actual tumor drug delivery is difficult to evaluate in the absence of direct analytical measurements performed in tumor tissues. The schedule of drug administration is often extrapolated from preclinical models, but the final dose must be confirmed by the safety and toxicity evaluation in clinical dose escalation trials. Traditionally, classical cytotoxic agents are administered in phase 2 trials at the maximal tolerated dose, based on the simplistic (but easily implemented) principle that more is better. However, for molecularly targeted therapies, it may not be desirable to treat patients at the brink of unacceptable toxicity. Rather, it may be desirable to define the optimal or minimally effective biological dose.

Defining the optimal or minimally effective biological dose for further clinical evaluation of a targeted treatment is not as straightforward as defining the MTD. For example, monoclonal antibodies may not generate dose-limiting toxicities at any practical dose. To assess whether a drug is hitting its target in cancer patients, pharmacodynamic biomarker assays previously tested in preclinical models must be applied in the clinical setting. This requires obtaining tissue specimens from patients enrolled in these early studies. In most solid-tumor phase 1 trials, routine collection of tumor biopsies during treatment is difficult, and investigators are often limited to monitoring surrogate tissues such as peripheral blood mononuclear cells (PBMC) or skin biopsies. These substitutes can determine if an investigational agent is modulating the target during dose escalation, but the relevance to drug effects in tumors is unproven. Less invasive tumor-specific assessments of drug action using functional imaging techniques (eg, PET or dynamic contrast enhanced MRI scans) or monitoring drug effects in circulating tumor cells may provide valuable pharmacodynamic information in early clinical dose escalation studies. However, most of these newer end points lack clinical validation.

As a drug progresses through clinical testing, the need for direct assessments of drug action in tumor tissue becomes extremely important. Clinical research centers that specialize in implementing, collecting, processing, and analyzing tumor biomarker end points will be in high demand. Finally, investigators will have to review all of the pharmacokinetic and pharmacodynamic data collected before making a best estimate of the optimal dose and schedule for further clinical evaluation.

This early analysis of a novel agent's pharmacokinetics, toxicities, and mechanistic pharmacodynamic profile must be carefully considered. Failure of an agent to generate expected drug concentrations or the lack of modulation of the intended target could lead to termination if the previously established critical performance criteria are defined with high levels of certainty.

Ultimately, the relationship between pharmacodynamic biomarker modulation and clinical outcomes must be addressed in a more homogeneous population than is normally studied in a phase 1 oncology trial. A more uniform group of phase 2 patients is required, while still allowing for the procurement of tissues specimens before and during treatment. This population is also the first opportunity to gather meaningful data related to drug-induced biomarker changes and important clinical end points such as tumor response, progression free survival, and overall survival. At this stage, the key hypothesis is whether the modulation of the molecular target produces the desired clinical outcome. A strong association confirmed in larger trials can potentially elevate a pharmacodynamic biomarker to the hallowed status of a surrogate end point.[74] Alternatively, successful target pathway modulation coupled with a failure to observe the desired clinical outcome could call into question the entire therapeutic strategy upon which the treatment is based.

Selecting the Right Patients

The fundamental premise of personalized medicine is that specific subgroups of patients can be selected that will derive optimal benefit from treatment with targeted therapies. Adopting this paradigm makes the discovery of predictive biomarkers associated with drug sensitivity or resistance a paramount goal. If a promising biomarker for drug sensitivity is identified, then further clinical testing might be narrowed to only include marker-positive patients using a target-enrichment strategy, with later testing conducted in general population-wide studies. Alternatively, efficacy evaluation can be initiated in an unselected population, with later clinical studies performed in a molecularly defined subset characterized by a predictive biomarker.[74] The approach selected will depend on the degree of confidence in the predictive biomarker. Either strategy will likely require greater time and resources spent in phase 2 testing to answer these questions. However, the payoff will be much smaller and focused phase 3 trials in a target-enriched population with a higher level of expected efficacy.

Full validation of a predictive biomarker must meet rigorous statistical criteria that are beyond of the scope of what can be achieved in clinical trials performed early in clinical development.[84] Such studies require randomization between marker-based and non-marker-based treatment arms.

The Regulatory Path

The implementation of personalized medicine in oncology depends on the coordinated development of a targeted therapeutic agent with a validated diagnostic test that identifies the optimal treatment population. This need to simultaneously develop a new drug with a companion diagnostic test presents unique challenges for all involved. From a regulatory perspective, this new paradigm raises several complex issues. First is the need to evaluate a predictive diagnostic test while simultaneously assessing the safety and efficacy of an experimental treatment in a coordinated manner. Second, diagnostic test kits are regulated by the FDA's Center for Devices and Radiologic Health, while therapeutics are evaluated by the Center for Drug Evaluation and Research or the Center for Biological Evaluation and Research. Furthermore, the FDA's legal mandate is to regulate therapeutic agents and diagnostic kits, but historically, the agency has refrained from placing major restrictions on physician judgment in the use of these tools in a variety of clinical settings.[85]

Despite these challenges, in personalized medicine drugs and their companion diagnostic tests are closely intertwined, and the safety and efficacy of a specific targeted agent may depend entirely on the coordinated use of a reliable and validated predictive diagnostic test. Industry sponsors have raised concerns about the early submission of pharmacogenomic data before their full validation. Many of the predictive tests relevant to personalized medicine are biomarkers based on pharmacogenomic data. Up to now, it has been unclear how the agency might use these data in the drug application process.

The FDA has responded proactively to these concerns by holding public meetings and workshops to address the challenges of simultaneously developing drugs and diagnostic tests.[86] The agency also released position documents that address these or closely related topics. In March 2005, the FDA issued guidance for industry entitled "Pharmacogenomic Data Submissions,"[87] and in April 2005, it released a draft concept paper on "Drug-Diagnostic Co-Development."[88] The latter paper specifically addressed various "issues related to the development of in vitro diagnostics ... for mandatory use in decision making about drug selection for patients in clinical practice."[88] The principal focus is on pharmacogenomic data used as predictive biomarkers for patient stratification and not on pharmacodynamic response biomarkers. Sponsors are encouraged to share relevant pharmacogenomic data with the agency on a voluntary basis as early as possible, even when such data are exploratory or purely research-based. These data would not be used in the final review of the relevant therapeutic agent. These documents clearly demonstrate the agency's endorsement of personalized medicine and it highlights the FDA's effort to accelerate the implementation of novel technologies into the drug development process.

In their co-development concept paper, the FDA offers specific examples and recommended timelines for the prospective coordinated development of a therapeutic agent with a diagnostic test.[88] This concept paper is designed to generate public discussion in preparation for a future guidance on this subject. It addresses both scientific and logistical issues related to the co-development of a single test in conjunction with a single drug undergoing simultaneous regulatory evaluation. The ultimate goal is to provide comprehensive information for the drug label on the status of the biomarker assay used for patient selection at the time of product approval. Because of the need for careful coordination, close communication between the agency and sponsor beginning at the early preclinical stage of development is recommended.

Key milestones in the co-development of a diagnostic assay include analytical test validation, clinical test validation, and clinical test utility. Analytical test validation is defined as the in vitro ability to quantify accurately the biomarker measurement of interest in well-defined test samples. Assay precision, accuracy, reproducibility, and hardware/software performance are important components of analytical test validation. Clinical test validation depends on the ability of a test to detect or predict the biomarker status of interest in biological specimens obtained from the target patient population. These issues can be evaluated in phase 1 and early phase 2 trials that demonstrate how the assay performs in real world situations. This should provide enough information about the test's operational characteristics to allow for formal testing in rigorously designed phase 2 and 3 trials. Finally, and most importantly, the test's clinical utility is demonstrated by improved clinical outcomes when it is used to select patients for treatment with a specific therapeutic agent. Thus, the implementation of personalized medicine in drug development encompasses scientific, clinical, and regulatory challenges. Despite these complexities, the FDA's position is clear; the rational development of novel therapeutics for specific segments of the population is in the public's best interest. At the behest of FDA, the American Association for Cancer Research convened a meeting of leaders from FDA, academics and industry to help formulate guidelines for predictive biomarker tests. This resulted in the AACR/NCI/FDA Biomarkers Consortium, which is producing a series of white papers that will help guide sponsors in preparing for submission of companion diagnostics.

Market and Economic Impact of Biomarkers

Government, academia, and industry share the view that successful biomarker research and development can lead to new targeted drugs, more productive development, and a realization of personalized medicine. However, biomarker programs are adding cost to the estimated $60 billion[89] that the pharmaceutical industry is investing annually in R&D. Less than one in ten cancer compounds entering phase 1 clinical trials are eventually approved for marketing.[90] Perhaps two to three biomarker targets will be explored early in development for many of these compounds. Most of these are unlikely to bear fruit, ie, they will not become part of clinical decision making, or be developed as a companion diagnostic test. Drug developers are asked to overcome the hurdles facing investigative compounds and in parallel to develop tests to predict which patients will benefit from a given compound.

Advocates of biomarker development need to understand and address the two sides of the equation that impact the sustainability of long-term investment. Biomarker development must improve R&D productivity and biomarker driven regimens must generate sufficient patient and market value. Organizations will need to prioritize biomarker development initiatives for greatest productivity and value. Public and private parties will need to work together to enable policies that support the reality of personalized medicine. This section will focus on selected issues facing private companies investing substantially in biomarker research and development.

Economic Value to R&D

In an era where it can cost more than one billion dollars[91] to bring a drug to market, biomarkers can potentially improve the productivity in R&D. Biomarker research can enhance understanding of risk and reduce reliance on empiricism in development decisions. PK/PD markers and surrogate end points can provide evidence-based rationale for dose and schedule and inform critical decisions in drug development. The ability and willingness to discontinue more compounds before large randomized trials are initiated allows resources and investment to be directed to more promising research.

Biomarker R&D adds cost, and possibly time, early in the drug development process. However, by enriching for likely responders, clinical trials can be powered to demonstrate a strong benefit with a greater probability of success. These benefits can be significant for phase 3 randomized trials that absorb the majority of clinical development budgets.

Consider a randomized phase 3 clinical trial powered to show a 25% benefit in survival over a benchmark survival of 12.5 months with a two-sided alpha *P*-value of 0.05. This trial might require 950 patients at a cost of >$75 million. This same phase 3 trial would be quite different with a biomarker that allowed enrichment for likely responders. If a biomarker identified that 35% of the population included all patients likely to benefit, the phase 3 protocols might then target a 50%, rather than 25%, improvement in survival. This trial would require only 300 patients and could save $50 million.

Biomarkers can also provide mechanistic data to guide the development of drugs that inhibit a new target; ie, first-in-class agents. The study of imatinib in patients with gastrointestinal stromal tumors (GIST) is an example of a drug used to treat a cancer that may have remained an unrecognized opportunity if it were not for the prediction that this drug would be active in tumors driven by the *c-Kit* oncogene. Biomarker supported compounds with single-agent activity also provide a starting point for rationally exploring combinations based on mechanism and biology.

Market Benefits

Predictive biomarkers have the potential to reduce uncertainty in clinical decisions, improve the cost effectiveness of a compound, and in many cases will provide a competitive advantage.

Predictive "class" biomarkers such as ER status and HER2 expression allow for exclusion of breast cancer patients not likely to benefit from drugs that inhibit these targets. This avoids unnecessary cost and toxicity and provides opportunity for alternative treatments. In breast cancer, patients who are ER(–) are not exposed to long-term estrogen modulation and the 70% of patients who are HER2(–) avoid the monthly cost of trastuzumab. As a result, in the United States, anti-estrogens and trastuzumab have earned dominant standard of care market shares in the eligible populations. In contrast, and more representative of the situation with most cancer compounds, a minority of NSCL cancer patients receive erlotinib for second line treatment with no validated biomarker to select either responders or the majority who will not benefit.

Biomarkers also improve the value proposition of compounds and thereby secure broader reimbursement. The value proposition reflects the willingness of doctors, governments and payers to provide access and pay for the benefit of the therapy. Value propositions are stronger when there is greater certainty related to efficacy, toxicity, and cost.

Strong value propositions do not just improve the willingness to pay but also can improve the market position of companies selling biomarker-defined regimens. First, appropriate patients are more easily identified. With uncertainty minimized, biomarker-supported compounds can achieve faster and higher market share. Second, because non-responders have been removed from the population, the average duration of treatment may be extended due to improved efficacy and fewer treatment interruptions. This increases revenue per patient. Finally, drugs with associated biomarkers have a stronger protection of their market position. A biomarker driven regimen has strong potential to become the reference therapy in its indication. Emerging therapies will tend to combine with this reference compound, further strengthening its market position.

Cost/Effectiveness of Biomarker-Driven Regimens

In most countries, cost effectiveness is currently not a dominant criterion for selecting cancer treatment. Many believe this will change as more drug approvals, competition, and budget constraints lead to a greater emphasis on cost as part of selection guidelines. A primary benefit of biomarkers is that they should result in greater cost-effectiveness by removing non-responders from the treatment population.

One surrogate for the cost-effectiveness of drug utilization is quality-adjusted life years (QALYs). With QALYs, the total benefit and harm of a treatment are converted into fractions equivalent to years of life. Incremental cost of the intervention is assessed and assigned a monetary value per QALY.

In the United Kingdom, cost effectiveness is already a criterion for government reimbursement of cancer regimens. The National Institute for Health and Clinical Excellence (NICE) in the United Kingdom uses incremental cost per QALY as one metric against which to determine eligibility for reimbursement. Thirty thousand pounds per QALY for end-stage renal disease patients on dialysis has been a generally accepted threshold for cost effectiveness for non-cancer treatments because it is universally reimbursed in developed countries.

As can be seen in Table 27-2, analysis of selected NICE assessments of cancer drugs reveals that the higher the cost per QALY the more likely is a negative appraisal in the United Kingdom. In this list, trastuzumab represents a compound where the presence of a biomarker has made a significant contribution to cost effectiveness. If trastuzumab were prescribed to a broader, but unselected population, its benefit would be diluted and its cost effectiveness reduced. For several other compounds (imatinib and rituximab) denoted as cost effective clinical use is determined by broader positive target expression—BCR-ABL, KIT, or PDGFr (imatinib) or CD20 (rituximab)—than is the case with HER2 (trastuzumab). Both imatinib and rituximab have demonstrated significant benefit. Even without a biomarker, the relative certainty of benefit and lack of competition creates a situation that supports broad market

Table 27-2 NICE Assessments of Selected Cancer Regimens Where Cost Effectiveness Is Key Factor

Regimen	Issue Date	Indication	QALY[a]	Outcome
Rituximab	September 2006[94]	Advanced Follicular lymphoma	17,000£	Positive
Imatinib	September 2006[95]	CML, chronic phase	26,000£	Positive
Docetaxel	September 2006[96]	Prostate, metastatic	32,700£	Positive
Trastuzumab + paclitaxel	August 2006[97]	Breast, metastatic	33,000£	Positive
Gemcitibine combinations	January 2007[98]	Breast, metastatic	45,800£	Positive
Pemetrexed	June 2006[99]	NSCLC, relapsed	50,000£	Negative
Cetuximab	January 2007[100]	CRC, relapsed	≥77,000£	Negative
Bevacizumab + 5-fluorouracil/ Leucovorin	January 2007[100]	CRC, metastatic	88,000£	Negative

[a] QALY, quality adjusted life years, in British pounds.

access. Biomarkers with strong positive predicative value would likely improve the cost effectiveness of all of the other compounds in the chart and could further support reimbursement by payers and governments.

Stratification and Market Success

Perhaps the most significant concern of manufacturers regarding biomarkers relates to revenue potential in increasingly stratified markets. Does a smaller biomarker-defined patient pool imply lower revenue? Does lower revenue always imply a poorer return on investment? The answer depends on the combined biomarker impact on revenue and R&D productivity.

The hypothetical product "Superlamycin" illustrates how a biomarker could create greater revenue for the manufacturer, even when the total eligible population is reduced. It is based on a basic formula for revenue:

Revenue = Price cycle
× Duration of treatment
× Market share

As shown in Table 27-3, 25 out of 100 patients will benefit from Superlamycin. However, in the second scenario 50% of eligible patients are eliminated from treatment consideration by a biomarker. In this example, the biomarker allows for a greater positive predictive value and stronger value proposition supporting price, a longer average duration of therapy, and a greater market share.

Superlamycin without a biomarker has a clinical benefit in 25% of the population but is prescribed (market share) to only 35% of 100 patients because there are other equally efficacious but uncertain alternatives. Its sales are $700,000.

Adding a biomarker for Superlamycin reduces the eligible population by 50%. The 25 responders remain in the smaller eligible population. This benefit can translate into greater cost effectiveness and a higher price supported by payers ($3000), longer median duration of treatment (15 cycles), and a greater share (70% of 50) of the remaining patients. Despite a smaller eligible population, the increased certainty of benefit leads to an increase in revenue.

In the example above, existing compounds for the treatment of the same disease(s) but without biomarkers would rapidly lose their market share in the biomarker defined segment or would be required to demonstrate benefit in combination with the biomarker-associated drug. Even in situations where net revenue is reduced, the return on investment can be positive where phase 3 costs and/or time to maximum share is reduced.

Some biomarker-defined regimens will not present the combination of value, reimbursement access, and a large enough patient population to create a positive return on investment. However, if markets become stratified by biomarkers, those compounds with the greater certainty of benefit have the greatest opportunity for sustainable market share and revenue, thereby providing the necessary incentive to explore biomarkers in clinical development.

Risks and Key Success Factors

An effective biomarker will not assure market success and may not even offer the best clinical alternative if it does not achieve a strong positive predictive value. Early in development there will be significant uncertainty regarding the eventual clinical and market impact of the biomarker. Developers will need to be rigorous in understanding the potential of their biomarker projects in order to prioritize and gain value from their resources.

In the new world of predictive biomarkers there will be three concurrent critical development paths: the compound, the biomarker, and the diagnostic tool. "Go/no go" decisions will be made for all three programs. To improve probability of success the developer should revisit the goals and feasibility of the program at each stage of development.

Is the Disease Optimal for Biomarker Development? ■ Some questions to consider:

- How will the biomarker improve upon the efficacy and safety benchmarks of emerging and current competing therapies?
- What specifically does the biomarker need to measure?
- Do we understand the epidemiology of the marker? How many patients will need to be screened to select the biomarker subset? If the hypothesized biomarker is expressed in a small proportion of patients, will sizing of clinical trails be feasible?
- Is biomarker testing practical? For example, if a biomarker were being developed for rapidly progressing refractory AML, the acute nature of the medical intervention would require immediate biomarker readouts. Time-delayed analytical reports may not be useful.
- In which indication does a biomarker provide the most value? Biomarker response may vary by pathway alterations in different cancers, leaving a compound with variable positive predictive values and value propositions. From a market perspective, the indication where the biomarker adds the greatest differentiation should be the first to launch.

Do We Understand the Investment and Impact on Timelines? ■ Biomarker programs require the same rigor as critical path clinical programs. The developer must anticipate operational requirements and impact on resources, trial size, timing, etc.

Will the biomarker program delay time to approval? Delay of launch has the greatest negative impact on investment. It delays revenue to offset development costs and increases probability that competitors will enter the market. In an economic analysis of the value of investment in biomarkers, Roberts has suggested that an anticipated delay of greater than 1½ years is a threshold for a negative return on investment in a biomarker program.[92]

- Will the biomarker be validated in time for product launch? If a biomarker is introduced at launch, the clinical and economic value can be presented as support for reimbursement. If a biomarker is introduced after the price of the drug has been set, there is currently no mechanism for resetting the price at a higher level in line with the new value proposition. The result, due to market stratification, will be a significant loss of revenue unless compensated by increased market share.

Will the Companion Diagnostic Test and Process Be Feasible and on Time? ■

- Can the developer access enough patient samples to discover and develop the biomarker? Will useful tissue samples be available during the clinical trials?
- What is the technical and commercial feasibility of developing a diagnostic test? Will the test be practical and standardized for use in the clinic? Will the diagnostic test be reimbursed?
- Is a diagnostic development partner needed to develop a test? Develop-

Table 27-3 ■ **Market Analysis of the Hypothetical Product "Superlamycin"**

	Price per Cycle	No. of Cycles	Total Eligible	Treated (Share of Eligible)	Revenue
Superlamycin	$2,000	10	100	35 (35% of 100)	$700,000
Superlamycin with biomarker	$3,000	15	50	35 (70% of 50)	$1,575,000

ers will need to understand and select from a range of potential testing platforms from basic urine or serum reference tests to biopsies, circulating cancer cells and plasma proteomics.

- What is the regulatory path for the biomarker and the diagnostic test? Regulatory pathways have not yet been optimized to encourage the codevelopment of diagnostics and therapeutics. Regulatory agencies may not have oversight of quality control of the test. This places burden on the drug developer to maintain market confidence in the validity of tests that are produced by a third party.

Will the Biomarker Offer Exclusivity? ■ Will the biomarker or testing platform be proprietary? While drugs normally have a period of intellectual or regulatory exclusivity, the drug manufacturer may not have exclusive rights to either test platforms or the biomarker/phenotypes. Competitors will quickly attempt to validate their same class compound with a biomarker that represents a drug class effect. This would be good for patients and payers, but the company that initially developed the biomarker may not gain the benefit.

As a compound moves through phase 2, the technical and market feasibility of a diagnostic test and the potential to improve the profile of the drug should become evident.

The commercial value of biomarker-defined regimens will be greatest when applied to regimens with moderate incremental benefits, with significant toxicities, or where there is substantial competition. Biomarkers will add less return on investment where the compound already has an extraordinary clinical benefit, the logistics of testing are impractical, or the biomarker comes to market after the compound has been launched and price cannot be adjusted to reflect value and loss of patients to stratification.

Conclusions

The promise of personalized medicine is profoundly influencing modern oncology drug development. Taking the most optimistic perspective, this shift is enhancing biomarker applications and translational science in clinical drug testing, resulting in an improvement in the efficacy and safety profiles of our next generation of cancer therapeutics. These changes also offer the promise of greater productivity and efficiency in pharmaceutical research and development. Not surprisingly, these advantages come at a cost, including an adjustment to the "one-drug-fits-all" thinking as an increasing number of niche-directed therapies are tailored to specific patient subsets. This requires a substantial reshaping of our clinical trial process and a reallocation of resources toward biomarker discovery in clinical development. Nonetheless, the inevitability of these changes makes this investment an essential step forward toward an increasingly bright future in oncology therapeutics.

Successful ideas often go through waves of initial hyperbole, disillusion as the theory is tempered by reality, and eventually, pragmatic implementation. Personalized medicine is no different. As such, personalized medicine is going through these same cycles triggered by the completion of the human genome sequence in 2001. This led to a peak of enthusiasm about how quickly the genomic sequence would impact medical practice. Years later we are in the trough with much questioning of the practical value of biomarkers in drug development and concern about the length of time required for meaningful clinical impact.[93] These concerns are reasonable and it is clear that while the $1000 genome is in view, it will take much longer to meaningfully interpret the data and justify the need to take our individual sequence with us to every physician appointment.

The examples in this chapter show that significant progress on predicting pharmacokinetic and pharmacodynamic variability has been made, and that treatment paradigms for CML, breast cancer, cardiovascular disease, acute lymphocytic leukemia, among others, have been greatly improved using pharmacogenomic analyses. In addition, the large number of targeted therapeutics in clinical development is significantly dependent on tools that "aim" at the appropriate patients who carry the specific molecular abnormality and will benefit from these therapies.

Ultimately, the potential of biomarkers is too great for drug developers to be on the sidelines. The potential clinical benefit to patients and the economic benefits to society and R&D organizations are numerous. But risks need to be mitigated by smart development, rigorous and transparent decision-making, and prioritization. Stakeholders will need to work together to align public policy—regulatory, intellectual property, and reimbursement policy—to continue to encourage investment in the innovation needed to realize the extraordinary promise of personalized cancer medicine.

Selected References

The complete reference list can be found at www.CANCERMEDICINE8.com

1. Johnston PG, et al. Thymidylate synthase gene and protein expression correlate and are associated with response to 5-fluorouracil in human colorectal and gastric tumors. *Cancer Res.* 1995;55(7):1407–1412.
2. Curt GA, et al. Unstable methotrexate resistance in human small-cell carcinoma associated with double minute chromosomes. *N Engl J Med.* 1983;308(4):199–202.
3. Gomez HL, et al. A phase II trial of pemetrexed in advanced breast cancer: clinical response and association with molecular target expression. *Clin Cancer Res.* 2006;12 (3 Pt 1):832–838.
4. Salmon SE. Human tumor clonogenic assays: growth conditions and applications. *Cancer Genet Cytogenet.* 1986;19(1–2):21–28.
5. Paik S, et al. A multigene assay to predict recurrence of tamoxifen-treated, node-negative breast cancer. *N Engl J Med.* 2004;351(27):2817–2826.
6. van de Vijver MJ, et al. A gene-expression signature as a predictor of survival in breast cancer. *N Engl J Med.* 2002;347(25):1999–2009.
7. Ma XJ, et al.. A two-gene expression ratio predicts clinical outcome in breast cancer patients treated with tamoxifen. *Cancer Cell.* 2004;5(6):607–616.
8. Lynch TJ, et al. Activating mutations in the epidermal growth factor receptor underlying responsiveness of non-small-cell lung cancer to gefitinib. *N Engl J Med.* 2004;350(21):2129–2139.
9. Paez JG, et al. EGFR mutations in lung cancer: correlation with clinical response to gefitinib therapy. *Science.* 2004;304(5676):1497–1500.
10. Han SW, et al. Predictive and prognostic impact of epidermal growth factor receptor mutation in non-small-cell lung cancer patients treated with gefitinib. *J Clin Oncol.* 2005;23(11):2493–2501.
11. Riordan JR, et al. Identification of the cystic fibrosis gene: cloning and characterization of complementary DNA. *Science.* 1989;245(4922):1066–1073.
12. A novel gene containing a trinucleotide repeat that is expanded and unstable on Huntington's disease chromosomes. The Huntington's Disease Collaborative Research Group. *Cell.* 1993;72(6):971–983.
13. Wilkinson GR. Drug metabolism and variability among patients in drug response. *N Engl J Med.* 2005;352(21):2211–2221.
14. Evans WE, McLeod HL. Pharmacogenomics—drug disposition, drug targets, and side effects. *N Engl J Med.* 2003;348(6):538–549.
15. McLeod HL, et al. Genetic polymorphism of thiopurine methyltransferase and its clinical relevance for childhood acute lymphoblastic leukemia. *Leukemia.* 2000;14(4):567–572.
16. Botstein D, et al. Construction of a genetic linkage map in man using restriction fragment length polymorphisms. *Am J Hum Genet.* 1980;32(3):314–331.
17. Litt M, Luty JA. A hypervariable microsatellite revealed by in vitro amplification of a dinucleotide repeat within the car-

diac muscle actin gene. *Am J Hum Genet.* 1989;44(3):397–401.

18. Weber JL, May PE. Abundant class of human DNA polymorphisms which can be typed using the polymerase chain reaction. *Am J Hum Genet.* 1989;44(3):388–396.
19. Hinds DA, et al. Whole-genome patterns of common DNA variation in three human populations. *Science.* 2005;307(5712):1072–1079.
20. Sachidanandam R, et al. A map of human genome sequence variation containing 1.42 million single nucleotide polymorphisms. *Nature.* 2001;409(6822):928–933.
21. Altshuler D, et al. A haplotype map of the human genome. *Nature.* 2005;437(7063): 1299–1320.
22. Venter JC, et al. The sequence of the human genome. *Science.* 2001;291(5507):1304–1351.
23. Lander ES, et al. Initial sequencing and analysis of the human genome. *Nature.* 2001;409(6822):860–921.
24. Hunter DJ, et al. A genome-wide association study identifies alleles in FGFR2 associated with risk of sporadic postmenopausal breast cancer. *Nat Genet.* 2007;39(7):870–874.
25. Easton DF, et al. Genome-wide association study identifies novel breast cancer susceptibility loci. *Nature.* 2007;447 (7148):1087–1093.
26. Wood LD, et al. The genomic landscapes of human breast and colorectal cancers. *Science.* 2007;318(5853):1108–1113.
27. Sjoblom T, et al. The consensus coding sequences of human breast and colorectal cancers. *Science.* 2006;314(5797):268–274.
28. Adams MD, et al. Complementary DNA sequencing: expressed sequence tags and human genome project. *Science.* 1991;252(5013):1651–1656.
29. Hanahan D, Weinberg RA. The hallmarks of cancer. *Cell.* 2000;100(1):57–70.
30. Ramaswamy S, et al. Multiclass cancer diagnosis using tumor gene expression signatures. *Proc Natl Acad Sci USA.* 2001;98(26):15149–15154.
31. DeRisi J, et al. Use of a cDNA microarray to analyse gene expression patterns in human cancer. *Nat Genet.* 1996;14(4):457–460.
32. Aebersold R, Mann M. Mass spectrometry-based proteomics. *Nature.* 2003;422(6928):198–207.
33. Anderson NL, Anderson NG. A two-dimensional gel database of human plasma proteins. *Electrophoresis.* 1991;12(11): 883–906.
34. Anderson NL, Anderson NG. The human plasma proteome: history, character, and diagnostic prospects. *Mol Cell Proteomics.* 2002;1(11):845–867.
35. Maguire PB, Fitzgerald DJ. Platelet proteomics. *J Thromb Haemost.* 2003;1(7):1593–1601.
36. Petricoin EF, et al. Use of proteomic patterns in serum to identify ovarian cancer. *Lancet.* 2002. 359(9306):572–577.
37. Wulfkuhle JD Liotta LA, Petricoin EF. Proteomic applications for the early detection of cancer. *Nat Rev Cancer.* 2003;3(4): 267–275.
38. Sorace JM, Zhan M. A data review and re-assessment of ovarian cancer serum proteomic profiling. *BMC Bioinformatics.* 2003;4:24.
39. Li J, et al. Proteomics and bioinformatics approaches for identification of serum biomarkers to detect breast cancer. *Clin Chem.* 2002;48(8):1296–1304.
40. Qu Y, et al. Boosted decision tree analysis of surface-enhanced laser desorption/ionization mass spectral serum profiles discriminates prostate cancer from noncancer patients. *Clin Chem.* 2002;48(10):1835–1843.
41. Adam BL, et al. Serum protein fingerprinting coupled with a pattern-matching algorithm distinguishes prostate cancer from benign prostate hyperplasia and healthy men. *Cancer Res.* 2002;62(13):3609–3614.
42. Petricoin EF 3rd, et al. Serum proteomic patterns for detection of prostate cancer. *J Natl Cancer Inst.* 2002;94(20):1576–1578.
43. Gianni L, et al. Gene expression profiles in paraffin-embedded core biopsy tissue predict response to chemotherapy in women with locally advanced breast cancer. *J Clin Oncol.* 2005;23(29):7265–7277.
44. van't Veer LJ, et al. Gene expression profiling predicts clinical outcome of breast cancer. *Nature.* 2002;415(6871):530–536.
45. Relling MV, et al. Prognostic importance of 6-mercaptopurine dose intensity in acute lymphoblastic leukemia. *Blood.* 1999;93(9):2817–2823.
46. McLeod HL, Siva C. The thiopurine S-methyltransferase gene locus—implications for clinical pharmacogenomics. *Pharmacogenomics.* 2002;3(1):89–98.
47. McLeod HL, Watters JW. Irinotecan pharmacogenetics: is it time to intervene? *J Clin Oncol.* 2004;22(8):1356–1359.
48. Zhang D, et al. In vitro inhibition of UDP glucuronosyltransferases by atazanavir and other HIV protease inhibitors and the relationship of this property to in vivo bilirubin glucuronidation. *Drug Metab Dispos.* 2005;33(11):1729–1739.
49. Rotger M, et al. Gilbert syndrome and the development of antiretroviral therapy-associated hyperbilirubinemia. *J Infect Dis.* 2005;192(8):1381–1386.
50. Sai K, et al. UGT1A1 haplotypes associated with reduced glucuronidation and increased serum bilirubin in irinotecan-administered Japanese patients with cancer. *Clin Pharmacol Ther.* 2004;75(6):501–515.

28 Cancer Genome Aberrations: Measures, Causes, and Consequences

Eric A. Collisson, MD ■ Anguraj Sadanandam, PhD ■ Paul T. Spellman, MD ■ Joe W. Gray, MD

Introduction

The last decade has seen an unprecedented explosion in knowledge about cancer genomes. Since Flemming and contemporaries reported the existence of chromosomes in the early 1880s, investigators have increasingly appreciated both the prevalence and complexity of genomic aberrations in cancer. Recurrent aberrations now known to contribute to oncogenesis, progression and response to therapy include mutations, increases and decreases in genome copy number, and structural rearrangements. These aberrations contribute to cancer pathophysiology by deregulating mRNA and miRNA expression levels, altering gene function, and/or creating gene chimeras. We summarize here mechanisms that give rise to these aberrations, review the evolving laboratory and bioinformatic technologies being used to discover and characterize cancer genome alterations, and summarize the dramatic impact these discoveries are having on our understanding of cancer pathogenesis, risk and management.

Mechanisms of Aberration Formation

Numerical and Structural Aberrations

Numerical and structural aberrations may occur via a variety of mechanisms. Breakage–fusion–bridge (BFB) cycles, first reported by McClintock,[1] generate both structural and numerical aberrations. During BFB cycles, broken chromosomes (resulting from diverse mechanisms) fuse via error prone nonhomologous end joining[2] to form dicentric chromosomes that frequently break during passage through mitosis, thereby restarting the BFB cycle. Daughter cells that inherit chromosome segments conferring a proliferative advantage will eventually overgrow the population so that the aberrations appear in most of the cells. The BFB cycles can be triggered by double-strand breaks[3] or by telomere erosion resulting from proliferation in the absence of telomerase that eventually culminates in end-to-end chromosome fusions.[4,5] Disruption of the mitotic apparatus through abrogation of mitotic spindle checkpoints[6] or deregulation of centrosome number[7] are mechanisms that likely to lead to changes in chromosome copy number. Formation of small circular DNA molecules physically separated from chromosomes such as episomes, minichromosomes, small polydispersed DNAs, or double minute chromosomes is another mechanism by which segments of the genome can be amplified.[8] Unequal partitioning of these extrachromosomal elements during cell division allows rapid selection for advantageous elements. Finally, some "fragile" chromosomal segments appear to be frequently lost or to nucleate amplification, probably as a result of deregulation of genes involved in DNA damage checkpoint response.[9]

Mutations

Mutation may be driven by the direct action of exogeneous DNA damaging agents such as radiation, environmental mutagens, and chemotherapy or may be mediated by endogenous- or exogenous-induced reactive oxygen or nitrogen species.[10] Mutations typically are single nucleotide substitutions, although it is becoming apparent that microdeletions may also be important.[11] The frequency and spectrum of mutations may be strongly influenced by the nature of the DNA damaging agents and can be enhanced by deregulation of aspects of DNA repair, DNA-damage signaling, DNA polymerase function, and/or DNA recombination and mismatch and repair.[12] For example, large-scale genome sequencing projects have now clearly demonstrated that breast and colorectal cancers show substantial differences in their mutation spectrum.[13,14] For example, C:G to T:A transitions predominate in colorectal cancers, whereas C:G to G:C transversions dominate in breast cancers. The impact of mutagen exposure is most apparent in cases of cancers exposed to chemotherapeutic agents. For example, glioblastoma multiforme (GBM) treated with alkylating agents that methylate the mismatch repair gene, MGMT, display a remarkable hypermutation phenotype,[11] providing a driving force to create diversity that eventually evolves to therapy resistance.

Technologies for Genome Anatomy Assessment

Molecular Cytogenetics and Microarrays

The detection of chromosomal abnormalities began with the ability to differentially stain human chromosomes with quinacrine mustard.[15] Since that time, numerous technologies have emerged to illuminate the anatomy of the cancer genome more fully. Assays relying on hybridization of DNA probes to the cancer genome began with fluorescence in situ hybridization (FISH) of locus or chromosome-specific probes[16] and evolved to allow genome-wide assessment of numerical and structural aberrations, at least in preparations of metaphase chromosomes, using multicolor FISH.[17,18] Comparative genomic hybridization[19] and microarray versions thereof[20] allowed genome-wide detection and accurate mapping of genome copy number changes. Today, some microarray version of CGH also allow allele-specific analysis.[21] Chromosome-based cytogenetic analyses were typically limited to about 5 Mbp resolution but today's CGH microarray technologies allow interrogation of cancer genomes with subgene resolution.[11,22] These methods reveal a genomic complexity and variation between tumors that are truly remarkable. For example, the genome copy number profiles for two different breast cancers shown in Figure 28-1A and B reveal stunning differences in genome aberration complexity, even within a single disease.

Large-Scale Sequencing

Hybridization protocols, although powerful, offer high-resolution information on genome copy number but so far have provided only cytogenetic (and not molecular) level resolution on structural changes. In addition, they do not easily link the copy number changes with structural changes in the genome. These limitations are now being overcome by DNA-sequence-based methods. The general approach is to generate DNA sequences from both ends of a DNA molecule of a known length and to map these onto a normal representation of the genome. Displays of the frequencies of mapped reads along the normal genome provides information on copy number, similar to

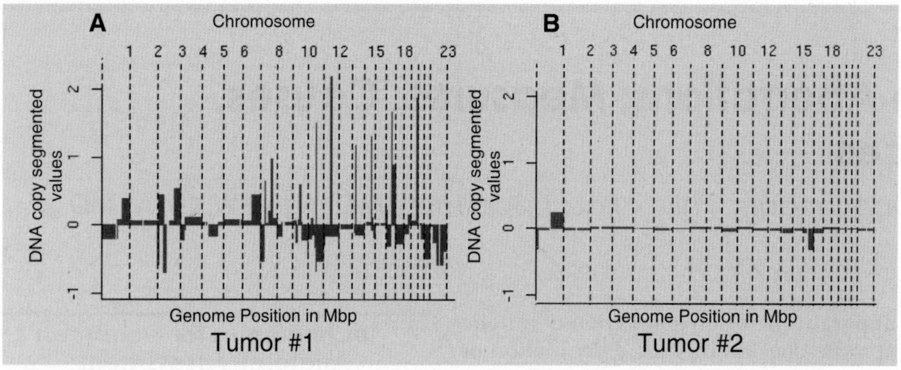

Figure 28-1 ■ Variation in genome copy number alterations in GBM. Segmented log2 copy number increases or decreases from normalized signal intensities of SNP array for two, individual breast tumors. (**A**) many aberrations and (**B**) few aberrations are plotted as a function of genome location. Positive values indicate gains and negative values indicate loss. The chromosome location is on the *x* axis.

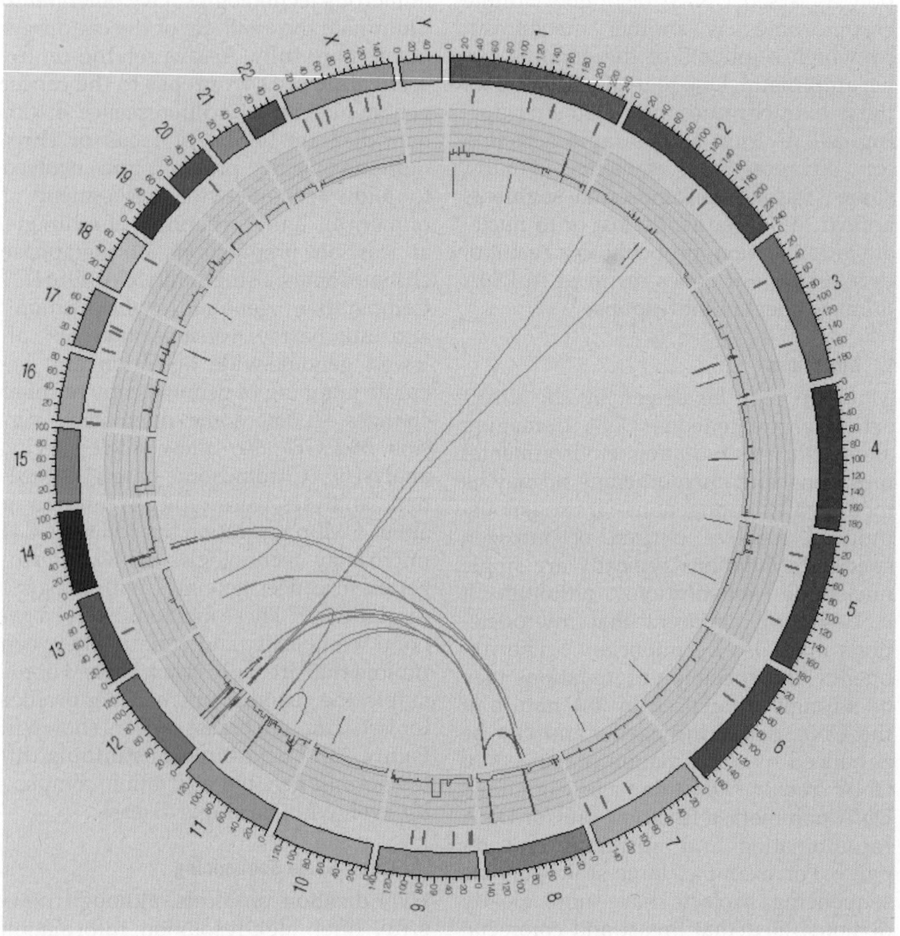

Figure 28-2 ■ Deep sequencing reconstruction of copy number and structure of NCI-H2171. The outer (first) ring represents each of the 22 autosomes, and the X and Y chromosomes based on their physical size. Point mutations are shown on the second ring as blue dashes. Estimated copy numbers are plotted on the third ring (blue line). Intrachromosomal structural aberrations are shown in the inner ring in red and interchromosomal structural aberrations are shown across the center of the diagram in green connecting the end points of the two fused chromosomes/segments. *Source*: Adapted from http://www.sanger.ac.uk/perl/genetics/CGP/cosmic?action=sample;id=688015

that obtained using CGH, although maps of the locations of sequence pairs allow identification of structural aberrations when the two end sequences do not map to the same chromosome or have an unexpected distance between them. This allows structural aberrations to be tied directly to copy number changes. First-generation technology, end-sequence profiling of bacterial artificial chromosomes (BACs), was informative but expensive.[2,23] The development of low-cost massively parallel sequencing is now making this integrated approach more practical.[24] A recent example of this work is shown in Figure 28-2, where data from the Stratton Group show copy number profiles and observed structural rearrangements in a single tumor cell line.[24] It now seems likely that continuing reductions in cost for massively parallel sequencing will allow this technology to supplant microarray technologies for analysis of genome copy number and genomic rearrangements (if gDNA is the input) and expression level and gene expression and gene fusions (if cDNA is the input).

A particularly interesting application of this technology is in the detection of novel fusion genes. Fusion genes, long known in sarcomas and hematopoietic tumors, are increasingly being discovered in carcinoma genomes, with prominent examples being the ETS fusions in prostate cancer[25] and the ALK fusion genes found in nonsmall cell lung cancer.[26] Campbell et al [24] and Raphael et al [2] have analyzed a small number of cancer cell lines using paired end sequencing approaches to find novel fusion genes and genomic rearrangements, not identifiable by assessment of CNA alone. The publication of whole exome sequencing of many breast and colorectal carcinomas[27] has recently been followed by the genomes of many GBM,[11,28] pancreatic adenocarcinomas,[29] and lung cancers.[30] Although these genomes have not yet been specifically mined for novel genomic rearrangements, the field eagerly awaits these analyses, as novel fusion genes or activating mutations could well be the new drug targets desperately needed in these currently poorly treated, lethal malignancies.

Finding Gene Aberrations that Contribute to Cancer Pathophysiology

The task of identifying the gene(s) in regions of genomic abnormality responsible for the aberration is critical but challenging. The CGH and molecular cytogenetic techniques have demonstrated that hundreds to thousands of genes may be deregulated by genome copy number changes.[31,32] DNA sequencing efforts have demonstrated the existence of hundreds of candidate cancer gene mutations[13,14,29,30] and the presence of tens to hundreds of mutations in individual tumors. A key question now is: Which of these many abnormalities play important roles in cancer progression?

Detection of significant copy number aberrations can be guided by algorithms such as Genomic *I*dentification of *S*ignificant *T*argets *i*n *C*ancer (GISTIC) that systematically compare the prevalence of aberrant events across samples, with weighting consideration given to frequency and magnitude of the aberration.[33] The GISTIC plots for genome copy number gains and losses in GBMs analyzed by the TCGA project is shown in Figure 28-3. Other algorithms such as *S*ignificance *T*esting for *A*berrant **Copy number** (STAC) utilize two complementary statistics in combination with a novel search strategy to identify nonrandom gains and losses across multiple experiments/samples using a multiple testing corrected permutation approach.[34] New high-resolution analyses are simplifying the identification of genes targeted for copy number gain or loss by more precisely defining the common aberration boundaries. That said, it is important to recognize that these and related algorithms tend to guide the observer to regions of highest amplification or homozygous deletion. This likely increases the chances of finding aberrant genes that contribute strongly to cancer genesis or progression, but may miss aberrant genes that influence the cancer phenotype less dramatically or that may do so through cooperation. Chin et al,[32] noted that low-level copy number aberrations may contribute to breast cancer pathophysiology by altering the expression of hundreds of genes that, in ensemble, contribute to increased metabolic activity. Likewise, work from our own group showing that the regions of amplification in breast cancer that encode ERBB2, MYC, and CCND1 loci each harbor 2–5 genes that provide amplification-dependent growth advantages to the tumors.[35] Thus, informatics algorithms finding minimal, common aberrations can only take us so far in finding the gene(s) "driving" amplification, and functional validation must be pursued in the wet lab. Several groups have employed cell line panels to this end, based on the understanding that cell lines retain most of the hallmark genomic abnormalities of a given malignancy. These cell line panels, annotated once with dense copy number data and coupled with siRNA technology, are a valuable inexhaustible proving ground for functional identification of gene aberrations that contribute to cancer pathophysiology.

As comprehensive catalogues of the mutations, copy number and structural changes and epigenomic modifications that influence cancers begin to emerge, it appears that deregulation of common cancer-related processes can occur through multiple, possibly more or less equivalent mechanisms. For example, activation of the PI3-kinase pathway leading to increased proliferation and reduced cell death may involve amplification or mutation of upstream receptor tyrosine kinases; amplification or mutation of the p110 α catalytic subunit of PI3K, *PIK3CA*; deletion or methylation of the negative regulator, PTEN; and/or amplification of one of the downstream AKT kinases.[36] Recent integrated analyses of glioblastoma illustrated in Figure 28-4, showed that important cancer-related pathways such as those involved in Ras/PI3K signaling, p53 signaling, and RB signaling are deregulated by "equivalent" events in almost 90% of gliomas. Similar high frequency, multiaberration deregulations of important cancer related pathways have been reported for cancers of the pancreas,[29] lung,[30] breast, and colon.[37] However, the actual functional equivalence of many of the aberrations that are integrated to "populate" these aberrant pathways has not been demonstrated, and are likely oversimplified in many cases. For example, activation of the Ras pathway is speculated to occur in 100% of pancreas and 88% of GBM tumors; however the spectrum of mutations differs dramatically, with ~90% of pancreas cancers harboring activating mutations in the KRAS gene compared to <2% in GBM (Fig. 28-4). Therefore, experimental verification of the pathway activation capacities of the aberrations now being discovered remains an important task for the future.

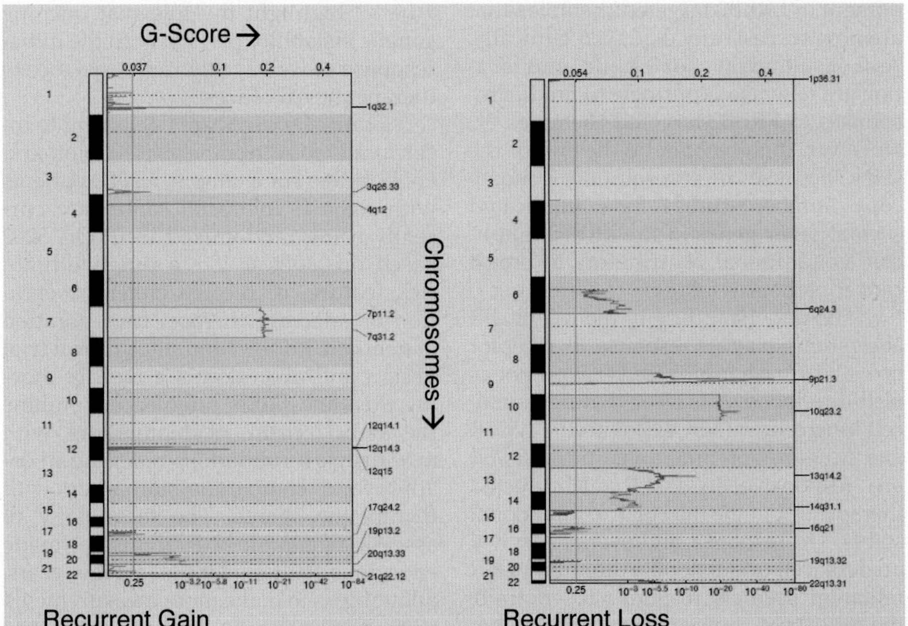

Figure 28-3 ■ Interpretation of copy number aberrations. Integrative analysis of copy number data from GBM in the TCGA study shows numerous regions of common gains and losses. Each gain or loss is identified by its position, focality, and the significance of the result. Note that many changes in GBM are very highly significant (log(q) < –10).

Epidemiology, Whole Genome Associations, and Copy Number Abnormalities

Microarrays that enable genome-wide interrogation of allelotype have ushered in a new paradigm in human genetics. In the last 3–4 years, investigators have identified genomic regions of heritable risk for a diverse set of cancers including breast,[38] colorectal,[39] lung,[40,41] and prostate[42] carcinomas. These genome-wide association studies (GWAS) have identified several regions associated with increased cancer risk, but in most cases the risk odds ratios are <2 so that very large populations must be screened to confidently identify the involved genes/regions. As an example of the challenges faced, several studies have identified a 136-kb region of human chromosome 8q24 associated with prostate and colon cancers. This region encodes several SNPs that confer an odds ratio of ~1.2–1.8 for colorectal and prostate cancers, but the region is devoid of protein coding genes. The c-MYC oncogene resides ~300 kb distal to this region; however, several large GWAS have revealed no evidence for linkage between genetic variants in the *MYC* gene and the loci associated with specific cancers,[43] and one study excluded differential expression of c-MYC mRNA in the prostate.[44] Thus, additional genomic approaches assessing transcriptional repercussions (at a distance) in *cis* or in *trans* may be needed to localize the genetic elements and the mechanisms responsible for the increased risk. One approach is to take advantage of the recent observations that polymorphisms associated with increased cancer risk are selectively increased in copy number during tumor evolution, whereas polymorphisms associated with decreased risk are eliminated.[45-47] With this in mind, it is intriguing that 8q24 is one of the most frequently amplified regions in cancer. However, the area is gene poor, and the amplicon structure varies both within and across diseases. So far, only one study has demonstrated

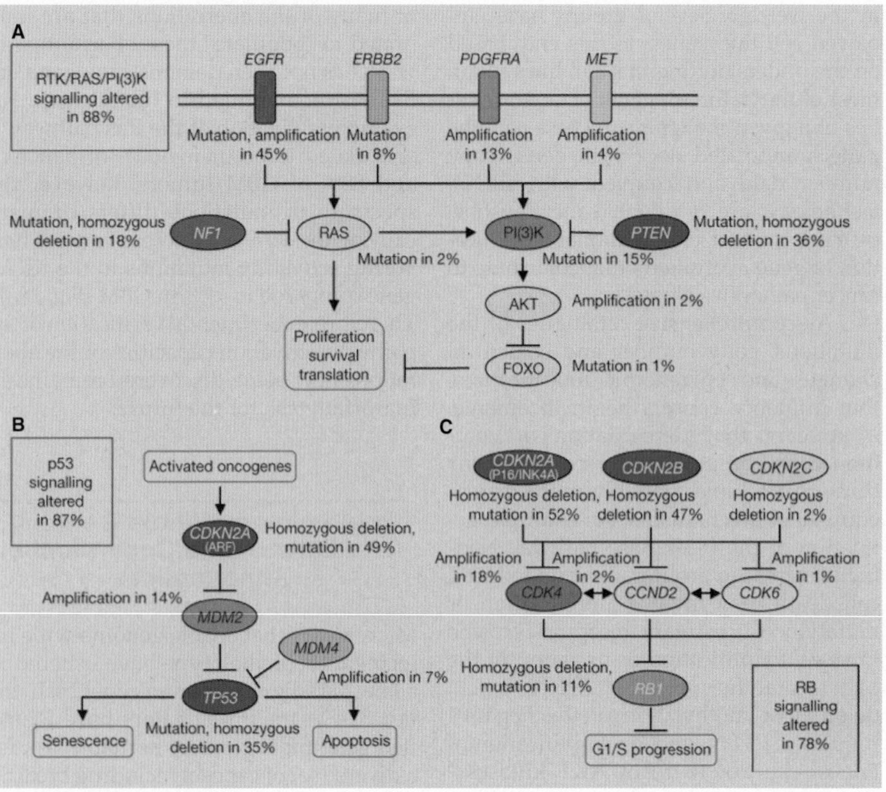

Figure 28-4 Integrated assessment of GBM aberrations. Frequent genetic alterations in three critical signaling pathways. Primary sequence alterations and significant copy number changes for components of the RTK/RAS/PI(3)K (**A**), p53 (**B**), and RB (**C**) signaling pathways are shown. Red indicates activating genetic alterations, with frequently altered genes showing deeper shades of red. In contrast, blue indicates inactivating alterations, with darker shades corresponding to a higher percentage of alteration. For each altered component of a particular pathway, the nature of the alteration and the percentage of tumors affected are indicated. Boxes contain the final percentages of glioblastomas with alterations in at least one known component gene of the designated pathway.[11] *Source:* From Ref. 11.

that a germ line genetic polymorphism at 8q24.21 (in this case G at *rs6983267*) is a target in the somatic amplification of 8q24 in *rs6983267* heterozygote colorectal patients,[48] supporting the concept that allele-specific amplification leads to growth advantage. Thus, the search continues. Perhaps future studies may need to focus on polymorphisms that influence aspects of genome function, such as expression of noncoding RNAs or that modulate aspects of genome vulnerability, such as susceptibility to epigenomic modification or amplification or deletion.

Genome Aberrations and Clinical Outcome

The prognostic importance of CNAs and specific rearrangements in hematopoetic malignancies is well known, and associations between aberrations and outcome are now being defined for solid tumors as well. The first successful translational genomic development derived from the discovery that ERBB2 amplification occurs in ~30% of breast cancer patients and is associated with poor outcome.[49] These observations and associated biological investigation inspired the development of ERBB2 targeted therapies that are now successfully deployed clinically. As a result, assays for ERBB2 amplification are now used routinely to predict responses to ERBB2-targeted therapies.[50,51] However, this may not be the end of the story because high-resolution genome copy number studies have implicated several other genes in the ERBB2 amplicon as additional contributors to breast cancer pathophysiology.[52]

The understanding of the role EGFR aberrations play in response to receptor tyrosine kinase inhibitors (TKIs) is not as well developed. It is clear that non-small cell lung cancer (NSCLC) with the L858R and Δ E746-A750 mutations in the EGFR are responsive to EGFR TKI-directed therapy,[53,54] but the interplay of mutational status, TKI response, and overall survival are less well understood. Although EGFR mutation predicts response to erlotinib, the BR21 trial showed no association between EGFR mutation and survival.[55] The EGFR copy number (by FISH) in NSCL carcinomas did seem to predict both response and a survival benefit with erlotinib in other settings[56] or gefitinib.[57] Furthermore in colon cancer, EGFR expression (as determined by IHC) is not required for cetuximab benefit,[58,59] and activating mutations in EGFR are exceedingly rare in this disease;[60] however, the differing mechanisms of action of antibodies and TKIs preclude direct comparisons.

The diagnostic and therapeutic relevance of structural genomic rearrangements in solid tumors is still being defined. The most well-studied structural aberration in solid tumors is the fusion of the 5′-untranslated region of the androgen responsive TMPRSS2 gene to the 3′ region of ERG in prostate cancer.[25] This, and similar translocations involving androgen-sensitive promoters and related ETS transcription factors are found in the majority of this highly prevalent disease, making this the most common genomic derangement in human cancer.[61] There is not clear agreement, however, as to the prognostic implications of these gene fusions, with some publications reporting more-[62,63] and some less-aggressive tumors.[64] Nonetheless, therapeutic strategies directed toward the fusion genes are now underway.[65]

Finally, in an elegant series of complementary experiments, investigators have shown the interplay that genomic rearrangements can play in the acquisition of resistance to an initially effective therapeutic compound. Based on the observation that cancer cells with defective DNA repair machinery (specifically defects in the *BRCA2* gene), investigators demonstrated that reversion of this initially sensitizing lesion to wild type BRCA2 lead to resistance to platinum compounds[66] and PARP inhibition.[67] These reports and others[68] highlight the role that ongoing genetic instability plays in both the initial response as well as acquired resistance to therapeutics in cancer.

Clinical trialists are beginning to incorporate copy number-based biomarkers in trials. For example, >3,000 patients with stage II colorectal cancer are currently being randomized in ECOG 5202 based on LOH at 18q, a putative high-risk feature, to receive either observation or adjuvant therapy. Incorporation of genomic information into clinical trial design and execution is a rapidly moving area and holds promise to combine the development of biomarkers with new drugs/formulations resulting in co-approval of companion biomarkers with therapeutic agents. The technology of assessing genomic aberrations has made enormous strides over the last few years, allowing us to make more measurements more precisely than we have ever done before. Applying these technologies to patient samples in real time takes an important step in realizing both a better understanding of the biology of cancer and the promise of personalized medicine.

Acknowledgments

This work was supported by the Director, Office of Science, Office of Biological & Environmental Research, of the U.S. Department of Energy under Contract No. DE-AC02-05CH11231, by the National Institutes of Health, National Cancer Institute grants P50 CA 58207, and by the U54 CA 112970

Selected References

The complete reference list can be found at www.CANCERMEDICINE8.com

1. McClintock B. Chromosome organization and genic expression. *Cold Spring Harb Symp Quant Biol.* 1951;16:13–47.
4. Artandi SE, Chang S, et al. Telomere dysfunction promotes non-reciprocal translocations and epithelial cancers in mice. *Nature.* 2000;406(6796):641–645.
5. Chin K, de Solorzano CO, et al. In situ analyses of genome instability in breast cancer. *Nat Genet.* 2004;36(9):984–988.
9. Albertson DG. Gene amplification in cancer. *Trends Genet.* 2006;22(8):447–455.
11. TCGA. Comprehensive genomic characterization defines human glioblastoma genes and core pathways. *Nature.* 2008;455(7216):1061–1068.
13. Sjoblom T, Jones S, et al. The consensus coding sequences of human breast and colorectal cancers. *Science.* 2006;314(5797):268–274.
14. Stephens P, Edkins S, et al. A screen of the complete protein kinase gene family identifies diverse patterns of somatic mutations in human breast cancer. *Nat Genet.* 2005;37(6):590–592.
15. Caspersson T, Lindsten J, et al. The nature of structural X chromosome aberrations in Turner's syndrome as revealed by quinacrine mustard fluorescence analysis. *Hereditas.* 1970;66(2):287–292.
16. Pinkel D, Landegent J, et al. Fluorescence in situ hybridization with human chromosome-specific libraries: detection of trisomy 21 and translocations of chromosome 4. *Proc Natl Acad Sci USA.* 1988;85(23):9138–9142.
17. Ried T, Baldini A, et al. Simultaneous visualization of seven different DNA probes by in situ hybridization using combinatorial fluorescence and digital imaging microscopy. *Proc Natl Acad Sci USA.* 1992; 89(4):1388–1392.
18. Padilla-Nash HM, Barenboim-Stapleton L, et al. Spectral karyotyping analysis of human and mouse chromosomes. *Nat Protoc.* 2006;1(6):3129–3142.
19. Kallioniemi A, Kallioniemi OP, et al. Comparative genomic hybridization for molecular cytogenetic analysis of solid tumors. *Science.* 1992;258(5083):818–821.
20. Pinkel D, Segraves R, et al. High resolution analysis of DNA copy number variation using comparative genomic hybridization to microarrays. *Nat Genet.* 1998;20(2):207–211.
21. Wang Y, Moorhead M, et al. Analysis of molecular inversion probe performance for allele copy number determination. *Genome Biol.* 2007;8(11):R246.
23. Volik S, Zhao S, et al. End-sequence profiling: sequence-based analysis of aberrant genomes. *Proc Natl Acad Sci USA.* 2003;100(13):7696–7701.
24. Campbell PJ, Stephens PJ, et al. Identification of somatically acquired rearrangements in cancer using genome-wide massively parallel paired-end sequencing. *Nat Genet.* 2008;40(6):722–729.
25. Tomlins SA, Rhodes DR, et al. Recurrent fusion of TMPRSS2 and ETS transcription factor genes in prostate cancer. *Science.* 2005;310(5748):644–648.
26. Soda M, Choi YL, et al. Identification of the transforming EML4-ALK fusion gene in non-small-cell lung cancer. *Nature.* 2007;448(7153):561–566.
27. Wood LD, Parsons DW, et al. The genomic landscapes of human breast and colorectal cancers. *Science.* 2007;318(5853):1108–1113.
28. Parsons DW, Jones S, et al. An integrated genomic analysis of human glioblastoma multiforme. *Science.* 2008;321(5897):1807–1812.
29. Jones S, Zhang X, et al. Core signaling pathways in human pancreatic cancers revealed by global genomic analyses. *Science.* 2008;321(5897):1801–1806.
30. Ding L, Getz G, et al. Somatic mutations affect key pathways in lung adenocarcinoma. *Nature.* 2008;455(7216):1069–1075.
31. Bergamaschi A, Kim YH, et al. Distinct patterns of DNA copy number alteration are associated with different clinicopathological features and gene-expression subtypes of breast cancer. *Genes Chromosomes Cancer.* 2006;45(11):1033–1040.
32. Chin K, DeVries S, et al. Genomic and transcriptional aberrations linked to breast cancer pathophysiologies. *Cancer Cell.* 2006;10(6):529–541.
33. Beroukhim R, Getz G, et al. Assessing the significance of chromosomal aberrations in cancer: methodology and application to glioma. *Proc Natl Acad Sci USA.* 2007;104(50):20007–20012.
37. Leary R J, Lin JC, et al. Integrated analysis of homozygous deletions, focal amplifications, and sequence alterations in breast and colorectal cancers. *Proc Natl Acad Sci USA.* 2008;105(42):16224–16229.
38. Easton DF, Pooley KA, et al. Genome-wide association study identifies novel breast cancer susceptibility loci. *Nature.* 2007;447(7148):1087–1093.
39. Zanke BW, Greenwood CM, et al. Genome-wide association scan identifies a colorectal cancer susceptibility locus on chromosome 8q24. *Nat Genet.* 2007;39(8):989–994.
40. Hung RJ, McKay JD, et al. A susceptibility locus for lung cancer maps to nicotinic acetylcholine receptor subunit genes on 15q25. *Nature.* 2008;452(7187):633–637.
41. Amos CI, Wu X, et al. Genome-wide association scan of tag SNPs identifies a susceptibility locus for lung cancer at 15q25.1. *Nat Genet.* 2008;40(5):616–622.
42. Yeager M, Orr N, et al. Genome-wide association study of prostate cancer identifies a second risk locus at 8q24. *Nat Genet.* 2007;39(5):645–649.
43. Yeager M, Xiao N, et al. Comprehensive resequence analysis of a 136 kb region of human chromosome 8q24 associated with prostate and colon cancers. *Hum Genet.* 2008;124(2):161–170.
44. Gudmundsson J, Sulem P, et al. Genome-wide association study identifies a second prostate cancer susceptibility variant at 8q24. *Nat Genet.* 2007;39(5):631–637.
45. Ewart-Toland A, Briassouli P, et al. Identification of Stk6/STK15 as a candidate low-penetrance tumor-susceptibility gene in mouse and human. *Nat Genet.* 2003;34(4):403–412.
47. Mao JH, Wu D, et al. Crosstalk between Aurora-A and p53: frequent deletion or downregulation of Aurora-A in tumors from p53 null mice. *Cancer Cell.* 2007;11(2):161–173.
48. Tuupanen S, Niittymaki I, et al. Allelic imbalance at rs6983267 suggests selection of the risk allele in somatic colorectal tumor evolution. *Cancer Res.* 2008;68(1):14–17.
49. Slamon DJ, Clark GM, et al. Human breast cancer: correlation of relapse and survival with amplification of the HER-2/neu oncogene. *Science.* 19/87;235(4785):177–182.
50. Pegram MD, Lipton A, et al. Phase II study of receptor-enhanced chemosensitivity using recombinant humanized anti-p185HER2/neu monoclonal antibody plus cisplatin in patients with HER2/neu-overexpressing metastatic breast cancer refractory to chemotherapy treatment. *J Clin Oncol.* 1998;16(8):2659–2671.
53. Lynch TJ, Bell DW, et al. Activating mutations in the epidermal growth factor receptor underlying responsiveness of non-small-cell lung cancer to gefitinib. *N Engl J Med.* 2004;350(21):2129–2139.
54. Pao W, Miller V, et al. EGF receptor gene mutations are common in lung cancers from "never smokers" and are associated with sensitivity of tumors to gefitinib and erlotinib. *Proc Natl Acad Sci USA.* 2004;101(36):13306–13311.
56. Zhu CQ, da Cunha Santos G, et al. Role of KRAS and EGFR as biomarkers of response to erlotinib in National Cancer Institute of Canada Clinical Trials Group Study BR.21. *J Clin Oncol.* 2008;26(26):4268–4275.
57. Cappuzzo F, Ligorio C, et al. Prospective study of gefitinib in epidermal growth factor receptor fluorescence in situ hybridization-positive/phospho-Akt-positive or never smoker patients with advanced non-small-cell lung cancer: the ONCOBELL trial. *J Clin Oncol.* 2007;25(16):2248–2255.
58. Chung KY, Shia J, et al. Cetuximab shows activity in colorectal cancer patients with tumors that do not express the epidermal growth factor receptor by immunohistochemistry. *J Clin Oncol.* 2005;23(9):1803–1810.
59. Lenz HJ, Van Cutsem E, et al. Multicenter phase II and translational study of cetuximab in metastatic colorectal carcinoma refractory to irinotecan, oxaliplatin, and fluoropyrimidines. *J Clin Oncol.* 2006;24(30):4914–4921.
60. Barber TD, Vogelstein B, et al. Somatic mutations of EGFR in colorectal cancers and glioblastomas. *N Engl J Med.* 2004; 351(27):2883.
62. Mehra R, Tomlins SA, et al. Comprehensive assessment of TMPRSS2 and ETS family gene aberrations in clinically localized prostate cancer. *Mod Pathol.* 2007;20(5):538–544.
63. Nam RK, Sugar L, et al. Expression of TMPRSS2:ERG gene fusion in prostate cancer cells is an important prognostic factor for cancer progression. *Cancer Biol Ther.* 2007;6(1):40–45.
64. Winnes M, Lissbrant E, et al. Molecular genetic analyses of the TMPRSS2-ERG and TMPRSS2-ETV1 gene fusions in 50 cases of prostate cancer. *Oncol Rep.* 2007;17(5):1033–1036.

29 Cancer Nanotechnology

Mauro Ferrari, PhD

Definition of Nanotechnology and Chapter Organization

The prefix "nano" denotes 10^{-9}, or a billionth of a quantity. Thus, a nanometer (nm) is a billionth of a meter, ie, a length comparable to interatomic distances in crystalline lattices. The shortest distance between potassium atoms is ~0.5 nm; sodium chloride has a lattice constant of about 0.6 nm; while the diameter of glucose molecules is 0.9 nm and a water molecule is 0.3 nm. Many biological molecules range from a few to several hundred nanometers, such as albumin (4-14 nm), gamma globulins (9-10 nm), and pentameric M globulins (30-40 nm). The diameter of an erythrocyte, the smallest of eukaryotic cells, is 5-7 μm, or 5000-7000 nm. The volume occupied by a spherical cell with a 10 μm diameter could contain hundreds of millions of particles of nanometer diameter, at maximum packing density. Subcellular organelles of nanometric dimensions include ribosomes (20-30 nm), endosomes (70-300 nm), and the nucleus itself (>500 nm). Viruses have dimensions in the range of tens to the hundreds of nanometers, with parvovirus (20-30 nm) and HIV (120 nm) in opposing extremes of the dimensional range.

Biology organizes hierarchically with atomic components comprising the building blocks of nanometer scale entities, which are further organized at the micron scale, like organelles into cells, and then assembled upward into functional tissues, organs, and organisms. Science and technology have developed greatly at the atomic scale, where chemistry and physics reign, and in the macroscopic domains of engineering practice. Micron-scale technology arose, with great success, from the challenges of the electronic age. The missing dimensional link, to which Nobel Laureate Richard Feynman prompted the community with his seminal 1959 address "There is Plenty of Room at the Bottom,"[1] has been at the nanoscale. Nanotechnology addresses this gap in human endeavor.

Nanotechnology pertains to man-made objects that are nanoscale in dimensions, and that possess special, "emergent" properties that arise specifically because of their nano size. This is a three-part definition, where each part is equally necessary for an object to be classified as nanotechnological. This definition captures the consensus components of the many definitions that are present in the literature.[2,3] By extension, we will also consider larger objects that comprise a critical functioning component at the nanoscale as "nanotechnological" in this chapter. Additional restrictions posed by some authors and agencies on the definition of nanotechnology include the requirement that the word "nanoscale" be interpreted to encompass the range of 1-100 nm, and that an object be nanoscale in at least two dimensions. Rather, we insist that the defining "emerging property" be accompanied by a constructive validation expressed in mathematical terms[4] in analogy to the need for a mechanism of action to accompany the presentation of a novel drug. The definition of nanotechnology adopted by the National Cancer Institute is: *The field of research that deals with the engineering and creation of things from materials that are less than 100 nanometers (one-billionth of a meter) in size, especially single atoms or molecules.*

Following a brief summary of significant time points in the evolution of nanotechnology and its applications to cancer, fundamental nanotechnology platforms are presented in this chapter. A simple taxonomy is employed, dividing these platforms into analytical and diagnostic laboratory applications, vs those for in vivo use in diagnostic imaging and site-directed therapy. Brief overview of nanotechnological implants for sustained release drug delivery, reconstructive medicine, tissue engineering, and nanostructured materials for improved biocompatibility is also presented.

A Historical Perspective on Nanotechnology and Cancer

Foundational events in nanoscience and nanotechnology were the discovery of carbon-60 molecules, or fullerenes, and the development of scanning tunneling microscopy. Nobel Prizes were awarded to Richard Smalley, Robert Curl, and Harold Kroto for the former (1996, Chemistry) and to Heinrich Rohrer and Gerd Binning (1986, Physics) for the latter, which gave rise to the ability to manipulate individual atoms one at the time.

While it is expected that its full import is still to be realized, nanotechnology has already been present for quite a few years in medicine, and in particular in oncology. The paradigmatic drug-delivery nanoparticle is the liposome.[5] Liposomally formulated doxorubicin was approved by the Food and Drug Administration in the United States in 1996 for use against Kaposi's sarcoma, and has since been approved for use in metastatic breast cancer and recurrent ovarian cancer. Together with hundreds of on-going clinical trials, these applications make liposomes the first broadly employed nanotechnology in cancer. Imaging contrast agents of common use comprise nanosized particles such as iron oxide for magnetic resonance imaging (MRI). Two classes of devices originally developed in the domain of microtechnology have now become truly nanotechnological, due to the evolution of the underlying technological foundations. The first comprises microarrays or DNA chips[6] and the second encompasses microfluidic systems or lab-on-chip approaches to diagnostics and molecular bioseparation procedures.[7] For both, the fundamental enabling technology was photolithography, which at the time of their origin in the mid-1980s allowed the writing of features on a chip with lateral resolution of about 10-100 nm. Photolithography now affords resolution in the 10-100 nm range. The potential information density on a chip has therefore increased by 1-100 million-fold, powerfully illustrating the power of nanoscale manufacturing control. Gold colloids, chromatographic nanoscale degassing membranes, and many other examples illustrate the use of nano-artifacts in many areas of medicine.

The state of nanotechnology for cancer applications has been reviewed in the literature.[3,8-10] Major funding programs currently support nanomedicine with applications to oncology. In 2005, the National Cancer Institute launched a $144 million Alliance for nanotechnology in cancer. The European community Framework Programme VII emphasizes cancer applications in its nanotechnology funding priorities.

Nanotechnology Platforms

Nanotechnologies for Laboratory Applications in Diagnostics and Research

Ultraviolet (UV) photolithography on silicon substrates is the basic technique that allowed the development of the integrated circuit and resulted in the microelectronic revolution. With the recognition that silicon possesses remarkable mechanical properties came the drive toward micro-electro-mechanical systems (MEMS), such as chemical sensors, and accelerometers for the deployment of air bags in the automotive industry. UV photolithography again provided the underpinning for the development of micro- and nanotechnologies for medicine, with the advent of Bio-MEMS, or MEMS for biomedical applications. Among these are microfluidic systems that have risen in the mid-1980s and offer the advantage of the precise handling of nanoliter amount of fluids and reagents in the laboratory for diagnostic and research applications.[7] Microfluidic systems have received a major impetus for their commercialization from the development of mass-fabrication approaches. Originating from the insight of George Whitesides,[11] soft lithography allows for the use of inexpensive polymers as base materials for fluidic disposable units. Functions that can routinely be performed on microfluidic chips include cell sorting, optical sensing, various types of biomolecular separation, PCR amplification, and controlled conjugation reactions.

A most creative combination of photolithographic techniques and nucleic acid chemistry[6] gave rise to the sequencing technology platforms known as "microarrays" (Fig. 29-1A). Many different approaches to DNA sequencing were developed[12] that are commonly found in cancer research laboratories and contribute to the diagnostic and therapy personalization platforms. The ability to reduce lithographic limit of resolution into the tens of nanometers, developed in recent years, affords a much greater information density per unit area, and opens new exploratory horizons for the postgenomic era, and in particular for proteomics.[13] In this context, photolithographically defined domains can be used on silicon chips to selectively capture and enrich the concentration of proteins and degradation peptides from biological fluids, as a prefractionation step for mass spectrometric analysis.[14,15] This approach is particularly aimed at the low molecular weight, low concentration proteome fractions, and is under development for cancer screening and early diagnostics from serum and plasma.[16] Innovative nanotechnological approaches to cancer biomarker detection include nanowires[17,18] and cantilever beams.[19] Nanowires are biologically gated transistors, which act on the principle that a quantitatively measurable electrical signal is transmitted (Fig. 29-1B) when a target biomolecular analyte adsorbs or binds upon their surface. With their typical diving-board configuration (Fig. 29-1C), cantilever beams transduce biomolecular conjugation of target analytes on their surface into two quantitative responses: a laser light-measurable deflection, and a shift in resonant frequencies. The overall advantages potentially offered by nanotechnological approaches to molecular sensing are: limit of detection in the pico and attomolar range, rapidity of analysis, quantitation, convenience of sample preparation, the use of very minute amounts of analyte and reagents, and most importantly the ability to perform a large number of measurements at the same time. One limiting consideration for the nanodevices that employ antibodies as recognition strategies is the purity and availability of suitable antibodies. Approaches that involve alternative recognition moieties such as aptamers are under development in many laboratories. Nanotechnological molecular diagnostic devices have been demonstrated to rival or outperform commercial approaches.[19] However, they have not yet translated into widespread clinical uses.

Many different strategies have emerged for the use of biologically targeted nanoparticles for selective staining in immunochemistry. The first one employed quantum dots for the simultaneous detection of multiple molecular targets. A particularly cogent and innovative amplification and detection approach employable for proteins and nucleic acids alike was developed by Chad Mirkin. His "bio-bar-code" approach uses magnetic microparticle probes that specifically bind a target of interest and DNA-encoded nanoparticle probes.[20] The method was recently employed to simultaneously detect three protein cancer markers (PSA, HCG, and AFP) at low femtomolar concentrations.[21]

Conceptual Overview of Nanovectors or Nanoparticulates for the Delivery of Therapy and Imaging Contrast

The utilization of nanoparticles as carriers of therapeutic agents and imaging contrast is based on the concurrent, expected advantages of drug localization at tumor lesion and the ability to bypass the biological barriers encountered between the point of administration and the intended target. Physical localization at lesion site is commonly referred to as "targeting" in the drug-delivery community. The word "targeting" has a different

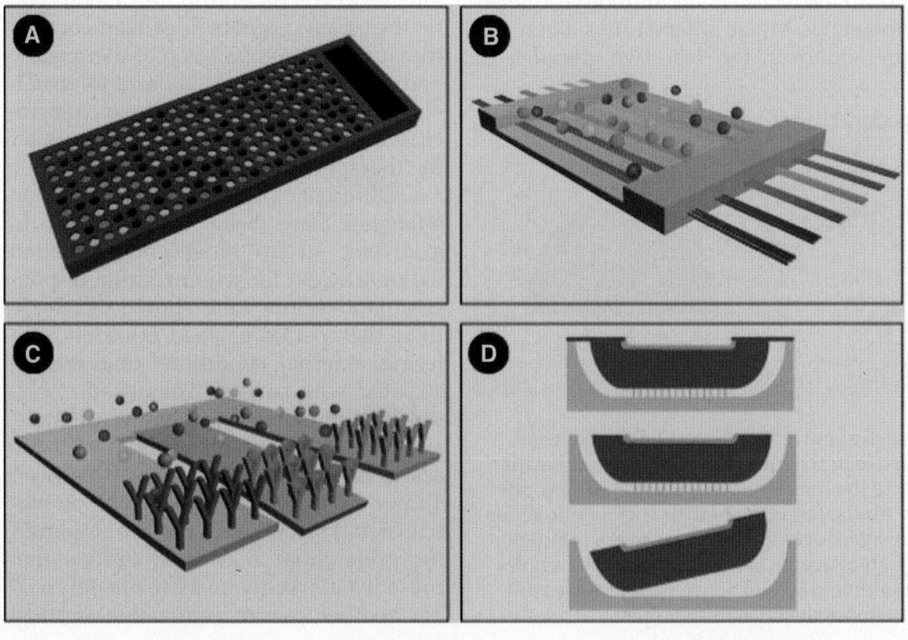

Figure 29-1 Ultraviolet photolithography is the key technology employed for the fabrication of electronic microchips and micro-electro-mechanical systems (MEMS). More recently, photolithography has been the cornerstone for the development of the following biomedical micro- and nanotechnologies: **(A)** nucleic acid microarrays[5]; **(B)** nanowires are biologically gated field effect sensors that send an electrical signal when contacted with a biomolecular analyte of interest, and can be used for the simultaneous detection of multiple cancer biomarkers[18]; **(C)** silicon cantilever beams for the quantitative detection of analytes including proteins and nuclei acids. The measured quantities are shifts in resonant frequencies, and optically measurable deflections[19]; and **(D)** nanoporous silicon microparticles manufactured with specific porosity, size, shape, and aspect ratio are used as delivery vectors for therapeutics and imaging contrast agents.[48]

meaning in the context of molecularly targeted therapeutics, where it signifies the preferential activity of the agent on tumor-associated biological pathways. In view of this difference, we will refer to nanoparticles that concentrate at desired lesion sites as "localizing" or "directed," rather than "targeted." We will occasionally use the term "targeting" when referring to antibody-mediated localization.

Nanoscale particles can act as contrast agents for all radiological imaging approaches. Iron oxide particle provides T2-mode negative contrast for MRI. Gold colloids and other metallic particulates offer enhanced contrast to x-ray and CT imaging in a manner essentially proportional to their atomic number. Mechanical impedence mismatch is the basis for the contrast in ultrasound imaging provided by the materials that are much stiffer (metals, ceramics) or much softer (microbubbles) than the surrounding tissue. The very existence of contrast agent can drive the development of new imaging modalities. The emergence of nanocrystalline quantum dots that do not photobleach and provide tunable emission properties based on their architecture and composition has generated great interest in novel optical imaging technologies. If they concentrate preferentially at tumor sites, nanoparticles comprising a contrast material can provide enhanced definition of anatomical contours, location, and extent of disease. If coupled with a biological recognition moiety, they can further offer molecular distribution information to the diagnostician.

A "nanovector" is a nanoscale particle for the delivery of therapeutic action or imaging contrast. In its simplest embodiment, a nanovector simply comprises the particle and the biologically active principle it carries (Fig. 29-2). Experience with liposomes and other particulates has shown that the nanovectors of dimensions between 10 and 1000 nm are cleared very rapidly from the blood stream, by means of uptake by the phagocytic cells of the reticuloendothelial system (RES).[5] To increase the clearance time, and thereby allow particles more time to localize at the desired target location, liposomes and other vectors are surface-decorated with polyethylene glycol (PEG) or other shielding moieties, that facilitate "stealth" delivery.[22] A nanoparticle comprising a drug and a stealth shielding layer is defined a "first-generation nanovector" (Fig. 29-2A), the paradigm for which are the current clinically available liposomal drug formulations. First-generation nanovectors localize at the tumor site by escaping the vascular compartment through the fenestrations that are typically present on tumor-associated, neovascular endothelia, and render the angiogenic vessels hyperpermeable. This passive localization mechanism is known as "enhanced permeation and retention" (EPR) (Fig. 29-3). EPR provides greater preferential tumor localization than the free drug. First-generation nanoparticulate contrast agents such as iron oxide nanoparticles are based on EPR. A different example of a first-generation nanovector is an albumin nanoparticle comprising paclitaxel. Approved in January 2005 for metastatic breast cancer with the trade name Abraxane,[23] this formulation does not require steroidal anti-inflammatory pretreatment, and allows administration of greater taxane dosages. The albumin acts as a trans-endothelial chaperone, increasing the likelihood of extravasation of the nanoparticle, but does not add tumor-targeting specificity.

Second-generation nanovectors by definition possess additional functionalities on individual particles (Fig. 29-2B). No nanovector of the second generation has secured FDA approval as yet, but many are currently engaged in clinical trials. A first example of second-generation nanovector is an antibody-targeted liposome. Much interest has been expressed over the last two decades in

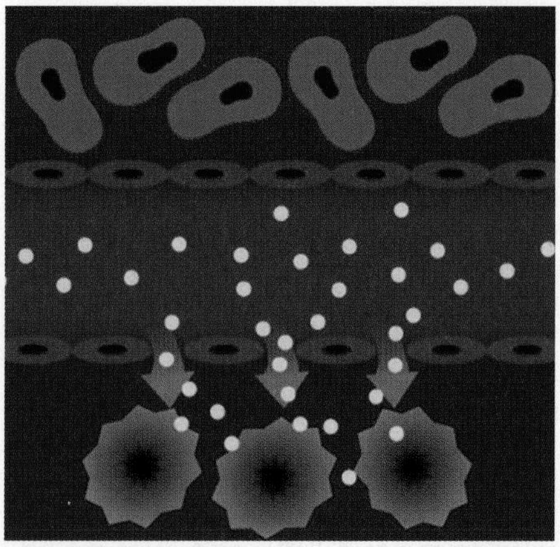

Figure 29-3 ■ Mechanism of passive tumor targeting by enhanced permeation and retention (EPR).

adding biological targeting capabilities to liposomes and many other vectors.[24] The dominant strategy involves the conjugation of targeting moieties to the surface of the nanovector, including antibodies,[25] ligands,[26] aptamers,[27] and small peptides.[28] Targeting has been directed to cancer cell surface markers and to molecules expressed in the tumor microenvironment, most notably on the tumor-associated vascular endothelium. A difficulty encountered with surface-bound biorecognition moieties is that they are typically much shorter than the PEG molecules used for evasion of the RES. Thus, they tend to be hidden inside the highly flexible PEG shield, resulting in a decrease in targeting efficacy. To avoid this problem, the targeting moiety has been attached at the distal end of the PEG chain. Different functionalities for second-generation nanovectors include the ability to attach two or more different moieties on the same nanoparticle. This strategy may be employed to provide local co-concentrations of synergistic therapeutic agents (localized cocktail therapy), or a combination of therapeutic and imaging moieties, in order to visualize the biodistribution of the active principle and to potentially monitor or alter the therapeutic course in real time.[29]

Different preferential localization strategies have been demonstrated in a diverse group of second-generation nanoparticles. Environmentally responsive nanovectors were shown to release their therapeutic payload upon encountering external conditions that are associated with cancers. For instance, pH-sensitive polymers will swell, degrade, and release drugs preferentially in the acidic environments of tumor lesions.[30] Tumor-associated enzymes such as matrix metalloproteinases may be employed for preferential release at lesions that present a markedly invasive phenotype.[31] Yet another cancer localization strategy

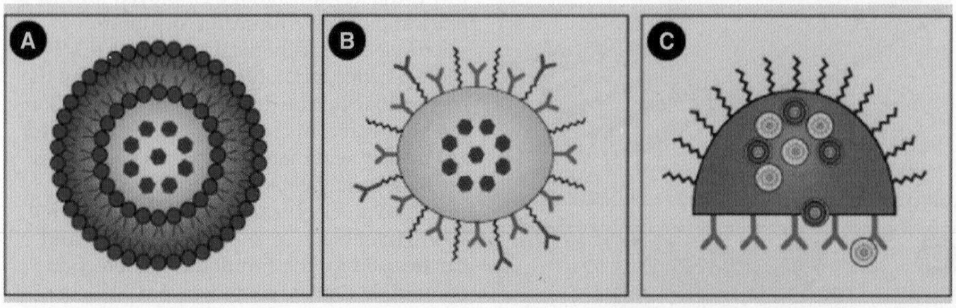

Figure 29-2 ■ **(A)** First-generation nanovectors such as currently clinical liposomes comprise a container and an active principle. They localize in the tumor by enhanced permeation and retention (EPR), or the enhanced permeability of the tumor neovasculature; **(B)** second-generation nanovectors further possess the ability for the targeting of their therapeutic action via antibodies and other biomolecules, remote activation, or responsiveness to environment; and **(C)** third-generation nanovectors such as multistage agents are capable of more complex functions, such a time-controlled deployment of multiple waves of active nanoparticles deployed across different biological barriers and with different subcellular targets.

involves the systemic administration of nanovectors, which discharge their therapeutic action only when triggered by an external stimulus. A diverse group of remote activation strategies has been demonstrated in vitro and in animal models. These include the activation of gold nanoshells by near-infrared (NIR) light. NIR radiation is harmless by itself, penetrates deeply into tissue, and upon irradiating suitably nanofabricated gold nanoshells causes the heating of the particles, which results in the thermal ablation of the surrounding cancer tissue.[32] The localization in this strategy is provided by the accurate pointing of the light beam onto the lesion, and in this sense it is similar to other photodynamic therapy approaches (PDT). The advantages in the nanoshell approach reside in the extent of cancer destruction, and the depth of tissue penetration. Another remote activation approach involves excitation of iron oxide nanoparticles with rapidly switching magnetic fields.[33] A further advantage of this approach is that the particles themselves are negative contrast agents for MRI, and therefore provide information on their biodistribution, and on the location and extent of the target lesion. Other remote activation strategies involve mechanical rupture of carriers by focused ultrasound,[34] the radiofrequency (RF) heating of carbon nanotubes for thermal ablation,[35] and the use of remotely induced heating not for thermal ablation per se, but as a triggering agent for the swelling of polymeric particle depots, with the concurrent release of drugs.[36]

Nanovectors have traditionally been considered passive carrier agents, limiting the analysis of their effect on cells to aspects of toxicity, biocompatibility, and clearance. However, recent developments on surface-derivatized metallic nanoparticles[37] have demonstrated the ability of nanoparticles to directly impact biological pathways of interest, such as apoptosis and proliferation through Akt and MAPK signaling. These interactions can be modulated by the design of the nanoparticle geometry as well as composition, and appear to be related to the redistribution and internalization of ErbB2 cell surface receptors associated with the uptake process of the herceptin-decorated nanovector. This observation opens the door to the development of nanovectors that will combine the effects of the bioactive principles they carry, with those induced, by design, through the control of their composition and geometry.[38]

Having briefly introduced the first two generations of nanovectors, in their great diversity, we can now reconsider their ability to penetrate biological barriers—ie, the fundamental advantages of nanovectored therapy—in a more comprehensive manner. Following parenteral administration, therapeutic agents encounter several biological barriers that impede their ability to reach cancer cells at effective concentrations.[3] The ability of nanovectors to penetrate these barriers is distinct from their ability to "recognize" the target, ie, by the use of antibodies, aptamers, or ligands. Despite high selectivity for cancer cells through recognition of distinctive molecular signatures, these agents invariably present with concentrations at target sites that are vastly inferior to what is expected on the basis of molecular recognition alone. Epithelial and endothelial barriers, such as the blood-brain barrier, are a prime example of biobarriers to therapeutic action. These are based on tight junctions that prevent or limit the paracellular transport of agents. Endo-/epithelial barriers are themselves multiplex and sequential in nature. The tight junctions owe their molecular discrimination to several structures made from distinctive proteins (occludin, claudin, desmosomes, zonula occludens). The selectivity of filtering is further enhanced by other biological barriers, such as the vascular endothelial basement membrane and the mucosal layer of the intestinal endothelium.

The interstitial oncotic pressure developed by cancers during their growth poses an entirely different biobarrier that prevents penetration of therapeutic agents, especially larger molecules and particles. Hemodynamics within the disordered tumor microvasculature also prevents nanoparticle localization in cancer cells due to lack of margination, firm adhesion, and endothelial cellular uptake.[39-41] Guided by mathematical simulations, it was shown that of all the geometries for drug-delivery nanoparticles, the worst possible is a spherical shape of about 50-100 nm diameter—which includes nearly all current nanoparticles in research, development, and clinical use. Spherical nanoparticles of these dimensions tend to stay in the center of the capillary blood flow, thus adversely impacting their extravasation through the fenestrations that are associated with the neovasculature, and limiting their ability to recognize specific molecular markers on the tumor-associated endothelium. Nanoparticulates of different, suitably designed shapes and sizes can offer a dramatic increase in therapeutic index, by optimizing their properties of margination, extravasation, firm adhesion to the vascular endothelium, and phagocytic uptake.

As a general observation, biological barriers present themselves sequentially to injected particulates and molecules. Mathematically, therefore, the probability of reaching the target lesion is obtained by multiplying the individual probabilities of passing through each of the different barriers. A nanovector with excellent properties of evasion of many barriers will not yield improvements in therapeutic index, even if a single barrier proves to be impassable. Localization, on the other hand, is the result of multiple concurrent mechanisms, including biological targeting using the specific surface moieties reviewed above, environmental triggering, site-specific remote activation, and passive EPR mechanisms, possibly enhanced by the design of the nanoparticles in suitable sizes and shapes. When multiple mechanisms are utilized, the probability of preferred localization of therapeutic action is once again the sum of the individual probabilities. Nanoparticles that utilize multiple, concurrent modalities to assure localization in cancer cells are therefore expected to exhibit superior localization efficacy. Many of the second-generation nanovectors utilize multimodal targeting, but have greater difficulty in passing through biological barriers due to their design.

Liposomes and other first- and second-generation nanotechnologies have proven successful for several specific indications, and will secure advances in an ever increasing number of clinical indications. However, based on the preceding considerations, it will be beneficial to develop a higher order of nanomanufacturing-based control over size, shape, multiparticle interactions, sequential activation, and other physicochemical controlling variables in order to attain the full benefit of nanomedicine.

In response to these requirements, third-generation nanovectors are here introduced as nanoscale particulates of higher complexity (Fig. 29-2C). By definition, they have the ability to perform a time sequence of functions that involve multiparticle cooperative coordination. An example of a third-generation nanovector is a "nanoshuttle,"[28] ie, a cluster of bacteriophage-entrapped metal nanoparticles. The envelopment by the networked phages provides for both the biological targeting, and the attainment of the critical mass that is required for therapeutic activity. Multistage systems were recently demonstrated,[42] and are another example of third-generation nanovector. As illustrated in Figure 29-4 these comprise a first-stage module that co-vectors multiple groups of different nanoparticles to a vascular endothelial site, deploys the second-stage nanoparticles in accordance with different time-release profiles, and degrades into elementary, biologically benign components. The different second-stage particles can be targeted to different tissue, cell surface, and ultimately to different subcellular locations. With their ability to perform time sequences of functions, third-generation

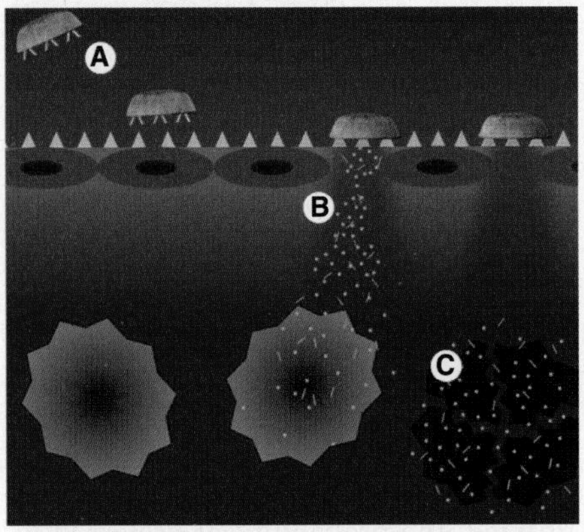

Figure 29-4 ■ The final stages of the intravenous journey with the arrival of a multistage vector and its payload of higher-stage nanoparticles anticancer medication. **(A)** shows the injected nanocarrier landing on the inner wall of a tumor-associated blood vessel, **(B)** the release of nanoparticles that penetrate both the blood vessel wall and the tumor cell membrane, and **(C)** the delivery to the tumor of doses of a cancer therapeutic agent.

nanoparticles offer opportunities to negotiate multiple, serially presented biological barriers, and therefore open new frontiers in drug delivery.

A Compendium of Therapeutic Nanovectors and Nanotechnological Imaging Contrast Agents

It is impossible to provide a full account of the very many different particle platforms in the rapidly evolving field of nanotechnology-enabled cancer imaging and therapeutics, and any attempt at taxonomy is inevitably marred by categorical overlaps. The major classes of nanovectors are based on lipids (eg, liposomes,[5] solid lipid nanoparticles[43]), polymers (eg, dendrimers, polymer-drug conjugates, biodegradable particulates[44]), metals (eg, colloidal gold, nanoshells, nanoshuttles[28]), carbon-60 nanovectors (fullerenes, nanotubes[35]), silicon-based particles,[42] biological nanoparticles (eg, engineered viral vectors,[45] bacterially derived nanoparticles[46]), magnetically activated oxides (eg, iron oxide[33]), and many others. Several nanovector systems include more than one class of materials.

First-Generation Therapeutic Nanovectors ■

Liposomes are the paradigmatic nanoparticles for drug delivery. The first-generation liposomes just employed EPR as a passive targeting mechanism to localize the delivery of anthracyclines such as doxorubicin (Myocet) and daunorubicin (DaunoXome) in order to reduce their cardiovascular toxicities in the treatment of recurrent and metastatic breast and ovarian cancers. Liposomal formulations of vincristine (OncoTCS) were approved for relapsed aggressive non-Hodgkins lymphoma. PEGylation was then introduced for the avoidance of RES uptake, giving rise to "stealth" liposome products of longer circulatory half-life (eg, Doxil/Caelyx for Kaposi sarcoma, breast and ovarian cancers). Liposomal formulations of amphoteracin B and ampicillin were approved for the treatment of cancer-related infections. Hundreds of clinical trials are currently underway, which investigate liposomal formulations in combination with chemotherapeutic and biotechnological agents for the therapy of many cancer types. EPR-based tumor targeting exploits the distinguishing characteristics of a biological barrier, the vascular endothelium, in a tumor-associated pathological presentation. Abraxane is a non-Cremophor-based, nanoparticle taxane formulation, which allows for higher dosing than paclitaxel since it does not require steroidal anti-inflammatory pretreatment. In a naked form, the taxane nanoparticles do not present the desired biodistribution, owing to the relative impermeability to the vascular endothelium. When encapsulated within an albumin shell, however, the taxane nanoparticles are chaperoned across the tumor vascular endothelium. Though it does not have molecular targeting capabilities, Abraxane was approved for the second-line treatment of metastatic breast cancer in 2005. The incorporation of RGD-targeting strategies on albumin nanocarriers was recently demonstrated in vitro.[47]

Polymer-drug conjugates are clinically available for hepatocellular carcinoma (Zinostatin/Stimalmer), acute lymphoblastic leukemia (Oncaspar), and the prevention of chemotherapy-associated neutropenia (Neulasta). PG-TXL comprises the conjugation of poly-l-glutamic acid to paclitaxel, and does not require Cremophor vehicle to address the limited solubility of the drug. Phase 2 clinical trials of PG-TXL on non-small cell lung cancer have yielded decreased collateral side effects and indication of improved efficacy for women with normal premenopausal estrogen levels.[48] Phase 3 studies in this patient group are currently underway.

EPR-based delivery strategies of any particle platform may be enhanced by the use of agents that increase the vascular permeability. For instance, low-dose delivery of an inhibitor of the transforming growth factor type I receptor was shown to reduce pericyte count in the vascular wall without reduction of the overall endothelial area. This led to increased therapeutic effectiveness of nanovectored doxorubicin for the therapy of intractable pancreatic and diffuse-type gastric cancers in murine models.[49] A mechanical approach to enhancing vascular and tissue permeability at target sites was introduced.[50] The method employed pulsed high-intensity ultrasound to allow for image-guided targeted delivery of macromolecular agents into the deep tissue.

Second-Generation Therapeutic Nanovectors ■

Vibrant research programs worldwide are dedicated to adding biomolecular recognition, targeting, and further functionalities to liposomal platforms.[51] The biomolecular targeting of liposomes through the RGD sequence or folate receptor are receiving particular interest. Neutral liposomes have emerged as a promising vehicle for biologically targeted delivery of siRNA, as demonstrated in vivo on a murine model of ovarian cancer.[52]

Dendrimers are polymers with repeatedly branched molecular structures.[53] They can be synthesized with exquisite control of sizes as small as a few nanometers, which affords their rapid clearance through the renal glomeruli. Dendrimers can host several cofunctioning moieties to provide biomolecular recognition, imaging contrast, and cytotoxicity. Methotrexate-containing polyamidoamine (PAMAM) G5 dendrimers were developed, which target tumor cells via the folate receptor. The formulation was administered to immunodeficient mice bearing KB tumors that overexpress the folic acid receptor, resulting in increased therapeutic efficacy and reduced adverse effects.[54] Biodegradable cationic amphiphilic copolymers were used to codeliver combinations of bioactive agents (paclitaxel, IL-12), genes, and siRNA complexes in 4T1 and MDA-MD-231 murine models of breast cancer.[55]

Remote triggering of EPR-targeted nanoparticles for the thermal ablation of tumors was demonstrated in a murine model by the groups of Naomi Halas and Jennifer West,[32] who employed silica-core gold nanoshells activated by deeply penetrating near-infrared (NIR) optical radiation. Biomolecular targeting by surface moieties was demonstrated in vitro. Heat from nanoshells or gold particles was also employed to trigger drug release from polymers.[36] Several alternative remote activation strategies have emerged, including the ultrasound-based release of fluorescent molecules from calcium carbonate particulates.[56] The laser-triggered release of fluorescent dyes within MDA-MB-435 cancer cells was demonstrated in vitro, employing polyelectrolyte-multilayer metallic capsules.[57]

PEGylated single-walled carbon nanotubes (SWNTs) were shown to concentrate at tumor sites, presumably by EPR, and to target tumor vasculature-expressed integrins via the RGD peptide sequence. Their biodistributions in murine models of human glioblastoma (U87MG cell line) and colorectal cancer (HT-29 cell line) were determined by microPET and confirmed by ex vivo Raman spectroscopy. The nanotubes are nondegradable, but they appear to be renally cleared over time, and may prove to support therapeutic delivery if concerns over adverse long-term effects are suitably addressed. The ability of SWNTs to deliver intracellularly both proteins and DNA in cell cultures was demonstrated.[58] Carbon nanotubes were remotely activated by noninvasive radiofrequency irradiation, leading to thermal ablation of gastrointestinal tumors in rabbit models.[35]

Thermal ablation of tumor cells was achieved by the heating of EPR-localized superparamagnetic iron oxide particle, through the application of rapidly switching magnetic fields. This approach is in clinical trials in Europe for glioblastoma multiforme.[59] The substitution of a superparamagnetic iron oxide core in the place of the silica core of the gold nanoshell affords for the particle itself to act as a MRI contrast agent, while retaining its thermal ablation properties.[60] Localization by surface decoration of nanoshells with guanylyl cyclase targeting surface moieties was presented as an innovative strategy for colorectal cancer treatment.[61] Similar approaches can be envisioned for other remotely activated nanoparticles.

Poly(ethylene oxide)-modified poly (beta-amino ester) nanoparticles are pH-sensitive, and degrade preferentially in the acidic environments, thereby leading to a tumor specificity of their therapeutic action. Such nanoparticles were loaded with paclitaxel and administered to mice bearing human ovarian adenocarcinoma (SKOV-3), resulting in enhanced therapeutic efficacy and safety.[62] General tumor-targeting strategies that employ pH- and thermally sensitive polymer particles were demonstrated in the literature. The combined use of PEG stealthing and pH sensitivity was shown to improve the biodistribution of liposomal cisplatin in a murine model of Ehrlich tumor.[63] Multifunctional polymeric nanoparticles ("nanoplatforms") with the ability to penetrate the blood-brain barrier for the imaging and treatment of brain cancers were recently reviewed.[64]

Third-Generation Therapeutic Nanovectors ■ Nanoparticle-aptamer conjugates are a first example of combination of two different nanotechnologies. The first implementation of this approach employed RNA aptamers that bind to prostate-specific membrane antigen to target prostate cancer epithelial cells with a drug model, and was followed by in vivo validation.[65] A multiplicity of different, site-specific nanoscale functionalities can be added to carrier particles, employing novel particle lithography techniques.[66] The approach was employed to demonstrate localized targeting on 3T3 fibroblasts in vitro by means of the RGD recognition sequence. Paclitaxel was incorporated with a self-assembly, layer-by-layer technique on polymeric cores, to form a new class of macromolecular nanoshell.[66] The therapeutic efficacy of the system was validated in vitro on MCF-7 breast cancer cells. Nanocells[67] are composite nanoparticles of ~200 nm diameters that comprise a phospholipid-based shell surrounding a biodegradable polymeric core. The core is synthesized to contain an antitumoral agent such as doxorubicin, while the outer shell provides evasion from RES uptake and comprises antiangiogenic compounds such as combrestatin. The system delivers the active compounds in temporal sequence to the tumor, and was demonstrated to reduce B16/F10 melanoma and Lewis lung carcinoma growth in murine models.[67] The staged delivery is directed at circumventing a conundrum of antiangiogenic treatment, namely the inability of chemotherapeutic agents to reach the tumor after its neo-vasculature has been shut down.

PEGylation increases the circulation time of nanoparticles, but adversely impacts biological recognition and targeting.[68] This simple observation has spurred research into therapeutic delivery systems that combine different nanocomponents, rather than replicate the paradigm of the PEG-covered nanovector. Spontaneous assemblies of gold nanoparticles and bacteriophage ("nanoshuttles") were developed and shown in melanoma cell cultures to convert NIR to heat, to provide biologically targeting through the phages via the 4C-RGD sequence, and to have the ability to serve as labels for enhanced fluorescence, dark field microscopy, and surface-enhanced Raman scattering.[28]

Multistage delivery particulates were introduced,[42] which comprise a nanoporous silicon first-stage microparticulate carrier (Fig. 29-2C). The first-stage particles are designed for optimal margination, adhesion to the vascular endothelium, and cellular uptake, in accordance with mathematical rational design prescriptions.[39-41] They were fabricated employing versatile photolithographic methods (Fig. 29-1D). The first-stage carriers are fully biodegradable, in a time-tunable fashion, with biologically benign degradation products. They release second- and higher-stage nanoparticles and bioactive agents which can penetrate into the stroma and the target cells. The multistage strategy, summarized in Figure 29-4, provides sequential release of different agents and carriers, so that the biological barriers to desired biodistributions can be sequentially addressed. The uptake and release of several second-stage nanoparticles was demonstrated, including the co-delivery of carbon nanotubes and quantum dots.[42]

Nanoparticle Contrast Agents ■ Much interest has been dedicated to the use of magnetic nanoparticles (MNP) as MRI contrast agents. Gadolinum-based T1-mode nanoparticles[69] and iron oxide T2-mode contrast nanoparticles[70] were demonstrated in animal models. The use of nanoparticles allows for dual-mode imaging, combining optical and MRI detection on a single platform[71] that can also be biomolecularly targeted. Dextran-based ferumoxytol was employed as bolus-administered T1 contrast to stage prostate cancer patients based on lymph node involvement.[72] The interest in lymph node metastases in nanotech-enabled imaging addresses the desire for nonsurgical node evaluation, and takes advantage of the fact that the nanoparticles are naturally drained via the lymphatics, and therefore can act as first-generation contrast, without need for additional biomolecular targeting.

The vascular endothelium may be a barrier for nanoparticle penetration into tumors, but by the same exclusion mechanisms a long-circulating nanoparticle may be advantageously used for targeting pathological vasculature. Under the combined leadership of M. Bednarski, D. Cheresh, and King Li, this approach was employed to image angiogenesis in animal tumor models.[73] The targeting of pathological vascular endothelium through overexpressed integrins was further demonstrated in imaging and targeted therapeutic applications in animal models by many groups. MRI nanoparticles were first employed to demonstrate the synergy between imaging and tissue analysis in vivo,[74] which can lead to targeted biomarker discovery and personalized therapeutic approaches.

Quantum dots have exceptional potential as optical imaging contrast since they do not photobleach and they can be manufactured in a broad array of different emission properties.[9,75] They were recently employed in animal models to differentiate cancer cells from their microenvironment, and in particular vessels, perivascular cells, and matrix.[76]

A concern with Cd-Se quantum dots is their potential cytotoxicity. In general, it may be expected that clinical deployment will be facilitated for nanoparticulates and nanovectors that are fully biodegradable, with no health-adverse residue at the administered dosages. Among these are liposomes, polylactic and polyglycolic acid-based nanopolymers, and nanoporous silicon particles. Quantum dots, gold nanoshells, and carbon nanotubes are among the non-biodegradable nanoparticles, which require careful scrutiny and addressing of toxicity and clearance concerns.

Nanotechnologies for Therapeutic Implants

The application of nanotechnologies for therapeutic implants is largely at the stage of laboratory research and preclinical development, yet it provides intriguing vistas on novel approaches to cancer care. Silicon nanotechnology has been used to demonstrate membranes with nanoscale channels manufactured with exquisite control over the nanochannel surface chemistry and its dimensions. Suitable tailoring of these control variables allows for the control of the release rate of therapeutic molecules from implants, achieving non-Fickian, constant release rates of biomolecular drugs for several weeks. The potential of these devices for the outpatient therapy of cancer has been discussed and illustrated in a murine model of melanoma. The application of electric fields across the nanochannel membranes gives rises to electro-osmosis, a nanoscale transport phenomenon that can be employed to modify the release rates from the implants. This opens the possibility of implanted devices that release therapeutic agents at a preprogrammed rate, or that can be remotely control to start, stop, or change release rates. An intriguing possibility is the development of implant devices that comprise sensors—biomolecular or physical—together with an intelligence-on-board processing chip, and active release mechanisms. Such devices could provide the release of cancer therapeutics in an intelligent, self-controlled fashion, for instance self-limiting the release when biomarkers of adverse reactions exceed a predetermined acceptability threshold.

The nanochannel technology was originally developed with the objective of providing immunoisolation for implanted cell bioreactors.[77] In this vision, the encapsulated cell xenografts would act as self-regulating providers of therapeutic agents. Therapeutic implants comprising a greater complexity of biological cells and engineered components were recently proposed.[78] A more near-term, yet high-impact envisioned use of nanotechnology is the development of biocompatible coatings for prosthetic implants as may be needed for cosmetic and functional reconstruction following cancer surgery. The principle underlying this approach is that the coatings can be made to comprise nanoscale domains which spatially alternate hydrophobic and hydrophilic characteristics. These oppose the extensive denaturing of proteins at the implant surface, which is the first step in the development of the cascade of molecular and cellular events that comprise inflammatory responses and decrease the body tolerance of the implant. In more advanced tissue-engineering scenarios, the implant nanomaterial itself could actively stimulate tissue regrowth and the recovery of compromised or lost functions.

Selected References

The complete reference list can be found at www.CANCERMEDICINE8.com

1. Feynman R. There is plenty of room at the bottom. *Eng Sci.* 1960;23:22-36.
2. Feature: nan′ o.tech.nol′ o.gy n. Nature Nanotechnology 2006;8-10.
3. Ferrari M. Cancer nanotechnology: opportunities and challenges. *Nat Rev Cancer.* 2005;5:161-171.
4. Ferrari M. The mathematical engines of nanomedicine. *Small.* 2008;4:20-25.
5. Gabizon A, Chisin R, Amselem S, et al. Pharmacokinetic and imaging studies in patients receiving a formulation of liposome-associated adriamycin. *Br J Cancer.* 1991;64:1125-1132.
6. Fodor SPA, Read JL, Pirrung MC, et al. Light-directed, spatially addressable parallel chemical synthesis. *Science.* 1991;251:767-773.
12. Ozkan M, Heller, M., Ferrari, M., eds. *Micro/Nano Technology for Genomics and Proteomics.* Springer; 2006.
13. Cheng MM, Cuda G, Bunimovich YL, et al. Nanotechnologies for biomolecular detection and medical diagnostics. *Curr Opin Chem Biol.* 2006;10:11-19.
16. Liotta LA, Ferrari M, Petricoin E. Clinical proteomics: written in blood. *Nature.* 2003;425:905.
17. Cui Y, Wei QQ, Park HK, Lieber CM. Nanowire nanosensors for highly sensitive and selective detection of biological and chemical species. *Science.* 2001;293:1289-1292.
18. Zheng G, Patolsky F, Cui Y, et al. Multiplexed electrical detection of cancer markers with nanowire sensor arrays. *Nat Biotechnol.* 2005;23:1294-1301.
19. Wu GH, Datar RH, Hansen KM, et al. Bioassay of prostate-specific antigen (PSA) using microcantilevers. *Nat Biotechnol.* 2001;19:856-860.
20. Nam JM, Thaxton CS, Mirkin CA. Nanoparticle-based bio-bar codes for the ultrasensitive detection of proteins. *Science.* 2003;301:1884-1886.
21. Stoeva SI, Lee JS, Smith JE, et al. Multiplexed detection of protein cancer markers with biobarcoded nanoparticle probes. *J Am Chem Soc.* 2006;128:8378-8379.
22. Harris JM, Chess RB. Effect of pegylation on pharmaceuticals. *Nat Rev Drug Discov.* 2003;2:214-221.
23. Gradishar WJ. Albumin-bound paclitaxel: a next-generation taxane. *Expert Opin Pharmacother.* 2006;7:1041-1053.
28. Souza GR, Christianson DR, Staquicini FI, et al. Networks of gold nanoparticles and bacteriophage as biological sensors and cell-targeting agents. *Proc Natl Acad Sci USA.* 2006;103:1215-1220.
29. Choi Y, Baker JR, Jr. Targeting cancer cells with DNA-assembled dendrimers: a mix and match strategy for cancer. *Cell Cycle.* 2005;4:669-671.
31. Sarkar N, Banerjee J, Hanson AJ, et al. Matrix metalloproteinase-assisted triggered release of liposomal contents. *Bioconjug Chem.* 2008;19:57-64.
32. O'Neal DP, Hirsch LR, Halas NJ, et al. Photo-thermal tumor ablation in mice using near infrared-absorbing nanoparticles. *Cancer Lett.* 2004;209:171-176.
33. Bergey EJ, Levy L, Wang XP, et al. DC magnetic field induced magnetocytolysis of cancer cells targeted by LH-RH magnetic nanoparticles in vitro. *Biomed Microdevices.* 2002;4:293-299.
34. Frenkel V, Etherington A, Greene M, et al. Delivery of liposomal doxorubicin (Doxil) in a breast cancer tumor model: investigation of potential enhancement by pulsed-high intensity focused ultrasound exposure. *Acad Radiol.* 2006;13:469-479.
35. Gannon CJ, Cherukuri P, Yakobson BI, et al. Carbon nanotube-enhanced thermal destruction of cancer cells in a noninvasive radiofrequency field. *Cancer.* 2007;110:2654-2665.
36. Owens DE, 3rd, Eby JK, Jian Y, Peppas NA. Temperature-responsive polymer-gold nanocomposites as intelligent therapeutic systems. *J Biomed Mater Res A.* 2007;83:692-695.
38. Ferrari M. Nanogeometry: beyond drug delivery. *Nat Nanotechnol.* 2008;3:131-132.
40. Decuzzi P, Ferrari M. Design maps for nanoparticles targeting the diseased microvasculature. *Biomaterials.* 2008;29:377-384.
41. Decuzzi P, Ferrari M. The receptor-mediated endocytosis of non-spherical particles. *Biophys J.* 2008:E Pub Ahead of print.
42. Tasciotti E, Liu X, Bhavane R, et al. Mesoporous Silicon particles as a multi stage delivery system for imaging and therapeutic applications *Nat Nanotechnol.* 2008;3:151-157.
43. Koziara JM, Lockman PR, Allen DD, Mumper RJ. Paclitaxel nanoparticles for the potential treatment of brain tumors. *J Control Release.* 2004;99:259-269.
44. Duncan R. Polymer conjugates as anticancer nanomedicine. *Nat Rev Cancer.* 2006;6:688-701.
46. MacDiarmid JA, Mugridge NB, Weiss JC, et al. Bacterially derived 400 nm particles for encapsulation and cancer cell targeting of chemotherapeutics. *Cancer Cell.* 2007;11:431-445.
49. Kano MR, Bae Y, Iwata C, et al. Improvement of cancer-targeting therapy, using nanocarriers for intractable solid tumors by inhibition of TGF-beta signaling. *Proc Natl Acad Sci USA.* 2007;104:3460-3465.
50. Bednarski MD, Lee JW, Callstrom MR, Li KC. In vivo target-specific delivery of macromolecular agents with MR-guided focused ultrasound. *Radiology.* 1997;204:263-268.
51. Torchilin VP. Recent advances with liposomes as pharmaceutical carriers. *Nat Rev Drug Discov.* 2005;4:145-160.
52. Halder J, Kamat AA, Landen CN, Jr., et al. Focal adhesion kinase targeting using in vivo short interfering RNA delivery in neutral liposomes for ovarian carcinoma therapy. *Clin Cancer Res.* 2006;12:4916-4924.
54. Kukowska-Latallo JF, Candido KA, Cao Z, et al. Nanoparticle targeting of anticancer drug improves therapeutic response in animal model of human epithelial cancer. *Cancer Res.* 2005;65:5317-5324.
59. Maier-Hauff K, Rothe R, Scholz R, et al. Intracranial thermotherapy using magnetic nanoparticles combined with external beam radiotherapy: results of a feasibility study on patients with glioblastoma multiforme. *J Neurooncol.* 2007;81:53-60.

30 Cancer Epidemiology

Michael J. Thun, MD, MS ■ Ahmedin Jemal, DVM, PhD

Introduction

The magnitude of the human and economic costs of cancer in the United States is enormous. Based on current incidence rates and the age structure of the population, approximately one in every two men and one in three women in the United States will be diagnosed with an invasive cancer during their lifetime.[1] Malignant diseases afflict two out of every three families. The annual cost of cancer is estimated to be $228.1-$93.2 billion for direct medical costs, $18.8 billion for lost productivity, and $116.1 billion for indirect mortality costs.[2]

This chapter describes the use of epidemiologic methods to monitor patterns of cancer occurrence and to identify factors that may increase or decrease the risk of cancer. By definition, epidemiologic studies examine the occurrence and determinants of disease in populations rather than in individual patients. This chapter also describes the measures used to characterize disease occurrence in epidemiologic studies, the role of surveillance and descriptive epidemiology to monitor temporal trends, geographic patterns, disparities, and the approaches used in analytic epidemiology to identify etiologic factors that influence cancer occurrence or progression.

Measures of Disease Occurrence

The primary measures of cancer occurrence are incidence and death rates, usually expressed per 100,000 persons per year. Incidence rates represent the number of newly diagnosed cases that occur each year in a population of specified size. Mortality rates represent the corresponding number of deaths, also generally expressed per 100,000 person years of observation. It is essential that rates be expressed based on a common person-time denominator if comparisons are to be made across populations of varying size and length of observation.[3]

Another measure of cancer occurrence, more familiar to the public, is the total number of newly diagnosed cancers or deaths that occur in a given year in a specified geographic area. Information on the current or projected count of cancer cases or deaths can be useful in determining health services needs for a region. However, numerator data alone do not allow valid comparisons of risk across populations that differ in size, duration of follow-up, or age. Thus, the number of cases or deaths in a given geographic area does not enumerate the average risk for individuals in the population.

Age and Age Adjustment

A fundamental characteristic of many cancers is that incidence and death rates increase exponentially with age during adulthood. The increase in the age-specific incidence rate of all cancers combined is so large that about 76% of all invasive cancers occur among the approximately 20% of the U.S. population 55 years of age or older.[1] Figure 30-1 shows that the death rate from all cancers combined increases progressively after age ten, and that the incidence rate increases with age except among persons age 85 and above. The decrease in cancer incidence rates in the oldest age group is predominantly an artifact of less complete diagnosis in the elderly and lower lung cancer incidence in the generations that preceded the peak of cigarette smoking in the United States. This downturn has occurred at progressively older ages over time as birth cohorts with substantial exposure to cigarette smoking populate progressively older age groups.

Rather than characterize all of the age-specific rates shown in Figure 30-1, vital statistics data and epidemiologic studies often present a single age-adjusted or age-standardized rate to compare cancer occurrence across populations with a different age composition. Age standardization serves a dual purpose: it summarizes the age-specific rates into a single number, and eliminates age differences between the populations by assigning them all a "standard" age distribution.[4] Age-specific rates are multiplied by the number of people within the corresponding 5-year age group in a "standard" population. The products or number of cases expected in each age group in the standard population, are then added across all age groups, and divided by the total number of people in the population to yield the age-standardized rate. Beginning with 1999 mortality and incidence data, U.S. cancer statistics have been standardized to the population estimates of year 2000

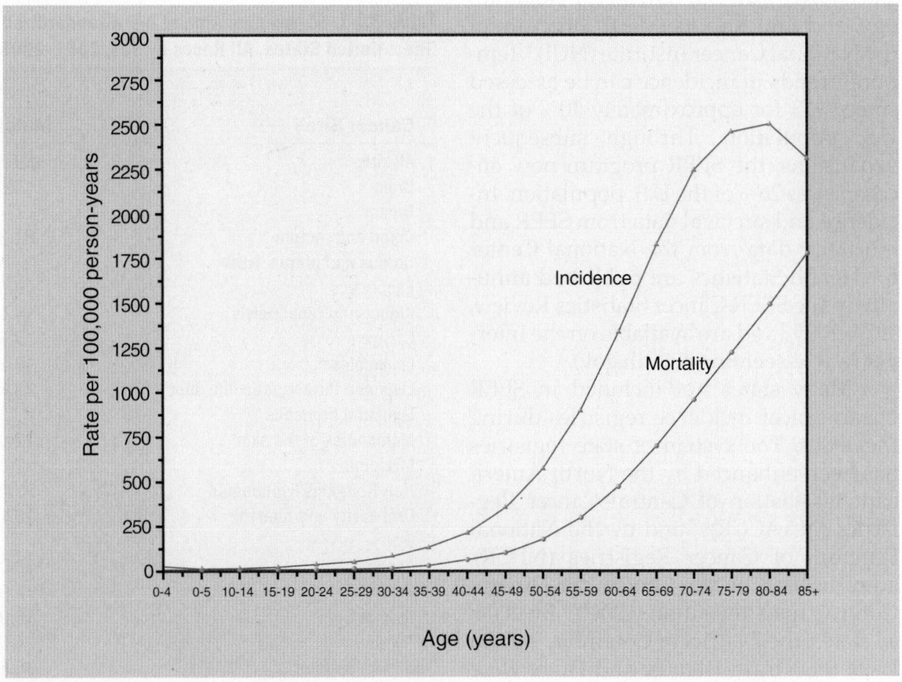

Figure 30-1 ■ Age-specific incidence and mortality rates from all cancers combined, United States, 1997–2001.

rather than to the 1970 U.S. age distribution. Valid comparisons of incidence or death rates from different populations or in different time periods can only be made when the rates have been standardized to the same age standard.

Cancer Surveillance

Descriptive epidemiologic studies measure the occurrence of cancer and other health-related factors in relation to person (eg, age, sex, race, social class, behavioral factors, etc.), place, and time. This section describes the systems that collect and report data on cancer incidence and mortality. It also discusses current patterns and trends in cancer occurrence, counts, individual lifetime probability of developing various cancers, and disparities in cancer occurrence and survival across subgroups of the population.

Date Collection and Reporting

Population-based statistics on cancer incidence and mortality are collected under several systems. Mortality data have been available nationally for most of the country since 1930.[1] Causes of death are reported on death certificates filed in the states. From these, the underlying cause of death is determined using criteria specified by the World Health Organization (WHO). Beginning with 1999, cancer deaths have been coded according to the tenth revision of the International Classification of Diseases (ICD-10).

Cancer incidence has been monitored since 1973 by the Surveillance, Epidemiology, and End Results (SEER) program of the National Cancer Institute (NCI).[5] Temporal trends in incidence can be assessed since 1973 for approximately 10% of the U.S. population. Through subsequent expansions, the SEER program now encompasses 26% of the U.S. population. Incidence and survival data from SEER and mortality data from the National Center for Health Statistics are published annually in the SEER Cancer Statistics Review, 1973–2005,[5] and are available on the Internet (www-seer.ims.nci.nih.gov).

Many states not included in SEER began cancer incidence registries during the 1980s. The system of state registries has been enhanced by the North American Association of Central Cancer Registries (NAACCR)[6,7] and by the National Program of Cancer Registries (NPCR), administered by the Centers for Disease Control and Prevention (CDC).[8] By 2004, 45 states, the District of Columbia, Puerto Rico, the Virgin Islands, and Palau were receiving appropriations from CDC to support their cancer registries.[6] State-specific cancer incidence and mortality data are available on the internet at http://statecancerprofiles.cancer.gov/. Incidence data for the combined SEER and NPCR registries are published annually.[7]

Many hospital registries also tabulate data on cancer care provided in their facility. Hospital registries are not population-based, yet they provide much of the primary data for state and other population-based registries. Hospitals that participate in the Approvals Program of the American College of Surgeons (ACoS) receive an annual report from the National Cancer Data Base (NCDB) that allows them to compare the cancer care statistics from their facility with those of other approved hospitals. The types and frequencies of cancers treated at a particular hospital may not be representative of the population as a whole due to distinctive referral patterns and catchment areas. The NCDB covers approximately 75% of cancer cases treated in the United States. It is currently the only registry that provides feedback on cancer care to participating hospitals.

International statistics on cancer occurrence are compiled by the International Agency for Research on Cancer (IARC), a division of the WHO. Nationwide incidence data are available from a few countries. More commonly, incidence data are collected in regional registries.[9] Where cancer incidence data are not available, the IARC uses age-, gender-, and cancer site-specific mortality statistics to estimate incidence. International data are available in both tabular[10,11] and map form through the IARC Globocan website, www.dep.iarc.fr. Mortality statistics reported to IARC derive mainly from the WHO mortality database.[11]

Age-Adjusted Incidence and Death Rates

Table 30-1 shows the average age-adjusted incidence and death rates from various cancers in the United States during the period 2001–2005. The death rates represent the entire United States; the incidence rates cover 40 states and the District of Columbia.[12] The rates in Table 30-1 are standardized to the age distribution of the U.S. population in the year 2000[12] and can be compared validly to any other rates that are age-adjusted to the same standard population. They cannot be compared to many international statistics, however, since vital statistics published by IARC are standardized to the world population, which is based on the international age distribution in approximately 1960.[10,11,13]

Estimated Number of Cases and Deaths From Cancer

Other widely cited indices of cancer occurrence are the estimates of new cases and deaths, published annually by the American Cancer Society (ACS).[1] Table 30-2 shows the estimated number of new cases and deaths predicted by ACS in 2008. The estimates of new cases are based on data from the SEER program, projected onto census information about the size and age-structure of the U.S. population.[14] The estimated number of deaths is based on the actual number of cancer deaths recorded annually in the United States from 1969 until the most recent year for which data are available, projected forward to the

Table 30-1 **Average Annual Age-Standardized Incidence and Death Rates[a] for Selected Cancer Sites: United States, All Races by Sex, 2001–2005**

Cancer Sites	Incidence Rates		Death Rates	
	Males	Females	Males	Females
All sites	562.3	417.3	234.4	159.9
Brain	7.9	5.7	5.4	3.6
Breast	–	123.6	0.3	25.0
Colon and rectum	61.2	44.8	22.7	15.9
Corpus and uterus, NOS	–	23.8	–	4.1
Esophagus	8.6	2.0	7.8	1.7
Kidney and renal pelvis	19.1	9.8	6.0	2.7
Larynx	7.3	4.0	2.3	0.5
Leukemias	16.2	9.7	9.9	5.6
Liver and intrahepatic bile duct	8.8	3.1	7.3	3.1
Lung and bronchus	87.3	55.4	72.0	41.0
Melanomas of the skin	22.0	14.2	3.9	1.7
Myeloma	7.0	4.6	4.6	3.0
Non-Hodgkins lymphomas	23.2	16.3	9.3	5.9
Oral cavity and pharynx	16.1	6.1	4.3	1.6
Ovary	–	13.3	–	8.8
Pancreas	13.0	10.1	12.2	9.3
Prostate	158.3	–	26.7	–
Stomach	10.3	5.0	5.7	2.9
Thyroid	4.6	13.4	0.5	0.5
Urinary bladder	38.4	9.8	7.5	2.3
Uterine cervix	–	8.5	–	2.5

[a]Rates are per 100,000 and are age-adjusted to the 2000 U.S. standard population.
Source: Jemal et al., *JNCI* 2008;100:1672–1694.

Table 30-2 ■ **Estimated Number of New Cancer Cases and Deaths by Sex: United States, 2008**[a]

	Estimated New Cases			Estimated Deaths		
	Both Sexes	**Male**	**Female**	**Both Sexes**	**Male**	**Female**
All sites	1,437,180	745,180	692,000	565,650	294,120	271,530
Oral cavity and pharynx	35,310	25,310	10,000	7,590	5,210	2,380
Tongue	10,140	7,280	2,860	1,880	1210	670
Mouth	10,820	6,590	4,230	1,840	1120	720
Pharynx	12,410	10,060	2,350	2,200	1620	580
Other oral cavity	1,940	1,380	560	1,670	1,260	410
Digestive system	271,290	148,560	122,730	135,130	74,860	60,280
Esophagus	16,470	12,970	3,500	14,280	11,250	3,030
Stomach	21,500	13,190	8,310	10,880	6,450	4,430
Small intestine	6,110	3,200	2,910	1,110	580	530
Colon[b]	108,070	53,760	54,310	49,960	24,260	25,700
Rectum	40,740	23,490	17,250	–	–	–
Anus, anal canal, and anorectum	5,070	2,020	3,050	680	250	430
Liver and intrahepatic bile duct	21,370	15,190	6,180	18,410	12,570	5,840
Gallbladder and other biliary	9,520	4,500	5,020	3,340	1,250	2,090
Pancreas	37,680	18,770	18,910	34,290	17,500	16,790
Other digestive organs	4,760	1,470	3,290	2,180	740	1,440
Respiratory system	232,270	127,880	104,390	166,280	94,210	72,070
Larynx	12,250	9,680	2,570	3,670	2,910	760
Lung and bronchus	215,020	114,690	100,330	161,840	90,810	71,030
Other respiratory organs	5,000	3,510	1,490	770	490	280
Bones and joints	2,380	1,270	1,110	1,470	820	650
Soft tissue (including heart)	10,390	5,720	4,670	3,680	1,880	1,800
Skin (excluding basal and squamous)	67,720	38,150	29,570	11,200	7,360	3,840
Melanoma-skin	62,480	34,950	27,530	8,420	5,400	3,020
Other nonepithelial skin	5,240	3,200	2,040	2,780	1,960	820
Breast	184,450	1,990	182,460	40,930	450	40,480
Genital system	274,150	195,660	78,490	57,820	29,330	28,490
Uterine cervix	11,070	–	11,070	3,870	–	3,870
Uterine corpus	40,100	–	40,100	7,470	–	7,470
Ovary	21,650	–	21,650	15,520	–	15,520
Vulva	3,460	–	3,460	870	–	870
Vagina and other genital, female	2,210	–	2,210	760	–	760
Prostate	186,320	186,320	–	28,660	28,660	–
Testis	8,090	8,090	–	380	380	–
Penis and other genital, male	1,250	–	1,250	–	290	290
Urinary system	125,490	85,870	39,620	27,810	18,430	9,380
Urinary bladder	68,810	51,230	17,580	14,100	9,950	4,150
Kidney and renal pelvis	54,390	33,130	21,260	13,010	8,100	4,910
Ureter and other urinary organs	2,290	1,510	780	700	380	320
Eye and orbit	2,390	1,340	1,050	240	130	110
Brain and other nervous system	21,810	11,780	10,030	13,070	7,420	5,650
Endocrine system	39,510	10,030	29,480	2,430	1,110	1,320
Thyroid	37,340	8,930	28,410	1,590	680	910
Other endocrine	2,170	1,100	1,070	840	430	410
Lymphoma	74,340	39,850	34,490	20,510	10,490	10,020
Hodgkin lymphoma	8,220	4,400	3,820	1,350	700	650
Non-Hodgkin lymphoma	66,120	35,450	30,670	19,160	9,790	9,370
Myeloma	19,920	11,190	8,730	10,690	5,640	5,050
Leukemia	44,270	26,180	19,090	21,710	12,460	9,250
Acute lymphocytic leukemia	5,430	3,220	2,210	1,460	800	660
Chronic lymphocytic leukemia	15,110	8,750	6,360	4,390	2,600	1,790
Acute myeloid leukemia	13,290	7,200	6,090	8,820	5,100	3720
Chronic myeloid leukemia	4,830	2,800	2,030	450	200	250
Other leukemia[c]	5,610	3,210	2,400	6,590	3,760	2,830
Other and unspecified primary sites[c]	31,490	15,400	16,090	45,090	24,330	20,760

[a]Rounded to the nearest 10; estimated new cases exclude basal and squamous cell skin cancers and in situ carcinomas except urinary bladder. About 67,770 female carcinoma in situ of the breast and 54,020 melanoma in situ will be newly diagnosed in 2008.
[b]Estimated deaths for colon and rectum cancers are combined.
[c]More deaths than cases suggests lack of specificity in recording underlying causes of death on death certificates.
Source: American Cancer Society, Cancer Facts & Figures 2008 (http://seer.cancer.gov/csr/1975_2005/index.html).

current year.[15] The value of the ACS projections is that they are current, readily understood by the public, and reasonably accurate when compared to the actual counts of cancer deaths, tabulated several years later. However, they represent projections rather than actual measurements. Because they estimate the absolute *number* of cancer cases and deaths rather than the *rates* shown in Figure 30-1, they increase with growth of the population and aging, even when age-specific rates remain constant.

Figures 30-2 and 30-3 show the percentage of all cancer cases or deaths contributed by the ten most common sites in U.S. men and women, for incidence and mortality respectively. The percentages are based on the ACS estimates for 2008.[1,16] Cancer of the lung and bronchus is the most common cancer site causing death in both sexes, whereas prostate cancer (in men) and breast cancer (in women) are the leading incident cancers. Four cancers (lung and bronchus, breast,

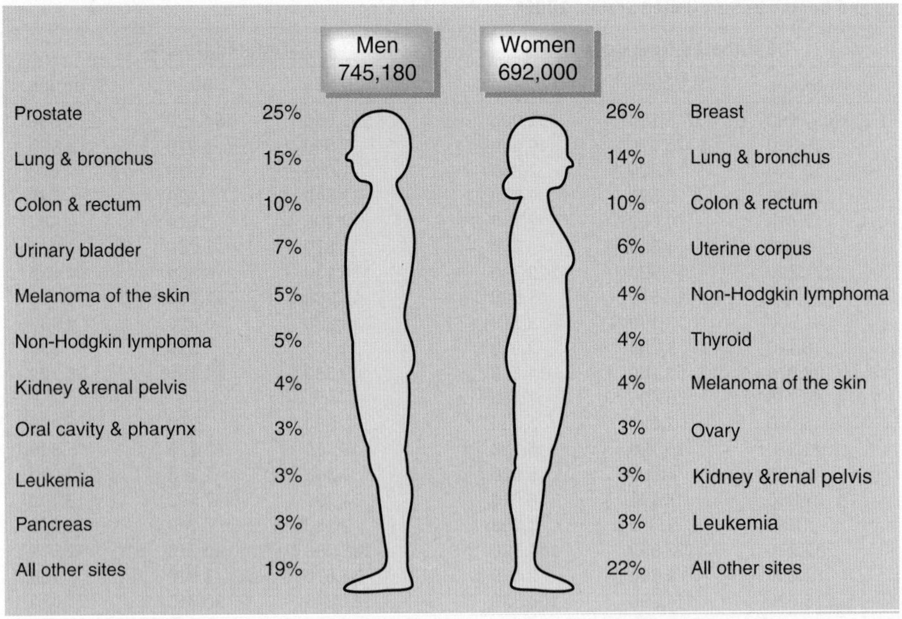

Figure 30–2 ■ Estimated percentage of new cancer cases for 10 leading sites by sex, United States, 2008. Excludes basal and squamous cell skin cancers and in situ carcinomas except urinary bladder. *Source*: American Cancer Society, Cancer Facts and Figures, 2008.

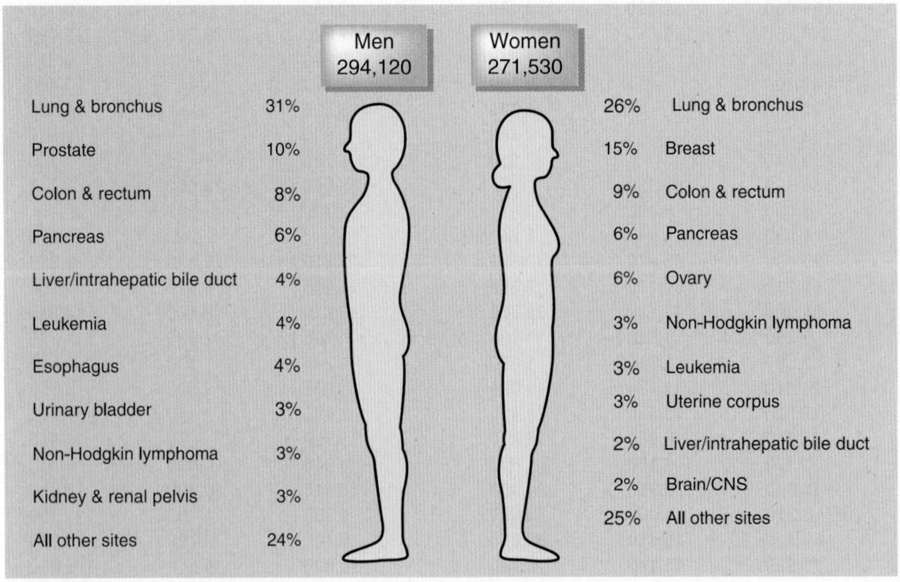

Figure 30–3 ■ Estimated percentage of cancer deaths for 10 leading sites by sex, United States, 2008. Excludes basal and squamous cell skin cancers and in situ carcinomas except urinary bladder. *Source*: American Cancer Society, Cancer Facts and Figures, 2008.

prostate, and colon and rectum) make up slightly over half of all incident invasive cancers and deaths in both sexes.[1]

Age affects the types of cancer that occur, as well as their frequency. Table 30-3 shows the ranking of the most common fatal cancers at different ages in males and females.[1] Before age 20 years, the five most common fatal cancers in both sexes include leukemia, brain and other nervous system (ONS), bones and joints, and non-Hodgkin lymphoma in males and soft tissues in females. In women age 20–39 and 40–59 years, breast cancer is the most common fatal cancer. At age 60 and above, the four most common fatal cancers are lung and bronchus, female breast, prostate, and colon and rectum.

Because the age-standardized death rates from heart disease have been decreasing more rapidly in the United States than the age-standardized death rate from cancer, it has become the most common cause of death among persons 40–74 years of age.[1]

Individual Risk of Cancer

Individuals frequently ask about their personal risk of developing cancer by a certain age or over a specific time period. Table 30-4 illustrates the average probability of a man or woman being diagnosed with an invasive cancer within certain age ranges.[1] It is important to note that these probabilities are based on population averages and may either over- or underestimate the risk for an individual. Personal factors that can cause an individual's risk to be greater or lesser than the national average include genetic susceptibility, lifestyle behaviors such as smoking, and competing causes of death. The average lifetime probability of developing cancer also increases with the longevity of the population. Nevertheless, the probabilities shown in Table 30-4 illustrate the average individual's risk of developing an invasive cancer at various ages.

One measure of disease frequency that is rarely used for cancer is prevalence, or the percentage of people alive during a particular time period, who have ever been diagnosed with cancer. Prevalence does not reflect disease occurrence; rather it reflects a combination of the incidence rate and survival. Prevalence imperfectly reflects the continuing burden of cancer in a population, because there is no reliable way to distinguish between people who have been free of disease for some specified period following cancer treatment and those who struggle with active disease.[17]

Validity of Cancer Surveillance Data

The quality of routinely collected medical information varies over time and across countries. Consequently, data quality can influence apparent temporal trends and international differences. Information on deaths from cancer derives from causes of death reported on death certificates that are coded systematically to indicate the probable underlying cause of death. Death registration is a statutory requirement in many countries. The accuracy of death certificate data depends on the disease under study (rapidly fatal diseases are more accurately recorded), the person completing the certificate (attending physician vs coroner), and the age of the patient (diagnoses are often less well documented in the elderly).[18] Despite the many well documented limitations of death certificates,[19] valid temporal comparisons of mortality rates have been possible in most developed countries in populations under age 75 since the 1960s.[20] Validation studies within SEER have found over 90% agreement between the clinical diagnosis and the underlying cause of death for 17 cancer sites that represent over two-thirds of cancers in the United States.[21,22] Major cancers such as lung, breast, prostate, pancreas, and ovary are included in this group. Other sites, such as cancers of the colon or rectum, can also be reliably classified from death certificates when selected sites are combined but not when

Table 30-3 **Reported Deaths for the Five Leading Cancer Sites by Age (in Years) and Sex, United States, 2005**

Male	<20	20–39	40–59	60–79	≥80
All sites 290,422	All sites 1,261	All sites 4,240	All sites 53,892	All sites 152,720	All sites 78,304
Lung and bronchus 90,141	Leukemia 382	Leukemia 571	Lung and bronchus 15,939	Lung and bronchus 54,692	Lung and bronchus 19,185
Prostate 28,905	Brain and ONS 298	Brain and ONS 524	Colon and rectum 4,994	Colon and rectum 13,525	Prostate 15,341
Colon and rectum 26,783	Bones and joints 121	Colon and rectum 400	Liver and bile duct 3,594	Prostate 12,378	Colon and rectum 7,850
Pancreas 16,147	Other endocrine system 109	Lung and bronchus 316	Pancreas 3,517	Pancreas 8,772	Urinary bladder 3,985
Leukemia 12,273	Non-Hodgkin lymphoma 78	Non-Hodgkin lymphoma 305	Esophagus 2,746	Leukemia 5,934	Pancreas 3,734
Female	**<20**	**20–39**	**40–59**	**60–79**	**≥80**
All sites 268,890	All sites 922	All sites 4,725	All sites 51,059	All sites 126,469	All sites 85,711
Lung and bronchus 69,079	Leukemia 258	Breast 1,170	Breast 12,198	Lung and bronchus 39,811	Lung and bronchus 17,648
Breast 41,116	Brain and ONS 246	Leukemia 421	Lung and bronchus 11,349	Breast 16,914	Colon and rectum 11,634
Colon and rectum 26,224	Bones and joints 91	Uterine cervix 416	Colon and rectum 3,791	Colon and rectum 10,468	Breast 10,834
Pancreas 16,613	Soft tissue 87	Colon and rectum 325	Ovary 3,448	Pancreas 7,934	Pancreas 6,217
Ovary 14,787	Other endocrine system 69	Brain and ONS 309	Pancreas 2,386	Ovary 7,231	Non-Hodgkin lymphoma 4,139

Note: Deaths within each age group do not sum to all ages combined due to the inclusion of unknown ages.
Source: Jemal et al. *CA Cancer J Clin*. 2008;58:71–96.
Abbreviation: ONS, Other nervous system.

Table 30-4 **Probability of Developing Invasive Cancers Within Selected Age Intervals (in Years) by Sex: United States[a]**

		Birth to 39 (%)		40–59 (%)		60–69 (%)		70 and Older (%)		Birth to Death (%)	
All sites[b]	Male	1.42	(1 in 70)	8.44	(1 in 12)	15.71	(1 in 6)	37.74	(1 in 3)	43.89	(1 in 2)
	Female	2.07	(1 in 48)	8.97	(1 in 11)	10.23	(1 in 10)	26.17	(1 in 4)	37.35	(1 in 3)
Urinary bladder[c]	Male	0.02	(1 in 4,448)	0.41	(1 in 246)	0.96	(1 in 104)	3.57	(1 in 28)	3.74	(1 in 27)
	Female	0.01	(1 in 10,185)	0.12	(1 in 810)	0.26	(1 in 378)	1.01	(1 in 99)	1.18	(1 in 84)
Breast	Female	0.48	(1 in 208)	3.79	(1 in 26)	3.41	(1 in 29)	6.44	(1 in 16)	12.03	(1 in 8)
Colon and rectum	Male	0.08	(1 in 1,296)	0.92	(1 in 109)	1.55	(1 in 65)	4.63	(1 in 22)	5.51	(1 in 18)
	Female	0.07	(1 in 1,343)	0.72	(1 in 138)	1.10	(1 in 91)	4.16	(1 in 24)	5.10	(1 in 20)
Leukemia	Male	0.16	(1 in 611)	0.22	(1 in 463)	0.35	(1 in 289)	1.17	(1 in 85)	1.50	(1 in 67)
	Female	0.12	(1 in 835)	0.14	(1 in 693)	0.20	(1 in 496)	0.77	(1 in 130)	1.07	(1 in 94)
Lung and bronchus	Male	0.03	(1 in 3,398)	0.99	(1 in 101)	2.43	(1 in 41)	6.70	(1 in 18)	7.78	(1 in 13)
	Female	0.03	(1 in 2,997)	0.81	(1 in 124)	1.78	(1 in 56)	4.70	(1 in 21)	6.22	(1 in 16)
Melanoma of the skin	Male	0.13	(1 in 780)	0.54	(1 in 184)	0.60	(1 in 166)	1.48	(1 in 67)	2.20	(1 in 45)
	Female	0.22	(1 in 453)	0.44	(1 in 227)	0.30	(1 in 332)	0.68	(1 in 146)	1.47	(1 in 68)
Non-Hodgkin lymphoma	Male	0.13	(1 in 763)	0.45	(1 in 225)	0.58	(1 in 171)	1.66	(1 in 60)	2.23	(1 in 45)
	Female	0.08	(1 in 1,191)	0.32	(1 in 316)	0.45	(1 in 223)	1.36	(1 in 73)	1.90	(1 in 53)
Prostate	Male	0.01	(1 in 10,002)	2.43	(1 in 41)	6.42	(1 in 16)	12.49	(1 in 8)	15.78	(1 in 6)
Uterine cervix	Female	0.15	(1 in 651)	0.27	(1 in 368)	0.13	(1 in 761)	0.19	(1 in 530)	0.69	(1 in 145)
Uterine corpus	Female	0.07	(1 in 1,499)	0.72	(1 in 140)	0.81	(1 in 123)	1.22	(1 in 82)	2.48	(1 in 40)

[a]For people free of cancer at beginning of age interval. [b]All sites excludes basal and squamous cell skin cancers and in situ cancers except urinary bladder. [c]Includes invasive and in situ cancer cases.
Source: DevCan: Probability of Developing or Dying of Cancer Software, Version 6.3.0. Statistical Research and Applications Branch, National Cancer Institute, 2008. www.srab.cancer.gov/devcan.

separate. While issues of data quality are fundamentally important, routinely collected data can be informative in both descriptive and analytic studies if appropriate consideration is given to data quality in relation to the cancer and research question of interest.

Temporal Trends in Cancer Occurrence in the United States

Cancer incidence and mortality rates continue to change over time in the United States. The largest increase occurred in the age-adjusted death rates from cancer of the lung and bronchus in men between 1930 and 1991 (Fig. 30-4).[23] This increase was followed by a decline in lung cancer death rates in men from 1992 to 2005. Lung cancer death rates did not increase sharply in U.S. women until after 1960, 30 years after the steep rise in men, because of the later uptake of cigarette smoking by U.S. women than men. The age-adjusted death rates from lung cancer have now begun to level off in U.S. women (Fig. 30-5), and are anticipated to show a steady decline. The gender differences in these temporal trends in lung cancer closely parallel sex-specific changes in smoking. They provide a remarkable record of how tobacco smoking has affected lung cancer mortality and incidence in the United States.

Two other large changes in cancer death rates since 1930 involve the decline in stomach cancer death rates in both sexes, and the decrease in uterine (cervix and corpus combined) death rates in women. The decrease in stomach cancer is largely attributed to the introduction of refrigeration (with reduced use of salted and smoked foods and increased

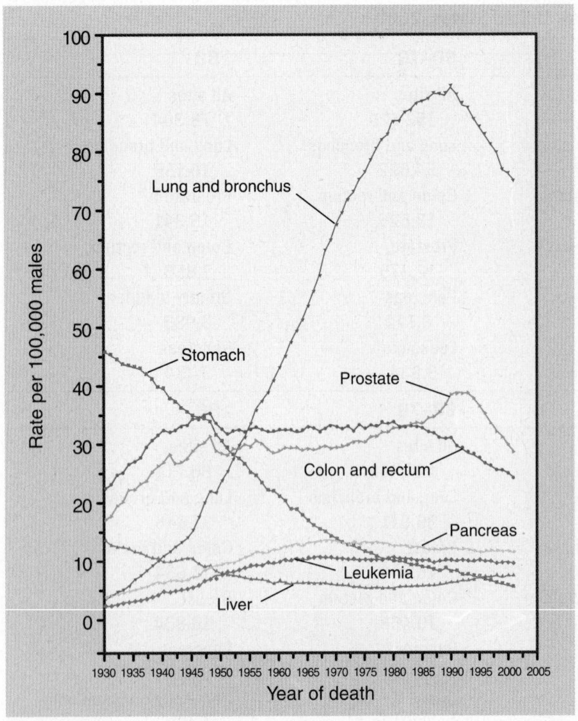

Figure 30-4 ■ Age-adjusted cancer death rates among males for selected cancer types, United States, 1930–2005. Rates are per 100,000 population per year and are age-adjusted to the 2000 U.S. standard population. *Note*: Due to changes in ICD coding, numerator information has changed over time. Rates for cancers of the liver, lung and bronchus, and colon and rectum are affected by these changes. *Source*: American Cancer Society, Surveillance Research, 2008. U.S. mortality public use data tapes, 1960–2005, U.S. mortality volumes, 1930–1959. National Center for Health Statistics, Centers for Disease Control and Prevention; 2008.

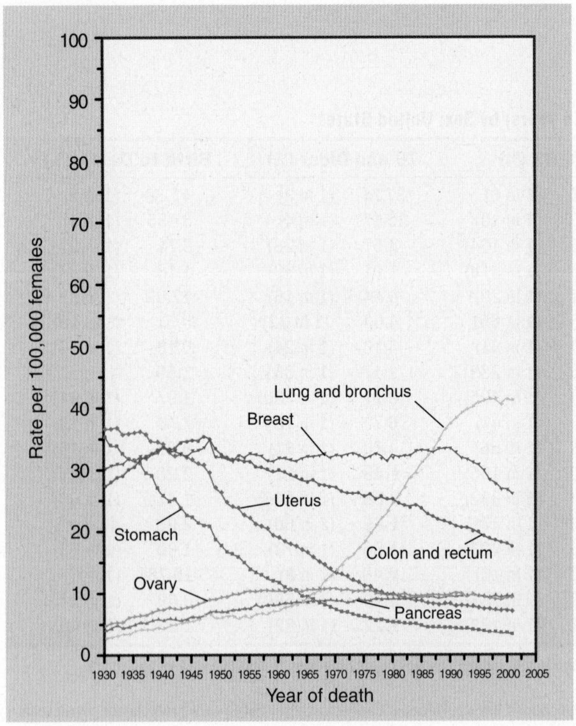

Figure 30-5 ■ Age-adjusted cancer death rates among females for selected cancer types, United States 1930–2005. Rates are per 100,000 population per year and are age-adjusted to the 2000 U.S. standard population. Note: Due to changes in ICD coding, numerator information has changed over time. Rates for cancers of the uterus, lung and bronchus, and colon and rectum are affected by these changes. Uterus cancer death rates are for uterine cervix and uterine corpus combined. *Source*: American Cancer Society, Surveillance Research, 2008. Data U.S. mortality public use data tapes, 1960–2005, U.S. mortality volumes, 1930–1959. National Center for Health Statistics, Centers for Disease Control and Prevention; 2008.

availability of fresh vegetables and fruit), and perhaps to improved living conditions that decreased chronic infection with *H. pylori* in childhood.[24] The decrease in the cervical cancer death rate is partly (but not entirely) attributable to early detection by PAP testing. The decline in death rates from cancer of the uterine cervix and corpus began well before 1945,[1] when the PAP test began to be introduced, and prior to widespread usage of PAP testing in the 1970s. It is unclear to what extent changes in surgical practice, nutrition, personal hygiene, or reproductive factors may also have contributed.

Temporal trends in the incidence of specific cancers, monitored in nine NCI SEER registries, are shown in Figure 30-6.[1] In men, the large increase in diagnoses of prostate cancer between 1989 and 1992 dominates the incidence trends in other cancer. This reflects the widespread introduction of screening for PSA in the late 1980s.[25] The prostate malignancies diagnosed by PSA represent real prostate cancer, but the apparent temporal increase is exaggerated by improved detection of tumors that would previously have gone undiagnosed. The shift towards earlier and more complete diagnosis of prostate cancer has had a much greater impact on prostate cancer incidence (Fig. 30-6) than mortality (Fig. 30-4).

When all cancers are combined in men and women (Fig. 30-7), the age-adjusted rate peaked in 1992 for cancer incidence and in 1991 for mortality. Both incidence and death rates subsequently decreased each year through 1996. If 1992 rates are used as a common baseline, the total decrease from 1992 through 2005 was 13.8% for mortality and 10.7% for incidence.[5] Much of the decline in cancer incidence was contributed by the large fall in prostate cancer incidence (Fig. 30-6), several years after the introduction of prostate specific antigen (PSA) testing, although sustained reductions in the lung cancer incidence in men and colorectal cancer in both sexes also contributed.

The temporal trend in cancer death rates for all sites combined is substantially different in men from that in women (Fig. 30-8, left panel). Whereas the combined death rate from all cases combined in men increased over most of 1930-1991, the rate in women has not changed markedly since the 1960s. This is because the decrease in death rates from cancers of the stomach, uterus, and colorectum has largely offset the increase in lung cancer mortality in women but not in men.

Whereas the death rate from all cancers combined decreased from 1991 to 2001, the total number of cancer deaths continued to increase, albeit more slowly than in earlier years (Fig. 30-8, right panel). As mentioned, the decrease in the death *rates* did not completely offset the aging and growth of the population. Future trends in the number of cases and deaths from cancer will continue to be influenced by aging of the "baby-boomer" generation for several decades. The demographic trends make it difficult to reduce the total number of cancer cases and deaths. It is therefore important to distinguish between trends in age-adjusted occurrence rates and trends in the number of people affected when discussing "progress" against cancer.

Variations Across Socioeconomic, Ethnic, and Racial Groups

The impact of socioeconomic status on cancer occurrence and survival is usually examined indirectly, through comparisons of racial and ethnic groups. Many analyses show that African-Americans experience disproportionately high cancer rates, but few studies have separated the impact of poverty and its attendant risk factors from genetic differences associated with race.[26]

Table 30-5 shows that incidence and death rates from all cancers combined and from the four most common cancers were generally higher in African

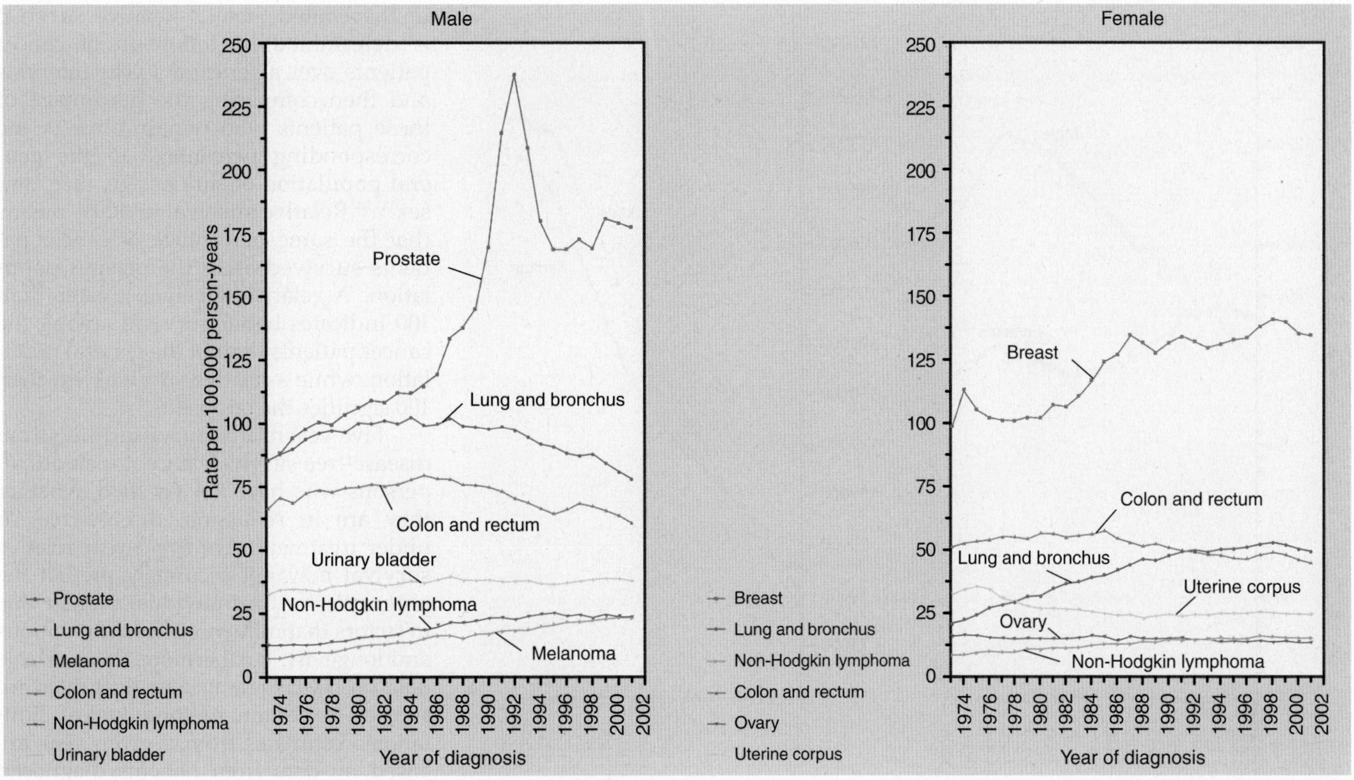

Figure 30-6 ■ Age-adjusted cancer incidence rates for males and females by site, United States, 1975–2005. Rates are per 100,000 population per year and are age-adjusted to the 2000 U.S. standard population. *Source:* American Cancer Society, Surveillance Research, 2009. Data NCI, Surveillance, Epidemiology, and End Results Program, Division of Cancer Control and Population Sciences, National Cancer Institute; 2009.

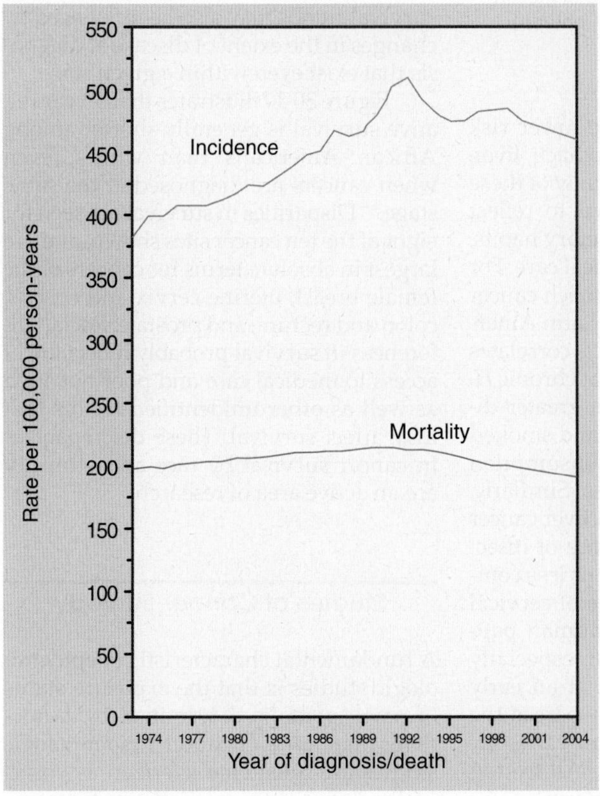

Figure 30-7 ■ Age-adjusted cancer incidence and mortality rates for males and females for all sites combined, United States, 1973–2004. *Rates are per 100,000 population per year and are age-adjusted to the 2000 U.S. standard population. *Source*: American Cancer Society, Surveillance Research, 2008. NCI, Surveillance, Epidemiology, and End Results Program, Division of Cancer Control and Population Sciences, National Cancer Institute, 2004. U.S. mortality public use data tapes, 1960–2001, US mortality volumes, 1930–1959. National Center for Health Statistics, Centers for Disease Control and Prevention; 2008.

Americans than other racial and ethnic groups during the years 2001–2005.[12] The one exception to this was breast cancer incidence in women, where the rate was highest in whites. Among men, the incidence rate of all invasive cancers combined (per 100,000) was 636 in African Americans, 560 in Whites, 440 in Hispanics, 340 in Asian/Pacific islanders, and 337 in American Indians. The high incidence in African American men involves cancers of the prostate, and lung and bronchus (shown) as well as oropharynx, larynx, esophagus, pancreas, and multiple myeloma (not shown in Table 30–5). The cancer incidence rate in African Americans has decreased from 1996 to 2005, as it has in other racial and ethnic groups.[12]

Table 30-6 shows the findings of one study that measured cancer death rates by race within strata of income and educational attainment, markers of socioeconomic status.[27] Although the death rate from the four most common cancers were generally higher in African Americans than in whites at each level of education, a much stronger gradient in risk was seen with education than with race (black vs white). The implication of this study is that many of the disparities in cancer mortality associated with race likely reflect lower educational and socioeconomic status, rather than inherited characteristics of race. Lower socioeconomic status limits educational attainment, reduces access to medical screening, and is often associated with greater exposure to tobacco, heavy alcohol consumption, poor nutrition, physical inactivity, overweight, and other risk factors.[28]

Cancer is frequently diagnosed at a later stage among persons with lower income and educational status, contributing to poorer survival.[29,30] This is reflected in Figure 30-9, where the percentage of cancers diagnosed at a localized stage (confined to the organ of origin) was lower for many cancer sites among

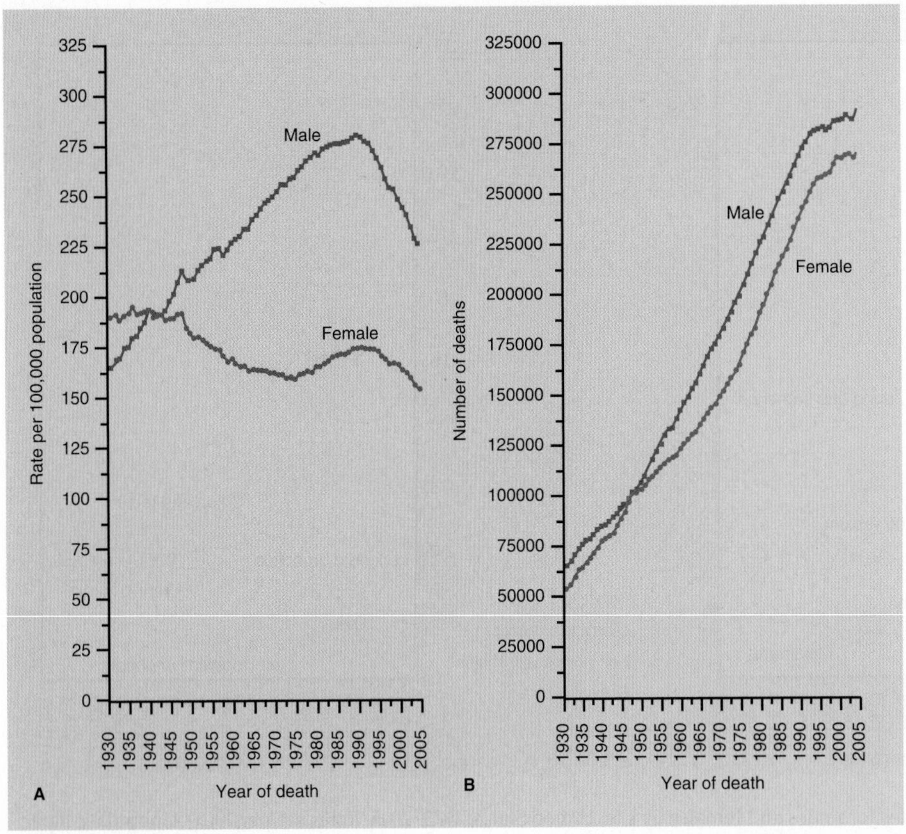

Figure 30-8 (A) Cancer death rates, all sites combined, all races, by sex, United States, 1930–2001. Age-adjusted to the 2000 U.S. population. (B) Number of cancer deaths, all sites combined, all races, men and women combined, United States, 1930–2001. *Source*: U.S. mortality public use data tapes, 1960–2001, U.S. mortality volumes, 1930–1959. National Center for Health Statistics, Centers for Disease Control and Prevention; 2004.

African Americans than whites between 1996 and 2005.[1] The difference in stage is largest for cancers of the female breast and uterine cervix and corpus. Lower utilization of mammography contributes to the racial disparity in stage at diagnosis for breast cancer.[31] The stage difference is more difficult to explain for cervical cancer, however, since utilization of PAP testing is actually higher in black than in white women.[31] PAP testing is underutilized in postmenopausal women of all races. It may be that the lack of PAP testing in older black women contributes particularly to their higher death rates from cervical cancer.

Other ethnic groups in the United States also have distinctive cancer patterns.[28,32] Relative to whites, age-adjusted incidence and mortality rates among Mexican-Americans (Hispanics) are higher for gallbladder, stomach, and cervical cancers; American Indian men and women have lower incidence rates of most cancers other than gallbladder, stomach, and cervix; Japanese Americans have higher rates of stomach and liver cancer; Chinese Americans have higher rates of nasopharyngeal, liver, and stomach cancer; Native Hawaiians have higher death rates from cancers of the esophagus, liver, pancreas, lung, breast, and uterine cervix; Filipino-Americans have lower risk of most cancers other than stomach, liver, oral cavity, and esophagus. Many of these ethnic differences are known to reflect differences in tobacco use, dietary habits, infectious exposures, or medical care. For example, the high rate of stomach cancer among recent migrants from Latin America, Asia, and parts of Africa correlates with their higher prevalence of chronic *H. pylori* infection in childhood, greater dietary consumption of salted and smoked preserved food, and lower consumption of fresh fruits and vegetables. Similarly, ethnic groups with increased liver cancer usually have higher prevalence of infection with chronic hepatitis B, or less commonly C virus. The incidence of cervical cancer reflects exposure to human papilloma virus types 16 and 18, especially when sexual activity begins at an early age with multiple partners, whereas the death rate from cervical cancer varies according to the utilization of PAP testing and early diagnosis and treatment.

Survival of Patients With Cancer

The survival of patients with cancer is monitored by the NCI SEER registries in the United States.[5] Relative survival is determined by follow-up of cancer patients over a series of 1-year intervals and then comparing the percentage of these patients who remain alive to the corresponding percentage in the general population of similar age, race, and sex.[33,34] Relative survival of 100% means that the same percentage of cancer patients survived as in the general population. A relative survival greater than 100 indicates better survival among the cancer patients than in the general population, while a relative survival less than 100 signifies the opposite.

Five-year relative survival differs from disease-free survival, since it includes all persons who have not yet died, whether they are in remission, disease-free, or under treatment. Average 5-year relative survival may not accurately predict the prognosis for an individual patient due to factors that influence treatment options and longevity. Furthermore, the available data on 5-year relative survival rates are subject to certain methodological limitations: estimates from a given year are based on data from patients diagnosed at least 8 years in the past, and may not reflect the most recent advances in treatment[35]; temporal changes in survival may be influenced by changes in screening and early detection as well as treatment; survival trends may also be influenced by changes in the extent of disease at diagnosis that exist even within a given stage.

Figure 30-10 illustrates that 5-year relative survival is generally shorter among African Americans than whites, even when cancers are diagnosed at the same stage.[1,5] Disparities in survival are seen for eight of the ten cancer sites shown, and are largest in absolute terms for cancers of the female breast, uterine cervix and corpus, colon and rectum, and prostate. Racial differences in survival probably reflect lower access to medical care and poor nutrition as well as other unidentified factors that may affect survival. These discrepancies in cancer survival by race and ethnicity are an active area of research.

Studies of Cancer Etiology

A fundamental characteristic of epidemiologic studies is that the exposure status of participants is determined by factors other than randomization. Epidemiologic studies are often characterized as observational to distinguish them from experimental studies where subjects are assigned randomly to either the exposure of interest or placebo. Because participants in epidemiologic studies make their own decisions regarding tobacco use, occupation, diet, place of residence, and other factors, such studies provide information

Table 30-5 Incidence and Mortality[a] by Site, Race, and Ethnicity: United States, 2001–2005

Incidence	White	African American	Asian American and Pacific Islander	American Indian and Alaska Native[b]	Hispanic/ Latino[c,d]
All sites					
Males	556.9	635.6	340.1	336.6	440.1
Females	423.4	389.9	276.3	296.4	331.7
Breast (female)	125.9	111.5	81.6	75.0	91.3
Colon and rectum					
Males	60.6	69.4	45.5	46.0	51.5
Females	44.0	52.4	33.6	41.2	36.2
Kidney and renal pelvis					
Males	19.3	20.0	8.7	19.5	17.9
Females	10.0	10.1	4.3	12.7	10.0
Liver and bile duct					
Males	7.8	12.5	21.5	14.4	15.6
Females	2.7	3.8	8.0	6.3	6.0
Lung and bronchus					
Males	86.9	106.8	51.9	54.3	50.9
Females	57.0	51.1	27.3	39.7	27.2
Prostate	149.8	236.0	84.7	73.3	134.9
Stomach					
Males	9.3	17.1	18.3	16.8	15.0
Females	4.3	8.8	10.2	7.7	8.8
Uterine cervix	8.1	11.9	7.8	6.9	13.4
Mortality	**White**	**African American**	**Asian American and Pacific Islander**	**American Indian and Alaska Native[b]**	**Hispanic/ Latino[c,d]**
All sites					
Males	230.7	313.0	138.8	190.0	159.0
Females	159.2	186.7	95.9	142.0	105.2
Breast (female)	24.4	33.5	12.6	17.1	15.8
Colon and rectum					
Males	22.1	31.8	14.4	20.5	16.5
Females	15.3	22.4	10.2	14.2	10.8
Kidney and renal pelvis					
Males	6.2	6.1	2.4	9.3	5.3
Females	2.8	2.7	1.2	4.3	2.4
Liver and bile duct					
Males	6.7	10.3	15.2	10.6	11.1
Females	2.9	3.9	6.6	6.6	5.1
Lung and bronchus					
Males	71.3	93.1	37.5	50.2	35.1
Females	42.0	39.9	18.5	33.8	14.6
Prostate	24.6	59.4	11.0	21.1	20.6
Stomach					
Males	5.0	11.5	10.1	9.9	8.7
Females	2.5	5.5	5.9	5.2	4.9
Uterine cervix	2.3	4.7	2.2	3.7	3.2

[a]Per 100,000 population, age adjusted to the 2000 US standard population. [b]Data based on Contract Health Service Delivery Areas (incidence, 1999–2004; mortality, 2001–2005), comprising about 55% of the US American Indian/Alaska Native population; for more information see Espey et al. *Cancer.* 2007;110:2119–2152 1975–2004, featuring cancer in American Indians and Alaska Natives. [c]Persons of Hispanic/Latino origin may be of any race. [d]Data unavailable from the Alaska Native Registry and Kentucky. [e]Data unavailable from Minnesota, New Hampshire, and North Dakota.
Source: Jemal et al. *JNCI* 2008;100:1672–1694.

about potentially deleterious exposures that cannot ethically be tested in randomized trials of humans. A disadvantage of observational studies, however, is that extraneous factors may be correlated with both the exposure and disease of interest.

Another distinction is often made between descriptive and analytic epidemiologic studies.[4] Descriptive studies usually characterize risk factor prevalence and/or disease occurrence based on aggregate data on the entire population. These studies identify personal characteristics, geographic locations, and time periods associated with unusually high or low risk of cancer, thereby generating hypotheses that can be tested elsewhere. Special caution is warranted in interpreting ecological studies that use aggregate statistics on populations to imply that a particular factor as causal. In contrast, analytic studies measure the exposure and disease status of individuals rather than aggregate statistics on the overall population. Analytic studies are more able to test pre-specified (*a priori*) hypotheses by measuring the association between individual exposure and subsequent disease.

Descriptive Studies

The huge geographic and temporal variation in many types of cancer provides strong evidence that cancer is not an intrinsic consequence of life, but is affected by lifestyle and environmental factors in addition to inherited genes. Doll and Peto, in 1981, compared the cumulative incidence (percent of people affected) by various cancers in countries with the highest and lowest risk around the world.[36] Figure 30-6 shows the range of cumulative incidence observed in 1976. It also shows the ratio of the highest to the lowest cumulative incidence in the age range 35–64 years, a range intended to reduce the reporting error in poorer countries. From the data in Table 30-7 and other lines of evidence, Doll and Peto inferred that approximately 75–80% of cancer deaths occurring in the United States in 1970 could theoretically be avoided.

Much of the enormous geographic and temporal variation in cancer rates is real rather than an artifact of incomplete registration of cases and deaths in economically developing countries. Some of the ranges shown in Table 30-7 have narrowed over time, yet high rates of cancer of the stomach persist in Japan, China, and parts of South America, nasopharyngeal cancer in southern China, colon cancer in Eastern Europe, Denmark, and New Zealand, cervical cancer in parts of South and Central America and Africa, liver cancer in much of Asia and sub-Saharan Africa, and melanoma in Australia.

The Doll and Peto analysis is descriptive only in that it uses routinely collected data on cancer incidence and mortality to demonstrate the large variation in cancer risk across countries.[36] It does not make inferences about why a particular cancer is common or uncommon in a certain region based on the descriptive data alone; rather, it considers all of the information available from analytic studies, clinical medicine, and basic research in estimating the fraction of cancers attributable to smoking, nutrition, alcohol consumption, and other factors.[36] Validity in epidemiologic studies depends partly on the conclusions being drawn as well as on the quality of the underlying data.

Studies in migrants who move from low- to high-, or high- to low-risk areas support the idea that many cancers are largely avoidable.[37] The change in cancer occurrence is seen more quickly after migration for some cancers than others. For instance, the low incidence of colon

Table 30-6 **Trends in Cancer Death Rates[a] by Education, Race, and Sex: United States, 1993 and 2001**

	Education	White Non-Hispanic			Black Non-Hispanic		
		1993	2001	APC[b]	1993	2001	APC[b]
Lung and bronchus							
Male	All[c]	48.81	36.43	−3.51[d]	88.54	60.17	−4.44[d]
	<12 years	88.06	87.32	−0.05	98.29	90.38	−0.24
	12 years	59.50	53.20	−1.50[d]	98.60	73.73	−3.16[d]
	13–15 years	32.73	24.19	−3.48[d]	45.58	32.21	−4.70[d]
	16+ years	20.73	13.68	−4.91[d]	38.32	20.95	−6.85[d]
	RR[e] (95% CI)	4.2 (4.1–4.4)	6.4 (6.2–6.6)		2.6 (2.5–2.8)	4.3 (3.9–4.8)	
Female	All[c]	28.44	25.07	−1.60[d]	30.49	26.90	−1.46[d]
	<12 years	45.48	55.39	2.39[d]	32.67	30.38	0.82
	12 years	32.11	33.09	0.12	37.26	35.72	−0.74
	13–15 years	19.84	16.64	−1.67[d]	20.07	19.30	−1.29
	16+ years	13.85	11.63	−2.88[d]	14.81	16.65	−2.17
	RR[e] (95% CI)	3.3 (3.1–3.5)	4.8 (4.5–5.0)		2.2 (1.8–2.7)	1.8 (1.6–2.1)	
Colon and rectum							
Male	All[c]	12.01	10.74	−1.64[d]	19.72	18.31	−0.67
	<12 years	14.12	16.04	0.87	17.40	20.93	2.73[d]
	12 years	14.58	13.90	−0.91	21.94	23.89	0.98
	13–15 years	9.16	8.13	−1.09[d]	15.43	11.72	−2.68
	16+ years	9.28	7.85	−2.35[d]	16.33	11.53	−4.84[d]
	RR[e] (95% CI)	1.5 (1.4–1.6)	2.0 (1.9–2.2)		1.1 (0.9–1.3)	1.8 (1.5–2.2)	
Female	All[c]	8.50	7.31	−1.82[d]	13.69	13.26	−0.68
	<12 years	9.54	10.37	1.43	11.03	10.25	−0.33
	12 years	9.71	9.19	−1.01[d]	16.13	17.79	−0.31
	13–15 years	6.44	5.45	−1.64[d]	9.40	10.03	0.68
	16+ years	6.75	5.43	−2.99[d]	15.55	12.18	−2.63[d]
	RR[e] (95% CI)	1.4 (1.3–1.6)	1.9 (1.7–2.1)		0.7 (0.6–0.9)	0.8 (0.7–1.0)	
Breast							
Female	All[c]	28.15	21.68	−3.50[d]	40.14	35.54	−1.53[d]
	<12 years	27.40	24.08	−1.43[d]	30.04	28.72	0.13
	12 years	30.62	25.41	−2.94[d]	45.29	43.38	−1.47
	13–15 years	23.20	17.28	−3.60[d]	35.30	29.97	−0.91
	16+ years	27.35	20.10	−4.32[d]	45.69	35.75	−3.75[d]
	RR[e] (95% CI)	1.0 (1.0–1.1)	1.2 (1.1–1.3)		0.7 (0.6–0.7)	0.8 (0.7–0.9)	
Prostate							
Male	All[c]	3.98	2.78	−4.71[d]	12.66	9.12	−3.60[d]
	<12 years	4.01	3.35	−1.62	10.36	9.59	−1.64
	12 years	4.27	3.34	−3.51[d]	16.17	12.68	−1.64
	13–15 years	3.42	2.29	−5.53[d]	10.31	5.31	−7.42[d]
	16+ years	3.77	2.25	−6.26[d]	7.64	4.76	−5.90
	RR[e] (95% CI)	1.1 (0.9–1.2)	1.5 (1.3–1.7)		1.4 (1.0–1.8)	2.0 (1.5–2.7)	

[a]Rates are for individuals aged 25–64 years at death, per 100,000 population, and age-adjusted to the 2000 US standard population.
[b]Annual percent change. [c]Includes persons with missing data for educational attainment. [d]The APC is statistically significant different from zero.
[e]Rate ratio comparing rate for <12 years education to 16+ years education for the indicated year.
Source: Kinsey et al. *JNCI* 2008;100:1003–1012.

cancer seen in Japan rises substantially in the first generation of Japanese who migrate to Hawaii or to the continental United States. In contrast, the low rate of breast cancer among women in Japan who migrate to the U.S. continues to rise into the second generation after migration. Ultimately, breast cancer incidence among Japanese American women rises to equal or exceed the rate among U.S. white women.[4]

Time trends within countries also illustrate the importance of exogenous, as well as genetic, factors on cancer occurrence.[38] Figure 30-11 shows the increase in death rates from colon, and to a lesser extent breast cancer, in Japan between 1955 and 1985.[39] Major changes in diet and other factors occurred in Japan after World War II. Figure 30-12 also shows the temporal increase in fat intake, based on per capita estimates of the total amount of fat in foods reportedly consumed in Japan during these years. These data alone do not establish that fat consumption caused the increase in death rates from colon and breast cancer. Certain other factors not shown in Figure 30-11 may also have contributed to the increase. These include increased consumption of total calories or meat, diminished consumption of fresh fruit and vegetables, and reduced physical activity. However, the temporal trends in Japan clearly show that mortality from breast and colorectal cancer is affected by external factors as well as by genetic inheritance.

Another example of how ecological studies have contributed to nutritional epidemiology is the correlation between per capita consumption (or disappearance) of various foods in selected countries and national cancer rates. Figure 30-12 shows the strong correlation coefficient (0.89) between per capita consumption of red meat in the late 1960s and the incidence of colorectal cancer in women.[40] These correlation studies do not measure the behavior or disease experience of individuals, nor can they separate other unmeasured risk factors such as physical inactivity, caloric intake, or abdominal obesity from the measured correlation with red meat consumption. Nevertheless, these ecological studies generate hypotheses that can be tested in other research including analytic epidemiologic studies as well as basic and clinical research.

Analytic Epidemiology

Analytic epidemiologic studies measure the association between a particular ex-

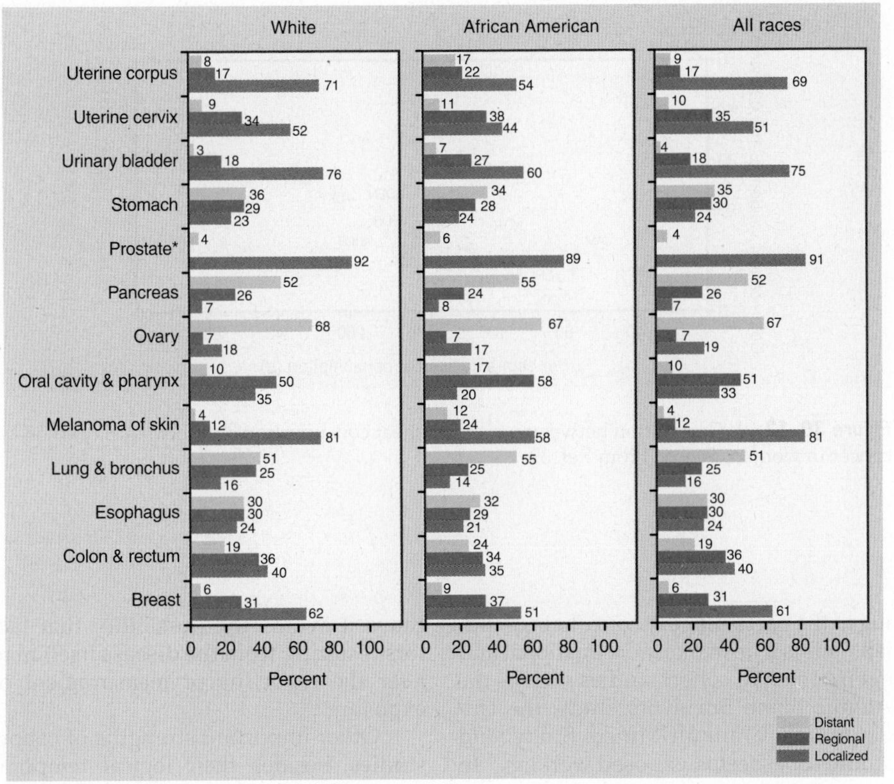

Figure 30-9 ■ Percent distribution of cancer cases by race and stage at diagnosis, United States 1995–2000. The rate for localized stage represents localized and regional stages combined. *Note*: Staging according to Surveillance, Epidemiology, and End Results (SEER) historic stage categories rather than the American Joint Committee on Cancer (AJCC) staging system. For each site and race, stage categories do not total 100% because sufficient information is not available to assign a stage to all cancer cases. *Source*: From Ref. 51.

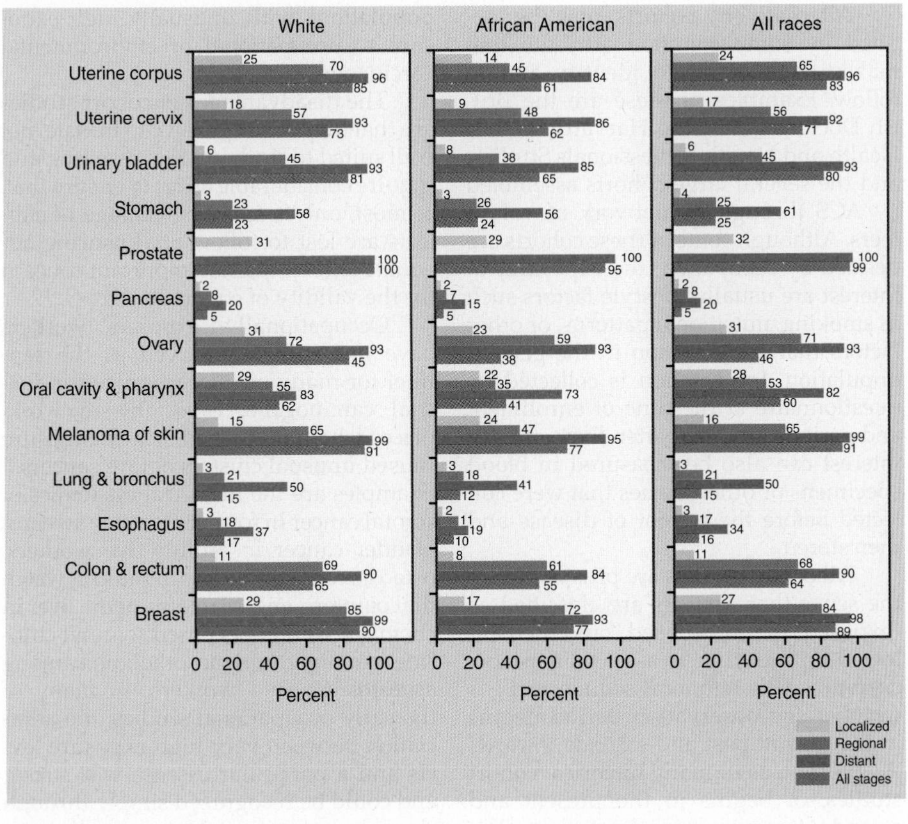

Figure 30-10 ■ Five-year relative survival from various cancers, by race and stage at diagnosis, United States 1995–2000. *Note*: Staging according to Surveillance, Epidemiology, and End Results (SEER) historic stage categories rather than the American Joint Committee on Cancer (AJCC) staging system. *Source*: From Ref. 51.

posure and a disease, using information collected from individuals, rather than from the aggregate population. The term "exposure" is defined broadly to include behavioral factors such as smoking or diet, environmental pollutants such as asbestos, personal characteristics such as obesity or tendency to sunburn, anthropometric measurements such as body mass index, and genetic traits and other measurable biological factors that may affect cancer.

The two most common study designs in analytic epidemiology are cohort and case-control, depending on whether the subjects are first identified based on characteristics other than disease status (see below). Both approaches measure the association between a particular exposure and a given disease; both provide a stronger basis for inference than do descriptive studies alone.

Measures of Association

The association between individual exposure and disease occurrence is most often expressed as the relative risk (RR or rate ratio) in a cohort study or odds ratio (OR) in a case-control study.[4] For example, a cohort study could measure the association between human papilloma virus (HPV) infection and cervical cancer by determining the incidence of cervical cancer among a defined group of women in a health maintenance organization who do or do not have chronic HPV infection. The increase associated with HPV infection could be expressed as the RR, representing the incidence rate among infected women divided by the incidence among the uninfected women. Alternatively, the association could also be estimated using the OR from a case-control study of women with cervical cancer, by comparing HPV infection among cases with the prevalence among non-cases or controls.

Both the RR and the OR characterize the association between the exposure and disease in relative terms. Both measures reflect the frequency of disease occurrence among exposed subjects as a multiple of the rate among unexposed persons. A second, less commonly used measure of association, however, is the absolute change in risk associated with exposure. This can be estimated in cohort but not usually in case-control studies. The absolute risk (or rate difference, RD) equals the rate among the exposed persons minus the rate in the unexposed. In our specific example of cervical cancer and HPV infection, the RD would reflect the absolute magnitude of the increase in cervical cancer incidence associated with HPV infection. The RD is informative because it describes the absolute impact of the exposure on dis-

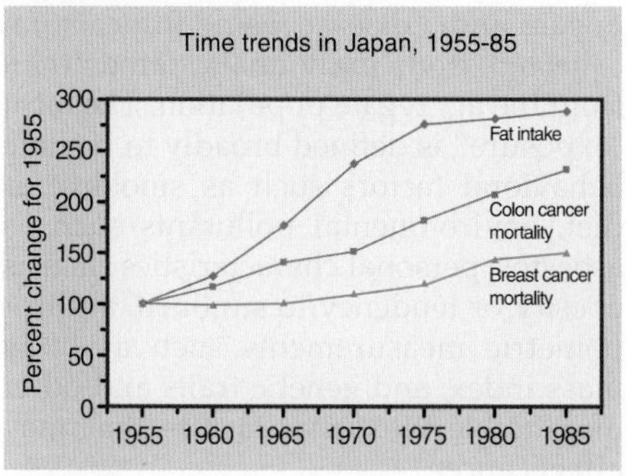

Figure 30–11 Time trends in per capita consumption of fat and death rates from colon and breast cancer in Japan, 1955–1985. *Source*: From Ref. 39.

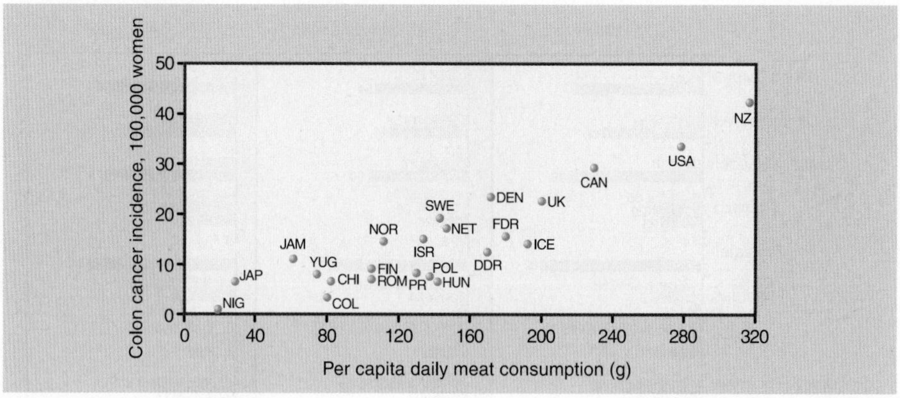

Figure 30–12 Correlation between per capita meat consumption and incidence of colon cancer in women. *Source*: From Ref. 39.

ease occurrence better than does the RR. This absolute impact is dependent on the background risk of disease in unexposed persons as well as on the RR. If the disease is rare, an exposure with RR = 10 will affect relatively few people. In contrast, if the disease is common, an exposure with RR = 1.5 would have a very large absolute impact on the population. The RD is less commonly measured in epidemiologic studies than is the RR, partly because it is only obtainable from cohort studies, and partly because it is more variable across different populations than is the RR.

Another measure of association is the attributable fraction (or risk), used to estimate the proportion of disease in the population caused by the exposure of interest. This may be expressed as either the percentage of disease caused by the exposure among exposed persons, or the corresponding percentage in the overall population, which includes both exposed and unexposed persons. In either case, estimates of the attributable fraction are based on the assumption that an association is causally related to the exposure of interest, rather than merely reflecting chance or correlated factors that have not been controlled.

Cohort Studies

Epidemiologic studies of various populations or cohorts have contributed to our understanding of how tobacco, radiation, and other occupational and environmental factors can increase cancer risk, and more recently, how nutritional and genetic factors may modify this risk. Two central characteristics of cohort studies are (a) participants are selected because of some common characteristic that precedes the disease being studied and are then followed forward for some specified time period (unlike case-control studies), and (b) participants are not randomly assigned to their exposure status by the researchers (unlike randomized clinical trials).

In some cohort studies, the population is defined based on records pertaining to the particular exposure being studied. This is true in many occupational and environmental cohort studies such as the Atomic Bomb Survivors study, the Underground Uranium Miners Study, and studies of asbestos-exposed workers.[41] In these, the historical records from workplaces and other places with unusually high level exposures are used to define the cohort and to estimate the degree of exposure. The health or vital status of the cohort is then followed forward for some specified time period, during which disease occurrence is measured.

Alternatively, cohorts may be defined by some common attribute that makes them easier to identify and to follow. Examples of these are the British Doctor's study, the Harvard Nurses' Health and Health Professionals Studies, and the several large cohorts assembled by ACS through its network of volunteers. Although some of these cohorts are defined by occupation, the exposures of interest are usually lifestyle factors such as smoking, nutritional patterns, or other factors that are common in the general population. Information is collected by questionnaire at the time of enrollment and periodically thereafter. Exposures of interest can also be measured in blood specimens or other tissues that were collected before the advent of disease and then stored.

All cohort studies are prospective in the sense that subjects are classified as "exposed" or "unexposed," and then followed-up over time to assess disease occurrence. This temporal sequence exists whether the observation period begins in the distant past and extends towards the present, as in many historical cohort studies, or begins in the present and extends forward into the future. The ability of cohort studies to document exposure status before the occurrence of disease is an important strength, because it avoids the possibility that factors resulting from the disease itself may alter the reporting or measurement of exposure.[21]

Other important strengths of cohort studies, besides their logical temporal progression from exposure to disease, are their ability to: (a) obtain biological specimens prospectively before the onset of disease; (b) measure absolute rates of disease occurrence (incidence and death rates) as well as relative risk; (c) study multiple disease endpoints simultaneously; and (d) identify and monitor populations with unusually high exposure to occupational or environmental carcinogens.

The disadvantages of cohort studies are that they are expensive to initiate, not well suited to studying rare diseases, and require considerable effort to ensure that, at most, only a small percentage of subjects are lost to follow-up. Ensuring adequate follow-up is an important concern for the validity of cohort studies.

Occupationally exposed workers have unfortunately served as the sentinel for many of the recognized industrial carcinogens, especially in workplaces where prolonged, heavy exposure caused unusual clusters of rare cancers.[41] Examples are the historical epidemics of scrotal cancer in former chimney sweeps, bladder cancer in aniline dye workers, osteosarcoma of the jaw in radium watch dial painters, angiosarcoma of the liver in chemical workers exposed to vinyl chloride monomer, and mesothelioma among asbestos-exposed workers. In many of the early occupational studies, the association between very high exposure levels and a particular disease was strong and could be recognized simply through clinical observation. More recently, systematic epidemiologic studies have been used to estimate the dose-response relationship at lower levels of exposure, or to assess whether smaller increases also occurred in more common cancers. For example, the association between lung cancer and employment in poorly ventilated underground uranium mines has been known for over a century. Efforts to quantify the dose-response relationship between lower exposures to radon and lung cancer continue to have important implications for the general population with domestic exposure to radon gas seeping into cellars. Occupational studies are most informative when records exist to quantify exposure, where there is a substantial range in the intensity and duration of exposure, and where the workforce is large.

Case-Control Studies

Subjects in case-control studies are selected based on whether they have (cases) or have not (controls) been diagnosed with the specific disease under study. Cases and controls may then be interviewed about past and ongoing exposures, and the proportion of cases with a particular exposure is compared to that of the controls to determine if there is an association between the exposure and the disease.[4,18]

The preferred approach in a case-control study is that cases and controls are drawn from the same population. Ideally, cases are identified from population-based cancer registry rather than a hospital, and controls are identified from the general population from the source. Moreover, cases should represent a single disease rather than a mixture of diseases with possibly diverse etiologies.

Advantages of case-control over cohort studies are that they are efficient for studying rare diseases, quicker and less expensive than cohort studies to initiate, and because of their smaller size, better able to collect detailed information on a wide variety of exposures of interest. Their disadvantages are that, because subjects are aware of their disease status, case-control studies are more susceptible to biased reporting of exposures. For instance the case-control approach is not well suited to studying the relationship between alcohol consumption and oropharyngeal cancer, since cases might report their alcohol consumption more honestly than the controls (reporting bias), and controls who drink heavily may be unwilling to participate in the study (selection bias). Misclassification of exposure can be random or systematic, and can cause the study to overestimate or to underestimate the differences in exposure between cases and controls. In this case, the association between drinking and oropharyngeal cancer may be exaggerated by both the reporting and selection bias.

Case-control studies are highly efficient in studying uncommon cancers such as brain cancer. The sample size can be much smaller, since only the cases and a sample of controls are studied, rather than the entire base population from which the cases arose. Case-control studies can also be situated in populations that broaden the range of the exposure of interest. For example, Whittemore et al. studied the relation of diet and physical activity to colorectal cancer among Chinese in North America and in China.[42] By including cases and controls from China as well as North America, this study took advantage of the far greater range in dietary fat and protein consumption between these two regions, compared to the range within each region. The OR (and 95% confidence intervals) between consumption of saturated fat and colorectal cancer among Chinese men in North America was 2.1 (1.6–2.7), similar to that among women in North America. However, among men in China the OR associated with saturated fat was smaller: 1.2 (0.84–1.7), as it was in women. By demonstrating a stronger association between saturated fat and colorectal cancer in North America than in China, the study adds to the aggregate evidence that fat consumption is correlated with and may contribute to the high incidence of colorectal cancer in the United States.

Use of Biomarkers in Epidemiological Research

Large-scale epidemiological studies have increasingly integrated biomarker research into studies of cancer etiology, susceptibility, prognosis, and treatment. Biomarker research has become possible because of rapid developments in high-throughput laboratory technology and the infrastructure to collect and preserve biospecimens on large numbers of people. Genome-wide association studies (GWAS) exemplify progress in high-throughput genetic analyses. GWAS are now commonly used to analyze the DNA from tens of thousands of cases and matched controls and to localize "common" inherited genetic variants (ie, those with minor allele frequency >1%) associated with a small to moderate increases or decreases in risk of the cancer under study. Germline DNA can be obtained from peripheral blood lymphocytes or from buccal cells collected in mouthwash samples. Only micrograms of DNA are needed to genotype a dense map of single nucleotide polymorphisms (SNPs) across the genome. The GWAS approach, optimally conducted in large consortia rather than in single studies to obtain a sufficient number of cases, identifies the general vicinity of the causal variant. It must be followed up by an intensive process of fine mapping and other studies to pinpoint the functional variant(s). The advantage of the GWAS approach, over traditional studies of candidate genes, is that it can detect associations in regions of DNA where one would not otherwise look. For example, GWAS studies have documented that prostate, breast, and colorectal cancer are all associated with various SNPs in 8q24[43]; this region contains no known genes and was previously considered to be "junk" DNA. Not only are GWAS findings accelerating the quest for susceptibility genes for common cancers but they are also transforming our understanding of the functions of DNA.

Biomarkers are used in other ways in epidemiological studies.[44] They provide a supplemental source of exposure data, help to identify steps in the causal pathway that links exposure to disease, serve as intermediate or proxy endpoints, and help to differentiate tumors into subtypes that may differ in their etiology, prognosis, or responsiveness to certain treatments.[45] In some cases, laboratory measurements based on stored serum, urine, or DNA may provide the only reliable data on exposure. For example, biological specimens are essential in determining the presence or absence of serum antigens to hepatitis B or C and the concentrations of various sex hormones among post-menopausal women not taking hormone replacement. Other markers, such as the measurements of aflatoxin metabolites in urine,[46] or cotinine in the serum or urine of persons exposed to second-hand smoke, supplement the data that can be obtained from questionnaires alone. Tumor markers such as hormone receptor status and HER2/neu, are used clinically for breast cancer to guide therapy, predict prognosis, and provide potential therapeutic targets. The same markers can be used in epidemiological studies of breast cancer by defining more homogeneous disease subgroups, which may differ in their etiology.

The recent study by Chan et al. of insulin-like growth factor-1 (IGF-1) in relation to prostate cancer in the Physician's Health Study is a example of how measurements of hormones, growth factors, nutrients etc. in blood can be informative about cancer.[47] This analysis found a strong positive association between IGF-1 in plasma collected from men and their subsequent development of prostate cancer. Plasma samples had been collected and stored on nearly 15,000 of the 22,000 male physicians who participated in this study. The fact that these blood samples preceded the diagnosis of prostate cancer, and that PSA levels were also measured on the stored specimens circumvented concern that prevalent prostate cancer might have affected the concentrations of IGF-1.

What Constitutes "Proof" in Epidemiological Studies?

There has been vigorous philosophic and scientific debate over what constitutes "proof" when epidemiologic and other evidence is evaluated with respect to policy. Cohort and case-control studies are, in principle, less definitive than are randomized clinical trials because they cannot control completely for unmeasured or incompletely measured risk factors that may be associated with both the exposure and disease of interest. However, the information from observational studies is often considered sufficient for public health action if chance, bias, or confounding can be reasonably excluded as alternative explanations for the findings.

Reliance on observational data as a basis for policy is inevitable in situations where randomized trials are unethical or infeasible. The criteria frequently used to make a judgment of causation were first proposed in the 1964 Surgeon General's report on Smoking and Health,[48] was subsequently expanded by Sir Austin Bradford Hill,[49] and later incorporated by organizations such as the IARC.[50] The inference that an association is causal is supported when:

(a) The association is strong (higher relative risks being more likely to indicate cause)
(b) Risk increases or decreases with exposure in a dose-response gradient
(c) Consistent findings are seen in multiple studies with different investigators, different study populations, and designs
(d) The exposure (cause) precedes the disease
(e) It appears biologically plausible that the exposure could cause the disease
(f) The association is specific between the exposure and a single disease
(g) The epidemiologic findings fit coherently with information from other types of research and other epidemiologic studies.

Certain of these criteria are considered more necessary than others. For example, an association that is reproducible in multiple epidemiologic studies and is consistent with other experimental and clinical research is far more credible than an association that meets only the criteria of specificity—one exposure causing one disease. In fact, the overwhelming evidence linking tobacco smoking with multiple types of cancer is strengthened, rather than diminished by the large number of cancers that it causes. In general, no single criterion from the above list should be considered necessary or sufficient to consider an exposure causally related to a disease.

IARC Classification of Carcinogens

Because it would be impossible for individual clinicians or even governments to evaluate the many substances suspected of carcinogenicity, IARC has established a formal process that systematically evaluates known and suspected carcinogens.[50] The evaluations are done by international working groups of experts who meet, ensure that all relevant and appropriate data have been collected, prepare accurate summaries of the data, and classify the evidence into one of four categories: (1) "Sufficient evidence" of carcinogenicity in humans (signifying that, in the opinion of the working group, a causal relationship has been established between the agent and human cancer in studies in which chance, bias, and confounding can be excluded with reasonable confidence); (2) "Limited evidence" of carcinogenicity (the agent has been associated with increased risk of human cancer, but that chance, bias, and confounding cannot be ruled out with reasonable confidence); (3) "Inadequate evidence" of carcinogenicity (available studies are of insufficient quality, consistency, or statistical power to permit a conclusion regarding the carcinogenicity of the agent, or no data on carcinogenicity in humans were available); and (4) "Evidence suggesting lack of carcinogenic activity" (several adequate studies of use or exposure are mutually consistent in not showing an increased risk for specified cancer sites, conditions, and levels of exposure). A complete list of the IARC monograph classification of agents, mixtures, and other substances is available on the Web at www.iarc.fr.

The same IARC website lists the various iatrogenic exposures that have been linked to cancer. These include diagnostic and therapeutic exposure to ionizing radiation, cancer treatment with alkylating agents such as melphalan, cyclophosphamide, busulfan, and mechlorethamine, immunosuppression (which increases risk of non-Hodgkin lymphoma and B-immunoblastic sarcomas), hormone medications (such as diethylstilbestrol, unopposed estrogen, and androgens), and antibiotics such as chloramphenicol.

Summary

Population research contributes to our understanding of cancer at many levels. Certain fundamental concepts such as individual risk, survival, and population-attributable risk are measurable only in populations, not individuals. In cancer surveillance, epidemiologic methods are used to measure cancer incidence, mortality, and survival, to identify high-risk subgroups, and to monitor progress (or lack of progress) against the disease. In etiologic research, epidemiologic studies have been crucial in identifying and characterizing the carcinogenicity of tobacco, radiation, and many other occupational, environmental, and infectious agents. Epidemiologic studies often provide conclusive information on effective strategies to prevent disease many decades before the precise causal mechanism is identified.

References

1. Jemal A, Siegel R, Ward E, et al. Cancer statistics, 2008. *CA Cancer J Clin.* 2008;58:71–96.
2. NHLBI. Factbook FY. Available at: http://www.nhlbi.nih.gov/about/factpdf.htm. Accessed January 30, 2009.
3. Rothman KJ, Greenland S, Lash TL. *Modern Epidemiology*, 3rd ed. Philadelphia: Lippincott Williams & Wilkins; 2008.
4. Hennekens C, Buring J. *Epidemiology.* Boston: Little, Brown; 1987.
5. Ries L, Melbert D, Krapcho M, et al. *SEER Cancer Statistics Review, 1975–2005.* Bethesda, MD: National Cancer Institute; 2008.
6. Cancer Registries: the Foundation for Cancer Prevention and Control, Centers for Disease Control and Prevention, 2005. Available at: http://www.cdc.gov/cancer/npcr/awards.htm. Accessed April 2, 2005.
7. U.S. Cancer Statistics Working Group. *United States Cancer Statistics: 2001 Incidence and Mortality.* Atlanta, GA: Department of Health and Human Services, Centers for Disease Control and Prevention, and National Cancer Institute; 2004.
8. MMWR. State cancer registries: status of authorizing legislation and enabling regulations-United States. *MMWR Morb Mortal Wkly Rep.* 1994;43:71–75.
9. Parkin D, Muir C, Whelan S, Gao Y, Ferlay J, Powell J. *Cancer Incidence in Five Continents.* Lyon (France): International Agency for Research on Cancer, IARC Scientific Publications No. 120; 1992.
10. Parkin D, Whelan S, Ferlay J, et al., editors. *Cancer Incidence in Five Continents, Vol. VII.* Lyon, France: IARC Scientific Publication; 1997:1028–1029.
11. World Health Organization. *World Health Statistics Annual, 1996.* Geneva: World Health Organization; 1998.
12. Jemal A, Thun M, Ries LA, et al. Annual report to the nation on the status of cancer, 1975–2005, featuring trends in lung can-

cer, tobacco use, and tobacco control. *J Natl Cancer Inst*. 2008;100:1672–1694.

13. Waterhouse J, Muir C, Correa P, Powell J, editors. *Cancer Incidence in Five Continents, Vol. III*. Lyon, France: IARC Scientific Publications No. 15; 1976.
14. Pickle LW, Hao Y, Jemal A, et al. A new method of estimating United States and state-level cancer incidence counts for the current calendar year. *CA Cancer J Clin*. 2007;57:30–42.
15. Tiwari RC, Ghosh K, Jemal A, et al. A new method of predicting US and state-level cancer mortality counts for the current calendar year. *CA Cancer J Clin*. 2004;54:30–40.
16. Jemal A, Murray T, Ward E, et al. Cancer statistics, 2005. *CA Cancer J Clin*. 2005;55:10–30.
17. Wingo P, Parkin D, Eyre H. Measuring the occurrence of cancer: impact and statistics. In: Lenhard R, Brady L, Osteen R, Gansler T, editors. *Clinical Oncology*, 3rd edn. Atlanta, GA: American Cancer Society; 2001, Chapter 1.
18. Kelsey J, Thompson W, Evans A. *Methods on Observational Epidemiology*. New York: Oxford University Press; 1986.
19. Messite J, Stellman S. Accuracy of death certificate completion. *JAMA*. 1996;275: 794–796.
20. Doll R, Muir C, Fraumeni J. Introduction. In: Sidebottom E, editor. *Trends in Cancer Incidence and Mortality, Vol 19/20*. Plainview: Cold Spring Harbor Laboratory Press; 1994:1–4.
21. Percy C, Miller B, Ries L. Effect of changes in cancer classification and the accuracy of cancer death certificates on trends in cancer mortality. *Ann NY Acad Sci*. 1990;609:87–98.
22. Percy C, Stanek E, Gloeckler L. Accuracy of cancer death certificates and its effect on cancer mortality statistics. *Nat Cancer Inst Monogr*. 1982;59:467–475.
23. Thun M, Henley S, Calle E. Tobacco use and cancer: an epidemiologic perspective for geneticists. *Oncogene*. 2002;21:7307–7325.
24. Shibata A, Parsonnet J. Stomach cancer. In: Schottenfeld D, Joseph F, Fraumeni J, editors. *Cancer Epidemiology and Prevention*. Oxford University Press; 2006.
25. Gann P. Interpreting recent trends in prostate cancer incidence and mortality. *Epidemiology*. 1997;8:117–119.
26. Baquet C, Horm J, Gibbs T, Greenwald P. Socioeconomic factors and cancer incidence among blacks and whites. *J Natl Cancer Inst*. 1999;83:551–557.
27. Kinsey T, Jemal A, Liff J, Ward E, Thun M. Secular trends in mortality from common cancers in the United States by educational attainment, 1993–2001. *J Natl Cancer Inst*. 2008;100:1003–1012.
28. American Cancer Society. *Cancer Facts & Figures 2003, Special Section on Cancer Disparities*. Atlanta, GA: American Cancer Society, Inc; 2004.
29. Singh G, Miller B, Hankey BF, Edwards BK. *Area Socioeconomic Variations in U.S. Cancer Incidence, Mortality, Stage, Treatment, and Survival*. Bethesda, MD: National Cancer Institute; 2003.
30. Howard J, Hankey B, Greenberg R, et al. A collaborative study of differences in the survival rates of black patients and white patients with cancer. *Cancer*. 1992;69:2349–2360.
31. Breen N, Wagener D, Brown M, Davis W, Ballard-Barbash R. Progress in cancer screening over a decade: results of cancer screening from the 1987, 1992, and 1998 National Health Interview Surveys. *J Natl Cancer Inst*. 2001;93:1704–1713.
32. Miller B, Kolonel L, Bernstein L, et al., editors. *Racial/ethnic Patterns of Cancer in the United States, 1988–1992*. Bethesda, MD: National Cancer Institution, NIH Pub. No. 96–4104; 1996.
33. Wingo P, Gloeckler-Ries L, Parker S, Heath C. Long-term cancer patient survival in the United States. *Cancer Epidemiol Biomarkers Prev*. 1998;7:271–282.
34. Ederer F, Axtell L, Cutler S. The relative survival rate: a statistical methodology. *Nat Cancer Inst Monogr*. 1961;6:101–121.
35. Jemal A, Clegg LX, Ward E, et al. Annual report to the nation on the status of cancer, 1975–2001, with a special feature regarding survival. *Cancer*. 2004;101:3–27.
36. Doll R, Peto R. The causes of cancer: quantitative estimates of avoidable risks of cancer in the United States today. *J Natl Cancer Inst*. 1981;66:1191–1308.
37. Kolonel LN, Wilkens LR. Migrant studies. In: Schottenfeld D, Joseph F, Fraumeni J, editors. *Cancer Epidemiology and Prevention*, 3rd ed. Oxford University Press; 2006.
38. Willett WC. Diet and nutrition. In: Schottenfeld D, Fraumeni J, Jr, editors. *Cancer Epidemiology and Prevention*. New York: Oxford University Press; 2006:405–421.
39. Willett W. The search for the cause of breast and colon cancer. *Nature*. 1989;338:389–393.
40. Armstrong B, Doll R. Environmental factors and cancer incidence and mortality in different countries, with special reference to dietary practices. *Int J Cancer*. 1975;15:617–631.
41. Siemiatycki JA, Richardson L, Boffetta P. Occupation. In: Schottenfeld D, Fraumeni J, Jr, editors. *Cancer Epidemiology and Prevention*. New York: Oxford University Press; 2006:322–354.
42. Whittemore A, Wu-Williams A, Lee M, et al. Diet physical activity and colorectal cancer among Chinese in North America and China. *J Natl Cancer Inst*. 1990;82:915–926.
43. Schumacher FR, Feigelson HS, Cox DG, et al. A common 8q24 variant in prostate and breast cancer from a large nested case-control study. *Cancer Res*. 2007;67:2951–2956.
44. Hunter DJ, Khoury MJ, Drazen JM. Molecular epidemiology of cancer. *CA Cancer J Clin*. 2005;55:45–54.
45. Garcia-Closas M, Vermeulen R, Sherman ME, Moore LE, Smith MT, Rothman N. Application of biomarkers in cancer epidemiology. In: Schottenfeld D, Fraumeni J, Jr, editors. *Cancer Epidemiology and Prevention*. New York: Oxford University Press; 2006:70–88.
46. Qian G, Ross R, Yu M, et al. A follow-up study of urinary markers of aflatoxin exposure and liver cancer risk in Shanghai, People's Republic of China. *Cancer Epidemiol Biomarkers Prev*. 1994;3:3–10.
47. Chan J, Stampfer M, et al. Plasma insulin-like growth factor-1 and prostate cancer risk: a prospective study. *Science*. 1998;279:563–566.
48. U.S. Public Health Service. Smoking and Health. Report of the Advisory Committee to the Surgeon General of the Public Health Service: U.S. Department of Health, Education, and Welfare, Public Health Service, Centers for Disease Control, PHS Publication No. 1103; 1964.
49. Hill A. The environment and disease: association or causation? *Proc R Soc Med*. 1965;58:295–300.
50. IARC. *IARC Monographs on the Evaluation of the Carcinogenic Risk of Chemicals to Humans: Chemicals, Industrial Processes and Industries Associated with Cancer in Humans*. Lyon: International Agency for Research on Cancer; 1982.

31 Tobacco-Induced Cancers and Their Prevention

Stephen S. Hecht, PhD ▪ Dorothy K. Hatsukami, PhD

Introduction

It is remarkable that tobacco use in the world continues to be so common, in spite of widespread knowledge of its disastrous health consequences. The marketing skills of wealthy multinational tobacco companies, which often target teenagers with enticing messages, together with the established addictive power of nicotine, make tobacco use the single largest cause of preventable cancer death in the world, where there are about 1200 million smokers and hundreds of millions of smokeless tobacco users.[1,2] China alone has ~300 million male smokers, quite close to the population of the United States.[1]

Approximately 5.5 trillion cigarettes were used annually in 1990-2000, about 1000 cigarettes for every person on our planet.[1] Over 15 billion cigarettes are smoked every day.[1] Other smoked products include *kreteks*, which are clove-flavored cigarettes popular in Indonesia, and "sticks" which are smoked in Papua New Guinea. *Bidis*, which consist of a small amount of tobacco wrapped in *temburni* leaf and tied with a thread, are popular in India and neighboring areas. *Chutta* are hand-rolled cigarettes used for reverse smoking by women in India. Cigars, including little cigars and cigarillos, as well as pipes are still used, and water pipes are increasing in popularity. A large amount of tobacco is consumed worldwide in the form of smokeless tobacco products, including the increasingly popular moist snuff, placed between the cheek and gum, and *pan* or betel quid, a product which often contains tobacco and is used extensively in India and other parts of southern Asia.

An Overview of Cancers Caused by Tobacco Products

It is estimated that cigarette smoking causes over 1 million cancer deaths annually worldwide,[2] amounting to 27% of cancer mortality in developed countries and 34% in the United States.[3] Lung cancer is the major cancer caused by cigarette smoking, with the total number of cases amounting to about 1.2 million annually. Ninety percent of lung cancer incidence and mortality is attributed to smoking.[4] Lung cancer was rare at the beginning of the 20th century, but incidence and death rates increased in parallel as smoking became more popular (Fig. 31-1), and smoking as a cause of lung cancer has been conclusively established.

The 2004 U.S. Surgeon General's Report and Volume 83 of the International Agency for Research on Cancer (IARC) Monographs on the Evaluation of Carcinogenic Risks to Humans provide recent authoritative summaries of the evidence for smoking as a cause of cancer, which is based on hundreds of epidemiologic studies carried out over the past 50-60 years.[4,5] Some of the important conclusions follow.[4]

The strongest determinant of lung cancer in smokers is duration of cigarette smoking, and the risk also becomes larger with the number of cigarettes smoked.[4] Smoking causes lung cancer in both men and women. The risk for all histologic types of lung cancer is increased by smoking: squamous cell carcinoma, small cell carcinoma, adenocarcinoma (including bronchiolar-alveolar carcinoma), and large cell carcinoma. Adenocarcinoma has now replaced squamous cell carcinoma as the most common type of lung cancer caused by smoking. Cessation of smoking at any age avoids the further increase in lung cancer risk caused by continued smoking. In ex-smokers, the risk for lung cancer remains elevated for years after cessation, compared to that of never smokers.

Cigarette smoking is a major cause of transitional cell carcinomas of the bladder, ureter, and renal pelvis. It causes cancer of the oral cavity including the lip and tongue. Alcohol consumption in combination with smoking greatly increases the risk of oral cancer. Cigarette smoking increases the risk of sinonasal and nasopharyngeal cancers and causes oropharyngeal and hypohpa-ryngeal cancers. It also causes cancer of the esophagus, particularly squamous cell cancer, but is also a cause of adenocarcinoma of the esophagus, which has been increasing in the United States. Laryngeal cancer is caused by cigarette smoking and the risk is greatly enhanced by alcohol consumption. Similarly, pancreatic and stomach cancers are caused by cigarette smoking.[4]

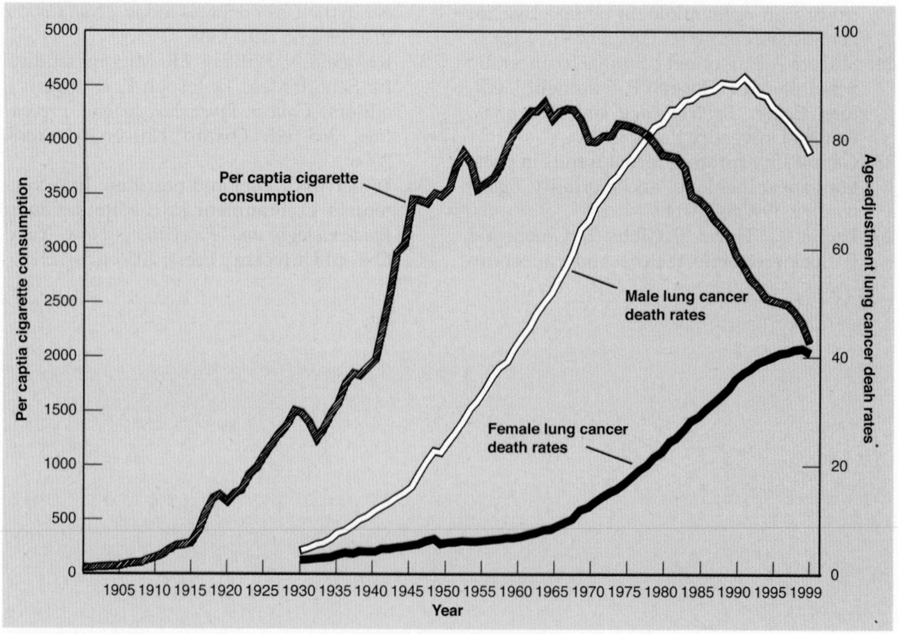

Figure 31-1 ▪ Tobacco use and lung cancer mortality, United States, 1900-1999. *Per 100,000 and age-adjusted to 2000 U.S. standard population. *Source:* Death rates from U.S. mortality public use tapes, 1960-1999, U.S. mortality volumes, 1930-1959, National Center for Health Statistics, Centers for Disease Control and Prevention, 2002. Per capita cigarette consumption: U.S. Department of Agriculture, 1900-1987, 1988, 1989-1997, 1998-1999. *Cancer Prevention & Early Detection Facts & Figures 2003*, American Cancer Society.[189]

Cigarette smoking is a cause of liver cancer, independent of the effects of hepatitis B and C virus infection and alcohol consumption. It causes cervical squamous cell carcinoma, after controlling for infection with human papilloma virus. Myeloid leukemia in adults is also causally related to cigarette smoking.[4]

Cigar and/or pipe smoking cause cancers of the oral cavity, oropharynx, hypopharynx, larynx, and esophagus, and the risk is similar to that of cigarette smoking. Dose-response relationships have been documented. Cigar and/or pipe smoking are causally associated with lung cancer and possibly with cancers of the pancreas, stomach, and urinary bladder.[4]

Secondhand smoke causes lung cancer in nonsmokers, although the risk is far less than that of a smoker. In spouses of smokers, the excess risk is about 20% in women and 30% in men. Workplace exposures to secondhand smoke also increase lung cancer risk in nonsmokers, by 12-19%.[4,6]

Epidemiologic studies from the United States, India, Pakistan, and Sweden provide sufficient evidence that smokeless tobacco is a cause of oral cancer in humans.[7] There is also sufficient evidence that smokeless tobacco causes pancreatic cancer in humans, based on studies from the United States and Norway,[7] and weaker but still persuasive evidence, including the results of a recent meta-analysis for smokeless tobacco as a cause of esophageal cancer.[8]

Table 31-1 Tobacco Smoke Carcinogens Recognized by the International Agency for Research on Cancer

Chemical Class	No. of Carcinogens	Representative Carcinogens
Polycyclic aromatic hydrocarbons (PAH) and their heterocyclic analogs	14	Benzo[*a*]pyrene (BaP) Dibenz[*a,h*]anthracene
N-Nitrosamines	8	4-(Methylnitrosamino)-1-(3-pyridyl)-1-butanone (NNK) *N'*-Nitrosonornicotine (NNN)
Aromatic amines	12	4-Aminobiphenyl 2-Naphthylamine
Aldehydes	2	Formaldehyde Acetaldehyde
Phenols	2	Catechol Caffeic acid
Volatile hydrocarbons	3	Benzene 1,3-Butadiene Isoprene
Other organics	11	Ethylene oxide Acrylonitrile
Inorganic compounds	9	Cadmium Polonium-210

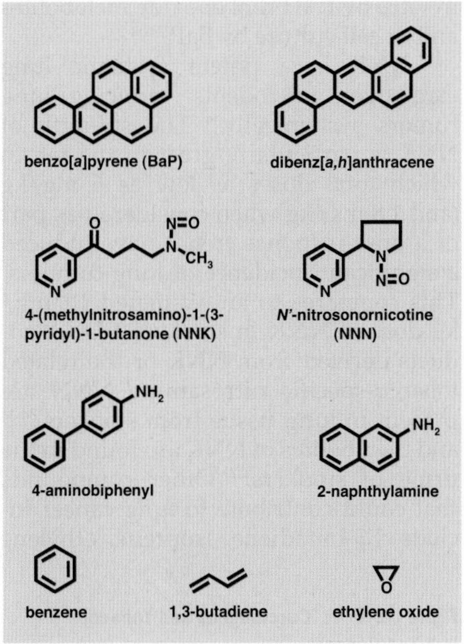

Figure 31-2 Structures of some representative tobacco smoke carcinogens.

Carcinogens in Tobacco Products

Cigarette smoke is a complex mixture containing over 4000 identified compounds. Of these, over 60 have been evaluated by IARC as having sufficient evidence for carcinogenicity in either laboratory animals or humans, with 16 of them being rated as carcinogenic to humans. The different classes of carcinogens and representatives of each are listed in Table 31-1.[2] Structures of some representative carcinogens in cigarette smoke are shown in Figure 31-2. There are other carcinogens in cigarette smoke that have not been evaluated by IARC. These include, for example, multiple polycyclic aromatic hydrocarbons (PAH) and aromatic amines with incompletely characterized occurrence levels and carcinogenic activities.[2,9]

In the early part of the 20th century, PAH were identified as carcinogenic constituents of coal tar.[10] They are products of incomplete combustion of all organic matter and occur always as complex mixtures, in tars, soots, broiled foods, vehicle engine exhaust and, of course, tobacco smoke. PAH are generally locally acting carcinogens, and some, such as benzo[*a*]pyrene (BaP), have strong carcinogenic activity on mouse skin and in rodent lung, as examples. BaP is considered carcinogenic to humans by IARC.[11] Heterocyclic analogs of PAH also occur in cigarette smoke.

Over 200 *N*-nitrosamines have been shown to be carcinogenic in at least 30 animal species.[12] They are potent systemic carcinogens that affect different tissues depending on their structures. Among these compounds are the "tobacco-specific *N*-nitrosamines," which are derived from, and structurally related to, alkaloids in tobacco leaf such as nicotine and nornicotine. Two of the most important *N*-nitrosamines in cigarette smoke are the tobacco-specific *N*-nitrosamines 4-(methylnitrosamino)-1-(3-pyridyl)-1-butanone (NNK) and *N'*-nitrosonornicotine (NNN).[13] NNK causes lung tumors in all species tested, and has particularly high activity in the rat. NNK can also induce tumors of the pancreas, nasal cavity, and liver. NNN produces esophageal and nasal tumors in rats and respiratory tract tumors in mice, hamsters, and mink.[14] NNK and NNN are carcinogenic to humans, according to IARC.[15]

Aromatic amines were first identified as human carcinogens due to industrial exposures in the dye industry in the early part of the 20th century. They include the well-known human bladder carcinogens 2-naphthylamine and 4-aminobiphenyl which, along with other isomers, are found in cigarette smoke.[16] Heterocyclic aromatic amines are also combustion products and are best known for their occurrence in broiled foods.[17]

Aldehydes such as formaldehyde and acetaldehyde occur widely in the human environment and are also endogenous metabolites found in human blood. Acetaldehyde is the major metabolite of ethanol. Concentrations of acetaldehyde and formaldehyde in cigarette smoke are far higher than those of PAH, *N*-nitrosamines, or aromatic amines, but their carcinogenic activities are weaker. Formaldehyde is considered carcinogenic to humans by IARC.[18]

Phenols such as catechol and caffeic acid occur in cigarette smoke and are relatively weak carcinogens in laboratory animals, but catechol is known to have potent cocarcinogenic activity with certain PAH.[19] Phenols have also been investigated as tumor promoters in cigarette smoke.[20]

The volatile hydrocarbons are 1,3-butadiene, a powerful multiorgan carcinogen in the mouse, with weaker activity in the rat; benzene, a known human leukemogen; and isoprene, a weaker carcinogen. 1,3-Butadiene and benzene are arguably the two most prevalent strong carcinogens in cigarette smoke, and both are considered carcinogenic to humans by IARC.[21,22]

Among the other carcinogenic organic compounds in cigarette smoke are the human carcinogens vinyl chloride, in low amounts, and ethylene oxide, in relatively large quantities. Ethylene oxide is associated with malignancies of the lymphatic and hematopoietic systems in both humans and experimental animals. Acrylonitrile, acrylamide, and acetamide are also present. Diverse metals such as the human carcinogen cadmium and the carcinogenic radionuclide polonium-210 are also found in cigarette smoke.[2]

Cigarette smoke also contains oxidants such as nitric oxide (up to 600 µg per cigarette) and related species,[23] and free radicals, which have been detected by electron spin resonance and spin trapping but are poorly characterized.[23] Other compounds may also be involved in oxidative damage produced by cigarette smoke. In addition, several studies demonstrate the presence in cigarette smoke of an as yet uncharacterized ethylating agent, which ethylates both DNA and hemoglobin.[24,25]

In summary, cigarette smoke contains multiple carcinogens. Based on various considerations, several of these carcinogens have been chosen for regulation under the Framework Convention on Tobacco Control, an international treaty of the World Health Organization. They are NNK, NNN, BaP, benzene, 1,3-butadiene, acetaldehyde, and formaldehyde. It should be noted that all of the carcinogens discussed earlier are also present in secondhand cigarette smoke, but human exposure is considerably less due to dilution with ambient air.

A variety of carcinogens have been detected in smokeless tobacco products.[26] The most abundant strong carcinogens are NNK and NNN, which are typically found in total amounts of 0.5-10 ppm in smokeless tobacco products, levels up to 1000 times higher than *N*-nitrosamines in other products designed for human consumption. Several other *N*-nitrosamines and *N*-nitrosamino acids are also present. Other carcinogenic compounds in smokeless tobacco include formaldehyde, acetaldehyde, crotonaldehyde, hydrazine, cadmium, nickel, and polonium-210.

Which Carcinogens Are Responsible for Which Cancers in Smokers?

Data from product analyses, carcinogenicity studies, and biochemical and molecular biological investigations support a role for certain carcinogens in specific types of tobacco-induced cancer, as summarized in Table 31-2. This represents a consensus view although proof remains elusive due to the complexity of the mixture.

Substantial evidence supports PAH and NNK as major causative factors in lung cancer. PAH can be potent locally acting carcinogens, and tobacco smoke fractions enriched in these compounds are carcinogenic to the lung.[27,28] PAH-DNA adducts have been detected in human lung, and the spectrum of mutations in the *p53* tumor suppressor gene isolated from lung tumors is similar to the spectrum of DNA damage produced in vitro by PAH diol epoxide metabolites and in cell culture by BaP.[29-32]

NNK is a potent systemic lung carcinogen in rodents, inducing lung tumors systemically.[14] The strength of NNK is particularly great in the rat, in which total doses as low as 6 mg/kg (and 1.8 mg/kg when considered as part of a dose-response trend) have induced a significant incidence of lung tumors.[33] This compares to an estimated 1.1 mg/kg dose of NNK in smokers.[14] DNA adducts derived from NNK or the related tobacco-specific nitrosamine NNN are present in lung tissue from smokers,[34-36] and metabolites of NNK are found in the urine of smokers.[37] Other compounds that could contribute to lung cancer include 1,3-butadiene, isoprene, ethylene oxide, ethyl carbamate, aldehydes, benzene, metals, and oxidants but the collective evidence for each of these is not as convincing as for PAH and NNK.[23,38]

Table 31-2 ■ Carcinogens and Tobacco-Induced Cancers

Cancer Type	Likely Carcinogen Involvement[a]
Lung	PAH, NNK (major) 1,3-butadiene, isoprene, ethylene oxide, ethyl carbamate, aldehydes, benzene, metals
Larynx	PAH
Nasal	NNK, NNN, other *N*-nitrosamines, aldehydes
Oral cavity	PAH, NNK, NNN
Esophagus	NNN, other *N*-nitrosamines
Liver	NNK, other *N*-nitrosamines, furan
Pancreas	NNK, NNAL
Bladder	4-Aminobiphenyl, other aromatic amines
Leukemia	Benzene

[a] Based on carcinogenicity studies in laboratory animals, biochemical evidence from human tissues and fluids, and epidemiological data, where available. NNAL, 4-(methylnitrosamino)-1-(3-pyridyl)-1-butanol; NNK, 4-(methylnitrosamino)-1-(3-pyridyl)-1-butanone; NNN, *N'*-nitrosonornicotine; PAH, polycyclic aromatic hydrocarbons. *Source:* Adapted from Surgeon General's Report 2008.

Cigarette smoke particulate phase causes larynx tumors in hamsters. This is most likely attributed to PAH,[9] and is consistent with *p53* gene mutations identified in tumors of the human larynx.[29] *N*-Nitrosamines, as well as acetaldehyde and formaldehyde, cause nasal tumors in rodents and are likely causes of smoking-associated nasal tumors.[12] Based on animal studies, PAH, NNK, and NNN are the most likely causes of oral cancer in smokers, while NNK and NNN are the most probable in smokeless tobacco users.[15,39] *N*-Nitrosamines are the most effective esophageal carcinogens known, and NNN, which produces tumors of the esophagus in rats, is the most prevalent *N*-nitrosamine carcinogen in cigarette smoke and smokeless tobacco.[15]

NNK and several other cigarette smoke *N*-nitrosamines are effective hepatocarcinogens in rats, as is furan.[12] NNK and its major metabolite 4-(methylnitrosamino)-1-(3-pyridyl)-1-butanol (NNAL) are the only pancreatic carcinogens known to be present in tobacco products, and biochemical data from studies with human tissues provide some support for their role in smoking-related pancreatic cancer, although DNA adducts were not detected.[40-42] The link between smokeless tobacco use and pancreatic cancer is also plausibly due to NNK and NNAL.[15]

4-Aminobiphenyl and 2-naphthylamine are bladder carcinogens in humans, and considerable data support the role of these and other aromatic amines as causes of bladder cancer in smokers.[43,44] The most probable cause of leukemia in smokers is benzene, which occurs in substantial quantities in cigarette smoke, and is a known cause of acute myelogenous leukemia in humans.[22]

Cigarette smoke causes oxidative damage, probably because it contains free radicals such as nitric oxide and mixtures of catechols, hydroquinones, semiquinones, and quinones that can induce redox cycling.[23,45] Smokers have lower levels of ascorbic acid, higher levels of oxidized lipids, and sometimes higher levels of oxidized DNA bases than nonsmokers, but the role of oxidative damage as a cause of specific tobacco-induced cancers remains unclear.[23,46]

Overview of Mechanisms of Tumor Induction by Tobacco Products

Figure 31-3 presents a conceptual model for the mechanisms by which cigarette smoke causes cancer.[23,47] A similar

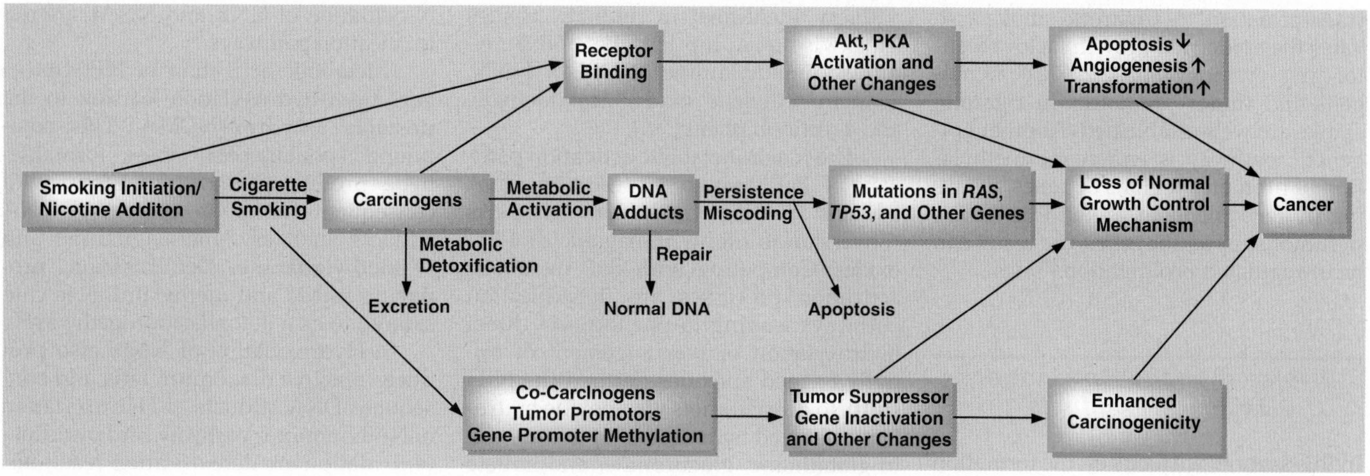

Figure 31-3 Conceptual model for understanding mechanisms of tobacco carcinogenesis.

model would apply to smokeless tobacco products, but there are less published data. The major established pathway by which cigarette smoke causes cancer is illustrated in the central track of Figure 31-3. Smokers are exposed to carcinogens which form DNA adducts, covalent binding products of the carcinogens, or their metabolites with DNA. These adducts cause miscoding resulting in permanent mutations in critical genes of somatic cells.

Most people begin smoking as teenagers and become addicted to nicotine. They cannot stop smoking in spite of their best efforts. The pathophysiology of nicotine addiction is discussed further, later in this chapter. Nicotine is not a carcinogen, but is accompanied in each puff by a mixture of the carcinogens listed in Table 31-1, along with many other compounds. Extensive data in the literature demonstrate the uptake of these carcinogens by smokers, and confirm the expected higher levels of their metabolites in urine of smokers than nonsmokers. Polymorphisms in nicotinic receptor genes are associated with increased lung cancer risk due to increased uptake of nicotine and carcinogens.[48-50]

The body responds to cigarette smoke constituents in a mode similar to its response to pharmaceutical agents and other "foreign compounds." Drug-metabolizing enzymes, usually cytochrome P450s (P450s), convert them to more water-soluble forms to facilitate excretion, but during this process some reactive (electrophilic) intermediates are formed. These intermediates covalently bind to DNA, forming DNA adducts.[51,52] P450s 1A1 and 1B1, inducible by cigarette smoke via interactions of smoke compounds with the aryl hydrocarbon receptor, are particularly important in the metabolic activation of PAH, while P450 2A13 is critical for the metabolism of NNK.[52,53] The inducibility of some P450s may be a critical aspect of cancer susceptibility in smokers. P450s 1A2, 2A6, 2E1, and 3A4 are also important in the activation of cigarette smoke carcinogens. Competing with metabolic activation is the intended detoxification, which results in harmless excretion of carcinogen metabolites, and is catalyzed by P450s and a variety of other enzymes including glutathione *S*-transferases and UDP-glucuronosyl transferases.[54,55] The balance between carcinogen metabolic activation and detoxification differs among individuals and is hypothesized to affect cancer susceptibility with those having higher activation and lower detoxification capacity being at highest risk. This is supported in part by evidence from molecular epidemiologic studies of polymorphisms, or variants, in the genes coding for these enzymes.[56]

DNA adducts are clearly critical in the carcinogenic process. Many investigations have examined the presence of DNA adducts in human tissues. There is massive evidence, especially from studies that use relatively nonspecific DNA adduct measurement methods, that DNA adduct levels in the lung and other tissues of smokers are higher than in nonsmokers, and some epidemiologic data link higher adduct levels with higher cancer risk.[4]

Cellular DNA repair systems can remove DNA adducts and restore the DNA structure to its normal state. DNA repair systems include direct base repair by alkyltransferases, excision of DNA damage by base and nucleotide excision repair, mismatch repair, and double-strand repair. If these repair enzymes are unsuccessful in removing the damage, then the DNA adducts will persist, increasing the probability of permanent mutations. There are polymorphisms in genes coding for some DNA repair enzymes and the resulting deficient DNA repair can increase the probability of cancer development.[57]

Persistent DNA adducts can cause miscoding during replication when DNA polymerase enzymes insert the wrong base opposite to an adduct. There is considerable specificity in the relationship between specific DNA adducts formed from cigarette smoke carcinogens and the types of mutations which they cause. G to T and G to A mutations have been frequently reported.[23] Mutations have been observed in the *KRAS* oncogene in lung cancer and in the *p53* tumor suppressor gene in a variety of cigarette smoke-induced cancers.[29,58] The cancer causing role of these genes has been firmly established in animal studies.[59,60] In addition, numerous cytogenetic changes are observed in lung cancer, and chromosome damage throughout the aerodigestive tract is strongly linked with cigarette smoke exposure. Gene mutations caused by DNA adducts can cause loss of normal cellular growth control functions, via a complex process of signal transduction pathways, ultimately resulting in genomic instability, cellular proliferation, and cancer.[61,62] Apoptosis, or programmed cell death, is protective, and can remove cells with DNA damage, thus serving as a counterbalance to these mutational events. The balance between mechanisms leading to apoptosis and those suppressing apoptosis will have a major impact on tumor growth.[62]

While the central track of Figure 31-3 is definitely a major pathway by which cigarette smoke carcinogens cause cancer, epigenetic pathways also contribute, as indicated in the top and bottom tracks.[47,63] Nicotine and tobacco-specific *N*-nitrosamines bind to nicotinic and other cellular receptors leading to activation of Akt (also known as protein kinase B), protein kinase A, and other changes, resulting in decreased apoptosis, increased angiogenesis, and increased transformation.[64,65] Cigarette smoke activates the epidermal growth factor receptor and cyclooxygenase-2.[66] Cocarcinogens and tumor promoters in cigarette smoke are well-established. Another epigenetic pathway is enzymatic methylation of promoter regions of genes, resulting in gene silencing. When this occurs in tumor suppressor genes, the result can be unregulated proliferation.[67]

Diverse Tobacco Carcinogens Form DNA Adducts

In this section, we focus on the formation of DNA adducts, which, as described earlier, are absolutely central to cancer causation in smokers and smokeless tobacco users. Many of the carcinogens listed in Table 31-1 require metabolic activation to intermediates, generally electrophiles, which react with nucleophilic sites in DNA resulting in the formation of DNA adducts, but some can form adducts without metabolism. Figure 31-a presents an overview of DNA adduct formation from eight tobacco smoke constituents that are implicated in the formation of DNA adducts identified in human tissues (clockwise from top left): BaP, NNK, *N*-nitrosodimethylamine (NDMA), NNN, acrolein, ethylene oxide, acetaldehyde, and 4-aminobiphenyl.

The major metabolic activation pathway of BaP known to result in DNA adducts identified in human tissues is conversion to highly mutagenic diol epoxides. Competing with BaP metabolic activation processes are detoxification pathways leading to phenols, via direct hydroxylation or rearrangement of initially formed epoxides (termed the NIH shift), to dihydrodiols via epoxide hydrolase catalyzed hydration of epoxides, and to glutathione, glucuronide, and sulfate conjugates. Quinone metabolites are also observed, resulting from initial hydroxylation at the six position followed by further oxidation.[68,69]

The major metabolic activation pathways of NNK and its metabolite, NNAL, occur by hydroxylation of the carbons adjacent to the *N*-nitroso group (α-hydroxylation) that leads, via diazonium ions, to the formation of DNA adducts.[14] Glucuronidation of NNAL, at either the hydroxyl group or the nitrogen of the pyridine ring, and pyridine-N-oxidation of NNK and NNAL are detoxification pathways.[14]

Metabolic activation of NDMA occurs by α-hydroxylation leading to the unstable α-hydroxyNDMA. This compound spontaneously loses formaldehyde producing diazonium ions with consequent formation of methyl DNA adducts such as 7-methylguanine and O^6-methylguanine. Denitrosation, producing nitrite and methylamine, is considered to be a detoxification pathway.[12]

α-Hydroxylation of NNN also produces reactive diazonium ions and consequent DNA adducts. β-Hydroxylation of NNN, a minor pathway, and pyridine-N-oxidation are detoxification reactions. NNN is also detoxified by denitrosation/oxidation to produce norcotinine, and by glucuronidation of the pyridine ring.[14,70]

Acrolein, ethylene oxide, and acetaldehyde react directly with DNA to form well-characterized adducts.[71-73] There are competing detoxification pathways involving glutathione conjugation and, in the case of acetaldehyde, oxidation.

4-Aminobiphenyl is metabolically activated by N-hydroxylation.[74] Conjugation of the resulting hydroxylamine with acetate or other groups such as sulfate ultimately

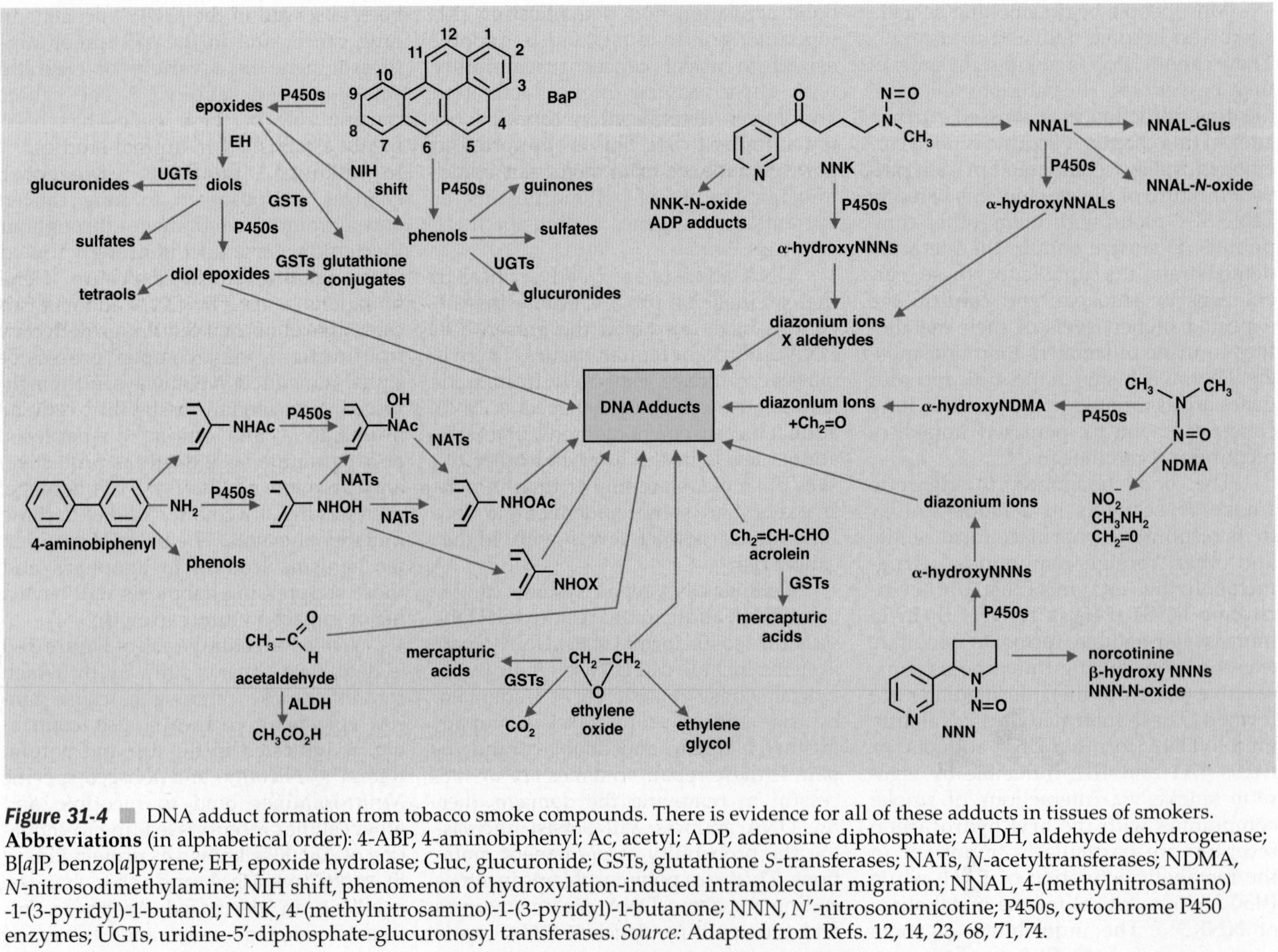

Figure 31-4 DNA adduct formation from tobacco smoke compounds. There is evidence for all of these adducts in tissues of smokers. **Abbreviations** (in alphabetical order): 4-ABP, 4-aminobiphenyl; Ac, acetyl; ADP, adenosine diphosphate; ALDH, aldehyde dehydrogenase; B[*a*]P, benzo[*a*]pyrene; EH, epoxide hydrolase; Gluc, glucuronide; GSTs, glutathione *S*-transferases; NATs, *N*-acetyltransferases; NDMA, *N*-nitrosodimethylamine; NIH shift, phenomenon of hydroxylation-induced intramolecular migration; NNAL, 4-(methylnitrosamino)-1-(3-pyridyl)-1-butanol; NNK, 4-(methylnitrosamino)-1-(3-pyridyl)-1-butanone; NNN, *N'*-nitrosonornicotine; P450s, cytochrome P450 enzymes; UGTs, uridine-5'-diphosphate-glucuronosyl transferases. *Source:* Adapted from Refs. 12, 14, 23, 68, 71, 74.

produces nitrenium ions, which react with DNA-producing adducts mainly at C-8 of guanine. Other aromatic amines as well as heterocyclic aromatic amines are predominantly metabolically activated in similar ways. Acetylation of 4-aminobiphenyl can be a detoxification pathway if not followed by N-hydroxylation. Ring hydroxylation and conjugation of the phenols results in detoxification.[74]

In summary, the major pathways of metabolic activation and detoxification of some of the principle carcinogens in cigarette smoke are quite well-established. Reactive intermediates that are critical in forming DNA adducts include diol epoxides of PAH, diazonium ions generated by α-hydroxylation of nitrosamines, and nitrenium ions formed from esters of N-hydroxylated aromatic amines. Other cigarette smoke compounds such as ethylene oxide, acrolein, and acetaldehyde react directly with DNA to form adducts. Glutathione and glucuronide conjugation play major roles in the detoxification of cigarette smoke carcinogens.

Tobacco Carcinogen Biomarkers

Tobacco carcinogen biomarkers are specific measurable compounds—usually adducts or metabolites—that come from particular carcinogens in tobacco.[47] Biomarker types include DNA and protein adducts, and tobacco carcinogens or their metabolites in breath, serum or plasma, saliva, hair, toenails, and urine. DNA adduct measurements can provide direct evidence concerning the extent of DNA damage in a person who uses tobacco products, and potentially could be the best indicator of risk. Protein adducts are frequently used as surrogates for DNA adducts because most carcinogens or their metabolically activated forms that react with DNA also react with proteins such as albumin and hemoglobin.[47] Metabolites or unchanged carcinogens in blood, saliva, hair, toenails, or urine can provide critical information on extents of carcinogen exposure and uptake as well as interindividual differences in carcinogen metabolism. The following are some examples of tobacco carcinogen biomarkers. Urinary 1-hydroxypyrene is a widely accepted biomarker of PAH dose.[37] It is a metabolite of pyrene, a compound that always occurs in PAH mixtures and is a constituent of cigarette smoke. Phenanthrene and fluorene metabolites are also being used as PAH biomarkers.[75,76] BaP diol epoxide-hemoglobin adducts are another biomarker of PAH uptake and metabolic activation.[30] For nitrosamines, the most widely used biomarker is "total NNAL," the sum of NNAL and its glucuronides, urinary metabolites of NNK.[37] Total NNAL has been applied in many studies to estimate NNK uptake in smokers, smokeless tobacco users, and nonsmokers exposed to secondhand smoke. For aromatic amines, hemoglobin adducts are consistently related to dose and have been extensively applied.[44] For benzene, 1,3-butadiene, acrolein, crotonaldehyde, and ethylene oxide, mercapturic acids of the parent compounds or their metabolites, excreted in urine, are useful biomarkers.[37] Benzene uptake has also been assessed by measuring unchanged benzene in urine and by quantifying urinary *trans, trans*-muconic acid.[37] Ethylene oxide hemoglobin adducts and ethyl hemoglobin adducts have been used to assess exposure to ethylene oxide and to an unknown ethylating agent in cigarette smoke.[24]

Tobacco carcinogen biomarkers are recognized as being critical in the study of tobacco and cancer.[77] It is now widely accepted that tobacco carcinogen biomarkers will be the best way to evaluate new tobacco products that come on the market, sometimes with claims of reduced carcinogenicity and toxicity.[77] Biomarkers could also be very important in the regulation of tobacco products, currently being considered by the U.S. Congress and the World Health Organization under the Framework Convention on Tobacco Control. Until now, tobacco products have been evaluated mainly by machine measurement of smoke components under standard conditions. While this is useful for comparing products under uniform conditions, it is recognized that machine measurements are misleading with respect to actual constituent delivery and to the health effects of tobacco products. Tobacco carcinogen biomarkers also are extraordinarily useful in evaluating the exposure of nonsmokers to secondhand smoke. Total NNAL has been particularly effective in this respect because of its tobacco specificity.[78]

Tobacco carcinogen biomarkers also have potential as measures of individual susceptibility to the effects of cigarette smoke. They could become part of an algorithm to predict which smoker will get cancer, information that is not presently available and could be very useful in cessation efforts.

Pathophysiology of Nicotine Addiction

Tobacco-related cancers are primarily a consequence of the persistent use of tobacco, ie, the addiction to nicotine. The addiction to nicotine is a consequence of the speed and magnitude of nicotine delivery, the clearance of nicotine, its effect on the brain and the development of physical dependence. Associative learning, where stimuli linked with smoking trigger craving and tobacco use, also plays an important role in the development of addiction. The speed and amount of nicotine delivery is dependent on the amount of nicotine in the product, the alkalinity of the product, and the route of administration. Nicotine is a volatile alkaloid in the tobacco plant and its absorption and renal secretion are highly pH-dependent.

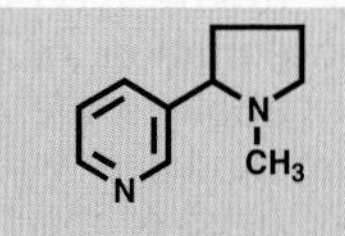

Nicotine

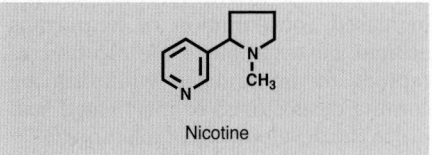

Higher alkalinity leads to a higher concentration of nonionized nicotine, facilitating crossing of cell membranes.[79,80] The fastest rate and greatest amount of nicotine delivery is through cigarettes. Nicotine, when inhaled, enters the lungs, undergoes dissolution in pulmonary fluid, is transported to the heart, and then immediately passes to the brain.[79,81]

Nicotine is metabolized to cotinine primarily by C-oxidation via P450 2A6. Cotinine is further hydroxylated to *trans*-3-hydroxycotinine also via P450 2A6 and other P450 enzymes. P450 2A6 activity varies significantly among individuals and may affect smoking behaviors.[82-87] Nicotine is also metabolized by two other pathways: glucuronidation and N-oxidation via UGT and FMO enzymes, respectively, which also may significantly influence the circulating levels of nicotine in a smoker and the amount of nicotine that reaches the brain.[88]

Nicotine targets various nicotinic acetylcholine receptor (nAchRs) subtypes, which are found in the periphery and in the central nervous system.[89,90] More specifically, nicotine targets neuronal nAchRs, such as α4β2,[91] α7,[92] and α3[93] containing receptors. Stimulation of these receptors results in the release of a number of neurotransmitters that are associated with the different effects from nicotine.[79,94] These neurotransmitters include dopamine that is critical for the reinforcing effects of nicotine,[95,96] glutamate, which is an excitatory neurotransmitter that stimulates the release of dopamine,[97] and endogenous opioid peptides.[98] In addition, nicotine has also been found to stimulate the release of γ-aminobutyric acid (GABA), an inhibitory neurotransmitter that reduces dopamine levels.[99] Because nAchRs on the GABA neuron are quicker to desensitize than the nAchRs on the glutamate neuron, a more prolonged release of glutamate occurs resulting in higher rather than lower levels of dopamine.[99] Nicotine administration also increases extracellular noradrenaline in various parts of the brain;[100-103] however, the effects of nicotine on neurotransmitters like serotonin or peptides, such as endocannabinoids, are less conclusive. The release of these various neurotransmitters leads to the arousal, mood modulation, performance enhancement, analgesic, and weight loss effects associated with tobacco use.[79,104]

With repeated administration of nicotine, neural adaptations occur to attain homeostasis resulting from the increased activity on the nAchR receptor sites and increased concentration of neurotransmitters. For example, some nicotinic receptors are upregulated while also becoming desensitized or inactivated leading to the development of tolerance.[79,105,106] Because the body develops a homeostatic response, upon abstinence from the drug, the smoker experiences withdrawal symptoms. These withdrawal symptoms include negative affect such as irritability, frustration or anger, anxiety, dysphoric or depressed mood. Withdrawal symptoms also include restlessness, difficulty concentrating, insomnia, decreased heart rate, and increased appetite.[107] More recently, constipation, cough, dizziness, increased dreaming, and mouth sores have also been described as potential withdrawal symptoms.[108]

With the exception of weight, withdrawal symptoms tend to peak during the first week of abstinence and then gradually decrease to baseline levels by 2-4 weeks.[108-110] However, recent studies have found some withdrawal symptoms to be persistent and elevated for several months after quitting.[111,112] Weight, on the other hand, may increase over the course of 6 months, and then decrease or be sustained.[113] Studies also show individual variations in the intensity, slope, and variability of symptoms.[114] Symptoms of greater intensity, positive slope, and variability have been observed to predict relapse to smoking[115,116] with craving and negative affect being the most likely symptoms to be associated with relapse.[117,118]

Behavioral or learning factors also sustain addiction. Stimuli in the environment become associated with the reinforcing effects of nicotine (eg, experience of pleasure, reduction of negative affect of withdrawal symptoms). Over time and through associative learning, these stimuli begin to control behavior, ie, these stimuli evoke craving for the drug or drug-seeking behavior. These stimuli can include the sensory aspects of smoking, smoking paraphernalia, people or situations associated with smoking, or mood states.[119-121] This associative learning has been considered to be as important a contributory factor to nicotine addiction as the direct effects of nicotine itself.[95,122-125] Nicotine has also been observed to enhance the reinforcing effects of stimuli or other reinforcers that are not directly paired with the administration of nicotine.[126-128] In other words, both stimuli paired with smoking and nicotine's enhancement of the reward value of other stimuli and reinforcers (eg, coffee, food, alcohol) not directly paired with smoking facilitates the development and maintenance of smoking behavior.

In summary, people become addicted to nicotine and persist in smoking because of the rewarding effects from nicotine, the development of neuroadaptation from repeated use, and the manifestation of withdrawal symptoms when they quit smoking. In addition, stimuli in the environment play a strong role in the urge for, and persistence of, cigarette use.

Susceptibility to Nicotine Addiction

Factors that contribute to an individual's susceptibility to nicotine addiction include the environmental culture (cost, access and availability of tobacco products, tobacco use bans, social acceptability, parental monitoring, and modeling) and the characteristics of the individual (eg, genes, comorbid psychiatry disorders, and personality features). With regard to the former factors, greater cost, less accessibility, smoking bans, less social acceptability, bans and restrictions on promotion and advertising on products, greater parental monitoring, and less parental and peer use are associated with less risk for uptake of tobacco products.[129,130] With regard to the latter factors, initiation of smoking behavior and transition to dependence (ie, persistent smoking) have been found to show strong heritability.[131] To date, the potential candidate gene variants include cholinergic nicotine receptor genes; dopamine D2 and D4 receptor and dopamine transport genes; tryptophan hydroxylase (associated with serotonin biosynthesis) and serotonin transporter (associated with serotonin reuptake) genes; monoamine oxidase (MAO-A) and dopamine β-hydroxylase genes affecting norepinephrine pathways; and genes involved in the metabolism of nicotine such as *CYPs*.[132-134] Individuals may be inheriting different attributes including responsiveness to nicotine, responsiveness of the various neurotransmitter pathways, or behavioral traits, such as novelty or sensation seeking, hostility, impulsivity, or harm avoidance.[132] Comorbid psychiatric disorders may also predispose a smoker to begin or persist in smoking. A population survey found that 41% of individuals with mental illness smoked cigarettes[135] and in another study, nicotine-dependent individuals with comorbid psychiatric disorder accounted for 34% of all cigarettes smoked in the United States.[136] Disorders that are particularly associated with daily or dependent smokers include alcohol and drug dependence, depression, and anxiety disorders.[137-142]

Prevention and Cessation of Tobacco Use

To significantly reduce the prevalence of tobacco use and the incidence of cancer, interventions include reducing environmental risk factors for tobacco use through policies and prevention efforts, providing interventions that assist the addicted smoker, and targeting the tobacco product.

The best way to reduce tobacco addiction is to prevent initiation of use and to provide effective treatments. Several policy and educational measures have been found to be effective in reducing the prevalence of smoking and to protect the lives of individuals who are exposed to smoking. The most effective means of reducing prevalence of tobacco use is a comprehensive tobacco control approach. In the most recent Institute of Medicine report, *Ending the Tobacco Problem: A Blueprint for the Nation*,[143] several recommendations were made and included the following:

- Increase state and federal excise tax rates to reduce the prevalence of smoking.
- Strengthen smoking restrictions and include nonresidential indoor locations, health-care facilities, correctional facilities, and residential complexes. Encourage parents to make their homes and vehicles smoke-free. Smoking bans have had a significant impact in protecting nonsmokers from health effects of secondhand smoke, reducing the amount and potentially the prevalence of smoking, and reinforcing nonsmoking social norms.[144]
- Limit youth access to tobacco products by requiring state licenses of all outlets that sell tobacco products. Obtaining and maintaining a license would include requirements that reduce the sale to minors (eg, verification of birth date, placing cigarettes behind the counter, banning the use of self-service displays and vending machines) and license suspension with repeated violations. Additionally, youth access should also be limited by banning the sale of tobacco products directly to consumers through mail order or internet sources or other electronic systems.
- Intensify prevention interventions by having school boards endorse a requirement for all middle and high schools to adopt evidence-based smoking prevention programs and funding ongoing national, youth-oriented

antismoking media campaigns. Furthermore, all health-care providers should screen and educate youth about tobacco use during clinic visits.
- Increase the demand and availability of evidence-based smoking cessation interventions through mass media and other public education programs and through comprehensive cessation polices that include the provision of effective cessation treatment through health-care systems and reimbursement for effective smoking cessation treatment as a lifetime benefit.
- Change the regulatory landscape to include such measures as giving the U.S. Food and Drug Administration broad regulatory authority over the manufacture, distribution, marketing, and use of tobacco products, as well as the authority to regulate the design and characteristics of the tobacco product to promote public health (see Tobacco Harm Reduction section for more details); strengthening and regularly updating and revising federally mandated warning labels for tobacco products, including information in or on tobacco packages on health effects from tobacco use and on products for quitting; and banning misleading terms or techniques that would lead a consumer to misperceive a product as being reduced risk (eg, terms such as "light," "ultralight," "mild").

Similar measures were proposed by the World Health Organization Framework Convention on Tobacco Control.[145] The objective of this Convention was to protect present and future generations from the devastating effects of tobacco consumption and exposure to tobacco smoke and to substantially reduce its use. This international treaty contained articles that described (a) increases in price and tax of tobacco products; (b) protection from exposure to tobacco smoke in indoor workplaces, public transport, indoor public places, and as appropriate, other public places; (c) education, communication, training, and public awareness of tobacco control issues (health risks, risk for addiction, benefits of cessation, economic consequences, development and implementation of tobacco control strategies and programs); (d) optimally, a comprehensive ban of all tobacco advertising, promotion, and sponsorship; (e) restriction on sales to youth and minors and reduction in accessibility of tobacco products to minors; and (f) demand reduction through promotion and provision of accessible and affordable evidence-based cessation. Provisions for regulation of tobacco advertising, promotion, and sponsorship, of content of tobacco products, of tobacco product disclosures, and of packaging and labeling of tobacco products were also described.

Treatment of Tobacco Use

Treatments are targeted toward dealing with the physical addiction to nicotine, the psychological reliance on the effects of nicotine, and the behavioral aspects of tobacco use. Many evidenced-based effective treatment interventions are available to assist smokers to quit smoking (www.cochrane.org/reviews/en/topics/94.html#topic_2).[146,147] According to the recent U.S. Department of Health and Human Services Clinical Practice Guideline on Treatment Tobacco Use and Dependence, these evidence-based treatments include both pharmacological treatments and counseling, with the combination of both treatments leading to the greater success than either alone.[148] With respect to pharmacological treatments, the U.S. Guideline recommends that all smokers should be provided pharmacotherapies unless medically contraindicated or if there is a lack of sufficient evidence to support their use (eg, among pregnant women, adolescents, smokeless tobacco users, and light smokers). The first-line therapies include nicotine replacement products (eg, nicotine patch, gum, lozenge, inhaler, nasal spray, and nicotine tablets in other parts of the world), bupropion, and varenicline. Second-line therapies include nortriptyline and clonidine. These drugs have different mechanisms of action, although all medications lead to reduction in craving and/or withdrawal symptoms. Nicotine replacement products are nicotine agonists, targeting the nicotinic acetylcholine receptors but delivering nicotine at a slower rate than most of the tobacco products. Varenicline is an α4β2 partial agonist, which means that it can provide relief of craving and withdrawal through its agonist effect and block the reinforcing effect of nicotine through its antagonist effect.[149,150] Bupropion and nortriptyline block the neuronal reuptake of specific neurotransmitters. This blockade results in the enhanced levels of neurotransmitters at the synapse: dopamine and norepinephrine from bupropion and norepinephrine and to lesser extent serotonin from nortriptyline. These effects are similar to those of nicotine. Bupropion is also considered to act as a noncompetitive nicotinic acetylcholine receptor antagonist.[151] Clonidine is an α2 adrenergic autoreceptor agonist that stimulates the α-adrenergic receptor and inhibits the production of norepinephrine, reducing sympathetic activity.[152] Decreasing sympathetic overactivity may be responsible for reducing the severity of some of the withdrawal symptoms; however, the mechanism is yet unclear.[153]

The odds ratio ranges from 1.5 (nicotine gum)- to 3.1 (varenicline)-fold greater efficacy of pharmacological products compared to placebo, with most medicinal products demonstrating a twofold increase in efficacy compared to placebo (see Table 31-3).[148] The efficacy of nicotine replacement products was questioned after some of them switched to over-the-counter availability[154]; however, meta-analysis of studies examining the efficacy

Table 31-3 **Meta-Analysis (2008): Effectiveness and Abstinence Rates for Various Medications and Medication Combinations Compared to Placebo at 6-month Post-Quit (n = 83 Studies)[a]**

Medication	No. of Arms	Estimated Odds Ratio (95% CI)	Estimated Abstinence Rate (95% CI)
Placebo	80	1.0	13.8
Monotherapies			
Varenicline (2 mg/day)	5	3.1 (2.5-3.8)	33.2 (28.9-37.8)
Nicotine nasal spray	4	2.3 (1.7-3.0)	26.7 (21.5-32.7)
High-dose nicotine patch (>25 mg) (this included both standard or long-term duration)	4	2.3 (1.7-3.0)	26.5 (21.3-32.5)
Long-term nicotine gum (>14 weeks)	6	2.2 (1.5-3.2)	26.1 (19.7-33.6)
Varenicline (1 mg/day)	3	2.1 (1.5-3.0)	25.4 (19.6-32.2)
Nicotine inhaler	6	2.1 (1.5-2.9)	24.8 (19.1-31.6)
Clonidine	3	2.1 (1.2-3.7)	25.0 (15.7-37.3)
Bupropion SR	26	2.0 (1.8-2.2)	24.2 (22.2-26.4)
Nicotine patch (6-14 weeks)	32	1.9 (1.7-2.3)	23.4 (21.3-25.8)
Long-term nicotine patch (>14 weeks)	10	1.9 (1.7-2.3)	23.7 (21.0-26.6)
Nortriptyline	5	1.8 (1.3-2.6)	22.5 (16.8-29.4)
Nicotine gum (6-14 weeks)	15	1.5 (1.2-1.7)	19.0 (16.5-21.9)
Combination therapies			
Patch (long-term; > 14 weeks) + ad libitum NRT (gum or spray)	3	3.6 (2.5-5.2)	36.5 (28.6-45.3)
Patch + bupropion SR	3	2.5 (1.9-3.4)	28.9 (23.5-35.1)
Patch + nortriptyline	2	2.3 (1.3-4.2)	27.3 (17.2-40.4)
Patch + inhaler	2	2.2 (1.3-3.6)	25.8 (17.4-36.5)

[a]Go to www.surgeongeneral.gov/tobacco/gdlnrefs.htm for the articles used in this meta-analysis.
Source: Adapted from U.S. Clinical Practice Guideline: Treating Tobacco Use and Dependence.

of over-the-counter nicotine replacement therapies and a recent "real-world effectiveness" study have continued to show a greater beneficial effect from these medicinal products than placebo or nonuse of these products.[148,155,156]

Very few studies have been conducted comparing the efficacy across products; however, of the few that have been conducted, bupropion led to greater treatment success than nicotine patch,[157] although this result has not been replicated; and varenicline led to greater treatment success than bupropion.[149,150] An a posteriori meta-analysis test comparing nicotine patch with various pharmacotherapies showed that varenicline (OR = 1.6, 95% CI = 1.3-2.0) is associated with significantly higher likelihood of long-term abstinence than patch alone.[148] One randomized study showed that varenicline is more effective than nicotine patch at the end of treatment (OR = 1.7, 95% CI = 1.26-2.28) and near significant for continuous abstinence at the end of 1 year (OR = 1.4, 95% CI = 0.99-1.99).[158]

Studies have been conducted to determine if efficacy rates can be enhanced. Higher doses of the nicotine gum and lozenge (4 mg compared to 2 mg) for highly dependent smokers improve cessation success rates,[159,160] but increasing the dose from one to two nicotine patches produces only a small benefit compared to the usual one patch among heavy smokers.[148,159] Compared to patch alone, long-term patch use (>14 weeks) plus ad libitum use (gum or spray; OR = 1.9, 95% CI = 1.3-2.7) is associated with higher long-term abstinence rates.[148] Although the patch plus bupropion, nortriptyline, or nicotine inhaler has also led to a greater than twofold increase in efficacy compared to placebo, it is unclear if higher rates of long-term abstinence are observed with these combination therapies compared to monotherapies. Studies have also examined the effects of increasing the duration of mono-nicotine replacement therapy, varenicline, nortriptyline, and bupropion. Longer treatment durations seem most promising for nicotine replacement therapy and for varenicline.[161] The meta-analysis for the U.S. Clinical Guideline showed that long-term use of nicotine gum (>14 weeks) led to a slightly higher odds ratio comparing nicotine gum to placebo than shorter use of the product (6-14 weeks), but as noted previously, longer-term use of the patch plus ad libitum gum or spray led to very high odds ratios (see Table 31-3).[148] For varenicline, smokers assigned to long-term use of this medication experienced higher cessation rates (37% vs 8% 7-day point prevalence).[162] Among quitters, those assigned to varenicline compared to placebo experienced fewer relapses, although the effect was somewhat modest (OR at 52 weeks = 1.3, 95% CI = 1.1-1.7).[163] In general, the choice of a pharmacological product is based on the tobacco user's history of quit attempts (success or lack of success with products), contraindications with the medication, consumer preference, and cost.

In addition to pharmacotherapies, group, individual, and proactive telephone counseling have also been found to be effective in assisting smokers quit smoking.[148] Effective counseling includes identifying high-risk situations, developing problem-solving and coping skills, and obtaining intra-treatment support (eg, support from individual providing treatment or members in treatment). The U.S. Clinical Guideline also noted that the greater the intensity of treatment, the higher the rate of success and recommended that sessions should be at least 10 min in duration and at least four sessions. Furthermore, the greater the number of clinicians involved in providing treatment, the greater the number of formats; and the more tailored the treatments are to the tobacco user, the higher the rate of abstinence. The provision of counseling via telephone-counseling quitlines has the particular advantage of being accessible to many people. Some of the quitlines provide free nicotine replacement therapy. The provision of free pharmacotherapies has been observed to increase calls to the quitlines[164] and the combination of medication and quitline counseling increases the odds of cessation compared to medication alone (OR = 1.3, 95% CI = 1.1-1.6).[148] Other promising vehicles for providing treatment include the Internet.[148,165]

The Guideline also states that those individuals who are not ready to make a quit attempt should be counseled using motivational interviewing techniques. Motivational interviewing has been found to be effective in increasing future quit attempts.[148] Motivational interventions are aimed at motivating the smoker to make future cessation attempts and include what has been described as providing the "5Rs." The 5Rs involve having the tobacco user: (1) indicate why quitting tobacco use is personally *relevant;* (2) identify *risks* associated with continued tobacco use; (3) identify personal *rewards* or benefits from quitting smoking; (4) identify *roadblocks* to quitting smoking and discuss ways to overcome these roadblocks. Finally, it is important to (5) *repeat* this intervention if the tobacco user continues to be unwilling to quit.

The dissemination of these evidence-based treatments is critical.[166] The U.S. Clinical Practice Guideline recommended developing an infrastructure in health-care settings, including hospitals, that facilitates the identification of all smokers, and trains and provides feedback to providers and dedicated staff to ensure delivery of effective interventions (eg, the provision of smoking cessation advice, assistance and arrangement for follow-up). Table 31-4 shows the 5 *A*s that health professionals are advised to follow. The Guideline also strongly recommended that health organizations and insurance companies provide coverage for smoking cessation to all of their members.

With a better understanding of the pathophysiology and behavioral/learning contributions of tobacco addiction and of the process of relapse or recovery, better pharmacological and behavioral treatments are likely to evolve. With the ever-expanding research on the interaction of genetic profiles or endophenotypes of addiction and response to treatment, matching treatments to patient profiles should also improve treatment efficacy.[132]

Tobacco Harm Reduction

One of the greatest threats, but also potentially a great opportunity, for reducing tobacco-related morbidity and mortality are efforts directed toward tobacco harm reduction. Tobacco harm reduction is defined as, "minimizing harms and decreasing total morbidity and mortality, without completely eliminating tobacco and nicotine use."[80] Harm reduction can

Table 31-4 ■ **The "5 As" Model for Treating Tobacco Use and Dependence**

Ask about tobacco use	Identify and document tobacco use status for every patient at every visit
Advise to quit	In a clear, strong, and personalized manner, urge every tobacco user to quit
Assess willingness to make a quit attempt	Is the tobacco user willing to make a quit attempt at this time?
Assist in quit attempt	For the patient willing to make a quit attempt, offer medication and provide or refer for counseling or additional treatment to help the patient quit For patients unwilling to quit at the time, provide interventions designed to increase future quit attempts
Arrange follow-up	For the patient willing to make a quit attempt, arrange for follow-up contacts, beginning within the first week after the quit date For patients unwilling to make a quit attempt at the time, address tobacco dependence and willingness to quit at next clinic visit

Source: From U.S. Clinical Practice Guideline: Treating Tobacco Use and Dependence.

be considered a threat because it may compromise effective tobacco control efforts if consumers believe "safer" tobacco products exist on the market, which might increase the overall prevalence of tobacco use. On the other hand, tobacco harm reduction can be considered an opportunity if manufacturers, through regulation, can develop and only market products that are less harmful than existing tobacco products. In the current unregulated market, tobacco companies have attempted to modify cigarettes to reduce one or more toxicants by various means and have introduced products that do not burn tobacco, but heat tobacco that vaporize nicotine. A few tobacco companies and public health scientists have advocated that smokers who cannot quit smoking substitute the use of smokeless tobacco products[167,168] or at a minimum inform the public about the relative toxicity across different tobacco products.[169] Unfortunately, major smokeless tobacco and cigarette companies have been marketing pouched smokeless tobacco products, which have lower tobacco-specific nitrosamines and varying levels of free nicotine,[170] to smokers as a substitute for cigarettes in situations where they cannot smoke, thus allowing continued smoking.

To date, research in this area of potential reduced exposure products (or PREPs) has not been comprehensive and methods and measures to assess these products are in various stages of development. However, the existing scientific literature would suggest that a combustible cigarette product is unlikely to result in any significant reduction in tobacco harm given the complex toxicant mixture that is delivered to the smoker. The only possible exception would be the reduced nicotine content cigarettes that are associated with significantly reduced addiction. These cigarettes would likely lead to reduction in harm by way of reducing initiation of smoking and facilitating smoking cessation.[171,172] Studies examining reduced nicotine content cigarettes have shown no compensatory smoking (compensating for low nicotine levels by smoking harder on the cigarette or smoking more cigarettes), no increase in toxicant exposure, and a reduction in nicotine dependence.[173] Heated cigarettes or electronic cigarettes that deliver nicotine vapor are more likely to result in reduced exposure and potentially risk for disease, but to date, there is insufficient evidence to support this claim. Smokeless tobacco products, particularly products with low tobacco-specific nitrosamines, are likely to result in reduced health risk if they completely substitute for cigarette smoking. However, recommending the use of smokeless tobacco as a substitute for cigarettes has raised concerns because of the extremely high levels of toxicants in these products in some countries, such as India and Sudan,[174] that are associated with premature mortality,[175] the potential for a gateway effect where smokeless tobacco users may graduate to cigarette smoking, the potential for dual use of tobacco products that may result in exposure to even greater levels of toxicants, and the concern over the population impact of the product if they are misperceived as safe.[176] The safest way to deliver nicotine is through medicinal nicotine products because the only main tobacco constituent delivered to the subjects is nicotine, which has minimal or reduced health consequences compared to tobacco.[177,178] Furthermore, unlike tobacco products, medicinal products are under strong regulatory control and undergo rigorous testing.[80]

In order to make significant strides in tobacco harm reduction, tobacco must be regulated. Tobacco regulation will require manufacturers to disclose all toxic constituents in both the product and product's smoke, will allow the promulgation of tobacco product standards including reducing nicotine and reducing or eliminating other constituents in all tobacco products, and will require evaluation of novel PREPs using specific standards and regulate and prohibit claims that will mislead consumers into thinking tobacco products are safer or safe without strong evidence to support such a claim.[179]

Chemoprevention of Tobacco-Induced Cancer

Prevention of initiation of tobacco use together with smoking cessation is the best way to avoid the deadly consequences of tobacco-induced cancer. But for those addicted individuals who cannot stop using tobacco products, and for ex-smokers, still at high risk for lung cancer for many years after quitting, chemoprevention remains a viable alternative. Clinical trials of chemopreventive agents against tobacco-induced cancers have to date targeted mainly cancers of the head and neck and lung. There are presently no validated clinically successful chemopreventive agents for these cancers.[180] This section will focus on lung cancer chemoprevention.

Potential chemopreventive agents must demonstrate efficacy in animal models before proceeding into further stages of development. Many agents have been tested in rodent models of lung tumor development, the most common of which is the A/J mouse. This mouse strain readily develops lung tumors upon treatment with DNA-damaging carcinogens such as NNK, BaP, and vinyl carbamate.[181] NNK and BaP are cigarette smoke carcinogens as discussed earlier in this chapter, while vinyl carbamate is a metabolite of ethyl carbamate (also known as urethane), an effective pulmonary carcinogen in A/J mice. Tumors have also been induced by exposure of A/J mice to secondhand cigarette smoke, but the tumor yield is low compared to that observed in mice treated with pure carcinogens, limiting its utility for this purpose.[182] Two types of study designs have been used. In one, the mice are treated with the potential chemopreventive agent before and/or during treatment with the carcinogen, in which case the chemopreventive agent is termed a "blocking agent," while in the other the chemopreventive agent is administered after the carcinogen, in which case it is called a "suppressing agent." In general, successful blocking agents would be more appropriate for people continuing to smoke, whereas suppressing agents would be targeted at ex-smokers. Some agents might be effective at both stages and therefore would be appropriate for smokers who were transitioning to cessation. A wide variety of agents, both naturally occurring and synthetic, has shown efficacy in lung tumor prevention in A/J mice. Agents which have shown promise in one or both of these types of protocols in A/J mice include isothiocyanates such as 2-phenethyl isothiocyanate (PEITC) and sulforaphane as well as their *N*-acetylcysteine conjugates, indole-3-carbinol, *myo*-inositol, dexamethasone and budesonide, dithiolethiones such as oltipraz, various nonsteroidal anti-inflammatory agents and COX-2 inhibitors, lipoxygenase inhibitors, chalcones, deguelin, rexinoids, and triterpenoids.[183-186] Some of these compounds have also been shown to prevent lung tumors in animal models other than the A/J mouse.

A second requirement for a successful chemopreventive agent is lack of toxicity. Chemopreventive agents will have to be taken regularly for a period of years, much like a vitamin pill. Any toxicity would be a severe detriment to compliance. Problems with agent toxicity have already arisen in clinical trials of retinoids as chemopreventive agents. It is sometimes prudent to investigate drugs with a known track record for indications other than chemoprevention, because potential side effects are already established.

Only a few specific agents have advanced to clinical trials for lung cancer prevention.[180,187,188] Such trials have been categorized as follows: primary prevention, the prevention of cancer in high risk individuals such as current or former smokers; secondary prevention, the prevention of cancer development in individuals with precancerous lesions such as dysplasia; and tertiary prevention, which is the prevention of second primary tumors in patients who have had a previous cancer.[180] Among the agents that have shown essentially no preventive activity in such trials carried out to date are retinoids, β-carotene alone or in combination with vitamin A or E, and *N*-acetylcysteine.[180] Some promising results have been obtained with anethole dithiolethione, inhaled corticosteroids, and *myo*-inositol, but these require confirmation.[187] Current clinical trials in various phases include tests of "polyphenon E" (a mixture of green tea catechins), PEITC, *myo*-inositiol, and a Chinese herbal preparation ACAPHA.[187]

Conclusions

Cigarette smoking represents the largest known voluntary exposure to multiple carcinogens and is the greatest preventable cause of cancer. This is a consequence of the addictive power of nicotine, a noncarcinogen, coupled with the simultaneous delivery of multiple carcinogenic compounds, a recipe for disaster that is perpetuated by a powerful industry that markets these products to teenagers. At least 14 types of human cancer are caused to varying extents by cigarette smoking, with lung cancer being quantitatively the most deadly among these. Cigar and pipe smoking are also causes of cancer. Smokeless tobacco, such as oral snuff, is a cause of oral and pancreatic cancers. The carcinogens in tobacco products that are responsible for these devastating effects have been well-characterized. In this respect, it is interesting to note that tobacco products are not held to the same standard for carcinogen exposure as other consumer products—a major regulatory failure.

Nevertheless, significant progress is being made in tobacco control, with the WHO Framework Convention on Tobacco Control now in place for ratifying nations. The decrease in cigarette smoking seen in countries like the United States results in a decrease in lung cancer and predicts a decrease in other tobacco-related cancers. These are encouraging developments, and the major successful methods of tobacco control—legislation to ban smoking in public places, increased taxation, and aggressive antitobacco advertising—must be continued. Effective treatment methods for nicotine and tobacco addiction are now available. However, tobacco use in the world continues to be pervasive and is unlikely to abate in the near future.

Research on mechanisms of nicotine addiction and tobacco-induced cancer has provided a strong framework for understanding the disastrous consequences of tobacco use. We have an excellent understanding of the carcinogens in tobacco products, their metabolism to DNA adducts that are central in the carcinogenic process, and their competing detoxification pathways. We have also achieved an ever-increasing appreciation of the complex pathways that lead to genomic instability and ultimately to cancer due to the persistence of unrepaired DNA adducts in tissues of people who use tobacco. These findings have provided new insights for blocking key steps in the nicotine addiction and cancer induction processes, knowledge that is being applied in the development of effective therapies. It is hoped that these insights will be translated into practical approaches for the prevention and cure of tobacco-induced cancer.

Selected References

The complete reference list can be found at www.CANCERMEDICINE8.com

1. Mackay J, Eriksen M. *The Tobacco Atlas*. Geneva, Switzerland: World Health Organization; 2002.
2. International Agency for Research on Cancer. *Tobacco Smoke and Involuntary Smoking*. IARC Monographs on the Evaluation of Carcinogenic Risks to Humans, vol. 83. Lyon, FR: 2004:53–119.
5. U.S. Department of Health and Human Services. *The Health Consequences of Smoking: A Report of the Surgeon General*. Rockville, MD: U.S. Department of Health and Human Services, Public Health Service, Centers for Disease Control, Center for Health Promotion and Education, Office on Smoking and Health; 2004.
6. U.S. Department of Health and Human Services. *The Health Consequences of Involuntary Exposure to Tobacco Smoke: A Report of the Surgeon General*. Washington, DC: U.S. Department of Health and Human Services, Centers for Disease Control and Prevention, National Center for Chronic Disease Prevention and Health Promotion, Office on Smoking and Health; 2006.
7. International Agency for Research on Cancer. *Smokeless tobacco and tobacco-specific nitrosamines*. IARC Monographs on the Evaluation of Carcinogenic Risks to Humans, vol. 89 Lyon, FR: 2007:363–370.
8. Boffetta P, Hecht SS, Gray N, Gupta P, Straif K. Smokeless tobacco and cancer. *Lancet Oncol*. 2007;9:667–675.
12. Preussmann R, Stewart BW. *N*-Nitroso Carcinogens. In: Searle CE, ed. *Chemical Carcinogens*. 2nd Ed. ACS Monograph 182, vol. 2. Washington, DC: American Chemical Society; 1984:643–828.
13. Hecht SS, Hoffmann D. Tobacco-specific nitrosamines, an important group of carcinogens in tobacco and tobacco smoke. *Carcinogenesis*. 1988;9:875–884.
14. Hecht SS. Biochemistry, biology, and carcinogenicity of tobacco-specific *N*-nitrosamines. *Chem Res Toxicol*. 1998;11: 559–603.
16. Luch A. Nature and nurture—lessons from chemical carcinogenesis. *Nat Rev Cancer*. 2005;5:113–125.
23. Hecht SS. Tobacco smoke carcinogens and lung cancer. *J Natl Cancer Inst*. 1999;91:1194–1210.
30. Boysen G, Hecht SS. Analysis of DNA and protein adducts of benzo[*a*]pyrene in human tissues using structure-specific methods. *Mutat Res*. 2003;543:17–30.
31. Phillips DH. Smoking-related DNA and protein adducts in human tissues. *Carcinogenesis*. 2002;23:1979–2004.
37. Hecht SS. Human urinary carcinogen metabolites: biomarkers for investigating tobacco and cancer. *Carcinogenesis*. 2002;23:907–922.
39. Hoffmann D, Hecht SS. Advances in tobacco carcinogenesis. In: Cooper CS, Grover PL, eds. *Handbook of Experimental Pharmacology*. 94/I ed. Heidelberg, Germany: Springer-Verlag; 1990:63–102.
47. Hecht SS. Tobacco carcinogens, their biomarkers, and tobacco-induced cancer. *Nature Rev Cancer*. 2003;3:733–744.
48. Thorgeirsson TE, Geller F, Sulem P, et al. A variant associated with nicotine dependence, lung cancer and peripheral arterial disease. *Nature*. 2008;452:638–642.
49. Hung RJ, McKay JD, Gaborieau V, et al. A susceptibility locus for lung cancer maps to nicotinic acetylcholine receptor subunit genes on 15q25. *Nature*. 2008;452:633–637.
50. Amos CI, Wu X, Broderick P, et al. Genome-wide association scan of tag SNPs identifies a susceptibility locus for lung cancer at 15q25.1. *Nat Genet*. 2008;40:616–622.
63. Schuller HM. Mechanisms of smoking-related lung and pancreatic adenocarcinoma development. *Nat Rev Cancer*. 2002;2:455–463.
64. West KA, Brognard J, Clark AS, et al. Rapid Akt activation by nicotine and a tobacco carcinogen modulates the phenotype of normal human airway epithelial cells. *J Clin Invest*. 2003;111:81–90.
68. Cooper CS, Grover PL, Sims P. The metabolism and activation of benzo[*a*]pyrene. *Prog Drug Metab*. 1983;7:295–396.
69. Conney AH. Induction of microsomal enzymes by foreign chemicals and carcinogenesis by polycyclic aromatic hydrocarbons: G.H.A. Clowes Memorial Lecture. *Cancer Res*. 1982;42:4875–4917.
78. Hecht SS. Carcinogen derived biomarkers: applications in studies of human exposure to secondhand tobacco smoke. *Tob Control*. 2003;13(Suppl 1):i48–i56.
79. Benowitz N. Nicotine addiction. *Prim Care*. 1999;26:611–631.
80. Stratton K, Shetty P, Wallace R, Bondurant S. *Clearing the Smoke: Assessing the Science Base for Tobacco Harm Reduction. Institute of Medicine*. Washington, DC: National Academy Press; 2001.
90. Paterson D, Norberg A. Neuronal nicotinic receptors in the human brain. *Prog Neurobiol*. 2000;6:75–111.

94. Watkins SS, Koob GF, Markou A. Neural mechanisms underlying nicotine addiction: acute positive reinforcement and withdrawal. *Nicotine Tob Res.* 2000; 2:19–37.
96. Picciotto MR, Corrigall WA. Neuronal systems underlying behaviors related to nicotine addiction: Neural circuits and molecular genetics. *J Neurosci.* 2002;22:3338–3341.
104. U.S. Department of Health and Human Services. *The Health Consequences of Smoking: Nicotine and Addiction. A Report of the Surgeon General.* DHHS Publication No. (CDC) 88-8406. Rockville, MD: 1988.
108. Hughes JR. Effects of abstinence from tobacco: Valid symptoms and time course. *Nicotine Tob Res.* 2007;9:315–327.
120. Rose JE. Nicotine and nonnicotine factors in cigarette addiction. *Psychopharmacology (Berl.).* 2006;184:274–285.
122. Caggiula AR, Donny EC, Chaudhri N, Perkins KA, Evans-Martin FF, Sved AF. Importance of nonpharmacological factors in nicotine self-administration. *Physiol Behav.* 2002;77:683–687.
125. Hyman S. Addiction: a disease of learning and memory. *Am J Psych.* 2005;162: 1414–1422.
126. Chaudhri N, Caggiula AR, Donny EC, Palmatier MI, Liu X, Sved AF. Complex interactions between nicotine and nonpharmacological stimuli reveal multiple roles for nicotine in reinforcement. *Psychoharmacology (Berl.).* 2006;184: 353–366.
129. Lynch BS, Bonnie RJ. *Growing Up Tobacco Free: Preventing Nicotine Addiction in Children and Youths.* Washington, DC: National Academy Press; 1994.
130. U.S. Department of Health and Human Services. *Preventing Tobacco Use Among Young People: A Report of the Surgeon General.* Atlanta, GA: U.S. Department of Health and Human Services, Public Health Service, Centers for Disease Control and Prevention, National Center for Chronic Disease Prevention and Health Promotion, Office on Smoking and Health; 1994.
131. Sullivan PF, Kendler KS. The genetic epidemiology of smoking. *Nicotine Tob Res.* 1999;1(Suppl 2):S51–S57.
132. Lerman C, Niaura R. Applying genetic approaches to the treatment of nicotine dependence. *Oncogene.* 2002;21:7412–7420.
133. Munafo M, Clark T, Johnstone E, Murphy M, Walton R. The genetic basis for smoking behavior: a systematic review and meta-analysis. *Nicotine Tob Res.* 2004;6:583–597.
135. Lasser K, Boyd JW, Woolhandler S, Himmelstein DU, McCormick D, Bor DH. Smoking and mental illness. *JAMA.* 2000;284:2606–2610.
143. Bonnie RJ, Stratton K, Wallace RB. *Ending the Tobacco Problem: A Blueprint for the Nation.* Washington, DC: The National Academies Press; 2007.
145. World Health Organization. *Framework Convention on Tobacco Control.* Geneva, Switzerland: WHO Document Production Services; 2005.
148. Fiore MC, Jaen CR, Baker TB, et al. *Treating Tobacco Use and Dependence: 2008 Update.* Rockville, MD: U.S. Department of Health and Human Services. Public Health Service. Clinical Practice Guideline; 2008.
161. Hatsukami D, Stead LF, Gupta PC. Tobacco addiction. *Lancet.* 2008;371:2027–2038.
166. NIH State-of-the-Science Conference Statement on Tobacco Use: Prevention CaC. *Ann Intern Med.* 2006;145:839–844.
174. Hatsukami D, Ebbert JO, Feuer RM, Stepanov I, Hecht SS. Changing smokeless tobacco products: New tobacco delivery systems. *Am J Prev Med.* 2007;33:S368–S378.
177. Benowitz N. *Nicotine Safety and Toxicity.* New York: Oxford University Press; 1998.
178. Royal College of Physicians. Harm reduction in nicotine addiction: helping people who can't quit. 2007. London, Royal College of Physicians of London. A report by the Tobacco Advisory Group of the Royal College of Physicians.
180. van Zandwijk N. Chemoprevention in lung carcinogenesis—An overview. *Eur J Cancer.* 2005;41:1990–2002.

32 Nutrition in the Etiology and Prevention of Cancer

Elizabeth M. Grainger, PhD, RD ▪ Edward L. Giovannucci, MD, ScD ▪ Steven K. Clinton, MD, PhD

Over the last two centuries, improvements in food production, processing, storage, and distribution have led to major changes in diet composition throughout the world. During this period, life expectancy also dramatically increased within economically developed nations because of a combination of factors, including public health measures, improved occupational safety, and major reductions in nutrient deficiency syndromes. As the population age, there has been a shift in the major causes of morbidity and mortality toward chronic diseases such as cancer and cardiovascular disease. These changes are associated with an increasingly overweight and sedentary population. Although nutritional deficiencies still plague subpopulations in developed nations such as the poor, the aged, alcoholics, and the chronically ill, we now recognize that the affluent diet contributes to the pathogenesis of chronic diseases that afflict the vast majority of the population. Efforts to understand the often complex etiologies of various cancers have led to epidemiologic and laboratory studies that strongly implicate certain dietary patterns and specific nutrients. In recent years, the interrelationships among diet, nutrition, and cancer have expanded to encompass support of patients undergoing therapy and during survivorship.

It is important to establish a conceptual framework for organizing data regarding diet, nutrition, and cancer that will help readers provide guidance to the public and patients. Organizations such as the National Cancer Institute, the American Cancer Society, and the American Institute for Cancer Research have published recommendations defining achievable dietary and nutritional goals for the entire population that may help reduce the overall cancer burden through primary prevention (Table 32-1). Some individuals, particularly those deemed to be at higher risk of specific types of cancer as a result of environmental exposures, family history, or the presence of premalignant conditions, are increasingly interested in the unique dietary and lifestyle interventions that may be tailored to lower their chances of developing cancer. Patients actively undergoing cancer therapy represent another group profoundly interested in the role of dietary and nutritional factors to enhance the efficacy of treatment while reducing the frequency and severity of side effects. Finally, as cancers are detected earlier and treatment interventions become more successful, the number of cancer survivors is increasing rapidly. Those completing cancer therapy are seeking information regarding diet and lifestyle interventions that will lower their risk of recurrence (secondary prevention) and reduce the severity of long-term complications of their cancer treatment, including therapy-related second malignancies and long-term organ dysfunction. Thus, those involved in cancer therapy and management of long-term health are increasingly being asked to provide evidence-based guidance in an area where scientific studies are few, and purveyors of alternative diet or nutrient-based interventions are allowed to market products in the absence of scientific data regarding efficacy and safety. We briefly review each of these categories of intervention and provide information that will assist in counseling individuals and groups interested in dietary and nutritional interventions. We believe this is a useful framework because it is likely that dietary variables may have unique effects during the prediagnostic phase, after diagnosis and during therapy, and following effective treatment.

The vast majority of research conducted in the field of diet, nutrition, and cancer focuses on etiology and prevention. Thus, this chapter emphasizes the public health model and focuses on the interventions that may reduce the overall cancer burden of large populations. We then consider the evidence for the prevention of the most commonly occurring cancers involving specific organs. Rather than detailing the complex, often incomplete, and occasionally contradictory literature concerning the role of diet in the etiology of specific cancers, this chapter provides a general guide with an emphasis on the major emerging concepts in the area. We conclude with a brief overview of the role of diet and nutrition to enhance therapy and survivorship.

Methodologic Issues in Diet, Nutrition, and Cancer Studies

It is valuable to briefly consider how dietary recommendations are established. The unbiased detection and quantification of risks that are associated with variations in diet and nutrient intake would ideally be achieved through randomized, prospective trials. Unfortunately, the enormous costs of long-term nutrition studies and the scientific difficulties in controlling or measuring nutrient intake limit their feasibility. Current nutritional guidelines for disease prevention are therefore based on the integration of information derived from a variety of different epidemiologic approaches and laboratory investigations. Thus, most guidelines are developed by committees convened by organizations such as the National Cancer Institute, the American Cancer Society, the American Institute of Cancer Research/World Cancer Research Fund, and the World Health Organization among others.[1-4] The evidence derived from epidemiologic studies, clinical investigations, and laboratory studies are reviewed and discussed by expert committees relative to criteria of causality. Causality is defined as a specific occurrence or outcome that is consistently preceded by a known set of circumstances or conditions. In nutritional sciences, clear representations of causality have been the demonstration of single-nutrient deficiency syndromes and their complete reversal by exposure to the nutrient. For example, the lack of fruits and vegetables in the diet leads to scurvy, which is readily reversed by vitamin C. Unfortunately, relationships between diet and cancer are much more complex than simple nutrient deficiency syndromes. To establish causality, conclusions about the occurrence of an event and its etiologic factor are based on several established criteria. These criteria have evolved over many years and include consistency, strength of association, biologic gradient, temporality, specificity, biologic plausibility, biologic mechanism, coherence, and experimental evidence.[5] Precisely quantitating risk has been difficult because the etiologies of most cancers are multifactorial and poorly understood. Human cancers show striking variations based on factors such as age, sex, race, socioeconomic status, and genetics as well as many occupational and lifestyle variables. The potential for complex interactions between these factors and diet is enormous, and this emphasizes the difficulties in demonstrating causal associations with the same clarity as is demonstrable for

Table 32-1 **Public Health Guidelines for Disease Prevention**

	American Institute of Cancer Research[3]	American Heart Association	United States Department of Agriculture[12]	American Cancer Society[1]
Body weight	Avoid being underweight or overweight and limit weight gain during adulthood to less than 5 kg (11 pounds).	Balance the number of calories you eat with the number you use each day.	Maintain body weight in a healthy range, balance calories from foods and beverages with calories expended.	Choose foods that maintain a healthful weight. Maintain a healthful weight throughout life. Lose weight if you are currently overweight or obese.
Physical activity	If occupational activity is low or moderate, take 1 hour brisk walk or similar exercise daily, and also exercise vigorously for a total of at least 1 h per week.	Maintain a level of physical activity that keeps you fit and matches the number of calories you eat.	Engage in regular physical activity and reduce sedentary activities to promote health, psychological wellbeing, and a healthy body weight	Adults: engage in moderate activity of ≥30 min, at least 5 days per week. Children and teens: ≥60 min per day of moderate-to-vigorous activity, at least 5 days per week.
Plant-based diet	Choose predominantly plant-based diets rich in a variety of vegetables and fruits, pulses (legumes), and minimally processed starchy staple foods.			Eat a variety of healthful foods, with an emphasis on plant sources.
Vegetable and fruit	Eat 15-30 ounces or 5 or more portions per day of a variety of vegetables and fruits, all year round.	Eat a variety of fruits and vegetables. Choose 5 or more servings per day.	Consume a sufficient amount of fruits and vegetables while staying within energy needs. Choose a variety of fruits and vegetables each day.	Eat 5 or more servings of a variety of fruits and vegetables each day.
Breads, grains, and cereals	Eat 20-30 ounces or more than 7 portions per day of a variety of cereals, grains, pulses (legumes), roots, tubers, and plantains.	Eat a variety of grain products, including whole grains. Choose 6 or more servings per day.	Consume 3 or more ounce-equivalents of whole-grain products per day, with the rest of the recommended grains coming from enriched or whole grain products.	Choose whole grains in preference to processed (refined) grains and sugars.
Animal products	If eaten at all, limit intake of red meat to less than 3 ounces daily. It is preferable to choose fish, poultry, or meat from nondomesticated animals in place of red meat.	Include fat-free and low fat milk products, fish, legumes (beans), skinless poultry, and lean meats.		Limit consumption of red meats, especially those high in fat, and processed meats.
Dietary fat	Limit consumption of fatty foods, particularly those of animal origin. Choose modest amounts of appropriate vegetable oils.	Limit foods high in saturated fat, trans fat and/or cholesterol. Choose fats with 2 g or less saturated fat per serving, such as liquid and tub margarine, canola oil, and olive oil.	Keep total fat intake between 20% and 35% of calories, with most fats coming from sources of polyunsaturated and monounsaturated fatty acids, such as fish, nuts, and vegetable oils.	Limit your intake of high-fat foods, particularly from animal sources. Choose foods low in fat.
Processed foods and refined sugar	Prefer minimally processed foods. Limit consumption of refined sugar.	Limit your intake of foods high in calories or low in nutrition, including foods like soft drinks and candy that have a lot of sugars.	Choose and prepare foods and beverages with few added sugars or caloric sweeteners.	
Salt and sodium	Limit consumption of salted foods and use of cooking and table salt. Use herbs and spices to season foods.	Eat less than 6 g of salt per day (2400 mg of sodium).	Consume less than 2300 mg (approximately 1 tsp of salt) of sodium per day. Choose and prepare foods with little salt.	
Alcohol	Alcohol consumption is not recommended. If consumed at all, limit alcoholic drinks to less than 2 drinks per day for men and 1 for women.	Have no more than 1 alcoholic drink per day if you are a woman and not more than 2 if you are a man.	Those who choose to drink alcoholic beverages should do so sensibly and in moderation defined as 1 drink/day for women and up to 2 drinks/day for men.	If you drink alcoholic beverages, limit consumption.
Food storage	Do not eat food which, as a result of prolonged storage, is liable to contamination. Use refrigeration and other appropriate methods to preserve perishable food as purchased and at home.		Chill (refrigerate) perishable food promptly and defrost foods properly.	
Food preparation	Do not eat charred foods. For meat and fish eaters, avoid burning of meat juices. Consume the following only occasionally: meat and fish grilled (broiled) in direct flame; cured, and smoked meats.		Clean hands, food contact surfaces, and fruits and vegetables. Meat and poultry should not be washed or rinsed. Separate raw, cooked, and ready-to-eat foods.	

(Continued)

Table 32-1 **Public Health Guidelines for Disease Prevention (*Continued*)**

	American Institute of Cancer Research[3]	American Heart Association	United States Department of Agriculture[12]	American Cancer Society[1]
Food additives	When levels of additives, contaminants and other residues are properly regulated, their presence in food and drink is not known to be harmful. However, unregulated or improper use can be a health hazard, and this applies particularly in economically developing countries.			
Tobacco	Do not smoke or chew tobacco			
Miscellaneous	For those who follow the above recommendations, dietary supplements are probably unnecessary, and possibly unhelpful, for reducing cancer risk.		Consume a variety of nutrient-dense foods and beverages within and among the basic food groups.	Increase access to healthful foods in schools, worksites, and communities.

high-risk environmental exposures, such as the impact of cigarette smoking on lung cancer.

Assessment of the Human Diet

Nutritional epidemiology poses some unique obstacles, in that food is a universal exposure, which is in stark contrast to many cancer-causing environmental exposures, such as cigarette smoke. Table 32-2 details the strengths and limitations of various types of study designs used in nutrition research. The critical limiting feature of most human studies is the imprecision of quantifying nutrient intake. Estimating the usual intake of foods or nutrients, as well as accounting for intraindividual variation over time, is a critical area of research.[6-8] An estimate of human nutrient intake is derived from a two-step process. First, interviews, questionnaires, or food diaries must determine the amounts and types of foods that are consumed.[9] This information can then be used to calculate nutrient intake if an accurate database has been established that quantifies the amount of each nutrient contained in the foods that are consumed by the population under investigation. Each step can be associated with significant error and contributes to the challenges in defining nutrient and cancer associations. The human diet is a complex array of foods that exhibits significant day-to-day and seasonal variations. The complexity of diet also differs widely among populations, cultures, and geographic areas. This often requires the development of different assessment methods for each population or subgroup. Future progress will depend, in part, on

Table 32-2 **Types of Studies Used to Assess Diet and Disease Relationships**

Study Type	Methods	Strengths	Limitations
Ecologic/correlational studies	The unit of observation is a population defined by a discriminator location (Japan v. United States, northern v. southern latitudes). Mortality or incidence among groups is compared with estimates of nutrient or food intake.	Large differences in cancer incidence and dietary patterns are often identified and hypotheses can be generated.	There are often many diet and lifestyle differences between populations, therefore correlations between disease incidence and dietary factors are confounded by known or unknown variables. Cancer incidence data and diet patterns may not be similarly quantitated among nations.
Case-control studies	Individuals experiencing a disease are identified and a similar group of matched subjects without the disease are identified. Information about past diet and nutrients is obtained from both the cases and controls for comparison.	Studies can be conducted over a relatively short period of time.	Selection bias can occur if a non-representative control group is selected. Recall bias can occur when subjects with a disease alter their perceptions and recall of past dietary habits. This often occurs when participants are familiar with a particular diet/disease hypothesis.
Prospective/cohort studies	A study population is identified and diet patterns assessed. The population is followed over time for disease outcome and changes in exposure to dietary risk factors.	Dietary intake can be monitored periodically over time. Diet assessment does not rely on long-term memory and is less affected by recall bias. Biochemical measures can be obtained periodically.	Long periods of time may be necessary for a disease to be diagnosed, therefore cohort studies often require many years of follow-up. A large number of subjects are required to compensate for subjects who drop out, are lost to follow-up, and the possibility that the frequency of the outcome of interest is low. Long term, large prospective studies are expensive.
Randomized controlled trials	Individuals are screened and a proper target population is identified, based on specific characteristics, and randomized to a control arm (standard of care) or an intervention arm. The subjects are followed for disease outcome or other biomarkers.	Especially useful for testing compounds (vitamins and minerals) that can be incorporated into pills or capsules and provided in a double-blind fashion over a period of years.	Difficult to implement for many nutrition and cancer hypotheses (weight loss, exercise, dietary fat, fiber, fruits and vegetables) because trials of dietary change cannot be blinded. Manipulation of single dietary components in large-scale intervention studies is difficult because foods are complex and contain many compounds. Compliance with food changes may be difficult to determine. Randomized, controlled trials can take a long time to complete and can be very expensive.

identifying biomarkers of nutrient exposure. Development of valid and reliable biomarkers of nutrient intake offers the promise of improved precision in epidemiologic studies because of reduced misclassification of participants according to intake estimates.[10] Finally, many of the bioactive compounds in foods that may impact cancer risk are not nutrients, for example, the vast array of phytochemicals derived from plants. Our ability to estimate exposure remains a challenge as databases regarding content in foods typically do not exist.

Laboratory Models

The effects of nutrients and their interactions on carcinogenesis can be rigorously tested in a growing array of animal models. Although the information derived from animal models must be extrapolated to humans with caution, it does provide important evidence for the biologic plausibility of relationships suggested by epidemiologic studies. The nutrient requirements of most laboratory animals have been precisely defined, and purified ingredients can be used to formulate diets for cancer studies. The rapid emergence of new animal models based upon transgenic and knockout technology has provided new opportunities to examine interactions between specific genetic targets and dietary variables.[11]

Public Health Guidelines for Cancer Prevention

We begin this section with a synthesis of public health dietary guidelines for cancer prevention and health published by several organizations including the American Cancer Society (ACS), American Institute of Cancer Research/World Cancer Research Fund (AICR/WCRF), and The American Heart Association (AHA).[1-3,12] The public health approach is a preventive strategy to decrease the overall disease incidence by reducing the adverse dietary habits of the entire population. Implementation of dietary recommendations requires cooperation among the media, food industry, nutritional scientists, public health personnel, medical practitioners, educators, and government agencies.[3] To achieve success, dietary recommendations must be clear as well as feasible and have minimal risk, low cost to society, and the potential to benefit many people.[3] Past efforts have been successful in the area of nutrition. For example, iron fortification of cereals benefits a large number of children and adult women, although risk is limited to a small number of individuals with hemochromatosis. Although much remains to be learned before the impact of the proposed recommendations on health can be precisely quantified, most experts agree that a number of dietary recommendations can be made with a reasonable degree of certainty, with the likelihood of minimal risk, and the potential for significant public health benefits.[3,4,13-15] The decision to formulate recommendations must take into account several factors, including strength of the evidence, potential benefits to society if the disease could be prevented, likelihood and severity of an adverse effect, and the feasibility of reducing exposure to the risk factor. In addition, economic issues, relative to the food and agricultural industry, are factors that may influence the decisions of committees to define nutritional guidelines. Table 32-1 summarizes current population-based dietary recommendations that together may lower the risk of chronic diseases, including cancer.[1-3,12]

Public Health Guidelines for Nutrition and Cancer Prevention

Maintain a Healthy Weight ■ Increasingly, studies are documenting that weight gain, overweight, and obesity are risk factors for human cancer.[1-3,16,17] Women with a body mass index (BMI) of greater than 25 kg/m^2, and men with a BMI greater than 27 kg/m^2 should make weight loss a priority. Weight loss of just 5-10% is associated with improved health and can reduce the incidence or severity of several diseases. Weight loss is best achieved by reducing total calorie consumption and increasing calorie expenditure to create a negative energy balance resulting in a modest, but consistent weight loss over time. Maximum weight loss of 1-2 pounds per week is appropriate for most people. Rapid weight loss achieved through fad diets does not encourage individuals to establish healthy eating patterns and weight loss is typically not maintained with these regimens. It is increasingly clear that maintaining a healthy weight throughout life may be one of the best ways to protect against many cancers.[1-3,16]

Participate in Physical Activity Daily and Moderate-to-Vigorous Intensity Exercise Several Days Each Week ■ The energy expenditure associated with physical activity is a critical component of maintaining a healthy body weight and preventing adult weight gain associated with risk of several types of cancer.[1,3,18] However, a combination of daily physical activity and regular bouts of moderate-to-vigorous intensity exercise has been shown in many studies to reduce cancer risk independent of weight and diet.[19-21] Physical activity should be incorporated into activities of daily living in combination with regular moderate-to-vigorous intensity exercise on most days of the week. There is general agreement that a daily minimum of 30 min of moderate-to-vigorous physical activity is recommended, but that 45-60 min of activity is preferred.[1,3]

Consume a Plant-Based Diet That Is Rich in Fruits, Vegetables, and a Variety of Whole Grains and Cereals ■ Several hundred studies have examined the relationships between fruit and vegetable intake and cancer risk.[3] The vast majority suggests a significant protective effect of a plant-based diet relative to cancer risk at many sites. Fruits and vegetables not only contain a diverse array of vitamins, minerals, fiber, and phytochemicals, but they are lower in calories and fat than most other foods. A variety of non-starchy fruits and vegetables should be included at every meal with a goal of consuming at least five servings (or at least 400-600 g) of fruits and vegetables per day. Additionally, emphasis should be placed on consumption of whole grain breads, cereals, and pastas that provide fiber, B vitamins, and a vast array of phytochemicals.

Minimize Consumption of Energy-Dense Foods and Sugary Drinks ■ This recommendation is vital to the overall prevention of weight gain and obesity. Foods supplies that are rich in processed foods are typically high in fat and/or high in refined sugars that contribute excess calories to the diet and do not provide a concentrated source of vitamins, minerals, and bioactive phytochemicals. Although a convincing role for dietary fat content in human cancer risk, independent of other factors, remains to be definitively demonstrated, the relationship between diets high in fat, especially saturated fat, and cardiovascular disease is well-established. Consumption of foods with added sugars has significantly increased and currently contributes over 15% of total calorie consumption.[22] The majority of this increase comes from the growing consumption of sugary beverages, especially soda.[3] Drinks containing added sugars have been associated with an increase risk of overweight and obesity in both adolescents and adults. For this reason, consumption of sugary beverages should be minimized.

For People Who Enjoy Red Meat, Moderate Portion Sizes and Avoidance of Highly Processed Red Meats Are Advisable ■ Specific populations consuming vegetarian diets are at lower risk for various diseases including some types of cancer; however, specific role for meat independent of other variables has not been possible. In addition, meat is an important source of many nutrients such as protein, iron, and vitamin B_{12}. Thus, modest meat consumption of 18 ounces or less of red meat (beef, lamb, and pork) per week probably does not significantly contribute to overall cancer risk, especially if meat does not displace consumption of fruits, vegetables, and whole grains. Choosing a variety of meats, including fresh chicken, fish, and turkey, is reasonable.[3]

Alcohol, if Consumed at All, Should Be Limited ■ The risks and potential benefits of modest alcohol consumption remain a subject of debate. Although the health effects of specific types of alcoholic beverages is an active area of research, chronic consumption of alcohol is strongly associated with cancers of the oropharynx, larynx, esophagus, and breast (both pre- and postmenopausal).[3] Smoking tobacco acts synergistically with alcohol in the pathogenesis of most of these cancers. Alcoholic beverages also probably contribute to liver and colon cancers.[3] Even a moderate amount of daily alcohol consumption may slightly, but significantly, increase the risk of breast cancer.[23] Because there is some evidence that alcohol in moderation may reduce the risk of heart disease, individuals need to consider their personal health history when deciding whether or not to consume alcohol. For those who choose to drink, alcohol intake should be limited to one drink per day for women and two drinks per day for men.[2,3]

Optimal Food Preservation, Processing, and Preparation ■ Salt is vital for human health but at levels much lower than typically found in most parts of the globe. Salt-preserved foods are associated with gastric cancer, a major malignancy worldwide. Although relationships remain uncertain, diets rich in processed meat are associated with risk of several cancers, and thus should be consumed in moderation.[3,24] Meat that is cooked at very high temperatures, grilled, and charred favors the formation of certain types of chemical carcinogens and should be consumed in moderation.[3] Microbial contamination of the food supply is a major problem globally. Most critically, the contamination of grains and legumes with fungal aflatoxins contributes significantly to the risk of liver cancer.

Dietary Supplements Are Probably Unnecessary in the Context of a Healthy Diet ■ An increasing proportion of the American population consumes some type of self-prescribed nutritional supplement on a regular basis. The public perceives nutrient supplements and alternative medications as an important form of self-therapy for the prevention and treatment of many ailments, including cancer.[3,18] Multivitamin and mineral supplements are usually inexpensive, easy to consume, relatively free of side effects when taken at the dosages approximating the recommended dietary allowance (RDA), and can be obtained without a prescription. There has been very little evidence in support of routine dietary supplements for population-wide cancer prevention. Although it is clear that Americans can achieve adequate nutrient intake by consuming a diet based upon the above recommendations, a standard multivitamin/mineral supplement providing the recommended dietary allowance may be beneficial to some and entails minimal risk. Increasingly, supplements are being aggressively marketed that contain high concentrations of specific nutrients combined with other components such as herbals, extracts, and concentrates. Consumers should be aware that regulations regarding implied health claims and requirements for demonstrating safety and efficacy are minimal and the buyer should maintain skepticism and caution.

Summary of Research Efforts Focusing on Specific Cancers

It is unlikely that any food, nutrient, or dietary pattern will influence all cancers uniformly.[1,3,18] Thus, in reviewing the relationships between nutrition and cancer risk, it is important to examine the data for each tissue or organ separately. It is clear that research will continue to improve our ability to identify individuals at high risk of specific cancers based upon genetic tests, family history, exposure to carcinogenic agents, and the presence of premalignant conditions. The future goal is to provide tailored dietary recommendations and chemopreventive strategies for individuals at risk. Additional research will define unique preventive strategies for various cancers. The following is a brief summary of the current understanding of relationships between diet, nutrition, and the risk of specific commonly occurring cancers.

■ Colon and Rectum

Colorectal cancer is the third most common cancer worldwide and the third leading cause of cancer death in the United States.[3,25] Genetic factors and premalignant conditions are being characterized that will define high-risk groups for chemoprevention and diet intervention studies that show promise in preclinical testing. The international variation in colorectal cancer is large (Fig. 32-1) and although diagnostic differences may account for some of the international variation, it is unlikely to account for the greater than tenfold variations that are observed between nations.[3] The lower rates in Japan suggest that cultural and lifestyle variables rather than industrialization are the critical factors.[3,26,27] Dramatic increases in incidence among Japanese and Chinese migrants to the United States[28] clearly indicate that international variations primarily result from environmental influences rather than genetic background.[29,30] Examination of time trends in colorectal cancer incidence, particularly in Japan since the 1940s, strongly suggests major contributions from lifestyle factors associated with westernization of their culture (Fig. 32-2).[3]

Energy Balance, Body Mass, and Physical Activity ■ Energy intake, metabolic efficiency, physical activity, and various measures

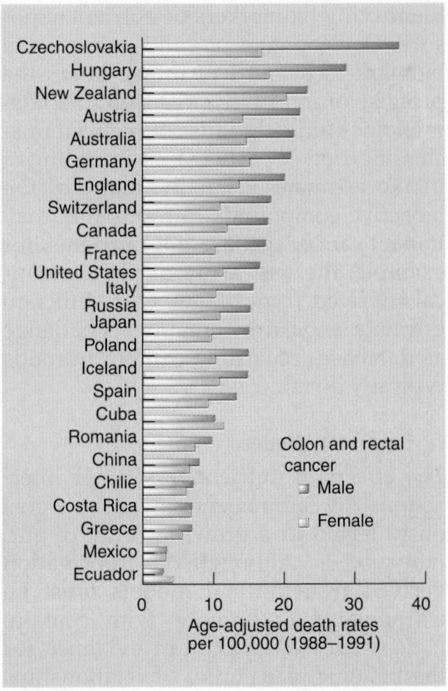

Figure 32-1 ■ Age-adjusted death rates per 100,000 population from colon and rectal cancer in selected countries. *Source*: Adapted from Ref. 138.

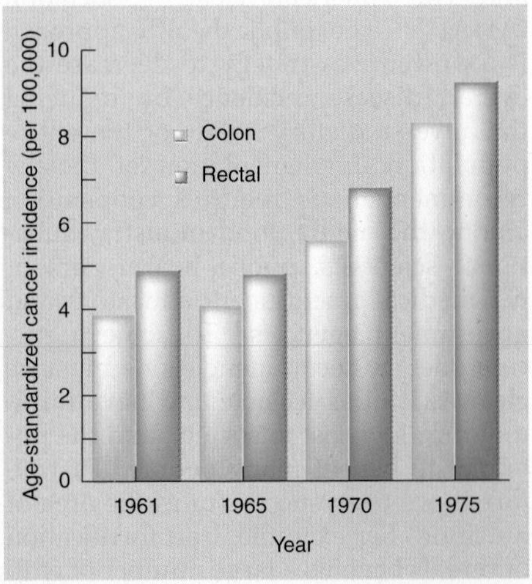

Figure 32-2 ■ Age-standardized colon and rectal cancer incidence per 100,000 men in Japan from 1960 through 1977.

of body size or obesity are intimately interrelated. It is difficult to quantitate or ascertain the role of each component in colon cancer risk without considering them as a group. A convincing inverse association between physical activity and risk of colon cancer has been consistently reported.[3,31,32] Several studies have found an association between BMI and elevated risk of colon cancer.[3,30,33-35] These associations between obesity and inactivity with risk of colon cancer have been observed in several countries (United States, China, Sweden, and Japan), among men and women, and for both occupational and recreational activities.[3] Obesity is also directly associated with risk of colon adenoma.[36] Some evidence suggests that height (perhaps a proxy of the net energy intake during childhood and adolescence) also is related to a higher risk of colon cancer.[37-39] Studies in rodent models of colon carcinogenesis have reported enhanced tumorigenesis with greater ad libitum intake[40] and reduced risk with restricted intake.[41] Overall, the evidence is convincing that physical activity and appropriate energy balance will decrease risk of colon cancer.[3]

Dietary Pattern ■ In general, a Western dietary pattern that is rich in red and processed meat, high in fat, and is low in fruits, vegetables, and fiber is associated with an increased risk of colon cancer.[3,42,43] The relationship between total fat intake, fat saturation, or different sources of fat and risk of colon cancer remains an active area of research, but definitive conclusions are not yet possible.[1,3,28,44-47] For example, Figure 32-3 illustrates a population-based case-control study suggesting that dietary fat accounts for 60% of colorectal cancer risk among Chinese migrants to the United States. Other cohort studies report that fat from red meats rather than total fat may increase colon cancer risk.[35,46,48-50] Dietary consumption of processed meats, which not only contain fat but also may contain suspected carcinogens, have emerged as a convincing risk factor for colon cancer.[3,51] Thus, moderation in consumption of red meats and processed meats should be considered for those at risk of colorectal cancer.

Fruits, Vegetables, and Fiber ■ Diets rich in plant products, particularly grains and vegetables, are often associated with a lower risk of colon cancer and many have postulated that the fiber content is a major mediating factor.[3,13,20,44,46,52-55] The chemistry of dietary fiber is exceptionally complex, and unfortunately, the quantitative and qualitative assessment of fiber intake in human studies is very difficult. However, the majority of stud-

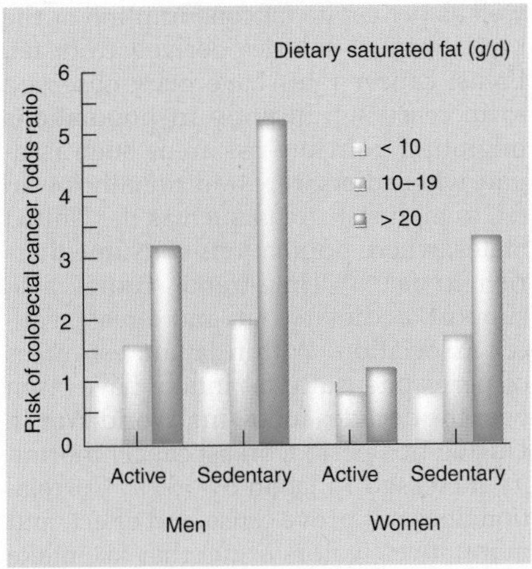

Figure 32-3 ■ The risk of colorectal cancer in Chinese migrants to the United States according to dietary fat intake and level of physical activity. *Source*: From Ref. 28.

ies suggest a diet rich in diverse fiber-containing foods may be beneficial. The European Prospective Investigation into Cancer (EPIC) study also found a 40% reduction in colon cancer risk for the highest quintile versus the lowest quintile of dietary fiber intake in over 500,000 individuals.[56] A few intervention trials have evaluated interventions focusing upon dietary fiber and colon cancer risk and thus far, the results are equivocal.[57-61]

Alcohol ■ A positive association between alcohol intake and risk of colon cancer is consistent among many ecologic, cohort, and population-based case-control studies.[1,3,62-64] Alcohol is also related to higher risk of colorectal adenoma.[1,3] Overall, the effects seem to be related more to total alcohol intake rather than to the source of alcohol.[1,3] Studies suggest that the elevated risk associated with alcohol occur predominantly in the rectum or distal colon.[50] Recent studies indicate that high intakes of folate or methionine, both of which are crucial for normal methyl group metabolism and, particularly, deoxyribonucleic acid (DNA) methylation, appears to mitigate the influence of alcohol.[62] This suggests that alcohol, which has a well-known adverse effect on methyl group metabolism, increases the risk of colorectal cancer via this mechanism; however, the role of folate during various stages of carcinogenesis remains to be clearly defined.

In summary, increased risk of colorectal cancer is strongly associated with a physically inactive lifestyle, and an affluent or Western dietary pattern, which is rich in high-fat foods (especially red meats and processed meats) and low in fruits, whole grain products, and vegetables, alcohol intake, and a high BMI.[1,3] The individual contributions of folate, methionine, meats, and specific fiber components require further investigation.[1,3] The potential interactions among these components and other factors contributing to risk, such as exercise and genetics, are numerous. At present, it is prudent to consider the combined impact of the total diet and physical activity when making recommendations for colon cancer prevention rather than focusing on a single factor.

Breast Cancer

Cancer of the breast is most common in the affluent nations of North America and Western Europe, and much less common in many parts of Asia and Africa[1,3,25]; and like colorectal cancer, we observe that migrants from low-risk nations show increasing risk after moving to a high-risk nation,[1,3,25,29] particularly in succeeding generations. This observation suggests that nutritional or other environmental factors active during youth and adolescence may have a long-term and major impact on subsequent risk of breast cancer.[1,3,25] The risk of breast cancer is reduced by early age of pregnancy and lactation.[3] A number of dietary and nutritional factors characteristic of an affluent culture have also been proposed to enhance risk of breast cancer and are briefly summarized.[1,3]

Alcohol Use ■ The accumulated evidence concerning alcohol intake and risk of breast cancer shows a positive and convincing association.[1,3] The relative risk (RR) from the consumption of one typical serving of beer, wine, or liquor (~12 g of ethanol) per day is estimated to be 1.4, whereas three drinks per day approximately doubles the risk. Recent analyses have reported a linear relationship between breast cancer risk and each 10 g increase in daily alcohol consumption and across different estrogen/progesterone hormone subtypes.[23,65]

Energy Balance, Weight, and Obesity ■ Evidence is accumulating that body fatness, adult weight gain, and a lack of physical activity are important risk factors for breast cancer.[1,3,66,67] The role of energy intake as a stimulator of mammary carcinogenesis has been well-established by rodent studies using diet or energy restriction,[68,69] or by regression analysis of ad libitum feeding.[40,70] Overall, higher levels of adult physical activity seem to be associated with a modest protection against breast cancer risk and the protective effect may also be independent of BMI or weight gain as an adult.[67,71,72] However, the precise relationships between energy intake, energy expenditure, anthropometrics, and risk of breast cancer must be examined for different critical periods in a woman's life cycle. The effects of these factors may vary during adolescence, the reproductive years, and the postmenopausal period.

Dietary Fat ■ The controversy concerning the contribution of dietary fat to risk of breast cancer can best be appreciated through examination of the representative data presented in Figure 32-4. Geographic studies show strong correlations between national rates of breast cancer and the estimated per capita fat consumption.[45,73] There are wide international variations in breast cancer rates as well as per capita fat consumption or the percentage of calories derived from fat. Breast cancer rates have been observed to increase significantly in populations migrating from low-risk areas, such as Japan, where diets were traditionally low in fat, to high-risk areas, such as the United States, where populations consume diets rich in fat.[29,74] Time-trend studies also support a dietary fat and breast cancer association. Within Japan, estimates of per capita daily fat intake have risen over the decades following World War II. During this period, breast cancer mortality increased in Japan by >30%. Correlation does not prove cause and effect, and many investigators argue that fat intake may be an indicator of some other unidentified combination of diet and environmental components that are the truly critical risk factors. The relationship between fat intake and risk of breast cancer has been examined in many case-control and cohort studies with inconsistent results.[75-78] Although the epidemiologic data have not provided definitive results concerning dietary fat and breast cancer, accumulated evidence from >100 animal studies using chemical carcinogens, hormones, irradiation, or viruses to induce breast cancer indicate that as a single variable, fat enhances mammary carcinogenesis (Fig. 32-5).[3,40,70,79] One randomized intervention study of women who had been treated for breast cancer suggested a 24% risk reduction in breast cancer recurrence among women who were able reduce their dietary fat consumption to ~33 g/day (vs 51 g per day for the control group).[80] Although not statistically significant, similar trends were observed in the very large, randomized Women's Health Initiative study.[75] Overall, the possibility that achievable reductions in fat intake during adulthood will cause an appreciable reduction in breast cancer risk remains uncertain and dietary patterns during adolescence and reproductive years may prove to be more critical to future breast cancer risk.[3]

Other Dietary Factors ■ Overall, plant-based diets rich in vegetables, fruits, and grains may have a role in decreasing the risk of breast cancer, but a specific role for selected fruits and vegetables has not been observed.[1,3,78,81] There are no consistent relationships for the consumption of specific vitamins or minerals and breast cancer risk, and recommendations regarding supplement use for prevention remain to be defined.[1,3] Other bioactive compounds found in the diet, such as soy

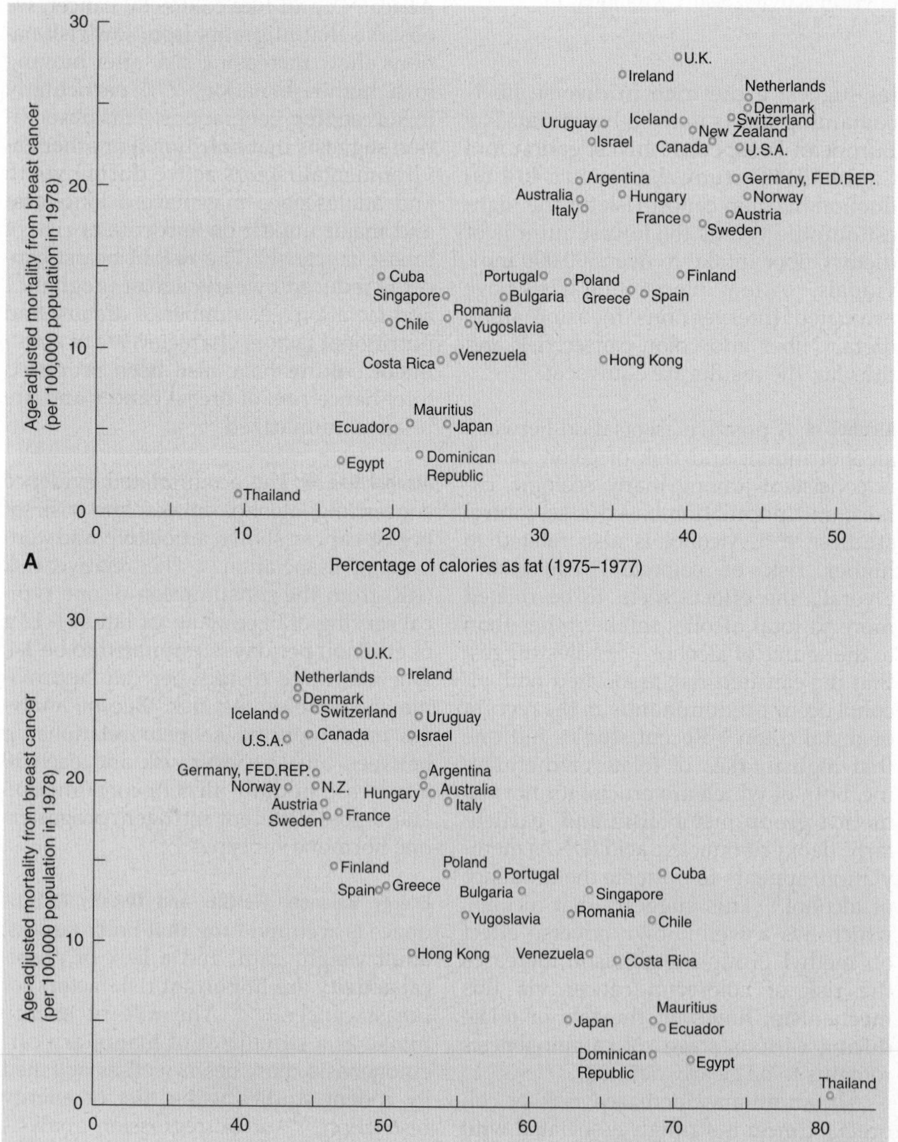

Figure 32-4 ■ International correlation of (**A**) estimated dietary fat intake (percentage of calories as fat) and (**B**) estimated carbohydrate intake (percentage of calories as carbohydrate) and age-adjusted breast cancer mortality. *Source*: From Carroll KK. Carbohydrate and cancer. In: Alfin-Slater RB, Kritchevsky D (eds.). In *Human Nutrition. A Comprehensive Treatise.* Vol 7. *Cancer and Nutrition*. New York: Plenum; 1991:97.

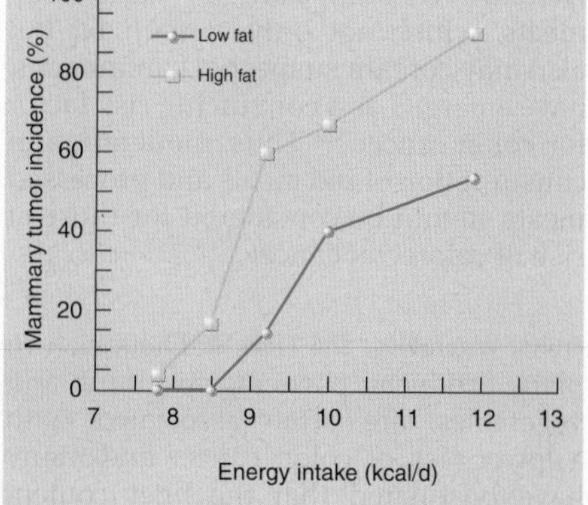

Figure 32-5 ■ The effects of low-and high-fat diets at different levels of caloric intake on spontaneous mammary tumorigenesis in C3H female mice. *Source*: Adapted from Ref. 69.

isoflavones, lignins, and fiber, may play a role in breast cancer, but evidence remains insufficient for recommendations.[1,3,78] In summary, the most well-established recommendations for breast cancer prevention are to engage in vigorous physical activity on a regular basis, avoid or limit intake of alcoholic beverages, and minimize lifetime weight gain and body fatness through physical activity and energy restriction.

Prostate Cancer

Cancer of the prostate is one of the most frequently diagnosed malignancies in American men, and it is especially common among the African American population.[3,25] Prostate cancer is a disease of aging men and the international distribution of prostate cancer is similar to that of colon and breast cancer; therefore, it correlates with affluent dietary patterns.[3,82] Relationships between diet and prostate cancer are not clearly defined and specific recommendations to prevent the disease remain speculative. A role for weight gain, energy balance, and activity is suggested by some human studies and clearly demonstrated in rodent studies.[3,16,82-85] International and intra-country correlational studies suggest associations between prostate cancer mortality and the per capita intake of total fat.[3,82] Similarly, several analytic epidemiologic studies and case-control studies have reported associations between total fat or the consumption of high-fat foods and prostate cancer, particularly saturated fats from animal products.[3,82-84,86,87]

Several studies suggest that specific nutrients such as vitamin E and selenium may influence prostate cancer risk.[88] A significantly lower risk of prostate cancer was noted among men randomized to vitamin E supplementation.[88] The possible role of selenium in the prevention of prostate cancer has been hypothesized based upon various lines of indirect evidence.[3,89-92] The largest prostate cancer chemoprevention trial to date, the Selenium and Vitamin E Chemoprevention Trial (SELECT), began randomizing 33,000 men in the fall of 2001. The study design was a 2 × 2 factorial of vitamin E, selenium, and a placebo. After a median follow-up of 5.4 years, selenium, vitamin E, or a combination of the two was not found to be protective for prostate cancer in a group of healthy men.[93]

The possibility that calcium and vitamin D are interacting components of a complex network of dietary and endocrine factors modulating prostate cancer risk is under investigation.[94] Several large cohort studies suggest that high dietary calcium consumption increases prostate cancer risk.[3,94-97] Endogenous production of the active form of vitamin D (1,25(OH)2) is suppressed with high calcium intake and with reduced exposure to sunlight. Prostate cells express vitamin D receptors and exposure to a ligand tends to induce differentiation pathways. These complex relationships have spurred many cell culture, animal and cohort studies with several suggesting an inverse relationship between vitamin D and prostate cancer risk.[98-100]

The overall consumption of fruits and vegetables has not shown a consistent reduction in risk of prostate cancer.[3,82] However, a reduced risk of prostate cancer associated with the consumption of tomatoes and processed tomato products has been observed in the prospectively evaluated Health Professional's Follow-up Study.[101-104] On the basis of these findings, it has been hypothesized that the carotenoid lycopene may account for some of the anticancer properties of tomato products, although other compounds found in tomato foods may also be important.[105-110] However, it is very premature to conclude that lycopene mediates a protective effect against prostate cancer or that lycopene is the only component of tomato products that may contribute to the association.[111] Interestingly, several interventions where subjects have been fed either tomato products or a lycopene supplement have reported modulation of both blood and prostate tissue biomarkers of prostate cancer.[112-114] Additionally, lycopene has been found to be the predominant carotenoid in human prostate tissue.[108]

In summary, epidemiologic studies and a limited number of laboratory investigations suggest a role for diet in prostate cancer. Rates of prostate cancer are higher in nations consuming an affluent dietary pattern and sedentary lifestyle, although the contributions of specific components are not well-defined and are being actively investigated.

Lung Cancer

Lung cancer is currently the most common worldwide malignancy and the leading cause of cancer-related death.[3] Cigarette smoking accounts for the vast majority of cases and incidence rates continue to climb in parallel with the globalization of cigarette manufacturing, marketing, and advertising.[3] Certain occupational exposures, such as to asbestos or radiation, may act synergistically with cigarette smoking to increase the risk.[3] Compared with the role of tobacco, the potential contribution of diet and nutrition is relatively trivial. However, the inverse relationship between the greater intake of fruits and vegetables and lower risk of lung cancer has been a frequent finding in human nutritional epidemiology.[3,115-117] Many hypothesized that beta-carotene found in fruits and vegetables or vitamin A derived from cleavage of beta-carotene may be the critical active agents in these foods.[3,118] However, two randomized controlled intervention trials in high-risk population found no reduction, and perhaps an increase, in the incidence of lung cancer among male smokers after several years of supplementation with beta-carotene at 20 or 30 mg/day.[119] These reports emphasize that protective benefits of diets rich in fruits and vegetables probably involve many interacting components and will not be reproduced by providing a single agent. A number of other nutrients including vitamin E, selenium, vitamin C, fat, soy, and retinoids are undergoing continuing evaluation regarding a protective role against lung cancer[3,120]; however, their roles remain uncertain. Overall, elimination of cigarette smoking and occupational risk factors will have the greatest impact on decreasing the incidence of lung cancer. Among high-risk individuals, the frequent consumption of a diverse array of fruits, vegetables, and other plant foods may provide some degree of protection against lung cancer.

Oral Cavity, Larynx, and Oropharynx Cancers

Like lung cancer, cancers of the oral cavity and the larynx are strongly related to the use of tobacco products.[2,3,18] Case-control studies completed over several decades have documented associations between the consumption of alcoholic beverages and cancers of these tissues. A dose-response relationship of alcohol and oral cancer, independent of tobacco usage, has been observed in a number of studies (Fig. 32-6).[121] Additional evidence is derived from studies of populations, such as alcoholics, who exhibit increased risk, and Seventh-Day Adventists and Mormons in the United States, who abstain from alcohol and have a much lower risk.[122,123] It is of interest that feeding pure alcohol as part of a nutritionally sound diet does not produce oral cancers in experimental animals. The extent that this represents biochemical differences between man and rodents, the lack of a direct carcinogenic effect of ethanol, the presence of carcinogens in alcoholic beverages consumed by man, the passive inhalation of ambient tobacco smoke in the places where ethanol is consumed, or the importance of other interacting carcinogens and nutritional deficits must be further evaluated. Both epidemiologic and laboratory studies provide convincing evidence supporting a protective role for diets rich in fruits and vegetables.[3,34,124] In addition, clinical and laboratory investigation has suggested that vitamin A and analogs or metabolites, as well as certain carotenoids, may serve as inhibitors of

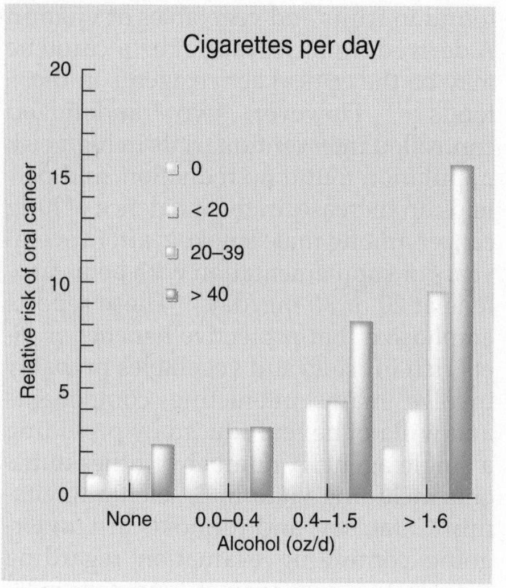

Figure 32-6 The interactions between alcohol intake and cigarette smoking on the relative risk of oral cancer. *Source*: Adapted from Rothman K, Keller A. The effect of joint exposure to alcohol and tobacco on risk of cancer of the mouth and pharynx. *J Chron Dis*. 1972;25:711–716.

carcinogenesis in the oral and respiratory epithelia. In summary, tobacco products are major contributors to cancers of the mouth and pharynx, especially in conjunction with the consumption of alcoholic beverages.[3] Further efforts to better define the role of vitamin A, synthetic retinoids, and other phytochemicals as possible chemopreventive agents for high-risk groups are warranted.

Esophageal Cancer

Squamous cell cancer of the esophagus is the eighth most common cancer worldwide and varies several hundredfold between nations and between geographic regions within nations.[3,124] In most developed nations, correlational analyses and case-control studies indicate that the major risk factors are ethanol and cigarette smoking for squamous-type esophageal cancer.[3] Risk increases in proportion to the amount of alcohol consumed.[3,125] A number of studies show an alcohol dose-response relationship after controlling for cigarette smoking, although the two factors may show a significant additive effect.[3] Increasing consumption of alcohol generally is associated with the marginal intake of many nutrients, which is thought to predispose individuals to greater risk. For example, alcohol may interact with folate, vitamin B12, and methyl group metabolism to modulate risk.[126] A number of studies suggest an inverse relationship between risk of esophageal cancer and the consumption of fresh fruits and vegetables.[3,116,127] In certain parts of Asia where alcohol consumption does not explain the high risk for esophageal cancer, there may be a relationship between esophageal cancer and the indigenous diet which is low in fresh fruits, vegetables, and animal products, and the estimated intakes of vitamin A, vitamin C, riboflavin, zinc, and several trace elements, such as molybdenum, frequently are cited as being low as well.[3,128,129] In summary, cigarette smoking and alcohol consumption are the most important etiologic factors. The possibility that marginal intakes of one or more nutrients may contribute to risk in affluent populations has been suggested but not firmly established. The most important protective dietary intervention is the frequent consumption of fruits and vegetables.[3]

Adenocarcinoma of the Esophagus and Gastric Cardia The incidence of adenocarcinoma of the distal esophagus and gastric cardia has been increasing rapidly over the last two decades in the United States and Western Europe.[130] Among white men, adenocarcinoma of the distal esophagus has increased >350% since the mid-1970s.[131] Current or past cigarette smoking may be one of the contributing factors.[131,132] However, one of the most consistent observations has been a positive association between risk and body mass index (BMI) and abdominal obesity.[133,134] As the prevalence of obesity has increased in the United States, a parallel trend can be observed in the incidence of adenocarcinoma of the esophagus and gastric cardia.[135] The mechanism remains under investigation; however, it has been speculated that obesity may predispose to gastroesophageal reflux disease. Other nutritional factors that have been investigated relative to the increased adenocarcinoma risk include diets high in animal sources of fat, low in fiber, and low in fruits and vegetables.[136,137] Additional efforts are needed to clarify the risk factors responsible for the dramatic increase in the incidence of adenocarcinoma of the esophagus and to devise effective intervention strategies.

Stomach Cancer

Gastric cancer is the fourth most common cancer worldwide.[138] The incidence varies dramatically among countries and is highest in parts of Asia (eg, Japan) and South America. A dramatic decrease in the incidence of stomach cancer in many affluent nations has been documented over the last century. In the United States, the current rate is among the lowest in the world, whereas in 1930 gastric cancer was the most frequently diagnosed malignancy in Americans. In recent years, investigators have identified a divergent incidence pattern for cancers of the gastric cardia and distal stomach, which suggests different etiologies. Adenocarcinomas of the cardia are typically grouped etiologically with those arising from the metaplastic distal esophagus showing a similar histology and may share risk factors. Convincing evidence for specific foods and nutrients is lacking. However, several variables under study are considered as likely related, including: (1) the protective role of diets rich in fruit and vegetables; (2) the protective effects of modern food processing and storage, thereby reducing spoilage; (3) increased risk due to the use of salt curing, pickling, and nitrates for preservation; (4) the role of *Helicobacter pylori* infection and interactions with dietary factors[139-141]; (5) identification of natural carcinogens or precursors such as nitrates, found in foods; (6) the production of carcinogens during grilling or barbecuing of meats; and (7) the synthesis of carcinogens from dietary precursors in the stomach.[3,132,139,140]

Liver Cancer

Primary hepatocellular carcinoma is very rare in the United States and Northern Europe. In contrast, it is one of the most frequent types of cancer in the developing nations of sub-Saharan Africa and Asia, and is now ranked as the sixth most common cancer worldwide.[3] Hepatitis B and C infections appear to be the major etiologic factors in many high-risk areas, where the carrier state imparts an RR of ~200-fold.[142] Contamination of foods with carcinogenic fungal products, such as certain aflatoxins, also likely contribute to risk in some populations.[3] Aflatoxins are found in geographic areas where food processing and storage are not optimal. Groups with high aflatoxin exposure often have high rates of hepatitis B infection, parasitic infections, and nutritional deficiencies, which may interact to determine risk. In low-risk nations, the regular and high consumption of alcohol is an important dietary factor in the pathogenesis of liver cancer.[3,44,84] The data also suggest that other cofactors may act in an additive or synergistic fashion.[143] It has been hypothesized that liver cancer primarily occurs in those whose cumulative experiences with alcohol, viral hepatitis, and toxin exposure lead to cirrhosis.

Pancreatic Cancer

Pancreatic cancer is frequently detected at an advanced stage and thus is highly lethal. Cigarette smoking has been firmly established as one etiologic factor.[18,144] The RR of smoking at least a pack per day is approximately fourfold, compared with that of nonsmokers.[3] Body fatness and excess energy intake are positively associated with pancreatic cancer risk,[3,145] and are supported by animal models where dietary restriction produces acinar cell atrophy, reduces DNA synthesis,[146] and inhibits experimental pancreatic carcinogenesis.[147] Furthermore, a diet high in glycemic load may increase risk of pancreatic cancer, particularly in those with elevated body mass index or with low physical activity.[148]

Endometrial Cancer

In general, endometrial cancer shows an international distribution similar to that of other cancers of affluence, such as breast, colon, and prostate cancers. Evidence for association between endometrial cancer and excess energy intake, lack of physical activity, and obesity continues to accumulate.[3,16,74,84,144] The role of fruits and vegetables in decreasing the risk of endometrial cancer is supported by data from some studies.[3,149] At the present time, the most appropriate guidance is to avoid obesity through reduced energy consumption and regular physical exercise coupled with a diet rich in fruits, vegetables, and grains.

Ovarian Cancer

There are considerable international and geographic variations in the incidence and mortality rates of ovarian cancer. The disease is more common in nations exhibiting Western culture, especially among the higher socioeconomic groups.[3,144] At present, no conclusive role for dietary components in the pathogenesis of ovarian cancer has been established, but additional studies are needed, particularly in conjunction with known risk factors of low parity and specific inherited genetic abnormalities.[3]

Bladder Cancer

Bladder cancer is more frequent in industrialized nations, especially among smokers and those in urban areas and of lower socioeconomic status.[3,44,116,150,151] The majority of epidemiologic and case-control studies support the hypothesis that the frequent consumption of fruits and vegetables will reduce risk.[3,116,150,152] A diet rich in cruciferous vegetables such as broccoli, but not other classes of fruits and vegetables, has been associated with a significantly reduced bladder cancer risk in both smokers and nonsmokers.[152] The role of fluid intake in bladder cancer risk has frequently been proposed.[3,153] The prospective evaluation of fluid intake found a significant inverse association between total daily fluid intake and bladder cancer risk, with no evidence for a benefit or risk from specific sources of fluid.[153] Laboratory studies have found that the nonnutritive sweeteners cyclamates and saccharine may be weak initiators or promoters of bladder carcinogenesis in rodents, but their contribution to human cancer probably is very small.[3]

Current Research

Specific Foods, Nutrients, and Dietary Components Frequently Associated with Cancer Prevention

Many people at risk of cancer focus their attention upon specific foods or nutrients in part because of the extensive marketing of products and publicity generated by the popular press. This tendency is facilitated by the news media when science reporters publicize results of single studies or preliminary findings, often confusing readers with contradictory and conflicting results. The following section briefly summarizes data regarding selected food components or nutrients and might assist the medical practitioner in responding to specific inquiries from individuals.

Vitamins

Vitamin A ■ Vitamin A is essential for the normal growth and development of epithelial tissues. Vitamin A deficiency is common in many parts of the developing world, but is extremely rare in Americans. Vitamin A is provided in the diet as retinol and its esters, primarily from milk and organ meats, and as beta-carotene and a few other provitamin A carotenoids in yellow and leafy green vegetables. A protective effect of consuming foods rich in vitamin A has been hypothesized for several types of cancer.[1,3,116] However, there is no clear evidence that vitamin A supplementation will decrease the risk of cancer in populations or individuals consuming a healthy diet. Although many studies in laboratory models indicate that vitamin A deficiency increases the susceptibility of tissues to chemical carcinogenesis, these observations do not support the concept that a lower risk will be observed by excessive supplementation in persons with adequate vitamin A status. The use of vitamin A and synthetic retinoids as pharmacologic agents in chemoprevention trials to determine their efficacy in specific high-risk populations is an important area of translational research.[154]

Vitamin D ■ Significant evidence has accumulated that suggests an important role of vitamin D in several cancer subtypes including colon, prostate, breast, and pancreatic cancers.[3,98] Vitamin D is a hormone-like nutrient obtained through the diet and it is endogenously produced with exposure to sunlight. Recent studies indicate that a vitamin D deficiency may be much more common than previously recognized and contribute to risk.[155] Cancer cells derived from many human tumors express the receptor for 1,25-dihydroxy vitamin D3 and respond to this agent in vitro, but the pathophysiologic significance in human cancer remains to be determined.[1,156] There are vitamin D analogs in development that do not have hypercalcemic effects but continue to interact with receptors on many cancer cells. These compounds may lead to the development of novel chemopreventive or therapeutic agents. However, it remains to be determined if increases in vitamin D exposure by individuals or populations can impact the risk of specific cancers.

Vitamin E ■ Vitamin E is a family of eight compounds that are collectively referred to as *tocopherols.* Vegetable oil, eggs, and whole grains are the major sources of dietary vitamin E. The antioxidant and free radical scavenger properties of vitamin E suggest a possible role as an antineoplastic vitamin.[156,157] However, few rodent, epidemiologic, or intervention studies provide strong evidence to support the consumption of vitamin E supplements to prevent cancer.[3,158]

Vitamin C ■ Vitamin C, which includes ascorbic acid and dehydroascorbic acid, functions as a water-soluble antioxidant and a component of several enzymatic reactions in intermediary metabolism. Citrus fruits, leafy vegetables, tomatoes, and potatoes are rich sources of vitamin C. Despite a large volume of publications, very little evidence supports a critical role of dietary vitamin C in the etiology of most human cancers, although several studies suggest that foods rich in vitamin C may be cancer protective.[1] Supplement studies, although few in number, have failed to show a reduced risk of cancer.[159] Some provocative evidence concerns the ability of vitamin C to inhibit the formation of carcinogenic nitrosamines, which ultimately may reduce the incidence of cancers that are thought to be associated with nitrosamines, such as gastric cancer.[160] At present, there is no evidence to suggest that consumption of vitamin C supplements at levels higher than that can be achieved in a well-balanced diet containing ample fresh fruits and vegetables is useful in the prevention or treatment of human cancer.[1,3]

Folate ■ Folate is an essential water-soluble B vitamin required for the normal metabolism of amino acids, methyl groups, and nucleotides. It is found in many vegetables, fruits, beans, and whole grains, and folic acid is also found in fortified grain products in the United States.[161] Folate plays a role in the methylation of DNA, which may be critical for the normal regulation of gene expression and tissue differentiation. Epidemiologic and laboratory studies are beginning to accumulate evidence suggesting that insufficient folate may relate to the risk of several malignancies, particularly colon and breast cancers. Cancer risk may also be higher among persons who consume alcohol regularly with a low-folate diet.[1,14,87,162] However, caution should be advised, as folate is critical for DNA metabolism and cell proliferation, thus additional studies are necessary.

Minerals

Calcium ■ Calcium is hypothesized to reduce the risk of colon cancer, but enhance the risk of prostate cancer.[1,3] For example, several prospective, cohort studies have found that those who develop colon cancer had a significantly lower intake of calcium and vitamin D.[1,3,163] Calcium supplementation of 1.2 g/day reduced the proliferative rate of colonic cells in patients who are considered to be at an increased risk of colon cancer.[164] Several clinical trials to determine the effects of calcium supplementation on polyp formation are currently ongoing with initial reports suggesting a modest benefit. Conversely, calcium from dietary sources and from supplements has been demonstrated in several prospective studies to be associated with an increased risk of prostate cancer,[94,97,165] particularly cancers with more aggressive characteristics. At this time, it is appropriate to target calcium intake at RDA levels from a variety of food sources. The RDA is currently 1000 mg/day for those ages 19-50 years and 1200 mg/day for people older than age 50 years.

Selenium ■ Selenium is a mineral required in the diet at very small concentrations with an RDA of 55 μg/day for both men and women. Grains, cereals, seafood, and meat are good sources of selenium. Selenium is an essential constituent of glutathione peroxidase, and it participates in the destruction of hydrogen peroxide and organic hydroperoxides, using reducing equivalents from glutathione. Selenium, thus, participates in cellular and tissue defense against oxidative damage. A major obstacle for epidemiologic studies is that estimates of dietary selenium intake are unreliable, especially in the developed nations where foods are extensively processed and shipped for long distances, because the selenium content of food is very sensitive to soil concentrations. An inverse association between the selenium levels in forage crops from different geographic areas or tissue selenium and mortality rates from certain cancers has been suggested.[1,3,89] A landmark human intervention trial reported that selenium supplements might reduce the risk of lung, colon, and prostate cancers.[89] However, larger randomized controlled trials are required to confirm and expand upon these findings. Overall, individuals choosing to consume a selenium supplement should be advised to consume the requirement of 55 μg/day and not more than 200 μg/day because there is a narrow margin between safe and potentially toxic dosages.[1,3]

Foods and Food Components

Soy Products ■ People living in countries such as Japan and China where soy foods are regularly consumed have a much lower risk of cancers of the breast, colon, and prostate than do people living in the United States where soy foods are not commonly consumed. However, many other variables in addition to soy probably contribute to the geographic variations. Soy foods contain several components, including soy protein, isoflavones, lignins, and saponins, which have been investigated for their anticancer effects in laboratory models.[166,167] Although many studies are currently underway, there is no convincing evidence that suggests the use of soy supplements, soy extracts, pure soy concentrates, or other soy components currently marketed will significantly impact human cancer risk. Some concerns have been raised about the risks and benefits for soy consumption relative to breast or endometrial cancer. Several soy isoflavones have a chemical structure similar to estrogen and may bind to the estrogen receptor and act as weak estrogen. It is plausible that high amounts of phytoestrogens may actually increase cell proliferation, although this remains controversial. At this time it is probably prudent for women at high risk of breast cancer to avoid concentrated isoflavone supplements, but it is unlikely that moderate amounts of soy foods as part of a plant-based diet will increase cancer risk.[168,169]

Beta-Carotene ■ Foods rich in beta-carotene, such as many fruits and vegetables, are associated with a lower risk of cancer. However, recent intervention trials with beta-carotene clearly question the validity of that hypothesis that the benefits of a plant-based diet can be produced through beta-carotene supplements. Two large intervention studies of beta-carotene demonstrated a higher risk of lung cancer in smokers.[119,170] Although beta-carotene is a potential antioxidant and source of vitamin A, supplements should be discouraged for cancer prevention and dietary sources should be encouraged.

Lycopene and Other Carotenoids ■ The bright red color of tomato products is caused by the non-provitamin carotenoid lycopene. Interest in lycopene has emerged because many studies demonstrate that the consumption of tomato products is associated with a lower risk of several cancers, particularly prostate cancer.[103,104,106] The recent American Institute of Cancer Research report concluded that there is a substantial amount of consistent evidence that tomatoes and tomato products are protective against prostate cancer.[3] However, at the present time it is prudent to consume tomatoes and tomato products as a source of lycopene and other phytochemicals rather than assume that the benefits will be achieved from the lycopene-enriched extracts currently being aggressively marketed.

Omega-3 Fatty Acids, Fish Oil, and Olive Oil ■ Diets rich in total fat have a high caloric density and contribute to excess energy intake and obesity. Thus, most healthy dietary patterns are lower in total fat than the current American pattern. However, the types of lipids may also have an impact upon cancer. Fish is a rich source of omega-3 fatty acids that can influence cell biology through a number of mechanisms including modulation in the production of bioactive lipids such as prostaglandins and leukotrienes. Animal models suggest some benefits for cancers of the prostate and breast.[171] Olive oil has generated interest because of its lack of association with cancers in studies where total lipids, saturated fats, and other measures of lipid intake demonstrate positive associations. Like other lipids, olive oil contributes to caloric intake and risk of obesity, but can be used in certain recipes to replace other types of lipid that may have a greater association with cancer and cardiovascular disease. Overall, very little definitive data are available regarding lipid sources and human cancer risk and specific recommendations are not possible at this time.[1,3]

Organic and Natural Foods

Government regulators will continue to evaluate information and provide updated standards and recommendations to consumers regarding expectations when the term "organic" is used in food labeling. In general, the term refers to foods grown without the use of synthesized pesticides or herbicides, and has been expanded to include nongenetically manipulated foods. At the present time, there are no studies demonstrating that consuming organic foods will substantially lower cancer risk when compared to the same foods produced by standard farming practices.[1,3]

Pesticides, Herbicides, and Environmental Contaminants in Food ■ Residues of pesticides and herbicides are found in low concentrations in fruits and vegetables. Overall, studies have not clearly defined cancer risks associated with exposure to these compounds at low concentrations and the preponderance of data supports the recommendation that fruits and vegetables should be consumed at greater concentrations. Additional concerns relate to the accumulation of some environmental toxins in meats, including fish, but without clear evidence of a cancer risk. Certainly, exposures to high concentrations of these compounds through industrial and agricultural exposures are associated with toxicity and concerns about cancer risk. Overall, regulatory agencies must continue to monitor agents and insure safety at expected exposure levels.[1,3]

Artificial Sweeteners (Aspartame and Saccharin) ■ Artificial sweeteners are the basis of many low-calorie foods currently marketed. No links between aspartame and cancer have been identified. Saccharin has been shown to slightly enhance the risk of bladder cancer in rodent studies when provided concentrations that would greatly exceed that consumed by humans. Human epidemiologic studies have not identified saccharin or aspartame consumption as a risk factor for human cancer.[1,3]

Sugar ■ Highly refined simple sugars provide calories but without the nutrients associated with whole foods. Diets containing large amounts of simple sugars are frequently nutrient poor and might also contribute to promoting obesity and hormonal changes that could potentially increase cancer risk. However, sugars *per se* are not carcinogens, and a diet with a modest amount of sweets should not be a concern in the context of a healthy dietary pattern.[1,3]

Tea ■ Investigations of green and black teas are currently underway to determine whether these products may have anticancer properties in humans to support data derived from laboratory studies. Thus far, tea has not been shown to lower the risk of any human cancer, but important studies are underway.[1,3]

Survivorship: Diet and Nutritional Guidance During and Following Cancer Treatment

Although the focus of this chapter is diet and nutrition in the etiology and prevention of cancer, we briefly introduce the emerging field of diet and nutrition during cancer survivorship. "Survivorship" is now accepted as beginning at the time of cancer diagnosis and continuing throughout the life of the individual. Diet and nutrition may have a role in several components of cancer survivorship, including (1) enhancing the benefits of treatment and reducing the frequency or severity of acute treatment-related toxicities; (2) promoting recovery during the immediate posttreatment phase; (3) support of patients suffering from cancer cachexia and during terminal phases of incurable or advanced cancers; and (4) promoting long-term survivorship by reducing the chance of recurrent disease, secondary prevention of cancer, and reducing the frequency and severity of late complications of therapy and enhancing overall health and longevity. At current rates, >1.2 million Americans are diagnosed with cancer each year and >10 millions are categorized as survivors. The need for scientifically based recommendations is now acute and has not kept pace with the desire of patients or survivors to obtain information on diet and nutrition. The American Cancer Society recently published a review of the field summarizing the state of nutrition and physical activity research and providing guidelines for communicating with survivors.[172]

Diet and nutrition represents, for many cancer patients, an opportunity to counteract the profound sense of loss of control that accompanies cancer treatment. Quality of life is improved when patients feel that they are active participants in the course of their care. Unfortunately, scientific evidence to help a patient choose optimal diet and nutritional information is insufficient in most areas. Cancer survivors are faced with a bewildering array of sources of dietary information ranging from well-intended family and friends, to alternative health-care providers, and those marketing products or selling publications touting dietary approaches. Coupled with the limited training and knowledge of nutrition by many health-care providers, such as physicians and nurses, a survivor is frequently confused or easily misled. Although definitive and detailed guidelines are not possible at the present, the following provides a framework for communicating with patients and directing future survivorship research.

Active Treatment Phase

Cancer treatment often includes surgery, radiation, chemotherapy, or biologic treatments, as well as combinations of approaches as multimodality interventions are established for a greater number of clinical scenarios. The key to guiding a patient undergoing therapy is to individualize the nutritional support. The care team should monitor individual needs through assessment of body weight, lean body mass, and the presence of eating or digestive impairments. Treatments for some cancers may compromise nutritional status caused by impairment of food intake, digestion, absorption, and metabolism of nutrients. For example, loss of appetite, nausea, vomiting, altered taste and smell perception, constipation, and diarrhea may transiently occur. Individually tailored interventions to nutritionally support a patient during these periods will enhance quality of life. In some patients, maintaining adequate energy intake is an obstacle and specific commercially prepared and tested nutritional products can easily be incorporated into a diet plan. Early referrals of patients at high risk for nutritional complications to a registered dietitian (RD) can prevent the development of more severe malnutrition that may limit the ability of the medical team to provide the optimal treatment intensity.[172]

The use of nutritional supplements during cancer therapy is controversial and few studies have been conducted to provide detailed guidance. For example, vitamin supplements with high dosages of antioxidants (vitamins C or E, selenium, etc.) during chemotherapy or radiation therapy are considered by some clinicians to potentially reduce the efficacy of treatments that may depend upon oxidative stress in the cancer cell as the mechanism of action. However, others suggest that antioxidant supplements may provide a benefit to patients by limiting damage to normal tissues such as bone marrow. In general, it is prudent for clinicians to advise patients undergoing chemotherapy or radiation therapy to limit antioxidants to levels that do not exceed the RDAs for specific nutrients and avoid other products that contain herbals or extracts enriched in antioxidant components. Folic acid is one nutrient where large dosages exceeding the RDA could influence the outcome of chemotherapy with agents such as methotrexate or 5-fluorouracil (5-FU) that target metabolic pathways involving folate. Daily supplements containing folate above the RDA should be discouraged for these patients.[172]

Recovery Following Treatment

The days and weeks following completion of intensive treatment are points in the cancer care continuum where many patients explore dietary and nutritional interventions to enhance survivorship. During this period, the frequency of contacts with health-care providers lessens and the patient is concerned about the efficacy of treatment and recovery from therapy. Diet and physical activity should be a component of the treatment plan with the goal of restoring muscle mass and functional status. Health-care providers must continue to question patients regarding supplements and alternative medical treatments and provide counseling as needed. Continuing individualized nutritional evaluation will identify those with more serious long-term nutritional complications of therapy, such as dysphagia, malabsorption, and bowel changes common in those treated for cancers of the oral pharynx, esophagus, stomach, pancreas, bowel, and others. A focus on energy balance and ensuring adequate intake of essential nutrients is critical. For example, gastric surgery or resection of the terminal ileum may lead to a vitamin B12 deficiency unless parenteral administration is initiated.[172]

Advanced Cancer

In general, progressive cancer is associated with a loss of appetite, and if a patient does not succumb quickly to a complication of the disease or co-morbid condition, progressive weight loss and other features of malnutrition will become evident. Unfortunately, many families and caretakers have the impression that reversal of the nutritional deficits will significantly prolong life. In reality, the failure to control the growth of the cancer, rather than malnutrition, is the critical issue. Frequently, the patient and caregivers experience conflict based upon loss of appetite and food consumption. The medical team should be alert and identify conflicts centering on food, help establish understanding, and provide guidance to families. In the setting of advanced disease, dietary and nutritional interventions can contribute to a sense of well-being and quality of life. Dietitians and the medical team can assist the patient in altering food choices and eating patterns and help maintain nutritional status in the setting of advanced disease often complicated by pain control issues and the resulting constipation caused by side effects of narcotic analgesics. Some medications can be coupled with limited physical activity to enhance appetite and improve bowel function. In some cases, additional nutritional support may be indicated.[172]

Prevention of Cancer Recurrence and Long-Term Complication of Therapy

The patient who achieves a complete remission from cancer is concerned about the reappearance of the primary cancer. In addition, survivors of certain cancers are at greater risk of second primaries, for example, survivors of oral or lung cancer may experience an ~10% chance of a second tobacco-related primary cancer yearly. Many cancer survivors are also at risk for cancers of other sites, often related to treatment, for example, secondary leukemia in cured testis cancer patients following treatment with etoposide-based chemotherapy or secondary breast cancer in survivors of adolescent lymphoma treated with mediastinal radiation. Very little research has been undertaken to establish optimal dietary patterns to prevent recurrent disease or second primaries at the same or different sites. In general, most experts will focus on the dietary recommendations summarized at the beginning of this chapter and by various groups for the prevention of cancer.[1,3,172]

As the population of cancer survivors expands, and physicians continue to monitor them over longer periods, long-term complications of treatments that are potential targets of dietary interventions are becoming apparent. For example, premature menopause in women treated with chemotherapy for breast cancer may contribute to accelerated osteoporosis[173] that may require alterations in dietary calcium and physical activity. Mediastinal radiation in young adults and children may contribute to premature coronary atherosclerosis. Medical caregivers should emphasize early interventions with dietary and exercise patterns that will maintain healthy blood cholesterol and triglyceride profiles. Although very little research concerning diet and nutrition has thus far been accumulated to provide clear guidance to cancer survivors, we anticipate that future efforts in this area will expand rapidly as a result of patient demands and the response of the National Institutes of Health through their support of survivorship issues.

Selected References

The complete reference list can be found at www.CANCERMEDICINE8.com

1. Kushi LH, Byers T, Doyle C, et al. American Cancer Society Guidelines on Nutrition and Physical Activity for cancer prevention: reducing the risk of cancer with healthy food choices and physical activity. *CA Cancer J Clin.* 2006;56:254–281; quiz 313–314.
2. Lichtenstein AH, Appel LJ, Brands M, et al. Diet and lifestyle recommendations revision 2006: a scientific statement from the American Heart Association Nutrition Committee. *Circulation.* 2006;114:82–96.
3. World Cancer Research Fund. *Food, Nutrition and the Prevention of Cancer: A Global Perspective.* Washington, DC: American Institute for Cancer Research; 2007.
4. World Health Organization. *Diet Nutrition and the Prevention of Chronic Diseases.* Geneva, Switzerland: WHO; 1990.
5. Weed DL, Greenwald P, Kramer BS, editors. *Cancer Prevention and Control.* New York: Marcel Dekker, Inc.; 1995.
6. Medlin C, Skinner JD. Individual dietary intake methodology: a 50-year review of progress. *J Am Diet Assoc.* 1988;88:137.
7. Block G. A review of validations of dietary assessment methods. *Am J Epidemiol.* 1982;115:492–505.
8. Willett W. *Nutritional Epidemiology,* Second Edition. New York: Oxford University Press; 1998.
9. Barnett-Connor E. Nutrition epidemiology: how do we know what they ate? *Am J Clin Nutr.* 1991;54:182S–187S.
10. Colditz GA, Willet WC. Epidemiologic approaches to the study of diet and cancer. In: Alfin-Slater RB, Kritchevsky D, editors. *Human Nutrition: a Comprehensive Treatise.* New York: Plenum; 1991:51.
11. Patel AC, Nunez NP, Perkins SN, Barrett JC, Hursting SD. Effects of energy balance on cancer in genetically altered mice. *J Nutr.* 2004;134:3394S–3398S.
12. U.S. Department of Health and Human Services and U.S. Department of Agriculture. *Dietary Guidelines for Americans.* Washington, DC: US Government Printing Office; 2005.
13. National Academy of Sciences Committee on Diet and Health Food and Nutrition Board. *Diet and Health: Implications for Reducing Risk of Chronic Disease.* Rockville, MD: Academy Press; 1989.
14. Willett WC. Goals for nutrition in the year 2000. *CA Cancer J Clin.* 1999;49:331–352.
15. National Academy of Sciences National Research Council. *Nutrient Requirements of Laboratory Animals.* Washington, DC: National Academy Press; 1978.
16. Calle EE, Rodriguez C, Walker-Thurmond K, Thun MJ. Overwieght, obesity, and mortality from cancer in a prospectively studies cohort of U.S. adults. *N Engl J Med.* 2003;348:1625–1638.
17. Renehan AG, Tyson M, Egger M, Heller RF, Zwahlen M. Body-mass index and incidence of cancer: a systematic review and meta-analysis of prospective observational studies. *Lancet.* 2008;371:569–578.
18. Eyre H, Kahn R, Robertson RM. Preventing cancer, cardiovascular disease, and diabetes. A common agenda for the American Cancer Society, the American Diabetes Association, and the American Heart Association. *Stroke.* 2004;35:1999–2010.
19. Peplonska B, Lissowska J, Hartman TJ, et al. Adulthood lifetime physical activity and breast cancer. *Epidemiology.* 2008;19:226–236.
20. Slattery ML, Caan BJ, Potter JD, et al. Dietary energy sources and colon cancer risk. *Am J Epidemiol.* 1997;145:199–210.
21. Sesso H, Paffenbarger RJ, Lee I. Physical activity and breast cancer risk in the College Alumni Health Study (United States). *Cancer Causes Control.* 1998;9:433–439.
22. Block G. Foods contributing to energy intake in the US: data from NHANES III and NHANES 1999-2000. *J Food Compost Anal.* 2004;17:439–447.
23. Smith-Warner SA, Spiegelman D, Yaun SS, et al. Alcohol and breast cancer in women: a pooled analysis of cohort studies. *JAMA.* 1998;279:535–540.
24. Cross AJ, Leitzmann MF, Gail MH, Hollenbeck AR, Schatzkin A, Sinha R. A prospective study of red and processed meat intake in relation to cancer risk. *PLoS Med.* 2007;4:e325.

33 Chemoprevention of Cancer

Scott M. Lippman, MD ■ Waun Ki Hong, MD, DMSc (Hon)

Clinical cancer therapy and prevention are progressing toward but have not yet succeeded in removing major epithelial cancers from the list of major threats to public health in the United States and worldwide. Cancer chemoprevention is beginning to add impressive clinical advances to the long list of advances resulting from cancer therapy. There have been many exciting developments in clinical chemoprevention, including, eg, the first two U.S. Food and Drug Administration (FDA) approvals specifically for cancer chemoprevention in the late 1990s—tamoxifen for reducing the risk of preinvasive and invasive breast cancer and celecoxib as an adjunct to therapy for controlling colorectal familial adenomatous polyposis (FAP)—and subsequent FDA approvals of raloxifene for reducing the risk of invasive breast cancer and of human papillomavirus (HPV) vaccine for reducing cervical neoplasia risk. More recently, a randomized controlled trial (RCT) of combined sulindac and difluoromethylornithine (DFMO) achieved an extraordinary 70% reduction in colorectal adenomas (>90% in advanced adenomas), and new findings from the Prostate Cancer Prevention Trial (PCPT) ease major concerns about finasteride raised by the primary report of the PCPT. The trial in colorectal adenomas highlights the chemoprevention focus on combined agents, signaling, perhaps, the near realization of this approach in standard clinical practice.

Biology of Chemoprevention

The entire field of cancer chemoprevention is underpinned by two phenomena of neoplasia: (1) field carcinogenesis, which is the multifocal development of intraepithelial neoplasia (IEN, or precancer) or the clonal spread of one or more IENs, and (2) multistep carcinogenesis, which is driven by genetic instability and accumulates progressive genetic and epigenetic changes.[1-4] These processes spur evasion of apoptosis, strong replicative potential, and sustained angiogenesis leading to IEN and cancer development. Multistep carcinogenesis allows chemopreventive interventions at step(s) of neoplasia that precede invasive cancer. Drugs developed for cancer therapy can be examined for cancer chemoprevention because of important commonalities—including genetic and epigenetic abnormalities, loss of cellular control, and certain phenotypic characteristics—between cancer and multistep IEN.[5] Field carcinogenesis makes approaches such as systemic agents attractive for controlling the neoplastic results of diffuse exposure to carcinogens throughout an epithelial field. The FDA has approved several treatments for IEN.

Cancer Risk Modeling

Accurate cancer risk models are critical to chemoprevention. Models based on clinical/demographic factors have been developed for breast cancer risk (Gail model) and lung cancer risk (Spitz model), and established identifiers of increased risk include precursor clinical/histologic lesions.[6,7] These risk models and lesions are useful on a population-wide basis but are less helpful in identifying individual or personalized risk. Breast ductal carcinoma in situ (DCIS) patients with expression of biomarkers of an abrogated response to cellular stress have a worse outcome.[8] A panel of methylation markers in sputum marked a high lung cancer risk in chronic smokers,[9] and recent work showed that clinical lung cancer risk models integrating genomic features (somatic gene expression arrays and host DNA-repair capacity) assessed risk more accurately than did the clinical models alone.[10,11] Barrett esophagus is a well-established but modest predictor of absolute esophageal cancer risk, whereas a striking model incorporating certain loss of heterozygosity (LOH) and DNA-content profiles with Barrett distinguished between populations with a high (79% in 6 years) and low (0% in over 6 years) esophageal cancer risk.[12] In oral leukoplakia, LOH at specific loci in chromosomes 3p and/or 9p confers a substantially increased risk of oral cancer (vs oral leukoplakia without such LOH),[13,14] especially in patients with a previously treated oral cancer.[15] A high cancer risk is associated with a specific cyclin D1 genotype (adenine/guanine single-nucleotide polymorphism at position 870 of exon 4 of the cyclin D1 gene)[16] in patients with dysplastic oral and/or laryngeal premalignant lesions. Recent work has shown that high cyclin D1 protein expression plus the high-risk cyclin D1 genotype further increased the cancer risk of laryngeal dysplasia patients.[17]

Many molecular factors marking risk and carcinogenesis may be targeted for chemoprevention. For example, agents targeting the epidermal growth factor receptor and mammalian target of rapamycin may downregulate the downstream target cyclin D1 (which marks oral and laryngeal cancer risk). One such agent is erlotinib, which is being tested in a phase III oral cancer prevention trial.[5] Clinical agents directly targeting cyclin D1 are not yet available. Another attractive chemopreventive approach is targeting methylation, particularly in people with epigenetic changes that increase cancer risk (eg, lung cancer, as mentioned above). The demethylating drugs 5-aza-2-(')-deoxycytidine and decitabine are currently in routine clinical use for treating the preleukemic disease myelodysplastic syndrome.[18]

Chemoprevention Trials

Head and Neck

Oral Premalignancy ■ Oral leukoplakia is a premalignant lesion that manifests with a white patch unclassifiable as any other disorder.[19,20] Current management ranges from observation to excision (discussed in detail in Chapter 77, "Neoplasms of the Head and Neck"), depending on the location, extent, and histology of the lesion. Chemoprevention may become standard systemic therapy in certain cases, such as those involving certain profiles of LOH or extensive multiple lesions.[21]

Oral leukoplakia is an excellent model system for clinical testing of chemopreventive agents with potential activity throughout the aerodigestive tract. This lesion is related to tobacco use and associated with squamous cell carcinoma. It is easily monitored clinically, cytologically, and histologically and is related to carcinogenesis in other aerodigestive tract sites.[20,21] The oral leukoplakia system has been used for clinical, laboratory, and translational studies of agent effects on histopathologic and other intermediate endpoint biomarkers of carcinogenesis.[21-24]

Early randomized testing involving the retinoid 13-*cis*-retinoic acid (13cRA) demonstrated that high-dose 13cRA was active but too toxic and reversible for sustained oral cancer prevention[3,25,26] and that lower, more tolerable doses did not translate into long-term oral cancer risk reduction. A long-term regimen of low-dose 13cRA (0.5 mg/kg/day for 1 year followed by 0.25 mg/kg/day for 2 years) was no more effective in reducing cancer risk than was β-carotene plus retinol or retinol alone in 162 randomized patients. 13cRA results in an RCT to prevent head and neck cancer-related second primary tumors (SPTs; discussed in detail below) further discouraged its use in the oral premalignancy setting.[27]

A recently reported randomized trial of celecoxib in oral premalignancy began as a two-arm trial of celecoxib at 200 mg bid versus placebo and later was expanded to include an arm of celecoxib at 400 mg bid.[28] The lower celecoxib dose was no better than was placebo in reversing oral premalignancy, and effects of the higher dose were uninterpretable because the arm was closed by cardiovascular toxicity concerns raised in colorectal adenoma prevention trials (discussed later). A recently reported phase II single-arm trial, however, suggested that celecoxib at 400 mg bid was biologically active because it suppressed prostaglandin E2 levels in premalignant oral tissue.

Adjunctive laboratory studies of retinoic acid receptors (RARs), *p53*, LOH, and cyclin D1 have been integrated into clinical retinoid trials in oral and laryngeal premalignancy. In a prospective 13cRA trial, RAR-β mRNA was detected via in situ hybridization with antisense RNA in only 21 (40%) of 52 premalignant oral lesions (p = .003). RAR-β mRNA expression increased significantly in response to high-dose 13cRA (from 40% to 90%, p < .001).[29] These translational data conform with strong preclinical data indicating that RAR-β is the nuclear receptor most highly regulated by retinoids.

p53 is another focus of translational research within head and neck cancer chemoprevention trials. Frequent alterations of the *p53* gene and its protein product occur in head and neck cancer and in adjacent normal appearing and premalignant tissue. A prospective study revealed a lack of *p53* modulation by 13cRA and a significant correlation between lesion resistance to 13cRA and levels of *p53* accumulation (p = .006).[30] Promising results in advanced oral IEN have been achieved by *p53* targeting. ONYX-015 is a replication-competent adenovirus that selectively replicates in and causes lysis of cells with deficient *p53* activity. A complete regression of dysplasia occurred in 7 of 19 advanced oral IEN patients who were taking ONYX-015.[31]

The molecular marker LOH (eg, at 3p and 9p) has been documented in oral premalignancy, providing evidence of genetic instability and clonal expansion in preinvasive head and neck lesions, and found to be a significant predictor of cancer development in this setting.[13,32,33] Complete resection did not statistically significantly reduce oral cancer in patients with molecular high-risk lesions defined by LOH patterns, unless the completeness was confirmed molecularly,[34] illustrating the importance of molecular confirmation of complete resection in this setting. The roles of optimal surgical margin width and molecularly confirmed complete resection in reducing cancer risk in high-risk LOH settings should be examined further. Topical supravital toluidine blue staining and fluorescence imaging may be helpful in identifying oral IEN with molecularly marked high cancer risk and in guiding surgical margin widths since these methods were found to be associated with the presence of LOH in dysplastic, minimally dysplastic, or nondysplastic oral IEN.[35,36] LOH also has been used to monitor molecular response to chemoprevention.

Prevention of SPTs ■ SPTs occur in a diffuse pattern throughout the aerodigestive tract and bladder, making them uncontrollable by local therapies. These tumors are a major cause of death following "cure" of head and neck cancer and are the leading cancer-related cause of death after resection of early-stage disease. SPTs develop at a constant rate of approximately 4-6% per year.[19]

The promising early results of retinoids in head and neck premalignancy[25] led to 2 RCTs, including a large-scale NCI Intergroup RCT of 13cRA in preventing head and neck cancer-related SPTs. The first of these trials (in patients with stages I-IV head and neck cancer) showed that adjuvant high-dose 13cRA had a significant shorter-term effect (median follow-up 32 months) in preventing all SPTs that persisted (median follow-up 55 months) for tobacco-related SPTs.[37,38] The second trial was a multicenter NCI intergroup effort (coordinated by M.D. Anderson Cancer Center) that accrued only patients with resected stage I or II head and neck cancer and used a lower dose of 13cRA[27]; low-dose 13cRA did not significantly reduce the rates of SPTs, recurrence or survival.

Investigators in France assessed the efficacy of the synthetic retinoid etretinate in preventing SPTs following definitive therapy of stage I-III squamous cell carcinomas of the oral cavity and oral pharynx.[39] By random assignment, patients received either etretinate or placebo at doses of 50 mg/day for 1 month, followed by 25 mg/day for 2 years. SPT rates in the two study arms did not differ significantly.

The Lung

Premalignancy ■ Clinical and translational chemoprevention trials, including 5 negative randomized trials of retinoids in smokers with metaplasia, have had little to no effect in reversing lung premalignancy.[40] These smoker-metaplasia trials did demonstrate that smoking cessation correlated with a reduction in metaplasia. Despite the generally negative data, encouraging phase IIb data have emerged from studies of 9-*cis*-retinoic acid modulation of RAR-β and Ki-67,[41,42] budesonide modulation of CT detected peripheral nodules,[43] and anethole dithiolthione modulation of bronchial dysplasia.[44]

Prevention of Primary Lung Cancer ■ The NCI-sponsored Alpha-Tocopherol, Beta-Carotene (ATBC) Cancer Prevention Study was a phase-III trial of α-tocopherol and β-carotene to prevent primary lung cancer. The ATBC study involved 29,133 male smokers between 50 and 69 years of age who had smoked an average of 1 pack of cigarettes a day for approximately 36 years.[45] This trial's 2 × 2 factorial design called for α-tocopherol (50 mg/d) and β-carotene (20 mg/d) to be given in a randomized, double-blind, placebo-controlled fashion. The factorial design allowed the study scientists to assess the individual effects of each agent. Significant increases in lung cancer incidence (18% increase, p = .01) and total mortality (8%, p = .02) occurred in the β-carotene-treated subjects after 6.1 years' median follow-up. α-Tocopherol had no significant impact on the lung cancer mortality rate, and there was no evidence of an interaction between α-tocopherol and β-carotene. The α-tocopherol group had a long-term nonsignificant trend of reduced lung cancer incidence and a significant positive secondary analysis in prostate cancer, a 32% decrease in incidence and 41% decrease in mortality.[46]

The Beta-Carotene and Retinol Efficacy Trial (CARET) is the other major NCI phase-III lung cancer chemoprevention trial. This trial tested the combination of β-carotene (30 mg/day) plus retinyl palmitate (25,000 IU/day) in 17,000 smokers and asbestos workers.[47] It confirmed the major finding of the ATBC study with its primary finding that the β-carotene combination increased lung cancer risk in this high-risk population. There was no evidence from either the ATBC study or the CARET that β-carotene increased lung cancer risk in nonsmokers, or former or moderate (less than 1 pack a day) smokers.

SPT Prevention ■ Based on encouraging high-dose retinoid data in the head and neck (see above) and lung,[48] two large-scale phase-III retinoid trials have been completed in the setting of SPT prevention; one in Europe, the other in the United States. The European trial, called the European Study on Chemoprevention with Vitamin A and N-Acetylcysteine (EUROSCAN),[49] was an open-label multicenter trial of 2 years of retinyl palmitate and N-acetyl-L-cysteine (NAC) in a 2 × 2 factorial design. Its aim was to prevent SPTs following definitive therapy of early-stage head and neck cancer (larynx Tis, T1-3, N0-1; oral cavity T1-2, N0-1) and non small cell lung cancer (pT1-2, N0-1, and T3 N0). Involving 2592 patients, EUROSCAN found that retinyl palmitate and/or NAC produced no improvement in event-free survival, survival, or incidence of SPTs. The U.S. multicenter phase III Lung Intergroup Trial (LIT) (NCI I 91–0001) involved low-dose 13cRA to prevent SPTs after definitive therapy of stage I non-small cell lung cancer.[50] Although LIT results were neutral overall, a provocative secondary finding of a drug interaction with smoking status was reported. Lung cancer recurrence and mortality were potentially increased in current smokers and decreased in nonsmokers.

Colon and Rectum

Colorectal trial designs have primarily employed the intermediate endpoints adenomatous polyp development and response and hyperproliferation markers. Many investigators believe that dysplastic aberrant crypt foci (ACF) are the earliest clonal precursor of colorectal cancer and thus are important surrogate endpoints for drug development in mice and humans. Unfortunately, ACF were not useful as a marker of synchronous or advanced adenomas or of celecoxib activity in the only prospective ACF analysis, a randomized placebo-controlled prespecified substudy of the Adenoma Prevention with Celecoxib (APC) trial, discussed in detail below.[51] Several nonsteroidal anti-inflammatory drugs (NSAIDs), calcium salts, fiber, folic acid, and vitamin micronutrient combinations and low fat/high fiber diets in the prevention of colon adenomas have been studied in RCTs.[3,4] NSAIDs' ability to inhibit colon carcinogenesis was suggested by preclinical and epidemiologic studies and led to substantial mechanistic research of these agents.[52-56] The eventual discovery of unexpected cardiovascular toxicity in large RCTs of cyclooxygenase-2 (COX-2)-selective NSAIDs in colorectal neoplasia (discussed below) has had a serious impact on NSAID research in colorectal and other settings of chemoprevention.

Sulindac and celecoxib can effectively treat (but not prevent) adenomas in FAP.[57,58] High-dose celecoxib (800 mg/d) reduced large-bowel polyposis by 28%[45] and duodenal polyposis, which is difficult to resect, by 14% (vs placebo).[59] Calcium (1200 mg/d) reduced the risk of sporadic adenomas by 15% overall[60] and even more in later-stage disease (vs placebo).

Four RCTs have tested the efficacy of aspirin in preventing sporadic adenomas, showing significant reductions in recurrent adenomas among patients treated for 1 or more years. Sandler and colleagues[61] randomized 635 colorectal cancer survivors to aspirin (325 mg/d) versus placebo. The aspirin group had a significant reduction in the number of patients with incident adenomas and a significant delay in the time to the first adenoma after a median follow-up of 12.8 months. Baron and colleagues[62] randomized 1121 patients with prior adenomas to aspirin (81 or 325 mg/d) versus placebo and reported a reduction in the adenoma risk in the low-dose aspirin group, especially in the risk of advanced adenomas (41% risk reduction). Benamouzig and colleagues[63] randomized 238 patients to lysine acetylsalicylate (160 or 300 mg/d) and found a similar, approximately 35% reduction in risk of adenomas with both doses. Most recently, Logan and colleagues[64] tested aspirin (300 mg/d) and folate (0.5 mg/d) in 853 patients; aspirin significantly reduced overall adenoma risk by 21% and reduced advanced adenoma risk by 37% (vs non-aspirin arms). There was no protective effect of aspirin on colorectal cancer risk in men and women in the Physician's Health Study and Women's Health Study. Recent pooled analyses of the British Doctors Aspirin Trial and the United Kingdom Transient Ischaemic Attack Aspirin Trial, however, found that aspirin was associated with a significant 26% reduction in colorectal cancer risk. The effect was greatest with at least 5 years treatment and did not appear for at least 10 years.[65] The latter results are consistent with a recent, very large cohort study involving over 47,000 men from the Health Professionals Follow-up Study, which found a significant dose- and duration-related reduction in colorectal cancer risk.[66]

Three RCTs assessed coxibs (vs placebo) in preventing sporadic adenomas in patients with a prior history of colorectal polyps. The Adenomatous Polyp Prevention on Vioxx (APPROVe) trial tested rofecoxib, and various doses of celecoxib were tested in the APC and Prevention of Colorectal Sporadic Adenomatous Polyps (PreSAP) trials. Interim cardiovascular event rates were unexpectedly higher in APPROVe and APC but not PreSAP.[67-69] The relevant data and safety monitoring committees stopped all three RCTs early because of these safety issues, despite significant activity against colorectal adenomas, and rofecoxib was withdrawn from the world market by the manufacturer. In APPROVe (2587 randomized subjects), rofecoxib reduced adenomas by 24%.[70] In the APC (2035 randomized patients), adenoma rates were significantly different at 37.5% (celecoxib, 400 mg twice daily), 43% (celecoxib, 200 mg twice daily) and 60% (placebo) ($p < 0.001$)[71]; serious cardiovascular adverse event rates significantly increased in a dose-dependant manner (3.4%, 2.6%, and 1%, respectively), and higher cardiovascular risk was associated with a previous history of cardiovascular disease. The PreSAP trial with 1561 randomized patients found incidences of adenomas of 33.6% (celecoxib, 400 mg once daily) and 49.3% (placebo) ($p < 0.001$).[67] The risk of cardiovascular events (defined as a composite endpoint of myocardial infarction, stroke, congestive heart failure, or death from cardiovascular causes) did not increase in the PreSAP trial. In a recent extension analysis of APC patients, it appeared that the serious cardiovascular event rate wore off 2 years after stopping the drug and that a repression of adenomas persisted (albeit diminished), particularly for advanced adenomas. Celecoxib activity was greater in advanced adenomas than overall, greatest in individuals at the highest risk of new adenomas, and similar in people who used or did not use aspirin. Results of a recent pooled analysis of the major celecoxib placebo-controlled trials (double-blind and planned follow-up of at least 3 years in nonarthritis disease settings) suggested that there was no increase in serious cardiovascular events at any studied dose (up to 400 mg b.i.d.) in people with a low-baseline cardiovascular risk (about 15-20% of people on these trials). These results strongly suggest that low baseline cardiovascular risk can improve risk-benefit and help in selecting patients for future COX-2-specific NSAID trials.[72]

Trials of vitamins and diet (low-fat, high fruits and vegetables and fiber) for reducing colorectal adenoma risk have had largely negative results.[73,74] Calcium reduced adenoma risk by a modest statistically significant 19%,[60] which persisted in long-term follow-up.[75] Two RCTs of folate showed no reduction in adenoma risk with a 0.5 or 1 mg/d dose; a subset analysis of one study suggested that folate (1 mg/d) may even increase the risk of advanced or multiple adenomas.[64,76]

Preclinical studies of low doses of DFMO and sulindac supported an RCT of combined oral DFMO (500 mg) and sulindac (150 mg; vs placebo) for 36 months in 375 patients with a history of resected (≥3 mm) adenomas (stratified by use of low-dose aspirin [81 mg] at baseline and clinical adenoma site).[77] Colorectal adenoma recurrence rates were as follows: one or more adenomas—41.1% placebo vs 12.3% (combination; RR 0.30; 95% CI, 0.18-0.49; $p < 0.001$); one or more advanced adenomas—8.5% (placebo) vs 0.7% (combination; RR 0.085; 0.011-0.65; $p < 0.001$); multiple adenomas—13.2% (placebo) vs 0.7% (combination; RR 0.055; 0.0074-0.41; $p < 0.001$). The rates of serious adverse events (grade ≥ 3) were favorable at 8.2% (placebo) vs 11% (combination; $p = 0.35$), and there was no significant difference between the arms in the proportions of patients reporting hearing changes (known to be associated with DFMO). Combination chemoprevention has been long believed to have great potential for enhancing the activity and reducing the toxicity of active single agents, a belief that is reinforced by the landmark advance of this combination trial.

The Breast

Based on highly significant positive results of the Breast Cancer Prevention Trial (BCPT), the selective estrogen-receptor (ER) modulator (SERM) tamoxifen became the first chemopreventive agent to earn FDA approval (longer term follow-up data on tamoxifen are discussed later in this section). Conducted by the National Surgical Adjuvant Breast and Bowel Project (NSABP), the BCPT compared tamoxifen with placebo in preventing breast cancer in 13,388 women at high-risk of this disease.[78] The major high-risk eligibility criteria were age >60 years and history of lobular carcinoma in situ (LCIS), or women from 35 to 59 years old with 5-year breast cancer risk of 1.66% based on the Gail model. The actual overall average, 5-year baseline, breast cancer risk was 3.2%.

At a median follow-up of 55 months, primary invasive breast cancer findings for the tamoxifen and placebo groups were 89 vs 175, respectively, for a 49% relative reduction ($p < .00001$). The relative breast cancer risk reduction was similar for all age and risk groups and was limited to ER-positive tumors. Relative risk reductions of invasive breast cancer were 56% and 86% for women with a history of LCIS and atypical hyperplasia, respectively. Tamoxifen achieved a 50% reduction (35 vs 69 cases) in noninvasive breast cancers. Tamoxifen nonsignificantly reduced overall and breast cancer mortality.

Beneficial secondary findings included 19% fewer fractures in the tamoxifen group. Secondary adverse findings associated with tamoxifen were increased endometrial cancers, vascular events and cataracts. Neutral secondary findings included coronary heart disease and depression of mental function.

Although the BCPT successfully completed testing its primary hypothesis, it also raised several key unresolved issues, such as effects on mortality, optimal tamoxifen duration, generalizability of results, and the issue of prevention versus treatment.

The FDA subsequently approved tamoxifen for breast cancer risk reduction in high-risk women.[4] The FDA recommendation is 20 mg/d for 5 years for high-risk women and warns of tamoxifen-associated risks. The FDA also approved tamoxifen for reducing the incidence of contralateral breast cancers, based on consistent secondary adjuvant data.[79]

Adverse tamoxifen effects make this agent's use a complex, highly individualized decision. In general, an improved tamoxifen risk-to-benefit ratio applies in (1) higher breast cancer risk at any age, (2) any breast cancer risk at lower age, and (3) hysterectomy at any breast cancer risk of women >50 years old. The risk of these adverse effects, especially endometrial cancer, however, has sharply limited the acceptance of tamoxifen for breast cancer risk reduction.

The NSABP B-24 study tested 5 years of tamoxifen (20 mg/d) versus placebo as adjuvant therapy after resection and radiation in 1804 patients with DCIS.[80] At 74 months median follow-up, 5-year incidences of all breast cancer events (invasive and noninvasive) were 8.2% and 13.4% in the tamoxifen and placebo groups, respectively, representing a 43% relative risk reduction ($p = .0009$). The cumulative incidence at 5 years of all invasive breast cancer events in the tamoxifen group was 4.1% versus 7.2% in the placebo group ($p = .004$). The FDA approved tamoxifen for risk reduction in the setting of locally treated (resection and radiation) breast DCIS.

The International Breast Cancer Intervention Study (IBIS-I) randomized 7410 women and showed a 32% reduction in breast cancer risk with tamoxifen.[81] The positive results in this trial and the BCPT (the two stronger RCTs in this setting) were limited to ER-positive cancers. A recent report of the long-term follow-up of IBIS-I suggests that the beneficial tamoxifen effects on breast cancer risk reduction persist for at least 10 years, but most side effects resolve after the 5-year treatment period, including all serious adverse events (eg, thrombotic events and endometrial cancer).[82] These long-term findings have important implications for the risk/benefit profile of tamoxifen for prevention.

The Study of Tamoxifen and Raloxifene (STAR) tested the SERM raloxifene against its fellow SERM tamoxifen for better efficacy and lesser toxicity in breast cancer prevention.[83] 19,747 postmenopausal women with an increased risk of breast cancer were randomized to tamoxifen (20 mg/d) or raloxifene (60 mg/d) for 5 years. The two arms had similar rates of invasive breast cancer, and raloxifene produced fewer cases of uterine cancer (23 cases) than tamoxifen (36 cases) (RR 0.62; 95% CI 0.35-1.08). Furthermore, the risks of thromboembolic events and cataracts were statistically significantly lower with raloxifene than with tamoxifen. Tamoxifen, however, had greater effects in reducing noninvasive breast cancer. Raloxifene was recently approved by the FDA for invasive breast cancer risk reduction in postmenopausal women at a high such risk or with osteoporosis.

Based largely on results of the Anastrozole, Tamoxifen Alone or in Combination (ATAC) trial, there is great interest in aromatase inhibitors for breast cancer prevention in postmenopausal women. Involving 9366 patients, ATAC found that the aromatase inhibitor anastrozole was more effective than was tamoxifen in reducing recurrence and contralateral breast cancer.[84] Anastrozole produced fewer vascular and endometrial events but more musculoskeletal events and fractures than did tamoxifen. These adjuvant ATAC data have led to international RCTs of anastrozole vs placebo in high-risk postmenopausal women and versus tamoxifen in resected DCIS.[85] Tamoxifen, raloxifene, and aromatase inhibitors are only active in reducing ER-positive breast cancer risk. Agents under development to prevent ER-negative breast cancer include RXR-selective retinoids, and inhibitors of COX-2 and epidermal growth factor receptor.[86]

Based on potent chemopreventive activity in breast carcinogenesis models and a favorable clinical toxicity profile, fenretinide (200 mg/d, with monthly 3-day drug holidays to avoid reduced night vision) was tested for 5 years in a large-scale, placebo-controlled Italian trial to prevent contralateral breast cancer (SPTs) in approximately 3000 women who had previously undergone resection for early-stage, node-negative breast cancer.[87] Contralateral breast cancers in this setting occur at a rate of approximately 0.8% per year. There was no significant overall effect of fenretinide in preventing contralateral breast cancer, but there was a trend toward benefit in premenopausal (but not postmenopausal) women. This trend was especially strong for women

40 years or younger and persisted for years after stopping the drug.[88]

The Prostate

Prostate carcinogenesis is an androgen-driven process, and a large-scale RCT, PCPT, tested finasteride (5 mg/d), which inhibits 5-alpha-reductase from converting testosterone into the more potent androgen dihydrotestosterone, vs placebo for 7 years in 18,882 men 55 years of age or older who had normal digital rectal exam (DRE) and prostate-specific antigen (PSA) level. Finasteride reduced the 7-year prostate cancer prevalence by 24.8%[89] but also appeared to increase high-grade disease—6.4% (finasteride) vs 5.1% (placebo). Finasteride also reduced the risk of high-grade prostatic intraepithelial neoplasia (PIN).[90] PCPT analyses also indicated a reduction in benign prostatic hypertrophy symptoms and an increase in sexual side effects, although a recent detailed analysis found that the effect of finasteride on sexual functioning was minimal.[91] Secondary PCPT findings indicated a high-risk of prostate cancer, including high-grade disease, among men with normal PSA levels[92] and differences in PSA screening performance in men taking or not taking finasteride.[93,94] The adverse high-grade (HG) disease finding has sharply limited public interest in finasteride for prostate cancer prevention, and another major concern is that intensive PSA/DRE screening and early detection of prostate cancer in the PCPT could mean that finasteride may have prevented more clinically "insignificant" than "significant" prostate cancer. Several analyses detailed in the following paragraph examined whether finasteride actually caused HG cancer or prevented mainly insignificant cancer.

Detailed analyses after the primary PCPT report found that finasteride biases toward improved prostate cancer detection and accuracy in prostate cancer grading at biopsy.[94,95] One multifaceted statistical modeling analysis accounted for these and other biases[96] in estimating the impact of finasteride on the risk of overall and HG prostate cancer.[97] In the first analytical step, the bias-adjusted prostate cancer rates were estimated to be 21.1% (4.2% HG; placebo) and 14.7% (4.8% HG; finasteride), a 30% risk reduction (RR =0.70, p <0.0001) and a nonsignificant 14% increase in HG cancer (p = 0.12) with finasteride. These investigators next incorporated grading information from radical prostatectomies in approximately 500 subjects diagnosed with cancer, finding estimated HG cancer rates of 8.2% (placebo) vs 6.0% (finasteride), a 27% risk reduction (p = 0.02). In the next analysis, there was a trend of reduced HG cancer risk with finasteride across a plausible range of biopsy sensitivity values (greater detection in finasteride vs placebo). This study found no evidence that HG disease was actually increased in the finasteride group. These findings were consistent with another, independent analysis using a different statistical modeling approach.[98] Both statistical modeling reports were consistent with an earlier pathology analysis based on samples from radical prostatectomies (n = 222, finasteride; n = 306, placebo) examined for tumor grade and extent, and, where possible, compared with grades at biopsy.[99] Degenerative hormonal changes in HG biopsies were equivalent in the finasteride and placebo groups, and prostate volumes were significantly reduced in the finasteride group (p <.001). Pathologic surrogates for tumor extent (including mean percentage of positive cores, mean tumor linear extent and aggregate, bilaterality and perineural invasion) were lower in the finasteride than placebo group. Increased HG disease (Gleason score ≥7) associated with finasteride at biopsy (42.7% finasteride vs 25.4% placebo, p <.001) was diminished at prostatectomy (46.4% finasteride vs 38.6% placebo, p = .10). More patients with HG disease at prostatectomy were detected initially by biopsy in the finasteride group than in the placebo group (69.7% vs 50.5%, p = .01). Based on these findings, effects on prostate volume and selective inhibition of low-grade cancer may have contributed to the initially reported increase in HG cancers and HG cancer may have been detected earlier and was less extensive in the finasteride versus placebo group. A concern that early detection by PSA and prevention by finasteride involved biologically inconsequential tumors was raised by PCPT results showing a risk of prostate cancer at PSA <4.0 ng/mL. This concern was carefully examined in a study of tumor pathology characteristics in biopsy specimens stratified by level of PSA for men in the placebo group who underwent radical prostatectomy.[100] The biopsy criteria for clinically significant tumors applied to 75% of all cancers and 62% of Gleason score (GS) ≤6 cancers in the PCPT. As mentioned above, surrogate measures for tumor volume and risk of perineural invasion were lower with finasteride (vs placebo). The PSA-associated risks of insignificant/HG (GS ≥7) cancer were as follows: 51.7%/15.6% for PSA 0-1.0 ng/mL; 33.7%/37.9% for PSA 1.1-2.5 ng/mL; 17.8%/49.1% for PSA 2.6-4.0 ng/mL; and 11.7%/52.4% for PSA 4.1-10 ng/mL. These findings indicate the effectiveness of finasteride in preventing prostate cancer, including GS ≤6 cancer, with meaningful rates of significant disease. The consensus of these study groups and others was that men undergoing regular prostate cancer screening or who express an interest in cancer prevention should be educated about finasteride for prostate cancer prevention.[101] The biology behind the provocative clinical results of the PCPT is being studied intensively in translational molecular epidemiologic studies based on the PCPT's invaluable repository of biological specimens and correlative patient data.

Another very large RCT, the Selenium and Vitamin E Cancer Prevention Trial (SELECT), recently discontinued supplements and reported results demonstrating that selenium or vitamin E, alone or in combination, did not prevent prostate cancer at the doses and formulations used in a heterogeneous population of 35,533 relatively healthy men. Accrued in the United States, Canada, and Puerto Rico, these men were eligible for select based on a DRE not suspicious for prostate cancer, PSA of ≤4 ng/mL, an age of 55 years or older (except African-American men, who were eligible at age 50 years or older), and other criteria.[102] The rationale for SELECT was based largely on secondary findings from the 2 large RCTs, the ATBC and Nutritional Prevention of Cancer studies.[103] There were 4 intervention groups: Oral selenium (200 µg/d from *L*-selenomethionine) and matched vitamin E placebo, vitamin E (400 IU/d of *all rac*-α-tocopheryl acetate) and matched selenium placebo, or the 2 combined or placebo plus placebo. A planned 7-year interim analysis found evidence that convincingly demonstrated no benefit from either study agent (p < 0.0001) and no possibility of a benefit to the planned degree with additional follow-up, leading the SELECT Data and Safety Monitoring Committee to recommend the early discontinuation of supplements. After a median follow-up of 5.47 years (range 4.17-7.33 years), hazard ratios for prostate cancer were 1.13 for vitamin E (n = 473 prostate cancers, 99% CI 0.91-1.41), 1.04 for selenium (n = 432 cancers; 99% CI 0.83-1.30), and 1.05 for the combination (n = 437; 99% CI 0.83-1.31) compared with placebo (n = 416 prostate cancers). Nor did any other prespecified cancer endpoint show a significant difference (all p-values >0.15). A nonsignificant increased risk of prostate cancer in the vitamin E arm (p = 0.06; RR 1.13; 99% CI 0.195-1.35) and of type 2 diabetes mellitus in the selenium arm (p = 0.16; RR 1.07; 99% CI 0.94-1.22) did not appear in the combination arm.

The Cervix

The characteristic multistep histologic evolution of cervical carcinogenesis, the well-documented rates of progression and spontaneous regression within each histopathologic grade (cervical intraepithelial neoplasia [CIN] 1, 2, and 3), and ease in monitoring make cervical carcinogenesis an excellent human model for studying chemoprevention agents. HPV infection is an established major risk factor for cervical cancer, and molecular targeting through immunization against infections related to neoplasia is a very successful way to prevent early steps of host cell damage that otherwise can lead to cancer. The proof of principle of vaccinating against infection-related cancer was provided in Taiwan, where vaccinating children against hepatitis B has dramatically reduced the incidence and mortality of liver cancer.[104] Vaccines against infections related to cancer development generate immune responses against very specific proteins (eg, the L1 HPV viral capside protein and hepatitis B surface antigen). A landmark advance of cancer chemoprevention was relatively recent RCTs of HPV vaccines to prevent HPV infection in girls and young women, and subsequent FDA approval of HPV vaccination in this setting.

The recent placebo-controlled (phase III) trial Females United to Unilaterally Reduce Endo/Ectocervical Disease (FUTURE) II found that a quadrivalent vaccine against HPV 6, 11, 16, and 18 reduced the risk of the primary composite endpoint (cervical IEN [grades 2 and 3], adenocarcinoma in situ, or cancer-related to HPV 16 or 18) by 98% in women between ages 15 and 26 years with no virologic evidence of HPV 16 or 18; the vaccine reduced this endpoint by 44% in an intent-to-treat analysis including women with previous HPV infection.[105] Another recent phase III trial tested a bivalent (HPV 16 and 18) vaccine in 18,644 girls and women aged 15-25 years. The primary endpoint, grade 2 cervical IEN associated with HPV 16 or 18, was reduced by 90% in women with no evidence of prior HPV infection.[106] A phase III trial of a quadrivalent vaccine (HPV 6, 11, 16, 18) was 100% effective in preventing the co-primary endpoints genital warts, vulvar or vaginal IEN or cancer, and cervical IEN, adenocarcinoma in situ, or cancer in 5455 females from 16 to 24 years old and with no virologic evidence on HPV infection through 7 months (which was the protocol specified primary analysis), or at 1 month after the 6-month treatment (3 doses of vaccine). An intent-to-treat analysis including disease unrelated to these HPV types and women with prevalent HPV infection showed that vaginal/vulvar lesions were reduced by 34% and cervical lesions by 20%.[107]

The striking results of these trials led to the U.S. FDA approval of HPV vaccine for use in girls and young women 9-26 years old for preventing cervical cancer, cervical adenocarcinoma in situ, and high-grade cervical, vulvar and vaginal IEN. HPV vaccines have not been shown to accelerate HPV clearance and so are unlikely to prevent cancer in already infected patients.[108]

Cervical dysplasia has been studied in over 10 randomized natural or synthetic agent trials,[109-118] including negative trials of locally applied interferon, folic acid and β-carotene. Only one of these trials was positive, and it involved the retinoid tretinoin.[117] The positive, randomized tretinoin trial used an intermittent schedule of locally applied tretinoin in 301 subjects—141 with biopsy-proved moderate (CIN 2) cervical dysplasia and 160 with severe (CIN 3) dysplasia.[117] Compared with placebo, tretinoin had significant activity in moderate dysplasia: complete regression rates of 43% vs 27%, respectively (p = .04). It had no activity in severe dysplasia. A subsequent RCT of topical tretinoin for a shorter duration was negative.[119]

The Skin

Premalignant skin lesions and skin cancer have been the endpoints of chemoprevention trials in this setting. Topical retinoid (tretinoin) had dose-related activity against actinic keratosis in nonrandomized and randomized trials.[120] Systemic retinoid therapy achieved significant activity against actinic keratosis in two placebo-controlled trials.[121,122] Topical eflornithine, colchicines, or 5-fluorouracil (5-FU) produced significant activity in suppressing or regressing actinic keratosis. Aminolevulinic acid HCl with photodynamic therapy and sodium diclofenac received FDA approvals for treating actinic keratosis.

13cRA reduced skin tumor incidence in a series of NCI-sponsored small trials. One of these trials was conducted in 5 xeroderma pigmentosum patients at extremely high-risk of developing nonmelanoma skin cancer.[123] This trial achieved a significant reduction in the number of skin cancers during the 2 years of high-dose 13cRA (2 mg/kg/d) treatment (p = .02). Subsequent studies showed that this chemopreventive effect was dose related and was lost after stopping treatment. A randomized placebo-controlled trial of the retinoid acitretin in 38 renal transplant recipients[124] showed significant (although reversible) reductions in premalignant lesions and skin cancers. 13cRA plus α-interferon had no benefit in a recent phase III trial to prevent skin SPTs and recurrences in 66 randomized patients with aggressive skin SCC.[125]

Several large-scale, long-term phase III chemoprevention trials have been conducted in subjects at much lower risk of developing skin cancer.[126-130] Only one of these trials was positive. In this trial, retinol (25,000 IU/day) significantly reduced the incidence of primary squamous cell (but not basal cell) skin cancer in patients with actinic keratosis.[138] The other trials, all negative, involved β-carotene, retinol, very low-dose 13cRA and selenium in patients with previous skin cancers. The study of selenium (200 μg/d in brewer's yeast) was negative in its primary end point of preventing squamous cell and basal cell carcinomas of the skin in 1312 patients having histories of nonmelanoma skin cancer and living in low selenium-intake regions of the United States.[126] This trial, however, produced provocative secondary findings of significant positive selenium effects on prostate, lung, and colon cancer incidence and of total cancer incidence and mortality, which were attenuated in the longer-term as shown by an analysis at the end of the blinded treatment period.

A novel randomized trial of a topical DNA-repair enzyme in xeroderma pigmentosum resulted in a reduction in the rates of actinic keratosis and basal cell carcinoma.[131]

Esophagus and Stomach

In the United States, esophageal carcinoma is strongly associated with tobacco and alcohol abuse. Causes of this cancer in other parts of the world, such as China, however, appear to include nutritional deficiencies and exposure to carcinogens, such as N-nitroso compounds. Several large placebo-controlled chemoprevention trials against esophageal or gastric carcinogenesis have been conducted. Subjects for most of these trials came from geographic regions with established high risks of esophageal or gastric cancers. Four trials were of multiple natural compounds. The applicability of the findings in developing countries to esophageal cancer in the United States and other developed countries with different epidemiologic risk profiles is not clear.

A placebo-controlled, randomized trial to reverse esophageal squamous carcinogenesis was conducted in Huixian, China.[132] This trial was based on several factors, including epidemiologic and endoscopic studies in high-risk geographic areas. Subjects received a combination of retinol, riboflavin, and zinc for 13.5 months. The intervention achieved no overall reduction in the occurrence of premalignant lesions. Two subset analyses revealed that (1) micronuclei frequency in the esophagus, but not in the oral cavity, decreased significantly in association with the chemopreventive regimen,[133] and (2) increased plasma micronutrient levels (primarily retinol) were associated with a reduction in dysplastic lesions, regardless of treatment arm.[134] This trial also illustrated an issue of concern to many investigators studying vitamins, minerals, and micronutrients. Plasma micronutrient levels in the Huixian trial increased substantially in about 50% of placebo recipients. Evidently these control subjects obtained readily available trial compounds via their diet or in over-the-counter preparations of vitamins and minerals. Poor study compliance, either in the form of drop-ins or dropouts, can greatly reduce the statistical power of a randomized trial.

A phase IIb trial was conducted in Uzbekistan. Retinol, β-carotene, and vitamin E with or without riboflavin were given in a factorial design to high- risk subjects with oral leukoplakia and/or chronic esophagitis.[135] As in the Huixian study, none of the vitamin regimens had a significant effect on esophageal premalignancy.

An RCT in Linxian, China, tested celecoxib (200 mg/bid) and selenomethionine (200 μg/qd) in a 2 × 2 factorial design for effects on moderate or mild esophageal squamous dysplasia. Celecoxib did not improve either moderate or mild dysplasia. Selenomethionine did not improve moderate dysplasia but did improve mild dysplasia ($p = .02$).[136]

There also have been trials in the prevention of esophageal adenocarcinoma, which has the fastest rising incidence of all cancers in Western countries.[137] Celecoxib (200 mg bid) did not suppress prostaglandin levels or prevent progression of Barrett dysplasia to cancer.[138] The adenocarcinoma precursor, Barrett esophagus, has been studied intensively. In 2003, the FDA approved a photosensitizing porphyrin mixture (Photofrin) in conjunction with photodynamic therapy (PDT) for the ablation of high-grade dysplasia in patients with Barrett esophagus who cannot or choose not to undergo esophagectomy. This approval was based on a multicenter RCT involving 138 patients randomized to Photofrin PDT plus omeprazole and 70 patients randomized to omeprazole alone (www.fda.gov/cder/foi/label/2003/20451s012_photofrin_lbl.pdf>). Follow-up ranging from 2 to 3.6 years showed that a complete and sustained eradication of high-grade dysplasia occurred in 77% of the patients treated with combination therapy vs in 39% of the patients treated with omeprazole alone ($p < .0001$). This chemopreventive approach involves intravenous injection of Photofrin, which is activated 40-50 hours later by endoscopically applied red light for a maximum of 3 treatment courses.

Two NCI placebo-controlled phase III trials of multiple vitamins and minerals were conducted in the high-risk area of Linxian, China. One trial employed a complex modified factorial design to test four different vitamin-mineral combinations given to 29,584 subjects for 5 years at doses of 1-2 times the U.S. recommended daily allowance (RDA).[139] The combination of β-carotene, α-tocopherol, and selenium was associated with 4% and 21% reductions in the esophageal cancer and gastric cancer mortality rates, respectively. The gastric cancer mortality reduction was significant ($p < .05$). In the other phase III trial, only higher risk subjects with esophageal dysplasia received either 26 vitamins and minerals (including β-carotene, α-tocopherol, and selenium, at 2-3 times the U.S. RDA) or placebo in a 2-arm design.[140] This intervention was associated with two nonsignificant changes: an 18% increase in mortality from gastric cancer and a 16% reduction in mortality from esophageal cancer. Interpretation of these 2 contrasting studies is made difficult by the many different interventions and end points.

A placebo-controlled study of 220 subjects in Venezuela reported no significant effect of bismuth and amoxicillin on *Helicobacter pylori* eradication rates.[141] The bacterium *H. pylori* has been implicated in the etiology of gastric carcinogenesis.

The Bladder

In vivo animal model, in vitro, and epidemiologic studies have shown that retinoids are active against bladder carcinogenesis.[142] The retinoid etretinate has been tested in three randomized clinical trials in patients following resection of superficial bladder tumors.[143-145] Two of these trials employed prolonged low-dose etretinate, which appeared to be effective.[80,145] Results of the 2 positive trials require confirmation, however, because of these trials' limited patient numbers and follow-up. A fourth randomized trial compared a multivitamin preparation at RDA levels alone or supplemented with 40,000 IU retinol, 100 mg pyridoxine, 2000 mg ascorbic acid, 400 IU of α-tocopherol, and 90 mg zinc. The estimated 5-year tumor recurrence rate was 91% in the RDA arm versus 41% in the megadose arm ($p = .0014$).

Fenretinide (200 mg/day) for 12 months was well tolerated but did not reduce time to recurrence in a recently reported phase III trial in 149 patients with resected nonmuscle-invasive bladder cancer.[146] A phase III trial of DFMO vs placebo for 12 months in 454 randomized patients did not prevent recurrence.[147] Celecoxib produced encouraging preliminary results in another recently completed RCT (final analysis of the data is in progress).

Overall Cancer

Two important large U.S. trials have tested the ability of β-carotene to reduce overall cancer incidence. The Physicians' Health Study was a 12-year test of β-carotene effects on overall cancer incidence.[148] β-carotene produced no significant differences in overall incidence of cancer (including lung cancer). Only 11% of this population were current smokers. Similar β-carotene results of the Women's Health Study were reported.[149]

Conclusions

Clinical cancer chemoprevention has matured with the FDA approvals of several agents to prevent cancer or to treat or prevent IEN, most recently raloxifene for preventing invasive breast cancer in high-risk women and HPV vaccine for cervical cancer prevention. The list of FDA approved agents for cancer prevention includes celecoxib, diclofenac, Photofrin (in conjunction with PDT), tamoxifen, hepatitis B vaccine, bacillus Calmette-Guerin, valrubicin, masoprocol, 5-FU, and aminolaevulinic acid (with PDT). Other agents with established activity in RCTs include finasteride in preventing high-grade PIN and prostate cancer, retinoids in preventing skin SCC, and celecoxib in preventing sporadic colorectal adenomas. Translational studies of cyclin D1 genotype and expression, LOH, clones and subclones, and many other biomarkers and signaling pathways are advancing cancer risk assessment and chemoprevention. Extension studies of the tamoxifen and celecoxib prevention trials are better defining risk/benefit profiles and optimal drug treatment duration.

Personalized approaches to identify patients most likely to benefit and least likely to be harmed by particular interventions are evolving from continued study of aspirin and celecoxib in colorectal neoplasia. For example, studies of single-nucleotide polymorphisms of the ornithine decarboxylase (*ODC*) gene suggest the possibility of selecting people most likely to benefit from aspirin.[150] Other studies suggest the possibility of identifying people least likely to be harmed by celecoxib.[72] Despite its ability to reduce adenoma risk by 15-25%, aspirin has not been accepted as standard prevention because of risk-benefit analyses. This outcome suggests that modest risk reductions, even with relatively innocuous agents, are not enough. Future studies need powering to detect a 50% or greater effect, to personalize selection for potential benefit[150] and adverse events,[72] and early efficacy assessments as, eg, in the APC trial, where celecoxib reduced adenoma risk similarly at 1 and 3 years.

One of the most promising current directions of cancer chemoprevention is combined agents. The concept that combinations can increase the ratio of benefit (activity) to risk (toxicity) for effective single agents received strong support from the stunning colorectal adenoma results of the DFMO-sulindac trial discussed earlier. Based on this trial, chemopreventive combinations may be at the threshold of becoming a standard clinical reality, and other active combinations should be moved into clinical trials.[151]

Selected References

The complete reference list can be found at www.CANCERMEDICINE8.com

1. Kelloff GJ, Lippman SM, Dannenberg AJ, et al. Progress in chemoprevention drug development: the promise of molecular biomarkers for prevention of intraepithelial neoplasia and cancer—a plan to move forward. *Clin Cancer Res.* 2006;12(12):3661–3697.
5. Lippman SM, Heymach JV. The convergent development of molecular-targeted drugs for cancer treatment and prevention. *Clin Cancer Res.* 2007;13(14):4035–4041.
7. Spitz MR, Hong WK, Amos CI, et al. A risk model for prediction of lung cancer. *J Natl Cancer Inst.* 2007;99(9):715–726.
9. Belinsky SA, Liechty KC, Gentry FD, et al. Promoter hypermethylation of multiple genes in sputum precedes lung cancer incidence in a high-risk cohort. *Cancer Res.* 2006;66(6):3338–3344.
13. Lee JJ, Hong WK, Hittelman WN, et al. Predicting cancer development in oral leukoplakia: ten years of translational research. *Clin Cancer Res.* 2000;6(5):1702–1710.
14. Rosin MP, Cheng X, Poh C, et al. Use of allelic loss to predict malignant risk for low-grade oral epithelial dysplasia. *Clin Cancer Res.* 2000;6(2):357–362.
16. Izzo JG, Papadimitrakopoulou VA, Liu DD, et al. Cyclin D1 genotype, response to biochemoprevention, and progression rate to upper aerodigestive tract cancer. *J Natl Cancer Inst.* 2003;95(3):198–205.
23. Mao L, Hong WK, Papadimitrakopoulou VA. Focus on head and neck cancer. *Cancer Cell.* 2004;5(4):311–316.
25. Hong WK, Endicott J, Itri LM, et al. 13-cis-retinoic acid in the treatment of oral leukoplakia. *N Engl J Med.* 1986;315(24):1501–1505.
26. Lippman SM, Batsakis JG, Toth BB, et al. Comparison of low-dose isotretinoin with beta carotene to prevent oral carcinogenesis. *N Engl J Med.* 1993;328(1):15–20.
27. Khuri FR, Lee JJ, Lippman SM, et al. Randomized phase III trial of low-dose isotretinoin for prevention of second primary tumors in stage I and II head and neck cancer patients. *J Natl Cancer Inst.* 2006;98(7):441–450.
29. Lotan R, Xu XC, Lippman SM, et al. Suppression of retinoic acid receptor-beta in premalignant oral lesions and its up-regulation by isotretinoin. *N Engl J Med.* 1995;332(21):1405–1410.
33. Mao L, Lee JS, Fan YH, et al. Frequent microsatellite alterations at chromosomes 9p21 and 3p14 in oral premalignant lesions and their value in cancer risk assessment. *Nat Med.* 1996;2(6):682–685.
37. Hong WK, Lippman SM, Itri LM, et al. Prevention of second primary tumors with isotretinoin in squamous-cell carcinoma of the head and neck. *N Engl J Med.* 1990;323(12):795–801.
44. Lam S, MacAulay C, Le Riche JC, et al. A randomized phase IIb trial of anethole dithiolethione in smokers with bronchial dysplasia. *J Natl Cancer Inst.* 2002;94(13):1001–1009.
45. The Alpha-Tocopherol, Beta-Carotene Cancer Prevention Study Group. The effect of vitamin E and beta-carotene on the incidence of lung cancer and other cancers in male smokers. *N Engl J Med.* 1994;330:1029–1035.
47. Omenn GS, Goodman GE, Thornquist MD, et al. Effects of a combination of beta carotene and vitamin A on lung cancer and cardiovascular disease. *N Engl J Med.* 1996;334(18):1150–1155.
50. Lippman SM, Lee JJ, Karp DD, et al. Randomized phase III intergroup trial of isotretinoin to prevent second primary tumors in stage I non-small-cell lung cancer. *J Natl Cancer Inst.* 2001;93(8):605–618.
53. Shureiqi I, Jiang W, Zuo X, et al. The 15-lipoxygenase-1 product 13-S-hydroxyoctadecadienoic acid down-regulates PPAR-delta to induce apoptosis in colorectal cancer cells. *Proc Natl Acad Sci USA.* 2003;100(17):9968–9973.
54. Shureiqi I, Wu Y, Chen D, et al. The critical role of 15-lipoxygenase-1 in colorectal epithelial cell terminal differentiation and tumorigenesis. *Cancer Res.* 2005;65(24):11486–11492.
58. Steinbach G, Lynch PM, Phillips RK, et al. The effect of celecoxib, a cyclooxygenase-2 inhibitor, in familial adenomatous polyposis. *N Engl J Med.* 2000;342(26):1946–1952.
60. Baron JA, Beach M, Mandel JS, et al. Calcium supplements for the prevention of colorectal adenomas. Calcium Polyp Prevention Study Group. *N Engl J Med.* 1999;340(2):101–107.
61. Sandler RS, Halabi S, Baron JA, et al. A randomized trial of aspirin to prevent colorectal adenomas in patients with previous colorectal cancer. *N Engl J Med.* 2003;348(10):883–890.
65. Flossmann E, Rothwell PM. Effect of aspirin on long-term risk of colorectal cancer: consistent evidence from randomised and observational studies. *Lancet.* 2007;369(9573):1603–1613.
67. Arber N, Eagle CJ, Spicak J, et al. Celecoxib for the prevention of colorectal adenomatous polyps. *N Engl J Med.* 2006;355(9):885–895.
68. Bresalier RS, Sandler RS, Quan H, et al. Cardiovascular events associated with rofecoxib in a colorectal adenoma chemoprevention trial. *N Engl J Med.* 2005;352(11):1092–1102.
69. Solomon SD, McMurray JJ, Pfeffer MA, et al. Cardiovascular risk associated with celecoxib in a clinical trial for colorectal adenoma prevention. *N Engl J Med.* 2005;352(11):1071–1080.
70. Baron JA, Sandler RS, Bresalier RS, et al. A randomized trial of rofecoxib for the chemoprevention of colorectal adenomas. *Gastroenterology.* 2006;131(6):1674–1682.
71. Bertagnolli MM, Eagle CJ, Zauber AG, et al. Celecoxib for the prevention of sporadic colorectal adenomas. *N Engl J Med.* 2006;355(9):873–884.
72. Solomon SD, Wittes J, Finn PV, et al. Cardiovascular risk of celecoxib in 6 randomized placebo-controlled trials: the cross trial safety analysis. *Circulation.* 2008;117(16):2104–2113.
74. Schatzkin A, Lanza E, Corle D, et al. Lack of effect of a low-fat, high-fiber diet on the recurrence of colorectal adenomas. Polyp Prevention Trial Study Group. *N Engl J Med.* 2000;342(16):1149–1155.
76. Cole BF, Baron JA, Sandler RS, et al. Folic acid for the prevention of colorectal adenomas: a randomized clinical trial. *JAMA.* 2007;297(21):2351–2359.
77. Meyskens FL, Jr, McLaren CE, Pelot D, et al. Difluoromethylornithine plus sulindac for the prevention of sporadic colorectal adenomas: a randomized placebo-controlled, double-blind trial. *Cancer Prev Res.* 2008;1(1):32–38.
82. Cuzick J, Forbes JF, Sestak I, et al. Long-term results of tamoxifen prophylaxis for breast cancer—96-month follow-up of the randomized IBIS-I trial. *J Natl Cancer Inst.* 2007;99(4):272–282.
83. Vogel VG, Costantino JP, Wickerham DL, et al. Effects of tamoxifen vs raloxifene on the risk of developing invasive breast cancer and other disease outcomes: the NSABP Study of Tamoxifen and Raloxifene (STAR) P-2 trial. *JAMA.* 2006;295(23):2727–2741.
88. Veronesi U, Mariani L, Decensi A, et al. Fifteen-year results of a randomized phase III trial of fenretinide to prevent second breast cancer. *Ann Oncol.* 2006;17(7):1065–1071.
91. Moinpour CM, Darke AK, Donaldson GW, et al. Longitudinal analysis of sexual function reported by men in the Prostate Cancer Prevention Trial. *J Natl Cancer Inst.* 2007;99(13):1025–1035.
92. Thompson IM, Pauler DK, Goodman PJ, et al. Prevalence of prostate cancer among men with a prostate-specific antigen level < or =4.0 ng per milliliter. *N Engl J Med.* 2004;350(22):2239–2246.
96. Goodman PJ, Thompson IM, Jr, Tangen CM, Crowley JJ, Ford LG, Coltman CA, Jr. The prostate cancer prevention trial: design, biases and interpretation of study results. *J Urol.* 2006;175(6):2234–2242.
98. Pinsky P, Parnes H, Ford L. Estimating rates of true high-grade disease in the prostate cancer prevention trial. *Cancer Prev Res.* 2008;1(3):182–186.
99. Lucia MS, Epstein JI, Goodman PJ, et al. Finasteride and high-grade prostate cancer in the Prostate Cancer Prevention Trial. *J Natl Cancer Inst.* 2007;99(18):1375–1383.
102. Lippman SM, Klein EA, Goodman PJ, et al. Effect of selenium and vitamin E on risk of prostate cancer and other cancers: the Selenium and Vitamin E Cancer Prevention Trial (SELECT). *JAMA.* 2009;301(1):39–51.
104. Powles T, Eeles R, Ashley S, et al. Interim analysis of the incidence of breast cancer in the Royal Marsden Hospital tamoxifen randomised chemoprevention trial. *Lancet.* 1998;352(9122):98–101.
125. Brewster AM, Lee JJ, Clayman GL, et al. Randomized trial of adjuvant 13-cis-retinoic acid and interferon alfa for patients with aggressive skin squamous cell carcinoma. *J Clin Oncol.* 2007;25(15):1974–1978.
128. Levine N, Moon TE, Cartmel B, et al. Trial of retinol and isotretinoin in skin cancer prevention: a randomized, double-blind, controlled trial. Southwest Skin Cancer Prevention Study Group. *Cancer Epidemiol Biomarkers Prev.* 1997;6(11):957–961.
138. Heath EI, Canto MI, Piantadosi S, et al. Secondary chemoprevention of Barrett's esophagus with celecoxib: results of a randomized trial. *J Natl Cancer Inst.* 2007;99(7):545–557.
147. Messing E, Kim KM, Sharkey F, et al. Randomized prospective phase III trial of difluoromethylornithine vs placebo in preventing recurrence of completely resected low risk superficial bladder cancer. *J Urol.* 2006;176(2):500–504.

34 Cancer Screening and Early Detection

Robert A. Smith, PhD ▪ Stephen W. Duffy, MSc ▪ Otis W. Brawley, MD

A feature common to most of the more prevalent cancers, that is, cancers of the skin, breast, cervix, endometrium, ovary, testis, colon and rectum, prostate, and lung, is that stage at diagnosis is the primary determinant of prognosis, and prognosis generally is better and treatment more successful if the disease is diagnosed while still localized. Secondary prevention of cancer is distinguished from primary prevention in that it is an intervention focused on: (1) detecting and treating early invasive disease and thus reducing the risk of death from cancer or (2) altering the natural history of the disease by identifying and treating precursor lesions known to be predictive of eventual malignancy, thus preventing progression to invasive disease. Cancer screening and early detection are secondary prevention strategies that have major importance in reducing morbidity and mortality from several high incidence cancers.

Key Criteria in the Decision to Screen

The observation that a particular cancer has more favorable survival if diagnosed at an early stage is important but only one element in the decision matrix used to determine whether to offer cancer screening to an asymptomatic population.[1] In general, the following criteria should be met.[2]

1. The disease should be an important health problem, as measured by morbidity, mortality, and other measures of disease burden.
2. The disease should have a detectable preclinical phase.
3. Treatment of disease detected before the onset of clinical symptoms should offer benefits compared with treatment after the onset of symptoms.
4. The screening test should meet acceptable levels of accuracy and cost.
5. The screening test and follow-up requirements should be acceptable to individuals at risk and to their health-care providers.

These criteria are important considerations prior to any decision to offer screening to a healthy population. However, although each criterion is important, there are no measurable thresholds to guide decision making; thus, the decision matrix requires considering the criteria collectively.[3,4] For example, a disease may not be an important cause of mortality but may account for significant morbidity. A high false-positive rate may be acceptable when screening for cancers at some organ sites but not at others due to the costs (financial, or harms to individuals) associated with diagnostic testing after an abnormal screening examination. A screening test may not meet the criteria very well, but the disease may be of great concern to the population at risk and the test will therefore be acceptable despite limitations. Values, in addition to scientific evidence, play a role in policy decisions about screening.[4]

Disease Burden

Diseases that are fatal or are the cause of significant morbidity are potentially suitable for screening. The International Agency for Research on Cancer (IARC) estimates that in 2002 there were 10.9 million new cases of cancer and 6.9 million deaths, excluding basal and squamous cell cancers of the skin and in situ cervix, breast, or melanoma lesions.[5] Lung cancer (1.35 million) is the most common cancer, followed by breast cancer (1.15 million), colorectal cancer (1 million), and stomach cancer (.93 million). Lung cancer also is the most common cause of death from cancer (1.18 million deaths), followed by stomach cancer (700,000 deaths), liver cancer (598,000 deaths), and colorectal cancer (529,000). There is considerable international variation in the incidence and mortality of these and other cancers, as well as disease-specific trends.

Characteristics of the Disease

If a disease is judged to be an important health problem, additional disease-specific criteria must be met to justify screening, specifically, knowledge of the natural history of the disease and the disease latency period, and the degree to which treatment before the onset of clinically apparent disease truly improves prognosis compared with later treatment.

Screening recommendations typically represent an interplay or balance between the age groups invited to screening and the screening interval. There needs to be a sufficient prevalence of detectable occult disease to justify screening large numbers of healthy individuals, and the screening interval must be set to ensure that most cancers will be detected at an early stage in a population adherent with screening recommendations. Most cancers have a long preclinical phase, which technically begins following the first reproduction of malignant cells. At a point late in the preclinical phase, a tumor may become detectable by a screening test before the onset of symptoms, hence the *detectable* period within the preclinical phase. The *detectable preclinical phase* (DPCP), also known as the *sojourn time,* is the estimated duration of time in which an occult tumor can be detected with a screening test before the onset of symptoms.[6] For screening to be successful, the *sojourn time* should be sufficiently long to insure that periodic screening provides the opportunity to detect most disease in the target population before the onset of symptoms. If the *sojourn time* is short, then the necessary screening interval may be so short that screening is impractical. Conversely, if the *sojourn time* is long, then screening too frequently will waste health-care resources. The screening interval should always be shorter than the estimated mean duration of the *sojourn time.* When a screening interval equals or exceeds the mean *sojourn time,* there will be higher rate of interval cancers (cancers that arise and present with clinical manifestations between regularly scheduled screening examinations) and thus poorer prognosis in that subset of the incident cases. The interrelationship between the *sojourn time* and the lead time is shown in Figure 34-1.

Treatment of screen-detected cancers should offer advantages compared with treatment of disease that presents with symptoms. These advantages may be measured by any single outcome or combination of outcomes: lower mortality, lower morbidity, and/or improved quality of life. However, it is important not to equate detection of occult disease with better outcomes since this may not always be the case, and the magnitude of the benefit may not be sufficient to warrant screening the population.

Is the Screening Test Effective?

The ultimate determinant of whether a screening test is effective in public health

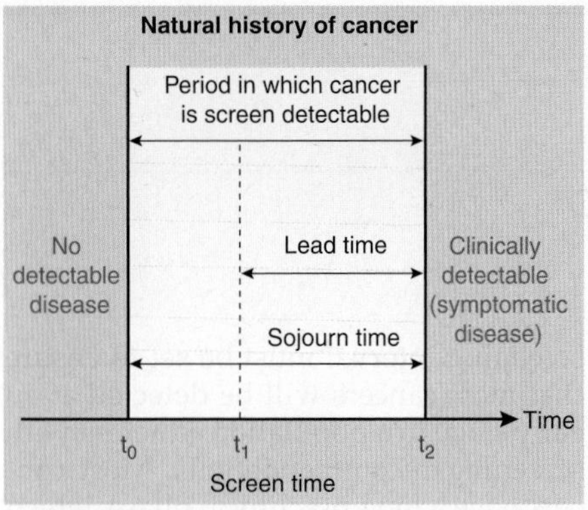

Figure 34-1 The natural history of cancer. In this figure, t_2-t_0 is the duration of the preclinical screen-detectable period, known as the "sojourn time"; t_2-t_1 is the amount of time by which the diagnosis is advanced by screening, known as the "lead time." Under the assumption of an exponential distribution of sojourn time, the expected lead time of a individual screen-detected case is equal to the mean of the distribution of the sojourn time.

terms is whether its routine use leads to a reduction in mortality or morbidity. In terms of its diagnostic effectiveness, the primary measures are sensitivity (S), specificity (Sp), positive predictive value (PPV), and negative predictive value (NPV).

Sensitivity and Specificity

The sensitivity is the probability that the test will have a positive result when applied to a person who truly has the disease. The specificity is the probability of a negative result when applied to a person who does not have the disease. The conventional formulas for calculating sensitivity and specificity are shown in Table 34-1. These are intuitively reasonable definitions, and they have obvious practical applications: A sensitive test will tend to catch disease cases and an insensitive test will miss them, possibly leading to false reassurance and actual delay in diagnosis; a specific test will tend only to catch disease cases, whereas a nonspecific test will raise suspicion of disease in normal subjects, leading to unnecessary further diagnostic investigations and possible treatments.

Clearly then, high sensitivity and high specificity are desirable features in a screening test. However, in general, they tend to be negatively correlated. For example, consider a blood test we class as positive if the value of a continuous assay exceeds a certain cutoff. A high cutoff will confer high specificity and low sensitivity, and vice versa. It should be borne in mind that there is a difference between screening and diagnosis. A positive screening test is not generally a definitive diagnosis of any condition: it merely indicates whether or not further diagnostic workup is necessary (thus, the ubiquitous use of the term "false-positive" for recalled subjects who are finally diagnosed normal is arguably misleading). Therefore, it is unreasonable to expect 100% sensitivity or specificity. In screening for cancer, one would prefer to avoid further diagnostic workup in >10% of truly disease negative subjects, and if at all possible one would not want to miss >10% of individuals who are disease-positive. These are arbitrary figures, but arguably reasonable targets.

Table 34-1 **Measures of Screening Performance**

	Disease Status	
Screening Test Results	Yes	No
Positive	a	b
Negative	c	d

Sensitivity = a/(a + c); specificity = d/(b + d); positive predictive value (PPV) = a/(a + b); negative predictive value (NPV) = c/(c + d).

Finally, we should not confuse test sensitivity with program sensitivity. The latter is the proportion of cases arising in individuals attending a screening program who are actually detected as a result of screening (as opposed to cases arising symptomatically between screens). Program sensitivity is measured over time, and is a function of test sensitivity, the duration of *sojourn time*, and the time interval between screens.

Positive and Negative Predictive Values

The positive predictive value is the probability that a subject with a positive screening result actually has the disease. For example, in mammography, it is not unusual to recall 5% of subjects screened for further investigation, and to finally diagnose only 0.5% of subjects screened with cancer. In this case the PPV is 10%. This figure seems low, superficially, but is acceptable to screened populations.[7] The benefit of early detection for the 10% with breast cancer is considered to outweigh the temporary inconvenience and anxiety for 90% who do not have cancer. The complement of the PPV is the proportion of screen-positive subjects who do not have disease. This should not be confused with overdiagnosis (see next section).

The NPV is the probability that a subject screened negative is truly free of disease, and is in some sense a quantification of the reassurance value of a negative test. It is arguably more important to have a high NPV, as this will mean that few disease subjects are missed and potentially have diagnosis and treatment delayed.

Overdiagnosis

In the context of screening, overdiagnosis is the diagnosis through screening of disease that would never have given rise to clinical symptoms during the lifetime of the case. Overdiagnosis is commonly applied to circumstances that, although quite disparate, results in the same lack of benefit from early detection. First is the theoretical possibility of diagnosis of lesions that have no biological propensity to progress. This clearly happens in the case of screen-detected premalignant lesions of the uterine cervix and large bowel, and possibly in cancers of the prostate. The issue is controversial in the case of mammography, as there are some in situ lesions with dubious potential for progression. These lesions are, however, likely to be a minority of ductal carcinoma in situ (DCIS) cases.[8] The second circumstance pertains to the early diagnosis and treatment of a cancer that would not have produced symptoms before a patient died from some other cause. This kind of overdiagnosis is of greatest concern when screening is offered to individuals who have very limited longevity due to life-limiting co-morbid conditions, with little possibility of benefiting from any preventive health measure.

Cost Effectiveness

The cost of screening extends far beyond the cost of the screening test. There are costs associated with diagnostic evaluations, which are influenced by the recall rate, and the cost of treatment for screen-detected disease that may never have become clinically apparent. For these reasons, decisions about screening should be made only after careful consideration of whether the implementation of a screening test not only meets well-defined criteria related to disease burden, benefit of early detection, test performance, and acceptability to the population, but also can be delivered at an acceptable cost. Put another way, does the potential exist for a favorable balance between the benefits of screening and the limitations and costs of screening?

There are two basic models for the evaluation of costs and outcomes: cost-benefit analysis (CBA) and cost-effectiveness analysis (CEA). In CBA, benefits are expressed in monetary terms whereas benefits in CEA are expressed as the unit cost for a particular health outcome.[9] Benefits in CBA may be based on a human capital model, in which case a life is assigned a monetary value, or alternatively, individuals are given an opportunity to establish what the benefit is worth to them. If costs exceed benefits, the intervention is judged to be not cost-beneficial and therefore not justified. In contrast, cost-effectiveness studies in medicine are focused on the unit or net cost of achieving a particular health-related outcome.[10] In cancer screening, CEA can be expressed in terms of the cost to detect one cancer, prevent one death, add a year of life, or add a quality-adjusted year of life.

At the most basic level, the most appropriate and intuitive estimate of the cost-effectiveness of cancer screening is an estimate of the marginal cost per year of life saved (MCYLS). The marginal costs of screening are the costs incurred by implementing a screening program minus the costs of case detection and management without screening. The marginal effectiveness is the years of life expected and gained in the screened group minus the years of life expected in the group not undergoing screening. The MCYLS is the fraction of the marginal costs of screening divided by the marginal effectiveness. In general, if a screening test achieves a benchmark of less than $50,000 per MCYLS, costs are judged to be within acceptable limits of cost-effectiveness.[9] This conventional benchmark, which has been applied for several decades, has not been subjected to any consexious adjustment for inflation or other value. In general, the greater advantage of CEA is comparing different disease control strategies rather than measuring all against an arbitrary benchmark.

Acceptability to Individuals at Risk and Health-Care Providers

No matter how effective a screening test may be, its potential to reduce disease burden is highly dependent on adherence with recommended screening intervals and follow-up procedures. Low participation in cancer screening among both providers (low rate of referral) and the public (low and irregular attendance) can be due to low awareness, low perceptions of individual risk, high costs, low access, and aversion to the test, learning test results, or follow-up. Probably the single most important factor related to screening participation, apart from having health insurance, is a recommendation from an individual's health-care provider.[11]

Methodologic Issues in the Evaluation of Early Detection Programs

Judging whether a screening intervention is effective may seem to be a simple matter. Theoretically, one only need observe whether persons have a lesser risk of dying from the disease in question as a result of application of a screening test. However, case reports or anecdotal evidence of good outcomes following cancer detection in asymptomatic persons cannot be trusted as evidence of screening effectiveness. Evaluations of screening tests done outside the context of a rigorous research design are subject to many biases that may (and usually do) invalidate the conclusions being drawn. Included among these complicating factors are lead-time and length biases, subject self-selection, and overdiagnosis.

Known Biases in the Evaluation of Screening Programs

Lead-Time Bias ■ As described earlier, the interval between the moment an occult condition is detected by screening and the moment that condition would have become known by patient awareness of signs or symptoms is known as the *lead time*. Unless lead time is accounted for, comparisons of survival rates in screened and unscreened populations will be misleading. There always is a bias toward better survival rates in the screened group because the length of the lead time moves the point at which survival begins to be measured forward by that amount of time. Thus, it is possible that earlier detection only moves forward the time of a patient's diagnosis, without moving backward the time of death (Fig. 34-2). If lead-time bias is present, screen-detected cancers appear to have better survival, but in fact death occurs at the same point it would have without screening. It is traditional to think of lead time and lead-time bias as synonymous, and thus as phenomenon that deceptively leads to falsely inflating the value of screening. In fact, while it can complicate data analysis, in clinical terms lead time is the essential benefit of screening. A screening test which does not advance the time of diagnosis will not improve the prognosis.

Length Bias ■ Because of variations in tumor growth rates and other biologic characteristics, more cancers with long preclinical phases will be detected when a population is screened. A tumor with a longer preclinical phase may also be a more indolent and less-threatening lesion. This bias toward detection of less-threatening cancers is *length bias* (Fig. 34-3). This form of potential bias complicates the interpretation of outcome differences between cancers detected by screening and those found outside the screening program because the cancers most likely to escape detection may be the very cancers that have the greatest likelihood of causing death.

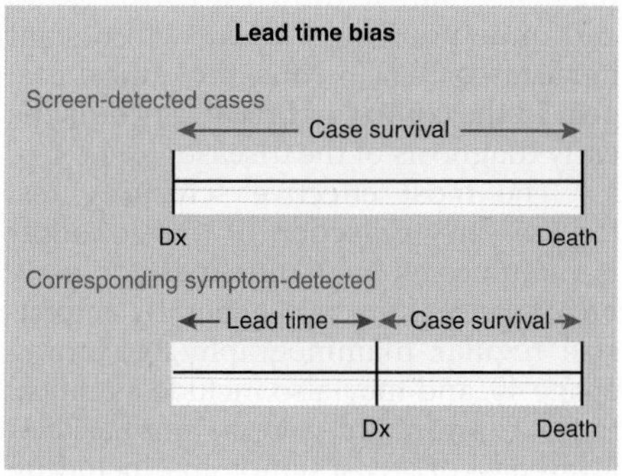

Figure 34-2 ■ Lead-time bias. In this figure, Dx is the time of diagnosis. Note that the screen-detected cases and the cases diagnosed with symptoms each die at the same time, but the survival time looks greater in the screen-detected case because of lead-time bias. *Source*: Adapted from www.3.cancer.gov/prevention/lss/vaslides.html

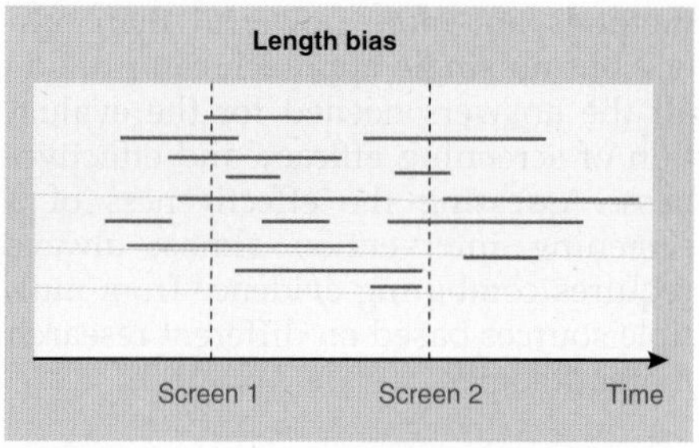

Figure 34-3 ■ Length bias. In this figure, the horizontal lines represent the sojourn times of individual tumors detected in a screening program. The two screening examinations detect six out of eight long sojourn time tumors, but only two out of six short sojourn time tumors.

Overdiagnosis ■ Overdiagnosis is an extreme example of length bias. Because early detection intervention is more likely than symptom recognition to yield lesions that might never become clinically significant cancers, survival statistics for screening detected cancers may be inflated. The occurrence of overdiagnosis may be suspected if an imbalance between the incidence rate in a screening program and the expected incidence rate in the absence of screening persists in a cohort after an extended period of follow-up. However, it is important not to confuse the enduring higher incidence rates after the introduction of screening with overdiagnosis, since higher incidence rates will always persist due to lead time and the year-to-year introduction of previously unscreened cohorts into the screening program.[12]

Patient Self-Selection ■ Individuals who elect to receive early detection tests may be different from those who do not in ways that could affect their survival or recovery from disease. For example, users of early detection services may be more health conscious, more likely to control risk factors such as smoking or diet, more alert to the signs and symptoms of disease, more adherent to treatment, or generally healthier.

Research Designs for Screening Evaluation

Researchers use several different approaches to study the efficacy and effectiveness of cancer screening, including descriptive studies, case-control studies, and randomized controlled trials (RCTs). Each of these strategies has certain strengths and weaknesses. Some methods are more powerful than others, but no single approach can provide all the answers needed for the evaluation of screening efficacy and effectiveness. Assessing the effectiveness of a screening intervention almost always requires combining evidence from multiple sources based on different research methodologies.

Descriptive Studies ■ Uncontrolled studies based on the experience of individual physicians, hospitals, and non-population-based registries can yield important information about screening. Indeed, the first evidence that screening may contribute to disease control often is reported from descriptive studies, as is evidence about the performance parameters of detection tests, such as sensitivity, specificity, and positive predictive values. Descriptive studies, however, do not establish efficacy, because of the absence of an appropriate control group and the influence of the potential biases described previously.

Case-Control Studies ■ Retrospective case-control studies can provide additional evidence on screening effectiveness. The advantage of this approach is that it is a low-cost strategy that may provide evidence more quickly than prospective studies when the screening procedure is already in clinical use.[13] Although mortality reduction can be an endpoint measured in these studies, case-control studies are subject to bias and confounding from uncontrolled factors.

Randomized Clinical Trials ■ The most rigorous assessment of screening is by RCTs that measure cancer-specific mortality reduction as the primary endpoint, with time measured from randomization as a healthy individual rather than from diagnosis, and using as the population denominator the entire population randomized. As a qualification to this, in a trial of cervical screening, where the object is to prevent invasive cervical cancer from occurring, a valid endpoint would be incidence of the disease. In an RCT, the distorting effects of self-selection are bypassed through random assignment to either an experimental group invited to receive screening or an uninvited group. The mortality endpoint is not subject to the effects of lead-time or length bias, or overdiagnosis. An RCT of screening evaluates the effect of an invitation to screening rather than screening per se, ie, end results are based on comparisons between invited and uninvited groups rather than screened and unscreened groups. The distinction is important since noncompliance to the invitation to screening in the experimental group, and contamination in the control group (ie, participation in screening outside of the trial), has an effect on the magnitude of the observed outcome. Although RCTs are the most desirable study design from a methodological perspective, the large sample sizes required, their expense, and their long duration have tended to limit the number of RCTs of screening that have been conducted.

All-cause mortality rather than disease-specific mortality has been proposed as a preferable endpoint in RCTs on the basis of possible biases in assignment of cause of death in experimental and control groups in a trial.[14] Cause of death committees generally build safeguards into the death ascertainment process so that these biases are avoided, or, at the least, minimized. These safeguards include blind review and a consensus process that referees disputes between multiple reviewers. Thus, although some level of misallocation may occur, there is little evidence that the rate of error approaches a level that would measurably bias end results.[15] It has been shown that in breast cancer screening, breast cancer mortality is an appropriate and reliable endpoint, and that all-cause mortality is inefficient and of little if any value.[16] This is also likely to be the case in evaluation of screening for other cancers, although investigators must always be sensitive to the possibility of associated deaths from other causes, in the near or long term, from diagnostic evaluations and therapy.

Breast Cancer

Breast cancer is the most common cancer diagnosed in women in the United States and in the world. Five-year survival is excellent when the disease is diagnosed while still localized (98%), but is poorer when the disease is diagnosed when the regional lymph nodes are involved (83%), and quite poor for women with distant metastases (34%).[17] Thus, the critical first goal in the control of breast cancer is the early diagnosis of the disease.

The most effective screening test for the early detection of breast cancer is mammography. Guidelines for early breast cancer detection generally emphasize regular mammography beginning at age 40, and may also include a clinical breast examination and an emphasis on awareness of breast symptoms, including the option (vs recommendation) of performing breast self-examination (BSE) if a woman chooses to do so.[18,19] After age 40, the principal roles of awareness of breast symptoms including the option of BSE and CBE are to identify masses that were not detected on mammography due to test limitations, rapid tumor growth, or human error. Increasingly, magnetic resonance imaging (MRI) and ultrasound are being added to mammography for women in certain risk groups due to the unique advantages of these technologies for imaging the dense breast.[20]

Mammography

Mammography is an x-ray examination of the breasts to detect abnormalities that may be breast cancer (Figs. 34-4 to 34-6). Modern mammography is done on dedicated imaging equipment, with either screen-film or digital image receptors, designed to produce a high-quality image of the breast at a minimum x-ray dose. Average breast dose per view has been reduced from several centigrays (rads) to 1-2 milliGray (0.1-0.2 rads) per view.[21] Image quality and interpretive skills have also been improved through

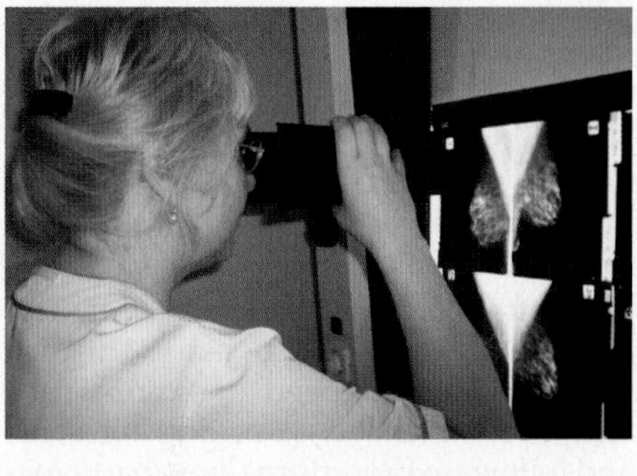

Figure 34-4 ■ Dr. Nadja Lindhe seen screening asymptomatic women using a multiviewer, Department of Mammography, Central Hospital, Falun Sweden. *Source*: Courtesy of Dr. Laszlo Tabar.

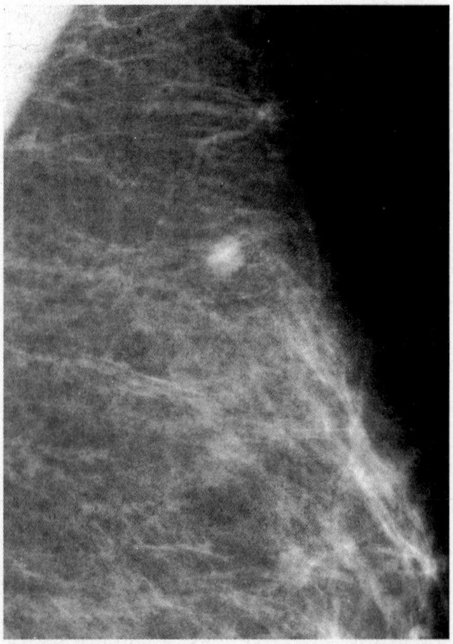

Figure 34-5 ■ Mediolateral oblique projection of the left breast of a 66-year-old asymptomatic woman. In the axillary portion of the breast a <10-mm solitary circular lesion is seen. *Source*: Courtesy of Dr. Laszlo Tabar.

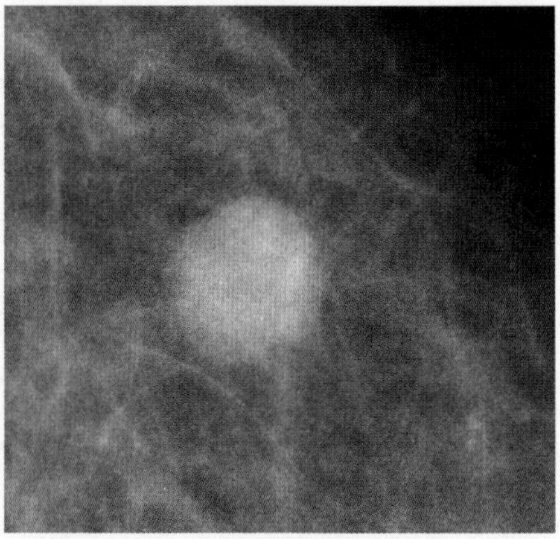

Figure 34-6 ■ Microfocus magnification image of the circular abnormality in Figure 34-5 shows an ill-defined, solitary, mammographically malignant lesion, later confirmed to be an invasive ductal carcinoma. *Source*: Courtesy of Dr. Laszlo Tabar.

early efforts by the American College of Radiology's Mammography Accreditation Program (ACRMAP), and subsequently, the passage of the Mammography Quality Standards Act (MQSA) of 1992, which requires a facility to meet a broad range of technical and personnel standards in order to be certified by the FDA.[22] Until recently, breast cancer screening was limited to dedicated x-ray equipment that produced images on x-ray film. The introduction of full-field digital units that capture the image electronically with solid-state detectors instead of film has been shown to offer similar diagnostic accuracy when compared with film-screen mammography,[23] but also appears to offer improved accuracy in pre- or perimenopausal women younger than 50 years who have dense breasts.[24]

A screening examination involves two views of each breast: a craniocaudal (CC) view and a mediolateral oblique (MLO) view. Prior to taking the x-ray, a radiology technologist positions a woman's breast on the image receptor and then applies pressure with a compression paddle to reduce breast thickness, which enhances image quality by reducing motion and x-ray scatter. After the examination, a radiologist examines the films for abnormalities. The rate of abnormal interpretations is generally higher for first screening examinations, but overall, the average range of initial abnormal interpretations is 5-10%.[25,26] In most instances, abnormalities are resolved through additional diagnostic mammography imaging with special views, or by ultrasonography. Abnormalities that cannot be resolved with additional imaging (including ultrasonography) generally will proceed to biopsy with fine needle aspiration, ultrasonographic or radiographically directed core needle biopsy, or surgical excision.

The sensitivity and specificity of mammography fall within acceptable parameters and vary somewhat by age, with sensitivity, specificity, and PPV improving with increasing age.[26] Historically, age-specific differences in mammographic sensitivity and specificity have been an issue in the debate over the value of screening women under age 50 (discussed below), leading to the mistaken impression that sensitivity, specificity, and PPV were uniform in postmenopausal women, but measurably poorer in premenopausal women.[27,28] More recent data examining sensitivity, specificity, and PPV by age have shown that there is a continuum of improvement with increasing age, and that performance in adjacent decades of life is more similar than different.[26,29,30]

No other cancer screening test has been studied as extensively as mammography.[31,32] There have been nine RCTs of breast cancer screening published to date. The most recently published results, excluding the U.K. Age Trial, are shown in Figure 34-7 indicating a 20% reduction in breast cancer mortality associated with an invitation to screening. An International Agency for Research on Cancer (IARC) in-depth review concluded that the benefits of actually receiving screening were higher, of the order of a 35% breast cancer mortality reduction.[33]

During the past two decades, the issue of breast cancer screening with mammography among women under age 50 dominated deliberations about breast cancer screening and has been a source of persistent debate in the United States and in Europe.[28,34-36] For the most part, the dispute over screening policy for women under age 50 was based on the lack of clear evidence from the world's RCTs that mammography screening for women aged 40-49 years was effective.

Prior to 1997, two trials (the Health Insurance Plan of Greater New York trial and the Swedish Two-County trial) had shown a statistically significant reduction in breast cancer mortality among women aged 50 years and older, but no statistically significant reduction in deaths from an individual trial had been observed for women aged 40-49 years.[37,38] More recent analyses of trial data have provided important insights about screening in different age groups of women and have helped explain why early trial results provided less favorable results in premenopausal women.[39,40] In the individual trials, a mortality benefit begins to appear relatively early (at about 5 years) for women aged 50 and over at randomization whereas it occurs much later for women ages 40-49 at randomization. With accumulating years of follow-up in the 40- to 49-year group, the RR of mortality steadily improves. Recent analysis of the Two-County data provides a clinically intuitive explanation for the delay in benefit observed in women under age 50, based on the interrelationship between tumor histology, sojourn time, and age.[41] As described earlier, the mean breast cancer sojourn time (ie, potential lead time) is shorter (1.7 years) in women under age 50 compared with women over age 50 (≥3.3 years).[42] Because the majority of the world's trials screened women aged 40-49 at randomization at an interval of 24 months, faster tumor growth rates in women in their 40s meant that these women were less likely to benefit from mammography when it is offered every 2 years compared with women aged 50 and older. Whereas a 2-year interval was equally effective in

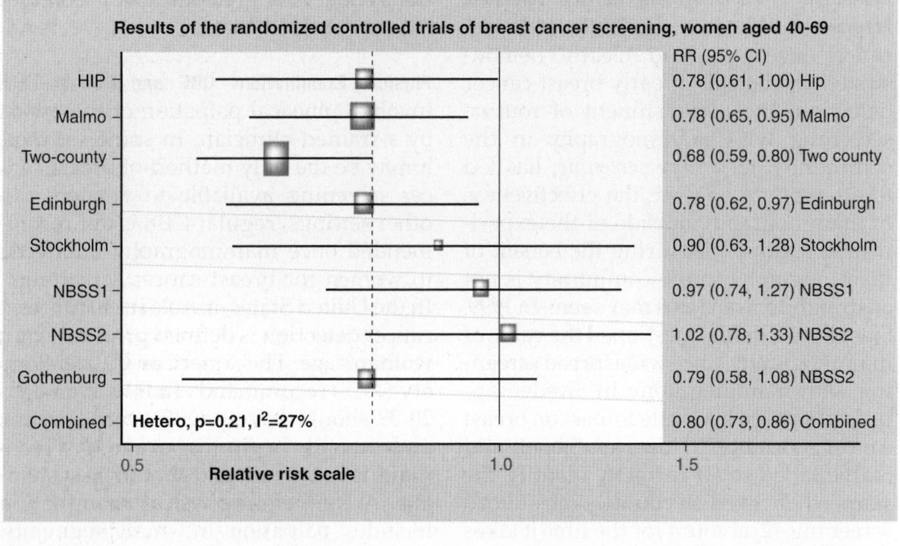

Figure 34-7 ■ Results of randomized controlled trials of breast cancer screening, women aged 40-69. Test for heterogeneity is non-significant, with only 27% of the variation between studies not due to chance.

both age groups for grade 2, medullary, and invasive lobular tumors, and was effective in reducing deaths among grade 3 tumors diagnosed in women aged 50 and older, it was not effective for grade 3 tumors diagnosed in women aged 40-49. The results from the Gothenburg trial, which screened women aged 39-49 at 18-month intervals, shows that the timing of the benefit, which appears at 6-8 years, is similar to that observed for women aged 50 and over.[43] In the Gothenburg trial, which screened women aged 40-49 every 18 months and showed a 44% reduction in breast cancer mortality, the proportional interval cancer incidence was 18% in the first 12 months after a negative screen and increased to >50% in the period of 12-18 months.[43] Data from service screening programs also support these observations. Tabar and colleagues compared breast cancer deaths occurring in 210,000 women aged 20-69 years in two Swedish counties during the 20 years before screening was introduced (1958-1977) and in the 20 years after the introduction of screening (1978-1997). Data were stratified into age groups, by invitation to screening, and by whether or not women had actually received screening. After adjustment for age, self-selection bias, and changes in breast cancer incidence in the 40-69 years age group, breast cancer mortality was reduced by 44% (0.56 [0.49-0.64]; $p < 0.0001$) in women exposed to screening compared with women not exposed to screening. Among women aged 40-49, breast cancer mortality was 48% (0.52 [0.4-0.67]; $p < 0.0001$) lower in women exposed to screening compared with women not exposed to screening.[44] In Sweden, women ages 40-54 are invited to screening every 18 months, and women ages 55-70 are invited every 24 months.

Evaluation of Mammography Service Screening Programs ■ Whereas the RCTs of breast cancer screening had clearly demonstrated the benefit of early breast cancer detection, the establishment of routine screening with mammography in the community, ie, *service screening*, has led to attempts to analyze the effectiveness of mammography outside of the experimental setting. Measuring the benefit of mammography in the community is not as straightforward as it may seem. In 1999, Sjönell and Stahle questioned the value of mammography since widespread screening with mammography in Sweden appeared to have had little impact on breast cancer mortality.[45] However, Sjönell and Stahle failed to (1) correctly identify the years when Swedish counties introduced screening, (2) account for the time it takes to introduce screening into a population, (3) consider that different counties would have different screening take-up rates, and (4) distinguish between screened and unscreened cohorts. For example, in any 10-year period after the introduction of screening, usually >50% of the breast cancer deaths will occur in women diagnosed before the introduction of screening, a group that clearly could not have benefited from the intervention.[46] For this reason, the analysis of service screening must be able to isolate screened and unscreened cohorts, and to classify women on the basis of whether or not they were invited to screening, attended screening (screen-detected and interval cancers), and whether or not they were non-attenders (not invited, or refusers). With these data, as well as information on access to screening, breast cancer mortality can be estimated for women who actually attend screening and for the population as a whole, the latter simulating a classic intention-to-treat analysis. Differences in mortality over time will be attributable to screening, improvements in therapy, and increased awareness, although distinguishing between screening and nonscreening factors is complex and can be only indirectly estimated.

Investigators from Sweden have been able to classify breast cancer cases before and after the introduction to screening on the basis of exposure to screening.[44,46,47] These studies typically show around a 30% reduction in breast cancer mortality associated with the policy of offering screening, and a 40% or higher reduction with individual exposure to screening.[48-51] The studies incorporate control for the various biases and estimation of the changes in mortality from other changes in addition to screening. The data demonstrate that organized screening with high rates of attendance in a setting that achieves a high degree of programmatic quality assurance can achieve breast cancer mortality reductions equal to or greater than observed in the randomized trials.

Physical Examinations CBE and BSE ■ CBE involves physical palpation of the breast by a trained clinician. In some settings, it may be the only method of breast cancer screening available to women.[52] In other settings, regular CBE is not recommended once mammography is offered to women for breast cancer screening.[53] In the United States, its role in early breast cancer detection is defined primarily by a woman's age. The American Cancer Society (ACS) recommends that women ages 20-39 should have a CBE every 3 years, and annually beginning at age 40.[19] Technique is important and should be systematic. A competent physical examination includes palpation in small segments, from the nipple to the periphery of the breast, including the axilla. Various techniques exist to organize the examination, and personal preference probably should be the deciding factor.[54]

There have been no randomized trials of the efficacy of CBE as a single screening modality. CBE has been included in some randomized trials of mammography, but any estimation of the sensitivity of CBE in these early studies must be interpreted in the historical context of the sensitivity of mammography at that time. The fact that some trials have examined the combined modality of mammography and CBE and the observation that a small percentage of palpable masses are not seen on mammography have led to guidelines that include routine CBE, ideally near to and prior to the timing of mammography, as part of the screening regimen, to increase sensitivity.[55] However, in a setting of high-quality mammography, and high adherence with regular mammography, routine CBE contributes very little to the detection of breast cancer.[56] Of course, if a patient has a palpable mass, then she is no longer asymptomatic and screening mammography is inappropriate.

BSE has obvious appeal as a screening test because it is simple and convenient, has no apparent financial cost to participants, is noninvasive, and is intended to lead to earlier awareness of the presence of breast cancer symptoms. However, recommendations for BSE have been controversial due to a lack of definitive evidence for its efficacy and to concerns about harms, including (1) the possibility that BSE promotion distracts from the importance of mammography, (2) false reassurance, (3) heightened anxiety about breast cancer, (4) anxiety during the examination, and (5) false-positives.[57] Results from two RCTs of BSE are now available, and neither has demonstrated a reduction in mortality in a group trained to do BSE compared with a group receiving usual care. The first RCT of BSE was conducted in St. Petersburg and Moscow in 1985, and showed no difference in mortality between the BSE instruction group and the control group, and also no difference in tumor size or stage between the two groups.[58] The second RCT was conducted in Shanghai, China. Thomas and colleagues randomized women employed by the Shanghai Textile Industry Bureau into two groups of ~133,000 women, in which one group received BSE instruction.[59] At 10-11 years of follow-up from the beginning of the study, there was no statistically significant difference in the mortality rate in the instruction group vs the control group, and no significant difference was observed in the proportion of Tis (in situ) and T1 lesions in the two groups.[60] However, close examination of the data from the Shanghai trial indicated that a significant proportion of the control group presented with tumors that were under 2 cm (45%) and not advanced at the time of diagnosis, suggesting that the combination of high awareness and access to health care in this region meant there was uncertain potential to improve on tumor characteristics at diagnosis through the initiation of BSE. In addition, the study group had nonsignificant reductions of around 10% in node-positive tumors and tumors at T2 stage or worse. Both studies have been criticized for methodological limitations,[61] and even the authors of the Shanghai study concluded that the findings from their study did not rule out the potential for BSE to be effective in a different setting.[60]

BSE and CBE potentially offer some advantage for the detection of palpable masses in women who have not reached an age when mammography is recommended, or to detect cancers missed by mammography or faster growing tumors among women in an age group in which mammography is recommended. However, the unique advantage of systematic physical examinations compared with self-detection during normal activities is unclear in a population that has gained heightened awareness of breast cancer symptoms and the importance of prompt reporting of new breast changes. while heightened awareness is key, it is also unclear whether that can be achieved through educational messages alone, or whether BSE instruction and periodic CBE reinforce heightened awareness, which likewise may be true for women undergoing regular mammography as well.[62] Because prognosis is very strongly influenced by tumor size, women should be continually educated about the importance of reporting any new breast symptom to a health-care professional.

Magnetic Resonance Imaging ■ Among the greatest challenges to breast cancer screening is meeting the needs of high-risk groups, specifically women with significant breast density and women who are known or suspected to be at elevated risk due to mutations on breast cancer susceptibility genes.[63,64] Studies comparing the effectiveness of mammography and magnetic resonance imaging (MRI) in high-risk women have shown that MRI is more sensitive than mammography in detecting breast cancer.[65] Based on the accumulation of data, the ACS now recommends that women at very high-risk of breast cancer due to carrying mutations on *BRCA1* or *BRCA2*, having a first-degree relative who has tested positive for a mutation on a *BRCA* gene, or having approximately 20-25% or greater lifetime risk based on family history, should begin annual mammography and MRI at age 30, or perhaps earlier if she and her physician believe it is prudent. Other high-risk conditions what warrant screening with MRI include other high-risk genetic syndromes, and women who have received high-dose mantle radiation to the chest.[20]

Ultrasound Screening ■ The sensitivity of mammography is strongly influenced by the radiographic density of the breast, with sensitivity as high as 98% in women with predominantly fatty breasts, and as 48% in women with extremely dense breasts.[63,66] Ultrasonic imaging has been used for many years in women with a suspicious abnormality that is not easily or fully seen on the mammogram, or to image an area of the breast that has such dense fibroglandular tissue that the ability of mammography to provide a clear image is limited. The limitations of mammography in imaging the dense breast have led to ongoing interest in using ultrasound for primary screening or as an adjunct to mammography.

In the fall of 2003, the ACR Imaging Network (ACRIN) initiated a multicenter trial to systematically evaluate screening ultrasound.[67] The trial enrolled women at higher than average risk for breast cancer due to family history and who also had significant breast density. Endpoints included measures predictive of screening performance and breast cancer mortality, ie, the cancer detection rate, tumor size, and nodal status. In the study 40 women were diagnosed with cancer: eight cases (20%) were suspicious on both ultrasound and mammography; equal numbers (30%, $n = 12$) were suspicious on either ultrasound alone or mammography alone; and in eight women, both ultrasound and mammography were normal. The breast cancer detection rate was 7.6 per 1000 for mammography alone, and 11.8 for the combination of mammography and ultrasound, increasing the yield by 4.2 breast cancers per 1000 women screened. However, while the addition of ultrasound to mammography improved the diagnostic yield in this high-risk cohort, the false-positive rate and negative biopsy rate were very high. The PPV of a biopsy recommendation after a full diagnostic workup was ~23% for mammography alone, 9% for ultrasound alone, and 11% for the combination of mammography and ultrasound.[67] While Berg and colleagues observed a significant improvement in the diagnostic yield of small, node-negative cancers in this higher-risk population, a number of questions remain about the potential for implementing routine screening ultrasound for some subpopulations of women.

■ Screening Recommendations

Screening guidelines for breast cancer generally are based on age-specific recommendations for periodic testing, and may include periodic regimens of BSE, CBE by a trained health professional, and mammography (Table 34-2). The ACS no longer recommends that women conduct monthly BSE, although the guidelines do stress that women may elect to do BSE irregularly or regularly, but what is most important for all women is to be educated about the importance of heightened vigilance about new breast symptoms.[19] The ACS recommends CBE every 3 years between ages 20 and 39, and annually thereafter. CBE should take place prior to mammography because if a mass is present, it can be brought to the attention of the radiologist, and a diagnostic evaluation can be considered. If CBE follows mammography and a mass that was not seen on the mammogram is detected, then the patient would need to return for additional directed imaging. CBE before mammography avoids potential waste of resources. Beginning at age 40, women should have annual mammography and CBE.[19] Guidelines from the American Medical Association and the American College of Radiology are equivalent to ACS recommendations.[68,69] In 2002, the United States Preventive Services Task Force (USPSTF) upgraded their breast cancer screening guidelines to recommend that women aged 40 years and older should receive mammography every 1-2 years with or without clinical breast examination.[70]

There is no upper age limit to ACS breast cancer screening guidelines as long as a woman is in good health. Women at significantly higher risk for breast cancer due to known mutation carrier status, or who have a first-degree relative who has tested positive for a *BRCA* mutation, or who have an approximately 20-25% lifetime risk based on pedigree analysis of both the maternal and paternal lineage should begin annual mammography and MRI at age 30, or earlier as determined by shared decision making. MRI and mammography screening also should begin earlier for women who have been treated with radiation to the chest or who are affected by rarer high-risk genetic syndromes.

Colorectal Cancer

Colorectal cancer is a leading cancer affecting both men and women. Cancers diagnosed at a localized stage have ~90% 5-year survival, while survival for regional disease (68%) and distant disease (11%) is significantly poorer.[17] Unfortunately in the United States. only about 40% of newly diagnosed colorectal cancers are diagnosed while still localized.[17]

The goal of screening for colorectal cancer is both the detection of early stage

Table 34-2 ■ **Recommendations for Early Detection of Cancer in Average-Risk Asymptomatic Individuals**

Cancer Site	Population	Test or Procedure	Frequency
Cervix[a]	Women, 3 years after first vaginal intercourse; no later than age 21	Pap test and pelvic examination	Age <30: Annual testing with conventional Pap tests or every 2 years using liquid-based Pap tests Age ≥30: After three normal test results in a row, screening every 2-3 years with cervical cytology (conventional or liquid-based Pap test) alone, or every 3 years with an HPV DNA test plus cervical cytology Age ≥70: Women who have had 3+ normal Pap tests and no abnormal Pap tests within 10 years Women who have had a total hysterectomy for benign reasons may choose to stop screening
Breast[b]	Women age 20+	Clinical breast examination (CBE)	Every 3 years on the occasion of a periodic checkup, age 20–39; annual, age 40+[c]
		Mammography	Annual, age 40+
Colorectal[d]	Men and women age 50+	Fecal occult blood test (FOBT)	Annual, age 50+
		Fecal immunochemical test (FIT)	Annual, age 50+
		Flexible sigmoidoscopy (FSIG)	Every 5 years, starting at age 50
		FOBT or FIT, and FSIG	Annual FOBT or FIT, and FSIG every 5 years starting at age 50
		Stool DNA	Interval uncertain
		Colonoscopy	Every 10 years starting at age 50
		CT colonoscopy	Every 5 years starting at age 50
		Double-contrast barium enema	Every 5 years, starting at age 50
Prostate[e]	Men age 50+	Digital rectal examination (DRE) and prostate-specific antigen test (PSA)	For those who seek regular testing, annual DRE and PSA starting at age 50

[a]Both the American College of Obstetricians and Gynecologists (ACOG) and USPSTF recommend the same algorithm for initiation of screening, and the screening interval. ACOG recommends annual pelvic examination after age 30; USPSTF recommends discontinuing screening at age 65.
[b]The American Cancer Society (ACS), American College of Radiology (ACR), and American Medical Association (AMA) endorse the guidelines shown. The United States Preventive Services Task Force (USPSTF) recommends mammography every 1–2 years for women aged 40 and older.
[c]Beginning at age 40, annual CBE should be done prior to mammography.
[d]The ACS, ACR, American College of Gastroenterology, American Gastroenterological Association, American Society for Gastrointestinal Endoscopy, have endorsed these guidelines for average-risk adults. The USPSTF also recommends screening for colorectal cancer beginning at age 50 with each of the tests listed above, excluding CT colonography and stool DNA testing.
[e]No organization recommends that average-risk men undergo routine testing for prostate cancer. Rather, the ACS, AMA, USPSTF, the American Academy of Family Physicians, the American College of Physicians-American Society of Internal Medicine, and the American Urologic Association recommend that clinicians (1) discuss the potential benefits and possible harms of PSA screening; (2) consider patient preferences; and (3) individualize the decision to test through a process of shared decision making.

adenocarcinomas and the detection and removal of adenomatous polyps, which are potential precursors for colorectal cancer. Reduction in colorectal cancer morbidity and mortality through screening is achieved through a combination of (1) a more favorable stage at diagnosis of occult disease and (2) disease prevention resulting from the removal of precursor lesions.

Polyps are common in adults over age 50. Since the majority of polyps will not develop into adenocarcinoma, histology and size determine their clinical importance as precursor lesions.[71-73] The most common and clinically important polyps are adenomatous polyps, which represent about one-half to two-thirds of all colorectal polyps and are associated with the greatest risk of colorectal cancer (Figs. 34-8 and 34-9). Other polyps, which include incidental hyperplastic polyps and mucosal tags, are not believed to have clinical significance in the development of colorectal cancer. The evidence for the importance of colorectal polyps in the development of colorectal cancer is largely indirect but is nonetheless convincing. First, adenomatous polyps and adenocarcinomas in the colon and rectum have a similar anatomic distribution, and the average age at which polyps begin to appear in adults precedes the age-incidence distribution of colorectal cancer,[74] with conventional estimates of

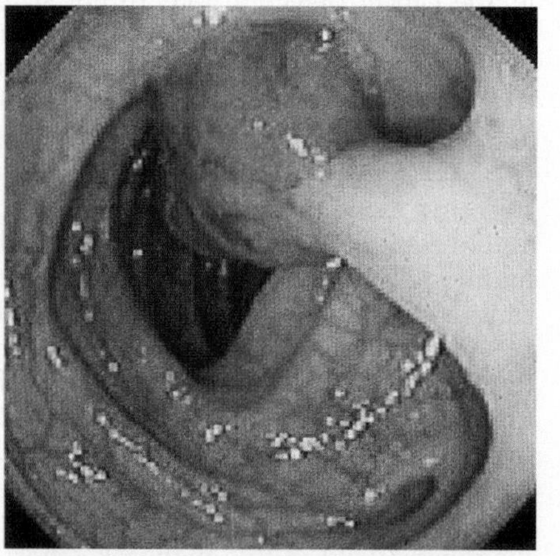

Figure 34-8 ■ Malignant pedunculated polyp without invasion of the stalk.

about 10 years for the time required for an adenomatous polyp <1 cm to become an invasive lesion.[75] Second, there is a strong association between polyp size and the grade of dysplasia, with higher-grade dysplasias more commonly observed in large polyps.[71] Third, epidemiologic evidence has shown higher risks of colorectal cancer after 14 years among individuals who had large polyps removed from the rectum or sigmoid colon and subsequently received no follow-up testing.[76] Fourth, individuals with familial adenomatous polyposis (FAP) have a nearly 100% probability of developing colorectal cancer and will experience earlier onset and extensive distribution of polyps throughout the colon and rectum.[77] Fifth, epidemiologic evidence has shown a lower incidence of colorectal cancer among individuals who have had large adenomatous polyps removed compared with the general population.[78,79] As will be seen below, the protection offered by screening and removal of adenomatous polyps extends only to the area of the bowel that has been examined.

There are a number of screening methods for colorectal cancer, and they fall into two general categories: stool tests, which include testing for occult blood or exfoliated DNA, and structural examinations, which include flexible sigmoidoscopy, colonoscopy, CT colonography (both 2D and 3D), and double-contrast barium enema. Stool tests principally are effective in detecting colorectal cancer, while the structural examinations are effective in the detection of both colorectal cancer and precursor lesions.[80] These tests may be used alone or in combination (to improve sensitivity, or in some instances, to insure a complete examination). Screening tests for colorectal cancer vary in terms of the degree of underlying evidence supporting their use, potential efficacy, cost-effectiveness, and acceptability among patients. Nevertheless, any one of these alternatives, applied in a program of regular surveillance, has the

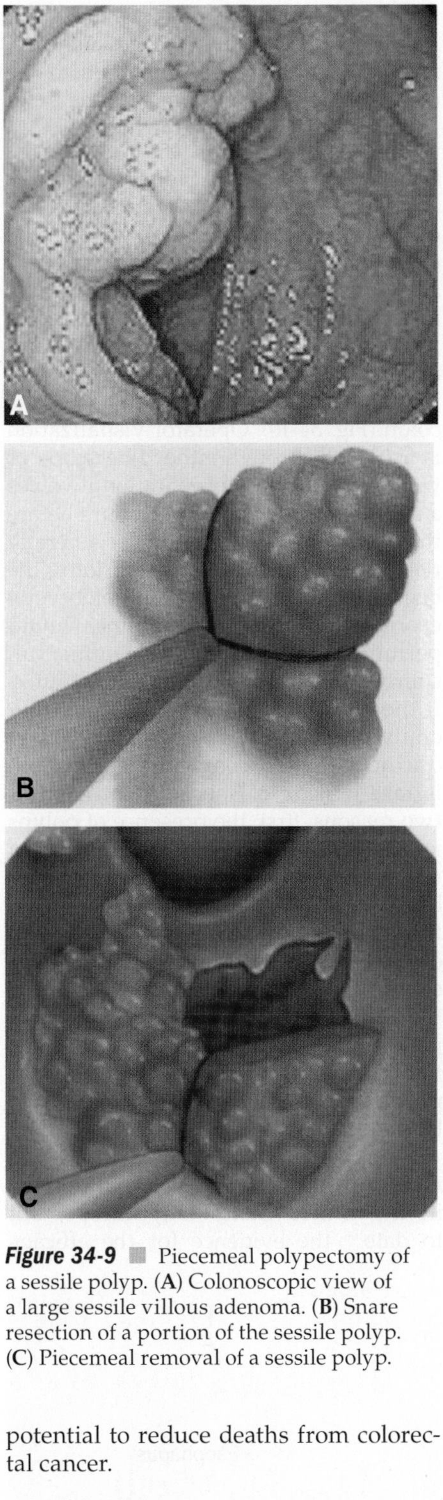

Figure 34-9 ■ Piecemeal polypectomy of a sessile polyp. (**A**) Colonoscopic view of a large sessile villous adenoma. (**B**) Snare resection of a portion of the sessile polyp. (**C**) Piecemeal removal of a sessile polyp.

potential to reduce deaths from colorectal cancer.

Stool Tests (gFOBT, FIT, and Stool DNA Tests) ■ Stool blood tests are conventionally known as fecal occult blood tests (FOBT) because they aim to discover the presence of occult blood in stool, which may derive from colorectal cancer or larger (>2 cm) polyps. The most common stool blood tests in use today are guaiac-based tests (gFOBT), followed by immunochemical tests (FIT). Guaiac-based tests detect blood in the stool through the pseudoperoxidase activity of heme or hemoglobin, but they also react with peroxidase in the diet, from sources such as red meat, cruciferous vegetables, and some fruits. Immunochemical tests (FIT) react to human globin, a protein which along with heme constitutes human hemoglobin. The FITs require no dietary restrictions, are not sensitive to upper gastrointestinal bleeding, generally rely on fewer samples with simpler collection methods, and can be processed with a particular threshold of fecal hemoglobin to balance sensitivity and specificity based on decisions about individual risk, or programmatic requirements.[81]

Because small polyps do not tend to bleed, and bleeding from cancers or large polyps may be intermittent, the proper use of stool blood tests requires serial specimens (2 or 3) per manufacturer's instructions during the occasion of testing, as well as annual testing.[82-84] While some gFOBTs can be processed in the physician's office, FITs are usually processed in a laboratory. For both types of FOBTs, laboratory processing insures great quality control and accuracy. Rehydration of some variants of gFOBTs improves sensitivity but remains controversial because it also increases the rate of false-positives. A positive gFOBT or FIT should be followed up with colonoscopy in order to rule out the presence of advanced neoplasia.

The observation that cancers detected through stool blood testing (gFOBT) had more favorable stages and better survival than cases diagnosed with symptoms led to prospective trials in Europe and the United States evaluating the efficacy of FOBT in reducing deaths from colorectal cancer. In the Minnesota trial, 46,551 asymptomatic participants aged 50-80 were randomly assigned to one of three groups: a group that would receive an annual invitation to screening, a group that would receive an invitation to biannual screening, and a control group that would receive usual care.[85] Participants with a positive gFOBT received a total colon examination with colonoscopy. After 14 years of follow-up, the 13-year cumulative mortality in the group offered annual screening was 5.33 per 1000, compared with 8.33 per 1000 in the biennially screened group and 8.83 in the usual care (control) group. Annual screening was associated with a statistically significant 33% reduction in deaths from colorectal cancer compared with usual care. The reduction in deaths associated with biannual screening compared with usual care was not statistically significant at the time of initial follow-up. Similar results with two yearly gFOBT have been observed in two other trials.[86,87] In a subsequent analysis of Minnesota trial data with 18 years of follow-up, Mandel and colleagues also observed a 20% reduction in incidence in the group invited to annual screening, and an 18% reduction in incidence in the group invited to biennial screening, likely attributable to detection and removal of advanced neoplasia.[88]

The sensitivity and specificity of a gFOBT can be influenced by the type of gFOBT (performance characteristics vary), whether or not the specimen is rehydrated (ie, adding a drop of water to the slide window before processing), and by variations in interpretation, specimen collection, number of samples collected per test, screening interval, and other factors.[89] In a review by Allison and colleagues, sensitivity for cancer ranged from 37.1% for unrehydrated Hemoccult II to 79.4% for Hemoccult Sensa, although considerable variation has been reported for these same tests by other investigators.[90] In a recent report by Lieberman and colleagues, sensitivity of a single, three panel gFOBT for cancer or high-grade dysplasia was 35.6%, and 23.9% for all advanced neoplasia.[91] However, the study by Lieberman and colleagues was carried out under controlled conditions in an experimental setting, and gFOBTs were rehydrated. In a more recent community study that compared gFOBT with sDNA, sensitivity of gFOBT for cancer was only 12.9%, and only 10.8% for advanced lesions.[92] These findings reinforce the importance of annual testing to achieve the program sensitivity observed in the randomized controlled trials.

FIT and high-sensitivity gFOBT have much better performance with one-time testing. Recent prospective studies comparing the performance of high-sensitivity gFOBT and FIT generally use posttest endoscopy as the gold standard. In a thousand ambulatory patients (with and without symptoms of colorectal cancer), Levi and colleagues sought to measure both sensitivity and specificity of a quantitative FIT and to measure fecal hemoglobin thresholds most predictive of advanced neoplasia and cancer.[81] The hemoglobin content of three bowel movements was measured. The sensitivity for cancer with three FIT samples with a hemoglobin threshold set at 75 ng/mL was 94.1%, and specificity for cancer was 87.5%. Allison and colleagues compared sensitive gFOBT (Hemoccult Sensa) with a FIT (Hemoccult ICT) for cancer and advanced adenomas in the distal colon in nearly 6000 average-risk subjects who had undergone flexible sigmoidoscopy.[93] Both the gFOBT and FIT showed superior sensitivity for cancer compared with the single-test performance of an unrehydrated gFOBT. While the sensitivity for colorectal cancer was higher for the FIT (81.8%) compared with the sensitive gFOBT (64.3%), the sensitive gFOBT showed superior performance for advanced adenomas (41.3%) compared with FIT (29.5%). The likely explanation for the different performance in sensitivity for cancer and advanced lesions between high-sensitivity gFOBT and FIT is the difference in specificity between the two tests, in which positive results from the stool test lead to diagnostic colonoscopy. In this study, the specificity for distal cancer and distal advanced lesions was higher for the Hemoccult ICT (96.9% and 97.3%, respectively) compared with the Hemoccult Sensa (96.9% and 97.3%). In studies to date, it appears that there is no clear pattern of superior overall test performance between a high-sensitivity guaiac-based test (Hemoccult Sensa) and a variety of FIT tests.

The performance of gFOBT is highly dependent on following a recommended protocol.[83,89,94] Although dietary restrictions have been recommended to reduce the rate of false-positives, recent data suggest that dietary restrictions do not influence the false-positivity rate in non-rehydrated tests, and they may reduce the compliance rate with testing.[95,96] Specimens should be collected over a 3-day period from successive bowel movements, with two samples placed on each test card. Once three samples have been collected, FOBT cards should be returned according to the provider's instructions, and the test should be processed without rehydration to reduce the rate of false-positives. Annual testing following this regimen is required in order to achieve the program sensitivity observed in the randomized controlled trials.

Recent data provide reason to be concerned that the quality of gFOBT testing in the United States is seriously deficient, and provide a good example the importance of strict adherence to recommended procedures for screening. In the recent comparison of stool DNA testing with gFOBT, Imperiale and colleagues observed that one-time gFOBT testing using the take-home method was only 12.9% sensitive for cancer, with poorer performance in part attributable to in-office processing of test results. Further, in the same study of veteran males reported earlier,[91] Collins et al. compared the performance of a single sample, in-office gFOBT following digital rectal examination (DRE) in the office. Keeping in mind that the sensitivity for advanced neoplasia of one-time gFOBT when done properly is very low, the sensitivity for advanced neoplasia with the in-office procedure was only 4.9%.[97] The observation that one-third of primary care physicians reported that this was the only method of stool blood testing that they conducted, and that an additional 41% reported using both the in-office and take-home methods, suggests that millions of gFOBTs done each year have limited value, and provides at least indirect evidence for one reason that colorectal cancer mortality has not dropped more despite the volume of stool blood testing.[98,99] Many physicians have difficulty bypassing the opportunity to do FOBT with stool acquired during DRE, having low confidence that the patient will complete the preferred at-home protocol. However, it is clear from the evidence that this kind of testing for occult blood not only is wasteful of time and resources, but a negative result also provides false reassurance. While convenient,[98] a one-sample gFOBT for colorectal cancer screening with stool collected during a digital rectal examination (DRE) is not recommended.[83,99] Additional data from Nadel et al. reveals further problems with stool blood testing, specifically that follow-up of positive gFOBTs commonly is inappropriate.[98] Nearly one in three physicians surveyed reported repeating the gFOBT if the first test was positive, and a higher percentage reported follow-up with flexible sigmoidoscopy rather than colonoscopy. One-third of adults in the National Health Interview Survey who reported having had a positive FOBT reported that they received no follow-up.[98]

Whereas conventional stool blood tests detect occult blood, a new approach to testing stool aims to detect molecular markers associated with colorectal neoplasia. Because the DNA mutations associated with colorectal cancer are relatively well understood, and because colorectal polyps and malignancies exfoliate cells into the lumen, it is possible to examine the stool for an array of mutations associated with colorectal cancer. Because no single gene mutation is present in cells shed by every adenoma or cancer, early efforts to develop sDNA tests focused on multitarget DNA stool assays in order to achieve high sensitivity. Early clinical studies in small numbers of patients with a multitarget DNA-based stool assay approach suggested high sensitivity and specificity for both colorectal cancer and premalignant adenomatous polyps.[100] More recent investigations in larger populations, utilizing a multiple marker panel that included 21 separate point mutations in the K-*ras* oncogene, a probe for BAT-26 (a marker of microsatellite instability), and a marker of DNA Integrity Analysis (DIA) have shown lower sensitivity (52%) for cancer than early studies (with similar specificity), but considerably better sensitivity for one-time testing compared with a non-rehydrated gFOBT.[92] Newer versions of sDNA tests evaluated in small experimental cohorts have shown improved sensitivity with simpler genetic analysis, further demonstrating the effectiveness of testing stool for molecular markers associated with advanced lesions.[101] Unlike gFOBT or FIT, sDNA requires a large single sample of stool, and presently collection kits are designed to collect the entire stool from a single bowel movement. One investigation showed that patients preferred the single sample method to the conventional method of sampling stool from consecutive bowel movements.[102]

Flexible Sigmoidoscopy ■ Sigmoidoscopy is a relatively simple procedure that requires minimal preparation prior to the examination.[103] Sigmoidoscopes used in screening may be rigid (25 cm) or flexible (35 or 60 cm) although the most common sigmoidoscope in use is flexible and about 60 cm in length, allowing for examination of somewhat less than half of the colon (Fig. 34-10). Operator visualization is achieved through either fiberscope or videoscope. Patient preparation involves a saline laxative enema 1-2 hours before the examination, and the test is generally performed without sedation. Prior to the beginning of a flexible sigmoidoscopy examination (FSIG), the examiner should perform a DRE.[104] A skilled examiner can complete the examination in <10 minutes. If the test is positive, the patient is generally referred for colonoscopy. Biopsy during sigmoidoscopy can be done, but is rare outside of specialty settings for two reasons: first, the presence of polyps in the distal bowel signals an elevated risk for polyps or cancer in the proximal bowel, and the patient may be referred for colonoscopy; second, biopsy with electrocautery poses the risk of explosion of ignited hydrogen or methane in the incompletely prepared bowel.[105] For patient safety and greater test sensitivity, total colon examination is generally postponed until a full bowel preparation can be done prior to colonoscopy.[84]

At present there are four ongoing randomized trials of FSIG underway in the United States and Europe, but to date[106] the evidence for the efficacy

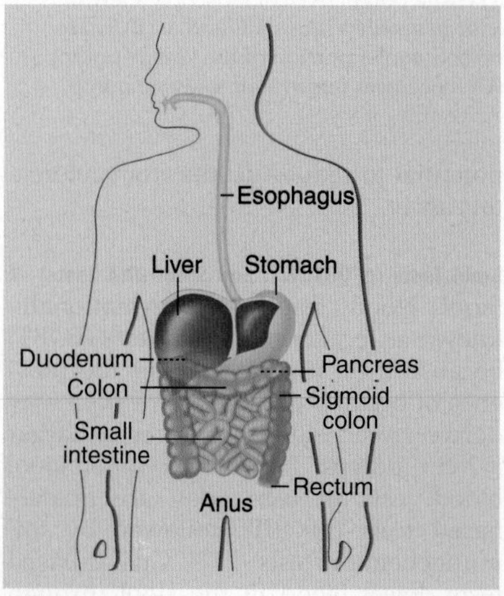

Figure 34-10 ■ Reach of flexible sigmoidoscopy (shaded area) in screening for colorectal cancer and adenomatous polyps. *Source*: Centers for Disease Control and Prevention.

of FSIG derives from case-control and cohort investigations. Selby and colleagues compared the screening histories of patients who died from colorectal cancer with those of controls matched for age and sex.[107] Evaluation of patient records revealed that a history of rigid sigmoidoscopy was associated with 59% fewer deaths from colorectal cancer lesions in the region of the bowel within reach of the sigmoidoscope. Consistent with this interpretation was the finding that there was no protective effect from sigmoidoscopy for death due to cancers that developed in the proximal colon, ie, that part of the colon outside the reach of the instrument. Newcomb and colleagues observed a 79% reduction in colorectal cancer mortality in patients who had a history of one or more sigmoidoscopies compared with patients who had never had sigmoidoscopy, and in subsequent analysis observed a long-term protective effect against incidence in the distal bowel.[108,109]

Additional evidence supporting the effectiveness of flexible sigmoidoscopy derives from colonoscopy studies that identify the detection rate of cancer and advanced lesions based in the depth of insertion of the scope. With insertion to the splenic flexure, and regarding any lesions in the distal colon to be an indication for follow-up colonoscopy, flexible sigmoidoscopy is 60-70% as sensitive for advanced adenomas and cancers in the colon compared with colonoscopy.[110,111]

In the United States, the recommended screening interval for FSIG is every 5 years. The shorter interval was recommended because of concerns about examination quality and completeness in most clinical settings, which tend to be low volume.[112] In clinics where endoscopists are experienced and perform complete examination on well-prepared patients and routinely achieve scope insertion beyond 40 cm, a 10-year interval between screening flexible sigmoidoscopy may be justified. Quality indicators for FSIG have been previously published, and emphasize: (1) appropriate training; (2) satisfactory examination rates to beyond 40 cm; (3) expected adenoma detection rates based on age and gender; and (4) ability to biopsy suspected adenomas.[113]

Combined Stool Blood Testing and FSIG ■ The combination of periodic FOBT (either gFOBT or iFOBT) and FSIG every 5 years is superior to either FOBT or FSIG alone insofar as the two examinations together constitute a quasi-total colon examination. FOBT provides for some surveillance in the proximal colon (outside of the reach of FSIG), and FSIG in the distal colon has higher sensitivity and specificity than FOBT and provides an opportunity to visualize cancer and polyps. Clearly, the advantage of adding FSIG to FOBT is far greater than the addition of FOBT to FSIG. The combination of FOBT and sigmoidoscopy was evaluated in a controlled trial that randomized asymptomatic individuals aged 40 and older into a group that would receive annual screening with rigid sigmoidoscopy and FOBT or with rigid sigmoidoscopy alone. After 5-11 years of follow-up, the investigators observed fewer colorectal cancer deaths in the group receiving annual FOBT and sigmoidoscopy compared with the group receiving sigmoidoscopy alone (0.36 vs 0.63 per 1000; p = .53).[114] Additional confirming evidence came from a simulation of combined FOBT and flexible sigmoidoscopy (based on findings from colonoscopy) suggested that the combined examination would achieve 76% sensitivity for advanced neoplasia.[91] Based on modeling, the USPSTF concluded that combining flexible sigmoidoscopy every 5 years with a high-sensitivity FOBT every 3 years was approximately equivalent in terms of life years gained to screening colonoscopy every 10 years.[115]

Barium Enema ■ Barium enema is an x-ray examination of the bowel that derives contrast from barium (a single-contrast study) or the combination of barium and instilled air (a double-contrast study, DCBE). DCBE is more sensitive than the single-contrast study for both malignancies and polyps. Because the addition of air into the colon can cause some discomfort, the single-contrast study may be used for patients who the physician anticipates would tolerate DCBE poorly. Bowel preparation for DCBE is similar to that required for colonoscopy since residual stool can mask lesions or lead to false-positives. Prior to the examination, a flexible tube is inserted into the rectum to introduce barium into the bowel. Fluoroscopic examination monitors the progress of the barium through the bowel (patients may be required to roll and assume various positions to insure bowel cavities will be coated with barium). Once the bowel is completely coated, x-rays are taken. If the patient has a positive test, the next step is a colonoscopy. The evidence for the efficacy of DCBE is largely indirect, based on the performance of DCBE in detecting small malignant lesions and polyps and on the known benefits of early detection and polypectomy for reducing mortality from colorectal cancer. Winawer et al. reported comparative results of DCBE and colonoscopy for 580 patients enrolled in the National Polyp Study who underwent surveillance following diagnosis of adenomatous polyps.[116] The proportion of examinations in which adenomatous polyps identified by colonoscopy also being detected by DCBE was significantly influenced by the size of the lesion, with DCBE sensitivity increasing with the size of the lesion. Although DCBE identified some lesions missed by colonoscopy, the number was comparatively much smaller. The authors concluded colonoscopy was a more effective method of surveillance than DCBE in patients who have undergone colonoscopic polypectomy. Among all currently recommended screening tests, DCBE is the least utilized. In a recent study of colorectal cancer screening among U.S. Medicare beneficiaries between 1979 and 1999, the median rate for DCBE was only 2.2%.[117]

Colonoscopy ■ Like DCBE, colonoscopy is a total colon examination (Fig. 34-11) and requires thorough bowel preparation. The modern colonoscope is capable of examining the entire bowel, with the examination terminating at the cecum. The instrument generally is far more complex than a sigmoidoscope since it must be capable of air insufflation, irrigation, suction, and the passage of biopsy forceps and polypectomy snares.[118] Like sigmoidoscopes, the tip of the instrument is equipped with a small video camera and light to provide high-resolution visualization of the wall of the bowel. Patients generally go on a liquid diet one or more days before the examination, followed by either ingestion of oral lavage solutions or saline laxatives to stimulate bowel movements until the bowel is clean. Proper bowel preparation is a critical element in the accuracy and cost-effectiveness of screening with colonoscopy.[119] It is common for the patient to receive a mild sedative prior to the procedure, but it is not essential for those who tolerate

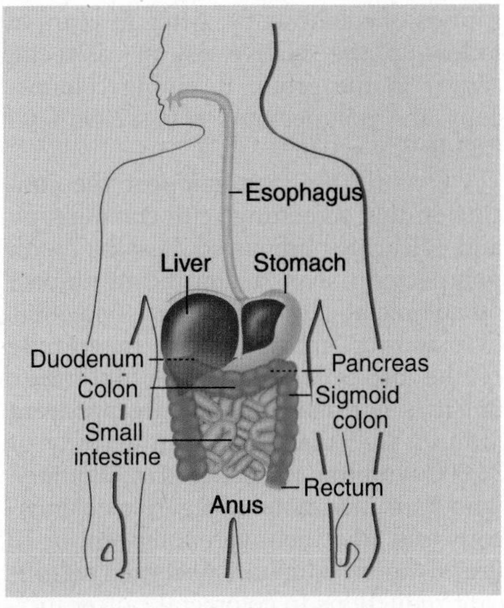

Figure 34-11 ■ Reach of colonoscopy (shaded area) in screening for colorectal cancer and adenomatous polyps. *Source*: Centers for Disease Control and Prevention.

the procedure with only mild discomfort.[120] Colonoscopy is commonly done in a hospital but can also be done in an outpatient setting. The examination is more complicated than sigmoidoscopy, with higher risk of complications, mostly due to the effects of sedation, biopsy, or polypectomy.[121,122] A skilled operator can complete an uncomplicated examination in ~30 minutes.[123]

Colonoscopy has a unique advantage among all screening tests for colorectal cancer in that direct visualization of the entire bowel is possible, and clinically significant adenomas can be identified and removed during the examination. Evidence for the effectiveness of colonoscopy is indirect in that no large trials with mortality endpoints have been conducted to evaluate the efficacy of screening. However, as with DCBE, the high sensitivity of the test to detect advanced neoplasia and to identify and remove high-risk adenomatous polyps has been regarded as sufficient for colonoscopy to be included among recommended screening tests. In the large majority of screening procedures (over 90%), the cecum can be visualized; when colonoscopy is incomplete, the examination may be repeated, or a total colon examination may be achieved with DCBE, or CT colonography.[84] In a case-control study of 32,702 veterans, patients who had undergone colonoscopy with polypectomy were significantly less likely to develop colorectal cancer (OR 0.48; 95% CI 0.35-0.66).[124] In the Telemark Polyp Study, 400 asymptomatic men and women aged 50-59 and 399 controls were randomly selected from the Telemark, Norway, and population registries. The experimental group was offered flexible sigmoidoscopy, and participants with detected polyps received colonoscopy with polypectomy, and two subsequent rounds of colonoscopy. After 13 years of follow-up, the relative risk of colorectal cancer in the group receiving colonoscopy and polypectomy was 0.2 (95% CI 0.03-0.95, $p = .02$).[79]

Overall, the data support the conclusion that screening with colonoscopy and clearing advanced lesions with polypectomy has a significant impact on colorectal cancer incidence and thus, by extension, mortality. The magnitude of the protective impact is uncertain, but it is not absolute, nor are apparent failures well understood. In a study of 35,000 symptomatic patients in Manitoba who had undergone a negative colonoscopy and who then were followed for 10 years, the investigators observed significant reductions in colorectal cancer incidence over time, with a reduction in the expected colorectal cancer incidence of 45% at five years, and 72% at 10 years.[125] These findings suggest detection failures during the initial apparently normal colonoscopy.

In the United States, a screening interval of 10 years is recommended based on the ability of colonoscopy to provide a clearing examination of the entire bowel, and estimated polyp growth time.[126] Imperiale and colleagues rescreened 1256 adults ~5 years after negative colonoscopy. While no cancers were detected, 201 (16%) of adults examined had one or more adenomas, of which only 16 had advanced adenomas. The findings support the conclusion that among individuals with no evidence of cancer or advanced adenomas at the time of screening, the 5-year risk of colorectal cancer is extremely low.[127]

The risk of postpolypectomy bleeding is higher when large polyps are removed, although bleeding from removal of small polyp is more common because small polyps are so numerous. Polyp removal in the proximal colon also is associated with a higher risk of bleeding. Risk of bowel perforation increases with increasing age, and also is higher in individuals with diverticular disease. Perforation rates were recently estimated to occur in 1 in 500 Medicare beneficiaries undergoing screening colonoscopy, and ~1 in 1000 screened patients overall.[122]

The long duration of reduced risk of colorectal cancer after colonoscopy must depend on quality of the examination and the complete removal of polyps. Quality assurance recommendations stress that high-quality colonoscopy depends on: (1) training and experience; (2) assessment and documentation of risk assessment; (3) complete examination to the cecum with adequate mucosal visualization and bowel preparation; (4) ability to detect and remove polyps safely; (5) documentation of polypoid lesions and methods of removal; (6) timely and appropriate management of adverse events; (7) appropriate follow-up of histopathology findings; (8) appropriate recommendation for surveillance or repeat screening based on published guidelines; and (9) continuous assessment and evaluation of performance, with corrective action when necessary.[123,128,129]

CT Colonography ■ CT colonography or virtual colonoscopy is an imaging procedure that uses computer programming to combine multiple helical CT scans in order to create two- or three-dimensional images of the interior of the colon. These images can be rotated for different views and even combined for a complete, "virtual" view of the colon that can be viewed in a manner that simulates the insertion and withdrawal of a colonoscope. The term "virtual colonoscopy" was coined in the mid-1990s by researchers at Wake Forest University who described this procedure as simulating conventional colonoscopy.[130]

Evaluation studies of CT colonography have typically used study designs that first performed the CT examination, which was then followed by optical colonoscopy, with the examiner blinded to the results of the CT examination. Although early results with 2D imaging were disappointing in terms of accuracy,[131] more recent back to back evaluations of CT colonography using faster scanners, updated 3D luminal displays, and oral stool tagging with digital subtraction have demonstrated sensitivities for large adenomas equivalent to colonoscopy.[132,133] Using these advanced techniques, Pickhardt et al. studied conducted back to back CT and optical colonoscopy examinations in 1233 asymptomatic adults and reported 94% sensitivity for large adenomas, with a per-patient sensitivity for adenomas ≥6 mm of 89%.[132] A collaborative American College of Radiology Imaging Network/NCI (ACRIN/NCI) trial comparing virtual colonoscopy with optical colonoscopy reported results in 2008. The trial was conducted in 15 centers, where investigators recruited 2600 asymptomatic adults aged 50 years or older who were scheduled for routine screening optical colonoscopy. Resulting images were randomly assigned to be interpreted on 2D display, or in 3D display in which the CT images were reconstructed to display a virtual image of the colon. After the CT examination, optical colonoscopy was performed according to the standard protocol at each participating center. CT colonography detected 90% of patients with large (≥9 mm) adenomas and cancers, with 86% specificity.[133] The per-polyp sensitivity for large adenomas and cancers was 84%, and the per-patient sensitivity for all colorectal lesions ≥6 mm was 78%. Thirty lesions ≥10 mm in size were detected by CT colonography in 27 patients that were not detected in the initial colonoscopy. Among 15 patients (18 reported lesions) that returned for follow-up colonoscopy, five lesions ≥10 mm were confirmed as true positives on the second colonoscopy.

Although the sensitivity of CT colonography is lower for lesions ≤6 mm, these lesions generally are regarded as clinically insignificant and raise questions as to whether or not there is actual value in test sensitivity for lesions that pose no real threat in the near term. With respect to lesions that are close to or exceed 1 cm in size, CT colonography has performance similar to optical colonoscopy.

CT colonography requires the same full cathartic bowel preparation and restricted diet as optical colonoscopy, and as an "imaging-only" evaluation of

Table 34-3 Guidelines for Screening and Surveillance for Early Detection of Colorectal Polyps and Cancer for Individuals at Greater Than Average Risk

Risk Category and Description	Recommendation	Age to Begin	Screening Interval and Recommendation
Moderate risk			
People with single, small (<1 cm) adenomatous polyps	Colonoscopy	At the initial polyp diagnosis	TCE within 3 years after initial polyp removal; if normal, follow recommendations for average-risk individuals
People with large (≥1 cm) or multiple adenomatous polyps of any size	Colonoscopy	At time of initial polyp diagnosis	TCE within 3 years after initial polyp removal; if normal TCE every 5 years
Personal history of curative-intent resection of colorectal cancer	TCE	Within 1 year after resection	If normal, TCE in 3 years; If second TCE is normal, TCE in 5 years
Colorectal cancer or adenomatous polyps, in first-degree relative younger than age 60 or in 2 or more first-degree relatives of any ages	TCE	40 years, or 10 years before the youngest case in the family, whichever is earlier	Every 5 years
Colorectal cancer in other relatives (not firstdegree)	Follow recommendations for age-risk individuals		
High risk			
Family history of FAP	Early surveillance with endoscopy, counseling to consider genetic testing, and referral for specialty care	Puberty	If genetic test is positive or polyposis is confirmed, consider colectomy; otherwise, continue endoscopy every 1–2 years
Family history of HNPCC	Colonoscopy and counseling to consider genetic testing	21 years	If untested, or if genetic test is positive, colonoscopy every 2 years until age 40; after age 40, colonoscopy every year
Inflammatory bowel disease	Colonoscopy with biopsies for dysplasia	8 years after the start of pancolitis; 12–15 years after the start of left-sided colitis	Colonoscopy every 1–2 years

Abbreviations: FAP, familial adenomatous polyposis; HNPCC, hereditary nonpolyposis colorectal cancer; TCE, total colon examination.

[a]TCE includes either colonoscopy, DCBE, or CT colonography. CT colonography or DCBE should be added to the colonoscopy examination in those instances when the entire colon can not be visualized by colonoscopy.

the colon, patients with polyps ≥6 mm in size should be referred to therapeutic colonoscopy for possible subsequent polypectomy.[126]

Screening Recommendations

Most organizations recommend that average-risk adults should be regularly screened for colorectal cancer beginning at age 50, although there are differences in recommended options for regular surveillance. As shown in Table 34-2, the ACS, USMSTF, and ACR recommendations for average-risk individuals include seven options for regular surveillance beginning at age 50, including annual high-sensitivity FOBT (gFOBT or FIT); sDNA (interval unknown); FSIG every 5 years, annual high-sensitivity gFOBT or FIT and flexible sigmoidoscopy every 5 years after initial screening with both tests; total colon (TCE) examination with DCBE every 5 years; or TCE with colonoscopy every 10 years. In reality, based on availability and preferences, most adults who undergo screening will undergo stool testing with gFOBT or FIT or colonoscopy, with CT colonography likely to increase in utilization once the test begins to be reimbursed by third party payers. Annual DRE is no longer recommended, due to low sensitivity, but DRE should be done prior to FSIG or colonoscopy. While there is strong consensus about the value of colorectal cancer screening in adults 50 years of age and older among U.S. organizations that issue guidelines, the USPSTF concluded in their recent guideline update that there was insufficient evidence to recommend for or against CT colonography or sDNA.[115] Guidelines for higher-risk individuals are also shown in Table 34-3. Higher-risk individuals include those with a family history of adenomatous polyps or colorectal cancer, a family history of familial adenomatous polyposis (FAP), a family history of hereditary nonpolyposis colorectal cancer (HNPCC), or a personal history of inflammatory bowel disease.[126] In general, colorectal cancer screening guidelines for higher-risk individuals recommend earlier onset of surveillance and more thorough examinations of the colon.

Cervical Cancer

Although rates of invasive cervical cancer declined dramatically during the 20th century, it is still a leading cause of cancer mortality in the world.[5] Five-year cervical cancer is excellent when the disease is diagnosed while still localized (92%), and poorer when invasive cervical cancer is diagnosed at a regional stage (56%), or when distant metastases are present (11%).[17]

The decline in cervical cancer mortality has been dramatic in United States women, declining >70% between 1930 and 1980. Similar declines in the incidence of invasive cervical cancer have been observed as well, and this same pattern of declining incidence and mortality has been observed in other countries that have introduced mass screening for cancer of the cervix.[134,135]

The relatively low incidence rate of invasive cervical cancer in Western countries compared with other cancers, and the long-term downward trend in incidence and mortality is a measure of the success of the Papanicolaou test, developed by Dr. George Nicolas Papanicolaou in the 1920s (Fig. 34-12) of the early detection of cancer and processor lesions, i.e., cervical intraepithelial neoplasia (CIN).[135] Rates of treatable precursor lesions are considerably higher than rates of invasive disease, due to the effectiveness of cervical cancer screening in advancing the stage at diagnosis from invasive cancer to lesions known to be precursors of cervical cancer. Although there is no sys-

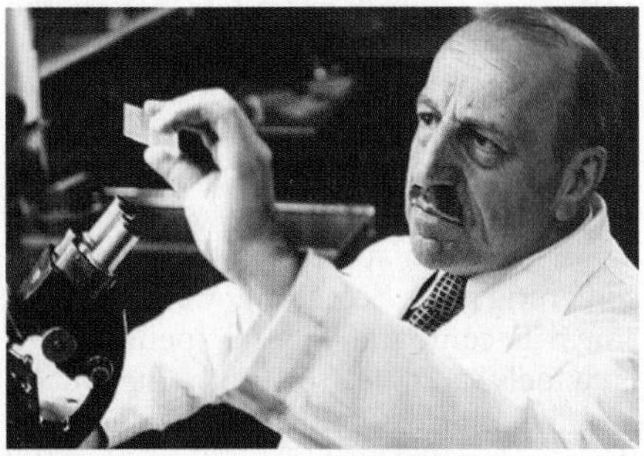

Figure 34-12 Dr. George Nicolas Papanicolaou (1883-1962) is credited with the development of the Pap test. *Source*: Reprinted with permission from the Telsa Memorial Society of New York.

tem for surveillance of precursor lesions, a report from the Centers for Disease Control and Prevention's (CDC) National Breast and Cervical Cancer Early Detection Program (NBCCEDP) summarizing findings from a broad spectrum of program participants throughout the United States showed an overall abnormality rate of 3.8% and a ratio of CIN III/carcinoma in situ (CIS) to invasive disease of 9:1 and a ratio of CIN II or worse to invasive disease of 18.5:1.[136]

Screening and Diagnostic Methods

It is generally accepted that screening for cancer of the cervix, but more specifically precancerous lesions of the cervix, is effective in reducing both the incidence and mortality from cervical cancer. Cervical cancer is characterized by a long *sojourn* time, with potentially cancerous lesions progressing through a succession of identifiable stages prior to invasive disease. If precursor lesions are detected prior to the point of progression to invasive disease, a variety of treatment options are available, the progression to invasive disease is prevented, and the disease is almost certainly curable. Age-specific incidence data previously available from NCI's Surveillance, Epidemiology, and End Results (SEER) program and from cross-sectional studies of small geographic areas or clinic populations are consistent with the following observations: (1) the prevalence of precursor dysplastic lesions is greater among younger women compared with older women; (2) a significant proportion of premalignant lesions will regress, especially in younger women; (3) carcinoma in situ (CIN) of the cervix peaks in the mid-30s; and (4) the incidence of invasive disease peaks in the mid-40s, remaining relatively constant among Caucasian women and continuing to rise among African American women.[17,137-139]

While there has never been a randomized trial of the efficacy of screening for cancer of the cervix, it has been observed that cytologic screening was an accepted part of medical care among both women and providers before the randomized trial with a mortality endpoint had become the standard by which the efficacy of a screening test is evaluated.[1] Even so, the logic of cytologic screening has always measured up well against criteria applied to the value of a screening test. Screening with the Pap smear is comparatively inexpensive and is widely accepted by both the public and health-care professionals. Perhaps the most widely cited evidence for the contribution of cytologic screening to the reduction in cervical cancer mortality is the long-term decline in the death rate from cervical cancer in the United States coincident with the introduction of the Pap smear, although it has been noted that death rates had begun to decline prior to widespread use of the test, perhaps due to other factors such as an increase in the hysterectomy rate, and trends in the underlying epidemiology of the disease.[140] However, there can be little argument that cytologic screening is the primary influence in the long-term trend in declining cervical cancer incidence and mortality rates. Scientific evidence for the efficacy of cervical cytology in reducing the incidence of invasive disease and mortality comes from observational studies and case-control studies. The best examples of observational studies are the evaluations of cervical cancer mortality rates in five Nordic countries before and after the introduction of screening programs.[134,141-144] Comparing mortality rates before and after the introduction of cytologic screening between two time periods (1963-1967 and 1978-1982), mortality reductions between 8% and 73% were observed. Factors underlying this wide range of mortality reductions are also consistent with a screening effect. In Norway, where participation rates were lowest, mortality remained comparatively unchanged whereas in Iceland, which organized an aggressive screening program that had high rates of participation, the mortality reduction (73%) was greatest among the five countries.[134,141,143] More recent investigations of population trends in the United Kingdom and the Republic of Ireland show similar associations with the organization and intensity of screening as was observed in the Nordic countries. Mortality in England, Wales, and Scotland has declined for over 30 years, with an accelerating rate since reorganization of the screening program in the 1980s, whereas in the Irish Republic, which has no screening program, mortality rates have been increasing at an average annual rate of 1.5% each year since 1978.[145] Numerous examples of case-control studies also show a benefit from cervical cancer screening, typically examining the screening histories of women diagnosed with invasive disease compared with matched controls.[146,147] Today, cervical cancer screening research focuses more on effectiveness and cost-effectiveness of various screening strategies than on issues of efficacy.

The Pap test is the most widely used cancer screening test in the world. At the most basic level, the Pap test involves the collection of exfoliating epithelial cells from the cervical squamocolumnar junction, or transformation zone. Both the ectocervix and endocervix should be sampled. Various collection tools (spatula, cotton swab, Cytobrush, Cervix brush, Cytopick, etc) are available for specimen collection. Boon and colleagues evaluated various approaches to specimen collection and found that the presence of endocervical cells varied considerably by sampling technique and tools. The combination of spatula and Cytobrush, or the Cytopick, had the best performance as measured by presence of endocervical cells, while the spatula alone or the combination of spatula and cotton swab gave poor performance.[148] Two samples should be applied to one side of a glass slide and quickly fixed (usually with a spray fixative) to prevent air-drying. The slide is then examined under a microscope by a cytotechnologist.

Although the Pap test is simple to conduct, its accuracy is greatly dependent on achieving a high level of quality in specimen collection, slide preparation, and microscopic examination and interpretation. Even under the best of circumstances, the Pap smear has a significant error rate.[149] Sampling error is estimated to account for about two-thirds of false-negative tests whereas errors in interpretation account for the remaining third.[150] A technology assessment of cervical cytology by the Duke University Center for Clinical Health Policy Research conducted for the Agency for Health Care Policy and Research concluded that conventional Pap smear screening had specificity of 98% but sensitivity of only 51%.[150] Sensitivity is lower when the threshold of a positive test is higher, ie, in the case of a high-grade squamous intraepithelial lesion (HSIL) versus a low-grade squamous intraepithelial lesion (LSIL) or atypical cells of undetermined significance (ASCUS).

In an effort to improve the accuracy and cost-effectiveness of the Pap smear, several new screening technologies have evolved, with each taking a somewhat different approach to resolving some of the shortcomings of the conventional Pap smear, specifically sampling error and interpretation error. Liquid-based cytology uses specimen collection techniques similar to the conventional Pap smear, and is equally dependent on collecting an adequate sample, but instead of directly placing the sample on a glass slide, the sample is suspended in a fixative solution, after which it is dispersed, filtered, and then distributed on a glass slide to achieve a monolayer of cells. Accuracy is supposedly increased because there are fewer artifacts (blood, mucus, etc.) and because cells, in particular nuclei, are not overlapping (Fig. 34-13). Presently there are conflicting data on whether the test achieves superior performance compared with conventional cytology. In some studies and reviews, liquid-based cytology has been shown to have higher sensitivity in populations with a lower prevalence of cytologic abnormalities.[150-152] More recent reviews applying more rigorous evidence-based

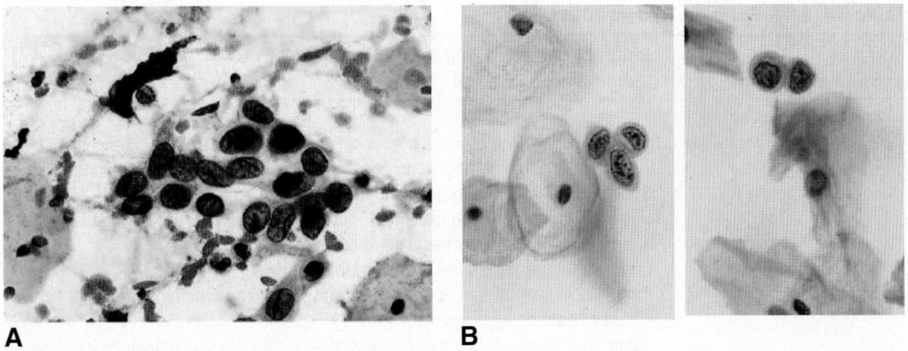

Figure 34-13 ■ Examples of conventional cervical cytology (**A**) and liquid-based cytology (**B**), interpreted as a high-grade squamous intraepithelial lesion (HSIL). *Source*: Centers for Disease Control and Prevention.

criteria both in terms of study design and adherence to standards for comparing diagnostic accuracy between two tests found no significant advantage in sensitivity or specificity for liquid-based cytology over conventional Pap testing.[153] It is clear, however, that numbers of inadequate specimens are considerably reduced with liquid-based cytology.

Computer-aided diagnosis applies neural-network technology to identify slides with areas of abnormal cells, and these targeted areas are reviewed by a cytotechnologist who then decides whether the slide should be further reviewed. Neural-network technology is being evaluated for primary screening in Finland in a prospective randomized trial, where early results revealed similar performance between conventional and automated screening.[154] Neural-network technology also has been used for rescreening slides with normal interpretation for the purpose of detection false negatives, where some studies have shown an improvement in sensitivity, but at a very high cost.[155] The National Health Service Health Technology Assessment Programme (NHS-HTA) conducted an evidence-based review of neural-network technology and concluded based on a limited number of rigorous studies that automated neural-network screening was approximately equivalent to conventional manual screening for cervical cancer, although slide processing times appeared to be significantly shorter.[156]

A comparative review of these new technologies concluded that their application was more cost-effective when incorporated into protocols of less frequent screening, and that cost-effectiveness was higher in populations with higher disease prevalence.[157] With annual screening, they offer little added advantage to life expectancy over the conventional Pap smear. In settings where conventional cytologic screening is well established, neural-network screening may offer an advantage if there is a persistent shortage of cytologists.

Because of the strong association between persistent infection with particular subtypes of human Papilloma virus (HPV) and cervical cancer, HPV testing is increasingly being used for surveillance and risk stratification, specifically as a strategy for risk assignment in order to distinguish a high-risk group for more aggressive surveillance, triaging women with low-grade Pap smear abnormalities [atypical cells of undetermined significance (ASCUS), atypical glandular cells of undetermined significance (AGUS), or low-grade squamous intraepithelial lesion (LSIL)], or for follow-up of women with confirmed CIN.[158-161] Moreover, HPV testing also is emerging as a potential strategy for primary screening, and along with HPV vaccines holds the potential for a comprehensive strategy for global cervical cancer control.[162] Current testing for HPV DNA is done with the hybrid capture test, which is the only test that has been approved by the FDA for commercial use. However, the hybrid capture test determines only the presence of 14 HPV subtypes, and does not identify specific subtypes, which requires polymerase chain reaction (PCR) techniques.[163] The value and the potential for HPV testing rest on the strong evidence that infection with particular subtypes of HPV—in particular, HPV type 16 and 18—is a necessary, not just sufficient, etiologic factor in nearly all cervical neoplasia.[164] At this time, HPV testing does appear to have value for triaging women with ASCUS and AGUS, specifically with regard to greater cost-effectiveness related to the management of the mildly abnormal Pap smear, and is increasingly used for that purpose compared with serial short-term follow-up examinations.[160] There is growing evidence that HPV testing may represent a lower-resource intense strategy for women at demonstrated lower risk, a more sensitive surveillance strategy when combined with cytology for women at elevated risk,[165-167] and as a strategy for routine screening for all women.[138] While the ACS endorses HPV testing with cytology every 3 years for women older than age 30,[168] a strategy for routine use of HPV testing, and management of abnormal test results, still is evolving. First, HPV infection may be active, latent, or transient; thus, the potential for misclassification from one-time testing is high. Second, exposure opportunities vary in individuals over time. Apart from the fact that a person may test negative because the infection is latent or the viral load low, they may also acquire an infection in the period after testing.[169] Third, since most HPV infections are cleared or suppressed by cellular-mediated immunity, it is important that positive test results in the presence of negative cytology are treated as an indication for surveillance rather than an indication for therapy. This is especially the case with younger women, which is why HPV testing is not endorsed before age 30.[168] Fourth, since HPV infection is common in adults who have had more than one sexual partner, and since most individuals with HPV infection do not develop cervical cancer, the public will need to be educated about the meaning of positive test results in order to mitigate feelings of stigma associated with testing positive for a sexually acquired infection.[170,171]

It is likely that the accumulation of additional evidence as well as a growing awareness in the public of the role of HPV in cervical cancer etiology will lead to the use of HPV information in testing and triaging, not only for screening and surveillance in specific groups, but also monitoring vaccine effectiveness.[172] Large trials examining primary HPV testing vs. conventional cytology are underway, and early results add additional supporting evidence that HPV testing in women ages 35-60 results in improved sensitivity for CIN 2+ lesions with only a small decrease in PPV, but that the increased sensitivity of HPV testing observed in women ages 25-34 compared with cytology alone suggests a significant rate of regression of CIN 2+ lesions in this age group.[138,173] Thus, strategies of triage or repeat testing will be needed to avoid overtreatment if HPV testing is a primary screening strategy in this younger age group.

After years of evolution in cytologic classification systems for Pap smear results, the NCI sponsored a meeting in 1988 to develop a new system, widely adopted, and revised twice since that time, to both standardize cytologic nomenclature and address shortcomings in the various systems in use. These shortcomings included uneven cytologic/histologic correlation, low reliability, and confusion in the communication with referring physicians by both the use of different systems and the inconsistent use of nomenclature within a system. This new system, known as the *Bethesda System*, was intended to provide "... a uniform format for cytopathology reports that is intended to communicate clinically relevant information using standardized terminology."[174] The current Bethesda System is shown in Table 34-4, and an online atlas is available at http://nih.techriver.net/index.php.[175,176]

Table 34-4 ■ **Bethesda System 2001**

Specimen Type	Indicate Conventional Smear (Pap Smear) vs Liquid-Based vs Other
Specimen adequacy	
Satisfactory for evaluation	Describe presence or absence of endocervical/transformation zone component and any other quality indicators, eg, partially obscuring blood, inflammation, etc
Unsatisfactory for evaluation	Specimen rejected/not processed (specify reason), or Specimen processed and examined, but unsatisfactory for evaluation of epithelial abnormality because of (specify reason)
General categorization (optional)	Negative for Intraepithelial lesion or malignancy Epithelial cell abnormality: See interpretation/result (specify "squamous" or "glandular" as appropriate) Other: See interpretation/result (eg, endometrial cells in a woman >40 years of age)
Automated review	If case examined by automated device, specify device and result
Ancillary testing	Provide a brief description of the test methods and report the result so that it is easily understood by the clinician
Interpretation/result	
Negative for intraepithelial lesion or malignancy	When there is no cellular evidence of neoplasia, state this in the General Categorization above and/or in the Interpretation/Result section of the report, whether or not there are organisms or other non-neoplastic findings)
Organisms	*Trichomonas vaginalis* Fungal organisms morphologically consistent with *Candida* spp Shift in flora suggestive of bacterial vaginosis Bacteria morphologically consistent with *Actinomyces* spp. Cellular changes consistent with herpes simplex virus
Other non-neoplastic findings (Optional to report; list not inclusive)	Reactive cellular changes associated with inflammation (includes typical repair) radiation intrauterine contraceptive device (IUD) Glandular cells status post hysterectomy Atrophy
Other	Endometrial cells (in a woman ≥ 40 years of age) (Specify if "negative for squamous intraepithelial lesion")
Epithelial cell abnormalities	
Squamous cell	Atypical squamous cells of undetermined significance (ASC-US) cannot exclude HSIL (ASC-H) Low grade squamous intraepithelial lesion (LSIL) encompassing: HPV/mild dysplasia/CIN 1 High grade squamous intraepithelial lesion (HSIL) encompassing: moderate and severe dysplasia, CIS/CIN 2 and CIN 3 with features suspicious for invasion (if invasion is suspected) Squamous cell carcinoma
Glandular cell	Atypical Endocervical cells (NOS or specify in comments) Endometrial cells (NOS or specify in comments) Glandular cells (NOS or specify in comments) Endocervical cells, favor neoplastic Glandular cells, favor neoplastic Endocervical adenocarcinoma in situ Adenocarcinoma Endocervical Endometrial Extrauterine Not otherwise specified
Other malignant neoplasms	Specify
Educational notes and suggestions (optional)	Suggestions should be concise and consistent with clinical follow-up guidelines published by professional organizations (references to relevant publications may be included).

Source: Adapted from Ref. 144

Screening Recommendations

The ACS updated guidelines for cervical cancer screening in 2002 (Table 34-2).[168] According to the ACS, cervical cancer screening should begin ~3 years after the onset of vaginal intercourse, but no later than 21 years of age. Cervical screening should be performed annually with conventional cervical cytology smears, or every 2 years using liquid-based cytology, until age 30, after which screening with the Pap test may continue every 2-3 years for those women who have had three consecutive, technically satisfactory normal/negative cytology results. Alternatively, for women aged 30 and over for whom less frequent screening is appropriate, cervical screening may be performed every 3 years using conventional or liquid-based cytology combined with a DNA test for from high-risk HPV types. Frequency of combined cytology and HPV DNA testing should not be more often than every 3 years. In 2004, a consensus conference of leading agencies further addressed the issue of HPV testing, and endorsed adding HPV DNA testing to cervical cytology for women 30 years and older, including guidance for women who test positive for high-risk HPV subtypes, but are negative on cytology should have the tests repeated in 6-12 months rather than being referred immediately for colposcopy, and if either test is subsequently positive, colposcopy should be performed.[167] Women who are age 70 and older with an intact cervix and who have had (1) three or more documented, consecutive, technically satisfactory normal/negative cervical cytology tests and (2) no abnormal/positive cytology tests within the 10-year period prior to age 70 may elect to cease cervical cancer screening. Women over the age of 70 should discuss their need for cervical cancer screening with a health-care professional, and make an informed decision about continuing screening based on the potential benefits, harms, and limitations of screening. Recommendations for cervical cancer screening from the USPSTF are similar. ACS guidelines also address screening recommendations for women a history of in utero exposure to diethylstilbestrol (DES), women who are immunocompromised (including HIV+), and women with a history of subtotal or total hysterectomy.

Historically, screening guidelines in the United States have recommended more aggressive surveillance than in those in Europe, with the organizations in the United States endorsing earlier ages to begin testing, more frequent testing, and not specifying an age to stop screening. While the new recommendations still endorse more aggressive screening than many European countries, they specify a more rational, cost-effective approach than earlier guidelines. Still, it is apparent that many United States clinicians are hesitant to embrace less frequent cervical cancer screening,[177] despite good evidence that overscreening is wasteful of resources and contributes to potential harms.[177-179]

Prostate Cancer

Prostate cancer is the most common cancer diagnosed in men in the United

States., and the second most common cancer among men in the world. Incidence varies considerably in the world's regions, with a six-fold difference between more developed regions compared with less developed regions, while mortality rates are only 2.5 times higher in developed vs. less developed regions.[180] In developed regions prostate cancer is sometimes observed to be a disease men are more likely to die "with" than "from," owing to the older average age at prostate cancer diagnosis and the typically slow progression of the disease. However, prostate cancer represents a significant clinical challenge for a number of reasons. It is exceeded only by lung cancer as a cause of cancer death in men, accounting for about 10% of all male cancer deaths.[181] While prostate cancer is commonly viewed as slow-growing and indolent, it is the usual cause of death for men with advanced disease. Prognosis is good if the diagnosis is made when the cancer is still localized to the prostate; but a significant percentage of prostate cancers are diagnosed after the tumor has spread locally, and in 4% of cases, the disease has distant metastases at diagnosis. The 5-year survival rate for men with distant disease is only 32%.[17]

Screening and Diagnostic Methods

Prostate cancer usually does not produce symptoms until it is locally advanced or metastatic. The principle methods that have been evaluated for early prostate cancer detection, both separately and in combination are the digital rectal examination (DRE), the prostate-specific antigen (PSA) blood test and variants, and transrectal ultrasonography (TRUS).

DRE ■ Palpable asymmetry of the prostate gland and, particularly, hard nodular areas sometimes indicate presence of prostate cancer. Palpation of the prostate gland with DRE was the earliest approach to detecting asymptomatic prostate cancer in the pre-serum marker era. Jacobsen and colleagues conducted a population-based case-control study on all men who died of prostate cancer in Olmsted County from 1976 to 1991.[182] They found case subjects were half as likely as control subjects to have had any DRE in the 10 years before diagnosis. In a more recent case-control study, Weinmann and colleagues observed that DRE was associated with a statistically significant 35% reduced risk of death from prostate cancer in white men, and a nonsignificant 14% reduction in African American men.[183] Two other case-control studies observed a smaller, although nonsignificant, protective effect.[184,185] Historical evaluations of DRE are subject to a number of potential biases, of which the most significant is the inability to determine if the patient was symptomatic. Schroder and colleagues evaluated the performance of DRE as a stand-alone screening test using data from the Rotterdam, Netherlands arm of the European Randomized Study of Screening for Prostate Cancer (ERSPC), and observed a detection rate of prostate cancer of 2.5% based on DRE results alone compared with 4.5% when men were screened with DRE, PSA, and TRUS.[186] The sensitivity of DRE was 37%, specificity was 91%, and the PPV was highly dependent on the underlying value of PSA. When PSA values were lower than a conventional threshold of 4.0 ng/mL, the PPV of a positive DRE averaged 12.8%, and averaged only 8.8% for PSA ranges between 0 and 2.9 ng/mL. Based on these findings, the ERSSPC dropped DRE and lowered the PSA threshold for indication for prostate biopsy to 3.0-4.0 ng/mL.[187] While the low predictive values observed in the ERSPC suggest that the DRE has limited value compared with stand-alone PSA testing, Basler and Thompson noted that between one-quarter and one-third of all prostate cancers are detected by DRE in the normal PSA range (<4.0 ng/mL), indicating that a considerable number of cases would be missed based on PSA testing alone.[188] Data from the first four rounds of screening in the Prostate, Lung Colorectal, and Ovarian Screening Trial (PLCO) showed that prostate cancer detection rate of 1.8-2.3 per 1000 in men with a PSA <4.0 ng/mL.[189]

The principal limitations of DRE are that the majority of palpable cancers are not early cancers and many clinically important cancers are located in regions of the gland that are inaccessible to digital palpation. In addition, the test is highly operator-dependent.[190] Although it has poor sensitivity, the DRE often is recommended as a component of prostate cancer screening because it may detect prostate cancers missed by other tests, it is an independent predictor of high-grade disease, it is a low-cost procedure, and it has value in evaluating other prostate abnormalities such as benign prostatic hyperplasia.[188,191]

PSA ■ PSA became widely used for screening and diagnosis following its commercial introduction as a test for monitoring prostate cancer patients. This pattern of use resulted in a marked increase in prostate cancer incidence rates in the United States in the late 1980s. This trend peaked in 1992, and subsequently declined, revealing a classic pattern of rise and decline in incidence consistent with the detection of a sizable prevalence of occult disease that without screening would potentially would have been detected in subsequent years, although some unknown fraction may never have been detected without screening. Over the reminder of the decade, the incidence rate rose to "catch up" with the earlier incidence trend.

The principal strengths of the PSA test are its sensitivity, reasonable cost, and high patient acceptance. The principal drawback of the test is its imperfect specificity, owing to the fact that common conditions such as benign prostatic hyperplasia and prostatitis can cause borderline or markedly abnormal test results. These false-positive results can lead to expensive further diagnostic evaluation and unwarranted patient anxiety. Conversely, the high sensitivity of the test may result in considerable overdiagnosis, with small indolent cancers, or less aggressive cancers that are not life threatening, being gathered in the same net as the aggressive, potentially life-threatening cancers. Current diagnostic algorithms are imperfect for distinguishing among these prognostic groups. However, while it is common to equate slow progression with overdiagnosis, a Swedish study with 21-year follow-up study of men with early stage, symptomatic disease who were initially untreated showed a significant decrease in disease-free survival after 15 years, with prostate cancer mortality increasing from 15 per 1000 person-years in the first 15 years of follow-up to 44 per 1000 person-years after 15 years.[192] These findings provide further support for current guidelines, which stress that expected longevity is an important consideration in decisions both about testing for early detection and therapy.

Another major concern about the utility of PSA is the lack of a dependable cutoff level. The PSA has been criticized for the lack of a good balance between sensitivity and specificity, and the fact that the conventional cutoff level (4.0 ng/mL) does not detect all prostate cancers. In fact, prostate cancer may be present even with very low levels of PSA. Recent results from the Prostate Cancer Prevention Trial showed that sensitivity measurably increased with successively lower PSA cutoff values, and for higher-grade disease, but that with each increment in sensitivity, specificity significantly declined.[193] These findings add to the evidence indicating that PSA levels lower than 4.0 ng/mL can not be assumed to be normal, and that the patient and physician will need to consider a number of factors in order to decide about further evaluation.

Evidence supporting the effectiveness (vs efficacy) of PSA testing alone or in combination with DRE and TRUS is available from several sources. Early comparative studies showed that prostate cancer detection in asymptomatic men could be increased by PSA and related testing.[186,194,195] In addition, it was demonstrated that the stage distribution of screen-detected cancers was much more favorable than that which occurred in the general, unscreened population diagnosed with symptoms. The American Cancer Society National Prostate Cancer Detection Project showed that after 5 years of annual testing by PSA, DRE, and TRUS, 92% of cancers detected were localized to the prostate, compared to 66% in a contemporaneous national database covering men of the same age.[196] In the report of the results of the first four rounds of screening in the PLCO, men with screen-detected prostate cancer in the second to fourth rounds of screening were significantly less likely to have Gleason 7-10 tumors and clinically advanced tumors (24.6-27.2%) than screen-detected cancers at baseline (34%), or the never screened group (37.9%).[189] More favorable Gleason score and clinical stage was also observed in the second round of screening in the ERSPC compared with the first.[197]

Transrectal Ultrasonography (TRUS) ■ TRUS uses a small rectal probe placed against the prostate gland to image the entire gland. Areas of the gland with differing morphology often yield different images. Unfortunately, prostate cancer has no unique and reliably assessed ultrasonographic signature, and TRUS has been shown to have poor sensitivity and specificity when employed as the sole screening modality, especially at low PSA levels.[195,198] It can, however, play an important role in the early detection process, since it is a means of accurately measuring gland dimensions and calculating total gland volume. This information is useful in evaluating borderline elevations in PSA using PSA density (PSAD). More importantly, TRUS is the means for directing needle biopsies of the prostate gland for diagnostic purposes. While endorectal MRI and other imaging approaches are being applied to the diagnostic process, innovations in ultrasound technology as well as limitations and costs associated with newer modalities have resulted in newer modalities having a complimentary role to TRUS in diagnostic evaluation.[199]

Population-based prospective, randomized trials of prostate cancer screening (described below) have been underway since 1993, but have not yet published findings on the efficacy of screening in the reduction of prostate cancer mortality. Since screening for prostate cancer increased significantly in the late 1980s in the United States and somewhat in other developed nations, there have been a number of non-experimental studies that have attempted to estimate the effectiveness of prostate cancer screening on mortality with very mixed results. Etzioni et al. have argued that decreases in prostate cancer mortality in the United States reported within the first decade after the onset of widespread PSA testing are unlikely to be due to PSA testing, given the long natural history of prostate cancer.[200] However, a decline in prostate cancer mortality could be due to the increased interest in early detection of prostate cancer with DRE that began prior to the PSA era, as manifested by trends in earlier stage at diagnosis and by increasing surgery rates for localized prostate cancer in the decade prior to the onset of widespread PSA testing. Another possible explanation for the decline in prostate cancer mortality is that there has been a shift in the tendency to classify prostate cancer as the underlying cause of death.[201] Alternatively, Tarone and colleagues have argued that stage-specific survival rates suggest that the rapid decrease in mortality was preceded by a large increase in the incidence of high-grade lesions diagnosed before metastasis.[202] Thus, rather than viewing the mortality trend in the context of the estimated average lead-time gained, it is reasonable to view the reduction in the incidence rate of advanced, metastatic disease as predictive of a subsequent reduction in prostate cancer mortality rates.[202] Based on the assumption that screening results in a shift from distant to local/regional disease, two separate modeling efforts within the NCI's Cancer Intervention Surveillance Modeling Network (CISNET) concluded that between 45% and 70% of the observed prostate cancer mortality decline in the United States could plausibly be attributed to screening-induced stage shifts.[203] Studies of regional differences in mortality trends associated with screening patterns have produced inconsistent results. For example, Lu-Yao and colleagues compared trends in prostate cancer mortality between 1987 and 1997 in the Seattle area and Connecticut to determine if more intensive screening activity in the Seattle area would be apparent in lower prostate cancer mortality rates.[204] They concluded that higher rates of prostate cancer screening and radical prostatectomy and radiotherapy were not associated with lower mortality rates over 11 years of follow-up. Shaw and colleagues examined PSA screening and prostate cancer mortality in nine geographic areas in the United States and applied different assumptions on treatment trends, measures of mortality, efficacy and lead-time assumptions, and time horizons to illustrate how different assumptions and omission of important cofounders could result in findings that lead to very different conclusions about efficacy. They observed a small association between increased screening activity and prostate cancer mortality reductions, but concluded that results of ecological analyses varied considerably based on the time horizon of the analysis and outcome measures used, and thus results of ecological analyses should be interpreted with caution.

Population-based results also are available from a natural experiment comparing prostate cancer mortality trends in the Federal State of Tyrol, Austria, where PSA testing had been made available at no cost since 1993, with the rest of the country, which did not have a screening program. Between 1993 and 2005, the cumulative PSA testing rate in men 45-74 exceeded 80%, with >50% of men having been tested by 1997.[205] After the introduction of the program, a significant shift toward more favorable stage at diagnosis was observed in Tyrol compared with the rest of Austria, followed by a much greater and statistically significant decline in the prostate cancer mortality rate.[206,207] In the most current analysis of mortality trends in Tyrol compared with the rest of Austria, standardized mortality ratios of observed to expected rates based on the pre-screening period (1986-1990) show a significant reduction in prostate cancer deaths in Tyrol of 54% (95% CI 34-69%) compared with 29% (95% CI 22-35%) in the rest of Austria, equivalent to an annual decline in prostate cancer mortality of 7.3% in Tyrol versus 3.2% in the rest of Austria. The authors acknowledge that it is not possible to segregate improvements in therapy and the influence of early detection, but conclude that the difference in mortality observed in Tyrol compared with the rest of Austria is unlikely to be artifactual.[205]

In addition to the case-control studies mentioned earlier, Agalliu and colleagues conducted a population-based case-control study to examine the relationships between PSA and DRE screening and fatal prostate cancer and other-cause mortality.[208] Study subjects were men aged 50-64 years (706 cases, 645 controls) from King County, Washington, who participated in a previous study of prostate cancer risk. Cases were men were diagnosed with prostate cancer from 1993 to 1996 and followed for vital status through June 2007. Controls were men without a self-reported history of prostate cancer and frequency age-matched to cases. Screening was defined on the basis of self-report of one or more PSA and/or DRE tests done during a checkup within the 5-year period prior to diagnosis or reference date for the case. The investigators examined two endpoints, prostate cancer as the underlying cause of death and death from any other cause. Among cases, men who reported a PSA or DRE within the 5-year period prior to diagnosis were significantly more likely to have been diagnosed with localized (84%) or regional disease (80%) compared with men diagnosed with distant metastases (54%). Further, controls were significantly more likely to have had one or more PSA and/or DRE screening tests within the 5-year period compared with men with fatal prostate cancer. After adjusting for age, race, first-degree family history of prostate cancer, education and co-morbid conditions, there were 62% fewer deaths from prostate cancer in the control group compared with the case group (95% CI 0.19-0.77). The investigators observed no association between PSA and/or DRE screening and other-cause mortality (OR 1.02; 95% CI 0.51-2.02).[208]

Ultimately, a definitive answer to the fundamental question of the efficacy of prostate cancer screening in the reduction of prostate cancer mortality requires evidence from a prospective randomized controlled trial, not only to control for known biases that can influence the findings in observational studies, but also to provide persuasive evidence for policy makers. Two large randomized trials of prostate cancer screening are also underway. The ERSPC trial is being conducted in seven European countries, and the United States NCI's PLCO trial is studying multimodality screening in men and women at ten locations in the United States.[187,189,209,210] The ERSPC and PLCO trials have entered into collaboration with the common goal of "sound and efficient evaluation of the screening programs."[211] The collaboration also provides an opportunity to increase statistical power, and carry out subgroup analysis that might not be possible in a smaller study.[211]

The discussion thus far has focused on the mechanics of screening, ie, the relative accuracy of the various frontline screening tests to detect prostate cancer at an early stage, and study designs that provide varying degrees of measurable confidence in outcomes that suggest a benefit, or lack thereof, from screening. One of the most fundamental questions related to prostate cancer screening is whether treatment is necessary and effective in early prostate cancer. In a study in Sweden, symptomatic men with localized prostate cancer (UICC stage T1b, T1c, or T2) were randomized to receive either radical prostatectomy or watchful waiting.[212] After an average 6.2 years of follow-up, there was a statistically significant difference in the rate of distant metastases (relative hazard 0.63, 95% CI 0.41-0.96), and disease-specific mortality (relative hazard 0.50, 95% CI 0.27-0.91) in the group randomized to radical treatment compared with the group randomized to watchful waiting. In an accompanying editorial, Walsh[213] applauded the results, and claimed that they were the first concrete evidence to answer Whitmore's often cited and fundamental question, "Is cure necessary in those in whom it may be possible, and is cure possible in those in whom it is necessary?"[214] However, Walsh also noted that while these results answered a fundamental question about the whether or not treatment reduced prostate cancer mortality, men still will be well served by careful consideration of treatment options based on tumor characteristics and expected longevity.[213]

Screening Recommendations

Over the years there has been considerable confusion about general guidelines related to prostate cancer screening in men at average and higher risk. This confusion has arisen due to different wording in the guidelines that distinguish between recommendations for population-based screening vs individualized decisions about testing for early detection. Further, in some cases advice has been vague with respect to the physician's responsibility to either initiate conversations about testing or simply be prepared to discuss testing if the patient raises the issue. Finally, it is also the case that a considerable volume of testing may take place in response to generalized symptoms related to voiding, etc., which increase in prevalence of testing with increasing age.[215] Although inferential evidence suggests a benefit from testing for early detection, the general state of evidence is insufficient to recommend for or against screening for prostate cancer with PSA and DRE, or to determine if benefits outweigh harms. Thus, the American Cancer Society, The United States Preventive Services Task Force The American Academy of Family Physicians, the American College of Physicians-American Society of Internal Medicine, the American Medical Association, and the American Urologic Association recommend that for men age 50 and older, and men at higher risk for prostate cancer, clinicians (1) discuss with patients the potential benefits and possible harms associated with PSA screening; (2) consider patient preferences; and (3) individualize the decision to screen (Table 34-2).[83,216-220] Both the ACS and American Urologic Association provide some additional guidance to help clinicians and men make informed decisions. For men at higher risk, including men of African descent (specifically, sub-Saharan African descent) and men with a first-degree relative diagnosed at a younger age, these discussion should begin at age 45.[221] Men at even higher risk of prostate cancer due to multiple first-degree relatives diagnosed with prostate cancer at an early age could have this discussion about testing at age 40. Discovery of genetic markers of prostate cancer risk may further refine the targeting of populations that may benefit most from screening interventions.[222] When genetic tests become available, it will be important to address which individuals are most suited for testing and how they are to be identified. In each instance, subsequent testing would depend on initial PSA results. In addition, these recommendations do not bypass the general recommendation related to informing patients about the potential benefits and possible harms of PSA screening as well as considering patient preferences.

While no upper age limit has been established after which PSA testing is not effective, there is some evidence that men with less than a 10-year life expectancy are unlikely to gain years of life from early detection, because of the long natural history of untreated localized prostate cancer and competing causes of death.[192,223] Thus, a significant proportion of men over the age of 70 are reaching an age when further PSA testing may not be beneficial in terms of life extension and when treatment may result in a net decrease in the quality of life. In 2008, the USPSTF recommended against testing for early prostate cancer detection in men 75 years and older.[218] Algorithms for estimating life expectancy and the likelihood of benefiting from preventive care have been proposed by Walter and Covinsky.[224] The implications from their estimates of projected longevity by age in the context of co-morbidity indicate that chronological age is a poor stand-alone measure for making determinations about whether or not an individual may benefit from cancer screening.

Lung Cancer

Lung cancer is the most common cause of cancer death in the United States and a leading and increasing cause of cancer mortality in other nations. Survival from lung cancer is very dependent on tumor size, even within stage groups. Compared with other cancers diagnosed at a localized stage, 5-year survival from lung cancer is significantly poorer (49.5%), while survival for regional (20.6%) and distant disease (2.8%) is very poor.[17]

Screening and Diagnostic Methods

The available technologies for detecting occult lung cancer include imaging modalities and cytologic and molecular evaluations of lung sputum. Chest x-ray has some, although likely limited, potential as a screening tool, especially in comparison with new imaging technologies

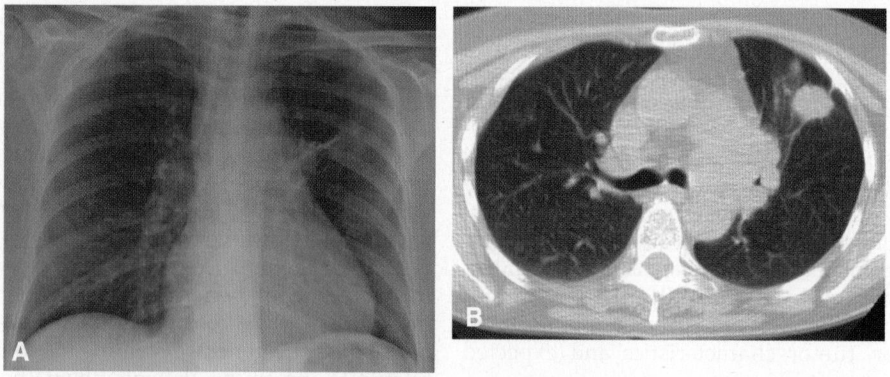

Figure 34-14 (A) Chest radiograph shows a 2-cm left upper lobe cancer. This is the median size of tumors detected in the Mayo Lung Project screening study initiated in 1971. **(B)** CT scan of the same left upper lobe cancer. *Source*: Courtesy of David Yankelevitz, M.D., New York-Presbyterian Hospital-Weill Cornell Medical Center, New York, NY.

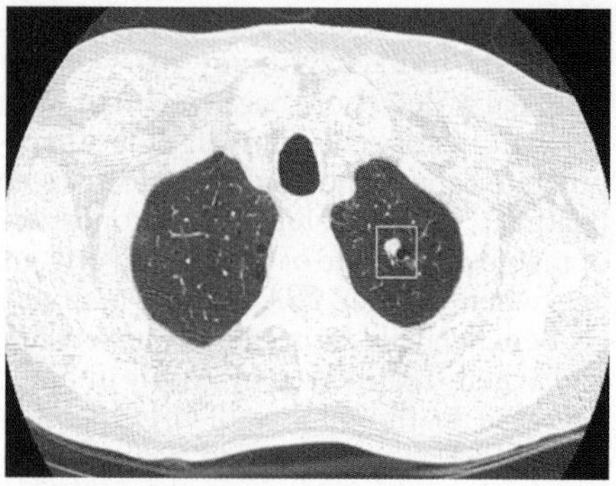

Figure 34-15 CT screen detected 7-mm left upper lobe cancer. This is the median size for cancers detected with CT screening. *Source*: Courtesy of David Yankelevitz, M.D., New York-Presbyterian Hospital-Weill Cornell Medical Center, New York, NY.

that achieve higher resolution (Figs. 34-14 and 34-15). With conventional chest x-ray, two images are normally taken: a posterior-anterior view and a lateral view. The sensitivity of chest x-rays is dependent on the size and location of the lesion, the quality assurance factors related to image quality, and the skill of the interpreting physician.[225] Failure to detect lesions at a favorable, or even larger, size can occur because the lesions can be obscured by the mediastinum and other aspects of chest structure, or as commonly occurs, due to errors in perception on the part of the interpreter.[226] To date, trials of lung cancer screening with chest x-ray have not shown sufficient evidence to conclude that chest x-ray is an effective screening tool,[227] although due to prior study limitations its potential still is being evaluated in two United States trials, one large prospective randomized trial where the experimental arm was invited to several rounds of screening compared with a control group that received usual care, and another more recently initiated prospective randomized trial that compares chest x-ray with low-dose spiral CT.[228,229]

Low-dose computed tomography (CT)—ie, spiral or helical CT—produces multiple images of the lung conventionally in 5-mm multiplanar slices that can produce a three-dimensional display of the lung. Low-dose CT is more sensitive than chest x-ray in the detection of small pulmonary nodules, is commonly used in diagnostic studies, and is regarded as having the greatest potential for early detection of lung malignancies.[230,231] Due to the higher resolution and the ability to image nodules under 1 cm in size, the high proportion of individuals undergoing screening will require short-term follow-up, which has led to concerted efforts to develop protocols for triaging those cases with clear malignant potential for further evaluation.[232]

Sputum cytology was believed to have potential for the early detection of lung cancer, but it showed little added advantage over chest x-ray in the NCI cooperative trials and was not associated with any reduction in deaths from lung cancer. However, further attempts to identify molecular markers from sputum associated with elevated risk or malignancy, as well as the application of autofluorescence bronchoscopy and positron emission tomography (PET), are potentially valuable new directions in the early detection of lung cancer.[233,234]

In the 1970s and 1980s four prospective trials of lung cancer screening were carried out, using combinations of chest x-ray and sputum cytology.[235-239] None of these studies showed a significant reduction in lung cancer mortality in the experimental groups associated with an invitation to screening, although some results were suggestive of a survival benefit.[240,241] While results of prospective trials were disappointing in the presence of such significant disease burden, these trials also were methodologically limited at inception in their ability to demonstrate a benefit from screening.[225] Although none of the studies showed fewer deaths in the experimental group compared with the control group, none of the studies compared disease outcome in a group offered screening with a group not invited to screening. In each of the trials, there was an element of early detection intervention in the control group. Further, chest radiography alone and in combination with sputum cytology improved the stage of diagnosis and was associated with more favorable survival, which has also been observed in case-finding series. In spite of limitations in study design and paradoxical findings in RCTs and case-finding series, for many years it has been widely accepted that lung cancer screening is not effective, whereas recent reevaluation of the trial data has led to the conclusion that these studies are an insufficient basis for recommending for or against lung cancer screening.[242,243]

From a policy basis, the net effect is the same, ie, population based screening for lung cancer cannot be endorsed; at this time however, the enormity of the disease burden in long-term smokers, both current and former, has kept interest alive in the possibility that an early detection strategy might eventually be identified that would satisfy conventional criteria required to endorse screening. In fact, based on concerns about a long list of shortcomings in the methodologies of the early trials, the NCI included randomization to receive chest x-ray screening in the PLCO trial that began in 1992. In the intervention group, current and former smokers received a baseline chest x-ray at the initial visit and then chest x-ray annually for 3 years. Never smokers also received a chest x-ray at study entry, and then annually for 2 years. Current or former smokers and never smokers in this arm received single-view posterior-anterior chest radiograph. At the initial screening examination, ~9% of adults screened had positive findings, with the highest positivity rates recorded among older adults with the greatest exposure to tobacco smoke. Among the 5991 adults with suspicious findings, 206 (3.4%) underwent biopsy, and 126 were diagnosed with lung cancer (PPV1 = 2.1%; PPV2 = 61.2%), for a detection rate of 1.9 lung cancers per 1000 screening examinations overall. Among current smokers the detection rate was 6.3 per 1000 screening examinations, and among former smokers the detection rate was 4.9 per 1000 screening examinations. Forty-four percent of lung cancers diagnosed at the initial screening examination were stage one, non-small cell lung cancers.[244]

Newer imaging technology for the early detection of lung cancer appears to be more promising than conventional chest x-rays. The Early Lung Cancer Action Project (ELCAP) is an observational study that was designed to evaluate lung cancer screening with low-radiation-dose CT.[245] In a report of the baseline experience with 1000 volunteers aged 60 and over with a smoking history of at least 10 pack-years and who would be acceptable candidates for thoracic surgery, low-dose CT significantly outperformed conventional chest x-ray in the detection of small pulmonary nodules. Low-dose CT identified 233 participants with noncalcified nodules and 27 malignancies, of which 26 were resectable and 23 were stage 1 disease. In contrast, conventional chest x-ray identified 68 noncalcified nodules, of which seven were malignant and four were diagnosed as stage 1 disease. Workup of positive CT results was based on the size of the nodule and change observed on repeat screening. Based on the average tumor size in the ELCAP study, the authors projected a significantly better 5-year survival for cases diagnosed using low-dose CT.[245]

The growing evidence that spiral CT may provide for a successful early detection strategy for adults at high risk for lung cancer, the NCI launched the National Lung Screening Trial (NLST) in September 2002.[229,246] The trial has enrolled 50,000 current and former smokers aged 55-74 who were randomized to an experimental group that were invited to receive annual spiral CT or a control group that were invited to receive annual chest x-ray. Study participants were scheduled to undergo three rounds of annual screening, and trial results are anticipated before 2010.[229]

A number of trials also were initiated in Europe and the two largest are still underway.[247] The Dutch-Belgian randomized CT lung screening trial (NELSON) is a prospective trial to determine whether 16-detector multislice computed tomography screening will decrease lung cancer mortality compared with no screening. The study was initiated in 2004, and is projected to be completed in 2015. The study population is mostly men aged 50-75 years who were current and former smokers (quit time ≤10 years ago) who smoked >15 cigarettes/day during 25+ years or >10 cigarettes/day during 30 + years. The investigators determined that a study with 17,300 subjects randomized to receive three rounds of annual screening and 27,900 controls would be needed to have 80% power to show a 20-25% lung cancer mortality reduction 10 years after randomization.[248] When pooling with Danish trial data (n = ~4000) the NELSON is the only prospective randomized trial without any screening in the control group, and is expected to have 80% power to show a lung cancer mortality reduction of at least 25% 10 years after randomization. Two trials are underway in Italy—the ITALUNG trial and the DANTE trial. In the ITALUNG trial, current or former smokers aged 55-69 years with 20+ pack/years were randomized in an active arm (n = 1613) invited to undergo a low-dose CT annually for 4 years and a control arm (n = 1593) receiving no invitation to screening.[249] Subjects in control (n = 1593) and active arm were balanced for age, gender, and smoking history. At baseline screening, 426 (30.3%) had positive test results and 21 lung cancers (prevalence = 1.5%) were detected. Among the 18 non-small cell lung cancers, 10 were stage I. The DANTE trial is randomized trial comparing screening for lung cancer with annual spiral CT versus a yearly clinical review. Study subjects are males aged 60-74 years old with a 20+ pack-years smoking history. Both study (n = 1276) and control (n = 1196) groups received a baseline chest x-rays (CXR) and sputum cytology upon accrual. Subjects randomized in the spiral CT arm received a spiral CT scan at baseline, and then were invited to yearly screening for the next 4 years; control subjects received a yearly clinical examination over the same period. Twenty-eight lung cancers were diagnosed in the group randomized to undergo spiral CT screening (13 lung cancers were visible on baseline chest x-ray). Among all lung cancers identified on baseline, 57% were stage 1, and 68% were resectable. In the control group, only eight cancers were detected, of which four were stage 1, and six were resectable.[250] While the ITALUNG and DANTE trials are underpowered to answer the question of efficacy of screening, the investigators of the European trials have indicated an intent to explore data pooling.[251]

Screening Recommendations

At this time, no organization recommends routine screening for lung cancer among the general adult population or among individuals who are at higher risk due to prolonged exposure to tobacco smoke or occupational exposures.[83,243] However, today, a growing number of institutions and facilities are promoting CT screening to asymptomatic individuals at risk for lung cancer, and some have argued that the current evidence is sufficient to promote screening to individuals at significant risk of lung cancer.[252] With greater interest in spiral CT testing among health-care providers and individuals at higher risk, the ACS determined that updated guidance about early lung cancer detection was needed, insofar as many adults at elevated risk seek testing for early lung cancer detection. Further, given the high rate of positive results that occur with CT screening for lung cancer and the complexity of the algorithm for working up small nodules,[253] there is reason to be concerned about broad dissemination of lung screening outside of experienced, multispecialty settings and prior to validation of this new technology.[83] The ACS recommends that individuals who seek testing for early lung cancer detection should be informed about what is currently known about the benefits, limitations, and risks associated with conventional and emerging early detection technologies, as well as the associated diagnostic procedures and treatment. Given the complexity of diagnostic and follow-up algorithms associated with positive test results, the ACS discourages testing in a setting that is not linked to multidisciplinary specialty groups for diagnosis and follow-up. Individuals who choose to undergo testing should have access to testing and follow-up that meets state-of-the-art standards, with informed decision making at every step of an ongoing process. The route to testing should be through an individual's primary care physician who can assist patients to understand their risks and reach informed decisions about testing and provide support if early detection tests are positive. If an individual seeks testing and does not have a referral from a primary care provider, the radiologist who provides testing is obliged to provide information about benefits, risks, and limitations of testing as described earlier, and must become the individual's physician of record until proper alternative care arrangements can be made. Individuals who are current smokers also should be informed that the more immediate preventive health priority is the elimination of tobacco use altogether, since smoking cessation offers the surest route at this time to reducing the risk of premature mortality from lung cancer.[254]

Testicular Cancer

Testicular cancer is relatively uncommon, although it is the most common cancer diagnosed in young men. Five-year survival for localized and regional disease is 99.3% and 95.7%, respectively, while survival for distant disease is still comparatively very good at 71%.[17]

Screening and Diagnostic Methods

There are no proven tests available to detect testicular cancer at an asymptomatic stage. Testicular cancer is generally detected through patient self-detection and physician palpation. Suspicious masses may be further evaluated through ultrasonography and biopsy.

There have been no randomized trials of the efficacy of testicular examination, either by a physician or by individuals. However, treatment of testicular cancer at an early stage has advantages in that survival is somewhat better and there is a reduced likelihood of undergoing toxic treatment or major surgery.[255] Due to the lack of an adequate evidence base to estimate the balance of benefits and harms associated with screening or self-examinations, no organization recommends either routine testicular self-examination, or examination of the testicles for lumps or nodules or any change in the size, shape, or consistency of the testes.[256] What is likely to offer greater advantage is health education to promote the seeking of medical care promptly, since patient delay after becoming aware of a testicular abnormality has been associated with poorer survival.[257] Khadra and colleagues investigated the degree to which a sample of men aged 18-50 in London were aware of testicular cancer and practiced testicular self-examination (TSE).[258] While ~90% of men reported that they had heard of testicular cancer, only one in four knew the age range most commonly affected, and only about 22% of respondents reported practicing monthly TSE. Similar findings have been reported by Ward et al.[259]

The issue of regular TSE by asymptomatic men is somewhat controversial. Self-palpation of the testes is simple and low cost, but has low specificity and predictive value, and performance of periodic self-examination is infrequent even by men educated about the technique.[260,261] Since self-examinations or clinical examinations result in additional provider encounters to have suspicious findings evaluated (nearly all of which, ultimately, are not cancer), false alarms do burden the health-care system and can be costly. Geczi and colleagues recently evaluated the impact of a 3-year program of public education about testicular cancer, TSE, and the importance of responding promptly to symptoms.[262] Based on the low yield of cancers detected and the high false-positive rate, the investigators concluded that the evidence did not justify screening programs for young men, and instead, efforts should focus on increased awareness for the population at risk and health-care professionals that typically see men in the commonly affected age group.

Screening Recommendations

No organization recommends routine screening for testicular cancer in average-risk men. The American Academy of Family Physicians recommends palpation of the testicles for men aged 13-39 who fall into a higher-risk group due to a history of cryptorchidism, orchiopexy, or testicular atrophy.[263] The USPSTF recommends against routine screening for testicular cancer in asymptomatic adolescent and adult males.[256]

Endometrial Cancer

Endometrial cancer is the most common malignancy diagnosed in women in the United States Five-year survival for localized disease is 95.5%, while survival for regional disease and distant metastases are 67.5% and 23.6, respectively. In the United States most endometrial cancer is diagnosed while still localized, but approximately one in four cases is advanced at the time of diagnosis.

Screening and Diagnostic Methods

Endometrial cancer may be detected through a variety of means; however, the efficacy of screening for endometrial cancer has never been evaluated in a prospective randomized trial. The Pap test may fortuitously identify endometrial abnormalities, but it is too insensitive to be used as a screening technique for detection of endometrial cancer.[264] Today, the endometrial biopsy is the most common technique used to obtain endometrial tissue, and evaluation of endometrial histology has been the gold standard of determining the status of the endometrium.[265] More recently, interest in screening for endometrial cancer with endometrial biopsy and transvaginal ultrasonography (TVU) has been stimulated due to increased risk of endometrial cancer in women at elevated risk for breast cancer who are taking tamoxifen for chemoprevention.[266] However, two studies of screening asymptomatic women for endometrial cancer with endometrial biopsy and transvaginal ultrasound reported disappointing results,[267,268] and each reported harms associated with diagnostic assessments, including unnecessary biopsies and in some cases uterine perforations. Recently, the ACS updated screening recommendations for endometrial cancer and concluded that a risk-based approach was reasonable only for women at high risk for endometrial cancer.[83] The population defined as at high risk for endometrial cancer includes women known to carry HNPCC-associated mutations (Lynch syndrome), women who appear to have a substantial likelihood of being a mutation carrier based on the presence of known mutation carriers in the family, and women from families with an autosomal dominant predisposition to colon cancer in the absence of genetic testing results.[269]

Screening Recommendations

At this time, no organization recommends routine screening for endometrial cancer in average-risk women. The ACS recommends at the time of menopause, all women should be informed about the risks and symptoms of endometrial cancer and strongly encouraged to report any unexpected bleeding or spotting to their physician. Women who are known or suspected of having Lynch syndrome should be offered endometrial screening annually beginning at age 35. Due to the absence of strong scientific evidence supporting the value of this recommendation, informed decision making following a discussion of options, including benefits, risks, and limitations of testing, is appropriate.[83]

Ovarian Cancer

Ovarian cancer has the highest mortality rate of all gynecologic cancers and it accounts for 6% of all cancer deaths in women in the United States About 46% of all ovarian cancer patients survive 5 years after diagnosis but prognosis for survival is largely dependent upon the extent of disease at diagnosis. Women diagnosed with local disease experience a 92.7% 5-year survival rate, while women with distant disease have only a 30.6% 5-year survival. Unfortunately, most women with ovarian cancer present with symptoms and only 19% of patients are diagnosed with localized disease.[17]

Screening and Diagnostic Methods

Screening tests for ovarian cancer include CA-125 antigen as a tumor marker, transvaginal ultrasound (TVU), and potentially bioinformatic analysis of proteomic patterns. CA-125 and TVU each has been evaluated as a stand-alone test, as a single test with serial measurements, and in combination. The sensitivity and specificity of pelvic examination for the detection of ovarian cancer are imprecisely defined but certainly poor, and thus cannot be regarded as a screening method. However, recent evaluations into presenting symptoms suggest that a more favorable diagnosis may be possible in some cases if early symptoms are evaluated. Goff and colleagues cited the prevailing belief that symptoms are not typically present until ovarian cancer has reached an advanced stage.[270] These symptoms include complaints of abdominal, pelvic, and back pain, bloating, and swelling, and urinary symptoms. While reports of symptoms are often dismissed as too nonspecific to evaluate, in a prospective case-control study, Goff et al. compared self-reported symptoms among ovarian cancer patients to a control group consisting of women seeking care in primary care clinics. Comparing cases to controls, significantly elevated odds were observed for abdominal size, bloating, urinary urgency, and pelvic pain. The authors concluded that the distinguishing features from the controls were rapid onset, frequency, and severity and that evidence supported that these symptoms were often present while the disease was still in an early, more curable stage.[270] While symptom reports have often been dismissed as recall bias, Smith and colleagues linked Medicare claims data to the California Surveillance, Epidemiology, and End Results data base to compare the prevalence of rates of symptom-related diagnoses and procedure codes during 3-month periods up to 36 months before diagnosis of ovarian cancer. Diagnoses and procedure codes were compared for 1985 women with ovarian cancer, 6024 women with localized breast cancer, and 10,941 age-matched, Medicare-enrolled women without cancer. Four target symptoms groups were evaluated: abdominal pain, swelling, gastrointestinal symptoms, and pelvic pain. Compared with cancer-free controls or breast cancer patients, ovarian cancer patients had elevated odds for all four symptom groups >6 months prior to diagnosis, and were more likely to have had abdominal imaging and gastrointestinal procedures than pelvic imaging or CA-125 testing.[271]

CA-125 ■ The most extensively studied ovarian cancer serum marker is CA-125. CA-125 is a tumor-associated antigen, and its main use is for surveillance in women who have already undergone surgery to remove an epithelial ovarian cancer.[272] The original CA-125 clinical assay only utilized the OC125 monoclonal antibody, whereas the current CA-125 II assay utilizes both the OC125 and MC11 antibodies.[273] CA-125 levels greater than 30-35 U/mL are regarded as abnormal. CA-125 levels are increased in many women with ovarian cancer, but noncancerous diseases of the ovaries can also increase the blood levels of CA-125.[274] Additionally, although CA-125 is elevated in large majority of advanced ovarian cancers, only half of early ovarian cancers produce enough CA-125 to cause a positive test.[275,276] Moreover, CA-125 levels can be influenced by the presence of other cancers, race/ethnicity, age, ever use of hormones, smoking status, and history of breast cancer.[273,277] Retrospective analysis has shown that patients with ovarian cancer had rising levels of CA-125 within the normal range,[278] which investigators have incorporated into clinical risk stratification algorithms, but even sequential measures are regarded as too insensitive to be used as a stand-alone test.[279]

Ultrasonography ■ Abdominal ultrasonography has been used in ovarian cancer screening with poor results, owing to low specificity.[280] TVU, however, is capable of detecting small ovarian masses and may distinguish some benign masses from some malignant adnexal masses. Even this more proximal examination, however, still only poorly predicts that masses are cancers and that are due to benign diseases of the ovary. As an independent test, ultrasound has shown poor performance in the detection of ovarian cancer in average- or high-risk women.[281] Color Doppler ultrasonography was believed to hold some promise for differentiating benign from malignant masses due to the influence of neovascularity on tumor features, but studies to date have not shown that the technology improves diagnostic accuracy.[282] At present, current data are insufficient to suggest that TVU or other imaging modalities are useful as stand-alone screening tools in average-risk asymptomatic women.

Combination CA-125 and Ultrasound ■ While neither CA-125 nor TVU are sufficiently accurate to be used as stand-alone screening tools, the use of both tests in tandem has shown improved performance compared with either test alone. Jabobs and colleagues assessed the performance of serial CA-125 and ultrasound in 22,000 postmenopausal women aged 45 years and older.[283] Three hundred forty five a CA-125>30 U/mL wew refered to ultrasound, and 41 also had positive ultrasound tests. Of 19 cancers detected, 11 were associated with elevated CA-125 and ultrasound. Eight women with negative CA-125 presented as interval cancers. In a report of baseline screening results in the PLCO, Buys et al. reported that among ~29,816 women who received at least one of the two tests, 1338 (4.7%) had a positive TVU, and 402 (1.4%) women had an elevated CA-125. The PPV for invasive ovarian cancer was 3.7% for an abnormal CA-125, 1.0% for an abnormal TVU, and 23.5% if both tests were abnormal. In an effort to further improve the predictive value of the two tests, the predictive value of changes in CA-125 levels from prospectively collected measurements has been investigated. Earlier findings had shown that preclinical CA-125 levels rose steadily in patients subsequently diagnosed with ovarian cancer, whereas stable levels, even if somewhat elevated, were not predictive of malignancy. In an effort to create a risk of ovarian cancer algorithm (ROC), Skates et al. evaluated CA-125 measurements from 9233 postmenopausal, average-risk women who had two or more serial samples with a median follow-up of 6.8 years.[284] Thus, this was a sample that excluded prevalent cases with CA-125 levels that exceed a threshold level for referral for diagnostic evaluation. The analysis used a Bayesian approach to compare the patient's serial measurements to the CA-125 patterns of known ovarian cancer patients at various levels of specificity. With a preset PPV of 2% and specificity of 98%, the ROC algorithm improved sensitivity for preclinical disease from 62% for the fixed cutoff CA-125 to 86%.[284] A PPV of 2% is based on the intent to use ultrasound as a secondary screening test. The algorithm is being used in the U.K. Collaborative Trial of Ovarian Cancer Screening (UKCTOCS), and by the United States Cancer Genetics Network for a pilot study for a trial of screening women at high risk for ovarian cancer.[280]

Proteomic Patterns ■ Investigators have applied intensive pattern recognition algorithms to identify a key subset of peptides that discriminate ovarian cancer cases from control subjects. After this algorithm was developed in "training" data, it was applied to the analysis of serum samples from 116 patients whose ovary cancer status was unknown to the investigators. They correctly identified all 50 patients with ovary cancer including 18 with localized disease yielding a sensitivity of 100%. Specificity was 95% having correctly classified 63 of 66 noncancer subjects. While encouraging, the suitability of this approach for general screening of women at risk has not yet been studied and, as is often the case, results achieved in select clinical series have yet to be duplicated in asymptomatic women.[285] In fact, a move to market a commercial test in 2003 was delayed by the United States FDA due to concerns about reliability and reproducibility.[286,287] At this time, the potential for either a stand-alone or adjunctive proteomic test for ovarian cancer screening is regarded as promising, but remains unrealized due to a number of enduring challenges that are common to the distance between promising early laboratory discoveries and population-based applications. First, if a test has been successful in identifying changes in the proteome in clinically confirmed cases, will it be as successful in identifying small changes associated with early stage cancer? Alternatively, could the test be overly sensitive, and identify a large number of cases that are nonprogressive among a smaller number that will progress? Second, can a test be developed that is reproducible within and between laboratories? Third, since clinical investigations often are conducted on enriched populations, there is a critical need to rule out the influence of non-disease-related factors on the proteomic signatures that could result in different performance in different population subgroups. To address these questions, very large and expensive studies will be required to have measurable confidence in a test that can be used in an average-risk population.[280]

Much of the evidence concerning the effectiveness of ovarian cancer screening in average- and high-risk women has come from nonrandomized cohort studies and pilot randomized controlled studies using TVU, CA-125, or a combination of the tests.[278,283,288-290] The common features of these investigations have been the limited sensitivity of CA-125 or ultrasound (abdominal or transvaginal) alone as a screening tool at an acceptable level of specificity, and the poor predictive value of a positive test. An emphasis on high specificity is important because laparoscopy or laparotomy, or both, is required to rule out the presence of ovarian cancer when either or both tests are positive. Over time, the development of multimodal approaches that include the combination of CA-125, ROC CA-125 algorithms, and the application of imaging has resulted in protocols that are now being evaluated in prospective randomized controlled trials. The PLCO trial (described earlier) recruited 78,237 women ages 55-74, of which 39,115 were randomized to be offered lung, colorectal, and ovarian cancers screening. Women were given a baseline CA-125 and TVU, and then were offered three additional annual rounds of TVU and five additional annual rounds of CA-125. The primary endpoint of the study is ovarian cancer mortality.[291,292] The UKCTOCS was initiated in 2001 and enrolled 200,000 average-risk, postmenopausal women aged 50-74 to be randomized to one of three groups: (1) a control group that will receive usual care (n = 100,000); (2) a group that will undergo annual multimodal screening with serum CA-125 as the primary test and CA-125 and ultrasound as the secondary test (n = 50,000); and (3) a group that will undergo annual ultrasound screening as the primary test and repeat ultrasound in 6-8 weeks as the secondary test (n = 50,000). Women in the experimental groups will undergo annual testing for 7 years. The primary endpoint of the trial is ovarian cancer mortality, with secondary objectives focused on the evaluation of alternative screening strategies, the determination of the feasibility and costs of screening for ovarian cancer, and an attempt to measure harms associated with screening.[293,294] Results of the UKCTOCS are expected in 2011. Several trials targeting women at high risk for ovarian cancer are also underway.[280]

Screening Recommendations

Although ovarian cancer clearly meets disease burden criteria in terms of suitability as a target for screening interventions at this time there are no screening interventions with sufficient sensitivity and specificity for use in the general population at risk of ovarian cancer. Neither the ACS or the USPSTF recommend ovarian cancer screening in average-risk women, and, in fact, the USPSTF specifically recommends against screening for ovarian cancer in average-risk women.[295] In 1994, a National Institutes of Health Consensus Panel concluded that all women should have a comprehensive family history taken, and that women with two or more first-degree relatives should be offered counseling about their ovarian cancer risk by a gynecologic oncologist (or other specialist qualified to evaluate family history and discuss hereditary cancer risks) since these women have a 3% chance of being positive for an ovarian cancer hereditary syndrome. Women with a known hereditary ovarian cancer syndrome, such as mutations on *BRCA1* and *BRCA2*, including breast-ovarian cancer syndrome, site-specific ovarian cancer syndrome, and HNPCC, should receive annual rectovaginal pelvic examinations, CA-125 determinations, and transvaginal ultrasonography until childbearing is completed or at least until age 35, at which time prophylactic bilateral oophorectomy is recommended.[296] Although women with these hereditary syndromes are estimated to represent only 0.05% of the female population, they have a 40% estimated lifetime risk of ovarian cancer.

Melanoma and Nonmelanoma Skin Cancer

Melanoma and nonmelanoma skin cancers together are the most common cancers, accounting for nearly half of all malignancies. Deaths from nonmelanoma skin cancer are rare, although significant morbidity can result from delay in diagnosis and treatment. Five-year survival of melanoma is very good when it is diagnosed while still localized (98.7%), and poor (15.5%) when distant metastases are present.[17]

Screening and Diagnostic Methods

Interest in the potential for screening for melanoma and nonmelanoma skin cancers has increased in recent years because the global incidence of skin cancers has been increasing.[297] The principle approach to detecting skin cancers early in their natural history is skin examinations, done either by a clinician or self-examinations. Skin cancer screening involves a 2- to 3-min visual inspection of the patient's entire body, including the scalp, hands, and feet. It also may involve questions to the patient regarding sun exposure, sun protection, and family history. A total examination of the skin is preferable to examining only the sunlight-exposed areas of the body because skin cancers often occur at anatomic sites that are not directly exposed to sources of risk. Evaluation of suspicious areas for melanoma has traditionally emphasized morphologic features and change over time, summarized as an ABCD algorithm that emphasizes asymmetry [A] of the lesion, uneven borders [B], changes in color [C], and changes in diameter [D].[298,299] A Cochrane Review of these criteria endorsed the addition of an "E" category—"evolving"—to emphasize the importance of change over time in the features of the lesion.[298] While the ABCD pattern describes the features that increase the probability of a malignant lesion, it appears most dermatologists rely on the overall pattern of appearance ("ugly duckling sign") versus a stepwise assessment of features.[300]

Self-examination of the skin has been evaluated for its role in the detection of melanoma at an earlier stage, both among individuals at higher risk for melanoma, and among melanoma patients, who are at elevated risk for a diagnosis of subsequent melanoma. Berwick and colleagues conducted a population-based, case-control study to examine whether detection of melanoma through skin self-examination was associated with either melanoma mortality or advanced disease. The study population consisted of 650 newly diagnosed melanoma patients and 549 controls matched for age and sex. Subjects were followed for 5 years, during which time 110 deaths from melanoma were identified. Skin self-examination was practiced by only 15% of subjects, but was associated with 34% reduction in melanoma incidence, a 42% reduction in the risk of being diagnosed with advanced disease, and a 63% reduction in death from melanoma; although due to the short duration of follow-up the magnitude of the mortality reduction could be influenced by lead-time bias.[301] In an accompanying editorial, Elwood was cautiously optimistic about these findings, but highlighted a number of inherent limitations in the case-control design, and noted in particular that the finding of a lower odds of incidence in the group practicing skin self-examination was paradoxical without collateral data on biopsy for the removal of precursor lesions prior to diagnosis with melanoma.[302] Hiatt and colleagues observed a significant increase in the rate of melanoma and skin biopsies associated with increased surveillance among employees at the Lawrence Livermore National Laboratory.[303] In an evaluation of the same cohort, Oliveria et al. observed that knowledge about melanoma and awareness of skin changes was associated with a significantly lower likelihood of delay in diagnosis and thinner lesions.[304]

In an effort to promote skin self-examination, Oliveria and colleagues evaluated the influence of a nurse-based intervention built around a photobook of the subject's whole body photographs accompanied by instruction in skin self-examination. The investigators concluded that the instruction and photobook was associated with a significant increase in reported skin self-examination in the follow-up period.[305] In New England, a randomized trial of monthly thorough skin self-examination was conducted to determine the effectiveness of a multicomponent intervention on performance of skin self-examination and outcome of skin surgeries. Among 1356 patients in primary care, the intervention group received instructional materials, counseling, and a follow-up phone call and letters. A control group received usual care and a dietary intervention. Medical records were examined to determine the occurrence of surgical procedures, and performance of skin self-examination was assessed by telephone interview. The authors observed that skin self-examination was increased in the intervention group compared with controls at 12 months (55% vs 35%, $p < 0.0001$), and a higher rate of skin surgeries in the first 6 months (8.0% vs 3.6%, $p = 0.0005$), but no difference in the 6-12-month period (3.9% vs 3.3%, $p = 0.5$).[306] The authors concluded that while self-examinations did result in an increase in biopsies, it was a short-term phenomenon.

Skin examinations by a health-care provider are uncommon in the U.S, although the practice is more common among dermatologists compared with primary care physicians.[307,308] Studies of high-risk populations report that patients routinely screened by dermatologists have mean tumor thicknesses of detected malignant melanoma that are thinner than that of historical or population-based controls.[309] The American Academy of Dermatology program of skin cancer screening has examined over 600,000 people of various risk categories between since 1985. In addition to the detection of over 35,000 nonmelanoma skin cancers, melanomas diagnosed by screening were more likely than historical controls to have lesions smaller than 1.5 mm.[310] The effectiveness of skin cancer screening may be increased if targeted to high-risk persons such as Caucasian patients older than age 20 with atypical mole syndrome or congenital melanocytic nevi, patients with specific phenotypic traits, or patients with a history of nonmelanoma skin cancer.[311]

In an update of an earlier USPSTF evidence review, Wolff et al. noted the continued lack of evidence to confidently address the question of screening efficacy, whether or not screening by primary care physicians or self-examinations accurately detects skin cancers, and whether or not screening or self-examinations detects melanomas or other skin cancers at an earlier stage.[312] Answers may come form a community-based randomized population trial of skin self-examination and examination by a clinician that is underway in Queensland Australia, with a primary outcome of melanoma mortality at study conclusion following 15 years of follow-up.[313]

Screening Recommendations

The ACS recommends an examination of the skin during the occasion of a periodic preventive health examination.[314] The American College of Preventive Medicine recommends periodic total cutaneous examinations for targeted populations at high risk for malignant melanoma.[315] Higher-risk groups include those with the following traits or conditions: Caucasian race, fair complexion, presence of pigmented lesions (dysplastic or atypical nevus), several large nondysplastic nevi, many small nevi, moderate freckling, or familial dysplastic nevus syndrome.[316,317] While recommending alertness to skin abnormalities, particularly in high-risk individuals, the USPSTF concluded that the evidence was insufficient to recommend for or against routine screening for skin cancer using a total-body skin examination for the early detection of cutaneous melanoma, basal cell cancer, or squamous cell skin cancer.[318]

Oral Cancer

Oral cancer is more common in men compared with women, and it occurs more frequently in African Americans compared with Caucasians. Incidence increases steadily with age until about age 65, when the rate levels off. Oral cancers diagnosed while still localized have 82% 5-year survival, but only 28% survival when diagnosed at an advanced stage. Only approximately one-third of oral cancers are diagnosed at a localized stage.[17]

Screening and Diagnostic Methods

Oral cancer occurs in a region of the body that is generally accessible to physical examination by the patient, the dentist, and the physician. Screening can be made more efficient by inspecting the high-risk sites where 90% of all squamous cell cancers arise: the floor of the mouth, the ventrolateral aspect of the tongue, and the soft-palate complex.[319] Leukoplakia and erythroplastic lesions are the earliest and most serious signs of squamous cell carcinoma. Symptoms include sores on the lip or the mouth, oral bleeding, persistent white or red patches in the mouth or on the gums, oral swelling and/or pain, sore throat, and difficulty swallowing. Although a number of new technological approaches to the detection of oral cancers are being evaluated and promoted, such as toluidine blue, brush cytology, tissue reflectance, and autofluorescence, none has been reliably shown to be superior to conventional oral examination.[320]

There is now significant evidence that visual inspection for oral premalignancies significantly reduces mortality from oral cancer in a high-risk population.[321] Using a cluster-randomized controlled trial design, Sankaranarayanan and colleagues randomized seven of 13 clusters in the Trivandrum district, Kerala, India to three rounds of oral visual inspection by trained health workers at 3-year intervals. Men and women aged 35 years and older were eligible to participate. In the intervention group, 87,655 (91%) were screened at least once; 63% of 5145 individuals who screened positive, complied with referral. There were 21% fewer oral cancer deaths in the intervention group compared with the control group (rate ratio = 0.79; 95% CI 0.51-1.22). Among male and female tobacco and alcohol users, there were 34% fewer oral cancer deaths in the intervention group compared with the control group (43% fewer oral cancer deaths in men).[321] The authors conclude that widespread application of visual oral examination has the potential to annually prevent 37,000 oral cancer deaths worldwide.

While some have advocated that an inspection of the oral cavity should be part of every physical examination in a dentist or physician's office,[322] the absence of a general recommendation for screening results in a low frequency of examinations. Further, evaluation of physician encounters by risk status has shown that groups at highest risk for oral cancers have a much lower frequency of physician and dental encounters than individuals at lower risk.[323] A simulation of various approaches to early detection of oral including general and targeted invitations and opportunistic screening in dental and general practitioner offices suggests that high-risk opportunistic screening may be the most cost-effective strategy.[324]

Screening Recommendations

At this time, no organization recommends routine screening for oral cancer, although the ACS recommends that on the occasion of a routine physical examination the oral cavity should be examined.[314] Insofar as oral cancer is easily detected and often curable in its early stages, recent evidence demonstrating the efficacy of screening for oral cancer will likely lead to renewed efforts to identify cost-effective strategies to identify an appropriate population for routine surveillance.

Conclusion

In the near term, the greatest potential for reducing deaths from cancer is through early detection. The adoption of healthier lifestyles, as well as risk identification and modification via genomics and proteomics, is believed to offer even greater potential in the long run, but at this time that potential is uncertain. However, it is also the case that the fullest benefit of applied early detection strategies remains unfulfilled in the United States and elsewhere due to limitations in access, insufficient resources, uneven quality, and lack of organized systems.[325-327] Screening under opportunistic conditions rather than through a system is inefficient at both the individual level and population level[326]; moreover, without a system, there is no readiness to implement any new early detection technology that could improve disease control. A comprehensive system of early detection potentially not only leads to high levels of participation but also can insure that all the elements of a program of early detection and intervention are highly competent, interrelated, and interdependent. A system has the potential not only to increase quality but also to reduce the volume of small errors that contribute to incremental erosion of efficiency, as well as the volume of gross failures that result in death when mortality is avoidable. While there are many practical barriers that must be overcome to establish true population-based screening programs, a system of organized screening holds the greatest potential to realize the benefits of reducing the incidence rate of advanced cancers, and subsequently avoiding premature mortality.

As outlined by Wilson and Junger, perhaps the most critical underpinning in the decision to implement screening policy is clear, unambiguous evidence in the efficacy of a screening test.[2] In this review of cancer screening, there are numerous examples of failures to promptly, or ever, conduct the necessary studies to determine whether or not screening for a particular cancer is efficacious, and properly consider the balance of benefits and harms. In general, failure to conduct these large trials typically is due to enormous costs and logistical requirements for these studies, which weighed against the opportunity costs leads national decision makers to either reject conducting the trial, or postponing decisions indefinitely. Ideally, new models of international cooperation in prevention and early detection trials could result in lower financial commitments per nation to support important studies, and faster accumulation of knowledge that can inform important public health policy decisions.[328]

Selected References

The complete reference list can be found at www.CANCERMEDICINE8.com

1. Morrison A. *Screening in Chronic Disease.* New York: Oxford University Press; 1992.
7. Schwartz LM, Woloshin S, Sox HC, et al. US women's attitudes to false positive mammography results and detection of ductal carcinoma in situ: cross sectional survey. *BMJ.* 2000;320(7250):1635–1640.
11. Fenton JJ, Cai Y, Weiss NS, et al. Delivery of cancer screening: how important is the preventive health examination? *Arch Intern Med.* 2007;167(6):580–585.
12. Duffy SW, Lynge E, Jonsson H, et al. Complexities in the estimation of overdiagnosis in breast cancer screening. *Br J Cancer.* 2008;99(7):1176–1178.
13. Cronin KA, Weed DL, Connor RJ, et al. Case-control studies of cancer screening: theory and practice. *J Natl Cancer Inst.* 1998;90(7):498–504.
16. Tabar L, Duffy SW, Yen M-F, et al. All-cause mortality among breast cancer patients in a screening trial: support for breast cancer mortality as an end point. *J Med Screen.* 2002;9:1–4.
19. Smith RA, Saslow D, Sawyer KA, et al. American Cancer Society guidelines for breast cancer screening: update 2003. *CA Cancer J Clin.* 2003;53(3):141–169.
20. Saslow D, Boates C, Burke W, et al. American Cancer Society guidelines for breast screening with MRI as an adjunct to mammography. *CA Cancer J Clin.* 2007;57(2):90–104 Available on line at http://caonline.amcancersoc.org.
24. Pisano ED, Hendrick RE, Yaffe MJ, et al. Diagnostic accuracy of digital versus film mammography: exploratory analysis of selected population subgroups in DMIST. *Radiology.* 2008;246(2):376–383.
29. Smith RA. Breast cancer screening among women younger than age 50: a current assessment of the issues. *CA Cancer J Clin.* 2000;50(5):312–336.
31. Humphrey LL, Helfand M, Chan BK, et al. Breast cancer screening: a summary of the evidence for the U.S. Preventive Services Task Force. *Ann Intern Med.* 2002;137 (5 Part 1):347–360.
32. Smith RA, Duffy SW, Gabe R, et al. The randomized trials of breast cancer screening: what have we learned? *Radiol Clin North Am.* 2004;42(5):793–806.
39. Organizing Committee and Collaborators. Breast cancer screening with mammography in women aged 40–49 Years. Report of the organizing oommittee and collaborators, Falun meeting, Falun, Sweden (21and 22 March, 1996). *Int J Cancer.* 1996;68:693–699.
42. Duffy SW, Day NE, Tabar L, et al. Markov models of breast tumor progression: some age-specific results. *J Natl Cancer Inst Monogr.* 1997;22:93–97.
46. Duffy S, Tabar L, Chen HH, et al. The impact of organized mammographic service screening on breast cancer mortality in seven Swedish counties. *Cancer.* 2002;95:458–469.
60. Thomas DB, Gao DL, Ray RM, et al. Randomized trial of breast self-examination in shanghai: final results. *J Natl Cancer Inst.* 2002;94(19):1445–1457.
61. Kearney AJ, Murray M. Evidence against breast self examination is not conclusive: what policymakers and health professionals need to know. *J Public Health Policy.* 2006;27(3):282–292.
83. Smith RA, von Eschenbach AC, Wender R, et al. American Cancer Society guidelines for the early detection of cancer: update of early detection guidelines for prostate, colorectal, and endometrial cancers. Also: update 2001—testing for early lung cancer detection. *CA Cancer J Clin.* 2001;51(1):38–75; quiz 7–80.
86. Hardcastle JD, Thomas WM, Chamberlain J, et al. Randomised, controlled trial of faecal occult blood screening for colorectal cancer. Results for first 107,349 subjects. *Lancet.* 1989;1(8648):1160–1164.
91. Lieberman DA, Weiss DG. One-time screening for colorectal cancer with combined fecal occult-blood testing and examination of the distal colon. *N Engl J Med.* 2001;345(8):555–560.
95. Cole SR, Young GP. Effect of dietary restriction on participation in faecal occult blood test screening for colorectal cancer. *Med J Aust.* 2001;175(4):195–198.
113. Levin TR, Farraye FA, Schoen RE, et al. Quality in the technical performance of screening flexible sigmoidoscopy: recommendations of an international multi-society task group. *Gut.* 2005;54(6):807–813.
124. Muller AD, Sonnenberg A. Prevention of colorectal cancer by flexible endoscopy and polypectomy. A case-control study of 32,702 veterans [see comments]. *Ann Intern Med.* 1995;123(12):904–910.
131. Cotton PB, Durkalski VL, Pineau BC, et al. Computed tomographic colonography (virtual colonoscopy): a multicenter comparison with standard colonoscopy for detection of colorectal neoplasia. *JAMA.* 2004;291(14):1713–1719.
136. Lawson H, Lee N, Thames S, et al. Cervical cancer screening among low-income women: results of a national screening program, 1991–1995. *Obstet Gynecol.* 1998;92(5):745–752.
143. Magnus K, Langmark F, Andersen A. Mass screening for cervical cancer in Ostfold county of Norway 1959–77. *Int J Cancer.* 1987;39(3):311–316.
160. Carozzi FM, Confortini M, Cecchini S, et al. Triage with human papillomavirus testing of women with cytologic abnormalities prompting referral for colposcopy assessment. *Cancer.* 2005;105(1):2–7.
163. Jenkins D, Sherlaw-Johnson C, Gallivan S. Assessing the role of HPV testing in cervical cancer screening. *Papilloma Report.* 1998;9(4):89–101.
174. Broder S. Rapid communication—the Bethesda system for reporting cervical/vaginal cytologic diagnoses—report of the 1991 Bethesda workshop. *JAMA.* 1992;267(14):1892.
185. Richert-Boe KE, Humphrey LL, Glass AG, et al. Screening digital rectal examination and prostate cancer mortality: a case-control study. *J Med Screen.* 1998;5(2):99–103.
191. Borden LS, Jr., Wright JL, Kim J, et al. An abnormal digital rectal examination is an independent predictor of Gleason > or =7 prostate cancer in men undergoing initial prostate biopsy: a prospective study of 790 men. *BJU Int.* 2007;99(3):559–563.
200. Etzioni R, Legler JM, Feuer EJ, et al. Cancer surveillance series: interpreting trends in

prostate cancer—part III: quantifying the link between population prostate-specific antigen testing and recent declines in prostate cancer mortality. *J Natl Cancer Inst.* 1999;91(12):1033–1039.

201. Feuer EJ, Merrill RM, Hankey BF. Cancer surveillance series: interpreting trends in prostate cancer—part II: cause of death misclassification and the recent rise and fall in prostate cancer mortality. *J Natl Cancer Inst.* 1999;91(12):1025–1032.
207. Horninger W, Berger A, Pelzer A, et al. Screening for prostate cancer: updated experience from the Tyrol study. *Can J Urol.* 2005;12(Suppl 1):7–13; discussion 92–93.
210. Standaert B, Denis L. The European Randomized Study of screening for prostate cancer: an update. *Cancer.* 1997;80(9): 1830–1834.
216. American Medical Association. Report 9 of the Council on Scientific Affairs (A-00). Screening and early detection of prostate cancer. Accessed March 1, 2001.
219. American Urological Association. Early detection of prostate cancer. http://www.auanet.org/content/guidelines-and-quality-care/policy-statements/e/early-detection-of-prostate-cancer.cfm. Accessed October 30, 2008, 2008.
222. Thompson I, Leach RJ, Pollock BH, et al. Prostate cancer and prostate-specific antigen: the more we know, the less we understand. *J Natl Cancer Inst.* 2003;95(14):1027–1028.
225. Black WC. Lung cancer. In: Kramer BS, Gohagan JK, Prorok PC, editors. *Cancer Screening: Theory and Practice.* New York: Marcel Dekker, Inc.; 1999:327–377.
240. Kubik A, Haerting J. Survival and mortality in a randomized study of lung cancer detection. *Neoplasma.* 1990;37(4):467–475.
243. Lung cancer screening: recommendation statement. *Ann Intern Med.* 2004;140(9):738–739.
254. Peto R, Darby S, Deo H, et al. Smoking, smoking cessation, and lung cancer in the UK since 1950: combination of national statistics with two case-control studies [see comments]. *BMJ.* 2000;321(7257):323–329.
278. Helzlsouer KJ, Bush TL, Alberg AJ, et al. Prospective study of serum CA-125 levels as markers of ovarian cancer [see comments]. *JAMA.* 1993;269(9):1123–1126.
304. Oliveria SA, Christos PJ, Halpern AC, et al. Patient knowledge, awareness, and delay in seeking medical attention for malignant melanoma. *J Clin Epidemiol.* 1999;52(11):1111–1116.
310. Geller AC, Zhang Z, Sober AJ, et al. The first 15 years of the American Academy of Dermatology skin cancer screening programs: 1985–1999. *J Am Acad Dermatol.* 2003;48(1):34–41.
319. Mashberg A, Samit A. Early diagnosis of asymptomatic oral and oropharyngeal squamous cancers. *CA Cancer J Clin.* 1995;45(6):328–351.
322. Smart CR. Screening for cancer of the aerodigestive tract. *Cancer.* 1993;72(3 Suppl):1061–1065.
324. Speight PM, Palmer S, Moles DR, et al. The cost-effectiveness of screening for oral cancer in primary care. *Health Technol Assess.* 2006;10(14):1–144, iii–iv.
325. Meissner HI, Smith RA, Rimer BK, et al. Promoting cancer screening: learning from experience. *Cancer.* 2004;101(5 Suppl):1107–1117.
326. Miles A, Cockburn J, Smith RA, et al. A perspective from countries using organized screening programs. *Cancer.* 2004; 101(5 Suppl):1201–1213.

35 Statistical Innovations in Cancer Research

Donald A. Berry, PhD

Statistics chapters in medical volumes are usually introductions to traditional statistical concepts. This chapter is different. Its goal is to introduce researchers and clinicians to recent innovations in the design and analysis of cancer experiments, especially clinical trials. Traditional statistical methods are not reviewed here for two reasons. First, many good biostatistics texts are available to readers. Second, the modern world of Internet search engines such as Google (Google, Mountain View, CA) allows the curious reader to find out as much as desired about any particular statistical method.

But the real motivation for the perspective of this chapter is that cancer research (and medical research more generally) is rapidly changing. The rigorous standards of modern statistics—including randomization—were developed for agricultural experiments. They have served us very well, taking medical research from case study and anecdote into a true science. When there were a few therapeutic regimens to investigate, the old-fashioned notion of equally randomizing thousands of patients to treatments A vs B may have been appropriate. But today, the number of possible cancer targets and cancer drugs is fast approaching the number of cancer patients. And there is no end in sight.

The old-fashioned approach leads to large phase III drug trials. The goal is to minimize the type II error while controlling the overall type I error rate. Too frequently, especially in oncology, phase III trials are initiated with less than a clear picture of the drug's effects. As a consequence, they frequently fail: "In the phase 3 trials, where a lot of money and a lot of hope, patient lives, and time have been invested, the failure rate is now reported to be about 50% [and substantially higher in oncology] ... [the time has come] to modernize the way we develop these products," said [Janet] Woodcock, Director of FDA's Center for Drugs and Experimental Research.[1]

The costs are huge, with estimates to bring each new drug to market in 2006 topping $1.3 billion. The biggest cost in bringing a new drug to market is human clinical trials, and these costs continue to grow.[2]

Recognizing the need to modernize drug development the FDA issued its Critical Path Opportunities Report in March 2006. The FDA identified two areas where changes were essential: "Our outreach efforts uncovered a remarkable consensus that the two most important areas for improving medical product development are biomarker development (Topic 1) and streamlining clinical trials (Topic 2)."[3]

Ideas of statistical methodology have been slow to change. To an extent this is understandable: we have achieved a high level of science and do not want to return to case study and anecdote. But it is possible to protect the baby while discarding the bath water. That is the approach of this chapter.

The principal goals of the innovations presented in this chapter are to (1) use information from clinical trials more efficiently in drawing conclusions about treatment effects, (2) use patient resources more efficiently while treating patients who participate in clinical trials as effectively as possible, and (3) identify better drugs and therapeutic strategies more rapidly, moving them more quickly through the development process. The underlying premise is to exploit all available evidence, placing information gleaned from an ongoing clinical trial into the context of what is already known. The innovations considered are intuitively appealing. But some are controversial. Some are being used in actual clinical trials while others are still being developed and evaluated for such use.

This chapter addresses two types of innovations. One is a natural extension of the traditional practice of statistics. The other type represents a sea change and is based on a Bayesian statistical philosophy. As not all readers will be familiar with the Bayesian approach, I will describe it and relate it to the more familiar frequentist approach. Readers who are familiar with Bayesian ideas may wish to skip "Bayesian Updating," provided later. An important distinction between the two approaches is one of attitude. The Bayesian approach is tailored to online learning (as data accrue), and the frequentist approach is tied to particular experiments and to the experiment's design. However, there is substantial overlap. Much of this chapter's development of clinical trial design employs the Bayesian approach as a tool for finding designs that tend to treat patients in the clinical trial more effectively and that identify better drugs more rapidly. But the frequentist properties (such as false-positive rate and power) of the design thus derived can always be found, sometimes requiring simulation. Ensuring that a design has prespecified frequentist properties means that the design is frequentist. But the Bayesian approach can serve as a tool for finding a good frequentist design.

In the early days of clinical trials, designs were not allowed to be complicated. For example, if the treatment assigned to the next patient were to depend on the currently available results of the patients previously treated in the trial, it would be difficult to evaluate the trial's false-positive rate. Such a calculation may be impossible using standard mathematical methods. But in the modern era, the availability of high-speed computers and sophisticated computational methods makes such calculations routine. For example, modern computers can be used to simulate trials having even the most complicated of designs and evaluate design properties such as power and false-positive rate. The basic requirement is that the design be specified prospectively.

Preliminaries

The basis of all experimentation is comparison. Evaluating an experimental therapy in a clinical trial requires information about the outcomes of these patients had they received some other therapy. The best way to address this issue is to randomize patients to the experimental therapy and to some comparison therapy. Although there are ways to learn without randomizing, there are limitations of approaches that do not employ randomization. And randomization does not require equal assignment probabilities to the therapeutic strategies, or "arms," being compared. Unbalanced randomization is possible, and so also randomization that is adaptive, ie, that assignment probabilities depend on accumulating data in the trial. (The latter possibility is the principal focus of this chapter.)

Most clinical trials are conducted in accord with a protocol. The traditional goal is science and not effective treatment of patients in the trial.[4] Protocols may refer to retrospective or sporadic collection of data, but they are usually prospective. A prospective protocol lays out how the trial is to be conducted, including how patients will be assigned to therapy and when the trial will end. Deviations from a protocol may make scientific inferences from the trial difficult or impossible (although they may be necessary to avoid exposing participants to unnecessary risks).

Bayesian Approach

This section is not essential for reading the remainder of this chapter. But the material covered will help readers understand some of the approaches and attitudes. The goals of this section are to show how Bayesian learning takes place and how the Bayesian approach relates to the more traditional frequentist approach. This introduction is necessarily superficial. In particular, I barely touch some philosophical issues. Further reading includes a comprehensive but elementary introduction to Bayesian ideas and methods,[5] discussions of their role in medical research[6] and of clinical trials in particular,[7,8] and an elegant and useful text describing more advanced Bayesian methods.[9]

Bayesian Updating

The defining characteristic of any statistical approach is how it deals with uncertainty. In the Bayesian approach, uncertainty is measured by probability. Any event whose occurrence is unknown has a probability. The frequentist approach uses probabilities as well, but in a more restricted fashion, as will be seen in the next section. Examples of probabilities in the Bayesian approach that do not have frequentist counterparts include the following: The probability that the drug is effective, the probability that patient Smith will respond to a particular chemotherapy, and the probability that the future results in the trial will show a statistically significant benefit for a particular therapy.

The Bayesian paradigm is one of learning. As information becomes available one updates one's knowledge about the unknown aspects of the process that is producing the information. The fundamental tool for learning under uncertainty is Bayes' rule. Bayes' rule relates inverse probabilities. An example that will be familiar to many readers is finding the positive predictive value (PPV) of a diagnostic test: In view of a positive test result, what is the probability that the individual being tested has the disease in question? The inverse probability is that of a positive test given the presence of the disease, which is called the test's sensitivity. PPV also depends on the test's specificity, which is the probability of a negative test, given that the individual does not have the disease. And PPV depends on the prevalence of disease in the population. In applying Bayes' rule to statistical inference, the analog of PPV is the "posterior probability" that a hypothesis is true, given the experimental results. The analog of disease prevalence is the "prior probability" that the hypothesis is true.

Consider an overly simplified numerical example, one with only two possible response rates (r): $r = 0.75$ and $r = 0.50$. If you are accustomed to thinking about PPV for diagnostic tests, consider one of these to be that the "patient has the disease" and the other to be that the "patient does not have the disease." The question is this: Is r equal to 0.75 or 0.50? Before any experimentation these two possibilities are regarded to be equally likely: $P(r = 0.75) = P(r = 0.50) = 1/2$.

The focus of the Bayesian approach is learning. Probabilities are calculated as new information becomes available, and is taken to be "given." Statisticians have a notation that facilitates thinking about and calculating probabilities as new information accrues. They use vertical bars to separate the event of interest from data or parameters that are regarded to be known (or taken to be given): $P(A|B)$ is read "probability of A given B." Assign R for tumor response and N for nonresponse. Using this notation, eg, $P(R|r = 0.75) = 0.75$. More interesting is the probability of $r = 0.75$ given a tumor response: $P(r = 0.75|R)$. These two expressions are the inverses of each other, with the roles of the event of interest and the event being assumed. Bayes' rule is the relationship between these two expressions. Namely, that the updated (posterior) probability of $r = 0.75$ is as follows:

$$P(r = 0.75|R) = P(R|r = 0.75)P(r = 0.75)/P(R)$$

The denominator on the right-hand side follows from the law of total probability:

$$P(R) = P(R|r = 0.75)P(r = 0.75) + P(R|r = 0.50)$$
$$= (0.75)(1/2) + (0.5)(1/2) = 5/8$$

That is, $P(R)$ is the average of the two response rates under consideration, 0.75 and 0.50, where the average is with respect to the corresponding prior probabilities—half each in this example. Substituting the numerical values into Bayes' rule, the posterior probability of $r = 0.75$ is as follows:

$$P(r = 0.75|R) = (0.75)(1/2)/(5/8) = 3/5$$

Therefore, the new evidence boosts the probability of $r = 0.75$ from 1/2 (or 50%) to 60%. As the total probability is 100%, the evidence in a single response lowers the probability of $r = 0.50$ from 50% to 40%.

Consider a second independent observation. The probabilities of the two values of r prior to this second observation are posterior to the first observation. If the second observation is also a response, then a second application of Bayes' rule applies to give $P(r = 0.75|R, R) = 9/13 = 69\%$, which is a further increase from the previous values of 50% and 60%. On one hand, if the second observation is a nonresponse then $P(r = 0.75|R, N) = 3/7 = 43\%$, a decrease from 60%. This process can go on indefinitely, updating either after each observation or all at once on the basis of whatever evidence available. The current probabilities of the various possible values of response rate r can be found at any time. These probabilities depend on the original prior probability and on the intervening data. This process of updating and online learning is an important advantage of the Bayesian approach to designing clinical trials.

The example mentioned previously considered only two possible values of r. More realistically, the response rate r may be any number between 0 and 1. The left-hand panel in Figure 35-1A shows a constant or flat curve that is a candidate for prior distribution. The flat curve indicates that the probability is spread equally over this range of values of r. This might be termed an "open-minded prior distribution" because the posterior distribution depends almost entirely on the evidence from the experiment at hand. After a single tumor response, Bayesian updating serves to change the probability distribution to the one shown in the right-hand panel of Figure 35-1A—ie, the right-hand panel is the posterior distribution after observing R when the prior distribution is the one shown in the left-hand panel. The shift in the distribution to larger values of r corresponds to the intuitive notion that larger response rates become more likely after observing R. Bayes' rule quantifies this intuition.

There are many candidate prior distributions other than the first one shown in Figure 35-1A. Three other prior/posterior pairs are shown in Figure 35-1B-D. The right-hand panel within each pair is the posterior distribution after observing R when the prior distribution is the one shown in the left-hand panel. Moreover, the left-hand curves in Figure 35-1B-D are themselves posterior distributions for the right-hand curves in Figure 35-1A-C, respectively, but in the situation when the observation is an N. Intuitively,

[a]For further explanation and examples, see chapter 5 of *Statistics: A Bayesian Perspective*.[5]

after a nonresponse the concentration of probabilities shifts to smaller values of r. Mathematically, observing R means to multiply the current distribution by r (the response rate) and renormalize it so that the area under the curve is 1. Similarly, observing an N means to multiply by $(1-r)$, the rate of nonresponse.

An implication is that moving left to right and top to bottom in Figure 35-1 corresponds to starting with the prior distribution in the left-hand panel of Figure 35-1A and observing RNRNRNR. The eight curves shown in Fig. 35-1 are proportional to the following respective functional forms: 1, r, $r(1-r)$, $r^2(1-r)$, $r^2(1-r)^2$, $r^3(1-r)^2$, $r^3(1-r)^3$, $r^4(1-r)^3$. Each observation of response increases the exponent of r by 1 and each observed N increases the exponent of $(1-r)$ by 1. As is evident in the figure, additional observations lead to narrower distributions. As the number of observations increases, the distribution tends to concentrate about a single point, which is the "true" value of r, the response rate that produces the observations.

The principal message of this section is not the numerical calculation defining the updated distribution, but the fact that updated distributions can be found using the Bayesian approach at any time during a clinical trial.

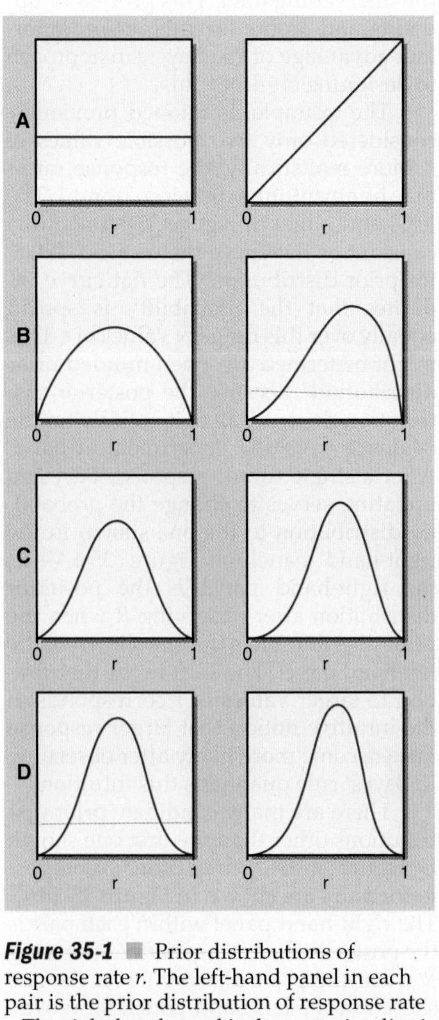

Figure 35-1 Prior distributions of response rate r. The left-hand panel in each pair is the prior distribution of response rate r. The right-hand panel is the posterior distribution of r after having observed a response in a single patient. The (predictive) probability of a response for each left-hand panel is 0.500, increasing in the right-hand panels to 0.667, 0.600, 0.571, 0.556 in cases **A** through **D**, respectively. Changes are greater and learning is more rapid when the prior distribution reflects greater uncertainty.

Prior Probabilities

Bayesian updating requires a starting point: a prior distribution of the various parameters. In the example, one must have a probability distribution for response rate r in advance of or separate from the experiment in question. This prior distribution may be subjectively assessed or based explicitly on the results of previous experiments. In some settings, such as some regulatory scenarios, an appropriate default distribution is noninformative or open-minded[5,8] in the sense that all possible values of the parameters are assigned the same prior probabilities. The left-hand panel of Fig. 35-1A is an example.

Noninformative or flat prior distributions limit the benefits of taking a Bayesian approach when they ignore information that is available from outside the experiment. However, the benefit of employing Bayesian updating may be substantial even if one starts with a flat distribution that does not reflect anyone's assessment of the prior information. Flat prior distributions serve some important roles. One is that it may be helpful to distinguish the evidence in the data in the experiment under consideration from that present before the experiment. Another is that the Bayesian conclusions that arise from using flat priors are often the same as the corresponding frequentist conclusions.

Prior distributions are usually based on historical data. Suppose that a similar drug (or the same drug in a possibly different patient population) gave a response rate of 50% in 20 patients: 10 responders and 10 nonresponders. The corresponding likelihood of response rate r (see "Frequentist/Bayesian Comparison" provided later) is $r^{10}(1-r)^{10}$. Given that there may be differences between the historical setting and that of the current trial, it would not be reasonable to use this as a prior distribution for r, but it would be appropriate to somehow exploit this relevant information. One possibility (another will be described in "Hazards over Time") is to discount the historical evidence as it applies to the context of the current trial. For example, weighing an historical observation as having the information equivalent of 30% that of a current observation would mean using a prior distribution proportional to $r^3(1-r)^3$. This is the distribution shown in Fig. 35-1D, left-hand panel.

Robustness Principle

In the presence of enough data, essentially all observers will have similar posterior distributions. This is the robustness principle. An implication is that the particular prior distribution assumed does not matter much when the sample size is moderate or large. As an example, consider the eight distributions shown in Fig. 35-1 and think each of them in turn as being the prior distribution of a different person. Parameter r is the response rate to a particular drug. Suppose that 40 patients are treated in a trial and 20 of them respond. Applying the robustness principle, the eight people in question will come to very nearly the same conclusion about the drug's response rate. The eight posterior distributions are shown in Fig. 35-2. The curves are nearly superposed. The eight 95% probability intervals will also be very similar. The data outweighs any of the prior distributions shown in Fig. 35-1.

If two prior distributions are markedly different, then the robustness principle still applies, but it could take a good deal of data to bring two disparate distributions close together.

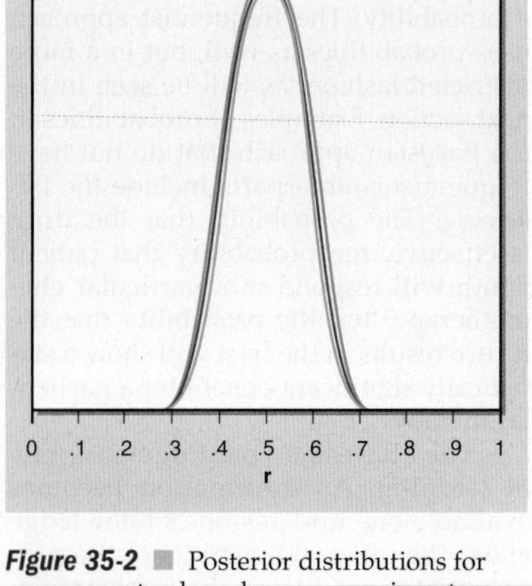

Figure 35-2 Posterior distributions for response rate r based on an experiment with 20 responses and 20 failures. The eight prior distributions considered are the eight distributions shown in Fig. 35-1. Except for proportionality constants these are 1, r, $r(1-r)$, $r^2(1-r)$, $r^2(1-r)^2$, $r^3(1-r)^2$, $r^3(1-r)^3$, and $r^4(1-r)^3$. The corresponding posterior distributions are proportional to $r^{20}(1-r)^{20}$, $r^{21}(1-r)^{20}$, $r^{21}(1-r)^{21}$, $r^{22}(1-r)^{21}$, $r^{22}(1-r)^{22}$, $r^{23}(1-r)^{22}$, $r^{23}(1-r)^{23}$, and $r^{24}(1-r)^{23}$. These eight posterior distributions are very similar, demonstrating the robustness principle.

Frequentist/Bayesian Comparison

In the frequentist approach, hypotheses and parameters do not have probabilities. Rather, probability assignments apply only to data, with particular values assumed for any unknown parameters in calculating these probabilities. For example, the ubiquitous *p*-value is the probability of data as or more extreme than the observed data assuming that the null hypothesis is true. In symbols:

- Frequentist *p*-value: *P*(observed or more extreme data | *H0*)
- Bayesian posterior probability: *P*(*H0* | observed data)

It is easy to confuse these two concepts. A *p*-value is commonly interpreted as the probability of no effect, and 1 minus the *p*-value as the probability of an effect. This interpretation is wrong. This is trying to have a Bayesian posterior probability without a prior probability, which is impossible.

There are two important differences between a frequentist *p*-value and a Bayesian posterior probability. One is the inversion of the conditions: what is assumed in the former has a probability in the latter. The second difference is that *p*-values include probabilities of results other than those observed in the experiment.

As an example, consider a single-arm phase II trial for testing *H0*: $r = 0.5$ vs *H1*: $r = 0.75$. Assuming a type I error rate $\alpha = 5\%$, a sample size of $n = 33$ gives 90% power. Suppose the final results are 22 responses of 33 patients, the (frequentist) one-sided *p*-value is the probability of 22 or more responses of the 33 patients assuming the null hypothesis, *H0*: $r = 0.5$. Under this assumption the probability of observing 22, 23, 24, . . . responses is 0.0225+0.0108+0.0045+ . . . = 0.0401. As this *p*-value is less than 5%, observing 22 responses is said to be "statistically significant."

The Bayesian measure is the posterior probability of the hypothesis that $r = 0.75$ (which is 1– the probability of $r = 0.5$) given 22 responses out of 33 trials. (As indicated earlier, the Bayesian calculation depends only on the probability of the data actually observed, 22 responses of 33, while the frequentist calculation also includes probabilities of 23, 24, etc, responses.) Using Bayes' rule:

$$P(H1|22 \text{ of } 33) = P(22 \text{ of } 33|H1)P(H1)/P(22 \text{ of } 33)$$

As mentioned in the equation, the denominator follows from the law of total probability:

$$P(22 \text{ of } 33) = P(22 \text{ of } 33|H1)P(H1) + P(22 \text{ of } 33|H0)P(H0) = (0.0823)(0.5) + (0.0225)(0.5) = 0.0524$$

Therefore,

$$P(H1|22 \text{ of } 33) = (0.0823)(0.5)/0.0524 = 0.785$$
$$P(H0|22 \text{ of } 33) = (0.0225)(0.5)/0.0524 = 0.215$$

The calculation considers just two hypotheses, $r = 0.5$ and $r = 0.75$. In considering other values of *r*, Bayes' rule weighs them by *P*(22 of 33|*r*), which is called the likelihood function of *r*. The likelihood function is pictured in Fig. 35-3. It indicates the degree of support for response rate *r* provided by the observed data. Values of *r* having the same likelihood are equally supported by the data. Only relative likelihoods matter. For example, conclusions about $r = 0.5$ vs 0.75 depend only on the ratio of their likelihoods, 0.0823 and 0.0225, values that are highlighted in Fig. 35-3. Because 0.0823/0.0225 = 3.66, the data lend 3.66 times as much support to $r = 0.75$ as they do to $r = 0.5$.

The conclusions of the two approaches are different conceptually and numerically. In the frequentist approach the results are statistically significant, with *p*-value = 0.0401. Some researchers interpret statistical significance to mean that *H0* is unlikely to be true. That is not what it means. The Bayesian posterior probability of *H0* addresses this question. This probability is 0.215. Although smaller than the prior probability of 0.50 (because the data point somewhat more strongly to *H1* than to *H0*), it is 5 times as large as the *p*-value.

Interval estimates also have different interpretations in the two approaches. In the Bayesian approach, one can find the probability that a parameter lies in any given interval. In the frequentist approach, confidence intervals have a long-run frequency interpretation for fixed and given parameters. So it is not correct to say that the probability is 95%, that the parameter in question is in a 95% confidence interval. Despite the different interpretations, there is a point of agreement between the two approaches. In other words, if the prior distribution is flat (eg, the left-hand panel of Fig. 35-1A), then the Bayesian posterior probability of a confidence interval is essentially the same as the frequentist level of confidence. For example, if the prior distribution is flat then the Bayesian posterior probability, indicating that a parameter lies in its 95% confidence interval, is in fact 95%. For prior distributions that are not flat the posterior probability of a 95% confidence interval may be greater than or less than 95%. If the historical data upon which the prior distribution is based are consistent with those from the current experiment then the posterior probability indicating that the parameter is in the 95% confidence interval will be greater than 95%. If the historical data are different from those in the current experiment then the probability of the 95% confidence interval will typically be less than 95%.

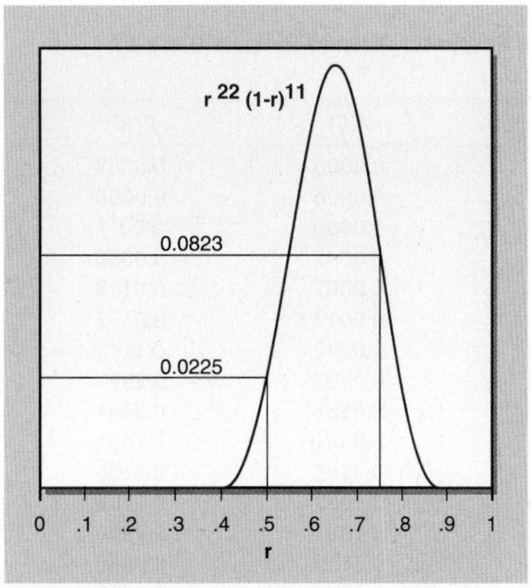

Figure 35-3 Likelihood of *r* for 22 responses out of 33 observations. The likelihood is *P*(22 of 33|*r*), which is proportional to $r^{22}(1-r)^{11}$. The likelihoods at $r = 0.5$ and 0.75 are highlighted. These values are used in the calculational example in the text.

Predictive Probabilities

The ability to predict the future—with the requisite uncertainty—is important for designing trials and for monitoring trials. The Bayesian approach allows for calculating probabilities of future results without having to assume that any particular hypothesis is true. The process is straightforward, at least logically if not mathematically. For a specified experimental design, one finds the conditional probabilities of the future data for each parameter value and averages them with respect to the current probabilities of the various parameter values. Predictive probabilities will be exploited extensively in this chapter.

Consider the 33-patient trial described earlier. Suppose that the first 16 patients have been treated, with 13 responses and 3 nonresponses. What will be the results after the full complement of 33 patients is available? The number of responses will be between 13 and 30, but it is possible to be more. In particular, it seems most unlikely that there will be no responses in the next 17 patients after having seen 13 in the first 16 patients, and it is.

It might seem reasonable to use an estimate of *r* (eg, the current rate, 13/16 = 0.81) and calculate the probabilities of the results of the next 17 patients assuming this value of *r*, but this could be wrong. Such a calculation incorporates the uncertainty in the future data for the given *r* but it fails to incorporate uncertainty in *r*. Bayesian predictive probabilities incorporate both types of uncertainty. Table 35-1 shows the results assuming just two values of r, 0.5 and 0.75. The first column (the leftmost column) lists the possible numbers (S) of responses after 33 patients. The second and third columns show the probabilities of the possible values of S for these two values of r. The corresponding probabilities without conditioning on r are shown in the fourth column. This is a weighted average of the second and third columns. The weights are the respective probabilities of the two values of r conditional on having observed 13 responses in the first 16 patients: 0.039 for $r = 0.5$ and 0.961 for $r = 0.75$. The fourth column evinces greater variability (greater standard deviation) than either of the previous two columns. Typically, including when all values of r between 0 and 1 are considered (ie, all values have positive probability), predictive probabilities reflect greater uncertainty about future results than when conditioning on a particular value of r. (The rightmost column of Table 35-1 will be discussed in the next section.)

For convenience in this example, equal prior probabilities are assumed: $P(H1) = P(H0) = 0.5$. Although there is no vertical bar "|" in these expressions, these probabilities can depend on other available evidence, such as results of earlier clinical and preclinical trials. There may be additional information from biological assessments, such as when considering targeted therapies. These overall conditions are taken to be understood in setting down $P(H0)$ and $P(H1)$.

Bayesian vs Frequentist Interim Analyses

There are numerous commonalties and a few differences between the Bayesian and frequentist approaches. This section addresses a principal difference. In the Bayesian approach, one makes an observation and updates the probabilities of the various hypotheses. This simple process implies a degree of flexibility that is difficult to mimic in the frequentist approach.

Consider the trial design described previously, with $n = 33$ patients and testing $H0$: $r = 0.5$ vs $H1$: $r = 0.75$. Observing 22 or more responses will be sufficient to reject $H0$ in favor of $H1$. However, assigning 33 patients to an experimental therapy without assessing interim results is ethically problematic and would likely be questioned by institutional review boards. If the results are conclusive (either positive, strongly suggesting $r > 0.5$, or negative, suggesting $r \leq 0.5$) part of the way through the trial, then the trial should be stopped. Suppose, eg, that after 16 patients, one finds that 13 respond and 3 do not, from a Bayesian perspective, the updated probability of $H1$ is 96.1% (assuming prior probability $P(H0) = 0.5$).

Whether this probability is "conclusive" is not clear. The decision as to whether to continue a trial is complicated. It depends on the consequences of the trial, given the current results and also given future results. In the Bayesian approach, the consequences of future results can be weighed by their predictive probabilities; eg, suppose the impact of the trial depends on whether the posterior probability of $H1$ is > 95% when the data from the full complement of 33 patients becomes available, then one can calculate the predictive probability of this event. The rightmost column in Table 35-1 shows the posterior probability of $H1$ assuming S responses of 33 patients. The shaded values are those having $P(H1|S/16) > 95\%$. To achieve > 95%, posterior probability requires at least 24 responses in the 33 patients. The predictive probability of this event is the sum of the predictive probabilities for $S \geq 24$ (the fourth column in Table 35-1), which is 0.8642. Although the current probability of $H1$ is > 95%, this characteristic will be lost with probability $1 - 0.8642 = 0.1358$. That this has moderate probability indicates the tentative nature of the current conclusion. The possibility that the current conclusion is moderately likely to change can be factored into the decision to continue the trial.

Alternatively, and mixing Bayesian and frequentist concepts, if the impact of the trial depends on achieving (one-sided) statistical significance then the Bayesian predictive probability of this event means adding the probabilities of 22 and 23 responses to 0.8642, the total being 0.9684.

If the predictive probability that the current conclusion will be maintained is sufficiently high, then one may reasonably decide to stop a trial. This is true for both claims of futility and superiority. The possibility of stopping a trial early on the basis of predictive probability should be stated explicitly in the trial's protocol.

The focus of the frequentist perspective is the type I error rate, α. This is the probability of rejecting $H0$ when $H0$ is true, which depends on the trial design. For a fixed sample size of 33 patients, the calculation is straightforward. Rejecting $H0$ for ≥ 22 responses means $\alpha = 0.0401$ (see the previous section). The calculation becomes more complicated when there is a possibility of stopping the trial early. In the example, if the trial is stopped and $H0$ is rejected, when there are 13 or more responses in the first 16 patients, then α is increased because there is additional opportunity for rejecting $H0$. Assuming $r = 0.5$, the probability of rejecting $H0$ is now 0.0712. (The possibility that r is different from its null value plays no role in calculating the type I error rate.) Because this is greater than 0.05, the convention is to modify the stopping and rejection criteria to reduce α to about 0.05. For example, rejecting only if there are 14 responses or more out of 16 patients treated, or if there are 23 or more responses after 33 patients are treated, gives an overall type I error rate of 0.0326.

It follows that it is more difficult to draw a conclusion of statistical significance when there are interim analyses. The reason is that the type I error rates are calculated assuming that a particular hypothesis (the null hypothesis of no effect) is true. In a sense, an investigator is penalized for interim analyses in the frequentist approach. There are no such penalties for interim analyses in a Bayesian perspective. The reason is that

Table 35-1 Predictive Probabilities of Number S of Responses After 33 Patients Given 13 Responses in the First 16 Patients

S(of 33)	$P(S\|r = 0.5)$	$P(S\|r = 0.75)$	$P(S)$	$P(HI)$
13	0.0000	0.0000	0.0000	0.0002
14	0.0001	0.0000	0.0000	0.0006
15	0.0010	0.0000	0.0000	0.0017
16	0.0052	0.0000	0.0002	0.0050
17	0.0182	0.0000	0.0007	0.0148
18	0.0472	0.0001	0.0019	0.0432
19	0.0944	0.0005	0.0042	0.1192
20	0.1484	0.0025	0.0082	0.2887
21	0.1855	0.0093	0.0162	0.5491
22	0.1855	0.0279	0.0341	0.7851
23	0.1484	0.0668	0.0701	0.9164
24	0.0944	0.1276	0.1263	0.9705
25	0.0472	0.1914	0.1857	0.9900
26	0.0181	0.2209	0.2129	0.9966
27	0.0052	0.1893	0.1820	0.9989
28	0.0010	0.1136	0.1091	0.9996
29	0.0001	0.0426	0.0409	0.9999
30	0.0000	0.0075	0.0072	1.0000

Note: Columns $P(S|r = 0.5)$ and $P(S|r = 0.75)$ assume the indicated value of r in calculating the probability. Column $P(S)$ is the weighted average of the two previous columns, where the respective weights are 0.039 and 0.961. The last column gives $P(HI)$, the probability of HI ($r = 0.75$), given S responses after 33 patients. The shaded cells are described in the text.

Bayesian probabilities do not condition on any particular hypothesis.

Although it is not a Bayesian quantity, the type I error rate of any Bayesian design, however complicated, can be evaluated. If the design has interim analyses, then such a calculation incorporates appropriate penalties. This calculation is straightforward in a simple example such as that given earlier. In more complicated settings it can require Monte Carlo simulations. To find α via simulation in the previous example, toss a fair coin 16 times. Make a tick mark if 13 or more "heads" result, and stop tossing. Otherwise, toss the coin an additional 17 times and make a tick mark if the total number of heads is 22 or more. Repeat the process thousands of times. (Program a computer to do the tossing!) Estimate α to be the number of tick marks divided by the number of times the process was simulated. Assuming that the random number generator works properly, the proportion with tick marks will be about 7%.

A recent breast cancer trial illustrates some advantages of a Bayesian design.[10] The trial randomized women at least 65 years of age who had breast cancer to receive either standard chemotherapy or capecitabine. The sample size was advertised as 600-1800. Starting after the 600th patient had enrolled in the trial, and following the protocol, predictive probability calculations were carried out. Calculations were made of the predictive probability of statistical significance given the present sample size and with additional patient follow-up at the present sample size. If that achieved a predetermined level, patient accrual would stop, but observations of the existing patients would continue. The predictive probability cutoff point was achieved at the first interim analysis and so accrual stopped (the final sample size was 633).

Indeed, with additional patient follow-up, the standard treatment was shown to be statistically superior to capecitabine.

Analysis Issues

The purpose of this section is to consider two types of analysis issues. The first is an extension of the previous section. The second is unrelated to the first and deals with a particular aspect of survival analysis.

Hierarchical Modeling: Synthesizing Information

When analyzing data from a clinical trial, other information is usually available about the treatment under consideration. This section deals with a method called hierarchical modeling. One of its uses is synthesizing information from different sources. The method applies in many settings, including meta-analysis and incorporating historical information. A hierarchical model is a random-effects model. In a meta-analysis, eg, one level of the experimental unit is the patient (within a trial) and the second level is trial itself. Hierarchical models also apply for design issues such as combining results across diseases or disease subtypes and for such seemingly disparate issues as cluster randomization. Design issues for hierarchical modeling will be considered in the next section.

Reconsider the phase II trial discussed previously, in which 21 of 33 patients responded. The one-sided p-value is 0.08 for the null hypothesis $H0$: r = 0.50, and so the results are not statistically significant at the 5% level. Now consider an earlier phase I trial using the same treatment in which 15 of 20 patients responded. This information seems relevant, even if the population being treated might have been somewhat different and the trial might have been conducted at a different institution. But it is not obvious how to incorporate the information into an analysis. The frequentist approach is experiment-specific, which requires imagining that the two trials are part of some larger experiment. If one assumes that the entire set of data resulted from a single trial involving 53 patients with 36 responses, then from a frequentist perspective this would lead to a p-value of 0.0063, which is highly statistically significant. But this conclusion is wrong because the assumption is wrong. And it is not clear how to make it right.

Any Bayesian analysis that assumes the same response rate applies in both trials would be similarly flawed. Response rate r may be reasonably expected to vary from one trial to another. Two response rates for the same therapy may be different even if the eligibility criteria in the two trials are the same. For one thing the eligibility criteria may be applied differently in the two settings. But even if the patients accrued are apparently similar, their accruals differ in time and place. Our understanding of cancer and its detection changes over time. Moreover, there are differences in the use of concomitant therapy and variations in the ability to assess clinical and laboratory variables. A way to repair the analysis is to explicitly consider two values of r, say $r1$ for the first trial and $r2$ for the second.

Recapitulating, there are two extreme assumptions that lead to analyses that are easy to carry out, but wrong. One is to assume $r1$ and $r2$ are unrelated and to base any inferences about $r2$ on the results of the second trial alone. The other is to assume that $r1 = r2$ and combine the results in the two trials.

The two r-values may be the same or different. In a Bayesian hierarchical model, both possibilities are allowed, but neither is assumed. In other words, $r1$ and $r2$ are regarded as having come from a population of r-values. The population may have little variability (homogeneity) or substantial variability (heterogeneity). The observed response rates give information concerning the extent of heterogeneity, with disparate rates suggesting greater heterogeneity. When the observed rates are similar, the precision of estimates of $r1$ and $r2$ will be greater than when the observed rates are disparate. In the former case there will be greater "borrowing of strength" across the trials. If it happens that the results of the trials are very different, then there will be little borrowing and the information from any one trial will not apply much beyond that trial.

More generally, there may be any number of related studies or databases that provide supportive information regarding a particular therapeutic effect. The studies may be heterogeneous and may consider different patient populations. The next example is generic but it is more complicated than the previous example because it includes nine studies.[11] The only commonalty in the studies is that all addressed the efficacy of the same therapy.

The response rates can take on any value between 0 and 1. The number S of responses and sample size n are shown for each study in Table 35-2 and Fig. 35-4.

Table 35-2 **Numbers of Responses S, Sample Size n, Observed Response Proportions (Including Its Standard Error) and Adjusted Estimates of Response Rates by Study**

Study No.	Responses S	Sample Size n	Observed Response Proportions (Standard Error)	Bayes Estimate (Standard Deviation)
1	11	16	0.69 (0.116)	0.69 (0.094)
2	20	20	1.00 (0.000)	0.90 (0.064)
3	4	10	0.40 (0.155)	0.53 (0.121)
4	10	19	0.53 (0.115)	0.57 (0.094)
5	5	14	0.36 (0.128)	0.48 (0.109)
6	36	46	0.78 (0.061)	0.77 (0.058)
7	9	10	0.90 (0.095)	0.80 (0.097)
8	7	9	0.78 (0.139)	0.73 (0.110)
9	4	6	0.67 (0.192)	0.68 (0.125)
Total	106	150	0.71 (0.037)	0.68 (0.064)

Note: The Bayes estimate column is described in the text.

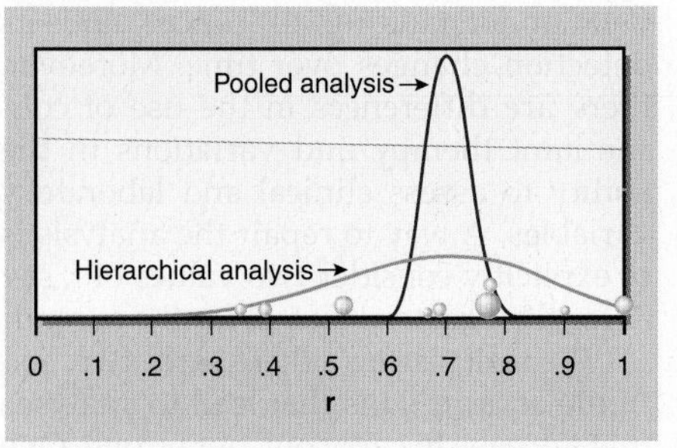

Figure 35-4 ■ Response comparisons. The dot plot on the *r*-axis shows the observed response proportions given in Table 35-2. The areas of the dots are approximately proportional to sample sizes *n*. The pooled analysis curve shows the distribution of response rate *r* assuming no study effect. The hierarchical analysis curve shows the Bayesian estimate of the distribution of response rates allowing for heterogeneity across the various studies.

There are nine response rates, *r*1, *r*2, up to *r*9, one for each study. Each of the nine sample response proportions *S*/*n* is an estimate of the corresponding *r*. There were 106 responses among 150 patients. If all nine of the response rates are assumed to be equal then the posterior distribution of the common response rate *r* (assuming a flat prior distribution) is that shown in Fig. 35-4, labeled "pooled analysis."

Even though this pooled analysis is wrong, the overall estimate of 106/150 may be quite reasonable. However, the precision associated with this estimate is too great (equivalently, its standard error is too small). In contrast, the "hierarchical analysis" curve in Fig. 35-4 is a Bayesian estimate of the distribution of the response rates in the population of studies. (This curve is the mean posterior distribution assuming a noninformative prior for the parameters in a particular class of distributions for *r*-values, called *beta distributions*.) As is typical of hierarchical analyses, this curve shows greater variability than does the analogous curve under the assumption of homogeneity.

In a hierarchical analysis, an individual study's *r* has a distribution that depends on the data from that study, but it also depends on the data from the other studies. The rightmost column in Table 35-2 shows the mean of the distribution of each study's response rate. This is also the predictive probability of the response for a future patient in that study. The individual study probabilities are shrunk toward the overall mean. This shrinkage is greater for smaller studies, and for studies with observed proportions further from the overall mean. Hierarchical borrowing is defensible because it does not make the assumption that all studies had the same true response rate, and because the extent of borrowing is determined by the data.

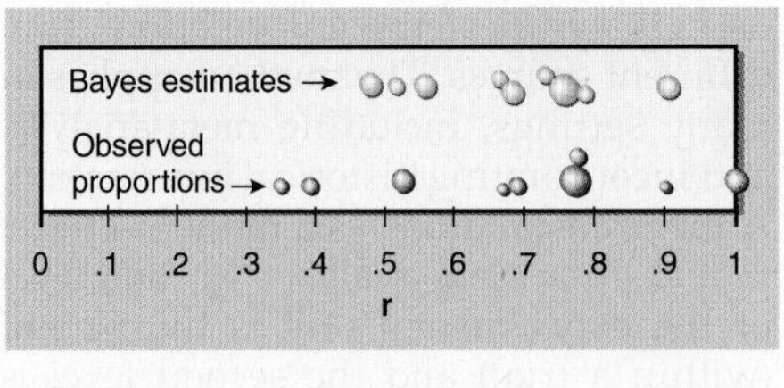

Figure 35-5 ■ Observed response proportions compared to the adjusted response rate estimates. Values are given in the two rightmost columns in Table 35-2. The dot plot on the *r*-axis shows the observed response proportions, just as in Fig. 35-4. The Bayes estimates assume a hierarchical model and show shrinkage toward the overall mean.

Fig. 35-5 provides a pictorial comparison of the rightmost two columns in Table 35-2, demonstrating shrinkage. The Bayesian estimates are intermediate between simple pooling (complete shrinkage) and each trial standing alone. The amount of shrinkage—including the two extremes mentioned previously—depends on the prior distribution of the population of trials. This aspect of the prior distribution should be set in advance, or varied to allow for assessing the sensitivity of the overall conclusion.

Shrinkage is a consequence of hierarchical modeling. The motivation for such modeling is to use the available information appropriately in improving precision or in decreasing the required sample size. Consider study number 1 in Table 35-2. Simply pooling the data from the other eight studies would greatly increase the precision of its estimated response rate. For example, the standard error would be reduced from 0.116 to 0.037. But in view of the possibility of heterogeneity in the studies, such pooling would not be justified. Borrowing hierarchically also strengthens the conclusion, but not as much. The standard deviation of the Bayes estimate is only about 20% smaller, from 0.116 to 0.094. Although smaller than the reduction with unabashed pooling, this reduction implies that >50% savings in sample size is necessary to carry out a clinical trial (in the setting of study number 1 in Table 35-2) with the same precision: $(0.116/0.094)^2 - 1 = 52\%$. For example, to achieve the same standard error in a stand-alone study would require 25 as opposed to 16 patients in study number 1 of Table 35-2.

Patient covariates can be incorporated into a hierarchical analysis, thus adjusting for known differences in the studies but still accounting for unknown effects. In this example and in more complicated hierarchical settings as well,[12] modeling allows for borrowing from other studies and databases. If the results are consistent across studies then the amount of borrowing will be greater. If the results are sufficiently different (after accounting for covariates) then this suggests heterogeneity among the studies and there is little borrowing.

Hierarchical Modeling in Trial Design

There are many settings in which trials can be set up to borrow strength from related, but not necessarily identical, experimental units.

Consider designing a trial for a therapy for a disease that has several subtypes, such as several different histologies that exist for one type of tumor. The response rates will likely differ for the different subtypes. The setting is essentially the same as that of the previous section. The focus is then the tumor response rate within the individual subtype. These have a distribution, just as in the previous section. Recognizing the possibility of borrowing across subtypes means greater precision for estimating each individual response rate and therefore that the sample size within each subtype can be smaller.

The extent of borrowing depends on the results, just as in the previous section. In other words, the savings in terms of sample size cannot be predicted with certainty. However, this is not a problem if the interim results can be monitored. The interim results can be used to determine the precision associated with the estimates of the various response rates. (This is a special case of an adaptive sample size to be described later in this chapter.) If interim results will not be available when the decision to stop the trial must be made, then the uncertainties regarding heterogeneity across subtypes can be assessed at the trial design stage and the sample size chosen accordingly, recognizing that the eventual precisions cannot be predicted perfectly.

Hazards Over Time

Time-to-event analyses are ubiquitous in cancer research. There are Bayesian analogs of the frequentist survival analyses with which the reader may be familiar. And there are hierarchical Bayesian analogs in which survival curves are allowed to depend on the category of patient or to vary with the study in a meta-analysis. However, the purpose of this section is not to extend the more traditional survival models and analyses to the Bayesian setting, rather, to focus on a narrow and relatively simple aspect of survival analysis, but one that enables greater understanding of cancer and its treatment, by using data from a clinical trial, protocol 8541 of the Cancer and Leukemia Group B (CALGB).[13]

This trial considered three different dose schedules of cyclophosphamide, Adriamycin (doxorubicin), and 5-fluorouracil (CAF) in the treatment of node-positive breast cancer: high, moderate (mod), and low. These are respectively, four cycles of CAF at 600, 60, and 600 mg/m^2, six cycles at 400, 40, 400, and four cycles at 300, 30, 300. The primary endpoint was disease-free survival, which is shown in Fig. 35-6 for the three dose groups using Kaplan–Meier plots. There are no *p*-values provided for the various comparisons (high vs moderate; high vs low) because whether these are statistically significant is immaterial to the purpose.

Time-to-event curves such as those in Fig. 35-6 are standard but they do not tell the whole story regarding any benefit of increasing dose and dose intensity. A clearer picture is contained in hazard plots over time. Hazards are the proportions of events within a particular time period as a fraction of those patients who are at risk at the beginning of the period. For example, suppose the event is a recurrence and there are 100 patients in a group that are at risk in the first year. If 10 of these patients experience a recurrence of the disease in the first year, then the first-year hazard is 10%. Going into the second year there are 90 patients at risk. If another 18 experience recurrences in the second year, then the second-year hazard is 18/90 = 20%. When calculating hazards from survival plots such as those in Fig. 35-6, one subtracts the current year's survival proportion from the previous year's survival proportion and divides by the previous year's survival proportion. The resulting yearly hazards are shown in Fig. 35-7.

A striking observation from Fig. 35-7 is that the hazards decrease over time (after the second year) for all three treatment arms. This is a reflection of the heterogeneity of this disease. The most aggressive tumors recur early, giving the high hazards evident in the first few years. Once their tumors have recurred, patients are

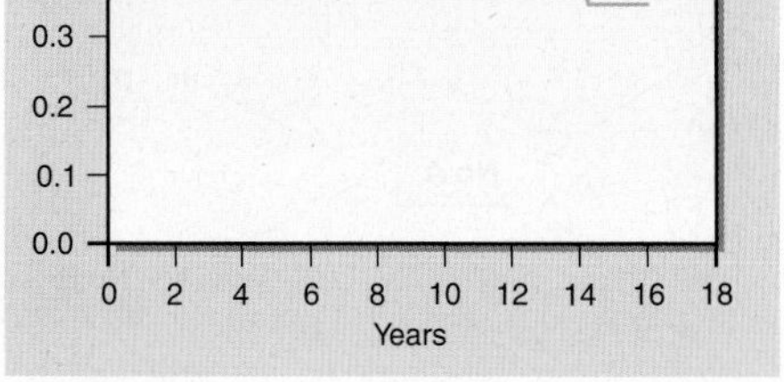

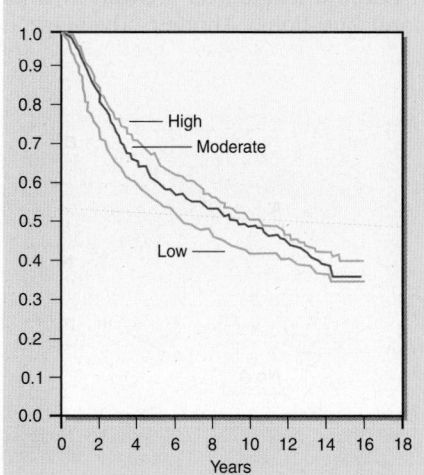

Figure 35-6 Disease-free survival proportions for the three CAF dose groups of CALGB 8541.

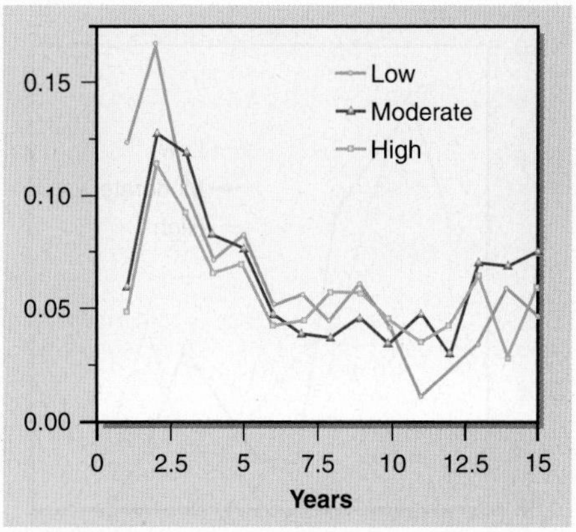

Figure 35-7 Hazards for the three CAF dose groups of CALGB 8541, derived from Fig. 35-6.

removed from the at-risk population. The remaining tumors are less aggressive and so they recur at a lower rate.

Regarding a treatment arm effect, the apparent benefit of the high-dose schedule is restricted to the first 5 years or so. Actually, the hazard for patients on the high-dose schedule is lower than those of the other two arms in each of the first 6 years. (Although it is not much lower in the last few of these 6 years, and it is not much lower than that of the moderate-dose schedule at any time.) This observation is impressive because each year is like a new study, with previous recurrences not counted when starting a new year.

Another observation from Fig. 35-7 is that after 5 years the risks of all three groups converge, with the annual risk of recurrence being approximately 5% in all three groups.

The reduction in hazard of recurrence for the high- vs low-dose schedules is 14% over the 18 years of follow-up (95% confidence interval: 6-22%). This is an average over these years (weighted over time because of the differences in at-risk sample sizes over time). But because there is no reduction at all in the later years, the overall reduction is being carried by the early years. Restricting to the first 3 years, the reduction is 24% (13-33%). A benefit of chemotherapy that is restricted to the first few years is typical in breast cancer trials. An implication is that a hazard reduction seen early in a trial, say one with a median of 3 years of follow-up, will deteriorate over time. This is because the comparison will eventually involve averaging over periods where there is no longer a treatment benefit.

In the later years, the hazards of about 5% are very similar to the annual hazard for patients with node-negative breast cancer. Interestingly, convergence to about 5% applies irrespective of the number of positive lymph nodes. Fig. 35-8 shows this effect. It gives hazard plots for

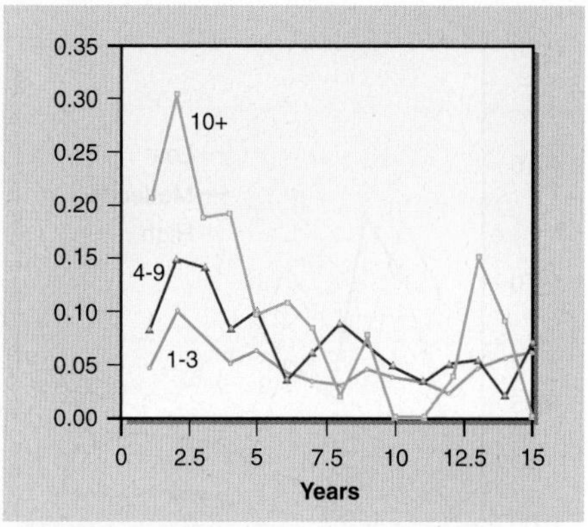

Figure 35-8 Hazards for the three categories of positive lymph nodes (1-3, 4-9, and 10 or more) for CALGB 8541. There are few patients at risk in the later years, especially in the 10+ group, and for two reasons. One is that this was the smallest group to start, with 174 of the 1,550 patients in the trial, and the other is that the disease recurred early for most in this group. At 13 years there were only 24 patients at risk, and 3 of these had disease recurrence in the 13th year.

three categories of positive nodes: 1-3, 4-9, and 10 or more (for the three dose groups combined). Early in the trial, patients with 10$^+$ positive nodes have a very high annual recurrence rate of 20-30%. However, after 5 years or so, the annual hazard is about 5% in all three groups. So, a woman with a large number of positive nodes who has not experienced disease recurrence in the first 5 years or so has the same updated prognosis as a woman with a small number of positive nodes, including no positive nodes. The effects of both the number of positive nodes and dose of CAF have worn off after 5 years.

An important aspect of CALGB 8541 is the role of tumor HER2/neu expression, and in particular its interaction with dose of CAF.[14] HER2/neu assessment was carried out for a subset of 992 patients from the original study. Its interaction with dose was shown to be significant in a multivariate proportional hazards model. But the manner of interaction is easiest to understand using hazards. Fig. 35-9 shows the effect of dose of CAF separately for patients with HER2/neu–negative (n = 720) and HER2/neu–positive (n = 272) tumors. HER2/neu–negative tumors (in the left-hand panel of Fig. 35-9) show no dose effect. The entire benefit of the high- over the moderate-dose treatment schedule and the high- over the low-dose treatment schedule that is observed in these patients is concentrated in those with HER2/neu–positive tumors. Moreover, this benefit occurs through a reduction in hazard in each of the first 3-4 years. Again, each year is a separate study and so each of these years provides a separate confirmation of the overall conclusion. The hazard reduction in the

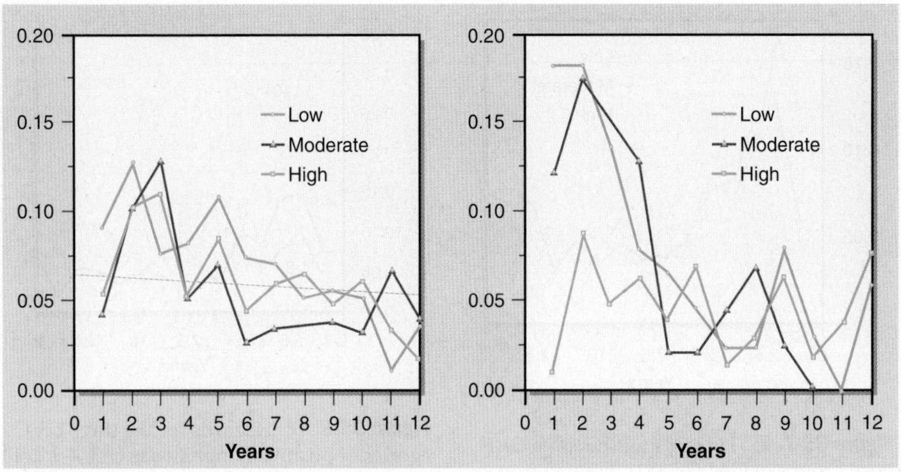

Figure 35-9 Annual disease-free survival hazards for a subset of patients (n = 992) in CALGB. The subset consists of patients for whom the expression of HER2/neu in the patient's tumor was assessed. The left-hand panel represents patients with HER2/neu-negative tumors and the right-hand panel patients with HER2/neu-positive tumors.

first 3 years for patients receiving the high-dose treatment schedule, as compared with the other two groups combined, was 65% among patients with HER2/neu–positive tumors. HER2/neu overexpression apparently conveys a poor prognosis for lower doses but not for higher doses—it might even provide a favorable prognosis for patients receiving higher doses.

Many of the conclusions in this section would have been difficult or impossible to make without considering hazards over time.

A final comment regarding hazards relates to the common problem of predicting survival results into the future for patients already accrued to a trial. This differs from the general problem of prediction discussed earlier in "Predictive Probabilities." Consider Fig. 35-6. Some of the patients have as little as 10 years of follow-up information. As more follow-up information becomes available, there will be no change in these curves prior to the 10-year time point. But the curves are subject to change beyond 10 years. Because the focus is on patients for whom the tumor has not yet recurred, the way the curves will change depends on the hazards beyond 10 years. The information available about these hazards is shown in Fig. 35-7. For predicting when and whether a patient's disease will recur, consider hazards 1 year at a time, always building on the patient's current year of follow-up. Each incremental hazard prediction depends on the data for the corresponding year.

Principles of Statistical Design: Factorial Experiments

Most comparative drug trials in oncology have two treatment arms. Typically, one uses an experimental agent and the other does not. The patients in both arms may receive additional therapy based on the current standard of care for the type and stage of their cancer, and on their prior treatment. They may have surgery and receive concomitant radiation and other chemotherapy, which may include several drugs. If the experimental drug is shown to be sufficiently effective, then it will be incorporated into the standard therapy.

This approach is simple and clean. It is sometimes called KISS: "Keep it simple, stupid!" But it has a number of drawbacks. One is that it is not possible to assess the individual contributions of the various components of polychemotherapy that are developed in this way. Another is that the approach provides a mechanism for adding drugs to standard regimens but not for subtracting them. An experimental agent's effectiveness may require all other components of the standard regimen. Adding an experimental drug to a standard regimen, however, may make other components of the regimen unnecessary. In the latter case, there is no way of identifying these components.

To some extent this conundrum is inevitable. Studying the possible removal of a component of standard chemotherapy is difficult, and for ethical reasons this is so, even if the component has never been proven to contribute to the overall effectiveness of the combination. However, better approaches for developing drugs would alleviate the problem and could lead to more rapid development of better therapies.

At any given time, various experimental agents are being studied by different clinical trial groups, in most cases by adding them to therapy that is standard for the disease in question. One group may be studying drug A and another drug B. If both are shown to be effective it will not be clear which is better and whether the combination of drugs A and B would prove better than, just as good as, or worse than using only one of the drugs.

A fundamental principle of optimal experimental design in statistics is in stark contrast with KISS: change the various contributing factors in such a way as to learn efficiently about their impact on outcome. This impact may involve interactions between the factors and it is important to learn about such interactions. What is required is to model relationships and exploit the available data to inform the model. From the perspective of optimal design, the KISS principle more appropriately stands for "Keep it simple AND stupid."

An alternative to varying one factor at a time in separate studies is using factorial designs. In the simplest example considered earlier, patients would be assigned to one of four regimens: A alone, B alone, A and B in combination, and neither. (The last of these does not mean "no therapy" because all patients receive standard therapy.) These four possibilities are shown schematically in Fig. 35-10 where "A" means that the patient receives A and "No A" means the patient does not receive A. The factors may be drugs, or other interventions (eg, "A" could be radiation therapy, or surgery before rather than after chemotherapy, or a high dose as opposed to a low dose of a drug). Reading from left to right in Fig. 35-10 may not indicate time. The two drugs may be given concurrently or sequentially, A before B or B before A. Indeed, sequential vs concurrent administration of drugs could be another factor in a factorial design (eg, see Citron and colleagues[15]).

An advantage of factorial designs is that they enable estimating the "main effects" of the individual drugs and therefore a single trial answers two (or more) questions. Another advantage is

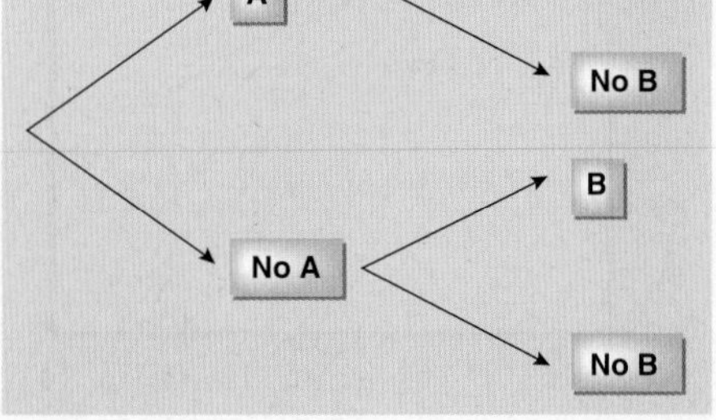

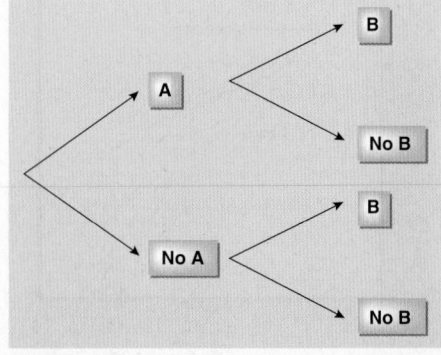

Figure 35-10 A 2×2 factorial design considering drugs A and B and their combination. There are 4 possible treatment combinations.

that factorial designs allow for assessing interactions between the factors. For example, comparing the difference between the top two cases in Fig. 35-10 with the difference between the bottom two cases addresses whether the effect of B is the same when it is given with drug A as when it is given without drug A. Table 35-3 shows the types of interactions that are possible for the four combinations of drugs A and B considered in Fig. 35-10, assuming that the endpoint is response rate. For negative interactions, the effect of the combination is less than the sum of the individual drug effects. For positive interactions, the effect of the combination is greater than the sum of the individual drug effects.

There are no compensating disadvantages in using factorial designs! In particular, the sample size is no greater than for a two-armed design that addresses the effect of just one of the two drugs. Each patient contributes equally to estimating the main effects of both factors. For example, assuming equal sample sizes in the four possible combinations, the estimated main effect of B is the simple average of the effect of B for those patients who also receive drug A and the effect of B for those patients who do not receive drug A.

A limitation of using factorial designs is that some treatment combinations may not be ethically or practically possible. For example, one of the combinations in Fig. 35-10 is neither of the two drugs. In some oncology settings it may not be possible to have such a treatment arm. Including only three arms in the trial is better than having only two, but then individual drug effects cannot be assessed and the sample size advantages of the factorial design are lost.

When a two-armed trial is designed to have a particular power, a second factor can be added without increasing the sample size. The power for assessing the interaction between the factors is not as great as for assessing a main effect, but there will be some information about interactions. The sample size can be increased if high power for assessing an interaction is required, but a reasonable and usually a more realistic alternative is to keep the sample size the same and accept modest power for assessing interactions. It may happen that the interaction is strong enough to show statistical significance. Moreover, any interaction that is clinically important is likely to show at least a hint of an interaction in the trial's results and this may lead to a follow-on trial to better quantify the degree of interaction.

Learning about interactions is essential, both clinically and scientifically, and interactions cannot be identified from a single two-armed trial. At best, three separate, two-armed trials would be required, and the likelihood of their being completed is not high. For example, one trial could compare A with No A, a second could compare B with No B, and a third could compare the combination with A alone. There are several disadvantages of this approach relative to factorial designs: (1) The total sample size is 3 times as large; (2) the third trial may not be possible if both the single-agent trials turn out to be effective as single agents; (3) neither drug may be effective on its own but the combination may be effective; and (4) outcomes of the clinical trials are heterogeneous even if they employ the same patient eligibility criteria. Therefore, treatment effects would be confounded with any trial effects. Possibility (3) that only in combination are the two drugs effective could happen in a variety of ways, one of which is when the two drugs target different but parallel metastatic pathways. In this circumstance (presented in the rightmost column in Table 35-3), both drugs would fail their respective two-armed trials and be abandoned, with the effectiveness of the combination never discovered.

Factorial designs can consider more than two factors and more than two levels per factor. For example, Henderson and colleagues[16] considered three dose schedules of doxorubicin and paclitaxel vs no paclitaxel in node-positive breast cancer using a 3 × 2 factorial design. This trial was noteworthy in answering two important clinical questions: increasing the dose of doxorubicin (in combination with 600 mg/m^2 of cyclophosphamide) from 60 to 75 to 90 mg/m^2 in four q3-week cycles did not improve either disease-free or overall survival, and adding four q3-week cycles of paclitaxel (75 mg/m^2) did improve both. Moreover, it answered a third question because there was not a hint of an interaction between the two factors.

Figure 35-11 shows a somewhat more complicated example, a 2 × 2 × 3 factorial design. Now there are three doses of drug C. (An application would be a modification of the aforementioned trial reported by Henderson and colleagues,[16] in which cyclophosphamide would have been used at two doses. A could be paclitaxel, B would then be cyclophosphamide, and C would be doxorubicin.) Again, data from every patient contribute in estimating the main effects of A, B, and C separately and so there is no increase in sample size. Estimating three-way interactions has less power than estimating two-way interactions, but the results from the factorial design in Fig. 35-11 will contain some information about the three-way interaction of drugs A, B, and C.

Factorial designs apply in both phases II and III. In phase II they are especially relevant in proof-of-concept trials involving multiple investigational agents. Such trials may involve many drugs, and many more possible combinations of the drugs. The number of drugs and their combinations may be so large that a balanced factorial design is not tenable. A modification is to use an adaptive randomization scheme, as discussed in a subsequent section of this chapter. The efficacy and toxicity of the various combinations could be explored using unbalanced assignments, favoring

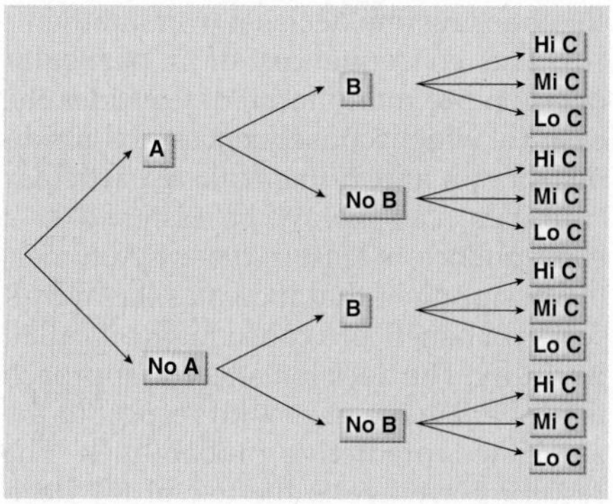

Figure 35-11 A 2×2×3 factorial design considering drugs A and B, three levels of drug C, and their combinations. There are 12 possible treatment combinations.

Table 35-3 **Response Rates (%) for the Four Treatment Combinations in a Factorial Design in Which Drugs A and B Are Added to Standard Therapy (Hypothetical Effects)**

Treatment Combination	Neither Effective	A Effective B Not	B Effective A Not	Additive Effects	Negative Interaction	Positive Interaction (Example i)	Positive Interaction (Example ii)
A and B	20	30	30	40	30	50	40
A, No B	20	30	20	30	30	30	20
B, no A	20	20	30	30	30	30	20
Neither	20	20	20	20	20	20	20

combinations that the accumulating data suggest are promising. If it turns out that one of the drugs is ineffective, whether used with or without the other drugs, it would be dropped.

In many oncology drug settings, toxicity is as important as efficacy. There are ways to incorporate them both in a factorial design. For example, one can establish the notion of *admissible combinations* based on toxicity. This involves allowing only certain of the full factorial combinations at the start of the trial. As experience accrues about toxicity, other combinations become admissible, or the number of admissible combinations shrinks. The assignment to treatment combinations within the set of admissible combinations can be made either randomly or adaptively based on accumulating information about efficacy (see Adaptive design of Clinical Trials).

Decision Analysis and Choosing Sample Size

Clinical practice and clinical research involve making decisions. An example of the latter is choosing the sample size of a clinical trial. It is impossible to precisely predict the result of making a particular decision, but one can list the possible results and associate (predictive) probabilities with each of the possibilities. Also associated with each possible result are the consequences of that result. A list of results, probabilities, and consequences characterizes each decision, and allows for choosing one decision over another.

The consequences of a particular decision are many faceted. Consider the case in which consequences are unidimensional, and numerical. A particular "number" can always be assigned to a consequence, at least in theory. A numerical assignment that indicates the overall worth or benefit of a consequence is called its utility. The decision analytic approach is to average the uses with respect to the associated predictive probabilities. The resulting average is the use of the decision in question, and the various possible decisions can be compared on the basis of their usage. The central role of predictive probabilities in this process makes the Bayesian approach ideally suited for decision making.

The terms decision making, decision analysis, and decision theory are used more or less interchangeably. Many references develop this subject more deeply than is possible to report here.[17-20]

A simple example will help fix the concept. One is offered an opportunity to win a prize that has a utility of 10. The utility of playing for the prize is –1. There are two decisions: play or not play. If one plays, then he will end up with a utility of either 9 or –1. Suppose that the probability of the former is r. (A class of decisions not considered here, performing an experiment to get information about r, is interesting and revealing.) The utility of playing is then $9r - (1-r) = 10r - 1$. The utility of not playing is 0. Playing is optimal if $r > 0.1$.

Averaging utilities to assess taking gambles is well and good. But it is less clear that it is appropriate when outcomes are health states or the results of clinical trials. Moreover, it may be difficult to assess the utilities of such outcomes. However, one must make a decision, and when faced with a list of outcomes and their associated probabilities for each available decision, reducing the lists to a single dimension greatly facilitates choosing among them. In addition, varying the probabilities and utilities assumed allows for assessing the sensitivity of the various aspects of the decision process.

Consider a decision-analytic approach for choosing a sample size in a two-armed clinical trial. The purpose of clinical trials is to learn about competing therapies. The benefit of learning about competing therapies is that it may affect the future treatment of patients having the disease in question. In a decision analysis one can consider delivering good medicine to all patients who have the disease. The utility of any particular design of a clinical trial is its consequent effect on patients who have the disease, including the patients in the trial as well as those outside the trial. This approach contrasts with the stark attitude of the Belmont Report[4] in which the knowledge derived from treating patients in the trial is distinguished from the treatment of patients who present after the trial.

Consider the patients who will benefit from the conclusions of the clinical trials being planned. Call this the "patient horizon" N. Its numerical value depends on the prevalence of the disease and the availability of alternative treatments. The population of patients with primary breast cancer who might benefit from an advance in therapy is very large. But N is small in a rare type of children's cancer. Experimentation has a greater value when N is large, whereas treating the current patients more effectively has a greater value when N is small. Therefore, these two extremes have different sample size implications. However, they are addressed in the same way when choosing sample sizes via power calculations. In the case of a small N, a substantial portion of the patients, perhaps all, may be in the clinical trial and so few if any subsequent patients will get to take advantage of the results obtained in the trial. In the case of a large N, a trial may be too small to enable an informed choice between the two treatments and so the very large number of patients outside the trial may receive inferior therapy. A conclusion of this section is that when the goal is treating as many patients as effectively as possible, the sample sizes of the clinical trials depend greatly on the magnitude of N.

The value of N is not usually precisely known. In particular, N depends on the effectiveness and side effects of both treatments, which are also unknown. However, a consequence of this section is that only the order of magnitude of N should be considered in choosing the sample sizes of clinical trials. Precision in fixing N is not very important. Considering the extremes, diseases or conditions that are very common (large N), call for larger trials than do rare diseases (small N). Moreover, when N is unknown, the results of this section rely on replacing N with its mean. So experts could assess the annual size of the patient population and the potential availability of other therapies over the next several years. Patients presenting in the future could be discounted by the probability that they will be treated using one of the treatments involved in the trial. This gives an expected value of N that can be used in designing the trial.

For convenience, consider dichotomous outcomes: response and nonresponse . The goal is to treat as many of the N patients as successfully as possible with one of two therapies. The utility of any trial is the number of responses over the patient horizon (including both those in the trial and those beyond). An optimal sample size maximizes the expected number of responses over the patient horizon N. By definition, patients in the horizon are those who present after the trial and who are given the therapy that performed better in the trial.

The optimal trial sample size has an order of magnitude the square root of N.[21] If there are two clinical trials (followed by implementation of the better performing therapy in clinical practice), then the first of the two should have a sample size with an order of magnitude the cube root of N. Table 35-4 considers a setting in which the optimal trial sample size for a common disease with N of about one million turns out to be 1000. The point of Table 35-4 is to compare this with the corresponding optimal sample sizes for more rare diseases. The table also shows the optimal sample size for the first of two clinical trials. The sample sizes are strikingly different for common vs uncommon diseases.

In a decision analysis one can explicitly consider asymmetry in information concerning the treatment arms under consideration. The allocation proportions

Table 35-4 **Optimal Sample Sizes of a Clinical Trial When the Patient Horizon Is *N***

Patient Horizon, *N*	1,000,000	100,000	10,000	1000	100
Single trial sample size	1000	320	100	32	10
Sample size for the first of two trials	170	78	36	17	8

Note: Sample sizes are given with two-digit accuracy. The optimal sample sizes for *N* = 1,000,000 are for a particular prior distribution of the unknown parameters. The ratios of optimal sample sizes within each row apply for arbitrary prior distributions. For example, if the optimal single-trial sample size for *N* = 1,000,000 were 2000 then that for *N* = 100 would be 20.

should also be asymmetric. As above, continue to assume a two-armed trial with the goal being to effectively treat as many patients in horizon *N* as possible. Consider the particular forms of prior information about the unknown rates of response that are shown in Fig. 35-12. Suppose the response rate for one of the arms, say arm 1, has distribution A and that for the other arm, arm 2, has either distribution A, B, or C.

Consider $N = 100$ or greater, as indicated in Table 35-5. The table shows the optimal sample sizes for each of the arms. As discussed above, these increase with *N* in proportion to the square root of *N* (approximately). Consider the case of $N = 1000$ and distribution A for both response rates. The table indicates that 21 patients should be assigned to one of the arms and 20 to the other. In view of symmetry, either arm 1 or arm 2 could get the extra patient. Using this assignment, the resulting response proportion among the 1000 patients in the horizon is 65%. Increasing either or both sample sizes decreases this response proportion. And decreasing either or both sample sizes decreases this response proportion. To consider the extremes, both not running a clinical trial at all and running a trial entering all 1000 patients have expected response proportions of 50%.

For the case distribution A vs B in Table 35-5, arm 2 is more promising than arm 1 and so it is assigned to more patients in the trial—about $\sqrt{3} - 1 = 73\%$ more for a large *N*. For distribution A vs C, the response rate for arm 2 is known to be 0.5. The response rate for arm 1 could be greater than 0.5 or less than 0.5. The trial's purpose—in addition to treating patients effectively—is to identify whether the arm 1 response rate is greater than or less than 0.5. To achieve this purpose it would be a waste to allocate patients to arm 2 because its response rate is known. Arm 2 is held in reserve and will be used after the trial should it turn out that arm 1's observed response rate is less than 0.5.

This section assumes no interim monitoring. There could be a substantial benefit in the response rate achieved if updating is possible during the trial. Such updating could be used to modify the proportions of patients allocated to the two arms, and it could be used to determine when the clinical trial should end. These possibilities and other related modifications are considered in the next section. However, the next section is not explicitly decision analytic, and in particular it does not address maximizing the overall response proportion in choosing a clinical trial design.

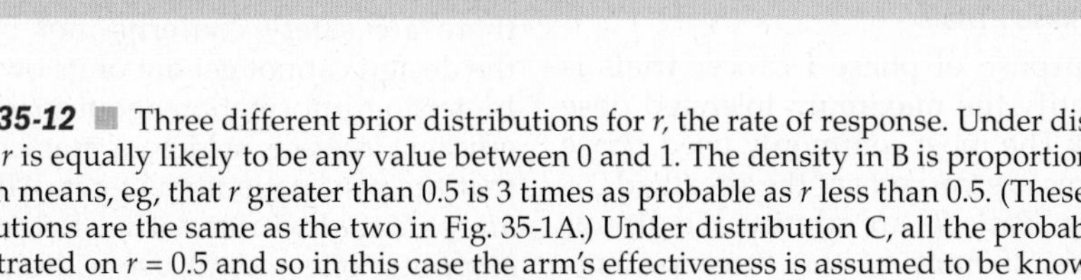

Figure 35-12 Three different prior distributions for *r*, the rate of response. Under distribution A, *r* is equally likely to be any value between 0 and 1. The density in B is proportional to *r*, which means, eg, that *r* greater than 0.5 is 3 times as probable as *r* less than 0.5. (These two distributions are the same as the two in Fig. 35-1A.) Under distribution C, all the probability is concentrated on $r = 0.5$ and so in this case the arm's effectiveness is assumed to be known.

Adaptive Designs of Clinical Trials

The first step in planning a trial is to assess the available evidence regarding the hypotheses and parameters of interest. In a Bayesian approach, the trial designer addresses the possibility of using this information in a prior distribution or incorporating it in a hierarchical model along with the results of the trial being planned.

At the planning stage it is important to consider the possible state of affairs when the trial is over. One consideration is the set of implications and consequences of each possible result. Another is the predictive probability of each possible result. The previous section presents an approach in which utilities are assessed for the former and weighed with respect to the latter. The present section deals with designs that are more flexible than the ones in the previous section. Although the designs in this section are not based on an explicit consideration of utilities, the goals are efficient learning and effective treatment of patients. For an explicit decision-analytic generalization of some parts of this section, see Bandit Problems: Sequential Allocation of Experiments.[22]

Consider a trial having a particular design. Calculating the predictive probabilities of the trial's results is always possible, even for the most complicated of designs (although the most complicated designs require simulations). These calculations allow for finding a variety of the design's attributes, including the probability of achieving a statistically significant benefit of one therapy over another, the expected number of patients in the trial, and the expected number of patients in the trial who successfully respond to their assigned treatment. Comparing the calculations for different designs facilitates choosing one design over another.

Designs of clinical trials are usually static in the sense that the sample size and any prescription for assigning treatment, including for randomization protocols, are fixed in advance. Results observed during the trial are not used to guide its course. There are exceptions. Some phase II cancer trials have two stages, with stopping after the first stage possible if the results are not sufficiently promising. And most phase III protocols specify interim analyses that determine whether the trial should be stopped early for sufficiently strong evidence of a difference between competing treatment arms. However, traditional early stopping criteria are very conservative and so few trials stop early.

The simplicity of trials with static designs makes them solid inferential tools. Their sample sizes tend to be large, at least in comparison with the alternatives to be discussed in this section. And they usually consider two therapeutic strategies, or arms, thus enabling straightforward treatment comparisons. That is not to say that static trials always give clear answers as to whether one arm is better than the other, but only that they usually allow for an unambiguous quantification

Table 35-5 Optimal Allocations of Sample Size to Arms 1 and 2 in a Two-Armed Clinical Trial Plus Response Proportion Among the N Patients for That Allocation

Patient Horizon, N	Prior Distributions of Rates from Figure 35-12; Optimal Success Proportion								
	1: A	2: A	Prop	1: A	2: B	Prop	1: A	2: C	Prop
100	6	5	0.63	4	8	0.71	9	0	0.60
1000	21	20	0.65	16	30	0.74	29	0	0.62
10,000	70	69	0.66	56	98	0.75	99	0	0.62
Large N	$\sqrt{N/2}$	$\sqrt{N/2}$	2/3	$\sqrt{N/3}$	$\sqrt{N}$	3/4	$\sqrt{N}$	0	5/8

For each value of N there are three pairings of prior distributions of the arm 1 and arm 2 response rates considered. The optimal asymptotic (large N) response proportion is the expected value of the maximum of the two response rates, where the expectation is with respect to the prior distribution.
Abbreviation: Prop, response proportion.

of the uncertainty regarding whether one arm is better.

Despite their virtues, static trials result in slow and unnecessarily costly drug development. Hundreds of millions of dollars and many years can be expended in developing a single cancer drug, one that may not make it to market. For a company developing a moderate number of drugs (say 20 or more), this circumstance is tolerated because costs are balanced by profits from other drugs. Smaller companies are at the mercy of the prevailing attitudes toward drug development and risk going bankrupt.

The tradition of drug development is one at a time. The number of cancer drugs available for development is increasing exponentially. It is inefficient to focus on a single drug when myriad others are sitting on the sidelines waiting to be evaluated. The standard types of errors in drug development are false positives and false negatives. These errors apply to drugs actually being tested. Another kind of error applies to drugs not under investigation: Every such drug is a false neutral. A drug not being developed has no chance of helping anyone. Finite resources limit the ability of the medical establishment to develop therapies. But when resources are limited we should approach their allocation in a more rational way. And what makes sense today may well be different from the ways of the past.

Pharmaceutical companies and medical researchers generally must be able to consider hundreds or thousands of drugs for development at the same time. Static trials inhibit the simultaneous processing of many drugs. And they cannot efficiently address dose-response questions when many drugs are under consideration. Dynamic designs that are integrated with the drug development process are necessary for reasonable progress in medical research.

The focus of this section is a family of designs that are dynamic in the sense that observations made during the trial can affect the subsequent course of the trial. The general class of designs is adaptive or sequential. The focus is clinical trials, but the ideas apply at least as forcefully in the preclinical setting. A main bottleneck of the drug development process occurs at the level of the preclinical animal toxicity/carcinogenicity studies. There are many opportunities for using adaptive designs in the preclinical area that will efficiently identify the best drugs to move forward in trials for humans.

Using an adaptive design means examining the accumulating data periodically, or even continually, with the goal of modifying the trial's design. These modifications depend on what the data show about the unknown hypotheses. Among the modifications possible are stopping early, restricting eligibility criteria, expanding accrual to additional sites, extending accrual beyond the trial's original sample size if its conclusion is still not clear, dropping arms or doses, and adding arms or doses. All of these possibilities are considered in the light of the accumulating information. Adaptive designs also include unbalanced randomization where the degree of imbalance depends on the accumulating data. For example, arms that give more information about the hypothesis in question or that are performing better than other arms can be weighted more heavily.[22]

Adaptation is not limited to the data accumulating in the trial. Information that is reported from other ongoing trials can also be used. This is easier to effect if one takes a Bayesian approach, possibly using hierarchical modeling as described in the previous section.

Adaptive designs are increasingly being used in cancer trials. This is true for trials sponsored by pharmaceutical companies, and more generally. For example, a variety of trials at The University of Texas M. D. Anderson Cancer Center (MDACC) are prospectively adaptive, as described below.

Continuous Reassessment Method (CRM) in Phase I Trials

The purpose of phase I cancer trials is to identify the maximum tolerated dose (MTD). The most commonly used phase I designs are variants of the so-called 3 + 3 design. Patients are admitted in groups of three. If none of the three patients experiences toxicity then the dose is increased one level for the next group of three. If two or three of the three patients experience toxicity then the next lower dose is the MTD. If one of the three experiences toxicity then three more patients are added at the same dose level. If two or more of the six patients at that dose experience toxicity then again the next lower dose is the MTD.[23]

This design is adaptive, but its adaptation is very crude. Such a design is likely to assign low doses and to select an MTD that is ineffective. Moreover, such a design ignores important information that is available in the trial. In particular, dose assignments are not based on sufficient statistics.[24] An alternative approach uses Bayesian updating: the continual reassessment method (CRM) of O'Quigley and colleagues.[25] In this method, updating takes place assuming a particular model of the relationship between dose and toxicity (such as the logistic function). The CRM too is adaptive. Each patient is assigned to the dose having the probability of toxicity closest to some predetermined target value. This is the Bayesian posterior probability calculated from the data available up to that point (and so it is based on sufficient statistics).

The CRM more effectively finds the MTD than does the 3 + 3 design. The CRM is the standard design used in phase I trials at MDACC. But it is rather crude and is being improved in a number of ways. One of these ways is based on the fundamental principle that ignoring information is wrong. (A catch, of course, is that taking information into account is work, and it can require modeling.) There is some information that accrues about efficacy in a phase I trial. This information is limited, especially regarding the dose-efficacy relationship. But at a minimum, in proceeding to phase II with a particular dose (usually the MTD), one should use the efficacy information from those patients in phase I who were assigned to that dose. This notion leads to using a phase I/II design that addresses safety and efficacy simultaneously, or one that focuses on efficacy after an initial focus on toxicity. Such an approach is efficient from the perspective of both time and patient resources.

A way in which both 3 + 3 and CRM designs are crude is the need to pause the accrual while waiting for toxicity information.[26,27] Such pauses are inefficient and they cause logistical problems. Trials should be paused or stopped if there are safety concerns, not because the design cannot get out of its own way. In getting information about toxicity (or efficacy), there is seldom a magical dose that the next patient must get. All doses are potentially informative. Rather than stopping, one should use a design that models dose response (toxicity and efficacy) and is able to assign a next dose even though patients previously treated are not yet fully evaluable.

Another way in which both 3 + 3 and CRM designs are crude is the assumption that toxicity is dichotomous. An approach that is better—again because of using all available information—would be to account for the severity of toxicity. Again, it would be better to consider both the severity of toxicity and the efficacy in a phase I/II design.[28] Assigning utilities to the various possible health states would lead to weighing these two conflicting desiderata in a decision analysis.

Adaptive Dose-Finding in Phase II Trials

In many diseases, the standard phase II dose-finding design is to allocate a fixed number of patients to each of a number of doses in a grid. Such questions are generally of less interest in cancer because of the MTD mentality: administer as much drug as the patient can tolerate. But with the increasing interest in biological agents, dose finding for efficacy is becoming important in cancer research.

After seeing the results of a dose-finding trial, the investigators usually wish they had assigned patients in some other fashion. Perhaps the dose-response curve was shifted more to the left or right than anticipated. If so, then the assignment of a bulk of the patients on one end or the other was wasted. Or perhaps the slope of the dose-response curve is greater than anticipated and the response of patients assigned to the flat regions of the curve would have been more informative if the doses assigned had been in the region where the slope is apparently greatest. Or perhaps the results for the early patients made it clear that the dose-response curve was flat over the entire range and therefore the trial could have stopped earlier. Or perhaps the results of the trial show that the standard deviation of the outcome of interest is greater or less than anticipated and so the trial should have been larger or could have been smaller.

The approach of Berry and colleagues[29] is to proceed sequentially, analyzing the data as it accumulates (see also the approach of Malakoff[30]). There are two stages of the trial, first dose ranging (phase II) and then confirmatory (phase III), if the latter is warranted. The dose-ranging stage continues until a decision is made that the drug is not sufficiently effective to pursue future development or that the optimal dose for the confirmatory phase III trial is sufficiently well known. (Switches to phase III can be effected seamlessly and without stopping accrual, and this is so even if the endpoint of interest is delayed, such as time to progression. See below.) The example trial of Berry and colleagues[29] involves a biological neuroprotective agent for stroke. But the same principles of trial design apply in cancer research. Each patient entering the trial is assigned the dose (1 of 16, including a placebo) that maximizes the information about the dose-response relationship, given the results observed so far. This dose could be in the region of the greatest apparent slope, or it could be the placebo or a high dose. But future patients are not assigned to doses in any region where accumulating evidence suggests that the dose-response curve is flat.

In the dose-ranging stage, neither the number of patients assigned to any particular dose nor the total number of patients assigned in this stage are fixed in advance. The dose-ranging sample size will be large when the data suggest that the drug has moderate benefit, when the dose-response curve is gently sloping, or when the standard deviation of the responses is moderately large. It will tend to be small if the drug has substantial benefit, if the drug has no benefit, if the dose-response curve rises over a narrow range of doses, or if the standard deviation of the responses turns out to be small. (In addition, and somewhat nonintuitively, the dose-ranging stage will be small if the standard deviation of the responses is very large. The reason is that a sufficiently large standard deviation means that a very large sample size would be required to demonstrate a beneficial drug effect. The required sample size may be so large that it would be impossible to study the drug and so the trial stops in the dose-ranging phase before substantial resources go down the drain.)

In the stroke trial considered by Berry and colleagues,[29] the ultimate endpoint is an improvement in the stroke scale from baseline to 13 weeks. If the accrual rate is large then the benefit of adaptive assignment can be limited by delays in obtaining the endpoint information. To minimize the effects of delayed information, each patient's stroke scale is assessed weekly between baseline and week 13. Within-patient measurements are correlated, with correlations greater if they are closer together in time. We incorporate a longitudinal model into the analysis of the trial and carry out Bayesian predictions of the ultimate endpoint based on the current patient-specific information, and we update the probability distributions of the treatment effect accordingly.

Adaptive dosing is more effective than is the standard design at identifying the right dose. And it usually identifies the right dose with a smaller sample size than when using fixed dose assignments. Another advantage is that many more doses can be considered in an adaptive design. (Even though some doses will be little used and some may never be used, these cannot be predicted in advance.) An adaptive design therefore has some ability to distinguish responses at adjacent doses and to estimate the nuances of the dose-response curve.

The circumstances of the stroke trial are similar to those in many other types of trials. Finding the right dose is a ubiquitous problem in pharmaceutical development, and it is seldom done well or efficiently. The adaptive nature of the stroke trial would be less advantageous if we had not exploited early endpoints. Cancer, too, is characterized by the availability of information about a patient's performance (local control of the disease, biomarkers, etc.) before reaching the primary endpoint. Finally, the possibility of moving seamlessly into phase III depending on the phase II results exists for many types of drugs. That issue leads naturally to the subject of the next section.

Seamless Phases II and III

The convention of categorizing drug development into phases is unfortunate. We proceed from one phase to the next when we think we know something: the MTD from phase I, or that a drug's impact on a phase II endpoint will translate into a benefit in phase III, and at the phase II dose. In the Bayesian approach one never takes a quantity to be perfectly known. Instead, the Bayesian perspective is to carry along uncertainty with whatever knowledge is available. Phases of drug development are arbitrary labels that describe a process that is, or should be, continuous.

One of the consequences of partitioning drug development into phases is that there are delays between phases. For example, there is a pause between phases II and III to set up one or more pivotal studies. As mentioned above in the context of the stroke trial, its design allows for avoiding such a hiatus. At each time point, say weekly, the algorithm that guides the conduct of the trial carries out a decision analysis and recommends either (1) continue the dose-ranging stage of the trial, (2) stop the trial for lack of efficacy (inadequate slope of the dose-response curve or, more accurately, evidence of a positive dose-response that is insufficient to justify continuing the trial), or (3) shift into a confirmatory trial. This shift can be made seamlessly, with no break in the accrual. Indeed, it is even theoretically possible to effect such a shift in a double-blind trial without informing the investigators: they simply continue to randomize doses, but unbeknownst to them, the only two being assigned are the phase III dose and the placebo.

Many trials designed at MDACC have encompassed both phases I and

II.[31,32] Such designs allow for addressing toxicity and efficacy throughout the trial. Only "admissible" doses or combinations of doses are used, and doses are escalated as others become admissible. All the while, the designs allow for learning about the relationship between dose and efficacy as well as about dose and toxicity.

Trials designed at MDACC have also encompassed both phases II and III, using a seamless switch to phase III.[33] The anticipated effect of the drug is on local control. Survival is modeled as it depends on local control and as it depends on treatment. (Although the possibility is remote, the design allows for the experimental drug to have a beneficial effect on survival that is not mitigated by local control.) So local control is a surrogate endpoint in a way similar to the way early stroke scale assessments are surrogate endpoints in the stroke trial. But the clear focus is on survival as the main endpoint and the utility of the surrogate endpoint must be demonstrated by the results actually observed in the trial. The trial exploits any relationships that exist, but does not assume such relationships. The data in the trial are analyzed frequently and the trial is adapted to the accruing evidence.

The seamless aspect is as follows. Initially, only MDACC patients are accrued to the trial. Think of this as phase II. If the accumulating data are sufficiently strong in suggesting that the drug has no effect on local control or survival, then the trial stops. If the data suggest that the drug may have an impact on local control and that this impact translates into a survival benefit, then the trial will be expanded to include other centers and the accrual rate will increase accordingly. During such an expansion, patients continue to accrue at MDACC so that there is no downtime in the local accrual while other centers gear up to join the trial. This is efficient use of patient resources because data from the patients who accrued early at MDACC contribute to the eventual inferences about survival. These patients are the most informative of all those enrolled because their follow-up times are the longest.

The trial continues until stopping occurs because (1) continuing would be futile, judged by predictive probabilities, (2) the maximum sample size is reached, or (3) the predictive probability of eventually achieving statistical significance becomes sufficiently large. If the third event occurs, the accrual ceases and the pharmaceutical company prepares a marketing application.

The sample size of a conventional phase III trial with the desired operating characteristics is 900. This is taken to be the maximum sample size in the seamless design as well. Actual accrual is very likely to be much less than this maximum sample size, and on average it will be about half as large. On the other hand, incorporating the same number of interim analyses in a conventional design using a conventional type of stopping boundary allows for only a slight decrease in the average sample size. Under any hypothesis, null or alternative, the Bayesian design occasionally leads to a relatively large trial (close to 900 patients). However, a pleasant aspect of the design is that the sample size is large precisely when a large trial is necessary. Conventional trials may well (and sometimes do!) come to their predetermined end with an ambiguous conclusion. In a Bayesian approach one may choose to continue such a trial to resolve the ambiguity, and this option has substantial utility. (Carrying this argument to the maximum sample size, there may be times for which stopping at 900 is ill advised, but for logistical reasons we specified a maximum size.)

Reductions in sample size result from two characteristics of the seamless design described above. First are the frequent analyses to assess the predictive probability of eventual statistical significance. The second is the explicit modeling of the possible relationship between local control and survival. Of the two, the second is more important.

A conventional drug development strategy involves running a phase II trial that addresses the local control, digesting the results, and if the results are positive, starting to develop phase III trials with survival as the primary endpoint. As indicated above, in comparison with such a strategy, a seamless approach can greatly reduce the sample size. In addition, a seamless design minimizes pauses between phases and so the total drug development time is greatly shortened.

Adaptive Allocation

The adaptive designs discussed so far are motivated by the desire to learn efficiently and as rapidly as possible. Another kind of adaptive design aims to treat patients in the trial as effectively as possible. These designs use adaptive allocation in which patients are more likely to be assigned to therapies that are performing better. In addition to making clinical trials more attractive to patients and thereby increasing participation in clinical trials, such strategies have the important side benefit of being efficient, and so they result in rapid learning.

More than a dozen trials at MDACC have been designed and are being conducted using adaptive allocation. The standard approach is to randomize the treatment assignment, but to shift the weights toward better performing arms as the trial proceeds and the results accumulate. Many of these trials have more than two arms. The arms are sometimes distinct therapies, and sometimes they are closely related. An example of the latter is an MDACC trial involving five doses (including 0) of a drug (pentostatin). The goal is to inhibit graft-vs-host-disease (GVHD) in leukemia patients who are receiving bone marrow transplants. The problem is that the drug may inhibit the successful engraftment of the transplant, which is necessary for survival. Such inhibition may be related to dose. A combination endpoint is used in the trial: survival at 100 days free of GVHD. The conflict between engraftment and freedom from GVHD means that the dose-response curve may not be monotone. In particular, it may increase for small doses and then decrease. Initially doses are assigned in a graduated fashion, climbing the dose ladder slowly. But as doses become admissible, patients are assigned to the doses that have been performing well.

Consider a patient who qualifies for the trial. To decide which pentostatin dose to assign, one calculates the current (Bayesian) probabilities that each admissible dose is better than the placebo. This calculation uses all the information from the patients treated to date. Doses are allocated randomly, with weights proportional to these probabilities. Other allocation algorithms are considered, including assigning in proportion to the powers of these probabilities. The assignments involve some degree of randomization, but all patients are more likely to receive doses that are performing better. Doses that are doing sufficiently poorly become inadmissible in the sense that their assignment weight becomes 0. When and if it is learned that the drug is effective, the trial is stopped. When and if it is learned that the drug is ineffective, then again the trial is stopped. Patients in the trial benefit from data collected in the trial. The explicit goal is to treat patients more effectively, but in addition learning is more efficient. Each design's frequentist operating characteristics are evaluated using Monte Carlo simulation, with possible modification of the parameters of the assignment algorithm to achieve desired characteristics.

Process or Trial? Evaluating Many Drugs Simultaneously Using Adaptive Allocation

The greatest need for innovation and the greatest room for improving drug development is the process of effectively dealing with the enormous numbers of potential drugs that are available for development. The notion of developing drugs one at a time is part of the pharmaceutical culture. It will change.

Companies that are able to screen many drugs simultaneously and effectively will survive and others will not.

Many different drugs should be evaluated in the same preclinical experiment or collection of experiments. Information should be updated frequently or even continually. The extent to which any particular drug is used and the order of drugs used will depend on the available data. Drugs that are apparently more promising will move faster through the preclinical setting. Drugs that give disappointing data will languish. And the sample sizes of patients treated with drugs that have promises and toxicities that are not clear will tend to be large so as to enable resolving uncertainties.

These ideas and imperatives apply as well to the clinical development of drugs. As an example, MDACC is building the foundation for a phase II trial for evaluating drugs that is more a process than a trial. The idea is an extension of the adaptive assignment strategies described in the previous section. A trial starts with a number of treatment arms plus a control—possibly a standard therapy. Patients are randomized to the arms and information is obtained about the relative efficacy of the arms as the trial proceeds. Arms that perform better get used more often. An arm that performs sufficiently poorly gets dropped. An arm that does well enough graduates to phase III, and if it does sufficiently well it might even replace the control. As more arms become available, they are added to the mix.

The result is that better arms (better treatments) move through quickly and poorer arms get dropped. Patients in the trial are provided with better treatment (when the arms are not equally good). Patients outside the trial get access to better drugs more rapidly.

Extraim Analyses

A common circumstance is that a clinical trial ends without a clear conclusion. For example, a statistical significance level of 5% in the primary endpoint may be required for drug registration, and the p-value may turn out to be 6%. The regulatory agency then suggests that the trial was "underpowered" and that the company should carry out another trial. It would be much more efficient to simply increase the sample size in the present trial. The problem is that the possibility of such an extension increases the type I error rate. The principle is identical to that for interim analyses.

The solution is to build into the design the possibility of continuing the trial depending on the results, and suitably adjusting the significance levels. In contrast to the adjustments for interim analyses, the adjustments for "extra-im" (extraim) analyses are reversed, with much of the overall significance level "spent" at the originally planned sample size. For example, taking equal significance levels at each possible termination point is preferable to O'Brien–Fleming stopping boundaries because the latter are too conservative for extraim analyses. Allowing for extending the trial increases the maximal sample size and also the average sample size. But a modest increase in the average sample size (such as 20%) comes with a substantial increase in statistical power (such as 80% increasing to 95%). The reason for this beneficial tradeoff is that the trial is extended only when such an extension is worthwhile.

The "penalty" in the significance level can be either partially or fully offset by including futility analyses as part of the design. Namely, the trial would be stopped for sufficiently negative results at preset interim time points. The reason such analyses offset the penalty for extraim analyses is that the null hypothesis is never rejected when the trial stops for futility. Decreasing the opportunity for a type I error also decreases the power of the trial. However, this decrease is usually quite modest and in any case is more than compensated by the increase in power due to the extraim analyses.

The increment in sample size depends on the available data at the time the decision is made to continue the accrual. It also depends on the number of possible extensions. In trials I have designed, I have based each extension on the predictive power. The usual definition of power assumes a particular value of the parameter of interest, say r. Predictive power considers all possible values of r. The data available at the time of the extraim analysis plays two roles. First, they count in the final results of the trial. Second, they are used to update the (Bayesian) probability distribution of r. Fix the total sample size n and calculate the power for detecting each possible value of r. Average this power with respect to the probability distribution of r to give the predictive power for sample size n. Extend the accrual by the minimum sample size that gives a total sample size having a pre-specified predictive power. If there is no such value of n, then continuing the accrual may be unwise.

There is an aspect of the development mentioned earlier that may be unrealistic. Namely, it assumes that the endpoints for those patients treated in the trial so far are available at the time of the extraim analysis. Even if the endpoint is tumor response, there is a delay in obtaining this information. There is no need to stop the trial just because some of the endpoint information is unavailable. Rather, these data can be predicted along with those from patients not yet accrued. If there is some early information (biomarkers, performance status, etc) that is correlated with the endpoint of interest then this can be used to inform the prediction. A special and important case is when the endpoint is the time to an event. The fact that a patient has not yet reached an event is useful information in predicting the time to that event. However, if there is no patient-specific early information, then patients treated but not yet assessed for response are treated in the same way as patients not yet treated. (This set of issues is sufficiently important that they deserve being addressed separately. See the next section.)

The process mentioned previously is complicated. But it can be completely and precisely described. That means it can be simulated. The simulations can be carried out under various assumptions about the parameter of interest. In particular, the false-positive rate can be calculated. If there is a target significance level (such as 5%), then the various inputs into the design (number and type of extraim analyses, number and type of futility analyses, etc) can be varied until that target is achieved. An advantage of simulations is that each iteration provides data from a fully accrued trial. Therefore, it is possible to check any characteristic of interest regarding the trial's design by calculating the proportion of the trials that have that characteristic. Characteristics of interest include the power, the actual sample size, and the probability of extending the accrual.

Auxiliary Variables and Biomarkers

The adaptive designs considered in the previous section are based on information on the primary endpoint that accrues during the trial. If the primary endpoint is delayed and the accrual is sufficiently fast, then adaptive methods are of limited value. This section addresses statistical procedures for designs that exploit information that accrues during the trial other than the primary endpoint.

Using Auxiliary Variables

Information that accrues during a trial has a broad interpretation. Suppose that the endpoint is time to progression and a patient has not yet progressed, then that can be called is information, and it can be used to update the distributions of whatever parameters are involved.

In addition, information accrues about each patient's circumstances and each patient's condition. Whether the patient's tumor has responded is information, and this is so even if response is not the endpoint of interest. Moreover, time to tumor response can be informative. A patient's performance status can change over time (or not!) and such information is important and the various possibilities can be used prospectively in designing a trial. There are many such variables that might be considered. They are auxiliary variables because they may contain information about the primary endpoint even though they are not themselves endpoints.

The critical issue is how to take advantage of the wealth of information that accrues in a trial. The answer is modeling. A model can relate the early information to the primary endpoint.

There are several benefits of modeling. One benefit was considered in the sections on adaptive dose-finding and on seamless phases. Waiting for long-term endpoints may rule out the ability to modify the design of a clinical trial during its course. Using auxiliary variables can make adaptation possible. Another benefit of modeling is that the relationship between the primary endpoint and auxiliary variables may allow for announcing the trial results earlier or for getting earlier regulatory approval of an experimental drug. For example, say that survival is the primary endpoint and that modeling its relationship with response was considered explicitly in the design of the trial. Suppose accrual to the trial has ended, all patients have been treated, and there is insufficient information to conclude drug benefit on the basis of survival alone. But the drug has a positive impact on tumor response. And it turns out that in both the experimental treatment and control groups there is a clear relationship between response and survival. A model can utilize this information to conclude a survival benefit.

The distinction between the auxiliary variable and surrogate endpoints is critically important. Surrogate endpoints are those that can substitute for the primary endpoint in the sense that the effect of a treatment on the primary endpoint is wholly explained by its effect on the surrogate endpoint. This is generally too high a hurdle. Auxiliary variables require a correlation and not a substitution. In the example mentioned earlier, tumor response is an auxiliary variable and it is not assumed to be a surrogate for survival. The focus of the definitive analysis is the primary endpoint and not the auxiliary variable. The conclusion of the trial is still that the drug improves survival or not.

A model incorporating early information can be arbitrarily complicated and, in particular, it can contain all the variables discussed earlier. However, one should tiptoe into model development and consider one auxiliary variable at a time. Especially important is in considering the possibility that any relationship between the auxiliary variable and the primary endpoint depends on treatment. Consequently, treatment must be explicitly considered in the equation. If it happens that there is an interaction between the auxiliary variable and treatment, such as that the tumor response is related to survival in the control group but not in the treatment group, then the model automatically discounts the auxiliary variable and relies on survival data alone.

Little is lost by modeling, and potential gains are large, as indicated in the seamless phase II/III trial design presented earlier. Moreover, as indicated previously, the gains and any losses can be assessed by simulation.

A special type of auxiliary variable is a biomarker. Models relating to primary endpoints can be based on longitudinal models that incorporate biomarker information that accrues over time. An example of a longitudinal model is described by Berry and colleagues[29] in the context of a stroke trial.

Biomarker Driven Clinical Trials

Biomarkers have at least three roles in cancer research. One is as a target of therapy; HER2/neu is an example.

The use of biological agents presents special drug development problems. Historically, oncology drug development has dealt primarily with cytotoxic agents, and drug activity has been judged by assessing tumor growth. An effective biological agent may well have an impact that slows tumor growth rather than killing the tumor. Or it may have little effect on local tumor growth, but may halt tumor spread. A possible strategy is to include stable disease with partial and complete tumor response as the phase II endpoint. Another is to use the time to progression of the disease as the phase II endpoint. The latter has the drawback that the sample size and length of the trial may increase, but not as much as when skipping phase II entirely. Both strategies may succeed. And both have the advantage that they do not involve a paradigm shift for the oncology research community. But there are better options.

A generic biological agent is one that may affect a disease through a variety of pathways. A targeted agent may be viewed as generic when assessing the expression of the target is subject to error. An example is trastuzumab, which may well benefit tumors that have normal levels of HER2/neu because laboratory tests are not perfect in assessing expression levels.[34,35]

All tumors are different and the differences can be measured by biomarkers. This second role of biomarkers is especially difficult and interesting. Different tumors respond differently to therapy. Understanding how different tumors respond to different therapies is a potential goal of cancer clinical trials. The statistical problems are enormous, and with many drugs and many categories of disease, the false positives will far outnumber the true positives. Controlling the false-positive rate is possible, however, and it is essential as these types of trials are being designed for "personalized medicine." Examples include the BATTLE trial[36] being conducted at MDACC, and the I-SPY 2 trial,[37] currently being designed through the Foundation of the National Institutes of Health.

The third possible role of biomarkers is as an indication of the extent of disease. CA125 and PSA are examples. These are candidates for "auxiliary variables" and are subject to longitudinal modeling as described in the previous section. If there is a target, think of it as a biomarker and develop a longitudinal model to relate its level with the primary endpoint, usually time to disease progression or overall survival. If there is no measurable target, then identify auxiliary variables (biological and otherwise) that may be correlated with the primary endpoint. Model the possibility of a relationship should one exist. Again, the goal is to learn early and quickly as to whether the drug has a benefit, and by which route that benefit travels.

Acknowledgment

The author thanks the Cancer and Leukemia Group B for permission to use data from CALGB 8541.

References

1. Hampton T. Targeted cancer therapies lagging: better trial design could boost success rate. *JAMA*. 2006;296:1951–1952.
2. DiMasi JA, Grabowski HG. The cost of biopharmaceutical R&D: is biotech different? *Managerial Dec Econ*. 2007;28:469–479.
3. US Department of Health and Human Services, Food and Drug Administration. *Innovation—Stagnation: Critical Path Opportunities Report*; March 2006:ii. Available at: http://www.fda.gov/oc/initiatives/criticalpath/reports/opp_report.pdf. Accessed February 12, 2009.
4. The National Commission for the Protection of Human Subjects of Biomedical and Behavioral Research (US). *The Belmont Report. Ethical Principles and Guidelines for the Protection of Human Subjects of Research*; 1979. Available at: http://ohsr.od.nih.gov/guidelines/belmont.html. Accessed February 12, 2009.

5. Berry DA. *Statistics: A Bayesian Perspective*. Belmont, CA: Duxbury Press; 1996.
6. Berry DA. A case for Bayesianism in clinical trials (with discussion). *Stat Med*. 1993; 12:1377–1404.
7. Berry DA. Introduction to Bayesian methods III: use and interpretation of Bayesian tools in design and analysis. *Clin Trials*. 2005;2:295–300.
8. Berry DA. Bayesian clinical trials. *Nat Rev Drug Discov*. 2006;5:27–36.
9. Speigelhalter DJ, Abrams KR, Myles JP. *Bayesian Approaches to Clinical Trials and Healthcare Evaluation*. Chichester, England: Wiley; 2004.
10. Muss HB, Berry DA, Cirrincione CT, et al; for the Cancer and Leukemia Group B. *Adjuvant Chemotherapy in Older Women With Early Stage-Breast Cancer. N Engl J Med*. 2009;360:2055–2065.
11. DuMouchel W. Bayesian metaanalysis. In: Berry DA, ed. *Statistical Methodology in the Pharmaceutical Sciences*. New York, NY: Marcel Dekker; 1989:509–529.
12. Thall PF, Wathen JK, Bekele BN, et al. Hierarchical Bayesian approaches to phase II trials in diseases with multiple subtypes. *Stat Med*. 2003;22:763–780.
13. Budman DR, Berry DA, Cirrincione CT, et al. Dose and dose intensity as determinants of outcome in the adjuvant treatment of breast cancer. *J Natl Cancer Inst*. 1998;90:1205–1211.
14. Thor A, Berry DA, Budman D, et al. *erb*B-2, p53 and efficacy of adjuvant therapy in lymph node-positive breast cancer. *J Natl Cancer Inst*. 1998;90:1346–1360.
15. Citron ML, Berry, DA, Cirrincione C, et al. Randomized trial of dose-dense vs conventionally scheduled and sequential vs concurrent combination chemotherapy as postoperative adjuvant treatment of node-positive primary breast cancer: First report of Intergroup C9741/Cancer and Leukemia Group B Trial 9741. *J Clin Oncol*. 2003;21:1431–1439.
16. Henderson IC, Berry DA, Demetri GD, et al. Improved outcomes from adding sequential paclitaxel but not from escalating doxorubicin dose in an adjuvant chemotherapy regimen for patients with node-positive primary breast cancer. *J Clin Oncol*. 2003;21:976–983.
17. Sox HC, Blatt MA, Higgins MC, Marton KI. *Medical Decision Making*. Boston, MA: Butterworth and Heinemann; 1988.
18. Clemen RT. *Making Hard Decisions*. Boston, MA: PWS-Kent; 1991.
19. Berry DA. Decision analysis and Bayesian methods in clinical trials. In: Thall PF, ed. *Recent Advances in Clinical Trial Design and Analysis*. New York, NY: Kluwer Press; 1995:125–154.
20. Lewis RJ, Berry DA. Decision theory. In: Armitage P, Colton T, eds. *Encyclopedia of Biostatistics*; vol 2. New York, NY: John Wiley & Sons; 1998:1109–1118.
21. Cheng Y, Su F, Berry DA. Choosing sample size for a clinical trial using decision analysis. *Biometrika*. 2003;90:923–936.
22. Berry DA, Fristedt B. *Bandit Problems: Sequential Allocation of Experiments*. London: Chapman-Hall; 1985.
23. Dixon WJ. The up-and down method for small samples. *J Am Stat Assoc*. 1965;60:967–978.
24. Berry DA, Lindgren BW. *Statistics: Theory and Methods*. 2nd ed. Belmont, CA: Duxbury Press; 1996.
25. O'Quigley J, Pepe M, Fisher L. Continual reassessment method: a practical design for phase I clinical trials in cancer. *Biometrics*. 1990;52:673–684.
26. Thall PF, Lee JJ, Tseng C-H, Estey E. Accrual strategies for phase I trials with delayed patient outcome. *Stat Med*. 1999;18:1155–1169.
27. Cheung YK, Chappell R. Sequential designs for phase I clinical trials with late-onset toxicities. *Biometrics*. 2000;56:1177–1182.
28. Thall PF, Russell KT. A strategy for dose-finding and safety monitoring based on efficacy and adverse outcomes in phase I/II clinical trials. *Biometrics*. 1998;54: 251–264.
29. Berry DA, Mueller P, Grieve AP, et al. Adaptive Bayesian designs for dose-ranging drug trials. In: Gatsonis C, Carlin B, Carriquiry A, eds. *Case Studies in Bayesian Statistics V*. New York, NY: Springer-Verlag; 2001:99–181.
30. Malakoff D. Bayes offers a "new" way to make sense of numbers. *Science*. 1999;286: 1460–1464.
31. Huang X, Biswas S, Oki Y, et al. A parallel phase I/II clinical trial design for combination therapies. *Biometrics*. 2007;63:429–436.
32. Biswas S, Liu DD, Lee JJ, Berry DA. Bayesian clinical trials at the University of Texas MD Anderson Cancer Center. *Clin Trial*. 2009;6:205–216.
33. Inoue LYT, Thall P, Berry DA. Seamlessly expanding a randomized phase II trial to phase III. *Biometrics*. 2002;58:264–272.
34. Paik S, Bryant J, Tan-Chiu E, et al. Real-world performance of HER2 testing—National Surgical Adjuvant Breast and Bowel Project experience. *J Natl Cancer Inst*. 2002;94:852–854.
35. Roche PC, Suman VJ, Jenkins RB, et al. Concordance between local and central laboratory HER2 testing in the Breast Intergroup Trial N9831. *J Natl Cancer Inst*. 2002;94:855–857.
36. Zhou X, Liu S, Kim ES et al. Bayesian adaptive design for targeted therapy development in lung cancer—a step toward personalized medicine. *Clin Trial*. 2008;5:181–193.
37. Barker AD, Sigman CC, Kelloff GJ, et al. I-SPY2: An Adaptive Breast Cancer Trial Design in the Setting of Neoadjuvant Chemotherapy. *Clin Pharmacol Ther*. 2009;86:97–100.

36 Outcomes Research in Oncology

James A. Talcott, MD, SM

Introduction

Because all medical research attempts to improve patient outcomes, clinical investigation is by definition outcomes research. However, this chapter describes a group of loosely related research strategies that complement traditional, biologically based clinical research. Outcomes research, as described here, borrows objectives and methodology from the social sciences. Compared to traditional clinical research, it studies nonbiological outcomes of potential interest to a broader range of stakeholders in medical care that comprises one-sixth of the US economy and the subject of ever more intensive public policy scrutiny.

Introducing a monograph produced by the National Cancer Institute's (NCI) Cancer Outcomes Measurement Working Group (COMWG), Lipscomb and colleagues indicated the field's scope. Outcomes research is "the scientific field devoted to measuring and interpreting the impact of medical conditions and health care on individuals and populations … and describes, interprets, and predicts the impact of various influences, especially (but not exclusively) interventions, on 'final' endpoints that matter to decision makers: patients, providers, private payers, government agencies, accrediting organizations and society at large."[1] Like traditional medical investigators, outcomes researchers seek interventions that delay death and neutralize disease symptoms. They also seek to preserve or improve patients' quality of life, support their decision-making autonomy, ensure consistent, high-quality medical care, and maximize economic efficiency. Acknowledging a central role played by biological processes, outcomes researchers ask additional questions using specialized, usually quantitative techniques developed by psychologists, sociologists, economists, and biostatisticians, including behavioral models, psychometric measurements, economic analyses, and decision analytical techniques (Table 36-1). When successful, these techniques address issues important to patients that physicians may have overlooked or undervalued, refine the objectives of treatment, rationalize its delivery, and incorporate additional perspectives from patients, physicians, payers, and policy makers.

Using basic scientists' studies of the complex processes that underlie human disease, translational medical researchers have brought new biological insights to bear on treatment. However, therapeutic innovation brings fresh challenges. Biologically powerful interventions may bring great benefits but also produce complex and unexpected consequences for patients, strikingly increased costs to society, and create powerful economic motivations for both overuse and misuse. Outcomes researchers, if successful, evaluate treatment innovations more comprehensively and help refine their use to meet patients' and society's needs more completely and with greater cost effectiveness.

History

Both historical circumstances and cancer's distinctive natural history combined to reduce oncology's role in the development of outcomes research. Oncologists, like other medical subspecialists, came late to a field developed largely by generalists, often in General Internal Medicine departments in medical schools. However, cancer's clinically discontinuous natural history, in contrast to that of other chronic diseases, was an additional obstacle. Low back pain, benign prostatic hyperplasia, degenerative joint disease, and other chronic diseases studied by early outcomes researchers share relatively straightforward and clinically evident natural histories that predispose to ongoing doctor-patient dialog. Typically, symptoms progress toward a definitive "fix," often a surgical procedure. Although specific diagnostic tests may be required to document clinical milestones that trigger treatment decisions, most patients experience progressive illness directly through increasing symptoms, provoking treatment discussions with their physicians.

By contrast, crucial developments in the natural history of cancer, a disease of an individual cell, its descendants and their microenvironment, are microscopic, unobservable, and often clinically silent. Primary cancers and metastases begin as single cellular events. Years of growth and dozens of cell divisions may be required to produce tumor masses large enough for symptoms or medical detection, even in skin or other easily observable sites. As a result, patients experience the clinical course of cancer as compressed and discontinuous, a sequence of crises rather than a unitary disease process. Despite many years of cancer growth in most cases, the discovery of a primary tumor or the first metastasis comes "out of the blue," presenting an often asymptomatic patient with a sudden, frightening prognosis and daunting treatment options. For patients with clinically localized cancers, whose potentially fatal disease may cause no symptoms, treatment offers a "high stakes" opportunity for cure that makes toxic, invasive interventions invoking the language and perspective of warfare[2]

Table 36-1 ■ Perspective, Goals, and Outcomes in Clinical Research

Perspective	Goal	Outcome Measured
Traditional (biological)	Define, measure, and modify the biological processes that underlie disease	Survival, other biological variables (eg, tumor "response" or shrinkage, blood pressure, cardiac arrhythmias, etc.). Physician-reported information about adverse effects, such as toxicity scales
Quality of life	Measure the impact of disease and medical interventions on the patient's experience of living	Patient-reported outcomes, including functional status, "bother" and preferences
Economics	Define and compare medical interventions' use of economic resources, both absolutely (cost minimization) and in terms of the benefit achieved (cost-benefit analyses)	Marginal costs and changes in quality-adjusted survival (or other indicators of health benefits)
Quality of health care	Identify and correct factors that produce medical harm	Medical error rates

acceptable. Unwarranted time pressure often ensues: patients experience the deliberate pace of the pretreatment workup as disconnected from the dire prognosis, compared to the emergency timeline of comparably life-threatening diseases like myocardial infarction and stroke. The discontinuous, emotionally charged natural history of cancer required outcomes researchers to overhaul methods developed for more typical chronic diseases. However, despite a late start, outcomes research in oncology is now firmly entrenched, and well in advance of other major disease groups, such as cardiovascular disease.[3]

The early impetus for medical outcomes research came from academia and society. Beginning in the early 1970s, Wennberg and colleagues found striking variations in medical practice patterns in adjacent small geographic areas, corresponding to hospital service areas.[4] While medical factors and patient preferences could explain part of the variation, much remained unexplained, forcing investigators to consider nonmedical explanations, including social and economic factors.[5,6] Documenting medical practice variation led directly to questions about the quality of medical care: if practitioners varied in their use of specific procedures and the overall treatment intensity, which practices were better, ie, most helpful to patients and economically efficient[7]? Using a systems approach, each of the three components of health care, *structure*, *process*, and *outcomes*, underwent scrutiny. Structure and process are easier to define and measure than outcomes, but in isolation, less relevant to the mission of medical care, ie, improving the health of patients. To weigh the structure and processes of alternative practice patterns requires measuring their outcomes, the output of medical care.[8]

As practice variability was appreciated, rapidly rising health care costs forced businesses and governments, the largest purchasers of health care, toward economic efficiency. The realization by officials of General Motors in the 1970s that health care was a greater cost component of automobile manufacture than steel, for example, impelled a closer examination of the quality of the health care it was purchasing.[9] Similarly, health care costs became the fastest-growing expenditure of the U.S. government, which, through the Medicare and Medicaid programs, is the largest single purchaser of medical care in the United States. The uneasy, dawning awareness of health care's relentlessly growing cost prompted the next major methodological steps for outcomes research.

Early studies examined the effect on utilization and costs of varying the structure of health care delivery. The variation in practice patterns documented by Wennberg and colleagues, as well as anecdotal evidence, suggested that a significant proportion of health care utilization was inappropriate, wasteful, and potentially harmful. Varying the payment structure of health care insurance was a potential corrective measure. Increasing financial disincentives, such as health insurance deductibles and other co-payments, was a potential lever to reduce inappropriate use of health care, control costs and, as a byproduct, protect patients from iatrogenic injury resulting from unnecessary medical interventions. The randomized RAND Health Insurance Study (HIS) compared utilization of health care provided free to patients to care requiring out-of-pocket co-payments or deductibles,[10] and found one-third lower expenditures when care required patient payments.[11]

However, the objective of the HIS was not to reduce health care utilization per se, but to reduce unnecessary care that produced expenditure without health benefits. To identify harmful underuse of care, investigators used both process and outcome measures. Applying process guidelines for medical appropriateness developed by physician evaluators, the study found that the apparent benefits of financial disincentives faded under close examination: increasing out-of-pocket costs reduced appropriate and inappropriate usage equally.[12] To address the more difficult task of measuring health outcomes, the HIS investigators developed health status measures, including the most widely used survey instrument in medical research, the Medical Outcomes Study Short Form 36-Item Health Survey (SF-36).[13,14] With these newly validated measures, they found sparse evidence that despite reduced medically appropriate care, patients with co-payments had worse health outcomes.[15] Other studies indicated the incomplete state of knowledge and fragile assumptions about improvements in health care. One found that HMOs reduced hospitalization rates without evidence of reduced patient health outcomes.[16] Another, using appropriateness criteria, found that inappropriate use of expensive medical procedures was common and ally variable, especially with complex and vague indications, such as cardiac catheterization, but accounted for only a small part of medically unexplained practice variation.[17,18]

These results put to rest the hope that financial disincentives could cleanly excise inappropriate health care utilization; patients were apparently unable to distinguish appropriate from inappropriate medical care. However, the results also left for future examination the implication that medically appropriate treatment may not offer measurable health benefits. If not left to patients under financial pressure, other decision-makers might identify unnecessary, costly health care; further work remained. The lingering experiments with insurance providers and primary care providers as gatekeepers are part of this contradictory intellectual legacy. However, the most obvious lasting benefit from the HIS was the methodological capacity to measure medical outcomes.

These pioneering investigations led directly to the creation of the Agency for Health Care and Policy Research (AHCPR) in 1989. The new Agency's goal, stated in its founding legislation, was "to enhance the quality, appropriateness, and effectiveness of health care services, and access to such services, through the establishment of a broad base of scientific research and through the promotion of improvements in clinical practice and in the organization, financing, and delivery of health care services." AHCPR devoted a substantial portion of its early research budget to funding a series of Patient Outcomes Research Teams (PORTs). These multidisciplinary teams were to address single, major clinical problems comprehensively, largely through existing data but also targeted new studies, to identify treatments that improved patient outcomes and promulgate them through evidence-based guidelines (vs expert opinion-based guidelines, an inferior, easily biased alternative). The first PORTs addressed nonmalignant chronic conditions, such as back pain, cataracts, hip fractures, and diabetes, although the benign prostatic hyperplasia (BPH) PORT also addressed localized prostate cancer. Later PORTs added local breast cancer and expanded prostate cancer research, as well as acute disease management and diagnostic technology. The policy aspect of the Agency's charge, issuing guidelines, proved troublesome. Guidelines produced by an early back pain PORT discouraged early surgical intervention, provoking a backlash of politically well-connected back surgeons that constrained Agency funding and eliminated the Federal Office for Technology Assessment. In late 1998, the Agency became the Agency for Healthcare Research and Quality (AHRQ), replacing the troublesome policy component with the implicit goal of outcomes research, improving quality of care. We explore this research objective in detail below.

During AHCPR's brief life, however, outcomes research established itself as a component, if still a bit player, in medical research funded by the US Federal Government, the most influential arbiter of noncommercial medical research. Perhaps the clearest indicator of its new status in oncology was the NCI's COMWG created in 2001 to evaluate the science of outcomes measurement and recommend approaches to improve its scientific quality and usefulness.[19] The Working Group report influenced the NIH Roadmap (RM)-funded initiatives designed to provide standardized patient-reported outcomes measures to clinical investigators, such as in the Patient-Reported Outcomes Measurement Information System (PROMIS).[20-22]

Outcomes Methods

Study Designs

Randomized Trials ■ Outcomes researchers use the gold standard clinical research design, randomized trials, while recognizing its limitations. Randomized trials' crucial design element is assignment of interventions through a chance-driven mechanism that is invisible to enrolling physicians, ensuring a valid answer to a single, focused research question for a homogeneous population under controlled circumstances. In sufficiently large studies, random assignment reliably balances measured and unmeasured prognostic factors, providing strong insurance against confounding. In addition, constraints on participating patients' characteristics and their physicians' responses to clinical contingencies limit the "noise" of clinical practice variation. Entry criteria exclude patients at increased risk of treatment toxicity, and the study protocol dictates diagnostic and treatment options. The resultant hothouse environment may produce results unrepresentative of broader clinical use of study interventions by physicians with less experience with treatments and unconstrained clinical options. Randomized trials assess the *efficacy* of medical interventions in research environments, in contrast to *effectiveness* in real-world conditions, where the results may be less gratifying. The randomized trial relinquishes authority on its usefulness under typical conditions and it is difficult to determine whether the experimental treatment can work under optimal conditions.

To this methodological limitation, randomized trials add another more troublesome factor for outcomes researchers. A patient undergoing treatment in a randomized trial must accept that no preferred treatment for her illness exists and, by extension, that her doctor's knowledge and experience are of little use. This position, *equipoise*, is especially difficult for patients with life-threatening diseases to accept. For cancer physicians, deeply committed to their patients and comfortable with the powerful, toxic therapies they routinely employ, achieving equipoise may be as difficult as for their patients. Patients' surprisingly strong interest in nonrandomized studies with little probability of benefit, such as phase 1 trials designed to define tolerable drug doses, suggests the emotional difficulty posed by randomization.[23] Patients report that their hope for clinical benefit motivates them,[24] and they expect it,[25] despite reliably contrary statements in consent forms.[26] While efforts to identify and overcome barriers to completing trials have stepped up,[27,28] outcomes researchers accept that while randomized trials are necessary to definitively document successful innovation, they have shortcomings when called on to study fundamental aspects of medical care. Decreasing the disparity between study treatments, by comparing two similar drugs, for example, may reduce the discomfort from randomization and ease patient recruitment, but at an important cost: more easily completed randomized trials address more trivial experimental deviation from current practice, while more fundamental questions remain unanswered, and increasingly unasked. For example, despite sparse comparative data on surgical or radiation treatments for clinically localized prostate cancer, especially the dramatically increased prostate-specific antigen (PSA) detected-cancers, ambitious trial efforts have stalled,[29,30] with a single exception, and are increasingly less relevant to contemporary patients.[31,32] However, resourceful investigators can overcome even such fundamental obstacles. Investigators for the ProtecT (Prostate testing for cancer and Treatment) trial informed prospective subjects for a randomized PSA screening and a nested treatment trial at the outset of the uncertain value of screening and treatment,[33] dramatically increasing study recruitment, and used qualitative research techniques to remove additional inadvertent barriers.[27,34] The study is a model for creative efforts to direct the most definitive research technique to fundamental medical questions.

Observational Studies ■ Observational research offers practical and cost advantages over randomized trials, but at a methodological cost. Because entering an observational study does not affect treatment, observational studies accrue more easily than randomized trials. Because observational studies need not use prospectively collected data, enrollment of individual patients is unnecessary if data recorded for other purposes, such as routine medical record keeping, disease registries, or even billing, is available for analysis. Observational studies using existing data may include hundreds of thousands of patients, producing extraordinarily powerful studies that produce very precise estimates of outcomes. These types of studies are usually more representative of the typical patient experience, particularly when the population is geographically based, than randomized trial populations consisting of the small proportion of patients willing to enroll in them. However, because treating physicians, not study procedures, determine the treatment patients receive, confounding is unavoidable, making causal inferences difficult. The power of observational studies based on large existing databases is so great that trivial clinical differences between groups regularly achieve statistical significance. In large observational studies, issues of potential confounding and bias, not statistical significance, are the main challenges for investigators. The Health Insurance Portability and Accountability Act (HIPAA) has made observational studies more difficult, since variables that identify patients even approximately, including the date of diagnosis, are in general inaccessible to investigators without patient consent.[35]

The major observational study designs are cohort studies and case-control studies. In a cohort study, investigators identify the characteristics and health status of a group of patients at a particular time point and evaluate subsequent outcomes. Large prospective cohort studies are costly to perform, but if carefully constructed, can produce rich research yields. The Nurses Health Study of women and the Health Professionals Follow-up Study of men have prospectively evaluated tens of thousands of medically trained subjects whose highly reliable survey responses permit omitting costly medical records corroboration. Regular participant surveys provide new and updated information about newly hypothesized risk factors, medical events, and other patient-reported information, such as quality of life.[36-39] Further, blood and other specimens permit study of biomarkers.[40-43]

Previously recorded information can retrospectively produce a cohort study. Administrative data collected for billing purposes, particularly for large, geographically based databases, such as national or regional health care authorities or the Medicare insurance program in the United States, permit massive cohort studies, providing data to determine both entry criteria and outcomes. However, the information from billing databases may not collect medically relevant data for many research questions, and the collected data may be ambiguous. Because it was recorded for other purposes, the data may have little relevance to the most interesting study hypotheses, sharply limiting both the range of research questions and alternative explanations for the results that can be explored. Further, the investigators do not control the procedures that ensure the quality of the collected data, resulting in possibly unreliable data.

These limitations assign observational studies a secondary role in treatment questions, particularly "close calls" easily overshadowed by confounding and bias. However, observational studies can make important contributions, especially when large databases are thoughtfully constructed with research purposes in mind, when the study explores novel relationships, and the effects of interest are large, or randomized trials are unethical, too expensive, or persistently unsuccessful.

However, Potosky and colleagues dramatically increased the value of the Medicare database for cancer research by merging it at the patient level with the NCI's Surveillance, Epidemiology and End Results (SEER) database, the population-based cancer registry maintained by the NCI that now includes about 15% of U.S. population.[44] The combined SEER-Medicare database has been exploited in scores of retrospective cancer cohort studies that document the relationships of a variety of factors, including sociodemographic characteristics such as age or race,[45,46] geographic location, treatment modalities, and provider characteristics, such as institution and provider procedure volume, or volume-outcome studies,[47-49], with survival. The combined SEER-Medicare database is also useful for economic studies.[50,51]

However, only patients 65 years or older are adequately represented in Medicare, limiting generalizability. Further, downstream events are sparsely documented and patient-reported information is absent in the SEER database and the power to explain observed associations is modest.[52] Strategies to enrich claims databases have arisen. Some investigators have used the Medicare or SEER-Medicare data to identify cancer patient groups to survey them directly to measure quality of life.[53] One large study, the Prostate Cancer Outcomes Study (PCOS), surveyed SEER prostate cancer patients at regular intervals up to 10 years after diagnosis,[54,55] providing a rich resource on the functional and quality-of-life outcomes of patients diagnosed with early prostate cancer. The NCI created a more ambitious research structure to investigate lung and colorectal cancers, the Cancer Care Outcomes Research and Surveillance (CanCORS) Consortium, a collaborative network of 8 patient populations to collect patient-reported and clinical information from patients with colorectal and lung cancer.[56] The Consortium's principal research aims are to "determine how the characteristics and beliefs of cancer patients and providers and the characteristics of health-care organizations influence treatments and outcomes" as well as "the effects of specific therapies on patients' survival, quality of life, and satisfaction with care." The consortium is addressing methodological issues[57] for which additional research funding is available.

Case-control studies, which compare patients with (cases) and without (controls) risk factors of interest, including interventions, are efficient research designs for uncommon conditions. Cancer is common, but many specific cancer diagnoses are not. The ratio of risk factors in the cases and controls is algebraically equivalent to the risk factor's relative risk. For example, the finding that patients with oral cancers have 10 times as often used chewing tobacco as those without the diagnosis is equivalent to a 10-fold increased risk of oral cancer associated with use of chewing tobacco. Like cohort studies, case-control studies are limited by available data that has been collected or may be collected by the investigators. Case-control studies arising from large cohort studies, or nested case-control studies, make efficient use of data already collected, limiting expensive new data collection.

While case-control studies are fundamental to cancer etiological research, they have been more recently used to address clinical questions. One pioneering study used a health maintenance organization's clinical database to assess sigmoidoscopy screening for colorectal cancer. Using fatal colorectal cancer patients as cases, the investigators found a more than 2-fold risk reduction in 10-year mortality from distal colon or rectal cancer (within the range of the procedure) from the procedure.[58] Because observed associations in observational studies are not causal, the authors were required to address other potential explanations, such as confounding by related health-conscious behaviors. A more definitive randomized trial would have required thousands of patients and 10 years of follow-up or introduced other design weaknesses to reduce costs, such as intermediate outcomes like cancer diagnosis or subsequent colonic polyps.[59,60] In principal, a case-control study could select cases based on good or bad quality-of-life outcomes, rather than cancer diagnosis or death. However, indicators of quality of life are far less likely to be recorded reliably in existing databases.

Modeling Studies ■ Mathematical models attempt to identify quantitative relationships between outcomes and factors of interest. Unlike mathematical models describing physical relationships, such as Einstein's archetypical equation $e = mc^2$, mathematical models in medicine are intended as shorthand descriptions of complex relationships. Using as few variables as possible, the model builder hopes to characterize the relationships between the most important factors in a clinical situation, understanding that the resultant understanding is approximate. Because a model built in a single *training* population may reflect idiosyncratic or chance relationships, it must be assessed in other *testing* populations to demonstrate validity. Put another way, all medical models are wrong, but some are useful.

Models are used to adjust for prognostic differences between patient groups in controlled trials, evaluate the information added by new diagnostic or prognostic tests, and create specific clinical decision rules.[61,62] One such model identified medically stable cancer patients with febrile neutropenia,[63] enabling trials of outpatient management.[64,65] An important branch of outcomes research, decision analysis, uses complex modeling procedures to evaluate complex medical situations flexibly and powerfully. Using working mathematical models of relationships between key factors in clinical populations, these models identify the intervention that on average produces the most desirable outcome, using information about currently available options, and test "what if" scenarios of altered existing parameters, such as efficacy or cost, or contemplated new approaches. The model outcomes can be survival, or alternatives such as quality of life, organ function, or survival adjusted for impaired quality of life, expressed as quality-adjusted life years, or QALYs.

QALYs, expressed as a cost-effectiveness analysis (CEA) "price," cost per QALY, are enormously appealing to policy makers and payers as a "common currency" unit, incorporating both the length and the quality of survival, for comparing medical interventions.[66] Accepting its assumptions discussed below (Outcomes, or Endpoints; Quality of Life), CEA can rank the universe of medical interventions in "league tables," with the interventions that produce health benefits (QALYs) most efficiently (lowest cost per QALY) at the top and progressively less efficient interventions lower. Using this list, health policy decision makers could simply proceed down the list, approving progressively less cost-effective interventions until the health care budget is exhausted, confident that they have purchased the most health benefit possible. In the most direct attempt to apply this method, the state of Oregon attempted to prioritize its Medicaid services as part of a plan to dramatically expand insurance coverage. The newly created Oregon Health Services Commission was charged with defining "basic" services that all health insurance must cover. However, the first pass produced alarmingly counterintuitive rankings, such as ranking orthodontic care above treatment for Hodgkin lymphoma. After a review, formal cost-effectiveness procedures were discarded in favor of subjective ranking of service categories by their value to individuals and whether they are essential to health care. Opinions differed on why the cost-effectiveness approach failed. Some argued that the cost-effectiveness approach fundamentally conflicts with the purposes of health care.[67] Most, however, held correctable errors in execution responsible and remain convinced that the rational framework of CEA is better than the existing approach.[68-70]

Quality of Care ■ Quality-of-care research arises from at least two major interacting research streams, studies of medical practice variability and studies of medical injury and patient safety. Wennberg and colleagues' studies, described above, documented small-area variation in medical practice patterns not explained by medical factors or by patient preferences. After validating their research methodology, they attempted to identify optimal practice patterns that exclude inefficient or harmful medical care. Using physician experts to define appropriate care and working through medical organizations, they undertook quality improvement campaigns to standardize care on optimal practice patterns.[71] They also used patient outcomes to assess practice patterns. Using claims data, they calculated risk-adjusted rates of mortality and other adverse outcomes, such as perioperative mortality, re-operation, or other salvage interventions, to define optimal treatment patterns.[72-74] More expansively, they compared mortality in regions in which health care was more or less intensive and thus costly. Surprisingly, they found that patient outcomes were not improved in higher cost regions, implying that most medical care could be eliminated without harm to patients.[75,76]

Studies examining the relationship between institutional and provider procedure volume and patient outcomes, known as volume-outcome studies, provided a methodology to compare providers and hospitals.[48,49,77] The volume-outcome relationship is strongest for the most complex cancer procedures, such as esophagectomy, compared to others performed in equally ill patients, such as pneumonectomy,[47] and influenced by both institutional and provider factors.[78,79] This research is politically thorny but potentially important for improving health care, since it could, for example, be used to justify restricting complex procedures to high-volume referral centers.[80]

The second research stream arose from political debate over malpractice litigation. For some, malpractice lawsuits provide humane compensation for patient injury from substandard medical care while discouraging negligent medical practice. For others, they punish irrationally, discouraging competent physicians from practice and provoking expensive, unnecessary "defensive medicine." The Harvard Malpractice Study, reported in 1991, examined New York state hospital records using explicit criteria to determine how often medical care injured patients or prolonged their hospitalization, called adverse events, and then determined their relationship to medical error, negligence and subsequent disability. They found that adverse events occurred in 3% of hospital admissions, 30% caused permanent injury or death, and negligence was responsible in about one-third of cases. Fewer than 5% of patients injured by negligence filed malpractice cases, and most cases filed involved no negligence. The results fundamentally altered thinking about patient safety.[81-83] After a series of high-visibility mishaps, primarily in cancer care, a United States Institute of Medicine report described systems, not individuals, that produce medical errors,[84] followed by a call for systematic efforts to improve cancer care.[85] Dramatically expanded efforts to reduce medical errors ensued, including a restructured AHRQ with quality of care replacing health policy in its research mission and a growing wave of research addressing quality of care in cancer.[86-88]

Outcomes or Endpoints

The starting point of any study is choosing the outcome of interest. For good reason, survival is the "gold standard" outcome for all medical researchers, including outcomes researchers; it is important and unambiguous. While traditional oncology researchers focus on "biological" disease-specific markers, such endpoints interest outcomes researchers largely as surrogate indicators of prolonged survival or fewer symptoms. However, other endpoints are better crafted to outcomes research questions.

Quality of Life ■ Both disease and its treatment may affect the length and the quality of life. Quality of life is daunting to define, much less measure. Outcomes researchers attempt to measure quality of life attributable to health, or health-related quality of life (HRQOL). Because of cancer's devastating potential and, in some circumstances, the possibility of cure, patients and physicians may accept treatment toxicity that is unacceptable for less frightening diagnoses. Therefore, quality-of-life assessment in oncology extends beyond the effects of cancer to its treatment. For cancer, like other serious illnesses, nonmedical consequences may affect quality of life, such as out-of-pocket costs or difficulties obtaining employment or medical insurance. Depending on the clinical situation or research objective, researchers may define HRQOL differently, and the patient's perspective may differ from that of the investigators. For example, researchers were surprised to document that radical prostatectomy causes substantial erectile dysfunction and urinary incontinence a year later but little measurable decrease in their HRQOL.[89,90] While survey instruments that are insufficiently sensitive to detect meaningful changes could explain these results, patients may adapt to dysfunction or simply consider treatment side effects irrelevant to their health.

Investigators may measure the quality-of-life impact of disease and its treatment as either specific symptoms, or dysfunction, or as the global impact on the patient, or utilities or preferences. Each approach has different uses, strengths, and weakness, although attempts to combine them have been described.[91,92] Measuring specific dysfunction usefully characterizes patient states, but the results lend themselves poorly to overall summaries, or global utility. Measures of global utility permit straightforward adjustment of survival to account for decreased quality of life, using the QALY, as the "common currency." However, they require daunting assumptions: that valid measures of the relationship between health states and self-assessed patient HRQOL are possible; that health states of sufficient complexity to represent clinical experience can be directly assessed or mathematically combined; that the measured relationship remains constant over time; and that averaged values do justice to individual circumstances. Each is subject to challenge.

Investigators have developed several ingenious techniques to quantify the quality-of-life adjustment for an impaired health state, but each can be challenging for patients, especially those who are "innumerate," or uncomfortable with numerical information.[93-95] The standard reference gamble (SRG) has the firmest theoretical underpinning. It requires that patients report the point at which they are indifferent to staying in the impaired health state or a theoretical gamble with 2 outcomes, death or "perfect health," with progressively more or less attractive odds. For example, a patient who reports indifference to losing speech from laryngectomy for a pharyngeal cancer[96] or accepting a gamble in which perfect health is 3 times more likely than death (odds 3:1) signals his quality adjustment for living without a larynx is 0.75; for this patient it is 75% as good as perfect health. Not surprisingly, for many people the standard gamble does not produce consistent, meaningful responses. Other approaches, such as the time-trade-off (TTO), in which patients report the number of years in perfect health they would be willing to trade for 10 years in an impaired health state, or simply a global assessment, in which patients are asked how they would rate the impaired health state on a scale of 100, where 0 is death and 100 perfect health, are less daunting mental tasks but are still very demanding to innumerate and theoretically less valid than the SRG. This measurement problem remains vexing despite the resourcefulness of thoughtful investigators mindful of the great potential usefulness of QALYs.

The nearly limitless potential permutations of organ dysfunction and other symptoms preclude direct assessments of all health states, requiring an accepted mathematical procedure to score combinations of health states. Patient circumstances affect their experience. The lowered health expectations of older age or a prior, more profound disability, may render a new dysfunction trivial by comparison, or even moot, while a similar condition might be highly distressful to a younger, healthier patient. For example, amputation to excise an osteosarcoma, even if curative, would profoundly alter an adolescent's life, while a diabetic older adult confined to a wheelchair by chronic respiratory failure might find an amputation due to diabetic vascular insufficiency a small hindrance and perhaps even relief from managing chronic, recurrent infections.

Models assume stable preferences, but patients adapt to reduced function, as patients develop strategies for addressing dysfunction and incremental age-related dysfunction contributes to evolving "new normal" expectations. The problem of adaptation does not disappear if one measures dysfunction instead of preferences. Because the individual response to disability varies, investigators distinguish dysfunction from the response to dysfunction, called bother, or distress. Empirical evidence suggests that adaptation may be a powerful factor, particularly over longer periods. For example, radiation doses increased sufficiently to delay detectable prostate cancer recurrence[97] produced no apparent long-term differences in patient-reported urinary, bowel, or sexual dysfunction.[98] Exquisite technique may render increased radiation doses sufficient to improve cancer control clinically harmless, or, more likely, long-term adaptation may render "new-normal" dysfunction irrelevant to the patient's perceived HRQOL, rendering inaccurate models that assign dysfunction a constant impact on QALYs. One useful and transparent method for evaluating cancer survival, Time Without Symptoms and Toxicity (TWiST), classifies cancer survival broadly into time with treatment-related toxicity, cancer-related symptoms or without either, or TWiST time.[99] The results can be expressed simply as time spent in the high-quality TWiST state,[100] or by applying quality weights to each interval (0-100% of the value of TwiST time), produce a straightforward approximation of QALYs.[101] While subject to the criticisms of other methods that quantify quality-of-life decrements, the TWiST method has a straightforward appeal to clinicians, who observe their patients' qualitatively different experiences on treatment, when the patients are in remission versus when in relapse.

The imperfect decision-analytic models offer a mechanism for examining the structure of a clinical problem, producing both the optimal decision on average situation under typical circumstances or in a specific situation of particular interest, and identify the factors with the greatest impact on the outcome. As a result, the exercise can illuminate whether adequate information on key factors is available to make authoritative decisions about the appropriate clinical strategy. A jarring result can shine a light on inadequately examined assumptions. A CEA was employed to evaluate the use of prophylactic intravenous immunoglobulins (IVIG) to prevent infectious complications of chronic lymphocytic leukemia. Despite a well-designed trial demonstrating the clinical efficacy of IVIG in this setting, the model's calculations found that under any plausible assumption, the cost-effectiveness of the therapy was over $1 million per QALY.[102]

The influence of the outcomes research agenda and of patient-reported outcomes on the practice of randomized trials has grown. While surrogates such as tumor shrinkage for the definitive endpoint, survival, are the response criteria of many randomized cancer trials, as recently updated by Response Evaluation Criteria in Solid Tumors (RECIST) criteria,[103-105] patient-reported quality-of-life outcomes have been the primary outcomes of some recent studies. In 2 pivotal drug trials, the required demonstration of "clinical benefit" supporting 2 indications awarded by the U.S. Food and Drug Administration (FDA) included patient-reported primary outcomes. The first study found that mitoxantrone palliated prostate cancer patients with painful bone metastases, based on reduced pain without offsetting increased narcotic use.[106] In the second, gemcitabine's clinical benefit in advanced pancreatic cancer was measured by a novel composite of pain (analgesic consumption and pain intensity), Karnofsky performance status, and weight. Benefit was defined as improvement lasting at least 4 weeks by at least one parameter without worsening in any other.[107] In these settings, patient-reported outcomes, particularly of pain, measured central clinical aspects of the patient experience of disease, and the measured outcomes were plausible clinical proxies for successful palliation. However, uncritical use of less focused patient-reported measures as trial endpoints can lead investigators and clinicians astray. Early studies reported that erythropoietin improved quality of life in patients with cancer and other diseases[108,109] were not supported by later studies[110,111] and may have increased mortality as well as expense.[112]

The techniques of outcomes research may play a role in oncology beyond drug trials. Since most advanced cancers are incurable by current methods, palliation is the goal when primary treatment fails, and quality of life, which improves with even marginal extension of patients' lives.[113] Further, cancer therapy, whether surgery, radiation, or medical, usually comes with toxicity, and treatment innovations increasingly aim to reduce it. Better treatments minimize treatment-related toxicity, and patient-reported outcomes are the most sensitive and valid measures of toxicity. Under increasing cost pressure, expensive technologies intended to reduce toxicity, such as proton radiation[114-116] or sphincter-sparing rectal cancer surgery, will require improved patient-reported outcomes as evidence of benefit. Further, the assumption that optimal treatment minimizes toxicity suggests that patient-reported outcomes may have a wider role in quality assessment and quality improvement of cancer therapies; disparate quality-of-life outcomes for nominally similar treatments implies that poorer-performing techniques or providers have measurable room for improvement.[79,117] The recently enacted American Recovery and Reinvestment Act allocates $400 million to Comparative Effectiveness Research (CER), suggesting that such formal evaluation may be on the near horizon. Methodological challenges to definitive measurement of quality of life remain, but as methodological progress addresses them, the role of quality-of-life outcomes in randomized cancer trials will continue to grow.

Costs ■ Measuring economic efficiency has long been a goal of outcomes research. In part because the major economic inputs in health care, specialized, highly skilled labor and complex technology, are difficult to monetarize.

Due to the highly regulated structure and complex payment schemes, the economic aspects of health care are difficult to study. The standard units of expenditure, costs, are not measured but calculated, based on ratios between billed amounts, or charges, and true economic costs. Medicare requires that each hospital report department-specific cost-to-charge ratios. Charges are determined through negotiations, which are in turn dependent on bargaining power. The largest purchasers, usually health care plans, negotiate the lowest charges, while those with the least power, such as individual uninsured patients in the United States have the highest charges. A third category is the record of actual economic activity, ie, charges paid, but is rarely the economic outcome of interest. Accepted procedures for economic analyses have also been published.[66,118-120]

As noted above, a common use of cost data in medicine is to arrive at a common measure of value for medical maneuvers, the cost-effectiveness ratio in QALYs. With such a "price," it is possible to rank the medical "efficiency" of various components of health care. The most straightforward use of CEA would be to rank potential interventions in a *league table* from the most to the least efficient (ie, from the lowest to the highest cost-effectiveness ratio), accepting all the interventions until the total expenditures exhaust the health care budget and rejecting the rest. That approach, in which each medical procedure is pitted against all others, has been rare in the United States. The most visible attempt, the Oregon Medicaid reform attempt, which failed, is described above. Far more common is analysis that asks only whether a procedure has an acceptably low cost-effectiveness ratio, either that of renal dialysis, an early procedure to which the US government made an early commitment to fund, or a range, often calibrated to dialysis, of $30,000-$70,000 per QALY. In this approach, *all* interventions meeting the threshold are recommended for acceptance by payers. Given the economic implications, many such analyses are performed by advocates of the intervention, often with a financial stake in the intervention, and use as the central or base case analysis the results of the most positive studies, which may be unrepresentative.

However, there is a further problem. Each additional procedure, whether or not it meets a cost-effectiveness criterion, adds to total health care expenditures. Only if each additional intervention is balanced by eliminating a less cost-effective intervention with the same total cost does this approach make medical care more efficient. If not, new technology adds to the total cost of health care. The latter situation holds today, accounting for the rapid increases in health care expenditures,[121] and the cost of cancer care is rising faster than any other area in medicine. It is easy to break a budget with cost-effective care. Controlling costs must be approached with the global budget in mind, not the absolute acceptance or rejection of individual interventions.

Measures of Quality ■ As noted above, the quality of care in medical care can be measured at three levels, structure, process, and outcomes, and each has been subject to analysis and evaluation by investigators. The quality field is in its early years, but some approaches deserve mention. In this brief discussion, references to the highly valuable quality improvement movement, a direct descendant of the approach that has been so successful in improving the safety of industries like commercial aviation, is not discussed.

Studies of structure have attempted to identify optimal institutional characteristics, such as for-profit versus non-profit, teaching versus non-teaching, and referral centers versus community institutions.[122] While these distinctions sometimes yield useful insights, the categories overlap and contain disparate institutions within them. Perhaps the most fertile current approach examines volume-outcome relationships. For most procedures, especially the most complex, providers and institutions that perform the most procedures have the best outcomes, no matter how the outcomes are assessed. Why the advantage occurs is not always evident, although one can imagine that staff experience, supporting structures, and specialized expertise might contribute. However, decisive factors may surprise. For example, much of the success of high-volume centers treating myocardial infarction has been attributed to more consistent prescription of beta-blockers on discharge.

Process is relatively easy to study, since procedures and many other interventions are regularly recorded for billing purposes. The highest quality providers would be expected to consistently use the best practice patterns. However, defining them requires reference to a standard. One approach developed by the RAND Corporation polls expert panels iteratively to rate candidate process and outcome indicators of quality care in terms of validity and feasibility. The approach brings to bear substantial weight of clinical expertise with the opportunity to interact, explore, and test the rationales of advocates. However, the process gives great sway to individual prejudices and idiosyncrasies. The larger difficulty with expert opinion-based results is that they tend to codify the currently accepted biases within the field.[80]

The alternative to guidelines based on expert opinion is evidence-based guidelines. Such guidelines are based on formal procedures to evaluate existing evidence, conform to strict methodological guidelines, and clearly indicate the strength of the conclusions and the supporting evidence.[123] Despite increasing support for the development of evidence-based guidelines from the Cochran Collaborative, medical authorities under financial pressure and pressure to choose between competing, high-cost interventions, and, more recently, ARHQ, may not choose the evidence-based approach because the process is time-consuming and can be performed successfully only when high-quality evidence is available. As a result, the process should be limited to settings in which the results are likely to be most useful; when practice variation is great, the clinical or economic implications are the most substantial, and adequate evidence is available. Attention must also be paid to the dissemination of guidelines. Presentations that obscure the key findings or present them so densely that the target audience is repelled are unlikely to influence practice. The American Society of Clinical Oncology has produced a long series of useful guidelines for the practice of oncology.[124,125]

Once guidelines are established, measuring compliance with them provides useful process indicators of quality. The value of such studies lies in determining not only the frequency of compliance with indicators but also the factors that depress it. Such studies find clinical factors, such as severity of illness and overriding contraindications, and structural factors, such as inadequate information systems support and other barriers, account for discrepancies more often then clinician resistance.

The ultimate endpoint for judging quality is patient outcomes. Because death (but not cause-specific mortality) is recorded reliably and its importance as a goal of therapy is unquestioned, many investigators have compared death rates to evaluate quality. When comparative trials are randomized, such comparisons produce unambiguous conclusions, since patients can be presumed to be similar clinically. However, for observational comparisons, adjustment for potential confounders is necessary. This process, risk adjustment, has proven the major barrier to accepting the results of quality comparisons based on patient mortality rates. Complicated patients are routinely referred to specialized centers, producing the belief that their patients have poorer prognoses that adjustment procedures cannot fully capture. Analyses that compare regions, not hospitals, sidestep that concern most successfully.[75,127] Other outcomes, more ambiguous and less well documented than mortality, are equally vexed by the problem of risk-adjustment.

Selected References

The complete reference list can be found at www.CANCERMEDICINE8.com

3. Krumholz HM, Peterson ED, Ayanian JZ, et al. Report of the National Heart, Lung, and Blood Institute working group on outcomes research in cardiovascular disease. *Circulation.* 2005;111:3158–3166.
16. Sloss EM, Keeler EB, Brook RH, Operskalski BH, Goldberg GA, Newhouse JP. Effect of a health maintenance organization on physiologic health. Results from a randomized trial. *Ann Intern Med.* 1987;106:130–138.
17. Chassin MR, Kosecoff J, Park RE, et al. Does inappropriate use explain geographic variations in the use of health care services? A study of three procedures. *JAMA.* 1987;258:2533–2537.
20. Cella D, Yount S, Rothrock N, et al. The Patient-Reported Outcomes Measurement Information System (PROMIS): progress of an NIH Roadmap cooperative group during its first two years. *Med Care.* 2007;45:S3–S11.
22. Garcia SF, Cella D, Clauser SB, et al. Standardizing patient-reported outcomes assessment in cancer clinical trials: a patient-reported outcomes measurement information system initiative. *J Clin Oncol.* 2007;25:5106–5112.
23. Joffe S, Cook EF, Cleary PD, Clark JW, Weeks JC. Quality of informed consent in cancer clinical trials: a cross-sectional survey. *Lancet.* 2001;358:1772–1777.
30. Langley S, Henderson A, Laing R. The SPIRIT of research: a new well-funded randomized study comparing brachytherapy with radical prostatectomy is about to open in the UK. *BJU Int.* 2004;93:6–7.
31. Bill-Axelson A, Holmberg L, Ruutu M, et al. Radical prostatectomy versus watchful waiting in early prostate cancer. *N Engl J Med.* 2005;352:1977–1984.
33. Donovan JL, Peters TJ, Noble S, et al. Who can best recruit to randomized trials? Randomized trial comparing surgeons and nurses recruiting patients to a trial of treatments for localized prostate cancer (the ProtecT study). *J Clin Epidemiol.* 2003;56:605–609.
45. Godley PA, Clark JA, Gellantly DD, Jackson ST, Talcott JA. Race and prostate cancer: attitudes toward diagnosis and treatment among newly diagnosed patients. *Proc Annu Meet Am Soc Clin Oncol.* 2004;23:A6056.
46. Sundararajan V, Hershman D, Grann VR, Jacobson JS, Neugut AI. Variations in the use of chemotherapy for elderly patients with advanced ovarian cancer: a population-based study. *J Clin Oncol.* 2002;20:173–178.
50. Ramsey SD, Berry K, Etzioni R. Lifetime cancer-attributable cost of care for long term survivors of colorectal cancer. *Am J Gastroenterol.* 2002;97:440–445.
52. Potosky AL, Warren JL, Riedel ER, Klabunde CN, Earle CC, Begg CB. Measuring complications of cancer treatment using the SEER-Medicare data. *Med Care.* 2002;40:IV-62-8.
55. Potosky AL, Davis WW, Hoffman RM, et al. Five-year outcomes after prostatectomy or radiotherapy for prostate cancer: the prostate cancer outcomes study. *J Natl Cancer Inst.* 2004;96:1358–1367.
56. Ayanian JZ, Chrischilles EA, Fletcher RH, et al. Understanding cancer treatment and outcomes: the Cancer Care Outcomes Research and Surveillance Consortium. *J Clin Oncol.* 2004;22:2992–2996.
57. Malin JL, Ko C, Ayanian JZ, et al. Understanding cancer patients' experience and outcomes: development and pilot study of the Cancer Care Outcomes Research and Surveillance patient survey. *Support Care Cancer.* 2006;14:837–848.
73. Wennberg JE, Freeman JL, Shelton RM, Bubolz TA. Hospital use and mortality among Medicare beneficiaries in Boston and New Haven. *N Engl J Med.* 1989;321:1168–1173.
74. Lu-Yao GL, Potosky AL, Albertsen PC, Wasson JH, Barry MJ, Wennberg JE. Follow-up prostate cancer treatments after radical prostatectomy: a population-based study. *J Natl Cancer Inst.* 1996;88:166–173.
76. Fisher ES, Wennberg DE, Stukel TA, Gottlieb DJ, Lucas FL, Pinder EL. The implications of regional variations in Medicare spending. Part 2: health outcomes and satisfaction with care. *Ann Intern Med.* 2003;138:288–298.
78. Schrag D, Panageas KS, Riedel E, et al. Hospital and surgeon procedure volume as predictors of outcome following rectal cancer resection. *Ann Surg.* 2002;236:583–592.
79. Hu JC, Gold KF, Pashos CL, Mehta SS, Litwin MS. Role of surgeon volume in radical prostatectomy outcomes. *J Clin Oncol.* 2003;21:401–405.
80. Talcott JA. Quality of care in prostate cancer: important to start and too important to stop here. *J Clin Oncol.* 2003;21:1902–1903.
81. Brennan TA, Leape LL, Laird NM, et al. Incidence of adverse events and negligence in hospitalized patients. Results of the Harvard Medical Practice Study I. *N Engl J Med.* 1991;324:370–376.
85. Hewitt M, Rowland JH, Yancik R. Cancer survivors in the United States: age, health, and disability. *J Gerontol A Biol Sci Med Sci.* 2003;58:82–91.
86. Weissman JS, Schneider EC, Weingart SN, et al. Comparing patient-reported hospital adverse events with medical record review: do patients know something that hospitals do not? *Ann Intern Med.* 2008;149:100–108.
87. Keating NL, Landrum MB, Guadagnoli E, Winer EP, Ayanian JZ. Surveillance testing among survivors of early-stage breast cancer. *J Clin Oncol.* 2007;25:1074–1081.
88. Earle CC, Neville BA, Landrum MB, et al. Evaluating claims-based indicators of the intensity of end-of-life cancer care. *Int J Qual Health Care.* 2005;17:505–509.
89. Clark JA, Rieker P, Propert KJ, Talcott JA. Changes in quality of life following treatment for early prostate cancer. *Urology.* 1999;53:161–168.
92. Furlong WJ, Feeny DH, Torrance GW, Barr RD. The Health Utilities Index (HUI) system for assessing health-related quality of life in clinical studies. *Ann Med.* 2001;33:375–384.
93. Peters E, Hibbard J, Slovic P, Dieckmann N. Numeracy skill and the communication, comprehension, and use of risk-benefit information. *Health Aff (Millwood).* 2007;26:741–748.
97. Zietman AL, DeSilvio ML, Slater JD, et al. Comparison of conventional-dose vs high-dose conformal radiation therapy in clinically localized adenocarcinoma of the prostate: a randomized controlled trial. *JAMA.* 2005;294:1233–1239.
98. Talcott JA, Slater JD, Zietman A, Rossi C, Shipley WU, Clark JA. Long-term quality of life after conventional-dose vs. high-dose radiation for prostate cancer: results from a randomized trial (PROG 95-09) *Proc Annu Meet Am Soc Clin Oncol.* 2008;26:A5058.
105. Therasse P, Arbuck SG, Eisenhauer EA, et al. New guidelines to evaluate the response to treatment in solid tumors. European Organization for Research and Treatment of Cancer, National Cancer Institute of the United States, National Cancer Institute of Canada. *J Natl Cancer Inst.* 2000;92:205–216.
107. Burris HA, 3rd, Moore MJ, Andersen J, et al. Improvements in survival and clinical benefit with gemcitabine as first-line therapy for patients with advanced pancreas cancer: a randomized trial. *J Clin Oncol.* 1997;15:2403–2413.
110. Gaston KE, Kouba E, Moore DT, Pruthi RS. The use of erythropoietin in patients undergoing radical prostatectomy: effects on hematocrit, transfusion rates and quality of life. *Urol Int.* 2006;77:211–215.
111. Casadevall N, Durieux P, Dubois S, et al. Health, economic, and quality-of-life effects of erythropoietin and granulocyte colony-stimulating factor for the treatment of myelodysplastic syndromes: a randomized, controlled trial. *Blood.* 2004;104:321–327.
112. Phrommintikul A, Haas SJ, Elsik M, Krum H. Mortality and target haemoglobin concentrations in anaemic patients with chronic kidney disease treated with erythropoietin: a meta-analysis. *Lancet.* 2007;369:381–388.
114. Zietman AL. The Titanic and the Iceberg: prostate proton therapy and health care economics. *J Clin Oncol.* 2007;25:3565–3566.
115. Tepper JE. Protons and parachutes. *J Clin Oncol.* 2008;26:2436–2437.
121. Bodenheimer T. High and rising health care costs. Part 1: seeking an explanation. *Ann Intern Med.* 2005;142:847–854.
125. Loblaw DA, Mendelson DS, Talcott JA, et al. American Society of Clinical Oncology recommendations for the initial hormonal management of androgen-sensitive metastatic, recurrent, or progressive prostate cancer. *J Clin Oncol.* 2004;22:2927–2941.

37 Principles of Cancer Pathology

James L. Connolly, MD ▪ Jeffrey D. Goldsmith, MD ▪ Helen H. Wang, Dr PH, MD ▪ Janina A. Longtine, MD ▪ Ann M. Dvorak, MD ▪ Harold F. Dvorak, MD ▪ Stanley R. Hamilton, MD

Pathologists are physicians who are concerned not only with the diagnosis and classification of disease at a cellular and molecular level but also with the study of disease in all its aspects including etiology, pathogenesis, molecular mechanisms, anatomic and biochemical features, progression, natural history, and prognosis and response to therapies. In many respects, therefore, pathologists are the "doctors' doctors," consultants with specialized knowledge who are helpful to other physicians with more direct care and treatment responsibilities for patients. *The majority of data and information upon which patient care decisions are made derive from laboratory testing.* Nowhere in medicine is the pathologist's knowledge base and skills more important than in the care of patients with cancer, especially in the era of personalized cancer care. Pathologists have custody of and responsibility for patients' tissues and body fluids that are sent to their laboratories for analysis, knowledge of and access to methodologies for evaluation of specimens, and expertise in validation, quality control and quality assurance of testing to drive high-quality individualized patient care.

Pathologists engage in several types of activity: *anatomic pathology*, which includes surgical pathology, cytology, and autopsy pathology; *clinical pathology*, also known as laboratory medicine, with laboratories for clinical chemistry, medical microbiology, hematology and coagulation, and blood banking and transfusion medicine; *hematopathology*, which is directed at blood, bone marrow, and lymph node evaluation; and *experimental pathology* that comprises basic investigations of the pathogenesis of disease including in vitro and animal models. Over the years, these distinctions have become increasingly blurred as advances in technology such as immunohistochemistry, in situ hybridization, flow cytometry, and molecular biologic approaches have moved from the research laboratory into the clinical laboratory for cancer diagnosis and classification.

This chapter reviews the basic principles of pathology as they apply to neoplastic diseases. The goal is to provide oncologists with a better understanding of what pathologists do, how we arrive at diagnoses, what tools are now at our disposal, and how the oncologist can interact most productively with the pathologist to achieve the greatest benefit for patients with cancer.

Definitions, Tumor Structure, and Tumor Stroma Generation

Although physicians know intuitively what they mean when they use the term "tumor," the definition is not simple, concise, and comprehensive. The generic word "tumor" is of Latin origin, meaning "swelling." But not all swellings are a tumor or neoplasm ("new growth") in the modern sense of the term, eg, the swellings of inflammation and repair. Tumors are classified as benign, borderline, or malignant based on their potential to invade and metastasize. The distinguished pathologist Wallace H. Clark[1] offered an excellent definition, paraphrased as follows: a malignant tumor (fully evolved) is a population of abnormal cells characterized by temporally unrestricted growth and the ability to grow in at least three different tissue compartments—the original compartment, the mesenchyme of the primary site (tumor invasion), and a distant mesenchyme (tumor metastasis). Clark's definition usefully emphasizes the progressive nature of cancer growth; the common (although not exclusive) origin of cancers as benign growths; their gradual acquisition of autonomy; and, at some stage, their ability to spread to and grow in new tissues distant from their site of origin—ie, to metastasize. More recently, Hanahan and Weinberg[2] identified six traits that cancers acquire including self-sufficiency in growth signals, insensitivity to antigrowth signals, evasion of apoptosis, limitless reproductive potential, sustained angiogenesis, tissue invasion and metastasis, and genomic instability.

Tumor Structure

Although some cancers (eg, leukemias and those in body cavity fluids such as ascites) grow as cell suspensions, most cancers grow as solid masses of tissue. Solid tumors have a distinct structure that mimics normal tissues[3–5] and that comprises two distinct but interdependent compartments: the parenchyma (neoplastic cells) and the stroma that the neoplastic cells induce and in which they are dispersed. In many tumors, including those of epithelial cell origin that are by far the most common, a basal lamina separates clumps of tumor cells from stroma. However, the basal lamina is often incomplete, especially at points of tumor invasion.

The neoplastic cells in tumors have received the lion's share of attention in cancer research, but all tumors have stroma that is required for nutritional support and for removal of waste products. In the case of leukemias, blood plasma serves as stroma, although an additional stromal response, ie, angiogenesis characterized by the formation of new blood vessels, occurs in the bone marrow.[6] When tumors grow in body cavities, a plasma exudate (eg, ascites) provides stroma.[7,8] In solid tumors, stroma includes connective tissue, blood vessels, and, very often, inflammatory cells, all of which are interposed between the malignant cells and normal host tissues. In all tumors, stroma is largely a product of the host and is induced as a result of tumor cell–host interactions. Solid tumors, regardless of their type or cellular origin, require stroma to grow beyond a minimal size of 1–2 mm.[9] By contrast, the stroma of solid tumors may also limit the influx of inflammatory cells or the egress of tumor cells ("invasion"). Stroma, therefore, simultaneously provides a lifeline that is necessary for tumor growth and imposes a barrier that inhibits and may regulate interchange of fluids, gases, and cells.

The importance of new blood vessel formation to tumor survival and growth has rightly led to an emphasis on tumor angiogenesis, but that emphasis has been accompanied by an unfortunate tendency to undervalue other tumor stromal components. In fact, in many tumors, interstitial connective tissue comprises the bulk of stroma, and blood vessels are only a minor component. In addition to being important in tumor biology, these nonneoplastic cells influence diagnostic interpretation and affect tumor–cell based assays by providing contaminating DNA, RNA, and proteins.

For the most part, tumor stroma is formed of elements that are derived from the circulating blood and from adjacent host connective tissues.[10] Plasma components include water and plasma proteins, together with various types and numbers of inflammatory cells. Almost any element found in normal connective tissue may be represented in tumor stroma, including even bone and cartilage in osseous and cartilaginous metaplasia. Generally speaking, the major components of tumor stroma include, in addition to new blood vessels, leaked plasma and plasma proteins, proteoglycans and glycosaminoglycans, interstitial collagens (primarily types I and III), fibrin (Fig. 37-1), fibronectin, and cells of two general types: connective tissue cells such as fibroblasts and inflammatory cells that are derived from the blood.[10]

Although all tumor stroma contains the same basic constituents, pathologists have long recognized that tumors differ markedly from each other in stromal content. Sometimes the differences are primarily quantitative. At one extreme are desmoplastic tumors, such as many carcinomas of the breast, stomach, and pancreas, in which as much as 90% or more of the total tumor consists of stroma with a minor component of malignant cells. At the other extreme are tumors such as medullary and lobular carcinomas of the breast and many lymphomas in which only minimal stroma develops. In other cases, differences in stromal content among various tumors are largely qualitative. For example, some carcinomas of the breast provoke the deposition of abundant elastic tissue and collagen. Others (eg, medullary carcinoma of the breast and colon) induce an extensive lymphocytic infiltrate and little else in the way of stroma. Even within a single tumor, there may be substantial variations in stromal composition from one area to another. Stromal heterogeneity should not be surprising in view of the well-recognized heterogeneity of the parenchymal cells present within individual tumors.

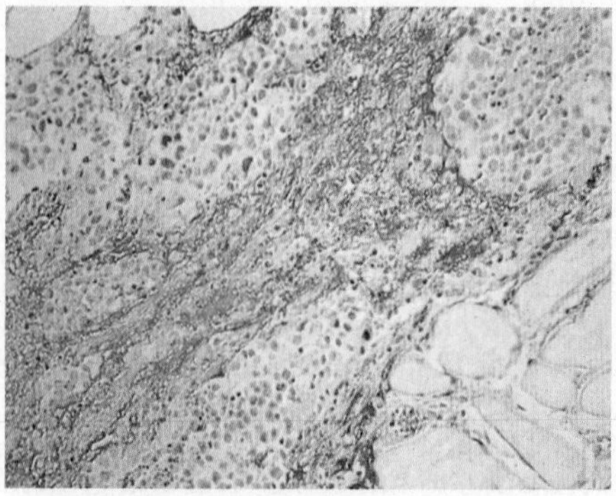

Figure 37-1 ■ Immunoperoxidase staining reaction of line 10 guinea pig undifferentiated bile duct carcinoma exposed to a monoclonal antibody specific for fibrin (supplied by Dr. Gary Matsueda). Tumor comprises nests of malignant cells interspersed in a stroma that stains heavily for fibrin. Immunoperoxidase stain; ×50 original magnification.

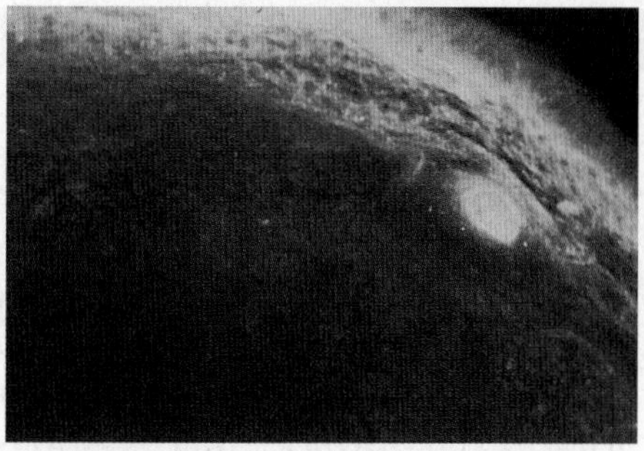

Figure 37-3 ■ Lewis lung carcinoma growing in flank of a syngeneic C57Bl/6 mouse that had received a macromolecular tracer, 70 kDa fluoresceinated dextran, 15 min previously. Bright-staining apple-green fluorescence forming a rim around the tumor represents extensive extravasation of tracer into surrounding normal connective tissue from leaky blood vessels at the tumor–host interface. The tumor itself is virtually unstained, appearing as a "black hole," because tracer at its periphery diffuses poorly into tumor. Fluorescence microscopy; magnification ×15.

Tumor Stroma Generation

Steps in the Process

Studies of transplantable tumors have yielded important information concerning the pathogenesis of tumor stroma generation (Figs. 37-2 and 37-3). Among the earliest steps in the process is local vascular hyperpermeability to circulating macromolecules. Increased vascular permeability is attributable to vascular permeability factor/vascular endothelial growth factor (VPF/VEGF, VEGF-A), a multifunctional cytokine that is synthesized and secreted by most animal and human tumors.[11]

Among other activities, VEGF-A renders the microvasculature hyperpermeable to plasma and plasma proteins extravasation with potency some 50,000 times that of histamine. It ranks among the most powerful vascular permeabilizing substances known (Figs. 37-2 and 37-3).[11,12] As with histamine, the primary target of VEGF-A action is postcapillary venules and small veins, whose lining endothelial cells express the two VEGF-A tyrosine kinase receptors VEGFR-1 (*FLT1*) and VEGFR-2 (*KDR*). Leakage of plasma proteins, including fibrinogen and other clotting factors, leads to activation of the coagulation system by a tissue factor–mediated mechanism[15] that results in formation of an extravascular gel of cross-linked fibrin (Figs. 37-1 and 37-2). Extravascular fibrin deposits transform the inert extravascular matrix of normal adult tissues into a proangiogenic provisional matrix that favors and stimulates inward migration of host mesenchymal cells.[13] Other plasma proteins (eg, plasma fibronectin) as well as locally synthesized structural proteins (eg, cellular fibronectins, tenascin), hyaluronan, and proteoglycans (eg, chondroitin sulfate–rich proteoglycan and decorin) also contribute to this new tissue.[13]

The fibrin gel deposited by tumors is modulated by proteases (Figs. 37-1 and 37-2) and gradually replaced by an ingrowth of fibroblasts and new blood vessels that give rise to loose connective tissue similar to the "granulation tissue" of healing wounds.[5] After an additional period, the granulation tissue is further transformed into the poorly vascularized, dense collagenous scar-like connective tissue characteristic of tumor desmoplasia. Simultaneously, tumor cells that break away from the original tumor site begin to recapitulate the same sequence of events at nearby sites, particularly at the tumor's invasive edge Thus, at any one time, growing desmoplastic tumors consist of older more centrally placed portions, comprising tumor cells that are encased in poorly vascularized dense collagenous stroma, and a more active newer

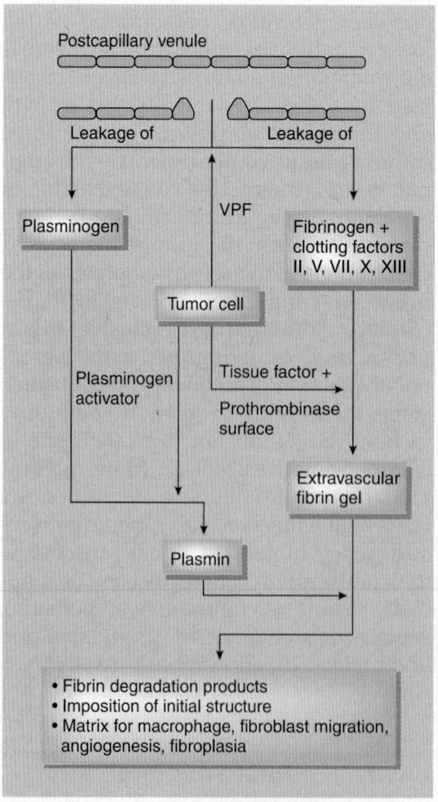

Figure 37-2 ■ Schematic diagram of tumor stroma generation.

fibrin-rich peripheral zone that interfaces with the surrounding host tissue.

Critical Role of VEGF-A in Stroma Formation

VEGF-A has a central role in tumor angiogenesis and stroma generation. It is expressed in several different isoforms as the result of alternative splicing of a single, highly conserved gene. VEGF-A is the founding member of a family of proteins whose members include placenta growth factor and VEGF-B, -C, -D, and -E. In addition to its potent function as an effecter of vascular hyperpermeability, VEGF-A stimulates endothelial cell division and migration, induces endothelial cells to express increased amounts of tissue factor, urokinase, tissue plasminogen activator, and matrix metalloproteases. Collectively, those endothelial cell products induce clotting and initiate fibrinolysis and degradation of collagen and other elements of pre-existing matrix.

A number of factors serve to stimulate VEGFA expression in tumor cells, ie, tissue hypoxia and low tissue pH in the tumor microenvironment. However, many tumor cells make substantial amounts of VEGF-A under normoxic or even hyperoxic conditions. Other factors that induce overexpression include cytokines (eg, epidermal growth factor, basic fibroblast growth factor), certain hormones (eg, thyroglobulin), and, perhaps of more general interest, various oncogenes (eg, *src*, *ras*) and tumor suppressor genes including the von Hippel–Lindau protein.

Relationship of Tumor Stroma Generation to Wound Healing and Other Examples of Pathologic and Physiologic Angiogenesis and Stroma Generation

The events of stroma generation in transplantable tumors closely mimic those of normal wound healing[5,14] with upregulation of VEGF-A expression, as in various analogous pathologic and physiologic processes that involve new blood vessel and stroma formation, including rheumatoid arthritis, psoriasis, delayed hypersensitivity, diabetic retinopathy, and corpus luteum formation. Tumors have preempted and subverted, for their own purposes, a fundamental host mechanism, the wound healing response, as the means to acquire the stroma they need to grow and spread.

Of course, some differences exist. Platelets, which play several critical roles in wound healing, seem not to participate to any great extent in tumor stroma generation; however, many platelet functions can be subsumed by tumor cells, which express similar or analogous cytokines and growth factors. Tumors differ from healing wounds in another important respect. At wound sites, overexpression of VEGF-A and consequent vascular hyperpermeability are limited to a period of a few days, presumably until oxygen tension has returned to normal.[15] By contrast, VEGF-A expression and vascular hyperpermeability are not limited in tumors; they persist indefinitely. Thus, tumors in some sense behave as wounds that do not heal.[5]

The analogy between wound healing and tumor stroma generation may be taken one step further. Except in lower vertebrates that are capable of regenerating normal tissues, wound healing does not recapitulate ontogeny but, instead, replaces injured parenchyma and stroma with connective tissue whose functional capacities fall well short of the original normal tissue. In the same manner, the stroma of a malignant tumor is generally a disorganized and poorly supportive parody of normal connective tissue. The vascular supply is often marginal. Tumor blood vessels are structurally and functionally abnormal, unevenly spaced, and often unequal to the task of supporting the growth and even the life of rapidly metabolizing tumor cells.[10,15] The result is irregular blood flow in leaky blood vessels, uneven perfusion, shifting zones of anoxia, low pH, and, commonly, necrosis and apoptosis.[10,16] In fact, the presence of necrosis is sometimes helpful to the pathologist in distinguishing malignant tumors from their benign counterparts and from certain nonneoplastic processes.

Role of the Surgical Pathologist in the Diagnosis and Management of Cancer Patients

Surgical pathologists have the definitive role in tumor diagnosis. No matter how high the index of clinical suspicion, a diagnosis of cancer is neither conclusively established nor safely assumed in the absence of a tissue diagnosis. With few exceptions, definitive therapy for cancer should not be undertaken in the absence of a tissue diagnosis. Policies supporting this practice are written into the bylaws of most hospitals and are regularly monitored by hospital tissue committees and by accrediting agencies.

The surgical pathologist has the task to provide an accurate, specific, and sufficiently comprehensive diagnosis to enable the clinician to develop an optimal plan of treatment and, to the extent possible, to estimate prognosis and response to therapies. Not many years ago, the simple designation "benign" or "malignant" provided the clinician with all of the information necessary to provide appropriate care for the patient. This is no longer the case. Tumors come in hundreds of distinct entities, variants, and patterns, some with characteristic biology. Moreover, tumors have a historical course of development and progression; in an individual, they may be first recognized at any stage along that course.

The tremendous advances in all fields of oncology require a great deal of additional information. In fact, to permit the most appropriate classification for research, prognosis, and therapeutic intervention, nearly every case requires a more complete understanding of the patient's particular tumor. Details of the type and origin of the tumor, its differentiation and level of invasion, the numbers of lymph nodes with and without metastatic tumor, the presence or absence of hormone receptors, the activity of specific enzymes, cytogenetic translocations, frequency of mitosis, and percentage of cells in the S-phase may all be relevant in the pathologic assessment of neoplasia. Molecular pathology, using nucleic acid probes with or without amplification by the polymerase chain reaction to detect expression of specific tumor genes or gene mutations, has become standard practice and promises an increasingly important role for pathology in the clinical management of cancer patients, eg, microsatellite instability in colorectal carcinoma as an indicator of hereditary nonpolyposis colorectal cancer syndrome,[17] as a prognostic marker and as a predictive marker.[18]

Surgical pathologists deal primarily with structure. Careful gross examination of excised tissue with the naked eye is followed by a more detailed histopathologic examination of tissue sections by light microscopy. Intraoperative examination may make use of frozen tissue sections, but in most instances, pathologists rely on the better preservation of structure afforded by permanent tissue sections stained with hematoxylin and eosin (H&E), and occasionally other dyes. Histochemistry, immunohistochemistry, and electron microscopy are helpful or necessary supplements for diagnosis in some solid tumors.

Surgical pathologists have evolved into organ–system specialists, especially with the increasing complexity of cancer diagnosis and treatment. They also collaborate closely with cytopathologists in diagnoses involving exfoliated cells or needle aspirates and with clinical pathologists, who make use of other techniques, such as culture for microorganisms, flow cytometry, and specialized laboratory tests of a biochemical, immunologic, or molecular nature. For most of these supplementary studies, the specimen must be specially processed while it is still fresh—ie, prior to tissue fixation. The surgical pathologist is responsible to coordinate these various activities and to synthesize the resulting information into a comprehensive diagnosis that is maximally informative to the clinician caring for the patient.

Methods for Obtaining Specimens

Tissues may be obtained in a number of ways. Each method has its appropriate place and uses, depending on the clinical circumstances. Sampling body fluids for exfoliated cells or scraping or brushing to obtain cells are rapid, efficient, and low-risk techniques. Those methods, and the related technique of fine-needle aspiration (FNA) biopsy, are discussed in greater detail later in this chapter.

For obvious reasons, those approaches do not always reveal the primary tumor site or the extent of disease. Cutting-needle biopsies, core-needle biopsies, and drill biopsies obtain tissue cores for histopathologic examination or for special studies that permit evaluation of architectural structure. Incisional biopsy (along with FNA) is often the method of choice for lesions that are inoperable or are too large for ready excision, or when excision could lead to functional or cosmetic impairment. Excisional biopsy with adequate margins is often favored because it provides generous amounts of tissue for diagnosis and may itself afford sufficient surgical therapy for some tumors—eg, small to medium-sized breast cancers.

Biopsy interpretation has many potential pitfalls. These include inadequate tissue sampling and artifacts induced by the procedure itself, such as thermal damage caused by an electrocautery or laser. Benign findings do *not* exclude the possibility that a tumor or other significant pathologic condition is present but was not included in the tissue submitted for examination because of the process of sampling. The clinician must be prepared to perform a second, often more extensive, procedure if the first does not yield sufficient diagnostic information.

Gross Handling of Specimens

The pathologist must regard a biopsy specimen as the definitive surgical specimen and properly triage each one, the excisional biopsy specimens in particular. To approach triage appropriately, the pathologist must be informed about the patient's clinical history, the differential diagnosis, relevant laboratory results, gross lesion examination that is usually done by the physician who obtains the specimen, gross examination of the specimen derived from the lesion, and frozen section findings, if any. Individually or together, these factors dictate whether special studies are required. Often, the tissue arrives in the pathology laboratory in formalin or another fixative. If a specimen has been fixed for preservation, some special studies are precluded (eg, microbiologic cultures) or will be suboptimal (certain types of immunohistochemistry, flow cytometry, and electron microscopy) although critical for diagnosis. To avoid the need for repeat biopsy, the surgeon should consult the pathologist in advance about initial tissue handling. Frequently, the goal of biopsy is to determine whether a lesion is benign or malignant, with the expectation of performing additional surgery if the lesion proves malignant. In this case, supplementary tests may properly be deferred to the subsequent, more definitive surgery, at which time larger amounts of tissue become available for analysis.

Specimens should be marked with clips, sutures, or ink to provide anatomic orientation for margins of excision, and the method of marking should be described in the pathology submission sheet. The gross specimen should also be described with regard to its appearance and characteristics, taking care to measure in three dimensions the size of the specimen and, if visible, the lesion itself and the distances between the lesion edges and the excision (resection) margins. Excision margins should be identified and marked with ink before any dissection, thus permitting accurate measurement of these distances in histopathologic section. Depending on the type of specimen and the clinical circumstances, margins can be evaluated by analysis of frozen sections. All lymph nodes associated with a cancer specimen need to be dissected out, described (including number submitted and location), and processed for histology.

Certain biopsy specimens require still more careful examination. Breast specimens with calcification also often require specimen radiography for comparison with preoperative mammogram. Ideally, therefore, a radiograph of the intact specimen should be obtained, then the margins should be inked, the specimen "breadloafed," and radiographs taken of each slice. Sections should then be coded, individually processed for histology, and correlated with the corresponding radiographs.[19,20]

Preparation of Microscopy Sections

Microscopy requires that tissues be cut with a microtome into thin sections that can be stained with dyes such as H&E, toluidine blue, and other stains for specific tissue components such as mucin, glycogen, cytoplasmic granules, collagen, bacteria, and fungi. The sectioning methods most commonly used are frozen sections and paraffin-embedded (permanent) sections.

Frozen Sections

These can be prepared rapidly (within minutes) during the course of surgery while the patient is under anesthesia. They are therefore of the greatest practical value when immediate information is required for an important clinical decision such as determining whether a lesion is a neoplasm and, if so, whether it is benign or malignant, to direct immediate surgical management. Frozen sections can provide information about the extent of regional tumor metastases that may govern decisions concerning a curative or palliative operation (eg, lymph node involvement in carcinoma of the pancreas). Following definitive cancer surgery, frozen sections allow the pathologist to determine whether the resection margins—eg, those of skin, gut, or pulmonary lesions—are adequate. If resection margins are inadequate, additional tissue can be removed immediately, without the need for a subsequent operation. Another common use of frozen sections is to determine, while the specimen is still fresh, the adequacy of the specimen and the appropriate additional work-up necessary for this particular tissue, especially in the era of personalized cancer care. For example, if the metastatic tumor found in a lymph node is recognized as a poorly differentiated carcinoma, special fixation for electron microscopy may be required for proper diagnosis. On the other hand, if the tumor is a lymphoma, an entirely different set of studies may be required, such as those for cell-surface antigen markers and gene rearrangement.

Permanent Sections

Most tumors, especially those arising in the soft tissues or breast, are best evaluated in permanent sections. In contrast to frozen sections, permanent sections are prepared from tissues that have been fixed, dehydrated, and embedded in paraffin wax as a supporting medium before sectioning. Although they require more time for preparation (generally 12–24 hours), permanent sections offer a number of important advantages over frozen sections. Permanent sections are generally thinner (typically 5 μm) and, because freezing artifacts are avoided, are of better overall quality, permitting greater certainty of interpretation. When consistent techniques are used, tissue characteristics are more consistent. Certain tissues, such as those containing fat or bone, cut poorly as frozen sections but are satisfactorily studied in well-fixed and well-processed permanent sections. As a general rule, if insufficient tissue is available for both frozen and permanent sections, only permanent sections should be prepared.

Microscopic Interpretation of Tissue Sections

In cases of suspected cancer, the first task of the surgical pathologist is to decide whether a neoplasm is present. Inflammation, repair, hypertrophy, and hyperplasia of tissues as well as choristomas (ectopic rests), and hamartomas (masses of mature cells that are appropriate to a given site but are arranged in a disorganized fashion as the result of aberrant differentiation) can masquerade as a neoplasm. The initial distinction is often easily made. For example, nasal polyps and skin tags are unlikely to be confused with true neoplasms. Sometimes, however, the task is less straightforward.

Not infrequently, tumors generate an extensive inflammatory response. It is not unusual, eg, in endoscopic biopsies of gastric carcinomas, to find only after a prolonged search rare individual cancer cells hidden in an extensive inflammatory cell infiltrate. Healing ulcerations of the gastrointestinal or cervical mucosa may sometimes closely resemble the carcinomas or premalignant lesions that arise in those tissues (eg, squamous intraepithelial lesions). Finally, atypical hyperplasia can be very difficult to distinguish from in situ carcinoma and, even when no evidence of tumor is found, may represent an important diagnostic finding. For example, patients whose breast biopsies show atypical hyperplasia have a fourfold to fivefold increased risk of developing breast cancer at a later time.[21]

Having decided, on the basis of criteria such as cellular abnormalities or invasion, that a neoplasm is present (see below), the pathologist's next task is to classify it. A number of classification schemes are possible, but the most important is based on the tumor's histogenetic or cytogenetic origin. The combination of histogenetic and cytogenetic classification is often supplemented by other useful descriptors such as those provided by the tumor's gross or microscopic appearance (eg, polypoid, papillomatous), by the degree of cellular differentiation (eg, well or poorly differentiated; Fig. 37-4), and, perhaps most important, by the expected biologic behavior (benign or malignant).

Nomenclature

Broadly speaking, tumors of epithelial cell origin are termed adenomas or papillomas when benign and carcinomas when malignant. Carcinomas account for approximately 80% of all malignant tumors. Their classification is often further qualified based on the type of epithelium present: eg, glandular (adenocarcinoma, Fig. 37-5), squamous cell carcinoma (Fig. 37-6), urothelial cell carcinoma. Addition of the suffix "-oma" to the cell of origin also describes benign tumors of mesenchymal origin (eg, lipomas, fibromas). Malignant tumors of mesenchymal origin are called sarcomas (eg, liposarcomas, fibrosarcomas).

Most tumors consist of a single type of neoplastic cell. However, a few tumors contain neoplastic cells of more than one type—for example, Wilms tumors. Even rarer are tumors that contain neoplastic cells deriving from more than a single germ layer—for example, teratomas (dermoid cysts). Certain tumors have long been identified with trivial names that do not follow any well-ordered classification scheme. Examples include seminomas (for carcinomas of testicular epithelial cell origin), and melanomas (Fig. 37-7). Other tumors, because of prolonged usage, continue to bear eponyms (eg, Hodgkin disease, Kaposi sarcoma).

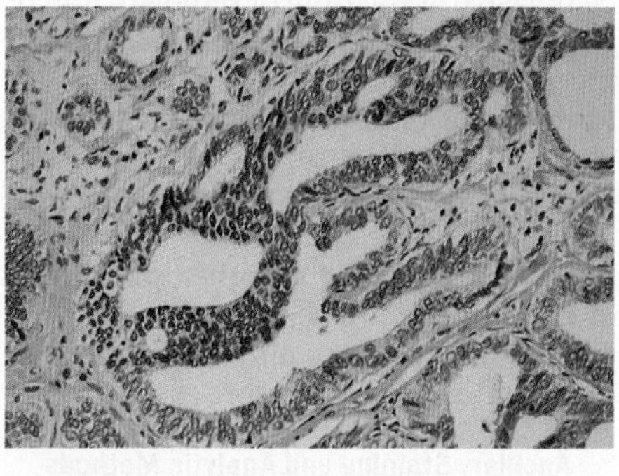

Figure 37-5 Adenocarcinoma of the breast. The tumor is arranged in the form of fairly well-differentiated glands separated by a fibrous connective tissue stroma. Moderate numbers of inflammatory cells, mostly lymphocytes, are present in the stroma. H & E; ×65 original magnification.

The pathologist must carry classification further still. Even within a single organ and within a single type of epithelium, several different tumor types may arise, each with its own special characteristics, prognosis, and response to therapy.

The distinction between tumors that are benign and those that are malignant is fundamental but sometimes complicated. In general, benign tumors share certain properties. The neoplastic cells that make up the tumor are usually well differentiated, closely resembling the corresponding cells of normal tissue. Benign tumors tend to expand uniformly in all directions unless impeded by surrounding structures. For example, compression by the bony skull often causes meningiomas to take on a flattened appearance. As expansile masses, benign tumors cause compression atrophy of surrounding normal tissues. As a result, a thin rim of fibrous connective tissue can form around the tumor. This enveloping connective tissue rim may serve as a "capsule" that renders benign tumors discrete, readily palpable, and easily movable. However, not all benign tumors have capsules. Some examples are leiomyomas of the uterus, hemangiomas, and adenomatous polyps in the lumen of the large intestine.

Malignant tumors, or cancers, are characterized primarily by the abnormality of their neoplastic cells. These cellular abnormalities are of two general types: those involving intercellular relationships and those affecting individual neoplastic cells. With regard to intercellular relationships, malignant tumors commonly exhibit increased cell numbers

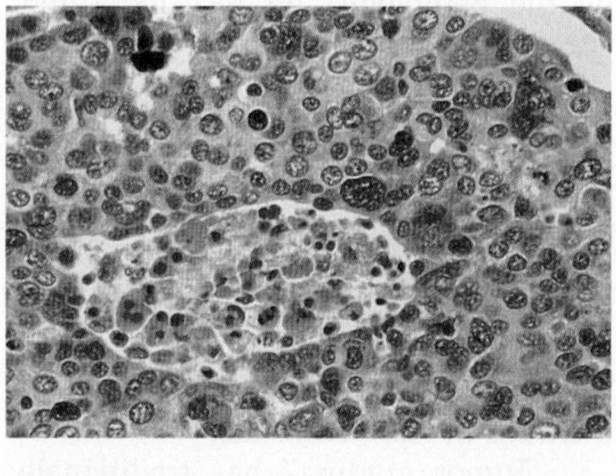

Figure 37-4 Undifferentiated carcinoma of lung. The tumor is composed of irregularly arranged pleomorphic tumor cells with large nuclei and prominent nucleoli. A central necrotic zone, typical of this type of tumor, is present. There is little stroma. H & E; ×100 original magnification.

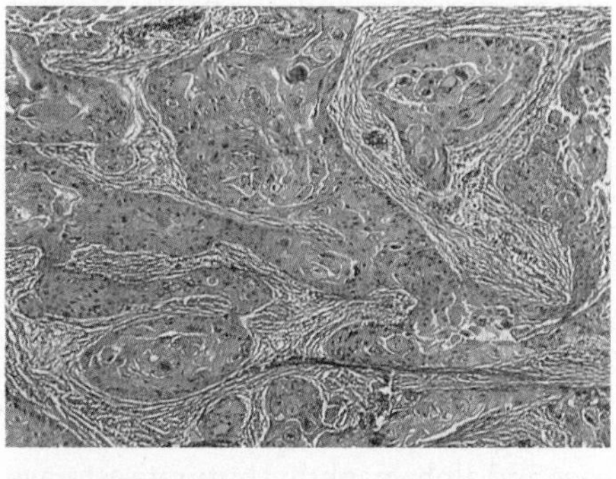

Figure 37-6 Squamous cell carcinoma of the skin of the face. Tumor consists of an island of well-differentiated squamous epithelium separated by fibrous connective-tissue stroma. Note that the epithelium forms "keratin pearls." H & E; ×60 original magnification.

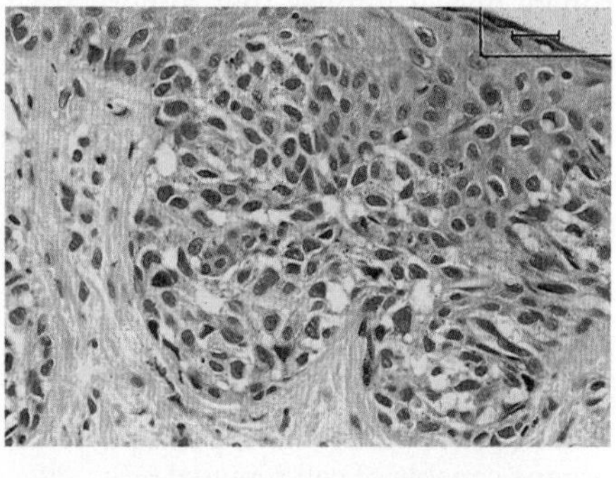

Figure 37-7 Malignant melanoma arising in skin. Tumor is composed of large, irregular cells with large nuclei, prominent nucleoli, and abundant, clear cytoplasm, peppered with dots and larger accumulations of melanin pigment. H & E; ×100 original magnification.

and altered orientation of both neoplastic cells and stroma that may be best described as "helter-skelter" or disorganized. For example, carcinomas of the skin may comprise squamous cells that differentiate and mature fairly normally; however, the cells are commonly organized into nests, in which the least differentiated cells are situated peripherally, and the most differentiated cells are positioned centrally, where they form keratin pearls (Fig. 37-6). Furthermore, these tumor cell nests are surrounded by disorganized stroma. Disturbed intercellular arrangements such as these are of great help to the pathologist interpreting a tissue section; much of tumor diagnosis depends on the pathologist's ability to recognize altered microscopic tissue patterns.

Abnormalities of individual neoplastic cells may also be helpful in diagnosis, particularly increased numbers of mitoses and cytologic features relating to the state of tumor cell differentiation. Cytologic features of malignancy include altered polarity, tumor cell enlargement, increased ratio of nuclear to cytoplasmic area (may approach 1:1 instead of the normal 1:4 or 1:6, although exceptions exist), pleomorphism (variation in size and shape) of tumor cells and their nuclei, clumping of nuclear chromatin and distribution of chromatin along the nuclear membrane, enlarged nucleoli, atypical or bizarre mitology (eg, tripolar), and tumor giant cells with one or more nuclei. However, some malignant tumors are well differentiated—so well differentiated, in fact, that their malignant cells cannot be distinguished from those of benign tumor or even from normal cells by any available diagnostic method. In such instances, the recognition of abnormal cellular relationships becomes especially important for correct diagnosis.

Anaplasia (from the Greek "to form backwards") is a term that describes the degree of tumor cell differentiation or, more correctly, the lack thereof. Although well entrenched, the term is an unfortunate one. It implies that tumors arise from mature, differentiated cells by a process of de-differentiation (ie, differentiation in reverse). Few pathologists hold that view today. Mammalian cells, once differentiated, generally lack the ability to reverse that process. Also, strong and growing evidence is providing support for the alternative explanation—namely, that tumors arise from populations of undifferentiated "stem" or "reserve" cells that are present in many, perhaps in all, organs capable of cell renewal.[22,23]

Stem Cells ■ Stem cells constitute a minority cell population that lacks differentiation markers, making them difficult to identify. However, positive recognition of stem cells has been achieved in several organs—eg, bone marrow, epidermis, liver, and gastrointestinal tract mucosa. Stem cells have a high capacity for cell proliferation but, unless stimulated, may divide infrequently. Stem cells alone have the capacity to regenerate normal tissues and, by extension, tumor cell populations. Oncologists have become increasingly aware that tumor stem cells may be the critically important target of cancer therapy. Destruction of differentiated tumor cells, without the simultaneous killing of tumor stem cells, may not lead to permanent tumor eradication.

Malignant tumors invariably lack a capsule. Instead they extend crab-like projections into the surrounding host tissues without respect for normal anatomic boundaries. This behavior is called "invasion." Malignant tumor cells often invade lymphatics and veins and are transported by lymph or blood flow to distant sites, opening the possibility of metastasis. Invasion is not a property confined to malignant tumor cells; placental trophoblasts, inflammatory cells, and many proliferations in fetal life also have the capacity to invade tissues. To be considered malignant, a tumor need not be invasive at the time of removal; it may have been "caught" before it had time to invade, or it may not yet have progressed to the point of acquiring the capacity to invade. Epithelial tumors that have not extended through the underlying basement membrane at the time of diagnosis but that exhibit all other properties of malignancy are described as "in situ carcinomas" and can almost certainly be cured by complete excision.

Ancillary Staining and Analytic Methods

Immunohistochemistry is the most commonly employed ancillary technique in surgical pathology (see "Role of the Immunohistochemist" later in this chapter), but special stains also aid in differential diagnosis and classification of tumors. Examples include the Van Gieson stain or the Masson trichrome method for distinguishing collagen and muscle, the Weigert stain for elastic tissue, silver stains for reticulin fibers, and special stains for mucins, amyloid, lipids, myelin, and glycogen—all substances whose identification may aid in the diagnosis of one type of tumor or another. In other instances, enzyme histochemistry may be essential for defining cell lineage, as in certain types of leukemia. Examples include chloroacetate esterase or endogenous peroxidase staining for cells of myelomonocytic lineage and alpha naphthyl butyrate esterase (called "nonspecific" esterase) staining for monocytes and macrophages.

Other techniques that may occasionally aid the surgical pathologist in tumor diagnosis are specimen radiography (for localizing and analyzing crystalline material such as calcium in breast biopsies) and morphometry.

Excision Margins ■ An important concern is the adequacy of tumor excision. Depending on the tissue, a decision about adequacy can be made from either frozen or permanent sections. If the tumor forms a discrete mass and the margins of the specimen are clearly recognizable, determination of excision margins is usually straightforward. Examples of tumors whose excision is likely to give clearly defined margins include those arising in the gastrointestinal tract, lung, and skin. The margins of tumors arising in soft tissues (eg, many sarcomas and breast carcinomas) and diffusely infiltrating tumors (eg, infiltrating lobular carcinoma of the breast, signet-ring-cell carcinoma tumors of the gastrointestinal tract, and nerve-invading tumors such as adenoid cystic carcinomas of the salivary glands and glioblastomas) may be much more difficult to define. In at least certain histologic patterns of breast carcinoma, factors such as the extent of intraductal growth must be considered when evaluating resection margins.[24] In patients treated with excision and radiotherapy for invasive breast cancer, the evaluation of excision margins in the context of an extensive intraductal component provides more prognostic information than does the evaluation of margins alone.[25]

Tumor Grading, Staging, and Prognosis

Pathologists are often called on to grade tumors or to participate in their staging to estimate tumor prognosis. Tumor staging (eg, the well-known tumor, nodes, metastasis [TNM] system) has proven to be of great value in estimating prognosis and indicating need for additional treatment. Staging tries to measure and to predict the extent of spread of a cancer within a patient. It uses parameters such as tumor size, lymph node involvement, and the presence of other metastases. Clearly, objective determinations made by the pathologist on resected tumor specimens have a critical impact on accurate tumor staging.

With rare exceptions, such as papillary carcinoma of the thyroid, the single most important risk factor in determining tumor prognosis is the presence of metastases to regional lymph nodes. Therefore, the pathologist must search diligently to find, examine, and prepare histologic sections from all lymph nodes included in resected tissue.

"Tumor grading" has traditionally referred to a pathologist's judgment as to a tumor's degree of differentiation and growth rate, often on a scale of I–III, where III represents the least differentiated, fastest dividing tumors (ie, the tumors presumed to have the worst prognosis).

Formal grading systems have improved in recent years with stricter standardization of criteria (Fig. 37-8).

Tumor grading does, however, have shortcomings. Each type of tumor requires a different scale, and scoring is subjective and poorly reproducible. Furthermore, tumors are typically heterogeneous; areas that vary significantly in differentiation and mitotic activity exist side by side, with the attendant risk of sampling error. Because prognosis is usually linked to the most malignant portions of a tumor, it follows that, for accurate diagnosis and grading, sufficient tissue and microscopic sections must be sampled to find the most malignant areas. Moreover, a regular (although not invariant) feature of malignant tumors is progression,[26] the property by which tumors become more and more malignant over time. Tumor progression is thought to result from genomic instability that leads to specific mutations of oncogenes or loss of tumor suppressor genes, from other genetic alterations such as gene amplification, and from epigenetic changes such as DNA hypermethylation that result in altered patterns of gene expression. Overt carcinogens, environmental promoters, and local factors such as hypoxia and nutrient deprivation may all contribute to those changes and therefore to tumor progression. Finally, the correlation between histologic appearance and biologic behavior is seldom perfect.

Pathologists are continuously on the lookout for more useful tumor-specific features that may be important independent predictors of tumor prognosis. For example, carcinomas of the prostate are usefully graded based on tissue architecture and neoplastic cell pattern in the

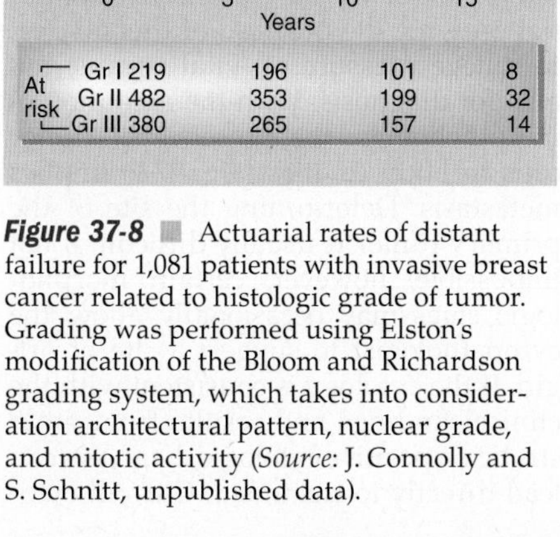

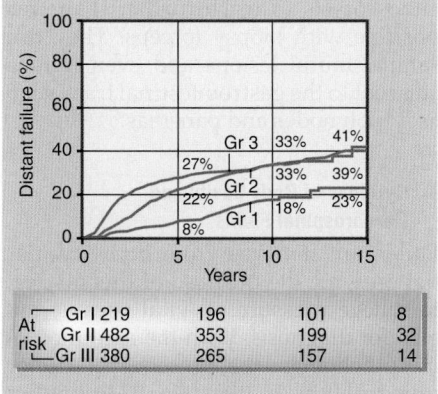

Figure 37-8 Actuarial rates of distant failure for 1,081 patients with invasive breast cancer related to histologic grade of tumor. Grading was performed using Elston's modification of the Bloom and Richardson grading system, which takes into consideration architectural pattern, nuclear grade, and mitotic activity (*Source*: J. Connolly and S. Schnitt, unpublished data).

Gleason classification.[27] A variety of criteria, including nuclear differentiation, degree of gland or tubule formation, and mitotic activity, have been usefully combined to grade breast carcinomas.[28–30]

Translation of tumor markers into clinical utilization has been problematical. The American Society of Clinical Oncology has convened a series of panels to prepare review literature and provide recommendations on the clinical use of markers based on levels of evidence.[31,32] For example, no tissue markers were recommended for routine use in gastrointestinal carcinomas despite decades of research and publications until the robust finding that mutation of the KRAS proto-oncogene abrogates response to antibodies directed against epidermal growth factor receptor (EGFR).[33] One of the most intensively studied and widely used measures of breast cancer evaluation is tumor expression of estrogen receptor (ER), progesterone receptor (PR), and HER2/neu. Those measures are, in fact, the only ones for which standardized quality control is currently available although after decades of research. The era of personalized cancer care is underway, and pathologists have an important role to predict prognosis and response to new and different therapeutic modalities.

Surgical Pathology Reports

Providing findings in understandable form to aid in patient management is the essential characteristic of surgical pathology reports. The results of analyses should be presented comprehensively, in terms that are understandable to both the pathologist and the clinicians caring for the patient. The report should provide enough information so that the clinicians can follow the thought processes of the pathologist, much as if they were viewing the case with the pathologist at a double-headed teaching microscope. The report should contain all the information to which the pathologist has access (ie, tumor size, grade, extent of spread, and nodal status) that is necessary to stage a patient with cancer. This information varies with tumor origin, type, and staging system employed. The report should include the results of all specialized tests performed, their interpretation, and the synthesis and coordination of all clinically useful information available to the pathologist that may be of aid in diagnosis and management.

A helpful method to standardize the reporting of malignancies has been the introduction of synoptic reporting. Both The Association of Directors of Anatomic Pathology and The College of American Pathologists Cancer Committee have produced synoptic reporting guidelines that are available on their Web sites. Use of these standardized reports in highly recommended.

Finally, reports should be issued in a timely manner. Failure to report results promptly may delay patient care (thus uselessly adding to the cost of medical care), lead to error and confusion, and at the very least prolong anxiety in patients who are often already distraught.

Role of the Cytopathologist

Cytology is used for both screening and diagnosis of lesions that may represent cancer or its precursors. Specific benefits include cost-effectiveness, rapid turnaround time, and diagnosis with minimal patient risk. Because cytology specimens usually consist of a very small quantity of cells or tissue fragments, optimal techniques for sample collection and slide preparation alike are crucial. Moreover, as in all areas of pathology, cytologic diagnosis should never be made "in a vacuum." Pertinent clinical data and clear communication between the cytopathologist and the clinician are essential to facilitate rapid, accurate, and definitive cytologic diagnoses.

Methods for Obtaining Specimens

The methods of obtaining cells for microscopy fall into two categories. In the first, a medium that contains naturally exfoliated cells (eg, urine, sputum, body cavity washings, and fluids) is obtained. In the second, cells of interest for examination are obtained using an instrument, such as a brush or a needle with a syringe in fine needle aspiration (FNA).

Preparation of Cytologic Specimens for Microscopy

The preparation of a cytologic specimen depends on the type of specimen. When cells are collected using an instrument, the cells can be either rinsed into a preservative solution or simply spread directly onto slides.[34–36] When the cells are collected in a medium, natural or artificial, the specimen needs to be processed to separate the medium from the cells. Possibilities include centrifugation, cytocentrifugation, filtering, or processing through a machine, such as a ThinPrep processor[37] or a PrepStain system.[38]

The optimal final product for every type of preparation is a slide holding a thin layer of evenly dispersed cells. Cells thinly spread on a slide dry out very easily; slides therefore need to be immediately fixed (using either 95% ethanol or a commercially available spray fixative) and then stained with Papanicolaou or H&E stain. Alternatively, slides allowed to air dry can be stained with a Romanowsky-type stain.

Microscopy Interpretation of Cytologic Specimens

In contrast to surgical pathologists, cytopathologists deal primarily with cells without regard to stroma. Although some architectural features are maintained in cytology specimens, many are lost in the process of specimen collection and preparation. Therefore, cytopathologists rely mainly on the cytologic features of malignancy and on residual structural features such as cohesion versus dyshesion to determine the benign or malignant nature of the lesion.

Cytopathologists usually report their result in one of four categories: "positive," "suspicious," "atypical," or "negative." A "positive" diagnosis indicates sufficient confidence in the malignant nature of the lesion that the pathologist is prepared to have the patient undergo definitive treatment such as surgical resection or chemotherapy based on the cytologic diagnosis alone.

Where doubt exists, the report should be less definitive and should fall into the "suspicious" category. Other diagnostic tests, such as a repeat cytology sample or a surgical biopsy, should be performed to determine with certainty the nature of the lesion before the patient undergoes definitive therapy. Occasionally, other evidence of malignancy, such as clinical and radiologic findings, is so strong that clinicians feel confident in implementing definitive therapy with a "suspicious" diagnosis. That must be a decision of the responsible clinician.

When cellular abnormalities whose clinical significance is not known are present, the report should be placed in the "atypical" category. Other diagnostic tests may be in order, depending on the clinical situation. Definitive therapy should never be initiated solely on the basis of atypia.

A "negative" cytology result means that no abnormal cells were found in the sample examined. All parties concerned must realize that a "negative" finding does not necessarily indicate absence of malignancy in the patient. False negative cytology results are often the result of sampling error. Laboratory error may produce both false negative and false positive results.

Exfoliative Cytology

Exfoliative cytology involves microscopic examination of cells exfoliated from the respiratory (sputum), urinary (urine), or female genital tracts. The use of the Papanicolaou (Pap) smear to screen for cervical cancer and its precursors in the general asymptomatic population has been instrumental in dramatically lowering the mortality rate from cervical cancer over the last four decades (see Chapter 98).

A problem inherent in all screening tests is the need to balance sensitivity and specificity. Lowering the threshold for a diagnosis of atypia means that fewer cases of neoplasia will be missed. However, the trade-off is that more patients without neoplastic disease will receive additional, expensive, and anxiety-provoking studies such as colposcopy to rule out the presence of cancer or its precursors. The importance of proper sample collection and preparation needs to be emphasized. Failure to fix samples immediately, to create a thin-enough smear, or to ensure the absence of significant amounts of blood may all result in specimens that are inadequate or suboptimal for diagnosis. Putting the sampled materials into a preservative medium and using a machine to make slides with a thin layer of cells can obviate most of the above pitfalls; however, the cost of preparation is significantly increased.[37,38]

Because human papillomavirus (HPV) was shown to be a necessary, although not sufficient, cause of cervical neoplasia,[39] testing for high-risk (oncogenic) types of HPV has now been added to the screening program for cervical neoplasia. Testing for high-risk HPV had initially been used to triage women with equivocal cytology results (ie, atypical squamous cells of undetermined significance [ASC-US]).[40] The US Food and Drug Administration has approved the use of the "high-risk" panel of Hybrid Capture 2 HPV DNA Test (HC2, which detects HPV types 16, 18, 31, 33, 35, 39, 45, 51, 52, 56, 58, 59, and 68) as an adjunct to cervical cytology screening in women aged 30 years or older.[41] In fact, for women in that age group, a strategy that uses HPV testing in combination with cytology for primary screening at 3-year intervals provides a greater reduction in cancer risk (91.9%) and is less costly (lifetime cost of $1647 US) than is annual conventional cytology (89.5% reduction, with lifetime cost of $2457 US).[42] Women who are negative both for cytology and for HPV can be screened every 3 years. Those whose cytology diagnosis is more serious than ASC-US, and those whose cytology diagnosis is ASC-US with positive HPV, should be referred promptly for colposcopy. Those who have negative cytology and positive HPV results should undergo both tests again at 6–12 months. Those whose cytology shows ASC-US, but negative HPV results, may repeat cytology at 12 months.

Cytologic examinations of sputum and urine are not currently used to screen the general population but are instead used to detect cancers in high-risk patients who either have had exposures that increase their risk of developing cancers or already have symptoms that may be caused by cancers in the lung or urinary bladder.[43,44] Similarly, patients with an increased risk of esophageal adenocarcinoma or squamous cell carcinoma can be surveyed by nonendoscopic sampling with balloon or encapsulated samplers.[45,46] A breast duct lavage technique has been proposed to detect cellular atypia for risk stratification in women at high risk for breast cancer.[47,48] For patients with symptoms or other clinical evidence of disease, more invasive procedures—such as bronchoscopy, cystoscopy, upper gastrointestinal endoscopy, colposcopy, and fine-needle aspirations or excisional biopsies—are called for if a diagnosis cannot be made on exfoliative cytology.

Endoscopic Cytology

In areas amenable to endoscopy, such as the bronchial tree and the gastrointestinal and urinary tracts, cytologic specimens obtained with brushing and washing techniques aimed at grossly identifiable lesions may serve a diagnostic function. Paired cytology and biopsy can improve the likelihood of diagnosing malignancy in a single procedure.[49,50] Because brush samples cover a wide area, they provide greater diagnostic sensitivity than biopsies, particularly in the case of early lesions that are not grossly obvious. However, endoscopic biopsies generally provide more information, particularly in determining tumor type and presence of invasion. Endoscopic FNA, either with the flexible needle used for injecting esophageal varices (sclerotherapy needle) or with a transbronchial aspiration needle, may make it possible to obtain samples from lesions lying deep to necrotic debris or to normal mucosa.[51] This technique is further enhanced by adding ultrasound guidance.[52] Endoscopic ultrasound-guided FNAs have enabled endoscopists to reach further than was possible with biopsy forceps. They can sample mural lesions and even lesions adjacent to the gastrointestinal tract, such as lymph nodes and pancreas.[53–55]

Cytology of Body Cavity and Cerebrospinal Fluids

Fluids are removed from body cavities not only for the purpose of therapy (eg, to relieve pressure on vital organs) but also for diagnosis. With the exception of mesotheliomas, the presence of tumor cells in body cavities (Fig. 37-9) implies metastasis. Determining the site of the primary tumor is usually difficult, if not impossible; however, certain morphologic clues may occasionally allow the cytopathologist to suggest a site of origin. If the cytology is consistent with the clinical findings and results from other studies, a positive cytologic diagnosis can lead directly to treatment. Current cyto-

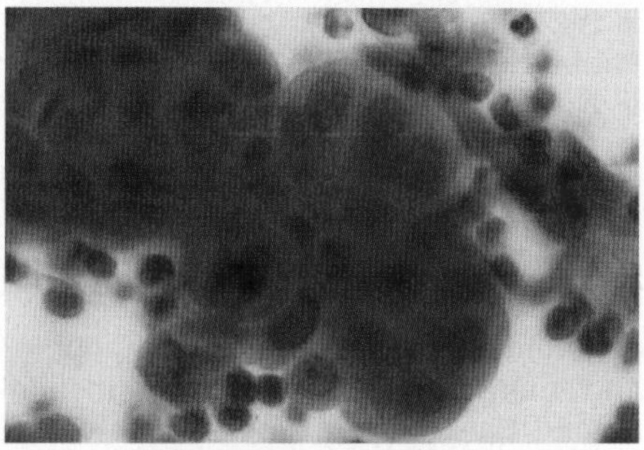

Figure 37-9 ■ Ovarian papillary serous adenocarcinoma in ascitic fluid. Cells are present in three-dimensional clusters with nuclear molding and irregular hyperchromatic nuclei. Papanicolaou stain; ×250 original magnification.

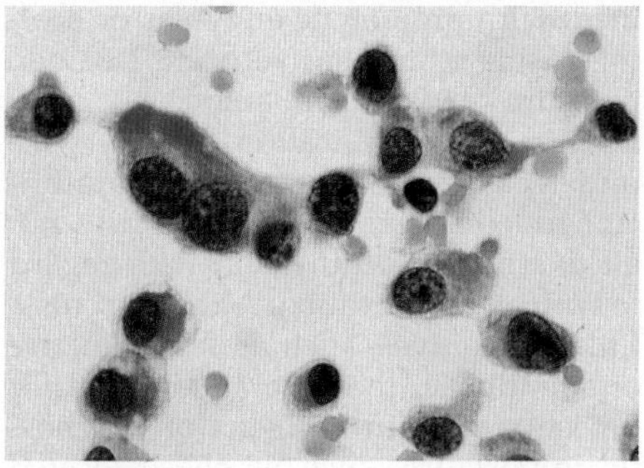

Figure 37-10 ■ Metastatic neuroendocrine tumor as seen in a fine-needle aspiration biopsy of liver. Note eccentric nuclei with "salt and pepper" chromatin and abundant granular cytoplasm. Immunocytochemical stains confirmed the diagnosis. Papanicolaou stain; ×250 original magnification.

logic specimens should always be compared to previous cytologic or histologic specimens, if available. Reactive mesothelial cells share certain characteristics with carcinoma cells, and the parallels should be considered in the differential diagnosis. Panels of immunocytochemical stains may prove useful (see "Role of the Immunohistochemist"). Sometimes (eg, in the case of mesotheliomas) tumor growth may be confined to the surfaces lining body cavities, without significant exfoliation of malignant cells. Under those circumstances, a biopsy of the cavity wall is required to establish the diagnosis. An alternative approach for future investigation may be to analyze tumor cell–free effusions for secreted products of malignant cells or other tumor-cell markers.

Aspiration Cytology

The earliest work on aspiration cytology was reported from Memorial Hospital in New York in the 1930s.[56] Subsequently, the impetus for this technique shifted to Europe and it was not "rediscovered" in the United States until the 1970s.[57] Cytopathologists, surgeons, and other clinicians can successfully perform an aspiration of a palpable lesion. In the case of nonpalpable lesions, a radiologist or clinician performs the aspiration under computed tomography, ultrasound, or fluoroscopic guidance. Deep aspiration procedures of this kind are expensive, time-consuming, and invasive. For these reasons, it is desirable that a cytotechnologist or cytopathologist attends the procedure to ensure specimen adequacy and optimal slide preparation. A further advantage of having experienced personnel on hand is effective triage of material for special studies such as immunocytochemistry (Fig. 37-10), electron microscopy, flow cytometry, and tissue culture. Definitive aspiration cytology diagnoses, rendered by an experienced cytopathologist, can provide the basis for definitive therapy. However, such diagnoses need to be viewed in the context of all other laboratory studies and clinical findings. Specific problems and pitfalls are associated with aspirations of various sites.

Thyroid ■ FNA biopsy is the first test used in most patients with a solitary thyroid nodule. The technique is safe and inexpensive and leads to a better selection of patients for surgery than does any other test.[58] FNA permits the accurate diagnosis of papillary, medullary, and anaplastic carcinomas; it is less useful in the diagnosis of follicular nodules. Certain cytologic features help to distinguish between the various types of follicular lesions,[59] but a definitive diagnosis is not possible by FNA. In that situation, FNA serves only to distinguish patients needing immediate surgery for thyroid disease from those who may be safely followed with or without hormonal suppression. However, even that limited information can eliminate many unnecessary surgeries.[60]

Breast ■ In the hands of an experienced cytopathologist, the diagnostic specificity of breast aspiration is very high, and a positive diagnosis may safely lead to mastectomy or other definitive treatment. Of course, atypical and suspicious cases require further workup. FNA of the breast may also be performed on nonpalpable lesions under the guidance of conventional or stereotactic mammography or ultrasonography.

Compared to core biopsy, breast cytology has certain inherent problems. These include an inability to distinguish infiltrating from in situ carcinoma and difficulty in rendering a specific benign diagnosis.[61,62] However, the needles used in FNA cost much less than core needles do, and they are more readily tolerated by patients. Most labs continue to show an increase in FNA of the breast, especially for palpable lesions, but that increase is much less than the increase in core biopsies of the breast.[63] Furthermore, there seems to be a tendency for clinicians to use FNA for lesions that are clinically benign and core biopsies for lesions that are clinically worrisome.[64]

Lungs ■ Aspiration cytology of the lungs may lead to diagnosis of both primary and metastatic tumors and of nonneoplastic lesions such as tuberculosis and fungal infections.[65] As in the case of histologic lung-tissue sections, distinguishing primary from metastatic carcinoma is not always possible.

Abdomen ■ Aspiration cytology is particularly useful in pretreatment diagnosis of malignancies in the liver, pancreas, kidney, and retroperitoneum. A diagnosis of metastatic tumor or lymphoma spares the patient major surgery and provides a basis for definitive therapy. Poorly differentiated tumors may be difficult to type, but the use of adjunct techniques is often helpful in establishing a definitive diagnosis.

Lymph Nodes ■ Some pathologists question the role of aspiration cytology in the diagnosis of lymph node lesions.[66] FNA can provide useful information to obviate the need for surgery in cases of suspected metastatic carcinoma or melanoma from a known primary to palpable lymph nodes. FNA can also help to identify infections. Lymph node aspirates may provide a diagnosis and classification of lymphoproliferative disorders, especially when used in conjunction with flow cytometry or another immunophenotyping technique.[67,68] If, on FNA, a lymphoproliferative lesion is suspected without a definitive diagnosis, the patient can proceed to have an excisional biopsy for diagnosis.

Application of Ancillary Studies on Cytologic Materials

Nearly all ancillary studies, such as those involving immunocytochemistry, electron microscopy, flow cytometry, and molecular biology, can be applied to cytologic materials (see "Role of the Immunohistochemist" for details).

Few of the diagnostic tests introduced into medicine have actually lowered the cost of high-quality patient care. Cytopathology is one of them. It offers the advantages of low morbidity, rapid turnaround time, and outstanding cost-effectiveness. The problems in cytology should not detract from its usefulness. All procedures have limitations, and the oncologist needs to be informed about the benefits and the pitfalls of this technique.

Role of Immunohistochemistry

Immunohistochemistry has become an important adjunct in the evaluation of human neoplasms. A detailed discussion of the technical aspects of immunohistochemistry is beyond the scope of this chapter, but the interested reader can consult several review articles and monographs.[69] The commercial availability of a broad range of reagents, including prediluted reagents in kit form, has made it possible for high-quality immunohistochemistry to be performed in most pathology laboratories. The most commonly employed immunohistochemical techniques are those in which enzymes, such as horseradish peroxidase or alkaline phosphatase, are used in conjunction with specific antibodies to provide color reactions at sites of antigen–antibody interactions. Variations of the avidin–biotin complex (ABC) technique are the most widely used in current practice.

The ABC procedure generally requires four sequential steps: an unlabeled primary antibody directed against the antigen of interest, a biotin-labeled anti-immunoglobulin secondary antibody, preformed avidin–biotin peroxidase complexes, and finally a chromogenic substrate (typically diaminobenzidine), which is enzymatically converted by the peroxidase moiety to a colored signal. One variation of the ABC method employs streptavidin, which has greater sensitivity than avidin and exhibits less nonspecific binding.

It should be noted that the sensitivity of any immunohistochemical procedure is, in large part, related to the tissue characteristics, reagents, and detailed procedures employed. As a consequence, comparing the results of immunohistochemical studies from different institutions that employ different reagents and methods is difficult, and this explains the paucity of validated immunohistochemical markers for prognosis and response to therapy. Almost any type of pathology specimen may be suitable for immunohistochemical staining, including fresh-frozen tissue, fixed tissue, and cytologic preparations. Unfortunately, however, not all antigens are equally well preserved after these various treatments, and the approach taken for immunohistochemical staining must depend on the antigen or antigens of interest. For example, although many cytoplasmic antigens are detectable in fixed, paraffin-embedded tissue, others, such as many cell surface–associated antigens, are destroyed or masked by common fixatives. They may be demonstrable only in fresh-frozen tissue or in cytologic preparations. Antigen retrieval methods, such as pretreatment with proteolytic enzymes or heating (using a microwave oven, steamer, pressure cooker, or autoclave), may permit the identification of otherwise undetectable antigens in fixed, paraffin-embedded tissue sections.[70] Finally, not all fixatives are equivalent with regard to antigen preservation. Although cross-linking fixatives, such as formalin, are often suitable, they are suboptimal for detecting certain antigens of diagnostic importance, such as those located on intermediate filaments that are best demonstrated in fresh-frozen or alcohol-fixed tissue.[71] Standardization of results is difficult even with standardization of methodologies, and quantitation is therefore problematical.

Applications

Despite its limitations, immunohistochemistry has widespread applicability in the evaluation of human tumors. Some of the more common applications are discussed in the following paragraphs.

Categorizing "Undifferentiated" Malignant Tumors

Not infrequently, a pathologist examining routine H&E-stained premanent sections recognizes the presence of a malignant tumor but is unable to characterize the tumor further because histologically undifferentiated tumors often lack visually recognizable characteristics that would permit more accurate classification. Yet further classification is often important in making clinical decisions about appropriate therapy and prognosis. Immunohistochemistry may be helpful in such situations (Fig. 37-11).

However, before performing immunohistochemistry, the pathologist must first develop a differential diagnosis, and that diagnosis will depend on the tumor's histologic appearance, anatomic location, radiologic characteristics, and the patient's clinical history. Only then is the pathologist in a position to select antibodies that will permit a more definitive diagnosis.

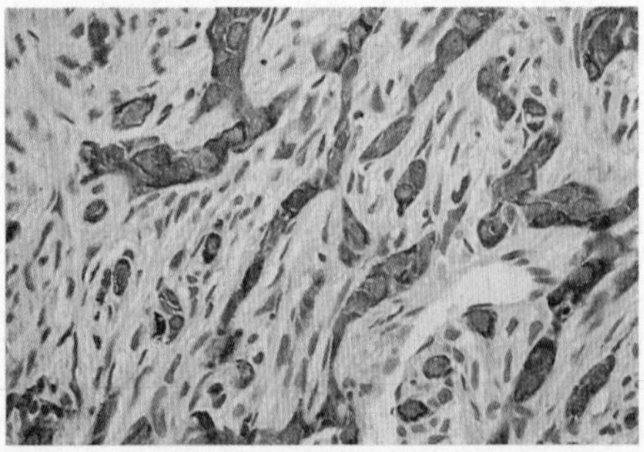

Figure 37-11 Immunoperoxidase staining of a monoclonal antibody specific for keratin in a poorly differentiated squamous cell carcinoma of skin. The "spindle cell" form of the tumor mimics tumors of connective-tissue origin, and its true nature can often be determined only by immunohistochemistry. Immunoperoxidase stain; ×100 original magnification.

The common problem of an undifferentiated tumor comprising large cells with an epithelioid appearance serves as an example. The differential diagnosis in such cases typically includes undifferentiated carcinoma, lymphoma, and malignant melanoma. Distinction among these tumor types can often be made using a panel of antibodies as illustrated in Table 37-1. Unfortunately, this table represents an ideal result that is not always achieved in practice. Some carcinomas show staining for vimentin or S100 protein, some melanomas show immunoreactivity for keratin, and some neoplasms other than melanomas express HMB-45.[72–74] Such results emphasize the need to use a panel of antibodies, rather than a single antibody, in evaluating tumors.

Determining Site of Origin of Metastatic Tumors

On routine microscopy examination, tumors may be classifiable with regard to general histologic type (eg, adenocarcinoma, squamous cell carcinoma). However, the site of origin may not be reliably determined using histologic cues alone. It would be highly desirable to have available antibodies specific for tumors arising in various sites. At present, however, very few organ- or tissue-specific antigens have been identified, thus limiting the ability of immunohistochemistry to resolve such problems in every instance.

Table 37-2 lists a number of useful antigens. It should be noted that antigens specific for some of the more common tumors—such as carcinomas of the colon, endometrium, and pancreas—are not currently available. Furthermore, some of the antigens listed in Table 37-3 have now been demonstrated in neoplasms other than those for which they were initially thought to be "specific." For example, the melanoma-associated antigen detected by one widely used antibody (HMB-45) has been found in some nonmelanocytic tumors.[72] A more recent approach for the subclassification of metastatic carcinomas exploits differences in the cytokeratin profiles of tumors from different primary sites.[75]

Subclassifying Tumors in Various Organ Systems

In some organs and tissue compartments, overlapping features may make it difficult to subclassify certain tumors solely on histologic grounds. Some of the distinctions are, at present, only of academic interest; eg, determining whether a high-grade sarcoma shows neural, myogenous, or fibrous differentiation. Other distinctions have therapeutic and prognostic significance.

Table 37-1 Idealized Immunohistochemical Evaluation of the "Undifferentiated" Malignant Tumor[a]

Antibody to	Tumor Type: Carcinoma	Lymphoma	Melanoma
Keratin	+	–	–
Epithelial membrane antigen	+	–	–
Vimentin	–	+ or –	+
Leukocyte common antigen	–	+	–
S100 protein	–	–	+
HMB-45	–	–	+

[a]In which the differential diagnosis includes carcinoma, lymphoma, and melanoma (see text).

Table 37-2 Antigens With Highly Restricted Specificity

Antigen	Tumor Specificity
Factor VIII–related antigen	Vascular tumors
Gross cystic disease fluid protein immunoglobin	Breast carcinomas; cutaneous tumors with protein apocrine differentiation
HMB-45	Melanoma, renal angiomyolipoma
Muscle-specific actin	Smooth muscle and skeletal muscle tumors
Myoglobin	Skeletal muscle tumors
Prostate-specific antigen	Prostatic carcinomas
Thyroglobulin	Thyroid follicular cell tumors
Ki+/CD117	Gastrointestinal stromal tumors

Table 37-3 Immunohistochemical Distinction Between Metastatic Adenocarcinoma and Malignant Mesothelioma Involving the Pleura or Peritoneum

	Adenocarcinoma	Mesothelioma
Keratin	+	+
Vimentin	+ or –	+ or –
Carcinoembryonic antigen	+ or –	–
Leu-M1	+ or –	–
B72.3	+ or –	–
Ber-EP4	+ or –	–
Calretinin	–	+

For example, in some cases, distinguishing with certainty an anaplastic seminoma from an embryonal carcinoma of the testis may be difficult or impossible by routine microscopy examination. Such a distinction has both therapeutic and prognostic implications. However, immunostaining for the intermediate filament keratin is often useful in such a case, because seminomas are typically keratin-negative, and embryonal carcinomas are usually keratin-positive.[76,77] Similar situations are encountered in other organ systems and tissue compartments.

Distinguishing Between Carcinomas and Malignant Mesotheliomas ■ A common problem encountered by the surgical pathologist is making the distinction between metastatic adenocarcinoma and malignant mesothelioma involving the pleura or peritoneum.[78,79] Immunohistochemical staining using a panel of antibodies is often useful in making this distinction (Table 37-3).

Categorizing Leukemias and Lymphomas ■ One of the most common uses for immunohistochemistry is the correct diagnosis and classification of leukemias and lymphomas. See Chapters 110–115 for additional details. In brief, immunohistochemistry is a useful adjunct to morphology and histochemistry in making the distinction between acute leukemias of the lymphoid and myeloid types and in distinguishing hairy-cell leukemia from other types of leukemic infiltrates in the bone marrow and at other sites. In addition, the technique is useful for subclassifying non-Hodgkin's lymphomas and Hodgkin's disease and in distinguishing the two conditions in problematic cases.

Detecting Antigens of Potential Prognostic or Therapeutic Significance ■ Immunohistochemistry can be used to detect a variety of antigens of possible prognostic and therapeutic importance, including estrogen and progesterone receptors in breast cancers, protein products of oncogenes (such as HER2/neu in breast cancers), antigens associated with tumor cell proliferation such as Ki-67 and the P-glycoprotein product of the multiple drug resistance (*MDR*) gene.

Ki-67 is of particular interest.[80,81] It is a nuclear antigen present in all proliferating cells; ie, it is present in the G1, S, G2, and M phases of the cell cycle but absent in G0 cells. Therefore, by staining for Ki-67, it is possible to measure the tumor growth fraction directly, simply, and in a manner more readily applicable to clinical specimens than are the ^{3}H–thymidine radiolabeling methods. Ki67 staining also yields results that are more reproducible than those obtained by counting mitotic figures.

Recognizing Invasive Carcinoma Using Myoepithelial Markers ■ The distinction between invasive adenocarcinoma of the prostate and its histologic mimics can be extremely difficult in core biopsies, the test of choice for the diagnosis of prostatic adenocarcinoma. Accurate diagnosis of invasive carcinoma in these small biopsies is extremely important because of the profound clinical and therapeutic consequences. The observation that benign lesions arising from glandular structures such as the prostate are invested with a layer of nonneoplastic myoepithelial cells has been exploited since the discovery of antibodies that are relatively specific for myoepithelial differentiation (eg, p63, calponin, and cytokeratin 903). The presence of myoepithelial cells surrounding nests of cells, as detected by immunohistochemistry, effectively excludes a diagnosis of invasive carcinoma; lack of such an investment strongly suggests invasive carcinoma (Fig. 37-12). These immunohistochemical markers of myoepithelial differentiation are also used extensively in the diagnosis of mammary carcinoma, in which markers such as p63 are useful for distinguishing in situ mammary carcinoma from the invasive form.

Limitations

An appreciation of the limitations of immunohistochemistry in tumor diagnosis is as important as an understanding of

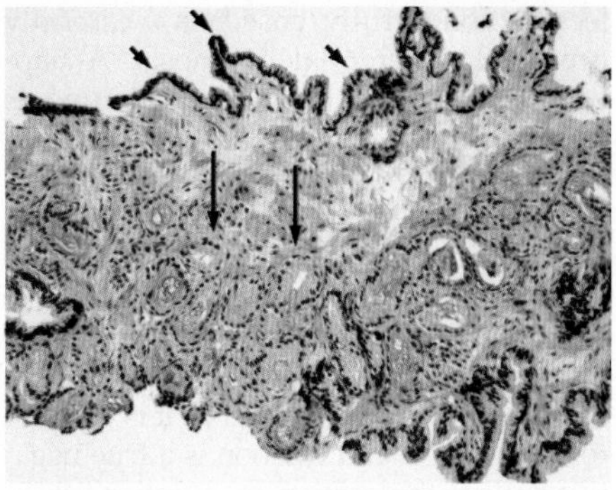

Figure 37-12 Immunoperoxidase staining for cytokeratin 903, a marker specific for prostatic myoepithelial cells. The absence of a rim of myoepithelial cells (*long arrows*) in the center of the photomicrograph confirms the presence of invasive adenocarcinoma. Note the surrounding benign glands (*short arrows*) that show expression of cytokeratin 903, which denotes the presence of myoepithelial cells, and, thus, the benign nature of these glands. Hematoxylin counterstain. Original magnification, 200×. *Source*: Courtesy of Dr. Elizabeth Genega.

its many useful applications. Potential limitations in the immunohistochemical evaluation of solid tumors can be broadly characterized as technical and interpretive.

Technical Limitations ■ Because demonstration of various types of antigens by immunostaining requires appropriate tissue preparation, advance planning for immunohistochemistry is essential so that the specimen may be handled appropriately. For example, if, on clinical grounds or at intraoperative examination (ie, frozen section or tissue imprint), an excised lymph node shows features suspicious for a lymphoma, a portion of the specimen may be snap-frozen to permit reliable demonstration of lymphocyte surface markers because some of those markers are not well demonstrated in fixed, paraffin-embedded tissue. In cases of suspected carcinoma in which demonstration of intermediate filament proteins is likely to be important, fixation of a portion of the tumor in an alcohol-based fixative may be advisable. As in any laboratory procedure, the use of appropriate positive and negative controls is mandatory in immunohistochemistry. Controls serve as a check on the technical adequacy of the procedure. If the appropriate controls are omitted or are suboptimal, the results of immunostaining must be viewed with caution.

Interpretive Limitations ■ Correct interpretation of immunohistochemical stains performed on tumor specimens depends not only on the technical adequacy of the procedure but also on interpretive factors. In most cases, a panel of antibodies is more useful than a single antibody. The antibodies that make up the panel must be selected thoughtfully, based on a carefully prepared differential diagnosis. A haphazard approach to immunostaining is strongly discouraged because it will only serve to compound diagnostic confusion.

Accurate interpretation of staining also requires familiarity with the sensitivity and specificity of the antibodies in question. Negative reactions are more difficult to interpret than are positive reactions. Even with the use of other controls, it is difficult to be certain that a reaction is a true negative unless the section in question stains positively for a complementary antigen. For example, in the analysis of an undifferentiated malignant tumor in which the differential diagnosis includes lymphoma and carcinoma, a negative reaction for keratin (the intermediate filament characteristic of many carcinomas) does not by itself rule out the possibility of carcinoma. However, if a negative keratin stain is accompanied by positive staining for the leukocyte common antigen (a marker present in most lymphomas), the likelihood of lymphoma is greatly enhanced. Some antibodies are of great diagnostic value in terms of both sensitivity and specificity—eg, the antibodies to prostate-specific antigen. Others are of limited diagnostic value even when used as part of a panel—eg, antibodies to the intermediate filament vimentin.

Pathologists who use immunohistochemistry must be experienced and aware of the limitations of the methodology, which is evolving at a rapid pace. An antigenic profile suitable today for diagnosing a particular type of tumor may tomorrow be shown to be suboptimal or less specific than was originally thought. Immunohistochemistry is a valuable tool for aiding in the diagnosis of difficult-to-identify tumors. However, it is only an adjunct to diagnosis, and the results must be interpreted in the context of other findings, particularly routine histologic sections and the clinical setting. Gene expression profiling of massage RNAs and noncoding RNA profiling of micro RNAs are under investigation.

Role of Electron Microscopy

Although it makes use of radically different technology, electron microscopy (EM) seeks the same type of information as that gleaned from immunohistochemistry—ie, detection of differentiated organelles ("markers" in the case of immunohistochemistry) that permit more accurate tumor identification and classification. EM is not useful in determining whether individual cells are malignant or benign. However, it is a powerful tool for recognizing subcellular structures not detectable under light microscopy. The presence of particular structures under EM permits confident identification of cells—eg, whether they are of epithelial or melanocyte origin.

Advances in immunohistochemistry have greatly reduced the need for EM in tumor diagnosis, although the method is useful in some cases.[82–84]

Technical Considerations

Appropriate tissue handling, fixation, and processing are of even greater importance in EM than in immunohistochemistry.[169] Advance planning and consultation between the clinician, the surgical pathologist, and the electron microscopist are therefore important. In many cases, having a pathologist or a knowledgeable technician in the operating room or at the bedside at the time of biopsy is advantageous. Tissue can then be fixed immediately and trimmed appropriately.

Tissue must be cut into small pieces because chemical fixatives penetrate slowly (taking minutes to hours), and the electron microscope glaringly exposes artifacts in poorly fixed tissues that are not detectable at the lower resolution afforded by light microscopy. In at least one dimension, the tissue must be no thicker than 1 mm. To achieve that small size, further trimming may be necessary after a brief preliminary fixation. Mixtures of glutaraldehyde and paraformaldehyde provide optimal fixation.[169] Vials of fixative can be frozen beforehand and thawed immediately before use, thereby avoiding the time-consuming need to prepare fresh fixative for each case. Tissues fixed in formalin or in other "routine" fixatives designed for light microscopy give inadequate tissue preservation for electron microscopy. Once tissues are fixed inappropriately, they generally cannot be recovered for adequate EM; and repeat biopsy becomes the best option. Peripheral blood, bone marrow, and cell-containing fluids (eg, pleural effusions and spinal or synovial fluid) are handled somewhat differently from samples of solid tissue.[84]

Applications

The great strength of EM lies in its exquisite resolution, which permits recognition of intracellular structures, organelles, or products that are undetectable under light microscopy.

EM is often helpful in the diagnosis of "undifferentiated" malignant tumors and in determining the origin of metastatic tumors of unknown primary site (Figs. 37-13 and 37-14). The recognition of cytoplasmic premelanosomes within tumor cells permits amelanotic malignant melanomas to be distinguished from the undifferentiated carcinomas and lymphomas with which they can be confused. Other ultrastructural features whose recognition may permit definitive diagnosis are the cytoplasmic granules characteristic of carcinoid tumors, the norepinephrine- and epinephrine-containing granules found in pheochromocytomas, the "terminal webs" characteristic of primary gastrointestinal carcinomas of absorptive epithelial cell type,[85] the lamellar (surfactant) bodies found only in type II pneumocytes (and therefore diagnostic of alveolar cell carcinomas of the lung),[86] the tonofilaments and desmosomes found in mesothelial cells and squamous cells, and the cytoplasmic glycogen aggregates and calligraphic nucleoli typical of germinomas. The presence of intercellular junctions permits the distinction of carcinomas from lymphomas, even if the carcinoma's primary site cannot be determined.

EM is also helpful in subclassifying tumors, an exercise that may have important therapeutic implications. The use of ultrastructural cytochemistry for endogenous peroxidase may allow the im-

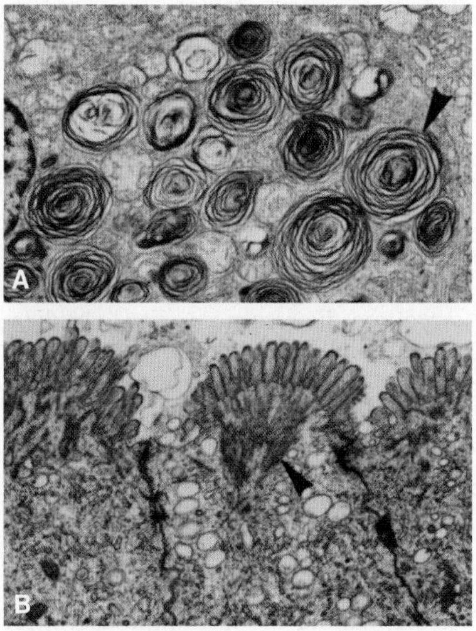

Figure 37-13 ■ **(A)** Electron micrograph from a lung mass shows typical surfactant-containing lamellar bodies ("surfactant bodies" [*arrowhead*]) that fill the cytoplasm of a tumor cell, allowing the specific diagnosis of primary alveolar cell carcinoma of the lung to be made. ×12,500 original magnification. **(B)** Electron micrograph from a lung mass shows apical cytoplasm of three tumor cells at high magnification. Note the short, blunt, surface microvilli and the dense terminal web (*arrowhead*) of cytoskeletal filaments that traverse the apical cytoplasm to enter individual microvilli. The tumor cells are joined by epithelial junctions and contain numerous apical cytoplasmic vesicles. The identification of the differentiated organelle, the terminal web, allows the specific diagnosis of metastatic adenocarcinoma of gut absorptive epithelial cell origin to be made. ×19,000 original magnification.

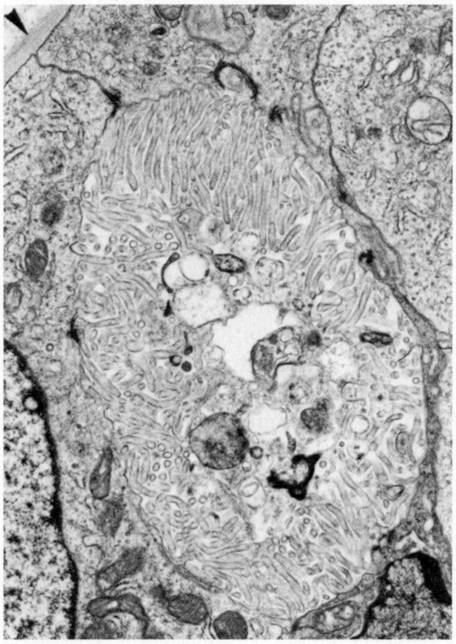

Figure 37-14 ■ High-magnification electron micrograph of pleural tumor shows three typical features of mesothelial cells: (1) numerous elongated, thick surface microvilli that (2) do not display evidence of terminal web differentiation, and (3) desmosomes that connect individual cells surrounding the extracellular acinar space and basal lamina (*arrowhead*). Another feature diagnostic of mesothelial cells—dense bundles of tonofilaments—is not seen in this high-magnification image. In concert, these four ultrastructural findings allow an ultrastructural diagnosis of mesothelioma to be made in the presence of light microscopy evidence of a malignant tumor proliferation of the pleura. ×22,000 original magnification.

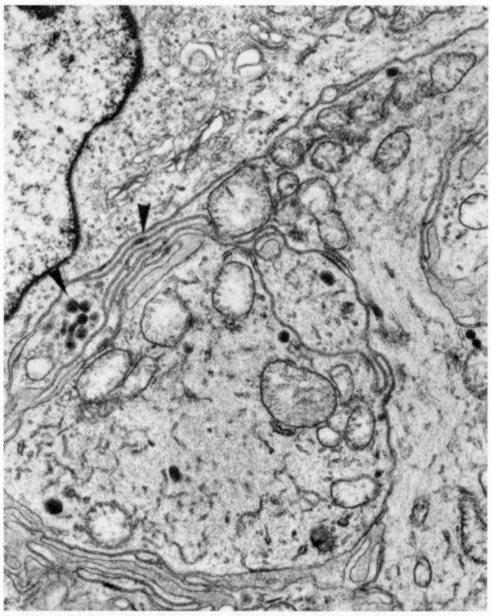

Figure 37-15 ■ This high-magnification electron micrograph of a gastric tumor shows tumor cells diagnostic for gastrointestinal autonomic nerve tumor/gastrointestinal stromal tumor (GIST). The elongated tumor cells are neurites, which contain numerous mitochondria and neurofilaments. Small numbers of dense core granules are present in larger cell processes adjacent to tumor plasma membranes and in Golgi areas (not shown). The number of dense core granules increases in smaller axons with synaptic connections to adjacent neurites (*arrowheads*). Basal lamina is absent from these cells, thus ruling out an origin from Schwann cells. ×19,000 original magnification.

portant distinction of acute myeloblastic leukemia from acute lymphoblastic leukemia. Histiocytosis X may be diagnosed by identification of Birbeck bodies characteristic of Langerhans cells. EM may also permit accurate diagnosis of lysosomal storage diseases and of bacterial, fungal, and viral infections.

Finally, EM is important in identifying the histogenesis of newly recognized neoplasms. One example (Fig. 37-15) was the recognition that certain spindle cell tumors of the gastrointestinal tract, previously thought to be of smooth muscle origin, in fact differentiate toward autonomic neurons (gastrointestinal tract autonomic nerve tumor/gastrointestinal stromal tumor (GIST)).[85]

Limitations

As in immunohistochemistry, the limitations of EM are both technical and interpretive. Technical limitations such as improper tissue handling and delayed or inappropriate fixation or processing have already been discussed. Another limitation is sampling, which is attributable to the very small size of the specimen that can be studied on an EM grid. Expense is also a limitation. Whereas the availability of commercial reagents, defined protocols, and relatively simple interpretation have permitted immunohistochemistry to be established in almost any hospital pathology laboratory, the same cannot be said for diagnostic EM. The costly electron microscope, the elaborate support equipment, the need for experienced technical and professional personnel, and the emergence of high-quality immunohistochemistry, in situ hybridization, and molecular assays have diminished the application of this methodology. Of particular importance is the need for a pathologist who is well trained in both surgical pathology and EM. Asking a basic science-oriented electron microscopist or an EM technician to take a few pictures of a tumor specimen is a prescription for error or futility.

Role of the Clinical Pathologist

The specific role of the clinical pathologist in the management of cancer patients is obvious and familiar to the oncologist and requires only brief mention here. Clinical pathologists are interested in measurements of body fluids that lead to the early detection and monitoring of cancer. The field of tumor antigens and tumor markers has generated a great deal of interest, and some of those antigens and markers are discussed elsewhere in this volume. At least in theory, tumor-specific antigens circulating in the plasma could be useful in tumor diagnosis and prognosis, assessment of tumor burden, prediction of recurrence, and guidance for treatment. These are discussed further in Chapter 26.

Properties of an ideal tumor marker include great sensitivity, specificity, and accuracy in reflecting total tumor burden. A tumor marker should also be prognostic of outcome and predictive of tumor recurrence. Unfortunately, none of the tumor markers discovered to date fulfills all of those criteria. In fact, none is uniquely produced by tumor cells. Normal cells of one sort or another make all of the tumor markers thus far recognized, and plasma or serum levels in tumor patients differ only quantitatively, not qualitatively, from those in normal control subjects or in patients with other diseases. A new concept has emerged—namely, that cancer may be diagnosed by testing a panel of serum proteins using proteomic methods, even when these proteins have not been identified.[87,88] Despite initial enthusiasm, proteomics are not as yet ready for routine use.

Role of the Hematopathologist

The laboratory evaluation of hematopoietic and lymphoid malignancies in clinical practice is far ahead of that for solid tumors and encompasses morphology, cytogenetics, flow cytometry, and molecular diagnostics in classification. For example, detection of gene rearrangements is important in differential diagnosis of clonal neoplasms from benign but highly reactive lymph nodes. In recent years, the cytogenetics laboratory has enjoyed a renaissance of activity in defining consistent chromosome abnormalities in a growing list of leukemias, lymphomas, and solid tumors. At present, specific chromosomal abnormalities are of greatest clinical importance in only a few tumors, primarily lymphomas, leukemias, and sarcomas. Cytogenetic information, including fluorescent in situ hybridization for translocations and genomic hybridization are likely to become increasingly useful in defining tumor progression and prognosis.

Role of the Molecular Pathologist

The molecular pathologist practices at the interface of anatomic pathology, clinical pathology, and hematopathology, using the principles, theories, and techniques of molecular biology to make or confirm diagnoses of cancer, to provide more specific classification of cancer, and to provide prognostic or therapeutic information.

Somatic mutations (ie, mutations that occur during the lifetime of an individual in tissue outside of the germline) are central to the development of cancer.[89] Neoplastic progression is characterized by a succession of mutations in critical genes. These mutations may be gene deletions, duplications, point mutations, or chromosomal translocations, in any combination, in the DNA of the tumor cells. The mutations affect regulation of the cell cycle, cellular differentiation, apoptosis, and cell–cell and cell–matrix interactions. They are associated with altered gene expression. Epigenetic alterations such as hypermethylation of cytosines in CpG dinucleotide islands in the promoter region of many genes and histone acetylation abnormalities also alter gene expression (cf. Chapter 6).

Different neoplasms have different combinations of genetic and epigenetic alterations, and those differences can be exploited in the laboratory for diagnostic, prognostic, or therapeutic purposes. Some genetic alterations are required for the development of specific tumor types. Those alterations are therefore discrete, objective indicators of the associated neoplasm. The best examples are the chromosomal translocations seen in some leukemias, lymphomas, and soft-tissue tumors (Table 37-4).[90] Other genetic alterations, such as *TP53* missense mutations that inactivate the protein's normal role in cell cycle control, seem to be common to many malignancies.[91] Still other genetic changes are seen in subsets of neoplasms—eg, the amplification of the HER2/neu gene that is present in 10–30% of breast carcinomas and that provides both prognostic information and targeted therapeutic options with trastuzumab.[92] HPV genotyping has proved to be a useful adjunct tool in the diagnosis of precancerous cervical dysplasias.[93]

Many cancer-related molecular pathology tests focus on genetic alterations that are markers of specific tumor types. The new World Health Organization classification of leukemias characterizes leukemia subtypes by specific chromosomal translocations.[94] For example, the Philadelphia chromosome, t(9;22)(q34;q11), juxtaposes the 5′ portion of the *BCR* gene to the 3′ portion of the *ABL* gene, creating a new chimeric *BCR–ABL* gene that is the sine qua non for chronic myelogenous leukemia (CML). The chromosomal breakpoints occur within the introns (noncoding regions) of the genes so that the exons (coding regions) remain intact and can be transcribed into mRNA and translated into a unique 210 kDa fusion protein that is an activated tyrosine kinase. It is this fusion protein that is oncogenic for hematopoietic cells and present in all cases of CML. The molecular pathologist can look for this specific marker of disease in a variety of ways, including complete cytogenetic analysis, fluorescence in situ hybridization on metaphase spreads or intact interphase nuclei, Southern blot hybridization on tumor DNA, reverse-transcriptase polymerase chain reaction (RT-PCR) on tumor mRNA, or Western blot on tumor protein. The most commonly used methods are karyotype, fluorescence in situ hybridization, and RT-PCR. All of these technologies are labor-intensive and expensive, which have limited their application. However, higher throughput technologies such as real-time RT-PCR have made more routine applications realistic.[95] RT-PCR assays have the added advantage of being sensitive as well as specific. As few as one abnormal cell in 100,000 can be detected, making the technique useful for following minimal residual disease post-therapy. RT-PCR has been adapted for use with formalin fixed paraffin embedded tissues, facilitating the performance of prognostic and predictive tests with routine clinical material.[96,97]

Molecular pathology assays are central not only to the accurate subclassification of neoplasms but also to treatment guidance, especially with targeted therapies, such as those employing small-molecule inhibitors. Imatinib mesylate, a tyrosine kinase inhibitor, blocks the tyrosine kinase activity of *BCR–ABL* and inhibits the proliferation of CML tumor cells. Most patients experience a significant hematologic and cytogenetic remission. Real-time RT-PCR assays offer a sensitive quantitative assessment of minimal residual disease by determining the amount of chimeric *BCR–ABL* mRNA expression relative to the expression of a control gene. Serial monitoring over time documents the kinetics of the leukemic clone, providing prognostic in-

Table 37-4 Examples of recurrent Chromosomal Translocations in Human Neoplasia

Malignancy	Chromosomal Translocations	Genes Involved
Acute myelogenous leukemia	(8;21)(q22;q22)	RUNX1/RUNX1T1
	inv(16)(p13;q22)	CBFB/MYH11
	t(15;17)(q22;q21)	PML/RARA
	t(9;11)(p21-22;q23)	MLL/MLLT3
Acute lymphoblastic leukemia	t(12;21)(p12;q22)	ETV6/RUNX1
	t(9;22)(q34;q11)	BCR/ABL
	t(1;19)(q23;p13)	TCF3/PBX1
	t(4;11)(q21;q23)	MLL/AF4
Chronic myelogenous leukemia	t(9;22)(q34;q11)	BCR/ABL
Follicular lymphoma	t(14;18)(q32;q21)	IGH@/BCL2
Chondrosarcoma, myxoid	t(9;22)(q22;q12)	TEC/ETS1
Clear cell sarcoma (MMSP)	t(12;22)(q13;q12)	ATF1/ETS1
Ewing sarcoma/PNET	t(11;22)(q24;q12)	FLI1/EWSR1
	t(21;22)(q22;q12)	ERG/EWSR1
Liposarcoma, myxoid	t(12;16)(q13;p11)	DDIT3/FUS
RhabdomyosarcomA, alveolar	t(2;13)(q35-37;q14)	PAX3/FOXO1A
	t(1;13)(p36;q14)	PAX7/FOXO1A
Synovial sarcoma	t(X;18)(p11,q11)	SSX1/SYT1 SSX2/SYT1
Prostate cancer	t(21;7)(q22,p21)	TMPRSS2/EVI1

Abbreviations: MMSP, malignant melanoma of the soft parts; PNET, peripheral neuroectodermal tumor.

formation and allowing for therapeutic intervention. Patients with a 3-log reduction in *BCR–ABL* transcripts compared to baseline have a significantly better progression-free survival than those who have a lesser response.[98] Rising levels of *BCR–ABL* can indicate the emergence of a clone resistant to imatinib, triggering a mutational analysis.[99]

Clinical resistance to imatinib is associated primarily with mutations in the kinase domain of *BCR–ABL*. The mutations lead to amino acid substitutions and conformational changes in the imatinib binding site. Different mutations predict different clinical outcomes and require different therapeutic strategies, from dose escalation to combined therapy to transplantation. Second generation *ABL* kinase inhibitors that are active in imatinib-resistant *BCR–ABL* mutants have been discovered and introduced into clinical practice.[100]

The interplay of the molecular pathologist and targeted therapy is not limited to hematologic malignancies. Clinical trials of gefitinib, a drug that binds to the ATP cleft of the tyrosine kinase domain of epidermal growth factor receptor (*EGFR*), showed that 10% of nonsmall cell lung carcinomas that overexpressed *EGFR* responded clinically.[101,102] Clinical response is correlated with the presence of specific heterozygous, gain of function, in-frame deletion mutations or point mutations associated with amino acid substitutions in the *EGFR* kinase domain.[103,104] Microdissection of relatively pure populations of nonsmall cell lung carcinoma from frozen tissue or paraffin-embedded sections, followed by DNA isolation and sequence analysis of the exons containing the clustered mutations, identifies the patients who are likely to respond to gefitinib or similar targeted drugs.

As the molecular basis of neoplastic transformation and progression for various cancers becomes clearer, more applications will become incorporated into the diagnostic laboratory. Recently, microarray technology has been successfully employed to stratify neoplasms by disease outcome. Pathologists will play a central role in determining the best way to incorporate these new biologic markers and technologies into the diagnostic laboratory. For example, chronic lymphocytic leukemia (CLL) is a heterogeneous disorder. It may follow an indolent course with no need for therapy or, alternatively, a rapidly progressive course that is resistant to treatment. Somatic mutation analysis of the immunoglobulin heavy chain gene variable region (mutated vs. unmutated) stratifies these two clinical groups but requires expensive and time-consuming sequencing techniques that are unlikely to be universally available.[105,106] Gene-expression profiling of CLL has shown differences in the expression patterns of several hundred genes.[107,108] The expression of one of these genes, *ZAP70* (a member of the Syk family of tyrosine kinases that normally plays a role in T cell receptor signaling, natural killer cell activation, and early B cell development), has emerged as a potential surrogate marker for risk stratification of CLL.[109] *ZAP70* expression can be analyzed by real-time PCR, flow cytometry, or immunoperoxidase staining. Pathologists will have to determine the most informative and cost-effective technique.

The chemotherapeutic agents used to treat cancer often have narrow therapeutic indexes with an inherent risk of toxicity. Pharmacogenetics—the study of the role of genetic inheritance in individual variation in drug response and toxicity—will affect the practice of oncology.[110] For example, thiopurine *S*-methyltransferase (*TPMT*) is a cytosolic enzyme that catalyzes the *S*-methylation of the cytotoxic thiopurine drugs, including 6-thioguanine and 6-mercaptopurine. Genetic polymorphisms in *TPMT* lead to variable in vivo activity of the enzyme. In the white population, 89% have high enzyme activity, 11% have intermediate activity, and 1 in 300 have undetectable activity. The latter are at risk of severe, and potentially fatal, myelosuppression after standard-dose thiopurine therapy.[111] Patients can be screened by phenotypic or genotypic assays to identify those who require a reduced dosage.

Role of the Autopsy Pathologist

Autopsies do not receive the respect they were at one time accorded, and the autopsy rate has declined precipitously throughout the United States from approximately 90% of hospital deaths in some teaching hospitals in the late 1960s to the current average rate of approximately 5%.[112] One widely voiced but erroneous reason for this change in attitude and practice is the belief that autopsies no longer yield much in the way of useful information. They are considered to have been preempted by new technologies, such as diagrophic imaging and other pathologic and biochemical tests performed on the patient during life. Clinicians' fear of malpractice suits resulting from new findings revealed at autopsy that had not been diagnosed during life may be a factor. Still another is the fact that the Joint Commission for the Accreditation of Health Care Organizations has greatly reduced its emphasis on the hospital autopsy rate for accreditation purposes. The cost in the current cost-obsessed environment is likely a major factor, and many pathologists are not proponents of autopsies. None—the pathologist, the hospital, or the oncologist—is reimbursed the cost in time, effort, and materials involved in performing an autopsy or in persuading a reluctant family to permit an autopsy.

In a series of cases from 1986 to 1995, clinically undiagnosed or misdiagnosed malignancies were found in 44% of autopsies—a rate similar to that reported in studies from 1923 to 1972. Among the undiagnosed cancers, 57% were felt to be directly related to the patient's death.[113] A recent paper indicates that, at a contemporary US institution, an autopsy could yield a major error rate of 8.4–24.4% and a class I error rate of 4.1–6.7%.[114]

Despite these objections, autopsy continues to have an important role in patient care. In fact, advances in technology have done little to change the incidence of unexpected, clinically significant findings at autopsy.

Psychological factors may also play a negative role. Because of the significant side effects that accompany the longer survivals achieved with modern cancer therapy, the family of the deceased may feel that the patient had "suffered enough." Also, the autopsy serves as a symbol of failure, reminding the clinician that a cure could not be effected. Finally, there is a negative economic incentive for performing autopsies. In our experience, it is most unusual for an unexpected autopsy finding to lead to litigation, and if an egregious error in patient management has occurred, it is the responsibility of the medical profession to discover this.

Autopsy has an important role in evaluating the care of the cancer patient who has succumbed to the illness. The autopsy will obviously not offer direct benefit to the decreased patient, but it may be essential for supporting or refuting clinical impressions, determining the extent of residual disease and the adequacy of therapy, evaluating new therapies, identifying the ultimate and proximate causes of death, and revealing unexpected findings that affected patient care. As a means of advancing knowledge, clinicians should regard an autopsy as the final contribution that they and the deceased patient can make to an understanding of disease. The usefulness of an autopsy is greatly enhanced when the clinician takes the time to address with the pathologist specific questions that need to be answered at postmortem examination.

Summary and Conclusions

Perhaps the most important theme of this chapter is its emphasis on the role of the pathologist as a member of the medical team caring for the patient with cancer.

The importance of close communication among the oncologist, surgeon, radiotherapist, other clinicians, and the pathologist cannot be overemphasized. Patient care will be optimized if the pathologist is consulted in advance of procedures designed to obtain tissue samples for definitive diagnosis and therapy. Only a single opportunity may exist to obtain tissue that will make a complete revolution possible, and it will be unfortunate if that opportunity is lost because portions of the specimen are not appropriately triaged for immunohistochemistry, electron microscopy, flow cytometry, culture, or other special procedures. Implementation of a high level of communication and cooperation between pathologists and clinicians has led to important contributions in the treatment and care of patients with malignant melanoma and breast cancer, among other examples. Those examples should serve as useful models for the study of other types of cancers, especially in the era of molecularly individualized therapy.

Selected References

The complete reference list can be found at www.CANCERMEDICINE8.com

1. Clark WH. Tumour progression and the nature of cancer. *Br J Cancer.* 1991;64:631–644.
2. Hanahan D, Weinberg RA. The hallmarks of cancer. *Cell.* 2000;100:57–70.
3. Kumar V, Fausto N, Abbas A. *Robbins & Cotran Pathologic Basis of Disease*, 7th edition, 2004.
4. Dvorak HF, Nagy JA, Dvorak AM. Structure of solid tumors and their vasculature: implications for therapy with monoclonal antibodies. *Cancer Cell.* 1991;3:77–85.
5. Dvorak HF. Tumors: wounds that do not heal. Similarities between tumor stroma generation and wound healing. *N Engl J Med.* 1986;315:1650–1659.
6. Dickson DJ, Shami PJ. Angiogenesis in acute and chronic leukemias. *Leuk Lymphoma.* 2001;42:847–853.
7. Nagy JA, Masse EM, Herzberg KT, et al. Pathogenesis of ascites tumor growth: vascular permeability factor, vascular hyperpermeability, and ascites fluid accumulation. *Cancer Res.* 1995;55:360–368.
8. Senger DR, Galli SJ, Dvorak AM, et al. Tumor cells secrete a vascular permeability factor that promotes accumulation of ascites fluid. *Science.* 1983;219:983–985.
9. Folkman J, Shing Y. Angiogenesis. *J Biol Chem.* 1992;267:10931–10934.
10. Dvorak HF. Rous-Whipple Award Lecture. How tumors make bad blood vessels and stroma. *Am J Pathol.* 2003;162:1747–1757.
11. Nagy JA, Dvorak AM, Dvorak HF.VEGF-A and the induction of pathological angiogenesis. *Annu Rev Pathol.* 2007;2:251–275.
12. Dvorak HF. Discovery of vascular permeability factor (VPF). *Exp Cell Res.* 2006;312:522–526.
13. Dvorak HF, Senger DR, Dvorak AM, et al. Regulation of extravascular coagulation by microvascular permeability. *Science.* 1985;227:1059–1061.
14. Brown LF, Yeo KT, Berse B, et al. Expression of vascular permeability factor (vascular endothelial growth factor) by epidermal keratinocytes during wound healing. *J Exp Med.* 1992;176:1375–1379.
15. Vaupel P, Kallinowski F, Okunieff P. Blood flow, oxygen and nutrient supply, and metabolic microenvironment of human tumors: a review. *Cancer Res.* 1989;49: 6449–6465.
16. Tannock IF, Rotin D. Acid pH in tumors and its potential for therapeutic exploitation. *Cancer Res.* 1989;49:4373–4384.
17. Frazier M, Su L-K, Amos CI, et al. Current applications of genetic technology in predisposition testing and microsatellite instability assays. *J Clin Oncol.* 2000;18: 70s–74s.
18. Ribic CM, Sargent DJ, Moore MJ, et al. Tumor microsatellite instability status as a predictor of benefit from fluorouracil-based adjuvant chemotherapy for colon cancer. *N Engl J Med.* 2003;349:247–257.
19. Connolly JL, Schnitt SJ. Evaluation of breast biopsy specimens in patients considered for treatment by conservative surgery and radiation therapy for early breast cancer. *Pathol Annu.* 1988;23:1–23.
20. Owings D, Hann L, Schnitt SJ. How thoroughly should needle localization breast biopsies be sampled for microscopic examination? A prospective mammographic–pathologic correlative study. *Am J Surg Pathol.* 1990;14:578–583.
21. Dupont WD, Page DL. Risk factors for breast cancer in women with proliferative breast disease. *N Engl J Med.* 1985;312: 146–151.
22. Beachy PA, Karhadkar SS, Berman DM. Tissue repair and stem cell renewal in carcinogenesis. *Nature.* 2004;432:324–331.
23. Reya T, Morrison SJ, Clarke MF, Weissman IL. Stem cells, cancer, and cancer stem cells. *Nature.* 2001;414:105–111.
24. Holland R, Connolly JL, Gelman R, et al. The presence of an extensive intraductal component (EIC) following a limited excision correlates with prominent residual disease in the remainder of the breast. *J Clin Oncol.* 1990;8:113–118.
25. Gage I, Schnitt SJ, Nixon AJ, et al. Pathologic margin involvement and the risk of recurrence in patients treated with breast-conserving therapy. *Cancer.* 1996;78: 1921–1928.
26. Hill RP. Tumor progression: potential role of unstable genomic changes. *Cancer Metastasis Rev.* 1990;9:137.
27. Gleason DF. Histologic grade, clinical stage, and patient age in prostate cancer. *NCI Monogr.* 1988;7:15–18.
28. Bloom HJG, Richardson WW. Histological grading and prognosis in breast cancer. *Br J Cancer.* 1957;11:359–377.
29. Scharf ERW, Hadley RS. Prognosis in carcinoma of the breast. *Lancet.* 1938;2:582–583.
30. Komaki K, Sano N, Tangoku A. Problems in histological grading of malignancy and its clinical significance in patients with operable breast cancer. *Breast Cancer.* 2006;13(3):249–253.
31. Locker GY, Hamilton S, Harris J, et al. ASCO 2006 update of recommendations for the use of tumor markers in gastrointestinal cancer. *J Clin Oncol.* 2006;24(33):5313–5327.
32. Harris L, Fritsche H, Mennel R, et al. ASCO 2006 update of recommendations for the use of tumor markers in breast cancer. *J Clin Oncol.* 2007;25:5287–5312.
33. Linardou H, Dahabreh IJ, Kanaloupiti D, et al. Assessment of somatic k-RAS mutations as a mechanism associated with resistance to EGFR-targeted agents: a systematic review and meta-analysis of studies in advanced non-small-cell lung cancer and metastatic colorectal cancer. *Lancet Oncol.* October 2008;9:962–972.
34. Crystal BS, Wang HH, Ducatman BS. Comparison of different preparation techniques for fine needle aspiration specimens. A semiquantitative and statistical analysis. *Acta Cytol.* 1993;37:24–28.
35. Ducatman BS, Hogan CL, Wang HH. A triage system for processing fine needle aspiration cytology specimens. *Acta Cytol.* 1989;33:797–799.
36. Wang HH, Sovie S, Trawinski G, et al. ThinPrep processing of endoscopic brushing specimens. *Am J Clin Pathol.* 1996;105: 163–167.
37. Linder J, Zahniser D. ThinPrep Papanicolaou testing to reduce false-negative cervical cytology. *Arch Pathol Lab Med.* 1998;122:139–144.
38. Bishop JW, Bigner SH, Colgan TJ, et al. Multicenter masked evaluation of AutoCyte Prep thin layers with matched conventional smears. Including initial biopsy results. *Acta Cytol.* 1998;42:189–197.
39. Walboomers JM, Jacobs MV, Manos MM, et al. Human papillomavirus is a necessary cause of invasive cervical cancer worldwide. *J Pathol.* 1999;189:12–19.
40. Wright TC Jr, Cox JT, Massad LS, et al. 2001 Consensus guidelines for the management of women with cervical cytological abnormalities. *JAMA.* 2002;287: 2120–2129.
41. Wright TC Jr, Schiffman M, Solomon D, et al. Interim guidance for the use of human papillomavirus DNA testing as an adjunct to cervical cytology for screening. *Obstet Gynecol.* 2004;103:304–309.
42. Goldie SJ, Kim JJ, Wright TC. Cost-effectiveness of human papillomavirus DNA testing for cervical cancer screening in women aged 30 years or more. *Obstet Gynecol.* 2004;103:619–631.
43. Patz EF Jr, Goodman PC, Bepler G. Screening for lung cancer. *N Engl J Med.* 2000;343:1627–1633.
44. Brown FM. Urine cytology. It is still the gold standard for screening? *Urol Clin North Am.* 2000;27:25–37.
45. Falk GW, Chittajallu R, Goldblum JR, et al. Surveillance of patients with Barrett's esophagus for dysplasia and cancer with balloon cytology [see comments]. *Gastroenterology.* 1997;112:1787–1797.
46. Leoni-Parvex S, Mihaescu A, Pellanda A. Esophageal cytology in the follow-up of patients with treated upper aerodigestive tract malignancies. *Cancer.* 2000;90:10–16.
47. Dooley WC, Ljung BM, Veronesi U, et al. Ductal lavage for detection of cellular atypia in women at high risk for breast cancer. *J Natl Cancer Inst.* 2001;93:1624–1632.
48. O'Shaughnessy JA, Ljung BM, Dooley WC, et al. Ductal lavage and the clinical management of women at high risk for breast carcinoma. *Cancer.* 2002;94:292–298.
49. Geisinger KR. Endoscopic biopsies and cytologic brushings of the esophagus are diagnostically complementary. *Am J Clin Pathol.* 1995;103:295–299.

38 Principles of Imaging

Edward F. Patz, Jr., MD

Imaging plays a fundamental diagnostic role in every aspect of clinical oncology. Radiological studies provide invaluable information in establishing a diagnosis and in guiding patient management. In some oncology patients, imaging studies can also be used to suggest appropriate treatment, determine prognosis, assess disease status following therapy, and guide interventional procedures.

The mainstay of imaging departments continues to be conventional radiological studies. Plain films are easy to perform, deliver a low dose of radiation, are relatively inexpensive, and provide a tremendous amount of diagnostic information. Cross sectional imaging studies, including computed tomography (CT) and magnetic resonance (MR) imaging, in addition to nuclear medicine scans, are also standard of care in the oncology patient and typically complement more traditional radiographs.

The type and frequency of radiological evaluation of the cancer patient depends on the tumor and the clinical situation. There is a wide spectrum of indications that includes screening, work-up of the symptomatic patient, further evaluation of an abnormality found on another imaging study, following progression of the disease, or complications of therapy. Each clinical scenario presents a different diagnostic problem, particularly in cancer patients. Before any imaging study is requested, it is imperative to understand the type of abnormality that is suspected, whether the test can provide the necessary information, and just as importantly, what can and will be done with the results to change the course of the disease.

While current imaging studies elucidate important information about the natural history of malignancies, cancer is a disease of the genes, which results in a complex interaction between the host and the tumor. In many situations, the intricacies of tumor biology will require diagnostic imaging to move beyond describing traditional anatomic and morphologic features, and incorporate fundamental molecular properties of the disease. Imaging studies that demonstrate these basic molecular events would certainly increase our understanding of malignancies, and eventually could be used to influence clinical practice.

The genesis of a molecular imaging initiative occurred in the early 1990s, with the use of positron emission tomography (PET) imaging and the glucose analog probe, [18F]-2-fluoro-2-deoxy-D-glucose (FDG). Over the last several years, FDG-PET imaging has become one of the most important tools to evaluate cancer patients. PET imaging has been used to differentiate benign from malignant lesions, to stage tumors, and to predict recurrent disease. As a move toward molecular imaging continues, the development of new targets, techniques, and tumor-specific imaging probes should provide more accurate diagnostic information. In the future, molecular imaging may be able to address many current, unresolved diagnostic issues in oncology. Although the technology is undergoing a dramatic expansion, it is also incumbent upon the radiologic community to carefully study new molecular imaging techniques and determine if they are truly useful and cost effective. The ability to create ever more spectacular images does not necessarily improve patient management and outcomes.

Hypothesis-driven, evidence-based studies are essential if noninvasive imaging is to have an impact on patient care. Because imaging is a fundamental part of diagnostic evaluation, understanding the utility of particular tests will guide a more efficient patient evaluation. This section's collection of chapters provides an overview of imaging principles, with a focus on the cancer patient. Imaging plays a central role in clinical management, and the information presented here provides general guidelines for using radiologic studies in everyday clinical practice.

Suggested Reading

Apolo AB, Pandit-Taskar N, Morris MJ. Novel tracers and their development for the imaging of metastatic prostate cancer. *J Nucl Med.* 2008;49:2031–2041.

Boss DS, Olmos RV, Sinaasappel M, Beijnen JH, Schellens JH. Application of PET/CT in the development of novel anticancer drugs. *Oncologist.* 2008;13(1):25–38.

Coleman RE, Delbeke D, Guiberteau MJ, et al. Concurrent PET/CT with an integrated imaging system: intersociety dialogue from the joint working group of the American College of Radiology, the Society of Nuclear Medicine, and the Society of Computed Body Tomography and Magnetic Resonance. *J Nucl Med.* 2005;46(7):1225–1239.

Fletcher JW, Djulbegovic B, Soares HP. Recommendations on the use of 18F-FDG PET in oncology. *J Nucl Med.* 2008;49(3): 480–508.

Gerstner ER, Sorensen AG, Jain RK, Batchelor TT. Advances in neuroimaging techniques for the evaluation of tumor growth, vascular permeability, and angiogenesis in gliomas. *Curr Opin Neurol.* 2008;21(6):728–735.

Heron DE, Andrade RS, Beriwal S, Smith RP, et al. PET-CT in radiation oncology: the impact on diagnosis, treatment planning, and assessment of treatment response. *Am J Clin Oncol.* 2008;31(4):352–362.

Hoh CK. Clinical use of FDG PET. *Nucl Med Biol.* 2007;34(7):737–742.

Hylton N. Dynamic contrast-enhanced magnetic resonance imaging as an imaging biomarker. *J Clin Oncol.* 2006;24(20): 3293–3298.

Kuehl H, Veit P, Rosenbaum SJ, Bockisch A, Antoch G. Can PET/CT replace separate diagnostic CT for cancer imaging? Optimizing CT protocols for imaging cancers of the chest and abdomen. *J Nucl Med.*, 2007;48(suppl 1): 45S–57S.

Kundra V, Silverman PM, Matin SF, Choi H. Imaging in oncology from the University of Texas M. D. Anderson Cancer Center: diagnosis, staging, and surveillance of prostate cancer. *AJR Am J Roentgenol.* 2007;189(4): 830–844.

McSheehy P, Allegrini P, Ametaby S, et al. Minimally invasive biomarkers for therapy monitoring. *Ernst Schering Found Symp Proc.* 2007;(4):153–188.

Schaefer JF, Schlemmer HP. Total-body MR-imaging in oncology. *Eur Radiol.* 2006;16(9): 2000–2015.

von Schulthess GK. Integrated modality imaging with PET-CT and SPECT-CT: CT issues. *Eur Radiol.* 2005;15(suppl 4):D121–126.

Tanvetyanon T, Eikman EA, Sommers E, Robinson L, Boulware D, Bepler G. Response by PET scan versus CT scan to predict survival after neoadjuvant chemotherapy for resectable non-small cell lung cancer. *JCO.* 2008. {AU: Please provide the volume number and page range for reference 6}

Veit P, Ruehm S, Kuehl H, et al. Lymph node staging with dual-modality PET/CT: enhancing the diagnostic accuracy in oncology. *Eur J Radiol.* 2006;58(3):383–389.

Wirth A, Foo M, Seymour JF, Macmanus MP, Hicks RJ. Impact of [18f] fluorodeoxyglucose positron emission tomography on staging and management of early-stage follicular non-hodgkin lymphoma. *Int J Radiat Oncol Biol Phys.* 2008;71(1):213–219.

Wong TZ, Paulson EK, Nelson RC, Patz EF Jr, Coleman RE. Practical approach to diagnostic CT combined with PET. *AJR Am J Roentgenol.* 2007;188(3):622–629.

Zafra M, Ayala F, Gonzalez-Billalabeitia E. Impact of whole-body 18F-FDG PET on diagnostic and therapeutic management of Medical Oncology patients. *Eur J Cancer.* 2008; 44(12):1678–1683.

39 Interventional Radiology for the Cancer Patient

Rony Avritscher, MD ■ Michael J. Wallace, MD

In the past decade, there has been a substantial expansion in the use of image-guided procedures for diagnosing and treating various types of cancer. There are several reasons for this increased use. Advances in cancer diagnosis and novel medical and surgical therapies have led to increased survival in this patient population. More patients now present with primary or metastatic disease confined to an organ and are consequently more likely to benefit from locoregional therapies than from systemic treatment. Thus, a neoplasm can be defined using standard imaging modalities, and then minimally invasive percutaneous techniques can be used to establish the diagnosis and to provide locoregional or palliative therapies to treat the cancer patient. Recent improvements in catheter/device technology, embolic agents and chemotherapy drugs, and delivery systems are associated with improved patient outcome and have sparked renewed interest in these approaches. In this chapter, we discuss hepatic vascular interventions, genitourinary interventions, thoracic interventions, several forms of palliative therapeutic procedures, and some additional image-guided procedures (vena cava filter placement, biopsy, and intratumoral gene therapy).

Hepatic Vascular Interventions

The liver has long occupied center stage in interventional oncology. Hepatic interventions for diagnosis and treatment are popular for a number of reasons, among them that this organ is a common site of metastatic disease and can be easily accessed percutaneously. However, the key feature that makes liver tumors particularly amenable to catheter-delivered therapies stems from the nature of their blood supply. Hepatic tumors derive most of their blood supply from the hepatic artery, whereas normal hepatic parenchyma derives most of its supply from the portal venous system. This unique arrangement allows the interventional oncologist to treat hepatic lesions while sparing the surrounding normal liver.

Arterial Infusion Therapy

The goal of arterial infusion is to achieve better tumor response by delivering chemotherapic agents directly into the artery that supplies the neoplasm. The rationale behind arterial infusion therapy is based on the first-pass effect, which occurs when a drug is given directly into the tissue that metabolizes it. The first-pass effect, compared with systemic administration, can lead to a severalfold increase in the drug concentration within the affected organ and, at the same time, a reduction in systemic concentration. Therefore, regional drug delivery is seen as a method of overcoming the limitations of the maximum-tolerated dose.[1]

Arterial infusion therapy has been primarily used for the treatment of metastatic colorectal cancer confined to the liver. A recent meta-analysis by Mocellin et al [2] summarized the results of 10 randomized controlled trials that compared hepatic arterial infusion (HAI) with systemic chemotherapy. Although the study revealed better tumor response to fluoropyrimidine-based HAI when compared with systemic fluoropyrimidine therapy, tumor response rates for modern systemic chemotherapy regimens using a combination of fluorouracil with oxaliplatin or irinotecan were similar or superior to those for HAI. Moreover, the meta-analysis showed no survival benefit associated with fluoropyrimidine-based HAI therapy. Further studies of the use of HAI for the delivery of novel anticancer agents will be instrumental in determining the role of this approach in future locoregional cancer therapy.

Arterial Embolization

The aim of transcatheter hepatic arterial embolization is to completely or partially occlude the arterial supply to the tumor. The rationale is that such occlusion will cause tumor ischemia, which in turn will lead to growth arrest and necrosis. After hepatic arterial embolization, collateral hepatic circulation comes into play immediately. This collateral circulation should be traced and occluded if it supplies the neoplasm. The more central the occlusion, the more abundant is the collateral flow. Therefore, to maximize ischemia, the most effective embolization should result in distal terminal vessel occlusion. Peripheral (segmental and subsegmental) vascular embolization is best accomplished with coaxial catheters and small particles.

Many different embolic agents have been used with success for hepatic embolization. The most common agents include absorbable gelatin sponge particles and powder, polyvinyl alcohol foam granules, fibrin glue, n-butyl cyanoacrylate, ethiodized oil, tris-acryl gelatin microspheres, and absolute alcohol. Gelatin sponge segments or stainless steel coils are used for central occlusion and not often used for tumor embolotherapy.

The most common complication after hepatic arterial embolization is postembolization syndrome. This syndrome consists of fever, nausea, fatigue, and elevated white blood cell count and liver function tests. These symptoms are usually self-limited. Complications resulting from nontargeted embolization include cholecystitis, pancreatitis, and gastrointestinal ulcers. Hepatic embolization may also lead to liver necrosis, liver failure, and hepatic abscess. Failure to recognize intrahepatic arteriovenous shunts during embolization may cause embolic material to reach the pulmonary circulation, which can in turn lead to respiratory failure. The complications of hepatic embolization in 284 patients who underwent 410 embolizations over a 10-year period were analyzed by Hemingway and Allison.[3] Minor complications occurred in 16% of patients, serious complications in 6.6%, and death in 2%.

Arterial Chemoembolization

Arterial chemoembolization consists of intra-arterial delivery of a combination of chemotherapy drugs and an embolic agent into a liver tumor. The rationale behind chemoembolization is based on the theory that tumor ischemia caused by embolization of the dominant arterial supply has a synergistic effect with the chemotherapeutic drugs. This technique has been the mainstay of interventional radiology since it was originally introduced by Yamada in 1977.[4] The introduction of iodized oil, an iodinated ester derived from poppy-seed oil, greatly advanced this technique. Iodized oil is well suited for chemoembolization because of its preferential tumoral uptake by hepatocellular carcinoma (HCC) and certain hepatic metastases; it acts simultaneously as an embolic agent and a vehicle for the chemotherapeutic agent.[5,6] These findings are partially explained by the concept of enhanced permeability and retention suggested by Maeda.[7] Newly formed tumor vessels are more permeable. This increased permeability coupled with a lack of lymphatics in the neoplasm, result in retention of molecules of higher molecular weight within the tumor interstitium for a more prolonged period. This retention may explain, in part, the accumulation of iodized oil or the increase in concentration of polymer conjugates of chemotherapeutic agents in neoplasms.

There are many different chemoembolization protocols. The most commonly used chemotherapy agent is doxorubicin. This agent is often combined with cisplatin and mitomycin C. Subsequently, these chemotherapeutic agents are mixed with iodized oil and slowly infused into the hepatic artery branch that feeds the tumor. Additional embolization with gelatin sponge or particles can be performed to enhance tumoral ischemia. The proximal arterial supply to the tumor should be preserved because increased response is observed with repeated procedures.

Transcatheter arterial chemoembolization has been used to treat, in addition to unresectable HCC, cholangiocarcinomas and hepatic metastases and has been used in conjunction with liver resection or tumor ablation. Two randomized clinical trials[8,9] showed a survival advantage when chemoembolization was performed in selected HCC patients. Recent advances in chemotherapy agents and embolic material suggest future potential for this technique. Incorporation of antiangiogenic agents into the mixture to be delivered to the tumor is currently being investigated.[10] In the realm of novel embolic material, drug-eluting beads have recently been developed. These beads, which contain chemotherapy agents (doxorubicin or irinotecan), can be administered by intra-arterial injection and show promising results for improved tumor control.[10,11] Moreover, advances in technology now allow intraprocedural acquisition of cross-sectional images using C-arm cone beam computed tomography (Fig. 39-1). This technique enables more selective embolization as multiplanar and three-dimensional images are used to understand the arterial anatomy and assess completeness of iodized-oil uptake.[12]

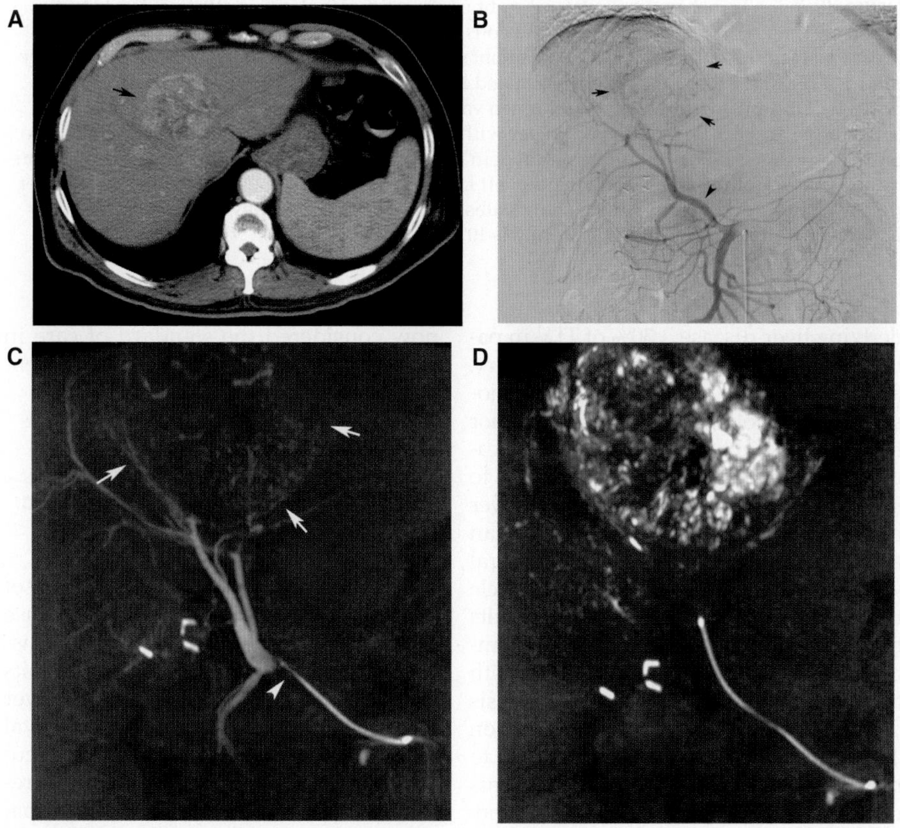

Figure 39-1 Transcatheter arterial chemoembolization performed in a 71-year-old man with unresectable hepatocellular carcinoma. **(A)** Contrast-enhanced CT scan obtained prior to chemoembolization shows a large, solitary, hypervascular mass in segment IV of the liver (*arrow*). **(B)** Anteroposterior digital subtraction angiography (DSA) of the abdomen shows a replaced right hepatic artery arising from the proximal superior mesenteric artery (arrowhead). This vessel supplies the hypervascular tumor in the left liver (*arrows*). **(C)** C-arm cone-beam CT images obtained during the procedure show tip of 3-French catheter in the distal replaced right hepatic artery (*arrowhead*) confirming origin of vascular supply to the hepatocellular carcinoma (*arrows*). **(D)** C-arm cone-beam CT images obtained after chemoembolization demonstrate retention of iodized oil throughout the lesion.

Hepatic Intra-arterial Brachytherapy

Radioembolization with yttrium-90 (^{90}Y) microspheres is a technique in which particles incorporating the isotope ^{90}Y are infused through a catheter directly into the hepatic arteries. Yttrium-90 is a beta emitter with a short half-life. The concept is similar to chemoembolization in that the injected particles are selectively distributed into the tumor arterial bed. This distribution is possible because the blood flow within the tumor is several times greater than the flow in the surrounding liver parenchyma. As a consequence, a much higher amount of radiation can be delivered to the lesion than with external-beam radiation, and at the same time the potential for radiation-induced hepatitis is reduced.

TheraSphere beads (MDS Nordion, Ottawa, Canada) are FDA approved for neoadjuvant treatment of unresectable HCC in patients with portal vein thrombosis or as a bridge to transplantation. SIR-Spheres (Sirtex Medical, Lane Cove, Australia) are approved for the treatment of metastatic colorectal cancer to the liver with concomitant use of floxuridine. Knowledge of the vascular anatomic variants in the celiac axis and superior mesenteric artery is critical to safely administering this therapy to avoid nontargeted embolization of the radioactive microspheres, which can have devastating consequences. Multiple studies have demonstrated the safety of radioembolization with yttrium-90 for the treatment of unresectable HCC and metastatic colorectal cancer.[13-15]

Local Tissue Ablation

Image-guided tumor ablation of focal hepatic malignancies can be accomplished using chemical agents or thermal energy. Chemical ablation options include direct intratumoral percutaneous ethanol injection (PEI) and ablation using hot water or saline, acetic acid, or chemotherapeutic agents that induce tumor cell death. Thermal ablation options include high-energy radiofrequency (RF), interstitial laser photocoagulation, microwave, cryotherapy, and high-intensity focused ultrasound that causes coagulation necrosis. These procedures can be performed under imaging guidance by interventional radiologists or by surgeons in the operating suite.

Ethanol is the most commonly used agent for chemical tumor ablation worldwide.[16] Once ethanol is injected into the tumor, it causes cytoplasmic dehydration, denaturation of cellular proteins, and small-vessel thrombosis.[17] PEI is well established for the treatment of HCC, but it is much less successful in the treatment of hepatic metastases; in metastases, thermal ablation methods are more promising. This distinction appears to stem from the way in which ethanol disseminates within the different tumors. The distribution of ethanol tends to be uniform in soft lesions surrounded by hardened cirrhotic liver parenchyma, as is the case in HCC. However, when the surrounding parenchyma is softer than the tumor, as is often the case with metastases, ethanol distribution is less uniform and the treatment less effective. Ebara and colleagues[18] reported on 20 years of experience with PEI for HCC lesions ≤3 cm in a total of 270 patients. The local recurrence rate at 3 years was 10%, with overall 3- and 5-year survival rates of 81% and 60%, respectively.

Livraghi and colleagues[19] studied RF ablation vs PEI in the treatment of small HCCs (≤3 cm in diameter). Complete necrosis was achieved in 47 of 52 tumors (90%) in an average of 1.2 sessions per tumor with RF ablation and 48 of 60 tumors (80%) in an average of 4.8 sessions per tumor with PEI. One major complication (hemothorax) and four minor complications (bleeding, hemobilia, pleural effusion, and cholecystitis) occurred with RF ablation, although there was none with PEI. Lencioni and colleagues[20] reported treatment of HCC with either RF ablation or PEI in a randomized series of 102 patients with hepatic cirrhosis. Although there was no overall difference in 1- and 2-year survival, there was a significant difference in 1- and 2-year local recurrence–free survival (98% for RF ablation vs 83% for PEI at 1 year and 96% vs 62% at 2 years). The study was limited to patients with either a single HCC ≤5 cm in diameter or a maximum of three HCCs ≤3 cm in diameter. However, up to 25% of the lesions in Ebara and colleagues' study[18] of PEI could not have been treated by RF ablation because of anatomic considerations, which emphasizes that there is still a role for PEI in small tumors despite results that overall favor RF ablation. Thermal ablation for hepatic metastases from colorectal cancer has also been reported to improve survival. Median survival time after thermal ablation was increased to 39 months from 21 to 25 months in a study reported by Gillams and Lees.[21]

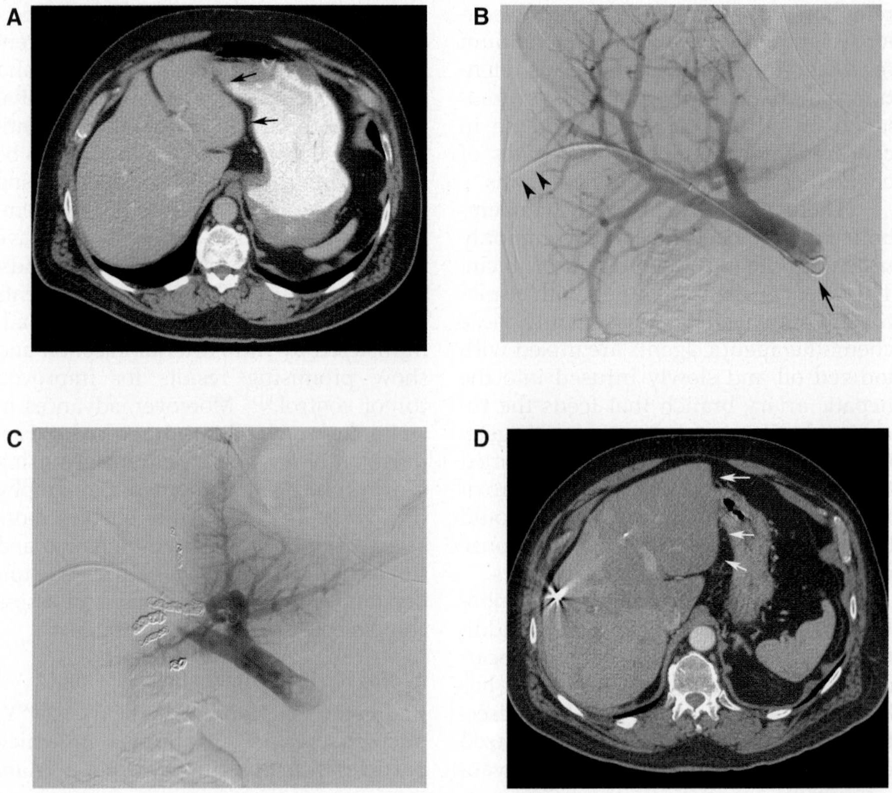

Figure 39-2 Transhepatic ipsilateral right portal vein embolization (PVE) extended to segment IV using tris-acryl particles and coils performed in a 52-year-old man with rectal cancer metastatic to the liver. **(A)** CT scan obtained prior to PVE shows marginal future liver remnant (FLR) (FLR-to-TELV (total estimated liver volume] ratio = 17%) (*arrows*). **(B)** Anteroposterior DSA portogram shows a 6-French vascular sheath in a right portal vein branch (*arrowheads*) and a 5-French flush catheter within the main portal vein (*arrow*). **(C)** Final DSA portogram shows occlusion of the portal vein branches to segments IV through VIII with continued patency of the vein supplying the left lateral liver. **(D)** CT scan obtained 1 month after right PVE extended to segment IV shows substantial FLR hypertrophy (FLR-to-TELV ratio = 27%) (*arrows*). The degree of hypertrophy is 10%.

Portal Vein Embolization

Successful resection of the liver depends on the function of the residual hepatic parenchyma. When the portal vein is occluded, hepatocyte growth factors (hepatopoietin A, insulin, and glucagon) are shunted into the liver segments supplied by nonembolized vessels.[22] The result is atrophy of the segments supplied by the occluded vessels and hypertrophy of the other areas of the liver. Thus portal vein embolization (PVE) is used preoperatively to induce liver hypertrophy in potential surgical candidates with anticipated marginal future liver remnant (FLR) volumes (Fig. 39-2).

PVE is performed if the FLR is estimated to be <20% of the estimated total liver volume (TLV) in patients without underlying liver disease, <30% of TLV in patients with underlying severe liver injury, and <40% of TLV in patients with cirrhosis.[23] For embolizations performed prior to extended right hepatectomy, modification of the preoperative embolization to include segment IV may optimize liver hypertrophy. The range of reported mean absolute FLR increase for PVE in general was 46-70%, depending on the particle type used for embolization. PVE results in hepatocyte apoptosis, so the postembolization syndrome associated with transarterial embolization and necrosis does not occur. Madoff et al.[24] reported on 44 patients who underwent PVE prior to major liver surgery. None of the patients developed liver failure after the resection.

Fibrin glue, gelatin sponge, thrombin, particles, coils, and absolute ethanol all have been used for PVE. In the United States, a combination of particles and embolization coils are the most common embolic agents.

Recent retrospective studies and meta-analysis suggest improved surgical outcomes after PVE.[23,25] For this reason, PVE prior to a major hepatectomy is now considered the standard of care in many comprehensive hepatobiliary centers worldwide.

Considerations in Hepatocellular Carcinoma

HCC is the fifth most prevalent type of cancer and the third most common cause of cancer death in the world.[26] This disease is common worldwide because of its strong association with underlying liver cirrhosis and hepatitis. Surgical removal of the tumor is the only potentially curative treatment. However, curative resection is possible only in 20-30% of patients.[27] Recurrence rates after surgical resection are high because of dissemination of primary disease, undetected hepatic micrometastases, or metachronous lesions. Five-year survival after partial hepatic resection is approximately 50%.[28] For patients with cirrhosis and unresectable disease, liver transplantation can potentially cure both the underlying liver disease and the tumor. Intra-arterial therapies (embolization, chemoembolization, and radioembolization) and ablative techniques are viable alternatives in patients who are not candidates for partial hepatectomy or transplantation. Systemic chemotherapy for HCC has been traditionally disappointing because of the low response rates. In recent times, sorafenib, a multikinase inhibitor with antiangiogenic, proapoptotic, and Raf kinase–inhibitory activity, has been shown to be well tolerated; it is the first agent to demonstrate a statistically significant improvement in overall survival for patients with advanced HCC.[29]

Local etiologic factors have to be evaluated when considering locoregional therapy, because HCC in Western countries is often different from the typical HCC treated by interventional radiologists in Japan.[30] Nodular HCC is seen in fewer than 25% of Western patients but in approximately 75% of patients in Japan. For patients with early to intermediate disease, ablative techniques are appealing, since the damage to the surrounding liver parenchyma is minimized, allowing for repeated treatments and serving as a bridge to transplantation. The current literature supports the use of percutaneous RF ablation in patients with HCC and either a single lesion <5 cm in diameter or up to three lesions <3 cm in diameter if partial hepatic resection or transplantation are not available.[31]

Chemoembolization is currently used for noncurative therapy for nonsurgical patients with large or multifocal HCC that has not spread extrahepatically. Two randomized studies have reported more favorable results for chemoembolization than for bland embolization, conservative therapy, or both. Llovet and colleagues[9] reported survival rates of 75% and 50% at 1 and 2 years, respectively, for 37 patients assigned to embolization alone, 82% and 63% for 40 patients assigned to chemoembolization, and 63% and 27% for 35 patients assigned to conservative treatment. The study was stopped early because of the proven survival benefit. Another study by Lo and colleagues[8] demonstrated a benefit in survival for patients with unresectable HCC treated with chemoembolization (iodized oil, cisplatin, and gelfoam) compared with a control group treated with symptomatic therapy only. Survival in the chemoembolization group was 57% at 1 year, 31% at 2 years, and 26% at 3 years, compared with 32%, 11%, and 3%, respectively, in the control group. Radioembolization with yttrium-90 is FDA-approved for neoadjuvant treatment of unresectable HCC in patients with portal vein thrombosis or as a bridge to transplantation, but randomized studies are needed to establish a wider role.

Considerations in Hepatic Metastases

Colorectal Metastases

The liver is often the first and only site of metastases from colon cancer. Many of these patients will die of their liver disease, thus local control can positively affect patient outcome. Although surgical resection is the first line of treatment for liver metastases, the majority of patients are not surgical candidates because of extent of disease or presence of medical comorbidities. Novel systemic chemotherapy agents are now available, which have been shown to effect significant improvement in patient survival.[32] In addition, local tissue ablation can be offered to patients who are not surgical candidates because of the presence of medical comorbidities or to patients with bilobar disease that can be completely treated with a combination of ablation and surgery. Recent series of patients with up to five lesions, each measuring ≤5 cm, showed 5-year survival ranges of 24-44%.[33,34] PVE may also be employed to increase the number of patients who can be converted into surgical candidates.[23] Palliative treatment can be offered in the form of arterial infusion therapy and radioembolization. The role of novel chemotherapy agents combined with arterial infusion is currently being investigated as an alternative viable palliative therapy. Radioembolization with SIR-Spheres (resin microspheres) is approved for the treatment of metastatic colorectal cancer to the liver with concomitant use of floxuridine.

Neuroendocrine Metastases

Hepatic artery embolization or chemoembolization is indicated for patients with multiple nonresectable, hormonally active tumors. The goal of treatment is to reduce tumor bulk and hormone secretion. The 5-year postembolization survival range is 50-60%, with symptomatic and biochemical response ranges of 40-80% and 50-60%, respectively.[35] Moertel and colleagues[36] reported their 10-year experience in 111 patients with neuroendocrine hepatic metastases, usually hypervascular, who received vascular occlusion therapy by a variety of methods. As many as 71 patients received subsequent alternating chemotherapy regimens (dacarbazine combined with doxorubicin, alternating with streptozotocin combined with 5-fluorouracil) also. Response rates of 60% with vascular occlusion alone and 80% with sequential therapy of vascular occlusion and chemotherapy were observed. Median survival times of 37 and 49 months were experienced in patients with islet cell carcinoma and carcinoid hepatic metastases, respectively. For the symptomatic treatment of hormonally active liver metastases, the use of repeated embolizations is preferred.

The best results for metastatic disease of the liver treated with hepatic artery embolization have been observed in patients with neuroendocrine tumors metastatic to the liver. Sequential and periodic embolization is required for effective palliation. Gupta and colleagues have reported on 81 patients with carcinoid syndrome who were treated with either bland embolization or chemoembolization.[37] Imaging was available for evaluation of a response in 69 patients. Partial response occurred in 67% of the patients, stable disease in 16%, and progression of tumor in 8.7%. The median response duration was 17 months in those patients with a partial response. A reduction of tumor-related symptoms occurred in 63%, with a median progression-free survival of 19 months and a median overall survival time of 31 months. In a subsequent study by Gupta and colleagues,[38] these 69 patients with carcinoid tumors were compared with 54 patients who had islet cell tumors with metastases to the liver. Patients with carcinoid tumors had a higher response rate and a longer progression-free survival than did patients with islet cell tumors (67% vs 35% and 23 months vs 16 months). Although chemoembolization, compared with bland embolization, did not prove to be beneficial for survival in patients with carcinoid tumors, it did result in improved overall survival and improved response (32 months vs 18 months and 50% vs 25) in patients treated for islet cell tumors.

RF ablation can be used to palliate symptoms associated with metastatic neuroendocrine tumors. In a series by Berber,[39] RF ablation provided complete symptomatic relief in 63% of 222 patients and partial relief in 95%. Radioembolization is another minimally invasive alternative to palliating a large burden of hepatic metastases from neuroendocrine tumors.

Other Hepatic Metastases

Other types of hepatic metastases are usually not as well suited for locoregional therapy as the tumor is likely widespread by the time of liver involvement. However, occasionally, certain types of hepatic metastases are amenable to local treatment because of the indolent nature of the primary disease. Such hepatic metastases that can sometimes be treated by chemoembolization include ocular melanoma, leiomyosarcoma, breast carcinoma, and renal cell carcinoma. In a group of 30 patients with metastatic ocular melanoma, chemoembolization with cisplatin produced a response rate of 46% and a median survival period of 11 months.[40] The longest survival was

5 years from the initial chemoembolization. In the past, such patients lived for 2-6 months after presentation with hepatic metastases. Additional studies have been reported using HAI of carboplatin-based chemotherapy and fotemustine, with response rates of 38% and 40%, respectively.[40] Hepatic artery immunoembolization has also been reported with variable responses. A group of 14 patients with metastatic leiomyosarcoma to the liver were treated with chemoembolization every 4 weeks with cisplatin and polyvinyl alcohol foam granules 150-250 μm in size, followed by vinblastine infusion.[41] The response rate was 70%, and responses lasted 4-19 months (median, 9 months). This rate compared well with the response rate of 15% obtained after systemic therapy with ifosfamide with doxorubicin. It should be noted that these are not common tumors and that most are treated on protocol studies. At MDACC, our approach to chemoembolization of hepatic metastases is similar to our approach to HCC; ie, a hypervascular tumor is more likely to benefit from the treatment than a hypovascular tumor. The goal of treatment, whether it is to provide symptomatic relief or to prolong survival, must be weighed against the risk of complications.

Genitourinary Interventions

Renal Arterial Embolization

Renal artery embolization for renal cell carcinoma may be performed preoperatively to decrease operative blood loss in patients with extensive local disease. A study by Zielinski et al.[42] showed a survival benefit to preoperative embolization, although previous studies have not demonstrated this advantage. Embolization of renal carcinoma can also be performed for palliative relief of symptoms in patients with extensive local tumor or as a cytoreductive measure when patients are not candidates for surgery.[43] Renal artery embolization has also been used in the management of congestive heart failure caused by arteriovenous shunting through the renal carcinoma and for hypertension, hypercalcemia, polycythemia, and hemorrhage caused by the renal neoplasm. Selective segmental embolization is especially necessary and effective in patients with impaired renal function or solitary kidney.

Renal Ablation

Thermal ablation plays an increasingly important role in the management of renal cell carcinoma. Although nephrectomy remains the gold standard for treatment of renal cell carcinoma, RF ablation is increasingly a viable alternative (Fig. 39-3). RF ablation for the treatment of renal tumors is minimally-invasive with a low morbidity rate.[44] Patients who are candidates for renal RF ablation include those with high surgical risk secondary to medical comorbidities; patients with a solitary kidney or multifocal disease, who are not candidates for nephron-sparing surgery; and patients who do not wish to undergo surgery. Patients with hereditary syndromes, such as von Hippel-Lindau disease, are at high-risk for multiple renal neoplasms over their lifetimes. These patients may be treated repeatedly with RF ablation, in an effort to preserve normal renal parenchyma adjacent to the tumors.

Gervais et al.[45,46] demonstrated that tumor size and location are directly related to ablation effectiveness. Exophytic lesions can be more effectively ablated because of surrounding fat, the presence of which makes lesions easier to target and provides heat insulation during ablation. Complete necrosis was achieved in 90% of tumors measuring less than 4.0 cm. Larger or central tumors may not be amenable to complete ablation and may require multiple ablations, or in some cases, multiple treatment sessions. This is in part owing to the proximity of medullary tumors to the renal hilar vessels resulting in an increased heat-sink effect, which affects ablation efficacy by lowering intralesional temperatures. A medullary tumor location also increases the risk of procedure-related complications. The most common complication of renal RF ablation is hemorrhage. This complication was observed in 5% of the patients in the series of 100 treated lesions by Gervais.[45,46] Hemorrhage can occur into the collecting system requiring stent placement for ureteral obstruction or it can be confined to the subcapsular space.

Ahrar and colleagues[44] described their experience with 29 patients with 30 renal tumors who underwent percutaneous RF ablation. The lesions had a mean largest diameter of 3.5 ± 0.24 cm. The primary tumor was completely ablated in 96% of patients. Mean and median follow-up intervals were 10 months and 7 months, respectively. Major complications were observed in 12% of the patients, including gross hematuria and urinary obstruction in three patients. All hemorrhagic complications were successfully treated. One patient had persistent weakness of the anterior abdominal wall. None of the patients in the study showed significant degradation of renal function after treatment.

Thoracic Interventions

Lung Ablation

Thermal ablation can be used to treat primary and metastatic lung cancers. Lung ablation is optimal for patients with early lung cancer, where complete ablation with curative intent can be attempted. In patients with large tumor burden, ablation may provide palliation of tumor-related symptoms.[47] Lung ablation is

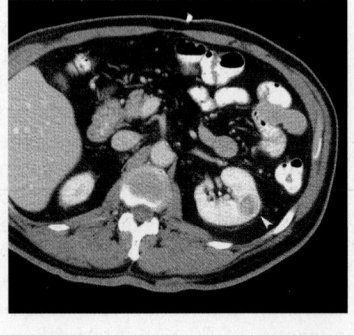

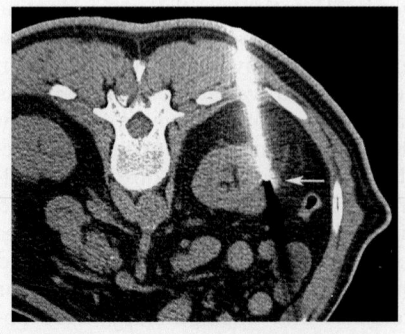

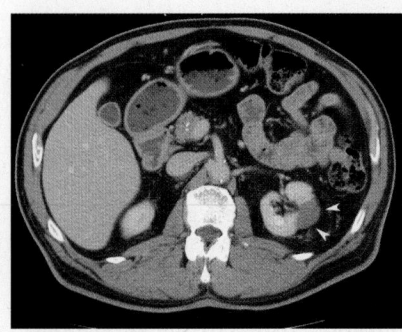

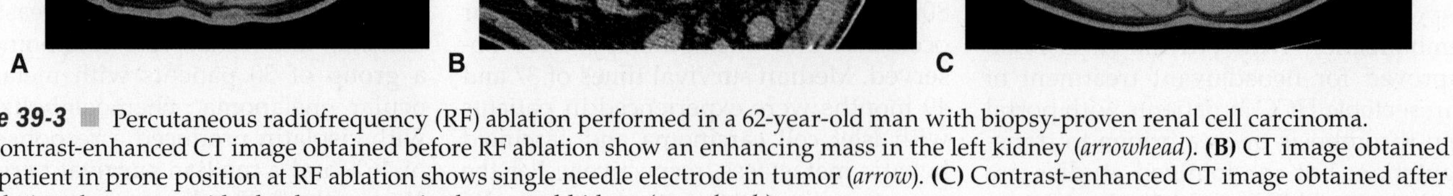

Figure 39-3 Percutaneous radiofrequency (RF) ablation performed in a 62-year-old man with biopsy-proven renal cell carcinoma. **(A)** Contrast-enhanced CT image obtained before RF ablation show an enhancing mass in the left kidney (*arrowhead*). **(B)** CT image obtained with patient in prone position at RF ablation shows single needle electrode in tumor (*arrow*). **(C)** Contrast-enhanced CT image obtained after RF ablation shows no residual enhancement in the treated kidney (*arrowheads*).

offered primarily to patients with lung cancer who are not operative candidates as well as to patients with pulmonary metastases.

Simon et al[48] reported a series of 153 patients with 189 primary or metastatic inoperable lung cancers treated with percutaneous pulmonary RF ablation. The overall 1-, 2-, 3-, 4-, and 5-year survival rates, respectively, for stage I non–small cell lung cancer were 78%, 57%, 36%, 27%, and 27%; rates for colorectal pulmonary metastasis were 87%, 78%, 57%, 57%, and 57%. The incidence of pneumothorax was 28.4%. Postablation pneumothorax may be treated conservatively, if the patient remains asymptomatic. In the patients with symptoms or progressively enlarging pneumothorax, placement of a chest drain is necessary. In the series by Simon et al.,[48] procedure-related 30-day mortality rate was 2.6%.

Pleural effusion is also a common complication after lung ablation. In their series of 60 patients, de Baere et al.[49] reported a minor pleural effusion in 9% of patients immediately after treatment and on 60% of CT scans obtained 24-48 h after treatment. Postprocedure hemoptysis was observed in 10% of the patients. The hemoptysis started 1-9 days after the ablation and lasted 2-13 days. These complications did not require any treatment.

Lung Chemoembolization

Lung chemoembolization can be used for the treatment of a multitude of lung tumors. The purpose of lung chemoembolization is to deliver chemotherapeutic agents to the tumor while blocking its blood supply. This is accomplished by simultaneously injecting embolic material and the chemotherapy into the pulmonary artery branches that supply the tumor. The embolization increases the chemotherapy dwell time within the lesion by slowing agent washout.

In 2005, Vogl et al.[50] examined transpulmonary chemoembolization with mitomycin C combined with iodized oil as an option for treatment of unresectable lung metastases in 23 patients. This study demonstrated that transpulmonary chemoembolization was feasible and well tolerated. No major complications were observed; 35% of patients had a partial response, 26% had stable tumor size, and 39% showed progression of disease.

Palliative Therapy

Percutaneous Biliary Drainage

Pancreatic carcinoma, cholangiocarcinoma, and ampullary carcinoma are the primary neoplasms that produce intrinsic biliary obstruction, whereas lymphadenopathy, HCC, and hepatic metastasis can produce extrinsic compression. Nonsurgical palliation of malignant biliary obstruction may be accomplished either endoscopically or percutaneously. The percutaneous methods include drainage by insertion of external or internal–external percutaneous biliary catheters.

The aims of palliative therapy are to provide relief of jaundice and pruritus as well as associated cholangitis and, most important, to prepare patients for anticancer therapy. Neither the endoscopic nor the percutaneous approach has an advantage with regard to influencing survival, and the choice of technique is often a team decision based on the available local expertise.

Internal drainage via endoscopy is preferable because of the inconvenience of an external catheter and the potential for pain at the tube entry site, bile leakage around the catheter, and sepsis from skin organisms. The percutaneous approach has the advantage of allowing prompt access to the biliary tree. Regardless of the approach, partial or complete jaundice relief can be achieved in 73-100% of treated patients.[51]

Percutaneous Biliary Stenting

Speer and colleagues[52] described 70 patients with malignant biliary obstruction who were randomized to undergo percutaneous vs endoscopic biliary stent placement. The success rate in relieving jaundice was 81% for endoscopically placed stents compared with 61% for the percutaneously placed stents. The complication rate was 19% vs 67%, in favor of the endoscopic approach. In addition, the 30-day mortality rate in the two groups was 15% for endoscopic stents vs 33% for the percutaneous method.

Cholangitis, hemorrhage, and bile leakage are the most common complications of stent placement. The incidence of cholangitis is lower in patients treated with a metallic stent than in patients treated with a plastic stent.[53] Plastic stents are also more prone to migration and remain patent on average for only 3-4 months.[53] Self-expanding metallic stents have longer patency but are more expensive. Metallic stents may be dislodged by balloon dilation immediately after deployment, but the incidence of spontaneous migration over the long term is negligible. These uncovered metallic stents cannot be removed. Despite advances in stent technology, occlusion secondary to tumor ingrowth or overgrowth remains a complex issue.

Musculoskeletal Ablation

The majority of patients with breast, prostate, and lung cancer show evidence of bone metastases at the time of death. These lesions are often accompanied by pain, and occasional fractures, which can dramatically decrease the quality of life of this patient population.[54] External-beam radiation therapy is the gold standard for localized pain secondary to osseous metastases. The majority of the patients will experience symptomatic relief after radiation therapy. However, in a substantial minority of patients, radiation therapy provides suboptimal response and durability of relief.[55]

Patients are candidates for ablative therapy of painful metastases when a patient reports moderate or severe musculoskeletal pain, the patient's pain is focal in nature and correlates with abnormality evident with radiological imaging, and the painful metastatic lesion is accessible to percutaneous treatment.[56]

Lesions that are amenable to ablative therapy are typically osteolytic or mixed osteolytic and osteoblastic in nature or otherwise composed of soft tissue. RF ablation and cryoablation are safe and effective treatments for the palliation of painful metastatic lesions that are refractory to standard therapies. Importantly, the quality of life for these patients is improved with this therapy. Goetz et al.[57] reported on 43 patients with painful bone metastases treated with RF ablation. As many as 95% of the patients experienced symptomatic relief that was considered clinically significant with decrease of opioid usage. A single ablative treatment is effective in most patients and appears to provide a long duration of pain relief.

Miscellaneous

Vena Cava Filter Placement

Cancer patients experience an increased incidence of thrombosis and pulmonary embolism (PE). The percutaneous placement of a vena cava filter is the optimal therapeutic approach for patients with PE, who have a contraindication to anticoagulant therapy or who develop recurrent emboli despite adequate anticoagulant administration. There are numerous filters currently in use, including devices that are retrievable and MRI compatible.

Wallace and colleagues[58] reported on the experience of vena cava filter placement in 308 patients with venous thromboembolic disease, in the setting of malignancy. Median survival times were 145 days and 207 days for 267 patients with solid tumors and 41 patients with liquid tumors, respectively. Patients with metastatic or disseminated disease were 3.7 times as likely to die as those with local disease, and patients with deep venous thrombosis and a history of hemorrhage were twice as likely to die as those with deep venous thrombosis and no history of hemorrhage. Major complications included pulmonary emboli, new caval thrombus, retroperitoneal hemorrhage, and filter incorrect deployment.

Stent Placement for Venous Stenosis

Vena caval syndrome is most frequently the result of intrinsic or extrinsic malignant disease.[59] In this syndrome, neoplasms, by their extension and localization or by causing mediastinal, retroperitoneal, and pelvic lymphadenopathy, create stenosis and obstruction by extrinsic compression of the vena cava. The complications of radiation therapy and chemotherapy for this syndrome include mediastinal fibrosis and thrombophlebitis.[59]

Superior vena cava syndrome symptoms have been grouped into four classes: (1) central nervous system symptoms, including headache, blurred vision, and cognitive dysfunction; (2) laryngopharyngeal edema, producing dyspnea and hoarseness; (3) nasal or facial edema; and (4) other signs of venous congestion and dilatation.[60] In addition to the stenosis or obstruction, there is frequently thrombosis complicating the mediastinal compression or intraluminal invasion by the tumor. Parish and colleagues[61] reported an average survival time of 7 months after the diagnosis of malignant superior vena cava obstruction. Vascular stents can effectively palliate symptoms of malignant vena cava stenosis in 68-80% of patients.[59]

Biopsy

Percutaneous biopsy has been traditionally a cost-effective modality to diagnose the patient with cancer. Almost all tissues, including the myocardium, are accessible to percutaneous biopsy. Varied needles (11-25 gauge) as well as biopsy forceps are efficient in obtaining representative specimens. Biopsy guns are available to automate the procedure. However, a negative biopsy result does not exclude the possibility of malignancy; it may merely represent an error in sampling. Most biopsies of lesions in adults are scheduled electively on an outpatient basis.

Guidance by fluoroscopy or CT is usually adequate for biopsy of the lung or mediastinum.[62] The reported accuracy of percutaneous transthoracic needle biopsy in patients with lung cancer and pulmonary metastases is 90-98%,[63] whereas the diagnostic yield for local pulmonary infection in immunocompromised patients is 73%.[64] Serious complications of lung and mediastinal biopsies include systemic air embolization, hemorrhage, pericardial tamponade, seeding of malignant cells into the needle track, and empyema. Pneumothorax is the most frequent complication with an incidence rate ranging from 5% to 61%,[65] when performed under fluoroscopy. CT-guided procedures may be associated with a higher incidence of pneumothorax, probably because it is commonly used on lesions with a smaller average size. The incidence of pneumothorax, when using CT guidance, is approximately 22-45%.[66] In a study described by Cox and colleagues,[67] when biopsies were done under CT guidance, smaller lesions (<2 cm) and the presence of emphysema strongly correlated with the occurrence of pneumothorax.

Abdominal biopsies guided by fluoroscopy, ultrasonography, CT, and MRI yielded adequate diagnostic material for cytologic analysis in 84-95% of patients. When a 20- to 23-gauge needle is used, biopsies of the liver, pancreas, kidney, adrenal gland, spleen, and ovary, among other organs, are performed with a sensitivity of 86%, a specificity of 98%, and an accuracy of 90%. The overall complication rate in a study of 63,180 biopsies was 0.16%. Seeding of malignant cells along the needle tract occurred in 0.05% of patients.[68-70]

The diagnostic accuracy of percutaneous skeletal biopsy is on average 80%. The overall diagnostic accuracy of 78% was reported in a series of 178 patients with primary skeletal tumors who underwent percutaneous needle biopsy.[71] The procedure was more accurate for malignant neoplasms (83%) than benign tumors (64%).

Transjugular Intrahepatic Portosystemic Shunt Placement

The formation of a transjugular intrahepatic portosystemic shunt (TIPS), by placing a metallic stent between the hepatic and portal venous systems, is an accepted means of decreasing certain sequelae associated with portal hypertension. Indications include gastrointestinal variceal bleeding, ascites, portal gastropathy, hepatic hydrothorax, and Budd–Chiari syndrome. Cancer patients with hepatic disease may be candidates for this procedure. Wallace and colleagues[72] have described 38 patients with malignancy and hepatic disease treated with TIPS placement. Technical success was achieved in 97% of patients. Recurrent variceal hemorrhage occurred in only 1 of 19 patients (5%), and ascites or hydrothorax resolved or significantly improved in 9 of 12 patients (75%). Intimal hyperplasia and occlusion of the TIPS stent is the most feared postprocedural complication. The 1-year patency rates for TIPS is reported at 25-66%.[73] Development of covered stents to prevent stenosis has shown dramatic promise, with two studies demonstrating identical 1-year primary patency of 84%.[74,75]

Selected References

The complete reference list can be found at www.CANCERMEDICINE8.com

1. Collins JM. Pharmacologic rationale for regional drug delivery. *J Clin Oncol.* 1984;2(5):498–504.
2. Mocellin S, Pilati P, Lise M, Nitti D. Meta-analysis of hepatic arterial infusion for unresectable liver metastases from colorectal cancer: the end of an era? *J Clin Oncol.* 2007;25(35):5649–5654.
3. Hemingway AP, Allison DJ. Complications of embolization: analysis of 410 procedures. *Radiology.* 1988;166(3):669–672.
4. Yamada R, Nakatsuka H, Nakamura K, et al. Hepatic artery embolization in 32 patients with unresectable hepatoma. *Osaka City Med J.* 1980;26(2):81–96.
5. Nakakuma K, Tashiro S, Hiraoka T, et al. Studies on anticancer treatment with an oily anticancer drug injected into the ligated feeding hepatic artery for liver cancer. *Cancer.* 1983;52(12):2193–2200.
8. Lo CM, Ngan H, Tso WK, et al. Randomized controlled trial of transarterial lipiodol chemoembolization for unresectable hepatocellular carcinoma. *Hepatology.* 2002;35(5):1164–1171.
9. Llovet JM, Real MI, Montana X, et al. Arterial embolisation or chemoembolisation versus symptomatic treatment in patients with unresectable hepatocellular carcinoma: a randomised controlled trial. *Lancet.* 2002;359(9319):1734–1739.
10. Liapi E, Georgiades CC, Hong K, Geschwind JF. Transcatheter arterial chemoembolization: current technique and future promise. *Tech Vasc Interv Radiol.* 2007;10(1):2–11.
11. Yoshizawa H, Nishino S, Shiomori K, Natsugoe S, Aiko T, Kitamura Y. Surface morphology control of polylactide microspheres enclosing irinotecan hydrochloride. *Int J Pharm.* 2005;296(1-2):112–116.
12. Wallace MJ, Murthy R, Kamat PP, et al. Impact of C-arm CT on hepatic arterial interventions for hepatic malignancies. *J Vasc Interv Radiol.* 2007;18(12):1500–1507.
13. Geschwind JF, Salem R, Carr BI, et al. Yttrium-90 microspheres for the treatment of hepatocellular carcinoma. *Gastroenterology.* 2004;127(5 Suppl):S194–S205.
14. Salem R, Lewandowski RJ, Atassi B, et al. Treatment of unresectable hepatocellular carcinoma with use of 90Y microspheres (TheraSphere): safety, tumor response, and survival. *J Vasc Interv Radiol.* 2005;16(12):1627–1639.
15. Stubbs RS, Cannan RJ, Mitchell AW. Selective internal radiation therapy (SIRT) with 90Yttrium microspheres for extensive colorectal liver metastases. *Hepatogastroenterology.* 2001;48(38):333–337.
16. Livraghi T, Giorgio A, Marin G, et al. Hepatocellular carcinoma and cirrhosis in 746 patients: long-term results of percutaneous ethanol injection. *Radiology.* 1995;197(1):101–108.
18. Ebara M, Okabe S, Kita K, et al. Percutaneous ethanol injection for small hepatocellular carcinoma: therapeutic efficacy based on 20-year observation. *J Hepatol.* 2005;43(3):458–464.
19. Livraghi T, Goldberg SN, Lazzaroni S, Meloni F, Solbiati L, Gazelle GS. Small

hepatocellular carcinoma: treatment with radio-frequency ablation versus ethanol injection. *Radiology.* 1999;210(3):655–661.

20. Lencioni RA, Allgaier HP, Cioni D, et al. Small hepatocellular carcinoma in cirrhosis: randomized comparison of radio-frequency thermal ablation versus percutaneous ethanol injection. *Radiology.* 2003;228(1):235–240.
21. Gillams AR, Lees WR. Survival after percutaneous, image-guided, thermal ablation of hepatic metastases from colorectal cancer. *Dis Colon Rectum.* 2000;43(5):656–661.
22. Yokoyama Y, Nagino M, Nimura Y. Mechanisms of hepatic regeneration following portal vein embolization and partial hepatectomy: a review. *World J Surg.* 2007;31(2):367–374.
24. Madoff DC, Abdalla EK, Gupta S, et al. Transhepatic ipsilateral right portal vein embolization extended to segment IV: improving hypertrophy and resection outcomes with spherical particles and coils. *J Vasc Interv Radiol.* 2005;16(2 Pt 1):215–225.
25. Abulkhir A, Limongelli P, Healey AJ, et al. Preoperative portal vein embolization for major liver resection: a meta-analysis. *Ann Surg.* 2008;247(1):49–57.
27. Yamada R, Kishi K, Sato M, et al. Transcatheter arterial chemoembolization (TACE) in the treatment of unresectable liver cancer. *World J Surg.* 1995;19(6):795–800.
28. Bruix J, Sherman M. Management of hepatocellular carcinoma. *Hepatology.* 2005; 42(5):1208–1236.
31. Chen MS, Li JQ, Zheng Y, et al. A prospective randomized trial comparing percutaneous local ablative therapy and partial hepatectomy for small hepatocellular carcinoma. *Ann Surg.* 2006;243(3):321–328.
32. Goldberg RM, Sargent DJ, Morton RF, et al. A randomized controlled trial of fluorouracil plus leucovorin, irinotecan, and oxaliplatin combinations in patients with previously untreated metastatic colorectal cancer. *J Clin Oncol.* 2004;22(1):23–30.
33. Lencioni R, Crocetti L, Cioni D, Della Pina C, Bartolozzi C. Percutaneous radiofrequency ablation of hepatic colorectal metastases: technique, indications, results, and new promises. *Invest Radiol.* 2004;39(11):689–697.
34. Gillams AR, Lees WR. Radio-frequency ablation of colorectal liver metastases in 167 patients. *Eur Radiol.* 2004;14(12):2261–2267.
35. Ramage JK, Davies AH, Ardill J, et al. Guidelines for the management of gastroenteropancreatic neuroendocrine (including carcinoid) tumours. *Gut.* 2005;54 (Suppl 4):iv1–iv16.
36. Moertel CG, Johnson CM, McKusick MA, et al. The management of patients with advanced carcinoid tumors and islet cell carcinomas. *Ann Intern Med.* 1994;120(4):302–309.
37. Gupta S, Yao JC, Ahrar K, et al. Hepatic artery embolization and chemoembolization for treatment of patients with metastatic carcinoid tumors: the M.D. Anderson experience. *Cancer J.* 2003;9(4):261–267.
38. Gupta S, Johnson MM, Murthy R, et al. Hepatic arterial embolization and chemoembolization for the treatment of patients with metastatic neuroendocrine tumors: variables affecting response rates and survival. *Cancer.* 2005;104(8):1590–1602.
44. Ahrar K, Matin S, Wood CG, et al. Percutaneous radiofrequency ablation of renal tumors: technique, complications, and outcomes. *J Vasc Interv Radiol.* 2005;16(5):679–688.
45. Gervais DA, McGovern FJ, Arellano RS, McDougal WS, Mueller PR. Radiofrequency ablation of renal cell carcinoma: part 1, Indications, results, and role in patient management over a 6-year period and ablation of 100 tumors. *AJR Am J Roentgenol.* 2005;185(1):64–71.
46. Gervais DA, Arellano RS, McGovern FJ, McDougal WS, Mueller PR. Radiofrequency ablation of renal cell carcinoma: part 2, Lessons learned with ablation of 100 tumors. *AJR Am J Roentgenol.* 2005;185(1):72–80.
48. Simon CJ, Dupuy DE, DiPetrillo TA, et al. Pulmonary radiofrequency ablation: long-term safety and efficacy in 153 patients. *Radiology.* 2007;243(1):268–275.
49. de Baere T, Palussiere J, Auperin A, et al. Midterm local efficacy and survival after radiofrequency ablation of lung tumors with minimum follow-up of 1 year: prospective evaluation. *Radiology.* 2006;240(2):587–596.
50. Vogl TJ, Wetter A, Lindemayr S, Zangos S. Treatment of unresectable lung metastases with transpulmonary chemoembolization: preliminary experience. *Radiology.* 2005;234(3):917–922.
52. Speer AG, Cotton PB, Russell RC, et al. Randomised trial of endoscopic versus percutaneous stent insertion in malignant obstructive jaundice. *Lancet.* 1987;2(8550):57–62.
56. Callstrom MR, Charboneau JW. Image-guided palliation of painful metastases using percutaneous ablation. *Tech Vasc Interv Radiol.* 2007;10(2):120–131.
57. Goetz MP, Callstrom MR, Charboneau JW, et al. Percutaneous image-guided radiofrequency ablation of painful metastases involving bone: a multicenter study. *J Clin Oncol.* 2004;22(2):300–306.
58. Wallace MJ, Jean JL, Gupta S, et al. Use of inferior vena caval filters and survival in patients with malignancy. *Cancer.* 2004;101(8):1902–1907.
59. Carrasco CH, Charnsangavej C, Wright KC, Wallace S, Gianturco C. Use of the Gianturco self-expanding stent in stenoses of the superior and inferior venae cavae. *J Vasc Interv Radiol.* 1992;3(2):409–419.
60. Kee ST, Kinoshita L, Razavi MK, Nyman UR, Semba CP, Dake MD. Superior vena cava syndrome: treatment with catheter-directed thrombolysis and endovascular stent placement. *Radiology.* 1998;206(1):187–193.
62. Gupta S, Seaberg K, Wallace MJ, et al. Imaging-guided percutaneous biopsy of mediastinal lesions: different approaches and anatomic considerations. *Radiographics.* 2005;25(3):763–786; discussion 86–88.
63. Westcott J. Lung Biopsy. In: Dondelinger RF Rossi P, Kurdziel JC, Wallace S, ed. *Interventional Radiology.* Stuttgart: Thieme; 1990:9–17.
66. Kazerooni EA, Lim FT, Mikhail A, Martinez FJ. Risk of pneumothorax in CT-guided transthoracic needle aspiration biopsy of the lung. *Radiology.* 1996;198(2):371–375.
67. Cox JE, Chiles C, McManus CM, Aquino SL, Choplin RH. Transthoracic needle aspiration biopsy: variables that affect risk of pneumothorax. *Radiology.* 1999;212(1):165–168.
69. Stewart CJ, Coldewey J, Stewart IS. Comparison of fine needle aspiration cytology and needle core biopsy in the diagnosis of radiologically detected abdominal lesions. *J Clin Pathol.* 2002;55(2):93–97.
71. Ayala AG, Zornosa J. Primary bone tumors: percutaneous needle biopsy. Radiologic-pathologic study of 222 biopsies. *Radiology.* 1983;149(3):675–679.
72. Wallace MJ, Madoff DC, Ahrar K, Warneke CL. Transjugular intrahepatic portosystemic shunts: experience in the oncology setting. *Cancer.* 2004;101(2):337–345.

40 Principles of Surgical Oncology

Raphael E. Pollock, MD, PhD, FACS ▪ Michael A. Choti, MD, MBA, FACS ▪ Donald L. Morton, MD, FACS

In spite of significant advances in various systemic approaches to the care of the cancer patient, surgical therapy of remains mainstay of treatment for most solid malignancies and plays a role in various components of the cancer care continuum, from prevention to diagnosis, curative therapy, survival prolongation, and palliation. To be maximally effective, the cancer surgeon must function as a member of the oncology team and is frequently the first oncology specialist that a patient will consult. The cancer surgeon is commonly charged with the responsibility to establish a tissue diagnosis for a suspicious lesion; this may either require an operative procedure or an image-directed or other biopsy approach. The cancer surgeon will usually bear the responsibility for communicating the biopsy findings to the patient, completing the procedures needed to stage the cancer, and initiating subsequent interaction between the patient and other members of the multimodality oncology team. Because of these responsibilities, it is most often the cancer surgeon who initially explains to the patient the sequence and rationale of the various treatment components that will be used to manage the specific malignancy. To be maximally effective, the cancer surgeon must therefore be aware of the different therapeutic options, the natural history of a given malignancy, and how these factors will be integrated into a well-conceived and appropriate multimodality treatment algorithm. It is also usually the surgical oncologist's responsibility to provide initial information about prognosis and to make decisions about follow-up care and surveillance to detect tumor recurrence. In these aspects, the surgical oncologist is unlike almost any other surgical specialist in that the commitment to a given patient is for both the acute and the long-term components of the patient's disease process.

Over the years, the practice of surgical oncology has come full circle. Originally, surgeons attempted to treat cancer conservatively by removing only the gross lesion. Unfortunately, this led to extremely high rates of local recurrence and subsequent patient mortality. In the late 19th century, surgeons began to undertake radical en bloc resections and amputations to treat patients with malignant disease. These techniques yielded improved results, but the procedures were often mutilating. With the advent of other complementary and effective treatment modalities, notably radiation therapy in the 1920s and chemotherapy after the 1940s, the orientation of surgical resection is once again becoming conservative with a focus on organ preservation and restoring the comorbid state when possible.

Adjuvant chemotherapy, alone or in combination with radiation therapy, has improved disease free survival and prolonged quality life for patients who have been rendered free of gross disease by surgery but who still have a high likelihood of recurrence as a consequence of microscopic residual metastases. Randomized clinical trials have demonstrated the benefit of adjuvant chemotherapy in a variety of tumors, including breast cancer, colorectal cancer, pancreatic cancer, osteogenic sarcoma, testicular cancer, ovarian cancer, and certain lung cancers.

Surgery is most effective in the treatment of apparently locoregionally confined primary disease. The principles of surgical resection include en bloc resection of the primary tumor that attempts to encompass gross and microscopic tumor in all contiguous and adjacent anatomic locations. For some tumor types, concomitant resection of regional lymph nodes make up an important component of the initial surgical management. In many cases, when disease is diagnosed and removed at an early stage, resection is the single therapeutic modality, often associated with a high rate of long-term success. Intuitively, it appears logical that surgery should have little role in disease management once a neoplasm has spread from the primary location to a distant site. However, surgical therapy is being applied with increasing frequency for metastatic disease as well. Prolonged survival can be seen in selected patients following resection of various metastatic sites, including in the liver, lung, or brain. In particular, complete resection of hepatic colorectal metastases results in 5-year survival rates in excess of 50% in most contemporary series. As more active systemic cytotoxic and targeted therapies are prolonging survival in patients with various tumor types, resection or ablation of residual metastatic sites are being utilized with increasing frequency.

Surgery operates by zero-order kinetics, in which 100% of excised cells are destroyed. In contrast, chemotherapy and radiation therapy operate by first-order kinetics, where only a fraction of tumor cells are killed by each treatment. It is for this reason that these therapies can be considered complementary. Surgical resection reduces the tumor burden, which hopefully increases the efficacy of nonsurgical adjuvant therapies intended to eliminate microscopic residual disease, thereby decreasing the risk of recurrence and prolonging survival.

During the past two decades, a significant reduction has been seen in the morbidity and mortality associated with many complex surgical cancer operations. These results, in part, can be attributed to improvements in surgical technique, patient selection, and regionalization to high-volume centers. For example, both perioperative risk and long-term survival after pancreaticoduodenectomy has been shown to be strongly influenced by hospital volume.[1] In addition, trends toward more limited cancer resections are being seen with comparable of improved oncologic outcome. Specifically, breast-preserving surgery has become an alternative to mastectomy in patients with breast carcinoma, limb salvage is often possible in patients with bone and soft-tissue sarcomas, and sphincter-preservation and sexual potency can frequently be preserved for patients with rectal cancer. Because surgery is increasingly combined with other treatment modalities, it is essential that most patients with solid neoplasms have their treatment planned by a multidisciplinary team, which includes radiation and medical oncologists as well as surgical oncologists. To retain a primary role in the management of the cancer patient, the successful surgical oncologist must be able to coordinate and integrate the efforts of the entire oncologic team.

The History of Surgical Oncology

Oncology (from the Greek words onkos, meaning mass or tumor, and logos, meaning study) is the study of neoplastic diseases. Early authors suggested that certain families, races, and working classes were predisposed to neoplastic transformations. In 1862, Edwin Smith, an American Egyptologist, discovered the apparently earliest recordings of the surgical treatment of cancer.[2] Written in Egypt circa 1600 bc, this treatise was based on teachings possibly dating back to 3000 bc. The Egyptian author advised surgeons to contend with tumors that might be cured by surgery but not to treat those lesions that might be fatal.

Hippocrates (460-375 B.C) was the first to describe the clinical symptoms associated with cancer. He advised against treating terminal patients, who would enjoy a better quality of life without surgical intervention.[3] He also coined the terms carcinoma (crab legs tumor) and sarcoma (fleshy mass). In the second century ad, Galen published his classification of tumors, describing cancer as a systemic disease caused by an excess of black bile.[4] Galen cautioned that as a systemic disease, cancer was not amenable to cure by surgery, which was often promptly followed by patient death. This strong admonition against surgery for cancer persisted for more than 1500 years until 18th-century pathologists discovered that cancer often grew locally before spreading to other anatomic sites. Prior to the advent of safe general anesthetics, surgery was used primarily to manage trauma or severe infectious problems such as abscess drainage. In that era, cancer surgery consisted primarily of amputation or cauterization of surface tumors of the trunk or extremities. Patients were usually unwilling to submit to the pain of tumor surgery, when there was little likelihood of improved survival.

During the 18th and 19th centuries, advances in anatomic pathology led to an increase in autopsies, which in turn resulted in a better understanding of human anatomy and physiology. The early work of Morgagni, Le Dran, and Da Salva established that there was an initial period of local tumor growth prior to distant dissemination. This led to the understanding that not all tumors spread systemically and that certain malignancies cause death solely by local invasive growth. Percival Pott (1714-1788) was the first to describe a specific etiologic factor associated with cancer development. In 1775, Pott demonstrated a high incidence of cancer of the scrotum in chimney sweeps who had reached puberty and recommended wide local resection for cure. In 1829, the French Surgeon Joseph Recamier (1774-1852) first described the complicated process of tumor dissemination. The first recorded elective tumor resection was performed in 1809 by Ephraim McDowell, an American surgeon. He successfully removed a 22-pound ovarian tumor from a patient, who subsequently survived 30 years. McDowell's work, which included 12 more ovarian resections, stimulated greater interest in elective surgery for cancer patients.

Surgeons were initially hindered by the extreme discomfort that patients experienced during surgical procedures as well as the lack of agents that could reduce the incidence of infection. Crawford Long (1815-1878) was the first to use ether for general anesthesia in 1842, but it was the reported work of John Collins Warren (1778-1856) and William T.G. Morton (1819-1868) that brought the potential of anesthesia to public attention. The surgical procedure in Warren's first published account of ether anesthesia (1846) was the elective removal of a tongue carcinoma for which submaxillary gland resection and partial glossectomy were performed. Warren was also responsible for the first American-authored textbook of tumor surgery, *Surgical Observations on Tumors*, published in 1838. Joseph Lister (1827-1912) was the first to report the successful use of antisepsis during elective surgery. In 1867, Lister applied Pasteur's concept that bacteria caused infection, when he introduced the use of carbolic acid as an antiseptic agent in conjunction with heat sterilization of surgical instruments. Lister is also credited with the introduction of absorbable ligatures as well as the placement of drainage tubes to control secretions and dead space in surgical wounds.

Even with the advent of antisepsis and general anesthesia, surgical oncology in the second half of the 19th and early 20th centuries was still associated with high mortality rates. Cancer was rarely diagnosed in the early stages; consequently, few patients were considered candidates for curative surgery. Those surgeons who did attempt surgical excision of malignant lesions were hindered by rudimentary anesthesia, which was also independently associated with high patient mortality. Antibiotics were not yet available, and surgical instruments were crude. The importance of the microscope to evaluate frozen tissues for surgical margins was not yet appreciated, and surgeons had great faith in their own unaided gross visual assessment of the tumor perimeter. However, several important developments in this era led to rapid advancements in surgical oncology. Emphasizing meticulous surgical technique, gentle tissue handling, and applications of listerian principles, pioneers such as Albert Theodore Billroth (first gastrectomy, laryngectomy, and esophagectomy), William Stewart Halsted (en bloc resection, radical mastectomy), and many other more contemporary surgeons defined and advanced the boundaries of surgical oncology (Table 40-1).[3,4]

Ongoing innovations to advance effective surgical primary tumor control have improved surgical outcomes and quality of life. Advances in microvascu-

Table 40-1 **Landmark Advances in Surgical Oncology**

Year	Event	Surgeon
1775	Etiologic basis of cancer	Percival Pott
1809	Elective oophorectomy	Ephraim McDowell
1829	Metastatic process	Joseph Recamier
1846	Ether as anesthesia	John Collins Warren
1867	Carbolic acid as antisepsis	Joseph Lister
1873	Laryngectomy	Albert Theodore Billroth
1878	Resection of rectal tumor	Richard von Volkman
1880	Esophagectomy	Albert Theodore Billroth
1881	Gastrectomy	Albert Theodore Billroth
1890	Radical mastectomy	William Stewart Halsted
1896	Oophorectomy for breast cancer	G.T. Beatson
1904	Radical prostatectomy	Hugh H. Young
1906	Radical hysterectomy	Ernest Wertheim
1908	Abdominoperineal resection	W. Ernest Miles
1909	Thyroid surgery (Nobel Prize)	Theodore Emil Kocher
1910	Craniotomy	Harvey Cushing
1912	Cordotomy for the treatment of pain	E. Martin
1913	Thoracic esophagectomy	Franz Torek
1927	Resection of pulmonary metastases	George Divis
1933	Pneumonectomy	Evarts Graham
1935	Pancreaticoduodenectomy	Allen O. Whipple
1945	Adrenalectomy for prostate cancer	Charles B. Huggins
1957	Isolated limb perfusion	Oliver Creech
1958	Organization of National Adjuvant Breast and Bowel Project (NSABP) to conduct prospective randomized trials	Bernard Fisher
1965	Hormonal therapy of cancer	Charles Huggins
1971	Free tissue transfer with microvascular anastomosis	Harry Buncke

lar surgery now permit the free transfer of complex autologous tissues, such as free jejunal grafts to reconstitute the upper aerodigestive system or osteomyocutaneous flaps to reconstruct extremities and other mobile body parts such as the jaw. Automatic stapling devices as well as laparoscopic instrumentation coupled with high-resolution optics have remarkably advanced minimally invasive cancer surgery resulting in less-morbid procedures that require significantly less patient discomfort and recuperation time (Fig. 40-1). Improvements in preoperative optimization of cormorbid disease and advances in perioperative critical care have made it possible to safely undertake increasingly complicated surgical procedures. A more sophisticated awareness of the patterns of tumor spread has also resulted in increasing opportunities for less-invasive surgical approaches. One example is the use of lymphatic mapping and sentinel node biopsy instead of formal lymphadenectomy in early-stage melanoma and breast carcinoma. In other cases, this better understanding of recurrence risk has led to more not less extensive surgical resections. An example of this includes the selected use of total hepatectomy and orthotopic liver transplantation for early-stage hepatocellular carcinoma.

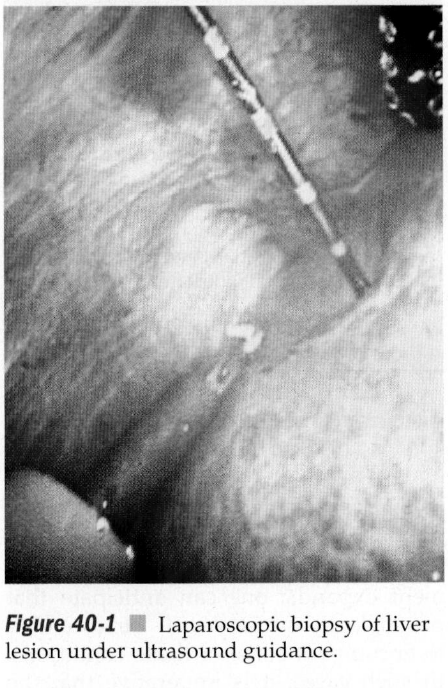

Figure 40-1 ■ Laparoscopic biopsy of liver lesion under ultrasound guidance.

Surgical Oncology in the Modern Era

Surgical oncologists are surgeons who devote most of their time to the study and treatment of malignant neoplastic disease. They must possess the necessary knowledge, skills, and clinical experience to perform both the standard and extraordinary surgical procedures required for patients with cancer. Surgical oncologists must be able to diagnose tumors accurately and to differentiate aggressive neoplastic lesions from benign reactive processes. In addition, surgical oncologists should have a firm understanding of radiation oncology, medical oncology as well as diagnostic and interventional radiology. They must also be capable of organizing interdisciplinary studies of cancer. Surgical oncologists should also be trained in pathology because they will be called on to excise appropriate tumor samples for pathologists and make decisions about adequacy of surgical margins. Surgical oncologists should have a shared role with medical oncologists as the "primary care physicians" of cancer treatment. Almost all cancer patients will initially be managed by one of these two specialists, who will bear the ultimate responsibility for coordinating appropriate multimodality care for the individual patient.

Given the complexity of contemporary multidisciplinary approaches to the cancer patient, cancer centers have developed facilities to provide the needed planning expertise, clinical care, patient support services, and access points to clinical trials. Comprehensive cancer centers are often affiliated with academic medical institutions and offer the complete spectrum of oncology therapies, clinical trials, rehabilitation, and social services as well as basic and translational research programs to move new knowledge from the laboratory bench to the patient bedside. In this contemporary understanding of the continuum of care of the cancer patient, the role of the surgical oncologist is taking on an ever-increasing importance.

Surgical oncology is more of a cognitive than a technical surgical specialty. With the exception of a small cluster of index operations, such as pancreatectoduodenectomy, limb salvage, retroperitoneal sarcoma surgery, isolated limb perfusion, and complex liver resection, most of the surgical procedures that are performed by surgical oncologists are similar to those performed by surgeons who are not oncologically trained. What frequently differentiates these two types of surgeons is not mere knowledge about how to do a specific operation but an awareness of how and when to do that operation; ie, the cognitive knowledge of contemporary multimodality cancer care. A broad knowledge of cancer in its presenting and recurring forms as well as an awareness of the mechanisms driving tumor proliferation and dissemination is an integral part of the special cognitive database of the surgical oncologist.

As part of the larger surgical community, the surgical oncologist is a critical conduit for the dissemination of cancer information to colleagues in general surgery and other surgical specialties. This individual makes academic presentations at large surgical meetings, directs hospital-based tumor boards, and consults on behalf of individual cancer patients. Because of their leading role in the initial diagnosis of cancer, it is not surprising that surgical oncologists are also frequently in leadership roles in cancer prevention and screening programs. Nationally based multimodality clinical trial groups also depend on surgical oncology expertise in helping the trial design; establishing the criteria of surgical quality control; educating trial participants regarding standards of surgical care (including indications for procedures); and assisting in accurate data collection, analysis, and presentation of trial results.

Multidisciplinary Management

Pediatric oncologists pioneered the use of combined modality therapy (radiation in combination with chemotherapy and surgery) as effective management of childhood neoplasms. Control of localized retinoblastoma in children has been dramatically increased by using multimodality therapy. The cure rate for patients with Wilms tumor is 75% and if surgical therapy is followed by chemotherapy and, in some cases, radiation, by an increase of 40% over operation alone. Embryonal rhabdomyosarcoma responds best to combinations of radiation, chemotherapy, and operation. Until recently, the effectiveness of multimodality therapy was only occasionally demonstrable for adult neoplasms. A striking example is the approach to skeletal and soft-tissue sarcomas. Surgical therapy, the accepted method for local management of most skeletal and soft-tissue sarcomas of the extremities, is associated with frequent treatment failure if used alone. In the past, approximately 50% of patients with soft-tissue sarcomas and 80% of those with bone sarcomas eventually succumbed to distant metastases, even after amputation of the extremity bearing the primary tumor. Consequently, multimodality treatment regimens were developed to improve these results. Preoperative chemotherapy with intra-arterial doxorubicin followed by radiation resulted in extensive tumor cell necrosis in as many as 75% of patients.[5] The effectiveness of this preoperative therapy permitted local resection of the sarcoma and salvage of a viable functional extremity. Local recurrence rates were as low as with amputation, and long-term results were functionally and psychologically superior. In addition, there was no decrease in overall or disease-free survival rates. Multimodality therapy is also effective for other solid malignancies, including colorectal cancer. Specifically, clinical trials have demonstrated improved efficacy and higher sphincter-preservation rates with the use of neoadjuvant chemoradiation therapy for stage II or III rectal cancer. Multimodality therapy has also been demonstrated to improve resectability rates and long-term survival in patients with hepatic colorectal metastases.[6]

Unlike surgery and radiation therapy, systemic therapies, such as chemotherapy, immunotherapy, and hormonal therapy, are treatments that can kill tumor cells that have already metastasized to distant sites. These systemic modalities have a greater chance of cure in patients with minimal (or even subclinical) tumor burden as compared with those patients with clinically evident disease. Consequently, surgery and radiation therapy may be useful in decreasing a given patient's tumor burden thereby maximizing the impact of subsequent systemic approaches. Whether the goals of therapy should be cure or palliation depends on the stage of a specific cancer. If the cancer is localized without evidence of spread, it may be possible to eradicate the cancer and cure the patient. When the cancer has spread beyond the possibility of cure, the goal is to control symptoms and maintain maximum activity and quality of life for as long as possible. Patients are generally judged incurable if they have distant metastases or evidence of extensive local infiltration of critical structures adjacent to tumor. However, some patients are potentially curable even though they have distant metastases. Specifically, patients with solitary hepatic or pulmonary metastases may still be curable by resection, and patients with disseminated germ cell or gastrointestinal stromal tumor may still be cured using systemic therapy alone. Histologic proof of distant metastases should be obtained before the patient is deemed incurable. Occasionally, an exploratory celiotomy or thoracotomy may be necessary to determine the histology of ambiguous lesions in the lungs or liver. In rare situations, the clinical situation may point so overwhelmingly to distant metastases that the patient may be considered incurable without biopsy. For each anatomic site, there are certain local criteria that place the patient unequivocally in an incurable status, whereas other anatomic constraints may imply a poor prognosis but are not an absolute indication of incurability per se. In equivocal situations where extensive studies fail to demonstrate metastatic or incurable local extension, the patient deserves the benefit of the doubt and should be treated for cure.

The selection of therapeutic modalities depends not only on the type and extent of cancer but also on the patient's general condition and the presence of any comorbid conditions. For example, surgery may be contraindicated in a patient who has significant emphysema or liver failure. A patient with preexisting diabetes will be much more susceptible to the toxic effects of hormonal therapy with corticosteroids. Renal disease may increase the toxicity of some of the chemotherapeutic agents, such as cisplatin or ifosfamide. Extensive staging procedures may indicate that a tumor is localized to a primary site and/or regional lymph nodes and hence potentially curable by locoregional therapy. However, approximately 60% of localized malignant tumors ultimately recur, suggesting that many such patients must have had subclinical metastases at the time of initial diagnosis. The probability of cure may be improved if systemic approaches are coupled with local treatment. Chemotherapeutic drugs must be given when the number of tumor cells is low enough to permit their destruction at doses that can be tolerated by the patient. The opportunity for cure is most likely during the early stage of disease or immediately after surgery when the tumor burden has been minimized. Adjuvant chemotherapy has remarkably improved surgical results in some malignancies, primarily because of cytocidal effects on clinically undetectable malignant cells outside the operative field. Neoadjuvant chemotherapy that is initiated prior to local and regional treatments also can affect micrometastatic distant disease while significantly cytoreducing the primary tumor.

Classically, surgical extirpation has been first in the sequence of therapies for resectable solid malignancies, but increasing evidence suggests that it may be more effective when used later in the treatment plan. Chemotherapy and radiation therapy both work by first-order kinetics. However, because of tumor cell heterogeneity, it can be anticipated that resistant clones of viable neoplastic cells may persist in the primary tumor after these therapies. Such clonal heterogeneity is more likely in large tumors that are both poorly perfused by chemotherapeutic agents and are also relatively hypoxic and therefore resistant to radiation therapy. Because surgery works by zero-order kinetics, it effectively removes the local residual primary tumor cells that are resistant to these other modalities.

From a practical management standpoint, the use of chemotherapy prior to surgical therapy can provide useful prognostic information regarding response to therapy. Presence of response to neoadjuvant therapy can aid in the planning of additional postoperative adjuvant chemotherapy. In addition, earlier administration of systemic therapy addresses the potential occult micrometastatic disease. In some cases, preoperative therapy (or "conversion" therapy) can be used to downsize a tumor from an unresectable to resectable status (Fig. 40-2).

A

B

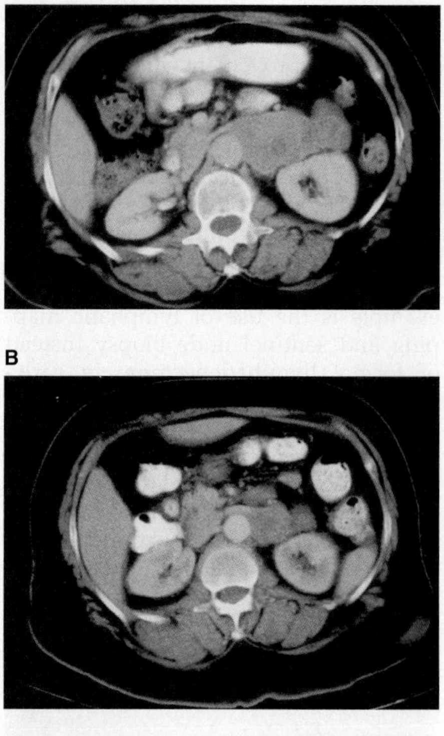

Figure 40-2 Downsizing of hepatic colorectal metastatic disease with preoperative chemotherapy **(A)** before treatment; **(B)** after 6 cycles of 5-fluorouracil/leucovorin and oxaliplatin. Note reduction in tumor size and regression from the left portal pedicle and hepatic veins. In addition, hypertrophy of the left liver occurred secondary to relative increased left portal blood flow.

Components of Surgical Management in the Care of the Cancer Patient

Surgical Prevention

As the role of genetic mutations that predispose to subsequent cancer development expands; one can anticipate that prophylactic surgery will be extended to encompass some of these conditions. In such cases, it is imperative that the surgical oncologist become intimately knowledgeable about the indications, limitations, and ethical considerations regarding genetic counseling, if only because it will be the responsibility of the surgeon to alert other family members at risk and arrange for appropriate testing. The above emerging indications are being added to an already established role for prophylactic surgery in the prevention of predisposing malignancies, including ulcerative colitis with dysplasia, familial adenomatous polyposis, multiple endocrine neoplasia syndromes, and hereditary breast cancer. Assessing the risk to benefit ratio of prophylactic surgery is critical but frequently inexact. The future advent of inexpensive and reliable genetic screening technologies, coupled with emerging insights derived from the new field of molecular epidemiology, should bring more definitive understanding of prophylactic surgery benefits in populations at risk.

Biopsy and Diagnosis

The diagnosis of solid tumors depends on locating and performing a biopsy of the lesion. The findings from biopsy specimens will be used to determine the histology and/or grade of a tumor, which is a prerequisite for planning definitive therapy. Significant therapeutic errors have been made when biopsy confirmation of malignancy was not obtained prior to treatment. Even when biopsy reports from another hospital are available, the slides of the previous biopsy must be obtained and reviewed prior to the institution of therapy. This is essential because all too often an erroneous interpretation may have been made in the initial pathology assessment.

Biopsy is easiest when the tumor is near the surface or involves an orifice that can be examined with appropriate visualizing instruments, such as the bronchoscope, colonoscope, or cystoscope. Carcinomas of the breast, tongue, or rectum can be seen or palpated and a portion can be excised for definitive diagnosis. In contrast, deep-seated lesions may grow to quite a large size before causing symptoms. Ultrasonography, computed tomography (CT), and magnetic resonance imaging (MRI) are all useful techniques for localizing such lesions at the time of invasive biopsy. However, although image-directed needle biopsy may be useful in some patients, exploratory surgery is occasionally required to obtain a definitive biopsy that establishes the exact histologic diagnosis. In some cases, tissue samples larger than that which is obtained by percutaneous biopsy may be required for tumor characterization, such as lymphoma, necessitating surgical biopsy. Fortunately, such procedures can now be frequently performed on an outpatient basis by using minimally invasive technology such as laparoscopic surgical approaches.

Three methods are commonly used to biopsy suspicious lesions: needle biopsy (fine needle aspiration or core), open incisional, or excisional biopsy. Regardless of the method used, the pathologic interpretation of the tumor mass will be valid only if a representative section of tumor is obtained. The surgical oncologist must be aware that a sampling error can occur with needle and incisional biopsies where only small portions of the total tumor mass are submitted for pathologic examination. It is the surgeon's task to provide adequate tissue for diagnosis. Orientation of the specimen, as may be necessary, is also the responsibility of the surgeon. It is axiomatic that adequate tissue can provide the basis for diagnosis by an adequate pathologist, whereas inadequate tissue will be insufficient for diagnosis by an adequate or inadequate pathologist.

Fine-needle aspiration (FNA) is a cytologic technique in which cells are aspirated from a tumor using a needle and syringe. The technique can be performed using image-directed guidance and is particularly helpful in the diagnosis of relatively inaccessible lesions such as deep visceral tumors. Because the aspirate consists of disaggregated cells rather than intact tissue, diagnosis of malignancy usually depends on detection of abnormal intracellular features, such as nuclear pleomorphism; thus the margin of error is higher than with other biopsy techniques. In addition, because of the lack of intact tumor architecture, FNA cannot distinguish invasive from noninvasive malignancy. Negative results do not rule out malignancy. Depending on the clinical context, such as distinguishing carcinoma in situ from an infiltrating malignancy, other types of biopsy may be more appropriate.

Core biopsy is the simplest method of histologic (as opposed to cytologic) diagnosis and may be useful for biopsy of subcutaneous masses and muscular masses as well as some internal organs, such as liver, kidney, and pancreas. The added benefit is that this method is inexpensive and causes minimal disturbance of the surrounding tissue. Cutting-core biopsies are performed with a large-bore needle, such as the Vim Silverman or Tru-Cut. This technique retrieves a small piece of intact tumor tissue, which allows the pathologist to study the invasive relationship between cancer cells and the surrounding microenvironment. The danger of implanting tumor cells in a needle track during biopsy is extremely small. This risk can be avoided altogether if the needle track is positioned so that it can be excised en bloc at the time of the definitive surgical procedure. Needle biopsy may be less appropriate if the specimen is small, which increases the likelihood of the needle missing the lesion or the biopsy not being representative of the entire tumor. Consequently, a needle biopsy report that is negative for malignant disease should be viewed with skepticism if it is inconsistent with the clinical presentation and should be followed by incisional or excisional biopsy.

Incisional biopsy for pathologic examination involves removal of a small portion of the tumor mass. It is best performed in circumstances where the incisional wound can be totally excised in continuity with the definitive surgical resection in the event that any tumor cells are spilled at the time of biopsy. Incisional biopsy is indicated for deeper subcutaneous or intramuscular tumor masses when initial needle biopsy fails to establish a diagnosis. An incisional biopsy is also appropriate when a tumor is so large that complete local excision would violate wide tissue planes and impair a subsequent wide local resection for curative purposes. If possible, an incisional biopsy should retrieve a deep section of tumor as well as a margin of normal tissue. Incisional biopsies suffer from the same disadvantages as needle biopsies in that the removed portion may not be representative of the entire tumor. Consequently, a negative biopsy does not preclude the possibility of cancer in the residual mass.

Excisional biopsy completely removes the mass of interest. It is used for small, discrete masses that are less than 3 cm in diameter, where complete removal will not interfere with a subsequent wider excision that may be required for definitive local control. Excisional biopsy allows the pathologist to examine the entire lesion. However, this method is contraindicated in large tumor masses because the biopsy procedure could scatter tumor cells throughout a large surgical field that would need to be widely and totally encompassed by the ultimate surgical resection. For this reason, excisional biopsy is usually contraindicated for skeletal and soft tissue masses when the diagnosis of sarcoma is being entertained. The excisional method is also used for polypoid lesions of the colon, for thyroid and breast nodules, lymph nodes, for small skin lesions, and when the pathologist cannot make a definitive diagnosis from tissue removed by incisional biopsy. An unbiopsied mass is also surgically removed when the suspicious character of the lesion, the need for its removal (whatever the diagnosis), and the nonmutilating nature of the operation render such an approach feasible. Examples of such procedures include hemithyroidectomy for thyroid nodules after an inconclusive FNA and a right hemicolectomy for a cecal mass that might be either inflammatory or neoplastic. In the latter instance, colonoscopic biopsy is informative only if positive for neoplasm. Surgeons should always mark the excisional biopsy margins with sutures or metal clips so that if removal is incomplete and further excision is needed the positive margin can be accurately identified in situ.

Orientation of biopsy incisions is also extremely important. Ill-conceived incisions can unnecessarily open up additional tissue planes, necessitating subsequent wider radiotherapy fields or more extensive ultimate surgical resections. For example, tumors of the extremities are best biopsied by using incisions that run parallel to the long axis of that limb. This facilitates a definitive en bloc resection that encompasses the biopsy track (Fig. 40-3). Biopsy incisions should be closed using meticulous hemostasis because a hematoma can lead to dissemination of tumor cells with contamination of tissue planes. Instruments, gloves, gowns, and drapes should be discarded and replaced with unused substitutes if the definitive surgical resection immediately follows the biopsy procedure.

Lymph nodes should be carefully selected for biopsy. Axillary nodes may be preferable to groin nodes if both are enlarged because of a decreased likelihood of postoperative infection. Other caveats are also noteworthy. For example, lymph node specimens preserved in formaldehyde cannot be analyzed for cytogenetics or flow cytometric immunophenotyping. The laboratory work-up for lymphoma usually requires unfixed sterile tissue. Cervical lymph nodes should not be biopsied until a careful search for a primary tumor has been made using nasopharyngoscopy, esophagoscopy, and bronchoscopy because enlargement of the upper cervical nodes by metastases is usually caused by laryngeal, oropharyngeal, and nasopharyngeal primary neoplasms. In contrast, supraclavicular nodes are more frequently enlarged as a result of metastases from primary tumors of the thoracic or abdominal cavities or breast.

The tumor specimen may be prepared for pathologic examination by either frozen or permanent sections. Frozen sections are made at the time of biopsy, and pathologic diagnosis can typically be obtained within 10 min. Frozen sections are used when the diagnosis is required to assess resectability at the time of major surgery or to check tumor margins intraoperatively. Frozen-section biopsy-proven carcinomatosis may mandate abandoning a procedure with a curative intent in favor of a palliative approach. Occasionally, mediastinoscopy, laparoscopy (peritoneoscopy), thoracoscopy, exploratory thoracotomy, or even laparotomy is necessary to obtain adequate representative tissue samples for microscopic examination to confirm diagnosis or tumor stage.

Staging

Tumor staging is a system used to describe the anatomic extent of a specific malignant process in an individual patient. Staging systems cluster relevant prognostic factors about the primary tumor, such as size, grade, and location, as well as information about dissemination to regional sites, such as lymph nodes or distant metastatic sites. Accurately staging a cancer is essential in designing an appropriate therapeutic program and advising on prognosis. Without accurate staging, it is impossible to meaningfully compare the results of therapies administered in different centers. New forms of therapy can be appropriately evaluated only by comparing the impact of current therapy of neoplasms of equivalent stage.

The recognized importance of staging has led to a variety of international and national attempts to standardize the staging of the patient with cancer. To date, no single system has been universally accepted. The American Joint Committee on Cancer (AJCC) has recommended a staging system ranging from stage I (small, localized malignancy) to stage IV (distant metastatic spread).[7] Both the AJCC and the Union Internationale Contre Cancer (International Union Against Cancer, UICC) have adopted a shared TNM system that defines a cancer in terms of the primary tumor (T), the presence or absence of nodal metastases (N), and the presence or absence of distant metastases (M). Increasing numerals after the T, such as T1, T2, T3, or T4, indicate lesions of increasing size or depth of penetration that are usually associated with a poorer prognosis. The absence of nodal metastasis is designated as N0, the presence of nodal metastasis is N1, and for more extensive nodal involvement, additional numbers may be used. Finally, distant metastases are indicated by adding the numeral 1 following M for metastases, or the numeral 0 signifying their absence. Thus, a small lesion that has neither spread to regional nodes nor metastasized to distant sites would be designated as T1 N0 M0. A larger lesion that involved regional nodes but not distant sites might be identified as T2 N1 M0. A large neoplasm associated with both regional and distant metastases would be designated T3 N1 M1. For some tumor types, such as soft tissue sarcoma, a G for grade of malignancy is added. High-grade tumors are less differentiated and tend to metastasize more readily.

The TNM system has four chronologic classifications. The clinical classification (cTNM or TNM) represents the extent of the disease prior to first definitive treatment as determined from physical examination, imaging studies, endoscopy, biopsy, surgical exploration, and any other relevant findings. The pathologic classification (pTNM) incorporates the additional information available

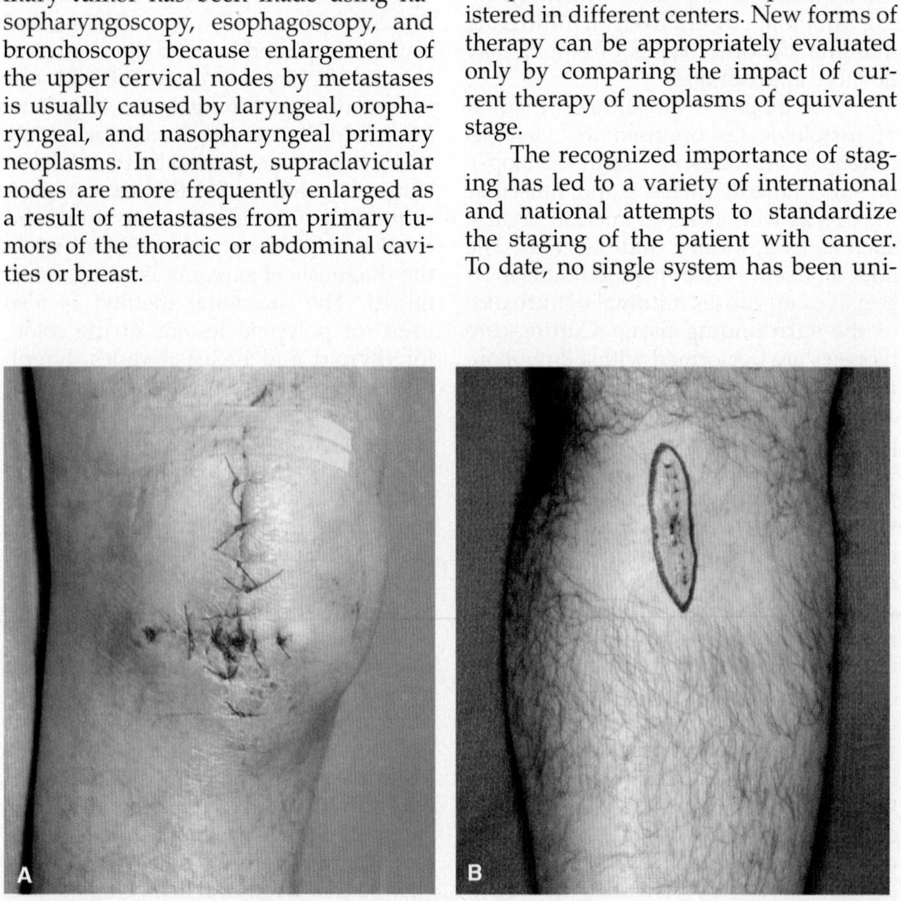

Figure 40-3 ■ Appropriate and inappropriate biopsy incisions. **(A)** A patient with a cruciate-shaped biopsy scar overlying the patellar tendon that contained a synovial sarcoma. Note the erythema in this infected incision. This ill-conceived biopsy scar would have required a wide-field soft tissue and osseous composite resection to encompass all of the violated tissue planes. Unfortunately, tumor was *intruded* into the joint space at the time of this biopsy, and this patient ultimately required an above-knee amputation to treat this small, otherwise limb-salvageable sarcoma. **(B)** An appropriately oriented incisional biopsy scar in the lower extremity. Note the alignment of the scar parallel with the long axis of the extremity and the meticulous placement of small biopsy wound sutures. The entire scar could be excised at surgery (blue ellipse) with minimal concomitant normal tissue sacrifice.

at the time of surgery or derived from pathologic examination of a completely resected specimen. This is especially useful in planning adjuvant therapy. The retreatment classification (rTNM) is used to stage a cancer that has recurred after a disease-free interval; it includes clinical and/or pathologic evidence of recurrence. Finally, the autopsy classification (aTNM) is based on postmortem examination.

Patterns of Tumor Spread

In general, a malignant tumor may spread (1) by direct extension into surrounding structures, (2) via the lymphatics, (3) by hematogenous spread, or (4) by implantation in serous cavities. However, many cancers spread by more than one route, and an orderly course of metastasis is not predictably certain. For example, patients with breast cancer or melanoma can manifest distant metastatic disease in the lungs, liver, or skeleton without ever developing evidence of lymph node metastases. Table 40-2 summarizes the metastatic patterns of various human tumors.

Table 40-2 Patterns of Neoplastic Spread for Common Human Malignancies

Neoplasms	Hematogenous	Lymphatic	Local Infiltration (Expressed as Local Recurrence)
Adenocarcinoma			
Breast	++++	+++	++
Endometrium	+	++	+
Ovary	++	+++	++++
Stomach	++++	++++	+++
Pancreas	++++	++++	+++
Colon	+++	+++	+
Kidney	++	++	++
Prostate	+++	+++	+++
Liver	+	+	++++
Epidermal carcinoma			
Lung	++++	+++	++
Oropharynx	++	+++	+++
Larynx	+	+++	++
Cervix	+	++++	+++
Transitional cell carcinoma			
Bladder	++	+++	++++
Cutaneous neoplasm			
Squamous cell carcinoma	+	++	+
Melanoma	+++	+++	++
Basal cell carcinoma	0	0	+
Sarcoma			
Bone	++++	+	+
Soft tissue	++++	+	+++
Brain neoplasm	0	0	++++

Key: Does not occur; 0, <1%; +, 1-5%; ++, 15–+++0%; 3, 30%; ++++, 50%.

Cancer cells may also spread by direct extension through tissue spaces and planes. Some neoplasms, such as soft tissue sarcomas and adenocarcinomas of the stomach or esophagus, may extend for a considerable distance (10-15 cm) along tissue planes beyond the palpable tumor mass. Other neoplasms, such as a basal cell carcinoma of skin, rarely extend for more than a few millimeters beyond the visible margin. Even though most central nervous system (CNS) tumors infrequently metastasize, they may penetrate nearby brain tissue, and their location can cause death by interfering with vital CNS functions.

Tumor cells can readily enter the lymphatics and extend through these channels by permeation or embolization to regional lymph nodes. Permeation is the growth of a colony of tumor cells along the course of the lymphatic vessel. This commonly occurs in the skin lymphatics in carcinoma of the breast and in the perineural lymphatics in carcinoma of the prostate. Lymphatic involvement is extremely common in malignant epithelial neoplasms of all types, except basal cell carcinoma of the skin, which metastasizes to regional lymphatics in less than 0.1% of cases, or mesenchymal neoplasms, such as sarcomas, which metastasize to lymph nodes in only 2-5% of cases.

Spread along the lymphatics by embolization to regional or distant lymph nodes is of great clinical importance. Tumor cells travel within local lymphatics and can spread to proximal nodal basins via the collateral lymphatic channels. Lymph node metastases are first confined to the subcapsular space; at this stage, the node is not enlarged and may appear grossly normal. Gradually, the tumor cells permeate the sinusoids and replace the nodal parenchyma, changing the shape and texture of the node. There is little direct spread from node to node because the nodal capsule is not penetrated until a late stage. However, when an involved lymph node is more than 3 cm in diameter, tumor has usually extended beyond the capsule into the perinodal fat.

Lymph from the abdominal organs and lower extremities drains into the cisterna chyli and then into the thoracic duct, which finally opens into the left jugular vein. By using this route, tumor cells can pass freely from the lymphatic system into the bloodstream. Oncologists originally believed that solid neoplasms first involved regional lymph nodes and then spread into the bloodstream by drainage into the thoracic duct and then to other parts of the body. An alternative explanation now favored by most oncologists assumes that the presence of cancer cells in regional lymph nodes indicates an unfavorable host–tumor relationship and the concomitant high likelihood of distant metastases.

Cancer cells may reach the bloodstream either through the thoracic duct or by direct invasion of blood vessels. Capillaries offer no resistance to tumor cell transgression. Small veins are frequently invaded, whereas thicker-walled arteries are rarely violated. Veins frequently form a plexus extending to the subendothelial regions, which provide a portal of entry through the thin vein wall. When the vascular endothelium is destroyed, a thrombus can form that is quickly invaded by tumor. This combination of thrombus and tumor may detach to form large tumor emboli. Vascular invasion is common in both carcinomas and sarcomas and is associated with a poor prognosis. Some types of neoplasms have a remarkable tendency to grow as a solid column along the course of veins. For example, renal cell carcinoma can grow into the renal vein and up the inferior vena cava extending to the right atrium. In this situation, a spectacular en bloc removal requiring cardiopulmonary bypass may still result in long-term survival or even cure.

Tumor cells occasionally gain entrance to serous cavities by growing through the wall of an organ. Many tumor cells can grow in suspension without a supporting matrix and may widely spread within the peritoneal cavity or attach to serous surfaces. Thus, widespread peritoneal seeding is common with gastrointestinal and ovarian cancers. Similarly, malignant gliomas may spread widely within the CNS via the cerebrospinal fluid.

Although much is known about the routes of tumor spread, the mechanisms underlying this process remain unclear. Some cancers are metastatic at the time of clinical discovery, whereas others of the same type and in the same organ tissue may remain localized for years. Metastases may dominate the presenting clinical picture although the primary tumor remains latent and asymptomatic or even undetectable. For example, cerebral metastases from silent cancers in the bronchus or the breast are often mistaken for primary benign CNS neoplasms.

Preoperative Preparation

Preparation of a patient for surgical cancer therapy is important in order to minimize perioperative complications, hasten recovery to premorbid state of health, and avoid delay in possible initiation of postoperative adjuvant therapy. Every effort should be made to correct nutritional deficiencies if present, restore depleted blood volume, and correct electrolyte imbalances prior to extensive surgical procedures. Total parenteral nutrition (TPN) can be used to prepare the malnourished patient for a major operation, although reconstitution is a slow process, and TPN may chiefly serve to interrupt further deterioration by restoring positive nitrogen balance. Surgical morbidity and mortality following extensive cancer operations will predictably be problematic if critical physiologic and biochemical deficiencies are not corrected in advance.

Determining the risk inherent in a given operation is a complicated and inexact assessment based on a number of factors. The physical status of the patient, including cardiopulmonary reserve, comorbid conditions, debility inherent to a specific operation, hepatic and renal function, and the intent of surgical procedure (curative vs palliative) are all pertinent to this assessment. The technical complexity of an operation, the type of anesthetic used, and the relative experience of the involved health care personnel can all impact on the complications of a procedure. Various schema for risk assessment, such as the five-level physical status classification of the American Society of Anesthesiologists (Table 40-3) and the Eastern Cooperative Oncology Group Five-Step Performance Scale (Table 40-4) may be useful in assessing the appropriateness of a given operation for a specific patient.

Operative mortality is defined as mortality that occurs within 30 days of an operative procedure. In cancer patients, the underlying disease is a major determinant of operative mortality. Although it is true that comparable operations are usually more morbid in the geriatric age group as compared with other adults, advanced age per se should not disqualify a patient from a potentially curative surgical procedure. Because of their high-risk nature, decisions about the indications for palliative surgical procedures are particularly difficult. For example, palliative surgery for extensive metastatic disease or symptomatic intestinal obstruction secondary to carcinomatosis has a 20- 30% perioperative mortality. In such circumstances, the risk to benefit ratio and ultimate surgical objectives must be defined as clearly as possible and accepted by patient, family, and surgeon.

Preoperative chemotherapy and or radiation therapy is being administered with increasing frequency in patients undergoing cancer operations. In some cases, these therapies can be associated with increased perioperative complications. For example, the antivascular endothelial growth factor antibody bevacizumab is associated with increased risk of wound healing complications when administered within several weeks before surgery.[8] As this targeted therapy has a 21-day half-life, discontinuation of bevacizumab is recommended at least 6-8 weeks prior to elective surgery.

Table 40-3 American Society of Anesthesiologists: Physical Status Classification

Class	Description
P-1	A normal healthy patient
P-2	A patient with mild systemic disease
P-3	A patient with severe systemic disease
P-4	A patient with severe systemic disease that is a constant threat to life
P-5	A moribund patient who is not expected to survive without the operation
P-6	A declared brain-dead patient whose organs are being removed for donor purposes

Source: Modified from Saklad M. Grading of patients for surgical procedures. *Anesthesiology*. 1941;2:281.

Table 40-4 Eastern Cooperative Oncology Group: Performance Scale and Corresponding Karnofsky Rating

Grade	Description
0	Fully active, able to carry on all predisease activities without restriction (Karnofsky 100)
1	Restricted in physically strenuous activity but ambulatory and able to carry out work of a light or sedentary nature, eg, light housework/office work (Karnofsky 80-90)
2	Ambulatory and capable of all self-care but unable to carry out any work activities; up and about more than 50% of waking hours (Karnofsky 60-70)
3	Capable of limited self-care; confined to bed or chair 50% or more of waking hours (Karnofsky 40-50)
4	Completely disabled; cannot carry on any self-care; totally confined to bed or chair (Karnofsky 30 or less)

Operative Considerations

Once a decision has been made to proceed with surgical therapy, the operative procedure itself must be carefully planned for the specific surgical patient. It is essential to realize that the best (and often the only) opportunity for cure is with the first resection, at the time of initial tissue plane, lymphatic, and blood vessel potential exposure to tumor cells that may be dislodged within the operative field. A subsequent recurrence may be difficult to distinguish from the normal postsurgical inflammatory reaction and scarring.

The principle of the "no touch technique" has maintained some traction in the surgical lore. This opinion is based on the theoretical concept that direct contact with and manipulation of the tumor during resection can lead to an increased risk in local implantation and embolization of tumor cells. Although little clinical evidence exists to support this principle, there may be some validity to this concept with respect to tumors that extend directly into the vascular system, such as hepatocellular or renal tumors with extension to the large veins or vena cava. Although not definitively proven to be detrimental, the general tenet of avoidance of forceful handling of the tumor and care to avoid any tumor disruption during surgical resection is sound technique.

Types of Cancer Operations

Wide local resection with removal of an adequate margin of normal peritumoral tissue may be adequate treatment of low-grade neoplasms that very rarely metastasize to regional nodes or widely infiltrate adjacent tissues. Basal cell carcinomas and mixed tumors of the parotid gland are examples of such tumors. In contrast, neoplasms that spread widely by infiltration into adjacent tissues, such as soft tissue sarcomas and esophageal and gastric carcinomas, must be excised with a wide margin of normal tissue. This wide tissue margin between the line of excision and the tumor mass may also act as a protective barrier against intraoperative tumor cell traversal into severed lymphatics and vessels. Tumor cells may have been implanted in the incision when an incisional biopsy alone had been previously performed. To encompass potentially contaminated tissues, it is extremely important to remove a wide segment of skin and underlying muscle, fat, and fascia beyond the limits of the original incision.

Malignant neoplasms are usually not truly encapsulated. The tumor is commonly encased by a pseudocapsule comprising a compression zone of normal tissue interspersed with neoplastic cells. This pseudoencapsulation offers a great temptation for simple enucleation in that the tumor may be easily dislodged from its bed. However, this approach must be resisted because microscopic extensions of tumor from the primary through the pseudocapsule will be left behind after simple enucleation, dooming the patient to a local recurrence. Ideally, the surgeon should operate through normal tissues at all times and never encounter or even directly visualize the neoplasm during its removal. Dissection should proceed with meticulous care to avoid tumor cell spillage. Many neoplasms metastasize via the lymphatics, and operations have been designed to remove the primary neoplasm and draining regional lymph nodes in continuity with all intervening tissues. Circumstances favor this type of operative approach when the lymph nodes draining the neoplasm lie adjacent to the tumor bed or when there is a single avenue of lymphatic drainage that can be removed without sacrificing vital structures. It is important to avoid cutting across involved lymphatic channels, which markedly increases the possibility of local recurrence.

At the present time, it is generally agreed that en bloc regional lymph node dissection is indicated for clinically demonstrable nodal involvement with metastatic tumor. However, in many cases, the tumor has already spread beyond regional nodes. Although the cure rates following resection in such circumstances may be quite low (20-50%), undue pessimism should not prevent such patients from receiving appropriate surgical treatment. En bloc removal of the involved lymph nodes may offer the only chance for cure and can at least provide significant palliative local control. Regional lymph node involvement should therefore not be viewed as a contraindication to surgery but as a possible indication for adjuvant therapies, such as radiation or chemotherapy.

The routine dissection of regional nodes in close proximity to the primary malignancy is recommended for most cancer types even when these structures are not clinically involved with tumor. This recommendation is based on the high rate of locoregional recurrence following surgical resection when multiple lymph nodes are microscopically involved and the high error rate when palpation alone is used to assess possible lymph node involvement with tumor. Microscopic tumor dissemination to regional lymph nodes can be detected in 20-40% of clinically node-negative carcinomas and melanomas.

The extent of lymph node dissection remains controversial. Sentinel lymphadenectomy is now a well-established technique for detection of early nodal disease in selected tumor types. First introduced by Morton et al for melanoma,[9] it is now being applied as well for the management of breast carcinoma[10] and other neoplasms.[11] Initially, the technique relied on the injection of a vital blue dye at the tumor site and visual tracking of this dye along the lymphatics draining to the nodal basin, sentinel node mapping has been facilitated by adding a radiolabeled isotope to the dye and monitoring its path using a handheld gamma probe.[12] Sentinel lymphadenectomy is a low-morbidity procedure that accurately stages the regional lymph nodes and identifies the 60-80% of melanoma and breast cancer patients who do not require complete lymphadenectomy.

Advances in surgical technique, anesthesia, and supportive care (blood transfusion, antibiotics, and fluid and electrolyte management) permit the more radical, extensive, and lengthy operative procedures to be done more safely. Such procedures offer a chance for a cure that cannot be achieved by other means and are justified in selected situations, if there is no evidence of distant metastases. For example, some slow-growing primary tumors may reach an enormous size and widely infiltrate locally without metastasizing to distant sites. Supraradical operative procedures should be considered for these extensive and nearly inoperable tumors because the occasional patient is cured. However, such operations should be undertaken only by experienced surgeons who can select those patients most likely to benefit. As an example of carefully indicated radical surgery, pelvic exenteration is a well-conceived operation capable of curing patients with radiation-treated recurrent cancer of the cervix and certain well-differentiated and locally extensive adenocarcinomas of the rectum. This operation removes all pelvic organs (bladder, uterus, and rectum) and soft tissues within the pelvis. Bowel function is restored with colostomy. Urinary tract drainage is established by anastomosis of the ureters into a segment of the bowel (ileum or sigmoid colon). The 5-year relapse-free survival is 25% when pelvic exenteration is used to manage these problems. It is also imperative that the surgical oncologist be willing to accept responsibility for helping to optimize the postoperative emotional and psychological rehabilitation of the patient prior to embarking on extensive resections, such as hemipelvectomy, forequarter amputation, mutilating operations for head and neck carcinomas, or total pelvic exenteration.

Although logic might suggest that once a neoplasm has metastasized to a distant site, it is no longer curable by surgical resection, experience shows otherwise. The removal of metastatic deposits within in the liver, lung, or other sites can occasionally result in log-term cure. In others, often with favorable biology and good response to systemic chemotherapy, metastatectomy can significantly prolong survival beyond that of chemotherapy alone, not infrequently turning advanced disease into a chronic condition. Prior to undertaking resection, an extensive work-up should be performed to rule out metastatic spread to other body sites outside of the proposed operative field.

Some patients with liver-only metastases may benefit from surgical resection, particularly when of colorectal origin. Advances in preoperative evaluation, surgical technique, and systemic therapies have all contributed to an increasingly aggressive approach to such patients. Although in the past, resectability was defined by the number, size, and distribution of hepatic metastases, more recently, resectability is defined by the capability to resect all disease with negative margins (R0) and have a sufficient functional remnant liver, regardless of the tumor number. Even patients with limited and resectable extrahepatic disease combined with liver metastases may be candidates for surgical therapy provided all disease can be safely removed. Moreover, when not initially optimally resectable, approaches to (1) reduce tumor size with preoperative chemotherapy, (2) expand the remnant liver with preoperative portal vein embolization or staged liver resections, or (3) application of thermal ablative approaches at time combined with resection, all can contribute to increasing the number of patients eligible for surgical therapy of liver metastases. Even with increasingly aggressive approaches, contemporary series are reporting 5-year survival rates following complete resection in excess of 50%.[6,13]

Surgical procedures are sometimes indicated to palliate symptoms without attempting to cure the patient, thereby prolonging a useful and comfortable life. A palliative operation may be justified to relieve pain, hemorrhage, obstruction, or infection when it can be done without untoward risk to the patient. Palliative surgery may also be applicable when there are no better nonsurgical means of palliation or when the procedure will improve the quality of life, even if it does not result in prolonged survival.

In contrast, surgery that only prolongs a miserable existence is not of benefit to the patient. Examples of indicated palliative surgical procedures include (1) colostomy, enteroenterostomy, or gastrojejunostomy to relieve intestinal obstruction; (2) cordotomy or celiac block to control pain; (3) hepaticojejunostomy to relieve biliary obstruction and pruritis; (4) amputation for intractably painful tumors of the extremities; (5) simple mastectomy for carcinoma of the breast, when the tumor is infected, large, ulcerated, and locally resectable (even in the presence of distant metastases); and (6) resection of obstructing colon cancer in the presence of disseminated metastatic disease. Surgery for residual disease is a special application of palliative surgery. In some patients, extensive yet isolated local spread of malignancy precludes gross total resection of all disease. In these patients, cytoreductive surgery may be of benefit, such as biologically indolent disease or that which is producing local or hormonal symptoms such as metastatic neuroendocrine tumors.

Problems with exsanguinating hemorrhage, perforated viscus, abscess formation, or impending obstruction of a hollow viscus, such as gastrointestinal organs, critical blood vessels, or respiratory structures, are sometimes amenable to emergency surgical intervention. Emergency surgery may also be indicated to decompress tumors that are invading the CNS or that are destroying critical neurologic components by exerting pressure in closed spaces. The cancer patient being evaluated for emergency surgery may be neutropenic or thrombocytopenic as a consequence of recent myelosuppressive chemotherapy. Sometimes a potential catastrophe can be avoided by operating on such patients expectantly just after they have gone through the nadir of their most recent myelosuppressive chemotherapy. Because of the high risks involved, each patient and the patient's family must be made aware of the dangers and benefits of the proposed surgery, as well as of other potentially effective treatments that might be available if the patient survives this emergency operation.

Reconstructive surgery after tumor resection has remarkably improved the quality of life for many cancer patients. The routine application of microvascular anastomotic techniques has enabled the free transfer of composite grafts containing skin, muscle, and/or bone to surgically created bodily defects. Breast reconstruction after mastectomy, tissue transfers as part of extremity surgery for sarcoma or mandible reconstruction, and aerodigestive reconstruction using jejunal-free grafts are examples of these dramatic improvements in the combined surgical management of complex cancer problems. In the future, applications of the new discipline of tissue engineering will remarkably extend the reconstructive armamentarium. Using these approaches in the future, it may be possible to custom-grow nerve, fat, muscle, bone cartilage, or other body components as replacements for tissues that will need to be resected as part of a composite cancer procedure.[14]

The Future of Surgical Oncology

Within the next decade, cancer is predicted to replace cardiovascular disease as the leading cause of death among Americans. The aging of the population will generate an enormous growth in demand for oncological procedures. By 2020, the number of patients undergoing oncological procedures is projected to increase by 24-51% (Table 40-5).[15] If a shortage of surgeons performing these procedures does occur, the result will inevitably be decreased access to care. To prevent this from happening, the ability of surgeons to cope with an increased burden of work needs to be critically evaluated and improved. Given that there are no more than approximately 50 surgical oncologists produced yearly in the United States, it is clear that the traditional surgical oncology educational roles in academic medical centers as well as in the larger health care community will continue and perhaps come under increasing pressure to expand.

As multimodality care grows in complexity and chemotherapy/radiotherapy move more prominently into the neoadjuvant position, surgical oncologists will have to become increasingly involved in clinical trial design. To be effective in this arena, understanding the natural history of specific malignancies will require an expanded knowledge base about the mutated genes and their cognate proteins that drive solid-tumor proliferation and metastasis. Surgical oncologists will have to become more knowledgeable about these factors, both during training and as a lifelong commitment to self education.

An important effort underway to strengthen the position of surgical oncology in medical community is the possibility of establishing board certification in surgical oncology. The past half-century has seen the unprecedented evolution of surgical specialties into their current status as discrete disciplines, with specialized knowledge, techniques, anatomic challenges, and diseases of focus. This is especially true in surgical oncology, which has attracted many owing to its strong allure as a combination of the technical and the cognitive. There is an emerging understanding that the surgical oncologist has specialized knowledge that is not acquired in general surgical training: knowledge of the natural history of malignant disease, knowledge of multidisciplinary care for the cancer patient, and certainly, knowledge of how to perform some very unusual and technically demanding oncological operative procedures. These factors, coupled with an awareness of the rapidly increasing manpower need, have led to an active interest in creating a board certification mechanism for surgical oncology. Board certification would strengthen the position and impact of surgical oncologists practicing in the community and might also aid in the development of comparable certification mechanisms in other countries.

TABLE 40-5 ■ Projected Numbers of Surgical Oncological Procedures: 2010 to 2020

Variable	2000[a]	2010[b]	2020[b]	Increase (2000–2020)
Breast (diagnostic)	364,800	416,100 (14.1%)	464,100 (27.2%)	99,300
Breast (excisions)	392,700	440,200 (12.1%)	485,600 (23.7%)	92,900
Outpatient total	757,500	856,300 (13.0%)	949,700 (25.4%)	192,200
Breast (mastectomy)	90,400	106,000 (17.3%)	123,700 (36.8%)	33,300
Colon resection	96,300	113,700 (18.1%)	141,100 (46.5%)	44,800
Rectal resection	27,800	33,300 (19.7%)	40,900 (47.0%)	13,100
Stomach resection	9400	11,100 (17.6%)	13,700 (45.1%)	4300
Pancreas resection	3900	4700 (19.7%)	5800 (47.4%)	1900
Esophageal resection	1400	1700 (24.0%)	2100 (51.2%)	700
Inpatient total	229,200	270,500 (18.0%)	327,100 (42.7%)	97,900

[a] Figures listed for inpatient procedures in 2000 are the numbers of procedures performed that year, based on NIS 2000. Figures for outpatient procedures (breast diagnostic and breast excisions) represent projections based on data from the NSAS 1996.

[b] Figures listed for 2010 and 2020 are projections; percentages listed indicate percent growth relative to the year 2000.

Source: From Etzioni et al. Ann Surg Onc, 2003.

References

1. Birkmeyer JD, Warshaw AL, Finlayson SR, et al., Relationship between hospital volume and late survival after pancreaticoduodenectomy. *Surgery.* 1999;126:178–183.

2. Breasted JH. *The Edwin Smith Surgical Papyrus.* Chicago: University of Chicago Press; 1930.
3. Hill GJ, II. Historic milestones in cancer surgery. *Semin Oncol.* 1979;6:409–427.
4. Antman KA, Eilber FR, Shiu MH. Soft tissue sarcomas: current trends in diagnosis and management. *Curr Prob Cancer.* 1989;13:339–367.
5. Eilber FC, Rosen G, Eckardt J, et al. Treatment induced pathologic necrosis: a predictor of local recurrence and survival in patients receiving neoadjuvant therapy for high-grade extremity soft tissue sarcoma. *J Clin Oncol.* 2001;19:3203–3209.
6. Choti MA, Sitzmann JV, Tiburi MF, et al. Trends in long-term survival following liver resection for hepatic colorectal metastases. *Ann Surg.* 2002 Jun;235(6):759–766.
7. Greene FL, Balch CM, Page DL, et al. eds. *American Joint Committee on Cancer (AJCC) Cancer Staging Manual.* 6th ed. New York: Springer-Verlag; 2002.
8. Scappaticci FA, Fehrenbacher L, Cartwright T, et al. Surgical wound healing complications in metastatic colorectal cancer patients treated with bevacizumab. *J Surg Oncol.* 2005 Sep 1;91(3):173–180.6.
9. Morton DL, Wen D-R, Wong JH, et al. Technical details of intraoperative lymphatic mapping for melanoma. *Arch Surg.* 1992;127:392–399.
10. Giuliano AE, Kirgan DM, Guenther JM, Morton DL. Lymphatic mapping and sentinel lymphadenectomy for breast cancer. *Ann Surg.* 1994;220:391–398.
11. Koch WM, Choti MA, Civelek AC, Eisele DW, Saunders JR. Gamma probe-directed biopsy of the sentinel node in oral squamous cell carcinoma. *Arch Otolaryngol Head Neck Surg.* 1998 Apr;124(4):455–459.
12. Krag DN, Meijer SJ, Weaver DL, et al. Minimal-access surgery for staging of malignant melanoma. *Arch Surg.* 1995;130:654–658.
13. Pawlik TM, Scoggins CR, Zorzi D, et al. Effect of surgical margin status on survival and site of recurrence after hepatic resection for colorectal metastases. *Ann Surg.* 2005 May;241(5):715–722.
14. Patrick CW, Jr, Mikos AG, McIntire LV. *Frontiers in Tissue Engineering.* 1st ed. New York: Pergamon Press; 1998.
15. Etzioni DA, Liu JH, Maggard MA, O'Connell JB, Ko CY. Workload projections for surgical oncology: will we need more surgeons? *Ann Surg Oncol.* 2003 Nov;10(9):1112–1117.

41 Principles of Radiation Oncology

Joseph K. Salama, MD ■ Mark W. Dewhirst, DVM, PhD ■ Ralph R. Weichselbaum, MD

Radiation oncology is the medical field in which malignant and nonmalignant diseases in both adults and children are treated with ionizing radiation (IR). Approximately 50% of all cancer patients will receive radiotherapy (RT) at some point during treatment for their disease. One-half of patients receive RT with curative intent, with the remainder receiving RT as an effective means of palliation. Reports of a wide variety of malignant tumors treated with RT began to appear shortly after the discovery of x-rays by Wilhelm Roentgen in 1895.[1-3] RT had relatively limited applicability until the introduction of high-energy (megavoltage) therapy in the 1950s, due to adverse normal tissue effects, most significantly cutaneous toxicity that limited dose delivered to deep-seated tumors. Over the past 20 years, advances in imaging and treatment delivery have improved targeting and increased sparing of normal tissues. Increased understanding of radiobiology has also provided a means to further reduce the risk of treatment sequelae while increasing treatment efficacy.

Physical Basis of Radiation Therapy

Types of Radiation

RT is delivered primarily with high-energy photons (gamma rays and x-rays) and charged particles (electrons and protons). The distinction between gamma rays and x-rays lies in their origin; gamma rays originate from excited and unstable nuclei, whereas x-rays are produced by electron energy transitions within the atom or through the deceleration of high-kinetic energy electrons (bremsstrahlung).[4,5] Gamma rays are typically produced by radioactive sources used in brachytherapy (see below), whereas x-rays are generated by linear accelerators and are used in external beam RT. Within a linear accelerator, a narrow beam of electrons is accelerated to nearly the speed of light before striking a tungsten target.[5] As the electrons decelerate, they emit bremsstrahlung radiation (x-rays) with a spectrum ranging from zero to their maximum kinetic energy. Beam quality is often expressed as the highest-energy photons produced in kVp (kilovolts peak) or MV (megavolts). Therapeutic beam energies range from 50 kVp to 25 MV or greater. In this energy range, the relevant interactions of photons with matter include the photoelectric effect, Compton effect, and pair production.[4,5] Compton effect is the predominant interaction in tissue for therapeutic beams, whereas for energies below 50 kVp, the photoelectric effect is the most important interaction. Pair production is the primary interaction at energies above 25 MV. As a result of these interactions, electrons are set into motion, causing ionization and excitation of other atoms in the medium. As an x-ray beam passes through matter, its intensity is reduced and can be expressed by the following formula:

$$I(x) = I_o e^{-\mu x}$$

where I_o is the initial intensity of the photon beam, I (x) is the intensity after traversing a depth x and μ is the material's linear attenuation coefficient. High-energy beams are less attenuated than low-energy beams and thus are used for the irradiation of deep-seated tumors. Radiation intensity from a point source also decreases as the inverse square of the distance from the source, a dependence known as the inverse square law.[4,5]

Unlike a photon beam, a charged particle travels a known range in tissue proportional to its energy. Tissues beyond the range of the charged particle are thus not irradiated. Electrons are the most common therapeutic charged particles and are also produced by a linear accelerator. Instead of striking a tungsten target, the beam passes through a series of filters that broaden and shape it. Charged particles interact with matter through three primary processes: soft collisions (coulomb force interactions with outer shell electrons), hard "knock on" collisions (direct interactions with electrons), and nuclear field interactions.[5] Typically, a 1 MeV electron will undergo 10^5 interactions before losing its energy.[4] Soft collisions account for approximately half the energy transferred to matter. The remaining energy is transferred primarily by the relatively fewer, but more energetic, hard collisions.

Other therapeutic modalities include neutrons[6,7] and protons.[8,9] Neutron beams are generated by bombarding a beryllium target with a cyclotron accelerated proton beam.[5] Like photons, neutrons are exponentially attenuated. Interactions with tissue include neutron–proton collisions and neutron–nuclei reactions, which set heavy charged particles in motion. Proton beams are also generated by a cyclotron. Unlike neutrons, protons primarily deposit their dose near the end of their range, a phenomenon known as a Bragg peak.[4,5] The Bragg peak can be modified to encompass the tumor without delivering high doses to more distal tissues.[8,9]

Radiation Absorbed Dose

The quantification of radiation has evolved over time. In the early 20th century, units of skin erythema and the roentgen, a measure of ionization produced in air, were used. Today, the accepted unit of measurement is "absorbed dose," which is the energy absorbed per unit mass. Physically, absorbed dose represents the energy deposited by secondary charged particles in the medium. The unit of absorbed dose is the Gray (Gy), which is defined as the absorption of 1 joule per kilogram (J/kg).[4,5] One Gray is equivalent to 100 centiGray (cGy) or 100 rads.

Treatment Planning and Delivery

External Beam Therapy

The goal of RT is to uniformly irradiate a specified target (usually a gross tumor, surgical bed, or areas at high risk for microscopic disease) while minimizing the dose to surrounding normal tissues.[10] The spatial distribution of the radiation delivered depends on a number of factors including patient anatomy, tissue density, beam energy, and the configuration of radiation portals. To maximize the therapeutic ratio of RT, pre-therapy planning is performed based on patient imaging in the treatment position. Because of complex tumor geometry, image-based three-dimensional (3D) planning is essential.[11-13] Both the concepts of treatment planning and the technical considerations related to 3D planning are described below.

Simulation and Target Delineation ■ Simulation is the process where the optimal patient position for treatment is decided, as well as the time when fabrication of custom immobilization devices and individual treatment aids takes place.[14] Specific positions are often used to minimize radiation dose delivered to neighboring normal tissues. Breast and lung cancer patients, eg, are simulated with their arms overhead to allow for the use of angled (oblique) beams that do not transverse the arms. Other specialized positions include the "frog leg" position (vulvar cancer) and the "chin tuck" position (pituitary tumors). Immobilization is accomplished with the aid of thermoplastics, foam cradles, bite blocks, and other accessories. The goal of immobilization is to minimize the day-to-day setup variability caused by patient movement. On a conventional simulator, field borders are chosen under fluoroscopic guidance on the basis of patient anatomy and knowledge of tumor spread. More commonly, computed tomography (CT) simulators allow for direct acquisition of CT data with the patient in the treatment position.

Imaging occupies a central role in RT planning, providing geometric information on external patient contour as well as tumor size, shape, and location relative to adjacent critical structures.[15,16] For 3D planning, the process begins during simulation with the acquisition of a CT scan of the patient in the treatment position. CT scanners dedicated to the purpose of simulation are often used for this process. Most of these scanners are capable of both axial (one slice at a time) and spiral scanning techniques. Spiral or helical CT allows data to be acquired, whereas the table and x-ray beam simultaneously translate and rotate, respectively. The spiral mode is preferred owing to its faster acquisition time. Multislice CT scanners have recently been adopted in CT simulation allowing for multiple slices to be acquired simultaneously. These scanners use multiple rows of detectors and acquire images faster and with a lower tube heat compared with conventional CT scanners. Multislice scanners are particularly useful for simulation of lung cancer patients as breathing artifacts can be minimized. Moreover, this technology can be used to simulate respiratory-gated treatments.

Routinely, a physician will delineate three volumes on each planning CT slice for RT planning[16]: the gross tumor volume (GTV), the clinical target volume (CTV), and the planning target volume (PTV). The GTV constitutes all known tumor visible on pretreatment imaging and clinical examination. Regions at risk for microscopic spread define the CTV. The PTV encompasses both the GTV and CTV with an added margin to account for the uncertainty in the day-to-day setup of patients as well as to account for the effects of organ motion. PTV expansion typically ranges from 3 to 10 mm.[17,18] Previously, larger margins had to be placed around tumors whose position varied with respiration. Lung tumor motion was often visualized fluoroscopically prior to treatment to ensure that it fell within defined target volumes. In recent times, multiple techniques have become available to compensate for respiratory motion during simulation and treatment delivery. A simple way to accomplish this is to obtain CT scans of the patient in the treatment position at maximum inspiration and maximum expiration, assuming that the tumor position at these points of the respiratory cycle represents the extremes of tumor motion. Target volumes contoured on each of these scans are fused to create and internal target volume (ITV) that is expanded for microscopic disease extension to form the CTV. Alternatively, techniques have been developed to acquire CT images at specific phases of the respiratory cycle with treatment delivery during the same phases. This technique of "respiratory gating" allows smaller margins to be used to account for respiratory motion.[19] Normal tissues are delineated as both acute and chronic RT toxicities have been related to the volume of organs receiving specific doses of RT. Once a physician delineates the target volumes to be irradiated, treatment planning commences.

Although CT is the primary imaging modality for simulation, magnetic resonance imaging (MRI) provides important complementary information,[20-22] especially for intracranial and head and neck tumors. In recent times, MRI simulators have been introduced into RT clinics. The MRI simulator consists of an open-MRI system, flat table top, and an external laser marking system. MRI simulators have been used to provide better delineation of the prostate for RT treatment planning. However, as this technology is relatively new, its clinical role is not fully defined. Other modalities, such as positron emission tomography (PET) and single photon emission computed tomography (SPECT), also provide complementary information.[23,24] Hybrid scanners, such as the PET/CT scanner have increasingly gained clinical acceptance. These devices provide both anatomical (CT) and functional (PET) imaging. Moreover, because these scans are obtained with the patient in the same position, the PET and CT data share a common coordinate system. Imaging data can also be cross-correlated to transfer regions of interest from one study to another.[25-27]

Treatment Planning ■ Treatment planning is performed interactively on a computer and is used to generate a dose distribution superimposed on CT images. Variables considered in planning include beam energy and modality, number of portals and beam angles, relative beam weights, and beam-modifying devices (wedges, compensators). Beam energy is chosen on the basis of patient anatomy. High-energy photon beams (6-25 MV) are used for deep-seated tumors; superficial tumors may be treated with orthovoltage-energy photon beams (100-250 kVp) or with electrons. Beam number is determined by a variety of factors including tumor size, shape, and location. Beam modifying devices are used to compensate for variations in external patient anatomy.

A number of tools have been developed that aid in the design and evaluation of a treatment plan.[28-30] Beam's eye view (BEV) allows the visualization of the tumor geometry relative to critical structures from the perspective of the radiation beam.[29] Beam orientations are chosen that encompass the PTV but spare adjacent critical structures. In addition, BEV also permits the design of customized shielding blocks. Quantitative evaluation of treatment plans is performed using dose volume histograms (DVH) and dose surface histograms (DSH).[28] DVH represents the volume of a particular organ irradiated as a function of dose. The surface area as a function of dose is represented by DSH and is used in the evaluation of hollow organs. Such quantitative evaluation assists in the selection of the optimal treatment plan. Other treatment planning tools include digitally reconstructed radiographs[30] and volume rendering.[31,32]

Treatment Delivery and Verification ■ Linear accelerators are used to administer external beam RT (Fig. 41-1). Most modern accelerators have dual photon energies ranging from 4 to 24 MV, and four to six electron energies (6-22 MeV). Accelerators are equipped with a gantry that rotates 360°, allowing treatment from any angle. Noncoplanar beams may be delivered through a combination of gantry and treatment table rotations. Linear accelerators are designed to produce rectangular shaped beams. Further beam shaping is accomplished with either Cerrobend blocks or a multileaf collimator (MLC). Cerrobend is a low-melting-point alloy that attenuates nearly all of the beam intensity.[4] Beam shaping is accomplished by inserting Cerrobend blocks into the path of the beam for each field manually. MLC, as the name implies, consists of a series of 0.5-1.0 cm leaves within the machine head.[33,34] An MLC increases the efficiency of treatment delivery by obviating the need for changing blocks between fields and offers the capability of delivering intensity-modulated radiation therapy (IMRT) (see below). An alternative treatment delivery approach is helical

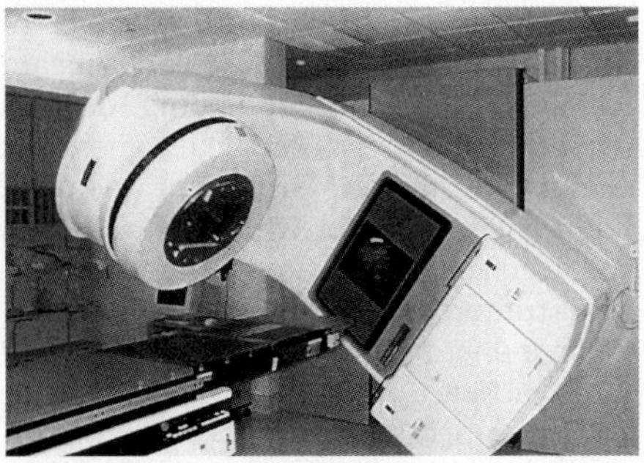

Figure 41-1 ■ Linear accelerator used for radiotherapy.

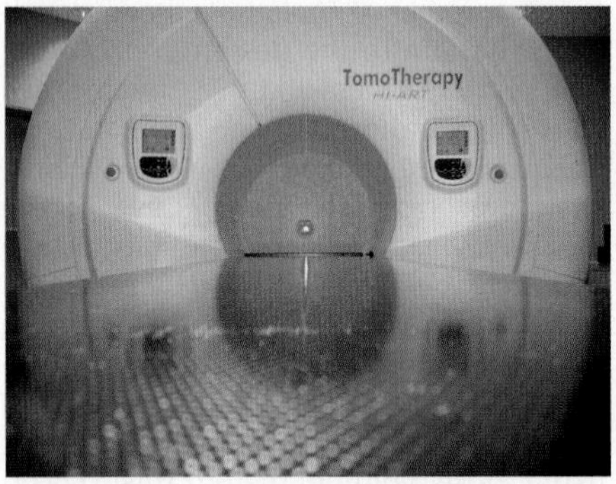

Figure 41-2 ■ A helical Tomotherapy unit.

Tomotherapy (Fig. 41-2) and volumetric arc therapy. On the outside, Tomotherapy units look like CT scanners. However, this device is equipped with a compact linear accelerator. Treatment is delivered as the beam rotates around the patient, whereas the couch moves continuously though the gantry. Simultaneously, a set of binary collimators open and close according to the treatment plan. Volumetric arc therapy utilizes a standard linear accelerator design, but treatment is delivered continuously during a single gantry rotation. A conformal dose distribution about the PTV is delivered by varying MLC position, gantry rotation speed, and dose rate.

RT is usually delivered with the patient placed on the treatment table in a customized immobilization device. On the first day of treatment, setup films are obtained and compared with those taken at simulation. The positions of anatomic landmarks are evaluated, and patient moves are made as needed. Films are also obtained at each treatment angle showing both the internal anatomy and the field aperture. Electronic portal imaging devices (EPIDs) have become standard in RT clinics.[35,36] EPIDs offer potential advantages over x-ray films, including online verification as well as the ability to monitor and compensate for patient motion during therapy.[37,38] Image-guided (IG) technologies have taken on an important role in RT, as they allow for daily treatment adjustments before and sometimes during therapy. Video, ultrasound, and kV x-ray devices allow physicians the unprecedented ability to monitor patient (and tumor) position in three dimensions on a daily basis. As IG technologies mature, daily modification of the treatment planning parameters (known as adaptive RT) based on the patient position as well as the size and location of the tumor will become commonplace.[39]

Intensity-Modulated Radiation Therapy ■ Conventional external beam RT is delivered with beams of uniform intensity. Recent advances, however, have made the use of beams of varying intensity possible. This approach, known IMRT, allows the high dose region to be better conformed to the shape of the PTV.[40-43] Better conformality translates to improved sparing of surrounding tissues, thereby allowing the delivery of higher radiation doses to the tumor. The beam intensity patterns used in IMRT are derived using an inverse process[41,43] and delivered using an MLC fitted on a linear accelerator. Beam intensity is varied by computer-controlled movement of the leaves of the MLC into and out of the beam's path. Delivery of IMRT requires accurate patient positioning and immobilization.[14] IMRT is now a routine part of clinical RT practice with 73.2% of surveyed physicians stating they had were using it in their clinics.[44]

IMRT has been shown to be a promising approach in several disease sites. In prostate cancer, IMRT is used to minimize the volume of the bladder and rectum irradiated, allowing higher doses to be delivered to the prostate.[45] IMRT has also been used to decrease xerostomia (dry mouth) in head and neck cancer patients by reducing the volume of parotid tissue irradiated.[46] IMRT also has shown promise in the treatment of pediatric tumors,[47] gastrointestinal,[48] and gynecologic malignancies[49] Some concern exists when using this technique for intrathoracic targets.

Figure 41-3 illustrates an axial CT image, with isodose lines superimposed in a patient with head and neck cancer. Note that the high-dose isodose lines conform to the shape of the target tissues minimizing dose to the neighboring parotid glands, reducing the risk of chronic xerostomia.

■ Brachytherapy

Brachytherapy involves the placement of radioactive sources either within an existing body cavity (eg, the vagina) in close proximity to the tumor (intracavitary) or directly within a tumor (interstitial). Intracavitary brachytherapy is accomplished with the aid of specialized applicators; the best known and most widely used is the Fletcher–Suit applicator for carcinoma of the cervix. A tube-like tandem is inserted into the uterus, and colpostats are positioned against the lateral fornices.

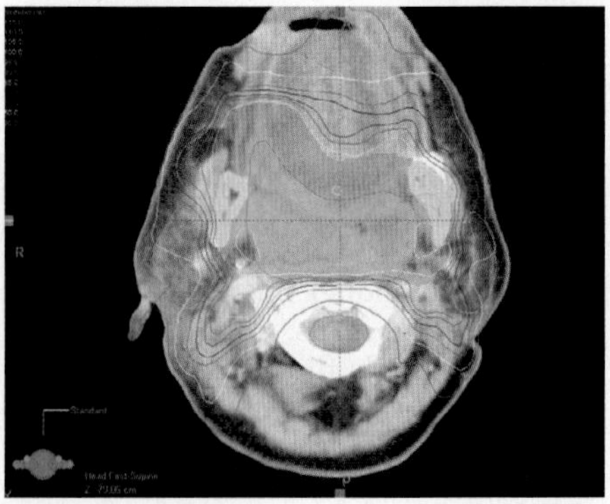

Figure 41-3 ■ An intensity-modulated radiation therapy treatment plan in a patient with head and neck cancer.

Other applicators include Heyman–Simon capsules (uterine cancer) and vaginal cylinders (uterine and vaginal tumors). Intracavitary brachytherapy may also be performed by inserting radioactive sources within a nasogastric tube (nasopharynx, esophageal tumors), biliary stents (cholangiocarcinoma), or directly within the lumen of a bronchus (lung cancer). Interstitial brachytherapy involves placing hollow needles within a tumor that can be replaced by flexible plastic catheters. Interstitial brachytherapy in gynecologic tumors uses a variety of treatment aids, eg, a Syed template.[50] In head and neck cancer, catheters are typically placed freehand via a submental approach.

At most centers, brachytherapy is currently performed with afterloading techniques that minimize exposure to the staff. Radioactive sources are placed either temporarily or permanently. Brachytherapy was initially instituted with the use of naturally occurring isotopes, such as radium or radon, but with the availability of artificially produced isotopes, it has been practiced more frequently with cesium 137, iridium 198, and iodine 125. Plans are generated by digitizing and reconstructing source positions from radiographs. Three-dimensional dose calculations are performed, and the dose is calculated to a limited number of normal, tissue points. Examples of intracavitary and interstitial brachytherapy in cervical and prostate cancer are shown in Figures 41-4 and 41-5. Brachytherapy has been traditionally delivered over 3-4 days as an inpatient procedure at a low-dose rate (LDR), eg, 40-70 cGy/h. In recent years, high-dose rate (HDR) techniques have been introduced using high-activity iridium sources with dose rates exceeding 200 cGy/min. Unlike LDR, HDR is an outpatient procedure requiring only minimal anesthesia. It is particularly appealing to the elderly and patients with multiple medical problems. Promising results have been reported in many sites, including the head and neck,[51] cervix,[52] endometrium,[5] and prostate.[54] HDR is

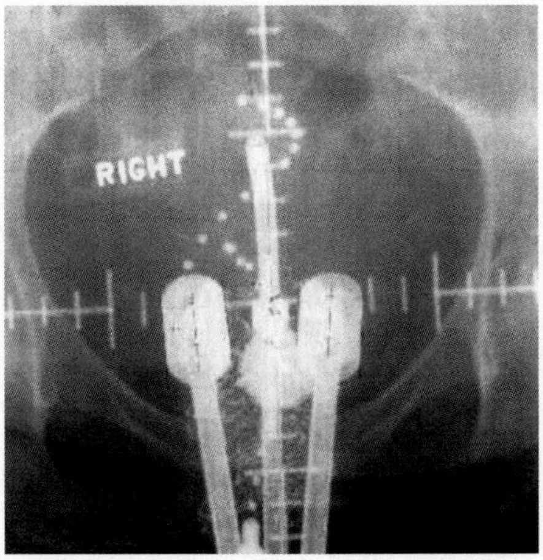

Figure 41-4 Intracavitary brachytherapy in a patient with early-stage cervical cancer.

beginning to replace LDR brachytherapy for many indications.

Stereotactic Radiosurgery, Stereotactic Radiotherapy, and Stereotactic Body Radiotherapy Stereotactic radiosurgery (SRS) is a technique used to precisely deliver a single, high-dose fraction of external beam radiation to a small, intracranial volume. It was first developed by Leksell in the early 1950s as an alternative to surgery.[55] The technique has since evolved to include heavy charged particles, gamma rays from Co-60 (gamma knife), and megavoltage beams from linear accelerators. The delivery of multiple fractions using the stereotactic process is known as stereotactic radiotherapy (SRT).[56] SRS and SRT have been used to supplement conventional external beam treatment in primary or metastatic brain tumors.[57] SRS is also used to treat benign conditions, such as arteriovenous malformations (AVMs),[58] pituitary adenomas,[59] trigeminal neuralgia,[60] and acoustic neuromas.[61] Both SRS and SRT involve the localization of a targeted lesion within a stereotactic frame. The stereotactic frame is either fixed (screwed into the cranium) (SRS) or relocatable (SRT). A stereotactic frame allows positioning of a patient with millimeter accuracy.[62] The goal of SRS/SRT is to conform the dose distribution to the targeted lesion while minimizing the dose to normal, surrounding brain parenchyma. In practice, this is accomplished with the use of multiple noncoplanar arcs or static fields. An example of an SRS treatment plan in a patient with a solitary brain metastasis from lung cancer is shown in Figure 41-6. This plan consists of five noncoplanar arcs and was delivered with 6 MV photons on a linear accelerator.

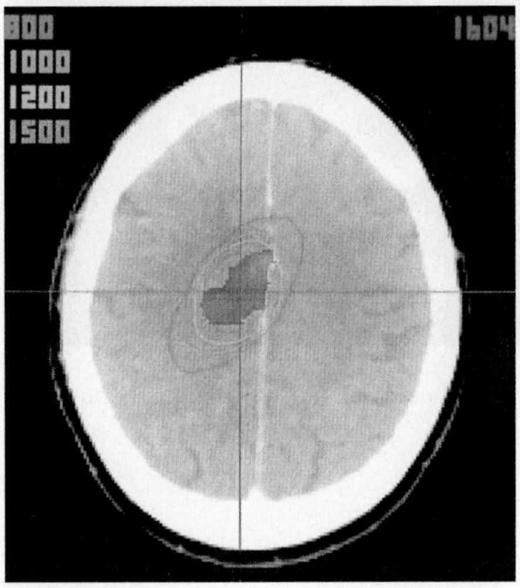

Figure 41-6 Stereotactic radiosurgery plan in a patient with a solitary brain metastasis from a lung cancer primary.

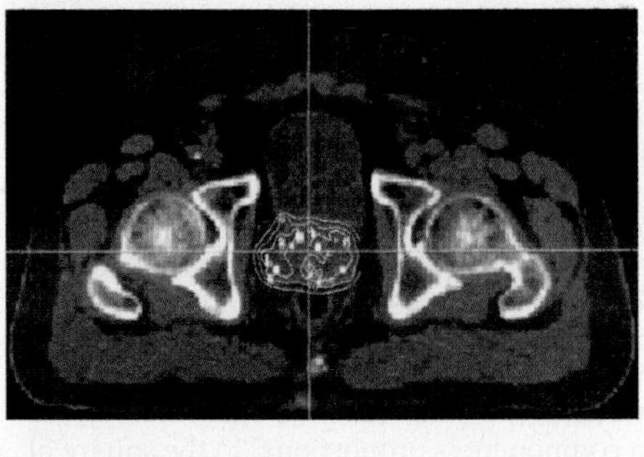

Figure 41-5 Interstitial brachytherapy in a patient with prostate carcinoma.

Stereotactic principles are now used to target extracranial tumors.[63] The lack of a rigid structure, such as the skull, makes immobilization for extracranial stereotactic radiation ablation difficult. Furthermore, respiratory induced tumor motion must be overcome. Typically, patients are immobilized for both simulation and treatment in a body frame, which also serves as reference for stereotactic coordinates. Respiratory motion is accounted for with various methods including external pressure, breath-hold techniques or respiratory gating. Stereotactic planning techniques are used to generate highly conformal dose distributions. This technique shows promise for treating early stage nonsmall cell lung cancer as well as metastases to the lung, liver, and abdominal sites.[64] Dose and fractionation schedules are not standardized for stereotactic body radiotherapy (SBRT). A dose of 60 Gy in three 20 Gy fractions has been shown to result in high rates of locoregional control for hepatic metastases, pulmonary metastases, and for peripheral lung targets,[64] but has been shown to have high rates of toxicity for centrally located thoracic tumors. Alternative schedules with single and multiple fractions are being developed to treat patients with low-volume metastatic disease.[65,66] A patient with limited metastatic disease treated with SBRT to four lung lesions is shown in Figure 41-7.

Another approach to improving the therapeutic ratio for patients with mediastinal tumors is the use of charged particles. Compared to conventional photon therapy, charged particles, such as protons and carbon ions, deposit a great deal of their energy at a given depth followed by a steep dose fall-off, with almost no dose deposition beyond forming the Bragg peak. This property can be exploited to deliver higher doses to the target without increasing toxicities to surrounding normal tissues. Protons have been shown to be a method by which radiation doses can be increased for prostate cancer. Current clinical indications for protons include ocular melanoma,[67] chordoma,[68] and some pediatric tumors.[69-71] The applicability of protons to common adult tumors is a subject of intense debate, especially because of the high cost of construction.[72-75]

Biologic Basis of Radiation Therapy

Cellular Response to Radiation

Radiation randomly interacts with molecules within the cell. Although the critical target for cell killing is deoxyribonucleic acid (DNA),[76] damage to cellular and nuclear membranes as well as other organelles may also be important. Radiation deposition results in DNA damage manifested by single- and double-strand breaks (DSBs) in the sugar-phosphate backbone of the DNA molecule. Cross-links between DNA strands and chromosomal proteins also occur. The mechanism of DNA damage differs among the various radiation types. For example, electromagnetic radiation is indirectly ionizing via short-lived, hydroxyl free radicals produced primarily by the ionization of cellular H_2O.[77] Protons and other heavy particles are directly ionizing and damage DNA directly.[78] Consequently, different types of radiation have varying relative biologic effectiveness (RBE). Directly ionizing radiation (eg, neutrons) has a greater RBE than indirectly ionizing radiation (photons or electrons).[6,79]

Radiation damage is primarily manifested in the loss of cellular reproductive capacity. Lethally irradiated cells are, thus, said to undergo a reproductive death, which is the result of aberrant cell mitosis or senescence. Some cell types do not show morphologic evidence of radiation damage until they attempt to divide. Alternatively, some cell types are killed via the induction of apoptosis.[80] A cell that has sustained lethal damage following radiation exposure may undergo one or more divisions prior to metabolic death and loss from the tumor population.

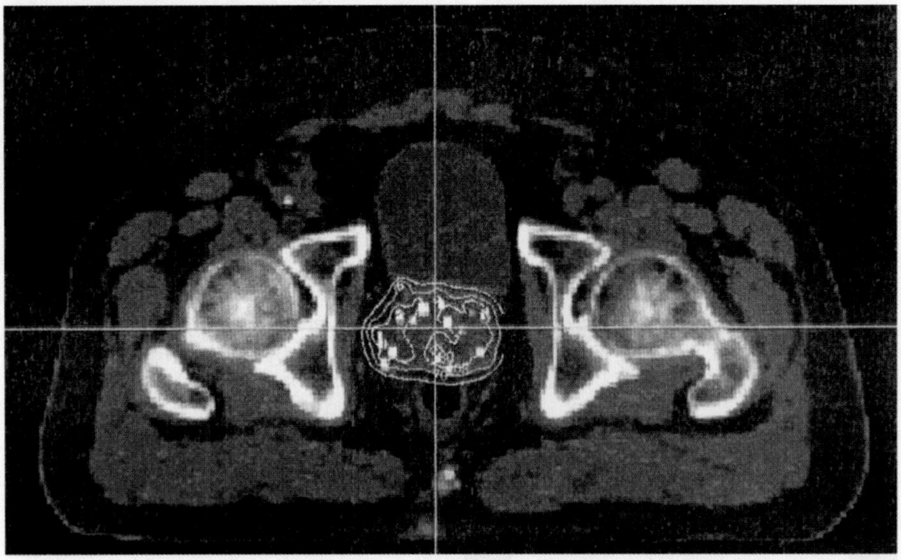

Figure 41-7 Hypofractionated image guided radiotherapy plan in a patient with four lung metastases from a melanoma primary.

The concept that cell death following radiation exposure may not be manifested until several cell divisions later has clinical relevance, such that tumors associated with very slowly proliferating cancers may persist for months and appear histologically viable. The histologic appearance may clear only after tumor cells have had the opportunity to attempt to divide. For example, prostate cancer may require up to 24 months after RT to obtain a normal biopsy.[81]

Radiation Survival Analysis

Radiation survival can be studied both in vitro and in vivo. In vitro experiments usually involve irradiating exponentially growing cells to known doses of radiation. Cells are plated, and after 2-3 weeks, colonies are stained. The surviving fraction is then calculated by dividing the number of colonies by the plating efficiency of unirradiated cells. A survival curve is then generated by graphing the log of the surviving fraction versus the absorbed dose (Fig. 41-8). Typically, survival curves are characterized by an initial shoulder, followed by exponential decrease in the fraction of surviving cells at higher doses.

In vivo models examine both the inherent radiosensitivity of tumor cells and environmental influences, such as hypoxia and host immunity. A model commonly used to study radiation effects is the growth delay assay, which measures the time interval required for a tumor exposed to radiation to regrow to a specified volume (Fig. 41-9).[82] An assay that analyzes the dose required to sterilize 50% of tumors is the TCD50 assay, which has been widely employed to study tumors in a variety of experimental systems.[83] Radiation survival parameters can be assayed for normal tissues, in vivo as well as for tumors. For acutely responding tissues, in vivo survival is measured by studying clones of normal tissues regrowing in situ (eg, skin, jejunal crypt cells) or cells transplanted to another site (bone marrow stem cells). To study radiation effects in late-responding tissues, such as the nervous system, functional assays, e.g. analysis and death, may be employed.

Models of Radiation Survival Curve Analysis

Two empirically derived mathematical models have been used to analyze radiation survival data (see Fig. 41-8). In the multitarget model, the reciprocal of the slope of the survival curve is defined as D_0, the radiosensitivity of the cell population or tissue under investigation. D_0 is the dose required to reduce the surviving fraction to 37% in the exponential portion of the survival curve. The width of the shoulder region is represented by the quantities n or Dq. Dq is the quasi-threshold dose, or the point at which killing becomes exponential.

The linear quadratic model (surviving fraction = $e^{\alpha D-\beta D2}$) fits radiation survival data to a continuously bending curve, where D is dose and α and β are constants. The linear component, a measure of the initial slope, termed alpha, represents single-hit killing kinetics and dominates the radiation response at low doses. The quadratic component of cell killing, termed beta, represents multiple-hit killing and causes the curve to bend at higher doses. The ratio of alpha to beta is the dose at which the linear and quadratic components of cell killing are equal. The more linear the response to killing of cells at low radiation dose, the higher the value of alpha, and the greater the radiosensitivity of the cells.[84] Neither model has a firmly established biologic

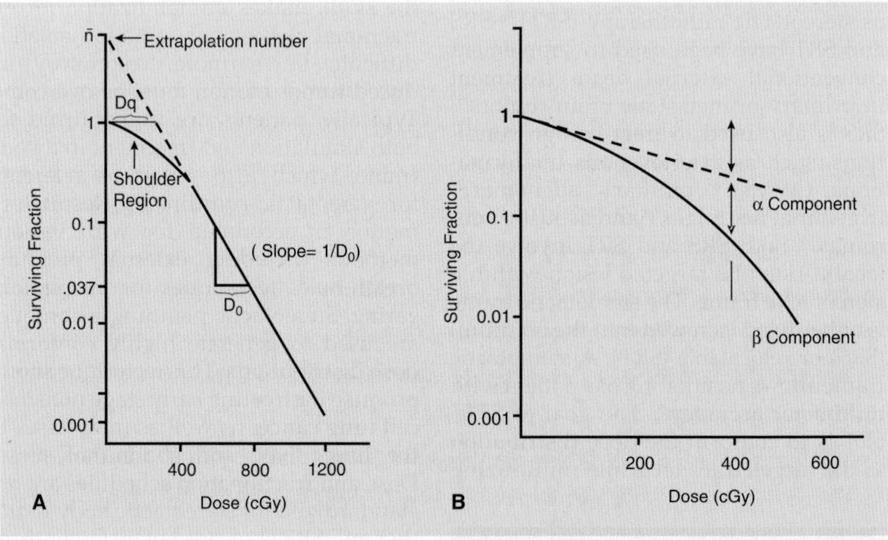

Figure 41-8 Models for survival curve analysis. Experimental data are typically shown as the fraction of cells surviving a dose of radiation plotted on a logarithmic scale, whereas the dosage of radiation is plotted on a linear scale (**A**). When using the multitarget model the shoulder region is quantified by the *y*-axis intercept. This point is referred to as *n* (extrapolation number), whereas a horizontal line drawn from 100% survival to the extrapolation line is referred to as Dq (or quasi threshold dose). Slope of the terminal portion of the survival curve is quantified by D_0, which is the inverse of the slope and designated as the radiosensitivity of the cell or tissue under study. (**B**) When using the linear-quadratic models for survival analyses there are two components for cell killing. The alpha component represents the initial slope and the beta component represents the terminal slope of the survival curve. The alpha component is proportional to dose while the beta component is proportional to the square of the dose. The dose at which the alpha and beta components are equal is referred to the alpha/beta ratio, which, for example, here is 400 cGy.

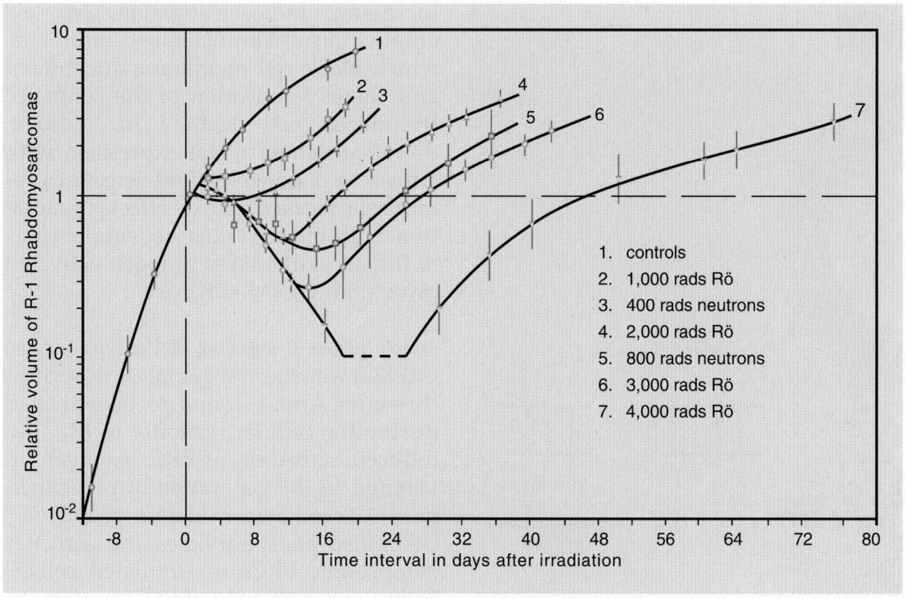

Figure 41-9 Data points represent volume changes observed in tumor animal models after irradiation. After an initial decrease in the volume size, tumors grow back to the original volume over a time interval referred to as the growth delay. Curve 1 is the growth of an unirradiated control tumor. Curves 2, 4, 6, and 7 represent the growth of tumors irradiated with 10, 20, 30, and 40 Gy photons. Curves 3 and 5 represent the growth of tumors irradiated with 4 Gy and 8 Gy of 152 MeV neutrons. Growth delay is prolonged with increasing dosage and more densely ionizing radiation such as neutrons.

basis. Therefore, both should be viewed as mathematical tools to describe the cellular radiosensitivity.

Molecular Events Following Cellular Exposure to Ionizing Radiation The ultimate fate of the irradiated cell is not only a function of the radiation dose but also an influence by the cell's natural defenses, including the ability to detect the DNA lesions and to repair them with high fidelity. Recent advances have revealed DNA is not the only cellular target that influences the radiation response. IR also interacts directly with lipid and protein signaling pathways and modulates gene expression through a variety of mechanisms including the direct activation of transcription factors. IR-induced activation of these signaling pathways can affect critical processes such as cell cycle regulation, DNA repair, apoptosis, and tissue repopulation. Figure 41-10 illustrates the current perspective on the interactions between IR-induced DNA damage and cell signaling.

Molecular Sensors and Effectors of Radiation-Induced DNA Damage As shown in Figure 41-10, components of the DNA-dependent protein kinase (DNA-PK) complex are involved in sensing DSBs as well as the repair of these breaks. DNA-PK consists of the 470 kDa catalytic serine/threonine kinase (DNA-PKCs) and the 70 and 80 kDa Ku heterodimer.[85-87] Ku binds directly to sites of DSBs,[88,89] and DNA-PKCs is recruited to sites of Ku/DNA complexes where it is activated.[87] The Ataxia Telangiectasia Mutated (ATM) protein is also involved in sensing DNA damage and is related to DNA-PKCs and other members of the phosphatidylinositol (PI) 3-kinase (PIK) family.

ATM proteins are involved in cell cycle regulation, recombination, telomere length control and the multiple steps in the cellular response to DNA damage.[90-92] Investigators have recently revealed that ATM phosphorylates a nuclease, Artemis, and directly affects radiation-induced DNA damage, independent of ATM-dependent cell cycle checkpoint arrest[93] and is likely important to repair DSBs critical to survival that are rejoined at relatively later time points. AT cells, like DNA-PKCs/Ku-deficient cells, are hypersensitive to IR.[94-96] AT cells that are deficient in ATM or express a nonfunctional mutant protein also exhibit defects in IR-induced growth arrest,[97-99] radioresistant DNA synthesis, and chromosome instability.[100,101] Because ATM is one of most widely studied components in the cellular response to DNA damage, it has been placed in the center of this figure. However, numerous other factors, such as the AT and Rad3-related (ATR) protein kinase, are essential for cell cycle modulation after the induction of other types of DNA damage.[100,101] The red bars indicate three main cell cycle checkpoints in late G1, late G2 and S; dashed lines show that the effect is of DSBs,[88,89] DNA-PKCs is recruited to sites of Ku/DNA complexes; and the question mark denotes links between G2 arrest and p53-mediated apoptosis currently under investigation. The p53 tumor suppressor gene plays a pivotal role in the cellular response to IR. Through its C-terminal domain, the p53 protein can bind directly to radiation-damaged DNA and to single-stranded DNA ends, suggesting that p53 can act as a sensor of DNA damage. Exposing cells to DNA-damaging agents or to restriction endonucleases that induce DNA breaks results in the stabilization and accumulation of p53 in the nucleus.[97,102] This increase in p53 is associated with transcription of p21 and BAX, leading to the induction of G1 arrest or apoptosis. ATM and CHK2, a mammalian homolog of Cds1/Rad53 that is activated by ATM, phosphorylates p53 and thereby prevents its degradation. DNA-PK interacts with the N-terminal region of p53 and contributes to its sequence-specific DNA binding, transactivation function, and stability.[103-106] Thus, p53 is an effector as well as sensor of DNA damage. c-Abl, a non-receptor tyrosine kinase, associates with p53[105, 107] to stabilize and induce its pro-apoptotic functions through a kinase-independent mechanism.[107] c-Abl also interacts with the p53-related protein p73 in the response to IR and other genotoxic agents.[108-110] c-Abl has been implicated in inhibiting the Mdm2 oncoprotein as well.[111] Mdm2 binds the transcriptional activation domain of p53 and blocks its ability to regulate target genes and to exert antiproliferative effects. Mdm2 also promotes the degradation of p53 via the ubiquitination/proteasome pathway. The role of p53 in cell cycle regulation is discussed later.

The Role of Growth and Stress-Signaling Pathways in the Radiation Response IR-induced activation of signaling pathways can have a variety of consequences, including increased or decreased radiosensitivity, induced proliferation, differentiation, or apoptosis, or affected biologic behavior (eg, invasiveness or metastases). Several of the key pathways that have been explored are summarized.

Ras, Raf, and Mitogen-Activated Protein Kinase Signaling The Ras/Raf signaling pathway mediates growth signals from receptors such as the epidermal growth factor receptor (EGFR), which is a member of the ErbB family. Overexpression of EGFR has been associated with uncontrolled proliferation, anchorage-independent growth, autocrine growth regulation, and increased radioresistance. IR activates the small G-protein Ras, which in turn activates c-Raf, a serine/threonine kinase that interacts with Ras.[112] Activating mutations in the Ras oncogene have been associated with radioresistance in certain cell lines.[113] Activation of c-Raf-1 has also been implicated in the development of radioresistance.[114,115] Ras and Raf thus represent potential targets for

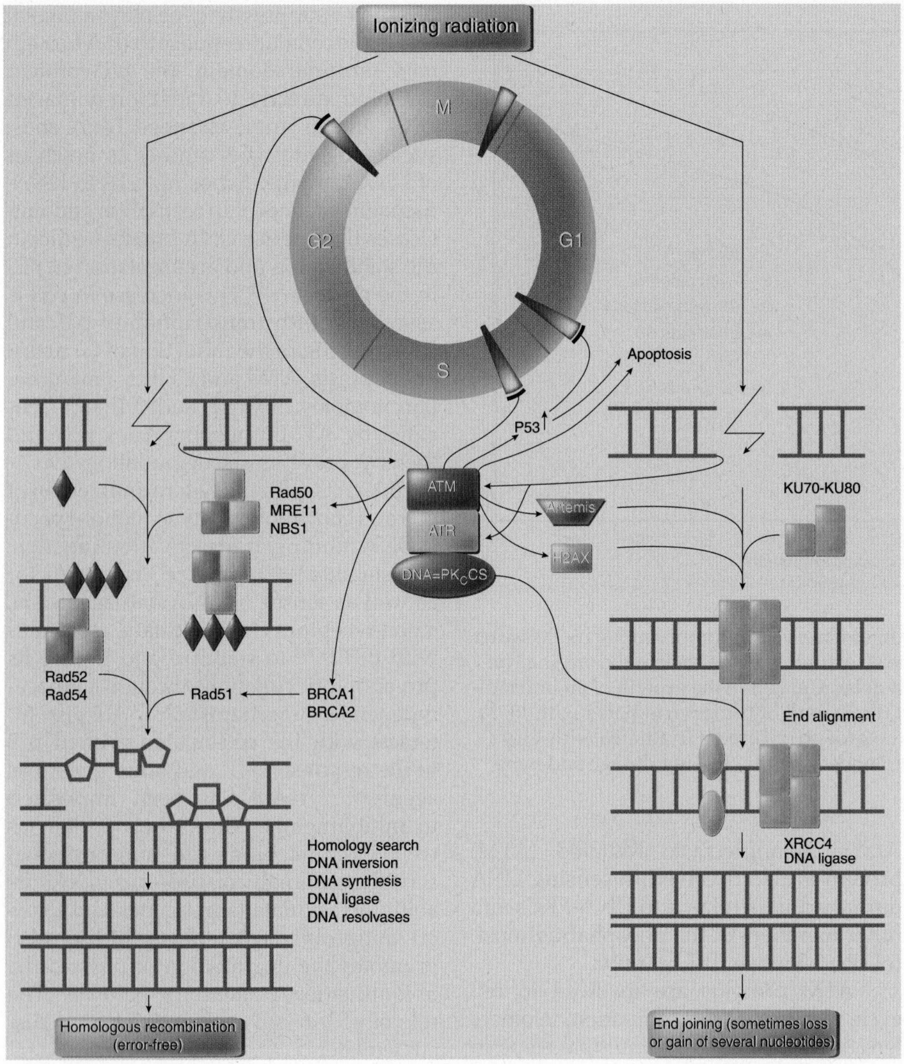

Figure 41-10 The DNA damage response to IR-induced DNA double-strand breaks in human cells. Irradiation induces a DSB on to which loads the MRN complex. Subsequent recruitment of the signaling kinases ATP or ATR-ATRIP results in phosphorylation of the histone variant H2AX. In addition, signaling by ATM or ATR leads to one of four responses. Signals can lead to checkpoint arrest or to induction of senescence or apoptosis depending on the cell type and conditions. Signaling can also induce the recruitment of DNA repair proteins on one of two DSB repair pathways: the end-joining pathway predominates in G1 cells while the homologous recombination pathway plays a major role in repairing breaks formed in S phase and G2. On the end-joining pathway, DNA protein kinase, consisting of the heterodimer Ku and the catalytic subunit are recruited to the break and coordinate subsequent recruitment of additional repair factors. If the DNA ends are intact, a ligation complex consisting of XRCC4/LIGASE4/XLF is sufficient for ligation. Otherwise, damaged DNA ends are processed by additional factors such as the nuclease Artemus and DNA repair polymerases before ends are ligated. End processing often uses regions of microhomology on the two ends to prime repair synthesis. In the homologous recombination pathway, DNA ends are resected by the action of the CtIP and other nucleases forming 3′ overhanging single-stranded ends. These ends serve as assembly sites for the recombinase RAD51. RAD51 filaments are assembled on 3′ single strand tails with help from BRCA1 and 2, the five RAD51 paralogues (RAD51B, RAD51C, RAD51C, XRCC2, XRCC3). Once assembled the RAD51 filament searches the sister chromatid for the corresponding sequence and then promotes strand invasion and exchange forming a heteroduplex joint with a free 3′ end. The 3′end is the substrate for polymerase which extends the end past the site of the DSB. After end extension the heteroduplex joint can be disrupted. The Werner (WRN) or Bloom's (BLM) helicases may contribute to this process. Once the extended end is released from the joint it can anneal with the partner end. This process is called "synthesis-dependent strand annealing". The annealed ends can then be "filled in" by polymerase and ligated. Another pathway for HR involves annealing of the second end to the joint formed by extension of the first end. This two-ended complex can be filled in by polymerase and ligated for form a so-called Double Holliday Junction. Double Holliday junctions can be unwound and "dissolved" by the combined action of the BLM helicase and topoisomerase III. Alternatively, the double Holliday junction can be cleaved by structure specific endonucleases. In this case, cleavage can form recombination products in which the chromosome arms flanking the site of the recombination event are reciprocally exchanged. Such reciprocal exchange, or "crossing over," can lead to loss of heterozygosity or chromosome rearrangement. *Source:* Figure and legend from Dr. Douglas Bishop.

increasing radiosensitization. For example, farnesyltransferase inhibitors, which block cell membrane attachment and thereby activation of Ras, enhance IR-induced cell death.[113] In addition, downregulation of Raf expression with antisense oligonucleotides sensitizes tumor cells to the cytotoxic effects of radiation.[116] IR-induced Ras activation leads to the upregulation of mitogen-activated protein kinase (MAPK).[117,118]

Protein Kinase C Signaling Protein kinase C (PKC) was the first cytoplasmic serine/threonine kinase found to be activated during the cellular response to IR.[119] IR-induced activation of PKC has been attributed to the generation of phospholipase A2-mediated oxidation products.[120] c-Abl also phosphorylates and activates cytoplasmic PKCs in irradiated cells.[121] IR-induced activation of PKCs is associated with translocation of PKCs to the nucleus.[121] PKC inhibitors block IR-induced activation of the early growth response 1 gene (EGR-1) and c-Jun.[119] In addition, PKC inhibitors such as calphostin C, PKC 412, and chelyrithine chloride, exhibit greater than additive antitumor effects in animal models when used in combination with IR.[122-124] Radioprotection of basic fibroblast growth factor (bFGF)-treated endothelial cells is also mediated by PKC activation.[125] Selective modulation of PKC could thus represent a strategy to enhance tumor cell killing or normal tissue survival. Inhibitors of EGFR block IR-induced activation of MAPK,[126] indicating that EGFR Ras, Raf, and MAPK all lie in the same IR response pathway. A recent phase III trial of a cetuximab, a humanized monoclonal antibody to EGFR has shown improvement in the overall survival of responses of head and neck cancer patients when added to RT.[127,128] Agents that target the intracellular tyrosine kinase region include small molecule tyrosine kinase inhibitors (TKIs), which act by interfering with ATP binding to the receptor, and various other compounds that act at substrate-binding regions or downstream components of the signaling pathway.[126] This group of compounds offers several advantages in cancer chemotherapy, including the possibility of inhibiting specific deregulated pathways in cancer cells while having minimal effects on normal cell function. They also have favorable pharmacokinetic and pharmacodynamic properties and low toxicity. Some TKIs, such as sunitinib,[129] sorafenib,[130] and erlotinib,[131] have been evaluated in phase III studies.

Lyn/c-Abl/SAPK Lyn, a member of the c-Src family of nonreceptor protein tyrosine kinases (PTKs), is activated in IR-treated cells[132,133] and is required for induction of the stress-activated protein kinase (SAPK), a member of the MAPK family, which is involved in the apoptotic response to genotoxic stress. Lyn inhibits the cyclin-dependent kinase Cdc2 in irradiated cells that is necessary for progression through the premitotic checkpoint[132] and inhibits DNAPKCs activity.[133] c-Abl activates MEKK-1, and thereby confers activation of the SEK1-SAPK pathway. In this context, SAPK induces the activation of transcription factors including c-Jun.

Early Response Genes ■ IR induces the expression of the *Egr-1* gene.[134] Its transcription is conferred by IR-induced activation of serum response (CArG) elements in the Egr-1 promoter.[134] As found for *c-Jun*, treatment with the free radical scavenger *N*-acetylcysteine (NAC) blocks the induction of the *Egr-1* gene in the IR response.[135] These findings showed that IR activates the *c-Jun* and *Egr-1* genes by ROS-mediated signaling mechanisms. The finding that IR activates gene transcription provided the experimental basis for the design of gene therapy strategies in which the spatial and temporal control of gene expression are regulated by high-energy x-rays. In this approach, a radio-inducible promoter, such as that from the *Egr-1* gene, is inserted upstream to sequences encoding a therapeutic protein. The CArG elements in the Egr-1 promoter have been used to activate IR-induced transcription of tumor necrosis factor (TNF) or the HSV-1 thymidine kinase (TK).[136-138] The TNF protein functions as a radiosensitizer, and in high local TNF concentrations, selectively increases the sensitivity of the tumor to IR treatment in the absence of systemic toxicity.[139] Several clinical trials are underway in which the Egr-1/CArG promoter–TNF construct is delivered to tumors in an adenoviral vector and activated by local RT.

Classic Aspects of DNA Repair in Radiotherapy

Irradiated cells that are not lethally damaged may undergo repair of the damage to their DNA. Sublethal damage repair (SLDR) is operationally defined as the enhancement in survival when a dose of radiation is separated over a period of time. SLDR may be represented by the extrapolation number (*n*) of the radiation survival curve when a multitarget survival model is employed.[140-144]

Sublethal damage has been studied in vitro and in vivo. In general, SLDR experiments divide a single dose into two relatively equal doses spaced at variable time intervals. Elkind and colleagues investigated this phenomenon in great detail.[141,145] Figure 41-11 shows results representative of splitdose experiments. An enhancement in survival, following two doses separated in time, is observed in exponentially growing Chinese hamster cells at 2 h. This enhancement in survival is due to the rapid repair of SLD and is followed by a subsequent decline in survival at 5 h and then another increase in survival at 8 h. This variability in survival is caused by synchronization of the exponentially growing cell populations by the first radiation dose and subsequent treatment with a second dose during the radioresistant S-phase (t = 2 h) or radiosensitive G2-M phase of the cell cycle (t = 6 h).[142-144]

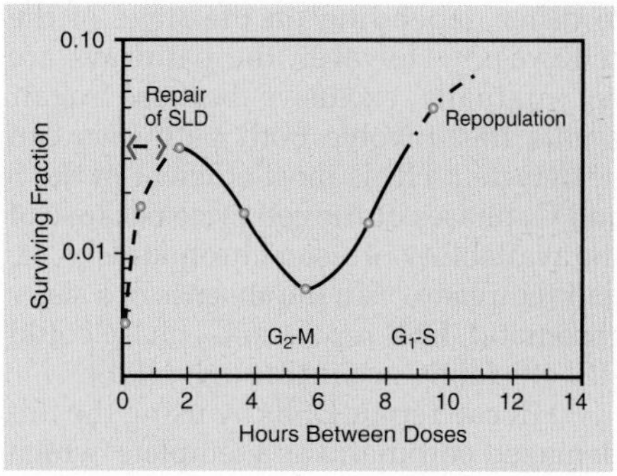

Figure 41-11 ■ The surviving fractions of Chinese hamster cells exposed to two doses of x-rays separated by various time intervals are shown. When the two doses are given together (time interval = 0 h), the surviving fraction is equal to that observed after the single larger dose of radiation. As the two doses are separated by time, an enhancement in survival occurs and is interpreted as the repair of sublethal damage (*dashed line*). Subsequent radiation doses result in a reduction of the surviving fraction. This reduction in survival occurs because of more sensitive phases of the cell cycle (G_2 and M). Later time points demonstrate increased surviving fractions due to radiation synchronization of cells and their entry into resistant phases of the cell cycle (G_1 and S).

The concept of SLDR is important during a course of fractionated RT because the shoulder region of the survival curve is recapitulated owing to SLDR.[140] Fractionation magnifies the surviving fraction after each treatment to an exponent equal to the number of treatments. Therefore, small differences in survival after each dose may have a great impact on treatment outcome. Most human tumor cell lines studied in vitro have relatively small shoulders[146,147]; however, a large capacity for SLDR has been reported for some human tumor cell lines.[82,148]

The ability of tissues to undergo SLDR has been demonstrated using a variety of normal tissue clonogenic or functional assays.[149-151] The capacity of different cell populations to repair SLD is reflected by the width of the shoulder (or initial slope) of their survival curve. An increase in the total dose required to give the same biologic damage when a single dose (D_1) is split into two doses (total dose D_2), with a time interval between the doses to obtain a single biologic end point, is the capacity of a normal tissue to repair SLD. The difference in the two doses, $D_2 - D_1$, is the measure of SLDR by the tissue, provided that the two doses are larger than those that generate the shoulder region of the survival curve.[84,150,152] (Fig. 41-12), $D_2 - D_1 = Dq$. If the D_0 is known, then n can be calculated from the equation:

$$\log n = Dq/D_0$$

Varying environmental conditions can influence cell survival after a dose of x-rays. Thus, damage that is potentially lethal under a given set of conditions may not be lethal if postirradiation conditions are altered.[153,154] The enhancement in survival seen following manipulation of postirradiation conditions is referred to as the repair of potentially lethal damage (PLD). PLD repair (PLDR) has been demonstrated in vitro[155,156] (Fig. 41-13). PLDR has also been shown to occur in vivo.[155,157,158] PLDR is reported to be more pronounced in large tumors, presumably because a large proportion of cells are in G_1 or G_0. PLDR has been described to occur principally in the G_1 phase of the cell cycle. Efficient PLDR occurs in a variety of human tumor cell lines in vitro.[159-161] Weichselbaum and colleagues[162-164] and Guichard and colleagues[165] have suggested that PLDR contributes to RT failure under certain circumstances.

PLDR and/or SLDR may not be expressed under all conditions in vivo. For example, cells must be genetically competent to repair these types of damages, and the tumor environment may affect the

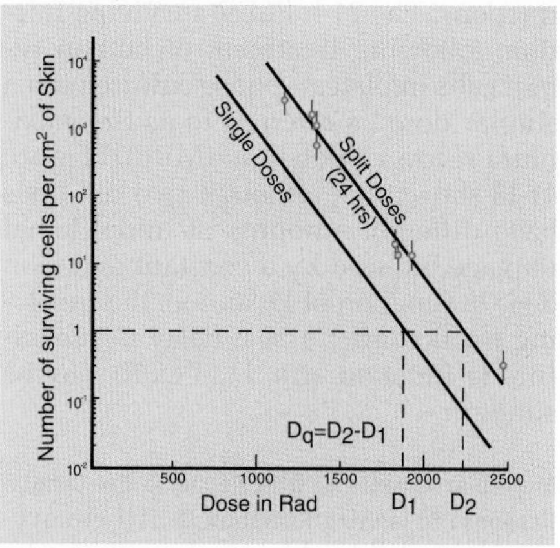

Figure 41-12 ■ Single-dose and two-dose survival curves for epithelial cells. The D_0 is 1.35 Gy. The ordinate is not the surviving fraction, as in survival curves for cells cultured in vitro, but is the number of surviving cells per square centimeter of skin (plating efficiency is obviously not known in vivo). In the two-dose survival curve, the interval between dose fractions is 24 h. Although the curves are paralleled (similar D_0), their graphical horizontal separation number (n) may then be calculated from D_0 and Dq.

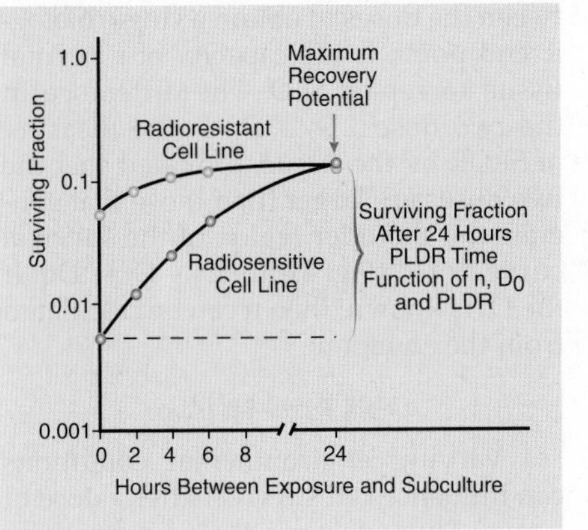

Figure 41-13 Maximum recovery potential (MRP) for radioresistant and radiosensitive cells. Confluent cell lines (noncycling) were irradiated and immediately subcultured, which resulted in an initial surviving fraction that is generally equal to or slightly less than the surviving fraction of exponentially growing cells in tissue culture. However, when these irradiated confluent cells are not subcultured for the indicated time intervals, an enhancement in survival interpreted as subtotal repair of potentially lethal damage (PLDR) occurs. The surviving fraction of cells after a 24-h delay in subculture (MRP) of confluent cells is dependent on n, D_0, and PLDR. The initial surviving fractions of cells at 0 h is dependent on n_0 and D_0 but not PLDR.

proliferative status of tumor cells.[154,164,166] Also, radiation (or chemotherapy) may induce tumor proliferation, which allows fixation of radiation damage before PLDR or SLDR is complete.[154,166] Therefore, PLDR is likely to be most important in tumor cells of intermediate or high radiosensitivity when cells are quiescent between fractions. The 24-h PLDR-surviving fraction, following treatment of human tumor cells in plateau-phase culture with a similar dose, is referred to as the maximum recovery potential (MRP).[83] Figure 41-13 shows that although two cell lines have different amounts of initial lethal damage induced by a constant radiation dose (a function of D_0 and n), the surviving fraction after a 24-h delay in subculture (a function of n, D_0, PLDR) may be similar.

Molecular Aspects of DNA Repair in the Cellular Response to Ionizing Radiation All eukaryotes have evolved several mechanisms to repair DSBs, which indicate the importance and difficulty of repairing this type of DNA injury. The two main pathways are homologous combination (HR) and nonhomologous end-joining (NHEJ). These two repair modes differ in their requirement for a homologous template DNA and in the fidelity of DSB repair. Whereas HR ensures accurate DSB repair, NHEJ does not. The contributions of these two DSB repair pathways are likely to differ depending on the stage of the cell cycle.[167] However, the pathways are not mutually exclusive because repair events that involve both pathways can be detected. HR is most efficient in the S and G_2 phases of the cell cycle because of the availability of sister chromatids as repair templates.[168] In the absence of a sister chromatid, DSB repair in G_1 phase could still efficiently occur through NHEJ.

HR can repair DSBs by using the undamaged chromatid as a template, which results in the accurate repair of the DSB. HR is mediated through the RAD52 family of proteins.[169] These proteins include RAD50, RAD51, RAD52, RAD54, and meiotic recombination 11 (MRE11). The initial cellular response to DSBs is mediated through ATM and Nijmegen breakage syndrome 1 (NBS1).[170] Subsequent steps of DSB repair through HR include DNA-end recognition, possibly by RAD52, and nucleolytic processing of the broken ends of DNA into 3′-end single-stranded DNA. This single-stranded DNA is bound by the RAD51 protein that mediates crucial steps in the reaction—the search for a homologous duplex template DNA and the formation of joint molecules between the broken DNA ends and the repair template. Other proteins, including replication protein A (RPA), RAD52, RAD5430, and several RAD51-related proteins (eg, RAD51B, RAD51C, RAD51D, XRCC2, XRCC3, and DMC1),[171] are thought to function as accessory proteins for RAD51 at various stages of HR. In mammalian cells, RAD51 forms nuclear foci in response to IR and decreased expression of RAD51 confers sensitivity to IR-induced DNA lesions.[121] The later steps of the process include polymerization of nucleotides to restore degraded DNA strands and resolution of the recombination intermediates. Mice with targeted disruption of the RAD51 gene exhibit an embryonic lethal phenotype.[172] Moreover, the failure to generate RAD51$^{-/-}$ stem cells has indicated that RAD51 is essential for cell viability. RAD51 interacts with Tp53[173] and BRCA1.[174] Although the breast cancer susceptibility proteins BRCA1 and BRCA2 are clearly implicated in HR, their roles are not well understood. Other studies have demonstrated that RAD51 is phosphorylated by c-Abl in IR-treated cells and that this response contributes to the downregulation of RAD51 activity in ATP-dependent DNA strand exchange reactions.[121] Treatment of cells with IR is also associated with inactivation of RAD51 by caspase-3- mediated proteolytic cleavage.[175]

In contrast to HR, NHEJ uses little or no homology to couple DNA ends. This pathway is not only used to repair DSBs generated by IR or other exogenous DNA-damaging agents but is also required to process the DSB intermediates that are generated during V(D)J recombination.[176] Several proteins that are involved in NHEJ have been identified. The Ku heterodimer, which consists of Ku70 and Ku80, has a high affinity for DNA ends, which indicates that it has an early role in the NHEJ process. Ku bound to at DNA end attracts the catalytic subunit of the DNA-dependent protein kinase (DNA-PKCs), a 470-kDa polypeptide with a protein kinase domain near its carboxyl terminus.[177] DNA-PKCs can subsequently phosphorylate several cellular target proteins, including p53, the Ku polypeptides and itself. At present, it is unclear which phosphorylation targets of DNA-PKCs are relevant in vivo. A complex that consists of DNA ligase IV and XRCC4 (x-ray-repair-cross-complementing defective repair in Chinese hamster mutant 4) accomplishes the final ligation step. Cell lines or animals that lack either of the genes encoding these proteins do not carry out V(D)J recombination and are sensitive to IR.[178] In addition to the involvement of the RAD50–MRE11-containing complex in HR, genetic experiments with yeast indicate that this complex also has a role in NHEJ.[179]

Although cells deficient in components of the NHEJ and HR pathways are more radiosensitive than their wild-type counterparts, few advances have been made in the development of inhibitors of IR-induced DSB repair. Initial attempts at inhibiting DNA repair in irradiated tumors were associated with increased normal tissue toxicity. A more recent strategy using antisense oligonucleotides to the RAD51 gene has resulted in enhancement of the effects of radiation on glioma cells in vitro and in animal models.[180] With improvements in the selective delivery of RT, the spatial targeting of IR-induced DSBs to tumors should theoretically establish inhibition of DNA repair as an attractive therapeutic approach.

Modulation of chromatin structure and function represents another novel strategy for biological targeting. Histone H2AX, a minor histone H2A variant, encodes a conserved Sr-Gln-Glu (SQE) motif in the carboxyl-terminal tail. IR induces phosphorylation of the Ser residue by ATM/ATR family kinases to form foci of H2AX immunoreactivity a DNA double-strand breaks. Weichselbaum and colleagues showed that peptides that mimic the H2AX carboxyl terminus block induction of H2AX foci and enhance cell death in irradiated radioresistant tumor cells.

Cell Cycle Checkpoints, Integration of Signaling, and DNA Repair

It is necessary for one phase of the cell cycle to be completed before initiating events associated with the following phase. Failure to achieve accurate completion of events may lead to genetic instability and/or cell death. Cells have evolved mechanisms to monitor genomic instability associated with DNA damage. The surveillance mechanisms and resulting inhibition of cell cycle progression are referred to as checkpoint controls. For example, a DNA damage checkpoint control communicates information between a DNA lesion and the regulatory components of the cell cycle. Radiation-induced single-strand breaks (SSBs) and DSBs are associated with the initiating signal that activates checkpoint controls. In general, the cell cycle is delayed at one of the checkpoints by inhibiting cyclin-dependent kinases (CDKs) until DNA repair is complete. Following exposure to IR, cells arrest at the checkpoints. Cell cycle regulation in irradiated and nonirradiated cells has recently been reviewed.[181,182]

DNA damage and its effect on cell cycle progression have been intensively studied in yeast and *Xenopus* oocyte as well as in mammalian cells. Studies show that the kinase activity of Cdc2–cyclin B complex is required for the G_2-to-M-phase (G_2/M) transition in the normal cell cycle and that tyrosine phosphorylation of Cdc2 inhibits its kinase activity.[183] Both inhibition of Cdc2 kinase activity and enhanced phosphorylation of Cdc2 have been observed following DNA damage. The phosphorylation state of Cdc2 is maintained by the kinases Wee1 and Myt1 and by the phosphatase Cdc25.[121,122,125,184] Cdc2 is inactivated by phosphorylation of Thr-14 and Tyr-15 in the ATP-binding domain by the Wee1 kinase.[185] Phosphorylation of Tyr-15 is also mediated in part by IR-induced activation of the Lyn tyrosine kinase.[132,186] Although checkpoint regulation of both sides exists, it is thought that regulation of Cdc25 activity is an important factor in the maintenance of G_2 arrest after DNA damage. In mammalian cells, two kinases, Chk1 and Cds1 (also known as Chk2), have been identified[120,187] and shown to phosphorylate Cdc25C and prevent it from dephosphorylating (Ser-216) and activating Cdc2.[88,120,187-189]

Phosphorylation of Cdc25 facilitates association with the 14-3-3 protein, resulting in its export from the nucleus; however, the mechanism of Chk1 and Cds1 activation following irradiation is not clear. Studies in Chk1-deficient cells have also shown that this kinase is required for initiating G_2 arrest[188,190] and is a downstream effector of ATM. The response of Cds1 to DNA damage has been shown to be dependent on the activity of ATM. The ATM-dependent DNA damage checkpoint pathway regulates both the G_1-S and G_2-M transitions in the response of mammalian cells to IR treatment. The IR-induced arrest at the G_1-S DNA damage checkpoint is mediated predominantly by p53-dependent induction of p21 expression and thereby inhibition of the Cdk2 kinase.[191]

p53 promotes arrest at the G0/G1 checkpoint. Following radiation exposure, p53 protein levels rise owing to posttranslational modifications that increase the p53 half-life. This rise is transient and is correlated with the presence of damaged DNA. DNA strand breaks are the most potent inducers of p53 following IR exposure.[180] Cell cycle arrest is induced by p53 when the protein acts as a transcriptional activator. One of the most important genes induced is p21waf-cip. The interaction of p21 with the cyclin E/CDK2 complex inhibits the progression of cells into the S-phase. p21 also binds directly to proliferating cell nuclear antigen (PCNA). In addition, p53 interacts with MDM2 and GADD45. As described above, MDM2 negatively regulates p53 and likely functions during the recovery phase in the late-G1 phase. GADD45 inhibits the progression of cells into the S-phase. A second mechanism of regulating the G_1 checkpoint by p53 is mediated by direct binding to proteins such as RPA. Bristow and colleagues[192] showed that rat fibroblast clones expressing increasing levels of transfected mutant p53 showed loss of the G1/S checkpoint and increasing levels of radioresistance. The increased survival was not associated with loss of apoptosis but consistent with observations of improved double-strand break repair.[193] This is not consistent with a "more time for repair" hypothesis for the G1/S checkpoint, because checkpoint abrogation would then be expected to sensitize and not protect. Interestingly, the radiosensitivity of p53 null fibroblasts remained unchanged, indicating a gain of function of mutant p53, possibly owing to improved damage sensing via the C-terminus of the protein that is known to bind to damaged DNA in a nonsequence-dependent manner.

Pharmacological agents that override the G2/M block often sensitize the cells to IR.[194] The classic inhibitor of the IR-induced G2 arrest response is caffeine. The precise mechanism for the effects of caffeine on G2 arrest is unresolved, although ATM has been proposed as the target.[195] Treatment of irradiated p53-deficient cells with caffeine is associated with activation of Cdc2 and hence mitotic cell death.[196] These findings are in concert with reports that demonstrate that abrogation of the G2 checkpoint results in differential radiosensitization of G1 checkpoint defective cells.[197] Caffeine and its analogues, however, have not proven to be effective radiosensitizers in the clinic, in part because of the toxicities associated with levels required for inhibition of IR-induced G2 arrest. The CHK1 inhibitors, UCN01 and SB-218078, block DNA damage–induced G2 arrest in human cells.[198-200] These findings and the demonstration that UCN01 does not inhibit hCHK2[198,200] have supported lack of involvement of CHK2 in the G2 arrest response. Whereas UCN01 is undergoing clinical evaluation as a radio- and chemosensitizer, other inhibitors of CHK1/2, such as debromohymenialdisine,[201] are under development. It is noteworthy that the concept of caffeine-induced override of G2-M block has been challenged by investigators who suggest this cell cycle perturbation and enhancement of the induced DNA damage associated with caffeine are attributed to inhibition of DNA repair and/or DNA synthesis.[202-204]

Both the initiation and elongation stages of DNA replication (S-phase checkpoint) are inhibited by IR. In budding yeast, the genes that regulate the S-phase checkpoint are *RAD17, RAD24, RAD53, MEC3* and *MEC1*. The sequence of gene interaction and function in mammalian cells is under investigation. The ATM gene product plays a role in replicon initiation and chain elongation. Both *MEC1* and *ATM* are members of the PI3K gene family.

Thousands of gene transcripts (RNA) can be analyzed by using RNA extracted from cells and hybridized to DNA embedded on chips. This DNA "micro analysis" was used by Amundsen et al to discover radiation responsive genes and radiation-inducible biomarkers from irradiated peripheral blood lymphocytes.[205] This technology has been broadly applied to gene discovery and radio-inducible genes have been discovered in the context of redox and mitochondrial genes that control apoptosis.[206] Khodarev et al demonstrated dose-specific and time-specific radio induction of genes in human tumor cells employing DNA array analysis that might have special applicability to the delivery of RT.[207] Most recently Amundsen et al analyzed the NCI 60 tumor cell lines and reemphasized the importance of p53 in the tumor response to radiation.[208] Because of the ability to analyze patterns of gene expression, DNA array analysis is broadly applied within radiobiology.

Importance of Tumor Hypoxia

Over the past 20 years, more than 125 clinical reports have been published showing that the presence of hypoxia is a poor prognostic sign in many types of human cancers, including head and neck, cervix, soft tissue sarcoma, and primary brain tumors.[209] In multivariate analysis hypoxia has often exhibited independent predictive power for local tumor control following RT.[210-212] Many of the molecular aspects of the hypoxic response not only predicts for local tumor control following RT, but also predict for disease progression and metastasis in tumors treated with chemotherapy and/or surgery. These clinical reports suggest that hypoxia influences tumor biology in ways independent of hypoxic radioresistance.[209] As described below, we now know that hypoxia causes profound changes in cellular metabolic machinery, angiogenesis, cell motility and invasion.

Thomlinson and Gray were the first investigators to suspect that human tumors were hypoxic, following elegant pathologic examination of patterns of necrosis in human lung tumor biopsies in which they found that the viable rim of tumor deposits rarely exceeded 200 μm[213] (Fig. 41-14). They modeled oxygen diffusion in tissue mathematically, coming to the conclusion that 200 μm likely represents the maximum diffusion distance for oxygen. By the time they performed this seminal work, it was already established by several investigators that hypoxic cells were relatively radioresistant. Thus, Thomlinson and Gray pointed out that viable tumor cells residing near the edge of necrosis in a tumor were likely hypoxic and radioresistant. Despite their prediction, it was over three decades before it was proven that human tumors were hypoxic. A handful of papers were published in the 1960s in which large polarographic needle electrodes were inserted into human tumors in an attempt to extract data on oxygen concentration. These sensors were susceptible to artifact because they consumed relatively large quantities of oxygen in the process of making the measurement; thus these results were suspect, but did suggest that human tumors might be hypoxic.[150]

Role of Hypoxia Inducing Factor-1 (HIF-1) ■ One of the major cellular responses to hypoxia is the upregulation of a transcription factor, known as HIF-1. This transcription factor upregulates over a hundred different proteins, referred to as endogenous hypoxia markers. More than 200 papers have been published regarding associations between expression of endogenous hypoxia markers and treatment outcome. Those that often correlate with outcome include CAIX, VEGF, HIF-1 itself, and PAI1. Other proteins that have been examined include Ephrin A1, lysyl oxidase, galectin-1, HIF-2, and dihyrofolate reductase.[214] Expression of endogenous hypoxia regulated proteins confers a poorer prognosis for local tumor control (following RT) as well as metastasis free and overall survival in studies that did not involve RT.

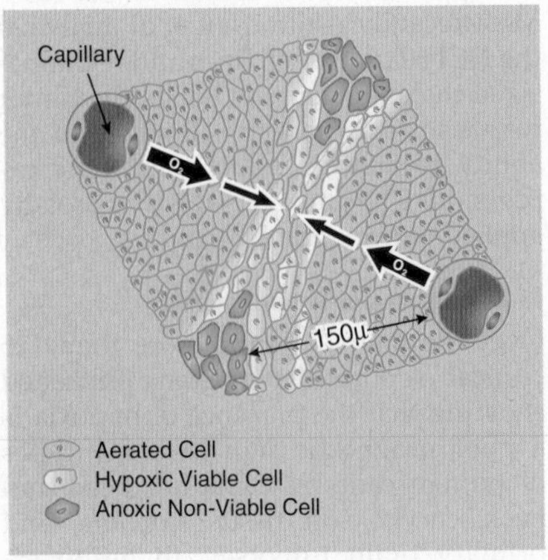

Figure 41-14 ■ Oxygen diffusion through tissue from a capillary resulting in hypoxic cells. Oxygen diffuses an average of 150 μm from the capillary. Cells beyond this region are anoxic and nonviable. Cells at the periphery of this region are hypoxic but viable.

Regulation of the HIF-1 Transcription Factor ■ HIF-1 is a heterodimeric transcription factor that has two subunits: HIF-1α and HIF-1β.[215] When the heterodimer forms, it binds to specific hypoxia regulatory elements (HRE) in the promoter regions of target genes, upregulating their transcription. Under normoxic conditions, HIF-1α is efficiently degraded by proteosomal degradation following hydroxylation and ubiquitination.[215] This process is very efficient in aerobic cells, rendering HIF-1α levels undetectable. There are many other points of regulation of HIF-1 transcriptional activity, including factors that influence the rate of synthesis of HIF-1 and cofactors that influence the binding of the heterodimer to DNA.[216,217]

Involvement of HIF-1 in Radiation Treatment Resistance ■ Until recently, the underlying rationale for the effect of hypoxia in influencing RT treatment outcome was attributed to hypoxic radioresistance. For RT, the rationale is based on the need for oxygen to confer types of DNA damage that are not easily repairable by the cell.[150] In the case of drugs, it has been suggested that hypoxic regions would be less proliferative and therefore resistant to cell cycle specific drugs and that cells farthest from the vasculature would be less accessible to drugs.[218] Whereas these factors may be important, the HIF-1 response to therapy is also an important cause for treatment resistance.

Moeller et al. found that treatment induced tumor reoxygenation after radiation treatment stabilizes HIF-1α. Two mechanisms were responsible. The first was tied to disaggregation of stress granules, aggregates of mRNA, and protein that form under stress conditions, including hypoxia. Upon reoxygenation, these granules disaggregate and release HIF-1–mediated mRNAs that go on to be translated. The second mechanism was linked to production of reactive oxygen/nitrogen species, formed after cell killing. Nitric oxide was shown to stabilize HIF-1 by nitrosylating a cysteine residue that prevented its degradation.[219] Inhibition of HIF-1 activation after RT was shown to greatly sensitize vascular endothelium, resulting in profound growth delay.[220-222] These results provided an explanation for the upregulation of VEGF that has been observed after RT.[223,224]

Rationale for Inhibiting HIF-1 in Combination With Radiation or Cytotoxic Drugs ■ The rationale for targeting HIF-1 in combination with radiation therapy is multifold. HIF-1 upregulation can activate both pro- and antiapoptotic genes; the balance between these opposing effects may influence the decision path taken by a particular cell under conditions of elevated HIF1 activity.[216] Knockdown of HIF-1 activity severely compromises viability of hypoxic cells because they cannot utilize anaerobic metabolism to produce ATP and glucose is their only energy source.[220] They are more likely to undergo necrosis and/or to remain in a G0 state. In addition to inhibiting anaerobic metabolism, HIF-1 inactivation leads to antiangiogenic effects because of reduced VEGF production and substantially increases the sensitivity of tumor vasculature to damaging effects of RT.[220-222] These observations play a major role in the rationale for targeting HIF-1, in that its inhibition not only results in an antiangiogenic effect, but it also selectively kills hypoxic cells by preventing anaerobic metabolism.

Several reviews have been written on the subject of inhibiting HIF-1 in cancer therapy.[215,217,225-227] Its dual effects in regulating angiogenesis and metabolism were predicted by examining the plethora of genes that are regulated by HIF-1.[215] One group has advocated blockade of HIF-1 as a means to accelerate respiration, thereby exacerbating hypoxia, which can then be targeted using hypoxic cytotoxins.[228] Several classes of drugs have been identified as HIF-1 inhibitors, including drugs that inhibit thioredoxin,[226] camptothecins,[229] drugs that inhibit the chaperone function of HSP90,[230] inhibitors of nitric oxide synthase[219,231] and superoxide dismutase mimetic compounds.[220-222]

Hypoxic cell sensitizers, including metronidazole, misonidazole, and etanidazole have been shown to modify the effects of IR.[232] These agents mimic oxygen and have been shown in vitro to increase cell kill of hypoxic cells.[233] Clinical experience, however, with these agents has been mixed. Only two prospective trials have demonstrated a benefit to their use in conjunction with RT.[234,235] Toxicity is common, particularly peripheral neuropathy. More promising results with less toxicity have been noted with the newest hypoxic sensitizer nimorazole.[236]

Modifiers of the Radiation Response

Other than hypoxic cell sensitizers, thymidine analogues iododeoxyuridine (IUdR) and bromodeoxyuridine (BudR), are incorporated into DNA in the place of thymidine and render DNA more susceptible to radiation damage. Although several nonrandomized trials have been promising,[237,238] no prospective trial has demonstrated a significant benefit to their use. Of note, both are associated with considerable acute toxicity.

Multiple chemotherapeutic agents sensitize cells to radiation including 5-fluorouracil, actinomycin D, cisplatin, gemcitabine, fludarabine, paclitaxel, doxorubicin, hydroxyurea, mitomycin C, topotecan, and vinorelbine. The mechanism of radiosensitization varies among the different agents. Cisplatin inhibits both SLDR and PLDR.[239] Inhibition of repair may also help explain the radiosensitizing properties of topotecan.[240] Doxorubicin increases cellular oxygen levels by inhibiting mitochondrial and tumor cell respiration.[241] Hydroxyurea is toxic to cells in the S-phase and inhibits entry of cells into the G1- from the S-phase.[242] Mitomycin C is preferentially toxic to hypoxic cells.[243] Paclitaxel synchronizes cells into the G2- and M-phases.[244]

Other drugs act as radioprotectors by protecting normal tissues from radiation damage while reportedly not affecting tumor radiosensitivity. The best-known radioprotector is amifostine, a derivative of cysteamine that acts as a free radical scavenger. Following administration, amifostine quickly penetrates into normal tissues but only slowly into tumors and thereby results in a preferential protection of normal tissues. Promising results have been reported in head and neck cancer patients undergoing RT.[245] Amifostine has also been used to reduce chemotherapy-related sequelae.[246] Various endogenous biologic response modifiers also act as radio protectors, including interleukin-1 and granulocyte macrophage colony stimulating factor (GM-CSF).[247] Neither is a classic radioprotector, since they do not directly scavenge free radicals but, rather, improve bone marrow tolerance compartment.

Radiation Exposure Growth and Regeneration Kinetics

The percentage of cycling tumor cells is called the growth fraction (GF). In human solid tumors, it is usually a small proportion of the total number of cells. If the GF remains constant with time, the growth rate of the tumor is proportional to the GF. If the GF decreases with time, the rate of the tumor growth slows. Solid tumors usually grow at a slower rate as they enlarge, and so growth is approximated by the Gompertz formula.[84,248] In circumstances of equilibrium in normal tissues, each mitotic division results in the average of only one new cell. Usually, one daughter cell is lost by desquamation or metastasis. By definition, the cell loss factor (CLF) in a steady state is 1. Maximum growth occurs if the CLF is reduced to 0. The only requirement for growth is a reduction from 1.0 in the CLF, ie, an average of <1 of two daughter cells of a division is lost. A CLF of <1 is characteristic of regeneration of both normal tissue and malignant growth. Tumor growth is usually characterized by CLFs that are closer to 1 than 0.

An index for the potential regeneration of tumors and normal tissue populations is the proliferative activity of the cell population.[84] One common measurement of tumor growth is the potential doubling time (PDT), which is defined as the time required to double the number of clonogenic cells if the CLF decreases to zero. In this concept, the doubling time is equal to the cell cycle time. Tumors with a high rate of both cell production and cell loss have the potential for early and rapid regeneration after irradiation or other cytotoxic treatment. Thus, even though a tumor may exhibit slow pretreatment growth, it may regenerate rapidly. Excessive protraction in the time of radiation fractionation or split-course regimens may give inferior local control results if accelerated proliferation occurs during the period when radiation is not given. Clonal proliferation during tumor regression after irradiation was demonstrated by Hermens and Barendsen, who showed an exponential increase in clonogen number in a rat rhabdomyosarcoma during a time of tumor shrinkage (Fig. 41-15).[248] Accelerated repopulation of irradiated tumors and tissues may be associated with the recruitment of quiescent cells into the cell cycle. This effect is associated with radiation-mediated induction of the immediate early genes c-Jun and EGR1.[249]

Cytokines and Growth Factors Following Radiotherapy ■ Although the induction of genes after DNA damage was well known in bacteria, it was only relatively recently that induction of transcription of the proinflammatory cytokine TNFα gene provided support for the theory that gene activation mediates the mammalian cell response to DNA damage.[249] TNFα is transcriptionally induced after irradiation of human tumor cells in vitro[248] and has paracrine and autocrine effects on tumor cell killing and might account for some of the systemic effects of localized RT. bFGF is induced in endothelial cells and mediates protection against apoptosis. The concept of the induction and release of growth factors after IR was initially reported in tumor cells and in normal endothelial cells.[250] Subsequent studies showed that IR induces the expression of genes encoding other growth factors, such as the platelet-derived growth factor, interleukin-1,[189] and bFGF.[184] IR induction of TGFO is proposed to mediate fibrosis after IR, and thereby to mediate some of the late effects of RT on normal tissues. Other cytokines have also been reported to be induced after radiation.[189] Potential applications of these observations are the use of TNFα or other cytokines as potential radio-enhancing agents in gene therapy combined with IR (see later). It has subsequently been discovered that bFGF protects some of the lung endothelium from radiation-mediated apoptosis and has potential as a radioprotector.[251] Also, secretion of growth factors and cytokines may be an important step in radiation carcinogenesis in normal cells. Inhibition of molecular mediators of deleterious late radiation effects on normal tissues may increase the therapeutic ratio and presents the possibility of genetic manipulation in clinical RT.

The recent demonstration of EGFR activation by IR makes this receptor and other members of ErbB receptor tyrosine kinase family important targets for radiosensitizing therapeutic interventions.[189] The radiation-induced activation of EGFR results in cytoprotective signaling dominantly involving MAPK and PI3K. The inhibition of EGFR by tyrphostin TK inhibitors or through overexpression of a dominant-negative (DN) EGFR inhibit the radiation-induced cytoprotective response and results in significant radiosensitization of xenograft tumors in mice. The monoclonal antibody, IMC-C225, cetuximab, which blocks the binding of EGF, exhibits antitumor activity in EGFR+ tumors and enhances radiation toxicity in cultured human squamous cell carcinoma; it also increases taxane-, platinum-induced cytotoxicity in nonsmall cell lung carcinoma xenografts.[252] In A431 head and neck squamous cell xenografts, cetuximab administered in conjunction with irradiation yielded a radiation enhancement factor of 3.62, attributable to both tumor necrosis and antiangiogenesis.[253] In phase I pharmacokinetic studies, cetuximab has a long half-life, lending itself to convenient weekly administration. The reported toxicity profile of cetuximab is limited to allergic and dermatologic reactions. A recently reported phase III international multicenter randomized study in locally advanced squamous cell carcinoma of the head and neck demonstrated that overall and disease-free survival was improved with the combination of cetuximab and radiation over radiation alone.[127]

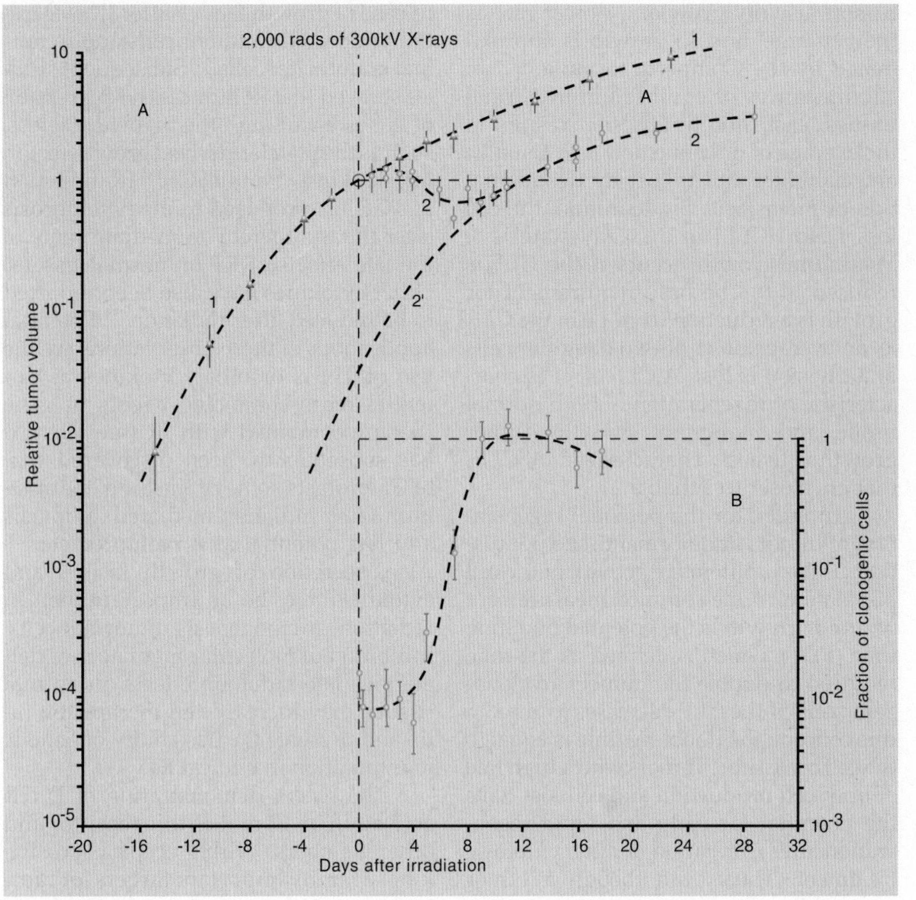

Figure 41-15 Growth curves of rat rhabdomyosarcoma tumors irradiated in vivo demonstrating accelerated repopulation **(A)**. Volume change in the tumor after a single dose of 20 Gy. Curve 1 is the growth of an unirradiated tumor. Curve 2 represents regression and regrowth of an irradiated tumor. **(B)** Exponential increase in the fractions of clonogenic cells as a function of time after irradiation. Cells were obtained from the tumors irradiated in A and the colony forming assay was used to determine clonogenic potential. This figure demonstrated that there is an exponential increase in the number of clonogenic cells within 6-10 days after irradiating a tumor in vivo and that clonogens can repopulate during tumor regression.

Induction of Apoptosis ■ The response of eukaryotic cells to IR and other DNA-damaging agents includes the induction of apoptosis. For more than 40 years, radiobiologists have been aware of cells in irradiated specimens that display the features of apoptosis. Despite this knowledge, the role of apoptosis in end points important in radiation therapy is not clear. The current model suggests that tumor cells with apoptotic propensity are more sensitive to radiation. If this hypothesis is confirmed, strategies can be envisioned that may restore apoptotic propensity to radioresistant tumor cells for therapeutic benefit.

Direct evidence for the activation of caspases in the induction of apoptosis comes from studies with peptide inhibitors,[254] the cowpox virus protein CRMA,[255] and the baculovirus protein p35.[256] Overexpression of CRMA inhibits the induction of apoptosis in diverse settings, including activation of the Fas receptor and treatment with TNFα.[257,258] Similarly, the p35 protein functions as an inhibitor of caspases and blocks apoptosis in insect and mammalian cells.[259] The recent finding that IR-induced apoptosis involves the activation of a CRMA-insensitive pathway has supported the existence of apoptotic signals that are distinct from those activated by Fas and TNK.[260] In this context, caspase-3 is inhibited by p35 but not CRMA in vitro, and IR-induced activation of caspase-3, similar to the induction of apoptosis, involves a p35-sensitive, CRMA-insensitive pathway.[260] Whereas caspase-3 is activated by IR, as well as Fas ligand and TNF, these findings are explained by the involvement of a CRMA-sensitive caspase in the Fas- and TNF-induced, but not the IR-induced cascade. IR-induced activation of caspase-3 is associated with the proteolytic cleavage of poly-(ADP-ribose) polymerase (PARP),[261] DNA-PK,[262] protein kinase C8,[263,264] and protein kinase C.[265] The activation of caspase 3 and the subsequent substrate cleavage in irradiated cells is regulated by the members of the Bc1-2/Bc1- x1 family.[266] Bcl-2 and Bcl-xL block the release of cytochrome *c* from the mitochondria of cells exposed to IR and other agents.[267-269] Whereas cytochrome *c* is not released from the mitochondria of cells induced to undergo apoptosis with Fas ligand,[85] this event upstream to activation of caspase-3[119] and the insensitivity of IR-induced caspase-3 activity to CRMA[260] support distinct apoptotic signals in Fas- and IR-treated cells.

IR-induced apoptosis is mediated at least in part by c-Abl-dependent activation of p53 and its homolog, p73.[270] IR also induces translocation of SAPK to mitochondria, interaction of SAPK and Bcl-xL, and thereby release of cytochrome c.[271,272] In turn, cytochrome *c* activates caspase-3 and the cleavage of diverse proteins that confer the apoptotic response.[273,274] Bcl-2 and Bcl-xL block IR-induced cytochrome *c* release and apoptosis.[271,275,276] These findings have supported the transduction of DNA damage-induced signals to mitochondria as a determinant of cell fate in the IR response.

Gene Therapy and Radiation Therapy

Experimental RT has been combined with gene therapy in a variety of different strategies. These include the use of various viral and nonviral vectors to transduce tumor cells with enzymes that convert specific prodrugs to radiosensitizers, cytotoxins, and/or immunomodulatory cytokines and other molecules that disrupt signaling pathways. Prodrug converting enzymes include herpes simplex virus (HSV), thymidine kinase, and bacterial cytosine deaminase. In another approach, the tumor suppressor gene p53 is employed to modulate radiation-mediated apoptosis in cells that lack p53. Limitations of gene therapy include the lack of transduction of the entire tumor cell population as well as the lack of control of gene expression. In an attempt to compensate for lack of uniform tumor transduction and to achieve spatial and temporal control of gene therapy, Weichselbaum and colleagues delineated a strategy whereby a radiation-inducible promotor is ligated to a therapeutic gene of interest.[136] Radiation-inducible DNA sequences from the EGR-1 promoter were ligated to a DNA encoding TNFα and cloned into a nonreplication competent adenoviral vector. Tumors treated with IR and EGR–TNFα (TNFerade; GenVec, Gaithersberg, MD) regressed more rapidly and to a greater extent than tumors treated with EGR–TNFα or radiation alone. TNFα was induced sevenfold over background levels in the tumor, but not in the blood, thus achieving control over gene expression. This approach to gene therapy overcomes some of the limitations of limited viral transduction by employing a diffusible cytokine. This strategy has been recently evaluated for safety in phase I clinical trials[277] and is currently being tested for efficacy in phase II trials in patients with rectal and esophageal cancer. A randomized phase III trial of TNFerade in combination with 50 Gy and 5-FU vs 5-FU and 50 Gy is ongoing.

In another strategy that targets gene therapy by IR, it has been demonstrated that genetically engineered herpes viruses can be induced to proliferate in irradiated tumors. Herpes virus can cause lethal encephalitis and has been modified to be less neurovirulent by one of two strategies. Herpes genes that encode enzymes necessary for viral DNA synthesis or the gamma1 34.5 gene are deleted. The 34.5 gene prevents host protein syntheses shut-off, which has evolved to defeat HSV proliferation. Advani and colleagues employed a herpes virus (with gamma 34.5 deleted) combined with radiation and demonstrated a superior antitumor effect when compared with radiation or herpes virus alone in a flank model of human gliomas.[278] These findings were extended and confirmed by Bradley and colleagues who employed IR and genetically engineered (GSE) herpes in an intracranial model of glioma and demonstrated a prolongation of survival in animals treated with the combination of herpes and IR.[279]

Cytotoxic applications of adenovirus have also been investigated. This virus exerts its control over host cell growth regulation by a complex set of proteins that facilitate viral replication. Adenoviral infection induces cellular p53 protein which is proapoptotic and therefore detrimental to the viral life cycle. The virally encoded E1B protein blocks p53 action, preventing apoptosis and allowing for viral replication to proceed. The ONYX-15 virus is an E1B deleted adenovirus that restricts lytic activity to cells expressing mutant p53. Freytag and colleagues have shown that ONYX-15 virus combined with radiation leads to enhanced tumor cell killing in tumors expressing mutant p53 in vivo.[280] DeWeese and colleagues used a prostate-specific antigen selective replication restricted adenovirus in a phase I dose escalation study in patients with locally recurrent prostate cancer. They showed that the highest dose levels of virus administered were associated with a decrease in PSA.[281]

Another strategy that has been used to improve the therapeutic ratio of RT by gene therapy has been to introduce genes that selectively protect normal tissue. An example of this is the delivery of manganese superoxide dismutase (MSOD) to normal cells to protect against radiation damage. Greenberger and colleagues have studied the delivery of liposome-MnSOD complexes for protecting both normal lung and bladder tissue in mice treated with IR.[282] Other investigators have shown that tissue levels of TGF-β1 can be reduced by soluble TGFβ type II receptor gene therapy and ameliorated radiation-induced pulmonary injury in rats.[283]

Another gene-based strategy is based on the overexpression of EGFR-CD533. This dominant-negative EGFR variant lacks the C-terminal 533 amino acids and forms nonfunctioning heterodimeric complexes with wt EGFR receptors.[284] Schmidt-Ullrich and colleagues have studied the potential therapeutic application of EGFR-CD533 in human tumor xenograft models.[285] These investigators demonstrated that the overexpression of EGFR-CD533 in mammary carcinoma cells abrogates the EGFR-mediated cytoprotective response induced by IR and enhances radiosensitivity.[286] They subsequently incorporated EGFR-CD533 into a replication-incompetent adenovirus (Ad) and showed that Ad-EGFR-CD533 delays growth of U-373 MG glioma xenograft tumors and overcomes the enhanced tumorigenic effects of EGFRvIII expression.[287]

Antiangiogenic Therapy Combined With Radiation Therapy

IR has been reported to mediate vascular collapse and thrombosis of very small tumor vessels. However, until recently, IR was not considered to target the tumor vessels. Tumor endothelial cells arise from host endothelium and are genetically stable, compared with tumor cells; they are therefore are less likely to become resistant to DNA-damaging agents. Additionally, one tumor vessel may supply up to 106 tumor cells with nutrients, thus amplifying the cytotoxic antitumor effects of IR. Teicher and colleagues conducted investigations combining radiation and synthetic antiangiogenesis compounds and demonstrated an increase in tumor cure and tumor growth delay.[288] In spite of potential toxicities of the antiangiogenesis drugs, these investigators validated the tumor vasculature as a potential target for RT. In concert with these findings, the synthetic angiogenesis inhibitor, TNP-470, has been found to potentiate the effects of RT in the treatment of human glioblastoma multiforme xenografts in the nude mouse.[289] Other studies have demonstrated that the endogenous angiogenesis inhibitor, angiostatin, enhances radiation-mediated tumor regressions without an increase in toxicity.[290] The potentiation of RT by angiostatin was observed in several human tumor xenografts, including a human glioma. A brief exposure to angiostatin enhances tumor regression when delivered at the same time as radiation.[291] These findings also showed that a prolonged course of angiostatin is not necessary for optimal therapeutic effects. The demonstration that endostatin similarly potentiates the antitumor effects of RT indicates that the interaction is broadly applicable to angiogenesis inhibitors.[292]

Another strategy has been to potentiate the effectiveness of RT with agents that function by directly blocking positive regulators of angiogenesis. For example, administration of antibodies against the vascular endothelial growth factor (VEGF) potentiates RT of murine and human tumor models, including that of a glioma xenograft.[291] In clinical trials, Willet and colleagues demonstrated that anti-VEGF antibody decreases tumor perfusion, vascular volume, and microvascular density in rectal cancer patients.[293] Similar findings have been corroborated in other studies using anti-VEGF antibodies or inhibitors (SU5416, SU6668, PTK787) of the VEGF-signaling pathway in combination with RT.[294-298] In addition, COX-2 inhibitors have been reported to enhance the antitumor efficacy of RT without increasing toxicity.[299-301] These findings collectively demonstrate that the inhibition of tumor angiogenesis potentiates the efficacy of radiation therapy.

Recently, investigators have suggested that vascular endothelial cell apoptosis represents a primary lesion in radiation-induced injury, at least in the GI tract. Fuks and colleagues demonstrated that bFGF increases survival of intestinal crypts and prevents GI syndrome in C57Bl/ 6 mice.[302] More recently, these authors suggested that microvascular damage regulates tumor cell response to radiation.[303]

Clinical Radiation Oncology

Dose Response and the Therapeutic Ratio Various levels of radiation yield different tumor control probabilities, depending on the size and anatomic extent of the lesion. The total number of surviving cells is proportional to the initial number and biologic characteristics of clonogenic cells and the total cell kill achieved with a specified dose of radiation. Dose-response relationships for local control of homogeneous tumor groups have been empirically determined. The higher the doses of radiation delivered, the more likely is tumor control (Table 41-1).

The dose of radiation that can be delivered to a tumor is limited by the probability of serious normal tissue complications. Therefore, the choice of a tumor dose is based on the relative probability of tumor control and normal tissue complications. The potential therapeutic gain can be estimated for an average group of patients on the basis of tumor size, histologic type, and the normal tissues that will be included in the treatment fields. Figure 41-16 shows a theoretic dose-response relationship for tumor control and normal tissue compli-

Table 41-1 Relationship Between Tumor Diameter and Dose to Percent Local Control

	% Control	
Dose (5 × 200 cGy/wk)	Squamous Cell Carcinoma	Adenocarcinoma
5000	>90% microfoci 50% 2-3 cm nodes	>90% subclinical
6000	80-90% T1 pharynx and larynx	
7000	90% 1-3 cm nodes 80% T3-T4 tonsil	90% axillary

cations. The therapeutic ratio is defined as the percentage of tumor cures obtained at a given level of toxicity for normal tissues. Figure 41-16A depicts a favorable therapeutic ratio and Figure 41-16B depicts an unfavorable therapeutic ratio. The greater the displacement between the two curves (in the favorable situation), the more radiocurable is the tumor.

Fractionation Early in the twentieth century, it became apparent that RT was equally efficacious but better tolerated when administered in divided doses,[304] a concept known as fractionation. Fractionation spares normal tissues by allowing time for repair and repopulation of normal cells. In addition, fractionation increases tumor cell kill due to reoxygenation and reassortment of tumor cells into sensitive phases of the cell cycle.[305] Conventional fractionation schemes involve a daily fraction of 1.8-2 Gy 5 days a week. Total treatment time depends on the total dose prescribed and thus ranges from 3 to 7 weeks. Various mathematical models have been proposed to equate total dose, time, and fraction size to achieve an isoeffective dose. However, clinical utility of these models remains controversial.

Clinical interest in altered fractionation has been resurrected due to recently reported improved outcomes in patients with advanced head and neck cancer. Hyperfractionation is defined as the use of reduced size fractions given twice or more per day such that a greater total dose is delivered by increasing the number of treatments (50–60 vs 30–35) in the same total treatment time. Thus, relatively rapidly dividing cell populations may have a higher proportion of cells in the most sensitive phases of the cell cycle at each treatment. Cells in late-responding normal tissues are slowly proliferating, and therefore, after a few fractions, many surviving cells will be concentrated in the more resistant phases. This strategy has been applied to a variety of tumors, including primary brain tumors[306] and head and neck cancer.[307,308]

Accelerated fractionation decreases the overall treatment time to diminish clonogenic proliferation between successive doses. Treatment is given 2-4 times per day, employing fraction sizes of 1.5-2 Gy per treatment with 4-6 h interfraction intervals.[84] The total daily dose is thus 3-6 Gy and the total dosage is given in 3-4 weeks. Although treatment interruptions are often necessary due to acute toxicity,[84] the total treatment time is substantially reduced. Hypofractionation is the use of larger than standard daily fractions. This approach is typically used when palliation is the goal. Treatment may involve 4-24 Gy fractions delivered weekly or several times a week as opposed to daily.

RT alone is used as curative therapy in a variety of tumor types. Treatment may consist of external beam alone, brachytherapy alone, or a combination of the two. Although combined modality chemoradiotherapy is more common today, definitive RT is still used in early-stage head and neck as well as gynecologic tumors. RT alone is associated with results comparable with that obtained with surgery for tumors of the oral cavity,[309] oropharynx,[310] supraglottic larynx,[311] and glottis.[312] Moreover, definitive RT is often associated with better long-term functional outcome than surgery. Definitive RT was recently compared in a large prospective randomized trial with radical surgery in women with early-stage operable cervical cancer. RT was associated with identical tumor control rates with less long-term sequelae.[313] Another tumor type that may be treated with RT alone is early-stage Hodgkin disease.[314]

RT alone is also the treatment of choice in elderly patients. A common belief is that the elderly are at higher risk of acute and chronic RT sequelae. However, numerous investigators have demonstrated that age per se is not associated with increased toxicity.[315] Instead, comorbidities present in the elderly may increase their risk.[316]

Adjuvant Therapy A more common use of RT is in combination with surgery and/or chemotherapy. When combined with surgery, RT may be given before (preoperative), after (postoperative), or during (intraoperative) surgery. Although common in the past, preoperative RT is less used today except in large borderline resectable tumors, eg, rectal cancer[317] and soft tissue sarcomas.[318] In contrast, postoperative RT is used in many tumor sites including tumors of the central nervous system,[319] head and neck,[320] breast,[321] lung,[322] genitourinary,[323] and gastrointestinal tract.[324] In patients with resectable disease, postoperative RT is preferred because it allows treatment to be tailored to the pathology findings, and higher doses are possible; moreover, there is reduced potential for interference in normal wound healing. Indications for postoperative RT include close/positive margins, residual disease, perineural invasion, lymphovascular space invasion, and lymph node involvement. Potential disadvantages of postoperative RT include delaying therapy until wound healing is complete and reduced vascularity of tissues following surgery. Intraoperative RT is the delivery of a single large fraction during surgery with either electrons or low-energy photons.[325] This is accomplished with either a

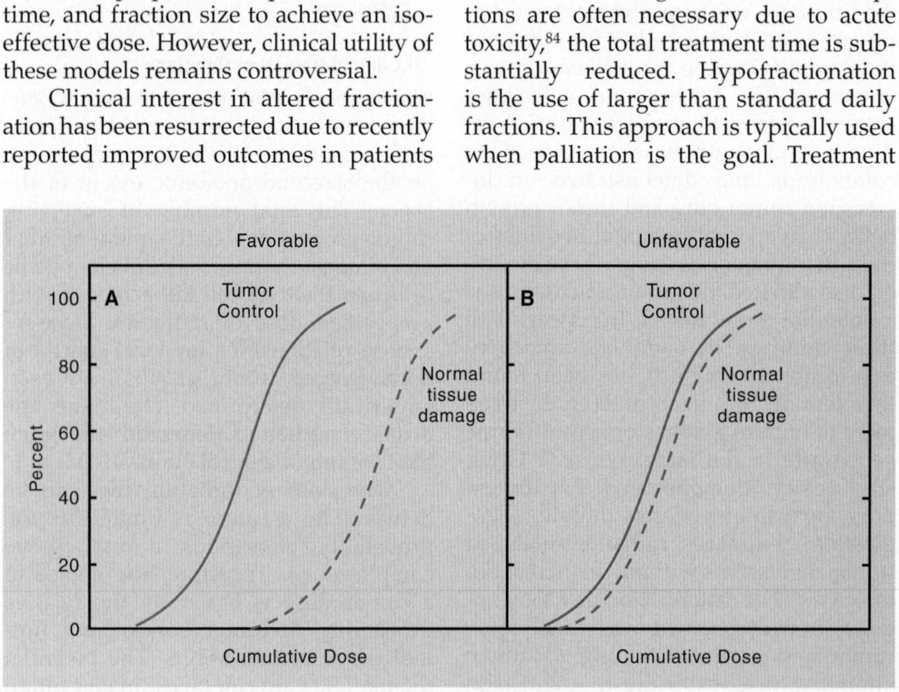

Figure 41-16 Dose control and complication curves in curable and incurable tumors treated with radiotherapy. The percentages of tumor control and normal tissue damage are sigmoidal. **(A)** In a radiocurable tumor, such as Hodgkin lymphoma, the dose required to control a tumor is less than the normal tissue tolerance. This results in a favorable therapeutic ratio. **(B)** The dosage required to control an unfavorable tumor such as pancreatic carcinoma is approximately that of normal tissue tolerance resulting in an unfavorable therapeutic ratio.

dedicated treatment machine in the operating room or by transporting the patient to the RT department during surgery. An important benefit is that normal tissues, eg, small bowel, can be displaced out of the treatment field. A disadvantage is that the total treatment is delivered in a single fraction, which obviates the benefit of fractionation. Promising results have been reported in retroperitoneal soft tissue sarcoma.[326] Brachytherapy has also been used at the time of surgery. It is imperative, however, to delay loading for several days to allow for adequate wound healing.[327]

When combined with radiation, chemotherapy may be administered before (neoadjuvant), during (concomitant), or after RT (maintenance). Chemoradiotherapy approaches have been shown to improve local control and eradicate micrometastatic disease. Neoadjuvant chemotherapy has been used in a number of sites including non-Hodgkin lymphoma[328] and advanced larynx cancer.[329] A potential advantage is that bulky disease sites can be cytoreduced allowing for smaller treatment volumes. However, increasing evidence suggests that concomitant chemoradiotherapy is preferable in a variety of disease sites. Concomitant chemoradiotherapy is used in locally advanced cancer of the lung,[330] head and neck,[331] esophagus,[332] bladder,[333] and cervix.[334] Possible interactions between chemotherapeutic drugs and radiation are summarized in Table 41-2.

In many sites, all three modalities are combined. A variety of schedules have been used. Examples include neoadjuvant chemotherapy, surgery, and postoperative RT (locally advanced breast cancer),[335] surgery followed by concomitant postoperative chemoradiotherapy (cancer of the pancreas, and stomach),[336,337] as well as neoadjuvant chemoradiotherapy followed by surgical resection.[338,339]

A disease state of "oligometastases" has been proposed.[340] In this paradigm, tumors early in the chain of metastatic progression may have metastasis limited in number and location based on a limited facility for metastatic growth (de novo oligometastases). Alternatively, with effective systemic therapy, patients with more widespread metastases may have the majority of their metastatic deposits eradicated, leaving behind few foci of residual tumor due to the presence of drug/hormone/targeted agent resistant cells (Induced oligometastases). In both classes of patients with oligometastatic disease, a window of opportunity may exist where focal therapy to known sites of gross disease may be beneficial. A recent analysis of nonsmall cell lung cancer patients supported this hypothesis revealing that 50% of nonsmall cell lung cancer patients had metastasis limited to three additional sites other than the primary tumor.[341] Therefore, metastatic cancer is not always widespread, and there may be a role for local therapy in these patients. The role of local therapy for long-term disease control of oligometastases is supported by reports indicating that surgery may be curative for a percentage of patients with limited lung,[342] liver,[343] synchronous lung and liver,[344] or adrenal metastasis.[345] Most patients who have several metastases to multiple organs have not generally been considered for curative surgical treatment. However, half of metastatic nonsmall cell lung cancer patients treated with systemic therapy do not progress or only progress at initially involved sites.[341] Recent reports have demonstrated that focal RT to all known sites of disease approximates the results of surgical metastasectomy with 21% of patients rendered disease free.[66] Further work is ongoing to integrate focused RT with systemic chemotherapy for the treatment of patients with oligometastatic disease.

Prophylactic Therapy ■ The most common example is the prophylactic treatment of regional, clinically uninvolved lymph nodes. Prophylactic cranial irradiation (PCI) is used in patients with limited and extensive stage small-cell lung cancer[346,347] and children with high-risk acute leukemia.[337,348] Other examples include breast irradiation in men with prostate cancer who receive diethylstilbestrol (DES).

Palliative Therapy ■ RT is an important means of providing rapid and effective palliation due to local and/or metastatic disease. Osseous metastases secondary to breast, prostate, and other cancers are treated with localized fields and short-course regimens, eg, 30 Gy in 10 fractions. Pain relief is achieved in more than 70% of patients.[349] The optimal fractionation schedule, however, remains unclear. Rapid large fractions, eg, 20 Gy over 5 days, are equivalent to more protracted regimens using smaller daily doses.[350] Such approaches are indicated in patients with symptomatic long-bone sites that are not in close proximity to critical organs. More rapid schedules are also possible. Many studies have compared large single fractions (6-10 Gy) vs more protracted schedules (30-40 Gy in 10-20 fractions). Pooled analyses of these studies as well as a recent Radiation Therapy Oncology Group (RTOG) study demonstrates that these schedules are equivalent in terms of symptomatic pain relief.[351] Large-field (hemibody) irradiation has been used in patients with widespread bone metastases.[352,353] Promising results have also been reported with intravenous 144Sr[353] and samarium.[354]

Whole-brain RT is indicated in patients with cerebral metastases. Treatment is typically delivered over 10 days to a total dose of 30 Gy. As with osseous metastases, controversy exists over the optimal treatment regimen in these patients. Borgelt and colleagues reviewed various regimens ranging from 20 Gy in 5 fractions to 40 Gy in 20 fractions on two randomized trials. No differences were seen in frequency or duration of response. Overall, 50% of patients had significant improvement in neurologic symptoms. However, the less protracted regimens resulted in more rapid overall response rates.[355] Protracted regimens are indicated, however, in patients with controlled primaries and solitary metastases.

Other indications for palliative RT include spinal cord compression,[356] liver metastases,[357] orbital metastases,[358] and carcinomatous meningitis.[359] Palliative RT is also used in symptomatic locally advanced lung[360] and ovarian cancer.[361] Brachytherapy can be used in palliative treatment as well, eg, bronchial,[362] biliary,[363] and esophageal[364] obstructions.

Therapy for Non-malignant Disease ■ RT is used in a wide variety of benign tumors and conditions, such as keloids[365] hemangiomas,[366] desmoids,[367] and pterygium.[368] Other indications include renal[369] and cardiac[370] transplant rejection, macular degeneration,[371] Grave's ophthalmopathy,[372] arteriovenous malformation, and heterotopic bone prophylaxis following arthroplasty.[373]

Radiation Sequelae

Acute Sequelae ■ Acute radiation sequelae, such as skin desquamation, mucosi-

Table 41-2 ■ Interaction of Radiotherapy and Chemotherapy

Chemotherapeutic drugs and radiation are active against different tumor cell subpopulations based on hypoxia, cell cycle specificity, and pH
Decreased tumor cell repopulation following fractionated radiation due to effects of chemotherapy
Increased tumor cell recruitment from G_0 into a therapy-responsive cell cycle phase
Increased tumor cell oxygenation following radiation with improved drug or radiation activity
Improved drug delivery with shrinkage of tumor
Early eradication of tumor cells preventing emergence of drug and/or radiation resistance
Eradication of cells resistant to one treatment modality by the other treatment
Cell cycle synchronization
Inhibition of repair of sublethal radiation damage or inhibition of recovery from potentially lethal radiation damage

tis, and diarrhea, occur during or immediately after treatment. Such sequelae are believed to be due to the interruption of repopulation in rapidly proliferating tissues.[374] The type of reaction is dependent on the site irradiated. The one exception is fatigue, which occurs in almost all patients. Most acute sequelae are self-limited and respond to pharmacologic management, such as diphenoxylate hydrochloride with atropine sulfate (diarrhea) and viscous lidocaine (esophagitis). It is imperative to control symptoms and avoid prolonged treatment breaks, since treatment protraction has been correlated with worse tumor control in several disease sites.[375,376] Prophylactic medication may also be helpful.[377] Promising results have been reported using sucralfate in patients undergoing thoracic irradiation to decrease the severity of esophagitis.[378]

The severity of acute sequelae is dependent on a variety of factors. Two major factors are fraction size and treatment volume. Whenever large treatment volumes are used, it is thus imperative to reduce the daily fraction size to minimize acute sequelae.

Chronic Sequelae ■ Chronic reactions, such as fibrosis, fistulae, and necrosis, occur months to years after treatment and are due, in part, to damage to slowly proliferating tissues. Other factors, including vascular damage, may also play a part in their development. Chronic reactions, like acute reactions, are dependent on the irradiated site. Chronic reactions, however, are often permanent. Sequelae vary widely in severity, ranging from mild fibrosis to small bowel obstruction, fistulae, and second malignancies. Overall, the risk of a second malignancy following RT is low. The notable exception is osteosarcoma arising in irradiated bones in children treated for retinoblastoma, particularly the hereditary type.[379] However, some are concerned that higher integral radiation doses required of such as IMRT may lead to an increase in second malignancies.

Select chronic radiation sequelae are responsive to medical management, eg, pneumonitis is managed with bronchodilators and, if necessary, a course of corticosteroids. Recent evidence supports the role of angiotensin II receptor antagonist in the treatment and prevention of radiation nephritis.[377] Prophylactic medications may also decrease the risk of select late sequelae. Promising results have been reported with pilocarpine in head and neck cancer to decrease the incidence of xerostomia.[380] Recently, zinc sulfate has been found to reduce the risk of significant taste alterations in patients with head and neck cancer.[381] The most important means of reducing the risk of chronic sequelae, however, is prevention. Strict attention to optimal technique is imperative. Soft tissue sarcoma patients, eg, should never receive treatment to the entire circumference of the extremity in order to reduce the risk of chronic edema. The risk of late sequelae is also reduced by avoiding the use of large daily fractions, since fraction size is a major determinant of late effects.[84] As noted earlier, new approaches including 3D CRT, IMRT, and inverse treatment planning should further aid in reducing the risk of late sequelae.

Selected References

The complete reference list can be found at www.CANCERMEDICINE8.com

1. Roentgen W. On a new kind of rays [preliminary communication]. Translation of a paper read before the Physikalische-medicinischen Gesellschaft of Wurzburg on December 28, 1895. *Br J Radiol.* 1931;4:32–36.
2. Coutard H. Roentgentherapy of epitheliomas of the tonsillar region, hypopharynx and larynx from 1920 to 1926. *AJR Am J Roentgenol.* 1932;28:313–332.
3. Paterson R. The radical x-ray treatment of carcinomata. *Br J Radiol.* 1936;9:671–679.
4. Attix F. *Introduction to Radiological Physics and Radiation Dosimetry.* New York: John Wiley & Sons; 1986.
5. Khan F. *The Physics of Radiation Therapy.* Baltimore, MD: Williams and Wilkins; 1994.
6. Laramore GE. The use of neutrons in cancer therapy: a historical perspective through the modern era. *Semin Oncol.* 1997;24(6):672–685.
7. Vynckier S, Schmidt R. The physical basis for radiotherapy with neutrons. *Recent Results Cancer Res.* 1998;150:1–30.
8. Bonnett DE. Current developments in proton therapy: a review. *Phys Med Biol.* 1993;38(10):1371–1392.
9. Miller DW. A review of proton beam radiation therapy. *Med Phys.* 1995;22(11 Pt 2):1943–1954.
10. Purdy JA, et al. State of the art of high energy photon treatment planning. *Front Radiat Ther Oncol.* 1987;21:4–24.
11. Graham MV, et al. Preliminary results of a prospective trial using three dimensional radiotherapy for lung cancer. *Int J Radiat Oncol Biol Phys.* 1995;33(5):993–1000.
12. Michalski JM, et al. Three dimensional conformal radiation therapy in pediatric parameningeal rhabdomyosarcomas. *Int J Radiat Oncol Biol Phys.* 1995;33(5):985–991.
13. Yang FE, et al. The potential for normal tissue dose reduction with neoadjuvant hormonal therapy in conformal treatment planning for stage C prostate cancer. *Int J Radiat Oncol Biol Phys.* 1995;33(5):1009–1017.
14. Bentel G. *Patient Positioning and Immobilization in Radiation Oncology.* New York: McGraw-Hill; 1999:1–38.
15. Austin-Seymour M, et al. Tumor and target delineation: current research and future challenges. *Int J Radiat Oncol Biol Phys.* 1995;33(5):1041–1052.
16. Purdy JA. Current ICRU definitions of volumes: limitations and future directions. *Semin Radiat Oncol.* 2004;14(1):27–40.
17. Roeske JC, et al. Evaluation of changes in the size and location of the prostate, seminal vesicles, bladder, and rectum during a course of external beam radiation therapy. *Int J Radiat Oncol Biol Phys.* 1995;33(5):1321–1329.
18. van Herk M, et al. Quantification of organ motion during conformal radiotherapy of the prostate by three dimensional image registration. *Int J Radiat Oncol Biol Phys.* 1995;33(5):1311–1320.
19. Giraud P, et al. Reduction of organ motion effects in IMRT and conformal 3D radiation delivery by using gating and tracking techniques. *Cancer Radiother.* 2006;10(5):269–282.
20. Levin DN, et al. The brain: integrated three-dimensional display of MR and PET images. *Radiology.* 1989;172(3):783–789.
21. Kooy HM, et al. Image fusion for stereotactic radiotherapy and radiosurgery treatment planning. *Int J Radiat Oncol Biol Phys.* 1994;28(5):1229–1234.
22. Hamilton RJ, et al. Functional imaging in treatment planning of brain lesions. *Int J Radiat Oncol Biol Phys.* 1997;37(1):181–188.
23. Nestle U, et al. 18F-deoxyglucose positron emission tomography (FDG-PET) for the planning of radiotherapy in lung cancer: high impact in patients with atelectasis. *Int J Radiat Oncol Biol Phys.* 1999;44(3):593–597.
24. Suga K, et al. 201Tl SPECT as an indicator for early prediction of therapeutic effects in patients with non-small cell lung cancer. *Ann Nucl Med.* 1998;12(6):355–362.
25. Kessler ML, et al. Integration of multimodality imaging data for radiotherapy treatment planning. *Int J Radiat Oncol Biol Phys.* 1991;21(6):1653–1667.
26. Pelizzari CA, et al. Accurate three-dimensional registration of CT, PET, and/or MR images of the brain. *J Comput Assist Tomogr.* 1989;13(1):20–26.
27. van Herk M, Kooy HM. Automatic three-dimensional correlation of CT-CT, CT-MRI, and CT-SPECT using chamfer matching. *Med Phys.* 1994;21(7):1163–1178.
28. Drzymala RE, et al. Dose-volume histograms. *Int J Radiat Oncol Biol Phys.* 1991;21(1):71–78.
29. McShan DL, et al. A computerized three-dimensional treatment planning system utilizing interactive colour graphics. *Br J Radiol.* 1979;52(618):478–481.
30. Sherouse GW, Novins K, Chaney EL. Computation of digitally reconstructed radiographs for use in radiotherapy treatment design. *Int J Radiat Oncol Biol Phys.* 1990;18(3):651–658.
31. Drebin R. Volume rendering. *Computer Graphics.* 1988;22:65–74.
32. Drebin RA, et al. Fidelity of three-dimensional CT imaging for detecting fracture gaps. *J Comput Assist Tomogr.* 1989;13(3):487–489.
33. Boyer AL, et al. Clinical dosimetry for implementation of a multileaf collimator. *Med Phys.* 1992;19(5):1255–1261.
34. Brahme A. Optimization of radiation therapy and the development of multi-leaf collimation. *Int J Radiat Oncol Biol Phys.* 1993;25(2):373–375.

35. Boyer AL, et al. A review of electronic portal imaging devices (EPIDs). *Med Phys.* 1992;19(1):1–16.
36. Meertens H, et al. First clinical experience with a newly developed electronic portal imaging device. *Int J Radiat Oncol Biol Phys.* 1990;18(5):1173–1181.
37. Dong L, Boyer AL. An image correlation procedure for digitally reconstructed radiographs and electronic portal images. *Int J Radiat Oncol Biol Phys.* 1995;33(5):1053–1060.
38. Michalski JM, et al. The use of on-line image verification to estimate the variation in radiation therapy dose delivery. *Int J Radiat Oncol Biol Phys.* 1993;27(3):707–716.
39. Court LE, et al. An automatic CT-guided adaptive radiation therapy technique by online modification of multileaf collimator leaf positions for prostate cancer. *Int J Radiat Oncol Biol Phys.* 2005;62(1):154–163.
40. Mohan R, Leibel S. Intensity modulation of the radiation beam. In: *Cancer: Principles and Practice of Oncology.* Devita V, Hellman S, Rosenberg S, eds. Philadelphia: Lippincott-Raen; 1997.
41. Stein J, et al. Number and orientations of beams in intensity-modulated radiation treatments. *Med Phys.* 1997;24(2):149–160.
42. Verhey LJ. Comparison of three-dimensional conformal radiation therapy and intensity-modulated radiation therapy systems. *Semin Radiat Oncol.* 1999;9(1):78–98.
43. Yu CX, et al. A method for implementing dynamic photon beam intensity modulation using independent jaws and a multileaf collimator. *Phys Med Biol.* 1995;40(5):769–787.
44. Mell LK, Roeske JC, Mundt AJ. A survey of intensity-modulated radiation therapy use in the United States. *Cancer.* 2003;98(1):204–211.
45. Teh BS, et al. Intensity modulated radiation therapy (IMRT) in the management of prostate cancer. *Cancer Invest.* 2004;22(6):913–924.
46. Chao KS, et al. Intensity-modulated radiation therapy reduces late salivary toxicity without compromising tumor control in patients with oropharyngeal carcinoma: a comparison with conventional techniques. *Radiother Oncol.* 2001;61(3):275–280.
47. Huang E, et al. Intensity-modulated radiation therapy for pediatric medulloblastoma: early report on the reduction of ototoxicity. *Int J Radiat Oncol Biol Phys.* 2002;52(3):599–605.
48. Salama JK, et al. Concurrent chemotherapy and intensity-modulated radiation therapy for anal canal cancer patients: a multicenter experience. *J Clin Oncol.* 2007;25(29):4581–4586.
49. Salama JK, et al. Intensity-modulated radiation therapy in gynecologic malignancies. *Curr Treat Options Oncol.* 2004;5(2): 97–108.
50. Syed A, Puthawala A, Neblett D. Transperineal interstitial/intracavitary "Syed-Neblett" applicator in the treatment of carcinoma of the uterine cervix. *Endocuriether Hyperther Oncol.* 1986;2:1–13.

42 Hyperthermia

Benjamin L. Viglianti, MD, PhD ▪ Paul Stauffer, MS, CCE ▪ Elizabeth Repasky, PhD ▪
Ellen Jones, MD ▪ Zeljko Vujaskovic, MD, PhD ▪ Mark Dewhirst, DVM, PhD

Introduction

The rationale for use of hyperthermia (HT) as a treatment for cancer rests on several mechanisms. HT is known to cause direct cytotoxicity and also act as a radiation (RT) and chemosensitizer. In addition, HT improves tumor oxygenation and delivery of novel drug carriers, such as liposomal agents. Recent developments in the field of gene therapy may also establish a role for HT as a strategy for targeted, localized induction of gene therapy using the heat shock promoter.

Despite the strong biological rationale, implementation of HT in the clinic presents significant challenges. The primary hurdle is to heat tumors to defined temperature ranges in a precise and reproducible manner. Ease of clinical application is critically important. Current techniques for measuring temperature are invasive and the definition and calculation of thermal dose has not been well defined. Further improvements in technologies to deliver HT and to measure thermal dose remain crucial, although significant progress has been made on these issues over the past 5 years.

Two recently published pivotal trials have demonstrated for the first time that prospective control of thermal dose, when HT is combined with RT, has an impact on tumor response and duration of local tumor control. A third key paper reports that measurement of thermal dose can be achieved using MRI-based noninvasive thermometry methods and that parameters derived from these measurements are prognostically important. Collectively, these trials set the stage for establishing methods for writing a prescription for HT and for controlling thermal dose in real-time.

In spite of the technical difficulties in delivering HT, however, there are many published randomized trials of HT in human cancer patients. The majority demonstrated a local control and/or survival advantage with the addition of HT to RT. Thus, even with the limitations of current technology, the promise of HT is emerging from clinical trials. As the technology improves, the benefits of this form of therapy will only become more visible.

The Biology of Hyperthermia

Definition of Hyperthermia

HT means elevation of temperature to a supra-physiological level. In this chapter, this refers to temperatures between 40°C and 45°C. Higher temperatures are used for thermal ablation but will not be discussed here.

Hyperthermic Cell Killing, the Arrhenius Relationship, and Thermal Isoeffect Dose

When cells are heated in vitro, they die exponentially and the rate of killing increases with temperature. The Arrhenius relationship has been used to define the temperature dependence of the rate of cell killing, which can then be used as a method for thermal dosimetry. This is done by plotting the log of the slope (1/Do) of cell survival curves as a function of temperature (Fig. 42-1). Typically, Arrhenius plots have a biphasic curve. The temperature at which the slope changes is referred to as a "breakpoint." Above the breakpoint for nearly all cell types, increase in temperature of 1.0°C doubles the rate of cell killing. The breakpoint for human cells is near 43.5°C; below the breakpoint the rate of cell killing drops by a factor of 2-4 for each 1.0°C drop in temperature. The change in slope below the breakpoint is due to development of thermotolerance during heating. The slopes of Arrhenius plots derived from in vivo and in vitro studies are virtually identical.[1] Collectively, these data provide a strong rationale for using the Arrhenius relationship as a basis for thermal dosimetry.

The recognition that there is a definable relationship between the rate of cell killing and temperature led Sapareto and Dewey[2] to propose using this relationship to normalize thermal data from HT treatments. The rationale came from observations that time-temperature histories vary from patient to patient and that temperatures within tumors were almost always nonuniform, thereby preventing the goal of reaching a uniform target temperature-time combination for therapy. The formulation takes the following form:

$$\text{CEM } 43^\circ\text{C} = tR^{(43-T)}$$

where CEM 43°C = cumulative equivalent minutes at 43°C (the temperature suggested for normalization), t = time of treatment, T = average temperature during desired interval of heating, and R is a constant. When above the breakpoint, R = 0.5; when below the breakpoint, R = 0.25.

For a complex time-temperature history, the heating profile is broken into short intervals of time "t" length (typically 1-2 minutes), where the temperature remains relatively constant. CEM 43°C is calculated for each interval and summed to give a final CEM 43°C for the entire HT treatment:

$$\text{CEM } 43^\circ\text{C} = \Sigma tR(43-T_{avg})$$

The CEM 43°C (thermal isoeffect dose) formulation has been used successfully in clinical trials to retrospectively assess heating efficacy.[3-6] This dosimetry concept has been evaluated prospectively

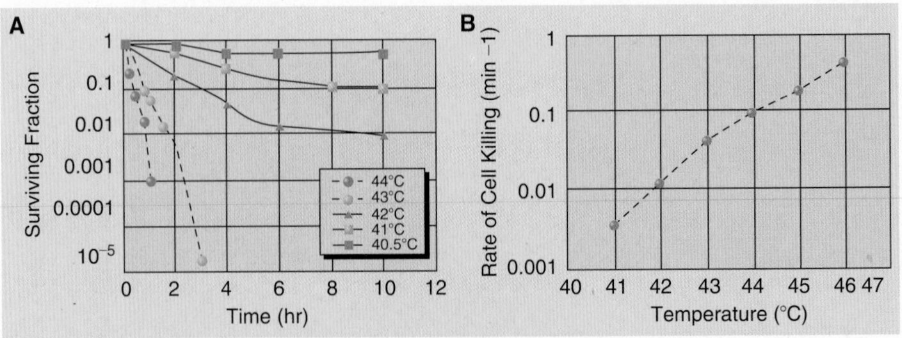

Figure 42-1 (A) Cell survival curves for V79 cells, plotted as log of surviving fraction as a function of time of heating at a defined temperature. *Source*: Data re-plotted from Reference 122. (B) Arrhenius plot from same data. Note change in slope of Arrhenius plot above and below 43°C.

in two recently published phase 3 trials (see below for details).[7,8] These trials have been critical for showing that prospective control of thermal dose delivery can affect probability for response and duration of local tumor control.

Mechanisms and Modifiers of Hyperthermic Cytotoxicity

Cellular and Tissue Responses to Hyperthermia

There are factors that are known to effect the position and slopes of the Arrhenius plot. These factors have potential clinical relevance (Fig. 42-2).

Targets for Hyperthermic Cytotoxicity ■ When cells are exposed to elevated temperatures (≥40.0°C), the predominant molecular target appears to be protein.[9] The heat of inactivation for cell killing and thermal damage is similar to the energy needed for protein denaturation (130-170 kcal/mole).[9,10] Additional evidence for proteins as being the primary target for cell killing is the importance of heat shock proteins (HSPs) in protecting thermotolerant cells from thermal damage. One of the primary functions of HSPs is to refold other proteins that have been denatured or damaged.[11] Two modes of death are induced by HT: apoptosis and necrosis.[12,13]

Some cellular organelles are especially important in thermal responses. Modification of cell membrane lipid content or use of membrane active agents, such as alcohols, can sensitize cells to heat killing, but the sensitization is probably related to destabilization of the membrane as it relates to lipid-protein interactions.[14] The cytoskeleton of cells, which controls many signal transduction pathways, is particularly heat sensitive.[15,16] Enzymes in the respiratory chain are more heat sensitive than enzymes in the glycolytic pathway.[9,17] Finally, the DNA repair process is heat sensitive and this may be one of the mechanisms that leads to heat-induced radio- and chemosensitization.[18,19] Chromosomal aberrations can occur if cells are in S-phase during the time of heating[20,21] or if centriolar damage occurs.[22]

Thermotolerance ■ Thermotolerance is a transient adaptation to thermal stress that renders surviving heated cells more resistant to additional heat stress. It is caused by upregulation of synthesis of HSPs within cells during and after thermal stress. Thermotolerance tends to shift the Arrhenius plot to the right and downward, indicating that higher temperatures are needed to achieve equivalent rates of cell killing in thermotolerant as compared with nonthermally tolerant cells. Generally, thermotolerance is avoided clinically by waiting 2-3 days between HT treatments to allow for its decay.

Acute Acidification ■ Acute acidification will sensitize cells to killing in two ways. The Arrhenius plot is shifted to the left and the breakpoint nearly disappears because thermotolerance induction is inhibited. Methods for achieving acute tumor-specific acidification have been studied extensively in pre-clinical models and in humans and are discussed in more detail in the Physiology section.[23-26]

Step-Down Heating ■ Step down-heating occurs when temperatures rise above the breakpoint and then drop below the breakpoint for the remainder of a treatment.[4] This occurs clinically when power is turned down after heating has started in response to pain or excessively high normal tissue temperatures, or when perfusion increases in response to increased temperatures. When step-down heating occurs, thermotolerance induction is prevented during that heating session.

Hyperthermia and Physiology

Tumor blood flow and metabolism have important influences on the efficacy of HT and conversely, the physiologic consequences of HT can influence the efficacy of other treatments that the patient may receive.

Physiologic Response to Hyperthermia

As temperatures are increased, the first tissue reaction is an increase in blood flow. The temperature threshold for this change is between 41°C and 41.5°C in skin.[27] Changes in vascular permeability also occur, leading to edema. At higher thermal doses, vascular stasis and hemorrhage develop. As a rough estimate, muscle and skin perfusion increase by at least 10-fold, whereas tumor perfusion may increase by 1.5-2-fold.[28] Mechanisms underlying vascular stasis may include arteriovenous shunting, thrombus formation, and leukocyte plugging.[29] It is rare to achieve temperatures high enough in the clinic to cause vascular damage, but there are physiologic changes in tumors at lower temperatures that are potentially beneficial (Fig. 42-3).

Taking Advantage of Physiological Response to Hyperthermia ■ ***Improvement in Macromolecular and Liposomal Drug Delivery*** ■ A liposome is a small lipid vesicle (≈100 nm diameter) that contains water or sa-

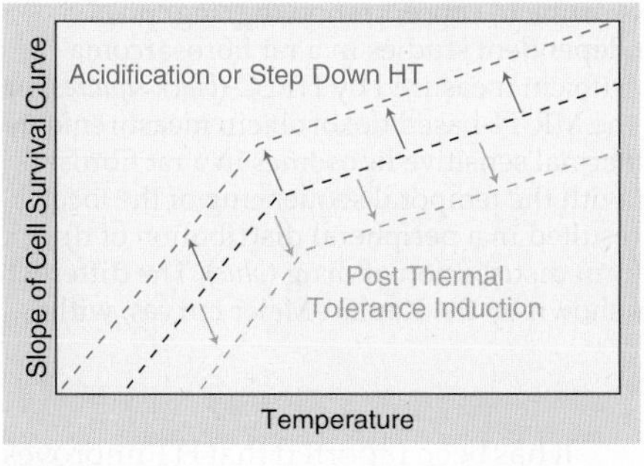

Figure 42-2 ■ Comparison of the effects of modifiers of the Arrhenius relationship (eg, thermal sensitivity).

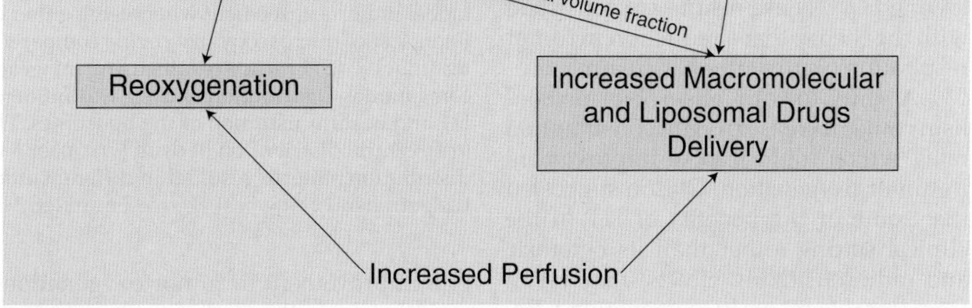

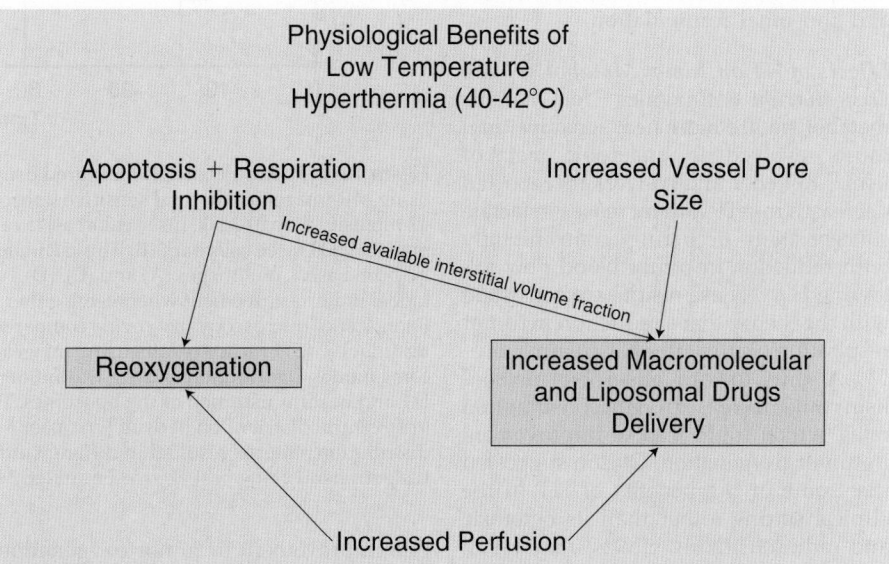

Figure 42-3 ■ Physiologic and therapeutic benefits to low- or mild-temperature HT (eg, 40-42°C).

line in the center. Drugs can be loaded into liposomes at high concentration. HT has been shown to augment liposomal drug delivery. Liposomes 100-nm in diameter do not extravasate at normothermia (34°C for mouse skin), but extravasate well at 40-42°C.[30,31] HT does not cause liposomal extravasation from normal vessels. When temperature sensitive liposomes are used, even better antitumor effects can be achieved, particularly using rapid drug release liposomes.[30,32] It has been recently reported that liposomal extravasation and release can be monitored and quantified noninvasively with MRI using a novel $MnSO_4$ Doxorubicin-loaded liposome[32,33] (Fig. 42-4a-d). Further work demonstrated that the distribution of the drug delivery was important in efficacy, with targeting of the neovascular rim leading to the best outcomes[34] (Fig. 42-4e). The mechanism of tumor cell killing with this formulation includes vascular destruction, occurring secondary to high drug concentrations that accumulate around vessels post HT.[35]

There is no physiologic advantage to using HT to augment transvascular delivery of small molecular weight drugs (<1,000 mw), although HT increases cellular drug uptake.[36] In contrast, for example, HT augments transvascular delivery of monoclonal antibodies.[37] Recently, polymeric peptides that can carry drugs or radioisotopes have been designed to undergo inverse phase transition in the typical HT temperature range. When this occurs, these peptides transition from a water-soluble state to form aggregates that accumulate in tumor tissue.[38] The available volume fraction (space between cells and stromal fibers) increases after heating as cells undergo either necrosis or apoptosis.[39] This may increase the space available for macromolecular and liposomal accumulation.

Effects of HT on Tumor Metabolism and Oxygenation ■ Enzymes for aerobic metabolism are more heat sensitive than those involved in anaerobic metabolism.[17] Kelleher and co-workers reported decreases in ATP and increases in lactate concentration occurring concomitantly with reduction in tumor blood flow following HT.[40] These results are consistent with the theory that a reduction in tumor respiration occurs after HT treatment.

A shift toward anaerobic metabolism could decrease oxygen consumption rates, which could lead to improvement in tumor oxygenation. Oleson suggested that some of the benefits of HT in the clinical setting (other than its cytotoxic and radiosensitizing effects) may result from improvements in oxygenation.[41] Results from several studies in rodent tumors and human tumor xenografts indicate improvement in tumor oxygenation resulting from thermal exposures below those which cause vascular damage (eg, 41-43°C, 60 minutes).[42,43]

It has been reported that HT improves tumor oxygenation in canine and human tumors.[44-46] In the human studies, failure to reoxygenate after the first HT fraction

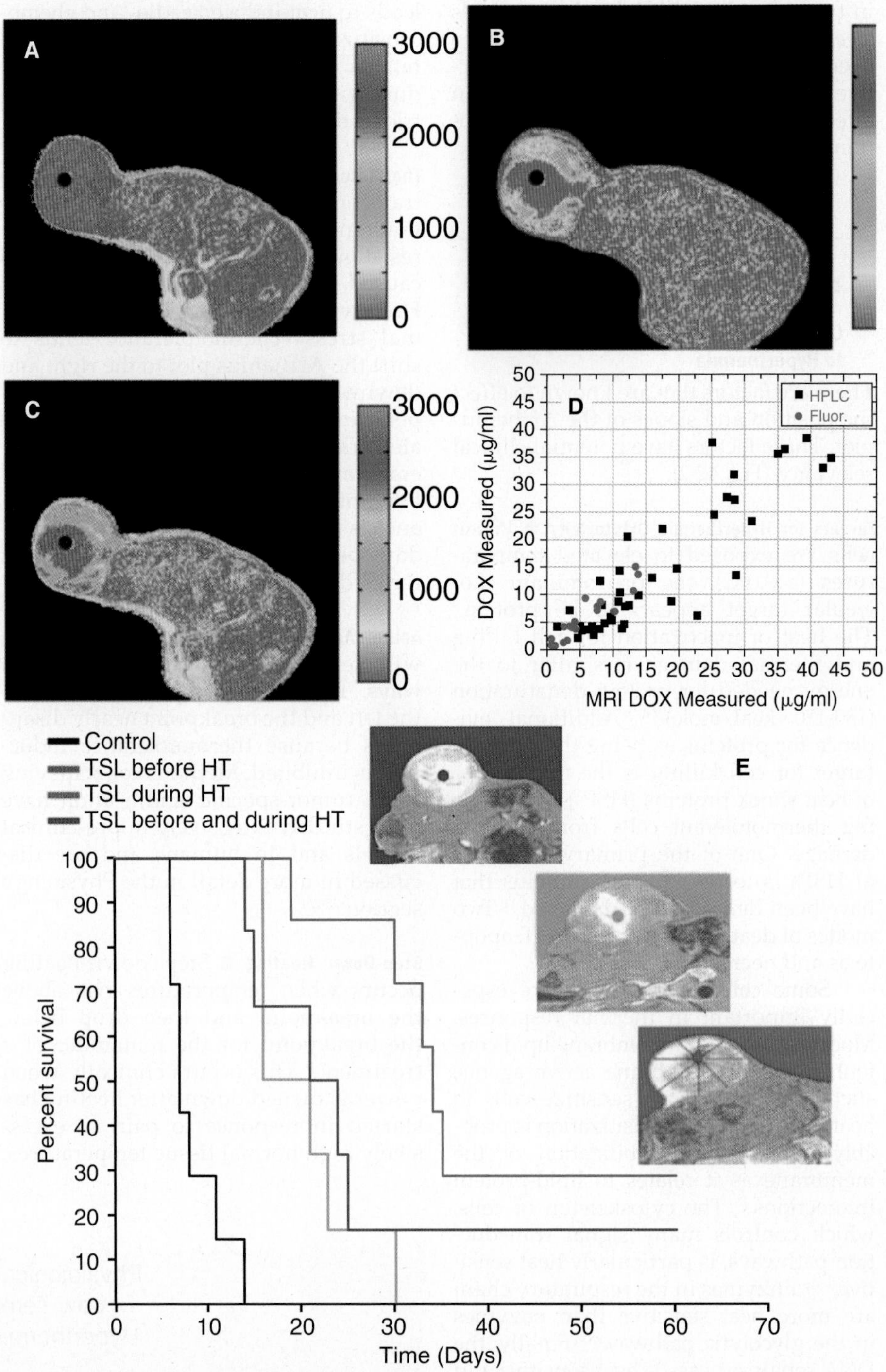

Figure 42-4 ■ Results of MR-measured drug concentration and effect on treatment therapy using MR-imageable thermal sensitive liposomes in a rat fibrosarcoma model. (**A**) The initial T1 intensity map (0-3,500 msec colorbar) is calculated. (**c**) Forty five minute posttreatment T1 map (0-3,500 msec colorbar). (**B**) The calculated doxorubicin concentration (ng/mg) pixel-by-pixel basis from images (**A**) and (**C**). (**D**) Two independent studies in a rat fibrosarcoma model indicate agreement when using either doxorubicin measured by HPLC (*black squares*) or fluorescence microscopy (*red circles*) compared to the MR T1-based doxorubicin measurements technique.[33] (**E**) Efficacy results using imageable thermal sensitive liposomes in a rat fibrosarcoma model. Distribution of drug was influenced with the temporal sequencing of the local HT and iv administration of the liposomes. This resulted in a peripheral distribution of drug (*red*), central distribution of drug (*green*), or a uniform distribution of drug (*blue*). The different distribution patterns resulted in different efficacy shown by the Kaplan-Meier curves, with the peripheral being best. *Source:* From Ref. 34.

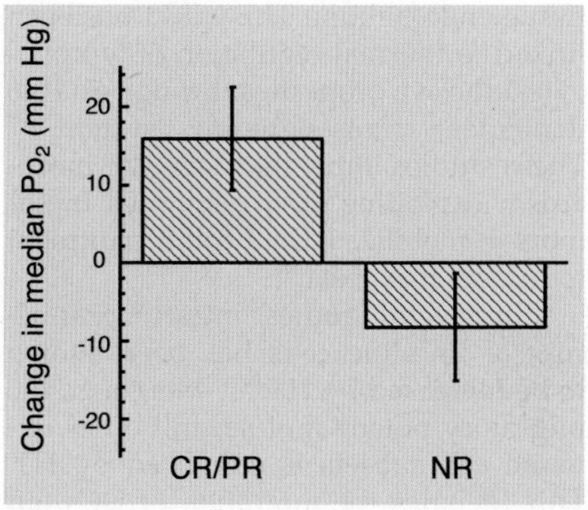

Figure 42-5 Relationship between change in Eppendorf electrode hypoxic fraction, as measured 24 hours post first HT, and clinical response in patients with locally advanced breast cancer. These patients were treated with a combination of Taxol, RT, and HT. Reoxygenation is clearly associated with those patients who achieved either a complete or a partial response. *Source*: From Ref. 45.

led to a significantly lower probability to achieve pathologic complete response at the time of surgery (Fig. 42-5).[44,45] Excessively high temperatures can decrease oxygenation, but this is not commonly observed in clinical treatments because such temperatures are difficult to achieve.

Normal Tissue Damage from Hyperthermia

Thermal damage to tissues is dependent on the severity of the injury and the tissue type being heated. Mild damage can merely lead to edema, whereas more severe injury can lead to massive necrosis and organ failure. This subject has been reviewed in detail recently.[19] When significant damage ensues, there is apoptosis, necrosis, and inflammatory reaction, with edema, focal hemorrhage, and granulocytic infiltrates within a few days following exposure. Chronic changes, seen after a few weeks, include fibrosis, parenchymal necrosis (death of tissue cells), and lymphohistiocytic infiltration. There is no clear ranking by tissue type of sensitivity/toxicity to HT.

There is no inherent difference in the thermal sensitivity between tumor and normal tissues. However, the microenvironment of tumors, which is often acidotic and nutritionally deprived, leads to an increase in thermal sensitivity.[47]

Physiologic Approaches to Enhance Thermal Cytotoxicity

pH Modification

It is well established that an acute reduction in extracellular pH can greatly enhance sensitivity to HT. Cells adapted to grow at low pH are relatively resistant to HT killing as a result of HSP upregulation.[48] Acute acidification of these cells below their resting pH leads to catastrophic cell death due to limited reserve to further increase proton pumping. Increased reduction in intracellular pH is responsible for increase in cytotoxicity.[24] Induction of hyperglycemia will shift tumor cells toward glycolysis increasing lactic acid production. Selectivity for tumors occurs because of alterations in respiratory pathways and a propensity toward sensitivity to the Crabtree effect.[49,50] The addition of the respiratory inhibitor, MIBG (metaiodobenzylguanadine) can further enhance selective acidification in tumors.[25,51,52] Pharmacologic agents that block the extrusion of hydrogen ions from cells have also been investigated.[26]

The use of hyperglycemia improves response to CT + HT and RT + HT in rodents.[53-55] One human study in a few patients suggested improvement in response with the use of hyperglycemia with RT + HT.[56] However, pH was not measured and the study was not randomized.

Immunologic Effects of Hyperthermia

The intriguing possibility that stimulation of the antitumor immune response by externally applied HT may influence improved patient survival, has not, until recently, been a predominant research theme in the field of hyperthermic oncology.[57] However, some of the earliest attempts to use immunotherapy are linked historically to the origins of hyperthermic oncology, since the most significant antitumor benefits were obtained in individuals who achieved the highest fevers in response to purposeful exposure to infectious products (eg, Coley's Toxins).[58] Further, there is a remarkable conservation in the fever response in association with inflammation or infection throughout nature,[59] and the development of febrile HT has been strongly correlated with improved survival in multiple species.[60,61] Several lines of recent experimental evidence reveal that externally applied HT may indeed have the potential to increase immunogenicity of tumors and stimulate the immune system, perhaps as an evolutionarily conserved response to increases in body temperature, and that strategically applied heat treatment may help to overcome barriers to more effective innate and adaptive antitumor immune responses in the treatment of cancer. The notion that HT, as well as radiation and chemotherapy, could serve to enhance immunotherapy is now recognized as a distinct possibility. While much more work is needed to test this assumption, the current evidence (briefly summarized below) includes: (1) enhanced immunogenicity of heated tumor cells, (2) increased immune effector cell activity following thermal exposure, and (3) enhanced vascular access and trafficking of immune effector cells in vivo following systemic thermal treatment (see schematic in Fig. 42-6). Current research goals in this rapidly growing field include definition of the thermally sensitive molecular components and signaling pathways associated with immune regulation and identification of the role of thermal stress-induced HSPs

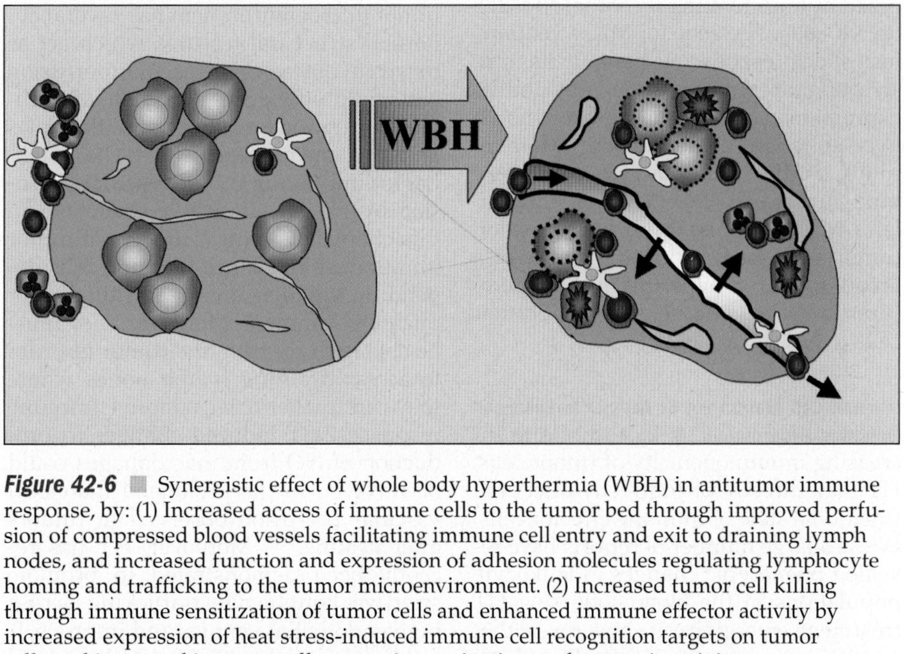

Figure 42-6 Synergistic effect of whole body hyperthermia (WBH) in antitumor immune response, by: (1) Increased access of immune cells to the tumor bed through improved perfusion of compressed blood vessels facilitating immune cell entry and exit to draining lymph nodes, and increased function and expression of adhesion molecules regulating lymphocyte homing and trafficking to the tumor microenvironment. (2) Increased tumor cell killing through immune sensitization of tumor cells and enhanced immune effector activity by increased expression of heat stress-induced immune cell recognition targets on tumor cells and increased immune cell maturation, activation, and cytotoxic activity.

in mediating enhanced tumor antigen recognition and antigen processing by dendritic cells. In addition, considerable research is being directed toward establishment of heating protocols in which thermally regulated immune effector mechanisms could be maximally exploited.

Tumor Cells Are Sensitized to Immune-Mediated Recognition and Destruction Following Hyperthermia

There is now strong evidence that exposure of tumor cells to HT can render them more sensitive to subsequent immune cell-mediated recognition and attack[62-65] and one potential mechanism appears to involve HSPs. In one study, heated tumor cells were unable to form tumors in syngeneic mice, whereas they do in nude mice,[62] suggesting a role for T lymphocytes in the improved immunogenicity of heated tumors. Exposure of dendritic cells (which are critical for driving adaptive immunity and development of long-term memory responses) to heated melanoma and colorectal carcinoma cells resulted in enhanced expression of surface molecules and cytokines critical for activation of T lymphocytes.[66,67] Members of the HSP family expressed on the surface of heated tumor cells have been proposed to activate NK cell proliferation and tumor cell cytotoxicity via receptor interaction and this may be an important mechanism by which heated tumor cells are rendered more immunogenic.[68-70]

Additional insight into the potential molecular mechanisms of thermally enhanced NK cell activity against heated tumor targets may come from studies of heat stress on inducible, nonclassical MHC class I ligand (MICA) on tumor cells, a cell surface protein which is recognized by an activating receptor (NKG2D) on NK cells. The gene for MICA contains heat shock response elements in its transcriptional regulatory sequences and its expression in tumor cells has been shown to be enhanced by heat shock.[71] More recently, studies have shown that even very mild (fever range) thermal stress upregulates MICA expression in human colon tumor cells[72] supporting the ability of a broad range of hyperthermic temperatures to increase the sensitivity of tumor cells to NK cell attack.

Immune Cell Maturation or Activity Is Enhanced Following Hyperthermia In addition to increasing immunogenicity of tumor cells, HT may directly or indirectly affect the functional state of immune effector cells. While a large number of reports have revealed phenotypic changes in leukocyte populations in the blood following HT treatment, emerging data now reveal that specific immune activity of cells of both adaptive and innate immunity is sensitive to externally applied HT. For example, the cytotoxic activity of macrophages, T cells, and NK cells (effects on NK cells reviewed in Refernece 73) against tumor targets is enhanced by their exposure to mild hyperthermic temperatures.[72,74-76]. HT treatment also appears to enhance the maturation and function of dendritic cells,[77-79] which could be critical for enhanced T cell responses against tumor antigens. Several lines of evidence suggest that HT may stimulate expression, or suppress expression, of pro-inflammatory cytokines from macrophages, causing either enhanced activation of host immunity or a reduction in damage from prolonged exposure to inflammatory cytokines, respectively.[80,81] Examples such as this reveal the potential complexity of body temperature changes on positive or negative regulation of immune responses.

An important mechanism by which HT may affect the cytotoxic activity of various immune effector cells is through the Fas/Fas ligand system.[74] Application of mild HT increases Fas-mediated T cell cytotoxicity of target cells and this depends on thermal activation of hsf-1. Upstream of this event, HT increases the expression and translocation of the AP-1 and NF-κB transcription factors, which regulates fas ligand expression HT also induces activation of certain protein kinase C (PKC) isoforms in T lymphocytes and is associated with the movement of PKC isoforms and receptor activated c kinase to the uropod. RACK 1, which is important for maintaining the activated T cell structure, also translocates to the cytoskeleton with HT treatment.[82]

Vascular Function and Immune Cell Trafficking Is Enhanced Following Hyperthermia The solid tumor microenvironment has several abnormal structural features which act as powerful obstacles to vascular perfusion and could effectively diminish solid tumor infiltration by blood-borne therapies and effector immune cells.[83] The potential for improving tumor vascular perfusion by HT (as discussed elsewhere in this chapter) is critical to the antitumor immune system, since immune cells depend on vascular access into the tumor microenvironment. Moreover, they must be able to drain from the tumor in order to access draining lymph nodes where they can further drive adaptive immune responses. HT induced changes in production of NO from macrophages could be involved in the prolonged increased vascular profusion observed in tumors after heating.[84,85] Moreover, HT has recently been demonstrated to promote selective lymphocyte trafficking across high endothelial venules and improve T-cell homing and trafficking to lymphoid tissue endothelium. This effect has been linked to thermal regulation of lymphocyte adhesive properties through an IL-6 dependent trans-signaling system.[86,87] These studies imply that a similar mechanism exploiting IL-6 responses in tumors to mobilize CD8 T cell recruitment to tumors may exist.[88]

In several studies, intratumoral access of immune cells has been shown to be increased by HT.[89-91] Moreover, the migratory potential of several other immune cell subsets is enhanced by HT. This includes the migration of DCs out of the skin into the lymph node[78,92] and increases in antigen specific lymphocyte homing in the contact hypersensitivity ear swelling response.[78]

Increased tumor immunogenicity, dendritic cell maturation, T cell and NK cell cytotoxicity, and the increase in vascular access and lymphocyte trafficking in response to HT may act in a concerted, or even synergistic, manner to effectively help overcome defective immune response against tumor antigens, and ultimately yield a more powerful and long-lasting protection against tumor recurrence or metastasis. These data also strongly support the testing of HT as an adjuvant for immunotherapy.

Defining Mechanisms by Which Thermal Stress Could Regulate Immune Activity The rapid upsurge in immunological studies associated with hyperthermic oncology has revealed several critical areas for additional research. Identification of the molecular basis for thermal sensitivity of the immune system will be essential for the design of clinical protocols that can best harness the immune potentiating benefits of HT in the cancer clinic. While some studies have noted effects on signaling molecules or expression of pro-inflammatory cytokines, the effects of HT on the lipid structure of the immune cell plasma membrane itself are also receiving considerable attention. Evidence in multiple immune effector cells suggests that decreased membrane fluidity is coupled with decreased cytotoxicity and phagocytic activity, impaired antigen uptake, and impaired activation potential.[93-96] Since it has been well documented that increases in temperature can influence plasma membrane fluidity in a variety of cells, including immune cells, it is likely that increasing the fluidity of the plasma membrane could be linked to the thermal activation of immune effector cells.[97,98] If HT affected the membrane lipid organization and/or composition of immune cell in vivo, there could be a favorable and temporary shift in the balance of immune activity against tumor target antigens.

As stated, a second mechanism by which HT could enhance immune activity is the resultant production of HSPs in the heated tumor cells. The well-known importance of inducible HSPs in regulating immune rejection of a variety of syngeneic tumor lines by chaperoning MHC class I epitopes could help to explain enhanced immunogenicity of heated tumor cells. While the exact nature of the complexed peptides and the dendritic cell surface receptors that may be involved in recognition of tumor-derived HSPs remains a topic of intense study and controversy, it is now clear that such interactions lead to a response capable of triggering cytokine release and increased expression of antigen-presenting cell surface molecules essential to development of effective adaptive immunity.[77,99-101] However, much more experimental data are needed. Heat-inducible HSPs (hsp110 and hsp70) from heat-treated tumors were found to be more immunogenic than those from nonheated tumors.[102] Thus, heating may change the antigenic profile chaperoned by HSPs by increasing the amount of tumor-specific antigens associated with HSPs. Induction of HSPs in immune cells could also play a critical role. HSP90 was shown to be upregulated in bone marrow-derived dendritic cells treated with fever-range thermal stress. HSP90 activates these cells to secrete IFN-γ, a pro-inflammatory cytokine that sustains NK cell activation.[77]

Finally, there is a great need for new research that can help define the optimal temperature range and heating protocols needed to exploit immunologic activity against tumors. While most HT applications utilize nonphysiologic temperatures of 40-45°C, or higher (as in ablation protocols), normal fever range body temperatures rarely exceed 40°C and are most often near 38-39°C. For this reason, there has been an increase in the number of in vivo studies using mild or fever range temperatures.[103,104] However, it should be kept in mind that even during thermal ablation, there are thermal gradients established at the margins of the tumor and in adjacent normal tissue where the temperature increase may be quite mild. Further, it would be expected that there are extended regions of normal tissue which receive heated blood from the region of locally heated tumors, and the blood may at an elevated temperature for sufficiently long period provoke at least some of the immunologic effects summarized here.[105]

Hyperthermia and Metastases

Pre-clinical data are mixed regarding whether local HT affects metastasis development. Local HT enhanced metastatic rates when the B16 melanoma was grown in the mouse foot pad.[106,107] Two other studies with different tumor models showed either a reduction in metastases following local HT[108] or no effect on the incidence of metastases, relative to controls.[109]

The question is difficult to answer in clinical trials unless the primary therapy has a high probability for local control. In a phase 3 trial of canine patients with primary malignant melanomas treated with the radiation ± HT, there was no difference in the likelihood for metastasis between the two arms.[110] However, local recurrence was a common event and its onset was frequently followed by appearance of distant metastases. In a phase 3 randomized trial of human melanomas treated in a similarly designed trial, there was significant improvement in the likelihood for survival when the local tumor was controlled. Since the radiotherapy + HT arm had improved local control, the combination therapy reduced the probability for metastases.[111,112] In a study comparing graded doses of radiation ± HT of canine soft tissue sarcomas, higher normal tissue temperatures surrounding tumor were correlated with lower likelihood for distant metastases.[113]

A large series of patients ($N = 95$) with previously untreated high-grade soft tissue sarcomas provides the most easily interpretable data because the local control rate following preoperative HT + RT was near 90%.[114] Fifty percent of these patients went on to develop distant metastases. This rate is essentially identical to that seen with preoperative RT alone.[115] The conclusion is that with the exception of one preclinical study with B16 melanoma, there is no evidence that local-regional HT causes an increase in metastases.

The results following total body HT are more provocative. In a randomized phase 2 study, dogs with soft tissue sarcomas received RT + local HT or RT + local HT + whole body HT.[116] The combination of local + whole body HT + RT did not improve local control over local HT + RT and it increased the likelihood for distant metastases. In a separate study, alteration in the location of metastases in dogs with primary osteosarcomas was seen following treatment whole body HT.[117] It has also been reported that patients who had a fever during or shortly after receiving brachytherapy for carcinoma of the cervix had an increased risk for developing distant metastases.[118]

Radiation and Hyperthermia

Rationale for Combining Hyperthermia with Radiotherapy

When radiation is combined with HT, complementary effects occur. Cells in S-phase of the cell cycle are relatively radioresistant, but they are most sensitive to HT. Hypoxic cells are three times more resistant to RT, as compared with aerobic cells. There is no difference in thermal sensitivity between aerobic and hypoxic cells. As discussed earlier, there is good evidence in human tumors (soft tissue sarcoma and locally advanced breast) that HT causes reoxygenation, which will further improve radiation response. Finally, HT inhibits the repair of both sublethal and potentially lethal damage, by inactivating crucial DNA repair pathways.[119-122]

Factors to Consider When Combining Hyperthermia With Radiotherapy

The interaction between RT and HT is described by the "thermal enhancement ratio" or TER, which is defined as the ratio of doses of RT to achieve an isoeffect for RT/(RT + HT). A number of murine studies compared TERs for tumor and normal tissues and in some cases it was possible to demonstrate therapeutic gain (ie, TERtumor > TERnormal tissue).[123] TERs for late tissue complications in feet and skin of mice were lower than TERs for moist desquamation.[124,125]

TERs for local tumor control have been estimated to be greater than 1 for several human tumor types.[126] TER values for normal tissue damage have been less than tumor in the same patient populations, suggesting potential for therapeutic gain for RT + HT compared with RT alone. Prospective randomized trials in dogs with spontaneous tumors have also shown evidence for improved local tumor control with RT + HT compared with RT alone[127-129] with no clinical increase in frequency of clinically relevant late normal tissue complications.

In summary, most available data from pre-clinical and clinical studies indicate that therapeutic gain is achievable for the combination of HT with RT. HT does not appear to enhance the incidence or severity of late normal tissue complications.

Hyperthermia and Chemotherapy

Rationale for Using Hyperthermia with Chemotherapy

Many chemotherapeutic agents have been shown to exhibit synergism with HT including cisplatin and related compounds, melphalan, cyclophosphamide, nitrogen mustards, anthracyclines, nitrosoureas, blyeomycin, mitomycin C, and hypoxic cell sensitizers.[36] The mechanisms that underlie the synergy may include: (1) increased cellular uptake, (2) increased oxygen radical production, and (3) increased DNA damage and inhibition of repair. Hypoxia and pH are also important in the thermochemotherapeutic response.[130-134]

Factors to Consider When Combining Hyperthermia with Chemotherapy

Reversal of Drug Resistance ■ An important factor in the potential use of HT with many drugs is its ability to reverse, at least partially, drug resistance. Examples of drugs for which this has been shown include cisplatin,[135] melphalan,[136] nitrosoureas,[137] and doxorubicin, when combined with the multiple drug resistance inhibitor, verapamil.[138]

In Vitro Results May Not Predict In Vivo Activity ■ Tubulin-binding agents, such as taxol, show no evidence for interaction in vitro,[139] but studies in combination with radiation therapy in vivo are more encouraging.[140] Generally speaking, most antimetabolites do not interact with HT when given concomitantly.[36] However, it is important to consider issues such as time of drug exposure and temperature, both of which may be important in determining where and when to expect a positive interaction. When 5FU has been given simultaneously with HT, there have been only additive effects.[141] However, 5FU has been shown to interact supra-additively with HT when simulated as continuous infusion. Heating to 39-41°C can lead to enhanced conversion to active metabolites thereby increasing drug cytotoxicity. In addition, continuous infusion protocols with this drug may lead to cell cycle block in S phase, a relatively HT sensitive part of the cell cycle.[142]

Sequencing ■ For most drugs (excluding 5FU and perhaps other antimetabolites), the optimal sequence between heat and drug is to administer them simultaneously or to give the drug immediately before the onset of heating. For platinum containing drugs, the tissue extraction rate of drug may be increased with HT, further substantiating the rationale for use of this sequence.[143]

Lack of Interaction ■ Etoposide and the vinca alkaloids have failed to show synergistic interaction with HT.[36]

Trimodality Therapies ■ The combination of HT, drugs, and radiation has been evaluated preclinically.[144,145] Limited but encouraging pilot human data based on the combination of the hypoxic cell sensitizer, etanidazole, radiation, and HT has been reported.[146] The combination of 5FU, HT, and radiation therapy has yielded favorable responses in patients with locally advanced colorectal cancer in a phase 2 study,[147] which has led to the current conduct of a randomized phase 3 trial of 5FU + radiation ± HT. Similarly, a pilot trial of HT + cisplatin + RT in patients with locally advanced cervical cancer[148] has led to initiation of a multinational multi-institutional phase 3 trial comparing cisplatin CT + RT with and without HT.

Hyperthermia and Gene Therapy

Several investigators have exploited the heat shock response as a means to perform gene therapy. The heat shock promoter is highly inducible and relatively quiescent under normothermic conditions.[149-151] The heat inducibility has been used to minimize therapeutic gene expression in normal tissues, by focusing the heat on the tumor bearing region only.[152]

Examples of therapeutic genes that have been investigated include interleukin 12 (as a modulator of immune function and angiogenesis),[153] thymidine kinase conversion of the prodrug gangcyclovir to a toxic chemotherapeutic agent,[154-156] and other cytokines such as TNFα, and restoration of wild-type P53 to induce apoptosis.[157-159] There are potential advantages to be gained through augmentation of immune function as well, by HSP70.[160]

Hyperthermia Physics

HT is usually delivered by exposing tissues to conductive heat sources, or nonionizing radiation, such as electromagnetic (EM) or ultrasound fields. Although these modalities deposit energy in tissue by different physical mechanisms, they have many similarities. They are sensitive to the heterogeneity of tissue properties, spatial and temporal variation of blood flow, and practical problems of coupling energy uniformly into a tissue target at depth in complex anatomical locations. HT can be delivered using either small implanted sources or noninvasively using externally applied power sources. An overview of most commonly used noninvasive methods is provided below and summarized in Table 42-1. More complete details of available technologies for superficial heating[161-163] and invasive interstitial heating approaches[164-166] are available elsewhere.

Electromagnetic Heating

When an electric field (E-field) is generated in tissue, heating results from resistive losses to the induced electric currents. For all tissue types the electrical conductivity increases as the EM frequency increases. This implies improved penetration for low frequency or long wavelengths. However, the ability to localize EM energy deposition is dependent on the wavelength. The longer the wavelength, the broader the focus of heating. Thus, there is a fundamental constraint on noninvasive heating by EM techniques that does not allow localized heating at depths greater than 1-4 cm. Utilization of EM techniques to achieve deep-heating results in regional energy deposition involving substantial volumes of tissue.

EM Heating Devices ■ A range of EM heating devices has been developed for external applications of HT. These devices can be separated into two categories: superficial applicators with effective penetration into tissue in the range of 1-4 cm and deep heating devices that have effective penetration greater than 4 cm. Examples of superficial devices include waveguides[167,168] and microstrip or patch antennas[169-175] that operate in the microwave band typically at 433, 915, or 2,450 MHz. Specialized dual purpose applicators are becoming available to deliver microwave heating simultaneously with radiation to maximize synergism.[163] Hence, devices are usually coupled into tissue through a deionized water bolus that is usually temperature controlled to maintain skin temperature below 43°C.

In order to heat at depths greater than 5 cm, one must use lower EM frequencies (5-200 MHz) with longer wavelength. There are three basic techniques for EM deep heating: magnetic induction, capacitively coupled conduction current, and radiative phased array fields.

Magnetic induction heating uses a time varying magnetic field to induce eddy currents within conductive tissue.[176] Although the magnetic field can penetrate deep in the body with little attenuation, the induced eddy current governed by paths of least resistance and separate eddy currents are produced in organs of different tissue conductivity. One way to selectively deliver power to tumor with this method is to use ferromagnetic needles or rods, implanted within the tumor volume[177,178] or ferromagnetic nanoparticles injected into the tissue.[179,180] These metals may be designed to undergo a Curie point transition, where their magnetic properties change with temperature, thereby providing self-regulated temperature control.[181,182]

Deep heating using the capacitive technique uses RF fields in the frequency range of 5-30 MHz.[183-185] Ion currents are driven between two or more conductive electrodes. Heating tends to be concentrated at the electrodes, so temperature-controlled saline pads or bolus are used to cool the skin and underlying high-resistance fat.[186] Varying the size of the respective electrodes can shift the current distribution toward the smaller electrode. RF capacitive heating is used almost exclusively in Asia, where patients tend to have a thinner layer of fat

Table 42-1

Method	Frequency	Coupling Medium	Invasive Thermometry	Power Focus in Tumor	Advantages	Disadvantages
Electromagnetic—Superficial						
Capacitive RF	5-30 MHz	Saline	High resistance lead thermistors or fiberoptics	Limited—higher SAR under smaller electrode	Simple to operate	Superficial fat heating, no SAR focus at depth
Microwave waveguide	433, 915, 2,450 MHz	Deionized water	High resistance lead thermistors or fiberoptics	Yes—by physical placement over tumor	Simple to operate	Limited size/depth, SAR not adjustable, poor coupling to contoured anatomy
Microwave Microstrip arrays	433, 915, 2,450 MHz	Deionized water	High resistance lead thermistors or fiberoptics	Yes—by physical placement over tumor	Conform to anatomy, Adjustable SAR, Larger Areas	Longer setup time for larger applicators
Electromagnetic—Deep Regional						
Magnetic induction	0.1-13.56 MHz	Air	Fiberoptics, shielded TC, high resistance lead thermistors	Yes—with interstitial implant ferrorods or ferroparticles	Simple to operate	Eddy currents in each organ, SAR not adjustable
Capacitive RF	5-30 MHz	Saline	High resistance lead thermistors or fiberoptics	No	Simple to operate	Superficial fat heating, no SAR focus at depth
Phased array RF/MW	75-200 MHz	Deionized water	High resistance lead thermistors or fiberoptics	Yes—SAR steering by phase and amplitude adjustment of antennae	Can steer heating into large focal regions	No precise control of size and location
Ultrasound—Superficial						
Planar ultrasound—single transducer or arrays	1-4 MHz	Degassed water	Metal encased thermistors or thermocouples	Yes—SAR steering in array with transducer power adjustments	Simple, highly directive SAR	Good coupling required, no air or bone in window, bone pain
Ultrasound—Deep Focus						
Electrically or physically scanned focused array	0.5-2 MHz	Degassed water	Metal encased thermistors or thermocouples	Yes—SAR focus in deep tumor by electric or scanning adjustments	Highly directive SAR, controllable tight focus	Large acoustic window with no air/bone, small focal heat volume

that can be cooled with aggressive surface cooling.

The third option for noninvasive deep heating is the RF phased array.[187-189] These devices consist of an array of RF antennae arranged in a geometric pattern surrounding the body region to be heated. Driven from a common source, the RF fields may be combined to form a moveable focal hot spot at depth depending on relative phase shifts of the antennae. In general, the phased array technique has more flexibility for adjusting the size and location of power deposition at depth than magnetic induction and capacitive techniques.

Ultrasound Heating

Energy transfer from an acoustic field is associated with mechanical viscous heating. Like EM waves, penetration of ultrasound also decreases with increasing frequency. However, because the wavelength of typical ultrasound fields is several orders of magnitude shorter, the problems of applicator size and focusing of ultrasound in deep tissue are greatly reduced. Since air reflects and bone absorbs US, anatomic geometry and tissue heterogeneity severely restrict the utility of US. The availability of an adequate "acoustic window" (a path unobstructed by bone or air proximal and distal to the target) is often a problem in clinical applications. The entry window size determines the size and depth of the target focal region.

Ultrasound devices are coupled into tissue using a temperature controlled degassed water bolus. Single and multiple transducer plane wave devices have been designed for superficial tumors (1-4 cm) heating, which typically operate in the 1-5 MHz range.[190,191] Specialized ultrasound arrays have been developed to facilitate simultaneous application of HT with RT, which will maximize the cytotoxic interactions between the two treatments.[192,193] Deep heating with ultrasound is accomplished by using scanned focused transducers, phased arrays, or multiple scanned focused ultrasound transducers.[194-196] Ultrasound frequencies for deep heating are in the 0.5-2 MHz range.

Measurement of Temperatures During Hyperthermia

The most commonly used method involves placing individual fixed position thermometry sensors into the tumor and/or on the tumor/skin surface. Invasive thermometry is accomplished by inserting blind-ended needles or catheters into a tumor and using either ultrasound or CT guidance to localize position relative to the tumor. Thermocouple, thermistor, or fiberoptic sensors are then placed inside the lumen to measure temperature at one or multiple fixed locations, or physically scanned within the catheter during heating. There are guidelines published for how these measurements should be taken.[197-200]

Invasive thermometry provides valuable information about the quality of a treatment. A number of clinical reports have correlated temperature-related parameters to treatment outcome[5,6,201] and two recent phase 3 trials used prospective control of thermal dose, as measured using noninvasive thermometry to increase tumor response and duration of local control following thermoradiotherapy (see clinical section for details).[7,8] While critical for verifying quality of HT, invasive thermometry also has a number of disadvantages: (1) patient discomfort, (2) risk of hemorrhage and/or infection, (3) requirement of physician time and image verification, and (4) small number of datapoints, which limits ability to assess temperature distribution or alter treatment.

Noninvasive Thermometry

The limitation of invasive techniques for characterizing temperature distributions has stimulated the development of noninvasive thermometry that should revolutionize the way HT is practiced because it can provide real-time adjustment of heating devices based on more complete 2D and 3D volumetric measures of temperature distribution rather than from a limited number of measured points. MRI is currently the preferred technology for volumetric thermometry.[202-205] Several MR parameters are temperature sensitive including the relaxation time T1, T2, bulk magnetization, and the proton resonance frequency. The latter has shown to provide the best temperature sensitivity and is most commonly used.[206] Several other methods are under investigation,[207,208] with microwave radiometry showing good promise for volumetric thermometry of both superficial[209] and deep tissues[210-214] with somewhat lower resolution than ultrasound and MRI based technologies.

Clinical studies in patients with extremity soft tissue sarcomas have reported resolution of 0.5-1°C (Fig. 42-7). Similar accuracy has been reported for pelvic malignancies.[202,215,216] There are significant issues to deal with that may limit the usefulness of MR thermometry, however. Drift in MR magnet coils, motion of the patient or parts of the patient, created by factors such as peristalsis must be corrected. Despite these concerns, recent clinical reports show that thermal dose parameters, derived from temperatures measured using MRI-based noninvasive thermometry, are correlated with treatment outcome in patients with locally advanced colorectal cancer, treated with thermochemoradiotherapy.[202,216]

Clinical Hyperthermia

General Considerations

HT alone has been studied in the treatment of superficial tumors. While an occasional response is noted, the duration is typically quite short.[217,218] Long-term tumor control has not been described with the use of HT as a sole treatment modality. HT alone remains widely practiced in certain alternative and complementary medicine clinics. Its use, however, is not supported by any peer-reviewed published scientific data.

A large number of phase 1/2 reports over the last two decades attest to the efficacy of HT + RT. The patients have been primarily those with superficial malignancies (and thus more amenable to heating) but present as a component of generalized disease. The most common clinical presentation has been local recurrence of breast carcinoma. With HT + RT, clinical response rates have doubled from 25% to 35% for RT alone to 50-70% with RT + HT.[219] The great majority of patients have had systemic disease as well; thus, survival data and long-term local control have infrequently been reported.

In addition to phase 2 studies, approximately 20-25 phase 3 trials have now been conducted worldwide with approximately two-third published in the English literature. These trials for the most part have been positive, lending additional validity to the information obtained from phase 2 studies.

Overall, HT is well tolerated and does not appear to significantly increase early or late toxicity of radiation.[123,127-129] The therapeutic ratio is thus improved by the addition of HT to RT. The most common side effect of HT is superficial or subcutaneous tissue burns, generally first or second degree in character and small in volume. Such burns occur in approximately 5% of patients treated in our clinic; characteristically they do not exceed 3-4 cm in maximum diameter. Third degree burns are rarely seen, in less than 1% of all patients treated. Complications (particularly infections) from the placement of thermometry catheters interstitially within the tumor have also been reported,[220] but are quite infrequent if thermometry catheters are removed following each HT treatment.[221] There are potential medical contraindications to HT, related to the physiologic stresses of heating. The latter has sometimes been compared to a moderately intense exercise workout. Guidelines for patient selection for deep HT have been developed by Radiation Therapy Oncology Group (RTOG).[198]

Published data on the efficacy of local-regional HT + CT is much less frequent. Both animal and human data have recently been reviewed.[219] Particularly encouraging phase 2 results have been reported for sarcomas[222] and breast carcinoma (Park et al., personal communication; Duke University Medical Center, unpublished data). Additionally, significant activity is seen when chemotherapy is administered to extremity tumors via perfusional or infusional methods where the perfusate is heated.[223]

Positive phase 2 results have also been reported for triple combinations of drug, HT, and radiotherapy. Examples include a phase 2 trial of of 5FU, leucovorin, HT, and radiotherapy for locally advanced rectal cancer[224] and a pilot phase 2 trial evaluating the combination of cisplatin + RT + HT for locally advanced cervix cancer.[148] No phase 3 data are as yet reported, but trials are underway for locally advanced rectal carcinoma, and cervical carcinoma.

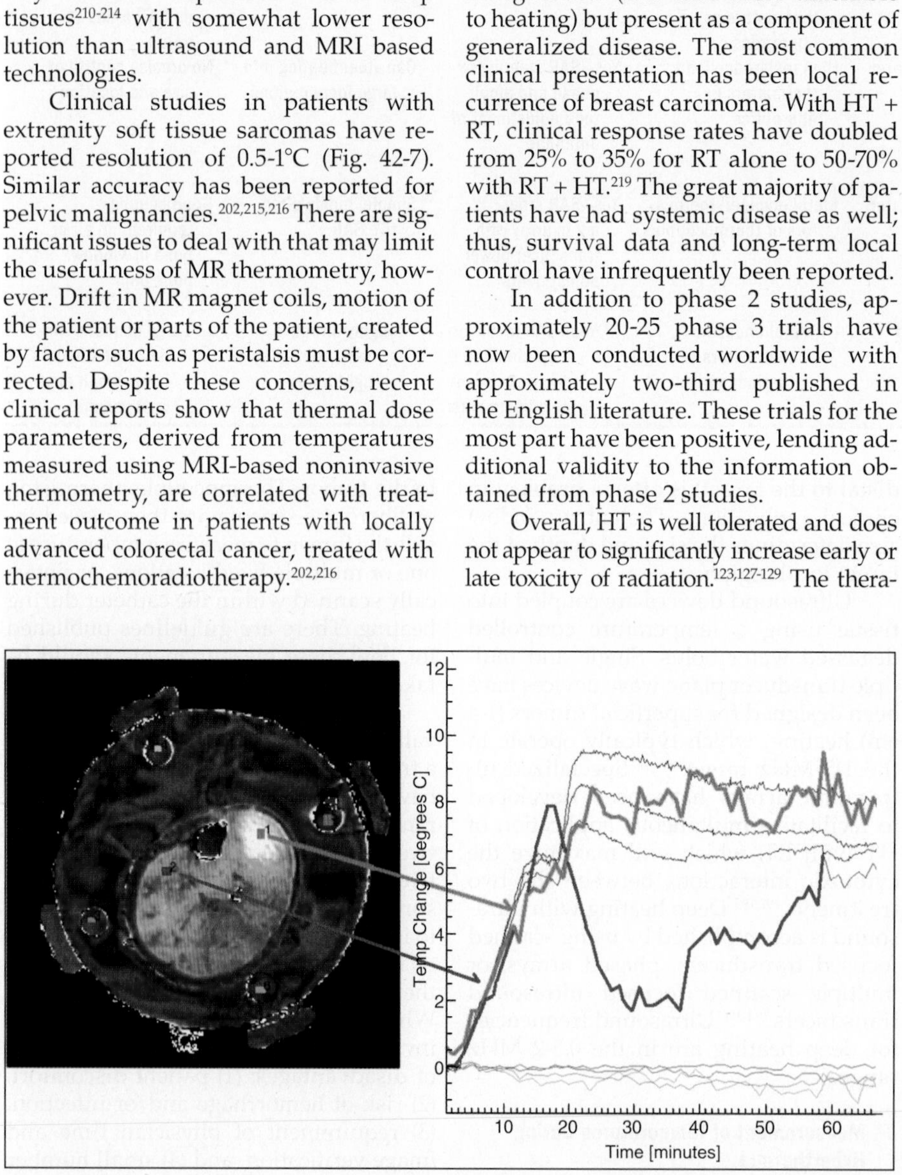

Figure 42-7 MR thermometry of lower leg sarcoma undergoing heat treatment. MRI with overlaid temperature rise (white = hot) shows effective localization of 140 MHz phased array heating in tumor at upper right. Quantitative display of temperature increase above initial baseline for three interstitially measured temperatures across tumor (*black lines*) and for MR PRFS-based measurements within small regions of interest around point 1 (*red line*) in tumor and point 2 (*blue line*) in contralateral normal tissue. Note the radical reduction in normal tissue heating achieved 18 minutes into heating in response to change in relative phase of the four heating antennae which led to improved focus of heating in tumor.

Relationship Between Thermal Dose and Outcome

The conduct of clinical trials and clinical practice of HT has been inhibited by difficulties in establishing quantifiable thermal dose parameters that correlate well with outcome in both tumor and normal tissue. As with any therapy, sound dosimetry is required to write a verifiable treatment prescription. Quality assurance standards have been established for treatment set up and invasive thermometry,[197,225,226] but a standard system for thermometry data reporting is still not established. A number of parameters have been described, based on simple descriptions of multipoint thermometry, such as minimum or average temperature. The tenth percentile of the temperature distribution, which is commonly referred to as the T90 (90% of measured points exceed this value), has often been used. To deal with variations in temperatures and times of heating between patients, clinical data have been converted to thermal dose, defined as CEM43°C at the minimum, average or T90 temperature point in order to permit comparative analysis.[4]

Many trials have shown positive relationships between such measures of thermal dose and treatment outcome.[4-6,201] In all of these studies, thermal analysis was performed retrospectively. It has been more difficult to demonstrate that prospective control of thermal dose relates to clinical outcome. Two studies compared various numbers of HT fractions, given in combination with fractionated RT,[227,228] using the assumption that more treatments would yield greater cumulative thermal dose. Neither study showed benefit with more HT fractions. This could be due to considerable overlap in thermal doses between arms because temperature is a stronger determinant of thermal dose than time of HT (see biology section). Thrall tested the hypothesis that RT combined with whole body HT + local HT would yield greater CEM43°C T90 than local HT alone and superior local control rates in dogs with soft tissue sarcomas.[116] This study failed to show any advantage for whole body + local HT even though thermal doses were higher in the whole body + local HT arm. Induction of thermotolerance during the whole body HT, which was administered prior to application of local heating may have reduced the overall effect of HT in the combined group.

The first attempt to prospectively control thermal dose, as prescribed by the CEM43°C T90, was a study of preoperative RT and HT for soft tissue sarcomas. The outcome variable was pathologic complete response (CR) assessed at the time of surgery. Even though the thermal goal was reached in the majority of patients the projected CR rate was not achieved.[229] A number of explanations are possible, but a major consideration is the limited number of tumor temperatures that were sampled with invasive thermometry and the small number of patients enrolled into the trial. Certain 31-MRS parameters were associated with pathologic outcome in this patient series, suggesting that mitigating features of tumor heterogeneity may have masked the thermal dose effect.[4]

Two additional phase 3 trials have recently been reported, however, showing that prospective control of thermal dose, when HT is combined with RT, has an effect on tumor response and duration of local control. Details of those trials are discussed below.

Clinical Trials Overview

In this section we focus on the major published phase 3 trials. These trials have involved a wide variety of disease sites: superficial malignancies and tumors deep within the body and palliative as well as potentially curative patients. The more important of these trials are summarized in Table 42-2. Several other important trials are still in progress.

Breast Cancer ■ Chest wall recurrences of breast cancer are well suited for strategies employing HT. They are difficult to control with conventional approaches, even when patients have not been previously treated.

Five separate phase 3 trials were conducted, which were subsequently combined in an international collaborative study.[230] Patients were randomized to either RT alone or RT + HT. A significant improvement in CR rate was seen for patients receiving HT + RT compared with RT alone, 59% in the former group, 41% in the latter with an odds ratio of 2.3 (95% CI 1.4-3.8). The greatest effect was observed in patients with recurrent lesions in previously irradiated areas where further irradiation was limited to low doses. Survival advantages were not apparent.

Other Superficial Malignancies ■ A prior study was conducted by the RTOG comparing RT versus RT + HT in superficial measurable tumors (RTOG 8104).[231-233] Three hundred seven patients were enrolled; approximately half had head and neck tumors, one-third breast carcinoma (chest wall recurrences), with the remaining patients having a variety of superficial malignancies. Patients treated with RT + HT had a CR rate of 32% compared with 30% for those receiving RT. Subgroup analysis revealed significant improvements in duration of local control in patients with tumors less than 3 cm and in those with breast and/or chest wall recurrences. For lesions greater than 3 cm there was no difference in outcome. It was postulated that the better outcome in smaller tumors was a consequence of better heating. This trial was characterized by highly variable HT techniques and inadequate thermal dosimetry. These issues led to the development of subsequent RTOG guidelines for performing HT.[197]

Duke University recently completed a single institution prospective randomized trial of radiation and HT for superficial tumors.[7] Patients who were about to receive a course of local RT for a superficial lesion less than 3 cm in thickness were eligible. Further, in recognition of the concept that the tumor must be "heatable" to potentially achieve a therapeutic gain, patients were assessed for heatability prior to randomization. Between July 1994 and July 2001, 122 patients were enrolled. The majority of patients (70/108) on this trial had chest wall recurrences. Based on a test dose criteria, 109 patients were deemed heatable, and were randomized to receive no additional heat (ie, radiation alone) versus additional HT with radiation. The HT dose CEM43°C T90 (CEM at 43°C for 90% of the measured target volume) was defined prospectively based on prior studies, and the HT arm received ≥ 10 minutes CEM43°C T90. This was the first study to employ the concepts of prospective dose/prescription to HT, and stringent quality assurance was used. The complete response rate in the HT arm was 66% versus 42% in the no HT arm. The odds ratio for complete response was 2.7 (95%CI [1.2-5.8], p = 0.02). These results are very similar to the meta-analysis results. Previously irradiated patients had the greatest incremental gain in complete response, 23.5% in the no HT arm versus 68.2% in the HT arm.

A recent seven-institution retrospective review of treatment for chest wall recurrence was presented at the American Society for Therapeutic Radiology and Oncology 2006 meeting.[24] Among 71 patients treated between 1993 and 2005, the complete response rate was 67% in those treated with HT and radiation versus 31% treated with radiation alone. While these are retrospective data, they are in agreement with the meta-analysis and recent randomized series.

Head and Neck Cancer ■ Two trials demonstrated an advantage to HT + RT. The first study randomized 65 patients to RT alone versus RT + HT.[234] RT doses consisted of 50 Gy in 5 weeks to the primary site and regional lymphatics followed by an additional 10-15 Gy to sites of gross disease in daily fractions of 2 Gy. HT was given twice a week with 72 hours between each session. HT + RT significantly improved response in patients with stage III and IV disease. Patients in stage III receiving RT + HT had a 58% CR compared with 20% in the RT group. Similarly patients with stage IV disease achieved a CR of 38% compared with 7% for those receiving RT alone. There was no benefit for patients with stage I and II disease, with greater than 90% achieving a CR with either treatment. This trial evaluated both the primary site as well as neck nodes despite difficulties of effectively heating most primary head and neck tumors.

A second trial restricted evaluation to metastatic cervical lymph nodes in 41 patients with advanced local regional squamous cell carcinoma of the head and neck randomized to treatment with either RT alone or RT + HT.[235,236] The CR rate was 41% for RT alone versus 83% for RT + HT. The 5-year actuarial probability of local control in the neck was 24% for RT alone versus 69% in the combined arm. Five year survival was 0 for RT alone and 53% in the RT + HT group. All of these differences were statistically significant. Two patients in the combined group developed late osteonecrosis of the mandible. Interpretation of normal tissue complications is difficult, however, since the only long-term survivors were in the combined group. Thermal parameters reported in this study included the Tmin, Tmax, T90, and CEM at 42.5°C. There was no clear relationship between thermal dose received and outcome. Nonetheless, this well-executed and well-described phase 3 trial, despite the relatively small number of patients, is an important component of the evidence suggesting the value of HT.

A trial of interstitial HT was carried out primarily in head and neck patients by the RTOG.[237] This trial entered 173 patients with persistent or recurrent tumors after prior RT and/or surgery that were amenable to interstitial RT. The lesion site was head and neck in approximately 45% of patients, the pelvis in approximately 40% with miscellaneous sites accounting for the rest. Patients were randomized to receive interstitial RT alone or combined with interstitial HT. There was no difference in CR rates or 2-year survival. There were major quality assurance issues with this trial. Only one patient was considered to have had adequate HT.

Esophagus ■ Two randomized studies demonstrated an advantage to the addition of HT to chemoradiotherapy or CT alone in neoadjuvant treatment of esophagus cancer. In the first study, 53 patients with squamous cell carcinoma of the thoracic esophagus were randomized to preoperative HT + RT + CT (bleomycin), compared with RT + CT alone.[238] HT + CT were given concurrently 1 hour prior to RT in a 3-week regimen with a total RT dose of approximately 32 Gy. Clinical complete responses as well as pathologic responses were significantly improved in the tri-modality arm, pathologic CR of 26% combined in the tri-modality group versus 8% in the chemoradiotherapy alone group.

In a follow-up study, an additional 40 patients were treated with CT alone (bleomycin and cisplatin) or combined with HT.[239] No RT was given in this trial. Again an improvement in histopathologic response was noted favoring the HT group (19% vs 41%).

Malignant Melanoma ■ A major multicenter trial was carried out in Europe in patients with metastatic melanoma. Seventy patients with 134 metastatic or recurrent malignant melanoma lesions were randomized to receive RT or RT followed by HT.[111] Overall there was a significant benefit for RT + HT with a 2-year local control of 46% in the combined group compared with 28% RT alone. Quality assurance was similarly an issue in this trial with only 14% of treatments achieving the objective of 43°C for 60 minutes. Despite this, positive benefits were seen.

Glioblastoma Multiforme ■ A University of California San Francisco study evaluated interstitial HT + brachytherapy RT boost for selected patients with glioblastoma multiforme.[221] Patients whose tumors were implantable following external beam RT and CT were randomized to receive brachytherapy RT alone or combined with HT. One hundred 12 patients were accrued and 79 qualified for brachytherapy and were randomized. The remaining patients were dropped from the protocol due to disease progression. Both time to tumor progression and survival were significantly improved for the HT patients compared with those treated with brachytherapy alone. Two-year survivals were 31% and 15%, respectively. Toxicity appeared to be slightly greater in the HT patients, with seven grade 3 toxicities reported compared with one in the brachytherapy alone group. Extensive thermal dose data were reported. Good heating was achieved in most patients, but no correlation found between thermal dose and response.

Carcinoma of the Cervix ■ Perhaps the most significant phase 3 trial is that of the Dutch group which explored the use

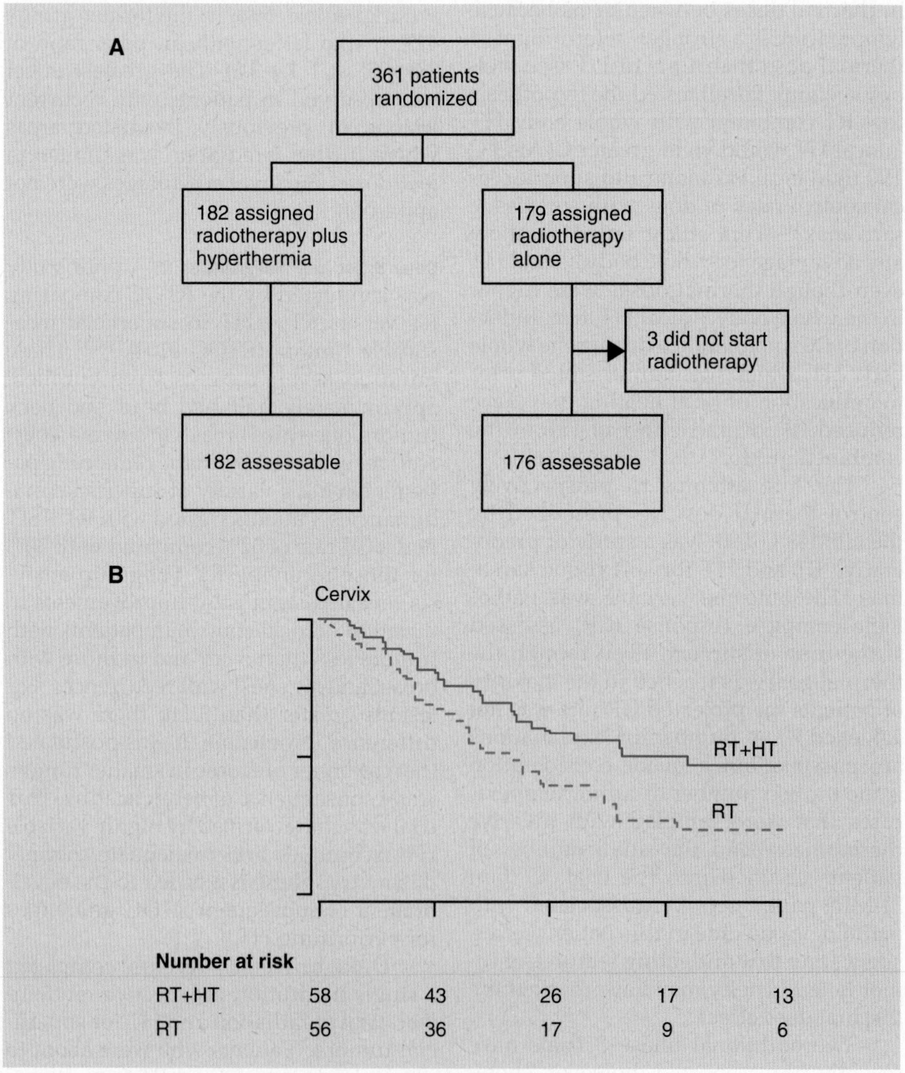

Figure 42-8 ■ Results of randomized phase 3 trial comparing radiotherapy ± HT for locally advanced cervix cancer. (**a**) Clinical trial design. (**b**) Overall survival following HT + RT versus RT alone for locally advanced cervix cancer. A distinct survival advantage was seen with the addition of HT ($p = 0.009$). Rectal and bladder cancer survival were not significantly affected by heat. *Abbreviations*: RT, radiotherapy; HT, hyperthermia. *Source*: From Ref. 240.

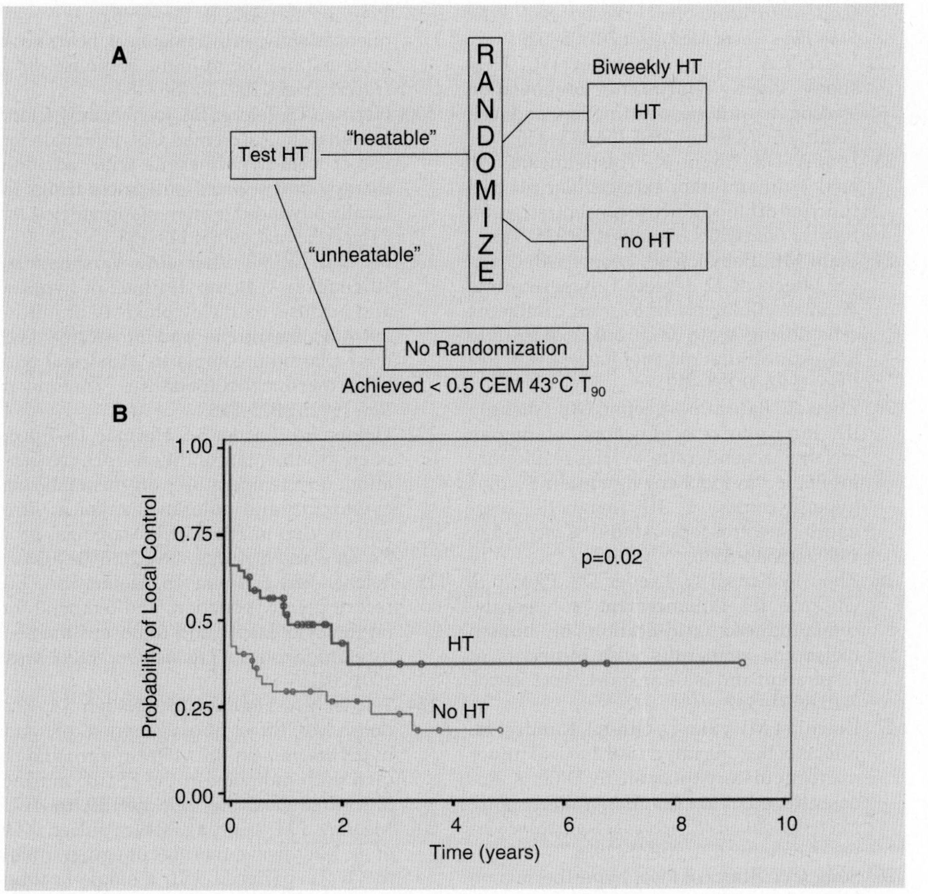

Figure 42-9 Results of a randomized phase 3 trial comparing efficacy of delivering a low versus high cumulative thermal dose in combination with radiotherapy for superficial tumors (primarily chest wall recurrences of breast cancer). (**a**) Clinical trial design. (**b**) Duration of local control in patients with superficial tumors treated with a low versus high cumulative thermal dose combined with RT. The difference in CR rate was significant as well as duration of local control following administration of a higher cumulative thermal dose. *Source*: From Reference 7.

of RT alone versus RT + HT in patients with locally advanced pelvic tumors.[240] This study randomized 361 patients with previously untreated locally advanced pelvic tumors to receive RT alone or RT + HT. There were approximately equal numbers of patients with rectal, bladder, and cervix carcinoma. No CT was given in this trial. CR rates were 39% after RT alone and 55% after RT + HT ($p \leq 0.001$). Duration of local control was also significantly improved with RT + HT compared with RT alone. Most of the benefit appeared to occur in patients with cervical carcinoma in whom the CR rate following RT + HT was 83% compared with 57% after RT alone. Three-year survival was 27% in the RT alone group of cervix cancer patients, 51% in the RT + HT group ($p = 0.003$) (Fig. 42-7). HT treatments were given once weekly for a total of five treatments. Generally, thermal goals were not achieved. Detailed thermal dose analyses were not published.

While the effect of HT in this study was fairly dramatic, it has been criticized for suboptimal therapy in the control arm, namely RT alone as opposed to RT + CT. At the time the trial was initiated in 1990, the role of CT in locally advanced cervix carcinoma was not established. Subsequently, a number of studies published in 1999/2000 have demonstrated a survival advantage for concurrent cisplatin + RT in cervical carcinoma.[241-245] Two new phase 3 trials have now been initiated comparing CT + RT + HT to CT + RT in the United States and the Netherlands. The control arm in the U.S. trial is CT + RT, while in the Netherlands it is RT + HT.

Adult Soft Tissue Sarcoma

The EORTC completed a randomized trial for sarcomas using neoadjuvant and adjuvant chemotherapy ± HT, and results demonstrating improvement in disease free survival were presented at ASCO 2007. We await reporting of the final trial results, which accrued over 340 evaluable patients.

Prospective Control of Thermal Dose Is Related to Superior Outcome Two recently completed phase 3 trials used extensive invasive thermometry to control the amount of HT delivered, as defined by CEM 43°C at the T90.[7,8] An important aspect of these trials was the requirement that patients were not randomized until it was determined that the tumors were heatable, using preset criteria. This was determined by performing a test HT. If the tumor was deemed heatable during that first HT, then they were randomized to receive either a low- or high-thermal dose, as accumulated over the course of thermoradiotherapy.

Superficial tumors were the subjects of the human trial. One hundred twenty patients were enrolled and 109 were deemed heatable and were randomized. Those patients who randomized to the low-HT dose group received no further HT, but received conventionally fractionated RT, with the total dose being determined by whether or not they had received prior RT. Those patients who were randomized to the high-HT group were targeted to receive more than 10 CEM 43°C T90, whereas the low-HT dose were targeted to 0.5-1 CEM 43°C T90 from the single HT treatment that they received. The CR rate in the high-HT dose arm was 66.1% versus 42.3% in the low-HT dose arm, with an odds ratio of 2.7 ($p = 0.02$; Fig. 42-9).

The canine trial involved pet dogs with spontaneous soft tissue sarcomas.[8] These animals were treated with conventionally fractionated RT, to a total dose of 52 Gy, combined with either low- or high-dose HT. This trial was different from the human trial in that animals that were randomized to low HT continued to be administered HT treatments, but the duration of HT was shortened so as to not exceed 2-5 CEM 43°C T90 over the entire treatment course. Animals in the high-HT dose group were targeted to receive 20-50 CEM 43°C T90. The endpoints in this trial were duration of local control, metastasis-free and overall survival. One hundred twenty two dogs were accrued into the trial and of these 109 met the criterion of having heatable tumors. The median duration of local control was not significantly different between the two arms, but after adjusting for other variables, such as tumor grade, volume, and institution where treatment was administered, thermal dose was found to be significantly important ($p = 0.023$). Other variables found to be important were tumor grade, volume, and HT treatment duration.

Summary of Clinical Trials

Results of the published phase 3 trials above are intriguing. Apart from the two early RTOG trials, they all appear to demonstrate substantial benefits for HT + RT. However, many of the trials were associated with significant design and implementation problems including relatively small numbers of patients, thermal dosimetry information that was highly variable in nature, thermal goals that were often not achieved, and control arms that may not have represented optimal standard therapy. Despite these difficulties, the generally positive nature of these trials suggest the future of HT is quite promising and that technological advances may well lead the way to even more positive results. The two positive thermal dose escalation trials provide strong rationale for implementing strict thermal dose requirements for future HT trials.

Selected References

The complete reference list can be found at www.CANCERMEDICINE8.com

2. Sapareto SA, Dewey WC. Thermal dose determination in cancer therapy. *Int J Radiat Oncol Biol Phys*. 1984;10:787–800.
3. Dewey WC. Arrhenius relationships from the molecule and cell to the clinic. *Int J Hyperthermia*. 1994;10:457–483.
4. Dewhirst MW. Thermal dosimetry. In: Seegenschmiedt M, Fessenden P, Vernon CC, eds. *Thermoradiotherapy and Thermochemotherapy*. Berlin: Springer Verlag; 1995:123–128.
5. Oleson JR, Samulski TV, Leopold KA, et al. Sensitivity of hyperthermia trial outcomes to temperature and time: implications for thermal goals of treatment. *Int J Radiat Oncol Biol Phys*. 1993;25:289–297.
6. Seegenschmiedt MH, Martus P, Fietkau R, Iro H, Brady LW, Sauer R. Multivariate analysis of prognostic parameters using interstitial thermoradiotherapy (IHT-IRT): tumor and treatment variables predict outcome. *Int J Radiat Oncol Biol Phys*. 1994;29:1049–1063.
7. Jones EL, Oleson JR, Prosnitz LR, et al. Randomized trial of hyperthermia and radiation for superficial tumors. *J Clin Oncol*. 2005;23:3079–3085.
8. Thrall DE, LaRue SM, Yu D, et al. Thermal dose is related to duration of local control in canine sarcomas treated with thermoradiotherapy. *Clin Cancer Res*. 2005;11:5206–5214.
9. Lepock JR. Cellular effects of hyperthermia: relevance to the minimum dose for thermal damage. *Int J Hyperthermia*. 2003;19:252–266.
10. Dewey WC, Hopwood LE, Sapareto SA, Gerweck LE. Cellular responses to combinations of hyperthermia and radiation. *Radiology*. 1977;123:463–474.
11. Morimoto RI, Kroeger PE, Cotto JJ. The transcriptional regulation of heat shock genes: a plethora of heat shock factors and regulatory conditions. *EXS*. 1996;77:139–163.
20. Dewey WC, Miller HH. Effect of temperature on x-ray induced cell lethality and chromosomal aberrations. *Int J Radiat Biol Relat Stud Phys Chem Med*. 1970;18:91–93.
21. Dewey WC, Westra A, Miller HH, Nagasawa H. Heat-induced lethality and chromosomal damage in synchronized Chinese hamster cells treated with 5-bromodeoxyuridine. *Int J Radiat Biol Relat Stud Phys Chem Med*. 1971;20:505–520.
22. Vidair CA, Doxsey SJ, Dewey WC. Heat shock alters centrosome organization leading to mitotic dysfunction and cell death. *J Cell Physiol*. 1993;154:443–455.
23. Leeper DB, Engin K, Thistlethwaite AJ, et al. Human tumor extracellular pH as a function of blood glucose concentration. *Int J Radiat Oncol Biol Phys*. 1994;28:935–943.
24. Wahl ML, Bobyock SB, Leeper DB, Owen CS. Effects of 42 degrees C hyperthermia on intracellular pH in ovarian carcinoma cells during acute or chronic exposure to low extracellular pH. *Int J Radiat Oncol Biol Phys*. 1997;39:205–212.
25. Zhou R, Bansal N, Leeper DB, Glickson JD. Intracellular acidification of human melanoma xenografts by the respiratory inhibitor m-iodobenzylguanidine plus hyperglycemia: a 31P magnetic resonance spectroscopy study. *Cancer Res*. 2000;60:3532–3536.
26. Zhou R, Bansal N, Leeper DB, Pickup S, Glickson JD. Enhancement of hyperglycemia-induced acidification of human melanoma xenografts with inhibitors of respiration and ion transport. *Acad Radiol*. 2001;8:571–582.
27. Dewhirst MW, Sim D, Gross J, Kundrat M. Effects of heating rate on normal and tumor microcirculatory function. In: Diller K, Roemer RB, eds. *Heat and Mass Transfer in the Microcirculation of Thermally Significant Vessels*. Anaheim, CA: ASME; 1986:75–80.
28. Song CW. Effect of local hyperthermia on blood flow and microenvironment: a review. *Cancer Res*. 1984;44:4721s–4730s.
49. Crabtree HG. Observations on the carbohydrate metabolism of tumours. *Biocheml J*. 1929;23:536–545.
50. Newsholme EA, Crabtree B, Ardawi MS. The role of high rates of glycolysis and glutamine utilization in rapidly dividing cells. *Biosci Rep*. 1985;5:393–400.
51. Biaglow JE, Manevich Y, Leeper D, et al. MIBG inhibits respiration: potential for radio- and hyperthermic sensitization. *Int J Radiat Oncol Biol Phys*. 1998;42:871–876.
52. Burd R, Lavorgna SN, Daskalakis C, et al. Tumor oxygenation and acidification are increased in melanoma xenografts after exposure to hyperglycemia and meta-iodo-benzylguanidine. *Radiat Res*. 2003;159:328–335.
53. Kozin SV, Zaitsev AV, Yarmonenko SP. Antitumour effect of irradiation followed by hyperglycemia and hyperthermia: the dependence on tumour size and blood flow. *Int J Hyperthermia*. 1996;12:147–156.
54. Mueller-Klieser W, Walenta S, Kelleher DK, Dinh H, Marx E, Vaupel P. Tumourgrowth inhibition by induced hyperglycaemia/hyperlactacidaemia and localized hyperthermia. *Int J Hyperthermia*. 1996;12:501–511.
55. van den Berg AP, van den Berg-Blok AE, Kal HB, Reinhold HS. A moderate elevation of blood glucose level increases the effectiveness of thermoradiotherapy in a rat tumor model II. Improved tumor control at clinically achievable temperatures. *Int J Radiat Oncol Biol Phys*. 2001;50:793–801.
56. Nagata K, Murata T, Shiga T, et al. Enhancement of thermoradiotherapy by glucose administration for superficial malignant tumours. *Int J Hyperthermia*. 1998;14:157–167.
57. Repasky E, Issels R. Physiological consequences of hyperthermia: heat, heat shock proteins and the immune response. *Int J Hyperthermia*. 2002;18:486–489.
130. Herman TS, Teicher BA, Jochelson M, Clark J, Svensson G, Coleman CN. Rationale for use of local hyperthermia with radiation therapy and selected anticancer drugs in locally advanced human malignancies. *Int J Hyperthermia*. 1988;4:143–158.
131. Herman TS, Teicher BA, Varshney A, Khandekar V, Brann T. Effect of hypoxia and acidosis on the cytotoxicity of mitoxantrone, bisantrene and amsacrine and their platinum complexes at normal and hyperthermic temperatures. *Anticancer Res*. 1992;12:827–836.
132. Holden SA, Teicher BA, Herman TS. Effect of environmental conditions (pH, oxygenation, and temperature) on misonidazole cytotoxicity and radiosensitization in vitro and in vivo in FSaIIC fibrosarcoma. *Int J Radiat Oncol Biol Phys*. 1991;20:1031–1038.
133. Teicher BA, Herman TS, Holden SA. Effect of pH, oxygenation, and temperature on the cytotoxicity and radiosensitization by etanidazole. *Int J Radiat Oncol Biol Phys*. 1991;20:723–731.
134. Teicher BA, Herman TS, Holden SA, Rudolph MB. Effect of oxygenation, pH and hyperthermia on RSU-1069 in vitro and in vivo with radiation in the FSaIIC murine fibrosarcoma. *Cancer Lett*. 1991;59:109–117.
207. Meaney PM, Fanning MW, Paulsen KD, et al. Microwave thermal imaging: initial in vivo experience with a single heating zone. *Int J Hyperthermia*. 2003;19:617–641.
208. Arthur RM, Straube WL, Trobaugh JW, Moros EG. Non-invasive estimation of hyperthermia temperatures with ultrasound. *Int J Hyperthermia*. 2005;21:589–600.
209. Jacobsen S, Stauffer PR. Can we settle with single-band radiometric temperature monitoring during hyperthermia treatment of chestwall recurrence of breast cancer using a dual-mode transceiving applicator? *Phys Med Biol*. 2007;52:911–928.
210. Bardati F, Brown VJ, Tognolatti P. Temperature reconstructions in a dielectric cylinder by multi-frequency microwave radiometry. *J Electronic Waves and Applications*. 1993;7:1549–1571.
211. Dubois L, Pribetich J, Fabre JJ, Chive M, Moschetto Y. Non-invasive microwave multifrequency radiometry used in microwave hyperthermia for bidimensional reconstruction of temperature patterns. *Int J Hyperthermia*. 1993;9:415–431.
212. Jacobsen S, Stauffer P. Non-invasive temperature profile estimation in a lossy medium based on multi-band radiometric signals sensed by a microwave dual-purpose body-contacting antenna. *Int J Hyperthermia*. 2002;18:86–103.
213. Mizushina S, Ohba K, Abe K, Mizoshiri S, Sugiura T. Recent trends in medical microwave radiometry. *IEICE Transactions on Communications*. 1995;E78-B:789–798.
226. Lagendijk JJ, Van Rhoon GC, Hornsleth SN, et al. ESHO quality assurance guidelines for regional hyperthermia. *Int J Hyperthermia*. 1998;14:125–133.
227. Engin K, Tupchong L, Moylan DJ, et al. Randomized trial of one versus two adjuvant hyperthermia treatments per week in patients with superficial tumours. *Int J Hyperthermia*. 1993;9:327–340.

43 Principles of Medical Oncology

William N. Hait, MD, PhD ■ James F. Holland, MD, ScD (hc) ■ Emil Frei III, MD ■ Donald W. Kufe, MD ■ Robert C. Bast Jr., MD ■ Waun Ki Hong, MD, DMSc (Hon)

Medical oncology evolved from a subspecialty of internal medicine whose hallmark was the ability to diagnose cancer and to safely administer dangerous drugs to the branch of medicine most directly linked to modern molecular biology; today it heralds in the era of personalized medicine. A medical oncologist understands the biologic basis of malignant transformation and applies this knowledge to the prevention, early detection, and treatment of cancer patients. An individual with cancer should be viewed in the context of the etiology, pathogenesis, pathology, and biochemistry of the neoplastic process and humanistically as a person struggling with a terrifying disease.

Training of medical oncologists originated in cancer institutes, divisions of hematology, and departments of pharmacology. The American Board of Internal Medicine established the subspecialty as a separate discipline in 1971. The Board in the subspecialty of medical oncology has further certified[1] approximately 8000 internists. There are over 25,000 members of the American Society of Clinical Oncology, and approximately one-third of the more than 26,000 members of the American Association of Cancer Research are physicians. Medical oncologists and hematologists have overlapping interests in neoplastic diseases of the hematopoietic tissues and share historic interests in training subspecialists in both fields. However, because each discipline became more complex, individual training programs are the preferred approach.

In this chapter, we introduce the subspecialty by attempting to define a set of principles that underlie the practice of medical oncology.

Principles

Principle n. An important underlying law or assumption required in a system of thought.

Certain principles underlie the practice of medical oncology and are listed in Table 43-1. These tenets, although not mathematically derived or subject to rigorous validation, should nonetheless serve the purpose of providing both the uninitiated young practitioner and the seasoned veteran with a perspective gleaned from the several vantage points of the authors.

The Treatment of Cancer Is Multidisciplinary, Requiring Consultation With Knowledgeable Colleagues in Related Subspecialties ■ The practice of medical oncology is dependent on highly productive interactions with cognate disciplines, particularly surgical oncology, radiation oncology, urology, orthopedic surgery, radiology, and pathology. Multiple other interactions occur with nursing oncology, psycho-oncology, neuro-oncology, gynecologic oncology, rehabilitation medicine, and, for young patients, pediatric oncology. Infectious diseases are common complications of cancers and their treatments, forming a natural alliance with specialists in infectious diseases. Today, with the gratifying number of long-term survivors, the medical oncologist must work closely with primary care physicians for follow-up surveillance and psychologists and psychiatrists, who may be required to address the existential complexities of survivorship and the sequelae of treatment.

The medical oncologist is often involved in the final decisions concerning management and is frequently the final common pathway through which decisions are implemented. The timing of surgery and radiotherapy, the decision whether to take a curative or a palliative approach, and the decision whether watchful waiting is the appropriate course or whether vigorous action is necessary are often entrusted to the medical oncologist.

Most patients have a relationship with other physicians before being diagnosed with cancer; a family physician or internist who referred the patient to a medical oncologist and other specialists may already have been involved with the patient before the recognition of a neoplastic disease. Medical oncologists must recognize their interest and continuing role in the management of patients with multisystem disease and communicate with them effectively. In the absence of such consultants, however, the medical oncologist must also attend to all aspects of internal medicine. Elsewhere, this book contains detailed descriptions of various diseases; the modalities used in their treatment; the pharmacologic, immunologic, neurologic, psychological, biochemical, epidemiologic, and molecular biologic aspects of cancers; and the complications that cancers cause. Oncologic emergencies, rehabilitation, and the oncologist's relationship to medical informatics and to government are also presented. Familiarity with these topics constitutes a foundation for medical oncology from which the principles derive.

Table 43-1 ■ Principles of Medical Oncology

The treatment of cancer is multidisciplinary, requiring consultation with knowledgeable colleagues in related subspecialties.
The suspicion of cancer is based on clinical acumen and the diagnosis on examination of tissue.
Prevention is more effective than treatment.
The medical treatment of cancer patients is based on a clear understanding of the mechanism of drug action, potential for harmful side effects, mechanisms of drug resistance, and the principles of therapeutics.
Early-stage cancers are more curable than late-stage cancers; the first treatment is more effective than the next.
The best treatment is often found through participation in clinical trials.
Cancer surveillance must be based on validated assumptions.
Oncologic care is for life.

The Suspicion of Cancer Is Based on Clinical Acumen and the Diagnosis on Examination of Tissue ■ Oncologists must be highly competent internists to diagnose, exclude, and treat cancer. Many diseases can mimic the signs and symptoms of cancer, but the medical oncologist must not miss a nonmalignant cause. Conversely, the internist and the medical oncologist must remember that cancer, like syphilis in the past, is the "great masquerader" and, thus, must be considered in every differential diagnosis.[2] A medical oncologist must understand the pathophysiology of cancer, the genetic predispositions, and the basic pharmacology that is the bedrock of effective cancer treatment. All cancers are not the same, and all patients with a given type of cancer do not behave in a similar manner. Increasingly, cancers are being segmented into a variety of distinct entities, each with subtle and not so subtle differences in prognosis and treatment. Just as the more precise classification of leukemias and lymphomas led to improvements in treatment in the past, the use of transcriptional profiling and other powerful molecular tools are identifying subsets of solid tumors that respond differently to treatment.

For complex new syndromes appearing in a patient who once had cancer, such as pulmonary insufficiency, meningoencephalopathy, or inexplicable pain, it is indispensable to establish by objective criteria that cancer is the proximate cause. Cancer patients are not protected from other symptomatic noncancerous diseases, such as pulmonary fibrosis and central nervous system disorders, or painful conditions, such as a herniated disk. No symptom should be attributed to cancer without persuasive evidence. Yet cancer must be suspected every time.

To ascribe a finding to cancer requires histologic proof. Modern medical oncologists will need to both understand the histologic appearance of malignant and premalignant lesions and be able to understand the interpretation of complex profiles of gene transcription and protein translation, as well as chromosomal abnormalities and gene sequences, to properly diagnose and manage their patients. These advances will lead to an even greater number of individuals who know that they are at risk of developing cancer, living with a diagnosis of cancer, or putatively cured of cancer but are concerned about recurrence. It is an exceptional case when a medical oncologist can consider treatment without a histologic diagnosis. Certain oncologic emergencies, such as spinal cord compression or superior vena cava syndrome, were once considered exceptions, but with modern imaging and biopsy techniques, a tissue diagnosis can usually be made rapidly and safely. Cytologic diagnoses may provide sufficient information in the presence of unambiguous clinical syndromes, but cytology of the bronchus, stomach, cervix, and body fluids has produced sufficient numbers of false-positive identifications to show that corroborating evidence is essential. Highly specific biochemical markers may be helpful when clinical and radiologic findings are characteristic and when a major intracavitary (cranial, thoracic, or abdominal) biopsy procedure would constitute an ominously serious event for a particular patient. Even elevation of human chorionic gonadotropin, alpha-fetoprotein, or cancer antigen (CA) 125 or CA 19-9 in the presence of compatible clinical manifestations is rarely sufficient, with the possible exception of relapsing disease. It is always preferable to have histologic evidence whenever possible.

The Management of Cancer Patients Requires an Understanding of the Genetics, Biology, and Pharmacology of Neoplasia and the Psychosocial Impact of a Cancer Predisposition or Diagnosis on Patient and Physician ■ The practice of medical oncology requires wisdom, sensitivity, and resourcefulness. For the patient in whom relatively asymptomatic findings lead to a diagnosis of cancer, it is useful to consider that the day before the discovery, the patient was living with cancer. It is a source of some encouragement to patients to know that a diagnosis of cancer does not lead immediately or inevitably to death. The medical oncologist may be able to stress the long-term evolution of a cancer, the several stages that intervene between the carcinogenic stimulus, genetic mutations, selection of cells with a survival advantage, and the appearance of an autonomous neoplasm. Because this process usually takes years and often decades, it is of value to place the neoplastic process in perspective (vide infra). This is particularly important when a patient is being urged to make an immediate decision regarding surgery, radiation, or chemotherapy. When one considers that, on average, it will take more than 5 years for a malignant cell to undergo the requisite 30 doublings to achieve a 1 cm (1 billion cell) mass required for most diagnoses, an additional week or two to gather information and opinions is unlikely to have a negative impact on the ultimate course of the disease.

Increasingly, individuals are recognized to harbor genetic predispositions to cancer owing to mutations or polymorphisms. The oncologist must combine an understanding of the impact of these changes on the probability of being diagnosed with cancer and weigh the risks and benefits of medical intervention while being sensitive to the emotional impact that this knowledge has on individuals and their families. In some, cancer or the prevention of cancer may become a chronic process requiring ongoing treatment analogous to the management of diabetes or hypertension. Similarly, oncologists must recognize environmental exposures that increase the risk of cancer and attempt intervention to mitigate that risk. An increasing number of patients who might have developed cancer will be at greater risk of dying from other diseases than of dying from cancer.

The medical oncologist must distinguish between a neoplasm in which a chance for cure exists versus one that is currently incurable ("precurable"). Most cancers are curable if detected early, and most cancers are incurable if detected late. Thus, a 1-cm tumor of 1×10^9 cells is often curable, whereas a tumor mass approaching 1×10^{12} cells is usually fatal. Whereas the former is likely to be driven by few genetic mutations and confined to one or two critical pathways, the latter is likely to harbor multiple mutations in several pathways that make successful treatment less likely. The medical oncologist must therefore appreciate the importance of prevention, screening, and early detection and must actively educate colleagues and patients.

Advances in our understanding of cancer biology encourage the belief that one day all cancers will be prevented or cured. It is axiomatic that the day before the first metastatic choriocarcinoma was cured with high-dose methotrexate,[3,4] metastatic cancer, in general, was considered incurable by most observers. Similar considerations apply to every neoplastic disease that is now curable (Table 43-2). Other neoplasms are currently not cured by medicines alone but require participation of surgery or radiotherapy as an intrinsic part of the therapeutic process (Table 43-3).

Patients are often influenced by their present state of subjective well-being. It is the responsibility of an oncologist to recognize the often pernicious behavior of cancer in its potential for recurrence and metastasis. In this context, the medical oncologist must interact directly with the patient and family, as well as with the medical record, films, slides, and other critical raw data. It is important to understand how patients make choices so as to present information in a way that does not bias an eventual decision. In addition, altering behaviors of patients and their families are likely to occur.[5] For example, following a "scare" that a lung nodule could have been malignant may be the best time to treat nicotine addiction in the patient and in members of the family. The diagnosis of cancer constitutes a serious emotional burden that may distort ordinary reason. By firsthand intimacy

Table 43-2 ■ **Cancers Curable With Chemotherapy**

Choriocarcinoma
Acute lymphocytic leukemia of childhood
Burkitt lymphoma
Hodgkin disease
Acute promyelocytic leukemia
Large follicular center cell lymphoma
Embryonal carcinoma of testis
Hairy cell leukemia

Table 43-3 ■ **Cancers Subcurable With Chemotherapy[a]**

With regional therapy
Wilms' tumor
Osteosarcoma
Ewing sarcoma
Embryonal rhabdomyosarcoma
Adenocarcinoma of breast
Small cell carcinoma of lung
Squamous cell carcinoma of upper aerodigestive tract[b]
Adenocarcinoma of ovary
Thymoma
Without regional therapy
Acute lymphocytic leukemia of adulthood
Acute myeloid leukemia
Lymphomas, some subsets

[a]By definition, <50% curable with chemotherapy alone; cure rates obtained with chemotherapy plus regional therapy are significantly superior to those with regional therapy alone (ie, chemotherapeutic cure of micrometastatic disease only).
[b]Cure rates <50% in most series.

with the diagnosis, the extent of the disease, and the patient's attitudes and infirmities, the medical oncologist can make rational recommendations to the patient and to the other physicians involved.

Explanations of disease, anticipated therapies, protocols in which there are randomization, and unknowns must be tailored to the intellectual and emotional levels of the particular patient. It is never permissible to lie, but it may be prudent not to deposit all of the truth at once on a patient who cannot accept the full details and ramifications of diagnosis and management. "Your patient has no more right to all the truth you know than to all the medicine in your saddlebags" was a humane and ethical tenet advanced by Oliver Wendell Holmes more than a century ago.[6] It is dishonest to twist facts or to deny specific features, such as the existence of metastases. By the same token, it is wrong to deny a patient an opportunity to make final dispositions with respect to self, family, religion, the law, and business by falsely stating that a disease is benign or cured. Families who assert that the patient must not know because the patient could not stand it are usually twice wrong: The patient often knows already or may be more distraught by being excluded from knowing, and the patient ordinarily incorporates the information into his or her life equation indistinguishably from other patients. A reading of Tolstoy's masterful *The Death of Ivan Ilyich* should convince any doubting oncologist about the terror of uncertainty and the value of direct and honest, yet humane, interactions with the patient. When a patient asks, "There is hope, isn't there?" the oncologist can always be positive. Hope is a uniquely human characteristic that sustains the will to continue, and all oncologists and all patients do hope for a better outcome.

The treatment of patients with life-threatening disease can take its toll on providers of care. A sense of frustration can affect anyone who encounters barriers to successful completion of an important task. This is particularly true of intellectual tasks and invisible barriers. When the barrier is a lethal disease about which the oncologist can do little that is effective, the frustration can be all consuming. Oncologists who encounter several instances of recrudescent or refractory disease in a short time (especially if punctuated by the deaths of young or favorite patients, uninterrupted by counterbalancing compensatory successes) may well experience frustration, a sense of inadequacy, and depression. Frequent repetition of this cyclic phenomenon may lead to burnout.

The medical oncologist knows that many of today's cancers are not yet curable. To the extent that the medical oncologist can be involved, actually and conceptually, in the solution to these complex mysteries, the frustration is lessened. Cancer research, whether at the basic or the clinical level, is held in high esteem by our fellow citizens. Group identity, "being one of the team," helps offset the self-deprecation when human tragedies mount despite one's best efforts. The camaraderie of other oncologists helps because they battle the same enemy with the same primitive weapons. Another oncologist can understand the trauma and the distress; it is an encounter on familiar terrain.

The appreciation that the horizon is distant, and that oncologists are all working intently to see beyond it, puts present frustration in a more appropriate perspective. Involvement in the systematized academic pursuit, whether in an academic setting, a medical school outreach, an oncology society, or a local collaborative group, provides the security of collegial support. A sound mind in a sound body implies rest, exercise, nutrition, and enjoyment. To ensure the last, the first three are prerequisites. Avocation and vacation are a portion of good mental health, included in the terms rest and exercise.

If these stratagems do not help the potentially burnt out oncologist find a new orientation and a more resilient response to the inevitable future traumas, the oncologist may well consider an alternative occupation. Many oncologists have moved honorably to laboratory, administrative, or pharmaceutical positions, where they are insulated from the difficulties of patients' illnesses.

Finally, all oncologists can benefit from the vast array of continuing medical education programs given at academic medical centers, on the World Wide Web, at national meetings such as the American Association for Cancer Research and the American Society of Clinical Oncology, and through textbooks such as *Cancer Medicine*.

Prevention Is More Effective Than Treatment ■ The seminal work of Dr. Bert Vogelstein of John Hopkins Medical School demonstrated that as a normal epithelium transforms through dysplasia, anaplasia, and, eventually, neoplasia, and that there is a progressive increase in genetic mutations, a process that may take many years.[7] Similarly, as chronic myelogenous leukemia progresses from the chronic phase, through the accelerated phase to blast crisis, more chromosomal and genetic abnormalities are acquired. Exposure to environmental carcinogens, most commonly through tobacco use owing to nicotine addiction, accelerates the oncogenic process most prominently in the bronchial mucosa. These mutations activate complex signaling pathways that favor cell viability and inactivate pathways that normally balance uncontrolled growth through programmed cell death. Not surprisingly, many of these molecular changes impart resistance to cancer treatment. It follows that the earlier a cancer is diagnosed and treated, the more effective the treatment. Furthermore, the oncogenic process provides substantial time for interventions that could prevent the formation of cancer in susceptible individuals.

Numerous studies now confirm that inhibition of cyclooxygenases within the intestinal epithelium with nonsteroidal anti-inflammatory drugs, including aspirin, naproxen, and ibuprofen, has prevented many cases of colorectal cancer.[8,9] Hepatitis B vaccines have dramatically reduced the incidence of hepatoma, once the Eastern world's most common malignancy, by preventing the chronic inflammation and cellular damage produced by chronic hepatitis.[10] Retinoic acid can decrease the appearance of second malignancies in heavy smokers[11]; tamoxifen and raloxifene can prevent breast cancer in patients at substantial risk.[12] Minor surgical interventions, such as colonic polypectomy[13] and loop electrosurgical procedure for carcinoma in situ of the cervix,[14] can prevent colon and cervical cancer, respectively.

Increasingly, the medical oncologist will be called on to decide whether medical or surgical prevention is indicated in individuals without cancer but for whom cancer is a significant risk. This will require a sophisticated understanding of medical genetics, genomics, and proteomics, which will ultimately extend to subtle genetic abnormalities, such as single nucleotide polymorphisms and circulating biomarkers. In addition, the use of preventive drugs will require long-term monitoring because they will likely be used each day for years. Currently, the medical oncologist is asked to decide who should receive tamoxifen for prevention of breast cancer, retinoids for prevention of head and neck cancer, and oral contraceptives for prevention of ovarian cancer. Medical oncologists frequently advise patients regarding the benefits of prophylactic oophorectomy and mastectomy in patients with *BRCA1* and *BRCA2* mutations. Similarly, oncologists must be aware that the hepatitis B vaccine will prevent hepatoma, and a vaccine against human papillomavirus will prevent many cases of cancer of the uterine cervix.[15] The oncologist must take a leading role in treating addiction to nicotine in all of its manifestations and must educate physicians and the public on the importance of early detection through appropriate screening.

Medical Oncologists Should Counsel Patients and Families About Good Nutrition and Healthy Sexual Practices as Well as Screening Tests Available for Some Cancer Types ■ Several chapters of this treatise deal with prevention and early detection, and numerous publications that deal with these topics are available for distribution to patients and families from the National Cancer Institute (NCI) and the American Cancer Society (ACS). The NCI Cancer Information Service (800-4-CANCER) and the ACS National Cancer Information Center (800-ACS-2345) will send available publications free of charge and publish this information on their Web sites (The medical treatment of cancer patients is based on a clear understanding of the mechanism of drug action, the potential for harmful side effects, mechanisms of drug resistance, and the principles of therapeutics. For a drug to be effective, it must hit its target, the target must be integral to the viability of cancer cells, and it must be present in the tumor being treated. The drug–target interaction must disable cancer cells better than normal cells. Modern methods of treatment adhere to these basic principles of cancer pharmacology and are important means by which one can predict a patient's response to treatment.

We have entered the era of "targeted therapies," broadly defined as the selective alteration of molecules that are essential to malignant cell growth. These new medications are likely to be less toxic than traditional cancer chemotherapy drugs that most commonly target DNA or microtubules. The proper use of the new-targeted therapies will require an understanding of the molecular pathways responsible for malignancy in general and possibly in each individual's tumor. Recent examples include imatinib to inhibit the transforming oncogenic protein in chronic phase chronic myelogenous leukemia (*Bcr-Abl*)[16]; gefitinib to effectively treat patients with non-small cell lung cancer by targeting those individuals whose tumors harbor activating mutations in the epidermal growth factor receptor[17]; erlotinib, which was shown to extend survival in patients with non-small cell lung cancer[18]; trastuzumab to treat metastatic breast cancer in patients whose cancers have amplification of the HER2/neu oncogene[19]; cetuximab to treat colorectal cancers by targeting the epidermal growth factor receptor[20]; and bevacizumab to treat colorectal cancer by targeting the vascular endothelial growth factor receptor and blocking angiogenesis.[21]

In addition, one must appreciate the importance of drug resistance and recognize it when it occurs. When choosing treatment for recurrent disease, one should consider the likely cross-resistance to several natural products owing to the multidrug resistance phenotype mediated by the adenosine triphosphate binding cassette family transporters (eg, P-glycoprotein, MRPs), the low probability of response to drugs of the same drug class (eg, taxanes), or sequential hormonal therapies when selecting drugs with the same mechanism of action (eg, aromatase inhibitors).

Treatment of cancer patients includes the use of drugs for host support. The effects of the tumor and its products on the structure and function of the patient's normal tissues, as well as the mind and emotions, define an understanding of the disease process and of the patient in whom it takes place. It is not sufficient to order a therapy with the appropriate dose and schedule. There must be a broad understanding of and attention to potential toxicities, which represent the drug's effects on normal tissues. A medical oncologist should understand the interaction of the administered drug with target molecules present in normal tissues and the potential for drug–drug interactions to avoid unnecessary toxicities.

The availability of effective antibiotics and the use of platelet transfusions were intrinsic to early cures of the acute leukemias. Colony-stimulating factors (filgrastim, sargramostim) have significantly altered the prospect of drug-induced granulocytopenia, and recombinant erythropoietin can diminish drug-induced anemia. Means to ameliorate thrombocytopenia, other than with platelet transfusions, are now available.

The use of cytokines to collect circulating hematopoietic progenitor (CD34) cells enabled the convenient collection of marrow-repopulating precursors, allowing autologous stem cell transfusions to substitute for autologous marrow transfusion. New antibiotics make granulocytopenia less ominous, and oral prophylaxis with antibiotics and antifungal agents has decreased hospital admissions. These assets allow chemotherapy to be given more safely at the intended dose and schedule without delay or dose reduction.

The availability of highly effective antiemetics makes cancer chemotherapy less dreaded than in the past. The emergence of psycho-oncology as a widely appreciated discipline has also made it possible for patients to strengthen their resolve to undertake approaches aimed at cure or to accept the unlikelihood of cure with greater serenity.

Intravenous medications that may be toxic to the venous wall, and vesicant if extravasated, require the use of central venous access. When venipuncture is difficult because of anatomy or obesity, repeated needle sticks and much time are wasted in attempting peripheral cannulation. Needle phobia is a perverse part of being under treatment; establishing permanent venous access can largely obviate it.

Most patients with cancer are over the age of 60 and are receiving treatment for comorbid conditions. Therefore, care must be taken when prescribing treatments that could have dire drug interactions, leading to untoward side effects. No modern physician should be without electronic tools, such as handheld computers, that contain a compendium of drug interactions, drug descriptions, and appropriate methods of monitoring for efficacy and toxicity. A medical oncologist benefits from using an electronic medical record system that saves time and prevents errors through online calculation of dosing and electronic ordering. These systems also allow the creation of databases that can be queried for identification of trends and unexpected results (see Chapter 138, "Oncologic Emergencies").

Therapies that are totally appropriate for someone whose disease might be cured by judicious application of surgery, radiotherapy, and/or chemotherapy might be totally inappropriate when applied to someone with widely metastatic disease for whom no known cure exists. Therapy with curative intent may be toxic but of relatively short duration. On the one hand, conservatism aims at saving a life, not avoiding toxicity; on the other hand, treatment for palliative purposes would not ordinarily condone similar risks and iatrogenic effects that diminish the quality of life, even temporarily. The same is true for therapies aimed at cancer prevention because these are often taken by asymptomatic individuals for prolonged periods of time. The recent experiences with high-dose cyclooxygenase II inhibitors over long periods, which caused increased cardiovascular side effects in patients participating in one of two cancer prevention studies, resulted in serious consequences for the pharmaceutical manufacturers.[22]

Certain principles govern the application of therapies, no matter what the disease. These were enunciated more than a half-century ago by Robert F. Loeb, Bard Professor of Medicine at Columbia University's College of Physicians and Surgeons. These simple rules have profundity and nearly universal applicability but must be tempered, however, by an understanding of the neoplastic process.

The first law is if what you are doing is "doing good," keep doing it. It is implicit that a physician measure the effects of any intervention on both the tumor and the host. The lessons learned from the treatment of acute lymphocytic leukemia of childhood are noteworthy. For example, vincristine plus prednisone is an excellent induction treatment, but in 1968, a question was raised: Why not keep administering this highly active induction regimen rather than shifting to antimetabolite management? A cohort of children who were induced into remission by vincristine and prednisone were randomized to continue the induction treatment or shift to the antimetabolite. They rapidly became resistant and relapsed, whereas those who were shifted to the antimetabolite experienced long-term sustained remissions and cures (Cancer and Leukemia Group B, unpublished data). Thus, the first law of therapeutics does not always apply to cancer for which sequential treatment regimens may have special importance. Much of curative oncology relates to the biology of the unseen tumor, for which the current clinical status may not be informative. The first law seems more applicable to clinically recognizable disease.

The second law of therapeutics states that if what you are doing is not "doing good," stop doing it. Most therapeutic regimens have little chance of success if after 8 weeks of treatment they have failed to elicit therapeutic benefit. Indeed, most patients show incipient tumor regression earlier. It is, nonetheless, advantageous to undertake a second month of treatment in most instances because a well-documented early increase in tumor diameter on radiographic examinations or increased pain can, indeed, be followed by tumor regression. If no symptomatic or objective benefit occurs after 2 months, a third month will not likely be beneficial. A few therapies work more slowly, however, and should be considered differently. New therapies that inhibit tumor growth that differentiate cancer cells may cause tumor stasis, however, and require different assessments of effectiveness. Before stopping treatment, corroborating information should be sought by direct measurements, radiography, or biochemical markers. Increased bony uptake of radionuclides can be a sign of bone healing, even of a previously unsuspected lesion, and is not a suitable end point. The appearance of a new metastatic deposit or the continued growth of a previously documented tumor despite chemotherapeutic treatment speaks against continuing that regimen. Always remember that it is not that the patient has failed the therapy but that the therapy has failed the patient.

Hippocrates' admonition, *Primum non nocere* (First do no harm), is also subject to reassessment in oncology.[23] Thus, the second law of therapeutics does not extend to toxic effects unless they are life-threatening or profoundly disabling. With many of the therapeutic agents available today, complete avoidance of toxicity would doom many patients to death from their neoplasm. Some patients can obtain cure, and more can achieve meaningful remission by accepting the transient effect of intensive therapy that kills tumor cells and normal cells alike. The patient almost always recovers, but the less resilient tumor may not. To treat a population of patients at so low a dose that it would avoid toxic harm (ie, lethal jeopardy) to any patient would surely exact a higher price in depriving others of adequate doses to achieve maximum benefit. Curative and subcurative cancer chemotherapy, as we know it today, is often toxic but rarely fatal. Attempts to abrogate toxicity for all by reducing the dose of an established regimen might compromise benefit for the majority.[24,25] Dose adjustment for an individual may be necessary and prudent but must always be considered with respect to other means of mitigating toxicity without dose reduction.

The third law of therapeutics—"if you do not know what to do, do nothing"—counsels against uninformed action. In many circumstances, a rush to judgment or, worse, a rush to do something, anything, can be disastrous. Aside from oncologic emergencies, there is rarely an occasion when observing the evolution of symptoms and findings or seeking consultation with another individual for a fresh viewpoint is contraindicated because of time pressure. In the presence of pain, one should not delay pain relief, but other therapy may be delayed to build an informed formulation. In the presence of a differential diagnosis that includes diseases other than cancer, particularly infections, one must be certain that delay does not risk mortality or morbidity from the other possible disorders. Thus, the time invested for observation and consultation should not be extravagant.

The fourth law of therapeutics is "never make the treatment worse than the disease." This relates to total life equation: the price the oncologist knows the patient may be obliged to pay in present side effects to attain future real effects. Often the patient's vision is foreshortened because today's symptoms caused by drug toxicity can be more severe than the original complaints related to the cancer. The medical oncologist must ascertain the patient's attitude toward quality of life versus duration of life. It is a medical oncologist's responsibility to counsel the patient concerning this weighty topic. With the rapid appearance of new oncology products and numerous new types of treatments available through clinical trials, it is becoming increasingly difficult to distinguish therapy with curative intent from a palliative orientation, except in the extreme situations of newly diagnosed, low-stage and grade disease versus palliative care for the terminally ill. In all cases, the proper goal is maximal life at maximal quality. It is a modification of the commentary that one should die young as late as possible. For some patients, the toxic effects of treatment outweigh the value of possible extension of life. This perception is often related directly to age. The treatments imperative for young patients may be inappropriate and unwise for patients in their eighties. Pain and disability from cancer may temper the desirability of certain therapies, which offer only temporary and partial relief. It is not a kindness to defer death only transiently by rescuing a dying patient back to a raft of suffering. Heroic efforts are justified only when a meaningful therapeutic option exists.

It is inappropriate for the medical oncologist to substitute professional judgment for a patient's ardent wishes when the patient strives to accomplish something that is a reasonable therapeutic goal. The medical oncologist must serve as a bastion of reality, however, advising the patient of what is possible and of what is likely. In the course of doing this, the laws of therapeutics and of humanity always include hope.

Early-Stage Cancers Are More Curable Than Late-Stage Cancers and the First Treatment Is More Effective Than the Next ■ Since no method of prevention is likely to be completely effective, medical oncologists must recommend appropriate tests to detect cancer at its earliest possible stage. They include mammography, colonoscopy, occult blood in the feces, digital rectal examination of the prostate, Papanicolaou smears, and examination of the skin and body orifices for signs of premalignancy, such as leukoplakia and dysplastic nevi. Soon, a variety of validated biomarkers will likely be available to identify early cancer or the presence of premalignancies, for example, ductal carcinoma in situ, prostatic intraepithelial neoplasia, colonic polyps, and cervical dysplasia. As described above, progression of cancer leads to the acquisition of mutations or changes in gene expression that select for cell survival over cell death. Many of these changes, such as the expression of the bcl-2 protein, mutation or deletion of the *TP53* or retinoblastoma tumor suppressor genes, and alterations in topoisomerases, allow tumor cells to exist in harsh environments characterized by hypoxia and a low pH. These same changes produce tumor cells that are increasingly resistant to cancer therapies.

Cancer cells that emerge following initial treatment often represent clones of cells with intrinsic resistance or cells in which the treatment has selected for drug resistance mechanisms. For example, the expression of P-glycoprotein increased severalfold in breast cancers following therapy, and this increase was associated with a markedly increased relative risk of failing to respond to chemotherapy.[26] This reality places a premium on getting it right the first time so that medical oncologists and their team must be certain that they have all of the requisite information at hand to allow the best choice for initial treatment. For example, treating a breast cancer patient without knowledge of the status of estrogen and progesterone receptors and the *HER2/neu* oncogene correctly measured would likely compromise the initial treatment of breast cancer patients. Similarly, embarking on the treatment of acute myelogenous leukemia without full genotyping and phenotyping risks making the wrong choice for initial treatment. Furthermore, resistance to imatinib is associated with both P-glycoprotein and specific mutations in the *BCR:ABL* gene. These changes are defined, and new drugs available to overcome these forms of resistance.

The advantage of treating early-stage patients who, by definition, have a lower body burden of cancer has proved so persuasive that the profession and patients have accepted the technique of postsurgical or adjuvant chemotherapy, acknowledging that this entails treating some if not the majority of patients whose risk of relapse and body burden of cancer are already zero. Adjuvant therapy after surgery has been demonstrated to be curative in several diseases for which surgery alone has low cure rates and chemotherapy alone cannot cure metastatic disease. Breast cancer, Wilms tumor, and osteosarcoma are the prime examples. In many diseases, there is evidence of prolonged disease-free survival and of longer survival, such as stage II and III breast cancer,[27,28] stage III ovarian cancer,[29] and stage III colon cancer.[30] Recent evidence suggests that transcriptional profiling of breast cancer specimens may help identify patients for whom adjuvant therapy is unnecessary.[31]

Because adjuvant treatment is aimed at micrometastatic disease remote from the primary tumor, exploration of chemotherapy before surgery ("neoadjuvant") has been undertaken in a few types of cancer. In addition to earlier exposure of the micrometastases, this approach has two more beneficial characteristics. First, regression of the primary lesion predicts that the micrometastases will also likely be sensitive.[32] Failure of the primary neoplasm to regress affords an opportunity to shift chemotherapeutic treatment while there is still a chance of affecting the micrometastases with a new regimen. Second, regression of the primary tumor may make primary surgery unnecessary, allowing curative radiotherapy, as in some head and neck cancers and as shown in a large series of patients with breast cancer.[33] In other instances, surgery after chemotherapy may be technically easier, although not always less radical, because there is no certainty that every cell has been eradicated at the original boundaries. Induction chemotherapy of sarcomas has allowed a major reduction in amputations, however, in favor of limb-sparing surgery. Induction chemotherapy often diminishes mastectomy for large breast cancers in favor of lumpectomy and radiotherapy. Induction or concurrent chemotherapy may also significantly enhance the effectiveness of radiotherapy for other tumors, such as anal carcinoma, thereby decreasing the need for surgery.

Treatment of recurrent disease is too often empiric. The response to these subsequent treatments predictably diminishes over time. For example, a breast cancer patient whose tumor strongly expresses the estrogen and progesterone receptor has a >50% chance of responding to first-line hormonal therapy, with a likely duration of response of ~18 months.[34] On relapse, that same patient's probability of response to second-line therapy is cut in half, as is the likely duration of response.[35] Similarly, patients with metastatic prostate cancer have a very high initial response to androgen ablation but limited response to further hormonal treatments once they relapse. Precisely why this occurs is an important area of cancer research, and one can anticipate that discoveries in this area will likely improve the treatment of cancer patients in the future.

The Best Treatment Is Often Found Through Participation in Clinical Trials ■ The most common and lethal cancers, including metastatic lung, colon, and breast, are often incurable by approved treatments. Relapsed, advanced disease is almost never cured and may not be effectively treated. Furthermore, most approved treatments have significant risks of side effects and produce limited prolongation of life. Yet, despite these facts, most patients receive standard rather than experimental therapies. For many, the best choice of treatment may be available only through clinical trials.

Patients are increasingly involved in decisions regarding the choice of therapy, having been empowered by information widely available through the Internet. Patients with cancer are often apprehensive that they may not receive the best treatment and will challenge us with appropriately tough questions before moving ahead. The medical oncologist can speak with greater authority when a deliberate comparison is being made because the goal of such studies is toward improvement on the standard, not toward finding treatments that are equally good.

A number of ethical issues are abrogated by the certainty that a specific patient's disease is not currently curable. For asymptomatic patients with indolent disease, precurability eliminates the need to rush to treatment. Many problems are initially best approached by masterful observation, particularly where age and comorbidity are factors. Where a rapid course portending symptoms or inquietude prevails, however, therapy is indicated. For metastatic disease for which no cure is known, it is not only ethical but also important that a systematically designed investigation of new treatments through participation in clinical trials be undertaken early in the course of the patient's disease. This allows assessment of a drug's activity before toxicity arises from conventional therapies that might limit dosing. Conventional therapies might also elicit resistance of one or another kind or immune system depression, which might foreclose the opportunity to recognize the activity of the candidate compound.

For diseases with an especially unfavorable outlook and rare therapeutic success, delays in introducing candidate compounds to ensure that they carry little or no risk of toxicity are an unwise investment of resources and time, let alone the patient's short-lived opportunity for possible benefit. The outcome of unsuccessfully treated cancer is more ominous than the hazards of clinical investigation.

Patients should be made aware of clinical trials as part of the initial discussions regarding treatment. Too often patients are not aware of clinical trials and discover this option through friends or the Internet rather than through their physicians. Heavily pretreated patients are usually precluded from phase II and III clinical trials, thereby depriving patients of their choice to receive potentially active drugs. A trial of candidate phase II agents prior to conventional chemotherapy for metastatic breast cancer has been conducted without significant compromise in response to the established regimen.[36] Today, therapies aimed at validated molecular targets may enter the clinic once proof of principle is obtained in cell lines and safety is confirmed in animal models. Although clinical activity was notoriously unpredictable from human xenografts, new mouse models based on manipulation of mouse embryonic stem cells to either knock in or knock out genes to produce tumors that mimic human cancers may be more promising. Major differences in pharmacokinetics exist between mouse and man, and the ultimate test remains the carefully designed, meticulously conducted clinical trial. The testing of new, targeted therapies is likely to change how we view early trials of anticancer drugs. For example, the phase I trial of imatinib did not reach a maximum tolerated dose. Rather, the dose was determined based on "maximum biological dose," that is, the dose in which the target enzyme was maximally inhibited.[37] Similarly, dynamic imaging techniques, such as positron emission tomography, predict the responsiveness to imatinib in patients with gastrointestinal stromal tumors well before changes occur in tumor size.[38]

Therefore, until the day arrives when all cancers are preventable or curable, enrollment of patients in clinical trials will be the hallmark of the practice of the best medical oncologists. No cancer is so well treated that an improvement in outcome or therapeutic approach cannot readily be imagined. Thus, research is imperative.

An individual in practice cannot devote the same time and energy to clinical research as one who serves full time on the faculty of a university, research institute, or hospital. However, the private practitioner has an opportunity to participate in clinical trials through cooperative groups or in collaboration with cancer centers; this opportunity should not be wasted. Every oncologist participated in clinical research during his or her training, and the oncologist's office should include the capacity to perform clinical research. It is the responsibility of the medical oncologist to discuss clinical trials with patients in a way that does not bias an ultimate decision.

Participation in Clinical Research Serves to Keep the Practitioner Current and Provides the Opportunity for Patients to Receive Therapy in a Setting in Which They May Be Most Comfortable ■ There is much reason to anticipate that progress would be more rapid if clinical research were accepted as an integral part of the practice of medical oncology, as it is in pediatric oncology. The technology exists in medical informatics for community oncologists to ally themselves with their alma mater or other academic centers to participate in diagnostic, preventive, and therapeutic research trials using the computer, electronic mail, and fax as expedient tools. The NCI has initiated an expanded participation project in which oncologists can access many important research protocols. Abundant resources can be found on the internet at <www.cancer.gov>. Those oncologists who have so heavy a workload that it prevents their devoting the necessary time to participate in clinical research risk depriving their patients of access to research advances. Sharing the workload with a newly recruited colleague would upgrade the practice. Clinical investigation should serve as the bridge to fundamental science and the excitement generated by the new molecular biologic understanding of cancer as a malignant tissue.[39]

Cancer Surveillance Must Be Based on Validated Assumptions ■ Following completion of curative therapy and attainment of a complete remission or following adjuvant therapy, surveillance for early signs of recurrence is based on the logical assumption that the earlier a recurrence is detected, the better the outcome of a therapeutic intervention. Although true in principle, in practice, this is rarely the case. There are several reasons for this illogical result, including the possibilities that surveillance tests are insensitive or nonspecific or that further treatment options are ineffective. Oversetting of patients at low risk of recurrence increases the probability of a false-positive result and the attendant morbidity, psychological or physical, associated with attempting to make a definitive diagnosis. In contrast, under testing in patients at risk of recurrence of a form of cancer for which effective salvage therapy is available (eg, germ cell tumors, large cell lymphoma, Hodgkin disease, osteosarcoma, breast cancer) is inexcusable. Thus, the oncologist must be aware of the predictive value of surveillance tests (tumor markers, imaging studies) in the context of specific malignancies and apply them accordingly.

Standards for quantifying diagnostic tests used frequently in surveillance have been adopted in most parts of the world (Système Internationale [SI] units), except the United States. It is impossible to read an international medical journal without being thoroughly familiar with SI units. They are presented in Table 43-4 so that readers can have ready access to a source for translation from the old nomenclature, characteristically American, which pervades this treatise.

Table 43-4 ■ **Representative Système International Units for Laboratory Tests of Importance in Oncology**

Component	Present Reference Interval	Present Unit	Conversion Factor	Intervals	Unit Symbols
Albumin	4.0-6.0	g/dL	10.0	40-60	g/L
Alpha-fetoprotein, radioimmunoassay	0-20	ng/mL	1.00	0-20	g/L
Bilirubin					
Total	0.1-1.0	mg/dL	17.10	2-18	μmol/L
Conjugated	0-0.2	mg/dL	17.10	0-4	mol/L
Calcium	8.8-10.3	mg/dL	0.2495	2.20-2.58	μmmol/L
Cholesterol	<200+	mg/dL	0.02586	<5.20	μmmol/L
Cortisol	4-19	g/dL	27.59	110-520	nmol/L
Creatinine	0.6-1.2	mg/dL	88.40	50-110	mol/L
Fibrinogen	200-400	mg/dL	0.01	2.0-4.0	g/L
Glucose	70-110	mg/dL	0.05551	3.9*6.1	μmmol/L
Hemoglobin					
Male	14.0-18.0	g/dL	10.0	140-180	g/L
Female	11.5-15.5	g/dL	10.0	115-155	g/L
Immunoglobulins					
IgG	500-1200	mg/dL	0.01	5.00-12.00	g/L
IgA	50-350	mg/dL	0.01	0.50-3.50	g/L
IgM	30-230	mg/dL	0.01	0.30-2.30	g/L
IgD	<6	mg/dL	10	<360	mg/L
IgE	20-1,000	ng/mL	1.00	20-1000	g/L
Iron	80-180	g/dL	0.1791	14-32	μmol/L
Iron-binding capacity	250-460	g/dL	0.1791	45-82	μmol/L
Lipoproteins					
Low density (LDL), as cholesterol	50-190	mg/dL	0.02586	1.30-490	mmol/L
High Density (HDL), as cholestrol	30-70	mg/dL	0.02586	.80-1.80	mmol/L
Magnesium	1.8-3.0	mg/dL	0.4114	0.80-1.20	mmol/L
	1.6-2.4	mEq/L	0.500		
Metanephrines (as normetanephrine)	0-2.0	mg/24h	5.458	0-11.0	μmol/d
Osmolality	280-300	mOsm/kg	1.00	280-300	nmol/kg
Phosphate (as inorganic P)	2.5-5.0	mg/dl	0.3229	0.80-1.60	mmol/L
Potassium	3.5-5.0	mEQ/L	1.00	3.5-5.0	mmol/L
Protein, total	6-8	g/dl	10.0	60-80	g/L
Serotonin	8-21	g/dl	0.05675	0.45-1.20	mol/L
Thyroxine, free (T_4)	0.8-2.8	ng/dL	12.87	10-36	pmol/L
Triiodothyronine (T_3)	75-220	ng/dL	0.01536	1.2-3.4	nmol/L
Urate (as uric acid)	2.0-6.0	mg/dL	59.48	120-360	μmol/L
Urea nitrogen	8-18	mg/dL	0.3570	3.0-6.5	mmol/L
Vanillylmandelic acid	<6.8	mg/24h	5.046	<35	μmol/d

Oncologic Care Is for Life ■ The relationship of a medical oncologist with patients is intimate and should not end once therapies aimed at controlling the spread of cancer are no longer effective. The medical oncologist must be skilled in the principles and practice of palliative care and collaborate actively with specialists in symptom control, for example, neurologists, psychiatrists, and hospice staff. No greater feeling of abandonment can occur than when a patient is abruptly released from care by an oncologist who fails to recognize this lifelong responsibility.

It is, however, also the responsibility of the medical oncologist to address end-of-life planning with the patient and the family. Advice regarding living wills, power of attorney, and resuscitation falls squarely within the purview of the medical oncologist. This responsibility is highlighted in states that require that do not resuscitate (DNR) orders be written on patient charts prior to death. In the absence of such orders, when a nurse finds a patient apparently dead, she must, by law, initiate emergency calls for resuscitative efforts.

When death comes from cancer as the expected final event of a gradual deterioration of vital forces, resuscitative efforts do not succeed. When we are unable to keep someone alive, the likelihood of bringing him or her back to meaningful life is infinitesimal. Resuscitative efforts should be applied to patients with cancer who were not expected to die because reversible phenomena, such as pulmonary emboli, cardiac arrhythmias, aspiration, and similar events, can provoke unexpected death in a patient with a neoplasm, just as in any other hospitalized or ambulatory patient. It is, however, in the circumstance of gradual decline and predictable disintegration of body functions that resuscitative efforts place great physical and emotional stress on the distraught family as well as on nursing and ancillary personnel, house staff, and attending physicians. Many patients, particularly the elderly and those apprised of the progress of their disease, can discuss the decision not to resuscitate with equanimity and, indeed, with a certain personal satisfaction of avoiding the fruitless anguish that such a procedure entails for the surviving family. Most patients sign living wills or appoint a health care proxy if these possibilities are presented to them.

Because of the legal implications involved, where particular religious scruples obtain or where families have emotionally uncontrolled members who cannot accept the anticipated death of a loved one, the medical oncologist should spend considerable time planning for an eventual death. Medical oncologists, through their organizations, should also invest effort to alter laws that place significant administrative burdens on them and their colleagues and that infringe on the appropriate professional practice of medicine. DNR forms are a technique of documentation and constitute further evidence that society has moved medicine onto a new plateau of accountability.

The medical oncologist should make known his or her intentions concerning the advisability of resuscitative efforts for each particular patient in advance to forestall unnecessary trauma to the patient, family, and staff; to forestall litigation; and to settle in advance any serious disagreements with the patient or family. An impasse might occasion a medical oncologist to find a suitable substitute physician if there is irresolvable conflict concerning the plans surrounding an anticipated death.

DNR orders do not imply that there be diminution of effort to control or palliate the disease before death. However, if good judgment indicates that continued efforts are fruitless and can only inflict suffering, with no prospect of benefit, discontinuation of active therapy should always be accompanied by DNR orders.

Summary

The medical oncologist stands at the crossroads of modern molecular biology and medical practice and often serves as the final common pathway for the application of cancer research to patients. A complex corpus of information is available that expands rapidly, both deeper into the nature of the cancer process and wider into new approaches that provide demonstrated effectiveness in therapy, prevention, or support.

The increasing appreciation that oncogenes and tumor suppressors act through usurpation of normal autocrine and paracrine signaling pathways and that cancer is in reality not merely a disease of cancer cells but of a cast of supporting characters that form a malignant tissue (blood vessels, fibroblasts, smooth muscle cells, macrophages, lymphocytes, etc) provides a variety of new targets for therapy. The realization that malignant transformation is a multistep process of accumulation of genetic abnormalities over long periods of time gives impetus for the design of rational preventive strategies and guidance to target patients at highest risk. These pathways have already led to effective targeted therapies that are less toxic than traditional cancer chemotherapy. Thus, the tide of fundamental discovery is washing away many of the unknowns and the flyspeck observations. It is axiomatic that certain cancers can be cured today without knowing the intimate nature of neoplasia. How better the day, perhaps soon upon us, when we know what we are doing!

Clinical accomplishments have similarly been exceptionally productive in the 49 years since the first cancer was cured with drugs.[3] A large assortment of drugs has since been provided. A new array of genetically engineered drugs support host function, and others that are still early in their development are on the way. Imaging technologies will continue to revolutionize the ability to detect, stage, treat, and monitor cancers. Biochemical markers of tumor behavior will provide increasing diagnostic and monitoring capacity and may offer new targets for therapy.

There is probably no cancer in which some progress in diagnosis or therapy has not been achieved in the last decade. Similar achievements for cancer prevention are materializing. Oncologists must assume greater responsibility for health preservation. Much could be accomplished by applying what is already known about lifestyle, diet, and exercise. Medical facts without political action were slow to change the tax on health that tobacco levies. A concerted effort within most states has begun, but a federal role in managing the tobacco plague has been thwarted.

The horizon has never been closer. Although still distant, there are enough promising paths to follow that one of them may prove considerably faster than even reasonable optimism would suppose. The information that serves as our foundation, its rate of accrual, its revelations, and the demonstrated success of translating science to clinical applications augur well for the future of medical oncology and for cancer patients.

References

1. Kennedy BJ, Calabresi P, Carbone PP, et al. Training program in medical oncology. *Ann Intern Med.* 1973;78:127–130.
2. Holland J. The diseases that cancer causes. *J Chron Dis.* 1963;16:635.
3. Hertz R, Li MC, Spencer DB. Effect of methotrexate therapy upon choriocarcinoma and chorioadenoma. *Proc Soc Exp Biol Med.* 1956;93:361–366.
4. Holland JF. Methotrexate therapy of metastatic choriocarcinoma. *Am J Obstet Gynecol.* 1958;75:195–199.
5. Mitka M. "Teachable moments" provide a means for physicians to lower alcohol abuse. *JAMA.* 1998;279:1767–1768.
6. Holmes O. Medical essays: the young practitioner.
7. Vogelstein B, Fearon ER, Hamilton SR, et al. Genetic alterations during colorectal-tumor development. *N Engl J Med.* 1988;319:525–532.
8. Thun MJ, Namboodiri MM, Heath CW Jr. Aspirin use and reduced risk of fatal colon cancer. *N Engl J Med.* 1991;325:1593–1596.

9. Koehne CH, Dubois RN. COX-2 inhibition and colorectal cancer. *Semin Oncol.* 2004;31:12–21.
10. O'Brien TR, Kirk G, Zhang M. Hepatocellular carcinoma: paradigm of preventive oncology. *Cancer J.* 2004;10:67–73.
11. Hong WK, Lippman SM, Itri LM, et al. Prevention of second primary tumors with isotretinoin in squamous-cell carcinoma of the head and neck. *N Engl J Med.* 1990;323:795–801.
12. Vogel VG, Costantino JP, Wickerham DL, et al. Effects of tamoxifen vs raloxifene on the risk of developing invasive breast cancer and other disease outcomes: the NSABP Study of Tamoxifen and Raloxifene (STAR) P-2 trial. *JAMA.* 2006;295:2727–2741.
13. Thiis-Evensen E, Hoff GS, Sauar J, et al. Population-based surveillance by colonoscopy: effect on the incidence of colorectal cancer. Telemark Polyp Study I. *Scand J Gastroenterol.* 1999;34:414–420.
14. Boardman LA, Steinhoff MM, Shackelton R, et al. A randomized trial of the Fischer cone biopsy excisor and loop electrosurgical excision procedure. *Obstet Gynecol.* 2004;104:745–750.
15. Koutsky LA, Ault KA, Wheeler CM, et al. A controlled trial of a human papillomavirus type 16 vaccine. *N Engl J Med.* 2002;347:1645–1651.
16. Druker BJ, Talpaz M, Resta DJ, et al. Efficacy and safety of a specific inhibitor of the BCR-ABL tyrosine kinase in chronic myeloid leukemia. *N Engl J Med.* 2001;344:1031–1037.
17. Lynch TJ, Bell DW, Sordella R, et al. Activating mutations in the epidermal growth factor receptor underlying responsiveness of non-small-cell lung cancer to gefitinib. *N Engl J Med.* 2004;350:2129–2139.
18. US Food and Drug Administration, 2004. Available at: www.fda. gov division.
19. Slamon DJ, Leyland-Jones B, Shak S, et al. Use of chemotherapy plus a monoclonal antibody against HER2 for metastatic breast cancer that overexpresses HER2. *N Engl J Med.* 2001;344:783–792.
20. Cunningham D, Humblet Y, Siena S, et al. Cetuximab monotherapy and cetuximab plus irinotecan in irinotecanrefractory metastatic colorectal cancer. *N Engl J Med.* 2004;351:337–345.
21. Hurwitz H, Fehrenbacher L, Novotny W, et al. Bevacizumab plus irinotecan, fluorouracil, and leucovorin for metastatic colorectal cancer. *N Engl J Med.* 2004;350:2335– 42.
22. Masters BA, Kaufman M. Painful withdrawal for makers of Vioxx: pulling of arthritis drug raises questions on marketing, safety risks. *Washington Post.* 2004;Sect. A:1, 8.
23. Holland JF. Ethics for a clinical investigator. Non primum non nocere. *Am J Med.* 1979;66:554–555.
24. Frei E III. Combination cancer therapy: presidential address. *Cancer Res.* 1972;32:2593–607.
25. Frei E III, Canellos GP. Dose: a critical factor in cancer chemotherapy. *Am J Med.* 1980;69:585–594.
26. Trock BJ, Leonessa F, Clarke R. Multidrug resistance in breast cancer: a meta-analysis of MDR1/gp170 expression and its possible functional significance. *J Natl Cancer Inst.* 1997;89:917–931.
27. Systemic treatment of early breast cancer by hormonal, cytotoxic, or immune therapy. 133 randomised trials involving 31,000 recurrences and 24,000 deaths among 75,000 women. Early Breast Cancer Trialists' Collaborative Group. *Lancet.* 1992;339:71–85.
28. Perloff M, Norton L, Korzun AH, et al. Postsurgical adjuvant chemotherapy of stage II breast carcinoma with or without crossover to a non-cross-resistant regimen: a Cancer and Leukemia Group B study. *J Clin Oncol.* 1996;14:1589–1598.
29. McGuire WP, Hoskins WJ, Brady MF, et al. Cyclophosphamide and cisplatin compared with paclitaxel and cisplatin in patients with stage III and stage IV ovarian cancer. *N Engl J Med.* 1996;334:1–6.
30. Moertel CG, Fleming TR, Macdonald JS, et al. Levamisole and fluorouracil for adjuvant therapy of resected colon carcinoma. *N Engl J Med.* 1990;322:352–358.
31. Paik S, Shak S, Tang G, et al. A multigene assay to predict recurrence of tamoxifen-treated, node-negative breast cancer. *N Engl J Med.* 2004;351:2817–2826.
32. Rosen G, Caparros B, Huvos AG, et al. Preoperative chemotherapy for osteogenic sarcoma: selection of postoperative adjuvant chemotherapy based on the response of the primary tumor to preoperative chemotherapy. *Cancer.* 1982;49:1221–1230.
33. Jacquillat C, Weil M, Baillet F, et al. Results of neoadjuvant chemotherapy and radiation therapy in the breast-conserving treatment of 250 patients with all stages of infiltrative breast cancer. *Cancer.* 1990;66:119–129.
34. Sawka CA, Pritchard KI, Shelley W, et al. A randomized crossover trial of tamoxifen versus ovarian ablation for metastatic breast cancer in premenopausal women: a report of the National Cancer Institute of Canada Clinical Trials Group (NCIC CTG) trial MA.1. *Breast Cancer Res Treat.* 1997;44:211–215.
35. Robertson JF, Osborne CK, Howell A, et al. Fulvestrant versus anastrozole for the treatment of advanced breast carcinoma in postmenopausal women: a prospective combined analysis of two multicenter trials. *Cancer.* 2003;98:229–238.
36. Costanza ME, Weiss RB, Henderson IC, et al. Safety and efficacy of using a single agent or a phase II agent before instituting standard combination chemotherapy in previously untreated metastatic breast cancer patients: report of a randomized study—Cancer and Leukemia Group B 8642. *J Clin Oncol.* 1999;17:1397–1406.
37. Druker BJ, Sawyers CL, Kantarjian H, et al. Activity of a specific inhibitor of the BCR-ABL tyrosine kinase in the blast crisis of chronic myeloid leukemia and acute lymphoblastic leukemia with the Philadelphia chromosome. *N Engl J Med.* 2001;344:1038–1042.
38. Demetri GD, von Mehren M, Blanke CD, et al. Efficacy and safety of imatinib mesylate in advanced gastrointestinal stromal tumors. *N Engl J Med.* 2002;347:472–480.
39. Weinberg RA.The biology of cancer. In: *Garland Science.* Taylor and Francis Group, LLC: New York NY, 2007.

44 Cytokinetics

Larry Norton, MD ■ Theresa Ann Gilewski, MD

Introduction

Kinetics is the study of movement or, more generally, changes in magnitude—size, shape, distance, velocity, or indeed anything quantifiable—over time. As a science, therefore, kinetics should be considered central to oncology. Cancer is, after all, all about changes in cancer cell numbers, sites of involvement, and tumor mass sizes as a function of time. Morbidity and mortality from cancer is a consequence of such changes, as measured by recurrence-free, progression-free, and overall survival times. Moreover, at the molecular level cancer is not a static process, but involves aberrations in gene integrity, copy number and expression, post-translational modification, and RNA and protein production and degradation that are time-dependent. Failure to analyze and interpret cancer biology with regard to changes over time, therefore, may miss the essences of phenomena and thereby lead to misinterpretations, both conceptual and clinical.

It is the purpose of this chapter to use recent results in cancer research to illustrate both the practical applications and theoretical implications of one aspect of kinetics—cytokinetics, the study of changes in cell number over time—for cancer medicine. While most examples will be drawn from breast cancer oncology, the principles so derived will be shown to be broadly relevant. After all, carcinogenesis, "stem cell" biology, cancerstroma interactions, metastasis, and drug scheduling are topics of wide-ranging importance in oncologic science, and all will be shown to be processes best understood within a kinetic framework.

Some Mysteries in Cancer Medicine

The study of cancer reveals many enigmas, sets of observations that are both true and seemingly incompatible. Identifying enigmas thereby indicates weakness in theories, creating opportunities for progress by hypothesis-testing experimentation. We will examine some of these and then seek their elucidation using kinetic science.

Polygenetic Etiology of Cancer

As our first example, let us consider the observation that cancer cells manifest myriad changes in gene morphology and copy numbers. This is consistent with the theory that malignancy results from accumulated abnormalities in diverse, somewhat independent genomic processes, the *polygenetic* concept of cancer. The functionalities associated with such changes include self-sufficiency in growth signals, insensitivity to antigrowth and pro-apoptotic signals, and the abilities to invade, to form metastases, to induce angiogenesis, and to replicate without limit. Yet how is this theory compatible with the equally well-documented observation that carcinomas in situ, which are clinically benign in that they do not metastasize and rarely grow to large sizes, are usually as aberrant genetically as the malignancies they spawn?

The concept of a polygenetic etiology of malignancy presents another mystery, which concerns the strong statistical association of histologic grade, tumor size, and propensity for traveling to regional (largely nodal) and distant sites. These traits are so commonly grouped together that we may forget that they are manifestations of distinct biologic processes: morphogenesis, regulation of mitosis-apoptosis, and metastasis respectively. Indeed, metastatic behavior presents many thought-provoking enigmas. Toward the end of the nineteenth century, Halsted used the prevailing mechanics of his time to hypothesize that the malignant spread of primary breast cancer could be halted by the meticulous removal of a whole breast containing the tumor in contiguity with the ipsilateral axillary contents. The idea behind the radical mastectomy was that cancer cells gain access to the rest of the body by invading lymphatic channels in the breast, channels that then traverse the axilla before connecting with the systemic circulation.

Many observations would seem to support Halsted's contention. Radical mastectomies did indeed cure some individuals, almost all of whom would have died of metastatic cancer had their breast cancers been left intact—a fact proven by observational studies in the nineteenth century. Also, lymphatic invasion is a powerful prognostic variable. Most compelling is the modern observation that sentinel lymph node mapping confirms a common flow pattern from the breast for lymph and cancer cells. Yet how would one invoke Halsted's theory to explain how some patients with uninvolved axillary lymph nodes at the time of radical local surgery still develop distant metastases?

Molecular Classification vs. Cancer Stem Cell Concept

Another enigma concerns the classification of tumors by RNA-expression profiling. It is unquestionably true that tumors differ in their patterns of gene expression, and that these differences correlate with clinically meaningful endpoints such as disease-free and overall survival and benefit from chemotherapy.[1] Hence, testing a small anatomic sample of a cancerous mass is informative regarding the behavior of the whole cancer, as if all of the cells in the cancer carry the critical information. Yet how can we reconcile this observation with the popular, experimentally-derived hypothesis that it is only a tiny minority of cancer cells—"cancer stem cells" or tumor-initiating cells—within the mass that have the capacity to form new tumors?

Cancer as a Local vs. Systemic Disease

That breast cancer is often a systemic disease early in its life-history is now clearly established by the impact of systemic adjuvant therapies like hormonal treatments and chemotherapy on cancer-free and overall survival. But how is this compatible with the equally venerable observation that better local control, as by radiation therapy to the remaining breast tissue following breast-conserving surgery, improves survival? Indeed, it seems that for every four cases of local recurrence prevented by radiation therapy one patient is saved from distant metastases and subsequent death. If the disease is metastatic early, why should local control make any difference at all? Part of the answer may be found in the observation that on detailed histopathogical analysis breast cancer cells are commonly found centimeters away from the clear margins of excised primary tumors. But this raises new questions. How did these cells get there, and what is the relationship between such cells and distant metastases?

Gompertzian Growth

Another enigma concerns growth patterns. It has been shown that the growth pattern of breast cancer cannot be explained by simple exponential or linear kinetics, but must follow an S-shaped curve intermediate between these two extremes (Fig. 44-1).[2] The evidence is not only from direct clinical observations but also from logical inferences based on clinical observations. For example, based on retrospective analyses of preexisting mammograms after the clinical diagnosis of breast cancer it has been estimated that an average tumor may take 2 years to grow in size from one cell to 10^9 or 10^{10} cells. This number of cells corresponds to a tumor volume of 1-10 cm^3 if all of the cells were packed tightly together, which for the sake of this argument is a rational size range for the diagnosis of a primary mass.

Now let us hypothesize that cancers grow in a linear pattern. This means that growth would be from one cell to two cells, then three cells, the four cells and so on in equal units of time. By this pattern, if it took a tumor 2 years to grow from one cell to this size range (10^9 or 10^{10} cells) it would take another 2 years for it to double in size to between 2-20 cm^3 and yet another 2 years to triple in size to 3-30 cm^3. This is clearly an unrealistically slow growth for an untreated primary cancer. Hence, it is extremely unlikely that cancers grow linearly.

Nor is exponential kinetics applicable. An exponential growth pattern involves constant doubling times. That is, if it takes a week for one cell to divide into two cells, by exponential kinetics it would take another week for those two cells to become four, an additional week for those four to divide into eight and so on. Many decades ago Howard Skipper and colleagues used exponential kinetics to explain the growth and response to therapy of a murine leukemia, laying the groundwork for much of the experimental and clinical chemotherapy to follow. But does exponential kinetics apply to human disease? Let us turn again to the case of a primary breast cancer growing from one cell to 10^9 or 10^{10} cells over 2 years. Were it to have grown exponentially to this point and continue to grow exponentially thereafter the mass would double in size every 22-24 days, which means that it would reach a size of 4-40 cm^3 in less than 7 weeks from diagnosis. This is an explosive growth rate that is just incompatible with general medical experience. Hence, exponential kinetics cannot apply. Yet, mitosis does produce two cells from one, so early malignant growth at the few-cell stage must be approximately exponential. This is truly an enigma.

The only way to resolve this mystery is to hypothesize that while growth may start in an exponential fashion there is a progressive deviation toward slower growth as the tumor becomes larger. Of the infinite number of possible decremented exponential curves, one type has been shown to accurately fit actual tumor growth curves.[3] This type was defined by Benjamin Gompertz in 1825 and has since been one of the most utilized mathematical formulas in all of biomathematics. It is illustrated in Figure 44-1 on two different scales of size: arithmetic and logarithmic. The "S" shape is apparent on the arithmetic scale but on the logarithmic scales the relative growth rate is seen to be continuously decreasing as the mass grows larger. As will be discussed in depth below, Gompertzian kinetics have proven very useful in designing improved regimens of anticancer chemotherapy, not only in breast cancer—where it was first explored—but also in malignant lymphoma, childhood sarcoma, and other malignant diseases. But if Gompertzian growth kinetics is ubiquitous in nature, what is its (necessarily ubiquitous) etiology?

In this chapter we will explore these issues—carcinogenesis, the behavior of tumorinitiating cells, pathohistologic grading, and patterns of metastatic spread—using the framework provided by the science of kinetics. We examine the fundamentals of cell proliferation as a cause of tumor growth and the development of cellular heterogeneity. We will seek in modem molecular science an etiology of Gompertzian growth. We will also illustrate the clinical relevance of growth kinetics in practical cancer medicine with a focus on the therapeutic implications of Gompertzian growth on the dose-scheduling of anticancer drugs. We will identify new areas for kinetic research that have implications for prognostication, choice of therapies, the discovery of new therapeutic targets, and the design of prevention strategies.

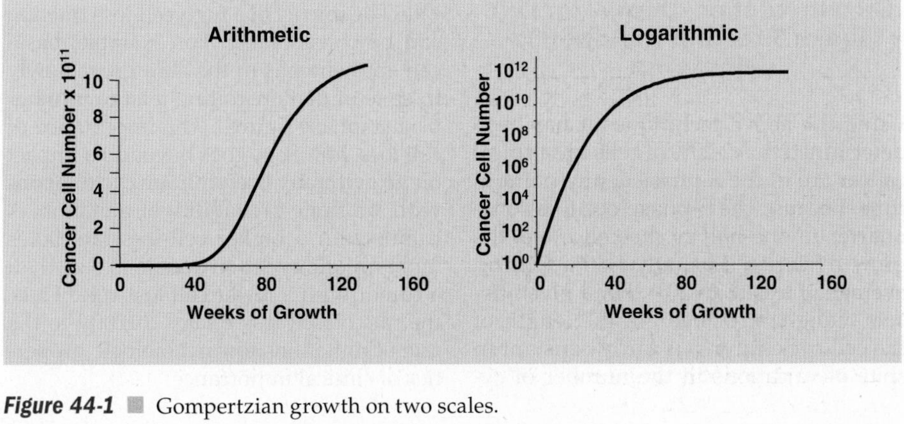

Figure 44-1 ■ Gompertzian growth on two scales.

The Kinetics of Cellular Proliferation

The study of how cancer cells divide provides some insight into these enigmas, but presents mysteries of its own, the contemplation which may provide further illumination. Since tumors are comprised of cancer cells with their supporting stroma, it is reasonable to start a discussion of tumor kinetics by considering the proliferative kinetics of cancer cells.

Assessing Growth Parameters

Mitosis, or cell division, is the basic biologic process that results in an increase in somatic cell numbers over time. The term *growth* applies to the increasing volume of a cellular population and is measured in units of volume (cubic centimeters) or weight (milligrams). Growth is largely the consequence of increasing numbers of cells but also can be influenced by the increasing size of the individual cells, edema, and changes in the context of the extracellular matrix, hemorrhage, and infiltration by host cells, such as leukocytes. The term *proliferation,* in contrast, applies specifically to an increase in the number of cells, which is measured as cell number as a function of time. Cells divide by progressing through a sequence of steps that are collectively called the mitotic or "cell" cycle.

It is important for the student of cell kinetics to understand the methods for assessing cell cycle phases since—as in all areas of science—concepts are inextricably confounded with their means of quantification.[4] At the simplest level, metaphase cells may be counted on a microscope slide. This *mitotic index* is a rough estimate of the percent of cells in M-phase. Experimentally, the mitotic index can be improved by a now seldom used method called the stathmokinetic technique, in which a mitotic poison is applied at a known time prior to counting. The proliferative activity of a tissue may also be estimated by examining microscopic slides after immunohistologic staining for the Ki-67 protein, present in all proliferating cells and absent in nonproliferating cells. While Ki-67 staining is now heavily used, historically the most productive technique is the thymidine labeling index (TLI). Here viable cells are exposed briefly in vitro to a radiolabeled precursor of DNA. The most common thymidine label is tritium, but carbon 14 has also been used. The percentage of tumor cells with autoradiographic grains over their nuclei estimates the fraction of cells that were in S-phase during the period of thymidine exposure.

Except for the stathmokinetic technique, all of the above are static assays, providing a snapshot rather than a movie of proliferation.[5] Nevertheless, the snapshot is of a concept called the *growth fraction*, the proportion of the cancerous mass that is actually involved in proliferation. In former years the growth fraction of human leukemias was assessed by the use of the TLI in vivo, now no longer permissible.

A kinetic extension of the TLI is the percentage of labeled mitoses (PLM) curve. This technique counts, as a function of time after exposure, the number of M-phases that contain radioactive label. This measures the cells currently in M-phase that had been in S-phase during the exposure to radioisotope. Hence, it is the only technique that actually measures cell cycle durations. Kinetic autoradiographic techniques of this type were used decades ago to divide the cell cycle into four phases: the synthesis of DNA occurs mostly in the S-phase and the actual division of the parent cell into two daughters during the M-phase; the time gap between cell division and DNA synthesis is gap number 1, or G1 and the time gap between DNA synthesis and cell division is gap number 2, or G2. Although the term *mitosis* is often used to refer to the M-phase, the adjective *mitotic* properly refers to all cells that are engaged in any portion of the whole process of self-replication: G1, S, G2, and M-phases. This distinguishes mitotic cells from cells that do not divide within a defined period of observation, called G0 cells. The M-phase is the least variable in length, lasting about one hour in most mammalian cells. The G2-phase is usually three hours in length. The total duration of the cell cycle varies considerably, but the average in human cancer is between 2 and 4 days. Most of this variability is accounted for my variability in the length of the G1 phase. The long mitotic cycle in adult humans is in marked contrast with the cell cycle duration in *Drosophila*, which may take minutes, or with that of mammalian embryos, which may take only hours.

In G1-phase a normal mammalian somatic cell contains a diploid number of chromosomes, and hence diploid (2N) DNA content. During the S-phase, a cell's DNA content should increase from 2N to 4N. (A very small number of so-called S0 cells may stop synthesizing DNA before completing the S-phase, and rarely a cell can rest in the G2-phase and not proceed into M-phase.) G0 cells tend to be smaller than G1-phase cells and have lower RNA and protein contents. The variations in cellular DNA content during the proliferative cycle can be exploited analytically by a collection of automated methods called *flow cytometry*. In fluorescence-activated cell sorting, a suspension of individual cells is automatically counted by being allocated into bins by DNA content, RNA content, cell size, antibody (such as Ki-67) label, uptake of bromodeoxyuridine and/or tritiated thymidine during the S-phase, or combinations of such markers. This can be performed on fresh tissue—leukemias, tumor cells in effusions or ascites, enzymatically dispersed solid tumors—or on cells recovered from paraffin-embedded specimens. By measuring DNA content per cell, flow cytometry can also identify cells with abnormal amounts of DNA in the G0-G1 peak, termed *aneuploid*. The S-phase fraction may be impossible to measure in the presence of marked aneuploidy, one limitation of this method.

Growth Fraction, Death Fraction, Tumor Size, and Therapeutic Response

Using the above techniques it has been determined that 2-20% of cells in a typical cancer are in the S-phase at any point in time. Because the S-phase occupies one-quarter to one-half of the cell cycle, the growth fraction is usually 4-80%, with an average of less than 20%. For a given tissue, malignant or benign, the length of the cell cycle in vivo is fairly constant in spite of variations in the number of cycling cells in that population. However, subtle changes in cycle kinetics have been seen in cancers in laboratory animals that are allowed to grow large and phase lengths can shift significantly as cells are cultured in vitro. This is in addition to changes in the growth fraction itself during tumor growth: One of the most robust, and mysterious, observations in cytokinetics is that the growth fraction decreases with increasing tumor size. Is this the etiology or the consequence of Gompertzian growth? We will further discuss this below.

It is relevant in this regard that the rate of decrease in the growth fraction as the mass gets larger is slower for malignant than for benign tissues. But this is one of the few quantitative differences between malignant and benign tissues in cytokinetic terms. Some normal tissues, such as bone marrow and alimentary mucosa, have larger growth fractions and shorter mitotic cycle times than many cancers, even cancers of those tissues. This is the second major enigma presented by cytokinetic data. But while the growth fraction of a malignancy may be no greater than that of normal tissues from which it sprang, within a given histologic type of cancer both a high S-phase fraction and the presence of aneuploidy are frequently associated with a growth rate that is relatively more rapid, a malignant behavior that is relatively more aggressive, and a therapeutic response that is relatively poorer. These observations amplify rather than solve the enigma mentioned above of the association between histologic grade, tumor size, and metastatic behavior.

A partial answer may perhaps be found in the important companion concept to the concept of the growth fraction: the *death fraction or cell-loss fraction*. This is simply the proportion of the cellular mass that is lost by cell death per unit of time. The cell-loss fraction is hard to estimate from actual measurements since apoptosis—a common path of cell death—can leave few anatomic traces. It is usually inferred by comparing the expected growth rate (calculated from the measured growth fraction) with the actual growth rate. The impact of a high cell-loss fraction can be considerable. For example, basal cell epitheliomas of the skin grow slowly in spite of demonstrating a large number of metaphase figures. The importance of cell loss, however, goes beyond its impact on growth rate. Each mitotic cycle carries with it a finite probability of mutation. A tumor with a higher cell loss rate takes more mitotic cycles to double in size than a tumor with a lower cell loss rate. Thus, the rate of cell loss relates directly to the rate of mutations toward biologic properties of clinical importance.

Indeed, high rates of cell turnover are implicated in carcinogenesis itself. Elevated levels of thyroid stimulating hormone predispose to thyroid cancer. Chronic thermal injury with compensatory hyperplasia and hyperplasia secondary to solar damage lead to skin cancer. Hyperproliferation of the bone marrow in dysmyelopoiesis and in chronic granulocytic leukemia are likely contributors to the development of acute leukemia. Hyperproliferation of benign colonic and breast epithelium are clearly associated with neoplastic transformation. Indeed, chemical carcinogenesis requires a growth promoter. It is even possible—based on studies of Hodgkin's lymphoma and gastrointestinal cancer—that the hyperproliferation of residual cancer cells in compensation for cell death secondary to antineoplastic drug treatment may predispose to the development of drug resistance.

But the concept of the cell-loss fraction is not free of its own enigmas. Chemotherapy is thought to shrink cancers by damaging cancer cells and thus inducing them to undergo apoptosis. Mitotic cells, especially those in S-phase, are thought to be especially vulnerable to this process, and indeed a great deal of experimental evidence supports this hypothesis. However, if the growth fraction of a typical tumor is less than 20%, meaning that the S-phase fraction is 5-10%, and if the spontaneous cell-loss fraction is already greater than zero even in the absence of chemotherapy, how does chemotherapy increase the cell-loss fraction further so that cytoreductions of more than 90% are routine? Furthermore, attempts to increase chemotherapy effects by recruiting breast cancer cells into S-phase by the use of estradiol have not yielded the expected large therapeutic benefits.

Another enigma concerns the effect of chemotherapy on normal host tissues. Chemotherapy is certainly toxic to rapidly dividing bone marrow, alimentary mucosa, and hair follicles. Yet, these tissues usually recover from the impact of chemotherapy. Some cancers, however, that are growing no more rapidly than these normal tissues may experience cytoreductions from which they never recover, that is, acute leukemias, malignant lymphomas, choriocarcinomas, and germ cell cancers may be cured by chemotherapy regimens that do not eradicate the patient's normal tissues that have comparable growth kinetics.

Hence, the study of cellular proliferation raises as many questions as answers. Why does the growth fraction decrease with population size, but less so in cancer than in normal tissues? How are the growth and cell-loss fractions related to histologic grade, tumor size, and metastatic potential? How does chemotherapy work given that so few cells, even in virulent cancers, are mitotic at the time of treatment? To approach an answer to these enigmas, we need to expand our focus from the kinetic behavior of cells to the kinetic behavior of cellular populations.

The Kinetics of Chemotherapy Response

We have already critically examined tumor growth and have concluded that the Gompertzian curve or patterns of growth closely approximating Gompertzian curves are the only tenable ways to explain clinical observations. Nevertheless, some concepts derived from non-Gompertzian laboratory models are useful and merit discussion. Foremost in this regard is the body of work associated with Howard Skipper and colleagues at the Southern Research Institute.[6] The experimental leukemia they studied grows exponentially and regresses exponentially in response to effective treatment. This means that the percentage of cells killed is always the same regardless of the tumor size at the time of treatment. When graphed on a logarithmic scale of cell number versus an arithmetic scale of time it would appear that the amount of cell death cause by the treatment is always the same in terms of logarithmic displacement: a log-kill of one means that 90% of the cells were killed, a log-kill of two means that 99% of the cells were killed etc. If a given dose of a given drug reduces 10^6 cells to 10^5, the same therapy applied against 10^4 cells will result in 10^3 survivors.

The second seminal observation associated with these scientists is that for many drugs the log-kill increases with increasing dose. Hence, it requires higher drug dosages to eradicate larger-sized transplanted tumors. Moreover, if two or more drugs are used, the log-kills are multiplicative: If drug A at a certain dose level causes a log-kill of one, and drug B at a certain dose level also causes a log-kill of one, then the combination of A plus B, each given at the same dose levels as when they were used as single agents, would cause a log-kill of two.

The third observation recalled the Nobel Prize winning work of Max Delbrück and Salvador Luria concerning mutations toward resistance to destruction.[7] While Delbrück and Luria worked on bacterial resistance to viral infection, Skipper and colleagues evaluated resistance to chemotherapy, based on Lloyd Law's demonstration of the applicability of the Delbrück-Luria model to this setting.[8] The concept is that genetic alterations for survival traits arise in the absence of selection pressure, rather than being in response to selection pressure. In fact, the concept is similar to Darwin's evolutionary theory of natural selection, but applied at the cellular rather than the organism level. A new way of stating this observation is as follows: If in one mitosis a bacterium or mammalian cell mutates toward a given property with small probability x, the probability of the unit not developing that property in one mitosis is $1 - x$. In y mitoses, the probability of no mutations occurring is $(1 - x)^y$. If each mitosis produces two viable cells (no cell loss), it takes $N - 1$ mitoses for one cell to grow into N cells. Hence, the probability of not finding any one unit with that property in N cells is $\exp[(N - 1)^* \ln(1 - x)]$, which is a very small number. Adding cell loss into the model, which increases the number of mitoses necessary to reach N cells, would make the probability of no mutations occurring even smaller. Hence, mutations toward drug resistance must be common in a clinical cancer, which has been shown in many experiments over many decades. The same mathematics would explain why aneuploidy, as a manifestation of genetic change, is so strongly associated with high cell turnover. It might also explain the positive association of primary tumor size with the probability of metastatic spread due to cells that mutated toward that property.

On the basis of this evolutionary model, some theoreticians suggested that when two equally active chemotherapy regimens were available, if they could not be given together at full dose levels they should be strictly alternated so as to kill cells as quickly as possible before they had a chance to mutate toward drug resistance.[9] Others argued that mutations had more likely occurred before diagnosis, so it was more important to achieve as high cell-kill as possible in each of the subpopulations of cells already present at the time of diagnosis.[10-12] While the former model argues that adjuvant treatment must be instituted as early as possible in the growth history of a cancer to be effective, many trials have failed to find an advantage to preoperative chemotherapy for primary breast cancer, which is more consistent with the latter model. Indeed, both points of view may be argued convincingly on theoretical grounds, but experimental evidence including large prospective clinical trials has strongly favored the latter. The latter model is also concordant with the observation that many cancers—malignant lymphomas, acute leukemias, and breast cancers specifically—that are not cured by chemotherapy often still retain sensitivity to the same chemotherapy when it is applied at a later time.[13] Hence, all chemotherapeutic failure cannot be attributed to permanent drug resistance, but

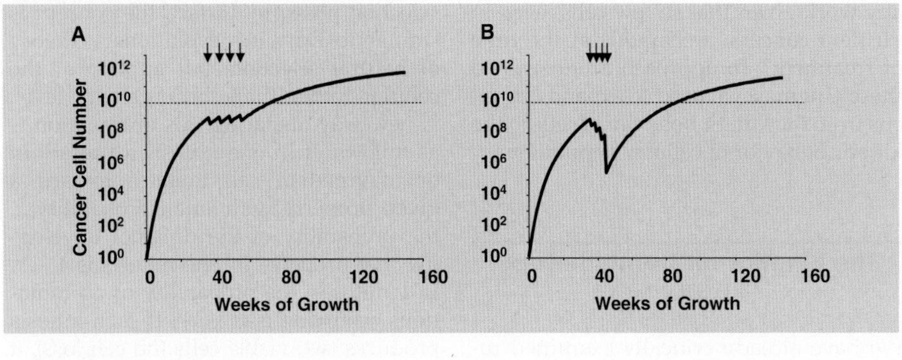

Figure 44-2 ■ Impact of dose density.

rather the persistence of cells that were not eradicated. A tumor may relapse because some of its cells, relatively but not absolutely insensitive to the agents applied, are not exposed to enough drug for a long enough time to be eradicated.[14] This is analogous to a bacterial infection relapsing because an insufficient dose intensity of an antibiotic is applied, even though the microorganisms are sensitive in vitro. In both infection and neoplasia, however, prolonged or repeated episodes of low-dose therapy can give rise to absolute resistance by the selection of cells that are biochemically resistant to treatment.

Can manipulations of dose level or schedule overcome this problem? As mentioned above, the strict alternation of agents or combinations of agents has not proven useful in this regard. Dose level escalations of a moderate degree have improved results in many common cancers including primary and metastatic breast cancer, childhood acute lymphoblastic leukemia, and adult germ cell tumors. Yet, results do not indicate a strictly rising dose-response relationship. For example, doses of cyclophosphamide over 600 mg/m^2 do not improve results in the adjuvant chemotherapy of breast cancer, nor do doses of doxorubicin over 60 mg/m^2. Neither has massive dose level escalation requiring autologous bone marrow rescue proven to be an advantageous strategy.

Yet schedule alterations are feasible and have provided some improvement in results. The principles established by Skipper and colleagues in the exponentially-growing murine leukemia have been translated into the Gompertzian setting.[15] The implications are illustrated in Figures 44-2 and 44-3, which are computer simulations of the mathematical model produced by this translation. In Figure 44-2A a tumor comprised of cells sensitive to therapy is shown to be growing in a Gompertzian fashion. In response to each administration of treatment, indicated by the arrows, the tumor volume shrinks because of the induced log-kill, and then regrows partially before the next administration for the first three cycles of treatment. After the fourth dose of chemotherapy the cancer is left untreated, eventually reaching 10^{10} cells, a clinically appreciable number, at the time indicated (dashed line) and continuing to grow thereafter. Figure 44-2B illustrates what would happen if the same tumor were treated with the same four cycles of chemotherapy, but with a shorter inter-treatment interval. Since there is less time for the tumor to regrow between cycles, the cancer cell number is smaller for each successive treatment after the first. It has been determined empirically that for Gompertzian populations the log-kill is proportional to the relative rate of growth at the time of treatment. Clearly, this may be because a greater percentage of the cells may be in S-phase and hence vulnerable. Because—in Gompertzian growth—the relative rate of growth is more rapid for smaller as compared with larger populations, the log-kill is greater for smaller populations as well. When, after the fourth dose of chemotherapy, the tumor grows in an unimpeded fashion, it is shown to take longer to reach 10^{10} cells (having started its regrowth at a smaller size), which translates to improved prognosis for the patient. Indeed, prospective, randomized clinical trials in primary breast cancer, then malignant lymphoma, then childhood Ewing's-family sarcoma have confirmed that the more frequent administration of chemotherapy improves overall survival time as predicted by this simulation.[16-18] The administration of CHOP chemotherapy for lymphoma each 14 days (as permitted by the use of granulocyte colony stimulating factor, G-CSF) rather than each 21 days, as was the old standard, is now widely used.[17]

Figure 44-3 extends this analysis to the case of a tumor that has developed heterogeneity in drug sensitivity prior to the time of initiation of therapy. This is illustrated by two growth curves, one black and one red, but the total tumor volume would be the sum of the two as the "black" cells and the "red" cells would be admixed in the tumor mass. The "black" cells are sensitive to the therapy symbolized by the black arrows, but are resistant to the therapy symbolized by the red arrows. In a parallel fashion, the "red" cells are sensitive to the therapy symbolized by the red arrows, but are resistant to the therapy symbolized by the black arrows. Figure 44-3A the black and red therapies are given in an alternating manner. In Figure 44-3B, the same therapies are given in sequence. It is clear that the log-kill from the sequential approach is greater in the "black" cancer cell population and not inferior in the "red" cells. Hence, the overall cytoreduction is greater, which results in a better prognosis for the patient—shown by increased time to 10^{10} cells. The reason for the greater log-kill is the increased

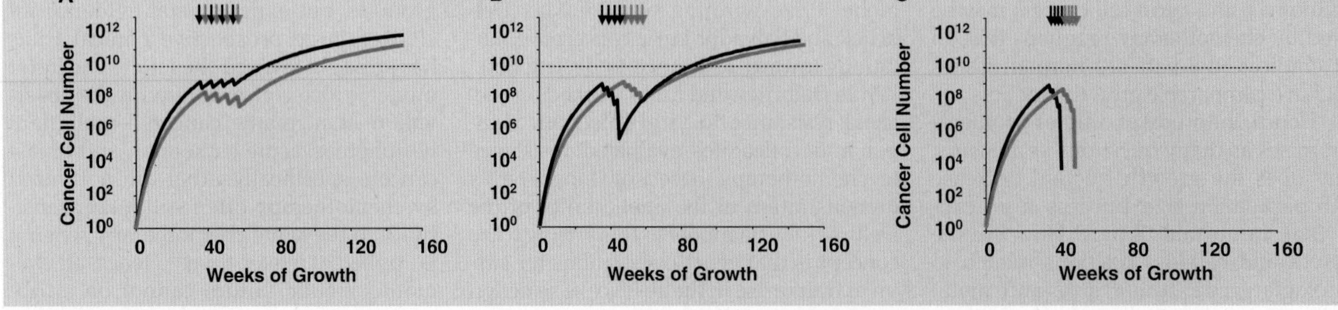

Figure 44-3 ■ Impact of sequential dose density.

density of the black treatment, as in Figure 44-2B. In the adjuvant chemotherapy of breast cancer the first use of doxorubicin—now a standard drug in this setting—was in such a sequential fashion.[19] The advantages of this approach have been shown in a prospective, randomized adjuvant chemotherapy trial conducted by the National Cancer Institute in Milan, Italy.[20] The administration of four cycles of doxorubicin followed by eight cycles of the three-drug combination CMF (cyclophosphamide, methotrexate, and 5-fluorouracil) was superior in disease-free and overall survival to a regimen giving the same drugs for the same number of cycles but in an alternating fashion. Similarly, the Breast International Group (Study 02-98) has published that taxane added benefit to doxorubicin only when used sequentially, not when used simultaneously at somewhat reduced dose levels.[21] (Both arms were followed by identical courses of CMF, which does not impact the conclusion that sequential therapy was superior to combination therapy.)

Figure 44-3C takes this concept further by reducing the inter-treatment time for both the black and red therapies. Here the log-kill is so much greater that regrowth may be precluded. This is the treatment plan tested in the breast cancer adjuvant setting by the North American Breast Intergroup in a trial (c9741) coordinated by the Cancer and Leukemia Group B. The use of G-CSF allowed for 14-day cycles of doxorubicin plus cyclophosphamide for four cycles followed sequentially by four, 14-day cycles of paclitaxel. Compared with the same chemotherapy given each 21 days, the dose-denser regimen not only improved disease-free and overall survival, but was less toxic by virtue of preserved granulocyte counts and perhaps other effects.[16] Corroborating results by other investigative teams have also been reported.

The concepts illustrated in Figure 44-3B are relevant to modern combinations of chemotherapy with biological agents. Figure 44-4 simulates the use of a prolonged, continuous treatment that inhibits cancer growth but does not interfere with the ability of chemotherapy to kill cancer cells. In Figure 44-4A the growth-inhibitory treatment (cross-hatched box) is started after the chemotherapy is completed. In Figure 44-4B the treatment is given simultaneously with the red chemotherapy. It is clear that the plan in Figure 44-4B is superior in time-to-10^{10}-cells for two reasons. The first is that the "black" cells, which are not sensitive to the red therapy, are inhibited earlier in their regrowth. The second is that because the growth of the "red" cells is inhibited by the growth-inhibitory therapy there is less regrowth between cycles of therapy, so fewer cells are present with each cycle after the first, meaning greater log-kill (as in Figure 44-3C). This may explain the efficacy of the HER2-modulating drug trastuzumab in adjuvant chemotherapy of HER2 over-expressing mode-positive primary breast cancer. In this trial (9831), coordinated for the North American Breast Intergroup by the North-Central Cancer Treatment Group, all patients received doxorubicin plus cyclophosphamide followed by weekly paclitaxel. The patients who received a year of continuous trastuzumab starting with the paclitaxel experienced fewer recurrences of breast cancer than those who started their trastuzumab after the paclitaxel was completed.[22] To build upon these results investigators at Memorial Sloan-Kettering Cancer Center have completed a phase II study proving the tolerability of a dose-dense chemotherapy regimen, following the concept in Figure 44-3C, with a year of trastuzumab starting simultaneously with the paclitaxel portion of the treatment.

However, it must not be assumed that growth-inhibitory therapy must always be given with chemotherapy. Figure 44-5 illustrates the impact of a growth-inhibitory treatment (cross-hatched box) that interferes with the action of chemotherapy. In Figure 44-5A this is given after the chemotherapy is completed and because it has no chemotherapy to disrupt it yields identical results to Figure 44-4A. However, in Figure 44-5B it is seen that the impact of the treatment on the "red" cells is complex. Because the growth-inhibitory treatment is started earlier on the "red" cells than in Figure 44-4A there is a greater effect. But also the impact of the chemotherapy, symbolized by the red arrows, is reduced, which is disadvantageous. The net effect—as measured by the time to 10^{10} cells—is neutral in this simulation. Should the growth-inhibitory drug be better at slowing growth or less interfering with chemotherapy the net effect would be beneficial to the patient as concerns the "red" cancer cells. But if the drug is less growth-inhibitory or more potent at interfering with chemotherapy then the net effect would not be beneficial. The other factor in this complex equation is the effect of earlier institution of the growth-inhibitory drug on the "black" cells. Hence, when one is dealing with a drug that might slow growth but also might interfere with the action of chemotherapy it would be difficult to predict if it would be better to use the drug during or after chemotherapy. This may explain why when the Southwest Oncology Group tested tamoxifen starting during or after chemotherapy for the adjuvant therapy of hormone-receptor positive primary breast cancer, it found that the sequential plan was superior.[23]

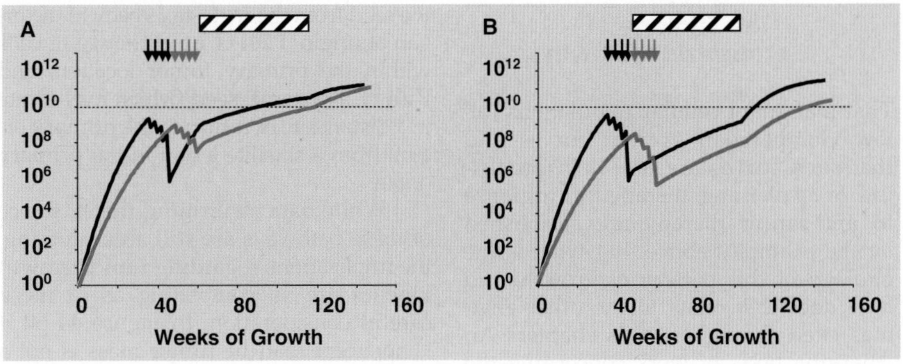

Figure 44-4 ■ Impact of growth-inhibitory therapy (that does not inhibit chemotherapy).

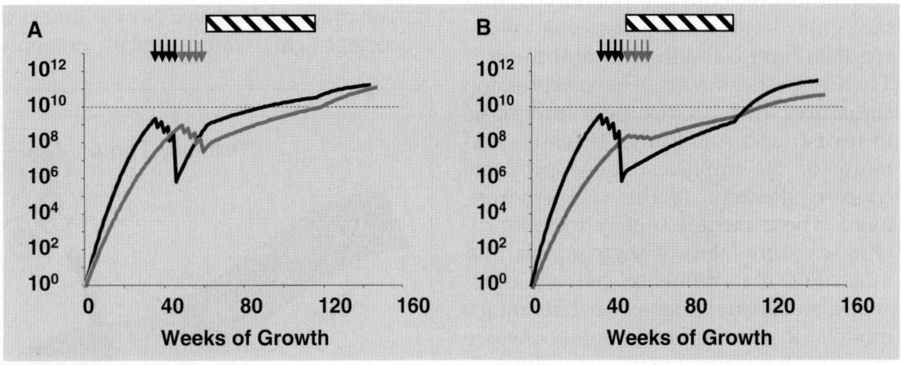

Figure 44-5 ■ Impact of growth-inhibitory therapy (that inhibits chemotherapy).

The Etiology of Gompertzian Growth

That malignant cellular populations follow Gompertzian growth curves and that such curves are useful in predicting or explaining therapeutic response to anti-cancer therapy are established by the examples above. But what is the etiology of this pattern of growth, and how does that relate to the other enigmas cited throughout this chapter? An emerging body of work concerning the molecular biology of metastases may provide insight in this regard.

One of the cardinal features of cancer cells is their abnormal mobility. This is manifest on both the phenotypic and molecular levels. Oncogenes often co-deregulate both cell adhesion and mitosis. There exist several sets of gene expression signatures that predict poor prognosis in breast cancer and other diseases, and many of the implicated gene products concern alteration of the microenvironment. These include matrix metalloproteinases, stimulators of angiogenesis, and molecules that influence cell adhesion, shape, and spatial orientation. Laboratory models of metastasis frequently involve genes of these functional classes. Indeed, a poor-prognosis signature in human breast cancer has been created that totally excludes genes associated with proliferation. Yet, in both the laboratory and clinic tumors with high levels of expression of environment-modifying genes tend to grow rapidly. This raises the question: How do environment-modifying genes, and genes associated with cell mobility, contribute to growth rate *independent* of aberrations in mitosis and apoptosis?

A working hypothesis that has recently been proposed this question is illustrated in Figure 44-6.[24] In Figure 44-6A we visualize a primary tumor as a collection of cohesive cells in the organ of origin. Some of these cells have the capacity, by virtue of the functions listed above, to move, either by direct extension into surrounding tissue (Path A) or into blood vessels in their vicinity (Paths B and C). We understand that these cells can extravasate in sites of potential metastases (Path B), but why cannot they also travel back to the primary site (Path C), with preference for locations close to the primary mass where growth factors secreted by cancer and stromal cells should be in abundance? We may term Path C *self seeding* as contrasted with the distant seeding via Path B. A later evolution of this process is shown in Figure 44-6B. Here the cells spread by Paths A, B, and C above have grown by mitosis into masses. In addition, new paths of seeding are now possible: Path D, direct extension into the tissue surrounding the metastasis; Path E, a self-seed from the metastasis to the metastasis; Path F, a seed from the metastasis back to the organ of origin; Path G, an exchange of cells within the primary tumor location; and Path H, a systemic seed (which may locate in a distant site or return to the primary organ) from a satellite lesion in the primary organ.

While data confirming the existence of these pathways are still accumulating, the implications regarding tumor growth kinetics are so compelling as to merit careful consideration. In Figure 44-6B it is apparent that the tumor mass is not a discrete, organized entity but rather a collection or conglomerate of smaller masses. Each, being independent, may induce its own blood supply, perhaps by attraction of marrow-derived circulating endothelial cell precursors as well as cytokine-rich leucocytes. This would explain not only the abundance of vessels in many cancers but the architectural disorganization characteristic of malignant anaplasia. Furthermore, since each of the component nodules of the conglomerate is relatively small, it is not unreasonable to expect that it would be relatively fast-growing, accounting for the rapid growth of neoplasia in spite of a growth fraction that—as we saw above—is not especially large compared with the tissue of origin.

The presence of self-seeded masses in the organ of origin (the progeny of Path C in Figure 44-6A) that can then send seeds back into circulation (Path H, Fig. 44-6B) would explain why it is necessary to irradiate residual "normal" tissue in organs after the "clean" excision of primary lesions from those organs. The exchange of seeds between sites in the primary lesion (Path

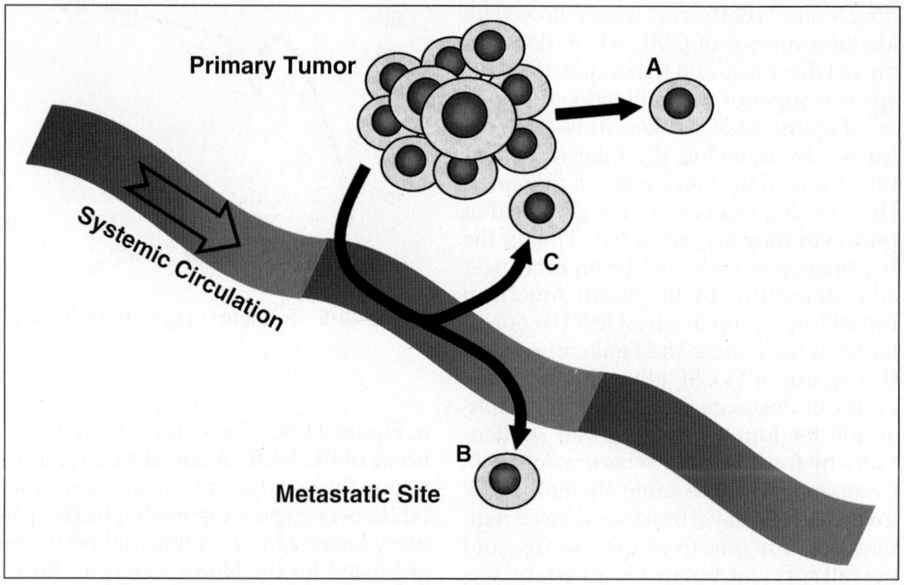

Figure 44-6A ■ Patterns of seeding—early.

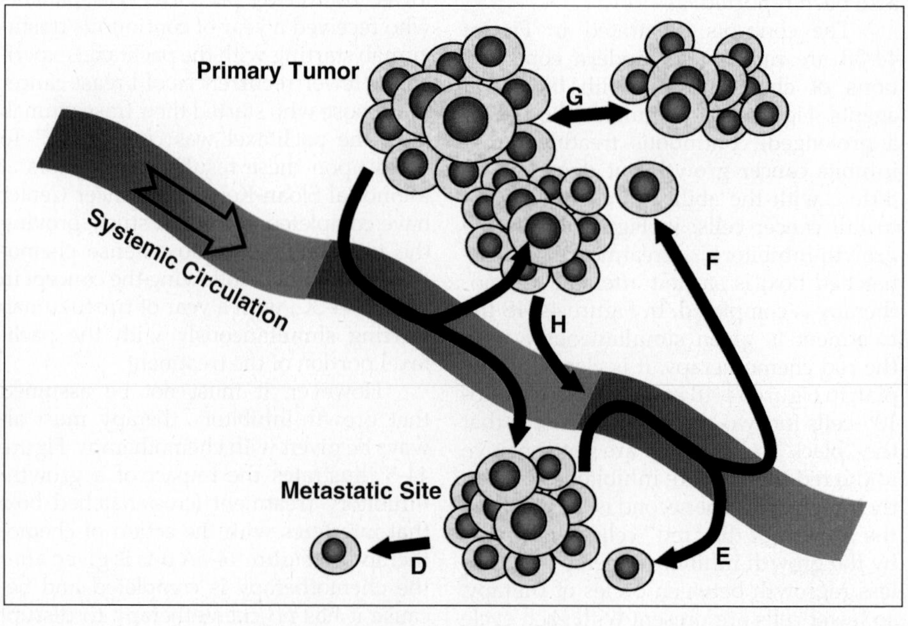

Figure 44-6B ■ Patterns of seeding—later

G) would explain how tumor-initiating or stem cells may become disseminated throughout a tumor mass, rendering sampling for expression profiling practical.

Moreover, growth of a primary mass from the outside-in (self seeding) as well as the inside-out (mitosis) provides a ready explanation for Gompertzian growth. In the simplest case, a sphere, the surface area is proportional to the square of its diameter while the volume is proportional to the cube of its diameter. As the mass and hence its diameter (d) grows larger, the ratio of surface area to volume drops proportional to 1/d. Since growth from outside-in happens at the surface, the growth fraction would be expected to fall proportional to 1/d. That is, the relative growth rate would fall as the mass grew large, which is exactly what is seen in Gompertzian growth. Now cancerous masses are not perfect spheres, so the surface area would not be proportional to the diameter raised to a power of two (that is, squared), but rather a power between two and three. The more aggressive the process of seeding, the more irregular would be the surface of the mass, and the closer the power would be to three. For example, if the self seeding is very prominent, the surface area may be proportional to $d^{2.9}$, so the growth fraction would fall proportional to $d^{2.9}/d^3$, which is very slowly compared with 1/d. This would account for the enigma, cited above, that the growth fraction falls more slowly with increasing population size than normal tissues with surface areas closer to a proportion of d^2.

This model would explain the association between anaplasia, growth rate, tumor size, and metastatic potential as follows: Many of the same gene functions that permit the movement of a cell into and out of the blood stream to form a self-seed should be involved in the formation of distant metastases. Hence, cancers that are more likely to involve regional lymph nodes are more likely to metastasize to distant sites because the genetic tool kits for both processes are similar, but not identical, accounting for discrepancies as well. Indeed, the genetic tool kit for preneoplasia may differ only slightly from that of invasive cancer, explaining the enigma of similar polygenetic abnormalities in both types of lesions. Ductal carcinoma in situ of the breast, for example, may be a frank neoplasia that is just not very efficient at self seeding, lacking, for example, the ability to enter or exit the circulation, alter the microenvironment in seeded locations, or attract marrow-derived stromal cells. This line of reasoning would also explain the observation above that cell cycle phase lengths are similar in cancer and normal tissues. The cells that seed the component masses of the primary-site conglomerate may be quite normal except for the fact that they are abnormally re-located because of their abnormal mobility. In this regard, a primary breast cancer could be thought of as a contiguous collection of dozens to thousands of embryonic breasts, each within itself close to normal.

That growth by seeding depends to such a large degree on supporting stroma, including or particularly marrow-derived cells that contribute to angiogenesis and matrix formation, would seem to make cancers vulnerable to interventions that attack these component in addition to the cancer cells themselves. This might explain how chemotherapy—which has profound effects on bone marrow—can be so effective against tumor in which five or fewer percent of the cells are in S-phase. How the self-seeding model relates to the very controversial but provocative concept of tumor dormancy and the impact of surgical debulking on such dormancy is a topic of active interest.[25]

Conclusion

We have in this chapter reviewed the kinetics of cellular proliferation and population growth, finding a theoretical basis for improved practices in cancer chemotherapy. Moreover, we have examined various clinical and laboratory-derived enigmas from a kinetic point of view, finding connections between molecular oncology and the behavior of malignancies on the macroscopic scale. This latter science is young but emergent, reinvigorating a mature field that has demonstrated practical worth at the same time as it promises future advances.

References

1. van't Veer LJ, Paik S, Hayes DF. Gene expression profiling of breast cancer: a new tumor marker. *J Clin Oncol*. 2005;8:1631–1635.
2. Norton LA. Gompertzian model of human breast cancer growth. *Cancer Res*. 1988;48:7067.
3. Laird AK. Dynamics of growth in tumors and normal organisms. *Monogr Natl Cancer Inst*. 1969;30:15.
4. Steel GG. Autoradiographic analysis of the cell cycle. Howard and Pelc to the present day. *Int J Radiat Biol*. 1986;49:227.
5. Frei E III, Whang J, Scoggins RB, et al. The stathmokinetic effect of vincristine. *Cancer Res*. 1964;18–25.
6. Skipper HE, Schabel FM Jr, Wilcox WS. Experimental evaluation of potential anticancer agents XIII. On the criteria and kinetics associated with "curability" of experimental leukemia. *Cancer Chemother Rep*. 1964;35:1.
7. Luria SE, Delbruck M. Mutations of bacteria from virus sensitivity to virus resistance. *Genetics*. 1943;28:491.
8. Law LW. Origin of resistance of leukaemic cells to folic acid antagonists. *Nature*. 1952;169:628.
9. Goldie JH, Coldman AJ. A mathematic model for relating the drug sensitivity of tumors to their spontaneous mutation rate. *Cancer Treat Rep*. 1979;63:1727.
10. Shapiro DM, Fugmann RA. A role for chemotherapy as an adjunct to surgery. *Cancer Res*. 1957;17:1098.
11. Schabel FM. Concepts for the systemic treatment of micrometastases. *Cancer*. 1975; 35:15.
12. Norton L. Implications of kinetic heterogeneity in clinical oncology. *Semin Oncol*. 1985;12:231.
13. DeVita VT. The relationship between tumor mass and resistance to treatment of cancer. *Cancer*. 1983;51:1209.
14. Holland JF. Clinical studies of unmaintained remissions in acute lymphocytic leukemia. In: The proliferation and spread of neoplastic cells. *21st Annual Symposium on Fundamental Cancer Research* 1967. Baltimore, MD: Williams & Wilkins; 1968:453–462.
15. Norton L, Simon R. Tumor size, sensitivity to therapy, and the design of treatment schedules. *Cancer Treat Rep*. 1977;61:1307.
16. Citron ML, Berry DA, Cirrincione C, et al. Randomized trial of dose-dense versus conventionally scheduled and sequential versus concurrent combination chemotherapy as postoperative adjuvant treatment of node-positive primary breast cancer: first report of Intergroup Trial C9741/ Cancer and Leukemia Group B Trial 9741. *J Clin Oncol*. 2003;21:1431–1439.
17. Held G, Schubert J, Reiser M, et al. Dose-intensified treatment of advanced-stage diffuse large B-cell lymphomas. *Semin Hematol*. October 2006;43(4):221–229.
18. Womer RB, West DC, Krailo MD, et al. Randomized comparison of every-two-week vs every-three-week chemotherapy in Ewing sarcoma family tumors. *J Clin Oncol*. 2008:abstr 10504.
19. Perloff M, Norton L, Korzun AH, et al. Postsurgical adjuvant chemotherapy of stage II breast carcinoma with or without crossover to a non-cross-resistant regimen: a Cancer and Leukemia Group B study. *J Clin Oncol*. 1996;1589–1598.
20. Bonadonna G, Zambetti M, Moliterni, et al. Clinical relevance of different sequencing of doxorubicin and cyclophosphamide, methotrexate, and Fluorouracil in operable breast cancer. *J Clin Oncol*. 2004;1614–1620.
21. Francis P, Crown J, Di Leo A, et al. Adjuvant chemotherapy with sequential or concurrent anthracycline and docetaxel: Breast International Group 02-98 randomized trial. *J Natl Cancer Inst*. 2008;121–133.
22. Baselga J, Perez EA, Pienkowski T, Bell R. Adjuvant trastuzumab: a milestone in the treatment of HER2-positive early breast cancer. *Oncologist*. 2006;4–12.
23. Albain KS, Green SJ, Ravdin PM, et al. Adjuvant chemohormonal therapy for primary breast cancer should be sequential instead of concurrent: initial results from Intergroup trial 0100 (SWOG-8814). *Proc Am Soc Clin Oncol*. 2002;21 (abstr 143).
24. Norton L, Massagué J. Is cancer a disease of self-seeding? *Nat Med*. 2006;875–878.
25. Demicheli R, Miceli R, Moliterni A, et al. Breast cancer recurrence dynamics following adjuvant CMF is consistent with tumor dormancy and mastectomy-driven acceleration of the metastatic process. *Ann Oncol*. 2005;1449–1457.

45 Principles of Dose, Schedule, and Combination Therapy

Joseph P. Eder, MD ■ William N. Hait, MD, PhD ■ Emil Frei III, MD ■ Louise B. Grochow, MD

Introduction

The identification of novel, clinically active agents has been central to progress in cancer chemotherapy. Table 45-1 presents examples of new agents and of cellular pathways and targets being explored for new therapeutic targets. Dose is a significant determinant of the antitumor activity and toxicology for the established, "classical" cytotoxic chemotherapeutic agents.[1] Higher doses (1.2 times to twice the baseline dose) made possible by growth factors (granulocyte-colony stimulating factor [G-CSF], granulocyte/macrophage-colony stimulating factor [GM-CSF]) are variably more effective. High-dose chemotherapy (4-10 times the baseline dose), made possible by hematopoietic stem cell transplantation, has proven curative for selected hematologic neoplasms. The effect of dose for biologically therapeutic agents such as the interferons, interleukins, monoclonal antibodies, hormones and for molecularly targeted tyrosine kinase inhibitors is complicated, and there is not the same unequivocal evidence for a dose–response effect with these agents.

The schedule of drug administration may be important to the therapeutic index independent of dose. Cytokinetic studies related to drug schedule have led to the improved use of agents such as cytosine arabinoside (cytarabine, ara-C) in both experimental and clinical leukemia (see "Cytokinetics of Bone Marrow" later in this chapter).[2,3] Most of the molecularly targeted agents, whether small molecules or monoclonal antibodies, are dosed to provide a continuous effect, which markedly changes the clinical toxicity profile.

Combination chemotherapy has been crucial in the development of curative regimens for hematologic malignancies, pediatric solid tumors, testicular cancer, and ovarian cancer, and for the adjuvant regimens for breast, lung, and bowel cancer, and for osteosarcomas.[4,5] The rationale for combination chemotherapy is discussed under the various topical headlines. The principal rationales include (1) the pragmatic, ie, almost all therapy that has proven curative in the clinic involves the use of agents in combination (Table 45-2); (2) the fact that genetic instability results in tumor cell heterogeneity, which manifests as drug resistance in cancer therapy;[6-8] and (3) selectively targeted molecular agents, with the exception of imatinib in chronic myelogenous leukemia (CML), must attack multiple pathways or be combined with DNA-damaging "classical" agents to have significant therapeutic benefit.[9] Although dose and combination chemotherapy are generally considered separately, they have an important and complex relationship.[10,11] There is an impressive increase in the number of putative molecular targets for cancer treatment in development (Table 45-1). A major clinical research challenge will be not only to maximize the effectiveness of individual agents but, particularly, to integrate drugs into optimal combination strategies.

Dose

In controlled experimental systems, such as established tumor cell lines in culture, the relationship between dose and tumor cytotoxicity may be close to linear-log (ie, exponential).[12] For example, a linear increase in the dose of selected chemotherapeutic agents causes a log reduction of MCF7 human breast cancer cells in culture.[13] In Figure 45-1, dose is expressed as multiples of the IC90 (ie, the dose or concentration that reduces the number of tumor cells by 90%), a very good response in terms of tumor regression in a patient. The estimated total tumor burden for patients with clinically evident cancer is $5 \times 10^{11} \pm 10^{1}$ (11 ± 1 logs). Thus, a dose that produces a good partial remission (eg, 50-90% tumor regression) produces at most a 1-log reduction, which is less than 10% of the "exponential iceberg." Numerous factors influence the dose effect. They are presented in the subsections that follow.[14,15]

Table 45-1 ■ **Molecular Targets for Cancer Treatment**

The cell cycle
• Cyclin-dependent kinases, cyclins, cyclin-dependent kinase inhibitors, mitotic tubule-associated proteins
Differentiation
• Retinoid and vitamin D nuclear steroid receptors
Apoptosis
• *BCL2*, NF-κB, *TP53*, *TNFSF10*, *FAS*
Angiogenesis
• *KDR*, the endothelial integrins, *PDGFRB*
Signaling cell surface receptors
• Insulin-like growth factor receptor (IGF), *ERBB* family of receptors, *KIT*
Metastasis
• Matrix metalloproteinases, chemokine receptors
Intracellular signaling elements
• *BCR-ABL1*, *ras*, *raf*, *MADD*, PI3 kinase, m-TOR, *src*, protein kinase C, focal adhesion kinase (*PTK2*: protein tyrosine kinase 2), anaplastic lymphoma kinase (*ALK*), the *STAT* family of proteins and the *MAP* family of protein kinases
Nuclear transcription factors
• eg, steroid hormone No. 4
Potential targets
• Telomerase
• DNA methylation (human DNA methyltransferase [MeTase]), proteasome 20S, farnesyltransferase, histone deacetylase, hsp90 (chaperone protein)
Cell surface antigens
• For example, CD20

Factors Influencing the Dose Effect

Class of Chemotherapeutic Agent

The ideal therapeutic agent would maintain a linear relationship between dose and log tumor cell reduction (log-TCR) down through multiple logs of tumor cell destruction (Fig. 45-1). Ionizing radiation comes closest to this ideal. As a group, alkylating agents are superior to the other chemotherapeutic agents in terms of maintained dose/log-TCR (Fig. 45-1). Alkylating agents exhibit major activity during the S and M periods of the cell cycle, but unlike other chemotherapeutic agents, they maintain activity throughout the cell cycle. Although comparative studies demonstrate a dose effect in chemotherapy-sensitive tumors such as the leukemias and lymphomas, the effect of dose is less evident in solid tumors, particularly those tumors of epithelial origin.[16,17] Antimetabolites are active mainly in proliferating cells, and therefore pharmacokinetic resistance occurs that is overcome less by increasing dose than by increasing the duration of exposure, thus allowing more cells to enter the proliferative compartment. This also applies to the DNA-damaging topoisomerase I and II directed agents and microtubule-interacting agents, where the target must be encountered in the setting of DNA synthesis or mitotic spindle assembly to produce antineoplastic cytotoxicity.[18,19]

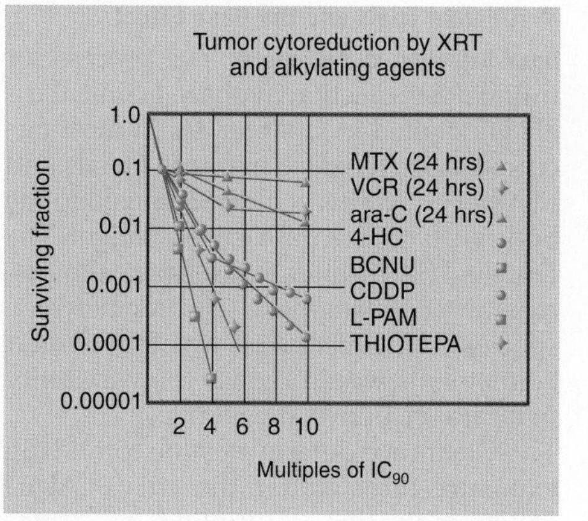

Figure 45-1 ■ Log kill in vitro: Effect of antitumor agent concentration expressed as multiples of the IC90 (ie, the dose or concentration that reduces the number of tumor cells by 90%), on the surviving fraction of human breast cancer (MCF7) cells in culture (colony assay). *Abbreviation:* 4-HC, 4-hydroxycyclophosphamide. *Source:* From Ref. 5.

Agents directed at hormone receptors, growth factor receptors and intracellular kinase signaling targets have a different relationship since once receptor/kinase interactions are saturated, further dose increases will produce no further effect.[20] Hence these agents are analogous to antimetabolites in that dose escalation once saturation levels of drug are achieved produces no further benefit. Higher doses of imatinib in chronic phase or accelerated phase CML with a suboptimal response to standard-dose can benefit a subgroup of patients, but the percentage is low and the duration of response brief.[21,22]

Tumor Factors

■ Intrinsic Tumor Cell Sensitivity

The more sensitive the tumor is to a given agent, the steeper the dose effect. Thus, if a unit dose produces a 0.5 log-TCR, then doubling that dose may produce up to a 1.0 log tumor cell kill—which clinically represents only a partial remission. In a chemotherapy-sensitive tumor, where a unit dose produces a 3 log-TCR, doubling the dose may produce up to a 6 log-TCR, depending on the degree of tumor cell heterogeneity and drug resistance (see "Drug Resistance" later in this subsection). A 6 log-TCR would produce a major clinical achievement in terms of complete response, duration of complete response, and, most important, an approach to tumor cure or eradication. Thus, for patients with a common epithelial tumor, such as breast cancer, the most that can be achieved with standard single-agent chemotherapy is a partial response (<1 log-TCR) in about 30% of patients. Combinations result in higher partial response rates and a low (10-20%) complete response rate. Alternatively, combination chemotherapy regimens in patients with chemotherapy-sensitive tumors (eg, non-Hodgkin lymphoma, Hodgkin disease, and testicular cancer) may achieve multilog-TCR as a result of combination chemotherapy.[23]

Tumor Burden ■ Tumor burden is a consistent adverse prognostic factor for response to chemotherapy. This finding was first demonstrated for transplanted tumors in mice; in these animals, macroscopic (ie, palpable) tumors often respond minimally to chemotherapy. The same tumor, at a microscopic tumor burden size, may be much more responsive and potentially curable.[23,24]

These observations in mice are consistent with the parallel observation that adjuvant cancer treatment can be curative for patients with breast cancer, but not for those with overt metastatic breast cancer. Postulates for the delay in growth of microscopic metastases include a balanced rate of cell loss (ie, apoptosis) and of cell production and inability to support tumor neovascularization (angiogenesis). Resistant microscopic tumor may persist in most long-term survivors, an observation that has major implications for therapeutic strategy (see "Cytokinetics of the Tumor" later in this subsection).

The study of microscopic metastases in patients may become increasingly possible with modern molecular techniques for detection and characterization of minimal tumor.[23] The kinetics of microscopic disease can be inferred from adjuvant chemotherapy studies (see "Adjuvant Chemotherapy").

Drug Resistance ■ In the laboratory, drug resistance is usually produced by "selection pressure"—ie, by exposing target cells to progressively increasing concentrations of the selecting agent. Drug resistance usually is expressed as the concentration of drug that is required to produce 50% inhibition in a colony or growth assay (IC_{50}) for the resistant cell line, divided by the concentration required (IC_{50}) for the parent sensitive cell line. For a detailed presentation of drug resistance, see "Combination Chemotherapy" later in this chapter and Chapter 48, "Drug Resistance and Its Clinical Circumvention."

Tumor Cytokinetics: Growth Fraction ■ The growth fraction (GF) of the tumor and the dose of cell cycle-specific agents has a major effect on the log-TCR of tumor cells. The generation time of cycling (ie, mitotically active) cells is much shorter than the volume doubling time.[25-29] Thus, many cells within tumors are dying or "noncycling"—ie, in G0/G1. The GF of a tumor is the ratio of the cycling cells to the total number of tumor cells.

For the common epithelial solid tumors, the GF is often less than 5%.[30,31] A solid tumor with a growth fraction of 5% would be minimally responsive to cell cycle-specific agents and variably sensitive to other chemotherapeutic agents. Repetitive treatments, however, might "recruit" cells into cycle by allowing dormant, noncycling cells access to necessary growth conditions and thus enabling them to be more effective. Prolonged exposure to cell cycle-specific agents might be effective in low-growth fraction tumors. In contrast, a high-growth fraction tumor such as Burkitt lymphoma might have a multilog response with the same treatment or even the same dose over a shorter period.[1] A recent challenge to the long-standing clonal evolution model of cancer evokes specific cancer stem cells (CSCs) as responsible for the continued proliferation of a tumor. By this hypothesis, self-renewing CSCs give rise to all progenitor and differentiated cells within a tumor, but remain a small proportion of all tumor cells.[32] CSCs, as with normal tissue stem cells, are extremely resistant to chemotherapy and radiotherapy. The difference between curative therapeutic regimens and those that are only palliative may be attributable to the rela-

Table 45-2 ■ **Number of Agents and Curative Treatment for Childhood Acute Lymphoblastic Leukemia (ALL)**

	No. of Chemotherapeutic Agents							
	1	2	3	4	5	6	7	8
Year	1948	1954	1956	1960	1965	1974	1985	1988
Agent	Methotrexate	MP	Prednisone	Vincristine	Methotrexate[a]	Adriamycin	Asparagine	ara-C
CR (%)	20-40	40-92	80-95	>95	>95	>95	>95	>95
Cure (%)	0	0	0	15	5-35	55	75	80

[a]Intrathecal methotrexate.

Abbreviations: CR, complete response; MP, 6-mercaptopurine.

tive sensitivities of CSCs and of the progenitor and differentiated cancer cells incapable of self-renewal. Identification of therapeutic targets within the CSC population should offer significant opportunities for more effective therapies.

Tumor Hypoxia ■ Hypoxia commonly occurs in both experimental and clinical solid tumors, a condition presumably resulting from inadequate angiogenesis and high metabolic activity (oxygen consumption). Oxygen distribution within tumors is heterogeneous and even a small fraction of hypoxic cells can profoundly affect chemotherapy responsiveness. The farther cells are from blood vessels, the lower the concentration of chemotherapeutic agents in those cells. Cellular proliferation decreases as a function of distance from blood vessels, with a significant fraction of nonproliferating cells conferring kinetic resistance to cell cycle-specific agents. Hypoxia selects for *TP53* mutants with a reduced apoptotic response to DNA damage or cell cycle arrest. Certain cancer chemotherapy agents require oxygen as an intermediate in toxicity or in metabolism. Finally, hypoxia produces altered gene expression. There may be increased expression of adenosine triphosphate–binding cassette (ABC) proteins such as p-glycoprotein (PgP) that may confer resistance to chemotherapeutic agents. Hypoxia-inducible factor-1 (*HIF1α*) stops proliferation and prevents apoptosis in the hypoxic fraction of cells by increasing angiogenesis. Hypoxia increases the production of hepatocytes growth factor (*HGF*) and its receptor *MET*, with a further increase in angiogenesis, and increased incidence of metastasis and drug resistance.[33,34] Exploiting hypoxia as a target in cancer therapy with bioreductive alkylating agents such as mitomycin C and the nitroimidazoles, which can serve as electron acceptors in lieu of oxygen, has been tried in numerous clinical circumstances with no or minimal benefit.[35,36] Radiotherapy in particular requires molecular oxygen for cytotoxicity.[37]

Oncogene Addiction-Growth Factor Signaling ■ The maintenance of the transformed state results in significant metabolic and genetic stress on cancer cells. Maintaining viability under these conditions requires positive antiapoptotic signaling factors and interfering with these survival pathways can result in tumor cell lethality. In particular, mutant oncogenes such as *BCR-ABL* in CML, or mutant growth factor receptors like *EGFR(ERBB1)* in lung cancer and *CKIT* in gastrointestinal stromal tumors (GIST) provide essential survival signals and interruption of these pathways produces significant clinical benefit in affected patient. Encouragingly, the emergence of diagnostic tests enables identification of patients and permits selection of appropriate therapy.

Host Factors

Cytokinetics of Bone Marrow ■ Because of the bone marrow's proliferative activity and relative lack of DNA repair capacity, myelosuppression is dose-limiting for many chemotherapeutic agents. Exploiting the cytokinetic difference between marrow and tumor has been a basis for the construction of selected clinical stratigies.[3,26-29]

Normal marrow recovers within 1-2 weeks after cytarabine, with little cumulative myelosuppression. For many patients, recovery of acute myelogenous leukemia (AML) cells as compared with normal marrow cells between courses of cytarabine is incomplete. AML cells in vitro are less susceptible to growth factors such as G- and GM-CSF than are the cells of the normal marrow. Thus, when marrow CSFs increase in homeostatic response to cytarabine-induced myelosuppression, the interval recovery of normal marrow may be more rapid than that demonstrated by the AML cells, a factor that should, with successive dosing, result in a cumulative effect—hence the therapeutic advantage.

Similar changes occur in other proliferative tissues, including the gastrointestinal tract, where drugs cause mitotic arrest with loss of epithelial surface cells, including cells involved in the adsorption of fluids. This requires a recovery periods just as the marrow does.[38]

Pharmacokinetics ■ Pharmacokinetic factors commonly affect the dose–response curve. For example, if an inactivating enzyme for the drug becomes saturated, both toxicity and antitumor effect may increase disproportionately, an effect observed with certain dose schedules of 5-fluorouracil (5-FU).[39,40]

The opposite effect may occur if a drug activation system becomes saturated. For example, ifosfamide, a prodrug, is activated by the cytochrome P450, oxygen-dependent, drug-metabolizing enzymes in the liver to the biologically active 4-hydroxyl derivative. The 3-day conventional dose of ifosfamide is higher (1200-2400 mg/m^2 daily) than that for cyclophosphamide (600 mg/m^2) because the rate of P450 activation of ifosfamide is relatively slow. With increasing doses of cyclophosphamide, a constant fractional conversion to active 4-hydroxyl cyclophosphamide occurs. However, for ifosfamide, once the P450 enzyme system becomes saturated, a decreasing proportion of ifosfamide is converted to the active form, with a consequent loss of antitumor effect at higher doses.

Clinical Trials and the Dose Effect

Dose Selection in Patients ■ The process for initial dose selection in phase I clinical trials is detailed in Chapter 46. In most circumstances, the dose in phase I trials and in other situations is individualized to the body surface area (BSA) of the patient. The Dubois BSA formula is useful in allometric scaling of drug-dose selection between species. The expectation was that similar adjustments would reduce the variability in clearance between patients.

Clearance determines the total drug exposure (area under the curve [AUC] of concentration multiplied by time), and AUC in mice correlates with toxicity in that species. This relationship of AUC with drug exposure and toxicity also holds true in humans and can be predicted from mouse data.[41] BSA may be helpful in selecting the dose of cytotoxic agents in childhood leukemia and was subsequently incorporated into standard usage.[42,43] Recent reviews of the literature and of individual institutional experience can find no significant correlation between BSA and clearance variability with investigational or commonly used anticancer drugs except for paclitaxel, oral busulfan, and possibly temozolomide.[44,45]

BSA may correlate with glomerular filtration rate, blood volume, and basal metabolic rate.[44] However, the variability in drug clearance introduced by these factors is small (<25%) compared with that induced by hepatic metabolic enzymes, and there is no correlation between BSA and metabolic activity.[44] Glomerular filtration rate as estimated from serum creatinine does correlate with toxicity for topotecan, etoposide, and carboplatin. Indeed, calculated AUC from serum creatinine (Calvert formula) is now used to dose carboplatin.[43]

Enzymatic pathways are responsible for the clearance of 5-FU and 6-mercaptopurine (6-MP) and for glucuronidation via *UGT1A1* for clearance of SN-38, the active product of irinotecan (see individual chapters). Each of these enzymes has a significant incidence of polymorphisms that affect drug disposition and correlate with toxicity. Persons with the UGT1A1*28 homozygous 7/7 genotype have a reduced capacity for glucuronidation as the major metabolic pathway of SN-38 and higher drug exposure (AUC). Several studies have confirmed a significant correlation between the SN-38 exposure, 1A1*28 genotype and severe neutropenia.[46] Pharmacogenetic profiling offers the prospect of individualized dose selection in the future and is a frequent component in early clinical drug development. These DNA-based tests are not commercially available yet and have no clinical role at the present time.

Cytochrome P450 3A4 (family 3, subfamily A, polypeptide 4) is the most prevalent metabolic enzyme in humans and is responsible for more than 55% of drug metabolic clearance.[47] Recent studies utilizing noncancer drugs as indicators of *CYP3A4* metabolic activity, such as the erythromycin breath test, suggest potential clinical utility with agents that are metabolized by this pathway—docetaxel.[48] At present, these alternatives (except for carboplatin AUC dosing) remain under investigation, and BSA-based dosing remains the standard of clinical practice.

All the molecularly targeted tyrosine kinase inhibitors approved for clinical use as well as the many more in clinical development are administered as a flat dose with no adjustment for weight or BSA.

Real-Time Pharmacokinetics and Patient Safety

Pharmacokinetic studies provide important information regarding the dose effect. Such studies indicate substantial variation in serum drug levels and in the AUC per given dose. For methotrexate and 6-MP in acute leukemia and for high-dose busulfan and carmustine (BCNU) in the transplant setting, the AUC level of drug or its active metabolites (or both) correlates with toxicity and therapeutic effect.[49-53]

Substantial variation in the AUC per given dose of paclitaxel was also observed in patients with solid tumors. Real-time adjustment of dose on subsequent days significantly reduced mucositis requiring morphine administration and decreased the duration of hospital stay.[54]

Dose Effect in Sensitive Tumors

Few clinical studies have included dose intensity as an independent, randomized variable. In a Cancer and Leukemia Group B (CALGB) study, 596 patients with AML were randomized to receive four 5-day courses of cytarabine at one of three dose schedules: (1) 100 mg/m^2 daily ("standard arm"); (2) 400 mg/m^2 by continuous-infusion; or (3) 3 g/m^2 in a 3-h infusion every 12 h (twice daily) on days 1, 3, and 5.[2] For patients 60 years of age or younger, the probability of remaining in continuous complete remission after 4 years was 24% in the 100 mg/m^2 group; 29% in the 400 mg/m^2 group; and 44% in the 3 g/m^2 group (p = .002), indicating a better response with increased dose. Elderly patients were less responsive. In acute lymphocytic leukemia (ALL), the dose rate of maintenance chemotherapy had a major impact on the duration of response.[55] Similarly, in studies of combination chemotherapy in small cell lung cancer, the dose effect was significant, albeit with outmoded therapy.[56]

Dose–response effects are less well studied in the new kinase inhibitors, which tend to be dosed at the maximum-tolerated daily dose, leaving little opportunity for significant increases. Increasing doses of imatinib in patients with chronic phase or accelerated phase CML show an increase in response rate in a subgroup of patients. In cases where resistance to imatinib is due to increased metabolic clearance, increased activity of PgP or amplification of the *BCR-ABL* gene, this might be expected although responses were seen even in patients with mutations in the *BCR-ABL* kinase itself.[21,22]

In treating individual patients, dose is a key factor if cure is possible. Thus, for leukemias, lymphomas, testicular cancer, childhood solid tumors, and conventional dose adjuvant treatment of breast cancer, dose should not be compromised even at the risk of significant toxicity. For more resistant tumors, where palliation is the goal, dose should be adjusted primarily on the basis of toxicity.

Peripheral-Blood Stem Cell and Marrow Transplantation

Allogeneic bone marrow transplantation produces disease-free survival (DFS) plateaus (ie, cures) in patients with acute and chronic leukemias and lymphomas, but because of the effect of graft versus leukemia, the component contributed by dose cannot be independently evaluated.

The most compelling evidence regarding dose–response is in high-dose, autologous stem cell rescue studies in patients with relapsed lymphoma.[57,58] Alkylating agents and total body radiotherapy-based regimens are commonly used because their dose-limiting toxicity is myelosuppression. Depending on the agent, dose can be escalated between 3 and 20 times baseline before non-myelosuppressive toxicity becomes dose-limiting. Given the considerable overlap of AUCs for serum levels of drugs at dose escalations of 2-4 times baseline, the escalations possible with stem cell support allow better comparisons of the effect of dose. High-dose therapy with autologous stem cell rescue produces high complete response rates and cures in non-Hodgkin's lymphoma and testicular cancer.[57,59] But because toxicity can be lethal, high-dose therapy should be limited to specialized centers.[60]

Adjuvant Chemotherapy

Randomized Studies ■ Cytokinetics provides an experimental basis for many therapeutic designs. A brief review of the related history follows.

Skipper and colleagues established the fundamental exponential relationship between drug treatment and surviving tumor fractions. It is the fractional tumor cell reduction that is constant for a given dose and drug.[12] Although this exponential relationship is modified by other factors, such as drug resistance and microenvironment, it remains the fundamental tenet of cytokinetics and chemotherapy. Norton and Simon applied Gompertzian theory and analysis to treatment during remission and demonstrated the potentially greater effectiveness of late intensification.[61] Goldie and Coldman introduced the mutation-to-resistance theory, relating tumor burden and inherent mutation rate to potential for cure.[62] Hryniuk and colleagues found a significant dose–response effect not only in the leukemias and lymphomas, but also in the relatively less chemosensitive tumors, such as breast cancer.[63-65]

The adjuvant setting, where the tumor burden is microscopic, should be ideal for demonstrating a dose effect. There, many factors that could reduce tumor cytotoxicity (tumor size, decreased and abnormal vascularity, low-GF, hypoxia, and increased tumor heterogeneity) and contribute to chemotherapy resistance are less evident in the microscopic tumor (adjuvant) setting. "Standard" combination chemotherapy with cyclophosphamide, methotrexate, and 5-FU (CMF) or with cyclophosphamide, doxorubicin (Adriamycin), and 5-FU (CAF), which produce only transient partial and a few complete responses in metastatic breast cancer, reduce relapse and mortality rates by 20-30% in the adjuvant breast cancer setting.[66] Similar effects are seen in colon cancer.[67]

Attempts to improve DFS by increasing the adjuvant chemotherapy dose in breast cancer have produced complicated results. The first statistically robust positive study was conducted by the CALGB.[16] Patients with node-positive breast cancer were randomized to one of three CAF regimens.[16] The high-dose arm involved 4 courses of CAF at doses of 600 cyclophosphamide, 60 doxorubicin, and 600 mg/m^2 5-FU every 3-4 weeks; in the low-dose arm, the doses were 300, 30, and 300 mg/m^2 respectively. A 10% difference in the relapse-free curve developed by 2 years and has persisted through 10 years. That result represents an approximately 20% reduction in mortality. The dose effect was seen most prominently in the 20% of patients whose tumors overexpressed *ERBB2* (*HER2/neu*). For tumors without *ERBB2* overexpression, no significant dose effect was seen.[17] This subset effect would not have been identified in the absence of the molecular marker.

Two other studies conducted by the National Surgical Adjuvant Breast and Bowel Project (NSABP) failed to show that a 2 or 4 times increase in the dose of cyclophosphamide alone affected response in terms of relapse or survival in adjuvant breast cancer.[68,69] Thus, in the comparative study of CAF, the dose of Adriamycin was probably important; however, in another study of adjuvant breast cancer, patients randomized to three doses of Adriamycin (60, 75, and 90 mg/m^2, all given with the standard-dose of cyclophosphamide) showed no difference in DFS or overall survival (OS). The 60 mg/m^2 is probably a threshold dose, above which no further benefit accrues.

The basis for the seemingly discordant results of dose in major clinical trials has been the subject of preclinical and mechanism-of-action studies, but it remains unexplained. We remain humble before the heterogeneity of human cancer, which permits such seemingly contradictory results. It can be speculated how often in the analysis of large comparative studies an important effect has been missed within a subset not known to exist at the time. That possibility is an important limitation in the interpretation of negative studies.

Dose-Dense Chemotherapy

The concept behind dose-dense chemotherapy is to increase the intensity of drug administration by shortening the interval between treatments without increasing the total dose of drug administered. This increase is accomplished by escalating the dose or the number of cycles in a given period of time. The use of neutrophil colony stimulating factors is an essential requirement for dose-dense therapy. Interim reports on the CALGB 9741 study, the use of dose-dense therapy with cyclophosphamide, doxorubicin, and paclitaxel in adjuvant breast cancer, either concurrently or sequentially in 2-week as opposed to the standard 3-week cycles significantly reduced the annual risk of recurrence or death. The DFS (risk ratio [RR] 0.74, *p* 0.10) and OS (RR 0.69, *p* 0.013) were prolonged in the dose-dense arms. There was no difference in either DFS or OS between sequential and concurrent therapy. There was no interaction between dose-density and sequence. This preliminary report supports the concept of dose-dense intensification as a means to enhance chemotherapy efficacy, albeit at a cost of increased toxicity.[70]

High-Dose Therapy Requiring Stem Cell Support

As mentioned earlier, the most compelling tests of dose escalation are the high-dose programs that require stem cell rescue. These programs have proven curative for a subset of hematologic neoplasms and have been investigated in epithelial solid tumors. The high-dose regimens generally involve combinations of alkylating agents, notably in breast cancer. Reports concerning five of the high-dose breast cancer studies showed survival benefit.[71-75] Two trials that have come to maturity have shown a reduced risk of relapse, but no improvement in OS—although for some patients with *ERBB2*-negative tumors, a trend toward a survival benefit was seen.[76,77] It is agreed that in patients with breast cancer treated in the adjuvant setting, the use of high-dose chemotherapy has no established role and that such endeavors should remain investigational.[78,79] Better identification of chemotherapy-sensitive subsets may select a more appropriate patient population for future studies.

Summary

In the clinic, the effect of dose correlates generally with the basic chemosensitivity of the tumor. Thus Burkitt lymphoma, ALL, and testicular cancer are all highly sensitive and highly responsive to dose intensity, including achievement of cure. On the other hand, relatively insensitive tumors such as gastrointestinal and lung cancers and melanoma respond poorly to chemotherapy and are therefore not significantly affected by dose. There are clearly unknown factors at work in the human cancer patient, with the complex milieu of the inherent genetic background in the particular cell type and patient in which cancer arises, the effect of somatic and nontransformed stromal cells, the emerging role of cancer stem cells and other unappreciated factors not accounted for by the reductionist in vitro and in vivo models on which cancer researchers depend that continue to defy simple explanation.

Schedule of Drug Administration

Schedule Effects of Individual Agents

Cytarabine ■ Skipper and colleagues performed elegant, quantitative studies of L1210 mouse leukemia of the prototype cell cycle phase-specific agent cytarabine.[3,12] Schedule "sensitivity" was marked, ie, cytarabine given in courses of appropriate duration and with intervals that allowed for recovery of normal bone marrow produced optimal therapeutic effects. Extrapolating their work to human AML, the investigators gave patients repeated courses of a continuous-infusion for 5-7 days separated by 2-3 weeks for recovery. In patients with AML, that schedule produced a 30-40% complete response rate as compared with 10% for other schedules, such as daily intravenous administration.[3,80,81] The addition of daunorubicin to cytarabine further increased the complete response rate. (For details, see "Cytokinetics of Bone Marrow," earlier in this chapter.)

Gemcitabine ■ The dose-limiting toxicity of gemcitabine, a nucleoside analog structurally related to cytarabine, is myelosuppression.[81] Unlike cytarabine, gemcitabine has activity in solid tumors, particularly in pancreatic, breast, and non-small cell lung cancer. Weekly or biweekly bolus treatments are well tolerated, with toxicity largely limited to the marrow. Clinically and in experimental animals, gemcitabine given by continuous-infusion necessitates a marked reduction in dose, particularly because of myelosuppression, but also because of gastrointestinal toxicity and, in some circumstances, hypotension.[82]

Methotrexate ■ Intermittent methotrexate (5-day bolus courses every 3-4 weeks), developed by Li and colleagues for gestational choriocarcinoma, proved to be curative.[83] Goldin and colleagues demonstrated in L1210 mouse leukemia that intermittent methotrexate was superior to continuous (daily) methotrexate.[84] In a randomized, comparative study of patients with ALL in complete remission, intermittent methotrexate was significantly superior to daily therapy.[85] This empiric observation is consistent with subsequent findings by Schimke and colleagues, indicating that continuous exposure to methotrexate in vitro produces drug resistance more effectively than does intermittent methotrexate.[86] Moreover, with continuous administration, resistance results from gene amplification as compared with a transport defect following intermittent methotrexate.[86,87] The kinetics of bone marrow recovery and mucosal cell replacement, important in cytarabine scheduling, may be important clinical determinants of scheduling with methotrexate as well.

Fluoropyrimidines ■ In clinical studies, 5-FU is commonly administered in daily pulse doses of 350-450 mg/m^2 for 5 days. Using that schedule, myelosuppression is dose-limiting. Twice that dose can be delivered by continuous-infusion over 5 days, in which case mucositis and diarrhea become dose limiting.[88]

Fluorodeoxyuridine (FUDR) is much more toxic when delivered by continuous infusion than by intermittent bolus dosing. For example, daily doses in the range 30-50 mg/m^2 produce toxicity. The biochemical basis for the schedule difference is speculative. Continuous-infusion FUDR may have a greater effect on DNA synthesis; other schedules have a relatively greater effect on host tissue ribonucleic acid (RNA) and RNA synthesis.[88] Data regarding the effect of these differences in schedule on the therapeutic index are few. (Modulation with leucovorin is discussed later in this chapter.) Longer durations of systemic administration currently are under study.[89]

Thus, mechanisms of action, resistance, and cross-resistance for 5-FU appear to differ depending on the analog chosen and the schedule of administration, among other factors.[90]

Alkylating Agents ■ The alkylating agents are a heterogeneous group of compounds that have in common interaction with DNA. That interaction leads to malignant transformation of mammalian cells in culture and to carcinogenesis in patients.

The alkylating agents are of equal potency in terms of antitumor effect. The difference is primarily host toxicity. This variation in toxicity is particularly true for the dichloroplatinum group of compounds, which closely resemble X-radiation in terms of antitumor effect. They are substantially different in toxicity depending on the nature of the *trans*-adducts. Most experimental data regarding alkylating agents suggest that they are schedule independent, ie, the antitumor and host effects are dose-related, independent of schedule.[91] (see "Pharmacokinetics" and "Adjuvant Chemotherapy" earlier in this chapter for discussions of specific aspects of cyclophosphamide and ifosfamides.)

There is evidence that specific scheduling of cancer chemotherapy agents, at lower doses but more frequently, may have an antitumor effect mediated by an antiangiogenesis effect that may result from a cell death mechanism that differs from the mechanism in high-dose or standard-dose chemotherapy. This may reflect the different growth kinetics within tumor associated endothelial cells versus normal endothelial cells or ability to fixate potentially repairable damage only in endothelial cells when used with an agent that disrupts specific survival signals in endothelial cells, such as VEGF.[92,93] This finding is consistent with evidence that resistance is much more difficult to produce experimentally in normal tissues than in tumor tissues. A popular and partial explanation is the greater DNA repair capacity of normal tissues. This difference between normal and tumor tissue has major implications for basic and clinical chemotherapy.[94,95]

Anthracyclines ■ Cardiotoxicity is an important delayed toxicity of anthracyclines. In experimental studies, peak concentrations produced more cardiotoxicity for an equivalent dose than did lower concentrations achieved by continuous-infusion schedules. Weiss and Manthel first demonstrated that weekly doxorubicin administration produced less cardiotoxicity per total dose administered than did standard tri-weekly regimens.[96] Legha and colleagues demonstrated that a 4-day, continuous-infusion of doxorubicin every 3 weeks is less cardiotoxic than bolus injections, an observation confirmed in randomized studies.[97-99] Infusion approaches allow a 30-50% increase in total cumulative dose before cardiotoxicity develops. In experimental and preliminary clinical studies, liposomal doxorubicin may be less cardiotoxic than doxorubicin.[100,101]

Etoposide ■ An inhibitor of topoisomerase II that produces DNA double strand breaks, etoposide is selectively active against cells in cycle. Etoposide is commonly used in combination chemotherapy of solid tumors, particularly with cisplatin. Preclinical studies showed that etoposide must be present both during and immediately following cisplatin to achieve optimal effect, consistent with a possible interaction with cisplatin involving inhibition of DNA repair. In small cell lung cancer, the optimal etoposide dose schedule of 5 daily doses every 3-4 weeks is consistent with the discussion earlier in this chapter of marrow and tumor cytokinetics and response to cell cycle-specific agents.[102]

Tubulin Binders ■ Although the *Vinca* alkaloids vincristine and vinblastine are cell cycle-specific, no schedule appears superior to standard weekly dosing.[103,104] On the basis of limited data, the same is true for vinorelbine. Paclitaxel schedule considerations have been dominated by acute histamine-like toxicity, probably related to the vehicle (Cremophor EL); this toxicity is relieved by antihistamines and corticosteroids. Practical and economic considerations favoring outpatient use have resulted in 1-3 h intravenous infusions, although some randomized trials suggest an advantage for infusions that are even longer.[104] Myelosuppression correlates with the duration of plasma concentrations of paclitaxel above the threshold of 0.1 mol/L.[104] Neutropenia appears to be related more to schedule than to dose, although neuropathy appears dose related.[105]

General Use of Intermittent Dosing

For most chemotherapeutic agents that directly or indirectly target DNA or the mitotic spindle used alone or in combination, intermittent courses (eg, four 5-day courses every 3-4 weeks) are generally superior to other schedules such as continuous (ie, daily) dosing. Such is the case for cyclophosphamide and methotrexate in Burkitt lymphoma, methotrexate and actinomycin D in choriocarcinoma, melphalan in myeloma, cytarabine in AML, and methotrexate in ALL.[106] It is also true for combination regimens for Hodgkin disease, ALL, and childhood solid tumors.[103,106,107] In experimental and clinical studies alike, intermittent intensive treatment for rapidly proliferating tumors is superior. The reason may be recruitment of resting G0/G1 cells into active cycle. Continuous treatment may be superior for more indolent, low-GF tumors, but more-definitive studies are needed.[108]

Advances in supportive care now allow a novel approach to intermittent intensive chemotherapy. Neutrophil colony stimulating factors in dose-dense adjuvant breast cancer therapy[109] or leukapheresis following marrow recovery from chemotherapy and treatment with G-CSF allow the harvest of sufficient peripheral-blood circulating stem cells to rescue as many as four courses of moderately intensive chemotherapy.[110]

Continuous Administration

Protracted infusions (6 weeks) of 5-FU combined with local radiotherapy in adjuvant rectal cancer demonstrated both a lower local recurrence rate in the irradiated field and a reduced incidence of metastatic relapse.[111] Capecitabine is an orally absorbable agent that undergoes biotransformation to 5-FU. Prolonged administration over 14 days of capecitabine as a single-agent, repeated at 21-day intervals, shows a response rate that is superior to that of intravenous 5-FU and leucovorin, although no survival benefit accrues.[112,113] Capecitabine is also active in refractory breast cancer as monotherapy or in combination. The role of continuous fluoropyrimidine administration with capecitabine is being explored in combination chemotherapy and with radiation. The treatment interruption every 3 weeks does seem to significantly reduce dose-limiting hand-foot syndrome toxicity with capecitabine.

For reasons related to the mechanism-of-action of new targeted therapies such as imatinib in CML and in GIST, continuous low-dose oral administration will likely become increasingly important in the future.[108,114] The continued suppression of proliferative growth factor signals and interruption of survival pathway signals in tumor cells or the tumor vascular network appears necessary in the clinic and in preclinical models. One clinical trial of a randomized discontinuation of the multitargeted tyrosine kinase inhibitor sorafenib in renal cell cancer patients with stable disease demonstrated a significant progression free survival advantage at 6 months for patients who continued to receive sorafenib versus placebo, which supports the preclinical modeling in the clinic.[115]

Combination Chemotherapy

Rationales

The most compelling rationales for combination chemotherapy are (1) tumor cell heterogeneity and its implication for drug resistance, and (2) the success of combination chemotherapy in the clinic. In practical clinical terms, the selection of specific combinations in particular types of cancer depends on the individual activity of the agents in the target cancer type and the absence of overlapping toxicities. The agents with the highest single-agent activity are preferred, particularly agents that produce complete responses (if any such agents exist), with different mechanisms of action to address the theoretical heterogeneity issue.

Combination Chemotherapy in the Clinic

Ample clinical precedent exists for using multiple agents. An example is the treatment of ALL in children, where eight active agents have been identified. A direct correlation is seen between the number of agents used and the cure rate (Table 45-2). In fact, essentially all curative chemotherapy involves combinations of two and usually three or more agents (Table 45-3).

Current studies have demonstrated evidence for synergy or an additive effect between established DNA/mitotic spindle targeted chemotherapeutic agents and agents representing other classes. When used in combination, tamoxifen is additive and sometimes synergistic. Molecularly targeted agents, whether monoclonal antibodies or small molecules, have been combined with both cytotoxic agents as well as with other similarly targeted agents. Herceptin, a monoclonal antibody to *ERBB2*, is synergistic with doxorubicin and paclitaxel. *ERBB2* is present on the cancer cell surface in 15-25% of patients with breast cancer and benefit is restricted to only those patients with amplification of the *ERBB2* gene[70,116] toxicities may be substantial, however. Herceptin in combination with doxorubicin increased cardiac toxicity. A lesser risk of cardiac toxicity exists when Herceptin is included in paclitaxel combinations. The addition of a complement-fixing monoclonal antibody, rituximab, to cyclophosphamide, hydroxydaunomycin, vincristine sulfate and prednisone chemotherapy in non-Hodgkin lymphoma increases response without an increase in toxicity. All-*trans*-retinoic acid (ATRA) and arsenic trioxide interact with acute progranulocytic leukemia cells with resultant differentiation and remission. Cure, however, requires the addition an anthracycline. This compatibility of new and old is not to be assumed, since combinations of cytotoxic chemotherapy with both erlotinib and gefitinib fail to produce significant benefit in lung cancer.[117]

The combination of multiple targets in a single molecule can be incorporated into novel molecularly targeted agents. Certainly, multiple targets within a single agent, such as VEGFR and PDGFR, in the angiogenesis pathways produces greater clinical benefit than targeting either alone, as the success, limited as it may be, of single-agent sorafenib and sunitinib demonstrate viz single-agent, including bevacizumab and many failed compounds limited to VEGFR2 alone.[9]

Tumor Cell Heterogeneity and Drug Resistance

Tumors are clonal in origin, but the increasing DNA instability that accompanies the onset of neoplasia leads to increased variation in the daughter cells, called "clonal evolution to tumor cell heterogeneity." This evolution is associated with selection for progeny with greater survival capacity, which is evident as higher proliferative capacity, resistance to apoptosis, greater metastatic or invasive potential, reduced dependence on normal cellular growth factors, and angiogenesis.[118] Heterogeneity among tumor cells increases the number and diversity of potential target sites for chemotherapy and the need to combine therapeutic agents.

Initially, resistance was thought to be limited to the selecting agent (monodrug resistance). The recognition of multidrug resistance required a reexamination of this rationale for combination chemotherapy.[119] The ABC family of transport proteins such as (*ABCB1*, PgP), the multidrug resistance proteins (*ABCC1*), and the breast cancer–related protein (*ABCG2*) confer multidrug resistance that relates almost exclusively to natural products. Prolonged exposure to low doses of substrate drugs such as doxorubicin may overcome resistance mediated by these transport proteins.[120] However, glutathione transferase, DNA repair capacity, and topoisomerase II alterations also may be associated with multidrug resistance.[121]

Recent studies of multicellular drug resistance indicate an altered set point for apoptosis.[122] Differences between in vitro and in vivo drug resistance are modifying the approach to combination chemotherapy.[123] Although prolonged drug exposure results in stable, resistant cell lines, acute exposure may induce short-term, reversible resistance. How the short-term resistance relates mechanistically to the long-term, presumably genetic, resistance is under study.

Cytokinetics ■ The discovery that solid tumors contain a large number of potentially clonogenic cells in G1 or G0—presumably because of tumor hypoxia and a low GF—provided a basis for combination chemotherapy.[24,25,30] Thus, cell cycle-specific agents were employed to kill mitotically active cells, and noncell cycle-specific agents (eg, alkylating agents) were added to damage the noncycling tumor cells. The use of repeated cycles allows normal tissues to recover, so that dose need not be compromised, and G0/G1 tumor cells can be recruited into the proliferating fraction by increased availability of nutrients, oxygen, and vascular access.

Synchronization ■ Synchronization of tumor or normal cells in vitro and in vivo with drugs that inhibit DNA synthesis or that arrest cells in mitosis can be achieved. Experimentally, the most impressive synchronization has been achieved with hormonal agents that affect tumor, but not essential normal cells.

Some degree of tumor cell synchrony follows this hormonal manipulation in experimental studies but the heterogeneity of human tumors with regard to the

Table 45-3 ■ **Cancer Chemotherapy—Number of Agents Required for Cure by Tumor Type**

Tumor	No. of Agents Required for Cure	Adjuvant or Neoadjuvant	No. of Agents Required for Cure
Acute lymphoblastic leukemia (children)	4-7	Wilms tumor	2-3
Gestational choriocarcinoma[a]		Embryonal rhabdosarcoma	2-3
Early	1-3	Osteogenic sarcoma	3
Advanced	2-4	Soft tissue sarcoma	3
Acute myeloid leukemia	3+	Ovarian cancer	3-4
Testicular cancer	3	Breast cancer	2-4
Burkitt lymphoma[b]	1-4	Colorectal cancer	2
Hodgkin disease	4-5	Non-small cell lung carcinoma, stage IIIA	2
Diffuse histiocytic lymphoma	4-5	Small cell lung carcinoma, limited	2-4

[a]One agent is curative, but a higher cure rate results with two or more agents.
[b]One agent cures state 1 African Burkitt lymphoma, but two or more agents are better.

time course of recruitment and synchronization has limited this approach, and it remains investigational.[124,125]

Modulation ■ Agents that are nontoxic may still improve the therapeutic index of an established chemotherapeutic agent, either by reducing normal-tissue toxicity, as leucovorin does for methotrexate, for example, or by preferentially enhancing antitumor efficacy, as 5-FU and leucovorin do in metastatic and adjuvant colon cancer studies.[126-137]

Biochemically, the product of 5-FU, fluorodeoxyuridine monophosphate (FdUMP), binds to the substrate site of thymidylate synthase (TS), thus inhibiting DNA synthesis and, therefore, cellular replication. The stability and duration of this inhibition directly relate to a third agent, 5,10-methylenetetrahydrofolate, which is a metabolic product of leucovorin that also binds to thymidylate synthase, producing the so-called ternary complex (FdUMP—TS—5, 10-methylenetetrahydrofolate). In preclinical systems, in vitro and in vivo alike, leucovorin favorably modulated the therapeutic index of 5-FU. A number of clinical trials comparing 5-FU to 5-FU with leucovorin indicated an advantage for 5-FU/leucovorin in patients with metastatic colorectal cancer at a cost of only moderately increased mucositis and diarrhea. The combination of 5-FU with leucovorin improved survival rates in two separate studies in metastatic and adjuvant colon cancers.[127,128,136,137]

Bevacizumab (Avastin) is a monoclonal antibody that depletes serum vascular endothelial growth factor (VEGF). VEGF is an essential mitogenic and antiapoptotic factor for endothelial cells (see Chapter 11). Signaling through the VEGF receptor-2 (KDR) and platelet-derived growth factor receptor beta (PDGFRB) act to increase endothelial cell permeability, which results in increased interstitial fluid pressure (IFP) within tumors. In colon, breast, lung, head and neck, cervix, and skin carcinomas, the IFP is significantly higher than in normal tissues.[138-141] Increased tumor IFP acts as a barrier for tumor transvascular transport; reduction of tumor IFP, or modulation of microvascular pressure, increases the transvascular transport of tumor-targeting antibodies or low molecular weight tracer compounds.[142,143] Growing evidence indicates that the PDGFRB and KDR tyrosine kinases play a crucial role in increased tumor IFP. That makes them candidate targets for pharmacologic intervention for tumor interstitial hypertension[144-147] and for a novel, possibly general, combination strategy that will enhance the therapeutic effects of standard chemotherapeutics. Bevacizumab reduced the IFP in patients with advanced colorectal cancer and increases the uptake of gadolinium in the tumors.[147] Combined with irinotecan, 5-FU, and leucovorin, bevacizumab produces a significant prolongation of survival in patients with metastatic colorectal cancer.[148] This modulation of IFP occurs only within tumors and provides a selective increase in drug levels to the tumor without increasing host toxicity, as was noted in both of the latter two studies. Those findings offer a general treatment strategy for solid tumors of any type.

Implications of Drug Resistance

Tumor cell heterogeneity in response to the potentially cytotoxic and antiproliferative effects of cancer chemotherapeutic agents has been the stimulus for a current novel approach to combination chemotherapy. Avoiding therapeutic resistance has been from the beginning a major rationale for combination chemotherapy.

Initial observations about resistance involved reduced drug levels at the site of action because of increased efflux, alteration or amplification of the target, and cellular inactivation. Recent investigations have focused on mechanisms of drug sensitivity or resistance operative after interaction of the drug and its target receptor, including apoptosis (programmed cell death). The varying cell damage caused by various chemotherapeutic agents has the common property of triggering the apoptosis cascade in an active process that requires energy, enzymes, and cytostructure for completion.[149]

In addition to apoptosis, under certain circumstances cells undergo necrotic cell death due to drug induced depletion of ATP.[150] Finally, autophagy, a highly conserved process of cell survival under conditions of nutrient and or oxygen deprivation can lead to a previously unappreciated form of drug resistance following treatment with cytotoxic drugs, hormonal agents and radiation.[151] Drug resistance must always be viewed in the context of therapeutic index. Resistance fundamentally means there exists no selective cancer cytotoxicity in relation to toxicity in the cancer-bearing host. This may be present at the outset or become apparent only during therapy. This narrow or lack of therapeutic index is present in most cancer therapeutic agents.

Reversal of Drug Resistance

Another approach to modulation involves reversal of drug resistance, the most studied of which is multidrug resistance mediated by PgP. Verapamil and several other lipid-soluble heterocyclic drugs, including cyclosporine analogs, can inhibit PgP and thus reduce the efflux of a number of natural antitumor products (doxorubicin, vincristine, taxanes, and others) from the cell, thereby increasing cytotoxicity. PgP is increased in B-cell tumors, AML, sarcoma, and tumors previously treated with drugs that led to multidrug resistance.[152] This approach has not yet produced significant clinical benefit in clinical trials or practice.[153]

The modulation of alkylating agents and cisplatin also is under study. Glutathione may combine chemically with alkylating agents, thus diminishing their activity. Amifostine, a thiol that quenches DNA-damaging species, reduces the nephrotoxicity of cisplatin and the mucositis of irradiated sites.[154,155]

Molecular Biology/Targeted Therapy

Implications for Dose and Schedule

The level of optimism among researchers has increased substantially as a result of recent "proof of concept" regarding the clinical effectiveness of more-targeted therapies. Evidence for unique molecular targets in cancer cells (eg, fusion genes, mutations, recombinations) and on their surfaces has led to synthesis of small molecules and monoclonal antibodies with a target specificity never before achieved in cancer therapeutics.[156-158]

Table 45-1 presents a sampling of combinations of molecules and biochemical pathways that are currently being evaluated as targets for selective antitumor agents. The magnitude of such activity and the number of active agents in preclinical systems offer remarkable opportunities for the use of agents in combination. The cumulative effect of these agents on a molecular level suggests an interaction that may result from the diversity of target interaction and a sequential or simultaneous attack on critical cell behavior.

Another important area of diversity relates to anticipated toxicity. Thus, as compared with classical chemotherapy agents, where dose-delineating toxicity usually relates to proliferating tissues and is relatively uniform, the molecular biologic agents will almost certainly express toxicity that varies from agent to agent and that largely differs from the classical antitumor agents. Molecular agents are under extensive study not only for their antitumor properties, but also most particularly for their interaction with each other and with other established antitumor agents.

Experimental Models of Combination Therapy

The classical antitumor agents are limited largely to those that directly or indirectly produce DNA damage; the products of the molecular biology era markedly extend the diversity of target mechanisms. Indeed, using experimental models, a number of interesting preclinical experiments have demonstrated an additive or synergistic effect. The literature on preclinical models and computer analysis has been superbly reviewed by Rideout and Chou.[159]

The future of combination chemotherapy will be influenced substantially by the number of these compounds and their interactions. Certainly, the strategy of combining drugs whose mechanisms of action vary has been successful, even in the curative treatment of hematologic, childhood, and embryonal neoplasms.

The terms "additive" and "synergistic" are commonly used in the clinic, but are not well defined. In considering these terms, selectivity for the tumor as compared to the host—the *therapeutic index*—is the key. If two agents with additive therapeutic effect have a differing dose-limiting toxicity, so that the toxicity is nonadditive, the overall antitumor effect should be described as additive. When the effects are greater than "additive," the term "synergism" may be appropriate.

Table 45-4 presents the properties and comparisons of combination chemotherapy and combined modality therapy. Incorporation of many more classes of agents will force more efficient experimental designs. Such designs may include, for example, a rolling phase-II/phase-III study design. Increasingly, quantitative molecular markers and "real-time" pharmacology will be integrated operationally into clinical studies. The effectiveness of such related approaches should markedly improve the efficiency and effectiveness of clinical trials.

Oncogenes and tumor-suppressor genes may operate by modifying or exploiting abnormalities in the cell cycle such as cyclin-D, which is commonly overexpressed in some of the epithelial solid tumors and mantle cell lymphoma, and by interfering with growth factors and angiogenesis, which are required in varying degrees for all tumors. Proteasomes, which facilitate the ubiquination of peptides and thus their removal from the cell, telomerase, and the cell cycle provide additional attractive targets for a pharmacodynamic modulatory approach. Opportunities for using such agents in combination represent major areas for preclinical and particularly clinical research.

In summary, targeted therapies provide an extension in our ability to apply and benefit from the use of cancer chemotherapeutic agents in combination.

An Integrated Approach to Cancer Chemotherapy (Holotherapy)

More than a half-century has elapsed since cancer chemotherapy began. The chemotherapy agents now in use originated as biologically targeted therapy. Hitchings and Elion developed specific inhibitors of purine synthesis such as 6-MP and 6-TG; Heidelberger targeted RNA synthesis with 5-FU; and Farber targeted the reduced folate pathway with aminopterin. These innovations not only provided the groundwork for cancer treatment, they also became tools for discovery of the basic workings of transformed cancer cells.

Natural products such as the *Vinca* alkaloids, anthracyclines, and taxanes were selected specifically for activity against cancer proliferation. These agents were combined with other classes of agents—eg, hormones, alkylating agents, and irradiation—that are active against proliferating cells. The optimal use of the new agents requires their integration into increasingly complex combinations so that a greater therapeutic index results. The same is true for the current classical chemotherapeutic agents, which largely inhibit proliferation.

Molecular biology particularly has expanded the number of classes. Thus, hormones, immunotoxins, and inhibitors of invasion and metastasis are available in addition to the classical antiproliferation compounds. Receptors of unique structure and quantity, capable of interactions with the more heterogeneous specific molecular site targets, have recently been described.[105,108,125]

It has become readily apparent that the vast majority of cancers will be treated successfully only with combinations of agents chosen for the highest possible individual activity against a specific type of cancer. Ideally, such drugs will have different dose-limiting toxicities. Empiricism was an essential component in the development of contemporary cancer therapy, but rational drug discovery, analog development, preclinical modeling, precise pathologic diagnosis, careful staging of disease, and clinical trial design are the foundation for the measure of success known today.

The breakthroughs in molecular biology have presented the cancer therapist with enormous opportunities and challenges. Based on these breakthroughs, a molecular diagnosis will be able not only to determine where and how cancer originates, but also the processes that are essential to its survival. The specific processes that initiate and propagate cancer have become the targets of unprecedented rational drug development (Table 45-1). Pharmaceutical technology provides not only small molecules, but also monoclonal antibodies, immunoconjugates, ribozymes, antisense RNA, and recombinant viruses.

The therapy of cancer now has the potential to combine agents with even more mechanisms of action to confront the heterogeneity of cancer with a wider array of therapeutics. Some of these combinations are now the standard of care, as improvements in response and survival demonstrate (Table 45-4). The challenges to be overcome include (1) clinical development of cytostatic agents without the expectation of significant acute toxicity; (2) combining of classes of targeted agents (Table 45-5) both molecular and biologic, with regard to dose and schedule; and (3) selection of the appropriate types of cancer and individual patients for a specific therapy.

With molecular biology playing an increasing role, the clinical and laboratory sciences that address the therapy of cancer will continue to accelerate toward cancer control.

Table 45-4 **Combination Chemotherapy vs Holotherapy**

Combination	Chemotherapy	Holotherapy
Diversity of agents	Drawn from one class, antiproliferative	Drawn from all classes[a]
Number of agents	2-5	4-12+
Toxicity	Bone marrow and gastrointestinal (steep dose), cardiac, neuralgic, pulmonary	Major diversity, including that relative to dose and toxicity; toxicity commonly nonadditive; limited, greater selection
Experimental design of clinical trials	Rigid, establishment	Flexible, innovative, semi-Bayesian; patient participation
Endpoints	Classical; R, dR, DFS, OS	MRT
Integration with basic science	Limited	Extensive, operational; PK, PD; targets

[a]Chemotherapy, immunotherapy, endocrinology, antiangiogenesis, antimatrix, gene therapy, control of cell cycle (anticyclins [*CDK* family], transcriptional control, antisense).

Abbreviations: DFS, disease-free survival; dR, duration of response; MRT, microbeam radiation therapy; OS, overall survival; PD, pharmacodynamics; PK, pharmacokinetics; R, response (partial or complete).

Table 45-5 Therapeutic Interaction Between Agents of Different Classes

Agent	Cancer Acted On
Chemotherapy + other systemic agent	
Chemo + immunotherapy	
Cisplatin + herceptin	Breast cancer
Taxol + herceptin	Breast cancer
CHOP + rituximab	Lymphoma
Chemotherapy → MRT → recovery of immunity → vaccine	
Minitransplant chemotherapy followed by allogeneic armed lymphocyte	
Chemotherapy + hormonal therapy	
Vincristine + prednisone	Acute lymphocytic leukemia
Chemotherapy + tamoxifen	Breast cancer
Chemotherapy + differentiation agent	
Daunorubicin + ATRA	Acute progranulocytic leukemia
Chemotherapy + antiangiogenesis	
IFL + bevacizumab	Colorectal cancer

Abbreviations: ATRA, all-*trans*-retinoic acid; IFL, irinotecan/5-fluorouracil/leucovorin; MRT, microbean radiation therapy.

Selected References

The complete reference list can be found at www.CANCERMEDICINE8.com

1. Frei E 3rd, Canellos GP. Dose, a critical factor in cancer chemotherapy. *Am J Med.* 1980;69:585–594.
2. Mayer RJ, Davis RB, Schiffer CA, et al. Intensive postremission chemotherapy in adults with acute myeloid leukemia. Cancer and Leukemia Group B. *N Engl J Med.* 1994;331:896–903.
3. Skipper HE, Schabel FM Jr, Wilcox WS. Experimental evaluation of potential anticancer agents. XXI. Scheduling of arabinosylcytosine to take advantage of its S-phase specificity against leukemia cells. *Cancer Chemother Rep.* 1967;51: 125–165.
4. Frei E 3rd. Combination cancer therapy. *Cancer Res.* 1972;32:2593–2607.
5. Frei E 3rd. Curative cancer chemotherapy. *Cancer Res.* 1985;45:6523–6537.
6. Tuberculosis Chemotherapy Trials Committee. Report to the British Medical Research Council. Various combinations of isoniazid with streptomycin or with PAS in the treatment of pulmonary tuberculosis. *Br Med J.* 1955;435:4911.
7. Law LW. Origin of the resistance of leukemic cells to folic acid antagonists. *Nature.* 1956;169:268–275.
8. Schnipper L. Clinical implications of tumor-cell heterogeneity. *N Engl J Med.* 1986;314:1423–1431.
9. LoRusso PM, Eder JP. Therapeutic Potential of novel selective-spectrum kinase inhibitors in oncology. *Expert Opin Invest Drugs.* 2008;17(7):1013–1028.
10. Frei E 3rd, Elias A, Wheeler C, et al. The relationship between high-dose treatment and combination chemotherapy. The concept of summation dose intensity. *Clin Cancer Res.* 1998;4:2027–2037.
11. Hryniuk W, Frei E 3rd, Wright FA. A single scale for comparing dose-intensity of all chemotherapy regimens in breast cancer: summation dose-intensity. *J Clin Oncol.* 1998;16:3137–3147.
12. Skipper HE, Schabel FM, Jary R, Wilcox WS. Experimental evaluation of potential anticancer agents. XIII. On the criteria and kinetics associated with "curability" of experimental leukemia. *Cancer Chemother Rep.* 1964;35:3–111.
13. Frei E 3rd, Cucchi C, Rosowsky A, et al. Alkylating agent resistance. In vitro studies of human cell lines. *Proc Natl Acad Sci USA.* 1985;82:2158–2162.
14. Frei E 3rd, Freireich EJ. Progress and perspectives in the chemotherapy of acute leukemia. *Adv Chemother.* 1965;2:269–289.
15. Bonadonna G. Karnofsky Memorial Lecture. Conceptual and practical advances in the management of breast cancer. *J Clin Oncol.* 1989;7:1380–1397.
16. Wood W, Budman D, Korzun A, et al. Dose and dose intensity of adjuvant chemotherapy for stage II, node-positive breast carcinoma. *N Engl J Med.* 1994;330:1253–1259.
17. Muss H, Thor A, Berry D, et al. c-*ErbB*-2 expression and response to adjuvant therapy in women with node-positive early breast cancer. *N Engl J Med.* 1994;330:1260–1266.
18. Eder JP Jr, Chan V, Wong J, et al. Sequence effect of irinotecan (cpt-11) and topoisomerase II inhibitors in vivo. *Cancer Chemother Pharmacol.* 1998;42(4):327–335.
19. Hennequin C, Giocanti N, Favoudon V. S-phase specificity of killing by docetaxel (Taxotere) in synchronized HeLa cells. *Br J Cancer.* 1995;71:1194–1198.
20. Dowsett M. Clinical development of aromatase inhibitors for the treatment of breast and prostate cancer. *J Steroid Biochem Mol Biol.* 1990;37(6):1037–1041.
21. Zonder JA, Pemberton P, Brandt H, Mohamed AN, Schiffer CA. The effect of dose increase in imatinib mesylate in patients with chronic or accelerated phase chronic myelogenous leukemia with inadequate hematalogic or cytogenetic response to initial treatment. *Clin Cancer Res.* 2003;9:2092–2097.
22. Kantarjian H, Pasquini R, Hamerschlak N, et al. Dasatinib or high-dose imatinib for chronic phase Chronic myelogenous leukemia after failure of first-line imatinib: a randomized phase 2 trial. *Blood.* 2007;109:5143–5150.
23. Gribben JG. Attainment of molecular remission. A worth-while goal? *J Clin Oncol.* 1994;12:1532–1534.
24. Norton L, Simon R, Brereton HD, Bogden AE. Predicting the course of Gompertzian growth. *Nature.* 1976;264:542–545.
25. Tannock I. Cell kinetics and chemotherapy. A critical review. *Cancer Treat Rep.* 1978;62:1117–1133.
26. Clarkson B, Ohkita T, Ota K, Fried J. Studies of cellular proliferation in human leukemia. I. Estimation of growth rates of leukemic and normal hematopoietic cells in two adults with acute leukemia given single injections of tritiated thymidine. *J Clin Invest.* 1967;46:506–529.
27. Clarkson B, Fried J, Strife A, et al. Studies of cellular proliferation in human leukemia. 3. Behavior of leukemic cells in three adults with acute leukemia given continuous-infusions of ^{3}H-thymidine for 8 or 10 days. *Cancer.* 1970;25:1237–1260.
28. Clarkson B, Strife A, Fried J, et al. Studies of cellular proliferation in human leukemia. IV.Behaviorofnormalhemotopoieticcellsin 3 adults with acute leukemia given continuous-infusions of 3H-thymidine for 8 or 10 days. *Cancer.* 1970;26:1–19.
29. Tannock I. Basic science of oncology. New York: McGraw–Hill; 1992:139–196.
30. Steel GG. The growth kinetics of tumors in relation to their therapeutic response. *Laryngoscope.* 1975;85:359–370.
31. Mendelsohn ML. The growth fraction. A new concept applied to tumors. *Science.* 1960;132:1496–1504.
32. Al-Hajj M, Clarke MF. Self-renewal and solid tumor stem cells. *Oncogene.* 2004;23: 7274–7282.
33. Dave S, Eder JP, Van de Woude GF, Boerner SA, LoRusso PM. The c-MET signaling pathway: its role in cancer and potential as a therapeutic target. *Clin Cancer Res.* 2009. 1567:2207–2214.
34. Engleman JA, Janne PA. Mechanisms of resistance to epidermal growth factor receptor tyrosine kinases in non-small cell lung cancer. *Clin Cancer Res.* May 15, 2008;14(10):2895–2899.
35. Brown JM, Wilson WR. Exploiting tumor hypoxia in cancer treatment. *Nat Rev Cancer.* 2004;4:437–447.
36. Leek RD, Stratford I, Harris AL. The role of hypoxia-inducible factor-1 in three-dimensional tumor growth, apoptosis, and regulation by the insulin-signaling pathway. *Cancer Res.* 2005;55:4147–4152.
37. Ward JF. DNA damage produced by ionizing radiation in mammalian cells: identities, mechanisms of formation, and reparability. *Prog Nucleic Acid Res Mol Biol.* 1988;35:95–98.
38. Ikuno N, Soda H, Watanabe M, Oka M. Irinotecan (CPT-11) and characteristic mucosal changes in the mouse ileum and cecum. *J Natl Cancer Inst.* December 20, 1995;87(24):1876–1883.
39. Collins JM, Dedrick RL, King FG, et al. Nonlinear pharmacokinetic models for 5-fluorouracil in man. Intravenous and intraperitoneal routes. *Clin Pharmacol Ther.* 1980;28:235–246.
40. Schaaf LJ, Dobbs BR, Edwards IR, Perrier DG. Nonlinear pharmacokinetic characteristics of 5-fluorouracil (5-FU) in colorectal cancer patients. *Eur J Clin Pharmacol.* 1987;32:411–418.
41. Baker SD, Verweij J, Rowinsky EK, et al. Role of body surface area in dosing of investigational anticancer agents in adults, 1991–2001. *J Natl Cancer Inst.* 2002;94:1883–1888.

46 Preclinical and Early Clinical Development of New Anticancer Agents

Daniel D. Von Hoff, MD ▪ Axcl-R. Hanauske, MD, PhD, MBA

Considering the rising death rates, it is obvious that there is a great need for development of new agents for treatment of patients with advanced cancer. There is also a newly perceived need for developing new agents that will be used to treat patients with "early cancer" (now referred to as intraepithelial neoplasia).[1-3] This latter approach for treating early cancer, referred to in the past as chemoprevention, represents a new concept that could have an enormous impact on the disease.[4-6]

In this chapter, we describe the fundamentals of development of new agents from discovery through the initial safety (phase 1) clinical trials. Along the way, we discuss a few studies that illustrate new methodologies introduced into drug development in recent years. This chapter largely concentrates on the development of new chemical entities and not on the development of biologic agents, although many of the principles outlined here also apply to the development of those agents.

As an overview, Figure 46-1 describes the classic stages in the development of a new agent. Using this basic process, there have been hundreds of agents developed for treatment of patients with a variety of malignancies as well as for treatment of early cancer. Although this is an impressive list of agents available to treat patients with a variety of cancers, it is—in the light of the biological diversity of the various types of cancer—obvious that we still need major additions to our armamentarium. Table 46-1 details all of the anticancer agents that are approved by the FDA and their officially approved indications. We provide that table because, as noted below, as new strategies are being developed for the proper testing of new agents, one has to be cognizant of the agents that are already approved for a specific indication. One must also be aware as to whether a new agent should be developed alone or in combination in a "front-line" setting or in a salvage or palliative setting. Only old agents have been approved with a broad label claim. Table 46-1 helps allow the design of pivotal clinical trials that will lead to approval by regulatory agencies and, most importantly, become available for the patients.

Evolution of the Discovery Process

Clinical Observation in the Discovery Process

As this chapter is being written, the process for discovery is changing rapidly. Initial anticancer drug discovery was based on important observations by clinicians and preclinical scientists. An example of such observations, where many feel the field of chemotherapy of cancer began, was the observation by Adair and Bogg in 1931 that troops in World War I exposed to sulfur mustard developed lymphoid and bone marrow hypoplasia.[7] They then used this very toxic agent, sulfur mustard, to treat a number of patients with cancer.. The agent had a limited effect. Further studies of the related nitrogen mustard (of World War II) demonstrated more substantial antitumor effects, particularly in patients with lymphoma.[8,9]

Another classic example of an astute observation by clinicians was when Farber and colleagues noticed that young patients with leukemia who were treated with liver extracts or folic acid had worsening of their leukemia.[10] They then treated the patients with folic acid antagonists and described the antileukemic activity of these antagonists.

Histocytotoxic Effects and Physiologic Observations

Just like the observation that mustard gases cause hypoplasia of lymph nodes, spleen, and bone marrow (with subsequent clinical activity of nitrogen mustard and other alkylating agents in patients with lymphoma), there have been a number of other correlations between specific histocytotoxicity (toxicity to a particular type of tissue) and clinical activity of an agent. One of the best examples is the finding that the agent streptozocin caused destruction of the islet cells in animals (leading to diabetes).[11] Streptozocin was tried and found to have clinical activity in patients with insulinomas (a histocytotoxic effect).[12]

In early animal toxicology studies, cisplatinum caused hypoplasia of the testes and ovaries in animals and was subsequently found to have substantial activity in patients with testicular or ovarian cancer.[13-15]

As an example of a physiologic observation leading to the development of a series of new anticancer agents, the physiologic observation that rat hepatomas incorporated more uracil than the surrounding normal liver led to the

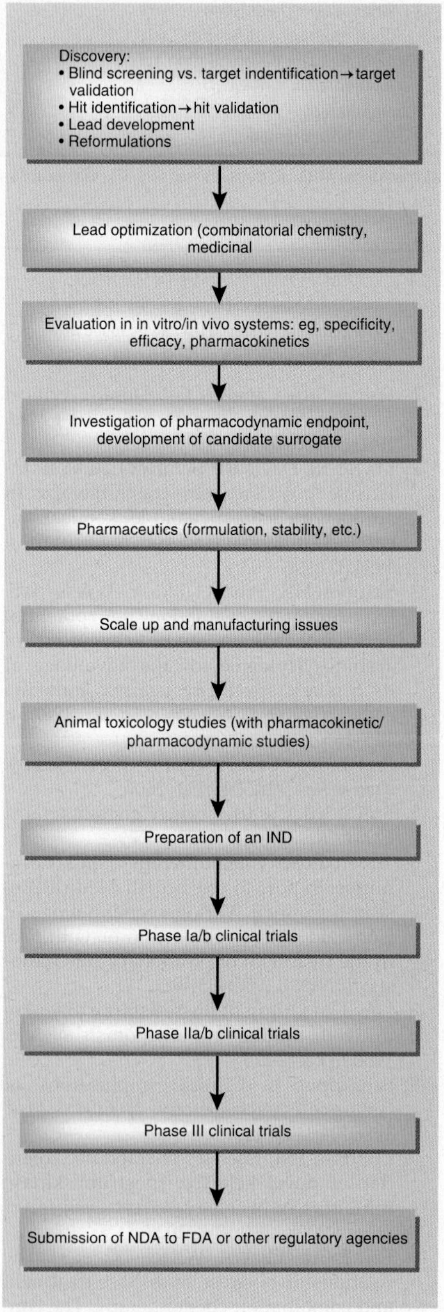

Figure 46-1 Classic stages in the development of a new anticancer agent. *Abbreviations:* IND, investigational new drug; NDA, new drug application.

Table 46-1 FDA-Approved Anticancer Agents and Their Indications[a]

Generic Name	Trade Name (Company)	Indication	Year[b]
Abarelix	Plenaxis depot (Praecis)	Advanced symptomatic prostate cancer, in whom LHRH agonist therapy is not appropriate and who refuse surgical castration, and have one or more of the following: (1) risk of neurological compromise due to metastases, (2) ureteral or bladder outlet obstruction due to local encroachment or metastatic disease, or (3) severe bone pain from skeletal metastases persisting on narcotic analgesia	2003
Aldesleukin	Proleukin (Chiron)	Adults with metastatic renal cell carcinoma Adults with metastatic melanoma	1992
Alemtuzumab	Campath (Berlex)	Treatment of B-cell chronic lymphocytic Leukemia (B-CLL) in patients who have been treated with alkylating agents and who have failed fludarabine therapy	2001
Alitretinoin	Panretin (Ligand)	Topical treatment of cutaneous lesions in patients with AIDS-related Kaposi sarcoma (KS), not indicated when systemic anti-KS-therapy is required	1999
Altretamine	Hexalen (MGI Pharma)	Single agent in the palliative treatment of patients with persistent or recurrent ovarian cancer following first-line therapy with a cisplatin and/or alkylating agent-based combination	1990
Aminolevulinic acid	Levulan Kerastick (Berlex)	Nonhyperkeratotic actinic keratoses of the face or scalp	1999
Anastrozole	Arimidex (Astra Zeneca)	First-line treatment of postmenopausal women with hormone receptor-positive or hormone receptor unknown locally advanced or metastatic breast cancer Advanced breast cancer in postmenopausal women with disease progression following tamoxifen therapy Adjuvant treatment of postmenopausal women with hormone receptor-positive early breast cancer	1995
Arsenic trioxide	Trisenox (Cell Therapeutics)	Second-line treatment of relapsed/refractory acute promyelocytic leukemia following ATRA plus an anthracycline	2000
Asparaginase	Elspar (Merck)	Acute lymphocytic leukemia, combination with other chemotherapeutic agents in the induction of remissions in pediatric patients	1978
Azacitidine	Vidaza (Pharmion)	Subtypes of myelodysplastic syndrome: refractory anemia (RA), RA with ringed sideroblasts (if accompanied by neutropenia or thrombocytopenia and requiring transfusions) RA with excess blasts RA with excess blasts in transformation, chronic myelomonocytic leukemia	2004
Bacille Calmette-Guérin (BCG) Live	Tice BCG (Organon)	Treatment of superficial bladder cancer	1998
Betamethasone	Celestone, Soluspan (Schering)	Celestone Hypercalcemia associated with cancer, Soluspan (Schering) mycosis fungoides, idiopathic thrombocytopenic purpura in adults, secondary thrombocytopenia in adults, erythroblastopenia, palliative management of leukemias and lymphomas in adults, palliative management of acute leukemia of childhood	1961
Bevacizumab	Avastin (Genentech/Roche)	Metastatic colon cancer First-line treatment of locally advanced, metastatic, or recurrent non-small cell lung cancer (NSCLC) in combination with platinum-based chemotherapy In combination with intravenous 5-fluorouracil-based chemotherapy for first-line treatment of patients with metastatic carcinoma of the colon or rectum	2006 2006 2004
Bexarotene	Targetin (Ligand)	*Oral*-cutaneous manifestations of cutaneous T-cell lymphoma in patients who are refractory to at least one prior systemic therapy *Topical*-patients with cutaneous t-cell lymphoma (stage IA and IB) who have refractory or persistent disease after other therapies or who have not tolerated other therapies	1999 2000
Bicalutamide	Casodex (Astra Zeneca)	Combination therapy with a luteinizing hormone-releasing hormone analog for the treatment of stage D2 metastatic carcinoma of the prostate	1995
Bleomycin	Blenoxane (Bristo-Myers Squibb)	Palliative treatment of squamous cell carcinoma: head and neck (including mouth, tongue, tonsil, nasopharynx, oropharynx, sinus, palate lip, buccal, mucosa, gingiva, epiglottis, skin, larynx), penis, cervix, and vulva Palliative treatment of lymphomas: Hodgkin's, reticulum cell sarcoma, lymphosarcoma Palliative treatment of testicular carcinoma: embryonal cell, choriocarcinoma, and teratocarcinoma Malignant pleural effusion and prevention of recurrent pleural effusions	1973 1996
Bortezomib	Velcade (Millennium)	Mantle cell lymphoma after at least one prior therapy Multiple myeloma patients after at least one prior therapy	2006 2005
Busulfan	Busulfex (IV formulation) (Orphan Medical) Myleran (oral formulation) (Glaxo SmithKline)	*Busulfex*-combination with cyclophosphamide as a conditioning regimen prior to allogeneic hematopoietic progenitor cell transplantation for chronic myelogenous leukemia *Myleran*-palliative treatment of chronic myelogenous (myeloid, myelocytic, granulocytic) leukemia	1999 1954
Capecitabine	Xeloda (Roche)	Metastatic breast cancer resistant to both paclitaxel and an anthracycline-containing chemotherapy regimen or resistant to paclitaxel and for whom further anthracycline therapy may be contraindicated Initial therapy of metastatic colorectal carcinoma when treatment with fluoropyrimidine therapy alone is preferred Combination chemotherapy has shown a survival benefit compared to 5-FU/LV alone A survival benefit over 5-FU/LV has not been demonstrated with Xeloda monotherapy In combination with docetaxel for metastatic breast cancer after failure of prior anthracycline containing chemotherapy Adjuvant treatment in patients with Dukes C colon cancer after complete resection when treatment with fluoropyrimidine therapy alone is preferred	1998 2001 2001 2001
Carboplatin	Paraplatin (Bristol-Myers Squibb)	Initial treatment of advanced ovarian carcinoma in established combination with other approved chemotherapeutic agents Palliative treatment of patients with ovarian carcinoma recurrent after prior chemotherapy, including patients who have been previously treated with cisplatin	1991 1989

(Continued)

Table 46-1 ■ **FDA-Approved Anticancer Agents and Their Indications[a] (Continued)**

Generic Name	Trade Name (Company)	Indication	Year[b]
Carmustine	BiCNU; BCNU (Bristol-Myers Squibb) Gliadel (MGI Pharma) Gliadel Wafer (Guilford Pharmaceuticals)	Palliative therapy as a single agent or in established combination therapy with other approved chemotherapeutic agents in: glioblastoma, brainstem glioma, medullo-blastoma, astrocytoma, ependymoma, and metastatic brain tumors Multiple myeloma—in combination with prednisone Hodgkin's disease—as secondary therapy in combination with other approved drugs in patients who relapse while being treated with primary therapy or who fail to respond to primary therapy Non-Hodgkin's lymphomas as secondary therapy in combination with other approved drugs for patients who relapse while being treated with primary therapy or who fail to respond to primary therapy Gliadel: Patient with malignant glioma undergoing primary surgical resection. Gliadel Wafer: Used in addition to surgery to prolong survival in patients with recurrent glioblastoma multiforme who qualify for surgery	1977 2003 1996
Celecoxib	Celebrex (Searle)	Reduction of polyp number in patients with the rare genetic disorder of familial adenomatous polyposis	1999
Cetuximab	Erbitux (Imclone)	In combination with Irinotecan for the treatment of EGFR expressing, metastatic colorectal carcinoma in patients who are refractory to Irinotecan-based chemotherapy Single agent: EGFR-expressing metastatic colorectal carcinoma in patients who are intolerant to irinotecan-based chemotherapy	2004
		In combination with radiation therapy (RT) for locally or regionally advanced squamous cell carcinoma of the head and neck (SCCHN) or as single agent for recurrent or metastatic SCCHN for whom prior platinum therapy has failed	2006
Chlorambucil	Leukeran (GlaxoSmithKline)	Chronic lymphatic (lymphocytic) leukemia, malignant lymphomas including lymphosarcoma, giant follicular lymphoma, and Hodgkin's disease	1957
Chromic phosphate P-32	Phosphocol P-32 (Mallinckrodt)	Peritoneal or pleural effusions caused by metastatic disease, and may be injected interstitially for the treatment of cancer	1974
Cisplatin	Platinol (Bristol-Myers Squibb)	Metastatic testicular tumors: in established combination therapy with other approved chemotherapeutic agents in patients with metastatic testicular tumors who have already received appropriate surgical and/or radio-therapeutic procedures Metastatic ovarian tumors: in established combination therapy with other approved chemotherapeutic agents in patients with metastatic ovarian tumors who have already received appropriate surgical and/or radio-therapeutic procedures; single agent is indicated as secondary therapy in patients with metastatic ovarian tumors refractory to standard chemotherapy who have not previously received cisplatin Advanced bladder cancer: single agent for patients with transitional cell bladder cancer that is no longer amenable to local treatments such as surgery and/or radiotherapy (Non–small-cell lung cancer: see gemcitabine, paclitaxel, vinorelbine)	1978
Cladribine	Leustatin, 2-cda (Ortho Bio-Tech)	Active hairy cell leukemia	1993
Clofarabine	Clolar (Genzyme)	Pediatric patients 1-21 years old with relapsed or refractory acute lymphoblastic leukemia after at least two prior regimens.	2004
Conjugated estrogens	Premarin (Wyeth-Ayerst)	Breast cancer (for palliation only) in appropriately selected women and men with metastatic disease Advanced androgen-dependent carcinoma of the prostate (for palliation only)	1938
Cortisone	Cortone (Merck)	Hypercalcemia associated with cancer, mycosis fungoides, idiopathic thrombocytopenic purpura in adults, secondary thrombocytopenia in adults, erythroblastopenia, palliative management of leukemias and lymphomas in adults, palliative management of acute leukemia of childhood	1950
Cyclophosphamide	Cytoxan, Neosar (Bristol-Myers Squibb)	Malignant lymphomas (Stages III and IV of the Ann Arbor staging system)	
	Neosar (Pharmacia)	Hodgkin's disease, lymphocytic lymphoma (nodular or diffuse), mixed-cell- type lymphoma histiocytic lymphoma, Burkitt lymphoma Leukemias: chronic lymphocytic leukemia, chronic granulocytic leukemia (it is usually ineffective in acute blastic crisis), acute myelogenous and monocytic leukemia, acute lymphoblastic (stem cell) leukemia in children (cyclophosphamide given during remission is effective in prolonging its duration) Multiple myeloma, mycosis fungoides (advanced disease), neuroblastoma (disseminated disease), adenocarcinoma of the ovary, retinoblastoma, carcinoma of the breast	1959
Cytarabine, liposomalDepoCyt (Chiron)		Intrathecal treatment of lymphomatous meningitis	1999
Cytarabine, ara-C	Cytosar-U (Pharmacia)	Combination with other approved anticancer drugs for remission induction in acute non-lymphocytic leukemia of adults and pediatric patients; it has also been found useful in the treatment of acute lymphocytic leukemia and the blast phase of chronic myelocytic leukemia; intrathecal administration of cytarabine is indicated in the prophylaxis and treatment of meningeal leukemia	1969
Dacarbazine	DTIC-Dome (Bayer)	Metastatic malignant melanoma Hodgkin's disease as a second-line therapy when used in combination with other effective agents	1975
Dactinomycin, actinomycin D	Cosmegen (Merck)	Wilms tumor, rhabdomyosarcoma, carcinoma of testis and uterus, palliative treatment of Ewing sarcoma and sarcoma botryoides	1964
Dasatinib	Sprycel (Bristol Myers Squibb)	Chronic myelogenous leukemia	2006
Daunorubicin	Cerubidine (Wyeth Ayerst)	Leukemia/myelogenous/monocytic/erythroid of adults/remission induction in acute lymphocyte leukemia of children and adults	1998

(*Continued*)

Table 46-1 ■ **FDA-Approved Anticancer Agents and Their Indications[a] (Continued)**

Generic Name	Trade Name (Company)	Indication	Year[b]
	Daunorubicin (Bedford Labs)	In combination with approved anticancer drugs for induction of remission in adult ALL	1998
Daunorubicin liposome	Dauno Xome (Nexstar)	First-line cytotoxic therapy for advanced HIV-associated Kaposi sarcoma	1996
Decitabine	Dacogen (MGI Pharma)	Myelodysplastic syndromes (MDS) including previously treated and untreated, de novo, and secondary MDA of all French-American-British subtypes and intermediate-1, intermediate-2, and high-risk International Prognostic Scoring System groups	2006
Denileukin difitox	Ontak (Ligand)	Patients with persistent or recurrent cutaneous T-cell lymphoma whose malignant cells express the CD25 component of theIL-2-receptor	1999
Dexamethasone	Decadron (Merck)	Hypercalcemia associated with cancer, mycosis fungoides, idiopathic thrombocytopenic purpura in adults, secondary thrombocytopenia in adults, erythroblastopenia, palliative management of leukemias and lymphomas in adults, palliative management of acute leukemia of childhood	1958
Diclofenac	Solaraze (SkyePharma)	Topical treatment of actinic keratoses	2000
Docetaxel	Taxotere (Aventis)	Locally advanced or metastatic breast cancer, which has progressed during anthracycline-based treatment or relapsed during anthracyclines-based adjuvant therapy	1998
		Locally advanced or metastatic NSCLC after failure of prior platinum-based chemotherapy	1999
		In combination with cisplatin for the treatment of patients with unresectable, locally advanced or metastatic NSCLC who have not previously received chemotherapy for this condition	2002
		In combination with prednisone as a treatment for patients with androgen independent (hormone refractory) metastatic prostate cancer	2004
		In combination with doxorubicin and cyclophosphamide for the adjuvant treatment of patients with operable, node positive breast cancer	2004
		In combination with cisplatin and fluorouracil for induction treatment of inoperable, locally advanced, squamous cell carcinoma of the head and neck	2006
Doxorubicin	Adriamycin (Pharmacia) Rubex (Bristol-Myers Squibb)	Acute lymphoblastic leukemia, acute myeloblastic leukemia, Wilms tumor, neuroblastoma, soft tissue and bone sarcomas, breast carcinoma, ovarian carcinoma, transitional cell bladder carcinoma, thyroid carcinoma, gastric carcinoma, Hodgkin's disease, malignant lymphoma, and bronchogenic carcinoma in which the small cell histologic type is the most responsive compared to other cell types	1974
		In combination with cyclophosphamide as a component of adjuvant therapy in patients with evidence of axillary node tumor involvement following resection of primary breast cancer	2003
Doxorubicin liposomal	Doxil (Alza, Sequus Pharmaceuticals)	Ovarian cancer that has progressed or recurred after platinum-based chemotherapy	2005
		Metastatic ovarian cancer refractory to both paclitaxel and platinum-based regimens	1999
		AIDS-related Kaposi sarcoma in patients with disease that has progressed on prior combination chemotherapy or in patients who are intolerant to such therapy	1995
Epirubicin	Ellence (Pharmacia) epirubicin hcl (Mayne)	Adjuvant therapy in patients with evidence of axillary node tumor involvement following resection of primary breast cancer	1999
Erlotinib	Tarceva (OSI)	Advanced or metastatic NSCLC after failure of at least one prior chemotherapy regimen	2004
		In combination with Gemcitabine as first-line treatment of locally advanced or metastatic pancreatic cancer	2005
Esterified estrogens	Estratab (Solvay) Menest (Monarch)	Breast cancer (for palliation only) in appropriately selected women and men with metastatic disease	1938
		Advanced androgen-dependent carcinoma of the prostate (for palliation only)	1938
Estradiol	Estrace (Bristol-Myers Squibb)	Breast cancer (for palliation only) in appropriately selected women and men with metastatic disease	1938
		Advanced androgen-dependent carcinoma of the prostate (for palliation only)	1938
Estradiol valerate	Delestrogen (Bristol-Myers Squibb)	Advanced androgen-dependent carcinoma of the prostate (for palliation only)	1938
Estramustine	Emcyt (Pharmacia)	Palliation of prostate cancer	1981
Estrone	Estrone (generic)	Breast cancer (for palliation only) in appropriately selected women and men with metastatic disease	1938
		Advanced androgen-dependent carcinoma of the prostate (for palliation only)	
Ethinyl estradiol	Estinyl (Schering)	Breast cancer (for palliation only) in Appropriately selected patients	1943
Etoposide	Toposar (Pharmacia) VePesid (Bristol-Myers Squibb)	Refractory testicular tumors in combination with other approved chemotherapeutic agents after appropriate surgical, chemotherapeutic, and radiotherapeutic therapy	1983
		First-line treatment of small-cell lung cancer in combination with other approved chemotherapeutic agents	1986
Etoposide phosphate	Etopophos (Bristo-Myers Squibb)	Refractory testicular tumors in combination with other approved chemotherapeutic agents.	1996
		First-line treatment of small-cell lung cancer in combination with other approved chemotherapeutic agents	1996
		Refractory testicular and small cell lung cancer	1998
Exemestane	Aromasin (Pharmacia)	Advanced breast cancer in postmenopausal women whose disease has progressed following tamoxifen therapy	1999
Floxuridine	FUDR (Roche)	Palliative management of gastrointestinal adenocarcinoma metastatic to the liver, when given by continuous regional intra-arterial infusion in carefully selected patients who are considered incurable by surgery or other means	1970
Fludarabine phsophate	Fludara (Berlex)	Patients with B-cell chronic lymphocytic leukemia (CLL) who have not responded to or whose disease has progressed during treatment with at least one standard alkylating-agent containing regimen	1991

(Continued)

Table 46-1 ■ **FDA-Approved Anticancer Agents and Their Indications[a] (Continued)**

Generic Name	Trade Name (Company)	Indication	Year[b]
Fluorouracil	Adrucil (Pharmacia)	Palliative management of carcinoma of the colon, rectum, breast, stomach, and pancreas	1962
Fluorouracil	Efudex (ICN)	Topical treatment of actinic or solar keratoses; in the 5% strength, it is also useful in the treatment of superficial basal cell carcinomas when conventional methods are impractical	1962
Fluorouracil	Fluoroplex (Allergan)	Topical treatment of multiple actinic (solar) Keratoses	1962
Fluoxymesterone	Halotestin (Pharmacia)	Palliation of androgen-responsive recurrent mammary cancer in women who are more than 1 year but less than 5 years postmenopausal or who have been proven to have a hormone-dependent tumor as shown by previous beneficial response to castration.	1956
Flutamide	Eulexin (Schering)	Combination with LHRH agonists for the management of locally confined stage B2-C and stage D2 metastatic carcinoma of the prostate	1989
Fulvestrant	Faslodex (IPR)	Hormone-receptor-positive metastatic breast cancer in postmenopausal women, progression following antiestrogen therapy	2002
Gefitinib	Iressa (AstraZeneca)	As monotherapy for the treatment of patients with locally advanced or metastatic NSCLC after failure of both platinum-based and docetaxel chemotherapies	2004
Gemeitabine	Gemzar (Eli Lilly)	In combination with cisplatin first-line treatment of patients with inoperable, locally advanced (Stage IIIA or IIIB) or metastatic (Stage IV)NSCLC.	1998
		First-line treatment for patients with locally advanced (nonresectable Stage II or Stage III) or metastatic (Stage IV), adenocarcinoma of the pancreas; Pancreatic cancer after treatment with 5-FU	1996 2004 2006
		In combination with paclitaxel for first-line treatment of patients with metastatic breast cancer after failure of prior anthracycline-containing adjuvant chemotherapy, unless anthracyclines were clinically contraindicated. Ovarian cancer.	
Gemtuzumab ozogamicin	Mylotarg (Wyeth-Ayerst)	CD33-positive acute myeloid leukemia in first relapse who are 60 years of age or older and who are not considered candidates for cytotoxic chemotherapy.	2000
Goserelin acetate	Zoladex (AstraZeneca)	Palliative treatment of advanced carcinoma of the prostate in combination with flutamide for the management of locally confined Stage T2b-T4 (Stage B2-C) carcinoma of the prostate.	1989
		Palliative treatment of advanced breast cancer in pre- and perimenopausal women	1995
Granisetron	Kytril (Roche)	Prevention of nausea and vomiting associated with initial and repeat courses of emetogenic cancer therapy, including high-dose cisplatin	1993
Histelin	Acetate (Valera) Histrelin Implant	Palliative treatment of advanced prostate cancer.	2004
Hydrocortisone	Cortef, Solu-Cortef (Pharmacia) Hydrocortone (Merck)	Hypercalcemia associated with cancer, mycosis fungoides, idiopathic thrombocytopenic purpura in adults, secondary thrombocytopenia in adults, erythroblastopenia, palliative management of leukemias and lymphomas in adults, palliative management of acute leukemia of childhood	1951
Hydroxyprogesterone	Hydroxyprogesterone (Schein)	Endometrial cancer	1956
Hydroxyurea	Hydrea (Bristol-Myers Squibb)	Melanoma, resistant chronic myelocytic leukemia, and recurrent, metastatic, or inoperable carcinoma of the ovary. Hydroxyurea used concomitantly with irradiation therapy is intended for use in the local control of primary squamous cell (epidermoid) carcinomas of the head and neck, excluding the lip	1967
Ibritumomab tiuxetan	Zevalin (IDEC Pharmaceuticals)	Relapsed or refractory low-grade, follicular or transformed B-cell non-Hodgkin's lymphoma, including patients with rituximab refractory follicular non-Hodgkin's lymphoma	2002
Idarubicin	Idamycin (Adria Laboratories, Pharmacia)	In combination with other approved antileukemic drugs for the treatment of acute myeloid leukemia in adults	1990
		In combination with other approved antileukemic drugs for the treatment of acute nonlymphocytic leukemia in adults	1997
Ifosfamide	Ifex (Bristo-Myers Squibb)	Third-line chemotherapy of germ cell testicular cancer in combination with certain other approved antineoplastic agents: it should ordinarily be used in combination with a prophylactic agent for hemorrhagic cystitis, such as mesna	1992
Imatinib mesylate	Gleevec (Novartis)	Philadelphia chromosome positive chronic myeloid leukemia (CML) in blast crisis, accelerated phase, or in chronic phase after failure of interferon-alpha therapy.	2001
		Pediatric patients with recurrent Philadelphia chromosome positive chronic myeloid leukemia (CML) after stem cell transplant or resistance to interferon-alpha.	2003
		Kit (CD117) positive unresectable and/or metastatic malignant gastrointestinal stromal tumors (GIST).	2002
Interferon alfa-2a	Roferon-A (Roche)	Hairy cell leukemia	1986
		AIDS-related Kaposi sarcoma in patients 18 years of age or older	1996
		Chronic phase, Philadelphia chromosome-positive chronic myelogenous leukemia patients who are minimally pretreated (within 1 year of diagnosis)	1995
Interferon alfa-2b	Intron A (Schering)	Paients 18 years of age or older with hairy cell leukemia	1986
		Adjuvant to surgical treatment in patients 18 years of age or older with malignant melanoma who are free of disease but at high risk for systemic recurrence, within 56 days of surgery	
		Initial treatment of clinically aggressive follicular non-Hodgkin's lymphoma in conjunction with anthracycline-containing combination chemotherapy in patients 18 years of age or older	1997
		Patients 18 years of age or older with AIDS-related Kaposi sarcoma	1988
Irinotecan	Camptosar (Pharmacia)	First-line therapy in combination with 5-fluorouracil and leucovorin for metastatic carcinoma of the colon or rectum	1996
		Metastatic carcinoma of the colon or rectum after recurrence or progression following initial fluorouracil-based Therapy	1998
Lapatinib ditosylate	Tykerb	Advanced or metastatic breast cancer with overexpression of HER2 (ErbB2) in combination with capecitabine after prior therapy including anthracyclines, a taxane, and trastuzumab	2007

(Continued)

Table 46-1 FDA-Approved Anticancer Agents and Their Indications[a] (Continued)

Generic Name	Trade Name (Company)	Indication	Year[b]
Letrozole	Femara (Novartis)	First-line treatment of postmenopausal women with hormone receptor positive or hormone receptor unknown locally advanced or metastatic breast cancer; It is also indicated for the treatment of advanced breast cancer in postmenopausal women with disease progression following antiestrogen therapy	1997
Lenalidomide	Revlimid (Celgene)	Multiple myeloma	2006
		Transfusion-dependent anemia due to low- or intermediate risk myelodysplastic syndromes associated with a deletion 5q cytogenetic abnormality with or without additional cytogenetic abnormalities	2005
Letrozole	Femara (Novartis)	Advanced breast cancer in postmenopausal women.	1997
		First-line treatment of postmenopausal women with hormone receptor positive or hormone receptor unknown locally advanced or metastatic breast cancer.	2001
		Extended adjuvant treatment of early breast cancer in postmenopausal women who have received 5 years of adjuvant tamoxifen therapy.	2004
Leuprolide acetate	Lupron, Lupron Depot (TAP) Viadur (Bayer) Eligard (QLT USA)	Palliative treatment of advanced prostate cancer	1985
Levamisole	Ergamisol (Jansen Research Foundation)	Adjuvant treatment in combination with 5-fluorouracil after surgical resection in patients with Dukes' Stage C. colon cancer.	1990
Levothyroxine	Unithroid (Jerome Stevens)	Pituitary TSH suppression—as an adjunct to surgery and radioiodine therapy in the management of thyrotropin-dependent well-differentiated thyroid cancer	2000
Lomustine	CeeNU (Bristol-Myers Squibb)	Single agent in addition to other treatment modalities or in established combination therapy with other approved chemotherapeutic agents in: Brain tumors (both primary and metastatic) in patients who have already received appropriate surgical and/or radiotherapeutic procedures; Hodgkin's disease: secondary therapy in combination with other approved drugs in patients who relapse while being treated with primary therapy or who fail to respond to primary therapy	1976
Mechlorethamine	Mustargen (Merck)	Palliative treatment of Hodgkin's disease (Stages III and IV), lymphosarcoma, chronic myelocytic or chronic lymphocytic leukemia, polycythemia vera, mycosis fungoides, and bronchogenic carcinoma and metastatic carcinoma resulting in effusion	1949
Medroxyprogesterone	Depo-Provera (Pharmacia)	Adjunctive therapy and palliative treatment of inoperable, recurrent, and metastatic endometrial or renal carcinoma	1959
Medroxyprogesterone	Provera (Pharmacia)	To reduce the incidence of endometrial Hyperplasia in nonhysterectomized postmenopausal women receiving 0.625 mg conjugated estrogen	1959
Megestrol acetate	Megace (Bristol-Myers Squibb)	Palliative treatment of advanced carcinoma of the breast or endometrium	1971
Melphalan	Alkeran (GlaxoSmithKline)	*Oral*-palliative treatment of multiple myeloma and nonresectable epithelial carcinoma of the ovary	1964
		Injection-palliative treatment of patients with multiple myeloma for whom oral therapy is not appropriate.	1992
Mercaptopurine	Purinethol (GlaxoSmithKline)	Remission induction and maintenance therapy of acute lymphatic leukemia Acute myelogenous (and acute myelomonocytic) leukemia.	1953
Methotrexate sodium	Methotrexate (Immunex)	Gestational choriocarcinoma, chorioadenoma destruens, hydatidiform mole. Acute lymphocytic leukemia: prophylaxis of meningeal leukemia and maintenance therapy in combination with other chemotherapeutic agents; methotrexate is also indicated in the treatment of meningeal leukemia. Alone or in combination with other anticancer agents in the treatment of breast cancer, epidermoid cancers of the head and neck, advanced mycosis fungoides, and lung cancer, particularly squamous cell and small cell types: Methotrexate is also used in combination with other chemotherapeutic agents in the treatment of advanced stage non-Hodgkin's lymphomas Methotrexate in high doses followed by leucovorin rescue in combination with other chemotherapeutic agents is effective in prolonging relapse-free survival in patients with nonmetastatic osteosarcoma who have undergone surgical resection or amputation for the primary tumor	1953
Methoxsalen	8-MOP (ICN) Uvadex (Therakos)	Photopheresis in the palliative treatment of the skin manifestations of cutaneous T-cell lymphoma in persons who have not been responsive to other forms of treatment	1954
Methylprednisolone	Depo-Medrol, Medrol, Solu-Medrol (Pharmacia)	Hypercalcemia associated with cancer, mycosis fungoides, idiopathic thrombocytopenic purpura in adults, secondary thrombocytopenia in adults, erythroblastopenia, palliative management of leukemias and lymphomas in adults, palliative management of acute leukemia of childhood	1957
Methyltestosterone	Android, Testred (ICN)	Secondarily in women with advancing inoperable metastatic (skeletal) mammary cancer who are 1-5 year postmenopausal	1939
Metrosyne	Demser (Merck)	Chronic treatment of patients with malignant Pheochromocytoma	1979
Mitomycin C	Mutamycin (BristolMyers Squibb)	Disseminated adenocarcinoma of the stomach or pancreas in proven combinations with other approved chemotherapeutic agents and as palliative treatment when other modalities have failed	1974
Mitotane	Lysodren (BristolMyers Squibb)	Inoperable adrenal cortical carcinoma of both functional and nonfunctional types	1970
Mitoxantrone	Novantrone (Immunex)	In combination with corticosteroids as initial chemotherapy for the treatment of patients with pain related to advanced hormone refractory prostate cancer	1996
		In combination with other approved drug(s) in the initial therapy of acute non-lymphocytic leukemia in adults	1987

(Continued)

Table 46-1 ■ **FDA-Approved Anticancer Agents and Their Indications[a] (Continued)**

Generic Name	Trade Name (Company)	Indication	Year[b]
Nandrolone phenpropionate	Durabolin-50 (Organon)	Secondarily in women with advanced inoperable metastatic (skeletal) mammary cancer who are 1 or 5 year postmenopausal	1959
Nelarabine	Arranon (GlaxoSmithKline)	T-cell acute lymphoblastic leukemia and T-cell lymphoblastic lymphoma that has not responded or has relapsed following treatment with at least two chemotherapy regimens.	2005
Nilutamide	Nilandron (Aventis)	Combination with surgical castration for the treatment of metastatic prostate cancer (stage D2)	1996
Octreotide acetate	Sandostatin, Sandostatin LAR Depot (Novartis)	Severe diarrhea and flushing episodes associated with metastatic carcinoid tumors	1988
		Profuse watery diarrhea associated with vasoactive intestinal peptide (VIP)-secreting tumors	
Oprelvekin	Neumega (Genetics Institute)	Prevention of severe thrombocytopenia and the reduction of the need for platelet transfusions following myelosuppressive chemotherapy in patients with nonmyeloid malignancies who are at high risk of severe thrombocytopenia	2002
Oxaliplatin	Eloxatin (Sanofi-Synthelabo)	In combination with infusional 5-FU/LV, is indicated for the treatment of patients with metastatic carcinoma of the colon or rectum whose disease has recurred or progressed during or within 6 months of completion of first-line therapy with the combination of bolus 5-FU/LV and Irinotecan	2002
		In combination with infusional 5-Fluorouracil (5-FU) and Leucovorin (LV) for the treatment of patients previously untreated for advanced colorectal cancer.	2004
		In combination with infusional 5-FU/LV, for the adjuvant treatment of Stage III colon cancer patients who have undergone complete resection of the primary tumor	2004
Oxymet	Holone	Anadrol-50 (Unimed) Myelofibrosis, hypoplastic anemias owing to the administration of myelotoxic drugs	1960
Paclitaxel	Taxol (Bristol Myers Squibb)	Treatment of patients with metastatic carcinoma of the ovary after failure of first-line or subsequent chemotherapy	1992
	Paxene (Baker Norton)	Treatment of breast cancer after failure of combination chemotherapy for metastatic disease or relapse within 6 months of adjuvant chemotherapy. Prior therapy should have included an anthracycline unless clinically contraindicated	1993
		Second-line therapy for AIDS-related Kaposi's sarcoma	1997
		First-line treatment in advanced carcinoma of the ovary in combination with cisplatin	1998
		In combination with cisplatin indicated for the first-line treatment of NSCLC in patients who are not candidates for potentially curative surgery and/or radiation therapy	1998
		Adjuvant treatment of node-positive breast cancer administered sequentially to standard doxorubicin-containing combination chemotherapy. The benefit has been demonstrated only in patients with estrogen and progesterone receptor negative tumors	1999
Paclitaxel, protein-bound particles	Abraxane (AM Bioscience)	Treatment of breast cancer after failure of combination chemotherapy for metastatic disease or relapse within 6 months of adjuvant chemotherapy. Prior therapy should have included an anthracycline unless clinically contraindicated	2005
Panitumumab	Vectibix (Amgen)	As a single agent for the treatment of EGFR-expressing, metastatic colorectal carcinoma with disease progression on or following fluoropyrimidine-, oxaliplatin-, and irinotecan-containing chemotherapy regimens	2006
Pegaspargase	Oncaspar (Enzon)	Patients with acute lymphoblastic leukemia who require L-asparaginase in their treatment regimen but have developed hypersensitivity to the native forms of L-asparaginase	1994
Pemetrexed	Alimta (Lilly)	Alimta in combination with cisplatin is indicated for the treatment of patients with malignant pleural mesothelioma whose disease is either unresectable or who are otherwise not candidates for curative surgery	2004
		Alimta as a single-agent is indicated for the treatment of patients with locally advanced or metastatic NSCLC after prior chemotherapy	
Pentostatin	Nipent (Parke-Davis Pharmaceutical Co.)	Single-agent treatment for both untreated and alpha-interferon-refractory hairy cell leukemia patients with active disease as defined by clinically significant anemia, neutropenia, thrombocytopenia, or disease-related symptoms	1991
Plicamycin	Mithracin (Bayer)	Hospitalized patients with malignant tumors of the testis in whom successful treatment by surgery and/or radiation is impossible Hypercalcemia and hypercalciuria associated with a variety of advanced neoplasms	1970
Polifeprosan	Gliadel (Aventis)	Adjunct to surgery to prolong survival in patients with recurrent glioblastoma multiforme for whom surgical resection is indicated	1996
Porfimer sodium	Photofrin (Axcan Scandipharm)	Palliation of patients with complete obstruction esophageal cancer or of patients with partially obstructing esophageal cancer who, in the opinion of their physicians, cannot be satisfactorily treated with Nd:YAG laser therapy	1995
		Microinvasive endobronchial NSCLC for which surgery and radiotherapy are not indicated	1998
		Reduction of obstruction and palliation of symptoms in patients with completely or partially obstructing endobronchial NSCLC	1998
		Microinvasive endobronchial NSCLC in patients for whom surgery and radiotherapy are not indicated Ablation of high-grade dysplasia in Barrett's esophagus patients who do not undergo esophagectomy	2003
Prednisolone	Prelone (Muro)	Hypercalcemia associated with cancer, mycosis fungoides, idiopathic thrombocytopenic purpura in adults, secondary thrombocytopenia in adults, erythroblastopenia, palliative management of leukemias and lymphomas in adults, palliative management of acute leukemia of childhood	1955
Prednisone	Deltasone (Pharmacia)	Hypercalcemia associated with cancer, mycosis fungoides, idiopathic thrombocytopenic purpura in adults, secondary thrombocytopenia in adults, erythroblastopenia, palliative management of leukemias and lymphomas in adults, palliative management of acute leukemia of childhood (Multiple myeloma see carmustine)	1955

(Continued)

Table 46-1 **FDA-Approved Anticancer Agents and Their Indications[a] (Continued)**

Generic Name	Trade Name (Company)	Indication	Year[b]
Procarbazine	Matulane (Sigma-Tau)	Combination with other anticancer drugs for the treatment of Stage III and IV Hodgkin's disease	1969
		Matulane is used as part of the MOPP (nitrogen mustard, vincristine, procarbazine, prednisone) regimen	
Progesterone	Prometrium (Solvay)	Prevention of endometrial hyperplasia in non-hysterectomized postmenopausal women who are receiving conjugated estrogen tablets	1939
Rituximab	Rituxan (Genentech)	Relapsed or refractory low grade or follicular, CD20 positive, B-cell non-Hodgkin's lymphoma	1997
		First-line treatment of low grade or follicular, CD20-positive B-cell non-Hodgkin's lymphoma	2006
Samarium-153 lexidronam pentasodium	Quadramet (Berlex)	Relief of pain in patients with confirmed osteoblastic metastatic bone lesions that enhance on radionuclide bone scan	1997
Sodium iodide I-131	Iodotope (Bracco) Sodium Iodide I-131 (CIS-US, Mallinckrodt)	Carcinoma of the thyroid	1957
Sodium phosphate P-32	Sodium Phosphate P-32 (Mallinckrodt)	Polycythemia vera, chronic myelocytic leukemia, chronic lymphocytic leukemia, and palliative treatment of selected patients with multiple areas of skeletal metastases	1952
Sorafenib	Nexavar	Advanced renal cell carcinoma	2005
		Unresectable hepatocellular cancer	2007
Streptozocin	Zanosar (Pharmacia)	Metastatic islet cell carcinoma of the pancreas	1982
Strontium-89 chloride	Metastron (Nyomed Amersham)	Relief of bone pain in patients with painful skeletal metastases	1993
Sunitinib	Sutent (Pfizer)	Gastrointestinal stromal tumor after progression on or intolerance to imatinib mesylate	2006
		Advanced renal cell carcinoma.	2007
Talc	Sclerosol (Bryan)	Prevention of recurrence of malignant pleural effusions in symptomatic patients	1997
Tamoxifen citrate	Nolvadex (AstaZeneca)	Metastatic breast cancer: tamoxifen is effective in the treatment of metastatic breast cancer in women and men; in premenopausal women with metastatic breast cancer, tamoxifen is an alternative to oophorectomy or ovarian irradiation; available evidence indicates that patients whose tumors are estrogen receptor positive are more likely to benefit from tamoxifen therapy	1977
		Adjuvant treatment of breast cancer: tamoxifen is indicated for the treatment of node-positive breast cancer in postmenopausal women following total mastectomy or segmental mastectomy, axillary dissection, and breast irradiation; tamoxifen is indicated for the treatment of axillary node-negative breast cancer in women following total mastectomy or segmental mastectomy, axillary dissection, and breast irradiation	
		Ductal carcinoma in situ (DCIS): in women with DCIS, following breast surgery and radiation, tamoxifen is indicated to reduce the risk of invasive breast cancer. Reduction in breast cancer incidence in high-risk women: tamoxifen is indicated to reduce the incidence of breast cancer in women at high risk for breast cancer	
Temozolomide	Temodar (Schering)	Adult patients with refractory anaplastic astrocytoma, ie, patients at first relapse who have experienced disease progression on a drug regimen containing a nitrosourea and procarbazine	1999
		Adult patients with newly diagnosed glioblastoma multiforme concomitantly with radiotherapy and then as maintenance treatment	2005
Teniposide	Vumon (Bristol-Myers Squibb)	Combination with other approved anticancer agents for induction therapy in patients with refractory childhood acute lymphoblastic leukemia	1992
Testolactone	Teslac (Bristol-Myers Squibb)	Adjunctive therapy in the palliative treatment of advanced or disseminated breast cancer in postmenopausal women when hormonal therapy is indicated; it may also be used in women who were diagnosed as having had disseminated breast carcinoma when premenopausal, in whom ovarial function has been subsequently terminated	1970
Testosterone enanthate	Delatestryl (Bio-Technology General)	Secondarily in women with advancing inoperable metastatic (skeletal) mammary cancer who are 1-5 year postmenopausal	1939
Thalidomide	Thalomid (Celgene)	Multiple myeloma.	2006
Thioguanine	Tabloid (GlaxoSmithKline)	Remission induction, remission consolidation, and maintenance therapy of acute nonlymphatic leukemias; although thioguanine is one of several agents with activity in the treatment of the chronic myelogenous leukemia, more objective responses are observed with busulfan, and therefore busulfan is usually regarded as the preferred drug	1966
Thiotepa	Thioplex (Immunex)	Adenocarcinoma of the breast and ovary	1959
		Intracavitary effusions secondary to diffuse or localized neoplastic diseases of various serosal cavities	
		Superficial papillary carcinoma of the urinary bladder. Although now largely superseded by other treatments, thiotepa has been effective against other lymphomas, such as lymphosarcoma and Hodgkin's disease	
Topotecan	Hycamtin (GlaxoSmithKline)	Metastatic carcinoma of the ovary after failure of initial or subsequent chemotherapy	1996
		Small-cell lung cancer-sensitive disease after failure of first-line chemotherapy	1998
		Cervical carcinoma	2006
Toremifene citrate	Fareston (Orion)	Metastatic breast cancer in postmenopausal women with estrogen-receptor positive or unknown tumors	1997
Tositumimab	Bexxarf (Corixa)	Treatment of patients with CD20 positive, follicular, non-Hodgkin's lymphoma, with and without transformation, whose disease is refractory to Rituximab and has relapsed following chemotherapy	2003
Tositumumab	Bexxar (Corixa Corporation)	CD20-positve, follicular non-Hodgkin's lymphoma with or without transformation when refractory to or have not received Rituximab and relapsed following chemotherapy	2003

(Continued)

Table 46-1 **FDA-Approved Anticancer Agents and Their Indications[a] (Continued)**

Generic Name	Trade Name (Company)	Indication	Year[b]
Trastuzumab	Herceptin (Genentech)	Single agent for the treatment of patients with metastatic breast cancer whose tumors overexpress the HER-2 protein and who have received 1 or more chemotherapy regimens for their metastatic disease	1998
		In combination with paclitaxel for treatment of patients with metastatic breast cancer whose tumors overexpress the HER-2 protein and who have not received chemotherapy for their metastatic disease	2000
		Early stage breast cancer after primary therapy	2006
Tretinoin	Vesanoid (Roche)	Induction of remission in patients with acute promyelocytic leukemia. French-American-British classification M3 (including the M3 variant), characterized by the presence of the t(15;17) translocation and/or the presence of the *PML/RARalpha* gene who are refractory to, or who have relapsed from, anthracycline chemotherapy or for whom anthracycline-based chemotherapy is contraindicated	1995
Triamcinolone	Aristocort (Fujisawa)	Hypercalcemia associated with cancer, mycosis fungoides, idiopathic thrombocytopenic purpura in adults, secondary thrombocytopenia in adults, erythroblastopenia, palliative management of leukemias and lymphomas in adults, palliative management of acute leukemia of childhood	1957
Triptorelin pamoate	Trelstar Depot (Pharmacia)	Palliative treatment of advanced prostate cancer	2000
Valrubicin	Valstar (Medeva)	Intravesical therapy of BCG-refractory carcinoma in situ of the urinary bladder in patients for whom immediate cystectomy would be associated with unacceptable morbidity or mortality	1998
Vinblastine	Velban (Eli Lilly)	Palliative treatment of frequently responsive malignancies: generalized Hodgkin's disease (Stage III and IV, Ann Arbor modification of Rye staging system), lymphocytic lymphoma (nodular and diffuse, poorly and well differentiated), histiocytic lymphoma, mycosis fungoides (advanced stages), advanced carcinoma of the testis, Kaposi sarcoma, Letterer-Siwe disease (histiocytosis X)	1961
		Less frequently responsive malignancies: choriocarcinoma resistant to other chemotherapeutic agents, carcinoma of the breast unresponsive to appropriate endocrine surgery and hormonal therapy	
Vincristine	Oncovin (Eli Lilly)	Acute leukemia	1963
	Vincasar (Pharmacia)	Combination with other oncolytic agents in Hodgkin's disease, non-Hodgkin's malignant lymphomas (lymphocytic, mixed cell, histiocytic, undifferentiated nodular, and diffuse types), rhabdomyosarcoma, neurblastoma, and Wilms tumor	
Vinorelbine	Navelbine (GlaxoSmithKline)	Single agent or in combination with cisplatin for the first-line treatment of ambulatory patients with unresectable, advanced NSCLC	1994
		In patients with Stage IV NSCLC, Navelbine is indicated as a single agent or in combination with cisplatin; in Stage III NSCLC, Navelbine is indicated in combination with cisplatin	2002
Vorinostat	Zolinza (Merck)	Cutaneous manifestations of cutaneous T-cell lymphoma (CTCL) in patients with progressive, persistent, or recurrent disease on or following 2 systemic therapies	2006

[a]Please refer to approved product label for exact language regarding the approved indications.
[b]Date first FDA approval was received (any indication).

Heidelberger group synthesizing the 5-fluoropyrimidines.[16,17] The observations by Elion and Hitchings, who surmised (based on the presumption that nucleic acids were in control of cell growth) that purine and pyrimidine analogs would be useful in treatment of cancers, led to the development of 6-mercaptopurine, 6-thioguanine, and many other useful anticancer agents.[18-20] Although there is still clearly room for important clinical, toxicologic, and physiologic observation, these observations will probably not dominate future drug discovery. However, readers are encouraged to keep their eyes open to clinical, histocytotoxic, and physiologic observations as described above as serendipity has historically been a pivotal step in successful drug development.

The National Cancer Institute's Drug Discovery Program as an Important Contribution in the Drug Discovery Process

In the early 1960s, the US National Cancer Institute (NCI) began a major leadership role in the discovery and development of new anticancer agents. This was critical at that time because industry felt that investment in this area would not be feasible financially and that the risks were high. The NCI began its leadership by establishing the National Service Center (NSC), which served as a clearinghouse and a bank for compounds for all chemists, biologists, and other interested investigators. Compounds could be submitted to the NSC, assigned an NSC number (eg, NSC 3101139 for mitoxantrone), and tested in a series of in vitro and in vivo preclinical models. Agents that passed certain hurdles of in vitro and in vivo antitumor activity were considered by a body at the NCI called the "Decision Network" to decide whether or not to bring them into toxicology studies and eventually into clinical trials.

The very early efforts of the NCI used the KB squamous cancer cell line, originally obtained from a patient with a carcinoma of the mouth, to screen a large numbers of compounds. Compounds that were active against that cell line were further evaluated in vivo in the two long-term murine leukemia cell lines P388 and L1210.[21,22] These in vitro and in vivo screens did lead to compounds with clinical activity against leukemia and lymphoma (eg, vinca alkaloids, nitrosoureas). Finding agents with antitumor activity against solid tumors was much less successful.[22]

In 1975, the NCI revisited their evaluation process to include in vivo evaluation of compounds against solid tumors (both autologous animal tumors and human tumors growing as xenografts in nude mice). A very important retrospective analysis of that big experiment was conducted by Staquet and colleagues.[23] The results of their analyses are detailed in Table 46-2. As seen in the table, the P388 and L1210 mouse leukemias continued to be predictive for activity of new agents in the clinic, as did the B16 mouse melanoma solid tumor autologous model growing in immunocompetent mice. The only human tumor xenograft that appeared to be predictive for clinical antitumor activity was the MXI mammary tumor xenograft growing in nude mice. The predictivity of these models was not tumor specific but rather in vivo activity

Table 46-2 **The Most Predictive Animal Models: The NCI Experience 1978-1982**

Reasonably Predictive[a]	Not Predictive
P388 leukemia (mouse)	Lewis lung (mouse)
L1210 leukemia (mouse)	CD8 breast
B16 melanoma (mouse)	Co38 colon
MX-1 mammary[b]	LX1[b] lung
CXI colon[b]	

[a]Especially with regression of established tumors.
[b]Xenografts.
Source: Adapted from Ref. 23.

in those systems predicted, in general, for clinical activity. Also of importance in the report by Staquet and colleagues was the finding that actual regression of established tumors in these models and the percentage of animals surviving for greater than 45 days were even stronger predictors of eventual clinical efficacy of the agents.[23] Of additional note in Table 46-2 is the finding that five models were judged as not predictive at all for clinical activity. Some of the models, such as the Lewis lung model, continue to be used to justify bringing many new agents into clinical trials. It is important that investigators who are contemplating bringing new agents into the clinic based on preclinical activity only in the Lewis lung, CD8, Co38, LX1, or CX1 models be mindful of the extensive prior experience demonstrating them not to be predictive for clinical activity.

To be most successful, however, it is important to remember the parameter Staquet and colleagues used for evidence of activity in the clinic (to make the correlation with the preclinical models): tumor shrinkage. Thus, their findings might not be applicable to the newer cytostatic agents being developed.[24,25]

A more recent study reported on the relationship between drug activity in NCI preclinical in vitro and in vivo models and clinical activity of a new agent.[26] It is of interest that of the 39 agents for which there were both xenograft and phase 2 clinical data available, clinical activity in at least some phase 2 trials was observed if there was activity in at least one-third of the xenograft models tested. Of particular note was that if there was preclinical activity in one-third or more of the xenografts tested there was a 45% chance the compound would have clinical activity. In that same study, only non-small cell lung cancer xenografts were predictive for the clinical activity against the same histology (eg, non-small cell lung cancer). Thus, although these in vivo evaluation systems are often maligned, when a systematic large-scale evaluation of them was examined, some models appeared to be reasonable predictors (although not tumor-specific predictors) for activity in the clinic.

The NCI made a further revision in their evaluation strategy in 1985 when they placed a large series of 60 human tumor cell lines in place for screening purposes.[22,27-31] They have attempted to make this a more tumor type-oriented approach with inclusion of breast, lung, colon, kidney, brain, ovary, prostate, and melanoma human tumor lines. At the time of introduction of this concept into the drug evaluation process, there was a great deal of discussion in the research community on how these cell lines were selected. Many investigators felt that cell lines with too rapid a doubling time were selected and did not represent the more slowly dividing solid tumors. However, this 60-cell line screening panel is the system that is currently in place. More can be learned about the 60-cell line success by visiting the website of the NCI at <http://dtp.nci.nih.gov/branches/btb/ivclsp.html>. Agents that are deemed active in the cell line screens (based on criteria outlined in references 22 and 29 and based on other criteria, such as disease-specific activity) are then evaluated in the traditional in vivo models to determine their therapeutic index. If they are found active, they are moved forward into preclinical toxicology studies (see below).[30,31]

The true predictivity of the NCI 60-cell line success is yet unknown as there are no published analyses as to the true predictivity of this approach for antitumor activity in the clinic. However, many excellent analyses of the results from the NCI 60 cell lines have led to some very provocative and useful research tools.[32,33]

As an initial example of a unique use of results from the 60-cell line screening, Paull and colleagues described a method (which they dubbed the COMPARE program) in which a compound evaluated in the 60-cell line screen is used as a seed and the COMPARE program is used to detect the compounds that have similar patterns (or fingerprints) of activity against the 60 cell lines.[34] A correlation coefficient is then calculated to describe the closeness of other agents to the pattern of activity of the seed compound. It appears that if two compounds have similar correlation coefficients this will predict for comparable mechanisms of action of the compounds or even the existence of a similar intracellular target, as described by Weinstein and colleagues.[35] If the correlation coefficient of a new, active compound is low compared with the compounds evaluated in the NCI screen, it might substantially increase interest in the new compound, as it is very likely to have a new (unique) mechanism of action.

Of additional importance and of great interest to the cancer research community is that the NCI 60 cell lines continue to be characterized for presence or absence of specific targets (kinases, telomerase, mismatch repair proteins, receptors).[36-40] The more precise characterization of these lines is relatively certain to help the evaluation of compounds in the lines. However, this assumes that there is no change in the parameters characterized over passages and/or time.

Other preclinical models explored by the NCI for evaluating compounds that deserve mention were models put in place to evaluate agents against tumors taken directly from patients. These are nicely summarized by Suggitt and Bibby.[41] There were two systems including the in vitro human tumor cloning assay (HTCA) and the in vivo subrenal capsule system (SRC). The NCI began a program using the HTCA to screen compounds for activity against tumors taken directly from patients and growing as colonies in soft agar.[42,43] Although initial correlations were promising between agents detected as active in the HTCA and having subsequent antitumor activity in the clinic, the HTCA was deemed as too logistically difficult to use as an upfront screen to evaluate the vast array of compounds. However, several groups of investigators continue to use the HTCA to determine whether an agent should be taken into the clinic against a particular histologic type of malignancy (eg, gemcitabine against pancreatic cancer) and to identify potentially predictive biomarkers to predict clinical outcome.[44-47] The SRC assay is a system in which tumors are taken directly from patients and are placed under the renal capsule in mice. New agents are administered to the mice to determine the effects of the agent against tumors growing under the renal capsule.[48] Once again, although initial correlations between activity in the SCR system and the clinical activity of the compound appeared promising, the logistics of evaluating a large number of compounds in this in vivo system were deemed too daunting. Thus, attempts using these two methods (the HTCA and the SRC systems) to evaluate large numbers of new compounds against tumors taken directly from patients (and thus not corrupted by in vitro passage in culture) were not pursued based on logistic problems (basically, the unavailability of tumors taken from patients and the technical challenges of the assays—ie, lots of manpower required). However, most investigators would agree that it would be helpful to have some way to evaluate a large number of compounds against tumors taken directly from patients.

Mechanism-Based Drug Discovery and Evaluation

With the explosion of molecular techniques and knowledge of cell biology, there is now an incredible array of new methods for discovery of potential targets present in tumor cells versus normal cells.

The most recent spectacular example of a mechanistically based approach to therapy is the development of the new agent imatinib, which has substantial activity against chronic myelogenous leukemia and against gastrointestinal stromal sarcomas. To put the timeline for development of imatinib into perspective, the basic biological ground work for the discovery and development of imatinib actually began with the discovery of the Philadelphia chromosome in chronic myeloid leukemias (CMLs) in 1960.[49] This was actually the first consistent chromosomal abnormality discovered in any type of cancer. The abnormality is a translocation involving chromosomes 9 and 22.[50] Work done from 1990 to 1993 documented that the translocation caused the *ABL* gene on the chromosome 9 (a non-receptor tyrosine kinase) to move next to the *BCR* (breakpoint cluster region) gene on chromosome 22. This translocation codes the BCR-ABL protein p210 BCR-ABL, which is a 210 kDa transforming protein tyrosine kinase constitutively expressed and responsible for the development of this disease in about 95% of patients with CML.[51,52] This abnormal tyrosine kinase does not exist in the normal cells of the patients. Therefore, it was an excellent target for development of an agent with activity against CML.

Screening was conducted to find compounds with specific activity against the BCR-ABL tyrosine kinase, and the agent (CGP57148, aka STI 571, imatinib) was found to be the most selective inhibitor by targeting the adenosine triphosphate binding site (ATP-pocket) of the enzyme.[53] The agent was further investigated in vitro and in vivo and was found to be toxic to BCR-ABL-positive cells.[53-55] Phase 1 and 2 trials in 1999-2000 documented marked clinical activity of Gleevec against CML, particularly in the chronic phase.[56,57] As noted above, this impressive example of drug development spanned nearly 40 years from identification of the chromosomal abnormality until documentation of clinical activity of a compound against the disease (10 years if one starts counting from the time of discovery of the target, the p120 BCR-ABL tyrosine kinase). Of note is that additional work has shown that imatinib also has substantial activity against gastrointestinal stromal sarcomas, which possess abnormalities in the c-kit oncogene.[58] However, subsequent work showed that imatinib is not such a selective inhibitor of BCR-ABL as thought earlier but that the compound inhibits among others the receptors for platelet-derived growth factor (c-sis) and macrophage colony-stimulating factor (c-fms) and that it appears to modulate diabetic nephropathy and liver fibrosis in preclinical models.[59-62] This paradigmatic example underlines that one should not be content with what is believed (and confirmed) to be the main mechanism of action but one must continue to carefully search for yet undetected potentials of new agents.[63]

The concept of mechanism-based drug development is not new and well introduced into clinical practice, eg, antiestrogens like tamoxifen. Although not within the scope of this chapter, a variety of other mechanism-based therapeutics has also demonstrated substantial clinical antitumor activity [antiandrogens, aromatase inhibitors, monoclonal antibodies to CD20, CD52, the HER-2/*neu* cell membrane receptor, the Epidermal Growth Factor Receptor (EGFR), and the vascular endothelial growth factor (VEGF), etc.]. However, at the time of the writing of this chapter, there are also some disappointments in the area of targeting. For example, the farnesyl transferase inhibitors that have been developed to target tumors with mutations in *ras* have not shown activity against pancreatic cancer, even though they have clear clinical activity against breast cancer and acute leukemias, where *ras* mutations are not thought to be critical to the development or progression of either disease.[64-66]

Another example of difficulties with targeting is the finding that despite the upregulation of the EGFR in a number of malignancies, the activity of small molecule inhibitors of the EGFR kinase or monoclonal antibodies to the EGFR do not appear to correlate with the increased expression of EGFR (at least by currently available methods of measuring the receptor/kinase).[67] However, some recent brilliant work has described the fact that specific receptor mutations may help differentiate between sensitive and resistant tumors.[68-71]

Clearly, there is a great deal of work to do if targeted therapy is to succeed in major tumor types. In a recent piece of work, Druker and Lydon outlined the lessons learned from the development of imatinib.[72] These lessons provide guidelines for thinking about improved mechanism-based approaches, including the following:

1. Identification of an appropriate target molecule for drug development. The identification of the BCR-ABL tyrosine kinase as the kinase to cause CML (ie, a single molecular defect as a target) was important. The kinase was a "disease gene." For success, one probably should have a target that is critical to the disease process.
2. Availability of a validated surrogate end point that can be easily measured in patients to ensure that the new agent is indeed interfering with the desired target and has the desired clinical effects. For CML, this is the Philadelphia chromosome, which is monitored in blood cells (and by blood counts).
3. Improvements in techniques that are important for drug designs (eg, crystallography, molecular modeling) to optimize the selectivity (specificity) of compounds.

There is no question that with improvements in understanding of the working of the cell, there will be continued efforts at developing mechanism-based agents.[72-76] However, given the terrific amount of work and substantial resources necessary to clinically develop a new agent, it is very critical that targets are selected wisely.[77,78] Bioinformatics support may be necessary to sieve through the large number of potential targets and identify promising approaches.[79]

In addition to targeting the tumor cells, it is now clear that targeting the environment of the tumor cells is taking on a completely new importance. The area of angiogenesis has given all clinicians a sense of optimism given the finding that the monoclonal antibody bevacizumab, directed against VEGF, has substantially improved (when used with chemotherapeutics) the survival of patients with colorectal cancer, non-small cell lung cancer, and breast cancer. It is clear the agent also has single agent activity against renal cell and ovarian cancer.[80-84] Small molecules which target VEGF or platelet-derived growth factor (PDGF) pathways to attack the angiogenic process are also being studied for their clinical antitumor activity.[85-88] Despite these unique mechanisms of action all new agents affecting the tumor environment will still require the normal drug development process as outlined in this chapter.

It also remains of unchallenged importance that mechanism-based drug development and clinical serendipity must continue to be integrated and that only the combination of both optimize drug development strategies.

Sources of Compounds to Evaluate Against Targets

There is no question that the most rational way to develop a new agent against a target is to understand the crystal structure of that target and rationally design an agent to interact with that target.[72,73,77] However, for a vast majority of these targets, a crystal structure is not identified. Fortunately, there is usually a method to aid in identifying inhibitors of targets using molecular screening.[89] Therefore, it is necessary for a drug development team to have access to major libraries of compounds to use against their target as well as to a high-throughput system.

The NCI has always been a key resource for libraries of compounds, including natural products.[90] Most recently, the NCI has made the NCI Diversity Library (http://dtp.nci.nih.gov/branches/dscb/diversity_explanation.html) available to investigators. In addition, there are a number of commercial libraries available for investigator use.

One of the most interesting new methods that has become available to find initial leads against a target is a new method developed by Kauvar and colleagues called the TRAP assay.[91,92] TRAP stands for Target Recorded Affinity Profiling (or affinity fingerprinting). The theory behind the TRAP assay is that the compounds are characterized by biologic properties (their affinities to a panel of 8-20 reference proteins) rather than chemical structures. With the TRAP method, the number of candidate drugs can be relatively reduced from tens of thousands to only a few hundred, which are then directly screened against the target-of-interest. If the early promise of the TRAP method is sustained, it will represent a considerable advance in rapidly finding leads against any new target. However, the overall impact on speed and quality of drug development by high-throughput assay has not yet been confirmed by structured analyses.

If one is developing a biologic agent against a cell surface receptor or against a small factor, the ability to produce a humanized monoclonal antibody appears to enable a straightforward approach with a higher likelihood of success compared to the development of a small molecule.

Preparation of Agents for Clinical Trials

Formulation

Pharmaceutics or the formulation of a compound for preclinical pharmacology, toxicology, and clinical trials is an often overlooked but very important aspect of drug development. It is very desirable to have the best formulation in place that you plan to use in clinical trials before proceeding with animal pharmacology and toxicology.[93]

Difficult formulations have often led to prolonged development programs that have occasionally caused great difficulties that development of the compound was nearly discontinued. This was certainly the case with paclitaxel, which requires solubilization of a difficult cremaphor-containing combination that may result in idiosyncratic reactions in some patients.[94] A multitude of anticancer agents (in addition to paclitaxel) have had significant formulation problems, including etoposide (solved by a formulation using 20 mg etoposide, 2 mg citric acid, 30 mg benzyl alcohol, 80 mg modified polysorbate 80/Tween 80, 650 mg polyethylene glycol 300, and 30.5% (V/V) alcohol, CPT-11 (topoisomerase I inhibitor) (solved by using a prodrug that is broken down by carboxylesterase in patients' serum and tumors), docetaxel (solved by using a formulation of polysorbate 80), geldanamycin, and several others. If one requires an exotic formulation for intravenous use, there may be a major delay in the start of clinical trials. In general, only formulations that have already been used in patients should be used to formulate a new agent.

Another major question that frequently arises in the formulation process is whether an oral route of administration would be preferable over an intravenous route. In general, for cytotoxic agents, there is a much greater chance for wide variability in the gastrointestinal absorption of orally administered agents. This variability could lead to unpredictable and potentially serious side effects in some patients and not in others. In addition, patient compliance with oral drug intake has been questioned, particularly if these drugs can cause nausea or vomiting. Therefore, in general, even if an agent can be formulated for both intravenous and oral use, it is deemed preferable to develop the intravenous formulation first. This allows one to carefully determine the pharmacology of the compound in a situation in which absorption is not an issue. An exception is when the compound has great schedule dependency in its preclinical activity work-up. In that situation, an oral formulation may be more desirable.[95] Also, if the drug is predicted to be taken repeatedly (eg, daily) for a prolonged period, development of an oral application may be advantageous. Finally, use of the oral route may also be desirable for some of the new, more "targeted" less toxic noncytotoxic agents.[96]

Development of an Assay for a Pharmacodynamic End Point (Surrogate Marker)

The development of new anticancer agents has, to date, for the most part been empiric. More specifically, there has not been a prior emphasis on ensuring that the new agent actually affected the target it was designed to hit. With more mechanism-based drug design, it has been recommended to try to have some assay in place to determine whether the agent is having the desired effect on the target (ie, a pharmacodynamic end point). Since it is plausible to assume that any compound exerts a variety of biological effects, such an assay of course may not reflect the totality of a drug's biochemical or clinical properties.

The philosophy of using surrogate biochemical markers from a patient's tumor that predict for treatment outcome in this patient is well established in Medical Oncology and has as hallmark example the determination of estrogen receptors in breast cancer tissue to predict the likelihood to respond to antiestrogen therapy.[96] However, with newer mechanism-based agents, this area is still in its infancy, but there are some examples of where assays for pharmacodynamic end points are being developed. For example, for the development of farnesyl transferase inhibitors, in the absence of monitoring farnesyl transferase activity in the serum or in tumor cells, there was an emphasis on analyzing inhibition of processing of farnesylated proteins such as prelaminin or HDJ2 in buccal mucosa cells or in blood mononuclear cells.[97,98] Hidalgo and colleagues have also measured phosphorylation of the EGFR in skin biopsies in patients receiving EGFR antagonists.[99] In addition, the likelihood to respond to pemetrexed has been linked to the expression level of thymidilate synthase and mrp-4 and the antitumor activity of the serin-threonine kinase inhibitor enzastaurin has been correlated with the expression GSK-3ß.[46,100] It is extremely important that these surrogate markers accompany mechanism-based drug development. Without these markers, their development will be confusing, and it will not be known whether it was an inappropriate target or whether the new agent just did not affect the target (for pharmacokinetic and a variety of other possible reasons) if the compound failed.

Animal Pharmacology

Animal pharmacology studies have rarely been a major part of the development of a new anticancer agent (at least in the preparation of an investigational new drug (IND) application). The exception to this is, of course, with oral anticancer agents for which bioavailability studies are required. Other important pieces of information that can be learned from pharmacology studies in animals can include (1) organ distribution of the agent including penetration and dwell time in tumors (particularly useful for compounds that are formulated in liposomes or are new compounds formulated in nanoparticles encapsulated in albumin) and (2) penetration into the central nervous system, or other sanctuaries.[101,102]

One other very powerful piece of information that can be gleaned from animal pharmacology was described by Collins and colleagues.[103] This often forgotten piece of work demonstrated that there was a direct relationship between the concentration × time (C × T) product at the LD10 in mice and the C × T product at the maximally tolerated dose (MTD) in patients.[103] Essentially (based on mg/m^2 basis), the C × T in mouse = C × T in humans. This important relationship appears to hold up across most animal species and can be used as a target for dose escalation in phase 1 trials with a new agent in patients (see below). Work by other researchers has confirmed the relationship and has documented how that relationship can be used to determine which serum concentrations of agents will be achieved in patients (and should therefore be used in in-vitro model systems).[104,105]

Animal Toxicology Studies

These studies are a critical part of any drug development program. In general, the models used for toxicology studies to date (mouse, rat, or beagle dog is used because of a biliary system closer to human) have given an excellent safety record for the development of new anticancer agents (eg, there essentially have been no catastrophes in the initial phase 1 clinical trials in patients). One area in which one must be a bit more careful is in the area of nucleosides and antimetabolites. As an example, the starting dose for the agent fludarabine phosphate was chosen too high and substantial bone marrow toxicity was noted in the first dose level in patients presumably owing to the fact that fludarabine requires activation by the enzyme deoxyctidine kinase and the levels of this enzyme are much higher in human cancer cells than they are in mouse and canine marrow cells.[106] Pemetrexed (MTA, LY231514). a multitargeted enzyme inhibitor recently approved for the treatment of patients with mesothelioma and non-small cell lung cancer, had a similar problem but with worse toxicities in animals than in patients.[107] Therefore, investigators should be alert about the possibility of discordance between animals and humans when examining results of animal toxicity studies with nucleoside analogs or other antimetabolites.

As noted above, the usual animal species required for formal toxicology studies is a mouse or a rat plus the beagle dog. For monoclonal antibodies and other biologics, a primate model is frequently required. An excellent review of toxicity requirements by the US Food and Drug Administration (FDA) has been published by DeGeorge and colleagues.[108] In Europe, there is a movement to use only two murine species (mouse and rat) as a toxicology package necessary to begin a phase 1 trial in patients.[109-111] However, if the tolerable doses in those species (based on a mg/m^2 basis) are widely divergent, additional toxicology studies in the dog are a necessity before beginning the phase 1 clinical trial in patients.

In general, the animal models used are reliable in predicting certain types of organ toxicities (such as myelosuppression).[112] However, the dog has been noted to be somewhat overpredictive for renal, hepatic, and gastrointestinal toxicities.[113] Neurologic, pancreatic, dermatologic, and pulmonary toxicities are generally not well predicted by the murine and canine models. The models are imperfect in predicting other organ toxicities, and occasionally, toxicities are noted in one species (eg, a murine species) but do not occur in another (eg, the dog). This is often attributable to a difference in metabolism of the agent between the species. If unacceptable toxicities are noted in mice, one should still strongly consider going into dogs or primates as they may not exhibit toxicities reported in murine models. This has been done for a few compounds that were cardiotoxic in the mouse toxicology program, but the dog correctly predicted that no serious cardiac toxicity would be noted in patients.[114] As will be outlined below, the animal toxicology package is most critical to help define the starting doses in patients beginning with the phase 1 trial of the agent. Since toxicity is one of the most important factor for drug attrition along the development process large-scale gene expression screening (called toxicogenomics) with the focus on toxicities is being studied for its value to identify toxic agents early.[115] Unfortunately there has been a unless <ill/> that to this impartial field.

Preparation of an IND (Investigational New Drug) Application

Before a clinical trial can begin in the United States and most other countries, it is necessary to prepare an IND application and to submit this document to a regulatory agency (eg, the FDA). The necessary components of the IND are as outlined in Table 46-3. The clinical trial can proceed with the new agent if 30 days goes by after filing the IND package and there is no comment by the FDA. Of course, if the FDA requires additional information before the 30-day waiting period expires, that information must be supplied and approved by FDA before the first phase 1 clinical trial can proceed.

Early Clinical Trials

Phase 0 Clinical Trial

Despite the unprecedented increase in potential targets and the subsequent advent of mechanism-based drug development the number of new drug approvals by the FDA has markedly decreased from 53 in 1996 to 20 in 2005.[116] This has prompted considerations to simplify the first-in-human dose and to the proposal of what is now called "Phase 0" trials by both the FDA and the European EMEA.[117,118] More details can be found using the following links for the FDA: http://www.fda.gov/cder/guidance/7086fnl.htm and for the EMEA: http://www.emea.curopa.

Table 46-3 **Content and Component of an IND Application**

1. Cover sheet – 1571
a) Name, address, and telephone number of sponsor, etc.
b) Phase of clinical investigation
c) Commitment not to begin clinical investigation until an IND is in effect
d) IRB commitment
e) Commitment to follow all regulation requirements
f) Name and title of person responsible for monitoring
g) Name and title of person responsible for safety
h) Any transfer obligations, ie, Clinical Research Organization
i) Signature of sponsor
2. Table of contents
3. Introductory statement and general investigational plan
4. Reserved for FDA
5. Investigator's brochure
6. Protocols
7. CMC information
8. Pharmacology and toxicology information
9. Previous human experience with the investigational drug
10. Additional information

More details can be found at the FDA website: <http://www.fda.gov/cder/regulatory/applications/ind_page_1.htm>
Abbreviations: CMC, chemistry, manufacturing, and control; IND, investigational new drug.

eu/pdfs/human/swp/259902en.pdf. The principle is to expose normal volunteers or cancer patients to very low doses of a new chemical entity in order to (1) obtain information on the pharmacokinetics, (2) obtain information whether the intended target is in fact inhibited in humans, (3) determine the optimal schedule when drug combinations are used. Supporters of this novel design argue that phase 0 trials help eliminate inactive drugs at a very early stage and thus save time and resources for more promising agents. However, the phase 0 trial design has not been applied widely to cancer drugs yet and has been critized as being ethically problematic and impractical for oncology because of the lack of validated assays for surrogate biomarkers.

Phase 1 Clinical Trial

Traditionally, this is the first trial of a new agent in patients (or in normal volunteers). Several excellent reviews have been written on phase 1 trial methodologies.[119-122] The objectives of the first phase 1 trial in humans differ as to whether the agent is first given to patients or is first given to normal volunteers.

Phase 1 Trial in Patients Versus Normal Volunteers

There is a growing interest in conducting initial phase 1 clinical trials of new anticancer agents in normal volunteers rather than in patients. The number one reason cited for this approach is that the normal volunteers have normal organ function not impaired by malignancy and by prior treatment of their malignancy, as is the case in patients. In addition, normal volunteers would not normally be on other concomitant medications (usually an average of 10 for patients on a phase 1 trial), which could complicate the pharmacokinetics and/or the side effect profile of a new agent.[123] However, clinicians caring for patients with cancer often view the conduct of the initial phase 1 trial in normal volunteers as a waste of precious time and a step that delays the administration of a promising agent to the very people who need it: patients with advanced cancer. However, with the development of many new cytostatics that are noncarcinogenic rather than cytotoxic agents, which are often carcinogenic, there is more and more interest in first trying the new agents in normal volunteers—just as is done in other areas of drug development such as cardiology.

For a new agent to even be considered for administration to a normal volunteer, it must be demonstrated to be non-carcinogenic and non-mutagenic in the appropriate preclinical systems. Then an initial trial in normal volunteers can begin.

The objectives of the initial clinical trial of a new anticancer agent performed in normal volunteers are more limited than if the initial clinical trial is performed in patients with advanced cancer. The objectives include the following:

1. To determine the clinical pharmacology of a *single dose* of the agent when given at the starting dose (and perhaps at 1 additional dose level, to ensure linear kinetics for the agent). This clinical pharmacology information would include peak plasma levels, half- lives of the agent, and the areas under the curve (AUC) for the agent. In addition, some pharmacodynamic data could be collected, for example, whether the agent hits a target in a particular normal tissue (such as white blood cells).
2. To determine the clinical pharmacology of *multiple daily doses* (usually not to exceed 5-7 days) of the new agent at the starting dose (and perhaps at one additional dose level) to ensure that no accumulation of the agent occurs. This clinical pharmacology of the agent would include peak plasma levels, trough levels, half-lives of the agent, AUCs for the agent, and steady-state plasma levels. In addition, some pharmacodynamic data could also be collected, for example, whether the agent was hitting a target in a particular normal tissue (such as white blood cells, buccal mucosal cells, saliva, hair, fingernails).
3. To determine if there are any *side effects* noted for these low doses of the agent in these volunteers. This is usually done by having a placebo control. This can be done by either a balanced randomization (one normal volunteer receives placebo for every one normal volunteer receiving the new agent) or by an unbalanced randomization (one normal volunteer receiving the placebo for every two or more normal volunteers receiving the new agent).

The idea of using the normal volunteer approach for the initial trials of a new antitumor agent is that the pharmacokinetic data obtained will have less variability than observed in patients with advanced cancer. It is felt that this solid information might actually shorten the phase 1 clinical trials for the new agent in patients and indeed allow patients with advanced cancer to actually receive more effective doses and schedules of the new agent. That information would give them a better chance of having drug activity against their tumor and subsequent clinical benefit.

There can, however, be problems with taking even a new cytostatic agent—even at low doses—into a normal volunteer population. There has been a recent instance in which a cytostatic agent (an EGFR antagonist) was given to normal volunteers and at low doses of daily administration caused a very severe cutaneous reaction (which had not been seen with the single dose). Although not life-threatening, it was cosmetically severe and actually delayed the administration of the agent to patients. A much more serious accident occurred with the first-in-human dose of a T-cell activating antibody, named TGN1412, in human volunteers. Potential indications for this antibody, which was well characterized in preclinical experiments, included B-cell chronic lymphocytic leukemia and autoimmune diseases. The antibody was injected in six normal volunteers at roughly the same time. Approximately 1 hour later, all six volunteers experienced an immediately life-threatening situation that was later described as cytokine storm and had to be treated for multiorgan failure in the intensive care unit.[124] This catastrophe has led to a reassessment of testing antibodies in normal human volunteers and to the development of new, stringent guidelines.[125]

In summary, the administration of new anticancer agents to normal volunteers remains somewhat controversial in oncology drug development circles.

The objectives for a phase 1 trial in patients with advanced malignancies include the following:

1. To determine the maximum tolerated dose (MTD) of the drug. The MTD is the dose recommended for subsequent phase 2 trials of the new agent.
2. To define the qualitative and quantitative toxicities of the new agent. In traditional studies, this is described by grading of toxicities according to internationally accepted tables and by observation of dose-limiting toxicities (DLTs). These tables are regularly updated and are published under <http://ctep.cancer.gov/forms/CTCAEv3.pdf>.
3. To obtain information on the clinical pharmacology of the new agent.
4. To obtain pharmacodynamic information on the new agent (eg, does a specific plasma level of the new agent interact/modulate a particular target). These studies can be done using tissue samples (normal and tumor), peripheral blood cells, skin biopsies, malignant effusions, serum proteins, buccal mucosal cells, hair, or new imaging techniques.
5. To anecdotally document clinical antitumor activity (eg. objective responses, tumor marker decline, clinical benefit).

Selection of Schedule and Route for a Phase I Trial

The schedules most commonly explored in phase 1 trials include (1) single dose repeated every 3 or 4 weeks, (2) daily × 5 administration repeated every 3 or 4 weeks, (3) weekly × 4 repeated every 6 weeks, (4) weekly × 3 repeated every 4 weeks, (5) 120 <ill/> continuous infusion, and (6) daily × 21 repeated every 28 days. Of course, as more information (eg, pharmacokinetic/pharmacodynamic information) becomes available on the new agent, it may become necessary to explore other schedules. The choice of what schedule to use (eg, the choice between a bolus vs a more frequent, eg, daily × 5 or daily × 21 schedule) is most frequently decided based on (1) the schedule—dependency for antitumor activity in the preclinical models, (2) the pharmacokinetics of the agent in the preclinical model (and eventually from data in patients), (3) very importantly, the mechanism of action and preclinical data regarding the mechanism of action (eg, dwell time for a drug to be "on target" to have an effect), (4) the practically for patients, (5) the clinical pharmacologic information (if available), (6) the planned clinical pharmacologic studies, (7) the pharmaceutical characteristics of the compound, and (8) the planned label indication. It is also a fact that market size and national reimbursement systems may influence the choice for a specific schedule. The reader is cautioned that decisions on schedule based on the most active schedule in the preclinical animal models need to take into account the fact that animal tumors have a more rapid doubling time and a much higher growth fraction than do most types of human cancers (other than leukemias or aggressive lymphomas).

As far as the route is concerned, the tried and true method for development of new agents (even if an oral route is possible with the new agent) is to proceed with the first phase 1 trial by the intravenous route. This intravenous trial could then be followed by the phase 1 oral trial. This has classically been done because (1) there is certainty of delivery of the agent with the intravenous route (patients with cancer may have abnormalities of their gastrointestinal tracts, they may have low-grade nausea from other medications (eg, pain medication), or swallowing might be difficult for them and compliance is an issue); (2) with the intravenous route, there is no question that the drug is delivered with a chance for the greatest peak plasma levels of the agent; and (3) having the correct intravenous dose first and then proceeding with the oral phase 1 trial of the agent allows one to assess the bioavailability of the oral form of the agent.

With the introduction of new cytostatic agents, which tend to have more schedule dependence, it is becoming more and more common to only develop an agent using the oral form of the agent (eg, tamoxifen, capecitabine, imatinib, erlotinib). With the oral form of the agent, there is more room for creativity in schedules (eg, daily × 5, 2 days off, daily × 5 and daily × 42). However, one must remember that the schedules used for the phase 1 trial cannot be greatly different than the schedules used in the animal toxicology package and should be manageable in a more uncontrolled clinical setting after approval of the new agent. One also needs to be cognizant of potential patient compliance issues with oral medications.[126,127]

Calculation of the Starting Dose for the Phase 1 Trial

The criteria for calculation of a starting dose include starting using either one-tenth the LD10 (or MTD) in the mouse or rat or one-third or one-sixth of the toxic dose low (TDL) in the dog. The TDL is defined as the dose in the dog that, if doubled, causes no lethality. The use of either the murine model or the dog to guide the starting dose is decided based on the dose, which will give the lower or more conservative starting dose on the schedule planned to be used.[128] Because animal toxicology studies frequently give data on a mg/kg basis, it is critical to scale all doses between animals und humans using a mg/m^2 basis.[129,130] Table 46-4 details the conversion factor suggested by Freireich and colleagues for mg/kg in an animal species to a mg/m^2 scale.[129]

To demonstrate how one would calculate the starting dose for a new agent, we could use the example of the development of the topoisomerase I inhibitor CPT-11.[131] In animal toxicology studies with CPT-11, the most sensitive animal species was the mouse using a weekly schedule. For CPT-11, the MTD in the mouse given CPT-11 on the weekly schedule was 70 mg/kg. Using the conversion factor of 3 (see Table 46-4), the MTD in the mouse on a mg/m^2 level would be 70 mg/kg × 3) 210 mg/m^2. Then, the starting dose in humans using the mouse information would be one-tenth of the MTD in mouse or one-tenth of 210 or 21 mg/m^2 given weekly. If the dog had been the most sensitive animal species to CPT-11, we would have used that dog toxicology information to determine our starting dose for CPT-11.

Table 46-4 **Conversion Factor for Changing mg/kg to mg/m^2 for Starting Dose in Humans**

Animal Model	Appropriate Conversion Factor for Converting mg/kg → mg/m^2
Mouse	3
Rat	6
Monkey	12
Dog	20
Human	37

Source: Adapted from Ref. 129.

Methods for Dose Escalation

The methods used for dose escalation in phase 1 trials had classically been the modified Fibonacci search scheme.[121,132] However, as can be seen in Table 46-5, there are now several other methods for escalation of dose in phase 1 trials that can be used.[133-139] Most of these other methods of dose escalation were developed to try to minimize the number of patients receiving very low, probably ineffective doses of a new agent to try to improve the ethics of the situation.[140-142]

The *modified Fibonacci* search scheme is the most often used method of dose escalation. However, it can result in the highest number of patients receiving ineffective doses, largely because whereas the initial dose escalation are substantial, there is eventually a tapering off of the percent dose escalation to just 33% escalations at each subsequent dose level. Table 46-6 details a classic modified Fibonacci dose escalation scheme. The real benefit of starting a phase 1 clinical trial with a new agent using the modified Fibonacci scheme is that it has a superb record of safety. It is particularly the preferred method when one has an agent that has a steep dose-toxicity curve

Table 46-5 **Methods for Dose Escalation in Phase 1 Trials**

Method	Proposed by
Modified Fibonacci	Hanson et al.[132]
Doubling method	Gottlieb[133] Freireich (personal communication)
Pharmacologically guided	Collins et al.[103]
2 × AUC method	Evans[134]
Geometric mean + extended factor of 2	Erlichmann[135]
Continual reassessment (and modified continual reassessment)	O'Quigley et al.[136,137] and Faries[138]
Accelerated titration design	Simon et al.[139]
Selection by patient method	Freedman[141,151]

Table 46-6 Modified Fibonacci Dose Escalation Scheme in Phase 1 Trials

n (Starting Dose)	% Increase Above Preceding Dose
n	-
2n	100
3,3n	67
5n	50
7n	40
12n	33
16n	33
etc.	33

in the animal toxicology studies with the new agent. With the modified Fibonacci method, there are generally three patients entered at each dose level. This must be done carefully. In general, the first patient (patient 1) at a new dose level is entered on study and observed for 3 weeks. If no toxicities are noted in patient 1, patient 2 on the same dose level is then entered and observed for at least 2 weeks (note that, by that time, patient 1 will be well into his/her second course). If no toxicities are noted in patient 2, patient 3 can be entered after patient 2 is observed for 2 weeks. Although there is always pressure from many quarters to enter patients more quickly into a phase 1 trial, following this methodology provides the highest degree of safety possible and provides added protection in cases in which the new agent (or its metabolites) has a particularly long half-life or a new agent has nonlinear kinetics. One must also be careful and probably use the modified Fibonacci method when one is dealing with an agent that is a prodrug (as was CPT-11) and limited information is available on the active metabolite.

If no DLT (see definition below) is reached at a dose level, the dose is escalated for the next cohort of patients. If only one of three patients at a particular dose level is noted to have a DLT, then up to three more patients can be entered onto that dose level. If two or more patients of three to six patients are noted to have DLTs, then one has exceeded the MTD of the drug. Then additional patients are entered on the preceding dose level to ensure that one has a correct MTD—the dose to be taken into phase 2 trials with the new agent. It is important to note that there is no real scientific basis for the three patients per dose level used in standard phase 1 trials.[143] The only rationale for the three patients per dose level is that, to date, it has provided a good safety record for phase 1 trials.

The next dose escalation method outlined in Table 46-5 is the *doubling method*. This was proposed to try to minimize the number of patients entered at ineffective dose levels. This method provides a more rapid dose escalation. Theoretically, it could lead to overshooting the dose with attendant severe toxicities (although one cannot find any examples of problems in the literature). This doubling method of dose escalation (*n*, 2*n*, 4*n*, 8*n*, 16*n*, ...) is probably now the most commonly used method of dose escalation in phase 1 trials. Once grade 2 toxicity is noted in a patient at a particular dose level, the dose escalation is reduced to a 50% increase at the next dose level.

The most aggressive concept introduced to try to minimize the number of patients receiving ineffective doses of a new agent is the *continual reassessment* method (CRM) proposed by O'Quigley and colleagues in 1990, repeatedly commented on, and modified by other authors.[136-138,144-146] In this modified continual reassessment method (MCRM), a group of clinicians estimates the lower and higher limits of where clinical toxicities might be noted (based on animal toxicology data). A Bayesian approach is then used to construct a dose-toxicity curve. The phase 1 trial is started at one-tenth, the LD10 or MTD in the mouse or at one-third or one-sixth of the TDL in the dog. However, the difference is that only one patient is entered at the first dose level. After the appropriate amount of follow-up (usually 2-3 weeks), it is judged whether the patient had toxicities (≥grade 1). If not, then the dose toxicities curve is consulted to determine the next dose escalation. Dose escalation usually can proceed by doubling the dose as long as the dose is below the estimated MTD (on the dose-toxicity curve). The CRM/MCRM methods have now been in use for some time. There have been a few reviews of the results of trials conducted using the MCRM.[147-149] In general, the MCRM does not save the time it takes to complete the phase 1 trial, nor does it actually substantially decrease the number of patients entered into the phase 1 trial. However, what it does do is shorten the time it takes to get to a dose that is close to the MTD for the study, and the MCRM helps decrease the number of patients who receive a potentially ineffective (<80% of the MTD) dose in the context of a phase 1 study (see response rate information below).

Another method for dose escalation introduced by Simon and colleagues that also uses one patient per dose level is the *accelerated titration* design.[139] They introduced two designs (designs I and II). With design I, cohorts of one patient per dose level are treated with 40% escalations between dose levels. With the first DLT, there is an expansion of the cohort to a total of three new patients. With design II, there is only one patient per dose level, but there are dose escalations of 100% between levels, and with the first DLT, the level is also expanded to three new patients. Then escalation proceeds by 40% increments. On both designs I and II, intrapatient dose escalation is allowed if patients had grade 0-1 toxicity on the prior course. It is of note that very few groups advocate dose escalation within patients.[150] Dose escalation within patients can be confusing, particularly if there are cumulative toxicities with an agent (as was seen with the nitrosoureas). What is generally agreed on in this area is that if an individual patient on a phase 1 trial is having a beneficial effect with a new agent and is still receiving a low dose of that new agent, the patient should at least be offered the opportunity to receive a higher dose of the agent which is one level below a dose that has been deemed as safe in the phase 1 trial. The key is keeping the phase 1 patient informed of where the study is and what the safety (and efficacy) has been at higher dose levels. Unfortunately, the reality of the situation is that the average number of courses that patients receive on a phase 1 trial is only about two courses before they have rapid progression of their disease. This rapid progression rarely permits intrapatient dose escalations.

Another phase 1 dose escalation methodology that is now infrequently used is the method proposed in 1990 by Collins and colleagues.[103] This method is also known as the *pharmacologically guided dose escalation* method. The method is based on an important piece of work showing that the area under the C × T plasma disappearance curve (AUC) at the LD10 (or MTD) in the mouse is equal to the AUC at the MTD in humans. This finding provides the investigators with a target AUC. In practice, at each dose level, an AUC is determined for patients receiving that dose of the new agent. The AUC at that level is then used to determine what the next dose escalation will be (if the agent has linear kinetics). Use of this method for pharmacologically guided dose escalation requires real-time pharmacokinetics, which is sometimes problematic in a clinical situation. However, it can lead to more aggressive dose escalations. There have been some suggested improvements in the methodology that have been implemented by some phase 1 clinical trial groups.[148]

The other dose escalation method outlined in Table 46-5 that is of interest is the method suggested by Freedman and followed up by Daugherty and colleagues in 1998.[141,151,152] Basically, with this method, patients who are considering entry into a phase 1 trial are given the range of doses that are to be explored (usually ranging between 0.1 and 1.0 times the LD10 in the mouse (or one-sixth to one-third of the TDL to 1.0 × TDL in the dog). Patients are then given the opportunity to select the dose that they feel they should be given.

This introduces the ability of *patients* (facing the certainty that their cancer will kill them) to take control of the situation and *select their own dose*. Once the patient has received that dose, the next patient could select a dose that is higher than that dose. Although this may appear to be a somewhat dangerous approach, at least in one reported clinical trial it has proven to be safe.[152] However, in that initially reported experience (using a phase 1 clinical trial of a combination of agents), the authors felt that this method actually resulted in too many patients receiving lower doses of the agent, (This was not because patients were not aggressive in selecting their doses but because a clinical response was noted at a low dose level, and patients, hearing that, opted to receive the lower dose, which, with additional experience, showed no additional activity. Therefore, eventually further dose escalations were needed.)[152]

Definitions of MTD and DLT

The classic definition of an *MTD* is the highest dose that causes one or less than six patients to have DLT. This MTD is the dose that is generally recommended as the dose to be used in single-agent phase 2 trials. However, there have been different definitions of the MTD used by European research groups and it is important to carefully review the MTD definition in a protocol before working with a new agent.

The definition of a *DLT* is ≥ grade 3 nonhematologic or grade 4 hematologic (absolute neutrophil count < 500/μL for ≥7 days) toxicities according to the NCI common toxicities criteria found at the following website: <http://ctep.cancer.gov/reporting/ctc.html>.

There are frequent discussions as to whether phase 1 trials should always seek to define the MTD and DLTs. This question is being increasingly asked in clinical trials with mechanism-based agents (eg, monoclonal antibodies, kinase inhibitors). Rather than define a MTD, there is an increasing emphasis (using pharmacodynamic measurements) on defining a biologically effective dose (BED). Of note is that in drugs later approved by the FDA often the BED and the MTD are actually quite close to each other. In addition, caution is urged at stopping the phase 1 trial at the BED. The phase 1 trials with imatinib may have stopped too early if only the BED was used as a basis for stopping dose escalation. There is new evidence that one mechanism of resistance of CML cells to imatinib may be attributable to leukeimic cells, which harbor less sensitive mutations.[153] It would be nice to know whether higher doses of imatinib could be used to kill these clones of tumor cells.

Selection Criteria for Patients for Phase 1 Trials

Table 46-7 details commonly used selection criteria for inclusion in a phase 1 trial. These are offered as guidelines only. A few points on the exclusion criteria are worthy of discussion.

One major question is whether older patients should participate in phase 1 trials. Of note is the study by Bowen and colleagues, which indicated that a patient's chronologic age did not impact on the toxicities experienced in phase 1 trials of a new agent.[154]

One of the most interesting new questions that is arising in the phase 1 trial arena (because of the development of more targeted agents) is whether only patients whose tumors exhibit the particular target should be entered into the phase 1 trial. This would seem to make sense because if the patient's tumor has the target (eg, estrogen receptor or HER2/*neu*, CD20 or CD52 positivity, or the Bcr-Abl rearrangement or mutated c-kit), the patient is more likely to respond to the new agent. It is clear that the presence of the target in the patient's tumor should be a criterion for entry into the study *if* the agent is certain to work only on tumors that possess the target and if one is certain that the mechanism of action for the new agent is only against that particular target. In addition, one must be certain that the assay used to measure that particular target is accurate and reproducible. The selection of patients for entry on the new agent trial based on presence of the target in their tumors is certainly an entry criterion that will become a more standard criterion as we can better pinpoint the precise mechanism(s) of action of a new agent. Until then, the use of an entry criterion of the patients' tumor having the target is a bit uncertain.

Another frequent issue in selection of patients for a phase 1 trial is whether only patients with a certain disease should be entered into the study (eg, only patients with prostate cancer some times referred to be a discore). Interestingly, this is not frequently done but will probably be done more frequently as more targeted disease-specific agents are brought into phase 1 trials. Until that is done, it is likely that most phase 1 trials will continue to allow entry of patients with a variety of malignancies.

Are Phase 1 Clinical Trials Therapeutic?

Studies have been done documenting that, indeed, conventional responses (complete and partial responses) can be seen in patients with advanced malignancies who are participating in single-agent phase 1 trials of a new agent.[155,156] In older reviews, the true response rate ranged from 5% to 7% (with about a 1%

Table 46-7 **Common Selection Criteria for Entry of Patients into a Phase 1 Trial**

1. Age ≥18 years
2. Pathologically confirmed diagnosis of any malignant solid tumor
3. Measurable disease not required
4. Life expectancy ≥12 weeks
5. Karnofsky Performance Status of ≥70% (ECOG ≤2)
6. Adequate organ function:
   a) Neutrophils ≥1,500/ μL, hemoglobin ≥ 9 g/dL
   b) Platelets ≥100,000/μL
   c) Serum bilirubin with normal limits
   d) SGOT ≤2 × ULN (except if owing to disease, then ≤5 × ULN is acceptable)
   e) Serum creatinine within normal limits and calculated creatinine clearance ≥60 mL/min
   f) No trial or ventricular arrhythmias requiring control by medication, no ischemic event experienced within the preceding 6 months
   g) No history of seizure disorder requiring active therapy, no clinical evidence of malignancy of the central nervous system
7. Must have exhausted all therapy, which has a better chance of working for the patients (including investigational therapy) or must be in a situation for which there is no standard therapy
8. Must not have received any chemotherapy within 4 weeks prior to entry (6 weeks for mitomycin C or nitrosoureas) with complete recovery from toxic effects of that therapy
9. Patients must not be receiving any concomitant radiation therapy
10. Patients must have recovered from the reversible toxicities of prior therapy
11. Female patients must be of nonchildbearing potential or nonlactating and using adequate contraception with a negative pregnancy test at study entry and prior to each course of therapy
12. Male patients must also be using adequate contraception
13. No other serious concurrent medical illness or active infection should be present that would jeopardize the ability of the patient to receive (with reasonable safety) the chemotherapy outlined in this protocol
14. An effort must be made to minimize concomitant medications to those necessary for pain control, patient comfort, or life-threatening problems
15. Patients must sign an informed consent form. The patient must be aware of the neoplastic nature of his/her disease and willingly consent after being informed of the procedure to be followed, the experimental nature of the therapy, alternatives, potential benefits, side effects, risks, and discomforts

Abbreviations: SGOT, serum glutamic-oxaloacetic transaminase; ULN, upper limits normal.

complete response rate).[155] However, there are also examples of considerably higher response rates, particularly in phase 1 combination trials.[56,157,158] Most responses are noted in a range of 80-120% of the MTD for the agent.[155]

There are two recent studies, which have again reviewed the benefits and risks of phase 1 trials.[159,160] Horstmann and colleagues reviewed all non-pediatric phase 1 studies sponsored by the NCI between 1991 and 2002 (460 trials with 11,935 patients). The overall response rate for the single agent phase 1 trials was 4.4%. The toxic death rate was 0.49%. Roberts and colleagues reviewed 213 studies (6,474 cancer patients) published in peer-reviewed journals. They noted an overall response rate of 3.8%. Of note is that they have found that response rates have decreased over the 12-year observation period (6.2% during the period from 1991 to 1999, 2.5% during the period from 1999 to 2002). During the time studied the toxic death rate declined steeply from 1.1% to 0.06%. From these data, the authors concluded that the ratio of risk to benefit for a patient participating in phase 1 trial probably has improved.

Of increasing relevance is whether the category of stable disease will become an increasingly used measure of antitumor activity (particularly stable disease lasting ≥ 4 months). There is interest in this category of non-progressing patients, and it is likely to be increasingly used as a criterion to determine whether a new agent is exhibiting some antitumor effect in a phase 1 and also in a phase 2 setting.[161]

Another method that is gaining interest to determine whether a new agent is having some antitumor activity in a phase 1 trial is the concept of using patients as their own controls.[162] In this method, one uses the time a patient who is about to enter a new agent phase 1 trial has been on their prior therapeutic regimen as a control period (period A in Fig. 46-2 below). If the patient remains on the new phase 1 agent for a period of time (period B) longer than he/she was on a prior therapy (period A), the agent is judged to have had some impact on the natural history of the patients' tumor. If 30% of patients on the phase 1 trial (who are at or near the MTD) have a period B that is longer than period A, the agent may be a promising one. Of course, this method has not been prospectively evaluated, but it is becoming a method used increasingly by many clinicians working in the phase 1 trial arena.

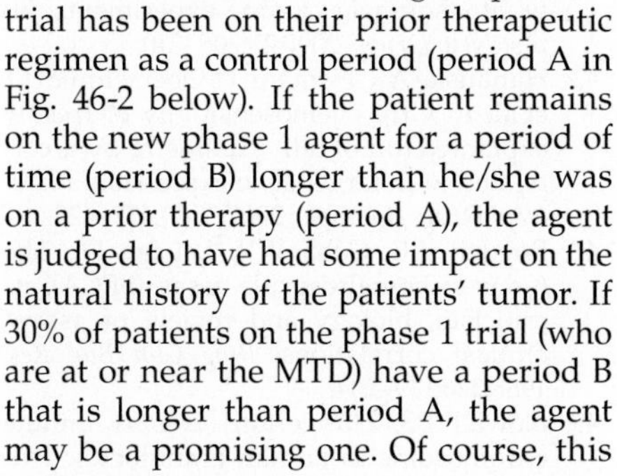

Figure 46-2 ■ The patient as his/her own control.

Combination of Agents in Phase 1 Trials

Conduct of phase 1 trials combining a new agent along with a standard already approved agent is a phase 1 trial in which the ethics are more straightforward (in that the patient will at least be getting one agent with proven clinical activity for some patients). There is an increasing amount of clinical trial activity in this area with initial experience, with at least the monoclonal antibodies (eg, trastuzumab, rituximab) demonstrating increased clinical activity when used in combination with standard chemotherapeutic agents. This is an area of active exploration with the recent addition of cytostatic agents such as signal transduction inhibitors used in combination with standard chemotherapeutic agents.[64] Of note is that to date, in randomized trials, the addition of a cytostatic small molecule to a cytotoxic agent has rarely added significant clinical activity to the cytotoxic agent.[163-165]

There are many issues in the design and conduct of these combination phase 1 trials. However, general guidelines include the fact that the standard agent should generally be administered at the dose and schedule that are usually used (eg, used at their approved dose and schedule) if possible. This improves acceptance by investigators and patients of the study design. Sequencing of the agents should be worked out in preclinical models (if possible), although the predictive value of these models is not well established. By starting with the recommended/acceptable dose of the standard agent, one can then start escalation of the new agent with a fixed dose of the standard agent. In general, the starting dose for the new agent would be 25% of the MTD for the new agent alone (if there are no overlapping toxicities with the standard agent). Depending on what is seen at that initial level, the next dose levels of the new agent would be 50% of its MTD, 75% of its MTD, and then 100% of its MTD (if possible). There are also some sophisticated models that have been reported to provide additional rationale for the dose escalations used in these combination phase 1 studies.[166]

Issues Regarding Phase 1 Trials in General

There are several publications about the ethics of patient participation in phase 1 trials.[141,167-169] Daugherty and colleagues noted that instead of the often quoted perception by many that patients were motivated by altruism, the motivation for patients participating in phase 1 trials included the following[170,171]:

1. Hope for improvement in their condition (high motivation)
2. Pressure exerted by relatives and friends (high motivation)
3. They felt they had no choice (high motivation)
4. Advice or trust of physicians (low motivation)
5. Altruism (low motivation)

These findings again emphasize how important it is for patients to have all the facts from the clinical development team so that they can make an informed decision as to whether or not to participate in a phase 1 trial. Two studies on the impact of a phase 1 trial on quality of life demonstrated that participation of a patient in a phase 1 trial increased a patient's level of hope and appetite (measures for quality of life).[172,173]

Future Technologies Likely to Impact on Phase 1 Trials

The rapid advances in functional imaging (eg, dynamic contrast magnetic resonance imaging, positron emission tomography, single-photon emission computed tomography) are likely to dramatically impact on the phase 1 clinical trial both by helping investigators assess pharmacodynamic end points as well as perhaps assess early evidence of an antitumor effect.

The above and other new technologies should help the phase 1 investigator determine more readily whether a particular new agent is helping a particular patient and improve the prospect for gain for patients who are willing to participate in phase 1 trials with new agents.

Selected References

The complete reference list can be found at www.CANCERMEDICINE8.com

1. O'Shaughnessy JA, Kelloff GJ, Gordon GB, et al. Treatment and prevention of intraepithelial neoplasia: an important target for accelerated new agent development. *Clin Cancer Res.* February 2002;8(2): 314–346.
2. Lippman SM, Heymach JV. The convergent development of molecular-targeted drugs for cancer treatment and prevention. *Clin Cancer Res.* July 15, 2007;13(14): 4035–4041.
3. Kelloff GJ, Sigman CC. Assessing intraepithelial neoplasia and drug safety in cancer-preventive drug development. *Nat Rev Cancer.* July 2007;7(7):508–518.

4. Bode AM, Dong Z. Targeting signal transduction pathways by chemopreventive agents. *Mutat Res.* November 2, 2004; 555(1–2):33–51.
5. Uliasz A, Spencer JM. Chemoprevention of skin cancer and photoaging. *Clin Dermatol.* May 2004;22(3):178–182.
6. Cohen V, Khuri FR. Chemoprevention of lung cancer. *Curr Opin Pulm Med.* July 2004;10(4):279–283.
7. Adair DS, Bogg HJ. Experimental and clinical studies on the treatment of cancer by dichloroethylsulfate (mustard gas). *Ann Surg.* 1931;93:190–199.
8. Goodman LS, Wintrobe MM, Damashek W, Goodman MJ, Gilman A, McLennan MT. Use of methyl-bis(beta-chloroethyl) amine hydrochloride and tris(beta-chloroethyl)amine hydrochloride for Hodgkin's disease, lymphosarcoma, leukemia and certain allied and miscellaneous disorders. *J Am Med Assoc.* 1946;132:126–132.
9. Rhoads CP. Nitrogen mustards in treatment of neoplastic disease. *J Am Med Assoc.* 1946;131:656–658.
10. Farber S, Diamond LK, Mercer RD, et al. Temporary remissions in acute leukemia in children produced by folic acid antagonist 4-aminopteroyl-glutamaic acid (aminopterin). *N Engl J Med.* 1948;238:787–793.
11. Rakieten N, Rakieten ML, Nadkarni MR. Studies on the diabetogenic action of streptozotocin (NSC-37917). *Cancer Chemother Rep.* May 1963;29:91–98.
12. Murray-Lyon IM, Eddleston AL, Williams R, et al. Treatment of multiple-hormone-producing malignant islet-cell tumour with streptozotocin. *Lancet.* October 26, 1968;2(7574):895–898.
13. Schaeppi U, Heyman IA, Fleischman RW, et al. cis-Dichlorodiammineplatinum(II) (NSC-119 875): preclinical toxicologic evaluation of intravenous injection in dogs, monkeys and mice. *Toxicol Appl Pharmacol.* June 1973;25(2):230–241.
14. Higby DJ, Wallace HJ, Jr, Albert D, Holland JF. Diamminodichloroplatinum in the chemotherapy of testicular tumors. *J Urol.* July 1974;112(1):100–104.
15. Wiltshaw E, Kroner T. Phase II study of cis-dichlorodiammineplatinum(II) (NSC-119875) in advanced adenocarcinoma of the ovary. *Cancer Treat Rep.* January 1976;60(1):55–60.
16. Rutman RJ, Cantarow A, Pasckis KE. Studies in 2-acetylaminofluorene carcinogenesis. III. The utilization of uracil-2-C14 by preneoplastic rat liver and rat hepatoma. *Cancer Res.* February 1954;14(2):119–123.
17. Heidelberger C. On the rational development of a new drug: the example of the fluorinated pyrimidines. *Cancer Treat Rep.* 1981;65(Suppl 3):3–9.
18. McGinn CJ, Zalupski MM, Shureiqi I, et al. Phase I trial of radiation dose escalation with concurrent weekly full-dose gemcitabine in patients with advanced pancreatic cancer. *J Clin Oncol.* November 15, 2001;19(22):4202–4208.
19. Elion GB, Hitchings GH, Vanderwerff H. Antagonists of nucleic acid derivatives. VI. Purines. *J Biol Chem.* October 1951;192(2):505–518.
20. Elion GB. Nobel Lecture. The purine path to chemotherapy. *Biosci Rep.* October 1989;9(5):509–529.
21. Driscoll JS. The preclinical new drug research program of the National Cancer Institute. *Cancer Treat Rep.* January 1984;68(1):63–76.
22. Boyd MR. Status of the NCI preclinical antitumor drug discovery screen. *Prine Pract Oncol Updates.* 1989;3:1–2.
23. Staquet MJ, Byar DP, Green SB, Rozeneweig M. Clinical predictivity of transplantable tumor systems in the selection of new drugs for solid tumors: rationale for a three-stage strategy. *Cancer Treat Rep.* September 1983;67(9):753–765.
24. Saijo N, Tamura T, Nishio K. Problems in the development of target-based drugs. *Cancer Chemother Pharmacol.* 2000;46(Suppl):S43–S45.
25. Gardner SN, Fernandes M. Cytostatic anticancer drug development. *J Exp Ther Oncol.* April 2004;4(1):9–18.
26. Johnson JI, Decker S, Zaharevitz D, et al. Relationships between drug activity in NCI preclinical in vitro and in vivo models and early clinical trials. *Br J Cancer.* May 18, 2001;84(10):1424–1431.
27. Skehan P, Storeng R, Scudiero D, et al. New colorimetric cytotoxicity assay for anticancer-drug screening. *J Natl Cancer Inst.* July 4, 1990;82(13):1107–1112.
28. Chabner BA. In defense of cell-line screening. *J Natl Cancer Inst.* July 4, 1990;82(13):1083–1085.
29. Grever MR, Schepartz SA, Chabner BA. The National Cancer Institute: cancer drug discovery and development program. *Semin Oncol.* December 1992;19(6):622–638.
30. Hodes L. Computer-aided selection of compounds for antitumor screening: validation of a statistical-heuristic method. *J Chem Inf Comput Sci.* August 1981;21(3):128–132.
31. Double JA, Bibby MC. Therapeutic index: a vital component in selection of anticancer agents for clinical trial. *J Natl Cancer Inst.* July 5, 1989;81(13):988–994.
32. Wang H, Klinginsmith J, Dong X, et al. Chemical data mining of the NCI human tumor cell line database. *J Chem Inf Model.* November 2007;47(6):2063–2076.
33. Covell DG, Huang R, Wallqvist A. Anticancer medicines in development: assessment of bioactivity profiles within the National Cancer Institute anticancer screening data. *Mol Cancer Ther.* August 2007;6(8):2261–2270.
34. Paull KD, Shoemaker RH, Hodes L, et al. Display and analysis of patterns of differential activity of drugs against human tumor cell lines: development of mean graph and COMPARE algorithm. *J Natl Cancer Inst.* July 19, 1989;81(14):1088–1092.
35. Weinstein JN, Myers TG, O'Connor PM, et al. An information-intensive approach to the molecular pharmacology of cancer. *Science.* January 17, 1997;275(5298):343–349.
36. Taverna P, Liu L, Hanson AJ, Monks A, Gerson SL. Characterization of MLH1 and MSH2 DNA mismatch repair proteins in cell lines of the NCI anticancer drug screen. *Cancer Chemother Pharmacol.* 2000;46(6):507–516.
37. O'Connor PM, Jackman J, Bac I, et al. Characterization of the p53 tumor suppressor pathway in cell lines of the National Cancer Institute anticancer drug screen and correlations with the growth-inhibitory potency of 123 anticancer agents. *Cancer Res.* October 1, 1997;57(19):4285–4300.
38. Scherf U, Ross DT, Waltham M, et al. A gene expression database for the molecular pharmacology of cancer. *Nat Genet.* March 2000;24(3):236–244.
39. Blower PE, Verducci JS, Lin S, et al. MicroRNA expression profiles for the NCI-60 cancer cell panel. *Mol Cancer Ther.* May 2007;6(5):1483–1491.
40. Shankavaram UT, Reinhold WC, Nishizuka S, et al. Transcript and protein expression profiles of the NCI-60 cancer cell panel: an integromic microarray study. *Mol Cancer Ther.* March 2007;6(3):820–832.
41. Suggitt M, Bibby MC. 50 years of preclinical anticancer drug screening: empirical to target-driven approaches. *Clin Cancer Res.* February 1, 2005;11(3):971–981.
42. Shoemaker RH, Wolpert-Defilippes MK, Kern DH, et al. Application of a human tumor colony-forming assay to new drug screening. *Cancer Res.* May 1985;45(5):2145–2153.
43. Hanauske A-R, Hanauske U, Von Hoff DD. The human tumor cloning assay in cancer research and therapy. *Curr Probl Cancer.* 1985;9:1–50.
44. Hanauske AR, Degen D, Marshall MH, Hilsenbeck SG, Grindey GB, Von Hoff DD. Activity of 2′,2′-difluorodeoxycytidine (Gemcitabine) against human tumor colony forming units. *Anticancer Drugs.* April 1992;3(2):143–146.
45. Hanauske AR, Degen D, Hilsenbeck SG, Bissery MC, Von Hoff DD. Effects of Taxotere and taxol on in vitro colony formation of freshly explanted human tumor cells. *Anticancer Drugs.* April 1992;3(2):121–124.
46. Hanauske A-R, Oberschmidt O, Hanauske-Abel H-M. Lahn MM, Eismann U. Antitumor activity of enzastaurin (LY317615. HCl) against human cancer cell lines and freshly explanted tumors investigated in *in vitro* soft-agar cloning experiments. *Invest New Drugs.* 2007;25:205–210.
47. Hanauske AR, Eismann U, Oberschmidt O, et al. In vitro chemosensitivity of freshly explanted tumor cells to pemetrexed is correlated with target gene expression. *Invest New Drugs.* October 2007;25(5):417–423.
48. Bogden AE, Cobb WR, Lepage DJ. The 6-day subrenal capsule assay (SRCA): its criticism, biology and review of assay/clinical correlations. *Prog Clin Biol Res.* 1988;276:139–204.
49. Nowell PS, Hungerford DA. A minute chromosome in human granulocytic leukemia. *Science.* 1960;132:1497.
50. Rowley JD. Letter: a new consistent chromosomal abnormality in chronic myelogenous leukaemia identified by quinacrine fluorescence and Giemsa staining. *Nature* June 1, 1973;243(5405):290–293.

47 Pharmacology

William K. Plunkett Jr., PhD ■ Mark Ratain, MD

This chapter will focus on the principles of clinical pharmacology as they apply to systemic anticancer therapy and will attempt to illustrate how an understanding of clinical pharmacokinetics and pharmacodynamics can optimize the therapeutic index of such agents.

General Mechanisms of Drug Action

The initial requirement for drug action is adequate drug delivery to the target site. This depends largely on blood flow in the tumor bed and the diffusion characteristics of the drug in tissue. However, delivery can also be influenced by the extent of plasma protein binding and, for orally administered drugs, by absorption, first-pass metabolism in the liver, and the requirement for activation by various mechanisms. Blood flow across a capillary bed is directly proportional to the arteriovenous pressure difference and inversely proportional to the geometric and viscous resistances. The geometric resistance to blood flow increases with increasing tumor size, a factor that may limit drug and oxygen delivery to large tumors, and thereby diminish the effectiveness of treatment with chemotherapy or radiation.[1] The most common route of drug administration for treatment of both localized and disseminated disease is by IV infusion, which by definition makes 100% of the drug available in the blood. Drugs may be administered by a number of routes in addition to IV infusions, however, to achieve specialized pharmacologic and therapeutic goals. Regional administration may be employed to more directly target the drug to the principal tumor site and to achieve a higher drug concentration in the vicinity of the tumor. Intraperitoneal infusion of cisplatin for ovarian cancers, intrapleural administration of bleomycin in the treatment of solid tumors, and intrathecal administration of cytarabine as a means of treating leukemias are examples of intracavitary drug delivery. alternatively, intravascular administration such as intra-arterial infusion of fluorodeoxyuridine into the hepatic artery for treatment of liver diseases has been used to achieve a pharmacologic advantage. Although oral administration is the most convenient and least expensive route of drug administration, it is associated with problems of inconsistent drug bioavailability among and within patients.[2] More consistent pharmacokinetic results are achieved with subcutaneous or intramuscular drug injections.

Delivery of the drug to the target cell is also dependent on the rate of removal from the blood. Excretion, either by the kidneys or by the biliary route, constitutes a major clearance mechanism. In addition, many drugs are cleared by metabolism to less effective or inactive metabolites as the blood passes through large body organs. Drug binding to plasma proteins can also effectively lower the concentration of free drug that is available for entry into target cells to a small fraction of the total concentration in blood.

Membrane Transport

In order to produce cytotoxicity, most anticancer drugs require uptake into the cell. A number of mechanisms exist for the passage of drugs across the plasma membrane, including passive diffusion, facilitated diffusion, and active transport systems. Passive diffusion of drugs through the lipid bilayer structure of the plasma membrane is a function of the size, lipid solubility, and charge of the drug molecule. If the extracellular drug concentration is constant, then drug accumulation by the cell will continue until the rate of drug uptake from the extracellular space is equal to the rate of drug efflux from the cell. At this point, a dynamic equilibrium is reached and intracellular and extracellular drug concentrations are equal. As the drug is cleared from the extracellular space, intracellular drug levels will decline if the drug is not bound or metabolized intracellularly. An important feature of the passive diffusion process is that it does not saturate; ie, as the extracellular drug concentration increases, influx into the cell increases proportionally and high intracellular drug levels can be achieved. Passive diffusion, however, is a highly inefficient and nonspecific process, although it may be a particularly important mechanism of drug uptake when carrier-mediated processes are nonfunctional, such as occurs in some cases of methotrexate resistance.

The passage of physiologically important hydrophilic compounds across the plasma membrane is usually mediated by a specific receptor, or carrier, in the plasma membrane that facilitates the translocation of the substance into or out of the cell. Carrier-mediated transport systems are distinguished from passive diffusion by having a higher degree of specificity and by being saturable at high extracellular drug concentrations owing to the presence of a finite number of receptor molecules within the membrane. Once all carrier sites become occupied, further increases in extracellular drug concentration will not produce further increments in drug influx unless a component of passive diffusion comes into play. The affinity of the carrier for the substrate can be estimated from the Km, the drug concentration at which the influx rate is one half maximal; the lower the Km, the higher the carrier affinity. Although carrier-mediated systems enhance the rate of influx into the cell, not all carriers are able to translocate compounds against electrochemical forces and ultimately develop gradients such that the intracellular concentration exceeds the extracellular drug level. To do so requires the expenditure of energy and the coupling of carrier-mediated transport to an energy requiring reaction, usually hydrolysis of adenosine triphosphate.

Many antineoplastic drugs, particularly those that are structural analogues of natural compounds, gain entry into the cell by carrier-mediated mechanisms. The functional and physiologic characteristics of several human nucleoside transporters have been characterized. However, substantial additional information is rapidly emerging as more of these molecules are cloned and their specificities are revealed.[3,4] Naturally occurring nucleosides are transported by both facilitated diffusion (equilibrative) and by concentrative mechanisms. Nucleoside analogues that are important in cancer therapy also use these transporters, but some specificity is emerging.[5] For instance, cytarabine, floxuridine, and pentostatin appear to use equilibrative transporters, whereas fludarabine, gemcitabine, and cladribine are also substrates for concentrative transport systems in addition to equilibrative pathways.[6–8] Antibodies with specificity for these membrane proteins are being developed and applied to answer questions that relate the prevalence of the proteins to clinical response to nucleoside analogue therapy.[9] Nucleobase transporters have also been identified, but their role in the entry of useful antimetabolites such as thiopurines and 5-fluorouracil (5-FU) into the cell has not been established.[3] Transport of reduced folates and methotrexate is an active energy-dependent process that can be mediated by two distinct mechanisms: a membrane carrier system capable of the rapid transport of reduced folates and of 4-amino analogues of folic acid,[10,11] and a group of membrane-bound folate receptors termed the folate binding proteins that are brought into the cell by endocytosis to release ligand before recycling back to the membrane.[12] The DNA sequences for genes performing this function have now been identified, and the expressed proteins have been evaluated in cells that otherwise lack the ability to transport methotrexate.[13,14] Altered methotrexate transport features have been described in acute lymphoblastic leukamia (ALL) blasts and in osteosarcoma as a mechanism of acquired resistance.[15] L-phenylalanine mustard uses at least two amino acid transport systems, and its influx can be inhibited by the amino acid substrates specific for these transport carriers.[16]

The importance of transmembrane movement of a drug to its pharmacologic effect depends on several factors including the rate of drug delivery to the tissue, the affinity of the transport process, and the nature of the intracellular biochemical events required for drug action. Though membrane transport can be the rate-limiting step in drug action if it governs the rate at which the drug reaches intracellular targets, this is not always the case. If drug delivery to a cell is slow relative to the influx rate, then the drug effect will be limited primarily by extracellular concentration, ie, blood flow and diffusion of the drug. Similarly, if a drug requires intracellular activation, such as phosphorylation of nucleoside analogues or polyglutamylation of methotrexate and other antifols, before they can exert a cytotoxic effect, then the rate-limiting step in drug action could be activation rather than transport.

Finally, it is important to recognize that membrane transport is frequently bidirectional with the final drug concentration in the cell representing the balance between drug influx and drug efflux. These processes may utilize different carrier systems and operate at different rates. Several efflux systems that appear to have importance in cancer chemotherapy mediate various forms of multidrug resistance. Although these have focused on efflux of complex biologically derived molecules, for example, anthracyclins and epipodophyllotoxins,[17,18] it is now clear that nucleotide analogues are also transported out of the cell by multidrug resistance-associated proteins, MRP4 and MRP5.[19,20]

Intracellular Activation

Many anticancer drugs require activation before they are able to exert a cytotoxic effect. The activation process may involve chemical or enzymatic reactions in either normal or tumor tissues (Table 47-1). Cisplatin, for example, undergoes a chemical reaction with water molecules intracellularly, resulting in the generation of a positively charged aquated species that attacks nucleophilic sites on DNA.[21] In contrast, the activation of cyclophosphamide is mediated primarily by CYP2B6 (one of the P-450 enzymes), resulting in the release of active alkylating species into the systemic circulation.[22]

Intracellular activation by tumor cells is a critical determinant of effect for most antimetabolites. Nucleoside analogues such as cytarabine, fludarabine, and gemcitabine require phosphorylation to active nucleotide triphosphate forms and incorporation into DNA before they are able to exert a cytotoxic effect.[23–26] Nucleobase analogues such as 6-mercaptopurine and 6-thioguanine undergo phosphoribosylation to the nucleoside monophosphate forms, which are active inhibitors of de novo purine nucleotide synthesis. Amination of 6-mercaptopurine to thioguanine monophosphate followed by phosphorylation, reduction to the deoxynucleotide, and a subsequent phosphorylation results in 2′-deoxythioguanine triphosphate, which is a substrate for incorporation into DNA. Phosphoribosylation also converts 5-FU to the monophosphate, which is then phosphorylated to the diphosphate, reduced to the deoxynucleotide and dephosphorylated to the active monophosphate F-dUMP that inhibits thymidylate synthase. Additionally, the drug may be cytotoxic after incorporation of either the ribosyl or deoxyribosyl triphosphate into RNA or DNA, respectively. Although methotrexate is an effective enzyme inhibitor in its native form, intracellular conversion of the drug to polyglutamate metabolites significantly increases its potency and facilitates its binding to a number of enzymatic sites.[27] Consistent with this is the finding of a more favorable clinical outcome in acute lymphocytic leukemia patients whose blasts accumulated higher levels of methotrexate polyglutamates.[28,29] It is important to note that phosphorylation of nucleic acid analogues and polyglutamylation of methotrexate produces charged molecules that are unlikely to diffuse or to be transported out of cells.

Table 47-1 **Activation of Anticancer Drugs**

Activation Reaction	Drug
Aquation	Cisplatin
Hydrolysis	Irinotecan
Polyglutamylation	Methotrexate
Phosphorylation	Cytarabine
	Fludarabine
	Gemcitabine
Phosphoribosylation	5-Fluorouracil
	6-Mercaptopurine
	6-Thioguanine
Microsomal oxidation	Cyclophosphamide
	Ifosphamide
	Procarbazine
Microsomal reduction	Bleomycin
Demethylation	Dacarbazine
	Hexamethylmelamine
Acetylation	Amonafide

The rate of formation of the activated drug species in the cell depends on the rate of transmembrane influx of the drug, the amount and affinity of the activating enzyme(s) in the cell, the extent of competition by the naturally occurring substrates of the activating enzymes, and the rate of degradation of the activated drug by catabolic enzymes. For many antimetabolites, membrane transport is rapid relative to enzymatic activation and is therefore not rate limiting. Once inside the cell, antimetabolites must compete with the natural substrates of metabolic enzymes for binding and activation. Finally, the activated drug then becomes a substrate for catabolic enzymes in the cell that tend to degrade it to the parent compound or to an inactive metabolite. Thus, the concentration of the active cytotoxic drug in the cell is the result of the interactions of all of these processes.

The pyrimidine nucleoside analogue, gemcitabine, provides an excellent example of these processes. Gemcitabine is a substrate for several transport systems, but likely gains entry to the cell by a high capacity equilibrative nucleoside transport system, the velocity of which is nearly proportional to gemcitabine concentrations, approaching millimolar.[30] This process is unlikely to limit gemcitabine transport into cells at the plasma concentrations (>60 μM) achieved by standard dose rates (>2000 mg/m^2/h). At such plasma concentrations, however, the transport systems provide cellular concentrations of gemcitabine that saturate the rate of gemcitabine phosphorylation by deoxycytidine kinase.[31] Recognition of this lack of linearity with increasing dose rate has prompted evaluation of strategies in which gemcitabine is infused at a fixed dose rate of 10 mg/m^2/min for several hours, which achieves plasma gemcitabine concentrations (~20 μM) that maximize the rate of gemcitabine phosphorylation.[32–34] Studies of circulating leukemia blasts have demonstrated that this approach increases the cellular accumulation of gemcitabine nucleotides.[35,36] Following the initial phosphorylation of gemcitabine, the monophosphate is metabolized by two successive phosphorylation reactions to the triphosphate, which, after its incorporation into replicating or repairing

DNA by various DNA polymerases is inhibitory to cell growth. The initial activating enzyme, deoxycytidine kinase, is present at the lowest specific activities in human leukemic blasts[37] and is believed to be the rate-limiting step in the formation of gemcitabine triphosphate,[32] and probably for incorporation of the drug into DNA. At each phosphorylation step, gemcitabine and its metabolites compete with endogenous deoxycytidine and its nucleotides for enzyme binding. Opposing the activation of gemcitabine are cytidine deaminase and dCMP deaminase that convert the nucleoside and its monophosphate, respectively, to inactive uracil derivatives.[38] In addition, the activity of phosphatases such as 5′-nucleotidase,[26] the activities of which differ among cell types, may be important determinants of the steady-state concentrations of gemcitabine nucleotides and the rate of elimination of the triphosphate at the end of gemcitabine infusion.[39] Thus, in the case of antimetabolites, the loss or diminished affinity of an activating enzyme or enhanced activity of a catabolic enzyme may tip the balance between clinical activity and drug resistance.

Drug Targets

Although cytotoxic anticancer drugs have traditionally been classified based on their mechanisms of action or their origins, they can also be grouped based on their targets. There are several major targets of drug action: nucleic acids, specific metabolic and signaling enzymes, and microtubules. When nucleic acids are the target, it is generally an action on the integrity or synthesis of DNA rather than of RNA that is presumed to cause cell death. There are several mechanisms by which drugs can bind DNA, the most well understood being alkylation of nucleophilic sites within the double helix. Most clinically effective alkylating agents have two moieties capable of developing a charged carbon that binds covalently to negatively charged sites on DNA such as the O^6 or N^7 positions of guanine. The cross-linking of the two strands of DNA produced by the bifunctional alkylating agents prevents the use of that DNA as a template for further DNA and RNA synthesis leading to inhibition of DNA replication and cell death.[40-42] Although alkylating agents are among the most widely used drugs in clinical oncology, the relationship of pharmacologic parameters to clinical effects has not been well defined for these agents. In part, this has been due to the lack of sensitive and specific techniques to detect drug-DNA binding in clinical specimens. Studies of chlorambucil-DNA binding in the tumor cells of patients with chronic lymphocytic leukemia have demonstrated considerable heterogeneity in drug-DNA binding among patient samples. However, no clear correlations have been demonstrated between the amount of drug bound and disease stage or sensitivity to treatment. In contrast, the formation of cisplatin adducts to DNA has been shown to correlate with cell kill in mammalian tumor cell lines.[43] Immunologic methods have been used to quantitate platinum-DNA adduct formation in peripheral white blood cells after cisplatin.[44] A separate study that used atomic absorption spectroscopy to quantitate total cell platinum in lymphocytes indicated a relationship between the levels of adduct after the first dose of either single-drug cisplatin or carboplatin and clinical response.[45] However, subsequent investigations have not found such a relationship between platinum-DNA adduct levels and clinical outcome.[46]

A second mechanism of drug binding to nucleic acids is intercalation, the insertion of a planar ring structure between two adjacent nucleotide bases of DNA. This mechanism is characteristic of many antitumor antibiotics. The antibiotic molecule is noncovalently, although firmly, bound to DNA and distorts the shape of the double helix, resulting in inhibition of RNA or DNA synthesis.[47,48] Many agents capable of classic intercalation, such as doxorubicin and mitoxantrone, are also inhibitors of topoisomerase II and may produce DNA strand breaks by inhibition of the re-ligation process of this enzyme.[49,50] Indeed, a direct correlation has been noted between DNA topoisomerase II activity and cytotoxicity in doxorubicin-sensitive and resistant P388 leukemia cells.[51] Although the epipodophyllotoxins, etoposide, and teniposide, do not intercalate in DNA, they are also effective topoisomerase II inhibitors that damage DNA. Topoisomerase I nicks a single DNA strand, which permits the rotation on the intact strand, after which the nick is closed. Blocking of the strand re-sealing function of topoisomerase I by topotecan and irinotecan can result in a double strand break when a DNA replication fork collides with the complex. Another of the drug-induced DNA to nucleic acids is illustrated by the mechanism of bleomycin. The amino terminal tripeptide of the bleomycin molecule appears to intercalate between guanine-cytosine base pairs of DNA. The opposite end of the bleomycin peptide binds Fe (II) and serves as a ferrous oxidase, able to catalyze the reduction of molecular oxygen to superoxide or hydroxyl radicals that produce DNA strand scission.[52,53] Predictably, the levels of antioxidant enzymes such as catalase, peroxidases, and superoxide dismutase in plasma and blood are inversely correlated with chromosomal damage.[54]

Enzymes represent the second general category of targets for chemotherapeutic agents. Antimetabolites function as inhibitors of key enzymes in the purine or pyrimidine biosynthetic pathways or as inhibitors of DNA polymerases. The triphosphate of fludarabine, for instance, is known to inhibit both ribonucleotide reductase[55] and DNA ligase I.[56] After incorporation into DNA it not only inhibits the function of multiple DNA polymerases,[57] DNA primase[58] and DNA ligase I,[56] it is also resistant to removal by the proof-reading exonuclease activities associated with DNA polymerases.[57] Since these enzymes are highly active during DNA replication, antimetabolites tend to be cytotoxic only when present in sufficient concentration during the vulnerable S phase of the cell cycle; these drugs are thus frequently referred to as S-phase specific. Nevertheless, because these enzymes are also required for repair of damaged DNA, it is likely that antimetabolites that inhibit these enzymes will be synergistic with agents which elicit an incision DNA repair response that requires re-synthesis of a DNA patch, regardless of cell-cycle stage. This has been a successful combination strategy for the treatment of chronic lymphocytic leukemia.[59]

Inhibition of oncogenic kinases with adenosine triphosphate (ATP) mimetics is an effective approach to targeting the pathophyisology of diseases. For instance, imatinib, dasatinib, and nilotinib are effective inhibitors of the Bcr-Abl kinase that drives chronic myelogenous leukemia. Imatinib is also effective against activated c-Kit kinase, which appears to have a major role in gastrointestinal stromal tumors. Sunitinib also inhibits c-Kit, as well as the receptor tyrosine kinases vascular endothelial growth factor receptor, and platelet-derived growth factor. Erlotinib, gifitinib, and lapatinib have a similar function against epidermal growth factor receptors expressed by several tumors.

The effectiveness of enzyme inhibitors also depends on the amount of the target enzyme, its affinity for the inhibitor, and on the extent of competition by natural substrates for enzyme binding. For example, complete saturation of all dihydrofolate reductase-binding sites is required before the enzyme is effectively inhibited. As methotrexate inhibits enzymatic activity, dihydrofolate, the natural substrate, accumulates behind the metabolic block and is able to effectively compete with methotrexate for further enzyme binding.[60] Thus, large amounts of methotrexate, well in excess of the enzyme binding capacity, are required to effectively inhibit dihydrofolate reductase activity. Similarly, in the case of 5-FU, the dUMP/F-dUMP value may be an important determinant of optimal inhibition of the target enzyme thymidylate synthase, and high ratios have been associated with lack of tumor response.[61] Also, the amount of thymidylate synthase expression or activity is an important determinant of 5-FU activity and correlates with therapeutic response.[62] Also, polymorphisims in the thymidylate synthase gene may have prognostic value.[63,64] In addition, high basal levels of thymidine phosphorylase have been associated with lack of response to 5-FU.[65] However, screening for thymidylate phosphorylase levels is an attractive approach to selecting patients for treatment with capecitabine or doxifluridine, nucleoside analogues that require the activity of this enzyme for release of 5-FU.[66,67]

The microtubule spindle structure provides a third target for chemotherapeutic agents, classically the vinca alkaloids, vincristine and vinblastine, but more recently vinorelbine. The vinca alkaloids exert their cytotoxic effects by binding to specific sites on tubulin inhibiting of assembly of tubulin into microtubules and ultimately dissolution of the mitotic spindle structure.[68] The microtubule system in cells performs a variety of other important functions, including transport of solutes, cell movement, and chromosomal separation, and provides structural integrity, any one of which could potentially be disrupted by tubulin binding agents.[69] The taxanes are a newer class of agents, consisting of the natural plant alkaloid paclitaxel and a semi-synthetic derivative docetaxel. These novel plant alkaloids inhibit cell division by stimulating tubulin polymerization, thus enhancing the formation and stability of microtubules[70] Paclitaxel-treated cells accumulate large numbers of microtubules, free and in bundles, that disrupt microtubule function, and which ultimately cause cell death.[71,72] Although docetaxel appears to be more potent than paclitaxel, the drugs appear to have similar toxicity profiles.[73] The epothilones are non-taxane agents that also are capable of stabilizing microtubules.[74,75] Early results indicate that these compounds are active in the clinic, but have a similar spectrum of toxicity as the taxanes.

Repair of Drug-Induced Injury

Cells that have been damaged by cytotoxic drugs exhibit a variety of repair mechanisms. Indeed the cytotoxic effects of a drug often represent the balance between injury and repair, and amplified repair mechanisms may account for cellular resistance to certain drugs. The cytotoxicity of alkylating agents reflects the balance between DNA adduct and cross-link formation and their removal by cellular repair processes.[76] Many cells contain specific enzymes that remove alkyl moieties from DNA, and thereby undergo direct repair of drug damage. A specific example is the protein O^6-alkylguanyltransferase that repairs DNA injury produced by chloroethylnitrosoureas. Cells containing large amounts of this protein tend to be relatively resistant to these chemotherapeutic agents. Depletion of alkyltransferase activity by exposure of cells to modified purine bases such as O^6 -benzyl guanine may be effective in circumventing this mechanism of resistance.[77–79] It is now clear that mammalian cells possess a family of such enzymes that are capable of repairing alkylation to specific nucleic acid bases, and that the abundance of these in a particular tissue may be responsible for conferring relative sensitivity or resistance to chemotherapeutic alkylating agents.[80–82]

Cells also contain a variety of free radical scavenging systems that protect them from the effects of ionizing radiation and drugs that generate oxygen free radicals intracellularly. Catalase, superoxide dismutase, and glutathione peroxidase, key enzymes in the detoxification of reactive oxygen species, may be deficient in some tissues, such as cardiac muscle, leading to excessive drug toxicity. Alternatively, an increase in these protective enzymes in tumor cells may be associated with resistance to drugs that act by generating reactive oxygen species.[83] For instance, some doxorubicin-resistant cells have been shown to increase activity of superoxide dismutase and sodium-dependent glutathione peroxidase; these cells exhibit diminished susceptibility to oxygen radical injury.[85] Recent investigations have indicated the potential for therapeutic approaches that target such protective mechanisms.[85] Other studies suggest that expansion of intracellular reduced glutathione pools or increased expression of glutathione transferase may be important mechanisms of alkylating agent resistance in animal and human tumors.[86–88]

Finally, cells may be able to circumvent drug-induced injury by increased production of target enzymes. In experimental models, exposure of cells to methotrexate or 5-FU can be shown to stimulate production of dihydrofolate reductase or thymidylate synthase, respectively.[89,90] New enzyme production occurs within minutes to hours of drug exposure and is presumed to represent enhanced translation of existing mRNA rather than transcription of additional message. Amplification of DNA also occurs, however, and may be a fundamental mechanism of acquired cellular resistance to antimetabolites and natural products because of increased constitutive production of target enzymes or P-glycoprotein.[91]

As mentioned earlier, a prerequisite to drug effect at the target tissue is adequate drug delivery. Pharmacokinetics describes the concentration-time history of a drug in the body and can be used to answer fundamental questions concerning the optimal route and schedule of drug administration. The remainder of this chapter will present the principles of pharmacokinetics and pharmacodynamics and illustrate their importance in cancer chemotherapy.

Principles of Pharmacokinetics

Definitions

Pharmacokinetics is the study of drug absorption, distribution, metabolism, and excretion (Fig. 47-1). A fundamental concept in pharmacokinetics is drug clearance, that is, elimination of drugs from the body, analogous to the concept of creatinine clearance. In clinical practice, clearance of a drug is rarely measured directly but is calculated as either of the following:

$$\text{Clearance} = \text{Dose}/\text{AUC} \quad (1)$$

or

$$\text{Clearance} = \text{Infusion rate}/C_{ss} \quad (2)$$

The area under the curve (AUC) represents the total drug exposure integrated over time and is an important parameter for both pharmacokinetic and pharmacodynamic analyses. As indicated in

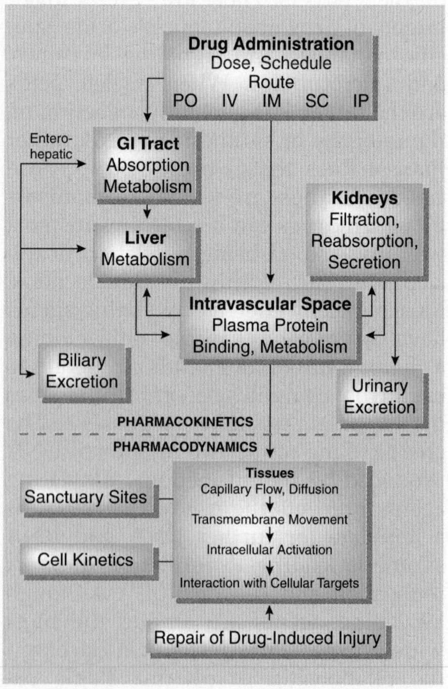

Figure 47-1 ■ Schematic representation of pharmacokinetics and pharmacodynamics. Pharmacokinetics represents the absorption, distribution, metabolism, and excretion of drugs from the body. Pharmacodynamics describes the interaction of drugs with target tissues. *Abbreviations*: GI, gastrointestinal; IM, intramuscular; IP, intraperitoneal; IV, intravenous; PO, by mouth; SC, subcutaneous.

Eq. 1, the clearance is simply the ratio of the dose to the AUC, so that the higher the AUC for a given dose, the lower the clearance. If a drug is administered by continuous infusion and a steady state is achieved, the clearance can be estimated from a single measurement of the plasma drug concentration (C_{ss}) as in Eq. 2.

Clearance can conceptually be considered to be a function of both distribution and elimination. In the simplest pharmacokinetic model,

$$\text{Clearance} = V\,K \quad (3)$$

where V is the volume of distribution, and K is the elimination constant. V is the volume of fluid in which the dose is initially diluted, and thus the higher the V, the lower the initial concentration. K is the elimination constant, which is inversely proportional to the half-life, the period of time that must elapse to reach a 50% decrease in plasma concentration. When the half-life is short, K is high and plasma concentrations decline rapidly. Thus both a high V and a high K result in relatively low plasma concentrations and a high clearance.

Linear Pharmacokinetic Models

Although pharmacokinetic analysis can be conducted without specifying any mathematical models (noncompartmental methods), it is helpful to use such models as guides in therapeutic decision making. There are several important characteristics of drugs that have linear pharmacokinetics (Table 47-2). The key feature of a linear pharmacokinetic model is that

$$dC/dt = -KC \quad (4)$$

This indicates that the instantaneous rate of change in drug concentration depends only on the current concentration. The half-life will remain constant no matter how high the concentration.

One implication of this principle is that the drug exposure (AUC) is not affected by changes in drug schedule. For example, the AUC after a 60 mg/m^2 bolus dose of doxorubicin equals the total AUC for 3 daily (or weekly) bolus doses of 20 mg/m^2, which equals the AUC for the same dose administered as a 96-h infusion. A second implication is that the AUC is proportional to the dose. Thus, if one measures the AUC for a 60 mg/m^2 dose, one can estimate the AUC for a 90 mg/m^2 dose in the same patient as being 50% greater.

Table 47-2 ■ **Characteristics of Drugs With Linear Pharmacokinetics**

Area under the curve (AUC) is directly proportional to dose
Half-life is independent of concentration
Clearance is independent of dose
Clearance is independent of schedule

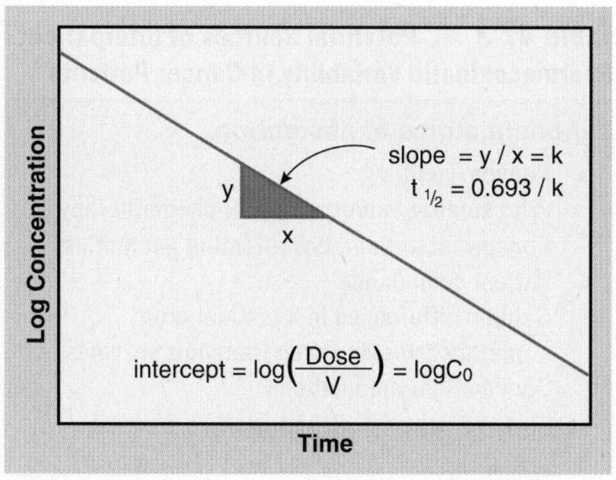

Figure 47-2 ■ Concentration-time plot for 1-compartment linear pharmacokinetic mode. C_0 represents the initial concentration, assuming instantaneous administration ad distribution. The half-life is $\log_e(2)/k$. *Abbreviation*: V, volume of distribution.

The simplest linear pharmacokinetic model, shown graphically in Figure 47-2, is

$$C(t) = \frac{\text{Dose}}{V}(e^{-kt}) \quad (5)$$

This model assumes that the drug is administered as an instantaneous bolus and that complete distribution of the drug is also instantaneous.

These assumptions are often not valid. If the drug is administered as a slow bolus or infusion, the model must be corrected for the infusion duration. During the administration of the drug, the concentration is increasing:

$$C(t) = \frac{\text{Dose}}{VKT}(1-e^{-kt}) \quad (6)$$

After the infusion is terminated, the drug concentration decays at the same rate as if it had been administered as an instantaneous bolus. Thus, if T represents the infusion time, then the postinfusion drug concentrations can be represented as

$$C'(t) = C\,(T)e^{-k(t-T)} \quad (7)$$

Often, the pharmacokinetic data are more complex than those shown in Figure 47-2 and may be optimally fitted to a multicompartment model, usually two or three compartments (Fig. 47-3). It must be emphasized that the compartments are theoretical and do not necessarily correlate with any anatomic space or physiologic process.

A large variety of computer software is available for pharmacokinetic analysis.[92–94] The interested reader is likely to benefit from hands on experience with such programs. Several caveats need to be emphasized for the casual reader. The validity of pharmacokinetic modeling depends to a large extent on the quality of the data entered into the model. Thus, drug infusions must be precisely timed, a sufficient number of plasma samples must be drawn, the samples must be obtained on schedule, and analytic methods must be sensitive and specific. The data must be properly weighted to avoid bias due to the increased probability of analytic errors at drug concentrations near the detection limit of the assay. Results obtained using a specific model should be compared with those using noncompartmental methods. Extrapolation of models outside the known time points must be done with great caution.

Nonlinear Pharmacokinetic Models

Nonlinear pharmacokinetic models imply that some aspect of the pharmacokinetic behavior of the drug is saturable. The mathematics of nonlinear models is beyond the scope of this chapter, but the principles are very relevant to several anticancer agents.[95–97] In contrast to the administration schedule of drugs with linear pharmacokinetics, alteration of the administration schedule of drugs that display nonlinear kinetics may markedly affect the AUC and potentially alter clinical effects.

Nonlinear pharmacokinetic behavior commonly occurs when there is saturation of a major metabolic or transport pathway. This results in decreased

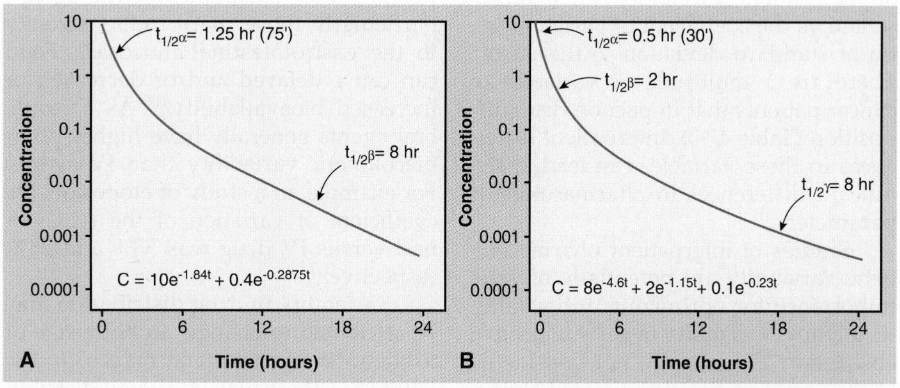

Figure 47-3 ■ Concentration-time plots for representative 2-compartment (**A**) and 3-compartment (**B**) linear pharmacokinetic models. The two curves are very similar, with $C_0 \sim 10$ for both models. Note that for each "compartment" there is one term, and the corresponding half-life equals t½ $\log_e(2)/k^n$, where k^n is the *n*th term.

clearance at higher doses, with a greater-than-proportional increase in the AUC. The AUC will also increase if the infusion duration is shortened because of slower clearance at the higher peak plasma concentrations. This is clearly the case for 5-FU, probably because of saturation of its conversion to dihydrofluorouracil by the enzyme dihydropyrimidine dehydrogenase.[98–100] Doubling of the 5-FU dose from approximately 7.5 mg/kg to 15 mg/kg (by IV bolus) resulted in a 135% increase in the mean AUC.[101] Since 5-FU is used on a variety of schedules, its nonlinear pharmacokinetic behavior may be one factor in its highly schedule-dependent effects. Paclitaxel has also been demonstrated to have nonlinear pharmacokinetics.[102–104] Thus, the AUC is higher, for a fixed dose, when administered by a shorter (3-h vs 24-h) infusion schedule, although this does not result in enhanced toxicity.[105]

The opposite situation arises when a drug's absorption from the gastrointestinal tract (or renal tubular reabsorption) is saturable. In this case, an increase in dose results in a less than proportional increase in the AUC. Gastrointestinal absorption of drugs that resemble natural compounds is frequently mediated by active transport processes that display saturable kinetics. Folate analogues such as methotrexate or leucovorin and amino acid analogues such as melphalan are examples of drugs with saturable absorption.[106–108] Cisplatin appears to have nonlinear pharmacokinetics owing to the saturation of its renal tubular reabsorption.[109,110] Free plasma platinum is increased by 42% when the drug is given as a 24-h continuous infusion, rather than as a 20-min infusion.[109] Prolonged infusion was also associated with a greater than threefold increase in the free platinum half-life.

Interpatient Pharmacokinetic Variability

In describing a drug's pharmacokinetics, it is important to consider the extent of interpatient variability, often represented as the coefficient of variation (ratio of standard deviation to the mean). There are a multitude of variables in cancer patients that impact on drug disposition (Table 47-3). Interpatient differences in these variables can lead to significant differences in pharmacokinetic parameters.[111]

Studies of interpatient pharmacokinetic variability are potentially of great importance for optimizing antineoplastic therapy. Variability in gastrointestinal absorption is generally not considered in the use of orally administered antineoplastic agents even though drugs such as cyclophosphamide, chlorambucil, melphalan, and etoposide are commonly administered orally for a variety of malignancies.[2] The fraction of an administered dose of drug that reaches systemic circulation is referred to as its bioavailability. Alternatively, it is the ratio of the plasma AUC after oral administration to the plasma AUC after IV administration of the same dose. Bioavailability is influenced both by absorption barriers and the first-pass effect, which is the reduction in available drug due to metabolism in the gastrointestinal tract and liver before an orally administered dose reaches systemic circulation. The bioavailability of the (6R) isomer of leucovorin, for example, is primarily limited by absorption. By contrast, (6S) leucovorin has limited bioavailability because of its rapid conversion to 5-methyltetrahydrofolate prior to reaching the systemic circulation.[112] Bioavailability is often highly variable and unpredictable[25,113–117] and may be accentuated by concomitant administration of other chemotherapeutic agents, particularly those that produce toxicity to the gastrointestinal mucosa.[107] Food can cause delayed and/or decreased or increased bioavailability.[118] As a result, oral agents generally have higher pharmacokinetic variability than IV agents. For example, in a study of etoposide, the coefficient of variation of the AUC for oral versus IV drug was 58% and 28%, respectively.[119]

Table 47-3 ■ Potential Sources of Interpatient Pharmacokinetic Variability in Cancer Patients

Abnormalities of absorption
Nausea/vomiting
Prior surgery, radiotherapy, or chemotherapy
Concurrent antiemetics affecting gut motility
Patient compliance
Genetic differences in intestinal drug metabolizing and drug transport enzymes
Concomitant medications
Abnormalities of distribution
Weight loss
Obesity
Decreased body fat (lipophilic drugs)
Pleural effusions or ascites (methotrexate)
Abnormalities of elimination
Hepatic dysfunction because of tumor replacement or prior (or concurrent) therapy
Renal dysfunction because of malignant involvement or prior (or concurrent) therapy
Genetic differences in drug metabolizing and drug transport enzymes
Concomitant medications
Abnormalities in protein binding
Hypoalbuminemia
Concomitant medications

Variability in drug distribution may be attributed to changes in body size or to the ratio of fat to total mass.[120] In the latter case, there may be altered distribution of lipophilic drugs, which includes most of the natural product anticancer drugs and their analogues. The terminal elimination half-lives of doxorubicin, cyclophosphamide, and ifosfamide are prolonged in obese patients.[121–124] In the case of doxorubicin and cyclophosphamide, this appears to be due to a reduction in clearance, whereas in the case of ifosfamide it is related to an increased volume of distribution of the drug.[122] Drug distribution can also be altered in the setting of "third-space" fluid. The best described example of this is the delayed clearance of methotrexate due to accumulation of drug in and slow release of the drug from ascites and pleural effusions.[125]

Many patients with advanced cancer have abnormalities of liver function tests or known mass lesions within the liver, often in association with significant malnutrition. Because many antineoplastic agents are metabolized or excreted by the liver, recognizing altered elimination by the liver becomes important in the optimization of chemotherapy dosing. Unfortunately, altered hepatic metabolism or excretion of drugs is not easily predictable. Clearly, patients with severe hyperbilirubinemia due to parenchymal replacement or obstruction are likely to have altered elimination.[126,127] However, it is not often recognized that many patients with normal serum bilirubin levels may have a low drug clearance resulting in a high AUC and corresponding toxicity as a result of other liver function test abnormalities. A decrease in serum albumin (in patients with normal serum bilirubin concentrations) has been associated with a decrease in the hepatic elimination of antipyrine, a commonly used marker drug, and of vinblastine and trimetrexate.[128–131] Thus, patients with a serum albumin less than 2.5 g/dL may be at increased risk of toxicity and are potential candidates for dose reduction of agents requiring hepatic metabolism or excretion.

In contrast, alterations in renal function generally correlate with renal clearance of drugs, since renal drug clearance tends to correlate with creatinine clearance. This has been well established for carboplatin, for which a firm relationship exists between renal function and carboplatin clearance. This relationship can be used prospectively to modify the carboplatin dose and avoid excessive toxicity.[132–134]

At present, dose adjustments for hepatic and renal dysfunction are most often made empirically and manufacturer recommendations are of limited use. This is illustrated by the recommended dose reduction for capecitabine in the setting of renal impairment.[135] In an editorial regarding this recommendation,[136] Ratain noted that the recommended 25% reduction was for patients with a creatinine clearance of 31–50 mL/min as estimated by the Cockcroft-Gault formula, which has been criticized as inaccurate.[137–141] This formula estimates a lower creatinine clearance for women and individuals with increased serum creatinine, low weight, and increased age. Furthermore, this definition of renal impairment is not adjusted for body surface area (BSA). As a result, it is possible that a small woman would receive a dosage reduction and a large man would not, even though their BSA-normalized creatinine clearances were the same. Also, before such a dose adjustment is recommended, there must be data supporting a correlation between creatinine clearance and drug pharmacokinetics or there is the potential for subtherapeutic dosing. Because of examples such as capecitabine, there is an increasing interest in performing dose-finding and pharmacokinetic studies in patients with hepatic and renal abnormalities. This is evidenced by the formation of the National Cancer Institute Organ Dysfunction Working Group and the recent publication of several trials in these subpopulations.[126,142–146]

Abnormalities of protein binding are common, but rarely have an impact on clinical outcome. Many anticancer drugs, such as the vinca alkaloids and etoposide, are highly bound to proteins such as albumin.[127,147,148] Changes in protein binding may affect drug clearance.[149,150] More importantly, abnormal protein binding must be considered in the interpretation of measured total plasma drug concentrations, since a decrease in protein binding will result in a relative increase in the pharmacologically active "free" drug[127,151] For a given dose, levels of unbound, active drug will be higher in the hypoalbuminemic patient as compared with the patient with normal albumin levels.

Identifying genetic differences in drug disposition (absorption, distribution, metabolism, and excretion) may be particularly important in understanding interindividual pharmacokinetic variability.[152–154] For example, SN-38 is the active metabolite of irinotecan and is primarily inactivated through biotransformation into SN-38 glucuronide (SN-38G) by UDP-glucuronosyltransferase 1A1 (UGT1A1).[155] Transcriptional efficiency of the UGT1A1 gene is inversely correlated with the number of TA repeats in the promoter TATA box of the gene.[156] Investigators have demonstrated that the AUC for SN-38 is directly correlated with the number of TA7 (7 TA repeats) alleles, so that individuals that are homozygous for TA7 have higher AUC values than those who are not.[157] Clinically, these patients are at higher risk of severe neutropenia. The observed pharmacokinetic variability of other anticancer agents, such as 6-mercaptopurine,[158,159] 5-FU, and amonafide,[160–162] can also be explained, in part, by pharmacogenetic variation. The importance of this source of interpatient variability is demonstrated by the incorporation into the product labels for irinotecan[163] 6-mercaptopurine[164] the recommendation that prescribers consider initial dosage reductions in the presence of reduced UGT1A1 and thiopurine methyltransferase (TPMT) activity, respectively.

Intrapatient Pharmacokinetic Variability

Although it is well established that interpatient pharmacokinetic variability may be significant, the importance of intrapatient variability (within a single patient) is less clear.[165] Oncologists are commonly faced with the clinical situation of increasing myelosuppression after repetitive dosing. This is generally assumed to be due to the cumulative effects of chemotherapy, making the patient more sensitive to subsequent doses. However, it is also possible that the patient's clearance of the drug(s) may have decreased, resulting in increased drug exposure.

Such a situation may arise when either hepatic or renal function changes. Renal function may change because of progressive disease (ureteral obstruction), complications of therapy (volume depletion), or as a direct toxic effect of therapy (cisplatin). Similarly, renal function may improve over time, reducing the actual drug exposure. Hepatic function may also change, producing changes in drug clearance that may result in the appearance of increased toxicity over time, as is the case for vinblastine administered by prolonged continuous infusion.[130] Thus, clinicians should carefully review the outcome of prior doses to minimize the risk of an undesirable outcome due to intrapatient pharmacokinetic variability.

Another potential source of intrapatient pharmacokinetic variability is an individual's circadian rhythm. The best studied drugs in this regard are 5-FU and 5-fluoro-2′-deoxyuridine. The circadian variability of 5-FU plasma concentrations during a 5-day infusion at a constant dose was twofold between maximum and minimum values.[166,167] An inverse correlation exists between plasma 5-FU concentration and the activity of dihydropyrimidine dehydrogenase, the major catabolic enzyme for 5-FU.[168] Investigators have explored the feasibility, toxicity, and activity of chronomodulated therapy with 5-FU, which takes advantage of the apparent circadian changes in drug clearance by increasing drug infusion during the time intervals when clearance is increased.[169–172]

Drug-Drug Interactions

Despite the fact that anticancer drugs are almost always given as combination chemotherapy, there have been relatively few studies in this area despite the risk of pharmacokinetic interactions. For example, with the combination of paclitaxel and cisplatin, an important regimen for ovarian cancer, cisplatin reduces paclitaxel clearance if given first.[173]

Studies of modulators of drug reactions have also demonstrated that inhibition of clearance may be an unexpected outcome. In a clinical study of the effects of oral cyclosporine on irinotecan pharmacokinetics, in which subjects received irinotecan both with and without cyclosporine, investigators found a marked reduction in irinotecan clearance (from 13.4 L/h/m^2 to 5.8 L/h/m^2) with the addition of cyclosporine.[174] Moreover, the AUC of the active metabolite SN-38 was significantly increased. Similar effects of cyclosporine on clearance have been demonstrated for etoposide,[175,176] doxorubicin,[177,178] and mitoxantrone.[176]

The oncologist must be aware of the patient's prescription medication list and consider the pharmacokinetic and therapeutic consequences when prescribing a new drug. A drug-drug interaction with potential therapeutic implications is that of tamoxifen and selective serotonin reuptake inhibitor (SSRI) antidepressants. Both are metabolized by CYP2D6, and SSRIs are commonly prescribed for the hot flashes associated with tamoxifen therapy. A prospective study of 80 breast cancer patients in which 29% were taking SSRI antidepressants after 4 months of tamoxifen therapy.[179] found that the mean plasma concentrations of endoxifen, an active metabolite of tamoxifen, decreased by 56% (p = .02) with paroxetine coadministration. There was also an interesting interaction between SSRIs and CYP2D6 genotype in that subjects who were homozygous for the wild-type CYP2D6 allele had a greater reduction in endoxifen concentrations as compared with those who were heterozygous (58% vs 38%). The precise clinical implications of a decrease in endoxifen concentrations is still under investigation, but these data do raise the question of whether concomitant administration of SSRI antidepressants to reduce the side effects of tamoxifen may jeopardize the efficacy of patient's anticancer therapy, and the U.S. Food and Drug Administration is currently considering incorporating the pharmacogenetic data into the product label for tamoxifen.

In recent years, the use of herbal medicines and nutritional supplements by cancer patients has been increasing.[180] The perceived low risk of these agents and lack of knowledge about their pharmacology can result in unexpected toxic and pharmacokinetic effects when they are used concomitantly with chemotherapy. For example, St. John's wort (*Hypericum perforatum*) is a known ligand for the pregnane X receptor (PXR).[181,182] It can therefore induce the transcription of PXR-regulated genes such as CYP3A and uridine diphosphate glucuronosyltransferases (UGTs).[181,183–185] The use of St. John's wort decreases plasma concentrations of SN-38 (active metabolite) in irinotecan-treated patients, prompting concerns that efficacy might be reduced.[186]

Principles of Pharmacodynamics

Definitions

In a general sense, pharmacodynamics is the study of dose-response relationships.[187] Thus, any laboratory or clinical study employing different doses of an agent is addressing a pharmacodynamic question. Examples include the exposure of tumor cells in vitro to varying doses of a new agent to evaluate its dose response relationship or a phase I clinical trial to define the maximally tolerated dose and dose-limiting toxicities in patients.

In the clinical setting, the results of treatment depend on both pharmacokinetics and pharmacodynamics (Fig. 47-1). A patient may have excessive toxicity at the "standard" dose for one of two reasons. If the patient's pharmacokinetics are different from those of the typical patient (eg, decreased renal clearance of carboplatin), there may be decreased total-body clearance resulting in a higher than expected drug exposure. The second possibility is that the patient might simply be more sensitive to an average drug exposure because of prior therapy, poor nutrition, or some other less well-defined reason. It is important to distinguish between these two possibilities. In the first case, lowering the dose will result in an "average" drug exposure, whereas in the second case, lowering the dose will result in a lower-than average drug exposure. Therefore, in the setting of dose reduction, there is a greater possibility of a response in the patient with abnormal pharmacokinetics than in the "sensitive" patient with abnormal pharmacodynamics.

General Pharmacodynamic Principles

In the most general sense, any drug may be considered to have a maximal effect and a median dose (the dose required for 50% of the maximal effect). Wagner proposed a generalized sigmoidal model of drug effect (Fig. 47-4), derived from the hypothesis that all drug effects require an initial interaction with a receptor.[188]

Most studies addressing pharmacodynamic modeling of anticancer agents have addressed phase-specific agents separately.[189,190] It may be adequate to use a simple log-linear model for nonphase-specific agents[189,190]

$$\text{Survival fraction (SF)} = \frac{\text{No. of treated cells}}{\text{No. of control cells}} = e^{-KC} \qquad (8)$$

This may be referred to as a steep dose-response curve, since the effect continues to increase proportionally as the concentration (C) increases. For any K (in Eq. 8), an increase in C by 2.3/K will result in a 1-log increase in antitumor effect (Fig. 47-5A).

The dose-response relationships for phase-specific agents, such as the antimetabolites, are much more complicated. By definition, some cells are out of "phase" and therefore not sensitive (or relatively insensitive) to the effects of the drug during the period of drug exposure. This is not necessarily overcome by increasing the dose, but could be overcome by increasing the duration of drug exposure. The result is the appearance of a plateau in the dose-response curve (Fig. 47-5B).

The effects of some antineoplastic agents depend on both the drug concentration and the duration of exposure to that concentration. For some agents, the effect is a function of the product of the concentration and exposure time, analogous to the AUC.[191] However, for antimetabolites and other phase-specific agents, the mathematical relationships are much more complex[189,190,192,193] and drug effect tends to be related to duration of exposure above a threshold concentration.

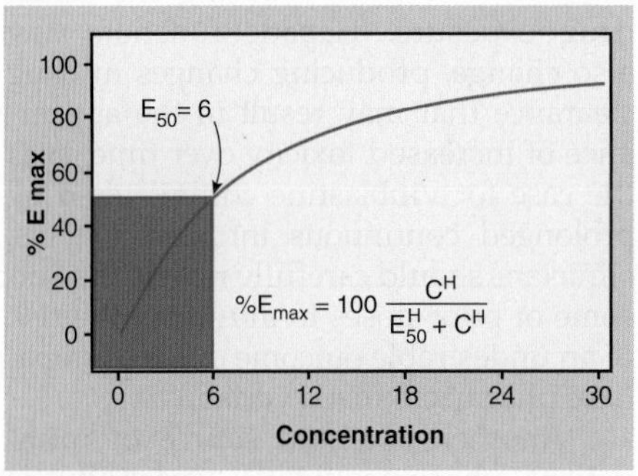

Figure 47-4 ■ Example of E_{max} model as proposed by Wagner. The maximum effect is 100%, and a concentration of six results in 50% effect. The exponent H, also known as the Hill constant, determines the shape of the curve and is usually between 1 and 2.

Plasma concentrations may be an inadequate predictor of clinical effect for those agents that undergo intracellular anabolism to active metabolites, such as is the case for cytarabine.[194] Plasma cytarabine concentrations do not appear to correlate with the rate of cellular cytarabine triphosphate (ara-CTP) accumulation or peak ara-CTP concentration in leukemia cells, although the intracellular concentration of ara-CTP is an important determinant of treatment outcome. Thus, knowledge of the plasma pharmacokinetics of cytarabine is not likely to be a useful predictor of treatment outcome for individual patients. For 6-mercaptopurine, pharmacogenetic evaluation may be potentially useful for modeling relationships between drug pharmacokinetics and clinical effects, as this drug's conversion to active intracellular 6-thioguanine metabolites by TPMT is genetically determined.[159] Studies in children with acute lymphoblastic leukemia suggest that intracellular levels of 6-thioguanine nucleotides may be an independent predictor of remission duration[158] and that heterozygosity for allelic variants of TPMT conferring lower enzyme activity correlates with a significantly lower rate of post-treatment minimal residual disease, an important prognostic factor.[195]

Pharmacodynamic Modeling of Cancer Chemotherapy

The introduction of pharmacodynamic modeling into clinical oncology has been a slow process. The relationship between toxicity subsequent to high-dose methotrexate and that of delayed methotrexate clearance has led to the routine use of therapeutic drug monitoring of plasma methotrexate concentrations to guide leucovorin dosing.[196] Studies of other drugs have not clearly resulted in a change in

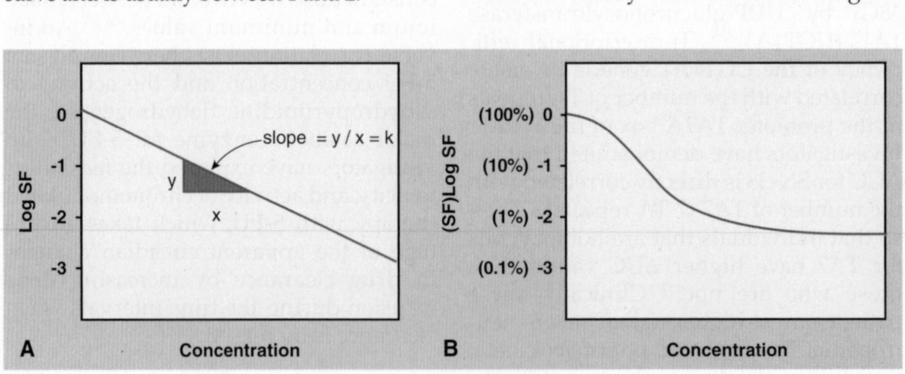

Figure 47-5 ■ Pharmacodynamic plots for drugs with **(A)** nonsaturable and **(B)** saturable effects. In the simplest pharmacodynamic model **(A)**, there is a linear relationship between dose and log kill. In **(B)** there is a maximal effect, resulting in a plateau in the dose-response curve. *Abbreviation:* SF, survival fraction.

clinical practice, although there has been an increase in clinical research in this area.[197]

Most early pharmacodynamic studies addressed relationships between measurements of drug exposure (AUC, C_{ss}) and toxicity. Such is the case for the leukopenia/neutropenia caused by etoposide.[151,198–204] More recently, investigators have modeled toxicity by using novel pharmacokinetic parameters, such as time above a threshold concentration for etoposide[205–207,221] and paclitaxel.[102,104,208,209] Other investigators have addressed the importance of active metabolites. This is of particular importance for irinotecan, a drug with both complex metabolism and toxicity patterns. Studies have suggested that irinotecan-induced diarrhea is due to direct intestinal damage by the biliary excretion of its active metabolite SN-38.[210,211] It has also been shown that neutropenia correlates strongly with SN-38 AUC.[157,212]

One of the best-characterized drugs is carboplatin, an analogue of cisplatin. Unlike cisplatin, the dose-limiting toxicity of carboplatin is thrombocytopenia, which is a function of drug dose, renal function, pretreatment platelet count, and prior therapy.[132] The platelet nadir produced by a dose of carboplatin is related to the carboplatin clearance, which is directly proportional to creatinine clearance. Thus, patients at high risk of severe thrombocytopenia following carboplatin therapy can be identified prospectively, and the drug doses can be modified by monitoring creatinine clearance. There is an expanding interest in trying to optimize cancer chemotherapy by individualizing dosing on the basis of measurements of plasma or tissue drug concentrations. Investigators have attempted to optimize the dosing of etoposide,[151,213] teniposide,[214] melphalan,[215] busulfan,[216,217] and 5-FU[218] by monitoring plasma drug concentrations during treatment, then using the information obtained to modify the total dose of chemotherapy administered in an attempt to avoid severe toxicity.

The targeted outcome with individualized dosing is most often toxicity. This is because of a lack of well-defined relationships between systemic exposure and efficacy for most anticancer agents. Such relationships, however, have been demonstrated for some drug/disease pairs. A prospective, randomized study of 182 children with acute lymphoblastic leukemia was conducted comparing standard fixed dosing versus individualized dosing of methotrexate-based therapy.[219] The latter was based on adjusting the doses to achieve plasma AUCs in the 50th to 90th percentile (based on historical controls). Researchers found that those receiving individualized therapy had an improvement in the rate of continuous complete remission (76% vs 66%) at 5 years. Pharmacodynamic relationships involving efficacy have also been found for carboplatin and ovarian cancer,[220] 5-FU and colorectal[221] and head and neck[191,222] cancer, and busulfan and allogeneic bone marrow transplantation.[223]

The Future Role of Anticancer Pharmacodynamics

Should the clinical oncologist care about pharmacodynamics? Will therapeutic drug monitoring of antineoplastics be as useful as monitoring of theophylline or aminoglycoside dosing? How will these studies improve the therapeutic index? These are important issues that are currently being addressed.

Our true understanding of the dosing of most antineoplastic drugs is primitive. BSA is generally the only value used to determine initial dosing; but this practice has come under increasing criticism because, for the vast majority of anticancer drugs, BSA does not correlate with pharmacokinetic or pharmacodynamic parameters.[224–229] Prior toxicity may be used to adjust dosing for subsequent cycles, although doses are more often reduced than escalated, and the magnitude of dose changes is determined empirically and often arbitrarily.

For drugs with a relatively broad therapeutic index and/or minimal interpatient pharmacokinetic or pharmacodynamic variability, individualized dosing strategies may not be necessary. However, when interpatient differences are significant, the implications on outcomes can be profound. As an example, individualized dosing of busulfan in the treatment of patients with advanced hematologic malignancies undergoing allogeneic bone marrow transplant may help to both minimize life-threatening toxicity (venoocclusive disease) and improve survival, since there is a relationship between drug exposure and successful engraftment.[224]

A particularly exciting area of current research is pharmacogenetics. As investigators discover drug disposition polymorphisms that impact absorption, metabolism, and transport of anticancer drugs, dose individualization based on a patient's genetics will become possible. Development of this dosing strategy will require collecting DNA samples for the genotyping of candidate polymorphisms and blood samples for pharmacokinetic data in the context of large phase II and/or III clinical trials. In this way, relationships can be developed that involve not only toxicity, but also efficacy. As studies of the pharmacodynamics of single agents are completed, the next challenge will be to optimize combination chemotherapy as most cancers are treated with combinations of anticancer agents. The importance of such studies is demonstrated by the example of carboplatin and paclitaxel, where the combination results in less thrombocytopenia than carboplatin as a single agent.[230,231] At a minimum, clinicians should understand the basic principles, realizing the limitations of our current approaches.

Selected References

The complete reference list can be found at www.CANCERMEDICINE8.com

2. DeMario MD, Ratain MJ. Oral chemotherapy: rationale and future directions. *J Clin Oncol.* 1998;16:2557–2567
10. McGuire JJ. Anticancer antifolates: current status and future directions. *Curr Pharm Des.* 2003;9:2593–2613.
11. Matherly LH, Goldman DI. Membrane transport of folates. *Vitam Horm.* 2003;66: 403–456.
12. Brigle KE, Seither RL, Westin EH, et al. Increased expression and genomic organization of a folate-binding protein homologous to the human placental isoform in L1210 murine leukemia cell lines with a defective reduced folate carrier. *J Biol Chem.* 1994;269:4267–4272.
18. Kvackajova-Kisucka J, Barancik M, Breier A. Drug transporters and their role in multidrug resistance of neoplastic cells. *Gen Physiol Biophys.* 2001;20:215–237.
19. Ritter CA, Jedlitschky G, Meyer zu Schwabedissen H, et al. Cellular export of drugs and signaling molecules by the ATP-binding cassette transporters MRP4 (ABCC4) and MRP5 (ABCC5). *Drug Metab Rev.* 2005;37:253–278.
24. Plunkett W, Gandhi V, Huang P, et al. Fludarabine: pharmacokinetics, mechanisms of action, and rationales for combination therapies. *Semin Oncol.* 1993;20:2–12.
25. Plunkett W, Huang P, Searcy CE, et al. Gemcitabine: preclinical pharmacology and mechanisms of action. *Semin Oncol.* 1996;23:3–15.
26. Galmarini CM, Jordheim L, Dumontet C. Pyrimidine nucleoside analogs in cancer treatment. *Expert Rev Anticancer Ther.* 2003;3:717–728.
30. Zhang J, Visser F, King KM, et al. The role of nucleoside transporters in cancer chemotherapy with nucleoside drugs. *Cancer Metastasis Rev.* 2007;26:85–110.
40. Ludeman SM. The chemistry of the metabolites of cyclophosphamide. *Curr Pharm Des.* 1999;5:627–643.
41. Cohen SM, Lippard SJ. Cisplatin: from DNA damage to cancer chemotherapy. *Prog Nucleic Acid Res Mol Biol.* 2001;67:93–130.
56. Yang SW, Huang P, Plunkett W, et al. Dual mode of inhibition of purified DNA ligase I from human cells by 9-beta-D-arabinofuranosyl-2-fluoroadenine triphosphate. *J Biol Chem.* 1992;267:2345–2349.
64. Danenberg PV. Pharmacogenomics of thymidylate synthase in cancer treatment. *Front Biosci.* 2004 1;2484–2494.
69. Pellegrini F, Budman DR. Review: tubulin function, action of antitubulin drugs, and new drug development. *Cancer Invest.* 2005;23:264–273.

73. Rowinsky EK. The development and clinical utility of the taxane class of antimicrotubule chemotherapy agents. *Annu Rev Med.* 1997;48:353–374.
76. Chaney SG, Sancar A. DNA repair: enzymatic mechanisms and relevance to drug response. *J Natl Cancer Inst.* 1996;88:1346-1360.
83. Doroshow JH, Locker GY, Myers CE. Enzymatic defenses of the mouse heart against reactive oxygen metabolites: alterations produced by doxorubicin. *J Clin Invest.* 1980;65:128–135.
87. Green JA, Vistica DT, Young RC, et al. Potentiation of melphalan cytotoxicity in human ovarian cancer cell lines by glutathione depletion. *Cancer Res.* 1984;44:5427–54231.
104. Sonnichsen DS, Hurwitz CA, Pratt CB, et al. Saturable pharmacokinetics and paclitaxel pharmacodynamics in children with solid tumors. *J Clin Oncol.* 1994;12:532–538.
111. Undevia SD, Gomez-Abuin G, Ratain MJ. Pharmacokinetic variability of anticancer agents. *Nat Rev Cancer.* 2005;5:447–458.
119. Singh BN, Malhotra, BK. Effects of food on the clinical pharmacokinetics of anticancer agents. *Clin Pharmacokinet.* 2004;43:1127–1156.
126. Raymond E, Boige V, Faivre S, et al. Dosage adjustment and pharmacokinetic profile of irinotecan in cancer patients with hepatic dysfunction. *J Clin Oncol.* 2002;20:4303–4312.
132. Egorin MJ, Van Echo DA, Tipping SJ, et al. Pharmacokinetics and dosage reduction of cis-diammine (1,1-cyclobutanedicarboxylato)platinum in patients with impaired renal function. *Cancer Res.* 1984;44:5432–5438.
134. Newell DR, Pearson AD, Balmanno K, et al. Carboplatin pharmacokinetics in children: the development of a pediatric dosing formula. *J Clin Oncol.* 1993;11:2314–2323.
137. Millward MJ, Webster LK, Toner GC, et al. Carboplatin dosing based on measurement of renal function: experience at the Peter MacCallum Cancer Institute. *Aust N Z J Med.* 1996;26:372–379.
153. Watters JW, McLeod HL. Cancer pharmacogenomics: current and future applications. *Biochim Biophys Acta.* 2003;1603:99–111.
154. Relling MV, Dervieux T. Pharmacogenetics and cancer therapy. *Nat Rev Cancer.* 2001;1:99–108.
166. Hrushesky WJ, von Roemeling R, Lanning RM, et al. Circadian-shaped infusions of floxuridine for progressive metastatic renal cell carcinoma. *J Clin Oncol.* 1990;8:1504–1513.
187. Mick R, Ratain MJ. Statistical approaches to pharmacodynamic modeling: motivations, methods, and misperceptions. *Cancer Chemother Pharmacol.* 1993;33:1–9.
204. Minami H, Ratain MJ, Ando Y, et al. Pharmacodynamic modeling of prolonged administration of etoposide. *Cancer Chemother Pharmacol.* 1996;39:61–66.
216. Grochow LB. Busulfan disposition: the role of therapeutic monitoring in bone marrow transplantation induction regimens. *Semin Oncol.* 1993;20(suppl 4):18–25.
219. Evans WE, Relling MV, Rodman JH, et al. Conventional compared with individualized chemotherapy for childhood acute lymphoblastic leukemia. *N Engl J Med.* 1998;338:499–505.
223. Bleyzac N, Souillet G, Magron P, et al. Improved clinical outcome of paediatric bone marrow recipients using a test dose and Bayesian pharmacokinetic individualization of busulfan dosage regimens. *Bone Marrow Transplant.* 2001;28:743–751.
224. Gurney H. Dose calculation of anticancer drugs: a review of the current practice and introduction of an alternative. *J Clin Oncol.* 1996;14:2590–2611.

48 Drug Resistance and Its Clinical Circumvention

Jeffrey A. Moscow, MD ■ Erasmus Schneider, PhD ■ Branimir I. Sikic, MD ■ Charles S. Morrow, MD, PhD ■ Kenneth H. Cowan, MD, PhD

Systemic therapy with cytotoxic drugs is the basis for most effective treatments of disseminated cancers. Additionally, adjuvant chemotherapy can offer a significant survival advantage to selected patients, following the treatment of localized disease with surgery or radiotherapy, presumably by eliminating undetected, minimal, or microscopic residual tumor. However, the responses of tumors to chemotherapeutic regimens vary, and failures are frequent owing to the emergence of drug resistance.

The phenomenon of clinical drug resistance has prompted studies to clarify mechanisms of drug action and to identify mechanisms of antineoplastic resistance. It is expected that through such information, drug resistance may be circumvented by rational design of new non-cross-resistant agents, by novel delivery or combinations of known drugs, and by the development of other treatments that might augment the activity of or reverse resistance to known antineoplastics. Multiple mechanisms of antineoplastic failure have been identified using in vitro (tissue culture) and in vivo (animal and xenograft) models of antineoplastic resistance (Table 48-1). These include anatomic and pharmacologic mechanisms that may be uniquely pertinent to individual patients as well as cellular mechanisms within tumor cells. Although mechanisms of drug resistance have been largely determined in experimental systems, many have been implicated in at least some examples of clinical studies of chemotherapeutic failure. Evidence that bears upon these mechanisms of resistance as well as strategies to circumvent them are discussed below.

General Mechanisms of Drug Resistance

Experimental selection of drug resistance by repeated exposure to single antineoplastic agents will generally result in cross-resistance to some related agents of the same drug class. This phenomenon is explained based on shared drug transport carriers, drug metabolizing pathways, and intracellular cytotoxic targets of these structurally and biochemically similar compounds.

Generally, the resistant cells retain sensitivity to drugs of different classes with alternative mechanisms of cytotoxic action.[1,2] Thus, cells selected for resistance to alkylating agents or antifolates will usually remain sensitive to unrelated drugs, such as anthracyclines. Exceptions include emergence of cross-resistance to multiple, apparently structurally and functionally unrelated drugs, to which the patient or cancer cells were never exposed during the initial drug treatment. Despite apparent differences in their presumed sites of action within cells, the drugs associated with multidrug resistance (MDR) phenotypes frequently share common metabolic pathways or efflux transport systems.

In this section, the processes related to drug resistance will be described. A more comprehensive discussion of mechanisms of resistance to specific classes of drugs will be discussed in subsequent sections.

Decreased Drug Accumulation

Decreased intracellular levels of cytotoxic agents is one of the most common mechanisms of drug resistance. Since polar, water-soluble drugs cannot penetrate the lipid bilayer of the cell membrane and require specific mechanisms of cell entry, resistance to these drugs is readily mediated by down-regulation of drug uptake mechanisms in tumor cells. For example, decreased influx via a high-affinity folate-transport system,[3] as well as via a reduced folate carrier,[4] are well described causes of methotrexate resistance.[5,6] For hydrophobic, nonpolar drugs that can easily diffuse across the cell membrane, decreased intracellular drug concentrations can be achieved by increasing the activities of drug efflux pumps. For example, overexpression of the P-glycoprotein (*MDR1/ABCB1*) drug efflux pump is an important example of this mechanism of resistance.[7,8]

Table 48-1 ■ **General Mechanisms of Drug Resistance**

Cellular and biochemical mechanisms
Decreased drug accumulation
Decreased drug influx
Increased drug efflux
Altered intracellular trafficking of drug
Decreased drug activation
Increased inactivation of drug or toxic intermediate
Increased repair of or tolerance to drug-induced damage to:
Deoxyribonucleic acid (DNA)
Protein
Membranes
Drug targets altered (quantitatively or qualitatively)
Altered cofactor or metabolite levels
Altered downstream effectors of cytotoxicity
Altered signaling pathway and/or apoptotic responses to drug insult
Altered gene expression
DNA mutation, amplification, or deletion
Altered transcription, post-transcription processing, or translation
Altered stability of macromolecules
Mechanisms relevant in vivo
Pharmacologic and anatomic drug barriers (tumor sanctuaries)
Host-drug interactions
Increased drug inactivation by normal tissues
Decreased drug activation by normal tissues
Relative increase in normal tissue drug sensitivity (toxicity)
Host-tumor interactions

Altered Drug Metabolism

Decreased drug activation, increased drug inactivation, or alterations in necessary cofactors can also confer resistance to selected antineoplastic agents. For example, decreased conversion of nucleobase analogs to their cytotoxic nucleoside and nucleotide derivatives by alterations in specific kinases and phosphoribosyl transferase salvage enzymes can lead to resistance to these anticancer drugs.[9,10] Another example associated with resistance is decreased levels of carboxyesterase—an activity necessary to convert a topoisomerase I inhibitor, CPT-11, to its active metabolite, SN-38.[11,12]

On the other hand, enhanced inactivation of pyrimidine and purine analogs by increased expression of deaminases is linked to resistance toward these agents.[13,14] Finally, alterations in cofactor levels can also modify drug toxicity. For example, optimal formation of inhibitory complexes between 5-fluorodeoxyuridine monophosphate (FdUMP) and its target enzyme, thymidylate synthase, require the cofactor 5,10-methylene tetrahydrofolate.[15] Alterations in the intracellular levels of this cofactor can lead to resistance to fluoropyrimidines.

Increased Repair or Cellular Tolerance to Drug-Induced Damage

Cells contain multiple complex systems involved in the repair of damage to membranes and deoxyribonucleic acid (DNA), and changes in these repair processes can influence drug sensitivity. For example, resistance to cisplatin, a drug whose cytotoxic action involves intrastrand DNA crosslinkages (see below), is associated with increased DNA repair. Conversely, defects in mismatch repair are associated with tolerance to cisplatin-induced DNA damage.[16] In this form of platinum resistance, the repair system is apparently unable to recognize platinum-DNA adducts and fails to activate the normal, appropriate, programmed cell death response.

Altered Drug Targets

Qualitative changes in the enzyme targets of antineoplastic drugs can compromise drug efficacy and have been associated with resistance to inhibitors of dihydrofolate reductase (DHFR),[17,18] thymidylate synthase,[19] and topoisomerases I and II.[20–25] Perhaps not surprisingly, alteration of the drug target has also been recognized as a mechanism of resistance to newer molecularly targeted chemotherapy. For example, clinical resistance to the BCR-ABL kinase inhibitor Gleevec (imatinib mesylate) results from the development of mutations in the kinase's drug binding site.[26]

Altered Gene Expression

Increased expression of target enzymes can also lead to drug resistance. These alterations may result from changes that occur at any point along the pathways of gene expression and regulation, including DNA deletion or amplification, altered transcriptional or post-transcriptional control of ribonucleic acid (RNA) levels, and altered post-translational modifications of proteins. In addition, the same molecular mechanisms that lead to oncogenesis can also lead to drug resistance through altered expression of drug targets.

For example, loss of function of the retinoblastoma (Rb) gene leads to accumulation of the transcription factor E2F, which, in turn, activates transcription of at least two genes involved in antifolate drug resistance, DHFR and thymidylate synthase (reviewed by Banerjee and colleagues[27]). Efforts to exploit these observations by using E2F as a marker of antifolate chemosensitivity have met with mixed results.[28–30]

Resistance to Multiple Drugs

De novo and acquired cross-resistance to multiple antineoplastic agents can result from several alternative factors and processes. Accordingly, we have grouped the major patterns of cross-resistance into several categories on the basis of their presumed underlying mechanisms (Table 48-2). First, MDR is frequently associated with decreased drug accumulation, usually because of increased drug efflux. MDR is generally thought to be caused by increased energy-dependent efflux of the anticancer drugs, mediated by the overexpression of ATP binding cassette (ABC) proteins. ABC proteins constitute a large family of 48 transport proteins organized into 7 subfamilies, ABCA–ABCG.[31] Of these, at least three have been directly shown to cause MDR, namely MDR1/P-glycoprotein (ABCB1), multidrug resistance-associated protein 1 (MRP1), (ABCC1), and BCRP/MXR/ABC-P (ABCG2). Classic MDR associated with resistance to drugs listed in Table 48-3 is mediated by P-glycoprotein (MDR1 or ABCB1). A similar but distinct MDR phenotype was attributed to the energy-dependent drug efflux activities of multidrug resistance protein (MRP) family members, including MRP1 or ABCC1.[32–35]

Table 48-2 ■ Mechanisms of Multidrug Resistance (MDR)

Resistance associated with decreased drug accumulation
ABC transporter-mediated resistance
• P-Glycoprotein/MDR 1/ABCB1-mediated classic MDR
• MRP family member-mediated MDR (currently at least 3 members, MRP1, 2, and 3 in ABCC1, ABCC2, ABCC3 implicated in MDR drug efflux and detoxification)
• BCRP (ABCG2)-mediated MDR (putative ABC half-transporter implicated in mitoxantrone and anthracycline resistance)
LRP (lung resistance protein, a major vault protein)
Alterations in topoisomerases

Table 48-3 ■ Cross-Resistance Pattern of Classic (P-Glycoprotein-Mediated) MDR

Class	Drug
Anthracyclines	Doxorubicin
	Daunorubicin
	Mitoxantrone
Antibiotics	Actinomycin D
	Plicamycin
Antimicrotubule drugs	Vincristine
	Vinblastine
	Colchicine
Epipodophyllotoxins	Etoposide
	Tenoposide

Another overlapping but discrete MDR phenotype is associated with increased expression of the recently isolated putative efflux transporter, breast cancer resistance protein (BCRP or ABCG2).[36,37] MDR has also been described in association with overexpression of the lung resistance protein (LRP). The mechanism of LRP-associated resistance is unclear, and whether LRP alone is sufficient to confer resistance is unknown. It is speculated that as a major vault protein, LRP is involved in nucleocytoplasmic transport and may be able to prevent entry of drugs into the nucleus.[38,39] Drug resistance defined by alterations in topoisomerases represents a third major category of MDR.[19–23,25,26]

Classic (MDR1/ABCB1-Mediated) MDR

A model of MDR was described by Biedler and Riehm 3 decades ago.[40] Exposure of cells to any of the drugs listed in Table 48-3 can generally result in a MDR phenotype.[7,8] Drug transport studies using parental and MDR cells demonstrate that the reduced cytotoxicity of these drugs is the result of decreased drug accumulation secondary to enhanced drug efflux.[41,42] The emergence of MDR was first associated with increased levels of a membrane-bound glycoprotein, P-glycoprotein. Although it is widely accepted that the MDR1 or *ABCB*1 gene encodes a protein (P-glycoprotein) that mediates an energy-dependent decrease in drug accumulation, there is considerable debate on the precise mechanism(s) involved.[8,43,44] Regardless of the mechanistic details, a great deal of evidence supports the consensus view that P-glycoprotein is an energy-dependent drug efflux pump responsible for the prevalent form of MDR. First, gene transfer experiments show that the *ABCB*1 gene expression is sufficient to confer drug resistance.[45,46] Second, *ABCB*1 belongs to a multigene family of transport proteins (ABC transporters), all of which share sequence homology with several bacterial transport proteins.[47,48] Third, photoaffinity labeling experiments demonstrate direct binding of drugs to P-glycoprotein.[49] Finally, the distribution of P-glycoprotein on the luminal surfaces of normal tissues, including renal tubules, colon, small intestine, and bile canaliculi is consistent with its proposed role in excretory transport.[50] Thus, P-glycoprotein appears to fulfill the requirements predicted of a membrane-bound energy-dependent drug exporter.

*MDR1/ABCB*1-mediated MDR displays significant phenotypic heterogeneity, and the relative degree of cross-resistance to the drugs listed in Table 48-3 varies based on the cell line and the selecting drug. Although the level of drug resistance is roughly correlated with the level of P-glycoprotein expression, *MDR1/ABCB*1 mutations or polymorphisms, as well as coselections of other mechanisms of resistance may also provide phenotypic diversity.[51]

Studies have shown that high levels of *MDR1/ABCB*1 expression are often associated with gene amplification and transcriptional activation.[7,8] Increased *MDR1/ABCB*1 expression can also be induced transiently by heat shock,[52] heavy metals, cytotoxic drugs,[53–55] regenerating liver,[53,54] differentiating agents,[56–58] and by repeated exposure to ionizing radiation. *ABCB*1 promoter activity can also be regulated by altered expression of oncogenes (raf and ras) and the tumor-suppressor gene, TP53.[59–63]

MDR1/ABCB1 expression has been detected in clinical samples from patients with acute and chronic leukemias,[64–68] ovarian cancer,[69] multiple myeloma,[70] breast cancer,[71–74] neuroblastoma,[75] soft tissue sarcomas,[76,77] renal cell carcinoma,[78] and others.[79] Although the numbers of patients with particular tumors in these studies were small, the results have tended to link increased *MDR/ABCB1* expression with a history of prior therapy (usually with MDR-associated drugs) and poorer treatment outcome. In general, the relationship between increased *MDR1/ABCB1* expression and adverse outcome in human cancers is strongest in hematologic malignancies. Recently, 3 prospective studies have shown that increased *MDR1/ABCB1* expression in patients with acute myelogenous leukemia (AML) is associated with decreased complete remission rates and reduced remission duration with use of conventional chemotherapy.[80–82] This correlation has also been demonstrated in adult multiple myeloma, lymphoma, and pediatric acute lymphoblastic leukemia (ALL).[83–86]

The relationship between *MDR1/ABCB1* expression and response to therapy in other cancers is less convincing.[87] In breast cancers, a meta-analysis found expression of *MDR1/ABCB1* in 30–40% of specimens at diagnosis, with a decreased rate of response to MDR-related cytotoxins, that is, anthracyclines and taxanes, in patients with positive tumors. Moreover, *MDR1/ABCB1* expression was more frequent in tumor specimens obtained after clinical resistance to therapy. In patients with advanced neuroblastoma, *MDR1/ABCB1* expression has been strongly associated with aggressive biologic behavior, poor treatment response, and poor outcome.[88] However, the significance of *MDR1/ABCB1* expression in neuroblastomas is controversial, as other data have suggested that increased *MDR1/ABCB1* expression is associated with more favorable clinical variables in patients with neuroblastoma.[89]

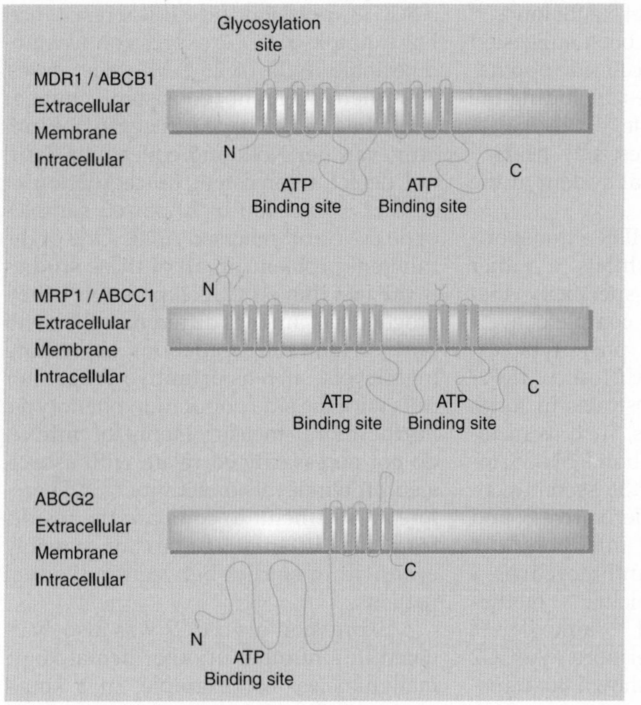

Figure 48-1 ■ Models of multidrug resistance transporters.

Multidrug Resistance Protein (MRP or ABCC1) Family

Similar phenotypes of multiple resistance to antineoplastic agents have been described that are associated with the expression of other membrane proteins, including MRP1 (or ABCC1, which was isolated from a doxorubicin-selected MDR lung cancer cell line.[90] ABCC1 encodes a 190 kDa transmembrane protein, whose structure is strikingly homologous to P-glycoprotein (*MDR1/ABCB1*) and other members of the ABC transmembrane transporter proteins.[90,91] Primary sequence analysis predicts the transmembrane structure shown in Figure 48-1. The structure, supported by immunochemical data, includes 11 plus 4 (or, alternatively, 11 plus 6) transmembrane domains with 2 cytosolic ATP-binding sites.[92] Increased *ABCC1* expression is associated with a MDR phenotype, while decreased *ABCC1* expression is associated with reversion to drug sensitivity. Gene transfer experiments establish that *ABCC1* can confer resistance to a variety of drugs, including anthracyclines, epipodophyllotoxins, and vinca alkaloids.[93–95] Transport studies indicate that MRP1 is involved in ATP-dependent efflux of some native natural product anticancer drugs. Additionally, MRP1 is an ATP-dependent transporter of a variety of anionic conjugates of drugs and other xenobiotics—conjugates that include glutathione conjugates, glucuronides, and sulfates.[96–101] Thus, MRP1 is an important xenobiotic-conjugate transport pump that is involved in efflux of a wide range of cellular poisons, including anticancer drugs and their conjugates. In contrast to P-glycoprotein, whose substrates are generally lipophilic neutral or cationic compounds, MRP1 preferentially recognizes amphiphilic organic anions. Although neutral, hydrophobic compounds such as vincristine are also substrates of MRP1, reduced glutathione is required for their transport.[99,102] Although no covalent linkage between glutathione and vincristine is observed, it is believed that both glutathione and the neutral drug must be simultaneously present to effect efflux, and they both may be co-transported by MRP1.

Nine human MRP isoforms have been identified.[103–106] Among them, MRP2 (*ABCC2*, cMOAT), and MRP3 (*ABCC3*) are also capable of supporting efflux detoxification of cancer drugs, including epipodophyllotoxins.[33,105] Recent results indicate that MRP1 (*ABCC1*), MRP2 (*ABCC2*), MRP3 (*ABCC3*), and MRP4 (*ABCC4*) can all act as methotrexate efflux pumps and can confer resistance to methotrexate.[105,107]

ABCG2 (MEDIATED MDR) ■ *ABCG2*-associated MDR was independently and almost simultaneously identified and described as placental ABC protein (ABC-P),[108] BCRP,[109] and mitoxantrone resistance (MXR) protein.[110] It is the second member of the *ABC*G subfamily of human ABC proteins and encodes a 72 kDa protein. Homologs have been found in mice,[111] rats,[112,113] pigs,[114,115] and rhesus monkeys.[116] The ABCG2 protein is a half-transporter, that is, it contains only 1 nucleotide-binding domain and 1 transmembrane domain, as opposed to the proteins encoded by *ABCB*1 and *ABCC*1, which contain 2 each of these domains (Fig. 48-1). In cells, ABCG2 protein is primarily localized to the plasma membrane,[117–119] where it forms a homodimer[120,121] or possibly a homotetramer,[122] with some evidence of even a higher order multimeric organization.[122] In the whole organism, ABCG2 protein has been found at the blood–brain barrier[113,115,123–126] and blood–testis barrier,[127] in the placenta,[108,128–131] on the luminal or apical side of many parts of the GI tract,[128] as well as in kidney tubules,[132] liver canaliculi,[128] mammary ducts,[128] and in venous and capillary, but not arterial, endothelium.[128] Thus, it has been proposed that one of the main functions of ABCG2 is to protect the organism from a variety of xenobiotics.[133] In addition, ABCG2 has been suggested as a marker for the stem cell side population in a variety of tissues, including the bone marrow,[134–137] muscle,[138] liver,[112,139,140] pancreas,[141,142] lung,[143] testis,[144] heart,[145] breast,[146,147] and the limbal system of the eye.[148–151]

Like the other MDR transporters, ABCG2 protein exhibits a rather promiscuous substrate specificity that shows some, though not complete, overlap with the resistance phenotype associated with *MDR1/ABCB1* and *MRP1/ABCC1*.[152] The list of substrates includes various anticancer drugs, such as irinotecan and its active metabolite SN-38, topotecan, and several of the second-generation camptothecin derivatives, and other topoisomerase I inhibitors,[153–158] mitoxantrone,[109] the anthracyclines—doxorubicin, daunorubicin,[109] methotrexate,[159–162] flavopiridol,[163] amoxifen,[164] and imatinib.[165] Furthermore, ABCG2 protein has also been shown to transport a number of other substances such as rhodamine[123,166] pheophorbide,[167] heme and orphyrins,[168,169] sulfated steroids and sterols,[164,170–172] and various HIV reverse transcriptase inhibitors.[173] The role of *ABCG2* in clinical MDR is not clear. Initial studies examined *ABCG2* in leukemias, especially AML.[174,175] For example, among a group of 40 adult patients with AML, *ABCG2* mRNA expression varied from 0 to 76 times the expression in control cells. Although there was no difference in expression between initial responders and nonresponders, among the subgroup of responders, those with the highest *ABCG2* expression had a significantly shorter overall survival (mean 38 months) compared with those with the lowest expression (mean 74 months, $p < 0.05$).[176] In another study of 149 adult patients with AML, *ABCG2* mRNA expression was a negative prognostic factor in patients treated with daunorubicin and mitoxantrone, but not idarubicin, which is consistent with idarubicin not being a substrate for ABCG2 protein.[177,178] A similar finding was reported by Sargent and colleagues,[179] who found that in 20 either pretreated or naïve patients with AML, ABCG2 protein expression correlated with resistance to daunorubicin, but not mitoxantrone, topotecan, or doxorubicin. In another study of 20 paired clinical AML samples, *ABCG2* mRNA expression was increased 1.7-fold at relapse compared with at diagnosis, whereas neither *MDR1/ABCB1* nor *MRP1/ABCC1* expression differed in the paired samples.[180] These results suggest that high *ABCG2* expression may be a negative prognostic factor in at least a subset of patients with AML.

In contrast, several other studies failed to detect a correlation between *ABCG2* expression and clinical resistance. For example, *ABCG2* expression was undetectable in 23 of 26 AML blast cases, and there were no consistent changes over the course of the disease.[181] Similarly, van der Kolk and colleagues[182] did not detect a consistent up-regulation of *ABCG2* expression in 20 paired samples of de novo and relapsed AML. One of the inherent problems in all of these studies is the fact that *ABCG2* expression is heterogeneous among different cells with only certain subpopulations expressing high levels, such as primitive progenitor cells with the side population phenotype. Furthermore, measurements of mRNA do not necessarily correlate with associated protein levels or activity.[183,184] Therefore, it is difficult to compare the results from the different studies, or possibly even within studies between individual patients.

Expression of *ABCG2* was also evaluated in a number of other hematologic malignancies. For example, in a small study of 30 adult patients with ALL, *ABCG2* expression was predictive of shorter disease-free survival ($p < .05$).[184] Another study of 46 patients with ALL showed that *ABCG2* expression and function was significantly higher in B-cell ALL than in T-cell ALL.[185] 2 other studies specifically investigated a possible role of ABCG2 in pediatric leukemias. In patients with T-cell ALL, there was generally a lower *ABCG2* expression then in B-cell ALL; however, there was no apparent relationship between *ABCG2* expression and clinical or in vivo resistance.[186] In contrast, *ABCG2* mRNA was more than 10 times higher in patients who failed to achieve complete remission. In this study of 59 children, higher levels of *ABCG2* expression were significantly associated with worse prognosis.[187] Furthermore, in a comparison of pediatric ALL subtypes, it was found that those with the TEL-AML1 translocation exhibited significantly higher *ABCG2* expression, which was accompanied by lower methotrexatepolyglutamate accumulation.[188]

In a study of 59 primary breast cancers, an association was observed between *ABCG2* expression and progression-free survival in a subgroup of patients with breast cancer treated with CAF, but not in those who received CMF therapy.[73] In contrast, another study reported that *ABCG2* RNA levels in 38 breast cancer patients who were treated with doxorubicin did not correlate with relapse or prognosis.[189] Similarly, there was no association of *ABCG2* expression with response to anthracycline therapy in a study of 25 primary breast carcinomas and 27 patients with preoperative therapy.[190] Interestingly, in that study, ABCG2 protein was detected only in blood vessels and normal epithelial cells, but not in tumor cells. In another study of 72 advanced-stage nonsmall-cell lung cancers that received platinum-based therapy, response to chemotherapy, progression-free survival, and overall survival were negatively correlated with ABCG2 positive staining by immunohistochemistry.[191]

In conclusion, it appears that *ABCG2* expression may contribute to poor chemotherapy response in AML, whereas its role in other leukemias or solid tumors is less clear.

MDR Associated With Topoisomerase Poisons

Topoisomerases are nuclear enzymes that catalyze the formation of transient single- or double-stranded DNA breaks, facilitate the passage of DNA strands through these breaks, and promote rejoining of the DNA strands.[192,193] As a consequence of these activities, topoisomerases are thought to be critical for DNA replication, transcription, and recombination. The cytotoxicity of many drugs that target topoisomerases, a class of drugs here termed "topoisomerase poisons" (Table 48-4), is thought to depend on the DNA cleavage activities of topoisomerases. There are 2 classes of mammalian enzymes, topoisomerases I and II.

Topoisomerase I catalyzes the formation of single-stranded DNA breaks, while topoisomerases II (α and β isoforms) catalyze both single- and double-stranded breaks. During the cleavage reactions, reversible DNA-topoisomerase complexes (cleavable complexes) can be stabilized by interactions with topoisomerase poisons. The formation of these stabilized DNA–topoisomerase–drug complexes is thought to initiate the production of lethal DNA strand breaks. Of the chemotherapeutic drugs that affect topoisomerase activities, the topoisomerase II poisons have been the most important clinically. A partial list of these agents, which include DNA intercalating and nonintercalating drugs, appears in Table 48-4. The topoisomerase I poisons topotecan and irinotecan are

Table 48-4 Topoisomerase II Poisons

	Class	Drug
Nonintercalators	Epipodophyllotoxins	Etoposide Tenoposide
Intercalators	Anthracyclines	Doxorubicin Daunorubicin Mitoxantrone
	Acridine	m-AMSA (amsacrine)
	Anthracenedione	Mitoxantrone
	Antibiotic	Actinomycin D
	Ellipticine	9-Hydroxy ellipticine

analogs of the natural plant-derived product camptothecin.

Several laboratories have described an MDR pattern characterized by resistance of cells to several or all of the drugs listed in Table 48-4.[194,195] It is readily apparent that many topoisomerase II–targeting drugs are also members of the classic MDR phenotype (Table 48-3). Hence, decreased drug accumulation via increased expression of *MDR1/ABCB*1, *MRP1/ABCC*1, or *ABCG*2 represent common mechanisms of resistance to topoisomerase II poisons. Another important mechanism of resistance to topoisomerase II poisons is thought to involve altered topoisomerase II expression or activity. Both qualitative and quantitative changes in topoisomerase II enzyme activity have been demonstrated in resistant cell lines. Reduced levels of topoisomerase activity are associated with decreased drug-induced DNA strand breaks, as well as reduced drug toxicity.[196,197] Other studies implicate intrinsic changes in drug-induced catalytic properties or associated cofactors as the basis of drug resistance in some cells.[22,198–200]

There are 2 mammalian isozymes of topoisomerase II, a 170 kDa form (topoisomerase IIa) and a 180 kDa form (topoisomerase IIß), either may be involved in clinical drug resistance.[201–203] These isozymes differ with respect to their regulation during the cell cycle[204] and their relative sensitivities to topoisomerase II poisons.[202,203] Hence, the relative levels of the specific topoisomerase II isozymes as well as the total topoisomerase II activity may be significant determinants of the sensitivity of tumor cells to topoisomerase II drugs.

Several reports suggest the molecular basis of drug resistance associated with qualitatively altered topoisomerase II.[205] Point mutations leading to amino acid substitutions in topoisomerase IIa isolated from cells selected for resistance to topoisomerase II drugs have been described. These mutations are clustered within the conserved ATP-binding consensus sequences[206–209] or near the Tyr 804 residue involved in covalent attachment of topoisomerase IIa to DNA.[208–210]

Although these topoisomerase IIa mutations are associated with drug resistance in intact cells and, in some cases, with altered enzymatic activities in vitro, the exact mechanism(s) of drug resistance and the relationship of these mutations to a specifically altered enzymatic property are incompletely understood. Moreover, the relevance for clinical drug resistance of these topoisomerase IIa mutations identified in experimentally drug-selected resistant cell lines is unknown. Indeed, 1 study of topoisomerase IIa derived from leukemic blasts of 15 relapsed patients failed to identify mutations in either of the above 2 regions implicated in experimental drug resistance.[208]

The camptothecin derivatives, topotecan and irinotecan, enhance topoisomerase I–mediated strand breaks. These drugs have important activity in several tumor types, including colorectal, ovarian, and lung cancers.[211] Consequently, the emergence of resistance to these agents has become an increasingly important consideration. There are reports of topoisomerase I mutations derived from cell lines selected for resistance to camptothecin or its derivative, irinotecan.[24,212,213] In 2 of these resistant cell lines, the mutant enzyme has altered topoisomerase I activity with a reduced capacity to mediate camptothecin-induced DNA strand breaks.[212–214]

MDR Associated With Altered Expression of Drug-Metabolizing Enzymes and Drug-Conjugate Export Pumps

The manner in which cells metabolize cancer drugs and other xenobiotics is often described as involving 3 phases of detoxification (Fig. 48-2).[215] Although none of these phases are obligatory steps in the metabolism of every drug, the concept illustrated in Figure 48-2 represents a useful framework with which to view cellular detoxification mechanisms. Alterations in any of these 3 phases can influence the sensitivity or resistance to a particular drug or xenobiotic toxin. Phase 1 drug metabolism is mediated by cytochrome P-450 mixed-function oxidases. Generally, the drug or xenobiotic is rendered into a more electrophilic, reactive intermediate—a process that may enhance toxicity. These metabolites may then be converted to a less reactive, presumably less toxic form in phase 2 reactions, which include the formation of drug/xenobiotic conjugations with glutathione (GSH), glucuronic acid, or sulfate—reactions that are catalyzed by multiple isozymes each of glutathione S-transferases (GSTs), uridine diphosphate (UDP)-glucuronosyl transferases, and sulfatases, respectively.[216–220] Phase 3 detoxification consists of export of the parent drug/xenobiotic or its metabolites by energy-dependent transmembrane efflux pumps, including MRP (ABCC) family members as described above.

Frequently, in cellular and animal models of drug or xenobiotic resistance, a coordinated down-regulation of phase 1 drug-activating enzymes and an up-regulation of specific phase II drug-conjugating enzymes is observed.[53,54,221,222] Such a programmed cellular stress response offers a versatile, generalized protective mechanism against exposure to a variety of exogenous toxins.

Of the phase 2 enzymes, the GSTs have been the most extensively studied. GSTs[219,220] comprise multiple soluble and membrane-associated isozymes, which catalyze the conjugation of electrophilic hydrophobic compounds (R-X) with the thiol, GSH:

$$\text{R-X} + \text{GSH} \xrightarrow{\text{GST}} \text{R-SG} + \text{HX}$$

Circumstantial evidence links the increase in specific GST isozymes or bulk GST activity in cells to resistance to alkylating agents and other drugs.[219,220,223–226] However, direct evidence that GSTs are responsible for altering drug sensitivities is limited. Another catalytic activity, selenium-independent glutathione peroxidase activity, has been attributed to some isozymes of GST:

$$\text{R–O–OH} + 2\text{GSH} \xrightarrow{\text{GST}} \text{R–OH} + \text{GSSG} + H_2O$$

This and other GST-mediated reactions are of interest because of their potential to detoxify oxidative damage to membranes and DNA.

Studies using cell-free preparations of GSTs have identified a limited number of antineoplastic drug substrates of these enzymes. Table 48-5 lists these drugs and other substrates that are possibly associated with drug-mediated oxidative damage. Whether GST levels in tumor cells are sufficient to detoxify antineoplastic drugs to a clinically significant extent is a matter of considerable debate. Several cancer drugs, particularly reactive electrophilic alkylating agents, can form conjugates with glutathione—both spontaneously and in enzyme-catalyzed reactions.[227–234] However, despite these catalytic activi-

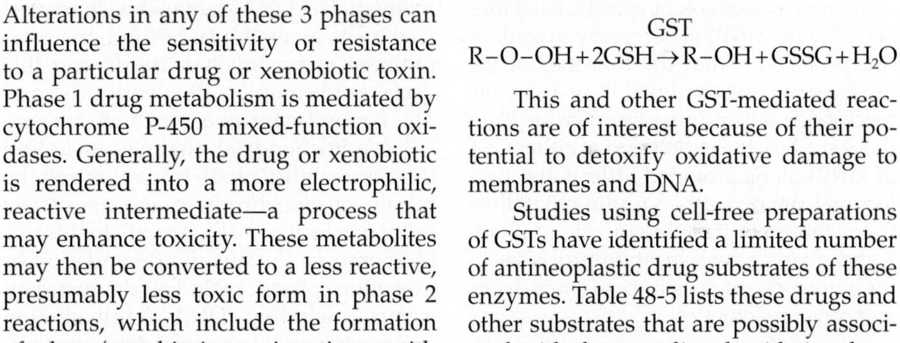

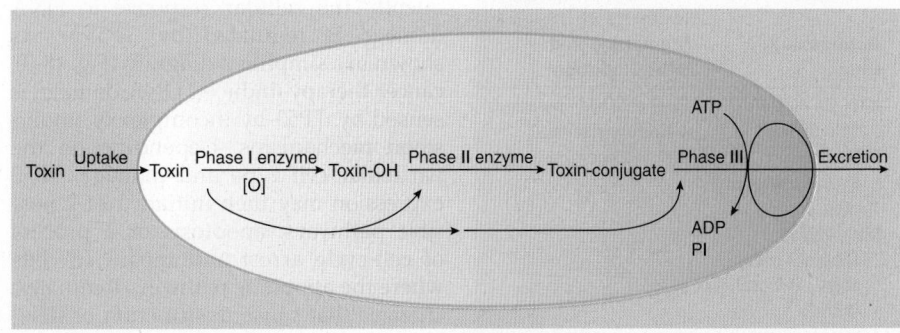

Figure 48-2 Phases 1, 2, and 3 of drug detoxification.

ties, the role of GSTs in drug resistance remains uncertain because of inconsistent results from different laboratories.[224,228,235–244] Indeed, some investigators have found an association between cellular resistance to some anticancer drugs and expression of a particular isozyme of GST, whereas others have found no such association.

The importance of drug/xenobiotic-conjugate transporters for cellular export and detoxification of certain compounds is increasingly appreciated. Conjugation frequently renders the parent drug more hydrophilic and less capable of diffusing through the plasma membrane—trapping the drug within the cell. Although conjugation with glutathionyl or glucuronosyl groups may render some drugs less toxic, these drug conjugates themselves may retain significant toxicity. For example, the glutathione conjugate formed with cisplatin is itself toxic and an inhibitor of protein synthesis.[245] Moreover, drug conjugates may inhibit their conjugating enzyme(s).[246] Thus, the relative resistance of cells expressing drug-metabolizing enzymes may depend on cellular levels of drug conjugate transporters, including the glutathione conjugate transporters,[215,247] such as the MRP (ABCC) family proteins.[35,100] Indeed, recent results using model cell lines demonstrate that combined expression of specific isozymes of GST with MRP1 is necessary to achieve full protection from the toxicities of the cancer drug chlorambucil,[248] or from the carcinogen 4-nitroquinoline 1-oxide.[249] In these studies, the expression of either GST or MRP1 alone provided little, if any, protection from toxicity—a finding that illustrates the synergistic interaction of phase 2 and phase 3 detoxification processes in the emergence of resistance to some drugs and other xenobiotics.

Multidrug Resistance Related to Suppression of Cell Death Pathways

Chemotherapeutic drugs initiate cytotoxicity through their interactions with a variety of molecular targets. For example, epipodophyllotoxins attack topoisomerases II, alkylating agents form adducts with the nucleophilic centers of DNA and proteins, and methotrexate inhibitsDHFR, resulting in reduced pyrimidine and purine synthesis. Despite these varied primary targets, most, if not all, cancer drugs affect cell death, at least partially, via downstream events that converge upon pathways mediating type 1 (apoptotic) or type 2 (autophagic) programmed cell death or apoptosis.

Table 48-5 ■ **Some Important Substrates of GSTs Related to Drug Detoxification and Repair of Drug-Mediated Damage**

Antineoplastic Drug	Products of Membrane and DNA Oxidation
Nitrogen mustards	Fatty acid hydroperoxides
Chlorambucil	4-Hydroxy alkenals
Melphalan	DNA hydroperoxides
Cyclophosphamide	
Thiotepa	
Nitrosoureas	
1,3-bis(2-chloro-ethyl)- 1nitrosourea (BCNU)	
Anthracenedione	
Mitoxantrone	

Apoptosis refers to an orderly cellular death program with predictable molecular and morphologic changes, including nuclear pyknosis and fragmentation, internucleosomal endonucleolytic DNA fragmentation, formation of cytoplasmic apoptotic bodies, and plasma membrane changes, such as transposition of phosphatidylserine to the extracellular surface.[250] Autophagy is a pathway for bulk degradation of subcellular constituents that occurs in response to stresses such as nutrient deprivation. It involves the creation of autophagosomes/autolysozymes[251] and can be inhibited by PI3 kinase inhibitors such as 3-methyladenosine and wortmannin.[251]

Apoptosis or type 1 programmed cell death is conveniently conceptualized in 3 phases. First, the initiation phase of apoptosis (eg, secondary to chemotherapy-mediated DNA damage) is characterized by its reversibility. Second, the commitment phase involves the irreversible decision to complete the death program. The commitment phase, which may involve mitochondrial changes including the permeability phase transition and the release of cytochrome c and apoptosis-inducing factor (AIF), are all hallmarks of apoptosis. Finally, the degradation or execution phase includes downstream events, including DNA fragmentation and morphologic changes. Prior to commitment, apoptosis can be modulated by regulatory elements, such as TP53 and the Bcl-2 family proteins.[250,252–254] Clearly, such regulation of the apoptotic response can have profound effects on the outcome of chemotherapy and is an area of active investigation germane to drug resistance and sensitivity.

Although apoptosis may be either TP53-dependent or -independent, frequently the cellular response to DNA damage is regulated by TP53.[252] As shown in a simplified diagram (Fig. 48-3), cancer therapy–induced DNA damage is sensed by TP53 by incompletely understood mechanisms. Depending on the particular cell type and damage, TP53 expression may then initiate 1 of 2 possible pathways: apoptosis or a process of cell-cycle arrest and repair. In cells where the apoptotic pathway dominates, changes that cause dysfunction or deletion of TP53 are likely to result in reduced apoptosis in response to DNA damage,

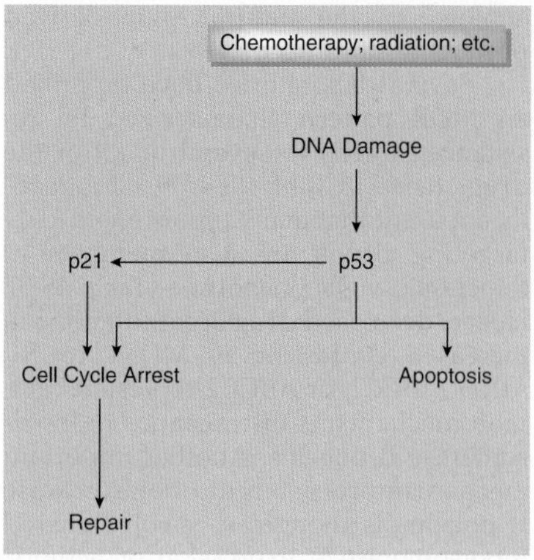

Figure 48-3 ■ Alternative cellular responses to cancer therapeutic stress.

leading to relative resistance and cell survival with damage. Indeed, TP53 is required for radiation- and etoposide-induced apoptosis in thymocytes, whereas lymphoma cell lines expressing mutant TP53 were relatively resistant to DNA-damaging agents.[255–257] In cells where the TP53-dependent cell-cycle arrest and repair response dominates, deletion or mutation of TP53 might be expected to result in decreased cell-cycle arrest and repair leading to accumulated DNA damage and hence sensitivity to the chemotherapeutic agent.[252]

The mitogen-activated protein kinase (MAPK)-signaling cascades are involved in the regulation of cellular response to exogenous factors, including geno- and cytotoxic cancer treatments.[258] The extracellular stimulus-regulated kinase (ERK1/2) pathway is implicated in the proliferative response to growth factors. In cells treated with potentially cytotoxic stressors, such as radiation or anticancer drugs, the p38 and stress-activated/c-Jun N-terminal protein kinase (SAPK/JNK) pathways are implicated in mediating cell-cycle arrest or apoptosis. Modulation of these interacting pathways can have a profound effect on whether a cancer cell responds to cytotoxin challenge by activation of apoptosis or by cell-cycle arrest and repair leading to resistance to treatment.[258,259]

The Bcl-2 family proteins comprise several important regulators of apoptosis. Although their mechanism(s) of action is incompletely known, the balance of expressed antiapoptotic family members (Bcl-2, Bcl-XL) and proapoptotic family members (Bax, Bak, Bad, and Bid) can influence the relative sensitivity of cells to toxic stressors.[253,254] Indeed, increased Bcl-2 and its antiapoptotic homologs are associated with increased resistance of lymphoid cells to the cytotoxic effects of corticosteroids, radiation, and DNA damage from chemotherapeutic drugs.[254,260–263] It has been proposed that increased levels of antiapoptotic proteins Bcl-2 or Bcl-XL may result in reduced sensitivity to DNA-damaging cancer drugs—a resistance phenotype characterized by cell survival and increased tolerance to DNA damage and genomic instability. This genomic instability may lead to further mutations activating additional resistance mechanisms and conferring more aggressive tumor behavior.[253] Although the role of Bcl-2 family proteins and the multidomain proapoptotic members of this family in the development of type 1 (apoptotic) programmed cell death has been extensively characterized, recent studies indicate that these proteins also control type 2 (autophagy) and nonapoptotic programmed cell death.[264] Thus, the expression of mutant and wild-type TP53, Bcl-2 family members, MAPK family members, and other proteins associated with the control of apoptosis and/or autophagy may contribute significantly to the clinical sensitivity of tumor cells. These proteins are the targets of investigational agents that may become important in future strategies to overcome clinical drug resistance.

Resistance Factors Unique to Tumor Cells In Vivo: Host-Tumor Interactions

The failure of chemotherapy to eradicate a tumor in vivo despite exquisite sensitivity to drug in vitro might be a result of anatomic or pharmacologic sanctuaries. For example, the failure to deliver adequate amounts of many drugs across blood–brain and blood–testicular barriers probably accounts for the relatively high frequency of acute lymphoblastic leukemia relapse at these sites.[265] In large solid tumors, chemotherapeutic failures are frequently attributed to decreased drug delivery to a tumor that has overgrown its vascular supply. Additionally, development of acidosis and hypoxia in poorly perfused areas of large tumors may interfere with the cytotoxicity of some drugs. Altered prodrug activation by liver or other normal tissues may profoundly influence the efficacy of drugs such as cyclophosphamide.

Studies by Teicher and Herman[266] suggest that tumor–host interactions may influence drug pharmacokinetics and tumor resistance in unexpected ways. In this study, tumor cells selected for cyclophosphamide and cisplatin resistance in vivo were normally sensitive to drugs in vitro. When the tumor cells were reimplanted into nude mice, in vivo drug resistance was restored. These results suggest that resistant tumors may harbor cellular resistance factors that are operative only in conjunction with host factors and, therefore, mediate resistance by altered drug pharmacokinetics in vivo only. If this novel host-dependent mechanism of tumor resistance proves common, these results would provide one explanation for the failure of conventional in vitro testing to predict clinical responsiveness in all cases.

Pharmacogenomics and Drug Resistance

Integration of the knowledge of mechanisms of drug resistance with the emerging field of pharmacogenomics, the study of genetic influence on all aspects of drug therapy, has been seen as having the potential for allowing clinicians to tailor therapy based on projected individual toxicity and intrinsic resistance of a tumor. Interest in the application of pharmacogenomics to the challenges of cancer drug resistance has been spurred by the success of the identification of genetic polymorphisms that can detect individuals with unusual sensitivities to drugs, such as the *TPMT* polymorphism that identifies patients with increased sensitivity to mercaptopurine.[267,268] The identification of genetic markers of drug resistance holds the promise of allowing clinical oncologists to practice individualized medicine, where the genetic profiles of patients and their tumors would reveal the most effective chemotherapy regimen with the fewest side effects for each patient.

However, the complexity of turning the vision of genomic medicine into a predictive tool for identifying intrinsic and acquired drug resistance creates a daunting challenge. In any predictive model, individual genetic characteristics of the host and the tumor would have to be considered. Characteristics of the host include factors that affect the classic aspects of pharmacokinetics—absorption, distribution, metabolism, and excretion of each anticancer agent. Characteristics of the tumor would include all mechanisms of pharmacodynamic interactions, including drug uptake and efflux, interaction with the site of drug action, and pathways of repair of drug damage and apoptosis.

Each aspect of pharmacokinetic and pharmacodynamic processes can involve the actions of the products of several genes, and the ultimate functional expression of these genes can be affected by hundreds of genetic factors. These genetic factors are both quantitative, usually assayed by differences in RNA or protein levels or function. Measurement of gene expression through DNA microarrays is a quantifiable surrogate for actual functional gene expression. Translational efficiency, post-translational modification, and modification of activity by other proteins all can affect ultimately quantitative function, but these parameters must be assayed separately. Using genetic analysis of SNPs to evaluate their potential or gene expression or protein function and correlating these genetic variants for drug resistance is also complex. Each gene with potential roles in drug resistance may have hundreds of SNPs, and the functional consequence of each SNP variation will require detailed analysis to determine its relevance in vitro and in vivo. Even though SNPs are often inherited in groups, in a phenomenon referred to as linkage disequilibrium, which can decrease the total number of variations present in the population, complete genetic and functional characterization of each gene is a great challenge. In addition, studies of the effect of a given SNP on drug disposition or patient outcome may not be consistent, leading to further complexity in developing predictive models based on pharmacogenomics.

For example, the *MDR1/ABCB1* gene encoding P-glycoprotein has a total of at least 216 identified SNPs.[269] Of these polymorphisms, 193 are located within introns, including 3 in the promoter region and 39 in the intron-exon border sequences, and 19 SNPs are located in the protein coding region, of which 8 result in a change of protein structure.[269] Because of linkage disequilibrium, these SNPs appear to be organized into 64 haplotypes, of which the 2 most common haplotypes account for 36% of all *MDR1/ABCB*1 genes. These haplotype frequencies can vary in different ethnic populations.[269]

The most widely studied *MDR1/ ABCB*1 SNP occurs at nucleotide 3435, and has 3 variations: homozygous CC, homozygous TT, and heterozygous CT. This C3435T SNP is located in an exon, but does not result in a change in the amino acid sequence of P-glycoprotein, so any effect of inheriting an allele containing a particular polymorphism at this site would have to be due to coinheritance of other SNPs in the allele. Several studies have shown that individuals with the TT genotype have a lower overall expression of P-glycoprotein in tissues and tumors,[270–275] although others have not.[276–283]

The potential role of *MDR1/ABCB*1 SNPs in drug resistance would be suggested by the selective expression of a particular allele during drug therapy. Again, studies are conflicting on this issue, with one study showing selective expansion of cells with a particular MDR1/ ABCB1 allele in heterozygous patients,[284] although another study was unable to demonstrate this effect.[285] The clinical role of *MDR1/ABCB1* polymorphisms would also be supported by evidence that a given SNP correlated with overall clinical outcome. Again, the evidence is conflicting, with one study showing that the C3435T SNP correlated with prognosis,[286] but another study unable to demonstrate such an effect.[283]

The pharmacogenomic characterization of the cellular metabolism of the anticancer drug methotrexate further illustrates the issues involved in developing predictive models of drug resistance.[287] Methotrexate enters cells through the reduced folate carrier, undergoes polyglutamylation resulting in intracellular accumulation, and inhibits the enzyme DHFR. The enzymes thymidylate synthase (TS) and methylene tetrahydrofolate reductase (MTHFR) interact in the DHFR metabolic pathway and can affect its function. Thus, there are multiple genes involved in methotrexate action, each with its own spectrum of expression levels and SNPs.

One frequently studied polymorphism is the A1298C SNP in the *MTHFR* gene. MTHFR enzyme regulates the relative levels of folate metabolites that are available for competing pathways for either nucleotide synthesis or DNA methylation. 2 SNPs in the *MTHFR* gene, C677T and A1298C, have an impact on the relative level of 5-methyl tetrahyofolate, and therefore on the sensitivity of cells to methotrexate. This polymorphism is a potential double-edged sword, since it might be expected to increase the sensitivity of tumor cells to the drug, but also increase the potential toxicity of the drug to normal tissues. The clinical analysis of the impact of genetic polymorphism is complicated by the fact that methotrexate is given in a multitude of different regimens employing a wide range of dosages. As with the pharmacogenomic studies of *MDR1/ABCB1*, clinical studies have yielded conflicting results regarding the effect of *MTHFR* polymorphisms on both efficacy and toxicity.[288–291] Polymorphisms of 2 other genes involved in methotrexate metabolism, deletions in the untranslated region of thymidylate synthase,[292,293] and the G80A SNP in the reduced folate carrier gene[291,294] also provide initial but conflicting evidence for a role of these polymorphisms in determining toxicity or outcome. In none of these genes have there been studies of allele selection in tumors, as has been attempted with *MDR1/ABCB1*, to determine a potential role of a given SNP in the development of drug resistance.

Similarly, polymorphisms in at least five genes affecting the efficacy and toxicity of irinotecan have been described.[295] Therefore, the complexity of applying pharmacogenomic information to the prediction of drug resistance and to strategies to overcome drug resistance presents an enormous challenge. New technologies may help speed the analysis of functional consequences of drug resistance–related genes.[296] However, unless truly phenotypically dominant polymorphisms are identified, such as is the case with *TMPT*, where activity is almost completely abrogated by an SNP, algorithms based on genetic profiles to determine optimal and nontoxic therapy are currently a potential but elusive goal.

Potential Clinical Application of Strategies to Avert or Overcome Drug Resistance

Approaches to overcome chemotherapeutic failures include efforts to prevent the emergence of drug resistance (Table 48-6). An appreciation of factors that induce resistance mechanisms may lead to the choice of more efficacious treatment regimens. For example, drugs that may have only sporadic activity against a specific tumor, yet are likely to select for cross-resistance to more active agents, would be avoided. It is hoped that aggressive combination chemotherapy with non-crossreacting drugs will eliminate tumor rapidly enough to prevent the selection of tumor cell clones with multiple resistance. Another approach is to develop therapies aimed at reversing or circumventing clinical drug resistance.

Reversal of *MDR1/ABCB1*, *MRP1/ABCC1*, AND *ABCG2*-Mediated Resistance

Prior to the original descriptions of *MDR1/ABCB1*, Tsuruo and colleagues noted that treatment with verapamil of leukemia cells made drug resistant by selection in vincristine or doxorubicin could partially restore antineoplastic drug sensitivity.[297] Furthermore, this verapamil-enhanced antineoplastic cytotoxicity was specific for drug-resistant but not-sensitive parental cells, was associated with increased accumulation of vincristine and doxorubicin. These results suggested that in the drug-resistant cells, vincristine and doxorubicin share a common transport system that is sensitive to modulation by verapamil. This transport system has now been identified as the P-glycoprotein drug efflux pump. Subsequently, numerous agents have been studied that can partially reverse the drug accumulation defects in classically multidrug-resistant cells, including several calcium channel blockers, calmodulin inhibitors such as phenothiazines, cyclosporin A, and cyclosporin derivatives, and other drugs.[298–304] Although the mechanism(s) by which these agents reverse MDR is incompletely understood, it is believed that direct interactions between these agents and P-glycoprotein interfere with antineoplastic drug efflux activity. Because a considerable clinical experience in the use of MDR-reversing agents has existed for the treatment of other disorders, these agents have been included in several clinical trials designed to enhance the antitumor activity of conventional cancer drugs in refractory human neoplasms.

Although there have been several encouraging studies showing the efficacy of P-glycoprotein inhibitors in murine models of MDR, most promising early clinical trials have been confined to those treating refractory or relapsed hematologic malignancies.[305–323] Studies involving the use of MDR-reversing agents in the treatment of solid human tumors have been generally disappointing.[323] Two recent phase 2 studies of P-glycoprotein reversal with PSC833 (valspodar),[303] a nonimmunosuppressant analog of cyclosporine A, in combination with paclitaxel and doxorubicin in refractory ovarian cancer failed to show a convincing benefit, with complete response rates of 0% and 3%, respectively, and partial response rates of 9% and 12%, respectively. A major problem with these studies is the lack of screening of patients for *MDR1/ABCB1* expression in tumors. Since only a minority of patients entered into these trials would be expected to have tumors positive for the target, P-glycoprotein, there would be a strong dilutional effect, reducing the power of the studies to demonstrate reversal of resistance.

Table 48-6 Approaches to Overcome or Circumvent Drug Resistance

Prevention	Aggressive multiple-agent therapy
	Appreciation of factors that induce resistance mechanism
Circumvention	Drug-screening programs and rational drug design
	Circumvention of drug uptake defects
	Dose escalation
	Drugs that use alternative transport mechanisms
	Agents that reverse increased efflux
	Cofactors that augment drug activation or efficacy
	Inhibition of drug inactivation
	Novel treatment modalities
	Immunotherapy
	Development of agents that target signaling and apoptotic pathways

The largest recent phase 3 studies of the potential benefit of P-glycoprotein reversal have focused on patients with refractory leukemia. One of these studies, in which 226 patients with AML were randomized to receive daunorubicin in a 72-hour infusion, with or without concomitant infusion of cyclosporine, showed that the addition of cyclosporine A improved relapse-free survival (34% vs 9% at 2 years; $p = 0.031$) and overall survival (22% vs 12%; $p = 0.046$).[311] It is of interest in this study that cyclosporine A did not significantly improve the remission rate and that survival improved with increasing daunorubicol concentrations in the cyclosporine-treated patients, but not in the controls, suggesting that the addition of cyclosporine enhanced the cytotoxicity of daunorubicin and eliminated resistant clones. This prospective clinical study of infusional cyclosporine and daunorubicin in AML by List and colleagues demonstrated for the first time a clear clinical benefit for the strategy of modulation of multidrug resistance.

In addition to their actions on P-glycoprotein - expressing tumor cells, MDR-reversing agents can also have profound effects on the pharmacokinetics and pharmacodynamics of cytotoxic drugs associated with MDR.[304,324] As noted above, marked increases in the area under the curve levels, decreased renal and nonrenal clearances, and increased volumes of distribution of etoposide have been observed in patients concomitantly treated with cyclosporins. These drug interactions are due in large part to inhibition of drug metabolizing enzymes and various drug transporters by cyclosporins in normal tissues, particularly the liver. Cyclosporine and its congener valspodar (PSC 833) are potent inhibitors of the mixed-function oxidase CYP 3A4, as well as the biliary drug transporter MRP2 (ABCC2, cMOAT). Toxicities of MDR-associated drugs, such as myelosuppression, are enhanced when administered with the cyclosporine reversing agents and require appropriate reduction in the dosage of cytotoxic drugs. Because MDR1/ABCB1 is expressed at high levels in central nervous system (CNS) endothelium and contributes to the blood–brain barrier,[325–327] concomitant administration of MDR-associated chemotherapeutic drugs and MDR1/ABCB1 inhibitors may also enhance neurotoxicities. These pharmacologic issues must be carefully considered in future clinical trials. The extent to which P-glycoprotein inhibition alone contributes to drug interactions with cytotoxins is currently being clarified by clinical trials with zosuquidar (LY335979), a potent and specific P-glycoprotein inhibitor that has no effect of CYP 3A4 and the MRP (ABCC) family of drug transporters.[328–334]

Alternative strategies for reversing P-glycoprotein -mediated MDR include the use of monoclonal antibodies directed against extracellular epitopes of P-glycoprotein,[335] anti–P-glycoprotein antibody–toxin conjugates that target P-glycoprotein expressing MDR tumor cells,[336,337] or anti-Pglycoprotein antibodies engineered to recruit activated T-lymphocytes for the cytolysis of MDR1/ABCB1-expressing tumor cells.[338] Other approaches to reversing MDR1/ABCB1-mediated MDR include antisense and ribozyme nucleotides directed against *MDR1/ABCB1* mRNA.[323] These approaches either do not result in substantial reversal of resistance or are faced with major technical obstacles in clinical application. Even with the reduced off-target effects and drug interactions on third generation MDR modulators, such approaches will be limited by the presence of other, redundant mechanisms of resistance in human tumor cell populations.[333,339]

Similar approaches for reversing MRP (*ABCC*) family–mediated MDR are possible. A number of compounds inhibit MRP1/ABCB1-mediated efflux activity, including the organic acids probenecid and sulfinpyrazone,[93] and the cyclosporin derivative, PSC 833.[340] Finally, MRP1/ABCC1-mediated transport of some drugs is dependent on intracellular glutathione either as a noncovalent cofactor,[99,341] or as a moiety covalently linked, nonenzymatically or by GST, to some electrophilic anticancer drugs.[248,342] Thus, depletion of tumor cell glutathione or inhibition of GST (see the section "Resistance to Free Radical–Mediated Drug Cytotoxicity" below) offer potential strategies for secondarily reversing MRP1/ABCC1-mediated drug resistance. Some substrates of MRP1 are glucuronide and sulfate derivatives of the parent drug.[96,97,343,344] Thus, selective inhibition of tumor cell UDP-glucuronosyl transferases or sulfotransferases could also represent a future avenue for secondary reversal of MRP1/ABCC1-associated drug resistance.

Several agents have also been described that act as inhibitors of ABCG2 protein and may be useful as reversal agents. The most widely used of these are fumitremorgin C (FTC),[345] which is, however, too toxic for clinical use, and GF120918 (Elacridar),[156,346] which is also an inhibitor of P-glycoprotein and is currently in phase 1 clinical trials.[347] Other inhibitors of ABCG2, and thus potential reversal agents, include biricodar (VX-710),[348] novobiocin,[349,350] gefitinib,[351] and imatinib[352] (although the latter has also been found to be a substrate of ABCG2165), the Her2 neu protein inhibitor CI10333,[353] several HIV protease inhibitors,[354] and some synthetic taxanes.[355,356] Interestingly, some reports have also shown that flavonoids, especially when given as an oral cocktail, may have ABCG2 reversing activity.[357–360]

Although fumitremorgin C and GF120918 are invaluable tools for the study of ABCG2 in vitro and are widely used for this purpose, it is too early to judge whether the use of ABCG2 inhibitors will also reverse MDR at the cellular level in a clinically useful way. In contrast, there is evidence that these agents can alter the oral bioavailability of drugs such as topotecan.[361,362] For example, when patients were treated with oral topotecan with coadministration of oral GF120918, the mean AUC of total topotecan more than doubled, as did the maximum plasma concentration, and the oral bioavailability increased from 40% to 97%, when compared with oral topotecan only. In contrast, coadministration of GF120918 with intravenous topotecan only had a small effect on the AUC, but no effect on the peak plasma concentration or the terminal half-life of topotecan.[361] Similar results, albeit so far only in mice, have been reported with gefitinib and irinotecan,[363] and with the fumitremorgin derivative Ko143 and topotecan.[364] These results are consistent with the apical localization of ABCG2 in the epithelium of the small intestine and colon and a possible role of ABCG2 in the protection of the organism from orally ingested xenobiotics.

Topoisomerase II Poisons

As discussed above, resistance to topoisomerase II poisons may occur as a consequence of MDR1/ABCB1, MRP1/ABCC1, or ABCG2 overexpression or altered topoisomerase II activities. However, none of these mechanisms will necessarily result in cross-resistance to all the topoisomerase II–directed drugs listed in Table 48-3. For example, resistance to pipodophyllotoxins and anthracyclines on the basis of increased *MDR1/ABCB1* expression is not usually associated with resistance to the acridine derivative, amsacrine. Conversely, resistance to amsacrine and other intercalating drugs caused by alterations in topoisomerase II protein is not always associated with resistance to the nonintercalating, epipodophyllotoxin class of topoisomerase II poisons.[200] Therefore, these in vitro studies suggest a rationale for administering an alternative class of topoisomerase II poison in selected cases of clinical resistance to another class of topoisomerase II–directed drug. Additionally, tumor cells resistant to classic topoisomerase II poisons (Table 48-4) frequently retain sensitivity to the cytotoxicities of the novel class of topoisomerase II–catalytic inhibitors (fostriecin, merbarone, aclarubicin, and bis [2,6-dioxopoperazines]).[205,365,366] This class of topoisomerase-directed drug offers an alternative for the treatment of topoisomerase poison–resistant tumors. Finally, structural analogs of parent topoisomerase II poisons may overcome resistance based on altered topoisomerase II.[367,368]

Resistance to Free Radical–Mediated Drug Cytotoxicity

Several pathways may contribute to protection of tumor cells from anthracycline-mediated free radical damage. First, superoxide anion formation is limited in poorly vascularized, relatively hypoxemic tissues, which may exist in the centers of large solid tumors. Second, increased intracellular levels of catalase and glutathione peroxidase (GSHPx) can deplete hydrogen peroxide, thus reducing the formation of toxic hydroxyl radicals. Indeed, in comparing parental and MDR MCF7 cells, Sinha and colleagues reported an association between increased GSHPx activity and reduced doxorubicin-stimulated hydroxyl radical formation.[369] Furthermore, lowering GSHPx activity by depleting the enzyme's cosubstrate, GSH, resulted in enhanced doxorubicin-dependent free radical formation and cytotoxicity.[370] Additionally, Kramer and colleagues found that GSH depletion with buthionine sulfoximine (BSO) could partially restore the doxorubicin sensitivity of MDR MCF7 cells, presumably by interfering with GSH-dependent reactions, including those catalyzed by GSHPx.[371] Although these results are consistent with the importance of hydrogen peroxide and hydroxyl radical formation in anthracycline cytotoxicity in MCF 7 cells, other investigators have noted that increased catalase, GSH, and GSHPx levels are not always protective of some cells from doxorubicin-mediated damage.[372]

The relative importance of free radical generation in tumor cell kill is unknown, and the protective mechanisms outlined above are speculative. Nevertheless, the GSH-dependent detoxification pathways are of particular interest because they are subject to pharmacologic manipulation. GSHPx and GST activities can be secondarily reduced by depleting tissue GSH with BSO treatment.[373,374] Furthermore, the activity of GSTs can be inhibited by the administration of competitive substrates, such as ethacrynic acid.[375] Such clinical manipulations may enhance tumoricidal activity of doxorubicin, but must be viewed cautiously as they may also potentiate drug toxicity toward normal tissues.

Alkylating Agents and Platinum Compounds

Resistance to alkylating agents and platinum compounds can be described by at least three broad mechanistic categories, including decreased drug accumulation, increased drug inactivation, and enhanced repair of DNA damage.[16,376–378] Additionally, the nature of the tumor cells' response to alkylating agent damage—whether primarily apoptosis, repair, or survival with damage—will contribute significantly to the outcome of alkylating agent treatment. Preclinical studies have indicated that all these mechanisms may be circumvented, at least partially, by pharmacologic manipulations. Reactions of electrophilic alkylating agents with thiol-containing compounds represent relatively general mechanisms of antineoplastic inactivation or detoxification. For example, GSH forms conjugates with a variety of alkylating agents in both nonenzymatic and in GST-dependent reactions.

Table 48-5 lists some of the compounds whose conjugation with GSH is catalyzed by GSTs in vitro.[224] Several laboratories have demonstrated an association between increased bulk GST levels or specific GST isozymes with resistance to drugs such as nitrosoureas,[379] chlorambucil, and other nitrogen mustards.[236,237,240,380,381] Additionally, increased GSH levels correlate with resistance to alkylating agents and cisplatin.[382,383] Although the electrophilic cisplatin compound can react directly with GSH, it is unknown whether GSTs can catalyze this reaction. This issue is unresolved because of conflicting results that show a correlation between elevated expression of the pi isozyme of GST and resistance to cisplatin in some cells,[384,385] but not others.[239] Perhaps more relevant to the issue of cisplatin resistance is the finding that glutathionylplatinum complexes, which are themselves toxic, are exported by an ATP-dependent pump, probably identical to one of the glutathione conjugate pumps described earlier.[245] Thus, these drug exporters should be considered in the design of treatments and formulation of strategies to enhance cisplatin efficacy.

The correlations between GSH or GST levels and drug resistance are variable. Indeed, some investigators have been unable to demonstrate a relationship between the overexpression of multiple isozymes of GST and antineoplastic resistance.[238,239,243,386] In studies that have compared paired parental and resistant cell lines, the magnitude of alkylating agent resistance associated with increased GST activity is often modest. As noted above, for some drugs such as chlorambucil, the coexpression of a glutathione conjugate efflux transporter appears to be required for the emergence of GST-mediated resistance in the MCF 7 cell model system.[248] Although the clinical importance of GST and GSH in alkylating resistance is, accordingly, debated, existing preclinical data have prompted phase 1 trials using GST inhibitors, or the GSH synthesis inhibitor BSO, in conjunction with alkylating agents. 3 phase 1 trials have been reported with the combination of BSO and melphalan. These trials demonstrate that it is possible to deplete glutathione levels by coadministration of BSO with alkylating agent chemotherapy. However, no phase 2 studies have yet been reported to demonstrate the antitumor efficacy of this approach.

Aldehyde dehydrogenase is another drug-metabolizing enzyme that is linked to cyclophosphamide-derivative resistance in murine and human models of drug resistance.[387–389] This enzyme converts aldophosphamide, a metabolite of cyclophosphamide, to the inactive compound, carboxyphosphamide, thereby preventing the decomposition of aldophosphamide to its cytotoxic derivative, phosphoramide mustard. Increased expression of aldehyde dehydrogenase is associated with resistance to cyclophosphamide in vitro. Whether inhibitors of aldehyde dehydrogenase, such as disulfiram and dimethylaminobenzaldehyde, can be used therapeutically to enhance the antitumor effect of cyclophosphamide without undue host toxicity remains to be explored.

Cisplatin toxicity is thought to be mediated primarily by the formation of lethal intrastrand DNA cross-links. Several reports suggest that either increased DNA repair or tolerance of DNA damage is associated with resistance to this compound. In a murine leukemia model, cells selected for cisplatin resistance showed enhanced ability to repair cisplatin-induced intrastrand DNA cross-links.[390,391] Aphidicolin can inhibit an enzyme implicated in DNA repair, DNA polymerase a. Treatment of ovarian carcinoma cells with aphidicolin potentiated the toxicity of cisplatin in resistant but not sensitive cells.[392] These results suggest that the coadministration of DNA polymerase a inhibitors with cisplatin may be useful in overcoming cisplatin resistance. Also implicated in platinum sensitivity and resistance are alterations in regulators of apoptosis, such as Bcl-2, Bax, or TP53.[16] Modulation of these pathways by therapeutic agents now in development represents an emerging strategy for overcoming resistance to platinum and other alkylating compounds.

Antimetabolites

The antimetabolites are a clinically important group of cancer drugs used in the treatment of a variety of solid tumors and hematologic malignancies. The cytotoxicities of the antimetabolites stem from their ability to interfere with key enzymatic steps in nucleic acid metabolism. The discussion that follows concerns 3 particularly well-studied compounds, the antifolate methotrexate (MTX) and the pyrimidine analogs 5-fluorouracil (5-FU) and cytosine arabinoside (ara-C, 1–0-D-arabinofuranosylcytosine, cytarabine). Strategies designed to overcome the multiple described mechanisms of cellular resistance to these compounds include dose escalation, pharmacologic manipulation of drug metabolism, and rational design of new antimetabolites.[393]

MTX, the clinically important antifolate, displays significant tumoricidal activity against a variety of human neoplasms, such as acute leukemia, osteogenic sarcoma, choriocarcinoma, breast cancer, head and neck cancers, and others.[394] Consideration of MTX metabolism and sites of action (Fig. 48-4) serves as the basis for understanding mechanisms of methotrexate resistance. Following uptake by the folate transport systems, MTX can bind avidly to and inhibit its primary enzyme target, DHFR. In the presence of adequate thymidylate synthase activity, inhibition of DHFR results in depletion of the reduced folate pools essential for thymidylate and de novo purine synthesis. The cytotoxicity of MTX is significantly influenced by intracellular polyglutamation. MTX polyglutamates are retained preferentially by cells and bind more effectively to DHFR. Additionally, these polyglutamyl derivatives can inhibit other folate-dependent enzymes, including thymidylate synthase and 5-aminoimadazole-4-carboxamide ribonucleoside (AICAR) transformylase,[395] enzymes involved in thymidylate and de novo purine synthesis, respectively. Therefore, resistance to MTX can result from a number of alternative mechanisms, including (1) reduced MTX uptake via a defective folate transport system,[5] such as decreased expression of the reduced folate carrier[4,396] or of the folate receptors; (2) increased export via MRP family proteins[107,397] or other exporters of polyglutamatable antifolates; (3) reduced polyglutamation leading to decreased drug retention as well as reduced inhibition of thymidylate synthase and AICAR transformylase[398]; and (4) either elevated levels of DHFR or reduced affinity of DHFR for MTX.[394,399–404]

The use of high-dose MTX (HDMTX) with subsequent rescue of normal tissues by administration of the reduced folate, leucovorin (N5-formyl tetrahydrofolate) has been advocated as an approach that could theoretically circumvent most mechanisms of MTX resistance. At high systemic drug concentrations, cytocidal levels can be achieved by passive diffusion of drug into transport-defective resistant cells. Furthermore, prolonged exposure of cells to high extracellular concentrations of drug can maintain cytotoxic intracellular drug levels in the face of a drug retention defect secondary to decreased polyglutamation. Finally, increased intracellular MTX delivered by HDMTX therapy can saturate DHFR in cells whose resistance is a result of amplification of the DHFR gene or of lowered affinity of DHFR for MTX. Although HDMTX is of proven value in the treatment of ALL and perhaps of osteogenic sarcoma, the rationale for the use of this modality in the treatment of other cancers was recently questioned.[405,406] Indeed, some tumors, as well as normal tissues, are rescued from HDMTX toxicity by leucovorin. In these and other cases, the use of HDMTX with leucovorin rescue offers no therapeutic advantage over regimens that use conventional MTX doses. Although early studies suggested that HDMTX improved response rates to chemotherapy of osteogenic sarcoma,[407] the contribution of HDMTX therapy to the success of recent multiagent adjuvant protocols is unclear. In contrast, HDMTX is indisputably efficacious in the treatment of ALL. The success of HDMTX in this setting is probably a result of the penetration of drug across anatomic and pharmacologic barriers into tumor sanctuaries, such as testes, and, at very high MTX doses, the CNS.[265]

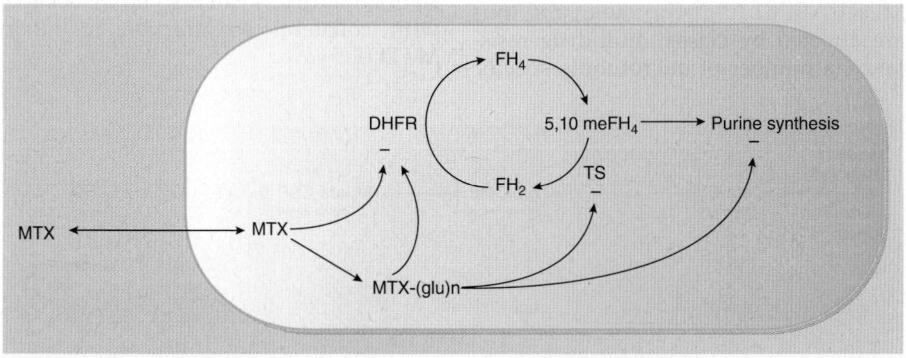

Figure 48-4 Methotrexate metabolism and toxicity. *Abbreviations:* DHFR, dihydrofolate reductase; FH2, dihydrofolate; FH4, tetrahydrofolate; 5,10 MEFH4, 5,10-methylene tetrahydrofolate; MTX, methotrexate; MTX-(glu)n, plyglutamate methotrexate; TS, thymidylate synthase.

In an effort to improve drug efficacy, other inhibitors of DHFR, such as trimetrexate and piritrexim, were developed.[408–410] These lipid-soluble drugs are taken up by cells independently of the folate-carrier system; consequently, their use might obviate transport-mediated antifolate resistance. However, cells that are resistant to MTX based on amplified DHFR will be cross-resistant to trimetrexate. The utility of trimetrexate is further limited by the association of classic MDR with cross-resistance to trimetrexate.[411] Cells can also overcome antifolate toxicity by increasing the salvage of nucleoside precursors. One mechanism of overcoming these mechanisms of resistance is the concomitant administration of the nucleoside transport inhibitor nitrobenzylmercaptopurine riboside (NBMPR) with antifolate drugs, which enhances antifolate cytotoxicity in rodent models.[411,412]

The pyrimidine base, 5-FU and its deoxynucleoside metabolite, 5-fluoro-2′-deoxyuridine (FdUrd) have been used in the treatment of gastrointestinal tumors, breast cancer, head and neck cancer, and some other malignancies. The metabolism of 5-FU is complex and is partially shown in Figure 48-5.[19] The best characterized mechanism of fluoropyrimidine cytotoxicity involves the inhibition of thymidylate synthase by 5-fluoro- 2′-deoxyuridine monophosphate (FdUMP). Additionally, the incorporation of the metabolite, 5-fluorouridine triphosphate (FUTP) into RNA correlates with cytotoxicity in some systems. Although 5-fluoro-2′-deoxyuridine triphosphate (FdUTP) can be incorporated into DNA, the relationship between this process and the cytocidal activity of fluoropyrimidines remains undetermined. Resistance to 5-FU may be conferred by alterations in enzymes involved in fluoropyrimidine metabolism, particularly those enzymes associated with the conversion of 5-FU to the thymidylate synthase inhibitor, FdUMP.[19] Furthermore, changes in thymidylate synthase level or its affinity for FdUMP are associated with 5-FU resistance.[413–415]

Several strategies to improve fluoropyrimidine efficacy and overcome resistance have been advanced. It has been suggested that tumor cell killing may be improved by prolonged or continuous exposure to drug.[416,417] Other studies advocate the coadministration of 5-FU with the reduced folate leucovorin. The efficacy of this combination stems from leucovorin-dependent increases in intracellular 5,10-methylene tetrahydrofolate (5,10-MTHF), a cofactor that stabilizes the FdUMP-thymidylate synthase inhibitor complex.[418,419] Synergy between 5-FU and other agents, which might be exploited clinically, has also been stud-

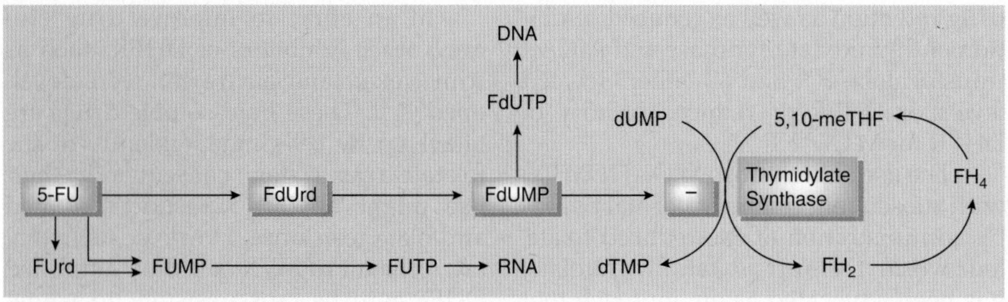

Figure 48-5 5-Fluorouracil metabolism and toxicity. *Abbreviations:* 5-FU, 5-fluorouracil; FdUMP and FdUTP, 5-fluoro-2′-deoxyuridine mono- and triphosphate; FdUrd, 5-fluoro-2′-deoxyuridine.

ied. For example, pretreatment of cells with methotrexate enhances the toxicity of 5-FU subsequently administered. Such pretreatment with methotrexate, an inhibitor of de novo purine synthesis (discussed above), increases the level of phosphoribosyl pyrophosphate (PRPP). Thus, the expanded pool of PRPP is available for conversion of 5-FU to FUMP and FUTP (Fig. 48-5). It has been suggested that the increased incorporation of FUTP into RNA that results is responsible for the improved cytotoxicity.[420,421] The inhibitor of de novo pyrimidine synthesis, N-phosphonacetyl-L-aspartatic acid (PALA), has been used with 5-FU in an effort to reduce pyrimidine metabolites that compete for the targets of fluoropyrimidine toxicity.[422] Finally, the synergistic interaction between interferon and halogenated pyrimidines has been investigated.[423]

Ara-C is an important nucleoside antineoplastic agent effective in the treatment of acute leukemias. Figure 48-6 presents the metabolism and mechanism of cytotoxicity of ara-C.[424] Following its uptake by the nucleoside transport system, ara-C is activated by a series of kinases to ara-CTP, a substrate of DNA polymerase that is incorporated into nascent DNA, causing premature chain termination and ultimately cell death. The rate-limiting step in ara-C activation is the S-phase specific reaction catalyzed by deoxycytidine kinase. The cytotoxic compound, ara-CTP or its precursors (ara-CMP and ara-CDP) can be catabolized by phosphatases or they (ara-C and ara-CMP) can be inactivated by deaminases. Several mechanisms of cancer cell resistance to ara-C have been demonstrated, including, but not confined to, the following. Because ara-C activation is cell-cycle dependent, quiescent cells or cells that fail to enter the S phase during the interval of treatment escape the cytotoxicity of ara-C. At suboptimal doses, otherwise drug-sensitive tumor cells located in pharmacologic or anatomic sanctuaries may survive ara-C treatment.[425] Decreased nucleoside transport has also been implicated in ara-C resistance.[426] Additionally, resistance may be conferred by altered drug metabolism, such as decreased activation by deoxycytidine kinase,[424] increased inactivation by cytidine deaminase,[14] or altered DNA polymerase affinity for ara-C.[427]

Administration of high-dose ara-C represents one approach to overcoming resistance to the drug and has been clinically useful in the treatment of some leukemias refractory to conventional doses of ara-C. Resistance based on diminished nucleoside transport and pharmacologic/anatomic sanctuaries can be circumvented with high-dose drug treatment.[425] In resistance secondary to increased drug inactivation by cytidine deaminase, coadministration of ara-C with a cytidine deaminase inhibitor such as tetrahydrouridine may reverse this mode of drug resistance.[428] Alternative pyrimidine analogs such as ara-AC (arabinofuranosyl-5-azacytosine, fazarabine) have shown activity against a broad range of tumor cells in preclinical testing and have been the subject of clinical trials.[429,430]

Resistance to Microtubule-Targeted Drugs

Since the discovery of the vinca alkaloids as anticancer agents over 40 years ago, microtubule-targeted drugs (MTTD) have become one of the most important class of anticancer agents.[431,432] However, as with any other drug, their long-term efficacy is limited by resistance. Although both the vinca alkaloids and the taxanes are substrates for the ABC transporter MDR1/ABCB1 (P-glycoprotein) and thus are affected by classic multidrug resistance, a number of microtubule-specific mechanisms have also been identified.[433] These include alterations in tubulin and tubulin-binding proteins, aberrant signal transduction, and cell death pathway, which will be further described in this section.

MTTDs are broadly divided into microtubule stabilizers (the taxanes, taxol and Taxotere; the epothilones; discodermolide; eleutherobin; the sarcodictyins; and the laulimalides) and microtubule destabilizers (the vinca alkaloids inblastine, vincristine, vindesine, vinorelbine, and vinflunine; colcemid; colchicines; halichandrins; dolastatins; and hemiasterlins).[431,434] As the classification implies, the microtubule destabilizers inhibit microtubule polymer assembly by binding to the a/ß-tubulin monomers, whereas the microtubule stabilizers facilitate microtubule stabilization by binding to the polymer. Accordingly, alterations in the MTTD binding sites have been found to confer resistance. For example, analysis of tubulin genes in 11 cell lines selected for resistance to vinblastine or colcemid revealed 5 different mutations in ß-tubulin and 4 mutations in a-tubulin.[435] Each of these genetic changes were found to make microtubules more stable, thus conferring resistance to the action of destabilizing MTTDs. Similarly, A549 and HeLa cells selected for resistance to epothilone were found to contain mutations in ß-tubulin.[436] Interestingly, these epothilon-eresistant cells are collaterally sensitive to vinblastine and colchicines, suggesting that alterations in tubulins negatively affected the stability of the microtubules following exposure to microtubule destabilizers. In another set of paclitaxel-selected Chinese hamster ovary cells, a cluster of ß-tubulin mutations was identified that resulted in destabilization of the microtubules, thereby conferring resistance to the stabilizer paclitaxel.[437] Thus, it appears that alterations that affect the stability of microtubules have a direct effect on a cell's sensitivity to MTTDs. Furthermore, it appears that destabilizing alterations in tubulins that can confer resistance to microtubule stabilizing drugs can also be associated with collateral sensitization to other MTTDs.

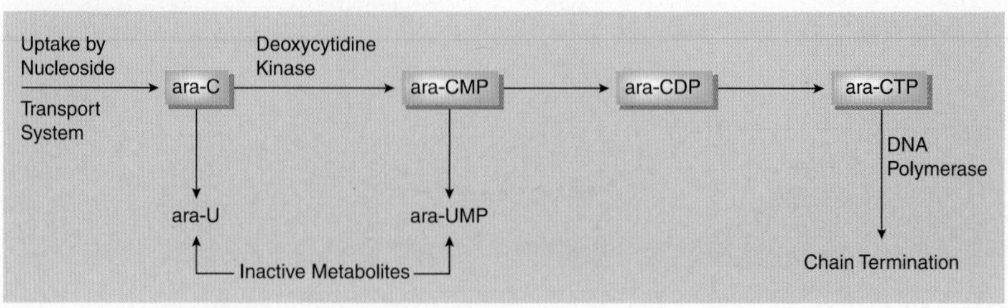

Figure 48-6 Cytosine arabinoside (ara-C) metabolism and toxicity.

In addition to tubulin mutations that alter the stability of the microtubules, several microtubule-interacting proteins have also been identified that affect sensitivity to MTTDs, including MAP-4, stathmin, and tau.[438–441] Whereas stathmin overexpression was found to decrease microtubule polymerization and stability, overexpression of MAP-4 had the opposite effect. Thus, changes in the levels of these proteins are expected to directly affect the sensitivity of cancer cells of MTTDs. Indeed, upregulation of stathmin in breast cancer cell lines was found to decrease the polymerization of microtubules and markedly reduce taxol binding, thus decreasing the cell's sensitivity to the drug.[438] Similarly, stathmin was found to be overexpressed in 2 taxol-resistant ovarian cancer cells, although these also have point mutations in their ß-tubulin genes.[439] Conversely to the effect of stathmin, up-regulation of MAP-4 expression was associated with increased resistance to vinca alkaloids and increased sensitivity to taxol.[441] Interestingly, both stathmin and MAP-4 activity are regulated by TP53. MAP-4 is transcriptionally repressed by wild-type TP53,[442] whereas inactivation of TP53 results in increased MAP-4 expression and a concomitant sensitization of cells to taxol and resistance to vinca alkaloids.[441] Similarly, cells expressing mutant TP53 were found to contain high levels of stathmin and were sensitive to taxol,[438] while other studies demonstrated that exposure of cells expressing wild-type TP53 to DNA-damaging agents resulted in increased sensitivity to vinblastine and increased resistance to taxol.[443] Furthermore, ectopic expression of mutant TP53 in J82 bladder cancer cells was associated with increased taxol cytotoxicity.[444] Similar findings were also reported with epothilone, another microtubule stabilizing agent that was more active in cells with mutant TP53.[445] Together, these observations indicate that the status of TP53 in cancer cells may have a profound influence on their sensitivity to MTTDs, suggesting that this can potentially be exploited when selecting antimicrotubule chemotherapy.

Conclusion and Future Directions

Through the kinds of studies done largely in vitro described in this chapter, many of the mechanisms of antineoplastic drug resistance have been identified. Although several of these processes operate in vivo, their relative clinical importance must be better clarified in controlled, prospective examinations of patient tumor specimens and correlations with therapeutic responses to chemotherapy. Nevertheless, these mechanisms suggest potentially useful approaches to overcoming clinical drug resistance. These approaches include the rational choice of conventional agents or design of novel drugs that are less likely to share resistance mechanisms. Additionally, many of the pathways of antineoplastic drug inactivation or transport are targets for pharmacologic manipulations that may reverse or circumvent the resistance of tumors to some drugs. Despite these efforts, many tumors will remain refractory to conventional chemotherapeutic drugs.

Selected References

The complete reference list can be found at www.CANCERMEDICINE8.com

1. Hill BT, Price LA, Goldies JH. The value of Adriamycin in overcoming resistance to methotrexate in tissue culture. *Eur J Cancer.* 1976;12:541–549.
2. Teicher BA, Cucchi CA, Lee JB, et al. Alkylating agents: in vitro studies of cross-resistance patterns in human cell lines. *Cancer Res.* 1986;46:4379–4383.
3. Antony AC, Kane MA, Portillo RM, et al. Studies of the role of a particulate folate-binding protein in the uptake of 5-methyltetrahydrofolate by cultured human KB cells. *J Biol Chem.* 1985;260:14911–14917.
4. Dixon KH, Lanpher BC, Chiu J, et al. A novel cDNA restores reduced folate carrier activity and methotrexate sensitivity to transport deficient cells. *J Biol Chem.* 1994;269:17–20.
5. Sirotnak FM, Moccio DM, Kelleher LE, et al. Relative frequency and kinetic properties of transport-defective phenotypes among methotrexate-resistant L1210 clonal cell lines derived in vivo. *Cancer Res.* 1981;41(11 Pt 1):4447–4452.
6. Hill BT, Bailey BD, White JC, et al. Characteristics of transport of 4-amino antifolates and folate compounds by two lines of L5178Y lymphoblasts, one with impaired transport of methotrexate. *Cancer Res.* 1979;39(7 Pt 1):2440–2446.
7. Endicott JA, Ling V. The biochemistry of P-glycoproteinmediated multidrug resistance. *Annu Rev Biochem.* 1989;58:137–171.
8. Gottesman MM, Pastan I. Biochemistry of multidrug resistance mediated by the multidrug transporter. *Annu Rev Biochem.* 1993;62:385–427.
9. Drahovsky D, Kreis W. Studies on drug resistance. II. Kinase patterns in P815 neoplasms sensitive and resistant to 1-beta-D-arabinofuranosylcytosine. *Biochem Pharmacol.* 1970;19:940–944.
10. Brockman RW. Mechanisms of resistance to anticancer agents. *Adv Cancer Res.* 1963;57:129–234.
11. Haaz MC, Rivory LP, Riche C, Robert J. The transformation of irinotecan (CPT-11) to its active metabolite SN-38 by human liver microsomes. Differential hydrolysis for the lactone and carboxylate forms. *Naunyn Schmiedebergs Arch Pharmacol.* 1997;356:257–262.
12. Kanzawa F, Sugimoto Y, Minato K, et al. Establishment of a camptothecin analogue (CPT-11)-resistant cell line of human non-small cell lung cancer: characterization and mechanism of resistance. *Cancer Res.* 1990;50:5919–5924.
13. Hunt SW 3rd, Hoffee PA, Amplification of adenosine deaminase gene sequences in deoxycoformycin-resistant rat hepatoma cells. *J Biol Chem.* 1983;258: 13185–13192.
14. Steuart CD, Burke PJ. Cytidine deaminase and the development of resistance to arabinosyl cytosine. *Nat New Biol.* 1971;233:109–110.
15. Houghton JA, Maroda SJ Jr, Phillips JO, Houghton PJ. Biochemical determinants of responsiveness to 5-fluorouracil and its derivatives in xenografts of human colorectal adenocarcinomas in mice. *Cancer Res.* 1981;41:144–149.
16. Perez RP. Cellular and molecular determinants of cisplatin resistance. *Eur J Cancer.* 1998;34:1535–1542.
17. Haber DA, Schimke RT. Unstable amplification of an altered dihydrofolate reductase gene associated with double-minute chromosomes. *Cell.* 1981;26 (3 Pt 1):355–362.
18. Haber DA, Beverley SM, Kiely ML, Schimke RT. Properties of an altered dihydrofolate reductase encoded by amplified genes in cultured mouse fibroblasts. *J Biol Chem.* 1981;256:9501–9510.
19. Armstrong RA. *Fluoropyrimidine Activity and Resistance at the Cellular Level.* Boca Raton, FL: CRC Press; 1989.
20. Vassetzky YS, Alghisi GC, Gasser SM. DNA topoisomerase II mutations and resistance to anti-tumor drugs. *Bioessays.* 1995;17:767–774.
21. Rubin EH, Li TK, Duann P, Liu LF. Cellular resistance to topoisomerase poisons. *Cancer Treat Res.* 1996;87:243–260.
22. Pommier Y, Kerrigan D, Schwartz RE, et al. Altered DNA topoisomerase II activity in Chinese hamster cells resistant to topoisomerase II inhibitors. *Cancer Res.* 1986;46:3075–3081.
23. Mirski SE, Evans CD, Almquist KC, et al. Altered topoisomerase II alpha in a drug-resistant small cell lung cancer cell line selected in VP-16. *Cancer Res.* 1993;53:4866–4873.
24. Kubota N, Kanzawa F, Nishio K, et al. Detection of topoisomerase I gene point mutation in CPT-11 resistant lung cancer cell line. *Biochem Biophy Res Commun.* 1992;188:571–577.
25. Hinds M, Deisseroth K, Mayes J, et al. Identification of a point mutation in the topoisomerase II gene from a human leukemia cell line containing an amsacrine-resistant form of topoisomerase II. *Cancer Res.* 1991;51:4729–4731.
26. Gorre ME, Mohammed M, Ellwood K, et al. Clinical resistance to STI-571 cancer therapy caused by BCR-ABL gene mutation or amplification. *Science.* 2001;293:876–880.
27. Banerjee D, Mayer-Kuckuk P, Capiaux G, et al. Novel aspects of resistance to drugs targeted to dihydrofolate reductase and thymidylate synthase. *Biochim Biophys Acta.* 2002;1587:164–173.

28. Banerjee D, Gorlick R, Liefshitz A, et al. Levels of E2F-1 expression are higher in lung metastasis of colon cancer as compared with hepatic metastasis and correlate with levels of thymidylate synthase. *Cancer Res.* 2000;60:2365–2367.
29. Belvedere O, Puglisi F, Di Loreto C, et al. Lack of correlation between immunohistochemical expression of E2F-1, thymidylate synthase expression and clinical response to 5-fluorouracil in advanced colorectal cancer. *Ann Oncol.* 2004;15:55–58.
30. Sowers R, Toguchida J, Qin J, et al. mRNA expression levels of E2F transcription factors correlate with dihydrofolate reductase, reduced folate carrier, and thymidylate synthase mRNA expression in osteosarcoma. *Mol Cancer Ther.* 2003;2:535–541.
31. Dean M, Rzhetsky A, Allikmets R. The human ATP-binding cassette (ABC) transporter superfamily. *Genome Res.* 2001;11:1156–1166.
32. Cole SP, Deeley RG. Multidrug resistance mediated by the ATP-binding cassette transporter protein MRP. *Bioessays.* 1998;20:931–940.
33. Cui Y, Konig J, Buchholz JK, et al. Drug resistance and ATPdependent conjugate transport mediated by the apical multidrug resistance protein, MRP2, permanently expressed in human and canine cells. *Mol Pharmacol.* 1999;55:929–937.
34. Kool M, de Haas M, Scheffer GL, et al. Analysis of expression of cMOAT (MRP2), MRP3, MRP4, and MRP5, homologues of the multidrug resistance-associated protein gene (MRP1), in human cancer cell lines. *Cancer Res.* 1997;57:3537–3547.
35. Loe DW, Deeley RG, Cole SP. Biology of the multidrug resistance-associated protein, MRP. *Eur J Cancer.* 1996;32A:945–957.
36. Doyle LA, Yang W, Abruzzo LV, et al. A multidrug resistance transporter from human MCF-7 breast cancer cells. *Proc Natl Acad Sci USA.* 1998;95:15665–15670.
37. Ross DD, Yang W, Abrusso LV, et al. Atypical multidrug resistance: breast cancer resistance protein messenger RNA expression in mitoxantrone-selected cell lines. *J Natl Cancer Inst.* 1999;91:429–433.
38. Kickhoefer VA, Rajavel KS, Scheffer GL, et al. Vaults are up-regulated in multidrug-resistant cancer cell lines. *J Biol Chem.* 1998;273:8971–8974.
39. Izquierdo MA, Scheffer GL, Flens MJ, et al. Relationship of LRP-human major vault protein to in vitro and clinical resistance to anticancer drugs. *Cytotechnology.* 1996;19:191–197.
40. Biedler JL, Riehm H. Cellular resistance to actinomycin D in Chinese hamster cells in vitro: cross-resistance, radioautographic, and cytogenetic studies. *Cancer Res.* 1970;30:1174–1184.
41. Juliano RL, Ling V. A surface glycoprotein modulating drug permeability in Chinese hamster ovary cell mutants. *Biochim Biophys Acta.* 1976;455:152–162.
42. Riordan JR, Ling V. Genetic and biochemical characterization of multidrug resistance. *Pharmacol Ther.* 1985;28:51–75.
43. Raviv Y, Pollard HV, Bruggemann EP, et al. Photosensitized labeling of a functional multidrug transporter in living drug-resistant tumor cells. *J Biol Chem.* 1990;265:3975–3980.
44. Higgins CF, Gottesman MM. Is the multidrug transporter a flippase? *Trends Biochem Sci.* 1992;17:18–21.
45. Gros P, Ben Neriah YB, Croop JM, Housman DE. Isolation and expression of a complementary DNA that confers multidrug resistance. *Nature.* 1986;323:728–731.
46. Ueda K, Cardarelli C, Gottesman MM, Pastan I. Expression of a full-length cDNA for the human "MDR1" gene confers resistance to colchicine, doxorubicin, and vinblastine. *Proc Natl Acad Sci USA.* 1987;84:3004–3008.
47. Chen CJ, Chin JE, Ueda K, et al. Internal duplication and homology with bacterial transport proteins in the mdr1 (P-glycoprotein) gene from multidrug-resistant human cells. *Cell.* 1986;47:381–389.
48. Gros P, Croop J, Housman D. Mammalian multidrug resistance gene: complete cDNA sequence indicates strong homology to bacterial transport proteins. *Cell.* 1986;47:371–380.
49. Safa AR, Glover CJ, Meyers MB, et al. Vinblastine photoaffinity labeling of a high molecular weight surface membrane glycoprotein specific for multidrug-resistant cells. *J Biol Chem.* 1986;261:6137–6140.
50. Gottesman MM, Pastan I. Resistance to multiple chemotherapeutic agents in human cancer cells. *Trends Pharmacol Sci.* 1988;9:54–58.

49 Folate Antagonists

Peter D. Cole, MD ■ Barton A. Kamen, MD ■ Joseph R. Bertino, MD

Introduction

Folic acid antagonists (antifols) are cytotoxic drugs used as antineoplastic, antimicrobial, anti-inflammatory, and immune-suppressive agents. Although several folate antagonists have been developed, methotrexate (4-amino-4-deoxy-10-*N*-methyl-pteroylglutamic acid; MTX; Fig. 49-1) is the antifol with the most extensive history and widest spectrum of use. MTX is an essential drug in curative chemotherapy regimens used to treat patients with acute lymphoblastic leukemia, osteosarcoma, and choriocarcinoma and is an important agent in the therapy of patients with lymphoma, breast cancer, bladder cancer, and head and neck cancer. In addition, it is used for patients with nonmalignant diseases such as rheumatoid arthritis, psoriasis, autoimmune diseases, and graft versus host disease. This chapter will review the clinical use of and metabolism of MTX and discuss several other folate antagonists that have been developed to overcome resistance or have alternate intracellular targets.

Historical Overview

In the early 1940s, the combined observations that patients with acute leukemia often have serum folate deficiency and that the bone marrow megaloblasts of folate-deficient patients morphologically resemble leukemic blasts prompted some investigators to postulate that leukemia might be a result of a deficiency of this B vitamin. However, it rapidly became apparent that administration of folic acid to patients with leukemia was not only ineffective but often accelerated the course of the disease.[1] Efforts to treat these leukemias thus turned to pharmacologically mimicking folate deficiency using folate analogs with effects antagonistic to those of the vitamin. Aminopterin (4-amino-4-deoxy PGA; AMT; Fig. 49-1) was the first of these analogs to produce temporary remissions in 5 of 16 patients with acute leukemia.[2] This report was a landmark in cancer chemotherapy as the first successful example of the power of rational drug design leading to an effective antineoplastic agent.

Since that initial study indicating the usefulness of AMT in the treatment of acute leukemia of childhood, there has been sustained interest in folate antagonists. Although known to be less potent, MTX supplanted AMT in the clinic in the early 1950s because the toxicity caused by AMT was greater and less predictable.[3-5] Newer antifols, rationally designed analogs of folate or MTX, have been synthesized either in an effort to overcome cellular resistance to MTX or to target alternative folate-dependent processes. Some of these newer antifols have been approved as antimicrobials or antineoplastic agents, and others are still in clinical trial.

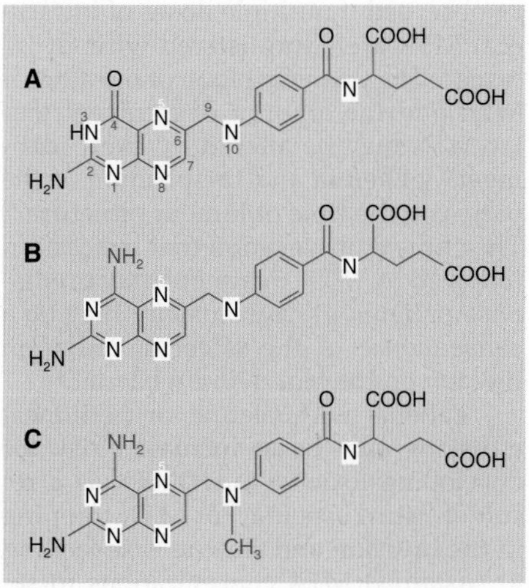

Figure 49-1 ■ Structure of folic acid and structurally related classic antifols, AMT and MTX. **(A)** Folic acid (pteroylglutamic acid; PGA). **(B)** Aminopterin (4-amino-PGA). **(C)** Methotrexate (4-amino-*N*-10-methyl PGA).

Mechanisms of Action of MTX

Folate antagonists function in several ways: by competing with folates for uptake into cells, by inhibiting the formation of folate coenzymes, or by inhibiting one or more reactions that are mediated by folate coenzymes. Thus far, the clinically important antineoplastic folate analogs appear to work primarily by inhibiting dihydrofolate reductase (DHFR) or thymidylate synthase (TS). The prototypic antifol DHFR inhibitor is a 4-amino-substituted pterin compound, such as MTX or AMT (Fig. 49-1). Substitution of an amino group for the 4-hydroxy moiety results in a folate analog with a several thousandfold increase in affinity for DHFR. The K_i of MTX for DHFR is less than 10^{-10} M, well below the K_m of the natural substrate, dihydrofolate, which is in the micromolar range. By stoichiometrically inhibiting DHFR at slightly acidic pH, MTX blocks the cell's ability to replenish a supply of reduced folates necessary for de novo thymidylate synthesis (Fig. 49-2).[6] In rapidly dividing cells, the inhibition of thymidylate biosynthesis leads to a decrease in thymidine triphosphate pools, a decrease in DNA synthesis, and eventually cell death.[7]

Intracellular metabolism of classical antifols such as MTX to polyglutamate species significantly impacts their function and mechanisms of cytotoxicity.[8] Folylpolyglutamate synthetase (FPGS), adds glutamate residues in γ-carboxyl linkage to both folate coenzymes and classical folate antagonists (those with a glutamate moiety). This addition of up to seven or eight additional glutamate molecules serves to add mass and negative charge, markedly reducing efflux and increasing total intracellular accumulation at steady state.[9] Both quantitative differences in FPGS expression and qualitative differences in FPGS function[10] exist between neoplastic and nonneoplastic

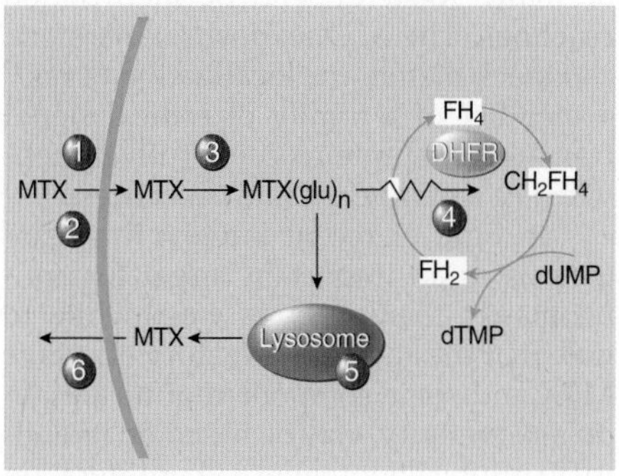

Figure 49-2 ■ Primary site of action of MTX and $MTX(glu)_N$. MTX enters cells by either the reduced folate carrier (1) or the membrane folate binding protein (2). MTX is then metabolized by the cytosolic enzyme folylpolyglutamate synthetase (3) to $MTX(glu)_N$, a potent inhibitor of dihydrofolate reductase (DHFR) (4). $MTX(glu)_N$ can be hydrolyzed to MTX by the lysosomal enzyme γ-glutamyl hydrolase (GGH) (5). *Abbreviations*: CH_2FH_4, N5, N10-methylene tetrahydrofolate; dTMP, deoxythymidine monophosphate; dUMP, deoxyuridine monophosphate/deoxyuridylate; FH_2, dihydrofolate; FH_4, tetrahydrofolate; MTX, methotrexate; $MTX(glu)_N$, MTX polyglutamates.

tissues, which may explain some of the selectivity of antifolates for neoplastic cells.[11] A relative lack of FPGS may explain the observation that a cell population with a large number of G_0 cells would be less affected by the same concentration and time of exposure to MTX than a population with more actively dividing cells.

The MTX polyglutamates are more potent inhibitors of DHFR than the parent compound because, although they bind to DHFR as tightly as does MTX, they dissociate less rapidly.[12] In addition, MTX polyglutamates are also potent inhibitors of other folate-requiring enzymes, including TS[13] and two of the rate limiting steps of de novo purine synthesis: glycinamide ribonucleotide (GAR) and aminoimidazole carboxamide ribonucleotide (AICAR) transformylases.[14] These two enzymes are also potently inhibited by DHF polyglutamates and 10-formyl-DHF polyglutamates, which increase after MTX inhibits DHFR.[15] As a result, inhibition of de novo purine synthesis may be at least as relevant as DHFR inhibition to the cytotoxic effects of MTX in cancer cells[16] and for the anti-inflammatory action of MTX in patients with rheumatologic diseases.[17,18]

Two other possible mechanisms by which MTX exerts antineoplastic or anti-inflammatory action are worth mentioning. First, by inhibiting folate-dependent methionine biosynthesis, MTX causes intracellular levels of the substrate, homocysteine (Hcy) to rise, resulting in a secondary elevation in *S*-adenosylhomocysteine (SAH), a potent inhibitor of many folate-dependent methylation reactions. The MTX exposure, therefore, can block membrane localization of ras,[19] a member of a family of critical signal transduction proteins constitutively activated in a number of human cancers.

In light of recent interest in angiogenesis as an important target for antineoplastic therapy, it is worthwhile to note that the anti-inflammatory effects of MTX and some component of its antineoplastic activity, may be based on its ability to inhibit endothelial cell proliferation at low concentrations.[20] Preclinical data confirm that low-dose methotrexate can inhibit the growth of microscopic metastatic disease through its antiangiogenic properties.[21]

Pharmacokinetics of MTX

The MTX is one of few anticancer agents for which pharmacokinetic data are routinely used in clinical practice to modulate the balance between efficacy and toxicity.[22] Retrospective analysis of children with ALL shows that lower MTX clearance[23] and higher MTX concentrations[24] are associated with lower risk of relapse. Even more intriguing are data from a prospective randomized trial in patients with ALL comparing dosing by BSA with individualized dosing based on pharmacokinetic data, which showed significantly improved complete continuous remission rates in the individualized therapy arm.[25] It is possible, however, that these results are protocol specific, because others have found that pharmacologically guided treatment intensification led to inferior outcomes for some subpopulations.[26]

Absorption

Following oral administration, peak plasma concentrations may occur 1–5 hours after a dose of 15–30 mg/m^2. Absorption can be relatively poor and unpredictable,[27,28] affected by food, nonabsorbable antibiotics, bile salts, and a shortened intestine transit time. Thus, it is suggested that the drug be taken on an empty stomach with clear liquids. Nevertheless, at a dose and schedule of 25 mg/m^2, given orally every 6 hours times four doses, plasma MTX concentration greater than 0.5 μM were seen in more than 85% of pediatric patients with ALL, indicating the reliability of this oral regimen.[29] Moreover, continued therapy with MTX in combination with mercaptopurine did not induce malabsorption over an 18-month period.

Distribution

After intravenous (IV) administration of MTX, the initial volume of distribution (Vd) is approximately 0.18 L/kg of body weight. Steady-state Vd is between 0.4 and 0.8 L/kg.[30] The initial distribution phase has a T½ of 30–45 min; the beta T½ is 3–4 hours.

After high doses of MTX (>3 g/m^2; HDMTX), peak serum concentrations in the range of 10^{-4}–10^{-3} M are achieved.[31] At these concentrations, transmembrane transport is saturated, limiting further influx of MTX to passive diffusion. Uptake of reduced folates, including leucovorin (LV), is inhibited. Studies of MTX metabolism in lymphoblasts in vitro have also shown that too high an extracellular concentration of drug can impede metabolism of MTX to a polyglutamate.[32]

Binding of MTX to plasma proteins, especially to albumin, is approximately 50%.[33,34] The 7-hydroxy metabolite of MTX is 90% bound to plasma proteins but apparently does not interfere with MTX binding to plasma proteins at clinically observed concentrations. The highest tissue-to-plasma concentrations found in humans are in the liver and kidney, followed by the gastrointestinal tract. Prolonged plasma levels after high-dose MTX infusions in humans have been attributed to decreased transit rate secondary to gastrointestinal obstruction.

Because of the blood–brain barrier and efflux mechanisms that actively remove MTX from the CNS,[35] cerebrospinal fluid (CSF) MTX concentrations are approximately 1% of those in the plasma. Cytocidal concentrations are therefore not obtained in the CSF after conventional doses but only with doses of 500 mg/m^2 and higher.[36] After HDMTX administration, lumbar CSF and ventricular CSF concentrations were similar. HDMTX was suggested as a possible alternative to intrathecal drug for the treatment of patients with nonleukemic leptomeningeal disease.[37] However, a recent meta-analysis of CNS-directed therapy for children with acute lymphoblastic leukemia concluded that efforts to increase CSF penetration using HDMTX have not produced the desired result of lowering the rate of CNS relapse in this population.[38]

Although MTX is accumulated poorly into the CSF, even small doses of LV given orally can increase CSF folates significantly. This systemic rescue, especially if given too early after MTX, may rescue cancer cells in the CSF compartment.[39]

When injected into an in-dwelling ventricular catheter, MTX reaches reproducible therapeutic drug concentrations (>10^{-6} M) for at least 48 hours.[40] In contrast, when MTX is given by the lumbar route into the CSF, it distributes unreliably into the ventricles. An improved dose schedule utilizing the administration of multiple small doses of intrathecal MTX has been suggested.[41] Following intrathecal administration, MTX slowly exits into the systemic circulation with a t½ of 8–10 hours.[35] Systemic toxicity can be observed if multiple doses of intrathecal MTX are administered without LV rescue. The pharmacology of intrathecal MTX and the amount of intraventricular MTX may be altered by overt meningeal leukemia and the position of the patient at the time of lumbar puncture.[42] The clinical observation that irradiation followed by MTX treatment may predispose patients to neurotoxicity may be a consequence of the effect of radiation therapy on the blood–brain barrier.[43]

Patients with pleural or peritoneal effusions may be at increased risk for developing toxicity to HDMTX as a result of "third spacing," or MTX trapping in the infusion and slow release leading to sustained MTX concentrations in serum.[44] In these circumstances, higher LV doses and prolonged LV rescue may be necessary, until the serum level of MTX decreases to less than 0.05×10^{-6} M.

Metabolism

The major metabolite of MTX, produced by the action of hepatic aldehyde oxidase, is 7-hydroxy MTX (7-OH MTX) (Fig. 49-3), which is only 1% as potent an inhibitor of DHFR as MTX.[45] It is also less water soluble than MTX and may contribute to renal toxicity after HDMTX.[46]

A second, less important pathway of metabolism of MTX occurs in the intestine. MTX is hydrolyzed by bacteria to the pteroate (4-deoxy-4-amino-*N*10-methyl pteroic acid; dAMPA) and glutamic acid (Fig. 49-3).[47] Like 7-OH MTX, dAMPA is also a relatively inactive metabolite with approximately 1/200th the affinity of MTX for DHFR. Excretion of dAMPA in the urine accounts for only a small percentage of the dose administered (<5%).

The third metabolic product of MTX is MTX polyglutamate. MTX polyglutamates are at least as potent inhibitors of DHFR as is MTX and have a slower rate of disassociation from DHFR than does MTX.[12] MTX polyglutamates are not found in plasma or urine because of the abundant activity of γ-glutamyl hydrolase(s) (GGH) in plasma that convert folyl- and MTX-polyglutamates to monoglutamates. Like MTX, 7-OH MTX is also polyglutamylated intracellularly, and retention of these polyglutamate forms could contribute to MTX cytotoxicity.[48]

It has been proposed that compliance with oral MTX regimens can be monitored by measuring MTX-polyglutamate concentrations within circulating erythrocytes (RBCs).[49-51] Nucleated RBC precursors within the bone marrow will accumulate and metabolize circulating MTX. The resulting MTX polyglutamates will remain within the mature RBC throughout its lifespan,[52] whereas unmetabolized MTX will gradually efflux.[53]

Excretion

The majority of administered MTX (and its metabolites 7-OH MTX and DAMPA) is excreted unchanged in the urine.[54,55] Because of active secretion in the proximal tubules, renal clearance of MTX can exceed creatinine clearance.[56] There is wide interpatient variability in MTX clearance, which does not correlate perfectly with renal function.[57] MTX excretion through organic acid transporters can be inhibited by probenecid or competitively blocked by other weak organic acids, such as aspirin or penicillin G. MTX elimination is increased by drugs that block distal tubular reabsorption, such as folic acid, some cephalosporins, and sulfamethoxazole.

Following IV administration of doses of 30–80 mg/m^2, 0.4–20% of the administered dose is excreted through the canalicular multiorganic acid transporter (cMOAT; ABCC2; MRP2) into the bile. Less than 10% of MTX is typically recovered in the feces.[58] Abnormal activity of ABCC2 may affect the pharmacokinetics and pharmacodynamic profile of camptothecins, CDDP and vinca alkaloids; overexpression of MRP2 has been shown to confer resistance to MTX in vitro by enhancing drug efflux.[59]

Drug Interactions

As indicated above, several drugs used in cancer patients, including antibiotics, may alter the renal excretion of MTX by increasing toxicity or decreasing efficacy. Deleterious and even fatal reactions have been reported between MTX and nonsteroidal anti-inflammatory drugs, in particular with naproxen and ketoprofen.[60,61] This increased toxicity may be owing to decreased renal elimination, possibly as a result of competition for renal secretion.[56] Other commonly used organic drugs may also potentiate MTX toxicity, such as phenylbutazone, salicylate, and probenecid.[62,63] Probenecid increased the efficacy of MTX in tumor-bearing mice, but it has not been used clinically with this goal in mind.[64]

Increased toxicity was also reported when the antibacterial agent trimethoprim was used together with MTX. Presumably this antifolate, with weak binding affinity to mammalian DHFR, lowers folate stores, especially in patients with subclinical folate deficiency, making marrow cells more susceptible to MTX-induced toxicity.[65] Alcohol should be avoided in patients receiving MTX because of the risk of hepatic fibrosis and cirrhosis.

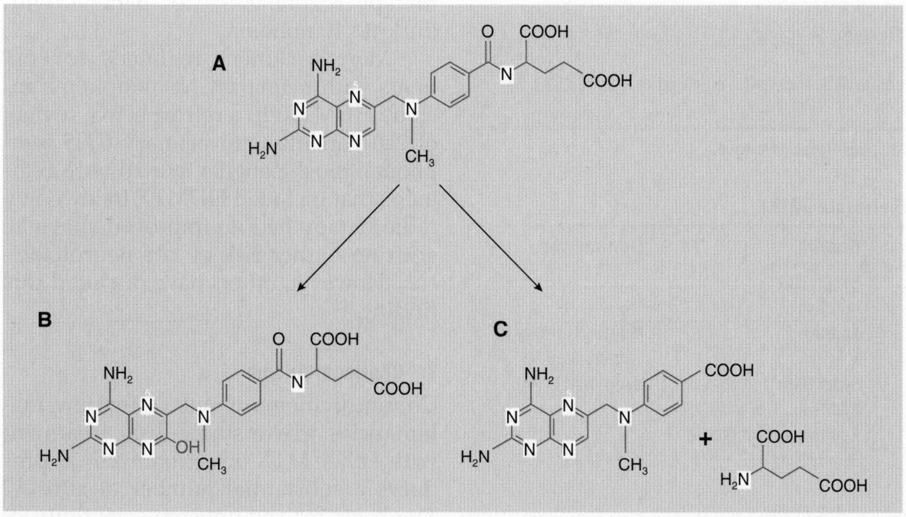

Figure 49-3 Catabolism of MTX. MTX (**A**) can be converted in the liver to 7-OH MTX (**B**). In addition, enteric bacteria will cleave the molecule to dAMPA plus glutamate (**C**).

Pharmacogenomics

A growing body of data implicates inherited variation in genes for enzymes responsible for folate metabolism in interpatient variability in antifolate response or toxicity. A more detailed discussion of these data is beyond the scope of this chapter but has been the subject of comprehensive reviews.[66-68] Briefly, functional polymorphisms have been described in either the promoter or coding regions of the genes for DHFR, methylenetetrahydrofolate reductase (MTHFR), aminoimidazole carboxamide ribonucleotide transformylase (ATIC), the reduced folate carrier (RFC), γ-glutamyl hydrolase (GGH), methionine synthase (MTR), methionine synthase reductase (MTRR), methylenetetrahydrofolate dehydrogenase (MTHFD), serine hydroxymethyltransferase (SHMT), and thymidylate synthase (TS). Many of these polymorphisms are present at significant frequency among the population, and some have been linked to higher rates of relapse or toxicity among patients with acute lymphoblastic leukemia[69-73] or rheumatoid arthritis.[74] If replicated in larger populations, these data suggest the potential for individualizing MTX therapy based on each patient's genotype.

However, gene–environment interactions may modulate the effects of genotypic variation on toxicity. To focus on one relevant example, some of the observed variation in serum homocysteine (a marker of functional folate deficiency) is explained by two common functional polymorphisms in the methylenetetrahydrofolate reductase (*MTHFR*) gene, C677T and A1298C, but only under conditions of decreased intake of dietary folate.[75,76] Adequate dietary folate in the current era of FDA-mandated folate supplementation could therefore erase the effects of genetic polymorphisms.

Clinical Application

Clinical Dosage Schedules

MTX has been administered on a variety of dosage schedules since its introduction into the clinic five decades ago (Table 49-1). In a trial of MTX in patients with head and neck cancer treated with 50, 500, or 5,000 mg/m^2 with LV "rescue," a trend toward dose responsiveness was seen (5 of 24, 5 of 16, or 9 of 18). Some responses were noted with the 5000 mg/m^2 dose regimen in patients who did not benefit at lower doses.[77]

The importance of dose scheduling was emphasized by an experimental study showing that resistance to high-dose pulse MTX may not extend to continuous low-dose exposure.[78] Determining the optimum dose schedule of MTX is complicated by the use of the drug in combination therapy (Table 49-2). Sequencing appears to be important when MTX is used with 5-fluorouracil (5-FU), with "L"-asparaginase and probably with cytosine arabinoside and 6-mecaptopurine or 6-thioguanine. Table 49-2 summarizes the use of some common drug combinations that include MTX, along with sequence specificity.

Current Uses for MTX in the Treatment of Neoplastic Disease

Acute Lymphoblastic Leukemia

MTX is a component of nearly all multiagent therapeutic regimens for patients with acute lymphoblastic leukemia postremission, and some protocols include MTX in remission induction. In addition to systemic use, MTX is administered intrathecally for the treatment of meningeal leukemia and for prophylaxis against CNS relapse.

During the intensive, early postremission phases, MTX can be administered orally or parenterally. Early studies showed that twice-weekly therapy (20 mg/m^2) was superior to continuous daily oral administration for treatment during remission.[79] The effectiveness of an oral divided dose (25–30 mg/m^2 given every 6 hours for 4–6 doses weekly) has also been shown.[29] Parenteral administration at intermediate dose (100–500 mg/m^2/dose) or high dose (µ1000 mg/m^2) has been incorporated in some protocols to increase accumulation of MTX-polyglutamates by blast cells,[80] to overcome mechanisms of resistance, and to increase penetration into protected sites including the CNS and testes.[81] Although the ability of HDMTX to prevent CNS relapse is not clearly proven,[38] the rate of isolated testicular relapse does appear to have decreased with the addition of intermediate or HDMTX.[82] With regard to marrow protection, randomized trials comparing escalating IV doses with oral MTX appear to give an edge to intermediate or HDMTX.[83-85] However, the marginal increase in event-free survival comes at the expense of increased hematologic and neurologic toxicity.[86-89]

During later maintenance phases, most current protocols rely on prolonged weekly administration of MTX at low doses (20–50 mg/m^2/dose) in combination with daily mercaptopurine.

Acute Myelogenous Leukemia

MTX has limited value in the current treatment of patients with acute nonlymphocytic leukemia. However, the combination MTX and "L"-asparaginase (the "Capizzi regimen") can result in remissions for patients with AML.[90,91] High-dose regimens with LV rescue have a transient but rapid effect on the peripheral blood count without producing marrow remissions in majority of these patients.[92] The lack of efficacy of MTX in this disease has been attributed to poor intracellular retention of the drug caused by a lack of polyglutamylation and an induction of the target enzyme DHFR following treatment.[93]

Lymphoma

Based on phase II studies that indicated that moderate to high doses of MTX (200 mg/m^2 to 3 gm/m^2) with LV rescue could produce transient regressions in patients with large cell lymphoma, MTX with LV rescue has been added to combination regimens for intermediate- and high-grade lymphomas. In some regimens (eg, M-BACOD), MTX is used with LV during the leukopenic phase of drug treatment, since the MTX/LV combination has little marrow toxicity.[94] Based on experimental studies showing that MTX and cytosine arabinoside produce additive and possibly synergistic effects,[95] this combination has also been utilized in regimens to treat this disease (eg, COMLA; cyclophosphamide, vincristine, MTX, cytosine arabinoside, and LV). Similarly, following documentation of responses among patients with Burkitt's lymphoma to therapy including MTX,[96,97] HDMTX with LV rescue has been added to CVAD, cytarabine, and intrathecal therapy as well as to other combination chemotherapy regimens[98-100] for patients with Burkitt's lymphoma.

Most treatment regimens for patients with primary CNS lymphoma include HDMTX. In a retrospective review of 226 patients with primary CNS lymphoma, those patients treated with regimens that included HDMTX followed by radiotherapy had an improved survival, with no higher risk of late neurotoxicity.[101] However, others have disputed this finding.[102]

Choriocarcinoma

Choriocarcinoma is one of the few malignancies where single-drug treatment with either MTX or actinomycin D produces a substantial number of cures.[103] The basis for the unusual sensitivity of this tumor to MTX is not very clear, but choriocarcinoma cells may accumulate

Table 49-1 Dosage Schedules Commonly Used for Methotrexate (MTX)

Schedule and Dose	Use/Comments
Oral:	
Weekly or biweekly (15–25 mg in single or divided doses)	Mainly for nonmalignant conditions, such as psoriasis or rheumatoid arthritis
Weekly or biweekly (20–30 mg/m^2)	Maintenance therapy for ALL
Parenteral:	
Pulse weekly (30–60 mg/m^2)	Choriocarcinoma, ALL
Intermediate dose (120–500 mg/m^2 weekly)	ALL, NHL; requires LV rescue, 10–15 mg/m^2 q6h × 6–8 doses
High dose (500–12,000 mg/m^2 weekly or every other week)	Osteosarcoma, ALL, neoplastic meningitis; requires LV rescue

Abbreviations: ALL, acute lymphoblastic leukemia; LV, leucovorin; NHL, non-Hodgkin lymphoma.

Table 49-2 Combination Chemotherapy With Methotrexate (MTX)

Used with	Schedule Notes	Result	Comments
5-FU	MTX must precede 5-FU by 24 h	Synergistic	
Anthracyclines		Additive	
Bleomycin		Additive	Mucosal toxicity is increased
Corticosteroids	Used together	Synergistic	Used in ALL
Cyclophosphamide	Used together	Additive	
Cytarabine	Used together	Additive or synergistic	
L-asparaginase	If MTX precedes l-asparaginase by 24 h	Synergistic	Used in ALL, AML
	If used simultaneously	Antagonistic	
Vinca alkaloids		Additive	

Abbreviations: ALL, acute lymphoblastic leukemia; AML, acute myelogenous leukemia; 5-FU, 5-fluorouracil.

and retain this drug effectively by synthesizing long-chain polyglutamates. The JAR (human choriocarcinoma) cell line was shown to have active-receptor-coupled uptake (potocytosis) of folates and antifolates.[104] Current programs for the treatment of this malignancy utilize MTX in combination with other drugs, especially for "poor-risk" patients.

Breast Cancer

MTX as a single agent causes regressions of breast cancer in approximately 30% of patients. When used with fluorouracil, sequential use of MTX followed by 5-FU improved response rates to 50% and improves disease-free survival when used as adjuvant therapy.[105] The adjuvant use of cyclophosphamide, MTX, and 5-FU (CMF) also significantly reduces the risk of relapse;[106] may allow more conservative surgery among women with localized disease when used as neoadjuvant therapy;[107] and has a role in the treatment for patients with inoperable, advanced disease.[108] The combination of MTX, 5-FU with vinorelbine (VMF) instead of cyclophosphamide has also shown activity among women with advanced breast cancer.[109] An additional advantage of this combination is the diminution of long-term toxicity (infertility, carcinogenesis) compared to regimens containing alkylating agents. Finally, it is interesting to note that "metronomic therapy" with low-dose oral MTX (2.5 mg BID × 2 day/week) plus daily oral cyclophosphamide has shown activity among heavily pretreated women with advanced metastatic breast cancer.[110]

Gastrointestinal Cancer

Antifolates have limited effectiveness in the treatment of gastrointestinal malignancies. Its role in the treatment of these diseases is mainly to modulate, and possibly improve, the effectiveness of 5-FU. By inhibiting purine synthesis, MTX pretreatment increases phosphoribosyl pyrophosphate, a precursor necessary for 5-FU nucleotide formation.[111] Data from recent trials using high-dose MTX followed by LV/5-FU in patients with colon cancer emphasize the need for a 7- to 24-hour interval between MTX and 5-FU administration.[112] Similar combinations also show activity for patients with advanced gastric cancer.[113,114]

Genitourinary Cancer

MTX alone (100 mg/m^2), or in high doses (≥500 mg/m^2) with LV rescue, is clearly active in the treatment of advanced bladder cancer. The response rate reported (~30%) is similar to the response rate of the other most active single drug, cisplatin. Combinations of drugs including MTX with cisplatin, vinblastine, and doxorubicin (M-VAC) have resulted in a substantial number of long-term clinical remissions.[115] A meta-analysis of randomized trials found that neoadjuvant treatment with MTX-containing regimens conferred a clear survival advantage.[116]

Head and Neck Cancer

MTX is an active agent for the treatment of patients with advanced carcinoma of the head and neck region. High-dose MTX regimens with LV rescue appear to improve response rates from 30% to 50%, but remission duration and survival are not improved.[117] MTX has also been used with 5-FU in this disease, with response rates as high as 60%.[118,119] The sequence and timing of drug administration have not been shown to affect the response rate, although different patterns of toxicity were observed.

Lung Cancer

MTX as a single agent in conventional doses, or in high doses with LV rescue, has only marginal activity in non–small cell lung cancer. This drug does have limited activity in small cell lung cancer and has been used in combination regimens to treat that disease.

Osteogenic Sarcoma

After studies were reported indicating that HDMTX with LV rescue could cause regressions in patients with advanced osteogenic sarcoma, the drug was tested as adjuvant therapy in patients with disease following resection of the tumor, with encouraging results.[120] Randomized trials demonstrated the beneficial effect of chemotherapy regimens that include HDMTX with LV rescue,[121] and showed that response may correlate with MTX dose density (defined as the amount of drug administered during a defined period).[122] However, a recent report demonstrated the paradoxical finding that higher MTX exposure (higher peak concentration and higher AUC) was associated with inferior outcome among patients with localized osteosarcoma.[123] Based on the effectiveness of platinum and doxorubicin and potential renal toxicity associated with use of both MTX and platinum, some centers are eliminating the use of HDMTX unless the tumor has a poor response to initial therapy.[124]

Neoplastic Meningitis

Intrathecal MTX is often a component of therapy for patients with solid-tumor neoplastic meningitis. HDMTX (8 g/m^2) given as the sole treatment with LV rescue may be a reasonable alternative,[37] as therapeutic antineoplastic concentrations of MTX can be achieved more easily in the presence of neoplastic meningitis.[125]

Adverse Effects

Hematologic Toxicity

Expression of many folate-dependent enzymes targeted by MTX are cell cycle specific, consistent with their role in DNA synthesis. Tissues that are self-renewing, with a higher S-phase fraction, are therefore at highest risk for damage by the folate antagonist. Bone marrow progenitor cells of all lineages are affected by MTX, but neutropenia usually predominates, with a nadir 10 days after drug administration and recovery typically between days 14 and 21. The effects on the marrow are dose related, but there is considerable variability among patients. Subclinical folate deficiency, impaired renal function, a damaged marrow owing to previous radiation therapy, chemotherapy, or infection, and the use of trimethoprim-sulfamethoxazole for *Pneumocystis carinii* prophylaxis may predispose patients to hematologic (and gastrointestinal) toxicity. Young patients usually tolerate MTX better than do older individuals, a fact presumably related to clearance of the drug by the kidneys. The administration of LV can prevent or lessen MTX toxicity and allow larger doses of the antifolate to be administered.

Gastrointestinal Toxicity

Nausea and vomiting, even with high doses of MTX, are usually mild to moderate. However, mucositis is a common side effect. Mucositis usually becomes manifest 3–5 days following exposure to the drug. This is an early sign of MTX toxicity, and the drug should be discontinued when it occurs. More severe gastrointestinal toxicity is manifest by diarrhea, which may progress to severe bloody diarrhea. When this occurs in association with neutropenia, patients are at high risk of typhlitis, sepsis and death. These severe side effects generally occur in a setting of renal damage, usually a consequence of high doses of MTX (≥500 mg/m^2/dose), but may also occur in patients treated with conventional doses. MTX blood levels and serum creatinine levels should be followed, and appropriate doses of LV administered, along with the supportive measures (see below).

Renal Toxicity

Renal toxicity occurs occasionally following high-dose regimens but is rare during treatment with lower doses of MTX. When it occurs, renal toxicity leads to delayed MTX clearance and subsequently to severe marrow and gastrointestinal toxicity, which can be fatal, especially in adults.[124] This toxicity is believed to be owing to precipitation of MTX and its less soluble metabolite 7-OH MTX (Fig. 49-3) in the tubules as well as to a possible direct effect of this drug on the renal tubule.[46] The use of vigorous hydration, often with osmotic diuresis and alkalinization of urine to increase solubility of MTX and 7-OH MTX, has markedly ameliorated this problem. Occasional patients, even with this regimen (Table 49-3), exhibit renal impairment. Through careful monitoring of MTX and creatinine serum levels, at-risk patients may be identified and larger doses and prolonged duration of LV employed to prevent toxicity.

Methylxanthines, such as caffeine or aminophylline, may be useful in the setting of delayed MTX clearance. MTX administration has been shown to increase serum adenosine concentrations, which will decrease glomerular filtration rate.[17] Adenosine receptor competitive antagonists, such as the methylxanthines, may therefore act as targeted diuretics to increase MTX elimination.[126]

Extremely high levels of MTX (>10^{-3} M) are difficult to rescue, even with high doses of LV.[127] Hemodialysis and peritoneal dialysis have proved ineffective in substantially lowering MTX plasma levels. Charcoal hemoperfusion columns have been used successfully in a small number of patients.[128] Oral charcoal and cholestyramine have also been used to bind MTX in the gut, thus limiting enterohepatic recirculation and toxicity.[129] Thymidine (1–3 g/m^2/day) is also capable of rescuing patients from MTX toxicity, but this metabolite is not generally available.[130] Carboxypeptidase G1 or more recently, the recombinant form, G2, an enzyme capable of cleaving the peptide bond in MTX resulting in glutamate and dAMPA (Fig. 49-3), has also been used to rapidly lower MTX levels, but dAMPA is even less soluble than MTX.[131] When given in combination with thymidine and LV, carboxypeptidase G2 is highly effective in patients at high risk for developing life-threatening MTX toxicity after intravenous[132,133] or intrathecal MTX administration.[134]

Table 49-3 ■ Supportive Care for High-Dose Methotrexate (MTX) Treatment

Pretreatment hydration and alkalinization:
8-12 h before treatment, patients should receive 1.5 L/m^2 of saline or 5% glucose with 100 mEq HCO3 and 20 mEq KCl/L. Continue hydration until urine pH is 7.0 or greater before MTX administration.
Monitoring:
MTX levels should be monitored at 24 h after completion of MTX infusion. Serum creatinine should be measured pretreatment, at 24, and at 48 h.
Additional LV rescue:
Required for an MTX level greater than 10-6 *M* at 24 h. Increase LV dose to 100 mg/m^2 q 6 h for levels above 10-6 *M* and 200 mg/m^2 q 6 h for levels above 5 × 10-6 *M*. Monitor MTX levels daily and continue LV until plasma MTX concentration is less than 10-8 *M*.

Abbreviation: LV, leucovorin.

Hepatotoxicity

Chronic low-dose weekly MTX treatment for patients with psoriasis, rheumatoid arthritis or ALL has been associated with portal fibrosis, and in some patients, with frank cirrhosis.[135] Among cancer patients, acute elevations of liver enzymes commonly occur within days after treatment with MTX but rapidly return to normal and do not appear to predict for chronic liver toxicity, even when elevated to 10–20 times the upper limit of normal.[136,137] Concurrent administration of dexamethasone may increase MTX-induced hepatotoxicity.[138] Alcohol and other hepatotoxic drugs should be avoided in these patient populations.

Central Nervous System Toxicity

Intrathecal MTX and intravenous administration of HDMTX have been associated with acute neurotoxicity, ranging from mild to severe. In cases of inadvertent overdosing (>100 mg intrathecally), fatalities have been reported. Greater understanding of the pathophysiology of MTX-induced neurotoxicity is now beginning to lead to therapeutic interventions to prevent or treat this complication of therapy.

The most common immediate side effect of intrathecal MTX administration, manifested by severe headache, fever, meningismus, vomiting, and CSF pleocytosis, is thought to be caused by a chemical arachnoiditis, or perhaps by the release of adenosine, which is a potent autocoid in the CNS. This effect of adenosine has been ameliorated by systemic administration of low doses of methylxanthines, such as aminophylline and theophylline, which act as competitive antagonists at adenosine receptors.[126] Dosage adjustment or switching to cytosine arabinoside may be required if these symptoms persist. Acute toxicity occurring several days after high-dose systemic MTX treatment manifests with headache, paresis, aphasia, or seizures. It is usually transient, resolving within 2–3 days.[139]

Subacute neurotoxicity (7–14 days after administration) has been observed in 5–18% of patients receiving intrathecal MTX and/or intravenous high-dose MTX. At its most severe condition, it presents with motor paralysis of the extremities, cranial nerve palsies, seizures, and even coma. Although the pathogenesis of subacute antifolate-induced neurotoxicity is likely multifactorial, increases in homocysteine may play a pivotal role. By inhibiting remethylation to methionine, MTX therapy leads to increased amounts of homocysteine in the plasma and CSF of patients treated with MTX.[140,141] Higher CSF homocysteine is observed among patients with symptoms of MTX-induced neurotoxicity than among asymptomatic patients receiving similar therapy.[142] As homocysteine and its metabolites are excitotoxic amino acids (glutamate analog) that activate the *N*-methyl-D-aspartate receptor (NMDA), it has been suggested that the subacute neurotoxicity of MTX can be ameliorated by an antagonist of the NMDA receptor, such as dextromethorphan.[142]

Delayed MTX-induced neurotoxicity may be associated with chronic demyelinating encephalopathy in as many as 80% of children with acute lymphoblastic leukemia, and the magnitude of the radiographic changes seems to correlate with number and the dose of IV MTX.[88,89] Computed tomography scans show cortical thinning, ventricular enlargement, and diffuse intracerebral calcifications. Although most commonly attributed to the combination of cranial radiation with intrathecal MTX, encephalopathy has been reported in patients treated only with HDMTX. The pathogenesis of delayed neurotoxicity may be a result of impairing folate dependent methylation of components of the myelin sheath.[143]

In patients who receive an MTX overdose intrathecally (>100 mg), immediate CSF removal with ventriculolumbar perfusion is indicated.[144] Intrathecal use of carboxypeptidase G2, an enzyme cleaves MTX to glutamate plus dAMPA, was shown to decrease mortality markedly in animals given a lethal dose of MTX intrathecally and may be the preferred treatment for this complication.[145] Intrathecal or systemic LV is not indicated in these cases, as it is unlikely that this toxicity is attributable to inhibition of DHFR.

Pulmonary Toxicity

Although uncommon, pulmonary toxicity owing to MTX has been noted in patients treated chronically with low-dose oral MTX.[146] The clinical picture usually consists of cough, dyspnea, fever, and hypoxemia. Chest radiograph findings are nonspecific, but may show patchy interstitial infiltrates. *P. carinii* must be ruled out, especially in patients also receiving steroids. Histologic examinations show diffused interstitial lymphocytic infiltrates, giant cells, and noncaseating granulomas. In some patients, a peripheral eosinophilia is observed, raising the possibility that this is an allergic pneumonitis. The process may progress to fibrosis, and it is important to discontinue MTX, although the pulmonary toxicity is reversible. Some patients have been retreated without recurrence of the problem.

Skin Toxicity

Skin toxicity to MTX occurs in 5–10% of patients. It manifests as an erythematous rash, characteristically noted on the neck and upper trunk. The rash may be pruritic and relatively insignificant and usually lasts for several days. A cutaneous vasculitis after intermediate-dose MTX has also been reported.[147] In the setting of severe systemic MTX toxicity following HD-MTX or overdose, the skin manifestations may progress to severe bullous formation and desquamation.[148]

Teratogenic and Mutagenic Effects

Folate deficiency alters gene expression by causing hypomethylation of DNA and increases DNA strand breaks by causing misincorporation of uracil instead of thymine. Consequently, folate deficiency can directly influence carcinogenesis.[149] MTX is known to be a potent abortifacient, especially if administered during the first trimester of pregnancy. Nevertheless, there is no direct evidence that MTX has any mutagenic or carcinogenic effects.

Miscellaneous Toxicity

Osteoporosis has been reported with chronic low-dose MTX administration[150] and may result from direct inhibition of osteoblastic differentiation.[151] Fever, seizures, radiation recall, phototoxicity, and anaphylactoid reactions have been reported with high-dose administration. Pleuritic and left-upper-quadrant pain, presumably attributable to splenic capsule inflammation, has been reported with a moderately high-dose regimen. An acute hemolytic anemia owing to an IgG-3 antibody that reacts with erythrocytes only in the presence of MTX has been described.[152]

Resistance to Antifolates

Although the development of effective chemotherapeutic regimens including MTX has significantly improved the therapy of a number of different malignancies, achieving prolonged disease-free survival is still difficult even in chemotherapy-sensitive diseases. The efficacy of MTX, as with other antineoplastic agents, is ultimately limited by either inherent resistance or resistance acquired during the course of therapy. Resistance to MTX has been documented as a result of changes at each of the following steps: decreased transport into the cell; decreased metabolism to polyglutamate forms; altered interaction with the target enzyme DHFR; increased expression of DHFR; increased breakdown of polyglutamates; and increased efflux from the cell. In addition, because both DHFR and FPGS activity fluctuate during the cell cycle, dysregulation of cell cycle genes may have a profound effect on antimetabolite resistance.

Intrinsic Resistance to MTX

Impaired ability to transport MTX into cells through the reduced folate carrier (RFC) results in intrinsic resistance in many tumor types. Decreased expression of RFC mRNA has been documented by quantitative RT-PCR in osteosarcoma samples at initial biopsy.[153] In other tumors, decreased expression can result from aberrant methylation in the promoter region.[154,155]

Mutations in the RFC gene corresponding to altered transport function have been documented both in resistant cell lines[156] and in leukemic blasts at diagnosis.[157] Single nucleotide polymorphisms in the gene for RFC can result in proteins with a decreased affinity for antifolates while maintaining sufficient affinity for folate to allow continued cell growth. Other known polymorphisms selectively increase affinity for folates and increase the intracellular folate pool. However, in one analysis of 246 pediatric leukemia patient samples, only 3 were found to have potentially functional RFC polymorphisms, suggesting they do not appear to play a major role in intrinsic MTX resistance in this population.[158]

Differing ability to form long-chain MTX polyglutamates to some degree explains the relative intrinsic resistance of AML to MTX, compared with ALL.[159,160] Similarly, tumor cells from patients with soft tissue sarcomas intrinsically resistant to MTX have a low capacity to form long-chain MTX polyglutamates.[161,162] Higher MTX-polyglutamate accumulation in B-lineage ALL blasts as compared to T-lineage blasts may be explained by the finding of higher FPGS activity in B-lineage blasts.[163,164] The possibility that different isoforms (splice variants) of FPGS are expressed in different tissues is supported by the finding of differences in FPGS affinity for MTX between AML and ALL cell lines and blast samples[165] and between resistant and sensitive sarcoma cell lines[166] as well as by differences between FPGS isolated from L1210 cells and murine liver in degree of inhibition by long-chain folylpolyglutamates.[10]

Increased expression of the target enzyme DHFR, a well-described mechanism of acquired MTX resistance, may also confer intrinsic resistance. A polymorphism in the 3' untranslated region that decreases binding of an inhibitory micro-RNA species (miR-24) leads to increased DHFR expression without prior MTX exposure.[167] This SNP was initially described as existing in 11–16% of a Japanese cohort;[168] therefore the prevalence of this SNP may be much lower in other populations.[169]

Lack of the retinoblastoma protein, frequently deleted or altered in many tumor types, may play a role in intrinsic MTX resistance. In the absence of retinoblastoma protein, levels of the transcription factor E2F increase, resulting in an increase in transcription of several genes involved in DNA replication, including DHFR.[170]

Overexpression of P-glycoprotein does not confer resistance to MTX. However, MTX is a substrate for the related proteins, multidrug resistance proteins 1–5 (ABCC1-5)[171,172] and the breast cancer resistance protein (ABCG2).[173] ABCC5[172] and ABCG2[174] are able to transport both MTX and MTX-diglutamate. Overexpression of these proteins has been shown to be associated with produce MTX resistance in vitro[172,175,176] and may affect the response to therapy among patients with leukemia.[177,178] It is not yet clear to what degree these proteins contribute to clinically relevant intrinsic resistance to MTX in other diseases.

Acquired Resistance to MTX

Four predominant mechanisms of acquired resistance to MTX have been described in experimental tumors and clinical samples: an increase in DHFR activity owing to amplification of this gene, altered binding of MTX to DHFR owing to DHFR mutations, decreased influx of MTX through the RFC, or a decrease of long-chain polyglutamate formation.

At the point of entry into the cell, either mutations or deletions in the RFC could result in decreased uptake of MTX and MTX resistance. Although polymorphisms in the gene for RFC do not seem to be a common mechanism of intrinsic resistance among patients with leukemia,[158] decreased transport of MTX through the RFC has been shown to be a common mechanism of acquired resistance to MTX in leukemic blasts from patients with relapsed ALL.[179]

Unstable or reversible resistance owing to gene amplification has usually been associated with the presence of "double minute" chromosomes containing the DHFR amplicon, whereas high-level stable resistance has been associated with an abnormal banding region, often referred to as a homogeneously staining region.[180-184] Point mutations in DHFR in several cell lines, including human cells, have been detected that cause a change in the binding of MTX to the enzyme and have usually involved amino acids that bind to the inhibitor by hydrophobic interaction.[185]

Although defects in polyglutamylation have been described in several MTX-resistant cell lines,[186] the resistance of these cells has usually been found to be attributable to a combination of mechanisms. Increased hydrolysis of MTX polyglutamates can result from increased transport of MTX-polyglutamates into the lysosome[187] or increased levels of GGH activity.[162,188] However, forced overexpression of GGH in cancer cell lines does not cause MTX resistance.[189]

Strategies to Overcome Resistance to MTX Using Antifols

The rational design of new folate antagonists is driven by an increasing understanding of the molecular basis of normal folate physiology, MTX cytotoxicity, and MTX resistance; it is guided by computer graphics using crystallographic data from the target enzymes.[185] Newer antifolates have been designed to have one or more of the following properties: increased transport into the cell by either increased affinity for the RFC or independence of the RFC, independence of polyglutamylation or increased polyglutamylation by virtue of increased affinity for FPGS, increased inhibition of DHFR or TS, or increased inhibition of enzymes responsible for purine synthesis.

Aminopterin (AMT)

Recent data support reevaluating an antifol older than MTX, 4-amino-pteroyl-glutamic acid (aminopterin; AMT; Fig. 49-1), the first antifolate to produce remissions among patients with leukemia.[2] AMT has several advantages over MTX, including 20–40 times greater clinical potency,[190] more efficient conversion (higher V_{max}:K_m ratio) by FPGS to polyglutamates[191] leading to greater accumulation by patients' leukemic blasts in vitro,[192] and complete oral bioavailability.[193] Twenty-seven percent of children with refractory ALL had clinically significant responses to oral AMT on the phase II trial,[194] and a phase IIb trial demonstrated that AMT can be safely substituted for MTX in multiagent therapy for children with newly diagnosed children with ALL at high risk of relapse without excessive toxicity.[195]

Newer Inhibitors of DHFR

Trimetrexate (TMTX; Fig. 49-4) is a nonclassical antifolate (lacking a glutamate moiety). Like MTX, it is a potent inhibitor of DHFR but crosses the cell membrane by passive or facilitative diffusion rather than through the RFC.[196] Consequently, TMTX and other nonclassical antifolates can still exert cytotoxic effects against MTX-resistant cells when the mechanism

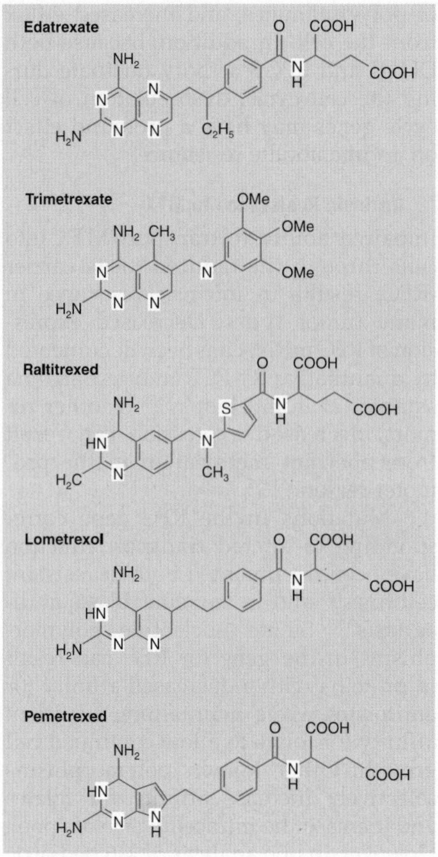

Figure 49-4 ■ Novel folate antagonists of clinical interest.

of resistance is impaired transport, decreased polyglutamylation, or even low-level amplification of DHFR.[197] Combined use of TMTX with LV rescue selectively targets tumors with intrinsic resistance to MTX owing to decreased transport through the RFC, as LV rescues normal host tissues that express RFC but not the tumor cells.[198] Cells resistant to MTX owing to a mutation in DHFR leading to decreased binding of the inhibitor may or may not be cross-resistant to TMTX, depending on the nature of the mutation.[185] Unlike MTX, however, TMTX is a substrate for the P-glycoprotein efflux pump so it may show cross-resistance to other P-glycoprotein substrate antineoplastic agents.[199]

TMTX has been under investigation as a modulating agent, based on preclinical data that TMTX followed by fluorouracil and high-dose LV led to synergistic cell kill, whereas MTX followed by fluorouracil and LV did not. Responses were noted in the phase II studies of this combination for patients with advanced gastrointestinal cancers, with manageable toxicity.[200,201] Two phase III studies have shown some evidence that this combination will delay tumor progression in patients with colorectal cancer, although there was no survival benefit when compared with 5-FU/LV treatment without TMTX.[202]

The agent 10-ethyldeazaaminopterin (edatrexate) Fig 48-4, was chosen for clinical trial after detailed structure activity studies demonstrated that hydrophobic substitutions at the N10 position of AMT resulted in improved uptake and retention (polyglutamylation) by tumor cells as compared with normal cells.[203] However, further development of edatrexate was stopped when a potentially more active analog, 10-propargyl-10-deazaaminopterin (pralatrexate; PDX), was shown to be more effective than edatrexate in preclinical models,[204] likely attributable to increased uptake by the RFC and greater intracellular polyglutamylation. PDX has shown activity for patients with previously treated nonsmall cell lung cancer[205] and T-cell lymphoma,[206] including cutaneous T-cell lymphoma.[207]

Inhibitors of Other Folate-Dependent Enzymes

Inhibitors of Purine Synthesis

5-10-Dideazatetrahydrofolate (DDTHF; Lometrexol; Fig. 49-4) is a potent inhibitor of GAR transformylase (GARFT), only after polyglutamation by FPGS. Its clinical utility has been hampered by delayed and prolonged marrow suppression, not predicted by rodent toxicity data.[208] This may be because of its rapid accumulation by folate receptor positive cells—and to the relatively folate-deficient state of patients in contrast to that of rodent models. DDTHF has been dropped from clinical development.

4-[2-(2-amino-4-oxo-4,6,7,8-tetrahydro-3H-pyrimidino[5,4,6][1,4]thiazin-6-yl)-(S)-ethyl]-2,5thienoylamino-l-glutamic acid (AG2034) is a second generation GARFT inhibitor, designed using knowledge of the X-ray crystal structure of GARFT. Phase I trials employing every 3-week dosing have been completed,[209,210] and its activity is being tested in phase II trials.

Inhibitors of Thymidylate Synthetase

Based on a series of structure–activity studies and toxicity studies in animals, the folate analog, *N*-(5-[*N*-(3,4-dihydro-2--methyl-4-oxoquinazolin-6-ylmethyl)-*N*-methylamino]-2-thenoyl)-l-glutamic acid (raltitrexed, Fig. 49-4), was chosen for further clinical trials and has shown clinical activity in colorectal carcinoma.[211,212] Raltitrexed primarily targets TS but is also a potent inhibitor of DHFR and GARFT. Of interest is that raltitrexed, even more so than MTX, is a "pro-drug," in that polyglutamylation increases cytotoxicity. Activity has been observed among 18 pediatric patients in a phase I trial[213] and among adults with colon cancer in phase III trials.[214] Raltitrexed has been licensed in Europe and Canada for use in the treatment of colon cancer. However, lack of superiority over standard 5FU/LV in one of three phase III trials led to disapproval by the FDA.

ZD9331 is a novel, nonpolyglutamatable antifolate inhibitor of TS. Like raltitrexed, it binds with high affinity to folate receptor alpha, suggesting it will have increased activity in tumors that highly overexpress this receptor, such as some ovarian cancers.[215]

Pemetrexed (Alimta) (*N*-[4-[2-(2-amino-3,4-dihydro-4-oxo-7H-pyrrolo[2,3-d] pyrimidin-5-yl)ethyl] benzoyl]-l-glutamic acid; Fig. 49-4) inhibits GAR and AICAR transformylases, DHFR and TS. Although initially promoted as a "multitargeted" antifolate, it is primarily a TS inhibitor, as indicated by its greater affinity for this enzyme and by end-product inhibition experiments.[216] Polyglutamylation appears necessary for pemetrexed to significantly inhibit TS and GARFT but not for inhibition of DHFR. Pemetrexed is rapidly polyglutamated by FPGS, with a K_m for the enzyme two orders of magnitude below that of MTX. Unlike MTX, pemetrexed is a substrate for both the proton-coupled folate transporter and RFC,[217] suggesting that loss of RFC alone would not result in resistance.

Early clinical trials showed that patients with even mild deficiencies of folate or cyanocobalamin experienced excessive toxicity from pemetrexed. Supplementation with these vitamins in all subsequent regimens reduced toxicity and allowed delivery of a greater number of courses, increasing response rates. Alone or in combination, pemetrexed has shown activity for patients with breast, gastric, cervical, bladder, colon and small cell lung cancer. Pemetrexed has FDA approval as second line treatment for patients with nonsmall cell lung cancer, based on a randomized comparison with docetaxel.[218] It also has approval in combination with carboplatin and bevacizumab as first-line therapy for patients with nonsquamous nonmall cell lung cancer and in combination with cisplatin for patients with malignant pleural mesothelioma.[219,220]

Selected References

The complete reference list can be found at www.CANCERMEDICINE8.com

2. Farber S, Diamond L, Mercer RD, et al. Temporary remissions in acute leukemia in children produced by folic acid antagonist, 4-aminopteroyl-glutamic acid (aminopterin). *N Engl J Med.* 1948;238:787.
6. Osborne MJ, Freeman MB, Huennekens FM. Inhibition of dihydrofolic reductase by aminopterin and amethopterin. *Proc Soc Exp Biol Med.* 1958;97:429–431.
13. Allegra CJ, Chabner BA, Drake JC, et al. Enhanced inhibition of thymidylate synthase by methotrexate polyglutamates. *J Biol Chem.* 1985;260:9720–9726.
16. Allegra CJ, Hoang K, Yeh GC, et al. Evidence for direct inhibition of de novo purine synthesis in human MCF-7 breast cells as a principal mode of metabolic inhibition by methotrexate. *J Biol Chem.* 1987;262:13520–13526.
17. Cronstein BN, Naime D, Ostad E. The antiinflammatory mechanism of methotrexate. Increased adenosine release at inflamed sites diminishes leukocyte accumulation in an in vivo model of inflammation. *J Clin Invest.* 1993;92:2675–2682.
22. Stoller RG, Hande KR, Jacobs SA, et al. Use of plasma pharmacokinetics to predict and prevent methotrexate toxicity. *N Engl J Med.* 1977;297:630–634.
24. Evans WE, Crom WR, Abromowitch M, et al. Clinical pharmacodynamics of high-dose methotrexate in acute lymphocytic leukemia. Identification of a relation between concentration and effect. *N Engl J Med.* 1986;314:471–477.
26. Schmiegelow K, Bjork O, Glomstein A, et al. Intensification of mercaptopurine/methotrexate maintenance chemotherapy may increase the risk of relapse for some children with acute lymphoblastic leukemia. *J Clin Oncol.* 2003;21:1332–1339.
27. Balis FM, Savitch JL, Bleyer WA. Pharmacokinetics of oral methotrexate in children. *Cancer Res.* 1983;43:2342–2345.
29. Winick N, Shuster JJ, Bowman WP, et al. Intensive oral methotrexate protects against lymphoid marrow relapse in childhood B-precursor acute lymphoblastic leukemia. *J Clin Oncol.* 1996;14:2803–2811.
31. Evans WE, Pratt CB, Taylor RH, et al. Pharmacokinetic monitoring of high-dose methotrexate. Early recognition of high-risk patients. *Cancer Chemother Pharmacol.* 1979;3:161–166.
32. Hum MC, Smith AK, Lark RH, et al. Evidence for negative feedback of extracellular methotrexate on blasts of acute lymphoblastic leukemia in vitro. *Pharmacotherapy.* 1997;17:1260–1266.
38. Clarke M, Gaynon P, Hann I, et al. CNS-directed therapy for childhood acute lymphoblastic leukemia: Childhood ALL Collaborative Group overview of 43 randomized trials. *J Clin Oncol.* 2003;21:1798–1809.
39. Thyss A, Milano G, Etienne MC, et al. Evidence for CSF accumulation of 5-methyltetrahydrofolate during repeated courses of methotrexate plus folinic acid rescue. *Br J Cancer.* 1989;59:627–630.
41. Bertino JR, Sawicki WL, Lindquist CA, et al. Schedule-dependent antitumor effects of methotrexate and 5-fluorouracil. *Cancer Res.* 1977;37:327–328.
49. Schmiegelow K, Schroder H, Pulczynska MK, et al. Maintenance chemotherapy for childhood acute lymphoblastic leukemia: relation of bone-marrow and hepatotoxicity to the concentration of methotrexate in erythrocytes. *Cancer Chemother Pharmacol.* 1989;25:65–69.
51. Kamen BA, Holcenberg JS, Turo K, et al. Methotrexate and folate content of erythrocytes in patients receiving oral vs intramuscular therapy with methotrexate. *J Pediatr.* 1984;104:131–133.
55. Calvert AH, Bondy PK, Harrap KR. Some observations on the human pharmacology of methotrexate. *Cancer Treat Rep.* 1977;61:1647–1656.
66. Relling MV, Dervieux T. Pharmacogenetics and cancer therapy. *Nat Rev Cancer.* 2001;1:99–108.
67. Robien K, Boynton A, Ulrich CM. Pharmacogenetics of folate-related drug targets in cancer treatment. *Pharmacogenomics.* 2005;6:673–689.
68. Krajinovic M, Moghrabi A. Pharmacogenetics of methotrexate. *Pharmacogenomics.* 2004;5:819–834.
78. Pizzorno G, Mini E, Coronnello M, et al. Impaired polyglutamylation of methotrexate as a cause of resistance in CCRF-CEM cells after short-term, high-dose treatment with this drug. *Cancer Res.* 1988;48:2149–2155.
80. Whitehead VM, Shuster JJ, Vuchich MJ, et al. Accumulation of methotrexate and methotrexate polyglutamates in lymphoblasts and treatment outcome in children with B-progenitor-cell acute lymphoblastic leukemia: a Pediatric Oncology Group study. *Leukemia.* 2005;19:533–536.
81. Jolivet J. Biochemical and pharmacologic rationale for high-dose methotrexate. *NCI Monogr.* 1987;5:61–65.
82. Dordelmann M, Reiter A, Zimmermann M, et al. Intermediate dose methotrexate is as effective as high dose methotrexate in preventing isolated testicular relapse in childhood acute lymphoblastic leukemia. *J Pediatr Hematol Oncol.* 1998;20:444–450.
83. Mahoney DH, Jr, Shuster J, Nitschke R, et al. Intermediate-dose intravenous methotrexate with intravenous mercaptopurine is superior to repetitive low-dose oral methotrexate with intravenous mercaptopurine for children with lower-risk B-lineage acute lymphoblastic leukemia: a Pediatric Oncology Group phase III trial. *J Clin Oncol.* 1998;16:246–254.
93. Bertino JR, Sawicki WL, Cashmore AR, et al. Natural resistance to methotrexate in human acute nonlymphocytic leukemia. *Cancer Treat Rep.* 1977;61:667–673.
111. Cadman E, Heimer R, Davis L. Enhanced 5-fluorouracil nucleotide formation after methotrexate administration: explanation for drug synergism. *Science.* 1979;205:1135–1137.
120. Jaffe N, Frei E, 3rd, Traggis D, et al. Adjuvant methotrexate and citrovorum-factor treatment of osteogenic sarcoma. *N Engl J Med.* 1974;291:994–997.
121. Link MP, Goorin AM, Miser AW, et al. The effect of adjuvant chemotherapy on relapse-free survival in patients with osteosarcoma of the extremity. *N Engl J Med.* 1986;314:1600–1606.
124. Ackland SP, Schilsky RL. High-dose methotrexate: a critical reappraisal. *J Clin Oncol.* 1987;5:2017–2031.
126. Bernini JC, Fort DW, Griener JC, et al. Aminophylline for methotrexate-induced neurotoxicity. *Lancet.* 1995;345:544–547.
137. Farrow AC, Buchanan GR, Zwiener RJ, et al. Serum aminotransferase elevation during and following treatment of childhood acute lymphoblastic leukemia. *J Clin Oncol.* 1997;15:1560–1566.
140. Quinn CT, Griener JC, Bottiglieri T, et al. Effects of intraventricular methotrexate on folate, adenosine, and homocysteine metabolism in cerebrospinal fluid. *J Pediatr Hematol Oncol.* 2004;26:386–388.

141. Cole PD, Beckwith KA, Vijayanathan V, et al. CSF folate homeostasis during therapy for acute lymphoblastic leukemia. *Pediatr Neurol.* 2009;40:35–42.
153. Guo W, Healey JH, Meyers PA, et al. Mechanisms of methotrexate resistance in osteosarcoma. *Clin Cancer Res.* 1999;5:621–627.
154. Ferreri AJ, Dell'Oro S, Capello D, et al. Aberrant methylation in the promoter region of the reduced folate carrier gene is a potential mechanism of resistance to methotrexate in primary central nervous system lymphomas. *Br J Haematol.* 2004;126:657–664.
157. Jansen G, Mauritz R, Drori S, et al. A structurally altered human reduced folate carrier with increased folic acid transport mediates a novel mechanism of antifolate resistance. *J Biol Chem.* 1998;273: 30189–30198.
160. Goker E, Lin JT, Trippett T, et al. Decreased polyglutamylation of methotrexate in acute lymphoblastic leukemia blasts in adults compared to children with this disease. *Leukemia.* 1993;7:1000–1004.
163. Barredo JC, Synold TW, Laver J, et al. Differences in constitutive and post-methotrexate folylpolyglutamate synthetase activity in B-lineage and T-lineage leukemia. *Blood.* 1994;84:564–569.
171. Kruh GD, Zeng H, Rea PA, et al. MRP subfamily transporters and resistance to anticancer agents. *J Bioenerg Biomembr.* 2001;33:493–501.
179. Gorlick R, Goker E, Trippett T, et al. Defective transport is a common mechanism of acquired methotrexate resistance in acute lymphocytic leukemia and is associated with decreased reduced folate carrier expression. *Blood.* 1997;89: 1013–1018.
185. Schweitzer BI, Dicker AP, Bertino JR. Dihydrofolate reductase as a therapeutic target. *FASEB J.* 1990;4:2441–2452.
188. Rhee MS, Wang Y, Nair MG, et al. Acquisition of resistance to antifolates caused by enhanced gamma-glutamyl hydrolase activity. *Cancer Res.* 1993;53:2227–2230.
190. Dameshek W, Freedman MH, Steinberg L. Folic acid antagonists in the treatment of acute and subacute leukemia. *Blood.* 1950;5:898–915.
198. Hum M, Holcenberg JS, Tkaczewski I, et al. High-dose trimetrexate and minimal-dose leucovorin: a case for selective protection? *Clin Cancer Res.* 1998;4:2981–2984.
215. Theti DS, Jackman AL. The role of alpha-folate receptor-mediated transport in the antitumor activity of antifolate drugs. *Clin Cancer Res.* 2004;10:1080–1089.
217. Zhao R, Qiu A, Tsai E, et al. The proton-coupled folate transporter: impact on pemetrexed transport and on antifolates activities compared with the reduced folate carrier. *Mol Pharmacol.* 2008;74:854–862.

50 Pyrimidine and Purine Antimetabolites

Giuseppe Pizzorno, PhD, PharmD ■ Sunil Sharma, MD ■ Yung-Chi Cheng, PhD

Development of pyrimidine and purine analogs as potential antineoplastic agents evolved from an early presumption that nucleic acids are involved in growth control. Among the first analogs produced and tested for biologic activity were the 5-halogenated pyrimidines. Although in original concept these agents were targeted toward the malaria parasite, Hitchings and Elion recognized that these compounds might be valuable in the treatment of cancer, which was correctly perceived as a disease of uncontrolled growth.[1,2] These early studies focused primarily on the incorporation of analog nucleic acid bases into ribonucleic acid (RNA) or deoxyribonucleic acid (DNA) of bacteria species.[3] Concurrent studies on the metabolic activation of these heterocyclic analogs and their biochemical targets for growth inhibition, as well as the study of resistance to them, afforded many new insights into the intermediary metabolism responsible for the synthesis of DNA and RNA precursors.[4] Subsequently, it was recognized that control of these biosynthetic pathways afforded additional targets for therapeutic intervention.

Further development of these analogs was stimulated by the demonstration of quantitative, but not qualitative, differences in the activity of these pathways between normal versus neoplastic tissue. It was also realized that rapid catabolism of these agents to inactive compounds could severely limit anabolic conversion to fraudulent nucleotides. This, in itself, affords targets for the modulation of cytotoxic activity on a tissue specific basis.

A virtually complete understanding of enzymes involved in the biosynthesis of purine and pyrimidine nucleotide precursors of RNA and DNA is now at hand.[5,6] This intricate matrix of metabolic reactions operates under a complex web of positive-feedback and negative-feedback controls. Most purine or pyrimidine analogs are active only after metabolic activation to the nucleotide form, so these fraudulent nucleotides not only may be incorporated, but also can mimic the natural effector compounds in regulatory pathways. Alternatively, they may deplete critical intermediates, thereby generating enlarged pools of the natural precursors behind a metabolic block, producing effects that can distort the balance of ribonucleoside and deoxyribonucleoside triphosphates. A target of even greater complexity is the incorporation of triphosphates into DNA or RNA and the subsequent modification of these macromolecules. Subtle differences in the specificity and function of the polymerases generate the selectivity of certain purine and pyrimidine nucleotides as anticancer and, more importantly, antiviral agents.

Pyrimidine Analogs

Pyrimidine analogs include 5-fluorouracil (5-FU), cytosine arabinoside, 5-azacytidine, and gemcitabine.

5-Fluorouracil

Background and Properties ■ A major motivation for the development of pyrimidine analogs of uracil was the early observation that preneoplastic rat liver and hepatomas incorporated uracil more actively than did the normal liver.[7] Although this may reflect a difference in the relative degradative capacity of these different tissues for uracil, it also provided a focus for the synthetic efforts of Duschinsky and colleagues that led to 5-FU (Fig. 50-1) and related ribosides and deoxyribosides.[8] This specific site of substitution on the pyrimidine ring was selected because it might block subsequent conversion of a uracil nucleotide to thymine nucleotides with consequent inhibition of DNA synthesis and, thus, growth.

As anticipated, the pKa of 5-FU (8.1) is more acidic than that of uracil (9.6); thus, under physiologic conditions, 5-FU partially exists as an anionic species. This is undoubtedly important to the metabolic activation to the nucleotide form via the orotidylate pyrophosphorylase reaction. This uridylate analog, 5-fluorouridine monophosphate (5-FUMP), can then substitute for uridine monophosphate (UMP) in a wide spectrum of intermediary reactions. The product of one of these reactions, fluorodeoxyuridine monophosphate (FdUMP), plays a major role by inhibiting displacement of

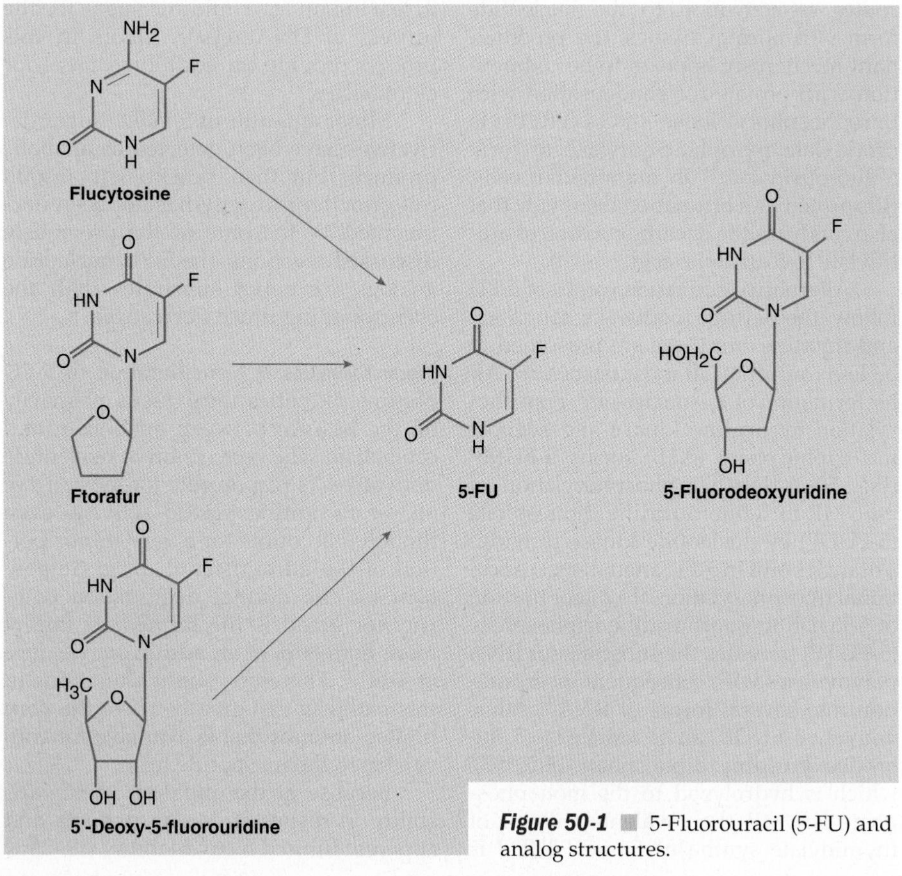

Figure 50-1 ■ 5-Fluorouracil (5-FU) and analog structures.

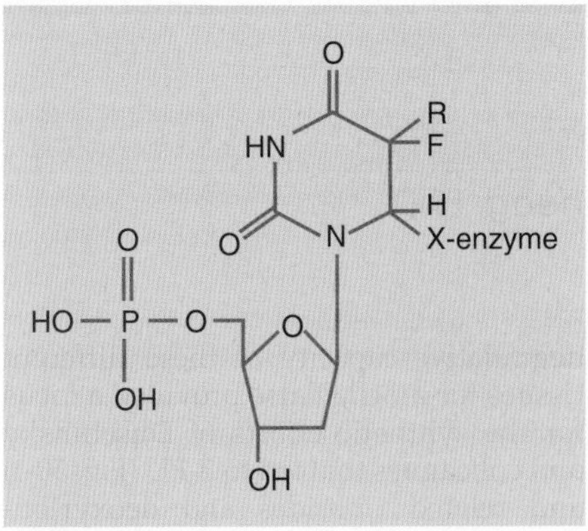

Figure 50-2 ■ Covalent thymidylate synthase-fluorodeoxyuridylate complex; R = H or CH2 FH4 = 5,10-methylene tetrahydrofolate.

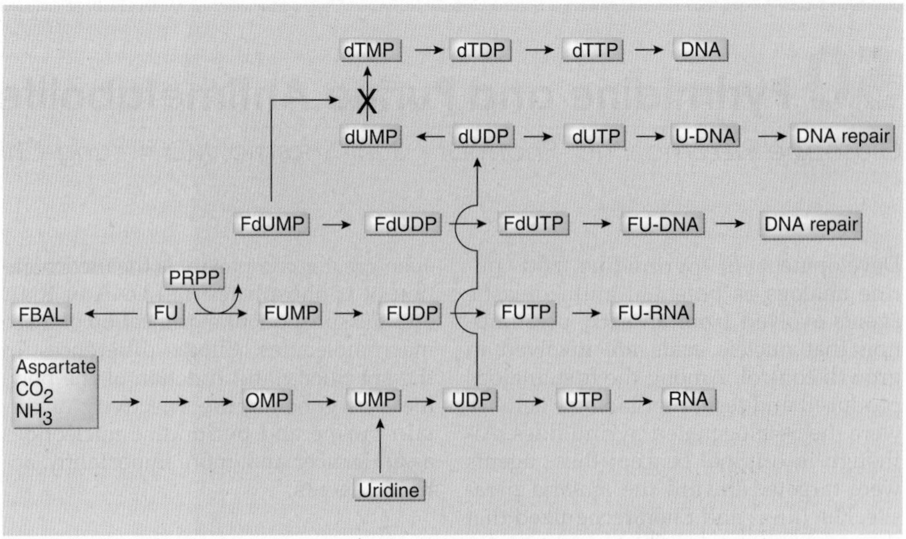

Figure 50-3 ■ Metabolic activation and targets of fluorinated pyrimidines. *Abbreviations*: CO_2, carbon dioxide; dT, thymidine (thymine deoxyriboside); dTMP also called thymidylate; dU, deoxyuridine; dUMP, deoxyuridine monophosphate; FBAL, fluoro-β-alanine; FdU, fluorodeoxyuridine; FdUMP, fluorodeoxyuridine monophosphate; 5-FU, fluorouracil; 5-FUMP, 5-fluorouridine monophosphate (also called fluorouridylate); MP, DP, TP, monophosphate, diphosphate, and triphosphate; NH_3, ammonia; O, orotidine; OMP also called orotidylate; PRPP, phosphoribosyl pyrophosphate; U, uridine (uracil riboside); UMP also called uridylate.

hydrogen from the 5-position of deoxyuridylate and replacing it with a methyl group via a tetrahydrofolate catalyzed reaction (Fig. 49–2).[9] Early clinical studies showed enough promise in colon cancer and other solid tumors to sustain 50 subsequent years of further development. A primary focus of this research has been to reduce its toxicity within a variety of normal tissues, while retaining its antitumor activity. Today, 5-FU remains an important component in the therapy of several of the most common solid tumors, not only as a single agent, but also in combination with other chemotherapy agents.

Anabolism ■ 5-FU has several possible routes of activation to the nucleotide form.[10] In normal tissues, the predominant mechanism appears to be competition with orotate for condensation with pyrophosphorylribose-5-PO 4 (PRPP) via orotidylate pyrophosphorylase to form 5-fluorouridylate.[11] In mammalian cells, this protein is a bifunctional enzyme that also catalyzes the decarboxylation of orotidylate to 5′-uridylic acid.[11]

Alternative activation routes of 5-FU follow the salvage pathways for uracil and thymine, but these are presumed to be less important in most tissues.[12–14] After formation of the nucleoside, phosphorylation by uridine kinase and adenosine triphosphate (ATP) forms 5-FUMP (Fig. 50-3). Further phosphorylation of 5-FUMP to 5-fluorouridine diphosphate (5-FUDP) by nucleotide kinase provides a branch point in 5-FU anabolism.[15] Additional phosphorylation of a major portion of 5-FUDP to fluorouridine triphosphate (5-FUTP) provides the substrate for RNA polymerases with consequent incorporation into several forms of RNA.[16] Alternatively, 5-FUDP can be reduced to 5-fluorodeoxyuridine diphosphate (FdUDP), which is hydrolyzed to the monophosphate FdUMP, the covalent inhibitor of thymidylate synthase.[9] Some FdUDP is phosphorylated to fluorodeoxyuridine triphosphate (FdUTP), which is an alternate substrate for deoxythymidine triphosphate (dTTP) in DNA polymerase reactions; however, high deoxyuridine triphosphate (dUTP) pyrophosphatase activity converts most of the FdUTP to FdUMP.[17] When 5-FU is incorporated into DNA, uracil N -glycosylase removes it, leaving an apyrimidinic sugar for the process of DNA repair. Errors in this process provide an additional basis for cytotoxicity.[18]

Minor amounts of 5-FUDP sugar derivatives have been detected as anabolic products, but their potential to inhibit cell growth or toxicity has not been documented.[19,20] In some of the previously discussed reactions, the 5-FU nucleotide analogs are better substrates than the corresponding uracil derivatives.

Pharmacokinetics ■ Consideration of 5-FU pharmacokinetics must focus primarily on the balance between anabolism and catabolism. The conversion to nucleotide derivatives is responsible for most, if not all, of its antineoplastic activity, even though it accounts for a very minor portion of the administered drug. Catabolism via the normal degradation pathway for uracil is the immediate fate of more than 80% of an administered dose of 5-FU.[21] Therefore, slight alterations in this pathway can greatly affect the very limited amount that is available for conversion to the nucleotide form.

Because of the apparent great variability in response among patients and apparent limited bioavailability (10–25%) via the oral route,[22] there has been a longheld recommendation that 5-FU should be administered intravenously (IV). Clinical studies in which 5-FU was administered orally together with ethynyluracil—a potent inactivator of the initial enzyme of the pyrimidine pathway, dihydropyrimidine dehydrogenase (DPD)—have demonstrated that 5-FU in fact has excellent absorption and bioavailability[23]; with the variability from patient to patient being due to the variability of DPD levels in the population.

Dosage used clinically in general depends on the schedule of administration.[24] The most common dosage schedules are a monthly course of one dose given on each 5 days as an IV bolus of 400–600 mg/m^2 or the same dosage given as a single bolus on a weekly basis.[25] The limiting toxic effect of these regimens is generally myelosuppression or mucositis. When continuous IV infusion is employed, higher doses are required (1000–2000 mg/m^2/d) to sustain steady state concentrations of 5-FU (1–5 μ M) in plasma, adequate to achieve therapeutic effects.[26] With this route, toxicity is most frequently mucositis, with minimal myelosuppression. Several studies have shown that this regimen is superior to the bolus regimen when 5-FU is given as a single agent.[26–28] Optimal treatment was a 48-h infusion at weekly intervals, which improved both response and survival. Prolonged infusion of 5-FU for up to 12 weeks at 300 mg/m^2/d also produced a better response than the bolus regimen.[29,30] The most prominent toxicity in this situation was a reversible hand-and-foot syndrome.[30] It was found that during continuous IV infusions, plasma concentrations of 5-FU varied by as much as 10-fold, and subsequent studies have demonstrated that variations in dihydropyrimidine dehydrogenase may be responsible for this effect.[31] Because 5-FU is most often used in combination with other agents such as leucovorin and methotrexate, it is important to modify the dosage in each case to limit, but not eliminate, host toxicity.

Administered 5-FU has a volume of distribution of 0.20–0.25 L/kg, which suggests distribution into the extracellular space.[32,33] Good penetration into the cerebrospinal fluid, lymph, and neoplastic effusions have been documented.[34] Since the drug apparently freely permeates cells in culture, it is not clear why the volume of distribution approximates the extracellular space.

The rate of plasma clearance is generally first order with a half-life of 10–20 min and ranges between 500 and 1500 mL/min.[21] Above a dosage of 800 mg/m^2, clearance may decrease rapidly. Because the primary fate of the drug is catabolism, this decreased clearance undoubtedly reflects saturation of these reactions.[35]

Intra-arterial infusion of 5-FU has been used with some success in patients with isolated hepatic metastases. As with systemic therapy, extensive single-pass clearance is achieved (19–51%), but saturation of catabolism occurs when doses are elevated.[36] Nevertheless, hepatic 5-FU concentrations considerably in excess of those tolerated systemically can be achieved. The limiting factor in high-dose regimens is cholestatic jaundice and evidence of chemical hepatitis.

The 2′-deoxyriboside of 5-FU, FdUrd, is a much more potent inhibitor of cell growth than 5- FU in cell culture.[37] This presumably reflects the ease with which this compound can be activated by thymidine kinase in a single step to FdUMP the titrating inhibitor of thymidylate synthase. In both humans and animals, IV bolus injection of FdUrd produces a dose response that is essentially that of 5-FU because it is cleaved rapidly to an equivalent amount of 5-FU that subsequently experiences the same metabolic fate as directly injected 5-FU. If, however, FdUrd is given by a 14-day continuous infusion, the maximum tolerated dose is approximately 100-fold less[36]; however, its therapeutic index is not significantly better than that of 5-FU. Even so, it can be used for isolated hepatic metastases of colon cancer by hepatic artery infusion because approximately 90% of the drug is cleared in a single pass by the liver, thus reducing systemic effects.[38] Using this route, major increases in the hepatic concentrations of intact drug are achieved relative to systemic targets of toxicity.

Catabolism ■ The primary clearance mode of 5-FU is via catabolism along the degradative pathway for uracil.[21] The initial reaction is reduction by dihydrouracil dehydrogenase. The liver is a major site of 5-FU metabolism, and this is particularly true when the drug is given orally, intraperitoneally, or by intrahepatic arterial infusion. It is now recognized, however, that metabolism in the lung and kidneys may be of equal, or even greater, importance after IV administration.[33]

Marked circadian variations in the metabolism of 5-FU have been detected related to 24-h cyclic variations in dihydrouracil dehydrogenase activity.[31,39] These changes are reflected in the inverse variations of plasma 5-FU concentrations during IV infusions in humans.[31,40] Means to employ these differences in the design of clinical protocols have been outlined.[41] Several clinical protocols comparing a continuous flat infusion with the circadian schedule have been conducted with 5-FU alone and in combination with leucovorin and/or platinum derivatives.[42–44] A clinical study using a 14-day continuous infusion of 5-FU and leucovorin suggests that circadian administration with a maximal infusion rate at 4 am increases the maximum tolerated dose (MTD) for both agents: 5-FU, 250 mg/m^2/d; leucovorin, 20 mg/m^2/d.[45] In patients who experienced grade 2 or higher toxicities with this schedule, the peak of their circadian infusion was moved from 9 pm to 10 pm. Decreased toxicity was observed (mostly diarrhea and stomatitis), and the MTD for 5-FU increased to 300 mg/m^2/d, a 50 mg increment over the MTD for a flat continuous infusion.[46]

Dihydropyrimidine dehydrogenase represents the initial rate-limiting step in the catabolism of the pyrimidines uracil, thymine, and 5-FU. More than 85% of an administered dose of 5-FU is metabolized with rapid formation of dihydrofluorouracil.[21] In a small percentage of the population, less than 3%, DPD activity is significantly below the average (below 50% of the control mean). This pharmacogenetic condition, which typically goes undetected until administration of 5-FU, can cause very serious life-threatening toxicity in patients following 5-FU-based chemotherapy; the toxicity is due to increased exposure to and activation of the anticancer agent.[47] The variability in DPD activity in normal tissues of the liver and gastrointestinal tract has been recently linked to the erratic oral bioavailability of 5-FU. DPD inhibitors, such as ethynyluracil, have been recently developed in an attempt to increase 5-FU efficacy and improve oral absorption; unfortunately, this has not been associated with an increase in the therapeutic index.[48–50]

The subsequent metabolic step, catalyzed by dihydropyrimidinase, yields β-fluoroureidopropionic acid. A wide variety of tumors apparently express high levels of this activity because they accumulate the subsequent degradation products β-ureidopropionic acid and β-alanine.[51]

α-Fluoro-β-alanine, the counterpart to the final product of uracil catabolism, β-alanine, is the major urinary excretion product of 5-FU.[52] In patients with cancer, this has been shown to be conjugated with bile acids and constitutes the primary biliary secretion product of 5-FU.[53] It has been suggested that the chenodeoxycholate conjugate may be responsible for the biliary toxicity seen after large-dose, intrahepatic infusion of 5-FU, and cholestasis associated with this conjugate has been demonstrated in isolated, perfused rat livers.[53] A summary of 5-FU metabolism is shown in Figure 50-3.

Mechanisms of Action ■ Experimental evidence has suggested numerous sites for the biologic action of 5-FU (Fig. 50-3). The relative importance of each varies widely among different normal tissues and neoplasms. Commonly, the effects are divided into RNA- or DNA-directed toxicity.

***RNA* ■** The predominant phosphorylated nucleoside of 5-FU, 5-FUTP, is as good a substrate as uridine triphosphate (UTP) for several RNA polymerase reactions. The degree of 5-FUTP incorporation into RNA bears a direct relationship to its concentration relative to that of the normal substrate UTP. In cell lines, greater incorporation is associated with reduced clonogenic survival.[54,55] Very substantial amounts of 5-FU replacement of uracil have been reported in each of the RNA species; the highest degree of incorporation is generally seen in the 4S-RNA.[16] Some evidence suggests that with a given cell type, the proportion of RNA incorporation in different species depends on the available form of the analog, 5-FU versus FdUrd. This result suggests compartmentalization or channeling of the analog en route to incorporation.[56]

What is less clear about incorporation into RNA is its contribution to cytotoxicity. Earlier studies indicated effects on transfer RNA acceptor activity, miscoding of protein synthesis, and inhibition of the maturation or processing of ribosomal RNA.[57] More recently, attention has focused on the inhibition of processing nuclear RNA to smaller molecular-weight species.[58] Other post-transcriptional effects of 5-FU include inhibiting polyadenylation of messenger RNA (mRNA) and effects on DNA primase. In some model tumors and tumor lines, there is persuasive evidence that these RNA-directed events can be associated with cytotoxicity, particularly when the effects of extended exposure are monitored.[59,60]

Thymidylate Synthase ■ The target site that can be defined most clearly is the covalent inactivation of thymidylate synthase by FdUMP.[61] Direct inhibition of the enzyme responsible for the 1-carbon transfer confirmed this site of action,[62,63] and subsequent research identified specific steps in the reaction in which a methylene group from 5,10-methylene tetrahydrofolate is transferred to the 5-position of 2′-deoxyuridylate.[9] These studies elegantly established the formation of a stable ternary covalent complex among the 5′-fluoro analog of deoxyuridylate, the reduced folate derivative, and thymidylate synthase.[64] The obvious consequence of this inhibition is an induced enzyme deficiency, depletion of dTTP, and the accumulation of deoxyuridine monophosphate (dUMP) behind the blockade.[61,65,66] More recently, it has been shown that in some tumors or normal tissues the rate-limiting factor in the formation of the abortive ternary complex with FdUMP is availability of the reduced folate derivative.[67,68] When this cofactor is limiting, it is possible to enhance inhibition by the administration of leucovorin.[69]

Other studies have analyzed a possible correlation between TS expression and therapeutic outcome in colorectal, head and neck, and breast tumors treated with infusional 5-FU, with evidence that patients with high level of TS are less likely to respond.[70–76] A likely explanation for the lack of correlation in these studies is that factors other than TS alone may be involved. Thus, more recent clinical studies have shown that tumor response and survival are likely determined by multiple factors including TS, DPD (which controls the amount of 5-FU available for anabolism), and various enzymes in the pyrimidine anabolic pathway that control the interconversions of 5-FU anabolites.[77]

DNA ■ Small quantities of 5-FU have been detected in internucleotide linkages within DNA.[78,79] Like dUTP, FdUTP, when it is available, is fully active as a substrate for the several DNA polymerases. But a very active glycosylase is present in most cells and excises any 5-FU or uracil that is incorporated in the place of thymine.[13,18] Mutants have been found that are relatively deficient in this editing function, and it may be that incorporation per se is not the cytotoxic event, but that the excision and repair involving a pyrimidine endonuclease generates opportunities for error-prone repair that might again reincorporate 5-FU or uracil instead of thymine nucleotides.[17,80,81] Because a considerable accumulation of dUMP occurs behind the blockade of thymidylate synthase, higher concentrations of dUTP are generated. These concentrations and any FdUTP increase the need for an editing function to remove incorporated uracil. Examination of the kinetics of this excision reaction indicates that uracil is removed as much as 30 times more rapidly than 5-FU.

It is not possible to rank the importance of these different potential mechanisms of cytotoxicity: RNA incorporation, dTTP depletion by thymidylate synthase inhibition, DNA incorporation, or damage to DNA consequent to excision of uracil or 5-FU. In fact, the relative importance of each of these sites may vary in different cell types. In some tumor lines, evidence for high sensitivity to RNA-directed effects is seen by the inability of thymidine to overcome growth inhibition, despite the presence of an active thymidine kinase.[82] In these same lines, uridine rescue is more successful than in others where thymidine effectively prevents cytotoxicity, presumably by repleting dTTP.

Resistance ■ As with most drugs, partial or complete responses of human cancer to 5-FU are generally followed by the eventual regrowth of tumor despite sustained, or even increased, dosages. Understanding some of the factors that contribute to natural or acquired resistance has stimulated several approaches to modulating 5-FU therapy. The most prominent mechanism seen in experimental tumors is reduced anabolism of the analog to nucleotide form.[83,84] This may reflect altered condensation with PRPP or activation via the two-stage salvage pathway involving ribose-1-phosphate or deoxyribose-1-phosphate and the appropriate nucleoside phosphorylase, with subsequent phosphorylation of the resultant nucleoside by uridine or thymidine kinase. Alternatively, lack of sensitivity has been correlated with an increased disappearance rate of 5-FU nucleotides, which were documented in one case to reflect enhanced nucleotide phosphatase activity.[85] Alterations in the catabolism of 5-FU appear to affect sensitivity and predict responsiveness to the drug. DPD, the rate-limiting enzyme in the catabolism of pyrimidines, regulates the amount of 5-FU available for the activation to nucleotide forms. In hepatocellular carcinomas inherently resistant to fluoropyrimidine-based chemotherapy, DPD activity was found elevated compared with that of normal tissue.[86] DPD activity was also found to predict response to 5-FU in head and neck tumors, and DPD mRNA levels predicted resistance to the drug in colorectal cancer patients.[87,88] Other well-documented mechanisms of resistance reflect changes in the thymidylate synthase, with reduced affinity for FdUMP,[89] or increases in the rate of synthesis and activity of the enzyme, possibly associated with gene amplification or altered enzyme turnover rates.[90] The mode of exposure to the drug can result in the selection of tumor cells with different mechanisms of resistance.[91–93]

Modulation of Therapy: Leucovorin ■ To improve the limited response rate to therapy with 5-FU, a rate of 10–25% in the most responsive cancers, various biochemical strategies have been investigated.[94] The degree of 5-FU activation by orotidylate pyrophosphorylase is affected by the available concentrations of PRPP. Because alterations of traffic along both the purine and pyrimidine nucleotide biosynthesis pathways affect the available concentrations of PRPP, several drug or metabolite combinations have been shown to modify the activation of 5-FU; presumably, by altering the concentration of this ribose-5′-phosphate donor.[95–97] Others have explored depletion of pyrimidine nucleotides by inhibitors of the de novo synthesis of pyrimidines. A major focus in this area has been enhancing the efficiency with which the covalent complex of FdUMP with the folate cofactor and thymidylate synthase is formed by supplementation with the reduced folate cofactor.[98]

Formation of the ternary complex of FdUMP, thymidylate synthase, and folate coenzymes may be limited by the availability of reduced folates in some cell lines and tumors.[64,99] To optimize formation of the covalent complex, large doses of leucovorin, or D,L-N-5-formyl tetrahydrofolate, have been employed to saturate target enzymes with L-5–10-methylene tetrahydrofolate via conversion of the l-isomer of leucovorin to 5-methyl tetrahydrofolate.[100]

5-FU cytotoxicity has been shown to be directly related to the quantity of the ternary complex formed within the cells.[59,98] Because of the enhanced inhibition of thymidylate synthase when prior supplementation with leucovorin is employed, the dose of 5-FU must be reduced by approximately 20%.[25] Under these conditions, diarrhea and mucositis remain the dose-limiting toxicities.

A wide range of clinical studies have generally confirmed the increased rate of response to 5-FU therapy in colorectal cancer when supplemented by leucovorin.[69,101,102] However, evidence for increased survival in these trials is limited.[25,101] In breast and stomach cancers, the response rate in patients who were not previously treated with 5-FU appears also to be increased by the addition of leucovorin; data for other diseases are insufficient to draw conclusions. The generally favorable results obtained in these studies have led to a rather universal addition of leucovorin to 5-FU trials in combination with other drugs. Particularly promising are three studies combining 5-FU–leucovorin with cisplatin in head and neck cancer.[69]

Oral Pro-drug of 5-Fluorouracil: Capecitabine ■ Meta-analysis of infusional versus bolus 5-FU has concluded that protracted low-dose infusion of 5-FU has resulted in a higher response rate, 22% versus 14%, with improvement in survival.[27] However, the long-term delivery requires a surgically implanted venous access and the use of an infusion pump. The administration of oral 5-FU could reduce the cost of treatment and be more convenient to the patient. Its oral use has been hampered by an incomplete and variable bioavailability. Over the past several years many oral fluoropyrimidines have been evaluated clinically. Although several had potentially desirable pharmacologic attributes, only capecitabine has received Food and Drug Administration (FDA) approval in the United States.

Capecitabine is an orally administered fluoropyrimidine carbamate prodrug (Fig. 50-4) that is activated to 5-FU by three sequential enzymatic steps. First, hepatic carboxyesterase hydrolyses the N-pentyl carbamate chain to form 5′-deoxy-5--fluorocytidine, which is then deaminated to 5′-deoxy-5-fluorouridine (5′-d5-FUR) by cytidine deaminase. Then thymidine and uridine phosphorylases hydrolyze 5′-d5-FUR to produce 5-FU. The higher phosphorolytic activity expressed in human tumor tissue compared with that of the surrounding normal tissue has been suggested to result in selective activation and an improved therapeutic index. A higher concentration of 5-FU (2.9-fold) has been demonstrated in colorectal tumor specimens when compared with adjacent normal tissue of patients who received oral capecitabine 5–7 days prior to surgical removal of the tumor.[103] Capecitabine is typically administered bid at a total daily dosage of 2000–2500 mg/m²/d over 14 days. This dosage generates plasma peak levels 2 h after administration, comparable with the ones achieved with a continuous IV infusion of 300 mg/m²/d of 5-FU. Toxicities were also similar to a continuous 5-FU infusion, with diarrhea, mucositis, and hand-and-foot syndrome.[104] The toxicities are for the most part tolerable, in particular at the 2000 mg/m²/d dosage, and reversible after a short interval off therapy.

Capecitabine was initially approved for the treatment of metastatic breast cancer resistant to chemotherapy containing both paclitaxel and anthracyclines. In this patient population, an 18.5% response rate was observed.[105]

Subsequently, capecitabine was approved for use in advanced and adjuvant colorectal cancer based on demonstrated equivalence in phase III studies to IV administered 5-FU-leucovorin (Mayo regimen).[106–108] It is of interest that coadministration of leucovorin was not required to obtain a comparable effect.

Most recently, capecitabine has been approved for combined use with docetaxel in advanced breast cancer.[109] The desirable effect of this combination may be due to upregulation of thymidine phosphorylase by docetaxel. Several other chemotherapy agents in addition to radiation are now recognized to upregulate thymidine phosphorylase, thereby increasing selective intratumoral activation of capecitabine.[110]

Cytosine Arabinoside

Background ■ Cytosine arabinoside (cytarabine or ara-C) is a nucleoside analog of deoxycytidine.[111] It represents one of the most important drugs in the treatment of

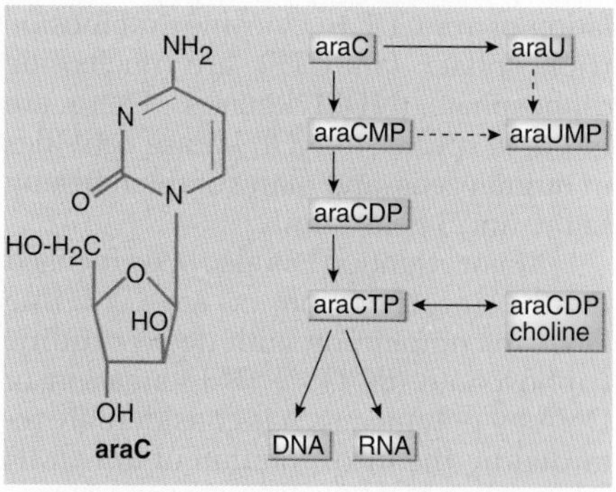

Figure 50-5 ■ Structure and metabolism of arabinosylcytosine (ara-C). *Abbreviations*: ara-CDP, cytosine arabinoside diphosphate; ara-CMP, cytosine arabinoside monophosphate; ara-CTP, cytosine arabinoside triphosphate; ara-U, arabinoxyluracil; araUMP, uracil arabinoside monophosphate; MP, monophosphate; DP, diphosphate; TP triphosphate.

acute myeloid leukemia. It is also active against acute lymphocytic leukemia and, to a lesser extent, is useful in chronic myelocytic leukemia and non-Hodgkin lymphoma.[112] It has not proven to be particularly useful in the treatment of nonhematologic neoplasms. Myelosuppression and gastrointestinal epithelial injury are the primary toxic effects of ara-C. Using high-dose ara-C regimens, additional toxic effects such as intrahepatic cholestasis and central nervous system (CNS) toxicity are frequently observed.[113]

Metabolism ■ Ara-C is rapidly deaminated by cytidine deaminase to a much less active compound, arabinosyluracil (ara-U).[114–116] Ara-C enters cells through a carrier-mediated process or by simple diffusion.[117,118] After entering the cells, it is metabolized primarily by the enzymes that normally metabolize deoxycytidine or, in some instances, cytidine (Fig. 50-5).

The enzyme that is responsible for cytosine arabinoside monophosphate (ara-CMP) synthesis is cytoplasmic deoxycytidine kinase. The amount of ara-CMP formed depends on the relative activity of cytoplasmic deoxycytidine kinase and cytidine deaminase. The enzyme responsible for conversion of ara-CMP to cytosine arabinoside diphosphate (ara-CDP) is cytidylate-uridylate-deoxycytidylate (CMP-UMP-dCMP) kinase. It has been suggested that ara-CMP could be deaminated to uracil arabinoside monophosphate (ara- UMP) by dCMP deaminase.[119] Whether this pathway is functional in cells is questionable, however, because ara-CMP is a very poor substrate for dCMP deaminase compared with dCMP. Several mammalian cell lines are partially resistant to ara-C because of an increased activity of dCMP deaminase.[120,121] Enzymes responsible for the phosphory-

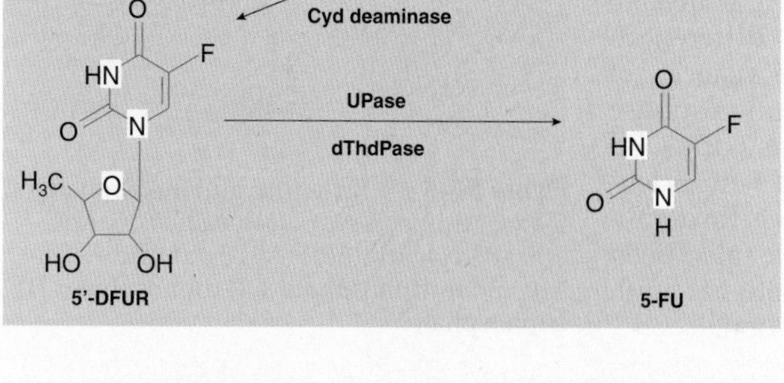

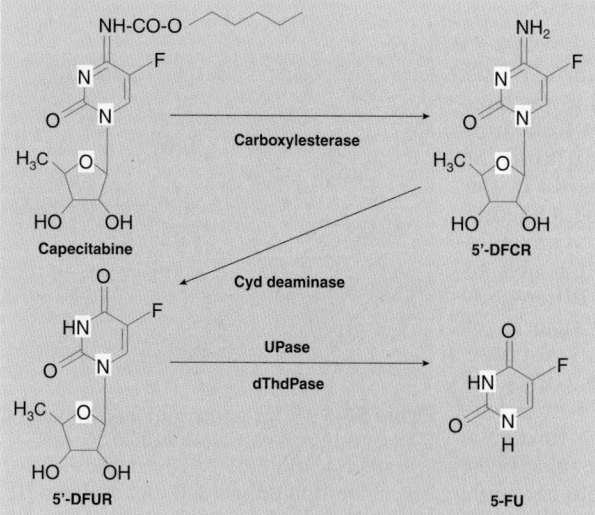

Figure 50-4 ■ Structure and activation of capecitabine. *Source*: Adapted from Xeloda product information, Roche USA. NHCO-(CH2)4CH3.

lation of ara-CDP to cytosine arabinoside triphosphate (ara-CTP) are nucleoside diphosphate (NDP) kinases. There are multiple species of NDP kinase activities in human cells, and many of them belong to the nm23 gene family.[122]

Major attention has also been focused on the incorporation of ara-CTP into DNA in competition with deoxycytidine triphosphate (dCTP).[123–125] Elongation of DNA by polymerase A is considerably retarded by the incorporation of ara-CMP, whereas no significant impact on elongation by DNA polymerase β could be seen after incorporation of a single ara-C nucleoside residue. However, neither polymerase alone could appreciably elongate the DNA if two consecutive ara-CMP residues were incorporated. Thus, the behavior of ara-CTP on DNA polymerase is not only polymerase dependent but also sequence dependent.[126,127]

Mechanism of Action ■ The primary action of ara-C is inhibition of nuclear DNA synthesis.[128,129] Mitochondrial DNA synthesis is not affected by ara-C, even at concentrations 10 times greater than that required to inhibit cell growth by 50%. The possibility remains, however, that the functional nature of mitochondrial DNA may be compromised through incorporation of ara-C internally.[115]

Three mechanisms have been suggested to account for the inhibition of nuclear DNA synthesis by ara-C. The relative importance of each mechanism may depend on the intracellular concentration of ara-CTP. The first mechanism is inhibition of the initiation of new replication units in chromosomes consequent to the incorporation of ara-C into the replicon-initiation primer.[130] The second mechanism is the retardation of DNA-chain elongation because of the incorporation of ara-C into DNA.[123,124] This effect is DNA polymerase and sequence dependent, as discussed earlier. Reactions catalyzed by DNA polymerase α, and perhaps DNA polymerase β, are more susceptible than other DNA polymerase activities. The third mechanism, which may become important only when a high-dose ara-C protocol is used, is the inhibition of DNA primase.[131]

In general, the inhibition of cell growth correlates well with the degree of the incorporation of ara-C into cellular DNA. The majority of incorporated ara-CMP is in internucleotide linkage in DNA. The relative ratio of ara-C in internucleotide, compared with chain-terminal positions, depends on the concentration of ara-C; the higher the concentration of ara-C to which the cells are exposed, the lower the relative amount of internucleotide ara-C residues. This could result from the higher probability of consecutive ara-CMPs being incorporated into DNA, which stops further DNA-chain elongation catalyzed by DNA polymerase α and DNA polymerase β. The amount of ara-CMP that is incorporated into DNA also depends on the relative ratio of ara-CTP to dCTP. Decreases in the intracellular pool of dCTP can increase the amount of ara-CMP that is incorporated. Exonucleases such as the recently identified TREX 1 and even TP53 could remove ara-C incorporated in terminal positions to limit the cytotoxic effects.

The mechanism of action for ara-C may be dosage dependent. At noncytotoxic concentrations, ara-C can cause human promyeloblast HL-60 cell lines to differentiate. It has been suggested that the success of low-dose ara-C therapy in patients with myelodysplastic syndrome may result from the differentiation effects of ara-C.[128] When given to patients with leukemia, high doses of ara-C cause rapid tumor-cell lysis.[132] Whether additional mechanisms of ara-C also play important roles in this protocol is unclear. In patients who receive high doses, the concentration of ara-U, the deamination product of ara-C, can exceed 100 μM in plasma.[133] The high concentrations of ara-U may act in concert with ara-C by inhibiting its metabolism, and it also may affect cell growth by mechanisms that have not yet been established.[134]

Mechanism of Resistance ■ Cells could become resistant to ara-C because of (1) decreased activities of the carrier for ara-C transport and for cytoplasmic deoxycytidine kinase; (2) increased catabolism of ara-C through the action of cytidine deaminase; (3) increased formation of dCTP by ribonucleotide reductase and NDP kinase; or (4) decreased activity of dCMP deaminase, which could lead to increased competition between dCTP and ara-CTP for incorporation into DNA. An increased activity of 3′ to 5′ exonuclease, which could remove ara-CMP from the DNA-chain terminus, has also been suggested.[135]

5-Azacytidine

Background ■ 5-Azacytidine (5-AC) was first synthesized in 1963, and it was later isolated as a natural product from fungal cultures.[136,137] The clinical utility of this cytidine analog is primarily in the treatment of acute myelocytic leukemia (AML) and myelodysplastic syndromes (MDS), where in low-dose, it is able to cause partial or complete differentiation in hematopoiesis in the majority of patients; occasionally, clinical response has been observed in patients with solid tumors. The major toxicity of 5-AC is leukopenia and, to a lesser degree, thrombocytopenia. Hepatotoxicity has also been reported, particularly in patients with pre-existing hepatic dysfunction.[112]

Metabolism ■ The replacement of carbon by nitrogen in position 5 of the cytidine heterocyclic ring results in a marked chemical instability. The product of the ring opening, N-formylamidinoribofuranosyl guanylurea, may recycle to form the parent compound, but it is also susceptible to further decomposition. This tendency to decompose not only may play a role in its mechanism of action, but also is troublesome in its clinical use.[138] Although 5-AC can be deaminated by cytidine deaminase to 5-azauridine (5-AU), a less toxic compound, the efficiency of this deamination by cytidine deaminase is less than that of cytidine. 5-AC enters mammalian cells by a facilitated nucleoside transport mechanism that is shared with other nucleosides.[139] The initial step in its activation is the conversion to 5-azacytidine monophosphate (5-ACMP) by uridine-cytidine kinase.[140] 5-ACMP is further phosphorylated to 5-AC diphosphate and triphosphate by CMP-UMP-dCMP kinases and nucleoside diphosphate kinases, respectively. 5-AC triphosphate can be incorporated into RNA, but its pathway for incorporation into DNA is not well defined. 5-Azacytidine disphosphate (5-ACDP) is likely reduced by ribonucleotide reductase to the corresponding deoxynucleotide diphosphate. This diphosphate is phosphorylated by nucleoside diphosphate kinases to 5-azadeoxycytidine disphosphate (5-AdCTP), which can be efficiently incorporated into DNA by DNA polymerases α and β. The incorporated 5-azadeoxycytidine monophosphate (5-AdCMP) at the 3′ terminus of DNA has less effect on subsequent DNA-chain elongation than the incorporated ara-CMP at the 3′ terminus of DNA. 5-Azadeoxycytidine (5-AdC) is also stabilized against hydrolytic degradation by incorporation into DNA, which could result, in part, from hydrophobic shielding of the triazine ring from water and other polar nucleophiles within the DNA double helix.[127,141]

A summary of 5-AC metabolism is shown in Figure 50-6. 5-AC is most

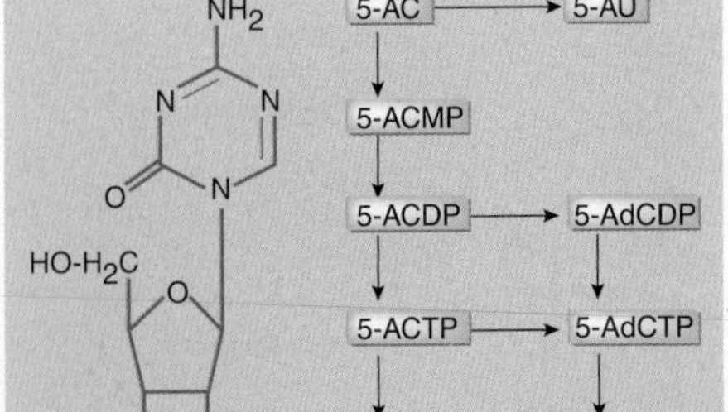

Figure 50-6 ■ Structure and metabolism of 5-azacytidine (5-AC). *Abbreviations*: 5-AdC, 5-azadeoxycytidine; 5-AU, 5-azauridine; MP; monotriphosphate; DP, diphosphate; TP, triphosphate.

cytotoxic to cells in the DNA-synthetic phase of the cell cycle, but the exact mechanism of its cytotoxic action has not been well established. It could inhibit both DNA and RNA synthesis. Incorporation into RNA can inhibit the processing of ribosomal RNA from higher-molecular-weight species, disassembly of polyribosomes, and markedly inhibit protein synthesis. Incorporation into DNA also could inhibit DNA synthesis.[142–145] One important, well-documented effect is the inhibition of DNA methylation because of stoichiometric binding with DNAmethyltransferase after incorporation. The nucleoside analog 5-azacytidine (Vidaza) and its derivative 5-aza-2'-deoxycytidine/decitabine (Dacogen) have been FDA-approved during the past 2–3 years for MDS treatment.[146,147] They appear to reduce hypermethylation and induce re-expression of key tumor suppressor genes in MDS.[148,149] Compared to supportive care, both agents show an improved overall response (60% vs 5%), a longer time to progression to AML or death, improvement of quality of life but still with limited overall survival advantage.[150] Recent studies have indicated that lower doses and longer administration of DNA methylation inhibitors may be more efficacious than previously studied higher dosing regimens with reduced toxicity.[151]

Mechanism of Resistance ■ Cells can become resistant to 5-AC by the reduction or elimination of uridine-cytidine kinase. Decreased nucleoside transport by the facilitated diffusion mechanism can also decrease sensitivity to 5-AC, and cytosine deaminase may play an important role in cell sensitivity as well. In animal models, tumor cells that are resistant to ara-C because of the deletion of cytoplasmic deoxycytidine kinase activity—a frequent mechanism of cellular resistance to ara-C—are more susceptible to 5-AC than is the parent tumor line.[152]

Gemcitabine

Background ■ 2′,2′-difluoro-2′-deoxycytidine (dFdC) is a deoxycytidine analog with two fluorine atoms in the 2′ position of the sugar moiety (Fig. 50-7). First synthesized in 1986, this molecule was initially developed as an antiviral agent because of its potent inhibitory activity against both DNA and RNA viruses.[153] Subsequently, its broad spectrum of activity in murine tumors and human tumor xenografts[154] led to evaluating this antineoplastic activity in clinical trials.

dFdC was approved by the FDA in 1996 as a first-line treatment of patients with locally advanced or metastatic adenocarcinoma of the pancreas.[155,156] Subsequently, dFdC has received FDA approval for the treatment of inoperable,

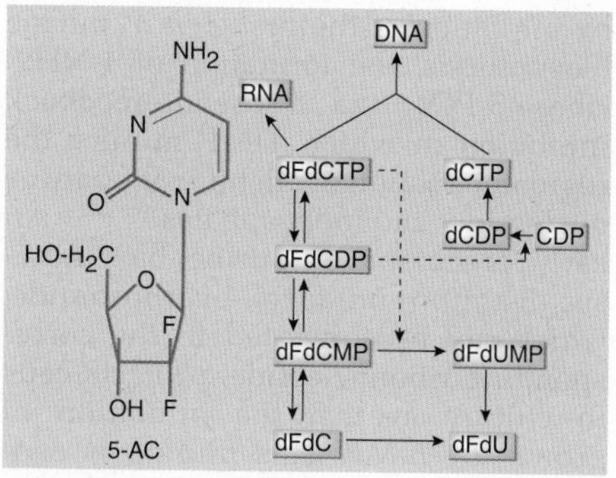

Figure 50-7 ■ Structure, metabolism, and actions of 2′, 2′-difluoro-2′-deoxycytidine (dFdC) and its nucleotides. Dashed lines indicate inhibitory actions. *Abbreviations:* CDP, cytidine diphosphate; dU, deoxyuridine; MP, monophosphate; DP, diphosphate; TP, triphosphate.

locally advanced or metastatic nonsmall-cell lung cancer, in combination with cisplatin.[157–160]

dFdC has been found active in the treatment of breast cancer when combined with cisplatin in patients pretreated with anthracycline and taxane.[161,162] It has also been found to have activity in breast carcinoma in combination with taxanes and was recently approved for therapy in first-line setting in combination with paclitaxel.[163] Activity has also been shown in bladder cancer[164–167] and in ovarian cancer.[168,169] dFdC was recently approved for second line treatment of advanced ovarian carcinoma in combination with carboplatin.[170] dFdC has demonstrated a promising effect in non-Hodgkin lymphoma,[171,172] in Hodgkin disease,[173] and in patients with relapsed or refractory cutaneous T-cell lymphoma.[174] The dose-limiting toxicity of dFdC in both single agent and combination studies is mild to moderate myelosuppression. The nonhematologic toxicity is mild, with nausea, vomiting, occasional skin rash, alopecia, and pneumonitis. Rare occurrences of hemolyticuremic syndrome have been reported.[175–177]

Metabolism ■ 2′-difluoro-2′-deoxycytidine requires phosphorylation by deoxycytidine kinase to exert its cytotoxic activity (Fig. 50-7). The major intracellular metabolite is 2′,2′-difluoro-2′-deoxycytidine triphosphate (dFdCTP); lesser amounts of the monophosphate (dFdCMP) and the diphosphate (dFdCDP) are also present.[178] Cellular elimination of dFdCTP follows a biphasic course, with a short initial half-life followed by a second, slower phase of degradation.[179,180] The biphasic elimination of dFd-CTP differs from the linear monophasic kinetic that is exhibited by the triphosphate of ara-C,[181] arabinosyladenine,[182] and arabinosyl-2-fluoroadenine.[183]

Deoxycytidine deaminase inactivates dFdC to 2′,2′-difluoro-2′-deoxyuridine (dFdU), which has no antitumor activity.[178] The monophosphate of dFdC also can be deaminated to the uracil derivative 2′difluoro-deoxyridine monophosphate (dFdUMP) by deoxycytidylate deaminase.[184]

Pharmacokinetic studies during phase 1 clinical trials have shown a very rapid half-life (8 min) for dFdC because of deamination over a wide range of dosages.[185] The concentration of dFdCTP in mononuclear cells increases in proportion to the dose of dFdC infused, up to 250 mg/m^2. Above this dose, the process shows saturation in accumulation of the triphosphate derivative.

Mechanism of Action ■ 2′,2′-difluoro-2′-deoxycytidine exerts its inhibitory activity on DNA synthesis through several distinct mechanisms. The accumulation of dFdCTP causes a reduction in the deoxyribonucleotide dCTP through direct inhibition of ribonucleotide reductase, caused mainly by dFdCDP.[186,187] Another important mechanism is the incorporation of dFdCTP into DNA. dFdCTP competes with dCTP for incorporation into the C sites of DNA as catalyzed by DNA polymerases α and ε. The primer extension pauses one deoxynucleotide after dFdCMP incorporation.[188] Moreover, the exonuclease activity of polymerase ε is unable to excise nucleotides from DNA containing dFdCMP at either the 3′ end or at an internal position.[188] The cytotoxic activity of dFdC strongly correlates with the amount of monophosphate that is incorporated into cellular DNA.

Incorporation of dFdC into RNA has been detected in tumor cell lines but the extent of this incorporation was 2-fold to 10-fold less than that into DNA.[189]

To date, two examples of resistance to dFdC have been reported.[190,191] Human ovarian carcinoma cells exposed to increasing concentrations of dFdC became highly resistant to the drug and are cross-resistant to ara-C and 2-chlorodeoxyadenosine, and modestly resistant to doxorubicin, vincristine, and cisplatin. Resistant cells did not possess deoxycytidine kinase activity; therefore, they were not able to phosphorylate dFdC as well as the other two nucleoside analogs. Another mechanism of resistance has been recently reported. Human KB tumor cells could become resistant to dFdC as the result of increased expression of the M2 unit of ribonucleotide reductase. Resistance leads to elevated activity of the same enzyme, as well as an augmented intracellular dCTP pool, which could prevent the phosphorylation of dFdC by deoxycytidine kinase.[191]

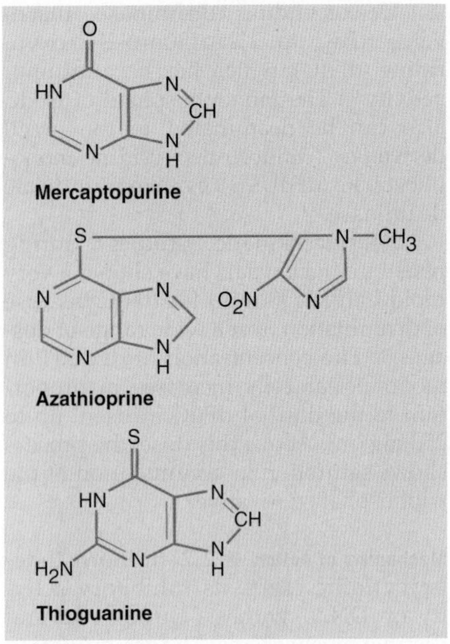

Figure 50-8 Purine antimetabolites.

Purine Analogs

6-Mercaptopurine

The original syntheses of purine antimetabolites focused on isosteric replacement of oxygen, carbon, or nitrogen in the purine ring, and they were predicated on the same logic as that used for pyrimidines.[2,3,192] The first clinically useful agent, however, was 6-mercaptopurine (6-MP),[193] in which the 6-OH of hypoxanthine was replaced with a thiol group (Fig. 50-8). Subsequently, the equivalent analog of guanine, 6-thioguanine, was prepared.[194]

By the identification of metabolites and characterization of resistance mechanisms, early studies with 6-MP in model systems quickly demonstrated the dependence of the inhibitory activity on metabolic conversion to the corresponding nucleotide analogs.[195] Equally important to the activity of many purine analogs has been an understanding of the catabolic reactions that limit their availability. Of particular relevance are xanthine oxidase, which inactivates 6-MP and thioguanine,[196] and adenosine deaminase,[197] which is the target for deoxycoformycin and limits the action of arabinosyl adenosine.

6-MP was among the first purine analogs that demonstrated antineoplastic activity, and it remains useful in the treatment of acute leukemia.[198] Metabolic activation primarily occurs by reaction with PRPP via hypoxanthineguanine pyrophosphorylase (HGPRT) to form 6-MP riboside 5′-phosphate, more properly called thioinosine monophosphate (TIMP).[199]

TIMP is believed to exert its major effect on purine nucleotide metabolism by inhibition of the first step in purine biosynthesis, the formation of 1-NH2-ribose-5-PO4, via a pseudo-feedback inhibition in which TIMP mimics the regulatory action of adenine or guanine nucleoside monophosphates.[200–202] An early precursor of purine biosynthesis, 5-amino imidazol-4-carboxamide, which can be converted to the corresponding ribonucleotide, protects cells in culture against the inhibition of growth by 6-MP. This finding is consistent with the view that the primary action is limitation of an early step in de novo synthesis. TIMP also blocks the subsequent metabolism of inosinic acid, the initial purine nucleotide, to adenylic acid by inhibiting adenosylsuccinate synthase.[199] Similarly, synthesis of guanine nucleotides is reduced by inhibition of the oxidation of inosinic acid to xanthylic acid. TIMP is not incorporated into nucleic acids as such, but minor amounts are converted to thioguanylic acid, which is incorporated into both RNA and DNA. It has not been established, however, that this incorporation is significant to the toxic or antineoplastic actions of 6-MP.[1] TIMP was recently shown to be a potent inhibitor of DNA exonuclease, which could excise ara-CMP from terminal DNA. This may partly explain the synergistic interaction of 6-MP and ara-C.[203] A summary of 6-MP metabolism is presented in Figure 50-9.

6-MP is generally administered orally (90 mg/m^2) for several weeks. Absorption is variable, incomplete, and associated with a half-life of 20–45 min in plasma, where it is minimally bound to serum proteins.[204] The rapid turnover largely results from oxidation by xanthine oxidase, which converts it to inactive thiouric acid, the primary urinary excretion product.[205] Another metabolite, the S-methyl derivative of 6-MP, is found in cells as methyl mercaptopurine ribonucleotide, where it inhibits purine metabolism. It is excreted in urine as methyl mercaptopurine riboside.

The dose-limiting toxicity of 6-MP is myelosuppression. It is slow in onset, 2–4 weeks, and rapidly reversed after the dose is either reduced or discontinued.[206,207] All formed elements (thrombocytes, granulocytes, and erythrocytes) can be affected. Although gastrointestinal mucositis or stomatitis is minimal, approximately 25% of treated patients experience nausea, vomiting, and anorexia. A small number display hepatotoxicity.[208]

Therapeutic action depends on the formation of the nucleotide 6-MP ribonucleoside monophosphate. In experimental tumor systems, resistance commonly is associated with a decreased rate of activation to the nucleotide form, resulting from deletion or modification of HGPRT activity. Limited studies in humans, however, suggest that resistance is caused by increased activity of a 5′-phosphatase that limits the concentration and duration of intracellular 6-MP ribonucleotide.[209]

6-MP is effective in combination with prednisone for inducing remission in children with acute lymphoblastic leukemia. Currently, it is a regular component of consolidation and maintenance

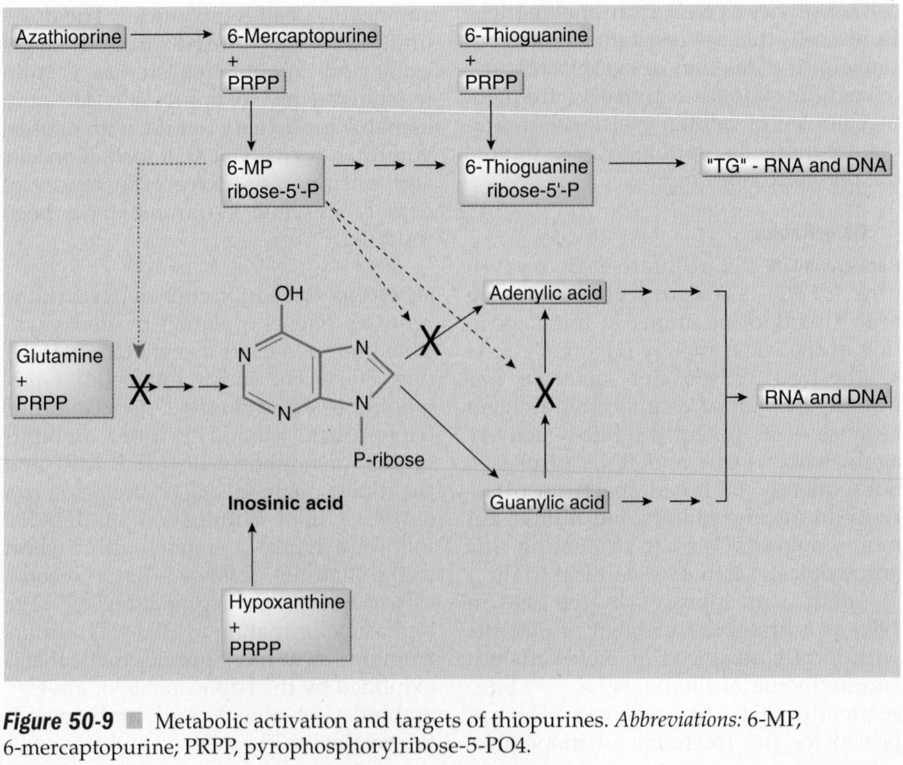

Figure 50-9 Metabolic activation and targets of thiopurines. *Abbreviations:* 6-MP, 6-mercaptopurine; PRPP, pyrophosphorylribose-5-PO4.

therapy for this disease. It is also of some value in adult acute lymphocytic leukemias. Thioguanine (Fig. 50-8) is the 6-thiol derivative of guanine corresponding to 6-MP and also depends on activation via HGPRT.[198] Unlike 6-MP, however, diphosphate and triphosphate of thioguanine ribonucleotide are formed and incorporated into RNA. After conversion to thioguanine deoxynucleotide triphosphate, it can substitute for deoxyguanosine triphosphate (dGTP) in DNA polymerase reactions.[210] This incorporation is thought to be the primary mechanism of cytotoxicity.[211]

Thioguanylate monophosphate is the predominant acid-soluble nucleotide, but it does not appear to exert the major effects on de novo purine synthesis that have been observed with 6-MP nor to deplete pools of normal purine nucleotides.

Like 6-MP, thioguanine, after deamination to thioxanthine by guanase, is readily catabolized to thiouric acid by xanthine oxidase. S-methylation is also observed, yielding S-methyl-thioguanine and thioxanthine.[212] Dethiolation contributes to metabolism as well, as evidenced by the urinary excretion of 35S-SO4 after administration of 35S-thioguanine. The primary use of thioguanine is in acute myeloid leukemia, where it may be combined with arabinosyl cytosine. However, recent studies question its value in this disease.[213,214] A summary of thioguanine metabolism is presented in Figure 50-9.

Allopurinol ■ 4-hydroxypyrazolo[3,4-d] pyrimidine is an important adjuvant to antineoplastic therapy (Fig. 50-10). This agent and its primary metabolite, oxypurinol, are potent inhibitors of xanthine oxidase.[215,216] As such, they limit the formation of uric acid from the degradation of purine nucleotides and nucleic acids. In addition to this mechanism, allopurinol has been shown to inhibit purine nucleotide biosynthesis by feedback inhibition of the first reaction in the pathway and to deplete pyrophosphoryl ribose-5-PO4, presumably by formation of the corresponding allopurinol and oxypurinol ribonucleotides.[217]

Although it was originally synthesized as an antineoplastic agent, allopurinol is widely used in the treatment of hyperuricemia that is associated with gout and other metabolic disorders.[218] Certain neoplastic states, particularly lympho- and myeloproliferative diseases, also generate hyperuricemia, and allopurinol is an effective means to avoid the associated episodes of gout or uric acid nephropathy.[219] This is particularly important in leukemias, lymphomas, and in patients with other bulky diseases when chemotherapy produces rapid tumor lysis and its attendant release of purine bases from the nucleic acids.

The elevation of hypoxanthine and xanthine concentrations in plasma by the inhibition of xanthine oxidase is less dangerous than elevated levels of uric acid. This is because these purines are more soluble and less likely to form stones or cause gout. Nevertheless, it is generally recommended that patients who are treated with allopurinol for hyperuricemia also be hydrated and alkalinized when uric acid concentrations rise significantly.

Oral dosages of 300–800 mg/d have been recommended and generally are well tolerated. Because allopurinol also reduces the rate of metabolic inactivation of oral 6-MP and azathioprine, doses of these purine antimetabolites must be reduced by 50–75% to avoid excessive toxicity.[204] Oxidation by xanthine oxidase is the primary route of allopurinol metabolism and the relevant site of action, but allopurinol can also inhibit the metabolism of drugs, such as cyclophosphamide, by the mixed function oxidases.[220]

Deoxycoformycin

Background ■ Deoxycoformycin (pentostatin) is a natural product first isolated in 1974 from the culture of *Streptomyces antibioticus* (Fig. 50-10).[221] Its structure mimics the transitional-state form of adenosine in an adenosine deaminase–catalyzed reaction, and it is one of the most potent inhibitors of adenosine deaminase.

The initial clinical development of deoxycoformycin centered on its activity as an adenosine deaminase inhibitor for the potentiation of adenosine arabinoside, which was also deaminated by adenosine deaminase to yield less toxic compounds. During early phase I studies, the profound lymphotoxic effect of deoxycoformycin was noted. Other studies described a congenital syndrome of severe combined immunodeficiency associated with low or undetectable levels of adenosine deaminase in lymphocytes.[222] These results suggested the importance of adenosine deaminase in lymphocyte function, leading to intensive development of deoxycoformycin as a single agent for the treatment of lymphoproliferative diseases.

The most responsive tumor identified is hairy-cell leukemia, in which durable remissions are achieved in over 90% of patients with a relatively brief course of treatment.[223,224] Other responsive lymphoid diseases include chronic lymphocytic leukemia and prolymphocytic leukemia, mycosis fungoides, and acute T-cell leukemia/lymphoma.[225,226] Considerable variation exists in the susceptibility of patients to deoxycoformycin toxicity. This includes immunosuppression,[227,228] CNS disturbances, impaired renal function, conjunctivitis, and muscle and joint pain. Impaired renal function and poor performance status place patients at high risk of toxicity, even with low dosages of this drug.

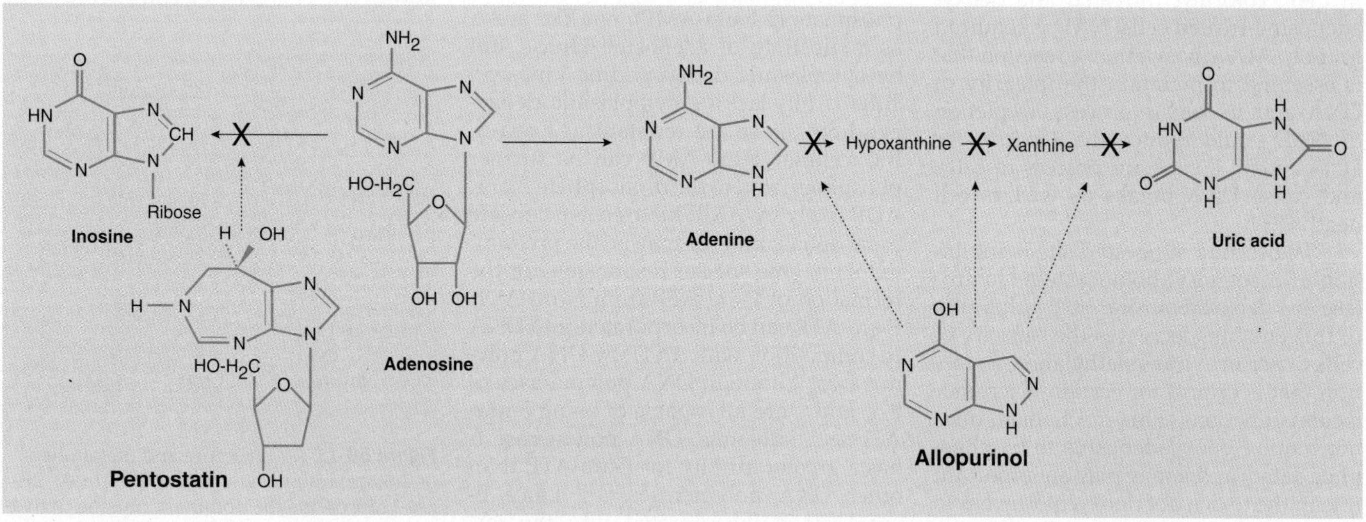

Figure 50-10 ■ Inhibitors of purine nucleoside catabolism.

Metabolism ■ Deoxycoformycin enters the cell through the facilitated-diffusion nucleoside carrier. It can be phosphorylated to monophosphate, diphosphate, and triphosphate nucleotides, and significant incorporation into DNA, but not RNA, has been observed.[223] Adenosine kinase and deoxycytidine kinase[221] do not appear to be responsible for the initial phosphorylation, but transphosphorylation with other purine nucleotide monophsosphates such as adenosine monophosphate (AMP) or inosine monophosphate (IMP) by 5′-nucleotidase reaction is a potential basis for nucleotide formation.

Mechanisms of Action and Resistance ■ The primary site of action is the inhibition of adenosine deaminase. Because of the inhibition of adenosine deaminase in vivo, deoxyadenosine and adenosine cannot be catabolized efficiently. Consequently, deoxyadenosine-phosphorylated metabolites accumulate in many types of cells.[229] This imbalance in deoxynucleotide pools is known to be toxic to cells, and the antitumor activity of deoxycoformycin may result from the combination of direct effects of deoxycoformycin and its metabolites as well as the expanded pools of deoxyadenosine.

The degree of deoxyadenosine triphosphate (dATP) accumulation correlated well with cell death caused by deoxycoformycin. Thus, dATP, which is known to be an allosteric inhibitor of ribonucleotide reductase, could result in growth inhibition by the generation of an imbalance of deoxynucleotide triphosphate pools. However, additional sites of action for both deoxycoformycin and deoxyadenosine are suggested by the observation that deoxycoformycin and deoxyadenosine are cytotoxic to nondividing cells, which do not require the function of ribonucleotide reductase. One potential site is the depletion of nicotinamide adenine dinucleotide (NAD) in deoxycoformycin-treated and deoxyadenosine-treated cells. NAD is required for poly-ADP ribosylation, a reaction that is essential to maintain the integrity of DNA and its repair process. Depletion of NAD could reduce the capacity for DNA repair, a constant process in cells, and cause DNA breaks as well as cell death.[230,231]

The second suggested site is inhibition of S-adenosyl homocysteine hydrolase by deoxyadenosine.[232,233] Inhibition of this enzyme decreases the capacity of cells to perform transmethylation, a reaction that is critical for certain macromolecular functions. This mechanism does not require deoxyadenosine to be phosphorylated, and it may play an important role in the toxicity of deoxycoformycin to nonproliferating tissues, such as in the liver and CNS. The activation of mitochondrial-dependent apoptosis through the interaction of Apf and dATP could also contribute to its activity.

Fludarabine

Background ■ In the search for more effective compounds than adenine arabinoside (ara-A, vidarabine), which has limited clinical usefulness because of its rapid deamination by adenosine deaminase, 2-fluoroadenosine arabinoside (9-β-D-arabinofuranosyl-2-fluoradenine) was synthesized. It has been found to be relatively resistant to adenosine deaminase and has impressive antitumor activity.[234] Its limited solubility and consequent difficulties in formulation led to the synthesis of a pro-drug, the 5′-monophosphate of 2-F-ara-A (Fludara IV).

Fludara IV entered clinical trials in 1982, and it is one of the most active agents in the treatment of chronic lymphocytic leukemia.[235,236] A high level of activity has also been observed in a variety of indolent lymphoproliferative neoplasms, including low-grade non-Hodgkin's lymphoma, cutaneous T-cell lymphoma, macroglobulinemia, and hairy-cell leukemia.[237–239] The dose-limiting toxicities during phase I trials were myelosuppression and leukopenia. Delayed onset of severe neurotoxicity was also noted with dosages of 96 mg/m^2/d for 5–7 days. Other toxicities noted during phase I trials included somnolence, mild to moderate nausea and vomiting, and rare but reversible interstitial pneumonitis. Fludara IV is converted by phosphatases to 2-F-ara-A within several minutes of injection; it is not further catabolized in plasma.[183]

Metabolism ■ Transport of 2-fluoroadenosine arabinoside (F-ara-A) appears to be mediated by nonconcentrative, high- and low-affinity systems.[240] Once 2-F-ara-A is taken up by cells, it is phosphorylated to 2-fluoroadenine arabinoside monophosphate (2-F-ara-AMP), not like ara-A as a substrate of adenosine kinase, but by cytoplasmic deoxycytidine kinase.[241] Tumor cells lacking cytoplasmic deoxycytidine kinase are resistant to F-ara-A. Intracellular F-ara-AMP can be further phosphorylated to the diphosphate F-ara-ADP likely by AMP kinases. Nucleoside diphosphate kinases may be the predominant enzyme species responsible for the formation of F-ara-ATP from F-ara-ADP. F-ara-ATP can be incorporated into DNA in competition with dATP by DNA polymerases. Although DNA polymerases α, β, ε, and γ. are all capable of using F-ara-ATP as a substrate, DNA polymerase α has a greater affinity for F-ara-ATP than other DNA polymerases.[242,243] Once F-ara-AMP is incorporated into the terminus of the growing DNA chain, the next step of elongation is retarded, regardless of which DNA polymerase is employed.[243,244]

In addition, F-ara-A has also been shown to be incorporated into RNA,[245,246] but which RNA polymerase is responsible has not been established. The incorporation of F-ara-A into poly (A1) RNA was 12-fold greater than that into poly (A) RNA. A summary of the metabolism of 2-F-ara-A is shown in Figure 50-11.

Investigations of F-ara-A as a modulator of ara-C therapy are currently underway. When F-ara-A is given before ara-C, an increase in the accumulation of ara-CTP occurs in leukemic lymphocytes.[247] This modulation of ara-C anabolism probably results from an indirect effect of F-ara-CTP on ribonucleotide reductase, which is also responsible for dCTP synthesis de novo or deoxycytidine kinase that relates to a reduction in the deoxynucleotide pools regulating the enzyme. It may also reflect a direct effect by F-ara-CTP on the activity of deoxycytidine kinase.[247,248] The in vitro accumulation of ara-CTP has also been shown in the lymphocytes of patients with chronic lymphocytic leukemia treated with this sequential combination.[241] The results of a clinical study in individuals who are refractory to F-ara-A therapy show partial or minor responses in approximately 35% of patients.[249]

Mechanism of Action ■ The major site of growth inhibition by F-ara-A is the inhibition of DNA synthesis. Treatment of cells with F-ara-A is associated with the accumulation of cells at the G1–S-phase boundary and in the S phase; thus, it is a cell-cycle S-phase–specific drug.[250] F-ara-ATP is also a potent inhibitor of ribonucleotide reductase, the key enzyme responsible for the formation of dATP. This causes a decrease of deoxynucleotides in 2-F-ara-A–treated cells, which enhances the incorporation of F-ara-ATP into DNA. This may be considered to be

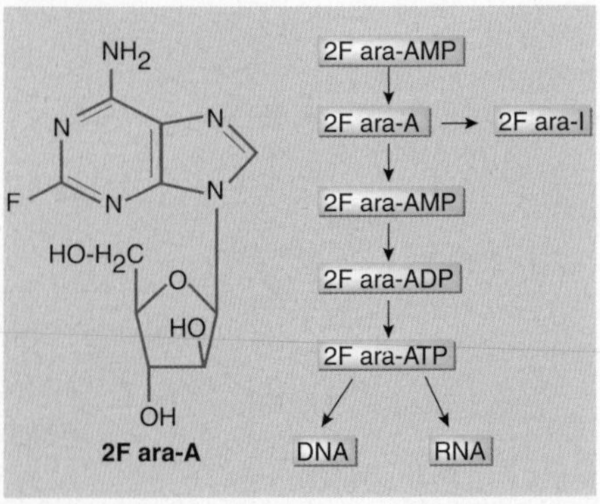

Figure 50-11 ■ Structure and metabolism of 2-fluoroarabinosyl-adenine (2F-ara-A). 2F-ara-I represents the dominant inosine derivative. *Abbreviations:* MP, monophosphate; DP, diphosphate; TP, triphosphate.

"self-potentiation" of the inhibition of DNA synthesis by F-ara-ATP. In addition, F-ara-ATP was found to be an inhibitor of DNA primase, which is responsible for Okazaki fragment synthesis,[130] another important step in DNA synthesis. The inhibition of RNA primer formation for DNA synthesis by F-ara-ATP was recently demonstrated as well,[251] but the inhibition of Okazaki fragment formation by F-ara-ATP could conceivably play a role in the inhibition of DNA synthesis by F-ara-A. In addition, F-ara-A can inhibit mitochondrial DNA synthesis at concentrations similar to those that cause cytotoxicity; however, such inhibition does not affect cell growth for several cell generations.[251] Thus, the cytotoxicity of F-ara-A, which is usually estimated by the continuous exposure of cells to drugs for three to four generations, likely does not result from the inhibition of mitochondrial DNA.

Resistance to F-ara-A may occur because of decreased uptake, lack of deoxycytidine kinase, increased intracellular concentration of dATP, decreased susceptibility to the activity of ribonucleotide reductase, decreased affinity of DNA polymerase for F-ara-ATP, or increased efficiency of the removal of F-ara-ATP from the 3′ terminus where incorporated into DNA. The potential role of the 3′ to 5′ exonuclease activities of DNA polymerase and other 3′ and 5′ exonuclease activities in removal of incorporated F-ara-AMP remains to be defined as a possible mechanism of resistance.

Cladribine

Background ■ The rationale for the development of 2-chlorodeoxyadenosine (Cl-dAdo, cladribine) was that the death of lymphocytes in patients with adenosine deaminase deficiency was associated with the accumulation of deoxynucleotides. This deoxyadenosine analog was selected for its resistance to adenosine deaminase. Its specific action on lymphoid cells is attributed to the high level of deoxycytidine kinase and low 5′-nucleotidase activity in these cells.[252–254] Cladribine was shown to have potent and lasting effects in the treatment of low-grade B-cell neoplasms, such as chronic lymphocytic leukemia, non-Hodgkin lymphoma, and hairy-cell leukemia.[255–257] In addition, Cl-dAdo has demonstrated clinical activity against acute myeloid leukemia in children, including those with leukemic blast cells in the CNS[258] and in T-cell lymphoproliferative disorders.[259] The spectrum of clinical activity is similar to that of Fludara IV; however, a few patients who do not respond to F-ara-A are sensitive to Cl-dAdo.[260] The major toxicity encountered is bone marrow suppression that is associated with severe infections. The degree of suppression relates to the rate of administration, cumulative dose, and tumor burden at the start of therapy.[255,261]

Metabolism ■ Cladribine is transported differently in different cell types.[262] Both nitrobenzyl thioinosine (NBT)-sensitive and NBTI-insensitive nucleoside transporters are involved. Once Cl-dAdo enters cells, it can be phosphorylated by deoxycytidine (dCyd) kinase to 2-chorodeoxyadenosine mono (2Cl-dAMP),[263] which subsequently is phosphorylated to 2-chorodeoxyadenosine diphosphate (2Cl-dADP) and then to 2CldATP. The enzymes involved, however, are not established. As 2Cl-dATP, it can be incorporated into DNA through the action of DNA polymerases by competing with dATP.[263] The structure and metabolism of 2-chlorodeoxyadenosine are shown in Figure 50-12.

Mechanism of Action ■ 2Cl-dAdo can inhibit DNA synthesis in growing cells as well as DNA repair in resting cells.[264] When growing cells were treated with 2Cl-dAdo, an accumulation of cells in the S phase was observed, suggesting that inhibition of DNA synthesis could be responsible for the cell-killing effect of the drug. The active metabolite is 2Cl-dATP, which can compete with dATP to be incorporated into the 3′-end of the growing DNA chain. Elongation beyond the incorporated analog was significantly retarded, and this could partly contribute to its inhibitory activity against DNA synthesis. Furthermore, 2Cl-dATP is a potent inhibitor of ribonucleotide reductase.[265] Levels of intracellular deoxynucleoside triphosphates were found to decrease in cells after exposure to 2Cl-dAdo,[263] which could also contribute to its antitumor activity.

Hydroxyurea

Background ■ Although hydroxyurea was first synthesized in 1869,[266] its biologic activity was not recognized until 60 years later, when it was discovered that hydroxyurea could produce leukopenia, anemia, and megaloblastic changes in the bone marrow of rabbits.[267] This simple molecule (Fig. 50-13) has been evaluated in a number of types of cancer, but its principal uses are in myeloproliferative diseases. Currently, it is an initial therapy of choice for chronic myelogenous leukemia; it also is used as therapy for polycythemia vera and hypereosinophilic syndrome. Activity against solid tumors has been demonstrated, but in these cases, it is generally used in combination with other anticancer agents or with radiation.[268]

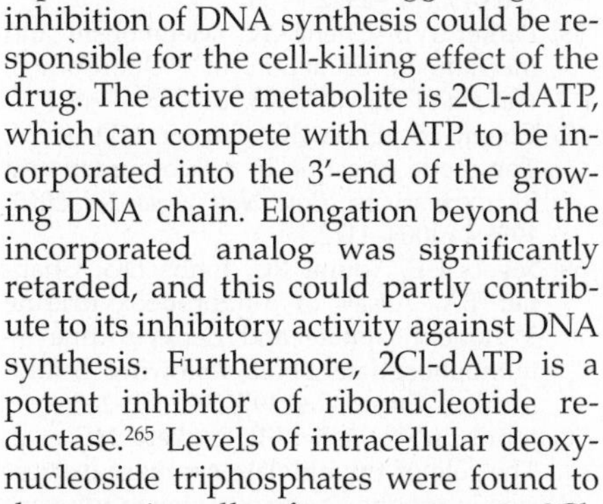

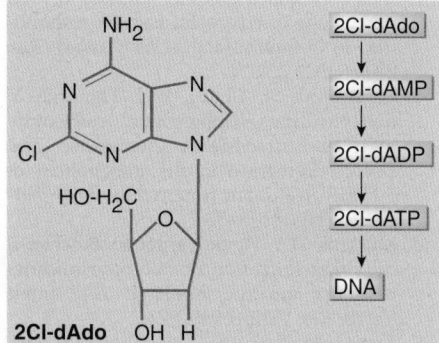

Figure 50-12 ■ Structure and metabolism of 2-chlorodeoxyadenosine (2C1-dAdo). *Abbreviations*: MP, monophosphate; DP, diphosphate; TP, triphosphate.

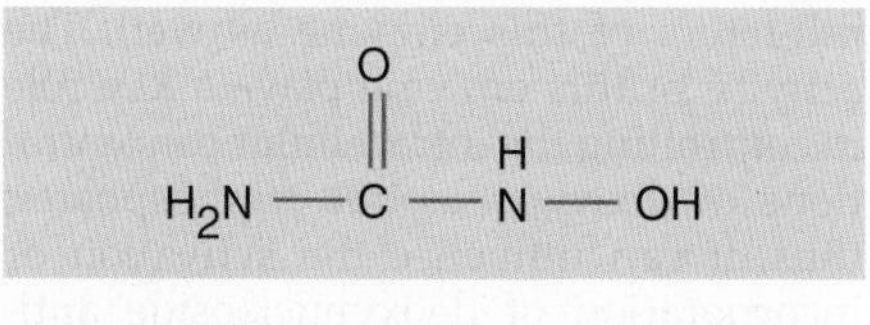

Figure 50-13 ■ Structure of hydroxyurea.

Hydroxyurea can be taken orally, and the half-life in plasma is approximately 4 h.[269] It readily crosses the blood-brain barrier. It is excreted predominantly in urine, but the interpatient variability is significant. The full extent and significance of hydroxyurea metabolism in humans has not been well established. It can be degraded by intestinal bacterial urease to form hydroxylamine, which can interact with acetylcoenzyme A to form acetohydroxamic acid; this metabolite is found in the plasma of patients receiving hydroxyurea therapy.[270]

The dose-limiting toxicity of hydroxyurea is myelosuppression. This results from inhibition of DNA synthesis in bone marrow. Toxicity begins within 2–5 days, and its duration is short once the drug is discontinued. Gastrointestinal side effects frequently are seen but rarely require discontinuation of therapy at the doses commonly used. Some dermatologic changes, such as hyperpigmentation, can also occur in patients after extended therapy.[268]

Mechanism of Action and Resistance ■ Hydroxyurea is considered to enter cells by passive diffusion.[271] It inhibits cellular DNA synthesis through the inhibition of ribonucleotide reductase, which is the key enzyme responsible for the synthesis of deoxynucleotides, the building blocks of DNA.[272] The activity of ribonucleotide reductase is highly regulated by the intracellular concentration of ribonucleoside and deoxyribonucleoside triphosphates. Two models, sequential and intercalating, have been proposed for the interplay of ribonucleotide reductase and deoxynucleoside triphosphates.[273] The metabolites of deoxynucleoside analogs, such as 2-F-ara-ATP and ara-ATP, are potent inhibitors of this enzyme as well. The activity of this enzyme plays a key role in controlling the intracellular concentrations of deoxynucleotide triphosphates; thus, it can influence the activation or incorporation of deoxynucleoside antimetabolites, such as ara-C, 5-FUdR, and 2-F-ara-A, into DNA.

Inhibition of ribonucleotide reductase by hydroxyurea would not affect the incorporation of these antimetabolites and, therefore, could potentiate their action. Ribonucleotide reductase is composed of two types of protein subunits, M1 and M2. M1 protein does not vary with cell cycle and is responsible for the interaction with nucleotides.[274,275] M2 protein fluctuates throughout the cell cycle, with peak activity in the S phase. The alteration of ribonucleotide reductase activity through the cell cycle is primarily controlled by the amount of M2 protein that binds a stoichiometric amount of iron and a stable organic free radical localized to a tyrosine residue.[276–278] Hydroxyurea inhibits ribonucleotide reductase through the inactivation of the tyrosyl free radical on the M2 subunit.

Because of the inhibition of ribonucleotide reductase by hydroxyurea, pools of deoxynucleotide triphosphates decrease, with concomitant inhibition of DNA synthesis. The cytotoxicity of hydroxyurea is dose and time dependent. Most cells are accumulated in the S phase and at the G1–S-phase boundary under the influence of hydroxyurea.[279,280]

Cells can become resistant to hydroxyurea because of increased ribonucleotide reductase activity, primarily resulting from increased levels of M2 protein. Levels of M1 protein increase only when high levels of resistance to hydroxyurea are generated. These increases of M1 or M2 proteins generally reflect the overexpression of the proteins because of gene amplification.[281–285]

Selected References

The complete reference list can be found at www.CANCERMEDICINE8.com

3. Elion GB, Hitchings GH, Vander-Werff H. Antagonists of nucleic acid derivatives. VI. Purines. *J Biol Chem.* 1951;192:505–518.
10. Madoc-Jones H, Bruce WR. On the mechanism of the lethal action of 5-fluorouracil on mouse L cells. *Cancer Res.* 1968;28:1976–1981.
14. Piper AA, Fox RM. Biochemical basis for the differential sensitivity of human T- and B-lymphocyte lines to 5-fluorouracil. *Cancer Res.* 1982;42:3753–3760.
21. Diasio RB, Harris BE. Clinical pharmacology of 5-fluorouracil. *Clin Pharmacokinet.* 1989;16:215–237.
27. Meta-Analysis Group in Cancer. Efficacy of intravenous continuous infusion of fluorouracil compared with bolus administration in advanced colorectal cancer. *J Clin Oncol.* 1998;16:301–308.
30. Lokich J, Bothe A, Fine N, Perri J. Phase I study of protracted venous infusion of 5-fluorouracil. *Cancer.* 1981;48:2565–2568.
33. MacMillan WE, Wolberg WH, Welling PG. Pharmacokinetics of fluorouracil in humans. *Cancer Res.* 1978;38:3479–3482.
37. Peters GJ, Lankelma J, Kok RM, et al. Prolonged retention of high concentrations of 5-fluorouracil in human and murine tumors as compared with plasma. *Cancer Chemother Pharmacol.* 1993;31:269–276.
44. Metzger G, Massari C, Etienne MC, et al. Spontaneous or imposed circadian changes in plasma concentrations of 5-fluorouracil coadministered with folinic acid and oxaliplatin: relationship with mucosal toxicity in patients with cancer. *Clin Pharmacol Ther.* 1994;56:190–201.
50. Levin J, Schilsky R, Burris H, et al. North American phase III study of oral eniluracil (EU) plus oral 5-fluorouracil (5-FU) versus intravenous (IV) 5-FU plus leucovorin (LV) in the treatment of advanced colorectal cancer (ACC) [abstract]. *Proc Am Soc Clin Oncol.* 2001;20:523.
54. Grem JL, Fischer PH. Augmentation of 5-fluorouracil cytotoxicity in human colon cancer cells by dipyridamole. *Cancer Res.* 1985;45:2967–2972.
58. Parker WB, Cheng YC. Metabolism and mechanism of action of 5-fluorouracil. *Pharmacol Ther.* 1990;48:381–395.
62. Cohen SS, Flaks JG, Barner HD, et al. The mode of action of 5-fluorouracil and its derivatives. *Proc Natl Acad Sci USA.* 1958;44:1004–1112.
66. Myers CE, Young RC, Johns DG, Chabner BA. Assay of 5-fluorodeoxyuridine 5′-monophosphate and deoxyuridine 5′-monophosphate pools following 5-fluorouracil. *Cancer Res.* 1974;34:2682–2688.
70. Johnston PG, Fisher ER, Rockette HE, et al. The role of thymidylate synthase expression in prognosis and outcome to adjuvant chemotherapy in patients with rectal cancer. *J Clin Oncol.* 1994;12:2640–2647.
74. Findlay MP, Cunningham D, Morgan G, et al. Lack of correlation between thymidylate synthase levels in primary colorectal tumors and subsequent response to chemotherapy. *Br J Cancer.* 1997;75:903–909.
77. Salonga D, Danenberg KD, Johnson M, et al. Gene expression levels of dihydropyrimidine dehydrogenase and thymidylate synthase together identify a high percentage of colorectal tumors responding to 5-fluorouracil. *Clin Cancer Res.* 2000;6:1322–1327.
80. Caradonna SJ, Cheng Y-C. The role of deoxyuridine triphosphate nucleotide hydrolase, uracil-DNA glycosylase, and DNA polymerase in the metabolism of 5-FUdR in human tumor cells. *Mol Pharmacol.* 1980;18:513–520.
83. Mulkins MA, Heidelberger C. Biochemical characterization of fluoropyrimidine-resistant murine leukemic cell lines. *Cancer Res.* 1982;42:965–973.
89. Bapat AR, Zarow C, Danenberg PV. Human leukemic cells resistant to 5-fluoro-2-′-deoxyuridine contain a thymidylate synthase with a lower affinity for nucleotides. *J Biol Chem.* 1983;258:4130–4136.
92. Pizzorno G, Sun Z, Handschumacher RE. Effect of clinically modeled regimens on the growth response and development of resistance in human colon carcinoma cell lines. *Biochem Pharmacol.* 1995;49:559–565.
100. Keyomarsi K, Moran R. Folinic acid augmentation of the effects of fluoropyrimidines on murine and human leukemic cells. *Cancer Res.* 1986;46:5229–5235.
105. Blum JL. Xeloda in the treatment of metastatic breast cancer. *Oncology.* 1999;57:16–20.
109. O'Shaughnessy J. Results of a large phase III trial of Xeloda/Taxotere combination therapy versus Taxotere monotherapy in metastatic breast cancer patients [abstract]. Xeloda Breast Cancer Study Group. *Breast Cancer Res Treat.* 2000:23a.
113. Calabresi P, Chabner BA. Antineoplastic agents. In: Gilman AG, Rall TW, Nies AS, Taylor P, editors. *The Pharmacological Basis of Therapeutics*, 8th ed. New York: Pergamon Press; 1990:1231–1232.
117. Paterson AR, Oliver UM. Nucleoside transport. II. Inhibition by p-nitrobenzylthioguanosine and related compounds. *Can J Biochem.* 1971;49:271–274.
121. De Saint Vincent BR, Dechamps M, Buttin G. The modulation of the thymidine triphosphate pool of Chinese hamster cells by dCMP deaminase and UDP reductase. *J Biol Chem.* 1980;255:162–167.
125. Valeriote F. Cellular aspects of the action of cytosine arabinoside. *Med Pediatr Oncol.* 1982;10(Suppl 1):5–26.
130. Fridland A. Effect of cytosine arabinoside on replicon initiation in human lymphoblasts. *Biochem Biophys Res Commun.* 1977;74:72–78.
134. Yang JL, Chang EH, Capizzi RL. Effect of uracil arabinoside on metabolism and cytotoxicity of cytosine arabinoside in 25178Y murine leukemia. *J Clin Invest.* 1985;75:141–146.
138. Beisler J. Isolation, characterization, and properties of labile hydrolysis product of the antitumor nucleoside 5-azacytidine. *J Med Chem.* 1978;21:204–208.
146. Silverman LR, Demakos EP, Peterson BL, et al. Randomized controlled trial of azacitidine in patients with the myelodysplastic syndrome: a study of the cancer and leukemia group B. *J Clin Oncol.* 2002;20:2429–2440.
151. Kantarjian H, Oki Y, Garcia-Manero G, et al. **Results of a randomized study of 3 schedules of low-dose decitabine in higher-risk myelodysplastic syndrome and chronic myelomonocytic leukemia.** *Blood.* 2007;109:52–57.
156. Rothenberg ML, Moore MJ, Cripps CM, et al. A phase II trial of gemcitabine in patients with 5-FU refractory pancreas cancer. *Ann Oncol.* 1996;7:347–353.
161. Carmichael J, Possinger K, Phillip P, et al. Advanced breast cancer: a phase II trial with gemcitabine. *J Clin Oncol.* 1995;13:2731–2736.
165. Stadler WM, Kuzel T, Roth B, et al. Phase II study of single agent gemcitabine in previously untreated patients with metastatic urothelial cancer. *J Clin Oncol.* 1997;15:3394–3398.
169. Friedlander M, Millward MJ, Bell D, et al. A phase II study of gemcitabine in platinum pre-treated patients with advanced epithelial ovarian cancer. *Ann Oncol.* 1998;9:1343–1345.

51 Alkylating Agents and Platinum Antitumor Compounds

Michael Colvin, MD ■ William N. Hait MD, PhD

The alkylating agents and the platinum antitumor compounds react with electron-rich atoms to form strong chemical bonds. In biological systems the primary cytotoxic reactions of these agents are with the atoms in proteins and DNA. The most important reactions for biological cytoxicity are with components of DNA, and to a lesser extent with RNA and proteins. Although monofunctional reactions with DNA, RNA, and proteins occur and have pharmacological effects (see below), including generating an antigenic site on a protein or, bending of DNA or RNA, the therapeutic effects and most of the toxicities of bifunctional alkylating agents are produced by reactions of these molecules to produce cross-links in DNA, which prevent separation of the DNA strands, and thus interfere with cellular replication.

The alkylating agents were the first nonhormonal compounds used successfully for the treatment of cancer. During World War I, poison gases were used as weapons, initially chlorine gas. At the battle of Ypres in Belgium, the German army released a new toxic gas, sulfur mustard, developed by a team of German scientists, whose structure is shown in Figure 51-1. Kaiser Wilhelm, the leader of Germany at the time of World War I, had built a major science facility in Berlin, Germany, and many of the most brilliant scientists in the country were attracted to the facility. A team from this group of scientists developed sulfur mustard, and several members of this team later received Nobel Prizes for their subsequent scientific discoveries after the war. The principal effect of sulfur mustard is to cross-link strands of proteins and DNA, since it has two reactive arms, which react with one strand of DNA, and then in a second reaction with the other strand of DNA to prevent cellular replication, as will be discussed below.

A major effect of sulfur mustard as a weapon was to produce lymphoid aplasia and bone marrow suppression. Because of the effects of sulfur mustard in inhibiting growth, the compound was evaluated as an antitumor agent in animals and in patients[1] and was found to have an antitumor effect. However, significant work on the medical applications of these compounds did not occur until the 1940s. At that time, the less reactive and less toxic compound nitrogen mustard (Fig. 51-2) was synthesized and used for the treatment of patients with lymphomas.

Most of this work was published after the end of World War II.[2-4] The clinical studies demonstrated that in patients with lymphoma, in particular, antitumor effects were seen with regression of tumors and improvement of symptoms.

$$ClCH_2CH_2\text{-}S\text{-}CH_2CH_2Cl$$

Figure 51-1 ■ Structure of sulfur mustard (bis[2-chloroethyl]sulfide).

Chemistry of the Alkylating Agents

As described above, the alkylating agents react with electron-rich atoms in biological compounds, mainly nitrogen and sulfur atoms. The more reactive agents are termed SN-1 reactors, and the less reactive agents are termed SN-2 agents, as shown in Figure 51-3. The terms refer to the kinetics of the reactions; the rate of reaction of an SN-1 agent is determined only on the concentration of the reactive molecule, as illustrated in Figure 51-3, whereas the rate of reaction of an SN-2 reagent is dependent on the concentration of the alkylating agent and of the biological target. This distinction is important because the SN-1 agents are more reactive and, in general, more toxic.

A large number of chemical compounds are alkylating agents, and many such agents have been and are used clinically. This chapter will describe the compounds that are currently used clinically or represent a type of alkylating agent.

$$RX \longrightarrow R^+ + X^- \xrightarrow{Y^-} RY + X^-$$

SN 1 Reaction

$$RX + Y^- \longrightarrow [\overset{\delta^-}{Y} \cdots R \cdots \overset{\delta^-}{X}] \longrightarrow RY + X^-$$

SN 2 Reaction

Figure 51-3 ■ SN-1 and SN-2 reactions of alkylating agents.

Types of Alkylating Agents

Nitrogen Mustards ■ The most frequently used alkylating agents are the nitrogen mustards, of which five are commonly used in cancer therapy currently. These compounds are mechlorethamine (the original "nitrogen mustard"), cyclophosphamide, ifosfamide, melphalan, and chlorambucil and are illustrated in Figure 51-2. The characteristic functional component of the nitrogen mustard is the bischloroethyl group, and all of the nitrogen mustards react through an aziridine intermediate,[5] as shown in Figure 51-4.

The remainder of the molecule is important in determining the physical properties of the molecule, which affect the stability, transport, distribution, and reactivity of the agent. The importance of the entire molecule is demonstrated by cyclophosphamide. Cyclophosphamide is not a reactive compound and undergoes metabolism and activation in the

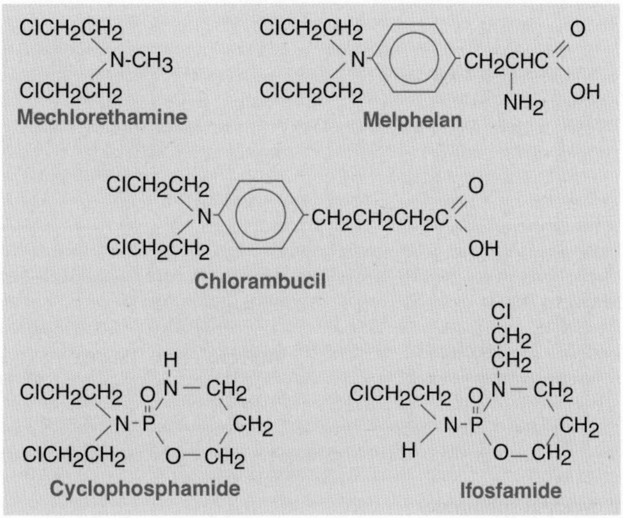

Figure 51-2 ■ Structures of nitrogen mustards currently used in therapy.

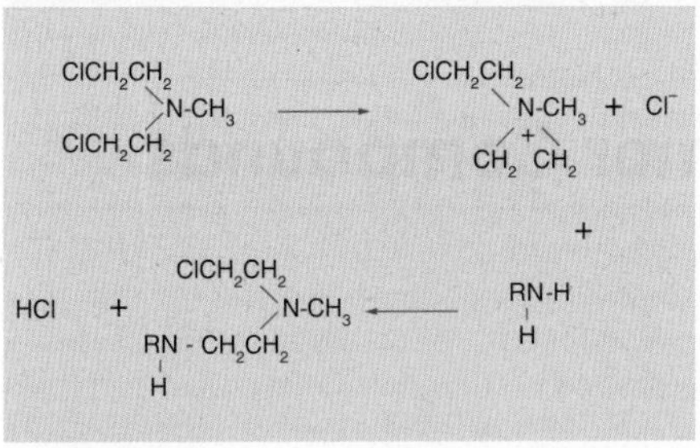

Figure 51–4 ■ Alkylation mechanism of nitrogen mustards.

body. Figure 51-5 illustrates the complex activation scheme.[6–11]

The initial activation reaction is by P-450-mediated microsomal oxidation in the liver to produce 4-hydroxycyclophosphamide, which is in spontaneous equilibrium with the open ring tautomer aldophosphamide.[6] At physiologic pH, this equilibrium is predominantly in the form of 4-hydroxycyclophosphamide.[7] This equilibrium mixture diffuses from the hepatocyte into the plasma and is distributed throughout the body. Because 4-hydroxycyclophosphamide is relatively nonpolar, it enters target cells readily by diffusion. Aldophosphamide spontaneously decomposes to produce phosphoramide mustard, which is the most reactive alkylating agent produced in the metabolism of cyclophosphamide. Although phosphoramide mustard is also produced extracellularly, this compound is polar and enters cells poorly, so that phosphoramide mustard in the plasma probably plays a minor role in the therapeutic and toxic effects of cyclophosphamide. Thus, 4-hydroxycyclophosphamide serves as an efficient mechanism to deliver the alkylating phosphoramide mustard into cells. Recent evidence indicates that after one of the chloroethyl groups of phosphoramide mustard cyclizes to form a chloroethylaziridinium moiety, the molecule cleaves to produce chloroethylaziridine.[8] It has been demonstrated that chloroethylaziridine is quite volatile and can diffuse between wells in in vitro studies and produce cytotoxicity in "control wells"[9] in such experiments.

The toxic compound acrolein was demonstrated to be produced by the metabolism of cyclophosphamide by Alarcon and Meienhofer,[10] but administration of didechloro-cyclophosphamide, a compound that can produce acrolein, but not cross-link, did not demonstrate antitumor activity in an animal model.[11] In 1992, Lee and colleagues[12] reported that a decrease in the enzyme O6-alkylguanine-alkyltransferase in circulating lymphocytes was produced by the administration of high doses of cyclophosphamide for bone marrow transplantation. Friedman and colleagues[13] reported that tumor cells with elevated O6-alkylguanine-alkyltransferase were sensitized to 4-hydroperoxycyclophosphamide by depletion of the enzyme. These and further studies indicate that acrolein released by cyclophosphamide metabolism forms an O6-guanyl adduct that can be removed by O6-alkylguanine-alkyltransferase. Thus, acrolein contributes to the antitumor activity and probably the carcinogenic effects of cyclophosphamide, and these effects are abrogated by the action of O6-alkylguanine-alkyltransferase.

Cyclophosphamide produces less gastrointestinal and hematopoietic toxicity than other alkylating agents. The parent compound (see Fig. 51-2) is inactive and is enzymatically activated (see Fig. 51-5). The basis for the decreased toxicity is the enzyme aldehyde dehydrogenase. This enzyme oxidizes aldophosphamide to carboxyphosphamide, an inactive product, which is excreted in the urine and accounts for approximately 80% of an administered dose of cyclophosphamide in any species. This enzyme is found in high concentration in the hepatic cytosol, in early hematopoietic cells, and in the stem cells and mucosal absorptive cells in the intestine.[11] Cyclophosphamide at high doses is also associated with an antidiuretic effect, which reduces urine output and produces systemic edema.[14] The dose-limiting toxicity of cyclophosphamide is a fatal cardiac lesion[15] that is now rarely seen, since the doses approaching this toxicity have been recognized and reduced.

Ifosfamide (see Fig. 51-2) is a structural isomer of cyclophosphamide that is used particularly in the treatment of testicular tumors and sarcomas.[16–19] Ifosfamide undergoes the same metabolic reactions as cyclophosphamide, but the location of the chloroethyl group on the ring nitrogen produces quantitative changes in the metabolism of the drug.[19] The primary metabolite, aldoifosfamide, is also a substrate for aldehyde dehydrogenase, so that the bone marrow and gastrointestinal tract sparing properties are similar to those of cyclophosphamide. However, the oxidation of the chloroethyl side chains to produce chloroacetaldehyde is a minor pathway for cyclophosphamide (~10% of dose), but is increased to as much as 50% for ifosfamide. The increased production of chloroacetaldehyde has been implicated in the neurotoxicity of ifosfamide[19] and may contribute to the greater renal and bladder toxicity of ifosfamide. The greater side chain oxidation of ifosfamide and the lesser reactivity of ifosfamide mustard are consistent with the higher doses of ifosfamide than cyclophosphamide that are used clinically.

Melphalan (see Fig. 51-2) is an alkylating agent that is used in the treatment of multiple myeloma,[20] ovarian cancer,[21,22] and breast cancer.[23] Melphalan is an amino acid analogue (see Fig. 51-2) that enters cells and crosses the blood-brain barrier through active transport systems. The natural substrates for the systems are amino acids,[24] and the entry of melphalan into cells and the central nervous system[25] can be modulated by the presence of amino acids in the extracellular fluid.

Chlorambucil (see Fig. 51-2) is used for the treatment of chronic lymphocytic leukemia,[26] ovarian carcinoma,[27] and lymphoma.[28] This agent is well tolerated by most patients and can be used in patients who have severe nausea and

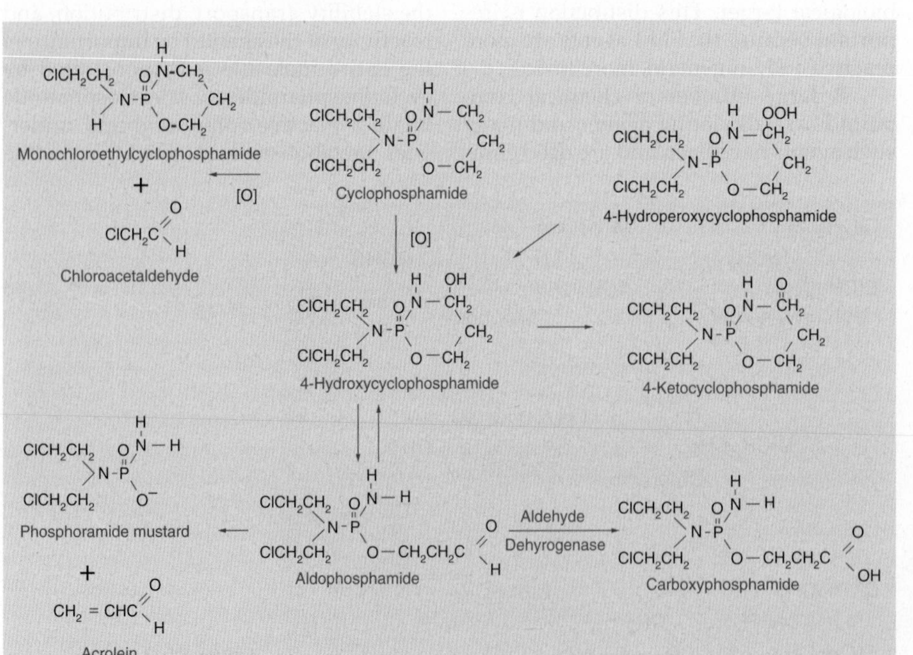

Figure 51–5 ■ Metabolism of cyclophosphamide.

vomiting with cyclophosphamide or melphalan.

Bendamustine (see Fig. 51-2) is structurally similar to chlorambucil and is indicated for the treatment of chronic lymphocytic leukemia in the United States, and multiple other hematological malignancies in Europe.[29] However, it is modified to include a benzimidazole ring with the aim of adding antimetabolite activity. In addition to inducing apoptosis, bendamustine can inhibit mitotic checkpoints and produce mitotic catastrophe, as well as activate nuclear excision base repair processes rather than DNA alkyltransferase reactions.

Aziridines and Epoxides ■ Closely related to the nitrogen mustards are the aziridines, which are represented in current therapy by N, N′, N″-triethylenethiphosphoramide (thiotepa) and mitomycin C, and are illustrated in Figure 51-6. These agents alkylate through the same mechanism as the aziridinium intermediates produced by nitrogen mustard, but the aziridine rings formed in these compounds are uncharged and less reactive than aziridinium compounds. The two aziridine agents that are frequently used clinically are thiotepa and mitomycin C (see Fig. 51-6). Like the nitrogen mustards, these compounds produce DNA interstrand cross-links. The diepoxide dianhydrogalactitol reacts with DNA in a similar fashion to the aziridines, but has been succeeded in clinical use by dibromodulcitol, which spontaneously generates dianhydrogalactitol in vivo (Fig. 51-7).

Thiotepa has been used in combination with other alkylating agents in high-dose therapy with stem cell support[30,31] for the treatment of breast cancer and for the intrathecal therapy of meningeal

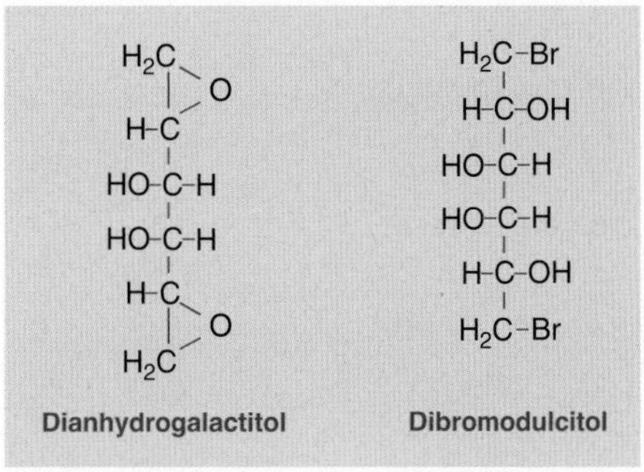

Figure 51-7 ■ Structures of an epoxide alkylating agent (dianhydrogalactitol) and an epoxide prodrug (dibromodulcitol).

carcinomatosis.[32] Thiotepa is oxidatively desulfurated by hepatic microsomes to produce triethylenethiophosphoramide (TEPA),[33] which is less reactive than thiotepa.

Mitomycin C is a natural product that has been used in the treatment of breast cancer,[34] cancers of the gastrointestinal tract,[35] and head and neck cancer.[36] This compound contains an aziridine ring and appears to exert its cytotoxic effect through the cross-linking of DNA.[37] Mitomycin C undergoes reduction in cells, with enhancement of the affinity of the carbon-1 atom of the aziridine ring for nucleophiles, such as the extracyclic nitrogen atom on guanylic acid in DNA. Following this alkylation there is displacement of the activated carbamate group on the 10-carbon atom of mitomycin C by an extracyclic amino nitrogen of a guanylic acid molecule on the complementary DNA strand to produce an interstrand cross-link.[38]

The epoxides, such as dianhydrogalactitol (see Fig. 51-7) are chemically related to the aziridines and alkylate through a similar mechanism of attack of a nucleophile, such an amino nitrogen, on a carbon of a strained three-membered ring in the agent. Dibromodulcitol is hydrolyzed to dianhydrogalactitol, and thus is a prodrug to an epoxide.[39] Dianhydrogalactitol and dibromodulcitol have been mainly used in Europe and have not been commonly used in the United States.

Alkyl Sulfonates ■ The alkyl alkane sulfonate busulfan (Fig. 51-8) was one of the first alkylating agents,[40] and for many years was the standard therapy for chronic myelogenous leukemia (CML), until being succeeded by the less toxic hydroxyurea and, more recently, by the molecularly targeted agent Gleevec, a specific inhibitor[41] of the *bcr-abl* oncogene expressed in CML. Busulfan has a most interesting, but not understood, selectivity and toxicity for early myeloid precursors.[42,43] Hepsulfam, an alkyl sulfonate analog of busulfan with a wider range of antitumor effects,[44] was not as active against CML. The current major use of busulfan is as a component of bone marrow ablative regimens for bone marrow and stem cell transplantation of patients with acute myeloid leukemia and other malignancies.[45] High doses of busulfan have been associated with liver damage, but this toxicity can be avoided by careful monitoring of the pharmacokinetics of the agent and appropriate dose adjustment.[46]

Nitrosoureas ■ The nitrosoureas are a class of alkylating agents that have received considerable attention and use during the past three decades.[47] The structures of the two most frequently used nitrosoureas, carmustine (BCNU) and lomustine (CCNU), are shown in Figure 51-9. BCNU was the first agent to demonstrate significant antitumor activity against a num-

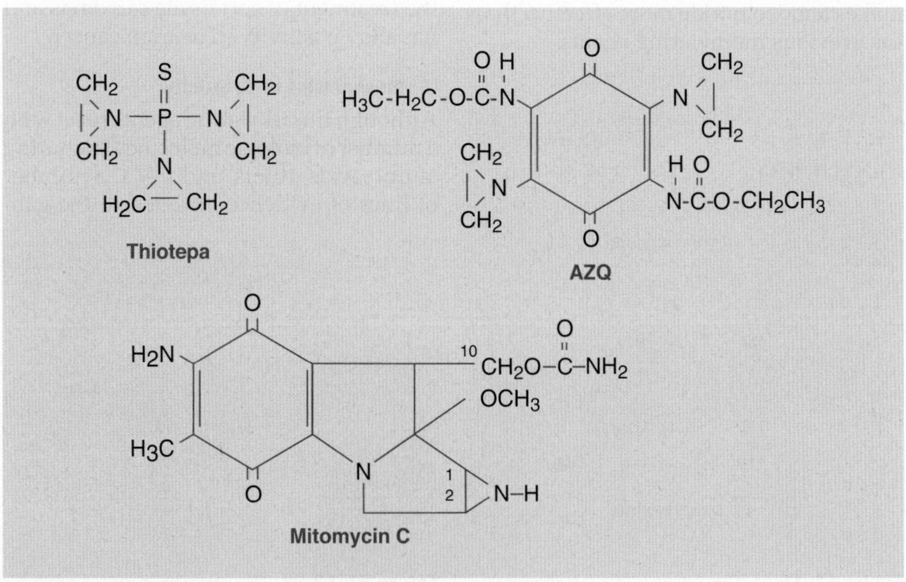

Figure 51-6 ■ Structures of aziridine alkylating agents.

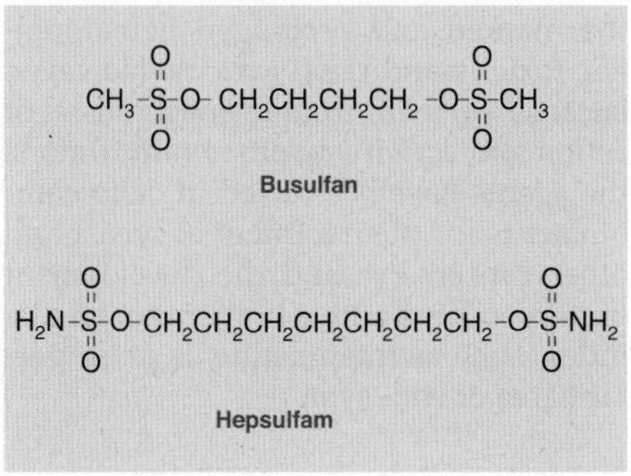

Figure 51-8 ■ Structure of alkyl sulfonate (busulfan) and alkyl sulfamate (hepsulfam) agents.

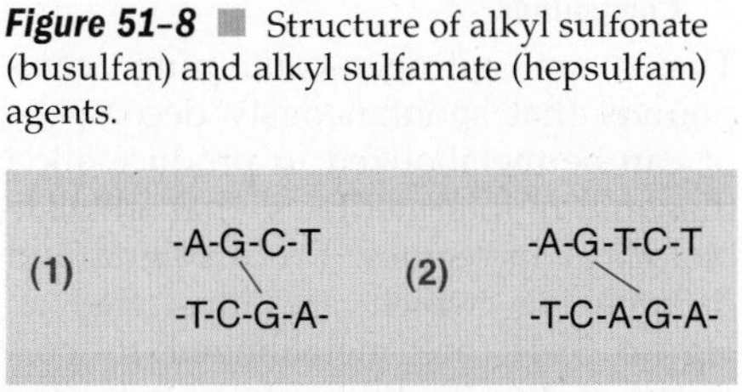

Figure 51-9 ■ Structures of nitrosoureas.

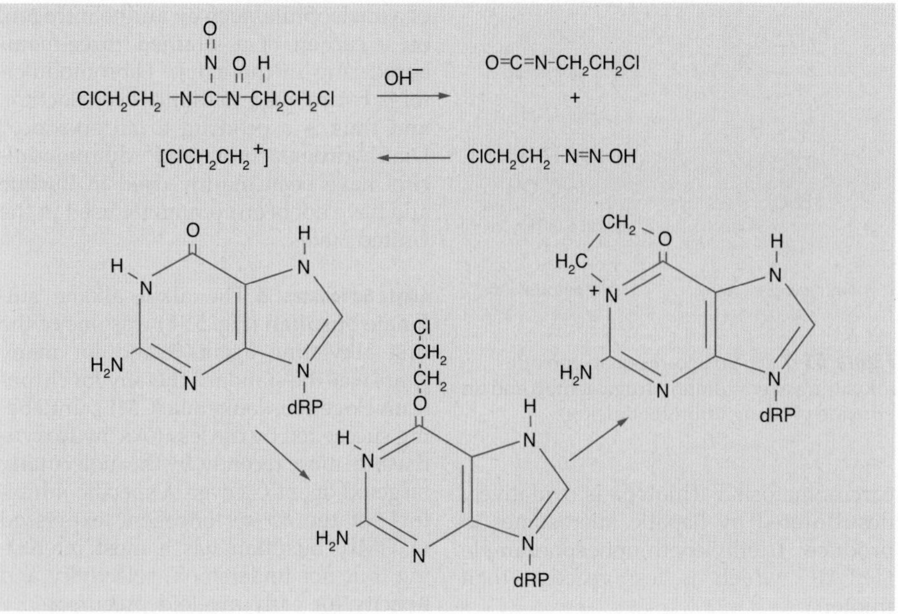

Figure 51-10 ■ Mechanism of nitrosourea activation and alkylation of deoxyguanylic acid.

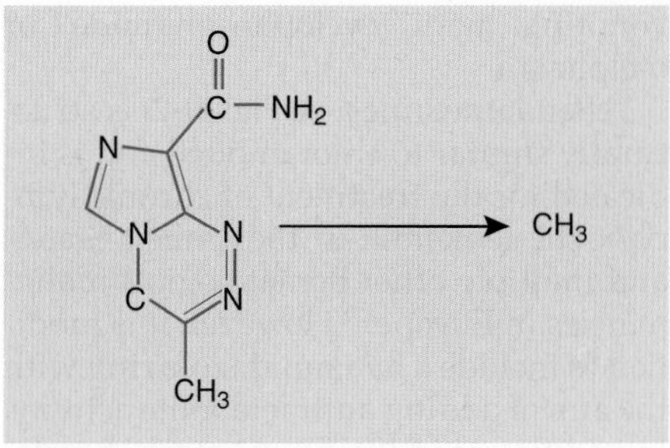

Figure 51-12 ■ The structure of temozolomide.

ber of preclinical brain tumor models,[48] was active in clinical trials, is currently used for the treatment of primary brain tumors, and has shown activity against multiple myeloma. Although there are several mechanisms through which the cytotoxic activity of the nitrosoureas may occur, the putative mechanism[49–52] is that shown in Figure 51-10, a base catalyzed decomposition to an alkylating chloroethyl diazonium moiety. CCNU and semustine (methyl CCNU) have demonstrated significant activity against solid tumors, including gastrointestinal tumors. Nimustine (ACNU) is more water soluble than the other nitrosoureas, and has been used for the intra-arterial and intrathecal treatment of central nervous system (CNS) tumors. The clinical use of the nitrosoureas has been limited by the marked and prolonged hematopoietic toxicity and renal toxicity. However, because of their unique mechanism of action and activity against brain tumors, the agents have been used in drug combinations for the treatment of breast and other cancers,[53–60] and the development of nitrosoureas with a higher therapeutic index, such as fotemustine, is an important area of endeavor.

Triazenes, Hydrazines, and Related Compounds

These are nitrogen-containing compounds that spontaneously decompose or can be metabolized to produce alkyl diazonium intermediates that alkylate biological molecules. Procarbazine and dacarbazine, which are illustrated in Figure 51-11, are metabolized to produce reactive methyl compounds that methylate DNA and alter its function. The metabolism of procarbazine is complex, and there are different pathways through which a reactive methyl group can be produced. The most likely pathway responsible for the DNA methylation and cytotoxicity is the generation of methylazoxyprocarbazine.[61–63] Both procarbazine and dacarbazine are used in the treatment of Hodgkin disease[64,65] and some refractory solid tumors.[66] Temozolomide (Fig. 51-12) spontaneously decomposes to generate a reactive methyl group,[67,69] which appears to produce more consistent concentrations of the reactive methyl group and has proven to be a useful agent for the treatment of brain tumors and other tumor types.[70,71] The spontaneous and the better time and spatially distributed release of the activated methyl group is probably what makes temozolomide more effective than the previous methylating agents.

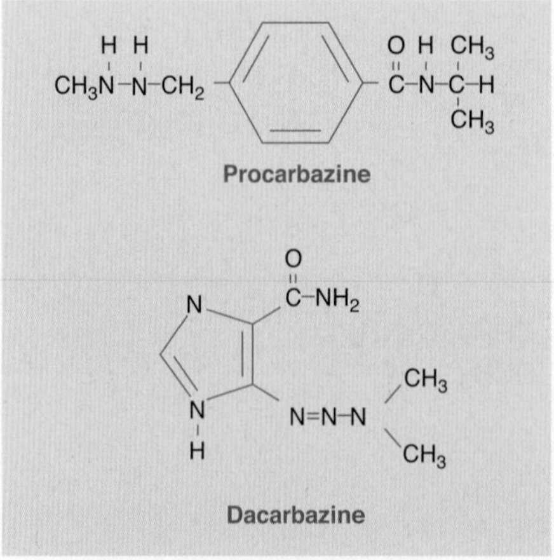

Figure 51-11 ■ Structures of monofunctional alkylating agents.

Hexamethylmelamine ■ Hexamethylmelamine is an active antitumor agent that is considered to be acting as an alkylating agent because the methyl groups are required for activity (Fig. 51-13). The methyl groups are hydroxylated with subsequent demethylation in vivo,[72] a reaction that generates a reactive methyl group. Analogues in which the methyl groups are hydroxylated are also active. The agent does have significant antitumor activity against ovarian cancer and is used primarily in the third-line treatment of that tumor.[73]

Trabectedin ■ Trabectedin (Ecteinascidin-743, Yondelis) is a tetrahydroisoquinoline alkaloid derived from the Caribbean marine tunicate or "sea squirt" (*Ecteinascidia turbinate*) (Fig. 51-14). It is now manufactured semi-synthetically from cyanosafracin B extracted after fermentation of *Pseudomonas fluorescens*, a marine bacterium.[74] Trabectedin preferentially binds to the minor groove and alkylates the N2 position on guanines. This results in bending of the DNA towards the major groove, recruiting nuclear excision repair proteins and trapping XPG (nuclear excision repair protein), which results in single stranded DNA breaks.[75] Trabectidin is approved outside of the United States for the treatment of soft tissue sarcomas and has shown activity in ovarian cancer.

Mechanisms of Cytoxicity

Although the alkylating agents react with a number of biologic molecules, including amino acids, thiols, and DNA, a number of lines of evidence have led to the gen-

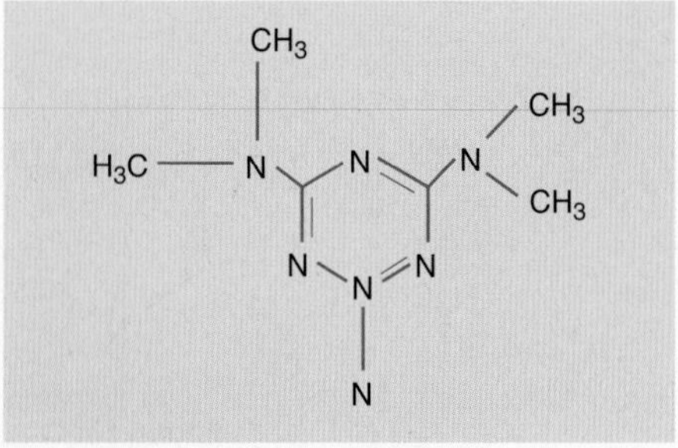

Figure 51-13 ■ The structure of hexamethylmelamine.

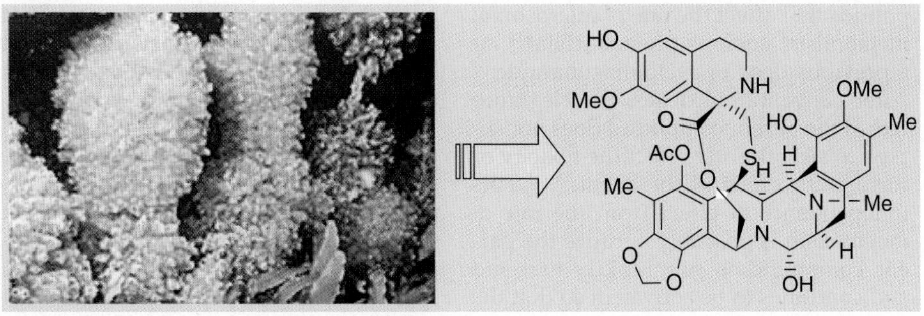

Figure 51-14 ■ Origin (*Ecteinascidia turbinate*) and structure of trabectidin.

erally accepted conclusion that the cytotoxic effects of the agents are a result of reactions with DNA. Bifunctional agents are more effective antitumor agents than monofunctional agents, but the addition of more than two alkylating groups does not further increase the cytotoxic activity. These observations[76] and the early studies of Brookes and Lawley[77,78] led to the postulation that interstrand cross-linking of DNA was responsible for the cytotoxic activity of the bifunctional alkylating agents. There is good correlation between cytotoxicity and the formation of interstrand cross-links by bifunctional alkylating agents.

Decomposition, Metabolism, and Cellular Resistance

The alkylating agents react with water and are inactivated by this hydrolysis. Cellular resistance to alkylating agents is an important determinant of the effectiveness of therapy. There are three general types of cellular resistance. These include: (1) decreased uptake[79] of agents into or increased export out of the cell, (2) increased inactivation of agents in the cell, and (3) enhanced repair of the DNA damage produced by the agents. Another mechanism of drug resistance, which only recently has been recognized, is the suppression of cellular mechanisms that produce cytotoxicity through the mechanism of apoptosis in response to cellular damage produced by antitumor agents.

The alkylating agents are inactivated by reaction with thiols such as glutathione.[80] The rate of reaction of alkylating agents with glutathione can be increased by the glutathione S-transferase enzymes,[80,81] and elevated glutathione concentrations in cells protects against the alkylating agents and may play a role in protecting normal cells from alkylating agents, but such resistance also occurs in tumor cells. Approaches to selectively increase glutathione concentrations in normal, but not tumor cells, have not been achieved.

Antitumor agents undergo microsomal and other types of xenobiotic metabolism. Such metabolism may activate agents, such as cyclophosphamide, inactivate them, or modify their physical properties without inactivating them. Nitrosoureas have been reported to be denitrosated and inactivated by microsomal metabolism.[82,83]

Chlorambucil is metabolized to bischloroethylphenylacetic acid, a less active alkylating agent, which probably continues to contribute to the therapeutic and toxic effects of chlorambucil.[84] The reactive aldophosphamide produced from cyclophosphamide is oxidized to carboxyphosphamide, an inactive metabolite (see Fig. 51-5), by the enzyme aldehyde dehydrogenase, as discussed earlier.[6] This mechanism has been shown to produce cellular resistance to cyclophosphamide.[85]

The cross-linking phosphoramide mustard produced from cyclophosphamide is hydrolyzed and inactivated by the hydroxyl moiety of water and other nucleophiles. Cellular repair of monoalkylations and DNA cross-links produced by alkylating agents are carried out by cellular resistance mechanisms, and the mechanisms of such repair have been studied extensively, as described below, but are still not completely elucidated.

The best defined DNA repair resistance to alkylating agents is resistance to the nitrosoureas and other compounds that alkylate the O-6-guanine position of DNA. The protein 06-alkylguanine-DNA-alkyltransferase (O6-AT) removes alkyl groups from the O-6 position of guanine,[86–94] preventing the formation of an interstrand cross-link from a chloroethyl adduct and subsequent cross-link. The removed alkyl group is covalently and irreversibly bound to the alkyltransferase, so that the protein can catalyze the removal of only one alkyl moiety and is then rapidly catabolized. It is now obvious that elevated O6-AT is a major mechanism of resistance to nitrosoureas in human gliomas and other tumors. However, the fact that O6-alkyltranferase is irreversibly inactivated by the attachment of an alkyl group provides an approach to counteracting this mechanism of resistance. If cells are treated with a monofunctional O-6 alkylating agent, such as streptozotocin, there follows a period when the O-6 alkyltransferase activity is decreased by its removal of the alkyl groups. Therefore, if therapy with alkylating agents is used during this period, the cell sensitivity has been restored. However, the bone marrow is also rendered more sensitive to alkylating agents during this period, so that lower doses of the alkylating agents should be used.

An association between increased cellular concentrations of metallothionein and resistance to platinum agents has been established,[95] which is due to binding of the agent to the multiple thiol groups of this cellular protein. Yu and colleagues have also described binding of melphalan[96] and Wei and colleagues have described phosphoramide mustard[97] to thiol groups in metallothionein, indicating that increased metallothionein in cells is another mechanism of sequestration and inactivation of alkylating agents.

The cytotoxicity of the bifunctional alkylating agents is due to a cross-link between guanylic acid nucleotides on opposite DNA strands.[98–102] The major mechanism of resistance to bifunctional alklyating agents is the excision of the cross-link.[103] Removal of interstrand cross-links from DNA in cells can be shown to occur in studies using alkaline elution and other techniques.[104] Friedman and colleagues[13] have described a human medulloblastoma cell that is resistant to cyclophosphamide on the basis of repair of the interstrand cross-link and have defined and modeled the structure of the cross-link[100] with the rationale that accurate molecular definition of the structure will enhance the development of a less reparable cross-link. Recently, cell resistance and survival after DNA damage have been demonstrated to occur in both tumor and normal cells by endogenous inhibition of the cellular death (apoptosis) pathway. Monofunctional alkylation of a purine base in DNA can result in depurination, cleavage of the DNA,[105,106] and cell death.

There is evidence that poly(ADP ribose) polymerase is involved in the repair of nitrogen mustard lesions.[107] Also, there is convincing evidence that cells that react to alkylation damage[108] by arresting in the G_2 phase of the cell cycle can repair DNA during this period and are more resistant to alkylating agents than cells that proceed through mitosis despite alkylation damage. Such cells have increased accumulation of phosphorylated (and inactivated) cdc2 kinase associated with G_2 arrest after nitrogen mustard treatment. This alteration allows repair of DNA damage before the cell enters mitosis. Inhibitors of DNA repair have been shown to enhance the cytotoxicity of alkylating agents.[101–104] It is very likely that increased understanding of the DNA repair process will allow more effective use of alkylating agents. Bendamustine is a bifunctional alkylating agent with antimetabolite properties. Its mechanism of cell killing differs somewhat from classical agents (see above). In addition, Trabectidin is a monofunctional alkylating agent with a particularly complex and somewhat unique mechanism of action. As described above, following binding to the minor groove and alkylating N2 positoins on guanine, the DNA distortion recruits the transcription-coupled nuclear excision repair apparatus, components of which are trapped and produce repetitive single strand breaks.[75]

In Vivo Resistance ■ Murine tumors that are resistant to alkylating agents in vivo, but not in vitro, have been reported.[109,110] Further studies of these tumors that are resistant to cyclophosphamide, cisplatin, and thiotepa in vivo demonstrate that the tumors are also resistant to the agents in three-dimensional in vitro culture, but not in two-dimensional in vitro culture.[111] Such resistance may be acquired rapidly after drug exposure[112] and may be associated with enhanced metastatic properties. The mechanisms responsible for this type of resistance have not yet been established. There may be differences between known cellular resistance factors or between membrane properties in the three-dimensional milieu, compared with the two-dimensional configuration, and adhesion molecules may alter drug sensitivity. Other potential mechanisms for drug resistance in vivo are poor perfusion of the tumor and changes in the intracellular pH.[113] Cell lines made resistant to classic alkylting agents remains sensitive to bendamustin, consistent with the complex mechanisms by which bendamustine appears to kill cells. Resitance to Trabectedin can be demonstrated in cell lines deficient in transcription-coupled nuclear excision repair.[114]

Clinical Pharmacology

Cyclophosphamide ■ After the administration of a systemic dose of 50 mg/kg, plasma concentrations of the parent compound of up to 400 mol/L can be achieved and decay with a half-life of 3–10 h.[115–117] The rate of metabolism of the parent compound varies considerably between individuals and can be modulated by the administration of compounds that affect the rate of microsomal metabolism, such as phenobarbital[118] or a previous dose of cyclophosphamide.[119] After conventional doses, the clearance rate of the parent compound does not appear to significantly affect the toxicity or therapeutic effect of the agent.[120,121] This independence of effect from the rate of metabolism is probably because the parent compound is not rapidly excreted and continues to be activated, so that the area under the curve (AUC) for systemic exposure to the active metabolite is similar after a given dose.

At the higher doses currently used in bone marrow transplantation regimens, however, the plasma concentrations of cyclophosphamide are close to the capacity of the microsomal activating enzymes. Grochow and colleagues[46] demonstrated that in patients receiving 4 g/m^2 of cyclophosphamide over 90 min and achieving initial plasma concentrations of greater than 500 μmol/L, saturable pharmacokinetics are seen. These investigators concluded that when the dosing rate equals or exceeds 4 g/m^2 in 90 min or the plasma concentration exceeds 150 μmol/L, nonlinear distribution may occur with variable exposure to the active metabolites. This study also confirmed previous reports that cyclophosphamide can induce its own metabolism.

Studies of the pharmacokinetics of the critical metabolite 4-hydroxycyclophosphamide were limited in the past by the difficulty of accurately measuring this labile molecule. However, more facile and specific methods are now available and the pharmacokinetics of this important metabolite are being elucidated. Anderson and colleagues measured 4-hydroxycyclophophamide in patient blood after cyclophosphamide administration by using a very specific gas chromatographic-mass spectrometric technique.[122] After a dose of cyclophosphamide of 110 mg/kg over 90 min, peak concentrations of 9–12 μmol/L and AUCs of 105–110 μmol/L h were measured; a cyclophosphamide dose of 170 mg/kg given as a continuous infusion over 4 days produced plasma concentrations 1–5 μmol/L with a total AUC of 98–110 μmol/L h.

Other studies found similar results.[123,124] All studies found a considerable patient variation in the exposure to 4-hydroxycyclophosphamide after the same dose of cyclophosphamide and differences in the exposure and ratios of cyclophosphamide/4-hydroxycyclophosphamide each day when short-duration infusions are given on subsequent days. These findings are most likely to be a result of differences in cytochrome P-450 complements in patients and the differing exposures to drugs that modulate the activities of these enzymes. These findings indicate that pharmacokinetically guided dose adjustment will be the best method to produce consistent patient exposures to the active metabolites of cyclophosphamide.

The majority of a dose of cyclophosphamide (ca 70%) is excreted in the urine as the inactive metabolite carboxyphosphamide. Renal function does not significantly affect the toxicity of cyclophosphamide[125] (most likely because spontaneous decomposition, and not renal excretion, determines the clearance of the principal active metabolites).

The clinical pharmacology of ifosfamide has been less studied than that of cyclophosphamide, but is similar to that of cyclophosphamide, except that microsomal activation is somewhat slower, and chloroethyl side chain oxidation plays a greater role in its metabolism.[126–130] Thus, for a dose of ifosfamide, lower systemic concentrations of the 4-hydroxy metabolite are achieved than for a similar dose of cyclophosphamide.[129] Both cyclophosphamide and ifosfamide are well absorbed after oral administration.[130]

Boddy and colleagues[19] demonstrated that ifosfamide, like cyclophosphamide, can induce its own metabolism. Because of the greater and more variable side chain of ifosfamide, differences in the P-450 drug metabolizing enzymes between individuals and the modulation of these enzymes by concomitantly administered agents may play a greater role in altering the clinical effects of ifosfamide than cyclophosphamide.[131,132]

Melphalan ■ Alberts and colleagues found that peak plasma levels of 4–13 μmol/L of melphalan were present after intravenous administration of a 0.6 mg/kg dose of melphalan, and the half-life ($t_{1/2}$ beta) was 1.8 h.[133,134] At this dose, the mean AUC for melphalan was 8 μmol/L h. Similar AUC per dose and pharmacokinetics have been demonstrated by other investigators after high intravenous doses of melphalan.[135] After conventional oral doses of 0.25 mg/kg, peak plasma levels of up to 0.625 μmol/L were measured.[136,137] There is variable systemic exposure after oral dosing, and it has been shown that oral administration of food with melphalan will inhibit absorption of the agent.[138] The half-life of melphalan is prolonged in anephric dogs,[139] and it has been reported that myelosuppression from melphalan is increased in patients with decreased renal function,[140] and significant renal clearance of the parent compound in patients has been shown by Reece and colleagues.[140]

Chlorambucil ■ After the oral administration of 0.6 mg/kg of chlorambucil, peak levels of 2–6 μmol/L of parent compound were found at 1 h by Alberts and colleagues.[141] Peak plasma levels of phenylacetic acid mustard of 2–4 μmol/L occurred at 2–4 h after chlorambucil administration. The plasma half-life of chlorambucil was 92 min, and that of phenylacetic acid mustard was 145 min. At the dose of 0.6 mg/kg of chlorambucil, the plasma AUC of chlorambucil was 3–9 μmol/L h.[142]

Bendamustine ■ The pharmacokinetics of bendamustine were originally determined by Preiss et al in 1985 in seven patients after both intravenous and oral administration.[143] Bendamstine is rapidly eliminated from the plasma after intravenous administration ($t_{1/2}$ alpha = 9.6 min, $t_{1/2}$ beta = 36.1 min). The AUC is 11.17 µg/mL h, the central distribution volume 11.15 L and the distribution volume in steady state 20.51 L. The mean total clearance was 528.9 mL/min. After oral administration, peak plasma concentrations were reached in less than 60 min. The mean oral bioavailability was 0.57 (range, 0.25–0.94). Bendamustine is metabolized in the liver where it is believed to be conjugated to glutathione. The monohydroxy-benzamine and dihydroxy-benzamine metabolites and parent compound are eliminated by the kidneys, whereas the N-dimethyl and gamma-hydroxy metabolites are eliminated in the bile.[144]

Thiotepa ■ The pharmacokinetics of thiotepa[145] were also studied by Henner and colleagues[146] after a continuous intravenous infusion of 12 mg/m^2. Peak plasma concentrations of about 5 μmol/L were achieved on the first day and were found to decay with a $t_{1/2}$ beta of 125 min. The mean AUC was 9 micromolar hours. Plasma concentrations of TEPA of up to 1 μmol/L were reached and remained in plasma longer than thiotepa. Wadler and colleagues[147] examined the plasma concentrations of thiotepa after intraperitoneal administration. Peak plasma concentrations of thiotepa of 7 μmol/L were attained on the first day, and then gradually decreased. Plasma AUC values of up to 600 μmol/L hours were achieved. When administered intraperitoneally, there was rapid loss of thiotepa from the intraperitoneal cavity and a concomitant increase in plasma concentrations to those associated with the same dose delivered intravenously. After intravenous injection, cerebrospinal fluid concentrations comparable with plasma concentrations were found.[148] Recent studies indicate that the simultaneous administration of thiotepa and cyclophosphamide will result in lower exposure to the active metabolite of cyclophosphamide, 4-hydroxycyclophosphamide, presumably because of competition for the P-450 enzymes (unpublished data, Colvin and Petros).

Nitrosoureas ■ Levin and colleagues have studied the pharmacokinetics of BCNU.[83] After the intravenous infusion of 60–170 mg/m^2, peak plasma concentrations of 5 μmol/L were present and decayed with an initial half-life of 68 min. Henner and colleagues[149] measured the pharmacokinetics of BCNU after intravenous doses of 600 mg/m^2. The peak plasma concentration of ultrafilterable BCNU was 23% of the total plasma BCNU. The pharmacokinetics of CCNU after administration of 130 mg/m^2 to patients have also been described.[150] The parent compound could not be detected in plasma, but the monohydroxylated metabolites, *trans*-4-hydroxy CCNU and *cis*-4-hydroxy CCNU, were found in a ratio of 6:4 and at total peak concentrations of about 3 μmol/L. The plasma clearance half-lives of the hydroxy-CCNU metabolites varied from 1 to 3 h between patients.

Busulfan ■ Because of its insolubility in aqueous solutions, busulfan was previously available only as an oral preparation. However, an intravenous preparation is now available in a DMSO solution (Busulfex), which is increasingly used, is well tolerated, and allows more reproducible dosing and better avoidance of veno-occlusive disease without the necessity for as extensive pharmacokinetic monitoring and dose adjustment, although some variability in exposure to the agent is still seen.

Trabectedin ■ When trabectedin is administered intravenously over 1 or 3 h at doses ranging from 800 to 1650 µg/m^2 repeated every three weeks the pharmacokinetic values are as follows: AUC (h.ng/mL) ranged from 23 to 71; the C_{max} (ng/mL) from 13 to 18, the clearance (L/h) from 25 to 100; the volume of distribution at steady state (L) from 910 to 2200 and; the terminal $t_{1/2}$ (h) from 33 to 50 after rapid disappearance from the plasma.[151] Other doses and schedules revealed generally similar pharmacokinetic profiles. Trabectedin is metabolized in the liver by Cyp3A4 and cleared by the kidneys.

■ Toxicities

The characteristic toxicities of the alkylating agents are hematopoietic, gastrointestinal, gonadal, and CNS toxicities. However, each of the agents has a characteristic set of toxicities, determined by the reactivity, metabolism, and distribution of the agent, and the clinician should be aware of the idiosyncrasies of each of the agents that he or she uses frequently.

Hematopoietic Toxicity ■ In general, the clinical dose-limiting toxicity for an alkylating agent is hematopoietic toxicity, particularly suppression of granulocytes and platelets. The nadir of granulocyte depression after alkylating agent treatment is usually 8–16 days, and granulocytes usually return to normal within 20 days after a single dose of alkylating agent. Cyclophosphamide and ifosfamide are less hematopoietically toxic than are the other alkylating agents, and granulocyte numbers return to normal more rapidly, platelets are affected less, and repeated doses of cyclophosphamide and ifosfamide do not produce cumulative damage and progressive deterioration of the hematopoietic elements. The decreased hematopoietic toxicity of cyclophosphamide is due to the presence of aldehyde dehydrogenase in the hematopoietic stem cells and in early megakaryocytes, as discussed earlier. In contrast, the nitrosoureas produce severe hematopoietic toxicity and nadirs of granulocytes and platelets occur as late as 45 days.[152] Busulfan also produces severe hematopoietic depression, with a selectivity for early myeloid precursors. The variations in the cellular patterns and time courses of hematopoietic suppression after the administration of different alkylating agents indicate that the individual agents have selectivity for different hematopoietic precursor cells (Fig. 51-15).

Peptide growth factors, such as granulocyte-macrophage colony-stimulating factor (GM-CSF) and granulocyte CSF (G-CSF), which stimulate the differentiation and proliferation of hematopoietic precursors are now used effectively. The degree and duration of granulocyte depression after antitumor drug administration can be reduced by the concomitant use of these growth factors. The use of these factors with the alkylating agents is particularly attractive because of the steep dose response curve of the alkylating agents and because a considerable increase in dose may be administered before another dose-limiting toxicity is reached. For these reasons, combinations of alkylating agents have been used in association with allogeneic and autologous bone marrow transplantation.

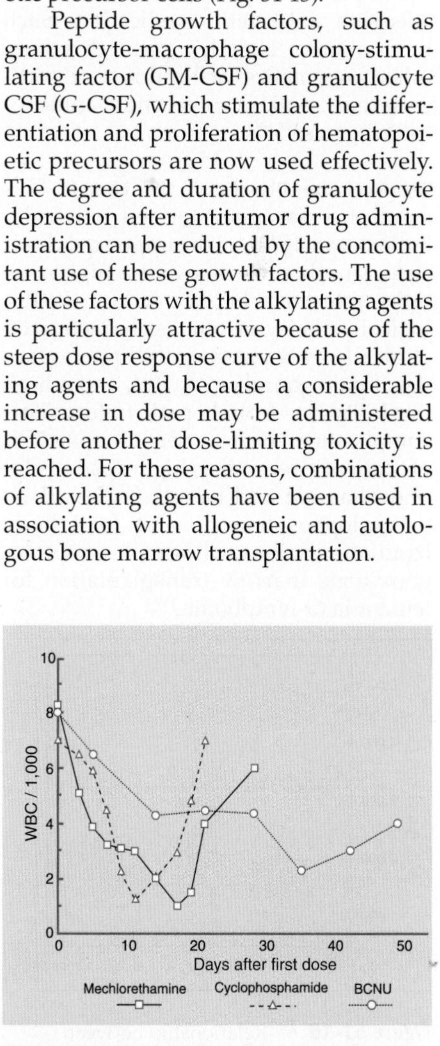

Figure 51-15 ■ Hematopoietic toxicity of alkylating agents. WBC, white blood cells.

Gastrointestinal Toxicity ■ Damage to the gastrointestinal tract is a toxicity that frequently occurs with high-dose regimens. Mucositis, stomatitis, esophagitis, and diarrhea occur with high doses of alkylating agents, particularly after high doses of melphalan and thiotepa or combinations of alkylating agents. Significant mucositis is unusual even after high doses of cyclophosphamide or ifosfamide. This lack of gastrointestinal toxicity is caused by the presence of the enzyme aldehyde dehydrogenase in the epithelial cells of the gastrointestinal tract, which inactivates the aldophosphamide metabolite produced from the metabolism of cyclophosphamide and ifosfamide.[11] The nausea and vomiting produced by alkylating agents are, at least in part, mediated through the CNS and not caused by direct gastrointestinal toxicity.[153,154] These effects are variable between patients in that some patients tolerate high doses of alkylating agents without nausea and vomiting, while other patients are incapacitated by even low doses of alkylating agents. The frequency of nausea and vomiting does increase as the dose of an alkylating is increased. Therefore, it is important to provide the patient with adequate antiemetic medication. Such medications include phenothiazines, other antiemetics, acute doses of corticosteroids, and, more recently, antiserotonin agents.[155,156]

Veno-occlusive Disease of the Liver ■ This syndrome is characterized clinically by hepatomegaly, right upper quadrant pain, jaundice, ascites, and a high mortality rate from hepatic failure. Pathologically, the syndrome is characterized clinically by hepatomegaly, upper quandrant pain, jaundice, ascites, and a high mortality rate from hepatic failure. This complication has been seen in up to 25% of patients receiving high-dose cyclophosphamide and busulfan (Fig. 51-16) or cyclophosphamide and total body irradiation prior to allogeneic or autologous bone marrow transplantation for leukemia or lymphoma.[157]

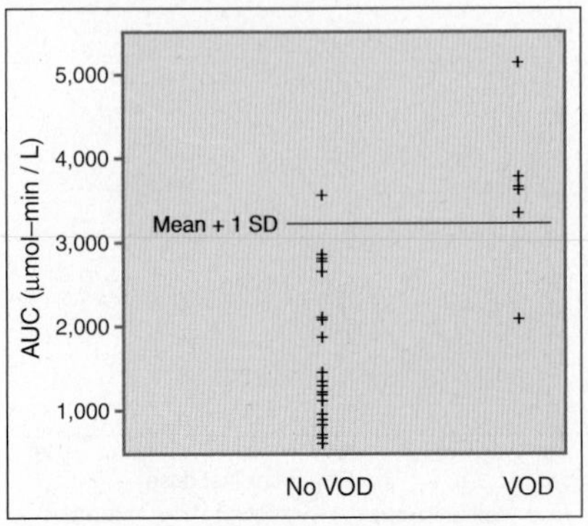

Figure 51–16 ■ Relationship between plasma AUC of busulfan and occurrence of veno-occlusive disease of the liver.

Gonadal Damage ■ A serious toxicity of the alkylating agents is gonadal damage. The characteristic lesion in men, depletion of testicular germ cells with preservation of Sertoli cells, was first described in 1948 in patients treated with mechlorethamine[158] and subsequently confirmed and better characterized[159–161] in men treated with many combinations of antitumor drugs, although the alkylating agents are probably the most potent agents in producing this effect, considering their mutagenic properties. Spermatogenesis and fertility may return after several years.[162,163] Amenorrhea, associated with disappearance of mature and primordial ovarian follicles, is seen in women treated with alkylating agents.[164,165] The frequency of this effect increases with the age of the woman and is more likely to be irreversible in older women.

Pulmonary Damage ■ Pulmonary damage in the form of interstitial pneumonitis and fibrosis is associated with the alkylating antitumor agents. Although the exact mechanism of the pulmonary toxicity is unknown, it is presumably caused by direct toxicity of the agents to pulmonary epithelial cells. The typical presentation of this toxicity is the onset of a nonproductive cough and dyspnea, which may progress to tachypnea and cyanosis, and to pulmonary insufficiency and death. This complication was first described in association with busulfan therapy,[166] but has subsequently been described after cyclophosphamide,[167] BCNU,[168,169] and melphalan[170] and appears to be a toxicity of all the alkylating agents. A significant incidence of pulmonary toxicity has been reported in patients receiving high doses of cyclophosphamide, cisplatin, and BCNU.[171]

Hemorrhagic Cystitis ■ The oxazaphosphorines cyclophosphamide and ifosfamide produce bladder toxicity, which is not seen with other alkylating agents. This toxicity is a hemorrhagic cystitis, which can progress to massive hemorrhage.[172] The metabolite principally responsive for this toxicity is acrolein,[173] although phosphoramide mustard and chloroacetaldehyde may contribute to the effect. Hemorrhagic cystitis is seen more commonly after ifosfamide therapy than cyclophosphamide therapy, probably because higher doses of this agent are used. Renal tubular damage has also been seen after ifosfamide, including a Fanconi-type syndrome with azotemia, elevated serum creatinine, and enzymuria.[174] The systemic administration of thiols can prevent or ameliorate the bladder damage from cyclophosphamide and ifosfamide because the thiols conjugate and inactivate the aldehyde functions of acrolein and chloroacetaldehyde. A widely used compound to prevent or ameliorate osazaphosphorine bladder toxicity is the sodium salt of 2-mercaptoethane sulfonate (Mesna). Mesna is usually administered to all patients receiving ifosfamide and to patients receiving high-dose cyclophosphamide. Subclinical renal toxicity has been observed in patients receiving ifosfamide,[16] despite Mesna administration, so that administration of Mesna does not eliminate the need for adequate hydration and careful observation of the patient.

Antidiuresis ■ An antidiuretic effect is commonly seen in patients receiving doses of cyclophosphamide of 50 mg/kg or greater.[175,176] This syndrome is characterized by a decrease in urine output 6–8 h after drug administration, weight gain, a marked increase in urine osmolality, and a decrease in serum osmolality and sodium concentration. Pericardial and pleural effusions may be seen, and seizures caused by hyponatremia have occurred with cyclophosphamide therapy,[177] especially if low-sodium replacement fluids are administered. This antidiuretic syndrome appears to be caused by an effect of cyclophosphamide metabolites on the distal renal tubule and is self-limited, with the excess fluid excreted over a period of about 12 h. Administration of furosemide promotes free water clearance and ameliorates the syndrome.[178]

Renal Toxicity ■ Renal toxicity is a serious toxicity of the nitrosureas.[179,180] This effect is dose related and can produce severe renal failure and death after administration of more than 1,200 mg of BCNU. Elevation of serum creatinine and other clinical evidence of renal toxicity may not be seen until after the completion of therapy. The histology of the kidneys in patients with renal nitrosourea damage is similar to that seen in radiation nephritis. A case of acute renal failure after melphalan therapy has also been reported,[181] indicating that adequate hydration of patients undergoing treatment with any alkylating agent therapy is very important. The histology of the kidneys in patients with renal nitrosourea damage is similar to that in radiation nephritis.

Alopecia ■ Although the association between an alkylating agent and alopecia was first described with busulfan therapy,[182] this toxicity is associated with most of the alkylating agents, and particularly with cyclophosphamide and ifosfamide therapy. The alopecia produced by these agents can be quite extensive, especially if the agent is given in combination with vincristine or doxorubicin. Regrowth of the hair occurs after cessation of therapy and may be associated with a change in the texture and color of the hair.[183] The structure-function studies of Feil and Lamoureaux[184] indicate that this toxicity is a result of entry of lipophilic metabolites into the hair follicles. This suggestion is consistent with the fact that busulfan, vincristine, and adriamycin are lipophilic and produce severe alopecia. It is important to recognize that the growing hair develops a nick, undoubtedly from inhibition of growth of the hair at the base of the follicle at the time of drug exposure, and the hair "breaks off," rather than "falls out." The practical implication of this fact is that patients should be advised not to brush their hair during and immediately after therapy administration to avoid the breaking off of the hair.

Allergic and Hypersensitivity Reactions ■ Because the alkylating agents react with many biologic molecules, it is not surprising that they serve as haptens and produce allergic reactions.[185–187] The most frequent reactions that have been reported have been cutaneous hypersensitivities. Anaphylactic reactions are rare, but have occurred.[188] Patterns of cross-reactivity have not been carefully defined, but cross-reactivity between agents of similar structure, such as the nitrogen mustards, have been described.[189]

Cardiotoxicity ■ The nonhematologic dose-limiting toxicity of cyclophosphamide is a fatal cardiac toxicity characterized by specific pathologic findings[15,190] in the heart and characterized clinically by fulminant cardiac failure. The hearts of these patients are dilated, with patchy transmural hemorrhage and pericardial effusion. The microscopic findings consist of interstitial hemorrhage and edema, myocardial necrosis and vacuolar changes, and specific changes in the intramural small coronary vessels. Decreased electrocardiographic voltage and a transient increase in heart size is seen in high-dose cyclophosphamide patients without clinical symptoms, and the characteristic pathologic findings are present in patients who die of other causes following high-dose cyclophosphamide. Age greater than 50 years and previous adriamycin exposure appear to increase the risk of cyclophosphamide cardiotoxicity.[190] To this author's knowledge, there have been no reports of pretherapy cardiac evaluation to correlate with cardiac clinical symptoms and outcome after high-dose cyclophosphamide.

Neurotoxicity ■ In preclinical studies of alkylating agents, severe neurotoxicity was seen.[191] At the usual clinical doses, including transplant doses, frank neurotoxicity is not often seen, but drowsiness and alterations of consciousness can be seen clinically, and changes in EEG findings were detected (unpublished experience of this author) after bone marrow transplantation doses of cyclophosphamide. At BCNU doses of 1,200 mg/m^2, severe CNS toxicity has been produced,[192] and the intracarotid administration of BCNU has produced severe eye pain and blindness.[193] High-dose busulfan therapy produces seizures, and anticonvulsants are often used prophylactically.[194]

Hepatoxicity ■ Trabectidin produces characteristic elevations in hepatic transaminases, whose magnitude decreases on subsequent dosing. The effects of Trabectidin on transaminase elevation and myelosuppression can be ameliorated by high-dose dexamethasone.[195]

Nitosoureas, particularly high-dose BCNU used in the setting of bone marrow transplantation, have been associated with veno-occlusive disease and hepatic failure. Risk factors included hepatic involvement with tumor and rate of infusion of BCNU.[196]

Teratogenicity ■ Studies carried out in vivo and in embryo cultures demonstrate that all of the alkylating agents are teratogenic.[197] The teratogenic effect is the result of cytotoxic effects on the embryo by the same mechanisms through which the compounds are toxic to tumor cells.[198,199] The available clinical information indicates that there is a definite risk of a malformed infant if the mother is treated during the first trimester of pregnancy.[200] However, the administration of alkylating agents during the second and third trimesters is not associated with an increased risk of fetal malformation.[201]

Carcinogenesis ■ Since the initial reports of acute leukemia occurring in patients treated with alkylating agents,[202,203] it has become increasingly obvious that this type of oncogenesis is a significant complication of alkylating agent therapy. Several studies indicate that the rate of acute leukemia may be 10% or higher in certain patients. Procarbazine and other methylating agents appear to be the most potent oncogenic agents.[204] Although sufficient data are not yet available to be certain, it appears that alkylating agent therapy administered over a relatively short period of time is less oncogenic than prolonged alkylating agent therapy.

Immunosuppression and Immune Enhancement ■ The immunosuppressive effect of alkylating agents was first described by Hektoen and Corper[205] for sulfur mustard. Cyclophosphamide is particularly immunosuppressive[206] and is used for the treatment of autoimmune diseases.[207] Low doses of cyclophosphamide can enhance the immune response by selectively inhibiting immune suppressor cells,[208] and moderate doses of cyclophosphamide have been used in conjunction with immunotherapy and biological response modifiers such as interleukin-2.[209,210]

The clinical significance of the immunosuppression produced by alkylating agents in their role as antitumor agents is not certain. The two major concerns are susceptibility to infection in the immunosuppressed host and the potential interference with a host immune response to the tumor. The available evidence indicates that most intermittent antitumor regimens do not produce a profound or prolonged immunosuppression.[211]

Platinum Antitumor Compounds

The platinum antitumor agents are complexes of platinum with ligands that can be displaced by nucleophilic (electron-rich) atoms to form strong bonds with covalent characteristics. Thus, like the alkylating agents, the platinum agents form strong chemical bonds with thiol sulfurs and animo nitrogens in nucleic acids and proteins.

The first antitumor platinum agent was discovered by Rosenberg and colleagues[212,213] while studying the effects of electric current on bacterial growth. The growth inhibition observed was found to be caused by a platinum complex of ammonia and chloride, which was produced in the medium from the platinum electrode. These investigators found several such compounds to have antitumor activity against murine tumors in vivo.[213] The most active of these compounds was the one now known as cisplatin (Fig. 51-17).

Cisplatin went into clinical trials in the early 1970s[214–216] and was found to have significant antitumor activity against testicular cancer, lymphoma, squamous cell carcinoma of the head and neck, ovarian cancer, and bladder cancer. Because of its significant therapeutic effect in these tumors and activity against a number of other solid tumors, it has become the most frequently used antitumor agent. Because of the renal and neurotoxicities of cisplatin, there were intensive efforts to devise analogs with fewer of these toxicities. This work led to the development of carboplatin, which produces primarily hematopoietic toxicity and has antitumor effects similar to those of cisplatin. Other platinum compounds have been developed and evaluated, as described later, but have not demonstrated significant advantages over *cis*-platinum and carboplatinum.

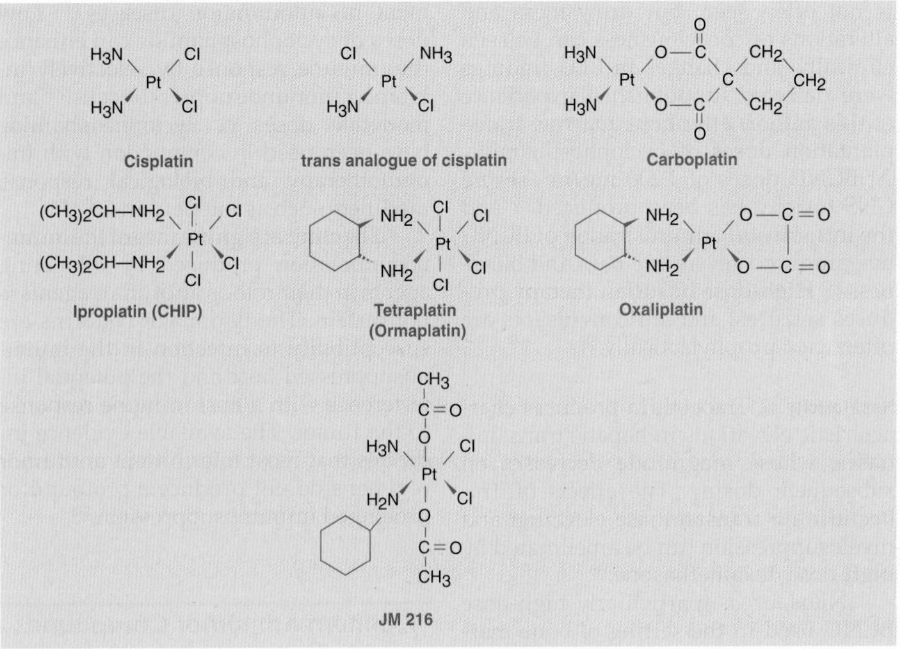

Figure 51-17 ■ Structures of platinum antitumor agents.

Chemistry

The platinum compounds that are active antitumor agents can have either four or six ligands (see Fig. 51-17) with a square planar or hexahedral configuration. Those with 4 ligands have an oxidation state of +2, and those with 6 ligands, an oxidation state of +4. The chloride ligands of cisplatin and the other complexes with the +2 oxidation state can be exchanged for nucleophilic atoms in the biologic milieu, including the nitrogens of the DNA bases. The chloride ligands of the +4 compounds are much less reactive than those of the +2 compounds,[217] and it is likely that the +4 compounds are reduced in vivo to produce the reactive +2 complexes.[218] The ligand substitution reactions of the square planar complexes occur with retention of the configuration of the platinum complex. Because the *trans*-platinum compounds are essentially inactive as antitumor compounds, the ability of the *cis* compounds to form certain stereospecific cross-links probably accounts for their antitumor activity, and specific intrastrand and interstrand cross-links have been identified.

In some *cis*-platinum compounds in clinical use, the chloride leaving ligands are replaced with carboxyl ester groups, as in carboplatin and oxaliplatin (Fig. 51-18). These ligands are less readily displaced; thus, these compounds require higher concentrations for cytotoxicity. The decreased renal and neuorlogic toxicity of these compounds is also probably a result of their being less chemically reactive than cisplatin. Substitutions on the amino groups alter the lipophilicity and distribution of the agent.

Cellular and Molecular Pharmacology

Although the chloride and carboxyester ligands can probably be directly displaced by biologic molecules, it is likely that, in the biologic milieu, the chloride or carboxy ligands are displaced by water to form the aquo ligand, which is a better leaving group than chloride or carboxy entities. The high chloride content of the extracellular fluid should maintain the platinum compounds in the chloride and less reactive form. However, in the lower chloride content of the cell, the more reactive aquo species is formed. The loss of a proton produces the hydroxyl ligand, which is unreactive. Figure 51-19 illustrates the proposed aquation pathway for cisplatin. The platinum compounds react with many biologic molecules; but here is considerable evidence that these compounds, like the bifunctional alkylating agents, exert their cytotoxic effect by interfering with DNA replication and cell division. Roberts and Pera[219] demonstrated that the amount of platinum bound to DNA was directly related to the degree of cytoxicity in rodent tumor cells. Zwelling and colleagues[220] demonstrated that the degree of DNA interstrand cross-linking in vitro and in vivo was directly related to the degree of cytotoxicity in rodent tumor cells.

The *cis*-platinum compounds, like the alkylating agents, react with nitrogen atoms of DNA and preferentially react with the N-7 atom of deoxyguanylic acid. Specific adducts of Pt compounds with DNA have now been characterized and studied and specific DNA intrastrand and interstrand cross-links identified.[219] The consensus of the studies is that the most frequent adducts are dGpdG and dApdG, which result from the *cis*-platinum complex linking adjacent deoxyguanylates or an adjacent deoxyadenylate and deoxyguanylate in a strand of DNA to produce an intrastrand cross-link, in both situations. A less common, but potentially more toxic lesion is one that results from binding of the platinum atom to the N-7 atom of a deoxyguanylate in the complementary strand of DNA, producing an interstrand cross-link, analogous to a nitrogen mustard interstrand cross-link. Repair of both lesions does occur, and the cytoxicity to the cell is determined by the resultant formation and repair of the lesions[221] by the cellular DNA mismatch repair complex. Cell resistance to cross-linking agents, including cisplatin-resistant cells, often have a deficiency in the mismatch repair complex, supporting the hypothesis that an intact mismatch repair system may render cells more sensitive to cross-linking agents in that the attempt to repair results in cell death.

Mechanisms of Cellular Resistance to Platinum Agents

Mechanisms of cellular resistance to platinum, which have been described, include decreased uptake of the platinum compound into cells, enhanced repair of the platinum- DNA damage, and increased efflux of the agent. Elevated cellular glutathione concentrations have also been associated with cellular resistance to platinum compounds. Although decreased cellular accumulation of the platinum compounds is a mechanism of cellular resistance, the mechanism of this type of resistance appears to be variable. Several investigators have shown that tumor cells can be sensitized to the platinum agents by depletion of cellular glutathione by treatment with butathione sulfoximine, an inhibitor of glutathione synthesis.[222] Eastman[223] has

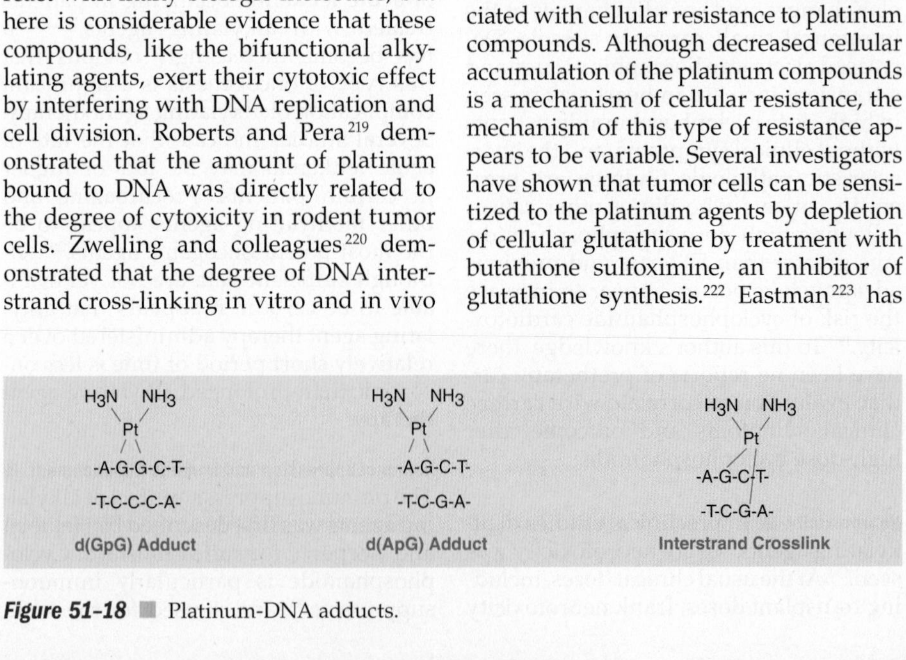

Figure 51-18 ■ Platinum-DNA adducts.

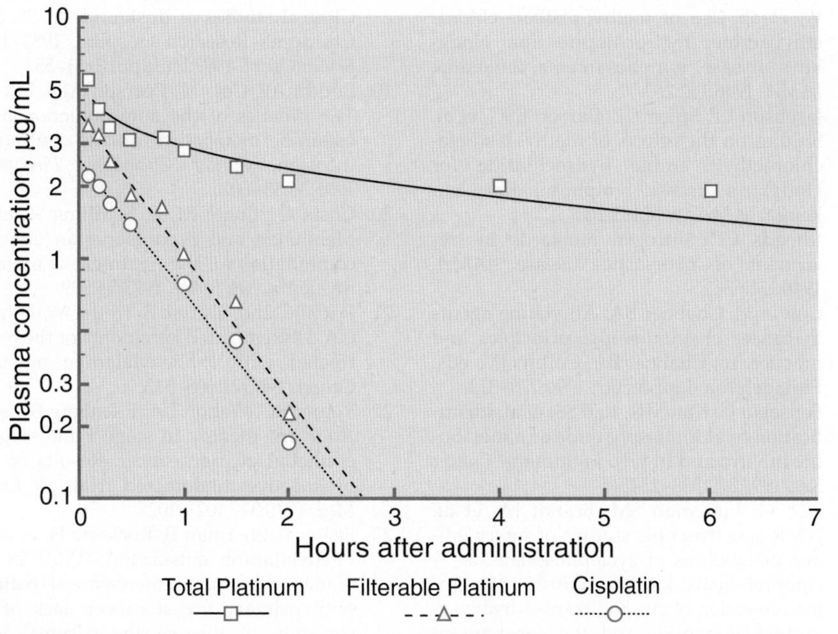

Figure 51-19 Clinical pharmacokinetics of cisplatin after single injection of 100 mg/m^2.

demonstrated that glutathione can react with monofunctional adducts on DNA to quench the second reactive ligand and prevent cross-link formation. Resistance to platinum agents has also been associated with elevation of glutathione transferase enzyme activity. Resistance to platinum agents has also been associated with another sulfhydryl-containing protein, metallothionein.[224] Decreased cellular uptake of cisplatin into cells has also been described, which is interesting in that the uptake of cisplatin into cells does not appear to be an active process.

Clinical Pharmacology

Pharmacokinetics The pharmacokinetics of platinum agents has been studied as total platinum, and more recently, the specific agents. In pharmacokinetic studies after cisplatin administration, total platinum in the plasma follows a triphasic pattern, with the first phase $t_{1/2}$ about 30 min, the second phase $t_{1/2}$ about 60 min, and the third phase $t_{1/2}$ greater than 24 h.[225,226] Carboplatin exhibits similar pharmacokinetics, except that the initial half-lives are somewhat longer, less of the total platinum is protein bound, and a greater percentage of the agent is excreted by the kidneys.[227] Decreased creatinine clearance results in higher plasma levels of both cisplatin and carboplatin with potentially greater toxicity.

Toxicities

Renal The most serious, and usually dose-limiting, toxicity of cisplatin is renal.[228,229] This toxicity presents clinically as elevated BUN and creatinine, is cumulative with continued cisplatin exposure, and is potentiated by other nephrotoxins.[230] Decreases in serum electrolytes have been associated with platinum renal toxicity, including symptomatic hypomagnesemia.[231] Although the toxicity may remain subclinical and the renal function return to normal, significant pathological damage may persist.[232] The pathology of the renal damage is characterized by focal acute tubular necrosis, dilation of convoluted tubules, thickened tubular basement membranes, formation of casts, and epithelial atypia of the collecting ducts.[232,233] High fluid intake with forced diuresis[234,235] can reduce the incidence and severity of the renal toxicity. Systemic administration of thiols can reduce renal toxicity of cisplatin in animal models, and in a clinical trial, systemic diethyldithiocarbamate appeared to reduce nephrotoxicity without affecting ototoxicity or myelosuppression.[236] The nephrotoxicity of the second generation platinum complexes, such as carboplatin iproplatin is markedly less than that of cisplatin.

Ototoxicity Ototoxicity has been a significant problem with cisplatin. This toxicity is characterized by tinnitus and hearing loss.[214,215,237] Since the higher frequencies are usually involved, the hearing loss may not be symptomatic. Vestibular toxicity does not usually occur, but can be seen.[238,239] The ototoxicity of cisplatin is dose related and is usually cumulative with subsequent courses of therapy.[240] Radiation prior to or simultaneous with the *cis*-platinum administration enhances the toxicity,[241] but the additive effect may be less if the cisplatin precedes the radiation.[242]

Neurotoxicity The neurotoxicity seen with the administraton of cisplatin consists principally of peripheral neuropathy involving both the upper and lower extremities, with paresthesias, weakness, tremors, and loss of taste.[243] Seizures and leukoencephalopathy have been described[244] and may progress after cessation of cisplatin therapy.

Particularly severe neurotoxicity has been reported after intra-arterial infusions for head and neck cancer. Since various pharmacologic maneuvers have been able to reduce the nephrotoxicity and severe nausea and vomiting produced by cisplatin, neurotoxicity has become the dose-limiting toxicity of cisplatinum. The observation has been made that treatment of animals with an ACTH analogue will prevent neurotoxicity from cisplatin and will facilitate the recovery of established nerotoxicity,[245] but does not interfere with the antitumor effect of the agent.

Gastrointestinal Toxicity Severe nausea and vomiting have been a significant problem with cisplatin, occurring in almost all patients receiving the agent.[229,246] The cause of this toxicity is not firmly established. Work in animal models indicates that abdominal visceral innervation and 5-hydroxytryptamine. Receptors on visceral afferent nerves play a role in this toxicity, but there is also evidence that the chemoreceptor trigger zone in the medulla plays a role. The use of a dopamine antagonist, metoclopromide, prior to and during cisplatin administration has been effective in controlling this toxicity.[247,248] Dexamethasone or methylprednisolone alone or in combination with metoclopromide have been useful. More recently, antiserotonin analogues such as ondansetron and granisetron have proven highly effective in controlling nausea and vomiting. The gastrointestinal toxicities of carboplatin and iproplatin are much less than those of cisplatin.

Immune Effects In contrast to the alkylating agents, many of which are significantly immunosuppressive, cisplatin appears to have no immunosuppressive effect at the usual clinical doses and may even augment immune effect.[249]

Other Analogues in Clinical Use: Oxaliplatin

Several other platinum analogues have been synthesized and evaluated clinically, including tetraplatinum and JM216. The greatest clinical impact has been observed with oxaliplatin that contains a diaminocyclohexane (DACH) carrier ligand (see Fig.

51-17). Among the platinum analogues, oxaliplatin is distinctive in its activity against colorectal cancer.[250] Oxaliplatin can inhibit growth of colorectal cancer cell lines that are resistant to cisplatin and carboplatin.[251] A combination of oxaliplatin, 5-fluorouracil (5-FU), and leucovorin (FOLFOX4) produced a higher response rate, longer time to progression and better overall survival than did irinotecan, 5-FU and leucovorin (IFL) in first line therapy for metastatic colorectal cancer,[252] resulting in U.S. FDA approval of the drug for this indication. Activity has also been observed with oxaliplatin containing regimens in nonsmall cell lung, breast, gastric, bladder, renal cell and ovarian cancers.

The dose-limiting toxicity of oxaliplatin is sensory neuropathy.[253] An acute, rapidly reversible neuropathy occurs in >90% of patients that can be aggravated by exposure to cold.[254] More problematic chronic neuropathy generally relates to the cumulative dose of drug. Neuropathy has been prevented in some studies by infusion of calcium and magnesium solutions, gabapentin, carbamazepine, amifostine, and glutathione. Existing neuropathy has been partially palliated by administration of calcium and magnesium solutions, gabapentin and alpha lipoic acid.[253]

As in the case of other platinum compounds, the antitumor activity of oxaliplatin is thought to relate to adduct formation that produces intrastrand and interstrand DNA cross-links, as well as the binding of DNA and protein. Oxaliplatin forms fewer DNA adducts, but more DNA single strand breaks than does cisplatin.[255] Whether the greater number of single strand breaks observed with oxaliplatin results from primary interaction with DNA or the rapid induction of apoptosis is not known. Greater efficiency for inducing apoptosis, despite the formation of fewer adducts, may relate to failure of DNA repair mechanisms to recognize the DACH moieties associated with oxaliplatin adducts.[255] Mismatch repair proteins and some damage recognition proteins bind to cisplatin-GG adducts with higher affinity than to oxaliplatin-GG adducts.[256] Recently described differences in conformation for the NMR solution structures of the two types of adducts provide an explanation for the differential recognition of cisplatin-induced and oxaliplatin-induced DNA damage.[256]

Selected References

The complete reference list can be found at www.CANCERMEDICINE8.com

1. Adair CPJ, Bogg HJ. Experimental and clinical studies on the treatment of cancer by dichlorethylsulfide (mustard gas). *Ann Surg*. 1931;93:190–199.
2. Goodman LS, Wintrobe MM, Dameshek W, et al. Use of methyl-bis(beta-chloroethyl)amine hydrochloride for Hodgkin's disease, lymphosarcoma, leukemia. *JAMA*. 1946;132:263.
3. Jacobson LP, Spurr CL, Barron ESG, et al. Studies on the effects of methyl-bis(beta-chloroethyl) amine hydrochloride for Hodgkin's disease, lymphosarcoma, leukemia. *JAMA*. 1946;132:263.
4. Rhoads CP. Nitrogen mustards in treatment of neoplastic disease. *JAMA*. 1946;131:656.
5. Colvin M, Chabner BA. Alkylating agents in cancer chemotherapy: principles and practice. In: Chabner BA, Collins JM, eds. Philadelphia: Lippincott; 1990:276–313.
6. Fenselau C, Kan MN, Rao SS, et al. Identification of aldophosphamide as a metabolite in vitro and in vivo in humans. *Cancer Res*. 1997;37:2538–2543.
7. Zon G, Ludeman SM, Brandt JA, et al. NMR spectroscopic studies of intermediary metabolites of cyclophosphamide. A comprehensive kinetic analysis of the interconversion of cis- and trans-4-hydroxycyclophosphamide and the concomitant partitioning of aldophosphamide between irreversible conjugation pathways. *J Med Chem*. 1984;27:466–485.
8. Shulman-Roskes EM, Noe DA, Gamcsik MP, et al. The partitioning of phosphoramide mustard and its aziridinium ions among alkylation and P-N bond hyrdrolysis reactions. *J Med Chem*. 1998;41:515–529.
9. Flowers JL, Ludeman SM, Gamcsik MP, et al. Evidence for a role of chloroethylaziridine in the cytotoxicity of cyclophosphamide. *Cancer Chemother Pharmacol*. 2000;45:335–344.
10. Alarcon RA, Meienhofer J. Formation of the cytotoxic aldehyde acrolein during the in vitro degradation of cyclophosphamide. *Nat New Biol*. 1971;233:250–252.
11. Russo JE, Hilton J, Colvin OM. The role of aldehyde dehydrogenase isoenzymes in cellular resistance to the alkylating agent cyclophosphamide. In: Weber G, ed. *Enzymology and Molecular Biology of Carbonyl Metabolism*, Vol. 2. New York: Liss; 1989:65.
12. Lee SM, Crowther D, Scarffe JH, et al. Cyclophosphamide decreases O6-alkylguanine-DNA transferase activity in peripheral lymphocytes of patients undergoing bone marrow transplantation. *Br J Cancer*. 1992;66:331–336.
13. Friedman HS, Pegg AE, Johnson SP, et al. Modulation of cyclophosphamide activity by 0–6-alkylguanine-DNA alkyltransferase. *Cancer Chemother Pharmacol*. 1999;43:80–85.
14. Bode U, Seif SM, Levine AS. Studies on the antidiuretic effect of cyclophosphamide-vasopression release and sodium excretion. *Med Ped Oncol*. 1980;8:295–303.
15. Slavin RE, Millan JC, Mullins G.M. Pathology of high dose intermittent cyclophosphamide therapy. *Hum Pathol*. 1975; 6:693–709.
16. Antman KH, Elias A, Ryan L. Ifosfamide and mesna: response and toxicity at standard and high dose schedules. *Semin Oncol*. 1990;17:68–73.
17. Loehrer PJ Sr, Lauer R, Roth BJ, et al. Salvage therapy in recurrent germ cell cancer: ifosfamide and cisplatin plus either vinblastine or etoposide. *Ann Intern Med*. 1988;109:540–546.
18. Pratt CB, Douglass EC, Etcubanas E, et al. Clinical studies of ifosfamide at St. Jude Children's Research Hospital, 1983–1988. *Semin Oncol*. 1989;16(Suppl 3):51–55.
19. Boddy AV, Cole M, Pearson ADJ, Idle JR. The kinetics of the auto-induction of ifosfamide metabolism during continuous infusion. *Cancer Chemother Pharmacol*. 1995;36:53–60.
20. Costa G., Engle RL Jr, Schilling A, et al. Melphalan and prednisone: an effective combination for the treatment of multiple myeloma. *Am J Med*. 1973;54:589.
21. Frick JC 2nd, Tretter P, Tretter W, Hyman GA. Disseminated carcinoma of the ovary treated with L-phenylalanine mustard. *Cancer*. 1968;21:508–513.
22. Young RC, Walton LA, Ellenberg SS, et al. Adjuvant therapy in stage I and stage II epithelial ovarian cancer. Results of two prospective randomized trials. *N Engl J Med*. 1990;322:1021–1027.
23. Fisher B, Sherman B, Rockette H, et al. L-Phenylalanine mustard (L-PAM) in the management of premenopausal patients with primary breast cancer: lack of association of disease-free survival with depression of ovarian function. *Cancer*. 1979;44:847–857.
24. Begleiter A., Lam H-YP, Grover J, et al. Evidence for active transport of melphalan by two amino acid carriers in L5178Y lymphoblasts in vitro. *Cancer Res*. 1979;39:353–359.
25. Greig NH, Momma S, Sweeney DJ, et al. Facilitated transport of melphalan at the rat blood-brain barrier by the large neutral amino acid carrier system. *Cancer Res*. 1987;47:1571–1576.
26. The French Cooperative Group on Chronic Lymphocytic Leukemia. A randomized clinical trial of chlorambucil versus COP in chronic lymphocytic leukemia. *Blood*. 1990;75:1422–1425.
27. Wiltshaw E. Chlorambucil in the treatment of primary adenocarcinoma of the ovary. *J Obstet Bynecol Br Commonw*. 1964;72:586–594.
28. Portlock CS, Fischer DS, Cadman E, et al. High-dosepulsechlorambucilinadvanced, low-grade non-Hodgkins lymphoma. *Cancer Treat Rep*. 1987;71:1029–1031.
29. Leoni LM, Bailey B, Reifert J, et al. Bendamustine (Treanda) displays a distinct pattern of cytotoxicity and unique mechanistic features compared with other alkylating agents. *Clin Cancer Res*. 2008;14:309–317.
30. Goncalves A., Brand AC, Viret F, et al. High dose alkylating agents with autologous hematopoietic stem cell support and trastuzumab in ERB-B2 overexpressing metastatic breast cancer: a feasibility study. *Anticancer Res*. 2005;25:663–667.
31 De Jonge ME, Mathot RA, Van Dam SM, et al. Extremely high exposures to thiotepa in an obese patient receiving high-dose cyclophosphamide, thiotepa and carboplatin. *Cancer Chemother Pharmacol*. 2002;50:251–255.
32. Gutin PH, Levi JA, Wiernik PH, Walker MD. Treatment of malignant meningeal disease with intrathecal thioTEPA: a phase II study. *Cancer Treat Rep*. 1977;61:885–887.
33. Ng SF, Waxman DJ. N,N',N"-triethylenethiphosphoramide (thio-TEPA) oxygenation by constitutive hepatic P-450 enzymes and modulation of drug metabolism and clearance in vivo by P450-inducing agents. *Cancer Res*. 1991;51: 2340–2345.

52 Drugs That Target DNA Topoisomerases

Eric H. Rubin, MD ■ William N. Hait, MD, PhD

Drugs that target topoisomerases represent some of the most active drugs in the oncology armamentarium. These drugs are active agents in the treatment of a wide variety a cancers, and they share a similar spectrum of untoward side effects that limit their therapeutic index. The epipodophyllotoxins, DNA intercalators, and camptothecins are considered together in this chapter because they share a common cellular target: DNA topoisomerases. Accordingly, mutations in topoisomerases can cause resistance to several drugs of unrelated structure.

Topoisomerase Biology

Double-stranded DNA can be too loosely wound (negatively supercoiled) or too tightly wound (positively supercoiled) relative to its lowest energy state. Protein complexes that track along DNA, such as transcription or replication complexes, produce alterations in DNA supercoiling that are regulated by ubiquitous topoisomerase enzymes.[1] The genomes of prokaryotes typically encode four topoisomerases. One of these enzymes, DNA gyrase, is the target of several antimicrobial agents, including the quinolone antibiotics.[2] The genomes of eukaryotes typically encode four or more topoisomerases, with the human genome currently known to contain five family members: topoisomerase I, topoisomerase IIα and IIβ, and topoisomerase IIIα and IIIβ. Topoisomerases are attractive therapeutic targets in that they share many of the characterisitics of "oncogenes": overexpression and gene amplification occur in cancer versus normal cells,[3,4] and overexpression confers genomic instability.[5]

Although the relative roles of these enzymes in mammalian DNA metabolism are not yet clear, loss of topoisomerase I, IIβ (and probably IIα), or IIIα is lethal, indicating that each enzyme serves an irreplaceable function.[6] Mice lacking topoisomerase IIIβ are viable, but have histologic lesions in multiple organs and a shortened lifespan.[7] Studies in both yeast and mammalian cells show that topoisomerase I is found in transcription and replication complexes, suggesting that topoisomerase I commonly provides the "DNA swivel" required for DNA tracking by ribonucleic acid (RNA) and DNA polymerases.[8,9]

By contrast, topoisomerase II enzymes seem to function predominantly after replication, during separation of daughter DNA strands or remodeling of chromatin structure.[10–13] Topoisomerase II enzymes also function in the decatenation cell cycle checkpoint.[14] Distinct roles for the IIα and IIβ isoforms of topoisomerase II are not yet known, although these enzymes differ in nuclear localization[15] and cell cycle regulation.[16]

Less is known regarding the role of topoisomerase III isozymes in mammalian cells. However, in yeast, topoisomerase III associates with Sgs1,[17] a protein homologous to the Bloom and Werner syndrome proteins, which are helicases involved in genomic stability and aging, respectively.[18,19] In addition, loss of the murine topoisomerase IIIβ enzyme results in aneuploidy in sperm and loss of fertility.[7]

Topoisomerases are also distinguishable biochemically. For example, topoisomerase I and III are classified as type I enzymes because they alter DNA supercoiling by cleaving a single-strand of the DNA duplex. The topoisomerase II enzymes are classified as type II enzymes and cleave both strands. Detailed structural and biochemical data have clarified the mechanisms by which these enzymes accomplish the seemingly treacherous task of breaking and then resealing DNA. In type I and II enzymes alike, a hydroxyl group in a tyrosine residue is used in a transesterification reaction involving the DNA phosphate backbone. The result is the formation of a transient reaction intermediate involving the covalent linkage of the protein to the DNA backbone. The topoisomerase–DNA link can be at the 3′ end of the DNA break (topoisomerase I), or at the 5′ end of the break (topoisomerase II). Based on data obtained from structural analyses of topoisomerase I–DNA complexes, a model of the cleavage of DNA by the enzyme has been proposed (Fig. 52-1).[20] In the covalent topo isomerase I–DNA complex, the 5′ end of the nick is not bound tightly by the enzyme, with rotation of the nicked strand around the noncleaved strand resulting in alterations in DNA supercoiling.[20]

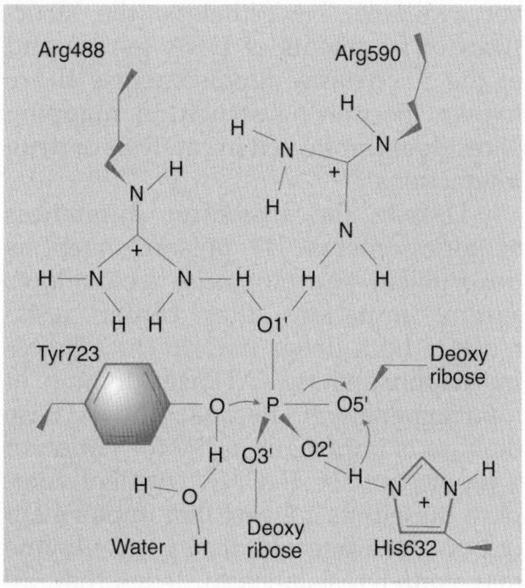

Figure 52-1 ■ Model of DNA strand cleavage by topoisomerase I. Formation of the covalent bond involving tyrosine 723 is shown, as are other active site amino acids believed to function in the cleavage process. *Source*: From Ref. 20.

In contrast to type I enzymes, type II enzymes function as homodimers or heterodimers (eg, IIα:IIβ) and require adenosine triphosphate (ATP) for catalysis. Type II enzyme catalysis involves binding of one DNA duplex by the dimer, followed by formation of an ATP-dependent clamp around another DNA duplex (Fig. 52-2).[21] Cleavage of the first duplex occurs in conjunction with, or after formation of, the clamp. Passage of the second duplex through the gap in the first duplex alters DNA topology. The clamp mechanism minimizes the risk of improper resealing of the transient double-strand break made by the enzyme.

How Drugs "Poison" Topoisomerases

Many organisms synthesize compounds that convert topoisomerases into DNA-damaging agents, thereby exploiting the toxic effects inherent in a reaction that requires breaking and resealing DNA. Currently, topoisomerase I and topoisomerase IIα and IIβ are known to be targets of naturally occurring plant alkaloids and yeast fermentation products. Similar targeting of topoisomerase III is likely but not yet proven.[22]

Elegant studies performed in the genetically tractable organism *Saccharomyces cerevisiae* indicate that topoisomerase-targeting compounds kill cells not simply by inhibiting topoisomerase

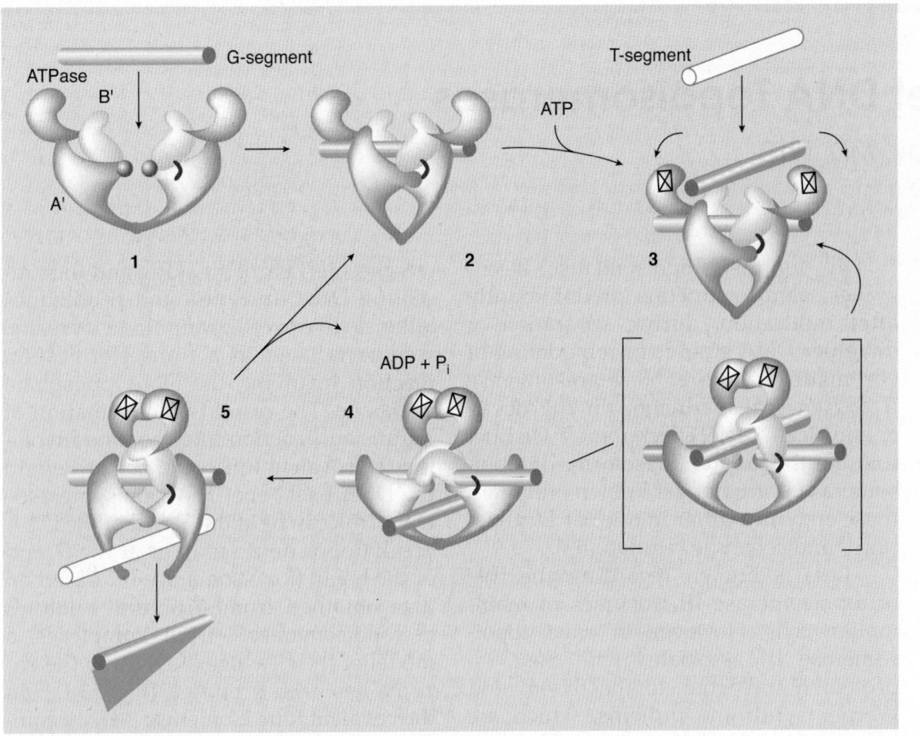

Figure 52-2 Model of topoisomerase II catalysis. The DNA duplex that undergoes cleavage is called the G-segment (for "gate") and the other DNA duplex is called the T-segment (for "transported"). Binding of the G-segment (step 1) results in a conformational change (step 2) in which the active-site tyrosines (shown as purple circles) are brought into position for cleavage of the G-segment. After binding of the T-segment and adenosine triphosphate (ATP), a "clamp" is formed around the T-segment (step 3), which is then transported though the gap in the G-segment (step 4). Subsequently, the G-strand is religated and the T-segment is released (step 5). After ATP hydrolysis, the "clamp" is opened, and the cycle can repeat. *Source*: Modified from Ref. 21.

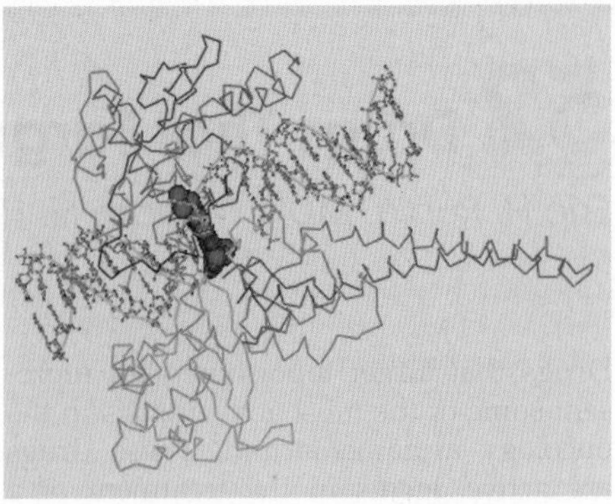

Figure 52-3 Structure of a topotecan–DNA–topoisomerase I covalent complex. The image was generated using iMol software (<http://www.pirx.com/iMol/>) and coordinates from Staker et al.,[26] obtained from the Protein Data Bank (<http://www.rcsb.org/pdb/>). The DNA duplex is shown in yellow, with topoisomerase I shown in wire format. The drug molecule (topotecan) is in the center of the figure and is shown as green and red spheres.

catalysis, but by stabilizing the normally transient reaction intermediate in which the enzyme is covalently linked to DNA.[23] Thus, these compounds are often called topoisomerase "poisons"[24] and either increase the rate of DNA cleavage or decrease the rate of DNA religation by the topoisomerase. Topoisomerase poisons are believed to bind to DNA, the topoisomerase, or both molecules concurrently at or near the region of the enzyme involved in the formation of the DNA–protein covalent linkage.

Many topoisomerase poisons, such as the anthracyclines and actinomycin D, are relatively planar hydrophobic compounds that bind to DNA with high affinity by intercalation, which involves stacking of the compound between adjacent base pairs. Nonintercalating DNA binders can also poison topoisomerases, exemplified by the effects of the DNA minor-groove ligand Hoechst 33358 on topoisomerase I.[25] However, DNA binding is neither necessary nor sufficient for topoisomerase poisoning. For example, neither camptothecin nor etoposide bind DNA stably, yet both are potent topoisomerase I and II poisons, respectively.

The crystal structure of a drug–topoisomerase I–DNA complex[26] provided insight into the mechanism of topoisomerase poisoning by anticancer drugs. In this complex, the drug mimics a DNA base pair and stacks into the DNA duplex at the topoisomerase I cleavage site (Fig. 52-3). The stacking prevents religation of the DNA by the enzyme.

Molecular models of topoisomerase II–DNA–drug ternary complexes are not yet available. Nevertheless, the structures of fragments of DNA gyrase and of the *S. cerevisiae* topoisomerase II are known, permitting structural mapping of residues implicated in catalysis or drug interactions.[27,28]

Despite the structural differences of topoisomerase II poisons such as doxorubicin and etoposide (see below), several mutations that confer resistance to both drugs map to the adenosine triphosphatase (ATPase) domain of topoisomerase II. Because the ATPase domain is important in the formation of a topoisomerase II–DNA covalent complex, these data suggest that impairment of DNA cleavage activity by the enzyme may confer resistance to drugs that, although structurally distinct, act by a common mechanism of trapping the covalent topoisomerase II–DNA complex.[29]

A novel mechanism of poisoning topoisomerase II was identified for bisdioxopiperazines, such as ICRF-187.[30] Rather than stabilizing the enzyme–DNA covalent bond, these compounds bind to a region of the enzyme that, in the presence of ATP, forms a circular clamp around DNA. By inhibiting the ATPase activity of the enzyme, these compounds prevent the topoisomerase II clamp from opening, resulting in a unique cytotoxic lesion in DNA.[31]

Although this chapter focuses on drugs that target topoisomerases, several types of natural or induced DNA damage can also poison topoisomerase I or II. For example, abasic sites, which occur frequently in cells, lead to stabilization of both topoisomerase I and II covalent complexes.[32,33] Base mismatches or other DNA structural alterations, such as pyrimidine dimers or platinum adducts, can also poison topoisomerases.[34–36] Incorporation of nucleoside analogues such as cytosine arabinoside[37] and 2′-deoxy-2′,2′difluorocytidine (gemcitabine)[38] induces topoisomerase I-mediated DNA cleavage, suggesting that topoisomerase I may be involved in the anticancer activity of these drugs. Oxidative stress may also poison topoisomerase II, either through oxidative DNA damage or perhaps by directly modifying the enzyme.[39]

Cellular Response to Topoisomerase-Mediated DNA Damage

The creation of drug-stabilized topoisomerase–DNA covalent complexes (ternary complexes) is not sufficient to kill cells. For example, treatment of cells with the DNA polymerase inhibitor aphidicolin protects cells from the cytotoxicity induced by brief exposure to either topoisomerase I or II poisons.[40] The effect is more pronounced for topoisomerase I poisons. Because topoisomerase I cleavage complexes involve single-strand breaks, whereas topoisomerase II cleavage complexes involve double-strand breaks, Hsiang and colleagues were led to propose a replication fork collision model for topoisomerase I poisons (Fig. 52-4).[41] In that model, replication forks generate lethal double-strand breaks upon encountering drug–topoisomerase I–DNA ternary complexes. A similar phenomenon likely occurs upon collision of RNA polymerase II transcription complexes with topoisomerase I–DNA–drug ternary complexes.[42] This transcription-based effect may explain the finding that camptothecins may also kill non S-phase cells.[43,44]

Certain DNA repair processes also determine the cytotoxic effects of topoisomerase poisons. Hypersensitivity to both topoisomerase I and II drugs occurs in cells in which repair of DNA double-strand breaks is defective.[45] Furthermore, cells lacking proteins involved in transcription-coupled DNA repair, such as in Cockayne syndrome, are specifically hypersensitive to topoisomerase I poisons.[46] Loss of proteins involved in DNA damage checkpoints, such as the ataxia telangiectasia or Chk1 proteins, also confers hypersensitivity to topoisomerase I poisons.[47,48] In addition, Nash and colleagues identified a tyrosyl–DNA phosphodiesterase that can hydrolyze the tyrosine–DNA phosphodiester bonds that link topoisomerase I molecules to DNA, suggesting that this phosphodiesterase is involved in the repair of topoisomerase-mediated DNA damage.[49] Indeed, overexpression of this protein was shown to reduce the DNA damage produced by treating cells with topoisomerase-targeting agents such as camptothecin or etoposide.[50] Topoisomerases are also modified in response to DNA damage. Those modifications include ubiquitination and conjugation to the small ubiquitin-like protein SUMO.[51–54] Ubiquitination of topoisomerases may lead to proteasome-mediated degradation, which by removing the target may limit the DNA damage produced by topoisomerase-targeting drugs.

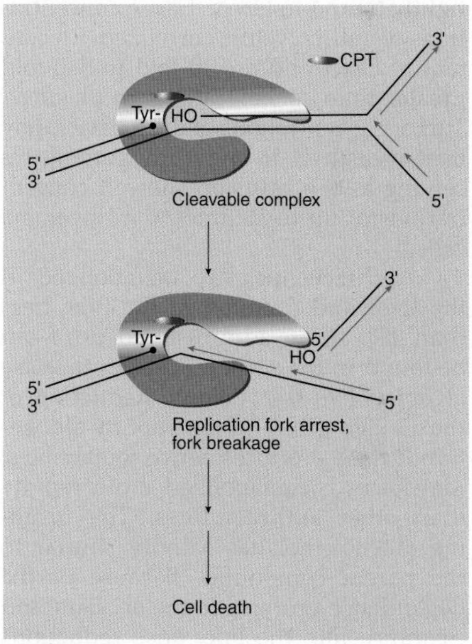

Figure 52-4 ■ Generation of DNA double-strand breaks from collision of a replication fork with a camptothecin–DNA–topoisomerase I ternary complex. The covalent linkage of the active site tyrosine (Tyr) with the cleaved DNA strand is shown, as is the presence of a 5′hydroxyl (HO) on the cleaved strand. *Source*: Courtesy of Li TK and Liu LF.

In addition to causing cell death, topoisomerase-mediated DNA damage may, under certain circumstances, lead to neoplastic transformation. Epidemiologic studies link etoposide therapy to secondary leukemias,[55] and in vitro studies demonstrate that both topoisomerase I and II can mediate illegitimate recombination as a result of incorrect ligation of a DNA strand to an enzyme-linked DNA break.[56,57] Furthermore, the 11q23 chromosomal translocation involving the *mll* oncogene that occurs commonly in leukemias occurring secondary to chemotherapy and childhood leukemias contains a breakpoint sequence that is a preferred topoisomerase II cleavage site.[58] Thus, it is possible that topoisomerase II is involved in leukemogenesis. Topoisomerase I was also found to be involved in a chimeric fusion protein that includes the nucleoporin gene *NUP98*, created by a t(11;20)(p15;q11) translocation.[59] This translocation is associated with secondary myelodysplastic syndromes; forced expression of the fusion protein confers a leukemogenic phenotype,[60] suggesting that topoisomerase I may also be involved in neoplastic transformation.

Mechanisms of Resistance to Topoisomerase Targeting

Resistance to topoisomerase-targeting drugs can involve alterations in drug accumulation, in the target topoisomerase, or in the response to topoisomerase-mediated DNA damage. Many topoisomerase-targeting drugs are natural products for which cellular efflux mechanisms exist. For example, several members of the ATP-binding cassette (ABC) family—including the Mdr1 (*ABCB1*), Mrp- (*ABCC1*), and Mrp-2 (*ABCC2*) gene products—produce resistance to certain topoisomerase II poisons through drug efflux.[61–63] Similarly, a variety of transporters have been implicated in resistance to the topoisomerase I-targeting camptothecins, most notably the ABC protein Bcrp (also known as Mxr and *ABCG2*).[64] Bcrp is widely expressed in normal human tissues, including the placenta, brain, small intestine, testis, ovary, colon, and liver.[65] Increased expression of Bcrp was implicated in resistance to induction therapy in children with acute myeloid leukemia.[66] Overexpression of Bcrp confers resistance to some, but not all, camptothecin analogues.[67]

Altered topoisomerases have been described in many drug-resistant cell lines. Those alterations include point mutations in a topoisomerase[68] and defects in topoisomerase phosphorylation—the latter having been implicated in the regulation of catalytic activity.[69,70] For both topoisomerase I and topoisomerase II, a single-point mutation can confer resistance to structurally distinct drugs. This phenomenon underscores the mechanistic similarity of topoisomerase-targeting drugs and is often called "atypical" multidrug resistance.[71]

Alteration of topoisomerase II localization by mutation or other mechanisms represents another resistance-conferring alteration.[72–76] In some of these cases, topoisomerase II localizes aberrantly in the cytoplasm, producing resistance by minimizing the possibility of drug-induced topoisomerase II–DNA complex formation. Similar resistance mechanisms may exist for topoisomerase I, because a change from a nucleolar localization to a diffuse nuclear localization of yeast topoisomerase I is associated with resistance to camptothecin.[77] Reduction of topoisomerase levels by increased ubiquitination and proteasome-dependent protein degradation has also been implicated as a drug-resistance mechanism.[52,78,79]

Resistance mechanisms that exist "downstream" from the formation of topoisomerase–DNA cleavage complexes also need to be considered. As discussed earlier, certain DNA repair enzymes may process topoisomerase-mediated DNA damage. Loss of proteins involved in the repair of DNA double-strand breaks results in hypersensitivity to topoisomerase I- and II-targeting drugs alike.[80] By contrast, overexpression of the DNA repair protein Xrcc1 confers resistance to camptothecins but not to topoisomerase II-targeting drugs.[81] Recently, Bond and colleagues identified a polymorphism in the *hdm2* promoter (SNP309) that increase susceptibility to a variety of cancers including breast, soft-tissue sarcomas, and non-Hodgkin lymphomas,[82] and Nayak and Hait found that this polymorphism can produce resistance to certain topoisomerase poisons.[83]

Intercalating Drugs That Target Topoisomerases

The Anthracyclines

History ■ The anthracyclines are fermentation products of *Streptomyces peucetius* var. *caesius* and were originally described as antitumor antibiotics. Daunomycin and doxorubicin were first shown to have antitumor activity in the 1960s.[84,85] Subsequently, a search for less-toxic derivatives identified additional drugs that have added to the repertoire available to the modern oncologist. Today, the anthracyclines constitute several of our most effective anticancer regimens.

Structure–Activity Relationships ■ Figure 52-5 shows the structures of the clinically used anthracyclines. The compounds consist of a planar, hydrophobic tetracycline ring linked to a daunosamine sugar through a glycosidic linkage. All drugs are positively charged at physiologic pH, favoring intercalation into DNA. In addition, the anthracyclines possess quinone moieties on adjacent rings that allow them to participate in electron-transfer reactions and to generate oxygen free radicals.

Daunomycin and doxorubicin differ by only a single hydroxyl at position C14, yet have distinct spectra of antitumor activity. Idarubicin is a semisynthetic derivative of daunomycin (4-demethoxydaunorubicin) lacking the 4-methoxy group present on the parent compound. Epirubicin is an epimer of doxorubicin, having the C4′ hydroxyl group on the amino sugar in the equatorial rather than the axial position, which increases lipophilicity as compared with doxorubicin. A liposome-encapsulated formulation of doxorubicin (Doxil) was approved for use in acquired immunodeficiency syndrome (AIDS)–related Kaposi sarcoma, multiple myeloma, ovarian cancer, and outside of the United States, breast cancer. Despite differences in the pharmacokinetics of Doxil and doxorubicin (eg, Doxil has a lower volume of distribution and greater area under the curve [AUC]), major differences in activity have not been seen between Doxil and conventional formulations of doxorubicin.

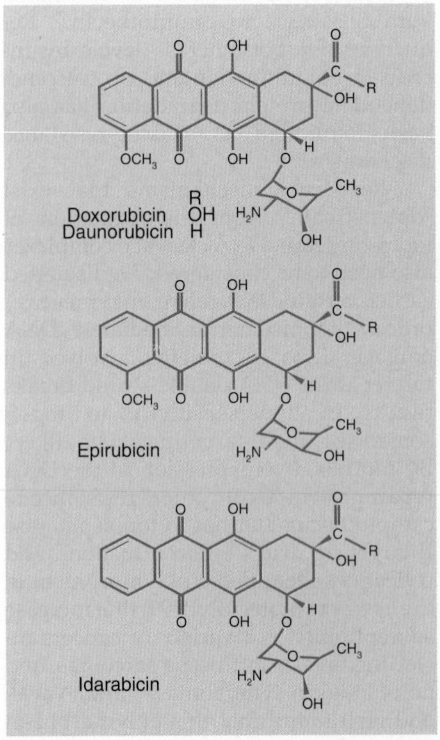

Figure 52-5 ■ Structures of anthracyclines.

Mechanism of Action ■ The anthracyclines are highly reactive in solution and create a panoply of effects on biologic systems. Much of their cytotoxicity results from topoisomerase II poisoning (see above). Anthracyclines also intercalate into double-stranded DNA and produce structural changes that interfere with DNA and RNA synthesis. Before the effects of the anthracyclines on topoisomerase II were fully appreciated, it was their ability to participate in oxidation and reduction reactions that was believed to produce cytotoxicity. Anthracyclines generate reactive oxygen species—including oxygen free radicals, hydroxyl radicals, and hydrogen peroxide—that damage DNA, messenger RNA (mRNA), proteins, and lipids. The peroxidation of lipids may account for much of the cardiac toxicity characteristic of these drugs.[86,87]

Clinical Pharmacology ■ ***Dose and Administration*** ■ Anthracyclines can be given at varying doses and schedules. Lower weekly doses or low-dose continuous infusions over 96 h result in decreased toxicity without adverse effects on efficacy.[88] Lower doses produce lower peak plasma concentrations that are believed to correlate with decreased cardiac toxicity. In contrast, efficacy correlates best with AUC. Changing the dose and schedule from a higher-dose bolus to a lower-dose continuous infusion increases the incidence and severity of mucositis but decreases myelosuppression, nausea, and vomiting. Most clinicians reduce the dose of anthracyclines by 50% and 75% in patients having plasma bilirubin concentrations of 1.2–3.0 mg/dL and 3.1–5.0 mg/dL, respectively.

As a single agent, doxorubicin (Adriamycin, Rubex) is given intravenously at a recommended dose of 40–75 mg/m^2. Care should be taken to avoid extravasation. Doxorubicin is indicated in the treatment of many solid tumors (eg, breast, sarcoma, bladder, thyroid, gastric, ovary, and small cell lung cancers) and in the treatment of Hodgkin and non-Hodgkin lymphoma, as well as in the treatment of acute lymphoblastic and myeloblastic leukemias. A liposomal encapsulation of doxorubicin (Doxil)[89] changes the Pharmaco/Kinetics. In this formulation, the liposomes are coated with polyethylene glycol to reduce clearance by the mononuclear phagocyte system. The liposomal formulation of doxorubicin may enhance accumulation of the drug at metastatic cancer sites as a result of alterations in tumor vasculature.[90]

Daunorubicin (Cerubidine) is given intravenously at a recommended dose of 30–60 mg/m^2 daily for 3 days. Care should be taken to avoid extravasation. Daunorubicin is indicated for the treatment of acute lymphocytic and myelogenous leukemias. It has limited activity against solid tumors and non-Hodgkin lymphoma.

Idarubicin (Idamycin) is given intravenously at a recommended dose of 12 mg/m^2 daily for 3 days in combination with cytosine arabinoside for the treatment of acute myelogenous leukemia.

Epirubicin (Ellence) is given intravenously at a recommended dose of 100–120 mg/m^2 by bolus injection every 3 weeks. It is a vesicant and must be given with caution. A variety of other schedules have been evaluated, including an intravenous injection of 40–50 mg/m^2 on 2 consecutive days.[91]

Following intravenous administration, anthracyclines are rapidly cleared from the plasma, where they reach all tissues except the brain and testes. Approximately 75% of the drug remaining in the plasma is bound to plasma proteins.[92] Within tissues, the drugs are tightly bound to DNA. Tissue concentrations of anthracycline correlate with content of DNA and are 10-fold to 500-fold greater than concentrations in plasma.[93] Tumor concentrations of drug have rarely been measured. In one study, patients receiving a 96-h infusion showed concentrations of up to 10 μmol/L in myeloma cells.[94]

Anthracyclines are metabolized in the liver and excreted in the bile. Less than 10% of an administered dose can be found in the urine, except in the case of epirubicin (see below). Reduction of the 13-keto group to the enol by aldoketoreductase produces active metabolites. Idarubicin is metabolized more rapidly than other anthracyclines. The resulting idarubicinol has activity similar to the parent compound. Because of the dependence on hepatic metabolism and clearance into the bile, dose reductions are recommended for patients with impaired hepatic function.

Epirubicin is conjugated with glucuronide on the 4′ equatorial hydroxyl and excreted in the bile. Ten percent of an administered dose of epirubicin is found in the urine as epirubicinol and as conjugates of the glucuronide aglycone.[95] Its metabolism is decreased in the presence of liver metastases, with or without hepatic dysfunction.[96]

Anthracyclines are eliminated primarily by biliary excretion and to a lesser extent through the kidneys. Disappearance of anthracyclines from the plasma is multiphasic. A rapid initial phase of redistribution is followed by prolonged 0-phase and y-phase terminal elimination. The prolonged terminal phase accounts for most of the AUC and results in sustained therapeutic concentrations in the plasma following a bolus injection.[92]

Anthracyclines produce myelosuppression, mucositis, alopecia, nausea, vomiting, and increased skin pigmentation. Myelosuppression is the acute dose-limiting toxicity. After administration of a bolus dose, the white blood cell count begins to fall in 7 days. The count reaches a nadir at 10–14 days and recovers 1–2 weeks later. Thrombocytopenia and anemia are less severe. Dose- and schedule-related toxicities include mucositis, nausea and vomiting, diarrhea, and alopecia. Erythema at the injection site ("flare reaction") is benign, in contrast to extravasation, which can lead to serious local complications such as severe necrosis of surrounding tissues. Inflammation at sites of previous radiation ("radiation recall") can lead to unanticipated complications, including pericarditis, pleural effusion, and skin rash. The incidence of nausea and vomiting, alopecia, and cardiac toxicity is less with epirubicin than with doxorubicin. Cardiac effects occur at higher doses, and congestive heart failure has been reported less frequently. Cardiac toxicity, manifested by arrhythmias, tachycardia, and congestive heart failure, is described in detail below.

Activity ■ The anthracyclines are indicated for use against both solid and hematologic malignancies. Doxorubicin has the broadest spectrum of activity. Its introduction in the 1960s and its incorporation into combination regimens led to curative treatments for non-Hodgkin lymphoma (cyclophosphamide, hydroxydaunomycin [doxorubicin], Oncovin [vincristine], and prednisone: CHOP) and less-toxic treatments for Hodgkin's disease (Adriamycin, bleomycin, vinblastine, dacarbazine: ABVD). Doxorubicin is also active against Ewing, osteogenic, and other soft-tissue sarcomas.

Doxorubicin is one of the most active agents in the treatment of breast cancer. Single agent activity is similar to that of paclitaxel[97] and is comparable with combination chemotherapy in patients with metastatic disease.[98,99] Also, in the adjuvant setting, doxorubicin-containing regimens are more active than are non-anthracyclinecontaining regimens.[100] Although this effect may be limited to those patients whose cancers overexpress Her-2/NEU.[101] Doxorubicin has limited but demonstrable activity against thyroid cancer, ovarian cancer, and small cell lung cancer. Finally, it has also demonstrated activity against endometrial carcinoma; cancer of the testis, prostate, cervix, and head and neck; and multiple myeloma.

Daunomycin is used mostly for the treatment of acute lymphocytic and myelocytic leukemias. Although it has some activity against pediatric solid tumors, it has little activity against adult solid malignancies. Idarubicin is used predominantly in the treatment of adult acute myelogenous leukemia.

Epirubicin has broad-spectrum antitumor activity in preclinical models. In the clinic, it has activity against melanoma; breast, colorectal, renal, gastric, pancreatic, hepatocellular, ovarian, and lung cancers; and soft-tissue sarcomas. In addition, it is part of active regimens against Hodgkin disease and non-Hodgkin lymphoma.[92] Epirubicin is indicated in the adjuvant treatment of breast cancer, where it has activity similar to that of doxorubicin.[102]

Amrubicin, a fully synthetic 9-amino anthracycline, is approved and marketed in Japan for the treatment of lung cancer. A recent randomized phase 2 study found that amrubicin was superior to topotecan in 60 relapsed small cell lung cancer patients in terms of response rates.[103]

Additional anthracyclines are in clinical development including aclarubicin, valrubicin, and zorubicin. All appear to share a similar mechanism of action in terms of topoisomerase 2 poisoning.

Cardiac Toxicity ■ All anthracyclines produce cardiac damage that can result in serious and even life-threatening complications.[104] Cardiac toxicity is more common with doxorubicin and daunorubicin than with epirubicin or idarubicin. Acutely, anthracyclines can produce arrhythmias and ST-T wave changes that are usually not serious and that resolve spontaneously. In rare cases, a syndrome resembling acute pericarditis myocarditis can occur. The syndrome is characterized by a fall in cardiac ejection fraction, conduction abnormalities, pericardial effusion, and congestive heart failure.

Congestive heart failure from congestive cardiomyopathy is more common and of greater clinical significance than are the acute cardiac effects. Mortality rates of more than 30% have been reported.[105–107] The anthracyclines produce myocardial damage by several mechanisms. Perhaps the most important is generation of reactive oxygen species during electron-transfer from the semiquinone to quinone moieties of the molecule. The generation of hydrogen peroxide and the peroxidation of myocardial lipids contribute to myocardial damage. The heart may be uniquely susceptible to cardiac damage from oxidation reactions. For example, the low activity of catalase in cardiac tissue renders the myocardium dependent on glutathione peroxidase for detoxification of hydrogen peroxide. Anthracyclines deplete glutathione, thereby leaving the heart vulnerable to oxidative attack.

The incidence of cardiomyopathy is related to both cumulative dose and schedule of administration. Cardiac toxicity is best correlated with peak plasma concentration of the parent drug rather than with the AUC. Greater cumulative doses of doxorubicin can be given to patients receiving low-dose continuous infusions than to those receiving higher-dose bolus injections every 3–4 weeks. Predisposition to cardiac damage includes a previous history of heart disease, hypertension, radiation to the mediastinum, age younger than 4 years, and prior use of anthracyclines or other cardiac toxins.[104,106] The addition of trastuzumab (Herceptin) to either epirubicin or doxorubicin produced an increase in congestive heart failure at cumulative anthracycline doses below those anticipated to produce cardiac damage.[108]

Table 52-1 lists the incidence of clinically detectable congestive heart failure when doxorubicin is given at doses of 40–75 mg/m^2 as a bolus injection every 3–4 weeks. When doxorubicin is given by a low-dose weekly regimen (10–20 mg/m^2/wk) or by slow continuous infusion over 96 h, cumulative doses of more than 500 mg/m^2 can be given.[109] However, careful monitoring of cardiac function is still required and should increase in frequency at higher cumulative doses. Doses of daunorubicin below 1000 mg/m^2 (equivalent to 550 mg/m^2 doxorubicin) are considered safe. Doses of idarubicin below 290 mg/m^2 do not produce clinical congestive heart failure despite changes in cardiac ejection.[110] Epirubicin appears to be as active as doxorubicin and has less cardiac toxicity.[111]

Cardiac function can be monitored during treatment with anthracyclines by electrocardiography, echocardiography, or radionuclide scans.[112] Numerous studies demonstrate the danger of embarking on anthracycline therapy in

Table 52-1 ■ **Incidence of Clinically Detectable Congestive Heart Failure as a Function of Cumulative Doxorubicin Dose**

Cumulative Dose (mg/m^2)	Incidence of Congestive Heart Failure (%)
<350	<1
550	7
600	15
700	30

patients with underlying cardiac disease (eg, a baseline left ventricular ejection fraction of less than 50%) and of continuing therapy after a documented decrease in ejection fraction by more than 10% (if this decrease falls below the lower limit of normal) or by 20% regardless of the absolute value.

Certain drugs may abrogate the damaging effects of anthracyclines on the heart. For example, dexrazoxane (ADR-529) is a metal chelator that decreases the myocardial toxicity of doxorubicin in breast cancer patients and has been approved for that use by the U.S. Food and Drug Administration (FDA).[113] Dexrazoxane chelates iron and copper, thereby interfering with the redox reactions that generate free radicals and damage myocardial lipids. The cardiac toxicity of liposomal doxorubicin appears to be less than that of the free compound. For example, in a phase III trial, cardiac toxicity from doxorubicin appeared at a cumulative dose of about 500 mg/m^2, whereas doses of up to 600 mg/m^2 of the liposomal compound were not associated with a significant change in left ventricular ejection fraction.[114] This finding is consistent with retrospective analyses in which median cumulative doses of liposomal doxorubicin ranging from 465 to 1700 mg/m^2 were not found to produce significant cardiac toxicity and confirms an earlier phase II trial.[115]

Mechanisms of Resistance ■ The general mechanisms of resistance to topoisomerase poisoning are covered above. The resistance of cancer cells to anthracyclines has received enormous attention.[116] Several plausible mechanisms exist, including decreased drug accumulation because of transport by P-glycoprotein, the *MDR1* gene product, and Mrp-1, the *ABCC1* (formerly *MRP1*) gene product. Both are members of the ATP-binding cassette family that includes *CFTR*, the gene implicated in cystic fibrosis. Additional mechanisms of resistance include downregulation of or mutations in topoisomerase II,[68] increases in drug-neutralizing species, such as glutathione or glutathione transferase,[117] mutations in *TP53*,[118] and overexpression of antiapoptotic molecules such as Bcl-2.[119] Attempts to reverse resistance to the anthracyclines with multidrug resistance modulatorshave had limited success.[120]

Recent attempts have been made to predict increased sensitivity to anthracyclines. Overexpression of topoisomerase 2 alpha has been suggested as a strong biomarker of response in patients with HER-2 positive breast cancer. However, these data have been confounded by the possibility that HER-2 amplification per se is predictive of response and that both topoisomerase amplification and deletion had equivalent predictive values in terms of both relapse-free and overall survival.[121] The hypothesis that topoisomerase 2 overexpression predicts sensitivity to anthracylines is supported by results obtained in the the neoadjuvant setting where overexpressin of topoisomerase 2α was predicted of pathological complete response.[122] In contrast Bartlett et al reported that a combination of normal expression of epidermal growth factor family members (HER1, HER2, and HER3) appeared to predict improved overall survival, and that overexpression of topoisomerase II or Ki67 did not demonstrate clear predictive value in this retrospective evaluation.[123]

The Anthracenediones

Mitoxantrone ■ *History* ■ A search for anthracycline analogues with less cardiac toxicity identified mitoxantrone, the most active compound in the anthracenedione series.[124] The antitumor spectrum of mitoxantrone is more limited than that of doxorubicin. Early clinical trials demonstrated significant differences from the anthracyclines in terms of spectrum of activity and cardiac toxicity.[125] Diminished cardiac toxicity is believed to be caused by the decreased ability of mitoxantrone to participate in the generation of oxygen free radicals. In addition, the potential for extravasation injury and nausea and vomiting is less.

Structure ■ Anthracenediones differ from anthracyclines by the lack of the glycoside substituents present in the latter. Figure 52-6 shows the structure of mitoxantrone, an amino anthracenedione.

Mechanism of Action ■ Mitoxantrone produces double-stranded DNA breaks by poisoning topoisomerase II.[126] Unlike the anthracyclines, mitoxantrone is less likely to participate in one-electron reduction reactions and is therefore less effective in forming free radicals.

Clinical Pharmacology ■ Mitoxantrone is given by intravenous injection at a dose of 12 mg/m^2 for 3 days with cytosine arabinoside to patients with acute myelogenous leukemia and at a dose of 12–14 mg/m^2 once every 3 weeks to patients with solid tumors. The drug is given over a period of 30 min and is rarely associated with extravasation injury.

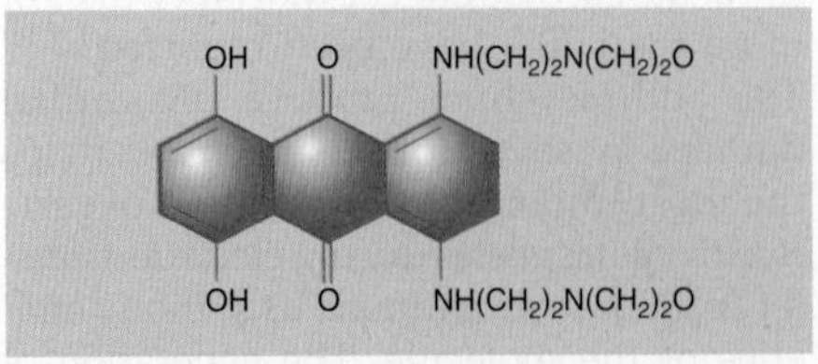

Figure 52-6 ■ Structure of mitoxantrone.

Following intravenous administration, mitoxantrone is rapidly cleared from the plasma. Its clearance is best described by a three-compartment model, with an initial α-phase $t_{1/2}$ of 2–15 min attributable to rapid uptake by formed elements of the blood; a 0 phase of between 17 min and 3 h that is the consequence of redistribution back into the blood and into most tissues of the body; and a terminal $t_{1/2}$ of 5–6 days.[127] As is the case with the anthracyclines, a high proportion of mitoxantrone is found in tissues tightly bound to DNA and in plasma bound to plasma proteins. Mitoxantrone is metabolized to the monocarboxylic and dicarboxylic acids formed by oxidation of the terminal hydroxyl groups on the alkyl side chain. Mitoxantrone may also be conjugated to glutathione.[128] Most of the drug is excreted in the feces, with less than 10% recovered in the urine. Dose reduction is recommended for patients with severe hepatic dysfunction (bilirubin > 3 mg/dL).

Myelosuppression is the dose-limiting side effect. Mucositis, nausea and vomiting, and alopecia are less common than with doxorubicin. Cardiac toxicity is seen at cumulative doses exceeding 160 mg/m^2 in patients not receiving prior therapy with an anthracycline or other cardiotoxic drug.[129]

Activity ■ Mitoxantrone is indicated for the treatment of acute leukemias. It is also used to treat breast and prostate cancer. When used in combination with cytosine arabinoside, response rates in acute myelogenous leukemia range from 50-70%.[130–132]

Mitoxantrone produces an overall response rate of 17-35% in metastatic breast cancer.[133] When used in combination with 5-fluorouracil and leucovorin, the response rate was 45-65%.[134] Mitoxantrone has activity similar to that of doxorubicin in patients with previously treated breast cancer but produces significantly less cardiac toxicity. In combination with prednisone, mitoxantrone had been considered the "gold standard" for the treatment of hormone-refractory prostate cancer, but newer docetaxel-containing regimens may be somewhat better.[135–137]

Pixantrone, a mitoxantrone derivative lacking the 5,8 dihydroxy substitution believed to be responsible for anthracendiione cardiac toxicity, is in clinical trials for both its antitumor and immunosuppressive activities.[138]

Mechanism of Resistance ■ Unlike the anthracyclines, mitoxantrone is not avidly transported by P-glycoprotein or Mrp1.[139] Resistance occurs through alterations in topoisomerase II, and the action of the breast cancer resistance protein (Bcrp/Abcg2).[140]

Actinomycin D (Dactinomycin, Cosmegen) ■ ***History*** ■ Actinomycins were the first antibiotics isolated from the culture broth of *Streptomyces* by Waksman in 1940, and they have activity against gram-positive and gram-negative bacteria and some fungi.[141] Toxicity precluded their use as anti-infection agents. Dactinomycin and other related antibiotics were subsequently found to have both antineoplastic and antibacterial activities.

Structure ■ The actinomycins are "chromopeptides," consisting of a planar phenoxazone actinocin ring (which produces the yellow-red color of the drug), attached to two peptide side chains (Fig. 52-7).

Mechanism of Action ■ Dactinomycin intercalates into DNA. Crystallographic radiography and nuclear magnetic resonance studies revealed that the inter-action between actinomycin D and DNA occurs between the drug and deoxyguanosine.[127–129,142–144] The phenoxazone ring intercalates between adjacent guanine–cytosine bases, and the polypeptide chains extend along the minor groove of the helix, thereby stabilizing the drug–DNA complex.

Although inhibition of DNA-mediated RNA polymerase is believed to be the primary mechanism of action, poisoning of topoisomerase II and the production of double-strand DNA breaks may also be important.[145] DNA breaks can also occur through the generation of free radicals.

Clinical Pharmacology ■ Dactinomycin is administered by intravenous injection or by isolation and perfusion of involved limbs or body areas. The usual adult daily dose is 10–15 µg/kg daily for 5 days, repeated at intervals of 4–6 weeks, or 400–600 µg/m^2 once weekly (maximum 2 mg/week) for 3 weeks. The usual pediatric dose is 10–15 µg/kg or 450 µg/m^2 daily (up to 500 µg/d) for a maximum of 5 days, or a total dose of 2.5 mg/m^2 in divided daily doses over a 7 day period. The dose can usually be repeated every 3–6 weeks. Dactinomycin can also be administered by isolation perfusion at 50 µg/kg for lower extremities or pelvis or 35 µg/kg for upper extremities.

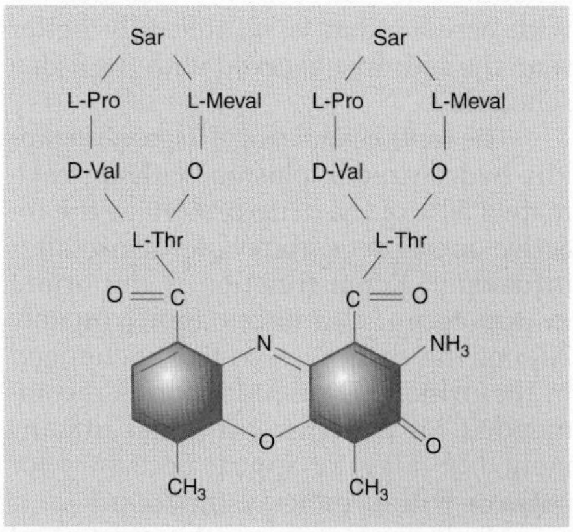

Figure 52-7 ■ Structure of actinomycin D.

Following intravenous administration, dactinomycin is rapidly bound to tissues. It undergoes minimal biotransformation and is found excreted unchanged in the bile and urine. The terminal $t_{1/2}$ is 36 h.[146] Dactinomycin does not cross the blood–brain barrier. Because of limited pharmacologic data, no firm guidelines have been established for using the drug in the presence of hepatic or renal dysfunction.

Myelosuppression occurs approximately 7–10 days following administration. Other important toxicities are mucositis (including esophagitis, ulceration, and proctitis), nausea, vomiting, alopecia, erythema, desquamation, and increased inflammation and pigmentation of skin in irradiated areas ("radiation recall"). Dactinomycin is a severe vesicant and must be administered with caution.

Activity ■ The most important indication for dactinomycin is in the treatment of Wilms tumor, where it is curative in combination with surgery, radiation, and vincristine.[147] It is also effective in the treatment of rhabdomyosarcoma in combination with cyclophosphamide and vincristine (VAC). Other uses include Kaposi sarcoma, sarcoma botryoides, gestational trophoblastic tumors, and testicular cancer.

Mechanism of Resistance ■ Dactinomycin was one of the first drugs shown to be transported by P-glycoprotein.[148] Other mechanisms of resistance remain poorly understood.

Nonintercalating Topoisomerase-Targeting Drugs

The Epipodophyllotoxins

History ■ The epipodophyllotoxins were synthesized in an effort to improve the activity of podophyllotoxin, an anti-microtubule agent that is present in mandrake plant extracts. A subtle structural change (the removal of a methyl group from the pendant aromatic ring of podophyllotoxin) abrogates tubulin binding, but confers the ability to poison topoisomerase II (Fig. 52-8).[149] The epipodophyllotoxins etoposide (VP-16) and teniposide (VM-26) were in clinical use long before their mechanisms of action were understood. Although early studies indicated that cells treated with these drugs exhibited DNA strand breaks,[150] topoisomerase II was not identified as the target until the early 1980s.[151,152]

Structure-Activity Relationships ■ A model for epipodophyllotoxin binding to the topoisomerase II–DNA complex does not yet exist, despite the availability of crystal structures for eukaryotic topoisomerase II[20] and the related prokaryotic DNA gyrase.[28] Nevertheless, the structure of the pendant aromatic ring is critical for activity; alterations in either the substituents of that ring or the stereochemical relationship between it and the tetracyclic ring system can greatly affect the topoisomerase poisoning activity of the drugs.[153] Subtle alterations in the tetracyclic ring may also significantly alter activity, but the glycosidic substituent can be replaced by a variety of other groups without affecting activity.[154] These data led to a model whereby the planar polycyclic component of epipodophyllotoxins stacks into the cleavage site of topoisomerase II–DNA complexes, with the pendant ring binding to either the enzyme or a DNA groove.[155]

Mechanism of Action ■ Epipodophyllotoxins are nonintercalating topoisomerase II poisons.

Etoposide and Etoposide Phosphate ■ ***Clinical Pharmacology*** ■ Etoposide is approved in the United States for the treatment of testicular and small cell lung carcinomas. Etoposide phosphate is more water soluble than etoposide and is a prodrug that is rapidly converted to etoposide in vivo.[156] Intravenous and oral formulations of etoposide and etoposide phosphate are both available. Schedules using prolonged or frequent intermittent dosing appear to be more effective than single-dose regimens.[157] Etoposide is commonly administered as a 1-h intravenous infusion using multiple daily doses of 100 mg/m^2. That dose is associated with a $t_{1/2}$ of about 9 h.[158] Approximately 96% of etoposide is bound to plasma proteins,[159] with a significant proportion of the drug excreted unchanged by the kidney.[160] A 30% dose reduction is recommended in patients with impaired renal function.[161] Although a small percentage of etoposide and etoposide metabolites are excreted in the bile, dose adjustment may not be required in patients with hepatic dysfunction.[162] When administered intravenously, etoposide should be infused slowly, because rapid infusion may result in hypotension. Etoposide phosphate can be administered more rapidly. When given orally, etoposide is often administered daily for 14–21 days. Bioavailability of oral etoposide is approximately 50%. Intestinal P-glycoprotein may efflux etoposide and is thus important in the intestinal absorption of the drug.[163]

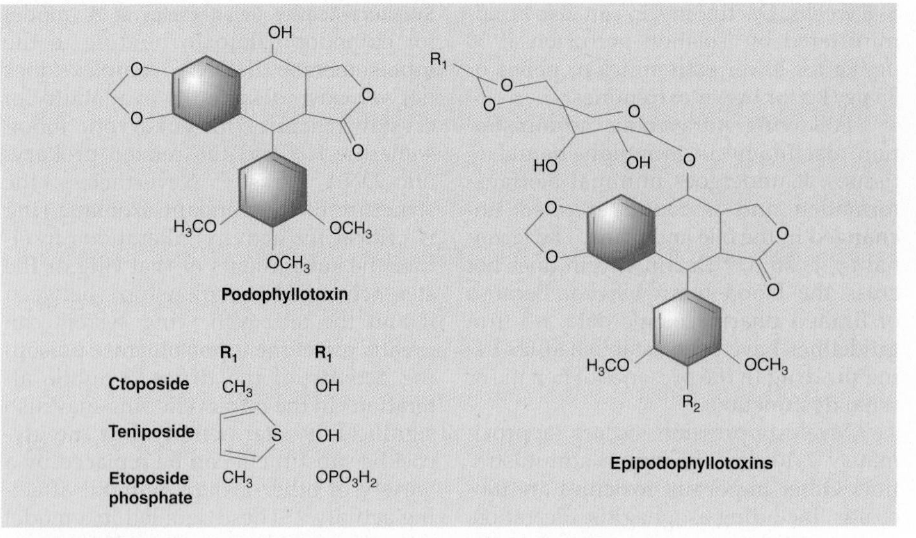

Figure 52-8 Structures of podophyllotoxin and epipodophyllotoxins.

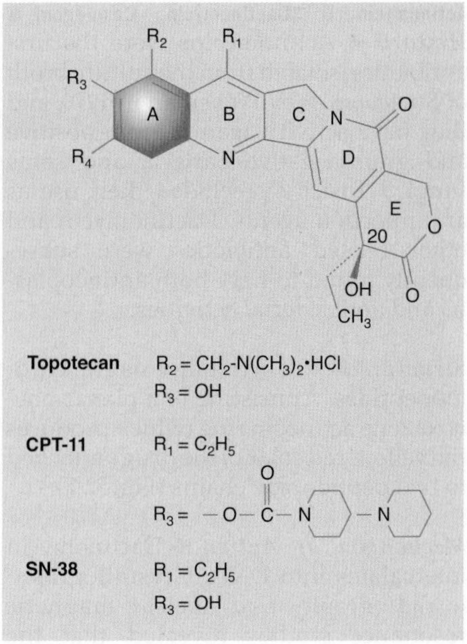

Figure 52-9 Structures of camptothecins.

Myelosuppression is the major toxicity associated with the administration of etoposide, either intravenously or orally. Infrequent toxicities include allergic or other infusional reactions manifested as fever, bronchospasm, and hypotension. Toxicities associated with oral etoposide include nausea, vomiting, and mucositis.

Activity ■ Etoposide is commonly used in combination with other drugs in the treatment of testicular cancer, small cell and nonsmall cell lung cancer, Hodgkin and non-Hodgkin lymphomas, acute myeloid leukemia, gastric cancer, and soft-tissue sarcomas.

Teniposide ■ *Clinical Pharmacology* ■ Teniposide is less commonly used than etoposide. It is approved for the treatment of refractory childhood acute lymphocytic leukemia. Teniposide is also used in the treatment of gliomas.[164] In teniposide, a thiophene group replaces the methyl group present on the glucose moiety of etoposide (Fig. 52-8). The alteration affects both the interaction with topoisomerase II and clinical pharmacology.

Teniposide is a more potent in vitro poison of topoisomerase II than etoposide is.[152] In addition, a greater fraction of teniposide is protein bound relative to etoposide,[165] and renal function is less relevant to teniposide clearance.[166] As is the case with etoposide, myelosuppression is the dose-limiting toxicity for teniposide. Cremophor is used in teniposide formulations, which may explain the greater frequency of hypersensitivity reactions observed with teniposide than with etoposide.[167]

Camptothecins ■ *History* ■ Camptothecin is an alkaloid (molecular weight: 348 kDa) produced by the Chinese tree *Camptotheca acuminata*. It was identified as an antineoplastic agent in the 1960s by Wall and Wani.[168] Early studies with camptothecin indicated that cellular exposure to the drug resulted in DNA breaks; the interaction with topoisomerase I was identified by Hsiang and colleagues in the 1980s.[169] Because the camptothecin alkaloid is relatively insoluble in aqueous solutions, initial clinical trials with camptothecin used a sodium salt derivative.[170,171]

Although responses occurred during those trials, severe myelosuppression or cystitis was frequently observed, and the drug was deemed too toxic for clinical use. Subsequently, it was discovered that, in the salt derivatives, the lactone at position 20 in camptothecin is hydrolyzed to a carboxylic acid. The resultant opening of the lactone ring significantly decreased the activity of the compound.[172] Further development of camptothecins led to two water soluble derivatives, topotecan and irinotecan, that can be delivered as lactones and that are currently approved for the treatment of cancer. Several other camptothecin analogues are in clinical development.

Structure–Activity Relationships ■ Camptothecin is a five-ringed heterocyclic alkaloid (Fig. 52-9). Certain substitutions in the A ring may augment topoisomerase poisoning, presumably by increasing drug binding to the topoisomerase I–DNA cleavage complex.[173] By contrast, substitutions in the E ring often abrogate activity. Indeed, the stereochemistry of C20 in the E ring is critical, with the *R*-isomer inactive.[174] Irinotecan is a prodrug; the piperidino group present at C10 is hydrolyzed by plasma or tissue carboxylesterases to SN-38, which is much more active than irinotecan in inducing topoisomerase I-mediated DNA damage.

Other notable derivation strategies have produced drugs currently in clinical testing:

1. 7 silyl congeners, designed to enhance lipophilicity and to stabilize the E ring lactone[175]
2. 20 esters, designed as prodrugs to prevent hydrolysis of the E ring[176]
3. homocamptothecins, which contain a seven-membered E ring that is less susceptible to hydrolysis in plasma[177]

Mechanism of Action ■ Camptothecins are topoisomerase I poisons that do not bind DNA in the absence of the enzyme.

Topotecan ■ *Clinical Pharmacology* ■ Topotecan is approved for the treatment of ovarian cancer[178] and small cell lung cancer.[179] Typically, it is administered intravenously at a dose of 1.5 mg/m^2 as a 30-min infusion daily for 5 days, followed by a 2-week period of rest. Several alternative dosing schedules have been explored, including a 1-month continuous intravenous infusion.[180,181] Those schedules do not seem to be associated with activity that is significantly better than the activity observed with the 5-day schedule.

The topotecan E ring[182] lactone is rapidly hydrolyzed in plasma, with approximately 50% of the drug present as the inactive open-ring carboxylate 15 min after infusion.[183] Renal function is important in topotecan clearance; approximately 30% of the drug is excreted unchanged in the urine.[184] Dose reduction is recommended for patients with renal impairment, but does not appear necessary for patients with hepatic dysfunction.[185]

Myelosuppression is the most common toxicity observed with daily administration of topotecan. Although severe nonhematologic toxicities are uncommon after administration of topotecan, mucositis was dose-limiting in trials that used a 5-day continuous infusion in patients with leukemia.[186]

Activity ■ Topotecan is active as a single agent in the treatment of ovarian cancer, small cell and nonsmall cell lung cancer, acute myelocytic leukemia, and myelodysplastic syndromes. The combination of topoisomerase I-targeting drugs with other cytotoxic agents was often additive or synergistic in preclinical models, and a variety of drug combination strategies are being investigated in the clinic.[187–189] Combinations of topotecan with topoisomerase II inhibitors or cisplatin have been studied and shown to have activity.[190–192] Topotecan crosses the blood–brain barrier and may be effective in treating brain metastases from a variety of primary cancers.[193]

Irinotecan ■ *Clinical Pharmacology* ■ Irinotecan is usually administered intravenously as a weekly infusion of 125 mg/m^2 for 4 weeks, with a 2-week rest period.[180,194,195] An alternative dosing schedule, commonly used in Europe, uses 90 min infusions of 240–350 mg/m^2 every 3 weeks.[196] Notably, xenograft studies suggest that the schedule of administration may be a critical determinant of efficacy for this drug, and it is not clear that either of these schedules is optimal for antitumor efficacy in patients.[197]

Irinotecan is rapidly metabolized by carboxylesterases to SN-38. Studies suggest that this metabolism may vary among body tissues (including malignant tissues).[198] With irinotecan, as compared with other camptothecins, a relatively greater proportion of SN-38 is maintained in plasma as the active lactone. This phenomenon may be related to stabilization of the SN-38 lactone by human albumin.[199]

In addition to being converted to SN-38, irinotecan is excreted in urine and bile. Biliary excretion of SN-38, following glucuronide conjugation in the liver (at least in part by the *UGT1A1* enzyme isotype), is a major clearance mechanism for this metabolite.[185,200] Reduction in the glucuronidation of SN-38 is associated with an increased risk of severe diarrhea following treatment with irinotecan.[201] Similarly, inherited defects in hepatic glucuronide transferases, which occur in patients with the Gilbert or Crigler-Najjar syndrome, may predispose to severe toxicity with conventional doses of irinotecan.[200,202] Patients with certain *UGT1A1* genetic polymorphisms are also at higher risk for developing diarrhea after irinotecan treatment.[200,203,204] Additional studies of irinotecan and SN-38 suggest that biliary excretion of both the conjugated and unconjugated forms of these drugs may depend upon the Mrp-2 (*ABCC3*) ATP-dependent transporter, which is defective in patients with Dubin-Johnson syndrome.[205]

The most common toxicities associated with weekly infusion schedules of irinotecan are diarrhea and myelosuppression. Two mechanisms are involved in irinotecan-induced diarrhea: (1) acute cholinergic effects produced by inhibition of acetylcholinesterase by the drug,[206] and (2) delayed mucosal cytotoxicity. The former toxicity may be treated by administration of atropine; the latter responds to early and aggressive administration of loperamide.[207]

Activity ■ Irinotecan is active in the treatment of several malignancies, including colorectal cancer,[208,209] small cell and nonsmall cell lung cancer,[210–212] gastric cancer,[213] and cervical cancer.[214]

Selected References

The complete reference list can be found at www.CANCERMEDICINE8.com

1. Wang JC. DNA topoisomerases. *Annu Rev Biochem*. 1996;65:635–692.
4. Tanner M, Isola J, Wiklund T, et al. Topoisomerase IIalpha gene amplification predicts favorable treatment response to tailored and dose-escalated anthracycline-based adjuvant chemotherapy in HER-2/neu-amplified breast cancer: Scandinavian Breast Group Trial 9401. *J Clin Oncol.* 2006;24:2428–2436.
12. Uemura T, Ohkura H, Adachi Y, Morino K, Shiozaki K, Yanagida M. DNA topoisomerase II is required for condensation and separation of mitotic chromosomes in S. pombe. *Cell*. 1987;50:917–925.
28. Morais Cabral JH, Jackson AP, et al. Crystal structure of the breakage-reunion domain of DNA gyrase. *Nature*. 1997;388:903–906.
31. Wessel I, Jensen LH, Jensen PB, et al. Human small cell lung cancer NYH cells selected for resistance to the bisdioxopiperazine topoisomerase II catalytic inhibitor ICRF-187 demonstrate a functional R162Q mutation in the Walker A consensus ATP binding domain of the alpha isoform. *Cancer Res.* 1999;59:3442–3450.
42. Wu J, Liu LF. Processing of topoisomerase I cleavable complexes into DNA damage by transcription. *Nucleic Acids Res.* 1997;25:4181–4186.
46. Squires S, Ryan AJ, Strutt HL, Johnson RT. Hypersensitivity of Cockayne's syndrome cells to camptothecin is associated with the generation of abnormally high levels of double strand breaks in nascent DNA. *Cancer Res*. 1993;53:2012–2019.
49. Pouliot JJ, Yao KC, Robertson CA, Nash HA. Yeast gene for a tyr-DNA phosphodiesterase that repairs topoisomerase I complexes [In Process Citation]. *Science.* 1999;286:552–555.
55. Ratain MJ, Rowley JD. Therapy-related acute myeloid leukemia secondary to inhibitors of topoisomerase II: from the bedside to the target genes [see comments]. *Ann Oncol*. 1992;3:107–111.
60. Gurevich RM, Aplan PD, Humphries RK. NUP98-topoisomerase I acute myeloid leukemia-associated fusion gene has potent leukemogenic activities independent of an engineered catalytic site mutation. *Blood*. 2004;104:1127–1136.
65. Doyle LA, Yang W, Abruzzo LV, et al. A multidrug resistance transporter from human MCF-7 breast cancer cells. *Proc Natl Acad Sci USA*. 1998;95:15665–15670.
74. Harker WG, Slade DL, Parr RL, Holguin MH. Selective use of an alternative stop codon and polyadenylation signal within intron sequences leads to a truncated topoisomerase II alpha messenger RNA and protein in human HL-60 leukemia cells selected for resistance to mitoxantrone. *Cancer Res*. 1995;55:4962–4971.
77. Edwards TK, Saleem A, Shaman JA, et al. Role for Nucleolin/Nsr1 in the Cellular Localization of Topoisomerase I. *J Biol Chem*. 2000;275:36181–36188.
84. Zunino F, Pratesi G. Camptothecins in clinical development. *Expert Opin Investig Drugs*. 2004;13:269–284.
89. Gordon AN, Tonda M, Sun S, Rackoff W. Long-term survival advantage for women treated with pegylated liposomal doxorubicin compared with topotecan in a phase 3 randomized study of recurrent and refractory epithelial ovarian cancer. *Gynecol Oncol*. 2004;95:1–8.
92. Greene RF, Collins JM, Jenkins JF, Speyer JL, Myers CE. Plasma pharmacokinetics of adriamycin and adriamycinol: implications for the design of in vitro experiments and treatment protocols. *Cancer Res.* 1983;43:3417–3421.
95. Weenen H, Lankelma J, Penders PG, et al. Pharmacokinetics of 4'-epi-doxorubicin in man. *Invest New Drugs*. 1983;1:59–64.
105. Bristow MR, Billingham ME, Mason JW, Daniels JR. Clinical spectrum of anthracycline antibiotic cardiotoxicity. *Cancer Treat Rep*. 1978;62:873–879.
110. Anderlini P, Benjamin RS, Wong FC, et al. Idarubicin cardiotoxicity: a retrospective study in acute myeloid leukemia and myelodysplasia. *J Clin Oncol*. 1995;13:2827–2834.
122. Orlando L, Del Curto B, Gandini S, et al. Topoisomerase IIalpha gene status and prediction of pathological complete remission after anthracycline-based neoadjuvant chemotherapy in endocrine non-responsive Her2/neu-positive breast cancer. *Breast*. 2008;17:506–511.
137. Tannock IF, de Wit R, Berry WR, et al. Docetaxel plus prednisone or mitoxantrone plus prednisone for advanced prostate cancer. *N Engl J Med*. 2004;351:1502–1512.
140. Ee PL, He X, Ross DD, Beck WT. Modulation of breast cancer resistance protein (BCRP/ABCG2) gene expression using RNA interference. *Mol Cancer Ther.* 2004;3:1577–1583.
143. Liu X, Chen H, PatelDJ. Solution structure of actinomycin-DNA complexes: drug intercalation at isolated G-C sites. *J Biomol NMR*. 1991;1:323–347.
147. Farber S. Chemotherapy in the treatment of leukemia and Wilms' tumor. *JAMA*. 1966;198:826–836.
150. WozniakAJ, RossWE. DNAdamageasabasis for 4'-demethylepipodophyllotoxin-9-(4,6-O-ethylidene-beta-D-glucopyranoside)

(etoposide) cytotoxicity. *Cancer Res.* 1983; 43:120–124.

155. Macdonald TL, Lehnert EK, Loper JT, Chow K-C, Ross WE. On the mechanism of interaction of topoisomerase II with chemotherapeutic agents. In: Potmesil M, Kohn KW, eds. *DNA Topoisomerases in Cancer.* New York: Oxford University Press; 1991:199–214.
162. Hande KR, Wolff SN, Greco FA, Hainsworth JD, Reed G, Johnson DH. Etoposide kinetics in patients with obstructive jaundice [see comments]. *J Clin Oncol.* 1990;8:1101–1107.
166. Clark PI, Slevin ML. The clinical pharmacology of etoposide and teniposide. *Clin Pharmacokinet.* 1987;12:223–252.
171. Moertel CG, Schutt AJ, Reitemeier RJ, Hahn RG. Phase II study of camptothecin (NSC-100880) in the treatment of advanced gastrointestinal cancer. *Cancer Chemother Rep.* 1972;56:95–101.
174. Wall ME, Wani MC, Natschke SM, Nicholas AW. Plant antitumor agents. 22. Isolation of 11-hydroxycamptothecin from Camptotheca acuminata Decne: total synthesis and biological activity. *J Med Chem.* 1986;29:1553–1555.
181. Markman M, Blessing JA, Alvarez RD, Hanjani P, Waggoner S, Hall K. Phase II evaluation of 24-h continuous infusion topotecan in recurrent, potentially platinum-sensitive ovarian cancer: a Gynecologic Oncology Group study. *Gynecol Oncol.* 2000;77:112–115.
186. Kantarjian HM, Beran M, Ellis A, et al. Phase I study of topotecan, a new topoisomerase I inhibitor, in patients with refractory or relapsed acute leukemia. *Blood.* 1993;81:1146–1151.
192. Crump M, Lipton J, Hedley D, et al. Phase I trial of sequential topotecan followed by etoposide in adults with myeloid leukemia: a National Cancer Institute of Canada Clinical Trials Group Study. *Leukemia.* 1999;13:343–347.
198. Ahmed F, Vyas V, Cornfield A, et al. In vitro activation of irinotecan to SN-38 by human liver and intestine. *Anticancer Res.* 1999;19:2067–2071.
203. Mathijssen RH, Marsh S, Karlsson MO, et al. Irinotecan pathway genotype analysis to predict pharmacokinetics. *Clin Cancer Res.* 2003;9:3246–3253.
206. Morton CL, Wadkins RM, Danks MK, Potter PM. The anticancer prodrug CPT-11 is a potent inhibitor of acetylcholinesterase but is rapidly catalyzed to SN-38 by butyrylcholinesterase. *Cancer Res.* 1999;59: 1458–1463.
209. Saltz LB, Cox JV, Blanke C, et al. Irinotecan plus fluorouracil and leucovorin for metastatic colorectal cancer. Irinotecan Study Group. *N Engl J Med.* 2000;343: 905–914.
212. Kudoh S, Fujiwara Y, Takada Y, et al. Phase II study of irinotecan combined with cisplatin in patients with previously untreated small-cell lung cancer. West Japan Lung Cancer Group. *J Clin Oncol.* 1998;16:1068–1074.

53 Microtubule-Targeting Natural Products

Eric K. Rowinsky, MD

The treatment of many diseases owes much to the importance of medicines that have been derived from natural sources, and the treatment of malignant disease is no exception. In essence, billions of years of evolutionary pressures have resulted in the natural selection of plants, fungi, and microorganisms that are capable of producing highly potent and specific protective toxins. After several plant-derived compounds and other natural products demonstrated prominent anticancer activity in patients with advanced malignancies in the 1950s and 1960s, the microtubule was recognized as a subcellular target of major strategic importance. The first widely used class of antimicrotubule agents, the vinca alkaloids, has been the mainstay of both palliative and curative regimens for treating both hematopoietic and lymphoid malignancies for several decades. The addition of the plant-derived taxanes, which possess a unique mechanism of action and antitumor spectra, to our therapeutic arsenal several decades later resulted in renewed interest in the microtubule as a target, as well as in the identification of other natural products, to treat cancers. More recently, a large number of plant-derived and marine-derived compounds with yet even more distinctive antimicrotubule and anticancer activities have been identified and are undergoing clinical evaluation. The epothilones are the most recent class of natural product antimicrotubules that have been added to our therapeutic armamentarium to treat cancer. This chapter focuses on the microtubule as a target for therapeutic development, relevant antimicrotubule agents that play a major role in cancer therapeutics, particularly the vinca alkaloids and taxanes, and several new classes of antimicrotubule agents, such as the epothilones and other agents targeting kinesins, mitotic kinases, and other critical microtubule elements.

Microtubules as Strategic Targets Against Cancer

Microtubules are highly regulated and integral components of the cellular cytoskeleton that can be disrupted by the vinca alkaloids, taxanes, epothilones, and an increasingly known number of natural products and synthetic compounds.[1-5] Although the most important functions of microtubules in proliferative cells are through their actions as components of the cytoskeleton and mitotic spindle apparatus, which is vital to cell division, they are also involved in many other essential functions throughout the cell cycle of both malignant and nonmalignant cells, including intracellular transport, locomotion, adhesion, anchorage of subcellular organelles and receptors, and signal transduction, and therefore antimicrotubule agents may disrupt many of these essential functions.[1-6]

Microtubules are composed of dimeric subunits made up of two globular subunits, α-tubulin and β-tubulin monomers, each of which consists of approximately 450 amino acids and has a molecular weight of 50 kD. The α-β-tubulin dimers assemble into microtubules by forming linear protofilaments.[1-6] Each microtubule is composed of 9-13 protofilaments that form a cylindrical wall around a hollow core, with the α-tubulin subunit of one dimer in contact with the β-tubulin subunit of the next, as shown in Figure 53-1. The microtubule has a distinct polarity, which is conferred by the alignment of protofilaments in parallel. At one end, termed the plus end, guanosine triphosphate (GTP) binding occurs, assembly is rapid, and net elongation occurs, whereas assembly is slow and net shortening occurs at the other negative end.

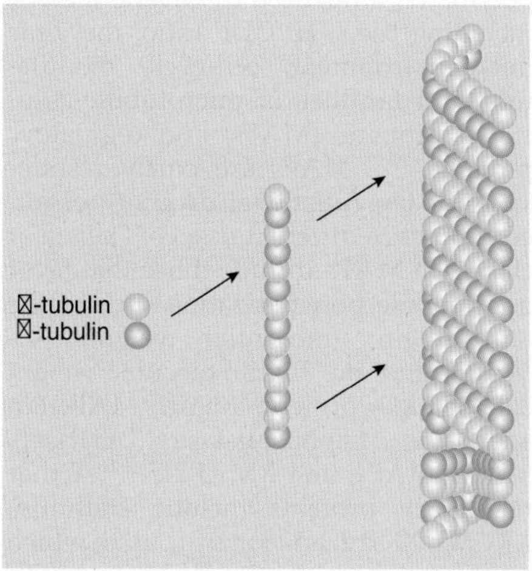

Figure 53-1 Schematic model of the α-β tubulin dimer with the monomers represented by shades of gray and white. The dimers associate linearly to form protofilaments that then in turn associate laterally to form the hollow cylindrical wall of the microtubule. Protofilaments can twist slowly around the microtubule axis, although these shown here are in parallel as in microtubles containing 13 protofilaments. Throughout most of the microtubule, lateral contacts involve α-α and β-β monomer interactions. Monomers of each type thus are in contact along a shallow spiral path around the microtubule.

The unique functions of microtubules are related to their polymerization dynamics, involving a complex and dynamic equilibrium between an intracellular pool of α-β-tubulin dimers and microtubule polymers, and simultaneous release of the α-β-tubulin dimers into the soluble tubulin pool.[1-7] Tubulin polymerization occurs by a nucleation-elongation mechanism, in which the slow formation of a short microtubule "nucleus" is followed by rapid elongation of the microtubule at its ends by the reversible, noncovalent addition of α-β-tubulin dimers. The dynamic equilibrium between free α-β-tubulin dimers and the microtubule occurs simultaneously at both ends of the microtubule.[1,2,4-7] Each tubulin molecule is associated with two molecules of GTP. The nucleoside bound to α-tubulin, at the N site, is nonexchangeable, whereas the one bound to β-tubulin, at the E site, can be exchanged with free guanosine diphosphate (GDP). The assembly process utilizes energy provided by the hydrolysis of GTP.[8] Tubulin binds GTP with high affinity, and as tubulin-GTP is added to the ends of growing microtubules, GTP is gradually hydrolyzed to GDP and Pi.[9] The Pi ultimately dissociates, leaving a microtubule core that consists of tubulin bound to GDP. The GDP nucleotide remains nonexchangeable until the tubulin subunit dissociates from the microtubule. Although tubulin polymerization and dissociation, and consequently microtubule elongation and shortening, occur simultaneously at each end, the net changes in length at the more kinetically dynamic plus end are much larger over time than those at the minus end. If the polymerization reaction is followed in vitro, an initial lag phase is noted, after which microtubules form rapidly until a plateau phase is reached. In the intact cell, the minus microtubule ends are often anchored at microtubule organizing centers (MTOCs), whereas the plus end is free in the cytoplasm radiating towards the cell periphery.

Two principal processes govern microtubule dynamics in vivo.[1-11] The first, known as *treadmilling*, is the net growth at one end of the microtubule and the net shortening at the opposite end.[8] Treadmilling plays a role in many microtubule functions, especially the formation of the mitotic spindle and chromosomal segregation during the anaphase stage of mitosis. The second dynamic process, termed *dynamic instability*, is a process in which the plus ends of microtubules switch spontaneously between states of slow sustained growth and rapid shortening.[8-11] Dynamic instability is dependent on a cycle of GTP hydrolysis and exchange. Mechanistically, the GTP cap model, in which a cap on the ends of the microtubule consisting of GTP or GDP with associated nonexchangeable Pi, stabilizes the microtubule, thus allowing growth at the plus end, likely explains the process of dynamic instability. In essence, the switch between growth and shortening depends on the end conformation of the microtubule where growing ends are stabilized by a layer of GTP-tubulin subunits (GTP cap), whereas shortening ends have lost their GTP, allowing terminal GDP-tubulin dimmers to dissociated from the microtubule lattice.[12]

At the onset of mitosis, the interphase array of microtubules, which are attached to the MTOC, disassemble and are replaced by a new population of spindle microtubules that are much more dynamic.[2,9,13,14] As the spindle-shaped array of newly assembled microtubules is organized, the nuclear envelope breaks down and releases the now condensed chromosomes, and the centrosomes, which were duplicated before mitosis, separate into the poles of the forming mitotic spindle. The rate of dynamic instability is accelerated during mitosis, resulting in the formation and attachment of the mitotic spindles to the chromosomes. In most cells, mitosis progresses rapidly and the highly dynamic microtubules that comprise the mitotic spindle render them sensitive to antimicrotubule agents that result in net depolyermization (eg, vinca alkaloids) and net polymerization (eg, taxanes and epothilones).[3,9]

Dynamic instability and treadmilling are vital to the assembly and function of the mitotic spindle, and the high dynamaticity of mitotic spindle microtubules is required for the precise alignment of the chromosomes and their attachment to the spindle during metaphase, as well as chromosome separation during anaphase. These processes enable the microtubules of the mitotic spindle to make vast growing and shortening excursions, essentially probing the cytoplasm, until they become attached to a chromosome at its kinetochore. If even a single chromosome is unable to achieve a bipolar attachment to the spindle, perhaps because of drug-induced suppression of microtubule dynamics, the cell will not traverse beyond a prometaphase/metaphase-like state, which eventually triggers apoptosis. Although mitotic spindles can form in the presence of low concentrations of antimicrotubule agents, mitosis cannot progress beyond the mitotic checkpoint at the metaphase/anaphase transition or is delayed in this stage.[9,13] Such perturbations in mitotic spindle dynamics may delay cell-cycle progression at critical mitotic checkpoints, ultimately triggering apoptosis.[7,9,13] In the unperturbed normal state, oscillations of the duplicated chromosomes, dynamic instability, and microtubule treadmilling, in which there is addition of tubulin to the spindle at the kinetochore and loss of tubulin at the spindle poles, exert considerable tension on the chromosomes in metaphase and facilitate progression to anaphase. In anaphase, microtubules that are attached to the chromosomes undergo shortening, while another subpopulation of microtubules, called interpolar microtubules lengthen, resulting in polar movement of the chromosomes. Suppression of spindle-microtubule treadmilling and dynamic instability by antimicrotubule agents reduce spindle tension and impede progression from metaphase to anaphase, thereby triggering cell death.[3,4,5,9,13-16]

The net direction of the dynamic equilibrium between the intracellular pool of tubulin and the microtubule polymer is influenced by several factors, including the GTP/GDP ratio, the ionic microenvironment, cell-cycle modulators, and families of microtubule-associated proteins (MAPs) and regulatory proteins.[1,4,5,17] MAPs are partly responsible for the functional diversity of microtubules in different tissues. The major classes of MAPs include those that favor microtubule polymerization such as the tau proteins (molecular weights, 40-60 kD) and the high-molecular weight (200-300 kD) proteins MAP1, MAPc (an adenosine triphosphatase [ATPase]), MAP2, MAP4, and XMAP215.[4,17,18] Other regulatory proteins include stathmin, XKCM1, XKIF2, and katanin, all of which favor depolymerization.[18] Most MAPs possess two binding domains, one of which binds to microtubules. Since this domain also binds to free tubulin molecules simultaneously, MAPs facilitate the initial nucleation step of tubulin polymerization. The other domain may be involved in linking the microtubule to other cellular constituents. Still, other MAPs, such as the dyneins (GTPases) and kinesins (ATPases), function as microtubule motor proteins, transmitting chemical energy to mechanical force and moving various solutes and subcellular organelles along the microtubule.[1,4,5,17,18] Motor proteins play critical roles in mitosis, premeiotic events, and organelle transport, and are being evaluated as strategic targets for anticancer therapeutic development.[19,20]

In addition to MAPs, the functional diversity of microtubules in various tissues is, in part, conferred by differences in tubulin isotypes and posttranslational modifications. There are at least six isotypes α-tubulin and β-tubulin each in human cells, which are distinguished by different C-terminal amino acid sequences and encoded by a large, multigene family that has been highly conserved throughout evolution.[4,21-24] Both forms of tubulin also undergo various posttranslational modifications, including phosphorylation, detyrosylation, polyglycylation, polyglutamylation, and others, which confer both structural and functional diversity, as well as cellular location.[25] Analysis of tubulin isotype expression in various tissues has demonstrated a complex, albeit highly conserved, pattern of isotype distribution, suggesting functional specificity.

Vinca Alkaloids: Introduction and Indications

The vinca alkaloids are naturally occurring or semisynthetic nitrogenous bases extracted from the pink periwinkle plant *Catharanthus roseus* G. Don.[26-28] The early medicinal uses of this plant led to the screening of these compounds for their hypoglycemic activity, which was ultimately of minor importance compared with their cytotoxic effects. Many vinca alkaloids have been extensively evaluated, but only vincristine (VCR), vinblastine (VBL), and vinorelbine (VRL) are approved for use in the United States. The vinca alkaloids have dimeric structures composed of two basic multiringed units (Fig. 52–2), an indole nucleus (catharanthine), and a dihydroindole nucleus (vindoline), joined together with other complex systems. Structurally, VCR and VBL are identical except for a single substitution on the vindoline nucleus, where VCR and VBL possess formyl and methyl groups, respectively. Although this minor difference does not fundamentally alter the mechanisms and tubulin-binding properties of these agents, the antitumor and toxicologic profiles of VCR and VBL differ significantly.[4,26-31]

VCR is used more commonly to treat pediatric malignancies, which is due, in part, to a generally greater level of intrinsic sensitivity of pediatric malignancies to VCR and better tolerance of therapeutic VCR doses in children. In

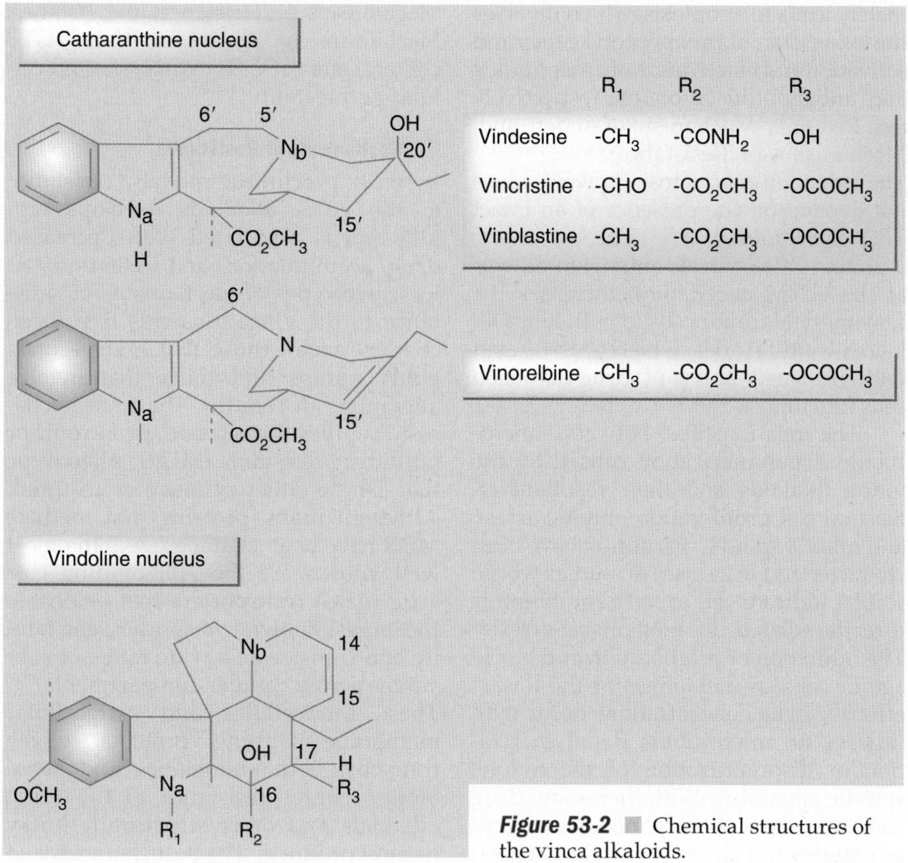

Figure 53-2 Chemical structures of the vinca alkaloids.

both children and adults, however, VCR is an essential component of the chemotherapy regimens used to treat acute lymphocytic leukemia, lymphoid blast crisis of chronic myeloid leukemia, and both Hodgkin and non-Hodgkin lymphomas. VCR also plays a role in some multimodality therapies of Wilms tumor, Ewing sarcoma, neuroblastoma, and rhabdomyosarcoma, as well as occasionally in the treatment of multiple myeloma, particularly as a component of the VCR, doxorubicin, and doxorubicin (VAD) regimen, small cell lung cancer, and soft-tissue and bone sarcomas.[28] The agent has also been used as a component of a combination regimen known as procarbazine, lomustine, and VCR (PCV) in the neoadjuvant, adjuvant, and advanced settings of anaplastic oligoastrocytoma and oligodendroglioma.[32] In addition, VCR and VCR-laden platelet transfusions have been reported to be effective in refractory autoimmune thrombocytopenia and VCR has been successfully used to treating other nonmalignant immunologically-mediated disorders such as, autoimmune hemolytic anemia, hemolytic uremic syndrome, thrombotic thrombocytopenia purpura, and steroid-dependent nephritic syndrome.[26-28,33]

VBL has been a mainstay component of chemotherapy regimens for germ cell malignancies and some types of advanced lymphomas.[28] Until recently, a regimen termed PVB, consisting of cisplatin, VBL, and bleomycin, was the standard therapy for advanced germ cell carcinoma. However, VBL has largely been replaced by etoposide in this setting because of the more favorable toxicity profile of the cisplatin-etoposide regimen. For Hodgkin lymphoma, VBL is often used in combination with doxorubicin, bleomycin, and dacarbazine (ABVD). This regimen is either administered alone or alternated with MOPP (nitrogen mustard, VCR, procarbazine, and prednisone), which is non cross-resistant to ABVD.[28] A MOPP/ABV hybrid regimen that includes both VCR and VBL has also been extensively studied. Antineoplastic activity is also observed with VBL as a single agent or in combination with other antineoplastic drugs in carcinomas of the breast, bladder, and lung, Kaposi sarcoma, choriocarcinoma, terminal phase of chronic myelogenous leukemia, mycosis fungoides, Letterer-Siwe disease (histiocytosis X), and drug refractory choriocarcinoma.[28] Infusions of VBL or VBL-laden platelets have been effective in some cases of refractory autoimmune thrombocytopenia because of its avidity to platelets.[28,33] VBL has also been used alone or in combination with other agents to treat Kaposi sarcoma and bladder, breast, and some types of central nervous system cancers.

The semisynthetic VBL derivative vinorelbine (5′-norhydro VBL; VRL), which is structurally modified on its catharanthine nucleus, resulting in much greater lipophilicity as compared with the other vinca alkaloids, is approved in the United States for treating non-small cell lung cancer as either a single agent or in combination with cisplatin, and has been registered elsewhere to treat patients with advanced breast cancer.[4,28,34-38] The agent has also demonstrated relevant clinical activity in advanced ovarian carcinoma and lymphoma, but a unique role in the treatment of these cancers has not been defined. VRL has also been demonstrated to confer favorable therapeutic indices to patients with advanced breast and lung cancers who are aged or have diminished performance abilities.[28,34-38]

Another widely studied vinca alkaloid, vindesine (VDS, desacetyl VBL caroxyamide), a semisynthetic derivative and human metabolite of VBL, was introduced in the 1970s.[28,30,31] In some reports, response rates in non-small cell lung cancer with combinations of VDS and cisplatin or mitomycin appear to be superior to those achieved with standard combinations or with either agent alone.[28,30,31] In addition, antineoplastic activity has been seen in acute lymphocytic leukemia, blast crisis of chronic myeloid leukemia, malignant melanoma, pediatric solid tumors, and metastatic renal, breast, esophageal, and colorectal carcinomas. More recently, vinflunine, which is a novel bifluorinated vinca alkaloid that appears to have unique antitumor and toxicity properties, has demonstrated notable clinical activity in bladder, breast, lung and other cancers, but, similar to VDS.[39,40] Despite these activities, unique roles for both VDS and vinflunine relative to other vinca alkaloids and anticancer agents has not yet been demonstrated.

Mechanism of Action

The vinca alkaloids principally induce cytotoxicity by disrupting microtubule function, particularly of microtubules that comprise the mitotic spindle apparatus, leading to metaphase arrest and cell death.[2-6,9,26-28,41-45] However, they are also capable of many other biochemical activities that may or may not be related to their effects on microtubules, including inhibiting synthesis of proteins and nucleic acids, elevating oxidized glutathione, altering lipid metabolism and membrane lipids, elevating cyclic adenosine monophosphate (cAMP), and inhibiting calcium–calmodulin-regulated cAMP phosphodiesterase.[28] Many of the effects that do not involve microtubule disruption occur only after treatment with superpharmacological concentrations that are not readily attained in vivo, whereas nanomolar concentrations, which are readily achievable in clinical practice, induce typical antimicrotubule effects. The vinca alkaloids also disrupt the structural integrity of platelets and other cells, which are rich in tubulin. In addition to mitotic disruption, the vinca alkaloids and other antimicrotubule agents perturb cells in nonmitotic cell-cycle phases, which is not surprising because microtubules are involved in many nonmitotic functions.[28,44,45]

The vinca alkaloids bind rapidly and reversibly to sites on tubulin (called the vinca domain), which are distinct from those of the taxanes, colchicine, podophyllotoxin, and GTP, but similar to those of maytansine and several other plant alkaloids.[2,4,6,7,27,28,39,41-43,46] The vinca alkaloids appear to bind to two binding sites with different affinities.[1,2,9,39,43,44,46-51] Binding of the vinca alkaloids to high-affinity sites (Kd, 1-2 µmol), which are at the ends of microtubule, is responsible for the potent suppression of tubulin exchange at low concentrations (<1 µ mol). At low vinca alkaloid concentrations, processes dependent on microtubule dynamics (treadmilling and dynamic instability) are disrupted, but microtubule mass is not affected. The overall result is a potent mitotic block at the metaphase/anaphase boundary. Binding of vinca alkaloids to low-affinity sites (Kd, 0.25-3.0 mmol) along the sides of microtubules, appears to result in reduced microtubule mass due to tubulin depolymerization and the splaying of microtubules into spiral aggregates or spiral protofilaments that form paracrystals, ultimately leading to microtubule disintegration. These effects occur at high drug concentrations (>1-2 µmol) by a self-propagated mechanism, initially involving drug binding to a limited number of sites, which progressively weakens the lateral interactions between the protofilaments, thereby exposing new sites.

The vinca alkaloids induce a potent block in mitosis at the metaphase/anaphase transition.[2,4,52] Following nuclear envelop breakdown, the vinca alkaloids block mitotic spindle formation and reduce the tension at the kinetochores of the chromosomes. Although chromosomes may condense, they remain scattered in the cells. The chromosomes separate along their lengths, but still remain attached at their centromeres.[2,4,9,14,16,44,45,53] Mitotic progress is delayed in a metaphase-like state, with chromosomes "stuck" at the spindle poles, unable to move to the spindle equator. The cell-cycle signal to the anaphase-promoting complex, which is required for the cell to transition from metaphase to anaphase, is blocked and apoptotic cell death ensues. Cell-cycle progression in the absence of anaphase or cytokinesis may occur, resulting in chromatin decondensation and formation of multilobed nuclei.[2,4,9,16] Disruption of spindle-microtubule dynamics without microtubule depolymerization ultimately leads to apoptosis, which involves the expression of proapoptotic genes and activation and inactivation of proapoptitoc and antiapoptotic proteins, respectively (see Taxanes, "Mechanism of Action, and; Mechanisms of Resistance).[2,4,9,14,15,16,39,53-58] The induction of apoptosis, however, does not depend on the presence of an intact TP53 checkpoint.[14,15,54,55,59] The loss of p21, a protein that controls entry into mitosis at the G2/M checkpoint, increases the sensitivity of tumor cells to both vinca alkaloids and taxanes, which is associated with hastened entry of drug-damaged cells into mitosis.[15,54-56]

The relationships between microtubule depolymerization caused by the vinca alkaloids and their resultant effects on cell proliferation, mitotic arrest, and mitotic spindle disruption have been characterized in a series of studies whose results indicate cell growth inhibition is directly related to metaphase arrest.[44] The inhibition of proliferation and blockage of cells in metaphase at the lowest effective drug concentrations occur with little or no microtubule depolymerization or disorganization of the mitotic spindle apparatus. With increasing drug concentrations, the organization of microtubules and chromosomes in arrested mitotic spindles deteriorates in a manner that is similar for most antimicrotubule agents.[2,3,4,9,10]

In addition to their direct cytotoxic effects on tumor cells, the vinca alkaloids, taxanes, and other antimicrotubule agents also appear to confer antitumor properties by inhibiting processes associated with malignant angiogenesis with surprising potency.[60] These antiangiogenic effects are most likely due to microtubule disruption. However, the relative contribution of these antiangiogenic effects to the clinical antitumor activity of the vinca alkaloids is unclear.

The disparate sensitivity of various tissues and tumors to the vinca alkaloids is multifactorial. One possible explanation is the differential sensitivity of tissues with varying tubulin isotype composition, which may affect intracellular drug accumulation and binding to tubulin binding.[4,23,61] In addition, differences in the type and concentration of MAPs and posttranslational tubulin modifications, which may influence drug interactions with tubulin, as well as variability in cellular permeability and retention, may affect the formation and stability of complexes formed between the vinca alkaloids and tubulin. Palmitoylation, a posttranslational tubulin modification, is directly inhibited by the vinca alkaloids, and depalmitoylation of tubulin may not only be a mechanism of action, but may also relate to drug sensitivity.[62] Other putative factors include differences in tubulin isotypes (see Vinca Alkaloids; Mechanisms of Resistance, and Taxanes; Mechanims of Resistance, tissue GTP content, rates of GTP hydrolysis, and cellular permeability.[61,63-67]

Mechanisms of Resistance

In most preclinical models, resistance to the vinca alkaloids develops rapidly and is associated with decreased drug accumulation and retention. At least two types of mechanisms of resistance to the vinca alkaloids have been characterized—those that involve drug efflux pumps and those that involve alterations in tubulin. The first mechanism typifies the "classic" pleiotropic or multidrug-resistant (MDR) phenotype that can be either primary or acquired. Although many proteins that mediate MDR have been characterized, the most well known are the ATP-binding cassette (ABC) transporters that belong to the largest known transporter gene family and translocate a wide range of substrates across cellular compartments.[68,69] These intracellular and extracellular membrane-spanning proteins, which transport both endobiotics and xenobiotics, confer resistance to the vinca alkaloids and other structurally bulky natural products. The best characterized ABC transporters are the permeability glycoproteins (Pgp) or the MDR1 encoded gene product MDR1 (ABC Subfamily B1) and the multidrug resistance protein (MRP; ABC Subfamily C2).[68]

MDR1 is a 170-kDa Pgp energy-dependent transmembrane pump that regulates the efflux of a wide range of bulky hydrophobic substances.[68] The protein is constitutively overexpressed in various normal tissues, which include renal tubule epithelium, colonic mucosa, and adrenal medulla, as well as tumors derived from these tissues. Pgp, an ATPase, functions to bind and extrude the vinca alkaloids from the tumor cell in a process that requires energy in the form of adenosine triphosphate (ATP). The MDR phenotype also confers varying degrees of cross-resistance to other structurally bulky natural products such as the taxanes, anthracyclines, epipodophyllotoxins, and colchicine. The specific Pgp associated with vinca alkaloid resistance shows slight antigenic and amino acid sequence differences and a different amino acid map after digestion than does Pgp from cells selected for resistance to colchicines or taxanes.[70-73] In fact, two forms of the protein have been demonstrated to be produced by a single clone of VCR-resistant cells, and these forms undergo posttranslational *N*-glycosylation and phosphorylation, which leads to further structural diversity and may explain the greater degree of resistance for the specific agent used compared with the resistance of other drugs conferred by MDR, and may also account for the variable patterns of resistance among MDR cells. The composition of membrane gangliosides in cancer cells resistant to the vinca alkaloids has also been shown to differ from that of wild-type cells. The clinical ramifications of these resistance mechanisms are not known. In one study in childhood acute lymphoblastic leukemia, however, VCR resistance measured in vitro did not correlate with Pgp overexpression.[74]

MRP1, a 190 kD membrane-spanning protein that shares 15% amino acid homology with MDR1, also confers resistance to the vinca alkaloids in vitro.[29,68,69,75-78] MRP1 expression has been found in many types of tumors and has been associated with the MDR phenotype in cancers of the lung, colon, breast, bladder, and prostate, as well as leukemia. MRP1 transports glutathione conjugates of alkylating agents and several types of xenobiotics such as etoposide and doxorubicin, but only confers resistance to the latter agents. The MRP1 resistance profile also includes the vinca alkaloids and methotrexate.[29,68,69,75-78] Although many other ABC transporters have been identified and several confer cellular resistance to the vinca alkaloids in vitro, their roles in conferring inherent or acquired drug resistance in the clinic are even less clear than those of MDR1 and MRP1.

Drug resistance conferred by MDR1 and MRP in vitro is reversible after treatment with agents that have distinctly different structural and functional characteristics, such as the calcium-channel blockers, calmodulin inhibitors, detergents, progestational and antiestrogenic agents, antibiotics, antihypertensives, antiarrhythmics, antimalarials, and immunosuppressives, which has been a source of clinical interest.[29,68,79,80] Those reversal agents bind directly to Pgp, thereby blocking the efflux of the cytotoxic drugs and increasing intracellular drug concentrations. However, clinical studies of resistance modulation have been confounded by the fact that MDR modulators, particularly MDR1 reversal agents, also enhance drug uptake in normal cells, decrease biliary elimination and drug clearance, and lead to enhanced toxicity.[29,68,79,80] Overall, clinical strategies aimed at reversing resistance to the vinca alkaloids with pharmacologic modulators of both MDR1 and MRP have been disappointing, most likely owing to the fact that the MDR1 expression is associated with overexpression of a large number of resistance proteins.[68] By characterizing the genetics and role of the ABC transporters in normal organ function and the disposition of chemotherapeutic agents, however, genetic polyporphisms that may impact upon pharmacokinetics and drug toxicity have been defined.

Structural and functional alterations in α- and β-tubulins due to either genetic mutations, posttranslational modifications, or differential expression of tubulin isotypes, particularly the β-III tubulin isotype, have been identified in tumor cells with resistance to the vinca alkaloids and taxanes in both preclinical and clinical studies.[81-92] In addition, these studies suggest that the β-III tubulin isotype could be both a prognostic and a predictive determinant of clinical benefit. Expression of β-II tubulin, which appears to depend on TP53 suppressor function, may also relate to vinca alkaloid resistance.[93]

Increased expression of MAPs, particularly MAP4, has also been associated with vinca alkaloid resistance.[94] This alteration, as well as alterations in α- and β-tubulin, promote resistance to agents that inhibit microtubule assembly by enhancing microtubule stability, possibly by promoting longitudinal interdimer and intradimer interactions and/or lateral interactions between protofilaments. Furthermore, these "hyperstable" microtubules are collaterally sensitive to the taxanes (see: Taxanes Mechanisms of Resistance). Although such tubulin modifications have been demonstrated repeatedly in tumor cells that are continuously exposed to the vinca alkaloids in vitro, the relevance of "hyperstable tubulin" caused by alterations in tubulins or MAPs is not known.

Variability in cellular permeation and retention may also influence the formation and stability of vinca alkaloid-tubulin complexes.[39,65,95-101] The vinca alkaloids are rapidly taken up into cells and then accumulate intracellularly, with intracellular to extracellular concentrations ratios as high as 5- to 500-fold, depending on the cell type.[66,67] In murine leukemia cells, the intracellular concentrations of VCR are 5- to 20-fold higher than the extracellular concentrations, and ratios ranging from 150- to 500-fold have been reported with other vinca alkaloids.[67,95,102] There are also marked differences in cellular uptake and retention between the vinca alkaloids, the latter of which may relate to potency and the duration of drug action. For example, VRL is more rapidly taken up and metabolized than other vinca alkaloids in isolated human hepatocytes,[101] and the greater potency of VCR during exposures of short duration compared with VBL was related to the greater cellular retention of VCR in another model system. An important determinant of drug accumulation and retention is lipophilicity. The differences in the catharanthine ring of VRL render it a more lipophilic agent and increase its retention in tissues, which may explain why it is more effective at disrupting the microtubules of the mitotic spindles compared with axonal microtubules.[100] The differential effects of the vinca alkaloids on axonal microtubules due to variable cellular retention and lipophilicity may explain why VRL treatment results in less neurotoxicity than other vinca alkaloids. The mechanisms responsible for the intracellular accumulation of the vinca alkaloids and other agents that bind to tubulin are not fully known, but may relate to their tubulin-binding properties and several other factors. Differential drug uptake among different tumor types may also relate to tubulin isotype expression, differential uptake and efflux, and intracellular reservoirs for drug accumulation.

Pharmacology

Cellular Pharmacology ■ Temperature-independent, nonsaturable mechanisms, analogous to simple diffusion, most likely account for most transport of the vinca alkaloids, and temperature-dependent saturable processes are less important.[101] Although the drug concentration and duration of treatment are important determinants of drug accumulation and cytotoxicity, the duration of drug exposure above a critical threshold concentration is perhaps the most important pharmacologic determinant of cytotoxicity.[66,103] Cytotoxicity is directly related to the extracellular concentration of drug when the duration of treatment is kept constant; for prolonged exposure to VCR, the concentration yielding 50% inhibition lies in the range of 1–5 nmol/L.[103]

Clinical Pharmacology ■ The clinical pharmacology of the vinca alkaloids, which were largely studied decades ago, largely reflect the fact that sensitive, specific, and reliable analytic assays capable of measuring the minute plasma concentrations resulting from the administration of milligram quantity doses were not available. The use of radiolabeled drugs and assay methods may have further confounded early results. The vinca alkaloids, particularly VCR and VBL, may undergo spontaneous degradation under mild conditions, forming degradative products that can be separated using high-pressure liquid chromatography (HPLC).[94] Radiolabeled compounds coupled to HPLC were later used for improved separation of the various chemical moieties. Radioimmunoassay (RIA) and enzyme-linked immunosorbent assay (ELISA) methods using can detect picomolar drug concentrations; however, these methods cannot distinguish between the parent compounds and related derivatives, and, therefore, may not provide sufficient quantitative information about degradation products and metabolites. To meet the challenge, more refined RIA and ELISA methods using monoclonal antibodies with considerably greater sensitivity and specificity have been developed. Furthermore, recent technical advances in extraction and detection methodologies have increased the sensitivity and specificity of chromatographic methods, particularly, tandem mass spectroscopy in conjunction with HPLC.

Table 53-1 summarizes the pharmacokinetic characteristics of the vinca alkaloids, which generally exhibit triphasic clearance from plasma following intravenous administration as a bolus infusion or brief injection. The pharmacokinetic behavior of these agents is typified by large volumes of distribution, high early clearance rates, long terminal half-lives, extensive hepatic metabolism, and biliary/fecal elimination. The relatively short α and β distribution phases, which are likely a result of rapid distribution and uptake into peripheral tissues and formed blood elements, are similar for all vinca alkaloids. However, the terminal (γ) phase, which is relatively long because of the avid tissue sequestration and slow release of drug, has been reported to vary by approximately 4-fold.

Vincristine (VCR) ■ VCR is rapidly distributed to the peripheral compartment following administration. There is extensive binding to both plasma proteins and formed blood elements, particularly platelets, which contain large quantities of tubulin. This served as the rationale for using VCR-laden platelets to treat disorders of platelet consumption such as refractory thrombocytopenia.[28,33] In contrast, penetration of VCR across the blood-brain barrier is poor, probably because of the molecule's large size and is an avid substrate for ABC transporter pumps that maintain the integrity of the blood-brain barrier. Following administration of conventional doses (1.4 mg/m^2), given as a brief intravenous infusion, peak plasma levels approach 0.4 μmol.[28,95,104,105-110] Total VCR clearance is slow, which reflects avid tissue binding and slow release, and terminal half-lives in the range of 23-85 h have been reported.[28,95,104,105-110] VCR is metabolized and excreted primarily by the hepatobiliary system. Seventy-two hours after the administration of radiolabeled VCR, approximately 12% of the radioactivity is recovered in the urine (50% of which consists of metabolites), and approximately 70% is recovered from feces (40% of which consists of metabolites).[28,95,103,104,105-112] As many as 6-11 metabolites have been detected in studies performed in both humans and animals.[113] The metabolites, 4-deacetyl-VCR, and both 4′-deoxy-3′-hydroxyVCR and 3′,4′-epoxyVCR *N*-oxide have been identified after incubation of VCR with bile.[28,95,103,104,94,105-113] The nature of the VCR metabolites identified to date, such as 4-deacetylVCR and *N*-deformylVCR, which have been isolated from human bile, and 4′-deoxy-3′-hydroxyVCR and 3′,4′-epoxyVCR *N*-oxide following incubation of VCR with bile, indicate that the agent is principally metabolized by hepatic cytochrome P-450 CYP3A. There has been conflicting, albeit sparse, evidence that peak plasma concentration and systemic exposure are the principal pharmacologic determinants of VCR-induced neurotoxicity.[114]

Vinblastine (VBL) ■ The pharmacologic behavior of VBL is similar to that of VCR.[28,95,104,115] Following rapid intravenous injection of VBL at standard doses, peak plasma drug concentrations are approximately 0.4 μmol/L. Tissue distribution is also extensive. Like VCR, binding of VBL to plasma proteins and formed elements of blood is considerable. Furthermore, distribution is rapid, with half-life values of approximately 4 min and 1.6 h for α and β phases, respectively. Terminal half-life values ranging from 20 to 24 h have been reported. Like VCR, VBL disposition is principally through the hepatobiliary system. The principal mode of VBL disposition is hepatic metabolism and biliary excretion. Fecal excretion of the parent compound is low, indicating that metabolism is substantial. The cytochrome P-450 CYP3A isoform appears to be principally responsible for its biotransformation.[101] At least one metabolite, 4-deacetylVBL, or VDS, which appears to be as active as the parent compound, has been identified in humans, and small quantities have been detected in both urine and feces.

Vinorelbine (VRL) ■ The pharmacologic behavior of VRL is similar to those of the other vinca alkaloids, and plasma concentrations decline in a biexponential or triexponential manner. Immediately following intravenous administration, plasma concentrations decline rapidly followed by much slower elimination phases ($t_{1/2}$, 18-49 h).[28,36,37,116,117] Plasma protein binding has been reported to range from 80% to 91%, with binding primarily to α1-acid glycoprotein, albumin, and lipoproteins.

VRL is widely distributed with extensive sequestration in virtually all tissues, except brain. The drug is also extensively bound to platelets. The wide distribution of VRL may reflect the agent's lipophilicity, which is among the highest of the vinca alkaloids. Tissue to plasma ratios range from 20 to 80, although VRL concentrations in human lung have been reported to be 300-fold greater than plasma concentrations and 3.4-13.8-fold higher than lung concentrations achieved with VDS and VCR, respectively. Hepatic metabolism and biliary excretion of metabolites and VRL are the predominant modes of drug disposition.[28,36,37,116-118] Approximately 33-80% of the administered dose of VRL is excreted into the feces, whereas urinary excretion represents only 16-30% of total drug disposition, the majority of which is metabolized VRL. Cytochrome P-450 isoform CYP3A is principally involved in biotransformation in humans.[36,38,118-124] The principal metabolites appear to be 4-*O*-deacetyl-VRL, 3,6-epoxy-VRL, and several hydroxy-VRL isomers. Most metabolites are inactive. Although 4-*O*-deacetyl-VRL may be as active as VRL,

Table 53-1 **Vinca Alkaloids: Comparative Pharmacokinetic and Toxicologic Characteristics**

	Vincristine	Vinblastine	Vindesine	Vinorelbine
Standard adult dose range (mg/m^2/wk)	1-2	6-8	3-4	15-30
Pharmacokinetic behavior	Triphasic	Triphasic	Triphasic	Triphasic
Plasma half-lives				
α (min)	<5	<5	<5	<5
β (min)	50-155	53-99	55-99	49-168
γ (h)	23-85	20-64	20-24	18-49
Clearance (L/h/kg)	0.16	0.74	0.25	0.4-1.29
Primary route	Hepatic metabolism and biliary elimination	Hepatic metabolism and biliary elimination	Hepatic metabolism and biliar elimination	Hepatic metabolism and biliary elimination
Principal toxicity	Neurotoxicity	Neutropenia	Neutropenia	Neutropenia
Other toxicities	Constipation, SIADH	Alopecia neurotoxicity, mucositis	Alopecia, neurotoxicity	Neurotoxicity vomiting, constipation, mucositis

Abbreviation: SIADH, syndrome of inappropriate secretion of antidiuretic hormone.

this finding is of minor importance since concentrations are minute.

The total body clearance of VRL (1.2 L/h/kg) and t1/2 values of approximately 26 h were found to be the same in elderly and younger patients with normal hepatic function in one study.[123] Clearance has been found to be adversely affected in patients who have liver metastases that involve more than 75% of the organ; clearance can be predicted in such patients by the monoethylglycinexylidide clearance test, which assesses CYP3A4 function.[124] Dexamethasone has also been used as a probe of CYP3A metabolism in the assessment of VRL pharmacokinetics.[118] Although VRL clearance is not accurately predicted by bilirubin concentrations in serum, markedly elevated levels have been associated with significant reductions in clearance in the few patients studied.

VRL is active when given orally. In animals, 100% of radioactivity is absorbed after the ingestion of tritium-labeled VRL, the bioavailability of the parent compound in human studies is 43% and 27% for the powder-filled and liquid-filled capsules, respectively; the bioavailability of the gel-filled capsule was negligibly affected by food.[116,125,126] C_{peak} values are achieved within 1-2 h after ingestion, and interindividual variability is moderate.

Drug Interactions

The vinca alkaloids, particularly VCR and VBL, have been demonstrated to enhance methotrexate accumulation in tumor cells in vitro, an effect mediated by a vinca alkaloid-induced blockade of drug efflux; however, the minimal VCR concentrations required to achieve this effect (0.1 μmol/L) are attained transiently in vivo.[127-129] The vinca alkaloids also inhibit the cellular influx and cytotoxicity of the epipodyllotoxins in vitro, but the clinical ramifications of this effect are unknown.[130] L-asparaginase may reduce the hepatic clearance of the vinca alkaloids, particularly VCR, which may result in increased toxicity. To minimize the possibility of this interaction, it is recommended that VCR be given 12-24 h before L-asparaginase.

Treatment with the vinca alkaloids has precipitated seizures associated with subtherapeutic plasma phenytoin concentrations, most likely due to the induction of CYP3A-mediated clearance of phenytoin.[131-134] Reduced plasma phenytoin levels have been noted from 1 to 10 days after treatment with both VCR and VBL. Administration of the vinca alkaloids with erythromycin, itraconazole, and other pharmacologic inhibitors of CYP3A may lead to severe toxicity.[131,135] Concomitantly administered drugs, such as pentobarbital and H2-receptor antagonists, may also influence VCR clearance by modulating hepatic cytochrome P-450 metabolic processes.[131,136] Another potential drug interaction may occur in patients who have Kaposi sarcoma related to acquired immunodeficiency syndrome and are receiving concurrent treatment with 3′ azido-3′-deoxythymidine (AZT) and the vinca alkaloids, as the vinca alkaloids may inhibit glucuronidation of AZT to its 5′-*O*-glucuronide metabolite.[137] Based on a report of a constellation of severe toxicities, including syndrome of inappropriate secretion of antidiuretic hormone (SIADH), bilateral cranial nerve palsies, peripheral neuropathy, cranial nerve palsies, heart failure, and cardiovascular effects following VCR treatment in children with acute lymphocytic leukemia who had been receiving treatment with nifedipine and itraconazole, it is possible that these medications may enhance the neurologic and cardiovascular effects of the vinca alkaloids.[136] Lastly, the significant interindividual and intraindividual variability of VCR pharmacokinetics in children has been attributed to the variable induction of P-450 metabolism due to concurrent use of P-450-inducing corticosteroids.[133,134]

The use of mitomycin C in combination with the vinca alkaloids has been associated with pulmonary toxicity as described in Toxicity: Miscellaneous.

Toxicity

The principal toxicities of the vinca alkaloids differ despite their structural and pharmacologic similarities. Peripheral neurotoxicity is the predominant toxicity of VCR, whereas myelosuppression predominates with VBL, VDS, and VRL. Nevertheless, peripheral neurotoxicity is often noted following cumulative treatment with VBL, VDS, and VRL, inadvertent high-dose treatment, and in patients who are inherently susceptible (see Neurotoxicity). Nevertheless, VCR can cause myelosuppression under the similar conditions.

Neurotoxicity ■ Although the vinca alkaloids are similar from a structural standpoint, their toxicologic profiles differ significantly. All of the vinca alkaloids induce a characteristic peripheral neurotoxicity, but VCR is most potent in this regard. The neurotoxicity is principally characterized by a peripheral, symmetric mixed sensory-motor, and autonomic polyneuropathy.[27,28,31,38,138-142] The primary pathologic effect is axonal degeneration and decreased axonal transport, most likely caused by a drug-induced perturbation of microtubule function. At onset, only symmetric sensory impairment and paresthesia in a length-dependent manner (distal extremities first) is often encountered. Neuritic pain and loss of deep tendon reflexes may develop with continued treatment, which may be followed by foot drop, wrist drop, motor dysfunction, ataxia, and paralysis. Back, bone, and limb pains may occur. Electrophysiologic studies typically reveal normal nerve conduction velocities; however, diminished amplitude of sensory and motor nerve action potentials and prolonged distal latencies, resembling axonal degeneration, may be noted.[27,28,31,38,128-132] Rarely, cranial nerves are affected, resulting in hoarseness, diplopia, jaw pain, facial palsies, and laryngeal paralysis.[143,144] The uptake of VCR into the brain is low, and central nervous system effects, such as confusion, mental status changes, depression, hallucinations, agitation, insomnia, seizures, coma, SIADH, and visual disturbances, may occur in rare situations.[38,145,146] Auditory effects, possibly secondary to disruption of the medial olivocochlear bundle, have also been reported.[147] Acute, severe autonomic neurotoxicity is uncommon, but may arise as a consequence of high-dose therapy (greater than 2 mg/m^2) or in patients with diminished drug clearance because of altered hepatic function.[140,141,145,146,148-151] Toxic manifestations of autonomic neurotoxicity include constipation, abdominal cramps, paralytic ileus, urinary retention, orthostatic hypotension, and hypertension.[130,131,133-138] Acute neurotoxic manifestations resembling Guillain-Barré syndrome have also been reported.[142]

In adults treated with VCR, the neurotoxic effects may begin with cumulative doses as little as 5-6 mg, and manifestations may be severe cumulative doses of 15-20 mg. Neurotoxic manifestations are generally cumulative and resolve slowly after treatment, often requiring many years. Neurotoxicity occasionally worsens for a short time following treatment.[152] Although it has been remarked that children are less susceptible to neurotoxicity than adults, and that the elderly are particularly prone, these apparent age-related differences may, in fact, be caused by previously inaccurate dose calculation using body weight in children and adults and using body surface area in infants.[143,153] In infants, VCR doses are calculated now according to body weight, which may be more accurate from a pharmacologic standpoint because of ubiquitous tissue distribution. Patients with antecedent neurologic disorders, such as Charcot-Marie-Tooth disease, hereditary and sensory neuropathy type 1, Guillain-Barré syndrome, and childhood poliomyelitis, are highly predisposed to neurotoxicity.[153-156] VCR treatment in patients with hepatic dysfunction or obstructive liver disease is associated with an increased risk of developing neuropathy because of impaired drug metabolism and delayed biliary excretion.[157]

The only known effective intervention for vinca alkaloid neurotoxicity is discontinuing treatment or reduction of the dose or frequency of drug administration.[148,157,158] Although a number of antidotes, including thiamine, vitamin B_{12}, folinic acid, pyridoxine, and neuroactive agents (eg, sedatives, tranquilizers, anticonvulsants), have been used, these treatments have not been clearly and consistently shown to be effective.[114,159-161] Folinic acid protects mice against otherwise lethal doses of the vinca alkaloids, and there are anecdotal reports of its successful use following VCR overdosage in man; however, prospective studies have never been performed.[160,161] Suggested dosages for folinic acid for the treatment of overdosage are 15 mg every 3-h for 24 h and then every 6-h for at least 48 h. There have been promising results with other neuroprotective agents. In one randomized, double-blind trial, coadministration of glutamic acid and VCR appeared to reduce neurotoxicity.[161] The adrenocorticotropin analogue ORG 2766 also demonstrated protection against VCR-induced neuropathy in an animal model, and in a double-blind, placebo-controlled pilot study in patients.[28] Several other agents, including nerve growth factor, insulin growth factor-I, and amifostine, appear to alter the natural course of neurotoxicity in experimental models, but there has been no definitive evidence that these agents may be effective in the clinic.

The manifestations of neurotoxicity are similar for all vinca alkaloids; however, severe neurotoxicity is observed less frequently with VBL, VDS, and VRL, as compared with VCR.[50,162] VRL has a lower affinity for axonal microtubules than either VCR or VBL, which seems to be confirmed by clinical observations.[28,26,38,100,162]

Myelosuppression ■ Neutropenia is the principal dose-limiting toxicity of VBL, VDS, and VRL. Thrombocytopenia and anemia are usually less common and less severe. The onset of neutropenia is usually 7-11 days after treatment, and recovery is generally by days 14-21. Myelosuppression is not typically cumulative. Although VCR is rarely associated with hematologic toxicity, severe myelosuppression has been observed in situations resulting in increased drug exposure, such as following inadvertent overdose, and hepatic insufficiency.

Gastrointestinal ■ GI toxicities, aside from those caused by autonomic dysfunction, may also occur.[27,28,31,38,114,163,164] GI autonomic dysfunction, as manifested by bloating, constipation, and abdominal pain, occurs most commonly with VCR, high doses of the other vinca alkaloids, or settings associated with high drug exposure (eg, hepatic dysfunction, overdosages). An initial manifestation of autonomic dysfunction due to poor intestinal transit may be impaction of stool in the upper colon. An empty rectum may be noted on digital examination or an abdominal radiograph may be useful in diagnosing this condition, which may be responsive to high enemas and laxatives. A routine prophylactic regimen to prevent constipation is therefore recommended for all patients receiving VCR. Severe autonomic toxicity may lead to paralytic ileus, particularly in children, intestinal necrosis, and even intestinal perforation. The ileus, which may mimic a "surgical abdomen," usually resolves with conservative measures after termination of treatment. Patients who receive high dosages of VCR or have hepatic dysfunction may be especially prone to develop severe gastrointestinal complications due to autonomic neurotoxicity. Although success with drugs used prophylactically to minimize toxicity, including lactulose, caerulein, metoclopramide, and the cholecystokinin analogue sincalide, has been reported anecdotally, these agents also may alter the pharmacokinetic behavior of the vinca alkaloids by affecting biliary excretion and/or enterohepatic recirculation, which may ultimately result in increased drug clearance.[28]

Mucositis, stomatitis, and pharyngitis occur more frequently with VBL than VRL or VDS, and are least common with VCR. Nausea, vomiting, and diarrhea may also occur to a lesser extent. Asymptomatic and brief elevations in serum levels of hepatic transaminases and alkaline phosphatase have been noted. Pancreatitis has also been reported rarely with VRL.[163]

Miscellaneous ■ The vinca alkaloids are potent vesicants and may cause profound tissue damage if extravasation occurs. If extravasation is suspected, treatment should be discontinued immediately and aspiration of any residual drug remaining in the tissues should be attempted.[165-170] In experimental studies, cold packs have been shown to increase toxicity, while heat appears to limit damage. The application of local heat immediately for 1-h four times daily for 3-5 days and the injection of hyaluronidase, 150-1500 units (15 units/mL in 6 mL of 0.9% sodium chloride solution) subcutaneously, through 6 clockwise injections in a circumferential manner using a 25-gauge needle (changing the needle with each injection) into surrounding tissues is the treatment of choice in minimizing both discomfort and latent cellulitis.[168-170] The use of leucovorin, diphenhydramine, hydrocortisone, isoproterenol, sodium bicarbonate, and vitamin A cream have been ineffective in animal models.[166] An immediate surgical consultation to consider early debridement is recommended. Discomfort and signs of phlebitis may also occur along the course of an injected vein, with resultant sclerosis, but phlebitis may be minimized if the vein is adequately flushed after treatment.

Mild and reversible alopecia occurs in approximately 10% and 20% of patients treated with VRL and VCR, respectively. Acute cardiac ischemia, chest pains without evidence of ischemia, fever without an obvious source, Raynaud's phenomenon, and palmar-plantar erythrodysthesia (hand-foot syndrome) have also been reported with the vinca alkaloids.[171-174]

Respiratory reactions, characterized by dyspnea, have been reported in approximately 5% of patients, particularly when vinca alkaloids are combined with mitomycin C.[175,176] The onset of pulmonary toxicity may be acute, with bronchospasm and dyspnea as the predominant manifestations, resembling an allergic reaction. The second type of toxicity is a subacute reversible reaction associated with cough and dyspnea and occasionally with interstitial infiltrates. This reaction typically occurs within 1-h after treatment. The use of steroids has been felt to be beneficial in severe cases, and several patients have been retreated without complications. There is no clear evidence that implicates VRL as a cause of chronic pulmonary toxicity.

All of the vinca alkaloids have been implicated as a cause of SIADH, and patients who are receiving intensive hydration are particularly prone to severe hyponatremia secondary to SIADH.[26-28,38,114] SIADH has also been associated with elevated plasma levels of antidiuretic hormone and usually remits in 2-3 days. Hyponatremia generally responds to fluid restriction. VBL may cause photosensitivity reactions, possibly due to corneal irritation, and muscular effects.[177]

The inadvertent intrathecal administration of the vinca alkaloids causes an ascending myeloencephalopathy that is usually fatal. Reports of immediate cerebrospinal fluid withdrawal and lavage with Ringer's lactate solution supplemented with fresh frozen plasma (15 mL/L) at a rate of 55 mL/h for 24 h has provided encouraging results, with two affected patients surviving with significant paraplegia, but intact cerebral function.[178] To prevent this mistake, intrathecal methotrexate and intravenous VCR setting should not be administered in the same setting, and the drugs should not be delivered together to staff.[179]

Administration, Dose, and Schedule

It is recommended that the vinca alkaloids be administered by rapid intravenous injection. Inadequate flushing following treatment may increase the risk of phlebitis and injection site reactions, and, therefore, the catheter should not be removed before the vein is flushed. VCR is commonly administered to children weighing more than 10 kg as a bolus intravenous injection at a dosage of 1.5-2.0 mg/m^2 weekly, although 0.05-0.65 mg/kg weekly is commonly used in smaller children. For adults, the conventional weekly dose is 1.4-2.0 mg/m^2. A restriction of the absolute dose of VCR to 2.0-2.5 mg in children and 2.0 mg in adults, which is often referred to as "capping," has been generally adopted based on early reports of gastrointestinal toxicity in small numbers of patients treated at higher doses. However, there is little pharmacologic or toxicologic evidence to support this practice, and available evidence suggests that it should be reconsidered, particularly in light of the wide interpatient variability in pharmacokinetic behavior and tolerance.[157,180,181] There is significant interpatient variability in the clearance of VCR (as much as 11-fold), and some patients are able to tolerate much higher doses with little or no toxicity. Moreover, the safety and efficacy of treatment regimens that do not employ capping at 2.0 mg have been documented in adults.[180] In any case, doses should not be reduced for mild peripheral neurotoxicity, particularly if VCR is being used in a potentially curative setting. Instead, doses should be modified for manifestions of more serious neurotoxicity, including severe symptomatic sensory changes, motor and cranial nerve deficits, and ileus, until toxicity resolves. In clearly palliative situations, dose reductions, lengthening dosing intervals, or selecting an alternative agent may be justified in the event of moderate neurotoxicity. A routine prophylactic regimen to prevent the serious consequences of severe autonomic toxicity, particularly severe constipation, is also recommended.

The most commonly used schedule for VBL in chemotherapy regimens uses a rapid intravenous injection at a dosage of 6 mg/m^2 weekly. Approved dosing recommendations for weekly dosing are 2.5 and 3.7 mg/m^2 for children and adults, respectively, followed by gradual escalation in increments of 1.8 mg/m^2 and 1.25 mg/m^2 weekly based on hematologic tolerance. It is recommended that weekly VBL doses of 18.5 mg/m^2 in adults and 12.5 mg/m^2 in children not be exceeded as a single agent; however, these doses are substantially higher than most patients can tolerate because of myelosuppression, even on less frequent schedules of administration. Because the severity of leukopenia that may occur with identical VBL doses varies widely, VBL should probably not be given more frequently than once each week. Five-day continuous infusions of VBL have been used at dosages ranging from 1.5 to 2.0 mg/m^2 per day, which achieves biologically relevant plasma concentrations of approximately 2.0 nmol/L, but the overall advantages of using protracted infusions for a drug that is widely distributed and avidly bound to peripheral tissues may be minimal.

VRL is usually administered at a dosage of 30 mg/m^2 on a weekly or biweekly schedule as a 6- to 10-min intravenous injection through a side-arm port into a running infusion (alternatively, a slow bolus injection followed by flushing the vein with 5% dextrose or 0.9% sodium chloride solutions) or as a short infusion over 20 min. It appears that the more rapid infusions are associated with less local venous toxicity. Oral dosages of 80-100 mg/m^2 given weekly are generally well tolerated, but an acceptable oral formulation has not yet been approved. Other dosing schedules that have been evaluated include chronic oral administration of low doses, intermittent high doses, and prolonged intravenous infusion schedules.

Because of their remarkable vesicant properties, the vinca alkaloids should not be administered intramuscularly, subcutaneously, intravesically, or intraperitoneally. Direct intrathecal injection of VCR and other vinca alkaloids, which has occurred as inadvertent clinical mishaps, induces a severe myeloencephalopathy characterized by ascending motor and sensory neuropathies, encephalopathy, and death (see Toxicity: "Neurotoxicity").

Although specific dosing guidelines for patients with hepatic dysfunction have not been thoroughly formulated, the major role of the liver in the disposition of the vinca alkaloids implies that dose modifications should be considered for patients with hepatic dysfunction, particularly hepatic excretory dysfunction.[181] A 50% dose reduction is often recommended for patients with total bilirubin levels between 1.5 and 3.0 mg/dL (50% dose reduction for bilirubin levels between 2.0 and 3.0 mg/dL is recommended for VRL), and at least a 75% dose reduction for plasma total bilirubin levels above 3.0 mg/dL. Dose reduction for renal insufficiency is not indicated.

Taxanes: Introduction and Indications

Although the taxanes affect microtubules, their principal mechanisms of action, pharmacology, clinical indications, and toxicities substantially differ from those of the vinca alkaloids. Interest in the taxanes began in 1963, when a crude extract of the bark of the Pacific yew tree, *Taxus brevifolia*, demonstrated broad activity in tumor models.[182] In 1971, Wall and colleagues identified paclitaxel as the active constituent of the bark extract, however, the limited supply of its primary source that was exclusively derived from the Pacific yew tree, the difficulties inherent in large-scale isolation, extraction, and preparation of bulk compound, and its poor aqueous solubility delayed its development.[182] Interest was maintained after characterization of its novel mechanism of action and the availability of an adequate supply for requisite preclinical and limited clinical studies. The early search for taxanes derived from more abundant and renewable resources led to the semisynthesis of docetaxel by the addition of a side chain to 10-deacetyl-baccatin III, an inactive taxane precursor found in the needles and other components of more abundant yew species.[183] The supply of paclitaxel is no longer preclusive of the development of a feasible semisynthetic process. A wide variety of taxane analogues, as well as paclitaxel formulations, have been evaluated. Recently, a protein-bound formulation (protein-bound paclitaxel particles for injection[PBPPI]), which is an albumin-bound form of paclitaxel, received regulatory approval in the United States and elsewhere.[184]

Figure 53-3 shows the structures of paclitaxel and docetaxel, which are complex esters consisting of a 15-member taxane ring system linked to an unusual 4-member oxetan ring. The taxane rings of both paclitaxel and docetaxel, but not 10-deacetylbaccatin III, are linked to an ester side chain attached to the C-13 position of the ring, which is essential for antimicrotubule and antitumor activity.[185] The structures of paclitaxel and docetaxel differ in substitutions at the C-10 taxane ring position and on the ester side chain attached at C-13, which render docetaxel slightly more water soluble and potent than paclitaxel. However, the clinical ramifications of these differences are not entirely clear.

Clinical Indications

Paclitaxel initially received regulatory approval in the United States and elsewhere for the treatment of patients with ovarian cancer after failure of first-line or subsequent chemotherapy.[182] Its use in combination with a platinum compound as primary induction therapy in suboptimally debulked stages III or IV ovarian cancer has demonstrated a survival advantage in randomized phase 3 studies.[186] In the United States, paclitaxel is also indicated for treatment of patients with metastatic breast cancer after failure of combination chemotherapy for

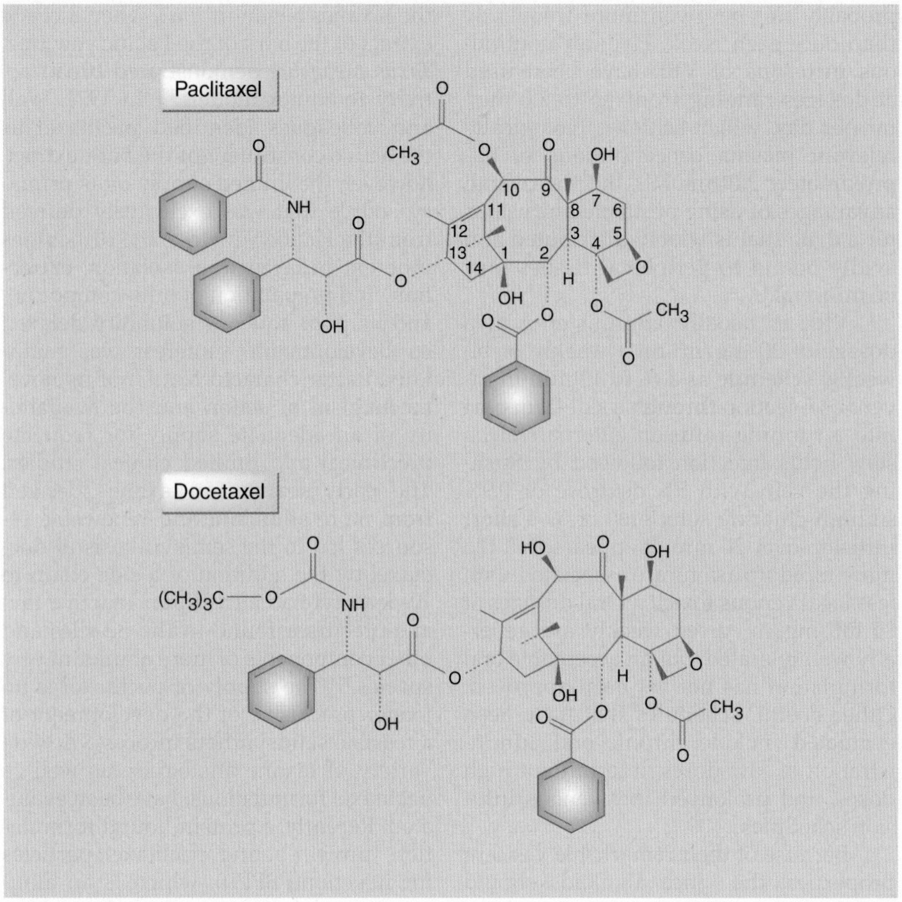

Figure 53-3 Chemical structures of the taxanes, paclitaxel and docetaxel.

metastatic disease or at relapse within 6 months of adjuvant chemotherapy, with prior therapy that includes an anthracycline unless clinically contraindicated.[187] In addition, it received regulatory approval for treating axillary lymph node-positive operable breast cancer following standard doxorubicin-based adjuvant chemotherapy after demonstrating improved disease-free survival, as well as overall survival in one of the studies.[188-190] Compelling early results have been noted following treatment of patients with high-risk early-stage breast cancer with alternative taxane-containing regimens, particularly "dose-dense" regimens, and weekly paclitaxel administration has demonstrated superiority over and every-3-week paclitaxel in women with axillary lymph node-positive or high-risk, lymph node-negative breast cancer.[188-190] Various other therapeutics have also received regulatory approval in specific indications as components of paclitaxel-based combination regimens. The combination of gemcitabine and paclitaxel demonstrated superior survival to paclitaxel alone in the first-line treatment of metastatic breast cancer, and gemcitabine received regulatory approval for use with paclitaxel in this setting.[191] Similarly, the combination of trastuzimab and paclitaxel demonstrated superior survival as first-line metastatic treatment in women with HER-2 expressing breast cancer, and the combination of bevacizumab and paclitaxel demonstrated superior survival over paclitaxel alone in the first-line treatment of women with metastatic breast cancer.[192,193] Paclitaxel has also received regulatory approval in the United States for second-line treatment of Kaposi sarcoma associated with the acquired immunodeficiency syndrome, and in combination with cisplatin as primary treatment advanced stage IIIB and stage IV non-small cell lung cancer patients who are not candidates for radiation therapy or potentially curative surgery.[194,195] Bevaciuzumab, in combination with paclitaxel and carboplatin, is approved for the treatment of stage IIIB and stage IV nonsquamous non-small cell lung cancer.[196]

Docetaxel initially received regulatory approval in the United States for patients with metastatic or locally advanced breast cancer after failure of anthracycline-based chemotherapy, which was later broadened to a general second-line indication.[183] Subsequently, the combination of capecitabine and docetaxel demonstrated superior survival over docetaxel alone after failure of an anthracycline in patients with locally advanced or metastatic breast cancer, and capecitabine as a component of this doublet received regulatory approval. Regulatory approval was also granted for docetaxel in combination with cyclophosphamide and doxorubicin in the adjuvant treatment of patients with local breast cancer following definitive local treatment.[197] In non-small cell lung cancer, docetaxel initially received regulatory approval for treatment of unresectable locally advanced or metastatic disease after demonstrating increased survival after failure of cisplatin-based therapy, and the combination of docetaxel and cisplatin was later granted regulatory approval as first-line treatment of such patients.[198] Both paclitaxel and docetaxel have demonstrated notable activity in patients with hormone-refractory prostate cancer (HRPC) and regulatory approval was recently granted for docetaxel in combination with prednisone for this indication as the regimen demonstrated superior survival over mitoxantrone and prednisone.[199] Similarly, the taxanes have notable activity in the treatment of squamous cell carcinoma of the head and neck, and docetaxel, in combination with cisplatin and 5-fluorouracil, has received regulatory approval in the United States in the neoadjuvant treatment of patients with locally advanced disease.[200] Docetaxel in combination with cisplatin and 5-fluorouracil has also been granted regulatory approval in the United States and elsewhere for untreated, advanced gastric and gastroesophageal junction adenocarcinoma.[201]

PBPPI, the newest taxane to receive regulatory approval in the United States and elsewhere for the treatment of breast cancer after failure of anthracycline-based chemotherapy for metastatic disease or relapse within 6 months of adjuvant therapy, is a formulation of paclitaxel in 3-4% human serum albumin, similar to the concentration of albumin in the blood, in contrast to earlier formulations of paclitaxel in polyoxyethylated castor oil.[184,202]

It is important to note that the antitumor spectra for paclitaxel and docetaxel are identical, with activity noted in many other diverse cancers including endometrial, bladder, small cell lung carcinoma, and germ cell carcinomas, and lymphoma and melanoma. Differences in clinical efficacy endpoints and regulatory indications between the various taxanes may, in part, reflect different regulatory strategies, study designs, and dose schedules, and not the inherent superiority of any specific taxane.

Mechanism of Action

The binding site for paclitaxel on microtubules is different from the binding sites for exchangeable GTP, colchicine, podophyllotoxin, and vinblastine. Paclitaxel binds to the N-terminal 31 amino acids of the β-tubulin subunit of tubulin polymers, however, other sites may be involved.[182,203-209] Paclitaxel binds in a pocket that is lined by several hydrophobic residues on the luminal side of the microtubule wall, roughly in the middle of the monomer along the protofilament direction.[7,209,210] Docetaxel, which most likely shares the same binding site as paclitaxel, appears to have a 1.9-fold higher affinity for the site, and the tubulin assembly process induced by docetaxel proceeds with a critical protein concentration that is 2.1-fold lower than that of paclitaxel.[208,211-215] However, it is not clear whether these differences translate into increased therapeutic indices for docetaxel in the clinic since higher potency may result in more severe toxicity at identical drug concentrations. Nevertheless, the results of both preclinical and clinical studies indicate that the taxanes may not be completely cross-resistant, but these results may reflect differences in delivered dose and schedule.

Although both the vinca alkaloids and taxanes produce similar disruptive effects on the mitotic spindle apparatus, their principal mechanisms of action differ. The taxanes alter the tubulin rate dissociation constants at both ends of the microtubules by reducing the critical tubulin concentration required for microtubule assembly and promoting both nucleation and elongation phases of the polymerization reaction, thereby stabilizing microtubules against depolymerization and enhancing polymerization.[2-6,41,214-220] Binding of the taxanes to polymerized tubulin strengthens the microtubule. At substoichiometric concentrations, the taxanes suppress microtubule dynamics without appreciably increasing the rate of formation of polymerized tubulin.[2-6,41,214-220] At much higher concentrations, which are readily achieved in the clinic, the taxanes induce tubulin polymerization and increase microtubule mass. The microtubules of taxane-treated cells are extraordinarily stable, resisting depolymerization by cold, calcium, GTP, and depolymerizing antimicrotubule agents. These actions result in the suppression of treadmilling and dynamic instability, which are essential for normal microtubule dynamics during both the mitotic and nonmitotic phases of the cell cycle.[2,3,9,13,16,211,217-220] Both stoichiometric and substoichiometric binding of the taxanes inhibit the proliferation of cells, principally by inducing a sustained mitotic block at the metaphase/anaphase boundary; however, morphologic changes, such as microtubule bundle formation during the nonmitotic phases of the cell cycle, suggest that the interphase microtubules are also affected. Nevertheless, perturbations in microtubule dynamics are most relevant during mitotic spindle formation, and therefore cells are most sensitive to the taxanes in mitosis.

Perturbations of mitotic processes and the induction of mitotic arrest by the taxanes trigger apoptosis; however, the precise mechanisms by which these perturbations result in cell death have not been determined. The taxanes do interact with numerous proteins that regulate the integrity of mitosis and several different mechanisms that potentially link the mitotic arrest induced by the taxanes and other antimicrotubule agents to the initiating event in the intrinsic pathway of apoptosis have been characterized.[59,219-234] For example, microtubule disruption induces the tumor suppressor gene TP53, inhibitors of cyclin-dependent kinases (eg, p21/Waf-1), and modulates several other protein kinases.[219,220,224] As a consequence, cells arrest in G2/M, after which time they may either undergo apoptosis or traverse through G2/M and divide.[231] The apoptotic initiating events include activation of the proapoptotic molecules Bax and Bad and inactivation of the antiapoptotic regulators Bcl-2 and BclxL.[232,233] Taxane-induced mitochondrial stress triggering apoptosis occurs through activation of both JNK and p38 pathways, and various kinases have been implicated in the phosphorylation of Bcl-2 induced by the taxanes and other antimicrotubule agents, including Jun N-terminal kinase (JNK) and its proapoptotic effector Bim, c-Raf, extracellular signal regulated kinase 1 and 2 (ERK1 and ERK2), apoptosis signal regulated kinase (ASK), cyclin-dependent kinase 1(CDK1), cAMP-dependent protein kinase A, and protein kinase C.[55,222,232-235] Phosphorylation (inactivation) of Bcl-2 family members and phosphorylation of proapoptotic molecules (activation) stimulate the intrinsic pathway of apoptosis and downstream effector caspases.[231,236] The antimitotic effects of the taxanes and other antimicrotubule agents may be linked to apoptosis through other modulatory events such as the phosphorylation of the proapoptotic protein Bad by activating CDK1.[234] The taxanes may also induce cell death independent of caspase activation.

The taxanes also perturb interphase microtubules in nonproliferating cells as manifested by the formation of microtubule bundles.[216,237] Paclitaxel has also been reported to induce transcription factors and enzymes that mediate proliferation, apoptosis, and inflammation.[224,234,238,239] In addition, these agents enhance the effects of ionizing radiation in vitro and in vivo, which may be related to the inhibition of cell-cycle progression in G2/M, which are the most radiosensitive phases of the cell cycle.[240-244] In angiogenesis inhibition assays, they inhibit parameters indicative of angiogenesis at concentrations below those that induce cytotoxicity, but the contribution of these effects to the antitumor actions of the taxanes is not clear.[230,245,246]

The taxanes have been demonstrated to induce many other cellular effects that may or may not relate to their disruptive effects on microtubule dynamics. Although the taxanes primarily block cell-cycle traverse in the mitotic phases, the agents prevent G0 to S-phase transition.[237,247] Explanations that have been proposed to account for the nonmitotic actions of the taxanes include disruptive effects on tubulin in the cell membrane, the interphase cytoskeleton, and microtubules that are involved in growth factor signaling, and vascular endothelial growth factor expression through reactive oxygen species production.[28,248]

The taxanes inhibit specific functions in nonmalignant tissues, which may be mediated through their disruptive effects on microtubule dynamics.[28] For example, paclitaxel inhibits relevant morphologic and biochemical processes in human neutrophils, including chemotaxis, migration, spreading, polarization, hydrogen peroxide generation, and killing of phagocytized microorganisms.[28] Paclitaxel also antagonizes the effects of microtubule-disrupting drugs on lymphocyte function, cAMP metabolism, and inhibits the proliferation of stimulated human lymphocytes.[28] Paclitaxel mimics the effects of endotoxic bacterial lipopolysaccharide on macrophages, which results in a rapid decrement in tumor necrosis factor-α (TNF-α) receptors and TNF-α release.[233,238,239] The agent also induces expression of the gene for TNF-α, but these activities are not related to paclitaxel's disruptive effects on microtubule assembly, which suggests the involvement of cytokine activation in the antitumor activities of the taxanes.[238] In addition, paclitaxel has been demonstrated to inhibit chorioretinal fibroblast proliferation and contractility in an in vitro model of proliferative vitreoretinopathy, as well as neointimal smooth muscle cell proliferation after angioplasty.[249,250] Cardiac arterial stents coated with paclitaxel received regulatory approval in the United States and elsewhere because of a significantly decreased incidence of restenosis from fibroblast proliferation and intimal hyperplasia.[251] Finally, paclitaxel inhibits secretory functions in many specialized cells, such as insulin secretion in isolated rat islets of Langerhans, protein secretion in rat hepatocytes, and the nicotinic receptor-stimulated release of catecholamines from chromaffin cells of the adrenal medulla.[28]

Althouth PBPPI likely affects malignant and nonmalignant tissues similar to conventional formulations of paclitaxel and docetaxel, the binding of paclitaxel to albumin may results in increased accumulation of paclitaxel molecules in tumor tissue via albumin-specific glycoprotein 60-mediated endothelial cell transcytosis of paclitaxel-bound albumin and accumulation in the area of tumor by alumin binding to secreted protein, acidic and rich in cysteine (SPARC).[252-255] This process may result in more rapid systemic distribution and clearance of paclitaxel than poloxyethylated castor oil formulations.

Mechanisms of Resistance

Two general types of mechanisms of acquired taxane resistance have been described in cells made resistant by prolonged drug treatment at low concentrations. The best characterized mechanism is the MDR phenotype, which can be mediated by several ABC multidrug transporter family members. The most important ABC transporter with respect to conferring taxane resistance is the 170-kDa Pgp efflux pump or the MDR1 encoded gene product MDR1 (ABC subfamily B1; ABCB1) and MDR2 (ABC subfamily ABCB4) (see Vinca Alkaloids: Introduction and Indications and Mechanisms of Resistance).[68,69,205,256,257] In addition, low-level taxane resistance appears to be conferred by the bile salt export protein (BSEP, also known as ABCC11).[68] Unlike the vinca alkaloids, ABCC1 (MRP1) and ABCC2 (MRP2) do not appear to be involved in transporting the taxanes.[258,259] In murine systems, the particular species of Pgp found in paclitaxel-resistant cells is similar, but not identical, to that found in VBL and colchicine-resistant cells derived from the same parental line.[68,224] These cells are cross-resistant with many other natural products, and resistance to both paclitaxel and docetaxel conferred by MDRl can be reversed by many classes of membrane-active drugs, including the calcium-channel blockers, tamoxifen, cyclosporine A, and antiarrhythmic agents.[68,224] Even the principal component of the vehicles used to formulate paclitaxel and docetaxel—polyoxyethylated castor oil and polysorbate-80, respectively, can reverse taxane resistance, but, whereas plasma concentrations of polyoxyethylated castor oil achieved with paclitaxel are sufficient to reverse MDR, sufficient modulatory concentrations of polysorbate-80 are not achieved with docetaxel in the clinic.[260,261] Strategies aimed at reversing resistance to taxanes and other MDR substrates in the clinic have not been successful to date, but most studies have been performed with MDR modulators that reduce taxane clearance and increase toxicity (eg, verapamil, cyclosporine A), thereby confounding interpretation of the inherent effects of these agents on MDR modulation. However, MDR modulators that do not affect taxane clearance and toxicity, such as the cyclosporine analogue PSC 833 and the MDR/MRP modulator VX-710, do not appear to enhance antitumor activity.[68,262,263]

Similar to the vinca alkaloids, several human cell lines rendered taxane-resistant by treatment with high drug concentrations for protracted periods have structurally altered α- and β-tubulins and an impaired ability to polymerize tubulin dimers into microtubules (see the section Vinca Alkaloids: Introduction and Indications and Mechanisms of Resistance).[82-84,264-267] These cells were found to lack normal microtubules in their interpolar mitotic spindles and have an inherently slow rate of microtubule assembly when grown in the absence of drug. The continuous presence of the taxanes is required for microtubule assembly to proceed. Furthermore, these mutants are also collaterally sensitive to the vinca alkaloids. In some experimental systems, paclitaxel-resistant cells had mutated β-tubulin alleles, with mutations involving the putative taxane binding sites; specifically, leucines at positions 215, 217, and 228 were mutated to histidine, arginine, or phenylalanine.[268,269] Low-level expression resulted in drug resistance, whereas, high-level expression of these mutations caused impairment of microtubule assembly, cell-cycle arrest, and failure to proliferate, all of which were reversed by incubation with paclitaxel.

There is increasing evidence that alterations in tubulin content, tubulin isotype profiles, and tubulin polymerization dynamics confer taxane resistance. For example, paclitaxel-resistant tumors have been shown to have high levels of class I, III, and IVa isotypes of β-tubulin[85,90-92,268-272] High intratumoral levels of the β_{III} isotype, which is a minor component of cellular β-tubulin and increases the dynamic instability of microtubules, impedes microtubule assembly, and confers resistance to the taxanes, has been demonstrated in tumor biopsies sampled from patients with taxane-resistant tumors and cell lines with acquired taxane resistance.[88,90-92,272-277] The absence of class III β-tubulin is associated with rapid microtubule assembly in vitro, whereas overexpression decreases the rate of microtubule assembly.[274] Higher levels of class β_{III} tubulin RNA levels have also been reported in non-small cell lung cancers of patients who did not respond to taxane-based treatment, which is in-line with in vitro findings. Mutations of tubulin isotype genes, gene amplifications, and isotype switching have also been reported in taxane-resistant cell lines.[59,82,224,225,267,269-278]

Aberrant proliferative signaling may contribute to taxane resistance by raising the cell's threshold for taxane-induced apoptosis. Insulin-like growth factor-I, for example, appears to protect responsive breast cancer cell lines from the cytotoxic effects of the anthracyclines and taxanes, possibly by activating the phosphatidylinositol 3-kinase (PI3K) pathway and inducing phosphorylation (inactivation) of antiapoptotic factors.[279] Other mediators that may influence the cell's threshold for drug-induced apoptosis include TP53, HER-2, auora 2-kinase, survivin, and BRAC1. The centromere-associated serine/threonine kinase, aurora 2- kinase, which is involved in centrosome separation, biopolar spindle formation, and chromosomal kinetochore attachment to the mitotic spindle, appears to override the mitotic assembly checkpoint and induce taxane resistance.[2] Also, overexpresssion of survivin, a member of the inhibitor of apoptosis family of proteins, inhibits caspase activity and apoptosis induced by antimicrotubule agents. The disruption of the tumor suppressor gene, BRAC1, which is implicated in maintaining genomic stability through DNA repair and appears to be involved in hereditary breast and ovarian cancers, appears to play a role in conferring resistance to paclitaxel and the inducible expression of BRAC1 may enhance paclitaxel-induced apoptosis.[2] The mutational loss of the TP53 tumor suppressor does not appear confer resistance to microtubule polymerizing agents in contrast to DNA-disruptive agents.[16]

MAPs have been implicated in mechanisms of resistance to apoptosis induced by the taxanes and other antimicrotubule agents, as illustrated by the observation that MAP4, which enhances microtubule polymerization and is negatively regulated by wild-type TP53, increases sensitivity to paclitaxel.[280,281] The suppression of dynamic instability by low concentrations of microtubule polymerizing agents may also enhance the nuclear accumulation of TP53 and the induction of proapoptotic TP53–up-regulated modulator of apoptosis.[2] This may represent a TP53-dependent mechanism of apoptosis induced by antimicrotubule agents in cells that harbor functional TP53.[16] Overexpression of p21, a downstream effector of TP53, also appears to impede cell-cycle traverse in G2, thereby blocking progression into the more drug-vulnerable mitotic phase and decreasing taxane sensitivity.[282,283] Finally, alterations in cytoskeletal components, particularly reduced γ-actin, has been related to chemotherapy resistance.[284]

Transfection of cells with HER-2, a member of the epidermal growth factor receptor family that is amplified and overexpressed, or both, in approximately 30% of breast cancers, increases taxane resistance, and high expression of HER-2 in vitro relates to taxane resistance.[282,283] Overexpression of HER-2 can also inhibit CDK1 either by inducing p21, which participates in the G2/M checkpoint and contributes to resistance to apoptosis induced by antimicrotubule agents, or directly phosphorylating (inactivating) CDK1, which may block taxane-mediated entry into mitosis and apoptosis.[2] Consistent with this relationship, downregulation of HER-2 by the anti–HER-2 antibody trastuzumab sensitizes breast cancer cells to the taxanes, and the combination of trastuzumab and either paclitaxel or docetaxel is associated with increased survival compared with the taxanes alone.[283,285] Nevertheless, the presence of HER-2 amplification does not adversely influence response to first-line paclitaxel-containing chemotherapy.[286] In one study, the expression or amplification, or both, of HER-2 is associated with benefit from the addition of paclitaxel after adjuvant treatment with doxorubicin plus cyclophosphamide in lymph node-positive breast cancer regardless of estrogen-receptor status, whereas women with HER-2 negative disease derived little, if any, benefit.[287]

Clinical Pharmacology

General ■ The taxanes are most commonly administered intravenously at dosages ranging from 175 to 225 mg/m² over 3 h (paclitaxel), 75 to 100 mg/m² over 1 h (docetaxel), or 260 mg/m² over 30 min (PBPPI) every 3 weeks, but other schedules, particularly weekly schedules, are commonly used (see the section "Administration, Dose, and Schedule" below). The oral bioavailability of both paclitaxel and docetaxel is poor, which is due, in part, to the constitutive overexpression of Pgp and P-450 metabolizing capability of enterocytes and/or first-pass metabolism in the liver and/or intestines. Congruent with this mechanism, oral bioavailability can be enhanced if the taxanes are administered orally following treatment with oral cyclosporine or other modulators of Pgp and cytochrome P-450 mixed-function oxidases.[288] As shown in Table 53-2, the taxanes share the following pharmacologic characteristics: large volumes of distribution, rapid and avid binding to all tissues except for the unperturbed central nervous system, long terminal half-lives and substantial hepatic metabolism, biliary excretion, and fecal elimination.

Paclitaxel ■ More recent pharmacologic evaluations of paclitaxel, which involved shorter administration schedules and highly sensitive analytical assays, indicate that its pharmacokinetic behavior is nonlinear or pseudo-nonlinear.[261,289-291] Nonlinear behavior is more apparent with shorter infusions that result in higher plasma paclitaxel concentrations and more effective saturation of both drug elimination and tissue distribution processes. Both saturable distribution and elimination processes may be, in part, responsible for paclitaxel's nonlinear behavior, with tissue distribution becoming effectively saturated at lower drug concentrations (achieved with paclitaxel dosages of less than 175 mg/m² over 3 h) as compared with elimination processes that are saturated at higher concentrations (achieved with paclitaxel dosages > 175 mg/m² over 3 h). A potential ramification of true nonlinearity is that dose escalation may result in a disproportionate increase in drug exposure and toxicity, whereas dose reduction may result in a disproportionate decrease in drug exposure. However, the use of shorter infusion schedules also results in higher plasma concentrations of paclitaxel's polyoxyethylated castor oil vehicle, which may simulate nonlinearity (pseudo-nonlinearity) by binding paclitaxel and inhibiting drug disposition.[292,293]

The pharmacologic behavior of paclitaxel in plasma appears to be triphasic and its volume of distribution is much larger than the volume of total body water, indicating extensive drug binding to plasma proteins or other tissue elements, possibly tubulin.[261] Plasma protein binding is high (>95%) and reversible. Albumin and α1-acid glycoprotein contribute equally to drug binding with a minor contribution from lipoproteins.[294-296] None of the drugs that are commonly administered with paclitaxel, including ranitidine, dexamethasone, diphenhydramine, doxorubicin, 5-fluorouracil, and cisplatin, significantly alter protein binding.[295] Drug binding to platelets is extensive and saturable, and animal distribution studies with radiolabeled paclitaxel indicate extensive uptake and retention by virtually all tissues, except for normal sanctuary sites such as the brain and testes, possibly due to xenobiotic efflux pumps in these tissues.[297,298]

Clearance is closely related to body surface area, providing a rationale for dosing based on this parameter. In humans, peak plasma concentrations achieved with 3-96-h schedules (more than 0.05-10 μmol/L) and drug concentrations in third-space fluid collections such as ascites (more than 0.1 μmol/L), are capable of inducing relevant biologic effects in vitro, but drug penetration into the unperturbed central nervous system is negligible.[261,298,299] The principal mode of paclitaxel disposition is hepatic metabolism and biliary excretion. The

Table 53-2 **Taxanes and Epothilones Comparative Pharmacokinetic and Toxicologic Characteristics**

Parameter	Paclitaxel	Docetaxel	PBPPI	Ixabepilone
Standard adult dose:				
Range (mg/m²/3 week)	175–225 (3-h infusion)	75–100 (1-h infusion)	260 (30-min infusion)	40 (3-h infusion); sshould be capped at 2.2 mg/m² for body surface areas exceeding this value
mg/m²/week	80	30–36	100–150	
Pharmacokinetic behavior (clinically relevant doses)	Triphasic	Triphasic	Biphasic	Multiexponential
(>175 mg/m²)	Saturable taxane elimination and distribution; pseudo-nonlinearity due to vehicle	Dose-proportional to 115 mg/m2	Dose-proportional	Dose-proporational
Plasma half-life (terminal)	10–20 h	10–20 h	27 h	52 h
Clearance	20–25 L/h[a]	36 L/h	15 L/h/m²	36–40 L/h
Primary route	Hepatic metabolism and biliary elimination	Hepatic metabolism and biliary elimination	Hepatic metabolism and biliary elimination	Hepatic metabolism and biliary elimination
Principal toxicity	Neutropenia	Neutropenia	Neutropenia	Neutropenia
Other toxicities	Alopecia, neurotoxicity, myalgia, arthralgia, hypersensitivity reactions, asthenia	Alopecia, skin and nail toxicity, asthenia, myalgia, arthralgia, fluid retention, neurotoxicity, hypersensitivity reactions	Alopecia, asthenia,myalgia, injection site reactions, hypersensitivity reactions	Neurotoxicity, hypersensitivity reactions

[a]175 mg/m² over 3 h (dose schedule).

liver metabolizes and excretes both paclitaxel and paclitaxel metabolites into the bile.[261,297,300-306] In rats treated with radiolabeled paclitaxel, 98% of radioactivity is recovered from feces collected for 6 days, and approximately 71% of an administered dose of paclitaxel is excreted in the feces over 5 days as either parent compound or metabolites in humans, with 6α-hydroxypaclitaxel being the largest component, accounting for 26% of the dose; unmetabolized paclitaxel accounts for only 5% of the dose. Renal clearance of paclitaxel and metabolites may account for up to 14% of the administered dose.[261] In humans, cytochrome P-450 mixed-function oxidases are responsible for the bulk of drug disposition, specifically the isoenzymes CYP2C8 and CYP3A4, which metabolize paclitaxel to 6α-hydroxypaclitaxel (major) and another hydroxylated metabolite, both of which are much less active than paclitaxel in vivo, possibly due to their greater polarity which precludes intracellular uptake.[261,300-304] There is considerable interindividual variability in paclitaxel metabolism that can be attributed to pharmacogenetic differences in P-450 metabolism and concurrent medications that alter metabolism.[261,303-306]

Pharmacodynamic studies demonstrated that several pharmacokinetic parameters indicative of drug exposure relate to the principal toxicities of paclitaxel, the most important and consistent of which is the relationship between the severity of neutropenia and the duration of drug exposure above biologically relevant plasma concentrations ranging from 0.05 to 0.1 μmol/L.[261,289,291,303] A prospective analysis of pharmacokinetic determinants of outcome in several hundred patients with advanced non-small cell lung cancer treated with the combination of cisplatin and paclitaxel at either 135 or 250 mg/m^2 over 24 h demonstrated that the magnitude of the steady-state plasma paclitaxel concentration correlates poorly with antitumor activity, disease-free survival, and overall survival.[307]

Docetaxel ■ The pharmacokinetics of docetaxel (1-h schedule) in plasma are triphasic and linear at doses of 115 mg/m^2 or less.[183,308,309] Terminal half-lives ranging from 11.1 to 18.5 h have been reported. In one population study, plasma concentration data revealed triphasic pharmacokinetics, and the following pharmacokinetic parameters: terminal half-life of 12.4 h, clearance of 1 L/h/m^2, and steady-state volume of distribution of 74 L/m^2.[183,308,309] The most important determinants of docetaxel clearance were body surface area, hepatic function, and plasma α1-acid glycoprotein concentration, whereas age and plasma albumin level had significant, albeit minor, influences on clearance. Like paclitaxel, plasma protein binding is high (>80-90%), and binding is primarily to α1-acid glycoprotein, albumin, and lipoproteins.[183,308,309] Like paclitaxel, docetaxel is widely distributed, but does not enter the unperturbed central nervous system.[310,311] In both dogs and mice treated with radiolabeled drug, fecal excretion accounts for 70-80% of total radioactivity, whereas urinary excretion accounts for 10% or less.[310] The hepatic cytochrome P-450 mixed-function oxidases, particularly CYP3A, the activity of which, in adults, is represented by the combined activities of CYP3A4, CYP3A5, CYP3A7, and CYP3A43, is responsible for most of docetaxel's metabolism.[312-314] In contrast to paclitaxel, the C-13 side chain, instead of the taxane ring, is metabolized.[312,313,315] These metabolites seem to be much less active than docetaxel.

The principal pharmacokinetic determinants of toxicity, particularly neutropenia, are drug exposure and the time that plasma concentrations exceed biologically relevant concentrations.[309] A population pharmacodynamic analysis of determinants of outcome in phase 2 trials of docetaxel revealed that the pretreatment plasma concentration of α1-acid glycoprotein is among the most important determinants of the time to progression in patients with metastatic breast cancer, whereas both drug exposure and the pretreatment plasma concentration of α1-acid glycoprotein were positive determinants of time to progression in patients with advanced lung cancer treated with docetaxel.[308,316] Conversely, the pretreatment plasma level of α1-acid glycoprotein was negatively, albeit significantly, related to the probability of experiencing both severe neutropenia and febrile neutropenia. The rate of docetaxel clearance has also been related to CYP3A4 activity, as assessed by the erythromycin breath test.[313]

PBPPI ■ In clinical studies following the administration of PBPPI doses ranging from 80 to 360 mg/m^2, paclitaxel pharmacokinetics were dose-proportional.[252-255,315,317] At the recommended dose of 260 mg/m^2, total clearance averaged 15 L/h/m^2 and the mean volume of distribution was 632 L/m^2. Approximately 89-98% of paclitaxel in PBPPI is protein-bound in vitro. In a phase 3 study in which the pharmacokinetics of PPBPI administered over 30 min was compared to 175 mg/m^2 paclitaxel injection over 3 h, the clearance of PBPPI was 43% larger than for the clearance of paclitaxel injection and the volume of distribution of PBPPI was also higher (53%). Differences in C_{max}, as well as C_{max} corrected for dose, is likely due to differences in total dose and rate of infusion. There were no differences in terminal half-lives. In a study that examined plasma pharmacokinetics and partitioning of radiolabeled paclitaxel from PBPPI and a polyoxyethylated paclitaxel formulation into red blood cells and tumor tissue for 24 h following tail vein injection of 20 mg/kg paclitaxel in a human breast cancer xenograft model, the distribution of PBPPI was rapid and extensive, as shown by a 5-fold larger volume of distribution and much lower values for both C_{max} and area under the concentration-time curve (AUC) compared with a polyoxyethylated castor oil formulation.[315,317] Furthermore, PBPPI demonstrated a lower plasma/blood ratio of paclitaxel across all time points and distributed more effectively into the tumors. Tumor AUC values of paclitaxel were 1.6-fold higher, on average, with PBPPI and terminal half-life values for PBPPI were significantly longer than from the polyoxyethylated castor oil formulation (17.1 vs 4.0 h) prolonged half-life for PBPPI could be attributed to red blood cell penetration and temporary storage of paclitaxel for PBPPI, releasing paclitaxel as plasma levels decrease.

The metabolic profiles of PBPPI and paclitaxel formulated in polyoxyethylated castor oil are similar.[252-255,315,317] Fecal and urinary excretion accounts for about 20% and 4% of the total dose of PBPPI administered, respectively. In vitro studies with human liver microsomes and tissue slices revealed identical CYP2C8- and CYP3A4-induced hydroxylated metabolites as with polyoxyethylated castor oil formulations.

Drug Interactions

Both sequence-dependent pharmacokinetic and toxicologic interactions between taxanes and other chemotherapy agents have been noted.[318] The most prominent sequence-dependent effects relate to the platinum compound and the taxanes, particularly with protracted taxane administration schedules. Sequence-dependence has been primarily reported with paclitaxel, which most likely relates to the fact that docetaxel has been evaluated on a shorter (1-h) schedule. The sequence of cisplatin followed by paclitaxel (24-h schedule) induces more profound neutropenia than the reverse sequence, which is explained by a 33% reduction in the clearance of paclitaxel following cisplatin.[319,320] The least toxic sequence, paclitaxel before cisplatin, was demonstrated to induce more cytotoxicity in vitro, and therefore it was selected for clinical development.[320] Sequence-dependence does not appear to be a clinically relevant phenomenon with the taxanes on shorter schedules. The modulation of cytochrome P-450-dependent paclitaxel-metabolizing enzymes by cisplatin may, in part, explain these findings. Treatment with paclitaxel on either a 3-h or 24-h schedule followed by carboplatin produces equivalent neutropenia and less thrombocytopenia as compared with carboplatin as a single agent, which is not explained by pharmacokinetic interactions.[308,321,322] Both neutropenia and mucositis are more severe when paclitaxel on a 24-h schedule is administered before doxorubicin, as compared with the reverse sequence, which is most likely caused by an approximately 32% reduction in the clearance of doxorubicin and doxorubicinol when the agent is administered after paclitaxel.[323-325] Neither sequence-dependent pharmacologic nor toxicologic interactions between doxorubicin and paclitaxel on a shorter (3-h) schedule have been noted; however, the doxorubicin clearance is reduced with both sequences, and the combination of paclitaxel (3-h schedule) and doxorubicin (bolus infusion) produces a much higher rate of congestive cardiotoxicity than would have been expected from an equivalent cumulative doxorubicin dose given without paclitaxel (see Toxicity, below, for a discussion of cardiotoxicity).[323,324] Although similar decrements in the clearance of epirubicin and its metabolites have been reported in studies of paclitaxel combined with epirubicin, an increased incidence of cardiotoxicity has not been observed.[326] The precise etiology for these interactions is unclear. The pharmacokinetic interactions may not be of sufficient magnitude to account for the enhanced cardiotoxicity of the combination, and there are experimental data indicating that paclitaxel enhances the metabolism of doxorubicin to cardiotoxic metabolites, such as doxorubicinol, in cardiomyocytes. Docetaxel does not appear to influence doxorubicin pharmacokinetics but, like paclitaxel, docetaxel can enhance the metabolism of doxorubicin to toxic species in the human heart.[327] Competition for the hepatic or biliary Pgp transport of the anthracyclines with paclitaxel or its polyoxyethylated castor oil vehicle (or both) is an alternate explanation.[260,318,319] Similar effects have not been noted with docetaxel, which is not formulated in polyoxyethylated castor oil.

Hematologic toxicity has been more profound with the sequence of cyclophosphamide before paclitaxel (24-h schedule) than with the reverse sequence.[328] Sequence-dependent cytotoxic effects have been reported when the taxanes are combined with 5-fluorouracil, etoposide, cytosine arabinoside, fludarabine, flavopiridol, and other antineoplastic agents in vitro.[288] In human tumor xenografts, both paclitaxel and docetaxel have been demonstrated to induce thymidine phosphorylase activity, which may increase the metabolic activation of the oral fluoropyrimidine prodrug capecitabine.[328,329]

Interactions between the taxanes and other classes of drugs, particularly those dependent on cytochrome P-450-dependent metabolism, have been documented.[329] Several inducers of cytochrome P-450 mixed-function oxidases, such as the anticonvulsants phenytoin and phenobarbital, accelerate the metabolism of both paclitaxel and docetaxel in human microsomes in vitro and in both children and adults who are concurrently receiving treatment with these anticonvulsants, as manifested by rapid drug clearance and tolerance of high drug doses.[261,300,302,304,318,330-334] There is preclinical evidence to suggest that docetaxel has a markedly reduced propensity to cause drug interactions that may entail hepatic CYP3A4 induction.[306] Conversely, many types of agents that inhibit cytochrome P-450 mixed-function oxidases, such as orphenadrine, erythromycin, cimetidine, testosterone, ketoconazole, fluconazole, midazolam, polyoxyethylated castor oil, and corticosteroids, interfere with the metabolism of paclitaxel and docetaxel in human microsomes in vitro; however, the inhibitory concentrations of these agents exceed those achieved in clinical practice, and the clinical relevance of these findings is not known. Besides the potent inhibitors of CYP3A listed above, other well-established inhibitors and inducers of CYP3A, including grapefruit juice and herbal products (eg, St. John's wort and Echinacea), may potentially induce pharmacokinetic interactions with the taxanes. Although there has been concern that the use of different H2-receptor antagonists with variable cytochrome P-450 inhibitory activities as components of premedication regimens may differentially affect drug clearance and hence toxicity, neither toxicologic nor pharmacologic differences between the agents were noted in a randomized clinical trial.[335] A review of early clinical trial results with docetaxel has not demonstrated significant alterations in docetaxel clearance by corticosteroids. In addition, interactions between warfarin and the taxanes, possibly due to protein-binding displacement effects, have been reported.[336]

The incidence of congestive heart failure has also been higher in breast cancer patients treated with the combination of trastuzumab and paclitaxel than with paclitaxel alone, but the explanation for this observation is not known.[337-339]

Although there has been less clinical experience with PBPPI compared to paclitaxel in polyoxyethylated castor oil, preclinical studies indicate that the prospects of drug interactions are likely to be similar. In vitro, the presence of cimetidine, ranitidine, dexamethasone did not affect the protein binding of paclitaxel in PBPPI. Although paclitaxel metabolism is inhibited by many agents, including ketoconazole, verapamil, diazepam, quinidine, dexamethasone, cyclosporin, teniposide, etoposide, and vincristine, the concentrations used in these studies exceeded those found in vivo following normal therapeutic doses. Testosterone, 17α-ethinyl estradiol, retinoic acid, and quercetin, a specific inhibitor of CYP2C8, also inhibited the formation of the principal metabolite, 6α-hydroxypaclitaxel, in vitro. Similar to paclitaxel in polyoxyethylated castor oil, paclitaxel pharmacokinetics following PBPPI administration may be altered as a result of interactions with compounds that are substrates, inducers, or inhibitors of CYP2C8 and/or CYP3A4.

Toxicity

General ■ Myelosuppression is the principal toxicity of the taxanes. However, despite similar structures, these agents possess modest differences in their toxicity spectra.

Paclitaxel ■ Neutropenia is the principal toxicity of paclitaxel.[340] The onset is usually on days 8-10, and recovery typically occurs by days 15-21. The main clinical determinant for the severity of neutropenia is the extent of prior myelosuppressive therapy; however, the neutropenia is typically noncumulative and the duration of severe neutropenia, even in heavily pretreated patients, is generally brief. Pharmacokinetic parameters of paclitaxel in plasma that reflect drug exposure, particularly the duration that plasma concentrations are maintained above biologically relevant levels (0.05-0.10 μmol/L; see Clinical Pharmacology) relate to the severity of neutropenia, which may explain why neutropenia is more severe with longer infusion schedules.[341,342] But because paclitaxel distributes widely and avidly even following treatment on short schedules, protracted schedules may not portend superior antitumor activity. At paclitaxel dosages exceeding 175 mg/m^2 on a 24-h schedule and 225 mg/m^2 on a 3-h schedule, neutrophil counts typically decrease to below 500/μL for fewer than 5 days in most courses, even in untreated patients. Even patients who have received extensive prior therapy can usually tolerate paclitaxel dosages in the range of 175-200 mg/m^2 administered over 3 h or 24 h. More frequent schedules, particularly weekly treatment with 80-100 mg/m^2, have resulted in less severe neutropenia than single-dosing schedules (Administration, Dose, and Schedule). Severe thrombocytopenia and anemia are unusual, except in heavily pretreated patients.

The incidence of major hypersensitivity reactions (HSRs) in early phase 1 trials approached 30%, but the incidence is approximately 1-3% following the advent and broad adoption of effective prophylaxis.[340,343-349] Most major reactions are characterized by dyspnea with bronchospasm, urticaria, and hypotension, which typically occur within the first 10 min after the first, and less frequently after the second, treatment. Major HSRs generally resolve completely after stopping treatment and occasionally after treatment with antihistamines, fluids, and vasopressors. Patients who have major reactions have been rechallenged successfully after receiving high doses of corticosteroids, but this approach is not always successful.[342,343,346-350] Patients who have experienced paclitaxel-related HSRs have also received docetaxel uneventfully.[351] Less severe manifestations of hypersensitivity phenomena, such as flushing and rashes, have been noted in as many as 40% of patients, and it is particularly important to note that minor HSRs do not portend the development of major reactions. The HSRs are most likely caused by a nonimmunologically mediated release of histamine or histamine-like substances in the polyoxyethylated castor oil vehicle, but the taxane moiety may also be contributory. In some cases, complement activation has been demonstrated.[348] Although the incidence of major HSRs is reduced with lower administration rates and longer infusion durations, the rates of major reactions are low on both 3- and 24-h schedules when patients are premedicated with corticosteroids and both Hl-histamine and H2-histamine antagonists (see Administration, Dose, and Schedule). In an assessment of the relative safety of two different paclitaxel schedules (24 h vs 3 h), the rates of major reactions were low and similar (2.1% vs. 1.0%) in patients receiving paclitaxel for 3 or 24 h, respectively, with premedication.[340,352]

A peripheral neuropathy dominated by sensory manifestations, such as numbness and paresthesia, in a glove-and-stocking distribution is the principal neurotoxic effect of paclitaxel.[340,353] There is often symmetric distal loss of sensation carried by both large (proprioception, vibration) and small (temperature, pinprick) fibers. Symptoms may begin as soon as 24-72 h after treatment with higher doses (≥250 mg/m^2), but usually occur only after multiple courses at 135-250 mg/m^2 every 3 weeks or 80-100 mg/m^2 weekly, and are cumulative thereafter. Severe neurotoxicity precludes chronic treatment with paclitaxel at dosages above 250 mg/m^2 over 3 h or 24 h, but severe neurotoxicity is uncommon at conventional doses (<200 mg/m^2) of paclitaxel alone even in patients who previously received other neurotoxic agents such as cisplatin. Patients treated with paclitaxel over shorter (eg, 3-h) schedules may be more prone to the neurotoxic effect of paclitaxel as compared with those treated with longer (eg, 24-h or 96-h) schedules, which argues that peak concentrations may be a principal pharmacologic determinant of neurotoxicity. The incidence of neurotoxicity has been particularly high in patients receiving paclitaxel as a 3-h infusion combined with cisplatin.

The distal, symmetric, length-dependent neurologic deficits suggest that paclitaxel causes a sensory and motor axonal loss similar to the dyingback neuropathies that may have their origin in the cell body or in axonal transport, but a few patients have the simultaneous onset of symptoms in the arms and legs, involvement of the face (perioral numbness), the predominance of large fiber loss, and diffuse areflexia suggestive of a neuronopathy. Both types of neuropathy depend on the dose of paclitaxel or its combination with cisplatin.[320,354] Motor and autonomic dysfunction may also occur, especially at high doses and in patients with preexisting neuropathies caused by diabetes mellitus and alcoholism. Although the administration of amifostine, glutamate, pyridoxine, sulfhydryl group scavenger drugs, and anticonvulsants, has been reported to reduce the neurotoxic effects of paclitaxel in some experimental models, anecdotal reports, or insufficiently powered randomized trials, there is no convincing evidence that any specific measure is effective at ameliorating existing manifestations or preventing the development or worsening of neurotoxicity.[355,356]

Optic nerve disturbances, characterized by scintillating scotomata, may also occur.[357] Acute encephalopathy, which can progress to coma and death, has been reported following treatment with high doses (>600 mg/m^2).[357,358,359] A transient acute encephalopathy following paclitaxel treatment in patients who receive prior cranial irradiation occurs rarely.[358-360]

Paclitaxel may produce transient myalgia without physical or biochemical evidence of myositis. Myalgia is typically experienced 2-5 days after treatment with doses above 170 mg/m^2.[361] A constellation of muscular and neuropathic effects often precludes continuous treatment with paclitaxel administered on a weekly schedule, requiring the institution of rest periods. In general, nonsteroidal anti-inflammatory agents are minimally effective at palliating or preventing symptoms, and the use of narcotics prophylactically on days 2-5 post-treatment may be useful in symptomatic patients. Antihistamines have been anecdotally reported to prevent acute myalgia. Treatment with corticosteroids, specifically prednisone 10 mg twice daily for 5 days beginning 24 h after treatment, may be effective at reducing myalgia and arthralgia, and gabapentin, glutamate, and antihistamines may be useful for management or prevention.

In the early studies, where routine cardiac monitoring was performed because of the high rate of major HSRs, paclitaxel was noted to cause cardiac rhythm disturbances, a overwhelming majority of which was not associated with symptoms or sequelae; therefore, the clinical relevance of these effects is not known.[340,362] The most common rhythm disturbance appears to be transient bradycardia. The cumulative experience to date suggests that isolated asymptomatic bradycardia without hemodynamic effects is not an indication for discontinuing paclitaxel. More important bradyarrhythmias, including Mobitz type 1 (Wenckebach syndrome), Mobitz type 2, and third-degree heart block, have been noted, but the incidence in a large National Cancer Institute database was only 0.1%.[363] Most documented episodes have been asymptomatic. Because such events were noted in patients enrolled in early trials that required continuous cardiac monitoring, second- and third-degree heart block are likely under-reported because cardiac monitoring is not usually performed. Interestingly, reports of similar disturbances in both animals and humans who ingested various species of yew plants and related taxanes affecting cardiac automaticity and conduction suggest that the bradyarrhythmias are caused by paclitaxel. Myocardial infarction, cardiac ischemia, atrial arrhythmias, and ventricular tachycardia have been noted, but whether there is a causal relationship between paclitaxel and these events is uncertain. There is no evidence that chronic, long-term treatment with paclitaxel causes progressive cardiac dysfunction. Routine cardiac monitoring during paclitaxel therapy is not necessary, but is recommended for those patients who may not be able to tolerate bradyarrhythmias, such as those with atrioventricular conduction disturbances or ventricular dysfunction. Although patients with a wide range of cardiac abnormalities and cardiac histories were broadly and empirically restricted from participating in early clinical trials, paclitaxel treatment has been reported to be well tolerated in a small series of gynecologic cancer patients with major cardiac risk factors.[364] On the other hand, repetitive treatment of patients with the combined regimen of paclitaxel on a 3-h schedule and doxorubicin as a brief infusion is associated with a higher frequency of congestive cardiotoxicity than would be expected to occur with the same cumulative doxorubicin dose given without paclitaxel (see Taxanes: Drug Interactions).[323] In one study in previously untreated women with advanced breast cancer treated with escalating doses of paclitaxel as a 3-h infusion and doxorubicin 60 mg/m^2 to a cumulative dose of 480 mg/m^2, which would be predicted to result in a less than 5% incidence of cardiotoxicity in patients treated with doxorubicin alone, the incidence of congestive cardiotoxicity was approximately 25%.[323] However, the incidence of cardiotoxicity was less than 5% when similar patients received identical schedules of paclitaxel and doxorubicin, but the cumulative doxorubicin dose did not exceed 360 mg/m^2.[365,366] Both experimental and early clinical results suggest that deferoxamine may reduce the cardiotoxicity of the doxorubicin paclitaxel combination.[296] The incidence of congestive heart failure was also significantly higher in breast cancer patients treated with the combination of trastuzumab and paclitaxel than in those treated with paclitaxel alone in a randomized phase 3 trial; consequently, careful monitoring of patients receiving this combination is warranted.[285,338-340]

Gastrointestinal toxicities, including nausea, vomiting, and diarrhea, are uncommon. Higher paclitaxel doses may cause mucositis, especially in patients with leukemia who may be more prone to mucosal barrier breakdown or in patients receiving protracted infusions. Rare cases of neutropenic enterocolitis and gastrointestinal necrosis have been noted, particularly in patients given high doses of paclitaxel in combination with doxorubicin or cyclophosphamide.[367,368] Severe hepatotoxicity and pancreatitis have also been noted, but these events are rare. Acute bilateral pneumonitis has been reported in less than 1% of patients treated on a 3-h schedule in one series, and both interstitial and parenchymal pulmonary toxicity have been reported, but clinically significant pulmonary effects are uncommon.[347,369]

Paclitaxel also induces reversible alopecia of the scalp, but all body hair is usually lost with cumulative therapy. Alopecia appears to be dose-related and occurs only following repetitive treatment with weekly administration schedules. Although the agent is often not considered a vesicant, extravasation of large volumes can cause moderate soft-tissue injury. Inflammation at the injection site and along the course of an injected vein may occur. Nail disorders have been reported, particularly in patients treated on weekly schedules.[370] Recall reactions in previously irradiated sites have also been noted. Taxane-induced taste alterations are common.

Docetaxel ■ Similar to paclitaxel, neutropenia is the principal toxicity of docetaxel.[183,371,372] At dosages ranging from 75 to 100 mg/m^2 administered as a 1-h infusion, neutrophil counts usually decrease to below 500/μL. The onset of neutropenia is usually noted on day 8 and complete resolution typically occurs by days 15-21. Neutropenia is significantly less when low doses are administered frequently, such as on a weekly schedule (see Administration, Dose, and Schedule). The most important determinant of neutropenia is the extent of prior therapy, but α1-acid glycoprotein and the duration of drug exposure above biologically relevant concentrations appear to be important determinants (see Clinical Pharmacology). Significant effects on platelets and red blood cells are uncommon.

Even though docetaxel is not formulated in polyoxyethylated castor oil, HSRs have been reported in approximately 31% of patients receiving docetaxel without premedications, but most are not severe.[166,336,337] Nevertheless, major reactions, characterized by dyspnea, bronchospasm, and hypotension, particularly during the first two courses and within min after the start of treatment, have been reported. Manifestations generally resolve within 15 min after cessation of treatment, and docetaxel is usually able to be reinstituted without consequences, occasionally after treatment with an Hl-histamine antagonist. Both the incidence and severity of HSRs appear to be reduced significantly by premedication with corticosteroids and both Hl- and H2-histamine antagonists (see Administration, Dose, and Schedule). Like paclitaxel, patients who experience major HSRs have been retreated successfully after resolution of symptoms and following treatment with corticosteroids and Hl-histamine antagonists. Although patients who have experienced HSRs following paclitaxel treatment have been retreated successfully with docetaxel, this strategy has not been studied in a rigorous fashion.

In early studies, a unique fluid retention syndrome, characterized by edema, weight gain, and third-space fluid collection (pericardial, pleural, ascites), has been noted in patients treated with multiple courses of docetaxel and appears to be related to the absolute cumulative dose.[183,371-374] Fluid retention did not appear to be related to hypoalbuminemia or cardiac, renal, or hepatic dysfunction, but to increased capillary permeability. Capillary filtration studies revealed a two-stage process with progressive congestion of the interstitial space by proteins and water, starting between the second and fourth course that progressed to insufficient lymphatic drainage. In early studies in which prophylactic medication was not used, fluid retention was not usually significant at cumulative docetaxel doses below 400 mg/m^2; however, the incidence and severity of fluid retention increased sharply at cumulative doses of 400 mg/m^2 or greater, and often resulted in the delay or termination of treatment. Prophylactic treatment with corticosteroids with or without H1- and H2-histamine antagonists reduces the incidence of fluid retention and increases the number of courses and cumulative docetaxel dose before the onset of this toxicity (see Administration, Dose, and Schedule).[373] In fact, drug-induced fluid retention has been uncommon following the broad adoption of corticosteroid premedication. Fluid retention resolves slowly after docetaxel is stopped, with complete resolution occurring several months after treatment in patients with severe toxicity. Aggressive and early treatment with progressively more potent diuretics, starting with potassium sparing diuretics, has been successfully used to manage fluid retention. The incidence of fluid retention appears to be lower in studies that used lower doses (60-75 mg/m^2) during each course, but this may be a result of the administration of lower overall cumulative doses, and the effects of lower doses on antitumor activity are unknown.

Although both neurosensory and neuromuscular effects due to docetaxel are similar to paclitaxel, they are less common and appear to be less severe compared with paclitaxel.[183,371-374] In a phase 3 trial, patients with advanced ovarian carcinoma receiving first-line treatment with docetaxel and carboplatin experienced significantly less severe and less total neurotoxicity than did those receiving treatment with paclitaxel and carboplatin.[375] Mild to moderate peripheral neurotoxicity is observed in approximately 40% of previously untreated patients. Previous treatment with cisplatin appears to increase the likelihood of developing neurotoxicity. The neurotoxicity is qualitatively similar to that of paclitaxel, with sensory effects predominating. Patients typically complain of paresthesia and numbness, but peripheral motor disturbances may also occur. Severe toxicity is unusual following repetitive treatment with docetaxel doses less than 100 mg/m^2, except in patients with antecedent disorders such as alcohol abuse.

Although cardiovascular effects, including angina, arrhythmia, conduction disturbances, congestive heart failure, hypertension, and hypotension, have been noted rarely in the pretreatment period, there is no convincing evidence that directly links docetaxel to these events. Stomatitis appears to occur more frequently with docetaxel than paclitaxel, particularly with prolonged infusions that are used rarely. Nausea, vomiting, and diarrhea have also been observed infrequently, but severe manifestations are rare. Empiric use of antiemetic premedication does not appear to be warranted. Phlebitis along the course of the infused veins and local inflammation at the injection site are occasionally noted; however, severe tissue damage following drug extravasation is not generally observed. Transient arthralgia and myalgia without inflammatory manifestations are occasionally noted within days following treatment. Malaise, often referred to as asthenia, has been a prominent complaint in patients who have been treated with large cumulative doses, particularly when docetaxel is administered on a continuous weekly schedule.[376,377]

Skin toxicity may occur in as many as 50-75% of patients,[150,151,183] however, premedication may reduce the overall incidence of this toxicity. An erythematous pruritic maculopapular rash that affects the forearms, hands, and/or feet is typical. Desquamation of the hands and feet, which is a component of a more general palmar-plantar syndrome that may respond to pyridoxine or cooling, and onychodystrophy characterized by brown discoloration, ridging, onycholysis, soreness, and brittleness and loss of the nail plate have been reported.[370,378,379] Skin and nail changes appear to be most prominent in patients treated frequently with low doses (ie, weekly schedules). Excessive lacrimation, occasionally due to cannicular stenosis, may also occur.[380] Other rare events that may or may not be related to docetaxel itself include confusion, erythema multiforme, neutropenic enterocolitis, hepatitis, ileus, interstitial pneumonia, seizures, pulmonary fibrosis, hepatitis, radiation recall, and visual disturbances.

PBPPI ■ The toxicity profile of PBPPI is similar to that of paclitaxel, with neutropenia as the principal dose-limiting toxicity.[202,255-258,317] Most other paclitaxel-related toxicities have also been observed with PBPPI. The rate of HSRs, particularly major reactions, appears less with PBPPI than that of paclitaxel formulated in polyoxyethylated castor oil. No premedication regimen to prevent HSRs is recommended. In a pivotal phase 3 trial in which in which the previously treated breast cancer were randomized to treatment with either 260 mg/m² PBPI administered over 30 min or 175 mg/m² paclitaxel in polyoxyethylated castor over 3 h, the frequencies of severe adverse events were similar. Potential important toxicologic differences (PBPPI vs. paclitaxel in poloxyethylated castor oil formulations) included neutrophils < 500/μL (9% vs. 22%), severe sensory neuropathic symptoms (10% vs. 2%), (severe arthralgia/myalgia [8% vs. 2%]), and severe asthenia (8% vs. 3%). Additional toxicities, most of which are noted with other taxane formulations, have been reported. These include increased lacrimation, conjunctivitis, radiation recall, Stevens-Johnson syndrome, toxic epidermal necrolysis, photosensitivity reactions, and palmar-plantar erythrodysaesthesia in patients previously treated with capecitabine.

Administration, Dose, and Schedule

Paclitaxel ■ Discerning the optimal dose and schedule for the taxanes, principally paclitaxel, has been a major focus of many evaluations over the last decade.[341] The collective results of these efforts indicate that paclitaxel has prominent antitumor activity on multiple schedules and that no particular schedule is superior from an efficacy standpoint across all tumor types; however, toxicity profiles are vastly different, and differences in efficacy have emerged in some disease settings. The earliest clinical studies of paclitaxel were limited to the 24-h schedule, largely as a consequence of an apparent increased rate of severe HSRs on shorter schedules, but the development of effective premedication regimens led to evaluation of a broad range of dosing schedules. Although paclitaxel 135 mg/m² on a 24-h schedule was initially approved for patients with refractory and recurrent ovarian cancer, regulatory approval was later obtained for paclitaxel 175 mg/m² on a 3-h schedule in these and other indications. In patients with advanced breast and ovarian cancer, the collective results of randomized studies indicate that response rates have occasionally been higher with more protracted (24-96 h) infusion schedules, but other indices of efficacy do not appear to be depend on infusion duration.[341,381,382] The extensive distribution of the taxanes to peripheral tissues, as well as the avid and protracted tissue binding of these agents, may explain the lack of substantial differences in antitumor activity between short and more protracted administration schedules despite substantial differences in vitro.

There has been considerable interest in intermittent schedules, particularly those in which paclitaxel is administered as a 1-h infusion weekly, which results in substantially less myelosuppression than every-3-week schedules.[376,377,383-386] Furthermore, there have been reports of impressive and superior activity of weekly compared with every-3-week schedules in several disease settings, particularly in treatment of both early-stage (adjuvant) and advanced breast cancer patients (see Clinical Indications).[383-387] However, there is no convincing evidence that weekly treatment results in robust activity in tumors unresponsive to the taxanes on every-3-week schedules. Nevertheless, the weekly schedule may be advantageous for patients who are at high risk of developing severe myelosuppression, but there appears to be a higher incidence of neuromuscular effects.

Paclitaxel is indicated and generally administered at a dosage of 175 mg/m² over 3 h or, less frequently, 135-175 mg/m² over 24 h every 3 weeks. Several randomized trials in patients with advanced lung, head and neck, and ovarian cancers have consistently failed to show that paclitaxel dosages above 135-175 mg/m² on a 24-h schedule are superior to conventional doses.[341,381] Nearly identical results have been obtained in a phase 3 study in patients with metastatic breast cancer, in which greater efficacy was not observed in patients treated with paclitaxel dosages above 175 mg/m² on a 3-h schedule.[388] The following dosages have been recommended on less conventional schedules: 200 mg/m² over 1 h as either a single dose or 3 divided doses every 3 weeks; 140 mg/m² over 96 h every 3 weeks; and 80-100 mg/m² weekly. The most common schedules evaluated in patients with Kaposi sarcoma caused by the acquired immunodeficiency syndrome are paclitaxel 135 mg/m² over 3 h or 24 h every 3 weeks and 100 mg/m² every 2 weeks.[195] Paclitaxel has also been administered into the pleural and peritoneal cavities. Biologically relevant plasma concentrations have been achieved with intraperitoneal administration, and concentrations in the peritoneal cavity are several orders of magnitude higher than plasma concentrations.

The following premedication is recommended to prevent major HSRs: dexamethasone 20 mg orally or intravenously, 12 and 6 h before treatment; an H1-histamine antagonist (such as diphenhydramine, 50 mg intravenously) 30 min before treatment; and an H2-histamine antagonist (such as cimetidine, 300 mg; famotidine, 20 mg; or ranitidine, 150 mg intravenously) 30 min before treatment. A single dose of a corticosteroid (dexamethasone 20 mg intravenously) administered 30 min before treatment also appears to confer effective prophylaxis of major HSRs.

Hepatic metabolism and biliary excretion are the principal modes of drug disposition, paclitaxel and dose modifications are required in patients with hepatic dysfunction. However, official recommendations have not been formulated, and study results are somewhat conflicting because of differences in the definitions of dose-limiting toxicity between various studies. Prospective studies indicate that patients with moderate to severe elevations in serum concentrations of hepatocellular enzymes and/or bilirubin are more likely to develop severe toxicity than patients without hepatic dysfunction.[389,390] Therefore, it is recommended that paclitaxel doses be reduced by at least 50% in patients with moderate or severe hepatic excretory dysfunction (hyperbilirubinemia) and/or substantial elevations in hepatic transaminases. Renal clearance contributes minimally to overall clearance (5-10%), and patients with severe renal dysfunction do not appear to require dose modification.[261,391] Based on the pharmacologic behavior, particularly the wide distributive properties of the taxanes, dose modifications are not required solely for peripheral edema and third-space fluid collections.

Contact of the paclitaxel-polyoxyethylated castor oil formulation with plasticized polyvinyl chloride (PVC) equipment or devices must be avoided because of the risk of patient exposures to plasticizers that may be leached from PVC infusion bags or sets. Paclitaxel solutions should be diluted and stored in glass or polypropylene bottles or suitable plastic bags (polypropylene or polyolefin) and administered through polyethylene-lined administration sets that include an in-line filter with a microporous membrane not greater than 0.22 microns.

Docetaxel ■ In the United States, docetaxel is indicated at a dosage range of 60-100 and 75 mg/m^2 over 1 h in patients with breast and non-small cell lung cancers, respectively, but most early clinical trials in advanced breast, ovarian, and non-small cell lung cancers evaluated doses at the higher end of this range (75-100 mg/m^2), with scant data available for patients treated with docetaxel 60 mg/m^2.[183] Although some untreated or minimally pretreated patients generally tolerate docetaxel at a dose of 100 mg/m^2, which is the only approved dose in many regions, 75 mg/m^2 appears to be more reasonable from a toxicologic perspective in more heavily pretreated patients.[392] Docetaxel 75 mg/m^2 is associated with a survival benefit in patients with non-small cell lung cancer following first-line treatment. Like paclitaxel, docetaxel has also been administered as a 1-h infusion weekly.[377] Although a clear benefit of chronic weekly drug administration over the conventional schedule in terms of antitumor activity has not been noted, hematologic toxicity is much less with weekly dose schedules than with conventional dose schedules. Both cumulative asthenia and neurotoxicity are the principal toxicities of docetaxel administered weekly, precluding administration of dosages exceeding 36 mg/m^2/week. Despite the use of a polysorbate-80 formulation instead of polyoxyethylated castor oil, which is used to formulate paclitaxel, a relatively high rate of HSRs and profound fluid retention in patients who did not receive premedication has led to the use of several effective premedication regimens, the most popular of which is dexamethasone 8 mg orally twice daily for 3 or 5 days starting 1 or 2 days, respectively, before docetaxel, with or without both H1- and H2-histamine antagonists given 30 min before docetaxel.[372,373] Administration of docetaxel without corticosteroids is not recommended, even in patients who do not develop HSRs, because drug-related fluid retention, which is a chronic toxicity, requires drug discontinuation.

A retrospective review of docetaxel pharmacokinetics in patients without hyperbilirubinemia demonstrated that docetaxel clearance is reduced by approximately 25% in patients with elevations in serum concentrations of both hepatic transaminases (1.5-fold or greater) and alkaline phosphatase (2.5-fold or greater), regardless of whether the elevations are a result of hepatic metastases.[316,393,394] Therefore, dose reductions by at least 25% are recommended for such individuals. More substantial reductions (50% or greater) may be required in patients who have moderate or severe hepatic excretory dysfunction (hyperbilirubinemia). Similar to paclitaxel (see Taxanes: Administration, Dose, and Schedule), there is no rationale for dose modification solely for renal deficiency and/or third-space fluid accumulation. Also similar to the case with paclitaxel (see Taxanes Administration, Dose, and Schedule), glass bottles or polypropylene or polyolefin plastic products should be used for preparation and storage, and docetaxel should be administered through polyethylene-lined administration sets.

PBPPI ■ PBPPI received regulatory approval in the United States for the treatment of patients with metastatic breast cancer after failure of combination chemotherapy for metastatic disease or relapse within 6 months of adjuvant chemotherapy.[202,252-255,313,314] The recommended dosage schedule for this indication is 260 mg/m^2 as a 30-min IV infusion, however, noteable anticancer activity have been observed with PBPPI doses of 100-150 mg/m^2 as a 30-min IV infusion weekly for 3 out of every 4 weeks following failure of previous taxane treatment. No premedication to prevent HSRs or edema is recommended prior to administration. The use of PVC-free containers and administration sets is not necessary, and the use of an in-line filter is not recommended. The most appropriate doses for patients with hepatic insufficiency (bilirubin $\geq$ 1.5 mg/dL) and renal insufficiency are not known, however, similar to the case with other taxanes, renal disposition is likely negligible. It is recommended that patients who experience severe neutropenia (neutrophil <500/µL for at least 7 days) or severe sensory neuropathy during PBPPI treatment should have the dosage reduced to 220 mg/m^2 for subsequent courses. Additional dose reduction should be made to 180 mg/m^2 in case of recurrences of severe neutropenia and/or sensory neuropathy. In cases of severe sensory neuropathy, it is recommended that treatment be discontinued until resolution to mild or moderate manifestions followed by a dose reduction for all subsequent courses.

Other Natural Products That Enhance Tubulin Polymerization

The success of the taxanes has led to a search for other drugs that enhance tubulin polymerization, yielding many promising compounds that may confer a therapeutic advantage over the taxanes, including the epothilones (isolated from myxobacterium *Sorangium cellulosum*), discodermolide (isolated from the Caribbean sponge *Discodermia dissoluta*), the sarcodictyins, eleutherobin (isolated from the soft coral *Eleutherobia sp*) and laulimalide (isolated from the marine sponge *Cacospongia mycofijiensis*), and sarcodictyins (isolated from the Mediterranean stoloniferan coral *Sarcodictyon roseum*) (Fig. 52–4). Some of these compounds compete with paclitaxel for binding to microtubules and appear to bind at or near the taxane site (epothilones, discodermolide, eleutherobins, and sarcodictyins), but others, such as laulimalide, seem to bind to unique sites on microtubules.[2,4,5,187,395] Because eleutherobin, epothilones A and B, and discodermolide, competitively inhibit paclitaxel binding to microtubules, a common pharmacophore was sought and identified, which may enable the development of hybrid constructs with more desirable biological characteristics.[187,395] Interestingly, discodermolide and paclitaxel have demonstrated synergistic cytotoxicity in vitro, suggesting that their tubulin-binding sites and microtubule effects are not identical.[368,369] However, unforeseen pulmonary toxicity has been seen in early clinical studies of a completely synthetic discodermolide (XAA296).[370] Most of the aforementioned compounds possess either low-level or no substrate affinity for ABC transporters, and retain various degrees of activity against taxane-resistant cells in vitro. Although the clinical implications of these characteristics are not entirely clear, the epothilones have demonstrated clinically relevant activity in patients who have been previously treated with taxanes, some of whom are clearly taxane-resistant. Of the non-taxane tubulin polymerizing agents, the epothilones are the furthest along in development, and one epothilone, ixabepilone has been ap-

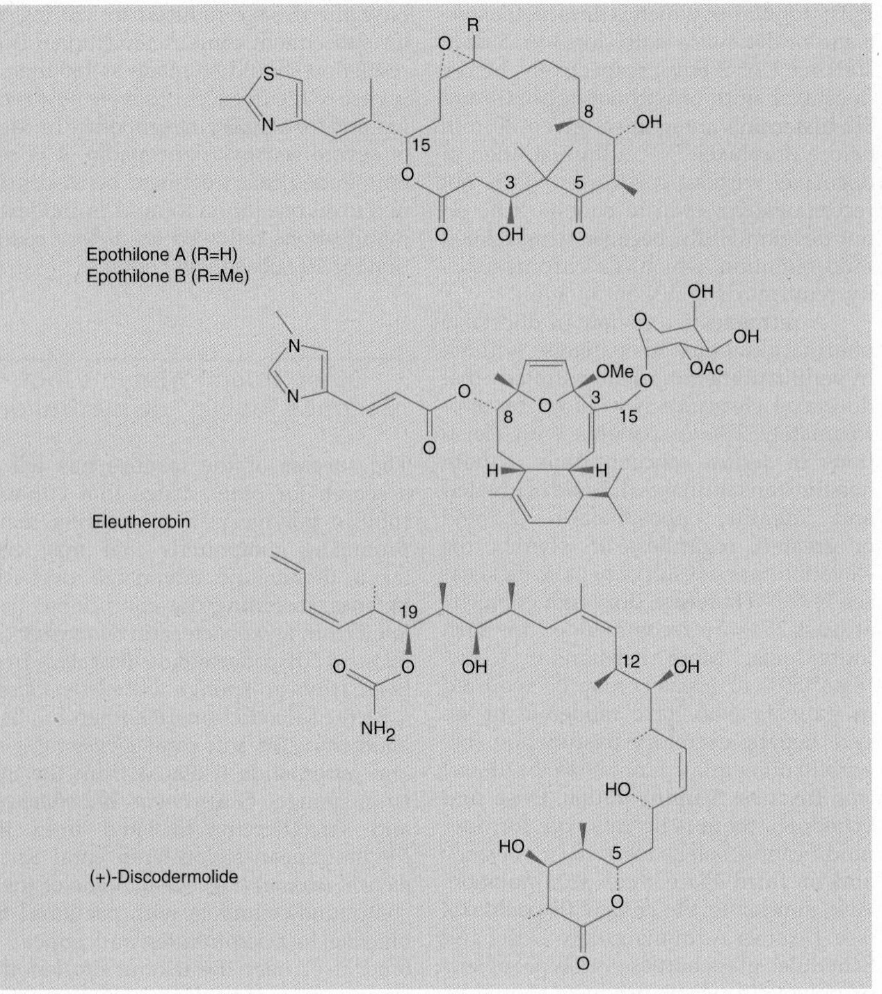

Figure 53-4 Chemical structures of epothilones A, B, C, and D.

proved for use in the United States for treatment of patients with breast cancer.

Epothilones

The epothilones A and B are 16-member polyketide macrolides with nearly identical structures, except that epothilone B has an additional methyl group at the C12 position (Fig. 53-4). The promising activities of epothilones A and B led to further modifications of the macrolactone ring, generating deoxyepothilone B (epothilone D), which possess a similar range of anticancer activity as epothilones A and B.

Clinical Indications

Ixabepilone, a semisynthetic analog of epothilone B, with a chemically modified lactam substitution for the naturally existing lactone, has received regulatory approval in the United States and elsewhere in combination with capecitabine for the treatment of patients with metastatic or locally advanced breast cancer resistant to treatment with an anthracycline and a taxane, or for patients whose cancer is taxane-resistant and for further anthracycline therapy is not indicated.[396,397] It is also indicated as monotherapy for the treatment of metastatic or locally advanced breast cancer that is resistant or refractory to anthracyclines, taxanes, and capecitabine.[396,397] In addition, both ixabepilone and epothilone B (patupilone) have demonstrated moderate antitumor activity in patients with non-small cell lung and prostate cancers.[398-400] Moderate to low-level activity has also been noted in tumor types in which the taxanes do not possess relevant levels of single agent activity including pancreatic, gastric, hepatobiliary, renal, urothelial, and colorectal cancers.[400] Epothilone D analogs possess anticancer activity in patients with breast and ovarian cancers.[400]

Both epitholones A and B competitively inhibit binding of paclitaxel to tubulin polymers in vitro, suggesting that the binding sites of the epothilones and taxanes overlap.[400-402] In fact, the epothilones and taxanes possess a common pharmacophore for microtubule binding.[208,212] However, the epothilones may occupy additional binding sites on tubulin. Both epothilones A and B promote tubulin polymerization in vitro with kinetics similar to paclitaxel, but epothilone B appears to be a more potent inducer than both epothilone A and paclitaxel.[400-402] Similar to the taxanes, the epothilones also induce tubulin polymerization in the absence of GTP and/or MAPs, resulting in microtubules that are long, rigid, and resistant to destabilization by cold temperature, and calcium, resulting in. enhanced microtubule stability and microtubule bundling.[400-406] Furthermore, the epothilones induce the formation of abnormal mitotic spindles, resulting in cell-cyle arrest in G2/M. At low concentrations, epothilone B does not induce mitotic arrest, but transforms proliferating cells into large anueploid cells, which undergo apoptotic cell death in G1. Thus, protracted mitotic arrest may not be essential for apoptotic cell death induced by these agents.[407]

Mechanisms of Resistance

A critical difference between the epothilones, taxanes and vinca alkaloids is that overexpression of the transporters Pgp and MRP-1 minimally affects the cytotoxicity of the epothilones which possess low-level or no substrate affinity for these transporters.[2,3,212,400-402,407-409] Epothilones A and B have strong antiproliferative activy in human cancer cells with high expression of P-glyocprotein (ABCB1), which are resistant to paclitaxel, and tumor samples obtained from patients with tumors responsive to ixabepilone showed significant expression of both MDR1 and MRP1 mRNA, also suggesting that these proteins may not confer resistance to ixabepilone in the clinic.[410,411]

In preclinical systems, cancer cells with various β-tubulin point mutations, which are critical for microtubule stabilization, appear to be resistant to the epothilones. Preclinical reports have also suggested additional mechanisms of resistance such as α-tubulin mutations, altered expression of tubulin isotypes, and altered MAP structure and function.[400,401,404,411]

Clinical Pharmacology

In cancer patients, ixabepilone exhibits dose-proportional pharmacokinetics in the range of 15-57 mg/m^2 (Table 53-2).[400,401,411] Following administration of a single 40 mg/m^2 dose, the mean Cmax was 252 ng/mL (coefficient of variation, 56%) and the terminal phase half-life averaged 52 h. Similar to the taxanes and vinca alkaloids, ixabepalone's volume of distribution at steady-state is large, with mean values exceeding 1000 Ls. Binding to human serum proteins has ranged from 67% to 77% in vitro, and the blood-to-plasma concentration ratios in human blood ranges from 0.65 to 0.85.

The principal mode of systemic disposition of ixabepilone is hepatic metabolism. Following intravenous administration of radiolabled ixabepilone, approximately 86% of the dose is eliminated within 7 days; fecal and urinary elimination accounted for 65% and 21% of the dose, respectively. The parent compound accounts for approximately 1.6% and 5.6% of the dose in feces and urine, respectively. In vitro studies have indicated that the principal metabolic pathway is oxidative metabolism via CYP3A4. More than 30 inactive metabolites are excreted into human urine and feces, but no single metabolite accounts for more than 6% of the administered dose.

Drug Interactions

In vitro studies using human liver microsomes have indicated that clinically relevant concentrations of ixabepilone do not affect the activities of CYP3A4, CYP1A2, CYP2A6, CYP2B6, CYP2C8, CYP2C9, CYP2C19, or CYP2D6 and therefore would likely not affect the phamacokinetics and metabolism of drugs that are substrates of these enzymes.[400,401,411] However, coadministration of ixabepilone with ketoconazole, a potent CYP3A4 inhibitor, increased ixabepilone AUC values by 79%, on average, compared to ixabepilone treatment alone. With regard to ketoconazole and similar agents, if alternative treatment cannot be administered, a dose adjustment should be considered. Since the effect of mild or moderate CYP3A4 inhibitors (eg, erythromycin, fluconazole, or verapamil) on exposure to ixabepilone has not been studied, caution should be exercised when administering such agents during ixabepalone treatment. Similarly, paitents receiving CYP3A4 inhibitors during treatment with ixabepilone should be monitored for toxicity. Potent inducers of CYP3A4, such as dexamethasone, phenytoin, carbamazepine, rifampin, rifampicin, rifabutin, and phenobarbital), may also decrease ixabepilone concentrations leading to subtherapeutic levels, and, therefore, agents with low CYP3A4 induction potential should be considered for coadministration with ixabepalone.

In studies involving cancer patients who received ixabepilone (40 mg/m^2) in combination with capecitabine (1000 mg/m^2), the effects of ixabepilone on the Cmax and AUC values of capecitabine and 5-fluorouracil, and visa versa, were modest and not clinically relevant, particularly since the rationale for the combination treatment is clearly supported by efficacy data.

Toxicity

Peripheral neurotoxicity is the most common serious toxicity observed with ixabepilone as both monotherapy and combined with capecitabine.[396-401,411] The most common symptoms include a burning sensation, hyperesthesia, hypoesthesia, paresthesia, discomfort, and neuropathic pain. Approximately 63% and 67% of breast cancer patients who had previously received taxane-based treatment develop peripheral neurotoxicity after treatment with ixabepilone alone and in combination with capectibine, respectively, however, severe (grades 3 and 4) toxicity was noted in 14% and 23% of patients, respectively. In heavily pretreated patients, the onset of neuropathy is early, with approximately 75% of new onset or worsening neuropathy occurring during the first three cycles and the most serious manifestations experienced after four cycles. In clinical trials, peripheral neuropathy was managed through dose reduction, dose delay, and treatment discontinuation (see Administration, Dose, and Schedule). Following treatment discontinuation and/or dose reduction, manifestations resolve rapidly relative to the taxanes and vinca alkaloids, with median times of 6 and 4.6 weeks for resolution of severe manifestation to grade 1 severeity. Patients who have hepatic insufficiency (see Administration, Dose, and Schedule) and diabetes mellitus are at increased risk of developing severe neuropathy. Although the presence of grade 1 neuropathy and prior therapy with neurotoxic chemotherapy do not predict for ixabepilone-induced neuropathy, it should be noted that patients with neuropathy of at least moderate severity were excluded from early clinical trials.

Dose-dependent myelosuppression, principally neutropenia, is common with ixabepilone treatment. Effects on platelets and red blood cells are less common. Grade 4 neuropenia (<500 cells/µL) occurred in 36% of patients treated with ixabepilone in combination with capecitabine and in 23% of patients treated with monotherapy, however, febrile neutropenia and infection with neutropenia were reported in 5% and 6% of patients treated with ixabepilone in combination with capecitabine, respectively, and 3% and 5% of patients treated with ixabepilone monotherapy. Myelosuppression does not generally worsen with successive treatment, suggesting that hematopoietic progenitor cells are not significantly affected. Dose reduction is recommended for patients experiencing severe neutropenia and dose modification is recommended for patients with moderate hepatic dysfunction (see Administration, Dose, and Schedule).

Since ixabepilone is formulated in polyoxyethylated castor oil, serere hypersensitivity reactions, largely secondary to this diluent, are noted. Manifestations of hypersensitivity include flushing, rash, dyspnea, and brochospasm. For this reason, it is recommended that all patients receive premedication with H1- and H2-histamine antagonists approximately 1 h before treatment (see Administration, Dose, and Schedule). In the case of severe hypersensitivity reactions, treatment should be stopped and aggressive supportive treatment (eg, epinephrine, corticosteroids) started. In clinical studies, approximately 1% of patients have experienced severe reactions despite various premedication regimens. There have been reports of successful retreatment of patients who had experienced prior reactions following the addition of a corticosteroid to H1- and H2-histamine antagonists, antagonists, and extension of the infusion time.

Patients treated with ixabepilone have experienced cognitive dysfunction, lethargy, and discoordinated movements in the peritreatment period, possibly due, in part, to the ethanol in the diluent. Myalgia and arthralgia have also been noted in the peritreatment period. A variety of cardiac disturbances, including myocardial infarction, supraventricular arrhythmia, left ventricular dysfunction, angina pectoris, atrial flutter, cardiomyopathy, myocardial ischemia, have also been observed, but these occurrences have not been directly attributed to ixabepilone. Ileus, colitis, impaired gastric emptying, esophagitis, dysphagia, gastritis, gastrointestinal hemorrhage, hepatic insufficiency, erythema multiforme, muscle spasms, trismus, and renal failure, have also been reported on rare occassion.

Administration, Dose, and Schedule

The recommended dosage of ixabepilone is 40 mg/m^2 intravenously over 3 h every 3 weeks.[396,397,400,401,411] The doses for patients with body surface areas greater than 2.2 m^2 should be calculated based on 2.2 m^2 since it was the method used to characterize dose-toxicity relationships. Although a range of intermittent dosing schedules have been evaluated, the preponderance of efficacy data relates to the 3-h every-3-week dosing schedule. Ixabepilone is intended for intravenous use only after constitution with the supplied diluent, which is a non-pyrogenic solution of 52.8% (w/v) purified polyoxyethylated castor oil and 39.8% (w/v) dehydrated alcohol, USP, and after further dilution with Lactated Ringers Injection, USP. To minimize the chance of occurrence of major hypersensitivity reactions, all patients should be premedicated approximately 1 h before treatment with both an H1-histamine antagonist, such as diphenhydramine 50 mg orally or equivalent, and an H2-histamine antagonist (eg, ranitidine 150-300 mg orally or equivalent. For patients who experience a hypersensitivity reaction, premedication with corticosteroids (eg, dexamethasone 20 mg intravenously, 30 min before infusion or orally, 60 min before infusion) in addition to pretreatment with H1-histamine and H2-histamine antagonists is recommended.

Dose modification and/or treatment delay are recommended for patients who develop clinically relevant grades of neuropathy and/or myelosuppression. Dose reduction by 20% is recommended for patients who develop neuropathic manifestions of grade 2 severity lasting at least 7 days or of grade 3 severity lasting less than 7 days. Discontinuation of treatment is recommended for more protracted grade 3 neuropathy or any grade 4 toxicity. Dose reduction by 20% is also recommended for patients who experience a neutrophil count < 500/μL lasting at least 7 days and/or associated with fever, a platelet count < 25,000/μL, or a platelet count < 50,000/μL with bleeding. A similar dose reduction (20%) is recommended for patients who experience other types of grade 3 (severe) toxicities, except fatigue, plantar-palmar erythrodysesthesia, and arthralgia/myalgia. Drug discontinuaiton is recommended for grade 4 (disabling) toxicity of any type.

In a study of ixabepilone in patients with mild to severe hepatic impairment, ixabepilone AUC values increased by 22% in patients with bilirubin vaues ranging from >1 to 1.5 times the upper limit of normal (ULN) or AST values exceeding the ULN with bilirubin <1.5 times the ULN, whereas AUC values increased by 30% in patients with bilirubin elevations ranging from 1.5 to 3 times the ULN and any AST level, and increased by 81% in patients with bilirubin values exceeding 3 times the ULN with any AST level. Doses of 10 and 20 mg/m^2 as monotherapy were tolerated in a small number of patients with severe hepatic impairment (bilirubin >3 times the ULN). It is recommended that the dose of ixabepilone as monotherapy be reduced to 32 mg/m^2 in patients with AST or ALT elevations up to 10 times the ULN and bilirubin up to 1.5 times the ULN. For patients with AST or ALT elevations up to 10 times the ULN and bilirubin ranging from 1.5 to 3.0 times the ULN of normal, ixabepilone monotherapy doses should be reduced to 20 mg/m^2. If tolerated, the dose can be increased up to, but not exceeding 30 mg/m^2 in subsequent cycles. Use of ixabepilone is not recommended in patients with severe hepatic dysfunction defined as ALT or AST values exceeding 10 times the ULN or bilirubin exceeding 3-times the ULN. Treatment with ixabepilone combined with capecitabine is not recommended for patients who have AST, ALT levels, and/or bilirubin levels exceeding the ULN. A standard dose of ixabepilone (40 mg/m^2) is recommended for patients who have AST and ALT less than 2.5 times the ULN and normal bilirubin values.

Ixabepilone is minimally excreted via the kidney, however, ixabepilone as monotherapy has not been evaluated in patients with creatinine >1.5 times ULN. In a population pharmacokinetic analysis of ixabepilone as monotherapy, there was no meaningful effect of mild and moderate renal insufficiency (creatinine clearance >30 mL/min) on the pharmacokinetics of ixabepilone. Ixabepilone in combination with capecitabine has not been evaluated in patients with calculated creatinine clearance <50 mL/min.

The use of concomitant strong CYP3A4 inhibitors (eg, ketoconazole, itraconazole, clarithromycin, atazanavir, nefazodone, saquinavir, telithromycin, ritonavir, amprenavir, indinavir, nelfinavir, delavirdine, or voriconazole) should be avoided. Grapefruit juice may also increase plasma concentrations of ixabepilone and should be avoided. Based on pharmacokinetic studies, if a strong CYP3A4 inhibitor must be coadministered, dose reduction to 20 mg/m^2, which should adjust the ixabepilone AUC to that observed without inhibitors, should be considered. If the strong inhibitor is discontinued, a 1-week washout period is recommended before the ixabepilone dose is increased to the indicated dose.

Other Natural Products That Enhance Tubulin Depolymerization

Other natural and semisynthetic agents under evaluation bind to the vinca or colchicine-binding domains of tubulin. Among the most potent are the dolastatins, which constitute a series of oligopeptides isolated from the sea hare, *Dolabela auricularia*.[409,412,413] Two of the most potent dolastatins, dolastatin-10 and -15 noncompetitively inhibit binding of vinca alkaloids to tubulin, tubulin polymerization, and tubulin-dependent GTP hydrolysis; stabilize the colchicine-binding activity of tubulin; and possess cytotoxic activity in the picomolar to low nanomolar range. Dolastatin-10 and semisynthetic dolastatin analogues (tasidotin [ILX-651] and TZT-1027), which binds in the vinca domain, are undergoing clinical evaluation.[2,4,408,413,414] Auristatin and related analogs, which are among the most potent derivatives of dolastatin-10, are being evaluated as cytotoxic "payloads" conjugated to therapeutic antibodies.[415] Phomopsin A, halichondrin B, homohalichondrin B, and spongistatin 1, which competitively inhibit vinca alkaloid binding to tubulin, are also in preclinical or early clinical evaluations.[416-418] Eribulin (E7389), a macrocyclic ketone analogue of the marine natural product halichondrin B originally isolated from the marine sponge *Halicondrin okadai*, and two less complex synthetic macrocyclic ketone analogues, ER-076349 and ER-086526 are in late stage clinical trials. Eribulin is currently in phases 2-3 evaluations in patients with advanced breast cancer and other malignancies. These compounds bind to tubulin, inhibit tubulin polymerization, disrupt mitotic spindle formation and centromere dynamics, induce mitotic arrest followed by apoptosis, and possess growth-inhibitory properties in the subnanomolar range and marked activity in preclinical studies.

Synthetic forms of hemiasterlin (HTI-286 and E7974), which is a natural product derived from marine sponges, are also in clinical development.[419] Hemiasterlin and its analogues bind to the vinca-peptide site in tubulin, disrupt normal microtubule dynamics, and, at stoichiometric amounts, depolymerize microtubules. They are much weaker substrate for Pgp than the vinca alkaloids and taxanes and have excellent activity in human xenograft models, including tumors that express Pgp.[420,421] They are also cross-resistant with other vinca peptide-binding agents, including hemiasterlin A, dolastatin-10, and vinblastine, and DNA-damaging drugs, but minimally cross-resistant with the taxanes, epothilones, and colchicine. In preclinical studies, resistance appears to be at least partially mediated by mutations of α-tubulin and/or an ATP-binding cassette drug pump distinct from P-glycoprotein, ABCG2, MRP1, or MRP3.[420,421]

Most efforts targeting the tumor vasculature are aimed at the development of agents that inhibit angiogenesis, but several antimicrotubule agents have been demonstrated to rapidly shut down existing tumor vasculature by inhibiting tubulin function in vascular endothelial cells.[422,423] Since the late 1990s, the combretastatins and *N*-acetylcolchicinol-*O*-phosphate, compounds that resemble colchicine and bind to the colchicine domain on tubulin, have undergone extensive development as antivascular agents. Several, including combretastatin-A-4 3-*O*-phosphate, combrestatin A-1-phosphate (CA-1-P), ZD6126 and AVE8062A are in clinical trials.[422,423] Although antitumor activity has been noted in the clinic, cardiovascular toxicity has also been observed.

Targeting Mitotic Kinesins and Kinases

Mitotic Kinesins ■ Although tubulin is the most abundant protein component of the mitotic spindle apparatus, many other proteins, such as mitotic kinesins, play critical roles in the mechanics of mitosis and in progression through the premitotic cell cycle checkpoint. Kinesins are motor proteins that convert energy released by the hydrolysis of ATP into mechanical force for movement along microtubules, transport of cargo, and the intracellular organization of the mitotic spindle and other microtubule-containing structures.[19,424,425]

The mitotic kinesins function exclusively in mitosis in proliferating cells.[19,424-426] During mitosis, different, highly specialized mitotic kinesins play critical roles in various aspects of mitotic spindle assembly, including the establishment of spindle bipolarity, spindle pole organization, chromosome alignment and segregation, and regulation of microtubule dynamics. The establishment of mitotic spindle bipolarity is among the earliest events in spindle assembly, and it requires the function of a specific kinesin motor protein KSP (also known as Eg5), which has no known role other than in mitosis. The expression profiles of KSP mRNA in normal tissues are consistent with preferential expression of KSP in proliferating cells relative to normal adjacent tissue and postmitotic neurons. As essential elements in mitotic spindle assembly and function, KSP and mitotic kinesins provide attractive targets for intervention into the cell cycle.[19,424-426] Ispinesib (SB-715992) a polycyclic, nitrogen-containing heterocycle and allosteric inhibitor of KSP motor domain ATPase with a Ki of 12 nM and a potent KSP inhibitor that causes mitotic arrest, is currently being studied in a wide range of soldi and hematologic cancers.[426] The compound, which is 10,000-fold more selective for KSP relative to other members of the kinesin superfamily, has been shown to block assembly of a functional mitotic spindle, thereby causing cell cycle arrest in mitosis and subsequent cell death.[426] In tumor-bearing mice, the agent exhibited antitumor activity comparable to or exceeding that of paclitaxel and caused the formation of monopolar mitotic figures identical to those produced in cultured cells.[426] In addition, more potent KSP inhibitor with apparently higher therapeutic indices than Ispinesib, SB743921, as well as several other Eg5 inhibitors, are in disease-directed evaluations. Other KSP inhibitors, some of which have increased potency and/or specificity for KSP, including MK-0731 and ARRY-649, are in early clinical trials.

Other mitotic kinesins in clinical development, such as GSK-923295, target centromere-associated protein E, (CENP-E), which plays an essential role in chromosome movement during early cell division or mitosis and integrates mitotic spindle mechanics with regulators of the mitotic checkpoint regulating cell-cycle transition from metaphase to anaphase.[427] Inhibition of CENP-E induces cell cycle arrest during cell duplication leading to subsequent apoptosis or cell death. In preclinical studies, GSK-923295 demonstrated a broad spectrum of activity against a range of human tumor xenografts grown in nude mice, including models of colon, breast, ovarian, lung and other tumors.

Mitotic Kinases ■ Mitotic kinases, particularly the aurora kinases, are being evaluated as strategic targets for anticancer therapeutic development.[428-430] The aurora kinases, which encompass three known family members known as aurora-A, aurora-B, and aurora-C, regulate chromosome segregation and cytokinesis during mitosis. Aberrant expression and activity of these kinases that may lead to aneuploidy and tumorigenesis, occur in many types of human cancer. Aurora-A and aurora-B kinases have distinct roles in mitotsis. Aurora-A kinase, which is typically found in the pericentrosomal region, recruits important components to the mitotic spindle, such as γ-tubulin, while the mitotic spindle is forming from the daughter centrosomes. Aurora-B kinase is localized to the interphase chromosomes proximal to the centromer, and as chromosome condensation occurs at the start of mitosis, both aurora-A and aurora-B kinases, share responsibility for phosphorylating histone H3.[428-430] Both kinases also have distinct roles in the function of the contractile ring that participates in the formation of two daughter cells. Aurora C kinase appears to have a highly specialized, albeit as of yet undetermined, role in mitosis. Recently, highly potent and selective small molecule inhibitors of aurora-A and aurora-B kinases, including VX-680 (also known as MK-0457), MLN-8054, AS703569, and AZD1152, which block cell-cycle progression and induce apoptosis in experimental models of human cancer, are undergoing clinical development. Neutropenia is their principal toxicity.

Like the aurora family of kinases, the polo-like, Nek, and other kinase families participate in the centrosome cycle and modulate spindle function, while Bub1, BubR1 and Mps1 kinases regulate the spindle assembly checkpoint.[428-430] Some members of these families, particularly the polo-like kinases, are being evaluated as potentially targets for therapeutic intervention. Small molecule inhibitors of polo-like kinase that are in early clinical development include BI2536 and ON01910.Na, which have demonstrated broad-spectrum antitumor activity against both solid and hematological malignancy in preclinical studies, as well as synergistic activity when combined with several types of cytotoxic agents.

Selected References

The complete reference list can be found at www.CANCERMEDICINE8.com

2. Jordan MA, Wilson L. Microtubules as a target for anticancer drugs. *Nat Rev Cancer.* 2004;4:253.
5. Jackson JR, Patrick DR, Dar MM, Huang PS. Targeted anti-mitotic therapies: can we improve on tubulin agents? *Nat Rev Cancer.* 2007;7:107.
13. Wilson L, Jordan MA. Pharmacological probes of microtubule function. *Biochemistry.* 1993;59:185.
15. Bhalla KN. Microtubule-targeted anticancer agents and apoptosis. *Oncogene.* 2003;22: 9075.
28. Rowinsky EK, Donehower RC. The clinical pharmacology and use of antimicrotubule agents in cancer chemotherapeutics. *Pharmacol Ther.* 1992;52:35.
31. Joel S. The comparative clinical pharmacology of vincristine and vindesine: does vindesine offer any advantage in clinical use? *Cancer Treat Rev.* 1996;21:513.
43. Himes RH, Kersey RN, Heller-Bettinger I, Sampson FE. Action of the vinca alkaloids, vincristine and vinblastine, and desacetyl vinblastine amide on microtubules in vitro. *Cancer Res.* 1976;36:3798.
46. Jordan MA, Thrower D, Wilson L. Mechanism of inhibition of cell proliferation by the vinca alkaloids. *Cancer Res.* 1991;51:2212.
47. Himes RH. Interactions of the Catharanthus (vinca) alkaloids with tubulin and microtubules. *Pharmacol Ther.* 1991;51:256.
56. Jordan MA, Thrower D, Wilson L. Effects of vinblastine, podophyllotoxin and nocodazole on mitotic spindles. Implications for the role of microtubule dynamics in mitosis. *J Cell Sci.* 1992;102:401.
68. Lockhart A, Tirona G, Kim B. Pharmacogenetics of ATPbinding cassette transporters in cancer and chemotherapy. *Mol Ther.* 2003; 2:685.
90. Gan PP, Pasquier E, Kavallaris M., et al. Class III beta-tubulin mediates sensitivity to chemotherapeutic drugs in non small cell lung cancer. *Cancer Res.* 2007;67:9356.
103. Jackson DV, Bender RA. Cytotoxic thresholds of vincristine in a murine and human leukemia cell line in vitro. *Cancer Res.* 1979;39:4346.
104. Rahmani R, Zhou XJ. Pharmacokinetics and metabolism of vinca alkaloids. *Cancer Surv.* 1993;17:269.
120. Rahmani R, Gueritte F, Martin M, et al. Comparative pharmacokinetics of antitumor vinca alkaloids: intravenous bolus injections of Navelbine and related alkaloids to cancer patients and rats. *Cancer Chemother Pharmacol.* 1986;16:223.
140. Quasthoff S, Hartung HP. Chemotherapy-induced peripheral neuropathy. *J Neurol.* 2002;249:9.
182. Rowinsky EK, Donehower RC. Drug therapy: paclitaxel (Taxol). *N Engl J Med.* 1995;332:1004.
183. Cortes JE, Pazdur R. Docetaxel. *J Clin Oncol.* 1995;13:2643.
186. McGuire WP, Hoskins WJ, Brady MF, et al. Cyclophosphamide and cisplatin compared with paclitaxel and cisplatin in patients with stage III and IV ovarian cancer. *N Engl J Med.* 1996;334:1.

204. Schiff PB, Fant J, Horwitz SB. Promotion of microtubule assembly in vitro by Taxol. *Nature*. 1979;22:665.
205. Horwitz SB, Cohen D, Rao S, et al. Taxol: mechanisms of action and resistance. *J Natl Cancer Inst Monogr*. 1993;15:55.
214. Ringel I, Horwitz SB. Studies with RP56976 (Taxotere): a semisynthetic analogue of Taxol. *J Natl Cancer Inst*. 1991;83:288.
220. Jordan MA, Toso RJ, Thrower D, Wilson L. Mechanism of mitotic block and inhibition of cell proliferation by Taxol at low concentrations. *Proc Natl Acad Sci USA*. 1993;90:9552.
224. Dumontet C, Sikic B. Mechanism of action and resistance to antitubulin agents: microtubule dynamics, drug transport, and cell death. *J Clin Oncol*. 1999;17:1061.
237. Rowinsky EK, Donehower RC, Jones RJ, Tucker RW. Microtubule changes and cytotoxicity in leukemic cell lines treated with Taxol. *Cancer Res*. 1988;48:4093.
243. Tishler RB, Geard CR, Hall EJ, Schiff PB. Taxol sensitizes human astrocytoma cells to radiation. *Cancer Res*. 1992;52:3595.
246. Klauber N, Paragni S, Flynn E, et al. Inhibitor of angiogenesis and breast cancer in mice by the microtubule inhibitors 2-methoxyestradiol and Taxol. *Cancer Res*. 1997;57:81.
254. Desai N, Trieu V, Yao Z, et al. Increased antitumor activity, intratumor paclitaxel concentrations, and endothelial cell transport of cremophor-free, albumin-bound paclitaxel, ABI-007, compared with cremophor-based paclitaxel. *Clin Cancer Res*. 2006;12:1317.
256. Orr, GA Verdier-Pinard P, McDaid H, Horwitz SB. Mechanisms of Taxol resistance related to microtubules. *Oncogene*. 2003;22:7280.
264. Cabral F, Wible L, Brenner S, Brinkley BR. Taxol-requiring mutants of Chinese hamster ovary cells with impaired mitotic spindle activity. *J Cell Biol*. 1983;97:30.
268. Giannakakou P, Sackett DL, Kang YK, et al. Paclitaxelresistant human ovarian cancer cells have mutant beta tubulins that exhibit impaired paclitaxel-driven polymerization. *J Biol Chem*. 1997;272:17118.
278. Verrills NM, Flemming CL, Liu M, et al. Microtubule alterations and mutations induced by desoxyepothilone B: implications for drug-target interactions. *Chem Biol*. 2003;10:597.
289. Huizing MT, Keung ACF, Rosing H, et al. Pharmacokinetics of paclitaxel and metabolites in a randomized comparative study in platinum-pretreated ovarian cancer patients. *J Clin Oncol*. 1993;11:2127.
290. Gianni L, Kearns C, Gianni A, et al. Nonlinear pharmacokinetics and metabolism of paclitaxel and its pharmacokinetic/pharmacodynamic relationships in humans. *J Clin Oncol*. 1995;13:180.
297. Walle T, Walle UK, Kumar GN, Bhalla KN. Taxol metabolism and disposition in cancer patients. *Drug Metab Dispos*. 1995;23:506.
301. Monsarrat B, Alvinerie P, Dubois J, et al. Hepatic metabolism and biliary clearance of Taxol in rats and humans. *J Natl Cancer Inst Monogr*. 1993;15:39.
303. Kearns CM, Egorin MJ. Considerations regarding the lessthan-expected thrombocytopenia encountered with combination paclitaxel/carboplatin chemotherapy. *Semin Oncol*. 1997;24(Suppl 2):S2.
340. Rowinsky EK, Eisenhauer EA, Chaudhry V, et al. Clinical toxicities encountered with Taxol. *Semin Oncol*. 1993;20(Suppl 3):1.
349. Weiss R, Donehower RC, Wiernik PH, et al. Hypersensitivity reactions from Taxol. *J Clin Oncol*. 1990;8:1263.
352. Eisenhower E, ten Bokkel Huinink W, Swenerton KD, et al. European-Canadian randomized trial of Taxol in relapsed ovarian cancer: high vs low dose and long vs short infusion. *J Clin Oncol*. 1994;12:2654.
353. Rowinsky EK, Chaudhry V, Cornblath DR, Donehower RC. The neurotoxicity of Taxol. *Monogr Natl Cancer Inst*. 1993;15:107.
376. Greco FA, Thomas M, Hainsworth JD. One-hour paclitaxel infusions: review of the safety and efficacy. *Cancer Sci Am*. 1999;5:179.
377. Hainsworth JD, Burris HA, Greco FA. Weekly administration of docetaxel (Taxotere): summary of clinical data. *Semin Oncol*. 1999;26(Suppl 10):19.
388. Winer EP, Berry DA, Woolf S, et al. Failure of higher-dose paclitaxel to improve outcome in patients with metastatic breast cancer: cancer and leukemia group B trial 9342. *J Clin Oncol*. 2004;22:2061.
393. Bruno R, Hille D, Riva A, et al. Population pharmacokinetic/pharmacodynamics of docetaxel in phase II studies in patients with cancer. *J Clin Oncol*. 1998;16:186.
398. Dawson NA. Epothilones in prostate cancer: review of clinical experience. *Ann Oncol*. 2007;18(Suppl 5):22.
404. Goodin S, Kane MP, Rubin EH. Epothilones: mechanism of action and biologic activity. *J Clin Oncol*. 2004;22:2015.
416. Jordan MA, Kamath K, Manna T, et al. The primary antimitotic mechanism of action of the synthetic halichondrin E7389 is suppression of microtubule growth. *Mol Cancer Ther*. 2005;4:1086.
424. Wood KW, Cornwell WD, Jackson JR. Past and future of the mitotic spindle as an oncology target. *Curr Opin Pharmacol*. 2001;4:370.
427. Kim Y, Heuser JE, Waterman CM, Cleveland DW.CENP-E combines a slow, processive motor and a flexible coiled coil to produce an essential motile kinetochore tether. *J Cell Biol*. 2008;181:411.

54 Interferons

Ernest C. Borden, MD

Interferons (IFNs) were the first biological and protein therapeutic to achieve regulatory approval for cancer patients. IFNs are now licensed worldwide not only for cancer but also as and antivirals for multiple sclerosis. As the first previously unavailable therapeutic produced by recombinant technology, approval of IFN-α2 for hairy cell leukemia little more than 20 years ago was a landmark event for the nascent biotechnology industry. IFNs have been a prototype for dissecting biologic actions, clinical effects, and development of other protein therapeutics.[1–7] Understanding of cellular effects, cloning, introduction, and clinical use has been a major advance in oncology—and indeed biomedicine—over the past three decades.

IFNs are a family of cytokines that come from >20 expressed genes coded on human chromosome 9 (except IFN-γ on chromosome 12). Cellular action follows binding to a relatively small number of high-affinity receptors. Regulatory proteins then transcriptionally regulate gene expression resulting in production of proteins that are not expressed constitutively or only at low levels. The products of these IFN-stimulated genes (ISGs) underlie the pleiotropic biologic effects: virus inhibition, immunomodulation, inhibition of cell proliferation, alterations in differentiation, increased apoptosis, and angiogenesis inhibition. However, which of the specific ISG products result in the various biologic and therapeutic effects remains undefined, as do the specific cellular mechanism(s) of antitumor action. In more than a dozen cancers, IFNs can result in regression or stability of the disease process. Suppression of the IFN system within malignant cells, however, contributes to cellular oncogenesis and the secreted cytokines are a critical component of the innate immune response to cancer. Although the spectrum of single-agent activity of IFNs compares favorably with other systemic antitumor modalities, its broad clinical use has now been superseded to a significant extent by other therapeutics targeting cell signaling (Table 54-1).

Molecules: Their Induction, Receptors, and Gene Regulation

Three major classes of IFNs (α, β, and γ) were initially defined on the basis of chemical, antigenic, and biologic differences. These major species and the more recently identified (κ, γ, and ω) families of human IFNs (the newer ones of as yet uncertain biological significance) have now been confirmed to have similarities in primary amino acid sequence, receptor structures, and/or activated signaling proteins.[3–7] All IFNs have the defining biologic effect of induction of intracellular resistance to replication of both RNA and DNA viruses. Secreted IFNs-α and IFN-β, members of the helical cytokine family, are 165-166 amino acids in length with an additional ~20 amino acid secretory peptide present on the amino-terminal end. Comparison of the sequences of IFNs-α and IFN-β has defined ~45% homology of nucleotides and 30% homology of amino acids. Each of the nonallelic, 12 human IFNs-α differ by 15% to 25% in amino acid sequence. Licensed for clinical use in cancer is IFN-α2. [IFN-α2a (Hoffmann-LaRoche) differs from IFN-α2b (Schering-Plough) by a single amino acid 23 (lysine in IFN-α2a; arginine in IFN-α2b) that seemingly does not influence function.] IFN-γ, which has only minimal sequence homology with IFN-α or IFN-β but also with a 20 amino acid secretory peptide, is 143 amino acids and functions in receptor binding as a dimer.[8–10]

Table 54-1 Interferons: Current Status

Regulation of gene transcription
Antiproliferative effects/apoptosis, antiangiogenesis, immunomodulation
Biologic response modulatory effects defined in man
Phase 2 antitumor activity confirmed in >12 human cancers
Randomized phase 3 improved survival in melanoma, renal carcinoma, CML, lymphoma

Induction

Conceptually, it is important to distinguish IFN production and action (Fig. 54-1). Viruses and their nucleic acids remain the prototypic inducers. Although all body cells probably have the capacity to produce IFNs-α and IFN-β, the primary cells of origin are plasmacytoid dendritic cells through activation of toll-like receptor (TLR) signaling.[4,11–13] IFN-γ, produced as part of the adaptive immune response by natural killer (NK) or activated T cells, was identified after exposure of lymphocytes to mitogens or sensitized lymphocytes to specific antigens.[8–10] Interleukin-2 (IL-2), tumor necrosis factors (TNFs), IL-12, IL-15, and other cytokines are also inducers of IFN-γ. IFNs are part of host defense mechanisms for resistance to neoplasia; experimental suppression of IFNs in mice results in increased lethality from tumors.[14,15]

As a component of the innate immune system, TLRs recognize distinct nucleic acids, lipids, polysaccharides, or proteins of microbes including bacteria and viruses and of damaged cells (Fig. 54-2). The first chemically defined inducers of IFNs were double-stranded polyribonucleotides, which, through binding to the endosomal TLR3, are potent IFN inducers in mice but not in humans. Single-stranded RNAs or DNAs bind to the endosomal TLRs 7, 8, and 9, as do the low-molecular-weight inducers that have been identified.[4,11–13,16,17] After TLR activation, adaptor proteins connect these receptor proteins to specific protein kinases that activate transcription factors including NFκB, IRF-3, IRF-7, and AP-1.[11–12,16–18] Several low-molecular-weight inducers have been introduced into clinical trials.[4–17] Oral activators of TLRs, such as the acridines, halopyrimidinones, or substituted quinolones, would be convenient and useful not only for therapeutic purposes but could also have benefit as chemopreventive agents.[19] Suggesting this latter clinical potential, halopyrimidinones are effective for low-grade transitional carcinomas of the bladder.[20]

Receptors

The cellular response to IFNs requires only a small number (<2000/cell) of ligands interacting with high-affinity, dimeric cell surface receptors. The receptors confer almost absolute species restrictions. Although engaging the receptor complex differently, IFNs-α and IFN-β share and compete for the same receptor.[3,4,21,22] Although some downregulation of receptors occurs with IFN-α2 administration, neither this event nor receptor number has correlated with therapeutic effects in hematologic malignancies.[23,24]

To elicit a cellular response, IFNs-α and IFN-β require two receptor subunits, IFNAR-1 and IFNAR-2. A 515 amino acid form of human IFNAR-2 has been identified as the universal ligand-binding subunit of IFNs-α and IFN-β.[1,4,5,7] The solution structure of other members of

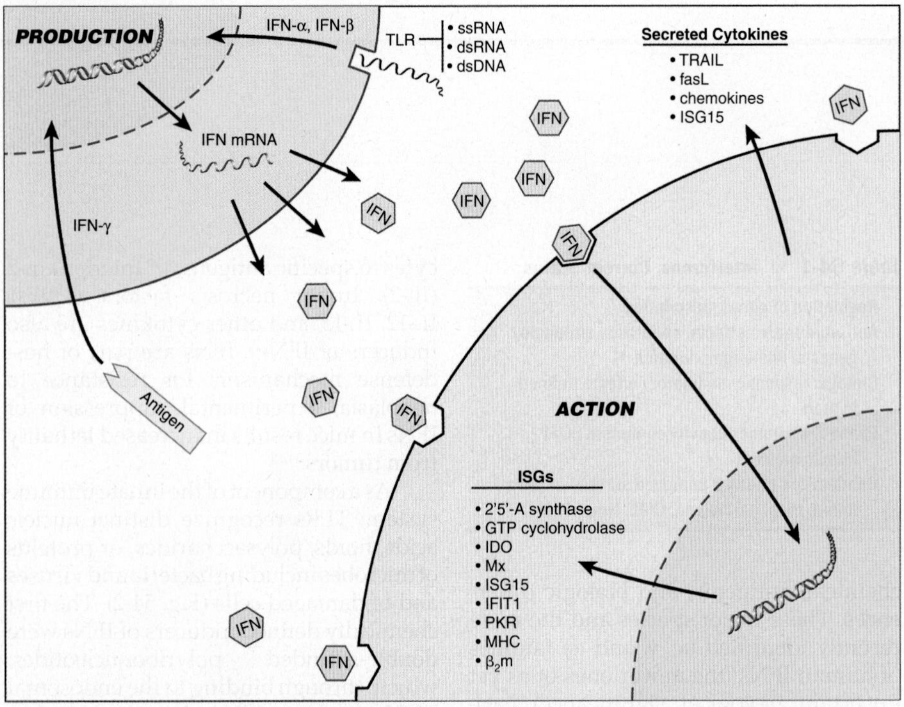

Figure 54-1 ■ Production of IFN-α or IFN-β is stimulated by nucleic acids through a final common pathway of double-stranded RNA or, in the case of IFN-γ, exposure to specific antigens. Action of IFNs is mediated via binding to a specific receptor on the cell surface with induction of secreted proteins (such as APO2L/TRAIL, fas ligand, interferon-stimulated gene-15 [ISG15], and many chemokines), cell surface proteins (such as MHC classes I and II, β2 microglobulin, tumor-associated antigens), and intracellular proteins (such as 2'5' synthease, protein kinase R, guanosine triphosphate [GTP] cyclohydrolase, indoleamine dioxygenase, and promyelocytic leukemia [PML]).

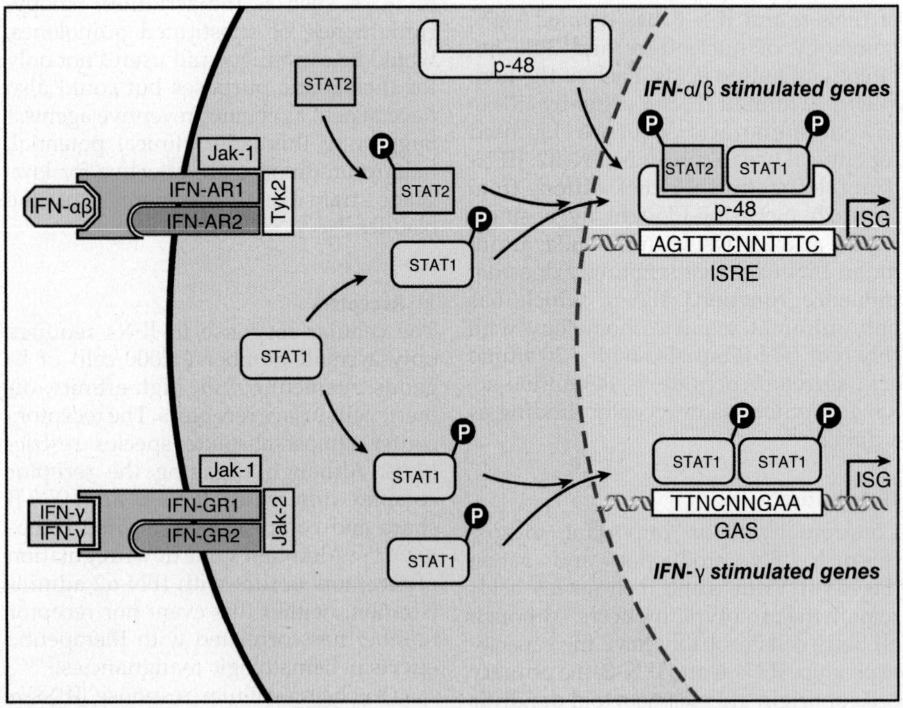

Figure 54-2 ■ Pathway of signal transduction by IFNs. After binding to specific receptors, tyrosine kinases (JAK-1, JAK-2, Tyk2) are activated. These tyrosine kinases phosphorylate inactive transcription factors (STAT-1α, STAT-1β, STAT-2), which form transcriptional factors, interferon-stimulated gene factor (ISGF)-3 or STAT-1 dimer. The interferon-stimulated response element (ISRE) or gamma-activation site (GAS) has shared nucleotides for all IFN-stimulated genes. *Abbreviations:* N, nucleotide; Y, pyrimidine.

the human cytokine receptor II family has enabled modeling of the three-dimensional structure of the extracellular domains of IFNAR-1 and IFNAR-2.[4,25] Receptor binding by IFN-β results in greater activation of subsets of genes through higher affinity, serine phosphorylation of STAT (signal transducers and activators of transcription)-1, and/or activation of other transcription factors.[26–31]

Signal Transduction

After receptor binding, cytoplasmic domains of two specific tyrosine kinases, tyk2 and JAK-1, are phosphorylated.[4,30–32] These activated tyrosine kinases activate the signal-transducing proteins (Fig. 54-3) and induce the formation of a complex of protein subunits (IFN-stimulated gene factor [ISGF]-3) consisting of STAT-1α or STAT-1β (alternatively spliced products of the same gene) and STAT-2 heterodimers or homodimers of STAT-1α. The phosphorylated ISGF-3 complex is translocated to the nucleus and forms (with the addition of a fourth subunit p48 or IRF-9) a DNA-binding complex specific for the IFN-stimulated response element (ISRE). IFN-γ receptor activation results in a similar sequence of events, although the transcriptional regulatory complex consists of a homodimer of STAT-1 that binds to DNA elements termed gamma-activated sites (GAS).[4,30,31,33] Other signaling cascades involving serine phosphorylation are also activated by IFNs, including activation of phosphatidylinositol-3-kinase and the mitogen-activated protein kinase cascades.[30,31,34,35] To add to the complexity of signaling by IFNs, several other STATs, such as STAT-3 and STAT-5, are also activated.[31,32] Thus, the global impact on gene induction is influenced by many factors, including cell lineage, exposure of the cells to other cytokines, and secondary cascades of signaling by gene products induced in the primary response.

Inhibitory for action at the receptor level are a family of suppressor of cytokine signaling (SOCS) proteins, effectors of a negative feedback mechanism following receptor stimulation.[36,37] Also inhibitory is a phosphatase, SHP-1, that influences receptor-activated tyrosine kinase signaling. Since both of these phosphatases are negative regulators of signaling by IFNs and other cytokines, inhibitors have been evaluated and proven effective in augmenting antitumor activities.[38,39]

Induced Genes and Antitumor Actions

Antitumor effects result from either a direct effect on viability and proliferation or antigenic expression of tumor cells,

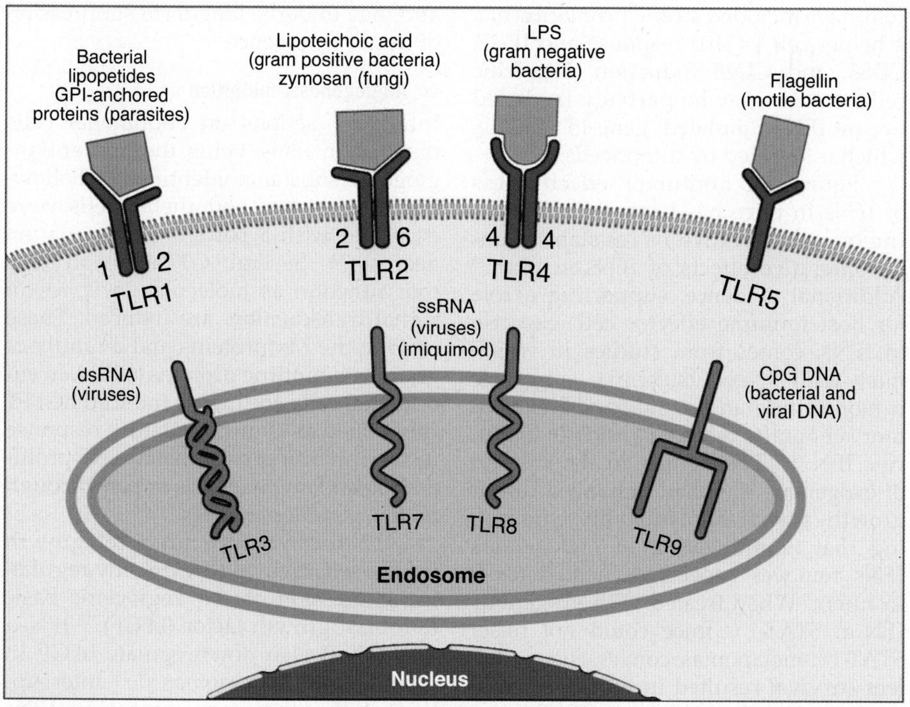

Figure 54-3 ■ Toll-like receptors (TLRs) and their ligands. TLR1, TLR2, TLR4, TLR5, and TLR6 are on the cytoplasmic membrane with extracellular domains that bind specific microbial ligands and then signal via specific cytoplasmic signaling proteins. Other TLRs, such as TLR3, TLR7/8, and TLR9, span the endosomal membrane with the ligand-binding domains in the lumen. They also function as dimers and recognize double-stranded (ds) RNA, single-stranded (ss) RNA, or dsDNA containing CpG sequences. *Abbreviations:* GPI, glycosylphosphatidylinositol; LPS, lipopolysaccharide.

or an effect on modulation of immune effector or endothelial cell populations (Table 54-2). IFNs regulate gene expression, modulate expression of proteins on the cell surface, and induce synthesis of new enzymes (Table 54-2). Alterations in gene expression result in modulation of receptors for other cytokines, concentration of regulatory proteins on the surface of immune effector cells, and activities of enzymes that control cellular growth and function. Attributing the effects of IFNs to specific gene products has been complicated by the hundreds of genes transcriptionally regulated across a diversity of cell types with quantitative and qualitative differences between IFNs-α, IFN-β, and IFN-γ[1,4,26,30–34] (Table 54-3). On a cellular basis, these effects translate into alterations of the state of differentiation, rate of proliferation and death, and functional activity of many cell types. Induced proteins and their products can be identified on cells and in serum of treated patients (Table 54-3). Their measurement or the quantitation of immune effector cell function can be used to define biologically active molecules, doses, schedules, and routes of administration.

■ Antiproliferative and Proapoptotic Effects

More than 100 ISGs can influence apoptosis including 2-5A synthetases, protein kinase R (PKR), promyelocytic leukemia (PML), RAP46/Bag-1, phospholipid scramblase, TNF-related apoptosis-inducing ligand (APO2L/TRAIL), and fas ligand.[4,27,40–46] Not only may these genes induce apoptosis themselves but also they may interact with other cytokines for augmented effects. Pretreatment with IFNs, particularly IFN-β, can enhance apoptosis from recombinant Apo2L/TRAIL or its receptor agonists, even in cells otherwise resistant to APO2L/TRAIL.[47] In IFN-sensitive but not IFN-resistant melanoma cells, TRAIL/APO2L was induced, as were other proteins implicated in apoptosis.[27,45] In chronic myelogenous leukemia (CML) and multiple myeloma, cellular induction by IFN-α of the death receptor Fas/CD95 resulted in apoptosis.[48] Intralesional administration of IFN-α into basal cell carcinomas increased Fas expression and led to regression.[49]

2'5'-A synthetases, a multiple isoform family, are relatively specific markers of IFN system activation.[40,50] A latent ribonuclease, RNaseL, is activated by oligonucleotides synthesized by 2'5'-A synthetase. The level of the RNaseL increased in growth-arrested cells and during cellular differentiation.[51] Apoptosis was suppressed in RNaseL null mice treated with different apoptotic agents.[52] Germ-line mutations in RNaseL are associated with familial prostate carcinoma and the infection of prostate stromal cells with a novel xenotropic retrovirus, further validating the postulate that influence on RNA levels by RNaseL may be important in oncogenesis.[40,53,54] Mutant variants of RNaseL may contribute to familial and sporadic pancreatic cancers and mutant of *RNASEL* corre-

Table 54-2 ■ **Pleiotropic Biologic Effects of Interferons**

Microbial inhibition	*Immunomodulatory*
RNA viruses	Cytotoxicity
DNA viruses	T cell
Intracellular pathogens	NK/LAK cell
	Monocytes/dendritic cells
Protein induction	
Adhesion proteins	Antibody dependent
Enzyme induction	Antigen processing
Chemokines	*Vascular*
Cell modulation	Angiogenesis inhibition
Oncogene depression	Lipoprotein reduction
Slow mitotic cycle	*Antitumor*
Differentiation	Mouse
Apoptosis	Man

Table 54-3 ■ **Modulation of Gene Expression by Interferons[a]**

Induced Proteins	
Antigen processing	Enzymes and other proteins
TAP	2-5A synthetase[a]
LMP-2	Protein kinase R (PKR)
HLA complex	Indoleamine dioxygenase[a]
Class I (A, B,C)[a]	Guanylate-binding proteins[a]
Class II (DR, DP, DQ)[a]	GTP cyclohydrolase[b]
B_2-Microglobulin[a]	Metallothionein II
Invariant chain	XAF1 (XIAP-associated factor)
Secreted proteins	ISG 15
APO2L/TRAIL	Phospholipid scramblase
Fas ligand	iNOS
Chemokines	PML
Depressed functional activities	IFITI (p56)
Ornithine decarboxylase	APO2LTTAIL
Oncogene	Transcription factors
C-MYC, H-RAS, C-FOS	IRF-1 (ISGF-2)
p450 microsomal enzymes	IRF2
	IRF-8 (ICSBP)
	STAT-1

[a] Representative of >100 genes transcriptionally augmented.[18]
[b] Modulation demonstrated after IFNs in patients.

lated with earlier age of onset of hereditary nonpolyposis colorectal cancer.[55,56]

A constitutive serine-threonine kinase, PKR, with a requirement for double-stranded RNA undergoes induction and activation and can induce apoptosis.[41,57,58] PKR and STAT-1 were both required for IFN-γ-mediated downregulation of C-MYC.[59] PKR expression may be partially controlled by an IFN-induced transcription factor, IRF-1.[60] Because IRF-1 increases rapidly in growth-arrested cells, it may influence expression of genes involved in negative control of cell growth and may mediate antiproliferative effects of IFNs.[61] A second transcription factor, IRF-2, has sequence homology to IRF-1, is a functional antagonist of IRF-1, and can result in cell transformation, which is inhibited by IRF-1.[61]

Several additional ISGs may influence apoptosis. Among these is the gene *PML*, a potential tumor suppressor gene.[43,62] $PML^{-/-}$ mice were used to demonstrate that PML is necessary for apoptosis by IFNs.[45] Phospholipid scramblase flips phosphatidylserine from the inner layer of the plasma membrane to the outer, a phenotypic change correlating with apoptosis.[63] These latter IFN-stimulated proteins can initiate the apoptotic cascade with alterations in mitochondrial membrane potential and changes in bcl-2 levels.[45,64,65] IFN-α reduction of transcription of *C-MYC* is at least in part a consequence of reduction in DNA binding of the transcription factor E2F, which binds to the *C-MYC* promoter.[66] Downstream of Rb and E2F, IFN-α reduced the amount of the cdc25 tyrosine phosphatase, resulting in the loss of activation of cyclin E–cdk2 and cyclin A–cdk2 kinase complexes.[67] Also, the cdk-inhibitor $p21^{WAF1}$ was induced,[68] which negatively regulated the cyclin E–cdk2 complex. Mouse 3T3 cells transformed with the human *HA-RAS-1* gene and cultured continuously in the presence of murine IFN-α/β, produced revertant colonies in which transcription of *RAS* was inhibited.[69]

Immune Effector Cells

Interferons have a role in augmenting effectiveness of all immune effector cell types that have the potential to kill tumor target cells. These include cytotoxic T cells, NK/lymphokine-activated killer (LAK) cells, and monocytes both in vitro and in vivo[4,15,71–80] (Table 54-2). In addition to augmenting expression of major histocompatibility complex (MHC) molecules (see below in this section), IFNs directly augment T-cell functions relevant to tumor cell cytotoxicity. Unique augmenting effects on dendritic cell maturation and function, differing from those of granulocyte–macrophage colony-stimulating factor (GM-CSF), have been identified.[13,81–86] These effects on dendritic cells have included strong promotion of a T helper cell 1 (Th1) response and IL-15, CD83, and CD25 induction. Dendritic cell function may be partially mediated by an IFN-stimulated gene-15 (ISG15), which is secreted by tumor cells.[87]

Equivalent antitumor effectiveness of IFNs in mice has been identified for tumor cells sensitive or resistant to antiproliferative effects of IFNs in vitro.[88] Additional evidence, supporting a role for host immune effector cell response to IFNs, comes from studies in which mice with Friend leukemia, syngeneic tumor, or human prostate and HeLa tumor xenografts received antibody to murine IFN.[89,90] These mice, in the absence of exogenous IFN, had enhanced tumor growth and transplantability, suggesting that neutralization of endogenous IFNs removes aspects of host defense to tumor. When treated with exogenous IFN-α, $STAT\text{-}1^{-/-}$ mice could not reject $STAT\text{-}1^{+/+}$ melanomas; conversely equivalent survival resulted in wild-type mice implanted with $STAT\text{-}1^{+}$ or $STAT\text{-}1^{-}$ tumors.[91] However, studies in nude mice with human tumor xenografts also demonstrate antitumor effects of exogenous human IFNs.[92–94] This finding demonstrates, in view of the strict species specificity of IFNs, that the direct effects can also limit tumor growth in vivo.

Induced gene modulation also underlies immune regulatory effects of IFNs (Table 54-3). IFNs enhance cell surface expression of MHC antigens, tumor-associated antigens (TAAs), and Fc receptors.[95–98] Enhancement of expression of TAAs, such as TAG72 and carcinoembryonic antigens (CEA), has both diagnostic and therapeutic implications.[99,100] Enhanced expression of TAA may lead to improved tumor cell recognition by host immune cells and could allow more directed therapy by using monoclonal antibodies as a carrier for radionuclides or cytotoxic agents. All IFNs augment MHC class I expression and IFN-γ enhances MHC class II expression on tumor cells as well.[96–98] Monocytes stimulated by IFNs have increased intracellular production of reactive oxygen species and have secreted colony-stimulating factor, TNF, and IL-1, as well as plasminogen activator, complement, and other cytotoxic mediators.[13,72,73,80,90,101] Other immunoregulatory ISGs include IL-12, the transporter associated with antigen processing (TAP) and lysosomal membrane permeabilization (LMP) proteins important for proteasomal antigen processing.[102,103] The chemokines CCL5 (RANTES), CSCL10 (IP-10), CCL2 (MCP-1), CCL3 (MIP-α), CXCL9 (MIG), and CXCL11(I-TAC), which are chemoattractive for both lymphocytes and monocytes, are all ISGs.[104–107] Thus substantial amplification of immune effector cell function can result from IFNs and may underlie long-term suppression of tumor emergence.[15]

Angiogenesis Inhibition

Inhibitory actions on endothelial cells resulted in IFNs, being the first antiangiogenic substance identified.[108] Following IFNs, tumor endothelial cells were damaged with a pattern of coagulation necrosis.[109] Several GTPases, proteins that function as molecular switches in signal transduction, are induced. These include the Mx proteins and a family of guanylate-binding proteins (GBPs). In endothelial cells, the highly induced hGBP1 functioned as an inflammatory response factor inhibiting endothelial cell proliferation and angiogenesis in part through matrix metalloproteases.[110–112]

IFN-α can reduce tumor cell growth in IFN-sensitive cells by directly regulating expression of the angiogenic basic fibroblast growth factor (bFGF).[113] IFN-α and IFN-β also downregulate bFGF in other human carcinomas.[114,115] Interruption of the angiogenic signal by IFNs precedes the antiproliferative effect and is detectable between 24 and 48 h after tumor inoculation.[109,116] IL-8, a potent mediator of angiogenesis and, consequently of tumorigenesis, can also be inhibited in production.[117,118] Other ISGs include angiogenesis inhibitory members of the chemokine family: CXCL9, CXCL10, and CXCL11.[119,120]

Clinically, IFN-α2 has successfully induced regression of bulky hemangiomas, tumors consisting of abnormal endothelial cells, and Kaposi sarcoma.[121,122] IFN-α2 was beneficial in life-threatening hemangiomas of infancy leading to regression in >80% of children. Not only did hemangiomas regress, but their life-threatening complications, including consumptive coagulopathy and high output cardiac failure, were controlled.[121] These preclinical and clinical observations have provided rationale for the assessment of IFN-α2 in angiosarcoma, giant cell tumor of bone, and renal carcinoma alone and in combination with bevacizumab.

Antitumor Effects in Humans

IFNs have achieved a role in clinical medicine well beyond that of the selective antiviral envisioned at discovery. Clinically beneficial therapeutic activity of IFN-α2 as a single agent has been demonstrated in more than a dozen malignancies (Table 54-4). The unique molecular and cellular effects of IFNs complement the mechanisms of actions of other therapies. In cell and animal models when combined with other therapies, IFNs have augmented effectiveness for malig-

Table 54-4 **Antitumor Effectiveness of Interferon Alpha in Phase 2/3 Trials**

Chronic leukemias	Melanoma[b]
Myeloid[a,b]	Carcinoids
Hairy cell[a,b]	Renal carcinomas[b]
Myeloproliferative syndromes[a]	Kaposi sarcomas[c]
Lymphomas	Ovarian carcinomas[c]
Follicular[a,b]	Basal cell carcinomas[c]
T cell[a]	Bladder carcinomas[c]
Myeloma	

[a] Response rates >40%.
[b] Improved survival in phase 3 trials.
[c] Intralesional or regional administration.

nancies of diverse histologies. Building upon these observations the single-agent clinical activity in hematopoietic malignancies and solid tumors, and upon the effects of second-generation IFNs or inducers, new IFN therapeutic applications will emerge.

Most gene and biologic response modulatory effects peak at 24 to 48 h, which contrasts with maximal serum levels of minutes to hours after intravenous or subcutaneous administration.[123–125] After intravenous bolus administration, the t½α of IFN-α2 is short (<60 min); mean terminal half-life is 4 to 5 h with no serum levels measurable at 12 h. After intramuscular or subcutaneous administration, peak levels are 3 to 8 h.[123] The pharmacologic hallmark of IFN-β is virtual absence of serum levels with subcutaneous or intramuscular administration; yet, biologic response modulatory and therapeutic effects occur.[125]

Pegylated IFNs have markedly different kinetics than do unmodified IFNs.[126–128] Once-weekly administration has resulted in measurable serum levels of IFN-α2 at 7 days—in excess of that required for gene induction and cellular effects in vitro. Pegylated IFN-α2 has resulted in tumor responses in metastatic renal carcinoma, CML, and melanoma.[128,129] Although pegylated IFNs may be slightly better tolerated, it is their greater therapeutic effectiveness that has resulted in regulatory approvals in chronic active hepatitis.[130,131] Clinical effectiveness against a hepatitis C virus serotype, previously unresponsive to unmodified IFN-α2,[130,131] suggests that the altered pharmacokinetics and pharmacodynamics result in a drug with different cellular and clinical actions. This activity may be important in decreasing frequency of development of hepatocellular carcinoma after hepatitis virus infections.[132,133]

Hematologic Malignancies

The degree of activity and improvement in quality of life of patients with hairy cell leukemia resulted in the first licensed approval for an IFN in the United States. More than 85% of patients had objective evidence of partial or complete hematologic response to IFN-α2.[134] Following IFNs, there was a gradual decrease in bone marrow infiltration with hairy cells as well as a normalization of peripheral hematologic parameters resulting in reduced morbidity from the disease process.[135,136] Although now replaced in clinical use by more effective drugs, FDA approval in hairy cell leukemia opened the way for expanded clinical trials of IFN-α2 in other malignancies.

In CML, IFN-α2 resulted in sustained therapeutic response in a majority (>75%) of newly diagnosed patients.[137,138] In addition to reduction in leukemic cell mass, a decrease occurred in frequency of cells bearing the underlying chromosomal translocation.[137] With continued treatment, ~25% of patients developed a major cytogenetic response. Equivalence and/or superiority of IFN-α2 to busulfan and hydroxyurea for CML was demonstrated.[139] Treatment resulted in 30% of all patients being alive for 8 or more years.[140] Median and 10-year survival data identified significant and cost-effective advantage for IFN-α2 when compared to chemotherapy.[141,142] Although with increased toxicity, an increase in cytogenetic response frequency occurred with addition of cytosine arabinoside in combination to IFN-α2.[143–145] Thrombocytosis associated with myeloproliferative disorders, whether Ph1 positive or negative, was also effectively controlled by IFN-α2, has been of polycythemia vera, hypereosinophilic syndrome, and chronic eosinophilic leukemia with chromosomal translocation.[146–151]

Clinical effectiveness in CML spurred investigations of potential mechanisms of action in that disorder. IFN-α restored defective adhesion of CML progenitors to bone marrow stroma, thereby allowing normal growth inhibitory signals to regulate stem cell and early precursor proliferation.[152] An IFN-induced transmembrane protein, associated with cell adhesion and antiproliferative effects, has been correlated with improved survival in CML.[153] Fas expression in vitro correlated with clinical response.[154–156] Loss in mice of expression of a transcription factor gene, IFN consensus sequence-binding protein (ICSBP), resulted in a myeloproliferative syndrome phenotypically similar to CML.[157] ICSBP expression was found to be low in patients with both acute and chronic myeloid leukemias.[157] Although the two modalities have synergistic effectiveness in inhibiting CML precursor proliferation,[158,159] whether IFN-α2 can in the future be used to clinical advantage with imatinib mesylate is only beginning to be assessed and considered.[160–162]

Response rates of 10% to 20% occur in patients with myeloma treated with various schedules.[163,164] However, patients who have had only limited prior therapies may have higher response frequency.[163,164] In patients who had a tumor response, levels of serum immunoglobulins were restored, an effect infrequently seen with chemotherapy.[164] Both induction and maintenance have repeatedly had shown to have therapeutic effectiveness in subsequent studies and analyses.[165–170] As molecular mechanisms of response and resistance are better defined, IFNs could be part of effective combination therapy for this disease.[64, 171–175]

In lymphomas of various histologies and of both B- and T-cell phenotypes, IFN-α can have a therapeutic role. IFNα2 was effective in 45% of patients with cutaneous T-cell lymphoma or follicular B-cell lymphomas, and even in patients previously treated with combination chemotherapy.[164,176,177] For B-cell lymphomas, the single-agent activity of IFN-α2 has been integrated into effective combined modality treatments for both low and intermediate grade lymphomas.[178–182] Because IFNs can increase both HLA class I and antibody-dependent cellular cytotoxicity, a relatively low dose of IFN-α2 was combined with rituximab in a Phase 2 trial with an increase in progression-free survival.[183]

Solid Tumors

Response rates for metastatic melanoma in patients who received IFN-α2 as a single agent have approximated 15%, comparable to cytotoxic agents used alone.[184–187] When combined with chemotherapy and IL-2, response rates can exceed 45% but with increased toxicity and with no marked prolongation in progression-free survival or overall survival.[187–192] Increase in disease-free survival with an impact in some trials on overall survival has, however, emerged from use of IFN-α2 as an adjuvant to surgery for melanoma for patients at high risk for disease recurrence (stage IIb or stage III).[193–197] A comparison to a ganglioside vaccine resulted in a 48% decrease in risk of death for those patients receiving IFN-α2 ($P < 0.01$).[196] Analysis of quality-of-life adjusted survival in the adjuvant setting has also identified an advantage for use of IFN-α2.[198] Thus, IFN-α2 has become a standard of care for patients with stage IIb or stage III melanoma in the United States, a use supported by meta-analyses.[198,199] A large European trial that used pegylated IFN-α2 for longer duration has confirmed benefit on disease-free survival in high-risk primary patients.[200]

Like other potent physiologic mediators, IFNs have toxicities when administered with pharmacologic intent (Table 54-5), which have led to analyses

Table 54-5 Clinical Side Effects of Interferons [202, 203]

Acute	Chronic
Fever	Fatigue
Chills	Anorexia
Malaise	Weight loss
Myalgias	Neutropenia
Headaches	Transaminase elevations
Nausea	Depression, mental slowing
	Infrequent: confusion, hair shedding, thrombocytopenia, diarrhea

Source: From Refs. 202, 203.

of quality adjusted survival in melanoma and other malignancies.[142,198,199,201] Side effects with the initial dose are constitutional, dominated by malaise, fever, and chills, subsiding after a few days.[202,203] Fatigue and anorexia are the dose-limiting toxicities with chronic administration; weight loss may necessitate dose reduction.[204] Chronic fatigue with the 1 year of administration for high-risk primary melanoma patients has hampered broad medical acceptance. Hematologic effects include mild granulocytopenia with a reduction in counts by 40% to 60% followed by rapid rebound to normal after discontinuation of therapy.

Pegylation has resulted in responses in metastatic melanoma leading to an innovative trial design of long-duration treatment with dose adjusted for fatigue and anorexia with confirmed increase in disease-free survival.[129,197,201,205] Another innovative approach has been investigation of high-dose IFN-α2 prior to surgery in patients with advanced nodal disease at diagnosis; 20 patients were treated with clinical response in 55% and pathological complete response in 15%.[206] Beneficial therapeutic effects of the high dose regimens, used in the United States, may result from an increasing the level of STAT-1 and decreasing the level of STAT-3 both in lymphocytes and tumor cells.[207]

Response rates from 4% to 26% have been reported in trials IFN-α2 in metastatic renal carcinoma, with a mean response of 15% in cumulative summary of several trials.[208] In two randomized trials comparing IFN-α alone or in combination with other treatments, a statistically significant increases in survival resulted.[209,210] Other randomized trials have suggested survival prolongations that may be the greatest for patients who have nephrectomies despite the presence of metastases and who then receive IFN-α.[211,212]

Carcinoids, although often behaving in an indolent fashion, produce symptoms, which may interfere with daily activities. In trials of IFN-α in midgut carcinoid tumors, a mean response rate of ~50% (improvement in symptoms or decrease in 5-hydroxyindoleacetic acid) resulted.[213,214] Objective tumor regression occurs less frequently but can include both primary tumors and hepatic metastases. Other solid tumors, such as ovarian, bladder, and basal cell carcinomas, have responded to IFN-α administered regionally, particularly in patients with lesser tumor bulk.[215–217]

Perspectives

IFNs have improved therapeutic outcomes for malignancies and viral diseases. They were the first human proteins to be effective as a cancer treatment modality. The full spectrum of actions and interactions, mechanism of antitumor effects, optimal dose, schedule, and type of IFN have still only been partially delineated. As the first clinical product of recombinant DNA technology for oncology, IFNs, both themselves and as a prototype for other therapeutic proteins, opened the use of biologic therapies for malignancies. Furthermore, their critical role in controlling emergence of malignancy through cellular control and augmentation of innate and acquired immunity is being increasingly defined.[4–7,15]

Suppression of the IFN system of the host in and by malignant cells is emerging as an important contributor to the development of the clinical disease. Mutation of a gene, *RNASEL*, in the IFN response pathway increases prostate cancer risk.[53,218] Gene expression profiling and cytogenetic analyses have identified decreases in ISGs in melanoma, colon, breast, and hematologic malignancies.[102,219–228] Epigenetic silencing of ISGs also likely influences tumor development.[227–229] In addition to being a primary source for production, dendritic cell maturation is also enhanced.[13,17,80,82,84–86] Activation of the IFN system, as has been used in experimental models and in chronic hepatitis to decrease risk of hepatocellular carcinoma, suggests that IFNs or inducers could play a role in chemoprevention.[19,230–232]

Second generation IFNs and inducers have begun to demonstrate potential clinical advantage. Phase 1 trials have identified better toleration and tumor responses for the only other recombinant IFN-α evaluated.[233,234] Pegylation of IFN-α2 has resulted in advantageous pharmacokinetics and improved outcomes for patients with chronic active hepatitis and has resulted in tumor response in renal carcinoma, melanoma, and CML. Agonists of TLRs can induce clinical tumor regression.[17,235,236] With further definition of the role of the pleiotropic molecular and cellular effects, innovative clinical studies of IFNs or IFN-induced proteins should result in improved therapeutic outcomes for a number of malignancies from IFNs or IFN inducers.

Selected References

The complete reference list can be found at www.CANCERMEDICINE8.com

1. Pfeffer LM, Dinarello CA, Herberman RB. et al. Biological properties of recombinant alpha-interferons: 40th anniversary of the discovery of interferons. *Cancer Res.* 1998;58:2489–2499.
4. Borden EC, Sen GC, Uze G, et al. Interferons at age 50: past, current and future impact on biomedicine. *Nat Rev Drug Discov.* 2007;6:975–990.
5. Chelbi-Alix MK, Wietzerbin J. Interferon, a growing cytokine family: 50 years of interferon research. *Biochimie.* 2007;89:713–718.
6. Pestka S. The interferons: 50 years after their discovery, there is much more to learn. *J Biol Chem.* 2007;282:20047–20051.
7. de Weerd NA, Samarajiwa SA, Hertzog PJ. Type I interferon receptors: biochemistry and biological functions. *J Biol Chem.* 2007;282:20053–20057.
8. Farrar MA, Schreiber RD. The molecular cell biology of interferon-gamma and its receptor. *Annu Rev Immunol.* 1993;11:571–611.
9. Schoenborn JR, Wilson CB. Regulation of interferon-gamma during innate and adaptive immune responses. *Adv Immunol.* 2007;96:41–101.
10. Young HA, Bream JH. IFN-gamma: recent advances in understanding regulation of expression, biological functions, and clinical applications. *Curr Top Microbiol Immunol.* 2007;316:97–117.
11. Kawai T, Akira S. Antiviral signaling through pattern recognition receptors. *J Biochem.* 2007;141:137–145.
12. Severa M, Fitzgerald KA. TLR-mediated activation of type I IFN during antiviral immune responses: fighting the battle to win the war. *Curr Top Microbiol Immunol.* 2007;316:167–192.
13. Liu YJ. IPC: professional type 1 interferon-producing cells and plasmacytoid dendritic cell precursors. *Annu Rev Immunol.* 2005;23:275–306.
14. Gresser I, Belardelli F, Maury C, et al. Injection of mice with antibody to interferon enhances the growth of transplantable murine tumors. *J Exp Med.* 1983;158:2095–2107.
15. Koebel CM, Vermi W, Swann JB, et al. Adaptive immunity maintains occult cancer in an equilibrium state. *Nature.* 2007;450:903–907.
16. Averett DR, Fletcher SP, Li W. The pharmacology of endosomal TLR agonists in viral disease. *Biochem Soc Trans.* 2007;35:1468–1472.
17. Krieg AM. Development of TLR9 agonists for cancer therapy. *J Clin Invest.* 2007;117:1184–1194.
18. Brikos C, O'Neill LA. Signalling of toll-like receptors. *Handb Exp Pharmacol.* 2008;183:21–50.
19. Borden E, Sidky Y, Erturk E, et al. Protection from carcinogen-induced murine bladder carcinoma by interferons and an oral interferon-inducing pyrimidinone, bropirimine. *Cancer Res.* 1990;50:1071–1074.
26. Der SD, Zhou A, Williams BR, Silverman RH. Identification of genes differentially regulated by interferon alpha, beta, or gamma using oligonucleotide arrays. *Proc Natl Acad Sci USA.* 1998;95:15623–15628.

27. Leaman DW, Chawla-Sarkar M, Borden EC, et al. Novel growth and death related interferon- stimulated genes (ISGs) in melanoma: greater potency of IFN-beta compared with IFN-alpha2. *J Interferon Cytokine Res.* 2003;23:745–756.
32. Brierley MM, Fish EN. Stats: multifaceted regulators of transcription. *J Interferon Cytokine Res.* 2005;25:733–744.
33. Stark GR. Cell type-specific signaling in response to interferon-gamma. *Curr Top Microbiol Immunol.* 2007;316:119–154.
34. van Boxel-Dezaire AH, Rani MR, Stark GR. Complex modulation of cell type-specific signaling in response to type I interferons. *Immunity* 2006;3:361–372.
35. Stark GR. How cells respond to interferons revisited: from early history to current complexity. *Cytokine Growth Factor Rev.* 2007;18:419–423.
36. Alexander WS. Suppressors of cytokine signaling (SOCS) in the immune system. *Nat Rev Immunol.* 2002;2:410–416.
40. Silverman RH. A scientific journey through the 2-5A/RNase L system. *Cytokine Growth Factor Rev.* 2007;18:381–388.
79. Dunn GP, Koebel CM, Schreiber RD. Interferons, immunity and cancer immunoediting. *Nat Rev Immunol.* 2006;611: 836–848.
80. Fitzgerald-Bocarsly P, Feng D. The role of type I interferon production by dendritic cells in host defense. *Biochimie.* 2007;89:843–855.
91. Lesinski GB, Anghelina M, Zimmerer J, et al. The antitumor effects of IFN-alpha are abrogated in a STAT1-deficient mouse. *J Clin Invest.* 2003;112:170–180.
92. Balkwill FR, Moodie EM, Freedman V, Fantes KH. Human interferon inhibits the growth of established human breast tumours in the nude mouse. *Int J Cancer.* 1982;30:231–235.
112. Lindner DJ. Interferons as antiangiogenic agents. *Curr Oncol Rep.* 2002;4:510–514.
140. The Italian Cooperative Study Group on Chronic Myeloid Leukemia. Interferon-alpha 2a as compared with conventional chemotherapy for the treatment of chronic myeloid leukemia. *N Engl J Med.* 1994;330:820–825.
144. Kantarjian HM, O'Brien S, Smith TL, et al. Treatment of Philadelphia chromosome-positive early chronic phase chronic myelogenous leukemia with daily doses of interferon alpha and low-dose cytarabine. *J Clin Oncol.* 1999;17:284–292.
170. Myeloma Trialists' Collaborative Group. Interferon as therapy for multiple myeloma: an individual patient data overview of 24 randomized trials and 4012 patients. *Br J Haematol.* 2001;113:1020–1034.
172. Cheriyath V, Glaser KB, Waring JF, et al. G1P3, an IFN-induced survival factor, antagonizes TRAIL-induced apoptosis in human myeloma cells. *J Clin Invest.* 2007;117:3107–3117.
181. Smalley RV, Weller E, Hawkins MJ, et al. Final analysis of the ECOG I-COPA trial (E6484) in patients with non-Hodgkin's lymphoma treated with interferon alfa (IFN-(α2a) plus an anthracycline-based induction regimen. *Leukemia.* 2001;15:1118–1122.
186. Masci P, Borden EC. Malignant melanoma: treatments emerging, but early detection is still key. *Cleve Clin J Med.* 2002;69:529, 529–545.
196. Kirkwood JM, Ibrahim JG, Sosman JA, et al. High-dose interferon alfa-2b significantly prolongs relapse-free and overall survival compared with the GM2-KLH/QS-21 vaccine in patients with resected stage IIB-III melanoma: results of intergroup trial E1694/S9512/C509801. *J Clin Oncol.* 2001;19:2370–2380.
200. Eggermont AM, Suciu S, Santinami M, et al. Adjuvant therapy with pegylated interferon alfa-2b versus observation alone in resected stage III melanoma: final results of EORTC 18991, a randomised phase III trial. *Lancet.* 2008;372:117-126.
205. Bottomley A, Coens C, Suciu S, et al. Adjuvant therapy with pegylated interferon alfa-2b versus observation in resected stage III melanoma: a phase III randomized controlled trial of health-related quality of life and symptoms by the European Organization for Research and Treatment of Cancer Melanoma Group. *J Clin Oncol.* 2009;27:2916-2923.
212. Flanigan RC, Salmon SE, Blumenstein BA, et al. Nephrectomy followed by interferon alfa-2b compared with interferon alfa-2b alone for metastatic renal-cell cancer. *N Engl J Med.* 2001;345:1655–1659.
218. Casey G, Neville PJ, Plummer SJ, Xiang Y. et al. RNASEL Arg462Gln variant is implicated in up to 13% of prostate cancer cases. *Nat Genet.* 2002;32:581–583.

55 Cytokines and Hematopoietic Growth Factors

Suhendan Ekmekcioglu, PhD ■ Razelle Kurzrock, MD ■ Elizabeth A. Grimm, PhD

Cytokines, a diverse family of signaling molecules, are produced by almost every cell in the body, including various cancer cells. In general, some cytokines are growth stimulatory and others are inhibitory. Cytokines with clinical relevance to cancer include those subclassified further as interleukins (ILs), monokines, chemokines, and hematopoietic growth factors. In cancer, certain cytokines act directly on the growth, differentiation, or survival of endothelial cells, while others act by attracting inflammatory cell types affecting angiogenesis, or by inducing secondary cytokines or other mediators regulating angiogenesis. Proinflammatory and chemotactic cytokines influence the tumor environment and control the quantity and nature of infiltrating hematopoietic effector cells, with inhibiting or enhancing effects on tumor growth. The important role of cytokines in regulating immune responses may permit an effective immune response against the tumors or suppress the function of antigen-presenting cells. Attempts to elicit immune activation in cancer patients using immunostimulatory ILs, and most notably IL-2, have provided some success in cancer therapy. Presuming antigens exist on tumor cells, various immunostimulatory cytokines, and particularly ILs, are now administered to patients in an attempt to initiate, augment, or otherwise stimulate a weak or previously nonexistent antitumor immune response. In addition to immune response stimulation, some ILs have been used to stimulate the growth and differentiation of various subpopulations of blood cells after chemotherapy or bone marrow transplantation (BMT) in a restorative role.

Interleukin designates any soluble protein or glycoprotein product of leukocytes that regulates the responses of other leukocytes. ILs produce their effects primarily through paracrine interactions. The cascades of ILs that are generated by both pathogen exposure and antigen-specific interactions are primarily local, with the functions of individual ILs mediated by paracrine interaction with specific receptors expressed differentially on different cell types, including hematopoietic and immunologic cells, but also including endothelial and other cells. It is now clear that the pleiotropic nature of many cytokines allows them to influence virtually all organ systems (Fig. 55-1). Cytokines may have their own private receptor but may also share a "public" receptor with other cytokines (Tables 55-1 and 55-2).[1]

The biologic characterization of the known clinically relevant ILs and selected cytokines, the rationale for their use in therapy for patients with cancer, and the accumulated clinical experience represent the subjects of this chapter.

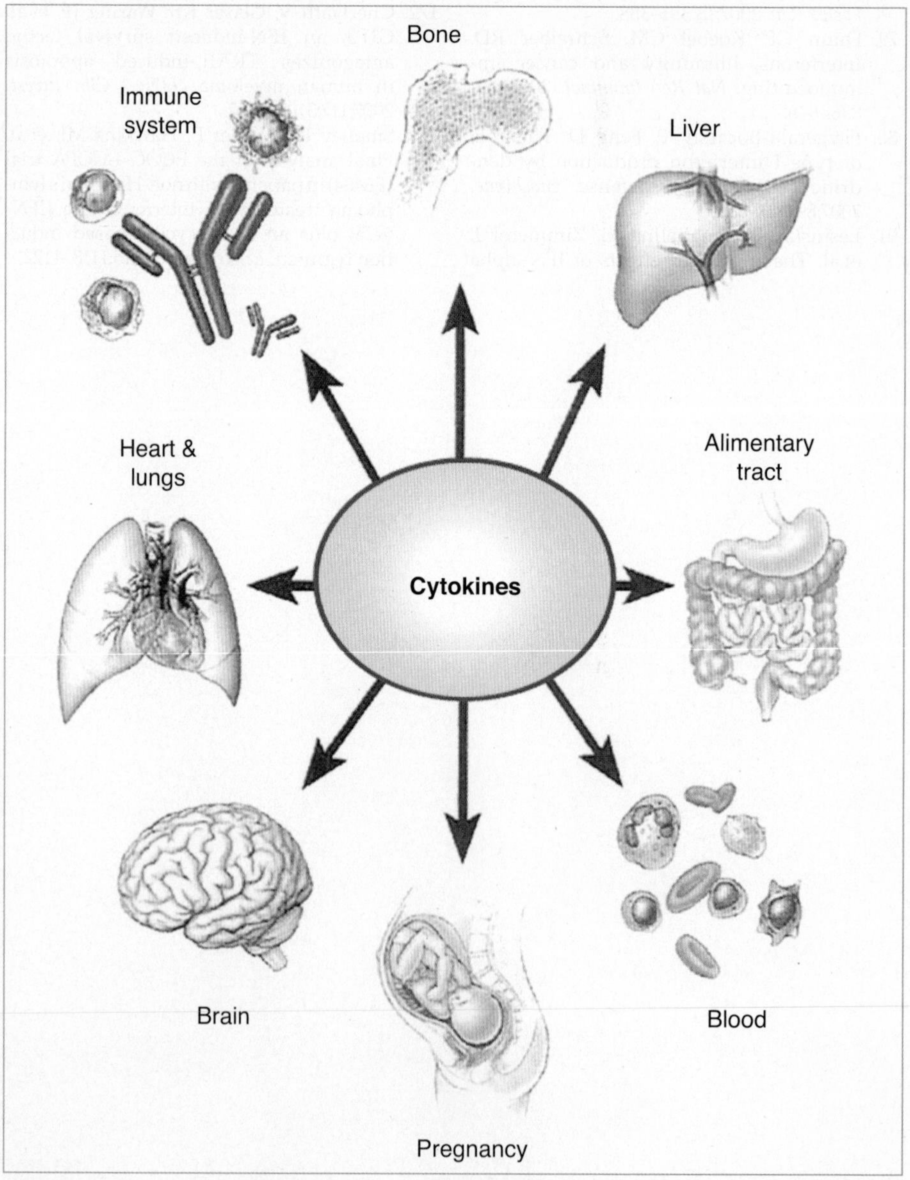

Figure 55-1 In addition to their effects on hematopoiesis and immunocompetence, "hematopoietic" growth factors influence multiple organ systems, including (but not limited to) bone remodeling, cardiorespiratory function, hepatic function, and the gastrointestinal tract.

Hematopoiesis and the Role of Growth Factors

Through a series of well-orchestrated divisions, hematopoietic stem cells give rise to all the blood cells. Functionally, these early progenitors are capable of self-renewal as well as proliferation and differentiation. Self-renewal occurs when a cell enters the cell cycle and undergoes one round of mitosis, giving rise to daughter

Table 55-1 **Types of Hematopoietic Growth Factor Receptors**

Type	Characteristics	Receptor Examples
Type I cytokine receptor	Does not possess intrinsic kinase activity. Receptor acts as docking site for adaptor molecules, which leads to phosphorylation of cellular substrates	IL-1, IL-2, IL-3, IL-4, IL-5, IL-6, IL-7, IL-9, IL-13, IL-18, IL-21, GM-CSF, G-CSF, EPO, TPO, leukemia inhibitory factor
Type II cytokine receptor	Contains extracellular fibronectin III type domain	Interferon and IL-10
Receptors with tyrosine kinase domains (type III)	Large extracellular immunoglobulin-like domain, single transmembrane spinning region, and a cytoplasmic tyrosine kinase domain(s)	fms (M-CSF receptor), FLT-3, c-kit (SCF receptor), PDGFR
Chemokine receptor	Seven transmembrane spanning G protein–linked regions	IL-8
Tumor necrosis factor family	Cysteine-rich repeats in the extracellular domain, and cytoplasmic 80 amino acid "death domain"	Tumor necrosis factor and Fas

Abbreviations: EPO, erythropoietin; G-CSF, granulocyte colony-stimulating factor; GM-CSF, granulocyte macrophage colony-stimulating factor; IL, interleukin; M-CSF, macrophage colony-stimulating factor; SCF, stem cell factor; TPO, thrombopoietin.
Source: From Ref. 1.

Table 55-2 **Receptor Subunits Shared Among Cytokines**

Some Cytokines Using Subunit	Receptor Subunit Shared
IL-3, IL-5, and GM-CSF	β subunit
IL-2, IL-4, IL-7, IL-9, IL-15, and IL-21	IL-2 receptor γc chain
IL-2 and IL-15	β chain of IL-2 receptor
IL-4 and IL-13	IL-4Rα and IL-13Rα1
IL-6, oncostatin M, leukemia inhibitory factor, IL-11, IL-27, IL-31	gp130
IL-10, IL-22, IL-28, IL-29	IL-10Rβ
IL-17, IL-25	IL-17BR
IL-19, IL-20, IL-24	IL-20Rα, IL-20Rβ
IL-20, IL-22, IL-24	IL-22Rα
IL-12, IL-23	IL-12Rβ1

Abbreviations: GM-CSF, granulocyte macrophage colony-stimulating factor; IL, interleukin.
Source: From Ref. 1.

cells at the same stage of development. Differentiation defines the sequence of events by which cells mature. There is a loss of self-renewal capacity as lineage commitment progresses, though some regenerative capacity may be maintained.

The development, homeostasis, trafficking, and response capacity of the hematopoietic system are tightly regulated by a complex communications network that is mediated by intercellular signals. These signals are triggered by direct cell-to-cell or cell-to-matrix contact or by the release of soluble cytokine mediators.

The identification and cloning of hematopoietic growth factors have revolutionized hematology practice. Raising white blood cell counts in neutropenic patients was unimaginable until the advent of granulocyte (G)-CSF and granulocyte macrophage (GM)-CSF. Today, growth factors are routinely used to alleviate neutropenia and, to a lesser extent, thrombocytopenia and anemia after chemotherapy. They can also help mobilize stem cells for transplantation, reverse cytopenias in a variety of nonmalignant illnesses, and may have the potential to mobilize the immune system against infection or cancer.

Erythropoietin

Erythropoietin (EPO) is the major hormone regulator of erythropoiesis. It has an established role in the treatment of anemia associated with a variety of illnesses (Table 55-3).

Biologic Activities of EPO EPO provides a proliferative signal to early erythroid progenitors (burst-forming unit erythroid [BFU-E]) and a differentiation signal to a later erythroid precursor (colony-forming unit erythroid [CFU-E]). EPO can also promote megakaryocyte differentiation, B-cell proliferation, and endothelial cell chemotaxis.

EPO and Human Disease On the one hand, high levels of endogenous EPO are often found in patients with anemia due to cancer, especially hematologic malignancies. On the other hand, in many patients with anemia, even anemia due to cancer, there is a relative deficiency in endogenous EPO. In other words, though the levels of this molecule are elevated, they are not as high as they should be for the degree of anemia. Certain cases of familial erythrocytosis have been attributed to the presence of EPO-hypersensitive cells. This heightened EPO response results from the formation of a truncated EPO receptor, which is missing a negative regulatory domain.[5]

Table 55-3 **Erythropoietin[a]**

	Characteristic[2-7]	Comment
Chromosomal localization[3]	7q21	Induced by hypoxia
Major production sites	Kidney, liver	
Selected biologic activities	Promotes the proliferation, differentiation, and survival of erythroid precursors	
Receptor	EPO receptor	Class I cytokine receptor encoded at 19p13 and utilizing JAK2 and STAT5 signaling
Natural antagonists	Soluble EPO receptor	
Major clinical indications	Anemia of renal failure	
	Anemia of zidovudine therapy of HIV (with endogenous EPO level < 500 mU/mL)	
	Anemia of cancer, especially after chemotherapy of solid tumors	
	Reduction of blood transfusions in elective surgery	
	Potentiation of autologous blood donation	
	Anemia of prematurity	
	Maximum quality-of-life improvement is at hemoglobin of 11–13 g/dL	
	Hyperglycosylated EPO (darbepoetin alfa) has prolonged half-life and can be administered less frequently	Correction of "functional iron deficiency" is important
	Postulated to offer neuroprotection after neurological damage since EPO/EOP receptors are present in the central nervous system	

[a]Reviewed in Cazzola M.[2]
Abbreviations: EPO, erythropoietin; HIV, human immunodeficiency virus.

EPO in the Clinic ■ EPO is most useful in those anemias where there is an absolute or a relative deficiency in endogenous EPO levels. First used successfully as replacement therapy to correct the anemia associated with chronic renal failure, EPO is also effective in increasing hemoglobin in some patients with both solid tumors and hematologic malignancies as well as in those with a variety of other conditions (see Table 55-3).[6]

EPO has generally been used for patients with significant anemia that is hemoglobin <10 g/dL. In addition, there have been several recent trials using EPO more liberally, in an effort to normalize hemoglobin. However, such efforts are now disfavored. Indeed, in light of recent data suggesting a negative impact of EPO on disease control, the U.S. FDA suggests that EPO be used conservatively to avoid transfusion, but not to normalize hemoglobin levels. In the case of cancer, however, not all patients respond, and those with the highest levels of endogenous EPO are probably less likely to benefit. Also, experience in patients with renal failure has revealed a state of "functional iron deficiency." Relative (or functional) iron deficiency occurs when erythropoiesis is stimulated to the point that iron cannot be mobilized rapidly enough from stores to adequately supply the erythron. Under these circumstances, percent transferrin saturation may decrease to <20% (though ferritin levels may be high), and hypochromic red blood cells/reticulocytes appear in the circulation despite the presence of normal or even increased iron stores. Whether or not, and to what extent "functional iron deficiency" complicates EPO therapy of the anemia of cancer is unclear.

Granulocyte Macrophage Colony-Stimulating Factor

GM-CSF was the first CSF to enter clinical trials. It has now been approved in many countries for treatment of neutropenia after chemotherapy or transplantation, for treatment of graft failure, and for peripheral blood stem cell mobilization (Table 55-4).

Major Biologic Activities of GM-CSF ■ GM-CSF stimulates proliferation of multilineage progenitors and the growth of BFU-E, granulocyte, macrophage, and eosinophil colonies. GM-CSF also enhances the functional activity of most phagocytes, including neutrophils, macrophages, and eosinophils.

GM-CSF in Human Disease ■ Autocrine expression of GM-CSF in myeloid leukemia cells and cell lines has been proposed to play a role in neoplasia.[9] Autonomous production by the tumor of GM-CSF (or G-CSF) has also been implicated as one possible pathophysiologic mechanism underlying leukemoid reactions in cancer patients.[10] In addition, the presence of GM-CSF biologic activity in synovial fluid from patients with rheumatoid arthritis suggests that it may enhance the tissue destruction associated with this disorder.

Clinical Indications for GM-CSF ■ GM-CSF has been shown to be safe and effective in the treatment of patients with acute myelogenous leukemia (AML) who are undergoing induction therapy. This molecule shortens the neutropenic period and decreases the rate of serious infections in older individuals. GM-CSF is also indicated for accelerating myeloid reconstitution after allogeneic BMTs. This molecule also enhances survival in patients who experience engraftment failure or delay after allogeneic or autologous transplantation. Finally, peripheral blood stem cells mobilized in the presence of GM-CSF yield significantly higher colony counts than those mobilized without this molecule and, after transplantation, recipients of GM-CSF-mobilized progenitors have quicker neutrophil, platelet, and red blood cell recovery and shorter hospital stays.

Granulocyte Colony-Stimulating Factor

Granulocyte colony-stimulating factor (G-CSF) has revolutionized the treatment of neutropenia and its sequelae (infection). It has been used worldwide and has been found to be remarkably effective and virtually devoid of side effects (Table 55-5).[12,13]

Biologic Activities of G-CSF ■ G-CSF is a relatively specific stimulator of the growth and differentiation of hematopoietic progenitor cells committed to the neutrophil lineage. It also protects neutrophils from apoptosis and enhances their function (chemotaxis, phagocytosis, oxidative responses, and microbicidal activity). Finally, G-CSF moves mature neutrophils from the marrow into the circulation.

G-CSF in Human Disease ■ In healthy persons, mean ± SD G-CSF levels are 25 ± 19.7 pg/mL. G-CSF levels increase by 30-fold in infection and by 10,000-fold in septic shock.[18] Some patients with solid tumors present with significantly increased leukocyte counts. In several of these individuals, elevated serum levels of G-CSF (or GM-CSF) have been demonstrated and probably account for the rise in white blood cell count.[10] Presumably, G-CSF (or GM-CSF) is produced by the tumor itself.

Point mutations in the gene for the G-CSF receptor have been described in patients with AML, which evolved from severe congenital neutropenia. These mutations truncate the C-terminal cytoplasmic region of the G-CSF receptor and hence are presumed to disrupt the maturation signal of the receptor.[14]

Clinical Indications for G-CSF ■ G-CSF promotes a rapid increase in neutrophilic leukocytes, which lasts about 24 h. Despite the multitude of patients who have

Table 55-4 ■ **Granulocyte Macrophage Colony-Stimulating Factor**

	Characteristic[8-11]	Comment
Chromosomal localization[3]	5q31.1	Located 9 kb downstream of IL-3
Forms	14–35 kDa	May be variably glycosylated. Removal of the carbohydrate increases the specific activity
Production sites	T and B cells, macrophages, mast cells, thymic epithelial cells, fibroblasts, endothelial cells, mesothelial cells, osteoblasts	
Selected biologic activities	Stimulates growth of multilineage progenitors, BFU-E, granulocyte, macrophage, and eosinophil colonies Induces migration and proliferation of vascular endothelial cells Activates mature phagocytes (neutrophils, macrophages, eosinophils)	
Receptor	Type I receptor with α and β subunits	α subunit = CD116 on Xp22.32 and Yp11.3 in the pseudoautosomal region β subunit = CDw131 at 22q12.2-13.1 β subunit shared by IL-3 and IL-5
Major clinical indications	Neutropenia due to myelosuppressive chemotherapy or BMT Peripheral blood stem cell mobilization Graft failure After induction therapy for AML	

Abbreviations: BFU-E, burst-forming unit erythroid; BMT, bone marrow transplantation.

Table 55-5 ■ Granulocyte Colony-Stimulating Factor

	Characteristic[12-21]	Comment
Chromosomal localization[3]	17q11.2-q12	
Major production sites	Stromal cells, endothelial cells, fibroblasts, monocytes	Induced by TNF-α and IL-1
Forms	Differential splicing produces two forms of biologically active G-CSF Two forms of G-CSF differ by three amino acids	
Selected biologic activities	Regulates production and function of neutrophils	
Receptor	G-CSF receptor	G-CSF receptor = CD114 on chromosome 1p35-34. Cytoplasmic region transduces proliferative and survival signals; C-terminal transduces differentiation signals
Major clinical indications	Neutropenia due to chemotherapy or BMT Chronic and cyclic neutropenia AIDS-related neutropenia Autoimmune neutropenia Peripheral blood stem cell mobilization G-CSF reduces morbidity from high-risk febrile neutropenia treated with antibiotics	PEGylated G-CSF is long-acting and requires only one dose per chemotherapy cycle

Abbreviations: AIDS, acquired immune deficiency syndrome; BMT, bone marrow transplantation; G-CSF, granulocyte colony-stimulating factor; TNF, tumor necrosis factor.

received G-CSF, few toxicities have been reported. Even very long-term G-CSF administration appears fairly innocuous; the most common side effect is bone pain.

Studies of G-CSF as an adjunct to standard-dose cytotoxic chemotherapy for solid tumors and lymphomas demonstrate that the duration of neutropenia, the number of days of hospitalization, and the number of days of antibiotic treatment are reduced significantly during G-CSF cycles. Placebo-controlled studies in patients with small-cell lung cancer showed a clinically significant protective effect of G-CSF against febrile neutropenia.[15] After high-dose chemotherapy, recovery from neutropenia and its associated complications is more rapid when patients receive G-CSF. These studies suggest that the dose intensity of nonmyeloablative chemotherapy can be increased with G-CSF support. In the transplantation setting, the administration of G-CSF results in reductions in neutropenia and infection.[16] G-CSF also mobilizes autologous peripheral blood progenitor cells; these cells are used to accelerate hematopoietic recovery in patients who have received myeloablative or myelosuppressive chemotherapy.[17] In patients with de novo AML, G-CSF administration is associated with reductions in the time to neutrophil recovery and the duration of fever.[19] However, there are no statistically significant differences between the G-CSF-treated and the placebo-treated groups, in terms of treatment outcome parameters—complete remission or relapse-free survival.

A new form of G-CSF has been developed; a conjugate of G-CSF and monomethoxypolyethylene glycol. PEGylated G-CSF has a prolonged half-life because of its reduced renal clearance. Serum clearance is directly related to neutrophil number. As a result, only a single SC dose of PEGylated G-CSF (Neulasta) is required after chemotherapy. Based on the results of randomized, blinded trials, this molecule is indicated to decrease the incidence of infection in patients with nonmyeloid malignancies receiving myelosuppressive chemotherapy with a significant incidence of febrile neutropenia.[21]

Macrophage Colony-Stimulating Factor

Although macrophage colony-stimulating factor (M-CSF) is known to affect a variety of organ systems, its cardinal effect remains its ability to influence most aspects of monocyte/macrophage development and function (Table 55-6).

Biologic Activities of M-CSF ■ M-CSF stimulates differentiation of progenitor cells to mature monocytes, and prolongs the survival of monocytes. It enhances cytotoxicity, superoxide production, phagocytosis, chemotaxis, and secondary cytokine production (G-CSF, IL-6, and IL-8) in monocytes and macrophages. In addition to stimulation of hematopoiesis, M-CSF also promotes differentiation and proliferation of osteoclast progenitor cells and has profound effects on lipid metabolism.

Table 55-6 ■ Macrophage Colony-Stimulating Factor

	Characteristic[22-26]	Comment
Chromosomal localization[3]	1p21-p13	
Forms	Three forms produced: soluble M-CSF, proteoglycan form, and membrane-bound form	Proteoglycan form binds to low-density lipoprotein
Major production sites	Monocytes/macrophages Fibroblasts Epithelial cells Vascular endothelium Osteoblasts	
Selected biologic activities	Influences most aspects of monocyte/macrophage development and function Stimulates hematopoiesis Induces osteoclast production Helps maintain pregnancies Lowers cholesterol levels Affects microglial function	
Receptor	Fms	Fms is a proto-oncogene product located at 5q33-34
Major clinical trials	Enhances hematopoietic recovery after chemotherapy or transplantation Attenuates neutropenia in chronic neutropenia Lowers serum cholesterol Lowers serum cholesterol	

M-CSF is important in pregnancy. Physiologically, a large amount of this molecule is produced in the placenta, and it is believed to play an essential role in trophoblast differentiation (see Table 55-6).[24] The elevated serum M-CSF levels of early pregnancy may participate in the immunologic mechanisms responsible for the maintenance of the pregnancy.[25]

M-CSF in Human Disease ■ M-CSF is intricately involved in atherosclerosis, but information about its role remains contradictory. For instance, M-CSF administration lowers cholesterol levels. Paradoxically, it appears that an absence of M-CSF protects against atherosclerosis even in the presence of hyperlipidemia.[25] M-CSF and Fms are expressed in the brain. This cytokine induces microglial proliferation, activation, and survival.

In malignancy, mutations in Fms (the M-CSF receptor) have been reported at codon 969 in about 10% of cases of human myeloid malignancies (including myelodysplasia and AML).

M-CSF in the Clinic ■ In a large-scale study, it has been shown that the administration of M-CSF to AML patients after consolidation chemotherapies shortens the periods of neutropenia and thrombocytopenia after chemotherapy and reduces the incidence and shortens the duration of febrile neutropenia.[24] Similar benefits have been reported after chemotherapy or BMT. M-CSF can elevate neutrophil counts in children with chronic neutropenia. Finally, preliminary results in uncontrolled trials suggest that this molecule may improve outcome after fungal infections.[26]

Stem Cell Factor

Stem cell factor (SCF) is also known as kit ligand, mast cell growth factor, or steel factor. It functions as a hematopoietic cytokine that triggers its biologic effect by binding to c-kit (the SCF receptor) (Table 55-7).[27]

Biologic Activities of SCF ■ SCF is constitutively produced by marrow stromal elements. It is now well established that SCF acts on hematopoietic stem cells and, in some lineages, mature cells.

SCF synergizes with other cytokines (including EPO, IL-3, GM-CSF, and G-CSF) to support the direct colony growth of BFU-E, CFU-GM, and CFU-granulocyte/erythroid/macrophage/megakaryocyte (GEMM) in semisolid media, and current data suggest that SCF can act on a more primitive cell (pre-CFU-C) capable of generating the direct colony-forming cells. SCF can also promote progenitor cell survival, accelerate stem cell entry into cell cycle, and function as a chemotactic and chemokinetic factor for these cells. Synergistic proliferative effects on megakaryocytic progenitor cells are observed when SCF is combined with thrombopoietin (TPO) or IL-3.[29] SCF is also involved in processes of cell adhesion and trafficking. SCF induces progenitor cell adhesion to fibronectin, a process that may involve alteration of integrin avidity through an inside-out signal initiated in response to c-kit receptor kinase activation after ligand binding. Alternatively, it is possible that the transmembrane form of SCF displayed on fibroblasts binds directly to the c-kit receptor on the surface of hematopoietic cells and, thus, helps to anchor the hematopoietic cells in the microenvironment.[29]

The effects of SCF when combined with G-CSF are even more pronounced.[34] Phase 1 clinical studies show that treatment with SCF increases the numbers of progenitor cells of many types (including BFU-E, CFU-GM, CFUMeg, and CFU-GEMM) in the marrow.[35]

SCF and c-kit in Human Disease ■ The concentration of SCF in normal human serum is, on average, 3.3 ng/mL. Serum SCF levels are not elevated in patients with aplastic anemia, myelodysplasia, chronic anemia, or after marrow ablative therapy.[29] Thus, the level of SCF in the circulation, unlike the level of EPO, is not inversely related to the hematocrit.

Alterations in the local distribution of SCF within the skin have been implicated in the pathogenesis of cutaneous mastocytosis.[29] Point mutations in the c-kit receptor cytoplasmic domain have been identified in murine and human mast cell lines and in hematopoietic cells from patients with mast cell disorders.[29] Activating mutations in kit characterize a type of leiomyosarcoma known as gastrointestinal stromal tumors.

Neoplastic human hematopoietic cells (in AML, anaplastic large-cell lymphoma, and Hodgkin disease) can also display the c-kit receptor. Receptor density is highest in erythroleukemia cell lines, which may express up to 50,000 to 100,000 c-kit receptors per cell. Solid tumor cell lines (including small-cell lung cancer, breast cancer, and neuroblastoma) as well as a variety of fresh human tumor tissues (particularly small-cell lung cancer, testicular seminoma, glioblastoma, and some breast cancers) also express c-kit receptor protein.[29]

SCF in the Clinic ■ Clinical trials of SCF in a number of situations have been undertaken. SCF factor seems to be reasonably well-tolerated, with the predominant side effects being transient local erythema and long-lasting hyperpigmentation at injection sites. The most worrisome toxicity is a mast cell effect resulting in allergic-like reactions characterized by urticaria, with or without respiratory symptoms.[29] The side effects of SCF, including the

Table 55-7 ■ **Stem Cell Factor**

	Characteristic[27-38]	Comment
Chromosomal localization[3]	12q22-12q24	
Natural forms of SCF	Transmembrane and soluble	Both forms are biologically active
Major sites of production	Marrow stroma Hematopoietic cells Gut epithelial cells Central nervous system Thymus Skin keratinocytes	IL-1 and TNF increase stromal SCF production
Selected biologic activities	Promotes hematopoiesis at multiple levels Influences primordial germ cell and melanocyte migration during embryonic life Affects immunoregulatory cells (B and T cells, mast cells, NK cells, dendritic cells) Influences hematopoietic cell adhesive properties	
Receptor	c-kit	Also known as CD117: Encoded on 4q11-q13 (piebald locus)
Natural antagonists	Soluble c-kit receptor	Kit is mutated in gastrointestinal stromal tumors
Major clinical trials	Peripheral blood progenitor mobilization (SCF + G-CSF better than SCF alone) Aplastic anemia (trilineage responses seen after SCF)	STI571 (Gleevec) targets the activated kit kinase activity and produces striking responses in gastrointestinal stromal tumors with kit mutations

Abbreviations: G-CSF, granulocyte colony-stimulating factor; IL-1, interleukin-1; NK, natural killer; SCF, stem cell factor; TNF, tumor necrosis factor.

allergic phenomenon, appear to be dose-dependent.

Clinical trials of SCF plus G-CSF are also underway. The incidence of allergic-like reactions was ~2% in 400 SCF-treated patients.[36] A randomized study in breast cancer patients demonstrated that SCF plus G-CSF is a more effective peripheral blood progenitor cell mobilization regimen than G-CSF alone.[37] Use of SCF alone and together with G-CSF has also resulted in trilineage responses in aplastic anemia patients.[38] Of special interest is the role of mutations in the SCF receptor (kit) in gastrointestinal stromal tumors. These mutations activate the kinase enzymatic activity of kit. A kinase inhibitor targeted against kit (STI571 or Gleevec) has been found to be dramatically effective in these notoriously chemotherapy-resistant tumors.[33]

Thrombopoietin

The humoral basis of megakaryocyte and platelet production has been more enigmatic than that of other lineages. Factors that have now been implicated in at least some aspects of thrombocyte development include IL-3, IL-6, IL-9, IL-11, G-CSF, GM-CSF, SCF, leukemia-inhibiting factor, and TPO. The latter molecule is believed to be of paramount importance in the physiologic regulation of platelet production. Unfortunately, however, compared with the striking effects of the granulopoietic factors in neutropenic patients, use of the thrombopoietic molecules in the clinic setting has met with less success. Of interest, a random-peptide-screening approach has permitted the identification of a 29-amino acid peptide that promotes megakaryocyte growth and platelet formation by stimulating the TPO receptor (Table 55-8).[39]

Biologic Properties of TPO ■ TPO participates in hematopoiesis in general, in addition to thrombopoiesis, is supported by experiments demonstrating that genetic elimination of TPO or its receptor causes a 65% to 95% reduction in the numbers of transplantable stem cells. The survival of TPO in the circulation is longer than that of other hematopoietic growth factors (half-life = 30 h).

TPO and Human Disease ■ High serum levels of TPO have been found in patients with autosomal dominant hereditary thrombocythemia.[43] Overproduction has been attributed to a splice donor mutation in the gene for TPO, which leads to a shortened 5'-untranslated region that is more efficiently translated than its normal counterpart.[43] Because platelets themselves regulate the level of circulating TPO, high levels of TPO are also found in patients with bone marrow failure states. Homozygous elimination of *c-mpl* (TPO receptor) results in congenital amegakaryocytic thrombocytopenia.

TPO in the Clinic ■ Two forms of TPO have entered clinical trials.[41,42] These forms are termed: TPO (the full-length polypeptide) and polyethylene glycol (PEG)-conjugated recombinant human megakaryocyte growth and development factor (PEG-rHuMGDF).

Because its biologic action is prolonged, parenteral administration of TPO for 7 to 10 days results in increased platelet production 6 to 16 days later.[44] Results of clinical trials of PEG-rHuMGDF or recombinant human TPO in patients with cancer who were receiving chemotherapy, albeit with regimens that produce only moderate thrombocytopenia, suggest that platelet counts return to baseline significantly faster and the nadir platelet counts are higher.[45,46] However, the effectiveness of these molecules in accelerating platelet recovery after myeloablative therapy has not been impressive.[47] Furthermore, in patients with delayed platelet recovery after peripheral blood stem cell or bone marrow transplantation, recombinant human TPO did not significantly raise platelet counts in most patients.[48] Because of the finding that platelets can remove TPO from the circulation, an issue that should be considered in future trials is the possibility that platelet transfusions may dampen the recovery of megakaryocytes after myelosuppressive therapy and may blunt response to exogenously administered TPO. Therefore, early treatment with this molecule may be more beneficial than treatment later during hematopoietic recovery.[41] Finally, TPO can result in multilineage mobilization of peripheral blood progenitor cells. The kinetics of progenitor release differs from that after G-CSF. Following G-CSF peripheral blood progenitors increase almost immediately, peak at day 5 to 6, and decrease with G-CSF cessation. In contrast, PEG-MGDF resulted in a late and sustained increase in progenitors, with levels first detected on day 8, and climbing on day 12, despite cytokine discontinuation.[50] Due to the development of neutralizing antibodies and subsequent thrombocytopenia in some patients, clinical studies with the PEGylated molecule have been terminated.

AMG 531 is another novel recombinant thrombopoiesis-stimulating peptibody showing impressive activity in the treatment of chronic immune thrombocytopenic purpura (ITP).[51] It targets megakaryocyte and platelet development

Table 55-8 ■ **Thrombopoietin**

	Characteristic[39-50]	Comment
Chromosomal localization[3]	3q27-q28	
Major sites of production	Liver Kidney Smooth muscle Marrow stroma Brain	
Selected biologic properties	Major regulator of platelet production Acts in synergy with EPO to stimulate growth of erythroid progenitors Acts in synergy with IL-3 and SCF to stimulate proliferation and prolong survival of hematopoietic stem cells	Homologous to murine myeloproliferative leukemia virus
Receptor	Mpl	Located on chromosome 1p34
Recombinant forms for clinical trials	TPO (the full-length polypeptide)	
Major clinical trials	Accelerates platelet recovery after chemotherapy Increases platelet yield from normal donors for platelet transfusions Enhances mobilization of peripheral blood progenitor cells by G-CSF Nonimpressive effects on platelet recovery after myeloablative therapy	Trials of PEG-conjugated recombinant human megakaryocyte growth and development factor have been suspended because of antibody formation

Abbreviations: EPO, erythropoietin; G-CSF, granulocyte colony-stimulating factor; IL-3, interleukin-3; PEG, polyethylene glycol; PEG-rHuMGDF, PEG-conjugated recombinant human megakaryocyte growth and development factor; SCF, stem cell factor; TPO, thrombopoietin.

through the same pathway as endogenous TPO (eTPO). However, it has no sequence homology with eTPO. Therefore, it has a low potential to elicit antibodies that can cross-react to eTPO. AMG 531 does not appear to affect the ongoing rate of platelet destruction. The study that has been conducted to evaluate the safety and efficacy of treatment with AMG 531 in patients with ITP has shown that it has caused no major adverse events and increased platelet counts.[52] The drug is also being evaluated for chemotherapy-induced thrombocytopenia and thrombocytopenia resulting from myelodysplastic syndrome (MDS). Researchers affiliated with The AMG 531 in MDS Study Group reported that it can reduce bleeding and transfusion events in patients with MDS.[53]

In conclusion, the issue of whether clinically relevant thrombocytopenia can be ameliorated after chemotherapy of solid tumors may be moot, since severe thrombocytopenia is not commonly encountered in this setting. In leukemias and after transplantation, future studies will need to address dose-timing issues. Finally, since thrombocytopenia is a major cause of morbidity and mortality in bone marrow failure states (myelodysplasia, aplastic anemia, graft failure), investigations of TPO in these illnesses are urgently needed. Several studies suggest that diverse hematopoietins can induce thrombopoietic responses in bone marrow failure that some of these responses are multilineage, and that recovery can be durable in a subset of individuals.[54] As reviewed in Ref 54, several molecules with putative thrombopoietic activity have entered the clinic. Each of these has been touted as a potent platelet growth factor, but initially, clinic results have been modest. However, recent results with AMG 531 appear to be more robust. For some other thrombopoietic factors, prolonged therapy may be necessary to achieve recovery.

Apoptosis-Based Therapies by TRAIL and Its Receptors

TNF-related apoptosis-inducing ligand (TRAIL) or Apo-2L is a type II membrane protein, which exerts major biologic activity in a trimeric form. In a quest for specific regulators of sensitivity to TRAIL, a broad family of receptor has been detected by numerous groups. TRAIL-R1 (death receptor 4; DR4) and TRAIL-R2 (death receptor 5; DR5) are type I transmembrane proteins exerting proapoptotic signals. Both receptors use signal transduction pathways very similar to that of the Fas system.[55] TRAIL appears to be a promising candidate for cancer therapy, because it specifically kills tumor cells while leaving normal tissues relatively unharmed.[56]

AMG 655 is a fully human monoclonal agonist antibody that binds human TRAIL-R2, activates caspases, and induces apoptosis in sensitive tumor cells. First-in-human study of AMG 655 in adult patients with advanced solid tumors has concluded that the administration of AMG 655 up to 20 mg/kg is well-tolerated in patients.[57] Antitumor activity was seen in non–small cell lung cancer. Recombinant human (rh) Apo2L/TRAIL protein designed to activate both proapoptotic receptors, DR4 and DR5. Phase 1 trials in patients with advanced tumors are currently underway and pharmacodynamic assays to monitor the activity shows the percentage of increase correlates with serum Caspase 3/7 levels and is dose-dependent.[58] Moreover, it is safe and well-tolerated up to 15 mg/kg as a single agent.[59] Antitumor activity has been seen in chondrosarcoma.

Apomab is another fully human antibody that is designed to specifically bind to a major receptor, DR5 which is found on the surface of various types of cancer cells.[60] Binding of Apomab to DR5 directly activates extrinsic apoptotic pathways. In preclinical models, Apomab selectively induces apoptosis in cancer cells while sparing normal cells.[61] Apomab is currently in Phase 1 studies.

Phase 1 studies with HGS-ETR2, which is a fully human agonist monoclonal antibody that targets TRAIL-R2, have revealed that it is a safe and well-tolerated drug for patients with advanced solid tumors, and supports further evaluation in Phase 2 trials.[62,63] In these studies, prolonged and stable disease was observed in a number of heavily pretreated and refractory patients. Preclinical studies designed to show its synergistic effects with other chemotherapeutic agents are further encouraging. Sequential treatment with paclitaxel followed by HGS-ETR1 or HGS-ETR2 results in markedly enhanced antitumor activity, in vivo.[64] Novel in vivo imaging techniques by scintigraphic imaging and autoradiography using radiolabeled receptor antibodies showed good tumor uptake, suggesting that sequential taxane treatment followed by TRAIL-R agonist antibodies could be applied in the clinic, and that novel imaging techniques could be exploitable to optimize sequence timing and patient selection.

Interleukin-1

IL-1 (IL-1α and IL-1β) is the prototypic pleiotropic cytokine (Table 55-9).[65,66] This molecule influences nearly every cell type. Because IL-1 is a highly inflammatory cytokine, the margin between salutary effects and serious toxicity in humans is exceedingly narrow. Compounds that attenuate the production and/or activity of IL-1 are therefore also being explored in clinical trials.

Biologic Effects of IL-1 ■ The basis for the protean effects of IL-1 is the ability of this cytokine to modulate the expression of a wide variety of genes and surface receptors. Indeed, IL-1 can increase the expression of itself as well as many other cytokines (including IL-1RA), cytokine receptors (including IL-2, IL-3, IL-5, GM-CSF, c-kit), inflammatory mediators (such as cyclooxygenase and inducible nitric oxide synthase), hepatic acute phase reactants, growth factors (including, but not limited to, fibroblast growth factor, keratinocyte growth factor, hepatocyte growth factor, nerve growth factor, insulin-like growth factor, activan), clotting factors, neuropeptides, lipid-related genes, extracellular matrix molecules, and oncogenes (eg, *c-jun*, *cabl*, *c-fms*, *c-myc*, *c-fos*).[65] Recent data on inflammation–cancer connection suggest that an inflammatory component is present in the microenvironment of most neoplastic tissues, including those not causally related to an obvious inflammatory process. Thus, as a proinflammatory cytokine, IL-1 may also be a major proangiogenic stimulus of both physiological and pathological angiogenesis.

IL-1 and Hematopoiesis ■ IL-1 is able to increase the production of various CSFs and SCFs, either by increasing their transcription or by stabilizing their mRNA. IL-1 may have protective effects after irradiation or cytotoxic drugs. In addition, IL-1 synergizes with CSFs for expansion of bone marrow. However, evidence in mice with specifically targeted gene deletions indicates that normal hematopoiesis can take place in the absence of IL-1-converting enzyme (ICE), IL-1β, or IL-1RI. Therefore, it appears that IL-1 is not necessary for normal hematopoiesis but plays a role in hematopoietic responses to disease states. In support of this contention is the observation that spontaneous expression of IL-1 in circulating blood cells from normal volunteers cannot be detected even using polymerase chain reaction methods.[69]

IL-1 in Human Disease ■ The IL-1 family has been implicated in the function and the dysfunction of virtually every human organ system. Indeed, increased IL-1 production has been reported in patients with infections (viral, bacterial, fungal, and parasitic), intravascular coagulation, cancer (both solid tumors and hematologic malignancies), Alzheimer's disease, autoimmune disorders, trauma, ischemic diseases, pancreatitis, graft-vs-host disease, transplant rejection, and in healthy subjects after exercise.[65]

Table 55-9 **Interleukin-1**

	Characteristic[65-77]	Comment
Chromosomal localization[3]	2q13	
Natural forms	IL-1α and IL-1β (extended family of 10 members)	
Selected biologic activities	Promotes acute phase response IL-1 acts on nearly every organ system50,51 Induces production of multiple cytokines Up-regulates cell-surface cytokine expression Synergizes with other cytokines to stimulate hematopoietic progenitor proliferation Influences immune regulation (T- and B-cell responses) Modulates endocrine function Affects bone formation IL-1R acts as a cofactor in neural transmission IL-1 is probably not critical for normal hematopoiesis; it is, however, central in disease states	Both pro-IL-1α and IL-1α are biologically active; function intracellularly; bind to the nucleus Pro-IL-1β is not fully biologically active; after cleavage by ICE, it is excreted extracellularly where it exerts its effects
Receptors	IL-1RI and IL-1RII (extended family of 10 members including IL-18R)	IL-1RI = CD121a at 2q12; IL-1RII = CDw121b at 2q12-q22 IL-1RI transduces a signal; IL-1RII does not
IL-1RI transduces a signal; IL-1RII does not		
Natural antagonists	Soluble IL-1RI and IL-1RII and IL-1RA	IL-1RA binds to IL-1 receptor but has not agonist activity (acts as antagonist). Intracellular pool of IL-1RA may compete for nuclear IL-1 binding sites. Soluble receptors can bind to IL-1α, IL-1β, and IL-1RA (thus antagonizing both IL-1 and its antagonist [IL-1RA])
Major clinical trials	IL-1α and IL-1β Modest reduction in post-chemotherapy neutropenia or thrombocytopenia; numerous side effects No significant antitumor activity in melanoma or renal cell carcinoma IL-1RA	IL-1α and IL-1β significant toxicities encountered IL-1RA well-tolerated

Abbreviations: ICE, interleukin-1-converting enzyme; IL-1, interleukin-1; IL-1R, interleukin-1 receptor; IL-1RA, interleukin-1 receptor antagonist of rheumatoid arthritis and graft-vs-host disease.

It has been suggested that it is really the balance between IL-1 and its naturally occurring antagonists that is most relevant to illness.[67] This balance may be altered in different ways, depending on the disease. For instance, after myocardial infarction or surgery, and in asymptomatic persons infected with human immunodeficiency virus (HIV)-1, markedly elevated levels of IL-1RA are present in the circulation without elevated IL-1β. On the one hand, in body fluids from patients with infectious, inflammatory, or autoimmune disease, the molar "ratio" of endogenous IL-1RA to IL-1β is often 10 to 100, and levels of IL-1RA may be a better indicator of disease severity than are levels of IL-1β. On the other hand, in AML, IL-10 is spontaneously expressed, but IL-1RA gene expression is suppressed even when stimulated with GM-CSF.[70,71] In chronic myelogenous leukemia (CML), patients with advanced disease and poor survival have suppressed IL-1RA accompanied by high IL-1β.[72] In AML and CML patients, IL-1β acts as an autocrine growth factor; exposure to molecules that decrease the activity of IL-1 suppresses leukemic proliferation.[73,74] Constitutive production of IL-lα, IL-1β, and/or IL-1RA in solid tumors (melanomas, hepatoblastoma, sarcomas, squamous cell carcinomas, transitional cell cancers, and ovarian carcinomas) has been described as well and may, in some cases, contribute to metastatic potential. However, the relationship between IL-1 and tumor growth is complex.

IL-1 in the Clinic ■ IL-lα and IL-1β have both been administered in clinical cancer trials.[65] In general, the acute toxicities of either isoform of IL-1 were greater after intravenous injection compared with subcutaneous injection. Subcutaneous injection was associated with significant local pain, erythema, and swelling. Dose-related chills and fever were observed in nearly all patients, and even a 1 ng/kg dose was pyrogenic. Nearly all patients receiving intravenous IL-1 at doses of 100 ng/kg or greater experienced significant hypotension, probably because of induction of nitric oxide.

IL-1 infusion into humans significantly increased circulating IL-6 levels and resulted in a rise in leukocyte counts, even at doses as low as 1 or 2 ng/kg. Increases in platelets were also observed in patients with normal marrow reserves. In addition, peripheral monocyte count and phorbol-induced superoxide production increased significantly. In contrast to the results in patients with good marrow function, patients with aplastic anemia treated with five daily doses of IL-lα (30-100 ng/kg) had no increases in peripheral blood counts or bone marrow cellularity.[75] However, after chemotherapy, two doses of IL-10 significantly shortened the duration of neutropenia,[76] and IL-lα (5 days) significantly reduced thrombocytopenia.[77] Overall, the benefits of IL-1 therapy were compromised by its toxicity.

IL-1RA has also been administered to humans. When given intravenously to healthy volunteers, it is without side effects or changes in biochemical, hematologic, or endocrinologic parameters. These studies support the concept that there is no role for IL-1 in the regulation of body temperature, blood pressure, or hematopoiesis in health.

Interleukin-2

Originally described as a T-cell growth factor, the function of IL-2 extends beyond lymphocyte activation and population expansion, though T cells still appear to be its major target (Table 55-10).[78]

Biologic Activities of IL-2 ■ IL-2 primarily acts as a T-cell growth factor, but B cells, NK cells, and lymphokine-activated killer cells are also responsive to this cytokine. Following binding of IL-2 with the trimeric receptor complex, internalization occurs and cell-cycle progression is induced in association with the expression of a defined series of genes.[83] A second functional response occurs through the IL-2β, dimeric receptor, also known as the intermediate affinity dimeric complex (kDa, 10^{-9}) and involves the differentiation of several subclasses of lymphocytes into lymphokine-activated killer (LAK) cells.[84] This response occurs in patients with cancer who receive IL-2[85,86] and was originally considered to be a critical part of the anticancer effect of IL-2. LAK cells recognize and kill tumor cells, irrespective of the histocompatibility expression status on fresh human tumor cells tested.[87] The multiple biologic effects of IL-2 on immune cells

Table 55-10 **Interleukin-2**

	Characteristic[78-82]	Comment
Chromosomal localization[3]	4q26-q27	
Production sites	T cells	
Selected biologic activities	Induces proliferation and activation of T cells, B cells, and NK cells	
Receptors	$\alpha\beta\gamma$ heterotrimeric complex	α chain (p55) = CD25 at 10p14-p15 β chain (p75) = CD122 at 22q11.2-q13 Ψ chain (p64) = CD132 at Xq13 β chain shared by IL-2 and IL-15 γ chain shared by IL-2, IL-4, IL-7, IL-9, and IL-15
Natural antagonists	Soluble IL-1RI and IL-1RII and IL-1RA	IL-1RA binds to IL-1 receptor but has not agonist activity (acts as antagonist). Intracellular pool of IL-1RA may compete for nuclear IL-1 binding sites. Soluble receptors can bind to IL-1α, IL-1β and IL-1RA (thus antagonizing both IL-1 and its antagonist [IL-1RA])
Major clinical indications	Antitumor activity in melanoma and renal cell carcinoma IL-2 diphtheria fusion toxin (DAB-IL-2) approved for use in cutaneous T-cell lymphomas	IL-2 use associated with significant toxicity

Abbreviations: IL, interleukin; NK, natural killer.

include the induced proliferation of antigen-stimulated T cells and induction of cytotoxicity in major histocompatibility complex (MHC)-restricted, antigen-specific T lymphocytes, NK cells leading to non-MHC-restricted LAK cell activity, and activation of tumoricidal monocytes; it is not clear what role any of these effector systems have in vivo.[88,89]

IL-2 in the Clinic ■ IL-2 has been used to treat several different cancers and have been approved by the FDA for the treatment of metastatic melanoma and metastatic renal cell cancer. In melanoma biochemotherapy, regimens combining IL-2 and interferon (IFN)-α with, for instance, cisplatin, vinblastine, and dacarbazine, produce response rates of up to 60%, but this has yet to be translated into a confirmed survival impact.[81] Overall response rates of renal cell cancer to IL-2 are in the range of 15% to 25% with a complete remission rate of 5% to 10%. Complete response rates and response duration appear to favor high- rather than low-dose regimens. Randomized phase 3 trials with high-dose IV bolus IL-2 showed that the treatment is one of the most effective treatments for either metastatic melanoma or renal cell carcinoma and imparts the chance for complete and durable response in a small subgroup of patients. Although a significant benefit is seen only in a minority of patients, long-term follow-up of patients treated in early high-dose IL-2 trials confirms that the benefit can be long-lasting. However, high-dose IL-2 can produce serious and toxic side effects and it is generally reserved for patients with preserved performance status and absence of major cardiovascular disease. IL-2 has also been given to leukemic patients in a variety of doses and schedules, with hints that it might be useful in remission maintenance.[81]

Development of second-generation IL-2 analogs that do not induce the same high levels of secondary cytokines provides promise for further reduction of the toxicities, providing that the efficacy is not dependent on these secondary effects.[90] Another approach to therapy has been to use IL-2 attached to a toxin to target and kill cancer cells bearing the IL-2 receptor. DAB389IL-2 is an IL-2 receptor (IL-2R)-specific fusion protein. It contains the enzymatic and translocation domains of the diphtheria toxin fused to human IL-2. This chimera is able to direct the cytocidal action of the diphtheria toxin enzymatic region only to cells that bear the IL-2R. DAB389IL-2 has been approved for therapy of cutaneous T-cell lymphomas. Antitumor effects may also be seen in patients with other lymphoid diseases bearing the IL-2 receptor.[82]

Interleukin-3

IL-3 was first described by Lee and Ihle as a T-cell product involved in the pathogenesis of Moloney leukemia virus–induced T-cell lymphomas.[91] This molecule is of interest because of its in vitro ability to stimulate multilineage hematopoietic progenitors (Table 55-11[91-98]).[92,93]

Biologic Properties of IL-3 ■ The multilineage response of normal hematopoietic progenitor cells to IL-3 has been demonstrated both in vitro and in vivo. In vitro, IL-3, in combination with other cytokines, such as SCF, IL-6, IL-1, G-CSF, GM-CSF, EPO, or TPO, induces the proliferation of CFU-GM, CFU-Eo, CFU-Baso, BFU-E, and CFU-GEMM in semisolid medium,

Table 55-11 **Interleukin-3**

	Characteristic[91-98]	Comment
Chromosomal localization[3]	5q31	
Major product sites	Activated T cells NK cells Stimulated mast cells	
Selected biologic activities	Stimulation of multilineage hematopoietic progenitors, especially when used in combination with other cytokines (SCF, IL-1, IL-6, G-CSF, GM-CSF, EPO, TPO)	
Receptor	IL-3 receptor (heterodimer of IL-3 specific α subunit and β subunit)	IL-3Rα = CDw123 at Xp22.3, Yp13.3 β subunit = CDw131 at 22q12-q13 β subunit used by receptors for GM-CSF and IL-5
Major clinical trials	Increases stem cell mobilization when used with G-CSF or GM-CSF In combination with GM-CSF, hastens bone marrow recovery after transplant Sequential IL-3 and GM-CSF produce multilineage responses in some marrow failure patients Induces occasional sustained remissions in Diamond-Blackfan anemia	

Abbreviations: EPO, erythropoietin; G-CSF, granulocyte colony-stimulating factor; GM-CSF, granulocyte macrophage colony-stimulating factor; IL, interleukin; NK, natural killer; SCF, stem cell factor; TPO, thrombopoietin.

and stimulates the proliferation of purified CD34+ cells in suspension culture.[92] Indeed, in combination with other cytokines, in particular SCF, IL-6, IL-1, FL, G-CSF, and/or EPO, IL-3 is included in almost all protocols to expand hematopoietic stem and progenitor cell in vitro.

IL-3 in Human Disease ■ In vitro data from supernatants of long-term bone marrow cultures suggest that marrow stromal cells produce reduced levels of IL-3 in patients with aplastic anemia.[95] IL-3 mRNA has been detected in allergen-induced type I responses in the nasal mucosa as well as in late-phase cutaneous reactions of atopic subjects, being coordinately expressed with GM-CSF, IL-5, and IL-4. The eosinophilia in tissues from chronic hyperplastic sinusitis was found to correlate with IL-3 and GM-CSF mRNA detected by in situ hybridization.[93]

Finally, IL-3 has also been implicated in acute lymphocytic leukemia (ALL) with a t(5:14)(q31;q32) translocation.[96] In two such patients, the translocation resulted in juxtaposition of the IL-3 gene and the immunoglobulin (Ig) heavy chain gene, and excess IL-3 transcripts were produced by the leukemic cells, perhaps explaining the eosinophilia seen in these patients.

IL-3 in the Clinic ■ IL-3 has been used in a variety of clinical trials; peripheral blood stem cell mobilization, post-chemotherapy and transplantation, and bone marrow failure states. The majority of studies show only modest effects of IL-3 by itself. However, in conjunction with other growth factors, significant salutary effects are demonstrated. For instance, in the mobilization studies, treatment with IL-3 did not mobilize by itself but significantly potentiated G-CSF-induced yield of all progenitor cell types used to restore hematopoiesis after high-dose chemotherapy. After transplantation, the combination of IL-3 and GM-CSF proved more efficient to support bone marrow engraftment than IL-3 or GM-CSF alone. The combination of IL-3 and GM-CSF was more efficient than G-CSF for supporting platelet recovery, but was of similar benefit for the reconstitution of myelopoiesis. Following chemotherapy, IL-3 was found to attenuate neutropenia and/or thrombocytopenia in some but not all clinical studies.

IL-3 protein levels have been shown elevated in myeloma patients' bone marrow samples, and IL-3 is both a growth factor for myeloma cells as well as a potent stimulator of osteoclast formation. Recently, it has been shown that IL-3 can also inhibit osteoblast differentiation and this differentiation could be inhibited by marrow plasma that had high levels of IL-3 in patients with myeloma and that this could be reversed by addition of a neutralizing antibody to IL-3. It has been suggested that IL-3 plays a dual role in the bone destructive process in myeloma, through directly stimulating osteoclast formation and indirectly inhibiting osteoblast formation. In addition, IL-3 can serve as a growth factor for myeloma cells further increasing the bone destructive process.[97]

Modest increases in platelets, hemoglobin, and neutrophil counts have also occasionally been seen in patients with myelodysplasia or aplastic anemia treated with IL-3.[98] Significantly better results have been observed in patients with bone marrow failure treated with IL-3 followed by GM-CSF. Although prolonged therapy was necessary to achieve maximal hematopoietic recovery, responses were durable for up to 4 years after discontinuation of treatment.[94,99] Side effects of IL-3 include dose-dependent fever, rash, fatigue, diarrhea, rigor, musculoskeletal pain, chills, headache, conjunctivitis, edema, chest pain, dyspnea, decreases in platelet counts, increase in basophilic counts, marrow fibrosis, and pulmonary edema. The tolerance to IL-3 appears to be several-fold better in patients with bone marrow failure states, as compared with those treated after chemotherapy.[94]

Interleukin-4 and Interleukin-13

IL-4 and IL-13 are closely related.[100-102] They share biologic and immunoregulatory functions on B cells, monocytes, dendritic cells, and fibroblasts. Both IL-4 and IL-13 genes are located in the same vicinity on chromosome 5. The major regulatory sequences in the IL-4 and IL-13 promoters are identical, thus explaining their restricted expression pattern in activated T cells and mast cells. Furthermore, the IL-4 and IL-13 receptors are multimeric and share at least one common chain—IL-4RA. This, together with similarities in IL-4 and IL-13 signal transduction, explains the striking overlap of biologic properties between these two cytokines (Table 55-12). The inability of IL-13 to regulate T-cell differentiation due to a lack of IL-13 receptors on T lymphocytes, however, represents a major difference between these cytokines. Therefore, despite the impact redundancy of these two molecules, regulatory mechanisms are in place to guarantee their distinct functions.

Biologic Activities of IL-4 and IL-13 ■ IL-13 elicits many, but not all, of the biologic actions of IL-4. IL-4 is, however, distinguished from IL-13 by its T-cell growth factor activity and its ability to drive differentiation of Th0 precursors toward the Th2 lineage. Th2 cells secrete IL-4 and IL-5 and lead to a preferential stimulation of humoral immunity. In contrast, Th1 cells, which produce IL-2 and IFN-γ, lead to a preferential stimulation of cellular immunity.

IL-4 and IL-13 in Human Disease ■ IL-4 and IL-13 play a key role in the development of the allergic reaction at the effector level by inducing the switch toward IgE. Atopic blood mononuclear cells display an increased capacity to produce IL-4 and allergen immunotherapy greatly

Table 55-12 ■ **Interleukin-4 and Interleukin-13**

	Characteristic[100-109]	Comment
Chromosomal localization[3]	5q31	The IL-13 gene is located 12 kb 5′ upstream to IL-4 and is linked to it in a "tail-to-head" fashion
Major production sites	IL-4 T cells (Th0 and Th2), basophils, mast cells, eosinophils IL-13 T cells (Th0, Th1, and Th2), basophils, mast cells, B cells	
Selected biologic activities	Both IL-4 and IL-13 are involved in allergic reaction (induce switch to IgE)	IL-4, but not IL-13, promotes T-cell growth and differentiation (perhaps because T cells lack IL-13 receptors)
Receptor	IL-4 and IL-13 receptors share subunits	IL-4Rα = CD124 at 16p11-p12; γc chain = CD132 at Xq13
	Type I IL-4 receptor (IL-4Rα and IL-2 receptor γc chain subunits) transduce IL-4; type II IL-4 receptor (IL-4Rα and the IL-13Rα1 subunits) transduce IL-4 and IL-13; IL-4Rα and IL-13Rα2 complex or two IL-13Rα transduce IL-13	IL-2 receptor γc chain is common to receptors for IL-2, IL-4, IL-7, IL-9, and IL-15
Natural antagonists	Soluble IL-4 and IL-13 exist	
Major clinical trials	Only minor antitumor activity has been seen in a variety of human cancers of IL-4	IL-4 is well-tolerated

Abbreviation: IL, interleukin.

reduces IL-4 production. Furthermore, spontaneous IgE synthesis in vitro by lymphocytes from patients with atopic dermatitis is partially inhibited by anti-IL-4 and anti-IL-13 antibodies.

IL-4 and IL-13 have anti-inflammatory effects, which have been demonstrated on synovium from rheumatoid arthritis. IL-4 can also inhibit the production of IL-6 and leukemia inhibitory factor. Finally, IL-4 can suppress stromal cell proliferation in vitro in long-term bone marrow cultures, suggesting its possible utility in myelofibrosis.[104]

IL-4 and IL-13 possess potent antitumor activity in vivo in mice.[105] It can inhibit the proliferation of some human cancer cell lines in vitro as well as in vivo in nude mice. A similar antiproliferative effect of IL-13 on human breast cancer cells has been described. Moreover, a chimeric protein composed of IL-13 and a truncated form of *Pseudomonas* exotoxin A exhibits specific cytotoxic activity toward human renal cell carcinoma, but not against normal hemopoietic cells.[106]

Clinical Trials of IL-4 ■ Despite the preclinical promise of IL-4, to date, clinical trials of this molecule in humans demonstrated that although the molecule is safe and nontoxic, only sporadic antitumor activity in a variety of cancers, including melanoma, lung cancer, and AIDS-related Kaposi's sarcoma, is observed.[107-109]

Interleukin-5

IL-5 is a T-cell-derived cytokine involved in the pathogenesis of atopic diseases. It specifically controls the production, activation, and localization of eosinophils. Eosinophils mediate allergic and asthmatic symptoms. T cells purified from the bronchoalveolar lavage (BAL) and peripheral blood of asthmatics secrete an elevated amount of IL-5. Therefore, agents that suppress either the production or the activity of IL-5 would be expected to ameliorate the pathologic effects of the allergic response (Table 55-13).[110]

Biologic Activities of IL-5 ■ IL-5 plays a central role in the control of eosinophilia. This cytokine affects the production and function of eosinophils and their tissue migration and localization. In addition, IL-5 promotes eosinophil survival by inhibiting their apoptosis.[112] IL-5 also enhances basophil numbers and can prime human basophils for histamine release, and leukotriene production and specific receptors have been shown on the cell surface.

Another target for IL-5 is the T cell itself. Interestingly, IL-5 enhances IL-2-dependent differentiation and proliferation of T cells, although no receptors for IL-5 have been demonstrated on these cells.

IL-5 in Human Disease ■ T cells in the bronchial alveolar lavage of atopic asthmatics show elevated expression of IL-4 and IL-5. In contrast, T cells purified from peripheral blood of nonatopic asthmatics secrete elevated amounts of IL-5, but not IL-4, as compared with normal controls. Monoclonal antibodies against IL-5 have been shown to reduce eosinophil influx and decrease bronchial hyperreactivity in animal models.[113] However, such an antibody failed to show responses in a clinical trial of allergen-induced airway diseases. The implications of these trials on the role of IL-5 and eosinophils in asthma are still being debated.[99] Interestingly, IL-5 secreted from Reed-Sternberg cells may be the cause of eosinophilia in patients with Hodgkin's disease.[114]

Interleukin-6

IL-6 was first cloned in 1986.[118] It is a typical cytokine, exhibiting functional pleiotropy and redundancy (Table 55-14).

Table 55-13 ■ **Interleukin-5**

	Characteristic[110-117]	Comment
Chromosomal localization[3]	5q31	Part of gene cluster encoding IL-3, IL-4, and GM-CSF
Structure	Structurally related to IL-3, IL-4, M-CSF, and GM-CSF	
Major production sites	Activated CD4+ T cells, mast cells, CD8+ T cells	Mostly produced by Th2 cells
Selected biologic activities	Regulates production, function, survival, and migration of eosinophils Enhances basophil number and function	
Receptor	Consists of IL-5Rα (IL-5-specific) and a β subunit β subunit is common to IL-3 and GM-CSF complexes	IL-5Rα = CDw125 located at 3p26-24 β subunit = CD2131 at 22q12-q13
Potential clinical application	IL-5 antagonists may be useful in treatment of allergy and asthma; however, trial of monoclonal antibody against IL-5 was not effective in asthma	

Abbreviations: GM-CSF, granulocyte macrophage colony-stimulating factor; IL, interleukin.

Table 55-14 ■ **Interleukin-6**

	Characteristic[118-134]	Comment
Chromosomal localization[3]	7p21	
Major production sites	Activated B and T cells Monocytes Fibroblasts Endothelial cells Keratinocytes Synovial cells	Inducers: IL-1, lipopolysaccharide, IFN-γ, platelet-derived growth factor, GM-CSF, and TNF Inhibitors: Glucocorticoids
Selected biologic activates	B- and T-cell development and function Thrombopoiesis Acute phase protein synthesis Inhibition of hepatic albumin excretion Osteoclastic bone resorption Neural differentiation	
Receptor	IL-6Rα together with gp130	-6Rα = CD126 at 1q21 gp130 = CD130 at 5q11 gp130 is also used by leukemia inhibitory factor and IL-11 Soluble IL-6 receptors exist but have agonist action. Can interact with cells that have gp130 but not IL-1Rα
Major clinical trials	Response rates = 8-14% in melanoma and renal cell carcinoma Modest platelet-enhancing ability post-chemotherapy or autologous transplant with significant toxicity Antibody to block IL-6 is entering clinical trial	

Abbreviations: GM-CSF, granulocyte macrophage colony-stimulating factor; IFN, interferon; IL, interleukin; TNF, tumor necrosis factor.

IL-6 is involved in the immune response, inflammation, and hematopoiesis. IL-6 is a 21- to 30-kDa glycoprotein of 212 amino acids that binds to a specific receptor that requires the same 130-kDa membrane glycoprotein for mediation of signal transduction, as has been described for several cytokines, including IL-2.[135,136] The biologic effects of IL-6 include synthesis of acute phase reactants in the liver, as well as effects on the hypothalamic–pituitary axis, bone resorption, and on both the humoral and cellular arms of the immune system.[137-141] As a major inducer of the acute phase response, this cytokine may play a role in the pathogenesis of sepsis.

Biologic Activities of IL-6 ■ IL-6 is a potent and essential factor for the normal development and function of both B and T lymphocytes.[121] This molecule is also involved in other biologic activities such as differentiation of myeloid leukemic cell lines into macrophages, megakaryocyte maturation, neural differentiation, osteoclast development, and acute phase protein synthesis in hepatocytes (see Table 55-14).[122]

IL-6 in Human Disease ■ IL-6 acts as a growth factor for myeloma/plasmacytoma, keratinocytes, mesangial cells, renal cell carcinoma, and Kaposi sarcoma and promotes the growth of hematopoietic stem cells. On the other hand, IL-6 also inhibits the growth of myeloid leukemic cell lines and certain carcinoma cell lines.

Significant correlations between serum IL-6 activity and serum levels of acute phase proteins have been demonstrated in a variety of inflammatory conditions. IL-6 may be involved in the abnormalities seen in patients with cardiac myxoma who show hypergammaglobulinemia. Abnormal IL-6 production may participate in the pathophysiology of rheumatoid arthritis and aberrant expression of the IL-6 receptor is seen in several autoimmune diseases.[124]

IL-6 has been implicated as a mediator of B symptoms in lymphoma.[125] Elevated serum IL-6 levels have also been associated with an adverse prognosis in both Hodgkin and non-Hodgkin lymphoma.[119,126-129] In diffuse large-cell lymphoma, IL-6 levels were found to be the single most important independent prognostic factor selected in multivariate analysis for predicting complete remission rate and relapse-free survival.[129] IL-6 levels may also be exploitable as a prognostic factor in renal cell carcinoma and multiple myeloma, and high levels are observed in prostate and ovarian cancers as well. IL-6 probably also plays an etiologic role in the systemic manifestations of the lymphoproliferative disorder Castleman disease.[130] High IL-6 levels are also an adverse prognostic factor in pancreatic cancer.[142]

IL-6 in the Clinic ■ In patients undergoing chemotherapy or autologous transplantation, IL-6 has minimal to no platelet-enhancing activity at tolerable doses. Toxicity includes fever and anemia.[131-133] IL-6 has also been tested as an antitumor agent in melanoma and renal cell carcinoma. Response rates have been low (<15%).[122] Because high levels of IL-6 correlate with an adverse outcome in many cancers and function as an autocrine/paracrine growth factor in some tumors, clinical studies of an IL-6 inhibitor may be worthwhile.

In summary, IL-6 is one of the most ubiquitously deregulated cytokines in cancer, and increased levels of IL-6 have been observed in virtually every tumor studied. As it has thoroughly reviewed in Ref. 143, a role for IL-6 has been implicated in almost every cancer, including breast, lung, colorectal, ovarian, prostate, pancreatic cancers, multiple myeloma, glioma, melanoma, renal cell carcinoma, leukemia, lymphoma, and Castleman' disease. Preclinical and translational findings support a role for IL-6 in diverse malignancies and provide a biologic rationale for targeted therapeutic investigations. Various compounds antagonize IL-6 production, including corticosteroids, nonsteroidal anti-inflammatory agents, estrogens, and cytokines. Targeted biologic therapies include IL-6 conjugated toxins and monoclonal antibodies directed against IL-6 and its receptor. As an example, a chimeric murine antihuman IL-6 antibody, CNTO 328, has been used in a phase 1 trial in subjects with B-cell non-Hodgkin lymphoma (NHL), multiple myeloma (MM) and Castleman's disease.[144] The treatment resulted in tumor response and disease control, especially in Castleman's disease, where striking responses have been seen.[145] Also, in Japan, an anti-IL-6 receptor antibody (Actemra®) has been approved for Castleman disease.

Interleukin-7

IL-7 was identified and cloned on the basis of its ability to induce proliferation of B-cell progenitors in the absence of stromal cells (Table 55-15[146-154]).[146] It is now known that this cytokine is secreted by stromal cells in the bone marrow and thymus and is irreplaceable in the development of both B and T cells.[147-149] Indeed, the nonredundant nature of IL-7 is underscored by the observation that ablation of IL-7 or parts of the IL-7 receptor in gene knockout mice ineluctably leads to a major defect in lymphocyte development.

Biologic Activities of IL-7/IL-7 Receptor ■ The major sites for the production of T and B cells are the thymus and the bone marrow, respectively. The T cells of the thymus are the progeny of progenitors initially generated in the bone marrow. Numerous cytokines play a role in B- and T-cell development. However, most single cytokine knockout mice show relatively normal B- and T-cell compartments, indicating that many cytokine functions are redundant. In contrast, IL-7-deficient mice present with striking lymphocyte depletion in both the thymus and bone marrow. Collectively, these genetic experiments identify clearly distinct in vivo roles for various lymphoid factors. IL-2 and IL-4 function by influencing mature lymphocyte populations during immune responses, whereas IL-7 plays a singularly dominant role for the production and expansion of lymphocytes.

All lymphocytes are derived from hematopoietic stem cells. The up-regulation of the IL-7R occurs at the stage of the clonogenic common lymphoid progenitor that can give rise to all lymphoid lineages at a single-cell level.[152] There are at least three principal means by which IL-7R-mediated signals act in lymphocyte development: enhancement of prolifera-

Table 55-15 ■ **Interleukin-7**

	Characteristic[146-154]	Comment
Chromosomal localization[3]	8q12-q13	
Major production sites	Stroma of thymus and bone marrow, keratinocytes, intestinal epithelium, liver, dendritic cells (not produced by lymphocytes)	
Selected biologic activities	Critical for T- and B-cell development	
Receptor	Composed of IL-7Rα (CD127) and the common γc chain subunits	IL-7Rγ = CD127 at 5p13 γc chain = CD132 at Xq13 γc chain is common to receptors for IL-2, IL-4, IL-7, IL-9, and IL-15

Abbreviations: IL, interleukin; IL-7R, interleukin-7 receptor.

Table 55-16 ■ **Interleukin-8**

	Characteristic[155-163]	Comment
Chromosomal localization[3]	4q12-q13	
Forms	8-kDa molecule. Four forms (79, 77, 72, and 69 amino acids) exist	Forms are tissue-specific
Major production sites	Monocytes, neutrophils, T cells, fibroblasts, endothelial cells, epithelial cells	Up-regulators IL-1α, IL-1β, TNF-α, IL-3, microorganisms, hypoxia, acidosis, nitric oxide Suppressors IL-4, TGF-β, glucocorticoids
Selected biologic activities	Potent chemoattractant agent for a variety of leukocytes, especially neutrophils Suppresses colony formation of immature myeloid progenitors Increases keratinocyte and endothelial cell proliferation Increases adhesiveness of melanoma cells	
Receptor	IL-8Rα and IL-8Rβ exist	IL-8Rα and IL-8Rβ reside at 2q35 IL-8 receptor is homologous to a gene encoded by HHV-8
Potential clinical application	Antibodies to block IL-8 are entering clinical trial	

Abbreviations: HHV-8, human herpesvirus-8; IL, interleukin; TGF, transforming growth factor; TNF, tumor necrosis factor.

tion, triggering of lineage-specific developmental programs, and maintenance of viability of appropriately selected cells.

IL-7 in Human Disease ■ High IL-7 levels are found in states of T-cell depletion and may, therefore, play a role in promoting T-cell expansion.[153] High levels of IL-7 are also found in chronic lymphocytic leukemia and in Burkitt lymphoma, and transgenic mice overexpressing the IL-7 gene show dramatic changes in lymphocyte development, which, in some instances, can result in the formation of lymphoid tumors.[154]

Interleukin-8

IL-8 was first identified in 1987 as a potent, proinflammatory chemokine that induces trafficking of neutrophils across the vascular wall (chemotaxis) (Table 55-16).[155] This molecule belongs to a chemokine superfamily whose members include neutrophil-activating peptide-2, platelet factor-4, growth-related cytokine (GRO) (also known as melanoma growth-stimulating activity), and IFN-inducible protein-10, all of which are responsible for the directional migration of various cells.[156] IL-8 receptor demonstrates strong homology to a gene encoded by human herpesvirus-8 (HHV-8).[157,158]

Biologic Activity of IL-8 ■ The chemotactic agents generated by inflammatory stimuli recruit the circulating leukocytes, in particular neutrophils, for defensive purposes and direct them to injury sites. The migration of circulating leukocytes is viewed as a multistep process, which consists of leukocyte rolling along the endothelial lining, accelerated activation of leukocyte integrins, adhesion of the cells to endothelial ligands, and diapedesis (migration across the vascular wall). The leukocytes follow the IL-8 concentration gradient and accumulate at the location of elevated concentration. These processes play a fundamental role in the host defense since activated leukocytes act to kill and engulf invading bacteria at the site of injury.

Among the neutrophil-affecting chemokines, IL-8 is one of the most potent.[160] On exposure to a chemokine, neutrophils are activated, and within seconds, their shapes are changed. The process of shape change is crucial. It is modulated by perturbations of cellular integrins and the actin cytoskeleton. The activation and up-regulation of integrins also permits the adherence of the neutrophils to the endothelial cells of the vessel wall so as to allow for subsequent migration into the tissues.

IL-8 in Human Disease ■ In the synovium of patients suffering from rheumatoid arthritis, IL-8 is part of the cytokine cascade. The production of IL-8 in large quantities has also been associated with other inflammatory diseases: asthma, leprosy, psoriasis, inflammatory bowel disease, atherosclerosis, cystic fibrosis, and in various respiratory syndromes.[156]

IL-8 can induce tumor growth, an effect attributed to its angiogenic activity, a property that promotes vascularization. On the one hand, the administration of anti-IL-8 to SCID mice bearing xenografts of IL-8-expressing human lung cancer has been shown to have beneficial effects.[162] On the other hand, antitumor effects of IL-8 have also been reported. Of interest in this regard is the fact that increased levels of IL-8 have been discerned in lung carcinomas and in melanomas. IL-8 may be a growth factor for pancreatic cancer and for melanoma.[156] In melanomas, IL-8 levels correlate with the growth and metastatic potential of the tumor cells, and exposure of the cells to IFN (an agent with known antitumor activity in melanoma) decreases IL-8 levels and cancer cell proliferation.[163] Blocking IL-8 or IL-8R has been suggested as a therapeutic strategy.[156]

Interleukin-9

Human IL-9 was initially identified and cloned as a mitogenic factor for a human megakaryoblastic leukemia.[164] Subsequently, IL-9 targets were found to encompass a wide range of cells (Table 55-17).[165,166]

Biologic Activities of IL-9 ■ Cellular elements responsive to IL-9 include erythroid progenitors, human T cells, B cells, fetal thymocytes, thymic lymphomas, and immature neuronal cell lines.[165]

IL-9 can support the clonogenic maturation of erythroid progenitors in the pres-

Table 55-17 ■ **Interleukin-9**

	Characteristic[164-167]	Comment
Chromosomal localization[3]	5q31.1	
Major production sites	Activated Th2 cells	
Selected biologic activities	Supports clonogenic maturation of erythroid progenitors Acts as a mast cell differentiation factor Protects lymphomas from apoptosis Cooperates with IL-4 in B-cell responses Enhances neuronal differentiation	Has more pronounced effect on fetal vs adult cells Transformed or activated T cells much more responsive to IL-9 than normal, resting T cells
Receptor	IL-9 receptor	Located on subtelomeric (pseudoautosomal) region of chromosomes X (Xq28) and Y (Yq12)

Abbreviation: IL, interleukin.

ence of EPO. In contrast, granulocyte or macrophage colony formation (CFU-GM, CFU-G, or CFU-M) is usually not influenced by IL-9. Experiments comparing the effects of IL-9 on fetal and adult progenitors have shown that IL-9 is more effective on fetal cells. Cells, which are activated, are also more likely to be responsive to this cytokine. In addition to its proliferative activity, IL-9 also seems to be a potent regulator of mast cell effector molecules.

IL-9 in Human Disease ■ There is an interesting paradox between the unresponsiveness of normal T cells to IL-9 and the potent activity of this molecule on lymphoma cells. This contrast is illustrated by the observation that murine T cells acquire the ability to respond to IL-9 after a long period of in vitro culture, while they simultaneously acquire characteristics of tumor cell lines. Observations made with transgenic mice also demonstrate the oncogenic potential of dysregulated IL-9 production since 5% to 10% of mice that overexpress this cytokine develop lymphoblastic lymphomas.[166] In line with these data, constitutive IL-9 production by human Hodgkin lymphomas and large-cell anaplastic lymphomas has now been clearly documented.[165] Even so, the pathophysiologic role of IL-9 remains elusive.

Interleukin-10

IL-10 is a pleiotropic cytokine discovered in 1989 as an activity produced by murine type 2 helper T cells (Th2) (Table 55-18).[168,169] It was initially designated as cytokine synthesis inhibitory factor because of its ability to inhibit the production of certain cytokines.[170] Of interest, IL-10 exhibits strong DNA and amino acid sequence homology to an open reading frame—BCRF1—in the Epstein-Barr virus (EBV) genome.[170] Indeed, the BCRF1 protein product displays many of the biologic properties of cellular IL-10 and has, therefore, been termed viral IL-10.

Biologic Activities of IL-10 ■ IL-10 inhibits the synthesis of Th1-derived cytokines, including IL-2, IFN-γ, GM-CSF, and lymphotoxin, and of monocyte-derived IL-1α and β, IL-6, IL-8, TNF-α, GM-CSF, and G-CSF. Exogenous IL-10 can also suppress expression of IL-10.[169] At the same time, IL-10 induces the synthesis of the IL-1 receptor antagonist by macrophages. IL-10 also suppresses the CD28 costimulatory pathway, and hence, acts as a decisive mechanism in determining if a T cell will contribute to an immune response or become anergic.

From the molecular standpoint, IL-10 suppresses cytokine expression at a transcriptional level and also at a post-transcriptional level.[171] Both these mechanisms appear to require new protein synthesis. At a cellular level, Th1 cytokines synthesis inhibition is mediated indirectly through the effect of IL-10 on antigen-presenting cells (APC), since suppression occurs when macrophages, but not B cells, are used as APC.[172]

In the presence of monocytes/macrophages, IL-10 inhibits proliferation of resting T cells, including Th0, Th1, and Th2 CD4+ T-cell clones. This inhibition can only be partially reversed by high concentrations of IL-2, suggesting that the reduced proliferation is only partially a reflection of reduced IL-2 production. IL-10 can also enhance the cytotoxic activity of CD8+ T cells. All these effects support an important role of IL-10 in regulating inflammatory responses.

In contrast to the inhibitory effects on other lineages, IL-10 has a stimulatory effect on B cells and mast cells.[173] For instance, IL-10 strongly stimulates proliferation and differentiation of activated B cells.

IL-10 in Human Disease ■ The protein product of BCRF1 (viral IL-10) exhibits properties similar to those of human IL-10. The ability of EBV to transform human B cells may be, at least in part, a ramification of the ability of viral IL-10 to stimulate B-cell proliferation. The *bcrf1* gene is transcribed late in the process of viral infection, when newly formed viral particles are produced.[174] Since IFN-γ is an important mediator of the antiviral activity of T cells and NK cells, the cytokine synthesis inhibitory activity of IL-10 may also contribute to tumorigenesis by allowing viral infection to proceed. Thus, IL-10 may have a role in the development of lymphoma through two mechanisms: its proliferation-stimulating properties on B cells, and its immunosuppressive properties that impair viral control and tumor immunosurveillance.

The role of IL-10 in cancer should be considered within the frame of a highly complex biological puzzle. It is known that IL-10 can have pleiotropic effects on adaptive and innate immunity cell mediators. Although several studies show that IL-10 can actively mediate immune suppression, some experimental models describe relatively opposite conclusions. Recent data on the relationship between IL-10 and anticancer immunity support an effective immune attack against malignant cells, which challenges the common belief that IL-10 acts as an immunosuppressive factor promoting tumor immune escape.

Interleukin-11

Originally characterized as a thrombopoietic factor, IL-11 is now known to be expressed and have activity in a multitude of other systems, including the gut, testes, and the central nervous system (Table 55-19).[181,182] Clinically, this cytokine has been approved by the FDA for amelioration of chemotherapy-induced thrombocytopenia.

Biologic Activities of IL-11 ■ IL-11 was originally isolated from cells derived from the hematopoietic microenvironment and may act as a paracrine or autocrine growth factor in this environment. IL-11 acts synergistically with other early- and late-acting growth factors to stimulate various stages and lineages of hematopoiesis.[181] In synergy with IL-3, IL-4, IL-7, IL-12, IL-13, SCF, FLT-3 ligand, and GM-CSF, IL-11 stimulates the proliferation of primitive stem cells and their

Table 55-18 ■ **Interleukin-10**

	Characteristic[168-180]	Comment
Chromosomal localization[3]	1q31-q32	
Structure	Strongly homologous to BCRF1 of the Epstein-Barr virus genome	BCRF1 protein is viral IL-10; IL-19, IL-20, IL-22, IL-24, and IL-26 are homologous to IL-10
Major production sites	CD4+ cells (Th0, Th1, and Th2), CD8+ cells, monocytes, macrophages, B cells	Th2 cells are main source
Selected biologic activities	Inhibits cytokine synthesis by Th1 cells and monocytes/macrophages Stimulates B-cell proliferation Involved in transformation of B cells by EBV and TNF receptors	Inhibits IL-1, IL-2, IL-6, IL-8, IL-10, IL-12, TNF, GM-CSF, G-CSF, IFN-γ, and lymphotoxin Up-regulates IL-1RA and soluble IL-1
Receptor	IL-10 receptor IFN receptors	Localized to 11q23
Clinical studies	Trend toward efficacy in rheumatoid arthritis, inflammatory bowel disease, and autoimmune diseases	Well-tolerated

Abbreviations: EBV, Epstein-Barr virus; G-CSF, granulocyte colony-stimulating factor; GM-CSF, granulocyte macrophage colony-stimulating factor; IFN, interferon; IL, interleukin; TNF, tumor necrosis factor.

Table 55-19 **Interleukin-11**

	Characteristic[181-189]	Comment
Chromosomal localization[3]	19q13.3-q13.4	
Major production sites	Gut, testis, central nervous system, stromal elements, osteoblasts, leukemic cell lines, melanoma cell lines	Can be induced by IL-1α and other cytokines
Selected biologic activities	Best known as a thrombopoietic factor Stimulates multilineage progenitors, erythropoiesis, myelopoiesis, and lymphopoiesis Decreases mucositis in animal models Stimulates osteoclast development Inhibits adipogenesis Stimulates proliferation of neuronal cells	
Receptor	IL-11Rα and gp130 subunits gp130 = CD130 on 5q11 IL-6, oncostatin M, and leukemia inhibitory factor also use gp130 subunit	IL-11Rα on 9p13
Major clinical trials	Approved for use to prevent chemotherapy-induced thrombocytopenia	Most common side effect is fluid accumulation

Abbreviations: IL, interleukin; IL-11R, interleukin-11 receptor.

commitment in to multilineage progenitors as well as their differentiation. The synergistic effects of IL-11 and TPO on multilineage cells may be mediated in part by SCF/c-kit interactions.

IL-11 acts synergistically with IL-3, TPO, or SCF to stimulate various stages of megakaryocytopoiesis and thrombopoiesis.[184,185] IL-11, alone or in combination with other cytokines (IL-3, SCF, or EPO), can stimulate multiple stages of erythropoiesis. IL-11 also modulates the differentiation and maturation of myeloid progenitor cells. IL-11 in combination with SCF stimulates myeloid colony formation. The combination of IL-11 with IL-13 or IL-14 can reduce the proportion of granulocytes and blasts in myeloid colonies, with a concomitant increase in macrophages. IL-11 in combination with SCF or IL-4 effectively supports the generation of B cells in primary cultures. IL-11 and IL-4 can also reverse the inhibitory effect of IL-3 on early B-lymphocyte development. The promotion of B-cell differentiation may be mediated by T cells.

IL-11 in Human Disease ■ IL-11 acts as a synergistic factor with IL-3, GM-CSF, and SCF to stimulate proliferation of human primary leukemia cells, myeloid leukemia cell lines, megakaryoblastic cell lines, and erythroleukemic cell lines and to stimulate leukemic blast colony formation. IL-11 mRNA expression in leukemic cells and inhibition of leukemic cell growth by IL-11 antisense oligonucleotides suggest that IL-11 may function as an autocrine growth factor in leukemic cell lines.[188] Although IL-11 stimulates the proliferation of murine plasmacytoma cells and murine hybridoma cells, the effect of IL-11 on the growth of human myeloma/plasmacytoma cells is controversial.[181]

Clinical Use of IL-11 ■ IL-11 was the second IL to receive FDA approval. It is indicated for the secondary prevention of chemotherapy-induced thrombocytopenia and for the reduction of the need for platelet transfusion in patients with nonmyeloid malignancies.

Interleukin-12

IL-12 was first identified as an NK-cell stimulatory factor.[190] Subsequently, it was demonstrated that IL-12 is crucial to the development of Th1 cells.[191] Indeed, there appears to be a common pathway leading from the innate immune response to adaptive immunity; intracellular pathogens stimulate macrophages to produce IL-12, which then promotes the development of Th1 cells from a naïve cell population. This pathway may be exploitable in the design of novel immunotherapies and vaccines (Table 55-20).

Biologic Activities of IL-12 and Role in Human Disease ■ IL-12 is a potent proinflammatory molecule, which is essential for resistance to bacterial, fungal, and parasitic infections. It is produced within a few hours of infection, activates NK cells, and, through its ability to induce IFN-γ production, enhances the phagocytic and bactericidal activity of phagocytic cells and their ability to release proinflammatory cytokines, including IL-12 itself. IL-12 is also a key immunoregulatory molecule, especially of Th1 responses. It is produced during the early phases of infection and inflammation and sets the stage for the ensuing antigen-specific immune response, favoring differentiation and function of the Th1 T cells, while inhibiting the differentiation of the Th2 T cells. IL-12 does not induce proliferation of resting peripheral blood T cells or NK cells; it does potentiate the proliferation of T cells induced by various mitogens and has a direct proliferative effect on preactivated T and NK cells.

IL-12 synergizes with other hematopoietic factors to promote survival and proliferation of early multipotent hematopoietic progenitor cells and lineage-committed precursor cells.[194] Although in vitro IL-12 has mostly stimulatory effects on hematopoiesis, in vivo IL-12 treatment results in decreased bone marrow hematopoiesis and both transient anemia and neutropenia, an effect mediated by IFN-γ.

Table 55-20 **Interleukin-12**

	Characteristic[190-196]	Comment
Chromosomal localization[3]	IL-12A: 3p12-q13.2 IL-12B: 5q31.1-q33.1	
Structure	Composed of IL-12A (p40) and IL-12B (p35)	IL-12A and IL-12B are encoded by two distinct genes
Major production sites	Macrophages Stimulated monocytes, neutrophils, and dendritic cells EBV-infected B cells	
Selected biologic activities	Proinflammatory cytokine important in resistance to infections Th1 development Stimulatory and inhibitory effects on hematopoiesis	
Receptor	IL-12Rβ1 and IL-12Rβ2 chains are related to gp130	IL-12Rβ1 at 19p13.1 IL-12Rβ2 at 1p31.2
Natural antagonists	IL-12 p40 homodimers	
Major clinical trials	Potential use in vaccine development No benefit in hepatitis C trial Modest antitumor activity with significant toxicity in melanoma and renal cell carcinoma	Significant toxicities may limit use

Abbreviations: EBV, Epstein-Barr virus; IL-12, interleukin-12; IL-12R, interleukin-12 receptor.

Table 55-21 **Interleukin-15**

	Characteristic[197-202]	Comment
Chromosomal localization[3]	4q31	
Major production sites	Monocytes/macrophages, fibroblasts, keratinocytes, epithelial cells, placenta, skeletal muscle, heart, lung, liver, kidney	Not expressed by resting or activated T cells
Selected biologic activities	Triggers proliferation and immunoglobulin production in preactivated B cells	Shares biologic effects with IL-2
	Number of CD8+ memory T cells may be controlled by balance of IL-15 (stimulatory) and IL-12 (inhibitory)	
	Stimulates proliferation of NK cells and activated CD4+ or CD8+ T cells Facilitates the induction of LAK cells and CTLs	
	Stimulates mast cell proliferation	
	Promotes proliferation of hairy-cell leukemia and chronic lymphocytic leukemia cells	
Receptor	High-affinity receptor requires IL-2Rβ and γ chains and IL-15Rα chain	IL-2Rβ = CD122 at 22q11.2-q13 IL-2Rγ = CD132 at Xq13 IL-15Rα at 10p14-p15

Abbreviations: CTL, cytolytic T lymphocyte; IL-2R, interleukin-2 receptor; LAK, lymphokine-activated killer; NK, natural killer.

IL-12 in the Clinic ■ IL-12 has potential for exploitation in allergy and as an adjuvant for infectious disease therapy.[195] Additionally, the ability of IL-12 to revert existing states of tolerance or anergy makes it a candidate for use in the composition of vaccines for infectious agents or tumors. Phase 1 clinical trials have been started in the last few years in oncology, as well as in the setting of HIV infection and chronic hepatitis B and C. To date, administration of IL-12 to patients with chronic hepatitis C does not appear advantageous.[196] What is more worrisome is in cancer patients treated with high doses of IL-12, acute hematopoietic, hepatic, and gastrointestinal toxicities were observed and several deaths were reported. In long-term treatments, toxicity was mostly pulmonary. It has been suggested that some of the severe toxicity of IL-12 can be attenuated if a single injection is administered 1 to 2 weeks before initiating daily dosing.[192]

Interleukin-15

IL-15 shares biologic activities with IL-2 (Table 55-21).[197]

Biologic Activities of IL-15 ■ Similar to IL-2, IL-15 is able to trigger both proliferation of and immunoglobulin production by normal B lymphocytes. These biologic functions may be acquired, however, only when B cells have been preactivated in vitro with polyclonal mitogens or when they are cultured in association with other stimuli. IL-15 also stimulates the proliferation of NK cells and activated CD4+ and CD8+ T cells, and facilitates the induction of cytolytic effector cells (such as lymphokine-activated killer cells). Finally, the numbers of CD8+ memory T cells is maintained in animals by a balance between the stimulatory effect of IL-15 and the suppressive effects of IL-12.[201]

IL-15 in Human Disease ■ High levels of IL-15 have been observed in rheumatoid arthritis, and IL-15 triggers T-cell growth in sarcoidosis. In addition, IL-15 responsiveness distinguishes malignant B cells from normal B lymphocytes. In contrast to normal B lymphocytes, which require preactivation in order to proliferate in response to IL-15, leukemic cells from patients with chronic B-cell malignancies proliferate in response to IL-15 regardless of in vitro preactivation, which is mainly related to the presence of the β and γ chains of the IL-2R system on the malignant B lymphocytes.[197] Even so, IL-15 cannot be considered an autocrine factor in these leukemias, since it is not produced by the leukemic cells themselves. Rather, the major reservoir of IL-15 in these patients is from cells belonging to the monocyte/macrophage lineage.[197]

Interleukin-16

IL-16 is a lymphocyte chemoattractant factor expressed by mitogen-stimulated human peripheral blood mononuclear cells (Table 55-22).[202]

Biologic Activities of IL-16 ■ IL-16 is a proinflammatory and immunomodulatory cytokine. It is a potent chemoattractant for all CD4+ cells including T cells, monocytes, and eosinophils and, as such, has been identified at inflammatory sites characterized by infiltrating CD4+ cells.[203] In addition to cell motility, IL-16 induces cell-cycle progression and cytokine synthesis in CD4+ T cells.

IL-16 in Human Disease ■ IL-16 may be involved in asthma because the airway epithelium from asthmatics produces IL-16 after histamine stimulation, although similar epithelium from normals does not.[202] Also, IL-16 may play a role in granulomatous inflammation. Since IL-16 is a T-cell chemoattractant, IL-16 inhibitors may have therapeutic implications in suppressing T-cell-mediated inflammation. In addition, IL-16 has antiviral effects on HIV-1 replication and, at the same time, can promote growth of CD4+ T cells. Both these activities are required for immune reconstitution in individuals infected with HIV-1 and suggest another possible clinical application for this molecule.[203]

Interleukin-17

Human IL-17 (Table 55-23) has 72% overall sequence identity at the amino acid

Table 55-22 **Interleukin-16**

	Characteristic[203,204]	Comment
Chromosomal localization[3]	15q26.1	
Forms	17-kDa peptide	Biologic activity requires cleavage of pro-IL-16 by caspase 3 and autoaggregation into tetrameric form
Major production sites	CD4+ and CD8+ T cells, airway epithelium (from asthmatics), eosinophils, mast cells	Main source is CD8+ cells
Selected biologic activities	Chemoattractant for CD4+ cells (T cells, monocytes, eosinophils)	
	May be involved in asthma and in granulomatous inflammation	
	Has antiviral effects on HIV-1	
Receptor	Requires CD4 for biologic activities	
Potential clinical trials	May have potential use in HIV infection	

Abbreviation: HIV, human immunodeficiency virus.

Table 55-23 ■ **Interleukin-17**

	Characteristic[205-213]	Comment
Chromosomal localization[3]	2q31	
Major production sites	CD4+ activated memory T cells (CD45+, Ro+)	
Selected biologic activities	May mediate, in part, T-cell contribution to inflammation	Homologous to open reading frame 13 of *herpesvirus saimiri*[189]
	Stimulates epithelial, endothelial, fibroblastic, and macrophage cells to express a variety of inflammatory cytokines	
	Promotes the capacity of fibroblasts to sustain hematopoietic progenitor growth	
	Promotes differentiation of dendritic cell progenitors	
	May be involved in the pathogenesis of rheumatoid arthritis and graft rejection	
Receptor	IL-17 receptor	Ubiquitously expressed on hematopoietic and epithelial cells. Located at 22q111.22-23

Abbreviation: IL-17, interleukin-17.

level with open reading frame 13 of herpesvirus saimiri.[206]

Biologic Activities of IL-17 ■ Although limited in number, studies suggest that IL-17 may be a soluble factor by which T cells induce or contribute to inflammation (see Table 55-23).[210] IL-17 can also stimulate epithelial, endothelial, and fibroblastic cells, and macrophages to express a variety of cytokines.[194] The cytokines released after exposure to IL-17 appear to be cell-specific. For instance, fibroblast cells produce IL-1, G-CSF, IFN-γ, IL-6, and IL-8 in response to IL-17, and macrophages produce TNF-α, IL-lβ, IL-1Rα, IL-6, IL-10, and IL-12.[212]

IL-17 also exhibits indirect hematopoietic activity by enhancing the capacity of fibroblasts to sustain the proliferation of CD34+ hematopoietic progenitors and their differentiation into neutrophils.[207,210] IL-17 can also promote the maturation of dendritic cell progenitors.[213]

IL-17 in Human Disease ■ In rheumatoid arthritis synovial tissue, high levels of IL-17 contribute to IL-6 production by synoviocytes and to local inflammatory reactions.[209] Because IL-17 acts to differentiate early dendritic cells, it has been implicated in host T-cell allostimulation and graft rejection.[213]

Interleukin-18

IL-18 (IFN-inducing factor) was first described as a serum activity that induced IFN-γ production in mouse spleen cells.[214] It is related to the IL-1 family of genes (Table 55-24). IL-18 has a molecular weight of 18-19 kDa and has homology to IL-1.[215,216] Like IL-1β, IL-18 is initially synthesized as an inactive precursor molecule (pro-IL-18) lacking a signal peptide and is cleaved by ICE to yield an active molecule.[217,218]

Biologic Activities of IL-18 ■ T lymphocytes, NK cells, and macrophages are primary targets for IL-18. For example, IL-18 directly stimulates production of TNF in human blood CD4+ T lymphocytes and NK cells and plays an important role in promoting a long-lasting Th1 lymphocyte response to viral antigens. IL-18 does not appear to be an endogenous pyrogen, but may nevertheless contribute to inflammation and fever because it is a potent inducer of TNF, chemokines, and IFN.[219] In the case of IFN-γ induction, IL-18 acts as a costimulant with mitogens or IL-2. Indeed, mice deficient in ICE, the molecule that cleaves pro-IL-18 to its mature form, fail to produce IFN-γ in response to endotoxin.

Table 55-24 ■ **Interleukin-18**

	Characteristic[68,214-221]	Comment
Chromosomal localization[3]	11q22.2-q22.3	
Structure	Shows homology to IL-1	ICE cleaves inactive pro-IL-18 to mature IL-18
Selected biologic activity	Promotes production of IFN-γ, TNF	
	Targets are T cells, NK cells, and macrophages	
	Promotes Th1 responses to virus	
Receptor	IL-18R	
Natural antagonists	IL-18-binding protein exists	Poxvirus carries a version of IL-18-binding protein, which blunts host response to infection

Abbreviations: ICE, IL-1-converting enzyme; IFN, interferon; IL-1Rrp, IL-1 receptor-related protein; TNF, tumor necrosis factor.

Table 55-25 ■ **Interleukin-19**

	Characteristic[222]	Comment
Chromosomal localization[3]	1q32	
Structure	Shows homology to IL-10	Belongs to IL-10 cytokine family
	Molecular weight ~21 kDa	
Selected biologic activities	Induces IL-6 and TNF-α	
Receptor	IL-20R1 and IL-20R2	
Major production sites	Monocytes and B cells at very low levels	No T-cell production has been found

Abbreviations: IL, interleukin; TNF, tumor necrosis factor.

Interleukin-19

IL-19 is one of the members of the human IL-10 family of cytokines (Table 55-25). IL-19 shares 21% amino acid identity with IL-10 and the exon/intron structure of IL-19 is similar to that of the human IL-10 gene, comprising five exons and four introns within the coding region of the IL-19 cDNA.[222] The expression of IL-19 mRNA can be induced in monocytes by LPS or GM-CSF.

Interleukin-20

IL-20 was discovered as another IL-10-related cytokine. It induces keratinocyte proliferation and causes aberrant epidermal differentiation in the skin.[223] IL-20 receptor complex is described as a heterodimer of two orphan class II cytokine receptor subunits named IL-20Rα and IL-20Rβ (Table 55-26). Recombinant IL-20 binds to its receptor on keratinocytes and stimulates a STAT3-containing signal transduction pathway.[225] Experimental evidence suggests a role for IL-20 and its receptor in psoriasis, a multigenic skin disease characterized by increased keratinocyte proliferation and differentiation. Clinical applications are currently under consideration.

Interleukin-21

IL-21, a cytokine most closely related to IL-2 and IL-15 (Table 55-27), is involved in the proliferation and maturation of NK-cell populations from bone marrow, as well as in the proliferation of mature B-cell and T-cell populations.[226] IL-21 has been implicated in the activation of innate immune responses and in the Th1 response. IL-21 also plays a critical role in regulating immunoglobulin production of B cells.[227]

Interleukin-22

IL-22 was originally described as an IL-9-inducible gene and called IL-TIF.[228] IL-22 activities include induction of the acute phase response in hepatocytes. These activities are mediated through a heterodimeric receptor composed of the IL-22R subunit and the β chain of IL-10R.[229] In addition to its cellular receptor, IL-22 binds to a secreted class II cytokine receptor family member that acts as a natural IL-22 antagonist (Table 55-28). To date, IL-22 has not been applied clinically.

Interleukin-23

IL-23 is a member of the IL-6 family of cytokines and is closely related in structure to IL-12. These cytokines are heterodimeric cytokines, which share the p40 subunit, and both have unique second subunits, IL-23p19 and IL-12p35 (Table 55-29). In addition to the close structural relationship between IL-23 and IL-12, their heterodimeric receptors share the IL-12Rb1 chain and these cytokines have been shown to have similar properties.[230,231]

Interleukin-24

IL-24 was originally named melanoma differentiation-associated gene-7 (*mda-7*) when it was discovered in 1995. It was identified by subtractive hybridization after the treatment of melanoma cells with IFN-β and mezerein, which caused their terminal differentiation and growth

Table 55-26 **Interleukin-20**

	Characteristic[223-225]	Comment
Chromosomal localization[3]	1q32	Belongs to IL-10 cytokine family
Signal transduction pathway	Activation of the JAK-STAT3 pathway	
Selected biologic activates	Induction of genes involved in inflammation such as TNF-α, MRP14, and MCP-1	
Potential clinical trials	May have potential for chronic inflammatory skin disease	Low levels of production have been seen in skin, trachea
Receptor	IL-20R1 and IL-20R2	

Abbreviations: IL, interleukin; JAK, janus-activated kinases; MCP, monocyte chemoattractant protein; MRP, myeloid-related proteins; STAT, signal transducer and activator of transcription.

Table 55-27 **Interleukin-21**

	Characteristic[224,226,227]	Comment
Chromosomal localization[3]	4q26-27	Belongs to IL-2 cytokine family
Structure	Shows homology to IL-15	They share about 25% amino acid identity
Selected biologic activities	Mainly, regulates T-cell proliferation and differentiation Regulates cell-mediated immunity and the clearance of tumors	In general, it modulates the proliferation and differentiation of not only T cells, but also B cells, NK cells, and dendritic cells
Signal transduction pathway	IL-21 binding stimulates activation of JAK1/JAK3 and the subsequent phosphorylation of STAT1, as well as STAT3 and STAT5	
Major production sites	Expressed preferentially in CD4+ T cells	
Receptor	IL-21R	
Potential clinical application	Since it controls adaptive immune responses, its use in a clinical setting may prove efficacious for the treatment of cancer and infectious disease	

Abbreviations: IL, interleukin; JAK, janus-activated kinases; NK, natural killer; STAT, signal transducer and activator of transcription.

Table 55-28 **Interleukin-22**

	Characteristic[228,229]	Comment
Chromosomal localization[3]	12q14	Belongs to IL-10 cytokine family
Structure	Shows homology to IL-10 Molecular weight ~25–40 kDa	
Selected biologic activities	Up-regulates the production of acute phase reactants Induces the production of ROS in resting B cells	Involvement in inflammatory and perhaps immune responses
Major production sites	Constitutive expression in thymus and brain	Cytokine can be induced by IL-9 in thymic lymphoma cells, T helper cells and mast cells
Receptor	IL-22R1 and IL-10R2	

Abbreviations: IL, interleukin; ROS, reactive oxygen species.

Table 55-29 **Interleukin-23**

	Characteristic[230,231]	Comment
Chromosomal localization[3]	12q13	Belongs to IL-12 cytokine family
Structure	Molecular weight ~40 kDa	
Selected biologic activities	A unique function of IL-23 is the preferential induction of proliferation of the memory subset of T cells	Its biological activities share many functions with IL-12. All induce T-cell IFN-γ production
Signal transduction pathway	JAK2 constitutively associates with IL-23 receptor, and ligand binding results in the activation of JAK2, TYK2, STAT1, STAT3, STAT4, and STAT5	
Receptor	IL-12Rb1 and IL-23R	The IL-23R is expressed at low levels on T cells, NK cells, monocytes, and DCs

Abbreviations: DC, dendritic cells; IFN, interferon; IL, interleukin; JAK, janus-activated kinases; NK, natural killer; STAT, signal transducer and activator of transcription; TYK, tyrosine kinases.

Table 55-30 ■ Interleukin-24

	Characteristic[224,233-237]	Comment
Chromosomal localization[3]	1q32	Belongs to IL-10 cytokine family
Structure	Shows homology to IL-10	
Selected biologic activities	Induces IL-6, TNF-α, IL-1b, IL-12, and GM-CSF Functionally it has opposite effects with IL-10 Infection with Ad-IL-24 results in down-regulation of Bcl-2 and Bcl-XL (antiapoptotic proteins) and up-regulation of Bax and Bak (proapoptotic proteins) in cancer cells	At low concentration, functions as a cytokine; however, overexpression induces apoptosis selectively in cancer cells
Major production sites	Human monocytes Its expression can be up-regulated in monocytes by LPS or in T cells by anti-CD3 MoAb	Expression could be induced in human PBMC Upon treatment with PHA or LPS
Receptor	IL-20R1 and IL-20R2 IL-22R1 and IL-20R2	

Abbreviations: IL, interleukin; GM-CFS, granulocyte macrophage colony-stimulating factors; LPS, lipopolysaccharide; PBMC, peripheral blood mononuclear cells; PHA, phytohemagglutinin; TNF, tumor necrosis factor.

arrest.[232] In 2001, it was discovered that *mda-7* encodes a secreted protein that exhibits significant homology to IL-10 as another member of the IL-10 family (Table 55-30). This molecule was officially designated as IL-24.[233] Human IL-24 is secreted by activated peripheral blood mononuclear cells and is the ligand for two heterodimeric receptors, IL-22R1/IL-20R2 and IL-20R1/IL-20R2.[234] IL-24 also acts as a tumor-suppressor gene and the protein product was found to be constitutively expressed by melanocytes, nevus cells, and some primary melanomas, but not metastatic lesions of melanoma.[218,219] This is possibly the first example of a tumor-suppressor gene exhibiting immune stimulatory properties.[237]

Biologic Activities of IL-24 ■ IL-24 has a number of interesting and unique properties, including direct cancer-killing activity, potent bystander antitumor activity, immune-modulating activity, and antiangiogenic properties. As an antitumor agent, *mda-7/IL-24* is truly unique, displaying selective antitumor activity in cancer cells and having the capacity to utilize diverse signaling pathways in mediating tumor cell death.

IL-24 in the Clinic ■ Based on its remarkable attributes and effective antitumor therapy in animal models, this cytokine has taken the important step of entering the clinic. In a Phase 1 clinical trial, intratumoral injections of adenovirus-administered *mda-7*/IL-24 (INGN 241) was safe, elicited tumor-regulatory and immune-activating processes, and provided clinically significant activity.[238,239]

Interleukin-25

IL-25 was recently identified as a cytokine that is structurally related to IL-17 and induces IL-4, IL-5, and IL-13 gene expression (Table 55-31). The induction of these cytokines results in Th2-like responses marked by increased serum IgE, IgG1, and IgA levels, blood eosinophilia, and epithelial-cell hyperplasia. As a newly discovered cytokine, little is known about IL-25 besides the fact that it is derived from Th2 T cells, and it is capable of amplifying allergic-type inflammatory responses by its actions on other cells.

Interleukin-26

Subtraction hybridization coupled with representational differential analysis identified IL-26/AK155 as a gene up-regulated in human T cells following infection with herpesvirus saimiri (HVS). It has the capacity to transform these cells in culture (Table 55-32). The IL-26 protein has 24.7% amino acid identity and 47% amino acid similarity with human IL-10. Structural analysis revealed that IL-26 contains six helices with four highly conserved cysteine residues, which are assumed to be relevant for dimer formation as is the case with IL-10. It was determined that IL-26 mRNA is specifically overexpressed by T cells after HVS transformation.

Interleukin-27

In 2002, Pflanz and colleagues[242] described a new heterodimeric cytokine, related to IL-12. This cytokine was designated IL-27. It acts together with IL-12 to trigger IFN- γ production by naïve CD4+ T cells (Table 55-33). They also identified IL-27 as the ligand for TCCR/WSX-1, a novel member of the class I cytokine receptor family shown to be important for Th1 development.[243] Recent studies revealed that IL-27 has the ability to induce tumor-specific antitumor activity and pro-

Table 55-31 ■ Interleukin-25

	Characteristic[240]	Comment
Chromosomal localization[3]	14q11	Belongs to IL-17 cytokine family
Structure	Shows significant homology to IL-17	
Selected biologic activities	IL-25 induces IL-4, IL-5, and IL-13 gene expression and protein production	
Clinical functions	Potent inflammatory activity and its association with various human disease states suggest this cytokine family as an important contributor to the pathophysiology of pulmonary diseases	
Receptor	IL-17BR	

Abbreviation: IL, interleukin.

Table 55-32 ■ Interleukin-26

	Characteristic[224,241]	Comment
Chromosomal localization[3]	12q14	Some cluster with IFN-γ and IL-22
Structure	Shows homology with IL-10 Molecular weight ~19 kDa	
Selected biologic activities	Immune-protective role against viral infection	
Major production sites	IL-26 mRNA is specifically overexpressed by T cells after HSV transformation	Expression could be induced in NK and T cells upon stimulation
Receptor	Unknown	

Abbreviations: HSV, herpesvirus saimiri; IFN, interferon; IL, interleukin; NK, natural killer.

Table 55-33 Interleukin-27

	Characteristic[242-244]	Comment
Chromosomal localization[3]	12q13	Belongs to IL-12 cytokine family
Structure	Shows homology to IL-12	
Selected biologic activities	Early Th1 initiation Synergizes with IL-12 in inducing IFN- γ production by T cells and NK cells	All IL-12, 23, and 27 induce T-cell IFN- γ production
Major production sites	IL-27 production is restricted to myeloid cells with the highest levels found in LPS-activated monocytes and monocyte-derived dendritic cells	
Receptor	TCCR/WSX-1 and GP130	WSX-1 is expressed mainly on T cells

Abbreviations: IFN, interferon; IL, interleukin; NK, natural killer.

tective immunity and that the antitumor activity is mediated mainly through CD8+ T cells, and IFN- γ.[244]

Interleukin-28 and Interleukin-29

The IL-28 family has been identified from the human genomic sequence, designated IL-28A, IL-28B, and IL-29. These molecules are distantly related to type I IFNs and the IL-10 family. IL-28 and IL-29 are induced by viral infection and show antiviral activity. Moreover, IL-28 and IL-29 interact with a heterodimeric class II cytokine receptor that consists of IL-10Rβ and an orphan class II receptor chain, designated IL-28Rα. This newly described cytokine family may serve as an alternative to type I IFNs in providing immunity to viral infection (Table 55-34).

Interleukin-31

IL-31 has been identified as a four-helix bundle cytokine that is preferentially produced by T helper type 2 cells. IL-31 signals through a receptor composed of IL-31 receptor A and oncostatin M receptor. Expression of IL-31 receptor A and oncostatin M receptor mRNA is induced in activated monocytes, whereas epithelial cells expressed both mRNAs constitutively (Table 55-35). More specifically, the data indicate that IL-31 may be involved in promoting the dermatitis and epithelial responses that characterize allergic and nonallergic diseases.

Interleukin-32

Although IL-32 does not share sequence homology with known cytokine families, IL-32 induces various cytokines, human TNF-α, and IL-8 in THP-1 monocytic cells as well as mouse TNF-α and MIP-2 in raw macrophage cells. IL-32 activates typical cytokine signal pathways of nuclear factor kappa B (NFκB) and p38 mitogen-activated protein kinase. IL-32 mRNA is highly expressed in immune tissue and exists as four splice variants. Induced in human peripheral lymphocyte cells after mitogen stimulation, in human epithelial cells by IFN-γ, and in NK cells after exposure to the combination of IL-12 plus IL-18, IL-32 may play a role in inflammatory/autoimmune diseases (Table 55-36).

Interleukin-33

IL-33 is a member of the IL-1 family cytokines and mediates its biological effects via IL-1 receptor ST 2, activates NFκB and MAP kinases, and drives production of Th2-associated cytokines from in vitro polarized Th2 cells. In vivo, IL-33 induces the expression of IL-4, IL-5, and IL-13 and leads to severe pathological changes in mucosal organs (Table 55-37).

Interleukin-35

IL-35 represents a new member of the heterodimeric IL-12 cytokine family. IL-35 is a novel inhibitory cytokine that is produced by Treg cells and contributes to their suppressive activity. Moreover, ectopic expression of IL-35 confers regulatory activity on naive T cells, whereas recombinant IL-35 suppresses T-cell proliferation. Because IL-35 may be secreted exclusively by Treg cells and other cell populations with regulatory potential, it represents a novel potential target for the therapeutic manipulation of Treg activity to treat cancer and autoimmune diseases (Table 55-38).

Table 55-34 Interleukin-28A, 28B, and 29

	Characteristic[245]	Comment
Chromosomal localization[3]	19q13	Distantly related to type I IFNs and IL-10 cytokine family
Signal transduction pathway	Can signal through ISRE regulatory sites	
Selected biologic activities	Antiviral activities	
Receptor	IL-28R1 and IL-10R2	
Potential clinical applications	Alternative therapeutic choice to type IFNs	

Abbreviations: IFN, interferon; IL, interleukin; ISRE, interferon stimulated response element.

Table 55-35 Interleukin-31

	Characteristic[246]	Comment
Chromosomal localization[3]	12q24	
Signal transduction pathway	Signals through STAT 1, 3, and 5	
Selected biologic activities	Responsible for promoting the dermatitis and epithelial responses that characterize allergic and nonallergic diseases	
Tissue distribution	Low expression of mRNA in testis, bone marrow, skeletal muscle, kidney, colon, thymus, small intestine, and trachea	
Major production sites	Activated CD4+ T cells and lower expression in activated CD8+ cells	
Receptor	IL-31RA and oncostatin M receptor	Homology of IL-31RA to gp130 places this cytokine in the gp130-IL-6 cytokine family

Abbreviations: IL, interleukin; STAT, signal transducer and activator of transcription.

Other Hematopoietic Growth Factors

Some of the growth factors discussed have already found their place in clinical medicine.[250-257] However, many other cytokines also have the ability to affect hematopoietic growth and development and are now being explored. These include early-acting, multipotential factors such as FLT-3 ligand, factors that may act indirectly such as TNF-α, and molecules such as insulin-like growth factors that were initially discovered by virtue of their effects on unrelated tissues (Table 55-39). In addition, because of its increasing importance, FLT-3 ligand will be discussed in depth in the following section.

FLT-3 Ligand

FLT-3 (Fms-like tyrosine kinase 3) is also known as FLK-2 (fetal liver kinase-2)

Table 55-36 ■ Interleukin-32

	Characteristic[247]	Comment
Chromosomal localization	16p13.3	
Signal transduction pathway	Activates NFκB pathway Induces the phosphorylation of p38 MAPK	
Selected biologic activities	Induces various cytokines, human TNF-α, and IL-8 in THP-1 monocytic cells Induces MIP-2 in Raw macrophage cells	It may play a role in inflammatory and/or autoimmune diseases
Major production sites	Highly expressed in immune tissues rather than other tissues Induced in human peripheral lymphocyte cells after mitogen stimulation, in human epithelial cells by IFN-γ, and in NK cells after exposure to the combination of IL-12 plus IL-18	Human IL-32 exist as four splice variants

Abbreviations: IL, interleukin; IFN, interferon; MAPK, mitogen-activated protein kinase; TNF-α, tumor necrosis factor-α; NFκB, nuclear factor kappa B; NK, natural killer.

Table 55-37 ■ Interleukin-33

	Characteristic[248]	Comment
Chromosomal localization	9p24.1	
Signal transduction pathway	Mediates its biological effects via IL-1 receptor ST2, activates NFκB and MAP kinases	It signals via ST2
Selected biologic activities	Induces TH2-associated cytokines, such as IL-5 and IL-13 Possible role in allergic disorders caused by eosinophilic tissue damage such as asthma	Belongs to IL-1 family cytokines Forms a complex with the orphan IL-1 Receptor, ST2
Major production sites	Activated dendritic cells and macrophages at low levels	

Abbreviations: IL, interleukin; MAP, mitogen-activated protein; NFκB, nuclear factor kappa B.

Table 55-38 ■ Interleukin-35

	Characteristic[249]	Comment
Selected biologic activities	Play a role in suppressing the inflammatory response by expanding Treg cells Functions in an inhibitory, rather than an immunostimulatory or proinflammatory manner	Member of the IL-12 family; two members of this family (IL-27 and IL-35) are immune suppressive, whereas the other two members (IL-12 and IL-23) activate immune responses
Major production sites	Regulatory T cells	

Abbreviations: IL, interleukin; Treg, regulatory T cells.

Table 55-39 ■ Other Hematopoietic Growth Factors

Molecule	Characteristics
TNF-α	Predominant effects may be indirect through induction of expression of other cytokines In vivo, stimulates granulopoiesis and inhibits erythropoiesis
IGF-1	Induces erythroid colony formation even in the absence of EPO
LIF	Induces differentiation of murine myeloid leukemia line Constitutively expressed by bone marrow stroma May enhance colony formation, especially if combined with other cytokines

Abbreviations: EPO, erythropoietin; IGF-1, insulin-like growth factor-1; IL, interleukin; LIF, leukemia inhibitory factor; NK, natural killer; TNF-α, tumor necrosis factor-α.

and STK-1 (human stem cell kinase-1) (Table 55-40).[258] The ligand for FLT-3 was cloned in 1993.

Biologic Activity of FLT-3 Ligand ■ Both the membrane-bound and soluble forms can activate the tyrosine kinase enzymatic activity of the receptor and stimulate growth of progenitor cells in the marrow and blood. However, like SCF, FLT-3 ligand does not efficiently induce proliferation of normal myeloid and lymphoid progenitors by itself, but rather strongly synergizes with other hematopoietic growth factors and ILs. FLT-3 ligand is a growth factor for immature myeloid cells and stem cells and can expand CD34+ cell populations.

FLT-3 Ligand in Human Disease ■ FLT-3 is expressed at high levels in a spectrum of hematologic malignancies, including subsets of patients with AML, B precursor cell, acute lymphoblastic leukemia (ALL), and a fraction of T-cell ALL and CML in lymphoid blast crisis. Interestingly, FLT-3 mutations have been described in about 30% of patients with AML, making these mutations the most common anomaly in AML. These have also been reported, albeit with lower frequency, in MDS but are rarely detected in ALL. The mutations result in activation of FLT-3 kinase enzymatic activity.

FLT-3 Ligand in the Clinic ■ Since FLT-3 can stimulate proliferation of early progenitors, its administration to leukemia patients will need to be undertaken with circumspection. However, FLT-3 ligand may also enhance antitumor immunity, and may be exploitable in this venue. Perhaps the most promising focus for development of the FLT-3 system relates to the advent of FLT-3 inhibitors, which suppress the enzymatic activity of the mutated receptor (FLT-3). This is especially pertinent to AML because, as mentioned earlier, activating mutations of FLT-3 are seen in about one-third of patients with this leukemia.

Clinical Use of Hematopoietic Growth Factors

The clinical use of hematopoietic growth factors has dramatically reduced the morbidity of chemotherapy and transplan-

Table 55-40 ■ FLT-3 Ligand

	Characteristics[258,259]	Comment
Forms	Soluble and membrane-bound	
Major production sites	Hematopoietic bone marrow microenvironment	
Selected biologic activities	Synergizes with other hematopoietins to promote progenitor growth Can expand CD34+ cells Increases dendritic and natural killer cells	
Receptor	FLT-3	
Potential clinical trials	FLT-3 inhibitors are being tested in AML	Activating FLT-3 mutations are found in ≈30% of AML

Abbreviations: AML, acute myelogenous leukemia; FLT-3, Fms-like tyrosine kinase 3.

tation. There are a multitude of studies that have addressed numerous questions in this field. The following recommendations are summarized from the 2006 Update for the *ASCO Practice Guidelines*.[251]

Hematopoietic Growth Factors and Chemotherapy of Solid Tumors

The use of hematopoietic growth factors as supportive care after chemotherapy revolves around several issues. These include the degree to which they are actually needed with standard-dose chemotherapy, whether or not high-dose chemotherapy with cytokine support is advantageous as compared with standard-dose chemotherapy, and the cost of the growth factors.[250] Primary prophylaxis is recommended for the prevention of febrile neutropenia in patients who have a high risk (over 20% risk) of this problem. Risk is assessed based on age, medical history, disease characteristics, and myelotoxicity of the chemotherapy regimen. In addition, prophylaxis may be appropriate in the presence of clinical factors that predispose to increased complications from prolonged neutropenia, even if the treatment regimen carries <20% risk of febrile neutropenia. These factors include being elderly (over 65 years), poor performance status, previous episodes of febrile neutropenia, extensive prior treatment including large radiation ports, administration of combined chemoradiotherapy, bone marrow involvement by tumor-producing cells, poor nutritional status, the presence of open wounds or active infections, more advanced cancer, as well as other serious co-morbidities. Secondary prophylaxis with CSFs is appropriate for patients who experienced a neutropenic complication from a prior cycle of chemotherapy (for which primary prophylaxis was not received), in which a reduced dose may compromise disease-free or overall survival or treatment outcome.

Hematopoietic Growth Factors and High-Dose Chemotherapy in Solid Tumors

At one time, it was taken as axiomatic that higher doses of chemotherapy would result in better responses, if toxicity could be avoided. This view was based on observations in animal models as well as published studies, which supported a dose threshold below which optimal responses are not seen.

Nearly all clinical trials have demonstrated an increased ability of patients to tolerate higher "dose intensities" of chemotherapy with equivalent toxicities, if adjunctive growth factor (usually G-CSF or GM-CSF) support is utilized. To date, reasonably good data have been generated to support the use of very high-dose therapy with stem cell support in leukemia, relapsed intermediate to high-grade lymphomas, and multiple myeloma. Even so, for the vast majority of the more common human solid tumors, dose escalation of chemotherapy to the degree requiring the routine support of hematopoietic cytokines has not yet been prospectively proven to be of worth. Therefore, dose- or schedule-based intensification of chemotherapy should be undertaken only in the context of clinical research trials.[251]

Use of Hematopoietic Growth Factors in Febrile and Afebrile Neutropenic Patients

CSFs should not be routinely used for patients with neutropenia who are afebrile nor should they be routinely given as adjunctive treatment with antibiotic therapy for patients with fever and neutropenia. However, they should be considered in patients with fever and neutropenia who are at high risk for infection-associated complications due to factors such as expected prolonged (over 10 days) or profound ($<0.1 \times 10^9$/L) neutropenia, age over 65, uncontrolled primary disease, pneumonia, hypotension and multiorgan dysfunction, invasive fungal infection, or being hospitalized at the time of the development of fever.

Hematopoietic Growth Factors in Leukemic Patients

Concern has been raised about the potential of growth factors to stimulate the proliferation of myeloid leukemia cells. Randomized trials have not, however, shown this to be clinically relevant. Indeed, the use of CSFs to support the intensive myelotoxic chemotherapy of leukemia has been one of the first "label expansions" for these agents on the basis of the strength of clinical trial data.[221] Overall, CSF use is appropriate after the completion of consolidation chemotherapy in AML. In this setting, CSFs appear to decrease the incidence of infection and eliminate the likelihood of hospitalization in some patients receiving intensive postremission chemotherapy. There seems to be more profound shortening of the duration of neutropenia after consolidation chemotherapy for patients with AML in remission than for patients receiving initial induction therapy. For acute myeloid leukemia in relapse, CSFs should be used judiciously, or not at all, since the expected benefit is only a few days of shortened neutropenia. Intermittent administration of CSFs is also reasonable in a subset of patients with myelodysplatic syndrome and severe neutropenia and recurrent infection. In ALL, CSF administration is recommended after the completion of the initial first few days of chemotherapy of the initial induction or first postremission course in order to shorten the duration of neutropenia.

Hematopoietic Growth Factors and Radiotherapy

CSFs should be avoided in patients receiving concomitant chemotherapy and radiation therapy, particularly involving the mediastinum. In the absence of chemotherapy, therapeutic use of growth factors may be considered in patients receiving radiation therapy alone if prolonged delays secondary to neutropenia are anticipated.

Hematopoietic Growth Factors and Children

As in adults, the use of G-CSF is reasonable for the primary prophylaxis of pediatric patients with a likelihood of febrile neutropenia. Similarly, the use of G-CSF for secondary prophylaxis or for therapy should be limited to high-risk patients. However, the potential risk for secondary myeloid leukemia or MDS associated with G-CSF represents a special concern in children with ALL whose prognosis is otherwise excellent. Therefore, G-CSF should be used in these patients only if clearly warranted for other reasons.

Hematopoietic Growth Factors and Older Adults

Hematopoietic growth factors are recommended for prophylaxis of adults over the age of 65 with lymphoma treated with curative chemotherapy. Age should be considered in other situations, but age alone is not a criterion for use of growth factors in other situations.

Hematopoietic Growth Factors and Lethal Irradiation

Prompt administration of CSFs is recommended for patients who might otherwise survive, if not for potential bone marrow failure.

G-CSF vs GM-CSF ■ Further trials are needed to compare the efficacy and cost-effectiveness of these two agents. Therefore, there are no clear guidelines for use of one vs the other.

Hematopoietic Growth Factors and Transplantation

CSFs are used to mobilize peripheral blood progenitor cells often in conjunction with chemotherapy, and their administration after autologous, but not allogeneic, peripheral blood progenitor cell transplantation is considered the standard of care.

Hematopoietic Growth Factors and Severe Chronic Neutropenia

G-CSF is indicated in patients with a diagnosis of congenital, cyclic, or idiopathic neutropenia. In congenital neutropenia, the recommended daily starting dosage is 6 μg/kg twice daily administered by subcutaneous injection. In idiopathic or cyclic neutropenia, the starting dosage is 5 μg/kg/day. Chronic daily administration is needed, with the target absolute neutrophil counts being 1500 to 10,000/μL.

Colony-Stimulating Factor Regimes (Timing and Duration)

Existing data suggest that for optimal neutrophil recovery, G-CSF or GM-CSF should be started between 24 and 72 h after chemotherapy. Growth factors are generally continued until an absolute neutrophil count of 2-3 × 10^9/L is attained. A PEGylated G-CSF (Neulasta) with a prolonged half-life has been approved for clinical use. Clearance of this molecule is via neutrophil receptor binding and, hence, is directly related to neutrophil counts. Therefore, a single dose of PEGylated G-CSF can be used after chemotherapy. In general, a dose of PEGylated G-CSF (6 mg SC) should be given at least 24 h after chemotherapy. It is indicated in patients with nonmyeloid malignancies receiving myelosuppressive drugs with a significant incident of febrile neutropenia.

Nonmyeloid Growth Factors

Currently, the only nonmyeloid growth factors approved for clinical use by FDA are EPO and IL-11. Given the difficulty in identifying patients who should receive G-CSF/GM-CSF, it is clear that the task is magnified significantly when other hematologic cell lineages are taken into account. Furthermore, the availability of blood components (red blood cells and platelets) for transfusion further complicates the issue.

The use of EPO and IL-11 has not been addressed in the *ASCO Clinical Practice Guidelines*. Since efficacy of IL-11 was demonstrated in patients who experienced marked lowering of platelet counts following the previous chemotherapy cycle; however, this molecule is approved in the United States for the prevention of severe thrombocytopenia following myelosuppressive chemotherapy in patients with nonmyeloid malignancies who are at high risk for this problem. Dosing with IL-11 should generally commence 6 to 24 h following the completion of chemotherapy. The recommended dosage is 50 μg/kg/day subcutaneously. Dosing is continued until the post-platelet nadir reaches 50,000 cells/μL (generally 10-21 days). Fluid retention is the most common side effect.

Erythropoietin

In regard to EPO, the potential to reduce red cell transfusion requirements and to increase quality of life has been therapeutic goal. EPO has been shown to increase hematocrit and decrease transfusion requirements after the first month of chemotherapy (months 2 and 3) in anemic cancer patients. On this basis, EPO has been FDA approved in the United States for the treatment of anemia in patients with nonmyeloid malignancies where the anemia is due to the effect of chemotherapy. Baseline endogenous serum EPO levels vary among such patients, and in general, individuals with lower baseline levels respond more vigorously. Although no specific serum EPO levels can be stipulated above which patients will not respond to EPO, those with levels above 200 mU/L are considered much less responsive. EPO has generally been used for patients with significant anemia, that is hemoglobin <10 g/dL. However, in light of recent data suggesting a negative impact of EPO on time to progression in cancer patients, FDA suggests that EPO be used conservatively to avoid transfusion, but not to normalize hemoglobin levels.

Thrombopoietic Agents in the Clinic: An Overview

Reliably raising platelet counts in thrombocytopenic humans has proven much more difficult than ameliorating neutropenia. Cytokines that stimulate platelet production may act on early progenitors promoting their commitment along the megakaryocytic lineage or may enhance survival of already committed megakaryocytes. During the 1990s, a series of molecules with thrombopoietic potential have been tested in clinical trials: IL-3, IL-6, SCF, IL-11, and TPO. Overall, the results have been disappointing.

Currently, the only thrombopoietic molecule approved for clinical use in the United States is IL-11. A phase 3 study of IL-11 in conjunction with a diuretic (to prevent fluid accumulation) demonstrated a reduction in thrombocytopenia after chemotherapy.[189] The favorable results of this trial prompted the FDA to approve the use of IL-11 for this indication (as discussed earlier). Even so, the effect of IL-11 on platelets appears to be much less dramatic than that of G-CSF on leukocytes and with considerably more side effects. However, the other thrombopoietic molecules have fared even worse in clinical trials.

Phase 1/2 studies of IL-3 given to cancer patients after chemotherapy or autologous BMT showed only modest augmentation of platelet recovery. Furthermore, these changes occurred at doses that were difficult to tolerate.[253-255] Interestingly, much higher doses of IL-3 were well-tolerated in patients with thrombocytopenia due to aplastic anemia, graft failure, or myelodysplasia.[98] Furthermore, though these patients rarely responded to IL-3 alone, over one-third had major trilineage recovery when IL-3 and GM-CSF were given sequentially for prolonged periods of time.[93] In some individuals, responses were durable even after discontinuation of therapy.[99]

SCF has also been administered after chemotherapy, again with modest salutary effects on neutrophils and platelet counts and a high incidence of transient allergic reactions.[233] Furthermore, though SCF, especially when combined with G-CSF, has shown efficacy at mobilizing stem cells (which were later reinfused), this regimen did not improve platelet recovery.[37] In aplastic anemia patients, however, use of SCF alone and together with G-CSF has resulted in trilineage responses.[38] As with the sequential IL-3/GM-CSF studies mentioned earlier, prolonged therapy was necessary to see responses, and recovery was durable in some individuals even after treatment was stopped.

PIXY321 is a fusion protein that consists of the active domains of GM-CSF and IL-3. Although attenuation of thrombocytopenia in PIXY321-treated sarcoma patients was reported in a phase 2 trial, several subsequent randomized studies have failed to confirm any benefit.

Clinical trials of IL-6 have also shown minimal to no platelet-enhancing activity when this molecule was administered to patients undergoing chemotherapy or autologous transplantation.[131-133] Combining this molecule with G-CSF also did not yield statistically significant improvements. It has been suggested that increased platelet counts require doses above the maximum tolerated level.

At the time of discovery of TPO, this molecule was trumpeted as the true platelet growth factor. However, it too has proven problematic. The PEGylated version of TPO (produced by Amgen Corp) resulted in significantly increased platelet yields in normal subjects[49] but was, nevertheless, abandoned because of the development of antibodies in some of the recipients.

An interesting new molecule that has been in clinical trials is AMG 531, which is a novel recombinant thrombopoiesis-stimulating peptibody showing impressive activity in the treatment of chronic ITP.[51] It targets megakaryocyte and platelet development through the same pathway as eTPO. However, it has no sequence homology with eTPO. Therefore, it has a low potential to elicit antibodies that can cross-react to eTPO. AMG 531 does not appear to affect the ongoing rate of platelet destruction. It has also been reported that it can reduce bleeding and transfusion events in patients with MDS.[53]

Future Perspectives

The inchoate understanding of cytokines of a decade ago has now emerged a complex picture of interacting stimulatory and inhibitory factors. Many of the molecules that govern this process have been cloned and have entered clinical trials. It is now clear that regulatory cytokines are characteristically pleiotropic and, at the same time, exhibit significant functional redundancy.

The history of medicine is replete with examples that show how innovative technologies improve clinical outcomes. The genetic engineering techniques that permitted the rapid cloning of newly identified cytokines and their translation into clinical therapies in hematology and oncology are an exciting example of this phenomenon.[250] However, it should be remembered that many, if not most, cytokines and their respective natural inhibitors are ubiquitously expressed and have myriad biologic properties that influence virtually every organ system (see Fig. 55-1). It is already apparent that these molecules may also be effective in allergic and inflammatory conditions. Furthermore, the emerging understanding of their role and the availability of recombinant molecules for therapeutics suggests that the clinical role of these agents will continue to grow and may ultimately impact most fields of medicine.

Selected References

The complete reference list can be found at www.CANCERMEDICINE8.com

1. Ozaki K, Leonard WJ. Cytokine and cytokine receptor pleiotropy and redundancy. *J Biol Chem.* 2002;277:29355–29358.
3. National Center for Biotechnology Information. *Online Mendelian Inheritance in Man: Gene Map.* http://www.ncbi.nlm.nih.gov/Omim/getmap.cgi. Accessed June 17, 2005.
6. Adamson JW. Epoietin alfa: into the new millennium. *Semin Oncol.* 1998;25:76–79.
21. Crawford J. Clinical uses of pegylated pharmaceuticals in oncology. *Cancer Treat Rev.* 2002;28(Suppl A):7–11.
22. Robinson WA, Stanley ER, Metcalf D. Stimulation of bone marrow colony growth in vitro. *Blood.* 1969;33:396–369.
23. Sherr CJ, Rettenmier CW, Sacca R, et al. The c-fms protooncogene product is related to the receptor for the mononuclear phagocyte growth factor, CSF-1. *Cell.* 1985;41:665–676.
27. Williams DE, Eisenman J, Baird A, et al. Identification of a ligand for the c-kit proto-oncogene. *Cell.* 1990;63:167–174.
29. Broudy VC. Stem cell factor and hematopoiesis. *Blood.* 1997;90:1345–1358.
30. Ullrich A, Schlessinger J. Signal transduction by receptors with tyrosine kinase activity. *Cell.* 1990;61:203–205.
45. Fanucchi M, Glaspy J, Crawford J, et al. Effects of polyethylene glycol-conjugated recombinant human megakaryocyte growth and development factor on platelet counts after chemotherapy for lung cancer. *N Engl J Med.* 1997;336:404–409.
52. Bussel JB, Kuter DJ, George JN, et al. AMG 531, a thrombopoiesis-stimulating protein, for chronic ITP. *N Engl J Med.* 2006;355(16):1672–1681.
54. *Kurzrock R. Thrombopoietic factors in chronic bone marrow failure states: the platelet problem revisited.* Clin Cancer Res. *2005;11:1361–1367.*
61. Fesik SW. Promoting apoptosis as a strategy for cancer drug discovery. *Nat Rev Cancer.* 2005;5:876–885.
73. Estrov Z, Kurzrock R, Estey E, et al. Inhibition of acute myelogenous leukemia blast proliferation by interleukin-1 (IL-1) receptor antagonist and soluble IL-1 receptors. *Blood.* 1992;79:1938–1945.
84. Grimm EA, Owen-Schaub LB, Londaon WG, Yagita M. Lymphokine-activated killer cells. induction and function. *Ann NY Acad Sci.* 1988;532:380–386.
87. Grimm EA, Mazumder A, Zhang HZ, Rosenberg SA. The lymphokine-activated killer cell phenomenon: lysis of NK-resistant fresh solid tumor cells by IL-2 activated autologous human peripheral blood lymphocytes. *J Exp Med.* 1982;155:1823–1841.
89. Owen-Schaub LB, de Mars M, Murphy EO Jr, Grimm EA. IL-2 dose regulates TNF-a mRNA transcription and protein secretion in human peripheral blood lymphocytes. *Cell Immunol.* 1991;132:193–200.
90. Heaton K, Ju G, Grimm EA. Human interleukin-2 analogs that preferentially bind the intermediate-affinity IL-2 receptor lead to reduced secondary cytokine secretion. *Cancer Res.* 1993;53:2597–2602.
98. Kurzrock R, Talpaz M, Estrov Z, et al. Phase I study of recombinant human interleukin-3 in patients with bone marrow failure. *J Clin Oncol.* 1991;9:1241–1250.
104. Wetzler M, Kurzrock R, Estrov A, et al. Suppressed formation of bone marrow adherent layers derived from acute myeloid leukemia patients after in vitro exposure to interleukin-4. *Leuk Res.* 1997;21:519–527.
119. Seymour JF, Kurzrock R. Interleukin-6: biologic properties and role in lymphoproliferative disorders. In: Kurzrock R, Talpaz M, editors. *Cytokines: Interleukins and Their Receptors.* Norwell (MA): Kluwer Academic Publishers; 1995:123–132.
143. Hong DS, Angelo LS, Kurzrock R. Interleukin-6 and its receptor in cancer. *Cancer.* 2007; **110(9):1911–1928.**
169. Cortes J, Kurzrock R. Interleukin-10 in non-Hodgkin's lymphoma. *Leuk Lymph.* 1997;26:251–259.
187. Kurzrock R, Cortes J, Thomas DA, et al. Pilot study of low dose interleukin-11 in patients with bone marrow failure. *J Clin Oncol.* 2001;19(21):4165–4172.
192. Trinchieri G, Scott P. Interleukin-1 basic principles and clinical applications. *Curr Top Microbiol Immunol.* 1999;238:57–78.
224. Pestka S, Krause CD, Sarkar D, et al. Interleukin-10 and related cytokines and receptors. *Annu Rev Immunol.* 2004;22:929–979.
226. Parrish-Novak J, Dillon SR, Nelson A, et al. Interleukin 21 and its receptor are involved in NK cell expansion and regulation of lymphocyte function. *Nature.* 2000;408:57–63.
228. Dumoutier L, Louahed J, Renauld JC. Cloning and characterization of IL-10-related T cell-derived inducible factor (IL-TIF), a novel cytokine structurally related to IL-10 and inducible by IL-9. *J Immunol.* 2000;164:1814–1819.
230. Oppmann, B, Lesley R, Blom B, et al. Novel p19 protein engages IL-12p40 to form a cytokine, IL-23, with biological activities similar as well as distinct from IL-12. *Immunity.* 2000;13:715–725.
233. Caudell EC, Mumm JB, Poindexter N, et al. The protein product of the tumor suppressor gene, melanoma differentiation-associated gene 7, exhibits immunostimulatory activity and is designated IL-24. *J Immunol.* 2002;168:6041–6046.
235. Ekmekcioglu S, Ellerhorst J, Mhashilkar AM, et al. Downregulated melanoma differentiation associated gene (*mda-7*) expression in human melanomas. *Int J Cancer.* 2001;94:54–59.
237. Chada S, Mhashilkar AM, Ramesh R, et al. Bystander activity of Ad-mda7: human MDA-7 protein kills melanoma cells via an IL-20 receptor-dependent but STAT3-independent mechanism. *Mol Ther.* 2004;10:1085–1095.
238. Cunningham CC, Chada S, Merritt JA, et al. Clinical and local biological effects of an intratumoral injection of mda-7 (IL24; INGN 241) in patients with advanced carcinoma: a phase I study. *Mol Ther.* 2005;11:149–159.
244. Hisada M, Kamiya S, Fujita K, et al. Potent antitumor activity of interleukin-27. *Cancer Res.* 2004;64:1152–1156.
245. Sheppard P, Kindsvogel W, Xu W, et al. IL-28, IL-29 and their class II cytokine receptor IL-28R. *Nature Imm.* 2003;4:63–68.
246. Dillon SR, Sprecher C, Hammond A, et al. Interleukin 31, a cytokine produced by activated T cells, induces dermatitis in mice. *Nature Imm.* 2004;5:752–760.
247. Kim S, Han S, Azam T, et al. Interleukin-32A Cytokine and Inducer of TNFα. *Immunity.*. 2005;22:131–142.
248. Schmitz J, Owyang A, Oldham E, et al. IL-33, an interleukin-1-like cytokine that signals via the IL-1 receptor-related protein ST2 and induces T helper type 2-associated cytokines. *Immunity.* 2005;23: 479–940.
249. Collison LW, Workman CJ, Kuo TT, et al. The inhibitory cytokine IL-35 contributes to regulatory T-cell function. *Nature.* 2007;450:566–569.
251. Smith TJ, Khatcheressian J, Lyman GH, et al. 2006 Update of Recommendations for the use of white blood cell growth factors: An Evidence-Based Clinical Practice Guidelines. *J Clin Oncol.* 2006;24:3187–205.
256. Kurzrock R, Talpaz M, Gutterman JU. Very low doses of GM-CSF administered alone or with erythropoietin in aplastic anemia. *Am J Med.* 1992;93:41–48.
259. Sawyers C. Finding the next Gleevec: FLT3 targeted kinase inhibitor therapy for acute myeloid leukemia. *Cancer Cell.* 2002;1:413–415.

56 Monoclonal Serotherapy

Robert C. Bast Jr, MD ■ Michael R. Zalutsky, PhD ■ Robert J. Kreitman, MD ■ Arthur E. Frankel, MD

Following the initial report of Kohler and Milstein,[1] the monoclonal antibody technology has exerted a prompt and substantial impact on laboratory investigation. Over the last three decades, the availability of monoclonal reagents has permitted the development of novel markers for in vitro applications, including monitoring response to treatment, detecting malignant cells histochemically, identifying subsets of patients with particularly favorable or unfavorable prognoses, and distinguishing some tumors of unknown origin. Application of monoclonal antibodies for the in vivo treatment of human cancer has been more gradual, but serotherapy with monoclonal antibodies and their conjugates now has an established role in the management of certain leukemias, lymphomas, breast cancers, lung cancers, head and neck cancers, and colon cancers.[2-5]

The United States Food and Drug Administration (FDA) has approved 21 monoclonal antibodies, radionuclide conjugates, or targeted toxins, for therapeutic indications, including transplant rejection, coronary thrombosis, respiratory syncytial virus infection, rheumatoid arthritis, Crohn disease, psoriasis, asthma, and cancer.[6] Nine of the 21 have been approved for the treatment of cancer (Table 56-1). Among the unmodified monoclonal antibodies, rituximab (Rituxan) is now marketed for relapsed or refractory low-grade non-Hodgkin lymphoma (NHL), trastuzumab (Herceptin) for breast cancers that overexpress HER-2 receptors, alemtuzumab (Campath) for B-cell chronic lymphocytic leukemia (B-CLL), cetuximab (Erbitux) for colorectal cancer and squamous cell cancer of the head and neck, panitumumab (Vectibix) for colon cancer, and bevacizumab (Avastin) for colon cancer, non–small cell lung cancer, and breast cancer. With the general availability of these agents, it appears that monoclonal serotherapy now has an established role in clinical oncology.

In an attempt to exert greater antitumor activity in vivo, monoclonal antibodies have been linked to cytotoxic drugs, radionuclides, and immunotoxins. Extensive preclinical and clinical studies have now been performed with each type of immunoconjugate. Gemtuzumab ozogamicin (Mylotarg), a conjugate of the cytotoxic antibiotic calicheamicin with a humanized anti-CD33 antibody, has received regulatory approval for the treatment of relapsed acute myelogenous leukemia (AML) in patients over 60 years of age. Ibritumomab tiuxetan (Zevalin), a conjugate of ^{90}Y with the murine monoclonal antibody from which rituximab was humanized, was the first radioimmunotherapeutic agent to be approved by the FDA based on its activity in relapsed or refractory follicular lymphoma, including lymphomas resistant to rituximab.[7] ^{131}I-tostuzumab (Bexxar) is a radioimmunoconjugate containing ^{131}I linked to another anti-CD20 antibody that has proven superior to anti-CD20 antibody alone and has also been approved for use in the United States. Several toxin-antibody conjugates appear promising. Although technically not a monoclonal antibody, denileukin diftitox (Ontak), a fusion protein that contains interleukin (IL)-2 and diphtheria toxin, is a targeted toxin that binds to the IL-2 receptor and has FDA approval for the treatment of cutaneous T-cell leukemia. This chapter considers some of the possibilities for, and limitations of, monoclonal reagents, radionuclide conjugates, and targeted toxins for the treatment of cancer patients.

Therapy with Unmodified Monoclonal Antibodies

Serotherapy of Lymphoma and Leukemia

With rare exceptions, murine monoclonal antibodies raised against human neoplasms recognize tumor-associated antigens, which are also expressed by normal adult or fetal tissues. Some antigens, however, are expressed by only a small number of normal cells that may not be essential to a patient's well-being.

Anti-idiotypic Antibodies ■ Some of the most convincing evidence for the clinical activity of monoclonal antibodies was provided in the early 1980s by Levy and colleagues, who prepared tumor-specific murine monoclonal antibodies against

Table 56-1 ■ **Monoclonal Antibodies, Radionuclide Conjugates, and Targeted Toxins Approved in the United States for Treatment of Cancer**

Antibody	Product Name	FDA Approved	Type	Antigenic Target	Indication
Rituximab	RituxRituxan	1997	Chimeric		Relapsed or refractory follicular and low-grade non-Hodgkin lymphoma
Trastuzumab	Herceptin	1998	Humanized	HER-2	Metastatic breast cancers that overexpress HER-2
Denileukindefitox	Ontak	1999	Humanized	CD25	Cutaneous T-cell leukemia
Gemtuzumab	Mylotarg	2000	Humanized	CD33	Relapsed acute myelogenous leukemia in elderly patients
Alemtuzumab	Campath	2001	Humanized	CD52	B-cell chronic lymphocytic leukemia
^{90}Y-ibritumomab tiuxetan	Zevalin	2002	Murine	CD20	Relapsed or refractory follicular and low-grade non-Hodgkin lymphomas in elderly patients and rituximab-resistant disease
^{131}I-tostuzumab	Bexxar	2003	Murine	CD20	Relapsed or refractory follicular and low-grade non-Hodgkin lymphomas in elderly patients and rituximab-resistant disease
Cetuximab	Erbitux	2004	Chimeric	EGFR	Metastatic colorectal cancer with irinotecan
		2006			Head and neck cancers with radiotherapy
Bevacizumab	Avastin	2004	Humanized	VEGF	Metastatic colorectal cancer
		2006			Non–small cell lung cancer
		2008			Advanced breast cancer
Panitumumab	Vectabix	2006	Human	EGFR	Colorectal cancer

the unique idiotopes associated with the cell surface membrane immunoglobulin present on human B-cell lymphomas, but expressed by, at most, a very small subset of normal B cells.[8,9] The original patient treated with a specific anti-idiotypic antibody remained in complete remission for 72 months and survived for >17 years.[6] Treatment of 18 lymphoma patients with anti-idiotypic antibodies alone produced an objective response rate of 67% with little toxicity.[6] In subsequent trials, anti-idiotypic antibodies were combined with interferon (IFN)-α, chlorambucil, or IL-2. Overall, a response rate of 63% was observed in 52 patients, with several complete responses extending beyond 10 years.[6] Most of the antibodies that produced responses in vivo were of the murine immunoglobulin G1 (IgG1) isotype, which is generally least efficient in fixing complement or participating in antibody-dependent cell-mediated cytotoxicity (ADCC). Anti-idiotypic antibodies that bind to the B-cell receptor complex appear to induce apoptosis (programmed cell death) by delivering a death signal. In a fraction of patients treated with anti-idiotypic antibodies, recurrence of lymphoma is associated with loss of the relevant antigen from the cancer cells. Genes encoding the cell surface membrane immunoglobulin continue to undergo point mutations, resulting in the loss of idiotypic determinants.[10] Use of anti-idiotypic antibodies has provided a critical proof of concept, but widespread application has been hindered by the logistic challenge of developing reagents for each patient.

Rituximab ■ Monoclonal antibodies against differentiation antigens that are shared by cancer cells from different patients have also been used to treat NHL, as well as acute and chronic leukemias. One target that has proven useful is CD20, a 35-kDa phosphoprotein calcium channel that is expressed on the surface of all normal B cells and in 80% of NHLs, but not on other normal tissues. Repeated weekly administration of a chimeric mouse/human IgG1 anti-CD20 antibody, rituximab, produced a 48% to 50% response rate in patients with relapsed low-grade follicular NHL, with a median time to progression of 10.2 to 13.2 months.[11,12] In 37 newly diagnosed patients, treatment with rituximab (375 mg/m^2 weekly for four infusions) produced an overall response rate of 72%, with 36% complete responses and median time to disease progression of 2.2 years.[13] Consequently, rituximab can be used to treat patients at relapse after chemotherapy, the indication for which it is currently approved, or it can be used as an alternative to observation in patients with a low tumor burden of indolent non-Hodgkin lymphoma, alone or in combination with chemotherapy.[14]

Since regulatory approval for the treatment of patients with recurrent or refractory follicular or indolent NHL, indications have been extended to provide eight rather than four weekly courses and to retreat patients who had previously responded.[15] After relapse, retreatment with a similar course of rituximab produced an overall response rate of 38% in 60 patients, with 10% complete remissions. Median time to progression exceeded 15 months.[16] Combination of rituximab with cyclophosphamide, doxorubicin, vincristine, and prednisone (CHOP) chemotherapy in 40 patients with low-grade follicular lymphoma, some of whom had been previously treated, resulted in an overall response of 100%, with 58% complete remissions and 42% partial remissions. Median time to progression exceeded 40.5 months.[17] In a meta-analysis of seven trials with 1943 patients with follicular lymphoma, other indolent lymphomas, and the more aggressive mantle cell lymphoma, the addition of rituximab to chemotherapy improved overall survival, although the statistical significance was higher with indolent lymphomas than with the mantle cell histotype.[18] The addition of rituximab to cyclophosphamide, vincristine, and prednisone (CVP) chemotherapy prolonged time to progression in patients with follicular NHL.[19] Maintenance therapy with rituxin has prolonged progression-free survival in four randomized trials, but overall survival has been extended in some but not all studies.[20] As 40% of patients will experience long-lasting remissions after retreatment with rituxin at relapse, an Eastern Cooperative Oncology Group Trial is underway to compare maintenance therapy with rituxumab until relapse with retreatment at relapse in patients with follicular lymphoma.[20]

More aggressive diffuse large-cell NHL has been less responsive to rituximab alone. Among 54 patients with disease in relapse, the overall response rate to eight cycles of rituximab was 31%, including 9% complete remissions with a median time to progression in responders of eight or more months.[21] A trial has been conducted by the Groupe d'Etude des Lymphomes de l'Adulte (GELA) in 399 elderly patients with more aggressive diffuse large-cell NHL who were randomized to receive CHOP plus rituximab or CHOP alone. A complete response rate of 76% was observed with the combination, compared with 60% with CHOP alone. Event-free survival ($P < 0.005$) and overall survival ($P < 0.01$) were significantly prolonged by the addition of rituximab. Similar results have been obtained in two confirmatory trials,[22,23] both in young and elderly individuals. Thus the addition of rituximab to CHOP has provided the first improvement in the systemic treatment of diffuse large-cell lymphoma in the last 20 years.

Treatment with rituximab, alone or in combination with fludarabine, has been extended to chronic lymphocytic leukemia (CLL).[24] In early studies, only a very modest response rate (15%) was observed with low standard doses of rituximab, possibly related to the lower concentration of CD20 on the CLL cell surface and to the shedding of soluble CD20, creating an "antigenic sink."[25] Treatment with higher doses of rituximab or thrice weekly administration has, however, achieved an overall response rate of 46% in CLL, with an even higher response rate in previously untreated patients.[25] A Cancer and Leukemia Group B (CALGB) trial of fludarabine and rituximab in 42 patients with CLL yielded a 100% response rate, with 48% of patients achieving a complete remission.[26] Rituxin has also been used with alkylating agents to treat Waldenstrom macroglobulinemia. One recent study reported a 74% response rate and 67% two-year progression-free survival with a combination of rituxamab, dexamethasone, and cyclophosphamide.[27]

Rituximab therapy has generally been well-tolerated. Most side effects are infusion-related and occur within the first few hours of treatment. Adverse events have generally lasted for minutes to hours and include chills, fever, nausea, vomiting, fatigue, headache, pruritus, and the sensation of throat swelling.[28] Although side effects are experienced by up to 77% of patients, they are severe in only 10%.[29] Normal B-lymphocyte counts can decrease to zero after the initial infusion; recovery begins by 6 months and completes by 9 to 12 months. As CD20 is not expressed on mature plasma cells, immunoglobulin levels are maintained, and intercurrent infections requiring hospitalization occurred in only 2% of patients during 1-year follow-up. Following approval by the FDA in 1997 and prior to 2002, >125,000 patients were treated with rituximab in the United States. Among these individuals, only eight deaths were associated with treatment related to the development of infusion reactions, paraneoplastic pemphigus, Stevens-Johnson syndrome, and toxic epidermal necrolysis.[30]

The mechanism(s) by which rituximab kills leukemia and lymphoma cells is not completely understood, but probably involves ADCC, complement-mediated cytotoxicity, and the direct effect of CD20 ligation.[31] In cancer cells, cross-linking CD20 can induce cell cycle arrest, inhibit DNA synthesis, activate caspases, and induce apoptosis.[26] Sensitization to chemotherapy may relate to inhibiting the constitutive activation of AKT, thus down-regulating the antiapoptotic protein Bcl-XL.[32] Both natural killer (NK) cells and polymorphonuclear leukocytes can be important effectors for ADCC,[26] and a correlation has been observed in some studies, but not all, between clinical response to rituximab and the presence of specific allelic polymorphisms in the FcgRIIIa and FcgRIIa receptors for IgG that are required to mediate ADCC.[33] Individual NK cells are capable of "serial killing" of multiple lymphoma cells, particularly in the presence of IL-2 and rituximab.[34] With regard to complement-mediated cytotoxicity, the response to rituximab is impaired in mice genetically deficient in C1q that lack the first component of the complement pathway, but that have intact ADCC.[35] Clinical resistance to rituximab treatment rarely involves loss of CD20 expression but can be associated with up-regulation of complement resistance proteins CD55 and CD59.[36] Interestingly, different patterns of gene expression have been observed in lymphoma cells obtained prior to treatment from responders and nonresponders to rituximab.[37] Gene expression in tumors that failed to respond resembled that in normal lymphoid tissues and exhibited higher expression of genes encoding certain complement components and genes involved in cytokine, T-cell, and tumor necrosis factor (TNF) signaling.

Antibodies Against Other Lymphocyte-Associated Cell Surface Proteins ■ Currently, phase 1-3 trials are being conducted to evaluate antibodies against CD22, CD23, CD40, CD74, and CD80 in patients with different B cell–derived cancers.[20] In early studies of CD10-positive acute lymphoblastic leukemia (ALL), anti-CD10 antibody induced prompt modulation of the common ALL antigen, preventing effective therapy.[38] Intravenous infusion of anti-CD5 also produced antigenic modulation and only transient, partial regression in a fraction of patients with T-cell leukemia/lymphoma and CLL.[39] In one of the first studies of serotherapy with monoclonal reagents, a serum-blocking factor was demonstrated that prevented binding of the monoclonal antibody to circulating lymphosarcoma cells, consistent with the presence of shed tumor antigen.[40]

Alemtuzumab ■ Other antigens have proven to be better targets for leukemic cells. CD52 is a 21- to 28-kDa nonmodulating cell surface glycophosphatidylinositol-linked glycoprotein that is abundantly expressed on most normal and malignant lymphocytes and monocytes. The Campath-1 family includes three monoclonal antibodies that bind to CD52 and that can mediate cell lysis with human complement and effectors for ADCC.41 Campath-1M is a rat IgM, Campath-1G is a rat IgG2b, and Campath-1H (alemtuzumab) is a humanized IgG1. Campath-1M has been used to purge normal T cells from human bone marrow prior to allogeneic transplantation, and Campath-1G has been administered to marrow recipients prior to transplantation to reduce subsequent graft-vs-host disease (GVHD).[42,43]

Alemtuzumab can be given intravenously or subcutaneously. An initial dose of 3 mg is recommended on day 1, 10 mg on day 2, and 30 mg on day 3 followed by 30 mg three times per week up to 12 weeks as tolerated.

In B-CLL, alemtuzumab produced responses in 30% to 42% of heavily pretreated patients.[44,45] Responses in previously untreated patients were durable, extending for some individuals beyond 2 years. Disease in the blood and bone marrow responded more frequently than did nodal disease.[46] In previously untreated patients with B-CLL, single agent alemtuzumab produced an overall response rate of 83% compared with 55% for single agent chlorambucil, extending time to alternative treatment from 15 to 23 months.[47] When consolidation with alemtuzumab was compared to observation, treatment with the monoclonal antibody produced a significantly longer disease-free survival.[48] As CLL cells can co-express CD52 and CD20, investigators have explored the combined use of anti-CD52 alemtuzumab and anti-CD20 rituximab. A combination of fludarabine, rituximab, and alemtuzumab has been associated with substantial toxicity in a community setting even for previously untreated patients.[49,50]

Although many T-cell neoplasms lack CD52 expression, alemtuzumab treatment produced 60% complete remissions and 13% partial remissions for an overall response rate of 73% in 15 patients with T-cell prolymphocytic leukemia (T-PLL).[51] In contrast, deoxycoformycin, the best available chemotherapeutic agent, achieved an overall response rate of 40%, with only 12% complete remissions among 25 historical controls. Sensitivity of T-PLL to alemtuzumab may relate to high levels of CD52 expression in this particular histotype or to the susceptibility of cells to damage by complement or ADCC. Responses to alemtuzumab were, however, relatively short-lived, with a median of 9 months. Consequently, alemtuzumab may be only one component of a successful plan for treatment of this disease. In 14 heavily pretreated peripheral T-cell lymphoma patients, alemtuzumab produced an overall response rate of 36% with three complete and two partial remissions.[52] The median duration of complete response was 6 months.

Treatment with alemtuzumab is associated with a "first-dose" reaction, consisting of fever, rigors, rash, nausea, vomiting, and dyspnea related to release of TNF-α and IL-6.[46] In contrast to rituximab, the prolonged depression of normal T- and B-lymphocyte levels produced by alemtuzumab predisposes to opportunistic infection with cytomegalovirus (CMV), herpesvirus, pneumocystis, and fungal pathogens. Infections are observed in 50% of patients with life-threatening disease in 25%.[20] Infections can be partly prevented by prophylaxis with acyclovir, cotrimoxazole, and itraconazole.[46] Close surveillance for CMV is also warranted. Cardiac toxicity has been reported with congestive heart failure and arrhythmias that improved when the drug was discontinued in patients with mycosis fungoides/Sézary syndrome.[53]

Serotherapy of Solid Tumors

The HER family of transmembrane tyrosine kinase growth factor receptors has provided targets for serotherapy in solid tumors. As outlined in Chapter 5, interaction of peptide growth factor ligands with HER family receptors triggers signaling through the Ras-mitogen-activated protein (MAP) kinase pathway and the phosphatidylinositol 3 (PI3)-kinase pathways, enhancing cell cycle progression, proliferation, and survival in normal cells and cancer cells. Of the four HER family receptors, most attention has been given to HER-1 (epidermal growth factor receptor or EGFR) and to HER-2.

Cetuximab ■ Several monoclonal antibodies have been prepared against the extracellular domain of the 170-kDa EGFR that is overexpressed in a number of carcinomas, including non–small cell lung cancer, head and neck cancers, pancreatic cancer, and colorectal cancers. Cetuximab is a chimeric monoclonal antibody that blocks the ligand-binding site of EGFR, preventing receptor activation, inducing internalization, and down-regulating receptor levels. In experimental systems, treatment of human cancer cells with cetuximab produces cell cycle arrest in G0-G1, induces p21, directs hypophosphorylation of Rb, inhibits proliferation, and blocks the production of angiogenic factors such as vascular endothelial growth factor (VEGF).[54] In addition, treatment with cetuximab potentiates the activity of doxorubicin, paclitaxel, topotecan, and irinotecan as well as radiation therapy in nude mouse heterografts of human cancer. Potentiation of cytotoxic chemotherapy and radiation therapy may relate to inhibition of MAP kinase and PI3 kinase with induction of BAX, activation of caspase 8, and down-regulation of BCL-2 and NFκB, rendering cancer cells more sensitive to apoptotic stimuli.[55] In addition, cetuximab can induce ADCC in the presence of peripheral blood mononuclear cells. Very little EFGR expression is required to mediate cancer cell death from ADCC.[56] As in the case of rituximab, FcγR polymorphisms correlated with progression-free survival after treatment with cetuximab, consistent with the importance of ADCC as an important mechanism of cancer cell killing.[57]

Weekly treatment with cetuximab alone produced partial remissions in 9% of 57 patients with chemotherapy-refractory colorectal cancer.[58] Side effects in a majority of patients included an acneiform rash, predominantly on the face and upper torso (Fig. 56-1), and a composite syndrome of asthenia, fatigue, and malaise or lethargy. Treatment with minocycline can reduce the severity of the acneiform rash.[59] Hypomagnesemia results from the direct effect of cetuximab on EGFR in distal renal tubules, producing magnesium wasting.[60] A small minority of patients have experienced severe anaphylactic reactions, often on the initial infusion of cetuximab, related to a preexisting IgE antibody against galactose-α-1,3-galactose oligosaccharide found on the Fab portion of the cetuximab heavy chain.[61]

In two trials, a combination of irinotecan and cetuximab was used to treat a total of 450 patients with documented metastases from EGFR-positive colorectal cancer that had previously received irinotecan.[62] A combination of cetuximab and irinotecan produced a partial response in 17% to 23% compared with 11% in patients retreated with irinotecan alone. In one study, progression-free, but not overall, survival was significantly prolonged from 1.1 to 4.1 months with the combination. In a subsequent phase 3 study, 1289 patients with recurrent EGFR expressing colorectal cancer who had been previously treated with first-line fluorouracil and oxaliplatin containing regimens were randomized to cetuximab plus irinotecan or irinotecan alone. Cetuximab significantly improved disease-free survival, but not overall survival, possibly related to cross over in 47% of patients.[63] Interestingly, the level of EGFR expression has not correlated with response to the cetuximab-based therapy. Consistent with this observation, four of 16 previously treated patients (25%) with EGFR immunohistologically negative cancers responded to a combination of cetuximab and irinotecan.[56] Consequently, patients should not be excluded from treatment based on immunohistochemical evaluation of EGFR. In contrast, in recent studies, colorectal cancers with *KRAS* mutations have failed to respond to cetuximab.[64] Based on the activity in patients with irinotecan-resistant disease, cetuximab has been approved by the FDA for use in patients with colorectal cancer.

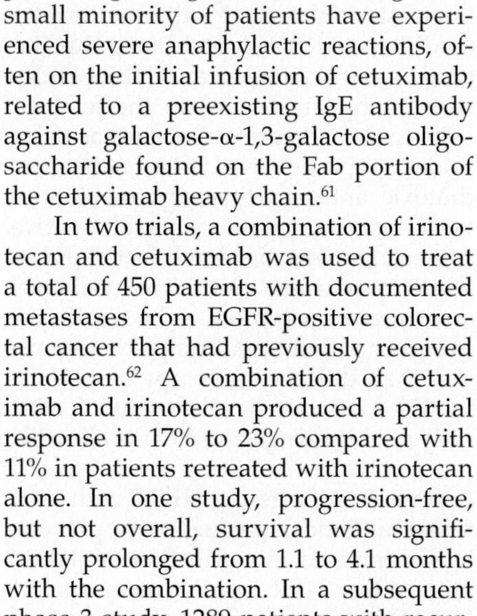

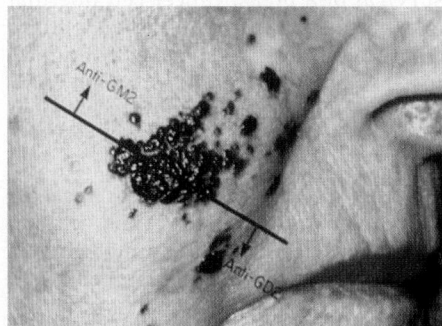

Figure 56-1 Recurrent melanoma, unresponsive to radiotherapy, prior to immunotherapy with intralesional injections of human monoclonal antibody to GM2 or GD2.

Cetuximab has also been approved by the FDA for use in squamous cell carcinoma of the head and neck. In a pivotal multinational, phase 3 study, 424 patients with locally advanced head and neck cancers were randomized to high-dose radiotherapy or to a combination of radiotherapy with cetuximab.[65] The addition of cetuximab increased the duration of locoregional control from 15 to 24 months and increased overall survival from 29 to 49 months. When cetuximab was administered to patients with recurrent squamous cell carcinoma of the head and neck who had progressed on platinum-based therapy, response rates of 10-13% were observed over three prospective trials (n = 103) with disease control rates of 46-56%.[66] The median time to disease progression ranged between 2.2 and 2.8 months, and the median overall survival ranged between 5.2 and 6.1 months.

Cetuximab has also been evaluated in patients with recurrent pancreatic cancer,[67] urothelial cancer,[68] ovarian cancer,[69] and non–small cell lung cancer.[70] A phase 3 study randomized 1125 patients with previously untreated non–small cell lung cancer to cetuximab plus cisplatin and vinorelbine (C/V) or to C/V chemotherapy alone. Addition of cetuximab increased response rate from 29.2% to 36.3% and prolonged median overall survival from 10.1 to 11.3 months. Interestingly, Caucasian patients fared better than Asian patients, despite the likely presence of a higher prevalence of EGFR mutations in the lung cancers of the latter population. In xenograft studies, cetuximab has shown activity against non–small cell lung cancer cell lines with wild-type and mutated EGFR.[71]

Panitumumab ■ Panitumumab is a fully humanized IgG2 anti-EGFR antibody that has been given accelerated approval by the FDA based on a trial in 463 patients with EGFR-positive colorectal cancer resistant to standard drugs who were randomized to single agent antibody therapy or best supportive care. Treatment with panitumumab produced an objective response of 10% compared to 0% in the supportive care control group and extended mean progression-free survival from 60 to 96 days.[72] As with cetuximab, responses were limited to patients with wild-type non-mutated Ras.[73] In previously untreated recurrent colorectal cancer, attempts to add panitumumab to bevacizumab plus FOLFOX-4 or FOLFIRI were discontinued when interim analysis of >1000 patients showed a statistically significant advantage in the control arm without panitumumab.[74]

A similar spectrum of side effects has been observed with panitumumab and cetuximab. Acneiform rash and hypomagnesemia have been most notable.[74] To date, fewer allergic reactions have been observed with panitumumab than with cetuximab.

Edrecolomab ■ Other monoclonal antibodies have been used to treat patients with colorectal cancer. Several clinical trials have used the 17-1A murine IgG2a antibody (edrecolomab), which reacts with human gastrointestinal carcinomas.[75-78] Responses have been reported in colorectal and pancreatic carcinoma, although evidence of tumor regression has often been equivocal and the role of the antibody difficult to define. Injection of 17-1A has evoked a human anti-murine immunoglobulin response, and some of the patients' antibodies have had anti-idiotypic specificity. Development of anti-murine immunoglobulin antibodies has generally been regarded as an undesirable consequence of injecting a foreign protein because they shorten the circulating half-life of the monoclonal antibody. Anti-idiotypic antibodies can, however, bear the internal image of the antigen and stimulate endogenous immunity in recipients.[79-82] Conflicting results have been obtained in large, randomized studies combining chemotherapy with edrecolomab in colorectal cancer patients.[83-86] At present, the role of edrecolomab in the management of colorectal cancer remains uncertain.

Trastuzumab ■ Approximately 20% to 30% of breast cancers overexpress the 185-kDa tyrosine kinase growth factor receptor c-erbB2 (HER-2).[87] While HER-2 lacks a functioning ligand-binding domain, it is the preferred dimerization partner for the other HER family members including EGFR, HER-3, and HER-4.[88] Overexpression of HER-2 by breast cancer cells is associated with a poor prognosis, particularly in node-positive disease, as well as with resistance to paclitaxel, CMF, and tamoxifen, but with an improved response to doxorubicin.[88,89] Resistance to systemic therapy, increased risk of recurrence, and shortened survival all reflect the biological consequences of HER-2 overexpression, including increased proliferation, increased cell survival, increased invasion and metastasis, and increased angiogenesis. Monoclonal antibodies directed against the extracellular domain of this receptor can inhibit growth of cancer cells that overexpress HER-2.[90,91] In addition, treatment with anti-HER-2 antibodies can increase the susceptibility of cancer cells to platinum compounds, taxanes, doxorubicin, and 4-hydroperoxy-cyclophosphamide.[92,93] Interestingly, binding of anti-HER-2 antibodies to the HER-2 receptors in the juxtamembrane region[94] can activate the tyrosine kinase[91] but may prevent ligand-driven interaction of HER-2 with HER-3 to activate the PI3 kinase pathway, decreasing the antiapoptotic activity of phospho-AKT.[91,95,96] Binding of trastuzumab to the extracellular domain of HER-2 can also down-regulate the HER-2 receptor. In vivo, inhibition of proangiogenic factors and mediation of ADCC may also play a role.

In clinical studies, the humanized murine anti-HER-2 IgG1 monoclonal antibody trastuzumab produced objective regression of recurrent breast carcinoma in 12% to 15% of 269 heavily pretreated women.[97,98] Although cisplatin has demonstrated marginal activity against breast cancer in previous studies, a combination of cisplatin and trastuzumab produced an objective clinical response in 24% of 37 patients, with a median duration of 8.4 months.[99] A critical international multi-institutional study was performed in 469 women with recurrent breast cancer.[100] Patients who had not previously received adjuvant therapy with doxorubicin were randomized to doxorubicin (or epirubicin) and cyclophosphamide, with or without trastuzumab. Women who had received adjuvant doxorubicin were randomized to paclitaxel with or without trastuzumab. The addition of trastuzumab to chemotherapy was associated with a longer time to disease progression (median 7.4 vs 4.6 months; $P < 0.001$), a higher objective response rate (50% vs 32%; $P < 0.001$), a longer duration of response (median 9.1 vs 6.1 months; $P < 0.001$), and longer survival (median 25.1 vs 20.3 months; $P = 0.01$). This study resulted in the approval of trastuzumab by the FDA in 1998 for the treatment of recurrent HER-2-overexpressing breast cancers. Subsequently, six large, multicenter adjuvant trials were undertaken (reviewed in Chapter 104) to test whether the addition of trastuzumab improved the ability of chemotherapy to prevent recurrence of primary HER-2-positive breast cancer. Interim analysis in five of the six trials demonstrated sufficiently dramatic improvement in disease-free survival to terminate the clinical studies and to recommend use of trastuzumab in this setting.[101-103] Addition of trastuzumab produced a 46-58% reduction in risk of recurrence, associated with an absolute reduction of 8-12% at 3 years in the five positive trials. Similarly, mortality was reduced 33-59%, producing an absolute decrease of 2-6% at 3 years.

Trastuzumab enhances the response rate to several other cytotoxic agents, including vinorelbine, gemcitabine, and platinum compounds.[104-108] A randomized trial in 81 patients with metastatic HER-2-positive breast cancer who had not received chemotherapy for recurrent disease demonstrated a 51% response rate to vinorelbine and trastuzumab compared to a 40% response rate with paclitaxel and trastuzumab.[109]

In most studies, only those breast cancers with strong expression of HER-2, driven by amplification of the gene, responded to the antibody alone or to a combination of antibody with chemotherapy. Immunohistochemistry can provide an initial screen for HER-2 overexpression, but 2+ to 3+ reactions should be confirmed with the more reliable fluorescence in situ hybridization assay.[110] HER-2 gene amplification can be acquired as breast cancers progress, arguing for repeated testing for HER-2 overexpression.[111] Because only a fraction of patients respond, overexpression of HER-2 is necessary, but not sufficient reason to ensure response to trastuzumab. Lack of response to trastuzumab correlated with lack of expression of the PTEN phosphatase, the enzyme that removes phosphate groups from PI3 and interrupts signaling through AKT.[112] Treatment with trastuzumab increased PTEN membrane localization and phosphatase activity by reducing PTEN tyrosine phosphorylation through inhibition of Src that could no longer dock on the HER-2 receptor.

Treatment with trastuzumab is well-tolerated and is associated with low-grade fever, chills, and fatigue that are generally observed with the first administration. In most studies, trastuzumab has been administered weekly, but it has been administered every 3 weeks at higher dosage with acceptable toxicity and trough levels.[113] When trastuzumab has been combined with doxorubicin or paclitaxel, increased cardiotoxicity has been observed. In the pivotal trial that demonstrated the efficacy of trastuzumab in recurrent breast cancer, American Heart Association class III and IV cardiac dysfunction occurred in 27% of the group given trastuzumab with anthracycline and cyclophosphamide compared to 8% of the group given anthracycline and cyclophosphamide alone.[114] A similar degree of cardiac dysfunction was observed in 13% of patients who received paclitaxel and trastuzumab compared with 1% who received paclitaxel alone. Long-term treatment of 218 breast cancer patients with trastuzumab-based therapy for at least 1 year was associated with an 11% incidence of class III cardiac dysfunction.[115] In the six adjuvant trials where trastuzumab was given either sequentially or concurrently with paclitaxel or carboplatin, but not doxorubicin, class III/IV cardiac dysfunction was observed in 0.5-4.1%.[101,102] Cardiac dysfunction generally responds to discontinuing trastuzumab and providing medical management.[114] Thus, the benefits of trastuzumab for recurrent disease or adjuvant treatment generally outweigh the risks in patients with normal baseline cardiac function. The mechanism for trastuzumab-induced cardiac dysfunction remains obscure. Only low levels of HER-2 are found on cardiac myocytes, but trastuzumab can localize to the myocardium, and the ligand heregulin that binds to HER-2-HER-3 and HER2-HER-4 dimers appears critical to the fetal development and survival of cardiac tissue under apoptotic stress.[116] Use of less cardiotoxic anthracyclines in combination with trastuzumab offers one alternative. A neoadjuvant trial has been reported where concurrent epirubicin, paclitaxel, and trastuzumab produced a significantly higher pathological complete response rate than did chemotherapy alone (67% vs 25%) without development of clinically evident congestive heart failure.[117]

Pertuzumab ■ Targeting HER-2 with a different antibody, pertuzumab, prevents ligand-induced dimerization of HER-2 with other HER family members.[118,119] Use of pertuzumab in combination with trastuzumab synergistically inhibited survival of a breast cancer cell line that overexpressed HER-2 associated with increased apoptosis and blockade of signaling through AKT, but not through MAP kinase.[120] Clinical trials are underway in breast and ovarian cancers.

Bevacizumab ■ Angiogenesis is critical for normal fetal growth and wound healing, but it is also required for tumor growth and metastasis.[121] Novel approaches to inhibiting angiogenesis have exploited the presence of antigens displayed on tumor-associated endothelium or the proangiogenic factors produced by tumor cells. Bevacizumab binds to the proangiogenic VEGF-A that has also been characterized as vascular permeability factor (VPF). Blockade of VEGF/VPF can inhibit tumor-driven angiogenesis in xenografts.[122] Expression of VEGF/VPF has correlated with formation of ascites in mice with ovarian cancer xenograft models.[123] Treatment with bevacizumab can completely inhibit ascites formation.[124] In addition, cancer cells themselves can express VEGF receptors. Autocrine stimulation with VEGF can enhance proliferation and resistance to chemotherapy.

Bevacizumab has received FDA approval for treatment of colorectal cancer, non–small cell lung cancer, and breast cancer, but its place in oncologic practice is still being defined.[125] In patients with previously untreated metastatic colorectal carcinoma, the addition of bevacizumab to irinotecan, fluorouracil, and leucovorin increased the overall response rate (34.8% to 44.8%) and significantly prolonged median progression-free survival (7.4 to 10.4 months) and median overall survival (15.6 to 20.3 months).[126] Two randomized phase 2 trials have demonstrated improved response rate, progression-free survival, and overall survival, when bevacizumab was added to 5-FU and leucovorin.[127-129] In phase 3 studies where bevacizumab has been added to more effective first-line regimens, including FOLFOX-4 and XELOX, response rate and overall survival were not significantly improved.[130,131] In second-line therapy, however, addition of a higher dose of bevacizumab (10 mg/kg for 2 weeks) to FOLFOX-4 significantly increased response rate (9 to 23%), progression-free survival (4.7 to 7.3 months), and overall survival (10.8 to 12.9 months).[132] Adjuvant studies are currently underway.

In previously untreated metastatic non–small cell lung cancer, two phase 3 trials have studied the addition of bevacizumab to carboplatin/paclitaxel[133] and to gemcitabine/cisplatin.[134] Modest, but significant, increases have been observed in response rate (15-20% to 34-35%) and in progression-free survival (4.5-6.1 to 6.2-6.7 months) or overall survival (10.3 to 12.3 months).

Addition of bevacizumab to paclitaxel in first-line treatment of patients with recurrent metastatic breast cancer significantly increased response rate (21% to 37%) and progression-free survival (5.9 to 11.8 months).[135] A modest, but significant, increase in progression-free survival (8.0 to 8.8 months) was observed when bevacizumab was added to docetaxel.[136] In second-line therapy, the addition of bevacizumab to capecitabine significantly increased the response rate (9 to 20%), but not progression-free survival (4.2 to 4.9 months) or overall survival (14.5 to 15.1 months).[137]

A majority of sporadic renal cell cancers exhibit inactivation of the von Hippel Lindau (VHL) gene with consequent overexpression of VEGF.[138] In a randomized phase 2 trial that compared two doses of bevacizumab (3 or 10 mg/kg every 2 weeks) with placebo in previously treated patients with renal cell carcinoma, a significant prolongation of progression-free survival was observed when high-dose bevacizumab was compared with placebo (2.5 to 4.8 months, $P < 0.01$).[139] IFN-α is a standard initial therapy for renal cell cancer with a modest response rate and a survival advantage demonstrated in randomized trials. Two phase 3 trials have compared treatment with IFN-α and bevacizumab to IFN-α alone in previously untreated patients with renal cell cancer.[140,141] Progression-free survival has been increased significantly from 5.2-5.4 to 8.5-10.2 months.

In heavily pretreated patients with recurrent ovarian cancer, administration of bevacizumab, alone[142,143] or in combination with daily oral low-dose cyclophosphamide to provide "metronomic" therapy,[144] has produced response rates of 16-24% with progression-free survival of 4.4 to 7.2 months. Stabilization of disease for 5-6 months has been observed in approximately half of ovarian cancer patients. Primary therapy with bevacizumab, carboplatin, and paclitaxel has been well-tolerated and phase 3 adjuvant studies are currently underway.

In patients with colorectal, non–small cell lung cancer, breast cancer, renal cell carcinoma, and ovarian cancer, bevacizumab administration has been well-tolerated by the majority. Grade 3 hypertension has been produced in a minority of patients who receive the anti-VEGF antibody, but has been readily managed in most cases. Nasal bleeding and proteinuria have also been observed. Greater risk for delayed wound healing and bleeding has been observed when bevacizumab was administered within 60 days of surgery.[145] Arterial thromboembolism has been observed in 2% of patients in large phase 3 trials. In patients with non–small cell lung cancer, major hemoptysis was observed, associated with four deaths among 35 patients in one early trial. Life-threatening hemoptysis occurred most frequently in elderly males with squamous cell histology, tumor necrosis, and cavitation, as well as disease close to major vessels. Patients with these characteristics have been excluded from many trials. In heavily pretreated patients with ovarian cancer, perforation of the bowel has been observed in 5-7% of cases, generally in the setting of partial small bowel obstruction and of treatment response in lesions that involve the bowel wall. Bowel perforation has occurred in only 1% of colorectal cancer patients when bevacizumab was administered with FOLFOX.[132]

To date, bevacizumab has demonstrated activity against a broad spectrum of human cancers, consistent with its antiangiogenic activity. Statistically significant prolongation of progression-free survival has been observed in colorectal, non–small cell lung, breast, and renal cell cancers, but the duration of response has ranged from 1 to 6 months in different settings. In general, treatment has continued until disease progression. Given the cost of prolonged administration of this agent, economic concerns have impacted on its availability.

Anti-CTLA4 Antibodies ■ Monoclonal antibodies have been used to intervene in immunoregulation. CD4+CD25+ T regulatory (Treg) cells express cytotoxic T-lymphocyte antigen 4 (CTLA4). The presence of Treg cells in tumor tissue has been associated with a poor prognosis in several human cancers and their elimination can potentiate antitumor responses in preclinical models.[145] In addition, effective activation of tumor immunity can be blocked by the interaction of CD80/86 on antigen-presenting cells with CTLA4 on T lymphocytes. Inhibiting this interaction with anti-CTLA4 antibody could enhance tumor-specific immunity.[146] Ipilimumab and tremelimumab are fully human monoclonal antibodies that react with CTLA4 and that are now in clinical trials. Administration of ipilimumab as a single agent has produced a 7-15% objective response rate in human melanomas and renal cell cancers.[147,148] Greater activity might be anticipated using these reagents to augment the effects of specific tumor vaccines.

Treatment with anti-CTLA4 antibodies has generally been associated with a grade 1 rash on the trunk and extremities, but occasional patients have developed colitis, hypophysitis, uveitis, or hepatitis,[145] possibly related to a failure of immunoregulation and the consequent development of autoimmune disease.

Barriers to Successful Serotherapy With Unmodified Monoclonal Antibodies

Antigen Specificity ■ Few, if any, monoclonal antibodies react only with tumor cells and fail to react with normal tissues. The remarkable efficacy and modest toxicity of anti-idiotypic antibodies reflect, at least in part, their limited reactivity with the vast majority of human B cells. The toxicity of Campath-1 reflects reactivity with normal lymphocytes and monocytes. To treat cancers in some organs, such as ovary or thyroid, tissue-specific antibodies rather than tumor-specific antibodies may suffice because all normal tissue is removed during primary therapy.

Antigenic Modulation ■ Antigens that modulate and are shed into the circulation, such as CD10 in ALL, have generally proven to be poor targets for serotherapy. An exception to this generalization has been observed with trastuzumab treatment of breast cancers that overexpress HER-2. The extracellular domain of HER-2 is cleaved and has been used as a marker for receptor overexpression.

Heterogeneity of Antigen Expression ■ Heterogeneity has been observed in antigen expression within and between cancers from different individuals. Cells that lack antigen expression cannot be effectively targeted. With unconjugated antibodies that lack "bystander" activity, a combination of several reagents may be required to target all cells. In the case of different breast cancers, a combination of five monoclonal reagents can target >90% of cells in >90% of cancers from different individuals.[149]

Effective Delivery of Antibody to Tumor Cells ■ Most attempts to develop effective serotherapy have utilized IgG antibodies with an Mr of 150 kDa. In contrast, most conventional cytotoxic drugs have a mass of <1 kDa. Consequently, monoclonal antibodies have slower kinetics of distribution and less tissue penetration than do conventional drugs.[150] For example, intravenous injection of an IgG2a murine monoclonal antibody against a 250-kDa melanoma-associated chondroitin sulfate proteoglycan core protein resulted in selective localization of antibody in metastatic nodules of malignant melanoma.[151] The greater the amount of antibody administered, the greater was the accumulation of murine immunoglobulin that could be demonstrated immunohistochemically in biopsied material. Even after the infusion of 500 mg of antibody, complete saturation of antigenic sites was not achieved in all patients, consistent with limited access of antibody to tumor cells outside the vascular compartment. The success of an antibody to localize to tumors depends on several factors. The ability of monoclonal antibodies to reach tumor cells can be limited by abnormal vascularity, elevated interstitial pressure, and relatively large distances for transport of immunoglobulins through the interstitium.[152,153] Disordered tumor vessels permit greater leakage of albumin and other plasma proteins into the interstitial space around cancer cells. Blockage of lymphatic outflow by tumor cells prevents clearance of interstitial protein, increasing oncotic pressure and fluid accumulation. Increased interstitial pressure impedes effective translocation of antibody. Biodistribution studies indicate that distance from blood vessels is an important factor affecting antigen recognition and binding. The central areas of bulky disease not only have increased fluid pressure, but are also poorly perfused, making these regions less accessible to antibodies.[154] In addition, large tumor masses can act as antigenic sinks, decreasing drug delivery to other tumor sites.[155] Modeling studies led Juweid and colleagues to formulate the hypothesis of the binding-site barrier, which postulated that antibody molecules could be prevented from penetrating tumors by the very fact of their successful binding to peritumoral antigen.[156] Subsequent experimental studies have supported this hypothesis. Intracavitary therapy has been used in an attempt to improve access of antibody to tumor cells, but antibody generally penetrates only a few millimeters beneath the serosal surface.

Immune Response to Foreign Immunoglobulin ■ Substantial effort has been expended on the development of human monoclonal antibodies that should be less immunogenic, but their titer, specificity, isotype, and affinity continue to limit the clinical utility of these reagents.[157–159] Because a large number of antibodies used clinically are derived from mice, they can induce the development of human antimouse antibodies (HAMAs). The presence of HAMAs can prevent effective delivery of murine monoclonal antibodies to tumor cells, particularly when multiple doses must be administered to obtain optimal antitumor activity. Genetic manipulation of murine monoclonal antibodies has been used to generate less immunogenic reagents. Chimeric (60% human) and humanized (95% human) antibodies have been engineered to retain the murine antigen-binding complementarity regions in association with human framework regions.[157] Although the immunogenicity of such antibodies can be substantially reduced and HAMA responses can be limited, their injection can still evoke an anti-idiotypic response. The availability of antibodies derived entirely from humans, isolated from combinatorial libraries using the process of phage display, has revolutionized therapeutic strategies.[159] Unlike murine antibodies, human or humanized antibodies that contain the human Fc antibody portion trigger ADCC and complement-dependent cytotoxicity. An array of novel affinity maturation techniques such as bacterial cell surface scFv display and cell-free ribosome display is emerging to isolate rare high-affinity clones.[160] Genetic engineering has also been used to produce single-chain antigen-binding proteins that may have more favorable pharmacokinetic properties than intact immunoglobulin or Fab fragments.[161]

Potency of Effector Mechanisms ■ To the extent that unmodified monoclonal antibodies inhibit tumor growth, several mechanisms may be important for antitumor activity, including direct growth inhibition, induction of apoptosis, inhibition of angiogenesis, complement-dependent lysis, and ADCC, in addition to possible intervention in the specific immunoregulatory network of the host. Antibodies that react with the EGFR or with HER-2 can inhibit the growth of tumor cells ex vivo in the absence of complement components or host effector cells.[162,163] Antibodies that block EGF binding to the EGFR such as cetuximab affect growth more readily than do antibodies that bind to other sites on the receptor. Inhibition of ligand binding appears important for the inhibition of anchorage-dependent, but not anchorage-independent, growth. Antibodies have been described that produce apoptosis in some lymphoid cell lines, activated T cells, and certain carcinoma cell lines.[164] Murine antibodies of the IgM, IgG2a, and IgG3 isotypes can fix human complement, but often rather poorly. The rat monoclonal antibody, Campath-1G, is an important exception to this generalization in that the antibody can mediate lysis of human cells that bear the appropriate antigen in the presence of human complement components.[165] Murine antibodies of IgG3, IgG2a, and IgG2b have been reported to mediate ADCC in which large granular lymphocytes (LGLs), monocytes, macrophages, or polymorphonuclear leukocytes are bound to tumor cells through Fc receptors after antibody has bound to specific antigenic determinants on the tumor cell surface. IgG3 appears to be particularly important for ADCC with LGLs, whereas IgG2a may interact more effectively with human monocytes.[166] In some instances, it has been possible to arm mononuclear leukocytes with antibody prior to interaction with tumor targets. In vivo, ADCC may be compromised in cancer patients due to a paucity of appropriate effector cells or to the presence of circulating immune complexes that occupy or down-regulate Fc receptors. Antibodies that react against GD3 on melanoma cells can also bind to GD3 on the surface of T cells, enhancing their cytotoxic and proliferative responses.[167] Hybrid antibodies have been generated with one binding site for T-cell-associated antigens and one binding site for tumor-associated antigens.[168] Such hybrid antibodies enhance tumor cell killing by IL-2-activated T cells, possibly by encouraging contact between effector cells and tumor targets.[169]

Therapy with Drug-Monoclonal Antibody Conjugates

Murine monoclonal antibodies have been coupled to a variety of conventional cytotoxic agents, including antifolates, anthracyclines, vinca alkyloids, and alkylating agents. Prepolymerization of some drugs such as doxorubicin prior to conjugation can achieve higher ratios of drug to antibody. Drugs can be bound to the amino side chains of lysine residues, provided that the most reactive residues are not found in the antigen-binding site. Linkage of drugs to antibody through the carbohydrate moieties of the murine immunoglobulin has provided site-specific conjugation that generally does not impair antibody binding.[170,171]

One concern raised by some investigators is based on the observation that many cell surface antigens have fewer than 10^5 copies per cell. Release of 1 to 3×10^6 drug molecules at the cell surface might or might not be sufficient to eliminate tumor. Another concern relates to the ability of large immunoglobulin carrier complexes to translocate across tumor capillaries. In preclinical studies, however, drug-monoclonal antibody conjugates proved substantially more effective than did the free drug. Only some of these conjugates are more potent, but many are less toxic, providing an improved therapeutic index. Therapeutic advantage may relate to different rates or patterns of drug uptake when linked with monoclonal reagents. In some instances, novel linkages have been devised that would release drug at low pH or only in the presence of lysosomal proteases. Not all drug-antibody conjugates must enter cells to provide effective antitumor therapy in nude mouse heterograft models. BR96-DOX used an anti-Lewis Y (LeY) antibody linked to multiple doxorubicin molecules with an acid-labile bond.[172] In phase 1 studies, upper gastrointestinal toxicity was noted consistent with the known distribution of LeY determinants and the ability of the Fc domain to activate immunologic effector mechanisms.

Gemtuzumab Ozogamicin ■ Calicheamicin has been conjugated with an anti-CD33 antibody.[173] CD33 is a 67-kDa glycoprotein expressed on the surface of >90% of AMLs and on early myeloid progenitor cells but not on normal pluripotent stem cells. Gemtuzumab ozogamicin, a conjugate of humanized anti-CD33 antibody and the cytotoxic antibiotic calicheamycin, is rapidly internalized by myeloblasts and induces apoptosis.[174] Three multicenter trials evaluated gemtuzumab ozogamicin in 142 patients with CD33 + AML in first relapse, administering two doses of 9 mg/m2 on days 1 and 15 by 2-h intravenous infusion.[175] Complete remission, with or without full platelet recovery, was observed in 30% of the patients. Because CD33 is expressed on hematopoietic precursors, grade 3 or 4 neutropenia and thrombocytopenia were observed in 99% of 101 patients aged 60 years or above. Infections (27%) and mucositis (4%) were less frequently observed.[176] Veno-occlusive disease occurred, however, in 14 of 119 patients (12%) who received gemtuzumab ozogamicin-based regimens, including five patients who had not previously undergone stem cell transplantation.[177] Current studies are incorporating gemtuzumab ozogamicin into frontline therapy.[178]

Other Agents ■ Investigators have explored the use of drug-containing liposomes coated with monoclonal antibodies to deliver larger aliquots of drug.[179,180] Stealth liposomes avoid deposition in normal liver, spleen, and lung after intravenous injection. In the future, antibody-coated nanoparticles might permit intravenous administration of targeted therapy.

Radioimmunotherapy of Cancer

Radioimmunotherapy (RIT) is a method of cancer treatment that involves the selective delivery of an antibody labeled with a radionuclide emitting cytotoxic radiation to tumor cells. While the concept of antibody-based targeting of radionuclides to cancer cells has long been appreciated, this approach did not become practical until the development of monoclonal reagents, which has permitted more specific targeting and the large-scale production of conjugates for clinical trials. The limited efficacy of unmodified monoclonal antibodies in most settings has prompted their use as carriers of radionuclides, drugs, or toxins. Drug conjugates and immunotoxins kill only the targeted cell, whereas radionuclide conjugates can exert a bystander effect, destroying adjacent cells that lack antigen expression. There are two types of bystander effects: physical and biological. The first relates to the fact that the range of therapeutic radiation is multicellular, with the result that cells not taking up the labeled molecule can still be hit. A second mechanism, the radiation-induced biological bystander effect, has been identified, in which cells not directly hit by radiation can also be killed via an as yet undefined mechanism.[181]

Requirements for Radioimmunotherapy

Choice of Radioisotope ■ With external beam therapy, only a limited area of the body is irradiated, with the dimensions defined to match the known limits of tumor location. Thus, occult metastatic disease beyond the margins of the radiation field generally escapes treatment. On the other hand, if the targeted antigen or receptor is also present on metastases, they can in principle also be irradiated even if their presence is unknown at the time of treatment. In RIT, the cytotoxic effect is mediated by deposition of energy from the emissions of the radionuclide in cancer cells, with cellular DNA considered to be the most sensitive cellular target. To take advantage of cell-specific tumor targeting, relatively short path lengths are desirable. Consequently, the vast majority of RIT studies have utilized radionuclides decaying by the emission of beta particles or alpha particles, which have tissue ranges of 1 to 10 mm and 50 to 90 μm, respectively. Recently, radionuclides that emit Auger electrons, which are only cytotoxic when localized in close proximity to the cell nucleus, also have been evaluated.[182] An advantage of RIT is the potential of matching the range of action of the radionuclides to the need to balance normal toxicity constraints vs the sesire to maximize homogeneity of tumor dose deposition for a given clinical application. Other factors that must be considered in the selection of radionuclides for RIT include: (a) compatability of physical half-life with antibody pharmacokinetics, (b) existence of labeling chemistry that provides acceptable stability, and (c) commercial availability of the radionuclide in a form suitable for clinical use.[183]

Beta Emitters ■ The vast majority of clinical RIT trials and the only two FDA-approved RIT products involve radionuclides that decay by the emission of beta particles. Given the length of their path, beta emissions are most appropriate for treating tumors >0.5 cm because under these circumstances, most of their decay energy will be absorbed by tumor and not neighboring normal tissues. In addition, not every cell needs to be targeted with a radionuclide conjugate. Bombardment of adjacent tumor cells by multiple beta particles results in enhanced killing through cross fire, partially compensating for a lack of homogeneity of antigen or receptor expression from cell to cell. In theory, one might choose among beta emitters based on the size of the tumor, or consider using a radionuclide cocktail consisting of radionuclides emitting radiation of a different range. Shorter range beta emitters such as ^{168}I, ^{147}Lu, and ^{99}Cu might be used to treat micrometastatic disease, in which a greater fraction of their decay energy would be deposited within small tumor cell clusters. Conversely, more energetic, longer range beta emitters such as ^{90}Y and ^{186}Re could destroy larger tumor deposits and eliminate tumor cells that had escaped direct targeting due to lack of antigen expression or poor vascularity.

The extent of heterogeneity of dose deposition in tumor is highly dependent on the characteristics of the antibody molecular target, tumor hemodynamics, and radionuclide properties. Radionuclide characteristics can affect the heterogeneity of dose deposition within viable and necrotic areas of a tumor. When ^{131}I- and ^{90}Y-labeled radioconjugates were compared directly, ^{131}I generally delivered a higher dose throughout the tumor; conversely, the instantaneous dose rate distribution for ^{90}Y was more uniform.[184] Although the long range of beta emitters can compensate for heterogeneous delivery of antibodies to malignant cell populations, this characteristic also increases the irradiation of normal tissues. Particularly problematic is the fact that beta decay from circulating radionuclide conjugates can irradiate bone marrow cells producing dose-limiting myelosuppression.[185]

Alpha Emitters ■ Alpha particles generally have higher energies than beta particles and exhibit very short path lengths (<100 μm) in tissue. Because of their short range, alpha emitters may be most effective in RIT directed against blood-borne tumor cells, micrometastatic disease, and cancer cells near the surface of cavities, such as ovarian carcinoma. They are considered to be radiations of high linear energy transfer (LET), which have a high probability of producing cytotoxic DNA double-strand breaks.[186] Alpha particle–emitting radionuclides that have been most widely investigated for use in RIT include 61-min ^{212}Bi, 46-min ^{213}Bi, 7.2-h ^{211}At, 10-day ^{225}Ac, and most recently, 18.7-day ^{227}Th.[187,188] The half-lives of ^{212}Bi and ^{213}Bi are so short that they create logistical problems in performance of antibody-labeling chemistry and in patient management. On the other hand, the much longer half-lives of ^{225}Ac and ^{227}Th, while advantageous in terms of logistics, present a major challenge from a radiochemistry perspective because strategies must be devised for maintaining a stable link between the radionuclide and the antibody over a multi-week time course. This is further complicated by the need to trap multiple alpha-emitting daughter radionuclides with diverse chemistries in the tumor and avoid dose-limiting toxicities to normal tissues. For these reasons, the most widely used alpha emitter for labeling antibodies has been ^{211}At.[189] Clinical trials with alpha emitters have begun and will be described in a later section of this chapter.

Radioimmunotherapy of Lymphoma

Hematological malignancies, particularly lymphomas, are particularly attractive targets for RIT because of their inherent radiosensitivity as well as the presence of differentiation antigens at the lymphoma cell surface that can be used for targeting. The only two RIT agents that currently have FDA approval have as their primary clinical indication the treatment of relapsed, refractory, or transformed non-Hodgkin lymphoma (NHL). These are ^{90}Y-ibritumomab tiuxetan and ^{131}I-tositumomab, which received clearance in 2002 and 2003, respectively. Both target the CD20 cell surface antigen that is expressed on about 95% of B-cell lymphoma but also is found on normal B cells. For this reason, an essential part of the treatment protocol is the administration of a relatively large dose of cold antibody in order to saturate normal B cell–binding sites before administration of the radiolabeled antibody. The properties of ^{90}Y-ibritumomab tiuxetan and ^{131}I-tositumomab and the manner in which they are utilized are summarized in Table 56-2. Despite their differing characteristics, both labeled antibodies have produced similarly impressive results. Which are even more encouraging when one considers that they have primarily been evaluated in patients who have failed conventional treatment with cytotoxic chemotherapy and, in some cases, external beam radiotherapy. As currently ongoing work suggests, the outcome of these trials may underestimate the potential of RIT that would be possible when the radioimmunoconjugate were used to treat minimal residual disease earlier in a patient's course. The current clinical status of ^{90}Y-ibritumomab tiuxetan and ^{131}I-tositumomab for the treatment of NHL as well as practical aspects of the use of these RIT agents can be found in a recent review.[190]

^{90}Y-Ibritumomab Tiuxetan ■ ^{90}Y-ibritumomab (Zevalin) consists of an anti-CD20 murine monoclonal antibody covalently linked to the pure beta-emitting radionuclide ^{90}Y via an MX-DTPA (tiuxetan) chelate.[191] The treatment protocol involves imaging the patient with ibritumomab labeled with another radiometal, ^{111}In, to document acceptable antibody biodistribution prior to treatment with ^{90}Y.[192] Generally, the therapeutic dose is administered about a week after the imaging dose, with the administered activity dependent on body weight and platelet count (Table 56-2). Calculation of dosimetry, either for tumor or normal organs, is not required. Although the antibody alone has some therapeutic effect, addition of the radionuclide significantly increases the therapeutic response. In a randomized trial that compared treatment with ^{90}Y-ibritumomab tiuxetan to treatment with rituximab in 143 patients with relapsed lymphoma, ^{90}Y-ibritumomab tiuxetan produced an 80% response rate compared with 56% with rituximab (P = 0.002).[191] Treatment of 54 patients with rituximab-refractory follicular NHL with ^{90}Y-ibritumomab tiuxetan resulted in an overall response rate of 74%, with 15% achieving a complete remission.[193] Particularly encouraging is the fact that extended follow-up of 211 patients has documented long-term responses of >12 months have been observed in 37% of patients.[194] The median time to progression in the long-term responder group was 29.3 months.

^{131}I-Tositumomab ■ Clinical experience with ^{131}I-tositumomab (Bexxar) has been summarized in a recent review.[195] In order to

Table 56-2 ■ **Approved Radioimmunotherapy Treatments for Non-Hodgkin Lymphoma**

Property	^{90}Y-Ibritumomab Tiuxetan	^{131}I-Tositumomab
Product Name	Zevalin	Bexxar
Antibody for labeling	Ibritumomab	Tositumomab
Form	Murine IgG1	Murine IgG2a
Antibody for blocking	Chimeric rituximab	Murine tositumomab
Dose	250 mg/m^2	450 mg
Therapy radionuclide	Yttrium-90 (^{90}Y)	Iodine-131 (^{131}I)
Half-life	2.7 days	8.1 days
Maximum beta energy	2.28 MeV	0.61 MeV
Maximum tissue range	11.3 mm	2.3 mm
Gamma ray emission	No	Yes
Labeling method	Bifunctional chelate (tiuxetan)	Electrophilic radiohalogenation
Imaging radionuclide	Indium-111 (^{111}In)	Iodine-131 (^{131}I)
Role of imaging	Demonstrate acceptable biodistribution	Determine whole-body clearance kinetics
Patient-specific dosimetry	No	Yrs
Administered activity	20-30 mCi	50-200 mCi
Parameter for dosing	mCi per kg body weight	Calculated whole-body dosimetry
Benchmark if platelets >150,000/mm^3	0.4 mCi/kg	75 cGy
Benchmark if platelets 100,000 to 149,000/mm^3	0.3 mCi/kg	65 cGy

minimize thyroid radiation dose resultant from dehalogenation of the radioiodinated antibody, a thyroid protective dose of a saturated solution of potassium iodide (or Lugol solution) is administered. Because of the widely variable kinetics of ^{131}I-tositumomab clearance in individual patients, an essential part of the treatment strategy is to determine whole-body clearance half-time from a series of three nuclear medicine scans obtained during ~1 week period after injection of a 5 mCi dosimetry dose of ^{131}I-tositumomab. The ^{131}I activity required to yield a total body dose of 65 or 75 cGy, depending upon whether the platelet count is above or below 150,000/mm^3, is then calculated.

In a pivotal study of 60 patients with chemotherapy-refractory low-grade or transformed low-grade NHL, treatment with ^{131}I-tositumomab was compared with the patients' last qualifying chemotherapy (LQC).[196] The overall response rate to a single course of ^{131}I-tositumomab was 65% compared with 28% with the patients' LQC ($P < 0.001$). Complete responses were observed in 20% after RIT and in 3% after the LQC ($P < 0.001$), with median durations of response of 6.5 and 3.4 months ($P < 0.001$), respectively. However, for complete responders, the median duration of response after the LQC was 6.1 months, whereas after RIT the median duration of response was >47 months. The results of an integrated analysis of five clinical trials indicate a 56% overall response rate and a 30% response rate for patients treated with ^{131}I-tositumomab.[197] Extension of this treatment strategy to newly diagnosed lymphoma patients is also being evaluated, and the results have been very encouraging with about 75% of patients achieving generally durable complete responses.[198]

Radioimmunotherapy of Solid Tumors

The successful treatment of solid tumors with RIT has been much more difficult to achieve and this is due to a number of factors. Compared with hematological malignancies, most solid tumors are considerably less radiation-sensitive, so considerably higher and sustained levels of labeled antibody are needed to achieve a similar effect. Because many patients have bulky disease at the time of presentation, the delivery of curative levels of radiation to all regions of the tumor is a difficult task. Trials involving patients with solid tumors, including breast,[199] colorectal,[200,201] renal cell,[202] and prostate[203] cancers, produced variable antitumor responses, but these were not as impressive as the responses observed in hematological malignancies. Some of the most encouraging results have been obtained in minimum residual disease settings, which are difficult to treat by conventional approaches.[204] Two notable examples are the treatment of colorectal cancer and brain tumors after surgical debulking.

Colorectal Cancer ■ Perhaps one of the most encouraging RIT trials in patients with solid tumors is a phase 2 study evaluating a radioiodinated anti-carcinoembryonic antigen (CEA) humanized monoclonal antibody labetuzumab as an adjuvant treatment after salvage resection of liver metastases in patients with colorectal cancer.[205] Iodine-131 was utilized as the radiolabel because the relatively short range of its β-particles were considered a good match for the dimensions of micrometastatic disease. Twenty-three patients received 40-60 mCi/m2 ^{131}I-labeled labetuzumab and 19 were evaluated for response in comparison to a contemporaneous control group that did not receive RIT. The median survival in patients receiving RIT was 58 months compared with 31 months for the control group.[206] An extension of this approach, which has shown promise in an animal model, is the use of locoregional adjuvant RIT after cytoreductive surgery in peritoneal carcinomatosis.[207]

Brain Tumors ■ Glioblastoma multiforme (GBM) is a malignancy with an extremely poor prognosis that generally kills through local invasion. Because brain tumors in adults rarely metastasize outside the cranium, locoregional approaches for RIT can be utilized, where the labeled antibody is injected directly into a surgically created tumor resection cavity. More than 500 brain tumor patients have been treated to date with radiolabeled antibodies that bind to tenascin-C, an extracellular matrix glycoprotein that is over expressed in >90% of GBM biopsies, with the level of expression increasing with advancing tumor grade. Encouraging responses have been reported in a series of phase 1 and 2 studies performed in both recurrent and newly diagnosed patients in whom ^{131}I-labeled antitenascin 81C6 antibody was administered on a fixed radioactivity basis, as mandated by the FDA.[208] In the most recent trial, the efficacy of ^{131}I-labeled 81C6 administered at the ^{131}I dose required to deliver an average radiation dose of 44 Gy to the 2-cm surgically created resection cavity was investigated.[209] The 44 Gy benchmark was based on analysis of the results of prior fixed activity level protocols that demonstrated that this dose provided maximum tumor control without accompanying radionecrosis.[208] A small dose of ^{131}I-labeled 81C6 was administered and imaged over time in order to determine the kinetics of clearance from the resection cavity, providing the data needed to calculate the patient-specific therapeutic dose. All patients received conventional external beam radiotherapy and chemotherapy after RIT. Median overall survival in these newly diagnosed patients (16 GBM, five anaplastic astrocytoma) was 97 and 91 weeks for all patients and GBM patients, respectively. A phase 3 randomizing patients to standard external beam therapy and temozolomide with/without patient-specific dosing of ^{131}I-labeled 81C6 has been approved by the FDA and is about to commence.

Strategies for Improved Radioimmunotherapy

The success of RIT in NHL has demonstrated the feasibility of this approach for cancer therapy. However, the more modest results to date in patients with solid tumors suggest that more sophisticated strategies may be needed to improve therapeutic outcomes for patients with these malignancies. Approaches under investigation for enhancing the effectiveness of RIT include dose fractionation, modification of tumor retention through the use of hyperthermia, external beam radiation, and compounds such as penetratin and combretastatin, and the use of genetically engineered multivalent constructs.[210,211] Two strategies that show particular promise for increasing the efficacy of RIT are pretargeting and the use of alpha particle–emitting radionuclides.

Pretargeting ■ An advantage of using intact antibodies for RIT is that their binding to tumor is both higher and more prolonged than that of antibody fragments, thereby resulting in higher tumor radiation dose. On the other hand, the larger molecular size of whole immunoglobulin decreases the rate of tumor accumulation, impedes diffusion within the tumor, and increases the likelihood of hematologic toxicity. Pretargeting approaches are attractive because they offer the possibility of obtaining the benefits of intact antibodies while minimizing the disadvantages. In pretargeting procedures, the antibody is administered first, and after a sufficient delay period to achieve sufficient uptake in the tumor and normal tissue clearance, a radiolabeled lower-molecular-weight compound is injected. By shifting the label from the antibody to a smaller molecule, enhanced tumor:normal tissue ratios and tumor radiation dose can be achieved.[212]

The most widely explored pretargeting strategy exploits the high-affinity (~10^{13} to 10^{15} M^{-1}) binding of the ~60-kDa proteins avidin and streptavidin to the 244-Da water-soluble vitamin, biotin. A number of different regimens have been investigated including injection of a radiolabeled biotin derivative after pretargeting of a streptavidin-antibody conjugate, and pretargeting of a biotinylated antibody, followed by streptavidin, followed by radiolabeled biotin. In some cases, a clearing agent is used before injection of the labeled biotin conjugate. Clinical investigations with streptavidin-biotin pretargeting have been performed in patients with lung, ovarian, and colorectal carcinomas, as well as other types of cancer.[212]

Encouraging results have been obtained with a three-step protocol—biotinylated antitenascin antibody, avidin and streptavidin, and finally, ^{90}Y-labeled biotin—all administered via a catheter placed in the surgical resection cavity of recurrent patients with anaplastic astrocytoma (AA) and GBM.[213] Patients received two cycles of treatment and the median survivals for AA and GBM patients were 19 and 11.5 months, respectively. The efficacy of this pretargeting RIT protocol has also been evaluated in an adjuvant setting in newly diagnosed patients.[214] All patients received surgery and external beam radiation; then, 19 patients received the three reagents in the sequence described earlier, with the remaining 18 patients serving as controls. In this trial, all reagents were administered via the intravenous route instead of directly into the surgical resection cavity. The median survivals estimated for GBM patients were 8 months in the control group and 33.5 months in the treated group. In a recent trial evaluating this pretargeting strategy in recurrent GBM patients, adding two cycles of temozolomide to the treatment regimen increased median overall survival from 17.5 to 25 months.[215]

A second pretargeting approach that has also entered the stage of clinical investigation involves the use of bispecific antibodies. In this method, one arm of the construct binds to a tumor-associated molecular target while the other is directed at a small molecule such as a radiometal-chelate complex.[216] An intriguing variation is to utilize a radiolabeled, stabilized peptide that contains two copies of the antigenic template.[217] In this way, it should be possible to promote binding to tumor cells, where antigen concentration is high, cross-linking two bispecific antibodies through a peptide bridge. The feasibility of this approach has been evaluated in patients with recurrent medullary thyroid carcinoma.[218] Patients first received a bispecific anti-CEA antibody and then after 4 days, ^{131}I-labeled peptide bearing two hapten groups. Tumor stabilization of >7 years was seen in 47% of 19 patients that compared favorably to that observed in a contemporaneous control group.

Recently, a third methodology for pretargeting has been investigated. The dock-and-lock method exploits the interaction between the regulatory subunits of protein kinase A and the anchoring domain of A kinase–anchoring proteins to generate multivalent and multifunctional proteins.[219] Clinical evaluation of this RIT strategy has not yet begun but results in animal models are highly encouraging.[220]

Alpha Particles ■ The most attractive feature of alpha particle–emitting radionuclides for RIT is their markedly increased potency compared with other types of radiation. Studies in cell culture have demonstrated that human tumor cells can be killed after only a few alpha particles traverse a cell.[221] Furthermore, the cytotoxicity of alpha particles is nearly independent of dose rate, oxygen concentration, and cell cycle stage. While the conceptual advantages of alpha particles for RIT were known for a long time, practical investigation in patients required developments in radionuclide production, protein-labeling chemistry, and radiation dosimetry.[187,189]

The first RIT agent labeled with an alpha particle–emitting radionuclide to be evaluated in patients was ^{213}Bi-labeled HuM195, a humanized antibody reactive with the CD33 antigen that is overexpressed on human leukemia cells.[186] A phase 1 trial was conducted in 18 patients with relapsed and refractory AML or chronic myelomonocytic leukemia. Because of the 46-min half-life of ^{213}Bi, the labeled antibody was administered in multiple doses (3–7) in order to achieve total administered activities ranging from 602 to 3515 MBq. Absorbed dose ratios between potential tumor sites (bone marrow, liver, and spleen) and whole body were about 1000 times higher than seen previously when this antibody was labeled with beta emitters. Large leukemia volume reductions were achieved in many patients; however, no complete remissions were observed. In large part because of the inconvenience associated with the short half-life of ^{213}Bi, these investigators have recently initiated a phase 1 trial of HuM195 labeled with the 10-day half-life alpha particle emitter ^{225}Ac.

A phase 1 trial has recently been reported to determine the pharmacokinetics and response to ^{211}At-labeled chimeric 81C6 antitenascin monoclonal antibody administered into surgically created glioma resection cavities in recurrent glioma patients.[222] The 7.2-h half-life alpha particle–emitting radiohalogen ^{211}At was produced at the Duke University Medical Center Cyclotron, and the antibody was labeled using *N*-succinimidyl 3-[^{211}At] astato benzoate.[223] Serial gamma camera imaging and blood counting demonstrated that the ^{211}At-labeled immunoconjugate was stable in vivo with 96.7 ± 3.6% of the decays occurring in the resection cavity. The median survival times for all patients, those with GBM and those with AA and oligodendroglioma, were 54, 52, and 116 weeks, respectively. For those with GBM, this represents a significant increase compared with conventional treatments (~25–30 weeks). A particularly encouraging result was that two patients with recurrent GBM survived for 151 and 153 weeks after ^{211}At-labeled 81C6 monoclonal antibody therapy.

Therapy with Targeted Toxins

Targeted toxins are hybrid protein drugs that contain tumor cell–binding domains and toxin domains. The tumor cell–binding domain delivers the drug to the tumor cell surface. After processing and/or internalization, the toxin domain triggers cell death (Fig. 56-2). The toxins may create cell surface pores (proaerolysin) or catalytically inactivate cytosolic protein synthesis (diphtheria toxin, *Pseudomonas* exotoxin, or saporin). In some cases, specificity is provided by protease-specific cleavage sequences added to the toxin. A major challenge in the construction of targeted toxins is to identify target receptors or proteases that permit tumor-selective cell killing. Most of the agents consist of a single polypeptide, although several compounds in development have separate cell binding and effector/toxin

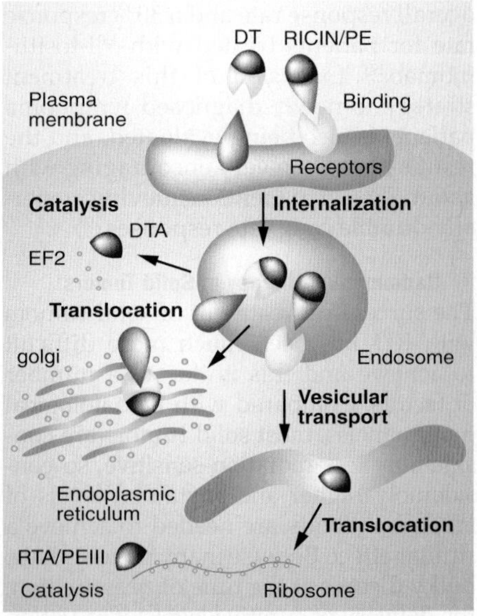

Figure 56-2 ■ Model of cell intoxication by toxins and targeted toxins. Receptors for targeted toxins differ from parent toxins, but post-binding steps appear to match between the targeted toxin and the parent toxin. Toxins bind cell surface receptors; the complex internalizes to endosomes; the toxin reaches a translocation-competent compartment (endosomes for *Diphtheria* toxin and endoplasmic reticulum for PE and ricin); the catalytic domain of the toxin crosses the membrane to the cytosol; cytosolic toxin inactivates protein synthesis.

peptides. Targeted toxins were designed to be clinically useful in patients with malignancies that have become resistant to standard cytotoxic agents. Since none of the targeted toxins are absolutely tumor-specific, different side effects are observed dependent on the binding or activation specificity and the particular toxin. While the synthesis of such complex protein compounds is challenging, several agents have shown excellent clinical benefit with mild-moderate side effects in a range of human cancers. We will discuss agents that have been approved or that are in middle-late clinical testing in cancer. Pharmacokinetics, immune response, toxicities, and response are described separately for each—though many share common pharmacologic and toxicologic properties.

Targeted Toxins for Leukemia and Lymphoma

Denileukin Diftitox ■ Diphtheria toxin is a 58-kDa Mr protein with three domains. An N-terminal domain catalyzes ADP-ribosylation of elongation factor-2 (EF-2) that inactivates cellular protein synthesis leading to cell death. The middle domain is a hydrophobic domain, facilitating transfer of the catalytic domain to the cell cytosol. The C-terminal domain is a beta sheet–rich region that causes cell binding. In the first FDA-approved targeted toxin, Murphy and colleagues replaced the normal cell-binding domain with human IL-2 (denileukin diftitox). The targeted toxin binds lymphoma cells and lymphocytes expressing intermediate or high-affinity IL-2 receptors and causes cell death. In the pivotal phase 3 study, patients with stage IB to IVA cutaneous T-cell lymphoma (CTCL) received 9 or 18 μg/kg/day IV drug for 5 days every 3 weeks for up to eight cycles.[224] The drug half-life was 30 min, and the side effects included an acute cytokine reaction (fever, chills, nausea, vomiting, myalgias, and arthralgias, chest pain, back pain), transient liver enzyme abnormalities (transaminasemia), and a vascular leak syndrome (hypotension, hypoalbuminemia, dyspnea, and edema). Most patients developed an immune response to the agent, but this did not correlate with toxicities or response. There were 30% clinical responses including 20% partial responses and 10% complete responses lasting a median of 6 months. Based on these results, denileukin diftitox was approved for refractory CTCL. In patients with non-CTCL relapsed/refractory T-cell non-Hodgkin lymphoma, the agent produced a 48% remission rate with 22% complete remissions and 26% partial remissions and median remission duration of 6 months.[225] Denileukin diftitox also produced remissions in CLL for a total of 27% overall response (4% complete remission and 23% partial responses) and a median response duration of 6 months.[226] Denileukin diftitox given for patients with relapsed or refractory B-cell non-Hodkgin lymphoma yielded an overall response rate of 25% (7% complete response and 18% partial response) with median response duration of 7 months.[227] There are case reports of denileukin diftitox-induced remissions in patients with systemic mastocytosis,[228] extranodal NK/T-cell lymphoma,[229] peripheral T-cell lymphoma,[230] subcutaneous panniculitis-like T-cell lymphoma,[231] and adult T-cell leukemia.[232] Among nonmalignant conditions, denileukin diftitox depletes autoimmune-activated T cells yielding a 71% response rate after 2-6 doses of 9 μg/kg in patients with steroid refractory acute graft-vs-host disease.[233] Additional studies evaluated the role of expression of the individual IL-2 receptor subunits in CTCL responses. The alpha subunit expression was measured by immunohistochemistry.[234] Denileukin diftitox responses occurred in both CD25-positive and -negative tumors, although patients with strongly CD25-positive tumors are more likely to respond. Responses were also more likely at 18 μg/kg vs 9 μg/kg.[224] Rare toxicities include thyrotoxicosis and vision loss.[235,236] Combination of denileukin diftitox with other agents including bexarotene, rituximab, and hyper-CVAD may enhance responses in CTCL, B-cell NHL, and adult T-cell leukemia, respectively.[237–239] The effect of denileukin diftitox on IL-2 receptor expressing Treg cells has been used to augment immune responses to poxvirus vaccine and melanomas.[240,241]

BL22 ■ Pseudomonas exotoxin is a 68-kDa Mr polypeptide with an N-terminal cell-binding domain followed by an amphipathic helix-containing translocation domain and a C-terminal ADP-ribosylation domain. Pseudomonas exotoxin was altered to eliminate normal tissue binding by deleting amino acid residues 1 to 252 and 365 to 380; a disulfide-stabilized anti-CD22 Fv was fused to the 38-kDa Mr modified toxin (PE38). The fusion protein, BL22, was given at doses of 3 to 50 μg/kg IV over 30 min every other day for a total of three doses every month for up to 14 cycles to patients with chemotherapy-refractory B-cell malignancies.[242] The drug was active in hairy cell leukemia (HCL) with 61% complete remissions and 19% partial remissions. Remissions were achieved after 1 to 14 cycles. Remissions were durable with only 27% of responders relapsing after 10 to 23 months. Retreatment produced second complete remissions. Responses were dose-dependent, and the maximal tolerated dose (MTD) was determined to be 40 μg/kg/dose. Neutralizing antibodies developed in 24% of patients. A reversible hemolytic uremic syndrome requiring plasmapheresis was observed in five patients. Other side effects included hypoalbuminemia, transminasemia, fatigue, and edema. BL22 immunotoxin appears to be the current best salvage treatment for relapsed hairy cell leukemia patients. An improved, higher affinity drug, HA22, has begun clinical testing in patients with refractory B-cell malignancies.[243]

LMB-2 ■ The catalytic and translocation domain containing fragment of Pseudomonas exotoxin (PE38) was fused to an anti-CD25 Fv to synthesize LMB-2. LMB-2 was administered to 35 patients with different lymphomas at doses of 2 to 63 μg/kg intravenously over 30 min every other day × 3.244 Dose-limiting toxicity at 63 μg/kg doses was reversible transminase elevation, diarrhea, and cardiomyopathy. The maximal tolerated dose was 40 μg/kg/dose. Other side effects were fever and mild transaminasemia. Seventeen percent of patients developed neutralizing antibodies after the first cycle. The drug half-life was 4 h. A complete remission was observed in one HCL patient that was ongoing at 20 months. There were seven partial remissions in patients with several different neoplasms, including HCL (three patients), CTCL (one patient), CLL (one patient), Hodgkin disease (one patient), and adult T-cell leukemia (one patient). Responders received at least 60 μg/kg total dose of LMB-2 per cycle. The median duration of remission has not been determined, but responses exceed 6 and 20 months in two patients. Responding patients had clearance of circulating malignant cells, improvement in skin lesions, and regression of adenopathy and splenomegaly. LMB-2 was also administered with the MART-1/gp-100 vaccine to patients with metastatic melanoma in an effort to augment anti-melanoma immunity via Treg depletion.[245] Similar to denileukin diftitox therapy, in vivo Treg cell depletion was confirmed but objective anti-melanoma responses were not seen.

DT388IL3 ■ The catalytic and translocation domains of diphtheria toxin (DT388) were fused via a Met-His linker to human IL-3. DT388IL3 was administered IV over 15 min every other day for up to six doses to 45 patients with poor-risk, relapsed, or refractory acute myeloid leukemia or myelodysplasia.[246] Half-life was 30 min and peak levels were dose-dependent. An inter-patient dose escalation schema was used with doses from 4 to 12.5 μg/kg/dose. Dose-limiting toxicity was not observed, but side effects included transient transaminasemia, hypoalbuminemia, and fever/chills/nausea/vomiting. Antifusion protein antibodies occurred between day 15 and day 30 in most patients. Responses included one complete remission lasting 8 months and two partial remissions of 3 and 4 months duration. A phase 1B inter-patient dose escalation study in acute myeloid leukemia and myelodysplasia patients with 10-40% blast marrow index (cellularity fraction times percent blasts) has begun examining five daily doses. A higher affinity variant, DT388K116W, is in final stages of testing and is expected to begin clinical trials in late 2008.[247]

Targeted Toxins for Solid Tumors

SS1P ■ The binding site–deleted *Pseudomonas* exotoxin PE38 fragment used to construct BL22 was fused to an anti-mesothelin disulfide-stabilized Fv to create the recombinant immunotoxin, SS1P. SS1P was given as 30 min IV infusions every other day for 3-6 doses to patients with advanced mesothelioma, ovarian cancer, and pancreatic cancer at 18-45 μg/kg/dose.[248] Dose-limiting toxicity was pleuritis and the maximal tolerated dose was 45 μg/kg on a three dose schedule. There were a few minor responses and over half of patients had stable disease. Phase 2 clinical studies are underway. Combinations with gemcitabine and paclitaxel are planned.[249,250] Novel constructs with releasable PEGylation have been tested in vivo and may maintain efficacy with reduced immunogenicity and toxicity.[251]

PRX302 ■ The furin cleavage site of proaerolysin was modified to a prostate-specific antigen (PSA)-selective cleavage site. Proaerolysin is a channel-forming bacterial protoxin that binds to ubiquitous cell surface receptors. The recombinant-modified proaerolysin, PRX302, was administered interstitially to 24 patients with locally recurrent prostate cancer after primary radiotherapy failure.[252] The drug was well-tolerated without dose-limiting toxicities at doses of 0.03-3 μg/g of prostate. Delivery was by a single multi-deposit, transrectal ultrasound-guided transperineal intraprostatic injection using a modified brachytherapy technique. PSA levels decreased in 63% of patients. The percentage of positive prostate biopsy cores post-therapy revealed a decrease in 75% of patients with three patients showing no positive biopsy cores at 30 days post-therapy. A phase 1B study has been initiated at multiple institutions to optimize the dose and delivery method.

TransMID ■ Diphtheria toxin S525F variant, CRM107, was covalently coupled to human transferrin. The conjugate TransMID was infused interstitially over 5 days via one or two catheters implanted into the tumor beds of patients with high-grade gliomas.[253] There was a 35% overall response rate by MRI criteria and a median survival of >71 weeks. Toxicity includes brain injury. TransMID is also being tested in low-grade gliomas, metastatic cancer to the brain.[254]

Cintredekin Besudotox ■ IL-13 was fused to PE38 with C-terminal QQR. IL-13-PE38QQR or cintredekin besudotox was administered by convection-enhanced delivery to recurrent glioblastoma multiforme tumors up to 6 days.[255] Optimal dose was 0.4 mL/h and 0.5 μg/mL over 50 h through two catheters with systemic corticosteroids. Toxicity was tumor necrosis and cerebral edema. Thirty-three percent of patients had remissions lasting from 7 to 117+ weeks. Response and survival depended upon optimal catheter placement. Unique characteristics of patient brain and tumor growth cause complex fluid distribution patterns after catheter placement and convection delivery. Both ^{123}I-labeled human serum albumin PET imaging and MR diffusion tensor imaging predict patient-specific drug distribution by convection-enhanced delivery and may improve prospective selection of catheter trajectories and targeted toxin efficacy.[256]

NBI-3001 ■ Circularly permutated IL-4 was fused to PE38. The recombinant immunotoxin, NBI-3001, was administered IV at dose levels of 0.008-0.027 mg/m^2 daily for 5 days every 28 days to patients with renal cancer and non–small cell lung cancer.[257] Dose-limiting toxicity was transient transaminasemia. Neutralizing antibodies were detected in 71% of patients after two cycles. No objective responses were seen. The same agent was administered with an inter-patient dose escalation of 6 μg/mL × 40 mL to 9 μg/mL × 100 mL intratumorally via 1-3 stereotactically placed catheters over 4-8 days to high-grade glioma patients resulted in central nervous system toxicity in 22% of patients at the maximal tolerated dose of 6 μg/mL × 40 mL.[258] MRI showed tumor necrosis following treatment. Median survival was 7 months. There was one unmaintained complete remission lasting over 18 months.

ScFv(FRP5)-ETA ■ The *Pseudomonas* exotoxin deletion mutant coding for domains II and III was fused to the scFv of the erbB-2-specific monoclonal antibody FRP5. ScFv(FRP5)-ETA was initially injected intratumorally once daily for 7-10 days with daily doses of 60 to 900 μg in patients with subcutaneous tumor nodules of metastatic breast cancer, colorectal cancer, and malignant melanoma.[259] Adverse reactions were restricted to local symptoms such as pain and inflammation at the injection sites. Partial regression or complete regression of injected nodules was seen in 20% and 40% of patients, respectively. Subsequently, patients with ErbB-2 expressing metastatic breast cancer, prostate cancer, head and neck cancers, non–small cell lung cancer, and transitional cell carcinoma were treated on an inter-patient dose escalation schedule systemically with 2-20 μg/kg bolus infusion daily for 5 days of each week for 2 weeks.[260] The dose-limiting toxicity was transient transaminasemia. The maximal tolerated dose was 12.5 μg/kg, and the peak drug level was ~100 ng/mL. Most patients developed anti-scFv(FRP5)-ETA antibodies after 8 days. There were no responses. Phase 2 studies are ongoing.

Toxicities of Targeted Toxins

In some instances, the receptor/antigen recognized by the targeted toxin is present on normal tissues and, in retrospect, predictable side effects have occurred. Pleuritis from SS1P is predictable based on pleural expression of mesothelin. The development of peritumoral focal brain injury in some patients after TransMID interstitial infusion may be due to the presence of transferrin receptor on normal brain capillaries.[261] Stereotypic changes were observed consisting of serpentine strips of increased signal in the peritumoral cortex evident on unenhanced T1-weighted MRI scans of TransMID-treated brains. Biopsy results confirmed thrombosed cortical venules and/or capillaries. By lowering the concentration of TransMID in the infusate and lowering the volume infused, toxicity to normal adjacent cortex was ameliorated.

Toxicities that are independent of ligand binding have been observed with most targeted toxins. These include either hepatocyte injury causing abnormal liver function tests or vascular endothelial damage with resultant VLS. Both the hepatic lesion and the vascular lesion may relate to nonspecific uptake of targeted toxins by normal human tissues. The normal tissue mediating these injuries may be the tissue showing the observed toxicity (liver or vascular endothelium) or may be macrophages that secondarily release cytokines, producing liver and blood vessel damage. Data support both hypotheses.

Hepatocytes have been exposed to targeted toxins in cell culture. Targeted toxins can bind to the hepatocyte cell surface dependent on the p*I* of the ligand in the conjugate.[262] Animals have been treated with toxins, and release of cytokines by macrophages has been demonstrated.[263] Cytokines, including TNF-α, can also directly injure hepatocytes. Which mechanism is more responsible for the transaminasemia in patients treated with fusion toxins cannot be determined from currently available data, but several mechanisms may operate simultaneously. Use of targeted toxins with lower nonspecific binding appears warranted as do efforts to block macrophage cytokine release.

Vascular leak syndrome (VLS) is characterized by weight gain, increased vascular permeability, hypoalbuminemia, myalgias, mild renal and pulmonary insufficiency, hypotension, and, in some cases, aphasias and pulmonary edema. The syndrome occurs transiently, but at times severely, after targeted toxin treatment. VLS usually occurs 4 to 6 days after initiating therapy and lasts 4 to 10 days. The cause of the endothelial lesion is unknown. Again, both uptake by vascular endothelium and macrophages have been postulated as triggering events. Several studies have shown apoptosis of endothelial cells in culture after toxin conjugate exposure.[264] Slight increase in loss of endothelial surface relative to replacement could lead to a significant leak. Endothelial cells may be uniquely sensitive due to exposure to high concentrations of the targeted toxin in the bloodstream. A correlation between AUC (blood concentration of conjugate × time) and VLS has been reported.[265] Smaller fusion toxins or recombinant immunotoxins with shorter circulating half-lives in vivo may yield less VLS at comparable doses. Vitetta and colleagues have identified a tripeptide disintegrin motif (*x*D*y*, where x = L, I, G, or V and y = V, L, or S) present on the surface of peptide toxins and IL-2 that can bind endothelial cell receptors and trigger increased vascular permeability.[266] Immunotoxins prepared with blocked disintegrin sites produce less VLS in vivo.[267] Clinical trials with such modified immunotoxins are eagerly anticipated. Alternatively, inflammatory cytokines released by toxin-ingested macrophages could also produce profound systemic alterations in vascular integrity. Although no animal model reproduces human VLS, a syndrome of hydrothorax, hypoalbuminemia, hemoconcentration, and neutrophilia developed in rats after intravenous injections of anti-LeY Fv-PE40.[268] Rats treated with PE40 alone or IL-6-PE4E also developed a VLS-like syndrome. The syndrome in rats was prevented by prophylaxis with steroids or nonsteroidal anti-inflammatory drugs (NSAIDs). This may result from the blocking of macrophage cytokine release by these agents. To date, however, no clinical data have documented an elevation in circulating inflammatory cytokines. However, it still appears prudent to select smaller targeted toxins. The role of steroid prophylaxis is less certain, as anecdotal reports suggest either protection or lack of protection in humans.

Other side effects have been reported with targeted toxins. Mild constitutional symptoms can occur when drug is infused rapidly (<30–60 min), including fever, chills, myalgias, headaches, chest discomfort, and transient hypotension. The infusion may be stopped and the patient treated symptomatically. The drug infusion can then be restarted at a slower rate, generally without complications. Corticosteroid prophylaxis appears to prevent these constitutional symptoms. Rarely, patients may have an anaphylactoid response to targeted toxin. As these are proteins, rare hypersensitivity reactions are not unexpected. However, the occurrence of this complication mandates administration of targeted toxins in a setting where diagnosis and treatment of anaphylaxis are routine. Therapy may include 0.3 mL of epinephrine, 100 mg of solumedrol, and 25 mg of diphenhydramine, all given intravenously along with supplemental boluses of intravenous normal saline, nasal prong or face mask oxygen, and continuous cardiac monitoring until resolution of signs and symptoms. Patients should not be retreated with the same targeted toxin, if anaphylaxis is due to the drug, because the reaction is likely to recur with further exposure.

Pharmacology of Targeted Toxins

Recent advances in disease selection and targeted toxin design have led to an improvement in tumor localization and reduced immunogenicity. However, there remain important pharmacologic barriers. The circulating half-life varies with the size of the molecule. Larger molecules have longer half-lives of hours. Smaller molecules, including the single-chain immunotoxins and the cytokine fusion toxins, have shorter half-lives of 30 min. Some of the clearance of the smaller molecules (near 60 kDa) may be through the renal glomerulus. However, most of the clearance of these foreign proteins is likely by the liver or reticuloendothelial system. No clinical protocols have been reported that comprehensively correlate the percentage of extravascular tumor cell saturation with the dose of targeted toxin. The assumption has been made that toxicities, including VLS, hepatotoxicity, or neurotoxicities, reflect the administration of sufficient doses to saturate extravascular tumor sites. In vitro studies with multicellular tumor spheroids and mathematical models using data from other proteins suggest that smaller-sized fusion toxins and permeability enhancers such as cisplatin or hyaluronidase may improve tumor uptake.[269] Clinical responses with targeted toxins in lymphomas and leukemias may be due in part to a significant fraction of circulating malignant stem cells in these diseases.

Targeted toxins have generated humoral immune responses in all recipients, with the exception of patients with CLL. Clearly, the development of neutralizing antibodies is detrimental to targeted toxin antitumor efficacy. In many trials, retreatment has been limited to a few cycles because of the development of neutralizing antibodies. Even when the antibodies generated are non-neutralizing, they may form immune complexes that accelerate clearance of the targeted toxin from the circulation, reducing clinical benefit. Rituximab was administered in combination with LMB-1 in an attempt to reduce the immune response to the immunotoxin.[270] Other methods include coadministration of 15-deoxyspergualin or anti-CTLA4 and have, to date, only been tried in animal models.[270] Immunodominant epitopes may be modified.[272] PEGylation has been tested in vitro and in animal models but not yet in man.[251,273] Finally, the use of human ribonuclease as a toxophore may be an additional method for reducing conjugate immunogenicity.[274]

Conclusions Regarding Targeted Toxins

The potential for targeted toxins, as postulated by Paul Ehrlich one century ago, has not been fully realized to date.[275] Over the last 30 years, with the advent of genetic engineering and advances in receptor physiology, we have progressed to the point where several targeted toxins have demonstrated clinical activity. Over the next decade, further ligand-receptor systems can be defined that extend the applications of targeted toxins to additional disease states. Control of the nonspecific toxicities and immune responses with various prophylactic maneuvers should further improve the therapeutic index of these molecules. Finally, combination therapy trials with cytotoxic chemotherapeutic agents are likely to yield even higher response rates with more durable responses. Combinations of radionuclide conjugates and targeted toxins have demonstrated synergy in heterograft models and deserve further evaluation in the clinic.[276] The next decade should see exciting advances in the development of these reagents and in their application to more effective treatment of patients with cancer.

Selected References

The complete reference list can be found at www.CANCERMEDICINE8.com

1. Kohler G, Milstein C. Continuous cultures of fused cells secreting antibody of predefined specificity. *Nature.* 1975;256:495–497.
4. Harris M. Monoclonal antibodies as therapeutic agents for cancer. *Lancet.* 2004;5:292–302.

5. Dalle S, Theiblemont C, Thomas L, Dumontet D. Monoclonal antibodies in clinical oncology. *Anticancer Agents Med Chem.* 2008;8:523–532.
6. Levy R. Karnofsky lecture: immunotherapy of lymphoma. *J Clin Oncol.* 1999;17:7–12.
7. Press OW. Radiolabeled antibody therapy of B-cell lymphomas. *Semin Oncol.* 1999;26(5 Suppl 14):58–65.
10. Raffeld M, Neckers L, Longo DL, Cossman J. Spontaneous alteration of idiotype in a monoclonal B-cell lymphoma. Escape from detection by anti-idiotype. *N Engl J Med.* 1985;312:1653–1658.
11. Maloney D, Grillo-Lopez A, White C, et al. IDEC-C2B8 (rituximab) anti-CD20 monoclonal antibody therapy in patients with relapsed low-grade non-Hodgkin's lymphoma. *Blood.* 1997;90:2188–2195.
14. Horning SJ. Optimizing rituximab in B-cell lymphoma. *J Clin Oncol.* 2005;23:1056–1058.
18. Schultz H, Bohlius J, Trelle S, et al. Immunochemotherapy with rituximab and overall survival in patients with indolent or mantel cell lymphoma: a systematic review and meta-analysis. *J Natl Cancer Inst.* 2007;9:706–714.
20. Cheson BD, Leonard JP. Monoclonal antibody therapy for B-cell non-Hodgkin's lymphoma. *N Engl J Med.* 2008;359:613–626.
29. Chung C. Managing premedications and the risk for reactions to infusional monoclonal antibody therapy. *The Oncologist.* 2008;13:725–732.
44. Keating M, Flinn I, Jain V, et al. Therapeutic role of alemtuzumab (Campath-1H) in patients who have failed fludarabine: results of a large international study. *Blood.* 1999;99: 3554–3561.
47. Hillmen P, Skotnicki AB, Robak T, et al. Alemtuzumab compared with chlorambucil as first-line therapy for chronic lymphocytic leukemia. *J Clin Oncol.* 2007;25:5616–5623.
54. Mendelsohn J. Targeting the epidermal growth factor receptor for cancer therapy. *J Clin Oncol.* 2002;20:1–13.
58. Saltz LB, Meropol NJ, Loehrer PJ Sr, et al. Phase II trial of cetuximab in patients with refractory colorectal cancer that expresses the epidermal growth factor receptor. *J Clin Oncol.* 2004;22:1201–1208.
62. Cunningham D, Humblet Y, Siena S, et al. Cetuximab monoclonal and cetuximab plus irinotecan in irinotecan refractory metastatic colorectal cancer. *N Engl J Med.* 2004;351:337–345.
64. Lievre A, Bachet JB, Boige V, et al. KRAS mutations as an independent prognostic factor in patients with advanced colorectal cancer treated with cetuximab. *J Clin Oncol.* 2008;26:374–379.
65. Bonner JA, Harari PM, Giralt J, et al. Radiotherapy plus cetuximab for squamous-cell carcinoma of the head and neck. *N Engl J Med.* 2006;354:567–578.
72. Giusti RM, Shastri K, Pilaro AM, et al. US food and drug administration approval: panitumumab for epidermal growth factor receptor-expressing metastatic colorectal carcinoma with progression following fluoropyrimidine-, oxaliplatin-, and irinotecan-containing chemotherapy regimens. *Clin Cancer Res.* 2008;14:1296–1207.
74. Mano M, Humblet Y. Drug insight: panitumumab, a human EGFR-targeted monoclonal antibody with promising clinical activity in colorectal cancer. *Nat Clin Pract Oncol.* 2008;5:415–425.
87. Slamon DJ, Godolphin W, Jones LA, et al. Studies of the HER-2/neu protooncogene in human breast and ovarian cancer. *Science.* 1989;244:707–712.
98. Cobleigh MA, Vogel CL, Tripathy NJ, et al. Multinational study of the efficacy and safety of humanized anti-HER2 monoclonal antibody in women who have HER2-overexpressing metastatic breast cancer that has progressed after chemotherapy for metastatic disease. *J Clin Oncol.* 1999;17:2639–2648.
100. Slamon DJ, Leyland-Jones B, Shak S, et al. Use of chemotherapy plus a monoclonal antibody against HER2 for metastatic breast cancer that overexpresses HER2. *N Engl J Med.* 2001;344:783–792.
102. Dinh P, Azambuja E. de, and Piccart-Gebhart MJ. Trastuzumab for early breast cancer: current status and future directions. *Clin Adv Hematol Oncol.* 2007;5(9):707–717.
112. Nagata Y, Lan KS, Zhou X, et al. PTEN activation contributions to tumor inhibition by trastuzumab, and loss of PTEN predicts trastuzumab resistance in patients. *Cancer Cell.* 2004;6:117–127.
126. Hurwitz H, Fehrenbacher L, Novotny W, et al. Bevacizumab plus irinotecan, fluorouracil, and leucovorin for metastatic colorectal cancer. *N Engl J Med.* 2004;350:2335–2342.
133. Sandler A, Gray R, Perry M, et al. Paclitaxel-carboplatin alone or with bevacizumab for non-small cell lung cancer. *New Engl J Med.* 2006;355:2542–2550.
135. Miller K, Wang M, Gralow J, et al. Paclitaxel plus bevacizumab versus paclitaxel alone for metastatic breast cancer. *N Engl J Med.* 2007;357:2666–2676.
139. Yang JC, Haworth L, Sherry RM, et al. A randomized trial of bevacizumab, an anti-vascular endothelial growth factor antibody, for metastatic renal cancer. *N Engl J Med.* 2003;349:427–434.
153. Jain RK. Physiological barriers to delivery of monoclonal antibodies and other macromolecules in tumors. *Cancer Res.* 1990;50:814s–819s.
175. Sievers EL, Larson RA, Stadtmauer EA, et al. Efficacy and safety of gemtuzumab ozogamicin in patients with CD33-positive acute myeloid leukemia in first relapse. *J Clin Oncol.* 2001;19:3244–3254.
181. Boyd M, Ross SC, Dorrens J et al. Radiation induced biological bystander effect elicited in vitro by targeted radiopharmaceuticals labeled with alph-, beta- and Auger Electron emitting radionuclides. *J Nucl Med.* 2006;47:1007–1015.
183. Zalutsky MR, Lewis J. Radiolabeled antibodies for tumor imaging and therapy. In: Welch MJ, Redvanly C., editors. *Handbook of Radiopharmaceuticals: Radiochemistry and Applications.* Chichester, UK: Wiley; 2003:685–714.
184. Jhanwar YS, Divgi C. Current status of therapy of solid tumors. *J Nucl Med.* 2005;46:141S–150S.
187. Mulford DA, Scheinberg DA, Jurcic JG. The promise of targeted α-particle therapy. *J Nucl Med.* 2005;46:199S–204S.
189. Zalutsky MR, Reardon DA, Pozzi OR, et al. Targeted α-particle radiotherapy with ^{211}At-labeled monoclonal antibodies. *Nucl Med Biol.* 2007;34:779–785.
190. Macklis RM, Pohlman, B. Radioimmunotherapy for non-Hodgkin's lymphoma: a review for radiation oncologists. *Int J Radiat Oncol Biol Phys.* 2007;66:833–841.
191. Witzig TE, Gordon LI, Cabanillas MS, et al. Randomized controlled trial of ytrium-90-labeled ibritumomab tiuxetan radioimmunotherapy versus rituximab immunotherapy for patients with relapsed or refractory, low grade, follicular, or transformed B-cell non-Hodgkin's lymphoma. *J Clin Oncol.* 2002;20:2453–2463.
194. Wiseman GA, Witzig TE. Yttrium-90 (^{90}Y) ibritumomab tiuxetan (Zevalin) induces long-term durable responses in patients with relapsed or refractory B-cell non-Hodgkin's lymphoma. *Cancer Biother Radiopharm.* 2005;20:185–188.
196. Kaminski M, Zelentz AD, Press OW, et al. Pivotal study of iodine 131-tositumomab for chemotherapy refractory low-grade or transformed low-grade B cell non-Hodgkin's lymphomas. *J Clin Oncol.* 2001;19:3908–3911.
197. Fisher RI, Kaminski MS, Wahl RL, et al. Tositumomab and iodine-131 tositumomab produces durable complete remissions in a subset of heavily pretreated patients with low-grade and transformed non-Hodgkin's lymphomas. *J Clin Oncol.* 2005;23: 7565–7573.
209. Reardon DA, Zalutsky MR, Akabani G, et al. A piolot study: ^{131}I-antitenascin monoclonal antibody 81C6 to deliver a 44-Gy resection cavity boost. *Neuro-Oncol.* 2008;10:182–189.
210. Jain M, Venkatraman G, Batra SK. Optimization of radioimmunotherapy of solid tumors: biological impediments and their modulation. *Clin Cancer Res.* 2007;13: 1374–1382.
212. Goldenberg DM, Sharkey RM, Paganelli G, et al. Antibody pretargeting advances cancer radioimmunodetection and radioimmunotherapy. *J Clin Oncol.* 2006;24:823–834.
218. Chatal JF, Campion L, Kraeber-Bodere F, et al. Survival improvement in patients with medullary thyroid carcinoma who undergo pretargeted anti-carcinoembryonic-antigen radioimmunotherapy: a collaborative study with the French Endocrine Tumor Group. *J Clin Oncol.* 2006;24:1705–1711.
222. Zalutsky MR, Reardon DA, Akabano G, et al. Clinical experience with α-particle-emitting ^{211}At: treatment of recurrent brain tumor patients with ^{211}At-labeled chimeric antitenascin monoclonal antibody 81C6. *J Nucl Med.* 2008:49:30–38.
224. Olsen E, Duvic M, Frankel AE, et al. Pivotal phase III trial of two dose levels of denileukin diftitox for the treatment of cutaneous T-cell lymphoma. *J Clin Oncol.* 2001;19:376–388.
227. Dang NH, Hagemeister FB, Pro B, et al. Phase II study of denileukin diftitox for relapsed/refractory B-cell non-Hodgkin's lymphoma. *J Clin Oncol.* 2004;22:4095–4102.
244. Kreitman RJ, Wilson WH, White JD, et al. Phase I trial of recombinant immunotoxin anti-Tac(Fv)-PE38 (LMB-2) in patients with hematologic malignancies. *J Clin Oncol.* 2000;18:1622–1636.
248. Hassan R, Bullock S, Premkumar A, et al. Phase I study of SS1P, a recombinant anti-mesothelin immunotoxin given as a bolus I.V. infusion to patients with mesothelin-expressing mesothelioma, ovarian, and pancreatic cancers. *Clin Cancer Res.* 2007;13: 5144–5149.
255. Kunwar S, Prados MD, Chang SM, et al. Direct intracerebral delivery of cintredekin besudotox (IL13-PE38QQR) in recurrent malignant glioma: a report by the Cintredekin Besudotox Intraparenchymal Study Group. *J Clin Oncol.* 2007;25:837–844.
260. von Minckwitz G, Harder S, Hovelmann S, et al. Phase I clinical study of the recombinant antibody toxin scFv(FRP5)-ETA specific for the ErbB2/HER2 receptor in patients with advanced solid malignancies. *Breast Cancer Res.* 2005;7:R617–R626.
267. Smallshaw JE, Ghetie V, Rizo J, et al. Genetic engineering of an immunotoxin to eliminate pulmonary vascular leak in mice. *Nature Biotech.* 2003;21:387–391.

57 Vaccines and Immunostimulants

James L. Gulley, MD, PhD, FACP ■ Philip M. Arlen, MD ■
James W. Hodge, PhD, MBA ■ Jeffrey Schlom, PhD

The use of therapeutic cancer vaccines for patients with human malignancies has reached several new milestones in scientific discovery. Areas of intense investigation include the development and characterization of (a) tumor-specific antigens (TSAs) or tumor-associated antigens (TAAs) selectively expressed or overexpressed by malignant cells as compared with normal adult tissues; (b) novel vaccine-delivery systems for the induction and/or enhancement of host antitumor immune responses; and (c) cytokines and other immunostimulants to further augment immunogenic properties of vaccine preparations. To date, no therapeutic cancer vaccine has been approved by the U.S. Federal Drug Administration (FDA). Evidence is mounting for patient benefit in the use of several new cancer vaccines and vaccine strategies, used alone or in combinatorial therapeutic approaches. This chapter will review the current status of the field of cancer vaccines and immunostimulants as well as the new approaches being evaluated.

Targets for Vaccine Therapy

Many potential targets for cancer immunotherapy have been identified. It is important to note that when an antigen is a target for vaccine therapy, the activated T cells induced by vaccination recognize peptide-major histocompatibility complex (MHC) complexes of the tumor antigen on the cell surface. T cells do not recognize the surface protein—only the TAA peptide-MHC complex. Thus, targets of vaccine therapy need not be cell-surface proteins. These targets can be grouped into two major categories: TSAs and TAAs.

Tumor-Specific Antigens

TSAs comprise gene products that are uniquely expressed in tumors, such as point-mutated *ras* oncogenes, p53 mutations, anti-idiotype antibodies (Abs), and products of ribonucleic acid (RNA) splice variants and gene translocations.

Three mutations at codon 12 represent the vast majority of *ras* mutations, which are found in ~20% to 30% of all human tumors.[1] Although the *ras* protein is not found on the cell surface, one can envision vaccine therapy directed against peptide-MHC complexes on the cell surface. Indeed, there are ongoing clinical trials in pancreatic carcinoma that target *ras*.[2,3]

B-cell lymphomas overexpress a single immunoglobulin variant on their cell surface; therefore, each B-cell lymphoma displays a unique target for immunotherapy.[4-6] The gene products of RNA splice variants and deoxyribonucleic acid (DNA) translocations also represent unique fusion proteins that can be specific targets for immunotherapy, including c-erb-B2 RNA splice variants and the bcr/abl product of DNA translocation of chronic myelogenous leukemia.

Tumor-Associated Antigens

TAAs can be categorized into four major groups: oncofetal antigens, oncogene products, tissue-lineage antigens, and viral antigens. Oncofetal antigens, normally found during fetal development, are greatly down-regulated after birth. This class of antigens, which includes carcinoembryonic antigen (CEA), the breast cancer mucin MUC-1, and prostate-specific membrane antigen (PSMA), is often overexpressed in tumors as compared with normal tissues. Two important considerations must be made when targeting oncofetal antigens with vaccines: (a) because these antigens are expressed in fetal tissue, a state of thymic and/or peripheral tolerance to them in the host may exist and (b) immunity to these antigens following vaccination may result in detrimental autoimmunity.

Oncogene and suppressor gene products, such as nonmutated HER-2/*neu* and p53, are analogous to oncofetal antigens in that they can be overexpressed in tumors and may be expressed in some fetal tissues. Similarly, telomerase, an enzyme important in cellular replication and chromosomal stability, is overexpressed in malignant cells as compared with most normal cells. Epitopes derived from human telomerase have been reported and presumably may be overexpressed by neoplastic cells.[7]

Tissue-lineage antigens such as prostate-specific antigen (PSA) and the melanocyte antigens such as MART-1/Melan A, tyrosinase, gp100, and TRP-1/gp75 are expressed in a tumor of a given type and the normal tissue from which it is derived. Tissue-lineage antigens are potentially useful targets for immunotherapy if the normal organ/tissue in which they are expressed is not essential, such as the prostate, breast, or melanocyte. Several viruses are associated with the etiology of some cancers. An excellent example of this is the connection between human papillomavirus (HPV) and cervical cancer. This has led to FDA approval of the preventive HPV vaccine for cervical cancer.

Types of Vaccines

Numerous vaccine-delivery systems have been analyzed in experimental models and many of these are now being evaluated in the clinic (Table 57-1). Each of these systems has advantages and disadvantages; moreover, some of these modalities may eventually prove to be the most beneficial when used in combination or in tandem.

Whole Tumor Cell Vaccines

The major advantage of using whole tumor cell vaccines is that several TSAs or TAAs, some identified and some as yet

Table 57-1 **Cancer Vaccine Modalities**

Tumor cells
• Allogeneic whole tumor cells (irradiated)
• Gene-modified allogeneic tumor cells (GM-CSF)
• In situ autologous whole tumor cell vaccine: direct injection of tumor with vector expressing cytokine or costimulatory gene
Protein-based
• Peptide
• Agonist peptide
• Anti-idiotype MAb
• Whole protein
Vector-based
• Viral vectors
Replication-competent: Vaccinia, adenovirus
Replication-defective: MVA, avipox: fowlpox, canarypox
• Yeast/bacterial vectors
• Saccharomyces cerevisiae
• Listeria
• Salmonella
Plasmid DNA
Antigen-presenting cells
• Dendritic cells
Protein/peptide pulsed
Loaded with tumor lysates
Fused with tumor cells

undefined, may be present in the vaccine preparation. The two types of whole tumor cell vaccine platforms being examined clinically are: (a) autologous (ie, manipulating the tumor from a patient into a vaccine for that patient) and (b) allogeneic, in which tumor cells from other patients, usually from established tumor cell lines, are used. Preparing an autologous tumor cell vaccine requires an enormous amount of effort, as fresh tumor needs to be obtained at surgery and prepared in a similar manner for each patient. Due to considerable variability of tumors among patients, and costs associated with custom vaccine production, most current whole tumor cell vaccine approaches have centered on the use of allogeneic cell lines and cell banks.[8-13]

Allogeneic tumor cell vaccines, which usually employ one or more tumor cell lines, are relatively easy to prepare compared with autologous vaccines. Moreover, the cell lines used in the preparations can be infected with vectors that express cytokine genes such as granulocyte-macrophage colony-stimulating factor (GM-CSF)[14] or other immunostimulatory transgenes[15] to enhance the immunogenicity of the tumor cell. A disadvantage of allogeneic vaccines is that because allogeneic cells are used, alloimmunity to nontumor components may develop, potentially skewing the desired immune T-cell response. However, this was not the case in early clinical trials, including studies using oncolysates (ie, tumor cell preparations that had been infected with vaccinia virus and then lysed in an effort to enhance their immunogenicity).[16] More recent studies used cell lines infected with GM-CSF with some success for pancreatic cancer, non–small cell lung cancer, and renal cell carcinoma.[11-14,17,18]

Direct Injection of Cytokine Genes or Costimulatory Molecule Genes into Tumor (In Situ Autologous Whole Tumor Cell Vaccines) ■ Two signals are required for the efficient activation of T cells. The first signal is mediated through a peptide-MHC complex on the cell surface of the antigen-presenting cell (APC), which binds to the T-cell receptor (TCR) on the surface of the T cell. The second signal involves the interaction of a T-cell costimulatory molecule on the surface of the APC with its ligand on the surface of the T cell. To date, the most studied of the T-cell costimulatory molecules is B7-1, which interacts with two ligands on the T-cell surface: CD28 for up-regulation of T-cell function and CTLA-4 for down-regulation of T-cell function. Numerous preclinical studies show that the addition of B7-1 to a weakly immunogenic tumor will make it more immunogenic.[15] This phenomenon has also occurred when other costimulatory molecules, such as intercellular adhesion molecule (ICAM)-1 and lymphocyte function-associated antigen (LFA)-3, have been added to tumors. Thus, one can envision the direct injection of a vector containing a costimulatory molecule into a tumor mass to induce an antitumor immune response. It should be pointed out that a costimulatory molecule must be on the surface of the tumor to induce an immune response, but it does not necessarily have to be present on the tumor for the T cell to kill the tumor cell. The advantage of this direct-injection approach is that the "vaccine" is the patient's own tumor, which may express a unique TSA or TAA profile. In clinical studies, vaccinia- and avipox-based recombinants expressing the B7-1 costimulatory molecule have been directly injected into melanoma or carcinoma lesions.[19] A clinical study has been reported with interesting findings in which recombinant vectors containing a triad of costimulatory molecules (B7-1, ICAM-1, and LFA-3; designated TRICOM) were directly injected into melanoma tumor lesions.[20] Cytokines can also be introduced into the tumor mass using vectors as delivery vehicles, as in the case of a recombinant vaccinia virus expressing GM-CSF directly injected into melanoma lesions.[21] Vectors encoding multiple costimulatory molecules as well as cytokines have been administered intratumorally in preclinical models[22,23] and in prostate tumor clinically.[24]

Peptides

Most peptides that are used to induce an immune response are from TSAs or TAAs and are ~8 to 11 amino acids in length. These peptides can bind with the appropriate class of the MHC molecule on the APC surface. These peptide-MHC complexes will then interact with the TCR to activate $CD8^+$ T cells. In experimental models, $CD8^+$ T cells, termed cytotoxic T lymphocytes (CTLs), are usually responsible for lytic destruction of tumors. These MHC-restricted responses are thus effective only if the appropriate MHC allele is present in a patient. The most studied MHC restriction element in the human population is the MHC class I allele, HLA-A2, which is found in ~50% of the Caucasian population. Many clinical trials are being carried out in individuals who possess the HLA-A2 allele; thus, T-cell responses to a particular defined peptide can be quantified.

Using peptides as immunogens has some advantages: (a) whole proteins may contain parts of the molecule that are shared with normal cellular proteins, and the use of peptides minimizes the potential for induction of autoimmunity; (b) preparation is relatively easy and affordable; (c) because the immunogen is extremely well-defined, the immune response can be analyzed in several ways and quantitated; (d) tetramers, which are molecules that contain specific peptides bound to MHC components, can be used to bind to, and isolate, antigen-specific T cells induced and amplified in the host; (e) tumors can be stripped of peptide-MHC complexes, and those peptides displayed on the surface of tumors can be identified; and (f) peptides can be modified to be more immunogenic in the generation of peptide agonists.

Agonist Peptides ■ Peptide agonists fall into two general categories. In the first category, amino acids of the peptide that bind to the MHC are modified. More vigorous MHC binding (ie, higher affinity for the MHC molecule) often leads to the generation of a more vigorous T-cell response. An example of this is the alteration in the gp100 melanoma peptide.[25] The second category of agonist has been termed a TCR agonist. In this case, an amino acid of the peptide that interacts with the TCR on the T cell is modified; this can also result in a more vigorous induction of the T-cell response. An example of this is the generation of the TCR agonist for CEA.[26]

The same property that makes a peptide vaccine attractive—its specificity—can also be a disadvantage. For example, a CTL epitope peptide may induce a CTL response that is short-lived because of the lack of help provided by helper peptides. Moreover, peptides are useful only in the vaccination of patients who have that specific allele (eg, for only ≤50% of the population who have the HLA-A2 allele for an HLA-A2-reactive peptide). Combinations of antigenic peptides with reactivities for multiple HLA alleles would circumvent this limitation. A large clinical experience in the use of peptides as cancer vaccines is now emerging. Some peptides under study include HPV,[27] *ras*,[28,29] HER-2/*neu*,[30] MAGE,[31] MART-1, tyrosinase,[32] gp100,[25,33] CEA,[34] MUC-1,[35] and PSMA,[36,37] among others.[38]

Anti-idiotypes

The idiotypic network is involved in the control of immune regulation. B-cell lymphomas present unique immunoglobulins on their cell surface, which make exquisite targets for immunotherapy. For this malignancy, anti-idiotype monoclonal Ab (MAb) vaccines have been quite successful clinically.[4,5,39-44] But the specificity inherent in these vaccine strategies is both an advantage and a disadvantage; different B-cell lymphomas will display unique idiotypes on their cell surface, making their preparation for each patient labor-intensive.

Vectors

Vectors are among the more flexible means of vaccine delivery. Several major categories of both viral and bacterial vectors are now in use in the clinic (Table 57-1). Each vector category and type has its own potential advantages and disadvantages. Review articles have been published on the potential merits of these vectors.[45–51]

In general, the advantages of a vector-based vaccine are that (a) either the entire tumor antigen gene or parts of that gene can be inserted; (b) multiple genes (including genes for costimulatory molecules and cytokines) can be inserted into some types of vectors; (c) the relative cost of production is low compared to the preparation and purification of proteins or whole tumor cell vaccines; and (d) many vectors have the ability to infect professional APCs so that the antigens they express can be processed. The disadvantage of some, but not all, vectors is the development of host-induced immunity to the vector itself, thus limiting its continued use.

Replication-Competent Vectors ■ One of the most studied groups of all vaccine vectors is the poxvirus group. Vaccinia virus, which was derived from a benign pox disease in cows, has been administered to >1 billion people and is responsible for the worldwide eradication of smallpox.[52] As a result, smallpox vaccinations in the United States and most Western countries were halted ~33 years ago. However, most cancer patients are older than 33 and, therefore, have some level of preexisting immunity to vaccinia virus. For this reason, recombinant vaccinia viruses cannot be given multiple times in vaccine protocols. Early studies of recombinant vaccinia viruses containing human immunodeficiency virus (HIV) transgenes showed that vaccinia virus–immune patients could not make as potent an immune response as vaccinia virus–naïve patients.[53] Subsequent studies show that when higher doses of recombinant vaccinia viruses are used, vaccinia virus–immune patients can mount a vigorous response to the transgene after vaccination. However, this response is greatly diminished at the second and third vaccination.[54] Thus, preclinical and recent clinical studies[38,55] show that optimal use of recombinant vaccinia viruses may be to prime the immune response, followed by boost vaccinations with other vectors such as replication-defective avipox vectors, peptides, or proteins. A major advantage of using vaccinia virus or the replication-incompetent avipox is that large amounts of foreign DNA can be inserted into the vector. Another major advantage is that proteins expressed in vaccinia virus are more immunogenic than the native protein, which is most likely a result of the inflammatory responses triggered against highly immunogenic vaccinia virus proteins. Other advantages of poxviruses such as vaccinia virus, modified vaccinia Ankara (MVA), and avipox viruses (see below) include wide host range, stable recombinants, accurate replication, and efficient posttranslational processing of the inserted gene. Several clinical trials with recombinant vaccinia containing TAAs such as CEA,[55] MUC-1, PSA,[56] and HPV[27,57] have been completed and others are ongoing.[38,58,59]

Adenovirus has also been proposed as a vector in recombinant vaccine design because its viral genome can be altered to accept foreign genes that are stably integrated. Furthermore, to produce recombinant adenovectors, endogenous viral DNA sequences are typically deleted from replication-competent regions, which results in an attenuated form of the virus with potentially improved safety. In preclinical studies, immunization of mice with a recombinant adenovirus expressing a model TAA led to the induction of an antigen-specific CTL response and regression of established pulmonary metastases. In clinical trials, recombinant adenoviruses encoding TAAs, TSAs, and/or cytokines are being utilized systemically and intratumorally.[60–63] Recombinant adenoviruses may eventually be combined in diversified prime-and-boost protocols.

Replication-Defective Viral Vectors ■ The poxvirus family contains the replication-incompetent MVA, a derivative of vaccinia virus.[45] A major attribute of this vector is its potential lack of toxicity, because it can infect mammalian cells but cannot replicate. This MVA is thought of as a safer alternative to the smallpox vaccine.[64] Recombinant MVA vectors encoding the tumor antigen MUC-1 along with the cytokine interleukin (IL)-2 are currently in phase 2 clinical trials.[65] Highlighting the safety of this vector system, MVA vectors encoding the tumor antigen 5T4 are being given concurrently with chemotherapy in colorectal cancer patients.[66]

Other replication-defective members of the poxvirus family are the avipox vectors (fowlpox and canarypox/ALVAC).[46] These avipox vectors infect human cells and express their transgenes for 2 to 3 weeks before undergoing cell death; they are incapable of reinfecting cells. Recent clinical studies have shown that avipox-based CEA vectors can be given to patients numerous times with a resulting increase in CEA-specific T-cell responses.[38,67] Avipox vectors encoding the melanoma antigen gp100 or MAGE are being examined in clinical trials.[68,69]

Yeast and Bacterial Vectors ■ One advantage of recombinant *Saccharomyces cerevisiae* as a vaccine vehicle is its lack of toxicity. Besides being inherently nonpathogenic, this particular species of yeast can be heat-killed before administration and has been shown to be safe in humans in several clinical trials, with maximum tolerated dose not reached.[51,70,71] *S. cerevisiae* can be easily engineered to express one or more antigens in large quantities, can be propagated and purified rapidly, and is very stable.[72] In addition, recombinant yeast has been shown to induce a robust host immune response to non-self-antigens.[51,72–74] These characteristics make *S. cerevisiae* a potential component of cancer immunotherapy protocols. Recombinant yeast vectors expressing the melanoma antigen MART-1,[75] the cancer testes antigen NY-ESO-1,[76] *ras*,[2] and CEA[77] are being examined preclinically and clinically.

Bacterial vectors, such as *Salmonella*[78,79] and *Listeria*,[50] have the advantage of tropism for professional APCs, such as macrophages. While these vectors are potentially virulent in humans, several attenuated strains have been developed for human use. From a clinical perspective, both recombinant *Salmonella*- and recombinant *Listeria monocytogenes*-based vectors may be administered orally.

Plasmid DNA ■ These vectors represent a potentially powerful vaccine-delivery system.[80] Polynucleotide vaccines are easy to prepare, but the mode of action of these vectors in inducing an immune response is not fully understood because most studies have involved intramuscular inoculations, and it is not known how antigens get to professional APCs. Many preclinical studies using infectious disease agents and cancer antigens have been carried out with DNA vectors. Clinical trials are under way using DNA vaccines encoding melanoma antigens such as MART-1,[81] gp100,[82] and PSA.[83]

Dendritic Cell Vaccines

The DC is considered the most potent APC and, therefore, one of the most attractive means of immunization.[84,85] DCs can be employed by (a) loading with a peptide, protein, or anti-idiotype Ab, (b) infecting with a viral vector, (c) loading with apoptotic bodies from tumor cells, or (d) fusing with a tumor cell.[86-89] The major disadvantages of this approach are the great cost and effort involved. Large amounts of peripheral blood mononuclear cells (PBMCs) must be obtained from patients via leukapheresis. The PBMCs must then be cultured for several days in the presence of cytokines such as GM-CSF, IL-4, and/or TNF-α, and then reinfused into the patient. This must be done for each patient. A particularly interesting strategy involves immunization with autologous DCs loaded ex vivo with a recombinant fusion protein consisting of the tumor antigen prostatic acid phosphatase (PAP) linked to GM-CSF.[90] This therapy is currently in late-stage phase 3 clinical trials.

Immunostimulants/Cytokines

An expanding principle in the field of immunology and immunotherapy is that DCs are central to the initiation of the adaptive immune response. But to be functionally useful for this essential role, DCs require prior activation by elements of the innate immune response. Thus, the DC is thought to be the cellular bridge linking innate and adaptive immunity. If therapeutic strategies can be developed to augment activation and maturation of DCs, it is conceivable that the immunogenicity of a weak TAA could be improved. One way to achieve this outcome is through the use of immunostimulants, which will likely play an important role in virtually all aspects of immunotherapy, especially cancer vaccine development.

TAAs and TSAs are by definition weak immunogens because tumors develop, persist, and grow in the presence of an intact immune system, as described earlier. This was originally thought to be due to tolerance mechanisms. However, there is considerable support for the idea that a danger signal is most important for initiating an immune response.[91] Evidence shows that a poor immunogen, such as a TAA, can be rendered more immunogenic by either its mode of presentation to the immune system or its use in combination with an immunostimulant. The term immunostimulant encompasses several classes of agents that can work in a variety of ways. Proteins and peptides rapidly dissipate from the injection site if administered alone. Conventional adjuvants, such as incomplete Freund's adjuvant (IFA), will allow the immunogen to be maintained at the injection site (the so-called depot effect) so that infiltrating APCs and effector cells can initiate a more vigorous immune response. Immunostimulants also work by crossing membrane barriers. In this case, proteins must be taken up by professional APCs and presented in the context of MHC molecules for effective presentation to the immune system. Adjuvants with lipophilic components and liposomes[92] facilitate this process.

Newer adjuvant-like molecules are also being evaluated. For example, chitosan is a nontoxic, biodegradable natural polysaccharide; in preclinical studies, it has been shown to both (a) enhance humoral and cell-mediated immune responses to protein vaccination and (b) enhance the immune-stimulating properties of GM-CSF.[93,94]

Microbial products such as those present in certain adjuvants (ie, IFA), BCG, and even poxviruses also are potent activators of DCs, partly because they contain agonists of toll-like receptors (TLRs). TLRs are expressed by DCs (and other innate immune cell types) and comprise a family of ~10 to 15 receptors that bind to a number of different microbial components, namely lipopolysaccharide (LPS), RNA species, and CpG motifs.[95,96] Activation of DCs via their TLRs augments expression of adhesion, chemokine, and chemokine receptor molecules, which, in turn, regulate cellular trafficking to sites of inflammation and pathogenic encounters. Thus, the biological consequences of TLR engagement lead to inflammation, characterized by the recruitment of key immune and nonimmune effector cells to mediate pathogen destruction. In regard to TLR agonists, CpG motifs constitute the most studied of these sequences.[97-100] Purified CpG sequences have been admixed with peptide immunogens to enhance immune responses in preclinical studies. Clinical studies are now in progress to explore their utility in cancer immunotherapy.[99] It is thought that some of the immunogenic properties of vectors such as BCG, poxviruses, and plasmid DNA constructs can be credited to the fact that they also contain numerous CpG motifs.

In addition, certain cytokines and chemokines have been shown to enhance the level of APC and/or effector cell function either locally or systemically. For example, GM-CSF has been reported to enhance antigen-specific T-cell responses, delayed-type hypersensitivity reactions, and antitumor responses.[101-108] It should be noted, however, that GM-CSF most likely acts indirectly by recruiting and activating host APC populations, such as macrophages and DCs.[109,110] Increased APC capacity correlates with heightened levels of MHC, adhesion, and costimulatory molecules, which seem to improve immune system interactions overall. Local GM-CSF at the vaccination site has been shown to increase the infiltration of DCs in regional lymph nodes.[103] Clinical studies using GM-CSF along with protein immunogens have shown an enhancement of the antigen-specific immune response.[39,111] Flt-3L administration has been shown to enhance the number of DCs systemically, both in animal models and clinically.[112,113] Finally, several cytokines and chemokines have been shown to play a critical role in enhancing T-cell function.[114-118] The most studied of these is IL-2.[119,120] When used as a single agent, IL-2 has been shown to have antitumor effects in melanoma and renal cell carcinoma patients[119,121] and, as recently reported, to enhance the effectiveness of melanoma-based peptide vaccines.[25] Other cytokines, such as IL-7, IL-12, and IL-15, have been shown to enhance T-cell responses and antitumor activity in experimental models and may have more potential clinical utility than IL-2.[115,122-124]

Vaccine Clinical Trials

It has been demonstrated that patients with advanced cancers can be administered vaccines directed against self-antigens, which are overexpressed on tumors as compared with normal tissues, and mount an immune response to those self-antigens. Overall, the actual method of presentation of the self-antigen to the immune system via the vaccine has proven to be an important factor in breaking tolerance. As described earlier, strategies employing modified whole tumor cells, peptide-pulsed DCs, recombinant vectors, altered peptides, and vaccines given in combination with cytokines and/or T-cell costimulatory molecules are now playing an important role in clinical trial design and development. Following is a partial description of previous and ongoing vaccine clinical trials.

Melanoma

The vast majority of vaccine clinical trials have been conducted in patients with melanoma because: (a) interferon (IFN) and IL-2 have both shown clinical responses in melanoma, indicating that the immune response to melanoma-associated antigens may be involved in therapeutic responses; (b) melanoma lesions often are readily accessible and thus can be studied for immune infiltrate; (c) cells from melanoma lesions can be grown in culture to obtain both tumor cells and tumor-infiltrating lymphocytes (TILs) for adoptive transfer; (d) numerous melanoma-associated antigens have been identified; and (e) of all solid tumor types, perhaps the most potent in vitro immune responses are directed against melanoma-associated antigens. Previous adoptive transfer clinical studies with TILs demonstrated that immune T cells directed against melanoma-associated antigens, in the presence of IL-2, can kill melanoma cells in situ.[125-130]

Clinical trials have been conducted using various peptides derived from melanoma-associated antigens, including tyrosinase, MART-1, gp100, Melan-A (a modified gp100 epitope[131]), and members of the MAGE family.[131-136] Vaccination-induced immune responses as well as clinical benefits were reported. Some of these reported strategies have not evidenced an ability to induce immune responses to the vaccine.[137] Newer approaches have combined these peptides with GM-CSF emulsified in Montanide ISA-51.[138] Another peptide approach is vaccination with autologous tumor-derived heat shock protein/peptide complexes.[139] Immune responses and clinical responses have also been observed using melanoma peptide vaccination in conjunction with anti-CTLA-4,[140] melanoma peptide-pulsed DCs,[85,133] tumor RNA–transfected DCs,[141] and intratumoral administration of autologous DCs.[142] A randomized phase 3 study showed no benefit using an autologous peptide-pulsed DC vaccine compared to dacarbazine in first-line treatment of patients with metastatic melanoma.[143]

Recombinant viral vectors encoding transgenes of melanoma TAAs have been utilized clinically, including an adenovirus encoding MART-1 and gp100[144] and an ultraviolet-inactivated nonreplicating recombinant vaccinia virus encoding epitopes from Melan-A, MART-1, gp100, and tyrosinase. Immunization with plasmid DNAs encoding either gp100[82] or tyrosinase[145] have not demonstrated significant clinical responses.

Several clinical studies have employed autologous melanoma cells as vaccine. Clinical responses were observed when these melanoma-cell vaccines were preceded by cyclophosphamide.[146,147] Clinical responses were also observed when autologous melanoma cells were transduced with GM-CSF and given as vaccine.[148,149] In addition, intratumoral administration of recombinant vaccinia encoding GM-CSF in patients with cutaneous melanoma has been reported to induce antitumor immune responses.[19,20,150]

Several randomized phase 2 trials have been carried out using either autologous[151,152] or allogeneic[153,154] melanoma vaccine in patients with resected melanoma (Table 57-2). In these trials, there is evidence of improved disease-free survival in the vaccine arm vs control or no-treatment groups.

Recent research indicates that immunization with hybrids of tumor cells and APCs can induce protective immunity and rejection of established tumors in various rodent models.[86,155,156] Novel clinical trial strategies incorporating DC-based vaccines have recently been reported.[157-159] Purified hybrids from the fusion of DCs and tumor cells (dendritomas) have been shown to be safe and to induce both immunological and clinical responses when combined with low-dose IL-2.[158]

Gastrointestinal Carcinoma

A prospective randomized-controlled phase 3 clinical trial was carried out in 254 patients with stage II and stage III colon cancer using autologous tumor cell vaccine with BCG post-surgery. A 5.3-year median follow-up showed 40 recurrences in the control group and 25 in the vaccine group. The vaccine showed a statistically significant recurrence-free survival in patients with surgically resected stage II colon cancer, but not stage III colon cancer.[160] Indeed, further follow-up demonstrated a significant survival benefit in the vaccine arm over surgery alone (Table 57-2).[161]

Several clinical trials have been conducted employing CEA-based vaccines. Results of vaccination of patients with recombinant vaccinia virus,[54] recombinant avipox virus,[67,162,163] or a prime with recombinant vaccinia (rV)-CEA and multiple boosts with avipox-CEA[38] have demonstrated the generation of CEA-specific immune responses in patients with advanced gastrointestinal (GI) carcinomas and other CEA-expressing carcinomas. A trial using both vaccinia- and avipox-CEA vaccines containing TRICOM has suggested improved survival in patients receiving the prime-and-boost regimen plus GM-CSF (Table 57-2); 40% had stable disease for at least 4 months.[38] CEA peptide-pulsed DCs have also been employed in clinical studies using a modified CEA agonist peptide.[164] Two of 12 patients with advanced cancers experienced tumor regression, one patient had a mixed response, and two had stable disease. Clinical responses correlated with the expansion of CEA-specific T cells.

Clinical studies have also been carried out using anti-idiotype antibodies directed against anti-CEA MAbs. These studies have demonstrated the induction of immune responses,[165,166] slowed disease progression, and prolonged survival.[167] Clinical studies are also ongoing in patients with GI carcinomas using a viral vector vaccine employing p53 as the target antigen.[168] MVA containing the gene for an oncofetal antigen found on many tumors (5T4) has been tested in a variety of cancers (TroVax, Oxford, UK). In a trial of 22 patients with metastatic colorectal cancer, immune responses appeared to correlate with disease control, which was seen up to 18 months in patients with immune responses.[66,169,170]

Allogeneic whole tumor cell vaccines modified to secrete GM-CSF have also been employed in a phase 1 trial in patients with pancreatic cancer. Evidence of vaccine-induced immune responses was observed as measured by delayed-type hypersensitivity.[12,171] A 60-patient phase 2 study of the same vaccine in the adjuvant setting showed that post-chemotherapy induction of mesothelin-specific CD8 cells correlated with progression-free survival.[172] The median overall survival was about 26 months compared with 21 months for chemotherapy alone in this same patient population at the same institution. A phase 1/2 telomerase peptide vaccine study also indicated that immune responses were correlated with prolonged survival.[173]

Breast Cancer

Several different breast cancer– and carcinoma-associated antigens have been employed as targets for vaccine clinical trials in patients with advanced breast cancer. sTn is a glycopeptide contained in carcinoma-associated mucin. Patients were randomized to receive vaccine (sTn coupled to keyhole limpet hemocyanin [KLH]) with or without cyclophosphamide. Patients treated with vaccine and cyclophosphamide were reported to have lived significantly longer[174] than those treated with the same vaccine without cyclophosphamide (12.6 months; $P = 0.017$) (Table 57-2). Additionally, sTn KLH vaccine has been administered to breast and ovarian cancer patients after an autologous stem cell transplant following high-dose chemotherapy. Vaccinated patients appeared more likely to survive and less likely to relapse, but further studies are required.[175] Several clinical trials have been carried out using MUC-1 as a target,[176] including the use of MUC-1 peptides,[177,178] recombinant vaccinia virus encoding MUC-1 and IL-2,[179] MVA expressing human MUC-1,[180] and mannan-MUC-1 fusion protein.[181] In other trials, this MUC-1 fusion protein induced greater immune responses when administered with cyclophosphamide.[182] In addition, a clinical trial is combining a MUC-1-containing vaccine with docetaxel.[183] In studies carried out with the HER-2/*neu* peptides with or without GM-CSF, patients with breast cancer were able to generate HER-2-specific immune responses.[184–186] Recent studies evaluating E75, an immunogenic HLA-A2-restricted peptide derived from the HER-2/*neu* protein, have demonstrated this vaccine's activity in patients with breast cancer.[187–192]

Fusion-cell (DCs and tumor cells) vaccination of patients with metastatic breast and renal cancers was shown to induce both immunological and clinical responses.[193] An anti-idiotype antibody that mimics the human milk-fat globule antigen has also been utilized as a breast cancer vaccine in conjunction with autologous stem cell transplantation. In that study, the 3-year overall survival rate was 48% (95% confidence interval [CI], 32-64%), whereas the progression-free survival rate was 32% (95% CI, 19-45%).[194]

Prostate Cancer

Prostatic acid phosphatase (PAP), which is expressed on over 95% of prostate cancer cells, has been used as a target of the vaccine sipuleucel-T (PAP-GM-

Table 57-2 ■ Cancer Vaccine Trials with Reported Evidence of Survival Benefit

Tumor	Vaccine Type	Comment	Trial Phase	(*n*)	Survival Benefit	Ref.
Prostate	Dendritic cell	APC loaded with PAP-GM-CSF	3	127	Median overall survival of 25.9 months in vaccine arm vs 22 months in placebo arm (*P* = 0.02). At 36 months 33% of patients in the vaccine arm were alive vs 11% of placebo patients (*P* = 0.003)	294
Prostate	Dendritic cell	APC loaded with PAP-GM-CSF	3	127	Median time to disease progression for vaccine was 11.7 weeks vs 10.0 weeks for placebo (*P* = 0.052)	195
Prostate	Vectors (viral)	rV/rF-PSA	2	64	78.1% clinical progression-free survival	295
Prostate	Allogeneic whole tumor cell	BCG included	2	28	Median time to disease progression was 58 weeks in the vaccine arm vs historical control values of 28 weeks	199
Prostate	Allogeneic whole tumor cell	GM-CSF modified	2	55	Median survival was 34.9 in the high dose vaccine arm vs 24.0 months in the control low dose vaccine arm	11
NSCLC	Autologous whole tumor cell	GM-CSF modified	1/2	83	Median survival of 17 months (95% CI) vs historical controls	296
NSCLC	Allogeneic whole tumor cell	B7-1 modified	2	19	Median survival for all vaccine patients is 18 months (90% CI vs control)	297
Colon	Vectors (viral)	MVA-5T4	1/2	17	Periods of disease stabilization ranging from 3 to 18 months were observed in 5 of 17 patients	169
Colon	Autologous whole tumor cell	BCG modified	3	254	5.8-year overall survival in Dukes stage II: significantly improved overall survival adjuvant to surgery vs surgery alone (*P* < 0.05)	161
Breast	Protein	STn (KLH modified)	1/2	40	Median survival of 19.7 months (vaccine with cyclophosphamide) vs 12.6 months (without cyclophosphamide; *P* = 0.017)	175
Ovarian	Anti-idiotypic antibody	CA125 antigen	1/2	119	Median survival: 19.4 months for vaccine arm vs 4.9 months for control arm (*P* = 0.0001)	229
CEA-expressing tumors	Vectors (viral)	Vaccinia-CEA avipox-CEA	1/2	57	Overall survival for patients in vaccine arm was 56% for patients in the vaccinia prime/avipox boost arm (VAAA) vs 11% for patients in the avipox arm (AAAV) (*P* = 0.05)	298
CEA-expressing tumors	Vectors (viral)	Fowlpox/vaccinia-CEA(6D)/TRICOM	1/2	58	60% of patients with stable disease for >6 months. Increased 2-year survival with patients in vaccine + GM-CSF arm	38
Pancreatic	Peptide	Telomerase peptide with GM-CSF	1/2	48	Median survival for the intermediate-dose group was 8.6 months, significantly longer for the low- (*P* = 0.006) and high- (*P* = 0.05) dose groups. One-year survival for evaluable patients in the intermediate-dose group was 25%	173
Melanoma	Allogeneic whole tumor cell	BCG modified	2	194	Median survival: 37 months for vaccine arm vs 17 months for no-treatment arm (*P* = 0.0277)	151
Melanoma	Vectors (viral)	Vaccinia cell lysates	3	700	10-year survival: 53.4% in vaccine arm vs 41% for no-treatment arm (*P* = 0.68)	299
Melanoma	Dendritic cell	DC loaded with autologous tumor	2	20	48% progression-free survival (interim analysis)	300
Melanoma	Dendritic cell	DC loaded with autologous tumor	2	19	Survival significantly increased over that noted with control patients (*P* < 0.001)	301
Melanoma	Autologous whole tumor cell	Unmodified	2	112	5-year overall survival: 39% in vaccine arm vs 19% for nonvaccine arm (*P* = 0.0009)	153
Melanoma	Autologous whole tumor cell	Unmodified	2	739	5-year overall survival stage III: 49% in vaccine arm vs 20% for nonvaccine arm (*P* = 0.0001)	302
Melanoma	Peptide	Unmodified	1/2	44	22% of patients relapse-free for >42 months	303
Renal	Autologous whole tumor cell	Unmodified	3	558	5-year survival: 78% in vaccine arm vs 67% for no-treatment arm (*P* = 0.02)	304
Renal	Autologous whole tumor cell	Lysate	2	236	5-year overall survival: 86% in vaccine arm vs 71% for no-treatment arm (*P* = 0.0059)	305
HCC	Autologous whole tumor cell	Unmodified	2	24	2-year recurrence of 29% in vaccine arm vs 54% in the control arm (*P* < 0.05)	306
Sarcomas	Autologous whole tumor cell	IFN-γ treated	1/2	20	Progression-free survival at 14 months: 95% in vaccine arm	307

Abbreviations: A, avipox-CEA; BCG, bacillus Calmette-Guérin; CA125, cancer antigen 125; CEA, carcinoembryonic antigen; CI, confidence interval; DC, dendritic cell; GM-CSF, granulocyte-macrophage colony-stimulating factor; HCC, hepatocellular carcinoma; IFN, interferon; MVA, modified vaccinia strain Ankara; NSCLC, non-small cell lung carcinoma; PAP, prostatic acid phosphatase; PSA, prostate-specific antigen; STn (KLH), sialyl-Tn (keyhole limpet hemocyanin); TRICOM, triad of costimulatory molecules; V, vaccinia-CEA.

CSF-pulsed APCs). A phase 3 trial of sipuleucel-T has recently been completed in patients with castration-resistant prostate cancer (CRPC). There was a trend to improve time to progression in patients treated with vaccine vs placebo ($P = 0.054$).[195] Moreover, there was statistically significant improvement in overall survival with vaccine (25.9 months in the treatment arm vs 21.4 months on placebo, $P = 0.01$). However, as overall survival was only a secondary end point in this trial, a confirmatory phase 3 study with overall survival as the primary end point is currently under way.

GVAX, a GM-CSF-secreting vaccine, is an admixture of prostate cancer cell lines PC-3 and LNCaP that have been transduced with a replication-defective retrovirus containing cDNA for GM-CSF. In two separate multicenter phase 2 trials, patients with asymptomatic CRPC given GVAX had a median survival of 26.2 to 35.0 months.[11,196] By estimating predicted survival based on a commonly used nomogram,[197] patients in both trials exceeded anticipated survival by >6 months.[198] However, two overall survival end point phase 3 trials in patients with metastatic CRPC failed to meet their primary end point.

A phase 2 trial of another whole tumor cell vaccine, Ony-P1, has been completed in nonmetastatic CRPC.[199] Eleven of 26 patients showed a statistically significant prolonged decrease in PSA doubling time, with no patient having a statistically significant increase in PSA doubling time post-vaccination. Mean time to metastatic disease was 58 weeks. Immunologic profiles correlated with PSA velocity responses by artificial neural network analysis. A multicenter randomized phase 2b trial has completed enrollment.

Clinical trials in patients with advanced prostate cancer and rising PSA have been carried out using recombinant vaccinia (rV) and recombinant fowlpox (rF) viruses expressing PSA. A randomized phase 2 study combining standard definitive radiotherapy with rV-PSA and a vector containing a single T-cell costimulatory molecule (rV-B7-1) followed by seven monthly boosts with rF-PSA in patients with localized prostate cancer has been completed. In that study, 13 of 17 patients had increases in PSA-specific T cells of ≥3-fold vs no detectable increases in the radiotherapy-only arm ($P < 0.0005$). A randomized phase 2 clinical trial in patients with nonmetastatic CRPC used the same prime-and-boost vaccine strategy.[200] The trial was randomized for second-line hormone therapy with nilutamide vs vaccine, with a crossover at disease progression so that each arm would receive combination vaccine plus hormone therapy. Time to treatment failure was prolonged in patients initially receiving vaccine alone and then receiving vaccine plus nilutamide.[201] Another study assessed the role of this same vaccine strategy combined with chemotherapy in patients with metastatic CRPC, based on preclinical studies showing that taxanes could potentiate immune response and augment the antitumor response seen with vaccines. Patients received either vaccine alone or vaccine plus docetaxel.[202] Of note, chemotherapy did not appear to blunt the immune response, as both cohorts demonstrated similar increases in PSA-specific T-cell precursors. Recent poxviral studies have added multiple costimulatory molecules to both priming and boosting vaccines.[58] These PSA-TRICOM vaccines are showing evidence of clinical benefit in terms of enhanced survival compared with predicted in patients with metastatic CRPC.[203]

Clinical trials have also been carried out using peptide-pulsed DCs loaded with peptides of human PSMA,[204-206] as well as DCs transfected with PSA tumor RNA.[207] In these studies, antigen-specific immune responses have been observed and some decreases in serum PSA have also been noted.

In addition to the numerous studies that have demonstrated the ability of patients to mount immune responses to prostate-associated self-antigens, it should also be pointed out that androgen withdrawal in patients with prostate cancer has led to the induction of T-cell infiltration in prostate tissue.[208] Thus, vaccine with androgen ablation may have implications for future immunotherapeutic treatment of prostate cancer.

Lung Cancer

BLP25 is a liposome-encapsulated peptide vaccine consisting of a synthetic peptide derived from the MUC-1 antigen. A phase 2b clinical study in patients with stage IIIb and IV non–small cell lung cancer (NSCLC) who had received first-line chemotherapy randomized patients to receive vaccine with best supportive care vs best supportive care alone. There was a trend in overall survival favoring the vaccine arm.[209] Other vaccine approaches include autologous and allogeneic vaccines genetically engineered to secrete GM-CSF.[13] A phase 2 study of belagenpumatucel-L, a transforming growth factor β-2 antisense gene-modified allogeneic tumor cell vaccine in NSCLC, has shown evidence of clinical benefit.[210] Active immunotherapy with an anti-idiotype vaccine has also been utilized in patients with small cell lung cancer.[211] An immune stimulant, talactoferrin (recombinant human lactoferrin) has also shown evidence of clinical benefit in randomized trials of patients with NSCLC.[212]

Leukemia/Lymphoma

The variable regions of B-cell receptor immunoglobulins on lymphomas are excellent targets for vaccines. These idiotypes have now been used successfully in the treatment of B-cell lymphomas.[39,213-216] An idiotype protein vaccine was used in 25 patients after a chemotherapy-induced second complete clinical remission. After vaccination, tumor-specific humoral or cellular immune responses were found in 20 of 25 patients.[215] All of the responders with enough follow-up maintained a second CR longer than the first CR, whereas the five patients who did not mount an immune response had a second CR that was, as expected, shorter than the first CR. Two large studies of anti-idiotype vaccines in lymphoma patients are ongoing. Clinical responses have also been observed using idiotype vaccine in patients with multiple myeloma.[41,217] For patients with chronic myelogenous leukemia, vaccination with bcr-abl oncogene breakpoint fusion peptides has generated specific immune responses.[218]

Other Tumor Types

Intravesical BCG has been used successfully in the treatment of bladder cancer, implicating immune mechanisms.[219] Intravesical administration of wild-type vaccinia virus has now been shown to be safe, and three of four patients treated were disease-free at 4-year follow-up.[220] The response of renal carcinoma to high-dose IL-2 and IFN-α also implicates immune mechanisms in therapeutic responses.[221] An autologous renal cell carcinoma tumor cell vaccine that was genetically modified to overexpress B7-1 to provide costimulation to tumor-reactive T cells was employed.[222] In this single-arm phase 2 study, 66 patients enrolled and 39 received at least one dose of vaccine and low-dose IL-2. Best responses were CR (3%), PR (5%), SD (64%), and PD (28%). A post-hoc analysis suggested that lymphocytic infiltration of the vaccine site determined by biopsy directly correlated with survival (28.4 vs 17.8 months, $P = 0.045$).

Vaccination of pediatric solid tumor patients with tumor-lysate-pulsed DCs has been shown to expand specific T cells and mediated some tumor regression.[223] In addition, clinical trials have examined vaccination of glioma patients with DC/glioma fusions and fusion-cell vaccination of patients with metastatic breast and renal cancers.[193,224] Early clinical trials in patients with primary brain tumors have shown immune responses and objective responses with DC vaccines,[225] autologous formalin-fixed[226] or TGF-β-modified[227] whole tumor cell vaccines. Clinical findings have also been reported in patients with advanced ovarian cancer using a vaccine consisting of an MAb directed against the tumor antigen CA125.[228] A phase 2 study examining an anti-idiotypic antibody vaccine that functionally imitated the CA125 antigen reported survival benefit; median survival of the vaccine group was 19.4 months vs 4.9 months for the control group (Table 57-2).[229] Heat shock proteins derived from patients' own tumors have been used as vaccines in a variety of cancer types with encouraging initial results.[230]

Considerations in the Analysis of Clinical Trial Results

It has now been demonstrated that appropriate vaccine-delivery systems and vaccine strategies can elicit immune responses to TAAs in patients with advanced cancer and, in some cases, can mediate prolonged survival, prolonged disease-free interval, drops in serum tumor markers, and/or regression of metastatic disease. The trials outlined in Table 57-2 provide only preliminary evidence of prolonged survival benefit; it is emphasized that only large-scale randomized phase 2 trials can prove the efficacy of such vaccines. As mentioned earlier, patients with advanced cancers are perhaps the least appropriate population to demonstrate the efficacy of a cancer vaccine; thus, future clinical trials should be carried out in patients with lower tumor burden metastatic disease or earlier in the disease process. Optimal use of vaccines would occur immediately prior to, during, or immediately following adjuvant therapy. Several such studies are ongoing.

The overall goal is the use of vaccine regimens in combination with frontline cancer therapies, thereby reducing the interval between disease diagnosis and the initiation of vaccine. This hopefully will bring the use of cancer vaccines closer to the original intention—use in patients with minimal disease.

Combination Therapies

Objective clinical responses (RECIST criteria) induced by cancer vaccines may be difficult to obtain in patients with large tumor masses for three different reasons: (a) tumor masses can produce large amounts of immunoregulatory molecules that have the potential to energize T cells, (b) large tumor masses are difficult to penetrate by T cells, and (c) the quantity of T cells generated by the host immune system would be far outnumbered by the cells in a large tumor mass. Vaccines would most probably show the greatest efficacy in the adjuvant or neoadjuvant setting or in the treatment of metastatic disease where tumor burden is minimal.[231] A great deal of effort is now being put into the use of vaccines with conventional therapies such as local radiation of tumor, chemotherapeutic agents, hormones, and MAbs.

Vaccine Plus Radiation

Radiation is the standard of care for many cancer types and has conventionally been exploited for its direct cytotoxic effect on tumors or palliative effects in patients. Local radiation of tumor has also been shown to alter tumor architecture, resulting in more effective drug delivery. Recently, it has been reported that local radiation of tumor cells given at doses insufficient to kill tumor will modulate numerous classes of genes and consequently alter the phenotype of the tumor cell.[232,233] Several genes that have been shown to be up-regulated in human tumor cells post-irradiation are Fas, MHC class I, ICAM-1, and the TAAs CEA, MUC-1, HER-2/*neu*, p53, and CA125. The up-regulation of any one of these genes has the ability to render a tumor cell more susceptible to T cell–mediated immune attack. For example, Fas, a member of the tumor necrosis factor (TNF) receptor family, is a death receptor that induces apoptosis on binding to FasL, its natural ligand. Fas-mediated apoptosis has been shown to play an important role in tumor cell destruction along with granzyme-mediated killing. Recent preclinical studies showed for the first time that the regulation of Fas expression in tumor cells via sublethal local tumor irradiation significantly improves the therapeutic efficacy of a recombinant anticancer vaccine in a preclinical model.[233] Subsequent studies also showed that sublethal doses of irradiation of human colorectal, lung, and prostate cancer cells altered numerous genes and led to the up-regulation of Fas and other molecules, rendering these tumor cells more susceptible to killing by human CTLs.[232] Although the mechanism of enhanced immunogenicity of irradiated tumor cells is not fully understood, it is also known that low doses of gamma rays can induce stress genes and increase reactive oxygen species. A recent clinical study has reported on the combined use of a recombinant cancer vaccine with standard definitive radiotherapy in patients with localized prostate cancer.[234] There is an excellent review on immune modulation by ionizing radiation and its implication for cancer therapy.[235]

Vaccine Plus Chemotherapy

If cancer vaccines are to be used early in the disease process, they would most likely need to be used in combination with certain chemotherapeutic agents. While counterintuitive, it has recently been shown that vaccine therapy may not only be compatible with certain chemotherapies, but also actually be synergistic.[231] It has been previously established that drugs such as interferon can up-regulate both MHC class I and numerous TAAs on the surface of tumor cells. It has also been shown that drugs commonly used in cancer chemotherapy can also up-regulate tumor antigens and/or histocompatibility antigens. For example, 5-fluorouracil treatment of tumor cells has been shown to up-regulate CEA and MHC class I. Systemic cyclophosphamide combined with local intratumoral injection of DCs (but not cyclophosphamide alone) led to complete tumor regression in an experimental melanoma model.[236] Adriamycin has also been shown to increase effector T-cell activity. In preclinical models, the chemotherapy agents cyclophosphamide, doxorubicin, paclitaxel, and docetaxel have been shown to enhance the antitumor immune response of a whole tumor cell vaccine.[237,238]

Several things are important in considering the use of chemotherapy with vaccine: (a) the combined use of vaccine and chemotherapy early in the disease process should not be confused with the use of vaccines following multiple regimens of different chemotherapeutic agents in the advanced disease setting, where the immune system would most likely be impaired; (b) not all chemotherapeutic agents will be compatible with vaccine; and (c) dose scheduling of vaccine when used with chemotherapy may be extremely important. Obviously, future studies will be required to optimize the combined use of vaccine and chemotherapy. An excellent review on combining antineoplastic drugs with tumor vaccines has been published.[239]

Vaccine Plus Hormone Therapy

The use of vaccines with antiandrogen therapy represents an intriguing possibility for the treatment of prostate cancer. It has previously been shown that androgen-ablative therapy induces profuse T-cell infiltration of benign glands and tumors in the human prostate. T-cell infiltration was readily apparent after 1 to 3 weeks of therapy. Also, T cells within the treated prostate exhibited restricted TCR usage consistent with a local oligoclonal response.[240] These studies thus have important implications for the potential use of vaccine in combination with androgen-ablative therapy in prostate cancer, as well as implications for other hormone-sensitive malignancies including breast cancer.[240] A clinical trial was recently carried out in prostate cancer patients who had received prior hormonal therapy but had an increasing serum PSA without radiographic evidence of metastases. The trial was randomized for second-line hormone therapy (nilutamide) vs vaccine with a crossover at disease progression so that each arm would receive combination vaccine plus hormone therapy. Time to treatment failure and survival at 4+ years[241] was prolonged in patients initially receiving vaccine alone and then receiving vaccine plus nilutamide. Further studies are obviously needed to validate such observations, but these studies clearly demonstrate the potential for the combined use of vaccine and hormone therapy.[201] An excellent review on the rationale for combining androgen deprivation therapy with prostate cancer vaccines has been published.[242]

Vaccine Plus Other Immunotherapies

There are several different ways in which vaccine and MAbs can be used in combination. These include (a) the use of therapeutic antibodies such as herceptin or rituxan in combination with vaccine, in which each acts independently, (b) the use of antitumor antibody cytokine fusion proteins such as antitumor antibody/IL-2 to enhance T-cell activity at the site of tumor,[243-247] (c) the use of MAbs such as anti-CTLA-4, which block negative regulatory immune signals and thus enhance immune responses,[140,248-251] and (d) the use of MAbs or fusion proteins directed against regulatory T cells.[252-254]

Vaccines can also be employed in combination with adoptive transfer of antigen-specific T cells. In preclinical studies, point-mutated ras-specific T cells were adoptively transferred into immuno-depleted hosts. Donor antigen-specific T-cell responses were greatest in recipient mice that received peptide boosts (with or without IL-2). These results indicate that a vaccine administration after T-cell transfer was more obligatory than exogenous IL-2 to sustain adoptively transferred T cells.[255]

Dose Scheduling of Vaccine With Other Therapies

Arguably the most unique feature of cancer vaccine therapy is a vaccine's ability to initiate a dynamic process of host immune responses that can be exploited in subsequent therapies. Several clinical studies have now provided evidence of this phenomenon.

In a phase 1 study, patients with advanced-stage progressive cancer received a vaccine directed against cytochrome P4501B1. Most patients who developed immunity to vaccine but required salvage therapy on progression showed marked responses to their next treatment regimen; most of these responses lasted >1 year.[256] In another study in patients with extensive-stage small cell lung cancer,[257] a high rate of objective clinical responses to chemotherapy immediately followed vaccine therapy. These clinical responses were also closely associated with induction or augmentation of immune response to vaccine.

Three randomized clinical trials in prostate cancer provided further evidence of this phenomenon. In the first trial, patients with metastatic CRPC were randomized to receive vaccine alone or vaccine plus weekly docetaxel.[202] Patients on the vaccine-alone arm were allowed to cross over to receive docetaxel at time of progression. After vaccine, median progression-free survival on docetaxel was 6.1 months compared with a progression-free survival of 3.7 months with the same docetaxel regimen and patient population at the same institution. Similar findings were observed using the sipuleucel vaccine.[258] In a randomized multicenter study, patients in both the vaccine and placebo arms received docetaxel at progression. There was a statistically significant ($P = 0.023$) increase in overall survival with docetaxel in patients who had prior vaccine vs placebo.

In a phase 2 trial,[201] patients with nonmetastatic CRPC and rising serum PSA were randomized to receive either vaccine or nilutamide, an androgen receptor antagonist (ARA). After 6 months, patients with rising PSA were allowed to cross over to a combination of both therapies. Median time to treatment failure was similar in the vaccine and ARA arms. However, for patients who received vaccine first and then received vaccine plus ARA, time to treatment failure was 13.9 months from the initiation of ARA and the time to treatment failure from the initiation of any therapy was 25.9 months. Of the initial randomized population, for those patients who first received nilutamide alone or nilutamide and then vaccine, 5-year overall survival was 38% vs a median overall survival of 59% for patients who first received vaccine alone or nilutamide plus vaccine.[259]

Each of the trials described earlier provided evidence of the same phenomenon: patients who receive vaccine and mount immune responses to vaccine, if monitored, have enhanced response to subsequent therapies. It is unlikely that this outcome is due to patient population selection, because three of the trials described were randomized. Rather, the subsequent therapies (a) may reduce suppressor cell populations, thus enhancing prior established T-cell responses, (b) may lyse some tumor cells that are then, as a consequence of cross priming, activating relatively dormant T cells to elicit an antitumor response, (c) may enhance host T-cell activity, and/or (d) may alter the phenotype of tumor cells.

Recent Innovations in Vaccine Design and Delivery

There have been numerous recent advances in our basic understanding of immune mechanisms, tumor immunology, and vaccinology.

Mechanism of T-Cell Activation

Recent studies have shown that a range of effector cells can be involved in antitumor effects. In most preclinical studies the $CD8^+$ CTL is involved in antitumor effects and the $CD4^+$ helper T cell is important for supplying help via cytokines to further activate the CTL. Other effector cells, however, can be involved, including macrophages and natural killer (NK) cells, and studies have also shown that in certain cases the generation of antitumor antibodies can mediate antitumor effects via antibody-dependent cell-mediated cytotoxicity.[260] T-cell activation has been shown to be a complex phenomenon involving the interaction of the peptide-MHC complex on the APC with the TCR on the T cell; for weak antigens such as TAAs, however, accessory molecules are necessary for efficient T-cell activation. These have been termed T-cell costimulatory molecules. At this time over a dozen such costimulatory molecules have been identified. Costimulatory molecules are found on professional APCs, such as DCs, but are not found on the vast majority of solid tumors. It has also recently been shown that combinations of these costimulatory molecules act synergistically to further enhance T-cell activation.[261] Preclinical and recent clinical studies have shown that either recombinant vaccinia virus or recombinant avipox vectors containing TRICOM (B7-1, ICAM-1, and LFA-3) can enhance T-cell responses and antitumor immunity to far greater levels than those recombinants containing only one costimulatory molecule or none at all.[261]

Recent studies have also shown that it is not necessarily the quantity of T cells generated that is essential, but their quality, or avidity.[262-264] This is measured by the ability of different populations of T cells to actually kill targets. It has recently been shown that the use of vaccines with T-cell costimulation and certain cytokines can actually enhance T-cell avidity.[263] T-cell activation has also been shown to be enhanced by the inhibition of regulatory signals through the use of reagents such as anti-CTLA-4 antibody.[265-267]

Regulatory T Cells

Several different types of regulatory T cells have now been identified.[268-271] The evolutionary reason for their existence is most likely to reduce autoimmune phenomena. Since TAAs for the most part are self-antigens, regulatory T cells appear to have a major role in reducing immune responses to TAAs. Three main types of regulatory T cells that have now been identified are: $CD4^+CD25^+FoxP3^+$ (Tregs), immature macrophages, and $CD4^+$ NKT^+ cells.[270,271] Studies are ongoing employing reagents that can potentially reduce the activity of these regulatory T cells, including the fusion protein Ontak,[272] cyclophosphamide,[174,182,273] and anti-CD25 Abs.[274,275] The inhibition of these cells will most likely be a part of cancer vaccine therapy in the future.

Antigen Cascade

The phenomenon of antigen cascade is now evolving as an important facet in the evaluation of cancer vaccines. This was first defined using the term epitope spreading, in which a given peptide was used as a vaccine and the host immune response post-vaccination was not only directed to that epitope, but also to other epitopes of the same tumor antigen.[233,275,276] This phenomenon has now been expanded using the term antigen cascade, in which a given antigen is used as a vaccine and the host immune response post-vaccination is not only directed against the antigen in the vaccine, but also to other antigens in the tumor. These phenomena can be explained that as a consequence of some tumor cell destruction induced by the vaccine, APCs will engulf tumor fragments and then cross-present those tumor fragments to T cells, thus initiating the antigen cascade phenomenon. This has now been observed in several preclinical models and in clinical trials[277] and may eventually be correlated with antitumor activity.

Diversified Prime-and-Boost Immunization Strategies

Although each of the various methods of immunization described has advantages and disadvantages, the most effective immunization protocol may involve priming with one type of immunogen and boosting with another. This method may be advantageous because (a) two different arms of the immune system may be enhanced by using two different modalities (ie, $CD4^+$ and then $CD8^+$ T cells); (b) one methodology may be more effective in priming naïve cells while another modality may be more effective in enhancing memory cell function; and (c) some of the most effective methods of immunization, like the use of recombinant vaccinia virus or adenoviruses, can be used only a limited number of times because of host antivector responses. These vectors may be most effective when used as priming agents, followed by boosts with other agents. Numerous preclinical studies demonstrate the advantages of diversified prime-and-boost protocols.[278-282] Recent clinical studies show that priming with a recombinant vaccinia virus and boosting with recombinant avipox viruses are more effective than using either recombinant vector alone.[38,55,67]

Route of Vaccination

Conventional vaccinations involve subcutaneous or intradermal inoculations. It has recently been shown in several preclinical models and some clinical studies that intratumoral and/or intranodal vaccination may be more efficacious in some cases. Indeed, a recent study has shown that the sequential use of primary subcutaneous vaccination followed by intratumoral booster vaccination is more efficacious in terms of antitumor effects than the sustained use of either route alone.[283]

Issues in Cancer Vaccine Development

An important issue involves the appropriate disease state at which to administer vaccines. Standard practice and medical ethics dictate that all new phase 1 immunotherapies and many phase 2 trials be administered to patients with advanced disease who have failed conventional therapy. A mind-set prevails in some that one must see the elimination of large tumor masses by traditional staging technologies (ie, radiography or computed tomography) before an immunotherapy can proceed to the adjuvant setting. However, as discussed earlier, a patient population with measurable disease may be the worst group in which to define the efficacy of a new vaccine because of (a) potential immunosuppressive factors produced by the tumor; (b) the potential presence of regulatory or suppressor cells that may exist in the circulation, lymphoid compartments, and at sites of tumor growth that might down-regulate productive antitumor immune responses[284-286]; (c) immunosuppression caused by previous therapy (ie, radiation, chemotherapy); and (d) tumor penetrance of the immunotherapeutic. It is hoped that the field will eventually mature to the point where, for example, vaccines that are shown to be safe and to elicit specific immune responses in advanced cancer patients will be more readily evaluated in patients in the adjuvant setting.

As a vaccine-mediated therapeutic T-cell response is developed, the possibility also exists for the development of undesirable immune reactions. For example, if vaccines are directed against a given TAA, the induction of immunity toward the tumor may also eventually lead to the induction of immunity to normal tissues also expressing that TAA. This has been the case in immune responses to some melanoma-associated antigens, where vitiligo has been induced in both experimental and clinical studies.[287,288] It is interesting to note that, in preclinical vaccine studies, the induction of antitumor immunity in transgenic mice expressing TAAs has not led to the induction of autoimmunity in normal tissues expressing those same TAAs.[87,289-293] Moreover, in the vast majority of clinical trials using vaccines directed against carcinomas, no autoimmunity has been observed, including those cases in which clinical antitumor effects have been demonstrated.[160]

Paradigm Shifts

The evaluation of cancer vaccines in clinical trials may well necessitate new paradigms.[231]

Vaccines vs Passive Therapies; ie, Drugs

Cancer vaccines and cytotoxic drugs act differently in terms of mode of action. Cytotoxic drugs either kill or do not kill tumor cells. Lack of efficacy is due to either drug resistance by tumor cells, inadequate amounts of drug delivered to the tumor, and/or drug-induced toxicity in the host. Thus, if a patient's disease is progressing on a cytotoxic drug, that drug is immediately withdrawn. The use of a cancer vaccine involves the initiation of a dynamic process in which the patient's own immune system is activated. It is clear from decades of preclinical studies and now clinical trials that to maximize the host immune response, one must give not only a primary vaccination but also multiple booster vaccinations over a period of weeks or months to further enhance the level of the immune response. Multiple vaccinations are especially important because factors may be given off by the tumor that will blunt the immune response. Thus it is not unusual to see disease progression following early vaccinations, but only then to see disease stabilization or a reduction in tumor burden following multiple vaccinations. Thus, the paradigm of "drug withdrawal upon progression" should be revisited with the use of cancer vaccines.

The Phase 1, 2, 3 Paradigm

Clinical trials with a new drug are traditionally evaluated in patients with advanced tumors (many times with a large tumor burden) who have failed prior cytotoxic therapies. Objective clinical responses are evaluated by RECIST criteria, looking for a sustained ≥30% reduction in the sum of the longest diameter of target lesions. Since generation of an immune response to a vaccine is a dynamic process in which T cells can be continually generated upon booster vaccines, a more appropriate end point for evaluation should be time to progression and, more importantly, survival. Since only a finite amount of T cells can be generated by a vaccine, it may be inappropriate to evaluate a cancer vaccine by its ability to drastically reduce a large tumor burden; this is especially true in patients whose immune system has been compromised due to numerous rounds of prior chemotherapy. A more appropriate setting would be the evaluation of cancer vaccines earlier in the disease setting in patients with either a small tumor burden or a high probability of disease progression. This should particularly be considered in light of the relatively low level of toxicity seen in the use of cancer vaccines. The scenario is all too familiar where claims of activity are made for cytotoxic drugs; there is a reduction of tumor burden by RECIST criteria in some patients, but no statistical difference in survival. Unfortunately, there is still a "paradigm paralysis" by some who hold on to the paradigm for the evaluation of cytotoxic drugs as the only means of evaluation of efficacy.

Combination Therapies

One of the major advantages of cancer vaccines is their reduced toxicity. One of the conventional thoughts now being reevaluated is that cancer vaccines cannot be used in combination with chemotherapy or radiation therapy. One should not confuse the potential reduced efficacy of a vaccine given to patients who have failed multiple rounds of prior chemotherapy vs administration of vaccine with or prior to chemotherapy. Preclinical studies, and now several clinical studies, have shown that patients can mount an immune response to cancer vaccine when given in combination with certain cytotoxic drugs, hormones, or local radiation of tumor. Indeed, recent preclinical studies have shown that when tumor cells are exposed to sublethal doses of radiation or certain chemotherapeutic agents, the phenotype of tumor cells is actually modulated to make them more susceptible to T cell–mediated killing.

Conclusion

Rapidly emerging achievements in the areas of molecular biology and immunology have led to the development of novel vaccines and vaccine strategies. Unraveling basic mechanisms of antigen recognition, antigen processing, antigen presentation, and tumor escape processes have led to the identification and exploitation of DCs, costimulatory molecules, and antigen-specific T cells for use in diverse aspects of immunotherapy. Although considerable knowledge has been acquired to this point, the steady influx of new information as a result of basic studies, translational studies, and clinical trials will most likely further translate the science of tumor immunology into clinical modalities for a range of human cancers and, perhaps, strategies for the prevention of certain neoplasms.

Acknowledgments

The authors gratefully acknowledge the assistance of Bonnie L. Casey and Debra Weingarten in the preparation of this chapter.

Selected References

The complete reference list can be found at www.CANCERMEDICINE8.com

3. Carbone DP, Ciernik IF, Kelley MJ, et al. Immunization with mutant p53- and K-ras-derived peptides in cancer patients: immune response and clinical outcome. *J Clin Oncol.* 2005;23:5099–5107.
11. Small EJ, Sacks N, Nemunaitis J, et al. Granulocyte macrophage colony-stimulating factor—secreting allogeneic cellular immunotherapy for hormone-refractory prostate cancer. *Clin Cancer Res.* 2007;13:3883–3891.
12. Jaffee EM, Hruban RH, Biedrzycki B, et al. Novel allogeneic granulocyte-macrophage colony-stimulating factor-secreting tumor vaccine for pancreatic cancer: a phase I trial of safety and immune activation. *J Clin Oncol.* 2001;19:145–156.
13. Nemunaitis J, Jahan T, Ross H, et al. Phase 1/2 trial of autologous tumor mixed with an allogeneic GVAX vaccine in advanced-stage non-small-cell lung cancer. *Cancer Gene Ther.* 2006;13:555–562.
20. Kaufman HL, Cohen S, Cheung K, et al. Local delivery of vaccinia virus expressing multiple costimulatory molecules for the treatment of established tumors. *Hum Gene Ther.* 2006;17:239–244.
38. Marshall JL, Gulley JL, Arlen PM, et al. Phase I study of sequential vaccinations with fowlpox-CEA(6D)-TRICOM alone and sequentially with vaccinia-CEA(6D)-TRICOM, with and without granulocyte-macrophage colony-stimulating factor, in patients with carcinoembryonic antigen-expressing carcinomas. *J Clin Oncol.* 2005;23:720–731.
39. Bendandi M, Gocke CD, Kobrin CB, et al. Complete molecular remissions induced by patient-specific vaccination plus granulocyte-monocyte colony-stimulating factor against lymphoma. *Nat Med.* 1999;5:1171–1177.
40. Kwak LW, Campbell MJ, Czerwinski DK, Hart S, Miller RA, Levy R. Induction of immune responses in patients with B-cell lymphoma against the surface-immunoglobulin idiotype expressed by their tumors. *N Engl J Med.* 1992;327:1209–1215.
43. Hansson L, Abdalla AO, Moshfegh A, et al. Long-term idiotype vaccination combined with interleukin-12 (IL-12), or IL-12 and granulocyte macrophage colony-stimulating factor, in early-stage multiple myeloma patients. *Clin Cancer Res.* 2007;13:1503–1510.
66. Harrop R, Drury N, Shingler W, et al. Vaccination of colorectal cancer patients with modified vaccinia Ankara encoding the tumor antigen 5T4 (TroVax) given alongside chemotherapy induces potent immune responses. *Clin Cancer Res.* 2007;13:4487–4494.
72. Stubbs AC, Wilson CC. Recombinant yeast as a vaccine vector for the induction of cytotoxic T-lymphocyte responses. *Curr Opin Mol Ther.* 2002;4:35–40.
84. Steinman RM, Dhodapkar M. Active immunization against cancer with dendritic cells: the near future. *Int J Cancer.* 2001;94:459–473.
85. Banchereau J, Palucka AK, Dhodapkar M, et al. Immune and clinical responses in patients with metastatic melanoma to CD34(+) progenitor-derived dendritic cell vaccine. *Cancer.* Res 2001;61:6451–6458.
87. Gong J, Chen D, Kashiwaba M, et al. Reversal of tolerance to human MUC1 antigen in MUC1 transgenic mice immunized with fusions of dendritic and carcinoma cells. *Proc Natl Acad Sci USA.* 1998;95:6279–6283.
90. Small EJ, Fratesi P, Reese DM, et al. Immunotherapy of hormone-refractory prostate cancer with antigen-loaded dendritic cells. *J Clin Oncol.* 2000;18:3894–3903.
91. Matzinger P. The danger model: a renewed sense of self. *Science.* 2002;296:301–305.
92. Alving CR, Koulchin V, Glenn GM, Rao M. Liposomes as carriers of peptide antigens: induction of antibodies and cytotoxic T lymphocytes to conjugated and unconjugated peptides. *Immunol Rev.* 1995;145:5–31.
94. Zaharoff DA, Rogers CJ, Hance KW, et al. Chitosan solution enhances both humoral and cell-mediated immune responses to subcutaneous vaccination. *Vaccine.* 2007;25:2085–2094.
96. Iwasaki A, Medzhitov R. Toll-like receptor control of the adaptive immune responses. *Nat Immunol.* 2004;5:987–995.
120. Dudley ME, Rosenberg SA. Adoptive-cell-transfer therapy for the treatment of patients with cancer. *Nat Rev Cancer.* 2003;3:666–675.
122. Waldmann TA, Dubois S, Tagaya Y. Contrasting roles of IL-2 and IL-15 in the life and death of lymphocytes: implications for immunotherapy. *Immunity.* 2001;14:105–110.
123. Fry TJ, Moniuszko M, Creekmore S, et al. IL-7 therapy dramatically alters peripheral T-cell homeostasis in normal and SIV-infected nonhuman primates. *Blood.* 2003;101:2294–2299.
124. Dranoff G. Cytokines in cancer pathogenesis and cancer therapy. *Nat Rev Cancer.* 2004;4:11–22.
125. Benlalam H, Vignard V, Khammari A, et al. Infusion of Melan-A/Mart-1 specific tumor-infiltrating lymphocytes enhanced relapse-free survival of melanoma patients. *Cancer Immunol Immunother.* 2007;56:515–526.
126. Dudley ME, Wunderlich JR, Yang JC, et al. Adoptive cell transfer therapy following non-myeloablative but lymphodepleting chemotherapy for the treatment of patients with refractory metastatic melanoma. *J Clin Oncol.* 2005;23:2346–2357.
132. Slingluff CL, Jr, Petroni GR, Yamshchikov GV, et al. Clinical and immunologic results of a randomized phase II trial of vaccination using four melanoma peptides either administered in granulocyte-macrophage colony-stimulating factor in adjuvant or pulsed on dendritic cells. *J Clin Oncol.* 2003;21:4016–4026.
155. Rosenblatt J, Kufe D, Avigan D. Dendritic cell fusion vaccines for cancer immunotherapy. *Expert Opin Biol Ther.* 2005;5:703–715.
169. Harrop R, Connolly N, Redchenko I, et al. Vaccination of colorectal cancer patients with modified vaccinia Ankara delivering the tumor antigen 5T4 (TroVax) induces immune responses which correlate with disease control: a phase I/II trial. *Clin Cancer Res.* 2006;12:3416–3424.
187. Peoples GE, Gurney JM, Hueman MT, et al. Clinical trial results of a HER2/neu (E75) vaccine to prevent recurrence in high-risk breast cancer patients. *J Clin Oncol.* 2005;23:7536–7545.
192. Salazar LG, Coveler AL, Swensen RE, et al. Kinetics of tumor-specific T-cell response development after active immunization in patients with HER-2/neu overexpressing cancers. *Clin Immunol.* 2007;125:275–280.
193. Avigan D, Vasir B, Gong J, et al. Fusion cell vaccination of patients with metastatic breast and renal cancer induces immunological and clinical responses. *Clin Cancer Res.* 2004;10:4699–4708.
195. Small EJ, Schellhammer PF, Higano CS, et al. Placebo-controlled phase III trial of immunologic therapy with sipuleucel-T (APC8015) in patients with metastatic, asymptomatic hormone refractory prostate cancer. *J Clin Oncol.* 2006;24:3089–3094.
196. Ward JE, McNeel DG. GVAX: an allogeneic, whole-cell, GM-CSF-secreting cellular immunotherapy for the treatment

of prostate cancer. *Expert Opin Biol Ther.* 2007;7:1893–1902.

197. Halabi S, Small EJ, Kantoff PW, et al. Prognostic model for predicting survival in men with hormone-refractory metastatic prostate cancer. *J Clin Oncol.* 2003;21:1232–1237.
202. Arlen PM, Gulley JL, Parker C, et al. A randomized phase II study of concurrent docetaxel plus vaccine versus vaccine alone in metastatic androgen-independent prostate cancer. *Clin Cancer Res.* 2006;12:1260–1269.
208. Mercader M, Bodner BK, Moser MT, et al. T cell infiltration of the prostate induced by androgen withdrawal in patients with prostate cancer. *Proc Natl Acad Sci USA.* 2001;98:14565–14570.
209. Butts C, Murray N, Maksymiuk A, et al. Randomized phase IIB trial of BLP25 liposome vaccine in stage IIIB and IV non-small-cell lung cancer. *J Clin Oncol.* 2005;23:6674–6681.
210. Nemunaitis J, Dillman RO, Schwarzenberger PO, et al. Phase II study of belagenpumatucel-L, a transforming growth factor beta-2 antisense gene-modified allogeneic tumor cell vaccine in non-small-cell lung cancer. *J Clin Oncol.* 2006; 24:4721–4730.
215. Inoges S, Rodriguez-Calvillo M, Zabalegui N, et al. Clinical benefit associated with idiotypic vaccination in patients with follicular lymphoma. *J Natl Cancer Inst.* 2006;98:1292–1301.
231. Schlom J, Arlen PM, Gulley JL. Cancer vaccines: moving beyond current paradigms. *Clin Cancer Res.* 2007;13:3776–3782.
233. Chakraborty M, Abrams SI, Coleman CN, Camphausen K, Schlom J, Hodge JW. External beam radiation of tumors alters phenotype of tumor cells to render them susceptible to vaccine-mediated T-cell killing. *Cancer Res.* 2004;64:4328–4337.
241. Madan R, Gulley J, Schlom J, et al. Analysis of overall survival in patients with non-metastatic castration-resistant prostate cancer treated with vaccine, nilutamide, and combination therapy: implications for vaccine clinical trial design. *Clin Cancer Res.* 2008, in press.
246. Schrama D, Straten P, Brocker EB, et al. Cytokine fusion protein treatment. Recent Results. *Cancer Res.* 2002;160:185–194.
251. Small EJ, Tchekmedyian NS, Rini BI, Fong L, Lowy I, Allison JP. A pilot trial of CTLA-4 blockade with human anti-CTLA-4 in patients with hormone-refractory prostate cancer. *Clin Cancer Res.* 2007;13:1810–1815.
252. Dannull J, Su Z, Rizzieri D, et al. Enhancement of vaccine-mediated antitumor immunity in cancer patients after depletion of regulatory T cells. *J Clin Invest.* 2005;115:3623–3633.
256. Gribben JG, Ryan DP, Boyajian R, et al. Unexpected association between induction of immunity to the universal tumor antigen CYP1B1 and response to next therapy. *Clin Cancer Res.* 2005;11:4430–4436.
260. Sondel PM, Hank JA. Antibody-directed, effector cell-mediated tumor destruction. *Hematol Oncol Clin North Am.* 2001;15: 703–721.
263. Hodge JW, Chakraborty M, Kudo-Saito C, et al. Multiple costimulatory modalities enhance CTL avidity. *J Immunol.* 2005;174: 5994–6004.
273. Lutsiak ME, Semnani RT, De Pascalis R, et al. Inhibition of CD4(+)25+ T regulatory cell function implicated in enhanced immune response by low-dose cyclophosphamide. *Blood.* 2005;105:2862–2868.
295. Kaufman HL, Wang W, Manola J, et al. Phase II randomized study of vaccine treatment of advanced prostate cancer (E7897): a trial of the Eastern Cooperative Oncology Group. *J Clin Oncol.* 2004;22:2122–2132.

58 Antiestrogens, Progestins, and Aromatase Inhibitors

Aman U. Buzdar, MD ▪ Shaheenah Dawood, MBBCh, MRCP (UK)MPH ▪
Harold A. Harvey, MD ▪ V. Craig Jordan, OBE, PhD, DSc

Introduction

The importance of the reproductive endocrine system in breast cancer treatment began to be appreciated at the turn of nineteenth century. It was around this time that it was realized that approximately one-third of premenopausal women with advanced breast cancer would respond to oophorectomy.[1] However, it was only when the estrogen receptor (ER) was discovered that it was possible to fully appreciate the mechanisms underlying the activity of ovarian ablation and other associated treatments for breast cancer such as ovarian irradiation, adrenalectomy, and hypophysectomy.[2] Research into the both the estrogen and progesterone pathways not only provided a deeper understanding of the underlying mechanism of the carcinogenic pathway involved in the development of breast cancer but also allowed identification of potential targets for therapeutic intervention.

This chapter discusses recent advances in the molecular biology and physiology underlying the ER and progesterone receptor (PR) pathways and potential targets for intervention. In addition it examines and compares the pharmacology and efficacy of the different endocrine agents used in the management of both early and advanced stage breast cancer (Fig. 58-1).

Biology Progestin Production and Action

Progestins are involved in the regulation of development and differentiation, proliferation, apoptosis, and metabolism in many target tissues with broad implications in neoplasia. In addition progestins serve as precursors to the estrogens, androgens, and adrenocortical steroids. Some of the progestin effects on target tissues are mediated by transcription, whereas other effects are more rapid and do not involve direct transcriptional effects. Progestins (Fig. 58-1A) include the naturally occurring hormone progesterone, 17α-acetoxyprogesterone derivatives in the pregnane series, 19-nortestosterone derivatives (estranes), and norgestrel and related compounds in the gonane series. In humans progesterone is the most important progestin.

Synthesis and Sites of Production

Progesterone is produced early in the scheme of the synthetic pathway involving the conversion of cholesterol to androgens, progestins, and estrogens. After menopause, in the absence of hormone replacement, the adrenal gland becomes the principal source of progestins (through the conversion of pregnenolone) as well as other sex steroids. In the premenopausal woman, progesterone is principally derived from the corpus luteum of the ovary, but in pregnancy after the eighth week of gestation, placental progesterone production greatly exceeds ovarian-derived progesterone. The placental trophoblast is the dominant cell responsible for progesterone production by the placenta. The development of a secretory endometrium in which the blastocyst can implant requires progesterone. Progesterone levels of 25 ng/mL are usual in the luteal phase of the menstrual cycle, where as levels up to 150 ng/mL are seen in late pregnancy.

Mechanism of Action

Progesterone functions in ribonucleic acid (RNA) transcription regulation through a complex series of interactions that is initiated by binding of the hormone to its cognate receptor. There are two isoforms of PR known as PR-A and PR-B that have distinct biological activities. PR-B has been shown to mediate the stimulatory activities of progesterone while PR-A functions to inhibit the action of PR-B as well as other steroid receptors.[3–5] Both isoforms are encoded by a single gene and their ratios vary in reproductive tissues as a consequence of developmental status, hormonal levels and tissue type. Both isoforms of PR contain AF-1 and AF-2 transactivation domains; PR-B contains an additional AF-3 domain, which contributes to its cell- and promoter-specific activity. The ligand for both isoforms of PR is identical.

In the absence of the hormone, PR is found in the nucleus in an inactive monomeric state associated with a complex of heat shock proteins (HSP-90, 70, 60, and 40) and is transcriptionally inactive.[6,7] Binding of progesterone to PR results in the dissociation of the heat shock proteins leading to the formation of receptor–ligand homodimers that remain localized in the nucleus and bind to highly selective progesterone response elements (PRE) located on target genes.[8] It is important to note that target cells must distinguish not only progesterone from other steroids present in small amounts, but also must distinguish progesterone from other hydrophobic molecules that are frequently found in 100-fold or greater excess. Such a high degree of discrimination is limited to differentiated cells that possess PR proteins and activatable PREs in their genome.[8,9] The next step in the process is the transcriptional activation by PR which results from the interaction with a number of coactivators including steroid receptor coactivator 1 (SRC-1), transcription intermediary factor 2, and retinoic acid coactivator 3, among others.[8–11] The SRC-1 interacts with the N-terminal AF-1 and the C-terminal AF-2 of the PR. This serves to emphasize that SRC-1 function to synergize the ligand-independent amino terminal AF-1 with the ligand-responsive carboxyl terminal AF-2 of the PR. The PR-coactivator complex then interacts further with additional proteins that have histone acetylase activity that causes chromatin remodeling serving to increase accessibility of transcriptional proteins to the promoter target.[10]

Physiologic Actions

Progestins are involved in a number of benign physiologic changes ranging from differentiated secretory activity to edematous changes in stromal tissues of the breast. They are also have implications on neoplastic processes being associated with both a decreased risk of endometrial neoplasms and a slightly increased risk of breast neoplasms when used in conjunction with estrogen replacement for menopause. Progestins have a critical role in the support of the products of conception: the differentiation of the endometrium and the promotion of the secretory phase of the endometrium; the maturation and cornification of the vaginal mucosal epithelium; the suppression of ovulation; the inhibition of gonadotropin release; the proliferation of breast epithelium and the induction of secretory activity in breast epithelium; and a natriuretic effect on the kidneys. A number of these biologic effects of progesterone are seen only in concert with priming of the target tissues with estrogen, whereas other effects appear to be interrelated with the actions of other steroid hormones, peptide hormones, and/or growth factors. Both progesterone and estrogen influence the response when superpharmacologic doses are used. Possible interactions between progesterone, estrogen, and growth factors must be taken into account when constructing treatment strategies.

Synthetic Progestins

Synthetic progestins are derivatives of the steroid structure of either progesterone or testosterone. The synthetic progestins most often encountered include 17-hydroxyprogesterone, medroxyprogesterone (Provera), medroxyprogesterone acetate, megestrol acetate (Megace), norethindrone, norethindrone enanthate, norethindrone acetate, norethynodrel, norgestrel, desogestrel, and gestodene. The two most widely used synthetic progestins are medroxyprogesterone acetate (MPA) and megestrol acetate (MA), which differs only by a single bond at C6-C7. MPA can be administered either as an oral or intramuscular preparation, while MA is administered as an oral preparation.

Synthetic progestins are used most frequently in contraception, in conjunction with estrogen in postmenopausal hormone replacement therapy (HRT) and in the endocrine treatment of uterine and breast cancer. In postmenopausal HRT, progestins are added to estrogen replacement principally to minimize the risk of uterine cancer associated with estrogen-only therapy, although the effects of adding progestins to estrogen on the risk of breast cancer have become of increasing concern.[12] In premenopausal women, progestins and anti-progestins are used predominantly in contraceptive preparations.[13] Progestins are often used alone in selected women with climacteric symptoms who are advised not to take estrogens.

Metastatic Breast Cancers

Progestins and PRs have been studied extensively in cancerous human breast tissue. Patients whose tumors are PR positive have a higher probability of responding to endocrine therapy (not necessarily progestins) and in most series show a somewhat better prognosis with respect to both survival and disease-free interval.[14] Both MPA and MA have been shown to produce similar reductions in serum estrogens levels and produce responses of approximately 30% in patients with metastatic breast cancer.[15] The principal progestin used for metastatic breast cancer has been MA. The response of metastatic breast cancer to MA is predicted not only by the presence of ERs and/or PR but also by the observation of an objective response to previous hormonal therapy. Randomized studies have shown comparable efficacy of progestins

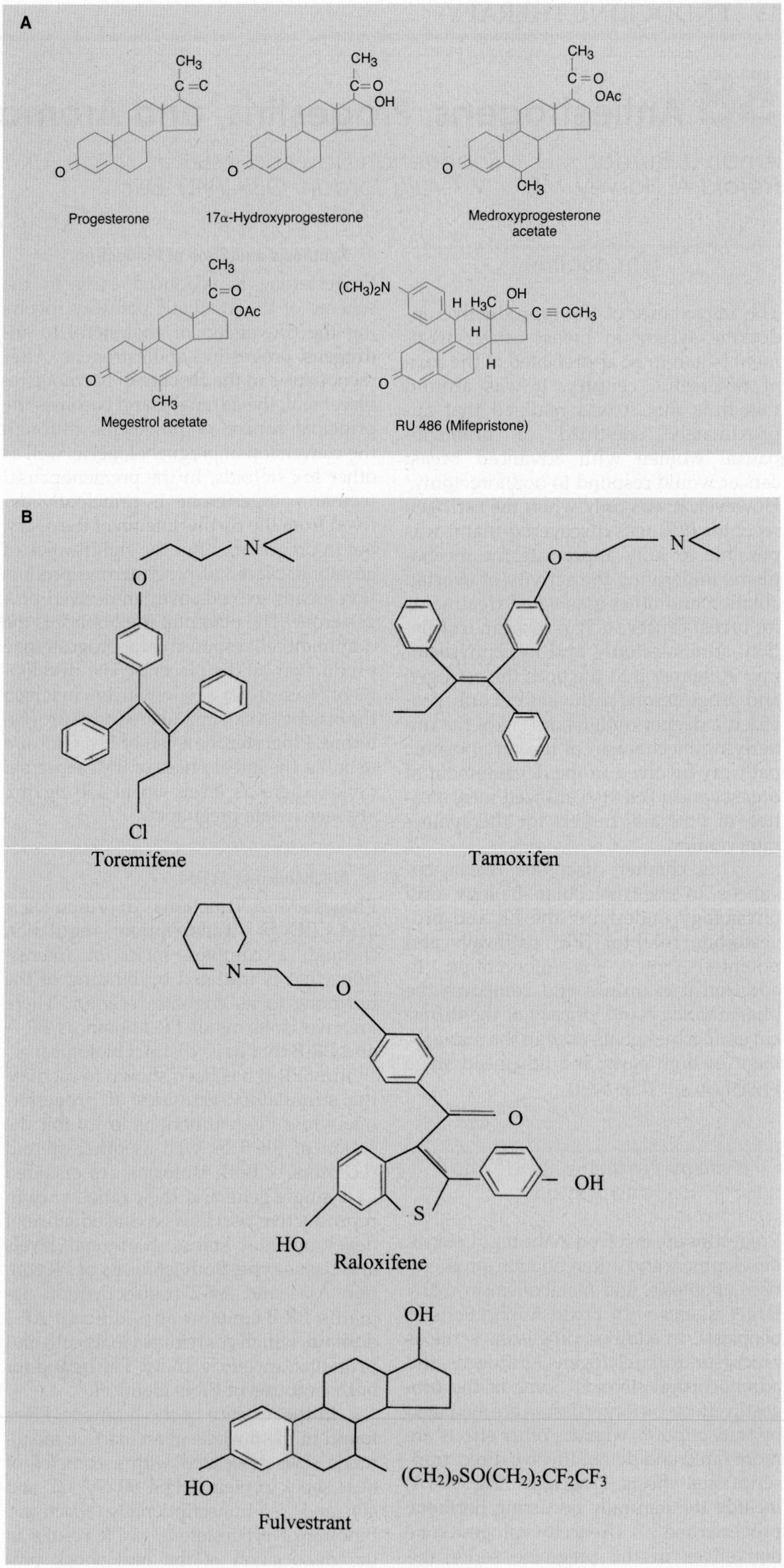

Figure 58-1 Endocrine agents for treatment or prevention of breast cancer. (**A**) Progestins; (**B**) antiestrogens. (*Continued*)

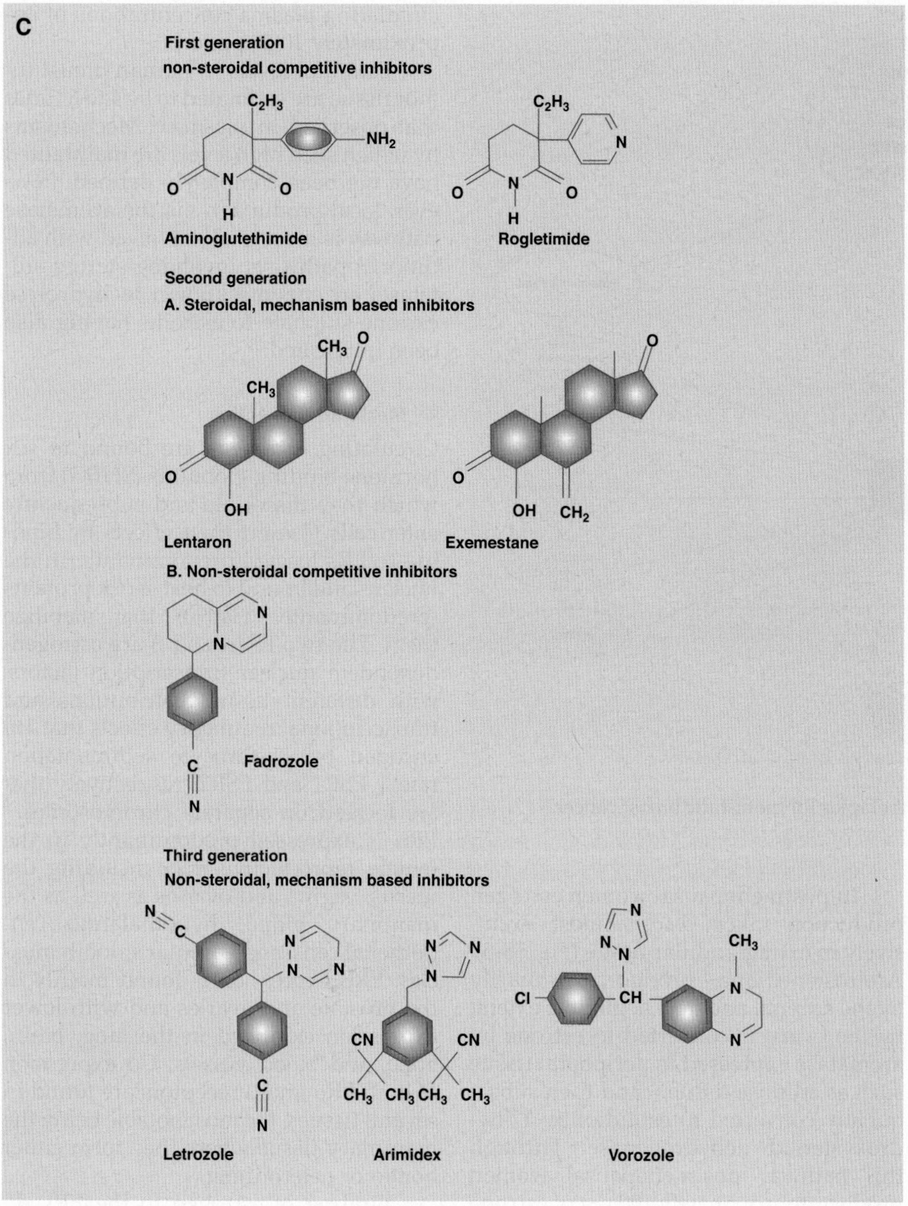

Figure 58-1 (*Continued*) (C) Aromatase inhibitors.

to tamoxifen, aminoglutethemide and aromatase inhibitors in the second and subsequent lines of treatment of metastatic breast cancer.[15,16] Currently progestin therapy for hormone receptor positive metastatic breast cancer is used principally after disease progression has been observed following use of selective ER modulators (eg, tamoxifen), aromatase inhibitors, and fulvestrant. As such a trial of progestins is commonly used as the third or subsequent line of therapy in patients with hormone receptor positive metastatic breast cancer (Fig. 58-2).

Uterine Cancer

The most common adverse effect of progestin is weight gain which occurs as results of increased appetite and fluid retention. Its appetite stimulating effect has frequently been used to treat cancer induced cachexia. Other reported side effects include hot flashes, sweating, vaginal bleeding, nausea, dyspnea, thromboembolism and rare cardiovascular events such as heart failure. Various dosing regimens of MA and MPA have been studied with a possible dose response effect observed. The recommended dose of MA is 160 mg/day and that of MPA is at least 400-500 mg/day.[17]

Progestins are also used in the treatment of endometrial carcinoma.[18] When diagnosed, adenocarcinoma of the uterus is cured by local therapy in 80% of cases. In the event of recurrence, exogenous progestin is an effective treatment in a significant fraction of cases: more than 30% of patients with recurrent disease demonstrate an objective response to exogenous progestins. ER and PR can be measured in these tumors, and the presence of these receptors correlates with differentiation of the tumor, prognosis for the patient, and response to progestins. The duration of response is not predicted by the presence of a receptor and varies from months to years. Tumors that lack ER and PR respond objectively to progestins in fewer than 10% of cases.

Anti-progestins

Anti-progestins have wide and varied therapeutic applications including uses as contraceptives, to induce labor and treatment of breast cancer, endometriosis, uterine leiomyomas and meningiomas.[19] The oldest and most widely used anti-progestin is RU 38486 or mifepristone that is a derivative of the 19-norprogestin norethindrone containing a dimethyl-aminophenol substituent at the 11β-position.[13,20] This compound is effectively absorbed orally and appears to bind with PR with high affinity and to effect altered co-regulatory protein interaction after binding. It has been shown to have both antagonist and some agonist activity and is thus considered to be a PR modulator. Together with prostaglandins it is used for the termination of early pregnancy.[20]

Biology of Estrogen Production and Action

A number of naturally occurring endogenous estrogens are produced in women with the most potent for both ERα- and β-mediated actions being estradiol followed by estrone and estriol. All three contain a phenolic A ring with a hydroxyl group at carbon 3 and a β-OH or ketone in position 17 of ring D with the phenolic A ring being the principle structural feature responsible for their selective high affinity binding to both ERs.

The principle role of naturally occurring estrogens is to modulate cell growth by causing an increase in stimulatory growth factors (eg, transforming growth factor-alpha [TGF-α]) and a decrease in inhibitory growth factors (eg, TGF-β).[21] These growth factors are thought to initiate, or prevent, progress through the cell cycle by interaction with their respective membrane receptors, with the regulatory mechanism functioning as an autocrine loop. There are also paracrine (cell-cell) influences of growth factors (eg, insulin-like growth factors-1 [IGF-1]) that can play a role in modulating the replication of epithelial cells.

Biosynthetic Pathway

The aromatase enzyme complex is located in the endoplasmic reticulum and consists of a cytochrome P450 hemoprotein (P-450 AROM, aromatase), and the flavoprotein nicotinamide adenine dinucleotide phosphate (NADPH) that is common to most cells types and whose

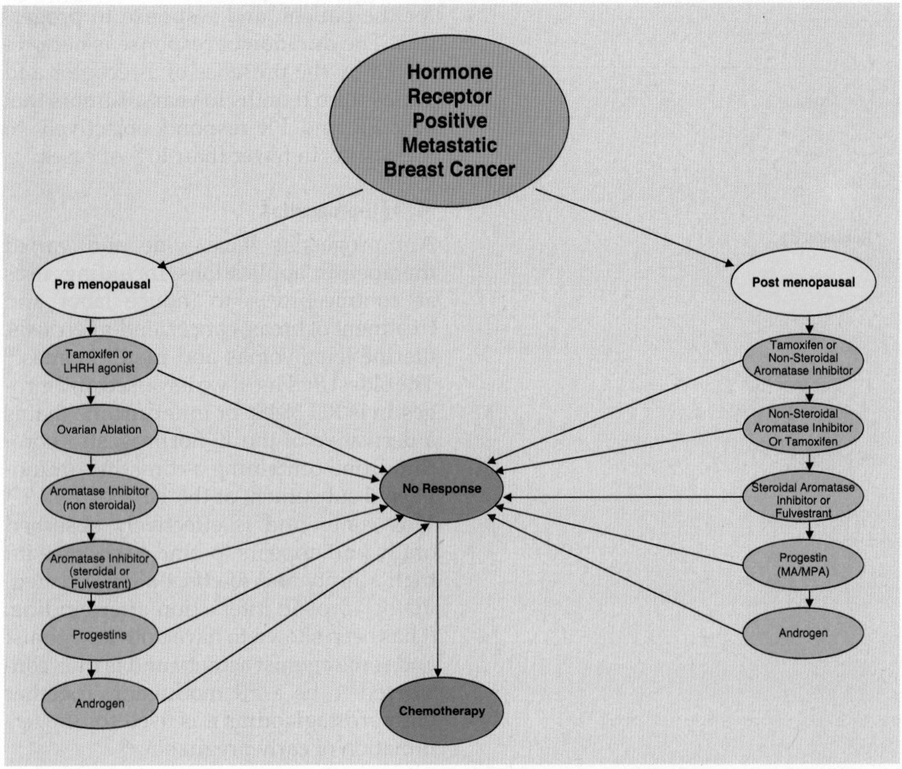

Figure 58-2 Schema of sequential endocrine therapies for metastatic breast cancer.

principle function is to donate electrons to cytochrome P450.[22] The principle enzyme involved in the conversion of androstenedione to estrone in the estrogen biosynthetic pathway is aromatase, a product of the CYP 19 gene that encodes a polypeptide of 503 amino acids with a molecular weight of 55 kilodaltons (KDa). Aromatase catalyzes three separate steroid hydroxylations involved in the conversion of androstenedione to estrone. The first two give rise to 19-hydroxy and 19-aldehyde structures, and the third, although still controversial, probably involves the C-19 methyl group with release of formic acid.[23]

Sites of Production

A number of tissues have the capacity to express aromatase and hence synthesize estrogens and these include the ovary, placenta, hypothalamus, liver, muscle, adipose tissue and malignant breast tumor tissue.[24]

In premenopausal women, the ovary is the most important site of aromatase and estrogen production. Luteinizing hormone (LH) controls production of androstenedione by the theca cell compartment, while follicle stimulating hormone (FSH) upregulates aromatase expression in granulose cells. Acting in concert, LH stimulates production of the substrate for aromatase; whereas, FSH increases the amount of aromatase so that estradiol production can increase by 8 to 10 fold at the time of ovulation.

In postmenopausal women estrogen production takes place almost exclusively in extraglandular tissue (Fig. 58-3). Androstenedione, produced primarily by the adrenal and, to a negligible extent, by the ovary is converted to estrone by aromatase expressed in peripheral tissue such as adipose tissue,[25] and then subsequently converted to estradiol by 17-hydroxysteriod dehydrogenase. Through this pathway postmenopausal women produce approximately 100 mg of estrone per day, with higher levels observed in obese women.[26] A fraction of estrone is also converted to estradiol to produce circulating plasma concentrations of approximately 10-20 pg/mL.

Estradiol levels in human breast tumor tissue are estimated to be 4 to 6 times that observed in plasma.[27] Mechanisms by which such high levels are maintained have not been completely defined: however, local production via the aromatase pathway is most likely involved with additional pathways involving steroid sulfatase, an enzyme known to hydrolyse estrone sulphate to estrone, having also been implicated.[28]

Mechanism of Action

Circulating estrogens are bound to sex hormone binding globulins (SHBG) from which they dissociate and subsequently enter cells to exert their effects by binding to ERs located predominantly in the nucleus and bound to heat shock proteins (predominantly Hsp90) that stabilize them. The two ERsα and β are estrogen-dependent nuclear transcription factors, with different tissue distributions and transcriptional regulatory effects that are encoded by erythrocyte sedimentation rate 1 ESR1 and ESR2, respectively that are located on separate chromosomes.[29] ERα is expressed predominantly in the female reproductive tract including the uterus, vagina and ovaries as well as the mammary gland, hypothalamus, endothelial cells, and vascular smooth muscles. ERβ expression is found mainly in the prostate and ovaries and with lower expression exhibited in the lung, brain, bone, and blood vessels. Co expression of both ERα and β receptors are found in several tissues, the most notable being the mammary tissue where they form either homo- or heterodimers.

Binding of estrogen to the ERs results in a conformational change in the receptor, leading to the release of ER from the stabilizing proteins. The estrogen-ER

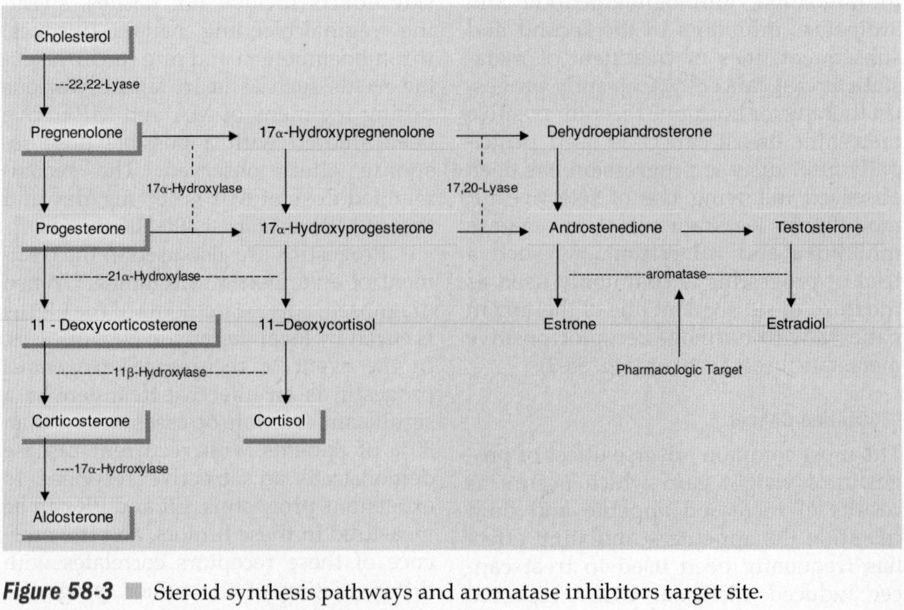

Figure 58-3 Steroid synthesis pathways and aromatase inhibitors target site.

homodimeric complex then binds to a specific sequence of nucleotides called estrogen response elements (ERE) that are located in the promoter region of various genes. This binding interaction also involves a number of nuclear proteins, co regulators as well as other components of the transcription machinery. Thus the genomic effects of estrogen are mainly the result of proteins synthesized from the regulation of transcription of a responsive gene. Two main modalities of treatment, the selective ER modulators (selective ER modulators [SERMS] tamoxifen or raloxifene) or aromatase inhibitors (exemestane, anastrozole, letrozole,[30] have been developed to treat estrogen responsive breast cancers that either target preventing its production or inhibiting its interaction with ERs for clinical purposes, the principal target for antihormonal therapeutic action in the breast tumor is ERα.[2]

Carcinogenic Effects

The major concern with the use of synthetic estrogens either alone or as a part of the preparation of oral contraceptives has been the development of cancer. Studies that reported the link between the intake of diethylstilbesterol (a synthetic estrogen) during the first trimester of pregnancy and the incidence of clear cell vaginal and cervical adenocarcinoma in later life of the offspring exposed in utero, established for the first time that developmental exposure to estrogens was associated with an increase in human cancer.[31,32] Studies have also shown that unopposed estrogen as part of the HRT in postmenopausal women increased the risk of endometrial cancer by 5 to 15 fold[33] with the increased risk prevented by the addition of a progestin.[34]

The relation of breast cancer risk and HRT in postmenopausal women has also been reported by two large trials. The Women's Health Initiative (WHI) was a large prospective trial that randomized women to either placebo or HRT. The investigators reported an increase in total risk of breast cancer of 24% among women who took an estrogen-progestin combination and a decrease of 23% among women without a uterus who took estrogen only compared to women who took placebo.[12,35] The Million Women Study (MWS) was a large cohort study that reported an increased relative risk of invasive breast cancer among women who did and did not take HRT.[36] Among women who took an estrogen-progestin combination the increased relative risk of invasive breast cancer was 2, and that for women who took estrogen alone was reported as 1.3.

Epidemiological studies have also linked high levels of natural estrogens to the development of cancer. High levels of natural estrogens are observed in women who are overweight. Among postmenopausal women who had never received HRT in the WHI those who were heavier (body mass index [BMI] >31.1) had an elevated risk of breast cancer compared to slimmer women (BMI < 22.6), relative risk [RR] 2.52; 95% CI 1.62-3.93).[33] High levels of natural estrogens were also found to be associated in a case-cohort study involving women with who had never received exogenous estrogens.[37] The investigators reported that compared to women with the lowest levels of circulating estradiol those with the highest levels (≥ 6.83 pmol/L or 1.9 pg/mL) had a RR of 3.6 (95% CI 1.3-10.0).

Bone mineral density has also been shown to be a surrogate marker of estrogen exposure. A high endogenous estrogen concentration has been reported to be associated with greater bone mineral density in elderly women.[38] Postmenopausal women with higher bone mineral densities have also been shown to have a higher incidence of breast cancer.[39] Such studies serve to indicate the potential benefit of circulating estrogens as a surrogate marker of breast cancer risk. However its reliability as a surrogate marker is controversial due to the low baseline line levels observed among postmenopausal women and the timing of circulating estrogen level measurement with relation to the menstrual cycle being important in premenopausal women. Regardless, enough evidence exist connecting estrogens to the development of hormone responsive breast cancer that has spawned a number of prevention trials that have used agents targeted either at blocking the production of estrogens or its interaction with its receptor.

SERMS and Antiestrogens

The first indication of the role of hormones in the development of breast cancer occurred more than a century ago when in 1896 Beatson observed that remission could be induced by removal of the ovaries in a subset of breast cancer patients.[1] Although not originally understood the observed effects occurred as a result of eliminating the primary source of estrogen in premenopausal women. This was confirmed in preclinical studies that demonstrated estradiol to promote proliferation of ER-positive breast cancer cells in culture[40] and numerous epidemiological studies that have linked estrogens to breast cancer risk.[35-39] With the realization of the important role estrogen played in the development and progression of breast cancer two groups of drugs were developed to counteract the action of estrogens. The first group essentially prevented the interaction of estrogen to its receptor and included the SERMS and antiesrtogens. SERMS including tamoxifen, raloxifene, and toremifene display unusual tissue selective pharmacology having estrogen agonist properties in some tissues (bone, liver, and cardiovascular system), estrogen antagonist properties in other tissues (brain and breast) and mixed agonist/antagonist estrogen properties in the uterus (Fig. 58-1B).[41] The antiestrogens which include fulvestrant are distinguished from SERMS in that they are uniformly estrogen antagonists. The second group of drugs blocks the production of estrogen by blocking the action of the aromatase enzyme and is known as aroamatase inhibitors (Fig. 58-1C). In this section we will review the various SERMS and antiestrogens used in clinical practice for the treatment and prevention of hormone receptor positive breast cancers.

Tamoxifen

Mode of Action ■ Tamoxifen is a nonsteroidal triphenylethylene compound[42] that exerts its effects by competitively inhibiting the binding of estradiol to ER thereby negating the stimulatory effects of estrogen causing the cell to be held at the G1 phase of the replication cycle.[43] Tamoxifen is an estrogen antagonist in the breast and an estrogen agonist in the endometrium and bone, and it is this balance in biological properties that is the key to the current strategies for the use of tamoxifen.

Clinical Pharmacology ■ The high therapeutic index of tamoxifen has permitted wide variations in dosage with schedules and dosage of treatment varying depending on the country and its initial clinical trials that evaluated efficacy of this drug. Schedules of 10 mg twice daily or 20 mg once daily are recommended in the United States, although 10 mg three times daily and 20 mg twice daily have been used in other countries.

Tamoxifen is administered orally and is rapidly absorbed, achieving a steady state serum levels within 4-6 weeks, and subsequently metabolized to N-desmethyltamoxifen (major metabolite) and 4-hydroxytamoxfien (minor metabolite) both of which have the potential to be further metabolized to 4-hydroxy-N-desmethyltamoxifen (minor metabolite).[44] Tamoxifen has a long serum half-life of 7 days, and the metabolite N-desmethyltamoxifen has an even longer half life of 14 days.[45] These long serum half lives are probably why a withdrawal response has not been routinely documented when tamoxifen therapy is discontinued. Although no clinical cases of teratogenesis has been documented with tamoxifen it is not recommended in pregnant women. Furthermore tamoxifen is known to cause ovarian stimulation in premenopausal women with ovulatory cycles and thus women taking tamoxifen who are at risk of getting pregnant should be counseled about various contraceptive options.[46]

Tamoxifen in Advanced Breast Cancer ■ Tamoxifen is an endocrine option for metastatic disease in postmenopausal women and those with ER-positive disease are more likely to benefit from this therapy.[47] Correlation of clinical response and ER status indicates that approximately 48% of patients with ER-positive disease achieve partial or complete responses, whereas only 13% of patients with ER-negative disease exhibit some form of response with endocrine therapy indicating the selective efficacy of endocrine therapy among patients with hormone receptor positive disease. More recent data suggests that aromatase inhibitors are a better option as first line treatment for this cohort of patients so long as resistance to the drug has not developed. This will be discussed in further detail in the section "Aromatase Inhibitors."

Tamoxifen is a first line endocrine therapy in premenopausal women with advanced breast cancer. In this group of patients small randomized clinical trials have demonstrated that tamoxifen produces a response rate and overall survival similar to what is seen after oophorectomy.[48] However, with the development of effective LH-releasing hormone (LHRH) agonists such as goserelin (Zoladex), which acts to reduce ovarian steroidogenesis by preventing LH release from the pituitary gland, the combination of goserelin and tamoxifen has become established as an effective therapeutic option.[49] Hence recent guidelines have suggested that the use of LHRH agonists and tamoxifen alone or in combination are appropriate therapeutic options for women for premenopausal women with advanced metastatic hormone receptor positive disease[50] (Fig. 58-3).

Tamoxifen in the Adjuvant Setting ■ Many randomized trials have addressed the question of tamoxifen efficacy in the adjuvant setting among women with early stage breast cancer. An overview and meta-analysis of the results from 145,000 women with early stage breast cancer who were randomized to 194 trials of adjuvant systemic therapy (chemotherapy and/or hormonal therapy) were recently updated by the Early Breast Cancer Trialists' Collaborative Group (EBCTCG).[51] The EBCTCG reported that 5-years of adjuvant tamoxifen among women with ER-positive disease resulted in reduction in the annual death rate by 31% regardless of age, PR status, menopausal status, or use of chemotherapy with benefits persisting up to 15-years of follow-up. In this report, 1-year of tamoxifen conferred little benefit; 5-years of tamoxifen was significantly more effective than 2-years, still requiring long term follow-up for assessing the benefit of more than 5-years of adjuvant tamoxifen treatment. However, results from the B-14 trial, a National Surgical Adjuvant Breast and Bowel Project (NSABP), in which women with lymph node negative ER-positive disease still in remission after receiving 5-years of tamoxifen were re randomized to receive either placebo or more prolonged therapy with tamoxifen have not shown any advantage from prolonged tamoxifen treatment through 7-years of follow-up.[52] Indeed, the longer duration of tamoxifen use was associated with shorter disease free survival (DFS) compared to the group who had stopped taking tamoxifen after 5-years (78% vs 82%, $p = .03$). Preliminary results from the Ajduvant Tamoxifen Longer Against Shorter (ATLAS) and Adjuvant Tamoxifen Treatment offer More (aTTom) trials, two large prospective trials that have randomized women with early stage breast cancer who completed five years of tamoxifen to either another five years tamoxifen, indicated a reduced risk of recurrence in the group that received continued tamoxifen beyond five years. Further follow-up is required to reliably assess the effects of tamoxifen on survival outcomes (both disease free and overall) as well as on any potentially associated side effects.[53,54] At present time, with the available evidence, current recommendations are that no more than five years tamoxifen therapy be offered as adjuvant therapy.[50]

Tamoxifen and Chemotherapy ■ In the latest update of the EBCTCG that addition of anthracyline based polychemotherapy regimens was reported to be associated with annual reduction of mortality of 38% and 20% among women aged <50 years and 50-69 years, respectively. The question however is whether the addition of an endocrine agent such as tamoxifen could further add to this benefit among women with ER-positive breast tumors. In the EBCTCG among 3330 women with ER-positive or ER unknown tumors 28.1% of women who received only chemotherapy experienced a recurrence compared to 17.5% who received chemotherapy and 5-years of tamoxifen with the difference being statistically significant.[51] Similarly among women with ER-positive or ER unknown breast tumors those who were less than 50 years of age and received chemotherapy and tamoxifen the EBCTCG reported a recurrence rate ratio of 0.64 (SE 0.08) and annual breast cancer mortality ratio of 0.65 (SE 0.10) compared to those who received tamoxifen alone with similar trends observed among women in the 50 to 69 years age group. When the sequence of chemotherapy and tamoxifen was explored among women 50 to 69 years of age a recurrence rate ratio and annual breast cancer mortality rate ratio of 0.80 (SE 0.03) and 0.90 (SE 0.03) among women treated with chemotherapy with tamoxifen compared to those who received tamoxifen alone with a recurrence rate ratio and annual breast cancer mortality rate ratio of 0.77 (SE 0.08) and 0.80 (SE 0.10) among women treated with chemotherapy followed by tamoxifen compared to those who received tamoxifen alone.[51] Therefore chemotherapy alone is not enough in women with ER-positive tumors with the clear data that the addition of tamoxifen is important. The data also indicate that sequential hormonal therapy maybe the better option. This is further strengthened by recent results from the South West Oncology Study Group (SWOG) 8814 study that reported improved disease free and overall survival outcomes when tamoxifen was given sequentially following cyclophosphamide, doxorubicin and 5-fluoruracil (CAF) compared with concurrent administration or tamoxifen alone.[55]

Prevention of Breast Cancer ■ Observations that long-term tamoxifen therapy reduced the incidence and risk of contralateral breast cancer in women with early stage breast cancer fueled interest in exploring the effect of tamoxifen in preventing the occurrence of breast cancer. An overview of the main outcomes from the five main breast cancer prevention trials, covering more than 28,000 patients, has shown that tamoxifen produced a 38% reduction in breast cancer incidence ($p < .0001$).[56] There was no effect on ER-negative disease ($p = .21$), but ER-positive cancers were reduced by 48% ($p < .0001$). However, endometrial cancer rates were increased (consensus RR 2.4; $p = .0005$) in patients receiving preventive tamoxifen, as were venous thromboembolic events (RR 1.9; $p < .0001$). As a result, tamoxifen cannot be used as a true preventive because the timing of the event is unknown and the unrestricted use of tamoxifen in young women of reproductive age would be unwise. An exception to this is when tamoxifen is used for the reduction of breast cancer risk in high-risk women, for which it is the first medicine to be approved by the U.S. Food and Drug Administration. Thus use of tamoxifen in preventive setting should be individualized to a woman's risk of developing breast cancer. As such women with a prior history of ductal carcinoma in situ, lobular carcinoma in situ, atypical hyperplasia or those with a deleterious mutation of (*BRCA*$_1$) or *BRCA*$_2$ are considered to be at higher risk of developing breast cancer and represent an ideal cohort to target where benefit out weights risk of adverse events associated with tamoxifen.[57–59]

Raloxifene

Raloxifene is a benzothiophene second generation SERM that is FDA approved for the treatment and prevention of osteoporosis and for the reduction of risk of invasive breast carcinoma in postmenopausal women with either osteoporosis or who are at high risk for invasive breast cancer respectively.[60–63] This agent has no significant anti-tumor activity in the metastatic setting and is not approved for the treatment of advanced metastatic breast cancer. Four large prospective trials have reported on the efficacy of raloxifene as a chemopreventive agent for breast cancer. The Multiple Outcomes and of Raloxifene Evaluation (MORE) trial that randomized 7705 postmenopausal women with osteoporosis to receive either raloxifene or placebo, whose primary end point was development of a fracture, was the first major trial to suggest raloxifene as a potential agent for chemoprevention of breast cancer.[60] In this trial following 4 years of treatment raloxifene reduced the risk of ER-positive invasive breast cancer by 84% (RR 0.16; 95% CI 0.09, 0.30). The Continuing Outcomes Relevant to Evista (CORE) trial was an extension of the MORE trial to examine the effect of four additional years of raloxifene therapy on the incidence of invasive breast cancer in women in MORE who agreed to continue on the trial.[61] Combining the 8 years of follow up of both the MORE and CORE trials the investigators reported that the incidences of invasive breast cancer overall and ER-positive invasive breast cancer were reduced by 66% (hazard ratio [HR] 0.34; 95% CI 0.22-0.50) and 76% (HR 0.24; 95% CI 0.15-0.40), respectively, in the raloxifene group compared with the placebo group. The goal of the Raloxifene Use for the Heart (RUTH) trial was to investigate the effect of raloxifene on the incidence of coronary events and breast cancer in 10,101 postmenopausal women.[62] The investigators found reductions in breast cancer similar in size to that seen for tamoxifen in other studies. The NSABP P-2 trial was a prospective, double-blinded, randomized clinical trial that compared the efficacy and safety of tamoxifen on the risk of developing invasive breast cancer in a cohort of 19,747 postmenopausal women.[63] The investigators reported similar efficacy of tamoxifen compared to raloxifene in reducing the risk of invasive breast cancer (RR 1.02; 95% CI 0.82-1.28). In terms of side effects compared to tamoxifen, raloxifene had fewer gynecological and thromboembolic events. Interestingly, raloxifene reduced the risk of invasive breast cancer but had no effect on the incidence of ductal carcinoma in situ.

Toremifene

Toremifene (Fareston) is a structural derivative of tamoxifen with similar antiestrogenic and estrogenic properties demonstrated in laboratory animals. In general, toremifene is highly protein bound, which could explain its long serum half-life. Toremifene is less potent than tamoxifen, and consequently, clinical studies have evaluated doses of toremifene up to 240 mg/day. Toremifene is cross-resistant with tamoxifen, but clinical trials have shown that it exhibits a similar efficacy and side effect profile to tamoxifen, and so may be used as an alternative to treat advanced breast cancer.[64,65] At this time, there is insufficient data to recommend its use in the adjuvant setting.

Trilostane

Trilostane (Modrenal) is an antiadrenal drug that is usually used for short-term adrenal suppression in the treatment of Cushing syndrome. However, trilostane's ability to modify the binding of estrogen to the ER has prompted interest in its potential to block breast tumor cell proliferation. A meta-analysis of several small studies investigating the use of trilostane in postmenopausal women with advanced breast cancer reported clinical benefit with this agent, and further trials are needed to evaluate its worth as an endocrine therapy for advanced breast cancer.[66]

Fulvestrant

Fulvestrant (Faslodex) is an antiesrtogen with no agonist properties and unlike tamoxifen has the following mechanism of action: it binds, blocks, and increases degradation of ER protein, leading to an inhibition of estrogen signaling through the ER together with dramatic loss of cellular ER levels, and is also associated with a significant reduction in PgR) expression.[67,68] A prospective, combined analysis of two phase 3 trials comparing fulvestrant (250 mg intramuscular injection once monthly) to anastrozole in a cohort of postmenopausal women with advanced breast cancer who had progressed on prior tamoxifen therapy indicated that, after a median follow-up of 15.1 months, fulvestrant was well tolerated and was at least as effective as anastrozole (median times to progression [TTP] were 5.5 months vs 4.1 months) with a similar and acceptable adverse event profile.[69] Subsequently fulvestrant as first line treatment of advanced breast cancer was compared to tamoxifen in a randomized clinical trial. At a median follow up of 14.5 months no significant difference for the primary end point of time to progression between the two groups was observed.[70] In the setting of a phase 3 randomized clinical trial fulvestrant has also been compared to exemestane for the treatment of postmenopausal women with hormone receptor positive advanced breast cancer who had progressed or recurred on a non steroidal aromatase inhibitor.[71] In this study overall response rate (7.4% vs 6.7%; $p = .736$) and time to treatment progression (3.7 months in both groups) were similar between the fulvestrane and exemestane groups suggesting that fulvestrant was no more effective than a steroidal aromatase inhibitor among women who had progressed on a non-steroidal aromatase inhibitor. Since fulvestrant can take 3 to 6 months to reach steady state plasma levels at the 250 mg/month dose (approved dosing schedule) there are currently ongoing trials that are evaluating the standard dosing regimen to a loading dosing schedule. Currently the fulvestrant is approved for the treatment of hormone receptor positive metastatic breast cancer in postmenopausal that had progressed on prior tamoxifen therapy.[72]

Side Effects of SERMS and Antiestrogens

Side effects related to the SERMS and antiesrtogens develop mainly as a result of the blockage of the stimulatory function of estrogen on a variety of tissues. The most frequent side effect encountered is hot flashes, night sweats and vaginal dryness similar to that seen in women undergoing menopause. Other less frequent but important side effects pertain to the bone, blood vessels and carcinogenic effects.

Osteoporosis ■ Estrogen is important in maintaining bone health in premenopausal women with HRT and often recommended to prevent the development of osteoporosis in postmenopausal women. Long-term administration of an antiestrogen has the potential to cause premature osteoporosis in premenopausal women. However, due to the partial estrogen agonist function of SERMS clinical studies have shown tamoxifen therapy to be not associated with a reduction of bone density[73] and raloxifene is an approved treatment for osteoporosis.[61]

Coronary Heart Disease ■ Estrogen lowers low-density lipoprotein (LDL) cholesterol levels and raises high-density lipoprotein (HDL) cholesterol levels and thus prolonged administration of an antiestrogen could produce a population at risk of premature coronary heart disease. However, the estrogen-like effects of tamoxifen has been shown to lower the circulating levels of cholesterol in female patients[74,75] with clinical studies reporting tamoxifen to be associated with either a significant or trend in reduction of risk of coronary heart disease.[76] Raloxifene has also been shown to reduce serum cholesterol levels[77]; however, has not been shown in a large randomized clinical trial to reduce the risk of coronary heart disease.[62]

Thromboembolism ■ A number of studies have demonstrated an association between the use of tamoxifen and subsequent thromboembolic episodes in both the treatment and preventive setting,[56,78] This is comparable with increases noted with HRT or raloxifene.[79] Patients with a known history of thromboembolic disorders should be carefully evaluated before a decision is made to use long-term tamoxifen therapy.

Endometrial Tumors ■ Research has demonstrated that increases in endometrial thickness, hyperplasia, and fibroids may follow treatment with tamoxifen.[80] Endometrial thickening is associated with the stromal component of the uterus rather than the epithelial component.[81] Clinical trials evaluating the efficacy of tamoxifen in the treatment and prevention of breast cancer have demonstrated an increased risk of endometrial tumors including carcinomas, and to a smaller extent, sarcomas.[82,83] Endometrial carcinoma that develops on tamoxifen therapy is not of high grade and as such is not associated with poor prognosis while endometrial sarcomas are generally associated with a poorer prognosis, seemingly because of less favorable histology and higher stage.[83] Thus when monitoring patients on tamoxifen treatment all cases of abnormal vaginal bleeding should be followed up with a gynecologic examination and an endometrial biopsy. It is important to note that this increased risk is restricted to postmenopausal women; premenopausal women are not at an increased risk of endometrial cancer. When raloxifene was directly compared to tamoxifen in the prevention of breast cancer (STAR trial), 36 cases of endometrial cancer were observed in the tamoxifen group compared to 23 cases in the raloxifene group (RR 0.62; 95% CI 0.35-1.08).[63]

Other Side Effects ■ Antiestrogens and SERMS have also been associated with ophthalmic side defects such cataracts and retinal changes.[84,85] Preclinical studies have also demonstrated tamoxifen to cause carcinogenesis in the liver; however an increase in human hepatocelluar carcinoma has not been demonstrated.[86]

Aromatase Inhibitors

In contrast to SERMs and antiesrtogens, aromatase inhibitors work by blocking the enzyme complex responsible for the final step in estrogen biosynthetic pathway and is thereby essentially preventing the production of the ER substrate. Moreover unlike tamoxifen aromatase inhibitors have no partial estrogen agonist function. Despite the ovaries being a rich source of aromatase, aromatase inhibitors are unable to sufficiently suppress ovarian estrogen production to postmenopausal levels, which may be due to compensatory rise in gonadotrophins which maintains adequate estrogen production, despite the presence of the inhibitor. In contrast aromatase inhibitors have been shown to adequately suppress estrogen production in postmenopausal women.

Aromatase inhibitors are classified into first-, second-, and third-generation aromatase inhibitors according to the specificity and potency with which they inhibit the aromatase enzyme (Fig. 58-1C). They are further subclassified according to their mechanism of action into steroidal (irreversible, type 1) and nonsteroidal (reversible, type 2) inhibitors. Type 1 inhibitors, including formestane and exemestane, function by irreversibly inhibiting the aromatase enzyme by covalently binding to it, resulting in permanent inactivation that persists even after discontinuation of the drug until the peripheral tissues synthesize new enzymes. Type 2 inhibitors, including anastrozole, letrozole and fadrozoel, in contrast bind reversibly to the active site of the aromatase enzyme and prevent product formation only as long as the inhibitor occupies the catalytic site. In this section we will focus on the newer third-generation aromatase inhibitors letrozole, anastrozole and exemestane that are in common clinical practice today. These aromatase inhibitors have challenged tamoxifen as the gold standard and are now the preferred first line treatment of postmenopausal women with hormone responsive breast cancer in either the early or advanced setting.

First-Generation Aromatase Inhibitors

Aminoglutethimide, a derivative of the sedative agent glutethimide, was initially introduced is an inhibitor of cytochrome P-450 N-mediated steroid hydroxylations.[87] The effects of this compound, however, are rather nonspecific because the drug affects a number of hydroxylation steps in the metabolic conversion of cholesterol to active steroid products, and overall, the use of aminoglutethimide plus glucocorticoid in women with breast cancer produces results similar to those expected from other forms of endocrine therapy. Side effects observed with standard doses of aminoglutethimide (1000 mg/day) include drug rash, fever, and lethargy.[87] With the development of more selective second- and third- generation aromatase inhibitors, aminoglutethimide is now rarely used for the treatment of breast cancer.

Second-Generation Aromatase Inhibitors

The two second-generation aromatase inhibitors on the market are fadrozole and formestane. Fadrozole (4-[5,6,7,8-tetrahydroimidazo-(1,5-a)-pyridin-5yl] benzonitrile)), a type 2 inhibitor, is a potent inhibitor of aromatase. Two large multicenter phase 3 trials have compared fadrozole with MA in patients who had received only tamoxifen as prior hormone therapy. No significant differences were observed between the two treatment arms of the trials with respect to time to treatment progression, overall response rate, response duration, or overall survival.[88] When compared to tamoxifen as a first line treatment among postmenopausal women with advanced breast cancer similar efficacy was observed between the two agents with fadrozole having a better tolerability profile.[89] Toxicity attributed to fadrozole is mild and consists mainly of nausea, anorexia, fatigue, and hot flashes. Fadrozole represents a major improvement over aminoglutethimide and the drug is approved in Japan for the treatment of patients with breast cancer.

Formestane (4-hydroxyandrostenedione, Lentaron), a type 1 inhibitor, is given by intramuscular injection and is thus associated with in-site reactions. It has been tested in clinical trials as second line treatment for postmenopausal women with metastatic disease and demonstrated similar efficacy to mestrol acetate among those who had progressed on tamoxifen[90] with clinical benefit also demonstrated in patients who have progressed on nonsteroidal aromatase inhibitors.[91]

Third-Generation Aromatase Inhibitors

Third generation aromatase inhibitors have now become the standard treatment for postmenopausal women with either advanced or early stage hormone responsive breast cancer having demonstrated superior efficacy and tolerability compared to tamoxifen. Third generation aromatoase inhibitors include exemestane, letrozole, and anastrazole.

Exemestane (6-methylene-androsta-1,4-diene-3,17-dione, AromasinS), a type 1 aromatase inhibitor, is an orally administered analog of the natural substrate androstenedione. It is rapidly absorbed from the gastrointestinal tract, reaching maximum plasma levels after 2 h and has been shown to lower estrogen levels more effectively than formestane. Single-dose administration of 25 mg/day inhibits aromatase activity by 97.9% and lowers plasma estrone and estradiol levels by about 90%.[92] The FDA approved dosing regimen for exemestane is 25 mg once daily.

Anastrozole (Arimidex), a type 2 inhibitor, is a potent and selective benzyltriazole derivative absorbed rapidly after oral administration with maximal plasma concentration occurring after 2 h, steady state plasma concentrations achieved after 7 days and has an elimination half-life in humans of approximately 32.2 h.[93] Anastrozole at doses of 1 or 10 mg administered once daily for 28 days has been shown to reduce total body aromatization by 96.7% and 98.1%, respectively. The FDA approved dosing regimen of anastrozole is 1 mg once daily.

Letrozole (4,4′-[(1H-1,2,4-triazol-1-yl) methylene] bis-benzonitrile, Femara), a type 2 inhibitor, is a highly potent inhibitor of aromatase in vitro, in vivo in animals and in humans, and is associated with greater suppression of estrogen than is achieved with other aromatase inhibitors. When administered orally to adult female rats at a dose of 1 mg/L/day for 14 days, letrozole decreased uterine weight to that observed after a surgical ovariectomy.[94] Clinical studies in normal healthy volunteers, as well as dose-seeking phase 1 trials in postmenopausal women with advanced breast cancer, showed that letrozole in a dose as little as 0.25 mg/day PO caused maximal suppression of plasma and urinary estrogens.[95] The FDA approved and recommended dosing regimen for letrozole is 2.5 mg once a day.

Vorozole (R83842; R76713; 6-[(S)4-Chlorophenyl)-1H-1,2,4-triazol-1-ylmethyl]-1-methyl-1H-benzotriazole) represents another specific type 2 aromatase inhibitor that has shown little toxicity in animal studies. However, despite results from phase 3 studies that have demonstrated the clinical efficacy of vorazole in postmenopausal women with metastatic disease,[96] this drug has been withdrawn from further clinical development.

Treatment of Metastatic Breast Cancer ■ Preclinical studies have shown aromatase inhibitors to be effective after initial treatment with tamoxifen.[97] Following demonstrated efficacy in phase 2 trials, a number of phase 3 trials have evaluated the efficacy of third generation aromatase (letrozole, anasztrozole, and exemestane) inhibitors as a second line agent compared to MA in the treatment of postmenopausal women with metastatic breast cancer who had previously been treated with tamoxifen (Table 58-1). In a cohort of 769 postmenopausal women with metastatic breast cancer, exemestane produced a statistically significant increase in median duration of overall clinical benefit (60.1 vs 49 weeks, $p = .025$), median time to tumor progression and median survival compared to MA.[98] In a similar cohort of 764 women from two pivotal phase 3 trials, patients randomized to either anastrozole (1 mg/day PO) or anastrozole (10 mg/day PO) had estimated hazards of progression of 0.97 (97.5% CI 0.75-1.24) and 0.92 (97.5% CI 0.71-1.19) respectively compared to patients receiving megastrol acetate.[99] No statistically significant dose-response differences were observed between the 1 mg/day and 10 mg/day dosage. With subsequent follow-up 2-year survival was 56.1% for the group of patients receiving anastrozole (1 mg/day), compared with 46.3% for patients treated with MA.[100] Similarly the efficacy of letrozole was evaluated in a pivotal trial of 555 postmenopausal women with metastatic breast cancer that had progressed on tamoxifen.[101] Letrozole (2.5 mg/day) yielded overall response rates of 36% and 35%, respectively, compared with 27% and 33%, respectively, for letrozole (0.5 mg/day) and 32% for MA. The median duration of response for letrozole (2.5 mg/day) was 33 months, compared with 18 months for both MA and letrozole 0.5 mg/day. A trend in time to tumor progression and survival that favored letrozole 2.5 mg/day was also observed.

Following the success of third generation aromatase inhibitors in the second line treatment of postmenopausal women with metastatic breast cancer focus shifted to first line treatment of this cohort directly comparing these agents with tamoxifen (Table 58-2). In a phase 2 study comparing exemestane (25 mg/day) with tamoxifen (20 mg/day) as first-line treatment for metastatic disease patients receiving exemestane had better objective response rates (complete response plus partial response) and median duration of response compared to tamoxifen.[102] The study was subsequently extended into a phase 3 trial where exemestane was reported to be well tolerated and was associated with a significantly longer progression-free survival compared with tamoxifen (10.9 vs 6.7 months, respectively).[103] In a combined analysis of two pivotal phase 3 trials that involved 1021 postmenopausal women with metastatic breast cancer first line treatment of anastrozole at a dose of 1 mg/day was compared to tamoxifen.[104] At a median follow-up of 18.5 months for patients with hormone receptor-positive tumors (59.8% of patients), median time to progression was significantly superior in the group receiving anastrozole compared to those receiving tamoxifen (10.7 months vs 6.4 months, $p = .022$). Similarly a large, multicenter, double-blind, first-line phase 3 clinical trial in 907 postmenopausal women with locally advanced or metastatic breast cancer compared letrozole (2.5 mg/day) with tamoxifen (20 mg/ day).[105] At a median follow-up of 32 months time to progression (median, 9.4 vs 6.0 months, respectively; $p < .0001$), time to treatment failure (median, 9 vs 5.7 months, respectively;

Table 58-1 **■ Combined Data From Phase 3 Trials Comparing Anastrozole, Letrozole, and Exemestane With Megestrol Acetate in Postmenopausal Women Previously Treated With Tamoxifen**

	Combined Data		Initial Trial		Second Trial		Initial Trial	
	Anastrozole	Megestrol Acetate	Letrozole	Megestrol Acetate	Letrozole	Megestrol Acetate	Exemestane	Megestrol Acetate
No. of patients	263	253	174	189	199	201	366	403
Objective response,[a] %	12.6	12.2	23.6	16.4	16.1	14.9	15	12
Clinical benefit,[b] %	42.2	40.3	34.5	31.7	26.7	23.4	37	35
Progression, %	57.4	59.3	53.4	56.1	51.3	50.7	48	53
Median TTP, months	5	5	5-6	5.5	3	3	5	5
Median duration of benefit, months	18.3	15.7	33	18	17.5	15.4	15	12
Median survival, months	28.7	21.5	25.3	21.5	28.6	26.2	NA	28

[a]Objective response = complete response + partial response. [b]Clinical benefit = complete response + partial response + stable disease for ≥ 6 months.
Abbreviations: NA, not available; TTP, time to progression.

Table 58-2 **Efficacy Data From Trials Comparing Anastrozole, Letrozole, and Exemestane With Tamoxifen in the First-Line Treatment of Postmenopausal Women With Metastatic Breast Cancer**

	Phase 2 Studies				Phase 3 Studies			
	Letrozole	Tamoxifen	Exemestane	Tamoxifen	Anastrozole[a]	Tamoxifen[a]	Anastrozole[b]	Tamoxifen[b]
No. of patients	453	454	61	59	170	182	340	453
Objective response, %	30	20[c]	41	14	21	17	33	30
Clinical benefit, %	49	38[c]	56	42	59	46[c]	56	56
TTP, months	9	6[c]	9	5	11	6[c]	8	8
TTF, months	9	6[c]	NR	NR	8	5	6	6

[a]North American Study. [b]European Study. [c]Difference is statistically significant.
Abbreviations: Nonprotocol analysis; NR, not recorded.

$p < .0001$) and overall objective response rate (32% vs 21%, respectively; $p = .0002$) were all reported to be significantly superior in the group receiving letrozole compared to tamoxifen. Median overall survival was 34 months for letrozole and 30 months for tamoxifen.

Current guidelines recommend the use of tamoxifen as first line therapy in premenopausal women with metastatic breast cancer.[50] Aromatase inhibitors are recommended as first line therapy of advanced breast cancer in postmenopausal women[50] (Fig. 58-3).

Adjuvant Studies ■ With the efficacy of third generation aromatase inhibitors established in the treatment of postmenopausal women with hormone responsive metastatic breast cancer focus then shifted to determine their efficacy in the adjuvant treatment of early stage breast cancer. With the recognized increased risk of endometrial carcinoma and thromboembolic events associated with the use of tamoxifen, aromatase inhibitors provided a reasonable alternative. Adjuvant studies evaluating third generation aromatase inhibitors have explored their efficacy both as upfront adjuvant treatment and following a course of adjuvant tamoxifen (Table 58-3). The following section will review results of the major trials that have explored these issues.

Upfront Treatment of Early Disease ■ The "Arimidex," Tamoxifen, Alone or in Combination (ATAC) trial is a randomized, double-blind study of 9366 postmenopausal women with early stage breast cancer that was designed to compare the efficacy and tolerability of 5 years of treatment with tamoxifen with that of anastrozole versus the combination of anastrozole and tamoxifen.[106] A planned analysis at a median follow-up of 33 months resulted in the combination arm being discontinued due to lack of superior efficacy or tolerability to tamoxifen alone. The primary endpoint for this study was DFS and secondary endpoints were time to recurrence (TTR), incidence of new contralateral breast cancer, time to distant recurrence (TTDR), and overall survival (OS). At a median follow-up of 100 months among women with hormone receptor positive disease DFS was significantly superior in the anastrazole group compared to the tamoxifen group (HR 0.85; 95% CI 0.76-0.94; $p = .003$) as were TTR, TTDR and incidence of contralateral breast cancer. No significant difference was noted in OS between the two groups (HR 0.97; 95% CI 0.86-1.11; $p = .7$).[107] Fracture rates were higher in the anastrozole group; however the risk of fracture was similar between the two groups once the endocrine therapy was discontinued. No difference in cardio vascular morbidity or mortality was noted between the two groups. There were significantly fewer cases of stroke in the anastrozole group compared to tamoxifen. Tamoxifen was noted to be associated with more hot flashes, endometrial cancers and thromboembolic events.[106]

The Breast International Group 1-98 (BIG 1-98) trial randomized 8,028 postmenopausal women with newly diagnosed hormone receptor-positive breast cancer. BIG 1-98 included two primary adjuvant arms comparing 5 years of letrozole with 5 years of tamoxifen, and two sequential treatment arms comparing 2 years of letrozole followed by 3 years of tamoxifen and 2 years of tamoxifen fol-

Table 58-3 **Efficacy Data From Studies of Aromatase Inhibitors in the Adjuvant Treatment of Postmenopausal Women With Early Breast Cancer**

	Initial Therapy	Post-Tamoxifen Therapy		
	ATAC Trial	MA 17 Trial	IES Trial	ITA Trial
	Anastrozole vs Tamoxifen	Letrozole vs Placebo	Exemestane vs Tamoxifen	Anastrozole vs Tamoxifen
Median follow-up:	68 months	2.4 years	30.6 months	24 months
No. of patients	9366	5187	4742	426
	DFS HR 0.87 (95% CI 0.78, 0.97; $p = .01$)	Death, recurrence or CLBC HR 0.61 (95% CI 0.47, 0.79; $p \leq .001$)	Risk of recurrence HR 0.68 (95% CI 0.56, 0.82; $p = .00005$)	Death HR 0.18 (95% CI 0.02, 1.57; $p = .07$)
	TTP HR 0.79 (95% CI 0.70, 0.90; $p = .0005$) CLCB OR 0.58 (95% CI 0.38, 0.88; $p = .01$)	Recurrence or CLBC HR 0.57 (95% CI 0.43, 0.75; $p = .00008$)	Survival free of distant metastases HR 0.66 (95% CI 0.52, 0.83; $p = .0004$) CLBC HR 0.44 (95% CI 0.20, 0.98; $p = .04$)	Relapse HR 0.36 (95% CI 0.17, 0.75; $p = .006$)

Abbreviations: CI, confidence intervals; CLBC, contralateral breast cancer; DFS, disease-free survival; HR, hazard ratio; OR, odds ratio; TTP, time to progression.

lowed by 3 years of letrozole.[108] Current analysis compared all patients who initially received letrozole to those that initially received tamoxifen with a primary end point of DFS. At a median follow-up of 51 months 352 DFS events among 2463 women receiving letrozole and 418 events among 2459 women receiving tamoxifen resulting in an 18% reduction in the risk of an event (HR 0.82; 95% CI, 0.71-0.95; p = .007) among women receiving letrozole compared to those receiving tamoxifen was observed.[109] There was a significantly greater incidence of bone fractures in patients receiving letrozole compared with those receiving tamoxifen (OR 1.44; p .0006). Patients in the tamoxifen group had significantly more grade 3-5 thromboembolic events (OR 0.38; $p < .0001$) than patients in the letrozole group.[108] There was a non significant trend towards an increased in cardiovascular events (myocardial infarction and cardiac deaths) in the letrozole group as compared to the tamoxifen group. At present time there are no data regarding direct comparison of these two aromatase inhibitors to accurately discern differences in safety and efficacy profiles between the different third generation aromatase inhibitors.

Post-Tamoxifen Treatment ■ The second issue to be explored was the sequential use of a third generation aromatase inhibitor following a period of adjuvant treatment of tamoxifen among postmenopausal women with early stage breast cancer. The MA 17 trial was a randomized, double-blind, extended adjuvant, placebo-controlled trial in 5187 postmenopausal women who had received 5 years of adjuvant treatment with tamoxifen with DFS as the primary end point.[110] Due to superior efficacy observed in the letrozole group compared to the placebo group at the first interim analysis the study was prematurely terminated. In an updated analysis, at a median follow up of 30 months the letrozole group had a significantly longer DFS compared to the placebo group (HR 0.58; 95% CI 0.45-0.76; $p < .001$).[111] Letrozole was found to be well tolerated and was associated with a lower incidence of vaginal bleeding and an increase in hot flashes, arthritis, arthralgia, and myalgia, compared with placebo. After premature termination of the study the group who were in the placebo of arm of the trial was offered letrozole. Women who elected to take letrozole did so at median of 2.8 years from completion of tamoxifen treatment with a recent update reporting improved DFS among those who elected to take letrozole compared to those who did not.[112]

The Intergroup Exemestane Study (IES) examined the efficacy and safety of exemestane therapy after 2 to 3 years of adjuvant tamoxifen therapy. The trial enrolled 4742 patients who were randomly assigned to continue with tamoxifen, or to switch to exemestane for the remainder of the 5-year treatment period. At a median follow-up of 30.6 months the data indicate that switching to exemestane was associated with a significant improvement in disease-free survival compared with continuing with tamoxifen (HR 0.68; 95% CI 0.56-0.82; $p < .001$).[113] At a median follow-up of 55.7 months switching to exemestane resulted in a 24% improvement in DFS (HR 0.76; 95% CI 0.66-0.88; p = .0001) and a 15% improvement in overall survival (HR 0.85; 95% CI 0.71-1.02; p = .08) as compared to the tamoxifen group.[114] The NSABP B-33 trial, similar to the MA17 trial, was a randomized trial that evaluated 5 years of exemestane to 5 years of placebo following the completion of 5-years of tamoxifen.[115] Due to the results of the MA-17 study the NASBP B-33 study was terminated early and unblinded. Despite a premature closure and cross over of patients an improvement in 4-year DFS was observed among the original cohort who received exemestane compared to the placebo group (91% vs 89%; HR 0.68; p = .07).[115]

Several other trials have also evaluated the sequential administration of aromatase inhibitors following tamoxifen therapy. The Italian Tamoxifen Anastrozole (ITA) and Arimdex Nolvadex 95/Austrian Breast cancer Study Group 8 (ARNO 95/ABCSG) have shown that switching to anastrazole after 2-3 years of tamoxifen significantly reduced the risk of recurrence.[116,117] In the ABCSG trial 6a postmenopausal women were randomized to either anastrozole or placebo following five years of adjuvant tamoxifen therapy.[118] At a median follow-up of 62.3 months women in the anastrozole group had a 38% risk reduction in recurrence compared to placebo (HR 0.62; 95% CI 0.40-0.96, p = .031).

Based on the evidence presented above, the author recommends that aromatase inhibitors be offered upfront as adjuvant therapy among postmenopausal women with hormone receptor positive early stage breast cancer (Fig. 58-4). The highest risk of recurrence is within the first 2 to 3 years of diagnosis. Despite no demonstrated overall survival benefit demonstrated at this time, the use of aromatase inhibitors have superior DFS rates compared to tamoxifen which with longer follow up may translate into a survival benefit. However, it is also important to note that current guidelines of adjuvant endocrine therapy for postmenopausal women recommend an aromatase inhibitor as either initial therapy or after an initial period of treatment with tamoxifen,[119] with the decision based on the risks and benefits of each agent for an individual patient. Longer term follow-up of the adjuvant trials described above are awaited to better define long-term efficacy results, side effect profile and delineate duration of required treatment for an aromatase inhibitor used in the adjuvant setting.

Neoadjuvant Studies ■ Neoadjuvant treatment is intended to downstage a tumor before primary locoregional therapy with surgery, thus allowing breast conserving surgery in a greater number of patients, or making surgery possible in cases that were considered inoperable. As the third generation aromatase inhibitors have demonstrated efficacy in the

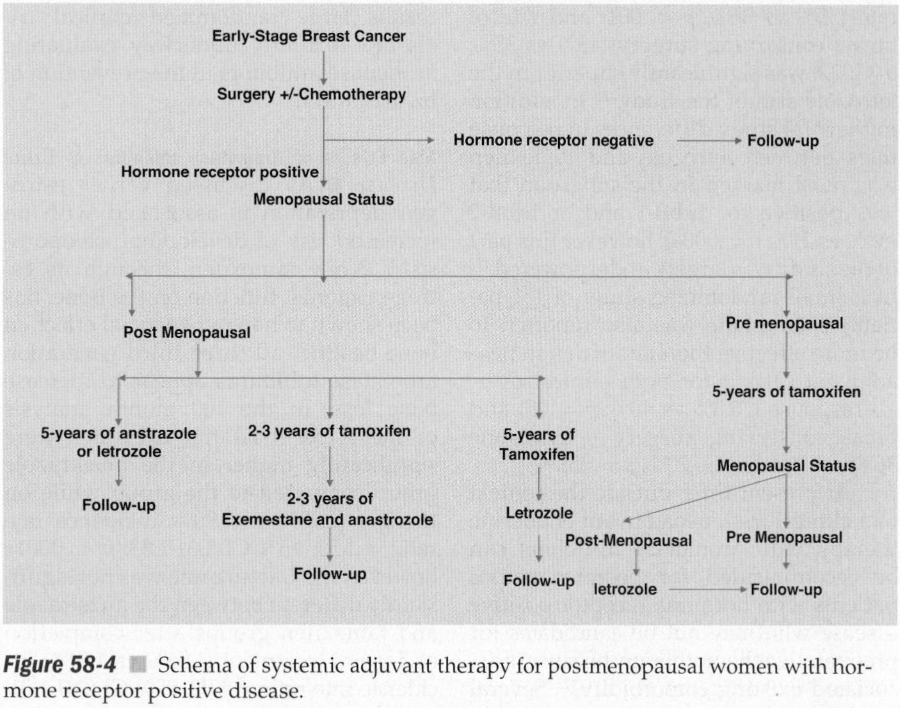

Figure 58-4 ■ Schema of systemic adjuvant therapy for postmenopausal women with hormone receptor positive disease.

treatment of advanced and early disease, it was important to examine the benefits these agents may bring to the pre operative setting.

Compared to neoadjuvant chemotherapy trials the neoadjuvant studies exploring the effect of endocrine therapy in the treatment of breast cancer have been smaller. Several trials have compared neoadjuvant tamoxifen to a third generation aromatase inhibitor postmenopausal women with hormone receptor positive breast cancer.[120–124] The Immediate Preoperative Arimidex, Tamoxifen, or Combined with Tamoxifen (IMPACT) trial compared 3 months of preoperative anastrazole with tamoxifen or a combination of both in 330 postmenopausal women with hormone receptor positive breast cancer.[36]No difference in overall response was noted in three groups (37% vs 36% vs 39%). However among the 124 women considered to require a mastectomy at baseline 46% treated with anastrozole were considered to be candidates for breast conserving surgery by their surgeon, compared with 22% receiving tamoxifen (p = .03).[120] Similarly in the PReOperative Arimidex Compared with Tamoxifen (PROACT) trial that randomized 451 postmenopausal women to either 3 months of neoadjuvant anastrozole or tamoxifen with or without chemotherapy reported that among the hormone therapy only group of patients who needed mastectomy, at baseline there was an improvement in breast conservation rates (43.0%) of patients receiving anastrozole compared to 30.8% receiving tamoxifen (p = .04).[121]

In the P024 study where 337 postmenopausal women were randomly assigned to either 4 months of neoadjuvant letrozole or tamoxifen overall response rate (55% vs 36%, p < .001) and rate of breast conserving surgery (45% vs 35%, p = .022) was significantly superior in the letrozole arm of the study.[122] In addition in the P024 study differences in response rates between letrozole and tamoxifen was most marked in the subgroup that was positive for ErbB-1 and/or ErbB-2 (88% vs 21%, p = .0004), however this part of the study was largely underpowered.[123] In a small randomized study of 151 patients exemestane was also reported to be more effective than tamoxifen in neoadjuvant setting for both clinical overall response (76.3% vs 40%; p = .05) and breast-conserving surgery (exemestane 36.8% vs tamoxifen 20%; p = .05).[124]

At present time, outside the context of a clinical trial, neoadjuvant endocrine therapy with aromatase inhibitors can be recommended for postmenopausal patients with hormone receptor positive disease who may not be candidates for preoperative chemotherapy because of associated existing comorbidity.[125] Several questions still remain to be addressed by future clinical trials including the appropriate duration of neoadjuvant endocrine therapy.

Chemoprevention of Breast Cancer ■ As discussed earlier the side effect profile of tamoxifen restricts its use in the prevention of breast cancer. Furthermore trials looking at tamoxifen and raloxifene in the prevention setting reduced the incidence of ER positive breast cancers by about 50% and thus looking for an agent that would reduce the incidence further is important. Aromatase inhibitors, with its proven efficacy in the treatment of hormone receptor positive breast cancers are a viable option. In the ATAC trial[107] at a median follow-up of 100 months, it was observed that the incidence of hormone receptor positive contralateral breast cancers was significantly lower in the anastrazole group compared to the tamoxifen group (HR 0.60; 95% CI 0.42-0.85; p = .004). Similarly in the BIG 1-98 trial[108,109] fewer cases of contralateral breast cancer were identified in the letrozole group than in the tamoxifen group (16 vs 27 cases). In the IES study[114] at a median follow-up of 55.7 months 17 cases of contralateral breast cancer were observed in the exemestane group compared to 35 cases in the tamoxifen group (HR 0.56; 95% CI 0.33-0.98; p = .04).

These trials data suggest that the third generation aromatase inhibitors can reduce the incidence of contralateral breast cancer by approximately ~40-50% above and beyond that observed by tamoxifen. By extrapolation this would be imply that these aromatase inhibitors, on their own, would reduce the incidence of ER positive contralateral breast cancer by ~70-80%.[126] With such encouraging results large randomized clinical trials are currently underway evaluating aromatase inhibitors in the prevention of breast cancer.

Side Effects of Aromatase Inhibitors ■ ***Bone Disease* ■** As discussed earlier estrogen deprivation is associated with an increased risk of developing osteoporosis.[127] While tamoxifen, through its estrogen agonist function on the bone, has been shown to have a beneficial effect on bone health,[73] all three third generation aromatase inhibitors appear to increase bone loss. In the 100 month analysis of the ATAC trial fracture rates were significantly higher in the anastrazole group compared to the group while on therapy (2.93% vs 1.90%; incidence rate ratio = 1.55; 95% CI 1.31-1.83; p < .0001); however, the fracture rate was not significantly different between the anastrazole and tamoxifen groups after completion of 5 years treatment (1.56% vs 1.51%; incidence rate ratio = 1.03, 95% CI 0.81-1.31, p = .79).[105] In BIG 1-98 trial at a median follow-up of 51 months the 8.6% of patients in the letrozole group experienced a fracture compared to 5.8% of patients in the tamoxifen group with the difference being statistically significant (p < .001).[109] Similar observations were also made in the IES trial where at a median follow-up of 55.7 months a significantly increased fracture rate of 7% was observed in the exemestane group compared to 5% in the tamoxifen group (OR 1.45; 95% CI 1.13-1.87; p = .003.[128] One method of preventing or reversing bone loss associated with aromatase inhibitors would be to use bisphosphonates. In the integrated analysis of two randomized Zometa-Femara Adjuvant Synergy Trials (Z-FAST and ZO-FAST) 1667 patients that were receiving adjuvant letrozole received either upfront zoledronic acid or received it only when bone mineral density decreased to below –2.[129] At month 12 patients the upfront group had lumbar spine bone mineral density that was 5.2% higher than the group of patients who received delayed zoledronic acid. Longer follow up will be needed to determine its effect on the bone fractures.

***Cardiovascular Disease* ■** Postmenopausal women with breast cancer may be at a higher risk of cardiovascular events due to their age, menopausal status, associated co morbid conditions and exposure to chemotherapeutic agents used in the treatment of breast cancer. As described earlier, tamoxifen, through its estrogen agonist function, has been shown to have a lipid lowering effect that has translated into modest reductions in cardiovascular events.[76] Anastrozole has not been shown to appreciably alter lipid profiles,[130,131] and in the adjuvant setting myocardial infarctions experienced by women taking anastrozole was similar compared to the group taking tamoxifen.[107] In the BIG 1-98 trial at a median follow-up of 51 months women in the letrozole group experienced a higher low grade cholesterol elevation and cardiovascular events (other than ischemic heart disease and cardiac failure) compared to women in the tamoxifen group.[109] The higher low grade cholesterol elevation in the letrozole group relative to that of patients in the tamoxifen group may be a reflection of the lipid lowering effect of tamoxifen as mentioned earlier. Studies with exemestane have shown that apart from a modest drop in HDL cholesterol,[132] exemestane has no appreciable effect on lipid levels. In the IES study, at a median follow-up of 55.7 months, among all patients the incidence of cardiovascular events (excluding thromboembolic events) did not seem to differ between the exemestane and tamoxifen groups with approximately 1.3% of exemestane-treated patients experiencing a myocardial infarction compared to 0.8% of tamoxifen-treated patients (p = .08). Longer follow-up will be required to assess the cardiovascular effects of the clinically used third generation aromatase inhibitors. Women with breast cancer are in general at higher risk of developing a cardiovascular event due to a multitude of factors and as such, and should be monitored and managed appropriately.

Other Adverse Events ■ Other side effects commonly associated with aromatase inhibitors include arthralgias, vaginal dryness, and dysparuenia. Although treatment with aromatase inhibitors increases the risk of vasomotor symptoms and vaginal bleeding/discharge large trials have shown that the incidence of these events were lower compared to those on tamoxifen treatment.[106–118] Furthermore these trials also reported that the incidence of thromboembolic events and endometrial carcinoma were also lower in women taking an aromatase inhibitor compared to those taking tamoxifen.

Resistance ■ In metastatic disease, the sequential utilization of hormonal agents can produce long-term palliation of hormone-dependent breast cancer. Eventually, however, the problem of hormone resistance is encountered. The mechanisms by which tumors become resistant to hormones, in general, are only partially understood.[133] Refractoriness to therapy with aromatase inhibitors is related not to the failure of these agents to suppress estradiol levels, but rather because of alterations in other cellular components, such as the growth factor receptor pathways and ability of then tumors to grow in estrogen deprived environments.[134] Our increasing understanding of these processes, and the development of target-orientated therapies such as trastuzumab (Herceptin), are interesting areas of future research that should make novel therapeutic approaches available for the treatment of endocrine resistance.

Conclusion

In summary a number of endocrine agents are now available for the management of both early and advanced stage hormone response breast cancer, each unique in its mechanism of action targeting different points in the ER and PR pathways. Tamoxifen has been ubiquitous as the front-line therapy for the treatment of all stages of breast cancer, and remains the central choice for the treatment of premenopausal women. Among postmenopausal women the introduction of the non-cross resistant aromatase inhibitors has changed recommendations being now at the fore front of treatment of both early and advanced staged breast cancers. However several questions regarding the use of aromatase inhibitors still remain including duration of use in the adjuvant setting and sequence of use with tamoxifen. Moreover among the three third generation aromatase inhibitors there are not head to head comparisons to support the superiority either in efficacy or safety of one aromatase inhibitor over another. Further more the use of aromatase inhibitors are not without side effects and clinical trials are underway to examine methods of preventing bone loss which can have a significant impact on quality of life. Antiestrogen (Fulvestrant) progestins including MA and MPA are useful agents to try when resistance to tamoxifen and aromatase inhibitors has developed.

Lastly, as more hormonal therapies become available, and our understanding of the molecular pathways underpinning resistance increases,[41,135] it is essential that the optimal sequence of endocrine agents be established in the treatment of breast cancer. This may prolong the time during which endocrine therapies can be used, so postponing the time when cytotoxic chemotherapy becomes a necessary option.

Selected References

The complete reference list can be found at www.CANCERMEDICINE8.com

10. Collingwood TN, Urnov FD, Wolffe AP. Nuclear receptors: coactivators, corepressors and chromatin remodeling in the control of transcription. J Mol Endocrinol. 1999;23:255–275.
12. Rossouw JE, Anderson GL, Prentice RL, et al. Risks and benefits of estrogen plus progestin in healthy postmenopausal women: principal results From the Women's Health Initiative randomized controlled trial. JAMA. 2002;288:321–333.
15. Lundgren S. Progestins in breast cancer treatment. A review. Acta Oncol. 1992;31:709–722.
16. Buzdar AU, Hortobagyi G. Update on endocrine therapy for breast cancer. [Review] [53 refs]. Clin Cancer Res. 1998;4:527–534.
17. Haller DG, Glick JH. Progestational agents in advanced breast cancer: an overview. Semin Oncol. 1986;13:2–8.
46. Sherman BM, Chapler FK, Crickard K, Wycoff D. Endocrine consequences of continuous antiestrogen therapy with tamoxifen in premenopausal women. J Clin Invest. 1979;64:398–404.
47. Jaiyesimi IA, Buzdar AU, Decker DA, Hortobagyi GN. Use of tamoxifen for breast cancer: twenty-eight years later [see comments] [Review]. J Clin Oncol. 1995;13:513–529.
48. Ingle JN, Krook JE, Green SJ, et al. Randomized trial of bilateral oophorectomy versus tamoxifen in premenopausal women with metastatic breast cancer. J Clin Oncol. 1986;4:178–185.
49. Klijn JG, Blamey RW, Boccardo F, et al. Combined tamoxifen and luteinizing hormone-releasing hormone (LHRH) agonist versus LHRH agonist alone in premenopausal advanced breast cancer: a meta-analysis of four randomized trials. J Clin Oncol. 2001;19:343–353.
51. Early Breast Cancer Trialists' Collaborative Group. Effects of chemotherapy and hormonal therapy for early breast cancer on recurrence and 15-year survival: an overview of the randomised trials. Lancet. 2005;365:1687–1717.
52. Fisher B, Dignam J, Bryant J, Wolmark N. Five versus more than five years of tamoxifen for lymph node-negative breast cancer: updated findings from the National Surgical Adjuvant Breast and Bowel Project B-14 randomized trial [see comments]. J Natl Cancer Inst. 2001;93:684–690.
53. Peto R, Davies C, and on behalf of the ATLAS Collaboration. ATLAS (Adjuvant Tamoxifen, Longer Against Shorter): international randomized trial of 10 versus 5 years of adjuvant tamoxifen among 11 500 women preliminary results. 30th Annual San Antonio Breast Cancer Symposium. 2007, Abstract.
54. Gray RG, Rea DW, Handley K, et al. and aTTom Collaborators. aTTom (adjuvant TamoxifenÑTo offer more?): Randomized trial of 10 versus 5 years of adjuvant tamoxifen among 6,934 women with estrogen receptor-positive (ER+) or ER untested breast cancerÑpreliminary results [Abstract]. J Clin Oncol. May 20, 2008;26(suppl).
56. Cuzick J, Powles T, Veronesi U, et al. Overview of the main outcomes in breast-cancer prevention trials [Review] [9 refs]. Lancet. 2003;361:296–300.
63. Vogel VG, Costantino JP, Wickerham DL, et al. Effects of tamoxifen vs raloxifene on the risk of developing invasive breast cancer and other disease outcomes: the NSABP Study of Tamoxifen and Raloxifene (STAR) P-2 trial. JAMA. 2006;295:2727–2741.
70. Howell A, Robertson JF, Abram P, et al. Comparison of fulvestrant versus tamoxifen for the treatment of advanced breast cancer in postmenopausal women previously untreated with endocrine therapy: a multinational, double-blind, randomized trial. J Clin Oncol. 2004;22:1605–1613.
71. Chia S, Gradishar W, Mauriac L, et al. Double-blind, randomized placebo controlled trial of fulvestrant compared with exemestane after prior nonsteroidal aromatase inhibitor therapy in postmenopausal women with hormone receptor-positive, advanced breast cancer: results from EFECT. J Clin Oncol. 2008;26:1664–1670.
107. Forbes JF, Cuzick J, Buzdar A, Howell A, Tobias JS, Baum M. Effect of anastrozole and tamoxifen as adjuvant treatment for early-stage breast cancer: 100-month analysis of the ATAC trial. Lancet Oncol. 2008;9:45–53.
109. Coates AS, Keshaviah A, Thurlimann B, et al. Five years of letrozole compared with tamoxifen as initial adjuvant therapy for postmenopausal women with endocrine-responsive early breast cancer:

59 Androgen Deprivation Strategies in the Treatment of Advanced Prostate Cancer

Samuel R. Denmeade, MD

Since the pioneering studies of Charles Brenton Huggins more than 60 years ago, it has been known that prostate cancer cells, like certain normal prostate epithelial cells, can be chronically dependent on a critical level of androgenic stimulation for their net continuous growth and survival.[1] It is on this basis that androgen ablation has been utilized as standard systemic therapy for metastatic prostate cancer. It has been estimated that in 2008, about 29,000 males in the United States will die from prostate cancer.[2] Undoubtedly, all these patients will have received treatment with a variety of androgen ablation techniques. Presently, there are a multitude of excellent means of ablating serum androgens, and these include surgical orchiectomy, chronic treatment with luteinizing hormone–releasing hormone (LHRH) analogues, alone and in combination with antiandrogens. In this chapter, a review of the present state of knowledge regarding the biology of androgen activity in prostate tissue and the use of new methods of androgen deprivation therapy to treat prostate cancer will be presented. Although androgen ablation therapy has been used to treat advanced prostate cancer for almost 60 years, debate continues to this day as to the optimal methods and timing of androgen deprivation therapy. This debate has become even more intensified with recent data demonstrating significant morbidity associated with the "metabolic syndrome" produced by androgen ablation therapy. In addition, new findings demonstrating continued expression of the androgen receptor in the majority of prostate cancer specimens from androgen-ablated patients has led to the reclassification of "hormone-refractory" disease as "castration-resistant prostate cancer" and has opened up new avenues of research into the function of the androgen receptor in the androgen-deprived state. These observations have also led to new classes of agents designed to inhibit the androgen axis, and several of these are now entering late-phase clinical testing in men with hormone-refractory disease. The controversial questions in this area that will be discussed in this chapter include the following: (1) Is intermittent androgen suppression a preferred alternative to continuous therapy? (2) Should androgen deprivation be initiated early in the course of the disease or delayed to minimize toxicities associated with the metabolic syndrome? (3) How should the toxicities of androgen blockade be properly managed? (4) What is the proper use of second-line hormonal therapies? (5) What is the status and anticipated role of new androgen deprivation agents under development? These topics will be explored in an attempt to provide information that will allow physicians to counsel patients to select the best available hormonal treatments.

Mechanism of Androgen Action in the Normal Prostate and Prostate Cancer

Androgens are the major regulators of proliferation and death for the normal prostate. This is because androgens regulate the total prostatic epithelial cell number by chronically stimulating the rate of cell proliferation (ie, agonistic ability of androgen), while simultaneously inhibiting the rate of cell death (ie, antagonistic ability of androgen) of specific subsets of epithelial cells and endothelial cells within the prostate sensitive to and dependent on androgen.[3-5] If a sufficient systemic androgen level is not chronically maintained (eg, following androgen ablation), then the subset of androgen-dependent prostatic epithelial and endothelial cells die rapidly via the activation of an energy-dependent cascade of biochemical and morphologic changes, collectively referred to as programmed cell death or apoptosis.

Studies at the molecular level have demonstrated that androgens function via binding to their cognate nuclear receptors inducing conformational changes in the occupied androgen receptor (AR). Androgen receptors exhibit a prototypic multi-domain structure containing an N-terminal activation domain, a C-terminal ligand-binding domain, and a centrally located DNA-binding region with two zinc finger motifs.[6-11] Specific interaction with androgenic ligands results in the conformational activation of AR. This allows the binding of the occupied AR with additional nuclear proteins (ie, coactivator proteins and general transcription factors) to produce transcriptional complexes, which can activate or repress specific gene expression by binding to the androgen-responsive elements present in the promoter regions in a series of androgen-regulated genes.[12] It does this by forming an active transcriptional complex, resulting in site-directed chromatin remodeling and enhancement of target gene expression.[12] The *src*-1 gene is a coactivator for AR; it functions in transcriptional activation through its histone acetyltransferase activity (HAT) and multiple interactions with agonist-bound receptors, other coactivators such as CBP or P300, other HAT, such as p/CAF, and some GTFs, such as TBP and TIFIIB.[12] And *src*-1 is a member of a gene family that includes *src*-1, *tif*-2 (also termed *grip*-1 and *src*-2), and p/*cip* (also termed *rac*-3, *actr*, *aibi*, and *src*-3).[12] Cell-free in vitro transcription and in vivo experiments have indicated that the *src*-1 family members enhance AR-dependent transactivation of nuclear genes.[12] It is the regulation of the expression of these genes that both stimulates prostate cell proliferation and inhibits prostate cell death.[3]

Overview of Regulation of Systemic Androgen Levels

The organs involved in the regulation of androgen production are the hypothalamus, pituitary, testes, and adrenal glands (Fig. 59-1). The peptide hormones, LHRH, and corticotropin-releasing factor (CRF) are produced by the hypothalamus. These releasing hormones reach the anterior pituitary via the hypothalamic–pituitary vascular network, where they stimulate, respectively, the release of luteinizing hormone (LH) and adrenocorticotropic hormone (ACTH) into the blood (Fig. 59-1). LH and ACTH, via the blood, stimulate the testes and adrenal glands, respectively. The Leydig cells of the testes under the influence of LH produce 95% of the circulating testosterone (T), while the adrenal, under the influence of ACTH, produces androstenedione and dehydro-epiandrosterone, which can be converted within prostatic tissues to more active androgens.[13] More than 95% of the circulating T is bound to T-estradiol-binding globulin and plasma albumin.[14] Feedback loops serve to modify the secretion of the anterior pituitary

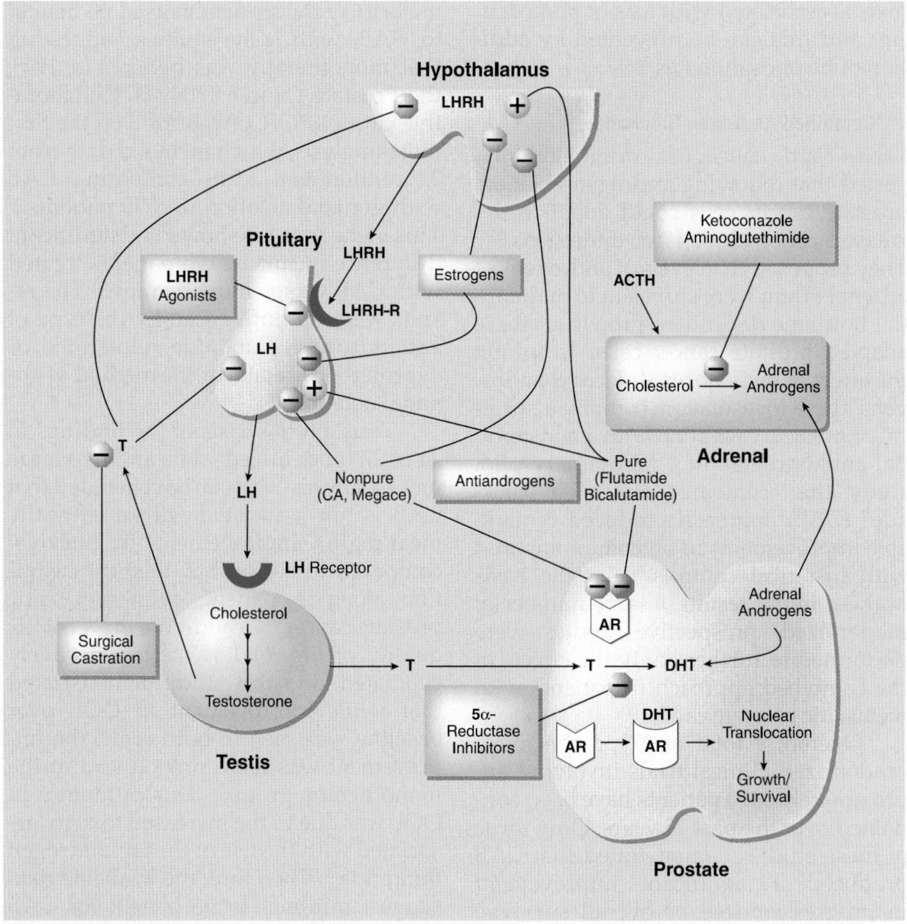

Figure 59-1 Regulation of androgen production and sites of blockade of angrogen action. *Abbreviations:* AR, androgen receptor; LH, luteinizing hormone; LHRH, luteinizing hormone-releasing hormone; DHT, dihydrotestosterone; T, testosterone; CA, cyproterone acetate.

and the hypothalamus. Thus, serum T exerts a negative feedback in both the hypothalamus and pituitary on the release of LHRH and LH, respectively. Serum cortisol feeds back on the hypothalamus and pituitary and inhibits further production of CRF and ACTH. Adrenal androgens appear to be quite weak and do not appear to exert any negative feedback on the hypothalamic–pituitary axis.[14]

The goal of androgen ablation therapy in prostatic cancer is to deprive the androgen-dependent cancer cells of androgenic stimulation. This can be achieved by one or more combinations of four mechanisms:

1. Surgical removal of the testes (ie, bilateral orchiectomy) to eliminate testicular androgens and by hypophysectomy or adrenalectomy to eliminate adrenal androgens
2. Suppression of pituitary LH release, thereby inhibiting T production by the testes (LHRH agonists/antagonists)
3. Inhibition of androgenic synthesis in the testes and adrenals
4. Inhibition of androgen action at the level of androgen-dependent prostatic cancer cells (antiandrogens, 5-α-reductase inhibitors)

At present the "gold standard" for androgen ablation therapy is bilateral orchiectomy.[1] Surgical removal of the testes results in a 95% reduction of circulating T.[13] The advantages of this surgical approach include efficacy, assurance of patient compliance, cost-effectiveness, minimal morbidity from the procedure, and rapidity of symptomatic response. The disadvantages include the permanent side effects of loss of libido, erectile impotence, hot flashes, occasional breast tenderness, possible psychological trauma of "disfiguring" surgery and metabolic syndrome. On the basis of these disadvantages, most men with metastatic prostatic cancer in the United States choose alternative pharmacologic approaches that produce androgen ablation. Presently, there are a large variety of pharmacologic agents to achieve androgen ablation. These agents can be divided into two basic groups. The first group of agents produces androgen ablation indirectly by lowering the extracellular supply of androgen to the prostatic cancer cells by means of lowering the level of androgen in the blood. These agents include LHRH agonists, estrogenic compounds, progestational agents, and androgen synthesis inhibitors of various types. The second group of agents produces androgen ablation by inhibiting the intracellular response to androgen within androgen-dependent prostatic cancer cells. Quantitatively, the major circulating androgen in the blood is T. Within prostate cancer cells, however, T is converted to a series of metabolites, the major one being 5α-dihydrotestosterone (DHT).[15,16] The enzyme responsible for the irreversible conversion of T to DHT is the membrane-bound nicotinamide-adenine dinucleotide phosphate (NADR)–dependent 5α-oxido-reductase (5α-reductase).[17] Once formed by the 5α-reductase enzymes, DHT binds to the intracellular AR.[18] It is this DHT–AR binding that results in the trophic stimulation of proliferation and blockage of death of the hormone-dependent prostatic cancer cells.[19] Thus, androgen ablation can be achieved at the prostatic cancer cell level either by inhibiting the production of DHT via 5α-reductase inhibitors or by preventing the binding of DHT to its receptor due to competitive inhibition by antiandrogen antagonists.

Androgen Deprivation Strategies for the Treatment of Recurrent and Metastatic Prostate Cancer

LHRH Agonists as Monotherapy

LHRH is a decapeptide that stimulates the release of LH protein by the anterior pituitary. LH stimulates the testes to release T (see Fig. 59-1). Substitutions at the sixth, ninth, or tenth positions of the decapeptide LHRH result in synthetic agonist analogues with prolonged half-life and potency. Initial administration of these agonist analogues results in stimulation on LH and follicle-stimulating hormone (FSH) production, such that T levels rise 140-170% within several days.[20,21] This rise in serum T can lead to a "flare" response in patients with metastatic prostatic cancer.[21,22] This flare response can result in increased bone pain, urinary obstruction, lymphedema, or spinal cord compression. The flare response can be blocked by administering an antiandrogen either before or concurrent with the start of LHRH agonist treatment.[23,24]

With chronic LHRH agonist administration (ie, after about 4 weeks of treatment), castrate levels of T are produced. This paradoxical T suppression by LHRH agonist analogues results from (1) alterations in the central feedback control of LH release; (2) desensitization of the testes to LH due to a decrease in LH receptor content; and (3) direct testicular steroid enzyme inhibition. In the United States, the most commonly used LHRH agonists are leuprolide acetate (Lupron) and goserelin acetate (Zoladex). These agents are available in depot forms that can be administered at intervals of 1, 3, or 4 months. Leuprolide acetate is formulated in microspheres for intramuscular injection, and goserelin acetate is formulated as a cylindrical plug for subcutaneous injection. A 12-month leuprolide acetate implant (Viadur) that requires surgical insertion is also now available.[25,26]

The LHRH agonists leuprolide and goserelin have been investigated in phase II and randomized phase III trials. These agents were found to be equivalent to DES and orchiectomy. Another LHRH agonist used outside the United States, buserelin, is also comparable with orchiectomy in response and survival. Overall, monotherapy studies with LHRH agonists, DES, or orchiectomy have been associated with objective and subjective improvement in 60-85% of patients, a median progression-free survival of 12-18 months, and a median survival of 24-30 months. While chronic use of these agents is considerably more expensive than orchiectomy, most patients now prefer the depot LHRH agonists because of the psychological implications of loss of the testicles.[27] In addition, the recent increased popularity of intermittent hormonal therapy, even though unproven as yet, has made orchiectomy an even less likely choice for most patients (Fig. 59-2). Long-term use of LHRH agonists is associated with loss of bone density and this can be prevented by addition of bisphosphonates.[28,29]

Combined Androgen Blockade

Labrie and colleagues originally suggested that following androgen ablation, prostate cancer cells could adapt to decreased concentrations of androgens.[30,31] They proposed that levels of androgens of adrenal origin were sufficient to maintain the hormone-dependent growth of these adapted prostate cancer cells. To inhibit the effect of these adrenal-derived androgens, these investigators combined surgical or medical castration with a nonsteroidal antiandrogen. In a preliminary pilot study, this "combined androgen blockade" (CAB) approach produced remarkable improvements in outcome compared with historical controls.[30] On the basis of these initial results, a large number of randomized, prospective studies were performed to further study the effects of the combined approach in patients with metastatic prostate cancer.[32]

Overall, a total of 27 prospectively randomized clinical trials involving approximately 8000 patients have been conducted over the past 15 years. Only three of these studies demonstrated that CAB produced a significant improvement in progression-free or overall survival, when compared with monotherapy. The majority of the studies showed no benefit to CAB, with some studies suggesting that monotherapy was better.[32] In 1995, the Prostate Cancer Trialists' Collaborative Group (PCTCG) reported on the first meta-analysis, which included data from 22 randomized trials comparing CAB with gonadal ablation in 5710 patients.[33] This meta-analysis showed no significant difference in survival in patients treated with CAB versus monotherapy.[33] The results were not influenced by the type of antiandrogens (flutamide, nilutamide, or cyproterone acetate) or the method of gonadal ablation.[33]

Thus, on the basis of the findings in 24 of 27 randomized trials and two large meta-analyses,[33,34] it can be concluded that CAB is not associated with a clinically meaningful improvement in survival compared to surgical or medical castration alone in patients with metastatic prostate cancer.[33] In addition, in INT-0015, quality of life (QOL) was prospectively evaluated, and this study demonstrated that while improvement in QOL over baseline was seen in both arms, the improvement was more pronounced in the monotherapy group.[35] This difference in QOL was due to the increased toxicity associated with the use of the antiandrogen flutamide.[35] Therefore, the available data suggest minimal to no benefit for CAB versus monotherapy.[33] On the basis of these results, monotherapy consisting of medical or surgical castration to achieve castrate levels of testosterone should be considered adequate first-line therapy in men with metastatic prostate cancer.[33] Antiandrogens can be used initially as short-term therapy to prevent the flare associated with LHRH agonists or added later as second-line agents.[33]

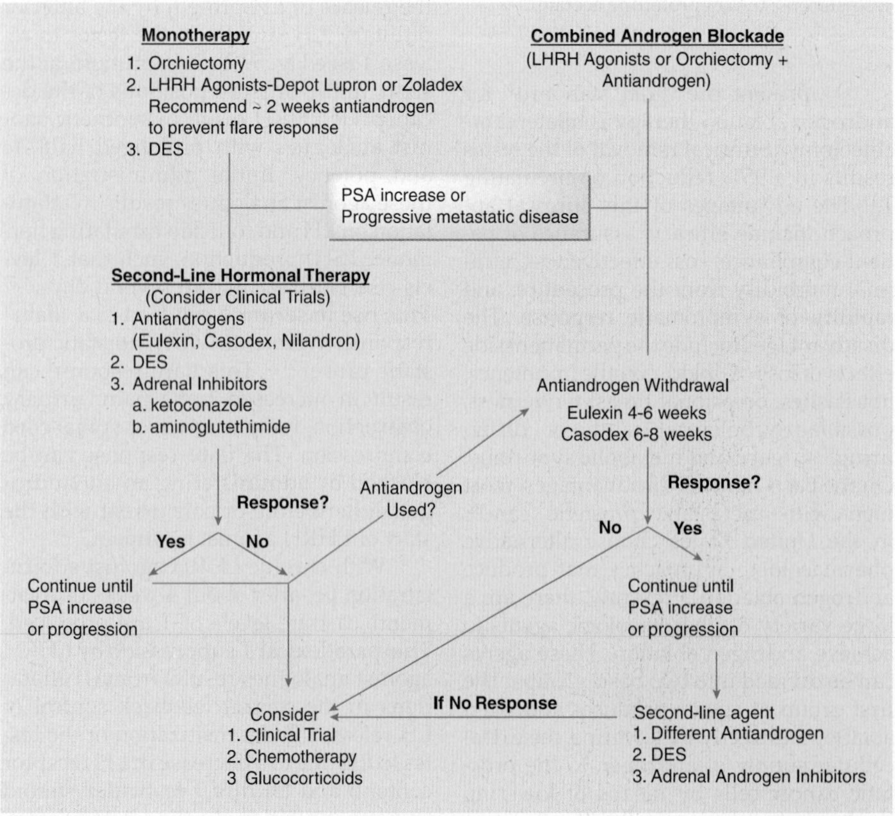

Figure 59-2 Algorithm for use of hormonal therapies in treatment of recurrent or metastatic prostate cancer. (See text for discussion of monotherapy versus combined androgen blockade and optimal timing of therapy initiation.)

Alternative Strategies for Androgen Deprivation

The reports of the benefit of neoadjuvant or adjuvant androgen ablation in combination with external beam radiation therapy in patients with high-risk or locally advanced prostate cancer probably explain the trend toward the increasing use of androgen ablation as primary or neoadjuvant therapy in men with localized prostate cancer reported recently by Cooperberg et al. through analysis of the CaPSURE database.[36,37] This increase in early and chronic use of androgen deprivation raises concerns regarding the short- and long-term consequences of androgen deprivation. Initial side effects to ADT are well-known and include loss of libido, erectile dysfunction, hot flashes, anemia, and depression.[38] Prolonged androgen deprivation in men is associated with decreased bone density.[39,40]

In addition, more recently, it has been demonstrated that ADT produces metabolic syndrome characterized by central obesity, insulin resistance, dyslipidemia, and hypertension with adverse effects on lipid levels, insulin levels, and arterial stiffness.[41,42] In several studies in which men received more than 3 months of ADT, increases in total cholesterol, triglyceride levels, and LDL and HDL cholesterol were observed.[41,43,44] These alterations in cardiac risk factors are consistent with epidemiological data linking hypogonadism with increased risk for coronary artery disease in the general population.[44-47] Recent data in men with prostate cancer have shown that the mortality from prostate cancer has declined such that by 1996 cardiovascular disease (CVD) had become a more likely cause of death than their cancer in these men.[48]

Due to the significant side effects associated with LHRH agonist-based gonadal suppression therapy, a number of alternative strategies are being tested with the goal of lessening the toxicity of medical castration while still depriving prostate cancer cells of androgen.

Parenteral Estrogen and Prostate Cancer: Is It Time for a Change?

When the blood level of estrogen rises to a pharmacologically sufficient concentration, inhibition of the release of LH from the pituitary results, thus decreasing T synthesis and release from the testes (Fig. 59-1). Therefore, chronic maintenance of pharmacologic blood levels of estrogen can depress serum T to the same minimal level as that observed following surgical orchiectomy.[49] When given orally, naturally occurring estrogens (ie, 17β-estradiol and estrone) are rapidly metabolized by the liver and are not able to sufficiently elevate the blood estrogen levels to depress serum T. DES is a synthetic compound that has potent estrogenic abilities and is capable of reaching sufficient blood levels following oral delivery to suppress LH release. In the 1940s Huggins and Hodges first reported on the use of surgical castration or oral estrogen as treatment for metastatic prostate cancer.[1] Bilateral orchiectomy produces rapid onset of symptomatic relief with minimal side effects and, therefore, has been the gold standard in prostate cancer therapy. As an alternative to surgery, DES was demonstrated to be as effective as orchiectomy in lowering testosterone to castrate levels.[1]

Unfortunately, the side effects of pharmacologic amounts of oral estrogen are numerous: nausea, vomiting, headaches, fluid retention, gynecomastia, impotence, pedal edema, thrombophlebitis, myocardial infarction, and stroke.[50-52] Because of the significantly increased risk of cardiovascular complications observed in earlier studies, oral estrogens are not used as first-line therapy for prostate cancer. Subsequent studies have shown that oral estrogen significantly increases the risk of thromboembolic complications, increases triglyceride levels, and raises levels of inflammatory markers in both women and men.[36] These results may explain the neutral or detrimental effects on cardiovascular and cerebrovascular disease previously reported from randomized trials of oral estrogen in men and women.[53-55]

The toxicity of oral estrogens appears to be due to "first-pass" effects on hepatic protein synthesis when absorption is via the portal route. These toxic effects can be ameliorated if estrogens are given parenterally, not orally. This has been clearly established by a large Finnish study of 477 men with prostatic cancer, which demonstrated that increased cardiovascular risks can be eliminated with parenteral depot estrogens.[56] This study demonstrated that when 160 mg/month of polyestradiol phosphate (PEP) (eg, Estradurin) is given as a slow-release intramuscular depot, the treatment is effective for prostate cancer control, and patients had significantly less cardiovascular deaths than those treated with orchiectomy or a combination intramuscular and oral estrogen therapy. In addition, in this study, parenteral PEP had a protective effect on cardiovascular deaths. This may be due to the fact that, when given as a once-monthly intramuscular injection, parenteral PEP caused a decrease in serum triglycerides and low-density lipoprotein (LDL) triglycerides.[56-58] Purnell et al. reported similar results in men with prostate cancer treated with transdermal estrogen.[36] In this study, transdermal estrogen treatment (0.6 mg/day) produced a decrease in total cholesterol, LDL cholesterol, and apolipoprotein B and an increase in HDL cholesterol.[36] No changes in C-reactive protein or other serum inflammatory markers were observed in this small study.

Finally, in a large, randomized study of 910 men, the Scandinavian Prostatic Cancer Group compared the effect on overall survival of combined androgen blockade (ie, orchiectomy or LHRH agonist and flutamide) (CAB) with that of parenteral estrogen (PEP).[59] This group recently published the final evaluation of the results of this study.[60] At this final evaluation 855 of 910 patients had died. There was no difference between the treatment groups in terms of biochemical or clinical progression-free survival or in overall or disease-specific survival.[60] There was no difference in cardiovascular mortality but a significant increase in nonfatal cardiovascular events in the PEP arm ($p < 0.05$), predominantly caused by an increase in ischemic heart and heart decompensation events.[60] There were 18 grave skeletal events in the CAD group but none in the PEP group ($p = 0.001$). The incidence of hot flashes was 30.1% in the PEP-treated group and 74.3% in the CAB-treated group, and the frequency and distress due to hot flashes were also significantly lower than in the CAB group.[61] Therefore, on the basis of this large randomized study these authors suggested that Estradurin could be used in the primary or secondary endocrine treatment of metastasized patients without prominent cardiac risk factors and especially those with osteoporosis.[60]

Thus, the use of parenteral estrogens given monthly as an intramuscular injection or via transdermal administration is an effective pharmacologic approach to androgen ablation that should be reconsidered as an effective alternative to LHRH agonists. In addition, the development of newer 3- to 4-month formulations of parenteral estrogen should be encouraged as an alternative to depot LHRH agonists.

Nonsteroidal Antiandrogens as Monotherapy

Because of the potential for preserving potency, antiandrogens have been tested as monotherapy. Several randomized studies have compared the antiandrogens with gonadal suppression. In one small study, flutamide was compared with DES and found to have an equivalent response rate but an inferior survival (28 versus 43 months).[62] A second study compared bicalutamide (50 mg daily) with surgical castration and found PSA normalization in 17% of the bicalutamide group and 47% in the castrate group. Even though survival was not significantly different between the two groups, the authors of this study concluded that standard-dose bicalutamide was not as effective as castration for treatment of patients with metastatic disease.[63]

Other studies have evaluated a higher dose of bicalutamide (150 mg) as monotherapy.[64] High-dose bicalutamide has been compared to gonadal suppression in two large open-label randomized studies. Combined data from these studies demonstrated that bicalutamide was inferior to castration in patients with metastatic disease with respect to time to progression and overall survival, although the median survival between the two groups was only 6 weeks.[65,66] For patients with rising PSA levels only, the two treatments were equivalent with respect to time to progression and overall survival.[65,66] Bicalutamide monotherapy was well tolerated, and patients had increased sexual interest and physical capacity when compared to the castrated group. In a small subgroup of one of these studies ($n = 29$) there was a no decrease in bone mineral density compared to age-matched controls, whereas clinically significant reductions in bone mineral density were seen in castrated patients.[67] This result needs to be confirmed in larger randomized studies. The incidence of gynecomastia in the bicalutamide-treated group was approximately 50%.[64] These data suggest that high-dose antiandrogen blockade may be a viable alternative in patients with nonmetastatic disease.

High-dose bicalutamide has also been evaluated as adjuvant therapy by the Early Prostate Cancer program, which consisted of three randomized, double blind, placebo-controlled trials prospectively designed for combined analysis.[68,69] In these combined trials a total of 8113 men with T1b-T4, M0, any N (N0 in 1 trial) prostate cancer were randomized to bicalutamide 150 mg/day (4052) or placebo (4061) in addition to standard care (radical prostatectomy, radiotherapy or watchful waiting). At median 5.4 years of follow-up (21.6% progression events) bicalutamide significantly improved progression-free survival (PFS) in the overall population, with positive results in two of the three trials.[69] Patients with locally advanced disease gained most benefit from bicalutamide in terms of PFS, irrespective of underlying therapy. Overall survival in these trials was similar in the bicalutamide and placebo groups, across the program and in each trial. Among watchful waiting patients survival appeared to be improved with bicalutamide in those with locally advanced disease, whereas survival appeared to be reduced with bicalutamide in those with localized disease. The most common adverse events with bicalutamide were gynecomastia and breast pain. The authors of these studies concluded from their analysis that bicalutamide may provide benefit in patients with locally advanced disease.[69] However, the current data from these trials suggest that early or adjuvant hormonal therapy for patients at low risk of disease progression, such as those with localized disease, is not appropriate.[69]

Intermittent Androgen Suppression

Intermittent androgen suppression (IAS) is being used with increasing frequency in an attempt to minimize the adverse effects associated with long-term androgen deprivation.[70] The rationale for this approach was initially based on the results of experiments in animal tumor models, which suggested that intermittent androgen suppression could delay, but not prevent, progression to androgen independence.[71,72] These studies also demonstrated that in both animal models and men with prostate cancer apoptosis could be induced multiple times with successive cycles of androgen withdrawal and replacement.

To date, 15 studies using IAS have been reported in the literature.[70] These studies had small patient populations distributed in different stages (ie, local, loco-regional, and metastatic).[70] In many of these studies, androgen ablation is achieved using combined androgen blockade with an LHRH agonist and an antiandrogen.[73-75] While treatment design has varied somewhat, in general, the approach has been to start patients on androgen deprivation and continue until the PSA level reaches a nadir or becomes undetectable. At this point, the androgen withdrawal is stopped and patients are followed up with serial PSA measurements. When the PSA reaches either a prescribed level (eg, 10 ng/mL) or returns to the patient's baseline level, the androgen suppression is reinitiated. In most patients treated in this manner, serum testosterone returned to the normal range within 5-20 weeks of discontinuing treatment.[76] The off-treatment periods in these studies have been associated with an improvement in the patient's sense of well-being and the recovery of libido and potency in those who reported normal sexual function before the start of therapy.[70] These preliminary studies, in aggregate, have demonstrated that repeated cycles of androgen suppression could induce repeated PSA responses. Daliani and colleagues[77] observed significant interpatient variability in the duration of the PSA response after each cycle of IAS in a small number of patients and concluded that due to this interpatient variability randomized studies will be needed to adequately explore the efficacy of individualized IAS.

These preliminary studies have led to several ongoing large, multi-institutional randomized studies comparing IAS with continuous androgen suppression. An NCI-sponsored study led by the Southwest Oncology Group (SWOG 9346) randomized approximately 1500 men with stage IV prostate cancer to either intermittent or continuous androgen deprivation with goserelin and bicalutamide. A second study sponsored by the National Cancer Institute of Canada (NCIC) randomized approximately 1300 men with PSA progression following radiotherapy to either intermittent or continuous androgen deprivation with an LHRH agonist (buserelin, goserelin, or leuprolide) and an antiandrogen (flutamide, bicalutamide, or nilutamide). Because of the potential improvement in quality of life, patient enthusiasm for IAS is understandable. These large randomized trials will provide the data needed to determine the role of IAS in the treatment of prostate cancer. Until this information is available, however, patients must be informed that the long-term safety and efficacy of this approach is unknown and should be considered experimental.[66]

Immediate Delayed Androgen Ablation

The question of when to initiate androgen deprivation therapy continues to be a topic of debate at national prostate cancer meetings. It will continue to be a topic of debate until the question is answered through a well-designed, adequately powered clinical trial puts the question to rest. Until that time, clinicians will have to decide the optimal timing of androgen deprivation with the help of very limited data.[78-84] A series of studies have been performed, which provide the background information that could be useful in the design and selection of patients for a randomized trial to answer this question. Walsh and associates characterized, in a retrospective analysis, the time course of disease progression in 1997 men with biochemical recurrence after radical prostatectomy.[85] Of the 1997 men, 315 (15%) developed biochemical PSA elevation, and 34% of these developed metastatic disease within the study period.[133] The median actuarial time to metastases was 8 years from the time of PSA level elevation and, once the patients developed metastatic disease, the median time to death was 5 years.[85] Prognostic factors associated with a high probability of remaining metastases free were a Gleason score of 5 to 7, PSA recurrence more than 2 years after prostatectomy, and a PSA doubling time of >10 months. In patients with all three good prognostic factors, the probability of remaining metastases free at 7 years was 82% In contrast, for patients with poor prognostic factors (ie, Gleason score 8-10 and PSA recurrence <2 years), the probability at 7 years was only 21% These authors provide an algorithm to help physicians counsel their patients on risks of recurrence based on these three factors.[85] These data suggest that for patients with good prognostic factors early hormonal therapy would unlikely be of benefit. In contrast, patients with poor prognosis would more likely benefit from early initiation of hormonal therapy.

These conclusions were further supported by recent reports from D'Amico et al.[86] This group evaluated outcomes in 8669 patients with prostate cancer treated with surgery (5918) or radiation (2751) and demonstrated that a short post-treatment prostate-specific antigen (PSA) doubling time of less than 3 months following radical prostatectomy or radiation therapy was significantly associated with time to prostate cancer-specific mortality.[86] On this basis, this group concluded that patients with PSA doubling time of less than 3 months should be considered for early initiation of androgen suppression therapy (or clinical trial) in order to delay the imminent sequelae of metastatic bone disease.[86]

However, until data from a randomized trial are available, the optimal timing for initiation of hormone therapy in PSA-only recurrences is unknown. Given the significant morbidity associated with ADT, the current approach in our practice is to delay initiation of ADT until patients have objective signs or symptoms of disease progression beyond a sustained elevation in PSA. Patients with rapid PSA doubling times receive counseling and information regarding the implications of a rapid doubling time, the lack of studies documenting survival benefit from early treatment with ADT, and the risks of chronic ADT in an effort to help them make informed treatment decisions.

Second-Line Hormonal Therapy

Eventually, all patients responding to initial androgen deprivation therapy will develop progressive disease as manifested by rising PSA levels, appearance of new lesions on imaging studies, or worsening symptoms. The treatment of androgen-ligand-independent prostate cancer remains a challenge for the clinician due to the lack of a clearly defined standard therapy. One important approach involves secondary hormonal manipulation, following failure of primary androgen deprivation (Fig. 59-2).[87,88]

Prostate cancer cells can be classified on the basis of responsiveness to androgen deprivation. Androgen-dependent cells are those that respond to androgen withdrawal by cessation of proliferation and activation of apoptosis. Within hormone-refractory metastatic sites, there is a heterogeneous collection of cells with relative degrees of androgen independence. One subset of cells consists of the androgen-sensitive cells, which have an increased proliferative rate in the presence of androgen. These cells are able to continue to proliferate, albeit more slowly, in the absence of androgen. These androgen-sensitive cells are also less likely to undergo apoptosis on androgen withdrawal. True androgen-independent cells do not alter their proliferative rates in the presence or absence of androgen.

Several studies have demonstrated that androgen-ligand-independent tumors progress in the castrated male; they maintain some degree of androgen responsiveness and can, therefore, derive a further growth advantage on reexposure to androgens.[89,90] The mechanisms for this continued sensitivity are not entirely clear and may be related to the continued expression of AR by prostate cancer cells in the androgen-deprived state. However, given this clinical observation, continued androgen suppression should be considered the standard of care for patients deemed "hormone refractory."[91]

AR is a key mediator of androgen function within normal and malignant prostate cells. AR is nearly universally expressed in primary and metastatic sites in untreated patients. In addition, AR continues to be expressed in the majority of androgen ablation recurrent patients, suggesting that AR is required for the progression of prostate cancer to the androgen-unresponsive metastatic stage.[92–94] This observation has led to the use of the term "castration-resistant prostate cancer" (CRPC) to characterize this stage of the disease. Molecular analysis demonstrated that amplification of the Xq11-q13 region where the AR gene is located is common in prostate cancer recurrence during androgen ablation therapy.[94,95] AR amplification has been detected in about 20-30% of recurrent prostate cancers but none in the specimens taken from the same patients prior to therapy.[94,95] These results taken together suggest that in approximately one-third of patients failure of androgen ablation therapy may be due to clonal outgrowth of prostate cancer cells with increased AR expression.

In addition to amplification, mutations in the gene can cause AR dysfunction, including alterations of androgen receptor specificity, binding affinity, and expression.[96–98] AR mutations occur in low frequency (ie, 5-15%) in primary prostate cancer.[99] In contrast, the cells in distant metastases and in recurrent prostate cancer with androgen ablation often contain AR mutations.[97–99] Functional studies indicate that in many cases these mutated receptors are not inhibited but rather can be stimulated by some antiandrogens.[97–99] These studies, which demonstrate AR amplification or mutation in patients failing primary androgen deprivation therapy, may explain, in part, the clinical benefit observed in a subset of patients treated with some form of second-line hormonal therapy.

Second-line hormone therapy can be divided into several categories as follows (Fig. 59-2)[88]:

1. Antiandrogen withdrawal
2. Addition of an antiandrogen in patients failing gonadal suppression
3. Inhibition of adrenal steroidogenesis
4. Use of glucocorticoids or other alternative steroids

Use of Antiandrogens

Antiandrogens compete with androgens for binding sites on the AR. Two classes of antiandrogens are used clinically: the "pure" and "nonpure" types.[100] A pure antiandrogen functions as an androgen antagonist by competitively inhibiting the binding of DHT or T with the ARs within target cells, without decreasing serum T systemically (see Fig. 59-1). The pure antiandrogens are used most commonly in the United States and include the nonsteroidal antiandrogens flutamide (Eulexin) and bicalutamide (Casodex) (Table 59-1). Nilutamide (Nilandron), a newer nonsteroidal antiandrogen, is also approved for use[100] (Table 59-1). Flutamide was initially approved because it blocked the flare from LHRH agonists, and bicalutamide was approved on the basis of a comparative trial showing antitumor equivalence and improved safety profile relative to flutamide.[101] Flutamide must be administered in multiple daily doses because of its short half-life, while bicalutamide and nilutamide have longer half-lives that permit once-a-day dosing. Toxicities of this class include diarrhea, elevations in serum transaminases, and gynecomastia (Table 59-1).

Most patients in the United States with advanced prostate cancer receive either medical or surgical castration, with or without an antiandrogen as primary hormonal therapy. On the basis of recent results demonstrating that combined androgen blockade is not superior to monotherapy, patients increasingly are treated with LHRH agonist until PSA levels begin to rise, and then they are given an antiandrogen as initial second-line hormonal therapy. Data from only a few studies are available, but existing evidence suggests that patients treated initially with gonadal suppression can benefit from the addition, later, of an antiandrogen, with response rates ranging from 15% to 50%.[102-105] The duration of decline in PSA observed with antiandrogens is typically between 4 and 8 months. No studies have been performed to document whether the use of antiandrogens or any other second-line therapy produces an improvement in overall survival.

In patients who demonstrate progression after primary therapy with combined androgen suppression, the recommended first maneuver is to withdraw the antiandrogen and assess response. Two clinical studies have investigated the effect of adding a bicalutamide following flutamide withdrawal. Scher and colleagues[104] reported on 10 of 26 patients (38%) who had prior flutamide therapy and had a greater than 50% decrease in PSA after high-dose bicalutamide. Responses were observed in patients with and without a prior withdrawal response to flutamide. Similarly, Joyce and colleagues[105] reported a 23% response rate to bicalutamide (150 mg/days), with the majority of responders having received prior flutamide. It appears, therefore, that bicalutamide may induce further responses in patients previously treated with flutamide.

Table 59-1 Hormonal Agents Commonly Used in Treatment of Prostate Cancer

	Agent	Dosage[a]	Toxicities
LHRH agonists	Leuprolide (Lupron)	7.5 mg/mo-22.5 mg/3 mo (IM)	For the class: hot flashes, decreased libido, impotence, gynecomastia, fatigue, edema, muscle waning, osteoporosis, anemia, disease flare
	Goserelin (Zoladex)	3.6 mg/mo-10.8 mg/3 mo (SC)	
Antiandrogens	Flutamide (Eulexin)	250 mg tid	For the class: decreased libido, gynecomastia, hot flashes, hepatotoxicity, diarrhea, Nilandron-impaired night vision
	Bicalutamide (Casodex)	50 mg daily	
	Nilutamide (Nilandron)	50 mg tid	
Adrenal enzyme inhibitors	Ketoconazole (Nizoral)	400 mg tid + HC 30 mg qday	Nausea, vomiting, requires acidic pH
Miscellaneous agents	Diethylstilbesterol (DES)	1 mg daily	DVT, stroke, cardiac ischemia (more common at higher doses), gynecomastia, fluid retention, weight gain,
	Megesterol acetate (Megace)	40 mg qid	DVT, impotence, gynecomastia, loss of libido side effects associated with hypercortisolism
	Prednisone	7.5-10 mg daily	

[a] Dosage from Swain SM, Lippman ME. Endocrine therapies of cancer. In: Chabner BA, Collins JM, eds. Cancer Chemotherapy: Principles and Practice. Philadelphia, PA: Lippincott; 1990:59-109.

Abbreviations: IM, intramuscular; SC, subcutaneous; tid, 3 times daily; qid, 4 times daily; HC, hydrocortisone; DVT, deep venous thrombosis.

Antiandrogen Withdrawal

Kelley and colleagues,[106] in 1993, were the first to observe that withdrawal of the antiandrogen flutamide from patients with hormone-refractory prostate cancer could result in symptomatic and objective improvement. These investigators termed this phenomenon the "antiandrogen withdrawal syndrome."[106] Although initially observed in patients on flutamide,[106-108] PSA declines and symptomatic benefits have also been described after withdrawal of both bicalutamide[109,110] and nilutamide.[111,112] Discontinuation responses have also been seen after removal of the steroidal antiandrogens megesterol acetate[113] and diethylstilbesterol.[114] In the studies reported to date, withdrawal responses have been observed in 15-30% of patients.[106-116] No particular clinical variable predicts likelihood of a withdrawal response.[115,117] With flutamide, the length of treatment seems to be associated with the likelihood of response, although this finding has not been seen in every study.[115,117] Patients treated with antiandrogen for as short a period as 2 months can have a withdrawal response.[117]

Most patients responding to flutamide withdrawal will experience a decrease in PSA within 4 weeks.[115,117] Responses may occur later (ie, 6-8 weeks) with bicalutamide and nilutamide due to their longer half-life.[116] The median duration of response to antiandrogen withdrawal is approximately 3-5 months, although prolonged responses have been observed.[115-117]

The recognition of the antiandrogen withdrawal response has significantly altered the treatment of hormone-refractory patients. A trial of antiandrogen withdrawal has become standard practice in patients on combined androgen therapy because it is nontoxic and can benefit a significant number of patients (Fig. 59-2). In addition, all clinical trials assessing response to new agents now require an adequate period of antiandrogen withdrawal prior to enrollment in order to avoid confusion in evaluating response rates.

Adrenal Androgen Synthesis Inhibitors

The adrenal gland is the source of 5-10% of peripheral testosterone.[16] Labrie and others have proposed that, following androgen ablation, a subset of prostate cancer cells can become hypersensitive to androgens.[30,31] Therefore, the low level of androgens produced by the adrenal glands may be sufficient to provide continued stimulation. The most commonly used agent to inhibit adrenal androgen production is ketoconazole. Ketoconazole inhibits the cholesterol side-chain cleavage enzyme and the 11β-hydroxylase enzyme, which converts progesterone to 17α-hydroxyprogesterone.[118] Ketoconazole also inhibits the 17α-hydroxylase and C17,20-lyase (CYP450c17) enzymes within the adrenal steroid synthetic pathway.[118] At the usual dose of 400 mg every 8 h, ketoconazole reduces serum T to castrate levels in less than 24 h in 75% of men.[118-121] High-dose ketoconazole (ie, 400 mg tid orally), although effective in lowering serum T, is not commonly used as first-line androgen ablation therapy. This is because of the necessity of a strict every-8-h regimen to compensate for the short duration of its action, coupled with poor compliance due to gastric intolerance. Additionally, because it also inhibits corticosteroid production by the adrenal gland, hydrocortisone must also be administered in combination with ketoconazole.

Multiple phase I and II studies have demonstrated a clinical response and a prostate-specific antigen (PSA) response in CRPC, which ranges from 15% to 80%.[122] On this basis, The Cancer and Leukemia Group B (CALGB) trial 9583 enrolled 260 patients with progressive disease who were receiving combined androgen blockade and was designed both to determine the single-agent efficacy of ketoconazole and to prospectively determine the frequency of the antiandrogen withdrawal (AAWD) response.[123] In this study patients were randomly assigned to either AAWD followed by ketoconazole at the time of PSA progression or AAWD with simultaneous ketoconazole. The PSA response proportion in the antiandrogen-withdrawal-alone arm was 13% compared with 30% in the combination arm ($p < 0.001$), and 14% of patients treated with ketoconazole/AAWD experienced objective responses.[123] Adrenal androgen levels (androstenedione, dehydroepiandrosterone, and dehydroepiandrosterone sulfate) were reduced after 1 month of therapy with ketoconazole and rose significantly above the nadir at the time of progression.[123] Further, analysis of baseline adrenal androgen data and clinical outcomes revealed that higher levels of circulating androgen, most notably androstenedione, corresponded to a higher likelihood of a response to ketoconazole and improved overall survival compared with patients with lower levels of circulating androgen.[124] Taken together, the results of this study confirmed that ketoconazole has clinical activity at the time of AAWD and strongly supported the hypothesis that the mechanism of action of ketoconazole is through a reduction in adrenal androgens. In a subgroup analysis, patients who experienced a >50% decline in PSA while receiving a secondary hormonal therapy had a significantly longer survival (41 months) compared with those who did not (13 months, $p < 0.001$).[122]

Other Second-Line Agents

Several other agents have been tested and may be useful as secondary therapy in hormone-refractory patients. Glucocorticoids have been used for some time as a palliative treatment in end-stage prostate cancer. Recently, Tannock and associates treated patients with 7.5-10 mg prednisone and observed that nearly 40% patients reported an improved quality of life at 1 month and that 20% maintained this improvement for 4 months.[125] In a larger randomized study comparing mitoxantrone and prednisone to prednisone alone, 21% of patients randomized to prednisone alone had improved quality of life and 22% had a greater than 50% decrease in PSA levels.[126] Smith and colleagues treated 21 hormone-refractory patients with low-dose DES (1 mg/day) and reported a 43% PSA response rate.[127] They concluded that oral DES should be considered an active second-line agent. Megace has also been tested as a second-line agent, but response rates in several studies have been lower than comparable studies using other second-line agents.[88] Withdrawal of megace may result in PSA decline, even in those receiving low-dose (20-40 mg daily) therapy for hot flashes.[128]

5α-Reductase Inhibitors

DHT is believed to be the active intracellular androgen in stimulating growth and inhibiting cell death of androgen-dependent normal prostatic cells and presumable prostatic cancer cells.[129] In prostate tissue, T is converted to DHT by the enzyme 5α-reductase. Inhibiting DHT production without decreasing systemic T levels could be advantageous. T itself, without conversion to DHT, is capable of maintaining the anabolic effects of androgen on muscle mass, male libido, as well as sperm maturation.[130] Theoretically, 5α-reductase inhibitors could inhibit the DHT-induced stimulation of androgen-dependent prostatic cancer growth, without negating the effects of T on muscle mass, libido, or erectile potency. Due to these quality-of-life issues, there is a great deal of clinical interest in developing effective and specific 5α-reductase inhibitors. The 5α-reductase family includes two isoforms each encoded by a distinct gene.[131] Type I 5α-reductase is expressed widely and is the major isoform expressed in tissues such as the liver and the skin.[131] The expression of 5α-reductase type II isoform is more restricted to the male sex accessory tissue such as the prostate.[131] While the type II isoform is expressed in prostate stroma, normal and malignant prostate cancer cells express the type I isoform.[131] Clinically, the two most commonly used 5α-reductase inhibitors are finasteride, which preferentially inhibits the type II isoform, and dutasteride, which inhibits both type I and II isoforms. Both of these agents have been demonstrated to inhibit prostate cancer growth and are under evaluation as both chemopreventive and second-line hormone therapies.

Finasteride was evaluated in the largest study of chemoprevention of prostate cancer, the Prostate Cancer Prevention Trial (PCPT), a prospective randomized study of 18,882 men, 55 years of age or older, with a normal digital rectal examination and a PSA level of <3.0 ng/mL.[132] Patients were given either finasteride or placebo for 7 years. Although a reduction of about 25% in prostate cancer diagnoses was reported, the enthusiasm for this chemopreventive approach could not be sustained because an increased rate of high-grade tumors was observed in the patients who received finasteride.[132] However, a recent reanalysis of the data from this study suggest that the increase in high-grade cancers may be due to the effects of finasteride on the prostate, leading to greater PSA sensitivity for detecting both cancer and high-grade cancer, better DRE sensitivity for cancer detection, and improved sensitivity of prostate biopsy for detecting high-grade prostate cancers.[133-135] These factors, examined by statistical modeling, appear to contribute to and might be the cause of the increase in detecting high-grade disease with finasteride.[136] It remains to be seen whether this recent reanalysis will lead to increased use of finasteride as a chemopreventive agent in men at higher risk of prostate cancer.

A second, large chemoprevention study, the Reduction by Dutasteride of Prostate Cancer Events (REDUCE) trial, was opened in 2004. It is a 4-year international, multicenter, randomized, double-blind, placebo-controlled, parallel-group study with the primary end point of biopsy-detectable prostate cancer at 2 and 4 years after initiation of treatment.[137]

New Approaches

The observation that AR expression and activation is maintained in the majority of "castration-resistant" prostate cancers has rekindled interest in the development of new agents directed at maximum suppression of the AR axis (Table 59-2).[122] More potent antiandrogens and new, less toxic adrenal androgen synthesis inhibitors are currently in clinical development. These include MDV3100, a small molecule antagonist of AR, which maintained its ability to block AR in experimental settings in which other antiandrogens functioned as agonists.[138]

The relatively high response rates but significant toxicity with ketoconazole as a second-line agent has stimulated interest in the development of novel adrenal androgen synthesis inhibitors. Abiraterone acetate specifically inhibits the 17α-hydroxylase and C17,20-lyase (CYP450c17) enzymes within the adrenal steroid synthetic pathway, with an inhibition constant of <1 nM.[139] Results presented in abstract form summarizing phase I and II trial results suggest that this agent has clinical activity in CRPC.[140,141] Currently, abiraterone acetate is being tested in combination with prednisone in phase III randomized trials in taxotere-failing patients with metastatic disease. Another agent in this class that is entering phase I testing for prostate cancer is BN83495, a steroid sulfatase inhibitor that prevents conversion of systemic DHEA-sulfate to DHEA.[142] Finally, the Brodie group has developed a novel steroidal agent that inhibits both AR and the C17,20-lyase, which is currently being tested in preclinical models.[143]

Conclusion

As reviewed, there are now a number of alternative pharmacologic approaches that can be used to produce androgen ablation. Recent shifts in treatment philosophy have caused a move from maximum therapy with combined androgen blockade toward strategies, such as intermittent androgen suppression, that try to minimize toxicities while still providing adequate treatment. Large randomized studies should answer several important treatment questions regarding the optimal timing of therapy, the role of intermittent androgen suppression, and the use of potential potency-preserving therapies, such as high-dose antiandrogens as first-line treatment. The discovery of the antiandrogen withdrawal response has also stimulated renewed interest in the use of second-line hormonal approaches and has forced us to rethink the term "hormone-refractory prostate cancer."

While these new androgen deprivation approaches offer expanded treatment options for patients with potentially less toxicity, it must be remembered that the annual death rate from metastatic prostate cancer has not changed significantly since androgen ablation was introduced as the standard therapy more than 50 years ago. Androgen deprivation provides excellent palliation for metastatic bone disease and may, in many cases, prolong survival. However, androgen-independent cells that are resistant to androgen deprivation therapy eventually develop, regardless of the pharma-

Table 59-2 Novel Androgen Axis Inhibitors in Clinical Development

Therapy	Target	Phase of Testing
Abiraterone acetate (Cougar Biotechnology)	C17, 20-lyase	Phase III
BMS-641988 (Bristol-Myers Squibb)	Androgen receptor	Phase I-II
BN83495 (Ipsen)	Steroid sulfatase	Phase I
MDV3100 (Medivation)	Androgen receptor	Phase I
CYP17/AP (Tokai Pharmaceuticals)	C17,20-lyase + AR	Preclinical
Ketocanazole + dutasteride (Glaxo)	5a-redictase type I and II	Phase II

cologic approach used.[144] Unfortunately, no treatment has proven effective as yet in prolonging the survival of patients whose disease progresses while they are on hormonal therapy. Significant progress is still needed in the development of non-androgen-ablative approaches for treating androgen-independent prostate cancer. Agents that can directly activate apoptosis, growth factor antagonists, antiangiogenesis agents, and immunomodulatory therapies are several promising areas currently being evaluated in the laboratory and in the clinic. Combinations of these new agents with androgen deprivation therapy need to be tested in well-designed clinical trials. Combination therapies may represent the next step toward the development of a curative therapy for prostate cancer.

Selected References

The complete reference list can be found at www.pmph-usa.cancermedicine.com

1. Huggins C, Stevens RE, Hodges CV. Studies of prostatic cancer: II. The effects of castration on advanced carcinoma of the prostate gland. *Arch Surg.* 1941;42:209–223.
19. Kyprianou N, English HF, Isaacs JT. Programmed cell death during regression of PC-82 human prostate cancer following androgen ablation. *Cancer Res.* 1990;50:3748–3753.
20. Tolis G, Menta A, Kinch R, et al. Suppression of sex steroids by an LH-Rh analogue in man. *Clin Res.* 1980;28:676–680.
21. The Leuprolide Study Group. Leuprolide versus diethystilbestrol for metastatic prostatic cancer. *N Engl J Med.* 1984;311:1281–1286.
22. Waxman J, Man A, Hendry WF, et al. Importance of early tumor exacerbation in patients treated with long acting analogues of gonadotropin releasing hormone for advanced prostatic cancer. *Br Med J.* 1985;291:1387–1388.
24. Kuhn J-M, Billebaud T, Navratil H, et al. Prevention of the transient adverse effects of a gonadotropin-releasing hormone analog (buserelin) in metastatic prostate carcinoma by administration of an antiandrogen (nilutamide). *N Engl J Med.* 1989;321:413–418.
25. Fowler JE Jr, Gottesman JE, Reid CF, Andriole GL Jr, Soloway MS. Safety and efficacy of an implantable leuprolide delivery system in patients with advanced prostate cancer. *J Urol.* 2000;164(3 Pt 1):730–734.
29. Lipton A, Small E, Saad F, et al. The new bisphosphonate, Zometa (zoledronic acid), decreases skeletal complications in both osteolytic and osteoblastic lesions: a comparison to pamidronate. *Cancer Invest.* 2002;20(Suppl 2):45–54.
30. Labrie F, Dupont A, Belanger A, et al. Combination therapy with flutamide and castration (LHRH agonists or orchiectomy) in advance prostate cancer: a marked improvement in response and survival. *J Steroid Biochem.* 1985;23:833–841.
31. Labrie F, Veillux R, Fournier A. Low androgen levels induce the development of androgen-hypersensitive cell clones in shionogi mammary carcinoma cells in culture. *J Natl Cancer Inst.* 1988;80:1138–1147.
32. Laufer M, Carducci M, Blumenstein B, Eisenberger MA. Combined androgen blockade (CAB) for the treatment of patients with metastatic prostate cancer: summary of 15 years of clinical research. Update Series Vol XVIII Lesson 29. AUA;1999.
33. Prostate Cancer Trialists' Collaborative Group. Maximum androgen blockade in advanced prostate cancer: an overview of 22 randomized trials with 3238 deaths in 5710 patients. *Lancet.* 1995;346:265–269.
34. Caubet JF, Tosteson TD, Dong EW, et al. Maximum androgen blockade in advanced prostate cancer: a meta-analysis of published randomized controlled trials using nonsteroidal antiandrogens. *Urology.* 1997;49:71–78.
35. Moinpour CM, Savage MJ, Troxel A, et al. Quality of life in advanced prostate cancer: results of a randomized therapeutic trial. *J Natl Cancer Inst.* 1998;90:1537–1544.
36. Purnell JQ, Bland LB, Garzotto M, et al. Effects of transdermal estrogen on levels of lipids, lipase activity, and inflammatory markers in men with prostate cancer. *J Lipid Res.* 2006;47:349–355.
37. Cooperberg MR, Grossfeld GD, Lubeck DP, Carroll PR. National practice patterns and time trends in androgen ablation for localized prostate cancer. *J Natl Cancer Inst.* 2003;95:981–989.
38. Higano CS. Side effects of androgen deprivation therapy: monitoring and minimizing toxicity. *Urology.* 2003;61:32–38.
39. Daniell HW, Dunn SR, Ferguson DW, Lomas G, Niazi Z, Stratte PT. Progressive osteoporosis during androgen deprivation therapy for prostate cancer. *J Urol.* 2000;163:181–186.
40. Berruti A, Dogliotti L, Terrone C, et al. Changes in bone mineral density, lean body mass and fat content as measured by dual energy x-ray absorptiometry in patients with prostate cancer without apparent bone metastasesgiven androgen deprivation therapy. *J Urol.* 2002;167:2361–2367.
41. Smith MR, Finkelstein JS, McGovern FJ, et al. Changes in body composition during androgen deprivation therapy for prostate cancer. *J Clin Endocrinol Metab.* 2002;87:599–603.
42. Braga-Basaria M, Dobs AS, Muller DC, et al. Metabolic syndrome in men with prostate cancer undergoing long-term androgen-deprivation therapy. *J Clin Oncol.* 2006;24:3979–3983.
45. Keating NL, O'Malley AJ, Smith MR. Diabetes and cardiovascular disease during androgen deprivation therapy for prostate cancer. *J Clin Oncol.* 2006;24:4448–4456.
47. Tsai HK, D'Amico AV, Sadetsky N, Chen MH, Carroll PR. Androgen deprivation therapy for localized prostate cancer and the risk of cardiovascular mortality. *J Natl Cancer Inst.* 2007;99:1516–1524.
55. Manson JE, Hsia J, Johnson KC, et al. Estrogen plus progestin and the risk of coronary heart disease. *N Engl J Med.* 2003;349:523–534.
57. Agardh CD, Nilsson-Ehle P, Lundgren R, Gustafson A. The influence of treatment with estrogens and estramustine phosphate on platelet aggregation and plasma lipoproteins in non-disseminated prostatic carcinoma. *J Urol.* 1984;132:1021–1024.
60. Hedlund PO, Damber JE, Hagerman I, et al. Parenteral estrogen versus combined androgen deprivation in the treatment of metastatic prostatic cancer: part 2. Final evaluation of the Scandinavian Prostatic Cancer Group (SPCG) Study No. 5. *Scand J Urol Nephrol.* 2008;42:220–229.
65. Chodak G, Sharifi R, Kasimis B, et al. Single agent therapy with bicalutamide: a comparison with medical or surgical castration in the treatment of prostate cancer. *Urology.* 1995;46:849.
66. Blackledge GRP. High-dose bicalutamide monotherapy for the treatment of prostate cancer. *Urology.* 1996;47:44.
69. Wirth MP, See WA, McLeod DG, Iversen P, Morris T, Carroll K; Casodex Early Prostate Cancer Trialists' Group. Bicalutamide 150 mg in addition to standard care in patients with localized or locally advanced prostate cancer: results from the second analysis of the early prostate cancer program at median followup of 5.4 years. *J Urol.* 2004;172:1865–1870.
71. Gleave M, Bruchovsky N, Bowden M, et al. Intermittent androgen suppression prolongs time to androgen-independent progression in the LNCaP prostate tumor model. *J Urol.* 1994;151:457A.
78. Veterans Administration Cooperative Urological Research Group. Treatment and survival of patients with cancer of the prostate. *Surg Gynecol Obstet.* 1967;124:1011.
79. Byar DP, Corle DK. Hormone therapy for prostate cancer: results of the Veterans Administration Cooperative Urological Research Group Studies. *NCI Monogr.* 1988;7:165–170.
80. The Medical Research Council Prostate Cancer Working Party Investigators Group. Immediate versus deferred treatment for advanced prostate cancer: initial results of the Medical Research Council trial. *Br J Urol.* 1997;79:235–246.
81. Medical Research Council Prostate Cancer Working Party Investigators Group. Immediate versus deferred hormone therapy for prostate cancer: how safe is androgen deprivation? *BJU Int.* 2000;86:2000.
83. Messing EM, Manola J, Sarosdy M, Wilding G, Crawford ED, Trump D. Immediate hormonal therapy compared with observation after radical prostatectomy and pelvic lymphadenectomy in men with node-positive prostate cancer. *N Engl J Med.* 1999;341:1781–1788.
85. Pound CR, Partin AW, Eisenberger MA, et al. Natural history of progression after PSA elevation following radical prostatectomy. *JAMA.* 1999;281:1591–1597.
86. D'Amico AV, Moul J, Carroll PR, Sun L, Lubeck D, Chen MH. Prostate specific antigen doubling time as a surrogate end point for prostate cancer specific mortality following radical prostatectomy or radiation therapy. *J Urol.* 2004;172:S42–S46.
90. Manni A, Bartholomew M, Caplan R, et al. Androgen priming and chemotherapy in advanced prostate cancer: evaluation of determinants of clinical outcome. *J Clin Oncol.* 1988;6:1456–1466.

60 Cancer Gene Therapy

Sunil J. Advani, MD ■ Ralph R. Weichselbaum, MD ■ Donald W. Kufe, MD

Advances in our understanding of the genetic alterations that accumulate in the progression to a malignant cell have provided unforeseen opportunities for the development of new therapeutic strategies. Cancer gene therapy is an emerging field that was initially received with unbridled enthusiasm as one such opportunity to take advantage of the genetic differences between normal and transformed cells. Limitations in our ability to deliver genes to every cancer cell, however, have dampened interest in developing approaches to inactivate oncogenes or replace nonfunctioning tumor suppressor genes. Nonetheless, other therapeutic strategies have emerged that exploit the presently available delivery systems and our understanding of alterations that distinguish the cancer cell. This chapter defines the principles of gene therapy and their application to the treatment of cancer.

Gene therapy can be broadly defined as the transfer of genetic material into a cell to transiently or permanently alter the cellular phenotype. Introduction of a nucleic acid or target gene (transgene) directly into cells is referred to as transfection. Alternatively, transduction refers to the introduction of a transgene into a cell through a viral vector system. Gene transfer can be performed by transfection or transduction of target cells in vitro and then administration of the modified cells to an animal or patient. In vivo gene transfer is accomplished by direct transfection or transduction of target cells in the patient. The introduction of genes that encode proteins with potential antitumor effects has been described as therapeutic gene transfer. The mechanistic effects of the therapeutic gene product and the stability of transgene expression are factors of importance to the different approaches that now constitute cancer gene therapy. Of equal importance is delivery of the therapeutic gene to the target cell. The delivery system, or vector, generally consists of a nucleic acid sequence or promoter that drives expression of the transgene and a polyadenylation signal that stabilizes the transcribed messenger ribonucleic acid (mRNA). The vector is usually inserted into a bacteriophage for propagation in vitro or integrated into a virus.

The delivery of therapeutic genes to cancer cells poses the greatest challenge to the successful application of cancer gene therapy in humans. As such, considerable effort is being devoted to the development of more selective and efficient vectors. In particular, vectors that target specific tumor cell populations, or that contain promoters that are selectively activated in tumor cells, are at the forefront of progress in the cancer gene therapy field. An extension of the cancer gene therapy paradigm is the use of replication-competent viruses (viral oncolysis). Replication-competent viruses are beginning to overcome some of the hurdles of inefficient delivery that plague other gene transfer methods. This chapter begins with a description of the available vector systems and then discusses the therapeutic genes that are presently under study. Although not involving the transfer of genes to cancer cells, certain other strategies, such as the administration of recombinant vaccines, indirectly target the tumor cell, and although considered in the context of cancer gene therapy, are described here and in the chapters on tumor immunology and active specific immunotherapy with vaccines.

Gene Delivery Systems

Viral and nonviral vector systems are being employed in gene therapy approaches to cancer. The following sections describe the RNA and DNA viruses and the nonviral vectors that are being used to deliver transgenes to tumor cells.

Retroviruses

Retroviruses are single-stranded RNA viruses that consist of the 5′ and 3′ long-terminal repeats (LTRs) and the *gag*, *pol*, and *env* structural genes. *Gag* encodes three proteins that form the shell of the virion. *Pol* encodes reverse transcriptase, integrase, and ribonuclease H (RNaseH), which are necessary for viral integration into host chromosomal DNA. The *env* gene encodes the envelope glycoprotein that extends from the lipid membrane of the virion and functions as a ligand for the cellular viral receptor.[1] When a transgene is inserted into an attenuated replication-defective virus and that virus infects a target cell, viral sequences containing the transgene integrate into the host genome and confer expression of both viral genes and the transgene. The deleted viral vector, however, is incapable of undergoing viral replication because the deleted structural gene that is necessary for this process is not expressed by the target cell. As such, the deleted viral vector transfers and expresses the transgene but is incapable of establishing an active infection in the host.

Retroviruses integrate into target cell DNA and thus achieve stable integration of the transgene. Theoretically, stable integration should provide long-term expression, although methylation of the LTR often results in downregulation of transgene transcription.[2] The receptor for the Moloney murine leukemia retrovirus (MoMuLV) is found on most human cells. Thus, although cell type is not limiting for vector transduction, a potential disadvantage is the ubiquitous distribution of the receptor, and thereby little target cell selectivity. To address this issue of selective target cell transduction, hybrid envelope proteins have been generated by fusing a portion of the env gene to a sequence encoding a ligand for a specific cell surface receptor. For example, fusions to the erythropoietin domain that binds to the erythropoietin receptor have generated recombinant retroviral vectors that selectively target those cells expressing the receptor. Identification of the crystal structure of the murine retroviral envelope protein should facilitate the development of vectors with modifications of this structure and restricted target cell tropisms.[3]

An important limitation of the MoMuLV-based retroviral vectors is that they integrate only into actively dividing cells. As most solid tumors have low growth fractions, it is unlikely that these retroviral vectors would transduce a significant proportion of the tumor. By contrast, the HIV type-1 replicates in nondividing cells,[4,5] and thus may represent a more effective vector for the transduction of tumors. In addition, retroviral vector-mediated insertional mutagenesis could result in transformation of the transduced target cell. On the basis of these limitations, MoMuLV-based retroviruses are considered best suited for in vitro transduction of specific target cells that can be isolated and stimulated to undergo proliferation. The eventual utility of retroviral vectors for in vivo transduction is uncertain.

Adenoviruses

Adenoviruses are nonenveloped, linear, double-stranded DNA viruses. Approximately 50 serotypes of adenovirus have been identified and grouped from A to F on the basis of genome size, composition, homology, and organization. The most studied adenoviruses are the group C serotypes 1, 2, 5, and 6. The prototype adenoviral vector for gene therapy is based on adenovirus type 5 (Ad5).

Adenoviral attachment to cells is mediated by fibers that extend from the 12 vertices of the outer capsid. The adenoviral genome is approximately 36 kilobases (kb) and is conventionally represented as 100 map units (1 map unit = 360 base pairs [bp]). Each end of the viral genome is flanked by 100-150 bp of repeated DNA sequence (inverted terminal repeat). Viral gene expression occurs in a sequential cascade. Adenoviral genes are grouped as early (E) genes whose expression precedes viral DNA replication and the transcription of late (L) genes at 6-8 hours after infection. The E genes encode regulatory proteins for viral replication and the L genes encode structural proteins necessary for assembly of progeny virions.

Adenoviral vectors have been based on the observation that deletion of the E1A and part of the E1B gene results in replication-deficient viruses. Such viruses can be propagated in helper cell lines that express the E1 gene products. For example, the 293 helper cell line was prepared from human embryonic cells stably transformed with Ad5 DNA fragments that constitutively express the E1 proteins.[6] The amount of DNA that can be effectively packaged into adenovirus virions is ~105% of the wild-type genome and thus allows for the insertion of ~2 kb of foreign DNA. With the E1A-deleted viruses, it has been possible to insert 5-6 kb of DNA. An additional 2 kb of DNA can be inserted by deletion of the E3 gene. The E3 gene product functions in abrogating the host immune response to the virus by preventing cytolysis mediated through cytotoxic T cells and tumor necrosis factor. E3 is not required for viral growth in tissue culture, and E3-deleted viruses appear to be fully infectious.

Adenoviral vectors have a number of potential advantages over retroviral vectors. Most human cell types are susceptible to adenoviral infection and are subject to efficient transduction. Additionally, adenoviruses can deliver transgenes to both dividing and nondividing cells. This property is of particular significance in the setting of tumors that contain a heterogeneous cell population of both cycling and noncycling cells. Because adenoviruses are relatively stable and resistant to physical manipulations, vectors can be concentrated to high titers (10^{11}-10^{12} PFU/mL) and frozen for use at later times (a property that is generally not possible with retroviruses because of their fragility under physical stresses such as freezing). Another advantage of adenoviral vectors is that the adenoviral life cycle does not require integration into the host cell genome. Because adenoviral DNA is episomal, insertional mutagenesis is much less a concern than it is for retroviral vectors. Also, a promoter of choice can be used to drive the inserted transgene, affording the opportunity for tissue selective expression or inducibility. By contrast, the use of heterologous promoters in retroviral vectors is often problematic because the promoter can be overridden by strong constitutive activity of the retroviral LTR.

A major disadvantage of current adenoviral vectors is the induction of a significant host immune response. A T-cell–mediated response against adenoviral proteins causes a local inflammatory reaction that can result in lysis of the transduced cells and a shorter duration of adenoviral mediated transgene expression. The immune response is partly a result of E1-deleted adenoviruses expressing other E and L genes and initiating viral DNA replication. As such, vectors are needed that exhibit silencing of viral gene expression and DNA replication and thereby prolong transgene expression. Adenoviral vectors are limited by the size of transgene insertion. With current vectors, 8.5 kb appears to be the limit of DNA that can be inserted. Also of concern in the propagation of E1-deleted viruses in helper cell lines is the generation of replication competent adenoviruses. In this regard, recombination can occur between the E1-deleted adenovirus and the E1 region present in the 293 helper cell line.

Herpes Simplex Viruses

Herpes simplex viruses (HSVs) are large, enveloped, double-stranded DNA viruses classified as either α, β, or γ, based on viral characteristics. HSV-1 is a herpes virus that is naturally neurotropic and also infects epithelial cells. A characteristic of HSV-1 infection is the establishment of a latent ("dormant") state in sensory neurons that, in the presence of certain stimuli, results in reactivation of the virus and entry into the lytic cycle.

HSV attachment to cells is mediated by binding of glycoproteins expressed at the viral envelope to cellular membrane receptors.[7] The HSV-1 genome is approximately 150 kb and encodes more than 90 proteins. The sequence is represented by two stretches of DNA, unique long and unique short, flanked by inverted repeat segments. Genes in the unique region are present as single copies, whereas those in the repeat segments are present as two copies. HSV-1 viral genes have been classified as either essential or nonessential depending on whether deletion of the gene allows for growth of the mutated virus in cell culture. Viral gene expression is coordinately regulated with the α genes (involved in regulatory functions) expressed first, followed by β genes (involved in nucleic acid metabolism and viral DNA replication), and then γ genes (encoding structural proteins).

Replication-deficient HSV-1–based vectors are categorized as helper virus dependent and independent. Helper virus-dependent vectors have also been termed amplicons. Amplicons are defective HSV genomes that arise spontaneously by recombination and are amplified by serial passage at high multiplicities of infection.[8] At a minimum, the defective genome (amplicon) consists of a terminal a sequence and an origin of viral DNA synthesis. A viral origin of DNA synthesis allows for propagation of the amplicon, and the a sequence is needed to cleave concatameric DNA and package the amplicon. As amplicons are largely devoid of coding sequences, viral structural proteins and those involved in viral DNA replication and exocytosis must be provided by a "helper" virus. One such helper virus was generated by deletion of an essential HSV-1 gene, α4. In this system, an α4-expressing complementary cell line is transfected with the amplicon and then superinfected with the α4-deleted HSV-1. In theory, amplicons could accommodate as much as 150 kb (the size of the HSV-1 genome) because the backbone of the amplicon is usually <15 kb. Moreover, amplicons efficiently express integrated transgenes for relatively long periods as there is no associated latency shutdown of viral gene expression.[9] Despite these advantages, there are certain problems that exist with the amplicon approach. First, because helper viruses are needed to encode the missing viral proteins, amplicons become contaminated with helper viral DNA. This problem has been solved in part by the generation of helper viruses that fail to package.[10] Second, the yields of amplicons are several orders of magnitude less than that achieved with wild-type viruses, and the ratio of amplicon to helper virus is low. Last, amplicons tend to be unstable with serial passage because there is a selective advantage for smaller amplicons.[11]

Helper virus-independent HSV-1 viral vectors have deletions in essential viral genes. Because of deletion of one or more essential genes, such viruses need to be grown in appropriate cell lines that complement the defects. These HSV-1 vectors replicate to high titers. In addition, up to 40 kb of foreign DNA can be inserted (at least fourfold greater than can be achieved with adenoviral vectors). HSV-1 vectors can also deliver genes to a wide range of cell types. With regard to disadvantages, many of the essential viral genes encode multifunctional proteins. For example, $\alpha 4$ is both a transcriptional activator and repressor. Thus, deletion of $\alpha 4$ may influence viral gene expression in a manner detrimental to a gene therapy vector. Also, as with E1-deleted adenoviruses, expression of the remaining viral genes in the infected cell may lead to the induction of an antiviral immune response. As found with defective viruses that are grown in complementing cell lines, there is the possibility of recombination and reversion to a wild-type phenotype. Given that wild-type HSV-1 infection is associated with neurologic sequelae, recombination is of concern in using the helper virus-independent HSV-1–based vectors. However, as the molecular basis for HSV-1 neurovirulence is better defined, such vectors may gain more widespread use.

Adeno-Associated Virus

Adeno-associated viruses (AAVs) are small, nonenveloped, linear single-stranded DNA parvoviruses that are naturally replication deficient. Four of the six known AAV serotypes are human isolates (AAV-2, AAV-3, AAV-5, and AAV-6), whereas AAV-1 and AAV-4 are of simian origin. AAV-2 is the predominant serotype used in gene therapy approaches. Infection with AAV results in either a latent or productive infection phase. Productive infection is dependent on the presence of a helper virus (adenovirus, herpes virus, or vaccinia) or on exposure to genotoxic stress. In the absence of a helper virus or genotoxic stress, AAV integrates into the long arm of chromosome 19 (q19.3-qter), known as the AAVS1 site, and enters a latent phase.

The genome of AAV is approximately 4.7 kb. The DNA is flanked by inverted terminal repeats (ITRs) of 145 bases. The ITRs serve as origins of DNA replication and are required for packaging recombinant AAV into infectious virus. Also, the ITRs are the only *cis* elements essential to the AAV replicative life cycle. Between the ITRs are two sets of open reading frames (ORFs), Rep and Cap. The Rep ORF encodes four nonstructural proteins that regulate AAV replication and site-specific integration. The Cap ORF encodes three structural proteins (VP1 to 3).

Recombinant AAVs (rAAVs) for gene therapy are constructed by deleting the Rep and Cap ORFs and replacing the deleted DNA with a transgene between the ITRs. To propagate rAAV in cell culture, rAAV vectors containing the ITRs and transgene are cotransfected with a plasmid expressing the Rep and Cap genes. The transfected cells are then infected with adenovirus to provide the helper function and thereby efficient rAAV replication. As such, the rAAV must subsequently be purified from the adenovirus in a setting in which the rAAV titers are often low relative to the adenovirus contamination. As the helper function of the adenovirus resides in the E1a, E1b, E2a, E4, and VA1 proteins, expression of these genes by 293 cells provides the requisite helper effect in the absence of adenoviral infection. This approach has also been reported to increase rAAV titers.[12,13]

rAAVs have certain advantages as gene therapy vectors. rAAVs are naturally replication defective and are considered nonpathogenic. Also, deletion of the Rep and Cap ORFs decreases immunogenicity. rAAVs have a broad tissue tropism (ie, lung, muscle, central nervous system, liver, and retina) as a consequence of attachment of AAV-2 to the ubiquitously expressed cell surface heparan sulfate proteoglycan (HSPG). Unlike retroviruses, rAAVs transduce both replicating and nonreplicating cells. Deletion of the Rep ORF, however, abolishes the site-specific integration of AAV into chromosome 19.[14,15] In addition, despite deletion of the Rep ORF, rAAV can accommodate only 4 kb of DNA insert.

Nonviral Gene Delivery

Viral vectors, having evolved to enter cells by receptor-mediated processes and to escape from endosomes with delivery of their DNA to nuclei, are highly efficient in gene transduction. Disadvantages of viral vectors include immune recognition of viral proteins with destruction of the infected cells and with an inability for repeated viral administration. Other limitations of viral vectors include the potential for insertional mutagenesis, restrictions in the size of the transgene, and difficulties encountered in large-scale production for clinical trials. Nonviral delivery systems have thus been explored to overcome some of these obstacles. Two commonly used laboratory techniques for transfecting plasmid DNA into cells involve calcium phosphate precipitation and electroporation. In calcium phosphate precipitation, plasmid DNA complexed to calcium phosphate crystals enters the cell by endocytosis and is then transported to the nucleus. In electroporation, brief high-voltage electrical pulses are applied to cells to induce the formation of transient pores in the cell membrane. DNA enters the cell through these pores. Both methods of transfection are restricted to cells in culture.

Direct microinjection of genes into nuclei of cells is another method of transfection that abrogates the exposure of DNA to the acidic conditions of endosomes. Although tedious, microinjection is particularly useful for delivering DNA to embryonic cells or oocytes. Direct injection of DNA into skeletal or cardiac muscle is associated with uptake by cells and expression of the transgene. Similar findings have been obtained following injection of DNA into solid tumors growing in nude mice. In this setting, reporter gene expression has been stable for 5 days and can persist for up to 10 days after injection.[16]

Direct DNA injection by the "gene gun" refers to particle-mediated gene transfer in which DNA is delivered by physical force. In this approach, DNA is commonly coated onto gold particles. Acceleration of the DNA-coated particles into tissues or target cells is followed by release of the DNA in the nucleus.[17] Gene gun delivery, like direct DNA injection, is limited by low transfection efficiencies and transfection of both tumor and normal cells.

Cationic liposomes form artificial membranes that complex with DNA and confer the transfection of DNA into cells by endocytosis.[18] Complexes of cationic liposomes and DNA have been used to deliver DNA into tumor cells in culture, into tumor xenografts in mice, and into tumors in patients.[19-22] Liposome-mediated gene transfer is limited by aggregation of the DNA in endosomes and thereby destruction in the acidic environment or by nuclease digestion during transfer of the DNA from the cytoplasm to the nucleus.[18]

"Synthetic viruses" were developed to exploit the efficiency of viral vectors and the advantages of liposomes.[23] DNA is condensed and packaged by poly-L-lysine and targeted to specific cells by conjugating a ligand for a cell surface receptor to the polylysine-DNA complex. Ligands include transferrin, basic fibroblast growth factor, and integrin-binding domains.[24,25] The polylysine-DNA complex is internalized by receptor-mediated endocytosis into endosomes. Fusogenic peptides have been incorporated into the complex to release the DNA from the endosomal compartment.[23,26] The N-terminal sequence of the influenza virus hemagglutinin subunit HA-2 induces destabilization of the endosomal membrane at acidic pH and releases internalized DNA from the endosomes. GALA, another fusogenic peptide, forms a random coil at pH 7.5 and an amphipathic helix at acidic pH. As such, in the acidic environment of the endosome, GALA destabilizes the endosomal membrane.[26] Thus, conjugation of the polylysine-DNA complex to both a ligand and a fusogenic peptide confers cell receptor-specific transfection and efficient transfer of DNA to the nucleus.

Virus-like coats have also been used to package and deliver DNA to cells. For example, an adenoviral-based dodecahedron has been constructed from the structural proteins, penton base, and fiber.[27] In this system, which is devoid of the viral genome, the penton base and fiber mediate efficient cell attachment, internalization, and release from the endosome.

In summary, although providing an alternative approach for cancer gene therapy, nonviral gene delivery is not as efficient as that achieved with viral vectors. Nonviral delivery systems, nonetheless, provide certain advantages in settings, such as immunomodulation strategies, in which transfection of only a fraction of the target cell population can be sufficient to achieve the requisite response. By contrast, more efficient transduction as achieved with viral vectors is necessary in the setting of treatment with therapeutic genes.

Therapeutic Genes

In cancer gene therapy, the replacement of mutated tumor-suppressor genes or other strategies to correct the transformed phenotype requires the transduction of every tumor cell. Given the limitations of the available gene transfer systems to achieve that goal, therapeutic approaches have been developed to exploit the potential for transduction or transfection of only limited populations of tumor cells. In this context, gene therapy for cancer has been focused on the delivery of genes that encode proteins that activate prodrugs and thereby induce cytotoxicity of both transduced and neighboring tumor cells. The delivery of genes that encode proteins that disrupt cell-cycle progression and induce apoptosis represents another area of focus. In addition, genes that modulate the immune response can be delivered to tumor or normal cell populations to induce antitumor immunity.

Virus-Directed Enzyme/Prodrug Therapy

Several cancer gene therapy strategies employ the delivery to tumor cells of genes encoding prodrug-converting enzymes and then treatment with systemic administration of nontoxic prodrug. This approach of expressing drug susceptibility genes in tumor cells has been termed "suicide gene therapy." Cells transduced to express the prodrug enzyme confer conversion of the prodrug to active metabolites and thereby selective cytotoxicity. In the setting of treatment with conventional chemotherapeutic agents, the achievement of high local tumor drug concentrations is limited by systemic toxicity. By contrast, virus-directed enzyme/prodrug improves the therapeutic ratio by administration of high systemic concentrations of the prodrug and conversion to the cytotoxic metabolite only within the transduced tumor microenvironment.

Essential to virus-directed enzyme/prodrug therapy is the identification of therapeutically effective converting enzyme/prodrug combinations. Transduction of tumor cells to express nonmammalian enzymes or to overexpress mammalian enzymes has been employed to selectively increase conversion of prodrugs to their toxic metabolites. Most of the strategies have employed transduction of genes encoding nonmammalian enzymes. Enzyme/prodrug combinations have been in large part based on the experience of treating tumors with conventional chemotherapeutic agents. For example, certain prodrugs have been converted to active antimetabolites that target replicating cells or to cell-cycle–active, phase-nonspecific, alkylating agents (Table 60-1).

HSV-Thymidine Kinase ■ In contrast to mammalian thymidine kinase, HSV-thymidine kinase (HSV-tk) preferentially phosphorylates the antiherpetic nucleoside analogs ganciclovir, acyclovir, and bromovinyl-deoxyuridine to monophosphates. In turn, cellular kinases phosphorylate the monophosphorylated nucleotides to triphosphates, which are then incorporated into replicating DNA by DNA polymerase α. Incorporation of the nucleotide analogs into DNA is associated with chain termination and the induction of DNA single-strand breaks. Compared with cells transduced to express HSV-tk, mammalian cells are relatively resistant to the toxic effects of these agents in vitro and in vivo.

Retroviral and adenoviral vectors have been used to directly transduce tumor cells with HSV-tk. Systemic administration of ganciclovir in the setting of HSV-tk–transduced tumor models is associated with substantial regressions.[28] Complete eradication of tumors is achieved despite transduction of only 10-70% of the tumor cell population. These observations contributed to identification of the "bystander effect."[29] Multiple mechanisms may be responsible for this effect. For example, studies have implicated the transfer of phosphorylated ganciclovir nucleotides from HSV-tk–transduced cells to surrounding cells via intracellular gap junctions.[30] Such a mechanism of eliciting a bystander effect is in concert with the finding in tissue culture of a requirement for cell-to-cell contact. In addition, interleukin (IL)-6 and IL-1 secreted by HSV-tk–transduced tumor cells treated with ganciclovir may function as paracrine factors in the induction of nontransduced cell death. The bystander effect has also been attributed to the transfer of signals from dying HSV-tk–transduced cells that induce apoptosis of adjacent cells. In this regard, the association of HSV-tk/ganciclovir treatment with aggregation of death receptors (CD95) and activation of caspases could transduce proapoptotic signals to neighboring cells.[31]

Cytosine Deaminase ■ Cytosine deaminase (CD) is expressed in bacteria and fungi but not in mammalian cells. CD deaminates cytosine to uracil and thereby converts the nontoxic prodrug 5-fluorocytosine (5-FC) to 5-fluorouracil (5-FU). 5-FU inhibits thymidylate synthase, and blocks methylation of uridylate to thymidylate. DNA synthesis is, in turn, inhibited by the decrease in thymidylate pools. Conversion of 5-FU to fluorouridine triphosphate (FUTP) and incorporation into RNA also disrupts ribosomal RNA and mRNA function. As 5-FU is an effective, but potentially toxic, anticancer agent, transduction of tumor cells to express CD and then administration of 5-FC can obviate normal tissue toxicity by increasing concentrations of 5-FU selectively within the tumor.

An advantage of the CD/5-FC combination is a substantial bystander effect that can compensate for the low transduction efficiencies of the available delivery systems. 5-FU readily diffuses in and out of cells by nonfacilitated diffusion

Table 60-1 ■ Enzyme/Prodrug Combinations

Converting Enzyme	Prodrug	Action of Drug
HSV-thymidine kinase	Ganciclovir, acyclovir, bromovinyl-deoxyuridine	Antimetabolite
E coli cytosine deaminase	5-Fluorocytosine	Antimetabolite
Human cytochrome P-450 2B1	Cyclophosphamide, ifosfamide	Alkylator
E coli XGPRT	6-Thioxanthine	Antimetabolite
E coli DeoD	6-Methylpurine-2′-deoxyribonucleoside	Antimetabolite
E coli nitroreductase	CB1954 (5-aziridin-1-yl)-2,4-dinitrobenzamide	Alkylator

mechanism. Cells near those transduced to express CD are exposed to a concentration gradient of 5-FU that decreases with increasing distance. Thus, with as few as 2% of the tumor cells transduced to express CD, significant tumor regressions are induced by administration of 5-FC.[32] Also, CD/5-FC therapy has been reported to be effective in tumor models (ie, gliomas) not sensitive to 5-FU.[33] A potential disadvantage of the CD/5-FC combination derives from diffusion of 5-FU into normal surrounding tissues. Nonetheless, 5-FU is predominantly toxic to dividing, as compared with quiescent, cells; thus, the CD/5-FC combination could be more effective against tumors, such as gliomas, hepatomas, and sarcomas, that reside in mitotically quiescent tissues. In addition, as 5-FU is a known radiosensitizer, the higher local tumor concentrations of this agent that are achieved with CD/5-FC therapy could provide a selective increase in sensitivity to irradiation.[34,35]

Cytochrome P-450 2B1 ■ Cyclophosphamide and ifosfamide are nontoxic to cells in the absence of conversion by cytochrome P-450 2B1 to their active metabolites. For example, cyclophosphamide is activated by hepatic cytochrome P-450 2B1 to 4-hydroxycyclophosphamide and thereby production of phosphoramide mustard (a DNA alkylator) and acrolein (a protein alkylator).[36] These metabolites circulate systemically to both tumor and normal tissue and result in toxicity to normal cell populations, such as hematopoietic cells and the gastrointestinal mucosa, with a high proliferative index. Cytochrome P-450 2B1 is expressed by hepatocytes and generally not by tumor cells. Thus, transduction of tumor cells to express cytochrome P-450 2B1 results in the direct intratumoral metabolism of cyclophosphamide or ifosphamide. This approach has been used to sensitize gliomas expressing cytochrome P-450 2B1 to cyclophosphamide.[37] In addition, this approach is associated with a bystander effect induced by diffusion of cyclophosphamide metabolites and is not dependent on cell-to-cell contact.[38]

Additional Suicide Genes ■ The *Escherichia coli gpt* gene encodes the xanthine-guanine phosphoribosyl transferase (XGPRT), which converts the xanthine analog 6-thioxanthine to 6-thioxanthine monophosphate by the addition of a ribose phosphate. Within the cell, 6-thioxanthine monophosphate is demethylated to 6-thioguanine monophosphate, a potent inhibitor of nucleic acid synthesis.[39]

The *E coli DeoD* gene encodes a purine nucleoside phosphorylase (PNP) that, in contrast to mammalian PNP, can hydrolyze the nontoxic 6-methylpurine-2′-deoxyribonucleoside to the toxic purine analog 6-methylpurine.[40]

The *E coli* nitroreductase (NTR) activates the prodrug CB1954, which is a weak mono-functional alkylating agent. CB1954 is bioreduced by NTR to the 4-hydroxylamino derivative, which is then converted by thioesters (ie, coenzyme A) into a potent bifunctional alkylating agent.[41] As bioreduction of CB1954 is more efficient with NTR than with the cellular DT diaphorase, transduction of tumor cells to express NTR confers sensitivity to the active CB1954 metabolite.

Gene Therapy Directed at Cell-Cycle Control and Apoptosis

The discovery of cellular proteins that regulate cell-cycle progression and the induction of apoptosis has provided opportunities to exploit their expression in cancer gene therapy strategies. The following are three such approaches that have been explored by transduction of tumor cells with cellular genes that, when constitutively expressed, disrupt proliferation and induce apoptosis.

p53 ■ The p53 tumor suppressor is induced in the cellular response to genotoxic agents, oxidative stress, hypoxia, and oncogene expression.[42] In response to DNA damage, p53 activates genes involved in (1) cell-cycle arrest (p21), (2) DNA repair (PCNA, GADD45), and (3) induction of apoptosis (Bax, IGF-bp3). p53 may also induce apoptosis independent of transcriptional activation. Whether p53 induces cell-cycle arrest and DNA repair or apoptosis is thought to be cell-type specific and dependent on the apoptotic threshold of the cell. Importantly, the induction of tumor cell apoptosis by cancer chemotherapeutic agents and radiation is dependent on normal p53 function.[43,44] In addition, the findings that p53 is mutated in approximately 50% of human tumors provide support for developing gene therapy strategies that confer expression of the normal p53 protein.

Several studies demonstrate that transduction of p53 into tumor cells induces cell-cycle arrest or apoptosis in culture and inhibits growth of tumor xenografts in mice.[45-47] Given the limitations of the available gene delivery systems, combining p53 gene therapy with conventional anticancer treatment may be important to achieving complete tumor cell kill. In this context, the combination of p53 gene therapy and cisplatin or radiation increases the apoptotic response of tumor cells and control of tumor xenografts.[12,48,49] Translation of these findings to clinical trials has demonstrated the feasibility of delivering p53 by replication-incompetent retroviral and adenoviral vectors into tumors of patients with non–small cell lung cancer (NSCLC). In a phase I study, adenovirus-mediated p53 gene transfer was accomplished by computed tomography-guided percutaneous fine-needle injection or by bronchoscopy in 28 NSCLC patients.[50] Evaluation of posttreatment tumor biopsy specimens demonstrated the adenoviral vector in 86% by polymerase chain reaction (PCR) and vector-specific expression of p53 in 46% by reverse transcriptase (RT)-PCR. These studies show that adenoviral mediated p53 gene therapy is feasible and that, given the safety of this approach, subsequent trials will be performed to assess efficacy.

E2F-1 ■ E2F-1 is a member of the E2F family of transcription factors that regulate the expression of gene products that are primarily involved in S-phase progression.[51] Although E2F-1 is oncogenic,[52] other evidence supports a role as a tumor suppressor. For example, overexpression of E2F-1 can result in apoptosis.[53] Also, E2F-1–deficient mice develop spontaneous tumors.[54,55] Based on these observations, an adenoviral vector was developed to deliver E2F-1 to glioma cells.[56] The results of these studies demonstrate that transduction of E2F-1 induces glioma cell apoptosis and inhibits glioma xenograft growth in nude mice. Thus, E2F-1 gene therapy, like that with p53, provides an approach to inhibit tumor cell growth and induce apoptosis.

p21 ■ *p21* is a cyclin-dependent kinase (cdk) inhibitor. By binding to and inhibiting the activity of cyclin/cdk complexes, *p21* blocks cell-cycle progression. Relevant to cancer gene therapy, transfer of the *p21* gene into tumor cells suppresses tumorigenicity[16,57] and induces apoptosis.[58]

Downregulation of Genes Involved in Tumor Progression

Another approach to suppress the malignant phenotype involves downregulation of oncogenes and other genes that contribute to tumor progression. Triple-helix formation, antisense oligonucleotides, ribozymes, and RNA-mediated interference (RNAi) have been developed to target the expression of specific genes. Although downregulation of genes to treat cancer is theoretically attractive, the available approaches are limited by the need to achieve sufficient suppression of the targeted gene to reverse the transformed phenotype or to induce cell death.

Triple-Helix Formation ■ Triple-helix–forming oligonucleotides (TFOs) bind to duplex DNA in a sequence-specific manner and, as a third strand, block gene transcription (Fig. 60-1). The polypurine or polypyrimidine TFO binds to the purine-

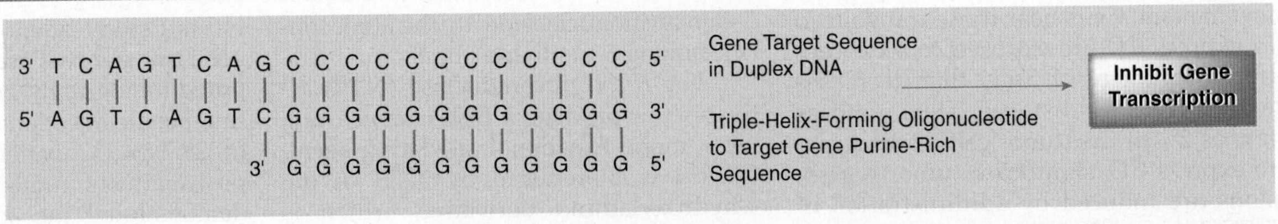

Figure 60-1 Triple-helix formation to block gene transcription.

rich strand in the major DNA groove through Hoogsteen hydrogen bonds.[59] A, C, or G in the TFO binds to G in the purine stretch of duplex DNA. Conversely, T or A in the TFO binds to A in the purine stretch of duplex DNA. To use TFOs as anticancer agents, a target sequence rich in purines must be identified that is involved in regulating the transcription of an oncogene. A complementary TFO is constructed that binds to the target sequence and thereby results in downregulation of oncogene transcription. TFO binding results in both conformational changes in the major groove and steric effects that block DNA-protein interactions. As a consequence of TFO binding, transcription factors, such as Sp 1 and NFκB, are unable to interact with the altered promoter elements. TFOs can also disrupt gene transcription by blocking transcriptional elongation.

The first use of a TFO to inhibit oncogene expression was directed at a 27-base–long purinerich sequence in the P1 region of the c-*myc* promoter.[60] The H-*ras*, *Her2/neu*, *IGF1-R*, *TNF*, and *GM-CSF* genes also have purine-rich sequences that serve as targets for TFOs.[61-66] Importantly, TFO-induced decreases in mRNAs of certain target genes are associated with suppression of growth factor-dependent cell growth (ie, *IGF1-R*, *TNF*, *GM-CSF*). Thus, although TFOs target specific gene sequences and, as such, require fewer molecules than when targeting RNA or protein, a requirement for purine-rich regulatory sequences limits this approach. Also, binding affinity needs to be improved to increase the stability of decreasing oncogene expression. In this context, free amino groups have been added to the 3′ end of the TFO to decrease susceptibility to nuclease digestion. Intercalating agents (ie, acridine) have been conjugated to TFOs to stabilize binding to duplex DNA. In addition, to ensure adequate intracellular levels of the TFO, these sequences have been incorporated into plasmids or vectors for transfection or transduction of the target cell.

Antisense ■ Antisense (AS) oligonucleotides and complementary DNAs (cDNAs) block translation of target mRNAs in a sequence-specific manner by the formation of complementary base pairing between the AS molecule and the mRNA (Fig. 60-2). AS molecules have been generated as single-stranded RNAs or DNAs with lengths as short as 15-20 bases (oligos) or as long as a sequence complementary to the entire mRNA. For AS oligonucleotides, the region of the mRNA to be targeted is crucial and is based on accessibility of that site to the AS molecule. RNA molecules are sensitive to nucleases and have half-lives of 15-30 minutes in serum. Therefore, most AS molecules are the more nuclease-resistant deoxynucleotides. To afford further protection against nuclease digestion, AS deoxyoligonucleotides are synthesized as phosphorothioates in which one of the nonbridging oxygens surrounding the phosphate group of the deoxynucleotide is replaced with a sulfur atom.[67]

AS molecules designed to bind to the entire mRNA are made by inserting the cDNA into the expression plasmid in the opposite or antisense orientation. AS molecules can function by blocking translation initiation factors from binding near the 5′ cap site of the mRNA or by interfering with interaction of the mRNA and ribosomes. In addition, binding of the AS deoxyoligonucleotide to the mRNA creates a hybrid that is sensitive to digestion by RNaseH and thereby degradation of the mRNA.[68]

A 13-base AS deoxyoligonucleotide complementary to Rous sarcoma virus sequences was used more than 20 years ago to inhibit viral translation and replication.[69,70] Since then, the *myb* protooncogene has been targeted by an 18-base AS deoxyoligonucleotide to inhibit the growth of hematopoietic and melanoma cells.[71,72] To target the c-*fos* protooncogene, a retrovirus encoding AS c-*fos* was used to transduce breast carcinoma cells and thereby decrease c-*fos* mRNA levels and inhibit growth.[73] This strategy with the AS c-*fos* retrovirus has been studied in clinical trials.[74]

Inhibition of tumor angiogenesis represents a promising target for AS therapy because the genetically stable endothelial cells rely on growth factors produced by the tumor cell. In this context, vascular endothelial growth factor (VEGF), an angiogenic factor that is produced by tumor cells, has been targeted for AS-mediated downregulation.[75-77] Transduction of tumor cells with a vector encoding an AS complementary to VEGF decreased VEGF mRNA and protein levels, decreased microvessel density, decreased tumor growth, and increased tumor necrosis.

Ribozymes ■ Ribozymes (RNA enzymes) are RNA molecules that catalyze site-specific cleavage of RNA (Fig. 60-3).[78,79] The activity of ribozymes is dependent on divalent cations, usually Mg2+, which contribute to folding and structural stability.[80] Most naturally occurring ribozymes function in a *cis* manner by cleaving intramolecular RNA. However, RNA in RNAseP, which is involved in transfer ribonucleic acid (tRNA) processing, acts intramolecularly by a *trans* mechanism.[81] The catalytic domains of the ribozymes are named after their secondary structure and include hammerhead, hairpin, axehead, and pseudoknot motifs. Hammerhead ribozyme, which is the most extensively studied ribozyme, consists of three helical stems with the core catalytic domain being adjacent to helix II and flanked by two targeting sequences (helix I and III) that bind to the complementary RNA. The hammerhead cleaves RNA at the 3′ end of a NUN triplet (N = any nucleotide) and prefers a G in the first position of the triplet (Fig. 60-3).

The therapeutic potential of ribozymes resides in their ability to cleave mRNA in a sequence-specific manner. For example, to target a certain oncogene, a GUN triplet and flanking sequences are identified in the corresponding mRNA. A hammerhead ribozyme is constructed to target the GUN site by linking the catalytic core and helix II to flanking sequences that are complementary to those in the oncogenic mRNA. Thus, the flanking sequences of the recombinant ribozyme form base pairs with the target RNA and thereby contact the ribozyme catalytic core with the mRNA GUN site.

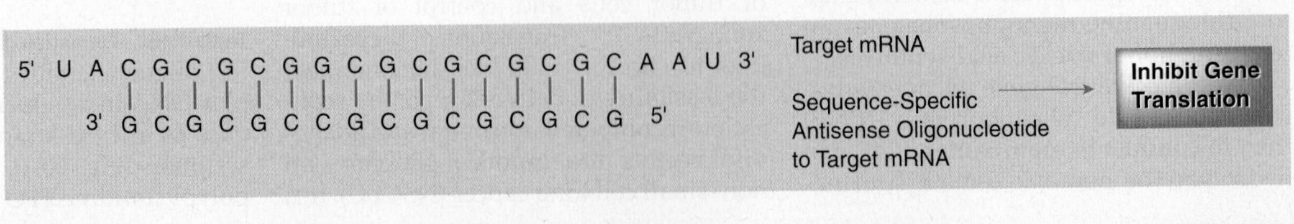

Figure 60-2 Antisense oligonucleotide to block mRNA translation.

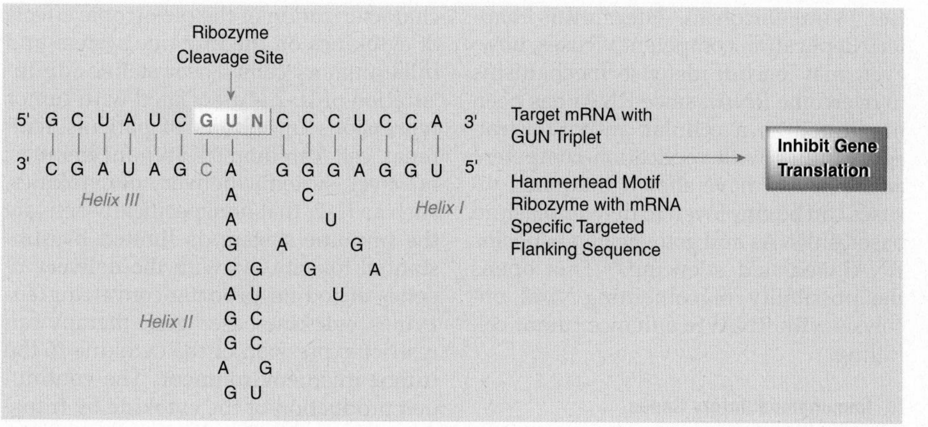

Figure 60-3 Ribozyme-mediated cleavage of mRNA.

Expression of the c-*fos* protooncogene is suppressed by a c-*fos* mRNA-specific ribozyme.[82] Another target for ribozymes is the multidrug resistance gene-1 (*MDR-1*) mRNA,[83] which has a GUC triplet at the –6 to –4 position (upstream to the translation start site). Ribozyme-mediated downregulation of MDR-1 expression increases the chemosensitivity of otherwise resistant tumor cells. These ribozyme-mediated approaches target both malignant and normal cells.

Tumor-specific mRNA targets include *bcr-abl*, H-*ras*, and the aberrantly spliced epidermal growth factor receptor. The *bcr-abl* fusion gene has a GUU triplet at the 3′ end of exon 3 of the *bcr* gene, which is adjacent to the fusion site in the *c-abl* exon 2.[84] As the flanking sequences of the GUU site reside in both the *bcr* and c-*abl* genes, the ribozyme specifically cleaves the *bcr-abl* fusion mRNA. Activating mutations of the H-*ras* gene have been identified in codons 12, 13, and 61. In codon 12, the normal GGU triplet is mutated to GUU, which serves as a cleavage site for the hammerhead ribozyme.[85] In gliomas, the epidermal growth factor receptor (EGFR) mRNA is aberrantly spliced such that the transcript lacks exons II-VI. Adjacent to the fusion site of exon I-exon VII is a GUA site that is cleaved by a hammerhead ribozyme containing flanking sequences that recognize exon I and exon VII.[86] Thus, this ribozyme can be used to specifically target the aberrantly spliced, but not the intact, EGFR transcript.

RNAi ■ RNAi is a posttranscriptional gene silencing mechanism conserved in nature from plants to mammals. The hints of such a process came from studies of transgenic plants in which overexpression of genes resulted in a paradoxical reduction in expression of the transgene. Such a mechanism was eventually elucidated in mammalian cells and has been developed as a powerful new approach to achieve gene-specific suppression. RNAi is a process in which small interfering RNAs (siRNAs) form double-stranded structures with complementary RNA molecules and mediate their degradation.[87] Cells produce siRNAs by degrading double-stranded RNA molecules (dsRNA) into 21-23 nucleotide base pairs with 2-3 nucleotide overhangs on the 3′ end through the action of a ribonuclease termed Dicer (Fig. 60-4). One strand of the siRNA then associates with an RNA-induced silencing complex (RISC). The siRNA serves as a template for complementary mRNA resulting in sequence-specific degradation of mRNA (transcriptional inhibition) by RISC. The target RNA is cleaved 10 nucleotides from the 5′ end of the antisense siRNA sequence. The nuclease activity of RISC is due to eIF2C, a member of the argonaute family of proteins.[88] It has also been reported that the RISC complex can block translation from mRNA. Viruses often produce dsRNA during the course of replication, and RNAi serves as a cellular antiviral mechanism. In principle, RNAi resembles antisense technology, however, RNAi results in more complete gene suppression than can be achieved with antisense approaches.

The ability to exploit RNAi for gene therapy was initially hampered by activation of interferon pathways after delivery of dsRNA molecules. RNA molecules greater than 30 nucleotides in length activate interferon-mediated signaling cascades resulting in global suppression of protein translation. However, transferring chemically synthesized 21-nucleotide base pair siRNAs into mammalian cells induced gene-specific suppression.[89] Delivering siRNAs for cancer gene therapy strategies may be limited by their degradation in blood and extracellular fluids as well as inefficient delivery methods to tumor cells of siRNA molecules. To overcome such obstacles, DNA vector-based approaches of RNAi have been developed.[90] Plasmids are constructed to express the target RNAi sequence as a palindromic sequence separated by a hairpin loop. These short hairpin RNAs (shRNA) are then processed by Dicer into siRNAs (see Fig. 60-4). Additionally, DNA-based RNAi vectors can be incorporated into more efficient viral-based delivery vectors. RNAi has proven to be a powerful technique in the laboratory to identify novel genes involved in the development of cancer, since gene-specific expression can be knocked "down" rap-

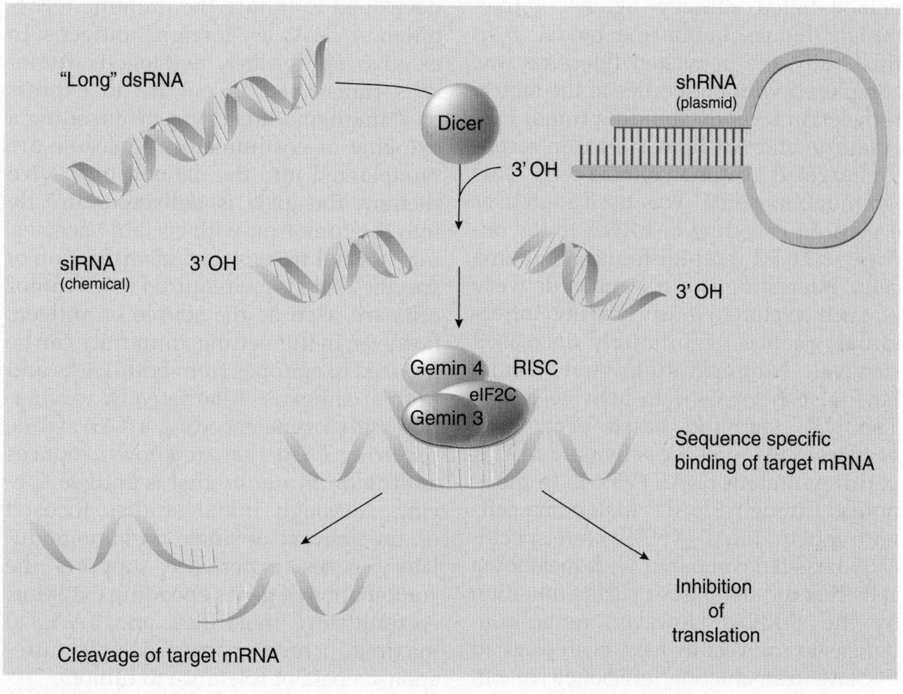

Figure 60-4 RNA interference. dsRNA or a short hairpin RNA (shRNA) is processed by the ribonuclease Dicer into siRNA molecules. siRNAs can also be chemically synthesized and bypass Dicer. siRNA binds to the RNA-induced silencing complex (RISC) to mediated sequence-specific degradation of target mRNA.

idly without the necessity of producing knockout cell lines.

Strategies have also been devised to employ RNAi as an anticancer therapy.[91] As with antisense, TFO and ribozymes, gain of function mutations (ie, oncogenes) need to be identified that can be targeted and blocked by RNAi. The last few years have seen a rapid expansion in the application of RNAi as a therapeutic agent in experimental tumor models. Here we will provide a few recent examples that demonstrate the different potential uses of RNAi in cancer gene therapy. Liposomal delivery of chemically synthesized siRNAs targeting fatty acid synthase was shown to induce apoptosis in prostate cancer cells, whereas no effect was noted on normal fibroblasts.[92] This study also validates fatty acid synthase as a therapeutic target for certain tumors. Transfection of multidrug-resistant (MDR) leukemic cells with plasmids encoding shRNA for the MDR P-glycoprotein resulted in reduced cell surface expression of P-glycoprotein as well as restored sensitivity to certain chemotherapy agents compared with parental therapy-resistant tumor cells.[93] Although these studies show siRNA can be potentially beneficial in cancer therapy, clinical situations require the ability to efficiently deliver and activate RNAi in preexisting tumors.

Plasmids encoding shRNAs have been delivered to tumor by different strategies, including viral and nonviral systems. Pegylated liposomes containing shRNA plasmids have been targeted to specific cell membranes and have demonstrated efficacy against intracranial gliomas in murine models.[94] In this study, the pegylated liposome was complexed with antibodies to the mouse transferrin receptor (binding tumor vasculature) and the human insulin receptor (targeted to human glioma cells). This "immunoliposome" was used to deliver a plasmid encoding a shRNA to the oncogenic EGFR receptor found on glioma cells. Interestingly, intravenous delivery of such vector to mice bearing intracranial gliomas significantly increased survival. Nonreplicating viral vectors have also been used to activate RNAi. The HIV lentiviral based vector has been used to target the activating MAPK pathway mutant BRAF (V599E) in melanomas through RNAi.[95] Melanoma cells with mutant BRAF (V599E) were specifically targeted compared with melanoma cells that did not harbor such a mutation by the shRNA. However, replication-deficient viral vectors have been plagued by low transduction efficiency of tumors. To overcome this barrier, replication-competent viral vectors have been investigated for cancer gene therapy (see "Viral Oncolysis" later in this chapter). Replication competent viruses, however, may encode defense mechanisms to overcome RNAi, since RNAi has been implicated as a cellular antiviral strategy. Studies with replication-competent adenoviruses have shown that such viruses can be employed to deliver plasmid based shRNAs and activate gene-specific RNAi-mediated silencing.[96] This opens the possibility of combining viral oncolysis with RNAi to enhance tumor cell killing.

Immunomodulatory Genes

The premise of cancer immunotherapy is based on the assumption that tumor-associated antigens (TAAs) exist and that the host immune system can recognize expression of these antigens by tumor cells. A significant advantage of immunotherapy is thus the ability to recruit the immune system to attack disseminated tumor cells and thereby eliminate both local and metastatic disease. In recent years, the identification of human TAAs and elucidation of the mechanisms responsible for the induction of antitumor immunity have provided the requisite background for bringing to bear the potential of immunotherapy in the treatment of cancer. Combining immunotherapy and gene therapy has provided an opportunity to induce immunity against specific TAAs and to selectively activate the immune response in the tumor microenvironment. Immunomodulatory genes include those encoding cytokines, costimulatory molecules, and TAAs.

Genetic immunotherapy has been developed to induce the immune recognition of TAAs as "foreign" antigens. In ex vivo approaches, autologous tumor cells transfected in culture to express an immunomodulatory gene encoding a cytokine or costimulatory molecule are reimplanted into the patient. In in vivo therapy, the gene is delivered directly into the tumor or, with certain vaccines, into normal tissues. The identification of specific TAAs is not required when tumor cells are used as the source of antigen; however, in this setting, immunity can be induced to epitopes from both TAAs and normal antigens. Alternatively, vaccination with a gene encoding a TAA, while requiring TAAs that are known, induces antitumor immunity that is antigen specific. Although initial studies focused on the delivery of single immunomodulatory genes, experience supports the combination of genes encoding cytokine, costimulatory molecules, and TAAs to maximally reverse immunologic unresponsiveness or tolerance to tumors.

Cytokine Genes ■ The identification and cloning of cytokine genes has enabled the characterization of the pleiotropic effects of cytokines on the immune system and inflammatory cells. The systemic administration of IL-2 is associated with tumor regressions in subsets of patients with renal cell carcinomas and melanomas; however, systemic delivery of cytokines, such as IL-2, that nonspecifically activate the immune system, is limited by substantial toxicity. As with the delivery of genes encoding prodrug-converting enzymes, cytokine-based gene therapy can restrict expression of the cytokine to the tumor microenvironment. The continuous production of the cytokine by transduced tumor cells also overcomes the disadvantages of circulating peak and trough cytokine levels associated with systemic administration.

Cytokine genes studied in the induction of antitumor immunity include IL-1, IL-2, IL-4, IL-6, IL-12, granulocyte-macrophage colony-stimulating factor (GM-CSF), tumor necrosis factor (TNF), IFN-α, and IFN-γ. The adoptive transfer approach involves transduction of cytokine genes into tumor explants and then lethal irradiation of the tumor cells. For example, prostate cancer tissue is excised, transduced in culture with a retrovirus expressing GM-CSF, irradiated, and then used to vaccinate the patient.[97] Production of GM-CSF recruits dendritic cells to the immunization site for presentation of tumor antigens to CD4+ and CD8+ T cells. Malignant melanomas have also been targeted by this approach using IL-2 as the cytokine.[98]

Direct in vivo delivery of genes into tumors represents an alternative approach. An IFN-γ encoding plasmid directly injected into tumors as naked DNA or in a cationic liposome has resulted in the production of IFN-γ for 7 days.[20] IFN-γ activates T cells, natural killer (NK) cells, and macrophages and induces major histocompatibility complex (MHC) class I and II expression. Gene gun mediated intratumoral delivery has been used for plasmids expressing IFN-γ, IL-6, TNF, and IL-2.[21] In addition, intramuscular injection of plasmid DNA encoding IFN-α is associated with reductions in tumor growth and in the development of metastases by a CD8+ T-cell–dependent mechanism.[99] IFN-α activates the immune system, decreases tumor cell proliferation, decreases angiogenesis, induces a T-helper pathway, and upregulates MHC class I expression. A variation on this approach is to add autologous irradiated tumor cells (as a source of antigen) to fibroblasts transfected to express cytokine encoding plasmids. This strategy is advantageous when tumor explants are difficult to culture and transfect ex vivo and has been employed in murine tumor models and phase I clinical trials.[22,100]

Costimulatory Genes ■ The effective activation of T cells is dependent on at least two signals. The first, mediated by MHC molecules, involves antigen-specific interactions with the T-cell receptor (TCR). The second involves costimulation provided by the interaction of B7 molecules (B7-1, B7-2) with CD28 or CTLA4 on the T cell surface. The antigen-TCR interaction can select antigen-specific cytolytic T cells (CTL); however, costimulation is needed for appropriate signaling and clonal expansion of a CTL population. Although most cells express MHC class I molecules for antigen presentation, costimulatory molecules are predominantly found on professional antigen-presenting cells (APCs), such as dendritic cells, Langerhan cells, B cells, monocytes, and macrophages. The lack of costimulatory molecules on tumor cells results in MHC class I presentation of tumor antigens in the absence of costimulation and thereby T cell anergy. Thus, one mechanism for generating antitumor CTL is through the delivery of costimulatory genes to tumor cells such that antigens are presented in the context for CTL activation.

Recombinant vaccinia virus has been used to transduce weakly immunogenic syngeneic murine tumor cells in vitro with genes encoding B7-1 or B7-2.[101] The finding that tumor growth is inhibited following implantation of the transduced tumor cells into immunocompetent mice indicated that costimulation by B7 molecules is sufficient to induce antitumor CTL activity. By contrast, mice immunosuppressed by irradiation failed to reject the B7-transduced tumor cells. Importantly, mice that rejected the transduced tumor also rejected a subsequent challenge with parental nontransduced tumor cells. Other studies demonstrate that B7 costimulation is needed to induce tumor-specific CTL in naive mice, but is not required for tumor rejection upon rechallenge.[102] These findings suggest that transduction of B7 genes into one tumor site could confer rejection of B7-negative tumors at other sites. Transduction of multiple myeloma cells with a recombinant AAV expressing B7-1 or B7-2 also induces specific antitumor CTL activity as measured by T-cell proliferation, production of IL-2 and IFN-γ, and lysis of target cells.[103]

CD40 ligand (CD40L) is selectively expressed on CD4+ T helper cells and stimulates APCs through binding to the CD40 receptor. As the interaction of CD40L with CD40 stimulates antigen-specific T-cell responses, transduction of tumor cells with the CD40L gene can confer more efficient presentation of TAA and enhanced antitumor immunity. For example, intratumoral delivery of an adenovirus expressing CD40L is associated with CD8+ T-cell–mediated antitumor immunity and inhibition of tumor growth in murine models.[104]

Activation of T cells is dependent on multiple factors. Thus, delivery of a single immunomodulatory gene will probably be insufficient to activate effective antitumor immunity. As certain cytokines are involved in expansion of T-cell clones, gene therapy strategies delivering both a cytokine and costimulatory gene could prove synergistic in inducing antitumor immunity. In this context, adenoviral-mediated transduction of both *IL-2* and *B7-1* genes has resulted in a greater than additive antitumor effect in a breast cancer model.[105]

Tumor-Associated Antigen Genes ■ Gene therapy with recombinant vectors that express a TAA has been developed as vaccines for the induction of active specific immunotherapy. Genes that express TAA can be distinguished as (1) endogenous, nonmutated genes that are often overexpressed in tumors; (2) endogenous genes that are mutated and thereby express an altered protein; and (3) exogenous genes. Examples of nonmutated genes associated with tumors include melanoma/melanocyte differentiation antigens (MART-1/ MelanA, gp100, tyrosinase, TRP-1, and TRP-2), testicular cancer/testes antigens (MAGE, BAGE, GAGE, and NY-ESO-1), carcinoembryonic antigen (CEA), PSA, and DF3/ MUC1.[21,106] TAAs expressed by endogenous mutated genes include p53, cdk4, caspase 8, and β-catenin.[107-109] TAAs from exogenous sources are often derived from viral transformation as exemplified in human papillomavirus-positive cervical cancer.

Gene therapy-based tumor vaccination induces immunity against specific TAAs and is distinguished from the nonspecific immune stimulation associated with transfer of cytokine or costimulatory genes. One method of vaccination involves delivery of the TAA-encoding gene directly into the patient by viral or nonviral systems. Another approach is accomplished through in vitro transfection or transduction of cells, generally APCs, with the TAA gene and reintroduction of these cells to the patient. Direct delivery of the TAA gene at subcutaneous or intradermal sites is used more widely than the ex vivo approach. Expression of the TAA in the epidermis is associated with processing of the TAA by Langerhans cells and thereby with presentation of TAA peptides to T cells.

Vaccination with genes encoding TAAs has been accomplished by transfection and viral transduction. For example, immunization of mice with naked DNA encoding a TAA was achieved by direct intramuscular injection.[110] The immunized mice are protected against challenge with tumor cells expressing the TAA. In clinical trials, recombinant vaccinia virus expressing CEA has been administered intradermally.[111] Peripheral blood lymphocytes from certain vaccinated patients responded to stimulation with CEA in vitro.[111,112] Genes encoding the melanoma/melanocyte differentiation antigens MART-1 and gp100 have been used to vaccinate patients with metastatic melanoma.[113] A long-term complete response was achieved in one patient vaccinated with an adenovirus expressing MART-1. Another phase I trial of a recombinant PSA expressing vaccinia virus vaccine (PROSTVAC) in men with advanced prostate cancer has demonstrated induction of anti-PSA immunity and stabilization of the disease course in certain patients.[114]

Multiple genes encoding TAAs can be constructed in a single plasmid or the genes can be coadministered in separate plasmids. In this context, a potential disadvantage of immunization against a single TAA is that expression of the antigen can be downregulated in tumors. Thus, immunization against multiple TAAs could decrease the potential for the development of immunologic resistance by the tumor cell. In this strategy, multiple TAAs for a tumor must be known; however, at present, there are few well characterized TAAs for most tumors. Another approach has been to co-deliver the B7-1 gene with the TAA gene to maximize the antitumor immune response. Recombinant vaccinia viruses encoding B7-1 or CEA have been coadministered to further stimulate the anti-CEA response.[115] Similar findings have been obtained following vaccination with mixtures of vaccinia viruses expressing B7-1 and MUC1.[116] More recently, recombinant poxvirus vectors have been created that encode for three costimulatory molecules B7-1, ICAM-1, and LFA-3 in addition to the transgene for a TAAs (CEA, PSA, or MUC-1). This strategy has been called TRICOM.[117] Selective Gene Expression

A major limitation of conventional cancer chemotherapy and radiotherapy is the toxicity of these agents to normal tissue. The nonselectivity of the available gene delivery systems also renders cancer gene therapy strategies potentially toxic to normal cell populations. Selectivity of gene therapy for tumors has been achieved to date largely by direct intratumoral administration of recombinant vectors. The ongoing cancer gene therapy clinical trials are, for the most part, limited to treatment of localized disease. As such, strategies are under development to increase selectivity of the available vectors by restricting transduction to tumor cells and by employing promoters that are activated in transformed, but not normal cell populations.

Tumor-Selective Retroviruses

Retroviruses are classified as either amphotropic or ecotropic on the basis of their species specificity. Amphotropic retroviruses infect most mammalian cells, whereas ecotropic viruses are restricted to murine cells because of specific interaction of a viral glycoprotein and a murine cell surface cationic amino acid transporter. Ecotropic retroviruses have been genetically altered to express a modified glycoprotein and thereby target retroviral gene delivery (Fig. 60-5).[118] In one approach to target human breast carcinoma cells with an envelope-modified ecotropic MoMuLV, heregulin, a ligand for the human epidermal growth factor receptor (HER) family, was inserted into the viral glycoprotein.[119] As HER-2 is overexpressed in 20-30% of human breast cancers,[120] virus expressing the heregulin chimeric glycoprotein is being developed to selectively target those cells.

Tumor-Selective Adenoviruses

Adenoviruses express trimeric fibers that extend from the vertices of the capsid. The fibers terminate into globular knob domains that interact with the cellular coxsackie-adenovirus receptor (CAR).[121] CAR is an integral membrane protein that is widely expressed on diverse cell types. After the fiber knob binds to CAR, internalization of the virus is mediated by arginine-glycine-aspartic acid (RGD) domains in the penton base of the virus that interact with integrins on the cell surface.

In the "adenobody" approach, an adenoviral neutralizing antibody is fused to a ligand of a specific cell receptor. The antibody–ligand fusion protein binds to the adenoviral fiber and blocks interaction with CAR. The ligand fused to the antibody then redirects the virus to cells expressing that ligand binding receptor (Fig. 60-6). For example, epidermal growth factor (EGF) has been linked to an adenoviral antibody to target viral infection of

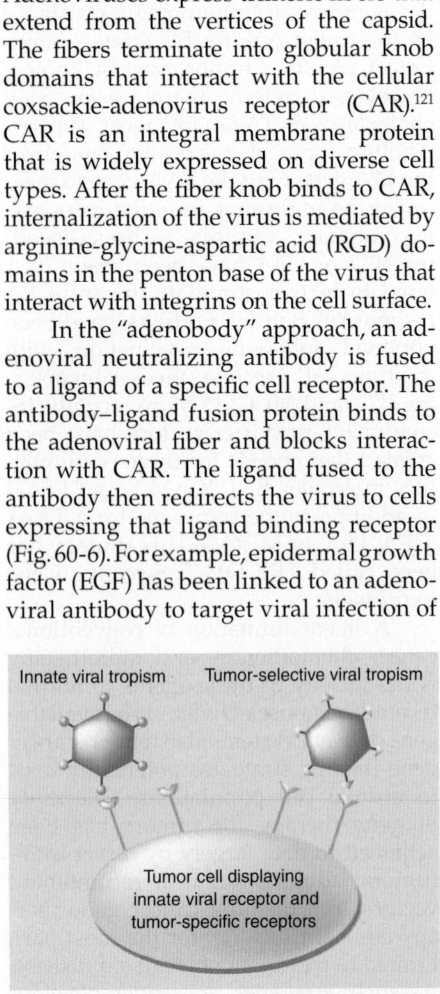

Figure 60-5 Genetic modification of viral receptor proteins to target tumor-specific receptors.

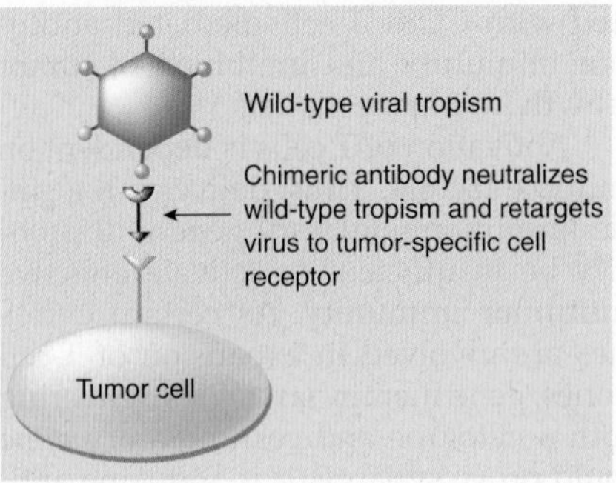

Figure 60-6 Chimeric antibodies to alter viral tropism for tumor cells.

cells that express the EGF receptor.[122] In addition, a bispecific antibody has been used that binds to both the adenovirus and the precarcinoma epithelial cell adhesion molecule (EpCAM).[123] EpCAM is expressed on breast, ovarian, lung, and colon carcinomas. As the adenobody approach is dependent on in vitro incubation of the fusion antibody and virus before tumor inoculation, a more appealing strategy is to genetically alter the adenoviral fibers to directly recognize receptors overexpressed on tumor cells. To this end, adenoviral chimeric fibers have been generated that alter adenoviral tropism,[124] and peptide epitopes have been inserted into the H1 loop of the adenoviral fiber domain.[125]

Certain tumors express low levels of CAR and are thereby resistant to adenoviral gene transfer.[126] To bypass CAR-dependent attachment, adenoviral vectors have been constructed that incorporate an RGD peptide within the H1 loop of the adenoviral fiber knob domain.[127] Certain tumors overexpress classes of RGD-binding integrins. For example, the α2β1 and α3β1 integrins are commonly overexpressed by squamous cell carcinomas of the head and neck. The RGD-containing adenoviral vectors have been reported to selectively target both head and neck cancer and ovarian cancer cells.[128,129]

Tumor-Selective Promoters/Enhancers

Viral vectors have been generated that infect a broad spectrum of cell types but only express the transgene in selected cells. Such selectivity of gene expression has been achieved by constructing these vectors with promoters/enhancers that confer tumor- or tissue-selective transcription (Fig. 60-7). Tissue-restricted

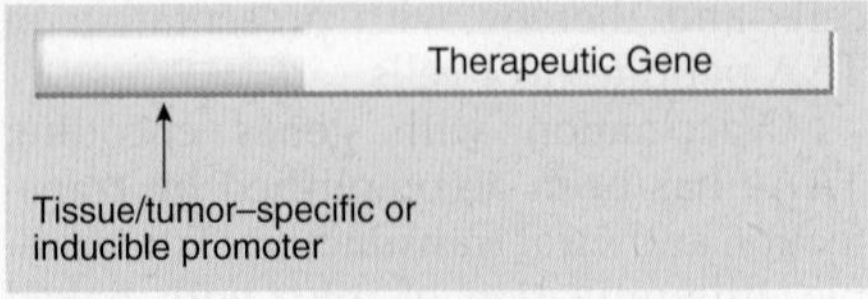

Figure 60-7 Transcriptional regulation of the delivered therapeutic gene through selective promoters and enhancers.

transcriptional control elements include the α1-antitrypsin and albumin promoters (hepatocyte-selective), tyrosine hydrolase promoter (melanocytes), villin promoter (intestinal epithelium), glial fibrillary acidic protein promoter (astrocytes), myelin basic protein (glial cells), and the immunoglobulin gene enhancer (B lymphocytes). If a tissue, such as the prostate, is nonessential, then tissue-selective promoters that target both tumor and normal cells can be used for cancer gene therapy. Alternatively, if only the tumor can be targeted and the surrounding normal tissue of an essential organ must be spared, then the approach necessitates use of tumor-selective promoters. Tumor-selective promoter elements have been identified in the following genes: α-fetoprotein (hepatoma), DF3/ MUC1 (breast and other carcinomas), thyroglobulin (thyroid carcinoma), prostate-specific antigen (prostate carcinoma), and carcinoembryonic antigen (breast, lung, and colorectal carcinomas). In this context, the DF3/MUC1 promoter has been incorporated into retroviral and adenoviral vectors to selectively drive the expression of transgenes in human carcinomas that overexpress the MUC1 gene.[130-133] The identification of new genes that are transcriptionally activated in tumor, as compared with normal, cells should be rapidly advanced by the recent developments in DNA microarray technologies and thereby the definition of new classes of tissue- and tumor-selective promoters for cancer gene therapy.

Inducible Promoters

Another strategy for regulating transgene expression is through the use of inducible promoters (Fig. 60-7). In the tetracycline repressor system, the bacterial tet operon mediates transcriptional repression of a heterologous promoter in the presence of the tet repressor (tetR) protein. The tetR gene is expressed by another vector or by another coding sequence in the same vector. Transcriptional repression is relieved by exposure to tetracycline, which binds to tetR and thereby prevents its interaction with the tet operon. Release from transcriptional repression in mammals is achieved at doses of tetracycline significantly lower than those used for antimicrobial purposes. This approach, although potentially amenable to regulating the level of transgene expression, activates transcription in both transduced tumor and normal cells and, thus, has no impact on selectivity. Another targeted gene therapy strategy has been developed with cancer therapy inducible promoters. One of the cellular responses to cancer therapeutic agents is transcriptional upregulation of genes.[134] Such genes products dictate the cellular response to the perceived insult. Upon delivery of ionizing radiation (IR) to cells, the early growth response-1 (Egr-1) gene is induced.[135] One implication of this result is that the promoter of Egr-1 can act as a "molecular switch" to activate a ligated transgene following IR (Fig. 60-8). TNFα is known to be tumoricidal, however, systemic toxicity of TNFα is a limiting factor. By placing the cDNA for TNFα upstream of the Egr-1 promoter, expression of TNFα can be placed under the control of IR.[136] This treatment paradigm has been incorporated with a replication defective adenovirus (designated TNFerade).[137] TNFα gene expression is restricted by 2 mechanisms. First, the replication-defective virus is delivered directly to the tumor bed via intratumoral inoculation and taken up by the surrounding tumor cells. Second, TNFα expression is activated in the targeted irradiated field (Fig. 60-9). An advantage of the radiation-inducible promoters is that transgene expression can be regulated in both a spatial and temporal manner. Both the location expression and the timing of transgene expression are restricted to the targeted irradiated field. Any plasmids delivered to cells located outside of the irradiated field, in principle, have low, if any, expression of the transgene. The replication-defective adenovirus containing the EGR-TNFα construct has entered phase III clinical trials in combination with radiation and chemotherapy for the treatment of locally advanced pancreatic cancer and head and neck cancer.[138,139]

While IR-mediated gene therapy is designed for improving local tumor control, the paradigm has been expanded to incorporate chemotherapy for systemic cancer therapy. IR activates the Egr-1 promoter through the production of free radical oxygen species ,and any agent capable of producing intracellular free radical oxygen species may activate the Egr-1 promoter (Fig. 60-10).[135] Recent studies demonstrated activation of the EGR-TNF construct by cisplatin and other genotoxic chemotherapeutic agents.[140,141] Another gene product activated by chemotherapeutic agents is mdr1.[142] In a similar vein to TNFerade, the chemotherapeutic response elements within the mdr promoter were ligated to TNFα.[143] In the above examples, not only is TNFα transcription regulated by IR/chemotherapy, but also the newly produced TNFα interacts synergistically with the inducing cancer agents for enhanced tumor cell kill (see Fig. 60-10). Importantly, the above combinations have been shown to target not only tumor cells, but in addition the surrounding tumor vasculature.[144] The advantages of this are at least twofold. First, the relative genetic stability of endothelial cells suggests that resistance to this therapeutic approach will not develop. Second, diverse histologic tumors may be amenable to such therapy by targeting the common vasculature instead of varied tumor types.

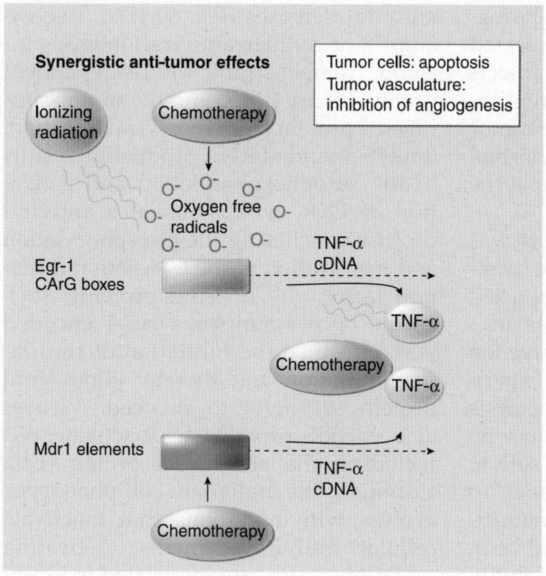

Figure 60-9 Spatial and temporal control of gene therapy by ionizing radiation (IR) is physically targeted to the tumor target volume. Intratumoral delivery of genetic constructs further restricts the spatial effects of combined therapy. In addition, temporal control of gene therapy is achieved by controlling the activity of gene therapy upon timing delivery of IR.

Viral Oncolysis

The use of a replicating virus as an antitumor agent is based on the premise that as a consequence of successful viral replication, multiple viral progeny are released from the destroyed cell to infect surrounding cells (viral oncolysis). Replication-competent viruses overcome one of the major limitations of replication-deficient viruses, distribution within the tumor. In principle, an initial infection of only a few tumor cells would initiate a chain reaction, such that surrounding tu-

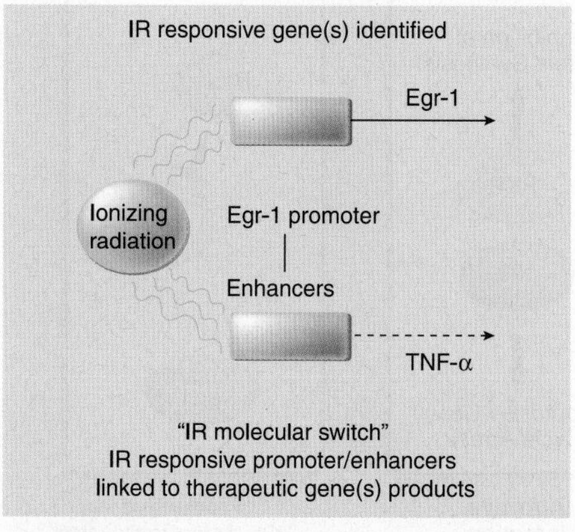

Figure 60-8 Creating ionizing radiation-activated therapeutic genes. Ionizing radiation (IR)-induced gene promoters are identified and then ligated to cDNA sequences whose gene products have antitumor activity.

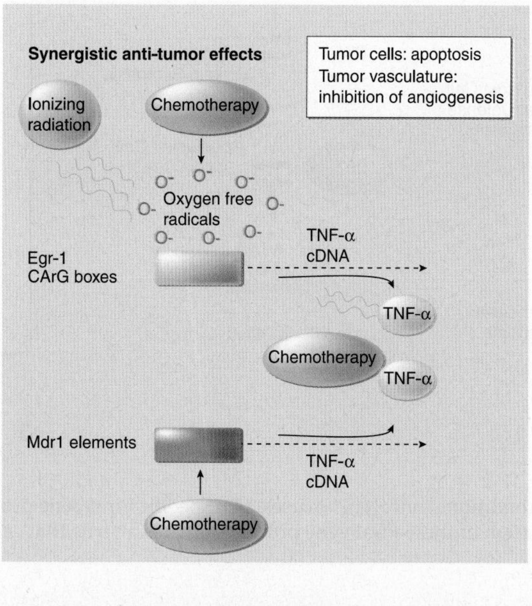

Figure 60-10 Local/systemic therapy to activate and synergize gene therapy. IR and chemotherapy activate gene expression through responsive promoter elements. Moreover, the transcribed therapeutic gene products interact synergistically with chemotherapy/IR to enhance tumor kill by targeting both tumor cells and the tumor vasculature.

mor cells become infected by viral progeny released from the initially infected cells. Once the virus reaches and infects the surrounding normal tissue, replication of a virus that is selective for tumor cells would be aborted, sparing normal tissue from the pathogenic effects of the wild-type parental virus.

The concept of viral oncolysis was introduced at the beginning of the twentieth century. In 1904, Dock reported a dramatic remission of leukemia in a woman following a presumed infection by influenza virus.[145] The first experimental demonstration of viral oncolysis is attributed to Levaditi and Nicolau, who showed that vaccinia virus was able to inhibit tumors in both mice and rats.[146] In the 1950s and 1960s, trials were conducted with multiple viruses that had been selected in tissue culture for their ability to replicate in tumor cells. However, no such clinically active viruses were identified and enthusiasm waned.

More recently, the replicative life cycle of many viruses has been elucidated at the molecular level, including the sequence of viral genomes and the functions of viral proteins. In a similar vein, mutations occurring in the transformation from wild-type to cancer cell have also begun to be unraveled. With such knowledge, the concept of viral oncolysis has reemerged with a more "rational" approach. A common theme emerging from studying the interaction of viruses with cells is the presence of viral proteins whose function is to overcome host-cell antiviral defenses (Fig. 60-11A). Two examples of cellular antiviral defenses include double-strand RNA-dependent protein kinase (PKR) and the tumor-suppressor protein p53. Upon viral infection, double-stranded RNA production results in the autophosphorylation and activation of PKR, which mediates antiviral defenses, including the phosphorylation and inactivation of the translation initiation factor, eIF-2α. Viral proteins, such as the herpes simplex virus-1 encoded γ134.5, reverse the inhibition of translation initiation and thereby allow viral protein synthesis to proceed. Viruses also encode proteins to inactivate p53 including the adenoviral protein E1B. Curiously, the malignant cell phenotype evolves with mutations that inactivate cellular antiviral proteins. Activating mutations in Ras are implicated in inhibiting PKR. Inactivation of p53 in tumor cells occurs by mutations in p53 itself or in the proteins regulating p53. In principle, attenuated replication-competent viruses could be constructed to target tumor cells that harbor such mutations by deleting the viral protein that corresponds to the mutated cellular protein (Fig. 60-11B). Such a mutant virus could replicate in tumor cells with disarmed cellular defenses and produce attenuated viral progeny to infect surrounding tumor cells. However, the mutant virus would be unable to grow in wild-type cells because it lacks the viral protein necessary to counteract a particular cellular antiviral defense. In general, this is the current paradigm for constructing replication competent tumor-selective viruses.

With the use of live, attenuated viruses for cancer therapy, certain safety considerations are warranted. The attenuated virus should be genetically stable such that mutants do not revert to wild-type phenotypes. Engineering multiple mutations into the therapeutic virus can minimize reversion of attenuated viruses to wild-type viruses. Employing nonintegrating viruses prevents untoward consequences of genetic mutations in the host cell. The pathology induced by the virus should be well characterized and minimal. Finally, effective antiviral drugs should be available in the event of toxicity from the viral therapy. The following are examples of oncolytic viruses currently being pursued in the laboratory and the clinic (Table 60-2).

Oncolytic Adenovirus

The basic biology of adenoviruses was briefly introduced above. Important in the development of replication-competent adenoviruses are two early adenoviral gene products, E1A and E1B. While both viral proteins are multifunctional, two well-characterized functions have played a pivotal role in the development of oncolytic adenoviruses. E1A binds to Rb pocket proteins and releases E2F proteins to induce Sphase gene synthesis, facilitating viral replication.[147] In response to adenoviral infection and the effects of E1A, p53 is activated and induces cell

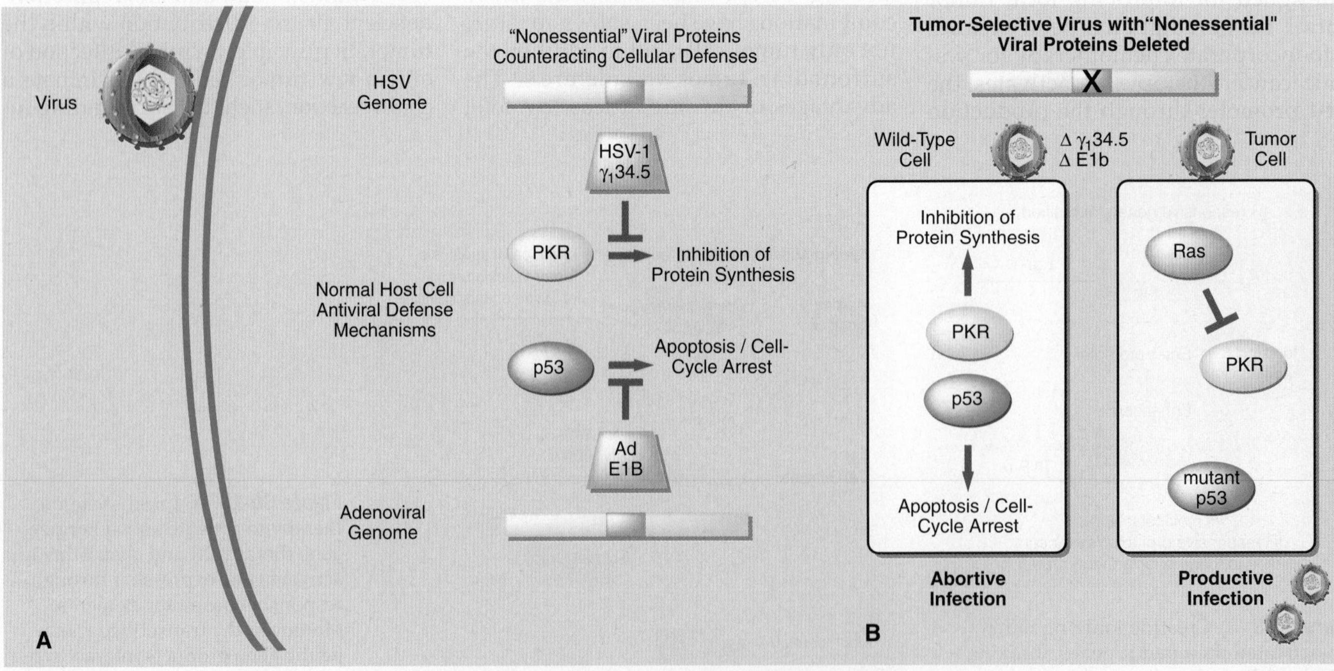

Figure 60-11 Creating replication-conditional oncolytic viruses. (**A**), Specific viral gene products are involved in counteracting host cell antiviral defense mechanisms. (**B**), Deletion of these viral gene products creates a virus that can only replicate in tumor cells with specific mutations.

cycle arrest or apoptosis, presumably as mechanisms to prevent viral replication. E1B is involved in transcriptionally silencing and degrading p53 and thereby blocks p53 antiviral effects. Because p53 is mutated or deleted in approximately 50% of human tumors, p53-mediated antiviral defense mechanisms are not available to those cells. To exploit this tumor cell phenotype, an adenovirus (*dl*1520; ONYX-015) with a deletion in the 55-kilodalton (kDa), E1B gene was created.[148] *dl*1520 was predicted to replicate preferentially in cells with nonfunctional p53, but not in cells expressing functional p53. As such, the virus would continuously replicate in and lyse tumor cells harboring nonfunctional p53. When the virus encounters normal tissue, replication is abrogated by p53-dependent defense mechanisms. Conflicting results, however, have been reported in the relationship between replication of the E1B-deleted virus and tumor cell p53 status.[149-151] A partial resolution to these apparently conflicting results lies in understanding the regulation of p53 stability and function by the p53-Mdm2 autoregulatory loop (Fig. 60-12).

In cells with wild-type p53 gene, p53 protein has a relatively short half-life in unstressed cells and is also functionally silent. A major regulator of p53 function and stability is the protooncogene Mdm2.[152] Mdm2 inhibits p53 function by blocking p53 transcriptional activity, exporting p53 to the cytoplasm, and acting as an E3 ubiquitin ligase to promote proteasome-dependent p53 degradation. Mdm2 could be thought of as a functional homolog of the 55-kDa E1B in terms of inactivating p53 (see Fig. 60-12). Also included in the regulatory pathway of p53 is p14ARF, a member of the INK4 tumor-suppressor proteins. p14ARF promotes the stability of p53 by binding to and blocking the E3 ubiquitin ligase activity of Mdm2. Mdm2 is amplified in 7% of human tumors and can further suppress the activity of p53. Deletion or inactivating mutations of p14ARF in tumor cells results in the unopposed action of Mdm2, again resulting in functionally inactive p53. Therefore, *dl*1520 may be able to preferentially replicate in tumor cells with inactivating mutations in p53 or p14ARF, as well as in cells with activating mutations in Mdm2. Mutations in any three of these proteins could result in the same phenotype, ie, nonfunctional p53. In support of this hypothesis, *dl*1520 was shown to replicate preferentially in colon carcinoma and mesothelioma cell lines that have loss of p14ARF.[153]

In creating *dl*1520, 827 base pairs were deleted from the E1B gene region. Because of their limited coding capacity, viruses have maximized the utility of their genome, with viral proteins encoding multiple functions. Deletion of the 55-kDa E1B, while done to target the p53 path-way, may also have unexpected consequences because of the knockout of functions that may be beneficial to viral replication and thereby reduce efficacy as an oncolytic agent. For example, the 55-kDa E1B also modulates the transport of mRNA during viral infection.[154] Point mutations within viral proteins may result in the ability to target specific functions, while sparing other functions of the viral protein. Such viruses may ultimately prove to be better oncolytic viruses. Specific mutations in the E1A protein have been introduced to test this principle.

The adenoviral E1A protein encodes at least two functions, S-phase induction and transactivation of adenoviral early genes. E1A induces S phase by binding to the retinoblastoma family of pocket proteins (Rb) and releasing the inhibition on E2F transcription factors. Mapping studies revealed amino acids 121 to 127 of the E1A protein are required to bind Rb.[155] E1A binding and inactivation of Rb permits adenovirus replication in either quiescent or cycling cells by inducing S-phase gene synthesis. Deletion of the E1A amino acids responsible for Rb binding blocks E2F transactivation and inhibits adenoviral replication in quiescent cells. Such a mutant virus preferentially replicates in cycling cells and it may replicate more efficiently in tumor cells, which routinely contain inactivating mutations of G1/S checkpoint proteins. Two groups created such an E1A

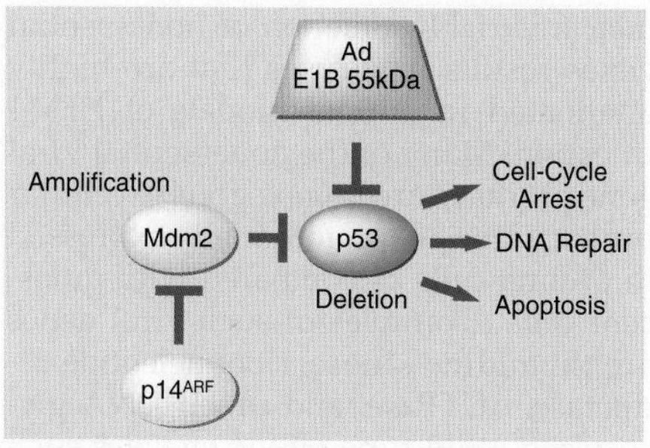

Figure 60-12 p53 and adenovirus E1B. The 55-kDa E1B adenoviral protein counteracts the antiviral effects of p53. In principle, an adenoviral mutant with E1B 55 kDa deleted can replicate in a tumor cell with (1) p53 deleted/nonfunctional, (2) Mdm2 amplified, or (3) p14ARF deleted/nonfunctional.

mutant virus with < 30 bp deleted from the E1A region, delta24 and *dl*922-947.[156,157] The *dl*922-947 virus appears to be a better oncolytic virus when compared directly with *dl*1520 (55-kDa E1B deleted). This result is explicable, given the nature of the deletions created in each virus. Whereas *dl*1520 is deleted of almost 900 bp in the 55-kDa E1B region (with loss of functions unrelated to p53 inactivation), *dl*922-947 is deleted in only a small portion of E1A (the Rb binding region). Importantly, *dl*922-947 mutant viruses encode the remainder of the E1A protein such that the virus can use the protein for its other known (ie, p300 binding and adenoviral early gene transactivation) and unknown functions.

Oncolytic HSV-1

HSV-1 is a relatively large double-stranded DNA virus that encodes at least 90 proteins, and these gene products are classified as either essential or nonessential. Essential proteins are required for viral replication to occur in tissue culture, and hence deletion of essential viral genes generates replication-deficient herpes viruses. Deletion of nonessential genes from HSV-1 genome creates viruses still capable of replicating in tissue culture, although usually with less efficiency than wild-type virus. The designation of nonessential for these gene products is something of a misno-

Table 60-2 **Representative Replication-Competent Tumor-Selective Viruses**

Parental Virus	Selective Virus	Viral Gene(s) Deleted/Mutated	Cellular Protein Target	Tumor Cell Selectivity
Adenovirus	*dl*1520 (Onyx-015)	E1B	Inactivates p53	Nonfunctional p53
	eg, *dl*922-947	E1A	Inactivates pRb	Disrupted G1S checkpoint
Herpes simplex virus-1	hrR3	UL39 (ribonucleotide reductase)	Creates deoxynucleotides	Cycling cells
	G207	γ134.5	Dephosphorylates eIF-2	? Activating Ras mutation
		UL39		
	R7020 (NV1020)	UL24	?	Attenuated neurovirulence
		UL56	?	Attenuated virulence
		Internal invert region (one copy of 134.5 0 and 4)	Dephosphorylates eIF-2	
Reovirus	Wild type	None		Activating Ras mutation

mer. Invariably, deletion of nonessential genes results in viruses that are highly attenuated in animal models of HSV-1 infection. Many of the nonessential viral gene products are homologous to cellular proteins that are preferentially expressed in cycling cells as compared with quiescent cells. Examples of such viral genes are thymidine kinase, ribonucleotide reductase, dUTPase, and uracil DNA glycosylase. Wild-type HSV-1 encodes such homologs because in the natural course of HSV-1 infection, the virus infects quiescent, postmitotic sensory neurons and requires a pool of nucleotides to replicate viral DNA. Elucidating the function of essential and nonessential genes of HSV-1 along with the virus' ability to infect both quiescent and cycling cells has resulted in the development of replication competent, tumor-selective attenuated HSV-1.

The first example of the creation of a genetically engineered, replication-competent HSV-1 exploited the differences of the intracellular environment of quiescent and cycling cells (ie, tumor cells) as an oncolytic agent for glioblastoma multiforme (GBM). Because GBM grow in an environment surrounded by quiescent terminally differentiated neurons, an attenuated replication competent HSV-1 was designed to infect replicating glioma cells, but not terminally differentiated noncycling cells (surrounding neural tissue). Deleting the HSV gene encoding thymidine kinase (tk, UL23) resulted in the viral mutant dlsptk.[158] To replicate efficiently, dlsptk requires a cellular pool of nucleotides created by cellular thymidine kinase. Cellular thymidine kinase functions in *trans* to complement the deletion within the virus. dlsptk replicates preferentially in actively cycling cells expressing thymidine kinase but not in terminally differentiated cells that do not have excess pools of nucleotides for DNA replication. A considerable disadvantage of dlsptk is that, by deleting HSV-1-tk, sensitivity to the common antiviral agents acyclovir and ganciclovir is lost in the event that it becomes necessary to treat patients with unacceptable viral toxicities. To retain sensitivity to acyclovir, viruses were developed by deleting other viral genes involved in DNA replication. Inactivating the viral gene UL39, encoding the large subunit of ribonucleotide reductase, resulted in the tumor-selective HSV-1 hrR3.[159] Similarly, deleting the HSV-1 gene UL2, encoding uracil DNA glycosylase, also created a virus (3616UB) that selectively replicates in cycling cells, which can complement for the function of the deleted viral protein.[160]

A major concern in the use of replication-competent HSV-1 in gene therapy is its neurovirulence with ensuing encephalitis. One HSV-1 gene involved in neurovirulence is γ134.5. Deleting both copies of the γ134.5 gene (virus R3616), present in the repeat regions, reduced HSV-1 neurovirulence by greater than five orders of magnitude in murine models.[161] The γ134.5 gene product (ICP 34.5) is involved in counteracting cellular antiviral machinery. A common innate host cell viral defense mechanism is activation of double-stranded RNA-dependent protein kinase, which phosphorylates the alpha subunit of translation initiation factor 2 (eIF-2α) and blocks translation of viral mRNA (see Fig. 60-13). ICP 34.5 effectively reverses the effects of PKR on eIF-2α by binding to cellular protein phosphatase-1 (PP1), dephosphorylating eIF-2α, and preventing protein synthesis shutoff.[162,163] R3616 is both safe and effective in the treatment of experimental gliomas in murine models.[164,165] How is R3616 capable of replicating in tumor cells when protein synthesis is shutoff by PKR in infected cells? Part of the answer may involve the Ras signaling pathway in tumor cells compared with normal cells.[166] Tumor cells routinely contain activating mutations in the Ras signaling pathway.[167] Thus, activated Ras in tumor cells may complement the deletion of γ134.5 in HSV-1 to allow tumor-selective viral replication (see Fig. 60-13).

G207 was generated by deleting the ribonucleotide reductase and γ134.5 genes of HSV-1.[168] With deletions in two genes, this virus has a lower probability of reversion to a wild-type phenotype, thereby increasing its safety profile. Also, there are two mechanisms of targeting tumor cells. The deletion of ribonucleotide reductase targets the virus to cycling cells, and deletion of the γ134.5 gene may target cells with an activated Ras pathway.

The attenuated herpes virus R7020 was designed as a potential vaccine for HSV-1 and HSV-2.[169] R7020 was constructed by deleting the internal inverted repeat sequence of HSV-1 and replacing this region with glycoproteins from HSV-2. Because R7020 was designed as a vaccine for healthy individuals, it underwent stringent safety studies followed by limited clinical trials. However, R7020 did not prove efficacious as a vaccine. Nonetheless, with the extensive safety profile, R7020 was studied as a potential antitumor agent. Studies demonstrate that R7020 (also known as NV1020) replicates efficiently in a variety of tumor xenografts, and there is no evidence for tumor resistance to repeated inoculation.[170,171]

Oncolytic Reovirus

Reovirus (respiratory enteric orphan virus) is a double-stranded RNA virus that is associated with mild upper respiratory infections or enteritis. No specific disease is associated with reovirus infection, and hence the designation of "orphan." Reovirus infection of permissive cells results in activation of transcription factors (NF1cB), MAP kinase pathways, and cell-cycle arrest, as well as apoptosis.[172] Being a double-stranded RNA virus, replication of the viral genome activates double-stranded RNA-activated protein kinase (PKR). As mentioned above, activated PKR phosphorylates the translation initiation factor, eIF-2α, resulting in the cessation of protein synthesis (Fig. 60-13). For reovirus replication to occur, the actions of PKR need to be inhibited. Important to the application of reovirus as an oncolytic agent was the observation that certain permissive cell lines (in which protein synthesis was not shut off) had activating mutations in the Ras signaling pathway. Cell lines resistant to reovirus infection in culture could be made sensitive to infection by transfecting genes encoding proteins that activate the Ras pathway, ie, EGFR, v-erbB oncogene, or SOS.[173-175] These data suggest the Ras pathway counteracted PKR and enabled reovirus replication. How Ras activation allows reovirus replication to proceed remains unclear; however, evidence suggests that Ras activation induces an inhibitor of PKR.[177]

The translation of these observations in employing reovirus as an oncolytic virus is coupled with the fact that 30% of human tumors have Ras-activating mutations.[181] Such mutations include

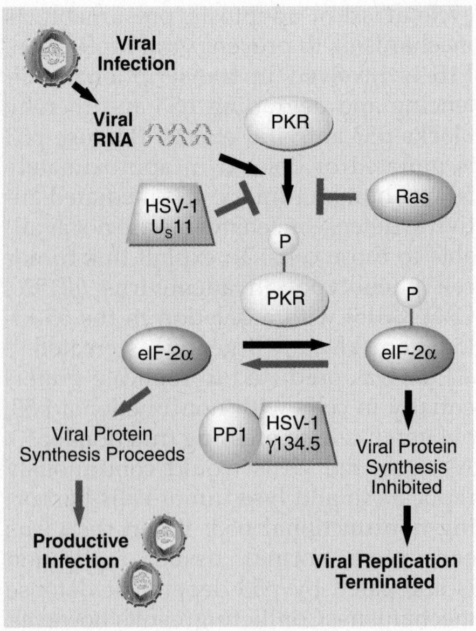

Figure 60-13 PKR and HSV-1. Activation of PKR by double-stranded RNA results in cessation of viral protein synthesis (gray arrows). The HSV-1 viral genes US11 or γ134.5 inhibit the action of PKR (black arrows). Activating mutations in Ras can also inhibit activation of the PKR pathway upon viral infection and thereby allow tumorselective HSV-1 to replicate.

activating mutations within Ras itself, or activating mutations in receptor tyrosine kinases (EGFR or platelet-derived growth factor receptor [PDGFR]). Tumors harboring such mutations would be predicted to permit reovirus replication. Initial results in tumor models appear to support such a hypothesis. Tumors with activated Ras (ie, gliomas, colorectal, and ovarian cancers) are sensitive to reovirus infection.[176-178] The interest in reovirus oncolytic therapy rests in its natural safety profile, with a lack of associated disease pathology upon wild-type reovirus infection.

Transcriptionally Targeted Oncolytic Viruses ■ Another technique to achieve tumor specific cytotoxicity with replication-competent viruses is to place viral essential genes under the transcriptional control of tumor specific promoter/enhancer sequences. Essential viral genes are absolutely required to be expressed for viral replication to proceed. Normally these genes are placed under the control of ubiquitous cellular transcription factors and/or viral transactivators (Fig. 60-14A). However, therapeutic gene constructs have been placed under the transcriptional control of tumor/tissue-specific or -inducible promoter sequences. Such a strategy restricts expression of the therapeutic gene to cell types that express requisite transcription factors for the promoter. In an analogous strategy, the replicating virus can be thought of as one large therapeutic gene construct. Placing the expression of a viral essential gene under the control of tumor/tissue-specific promoter/enhancer elements restricts viral replication to the targeted tumor/tissue type (Fig. 60-14B). Viral infection of cells not expressing the necessary transcription factor(s) results in nonexpression of the essential gene and an abortive infection without progeny virus. Transcriptionally targeted replicating viruses have been created using either adenovirus or HSV-1.

The E1 region (E1A and E1B) of adenovirus encodes proteins required for viral gene expression. By controlling expression of the E1 region with a tumor-selective promoter, viral replication can be restricted to tumor cells. For example, to target hepatocellular carcinoma cells, the promoter/enhancer of the α-fetoprotein gene has been placed upstream to the E1 sequences.[179] This virus replicates selectively in hepatocellular carcinoma cells that overexpress α-fetoprotein, but not in α-fetoprotein–negative tumor cells. Similarly, an adenovirus was generated to specifically target prostate cancer cells. The engineered adenovirus, CN706, was constructed by placing the promoter/enhancer region of the PSA gene upstream of the E1A gene.[180] This virus replicates to

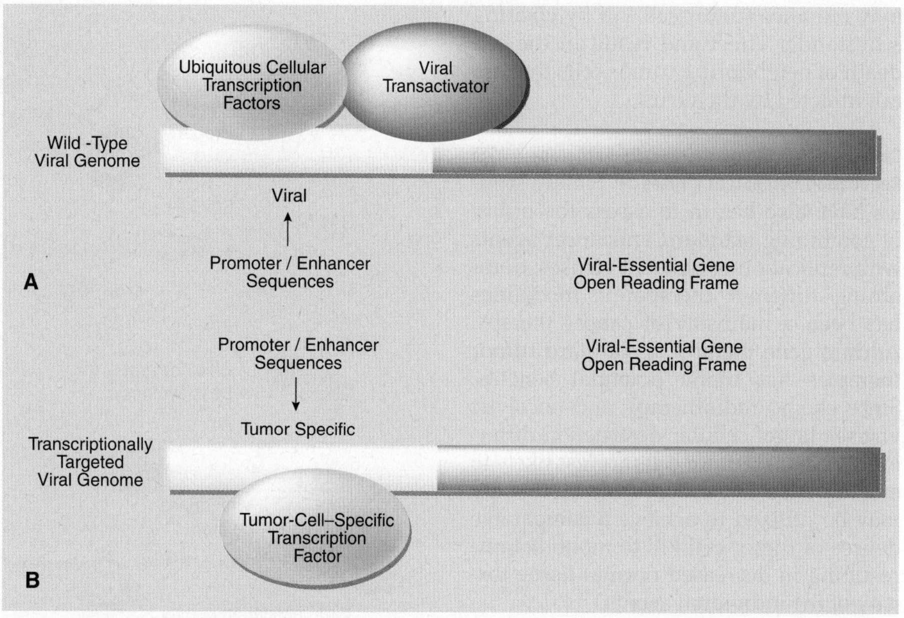

Figure 60-14 ■ Transcription-targeted oncolytic viruses. (**A**) In wild-type viral genomes, viral-essential genes are under the control of ubiquitous cellular transcription factors that allow replication to proceed in multiple cell histologies. (**B**) In transcription-targeted tumor viruses, viral-essential genes are placed under the control of tumor-specific transcription factors that allow replication to occur only in specific tumor histologies.

high titers in prostate cancer cells overexpressing PSA and not in cancer cells that do not express PSA. To target MUC1-positive tumor cells (ie, breast tumor), the E1A gene has been placed under the control of the DF3/MUC1 promoter/enhancer sequences described above.[181]

The transcriptionally targeted HSV-1 G92A was created by placing the essential HSV-1 α4 gene under the transcriptional control of the albumin enhancer/promoter elements and restricted viral replication to albumin expressing cells.[182] Wild-type HSV-1 replicated efficiently in cells irrespective of albumin expression, while virus G92A replicated more efficiently in albumin expressing cell lines compared to nonalbumin expressing cell lines. The calponin promoter has also been used to control expression of HSV-1 α4.[183] Calponin mRNA is overexpressed in soft-tissue/bone tumors, thereby providing a means to target such tumors with replication-conditional viruses.

The drawback of the above-mentioned transcription-targeted approaches is that individualized viruses have to be created for each tumor type. Also, tumors within a given tissue type also can vary in their expression of specific transcription factors, limiting the utility of such viruses for broad tissue types. To circumvent these problems, an adenovirus was constructed that targets tumor endothelial cells.[184] The benefits of targeting the tumor vasculature are twofold: genetic stability and a common process among multiple solid tumors. The process of angiogenesis by endothelial cells involves the upregulation of multiple endothelial cell receptor complexes such as VEGF and transforming growth factor (TGF)- β. By placing the adenoviral E1A and E1B genes under the transcriptional control of the Flk-1 (VEGFR-2) and endoglin (CD105/TGF-β receptor component) promoter/enhancer sequences, the adenovirus preferentially replicates in dividing endothelial cells compared with tumor cells.

Therapeutic Gene Delivery With Replication-Competent Viruses ■ Previously the delivery of therapeutic gene products with replication defective viral vectors was discussed. Strategies described earlier in "Therapeutic Genes" have also been employed with replication-selective tumor viruses as well. These strategies have included the delivery of immunomodulatory genes, prodrug-converting enzymes (suicide gene therapy), and cytotoxic genes. Replication-competent HSV-1 has been created to express the immunostimulatory IL-12 gene and the prodrug-converting enzyme cytosine deaminase gene.[185,186] Conditionally replicating adenoviruses have been created that express the cytotoxic TNF-α gene and the genes encoding the prodrug-converting enzymes cytosine deaminase and thymidine kinase.[181,187] Delivery of a cytotoxic gene in combination with a replication-competent virus seems counterintuitive. However, these gene-delivery approaches appear to enhance the therapeutic effect of antitumor therapy schedules in murine experimental tumor model systems. The therapeutic gene delivered may enhance tumor cell kill by eliciting a bystander effect and result in the cell death of neighboring tumor cells that are not infected by the virus.

Combination Chemotherapy/Radiotherapy With Replication-Competent Viruses ■ Finally, studies have also begun to assess the utility of combining standard anticancer agents with replication-competent viruses. Combining different therapeutic modalities has been a mainstay of cancer therapy. Adding gene therapy to standard tumor therapies has many potential benefits. Since chemo/radiotherapy and oncolytic viruses target cellular destruction differently, resistant tumor cells are less likely to emerge. Also, lower doses of each therapy may be utilized to achieve a comparable degree of tumor cell kill to monotherapy, resulting in decreased normal tissue toxicity of the individual agents.

Of greater interest is the combination of oncolytic viruses with ionizing radiation (IR)/chemotherapy resulting in synergistic tumor cell kill. IR enhances the therapeutic potential of mutant oncolytic adenoviruses and HSV-1 in part by increasing the replication potential of the viruses.[187-190] A variety of chemotherapeutic agents have also been reported to augment the efficacy of replication-conditional adenovirus and HSV-1.[191-194] Especially intriguing in this treatment paradigm are results of a phase II clinical trial for recurrent head and neck cancer treated with E1B-deleted adenovirus (ONYX-015) in combination with 5-FU and cisplatin.[195] Preliminary results suggest that the chemotherapy augments the therapeutic effect of replicating-conditional adenovirus in patients' tumors.

Studies have begun to address how chemotherapy/IR enhance the ability of viruses to replicate. In creating oncolytic viruses, viral genes are deleted, resulting in relative tumor specificity of the mutant virus (see Fig. 60-11). One way to enhance viral replication is to provide the deleted viral function in *trans* by a cellular protein homologue. For the HSV-1 mutant G207 (see Table 60-2), both deleted viral genes (ie, large subunit of ribonucleotide reductase [RR] and γ134.5) have cellular counterparts that are upregulated by IR/chemotherapy.[196,197] IR induces cellular RR activity that complements the viral RR deletion.[198] Also, IR induces the growth arrest and DNA damage inducible genes, Gadd.[199] One of these genes, Gadd34, shares significant homology to the carboxy terminus of γ134.5.[200,201] As the name implies, Gadd34 is induced by genotoxic agents, including IR and chemotherapy. Therefore, IR and chemotherapy may be able to increase transcomplementation of virally deleted gene functions (Fig. 60-15). One other implication of these observations is that

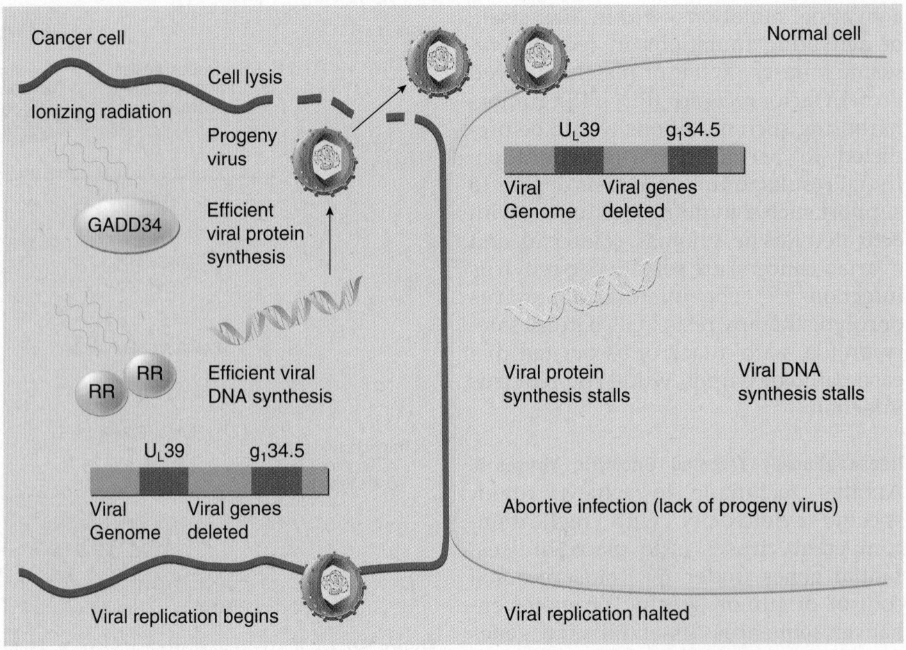

Figure 60-15 ■ IR enhancing the oncolytic capacity of attenuated, replication-competent viruses. IR activates cellular genes/proteins that provide transcomplementation to virally deleted genes. Spatial restriction of IR to cancer cells provides a mechanism by which attenuated viruses can replicate more robustly in tumor cells compared with normal cells outside of the targeted irradiated volume.

viral oncolysis may also be regulated in a spatial and temporal manner by IR (see Fig. 60-9). Cellular homologues can be induced within the targeted irradiated tumor field enhancing viral replication and tumor kill. However, when the mutant virus reaches nonirradiated, normal cells, there is a lack of transcomplementation and viral replication ceases.

These examples demonstrate how knowledge of cell and viral molecular biology has provided the basis for the construction of genetically engineered viruses that selectively replicate in tumor cells. Other replication-competent viruses under study include Newcastle disease virus and parvoviruses. Multiple clinical trials are underway to determine the therapeutic efficacy of the current generation of replication-conditional viruses. At the same time, further basic science research in both tumor and viral biology is providing means to create more potent oncolytic viruses with increased safeguards to specifically target the tumor. The majority of current studies have focused on the use of replication-conditional viruses for regional therapy (ie, direct tumor inoculation); however, studies are also evolving that use the virus as a systemic therapeutic agent that could target metastases. This would involve the virus surviving the systemic circulation and then homing in on malignant cells. Such viruses could bind selectively to tumor-cell–specific receptors to gain entry and have their gene expression driven by tumor cell–specific transcription factors.

Selected References

The complete reference list can be found at www.CANCERMEDICINE8.com

1. Miller A. Retroviral vectors. *Curr Top Microbiol Immunol*. 1993;158.
15. Flotte T, Carter B. Adeno-associated virus vectors for gene therapy. *Gene Ther.* 1995;2:357–362.
29. Freeman S, Abboud C, Whartenby K, et al. The "bystander effect": tumor regression when a fraction of the tumor mass is genetically modified. *Cancer Res.* 1993;53:5274–5283.
32. Huber B, Austin E, Good S, et al. In vivo antitumor activity of 5–fluorocytosine on human colorectal carcinoma cells genetically modified to express cytosine deaminase. *Cancer Res.* 1993;53:4619–4626.
34. Hanna N, Mauceri H, Wayne J, et al. Virally directed cytosine deaminase/5–fluorocytosine gene therapy enhances radiation response in human cancer xenografts. *Cancer Res.* 1997;57:4205–4209.
43. Lowe SW, Ruley HE, Jacks T, Housman DE. p53–dependent apoptosis modulates the cytotoxicity of anticancer agents. *Cell.* 1993;74:957–967.
50. Swisher S, Roth J, Nemunaitis J, et al. Adenovirus-mediated p53 gene transfer in advanced non-small-cell lung cancer. *J Natl Cancer Inst.* 1999;91:763–771.
56. Fueyo J, Gomez-Manzano C, Yung W, et al. Overexpression of E2F-1 in glioma triggers apoptosis and suppresses tumor growth in vitro and in vivo. *Nat Med.* 1998;4:685–690.
67. Stein C, Cohen J. Oligodeoxynucleotides as inhibitors of gene expression: a review. *Cancer Res.* 1988;48:2659–2668.
77. Oku T, Tjuvajev J, Miyagawa T, et al. Tumor growth modulation by sense and antisense vascular endothelial growth

factor gene expression: effects on angiogenesis, vascular permeability, blood volume, blood flow, fluorodeoxyglucose uptake, and proliferation of human melanoma intracerebral xenografts. *Cancer Res.* 1998;58:4185–4192.

79. Scanlon K, Ohta Y, Ishida H, et al. Oligonucleotide-mediated modulation of mammalian gene expression. *FASEB.* 1995;9:1288–1296.
81. James H, Gibson I. The therapeutic potential of ribozymes. *Blood.* 1998;91:371–382.
86. Yamazaki H, Kijima H, Ohnishi Y, et al. Inhibition of tumor growth by ribozyme-mediated suppression of aberrant epidermal growth factor receptor gene expression. *J Natl Cancer Inst.* 1998;90:581–587.
87. Fire A, Xu S, Montgomery MK, et al. Potent and specific genetic interference by double-stranded RNA in Caenorhabditis elegans. *Nature.* 1998;391:806–811.
89. Elbashir SM, Harborth J, Lendeckel W, et al. Duplexes of 21–nucleotide RNAs mediate RNA interference in cultured mammalian cells. *Nature.* 2001;411:494–498.
90. Sui G, Soohoo C, Affar E, et al. A DNA vector-based RNAi technology to suppress gene expression in mammalian cells. *Proc Natl Acad Sci U S A.* 2002;99:5515–5520.
91. Pirollo KF, Chang EH. Targeted delivery of small interfering RNA: approaching effective cancer therapies. *Cancer Res.* 2008;68:1247–1250.
96. Carette JE, Overmeer RM, Schagen FH, et al. Conditionally replicating adenoviruses expressing short hairpin RNAs silence the expression of a target gene in cancer cells. *Cancer Res.* 2004;64:2663–2667.
97. Simons J, Mikhak B, Chang J, et al. Induction of immunity to prostate cancer antigens: results of a clinical trial of vaccination with irradiated autologous prostate tumor cells engineered to secrete granulocyte-macrophage colony-stimulating factor using ex vivo gene transfer. *Cancer Res.* 1999;59:5160–5168.
101. Hodge JW, Abrams S, Schlom J, Kantor JA. Induction of antitumor immunity by recombinant vaccinia viruses expressing B7–1 or B7–2 costimulatory molecules. *Cancer Res.* 1994;54:5552–5555.
106. Rosenberg S. A new era for cancer immunotherapy based on the genes that encode cancer antigens. *Immunity.* 1999;10:281–287.
113. Rosenberg S, Zhai Y, Yang J, et al. Immunizing patients with metastic melanoma using recombinant adenovirus encoding MART-1 or gp100 melanoma antigens. *J Natl Cancer Inst.* 1998;90:1894–1900.
117. Arlen PM, Gulley JL, Madan RA, Hodge JW, Schlom J. Preclinical and clinical studies of recombinant poxvirus vaccines for carcinoma therapy. *Crit Rev Immunol.* 2007;27:451–462.
118. Kasahara N, Dozy A, Kan Y. Tissue-specific targeting of retroviral vectors through ligand-receptor interactions. *Science.* 1994;266:1373–1376.
124. Krasnykh V, Mikheeva G, Douglas J, Curiel D. Generation of recombinant adenovirus vectors with modified fibers for altering viral tropism. *J Virol.* 1996;70:6839–6846.
132. Chen L, Chen D, Manome Y, et al. Breast cancer selective gene expression and therapy mediated by recombinant adenoviruses containing the DF3/MUC1 promoter. *J Clin Invest.* 1995;96:2775–2782.
134. Weichselbaum RR, Kufe DW, Hellman S, et al. Radiation-induced tumour necrosis factor-alpha expression: clinical application of transcriptional and physical targeting of gene therapy. *Lancet Oncol.* 2002;3:665–671.
136. Hallanhan D, Mauceri H, Seung L, et al. Spatial and temporal control of gene therapy using ionizing radiation. *Nat Med.* 1995;1:786–791.
137. Rasmussen H, Rasmussen C, Lempicki M, et al. TNFerade Biologic: preclinical toxicology of a novel adenovector with a radiation-inducible promoter, carrying the human tumor necrosis factor alpha gene. *Cancer Gene Ther.* 2002;9:951–957.
138. Senzer N, Mani S, Rosemurgy A, et al. TNFerade biologic, an adenovector with a radiation-inducible promoter, carrying the human tumor necrosis factor alpha gene: a phase I study in patients with solid tumors. *J Clin Oncol.* 2004;22:592–601.
139. Advani SJ, Weichselbaum RR, Chmura SJ. Enhancing radiotherapy with genetically engineered viruses. *J Clin Oncol.* 2007;25:4090–4095.
141. Park JO, Lopez CA, Gupta VK, et al. Transcriptional control of viral gene therapy by cisplatin. *J Clin Invest.* 2002;110:403–410.
143. Walther W, Wendt J, Stein U. Employment of the mdr1 promoter for the chemotherapy-inducible expression of therapeutic genes in cancer gene therapy. *Gene Ther.* 1997;4:544–552.
144. Mauceri HJ, Hanna NN, Wayne JD, et al. Tumor necrosis factor alpha (TNF-alpha) gene therapy targeted by ionizing radiation selectively damages tumor vasculature. *Cancer Res.* 1996;56:4311–4314.
148. Bischoff J, Kirn D, Williams A, et al. An adenovirus mutant that replicates selectively in p53–deficient human tumor cells. *Science.* 1996;274:373–376.
157. Heise C, Kirn DH. Replication-selective adenoviruses as oncolytic agents. *J Clin Invest.* 2000;105:847–851.
158. Martuza R, Malick A, Markert J, et al. Experimental therapy of human glioma by means of a genetically engineered virus mutant. *Science.* 1991;252:854–856.
159. Mineta T, Rabkin S, Yazaki T, et al. Attenuated multimutated herpes simplex virus-1 for treatment of malignant gliomas. *Nat Med.* 1995;1:938–943.
170. Advani SJ, Chung SM, Yan SY, et al. Replication-competent, nonneuroinvasive genetically engineered herpes virus is highly effective in the treatment of therapy-resistant experimental human tumors. *Cancer Res.* 1999;59:2055–2058.
174. Strong J, Coffey M, Tang D, et al. The molecular basis of viral oncolysis: usurpation of the Ras signaling pathway by reovirus. *EMBO J.* 1998;17:3351–3362.
176. Coffey M, Strong J, Forsyth P, Lee P. Reovirus therapy of tumors with activated Ras pathway. *Science.* 1998;282:1332–1334.
180. Rodriguez R, Schuur E, Lim H, et al. Prostate attenuated replication competent adenovirus (ARCA) CN706: a selective cytotoxic for prostate-specific antigen-positive prostate cancer cells. *Cancer Res.* 1997;57:2559–2563.
185. Parker JN, Gillespie GY, Love CE, et al. Engineered herpes simplex virus expressing IL-12 in the treatment of experimental murine brain tumors. *Proc Natl Acad Sci U S A.* 2000;97:2208–2213.
187. Rogulski KR, Wing MS, Paielli DL, et al. Double suicide gene therapy augments the antitumor activity of a replication-competent lytic adenovirus through enhanced cytotoxicity and radiosensitization. *Hum Gene Ther.* 2000;11:67–76.
190. Advani SJ, Sibley GS, Song PY, et al. Enhancement of replication of genetically engineered herpes simplex viruses by ionizing radiation: a new paradigm for destruction of therapeutically intractable tumors. *Gene Ther.* 1998;5:160–165.
192. Heise C, Sampson-Johannes A, Williams A, et al. ONYX-015, an E1B gene-attenuated adenovirus, causes tumor-specific cytolysis and antitumoral efficacy that can be augmented by standard chemotherapeutic agents. *Nat Med.* 1997;3:639–645.
195. Khuri FR, Nemunaitis J, Ganly I, et al. A controlled trial of intratumoral ONYX-015, a selectively-replicating adenovirus, in combination with cisplatin and 5–fluorouracil in patients with recurrent head and neck cancer. *Nat Med.* 2000;6:879–885.
197. Bennett JJ, Delman KA, Burt BM, et al. Comparison of safety, delivery, and efficacy of two oncolytic herpes viruses (G207 and NV1020) for peritoneal cancer. *Cancer Gene Ther.* 2002;9:935–945.

61 Hematopoietic Cell Transplantation

Roy Jones, PhD, MD ■ Elizabeth Shpall, MD ■ Richard Champlin, MD

Hematopoietic cell transplantation involves engraftment of stem cells which can be collected from the bone marrow, peripheral blood, or umbilical cord blood. Allogeneic transplants are obtained from another individual. Autologous transplants involve use of a patient's own hematopoietic cells, usually after cryopreservation. Syngeneic transplants are between genetically identical twins.

Hematopoietic transplantation is an effective treatment for many life-threatening hematologic, immune, metabolic, and neoplastic diseases (Table 61-1).[1,2] Hematopoietic transplantation has been studied in animal models since the late 1940s as a means to rescue recipients exposed to lethal irradiation or myeloablative drugs. Allogeneic transplantation was first successfully used in humans for treatment of children with severe combined immune deficiency.[2] Allogeneic transplants are used for treatment of bone marrow failure states, hemoglobinopathies, immune deficiencies, and inborn errors of metabolism by establishing a new, normally functioning hematopoietic and immune system.

Donnall Thomas was awarded the Nobel Prize for his pioneering work in the development of hematopoietic cell transplantation, particularly for acute myelogenous leukemia.[3] Over time the use of transplantation has expanded to include at least the variety of indications included in Table 61-1 and its scientific basis has been more clearly refined to emphasize intensive chemoradiotherapy treatment of malignancy, immune replacement or augmentation for a variety of conditions, or genetic replacement.[4-7]

Table 61-1 ■ Diseases Treated With Hematopoietic Transplantation

Malignant
- Acute myelogenous leukemia
- Myelodysplastic syndromes
- Acute lymphoblastic leukemia
- Chronic myelogenous leukemia and myeloproliferative disorders
- Chronic lymphocytic leukemia
- Non-Hodgkin lymphoma
- Hodgkin disease
- Multiple myeloma and amyloidosis
- Solid tumors: breast, testicular, ovarian, and small cell lung cancer
- Pediatric solid tumors: neuroblastoma, Ewing sarcoma, medulloblastoma, renal cell cancer, melanoma

Nonmalignant
- Aplastic anemia and related bone marrow failure states
- Hemoglobinopathies: thalassemia, sickle cell anemia
- Congenital disorders of hematopoiesis:
- Fanconi anemia and related syndromes
- Congenital immune deficiencies: severe combined immune deficiency, Wiskott-Aldrich syndrome, chronic granulomatous disease, and related syndromes
- Inborn errors of metabolism
- Autoimmune disorders

The basis for autologous hematopoietic cell transplantation is to use patient-derived hematopoietic stem cells to prevent otherwise lethal myelosuppression from intensive treatment. The primary use of this technique is to eradicate malignant cells or tumors resistant to less intense treatment. Recently, this technique is being explored as a method to deplete autoimmune cells associated with diverse diseases such as multiple sclerosis[8] or scleroderma.[9]

The basis of allogeneic hematopoietic transplantation is the engraftment of donor-derived stem cells; in the recipient these cells reconstitute hematopoiesis and immunity. Following successful transplantation, recipients are considered chimeras with hematopoietic and immune cells derived from the donor. Mesenchymal and epithelial tissues remain predominantly host derived. Recently, it has become established that bone marrow stem cells are capable of limited differentiation into nonhematopoietic tissues[10] including mesenchymal cells,[11,12] liver,[13,14] cardiovascular tissues,[15] and, possibly, neural tissue.[16] There is considerable interest in stem cell transplantation for restoration of damaged or diseased organs and tissues.[17,18]

Methods of Transplantation

In most cases, transplanted hematopoietic cells are infused following intensive chemotherapy, irradiation, or other therapies such as antibodies. In the case of autologous transplantation, intensive treatment is the critical therapeutic principle and always precedes the cell infusion. As initially designed by Thomas[19-21] and Santos,[22] allogeneic transplantation utilized intensive chemotherapy with or without irradiation in a manner similar to autotransplants. This treatment was conceived with three goals in mind: (1) eradication of malignancy, (2) host immune ablation to allow acceptance of foreign cells, and (3) creation of "space" to allow engraftment. Over time a variety of chemotherapeutic agents has been explored for use in transplantation, emphasizing the alkylating agents cyclophosphamide, busulfan, melphalan, thiotepa, and carmustine (BCNU). The goal was to administer the highest doses of treatment that produced tolerable extrahematopoietic toxicity and, hopefully, maximal antitumor effect. It was established that total body irradiation could be delivered in a maximal dose of 1200-1400 cGy.[20,23]

More recently, the existence of graft-versus-malignancy (GVM) effect has been shown and established a therapeutic activity for allotransplantation independent of the pre-cell infusion treatment.[24] As with any treatment, GVM activity produces its own toxicity, immunosuppression, because of its close association with graft-versus-host disease (GVHD). With this new activity, reduced-intensity treatment (nonmyeloablative allotransplantation) has been explored as a means of reducing the risk of allotransplantation. In addition, donor lymphocyte infusions (DLI) following transplantation can be used to augment the GVM effect.[25]

Hematopoietic Transplantation as Treatment for Malignancies

Most hematopoietic transplants have been performed for treatment of hematologic malignancies.[25] Many chemotherapy drugs (predominantly alkylating agents[26]) and irradiation produce a dose-dependent antitumor response. Higher doses produce greater cytoreduction and may overcome drug resistance. Myelosuppression is the dose limiting toxicity of many chemotherapeutic agents and whole body irradiation. Doses of some agents can be markedly escalated three to five-fold above conventional maximally tolerated dose if followed by autologous or allogeneic transplantation to restore hematopoiesis (Figure 61-1).

Autologous Transplantation

Autologous transplantation is generally designed to exploit the concept of dose intensity as described, and has been used to produce killing of tumor following relapse from conventional treatment or in

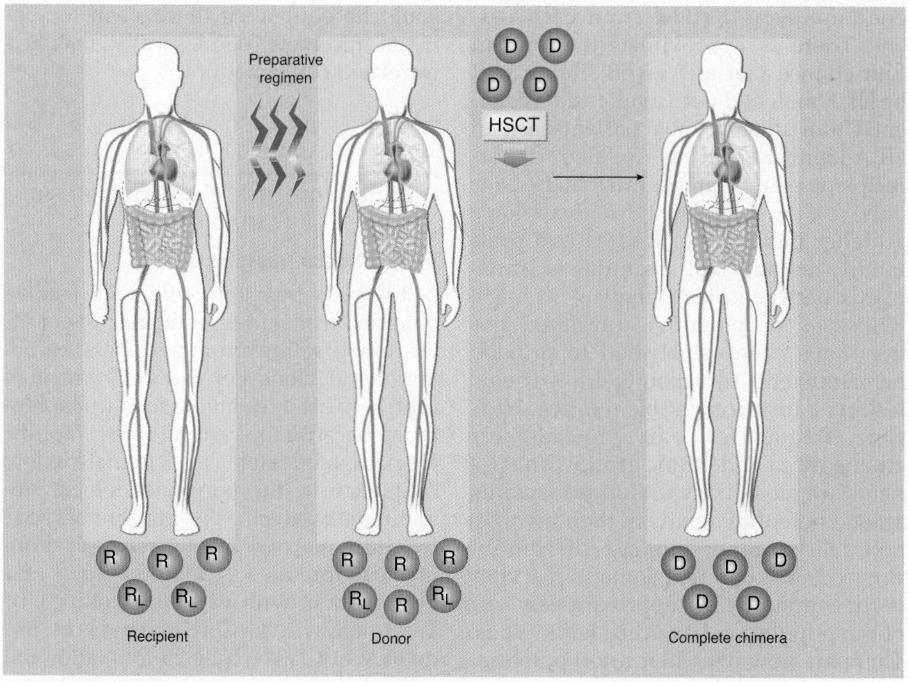

Figure 61-1 Scheme of allogeneic hematopoietic transplantation. The recipient receives a myeloablative preparative regimen designed to eradicate malignant and normal cells. The recipient then receives donor hematopoietic cells that restore hematopoiesis. *Abbreviations:* D, donor hematopoietic cells; HSCT, hematopoietic stem cell transplant; R, recipient's normal bone marrow cells; RL, recipient's leukemia cells in bone marrow.

a setting where conventional treatments are known to have little or no probability of tumor eradication. As a general rule, autologous hematopoietic transplantation is most effective in patients with malignancies shown to be responsive to conventional treatment immediately prior to the transplant regimen.[27] Other factors known to predispose to treatment failure include higher volume residual tumor[28,29] tumor types not known to exhibit a steep dose-killing relationship,[30] or treatment of patients at high risk for toxicities from the proposed treatment regimen.

During and for months following the transplant process significant immune suppression occurs as a result of depletion of immune cells from the patient and slow regrowth of the transplant.[31,32] The extent to which antitumor immunity aids in control of minimal tumor is controversial. Immune augmentation strategies used in the post-transplant setting are being actively explored to avoid this potential weakness.[33] An additional factor which might predispose to relapse using this technique is contamination of the harvested cells with tumor. Although limited investigation using gene-marked tumor cells has shown that cryopreserved tumor cells can engraft and contribute to relapse, the clinical importance of this phenomenon is unclear.[34] Numerous studies have failed to demonstrate benefit from partial depletion of tumor cells from grafts.[35] Further researches await development of high-level tumor depletion technologies.

Malignancies shown to be cured by autologous hematopoietic cell transplantation include intermediate grade lymphoma,[36] Hodgkin disease,[37] acute lymphoblastic leukemia,[21,38] and acute myelogenous leukemia.[39,40] Although not proven to be curative, major improvement in survival in myeloma patients receiving autologous transplantation have made the technique a standard treatment for appropriate patients with this condition.[41,42] Benefit for patients with germ cell cancers,[43] low grade lymphomas,[44] and a variety of pediatric solid tumors[45] are more controversial but are being actively studied.

Allogeneic Transplantation

Allogeneic hematopoietic transplants also confer an immune mediated GVM effect. Donor-derived lymphoid cells may react against and eradicate malignant cells that survive high dose cytotoxic therapy.[46,47] The risk of relapse of the malignancy after high-dose therapy and hematopoietic transplantation is increased in syngeneic transplants compared to allogeneic transplants.[48,49] Relapse risk is also increased if the putative effector cells, T lymphocytes, are depleted from an allogeneic transplant for prevention of GVHD.[50] Patients with acute or chronic GVHD have reduced risk of relapse, suggesting a relationship between GVM and GVHD.[51,52] High doses of immunosuppressive therapy have been associated with an increased risk of relapse, and withdrawal of immunosuppressive treatment can occasionally produce remission in patients relapsing after transplantation.[53] The most direct evidence for GVM comes from the observation that DLI can reinduce remission in patients who relapse post-transplant.[54,55]

There are major differences among malignancies in their susceptibility to GVM effects. Indolent myeloid and lymphoid malignancies are highly sensitive to this process, as evidenced by durable remissions after modulation of immunosuppression or donor lymphocyte infusions in patients who have relapsed after an allogeneic transplant. GVM effects have been best documented in patients with chronic myelogenous leukemia. The majority of patients who relapse into chronic phase following an allogeneic transplant achieve durable complete remission with donor lymphocyte infusions.[53] Follicular lymphomas, mantle cell lymphoma, and chronic lymphocytic leukemia (CLL) also appear very sensitive to graft-versus-malignancy effects.[56,57] Allogeneic transplants are associated with a substantially lower relapse rate than purged autologous transplants. Selected patients with CLL or low-grade lymphoma have responded to donor lymphocyte infusions or modification of immunosuppressive therapy.

GVM effects also occur but with lesser intensity against other hematologic malignancies including acute myelogenous leukemia (AML), multiple myeloma, Hodgkin disease and intermediate-grade lymphoma. In these diagnoses, allogeneic transplants produce a greater frequency of durable remissions than syngeneic or autologous transplants, but these disorders respond less frequently to DLI and responses are usually transient. Acute lymphoblastic leukemia and high-grade lymphoma appear relatively insensitive to graft-versus-leukemia (GVL) effects,[58] although patients with GVHD do have a reduced risk of relapse.[51]

GVM effects may be directed against a number of potential target antigens. Development of methods to separate GVM effects and GVHD, and generate antigen-specific antitumor responses is a major goal of ongoing research.

Donor Selection

Autologous Transplantation

Autologous transplants use the patient as their own donor. In the closely related special case, syngeneic transplants are donations from a genetically identical twin. Autologous transplants require no histocompatibility matching but often come from patients who have received extensive prior chemotherapy. This treatment often produces compromise of marrow stem cell function. The general rule is that the more extensive the pre-harvest chemotherapy, greater the probability that the harvest will be unsatisfactory. Because the harvested patient has already been screened for suitability as a transplant patient, comorbid factors preventing the patient from being harvested are unlikely. Thus, adequacy of the harvested cells is the single critical factor in this process. Two factors limit suitability of harvested cells: (1) engraftment potential, and (2) extent of tumor contamination. Both of these factors are discussed later in the chapter. Patients undergo collection of bone marrow or peripheral blood progenitor cells that are then cryopreserved in a viable state. Patients subsequently receive high-dose myelosuppressive therapy to eradicate the malignancy, followed by reinfusion of the stored autologous cells to reconstitute hematopoiesis. Autologous transplants have the advantage that the hematopoietic cells will not be rejected or produce GVHD. However, autologous transplants may be contaminated by malignant cells and do not confer a GVM effect. Unmodified autologous transplants cannot be used for genetic or acquired diseases in which the hematopoietic cells are injured or defective, although autologous hematopoietic cells can potentially be used as vehicles for gene therapy designed to correct deficiency states.

Certain families at high risk for a transplant-sensitive disease elect to have umbilical cord blood stored at the time of delivery. If the child develops the disease, the cord blood could be used for transplantation.[57]

Allogeneic Transplantation

Allogeneic transplants are collected from a related or unrelated donor. The human leukocyte antigen (HLA) system is the major histocompatibility complex (MHC) in man, and the results of allogeneic transplantation depend on the histocompatibility between donor and recipient. The HLA system is encoded by several closely linked loci on the short arm of chromosome 6.[59,60] Class I loci include HLAA, -B, and -C alleles. The class II region includes DR, DQ, and DP loci. Compatibility was initially defined by serologic assays. The serologic groups have recently been further divided into specific alleles by molecular oligonucleotide typing.

Most transplants have been from HLA-identical sibling donors. The HLA genes are inherited as a haplotype with one haplotype derived from each parent. There is approximately a one in four chance that any given sibling will be HLA matched with a potential recipient. Unfortunately, most patients lack an HLA-identical sibling. Related donor-recipient pairs that are mismatched for only one A, B, or DR HLA locus have a higher incidence of GVHD and graft failure, but survival is similar to transplants between HLA-identical siblings. Registries of potential unrelated donors have been established to provide hematopoietic transplants for patients lacking a histocompatible relative. HLA gene frequencies vary considerably among racial and ethnic groups, and patients are most likely to find transplants among potential donors of their own genetic background. Linkage disequilibrium occurs such that some haplotypes occur commonly, but approximately half of the population have rare haplotypes. There are now over 10 million potential unrelated bone marrow donors accessible in registries worldwide, and approximately half of patients can access an HLA-A, -B, -C, -DR–, and -DQ identical donor. Unrelated donor transplants are often successful, although the incidence and severity of graft-versus-host disease is increased, compared to transplants from HLA-identical siblings.[61,62] This is related in part to greater genetic disparity for non-HLA antigens among unrelated individuals; these pairs are also more likely to be mismatched for HLA molecular variants. Recent studies in which unrelated donors were selected using molecular allele typing methods have had a reduced risk of GVHD, and results are approaching those seen with transplants from HLA-identical siblings.[63-66]

Transplant recipients who are mismatched for two or more loci have relatively poor results, with a high risk of graft rejection, GVHD, and associated complications. Haploidentical donors are readily available for most patients. Aggressive Tcell depletion (4-5 log reduction) of the donor hematopoietic cells can prevent GVHD, but results in a higher rate of graft failure.[67] Delayed immune reconstitution and a high frequency of opportunistic infections remain major complications. Because these difficulties have resisted substantial improvement, umbilical cord blood (UCB) is now frequently used.[68,69] Constraints for HL-A matching of UCB are much less than that for other cell sources, with mismatches at 2 of 6 HL-A A, B, and DR loci acceptable.[70] Owing to the size of the units, cord blood transplants have been most successful in children, but are also under investigation in adults.[71] Recent data suggest that outcomes may be improving rapidly, and could be equivalent to survival for patients receiving serologically matched unrelated cell donations.[68]

Engraftment of Hematopoietic Transplants

Autologous Transplants

Autologous hematopoietic cells can be obtained from either bone marrow or after "mobilization" from peripheral blood. Peripheral blood-derived cells are now routinely used for autologous transplantation because they engraft more rapidly. Hematopoietic stem cells circulate in low frequency in the peripheral blood Hematopoietic stem cells are "mobilized" from the marrow during recovery from myelosuppressive chemotherapy and by treatment with various cytokines.[72-74] Treatment with G-CSF increases the frequency of CD34+ cells 25-fold, allowing collection of an adequate dose for transplantation by apheresis.[75]

The combination is more time consuming and requires doses of chemotherapy that produce transient pancytopenia and risk of infection. Human repopulating stem and progenitor cells express the CD34 cell surface antigen that comprises <1% of the bone marrow. Highly enriched CD34 positively selected cells have been used for autologous or allogeneic hematopoietic transplantation, resulting in rapid hematologic recovery.

Hematopoietic stem cells reside primarily in the bone marrow, and initially, hematopoietic transplantation used unfractionated bone marrow cells. Donors undergo general or regional anesthesia. One to 1.5 liters of marrow is harvested by multiple aspirations; usually from the posterior superior iliac crests.[75] Adequate collections include 2-5 × 10^8 nucleated cells/kg and 0.5-3 × 10^6 CD34+ cells/kg. Hematopoietic cells are rapidly regenerated and there are no long-term adverse consequences for the donors. Rare complications may occur, primarily relating to general anesthesia and to infection or injury at the site of marrow aspirations.

The rate of hematopoietic recovery post transplant correlates with the number of CD34+ cells/kg infused. The minimum number of cells necessary for transplantation is not well defined, but optimal hematopoietic recovery with peripheral blood progenitor cell (PBPC) requires > 5 × 10^6 CD34+ cells/kg.[73] After the therapy is completed, the hematopoietic cells are infused intravenously. The cells circulate transiently and sufficient numbers of stem cells home to the bone marrow to restore hematopoiesis. Peripheral blood counts are profoundly suppressed following high-dose chemotherapy, but generally recover within 10-15 days,[72] following bone marrow transplantation. The date of engraftment is generally defined as the first of three consecutive days with an absolute neutrophil count > 0.5×10^9/L. Hematopoietic growth factors granulocyte colony-stimulating factor (G-CSF) or granulocyte-macrophage colonystimulating factor (GM-CSF) accelerate recovery of granulocyte counts, but have no effect on erythrocytes or platelets. Transplantation of PBPC generally produces more rapid hematopoietic recovery than bone marrow, and they accelerate recovery of platelets as well as granulocytes.

Tumor Cell Contamination and Purging

For autologous transplantation, the patient must first undergo collection of hematopoietic stem cells and cryopreservation.[75] Cryopreservation can be reliably performed, and the stored cells remain viable for more than 5 years. Hematopoietic cell collection should ideally occur at a time when the bone marrow is normally cellular and the blood and marrow do not contain malignant cells. Malignant cells may contaminate autologous stem cell products; the likelihood varies with the diagnosis and disease stage. Mobilized peripheral blood stem cells tend to have a lower frequency of tumor cell contamination than bone marrow harvests.[76-80] Peripheral blood stem cell transplants can be performed in patients in whom marrow harvesting is not feasible, such as those with prior pelvic radiotherapy.

Numerous clinical studies have shown that tumor cell contamination of the autograft is associated with shortened disease-free survival.[81-83] Purging methods have been developed to deplete the autograft of tumor cells in an attempt to improve outcomes.[83] Purging methods often use monoclonal antibodies combined with complement, immunomagnetic beads, or conjugated toxins. Positive selection of CD34+ cells is another widely used approach, and combined methods are investigated as a potentially better purging strategy. Pharmacological purging include ex vivo treatment of the autograft with chemotherapeutic agents such as 4-hydroxycyclophosphamide.[83]

The clinical benefit of purging is not well documented. Successful purging of marrow harvests of patients with follicular lymphoma or with breast cancer was associated with superior outcome.[77] However, the presence of tumor cells in the autograft may correlate with the extent of systemic residual disease, and this is not direct evidence that reinfused tumor cells caused relapse. Most patients relapse in sites of prior disease, and inadequate systemic cytoreduction is believed to be the major cause of relapse postautologous transplantation. An alternative explanation is that tumor cells in the graft home preferentially to sites of prior disease where the microenvironment supports their growth. There are no randomized studies documenting reduced relapse rates using purged versus unpurged autologous transplants, and the role of purging remains controversial.

Allogeneic Transplantation

A pretransplant immunosuppressive treatment often termed the "preparative regimen" or "conditioning," is necessary to prevent rejection of an allogeneic hematopoietic transplant. The immunosuppressive preparative treatment administered prior to transplantation must markedly suppress the recipient's T lymphocyte and natural killer (NK) cell function. The intensity of immunosuppressive therapy required for engraftment varies depending on the immunocompetence of the recipient and the composition of the transplanted cells. High doses of donor stem cells and T cells present in the allograft also enhance engraftment by an alloreactive graft-versus-host hematopoietic effect.[84,85]

Allogeneic engraftment of donor cells can be documented by acquisition of donor-type cell surface antigens, isoenzymes, chromosome markers, or DNA–restriction fragment length polymorphisms. Following successful transplantation, cells of the hematologic and immunologic systems are primarily derived from the donor, although in some cases mixed chimerism occurs in which both donor and recipient derived cells are present. Mixed chimerism is more frequent after T-cell depletion of the donor graft and after nonmyeloablative conditioning.

Granulocyte recovery after PBPC or bone marrow allotransplantation occurs with timing similar to autologous transplantation. PBPC contain approximately one log more T cells than a bone marrow harvest which affects the immunologic effects after allogeneic transplantation. In some studies, the incidence and severity of acute GVHD is unchanged with PBPC compared to bone marrow,[86-88] but the rate of chronic GVHD has generally been increased.[89] The effect on survival is being actively studied.

Umbilical cord blood has recently been proposed as an alternative source of hematopoietic stem cells for transplantation from related or unrelated donors. The umbilical cord contains 50-100 mL of fetal blood, which can be collected after delivery of the placenta and separation from the fetus. Cord blood is a rich source of hematopoietic stem and progenitor cells.[90,91] The major limitation is the small number of hematopoietic cells that can be collected from a single umbilical cord, less than 10% of the cell dose administered in a typical bone marrow transplant. The advantage with cord blood transplantation is that the rate of GVHD is reduced compared to bone marrow transplantation[91-95]; this reduction allows transplantation into partially HLA-mismatched, related and unrelated recipients. Many unrelated cord blood registries and collection centers have been established. Transplant results have been related to the cell dose transplanted per kg recipient body weight, with the best results if >3×10^7 nucleated cells/kg are infused. The time to engraftment and hematologic recovery after cord blood transplantation depends on the cell dose administered and may be very prolonged, >6 weeks in some patients. Recent data suggests that simultaneous use of two cord blood transplants or perhaps exvivo cord blood expansion strategies shorten the engraftment time.

Nonablative Hematopoietic Transplant

The recipient (R), a patient with normal and malignant leukemia cells (RL) in the bone marrow, receives a nonmyeloablative preparative regimen designed to prevent rejection of the transplant. The patient receives hematopoietic cells from the donor, which, after engraftment, produces a state of mixed chimerism in which both donor and recipient derived cells coexist (Fig. 61-2). A subsequent graft-versus-hematopoietic effect may then occur which eradicates residual normal and malignant cells of host origin, resulting in complete chimerism (presence of only donor derived hematopoietic and immune cells). A DLI may be administered to augment the graft-versus-malignancy effect.

Selection of Autologous or Allogeneic Transplantation

Selection of the type of transplantation for a patient, autologous or allogeneic, depends on the type of malignancy, age of the recipient, availability of a suitable donor, the ability to collect a tumor-free autograft, the stage and status of disease (bone marrow involvement, bulk of disease, chemosensitivity to conventional chemotherapy), and the malignancy's susceptibility to GVM effects.

Autologous transplantation is readily available, and there is no need to identify an HLA-matched donor. Autologous transplants have a lower risk of life-threatening complications; there is no risk of GVHD and no need for immunosuppressive therapy to prevent GVHD and graft rejection. Immune reconstitution is more rapid than after an allogeneic transplant and there is a lower risk of opportunistic infections. Graft failure occurs rarely. Treatment-related mortality is lower than 5% in most studies, and elderly patients can tolerate treatment relatively well.[96-100] However, autologous transplants have several drawbacks. Since malignant cells may involve the blood and bone marrow, the autograft may be contaminated with clonogenic tumor cells that can contribute to relapse. Autologous transplantation relies solely on the effect of high-dose cytoreductive treatment and lacks the immune-mediated GVM effect resulting after allogeneic transplantation. In most malignancies, relapse rates are higher after autologous transplants than after allogeneic transplantation, although this is often offset by a lower rate of treatment-related mortality. Prior therapy, especially with multiple courses of alkylating agents or purine analogs, produces cumulative myelosuppression and may result in poor stem cell collection and persistent pancytopenia after transplant.[98] Patients with extensive prior therapy are at high risk for developing myelodysplasia and secondary acute leukemia after autologous hematopoietic transplantation.[99-101]

Allogeneic transplantation has the advantage that the graft is free of contaminating tumor cells. The graft also includes donor-derived immunocompetent cells, which may produce an immune GVM effect. There is generally a lower risk for disease recurrence after allogeneic transplants compared to autologous transplantation. However, allogeneic transplants may be associated with a number of potentially fatal complications such as regimen-related organ toxicity, graft failure, and GVHD. Immune reconstitution is slower after allogeneic transplantation and opportunistic infections are more frequent. Treatment-related mortality is significantly higher than with autologous transplantation and is increased with mismatched or unrelated allogeneic transplants compared to transplantation from an HLA-identical sibling donor.

Allogeneic hematopoietic transplantation has usually been restricted to younger patients in good general condition because of the increased risk of regimen-related toxicity and GVHD with advanced age. Most malignancies that are effectively treated by allogeneic transplantation are more common in elderly patients. The development of nonablative preparative regimens, as well as improvement in supportive care, infection control, and immunosuppressive therapy now enable many centers to treat older patients, >65 years of age.[102-104]

In general, allogeneic transplants have been used in the treatment of leukemias and myelodysplastic syndromes. Autologous transplants have been used more often in solid tumors, lymphoma, and myeloma, although nonablative allogeneic transplants are under evaluation in these disorders as a means to induce GVM effects.

The outcome of transplantation relates to the selection of patients and timing of transplant during the natural history of the malignancy. The best results occur when the transplant is performed early in the disease course, when the malignancy is still sensitive to chemoradiotherapy treatment, and when the tumor burden is low. Conversely, transplants done as a last resort are associated with high rates of both relapse and treatment related toxicity. These transplants may also be complicated by development of infections, organ toxicity, or poor performance status over time, which markedly increases the risk of transplant related complications. Many malignancies can be initially controlled with relatively less toxic standard forms of chemotherapy, and transplants are best employed after failure of initial treatment. In general, transplantation should be offered early in the course to patients with diseases that are at high risk for relapse or transformation to aggressive form, or to patients with early disease recurrence. The possibility of future transplant should be considered early in the course of appropriate malignancies, and early identification of a potential donor is advisable so that a transplant can be promptly performed should the disease recur.

Responsiveness to conventional-dose chemotherapy is a major predictive factor for the outcome of hematopoietic transplant. The best results have been achieved in patients with chemosensitive relapse or when transplant is performed in high risk patients as consolidation of response, particularly in patients with minimal disease at the time of transplant. Patients with partial response to initial chemotherapy are also good candidates. Primary resistance can sometimes be overcome by dose intense treatment, such as in patients with acute leukemia, Hodgkin disease, or multiple myeloma who have failed to achieve an initial remission. However, patients with bulky disease, refractory relapse, or multiple relapses of their malignancy have a poor prognosis.

Pretransplant Therapy

Autologous Transplantation

Early autologous treatment regimens were copied from the allogeneic experience and utilized cyclophosphamide plus either total body irradiation (TBI) or busulfan. TBI has the advantage of being able to be delivered in precise dose and with protection of vulnerable organs such as lungs and kidneys. TBI is suboptimal for the treatment of bulk tumor masses where hypoxia and resistance may characterize deep-seated tumor cells. In contrast, chemotherapy agents such as busulfan penetrate tumor vascularity and reach deep-seated tumors more effectively. Thus, although TBI is still used in autotransplantation and can be very effective in patients with leukemia or non-bulky tumor, regional radiotherapy is used increasingly as an adjunct to chemotherapy treatments to areas of bulk tumor.

Alkylating agents are the most commonly used drugs in transplant regimens because they usually kill tumor cells in proportion to increasing dose.[1] Ironically cyclophosphamide, the first agent used in transplantation, only does so if the rate of drug dosing is less than the activating capacity of the liver, as cyclophosphamide is a prodrug incapable of killing tumor without activation. The other most commonly used alkylating agents include melphalan, busulfan, BCNU, and thiotepa. The platinum derivatives carboplatin,[105] and cisplatin,[106] are also used extensively. Other commonly used nonalkylators are etoposide (VP-16), cytosine arabinoside, and fludarabine. As a general rule, drugs explored for use with transplantation must be able to have their doses escalated several fold above conventional dose range.

The most frequently used chemotherapy regimen is BCNU, etoposide, Ara-C, and melphalan (BEAM), commonly used for Hodgkin disease and lymphomas.[107] The isosfamide, carboplatin, etoposide (ICE) regimen is also used for these diseases.

In recent years, monoclonal antibodies have proven to be useful when added to standard treatments for leukemia and lymphoma. Gemtuzumab (Mylotarg) is being studied as part of transplant regimens.[108] Rituximab, shown to improve the survival of patients with intermediate grade lymphoma when combined with cyclophosphamide, doxorubicin, vincristine, and prednisone (CHOP) chemotherapy, appears to improve the effectiveness of BEAM.[109] Radiolabeled monoclonal antibodies are also being explored in this setting as are radioisotopes chelated by bone-seeking small molecules capable of targeted treatment to tumor involving bone and bone marrow.[110]

Allogeneic Transplantation

For the treatment of malignancies, the preparative regimen may be directed to eradicating the malignancy or the defective hematopoietic tissue. The preparative regimen generally involves chemotherapy drugs alone, perhaps using newer agents as previously described for autotransplants, or combined with TBI. The classical "myeloablative" regimens used in the treatment of leukemia are designed to ablate both hematopoiesis and immunity in the recipient and typically involves the combination of high dose cyclophosphamide with either TBI,[111,112] or

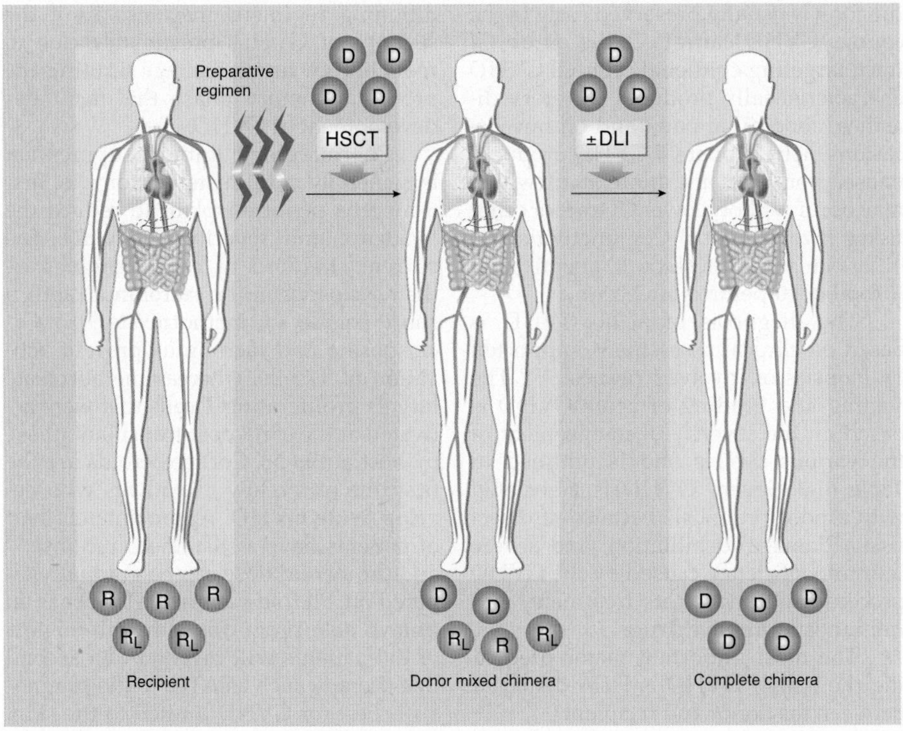

Figure 61-2 ■ Scheme of nonablative allogeneic hematopoietic transplantation. *Abbreviations:* D, donor hematopoietic cells; DLI, donor lymphocyte infusion; HSCT, hematopoietic stem cell transplant; R, recipient's normal bone marrow cells; RL, recipient's leukemia cells in bone marrow.

Table 61-2 ■ Complications After Hematopoietic Transplantation

Immune Complications
- Graft rejection
- Acute and chronic graft-versus-host disease
- Regimen-related toxicity of the preparative regimen
- Mucositis and gastroenteritis
- Veno-occlusive disease of the liver
- Diffuse alveolar hemorrhage and interstitial pneumonitis

Hemorrhagic cystitis
- Hematologic Complications
- Hemolytic anemia
- Thrombotic thrombocytopenic purpura and hemolytic disorders
- Infections and immunodeficiency
- EBV associated lymphoproliferative disease
- Late complications
- Growth disturbances
- Hypothyroidism
- Sterility and hypogonadism
- Cataracts
- Avascular necrosis
- Secondary malignancies

Abbreviation: EBV, Epstein–Barr virus.

high-dose busulfan.[113,114] These regimens are sufficient to produce engraftment of >98% of allogeneic transplants from HLA-identical siblings. More intensive immunosuppression is necessary for transplants from HLA-nonidentical siblings or if T cells are depleted from the allograft in order to prevent GVHD; addition of other myelosuppressive or immunosuppressive drugs such as antithymocyte globulin (ATG) have been employed to enhance engraftment in these settings.

The toxicity of high-dose myeloablative therapy limits the use of this modality to relatively young patients in good medical condition. The discovery of the curative potential of the immune mediated GVM effect has led to a novel approach using lower-dose, nonablative preparative regimens as a means to reduce the toxicity of allogeneic hematopoietic transplantation. These nonmyeloablative conditioning regimens have been designed not to eradicate the malignancy, but rather to provide sufficient immunosuppression to achieve engraftment and to allow induction of GVM (Fig. 61-2).[115,116] These regimens can be tolerated by older patients and those with co-morbidities who are not eligible to receive an ablative preparative regimen. Nonablative regimens are now being investigated as an alternative strategy to reduce transplant-related morbidity in a variety of settings. Most nonablative regimens include a purine analog, such as fludarabine, combined with an alkylating agent (cyclophosphamide, melphalan, or busulfan), or low-dose total body irradiation. Engraftment has been achieved in most patients, and this approach is effective against a range of hematologic malignancies.

Complications of Hematopoietic Transplantation

Intensive chemoradiotherapy and hematopoietic transplantations may be associated with a number of serious complications as listed in Table 61-2. These include immune-mediated processes such as graft rejection and GVHD, toxicities resulting from the pretransplant conditioning regimen, infections due to neutropenia, and post-transplant immune deficiency.

Graft Rejection and Graft Failure

Graft failure is defined as the failure to establish hematopoietic engraftment (primary graft failure) or loss of an established graft (secondary graft failure). Graft failure after autologous transplant occurs rarely and is most often related to infusion of an inadequate number of viable stem cells. Purging techniques, which may injure or reduce the numbers of hematopoietic stem cells, increase the risk of graft failure. It is recommended that an untreated, autologous backup marrow or peripheral blood stem cell collection be stored for patients receiving purged grafts; this backup collection can be infused to rescue patients if poor hematologic recovery or graft failure occurs.

Graft failure after allogeneic transplantation is most commonly due to immunologic rejection. Graft rejection is caused by host-derived cytotoxic T lymphocytes, NK cells, or antibodies directed against donor hematopoietic cells.[117,118] With current regimens, rejection occurs in fewer than 2% of transplants from an HLA-identical sibling. The risk is increased in recipients of HLA-mismatched or matched unrelated donor transplants.[118,119] Donor CD8+ T lymphocytes provide a graft-facilitating effect, and T lymphocyte depletion from the allogeneic graft increases the risk of graft failure.[120-122] Cord blood transplants containing a lower number of CD34+ and CD8+ cells are more prone to engraftment failure.

Graft failure or poor graft function may be caused by administration of myelosuppressive drugs, GVHD, and infections in the early post transplant period. Ganciclovir, given for prevention or treatment of cytomegalovirus infections, is the most common drug producing graft failure; this is generally reversible when the drug is discontinued. Trimethoprim-sulfamethoxazole given to prevent *Pneumocystis carinii* infections is modestly myelosuppressive and only rarely produces graft failure. Cytomegalovirus,[123] parvovirus,[124] human herpesvirus,[6,125] and mycobacterial and fungal infections may also compromise the graft. Poor engraftment may also result from microenvironment or marrow stroma dysfunction related to the patient's underlying disease or prior therapy.

Graft failure that is not due to rejection can often be successfully treated with growth factors G-CSF or GM-CSF,[126] or second hematopoietic stem cell infusion from the same donor or an alternative donor.

Graft-versus-Host Disease

Graft-versus-host disease is a major, potentially life threatening complication of allogeneic hematopoietic transplantation. Acute and chronic GVHD are distinct, but interrelated syndromes. Acute GVHD typically occurs within the first 100 days post-transplant and results from reactivity of mature donor T lymphocytes present in the graft directed against disparate major or minor histocompatibility antigens of the recipient (the host). Chronic GVHD is a syndrome of disordered immune regulation that resembles a number of autoimmune diseases. The classical manifestations of chronic GVHD generally develop between day 80 and 2 years post-transplant.

The pathophysiology of acute GVHD involves three phases.[127] The first involves conditioning-regimen–related tissue injury resulting in cytokine release, upregulation of HLA molecules, activation of macrophages, and generation of a pro-inflammatory state. In the second phase, alloreactive T cells recognize allogeneic antigens presented on host dendritic cells, become activated, and expand. The third phase involves generation of effector cells and cytokines that produce tissue injury. Acute GVHD requires donor T lymphocytes and recipient antigen-presenting cells to occur. A corollary of these activation mechanisms is that conditioning regimens producing greater tissue injury may produce more intense GVHD.

Acute GVHD involves the skin, gastrointestinal (GI) tract, and liver as the primary target tissues. The hematopoietic and immune systems are also involved. It is unclear why other tissues are not directly affected by GVHD. A maculopapular rash is usually the first presentation and is typically pruritic and confluent. When severe, generalized erythroderma, bullae, and desquamation may occur. Acute GVHD of the liver targets the biliary epithelium and produces cholestatic hepatitis with marked elevation of bilirubin and alkaline phosphatase. Synthetic function is usually preserved early in the course. GVHD can affect the entire GI tract, targeting epithelial cells. GI GVHD characteristically produces secretory diarrhea, abdominal pain, and on rare occasions, ileus. Upper GI GVHD produces nausea, vomiting, and anorexia, all which may occur without lower GI tract or other tissue involvement.[128] Conjunctivitis and other ocular manifestations, anemia, and thrombocytopenia often occur.

The diagnosis of acute GVHD is based on clinical assessment, supported by biopsies of involved tissues.[129,130] The staging and grading of acute GVHD is based on the severity of involvement of the various tissues and is outlined in Table 61-3. Severe GVHD is associated with a poor prognosis because of direct tissue damage, debilitation, and severe immunodeficiency caused by the GVHD process itself and by its treatment with immunosuppressive drugs.

The most important factor predicting the risk of GVHD is HLA disparity between the donor and recipient.[65,130,131,138] With current immunosuppressive prophylaxis, acute GVHD occurs in 25-50% of patients after transplants from an HLA identical sibling; this may be related to disparity between minor histocompatibility antigens. A higher incidence, up to 61-90% has been reported following transplants from mismatched and unrelated donors. Results are improving for unrelated donor transplantation with the use of more precise molecular histocompatibility typing to identify donors. Older age is associated with an increased incidence of acute and chronic GVHD. Less intensive, nonmyeloablative conditioning regimens may also limit the severity of GVHD, presumably due to reduction in tissue damage limiting the pro-inflammatory phase that facilitates development of GVHD.

Pharmacologic immunosuppression is generally administered for the first 6 months post-transplant to reduce the incidence and severity of GVHD. The current standard of care combines either cyclosporine or tacrolimus with a short course of methotrexate.[132-134] Cyclosporine and tacrolimus prevent activation of T cells, whereas methotrexate targets proliferating T cells that were activated at the early post-transplant phase by host antigens. Corticosteroids are the first line of therapy in patients who develop acute GVHD. Approximately half of patients have a sustained response,[135] and the steroid dose can be gradually tapered off. Steroid-resistant GVHD has an unfavorable prognosis although 30-40% of the patients will respond to a second line therapy such as ATG.[136] The prognosis is best for GVHD limited to the skin. Acute GVHD involving the liver or multiple organs has a poorer prognosis than other sites. A number of other immunosuppressive agents are being studied.The most effective method for prevention of GVHD is depletion of T lymphocytes from the graft.[50] This approach is primarily used for haploidentical transplants where the risk of GVHD is very high.

Chronic GVHD is a related syndrome affecting 25-60% of recipients of allogeneic transplantation who survive more than 6 months after transplant.[137] It most often occurs between 80 and 200 days after transplant, but the onset may be

Table 61-3 **Clinical Staging and Grading of Graft-versus-Host Disease (GVHD)**

Acute GVHD

Stage	Skin[a]	Liver[b]	Gut[b]
1	Mmaculopapular rash <25%	Bbilirubin 2-3 mg/dL	Diarrhea 500-1000 mL or persistent nausea[c]
2	Maculopapular rash 25-50%	Bilirubin 3-6 mg/dL	Diarrhea 1000-1500 mL
3	Generalized erythroderma	Bilirubin 6-15 mg/dL	Diarrhea >1500 mL
4	Desquamation and bulla	Bilirubin >15 mg/dL	Severe abdominal pain or ileus

Overall Grade[d]	Severity	Skin		Liver		Gut
0	None	0		0		0
I	Mild	1-2		0		0
II	Moderate	3	*or*	1 or	*or*	1
III	Severe			2-3 or		2-3
IV[e]	Life threatening	4	*or*	4 or	*or*	4

Chronic GVHD

Limited	Localized skin involvement *and/or* hepatic dysfunction
Extensive	1. Generalized skin involvement *or* 2. Localized skin involvement *and/or* hepatic dysfunction, *plus* any of the following: a. liver histology showing chronic aggressive hepatitis, bridging necrosis or cirrhosis b. eye involvement (Schirmer test <5 mm wetting) c. involvement of mucosalivary glands or oral mucosa d. involvement of any other target organ

[a] Extents determined by rule of nines or burn chart; [b] downgrade one stage for additional causes of elevated bilirubin or diarrhea; [c] requires histologic evidence of GVHD in the stomach or duodenum; [d] minimal organ stage required to determine grade; [e] grade IV may also be determined with lower organ involvement with extreme decrease in performance status.

Sources: From Ref. 117, 118, 137.

delayed to the second year. Chronic GVHD is more common in older patients and in patients with prior acute GVHD although approximately one third of affected patients have a de novo presentation without prior acute GVHD.[138] Chronic GVHD is more prevalent after transplants with peripheral blood stem cells than with marrow transplantation.[139]

Chronic GVHD has multiple clinical manifestations similar to those seen in several autoimmune disorders such as progressive systemic sclerosis, Sjögren syndrome, and primary biliary cirrhosis.[137] It is a syndrome of immune dysregulation with generation of autoreactive T cells and autoantibodies. Chronic GVHD is associated with thymic dysfunction and failure of the thymus to delete autoreactive cells and induce tolerance. Chronic GVHD is associated with profound immunosuppression and the major risk to the patients relates to high incidence of opportunistic infections.

Chronic GVHD most frequently involves the skin, liver, oral cavity, and eyes. Skin involvement consists of erythema, hyperkeratosis, and desquamation. Its onset is often insidious with gradual thickening and tightness of the subcutaneous tissues and limitation of joint flexibility. Additional symptoms include sicca syndrome with dry eyes, dry mouth, and lichenoid changes in the mouth. Liver involvement is characterized by cholestatic changes. Bronchiolitis obliterans may occur without other major manifestations of chronic GVHD. Intestinal involvement with anorexia, dysphagia, malabsorption, and wasting may occur. Polymyositis, serositis, and autoimmune manifestation occur rarely. Secondary infections are common causes of morbidity and mortality, and antimicrobial prophylaxis is warranted. Chronic GVHD may become a chronic debilitating disease affecting quality of life and remains the major determinant of late transplant-related morbidity. Chronic GVHD is classified as "limited" if only minor skin or liver involvement occurs, or "extensive" if there is diffuse involvement of the skin or multiple organs or when the liver histology indicates advanced changes. Progressive onset of extensive chronic GVHD from acute GVHD and the presence of thrombocytopenia are poor prognostic factors.[140]

Corticosteroids are the first line of therapy for chronic GVHD.[148] The chronic nature of this syndrome requires long-term therapy for at least 6-9 months, using the lowest steroid doses, which control symptoms. Alternate day dosage may be preferable to minimize the complications resulting from chronic steroid therapy. Cyclosporine or tacrolimus may be used in combination with corticosteroids in high-risk patients.[141-143] Combinations of immunosuppressive agents may improve control of the direct manifestations of chronic GVHD, but they increase the risk of infectious morbidity and mortality. Mycophenolate mofetil has some efficacy and can be employed as a steroid-sparing agent.[144-146]

Regimen-Related Toxicity

Myeloablative preparative regimens used to cytoreduce the malignancy approach the limit of tolerance for several tissues. The gastrointestinal tract, kidneys, lungs, and liver are the most susceptible to toxic damage, but severe toxicity may also involve the heart, bladder, nervous system, and other tissues. The actual risk for toxicity varies among regimens and their relative dose intensity. Specific determinants include the toxicity profiles of the involved agents and their interactions that are affected by coexisting organ dysfunction, the effects of the diseases and prior therapy, and infections. Most toxicities are experienced during the first 30 days post-transplant, but regimen-related hepatic injury (hepatic veno-occlusive disease), pulmonary toxicity, and neurologic effects may be delayed for several months.

Veno-occlusive disease (VOD) of the liver frequently occurs after TBI, busulfan, BCNU, thiotepa, carboplatin, and etoposide-containing regimens.[147] The relative incidence varies widely but may approach 40-50% with very intensive treatments. VOD involves an injury to hepatic venules and hepatocytes, which is characteristic and can be diagnosed by transvenous liver biopsy even in the presence of thrombocytopenia. The clinical syndrome is characterized by painful hepatic enlargement, ascites, generalized fluid retention, and striking elevation of serum bilirubin. There is no proven treatment other than supportive care, and factors predicting the probability of a fatal outcome from VOD have been described.[148] Pulmonary toxicity directly related to drug injury is most commonly caused by BCNU, the frequency varying from 5% to 60% with increasing dose.[149] Virtually every alkylating agent used in transplantation has been associated with pulmonary toxicity, though much less commonly than with BCNU. This injury typically occurs between 3 and 12 weeks following transplant and usually produces progressive shortness of breath, cough, and diffuse interstitial abnormalities on chest radiograph or CT scan. If infection is excluded, steroid treatment can produce total reversal of this side effect.[149] Central neurotoxicity, most commonly manifest by subtle cognitive dysfunction, has been frequently reported. Severe nonfocal toxicity, including stupor and coma, has been associated with regimens containing high doses of BCNU and thiotepa, both of which penetrate the central nervous system (CNS) well. In addition, the immunosuppressives cyclosporine and tacrolimus can cause both focal and nonfocal CNS dysfunction that often responds to temporary discontinuation of the drug.[150] These agents also produce sporadic peripheral neuropathy, which is slow to resolve after drug discontinuation. Cardiac toxicity, usually manifests temporary myocardial injury and decline in cardiac ejection fraction, is also produced by a variety of alkylating agent regimens. Although most commonly asymptomatic and lasting only 1-3 months, it can occur in 20-40% of patients in selected regimens.[151] Irreversible cardiac failure can be seen but is much less common.

Hematologic Complications

Hemolytic reactions may result from ABO blood group incompatibility between the donor and recipient.[152] The incompatibility may be major when the recipient plasma contains isohemagglutinins against donor red blood cells (RBC) or minor when the donor plasma contains isohemagglutinins against recipient RBC. ABO incompatibility is not a contraindication for allogeneic transplant. Red blood cells should be removed from the donor graft to prevent acute hemolytic reaction in cases with major ABO incompatibility and plasma should be removed in pairs with minor ABO incompatibility.

Thrombotic thrombocytopenic purpura (TTP) may occur after hematopoietic transplantation and is more common after allogeneic than autologous transplants.[153] Factors implicated in initiating endothelial injury include chemotherapeutic agents, irradiation, cyclosporine and tacrolimus, cytomegalovirus (CMV) and fungal infections, and cytokine-release syndromes. TTP occurring post-autologous or -allogeneic hematopoietic transplantation has a poor prognosis. Treatment with plasma exchange results in response in some patients.[154,155]

Immunodeficiency and Infections

Recipients of hematopoietic transplants have a severe immunodeficiency involving both T and B cells.[156-158] Intensive preparative regimens ablate the host immune system. Myeloid cells, macrophage/monocytes, and lymphocytes are subsequently produced from precursor cells present in the graft. The most profound abnormalities occur within the first 6 months followed by slow recovery over the first year.[159] HLA-mismatched or unrelated donor transplants have a more severe immunodeficiency and risk for opportunistic infections, particularly if T-cell depletion is used to prevent GVHD.[160] Patients receiving umbilical cord blood transplants are at particular risk for profound and prolonged immunodeficiency because of the immature nature of the infused cells and the small size of the graft. Recipients of autologous and syngeneic transplants also have a period of immunodeficiency, but their recovery is usually more rapid and post-transplant infections are less frequent and severe than after allogeneic transplantation. Patients with acute and chronic GVHD have a profound immunodeficiency state for prolonged periods.[161] Recipients of hematopoietic transplants may be susceptible to unusual opportunistic infections and also to acute overwhelming infections. Prophylactic strategies against an array of potential infections and rapid recognition and treatment of infections are an essential part of successful management of transplant recipients.[162] Immunoglobulin replacement therapy should be considered in patients with documented immunoglobulin deficiency. Revaccinations should be performed upon immune recovery and are typically carried out 1 year post-transplant.[163] Isolation measures and especially meticulous hand washing are important in prevention of nosocomial acquisition of infections.

Post-transplant lymphoproliferative disease (PTLD) is a life-threatening complication of allogeneic transplantation.[164] It is more prevalent in recipients of T-cell depleted marrow grafts, transplants from unrelated donors, in patients with GVHD, and especially in those treated with aggressive immunosuppressive treatment including ATG. PTLD in hematopoietic transplant recipients arises from the transformation of donor-derived B-lymphocytes by Epstein-Barr virus (EBV) infection. PTLD presents with systemic symptoms, adenopathy, and frequently with extranodal lesions in the GI tract, liver, and CNS. Treatment includes withdrawal of immunosuppression and administration of the antiCD20 monoclonal antibody, rituximab. Cellular therapy with donor lymphocyte infusion, at relatively low cell numbers, can have dramatic results in controlling PTLD.[165] More recently methods have been developed to generate EBV-specific cytotoxic lymphocytes for the treatment of this complication.[166] Patients with increasing levels of EBV deoxyribonucleic acid are at highest risk for lymphoproliferative disease and are candidates for preemptive immunotherapy.

Late Effects

Late complications of hematopoietic transplantation include delayed effects of high-dose therapy, indolent infections, transfusion-related complications, and chronic GVHD. Late toxicity of high-dose therapy can produce cataracts, pulmonary fibrosis, dental abnormalities, hypothyroidism, and hypogonadism, growth retardation, osteoporosis, and avascular necrosis of the hip or other bones. Permanent sterility occurs in most patients. There is an increased risk of solid and hematologic secondary tumors after hematopoietic transplantation. Solid tumors such as head and neck cancers, squamous cell carcinomas, melanomas, and brain, breast, and thyroid cancers may be more common in recipients of TBI-containing regimens and the cumulative incidence is up to 7-10% at 15 years. Myelodysplasia and secondary leukemia occur more commonly after autologous transplant, occurring in 4-18% of patients within 2.5-8.5 years of transplant.[167,168] There are data to suggest that myelodysplasia is associated more with extensive prior therapy than with the high-dose chemotherapy given prior to the transplant.

Indications for Hematopoietic Transplantation

Acute Myeloid Leukemia

Hematopoietic cellular transplantation has been extensively evaluated for the treatment of patients with AML.[169,170] Myeloablative transplants have been used in younger patients. AML is more common with advanced age, but about 30% of the patients are younger than 55 years. Most patients have received preparative regimens involving high-dose cyclophosphamide and total body irradiation or the combination of busulfan and cyclophosphamide and, more recently, busulfan and fludarabine. Most studies showed no difference in outcome between the first two regimens, but one randomized study showed an advantage for TBI.[171,172] Most patients achieve complete remission after highdose therapy and hematopoietic transplantation. The major causes of treatment failure are GVHD, regimen-related toxicity, infections, and recurrent leukemia. More intensive regimens designed to have greater antileukemic activity by increasing the TBI dose or adding additional chemotherapeutic agents have produced additional toxicity, and overall survival has not improved.[173] The outcome after allogeneic transplantation is primarily dependent on the disease status (remission versus relapse), cytogenetic abnormality of the leukemia, patient age, and histocompatibility between donor and recipient.[174]

Nonmyeloablative regimens have also been investigated as a means to decrease regimen-related toxicity. This has been effective in patients transplanted while in remission, but there is a high relapse rate in patients with overt leukemia.[115] Novel approaches include the inclusion of antimyeloid monoclonal antibodies, which are often radiolabeled or conjugated to toxins that can target the malignant cells with little systemic toxicity.[175]

Autologous bone marrow transplantation has also been evaluated as treatment for AML.[176,177] Patients undergo procurement and cryopreservation of bone marrow cells while in remission. They may then receive similar marrow ablative chemoradiotherapy followed by reinfusion of the cryopreserved hematopoietic cells to restore hematopoiesis. A major limitation is the high likelihood that the "remission" bone marrow may be contaminated by small numbers of leukemic cells, which would be cryopreserved and reinfused with the autologous marrow. Additionally, no GVL effect accompanies this treatment. Nonetheless, 30-50% of patients have achieved prolonged remissions after autologous transplants performed in first or second remission. A number of techniques have been explored to deplete occult leukemic cells from the harvested bone marrow in vitro prior to cryopreservation. Immunologic approaches using anti-AML monoclonal antibodies,[178] or pharmacologic agents, such as *cis*-4-hydroperoxycyclophosphamide[83] or mafosfamide[82] have been studied. Although some of the best results are reported in series using purged marrow, no controlled studies have been done, and the efficacy of purging remains to be determined.

The best results are achieved when allogeneic or autologous transplantation is given to patients in first remission where long-term disease-free survival is 40-60%.[179,180] It remains an unresolved question whether patients with a sibling donor should receive allogeneic transplant while in first remission or at the time of relapse. There are numerous studies comparing allogeneic hematopoietic transplantation with autologous transplantation and consolidation chemotherapy in patients with AML in first remission.[181,182] Results have been conflicting, in part because of various regimens used, different type, intensity, and number of consolidation cycles prior to transplant, and because only a portion of patients received the assigned treatment in each study. In general, most studies have shown a significantly lower relapse rate in patients receiving allogeneic transplantation. Relapse rates after autologous transplantation is higher, but still superior to chemotherapy in many studies. Survival has not been significantly improved in most studies in adults, because some patients may be salvaged with allogeneic transplantation after relapse. Most centers recommend allogeneic transplants in first remission for patients with intermediate or high-risk cytogenetic abnormalities and clinical features, but not for patients with a favorable prognosis, such as those with $t^{8;21}$, inv 16, or $t^{15;17}$ abnormalities.

Elderly patients have a higher rate of regimen-related toxicity and GVHD. Most centers have limited transplantation to patients less than 55-60 years of age who have an HLA-identical sibling donor. However, AML is more common with advanced age. Elderly patients are more likely to have adverse cytogenetics and antecedent hematologic disorders and thus an unfavorable outcome. The use of nonmyeloablative regimens for induction of GVL as the main goal of treatment has opened the option of allogeneic transplantation to patients up to 75 years of age with chemotherapy-sensitive disease.

The risks of allogeneic transplantation are increased in patients without an HLA-identical sibling donor. Some studies suggest that unrelated donors fully matched using molecular methods have outcomes similar to patients having HLA sibling donors. Transplants from a matched unrelated donor or related mismatched donor should generally be considered in patients after relapse, those with poor-risk cytogenetic abnormalities, or patients with an antecedent hematologic disorder.[183,184] Haploidentical transplants or umbilical cord blood transplants can also be considered for younger patients in second or subsequent remission and lacking a matched donor, but with increased risk.

Myelodysplastic Syndromes

Myelodysplastic syndromes (MDS) are a group of clonal hematologic disorders, manifested by peripheral cytopenias and a high risk of transformation to AML. They may occur de novo or secondary to prior chemotherapy for another malignancy. MDS most often occur in elderly patients, but about 10% of patients are young. Outcome is determined by the French-American-British morphological classification. Patients with refractory anemia or refractory anemia with ringed sideroblasts have longer survival than patients with refractory anemia with excess myeloblasts or chronic myelomonocytic leukemia (advanced MDS). The International Prognostic Score (IPPS) score defines low-, intermediate-, and high-risk groups based on marrow blast percentage, cytopenias, and karyotype.[185] The median survival of patients with low-risk IPPS scores is 5.7 years, but it is only 0.4 years for high-risk patients.

Allogeneic transplantation is a potentially curative treatment for MDS[186-189]; however the timing of transplantation is controversial. Patients with high-risk disease, excess blasts, severe neutropenia, transfusion dependency, and high-risk cytogenetic abnormalities are considered candidates. Stable patients with low-risk disease may have extended survival with conservative therapy and should generally not be offered transplant until disease progression. The conditioning regimens used are similar to those used for AML. Nonmyeloablative transplants have been successful in some patients, and DLI can restore remission in some patients with post-transplantation relapse.

The outcome is related to the MDS morphology or IPPS score.[190] The relapse rate after transplant for early MDS is less than 10%, and long-term disease-free survival is 50-60%. The risk of relapse for patients with RAEB/RAEB-T is approximately 30% with 30-40% long-term survival. Survival is better for young patients and when transplant is given early after diagnosis, but is worse after transplants from an unrelated donor. The relapse rate after transplant for therapy-related MDS is similar to de novo MDS, but treatment-related complications occur more often, probably because these patients are usually heavily pretreated for their primary malignancy.[191,192]

Acute Lymphoblastic Leukemia

Hematopoietic transplantation is an effective treatment for acute lymphoblastic leukemia (ALL).[193-197] Intensive chemotherapy regimens have resulted in cure of approximately 70% of children with ALL. There has also been a substantial improvement in the treatment of adult ALL with similar regimens; 80-90% achieve complete response (CR) with induction regimens and 30-35% can be cured.[198] Consequently, hematopoietic transplantation has generally been reserved for patients after relapse, patients who fail to achieve remission with initial chemotherapy, and for a subset of patients in first remission with a high risk for recurrence of the disease. Transplantation in first remission is controversial.[199,200] Most studies have shown no survival advantage for such patients having hematopoietic transplantation because a reduced relapse rate is offset by treatment-related mortality. Patients with Philadelphia chromosome positive ALL have an extremely poor prognosis, with <10% achieving long-term disease-free survival. Allogeneic transplantation in first remission can cure 30-40%, and should be considered a standard of care for these patients.[201,202] The use of other adverse prognostic factors to select patients for transplantation in first remission is controversial.

Hematopoietic transplantation is indicated for most patients with relapsed disease.[203,204] Children with relapse occurring more than 36 months after first remission, or more than 12 months after completion of maintenance chemotherapy may still be cured with chemotherapy.[205] The outcome of most adults with relapsing disease is dismal, and they should be considered for hematopoietic transplantation.[206] About 20-30% of patients with primary refractory ALL can be salvaged with allogeneic transplant. The prognosis of patients with chemotherapy resistant relapse is poor.

The most common preparative regimen used for transplants in ALL includes high-dose cyclophosphamide and total body irradiation with or without other chemotherapeutic agents. TBI-containing regimens may be associated with improved disease-free survival, in comparison to non–TBI-containing regimens.[207] Intensification of irradiation or addition of other agents to TBI has generally not improved overall outcome, and development of more effective regimens would be desirable.

Autologous hematopoietic transplantation has also been evaluated in patients with ALL, mostly in children.[208-210] A number of monoclonal antibodies to leukemia-associated antigens are available in ALL; these antigens are nonreactive with normal hematopoietic progenitors. These include antibodies to the common ALL antigen (CD10) or a number of T-cell antigens. A number of patients have received autologous transplants using bone marrow that was treated ex vivo with one or more of these antibodies and complement. Limitations to this technique include probable antigenic heterogeneity among neoplastic cells, and it is unclear if leukemic stem cells express these cell surface antigens. Although selected patients with ALL in second remission have achieved prolonged remissions after receiving intensive chemotherapy, total body irradiation, and autologous transplantation using antiCD10 antibody and complement-treated marrow, longterm disease-free survival is <20% in most series. These data are difficult to interpret because many of the successful cases involved patients having a relatively good prognosis with conventional treatment.

Chronic Myeloid Leukemia

Chronic myeloid leukemia (CML) is a hematologic malignancy characterized by excessive clonal proliferation of myeloid cells and their progenitors. In greater than 90% of cases, the Philadelphia chromosome, t[9;22] is a marker of the malignant clone and results from rearrangement of the BCR and ABL genes, producing a fusion protein with abnormal tyrosine kinase activity. CML is more common with advanced age, and the median age of onset is 60 years.

The disease can be divided into two phases: an initial chronic phase in which cell maturation is normal followed by transformation to accelerated or acute phase (blast crisis). Blast crisis is characterized by maturation arrest at the level of the myeloblast or lymphoblast and resembles acute leukemia.

CML has been treated with chemotherapy, interferon-based therapies, and hematopoietic transplantation. The recent development of imatinib mesylate, a selective inhibitor of the BCR-ABL tyrosine kinase, has changed the standard of care for this disease.[211] Imatinib mesylate has produced a high rate of cytogenetic complete remissions in initial trials[212] and followup exceeding 5 years now indicates that >80% of patients remain in cytogenetic remission. Responding patients typically still have minimal residual disease detectable by polymerase chain reaction assays and the impact of this agent after longer folllowup periods remains to be determined. Additional tyrosine kinase inhibitors have been developed and can produce responses in CML following imatinib failure or detection of specific mutations in CML cells, which correlate with imatinib resistance. The role of hematopoietic transplantation is being reevaluated as long-term data with tyrosine kinase inhibitors become available.

Allogeneic hematopoietic transplantation is a highly effective treatment for CML, capable of producing cure of the disease.[213,214] Most patients have received busulfan and cyclophosphamide or cyclophosphamide and total body irradiation as the preparative regimen. Both regimens appear equally effective.[215,216] The oral busulfan formulation is erratically absorbed; toxicity and antileukemic effects are dependent on the levels of busulfan achieved.[217,218] Intravenous busulfan has more reliable pharmacokinetics and appears to have less toxicity.

The major determinants of transplant outcome are the stage of the disease at the time of transplant, age of recipient, type of donor, and interval from diagnosis to transplantation. Hematopoietic transplantation is the only treatment that potentially allows long-term survival in accelerated or blastic CML. Patients who are in an accelerated phase have a 35% chance of prolonged survival. For patients undergoing transplantation during blast crisis, only 10-20% approximately become long-term survivors. Most commonly, patients in blast crisis are treated with conventional therapy attempting to return the patient to chronic phase and then proceeding rapidly to transplant. The major cause of treatment failure in advanced CML is leukemia relapse.

The high dose preparative regimen may not completely eliminate all malignant cells and a graft-versus-leukemia effect is necessary to prevent relapse. Many patients may still have small numbers of Philadelphia chromosome positive cells identified by cytogenetics or polymerase chain reaction analysis up to 6-12 months post-transplant[219]; typically, these cells are gradually eliminated due to the GVL effect. Relapse after transplant can be clinically overt or diagnosed only by cytogenetic or molecular analysis. CML is the most sensitive malignancy to graft-versus-leukemia effects; infusion of additional donor T lymphocytes can reinduce durable remission in 80-90% of patients with early relapse.[220,221] Relapse in advanced phase is less likely to respond to DLI. Patients receiving DLI may become pancytopenic at the time of response. This is more common in patients with a high percentage of host-derived hematopoiesis at the time of DLI.[220] Recovery of donor-derived hematopoiesis usually follows, but some patients require infusion of additional donor stem cells to support hematopoietic recovery. GVHD is a major risk after DLI; its risk can be minimized by starting with a low T-cell dose of 5-10 × 106/kg and subsequently escalating the dose until response occurs.

Hematopoietic transplantation has been used for the treatment of other myeloproliferative disorders.[223-225] The appropriate timing of transplantation is not well defined. Most researchers require the patient to be transfusion-dependent to justify the risks inherent with hematopoietic transplantation.[225]

Chronic Lymphoctic Leukemia

CLL is an indolent lymphoid malignancy; median survival exceeds 10 years.[226,227] Chronic lymphocytic leukemia is a clonal disorder of B cells, characterized by the accumulation of small mature-appearing lymphocytes, although rare Tcell variants also occur. The Rai and the Binet systems separate CLL patients into prognostic groups.[228] The National Cancer Institute-sponsored Working Group recommends use of the "3-risk group" modification of the original five-stage Rai staging system.[229] The median survival is >14 years for the low-risk group, 8 years for the intermediate group, and 4 years for the high-risk group. Adverse prognostic factors are recent absence of immunoglobulin gene rearrangement, expression of CD38, and higher levels of beta2-microglobulin.[230]

Chemotherapy is generally recommended if the disease causes symptoms or impaired performance status.[231] Chemotherapy involving fludarabine combined with alkylating agents such as cyclophosphamide is effective to control symptoms, reduce bulk of disease, and has palliative benefit. More recent trials have employed rituximab as well, and complete clinical response of high-risk CLL are becoming more frequent.[232] Responses are transient, however, and overall survival has not been substantially improved; this disease is considered incurable. The prognosis is poorer once disease progression occurs after initial chemotherapy. Results depend on the response to salvage chemotherapy. The overall survival is 2.5-4 years.

Several studies of high-dose chemoradiotherapy with autologous hematopoietic transplantation have been reported using marrow collected after a fludarabine induced remission.[233,234] The autograft can be purged by monoclonal antibodies directed against B lymphocytes, and elimination of detectable systemic malignant cells is associated with improved survival.[235] The role and optimal timing of autologous transplantation is controversial. The results of autologous transplants have been best when performed early in the disease, but the impact on survival in this selected group of lower-risk patients is unknown. Only transient remissions have been achieved in heavily pretreated patients with advanced disease.

Allogeneic transplantation has been studied predominantly in younger patients with advanced disease and poor prognosis.[236-238] Patients with chemosensitive disease have better outcome following transplant. An International Bone Marrow Transplant Registry (IBMTR) analysis showed a 3-year survival of 46%, but also a high risk for transplant-related mortality.[239] A graft-versus-leukemia effect has been shown in this disease,[240] and this has led to studies using nonmyeloablative conditioning to reduce toxicity and to extend the use of allogeneic transplantation options to the treatment of patients up to age 75. Encouraging preliminary results have been reported by many groups using this strategy.

The optimal timing of allogeneic transplantation is controversial. Given the risks of allogeneic transplantation and the indolent course of newly diagnosed patients, it is generally recommended that the procedure be considered only after failure of initial therapy. The prognosis is relatively poor if the procedure is delayed until after multiple relapses or after development of refractoriness to chemotherapy.

Non-Hodgkin Lymphoma

The non-Hodgkin lymphomas are a heterogeneous group of malignancies with indolent to highly aggressive natural histories. Treatment with both standard and transplant-based therapies depends on the histologic subtype and prognostic factors operative in each patient. A number of classification systems have been proposed. A Revised European-American Lymphoma classification is widely used and incorporates immunophenotype as well as morphologic criteria,[241] and a World Health Organization classification has recently been proposed.[241] These disorders result from malignant transformation and clonal proliferation of lymphoid cells and their progenitors. Each histologic type is associated with characteristic cytogenetic and molecular abnormalities.

Lymphomas can be grouped into major categories: low-, intermediate-, and highgrade. The low-grade lymphomas—small lymphocytic lymphoma, follicular small cleaved cell lymphoma, and follicular mixed cell lymphoma—are indolent diseases but incurable with standard forms of chemotherapy. Follicular small-cleaved cell lymphoma and follicular mixed cell lymphoma are the most common categories included among low-grade lymphomas. These diseases are associated with the $t^{14;18}$, resulting in rearrangement of the BCL2 gene. Low-grade lymphoma patients have a median survival of 7-15 years.[242] The major factors influencing prognosis include stage, lactic dehydrogenase, and beta2-microglobin level.

High-dose chemotherapy with autologous hematopoietic transplantation has been extensively evaluated for low-grade lymphoma, producing rates of complete remission over 80%. Since these disorders characteristically involve the bone marrow, many studies have used marrow or blood stem-cell autografts depleted of malignant cells by using anti–B-cell monoclonal antibodies, a process which may achieve prolonged remissions.[243,244] Achievement of molecular complete remissions in which BCL2 rearrangement is undetectable by polymerase chain reaction analysis has been associated with prolonged disease-free survival. There is controversy, however, regarding the role of autologous transplantation in this disease. Long-term survival is similar after autologous hematopoietic transplantation and with conservative forms of standard-dose chemotherapy.[245] There is a risk of secondary myelodysplasia and acute leukemia after autotransplants in this disease, particularly in heavily pretreated patients.[246,247]

Allogeneic bone marrow transplantation has also been evaluated in patients with low-grade lymphoma. High-dose cyclophosphamide and TBI, with or without other agents, or BEAM are the most commonly used preparative regimens. Several groups have reported extended disease-free survival in patients with far advanced disease. Relapse rates after allogeneic transplants have been substantially lower than with transplantation of purged autologous transplants, most likely due to the graft-versus-lymphoma effect.[248,249] The recent encouraging results using nonmyeloablative preparative regimens for allogeneic transplantation may reduce the risk of treatment-related mortality; approximately 85% were alive and disease free.[116] This option can be considered for patients after failure of initial chemotherapy.

Mantle cell lymphoma is associated with a poor prognosis. Autologous hematopoietic transplants may be effective in chemoresponsive patients in first remission, but patients with resistant or recurrent disease have a high rate of treatment failure.[250] Allogeneic hematopoietic transplants have been promising in this disease.[251-253] Khouri and colleagues reported a series of 16 patients treated with allogeneic blood or marrow transplantation achieving 55% disease-free survival at 3 years. These preliminary data indicate that allogeneic hematopoietic transplantation using an ablative or nonmyeloablative regimen can induce durable remission in patients with mantle cell lymphoma. Allogeneic transplantation appears promising in patients who fail to respond to initial chemotherapy or relapse; its role in newly diagnosed patients needs to be determined. Further clinical trials are needed.

Intermediate- and high-grade lymphomas are aggressive malignancies with a short natural history in the absence of effective therapy. These disorders are responsive to combination chemotherapy, and a fraction of patients achieve durable remissions. Standard chemotherapy for large cell lymphoma results in cure in approximately 40-60% for newly diagnosed patients with diffuse large cell lymphoma. High-, intermediate- and low-risk groups have been defined.

High-dose chemotherapy and autologous transplantation improve cure rates for patients with recurrent large cell lymphoma who respond to salvage chemotherapy.[254,255] The Parma study randomized patients younger than 60 years, with chemosensitive relapse and no marrow or CNS involvement, either to continued salvage chemotherapy or to high-dose chemotherapy and autologous bone marrow transplantation.[256] The 5-year event-free survival was 46% in the transplant group, and 12% in the standard chemotherapy group; overall survival was also improved. Autologous hematopoietic transplantation can therefore be considered the preferred treatment for that group of patients. Patients with chemotherapy resistant disease and those with multiple relapses have poor results, with less than 20% durable remissions.

Patients achieving only a partial response to initial chemotherapy are rarely cured with chemotherapy and are appropriate candidates for autologous HCT; however, patients who continue to progress through initial treatment only rarely achieve prolonged remission if autologous hematopoietic transplantation is attempted at that time.[257] One study showed that patients with a slow antitumor response might do as well with continuing induction chemotherapy as those with early hematopoietic transplant.[258]

High-dose chemotherapy with autologous hematopoietic transplantation has also been studied in high-risk patients with intermediate-grade lymphoma in first remission. Two studies reported that high-dose chemotherapy with autologous hematopoietic transplantation improved event-free survival of patients with intermediate or high-risk prognostic features,[259,260] but other studies failed to confirm this benefit.[261] Ongoing clinical trials are addressing this issue.

High-dose therapy with allogeneic transplantation has been examined in a number of phase 1 and 2 studies in patients with intermediate- or highgrade lymphoma. Several studies reported a decreased recurrence rate compared to autologous transplants, but the benefit is off-set by higher rates of treatment-related mortality.[261] Many physicians have reserved allotransplantation for patients having a poor prognosis with alternative modalities, such as a relatively poor response to chemotherapy, or patients in which autologous transplants were not feasible.

Hodgkin Disease

Hodgkin disease is a chemotherapy responsive malignancy, but 20-30% of patients with advanced disease may fail to achieve complete remission and approximately one-third of responders will subsequently relapse. For patients with recurrent Hodgkin disease, high-dose chemotherapy and autologous hematopoietic transplantation results in a complete remission rate of 50-80% and a 40-60% disease-free survival at 3-5 years post-transplant.[263-265] The BEAM and cyclophosphamide carmustine etoposide preparative regimens have been most frequently used. Numerous phase 2 studies have suggested that high-dose chemotherapy improves disease-free survival and possibly overall survival compared to standard chemotherapy in this setting.

Patients recurring after an initial remission that is shorter than 1 year have superior disease-free survival with high-dose chemotherapy compared to standard dose-salvage treatment, and most researchers recommend high-dose therapy for those patients. Controversy remains regarding patients with a long first remission. For patients in second or subsequent relapse and considered incurable with standard dose chemotherapy, autologous transplantation is recommended.

Patients who fail to achieve complete remission with initial chemotherapy have a poor outcome; however, 20-40% can be salvaged by autologous transplant. Patients with partial response fare better than patients with bulky progressive disease.

Late relapses and a high incidence of secondary myelodysplasia (approximately 15%) continue to be major problems among long-term survivors. Late infections and cardiac and pulmonary toxicity may also occur.

Relatively few allogeneic transplants have been performed in patients with Hodgkin disease.[266] High-dose therapy with allogeneic transplantation is associated with a high treatment-related mortality in patients with Hodgkin disease, exceeding 50% in some studies. Studies of patients with advanced disease not suitable for autologous transplant have shown a 15-20% salvage rate with HLA-matched sibling trans-plantation. Use of nonmyeloablative regimens to reduce treatment-related mortality is currently being investigated, and the preliminary results are encouraging.[267,268]

Multiple Myeloma

Multiple myeloma is a common hematologic malignancy that occurs in increasing frequently with advancing age. Standard chemotherapy can control the disease for variable periods, but even with newer regimens containing thalidomide and bortezimib only 20-30%% achieve complete remission, and the median survival is approximately 6 years.[269] In a randomized study of newly diagnosed multiple-myeloma patients, high-dose chemoradiotherapy with autologous hematopoietic transplantation was superior to standard chemotherapy[270]; 52% of the patients randomized to the transplant were alive and 28% were progression free at 5 years, compared to 12% and 10%, respectively, for the standard chemotherapy group. High-dose chemotherapy with autologous hematopoietic transplantation is now considered standard treatment for patients with intermediate or high-tumor-mass multiple myeloma. High-dose therapy and autologous transplantation delays relapse, but is not curative, and almost all patients ultimately develop recurrent disease.

Chemosensitivity of the tumor is a major determinant of transplant outcome. Patients with chemosensitive disease who received transplants within the first year had a more favorable outcome, and 40-50% may achieve CR. Encouraging results have also been achieved in patients with primary refractory disease if transplanted early in the course of disease,[271,272] but treatment is of only limited value in advanced resistant disease, and especially in patients with refractory relapse.[273] Advanced age, high beta2-microglobulin level, and cytogenetic abnormalities involving chromosome 13 are the most prominent adverse prognostic factors.[274,275]

With the introduction of peripheral blood progenitor cell transplants and better supportive care, autologous hematopoietic transplants have become considerably safer. Treatment-related mortality is typically less than 1-2%, even for elderly patients up to 70 years of age. The most common regimen used includes high-dose melphalan. A recent randomized trial failed to demonstrate any advantage with the addition of TBI to high-dose melphalan. The use of two sequential (or tandem) transplants has been explored in a French study. Patients randomized to one transplant had poorer relapse-free and overall survival than patients treated with the tandem method.[276] Unplanned subgroup analysis suggests that the tandem technique primarily benefited patients achieving a partial but not complete remission with the first transplant.

The timing of autologous transplant remains controversial. Most studies have suggested a better outcome when autologous hematopoietic transplantation is performed early, within 1 year of diagnosis. Others advocate early collection of stem cells, but delaying high-dose chemotherapy itself to subsequent progression. A randomized French study of early versus late transplant did not show any survival difference, but patients randomized to early transplant enjoyed longer periods of time without a need for chemotherapy.[277] Improved treatment for cytoreduction is needed. Novel approaches include investigation of tumor vaccines,[278] and post-transplant maintenance treatment.

Allogeneic hematopoietic transplants using full-intensity treatment have been studied, primarily in young patients with myeloma who have relapsed or progressed during standard chemotherapy.[279] Allogeneic transplantation provides a tumor-free graft and also an immune graft-versus-myeloma effect. Relapse occurs almost invariably after autologous HCT, but may be less common after allogeneic transplant. Donor lymphocyte infusions have reinduced remission in a few patients relapsing after allogeneic transplant, consistent with the presence of a graft-versus-myeloma effect.[280,281] However, the reduced relapse rate is offset by a high treatment related mortality rate approaching 50% in heavily pretreated myeloma patients. Three-year progression-free survival is approximately 30-40%. Most comparative studies have shown that autologous transplants have a better overall survival than allografts, at least during the first few years after transplant.[282,283] Encouraging results have recently been reported using an autologous transplant for tumor cytoreduction followed by an nonablative allogeneic transplant several months later to induce an immune graft-versus-myeloma effect. A recent randomized trial comparing sequential auto-auto transplants to auto-allo transplant (the latter using nonablative treatment) suggests superiority of the auto-allo technique for younger patients.[284] Other plasma cell dyscrasias have also been effectively treated with high-dose melphalan and autologous hematopoietic transplantation. Amyloidosis may benefit, but results of recent studies are conflicting.[285]

Solid Tumors

High-dose chemotherapy with autologous hematopoietic transplantation has been studied in a number of chemotherapy responsive solid tumors to exploit the dose-response effects of many chemotherapeutic agents. Breast cancer has been the most common disease treated by high-dose chemotherapy and autologous transplantation. There remains, however, considerable controversy regarding the efficacy of high-dose therapy in this disease and the role of hematopoietic transplant based therapies and their use at this time should be considered investigational. Patients with metastatic breast cancer achieve a higher complete remission rate following autologous transplantation than with reported conventional treatments. Whether additional treatments can prolong the complete response duration is the subject of ongoing research.

Relapse remains a major problem and use of biologic or immunologic therapies for minimal residual breast cancer after autologous transplantation needs to be evaluated.[35] Clinical studies using allogeneic transplantation are exploring the potential of graft-versus-malignancy effect in this disease.

Dose-intensive chemotherapy has been explored for treating ovarian cancer.[286-288] Like breast cancer, this tumor is sensitive to alkylating agents, platinum-based chemotherapy agents, taxanes, and topoisomerase I inhibitors. Transplants have not been used commonly in the adjuvant setting, but may have a role for patients with low-bulk disease after a second-look laparotomy and for patients with chemotherapy-sensitive low-bulk relapsed disease. Randomized trials haved failed to demonstrate benefit in several clinical settings, but most have tested regimens that would be considered suboptimal by modern standards.

A similar approach with autologous transplantation has been used for the treatment of other chemotherapy-responsive solid tumors in adults, including testicular or germ cell carcinomas, and small cell carcinoma of the lung. Testicular carcinoma is a chemotherapy-responsive malignancy that is frequently cured using standard chemotherapy. Patients failing first- and secondline chemotherapy regimens have received highdose chemotherapy and autologous transplants. Response rates are high, and a fraction have achieved long-term remissions.[289]

Autologous transplants have been 24 studied in small cell lung cancer.[290] Patients with extensive disease or relapsed carcinoma have generally had only brief responses and modest clinical benefit. Better results have been obtained as consolidation therapy for patients with limited small cell lung cancer with prolongation of remission duration in some studies. Few patients are long-term survivors, and the efficacy of this approach remains to be established.

Autologous transplants have been studied in a range of pediatric solid tumors such as neuroblastoma and Ewing sarcoma, tumors that are highly sensitive to chemotherapy and irradiation, yet have a poor prognosis in patients with advanced disease.[291,292]

Allogeneic hematopoietic transplants have recently been studied in renal cell carcinoma. Nonablative allogeneic transplantation has been studied as a means to induce the immunotherapeutic graft-versus-tumor effect and approximately 40% of patients with metastatic disease have achieved complete and partial responses.[293]

Most responses have occurred in patients with graft-versus-host disease and after withdrawal of immunosuppressive therapy. Ongoing research is directed at identifying the target antigens for this graft-versus-tumor effect.

Nonmalignant Indications

Aplastic anemia (AA) is an uncommon disease producing primary bone marrow failure with pancytopenia and hypocellular bone marrow. Severe aplastic anemia is defined as marrow cellularity of less than 25%, with either neutrophil count <0.5 × 10^9/L, platelet count <20 × 10^9/L, or total reticulocyte count <40 × 10^9/L. Without effective therapy, more than 50% of patients with severe AA may die within 6 months of diagnosis. Effective treatments for AA include immunosuppressive therapy (such as cyclosporine and ATG)[294] and hematopoietic transplantation.

Historically, graft rejection was a major complication of allogeneic transplantation for AA, occurring in up to 30% of recipients.[295] Multiple blood transfusions may sensitize the recipient against the donor and increase the risk of rejection. Cyclophosphamide alone or in combination with ATG is the most commonly used preparative regimen for bone marrow transplantation from a matched sibling donor.[296] Late graft rejection may occur after the post-transplant immunosuppression is withdrawn. With current regimens, early transplant, a judicious transfusion policy, and improved supportive care systems, less than 10% reject the grafts and long-term survival can be achieved in 80-90% of recipients of marrow from an HLA-matched sibling donor.

Hematopoietic transplantation from a partially matched related donor or a phenotypically matched unrelated donor requires additional immunosuppression for prevention of rejection, but the mode and dose have not been established.[297,298] Fewer than 50% are long-term survivors.[299,300]

Several studies have compared the effectiveness of allogeneic transplantation and immunosuppressive therapy. Most studies have shown a survival advantage for patients younger than 40 who have allogeneic transplantation from an HLA-matched sibling. Immunosuppressive therapy has a higher risk for late complications, such as relapse or development of myelodysplasia or AML. However, for patients above age 40-50, there is a higher risk of complications with allogeneic transplantation, and it should be reserved for those who fail immunosuppressive therapy. Patients lacking an HLA-identical related donor should receive a trial of immunosuppressive therapy; alternative donor transplants should be considered only in those who fail to respond.

Allogeneic bone marrow transplantation is also an effective treatment for paroxysmal nocturnal hemoglobinuria and other nonmalignant bone marrow failure states.[301]

Congenital Metabolic and Immune Disorders

■ Allogeneic transplantation is a potentially curative treatment in a number of congenital disorders of the hematopoietic and immune systems. Thalassemia[302] and sickle cell anemia[303] are among the most common nonmalignant hematological disorders curable with transplant. Results in patients with thalassemia have been more favorable when performed early, and in patients who are not heavily transfused and with no sign of severe hepatic iron overload or portal fibrosis. Most patients received busulfan and cyclophosphamide to avoid the many toxic effects of TBI in young children. Fanconi anemia has been treated similarly to aplastic anemia, but with very low-dose conditioning regimen due to the known sensitivity of these patients to the effects of irradiation and alkylating agents.[304,305] Patients are not cured of the non-hematologic manifestations of the disease, and many develop secondary solid tumors.

Allogeneic transplantation has been the treatment of choice for infants with severe combined immunodeficiency.[306] Engraftment can be achieved in many patients even without conditioning in this disorder. Allogeneic transplantation has been able to reverse the bone sclerosis in osteopetrosis.[307] The results in storage diseases have been inconsistent.[308] T-cell depletion may be useful in preventing GVHD. For patients without a matched sibling, both unrelated donor transplants, or mismatched related transplants have been successful.[309] In most disorders outcome was better when transplants were given early, and promising results have been reported for transplants in utero.[310] In the future, gene modification of autologous cells may be a curative approach for some of these disorders.[311]

There has been increasing interest over the last few years in autologous transplantation with or without T-cell depletion of the graft for the treatment of autoimmune disorders.[312] The goal is to ablate the abnormal immune response and reconstitute immunity from hematopoietic stem cells and progenitors. Encouraging results have been reported in a limited number of patients with rheumatoid arthritis, systemic lupus erythematosus, multiple sclerosis, myasthenia gravis, and other disorders.[5]

Future Directions

Over the last decade hematopoietic transplantation has become a much safer procedure, applicable to a larger patient population in a variety of disease processes. The use of hematopoietic transplantation is likely to evolve with the development of molecularly directed anticancer therapies and with improved methods to selectively target and modulate immunity. Targeted radiation therapies, such as monoclonal antibody–radionuclide immunoconjugates and bone-seeking isotopes, are under active evaluation as a means to target radiotherapy to the tumor; this approach has little systemic toxicity other than myelosuppression. It may be possible to further improve results by using strategies to overcome drug resistance mechanisms, strategies such as administration of inhibitors DNA repair processes, glutathione conjugation, or other mechanisms of drug resistance.

The graft-versus-malignancy effect associated with allogeneic transplants illustrates the capability of the immune system in eradicating cancer. Strategies to enhance immune antitumor mechanisms with both allogeneic and autologous transplants are under active investigation. The major goal is to separate the beneficial graft-versus-malignancy effect from the graft-versus-host disease. Tumor vaccines have been generated by ex vivo transfection of tumors with genes (to improve presentation of antigens), costimulatory molecules, and various cytokines to enhance the immune response directed against the tumor. Autologous antigen-presenting cells either pulsed with tumor antigens or used by themselves when they originate from the malignant clone, have also been used in vitro or in vivo to stimulate and expand cytotoxic T lymphocytes and other effectors for cellular immunotherapy. Ongoing research efforts seek to generate antigen-specific immune cells directed against tumors and major pathogens, but sparing normal donor tissues.

In the allogeneic transplant setting, efforts are directed at expanding the donor pool, reducing the toxicity of the procedure, and improving the methods to deliver immunotherapy. The majority of patients who are candidates for allogeneic transplant do not have an HLA-matched sibling donor. Further development of international unrelated donor registries for bone marrow, blood stem cells, and cord blood will increase the likelihood of finding a well-matched donor. Special attention is given to representation of ethnic minorities in these registries. New molecular methods to improve the precision of histocompatibility matching may decrease the risk of rejection and GVHD. Another approach is to use related partially matched donors. The risk of graft failure and GVHD can been minimized by infusions of large numbers of stem cells and aggressive T-cell depletion, but this type of transplant is still limited by delayed immune reconstitution after transplant and high risk of infections. Strategies are being investigated to find ways to delete alloreactive T-cell subsets, but retain subsets that contribute to graft facilitation, GVL, and infection control. Methods to improve the engraftment speed of umbilical cord blood transplants hopefully will decrease the risk of this procedure.

Considerable progress has been achieved in supportive care to make allogeneic transplants increasingly safe over time by preventing infections and transplant-related complications. The finding that GVL is responsible for much of the therapeutic potential of allogeneic transplants has opened the way for the use of nonmyeloablative regimens as a means to allow engraftment of donor cells with reduced toxicity. Providing GVL as the primary treatment requires carefully planned prospective clinical trials to define the role of this strategy, the diseases, and the patient population for which it will be useful.

Selected References

The complete reference list can be found at www.CANCERMEDICINE8.com

1. Thomas ED, Storb R, Clift RA, et al. Bone-marrow transplantation (second of two parts). *N Engl J Med.* 1975;292:895902.
3. Thomas ED, Buckner CD, Banaji M, et al. One hundred patients with acute leukemia treated by chemotherapy, total body irradiation, and allogeneic marrow transplantation. *Blood.* 1977;49:511–533.
5. Burt RK, Traynor AE, Pope R, et al. Treatment of autoimmune disease by intense immunosuppressive conditioning and autologous hematopoietic stem cell transplantation. *Blood.* 1998;92:3505–3514.
17. Korbling M, Katz RL, Khanna A, et al. Hepatocytes and epithelial cells of donor origin in recipients of peripheralblood stem cells. *N Engl J Med.* 2002;346:738–746.
24. Slavin S, Morecki S, Weiss L, Or R. Donor lymphocyte infusion: the use of alloreactive and tumor-reactive lymphocytes for immunotherapy of malignant and nonmalignant diseases in conjunction with allogeneic stem cell transplantation. *J Hematother Stem Cell Res.* 2002;11:265–276.
41. Attal M, Harousseau J-L, Stoppa A-M, et al. A prospective, randomized trial of autologous bone marrow transplantation and chemotherapy in multiple myeloma. *N Engl J Med.* 1996;335:91–97.
49. Gale RP, Horowitz MM, Ash RC, et al. Identical-twin bone marrow transplants for leukemia. *Ann Intern Med.* 1994;120:646–652.
53. Collins RH Jr, Rogers ZR, Bennett M, et al. Hematologic relapse of chronic myelogenous leukemia following allogeneic bone marrow transplantation: apparent graft-versus leukemia effect following abrupt discontinuation of immunosuppression. *Bone Marrow Transplant.* 1992;10:391–395.
54. Kolb HJ, Schattenberg A, Goldman JM, et al. Graft-versus leukemia effect of donor lymphocyte transfusions in marrow grafted patients. European Group for Blood and Marrow Transplantation Working Party Chronic Leukemia. *Blood.* 1995;86:2041–2050.
58. Collins RH Jr, Goldstein S, Giralt S, et al. Donor leukocyte infusions in acute lymphocytic leukemia. *Bone Marrow Transplant.* 2000;26:511–516.
63. Petersdorf EW, Mickelson EM, Anasetti C, et al. Effect of HLA mismatches on the outcome of hematopoietic transplants. *Curr Opin Immunol.* 1999;11:521–526.
67. Aversa F, Tabilio A, Terenzi A, et al. Successful engraftment of T-cell-depleted haploidentical "three-loci" incompatible transplants in leukemia patients by addition of recombinant human granulocyte colony-stimulating factor mobilized peripheral blood progenitor cells to bone marrow inoculum. *Blood.* 1994;84:3948–3955.
70. Laughlin MJ, Eapen M, Rubinstein P, et al. Outcomes after transplantation of cord blood or bone marrow from unrelated donors in adults with leukemia. *N Engl J Med.* 2004;351:2265–2275.
75. Rowley SD, Bensinger WI, Gooley TA, Buckner CD. Effect of cell concentration on bone marrow and peripheral blood stem cell cryopreservation. *Blood.* 1994;83:2731–2736.
77. Gribben JG, Freedman AS, Neuberg D, et al. Immunologic purging of marrow assessed by PCR before autologous bone marrow transplantation for B-cell lymphoma. *N Engl J Med.* 1991;325:1525–1533.
93. Rubinstein P, Carrier C, Scaradavou A, et al. Outcomes among 562 recipients of placental-blood transplants from unrelated donors. *N Engl J Med.* 1998;339:1565–1577.
99. Bensinger W, Appelbaum F, Rowley S, et al. Factors that influence collection and engraftment of autologous peripheralblood stem cells. *J Clin Oncol.* 1995;13:2547–2555.
104. Champlin R, Khouri I, Komblau S, et al. Reinventing bone marrow transplantation. Nonmyeloablative preparative regimens and induction of graft-vs-malignancy effect. *Oncology (Huntingt).* 1999;13:621–628.
107. Chopra R, McMillan AK, Linch DC, et al. The place of highdose BEAM therapy and autologous bone marrow transplantation in poor-risk Hodgkin's disease. A single-center eight-year study of 155 patients. *Blood.* 1993;81:1137–1145.
115. Giralt S, Estey E, Albitar M, et al. Engraftment of allogeneic hematopoietic progenitor cells with purine analog-containing chemotherapy: harnessing graft-vs-leukemia without myeloablative therapy. *Blood.* 1997;89:4531–4536.
117. Kernan NA, Bordignon C, Heller G, et al. Graft failure after T-cell-depleted human leukocyte antigen identical marrow transplants for leukemia: I. Analysis of risk factors and results of secondary transplants. *Blood.* 1989;74:2227–2236.
127. Ferrara JL, Deeg HJ. Graft-versus-host disease. *N Engl J Med.* 1991;324:667–674.
134. Storb R, Pepe M, Deeg HJ, et al. Long-term follow-up of a controlled trial comparing a combination of methotrexate plus cyclosporine with cyclosporine alone for prophylaxis of graft-versus-host disease in patients administered HLA-identical marrow grafts for leukemia. *Blood.* 1992;80:560–561.
147. Schulman HM, Hinterberger W. Hepatic veno-occlusive disease- liver toxicity syndrome after bone marrow transplantation. *Bone Marrow Transplant.* 1992;10:197–214.
149. Jones RB, Matthes S, Shpall EJ, et al. Acute lung injury following high-dose cyclophosphamide, cisplatin and BCNU. Pharmacodynamic evaluation of BCNU. *J Natl Cancer Inst.* 1993;85:640–647.
161. Brochu S, Rioux-Masse B, Roy J, et al. Massive activation induced cell death of alloreactive T cells with apoptosis of bystander

post-thymic T cells prevents immune reconstitution in mice with graft-versus-host disease. *Blood*. 1999;94:390–400.

168. Armitage JO. Myelodysplasia and acute leukemia after autologous bone marrow transplantation. *J Clin Oncol*. 2000;18:945–946.
169. Clift RA, Buckner CD. Marrow transplantation for acute myeloid leukemia. *Cancer Invest*. 1998;16:53–61.
188. Deeg HJ, Shulman HM, Anderson JE, et al. Allogeneic and syngeneic marrow transplantation for myelodysplastic syndrome in patients 55 to 66 years of age. *Blood*. 2000;95:1188–1194.
191. Yakoub-Agha I, de La SP, Ribaud P, et al. Allogeneic bone marrow transplantation for therapy-related myelodysplastic syndrome and acute myeloid leukemia: a longterm study of 70 patients-report of the French society of bone marrow transplantation. *J Clin Oncol*. 2000;18:963–971.
206. Champlin R, Gale RP. Acute lymphoblastic leukemia: recent advances in biology and therapy. *Blood*. 1989;73:2051–2066.
214. Thomas ED, Clift RA. Indications for marrow transplantation in chronic myelogenous leukemia. *Blood*. 1989;73:861–864.
220. Dazzi F, Szydlo RM, Craddock C, et al. Comparison of single-dose and escalating-dose regimens of donor lymphocyte infusion for relapse after allografting for chronic myeloid leukemia. *Blood*. 2000;95:67–71.
223. Przepiorka D, Giralt S, Khouri I, et al. Allogeneic marrow transplantation for myeloproliferative disorders other than chronic myelogenous leukemia: review of forty cases. *Am J Hematol*. 1998;57:24–28.
236. Khouri I, Champlin R. Allogenic bone marrow transplantation in chronic lymphocytic leukemia. *Ann Intern Med*. 1996;125:780.
240. Rondon G, Giralt S, Huh Y, et al. Graft-vs-leukemia effect after allogeneic bone marrow transplantation for chronic lymphocytic leukemia. *Bone Marrow Transplant*. 1996;18:669–672.
245. Johnson PW, Rohatiner AZ, Whelan JS, et al. Patterns of survival in patients with recurrent follicular lymphoma: a 20-year study from a single center. *J Clin Oncol*. 1995;13:140–147.
251. Khouri IF, Lee MS, Romaguera J, et al. Allogeneic hematopoietic transplantation for mantle-cell lymphoma: molecular remissions and evidence of graft-versusmalignancy. *Ann Oncol*. 1999;10:1293–1299.
256. Philip T, Guglielmi C, Hagenbeek A, et al. Autologous bone marrow transplantation as compared with salvage chemotherapy in relapses of chemotherapy-sensitive non-Hodgkin's lymphoma. *N Engl J Med*. 1995;333:1540–1545.
263. Bierman PJ, Vose JM, Armitage JO. Autologous transplantation for Hodgkin's disease: coming of age? *Blood*. 1994;83:1161–1164.
276. Moreau P, Hullin C, Garban F et al. Tandem autologous stem cell transplantation in high-risk de nove multiple myeloma: final results of the prospective and randomized IFM 99-04 protocol. *Blood*. 2006;107(1):397–403.
284. Bruno B, Rotta M, Patriarca F, et al. A comparison of allografting and autografting for newly diagnosed myeloma. *N Engl J Med*. 2007;356(11):1110–1120.
289. Nichols CR, Rosti G. Dose-intensive therapy for germ cell neoplasms. *Semin Oncol*. 1992;19(1 Suppl 2):145–149.
291. Matthay KK, O'Leary MC, Ramsay NK, et al. Role of myeloablative therapy in improved outcome for high risk neuroblastoma: review of recent Children's Cancer Group results. *Eur J Cancer*. 1995;31A:572–575.
293. Childs RW, Clave E, Tisdale J, et al. Successful treatment of metastatic renal cell carcinoma with a nonmyeloablative allogeneic peripheral-blood progenitor-cell transplant: evidence for a graft-versus-tumor effect. *J Clin Oncol*. 1999;17:2044–2049.
294. Bacigalupo A, Bruno B, Saracco P, et al. Antilymphocyte globulin, cyclosporine, prednisolone, and granulocyte colony-stimulating factor for severe aplastic anemia: an update of the GITMO/EBMT study on 100 patients. European Group for Blood and Marrow Transplantation (EBMT) Working Party on Severe Aplastic Anemia and the Gruppo Italiano Trapianti di Midolio Osseo (GITMO). *Blood*. 2000;95:1931–1934.
301. Saso R, Marsh J, Cevreska L, et al. Bone marrow transplants for paroxysmal nocturnal haemoglobinuria. *Br J Haematol*. 1999;104:392–396.
303. Walters MC, Storb R, Patience M, et al. Impact of bone marrow transplantation for symptomatic sickle cell disease: an interim report. Multi-center investigation of bone marrow transplantation for sickle cell disease. *Blood*. 2000;95:1918–1924.
308. Krivit W, Lockman LA, Watkins PA, et al. The future for treatment by bone marrow transplantation for adrenoleukodystrophy, met achromatic leukodystrophy, globoid cell leukodystrophy and Hurler syndrome. *J Inherit Metab Dis*. 1995;18:398–412.

62 Principles of Psycho-Oncology

Jimmie C. Holland, MD ▪ Talia R. Weiss, BA

We are not ourselves when nature, being oppressed, commands the mind to suffer with the body.

King Lear, Act II, Sc. IV

Introduction

Quality-of-life (QOL) and patient-reported outcomes (PROs), have received increasing attention in recent years. More concern has also been directed toward recognizing and treating the distressed patient or family member. Stresses on oncologists have also been identified, particularly the effect of constant confrontation with serious illness and death. Research is more actively exploring social, behavioral, and psychological contributions to cancer prevention, early detection, survival, and palliative care. Psycho-oncology has emerged since 1975 as a subspecialty of oncology. An extensive body of literature and information is now available, training programs exist, a research agenda has been formulated, and evidence-based clinical practice guidelines have been developed through the National Cancer Center Network.[1] In 2006 the National Institutes of Health (NIH) requested the Institute of Medicine (IOM) of the National Academies of Sciences to "empanel a committee to conduct a study on the delivery of psychosocial services to patients with cancer in the community and barriers to access." It noted that American medical treatment for cancer is arguably the best in the world, however, psychosocial services have lagged significantly behind. In November 2007 the IOM published an independent evidence-based report stating that quality cancer care today must integrate the psychosocial domain into routine cancer care. This report titled *Cancer Care for the Whole Patient: Meeting Psychosocial Health Needs* gives new credibility to the field and its clinical interventions.[2-4] (For a free online summary of the report go to http://www.nap.edu/catalog.php?record id=11993.)

Psycho-oncology addresses the two psychological dimensions of cancer: first, the psychological response to cancer at all stages of disease, of patients, their families, and the medical team. The patient and physician relationship, dependent on effective communication, impacts the care of all patients, at every visit, at all sites and stages of cancer, and during all treatments. The second dimension addresses psychological, behavioral, and social factors that influence cancer risk, detection, treatment adherence and survival. Clinicians and clinical investigators, from psychology, psychiatry, social work, nursing and clergy, comprise the multidisciplinary psychosocial teams existing in many cancer centers and hospitals. These teams provide consultation, teach psychosocial issues to oncology staff, raise awareness of this dimension of care, and collaborate in studies in which QOL is important. Also, the biopsychosocial model incorporates the active research which is presently examining the role of cytokines in producing "sickness behavior" which provides a biological basis for several common symptoms of fatigue, depression, anxiety, weakness, and cognitive changes in cancer patients.[5-8]

Most cancer centers and oncology divisions now have a psycho-oncology or psychosocial unit whose role is to treat distressed patients and family members, and to serve as a psychosocial resource for oncology staff. Only a few centers have programs that include research and training. Trained volunteers, particularly those who have had a personal experience with cancer, often play an important role. Advocacy organizations, such as the National Coalition for Cancer Survivors (NCCS) and disease-specific organizations are collaborating with the American Psychosocial Oncology Society (APOS), the only multidisciplinary national organization representing this subspecialty of oncology, to address health policy barriers to quality care which integrates the psychosocial component in routine care (website: www.apos.org).

This chapter describes the development of psycho-oncology, the psychiatric disorders and common psychosocial problems experienced by cancer patients, the range of therapeutic interventions available, and the research directions to improve the quality of science and clinical practice of psycho-oncology.[9]

Historical Perspective

The stigma that cancer equals death, which has been attached to the disease for centuries, led to the longstanding custom of not revealing the diagnosis of cancer to patients. To tell the cancer diagnosis was considered cruel and was viewed as robbing the patient of hope (Table 62-1). For centuries, lack of available or effective treatment resulted in a sense of futility and helplessness as physicians and patients awaited the inevitable outcome of death. The advent of anesthesia and antisepsis led to surgical resection of some tumors which resulted in cure of early lesions. Near the end of the nineteenth century, and early in the twentieth century, it became important to counter the public's fatalistic attitudes since surgical cure was possible, if the cancer was detected in an early stage. The American Cancer Society was formed in 1913 to educate the public of the warning symptoms of cancer and to reduce their immobilizing fears. The combination of radiation and surgery achieved more definitive cures. The establishment of the National Cancer Institute (NCI) in 1937 reflected new enthusiasm for seeking a cause and cure of cancer. The addition of chemotherapy to the combined modalities beginning in the 1950s resulted in the cure of several tumors of childhood and early adulthood. By 1975, there was an increased interest in medical and psychological outcomes of long-term survivors of cancer which provided the first opportunity for exploring patients' psychological responses to cancer. Around the same time, physicians began to tell patients their diagnosis and discuss their treatment options.

By the early 1970s, as survival improved and patients became more willing to reveal their cancer diagnosis physicians became more comfortable discussing the diagnosis with patients, and the importance of a doctor-patient dialogue became clearer. Concurrently, concern for more humane care of patients at the end-of-life was seen, with the development of the hospice movement with greater interest in pain management and palliative care. Greater openness in revealing the diagnosis, increased concern for

Table 62-1 Historical Attitudes About Cancer and Development of Psycho-Oncology

1800s	Prevailing attitude was cancer equals death; fatalistic acceptance of diagnosis; diagnosis never revealed to patient
1900–20	American Cancer Society formed to fight fatalism and educate public that early treatment by surgery could be curative
1937	National Cancer Institute formed to seek a cure for cancer
1950s	First studies of psychological response to cancer reported
1960s	Combined modalities lead to increased survival in Hodgkin disease, ALL and childhood tumors
1960–70	Debate about telling or not telling diagnosis and change to revealing the diagnosis; federally mandated guidelines for informed consent
1979	*Handbook of Psycho-oncology*, Oxford University Press
1980	Prevalence studies of psychiatric and psychological sequelae in cancer Psycho-oncology units develop in larger cancer centers Education of public about lifestyle and cancer prevention; behavioral research in changing habits (eg, smoking), diet, and lifestyle Development of the International Psycho-oncology Society (1984) Establishment of the American Psycho-oncology Society (1986) (made a multidisciplinary organization in 2002)
1989	*Oxford Textbook of Psycho-oncology*
1990	Health-related Quality of Life assessment was accepted as an outcome measure in clinical trials Intervention studies undertaken to impact quality of life and reduce distress
1992	*International Psycho-oncology Journal began*
2000	Standards for psychosocial care developed and clinical practice treatment guidelines for management of common types of psychiatric disorders and psychosocial forms of distress Exploration of genetic factors in vulnerability to fatigue; and cognitive dysfunction with chemotherapy; biologic contribution of proinflamatory cytokines to symptoms of fatigue, depression, and cognitive problems
2006	Quick reference for oncology clinicians: psychiatric and psychological dimensions, IPOS Press
2007	Publication of the Institute of Medicine Report: cancer care for the whole patient: meeting psychosocial health needs
2008	Formation of the Federation of Psycho-oncology National Societies in the International Psycho-oncology Society (IPOS)

palliative care, and enhanced concern about QOL and patient-centered medicine led to more attention for the supportive and psychologic aspects of care. Evidence of the link between cigarette smoking and lung cancer gave new impetus to examine the role of psychological and behavioral factors in cancer prevention.

Around this same period, psychosomatic medicine developed within the field of psychiatry, leading to a powerful movement that sought to identify psychological factors as the major cause of several chronic diseases, particularly asthma, peptic ulcer, rheumatoid arthritis, and cancer. Although these suppositions were not substantiated, attitudes of the public led cancer patients to fear they had "caused their own cancer." Beliefs such as this led to "blaming the victim" which made coping with cancer more difficult.

By 1980, researchers were prepared to study the psychological challenges of patients with cancer. Valid tools to assess these variables were few, however, early investigators needed to develop new instruments or to modify tools originally developed to assess patients with major psychiatric disorders. Investigators with knowledge of research methods in both cancer and social science were limited. Nevertheless, a small group of investigators largely associated with a few cancer centers around the world, primarily in the United States, the United Kingdom, and Sweden, began to study prevalence of psychiatric comorbidity in cancer, and to address key psychosocial questions. The first national meeting of psycho-oncology researchers was sponsored by the NCI in 1976.[10] The field continued to grow as these groups developed training programs for young clinicians and investigators. Today, there are approximately 5000 professionals internationally who network through the Federation of Psycho-oncology Societies of the International Psycho-oncology Society (www.ipos-societv.org). This brief history underscores the relative youth of psycho-oncology and exhibits the degree to which historical attitudes and stigma toward both cancer and mental disorders have contributed to the reluctance of patients to identify their emotional problems to their oncologists, even today.

Common Psychological Responses

Reactions to Diagnosis of Cancer

Patients often respond with anxiety and dread when they recognize that tests are being done to rule out cancer. If the doctor delivers the news that the diagnosis *is* cancer, an existential crisis occurs which requires an individual to call upon all inner psychological resources to cope. The common concerns can be remembered as 4 Ds: death (with pain), disability, dependence on others, and disfigurement (physical changes in body). *How* the doctor delivers the bad news is a factor in the patient's response. Insensitivity or lack of empathy in giving bad news is often recalled years later by patients and their caregivers. The importance of good communication skills is a critical aspect of quality cancer care.[11] Research has given rise to practice guidelines to optimize the delivery of distressing information, to develop empathetic listening and response skills, and to present a treatment plan that reflects an understanding of an individual patient's needs.[12-16]

Our society avoids thinking about death, but the first thought on learning a cancer diagnosis is frequently, "I could die of this." This creates both a psychological and an existential crisis. The person seeks to cope with the challenge and to maintain emotional control. This is often done by trying to put the information in a context that yields a tolerable meaning.[17-19] Park and Folkman (1997) described how stressful information is processed cognitively by individuals, first by confronting the situation and changing it if possible. When the diagnosis is cancer and it cannot be changed, the person searches all alternatives and finally chooses a course of treatment that is consistent with his or her own values and life goals.[17] For some, searching for meaning in the situation may result in exploring prior religious, spiritual, or philosophical beliefs that give a context in which the threat to life and the possibility of death can be more readily accepted.[17,20]

The diagnosis creates a period of expected crisis and normal emotional upheaval (Table 62-2).[2] The initial phase is often characterized by disbelief and denial that the news is true: "They must have mixed up the slides." High anxiety levels make it hard to process information, at the very time that critical treat-

Table 62-2 Normal Responses to Crises Encountered With Cancer

Phase	Symptoms	Time Interval
Phase I: initial response	Disbelief or denial or despair ("I knew it all along")	Usually less than 1 week
Phase II: dysphoria	Anxiety, depressed mood, anorexia, insomnia, poor concentration, inability to function	Usually 1-2 weeks, but varies
Phase III: adaptation	Accepts validity of information and begins dealing with treatment options available. Finds reasons for optimism and resumes usual activities	Usually by 2 weeks, but adaptation continues over months; may or may not be successful

ment decisions must be made. Feeling "numb" and being unable to concentrate may require that information must be repeated several times.

Phase II of response to the diagnosis is usually characterized by emotional turmoil and dysphoria during which the reality is slowly acknowledged. The person is anxious and depressed, has a short attention span, anorexia and insomnia, and inability to maintain daily activities. Thoughts of illness and death intrude repeatedly and cannot be dispelled. This period may last 1-2 weeks, ordinarily diminishing as the person begins treatment, which leads to a sense of regaining control. A therapeutic alliance with the doctor and a definitive treatment plan restores hopefulness.

Phase III represents the longer-term adaptation to illness, lasting from weeks to months, during which the patient adjusts to the diagnosis and treatment, finds reason for optimism, and returns to normal routines and ways of coping that were successful in the past. The quality of adaptation depends on the patient's prior level of adjustment and emotional maturity. It is important that family, friends, and staff be aware that there is no single *best* way to cope. Individuals have developed their own coping styles that, for better or worse, have sustained them through prior life crises. Society's attitudes often seem to demand that individuals with cancer maintain a "positive attitude to beat their disease." Many patients are inappropriately made to feel guilty if they do not cope in this way, and they often are told that the absence of a positive attitude will lead to worse outcomes. While a "positive thinking" strategy works well for some individuals, it does not for others. The doctor's understanding of and respect for each individual's way of coping is critically important.[21,22] This sequence of disbelief, turmoil, and adaptation reappears with each new crisis in the course of illness. Depression becomes more prominent at time of progression or treatment failure.

Factors in Adaptation to Cancer

It is important to recognize psychological and social factors that predict good (effective) or poor (ineffective) adjustment, enabling early identification of vulnerable individuals. Factors that contribute to adaptation derive from three areas: (a) society-derived, the social attitudes and beliefs about cancer that impact the patient, (b) patient-derived, the individual attributes the person brings to illness, and (c) cancer-derived, which represent the clinical reality of the specific illness to which the patient must adapt (Table 62-3).

Table 62-3 Factors That Determine Psychological Adjustment to Cancer

Society-derived
Open discussion of diagnosis vs unrevealed secret
Knowledge of treatment options, prognosis, and participation as partner in treatment
Popular beliefs (stress causes cancer)
Patient-derived
Intrapersonal
Developmental stage at time of cancer and meaning of curtailed goals (eg, marriage, children)
Coping ability and emotional maturity at time of cancer; philosophic, spiritual, or religious beliefs that give meaning to illness
Interpersonal
Spouse, family, friends (social support)
Socioeconomic/social class
Cancer-derived
Site, stage, symptoms (especially pain), and prognosis
Treatment required (surgery, radiation, chemotherapy) and sequelae (immediate and delayed)
Temporary or permanent altered appearance or function; rehabilitation/restoration possible
Psychologic management by the treating staff

Society-Derived Factors

The society-derived factors are continually evolving since they reflect society's attitudes toward cancer and its treatment, as well as perceptions and knowledge of particular cancers at a given time. Long feared and stigmatized, many cancers are somewhat less frightening today. The diagnosis is routinely given in the United States, and the public is better informed about treatment options; they are justifiably more optimistic about outcome. Coupled with current standards of informed consent and legal mandates for patients' knowledge of treatment options, better communication between doctor and patient has been a positive by-product. This has resulted, however, in an added burden for the patient because of the fuller knowledge of the realistic expectation associated with each treatment option. In addition, patients who have finished cancer treatment are followed far more carefully today with frequent scans and markers to detect recurrent cancer. Follow-up visits and scans are preceded by a period of increased anxiety and fears. Uncertainty about the future is still a major component of the challenge for most patients.

Diseases about which little are known of cause or cure tend to be irrationally feared and myths may grow up about their causes, particularly psychological causes. Some patients mistakenly feel that grief, depression, a stressful event, or flaws in their personalities caused their cancer. Repeated reassurance that this is not true is necessary. Johansen's group in Denmark, using the extensive data from the Danish national cancer registry regarding physical and mental health of its citizens over time, unambiguously demonstrated that depression, personality, and grief do not increase risk of cancer.[23,24]

Patient-Derived Factors

The patient-derived factors that affect adaptation come from three sources: the intrapersonal (developmental stage and coping ability), interpersonal (the social support from others), and socioeconomic and social class (the material resources available).

The developmental stage of the person at the time that cancer is diagnosed determines in part the meaning of an illness- or treatment-related loss. Jeopardy to fertility or altered appearance, such as hair loss, may impact patients differently, depending upon the time of life when the event occurs. An awareness of the individual's developmental stage and the biologic, psychologic, and social tasks that typically pertain to it help to understand the impact of cancer and to derive interventions for each age. Table 62-4 outlines the developmental stages, the normal tasks that ordinarily should be achieved at each age, the disruption in achieving expected life goals, and the interventions to minimize the deleterious effects of illness.[25] It is particularly important in treating childhood and adolescent cancer to assure that, as nearly as possible, normal developmental milestones are reached and maintained.[26] Data also show that young adults have greater distress (anger, depression) than older patients, likely due to the sense of "a life not to be lived."[27] Older adults, perhaps because of coping with a lifetime of difficult events, have "psychological inoculation" to adverse events.[28] However, symptoms of minor or subsyndromal depression is seen often in older patients with cancer.[29-39]

The strategies that patients use to cope with cancer must accomplish several goals: (a) to keep distress within manageable levels, (b) to maintain a sense of personal worth, (c) to restore or maintain relations with significant others, (d) to enhance recovery and physical function, and (e) to work out a socially acceptable postillness emotional state with maximal physical function.[18] Effective coping strategies are important in maintaining a sense of control, optimism, humor, while acknowledging an uncertain future. Philosophic, spiritual and religious beliefs that provide a meaning to confronting life, death, and illness are positive assets, especially in later stages of illness.[20,40]

Patients who are at greater risk of poor coping are well known and they

Table 62-4 **Developmental Stages and Cancer**

Stage	Tasks	Disruption	Intervention
Childhood (early)	Motor	Developmental	Physical/social
	Speech	Slowing	Stimulation
	Cognition	Regression	Structured play
	Family bonding	Separation anxiety	Increasing family contact
	Socialization	Withdrawal	Continuity of staff
	Confidence	Increasing fears (pain)	Trust of staff
Childhood (late)	Prepubertal	Being "different"	Maintain appearance
	Peer relations	School phobia	Minimize absences
	Intellectual and physical prowess	Death fears	Discuss illness and monitor responses
Adolescence	Menarche/puberty	Alopecia/amputation "differentness"	Maintain appearance
	Peer acceptance	Decreasing school/physical performance	Maintain peer contact
	Increasing independence	Increasing dependence	Support independence
	Sexual experimentation	Conflicts about self and sexuality	Counseling
Young adult	Formation of identity	Impact of illness	Counseling
	Intimacy	Decreasing attractiveness	Maintain appearance
	Marriage	Sterility/impotence	Sex counseling
	Parental role	Decreasing family role	Homemaker Support children
	Work role	Disruption of job performance	Decreasing job interruptions
Adult (middle)	Changing hormonal status/menopause	Altered appearance	Maintain appearance
	Older children "Empty nest"	Disrupted marital/family role	Counseling (patient and family)
	Peak of career	Disrupted achievements	Financial planning
Adult (old)	Aging changes	Increasing physical/emotional	Health-related care of self
	Physical limitations	Services to maintain health	
	Adjustment to increasing losses	Increasing dependence on others	Provide adequate social support system
	Increasing social support needed	Increasing isolation	Promote social/familial contacts
	Retirement	Decreasing financial security	Financial planning

Source: Adapted from Ref. 26.

Table 62-5 **Predictors of Poor Coping With Cancer**

Social isolation
Younger age (sense of life not to be lived)
Low socioeconomic status
Alcohol or drug abuse history
Prior psychiatric history
Recent losses/bereavement
Inflexibility and rigidity of coping
Pessimistic personality
Absence of a philosophy of life from which to view life and death
Multiple obligations

Source: Adapted from Ref. 26.

should be identified for early intervention (Table 62-5). Being younger, socially isolated (especially elderly), prior substance abuse or alcohol history, other stressors and personality factors are all signs of vulnerability.

The patient's social environment provides the important interpersonal resources of a spouse or partner, family, and friends. Increasing evidence suggests the central role that social support plays in both coping and survival. Isolated individuals have more trouble coping with illness, and have a higher age-matched mortality.[41-43] Recent research suggests that social capital, which is the nature of one's community in terms of safety, resources and cohesion, may be an important factor in the health disparities seen in cancer care: at community level (the macro-system); the individual's social networks (mezzo-system); one's social support (micro-system). Social capital is thus the total of the cohesion and integrates of social system.[44,45]

A third patient-derived factor is that of socioeconomic resources and social class. Increasing evidence points to impact on both morbidity and mortality, not only by limited access to appropriate care but also because of poorer education and fewer resources that affect cancer treatment availability and outcome.[46,47] Research points to a social class gradient across the five social classes, based on education and income, in which higher mortality correlates with lower social class.[46,48]

Cancer-Derived Factors

The cancer-derived factors are the clinical facts themselves of stage of disease at diagnosis; site; presence of symptoms (especially pain); prognosis; the type(s) of treatment required and their immediate and long-term impact on function; and the rehabilitation available. These factors are the "givens," along with the psychologic management by the oncology team. The sensitive and empathic oncologist and nurse are key sources of psychological support for the patient and family. Concern, compassion, listening thoughtfully, and "caring" in the context of professional ministrations are invaluable aids to the patient's ability to cope with illness. The NCI has published a monograph giving the strong evidence base for adequate communication as the key to both medical and psychosocial care.[49,50]

Psychological Issues by Stage of Disease

Psychological issues are different in each stage of disease: (a) patients receiving active treatment with cure as a goal, (b) patients receiving palliative care, with the treatment of cancer aimed at control, not cure, and (c) patients who have completed active treatment and who are survivors.

Increasingly, asymptomatic, healthy individuals are recognized as having enhanced risk of cancer by positive tumor markers, family history or genetic testing. Their psychological concerns are a part of emerging psycho-oncology research.[51-61]

Adaptation to Active Treatment

In patients undergoing treatment aimed at cure, the goal of psychosocial intervention is to support the ability to cope with the demands of treatment and side effects, to reduce distress, and to assist with symptom management (eg, anxiety, nausea and vomiting, pain).[62-67] Some sites of cancer, particularly pancreatic, are associated with greater physical symptoms and depression, anxiety and cognitive problems. The role of proinflammatory cytokines increasingly being explored as a major contributing factor.[5,6,68]

Oncologists often underestimate levels of anxiety and depression.[69] Hospitalized patients who are more acutely (and often chronically ill) have higher frequency of both psychosocial problems and psychiatric disorders related to illness.[70,71] Among almost 5000 ambulatory patients screened at Johns Hopkins on their initial visit, a mean of 35% scored above a cutoff for significant distress. Lung cancer patients scored highest at 45%. Using the Brief Symptom Inventory Scale the screening data showed that at least one-third of patients screened should be referred to a mental health professional.[72-75]

The goal of cure encourages most individuals to tolerate the temporary discomfort and side effects of surgery, chemotherapy, and radiation, and to adapt to the permanent physical changes necessary to achieve a cure.[76] Effective management of anxiety, depression, delirium, pain, nausea and vomiting helps patients to adhere to treatment. McQuellon and colleagues have utilized an orientation program for new patients that provided them with added information about what to expect during treatment.[77] Anxiety and depression symptoms were reduced as compared to the usual care group. Counseling, support groups, cognitive-behavioral interventions, and psychopharmacologic agents all are useful to reduce distress. The status of psychosocial and psychopharmacologic interventions was reviewed in the 2007 IOM monograph.[78] Data from meta-analyses and controlled clinical trials of the interventions revealed the efficacy has been established based on evidence from the literature. Clinical practice guidelines can be developed based on them.[79,80]

Adaptation to Palliative Care

The transition from curative treatment to palliative care is extremely difficult for the patient, family, and the oncologist who has often worked with and has supported the patient through months of arduous treatment. The combination of physical symptoms, psychological distress and the existential crisis of confronting death constitutes the "suffering" associated with advanced cancer.[70,81] Patients have a period of heightened distress upon learning that the therapeutic goal has shifted from cure to control of their cancer. However, with support, most patients adapt remarkably well to the altered goal. Today, the perception that recurrent cancer can be a chronic disease, particularly in those living with advanced prostate, colon and breast cancer, helps to maintain hope for long control. This phase may last for years. In older patients, the need for support is particularly apparent. A group psychoeducational intervention developed at Memorial targets this cohort by addressing the social isolation and need to encourage successful coping.[82] It is only when treatments and investigational therapies begin to fail that end-of-life issues more clearly emerge.

Assurance of the physician's commitment to continued care and symptom control becomes more important. Appointing a health proxy and discussion of wishes about resuscitation and life-sustaining measures are best discussed early in the course of illness rather than later on. Decisions about where continuing care will be given must be discussed, as well as assessing whether end-of-life care can be managed at home with hospice or if inpatient hospice is more appropriate. When it is possible, both patient and family benefit psychologically from this conversations.[83-85] Considerable information exists today about symptom control in advanced stages of illness, with better control of pain, anorexia, nausea, constipation, dyspnea, weakness, cachexia, and suffering (distress).[86-89] Portenoy and colleagues studied prevalence of symptoms in patients with advanced cancer and found fatigue, weakness, pain, and emotional distress present in over two-thirds of patients.[76] Palliative care in children is also better defined.[90]

There are growing numbers of controlled trials utilizing medication, behavioral, and psychological interventions. These include clinical practice guidelines and their use at end-of-life to treat the psychosocial and psychiatric disorders common in advanced illness: anxiety, depression, and confusion (delirium).[84,86,91,92] Psychotherapeutic approaches have been devised for patients facing the existential crisis of the end-of-life. Chochinov has described "dignity-conserving" psychotherapy to help the person feel valued and esteemed: "It targets maintenance of dignity as a therapeutic objective and as a principle of bedside care for patients nearing death."[93] Breitbart and colleagues have developed a "meaning-centered" therapy, based on the principles of logotherapy developed by Viktor Frankl.[94] Other studies have identified the role of the psychiatrist in managing psychiatric disorders associated with terminal cancer, particularly depression.[81,95,96] Requests for physician-assisted suicide require careful consideration in the context of control of the physical, psychological and spiritual aspects.[96-100] Concern for family, especially the caregiver and children must be a part of palliative care. Rauch and Muriel have described a clinical consultation for parents during treatment to guide them in talking with their children. Table 62-5A shows what children can understand at different ages and Table 62-5B provides ways the oncologist can advise and facilitate children's coping when a parent has cancer.[101-102]

Adaptation to Being a Survivor

Common concerns of survivors are fears of recurrence, worry about delayed physical effects, risk of developing secondary cancers, and sterility.[103] Cancer survivors are important advocates for improving cancer care, representing the 10 million US survivors. Patient advocates are now members of committees in the NCI's policy bodies, cooperative groups and increasingly in cancer center committees. An Institute of Medicine monograph on childhood survivors presents the current status of our knowledge[104]; a similar report on adult survivors is published.[105]

Cognitive deficits occur with radiation to the brain and with several types of chemotherapy in adults and in children. Recent reviews by Ahles and others suggest that even adjuvant chemotherapy for breast cancer produces subtle cognitive deficits that are apparent months and even years after treatment.[106,107] These cognitive changes, long identified by patients as "chemo-brain," are the subject of greater investigation currently. Ahles has proposed, from preliminary data, that the presence of the APOE4 allele, known to be associated with Alzheimer, may predispose patients after chemotherapy to greater cognitive problems in the spa-

Table 62-5A Child Development and Experience of a Parent's Illness

Infancy (0-2 years)
• Does not understand the meaning of illness
• Experiences parental absence, distracted mood of caretakers, and changes in environment and schedule
Preschool age (3-6 years)
• Combination of egocentric perspective and associative, idiosyncratic logic leads the child to believe s/he caused the cancer or can get the cancer
• Misplaced feelings of blame/guilt can lead to behavioral outbursts or increased anxiety
• Fantasy/imaginative play helps children work through worries
• Children may be reactive to inconsistent rules about bedtime, food choices, attending preschool
Latency (7-12 years)
• Simple cause and effect logic may lead the child to assume a specific cause of the cancer (eg, cigarette smoking or cancer is contagious)
• Normal school-age emphasis on rules and fairness may lead to the expectation that if a parent follows all the treatment recommendations, they will automatically be cured
• Importance of "fitting in" may cause discomfort with the parent's appearance in front of peers (eg, a mother without hair)
Adolescence (13-21 years)
• Abstract thinking enables the child to reflect on the possible outcomes of a serious illness and its impact on different family members, yet a child may continue to be largely self-centered
• Normal teenage wishes for greater independence are complicated by parental needs and expectations in the context of the illness
• Mood symptoms, risk-taking behavior, and substance abuse may be veiled responses to the parental illness

Source: Adapted from Refs. 101, 102.

Table 62-5B Maximizing Childhood Coping When a Parent Has Cancer

Support the child
• Maintain usual daily routines
• Utilize a small number of familiar caretakers as much as possible
• Ask about the details of a child's day
• Allow children who want to visit a sick parent in the hospital to do so, but prepare the child for what he or she will see
• For hospital visits, bring a familiar adult who is willing to leave the hospital room with the child when the child is ready to leave
Protect family time
• Continue family rituals and activities
• Designate a close friend or relative to organize community and neighborhood support
• Encourage adult friends and family not to call to ask about the parent's illness during family time
Facilitate parent and child communication
• Use simple, developmentally appropriate language to describe the cancer, but be honest. Euphemisms lead to confusion and more anxiety
• Give news bulletins about any new information that might be overheard
• Welcome all questions warmly
• Take the time to understand what underlies a child's question
• Questions need not be answered immediately
• Remind children not to worry alone
• Note the settings that most often facilitate questions and discussion
• Respect a child's wish not to talk

Source: Adapted from Refs. 101, 102.

tial and visual memory and executive function.[108]

Another area for potential psychological translational research is the discovery of a genetic pattern which predicted greater fatigue and poorer QOL in patients who were tested before beginning treatment for stage IV colon cancer. The overexpression of DP4D gene, the only endogenous source of neurotransmitter B-alanine, was significantly associated with greater patient-reported fatigue (p = .008).[109] This finding demands further translational research in children and adults since fatigue is a troubling and common symptom.

Studies of young adult survivors of Hodgkin disease,[110] acute leukemia, and testicular cancer reveal several psychosocial issues that apply to survivors in general.[110,111] Most psychologically healthy individuals emerge from cancer treatment without serious psychologic sequelae or significant psychiatric disorders. However, a subset of survivors, (approximately 15-20%) demonstrates significant psychopathology including posttraumatic stress disorder (PTSD) symptoms. Usually, these patients are younger and report greater physical sequelae.

Survivors report persistent fears of recurrence and death (Damocles syndrome), a greater sense of uncertainty and vulnerability about the future, and lower self-esteem. Minor physical symptoms are frequently interpreted as a sign of recurrent cancer; anxiety and even panic is common before follow-up visits. Anxiety diminishes over time, but it continues to exacerbate at times of medical visits.

Gonadal toxicity results in infertility in both sexes. Pretreatment sperm banking for men is very important to reduce stress about fertility. Women may experience symptoms of premature menopause and sexual dysfunction. Even when no treatment-related gonadal toxicity is present, there often is lower sexual desire and poorer sexual satisfaction and performance for both men and women.[112-115]

Career goals may suffer from difficulty in changing jobs and pursuing a chosen career, based in part on realistic concerns about health insurance and prejudice about having had cancer. Many survivors report subtle forms of discrimination.[110] However, a study by Maunsell and colleagues in Quebec found that 646 women, 3 years after breast cancer, were only slightly more often unemployed than an equally large (890) comparison group.[116] The data suggest that working women complete primary treatment and return to an unchanged job situation, which provides a more optimistic perspective.[117]

Chemotherapy may result in long-lasting, conditioned, Pavlovian responses to cues/reminders of the original treatment context where nausea and vomiting occurred with cyclic chemotherapy.[62,118] Cella and colleagues found that smells, tastes, and sights that were reminders of treatment evoked anxiety and nausea (but rarely vomiting) up to 11 years later.[119]

Recently there has been increased interest in the salutary effects of exercise on both physical and psychological health of cancer patients, particularly for survivors.[120] Well-designed, randomized controlled trials are needed to provide a stronger evidence base.

Anxiety disorders such as PTSD may develop after aggressive cancer treatment, particularly stem cell transplant. Symptoms of hypervigilance, flashbacks, anxiety, depressive symptoms, poor self-esteem, and poor concentration have been reported.[121-124] Studies suggest that 10-15% of survivors of transplant meet diagnostic criteria for PTSD, and another 10-15% experience some of the symptoms of PTSD that do not meet full criteria for diagnosis. Kornblith and colleagues in CALGB reported that women who were long-term breast cancer survivors (up to 20 years) experienced low levels of anxiety about cancer; however, a significant subgroup (20%) suffered from PTSD symptoms related to memories of treatment.[125] Cognitive-behavioral therapy with or without medication, is the current treatment.

Adaptation to Increased Risk of Cancer

Healthy individuals increasingly recognize enhanced risk of developing a particular type of cancer based on family history.[51,52,126] Family members are more informed today of increased risk of breast, colon, ovarian, pancreatic, endometrial, ureteral, gastric, and prostate cancer among first-degree relatives as well as of melanoma and endocrine tumors (MENS I and II).[127] The psychologic impact of this knowledge results in an increasing number of individuals who are physically healthy but constitute the "worried well": they must deal with knowledge of enhanced risk despite good health. Some perceive themselves as "walking time-bombs." Studies have been conducted to explore how to counsel those at risk.[53,54] People usually overestimate their actual risk, and genetic counseling is helpful to give them accurate information about actual risk.

Most studies have explored psychological responses to breast, ovarian, and colon cancer genetic risk.[51,53-61,126-128] The potential for discrimination in the workplace, health and life insurance, and breach of privacy regarding this information are concerns for the patient and for family members. In addition, because many unidentified genetic mutations exist, testing results may be uninformative or incomplete. Genetic testing of minors is controversial, except when therapeutic interventions exist, The potential harm to minors is particularly worrisome, except when an intervention could be life-saving, as in MENS I and II or familial polyposis coli, when it is appropriate to involve minors in the information. Pretest counseling ideally is designed to identify the psychologically vulnerable individuals for additional attention and therapeutic intervention. Severe psychological sequelae have not been reported and most individuals who learn their genetic results, whether positive or negative, tolerate the information well, even when the clinical significance of results are ambiguous. More studies are needed of the impact on family members who indirectly learn of their own risk through a relative's test results as well as handling family conflicts which sometimes follow disclosures. The Institute of Medicine and the Human Genome Project is examining these social policy issues.

Screening for Distress and Clinical Practice Guidelines

As delivery of oncology care shifted to ambulatory settings and managed care mandated shorter visits, underrecognition and undertreatment of psychiatric and psychosocial problems has increased.[129] The Panel for Management of Psychosocial Distress, appointed by the National Cancer Centers Network (NCCN), has addressed this issue by developing standards and guidelines of care over the past 10 years.[3] The United States followed Australia's lead in developing national guidelines for psychosocial care.[130] The NCCN Panel identified the barriers to effective recognition of distress that come from both patients' and physicians' attitudes about psychological issues. Patients with cancer are reluctant to ask for help for fear of the "psychiatric" or "psychological" label. The panel comprised of psychiatrists, psychologists, oncologists, nurses, social workers, clergy, and patient advocates, proposed that the word "distress" be used as a more acceptable and nonstigmatizing "umbrella" word. The assumption is that a level of distress is normal if one has cancer, but severity can increase until it reaches a level of disabling symptoms of anxiety or depression.[3,73] The Panel defined distress as: "An unpleasant emotional experience of a psychological (cognitive, behavioral, emotional), social, and/or spiritual nature that may interfere with the ability to cope effectively with cancer and its treatment. Distress extends along a continuum, ranging from common normal feelings of vulnerability, sadness, and fears to problems that can become disabling, such as depression, anxiety, panic, social isolation, and spiritual crisis."[3]

The panel developed standards for psychosocial care, similar to those developed to improve pain management (Table 62-6). The goal is to rapidly screen and identify patients with distress using a single item or short screening tool in the waiting room, using pencil and paper or a touch screen. At Johns Hopkins Cancer Center, all patients fill out a short questionnaire that identifies patients with high distress. These patients are scheduled for an appointment with the social worker.[27] The NCCN Panel proposed use of a simple item Distress Thermometer, a

Table 62-6 ■ Standards of Care for Management of Distress

- Distress should be *recognized, monitored, documented* and *treated* promptly at all stages of disease
- All patients should be screened for distress at their initial visit and as clinically indicated
- Screening should identify the level and nature of the distress
- Distress should be assessed and managed by clinical practice guidelines

Source: NCCN Practice Guidelines.

0-10 scale, asking, "How distressed have you been this week?"; the patient marks the level (Fig. 62-1). This is based on the successful use of the 0-10 scale used extensively to ask patients to rate their pain. Studies by several investigators have validated the Distress Thermometer and recommended that patients with a score of 4 or greater receive further evaluation and intervention.[72,74] A score of 4-5 provides the "trigger" for further questioning by the nurse or social workers, as the first stage of a two-stage screening with a fuller evaluation done at a second stage.[3] The Thermometer includes a Problem List, which allows patients to indicate the major sources of distress: physical, psychological, social, practical (eg, finances) or spiritual problems (Fig. 62-1). The type of problem identified indicates the psychosocial resource needed and generates appropriate triage or referral to the source able to provide support. If the problem is physical, then it is addressed by the oncologist, as well as mild psychosocial problems. Figures 62-1 and 62-2 provide the Distress Thermometer, Problem List,

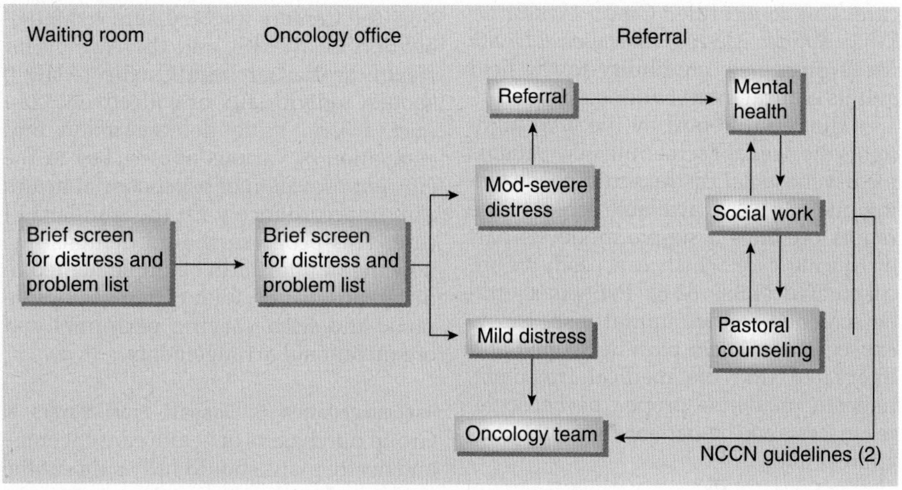

Figure 62-1 ■ Evaluation/treatment guideline in oncology clinic.

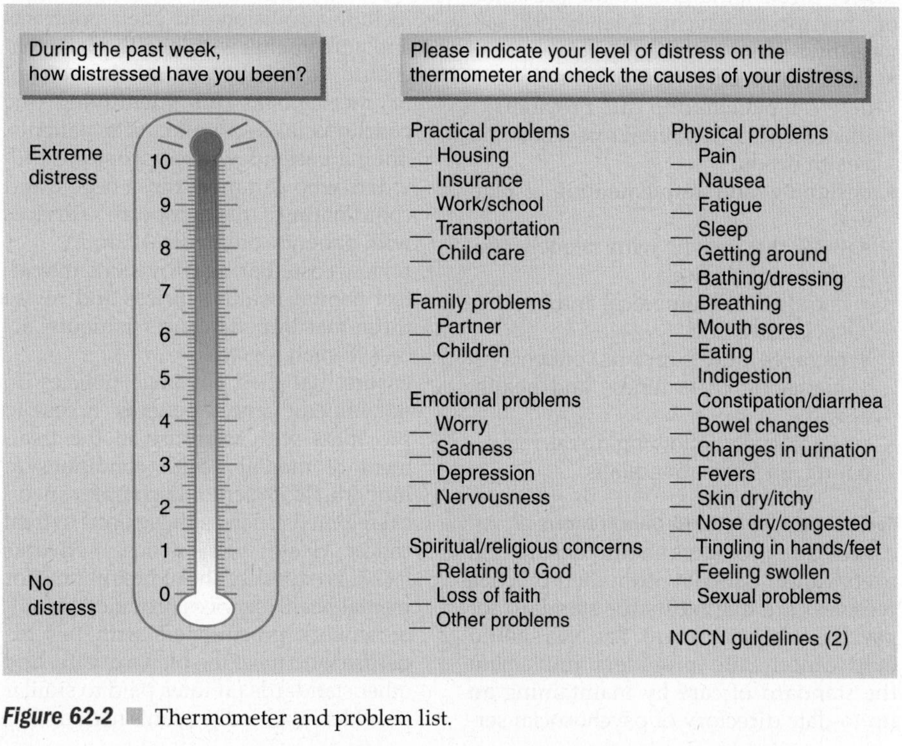

Figure 62-2 ■ Thermometer and problem list.

and recommended triage guidelines. (For additional studies see references.[75,131-133]) This provides a model in which counseling is integrated into total care.

However, oncologists often note the difficulty in identifying mental health professionals in their communities who are skilled in working with patients who have cancer. The APOS has addressed this need by developing a directory of counselors who are trained in psycho-oncology. The directory can be accessed by a call to the help line: 1-866-APOS-4-HELP or through the APOS Web site at www.apos-society.org.

Institute of Medicine (IOM) Report: 2007

New Credibility for the Field ■ In November, 2007, the IOM published an independent evidence-based report stating that quality cancer care today must integrate the psychosocial domain into routine cancer care. This report titled *Cancer Care for the Whole Patient: Meeting Psychosocial Health Needs* gives new credibility to the field and its clinical interventions.[3,4]

The recent report by the IOM highlights the need for screening new patients for psychosocial distress and needs, using one of several available screens. The report provides a simple model as part of routine care which can easily be incorporated (Table 62-6). Patients should be screened at their initial visit, a psychosocial treatment plan developed and integrated into the medical treatment, referrals made to proper psychosocial resources and the patient reevaluated as appropriate.

IOM's 10 Recommendations

Recommendation 1: Standard of Care ■ All cancer care should ensure the provision of appropriate psychosocial health services by
- facilitating effective communication between patients and care providers;
- identifying each patient's psychosocial health needs;
- designing and implementing a plan that
  - links the patient with needed psychosocial services,
  - coordinates biomedical and psychosocial care, and
  - engages and supports patients in managing their illness and health; and
- systematically following up on, reevaluating, and adjusting plans.

Recommendation 2: Health Care Providers ■ All cancer care providers should ensure that every cancer patient within their practice receives care that meets the standard for psychosocial health care. The NCI should help cancer care providers implement the standard of care by maintaining an up-to-date directory of psychosocial services available at no cost to individuals/families with cancer.

Recommendation 3: Patient and Family Education ■ Patient education and advocacy organizations should educate patients with cancer and their family caregivers to expect, and request when necessary, cancer care that meets the standard for psychosocial care. These organizations should also continue their work on strengthening the patient side of the patient–provider partnership. The goals should be to enable patients to participate actively in their care by providing tools and training in how to obtain information, make decisions, solve problems, and communicate more effectively with their health care providers.

Recommendation 4: Support for Dissemination and Uptake ■ The National Cancer Institute, the Centers for Medicare & Medicaid Services (CMS), and the Agency for Healthcare Research and Quality (AHRQ) should, individually or collectively, conduct a large-scale demonstration and evaluation of various approaches to the efficient provision of psychosocial health care in accordance with the standard of care. This program should demonstrate how the standard can be implemented in different settings, with different populations, and with varying personnel and organizational arrangements.

Recommendation 5: Support From Payers ■ Group purchasers of health care coverage and health plans should fully support the evidence-based interventions necessary to deliver effective psychosocial health services. Group purchasers should

- include provisions in their contracts and agreements with health plans that ensure coverage and reimbursement of mechanisms for identifying the psychosocial needs of cancer patients, linking patients with appropriate providers who can meet those needs, and coordinating psychosocial services with patients' biomedical care.
- review cost-sharing provisions that affect mental health services and revise those that impede cancer patients' access to such services.
- ensure that their coverage policies do not impede cancer patients' access to providers with expertise in the treatment of mental health conditions in individuals undergoing complex medical regimens such as those used to treat cancer. Health plans whose networks lack this expertise should reimburse for mental health services provided by out-of-network practitioners with this expertise who meet the plan's quality and other standards (at rates paid to similar providers within the plan's network).
- include incentives for the effective delivery of psychosocial care in payment reform programs—such as pay-for-performance and pay-for-reporting initiatives—in which they participate.

Recommendation 6: Quality Oversight ■ The National Cancer Institute, CMS, and AHRQ should fund research focused on the development of performance measures for psychosocial cancer care. Organizations setting standards for cancer care (eg, NCCN, ASCO, American College of Surgeons' Commission on Cancer, ONS, APOS) and other standards-setting organizations (eg, National Quality Forum, National Committee for Quality Assurance, URAC, Joint Commission) should
- create oversight mechanisms that can be used to measure and report on the quality of ambulatory oncology care (including psychosocial health care).
- incorporate requirements for identifying and responding to psychosocial health care needs into their protocols, policies, and standards.
- develop and use performance measures for psychosocial health care in their quality oversight activities.

Recommendation 7: Workforce Competencies ■
- Educational accrediting organizations, licensing bodies, and professional societies should examine their standards and licensing and certification criteria with an eye to identifying competencies in delivering psychosocial health care and developing them as fully as possible in accordance with a model that integrates biomedical and psychosocial care.
- Congress and federal agencies should support and fund the establishment of a Workforce Development Collaborative on Psychosocial Care during Chronic Medical Illness. This cross-specialty, multidisciplinary group should comprise educators, consumer and family advocates, and providers of psychosocial and biomedical health services and be charged with
  - identifying, refini ng, and broadly disseminating to health care educators information about workforce competencies, models, and preservice curricula relevant to providing psychosocial services to persons with chronic medical illnesses and their families;
  - adapting curricula for continuing education of the existing workforce using efficient workplace-based learning approaches;
  - drafting and implementing a plan for developing the skills of faculty and other trainers in teaching psychosocial health care using evidence-based teaching strategies; and

Table 62-6 Institute of Medicine Model for Meeting Psychosocial Needs

IOM Report Recommendations for Action

1: The standard of psychosocial care
- Facilitate effective communication between patients and care providers;
  - Identify each patient's psychosocial health needs;
  - Design and implement a plan that
    - links the patient with needed psychosocial services,
    - coordinates biomedical and psychosocial care,
    - engages and supports patients in managing their illness and health; and
  - Systematically follows up on, reevaluate, and adjust plans.

2: Health care providers' responsibility
To ensure that every cancer patient within their practice receives care that meets the standard for psychosocial health care.

3: Patient & family education and advocacy organizations' responsibility
- To educate patients with cancer and their family caregivers to expect, and request when necessary, care that meets the standard for psychosocial care.
- To continue to work on strengthening the patient side of the patient–provider partnership by enabling patients to participate actively in their care by providing tools and training in how to:
  - obtain information, make decisions, solve problems, and communicate more effectively with their health care providers.

4: Support for dissemination and uptake
The NCI, CMS, and the AHRQ should conduct a large-scale evaluation of various approaches to the efficient provision of psychosocial health care in accordance with the standard of care. This program should demonstrate how the standard can be implemented in different settings, with different populations, and with varying personnel and organizational arrangements.

5: Support from payers
Group purchasers of health care coverage and health plans should fully support the evidence- based interventions necessary to deliver effective psychosocial health services. Group purchasers should:
- Ensure coverage and reimbursement of mechanisms for identifying the psychosocial needs of cancer patients and linking them with appropriate providers who can meet those needs, and coordinating psychosocial services with patients' biomedical care.
- Review cost-sharing provisions that affect mental health services and revise those that impede cancer patients' access to such services.
- Ensure that their coverage policies do not impede cancer patients' access to providers with expertise in the treatment of mental health conditions in individuals undergoing complex medical regimens such as those used to treat cancer.
- Include incentives for the effective delivery of psychosocial care in payment reform programs—such as pay-for-performance and pay-for-reporting initiatives—in which they participate.

6: Quality oversight
- The NCI, CMS, and AHRQ should fund research focused on the development of performance measures for psychosocial cancer care. Organizations setting standards for cancer care and other standards-setting organizations should:
- Create oversight mechanisms that can be used to measure and report on the quality of ambulatory oncology care (including psychosocial health care).
- Incorporate requirements for identifying and responding to psychosocial health care needs into their protocols, policies, and standards.
- Develop and use performance measures for psychosocial health care in their quality oversight activities.

7: Workforce competencies
- Educational accrediting organizations, licensing bodies, and professional societies should develop their standards for licensing and certification criteria as fully as possible in accordance with a model that integrates biomedical and psychosocial health care.
- Congress and federal agencies should support and fund the establishment of a workforce development collaborative on psychosocial care during chronic medical illness. This cross-specialty, multidisciplinary group should comprise educators, consumer and family advocates, and providers of psychosocial and biomedical health services and be charged with
  - identifying, refining, and broadly disseminating to health care educators information about workforce competencies, models, and preservice curricula relevant to providing psychosocial services to persons with chronic medical illnesses and their families; adapting curricula for continuing education of the existing workforce using efficient workplace-based learning approaches; drafting and implementing a plan for developing the skills of faculty and other trainers in teaching psychosocial health care using evidence-based teaching strategies; and strengthening the emphasis on psychosocial health care in educational accreditation standards and professional licensing and certification exams by recommending revisions to the relevant oversight organizations.
- Organizations providing research funding should support assessment of the implementation in education, training, and clinical practice of the workforce competencies necessary to provide psychosocial care and their impact on achieving the standard for such care.

8: Standardized nomenclature
To facilitate research on and quality measurement of psychosocial interventions, the NIH and AHRQ should create and lead an initiative to develop a standardized, transdisciplinary taxonomy and nomenclature for psychosocial health services. This initiative should aim to incorporate this taxonomy and nomenclature into such databases as the National Library of Medicine's MeSH, PsycINFO, CINAHL and EMBASE.

9: Research priorities
Organizations sponsoring research in oncology care should include the following areas among their funding priorities:
- Further development of reliable, valid, and efficient tools and strategies for use by clinical practices to ensure that all patients with cancer receive care that meets the standard of psychosocial care. These tools and strategies should include:
  - approaches for improving patient–provider communication and providing decision support to cancer patients; screening instruments that can be used to identify individuals with any of a comprehensive array of psychosocial health problems; needs assessment instruments to assist in planning psychosocial services; illness and wellness management interventions; and approaches for effectively linking patients with services and coordinating care.
- Identification of more effective psychosocial services to treat mental health problems and to assist patients in adopting and maintaining healthy behaviors, such as smoking cessation, exercise, and dietary change. This effort should include:
  - identifying populations for whom specific psychosocial services are most effective, and psychosocial services most effective for specific populations; and development of standard outcome measures for assessing the effectiveness of these services.
- Creation and testing of reimbursement arrangements that will promote psychosocial care and reward its best performance.

10: Promoting uptake and monitoring progress
The NCI/NIH should monitor progress and report its findings on at least a biannual basis to:
  - oncology providers, consumer organizations, group purchasers and health plans, quality oversight organizations, and other stakeholders.

These findings could be used to inform an evaluation of the impact of the report and each of its recommendations. Monitoring activities should make maximal use of existing data collection tools and activities.

- strengthening the emphasis on psychosocial health care in educational accreditation standards and professional licensing and certification exams by recommending revisions to the relevant oversight organizations.

- Organizations providing research funding should support assessment of the implementation in education, training, and clinical practice of the workforce competencies necessary to provide psychosocial care and their impact on achieving the standard for such care set forth in recommendation 1.

Recommendation 8: Standardized Nomenclature ■ To facilitate research on and quality measurement of psychosocial interventions, the NIH and AHRQ should create and lead an initiative to develop a standardized, transdisciplinary taxonomy and nomenclature for psychosocial health services. This initiative should aim to incorporate this taxonomy and nomenclature into such databases as the National Library of Medicine's Medical Subject Headings (MeSH), PsycINFO, Cumulative Index to Nursing and Allied Health Literature (CINAHL), and EMBASE.

Recommendation 9: Research Priorities ■ Organizations sponsoring research in oncology care should include the following areas among their funding priorities:

- Further development of reliable, valid, and efficient tools and strategies for use by clinical practices to ensure that all patients with cancer receive care that meets the standard of psychosocial care set forth in recommendation 1. These tools and strategies should include
  - approaches for improving patient–provider communication and providing decision support to cancer patients;
  - screening instruments that can be used to identify individuals with any of a comprehensive array of psychosocial health problems;
  - needs assessment instruments to assist in planning psychosocial services;
  - illness and wellness management interventions; and
  - approaches for effectively linking patients with services and coordinating care.
- Identification of more effective psychosocial services to treat mental health problems and to assist patients in adopting and maintaining healthy behaviors, such as smoking cessation, exercise, and dietary change. This effort should include
  - identifying populations for whom specific psychosocial services are most effective, and psychosocial services most effective for specific populations; and
  - development of standard outcome measures for assessing the effectiveness of these services.
- Creation and testing of reimbursement arrangements that will promote psychosocial care and reward its best performance.

Research on the use of these tools, strategies, and services should also focus on how best to ensure delivery of appropriate psychosocial services to vulnerable populations, such as those with low literacy, older adults, the socially isolated, and members of cultural minorities.

Recommendation 10. Promoting Uptake and Monitoring Progress ■ The NCI/NIH should monitor progress toward improved delivery of psychosocial services in cancer care and report its findings on at least a biannual basis to oncology providers, consumer organizations, group purchasers and health plans, quality oversight organizations, and other stakeholders. These findings could be used to inform an evaluation of the impact of this report and each of its recommendations. Monitoring activities should make maximal use of existing data collection tools and activities.

Psychiatric Disorders

The key clinical question for the oncologist is how to identify the point at which the normal distress associated with cancer (eg, fear, worry, and sadness) has become a treatable psychiatric disorder. Most psychiatric disturbances in patients with cancer relate to illness or treatment side effects.[134] Taken overall, about one third of patients will experience distress that requires evaluation and treatment.[78,134-136] The prevalence is greater among younger patients; those with sites of cancer with poorer prognosis, eg, brain, pancreas, lung; and those who are hospitalized with greater level of illness causing confusional states and greater anxiety and depression.[27,137]

Anxiety Disorders

Anxiety is the most common form of distress experienced by patients in the oncology setting (Tables 62-7 and 62-8). Medical etiologies include hypoxia, pulmonary embolus, sepsis, delirium, bleeding, cardiac arrhythmia, and hypoglycemia. Hormone-secreting tumors which produce anxiety are: pheochromocytoma, thyroid tumors, carcinoid, parathyroid adenoma, ACTH-producing tumors, insulinoma, and paraneoplastic disorders (remote CNS effect).

Table 62-7 ■ **Causes of Anxiety in Patients With Cancer**

Situational
Diagnosis of cancer, prognosis discussion
Crisis, illness/treatment
Conflicts with family or staff
Anticipating a frightening procedure
Awaiting results of tests
Fears of recurrence *after* completing treatment
Disease-related
Poorly controlled pain
Abnormal metabolic states
Hormone-secreting tumors
Paraneoplastic syndromes (remote CNS effects)
Treatment-related
Frightening or painful procedures (MRI, scans, wound debridement)
Anxiety-producing drugs (antiemetic neuroleptics, bronchodilators)
Withdrawal states (opioids, benzodiazepines, alcohol)
Conditioned (anticipatory) anxiety, nausea, and vomiting with cyclic chemotherapy
Exacerbation of preexisting anxiety disorder
Phobias (needles, claustrophobia)
Panic or generalized anxiety disorder
Posttraumatic stress disorder (Holocaust survivors, Vietnam veterans, recall of the death of a relative with cancer)
Obsessive-compulsive disorder

Several drugs can produce symptoms of anxiety: corticosteroids, neuroleptics, bronchodilators, thyroxine, and psychostimulants. Metoclopramide or other neuroleptics given for the control of chemotherapy-related nausea and vomiting can produce restlessness, akathisias, and dystonias. A benzodiazepine promptly reduces the restless movements, anxiety and agitation. Withdrawal states from alcohol, narcotic analgesics, and sedative-hypnotics often produce anxiety as a prominent symptom.

Some patients undergoing cyclic chemotherapy using an emetogenic regimen begin to develop anticipatory anxiety, nausea, and vomiting by about the third cycle, a few days to hours in advance of receiving the next cycle of treatment.[62,138,139] This is a learned, conditioned, Pavlovian autonomic response to the repeated chemotherapy-related experience of nausea and vomiting (described earlier in survivors). More effective antiemesis regimens have reduced the frequency and severity of this problem; however, it persists in some patients.

Patients who have preexisting phobias, panic attacks, generalized anxiety, PTSD or obsessive-compulsive disorder (OCD) are at risk of their symptoms exacerbating during cancer treatment (Table 62-7).[140] Phobias of needles, blood, hospitals, claustrophobia, or agoraphobia complicate a patient's ability to tolerate hospital procedures or adhere to recommended treatments. Panic attacks often occur in patients who already have shortness of

Table 62-8 **Anxiety Related to Common Medical Problems in Cancer**

Medical Problems	Examples
Poorly controlled pain	Unresponsive or under-treated pain
Abnormal metabolic states	Hypoxia, pulmonary embolus, sepsis, fever, delirium, hypoglycemia, hypercalcemia, bleeding, coronary occlusion and heart failure, cardiac arrhythmia
Hormone-secreting tumors	Pheochromocytoma, thyroid tumors, carcinoid, parathyroid adenoma, ACTH-producing tumors, insulinoma
Anxiety-producing drugs	Corticosteroids, neuroleptics used as antiemetics, thyroxine, bronchodilators, β-adrenergic stimulants, antihistamines, (paradoxic reactions), withdrawal states (alcohol, narcotic analgesics, sedative-hypnotics)
Side effects of treatment	Allergic skin rash to antibiotics, unexpected toxicity (eg, diarrhea)

Table 62-9 **Treatment of Anxiety Disorders**

Treatment Modality	Components
Supportive psychotherapy	Providing information, rehearsal of feared events, reassurance
	Individual therapy
	Support group
Behavioral	Relaxation, hypnosis
	Systematic desensitization
Psychopharmacologic	Benzodiazepines
	Short acting (alprazolam, lorazepam, oxazepam)
	Long acting (diazepam, clorazepate, clonazepam)
	Selective serotonin-reuptake Inhibitors (SSRIs) (paroxetine, sertraline, citalopram, escitalopram, fluoxetine)
	β-Blockers (propranolol)
	Antihistamines
	Neuroleptics (thioridazine, trifluperazine, haloperidol)
	Buspirone
Combinations of the above	

breath or tachycardia for medical reasons, complicating the management of these physical symptoms.[134,141] Patients who have had prior traumatic events may have flashbacks of painful memories which have been quiescent for many years.[25,121]

OCD is a complicating psychiatric disorder during cancer treatment, which leads to indecisiveness about treatment decisions and difficulty with the inability to control the situation. Fears of the future, phobias, and rigidity, make it difficult for patients with OCD to cope with illness and they often reject psychotropic drugs.

Anticipatory anxiety responds to empathetic validation of the fear, good communication and adequate information, allowing the person to "rehearse" the feared event (Table 62-9). Enlisting the assistance of the oncology nurse or social worker is often helpful in giving additional information and offering reassurance.

For persistent or distressing anxiety, three types of treatment are available, often used in combination: (1) psychotherapy and counseling, (2) cognitive-behavioral interventions, and (3) psychopharmacologic medications. Counseling or formal psychotherapy using a psychoeducational, cognitive-behavioral or supportive intervention model is helpful[142-145] (Table 62-9). A meta-analysis of randomized controlled trials showed that a range of interventions are efficacious in improving QOL and decreasing distress, but data do not show an effect upon survival.[4,146]

Several forms of psychotherapy have demonstrated benefit, and more trials are in development including psychoeducational, interpersonal psychotherapy (IPT), supportive, cognitive-behavioral, and existential or meaning-centered therapies. Several behavioral interventions are effective. Relaxation exercises with guided imagery and hypnosis are most frequently employed. These methods are particularly helpful to patients who wish to maintain and enhance their beleaguered sense of control. Relaxation and meditation are useful adjunctive treatments for anxiety related to pain and for control of conditioned chemotherapy-related nausea and vomiting.[138,147,148]

Table 62-10 **Common Antianxiety Agents**

Drug	Brand Name	Starting Dose/Day	Theraputic Dose (mg)/Day
SSRIs			
Sertraline	Zoloft	25-50 mg AM	50-150
Fluoxetine	Prozac	10-20 mg AM	20-60
Paroxetine	Paxil	10-20 mg	20-60
Citalopram	Celexa	10-20 mg	20-60
Escitalopram	Lexapro	10-20 mg	10-20
Benzodiazepines			
Alprazolam, XR	Xanax	0.25-1 mg	0.5-2.0
Clonazepam, wafers	Klonopin	0.25-0.5 mg	0.5-2.0
Lorazepam[a]	Ativan	0.5-2 mg	0.5-2.0
Diazepam[a]	Valium	2-10 mg	5-20
Hypnotics			
Temazepam	Restoril	15 mg	15-45
Zolpidem	Ambien	5 mg	5-20
Eszopiclone	Lunesta	1 mg	1-3
Oxazapam	Serax	10 mg	10-20
Zaleplon	Sonata	5 mg	5-10

[a] Also IV, IM.

Significant anxiety symptoms are most often treated pharmacologically by sedative-hypnotics from the benzodiazepine class of drugs, by the selective serotonin-reuptake inhibitors (SSRIs), by antidepressants which impact upon depression and anxiety (often present together), as well as by antihistamines, beta-blockers, and neuroleptics in low dose. Table 62-10 outlines the benzodiazepines commonly used and their starting and therapeutic doses. A shorter half-life provides better control and less likelihood of poor elimination and oversedation. Insomnia responds to a bedtime dose of temazepam 15 mg, clonazepam 1 mg, or zolpidem 5 mg. The antidepressants trazodone 50 mg and mirtazapine 15 mg are also useful for bedtime sedation (see Table 62-14). Daytime anxiety responds to lorazepam, 0.5 mg; alprazolam, 0.25-0.50 mg tid or qid, clonazepam, 0.5 mg bid, or diazepam 5 mg bid are longer acting. It is important to taper these medications to prevent a mild rebound in anxiety or withdrawal symptoms. Buspirone is useful, because it has no sedating effects and no addictive qualities. Low-dose neuroleptics are useful to control anxiety in older patients, using resiperdone, olanzapine or quetiapine during the day or at bedtime.

Mood Disorders

It is important to keep in mind that depression does respond to treatment and should not be left untreated because it is "based on reality" in patients with cancer. Depressive symptoms occur as depression reactive to illness (often with anxiety); preexisting dysthymia (chronic); minor or subsyndromal depression; major depression and bipolar disorder. A common presentation in illness, especially in older patients is minor depression not reaching severity of major depression, yet with troubling similar symptoms of anhedonia and sadness.[34-36]

Depression is difficult to diagnose in patients with cancer because the neoplastic disease itself may produce the vegetative symptoms of cancer: fatigue, weakness, loss of libido, insomnia, loss of interest, poor concentration and motivation.[149,150] The oncologist must depend on the psychological symptoms of dysphoric mood, helplessness, hopelessness, worthlessness, loss of pleasure (anhedonia) and suicidal thoughts.[151] Table 62-11 outlines the common symptoms in major depression. A personal or family history of depression or bipolar illness suggests increased risk during illness as well as having poor social support, being socially isolated and having experienced a recent loss. Evaluation should explore mental status, mood, hopelessness, feeling of being a burden, and suicidal ideation. Insomnia, anorexia, fatigue, agitation, or psychomotor retardation may relate to illness and must be interpreted in light of that fact. In fact, all these symptoms are being studied as a possible consequence of proinflammatory cytokines, suggesting a possible biologic contribution.[5,6]

Table 62-12 outlines the medically related risk factors for developing depression: greater level of debilitation, advanced disease and presence of another chronic illness or disability. Several medications frequently contribute: steroids (dexamethasone and prednisone), some chemotherapeutic agents (interferon, interleukin-2, vincristine, procarbazine, L-asparaginase), and supportive medications.[151] Depression may relate to organ failure or nutritional, endocrine, and neurologic complications of cancer. Depression is a common symptom of pancreatic cancer, which has led to speculation about a tumor-induced mood change, possibly though alteration of brain serotonergic function through the effect of proinflammatory cytokines.[68,152,153] These disease-related major depressions are called mood disorder related to medical condition.

Table 62-12 **Medical Related Risk Factors for Depression in Patients With Cancer**

Poorly controlled pain
Other chronic disease/disability; advanced stage
Medications
Corticosteroids
Prednisone, dexamethasone
Inteferon and interleukin-2
Chemotherapeutic agents: Vincristine, vinblastine, procarbazine, L-asparaginase
Other medications
Cimetidine
Indomethacin
Levodopa
Methyldopa
Pentazocine
Phenmetrazine
Phenobarbital
Propranolol
Rauwolfia alkaloids
Tamoxifen
Antibiotics (amphotericin B)
Other medical conditions
Metabolic (anemia; hypercalcemia)
Nutritional (B12 or folate)
Endocrine (hyper-hypothyroidism; adrenal insufficiency)
Neurologic (paraneoplastic syndrome)
Sites of cancer
Pancreas, small cell lung, breast, lymphoma (producing remote CNS effects)

Depression is managed first by establishing good rapport with the patient and suring support from available family or friends. Supportive psychotherapeutic, behavioral interventions, and psychotropic agents are often combined in treatment.[154,155]

Depression is especially prevalent in older patients with cancer. By the year 2030, 20% of the U.S. population will be over the age of 65.[156] Cancer is a disease primarily of this age group. The elderly comprise 61% of cancer survivors.[157] People in this cohort experience increasing physical losses of mobility, vision, hearing, mental acuity, and stamina, usually along with one or more comorbid medical problems (arthritis, hypertension, diabetes, kidney and cardiovascular disease). Personal losses, such as the death of a spouse, family members and friends of a similar age isolate older adults even more, often forcing them to deal with illness alone. This sense of isolation can be further exacerbated by retirement and geographic scattering of families. Addressing the psychological issues in the elderly, even physically healthy older individuals experience a significant level of depression (10-20% in the community and primary care settings[158]). Older adults often have minor subsyndromal depressions that do not fit the major categories of major depression or dysthymic disorder, suggesting they are part of a spectrum of depressive illness in the elderly.[158] Among the elderly with chronic illness, the frequency of depression (15-25% or greater in medically ill groups[158]) often interferes with the ability to make treatment decisions and adhere to lengthy treatment regimens.[159-163]

Despite the prevalence of cancer in older age patients, they have systematically been underrepresented in research studies (Aapro et al 2000). Kua[35] suggests that as many as a third of elderly cancer patients may experience some form of psychological distress.[35] What research there is has largely focused on depression. In older patients with cancer, the estimates of depression range from 17% to 25%.[34-36,38,156,164] In a longitudinal study of patients with breast, prostate, colon, and lung cancer, the prevalence of depression was 26% early after the diagnosis; and this rate still remained high (16%).[34,38] In another longitudinal study of depression in elderly patients with colorectal cancer, the prevalence was 18%.[37] While several studies have reported lower rates of depressive disorders in elderly cancer patients compared to younger ones, this may reflect the scales used, phenomenological presenting symptoms, and a tendency to underdiagnose.[39,165] While older people are generally thought to cope better with illness and loss than younger individuals,[157,166-169] the presence of physical aging-related problems, comorbid medical conditions and their symptom burden can overwhelm their strong coping ability, leading increased vulnerability to distress, anxiety, and depression.[36,170]

Erik Erikson, a developmental psychologist who studied aging through the life span described the psychosocial goals at different life stages of normal aging.[171] Stage 7, which is called middle adult stage, is characterized by the developmental task of generativity: moving from primary interest in oneself to con-

Table 62-11 **Evaluation of Depression and Predisposing Factors**

Evaluative category	Findings
Family history	Depression; suicide
Personal history	Previous depression, bipolar disorder, suicide attempt, alcoholism, substance abuse
	Recent bereavement
Signs and symptoms	Psychologic
	Dysphoric mood (eg, sad, depressed, anxious, crying, diurnal mood change)
	Feelings of hopelessness; helplessness
	Loss of interest and pleasure; anhedonia
	Guilt, burden on others, worthlessness
	Poor concentration
	Mood incongruent to disease outlook
	Suicidal thoughts or plans
	Delusional thoughts (psychotic symptoms rare, except in organic affective syndrome)
	Somatic (less interpretable in more physically impaired patients)
	Insomnia
	Anorexia and weight loss
	Fatigue
	Psychomotor retardation or agitation
	Constipation
	Decreased libido

cern for others and mentoring the next generation. George Vaillant, a Harvard psychiatrist who has conducted longitudinal studies of aging, has extended the description to include being Keeper of Meaning, namely becoming engaged in preserving the culture and being a link between the past and future.[172] When this is accomplished well, the person has achieved generativity; when it is not, Erikson described stagnation, which is characterized by a rejection of others and authoritarian rigid views that do not allow for the normal interpersonal connection with others. In the 8th and final stage, the psychosocial task is to achieve ego integrity—a sense of "making peace" with one's life (Table 62-13).[173] Achieving integrity is equated with achieving wisdom; the absence of integrity is despair and disdain. The absence of achieving these goals, resulting in stagnation and despair, suggests that they are vulnerable to developing depressive symptoms, loneliness and isolation. Only a portion of elderly successfully reach these last goals of generativity and wisdom. Elderly, who, for many reasons, may fall short of those goals, have fewer personal and interpersonal resources for facing cancer. They are vulnerable to developing depressive symptoms along the spectrum from minor to major depression. These concepts serve as the basis for both groups and individual interventions to enhance coping strategies.[156,159-162,165,174-184]

Psychotropic drugs are effective in controlling depressive symptoms with cancer.[155] Table 62-14 lists the most frequently used antidepressant medications in patients with cancer and their starting and maintenance doses. The antidepressants commonly used today are SSRIs. Today, tricyclic antidepressants and duloxetine are used primarily for adjuvant pain management and peripheral neuropathy. Psychostimulants (dextroamphetamine, methylphenidate, and modafinil) are widely used to rapidly promote well-being and counteract the fatigue from advanced illness and opioids, as compared to SSRs which have a slow onset of effect. All antidepressants should be started in low dose in elderly and debilitated patients and titrated upward as tolerated provides similar benefits, but over a longer period of time.

Table 62-14 ■ Commonly Used Antidepressants in Cancer

Drug	Brand Name	Starting Daily Dose PO (mg)	Therapeutic Daily Dose PO (mg)
Selective serotonin-reuptake inhibitors			
Sertraline	Zoloft	25-50 mg AM	50-150
Fluoxetine	Prozac	10-20 mg AM	20-60
Paroxetine	Paxil	10-20 mg AM	20-60
Citalopram	Celexa	10-20 mg AM	20-60
Escitalopram	Lexapro	5-10 mg	10-20
Tricyclics (neuropathic pain management primarily)			
Nortriptyline	Pamelor	25-50 mg	50-200
Amitriptyline	Elavil	25-50 mg	50-200
Desipramine	Norpramin	25-50 mg	50-200
Other agents			
Venlafaxine	Effexor	18.75-37.5 mg	75-225
Trazodone	Desyrel	50-100 mg	100-200
Bupropion (XL, SR)	Wellbutrin, Zyban	50-75 mg	150-400
Mirtazapine	Remeron	15 mg HS	15-45
Psychostimulants			
Methylphenidate	Ritalin	5-10 mg (8 AM & noon)	10-30
Modafinil	Provigil	50-100 mg (8 AM & noon)	100-400
Dextroamphetamine	Dexedrine	5-10 mg (8 AM & noon)	10-20

Note: Lithium and mood stabilizers only for bipolar disorder; MAOIs not recommended.

Suicide and Cancer

The incidence of suicide is increased in patients with cancer compared to the general population, but it is not as high as often is assumed. Suicide by overdose at home during the terminal stages of cancer is certainly under-diagnosed and under reported due to stigma.[185-187] Suicide is more likely to occur in advanced disease as depression, hopelessness, and the presence of poorly controlled symptoms (especially pain) escalate. Table 62-15 outlines risk factors, Table 62-16 outlines assessment of suicidal risk, and Table 62-17 outlines suicide in relation to stage of disease. Key questions are the nature of suicidal thoughts (passive or active); past history of psychiatric problems, particularly depression or suicide attempts; recent bereavement; family history of depression or suicide; and poorly controlled pain. Availability of family and social support are integral to assume adequate surveillance at home.

Almost all patients who receive a diagnosis of cancer, even when the prognosis is good, carry a "secret" thought that "I won't die in pain with advanced cancer–I'll kill myself first." Some patients maintain a hidden supply of a drug, which is kept for this purpose. It usually serves as a "steam valve" with which the person is able to maintain a sense of ultimate control over the disease and feared intolerable pain. The thought actually serves as a protective coping device.

Table 62-15 ■ Risk Factors for Suicide in Cancer

Personal
Prior history of depression or suicide attempt (personal or family)
Prior psychiatric disorder
Prior alcohol or drug abuse
Depression and hopelessness
Recent loss/bereavement
Socially isolated
Medical
Pain
Delirium with poor impulse control
Advanced illness
Debilitation, exhaustion, fatigue

Table 62-16 ■ Evaluation of Suicidal Risk

Establish rapport
Ask about symptoms (pain, discomfort, and adequacy of their control)
Ask about depression and suicidal thoughts at present or in the past
Ask about suicidal thoughts (Are they passive ["I wish I could die"] or active ["I am thinking of ways to do it"])
Ask about family or friends and sense of support from others
Ask about any recent loss of close person, especially if by cancer
Ask about understanding of illness, presence of confusion, fatigue
Asking does not cause suicidal thoughts; the patient is usually relieved to express them

Table 62-13 ■ Erikson's Psychosocial Tasks in Older Years

Middle Adult (50s-60s)	Older Age (70s-onward)
Developmental Task: *Generativity* • Capacity to unselfishly guide the next generation • "Care" for younger as mentor, guide, consultant 'Keeper of Meaning': • Preserving the culture in which one lives • Link between the past and future Life lessons: care	Developmental Task: *Integrity* • Making peace with one's life as a unified whole • Achieve a sense of wisdom through life's experience and lessons • Concern with life in the face of death & teaching the young not to fear death • Struggle to accept inalterability of past & unknowable future Life Lessons Wisdom

Source: Adapted from Erikson, 1950

Table 62-17 ■ Suicide in Relation to Stage of Disease

Patients at all stages of cancer
Suicidal thoughts are common and serve as a means to maintain a sense of control over the disease
Carrying out the act is viewed as for "the future when I need to do it"
Some maintain a means of suicide (eg, drugs) to assure ultimate control over feared intolerable symptoms
Patients in remission, with good prognosis
Serious suicidal thoughts represent underlying psychiatric disorder (depression, substance abuse)
Unlikely to appear "rational"; treat aggressively, including hospitalization
Patients with poor prognosis and poorly controlled symptoms
Thoughts of suicide often appear "rational"
May request advice about physician-assisted suicide
Need evaluation for presence of treatable depression
Need attention to quality-of-life issues and comfort
Suicidal wishes usually diminish with control of distressing symptoms
Adequate symptom control by physician may hasten death (dual effect) but is not actual physician-assisted suicide
Patients in terminal stage
May request euthanasia by lethal injection from physician
Request often reflects poor quality of life, hopelessness, and depression
Need for control of symptoms, even when hastens death

Serious ruminating about suicide in a patient for whom the disease is in remission or in whom a good prognosis exists requires careful evaluation.[187]

Patients with a poor prognosis, advanced disease, and poorly controlled symptoms often have thoughts of suicide that are more likely to be viewed as rational.[188] They may request help from a physician to write a prescription for a drug to use to commit suicide. A treatable major depression may be fueling their suicidal ideation. A persistent desire for death may relate to depression but hopelessness is another important predictor.[98,100,187]

Attention to any uncontrolled physical symptom, especially pain, is crucial. Adequate pain control may have the dual effect of hastening death while ameliorating suffering. Most physicians feel comfortable providing comfort and relieving distress. Increasing numbers of physicians do not regard this as assisted suicide but as best medical care geared to maximal comfort.[93]

Patients who are in the terminal stages and are too weak to carry out a suicidal act are those most likely to request euthanasia. Despite intense societal debate, support for legalized euthanasia has not occurred. Even in the state of Oregon, which legalized physician-assisted suicide, few patients request assistance. Controversy continues over individual state's rights to legalize this practice, despite continued federal legislation that prohibits the use of FDA controlled substances for this specific purpose.

Poorly controlled pain in patients with beginning organ failure and a mild metabolic encephalopathy results in poor judgment and poor impulse control and may lead to an impulsive and unpredictable suicide attempts.[70] Such patients in the hospital should be given a 24-hour companion, a nurse, or a family member who understands the patient's compromised state.

Delirium

Delirium, or encephalopathy, is a nonfocal global cerebral dysfunction characterized by waxing and waning levels of consciousness, disordered thinking, mood change, disorientation and confusion, psychomotor slowing or agitation, altered behavior, judgment and altered sleep-wake cycles. It is often worse at night, hence the term "sundowning." It is distinguished from dementia in part by its reversibility. However, in advanced stages of cancer, due to organ failure and metabolic derangements, delirium is often not reversible. The primary goal is to control behaviors that may be harmful to the patient or others (eg, pulling out lines, combative behavior). Care providers and family members should be told that the cause of the behavior is brain dysfunction, not a mental aberration, and given guidance in understanding the patient's states.

In patients with cancer, especially those in advanced stages, a sudden change in mood or behavior is most often related to a change in neurologic, vascular, or metabolic status; a psychological basis is far less likely. In fact, up to three-quarters of terminally ill patients may develop a delirium before death. Common causes of delirium in cancer are outlined in Table 62-18. A change in behavior in which the person becomes irritable, uncooperative, agitated or somnolent, and misinterprets sounds or objects is apt to represent early signs of delirium. This picture may be followed by delusions, usually paranoid ("there are people here trying to hurt me"), frank hallucinations, and difficulty in being maintained in bed or hospital rooms (Table 62-19). Mood can change markedly with irritability or depression with suicidal ideation. Patients may present with a hyperactive delirium as described above, or a hypoactive delirium with a quiet, withdrawn state.

Management begins with attention to the patient's safety. It is important to have one-to-one observation, preferably by a person present who can correct

Table 62-18 ■ Common Causes of Delirium in Cancer

Causes	Examples
Metabolic encephalopathy because of vital organ failure	Liver, kidney, lung (hypoxia), thyroid, adrenal
Electrolyte imbalance	Sodium, potassium, calcium, glucose
Treatment side effects	Narcotic/analgesics
	Anticholinergics
	Phenothiazines
	Antihistamines
	Chemotherapeutic agents
	Steroids
	Radiation therapy to brain
Infection	Septicemia
Hematologic abnormalities	Microcytic and macrocytic anemias, coagulopathies
Nutritional	General malnutrition, thiamine, folic acid, vitamin B12
Paraneoplastic syndromes	Remote effects of tumors
Metastatic or primary brain tumor	Hormone-producing tumors

Table 62-19 ■ Behavioral Symptoms of Delirium in Patients With Cancer

State	Symptom
Early, mild	Change in sleep pattern with restlessness, attempts to get out of bed, transient periods of disorientation
	Unexplained anxiety and sense of dread
	Increased irritability, anger, temper outbursts
	Withdrawal, refusal to talk to staff or relatives
Late, severe with behavioral changes	Forgetfulness, not previously present
	Refusal to cooperate with reasonable requests; pulling out tubes and lines
	Angry, swearing, shouting, abusive
	Demanding to go home, pacing corridor
	Illusions (misidentifies staff, visual and sensory clues)
	Delusions (misinterprets events, usually paranoid, fears of being harmed)
	Hallucinations (visual and auditory)

misinterpretations of what is happening. Limiting the number of new faces and experiences is useful while enhancing awareness of time and place. Older patients are most prone to become confused, and delirium may be superimposed on early mild dementia. Physical restraints must sometimes be used to prevent removal of vital IV lines and bandages, and to prevent falls. Chemical restraint may be necessary. The management regimen is low-dose haloperidol, a potent dopamine blocker, 0.5-1.0 mg bid to qid oral or IV. Lorazepam given with a neuroleptic reduces agitation in doses of 0.5-1.0 mg tid to qid oral or IV; however, given alone, it may increase confusion. Haloperidol and lorazepam often are given together to reduce confusion and diminish agitation.[189] Olanzapine is a highly effective antidelirium drug given by mouth. Table 62-20 outlines the drugs which are useful and their route of administration. Correcting the underlying metabolic or neurologic problem is not always possible, however, and comfort for the patient and family may depend materially on being able to control the symptoms of confusion and agitation. Patients with psychomotor slowing may safely be observed without treatment, but significant degrees of confusion with agitation must be treated.[95,190]

Psychiatric and Psychosocial Interventions

The literature provides an increasing number of randomized controlled trials of well defined specific psychotherapies that demonstrate sustained efficacy in reducing distress and improving QOL.[144,145,191,192] This evidence is well-reviewed in the 2007 IOM Report.[4] Brief crisis counseling[193] combined with psychosocial and educational interventions has demonstrated effectiveness in enhancing coping.[194]

The widespread use of supportive groups has led to questions of whether psychosocial interventions prolong survival. Early enthusiasm for impact beyond effect on QOL has been diminished by the controlled trials by Goodwin and colleagues[195] and Kissane, Coyne, and Speigel.[196-198] They confirmed the reduction of distress and enhanced QOL, but they did not show a survival advantage. Kissane has raised the issue that the women in the intervention group actually received a greater amount of chemotherapy, suggesting they adhered to treatment at a higher rate.[199] It is possible that group interventions improve treatment adherence and could improve survival based on better adherence.

A meta-analysis conducted by Petticrew and colleagues[200] found little support for any association between psychological coping styles and recurrence and survival from cancer.

Behavioral interventions have demonstrated efficacy in cancer patients. Relaxation, meditation, and systematic desensitization are all effective in reducing anxiety, conditioned responses from chemotherapy-induced nausea and vomiting, and pain.[120] These behavioral interventions are often coupled with cognitive therapy approaches.[147] The value of art therapy in helping patients cope has also been shown in both hospitalized and ambulatory patients.[201]

Cancer centers have integrated complementary/alternative medicine (CAM), services that provide adjunctive symptom management with a tendency to overlap with behavioral interventions.[202] These interventions are utilized by many patients, both children and adults. They are often more acceptable and less stigmatizing than psychotherapeutic approaches for many patients. The wide range of interventions offers some type that fits each person's preference.

Quality-of-Life Assessment

The definition of health-related QOL is the level of performance in the major domains of life function as reported by patient-self-report.[83,147] In the 1990s, clinical trials have increasingly included the assessment of QOL. Interest in QOL grew after 1984, when the U.S. Food and Drug Administration demanded that the efficacy of new anticancer agents be demonstrated by improved survival or evidence of enhanced QOL. This mandate led to the development of valid measurement tools. Karnofsky and Burchenal described in 1949 that, in addition to survival, subjective improvement was equally important in the evaluation of patients' responses to treatment.[203] QOL was thus included as an outcome. Despite that early observation, however, only selected trials assess QOL, usually when there is a small likely treatment advantage (eg, trials of chemotherapy agents in pancreatic cancer) or when a highly effective new treatment has significant side effects (eg, stem cell transplant). PRO, which is a much more descriptive and accurate term has been proposed to replace quality of life.[204]

Six domains are included in multidimensional QOL measures: physical, functional, psychologic, social, sexual, and occupational (Table 62-21). No "gold standard" of measurement currently exists, however the EORTC instruments in Europe and the Functional Assessment of Cancer Therapy (FACT) developed by Cella in the US[205] are widely used and available in many languages.

In development of the FACT, which added an aspect of patient assessment regarding the discrepancy between prior and present function. In addition to the FACT-General, Cella core set of questions, he developed modules for the specific cancer sites and for common problems such as nausea, vomiting, pain, spiritual beliefs, and fatigue. In addition to the Karnofsky Performance Rating Scale, Spitzer and colleagues' QOL Index (QL-index) is the major observer-rated measure of QOL that is used with any frequency.[206] The Medical Outcomes Study (MOS) General Health Survey instruments have the advantage of being used with other diseases, and short and longer valid forms are available.[207]

Recent efforts in QOL research have concentrated on development of a unitary measure that combines length of survival and QOL, referred to as "quality-adjusted life years" or QALY. Time Without Symptoms or Toxicity (TWIST), is another QALY method. These meth-

Table 62-20 **Medications for Managing Delirium in Cancer Patients**

Drug	Brand Name	Approximate Daily Dose
Neuroleptics		
Haloperidol	Haldol	0.5-5 mg every 2-12 h, PO, IV, SC, IM
Chlorpromazine	Thorazine	12.5-50 mg every 4-12 h, PO, IV, IM
Risperidone	Risperdal	1-3 mg every 12 h, PO
Olanzapine	Zyprexa	2.5-5 mg every 6-8 h, PO
Quetiapine	Seroquel	12.5-50 mg every 12 h, PO
Benzodiazepines		
Lorazepam	Ativan	0.5-2.0 mg every 1-4 h, PO, IV, IM
Midazolam[a]		30-100 mg every 24 h, IV, SC
Anesthetics		
Propofol[a]		10-50 mg every hour, IV

[a]Usually IV continuous infusion in intensive care setting.

Table 62-21 **Quality-of-Life Measurement: Functional Areas of Living Assessed**

Physical	Symptoms of disease and treatment of side effects
Functional	Ability to perform usual activities
Psychologic	Mood, sense of well-being
Sexual	Desire, performance
Social	Family, friends, leisure
Work	Usual level of activity

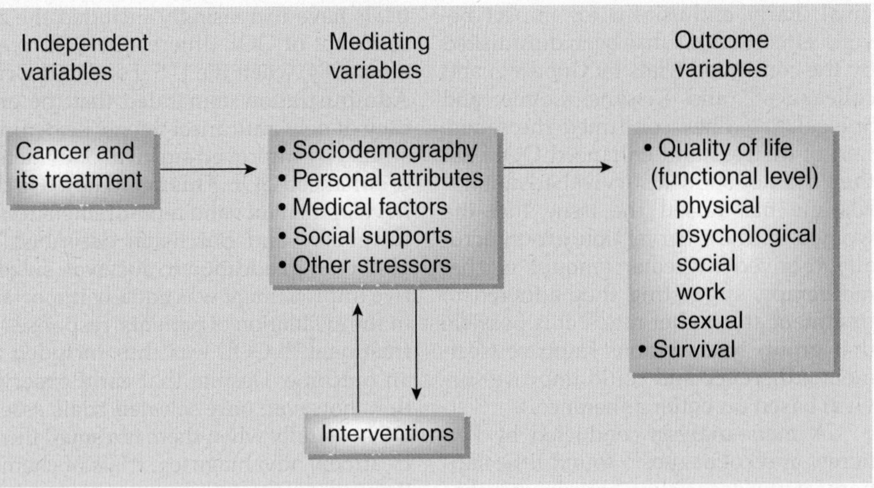

Figure 62-3 ■ Research model for psychiatric and quality-of-life research in oncology.

ods, coupled with economic analysis, are providing increasing information to assist patients and doctors in making decisions about cancer treatments.

Family Issues and Bereavement

Families have emerged as a significant overburdened and under-recognized component of health care today. Families of patients often feel the doctors view them as "difficult."[208] Yet, families must care for patients at home today with high levels of illness. The demand for family members to provide nursing care and carry out medical procedures is greater than ever. An estimated 25 million households are caring for a chronically ill family member—many in homes of the economically deprived.[209]

Attention is slowly being given to the greater needs of families today by health policy planners. In addition to economic burdens, there are profound stressful psychological and social consequences. These issues are compounded when the care delivered at home is provided for advanced and terminal stages of cancer.[85] Oncologists' responsibility to the patient extends to evaluation of the caregiver as well, and the ability of that key person to cope with the demands. Children in the household also require attention. Providing guidance for the adult caregiver about answering children's questions is important (Tables 62-5A,B).[101,102]

Grief in Surviving Family Members

Oncologists who treat patients with cancer often come to know family members well, especially during terminal stages of illness. They are in a unique position to support the family when the patient dies and to assure care for grief in the surviving family members, especially children.[210] They need to recognize abnormal reactions and refer the grieving relative for bereavement counseling. Hospice programs include this as part of their services. It is important to be aware of resources in one's community including support groups for the bereaved and mental health professionals who offer bereavement counseling. Caregivers at risk of severe, protracted or complicated grief reactions require treatment to relieve distress and prevent progression of major depression. They also tend to neglect physical symptoms and seeking appropriate medical care. Overall, 80% of people experience normal bereavement but around 20% will have complicated or abnormal grief, which will require intervention for symptoms of significant distress, inability to function, and suicidal ideation.

There has been much interest in the question of whether grief results in increased risk of cancer or progression. Studies did not demonstrate an increase in mortality from cancer among parents in Israel who lost a child by accident or war 10 years earlier,[211] or in parents in Denmark who had experienced death of their child secondary to cancer.[24]

These findings suggest that, based on epidemiological data, grief does not increase risk of cancer or lead to its recurrence or progression in survivors. This information is reassuring for individuals who fear that experiencing a loss makes them more vulnerable to initiation of cancer or progression of disease.

Stress and Burnout in Oncology Staff

A topic of increasing concern is the impact of repeated loss and stress on oncologists and nurses resulting in burnout. The newer term used is "compassion fatigue." Nurses experience more burnout and job dissatisfaction when their work load is excessive.[212] The daily impact of giving bad news to patients and families accumulates.[213] In 1991, Whippen and Canellos did a survey of ASCO oncologists. Approximately 60% expressed feelings of burnout and stress related to excessive paper work, administrative matters, inadequate time for family, heavy workloads, and caring for patients receiving palliative care.[214] A second unpublished survey conducted in 2001 confirmed the continuing concern.

A study at Memorial Sloan-Kettering Cancer Center found that the house staff with the highest burnout scores had greater emotional exhaustion, (eg, felt "distanced" from patients), and experienced a sense of diminished professional accomplishment.[215] Possessing effective communication skills, having religious beliefs and good patient relationships appeared to counter burnout development, as did having a "hardy" personality characterized by maintaining a sense of control, challenge, and commitment despite stresses of work.[215] Continuing examination of the impact of clinical practice on oncologists and their primary team is necessary.

Summary

The subspecialty of psycho-oncology began in the last quarter of the twentieth century, reflecting the increased interest in psychiatric, psychologic, and social factors in cancer prevention, the "human" side of the care of patients with cancer at all stages, and the impact of cancer on family members and on medical and nursing staff. Early of vulnerable patients is important through a rapid screen which can lead to a second-stage evaluation to recognize and diagnose the common psychiatric disorders of anxiety, depression, and delirium, the latter often caused by medications and metabolic complications of cancer. The modalities available to treat these symptoms are psychotherapeutic, behavioral, pharmacologic, and complementary therapies.

The Institute of Medicine's Report in 2007 has as its major tenet that quality cancer medicine must integrate psychosocial care into routine oncology care. The report provides a model for use in all sizes and types of oncology practices and offices, to assure that psychosocial care is available to all patients, in communities of all sizes. The model requires a psychosocial evaluation on the initial visit, develop a treatment plan that incorporates it into medical care, finds appropriate psychosocial resources needed, and reevaluates at appropriate intervals, incorporating family as needed. The model has equal application in the care of any chronically ill patient.

The successful development of psycho-oncology over almost 30 years as an integrated part of oncology suggests that it is a model for treating chronic diseases in other medical specialties such as cardiology, nephrology, and neurology.

Selected References

The complete reference list can be found at www.CANCERMEDICINE8.com

1. NCCN. Distress management. In *The Complete Library of NCCN Clinical Practice Guidelines in Oncology.* Version 1. Jenkintown, Pennsylvania: National Comprehensive Cancer Network; 2007.
2. Holland J. *Psycho-Oncology.* New York, NY: Oxford University Press; 1998.
3. Holland J, Andersen B, Booth-Jones M, et al. NCCN distress management clinical practice guidelines in oncology. *J Natl Compr Canc Netw.* 2003;1:344-374.
4. IOM. *Cancer Care for the Whole Patient.* Washington, DC: The National Academies Press; 2007.
5. Cleeland CS, Bennett GJ, Dantzen R. Are the symptoms of cancer and cancer treatment due to a shared biologic mechanism? *Cancer.* 2003;97:2919-2925.
6. Musselman DL, Miller AH, Porter MR, et al. Higher than normal interleukin-6 concentrations in cancer patients with depression: preliminary findings. *Am J Psychiatry.* 2001;158:1252-1257.
7. Menzies H, Chochinov H, Breitbart W. Cytokines, cancer and depression: connecting the dots. *J Support Oncol.* 2005;3:55-57.
8. Illman J, Corringham R, Robinson D Jr, et al. Are inflammatory cytokines the common link between cancer-associated cachexia and depression? *J Support Oncol.* 2005;3:37-50.
9. Holland J. History of psycho-oncology: overcoming attitudinal and conceptual barriers. *Psychosom Med.* 2002;64:206-221.
11. Hagerty RG, Butow PN, Ellis PM, et al. Communicating with realism and hope: incurable cancer patients' views on the disclosure of prognosis. *J Clin Oncol.* 2005;23:1278-1288.
17. Park C, Folkman S. Meaning in the Context of Stress and Coping. *Review of Gen Psych* 1997;1:115-44.
22. Holland J, Lewis S. *The Human Side of Cancer.* New York, NY: Harper Collins; 2000.
23. Jiong Li, Christoffer Johansen, Dorthe Hansen, Jørn Olsen. Cancer Incidence in Parents After Loss of a Child: A Nationwide Study. *Cancer* 2002;95:2237-42.
24. Dalton SO, Boeson EH, Ross L, Schapiro IR, Johansen C. Mind and cancer: do psychological factors cause cancer? *Eur J Cancer.* 2002;38:1313-1323.
27. Zabora J. The prevalence of psychological distress by cancer site. *Psychooncology.* 2001;10:19-28.
31. Deimling GT, Bowman KF, Sterns S, Wagner LJ, Kahana B. Cancer-related health worries and psychological distress among older adult, long-term cancer survivors. *Psychooncology.* 2006;15:306-320.
34. Holland J, Evcimen Y. Common psychiatric problems in elderly patients with cancer. In: Ramaswamy G, MD ed. *American Society of Clinical Oncology Educational Book.* Alexandria, VA: ASCO (American Society of Clinical Oncology);2007:307-311.
44. Kroenke CH, Kubzansky LD, Schernhammer ES, Holmes MD, Kawachi I. Social networks, social support, and survival after breast cancer diagnosis. *J Clin Oncol.* 2006;24:1105-1111.
45. Bloom JR. Improving the health and well-being of cancer survivors: past as prologue. *Psychooncology.* 2008.
46. Marmot M. *Status Syndrome: How Your Social Standing Directly Affects Your Health & Life Expectancy.* London: Bloomburt & Henry Holt; 2004.
50. *Epstein RM, Street RL Jr. Patient-Centered Communication in Cancer Care: Promoting Healing and Reducing Suffering. National Cancer Institute, NIH Publication No. 07-6225.* Bethesda, MD, 2007.
53. Lerman C, Kash K, Stefanek M. Younger women and increased risk for breast cancer: perceived risk, psychological well-being and surveillance behaviors. *Monogr Natl Cancer Inst.* 1994;16:171-177.
57. Audrain J, Schwartz MD, Lerman C, et al. Psychological distress in women seeking genetic counseling for breast-ovarian cancer risk: the contributions of personality and appraisal. *Ann Behav Med.* 1998;19:370-377.
62. Jacobsen PB, Bovbjerg DH, Schwartz M, Hudis CA, Gilewski TA, Norton L. Conditioned emotional distress in women receiving chemotherapy for breast cancer. *J Consult Clin Psychol.* 1995;63:108-114.
68. Ebrahimi B, Tucker SL, Li D, Abbruzzese JL, Kurzrock R. Cytokines in pancreatic carcinoma. *Cancer.* 2004;101:2727-2736.
69. Newell S, Sanson-Fisher R, Girgis A, Bonaventura A. How well do medical oncologist's perceptions reflect their patients' reported physical and psychosocial problems? *Cancer.* 1998;83:1640-1651.
79. Pirl W. Evidence report on the occurrence, assessment, and treatment of depression in cancer patients. *J Natl Cancer Inst Monogr.* 2004;32:32-39.
81. Lee V, Cohen R, Edgar L. Clarifying "meaning" in the context of cancer research: a systematic literature review. *Palliat Support Care.* 2004;2:291-303.
82. Poppito S, Weiss T, Holland J, Roth A, Nelson C. Learning to cope with aging and loss: development of a geriatric-specific educational support program with participation from an expert panel of older cancer patients. *Psychooncology.* 2007;16: S1-S288.
84. Goldenberg D, Holland J, Schacter S. Palliative Care in the Chronically Mentally Ill. In: Breibart W, Chochinov H, eds. *Psychiatric Issues in Palliative Care.* New York: Oxford University Press; 1999:91-6.
90. IOM. *When Children Die: Improving Palliative and End-of-Life Care of Children and Their Families.* Washington, DC: National Academy Press; 2003.
93. Chochinov HM. Dignity-conserving care—a new model for palliative care: helping the patient feel valued. *JAMA.* 2002;287:2253-2260.
96. Block SD, Billings JA. Patient request for euthanasia and assisted suicide in terminal illness. The role of the psychiatrist. *Psychosomatics.* 1995;36:445-457.
98. Chochinov HM, Wilson KG, Enns M, et al. Desire for death in the terminally ill. *Am J Psychiatry.* 1995;152:1185-1191.
101. Rauch PK, Muriel AC, Cassem NH. Parents with cancer: who's looking after the children? *J Clin Oncol.* 2003;21:117s-121s.
103. Kornblith AB. Psychosocial adaptation of cancer survivors. In: Holland JC, ed. *Psycho-Oncology.* New York, NY: Oxford University Press; 1998:223-256.
104. Hewitt M, Weiner S, Simone JV. *Childhood Cancer Survivorship: Improving Care and Quality of Life.* Washington, DC: Institute of Medicine, National Academies Press; 2003.
106. Ahles TA, Saykin AJ, Furstenberg CT, et al. Neuropsychologic impact of standard-dose systemic chemotherapy in long-term survivors of breast cancer and lymphoma. *J Clin Oncol.* 2002;20:485-493.
114. Syrjala KL, Roth-Roemer SL, Abrams JR, et al. Prevalence and predictors of sexual dysfunction in long-term survivors of marrow transplantation. *J Clin Oncol.* 1998;16:3148-3157.
117. Schover LR. Myth-busters: telling the true story of breast cancer survivorship. *J Natl Cancer Inst.* 2004;96:1800-1801.
118. Morrow G, Roscoe J, Hickok J. Nausea and vomiting. In: Holland J, ed. *Psycho-Oncology.* New York, NY: Oxford University Press; 1998:476-484.
122. Andrykowski MA, Cordova MJ. Factors associated with ptsd symptoms following treatment for breast cancer: test of the andersen model. *J Trauma Stress.* 1998;11:189-203.
129. Hoffman B, Zevon M, D'Arrigo MC, Cecchini TB. Screening for distress in cancer patients: the NCCN rapid screening measure. *Psychooncology.* 2004;13:1-8.
130. Turner J, Zapart S, Pedersen K. Clinical practice guidelines for psychosocial care of adults with cancer. *Psychooncology.* 2005;14:159-174.
150. *Quick Reference for Oncology Clinicians: The Psychiatric and Psychological Dimensions of Cancer Symptom Management.* Charlottesville, VA: IPOS Press; 2006.
151. Coups E, Winell J, Holland J. Depression in the context of cancer. In: Lucinio J, MaLeWong W, eds. *Biology of Depression: From Novel Insights to Therapeutic Strategies.* Weinheim, Germany: Wiley; 2005:365-385.
154. Breitbart W, Payne D. Psychiatric aspects of pain management in patients with adrenal cancer and AIDS. In: Chochinov H, Breitbart W, eds. *Handbook of Psychiatry in Palliative Medicine.* New York, NY: Oxford University Press; 2000:131-161.
157. IOM. *From Cancer Patient to Cancer Survivor: Lost in Transition.* Washington, DC: The National Academies Press; 2007.
159. Katon W, Lin, E, Kroenke, K. The association of depression and anxiety with medical symptom burden in patients with chronic medical illness. *Gen Hosp Psychiatry.* 2007;29:147-155

63 Principles of Cancer Rehabilitation Medicine

David C. Thomas, MD ■ Kristjan T. Ragnarsson, MD

Medical advances in the diagnosis and management of cancer have markedly increased survival rates. Although the treatment for some patients may now result in complete cure and no perceived physical deficits, for others, an aggressive definitive treatment may result in significant physical impairment or disability. To ensure quick restoration of optimal function, early and continued aggressive rehabilitation interventions should be provided, including physical and occupational therapy, prosthetic and orthotic devices, and assistive equipment. Application of rehabilitation techniques frequently results in a swift functional improvement and a reduction in subjective complaints, even when the prognosis for life is poor. It has always been difficult to predict with a degree of certainty the life expectancy of an individual with cancer. Modern diagnostic techniques and effective treatment of malignant neoplastic diseases have invalidated old statistics and dogmas regarding life expectancy and thus made accurate prognostication even more difficult for the clinician. No cancer patient, even one with widespread metastases, should be denied the benefits of aggressive treatment, including appropriate surgical intervention, chemotherapy, radiation, and comprehensive rehabilitation. These interventions, when offered in an integrated and timely fashion, prolong life, protect organs and residual healthy tissue, reduce pain, and maximize self-care and mobility skills, helping reduce the stigma of cancer and physical impairment while providing dignity and a better quality of life for the cancer patient.

Early referral for rehabilitation services and good communication among the oncologist, the surgeon, the rehabilitation specialist (physiatrist), and the other members of the cancer rehabilitation team are essential to the patient's successful return to optimal function. A comprehensive and well-coordinated rehabilitation approach that concurrently deals with the physical, psychological, and social problems caused by the malignancy and the consequent disability usually yields the best results. Most important for success, however, is the patient's personal interest and ability to participate in the rehabilitation program and to pursue the established functional goals, supported by family, friends, and caregivers.

Application of Rehabilitation Concepts

Many persons afflicted by cancer develop some form of functional impairment or disability that will interfere with self-care, mobility, and a smooth transition to their former lifestyle. Cancer rehabilitation can be broadly defined as the maximum restoration of physical, psychological, social, vocational, recreational, and economic functions within the limits imposed by the malignancy and its treatment. To make a significant and timely impact on such a wide variety of functions and needs, the efforts of a well-coordinated and goal-oriented multidisciplinary cancer rehabilitation team are required (Table 63-1). Because of the patient's often uncertain prognosis, most cancer rehabilitation programs focus on quick gains in mobility and self-care skills and the provision of psychosocial support to the patient and family. Flexibility in goal setting is unavoidable because of the patient's changing needs, stamina and medical status.

Several studies show that cancer rehabilitation programs result in measurable benefits when individualized, specific, and realistic goals are set.[1-3] Comprehensive inpatient rehabilitation services may be economically provided for disabled cancer patients who are considered "cured or controlled," but precise short-term rehabilitation interventions may enable even those with a poor prognosis to gain the mobility and self-care skills that facilitate early hospital discharge.[4]

The physical impairment experienced by cancer patients may result from tissue destruction caused by the cancer itself, prolonged bed rest, and inactivity or from definitive treatment, such as surgery, radiation, or chemotherapy. The exact nature of the impairment may vary, but, in essence, it is no different from impairment caused by trauma or noncancerous disease that is customarily managed by the rehabilitation team. A specific rehabilitation goal must be established for each patient and an individualized program prescribed that is designed to obtain measurable early results. The main rehabilitation goals for all people with physical disabilities are, first, to develop maximum skills in the activities of daily living (ADL) (Table 63-2) allowed by the disability and, second, to obtain independent mobility with or without assistive devices, such as wheelchairs, prostheses, orthoses, walkers, crutches, or canes. To reach these goals, the therapist uses physical exercise to improve muscle strength, endurance, joint flexibility, and self-care skills, as well as to apply physical modalities to decrease pain and swelling. Prescription, fabrication, and fitting of prosthetic and orthotic devices and other assistive equipment, followed by training in their use, are essential for amputees and individuals with significant muscle weakness, paralysis, or unstable skeletal structures.

It is essential to provide rehabilitation interventions that also aim at the profound psychological, sexual, social, and vocational consequences of the cancer and the physical impairment. Preferably, the anticipated guidance of the psychosocial difficulties should be addressed when the initial diagnosis is made and when treatment is begun. The goal of cancer care is not just to eradicate or control the malignancy and extend the patient's life but also to maintain or reestablish a life of quality.[5]

The rehabilitation goals of cancer patients may be broadly classified according to the different stages of the disease. *Preventive rehabilitation therapy* is started early after the diagnosis of cancer, that is, before or immediately after surgery, radiotherapy, and/or chemotherapy. At this stage, no significant physical impairment exists, but therapy is started to prevent func-

Table 63-1 ■ Interdisciplinary Cancer Rehabilitation Team

Physician (physiatrist)	Speech-language pathologist
Rehabilitation nurse	Social worker
Physical therapist	Psychologist
Occupational therapist	Chaplain
Prosthetist-orthotist	Vocational counselor
Nutritionist	Recreational therapist

Table 63-2 ■ Activities of Daily Living[a]

Eating and drinking	Moving in bed
Dressing and undressing	Changing position
Bathing and grooming	Walking
Toileting	Climbing stairs
Managing bladder and bowel functions	General wheelchair skills
Manipulating small objects	Using a manual wheelchair
Caring for health and fitness	Using a powered wheelchair

[a]Rehabilitation indicators: skill indicators.

tional loss. *Restorative rehabilitation therapy* is directed at the comprehensive restoration of maximum function for patients considered "cured or controlled" but who have a residual physical impairment and disability. *Supportive rehabilitation therapy* attempts to increase the self-care skills and mobility of the cancer patient with growing cancer and progressive impairment and disability by the application of quick, effective methods, for example, providing appropriate assistive devices and the teaching of simple techniques for self-care.[6] *Supportive rehabilitation therapy* also includes physical exercises to prevent the effects of immobilization, such as joint contractures, muscle atrophy, weakness, and pressure sores. *Palliative rehabilitation therapy* aims to increase or maintain the comfort and function of patients with terminal cancer by using physical modalities, simple orthotic devices, and assistive equipment to manage pain, joint contractures, and pressure stores and to provide at least partial self-sufficiency.[6]

Cancer Rehabilitation and Adaptation Team

Organized cancer rehabilitation programs can significantly improve a patient's physical function and community reintegration.[4,7] An integral part of such programs is an interdisciplinary cancer rehabilitation and adaptation team (Table 63-1). The exact composition of the team may vary considerably, depending on the program's philosophy and size, the type of institution, and the range of disabilities encountered. The team is led by a physician who is either an oncologist or, more commonly, a physiatrist.[7] (An oncology nurse, social worker, psychologist, physical therapist, occupational therapist, vocational counselor, chaplain, and nutritionist are present on most teams.) Other rehabilitation professionals may contribute to the rehabilitation of cancer patients, depending on each patient's specific physical impairment, including a prosthetist, an orthotist, a speech-language pathologist, a driver's trainer, and a recreational therapist. The roles of the various team members are described below.

The physiatrist, the medical specialist who usually directs the cancer rehabilitation team, needs to be knowledgeable in oncology in addition to having expertise in the field of physical medicine and rehabilitation. To establish realistic goals and prescribe an appropriate rehabilitation program, the physiatrist needs to know (1) details of the cancer diagnosis with respect to organ site, histology, and grade of anaplasia; (2) the cancer's anatomic staging (primary site only, involvement of regional nodes, or metastases); (3) the patient's life expectancy, that is, whether the patient is "cured or controlled" and, if not, the anticipated rapidity of the cancer's progression; and (4) the definitive treatment plan for the cancer, that is, the timing of surgery, chemotherapy, or radiation and its anticipated efficacy and potential side effects. The physiatrist discusses this information with the rehabilitation team as the basis for developing a specific and realistic plan of preventive, restorative, supportive, and palliative therapies. The physiatrist introduces the patient and caregivers to the goals of the cancer rehabilitation team and meets regularly with the team, as well as with the patient and caregivers, to identify rehabilitation needs and to direct and coordinate etc. their efforts while taking into account the patient's progress and changing needs.[8] The rehabilitation oncology nurse serves primarily as an easily accessible resource to the nursing staff, giving care to the cancer patient, as well as to the patient and the caregivers. The nurse evaluates the patient's specific nursing needs, plans the patient's care, helps obtain nursing supplies, and educates other nurses, the patient, and their caregivers about nursing techniques and the principles of cancer treatment while monitoring and assisting in the discharge process.

The physical therapist teaches the patient to perform specific exercises to strengthen muscles, increase stamina, and maintain or improve joint range of motion and trunk flexibility. When indicated, training is provided to improve balance and coordination, as well as functional skills: transfers into and out of bed, wheelchair locomotion, and ambulation with or without assistive devices. Task-oriented exercises, such as ambulation or training in self-care, may improve function and safety by repetition and prolonged therapy.

The occupational therapist focuses on upper extremity exercises and training in self-care activities (Table 63-2). Different adaptive equipment may be provided to make the patient more proficient in self-care and activities related to work and recreation.

The nutritionist evaluates the patient's nutritional condition, assesses the additional metabolic demands that the cancer places on the body, and recommends the optimal diet with respect to specific clinical condition, caloric intake, food ingredients of choice, optimal consistency for easy swallowing, and the individual's tastes.

The prosthetist or orthotist makes artificial limbs (prostheses) or special braces (orthoses) for patients in need of such devices.

The speech-language pathologist evaluates and provides therapy for impaired oral communication and works closely with the occupational therapist and nutritionist in the assessment and care of swallowing disorders.

The social worker has many important roles in the rehabilitation of the cancer patient, but especially with respect to discharge planning, facilitating a smooth transition from the hospital to the community, ensuring continuity of care, and securing appropriate follow-up services after discharge. The psychologist assesses the patient's cognition and behavior, including intelligence, personality (ie, ideational, emotional, behavioral, and character patterns), personal history, motivation, and reaction to the illness, and assists the patient and the caregivers in coping.[9-11]

A chaplain or religious counselor is often included in the cancer rehabilitation team. A vocational counselor should participate in the care of physically impaired cancer patients who have any potential of returning to work.

The recreational therapist offers activities to meet the different needs and interests of disabled individuals both in and out of the hospital, such as art therapy, music therapy, attending art shows and sports events, going to theaters, eating at restaurants, and shopping.

Functional Assessment

Unlike other fields of medicine, the outcome of rehabilitation interventions cannot be measured by survival or by the disappearance of symptoms. The effectiveness of rehabilitation interventions is judged by the patient's degree of functional independence. The revised International Classification of Functioning and Disability (ICIDH-2) offers a framework for understanding the complex interaction between disease and disability.[12]

To assess and monitor function accurately, the performance in different activities of self-care, mobility, and communication must be numerically rated according to the patient's level of independence: completely independent, independent with devices, requires assistance (supervision, "spotting," reminding, physical help), or completely dependent. This requires the collection of numerous diverse data by various means, including physical examination, observation, and a review of records and reports from the various rehabilitation team members, as well as the gathering of information directly from the patient and caregivers. The functional evaluation scale that currently is gaining the widest acceptance by rehabilitation professionals is the Functional Independence Measure (FIM) (Table 63-3),[13-15] but for cancer patients, the Karnofsky performance Status Scale is the most widely used evaluation scale (Table 63-4).[16]

Table 63-3 ■ **Functional Independence Measure (FIM)**

L E V E L S	Seven Complete Independence (Timely, Safely) Six Modified Independence (Device)	NO HELPER
	Modified Dependence Five Supervision Four Minimal Assist (Subject = 75%+) Three Moderate Assist (Subject=50%+) Complete Dependence Two Maximal Assist (Subject = 25%+) One Total Assist (Subject = 0%+)	HELPER

Self Care	ADMIT	DISCHG	FOL-UP
A. Eating			
B. Grooming			
C. Bathing			
D. Dressing-Upper Body			
E. Dressing-Lower Body			
F. Toileting			
Sphincter Control			
G. Bladder Management			
H. Bowel Management			
Mobility			
Transfer:			
I. Bed, Chair, Wheelchair			
J. Toilet			
K. Tub, Shower			
Locomotion			
L. Walk/wheel Chair	w c	w c	w c
M. Stairs			
Communication			
N. Comprehension	a v	a v	a v
O. Expression	v n	v n	v n
Social Cognition			
P. Social Interaction			
Q. Problem Solving			
R. Memory			
Total F/M			

Note: Leave no blanks; enter 1 if patient not testable due to risk.
Source: Copyright 1990 Research Foundation-State University of New York.

Table 63-4 ■ **Karnofsky Performance Status Scale**

General	Index	Specific Criteria
Able to carry on normal activity; no special care needed	100	Normal; no complaints; no evidence of disease
	90	Able to carry on normal activity; minor signs or symptoms of disease
	80	Normal activity with effort; Signs or symptoms of disease
Unable to work; able to live at home and care for most personal needs; varying amount of assistance needed	70	Cares for self; unable to carry on normal activity or to do work
	60	Requires occasional assistance from others, but able to care for most needs
	50	Requires considerable assistance from others; needs frequent medical care
Unable to care for self; requires institutional or hospital care or equivalent; disease may be rapidly progressing	40	Disable; requires special care and assistance
	30	Severely disable; hospitalization indicated; death not imminent
	20	Very sick, hospitalization necessary; active supportive treatment necessary
	10	Moribund
	0	Dead

The Cancer Rehabilitation Evaluation System (CARES) is another scale developed specifically to measure quality of life and functional outcome for patients with cancer. It is valid, reliable, and sensitive to changes in status. Recent investigators have looked at specific populations, namely the older patient, and specific assessments, which could be used to follow their course of treatment.[17-20]

Rehabilitation Process

Rehabilitation services are frequently requested too late in the care of the cancer patient. The physiatrist should be consulted as soon as it may be anticipated that the cancer will result in a physical disability. The rehabilitation interventions may thus be planned and explained to the patient before, during, or immediately following definitive treatment. Physical and occupational therapy is initially provided at the bedside, but the patient should be mobilized out of bed as soon as possible and escorted to the rehabilitation area, where facilities and equipment are conducive to better performance. Other members of the rehabilitation team become involved in the care of the disabled cancer patient as deemed appropriate by the physiatrist. If these interventions allow the patient to become self-sufficient and ambulatory, then the patient should be discharged home directly from the acute service, when medically indicated, having received proper instructions, equipment, and referrals for specific nursing interventions.

A more comprehensive and intensive rehabilitation program on an inpatient rehabilitation service is provided for physically disabled cancer patients who do not swiftly gain independence in ADL and mobility with daily therapy on the acute service, who are medically capable of actively participating in the program for at least 3 hours daily, and who are motivated and mentally capable of following instructions and learning the different tasks.

The inpatient rehabilitation unit should be in a hospital with an in-house physician on call and the various medical and surgical consultation services available at all times. Here the disabled cancer patient is reevaluated by the physiatrist, who obtains a detailed medical and social history and performs a careful physical examination to assess the general medical and precise musculoskeletal and neurologic condition, as well as the current functional ability. The physiatrist writes the routine medical orders for nursing care, medications, and disability-specific diagnostic tests, including radiologic studies, urologic evaluation, pulmonary function tests, and electrodiagnostic studies. The physiatrist prescribes the specific exercises and training methods to be given by the physical and occupational therapists, as well as interventions by the other members of the interdisciplinary team.

The rehabilitation program begins promptly after transfer to the inpatient rehabilitation service. Several hours each day are spent in an active therapy program in addition to different ward activities, such as self-care training, management of bowel and bladder dysfunction, and educational and recreational activities. When serious medical complications arise during the course of rehabilitation that interfere with the patient's ability to attend the rehabilitation program for at least 3 hours a day for more than 3 consecutive days, the patient should be transferred to the appropriate medical or surgical service for definitive care.

Within 1 week of admission, an initial team conference is held at which the patient's medical, functional, psychologic, social, vocational, and recreational status, as well as the rehabilitation potential and prognosis, are presented. Moreover, adaptive gait aids (ie, canes, crutches, or a walker and wearing of proper shoes) that may help the patient ambulate functionally again are also provided.

Cancer of the Brain

Brain damage may result from primary tumors of the brain, metastatic disease, or treatment of the cancer—surgery, radiation, or, more rarely, chemotherapy. The symptoms and disability that may result vary extensively but, in essence, are similar to those that are seen in patients who have sustained traumatic brain injury or a stroke involving different parts of the brain (Table 63-5). The main difference, however, is the potentially progressive or recurrent nature of the brain cancer and its uncertain prognosis. The greatest deficits are frequently seen immediately after surgery or during radiation and chemotherapy, after which remarkable improvement may occur. Late brain injury from radiation with infarction or necrosis also may occur, but the resulting disability has a less favorable prognosis for recovery. All patients with brain cancer and impaired function in mobility or ADL should be referred for rehabilitation services. Many, regardless of tumor type, can be helped with simple rehabilitation measures, whereas others may require comprehensive in patient rehabilitation, which should be provided when longer life expectancy allows.[21,22] Following definitive treatment of primary brain tumors in children, rehabilitation significantly improves outcome in self care activities, transfers into and out of bed, and locomotion by a wheelchair or walking.[23]

Most commonly, the rehabilitation intervention starts after surgical resection or removal of the brain tumor. When medically stable, the patient should be helped to sit up, get out of bed, and start on an active restoration program that is designed according to the patient's general condition. The location and size of the cerebral lesion clearly determine the clinical symptoms encountered. The variability of the symptoms precludes a standard rehabilitation approach but demandsan individual evaluation and treatment plan. Broadly, the problems of patients with cancer of the brain are physical, psychological, social, and vocational. Table 63-5 lists the most common problems, which are briefly discussed below. Paralysis, often in the form of hemiplegia, can be a conspicuous consequence of brain cancer. Although the paralysis is most profound just after the brain surgery, a certain return of motor power is common and may continue for several weeks or months. Mobilization training starts when the patient is ready to be transferred out of bed. Depending on the extent of the paralysis, the patient may be taught to ambulate with assistive devices or tomaneuver a wheel chair. As the body balance improves and the patient has learned to lean consistently to his or her good side, ambulation out-side the parallel bars can begin, with the patientusing an appropriate ambulation aid carried in the unaffected upper extremity. Usually, some knee extens or strength returns, providing the patient with adequate knee support, but the ankle dorsiflexors and invertors still may be weak. Here aplastic ankle-foot orthosis (AFO) may be pre-scribed to prevent the foot dragging during the swing phase of gait. This orthosis is easily inserted into most shoes. It is cosmetically superior to the old metal orthoses and usually provides equal or better function. If knee extens or strength does not return, fabrication of a knee-ankle-foot or thosis may be considered, but the prognosis for functional ambulation with such a device is poor.

The major goal in the rehabilitation of the patient with cancer of the brain is independence in ADL, which may be obtained through training, prescription of proper assistive devices, and possibly modification of the patient's clothing and the architecture of the patient's home. Spasticity frequently interferes with mobility and performance of ADL. Factors that may aggravate the spasticity (eg, skin lesions, infections, and anxiety) need to be identified and treated. Thorough stretching of all joints should be performed daily. Medications (ie, dantrolene sodium, baclofen, or diazepam) may be of some benefit but should be used sparingly in view of their potential side effects. Selected nerve blocks with-dilute solutions of phenol or motor point blocks with botulinum toxin are usually effective in reducing local spasticity, but surgical procedures for reduction of spasticity in patients with cancer of the brain are rarely indicated.

Joint contractures, whether owing to muscle imbalance, spasticity, improper bed positioning, or an inadequate exercise program, may change there habilitation prognosis significantly. A 10° flexion contracture of the knee, for example, will greatly increase oxygen consumption during ambulation and thus markedly reduce endurance. Knee contractures that exceed 15° will usually make functional ambulation impossible for the patient with brain cancer and hemiplegia. Development of a frozen shoulder may make independent dressing impossible. Prevention of contractures by proper joint range of motion exercises is imperative from the onset of the disability because treatment of contracture is relatively ineffective.

Pain in different parts of the body may be experienced in patients with neurologic deficits caused by cancer of the brain. Dysesthetic thalamic pain is notably refractory to treatment, although various centrally acting agents may be helpful. Pain with motion of the hemiplegic shoulder is common, perhaps owing to muscle imbalance at the shoulder girdle and recurrentminor trauma to the periarticular structures. Shoulder support by an arm sling or a lapboard, administration of analgesics, application of heat or cold modalities, and gentle range of motion and strengthening exercises may all help reduce the pain and improve shoulder function. Complex regional pain syndrome, formerly known as reflex sympathetic dystrophy, may occur and requires similar treatment, but more effective relief may be obtained by simply administering oral steroids, for example, prednisone 5 mg four times a day for 2 to 3 weeks.[19] Sympathetic nerve blocks may be performed when symptoms are more persistent.

Sensory deficits of varying degrees are commonly seen in patients with brain cancer, either in the distribution of the cranial nerves or on one or both sides of the body. Cancer affecting the parietal lobes of the brain may cause severe sensory loss with little muscle weakness. This may interfere with balance and mobility because the patient who cannot feel motion is unable to control it. Although physical exercise cannot decrease the sensory loss, training with adaptive gait aids (ie, canes, crutches, or a walker and wearing of proper shoes) may help the patient ambulate functionally again.

Visual deficits, such as double vision or visual field deficits, are commonly seen as a result of cancer in the lower brain or above the tentorium, respectively. Although double vision may improve spontaneously, the use of unilateral or alternating eye patches or special prism glasses may be helpful. The value of exercises for retraining the eye muscles is uncertain. Homonymous hemianopsia—blindness to the affected side of the body caused by a contralateral brain tumor—rarely resolves spontaneously. Whereas a patient with a left brain lesion usually learns easily to compensate for hemianopsia through scanning of the environment, the patient with a right brain lesion may experience severe difficulties owing to accompanying anosognosia, that is, lack of awareness of the affected left side of the body and of the surroundings. Specialized programs of cognitive remediation have been found to be effective with these patients.[25]

Aphasia may be seen in patients with cancer in the left dominant hemisphere of the brain. This is an impairment of the central language process, with reduced capacity for interpretation and formulation of the symbols for communication. Although all components of language—listening, speaking, reading, and writing—are usually affected, they are not affected to an equal extent; thus, several types of aphasia are recognized.[26,27] Expressive or nonfluent aphasia is caused by lesions in the Broca area of the brain and is characterized by reduced language production, vocabulary, and use of grammar. The patient is well aware of these difficulties and becomes very frustrated. Less well known is receptive or fluent aphasia, which is caused by lesions in the Wernicke area of the brain. Here the patient primarily has difficulty in understanding language, both his or her own and that of others. The patient thus may be able to speak continuously at normal speed and with normal intonation without giving any pertinent information or being aware of the errors. The efficiency of speech therapy is debated because most patients will have a degree of spontaneous improvement. Nonetheless, speech therapy is indicated, whenever available, not only for psychological support but also to provide the necessary stimulation for the patient to use his or her maximum speech ability, to adjust to new circumstances, and to instruct the caregiver in proper communication with the patient by using short, simple sentences at a normal voice volume, gestures, and facial expressions, always with respect, optimism, patience, and encouragement.

Dysarthria is a motor disturbance of speech, which implies weakness, slowness, or incoordination of the muscles that produce speech. Understanding written or spoken language is, therefore, never a problem. Articulation is usually the main problem, but speed, rhythm, sound, and intonation may also be disturbed. Mild dysarthria accompanies many brain cancers that involve cranial nerves and the cerebrum and affect the facial musculature, but dysarthria is particularly prominent in brainstem tumors. If speech remains completely unintelligible, other communication methods are introduced, such as writing, typing, sign language, or pictures.

Dysphagia, or impaired swallowing, is frequently seen in patients with brain cancer, especially when the brainstem is involved. In its most severe form, the patient may be unable to swallow, but in milder cases, there may only be difficulty with the swallowing of liquids. Serial radiographic swallowing studies should be done for proper monitoring of the condition until it is resolved or until other safer means of nutrition are established. A swallowing training program may be instituted by the speech or occupational therapist in which the patient attempts to swallow food of different consistency using different techniques and positions. A nasogastric tube may be used for a week or so while waiting for spontaneous recovery, but a more persistent dysphagia warrants insertion of a gastrostomy tube for prolonged feeding.

Neuropsychological changes may be prominent when cancer affects the cerebral hemispheres. Reduced memory and judgment frequently make successful rehabilitation impossible because the patient may be unable to remember instructions. Visual perceptual deficits, caused by a central disturbance in organizing visual stimuli from the environment, frequently accompany right brain damage even when visual field and acuity are normal. These patients may experience difficulty in recognizing the 3 dimensions: depth and distances, the relationship of lines and objects, and vertical and horizontal lines. Patients with lesions in the left hemisphere, on the other hand, usually act and learn slowly, make few mistakes, and are aware of their deficits, which frustrate them severely. In recent years, neuropsychological training programs designed to help patients overcome the visual, perceptual, and cognitive deficits have been reported as being successful.[28,29] In addition, repeated neuropsychological evaluations have been found to be sensitive indicators of recurrence.[30]

Cancer of the Spine

The spine is the most common site for skeletal metastases.[31] At autopsy, 70% of patients who die from cancer demonstrate vertebral metastases[32] and more than 5% have evidence of metastatic compression of the spinal cord.[33] This is usually an extradural anterior mass that involves bone. Intradural extramedullary tumors are usually histologically benign meningiomas or neurofibromas. Gliomas (ie, ependymomas, astrocytomas, and medulloblastomas) are usually intramedullary, although occasionally they are also found in an extramedullary site. Although the response to treatment is quite different for all of these histologically distinct tumors, the neurologic symptoms, signs, and rehabilitation interventions are quite similar.

Injury to the spinal cord and peripheral nerves is a recognized risk of therapeutic radiation that may not become manifest for many months or even years.[34] A transient radiation myelopathy primarily involving sensory neurons may occur in 10-15% of patients receiving mantle radiation for Hodgkin's disease.[30] This condition is usually associated only with sensory symptoms, such as paresthesias and Lhermitte's sign, and resolves in 1-9 months.[35] Delayed radiation myelopathy is an irreversible and progressive neurologic condition that may affect motor, sensory, and sphincter functions and has a reported incidence of 1-12%.[36]

Clinical Presentation

By far the most frequent presenting symptom of a tumor of the spine is pain. The pain may be localized, diffuse, or radicular in nature. It is characteristically made worse by activity and by straining. Different from more benign back pain, the pain caused by tumors tends to be persistent, tends to be present or even worse at night, and is not relieved by rest. Additional symptoms at presentation may be weakness of the legs, difficulty in walking, and urinary sphincteric problems leading to incontinence.

Neurologic deficits may develop insidiously or occur suddenly, depending on the tumor's rate of growth and location or on the occurrence of a sudden pathologic fracture. Slowly progressive neurologic dysfunction is often seen with tumors of the lower spine that encroach on the cauda equina, whereas tumors of the thoracic spine may cause the sudden collapse of the vertebral body with direct compression of the spinal cord or of its blood supply. Although only half of all tumors of the spine are located in the thoracic region, these cause 70% of all spinal cord compressions that result in paraplegia. Frequently, the neurologic lesion is incomplete, with sensation and motor function preserved to varying degrees, and may be rated by the American Spinal Injury Association (ASIA) Impairment Scale.[37] Impaired bladder and bowel control at first may present clinically as urinary urgency or hesitancy, but with progressive cord compression, urinary retention or bowel and bladder incontinence may occur.

Treatment

Proper rehabilitation management planning and intervention depend on an accurate diagnosis and staging of the tumor, just as does medical and surgical management. The Tokuhashi scale has been shown to have over 80% reliability in predicting prognosis in persons with spinal metastases.[38] It has been shown that rehabilitation improves functional outcomes in persons with spinal metastases and may even increase survival in those with high Tokuhashi scores.[39] Most patients with spinal metastases can and should be managed nonsurgically with radiation, chemotherapy, vetebroplasty (Chapter 126), and orthotic stabilization of the spine because it has been demonstrated that radiation alone provides results that are similar to those of surgery followed by radiation.[40] In general, laminectomy with decompression is of limited use compared with radiation because the compressive lesion is usually located anteriorly to the cord and the surgical procedure itself contributes to spinal instability. However, profound neurologic deficits, especially when occurring rapidly, may warrant surgical decompression, which preferably should be done by an anterior approach followed by surgical stabilization of the spine. Surgical decompression of the spinal cord is not very effective once the patient has become completely paraplegic. Surgical stabilization may often be indicated when gross spinal instability is present because 2 of the 3 "columns" (anterior, middle, and posterior) of the spine have been destroyed by the tumor.[41]

Spinal metastases and myelomatous lesions, even when accompanied by compression fractures and minor or modest spinal instability, can be successfully managed by spinal orthotic support and radiation. Both modalities may significantly decrease pain. Lesions in the cervical spine are most rigidly immobilized by a halo brace (Fig. 63-1) but also may be adequately supported by a sternal-occipital-mandibular immobilizer (SOMI brace) (Fig. 63-2). When such lesions are present in the upper thoracic spine, spinal orthoses may not be necessary because this part of the spine is stabilized inherently by the rib cage. Lesions in the more mobile lower thoracic and lumbar spine are often associated with severe pain. An adjustable thoracolumbosacral orthosis (TLSO) (Fig. 63-3) with posterior stays may provide sufficient support for less severe lesions, decrease pain, and allow greater mobility. Larger lesions and postoperative conditions may require fabrication of a custom-molded plastic TLS brace, a 2-piece removable orthosis (Fig. 63-4) that firmly grabs the pelvis below and the chest above.

When neurologic loss has occurred, the rehabilitation therapy must be carefully individualized, based on the extent of the neurologic dysfunction, the medical or surgical condition, and the patient's

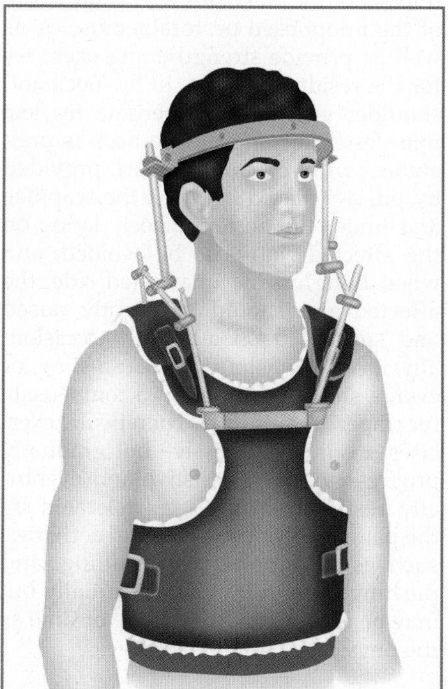

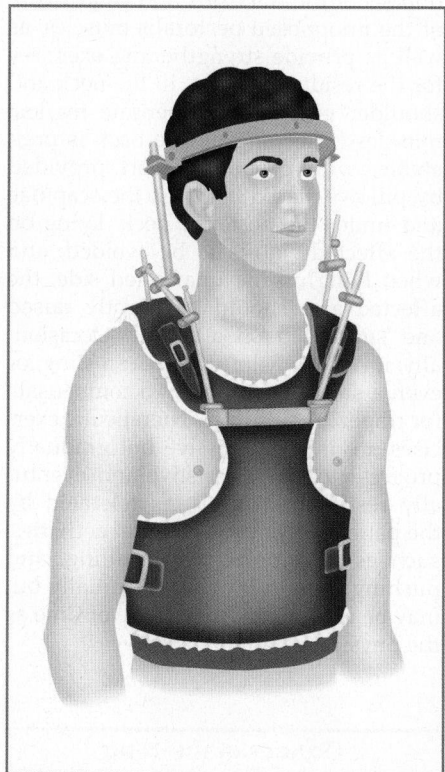

Figure 63-1 ■ Halo-orthosis. *Source*: Reproduced with permission from Ragnarsson KT. Orthotics and shoes. In: DeLisa JA, ed. *Rehabilitation Medicine: Principles and Practice*. Philadelphia: Lippincott; 1988:326.

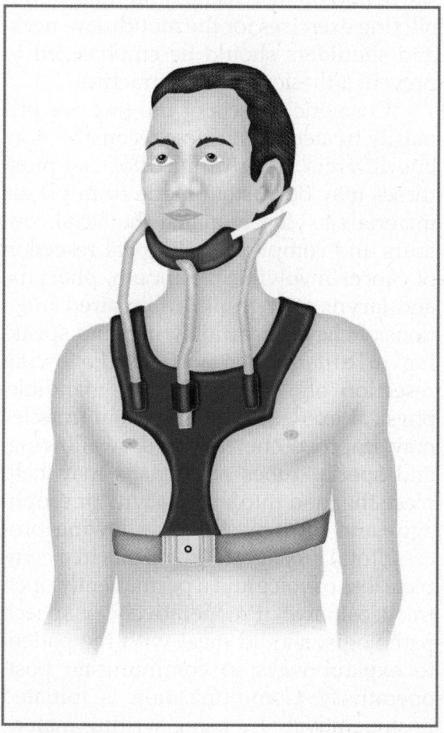

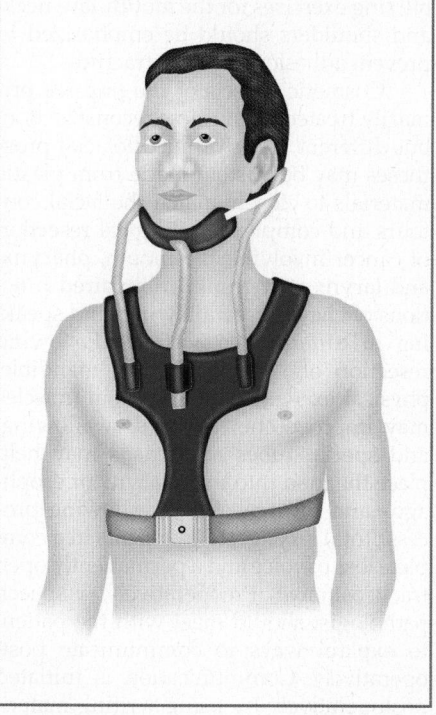

Figure 63-2 ■ Sternal-occipital-mandibular immobilizer (SOMI orthosis). *Source*: Reproduced with permission from Ragnarsson KT. Orthotics and shoes. In: DeLisa JA, ed. *Rehabilitation Medicine: Principles and Practice*. Philadelphia: Lippincott; 1988:326.

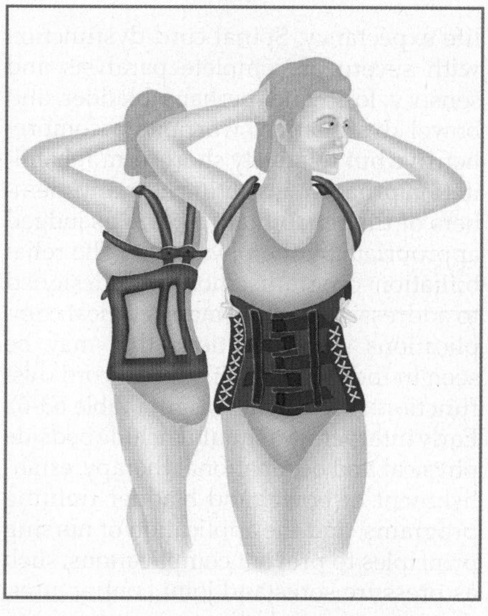

Figure 63-3 ■ Thoracolumbosacral orthosis (Knight-Taylor brace). *Source*: Reproduced with permission from Ragnarsson KT. Rehabilitation of patients with physical disabilities caused by tumors of the musculoskeletal system. In: Lewis MM, ed. *Musculoskeletal Oncology: A Multidisciplinary Approach*. Philadelphia: WB Saunders; 1992:463.

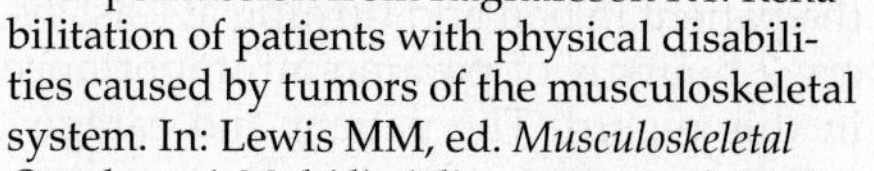

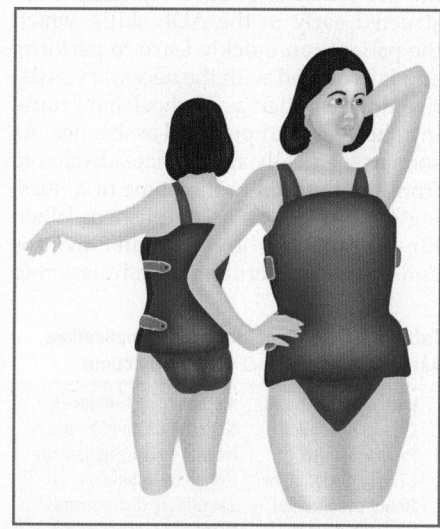

Figure 63-4 ■ Custom-molded thoracolumbosacral orthosis (TLSO), a two-piece removable plastic orthosis ("body jacket"). *Source*: Reproduced with permission from Ragnarsson KT. Rehabilitation of patients with physical disabilities caused by tumors of the musculoskeletal system. In: Lewis MM, ed. *Musculoskeletal Oncology: A Multidisciplinary Approach*. Philadelphia: WB Saunders; 1992:463.

Table 63-5 ■ Rehabilitation Problems Associated With Cancer of the Brain

Paralysis	Dysarthria
Spasticity	Aprosodia
Joint contractures	Dysphagia
Pain	Ataxia
Sensory deficits	Visual-perceptual deficits
Visual field deficits	Cognitive and behavioral deficits
Diplopia	Psychosocial-vocational problems
Aphasia	

life expectancy. Spinal cord dysfunction with severe or complete paralysis and sensory loss, and perhaps bladder and bowel dysfunction, warrants a comprehensive but relatively short-term rehabilitation program involving as many members of the rehabilitation team as judged appropriate by the physiatrist. The rehabilitation programs should be designed to address each of the many clinical complications and conditions that may be seen in individuals with spinal cord dysfunction of traumatic origin (Table 63-6). Early intervention should include bedside physical and occupational therapy, establishment of bowel and bladder training programs, and the application of nursing principles to prevent complications, such as pressure sores and joint contractures, that increase morbidity, worsen the functional prognosis, and prolong the rehabilitation phase. Proper positioning of the patient in bed and turning at least every 2 hours is of paramount importance in this regard. The patient and caregivers are given emotional support and are educated in the medical aspects of spinal cord dysfunction and management. If the prognosis is poor, the patient is instructed early in the ADL skills, which the patient can quickly learn to perform, and is provided with the necessary assistive devices, such as a wheelchair, nursing supplies, and personal assistance. As soon as medically appropriate, discharge from the hospital to the home or a nursing facility can be accomplished. When life expectancy is greater than 3 months and the general criteria for admission to the inpatient rehabilitation service are met, the patient should be transferred there for a more comprehensive and intensive rehabilitation program to improve mobility and self-care skills.[42,43]

Table 63-6 ■ Conditions and Complications Associated With Spinal Cord Dysfunctions

Loss of motor power	Metabolic disturbances
Loss of sensation	Negative calcium balance
Pressure sores	Negative nitrogen balance
Urinary dysfunction	Hormonal imbalance
Bowel dysfunction	Circulatory disturbances
Sexual dysfunction	Orthostatic hypotension
Autonomic hyperreflexia	Edema
Pain	Deep vein thrombophlebitis
Spasticity	Respiratory disturbances
Joint contractures	Psychological problems
Heterotopic ossifications	Social problems
Vocational problems	

Cancer of the Head and Neck

Definitive treatment of cancer that arises from the skin of the face and neck or tissues of the nose, mouth, throat, and larynx may result in impairments in cosmesis, oral communication, feeding, and respiration, as well as affect the senses of sight, hearing, taste, and smell.[44] These functional deficits may have major psychological, social, and vocational consequences if not adequately addressed early and managed properly. Sensory deficits and radiation-induced skin changes require careful grooming and hygiene to prevent further skin damage by using nonirritating soaps and cosmetic products, an electric razor instead of a blade, lukewarm water for washing, loose-fitting garments, and similar measures. Meticulous oral hygiene is essential, and the patient should frequently use diluted mouthwash with 3% hydrogen peroxide but avoid all irritating agents (ie, alcohol, tobacco, and astringent toothpaste) and should limit denture wear. A noxious taste and dry mouth may be reduced by the use of artificial saliva and by increasing fluid intake. Mobilizing exercises for the mouth, jaw, neck, and shoulders should be emphasized to prevent adhesions and contractures.

Cosmetic defects of the face are primarily treated by surgical reconstruction, but different types of maxillofacial prostheses may be custom-made from plastic materials to closely match the facial contours and complexion. Surgical resection of cancer involving the mouth, pharynx, and larynx may result in impaired functions of chewing, swallowing, and speaking in different proportions. Following resection of the tongue and mandible, physical exercise of the residual muscles may improve chewing and swallowing, and special tubes or utensils may help place the food into the pharynx or esophagus and thus ease the swallowing process. Total laryngectomy results in a complete loss of voice and a permanently open tracheostomy.[45] Preoperatively, a speech pathologist should meet with the patient to explain ways to communicate postoperatively. Communication is initiated postoperatively by using writing materials, communication boards, or electronic typing gadgets, but as early as possible, the patient is instructed in the use of an artificial electrolarynx. Here a handheld battery-powered "diaphragm" is placed firmly against the neck to transmit sound waves through the tissues into the mouth, where it resonates and may be articulated with relative ease as comprehensible speech. Greater training, however, is required to become proficient in esophageal speech, which is generated by trapping air in the upper esophagus by the tongue and releasing it suddenly into the pharynx, thus producing a "burp-like" low-pitched sound that may be articulated into words. In some cases, a tracheopharyngeal shunt may be surgically reconstructed to restore a more normal voice.[46] Because of the open tracheostomy, the laryngectomized patient is unable to strain during lifting, pushing, or defecation, except by manually closing the stoma. The permanent tracheostomy requires not only good local care but also inhalation of humidified air through a stoma cover made of a piece of gauze that acts as a sieve for dust and other foreign materials.

Radical neck dissection may involve the removal of several neck muscles and temporary or permanent damage of the spinal accessory nerve that supplies the sternocleidomastoid and the trapezius muscles. This is likely to result in gross asymmetry of the neck and shoulders, restriction of motion, overstretching of remaining muscles, and persistent pain if not treated early.[47] During the rehabilitation of these patients, it is of primary importance to unload the shoulder immediately postoperatively, reduce shoulder and neck pain, and prevent stretch fibrosis of the trapezius and contracture of the unopposed pectoralis muscles, as well as provide strengthening exercises for the residual muscles in the neck and shoulder girdle to compensate for lost muscles.[48] Sleeping on the back is preferable, with proper support provided by pillows placed between the scapulae and under the posterior neck. Lying on the affected side is to be avoided, and when lying on the unaffected side, the affected arm should be slightly raised and supported on a pillow. Occasionally, it may be helpful to wear a sling, or even a shoulder orthosis, to compensate for trapezius paralysis. Therapeutic exercises are initially passive but gradually progress to active-assistive and eventually resistive exercises, as tolerated by the patient. Strenuous physical activities, such as lifting, carrying, pulling, and pushing, should be avoided initially but may be resumed in the course of time as the physical condition improves.[49]

Cancer of the Lung

The physical disabilities associated with lung cancer and its treatment include respiratory insufficiency, shoulder pain and stiffness, scoliosis, and the remote effects of certain lung cancers that cause a neuromuscular disorder that becomes manifest as weakness and incoordination. However, the functional limitations associated with lung cancer frequently do not receive adequate attention and intervention because of the high mortality and short life expectancy associated with the disease.

Reduced respiratory capacity after lung resection or pneumonectomy, especially when combined with preexisting chronic obstructive pulmonary disease, may result in respiratory complications and insufficiency during both the postoperative period and the long-term follow-up. As the patient recuperates and becomes ambulatory, shoulder range of motion, general strengthening, and endurance exercises, as well as postural training, are added to the therapy program to increase strength and stamina and prevent post-thoracotomy scoliosis and scapulohumeral displacement.[50]

Cancer of the Breast

Breast cancer that is treated with mastectomy or with lumpectomy followed by radiation, and/or with chemotherapy may result in considerable physical disability. Radical mastectomy with removal of the pectoralis muscles, although now rarely performed, may cause shoulder weakness and, together with axillary node dissection, may produce swelling of the ipsilateral arm. Stiffness of the shoulder and hand may limit reach and manual dexterity. Fortunately, the recent trend of performing modified radical mastectomies or lumpectomies and routinely providing proper postoperative rehabilitation therapy has reduced the frequency and severity of these problems.

Postoperative rehabilitation has three main goals: prevention of physical disability, restoration of cosmetic appearance, and psychosocial and vocational readjustment. Physical rehabilitation aims at improving muscle strength and mobility at the shoulder, minimizing arm swelling, and facilitating resumption of all functional activities—ADL, recreation, and work. Following radical mastectomy, the arm should be kept slightly elevated, with the shoulder abducted to 80°-90° and externally rotated, keeping the elbow free.[51] The entire arm is compressed by a well-wrapped elastic Ace bandage, which is reapplied every 8 hours to reduce the swelling. Substantially less physical rehabilitation is necessary following modified radical mastectomy and axillary dissection, an operation that spares the pectoralis major and usually the pectoralis minor. Lumpectomy with sentinel mode sampling or axillary dissection requires even less physical rehabilitation, which may proceed at a more rapid pace. Depending on the extent of the mastectomy, physical exercises may be started within 2-5 days postoperatively. Gentle exercises are started at this time, with the patient actively moving all of the unaffected limbs, as well as the elbow, wrist, and hand on the affected side, and isometrically contracting the distal muscles (hand squeezing) while supine and with the affected arm elevated. When the drains have been removed from the surgical site, the exercises may become more demanding. The patient starts performing gentle active exercises of the affected shoulder while still in a supine position. Approximately 10 days postoperatively, when the sutures are removed, active or active-assistive shoulder exercises in the upright position are begun, that is, "wall climbing" exercises using the uninvolved arm or an overhead pulley system to ease the task. On discharge, the patient receives a series of exercises to perform at home to ensure that full shoulder mobility and maximum strength is regained.

Lymphedema of the arm after radical mastectomy is seen in approximately 10-15% of patients, although relatively mild or moderate arm swelling is much more common, especially in the early postoperative days. Lymphedema is less common after modified radical mastectomy and rare after lumpectomy, even though both procedures do have axillary dissection. When lymphedema is severe, it may result in both a significant disability and a disfigurement. Although surgical removal of lymph nodes and lymph vessels or their destruction by radiation undoubtedly is the major etiologic factor, a number of other contributing factors may play a role, including infection, inflammation, scar formation, obesity, thrombophlebitis, arm dominance, and habitual dependent position of the arm. The greatest incidence of lymphedema has been noted among those who received high-dose radiation or had a history of one or more infections.[52,53] Prevention of lymphedema with proper postoperative care and initiation of an exercise program, referred to as complex decongestive physiotherapy, is most important because treatment of persisting lymphedema is relatively ineffective. Such treatment usually involves different physical interventions: performing, several times a day, sets of isometric exercises of all of the arm muscles while the arm is maintained in an elevated position, compression bandaging, manual massage, and skin care with patient education. These modalities help pump the fluid from the hand and distal arm toward the body. Compression therapy by manual massage of both the edematous[54-57] and the contralateral arm[46] has also been advocated but is considered by some to be time-consuming and inefficient.[47] Between periods of use, the arm should be carefully wrapped with elastic bandages, and when maximum reduction of the edema has been obtained, a custom-fitted elastic support sleeve should be fabricated and worn continuously. The entire limb should be guarded against even trivial trauma, which may be caused by constricting garments and excessive heat or exercise, to minimize swelling. Treatment with these physical modalities and exercise benefits the majority of patients with postoperative lymphedema and is more effective than diuretics, salt restriction diets, benzopyrones, or surgical procedures.[58-61] Benzopyrone reportedly causes a slow but safe reduction of high-protein lymphedema of the extremities by stimulating proteolysis *by* macrophages.[62]

Cancer of the Gastrointestinal Tract

The cancer rehabilitation team is involved in the care of the patient who has cancer limited to the gastrointestinal tract when the definitive surgical treatment has resulted in an ostomy. The enterostomal therapist (ET nurse) plays a major role in helping the cancer patient with an ostomy (ie, colostomy, ileostomy, or urostomy) understand the principles of ostomy care, learn the different aspects of ostomy management, and adjust to the altered self-image.

Colostomy

The surgical treatment of cancer of the rectum often mandates the creation of a colostomy by using the sigmoid colon. A cancer higher in the colon can frequently be resected and the bowel reconnected by anastomosis. Before undergoing a surgical procedure for cancer that will result in a colostomy, the surgeon needs to discuss the plans carefully with the patient. Subsequently, the ET nurse should meet with the patient and family members to explain in simple but clear terms the nature of the colostomy, for example, where the stoma will be located on the abdominal wall, how it will look, what coverings and collection appliances will be needed, how evacuation will occur, and so on. A positive attitude on the part of the medical and nursing staff is important at this time, although the patient's fears and concerns regarding function, appearance, and sexual activity need to be acknowledged and discussed. A visit by a person who is successfully managing his or her colostomy may be very helpful. Good preoperative preparation reduces the patient's fears and builds confidence, both of which will facilitate postoperative rehabilitation.

Postoperatively, protecting the skin and collecting the drainage should be the primary goals. This is accomplished by a properly fitted appliance. Modern appliances with protective skin barriers cut to fit the exact size of the stoma will avoid postoperative peristomal skin excoriation and keep the patient dry and odor free. A person with a colostomy has a choice of allowing the bowels to function normally or to irrigate as a method of attempting to control bowel movements. Often the bowel habits return to normal patterns, and a well-fitting appliance may be emptied or changed as needed.

Numerous clinical problems may arise at any time after the creation of a colostomy. These may include constipation, diarrhea, odor, skin excoriation and maceration, skin infections (fungal or bacteria), and stomal bleeding. Sexual dysfunction after abdominoperineal resection is common, not owing to the colostomy per se but to damage to the autonomic nerves in the pelvis sustained during extensive surgery. The altered self-image often associated with the colostomy can cause temporary sexual dysfunction, although sexual desire is not lessened.[63] Sexual counseling for both partners, good communication, and the teaching of new techniques for mutual gratification can do much to restore successful sexual activity. The colostomy patient may experience a reactive depression or grief and subsequently go through the different stages of adaptation that are associated with any kind of major personal loss. The colostomy's negative influence on the patient's self-image is best counteracted by the physician and the ET nurse when they are able to make an accurate assessment of the patient's complaints and condition, plan actions and interventions accordingly, and provide supportive counseling on an individual basis.[64]

Ileostomy

The principles and techniques of ileostomy care or similar to those of colostomy. The stools are of a loose consistency and drain continuously from the ileostomy. It is, therefore, necessary that the collecting pouch be worn at all times and that it be properly fitted by an ET nurse. Small bowel contents contain active digestive enzymes, which can cause severe peristomal skin excoriation if leakage occurs. Because the fluid loss through ileostomy is greater than with colostomy, fluid intake must be increased to prevent dehydration. In general, the psychosocial adjustment and rehabilitation outcome for an individual with ileostomy are similar to those after any surgery that requires alteration of elimination habits and results in living with a stoma.

Cancer of the Genitourinary System

Invasive cancer of the bladder frequently requires radical cystectomy and the creation of a new outlet for urine. More than 40 years ago, Bricker developed the ileal conduit procedure by connecting the ureters to an isolated segment of ileum, which is surgically closed at one end but opens at the other as a stoma on the abdominal wall, allowing free elimination of the urine. This procedure has become the traditional form of long-term urinary diversion. The management principles of ileal conduit stoma care are similar to those of colostomy and ileostomy. Because urine flows continuously from the stoma, the collecting system must be well fitted and watertight to prevent leakage. Skin or stoma problems from the urine are not uncommon and may be caused by alkaline urine. Many physicians prescribe vitamin C, 1,000 mg daily, to keep the urine slightly acidic. The intake of 8-10 glasses of fluid daily is important. In recent years, the continent urostomy has gained considerable popularity when used with compliant patients. The Kock pouch and the Indiana pouch, with several modifications of both procedures, result in an internal reservoir.[65-70] The patient inserts a catheter into the stoma every 4-6 hours to empty the internal pouch contents. This procedure eliminates the need for external devices.

Genital Cancer

The cancer rehabilitation team may occasionally be asked to provide care for a patient with cancer involving the genital organs or when the cancer and its treatment have caused sexual dysfunction. Rehabilitation interventions usually involve carefully planned reconstructive surgery and psychological and sexual counseling. The form of surgical reconstruction varies, depending on the type of the cancer and the extent of the surgical resection but also on the specific needs of the patient. The woman who has undergone radical gynecologic surgery with resection of the vagina may benefit from vaginal reconstruction that allows resumption of sexual intercourse.[71] The man who is unable to achieve penile erection can be prescribed medications (ie, sildenafil), taught intrapenile injection of vasodilating drugs to cause erection when desired, use of a vacuum-assisted erection device, or, rarely nowadays, have a penile prosthesis implanted.[72,73] The choice of prosthesis is between semirigid silicone rod implants and a system of inflatable cylinders implanted into the shaft of the penis, with the scrotal pump and fluid reservoir placed in the abdominal wall.[74-76] The implantation of the semirigid rod is a relatively simple surgical procedure with few mechanical problems, but the penis stays semierect permanently. The inflatable prosthesis provides a more normal appearance of the penis both when flaccid and erect, but mechanical problems with the system often arise.

Cancer of the testes is usually treated with prompt surgical excision of one or both of the testicles, followed by radiation and/or chemotherapy. Surgical implantation of a prosthetic testicle may be gratifying for patients concerned about their appearance and self-image.

Sexual Rehabilitation

Sexual rehabilitation is not limited to those who have cancer affecting the genital organs but should be available for anyone who experiences sexual dysfunction for physical or psychological reasons as a result of cancer and its treatment. Different members of the rehabilitation team collaborate in providing sexual counseling for patients with different forms of cancer, both on an individual basis and by organizing courses and seminars on the physiology and anatomy of sexual function, on human sexuality, and on ways of adjusting to sexual dysfunction. Male sexual impotence compounds the reactive depression associated with the diagnosis of cancer and adds to the stigma of any physical disability. This condition is frequently met with prejudice and poor understanding on the part of both the patient and the patient's sexual partner. Sexual rehabilitation emphasizes that sexuality is considered part of the whole person and cannot be lost because of an illness or injury. Physical disability, in contrast to a physical illness, does not decrease sexual drive, although it may affect sexual function both physically and psychologically. The anatomy and physiology of sexual function should be carefully explained to the patient and his or her partner and general guidelines for success are to be specified . Good communication and strengthening of relationships between sexual partners are emphasized. The different physical aspects of sexual performance are explained to make expectations compatible with performance capability. For most cancer patients with a physical disability, impairment of mobility, sensation, continence, and erection should not interfere with building a solid personal relationship, with having sensitivity to the partner's desires, or with being able to please and enjoy. Sexual rehabilitation is built on the concept that if sexual comfort is taught, sexual competence may result.[77] Manual and oral sexual acts may be appropriate for both sexes. No treatment or rehabilitation of the patient with cancer can be considered complete until the clinician has adequately addressed the impact of the condition on sexual function. Sexual health cannot be separated from total health. The extra time spent considering sexual adequacy and providing guidelines for help can benefit the patient for years.

Cancer of the Limbs

Primary malignant tumors of the limbs require surgical treatment. The main surgical goal is to remove the tumor, either by an excision with wide margins through a site well clear of any malignant growth or by radical removal of the entire bone or the compartment afflicted by the tumor. A subsequent surgical goal is to reconstruct the resulting defect for optimal function and cosmesis. Although limb amputation has been practiced for centuries, in recent years, limb salvage by extended local or regional excision and reconstruction has been the principal goal. The survival and disease-free survival after both types of surgical approaches are similar and have been vastly improved in recent years by the use of chemotherapy, radiation, or both. The return to optimal function can best be ensured by a multidisciplinary rehabilitation team approach that includes the surgeon, the medical and radiation oncologists, the physiatrist, and all of the members of the rehabilitation team.[78]

Skeletal metastases are more common than primary bone tumors.[79] Metastases to the limb bones are less common than those to the spine. Although some patients may complain of localized pain, others are essentially asymptomatic until a pathologic fracture occurs. Such fractures occur in approximately 10-15% of patients who have radiographic evidence of skeletal metastasis. Pathologic fractures are most debilitating and often result in diminished survival for otherwise stable patients.[31] At particular risk of pathologic fractures are women with metastatic breast cancer, patients with advanced metastatic disease, and those with a large single lytic lesion eroding the bony cortex.[80] Active rehabilitation and physical mobilization do not seem to increase the fracture risk significantly. When prognosis suggests many months of anticipated function, prophylactic surgery for impending fracture of the femoral neck or shaft often diminishes the total disability consequent to pathologic fracture and more difficult surgical repair. Prophylactic surgery is otherwise generally not warranted, but radiation may have some effect in reducing pain and limiting tumor growth.[81] If pathologic fracture occurs, open surgical treatment with adequate internal fixation and conjunctive use of methylmethacrylate may be employed successfully to relieve pain, restore mobility, ease nursing care, and provide psychological reassurance.[82] Postoperative immobilization should be brief, and aggressive physical therapy should be started early to return the patient swiftly to previous function and to minimize hospitalization.

Preoperative Rehabilitation

Preoperative rehabilitation care should start immediately after the diagnosis of primary cancer of a limb is established, regardless of whether amputation or limb-sparing surgery is planned for cancer removal or whether chemotherapy and radiation are to be instituted pre- or postoperatively. The implications of surgery and the postoperative course should be discussed at this time with the patient and caregivers. Simultaneously, an appropriate physical exercise program should begin. Although it is important that the positive aspects of the surgical treatment be explained (ie, that it is a swift, lifesaving technique and that modern technology and training allow significant restoration of function), it is best for the physician to resist overly optimistic predictions and to discourage unrealistic hopes until postoperative rehabilitation success has been ensured. On the other hand, pessimistic statements as to what the patient will never be able to do are needless and are usually inaccurate. Peer counseling by a successfully rehabilitated amputee may further help the patient anticipate postoperative events and function.

When amputation or limb-sparing surgery is planned, the exact level of amputation and the surgical approach should be thoughtfully chosen, taking into account not only the location and type of cancer but also the probability of good wound healing and the successful fitting of a prosthesis when required. It may be helpful for the surgeon to consult with the physiatrist and prosthetist for this purpose.[83] Preoperatively, strengthening exercises should be started for muscles in the uninvolved extremities and the trunk, as well as for muscles to be spared in the affected limb. Specifically, the patient should learn to perform isometric exercises for the quadriceps and gluteal muscles. Strengthening exercises for the unaffected limbs should focus specifically on shoulder depressors and elbow extensors, which are critical for ambulation with crutches or walkers. Trunk-strengthening and balancing exercises may further ensure postoperative ambulation success. Ambulation with a walker or a pair of crutches, non-weight bearing on the affected limb, should be practiced preoperatively while the patient has no fear of falling because of a lack of limb support and is not impaired by incisional pain, medications, or postoperative complications. Such preoperative therapy not only will help the patient succeed swiftly in postoperative ambulation and self-care activities, but a quick restoration of function will ease the emotional adjustment to the disability, whether it be amputation or limb sparing with an internal prosthesis.

Limb Amputation

Limb amputation for cancer at one time was discouraged because the prevailing opinion was that poor life expectancy did not justify the expense of surgery and prosthetic fitting. However, the 5-year survival rate for patients who have undergone amputations for limb cancer (now7,509) compares favorably with the survival rate of patients with amputations for limb ischemia,[84] and the functional skills of cancer amputees are reportedly better than the skills of those patients who have had amputations for other reasons.[85]

In the past, amputations for cancer were done in a radical fashion and left little, if any, residual limb, except when amputating for very distal limb tumors, because the basic clinical rule was to amputate proximally to the joint immediately above the tumor site. Lower limb amputations for cancer involving the knee joint or thigh thus were frequently performed by a hip disarticulation or hemipelvectomy and upper limb amputations by shoulder disarticulation or interscapulothoracic (forequarter) amputations. Modern diagnostic techniques now can demonstrate the presence or absence of metastases with a high degree of accuracy. A survey showed that because of the use of adjuvant chemotherapy, sarcomatous metastases are not as common as was previously thought.[86] Thus, less extensive amputation techniques can now be employed such as cross-bone amputations with 3-4 inches of normal bone left as the margin. Greater residual limb length thus results, and functional outcome is better for most patients. Accordingly, primary cancer in the distal femur now permits an amputation through the proximal femur, a cancer in the proximal tibia permits amputation in the mid- or distal femur, and cancer in the distal tibia allows a below-knee amputation (BKA). Analogous amputation levels may be appropriately considered for cancer of the upper limbs.

Although maximum preservation of limb length compatible with eradication of the cancer is desirable, certain amputation levels may result in residual limbs that are difficult to fit and, therefore, best avoided, such as the hind foot, the distal third of the leg, and the femoral supracondylar region. It is critical to preserve the knee joint, if possible, to ensure smoothness of gait, lower energy cost, and better function. Whenever possible, 12-18 cm of tibia should be retained for optimal prosthetic fitting, but even a very short BKA that retains the tibial tubercle will preserve knee extension by the quadriceps muscle, and preservation of the knee joint will provide the needed position sense. This amputation level is, therefore, better than amputating above the knee. When the fibula is retained, it should be cut slightly shorter than the tibia. Disarticulation at the knee is also preferable to above-knee amputation (AKA) because it provides a wide weight-bearing surface, a long lever arm, and proprioception. Unfortunately, this level often cannot be chosen owing to intra-articular spread of cancer located in the mid- or proximal tibia. It is preferable to have the AKA residual limb as long as possible to preserve maximal adduction power. Prosthetic knee joints can accommodate any length of femur. A residual femoral length that is less than 8 cm from the greater trochanter to the tip functions poorly. As a rule, hip disarticulation is preferred to an amputation level above the lesser trochanter. Hip disarticulation and hemipelvectomy need reconstruction with a long posterior flap to create a proper sitting area on the prosthesis.[87] When provided with a well-fitting plastic laminated socket and an endoskeletal modular-design prosthesis, persons with hip disarticulation are able to stand, walk, and sit quite comfortably. Hemicorporectomy (translumbar amputation) has been performed on rare occasions on patients with widespread cancer of the pelvis but without metastases elsewhere. This procedure is a challenging alternative to the nonsurgical approach and has been shown to have a good rehabilitation outcome.[88] Cancers in the upper limbs unfortunately are primarily found in the proximal humerus and may require shoulder disarticulation or interscapulothoracic amputation. Here it is important to retain quality skin and maximum muscle mass for padding the shoulder, but retention of the humeral head, if possible, will result in better prosthetic fitting. Successful prosthetic use depends to a large extent on proper surgical techniques of amputation.[89] It is not adequate to provide only a long residual limb, although this is important for both leverage and large total contact area for weight bearing. Optimally, the residual limb should be firm and tapered or cylindrical in shape, with all bone ends well padded. The skin must have good innervation and vascular supply and not be adherent to bone or have sensitive scars.

Postoperative care should ensure optimal wound healing, minimize limb swelling, prevent joint contractures, and improve muscle strength and function. Application of appropriate dressing and external pressure on the residual limb is very important.[90] Wrapping with the customary elastic bandages must be done skillfully with frequent reapplications to maintain maximum sustained pressure and to avoid a tourniquet effect. Different forms of semirigid dressings have been used, such as Unna paste dressings, custom-made elastic "socks," plastic films, and inflatable air splints, each of which has advantages and disadvantages. Inflatable and removable air splints, recently popularized, are made of clear plastic and have a zipper, which allows easy inspection, attachments, and removal. If immediate surgical fitting is done with a semirigid dressing and prosthetic pylon and foot attached, full weight bearing is possible in 3-4 weeks.[91] There are several advantages and disadvantages to using this technique.[92,93]

Postoperative Exercise Program

Physical and occupational therapy should be initiated within 2 days after amputation. The preoperative exercise program is resumed for muscle strengthening and joint mobilization. Knee flexion contractures may easily develop after BKA, whereas hip flexion and abduction contractures are frequently seen with short AKA. Mobilization is started at the bedside, but within a few days, the patient is taken to the therapy area and ambulation in parallel bars or with a walker is started. The skillful amputee is subsequently provided with an ambulation device; however, when prosthetic fitting has been completed, a single cane may suffice. Different types of ready-made or prefabricated temporary prosthetic devices exist for the earliest ambulation efforts, but a custom-fitted provisional prosthesis should be provided as soon as the surgical incision has healed. The amputee, however, may be discharged from the hospital even without prosthesis if the patient is ambulating safely with assistive gait devices and is independent in ADL. Transfer to the inpatient rehabilitation unit for more intensive therapy may be advisable at any time before these two goals are reached if the amputee is otherwise medically stable.

Prescription of an Artificial Limb

The physician needs to consider multiple factors when prescribing limb prosthesis. The amputation level and limb condition clearly are of primary importance, but prosthetic candidacy may be affected by numerous other factors, including associated medical conditions, other physical disabilities, life expectancy, muscle strength and coordination, stamina, various psychological factors (ie, motivation, emotional adjustment, and cognition), and individual lifestyle factors (ie, age, weight, family support, recreational interest, environment, and type of work). The extent of prosthetic use is, to some degree, predictable because each symptomatic medical problem adversely affects functional prognosis. The ability of the patient to ambulate with a walker or a pair of crutches but without a prosthesis strongly suggests prosthetic candidacy. After carefully considering these different factors, the physiatrist may have to choose between a prosthesis that provides relatively greater safety with stability and one with greater function and mobility and between durability and low prosthetic weight, besides considering differences in cost and cosraesis. In recent years, prosthetic techniques for all types of amputations have advanced significantly, especially with respect to evaluation methods, socket design, ankle-foot components, and cosmesis.[94-99]

Most prostheses are currently fabricated from metals and plastics. The customary BKA prosthesis consists of a socket, shank, and ankle-foot components, as well as a suspension system. The socket usually has a patellar tendon-bearing design and total contact with the residual limb for maximum pressure distribution.[80] Modern liners that add comfort and protect sensitive skin are usually made of silicone gel may be designed to provide a suction suspension system with an attached distal pie that locks into a receptacle in the bottom of the socket or shank.[95] The shank is either of an endoskeletal design with an internal metal pylon or an exoskeletal structure made from laminated plastic. The solid-ankle cushioned heel foot is simple, durable, lightweight, and cosmetic and is still most commonly prescribed, despite the arrival of a variety of new energy-storing prosthetic feet, such as the Seattle and FLEX feet designs. The below-knee prosthesis is usually attached to the residual limb by a supracondylar cuff, although several other alternatives exist. The AKA traditionally obtains a prosthesis with a rigid quadrilateral socket and a posterior ischial seat for additional weight bearing. More modern socket designs promise greater comfort in sitting and better control during ambulation.[96] The popular single-axis knee joint with constant friction is simple and durable, whereas the more costly and complex polycentric or hydraulic knee units can provide better function for young, physically active amputees. Stability of the knee joint during stance may be increased by posterior placement of the knee axis, but for maximum safety, manual or automatic knee locks may be added. The above-knee prosthesis optimally is suspended total suction or by partial suction and a Silesian bandage or a pelvic band. An endoskeletal pylon connects the knee unit above to the prosthetics foot below. After a hip disarticulation, the amputee receives the Canadian-type prosthesis, which has a plastic laminated socket encircling the pelvis. This provides a resting surface for the ischial tuberosity for weight bearing. With proper molding, it is suspended from the iliac crest. A similar prosthesis is worn after hemipelvectomy, with the rib cage providing the weight-bearing surface.

Cancer in the upper limb may require shoulder disarticulation or interscapular thoracic amputation, which make fitting the patient with a functional body-powered prosthesis difficult or impossible. Myoelectrically controlled and externally powered prostheses may provide some gross function, but such prostheses are relatively expensive and heavy, and require repair more often than body-powered prostheses. In recent years, prosthetic techniques for all types of amputations have advanced significantly, especially with respect to evaluation methods, socket design, ankle-foots components, and cosmesis.[97,98]

Prosthetic Fitting and Training

Before completion of the prosthesis, the amputee needs to visit the prosthetist several times to ensure optimal fit, function, and comfort. When fabrication has been completed, the prescribing physician checks the prosthesis for fit and comfort, socket stability, joint motions, appearance, and function. The lower limb amputee receives gait training, with or without gait aids, depending on motor skills, instructions in attachment and removal techniques, and exercises to increase muscle strength, joint range of motion, balance, and posture. The upper limb amputee learns to open and close the terminal device, position the arm, manipulate objects, and perform self-care tasks. Initially, a prosthesis may not be worn comfortably for more than 15-30 minutes at a time. The amputee thus requires frequent rest periods and short therapy sessions. After each wear, the skin of the residual limb must be examined for signs of excessive pressure or poor socket fit. At the beginning of prosthetic wear, confrontational situations may develop between the amputee and the health professional, especially when the patient's expectations do not match the actual situation.

Lower limb amputees ambulate at greater energy costs than do persons with no disability.[100,101] The BKA expends 23-68% more energy per unit distance than does a person without amputation, and the AKA expends 52-124% more.[102] However, to save energy, most amputees decrease their speed of ambulation, which is approximately 2.0-2.5 mph for BKA and 1.0-1.5 mph for AKA compared with a normal speed of 3-4 mph for persons without amputation. The lower energy cost and greater speed of ambulation for the BKA clearly show the importance of sparing the knee joint whenever possible. Patients with hip disarticulation or hemipelvectomy ambulate with lower energy expenditure if they use axillary crutches without a prosthesis compared with prosthetic use.[102]

Various clinical problems may occur as the result of the amputation and consequent prosthetic wear, including pain, skin lesions, swelling, joint contractures, and depression. Most amputees experience phantom sensation, which is a painless awareness of the amputated part. In contrast, phantom pain may be described as burning, crushing, cramping, or shooting sensations in the amputated phantom limb. The reported incidence of phantom pain has varied between 10% and 85%.[103] This variation may be due to differences in classification of the types of pain,[104] the fear of presumed mental illness if a phantom pain is reported,[103] and the time delay since surgery.[105] The pain may be aggravated by limb contact and different physical activities, but the exact cause remains unknown because no detectable pathology is usually discovered. Phantom pain[106] may be preventable or effectively managed by careful preoperative explanations of the nature of the phantom phenomenon, good surgical techniques, regular examinations postoperatively, and frequent manual handling and good care of the residual limb, as well as by effective treatment of infections and early provision of a functional prosthesis. Definitive treatment, however, is difficult, but symptoms usually improve when a relatively normal situation has been restored. Other beneficial interventions include desensitization by frequent self-inspection and manipulation of the residual limb, application of superficial heat or cold, deep heating with diathermy, massage, vibration, transcutaneous electrical nerve stimulation, imaginary exercises of the phantom limb, active exercises of the entire body, local anesthesia, and psychological interventions. Analgesic medications are relatively ineffective, but agents acting on the central nervous system may be helpful.

Limb-Sparing Surgical Reconstruction

Local resection of cancer with limb-sparing reconstruction may result in survival, disease-free survival equal to that for amputation, and function that may be superior to that for amputation.[107-109] Amputation, however, is still a primary treatment for many limb tumors because it may, at times, be impossible to perform a proper resection while preserving key nerves and vessels and to reconstruct a functional limb.

Limb-sparing reconstructive surgery obviously is an attractive alternative to amputation for both cosmetic and emotional reasons, but it should be undertaken only if it would restore better and longer lasting function than amputation with subsequent prosthetic fitting.[110] Depending on the location and size of the tumor, it may be a difficult procedure in which muscles, bone, and even joints are removed with the tumor. The cancerous bone may be replaced by transplanting a fresh-frozen cadaveric bone allograft or an autologous graft but more commonly by installing a synthetic metallic prosthetic implant.[111-113] An expandable and adjustable prosthesis may now be installed in growing children, who formerly were felt to fare better with amputation.[114] Rehabilitation interventions preferably should begin preoperatively when physical and/or occupational therapists first teach the patient the muscle-strengthening, range of motion, and ambulation exercises that will be resumed postoperatively. Following lower limb- sparing surgery, the patient may begin exercising the uninvolved limbs on the first postoperative day, but the initiation, pace, and intensity of exercises and the amount of weight bearing for the affected limb depend on the exact mode of reconstruction and the postoperative course. In recent years, more information has been published regarding the functional outcomes from limb-sparing surgeries. Many indicate that with improved surgical procedures and adjuvant therapy, patients experience good to excellent function.[115] The functional outcomes have implications for the patients' quality of life. One study found that although an impairmant can affect ADL it was the restriction in life roles that had the most impact on patients' quality of life.[116] Following upper limb-saving surgery, active hand and isometric shoulder muscle exercises are started on the first postoperative day, but if humeral resection is performed, active elbow and shoulder exercises should not begin for 2 or 8 weeks postoperatively, depending on whether a metallic implant or allografts or autografts, respectively, are used.[117] It is thus of primary importance that the rehabilitation staff know exactly which muscles, nerves, and bones were resected and what the reconstruction entailed to plan a safe and effective rehabilitation program. The patient should be counseled on their potential functional recovery based on their current condition.[118] Training in ADL is initiated approximately 1 week postoperatively.

Conclusion

Management of cancer appropriately focuses on prevention, early diagnosis, and cure, but following effective treatment, many cancer patients experience some physical impairment that results in a physical disability or a handicap. As the prognosis for cancer improves, it becomes more important to ensure that all cancer patients regain maximum function in the broadest sense to ensure return to all former roles. Multidisciplinary rehabilitation, therefore, is an integral part of the total management of the cancer patient. The exact functional deficits need to be identified for each patient and proper rehabilitation interventions started promptly or at the same time as other treatments.

Selected References

The complete reference list can be found at www.CANCERMEDICINE8.com

3. DeBacker IC, Van Brend F, Vreugdenhil A, et al. High intensity strength training improves quality of life in cancer survivors. *Acta Oncol*. 2007;30:1-9.
8. Movsas SC, Chang VT, Tunkel RS, et al. Rehabilitation needs of an inpatient medical oncology unit. *Arch Phys Med Rehabil*. 2003;1642–1646.
11. Holland JC. *Psychooncology*. New York and London: Oxford University Press; 1998.
16. Mor V, Laliberte L, Morris JN, Wiemann M. The Karnofsky Performance Status Scale: an examination of its reliability and validity in a research setting. *Cancer*. 1984;53:2002–2007.
20. Thomas DC, Kreizman IJ, Melchiorre P, Ragnarsson KT. Rehabilitation of the patient with chronic critical illness. In: Nierman D, Nelson J, eds. *Critical Care Clinics*. Philadelphia: WB Saunders; 2002: 695–715.
22. Giordana MT, Clara E. Functional rehabilitation and brain tumor patients. A review of outcome. *Neurol Sci*. 2006;27:240–244.
29. Gordon WA, Hibbard MR, Kreutzer J. Cognitive remediation issues in research and practice. *J Head Trauma Rehabil*. 1989;4:76–85.
33. Barron KD, Hirano A, Araki S, Ferry RD. Experiences with metastatic neoplasms involving the spinal cord. *Neurology*. 1959;9:91–106.
34. Garden FH. Radiation injuries to the spinal cord and peripheral nerves. *Phys Med Rehabil State Art Rev*. 1994;8:405–411.
36. Dropcho EJ. Central nervous system injury by therapeutic irradiation. *Neurol Clin*. 1991;9:969–988.
38. Tokuhashi Y, Matsuzaki H, Oda H, Oshima M, Ryu J. A revised scoring system for preoperative evaluation of metastic spine tumor prognosis. *Spine*. 2005;30:2186–2191.
39. Tang V, Harvey D, Dorsay JP, Jiang S, Rathbone MP. Prognostic indicators in metastatic spine cord compression: using functional independence measure and Tokuhasi scale to optimize rehabilitation planning. *Spinal Cord*. 2007;45:671–611.
47. Terrell JE, Welsh DE, Bradford CR, et al. Pain, quality of life, and spinal accessory nerve status after neck dissection. *Laryngoscope*. 2000;110:620–626.
49. Shimado Y, Chida S, Matsunaga T, et al. Clinical results of rehabilitation for accessory nerve palsy after radical neck dissection. *Acta Otolaryngol*. 2007;127:491–497.
54. Cheville AL, McGarvey CL, Petrek JA, et al. Lymphedema management. *Semin Radiat Oncol*. 2003;13:290–301.
56. Moseley AL, Carati CJ, Filler NB. A systematic review of common conservative therapies for arm lymphedema secondary to breast cancer treatment. *Ann Oncol*. 2007;18:639–646.
61. Casley-Smith JR, Boris M, Weindorf S, Lasinski B. Treatment for lymphedema of the arm, the Casley-Smith method: a noninvasive method produces continued reduction. *Cancer*. 1998;83(12 Suppl Am):2843–2860.
64. Brogna L. Self-concept and rehabilitation of the person with an ostomy. *J Enterostomal Ther*. 1985;12:205–209.
65. Brogna L, Lakaszawski M. Nursing management. The continent urostomy. *J Enterostomal Ther*. 1986;13:139–147.
71. Edwards CL, Loeffler M, Rutledge FN. Vaginal reconstruction. In: Von Eschenbach AC, Rodriguez DB, eds. *Sexual Rehabilitation of the Urologic Cancer Patient*. Boston: Hall; 1981:250–265.
74. Finney RP. The treatment of erectile impotence with semirigid penile prosthesis. In: Von Eschenbach AC, Rodriguez DB, eds. *Sexual Rehabilitation of the Urologic Cancer Patient*. Boston: Hall; 1981:228–229.
77. Comfort A. *Sexual Consequences of Disability*. Philadelphia: Stickley; 1978.
81. Schocker JD, Brady LW. Radiation therapy for metastasis. *Clin Orthop*. 1982;169:38–43.
85. Kegel B, Carpenter ML, Burgess EM. Functional capabilities of lower extremity amputees. *Arch Phys Med Rehabil*. 1978;59:109–120.
89. Burgess EM, Zettl JH. Amputations below the knee. *Artif Limbs*. 1969;13:1–12.
94. Edwards ML. Below knee prosthetic socket designs and suspension systems. *Phys Med Rehabil Clin N Am*. 2000;11:585–593, vi.
98. Huang ME, Levy CE, Webster JB. Acquired limb deficiencies. 3. Prosthetic components, prescriptions and indications. *Arch Phys Med Rehabil*. 2001;82(3 Suppl 1):S17–S24.
103. Davis RW. Phantom sensation, phantom pain, and stump pain. *Arch Phys Med Rehabil*. 1993;74:79–91.
106. Harwood DD, Hanumanthu S, Stoudemire A. Pathophysiology and management of phantom limb pain. *Gen Hosp Psychiatry*. 1992;14:107–118.
109. Heller L, Kronowitz SJ. Lower extremity reconstruction. *J Surg Oncol*. 2006;94:479–489.
113. Mankin HJ, Gebhardt MC. Allografts in the management of bone tumors: part II. *Surg Rounds Orthop*. 1988;24–40.
115. Serlett JM, Carras AJ, O'Keefe RJ, Rosier RN. Functional outcome after soft-tissue reconstruction from limb salvage after sarcoma surgery. *Plast Reconstru Surg*. 1998;102:1576–1583.
118. Davis AM, Sennik S, Gruffin AM, et al. Predictors of functional outcomes following limb salvage surgery for lower-extremity soft tissue sarcoma. *J Surg Oncol*. 2000;73:206–211.

64 Multidisciplinary Management

James F. Holland, MD, ScD(h.c.) ▪ Emil Frei III, MD ▪ Waun Ki Hong, MD ▪ Donald W. Kufe, MD ▪ Robert C. Bast Jr., MD ▪ Raphael E. Pollock, MD, PhD ▪ Ralph R. Weichselbaum, MD ▪ William N. Hait, MD, PhD

Most cancer patients, and society in general, would like to think that the entire team of doctors, nurses, and specialists are cooperatively involved in solving their medical problems. Patients have little awareness of turf battles, professional egos, personal animosities, or medical fads, but if they knew of their existence, they would have little tolerance for them. Oncologists of all disciplines and health professionals who interact with them are human beings, not unemotional automatons. Happily, the energies they squander in picayune or counterproductive activities are small compared to their constructive, positive efforts to seek improved (not just new) approaches to cancer.

The keystone for a successful interdisciplinary management team is attitude: humility, tolerance, adaptability, and appreciation for alternative approaches. None of us is so skilled that he or she can be as expert in every discipline as a highly competent exponent of that particular specialty. No one is omniscient. We are, and must be, interdependent, so it is important to work with individuals who are trustworthy and friendly. More failures of interdisciplinary management teams seem to occur because of personality conflicts than because of intellectual disagreements. In the heat of confrontational oratory, emotional preferences may win out over reasoned accord. Resorting to the literature should shed more light on a problem, not more heat. A selective literature survey can often be construed to support either side of an acrimonious dispute. Facts trump opinions.

In actual clinical practice, decisions are often implemented by the oncologic specialist who first encounters the patient. A much better way is to work with trusted colleagues and consultants whose opinions, where appropriate, are solicited before the first irreversible step is taken. Actions already taken can seldom be undone. A formal tumor conference (never really possible or necessary for every patient) serves the purpose of institutionalizing a forum for discussion, thereby diminishing the impact of bias and prior anecdotal experience. A conference serves the additional function of allowing oncologists of several disciplines to recognize individuals of other disciplines whose opinions and consultations appear to be the most learned and whose personalities are compatible. A tumor conference occasionally alters the primary oncologist's opinions and plans and, thus, the therapeutic approach for a specific patient. A conference may surface unfamiliar data, with references, that can change the course. Increasingly, tumor characteristics deduced from biopsy specimens by pathologic and molecular techniques may determine chemotherapeutic or endocrine treatments that are administered as primary therapy before surgery or radiation. An important contribution of a conference is the establishment of dialogue, which impacts on the future disposition of similar clinical problems. Managed-care programs undeniably intrude on this concept, however, with limitation of referrals to plan members and the pressure of economic constraints to spend less time with and on each patient.

A second oncologic specialist of a different discipline, whose encounter with the patient occurs after the first oncologist has already changed the tumor and the patient, may rightly point out a better approach for the future. A medical oncologist or radiation oncologist can better know and eventually better treat a patient who has been seen before definitive surgical treatment rather than after. A surgical oncologist (and the patient) would be ill-treated if a patient were prepared for surgery with chemotherapy or radiation therapy without the surgeon's examining the tumor and the patient beforehand. In diseases where radiotherapy and chemotherapy both play a role, joint planning is mandatory.

In the absence of absolute oncologic truths, there is much room for diverse opinions. Interdisciplinary oncology implies that each discipline performs a complementary function. The best analogy is to a symphony: each instrument is played harmoniously on the same score, rather than all on the same note, or each to a different tune. And as in a symphony's output of music, interdisciplinary oncology requires belief in the probability that better outcomes will result, thus validating the extra commitment in time.

The Primary Physician

No universal blood or urine tests exist that can diagnose asymptomatic cancer. Occasional patients may present abnormal protein patterns or marker alterations, but except for the prostate-specific antigen (PSA) such tests are not yet sufficiently sensitive or specific to justify their use for screening. Many cancers can be found in asymptomatic status by periodic, careful physical examinations. These are cancers of the skin, subcutaneous tissues, oral cavity, thyroid, lymph nodes, breast, gynecologic tract, penis, testes, anus, prostate, and rectum. Some asymptomatic cancers are announced by conditions revealed through simple laboratory tests often done for other purposes: leukocytosis, anemia, microscopic hematuria, hyperglobulinemia, and chest radiography or computed tomography (CT). Specific examinations proved to be of value in screening for cancer, such as cervical cytology, fecal occult blood testing, regular mammography, systematic colonoscopy, and PSA are discussed in detail in Chapter 34 "Cancer Screening and Early Detection." Furthermore, some diagnoses can be made before cancer cells invade. Asymptomatic cancers tend to be smaller than symptomatic ones and often imply a better prognosis. Regrettably, for most sites diagnosis when the cancer is asymptomatic is still uncommon.

Until reliable diagnostic blood tests for visceral cancers are invented, probably tumor-by-tumor history-taking remains the most important diagnostic tool. Most cancers are discovered when the patient no longer has other simple explanations and remedies for a new significant symptom and finally seeks medical attention. Most such symptoms of cancer are readily confused with symptoms of common benign diseases. By attentive consideration of every minor symptom, a good primary doctor must sift out the symptom that could be due to cancer from that which is not likely to be. It is the constellation of symptoms, their duration, and associated findings that lead the alert physician to consider cancer. Cough, dyspepsia, anorexia, hoarseness, constipation, diarrhea, menorrhagia, weight loss, fever, fatigue, a lump, or pain, any one of which persists for 2 weeks, even if intermittently, and cannot be readily explained, requires consideration of cancer in the differential diagnosis. Other possible causes may exist and lead to other diagnoses, but cancer that is not thought of early is always diagnosed too late. It is the physician's job to be suspicious and to exclude the diagnosis of cancer, rather than to be complacent, and finally arrive at the diagnosis of cancer when the patient's complaints are severe and unambiguous. Suspicion is a virtue when looking for cancer. Early cancer symptoms are usually intermittent. Any pain at the outset is ordinarily not constant and may be poorly localized or even migratory. Subcutaneous masses and nodes can even seem to regress temporarily. Systemic dysfunction may be so mild as to be easily rationalized or overlooked by the patient.

Histories that are taken are more valuable than histories that are given. On suspecting cancer, the primary physician is often able to order the appropriate tests for radiologic, histologic or cytologic confirmation of that suspicion. It is at this point that the interdisciplinary process should start. Studies that do not establish a diagnosis of cancer could be the wrong studies. Oncologic consultation might suggest other procedures of value. The primary physician often sends a patient to a surgeon for biopsy, which, when positive, may be followed by resection without further consultation. We believe that the proper time for discussion with representatives from the many disciplines who might eventually become involved is after a diagnosis is suspected or after it is proved, but before the inauguration of definitive therapy. Psycho-oncologic consultation and formal rehabilitation may not be necessary for every patient but, when needed, should be arranged before the therapeutic program is initiated. Pathology consultation is always needed and is best obtained in person at the pathologist's double-headed microscope with the slide in view.

The surgeon, medical oncologist, and radiation oncologist should, in many cases, have protocols for therapy of common cancers. Where possible, these protocols should be part of designed studies that will accumulate sufficient numbers from which conclusions can be drawn. Sometimes this involves a single institution (or even a single practice); whenever possible, it should be part of institutional or national protocols designed to answer fundamental questions concerning the management of cancer. When multiple protocols exist, a consensus must be reached to prioritize the sequence in which they will be offered to patients. Where no protocol exists, agreement that defines the procedures and the sequence for a particular patient should be sought ahead of time. The family physician should be a full partner in all of these decisions.

The primary physician may also be a principal member of the follow-up team for a cancer patient and can identify any change from well-being that signals possible tumor activity. At this point participation of an oncologist is called for. Alternatively, oncologic surveillance can fall to the medical oncologist. The primary physician must also assess the possible familial risk and supervise the appropriate survey of family members in conjunction with the medical oncologist.

The Radiologist

Imaging specialties are essential in the diagnosis and staging of cancer. An oncologist should review all relevant imaging studies with the appropriate radiologist, sonographer, or nuclear medicine physician. A written report is mandatory, but it is much increased in value by the oncologist's personal viewing of the images with the radiologist. Although it is commonplace to order standard menus (a CT or magnetic resonance imaging [MRI] scan), a radiologist can suggest the best techniques for particular problems. MRI with and without gadolinium enhancement is the preferred technique to visualize brain tumors. MRI of the breast may be more discriminating than other techniques in evaluating complex lesions of the breast.

Positron emission tomography-computerized tomography (PET-CT) has become an extremely valuable diagnostic and staging tool. In addition to anatomic structure, the avidity of a lesion (sometimes otherwise unrecognized) for radioactive fluorodeoxyglucose has significantly sharpened the diagnosis of small primary cancers and has much improved the detection of metastases. Therapeutic planning that might involve surgery or radiotherapy is made more robust in many areas where PET-CT could delineate regional or distant metastases. PET-CT is of great value in follow-up examination of patients whose tumor recurrence or metastases could not be readily detected by physical exam, serum marker abnormalities, or standard radiologic techniques. Special CT scans with thinner slices can provide better definition of small lesions, or special MRI views with or without fat suppression or gadolinium may provide optimal visualization. Follow-up examinations using dynamic flow scanning, sonographic or CT-guided needle biopsy, and similar procedures always require the professional input of an imaging specialist. Increasingly the interventional radiologist is called upon to make the definitive biopsy of suspect lesions in the parachymetous organs: lung, liver, pancreas, and spleen. Mammographers are usually the agents who diagnose breast cancer, first visually and then by fine needle or mammotome biopsy or by localization for a surgical procedure. Studies on these biopsied tissues and/or cells may specify specific therapies before surgery or radiation.

The interventional radiologist has a major therapeutic role, too, in metastatic disease of the axial skeleton. Intravertebral injection of a polymerizing cement can prevent or stabilize vertebral collapse and diminish or even relieve back pain.

Oncologists can request that the imaging specialist not give an interpretation directly to the patient. Reporting radiologic findings to patients before they are known by the responsible oncologist can sometimes cause significant difficulty in management, for both oncologist and patient. The radiologist is a consultant to the oncologist, not to the patient. The responsibility for the interpretation of findings to the patient, and for the support that often must go with it, rests with the oncologist.

The Endoscopist and the Sonographer

As endoscopy has largely replaced barium sulfate contrast radiography for diagnosing gastrointestinal cancers, the endoscopist is often the first individual to recognize and biopsy neoplasms of the alimentary canal. In the presence of negative upper and lower gastrointestinal (GI) tract inspections yet persistent symptoms or occult bleeding, small intestinal capsule endoscopy may discover primary or metastatic lesions of the jejunum or ileum. Endoscopic ultrasound is helpful in determining penetration of muscle layers of esophagus and rectum, and of detecting nearby nodes in those locations and around the pancreas. Endoscopic examination of the upper airway and tracheobronchial tree may be the preferred route for diagnosis and biopsy. Colposcopy, and in specific instances hysteroscopy are additional instances where visualization permits definitive biopsy. Vaginal sonography visualizes ovaries and endometrium better than external exams. Breast ultrasonography supplements mammography, and is particularly useful in young women.

The Pathologist

The pathologist is an indispensable member of every interdisciplinary team. The function of the entire team is dependent on a proper diagnosis, and therefore pathology is a defining control. When the team pathologist is uncertain of a diagnosis, other local pathologists can be consulted for their opinions. Furthermore, the Armed Forces Institute of Pathology and several prominent universities and cancer centers are justly famed for their consultations.

The ready access of most of the GI tract to endoscopic inspection and biopsy, easy access to the genitalia in both sexes, the accessibility of the tracheobronchial tree to fiberoptic bronchoscopy, mediastinoscopy, image-guided needle biopsies, and safe intraoperative biopsies mean that preoperative or intraoperative pathologic confirmation of diagnosis should be available for nearly every tumor. Based on clinical studies and the presence of tumor-associated markers, renal and testicular masses are typically removed without first establishing histologic proof. This is justified by the desire to avoid tumor spillage that can occur during a biopsy. For other diseases, radical surgery without preceding pathologic diagnosis is unnecessary and dangerous. Similarly, an inadequate surgical procedure performed because the nature of the pathologic process was not appreciated suggests insufficient or mistaken intraoperative consultation. Amputation of a breast or an extremity without preoperative or intraoperative pathologic diagnosis of cancer constitutes malpractice. However, in the presence of cancer, a surgeon may conscientiously and competently sacrifice adjacent, dispensable, normal tissue—organs such as the spleen, kidney, and adrenal, or a segment of gut, diaphragm, bladder, or vaginal wall—which appears to be involved by cancer, without histologically establishing invasion. In other circumstances, the pathologist's imprimatur is necessary to justify cancer therapies. The same restrictions apply to primary radiation therapy or chemotherapy.

The pathologist is responsible for giving as definitive a description of the tumor as determined effort can provide: its extent, its relationship to surgical margins and normal structures, and the involvement of lymph nodes, lymphatics, and blood vessels. Wherever possible, a specimen of fresh tissue should be maintained frozen, since, increasingly, new immunodiagnostic, molecular biologic, and biochemical techniques allow classification of tumors for receptors, oncogenes, tumor suppressor genes, and antigens that may some day provide prognostic information of great value. In selected circumstances, fresh tissue can be utilized for assays that predict chemotherapeutic or immunotherapeutic sensitivity for application in real-time before surgery or radiation therapy.

In addition to tissue preservation for more sophisticated studies, pathology now allows better classification of tumors. Immunopathology and cytochemistry should be able to distinguish among most anaplastic neoplasms by studies of markers such as common leukocyte antigen, cytokeratins, vimentin, mucin, neuron-specific enolase, and S-100 protein often used as panels of reagents to decide whether the tumor is a lymphoma, squamous cell carcinoma, sarcoma, adenocarcinoma, neuroectodermal tumor, or melanoma. Communication ahead of time with the pathologist can refine the choice of reagents, and can provide extant or ancillary pathologic materials and information to aid in reaching the correct diagnosis. In their anaplastic state, all the tumors mentioned may resemble one another in hematoxylin and eosin staining. If any suggestion exists that pathologic classification might be elusive, in addition to a specimen for freezing (which could later be subjected to molecular biologic study and possible genetic classification) a small fresh sample of representative neoplasm should be placed in glutaraldehyde fixative in the operating room for eventual electron microscopy. Today's research classifications may well become tomorrow's standard rubric and nomenclature. Oncologists should encourage the most discriminating description and classification of tumors, since new therapeutic considerations may prove to be applicable as discoveries are made.

When doubt exists concerning the nature of a neoplasm, additional opinions are always appropriate. Pathologic uncertainty is a shaky foundation on which to build a therapeutic strategy.

The Surgical Oncologist

The surgical oncologist is most often the first among oncologic specialists to see the patient. The primary physician most commonly pursues a diagnosis, and in circumstances where this requires biopsy, the interventional radiologist, endoscopist, or surgeon is called. For decades, any surgeon was considered competent to exercise all surgical skills, including cancer surgery. Indeed, although most surgeons may be acceptably competent, the specialty of surgical oncology has increasingly become recognized. Surgical oncologists are clinical scientists with knowledge of and experience in cancer surgery that come from additional training, limitation of the scope of general surgical practice, familiarity with the biology and natural history of cancers, and familiarity with the role of the other oncologic specialties in their diagnosis and management. Increasingly, surgical oncologists are performing many cancer operations by thoracoscopic or laparoscopic minimally invasive techniques and by robotic instruments for certain sites. Such advances require special training and expertise. Until surgical oncology becomes recognized by the proper accrediting agencies, other oncologists must exercise their judgment about the oncologic qualifications of their surgical confreres. Some of the appropriate criteria are membership in the Society of Surgical Oncology, postgraduate training in a cancer institute or university program under a mentor known for cancer surgical expertise, concentration of surgical practice on cancer and related diseases, and published work.

Since an interventional radiologist, endoscopist, or general surgeon may perform the biopsy, a surgical oncologist is often called upon to supersede the first operator. Herein lie some of the problems, because the primary cancer operation is of utmost importance for proper staging and for achieving surgical cure. In this regard, biopsy of any mass should be considered in the context of whether the operating surgeon will be the best choice for eventual definitive surgical therapy. Since a considerable portion of their activity deals with neoplasia, thoracic surgeons, urologic surgeons, and neurosurgeons must be chosen for their specific interest and general expertise because there is not likely to be an oncologic subspecialty in the near future for those specific organ systems. On the other hand, gynecologic oncology, orthopedic oncology, otorhinolaryngologic oncology, and surgical oncology are well defined, and the general gynecologist, orthopedist, otorhinolaryngologist, or surgeon is unlikely to be as well qualified as the oncologist within the specialty.

Because the implications for a potentially resectable neoplasm entail many other considerations to optimize curability, the prudent surgical oncologist surveys the potential contributions of medical oncology, radiation oncology, and other specialties before proceeding with the operation.

Where appropriate and possible, patients should be entered into clinical investigative trials. There is so much that is unknown about cancer that investigative activities should still be of prime concern to all oncologists. In institutions where investigative programs are not employed, sober consideration of joining in this effort through a community oncology program or in alliance with some other active institution should be considered.

In the absence of a structured protocol, joint assessment is appropriate to determine whether chemotherapy or radiotherapy prior to surgery may improve outcome. Most often, this entails direct consultation with the medical and radiation oncologists. An opportunity for the three specialties to see the patient in the native unaltered state is of great value for subsequent planning. The treatment of breast cancer, rectal cancer, head and neck cancer, lung cancer, esophageal cancer, bone and soft tissue sarcoma, and brain tumors are most often best approached by multidisciplinary components from all three specialties. Often chemotherapy and radiotherapy before surgery can improve outcome. Whereas specific diseases may be treated well by single-modality approaches, bi-disciplinary or tri-disciplinary opinion is usually advantageous. Sentinel node biopsy in breast cancer and melanoma is a surgical innovation requiring nuclear medicine and pathologic collaboration. Surgical oncologists must work collaboratively with plastic surgeons to undertake breast reconstruction, and sometimes to effect facial reconstruction.

Surgical oncologists must also be available for surgical aspects of management later in the course of disease. Venous access devices may be required, depending on the drugs to be used and the status of peripheral veins. End-staging laparoscopy or laparotomy may, in many instances, make more sense than earlier operation so that the medical oncologist may be certain that a complete clinical remission is pathologically confirmed, rather than waiting for a lymphoma or ovarian cancer to relapse. Intestinal obstruction in the course of cancer may require operative surgical management. A medical or radiation oncologist may discover a suspicious mass or infiltration that needs biopsy and pathologic assessment.

Palliative surgery is an area where medical and radiation oncologists often present problems to the surgeon in hopes of potential operative remedy. Debulking, diverting, and pain-relieving operations may all be appropriate procedures in the proper circumstance.

Surgical oncologists also have legitimate interests in adjuvant chemotherapy and immunotherapy. For those willing to devote the time required for this undertaking, use of established drugs in adjuvant programs can be an improvement over surgical procedures alone. Indeed, the National Surgical Adjuvant Breast and Bowel Project has contributed significantly to our knowledge of adjuvant and neo-adjuvant therapy for these diseases. Surgical oncologic investigators have also been among the pioneers of immunologic cancer research. The rarity of surgical oncologists in practice, however, ordinarily precludes these activities for surgeons, since so much of their time is ordinarily invested in preoperative and postoperative care and in actual surgery. Medical oncologists must stand ready to assume primary responsibility for subsequent oncologic management. Orthopedic oncologists, otorhinolaryngologic oncologists, and neurosurgical oncologists ordinarily ally themselves with a medical oncologist who has specialized interests and expertise in the treatment of neoplasms of their particular discipline.

The Anesthesiologist

Intraoperative management of a cancer patient is similar to that for any major surgery. Since anesthesiologists often manage recovery rooms and even surgical intensive care units, their role has expanded. Assurance of effective pain control in the immediate postoperative period is fundamental. Patient-controlled epidural analgesia postoperatively is the province of anesthesiology. Epidural block by continuous administration of narcotic and anesthetic solutions or nerve block may also be indispensable for refractory pain in the course of metastatic cancer. Patient-controlled analgesia by intravenous or subcutaneous narcotics at other times for efficient pain control is a technique of importance to all branches of oncology, however, and should not be considered a proprietary anesthesiologic exclusive. Most patients can achieve pain control on oral medications.

The Medical Oncologist

The medical oncologist usually serves the traditional role of internist in the interdisciplinary management of cancer. Whereas the surgical procedure or the radiotherapeutic treatment course is of short duration, the medical oncologist has continuing responsibility that may stretch over months or years of therapy and decades of follow-up, depending on the neoplasm.

There is an understandable but regrettable tendency for every specialist who has interacted with a patient to schedule follow-up appointments, which may entail many more visits and much greater expense than is necessary or prudent. A combined modality follow-up clinic avoids this problem, but may not be adaptable to most office practices. Each therapist is entitled to see the results of the particular treatment regimen that has been applied. The region of prior disease is only a portion of the patient's overall health concerns, however. The search for remediable disease in regional and distant areas and a continuing assessment of the impact of the disease and its treatment on the patient as a whole are ordinarily considered medical tasks. A useful approach for medical oncologists is to send the findings at a follow-up visit, including laboratory and radiologic results, to the primary physician, surgeon, and radiation oncologist (or other appropriate specialist) so that what is going on is communicated to all. The medical oncologist is also most often the conduit to the patient for announcing program change, such as the appearance of metastases, the necessity for more therapy of whatever kind, and sometimes the shift to a palliative approach. The medical oncologist may also superintend both the medical activities of the patient that are not addressed by the primary physician and the general oncologic assessments that are of importance to the surgeon, radiation oncologist, and medical oncologist alike. When regional concerns arise that are in the purview of the other specialties, the medical oncologist should facilitate early real-time consultation.

The medical oncologist should participate in the decisions concerning choice of therapy as well as in the clinical staging which may determine operability. The medical oncologist should be responsible for evaluating the potential for induction (primary, neo-adjuvant) chemotherapy and for the choice of regimen for postoperative chemotherapeutic or immunotherapeutic management.

Since our knowledge base is still incomplete, wherever possible, patients should enter research protocols. Data are emerging that emphasize the value of neo-adjuvant (primary or induction) chemotherapy in the care of tumors classically considered first for regional surgical or radiotherapeutic approaches. Osteosarcoma and several pediatric tumors, stage III breast cancer, stage III nonsmall-cell lung cancer, advanced head and neck carcinoma, esophageal cancer, rectal cancer, and arguably some other cancers have benefited from chemotherapeutic impact on the presumptive micrometastases and on the primary tumor. Chemotherapeutic effect on the primary tumor serves as an in vivo bioassay of drug effect, allowing shift to a different regimen, if ineffectual. Complete pathologic regression of primary tumors from chemotherapy has been associated with improved results for osteosarcoma, breast cancer, and head and neck cancer and of chemoradiotherapy for esophageal, rectal, and bladder cancer. Treatment of the primary neoplasm may be simplified, and lesions once considered inoperable are now potentially curable. This changing paradigm may increase the applicability of radiotherapy and surgery with intent to cure.

The medical oncologist is most often the physician to reassure the patient when there is no evident cancer. Although the absence of tumor may in fact be tumor in eclipse, the medical oncologist must keep the patient from dwelling incessantly and anxiously on imminent relapse. Reassurance should never involve a lie, just a reasoned basis for hope that relapse will not occur. Osler's admonition to live life in day-tight packages is helpful.

The medical oncologist is the responsible physician when therapeutic options for disease control become progressively restricted as a cancer patient approaches death. Though selective interventions by surgical or radiation oncologists or other specialists may be required, the overall responsibility for the patient's palliative care, pain control, nutrition, psychosocial adaptation, and coping with the actual dying process falls on the medical oncologist. A competent medical oncologist is expert at palliative care.

The Radiation Oncologist

Radiation oncology is entirely devoted to the study of cancer since radiation is no longer used in the treatment of benign diseases. The radiation oncologist must, therefore, be in a position to make an overall oncologic evaluation, as well as specific recommendations for radiotherapy.

In the case of diseases where radiotherapy can often cure, such as localized lymphomas, cancer of the tongue and oral cavity, cancer of the cervix, and cancer of the prostate, the radiation oncologist must have equal early access to the patient to set forth the possible indications for and accomplishments of radiation therapy for such tumors. Cordial interactive liaison with surgical and medical oncologists is crucial to allow this delineation of options before the patient is committed to and is changed by another treatment approach.

Controversy exists over the relative debilities and late toxicities of surgery and radiotherapy. Where equal curative potential exists, there is additional reason to assess the disruption of anatomy and the dysfunction that might occur from surgery or from radiotherapy. There is no consensus because each discipline often champions its own approach. The major improvement in immediate reconstructive techniques has made surgery around the face much less disfiguring. Surgeons point out dry mouth and dysgeusia as late undesirable toxicities of radiation whereas radiotherapists decry the organ loss, physiologic distortions, and cosmetic problems of surgery. Similar controversy attends vaginal dysfunction after radiation treatment for early carcinoma of the cervix, compared to total hysterectomy. In carcinomas of the bladder, the discordance is even greater because total cystectomy diminishes the quality of life, but American urologists often question whether radiation therapy is equally effective, stage for stage. Although radiotherapy for T2 and T3 bladder cancers is reportedly highly effective in Europe, there has been little clinical investigation of this approach in the United States. Surgery for carcinoma of the prostate, now improved by laparoscopic and robotic techniques, but with problems of capsular invasion, impotence, and incontinence, has not been directly compared with interstitial radiotherapy and teletherapy, which have complications of their own. A definitive comparison in early-stage prostate cancer is overdue, once there is consensus about which patients with biopsy proven prostate cancer do not need treatment at all.

For operable oral, pharyngeal, laryngeal, cervical, bladder, and prostate cancer, closer cooperation of the radiation oncologist and surgeon before decisions are finalized might provide for greater organ preservation and less dysfunction when therapy is equivalent stage for stage. The great problem, however, is to overcome the prejudice that the results will not be the same, with each specialty nearly equally unpersuaded and equally unpersuasive. Randomized clinical trials are sorely needed but may never be done because of the evolution of the combined modality approaches.

In combined modality approaches, chemotherapy is a major component, together with radiotherapy and surgery. Many reports indicate that chemotherapy induces major regressions when used as primary therapy for head and neck cancer, bladder cancer, breast cancer, pediatric sarcomas, and lymphomas. So, too, does hormonal therapy for prostate and breast cancer. Primary chemotherapy, with its major theoretical advantage of decreasing the number of cells to be killed by radiation or to be removed by surgery is under active study. Until proven otherwise, radiation field sizes and surgical boundaries cannot be safely reduced below the original extent of the tumor, where residual cells may remain after medical therapy. A major advantage of primary chemotherapy, in addition to a decrease in primary tumor burden, is an early attack against undetected micrometastatic disease. Furthermore, when the primary tumor vasculature is intact, unimpaired by radiation angiopathy or surgical disruption, there is a greater chance of delivering a chemotherapeutically effective dose. Lastly, the regression of tumor seen in the primary neoplasm reinforces confidence in using the same chemotherapeutic regimen for presumed micrometastases during the adjuvant period. Indeed, when complete regression of tumor occurs, as demonstrated pathologically, outcomes are much improved in osteosarcoma and in breast cancer and probably in other cancers.

For tumors that are regionally invasive beyond resectability in the pharynx, esophagus, pancreas, cervix, and prostate, radiation is usually employed as primary therapy, often with chemotherapy or hormone therapy. The dismal results often seen in these advanced tumors unfairly taints the potential contributions of radiation oncology in the treatment of less advanced tumors. Pilot efforts are needed to construct combined modality approaches for tumors that are regionally inoperable at first encounter but which might become resectable after chemotherapy and/or radiation therapy.

Primary brain tumors are usually best treated by primary surgery followed by radiotherapy, often with chemotherapy. When surgery is unfeasible, stereotactic radiotherapy, delivering precisely localized radiation so as to spare normal brain, offers promise. Sterotatctic radiation has been used in other sites. Intensity modulated radiation therapy (IMRT) is a computer-dependent technique of minimizing exposure of normal tissues during treatment.

Radiotherapy can cure localized and regionalized lymphomas of certain types. The advantages and disadvantages of combined modality therapy or of the use of chemotherapy alone are presented in detail in the specific diseases chapters. A clear indication for combined chemotherapy and radiotherapy exists in patients whose localized lymphomas are large and where there if no certainty of tumor eradication by either modality alone. Radiotherapy may be a critical component in salvage regimens for relapsed leukemias and lymphomas, where maximal chemotherapy together with autologous stem cell rescue or allogeneic stem cell transplantation is undertaken.

For palliation and pain relief, radiation therapy is indispensable to the practice of oncology. Radiotherapy can usually offer relief from the pain of tumor infiltration in bone, regardless of tumor type. Although the extent of tumor regression (as a measure of radiosensitivity) varies, this may determine duration of effect rather than initial pain relief.

The Gynecologic Oncologist

Gynecologic oncologists as a class may belong to the most integrated oncologic specialty. They are fully qualified to diagnose and treat neoplasia of the female genital organs by surgery and chemotherapy and to share in radiotherapeutic planning and execution to a considerable degree, particularly for brachytherapy. Highly skilled gynecologic oncologists are divided on whether gastrointestinal complications of ovarian or other cancers should be handled by surgical oncologists, general surgeons, or gynecologic oncologists. Much of this depends on local custom rather than expertise at performing lysis of adhesions or enteroenterostomies. The preoperative preparation for and execution of procedures that involve urinary tract manipulation are almost invariably conducted cooperatively with urologists.

Many medical oncologists treat gynecologic neoplasms with chemotherapy in investigational and clinical settings. This is true for adjuvant therapy as well as treatment of manifest clinical metastasis. In many academic institutions medical and gynecologic oncologists have collaborated in the study of the biology and treatment of gynecologic cancers. Local custom, the surgical obligations of gynecologic oncologists, and collaborative undertakings involving both specialties determine the allocation of work. Medical oncologists should be actively involved when a gynecologist without specific oncologic expertise or interest has undertaken to perform the surgery.

The Neurosurgeon

Primary brain tumors increasingly require multi-modality therapy, involving surgery, chemotherapy, and radiation, often stereotactic. The longer survival of patients with many types of systemic cancers has led to a higher frequency of patients presenting with one or two brain metastases that can be resected. Metastases to vertebral bodies with pain, vertebral collapse or impending cord compression also appears to be more common. In each such instance, surgical correction or vertebral stabilization must be considered, as well as radiation therapy. Neurosurgical procedures for pain control are crucial as last-resort measures, although they have largely been replaced by systemic and regional narcotics.

The Pediatric Oncologist

Pediatric oncologists generally maintain independence from adult oncologic specialties. Radiotherapists and surgeons in major centers subspecialize in pediatric neoplasms. Some gynecologists and urologists have particular interests in pediatric diseases. Orthopedic oncologists devote much of their time to pediatric sarcomas, and thus there is no specialized subset for pediatric neoplasms. In major centers, pediatric counterparts to all the medical oncologic resources, such as pediatric neurologists, radiologists, and even pathologists illustrate the specificity of pediatric oncologic information. Nearly every child in the United States can have access to programs of the Children's Oncology Group. The dramatic progress in cancer therapeutics in children derives, in part, from the universal recognition that childhood cancer is a terrible tragedy, and that every effort must be made to derive all possible information from every case. This allows the child with cancer to benefit from all the information that has gone before and creates a new database for those who will come after. The unique features of pediatric oncology are summarized in Chapter 121, but detailed coverage is best sought in other works.

The Psycho-Oncologist

The mind is the only organ system that is affected in every patient with cancer. Nonetheless, all patients do not need formal psychiatric help. Because general psychiatrists often lack full understanding of the organic aspects of cancers and the therapeutic procedures that are commonly employed, their effectiveness in dealing with these real-life problems is lessened. Psycho-oncologists have, by dint of special education and experience, a better foundation from which to undertake supervision of those patients whose psychiatric problems are too pervasive for oncologists of other disciplines to manage. Psycho-oncologists implement much of their influence by interaction with staff in addition to patients.

Helping train oncologists to deal sensitively and empathically with patients is a continuing task for psycho-oncologists. It is important for oncologists to recognize the fact that a patient's cancer is usually the greatest challenge that he or she has ever faced. Staring into the abyss, often for the first time, requires more equanimity and fortitude than many patients can muster. There are sensitive and insensitive ways to communicate bad news to a patient. Training can make a difference. Psycho-oncology's best offerings teach doctors how to handle their own inadequacies, how to tolerate their own frustrations and failures, and how to convey a humanitarian dimension to the grim reality of many cancer treatments. Not all the medicine comes in a bottle.

Psycho-oncologists have stressed objective methods of quantifying emotions and subjective judgments that determine the quality of life. The pain thermometer has been paralleled by the distress thermometer, which may serve as a triggering indicator for medication to allay anxiety or depression. Major elevation of the stress thermometer indicates need for psychiatric or psychologic intervention. See Chapter 62.

The Rehabilitation Specialist

Rehabilitation specialists provide patients with the opportunity for self-reliance. Cutting the bonds of dependency can be the best of all remedies. Whether in speech, ambulation, ostomy care, physical performance, occupational rehabilitation, or sexual expression, oncologists must maintain as a goal that patients should lead pain-free lives with minimal, if any, deficits in normal function. Early and vigorous rehabilitation efforts can make life more worth living. Oncologists could and should consult rehabilitation medicine specialists earlier and more often. See Chapter 62.

The Oncology Nurse

An oncology nurse has become one of the team's indispensable specialists. An oncologist's nightmare is to have a complex cancer patient admitted to a general service floor. The unique medications, procedures, and tests for oncology patients are themselves adequate justification for the specialty of oncology nursing. Oncology nurses have a greater than ordinary understanding of cancer pain and a perception of the psychologic stresses that cancer patients suffer. These two precious insights allow a much more aggressive advocacy for pain control and a humanistic and realistic support of patients and families during their crises. Oncology nurses in ambulatory settings become telephone specialists in patient management and triage, to the great advantage and comfort of cancer patients—and to the great advantage, and efficiency, of physician oncologists.

Oncology nurses have become the prime movers in home care, rendering active therapy or supervision of palliative measures. Because of them, home hospice care has become more common, more economical and more desirable.

The Nutritionist

Although it is reasonable to associate nutritional practices and certain foods with cancer risk, there is less evidence that dietary change after a cancer appears can change outcome. A recent observational study did show, however, that those who chose a prudent diet emphasizing fruits, vegetables, poultry, and fish had significantly fewer recurrences of surgically-resected and chemotherapeutically-treated stage III colon cancer than those who ate a typical Western diet of meat, fat, refined grains and desserts.

It has been known for decades that undernourished mice live longer and develop less cancer. Obesity in humans is a risk factor for many different cancers. There is wisdom in the folk saying that you can't be too rich or too thin. But matching the stringent dietary restriction that is effective in mice eludes most human attempts. Maintaining a diet that provides appropriate calories, proteins, and incentives to consume them can be a challenge for many cancer patients. A nutritionist can be helpful.

Fad diets for cancer patients substitute hope for data. When upper digestive tract disease or toxicity mandates enteral feedings by percutaneous gastrostomy or jejunostomy, the nutritionist is an indispensable member of the oncology team. Temporary parenteral nutritional support during severe stomatitis, esophagitis, or correctable small bowel obstruction may be helpful, but chronic parenteral nutrition in cancer patients has not improved quality of life or outcome.

The Oncology Pharmacist

The very nature of oncologic drugs imparts a special responsibility for their appropriate and safe use. The special postgraduate training of an oncology pharmacist and the conscientious practice of his or her profession significantly benefits every cancer patient. Knowledge of appropriate doses, pharmacokinetics, incompatibilities, special administration procedures, acute and cumulative toxic manifestations, unique databases, alternative drugs and routes of administration, and avoidance of personal exposure are all attributes brought to the interdisciplinary team by an oncology pharmacist. Meticulous record-keeping in computerized files is an indispensable backup for the clinical chart. Any installation treating several patients each day can ill afford not to have a specialized oncology pharmacist. For the smaller practice, premixed drugs prepared by a central oncology pharmacist adds a layer of convenience and security.

The Social Worker

A few additional people are crucial in the oncologic approach to advanced cancer at home. A social worker familiar with the great stresses of cancer on every member of the family is a treasured asset. The complexities in social, insurance, economic, and service spheres can be greatly simplified by the compassionate and professional interest of an oncology social worker. Additional, often critical, community resources, such as the American Cancer Society, Cancer Care, veteran patient support groups, Meals on Wheels, companion visits, and home health care aides, may seem to be effortlessly mobilized by a social worker.

The Clergy

For those who have been guided by religious tenets and who have practiced their religion, the clergy can be extremely helpful. Religious practices can be strengthening; however, death-bed conversions are uncommon. For those who have not made religion a significant portion of their lives, visits of the clergy or allusions to an afterlife provide little comfort.

The Business Person

Competent business associates who manage the complexities of third-party payers, precertifications, collections, write-offs, and purchases can be worth their weight in gold. Indeed, the success or failure of an oncology practice depends in large part on an undiscounted revenue stream and prudent cost control.

Family Members

The principal support throughout the cancer experience comes from a loving family. All else may pale in comparison to the radiant affection of a spouse or other family member. The loving one who recognizes that all the good that can be done must be done creates the palpable substance for the patient of being loved. In addition to benefit for the patient, such behavior creates comforting memories for the doer and future self-satisfaction that in the ultimate crisis he or she was steadfast.

65 Cancer and Pregnancy

Jennifer K. Litton, MD ▪ Richard L. Theriault, DO, MBA, FACP

The diagnosis of cancer during pregnancy presents a complex set of challenges for the patient, family members, and physicians. Often, the welfare of the mother is perceived to be threatened by the pregnancy due to concerns regarding the disease, diagnostic and therapeutic procedures required for treatment, and a desire to avoid harm to the fetus during treatment for the mother's malignancy. A frequent recommendation in the past has been to terminate the pregnancy. For those patients wishing to maintain the pregnancy, concern for the welfare of the fetus and neonate dominates the process of diagnosis and treatment. Many have perceived that treatment may require compromise of the wellbeing of either the mother or the fetus. In some circumstances, fetal death may be an unavoidable consequence of cancer treatment. Frequently, however, judicious decision making not only can provide cancer care for the pregnant woman but also will preserve the pregnancy through successful labor and delivery.

Many issues arise in the realm of concurrent cancer and pregnancy (Table 65-1). The data for specific tumor types, diagnostic procedures, therapeutic interventions, and long-term cancer outcomes have been derived primarily from case reports, small case series, and retrospective reviews. Controlled studies are rare, and prospective data is even rarer. Data on labor and delivery outcomes for patients completing pregnancy remains scarce, as are long-term data on growth and development of children exposed to cancer treatment in utero. Decision making for patients and physicians is complex and must take into consideration not only medical issues but also moral, religious, ethical, and legal concerns.[1,2] Informed decisions are difficult when little information is available. The historical record, as imperfect as it may be, serves as the basis for patient care in the unusual circumstance of the concurrent diagnosis of cancer and pregnancy.

Table 65-1 ▪ **Issues (A Few) Related to Cancer and Pregnancy**

Impact of cancer on pregnancy
Impact of pregnancy on cancer
Termination of pregnancy/fetal death with cancer treatment
Diagnostic procedures and staging during pregnancy
Cancer treatment, maternal effects
Cancer treatment, fetal effects
Placental metastasis
Transplacental malignancy
Long-term outcome for children
Ethical, moral, legal concerns
The UNKNOWN

Cancer and Pregnancy Epidemiology

The diagnosis of cancer during pregnancy is rare. For example, the published data for breast cancer estimate 1:3000-3:10,000 deliveries occur in women with a diagnosis of breast cancer.[3-6] The most frequent cancer diagnoses, in association with pregnancy, have been reported by Smith and colleagues in a retrospective review of 3,168,911 deliveries in California from 1992 to 1997.[7] In this review, 2247 cases of primary malignancy were reported. They found 7.1 cases per 10,000 live singleton births; among these cases, the cancer diagnosis occurred in the prenatal period, at the time of delivery, or up to 12 months postpartum. There were 1.8 cases per 10,000 live singleton births for the prenatal period. Per 10,000 live singleton births, the most common tumor types were breast (1.3), thyroid (1.2), cervix (0.8), Hodgkin disease (0.5), ovarian (0.5), acute and chronic leukemia (0.37), and lymphoma (0.28). As the trend towards delayed childbearing continues, it has been surmised that cancers whose incidence increases with age may be more frequently seen concurrent with pregnancy.[7-9]

In a retrospective review spanning 24 years, Sayedur and colleagues reported an ovarian cancer incidence of 0.08/1000 deliveries.[10] Komurcu and colleagues reported a slightly greater incidence of colorectal carcinoma in association with pregnancy, with an estimated 1 case per 13,000 live born deliveries.[11] The rate of cervix cancer during pregnancy is 1 per 1200-10,000 pregnancies and presents difficult management choices with regard to surgical and radiation treatment. Similar to the California study, Kaiser and colleagues estimated the incidence of cancer in pregnancy as 1 in 1000, with cervix cancer being most frequent.[12] This finding is consistent with the observations of Allen and colleagues, who reported an incidence of 0.26 per 1000 pregnancies for cervix cancer, noting that cervix cancer was the most common malignancy to complicate pregnancy.[13] However, cancer from nearly any anatomic location can occur with pregnancy (Table 65-2).

Diagnosis and Staging

A biopsy, with review of cytologic and histologic material, is required for the diagnosis of any malignancy during pregnancy. The type of biopsy is determined by the accessibility of the disease site and the quantity of material required.

If a surgical biopsy is required, the anatomic location of the biopsy and the gestational age of the fetus are factors to be considered prior to proceeding. A surgical biopsy can be performed safely.[14,15] It is imperative that adequate material for pathologic diagnosis and required studies be obtained; for example, hormone receptors and *HER-2/neu* status are necessary for the proper evaluation of breast cancer and morphologic and immunophenotyping of lymphomas and leukemias is essential to their optimal assessment and treatment.

Staging provides guidance for discussions regarding cancer prognosis, recommended loco-regional and/or systemic therapies, and potential risks of treatment in relation to benefit and outcome for the patient. Frequently, staging assessment in the non-pregnant patient involves exposure to ionizing radiation, which is to be avoided whenever possible during pregnancy. The impact of radiation upon the fetus varies with respect to fetal gestational age. Preimplantation and fetal organogenesis are most sensitive to the negative effects of radiation exposure.[16] Fetal exposures of <5 cGy are not thought to be harmful.[17] With a number of procedures, exposure to radiation is negligible; examples are the chest radiograph (2.6 millirads) and IV pyelogram (500-800 millirads).[18] With chest computed tomography (CT), radiation exposure increases up to 3000 millirads; for abdominal computed tomography (CT), exposure may be as high

Table 65-2 Tumor Types Reported During Pregnancy (Partial List)

Acoustic neuroma[170]	Hepatocellular[171]
Acute leukemia-lymphoid and myeloid[132,172]	Hodgkin disease[32,107,108]
Adenocarcinoma of cervix[173]	Melanoma[174]
Adenocarcinoma of the papilla of Vater[175]	Multiple myeloma[176]
Bladder[177]	Mycosis fungoides[178]
Breast[179,180]	Neuroectodermal[181]
Burkitt lymphoma[119,120]	Non-Hodgkin lymphoma[105,111,112]
Cervix[13,92,96]	Non-small cell lung[182]
Chronic lymphocytic leukemia[137,138]	Ovary[10]
Chronic myelogenous leukemia[141-144]	Pancreas[175]
Colon[11]	Pheochromocytoma[183]
Craniopharyngioma[184]	Rectal[185]
Endometrial[186]	Renal[187]
Fallopian tube carcinoma[188]	Sarcoma[189]
Gastric[190]	T-cell leukemia[191]
Hairy cell leukemia[192]	Thyroid[84,86,193,194]
Head/neck[195]	Vulvar[196]

as 9000 millirads.[18] As a consequence of known fetal toxicity associated with exposure to ionizing radiation during pregnancy, abdominal shielding and non-ionizing techniques should be used whenever possible during these imaging procedures.[19,20] Ultrasonography for breast, liver, and other abdominal organ imaging can also contribute to the staging evaluation.[18] Magnetic resonance imaging (MRI) can be used to assess for bone and liver disease, as well as fetal abnormalities, if required.[21-27] Use of gadolinium as a contrast agent for MRI during pregnancy remains controversial. Although multiple case reports have not demonstrated a known increase in adverse effects to the fetus, gadolinium is often avoided if possible due to lack of toxicity information.[28-30] As more data accumulate, this recommendation may change. Accurate determination of disease stage is essential in ensuring accurate cancer treatment decisions, and findings during the staging process also may influence the woman's decision regarding the maintenance of her pregnancy.

Cancer Treatment During Pregnancy

The optimal treatment of cancer during pregnancy requires a meticulously coordinated multidisciplinary approach. Careful and repeated consultation with the obstetrician and/or maternal fetal medicine specialist is essential during the course of the pregnancy. Accurate assessment of fetal age, maturation, and the expected delivery date must be performed prior to treatment planning. The therapeutic options for the pregnant patient do not differ from those of the non-pregnant patient with cancer, but the application of treatment may be more complex.

Surgery

Surgery remains the mainstay for treatment of solid tumors, and pregnancy is not a contraindication for cancer surgery. Mazze and Kallen have reported on a registry series of 5405 pregnant patients on whom surgery was performed.[14] They did not observe an increased incidence of congenital malformations or stillbirths in women who had surgical procedures while pregnant.[14] An increased frequency of low- and very low birthweight infants was noted and attributed to prematurity and intrauterine growth retardation. No specific type of surgical procedure or anesthesia was associated with an increase in adverse reproductive outcomes. In a case-control study, Duncan and colleagues did not observe an increase in congenital anomalies in 2565 pregnant women who had surgery while pregnant, when compared to control patients who did not have surgery.[15] If warranted by tumor type and disease stage, surgery should proceed and should be coordinated with the obstetrician, anesthesiologist, and neonatal specialist.

Radiation

Pregnancy has been considered an absolute contraindication to radiation therapy for cancer. Radiation therapy for cervix cancer during pregnancy usually leads to fetal death and spontaneous abortion.[31] The fetus is most sensitive to malformation from radiation exposure 2-8 weeks after conception, whereas exposure from 8 to 25 weeks of gestation has the greatest risk of mental retardation.[16] Nevertheless, successful radiation therapy of pregnant women with Hodgkin disease has been reported.[32] If radiation is warranted, appropriate fetal shielding, careful dosimetry calculations, and estimates of fetal dose exposure are necessary.[33-37] Radiation therapy for breast cancer, following mastectomy or breast conservation surgery, can usually be delayed until the postpartum period. The National Commission on Radiation Protection has established recommended guidelines for total radiation exposure during pregnancy.[17] Less than 5 cGy is considered safe. If fetal exposure exceeds >15 cGy, termination of pregnancy has been recommended.[17]

Systemic Therapy

For many malignancies systemic therapy is used as primary or adjuvant treatment. Many different agents have been reported to have been used in pregnancy. Representative chemotherapeutic, hormone, and biologic agents are listed in Table 65-3.

Systemic therapy is of concern because of the potential deleterious effects on the fetus. Physiological changes associated with pregnancy (elevated blood volume, increased cardiac output, amplified glomerular filtration rate, and changes in circulating protein levels) make predictions about drug pharmacokinetics uncertain at best.[38] In addition, systemic agents are designed to be anti-proliferative compounds, and their administration during pregnancy poses genuine risk to the developing fetus. Potential concerns include stillbirth, spontaneous abortion, fetal malformations/teratogenesis, organ-specific toxicities, intrauterine growth retardation with low birth weight, and premature delivery.[39]

The fetal risks related to chemotherapy appear to be greatest during the first trimester of pregnancy. Doll and colleagues reviewed antineoplastic agents and fetal malformations in relation to the trimester of pregnancy.[39] They reported in utero exposure to systemic agents was associated fetal malformation risks of 14% and 19% for alkylating agents and antimetabolites, respectively. A similar review of second- and third-trimester exposure demonstrated a 1.3% incidence of fetal malformation. Thus, they concluded that single-agent or combination chemotherapy could be given during the second and third trimesters with low risk of fetal malformation, but these agents should be avoided during the first trimester of pregnancy. Similarly, in a review of cytotoxic agents used during pregnancy, Ebert and colleagues collected 217 cases from the literature published between 1983 and 1995.[38] They classified the use of the agents by disease category and analyzed outcome of pregnancy in relation to agent, dose, and gestational age at ex-

Table 65-3 Drugs Reported to Have Been Used During Pregnancy

MACOP-B	Hydroxyurea	α Interferon	Prednisone
MOPP-ABVD	All-trans retinoic acid	Rituximab	Tamoxifen
FAC	Methotrexate	Erythropoetin	
CMF	Doxorubicin/epirubicin	Filgrastim	
AC	Cyclophosphamide, nitrogen mustard	Trastuzumab	
VACOP-B	Vincristine, triethylene melamine	Lapatinib	
	Bleomycin	Imatinib	
	Cisplatin		
	Vinorelbine, vinblastine, vincristine		
	Paclitaxel		
	Docetaxel		
	Etoposide		
	Idarubicin, daunorubicin		
	Cytosine-arabinosine		
	5-fluororucil, busulfane		
	Teniposide		
	6-mercaptopurine		
	Dacarbazine		
	Aminopterin		
	Actimomycin D		
	Procarbazine		
	Amsacrine		
	L-asparaginase		

Abbreviations: ABVD, Adriamycin (doxorubicin), bleomycin, vinblastine and dacarbazine; AC, Adriamycin (doxorubicin) and cyclophosphamide; CMF, cyclophosphamide, methotrexate and 5-fluorouracil; FAC, 5-fluorouracil, Adriamycin (doxorubicin) and cyclophosphamide; MACOP-B, methotrexate, Adriamycin (doxorubicin), cyclophosphamide, Oncovin (vincristine), prednisone and bleomycin; MOPP, mechlorethamine, Oncovin (vincristine) procarbazine, and prednisone; VACOP-B, VePesid (etoposide), Adriamyicn (doxorubicin), cyclophosphamide, Oncovin (vincristine), prednisone and bleomycin.

posure. There were 94 cases of leukemia, 57 cases of lymphoma, 26 cases of breast or ovarian cancer, 16 cases of cytotoxic therapy used for rheumatic diseases, and the remainder of the malignancies. Eighteen newborns were reported to have congenital developmental abnormalities. Of these 18 newborns, 15 neonates had been exposed to cytotoxic drugs during the first trimester. Chromosomal abnormalities were noted in two neonates who had experienced exposure to cytotoxic agents during the first trimester.[38] Antimetabolite use was found in 50% of the neonates with congenital abnormalities following first-trimester exposure to chemotherapy. Of the reviewed cases, 82.3% of leukemia patients, 75.4% of lymphoma patients, and 75% of breast or ovary cancer patients with associated pregnancies were reported to have live births with normally developed neonates. Germann et al. collected data involving 160 patients who received anthracyclines during pregnancy.[40] In this group five cases of fetal malformations (3%) were found, with three cases occurring with the use of chemotherapy in the first trimester. The remaining two cases of fetal malformation occurred after chemotherapy administration in the second trimester; one involved Down syndrome unrelated to chemotherapy, and the other involved a congenital adherence of the iris to the cornea that demonstrated no clinical consequence. The combination chemotherapy regimens associated with fetal malformations included cytosine arabinoside or cyclophosphamide. Systemic treatment, especially with antimetabolites, should be avoided during the first trimester of pregnancy except in circumstances in which delay in cancer treatment would jeopardize the life of the patient, such as acute leukemia.

Erythropoietin use during pregnancy was reported by Scott and colleagues. No maternal or fetal toxicities have been noted.[41] Recent FDA Black Box warnings about the use of erythropoietin in cancer patients would apply to the pregnant patient as well, even in the absence of specific risk data in these patients. Dale and colleagues found that use of filgrastim during pregnancy was not associated with a change in neonatal outcome, when compared to untreated patients.[42] There are no data regarding pegfilgastrim in pregnancy. The U.S. FDA lists this as a Class C drug and the Australian FDA as Class B3.

Specific Cancers

Breast Cancer

The diagnosis of breast cancer during pregnancy is often delayed, presumably due to the anatomical and physiological changes in the pregnant breast.[43,44] However, women with breast cancer during pregnancy have demonstrated the same survival rates, stage for stage, as non-pregnant patients with breast cancer.[45,46] Imaging of the breast in women with a palpable mass or thickening is warranted. Mammography and ultrasonography may confirm the presence of a malignant mass. Although Max and Klamer reported normal mammograms in six of eight women with breast cancer during pregnancy, others have reported abnormal mammograms in the majority of women with pregnancy and breast cancer (18 of 23 and 5 of 8).[47-49]

There are limited data on ultrasonography; Liberman reported positive findings in six of six patients, and Samuels found positive findings in two of four patients.[47,48] Yang et al. diagnosed 100% of the masses as well as axillary metastases in 18 of 20 women.[50] Ultrasound was also shown to be effective for restaging to evaluate response to pre-operative chemotherapy in the pregnant breast.[50] Ultrasonography may be useful for guiding either fine needle aspiration (FNA) or core biopsy in order to confirm a diagnosis of malignancy.[51-53]

The use of positron emission tomography/computed tomography (PET/CT) scanning has become standard in the treatment and evaluation of lymphomas and has had an increase in use in evaluation of metastatic disease in solid tumors as well. There are very limited data regarding the use of PET/CT in the pregnant breast cancer patient. Evidence that fluorodeoxyglucose (FDG) crosses the placenta and can accumulate in fetal brain, bladder and cardiac tissue has been demonstrated in animal studies.[54] Zanotti-Fregonara et al. estimated the F-FDG uptake by embryo tissues in early pregnancy is at least 3.3E-2mGy/MBq in a patient found to be pregnant at the time of scanning [55]; few other case reports exist. Hove et al. describe an 18 year-old woman with Hodgkin disease who underwent PET/CT. There was significant uptake in the fetal myocardium. The patient developed hemolytic anemia, elevated liver enzymes and low platelet count (HELLP) syndrome and the child was delivered at 31 weeks by caesarian section.[56] Therefore, there was insufficient safety data to support the use of PET/CT scanning during pregnancy and it should be delayed until after delivery whenever possible.

Staging evaluation can be tailored to clinical findings. If clinically suspicious regional nodes are identified on physical examination or by imaging techniques, an FNA that is guided by palpation or ultrasonography can be utilized to confirm metastases. Chest radiography, liver ultrasound and MRI of the thoracic/lumbar spine can be used to assess for extant organ metastasis.[18,21,22] The theoretical dosage of radiation that would be absorbed by the fetus following sentinel lymph node biopsy has been calculated to be less than 5 cGy.[57,58] Khera et al. recently reported their experience with sentinel node procedures in the pregnant patient.[59] Ten patients had sentinel node procedures, six with blue dye and Tc99m, two with Tc99m alone and two with blue dye alone. No adverse sequelae were reported for nine neonates. One woman chose elective termination of pregnancy.

Local regional treatment with mastectomy and axillary lymph node dissection, has been considered standard.[60] Breast-conserving surgery is possible with postpartum breast irradiation.[61] Pre- or postoperative chemotherapy is used with the same criteria for selection of therapy as in the non-pregnant patient. Hahn and colleagues have reported on a prospective cohort of 57 breast cancer patients using 5-fluorouracil, doxorubicin, and cyclophosphamide during pregnancy.[62] No spontaneous abortions, stillbirths, or congenital malformations were noted. Complications for the neonate included: prematurity, neutropenia, tachypnea of the newborn, and respiratory distress syndrome. One case of spontaneous cryptogenic intracranial hemorrhage occurred. These have all resolved. There were three congenital abnormalities reported which included Down syndrome (1), congenital ureteral reflux (1) and clubfoot (1).[62]

A retrospective survey of breast cancer treated during pregnancy has been reported by Giacalone and colleagues. They reported 17 live births, 2 spontaneous abortions, and 1 stillbirth in 20 patients. A variety of chemotherapy agents was used, including alkylating agents and anthracyclines. Complications of labor and delivery were not reported.[63]

Other agents have been described in the literature including vinorelbine, paclitaxel, docetaxel and cisplatin.[64] One report could be found for cisplatin therapy for a squamous cell breast cancer.[65] Paclitaxel has been described in at least four cases of breast cancer[64,66-68] and docetaxel in six cases[69-71] with all available follow-up data reported healthy children.[64] Vinorelbine has been reported to be used at least 6 times in both adjuvant and metastatic settings, with 5 of the 6 children reporting healthy at 6-35 months of follow-up. Information on one of the children was not available in the literature. Neonatal complications included one episode of grade 4 neutropenia and transient cytopenia at day 6 of life.[69,72,73]

At least eight reports of trastuzumab administered during pregnancy have been identified. No fetal abnormalities have been reported; however, anhydramnios with its use was described in 6 of the case reports.[67,72,74-76] One case was of reversible heart failure in the mother with no anhydramnios in the fetus.[77] One of the children born developed respiratory failure, capillary leak syndrome, infections and necrotizing enterocolitis, dying from multiple organ failure 21 weeks after delivery.[75] Additionally, Bader et al. described a case of reversible renal failure in the fetus.[67] One recent report describes the use of lapatinib; the patient conceived while on lapatinib. Despite approximately 11 weeks of exposure, the pregnancy was otherwise uncomplicated with the delivery of a healthy baby.[78] Routine administration of biologic agents is not recommended during pregnancy given these very limited data.

Tamoxifen is a standard treatment for hormone receptor positive tumors in premenopausal women. Although some case reports of tamoxifen fetal exposure demonstrated no effect on the newborn, there are other reports including Goldenhar syndrome (microtia, preauricular skin tags and hemifacial microsomia),[79] ambiguous genitalia and other birth defects. Additionally vaginal bleeding and spontaneous abortion have also been reported.[79-83] Aromatase inhibitors are not indicated in premenopausal women and should not be used.

Thyroid Cancer

In pregnant women, thyroid cancer presents most often as an asymptomatic nodule in the neck. Ultrasound evaluation can confirm the size and solid character of the nodule. FNA biopsy is the most reliable diagnostic test and is safe and accurate during pregnancy.[84-86] Most often, pregnancy-associated thyroid cancers are well-differentiated tumors. Radioiodine scans and therapeutic radioiodine should not be given during pregnancy and can be safely delayed until after delivery.[87] Thyroid surgery can be delayed until after delivery for many patients, especially if the diagnosis is made during the third trimester of pregnancy.[87,88] If warranted, thyroid resection can be done under local anesthesia.[89] Moosa and Mazzaferi reported on 61 pregnant patients with thyroid cancer and 528 age-matched non-pregnant controls.[90] They reviewed diagnosis, treatment, and outcome for the two cohorts. Seventy-four percent of the pregnant patients had been discovered to possess an asymptomatic thyroid nodule during routine examinations. Twenty percent of the pregnant patients underwent thyroid surgery during the second trimester, while 77% of patients underwent surgery following delivery. Thirty percent of the patients received postoperative iodine-131 therapy; all of these treatments were administered postpartum. The presence of pregnancy or delayed surgery did not result in differences in cancer recurrence, distant recurrence, or death. Based upon these findings, Moosa and Mazzaferi concluded that treatment for thyroid cancer during pregnancy may be delayed until after delivery in most patients.[90] Additionally, Yasmeen et al. reviewed data from the California Cancer Registry of 595 women diagnosed with thyroid cancer within 9 months antepartum to 12 months postpartum, compared to matched non-pregnant counterparts, and no significant differences were found in overall survival, maternal or fetal outcomes.[91]

Cervix Cancer

In the California series, cervix cancer was the third most common cancer diagnosed during pregnancy and the postpartum period.[7] Nguyen and colleagues have stated that all pregnant women should have cytologic screening of the cervix and, as appropriate, colposcopy, biopsy, and selective conization.[92]

Evaluation of extent of disease for diagnosed cervix cancer includes physical examination and assessment of pelvic anatomic structures by MRI. A report of laparoscopic lymph node staging at 16 weeks of pregnancy demonstrates the feasibility of this technique.[93] Treatment options vary with disease stage, gestational age at diagnosis, and the desires of the patient. For stage I disease, Sorosky and colleagues have reported a favorable outcome with only planned follow-up observation until the third trimester.[94] They followed eight women with stage I disease, <2.5 cm in dimension, for a mean interval of 109 days. All patients underwent delivery via caesarean delivery, followed by radical hysterectomy. Serial MRIs was used to follow the disease for two patients, and no clinical disease progression was noted. After treatment, all patients were alive and free of disease at a mean follow-up of 37 months.

In a review of 22 patients with cervix cancer diagnosed during pregnancy or within 12 months postpartum, Allen and colleagues noted twenty live deliveries and only one disease recurrence.[13] Nine of eleven patients with microinvasive disease were treated with core biopsy only. Ten patients with stage IB or IIA disease were treated with radical hysterectomy, and one patient with stage IIIB disease received chemotherapy, radiation therapy, and simple hysterectomy as treatment. Allen recommended all pregnant women undergo cervical cytologic evaluation. Cone biopsy is safe in pregnancy and may be adequate treatment for microinvasive disease.[13]

Outcome and recurrence risk have been assessed in relation to method of delivery for women diagnosed with cervix cancer during pregnancy or within 6 months postpartum. Sood and colleagues followed 83 pregnant women with cervix cancer; 56 of these patients were diagnosed during pregnancy, and 27 patients were diagnosed postpartum.[95] Since the risk of recurrence was increased in those diagnosed postpartum who delivered vaginally, Sood et al. concluded that women with cervix cancer should be delivered by caesarean.[95] However, van der Vange and colleagues, in a case-control study, reported that mode of delivery had no effect on survival.[96] Overall, they noted no difference in survival of pregnant patients with cervix cancer compared to the non-pregnant group. For cervix malignancies diagnosed at delivery and during the immediate postpartum period, episiotomy site recurrence of cancer has been reported.[97] Systemic chemotherapy for cervix cancer can be effective when given during pregnancy, although the role of neoadjuvant therapy has not been established. For example, Marana and colleagues reported on a 26-year-old patient with stage IIB cervix cancer diagnosed at 14 weeks of gestation.[98] She was treated with cisplatin and bleomycin, and delivered a normal infant at 38 weeks gestation. Indeed, cisplatin has been the most frequently used agent in case reports of cervix cancer chemotherapy. In addition, one case report describes the delivery of a normal infant following systemic treatment of a pregnant patient with a combined regimen of cisplatin and paclitaxel.[99] There are several case reports describing the use of neoadjuvant cisplatin-based regimens with either taxane or vinorelbine used in order to preserve the pregnancy until the fetus is viable with good maternal and fetal outcomes.[100-102]

Treatment of the pregnant patient with cervix cancer requires careful consideration of disease stage and gestational age. Early in pregnancy with early stage disease, pregnancy termination followed by cancer treatment may be appropriate. Alternatively, planned delay in cancer treatment with careful monitoring of disease may allow for successful completion of the pregnancy.[94] Radiation therapy will cause fetal death and usually results in spontaneous abortion.[31]

Since a significant population of patients is diagnosed with cervical cancer while in childbearing age, the concern for preservation of fertility has led to the utilization of radical vaginal trachelectomy with pelvic lymphadenectomy, instead of radical hysterectomy, in select patients with stage I cervical cancer. Burnett and colleagues made this procedure available to 21 patients over a period of 6 years.[103] Following the procedure, eight patients demonstrated no residual cervical disease. Eight patients had minimal residual cancer without lymph vascular space invasion (LVSI). Two patients demonstrated LVSI, but negative margins and lymph nodes. Two patients required completion of radical vaginal hysterectomy in order to successfully obtain negative margins. The last patient had lymph vascular space invasion and a positive margin present within the surgical specimen. The latter three patients underwent postoperative pelvic radiation therapy. Therefore, 18 of 21 patients received radical trachelectomy in order to preserve fertility. Within this group, one patient gave birth to healthy twins, delivered at 24 weeks, following superovulation treatment. One patient delivered a singleton term infant via caesarean hysterectomy; no residual disease was found in the cervix. The last patient most likely became pregnant in the week prior to the radical vaginal trachelectomy. She had spontaneous rupture of membranes at 20 weeks gestation, requiring hysterotomy for evacuation of the uterus with subsequent neonatal demise.

No prospective studies have assessed the impact of pregnancy neither on the prognosis of cervix cancer nor on pregnancy outcome. Nguyen and colleagues concluded that tumor characteristics and maternal survival were not adversely affected by pregnancy, nor was pregnancy adversely affected by cervix cancer.[92] Similar conclusions were reached by van der Vange and colleagues in a case-control study. They reported on 23 patients diagnosed during pregnancy and 24 patients diagnosed within 6 months postpartum. Thirty-nine patients had early stage disease. No difference in survival was noted for cases compared to controls. They noted that the delivery method had no effect on survival, thus concluding that prognosis for early stage cervix cancer is similar in pregnant and non-pregnant women.[96] Zemlickis and colleagues reported on a long-term follow-up of cervix cancer outcome in a case-control study of pregnant women. No survival differences were observed. When compared to matched controls, patients with invasive cervix cancer were more likely to give birth to children who had lower birth weights. No adverse impact of pregnancy on cervix cancer outcome could be demonstrated.[104]

Hodgkin Disease and Non-Hodgkin Lymphoma

The presentation of Hodgkin disease during pregnancy does not differ from that of the non-pregnant patient, with lymphadenopathy being the most common method of presentation.[105] The diagnosis is established by lymph node biopsy, obtaining sufficient material to confirm specific type of disease.[106] Staging assessment, in addition to medical history and physical examination, can include an abdominal shielded chest radiograph, abdominal ultrasonography, and MRI to document disease location and extent in order to assist treatment planning. For supradiaphragmatic disease, radiation therapy can be completed successfully while maintaining the pregnancy with uterine/fetal shielding.[32,34,106-108] Radiation therapy during pregnancy for stage IA and IIA Hodgkin disease has been reported by Woo and colleagues.[32] Sixteen patients received radiation to the neck (2), neck and mediastinum (3), or mantle (11). Fetal radiation dose estimates were determined for nine patients. Reported doses ranged from 1.4 to 5.5 cGy for photon therapy and 10-13.6 cGy for cobalt therapy. There were 16 normal full-term infants, and the 10-year patient survival rate was 71%.[32] This outcome is similar to an earlier report by Jacobs and colleagues, who reported on the use of radiation therapy involving the neck and mediastinum during the second and third trimesters of pregnancy.[108] Supradiaphragmatic radiation therapy can be accomplished while maintaining a viable pregnancy. There are limited data regarding the impact of Hodgkin disease on pregnancy, and the effects of pregnancy upon disease prognosis. Anselmo and colleagues concluded that the prognosis of Hodgkin disease was not affected by pregnancy.[109] Tawil and colleagues, reporting on their experience with 12 patients with Hodgkin disease and pregnancy, concluded that pregnancy did not significantly affect the course of the malignancy, and the presence of this malignancy did not affect pregnancy outcome.[107] Examining pregnancy outcome, Zuazu and colleagues found no increase in the complication rate of pregnancy in 56 patients with leukemia or lymphoma. In those patients treated with systemic chemotherapy, there was no increase in incidence of fetal malformations.[110] In the Gelb series, patients were treated with a variety of systemic chemotherapy agent combinations, including mechlorethamine, vincristine, procarbazine, prednisone(MOPP), doxorubicin, bleomycin, vinblastine (ABV), cyclophosphamide, vincristine, prednisone (COP), and cyclophosphamide, doxorubicin, vincristine, prednisone (CHOP).[105] No fetal malformations were reported. Fifteen patients were alive and disease free. Gelb and colleagues concluded that otherwise indicated systemic therapy should not be delayed because of pregnancy.

Non-Hodgkin lymphoma during pregnancy presents at more advanced stage and has more aggressive biologic behavior than Hodgkin disease during pregnancy.[105,111,112] The clinical behavior of non-Hodgkin lymphoma appears to be the same with or without pregnancy.[105] Because the majority of patients present with advanced stage disease, systemic chemotherapy is warranted. Combination chemotherapy has been reported to be used with some success. Agents used have included epirubicin, vincristine, prednisone, etoposide, cyclophosphamide, doxorubicin, and bleomycin in various combinations (VACOP-B, MACOP-B).[113-115] Two separate publications have reported the use of rituximab in the treatment of non-Hodgkin lymphoma (NHL) during pregnancy. Herold and colleagues utilized a combination of rituximab, doxorubicin, vincristine, and prednisolone to treat a female with bulky stage IIA NHL.[116] At the time of initiation of therapy, the patient was in her 21st week of pregnancy. She demonstrated an excellent response to the regimen, with good tolerance. The patient then delivered a healthy infant at 35 weeks via caesarean section; the child demonstrated a normal B cell population. Kimby and colleagues treated a patient with Stage IIB NHL with weekly rituximab for four cycles.[117] The patient reported conception occurrence between the first and second infusions of rituximab. She delivered a healthy baby girl at 40 weeks. The infant demonstrated a low granulocyte count at birth, but her hematologic parameters had recovered by 18 months of age.

Aviles and colleagues reported the out-come of 16 patients treated for NHLHodgkin during pregnancy, including eight during the first trimester.[118] No congenital malformations were noted, and normal deliveries were reported. They concluded that pregnancy was not a contraindication to treating NHLHodgkin and that long-term remission was possible. Burkitt lymphoma, anaplastic large cell lymphoma, and T-cell lymphoma have all been reported in association with pregnancy.[119-124]

Ovarian Cancer

Ovarian cancer during pregnancy is rare. In a review of adnexal masses during pregnancy, one ovarian cancer was found in 125 patients.[125] There were 40 dermoids, 15 endometriomas, 14 cysts, 13 cystoadenomas, 9 tubal cysts, and 4 fibroids, a 0.8% malignancy rate.[125]

In a retrospective review, Sayedur and colleagues identified nine cases of ovarian cancer and pregnancy over 24 years, an incidence of 0.08/1000 pregnant women. For pregnant women, adnexal masses are more frequent, likely to be benign and management decisions are becoming more complex.[10] Ultrasonography, percutaneous aspiration, and surgical intervention are possible.

In a study by Platek and colleagues, 31 patients of 43,372 deliveries were found to have adnexal masses >6 cm persistent beyond 16 weeks of gestation.[126] No ovarian cancers were diagnosed. When malignancies have been found, germ cell tumors and epithelial cancers of low malignant potential were most common.[127] The pathology of ovarian cancer during pregnancy was reviewed by Dgani and colleagues.[128] They recorded data on 23 patients over a 24-year period. Borderline carcinomas were most frequent (35%), followed by invasive epithelial tumors (30%), dysgerminomas (17%), and granulosa cell tumors (13%). Early stage disease was common; 74% of patients were stage I.

In the series of Sayedur and colleagues, seven of the nine patients had stage I epithelial tumors.[10] Five patients were treated with salpingo-oophorectomy, three with total abdominal hysterectomy and bilateral salpingo-oophorectomy with omentectomy. They reported 100% survival for stage I disease and 78% 5-year survival overall.

Conservative surgery for early stage disease and low malignant potential tumors may preserve fertility. In the Dgani series, 14 of the 23 patients delivered live neonates.[128] Dgani concluded that the overall prognosis for ovarian cancer during pregnancy is better than ovarian tumors in general because of early stage at diagnosis and tumors of low malignant potential.[128]

Chemotherapy for more advanced-stage disease has been reported primarily as case reports. Cisplatin, carboplatin, doxorubicin, bleomycin, cyclophosphamide, and, most recently, paclitaxel have all been given for treatment of ovarian cancer during pregnancy.[99,129,131]

Acute and Chronic Leukemia

Acute Leukemia

Acute leukemia occurring during pregnancy presents unique circumstances because of bone marrow failure and the attendant cytopenias that may occur. Myeloid leukemias are more common than lymphoid. The presenting signs and symptoms are not different from those of the non-pregnant patient. The diagnosis is made by bone marrow aspiration, and standard classification is used for sub-typing. In a series from the Mayo Clinic, 17 pregnant patients with acute leukemia were seen in a 37-year period. Fifteen of the 17 patients were diagnosed with acute myeloid disease. The majority of these individuals presented during the first or second trimester of pregnancy. Five of nine patients treated with chemotherapy during pregnancy had long-term complete remissions, whereas three of four patients who delayed treatment until after delivery died of disease. No fetal malformations were noted in those treated with chemotherapy during pregnancy.[132]

Cardonick and Iacobucci performed an analysis of 152 patients who were treated for acute lymphoblastic leukemia (63 cases) or acute myelogenous leukemia (89 cases).[133] They found that six neonates developed congenital abnormalities and 12 neonates demonstrated intrauterine growth retardation. There were 11 cases of intrauterine fetal death and 2 neonatal deaths. All cases of abnormalities occurred in association with first trimester usage of cytarabine or thioguanine, as monotherapy or in combination with an anthracycline. However, combinations of vincristine, mercaptopurine, doxorubicin or daunorubicin, cyclophosphamide, prednisone, and methotrexate were used in all trimesters without anomalies.

Acute promyelocytic leukemia (APL) is of special interest because of the use of all-transretinoic acid (ATRA) in the treatment program. Retinoids have known teratogenic effects.[134] However, a number of case reports have documented fetal safety and favorable patient outcome with the use of ATRA for APL.[135,136]

Chronic Leukemia

Pregnancy and chronic lymphocytic leukemia (CLL) is extraordinarily rare.[137,138] Welsh and colleagues reported a case of CLL with pregnancy and noted a substantial decrease in white blood cells after delivery.[138] They noted this apparent hematologic remission was not accompanied by clonal remission. Gurman described a case of a patient who became pregnant shortly after her diagnosis of CLL. She received no cytotoxic therapy, and she delivered a healthy infant at 39 weeks gestation.[139] Her third trimester was complicated by gestational diabetes and pre-eclampsia. Unlike the Welsh report, which demonstrated elevated numbers of lymphocytes in the intervillous space, the latter case demonstrated no lymphocytic infiltration of the placenta. Ali and colleagues treated a patient who was diagnosed with CLL during her 17th week of gestation.[140] She received three courses of leukopheresis at the 25th, 30th, and 38th week of gestation in order to maintain her WBC count below $100 \times 10^9/L$. She delivered a normal infant at 39 weeks of gestation.

Chronic myeloid leukemia has been treated during pregnancy with interferon α, hydroxyurea and leukapheresis, and leukapheresis alone.[141-144] No untoward effects of treatment on fetal growth, nor development or complications of labor and delivery have been reported.

Sustaining the pregnancy until delivery is feasible. No fetal malformations with the use of interferon or hydroxyurea have been reported. Limited data suggest that pregnancy has no effect on CML long-term outcome; however there are no case-control studies. Although limited data from animal studies suggest imatinib may have teratogenic properties, there is increasing but conflicting data on imatinib use during pregnancy. Yilmaz et al. described three patients exposed to imatinib during pregnancy, all with healthy neonates at delivery.[145] Prabash et al. describes two cases of normal births after imatinib exposure and continuation of imatinib therapy throughout the pregnancy.[146] Ault et al. described 19 pregnancies involving 18 patients who conceived while receiving imatinib. All female patients discontinued therapy at the time the pregnancy was discovered. Three pregnancies ended in spontaneous abortion and one with an elective abortion. Two of the 16 babies had abnormalities; one with hypospadias and another with rotation of the small intestine. The authors concluded that patients should use contraception as the discontinuation of imatinib may lead to loss of disease response. Another case report describes the development of a meningocele and death of the fetus exposed to imatinib.[147] Therefore, patients should be encouraged to continue with contraception while on imatinib given these scant and conflicting reports; however, some patients have maintained imatinib therapy during pregnancy. This may be an option for some women, only after detailed and deliberative discussion with the treating team regarding risks and the limits of available information.

Transplacental Malignancy and Placental Metastasis

A number of case reports have noted transplacental passage of malignancy from mother to neonate (Table 65-4).[148-155] Catlin and colleagues reported a neonatal death related to the transplacental passage of maternal natural killer cell lymphoma.[148] Successful treatment of maternal transplacental small-cell lung cancer has been noted.[155] Teksam presented a striking case of a 33-week neonate who was emergently delivered after her mother was diagnosed with lung cancer. Due to the presence of placental metastases, the infant underwent initial screening with brain MRI and chest/abdomen CT, both of which were apparently normal. Unfortunately, serial examinations demonstrated development of a cerebellar tumor that significantly improved after chemotherapy, but the mass progressed a few months afterwards. Biopsy and resection confirmed that the neoplasm was metastatic lung cancer. Additional metastatic lesions were identified in the frontal and temporal lobes on follow-up MRI.[156]

Leukemia cell identification in circulation in a neonate born to a mother with ALL has also been reported. However, leukemic cell engraftment and neonatal disease was not observed.[157] Acute monocytic leukemia transmission from mother to fetus has been documented.[151]

Alexander and colleagues reviewed 87 cases of fetal or placental metastases; they found that malignant melanoma affected 31% of these patients, making melanoma the most common malignancy to involve both the fetus and placenta.[152]

Dildy and colleagues reviewed placental metastases and reported 52 cases in 1989. Solid tumors and hematologic malignancies have been noted to involve the placenta (Table 65-5).[121,158-166] Systematic evaluation of the placenta at the time of delivery of the pregnant woman with cancer has not been routine.[166]

Table 65-4 Transplacental Malignancy (Partial List)

Tumor
Choriocarcinoma[154]
Leukemia[151,197]
Melanoma[150]
Natural killer cell lymphoma[148]
Small cell lung cancer[155]

Table 65-5 Placental Metastases

Tumor Type
Small cell lung cancer[155]
Melanoma[158]
Pancreas[160]
Breast[162]
Medulloblastoma[159]
Large cell lung cancer[161]
B-cell lymphoma[164]
T-cell lymphoma[165]
Non-Hodgkin lymphoma[166]
Large cell lymphoma[121]
Hodgkin Disease

Outcome of Children Exposed to Cancer Therapy In Utero

There is a paucity of data regarding long term follow-up in children exposed to chemotherapy in utero. Little long-term data have been reported other than anecdotal reports noting "normal" development.[62] Delayed effects on cognitive function and on neurological and behavioral development are lacking.[167] A long-term report on children exposed to chemotherapy in utero during treatment of mothers for a variety of hematologic malignancies has been presented by Aviles and Neri.[168] They described 84 children followed a median of 18.7 years. Thirty-eight had been exposed to chemotherapy in utero during the first trimester of pregnancy. Fertility was reported to be preserved, some of the chemotherapy-exposed children having become parents. No learning, neurologic, or psychological problems were reported for any of the in utero chemotherapy–exposed subjects. Van Calsteren et al. report on ten children from nine pregnancies exposed to chemotherapy in utero for differing primary cancers. The children who were born prematurely had multiple abnormalities ranging from speech delay to mental and motor retardation. These were children born at less than 33 weeks gestation. Echocardiograms were also obtained demonstrating a tendency towards a thinner ventricular wall.[169]

Table 65-6 Multidisciplinary Approach to the Pregnant Patient With Cancer

Diagnosis and Treatment Planning	Considerations
Confirm diagnosis	Cytology, histology
Assess extent of disease	Staging, physical exam, organ function, metastatic disease
Disease related prognosis independent of pregnancy	
Assess pregnancy	Comorbidities: age, diabetes, cardiac function
	Gestational age
	Expected delivery date
Review treatment options	Patient
	Anticipated benefits for the patient
	"Cure," prolongation of life, improve or delay symptoms
Anticipated risks for the patient	
Review treatment options	Fetus
	Anticipated outcome
	Maintaining pregnancy
	Anticipated risks for fetus
Plan and implement treatment plan	
Reevaluate patient and fetus at frequent intervals	
Multidisciplinary treatment team members	Patient
	Obstetrician
	Oncologists: surgical, radiation, medical, gynecologist, radiation physicist
	Nurses
	Ethicists
	Social services
	Pastoral care

Conclusion

Cancer and pregnancy presents a unique opportunity for multispecialty oncologic and prenatal care. The gathering and discussion of data to be utilized in treatment planning requires careful coordination with obstetrical, surgical, and anesthesiology colleagues. Given the concern for the well-being of both the mother and fetus, support for and reassurance of the patient during the decision process becomes a paramount duty for physicians. It is possible to have a favorable outcome for mother and child. An outline of a sequential approach to multispecialty management for cancer and pregnancy is presented in Table 65-6.

Selected References

The complete reference list can be found at www.CANCERMEDICINE8.com

1. Minkoff H, Paltrow LM. The rights of "Unborn children" and the value of pregnant women. *Hastings Cent Rep.* 2006;36:26–28.
2. Chervenak FA, McCullough LB, Knapp RC, Caputo TA, Barber HR. A clinically comprehensive ethical framework for offering and recommending cancer treatment before and during pregnancy. *Cancer* 2004;100:215–222.
7. Smith LH, Dalrymple JL, Leiserowitz GS, Danielsen B, Gilbert WM. Obstetrical deliveries associated with maternal malignancy in California, 1992 through 1997. *Am J Obstet Gynecol.* 2001;184:1504–1512.
14. Mazze RI, Kallen B. Reproductive outcome after anesthesia and operation during pregnancy: a registry study of 5405 cases. *Am J Obstet Gynecol* 1989;161:1178–1185.
15. Duncan PG, Pope WD, Cohen MM, Greer N. Fetal risk of anesthesia and surgery during pregnancy. *Anesthesiology.* 1986;64:790–794.
24. Gosfield E, Alavi A, Kneeland B. Comparison of radionuclide bone scans and magnetic resonance imaging in detecting spinal metastases. *J Nucl Med.* 1993;34:2191.
28. De SM, Straface G, Cavaliere AF, Carducci B, Caruso A. Gadolinium periconceptional exposure: pregnancy and neonatal outcome. *Acta Obstet Gynecol Scand.* 2007;86:99–101.
30. Marcos HB, Semelka RC, Worawattanakul S. Normal placenta: gadolinium-enhanced dynamic MR imaging. *Radiology.* 1997;205:493–496.
32. Woo SY, Fuller LM, Cundiff JH, et al. Radiotherapy during pregnancy for clinical stages IA-IIA Hodgkin's disease. *Int J Radiat Oncol Biol Phys.* 1992;23:407–412.
38. Ebert U, Loffler H, Kirch W. Cytotoxic therapy and pregnancy. *Pharmacol Ther.* 1997;74:207–220.
39. Doll DC, Ringenberg QS, Yarbro JW. Antineoplastic agents and pregnancy. *Semin Oncol.* 1989;16:337–346.
40. Germann N, Goffinet F, Goldwasser F. Anthracyclines during pregnancy: embryo-fetal outcome in 160 patients 3. *Ann Oncol.* 2004;15:146–150.
50. Yang WT, Dryden MJ, Gwyn K, Whitman GJ, Theriault R. Imaging of breast cancer diagnosed and treated with chemotherapy during pregnancy. *Radiology.* 2006;239:52–60.
51. Gupta RK, McHutchinson AGR, Dowle CS, Simpson JS. Fine-needle aspiration cytodiagnosis of breast masses in pregnant and lactating women and its impact on management. *Diagn Cytopathol.* 1993;19:156–159.
57. Keleher A, Wendt R, III, Delpassand E, Stachowiak AM, Kuerer HM. The safety of lymphatic mapping in pregnant breast cancer patients using Tc-99m sulfur colloid 1. *Breast J.* 2004;10:492–495.
61. Kuerer HM, Gwyn K, Ames FC, Theriault RL. Conservative surgery and chemotherapy for breast carcinoma during pregnancy. *Surgery.* 2002;131:108–110.
62. Hahn KM, Johnson PH, Gordon N, et al. Treatment of pregnant breast cancer patients and outcomes of children exposed to chemotherapy in utero. *Cancer.* 2006;107:1219–1226.
64. Mir O, Berveiller P, Ropert S, et al. Emerging therapeutic options for breast cancer chemotherapy during pregnancy. *Ann Oncol.* 2008;19:607–613.
67. Bader AA, Schlembach D, Tamussino KF, Pristauz G, Petru E. Anhydramnios associated with administration of trastuzumab and paclitaxel for metastatic breast cancer during pregnancy. *Lancet Oncol.* 2007;8:79–81.
70. Sekar R, Stone PR. Trastuzumab use for metastatic breast cancer in pregnancy. *Obstet Gynecol.* 2007;110:507–510.
77. Shrim A, Garcia-Bournissen F, Maxwell C, Farine D, Koren G. Favorable pregnancy outcome following Trastuzumab (Herceptin) use during pregnancyÑcase report and updated literature review. *Reprod Toxicol.* 2007;23:611–613.
80. Cunha GR, Taguchi O, Namikawa R, Nishizuka Y, Robboy SJ. Teratogenic effects of clomiphene, tamoxifen, and diethylstilbestrol on the developing human female genital tract. *Hum Pathol.* 1987;18:1132–1143.
83. Loibl S, von Minckwitz G, Gwyn K, et al. Breast carcinoma during pregnancy. International recommendations from an expert meeting. *Cancer.* 2006;106:237–246.
88. Nam KH, Yoon JH, Chang HS, Park CS. Optimal timing of surgery in well-differentiated thyroid carcinoma detected during pregnancy. *J Surg Oncol.* 2005;91:199–203.
92. Nguyen C, Montz FJ, Bristow RE. Management of stage I cervical cancer in pregnancy. *Obstet Gynecol Surv.* 2001;55:633–643.
95. Sood AK, Sorosky JI, Mayr N, Anderson B, Buller RE, Niebyl J. Cervical cancer diagnosed shortly after pregnancy: prognostic variables and delivery routes. *Obstet Gynecol.* 2000;95:832–838.
96. Van Der Vange N, Weverling GJ, Ketting BW, Ankum WM, Samlal R, Lammes FB. The prognosis of cervical cancer associated with pregnancy: a matched cohort study. *Obstet Gynecol.* 1995;85:1022–1026.
98. Marana HRC, deAndrade JM, Mathes A, Duarte G, daCunha SP, Bighetti S. Chemotherapy in the treatment of locally advanced cervical cancer and pregnancy. *Gynecol Oncol.* 2001;80:272–274.
100. Caluwaerts S, VAN CK, Mertens L, et al. Neoadjuvant chemotherapy followed by radical hysterectomy for invasive cervical cancer diagnosed during pregnancy: report of a case and review of the literature. *Int J Gynecol Cancer.* 2006;16:905–908.
105. Gelb AB, van de Rijn M, Warnke RA, Kamel OW. Pregnancy-associated lymphomas: a clinicopathologic study. *Cancer.* 1996;78:304–310.
111. Lishner M, Zemlickis D, Sutcliffe SB, Koren G. Non-Hodgkin's lymphoma and pregnancy. *Leuk Lymphoma.* 1994;14:411–413.
116. Herold M, Schnohr S, Bittrich H. Efficacy and safety of a combined rituximab chemotherapy during pregnancy. *J Clin Oncol.* 2001;19:3439.
118. Aviles A, Diaz-Maqueo JC, Torras V, Garcia EL, Guzman R. Non-Hodgkin's lymphomas and pregnancy: presentation of 16 cases. *Gynecol Oncol.* 1990;37:335–337.
132. Greenlund LJ, Letendre L, Tefferi A. Acute leukemia during pregnancy: a single institutional experience with 17 cases. *Leuk Lymphoma.* 2001;41:571–577.
133. Cardonick E, Iacobucci A. Use of chemotherapy during human pregnancy. *Lancet Oncol.* 2004;5:283–291.
136. Hansen WF, Fretz P, Hunter SK, Yankowitz J. Leukemia in pregnancy and fetal response to multiagent chemotherapy. *Obstet Gynecol.* 2001;97:809–812.
141. Celiloglu M, Altunyurt S, Undar B. Hydroxyurea treatment for chronic myeloid leukemia during pregnancy. *Acta Obstet Gynecol Scand.* 2000;79:803–804.
146. Prabhash K, Sastry PS, Biswas G, et al. Pregnancy outcome of two patients treated with imatinib. *Ann Oncol.* 2005;16:1983–1984.
154. McNally OM, Tran M, Fortune D, Quinn MA. Successful treatment of mother and baby with metastatic choriocarcinoma. *Int J Gynecol Cancer.* 2002;12:394–398.
156. Teksam M, McKinney A, Short J, Casey SO, Truwit CL. Intracranial metastasis via transplacental (vertical) transmission of maternal small cell lung cancer to fetus: CT and MRI findings. *Acta Radiol.* 2004;45:577–579.
158. Baergen RN, Johnson D, Moore T, Benirschke K. Maternal melanoma metastatic to the placenta: a case report and review of the literature. *Arch Pathol Lab Med.* 1997;121:508–511.
168. Aviles A, Neri N. Hematological malignancies and pregnancy: a final report of 84 children who received chemotherapy in utero. *Clin Lymphoma.* 2001;2:173–177.
171. Lau WY, Leung WT, Ho S, et al. Hepatocellular carcinoma during pregnancy and its comparison with other pregnancy-associated malignancies. *Cancer.* 1995;75:2669–2676.
179. Berry DL, Theriault RL, Holmes FA, et al. Management of breast cancer during pregnancy using a standardized protocol. *J Clin Oncol.* 1999;17:855–861.

66 Cancer and Aging

Arti Hurria, MD ▪ Hyman B. Muss, MD ▪ Harvey J. Cohen, MD

Cancer is a disease that disproportionately affects older patients. Sixty percent of all cancers occur in people 65 years of age. People age 65 and older have an 11-fold increase in the incidence of cancer and a 15-fold increase in cancer mortality in comparison to people younger than age 65 (Tables 66-1 and 66-2).[1,2] The number of older people with cancer is continuously growing as the population is aging. In the United States, in 1900, 3.1 million people were age 65 and older. Over the century, this number increased ~10-fold, so that in the year 2000 there were 35 million people age 65 and older. This number is expected to double yet again; thus in 2030, it is projected that there will be 70.2 million people over the age of 65, accounting for 20% of the population (Table 66-3).[1,3]

Among those over age 65, there has been an age shift over time, leading to an increase in the older segment of the population. For example, during the 1990s the number age 85 and older increased by 38%, the number age 75-84 increased by 23%, and the number age 66-74 increased by <2%.[3] By 2030, the number ≥age 85 is expected to double.[1] Those who live to age 100 and beyond, the "centenarians," are the fastest growing segment of the older population. Based on these statistics, oncologists inevitably care for a large number of older patients. There is no standard chronological age at which a person is considered "older." Historically, aged ≥65 was used for two reasons:

1. This was the traditional age for retirement.
2. People in the United States become eligible for entitlement programs (Social Security, Medicare).

As our population ages, we see much heterogeneity in the ≥65 years population, with many individuals continuing to work and function similarly to younger counterparts. Therefore, this chapter will focus on defining characteristics to understand "functional age," rather than "chronological age" to distinguish the "older" patient. This chapter will also be dedicated to discussing the unique issues and considerations in caring for an older patient with cancer.

Life Expectancy and Aging

Statistics regarding average life expectancy are useful to consider when caring for an older patient. The average life expectancy at birth is 76.5 years. As an individual ages, the average projected life expectancy increases. For example, a person who lives to 65 years of age has an average life expectancy of 17.7 years, placing their projected age of death at 82.7 years. A person, who lives to 80 years of age, has an average projected life expectancy of 8.5 years, placing the projected age of death at 88.5 years. Even the 100-year-old person has an average life expectancy of 2.5 years, placing their average projected age of death at 102.5 years. One may think of this as a "survival of the fittest" phenomenon, in which the absolute life expectancy increases as one ages (Table 66-4).[4] In addition, this projected life expectancy will be impacted by other co-morbid (coexisting) medical problems (Table 66-5).

The Biology of Cancer and Aging

Aging can be defined as "the process that converts healthy adults into frail ones with diminished reserves in most physiologic systems and an exponentially increasing vulnerability to disease and death."[5] Despite the universality of

Table 66-1 **11-Fold Increase in Cancer Incidence and 15-Fold Increase in Cancer Mortality With Age ≥65**

Age	Incidence (Per 100,000)	Mortality (Per 100,000)
Age <65	204.1	73.3
Age ≥65	2255.1	1080.3

Table 66-2 **Incidence of 10 Major Tumors in Patients Under and Over 65 Years of Age**

Tumor site	Patients Aged Under 65 Years (%)	Patients Aged Over 65 Years (%)	No. of Cases
Prostate	23.1	76.9	179,300
Colon	26.1	73.9	94,700
Pancreas	27.0	73.0	28,600
Urinary bladder	28.6	71.4	54,200
Stomach	30.4	69.6	21,900
Lung	34.2	65.8	171,600
Rectum	34.6	65.4	34,700
Non-Hodgkin lymphoma	49.0	51.0	56,800
Breast (women)	52.5	47.5	175,000
Ovary	54.1	45.9	25,200

Source: From Ref. 2.

Table 66-3 **The Growing US Population Age 65 and Older**

Year	Million	% of Population
1900	3.1	4.1
2000	35	12.4
2030	70.2	20.1

Source: From Refs. 1, 2.

Table 66-4 **Average Life Expectancy**

Age Now	Life Expectancy	Age of Death
65	17.7	82.7
70	14.3	84.3
75	11.2	86.2
80	8.5	88.5
85	6.3	91.3
90	4.5	94.5
95	3.3	98.3
100	2.5	102.5

Source: Data derived from Ref. 4.

Table 66-5 **Baseline Life Expectancy for Patients With Various Ages and Co-morbidity Levels**

Age	Healthy	Average	Sick
65	20.0	18.5	9.7
70	15.8	14.8	8.6
75	12.1	11.5	7.3
80	8.8	8.4	5.9
85	6.1	5.9	4.5

Source: From Ref. 59.

this definition, aging is clearly a heterogeneous process. Each individual ages at a unique pace and demonstrates varying manifestations of vulnerability. The mechanisms of both aging and neoplasia are incompletely understood and therefore theories about the association of these two processes are an area of active research.

Several theories of the association with aging and neoplasia have been described.[6,7] They include: longer duration of exposure (time) and possibly increased susceptibility to oxidative stress and carcinogens; age-induced increase in DNA instability resulting in higher mutation potentialÑthis could result in both oncogene activation or amplification or tumor suppressor gene defects; a decrease in DNA repair with age that might enhance the predisposition to the genetic defects; age-related telomere shortening that might increase the above mentioned DNA instability; immune dysregulation that may decrease immune surveillance and allow the emergence of malignant clones, but that may also create a proinflammatory environment favoring the growth of malignant cells; and finally an altered microenvironment, including the presence of senescent cells that may secrete proinflammatory and carcinogenic cytokines.

Although each of these theories is plausible, they do not explain why an individual is more or less susceptible to the development of neoplasia, especially in the absence of carcinogen exposure. In addition, these theories do not explain why there may be a decrease in cancer incidence in the oldest segment of the population. Autopsy studies have suggested that among older patients, there is a difference in the incidence of cancer in the centenarians in comparison to younger patients. In a study of 507 patients over 75 years of age, the prevalence of cancer at the time of autopsy decreased with increasing age (35% age 75-79, 20% age 95-99, and 16% in centenarians). Cancer was the cause of death in fewer older patients (67% of patients aged 75-90 and 41% of patient aged 95 and older), and there was a decreased incidence of metastatic disease, with increasing age.[8]

Physiologic Changes With Aging

Physiologic changes occur in each organ system with aging, independent of disease. Most organ systems show a linear physiological decline beginning at 30 years of age. This decline occurs at variable rates between individuals and across organ systems. The consequence of these changes during normal activity is minimal; however, during times of stress the decreased reserve becomes more apparent.[9]

As the cardiovascular system ages, there is a decrease in cardiac output, decrease in maximal heart rate, and prolonged recovery following exertion. During times of stress, there is a decreased response to catecholamines. As the pulmonary system ages, there is a decreased response to hypoxemia or hypercapnia, decreased elasticity in the lung tissue, increased ventilation-perfusion mismatch, and decreased forced expiratory volume. Endocrine changes with aging include a decrease in certain hormone levels and an increase in others. For example, there is a decrease in insulin-like growth factor, growth hormone, renin, aldosterone, dehydroepiandrosterone, and sex steroids, and increase in insulin, norepinephrine, parathyroid hormone, vasopressin, and atrial natriuretic peptide. Changes to the neurological system with aging include neuronal loss, decrease in brain weight, decreased vision, loss in high frequency and low frequency hearing, and alterations in both taste and smell. Changes in the immune system manifest as decrease in thymic mass, decrease in production of thymic hormones, decrease in naive lymphocytes, and a decrease in antibody response.[9]

There is a decrease in hepatic and renal mass with aging. Autopsy studies demonstrate a decrease in liver volume with aging by ~25-50%. In addition, there is decreased hepatic blood flow, estimated at a 10-15% decrease in liver perfusion, even after taking into account the decrease in liver volume.[10-12] Renal mass decreases by 25-30% over the lifespan, leading to a decreased number of functional nephrons. Renal blood flow decreases by 1% per year after 50 years of age and glomerular filtration decreases by 1 mL/min/year after the age of 40.[10,12]

Hematopoietic changes with aging include a decrease in bone marrow mass and increase in bone marrow fat. Despite this, peripheral blood cell concentrations in healthy older patients are similar to those of younger patients.[13]

The Frail Older Patient

The term "frail" is used to describe a subset of older patients with a critically reduced functional reserve that places them at risk for dependency, institutionalization, illness, hospitalization, and mortality.[14] A proposed definition of frailty is "a state of age-related physiologic vulnerability resulting from impaired homeostatic reserve and reduced capacity of the organism to withstand stress." Therefore, the clinical syndrome of frailty is proposed to be a dynamic consequence of a negative energy balance; for example, starting with undernutrition that leads to loss of muscle and bone mass and contributes to further decline in activity level and strength. This, in combination with decreased reserve, contributes to the increased vulnerability of the frail patient. The end result is failure to thrive, which is a syndrome of unexplained weight loss, decreased muscle mass, and metabolic abnormalities including a decrease in albumin, creatinine, cholesterol, and hemoglobin. Immune dysfunction and chronic inflammation may play a role in frailty. Markers of inflammation are associated with aging and frailty including the cytokine interleukin 6 (IL-6) and the acute phase reactant, C-reactive protein (CRP).[15-17] In addition, elevations in plasma D dimer have been associated with age. Both IL-6 and D dimer have been predictive of mortality and functional decline.[14,18,19]

A phenotype for frailty was developed in a prospective observational study of 5317 community-dwelling men and women age ≥65. The "frailty phenotype" was defined as a clinical syndrome in which three or more of the following criteria are present: (1) unintentional weight loss ≥10 lbs in past year; (2) self-reported exhaustion; (3) weakness defined as the lowest 20th percentile in grip strength adjusted for gender and body mass index; (4) slow walking speed defined as the lowest 20th percentile on a timed walk of 15 ft; and (5) low physical activity defined as the lowest quintile of kilocalories per week. Individuals with one or two of the criteria were categorized as an "intermediate or pre-frail phenotype." Patients defined as frail or pre-frail, compared with non-frail, had a higher incidence of 3- and 7-year mortality, hospitalization, incident falls, progressive decline in ability to complete activities of daily living, and decreased mobility. Based on these criteria, 7% of community-dwelling individuals age 65 and older were frail and 47% were pre-frail. The prevalence of frailty and pre-frailty was greater in women than men and increased with age.[20] Frailty is also associated with an increased risk of recurrent falls, hip fracture, and any non-spine fractures.[21]

Frail older patients with cancer represent a unique subset of patients that pose challenging therapeutic decisions.

An important initial step in evaluation of the frail patient is to determine whether the cancer is likely to decrease the patient's life expectancy. In a model proposed by Balducci and Stanta, one would consider treatment of the cancer if it was impacting the patient's life expectancy or if it was causing a compromise in quality of life. The goal of treatment must be determined: life prolonging verses palliation. Treatment decisions involve weighing the risks and benefits with the patient and caregiver. As the nation is aging, there will be a rise in the number of frail older patients with cancer. Clinical trials focusing on efficacy and tolerability of treatment within this patient population are needed.[22]

Evaluation of the Older Patient: Geriatric Assessment

The term "geriatric assessment" was defined at a consensus conference in 1989, as "a multidimensional interdisciplinary patient evaluation that leads to the identification of patient's problems."[23] The assessment includes an evaluation of the older person's functional status (ability to live independently at home and in the community), co-morbid medical conditions, cognition, psychological status, social functioning and support, medication review, and nutritional status (Table 66-6). This comprehensive assessment allows for identification of areas of vulnerability and a multidisciplinary plan to address these areas. In addition, geriatric assessment provides valuable information regarding prognostic factors for morbidity and mortality in the older patient. Each domain of a geriatric assessment will be reviewed below.

Functional Status

Assessment of functional status includes an evaluation of an individual's ability to live independently at home and in the community. Traditional assessment measures are "activities of daily living" (ADL) and "instrumental activities of daily living" (IADL) (Table 66-7). Activities of daily living are basic self-care skills, such as ability to bathe, dress, toilet, transfer, maintain continence, and feed oneself. These activities are essential in order for one to maintain independence in the home. The need for assistance with activities of daily living has been predictive of survival, nursing home placement, prolonged hospital stay, worsening of function in the hospital, and greater home care use.[24,25] An individual who requires assistance for one or more activities of daily living has an average life expectancy of <3 years.[26]

Table 66-6 Key Components of a Comprehensive Geriatric Assessment

- Functional status
- Co-morbid (coexisting) medical conditions
- Cognition
- Psychological status
- Social functioning and support
- Socioeconomic issues
- Medication review
- Nutritional status

Table 66-7 Functional Status Assessment

Activities of Daily Living	Instrumental Activities of Daily Living
Bathing	Telephone
Dressing	Traveling
Toileting	Shopping
Transfer	Preparing meals
Continence	Housework
Eating	Medication management
	Money management

Instrumental activities of daily living include those self-care skills that allow one to live independently in the community. These include ability to telephone, shop, travel, prepare meals, do housework, take medications, and manage one's finances. In a study by Reuben and colleagues of 282 patients aged 64 and older, dependence in instrumental activities of daily living (such as housework, shopping, and driving, scored as a continuous variables) was an independent predictor of mortality ($p < .0001$).[27] The need for assistance with instrumental activities of daily living is predictive of risk of cognitive impairment.[28] Individuals who require assistance with instrumental activities of daily living often need assistance to maintain independence in the community.

Cancer in an older patient is associated with an increased need for assistance in daily activities. In a large study of older patients, individuals with cancer had more limitations in activities of daily living and instrumental activities of daily living than individuals without cancer and required more health-care use.[29] Independence in performing instrumental activities of daily living and better quality of life are associated with improved overall survival among older adults with lung cancer.[30] In a study of older adults with ovarian cancer, predictors of chemotherapy toxicity included a poor performance status (Eastern Cooperative Oncology Group performance status of <2) and functional dependence (defined as living at home with assistance or living with assistance in a specialized institution).[31]

Co-morbid Medical Conditions

Co-morbidity is defined as a concurrent medical problem that is a competing source of morbidity or mortality. In a study by Yancik and colleagues, summary data on co-morbidity were collected on 7600 patients aged ≥55 years. The most common concurrent medical problems included hypertension (42.9%), heart-related conditions (39.1%), and arthritis (34.9%). The number of co-morbid conditions increased with age. Patients aged 55-64 had an average of 2.9 co-morbid conditions, patients aged 66-74 had 3.6 co-morbid conditions, and those 75 and older had 4.2 medical conditions (Table 66-8).[1] In a study by Extermann and colleagues of 203 patients with cancer (median age 75; range 63-91), co-morbidity and functional status were found to be independent.[32] Therefore, each is an important domain to assess.

The level of co-morbidity has been shown to affect functional recovery following surgical treatment for breast cancer. In a study of older women with breast cancer, women with more than two co-morbid conditions were less likely following surgery to become independent in completing instrumental activities of daily living and more likely to experience difficulty completing tasks requiring upper body strength.[33]

Co-morbid medical conditions also impact the likelihood of receipt and tolerance of chemotherapy. Data from the Surveillance, Epidemiology, and End Results-Medicare database demonstrate that older patients with colon cancer, who have a history of heart failure, diabetes, or chronic obstructive pulmonary disease, are less likely to receive adjuvant chemotherapy.[34] In a clinical trial of older adults with lung cancer, patients with higher levels of co-morbidity were more likely to discontinue chemotherapy.[35]

The impact of co-morbidity on overall survival has been demonstrated. In a

Table 66-8 Rank Order of Major Condition, >10% of Study Sample

Condition	Percent
Hypertension	42.9
Heart-related conditions	39.1
Arthritis	34.9
Gastrointestinal problems	31.0
Anemia	22.6
Eye problems	19.0
Urinary tract	18.0
Previous cancers	15.4
Gallbladder problems	14.9
Chronic obstructive pulmonary disease	14.5
Diabetes	12.8
Fracture	10.8
Gland disorders	10.6

Source: From Ref. 1.

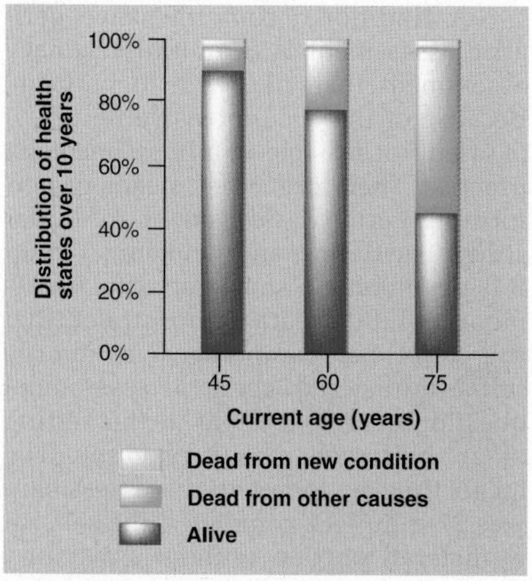

Figure 66-1 ■ This example considers the distribution of health status over 10 years for women newly diagnosed with a disease for which the 10-year disease-related mortality is 10%. *Source:* From Ref. 37.

study by Satariano and colleagues, patients with breast cancer who had three or more of seven selected co-morbid conditions had a 20-fold higher rate of mortality from a co-morbid medical condition than from breast cancer. These findings were independent of a number of other factors including age, race, treatment, tumor stage, tumor histology, tumor size, and social or behavioral factors. Patients with three or more co-morbid conditions had a fourfold increase in mortality in comparison to those with no co-morbid medical conditions.[36] The impact of age on the relative risk of mortality from a concurrent, co-morbid illness in comparison to a newly diagnosed illness is illustrated in Figure 66-1.[37]

The potential impact of a new disease as a competing cause of mortality decreases with increasing age secondary to the decrease in absolute projected life expectancy. For example, consider the impact of a disease with a projected 50% mortality over 5 years in a 65-year-old person in comparison to an 85-year-old person. This disease will decrease the 65-year-old average life expectancy by ~10 years, whereas because the absolute projected life expectancy of an 85-year-old person is less than that of a 65-year-old person it will decrease an 85-year-old person's average life expectancy by only about 2 years.[37]

Nutrition

Poor nutritional status is an independent predictor of functional dependency and survival. In a prospective cohort study of 214 older community-dwelling adults, a low body mass index, defined as a body mass index <22 kg/m^2, was associated with dependency in activities of daily living (odds ratio 1.21; 95% confidence interval [CI] 1.01-1.45). After adjusting for potential confounding factors including age, gender, mental status, co-morbidity, and functional dependency, body mass index <22 kg/m^2 was associated with decreased 1-year survival (relative risk [RR] 0.85, 95% CI 0.74-0.97).[38]

Weight change over a 3-year period was recorded in a study of 4714 community-dwelling adults, aged 65 and older. Weight change, defined as a 5% or greater loss or gain in weight over a 3-year period, occurred in 34.6% of women and 27.3% of men. A higher proportion of participants lost weight, than gained weight. Weight loss, and not weight gain, was associated with an increased risk of mortality (hazard ratio 1.67; 95% CI 1.29-2.15).[39]

The prognostic effect of unintentional weight loss in patients with cancer was evaluated in a study of 3047 patients enrolled in Eastern Cooperative Oncology Group chemotherapy trials. Weight loss during the 6 months prior to chemotherapy was associated with poorer survival (statistically significant in 9 out of 12 tumor types). In addition, weight loss was associated with lower chemotherapy response rates (significant only in patients with breast cancer). Decreasing weight correlated with decreased performance status in all tumor types except pancreatic and gastric cancers.[40]

Cognition

The presence of dementia is an independent prognostic indicator of survival.[41,42] In a study by Wolfson and colleagues, 10,263 people aged 65 and older were screened for dementia. Of these 821 people had a diagnosis of probable Alzheimer disease, possible Alzheimer disease, or vascular dementia. The median survival of these patients was 3.3 years (3.1 years if a diagnosis of probable Alzheimer disease, 3.5 years if possible Alzheimer disease, and 3.3 years if vascular dementia).[42]

A baseline assessment of cognition in an older patient with cancer is important for several reasons. First, if a person has a rapid change in memory or new cognitive deficits, metastatic disease to the brain should be excluded. Second, the degree of cognitive impairment will need to be considered when devising a treatment plan. For example, all oral medications and especially chemotherapy drugs should be used with caution in patients with cognitive impairment. Correct dosing for oral chemotherapy is as important as with intravenous chemotherapy, so that if the patient takes an incorrect dose, the side effects could be serious or even fatal. The role of the patient's family or caregiver is critical in maintaining safety. A patient with cognitive impairment will need assistance in remembering instructions regarding use of supportive medications such as antiemetics. A caregiver will need to be aware of potential side effects of treatment that would necessitate medical attention.

Psychological State and Social Support

Older patients with cancer often demonstrate better psychological functioning in comparison to younger patients. Following a diagnosis of breast cancer, older women demonstrate better mental health and well-being in comparison to younger patients.[43] In women aged <65, a recent diagnosis of breast cancer produced a marked increase in anxiety and depression and decreased morale in comparison to people of the same age who had a diagnosis over 5 years prior. In comparison, for women ≥65 years of age, a more recent diagnosis did not affect their level of anxiety, depression, or morale in comparison to age counterparts with a diagnosis greater than 5 years ago.[44]

The presence of social support plays an important role in the psychological functioning of the older patient. Significant predictors of severe psychological distress in women of breast cancer of any age include being divorced or separated and having less social support.[45] Therefore, social support can serve as a buffer against the psychological impact of a stressful life event.

In addition, social isolation is an independent predictor of mortality. This was demonstrated in a study by Seeman and colleagues in which they examined the importance of four measures of social support: (1) marital status, (2) close contact with two or more close friends/relatives, (3) regular church attendance, and (4) membership in other types of groups. The presence of social ties was related to survival, independent of age. The relative hazard for increased 5-year mortality among men and women in three community-based cohorts ranged from 1.97 to 3.06 for participants with no social ties in comparison to those with all four social ties.[45] In another study of 282 patients aged 65 and older, living alone was independently predictive of risk of death.[27]

Medication Review: Evaluation for Polypharmacy

A review of the patient's medication list is an important part of the geriatric assessment. In addition, one must consider whether newly prescribed medications may cause an adverse effect or drug interaction. Older patients are more vulnerable to adverse drug events than younger patients. Approximately one-fifth of hospital admissions in older patients are secondary to adverse drug events.[10] This is partly because older patients use threefold more medications than younger patients. The average number of medications taken by an older patient is four drugs. Ninety percent of older patients take at least one drug.

Contributing to the risk of adverse drug events are the changes in pharmacokinetics and pharmacodynamics that occur with aging. These changes should be considered with the dosing of any medication, including chemotherapy. There are age-related changes in the gastrointestinal tract such as decreased acid secretion and fewer villi in mucosal surfaces. There are significant changes in volume of distribution including increased body fat (leading to slower metabolism of lipid-soluble drugs), decrease in total body water (leading to an increase in the plasma level of water-soluble drugs), decrease in lean body mass, decrease in serum albumin, and decrease in hemoglobin.[11] Hepatic metabolism changes with aging, secondary to decreased liver volume and decreased hepatic blood flow. Phase I hepatic reactions (oxidation, deamination, hydroxylation) decrease with aging. These include reactions mediated via cytochrome P-450, decreasing by ~30% in older patients. There is no significant change in phase II hepatic reactions (conjugation: acetylation, glucuronidation, sulfation) with aging.[10-12] Renal mass decreases by 25-30% over the lifespan, leading to a decreased number of functional nephrons. Consequently there is a decrease in glomerular filtration, tubular secretion, and reabsorption with aging. Therefore, drugs dependent on renal clearance have a longer half-life in older patients and drug dosing may need to be adjusted based on creatinine clearance.

Comprehensive Geriatric Assessment

Geriatric assessment is a comprehensive approach to the evaluation of the older patient, with an evaluation of the domains described earlier: functional status, co-morbidity, cognition, nutritional status, psychological state and social support, and medication review. Studies regarding the value of this assessment have been conflicting; however, a meta-analysis of the controlled trials by Stuck and colleagues suggests a benefit to geriatric assessment. This meta-analysis of 28 controlled trials comprising 4959 participants and 4912 controls randomized to one of five comprehensive geriatric assessment programs demonstrated that a geriatric evaluation and management unit (inpatient unit for geriatric assessment and rehabilitation) reduced mortality by 35% at 6 months and a home assessment service (in-home geriatric assessment) reduced mortality by 14% at 36 months via early identification and treatment of problems.[46] A more recently published multisite randomized, controlled trial of inpatient and outpatient geriatric evaluation and management demonstrated that geriatric evaluation and management reduced functional decline and improved mental health but had no effect on survival.[47]

The role of geriatric assessment in care of the older cancer patient is an area under active research. Balducci and colleagues studied geriatric assessment in the evaluation of the older patient with cancer and found that this assessment helped to characterize patients of the same chronological age by identifying impairment in the following areas: dependency in functional status (18% ADL, 72% IADL), serious co-morbidity (36% by Charlson scale, 94% by Cumulative Illness Rating ScaleÑGeriatrics), memory impairment (22%), poor nutrition (19%), and polypharmacy (41%).[48] Garman and colleagues performed a retrospective chart review of older patients with cancer admitted to an inpatient Geriatric Evaluation and Management Unit, in which a comprehensive geriatric assessment was used to identify goals of care. These goals were accomplished in over 75% of cases: 73% in symptom management, 79% in functional improvement, and 100% in disposition and caregiver support.[49] Other studies have demonstrated that domains of a geriatric assessment can predict survival and toxicity to chemotherapy in older adults with cancer.[30,31] Geriatric assessment and intervention can lead to improve pain control, mental health, and emotional well-being among older adults with cancer.[50]

The information derived from a geriatric assessment could be potentially valuable to oncologists for several reasons. First, it would help the clinician get a sense of the "functional age" of the patient. Second, it would identify patients at high risk for functional decline or toxicity to treatment, for whom targeted intervention may be beneficial. Third, it would provide valuable information regarding older patients in clinical trials, allowing us to standardize patient characteristics across studies and to control for possible confounding factors contributing to mortality.

A traditional comprehensive geriatric assessment is a multidisciplinary assessment that takes 2 h to perform. Because of the time-intensive nature, it is often not feasible in a busy oncology practice. Therefore, other means of performing geriatric assessment are under study. The Cancer and Leukemia Group B is developing a short geriatric assessment tool. Pilot data demonstrated that this brief but comprehensive, mainly self-administered geriatric assessment questionnaire is feasible in the setting of an outpatient oncology clinic. The mean time to complete the assessment was 27 min; 78% completed the self-administered portion without assistance. The majority of participants stated that the assessment was easy to understand (83%) and were satisfied with the length of the questionnaire (90%).[51] This geriatric assessment will be collected as baseline information in subsequent clinical trials. Other authors have reported on the feasibility of an abbreviated geriatric assessment screening tool[52] or a geriatric assessment that is mailed to the patient to complete prior to the office visit.[53,54]

A proposed framework depicting the factors to consider in decision making for an older patient with cancer is described in the Comprehensive Geriatric Model, developed by Cohen and DeMaria (Fig. 66-2).[55] This model summarizes the key aspects critical to the care of the older patient including social, psychological, and biological factors that may impact on the host, the disease, and the outcomes from treatment. In this model, chronological age plays a role by defining the decreased functional reserve that can occur with aging, but subsequent factors including biological, social, and psychological factors unique to the individual patient are factored into decision making. This is a dynamic process in which alterations in one domain can subsequently impact upon the other domains within the model.

Knowledge About Older Cancer Patients: Underrepresentation on Clinical Trials

Despite the aging population and the association of cancer with aging, data regarding the benefits and risks of treatment of the older cancer patient are limited. This is secondary to limited involvement of older patients on clinical trials. The Southwest Oncology Group analyzed 164 clinical trials from 1993 to 1996, comprised of 16,396 patients. They found that only 25% of the patients on clinical trial were aged 65 and older. This underrepresentation was across 15 cancer types, except lymphoma. Older

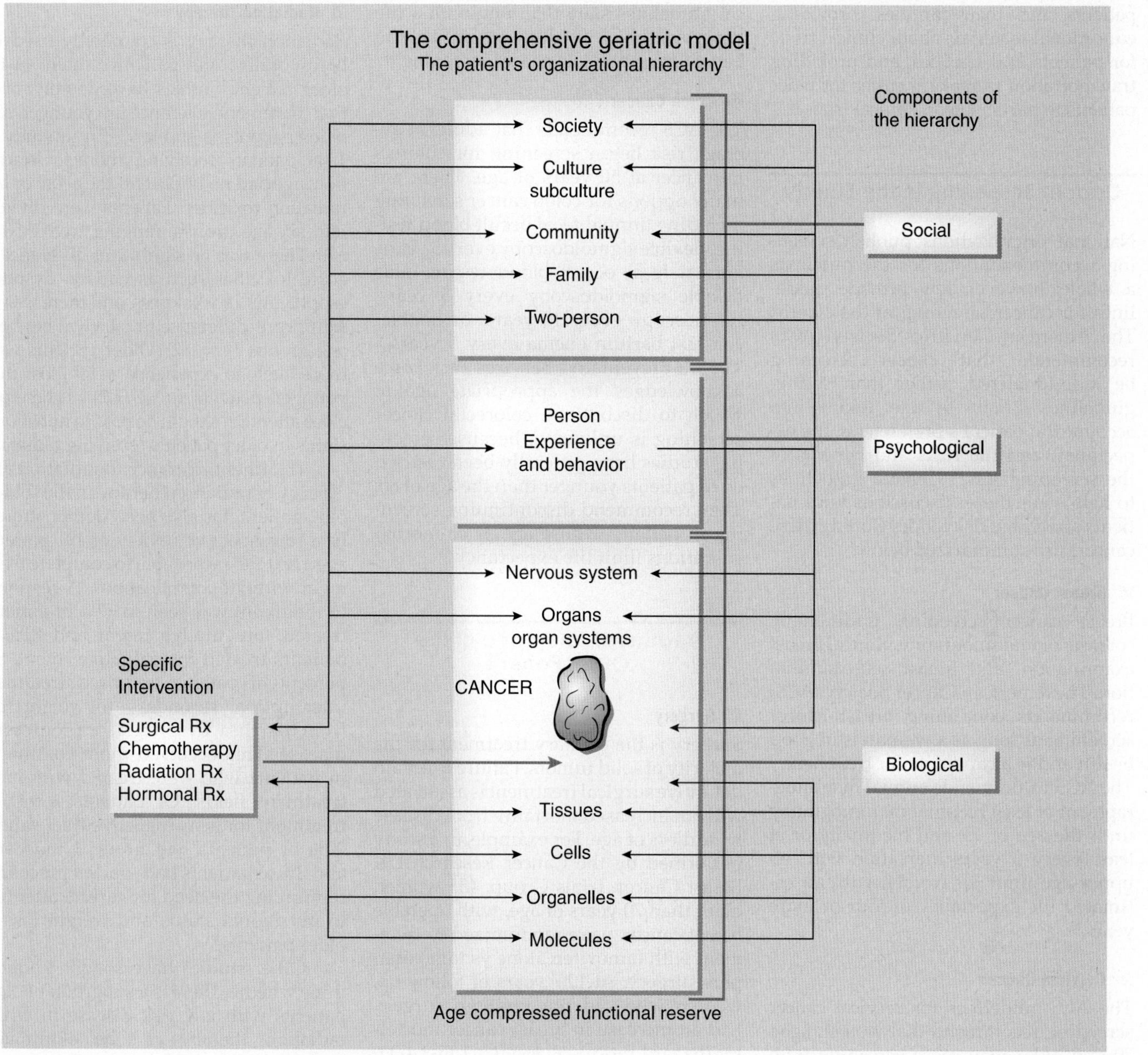

Figure 66-2 The Comprehensive Geriatric Model. *Source:* From Ref. 55.

patients with breast cancer were the least represented, with only 9% of patients over the age of 65.[56]

Similar data regarding the underrepresentation of the older patient are seen in Canadian trials. Enrollment on clinical trials by age was analyzed from 1993 to 1996. Fifty-eight percent of the Canadian population with cancer is of age ≥65, whereas only 22% of patients enrolled on trial were of age ≥65.[57]

The representation on clinical trials worsens with increasing age. The National Cancer Institute analyzed enrollment of patients aged ≥65 and patients aged ≥75. Data from 23,000 patients across 500 therapeutic trials were analyzed. They found an underrepresentation of patients over the age of 65 on clinical trial; however, this was even more pronounced for patients aged ≥75. Only 11% of men on clinical trial were over the age of 75 and only 5% of women were over the age of 75. There was a striking underrepresentation of older patients with breast cancer, with only 2.7% being over the age of 75. This study demonstrated that with increasing age, there is even less representation on clinical trial.[58]

Understanding Barriers to Clinical Trial Enrollment

The Cancer and Leukemia Group B (CALGB) Committee on Cancer in the Elderly developed a study to understand barriers to participation of older patients on cancer treatment trials. Women with breast cancer, aged <65 and ≥65, were paired by physician and stage. The trial sought to determine the frequency with which each group was offered enrollment on clinical trial and likelihood of accepting treatment on trial. The results demonstrated that older women were less likely to be offered enrollment onto clinical trial than younger women (51% aged <65 vs 35% aged ≥65; $p = .06$); however, if offered, older women would be as likely to accept enrollment on trial as younger women (56% aged <65 vs 50% aged ≥65; $p = .67$). Physicians did not offer a clinical trial to older patients because: (1) physicians were concerned about the toxicity of treatment in older patients and (2) physicians were concerned regarding the impact of co-morbid diseases.[59] The most common physician recommendations of ways to improve accrual of older patients to clinical trials include providing clinic personnel to explain trials to older patients and their families, providing educational materials about clinical trials for patients and families, and providing transportation to make it easier for older patients to participate in clinical trials.[60]

Cancer Screening in the Elderly

National organizations publish screening recommendations for the public as a whole; however, few provide guidelines for cancer screening in the elderly. The American Geriatrics Society (AGS) recommends that cancer screening be individualized, rather than setting guidelines strictly by age, taking into account the patient's preferences, life expectancy, and the risks and benefits of the screening test.[61] General guidelines to help steer these discussions with patients at average risk for developing these cancers are summarized below.

Breast Cancer

Breast cancer screening traditionally consists of mammography, clinical breast examination, and breast self-examination. The American Cancer Society (ACS) recommends continuing breast cancer screening as long as a woman is in good health and is a candidate for treatment.[62] The AGS recommends annual mammography or at least biennial mammography until the age of 75, and biennially or at least every 3 years thereafter, with no upper age limit for women with an estimated life expectancy of four or more years.[63]

Cervical Cancer

The ACS guidelines for cervical cancer screening recommend that women aged 70 and older may cease screening with the Papanicolaou (Pap) smear if there are three or more documented, consecutive, normal Pap smears and no abnormal smears within the 10-year period before the age of 70.[62] The US Preventative Service Task Force recommends discontinuing cytologic screening for women aged 65 and older who have had adequate screening with normal results.[62]

Prostate Cancer

Screening for prostate cancer consists of a digital rectal examination and prostate-specific antigen (PSA) test. The ACS recommends offering annual screening for prostate cancer, with digital rectal examination and PSA test, beginning at the age of 50 in patients at average risk and continued in men who have a life expectancy of at least 10 years. The benefits and limitations of testing should be discussed with the patient so that an informed decision regarding screening is made.[62] The US Preventative Service Task Force clinical guidelines state that men with a life expectancy of <10 years are unlikely to benefit from prostate cancer screening.[64]

Colon Cancer

The ACS recommends that adults at average risk begin screening for colorectal cancer at 50 years of age. There are many options for colon cancer screening including annual fecal occult blood testing, flexible sigmoidoscopy every 5 years, annual fecal occult blood testing plus flexible sigmoidoscopy every 5 years, colonoscopy every 10 years, or double-contrast barium enema every 5 years.[62] The US Preventative Services Task Force acknowledges the appropriate age at which to discontinue colorectal cancer screening is unknown, because screening studies have generally been restricted to patients younger than the age of 80. They recommend discontinuing screening in patients whose age or co-morbid conditions limit life expectancy.[65]

Treatment Tolerance of the Older Patient

Surgery

Surgery is the primary treatment for the majority of solid tumors. Failure to obtain definitive surgical treatment is associated with an increased mortality from disease regardless of age. For example, in a study performed by the Cancer Research UK Breast Cancer Trials Group, 455 women older than 70 years of age, with operable breast cancer, were randomized to treatment with tamoxifen alone vs tamoxifen plus surgery. At 12.7 years of follow-up, women who did not undergo surgery had an increase in breast cancer mortality (hazard ratio 1.68; 95% CI 1.15-2.47).[66] Therefore if possible, older women should undergo primary surgical removal of breast cancer in order to decrease their risk of breast cancer mortality.

Several studies have demonstrated that advanced age alone should not be a reason to deny surgical treatment for colorectal cancer.[67-70] Risk of surgical morbidity and mortality is increased with intra-abdominal surgery or those performed under an emergency situation; however, even in these high-risk situations, older patients benefit from surgical management. In a study of emergency colorectal surgery, older and younger patients had a similar primary resection rate (95% > age 70, 89% ≤ age 70; p = .70) and primary anastomosis rate (84% > age 70, 78% ≥ age 70; p = .64). Older patients had a higher incidence of postoperative cardiopulmonary complications, but no statistically significant difference in mortality (9% < age 70, 5% ≥ age 70; p = .48).[67]

Radiation Therapy

Radiation therapy is commonly used for both curative and palliative intent in the older patient. Studies have demonstrated that treatment tolerance in younger and older patients is similar.[71,72] In a study of 1208 patients receiving thoracic irradiation, age had no impact on the acute or late radiation toxicities. Patients were divided into six age groups, ranging from <50 to >70. There was no significant difference in acute toxicities such as nausea, dyspnea, esophagitis, or weakness, and there was no significant difference in survival between age groups (p = .82). Older patients were more likely to experience weight loss than younger patients (p = .002).[72] Therefore, close attention should be paid to nutritional status in older patients receiving radiation.

Treatment tolerance to radiation and efficacy of radiation therapy in the "oldest old" patient has also been demonstrated. In a retrospective review of 191 patients aged ≥80, 94% were able to complete treatment without complications. A response to treatment was seen in 77% of patients treated for curative intent and 81% of patients treated for palliative intent. Six percent of patients required treatment interruption, secondary to weight loss from diarrhea, dysphagia, or progressive disease. This occurred more commonly in patients who were treated with large treatment fields. Of patients receiving treatment for aero-digestive tract cancer, 20% of patients had grade 3 mucositis and 2% of patients had grade 4 mucositis, reinforcing the need for careful attention to nutritional status and weight loss in older patients.[73]

Other studies have sought to determine whether there is a subgroup of older patients with low risk disease in which radiation therapy can be eliminated. A study performed by the Cancer and Leukemia Group B randomized 636 women aged 70 and older with clinical stage I, estrogen receptor–positive breast cancer who underwent a lumpectomy to treatment with radiation to the affected breast and tamoxifen, or tamoxifen alone. The women treated with tamoxifen alone had more locoregional recurrences at 5 years of follow-up: 4% in the tamoxifen alone arm verses 1% in the tamoxifen and radiation arm (p < .001); however, there was no difference in breast cancer–specific mortality or 5-year rates of overall survival.[74]

Chemotherapy

Several studies have sought to determine whether treatment on chemotherapy trials is more toxic for older patients.[75] A study by the Piedmont Oncology Association was a case-control study of women with metastatic breast cancer enrolled on clinical trials. The women were divided into three groups, by age: <50,

50-69, and >70. The study demonstrated that older women receiving treatment on clinical trial had no significant difference in the incidence of toxic effects, dose delivery, or dose delays in comparison to younger women. In addition, there was no difference in response, time to disease progression, or survival. Therefore, older women who received treatment on clinical trial not only tolerated the treatment as well, but also equally benefited from this treatment.[76] An analysis of phase II trials at Illinois Cancer Center found similar results. Older and younger patients had no difference in toxic effects, need for dose reduction, or need for treatment interruption or delay. In addition, there was no difference in response to treatment.[77] In contrast, an analysis of three Cancer and Leukemia Group B clinical trials for the adjuvant treatment of patient with node positive breast cancer demonstrated that older adults were more likely to experience a grade 4 hematologic toxicity and were more likely to discontinue therapy because of toxicity. In addition, older adults were more likely to die of acute myelogenous leukemia or myelodysplatic syndrome.[78]

A limitation in interpreting these studies is that geriatric assessment information was not collected. Therefore, it is not clear that whether the older patients who enrolled on these clinical trials are representative of the patients cared for in everyday practice. Since so few older patients are offered entry on clinical trial, the older patients represented on clinical trials may have a younger "functional age." Therefore, incorporating geriatric assessment into clinical trials would be a valuable way of standardizing possible confounding factors across patients of the same chronological age, helping to determine the "functional age" of the patients represented. Clinical trials focusing on the older patient are needed in order to optimize care of this patient population. Developing a registry of older patients with selected diseases (breast cancer, colon cancer, intermediate grade lymphoma, etc.) and treating with chemotherapy with curative intent would provide a database to evaluate patterns of care and outcomes.

Conclusions

Cancer is a disease that disproportionately affects older patients. Data regarding the care of these patients are limited secondary to the underrepresentation of older patients on clinical trials. In moving forward, an effort should be made to include older patients on clinical trial, in order to increase our understanding about the optimal way to care for this growing population. Incorporation of geriatric assessment in the care of the older patient will provide information regarding prognostic factors that distinguish two individuals of the same chronological age, thereby helping us understand "functional age." Brief, comprehensive geriatric assessment screening tools for older oncology patients are currently under development.

Selected References

The complete reference list can be found at www.CANCERMEDICINE8.com

1. Yancik R. Cancer burden in the aged: an epidemiologic and demographic overview. Cancer. 1997;80(7):1273–1283.
2. Yancik R, Ries LA. Aging and cancer in America. Demographic and epidemiologic perspectives. Hematol Oncol Clin North Am. 2000;14(1):17–23.
3. US Census Bureau. The 65 Years and Over Population: 2000. In: Census 2000 Summary File 1; 1990 Census of Population, General Population Characteristics, United States (1990 CP-1-1); 2000.
6. Irminger-Finger I. Science of cancer and aging. J Clin Oncol. 2007;25(14):1844–1851.
7. Rao A, Cohen HJ. Oncology and aging: general principles of cancer in the elderly. In: Hazzard W, Blass J, Ettinger W, Halter J, Ouslander J, eds. Principles of Geriatric Medicine and Gerontology. New York: McGraw-Hill; 2008.
8. Stanta G, Campagner L, Cavallieri F, Giarelli L. Cancer of the oldest old. What we have learned from autopsy studies. Clin Geriatr Med. 1997;13(1):55–68.
9. Cohen HJ. Cancer Care in the Older Population: Physiology of Aging. In: American Society of Clinical Oncology Curriculum; 2002.
10. Vestal RE. Aging and pharmacology. Cancer. 1997;80(7):1302–1310.
11. Avorn J, Gurwitz JH. Principles of pharmacology. In: Cassel C, Cohen H, Larson E, Meier D, Resnick N, Rubenstein L, eds. Geriatric Medicine, 3rd ed. New York: Springer-Verlag; 1997:55–70.
12. Lichtman SM, Villani G. Chemotherapy in the elderly: pharmacologic considerations. Cancer Control. 2000;7(6):548–556.
21. Ensrud KE, Ewing SK, Taylor BC, et al. Frailty and risk of falls, fracture, and mortality in older women: the study of osteoporotic fractures. J Gerontol A Biol Sci Med Sci. 2007;62(7):744–751.
22. Balducci L, Stanta G. Cancer in the frail patient. A coming epidemic. Hematol Oncol Clin North Am. 2000;14(1):235–250, xi.
23. Repetto L, Comandini D. Cancer in the elderly: assessing patients for fitness. Crit Rev Oncol Hematol. 2000;35(3):155–160.
24. Naglie G. Oxford Textbook of Geriatric Medicine. New York: Oxford University Press, Inc.; 2000.
25. Narain P, Rubenstein LZ, Wieland GD, et al. Predictors of immediate and 6-month outcomes in hospitalized elderly patients. The importance of functional status. J Am Geriatr Soc. 1988;36(9):775–783.
34. Gross CP, McAvay GJ, Guo Z, Tinetti ME. The impact of chronic illnesses on the use and effectiveness of adjuvant chemotherapy for colon cancer. Cancer. 2007;109(12):2410–2419.
35. Frasci G, Lorusso V, Panza N, et al. Gemcitabine plus vinorelbine versus vinorelbine alone in elderly patients with advanced non-small-cell lung cancer. J Clin Oncol. 2000;18(13):2529–2536.
36. Satariano WA, Ragland DR. The effect of comorbidity on 3-year survival of women with primary breast cancer. Ann Intern Med. 1994;120(2):104–110.
37. Welch HG, Albertsen PC, Nease RF, Bubolz TA, Wasson JH. Estimating treatment benefits for the elderly: the effect of competing risks. Ann Intern Med. 1996;124(6):577–584.
38. Landi F, Zuccala G, Gambassi G, et al. Body mass index and mortality among older people living in the community. J Am Geriatr Soc. 1999;47(9):1072–1076.
39. Newman AB, Yanez D, Harris T, Duxbury A, Enright PL, Fried LP. Weight change in old age and its association with mortality. J Am Geriatr Soc. 2001;49(10):1309–1318.
40. Dewys WD, Begg C, Lavin PT, et al. Prognostic effect of weight loss prior to chemotherapy in cancer patients. Eastern Cooperative Oncology Group. Am J Med. 1980;69(4):491–497.
49. Garman KS, McConnell ES, Cohen HJ. Inpatient care for elderly cancer patients: the role for Geriatric Evaluation and Management Units in fulfilling goals for care. Crit Rev Oncol Hematol. 2004;51(3):241–247.
50. Rao AV, Hsieh F, Feussner JR, Cohen HJ. Geriatric evaluation and management units in the care of the frail elderly cancer patient. J Gerontol A Biol Sci Med Sci. 2005;60(6):798–803.
51. Hurria A, Gupta S, Zauderer M, et al. Developing a cancer-specific geriatric assessment: a feasibility study. Cancer. 2005;104(9):1998–2005.
57. Yee KW, Pater JL, Pho L, Zee B, Siu LL. Enrollment of older patients in cancer treatment trials in Canada: why is age a barrier? J Clin Oncol. 2003;21(8):1618–1623.
58. Trimble EL, Carter CL, Cain D, Freidlin B, Ungerleider RS, Friedman MA. Representation of older patients in cancer treatment trials. Cancer. 1994;74(7 Suppl):2208–2214.
59. Kemeny MM, Peterson BL, Kornblith AB, et al. Barriers to clinical trial participation by older women with breast cancer. J Clin Oncol. 2003;21(12):2268–2275.
60. Kornblith AB, Kemeny M, Peterson BL, et al. Survey of oncologists' perceptions of barriers to accrual of older patients with breast carcinoma to clinical trials. Cancer. 2002;95(5):989–996.
61. AGS Ethics Committee. AGS Position Paper: Health Screening Decisions for Older Adults. (Accessed December 24, 2004, at Available at: http://www.americangeriatrics.org/products/positionpapers/stopscreeningPF.shtml)
62. Smith RA, Cokkinides V, Eyre HJ. American Cancer Society guidelines for the early detection of cancer, 2004. CA Cancer J Clin. 2004;54(1):41–52.
75. Muss HB, Cohen HJ, Lichtman SM. Clinical research in the older cancer patient. Hematol Oncol Clin North Am. 2000;14(1):283–291.
76. Giovanazzi-Bannon S, Rademaker A, Lai G, Benson AB, 3rd. Treatment tolerance of elderly cancer patients entered onto phase II clinical trials: an Illinois Cancer Center study. J Clin Oncol. 1994;12(11):2447–2452.

67 The Role of Integrative Oncology in Cancer Care

Lorenzo Cohen, PhD ■ Nancy Russell, PhD ■ Kay Garcia, RN, LAC, DrPH ■ Moshe Frenkel, MD

Introduction

Integrative medicine seeks to combine conventional medicine with the safest and most effective complementary therapies. Although applying the concept of integrative medicine to cancer care is still in its infancy, a number of comprehensive cancer centers in the United States are trying to put this concept into practice under the term *integrative oncology*. As a result of this growing interest in integrative medicine in cancer care, the National Cancer Institute formed the Office of Cancer Complementary and Alternative Medicine, the American Cancer Society dedicated a portion of its web site to assessment of complementary therapies, the Consortium of Academic Centers for Integrative Medicine formed an oncology working group, and the Society for Integrative Oncology (SIO) was formed. The SIO mission is to study and facilitate cancer treatment and recovery through the use of integrated complementary therapeutic options, including natural and botanical products, nutrition, acupuncture, massage, mind-body therapies, and other complementary modalities (www.integrativeonc.org). This chapter will review the role of integrative medicine in cancer care with an emphasis on effective communication, an overview of the evidence, integrative-based resources to guide health care providers and patients, and an example of how to effectively incorporate integrative medicine within cancer care.

Definitions

Complementary and alternative medicine (CAM) has been defined by the National Center for Complementary and Alternative Medicine and major U.S. surveys as "... diverse medical and healthcare systems, practices, and products that are not presently considered to be part of conventional medicine."[1] Although evidence may exist for some of these modalities, it may not be sufficient to bring them into the realm of *conventional* medicine, and other CAM modalities may have no support for their use. Strictly speaking, *alternative* medicine by definition is when a patient makes use of a nonconventional treatment modality in place of conventional medicine whether or not there is evidence for its efficacy. *Complementary* medicine, on the other hand, is when a patient makes use of a CAM modality in combination with conventional medicine. The use of *alternative* or *complementary* medicine outside the context of research is ill-advised and patients need to be appropriately counseled on the risks and benefits of such choices as will be discussed in the section on communication.

The terms *alternative, complementary,* and *conventional* focus on types of treatment modalities. In the last few years, the term *integrative* medicine or complementary and integrative medicine (CIM) has become more prevalent in medical settings. CIM is more about a philosophy of medical practice that utilizes both conventional and complementary medicine. The Consortium of Academic Health Centers for Integrative Medicine has defined this term as "the practice of medicine that reaffirms the importance of the relationship between practitioner and patient, focuses on the whole person, is informed by evidence, and makes use of all appropriate therapeutic approaches, healthcare professionals and disciplines to achieve optimal health and healing."[2] In this way, integrative medicine makes use of both conventional and complementary treatment modalities using a multidisciplinary approach to health care. Practitioners of all disciplines should be knowledgeable and aware of all treatment options and open to communication with other types of practitioners. When this is done effectively, patients receive complementary treatment modalities using an integrative medicine approach, versus simply receiving two different treatment modalities (conventional and complementary) with fractionated medical care. Throughout this chapter we will use the term CIM in favor of CAM or other terms.

Complementary therapies include mind-body approaches such as meditation, guided imagery, music, art, other expressive arts and behavioral techniques; energy-based therapies such as yoga, tai chi, qigong, Reiki, and healing touch; body-manipulative approaches such as massage and reflexology; whole medical systems such as traditional Chinese medicine, homeopathy, and Ayurveda; and biologically based approaches such as those centered on nutrition, herbs, plants, animal, mineral, or other products. Several different types of specialty health care providers offer CIM therapies and these may include physicians, nurses, physical therapists, psychiatrists, psychologists, chiropractors, massage therapists and naturopaths who are operating within the guidelines of their licenses or accrediting organizations.

Utilization

The World Health Organization (WHO) estimates that up to 80% of people in developing countries rely on nonconventional traditional medicines for their primary health care. People in more developed countries also seek out complementary medicine and practices. A 1997 survey of U.S. adults found CIM use (excluding self prayer) varied from 32% to 54%.[3] A 2002 survey by the U.S. Centers for Disease Control found that 36% of adults had used CIM therapies (62% when prayer was included) during the past 12 months.[4]

Among patients and families touched by cancer the use of CIM is even higher than in the general population. An estimated 48-69% of U.S. patients with cancer use CIM therapies[5,6] and percentages increase if spiritual practices are included.[6] Complementary therapies are used in 70% of all oncology departments engaged in palliative care in Britain.[7,8] A survey of five clinics within a U.S. comprehensive cancer care center found that CIM therapies were used by 68.7% of patients (excluding psychotherapy and spiritual practices).[6] A later survey in the breast and gynecologic clinics within that same center found that CIM therapies (defined as herbs, supplements, and mega doses of vitamins) were used by 48% of patients.[5] Most estimates are that at least 50% of patients utilize CIM at some point in their journey.

In most cases, people who use CIM are not disappointed or dissatisfied with conventional medicine but want to do everything possible to regain health and to improve their quality of life.[9-16] Patients use CIM to reduce side effects and organ toxicity, to improve quality of life, to protect and stimulate immunity, or to prevent further cancers or recurrences. Whether or not patients use CIM therapies to treat cancer or its effects, they may use them to treat other chronic conditions such as arthritis, heart disease, diabetes, chronic pain, and other conditions.

The Mind-Body Connection

The belief that what we think and feel can influence our health and healing dates back thousands of years.[17] The importance of the role of the mind, emotions, and behaviors in health and well being was part of traditional Chinese, Tibetan, and Ayurvedic medicine and other medical traditions of the world. Many patients with cancer turn to CIM therapies as a way to reduce stress due to the now substantial evidence showing the negative health consequences of sustained stress on health and well being through profound psychological, behavioral, and physiological effects. These psychological and behavioral effects of stress may include increased negative affect, post-traumatic stress disorder, increased health-impairing behaviors (eg, poor diet, lack of exercise, or substance abuse), poor sleep, and decreased quality of life (QOL).[18-22] Research has shown that stress can also decrease compliance with health-screening behaviors.[23,24]

Stress-induced physiological changes that can have a direct effect on health include persistent increases in sympathetic nervous system activity and the hypothalamic-pituitary-axis that can cause increased blood pressure, heart rate, catecholamine secretion, and platelet aggregation.[25-30] Further, recent research suggests that stress is associated with increased latent viral reactivation, upper respiratory tract infections, and wound-healing time.[31-35] Stress also deregulates a variety of immune indices, as has been found in both healthy subjects and people with cancer.[32,36-47] Such stress-induced physiological changes may affect cancer progression, treatment, recovery, recurrence, and survival.[46-56] For example, several studies have linked stress and other psychosocial factors to the incidence and progression of cancer.[57-59] In addition, research has shown that depression, which is a common psychological response to stressful life events or circumstances, is linked to an increased risk of cancer, progression of disease, and decreased survival.[60-64] Extensive research has also now established that stress and depression cause the suppression of cell-mediated immunity.[37,65] Studies in cancer patients have linked immune function, including NK cell function and T-lymphocyte proliferation, to prognosis, recurrence, and survival time.[48-53,56,64,66,67] Recent laboratory research has also linked stress directly to changes in the tumor micro-environment and stress was found to be directly responsible for progression of disease and survival.[68] The clinical significance of stress-related immune and endocrine system changes and changes in the tumor micro-environment has not been widely studied. However, these changes may be significant enough to affect not only the immediate health of the patient, but also the course of the disease and thus the future health of the patient.[44,47,69-71] Decreasing distress and maintaining the functional integrity of the immune system and other physiological systems are therefore important in helping patients adjust to cancer treatment, recovery, treatment complications, and possibly metastatic growth. Although this area of research is relatively new, it has been demonstrated that psychological factors can result in behavioral and regulatory system changes that, in turn, may affect future health.[44,46,47,71,72] This has helped to legitimize what is called the mind-body connection and mind-body medicine research.

Thus, the mind-body connection is an important aspect of integrative oncology as emphasized in the recent Institute of Medicine (IOM) report *"Cancer Care for the Whole Patient."*[73] In this comprehensive report it is mentioned that "cancer care today often provides state-of-the-science biomedical treatment, but fails to address the psychological and social (psychosocial) problems associated with the illness. These problems—including … anxiety, depression or other emotional problems … —cause additional suffering, weaken adherence to prescribed treatments, and threaten patients' return to health." Extensive research has documented that mind-body interventions appear to address many of the issues mentioned in the IOM report. Some techniques will be discussed below.

Communication

The extensive use of CIM can be a challenge to health care professionals who typically have limited knowledge of this "new" area and limited time to reeducate themselves. At the same time, patients can become frustrated if they cannot discuss CIM with their physician. This bilateral frustration can result in a communication gap, which damages the patient–physician interaction. The most common reason patients give for not bringing up the topic of CIM even if they have questions or are taking CIM is that it just never came up in the discussion, that is, no one asked them, and they did not think it was important. Patients may also fear that the topic will be received with indifference or dismissed without discussion[16,74] and health care professionals may fear not knowing how to respond to questions or not want to initiate a time-consuming discussion. As a result, it is estimated that 38-60% of patients with cancer are taking complementary medicines without informing any member of their health care team.[5,6] This lack of discussion is of grave concern, especially for ingestible substances.

The failure of physicians to communicate effectively with patients about CIM may result in a loss of trust within the therapeutic relationship. In the absence of physician guidance, patients may choose harmful, useless, ineffective, and costly complementary therapies when effective CIM therapies may exist. The erosion in trust due to lack of communication can also lead to decreased compliance with conventional medicine and certainly to not following the physicians advice about CIM use. Poor communication may also lead to a diminishment of patient autonomy and sense of control over their treatment, thereby interfering with potential self-healing responses.[16,74]

While scientific and evidence-based thinking is fundamental to contemporary medical practice, patients often do not base their decisions in the same scientific processes, and often rely instead on preliminary laboratory research, poorly designed studies, case reports or testimonials from family and others. A physician's failure to recognize this difference interferes with their ability to address the unspoken needs of patients. Psychological, social, and spiritual dimensions of care may be ignored if physicians cannot adapt to the individual needs of the patient or if they provide care without sensitivity. When physicians are faced with unfamiliar information about CIM therapies, they may feel "de-skilled" by being forced outside their medical specialty. This discomfort can lead to defensiveness and a breakdown in communication with the patient. In contrast, the physician who is receptive to patient inquiries and aware of subtle, nonverbal messages can create an environment in which a patient feels protected and can openly discuss potential CIM choices.[74,75] Even when similar understanding of scientific processes exists, patients may recognize that the economics of research interfere with progress concerning proposed CIM therapies that typically do not have powerful companies supporting research. In some cases, complementary therapies may even be held to higher standards of evidence than currently accepted conventional therapies.

Existing research suggests that the majority of cancer patients desire communication with their doctors about CIM[76] and there is general agreement within the oncology community that oncologists must be aware of CIM use and be able to guide their use of all therapeutic approaches in order to provide effective patient care.[77,78] It is the health care professional's responsibility to ask patients about their use of complementary medicines. Optimally, the discussion should take place before the patient starts using a complementary treatment whether it is a nutritional supplement, mind-body therapy or other approach. A number of strategies can be used to increase the chance of a worthwhile dialogue. Underlying these specific strategies should be an open attitude combined with a willingness to review evidence-based references and consult with other health care professionals.[79]

Integrating complementary therapies with conventional treatments is dependent upon many different aspects of effective communication. Communication is defined as the giving or exchange of information, but patient-physician communication is not unilateral and is not limited to the transferring of information. This type of communication is an interactive process and usually more than a concise, focused dialogue of questions and answers. Patient-physician dialogue has a much broader meaning that involves not just "words," but also tone of voice, meaningful looks and gestures. Understanding nonverbal patterns, which include voice tone, pitch, timbre and tempo, together with symmetry and asymmetry of posture and breathing, is vital to communication. For example, sarcasm in a physician's voice or raised eyebrows can undo the surface intent of any words and shut down future communication from the patient. Role playing with professional coaches is one way to detect unintended voice and body language reactions.

When physicians pay particular attention to incongruence's, in which the verbal and nonverbal aspects are not aligned, it can yield valuable information about the underlying concerns, beliefs, emotions, and expectations of patients. This kind of information gets to the root of problems and facilitates their resolution. Unfortunately, although these skills are easily learned, they are generally either not taught or only superficially addressed in the medical curriculum.[80] The Toronto consensus statement on doctor patient communication clearly showed that communication problems in clinical practice are important and common. It also showed that the quality of communication is related to health outcomes for patients.[81]

Communication relating to complementary therapy use can be introduced related to previous visits, family and caregiver involvement, other healthcare providers, and personal and professional experiences of the physician and the patient. Family, employment, emotions, desires and wants, hidden wishes and concerns, health beliefs, and social, religious and spiritual issues may all be a necessary part of this communication.

A survey of patients and staff at a large oncology center in Israel found that patients believed CIM practices addressed psychological distress and spiritual and religious issues more than staff members did. On the other hand, staff members attributed CIM use more to a patient's disappointment with conventional medicine than did the patients.[82] A study of patients and physicians in the U.S. found that patients were using CIM as a source of hope and control and a nontoxic approach to treatment. Both physicians and patients agreed that CIM could relieve symptoms and side effects, but physicians were less likely than patients to expect CIM to improve immunity or quality of life, cure disease, or prolong life.[10]

Communication is crucial to establishing trust with the patient, gathering information, addressing patient emotions, and assisting patients in decisions about care. The quality of communication in cancer care has been shown to affect patient satisfaction, decision making, patient distress, and even malpractice litigation. Communication is now recognized as a core clinical skill in medicine and in cancer care.[83] A review of the literature has shown that healthcare professionals' effective communication improves patient health by positively influencing emotional health, symptom resolution, functioning, and pain control.[84] Effective communication positively influences not only the patient's outcomes but also the healthcare professional's function. Cancer clinicians who feel inadequately trained to respond to patients' emotional needs are at an increased risk of burnout.[85] Patients react to physicians in multiple ways that can inhibit or enhance the relationship. Physicians may become overly distant, leading to both physician and patient dissatisfaction, or they can become overly involved emotionally, which can have serious psychological and clinical consequences.[86]

Another issue that needs to be addressed is appropriate response to patient emotions. One of the most challenging tasks in cancer care is determining how to provide adequate emotional support.[87,88] An approach that incorporates empathy, hope, friendliness, listening, and humor, that encourages questions, and that checks a patient's understanding of the answers can be helpful.

The issue of CIM use among patients' surfaces quite frequently, and clinicians need to develop an empathic communication strategy that addresses patients' needs, while maintaining the health care professional's understanding of the current state of the science. That is, this strategy needs to be balanced between clinical objectivity and bonding with the patient so that it can benefit both the patient and the healthcare provider. Because of the threat posed by cancer and the uncertain outcome of treatment, most patients require much information about their disease and its treatment.[89] As such, patients need reliable information on CIM, require adequate time to discuss this information and easy access to reliable resources that they can easily refer to.

Patient-physician communication is complicated and the use of CIM by the patient may cause additional confusion. Some CIM therapies are being administered by a CIM practitioner which can complicate communication even more because of a triangular relationship: the patient and their physician, the patient and his CIM practitioner, and the physician and the CIM practitioner. A productive and fruitful communication process requires all three relationships to be addressed.[90]

The Evidence

The field of integrative oncology is a constantly evolving set of disciplines. As such, the evidence at any point in time becomes dated as quickly as new modalities for specific conditions are found to either be effective or ineffective and either incorporated into conventional medicine or dismissed. There has been a dramatic increase in research in integrative oncology within conventional scientific journals, including two journals specifically dedicated to integrative oncology: the *Journal of the Society for Integrative Oncology* and *Integrative Cancer Therapies*, both of which are peer-reviewed, MEDLINE indexed journals dedicated to publishing original research and to education within the field of integrative oncology.

Although scientific evidence for the efficacy of a treatment is necessary to gain acceptance within the conventional medical arena, it is usually not sufficient and several political steps are often necessary. An example of this is the role of acupuncture in treating chemotherapy induced nausea and vomiting. A National Institutes of Health (NIH) consensus statement in 1997 supported this use, stating that the level of evidence was sufficient.[91] Further research has substantiated this claim and the American Cancer Society now states that clinical studies have found acupuncture may help treat nausea caused by chemotherapy drugs and surgical anesthesia.[92] In addition, specific research using neuroimaging of patients while undergoing acupuncture treatments of nausea points has delineated the neural mechanisms of action.[93] Even so, acupuncture has still to be accepted into the standard of care for chemotherapy-induced nausea and vomiting.

Below we list some of the key findings to date in integrative oncology in the main areas of CIM where there is sufficient evidence to recommend the therapies: mind-body treatments, massage, and acupuncture. The important role of physical activity, exercise, and energy-balance/nutrition is discussed thoroughly in Chapter 32. Although there is ongoing research in many other areas such as healing touch, homeopathy, natural products, and special diets there is insufficient evidence to recommend these at this point in time. The SIO Integrative Oncology Practice Guidelines state that "... until there is evidence for the safety and efficacy of the substance, they should not be used as alternatives to mainstream care. Clinical trials of some herbs and other botanicals aside, most complementary therapies are not specific to a particular cancer diagnosis. Instead, they are used typically to treat symptoms shared by patients across many cancer diagnoses."[94]

Reviewing the current literature is often not sufficient to answer questions about CIM use with a high level of certainty from the perspective of evidence-based medicine. So the challenge for the clinician is how to deal with an issue that has a high level of uncertainty. Physicians urgently need to approach CIM use in cancer in a systematic way. When limited scientific data in the medical literature support the use of a particular CIM, these data cannot be considered proofs of efficacy, but they do offer clinical clues that support the use or avoidance of the therapy. Such clues can provide a basis for honest and open discussion with the patient. When physicians use a patient-centered approach, they can promote informed decision making by the patient in collaboration with the physician. This combined effort can provide a base for an improved patient-doctor relationship and can empower the patient in his/her own healthcare.

We suggest a rational strategy for approaching CIM use by patients that suffer from cancer. The first step is to increase one's knowledge about the therapy in question, mainly by searching reliable websites as well as Medline. In this step, one has to examine two main issues: safety and efficacy. The most crucial elements are the *safety* of the therapy in question, side effect profile, and possible interactions with other nutrients and medications. *Primum non nocere* is the dictum of physicians: first of all, to do no harm. Ignorance of information on CIM is no longer excusable, as it is widely available in medical journals, texts, reliable websites, and databases. A corollary to this dictum may be stated as "prevent the patient from harming them self." Frank, nonjudgmental discussion with the patient is necessary to inform the patient effectively about the known risks and benefits of the therapies.

No matter how safe a therapy is, if it is ineffective the patient must be so informed. Complementary therapies, by definition, have generally not reached the level of evidence of many conventional therapies. They exist at the interface of science and healing. However, note that many cancer therapies, including chemotherapy, radiation therapy, and a number of plant-based agents, were considered "alternative" before they were accepted as the standard of care. Moreover, arguing with the patient that they should not try an unproven therapy, which they are convinced will help them is not very productive; it is likely to damage the therapeutic relationship and drive the communication process underground. It may even be considered cruel; if no better conventional therapy is available.

If it seems that the therapy is safe and there are clinical clues that it may have some effectiveness, the next step is to discuss the level of uncertainty of the product with the patient. A realistic view may be that more complete information will not be available in the near future and that we may need to make a decision that balances risk and benefit. The higher the patient's expectations, the higher degree of disappointment will be, when the course of care does not go as expected. An informed discussion should give basic hard data on the therapy in question in order to minimize unrealistic expectations. This discussion can also be used as a tool to improve the doctor-patient communication and empower the patient in his/her own care at a critical juncture in the cancer care journey.

If a decision is reached to add a complementary therapy to the treatment of cancer, the physician's role has not ended. The physician still has the responsibility of verifying, with some degree of certainty, the reliability of the specific therapy in question. A physician with some market knowledge can verify a therapy's reliability by referencing independent websites. Once a plan is determined, regular follow up is needed to monitor adverse effects and effectiveness, and make adjustments, as with any other conventional treatment.[95]

Many natural products are safe for patient use and some physicians may be comfortable with the preponderance of evidence for some in terms of quality of life or even disease-related outcomes. St. John's wort has been found to be effective for moderate mood regulation, ginger for nausea, and valerian for sleep problems. However, more studies in humans are needed and important contraindications need to be observed with these herbs; eg, St. John's wort increases metabolism of certain drugs. Patients and health care professionals need to seek out information from reputable and reliable resources and make shared decisions on what to incorporate or not incorporate into treatment plans based on each person's level of comfort.[94,96-98]

Mind-Body Practices

Mind-body practices are defined as a variety of techniques designed to enhance the mind's capacity to affect bodily function and symptoms.[1] Mind-body techniques include relaxation, hypnosis, visual imagery, meditation, biofeedback, cognitive-behavioral therapies, group support, autogenic training, and spirituality and expressive arts therapies such as art, music, or dance. Therapies such as yoga, tai chi, and qigong often fall into the CIM category of energy medicine, as they are intended to work with bodily "energetic fields" (eg, meridians and *qi* [pronounced chee—China], *lung* [pronounced loong—Tibet], *prana* [India], and *ki* [pronounced kee—Japan]). However, they are also likely to exert strong effects through a mind-body connection and as such fall into the mind-body medicine category. Some of these therapies are no longer considered "alternative" and they are well integrated into conventional medicine and most medical settings (hypnosis, biofeedback, cognitive-behavioral therapy, and group support). As research continues, the treatments that are found beneficial will hopefully become integrated into conventional medical care.

Research has shown that after being diagnosed with cancer, patients try to bring about positive changes in their lifestyles, indicating a tendency to take control of their health care.[99] Techniques of stress management that have proven helpful include progressive muscle relaxation,[100,101] diaphragmatic breathing,[102,103] guided imagery,[104-106] social support,[107,108] and meditation.[109,110] Participating in stress management programs prior to treatment have enabled patients to tolerate therapy with fewer reported side effects.[111-114] Supportive expressive group therapy has also been found to be useful for patients with cancer.[115-117] Psychosocial interventions have been shown to specifically decrease depression and anxiety and to increase self-esteem and active-approach coping strategies.[118-121]

A meta-analysis of 116 studies found that mind-body therapies could reduce anxiety, depression and mood disturbance in cancer patients, and assist their coping skills.[122] Newell and colleagues[123] reviewed psychological therapies for cancer patients and concluded that interventions involving self-practice and hypnosis for managing nausea and vomiting could be recommended, but that further research was suggested to examine the benefits of relaxation training and guided imagery. Further research was also warranted to examine the benefits of relaxation and guided imagery for managing general nausea, anxiety, quality of life, and overall physical symptoms.[123] More recently, Ernst et al.[124] examined the change in the state of the evidence for mind-body therapies for various medical conditions between 2000 and 2005 and found that there is now maximal evidence for the use of relaxation techniques for anxiety, hypertension, insomnia, and nausea due to chemotherapy.

Research examining yoga, tai chi, and meditation incorporated into cancer care suggests that these mind-body practices help to improve aspects of quality of life including improved mood, sleep quality, physical functioning, and overall well being.[121,125] Hypnosis, and especially self-hypnosis, has been found to be beneficial to help reduce distress and discomfort during difficult medical procedures.[126] An NIH Technology Assessment Panel found strong evidence for hypnosis in alleviating cancer-related pain.[127] Hypnosis effectively treats anticipatory nausea in pediatric[128] and adult cancer patients,[129] reduces post-operative nausea and vomiting,[130] and improves adjustment to invasive medical procedures.[131-133]

Massage

Massage for relaxation and to help manage pain and discomfort has been used for thousands of years. There are various forms of massage and they all typically apply some degree of pressure to muscle and connective tissue and in some cases work with specific pressure points. A clinical form of massage know as manual lymph drainage has been shown to decrease lymphedema when combined with elastic sleeves or bandaging for patients with arm edema after breast cancer surgery.[134] However, this is a detailed and lengthy process and self-massage with this technique has not been found to be as effective as either that done by a trained therapist or simulation by a specially designed pump.

Research to date suggests that massage is helpful at relieving pain, anxiety, fatigue, distress and increasing relaxation.[135-138] A challenge of course in conducting massage therapy research is having a placebo control group. It is therefore not clear what the exact mechanisms are for the benefits of massage in an oncology setting. Regardless of some of the imperfections in research design, the finds are encouraging and there is no question that patients derive benefit from this treatment. Moreover, massage is generally safe when it is conducted by a licensed practitioner who has also had some training in working with cancer patients. In general, cancer patients should not receive deep tissue massage and patients with bleeding tendencies should only receive light touch. Obviously, areas that have recently had surgery or radiation should be avoided. Therapeutic benefit can also be derived from simply receiving a massage to the feet, hands, and head as these areas are especially sensitive to tactile stimulation and can result in providing relaxation and an increase in general well being.[139,140]

Acupuncture

Acupuncture is a common treatment modality that is part of traditional Chinese medicine (TCM) and has been practiced in China for thousands of years. Acupuncture is the most popular TCM treatment around the world and is used in at least 78 countries.[141] The theory behind the benefits of acupuncture is that the placement of needles, heat, or pressure at specific places on the body can help to regulate the flow of Qi (vital energy) within the body.

The most common form of acupuncture involves the placement of solid, sterile, stainless steel needles into various points on the body that are known to have reduced bioelectrical resistance and increased conductance.[142,143] Different techniques can be used to stimulate the needles including manual manipulation or electrical stimulation.[142-144] Stainless steel or gold (semipermanent) needles, or "studs," are also sometimes placed at specific points on the ears and left in place for 3-5 days. Heat or pressure can also be applied at acupoints on the body instead of puncturing the skin. However, the therapeutic benefit is higher when needles are actually inserted.

The strongest evidence for the efficacy of acupuncture in cancer care is for symptom management for nausea, vomiting, and pain based on good evidence to support its use in the management of nausea and vomiting from multiple causes (ie, chemotherapy-induced nausea and vomiting [CINV], postoperative nausea and vomiting, and pregnancy).[91,145-148] In one systematic review,[147] stimulation of acupoint P6 reduced the risk of nausea but not vomiting, when compared with antiemetics. Although there is good evidence for the use of acupuncture to control pain, there is still limited research in a cancer setting. However, one well controlled randomized, blinded, placebo controlled trial found acupuncture decreased pain scores by 36% and the scores remained stable in the placebo groups (acupuncture or pressure at nonacupuncture points).[149]

Another area for which there is good evidence for the role of acupuncture is in the treatment of radiation induced xerostomia.[150,151] Although there have been a number of clinical trials, both controlled and uncontrolled, methodological rigor is still lacking and a large definitive randomized clinical trial is needed. However, this initial research suggests acupuncture is beneficial and in some cases can have a lasting effect.

For the management of other treatment- or cancer-related symptoms the evidence is not as strong as that for pain and nausea. Nevertheless, there is some evidence to suggest that acupuncture may be useful in treating or helping to manage: constipation, loss of appetite, peripheral neuropathy, hot flushes, fatigue, insomnia and sleep disorders, dyspnea, anxiety/depression, and leucopenia.[152,153] However, the quality of the research for these symptoms remains weak and further research is needed.

When performed correctly, acupuncture has been shown to be a safe, minimally invasive procedure with very few side effects. The side effects most commonly reported are fainting, bruising, and mild pain. Infection is also a potential risk, although very uncommon.[154,155] Acupuncture should only be performed by a health care professional with an appropriate license and preferably one who has had experience in treating patients with malignant diseases.

Although the mechanisms of acupuncture are not well understood, for symptoms such as chemotherapy-related and postoperative nausea, vomiting, and pain, there is clear evidence to support the use of acupuncture. Although data are currently lacking for the control of other cancer-related symptoms and cancer treatment-related symptoms, as a very low risk and cost effective treatment option, acupuncture may be a helpful adjunct to conventional treatment for patients suffering from uncontrolled treatment-related side effects or for those in whom conventional treatment approaches have failed.[156]

Educational Resources

The rapidity with which a comprehensive review can become out-of-date and the ease of Internet publishing have fostered the growth of comprehensive scientific review organizations that provide electronic access to their reviews. An assessment of websites with reviews of CIM therapies for patients with cancer was published in 2004 by Schmidt and Ernst.[157] They used eight popular search engines to search for the terms "complementary" or "alternative medicine" and "cancer" and identified the first 50 websites that appeared on at least three engines. Their final list of 32 websites was evaluated for: (1) quality based upon a Sandvik score of 0-5 points as "poor," 6-10 points as "medium" and 11-14 points as "excellent"; (2) reliability based on whether it displayed the Health on the Net (HON) code; and (3) risk to patients based on an overall score and type of CIM discussed (curative, preventative, or palliative). Each website was also downgraded for discouraging the use of conventional medicine or clinician's advice, and providing commercial details. Ten websites received a score of 12 or better. Seven of these top ten websites were sponsored by either government or academic institutions and three were sponsored by individuals or private businesses.[157]

For recommendation to health professionals, we evaluated 15 websites: the ten websites recognized by Schmidt and Ernst (1) Quackwatch[158]; (2) Oxford University's Bandolier[159]; (3) the National Cancer Institute (NCI) Fact Sheets[160]; (4) Rosenthal Center of Columbia University[161]; (5) Holistic online[162]; (6) International Health News–yourhealthbase[163]; (7) Oncolink sponsored by the Abramson Cancer Center of the University of Pennsylvania[164]; (8) University of Virginia Medical Center[165]; (9) NCI Office of Cancer Complementary and Alternative Medicine (OCCAM) PDQ summaries[166]; and (10) The University of Texas M. D. Anderson Cancer Center Complementary/Integrative Medicine Education Resources (CIMER)[97]; plus five others that were not identified by Schmidt and Ernst as being within in the top 32 websites: (11) American Cancer Society[167]; (12) Memorial Sloan-Kettering Cancer Center[96]; (13) the Cochrane Review Organization,[168]; (14) Natural Standard[169] and; (15) Natural Medicines Comprehensive Database.[170]

Eight of these fifteen complementary/alternative websites provide generally reliable information for patients and the general public, but are not adequate for health professionals. Quackwatch[158] can be useful for checking on the reliability of proprietary sources and status with regulatory agencies, but has a predominantly negative bias consistent with its mission to "combat health related frauds." In contrast, Holistic online[162] provides a generally positive bias about the healing and disease prevention properties of an extensive set of herbs and other therapies (both alternative and conventional), but it does not provide professional documentation or descriptions of their review process. The Rosenthal Center at Columbia University provides links to information resources at Columbia University and elsewhere compiled between 1994 and 2007. It is now an archived set of resources not further updated as of June, 2007.[161] One of this center's featured databases, HerbMedPro, previously compiled by the Alternative Medicine Foundation, is now managed by the American Botanical Council. HerbMedPro provides links to abstracts of published studies of herbs, but not systematic reviews. The University of Virginia Medical Center[165] describes opportunities for research at their center on pain, pain-related symptoms and physiological mechanisms underlying the beneficial effects of selected CIM modalities, but it does not provide reviews or study results. The University of Pennsylvania's Oncolink provides an overview about complementary therapies and short list of dangerous herbs.[164] International Health News provides summaries of individual articles on a variety of topics not limited to complementary therapies.[163] The American Cancer Society (ACS) provides authoritative reviews suitable for patients and the general public on a wide variety of complementary therapies.[167] The National Cancer Institute provides factsheets on general issues concerning complementary therapies.[160] It also provides links to "PDQ" reviews of the evidence for specific complementary treatments for patients and the public that are now posted alongside professional reviews described in the next section.

Seven remaining websites provide valuable resources for healthcare professionals (see Table 67-1). Natural Medicines Comprehensive Database (www.naturalmedicinedatabase.com) provides the largest number of evidence-based reviews of complementary therapies (over 1000).[170] The majority of its authors and editors are doctors of Pharmacy and their reviews include scientific names, uses, safety, effectiveness, and mechanisms of action, adverse reactions, interactions, dosage and administration. Full access requires an individual or institutional subscription. It has received top ratings in comparative evaluations for answering questions about herbal and dietary supplements.[171-173] However, these one to two page reviews do not provide background or in-depth assessments of the evidence on which their conclusions are based.

The oldest and most comprehensive of the scientific review organizations for conventional therapies is the Cochrane Review Organization (www.cochrane.org).[168] Founded in 1993 as an international non-profit independent organization, it now provides over 2000 systematic reviews and has recently added the complementary therapies of massage, acupuncture and chiropractic. Its review process includes searches of multiple bibliographic databases by professional librarians. At least two blinded independent reviewers evaluate studies according to standard sets of questions with discrepancies resolved through conferences with attempts to contact authors for resolution of remaining questions. A statistician and an editorial board join with reviewers for development and summation of final conclusions. Abstracts of Cochrane reviews are free, but completed reviews require either individual or institutional subscription.[168,174]

Modeling itself upon the Cochrane organization, Natural Standard (www.naturalstandard.com) formed a multidisciplinary, multi-institutional initiative dedicated to the review of complementary and alternative therapies.[169] It follows a similar process to build in-depth evidence and consensus-based analysis of scientific data in addition to historic and folkloric perspectives. It now provides several hundred authoritative reviews. Access requires an institutional subscription, but some subscribing institutions have also purchased summaries of reviews for public access.

The NCI Office of Cancer Complementary and Alternative Medicine (OCCAM) has reviewed about a dozen complementary therapies (http://www.cancer.gov/cam).[166] These "PDQ" Cancer Information Summaries provide extensive details and citations for health professionals including background, history of development, proposed mechanisms of action, and relevant laboratory, animal and clinical studies.

Table 67-1 **Recommended Web Sites for Evidence-Based Resources**

Organization/Web Site (Alphabetical Order)	Address/URL
Bandolier	http://www.jr2.ox.ac.uk/bandolier/booth/booths/altmed.html
Cochrane Review Organization	www.cochrane.org
Memorial Sloan-Kettering Cancer Center	http://www.mskcc.org/aboutherbs
Natural Medicines Comprehensive Database	http://www.naturaldatabase.com/
Natural Standard	http://www.naturalstandard.com/
NCI Office of Cancer Complementary and Alternative Medicine (OCCAM)	http://www.cancer.gov/cam
University of Texas MD Anderson Cancer Center Complementary/Integrative Medicine Education Resources	www.mdanderson.org/CIMER

Memorial Sloan-Kettering Cancer Center (www.mskcc.org/aboutherbs) provides over 200 evidence-based reviews.[96] These are written either by an oncology-trained pharmacist with expertise in botanicals or a cancer nutrition specialist with secondary reviews by at least two other editors or panel advisors.

Bandolier, a monthly journal about evidence-based healthcare produced by scientists at Oxford University, provides a subset of complementary therapy in-depth analyses, commentaries and meta-analyses found in searches of the Cochrane Library and Pub Med (www.jr2.ox.ac.uk/bandolier/booth/booths/altmed.html).[159]

The University of Texas M.D. Anderson Cancer Center's website for complementary/integrative medicine (www.mdanderson.org/cimer) provides over 90 reviews that include in-depth assessments of the background and evidence by their own staff plus purchased summaries of some of the previously described reviews by Natural Standard and the Cochrane Library and access to all reviews by the NCI OCCAM and Memorial Sloan-Kettering.[97] Their own methodology includes searches by library personnel, reviews by staff with expertise in laboratory, clinical and population studies, and secondary reviews by appropriate faculty members or outside advisors.

Searching these seven websites may be efficiently accomplished by physicians or delegated to appropriate clinic personnel. Patients or caregivers can then be given specific recommendations, printed summaries, or the names of these or other pre-screened websites. Questions generated from this information can then be brought back for discussion with the physician or other clinic professional.

Although the National Cancer Institute, the American Cancer Society and the MD Anderson Cancer Center websites also provide links to other reliable websites, patients or caregivers may wish to investigate independently. If so, they should be encouraged to look for websites that subscribe to the principles of the Health on the Net Foundation and carry its "HonCode" seal. This nongovernmental organization is supported by the State of Geneva in Switzerland, the Swiss Institute of Bioinformatics and the University Hospitals of Geneva. It screens websites for compliance with its eight principles of authority: medically trained and qualified professionals, support of the patient/site visitor and his/her physician, confidentiality, clear references to source data, claims supported by appropriate and balanced evidence, transparency of authorship, transparency of ownership, and honesty in advertising and editorial policy.[175] The HonCode is displayed by two of the above seven websites for health care professionals: the National Cancer Institute and the MD Anderson Cancer Center.

Effective Integration

In order to provide patients with appropriate services for the management of their cancer and cancer-related morbidity, it is likely that complementary medicine treatment modalities will need to be integrated into the treatment plan. This makes clinical sense when the evidence for safety and efficacy is strong. Conversely, it makes clinical sense to avoid therapies and discourage therapies when the evidence for safety and efficacy is weak.[176] This will result in a safer method for the delivery of medicine as a whole. When patients receive their conventional medical treatments fractionated from their complementary medicine treatments the risk of adverse events increases as there is a lack of communication between patient and conventional practitioner and even between the conventional and nonconventional practitioners.

Most major medical centers now offer some complementary medicine treatment modalities along side the conventional care. When both the conventional and nonconventional health care professionals are aware of each other and there is open communication between patient and practitioner, then the practice of integrative medicine has been established and can be more effective. Many comprehensive cancer centers have integrative medicine established within their conventional system as is the case at the Dana Farber Cancer Institute, Memorial Sloan-Kettering Cancer Center, University if Texas MD Anderson Cancer Center, and others.[177]

The Integrative Medicine Program at MD Anderson is an important component of the mission to treat the whole person—from prevention and treatment—through survivorship.[178] Ongoing research is examining intervention programs and treatments that can improve quality of life and clinical outcomes. Educational programs provide authoritative, accurate and current information to the faculty, staff, students, trainees, and the public about complementary and alternative approaches. The integrative medicine clinic offers consultation with a physician on the appropriate use of complementary therapies. Many complementary therapies are provided through the *Place ... of wellness* where therapies known to be safe and effective are used alongside conventional care.

Clinical delivery of integrative medicine is provided in three locations: *Place ...of wellness* (at two locations), inpatient services, and the Integrative Medicine Clinic where individual consultations take place with a physician on the proper integration of CIM in all stages of cancer care. This clinic offers professional guidance to assist patients regarding complementary treatments. The clinic medical director meets regularly with a team of professionals who have experience in conventional and integrative treatments. This experience ranges from researching reliable information sources related to CIM therapies to providing expertise in natural products, including nutritional supplements, vitamins and herbs, and the interactions these substances may have with each other and conventional medications. The use of diet and food as a medicinal element in the treatment of cancer is also discussed. Other therapists focus on managing pain, stress and anxiety, and other symptoms resulting from illness and/or treatment side effects.

The *Place ... of wellness* is a clinical center providing therapies to patients and caregivers. Therapies offered can enhance patients' quality of life through programs that complement medical care and focus on the mind, body, and spirit such as guided imagery, meditation, yoga, tai chi, music therapy, acupuncture, massage, and cooking classes. Faculty, staff, and community practitioners credentialed in their respective areas of expertise facilitate the programs. Most programs are offered free of charge, except acupuncture and full body massage, which are provided for a nominal fee.

Integrative oncology is a rapidly expanding discipline that holds tremendous promise for additional treatment options and more effective symptom control. An integrative approach also provides patients with a more personalized system of care for meeting their needs. The majority of patients are either using complementary medicines or want to know about them so it is incumbent on the conventional medical system to provide appropriate education and clinical services. The clinical model for integrative care requires a patient-centered approach with attention to patient concerns and enhanced communication skills. In addition, it is essential that conventional and nonconventional practitioners work together in developing an integrative model. In this way, cancer patients will be receiving the best medical care making use of all appropriate treatment modalities.

Selected References

The complete reference list can be found at www.CANCERMEDICINE8.com

1. NCCAM. National Center for Complementary/Alternative Medicine of the National Institutes of Health. What is complemen-

tary and alternative medicine? http://nccam.nih.gov/health/whatiscam/. (Accessed June 24, 2008).

2. CAHCIM. http://www.imconsortium.org/cahcim/about/home.html. (Accessed June 24, 2008).
5. Navo MA, Phan J, Vaughan C, et al. An assessment of the utilization of complementary and alternative medication in women with gynecologic or breast malignancies. *J Clin Oncol*. 2004;22(4):671–677.
6. Richardson MA, Sanders T, Palmer JL, Greisinger A, Singletary SE. Complementary/alternative medicine use in a comprehensive cancer center and the implications for oncology. *J Clin Oncol*. 2000;18(13):2505–2514.
10. Richardson MA, Masse LC, Nanny K, Sanders C. Discrepant views of oncologists and cancer patients on complementary/alternative medicine. *Support Care Cancer*. 2004;12(11):797–804.
16. Wyatt GK, Friedman LL, Given CW, Given BA, Beckrow KC. Complementary therapy use among older cancer patients. *Cancer Pract*. 1999;7(3):136–144.
24. Lerman C, Daly M, Sands C, et al. Mammography adherence and psychological distress among women at risk for breast cancer. *J Natl Cancer Inst*. 1993;85(13):1074–1080.
40. Cohen S, Herbert TB. Health psychology: Psychological factors and physical disease from the perspective of human psychoneuroimmunology. *Annu Rev Psychol*. 1996;47:113–142.
46. Antoni MH, Lutgendorf SK, Cole SW, et al. The influence of bio-behavioural factors on tumour biology: pathways and mechanisms. Nature Reviews. *Cancer*. 2006;6(3):240–248.
47. Glaser R, Kiecolt-Glaser JK. Stress-induced immune dysfunction: implications for health. Nature Reviews. *Immunology*. 2005;5(3):243–251.
61. Watson M, Haviland JS, Greer S, Davidson J, Bliss JM. Influence of psychological response on survival in breast cancer: a population-based cohort study. *Lancet*. 1999;354(9187):1331–1336.
62. Strommel M, Given BA, Given CW. Depression and functional status as predictors of death among cancer patients. *Cancer*. 2002;94:2719–2727.
65. Rabin BS. *Stress, Immune Function, and Health: The Connection*. New York: Wiley-Liss & Sons; 1999.
67. Ader R, Cohen N, Felten D. Psychoneuroimmunology: interactions between the nervous system and the immune system. *Lancet*. 1995;345(8942):99–103.
68. Thaker PH, Han LY, Kamat AA, et al. Chronic stress promotes tumor growth and angiogenesis in a mouse model of ovarian carcinoma. *Nat Med*. 2006;12(8):939–944.
69. Redd WH, Silberfarb PM, Andersen BL, et al. Physiologic and psychobehavioral research in oncology. *Cancer*. 1991; 67(3):813–822.
71. Bovbjerg DH. Psychoneuroimmunology. Implications for oncology? *Cancer*. 1991; 67:828–832.
73. IOM. Institute of Medicine: Cancer Care for the Whole Patient: Meeting Psychosocial Health Needs. The National Academies Press 2008 Prepublication available on line. http://www.nap.edu/catalog.php?record_id=11993 (accessed Februrary 25, 2008).
74. Tasaki K, Maskarinec G, Shumay DM, Tatsumura Y, Kakai H. Communication between physicians and cancer patients about complementary and alternative medicine: exploring patients' perspectives. [see comment]. *Psychooncology*. 2002;11(3):212–220.
77. Berk LB. Primer on integrative oncology. *Hematol Oncol Clin North Am*. 2006;20(1): 213–231.
79. Cohen L, Cohen MH, Kirkwood C, Russell NC. Discussing complementary therapies in an oncology setting. *J Soc Integr Oncol*. 2007;5(1):18–24.
81. Simpson M, Buckman R, Stewart M, et al. Doctor-patient communication: the Toronto consensus statement. *BMJ*. 1991;303(6814): 1385–1387.
82. Ben-Arye E, Bar-Sela G, Frenkel M, Kuten A, Hermoni D. Is a biopsychosocial-spiritual approach relevant to cancer treatment? A study of patients and oncology staff members on issues of complementary medicine and spirituality. *Support Care Cancer*. 2006;14(2):147–152.
90. Frenkel M, Ben-Arye E. Communicating with patients about the use of complementary and integrative medicine in cancer care. In: Cohen L, Markman M, eds. *Incorporating Complementary Medicine into Conventional Cancer Care*. Totowa: Humana Press; 2008: 33–46.
91. Acupuncture. NIH Consensus Statement. November 3–5, 1997;15(5):1–34.
94. Deng GE, Cassileth BR, Cohen L, et al. Integrative oncology practice guidelines. *J Soc Integr Oncol*. 2007;5(2):65–84.
95. Frenkel M, Ben-Arye E, Baldwin CD, Sierpina V. Approach to communicating with patients about the use of nutritional supplements in cancer care. *South Med J*. 2005;98(3):289–294.
96. Memorial Sloan-Kettering Cancer Center: About Herbs. http://www.mskcc.org/aboutherbs (accessed June 15, 2008).
97. The University of Texas M.D. Anderson Cancer Center: Complementary/Integrative Medicine Education Resources (CIMER). http://www.mdanderson.org/cimer (accessed June 15, 2008).
104. Spiegel D. Psychosocial aspects of breast cancer treatment. Semin Oncol. 1997;24(1): 36–47.
106. Wallace KG. Analysis of recent literature concerning relaxation and imagery interventions for cancer pain. Cancer Nurs. 1997;20(2):79–87.
121. Gordon JS. Mind-Body Medicine and Cancer. In: Cohen L, Frenkel M, eds. Integrative Medicine in Oncology: Hematology/Oncology Clinics of North America. 2008.
122. Devine EC, Westlake SK. The effects of psychoeducational care provided to adults with cancer: meta-analysis of 116 studies. Oncol Nurs Forum. 1995;22(9):1369–1381.
123. Newell SA, Sanson-Fisher W, Savolainen NJ. Systematic review of psychological therapies for cancer patients: overview and recommendations for future research. J Natl Cancer Inst. 2002;94(8):558–584.
124. Ernst E, Pittler MH, Wider B, Boddy K. Mind-body therapies: are the trial data getting stronger? Altern Ther Health Med. 2007;13(5):62–64.
125. Bower JE, Woolery A, Sternlieb B, Garet D. Yoga for cancer patients and survivors. Cancer Control. 2005;12(3):165–171.
129. Morrow GR, Morrell C. Behavioral treatment for the anticipatory nausea and vomiting induced by cancer chemotherapy. N Engl J Med. 1982;307:1476–1480.
132. Lang EV, Berbaum KS, Faintuch S, et al. Adjunctive self-hypnotic relaxation for outpatient medical procedures: a prospective randomized trial with women undergoing large core breast biopsy. Pain. 2006;126(1-3):155–164.
133. Montgomery GH, Bovbjerg DH, Schnur JB, et al. A randomized clinical trial of a brief hypnosis intervention to control side effects in breast surgery patients. J Natl Cancer Inst. 2007;99(17):1304–1312.
139. Russell NC, Sumler SS, Beinhorn CM, Frenkel MA. Role of massage therapy in cancer care. J Altern Complement Med. 2008;14(2):209–214.
140. Myers CD. The value of massage therapy in cancer care. In: Cohnen L, Frenkel M, eds. Integrative Medicine in Oncology: Hematology/Oncology Clinics of North America. 2008.
145. Ezzo J, Vickers A, Richardson MA, et al. Acupuncture-point stimulation for chemotherapy-induced nausea and vomiting. J Clin Oncol. 2005;23(28):7188–7198.
152. Filshie J, Hester J. Guidelines for providing acupuncture treatment for cancer patients—a peer-reviewed sample policy document. Acupunct Med. 2006;24(4):172–182.
153. Lewith G, Berman B, Cummings M, Filshie J, Fisher P, White A. Systematic review of systematic reviews of acupuncture published 1996–2005. [comment]. Clin Med. 2006;6(6):623–625.
156. Lu W, Dean-Clower E, Doherty-Gilman A, Rosenthal D. The value of acupuncture in cancer care. In: Cohen L, Frenkel M, eds. Integrative Medicine in Oncology: Hematology/Oncology Clinics of North America. 2008.
157. Schmidt K, Ernst E. Assessing websites on complementary and alternative medicine for cancer. Ann Oncol. 2004;15:733–742.
177. Cohen L, Markman M. Integrative Oncology: Incorporating Complementary Medicine into Conventional Cancer Care. Totowa: Humana Press; 2008.
178. Frenkel M, Cohen L. Incorporating complementary and integrative medicine in a comprehensive cancer center. In: Cohen L, Frenkel M, eds. Integrative Medicine in Oncology: Hematology/Oncology Clinics of North America. 2008.

68 Palliative Care

Cardinale B. Smith, MD ■ Gabrielle R. Goldberg, MD ■ Diane E. Meier, MD

Palliative Care

Palliative care is medical care focused on relief of suffering and support for the best possible quality of life for patients facing serious, life-threatening illness and their families. It aims to identify and address the physical, psychological, and practical burdens of illness.[1] Palliative care is delivered simultaneously with all appropriate curative and life-prolonging interventions. Palliative care practitioners provide assessment and treatment of pain and other symptoms; employ communication skills with patients, families, and colleagues; support complex medical decision making and goal setting based on identifying and respecting patient wishes and goals; promote medically informed care coordination, continuity, and practical support for patients, family caregivers, and professional colleagues across healthcare settings and through the trajectory of an illness.[1] Palliative care in cancer patients should begin at the time of diagnosis. The emphasis of care will vary over the course of illness, with anti-cancer therapy provided concomitantly with supportive care and symptom management. For many patients, antineoplastic therapy and symptom management will be provided with the expectation of cure. For the remainder of patients the focus of care will shift from primarily antineoplastic therapy to solely supportive care and symptom management as cancer progresses. Palliative care specialists provide care with an interdisciplinary team consisting of physicians, nurses, social workers, psychologists, pharmacists, chaplains, and other professionals as necessary. Each discipline brings a unique set of skills which together provide coordinated patient and family centered care. The clinical provision of palliative care can be psychologically and emotionally draining; practice as a team serves as an outlet for shared burden and professional self-care.[1]

History of Palliative Care

Palliative care evolved out of the hospice movement. The modern hospice is a relatively recent concept that originated and gained momentum in the United Kingdom after the founding of St. Christopher's Hospice in 1967 by Dame Cicely Saunders. Dame Saunders's goal was to provide compassionate care for the dying by developing an interdisciplinary approach to care acknowledging that pain and suffering are not only physical, but also includes psychological, spiritual and social components.

The need for medical care focused on the total care of patients and families was highlighted in the 1990s by the Study to Understand Prognoses and Preferences for Outcomes and Risks for Treatment (SUPPORT) trial.[2] The SUPPORT trial, a pivotal two phase study which enrolled nearly 10,000 patients from 1989 to 1994 at five major U.S. hospitals, revealed serious limitations in providing care for patients with life-threatening illness. The trial demonstrated that patient and family communication with healthcare professionals at the end-of life was poor with less than 50% of physicians aware that their patients preferred a do-not-resuscitate order (DNR), that 46% of DNR orders were written within 2 days of death, and that 50% of patients, the majority with advanced cancer, reported moderate to severe pain in the last 3 days of life.[2]

Palliative care has had a rapid growth in the last two decades in response to the increasing number of patients living with serious, chronic conditions and as a result of a demand for high-quality symptom control, coordination of care across settings and advanced care planning. In 1998, the American Society of Clinical Oncology (ASCO) published a consensus statement on providing quality cancer care and stated that to do so requires effective pain management, including the use of opioid analgesics and other supportive care, for conditions induced by cancer treatment or by the disease itself and when effective cancer therapy is no longer available, patients should have access to optimal palliative care and counseling with respect to end-of-life issues.[3] ASCO also recommends that optimal cancer treatment requires a multidisciplinary team that should include palliative care specialists.

Although palliative care originates from the hospice movement, it has evolved over the last several decades. The initial WHO definition of palliative care in 1990 was "the active total care of patients whose disease is not responsive to curative treatment." In 2000 the WHO amended their definition: "Palliative care is an approach that improves the quality of life of patients and their families facing the problems associated with life-threatening illness, through the prevention and relief of suffering."[4] In 2006, palliative medicine became an official medical subspecialty of the American Board of Medical Specialties (ABMS) and the Accreditation Council for Graduate Medical Education (ACGME), receiving unprecedented support from 10 medical specialties.[5,6]

There are several core components involved in providing quality palliative care for oncology patients. These include the following:

- Whole patient assessment
- Effective communication
- Advanced care planning
- Symptom management
- Care at the end of life
- Grief and bereavement support

Whole Patient Assessment

The whole patient assessment involves a complete assessment of a patient's medical, psychological, spiritual and social history. It begins with the standard assessment of chief complaint, history of the present illness, past medical, surgical and social history and continues in exploring patients social and community support, impact of the cancer diagnosis and treatment on patients' quality of life, spiritual and social well-being, as well as patients' expectations of therapy and goals of care. The whole patient assessment improves patient physician communication and assists the physician in understanding potential barriers to patient compliance with treatment plans. This assessment is optimized by utilization of the interdisciplinary team to attend to all medical and psycho-social aspects of diagnosis, treatment and to assist with patient and family distress.

Communication

Effective communication is an important component of the oncologist–patient relationship and assists in providing the highest quality cancer care. In an ASCO survey conducted in 1998, approximately

60% of respondents indicated that they broke bad news to patients from 5 to 20 times per month and 14% of respondents reported they broke bad news more than 20 times per month.[7] When asked to identify the most difficult task, 55% ranked "how to be honest with the patient and not destroy hope" as most important, whereas 25% reported "dealing with the patient's emotions." Despite these challenges, less than 10% of respondents received formal training in breaking bad news and only 32% had the opportunity during training to regularly observe interviews where bad news was delivered. In a similar survey at the 2004 ASCO Annual Meeting, oncology fellows reported that they were more likely to have received observation and feedback on bone marrow biopsies than on end of life discussions.[8]

There are established guidelines for communicating bad news and addressing goals of care (Table 68-1).[9,10] Buckman describes the process of breaking bad news as an attempt to achieve four main goals: gathering information from the patient to elicit their readiness to hear the news; provide information in accordance with the patient's needs and desires; reduce the emotional impact and isolation experienced by the recipient of the bad news; and develop a treatment plan with the input of the patient.[9] These same four goals can also be applied to discussing goals of care. It is best to use open ended questions to help facilitate discussing goals of care. Examples include, "What are your most important hopes?," "What are your biggest fears?," and "What makes life worth living for you?"[10] Try to avoid language with unintended consequences such as "I think we should start pulling back," "Do you want us to do everything possible?," and "There's nothing more we can do for you."[10] Instead, try using language like "We will concentrate on improving your quality of life and minimizing your symptoms," "I want to give you the best care possible," and "Let's discuss what we can do to meet your goal of …." Once the goals of care are established, it becomes much easier to construct a plan of care centered on those preferences.

Table 68-1 Protocol for Breaking Bad News and Addressing Goals of Care

Recommendation	Comments
Create the proper setting	• Prior to the meeting determine the most appropriate participants (family members, and other healthcare providers). • Allow adequate time. • Determine what to say prior to the meeting.
Clarify what the patient and family already know	• "What have you been told about your medical situation so far?" • This allows you to correct any misinformation and tailor the conversation based on their prior knowledge.
Explore hopes and expectations of patient and family	• Allows you to distinguish between attainable and unattainable goals.
Suggest realistic goals	• Suggest attainable goals based on the present clinical scenario and how they can best be achieved. • Review appropriateness of disease-modifying treatments. • Try to explain using simple language why unrealistic goals can not be met.
Use empathic responses	• Very important to allow silence and to listen. • Let patient and family express emotions. • Once emotions are expressed use a connector such as "I can see how upsetting this is to you."
Make a plan and follow through	• Summarize the plan to ensure that your interpretation of the conversation and decisions is in concordance with patient and family and how the plan of care will meet their goals. • Make a plan for continued follow-up. • Inform the patient and family how to contact you if they have further questions or concerns. • Continue to review and revise the plan as needed.

Source: Adapted from Refs. 9 and 10.

Goals of Care

Once the patients' goals of care are established, they should be documented in the form of advanced directives. It is important for every cancer patient to have advanced directives to help avoid confusion and conflict, to prepare for future medical care and to ensure that the patients' wishes will be followed. Advanced directives include a durable power of attorney for health care or health care proxy and living wills. It is important that the patient communicate with their proxy about wishes for medical treatment. These discussions should focus on the use of artificial nutrition and hydration as well as the desire for life-sustaining treatments.

Symptom Management

Patients with cancer experience many physical and psychosocial symptoms either as a consequence of therapy or as a result of advanced disease. The essential components of symptom management include: (1) routine and repeated formal assessment, (2) expertise in prescribing medications, including the safe use of opioid analgesics, adjuvant approaches to pain management, and management of a wide range of other common and distressing symptoms and syndromes, and (3) skillful management of treatment side effects.[11] Currently there is no gold standard for symptom assessment in palliative care. One of the most commonly used instruments to assess for the presence of multiple symptoms is the Edmonton Symptom Assessment System (ESAS) which consists of nine visual analog scales (VAS) or numerical rating scales (NRS) that evaluate a combination of the most common physical and psychological symptoms.[12] The ESAS has been validated for internal consistency, criterion validity, and concurrent validity.[13] The most common symptom experienced by cancer patients is pain,[14] the management of which is thoroughly detailed elsewhere. The most frequent non-pain symptoms are constipation, nausea and vomiting, anorexia/cachexia, fatigue, dyspnea, delirium, and anxiety.[14] The management of these symptoms will be discussed in the following sections.

Constipation

Constipation is defined as the infrequent and difficult passage of hard stool. There are many factors that contribute to constipation. It is a common cause of morbidity in the palliative care setting, occurring in approximately 40% of patients referred to a palliative care service,[14] and affects more than 95% of patients who are treated with opioids for cancer related pain.[15] The two most common etiologies are related to the side effects of opioids and the effects of progressive disease. Severe constipation can lead to bowel obstruction, perforation and can be a cause of severe morbidity. In patients who are neutropenic, severe constipation can lead to bacterial transfer across the colon, resulting in bacteremia and potentially sepsis. The Rome criteria[16] defines constipation as the presence of two or more of the following symptoms for at least 3 months:

- Straining at least 25% of the time
- Hard stools at least 25% of the time
- Incomplete evacuation at least 25% of the time
- ≤2 bowel movements per week

Assessment of constipation should involve a history of the patient's bowel pattern, fluid intake, recent dietary changes, review of current medications and a thorough physical examination, including a rectal exam–with caution in patients with neutropenia. In addition, abdominal radiography can be performed to look for the presence of stool if the diagnosis remains unclear.

Constipation can be managed with non-pharmacologic measures as well as pharmacologic interventions. Non-pharmacologic measures include increasing fluid intake if possible and regular toileting as colonic activity is highest early in the morning, after walking, and 30 min after meals. Pharmacologic interventions for the management of constipation may be administered orally or rectally and are summarized in Table 68-2. There is no single correct management approach to laxative prescribing. There have been a small number of randomized studies with conflicting results.[17-19] Initial regimens often include a stool-softening agent, such as docusate, combined with a stimulant, such as senna, given once or twice per day and titrated according to response.[20] Whichever bowel regimen is initiated should be individualized and titrated to response. It is important to note that the best treatment of constipation is prevention. A prophylactic bowel regimen should be initiated at the time opioids are initially prescribed and should be continued for as long as the patient remains on opioids.

Nausea and Vomiting

Nausea and vomiting is reported to affect between 40% and 70% of patients with cancer.[21,22] Nausea and vomiting can cause substantial psychological distress for patients and families and impact overall quality of life.[23] Nausea is subjective and is defined as an unpleasant sensation of the need to vomit and can be associated with autonomic symptoms, including pallor, cold sweats, tachycardia and diarrhea. Vomiting is the forceful discharge of gastric contents via the mouth resulting from the contraction of the abdominal musculature and diaphragm. The pathophysiology of nausea and vomiting is complex and involves four pathways which when stimulated can induce nausea and vomiting[24-26]:

1. *Chemoreceptor trigger zone (CTZ)*: Functionally outside the blood-brain barrier, the CTZ is exposed to toxins in the bloodstream and cerebrospinal fluid that can stimulate vomiting. The principal receptors are dopamine (D2), serotonin (5HT3), acetylcholine (ACH) and opioids (MU2).
2. *Cortex*: Thought to cause nausea due to input from the 5 senses, anxiety, meningeal irritation, and increased intracranial pressure, the cortex supplies many afferents to the vomiting center in the brainstem. The principal receptors are ACH and histamine type 1 (H1).
3. *Peripheral pathways*: The main emetogenic input from the periphery, these are triggered by mechanoreceptors and chemoreceptors in the GI tract, serosa, and viscera and transmitted via the D2 receptors of the stomach wall, and 5HT3 receptors.
4. *Vestibular system*: Mediated through labyrinthine inputs into the vomiting center via the vestibulocochlear nerve. Nausea and vomiting are triggered by motion. The principal receptors are H1 and ACH.

The etiology of nausea and vomiting are varied, but it is important to determine the exact cause in order to select targeted and effective treatment. The most common etiologies in patients with cancer are chemotherapy induced nausea and vomiting (CINV), opioid-induced, bowel obstruction and

Table 68-2 ■ Laxatives Commonly Used to Treat Constipation

Type of Laxative	Preparation	Starting Dose	Mechanism of Action	Comments
Oral:				
Lubricant	Mineral oil	5-10 mL/day	Lubricates stool surface, allows easier passage	Adverse effects include lipoid pneumonia, leakage of oily fecal material. 255 paraffin and magnesium hydroxide considered safest.
Surfactant	Docusate sodium	100-300 mg in divided doses	Ionic detergent softens stool by increasing water penetration	Can be used alone or in combination with senna or bisacodyl.
Bulk-forming agents	Methycellulose, bran, psyllium	Bran 8 g daily Others 3-4 g daily	Increases stool bulk, stimulating peristalsis	Good for mild constipation. Caution as needs to be taken with at least 200-300 mL of water. May precipitate obstruction in a debilitated patient by forming a viscous mass. May cause flatulence and bloating.
Osmotic (poorly absorbed sugars)	Lactulose	15 mL daily	Retention of water in the lumen via osmotic effects	Sweet taste which may not be well tolerated. Bloating, abdominal cramping and flatulence are common.
Saline	Magnesium hydroxide Sodium bisposphonate	2-4 g daily	High osmolarity compounds causes retention of water in the lumen throughout the entire gut. Directly stimulates peristalsis.	Strong cathartic. Mostly used as a bowel prep for endoscopic procedures. May alter fluid and electrolyte imbalance. Caution in patients with heart failure or renal insufficiency.
Anthraquinones	Senna	187 mg daily	Direct stimulation of myenteric plexus causing induction of peristalsis.	Often combined with docusate. May cause abdominal cramping. Do not use if obstruction is suspected.
Polyphenolic	Bisacodyl	10 mg daily	Stimulates secretion and motility of small intestine and colon.	May cause abdominal cramping.
Rectal:				
Lubricant	Mineral oil enema	One enema	Used as retention enema to allow evacuation or manual removal of impacted stool	Efficacy is dependent on ability to retain the oil.
Osmotic	Glycerin	One suppository	Softens stools via osmosis	
Saline	Sodium phosphate	One enema or suppository	Releases bound water from feces May stimulate rectal or distal colonic peristalsis.	May alter fluid and electrolyte balance. Caution in patients with heart failure or renal insufficiency.
Polyphenolic	Bisacodyl	10 mg suppository	Promotes colonic peristalsis	Activity depends on bisacodyl reaching the rectal wall.

constipation. A complete history including, current medications, previous or current radiation therapy, the type of malignancy and its site of disease, including location of metastases and psychological state, can help establish a potential etiology. A physical exam should include an eye exam looking for the presence of papilledema indicating raised intracranial pressure, an abdominal examination, as well as a rectal examination to rule out fecal impaction. Laboratory tests include evaluation of liver function, renal function, serum electrolytes glucose, and calcium levels as metabolic abnormalities are a cause of nausea and vomiting. Abdominal x-rays may show bowel obstruction or fecal impaction. CT scan or MRI of the brain is indicated when brain metastasis is suspected.

Once the likely etiology of nausea and vomiting is identified, directed therapy can begin. Due to the lack of well-designed studies, there is a paucity of data and current management is based on expert opinion. The most commonly used approach is based on identifying the etiology and administering the most potent antagonist targeted towards the implicated receptors. This strategy has been shown to be effective in up to 80-90% of patients.[27,28] Some practitioners recommend starting an empirical antiemetic regimen, typically with a D2 antagonist, regardless of the presumed etiology.[29-33] No direct comparisons currently exist between mechanism-based and empirical therapy. Therapy should consist of non-pharmacologic and pharmacologic measures aimed at alleviating the cause of the symptoms. Non-pharmacologic measures include avoiding strong smells or other nausea triggers, eating small, frequent meals, limiting oral intake during periods of extreme emesis,[34] relaxation techniques,[35] acupuncture and acupressure.[36] Progressive muscle relaxation and guided mental imagery during periods of chemotherapy have also shown beneficial effects.[35,38-39] The most commonly used antiemetics worldwide are metoclopramide, dexamethasone, haloperidol, hyoscine butylbromide, and cyclizine.[40] Antiemetics are available in the form of pills, orally dissolvable tablets, intravenous infusion, rectal suppositories, and subcutaneous infusions. Thought should be given to selection of the appropriate route of administration of the antiemetic to ensure maximum efficacy. A list of antiemetics, routes of administration and their properties can be found in Table 68-3.

Anorexia/Cachexia Syndrome (ACS)

Cachexia is the involuntary loss of more than 10% of premorbid weight and is a marker for poor prognosis.[41] It is associated with anorexia which is defined as a loss of appetite and reduced caloric intake. Anorexia/cachexia syndrome (ACS) is characterized by disproportionate and excessive loss of lean body mass. ACS may occur in up to 80% of patients with advanced cancer.[42] The mechanisms that lead to ACS are complex. Possible contributing mechanisms include immune alterations resulting in the production of pro-inflammatory cytokines, metabolic alterations with synthesis of acute phase proteins in the liver at the expense of muscle protein,

Table 68-3 Antiemetics Commonly Used to Treat Nausea and Vomiting

Receptor Site of Action	Drug Name	Dosage/Route	Adverse Effects
Dopamine antagonists (D_2)	Chlorpromazine	10–25 mg PO every 4 h, 25–50 mg IM/IV every 4 h, or 50–100 mg rectally every 6 h 0.5–2 mg PO, IV/SQ every 6 h (up to 20 mg/day)	Dystonia, akathisia, sedation and postural hypotension
	Haldol	10–20 mg PO, IV/SQ before meals and at bedtime or every 6 h	Dystonia and akathisia
	Metoclopramide	10–20 mg PO every 6 h, 5–10 mg IV every 6 h or 25 mg rectally every 6 h	Dystonia, akathisia, abdominal cramping in obstruction
	Prochlorperazine	250 mg PO every 6–8 h or 200 mg rectally every 6–8 h	Dystonia, akathisia, and sedation
	Trimethobenzamine		Dystonia, akathisia, and sedation
Histamine antagonists (H_1)	Cyclizine	25–50 mg PO/SQ or rectally every 8 h	Dry mouth, sedation, skin irritation at SQ sites may occur
	Diphenhydramine	25–50 mg PO/IV/SQ every 6 h	
	Promethazine (also has activity on D_2 and ACH)	12.5–25 mg PO,IV every 4–6 h or 25 mg rectally every 6 h	Sedation, dry mouth, and urinary retention Dry mouth, dystonia, akathisia, and sedation
Acetylcholine antagonists (ACH)	Glycopyrrolate	0.2 mg IV/SQ every 4–6 h	Dry mouth, blurred vision, confusion, urinary retention, ileus
	Hycosamine	0.125–0.25 mg PO/SL every 4 h or 0.25–0.5 mg IV/SQ every 4 h	Dry mouth, blurred vision, confusion, urinary retention, ileus
	Scopolamine	0.1–0.4 mg IV/SQ every 4 h or 1.5 mg transdermal patch every 72 h	Dry mouth, blurred vision, confusion, urinary retention, ileus
Serotonin antagonists ($5HT_3$)	Dolasetron	100 mg PO/IV daily	Headache, diarrhea
	Granisetron	1 mg PO daily or twice a day or 1 mg IV daily	Headache, constipation, weakness
	Ondansetron	4–8 mg PO/IV or dissolvable tablet IV every 4–8 h	Headache, constipation, weakness
		0.25 mg IV on day 1 of chemotherapy[a]	Headache, constipation
	Palonosetron		
Substance P antagonist	Aprepitant	125 mg PO or 115 mg IV on day 1 of chemotherapy 80 mg PO on days 2 and 3[a]	Headache, infusion site pain
Other			
Corticosteroids	Dexamethasone	2–10 mg PO/IV every 6 h	Hyperglycemia, GI Bleeding, insomnia, psychosis
Cannabinoids	Dronabinol	2–20 mg PO daily in divided doses	Dizziness, euphoria in the young and dysphoria in the elderly, paranoid reaction, somnolence
Benzodiazepines	Lorazepam[b]		
Somatostatin analogue	Octreotide[c]	0.5–2 mg PO/IV every 4-6 h 100 mcg every 8–12 h IV/SQ or 100 mcG/h as continuous IV infusion	Sedation, respiratory depression Bradycardia, headache, malaise, hyperglycemia

[a]Have not been shown to be effective in terminating nausea or vomiting once it occurs and should not be used for this purpose.
[b]Best used for anticipatory nausea and vomiting.
[c]Efficacious for patients with bowel obstruction.

increased proteolysis, lipolysis, insulin resistance, decreased lipogenesis, and neuroendocrine alterations.[42] ACS is usually a marker of disease progression. In a multicenter retrospective review of 3047 cancer patients enrolled on clinical trials from the Eastern Cooperative Oncology Group, weight loss of more than 5% of premorbid weight prior to the initiation of chemotherapy was predictive of early mortality.[41] Weight loss was independent of disease stage, tumor histology, and patient performance status in its predictive value.[41]

In patients with cancer there are several factors other than ACS that can lead to anorexia and weight loss. It is important to identify and treat potentially reversible causes. Secondary causes include malnutrition due to impaired oral intake and impaired gastrointestinal absorption, loss of muscle mass due to prolonged inactivity as a result of deconditioning, and other catabolic states such as infections.

Management of this syndrome should first focus on trying to treat any of the contributing secondary causes. Because anorexia is a prevalent and distressing symptom suffered by most cancer patients, the basis of pharmacologic treatment has focused on alleviating this symptom. The two classes of drugs that have been shown to be effective in phase III clinical trials are corticosteroids and progestational agents.[44-50] These drugs do not appear to improve survival, but may improve quality of life. Corticosteroids, usually in the form of dexamethasone at a dose of 4 mg/day (although doses of 2-20 mg/day can be used), has been shown to alleviate cancer anorexia on a short-term basis.[44] This finding has been replicated by other studies and both prednisolone and methylprednisolone have been shown to be effective.[45,46] As the duration of appetite stimulation is short lived, and the side effects increase over time, it is most useful for patients with a life expectancy of less than 6 weeks. Megestrol acetate has been shown to result in dose dependent improvements in appetite which usually occur in about 1 week. Improvement in overall well being has been demonstrated in more than 60% of patients starting at doses of 160 mg per day.[47-49] The optimal dosing for weight gain appears to be between 480 and 800 mg per day. Effects are seen after several weeks in only 25% of patients.[47] It is important to start at a lower dose and titrate upwards as adverse events are dose related.[50] Adverse events include deep vein thrombosis, especially in those concomitantly on chemotherapy,[51] edema, hyperglycemia and elevated liver enzymes. Cannabinoids, in its synthetic form of dronabinol, may have some limited effects on improving appetite, but does not contribute to significant weight gain.[52,53] In a randomized trial comparing dronabinol to megestrol acetate significantly more patients had improvement in appetite and weight gain with megestrol acetate.[54] Combined therapy with both megestrol acetate and dronabinol had no benefit beyond that obtained with megestrol acetate alone. Adverse events with dronabinol include sedation, confusion and perceptual disturbances.

Fatigue

Fatigue is a subjective sensation, which manifests with a wide array of impaired physical, cognitive, and affective functioning.[55] Major manifestations include: easy tiring, reduced capacity to maintain performance, and generalized weakness and mental fatigue, that is defined as the presence of impaired concentration and loss of memory.[56] Cancer-related fatigue (CRF) occurs as a result of cancer, cancer treatment and is commonly seen in cancer survivors.[57] The prevalence of CRF, which varies greatly depending on the diagnostic criteria used and the patient populations studied, is reported to be 60-90%.[58] Assessment should involve evaluation of the severity of fatigue, level of interference with everyday life, associated psychological problems and possible underlying causes (Table 68-4). Currently there is no "gold standard" tool for the assessment of CRF. The National Comprehensive Cancer Network (NCCN) suggests the use of the numeric Brief Fatigue Inventory, with 0 representing no fatigue, and 10 the worst imaginable fatigue.[59] Mild, moderate, and severe fatigue are represented by scores of 1 to 3, 4 to 6, and 7 to 10, respectively. A decrease in physical functioning occurs when fatigue levels are 7 or higher.[60]

Management of CRF can be directed towards addressing contributing factors or using non-pharmacologic and pharmacologic based approaches. Non-pharmacologic measures include conserving energy for important tasks, rearranging schedules within the day depending on fatigue patterns and the use of exercise programs which have been shown to be effective in the treatment of CRF.[61-64] Most importantly patients and their families should be educated about the nature of fatigue and outcomes so they can set realistic expectations.

Pharmacologic treatments that have been shown to have some improvement in CRF include the use of psychostimulants and corticosteroids. The most commonly used psychostimulant in the treatment of CRF is methylphenidate. A meta-analysis performed to assess the efficacy of pharmacologic agents for the management of CRF showed a small but significant improvement with methylphenidate over placebo; however, it was not possible to determine optimal dosing.[65] In clinical practice starting doses are usually 2.5-5 mg taken at 8 A.M. and noon with a maximum dose of 20 mg per day. Methylphenidate has also been used in cancer patients to treat opioid induced somnolence, reduce pain intensity, treat depression, and improve cognition.[66] Adverse events related to methylphenidate include tremulousness, tachycardia and insomnia. Modafinil, which is licensed for the treatment of narcolepsy, is a novel psychostimulant that has been shown in a pilot study to improve CRF in patients with primary brain tumors.[67] Corticosteroids have been shown to be beneficial for some patients with CRF, but, side effects limit their long-term use.[45] Steroids may be most helpful for patients with CRF who are in the terminal phase of advanced cancer.

Table 68-4 Contributors to Fatigue in Cancer Patients

Anemia	Hypoxia
Pain	Metabolic abnormalities
Infection	Endocrine abnormalities
Dehydration	• Hypothyroidism
Cancer therapy	Medications
• Chemotherapy	
• Radiation therapy	
• Surgery	

Dyspnea

Dyspnea is the awareness of an uncomfortable or unpleasant sensation of breathing. The prevalence of dyspnea varies greatly and ranges from 21% to 79% depending on primary disease site, stage of disease, and location of metastasis.[69-71] Dyspnea most commonly occurs in those with primary lung cancer or pulmonary metastasis[70] but also occurs in cancer patients without direct cardiac or pulmonary involvement. The sensation of dyspnea is a subjective experience with numerous etiologies. The presence of tachypnea and hypoxia does not adequately reflect the severity of symptoms felt by the patient.[71] It is not uncommon that patients with moderate to severe tachypnea will not complain of dyspnea. In contrast, patients who are not tachypneic may report severe dyspnea. It is therefore of utmost importance that assessment be based on patient report. The goal of treatment is symptomatic relief of the patient's expression of dyspnea, rather than the correction of objective variables (tachypnea, low oxygen saturation).

The first step in management is to identify the underlying cause. The causes of dyspnea other than those related directly to the cancer itself are shown in Table 68-5 along with potential treatment modalities. The most common modali-

Table 68-5 Treatment of Specific Causes of Dyspnea

Cause of Dyspnea	Potential Treatment
Airway obstruction	Radiation therapy Interventional bronchoscopic procedures • Endobronchial stents • Photodynamic therapy • Cryotherapy
Anemia	Transfusion
Anxiety	Benzodiazepines • Lorazepam 0.5-2 mg PO every 4-6 h • Diazepam 5-10 mg PO/IV every 6-8 h • Clonazepam 0.25-2 mg PO every 12 h
Ascites	Paracentesis
Bronchospasm	Bronchodilators
COPD exacerbation	Oxygen, bronchodilators, steroids (inhaled, PO, IV)
Pericardial effusion	Pericardiocentesis, Pericardial window
Pleural effusion	Thoracentesis
Pneumonia	Antibiotics, antivirals or antifungals
Pneumothorax	Chest tube
Pulmonary edema	Diuretics
Pulmonary embolus	Anticoagulation
Treatment related • radiation pneumonitis • pulmonary toxicity from chemotherapy	Corticosteroids

ties used to treat dyspnea include oxygen therapy and opioids. Three randomized controlled crossover studies have evaluated the use of oxygen (4 or 5 L/min) vs air in advanced cancer patients with dyspnea.[72-74] Two of these studies evaluated patients with hypoxemia on room air and found that oxygen therapy was more beneficial.[72,73] The third evaluated nonhypoxemic cancer patients and found that there was no difference between oxygen therapy and air in reducing the intensity of dyspnea.[74] Opioids are the pharmacologic treatment of choice in the management of dyspnea. Several randomized controlled trials in cancer patients with dyspnea have demonstrated their benefit.[75,76] In opioid-naive patients, a starting dose of morphine sulfate 2.5-5 mg orally or its equivalent intravenously or subcutaneously every four hours can be effective. In those patients already on opioid therapy an increase of 25% in the baseline dose may provide relief.[77]

Delirium

Delirium is a transient syndrome of disordered attention characterized by an acute onset and fluctuating course. The essential core criteria are derived from the *Diagnostic and Statistical Manual for Mental Illness* (DSM-IV). The three subtypes of delirium are hyperactive, hypoactive and mixed. The prevalence rates for delirium in patients with cancer admitted to acute care hospitals are varied and range from 28-48%[78-80] with 85-90% of all patients experiencing delirium in the hours or days before death.[80-82] There are several assessment tools available to aid in the diagnosis of delirium including the Memorial Delirium Assessment scale (MDAS)[83] and the Confusion Assessment Method (CAM).[84] The MDAS consists of a 10-item, four-point observer-rated scale that was designed to assess the severity of delirium. It includes assessment of disturbances in awareness, orientation, short-term memory, digit span, attention, organized thinking, perception, delusions, psychomotor activity, and arousal in a way that reflects all the main diagnostic criteria according to the DSM. The CAM is a diagnostic tool used to apply the DSM criteria and consists of an algorithm that requires the presence of an acute onset fluctuating course, inattention, and either disorganized thinking or altered level of consciousness. Many factors can contribute to the development of delirium (Table 68-6).

Treatment should be aimed at the symptoms of delirium while simultaneously attempting to treat reversible causes. Although delirium is most often associated with the last hours to days of life, in some episodes it may be reversible with therapeutic intervention.[85,86] Neuroleptic agents are the mainstay of pharmacologic treatment as they are effective in both hypoactive and hyperactive delirium. Of these agents, haloperidol is the agent of choice as it has lower sedating properties, less anticholinergic and cardiovascular effects. Delirium in patients with cancer commonly requires the use of more than one agent[87] (Table 68-7).

Table 68-6 Factors Contributing to the Onset of Delirium in Patients With Cancer

Drugs
• Opioids
• Anticholinergics
• Benzodiazepines
• Alcohol withdrawal or intoxication
• Chemotherapy (methotrexate, cisplatin, aspariginase, 5-FU, ifosfamide)
• Corticosteroids
Infection
Dehydration
Metabolic abnormalities
• Hypercalcemia
• Hypo- or hypernatremia
• Renal failure
Endocrine abnormalities
• Hypothyroidism
• Hypo- or hyperglycemia
Paraneoplastic syndromes
CNS tumors or metastasis

The Terminal Phase

Death is a natural process that will occur for every patient. About 10% of people will die suddenly and unexpectedly while the other 90% die after a period of illness with gradual deterioration until an active dying phase occurs signifying the end of life.[88] There are "two roads to death,"[89] the usual road which occurs in most patients and presents as decreasing level of consciousness that leads to coma and death, and the difficult road. The difficult road is marked by terminal delirium which can manifest as restlessness, confusion, and agitation; it can be a source of great distress for patients, family, and loved ones.[89] The exact prevalence of symptoms encountered in the terminal phase varies among different studies (Table 68-8). The most common symptoms reported by families in the last week of life are fatigue, dyspnea, and dry mouth, while the most distressing are fatigue, dyspnea, and pain.[90] It is important for families to know what to expect when the patient is imminently dying. The Clinical Practice Guidelines for Quality Palliative Care emphasize that families should be educated regarding the signs and symptoms of approaching death in a manner that is developmentally, age, and culturally appropriate.[91] A variety of physiologic changes occur in the last hours to days of life and the following is a summary of the most common changes that occur[92]:

1. **Weakness and fatigue:** Weakness and fatigue usually increase as the patient is approaching death. Patients will begin to spend all of their time in bed and will be less interested in participating in usual activities, including visiting with others.
2. **Decreased oral intake:** Most dying patients lose their appetite and stop drinking. Many caregivers interpret this as a patient "giving up" or "starving to death." It is important to explain to patients and their family members that there is a decreased need for food and drink during this phase. There is some evidence suggesting that prolonged anorexia is not uncomfortable. One study found that 97% of dying patients who stopped eating experienced no hunger or hunger only initially.[93] It has been proposed that terminal anorexia induces a ketosis that contributes to a sense of wellbeing and diminished discomfort and may in fact be beneficial to dying patients.[92,94] Two meta-analyses of studies of both parenteral[95] and enteral[96] nutrition in patients with metastatic cancer found that neither therapy resulted in an improvement in morbidity or mortality and actually resulted in an increased total complication rate. The evidence

Table 68-7 ■ Pharmacologic Therapy of Delirium

Drug Name	Dosage/Route	Comments
Haloperidol	0.5–5 mg PO/IV/IM/SC every 6–12 h	Most commonly used agent. Can prolong QT interval.
Chlorpromazine	12.5–50 mg PO/IV/IM every 8–12 h	Has similar efficacy to haloperidol, but more sedating, anticholinergic and hypotensive effects.
Lorazepam	0.5–2 mg PO/SL/IV every 4–8 h and titrate as needed	Most commonly used as a second agent in combination with haloperidol. Can also be used as a continuous infusion for refractory cases where deep sedation is needed. May worsen delirium in the elderly. Caution with liver failure.
Risperidone	Start at 0.5–1 mg/day PO and titrate up to 4–6 mg/day	In one study shown to have no differences in side effects when compared to haloperidol.[95] Limited use as only available in oral route.
Olanzapine	5 mg PO qhs and titrated to effect (max 20 mg/day)	Risk factors for a poor response to olanzapine in cancer patients are[87]: • Age >70 • History of dementia • CNS metastases • Hypoxia • Hypoactive delirium
Midazolam	1 mg/h IV and titrated to effect	Most commonly used for refractory cases where sedation is needed.

Table 68-8 ■ Commonly Encountered Symptoms in the Terminal Phase

	Coyle et al.[103]	Kutner et al.[104]	Conill et al.[105]
Estimated time until death	1 week	17 days	1 week
No. of patients	90	86	319
Symptoms (%)			
Anorexia	6	70	80
Confusion	57		68
Constipation	7		55
Dry mouth		75	70
Dyspnea	28	73	47
Fatigue	52	92	82
Nausea	13		13
Pain	34	82	30

with respect to hydration in dying patients is less straightforward with many differing expert opinions.[92,97-99] Some studies suggest that parenteral hydration prevents and treats some cases of terminal delirium[97,98,102] and others correlate dehydration with adverse symptoms such as thirst.[99-101] Still others believe that the data does not support a correlation between dehydration and symptoms and that rehydration does not improve patient comfort.[93,102] It is important that each individual patient be evaluated to determine the risk benefit ratio. Attention should be placed on minimizing the sense of thirst and maintaining patient comfort even when dehydration is present, with oral hygiene. This can be achieved by using lollipop sponges dipped in cold fluids such as water, a lemon flavored drink or sorbet.

3. **Respiratory changes:** Most commonly, breaths become shallow and frequent periods of apnea and/or Cheyne-Stokes respirations develop, and accessory respiratory muscle use becomes prominent. These breathing changes can be very distressing for family and caregivers, who may fear the patient is suffocating.[92] It is important to explain these changes as a natural part of the dying process. If patients' appear to be uncomfortable, the same principles as discussed previously for the treatment of dyspnea apply.
4. **Loss of ability to swallow:** With decreasing levels of consciousness, patients at the end of life often lose the ability to swallow. This results in the accumulation of saliva and respiratory tract secretions. This often manifests as a gurgling noise, often referred to as the "death rattle," and can cause severe distress for families. Once the ability to swallow is lost, all oral intakes should be stopped. The use of anticholinergic medications, such as scopolamine (can be given via transdermal route, IV or SC), glycopyrrolate (can be given IV or SC) or atropine ophthalmic drops (administered orally) may minimize or eliminate the gurgling and crackling sounds, and may be used prophylactically in the unconscious dying patient.
5. **Terminal delirium:** While reversible factors may be identified in up to half of cases, terminal delirium management typically focuses on symptom control with medications.[80] The same principles as discussed previously for the treatment of delirium apply (Table 68-7).

Medications should be reassessed to ensure the patient is taking only those that are essential to providing comfort. The least invasive route of administration should be used for the administration of medications to manage the patient's symptoms.

Grief and Bereavement

Bereavement is the state of loss as a consequence of death.[106] Grief is defined as the emotional response to loss and mourning, and often refers to social expressions associated with loss.[106] Several types of grief exist: anticipatory grief, uncomplicated grief and complicated grief. Anticipatory grief refers to the mourning that occurs in patients and families prior to death and is a way to facilitate the adjustment to bereavement. Uncomplicated grief is the most common type of grief reaction and is socially perceived as normal. Complicated grief involves the persistence of grief reactions over a long period of time and is characterized by an inability to return to the pre-loss level of functioning.[107] Palliative care provides grief and bereavement services to patients and their caregivers before, during and after death to help promote healthy grieving.

Caregivers report significant benefits of receiving comprehensive information to prepare them for the death of a loved one. In one study, preparation for life's end—life review, resolving conflicts, and saying goodbye was very important or extremely important in close to 90% of patients and their caregivers.[108] Despite this, about 25% of caregivers report that death of a loved one was unexpected, generally due to lack of preparedness by the primary treating physician.[109] Being unprepared for the death of a loved one is associated with greater depression, anxiety, and complicated grief.[110,111]

Both hospice and palliative care have been shown to provide effective pre-loss interventions for preventing complicated bereavement. These interventions are associated with a reduced risk of major depressive disorder in caregivers.[112] The multidisciplinary palliative care team including physicians, social workers, nurses, psychologists and chaplains performs a psychosocial assessment of the patient and caregiver in order to identify those that may be high risk for complicated grief. The palliative care team can provide basic practical help before death such as assisting with advanced directives, assistance with financial matters and encouraging individual medical care of the caregiver as well as providing assistance after death by offering counseling or referral to other support services.

Hospice

Hospice is a philosophy of care. The goal of hospice is to focus on maintaining the best quality of life rather than length of life in patients who have a life expectancy of 6 months or less. It is different from palliative care in that palliative care is given simultaneously with other curative and life-prolonging therapies. Hospice services have been available in the United States since 1974 and have been funded by Medicare as part of the Medicare hospice benefit since 1982.[113]

Hospice is the only Medicare benefit that includes medications, durable medical equipment, and continuous around-the-clock access to care and support. Bereavement services are also offered to family members after a patient's death. The Medicare hospice benefit covers all care related to the cancer diagnosis. The patient can still receive Medicare benefits for the treatment of other illnesses.

Most hospice care is delivered at home. It is also provided in other settings such as inpatient hospice facilities, nursing homes, assisted living facilities, and hospitals. It is estimated that approximately 36% of all people who died in the United States in 2006 were under the care of a hospice program and of all patients enrolled, 44% had a diagnosis of cancer.[114] In a study comparing survival of hospice to non-hospice patients, hospice care prolonged the lives of some terminally ill cancer patients.[115] The mean survival period was significantly longer for hospice patients with lung cancer (39 days longer) and pancreatic cancer (21 days), while marginally significant for colon cancer (33 days).[115]

Barriers to Providing Palliative Care

Despite the recognition of the importance of providing high-quality symptom control and end-of-life care to patients with cancer, many barriers to receiving palliative exist. Inadequate training of physicians in symptom management, communication skills, prognostication, and palliative care principles remain a major obstacle.[116-119] On average, nearly 16% of Medicare patients are being treated with chemotherapy within 2 weeks of their death, and 16% are being referred to hospice within 3 days of their death.[120] This trend appears to be significantly increasing over time.[120] Physicians tend to substantially overestimate, by a factor of 5, the survival of patients with advanced cancer.[121] Patients with metastatic cancer have been found to overestimate their survival, which may lead them to choose aggressive therapy rather than focusing on symptom control and maximizing quality of life.[122,123] This has been attributed to unrealistic expectations created by physicians[124] and poor patient-physician communication.[2] The unrealistic hope about longer survival may contribute to late referral for palliative and hospice care services. According to the National Hospice and Palliative Care Organization, of those patients admitted to hospice, 35% die within the first week.[114]

Summary

Palliative care is patient and family-centered interdisciplinary care that focuses on relieving suffering and providing the best quality of life for patients undergoing curative and life prolonging treatments as well as for patients in whom cancer specific treatments are no longer available. It is estimated that 38.7% of patients with cancer will die from their disease.[125] Increasing attention has been given to improvements in quality-of-life issues in oncology, for patients undergoing chemotherapy, patients at the end of life as well as cancer survivors. Prevalence of symptoms during cancer treatment can be substantial. Palliative care is an integral part of comprehensive cancer care. Palliative care is most effective when initiated at the time of diagnosis allowing for patients to be followed through the trajectory of illness. The oncologist plays a key role in discussing treatment options, curative or palliative, from the outset of the diagnosis. Assessing the patients' goals is equally as important. Patients should be made aware that receiving anticancer treatments does not preclude them from access to palliative care services. Increasing the emphasis on palliative care in oncology should improve patient outcomes and can diminish some of the oncologist's stress of caring for patients with serious and life-threatening illness.

As of 2008, nearly 1300 U.S. hospitals provide palliative care programs compared to just 632 programs in 2000.[126] Expansion of palliative medicine education is supported by the Liaison Committee on Medical Education (LCME), which has mandated medical school education in palliative medicine and the ACGME which requires oncology fellow training in palliative medicine. There is an array of internet based resources that provide physicians in practice with access to further information and education on palliative care (Table 68-9).

Table 68-9 Palliative Care Internet Resources

- www.epeconline.net: Education on Palliative and End of Life Care (EPEC): Comprehensive curriculum covering fundamentals of palliative medicine; free downloadable power point and teaching guides.
- www.eperc.mcw.edu: End of Life/Palliative Education Resource Center (EPERC): Medical educator resources for peer-reviewed palliative care teaching materials.
- www.StopPain.org: Department of Pain Medicine and Palliative Medicine at Beth Israel Medical Center: Clinical, educational, professional, and public resources.
- www.palliativedrugs.com: Extensive information on pharmacologic symptom management.
- www.aahpm.org: American Academy of Hospice and Palliative Medicine: Physician membership organization; board review courses, publications.
- www.hms.harvard.edu/cdi/pallcare: Center for Palliative Care at Harvard Medical School: Faculty development courses, other educational programs.
- www.nationalconsensusproject.org: National Consensus Project for Quality Palliative Care: Clinical practice guidelines.
- http://endoflife.stanford.edu/: Joint project of the US Veterans Administration and SUMMIT, Stanford University Medical School. Curriculum covering fundamentals of palliative medicine.
- www.capc.org: Center to Advance Palliative Care: Technical assistance for clinicians and hospitals seeking to establish or strengthen a palliative care program.

Selected References

The complete reference list can be found at www.CANCERMEDICINE8.com

1. Morrison RS, Meier DE. Clinical practice: palliative care. *N Engl J Med.* 2004;350: 2582–2590.
2. The SUPPORT Principal Investigators. A controlled trial to improve care for seriously ill hospitalized patients: the Study to Understand Prognoses and Preferences for Outcomes and Risks of Treatments (SUPPORT). *JAMA.* 1995;274:1591–1598.
3. ASCO-ESMO Consensus Statement on Quality Cancer Care. *J Clin Oncol.* 2006;24: 3498–3499.
7. American Society of Clinical Oncology. Cancer care during the last phase of life. *J Clin Oncol.* May 1998;16(5):1986–1996.
8. Buss MK, et al. A study of oncology fellows' training in end-of-life care. *J Support Oncol.* May 2007;5(5):237–242.
9. Baile W, Buckman R, Lenzi R, Glober G, Beale E, Kudelka A. SPIKES A six-step

protocol for delivering bad news: application to the patient with cancer. *Oncologist.* 2000;5:302–311.

10. The EPEC Project: Education on Palliative and End-of-life Care. (Accessed March 16, 2008, at http://www.epec.net)
11. Ripamonti C, Bruera E. Pain and symptom management in palliative care. *Cancer Control.* 1996;3:204–213.
12. Bruera E, Kuehn N, Miller MJ, Selmser P, Macmillan K. The Edmonton Symptom Assessment System (ESAS): a simple method for the assessment of palliative care patients. *J Palliat Care.* 1991;7:6–9.
14. Curtis EB, Krech R, Walsh TD. Common symptoms in patients with advanced cancer. *J Palliat Care.* 1991;7:25–29.
15. Mancini I, Bruera E. Constipation in advanced cancer patients. *Support Care Cancer.* 1998;6:356–364.
27. Stephenson J, Davies A. An assessment of etiology-based guidelines for the management of nausea and vomiting in patients with advanced cancer. *Support Care Cancer.* 2006;14(4):348–353.
29. Glare P, Pereira G, Kristjanson LJ, Stockler M, Tattersall M. Systematic review of the efficacy of antiemetics in the treatment of nausea in patients with far-advanced cancer. *Support Care Cancer.* 2004;12(6):432–440.
31. Bruera E, Belzile M, Neumann C, Harsanyi Z, Babul N, Darke A. A double blind crossover study of controlled release metoclopramide and placebo for the chronic nausea and dyspepsia of advanced cancer. *J Pain Symptom Manage.* 2000;19:427–435.
32. Mystakidou K, Befon S, Liossi C, Vlachos L. Comparison of the efficacy and safety of tropisetron, metoclopramide, and chlorpromazine in the treatment of emesis associated with far advanced cancer. *Cancer.* 1998;83:1214–1223.
35. Burish TG, Tope DM. Psychological techniques for controlling the adverse side effects of cancer chemotherapy: findings from a decade of research. *J Pain Symptom Manage.* 1992;7(5):287–301.
38. Contach PH. Use of nonpharmacological techniques to prevent chemotherapy induced nausea and vomiting. *Recent Results Cancer Res.* 1991;121:101–107.
39. Dickerson D. The 20 essential drugs in palliative care. *Eur J Palliat Care.* 1993;6:130–135.
40. DeWys WD, Begg D, Lavin PT. Prognostic effect of weight loss prior to chemotherapy in cancer patients. *Am J Med.* 1980;69:491–499.
43. Bruera E, Roca E, Cedaro L, et al. Action of oral methylprednisolone in terminal cancer patients: a prospective randomized double-blind study. *Cancer Treat Rep.* 1985;69:751.
44. Popiela T, Lucchi R, Giongo F. Methylprednisolone as an appetite stimulant in patients with cancer. *Eur J Cancer Clin Oncol.* 1989;25:1823.
47. Bruera E, Ernst S, Hagen N, et al. Effectiveness of megestrol acetate in patients with advanced cancer: a randomized, double-blind, crossover study. *Cancer Prev Control.* 1998;2:74–78.
52. Jatoi A, Windschitl HE, Loprinzi CL, et al. Dronabinol versus megestrol acetate versus combination therapy for cancer-associated anorexia: a North Central Cancer Treatment Group study. *J Clin Oncol.* 2002;20:567–573.
57. Mock V, Atkinson A, Barsevick A, et al. NCCN Practice Guidelines for Cancer-Related Fatigue. *Oncology.* 2000;14:151.
60. Mock V. Fatigue management: evidence and guidelines for practice. *Cancer.* 2001;92: 1699–1707.
62. Dimeo FC. Effects of exercise on cancer-related fatigue. *Cancer.* 2001;15(Suppl 6): 1689–1693.
63. Minton O, Stone P, Richardson A, Sharpe M, Hotopf M. Drug therapy for the management of cancer related fatigue. *Cochrane Database Syst Rev.* January 23, 2008;(1):CD006704.
64. Rozans M, Dreisbach A, Lertora JJ, Kahn MJ. Palliative uses of methylphenidate in patients with cancer: a review. *J Clin Oncol.* 2002;20:335–339.
70. Bruera E, Schoeller T, MacEachern T. Symptomatic benefit of supplemental oxygen in hypoxemic patients with terminal cancer: the use of the N of 1 randomized controlled trial. *J Pain Symptom Manage.* 1992;7:365–368.
71. Bruera E, Sweeney C, Willey J, et al. A randomized controlled trial of supplemental oxygen versus air in cancer patients with dyspnea. *Palliat Med.* 2003;17:659–663.
72. Abernethy AP, Currow DC, Frith P, Fazekas BS, McHugh A, Bui C. Randomised, double blind, placebo controlled crossover trial of sustained release morphine for the management of refractory dyspnoea. *BMJ.* September 6, 2003;327(7414):523–528.
74. Allard P, Lamontagne C, Bernard P, Tremblay C. How effective are supplementary doses of opioids for dyspnea in terminally ill cancer patients? A randomized continuous sequential clinical trial. *J Pain Symptom Manage.* April 1999;17(4): 256–265.
77. Lawlor PG, Gagnon B, Mancini IL, et al. Occurrence, causes, and outcome of delirium in patients with advanced cancer: a prospective study. *Arch Intern Med.* 2000;160:786–794.
81. Inouye SK, van Dyck CH, Alessi CA, et al. Clarifying confusion: the Confusion Assessment Method, a new method for detection of delirium. *Ann Intern Med.* 1990;113:941.
89. Ferris FD, von Gunten CF, Emanuel LL. Competency in end-of-life care: last hours of life. *J Palliat Med.* 2003;6:605–613.
90. McCann RM, Hall WJ, Groth-Juncker A. Comfort care for terminally ill patients: the appropriate use of nutrition and hydration. *JAMA.* 1994;272:1263–1266.
92. Koretz RL, Lipman TO, Klein S. AGA technical review on parenteral nutrition. *Gastroenterology.* 2001;121:970.
93. Koretz RL, Avenell A, Lipman TO, et al. Does enteral nutrition affect clinical outcome? A systematic review of the randomized trials. *Am J Gastroenterol* 2007;102:412.
96. Morita T, Tei Y, Tsunoda J, Inoue S, Chihara S. Determinants of the sensation of thirst in terminally ill cancer patients. *Supp Care Cancer.* 2001;9:177–186.
99. Coyle N, Adelhardt J, Foley KM, Portenoy RK. Character of terminal illness in the advanced cancer patient: pain and other symptoms during the last four weeks of life. *J Pain Symptom Manage.* 1990;5:83–93.
100. Kutner J, Bryant L, Beaty B, Fairclough D. Time course and characteristics of symptom distress and quality of life at the end of life. *J Pain Symptom Manage.* 2007;34:227–236.
101. Conill C, et al. Symptom prevalence in the last week of life. *J Pain Symptom Manage.* 1997;14:328–331.
104. Heyland DK, et al. for the Canadian Researchers, End-of-Life Network (CARENET). What matters most in end-of-life care: perceptions of seriously ill patients and their family members.
105. Teno JM, Clarridge BR, Casey V, et al. Family perspectives on end-of-life care at the last place of care. *JAMA.* 2004;291:88–93.
108. El-Jawahri A, Prigerson HG. Update on bereavement research evidence-based guidelines for the diagnosis and treatment of complicated bereavement. *J Palliat Med.* 2006;9:1188–1203.
111. Connor SR, Pyenson B, Fitch K, Spence C, Iwasaki K. Comparing hospice and non hospice patient survival among patients who die within a three-year window. *J Pain Symptom Manage.* March 2007;33(3):238–246.
116. Earle CC, Neville BA, Landrum MB, Ayanian JZ, Block SA, Weeks JC. Trends in the aggressiveness of cancer care near the end of life. *J Clin Oncol.* 2004;22:315–321.
117. Christakis NA, Lamont EB. Extent and determinants of error in doctors' prognoses in terminally ill patients: prospective cohort study. *BMJ.* 2000;320:469–473.
118. Weeks JC, Cook F, O'Day SJ, et al. Relationship between cancer patients' predictions of prognosis and other treatment preferences. *JAMA.* 1998;279:1709–1714.
120. Smith TJ, Swisher K. Telling the truth about terminal cancer. *JAMA.* 1998;279:1746–1748.

69 Management of Cancer Pain

Natalie Moryl, MD ▪ Alan C. Carver, MD ▪ Kathleen M. Foley, MD

The International Association for the Study of Pain defines pain as "an unpleasant sensory and emotional experience associated with actual or potential tissue damage or described in terms of such damage" (IASP, 1979).

The evaluation and treatment of pain is an essential skill for an oncologist who is responsible for pain management in most cancer patients, with only a minority of patients with complex pain syndromes or significant side effects of treatment requiring a referral to a pain specialist. The armamentarium of an oncologist includes current knowledge of the common pain syndromes in patients with cancer as well as their postulated neurophysiologic mechanisms,[1,2] methodologies to measure pain, pharmacokinetic, and pharmacodynamic data that correlate drug therapy with pain relief,[3-6] the psychological factors that contribute to and alter the pain complaint,[7-9] and management of side effects of the analgesics.

Pain management for the patient with cancer has, as its primary goal, effective symptom control for improving the patient's and caregiver's quality of life, and allowing patients to participate in diagnostic and therapeutic interventions.

Scope of the Problem

Cancer is a major world health problem.[10] Every year, about 17 million new cases of cancer are diagnosed; half in developing countries, and 5 million patients die from these diseases annually. In Europe alone nearly 2.9 million new cases of cancer and more than 1.7 million cancer deaths were registered in 2004. Prevalence data indicate that there are currently about 14 million people worldwide with cancer. Published reports indicate that between 30% and 50% of such cancer patients are in active therapy, and that 70-90% of patients with far-advanced disease suffer significant pain.[10] The prevalence of pain increases with disease progression and varies according to the primary site. Other factors correlating with pain include the presence of metastases, the proximity of tumor to neural structures, and patient psychosocial characteristics.

Several studies have demonstrated that cancer patients experience more than one type of pain.[11-14] In one survey, 81% of patients reported two or more distinct pain complaints, and 34% of these patients reported more than three types.[13] Patients' fear of cancer is directly related to their fear of severe pain.[15-17] Around 69% of patients with cancer who were surveyed, reported that severe pain from cancer might lead them to consider suicide, and 57% perceive death from cancer as painful.

In addition to the adverse effect on the patient's quality of life, pain is a common presentation of cancer progression and the importance of a comprehensive evaluation cannot be overstated. In a study of 276 consecutive pain consultations at Memorial Sloan-Kettering Cancer Center (MSKCC) the consultation identified a previously undiagnosed etiology for the pain in 64% of patients resulting in 18% of patients receiving previously unplanned radiotherapy, surgery, or chemotherapy.[18]

Barriers to Cancer Pain Management

Despite the publication of numerous national and international guidelines on how to manage cancer pain effectively,[6,10] undertreatment of pain remains a significant problem. Barriers include poor physician's training, inadequate knowledge of pharmacologic and other management strategies, and negative physician and patient attitudes toward opioid use for pain.[15]

The Study to Understand Prognoses and Preferences for Outcomes and Risks of Treatments (SUPPORT) showed that 50% of adults who die in hospital experience moderate to severe pain in the immediate period prior to death.[19] Over 20 years later, a large meta-analysis using 52 studies demonstrated that the prevalence of pain in cancer patients remains above 50%.[20] After curative treatment 33% of cancer patients had pain; among patients undergoing anticancer treatment 59% had pain; and among patients with advanced, metastatic, or terminal disease, 64% had pain. Of the patients with pain, more than one-third graded their pain as moderate or severe. Based on these and other data, pain remains a big component of quality cancer care that has not improved significantly despite increasing awareness among patients and clinicians.

In the past several years, there have been important developments in the legal status of palliative care. In 2001 and 2002, two cases in California held the undertreatment of pain to be elder abuse. In *Bergman v. Eden Medical Center*, a jury found that by failing to relieve the pain of a patient dying of lung cancer, a doctor committed reckless negligence and elder abuse. In *Tomlinson v. Bayberry Care Center*, a lung cancer patient died after 20 days of severe and undertreated pain. His family filed a civil suit, as well as complaints with the Medical Board of California, the California Department of Health, and the Center for Medicaid and Medical Services. The Medical Board filed charges against Mr. Tomlinson's physician, and the Department of Health sanctioned the facility where he died. When the civil suit was settled, the hospital agreed to implement a palliative care education program for its staff. In 2002, more state attorneys general became further involved in palliative care policy when the National Association of Attorneys General (NAAG) launched the End-of-Life Healthcare Project. The NAAG End-of-Life Healthcare Project has provided an invaluable resource for attorneys general working to improve palliative care for their constituents.

A large multicenter study to address knowledge and attitudes of physicians regarding cancer pain management demonstrated that 86% of physicians felt that the majority of patients were undermedicated.[21] Only 51% believed pain control in their own practice setting was good or very good, and 31% would wait until the patient's prognosis was 6 months or less before they would start maximal analgesia. The study also identified critical barriers to effective pain management (Table 69-1). In addition to the lack of education about palliative care, fear among providers that prescribing opioids, even when they are the only way to relieve a patient's pain, may result in regulatory and legal consequences. This educational deficit and fear remain among the main barriers

Table 69-1 **Barriers to Cancer Pain Management**

Inadequate assessment
Patient reluctance to report pain
Patient reluctance to take opioids
Physician reluctance to prescribe opioids
Inadequate staff knowledge about pain management
Nursing staff reluctance to give opioids
Excessive state regulation of analgesics

Source: Adapted from Ref. 21.

to successful pain management. Ongoing educational programs of the fundamental principles of cancer pain management need to be incorporated in the different phases of the clinicians' training, starting with medical school. Institutional commitments to provide improved pain management are essential in terms of education, resources, and establishing scientifically based guidelines.[22-24]

Mechanisms of Cancer Pain

Pain associated with cancer most commonly results from tumor infiltration of pain-sensitive structures such as bones, soft tissue, nerves, viscera, and blood vessels. Pain may also be caused by surgery, chemotherapy, or radiation therapy. Although the cause of the pain and the type of injury vary, the constellation of complex neurophysiologic phenomena of pain includes two broad categories, nociceptive pain, which include both somatic and visceral pain, and neuropathic pain.[25]

Neurophysiology of Pain

There are sensory receptors preferentially sensitive to noxious stimuli. These nociceptors are primary afferent nerves with peripheral terminals that respond differentially to noxious stimuli. These nociceptors serve two major functions, defined as transduction and transmission. A series of chemical, mechanical, or thermal factors can produce receptor activation, producing an electrochemical nerve impulse in the primary afferent. The information is then transmitted to the central nervous system (CNS), where pain perception occurs. Both myelinated and unmyelinated nociceptors convey pain sensation to the CNS. The myelinated nociceptor responds to noxious mechanical stimuli almost exclusively and has a rapid conduction over A delta fibers, causing a sharp stinging pain. Unmyelinated nociceptors are polymodal, responding to mechanical, thermal, and chemical stimuli, have a slower rate of conduction in a C fiber range, and are associated with a dull, burning, or aching pain. Once activated, pain is transmitted over A delta and C fibers and enters the spinal cord laterally, synapsing in the superficial dorsal horn to activate ascending nociceptive systems. Sensory transmission is then mediated through neuropeptides, substance P, calcitonin gene-related peptides, and the excitatory amino acids glutamate and aspartate.[26]

In general, unmyelinated nociceptors are not spontaneously active but become sensitized with any tissue injury. A variety of substances can mediate this sensitization, including potassium ions, adenosine triphosphate, bradykinin, prostaglandins (especially prostaglandin E2), and leukotrienes. The activation of the NMDA receptor and the α-amino-3-hydroxy-5-methyl-4-isoxazolepropionic acid (AMPA) receptor contribute to the establishment of central sensitization and neuronal windup that underlie hyperalgesia, allodynia (pain resulting from a nonpainful stimulus), and persistent pain states. Primary hyperalgesia or accentuated pain response to painful stimulus occurs by nociceptor sensitization at the site of tissue injury. Secondary hyperalgesia refers to the expansion of the area of cutaneous hyperalgesia beyond the area of injury.[25]

Two physiologically distinct pathways ascend in the anterolateral quadrant of the spinal cord. The neospinothalamic pathway projects to the ventrobasilar thalamic complex, and from there, axons project to the somatosensory cortex in the parietal lobe. This pathway mediates sensory-discriminative aspects of pain perception (stimulus localization and intensity). The paleospinothalamic tract ascends, projecting to the reticular formation, posterior thalamic nucleus, intralaminar thalamic nuclear complex, and to the cortex. This pathway mediates the arousal, emotional, and affective/suffering components of pain.

The existence of a specific nucleus in the posterior thalamus responsible for pain and temperature sensation has recently been elucidated.[27] There is an endogenous pain suppression pathway that arises in the periaqueductal grey (PAG) of the midbrain and descends to the nucleus raphe magnus (NRM) in the medulla. From the NRM, there are projections to the dorsal horn of the spinal cord through the dorsal longitudinal fasciculus. This pathway modulates afferent nociceptive impulses. Electrical stimulation of the PAG, NRM, or dorsal horn or microinjection of morphine at these sites produces analgesia without concomitant motor, sensory, or autonomic blockade. Serotonin and norepinephrine are the putative neurotransmitters in these areas. Endogenous opioid compounds are also involved as modulators in this pain suppression system. Enkephalin, β-endorphin, and dynorphin are the most potent inhibitors of nociceptive activity. These three peptides are derived from three precursor molecules: (1) pro-opiomelanocortin is the common precursor for β-endorphin, (2) proenkephalin A is the common precursor for met-enkephalin and leu-enkephalin, and (3) proenkephalin B is the precursor for dynorphin. Enkephalin is distributed in specific nuclei in the brain stem and spinal cord. β-Endorphin is found in the arcuate nucleus of the hypothalamus and in the pituitary. These endogenous opioid peptides produce analgesia by binding to specific receptors that are found in high concentration in cortical, brain stem, and spinal cord sites. β-Endorphin binds to the μ-receptor, enkephalin to the delta receptor, and dynorphin to the κ receptor. Morphine and the commonly used opioids exert their effects through mu-opioid receptors mimicking the action of endogenous opioid peptides.

Assessment of Pain

Critical to the development of a successful therapeutic strategy is the physician's ability to establish a trusting relationship with the patient (Table 69-2).

Assessment of pain and its impact on the patient's quality of life may be viewed as a promise to provide total care with attention to the symptoms of cancer that are feared the most. Cancer history should include description of the pain complaint, including the patient's description of pain and intensity; its quality, exacerbating, relieving factors, and its radiation if any; its exact onset and temporal pattern. Impact of pain on the activities of daily living, sleep, mood, and affect should be assessed. Multiple pain complaints, particularly common in patients with advanced disease, need to be prioritized and classified. Physical examination including neurological assessment and imaging studies' review helps to provide the necessary data to substantiate the clinical pain diagnosis.[28,29] For instance, complaints of back pain, the most common symptom for neurological

Table 69-2 **Algorithm for the Clinical Assessment of Pain**

1. Believe the patient's complaint of pain.
2. Take a careful history of the pain complaint to place it temporally in the patient's cancer history.
3. Assess the characteristics of each pain, including its site, its pattern of referral, and its aggravating and relieving factors.
4. Clarify the temporal aspects of the pain: acute, subacute, chronic, episodic, intermittent, breakthrough, or incident.
5. List and prioritize each pain complaint.
6. Evaluate the response to previous and current analgesic therapies.
7. Evaluate the psychological state of the patient.
8. Ask if the patient has a past history of alcohol or drug dependence.
9. Perform a careful medical and neurologic examination.
10. Order and personally review the appropriate diagnostic procedures.
11. Treat the patient's pain to facilitate the necessary work-up.
12. Design the diagnostic and therapeutic approach to suit the individual.
13. Provide continuity of care from evaluation to treatment, to ensure patient compliance, and to reduce patient anxiety.
14. Reassess the patient's response to pain therapy.
15. Discuss advance directives with the patient and the family.

referral at MSKCC, may lead to diagnosis of a number of the neurologic complications of cancer, including epidural spinal cord compression with resultant paraplegia. Another example is postmastectomy pain syndrome that is quite characteristic and can be diagnosed by its temporal relationship to the surgery, the site of pain in the distribution of the intercostobrachial nerve, and the pain description.[2] Patient's beliefs and attitudes about pain medications, goals, and expectations of therapy are important in setting the treatment goals and developing the treatment plans. Of greatest importance, no patient should be inadequately evaluated because of patient's experiencing "too much pain." Immediate treatment of pain concurrently with pain assessment will enable the patient to cooperate with examination and treatment.

Psychological factors accounting for differences in pain experiences in patients with cancer must be recognized.[3,30,31] In a study of the incidence of psychiatric disorders in patients with cancer, 39% of patients with psychiatric comorbidity had significant pain. In contrast, only 19% of patients who did not have a psychiatric diagnosis had significant pain. Among patients with cancer pain, the psychiatric diagnoses included adjustment disorders with depressed or mixed mood or major depression occurring in as many as 25% of patients.[32,33] As depression is often a treatable disorder, patients may experience significant pain relief if their psychiatric symptoms are promptly recognized and managed appropriately.[5] Psychiatric symptoms in patients with cancer pain without a psychiatric diagnosis usually are a consequence of uncontrolled pain. This has been documented in both adults and children.[31]

The National Comprehensive Cancer Network has provided important guidelines for the management of psychiatric symptoms in the cancer population (see Chapter 62, "Principles of Psycho-Oncology").

Meaning of pain can be an important contributor to the pain report. It is not uncommon for patients during active therapy to endure significant pain for the promise of a successful outcome. With advanced disease, when active antitumor therapy is no longer effective, it is common for patients and families to request that if nothing else can be done that at least their pain should be adequately managed.[34-36]

Social support is a very important factor as well. Uncontrolled pain, as well as low family support and depression are major factors in cancer-related suicide.[37,38]

To determine the degrees of emotional and physical pain as well as contribution of the emotional distress to the pain report, a repetitive measurements of mood and pain using validated scales such as the Brief Pain Inventory, the McGill Pain Questionnaire, the Memorial Pain Assessment Card (MPAC), and the Memorial Symptom Assessment Scale (MSAS) may be helpful.[4,5] Using the MPAC, pain relief and mood can be evaluated in 20 seconds. Recording pain intensity on the daily chart of each inpatient at MSKCC receiving intravenous opioids not only establishes pain intensity as a fifth vital sign but also underscores a critical institutional commitment to pain management.[34]

Types of Pain

Somatic Pain ■ Somatic pain is the most common type of pain in patients with cancer, and bone metastases are the most prevalent cause. Somatic pain is characterized as well localized, intermittent, or constant, and is described as aching, gnawing, throbbing, or cramping. Bone metastases are characterized by bone destruction with concurrent new bone formation. Prostaglandins sensitize nociceptors and produce hyperalgesia and pain as osteolysis and osteoclast formation occur.[28] Vertebral compression fractures add mechanical factors to pain causation. Other factors, such as osteoclast-activating factor, also sensitize nociceptors and produce increased pain perception.[35] Drugs that interfere with prostaglandin synthesis and osteoclast formation inhibit bone pain by inhibiting this sensitization and may also inhibit tumor growth. This partially explains relatively high potency of nonsteroidal analgesics (NSAIDs) in bone pain. The widespread use of bisphosphonates has resulted in improved analgesia and a significant reduction of skeletal complications in patients with malignant bone pain (see "Adjuvant Drugs" section). However, recently, the FDA issued a warning that a variety of bisphosphonates have been linked to severe and sometimes incapacitating bone, joint, and muscle (musculoskeletal) pain. The association between bisphosphonates and severe musculoskeletal pain may be overlooked, delaying diagnosis, prolonging pain and impairment. Steroids and radiopharmaceuticals are the other two groups of analgesics that add to the traditional analgesic regimen in cancer pain management.

Visceral Pain ■ Visceral pain is mediated by discrete nociceptors in the cardiovascular, respiratory, gastrointestinal, and genitourinary systems. It is usually described as deep, squeezing, or colicky, and is commonly referred to cutaneous sites, which may be tender. Shoulder pain, resulting from diaphragmatic irritation from a pleural disease, similarly to left jaw or arm pain with myocardial infarction, is an example of a cutaneous referral of a visceral pain. This referral pattern is thought to be related to the fact that somatic and visceral structures have dual innervation by the fibers that converge in the dorsal horn in the spinal cord. Visceral pain results from mechanical or chemical activation of nociceptors by tumor compression or visceral distension and responds to a wide variety of pain management approaches including pharmacologic, anesthetic, and neurosurgical procedures.[35,36,39] Recent experimental data in animals suggest that kappa-opioid receptor agonists may be uniquely efficacious in the treatment of visceral pain.[40-42] The role of such agents in the management of human cancer pain requires further investigation. The only clinically used opioid, which in addition to the mu-opioid activity is thought to be a kappa-opioid agonist, is oxycodone.

Neuropathic Pain ■ The second category of pain common in cancer patients is neuropathic pain, which results from injury to the peripheral receptor, afferent fiber, or CNS. Such injury is associated with spontaneous and ectopic firing in the peripheral nerve, at the level of the dorsal horn or brain, including thalamus. Neuropathic pain is clinically described as a burning, dysesthetic, squeezing sensation with paroxysms of shock-like pain. Chemotherapy-induced peripheral neuropathy is the most common cause of cancer-associated neuropathic pain. Tumor infiltration of the brachial and lumbar plexus are common in cancer patients as well.[43] Neuropathic pain may result from injury to the peripheral nerve as occurs in postmastectomy and post-thoracotomy pain.

Tricyclic antidepressants, selective serotonin reuptake inhibitors, anticonvulsants, local anesthetics, NMDA antagonists, opioids, intrathecal, and epidural opioids with local anesthetics and other adjuvant analgesics, as well as some neurostimulatory procedures have improved the outcome for cancer patients with neuropathic pain (see later).

Common Pain Syndromes in Patients With Cancer

Over the last 15 years, a series of well-defined pain syndromes have been described in patients with cancer pain. Many of these pain syndromes are unique to cancer and may be misdiagnosed if health care professionals are unfamiliar with their clinical presentation.[1,2,44] Knowledge of the common pain syndromes, essential in an oncologist's training, facilitates pain diagnosis and improves treatment of cancer pain. The major categories of pain syndromes are listed in Table 69-3.

Table 69-3 ■ Cancer Pain Syndromes

Pain syndromes associated with tumor infiltration
Metastatic bone pain
Retroperitoneal lymphadenopathy pain
Liver capsule pain
Headache
Cranial neuralgias
Glossopharyngeal neuralgia
Trigeminal neuralgia
Perineal pain
Pain syndromes associated with cancer therapy
Postchemotherapy myalgias, arthralgias, peripheral neuropathy
Steroid pseudorheumatism
Aseptic necrosis of bone
Headache
Postsurgical pain syndromes
Postmastectomy pain
Postradical neck dissection pain
Post-thoracotomy pain
Phantom limb and stump pain
Postradiation pain syndromes
Radiation fibrosis of brachial plexus
Radiation fibrosis of lumbosacral plexus
Radiation myelopathy
Radiation-induced peripheral nerve tumors
Acute herpetic and postherpetic neuralgia
Pain syndromes unrelated to cancer or cancer therapy
Lumbar disk disease
Osteoarthitis

One of the biggest challenges is metastatic bone pain. Most common cancers associated with painful bone metastases are lung, breast, prostate, colon, and renal metastases. Rapid escalation of pain escalating with movement may require opioid dose that may be excessive for the patient at rest. Balance between suboptimal analgesia of incident pain and sedation at rest may be a challenge. Transcitoneous vertebroplasty with methyl methacrylate may immobilize bone fragments in vertebral metastases with major relief. Similarly, orthopedic or radio-therapeutic procedures for painful appendicular metastases may be very helpful (see Chapter 126).

Vertebral metastases cause up to 90% of cases of spinal cord compression. Para vertebral metastases may cause spinal cord compression by tumor extension through neural foramen. They are seen mostly in lymphoproliferative disorders. Spinal cord compression usually presents with local vertebral pain associated with radicular pain, progressing weakness below the lesion, followed by sensory loss, reflex abnormalities, bladder, and bowel dysfunction.

Multiple new sites of pain with numerous symptoms may be seen in leptomeningeal metastases. Headache, facial pain, back, and radicular pain may be associated with nausea, vomiting, lethargy, seizures, visual and hearing loss, extremities weakness, and bladder and bowel incontinence or pain may be the only presenting symptoms without any physical findings.

Postthoracotomy and postmastectomy pain, as well as phantom limb pain are neuropathic pain syndromes that often require polypharmacy. Postthoracotomy pain is usually localized to the area of the incision. Chronic postthoracotomy pain may be complicated by the adhesive capsulitis of the shoulder if pain in not rapidly controlled. Postmastectomy pain can start up to 6 months after mastectomy or lumpectomy. It is caused by the injury of the intercostobrachial nerve (T1–T2 distribution) or a neuroma. It may occur in up to 15% of all mastectomies. Pain is neuropathic, burning and constricting, associated with severe allodynia of the axillary area and the anterior chest wall. Adhesive capsulitis of the shoulder is a common comorbidity.

Brachial plexopathy and lumbosacral plexopathy may present with pain in the plexus distribution. It is usually associated with a burning sensation and dysesthesia; pain is usually followed by progressive weakness, and later by atrophy. Predominantly upper brachial plexus involvement and ipsilateral Homer syndrome are suggestive of epidural tumor extension. Plexopathy may be tumor or radiation related. Chemotherapy may worsen preexisting plexopathy. Autoimmune plexitis is a self-limiting plexopathy that is clinically almost indistinguishable from the tumor-associated plexopathy, except for a relatively rapid onset of atrophy.

Of painful conditions related to chemotherapy, peripheral neuropathy is most common. Pain and usually burning, may be associated with numbness, paresthesia, and allodynia mostly in the fingers and toes. Decreased vibration sense is the earliest physical finding, followed by absent ankle reflex and weakness in the distal muscle groups.

One of the big challenges in cancer pain management is a postherpetic neuralgia (PHN) that is not uncommon in patients undergoing chemo or radiation therapy.

Strategy for Assessment and Treatment

In developing a strategy to manage the pain in a cancer patient, establishing the cause of the pain and the specific pain syndrome are paramount (Table 69-3).

General guidelines of cancer pain treatment are listed in Table 69-4.

The guiding principles of a therapeutic strategy for cancer pain must include: (1) detailed assessment of the patient's pain, (2) making a pain diagnosis, (3) understanding the goals of care and the patient's preferences, (4) developing and implementing the best therapeutic and diagnostic strategy, (5) continual reassessment of the degree of pain and analgesia, (6) assurance of institutional resources and (7) expertise to provide alternative therapeutic strategies.

A series of algorithms have been developed for the management of cancer pain.[28,45,46] The WHO Cancer Pain and Palliative Care Program advocates the three-step approach shown in Figure 69-1.[10,43]

Validation studies of the WHO guidelines reveal successful treatment of cancer pain in 69-100% of patients.[47-51] Such an approach advocates the use of nonopioid, opioid, and adjuvant analgesics alone and in combination, titrated to the needs of the individual patient. The Agency for Health Care Policy and Research (AHCPR) has developed guidelines for the treatment of cancer pain.[3] A randomized, controlled clinical trial implementing a treatment algorithm based on the AHCPR guidelines for cancer pain management revealed that patients in the treatment algorithm group experienced a significant reduction in pain intensity compared to the control group.[52] Furthermore, reduction in pain intensity correlated with the patients' adherence to analgesic therapies.

NCCN pain management guidelines provide an algorithm of a stepwise approach to the treatment of mild, moderate, and severe pain and strategy of rapid but safe opioid titration to provide analgesia.[53]

Use of other guidelines and protocol also appear to improve the patient's access to analgesics and improve pain control. In an intergroup study of 129 randomized patients with cancer pain coordinated by the Eastern Cooperative Oncology Group, Cleeland et al demonstrated that an oral analgesic protocol implemented in oncology practices improves pain control.[54] In particular, the proportion of lung and prostate cancer patients with no or mild pain increased significantly among the patients treated according to the "analgesic protocol" as compared to the sites treated as per "physician discretion."

Standard guidelines may need to be adapted to match the clinical practices and resources of particular institutions. Such institutional guidelines are important for resource allocation both of staff time, facilities, and medication availability. They enable rapid and safe titration of the analgesics and frame a standard of care, informing both the patient and the health care professionals of a recommended approach, and help to distinguish the appropriate use of rapidly-escalating high-dose opioids and other agents in a dying patient from inappropriate strategies of euthanasia and physician-assisted suicide (illegal in all states except Oregon).

Table 69-4 **Guidelines for the Use of Analgesic Drugs in Cancer Pain Management**

Start with a specific drug for a specific type of pain

1. Clarify the patient's pain, its nature, site, duration, and intensity, and the degree of pain relief from prior nonopioid and opioid drug use.
2. Complete a careful medical and neurologic history and examination. Assess the potential role of radiotherapy, surgery, and/or chemotherapy in pain control.
3. Assess the psychological factors contributing to the pain complaint, and understand the meaning of the pain for the patient.
4. Choose the route of administration to fit the needs of the individual patient.
   i. Choose the oral route as the simplest approach.
   ii. Consider the buccal or rectal routes for patients who cannot tolerate oral drugs and refuse parenteral routes. Start intravenous intermittent boluses or continuous infusions in patients requiring rapid escalation of opioids for pain control.
   iii. Use intermittent boluses or continuous subcutaneous infusions for patients without venous access or in patients at home.
   iv. Choose the epidural or intrathecal route in patients who develop limiting side effects from systemic opioids.
   v. Use PCA pumps for selected patients in hospital and at home.
5. Know the pharmacology of the available opioid drugs. Titrate the dose to the individual needs of the patient.
   i. Start with a dose that is at least equivalent or slightly greater than the equianalgesic dose of the previous analgesic used.
   ii. Order the medication on a regular basis (oral—every 3-4 h, intravenous—every 15-60 min as needed).
   iii. Instruct the patient to take the medication on a PRN basis if the patient is opioid naive.
   iv. Order "rescue medication" equivalent to 1/2 the standing dose to begin with on a PRN basis.
   v. Inform the patient of options in taking the medication, and request that he or she report side effects of excessive sedation or confusion. Monitor the side effects closely.
6. Use a combination of drugs to provide additive analgesia to reduce side effects or to control other symptoms.
   i. Know the various adjuvant drugs that provide additive analgesia, eg, anticonvulsants, corticosteroids.
   ii. Use neurostimulants to reduce sedative effects, eg, caffeine, dextroamphetamine, methylphenidate, modafinil.
   iii. Use antidepressant, anticonvulsant, and other analgesics to manage neuropathic pain.
7. Anticipate and treat side effects.
   i. Watch for respiratory depression, and use naloxone if needed (in diluted doses to prevent acute withdrawal).
   ii. Counteract sedation with neurostimulants.
   iii. Use antiemetics to suppress the emetic effect of opioids.
   iv. Define an individualized bowel regimen to prevent and manage constipation.
   v. Treat myoclonus by switching to an alternative analgesic, or suppress it with anxiolytic drugs.
8. Watch for the development of tolerance
   i. Distinguish tolerance from progression of tumor.
   ii. Recognize that there is no limit to tolerance.
   iii. Switch to an alternative opioid if the dose of the current opioid cannot be escalated.
   iv. Use epidural local anesthetics to control localized pain.
   v. Consider cordotomy in a patient with chronic unilateral pain below the waist with stable pulmonary function.
   vi. Consider opioid rotation if one or more intractable side effects are noted.
9. Differentiate physical and psychological dependence.
   i. Prevent withdrawal by administering 25% of the opioid daily dose and tapering the dose in decrements of 10%.
   ii. Use diluted doses of naloxone to reverse respiratory depression without reversing analgesia.
   iii. Assess the risk of substance abuse in the individual patient.
10. Reassess the patient's pain, mood, and quality of life
   i. Reevaluate the pain symptoms.
   ii. Evaluate the patient's goals of care and quality of life.
   iii. Assess the patient for psychiatric disorders and suicidal ideation.
   iv. Clarify the patient's DNR status.

Abbreviations: DNR, do-not-resuscitate; PCA, patient-controlled analgesia; PRN, pro re nata (according as circumstances may require).

Therapeutic Approaches to Cancer Pain

Pharmacological Approaches

Pharmacological approaches are the most commonly used method for managing cancer pain. The effective use of analgesic drugs should be a major part of every physician's armamentarium in managing cancer patients.

The brief outline of pharmacologic approach is detailed in Tables 69-3 and 69-4. The fundamental concept that underlies this approach is individualization of pharmacotherapy. The selection of the right analgesic to maximize pain relief and minimize adverse effects begins with the use of nonopioids for mild pain. In patients with moderate pain that is not controlled with nonopioids such as acetaminophen, nonsteroidal, anti-inflammatory drugs (NSAIDs), and adjuvant medications (WHO step 1), the so-called weak opioid-agonists (codeine, hydrocodone, oxycodone, and tramadol) alone or in combination are prescribed (step 2). In patients with severe pain, a strong opioid (morphine, hydromorphone, fentanyl, methadone, oxycodone, oxymorphone, or levorphanol) is the drug of choice (step 3). At all levels, certain NSAIDs and adjuvant drugs may be used for specific indications. It is critical that patients presenting in severe pain should generally be treated with a strong opioid immediately.

Aspirin and the other NSAIDs have analgesic, antipyretic, anti-inflammatory, and antiplatelet actions all levels, certain NSAIDs and adjuvant drugs may be used for specific indications. It is critical that patients presenting in severe pain should generally be treated with a strong opioid immediately.

Aspirin and the other NSAIDs have analgesic, antipyretic, anti-inflammatory, and antiplatelet actions (Table 69-4). These drugs produce analgesia by inhibiting the arachidonic acid cascade that follows nociceptive tissue injury and serves as a substrate for the cyclooxygenase (COX) pathway. Affecting prostaglandin E2 (PGE2) and prostacyclin production, NSAIDs are said to decrease hyperalgesia as well. In addition to this peripheral action, a recent study indicates that they may also interfere with the action of glutamate and substance P in the CNS when cyclooxygenase is inhibited.[55] Two isoforms of the cyclooxygenase enzyme have been identified. cyclooxygenase 1 is a normal constituent of blood vessels, stomach, and kidney. Cyclooxegenase-2 (Cox-2) is induced in the setting of peripheral inflammation and acts as an attractant of inflammatory mediators. These compounds are most commonly used orally. Intravenous ketorolac is the only NSAID available in the United States for intravenous use. Although very useful as an opioid-sparing or opioid-reducing agent in cancer patients who are difficult to manage with morphine alone, its use is limited to a 5-day course due to gastrointestinal toxicity.[56,57] In clinical experience, some patients respond better to one NSAID than to others, and each patient should therefore be given an adequate trial of one drug on a regular basis before switching to another.

Absence of tolerance and physical dependence with repeated administration of NSAIDs is of great therapeutic value. When used short-term their side effects profile compares favorably with opioid analgesics, unless specific contraindications are present.

Limitation of NSAIDs as a group is a ceiling effect, that is, increasing the dose beyond a certain level (eg, 900-1,300 mg

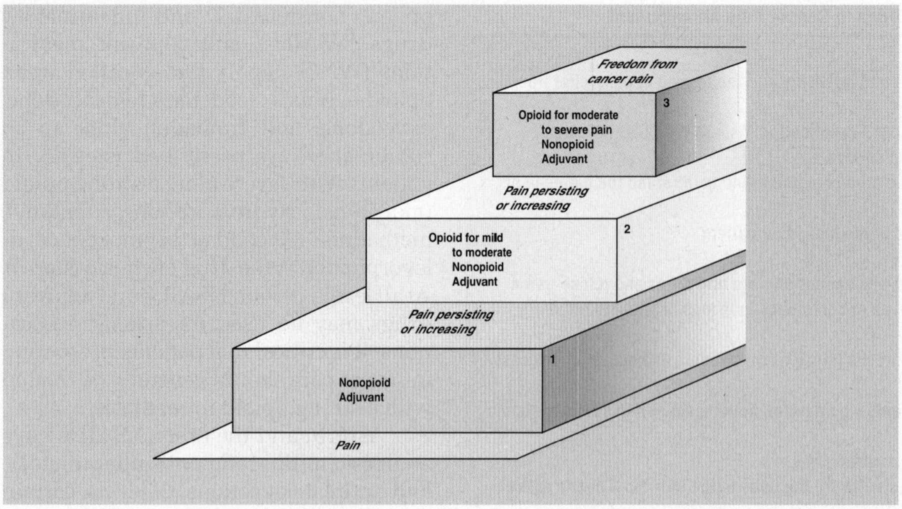

Figure 69-1 The World Health Organization three-step analgesic ladder for cancer pain.

per dose of aspirin and 300-400 mg of acetaminophen) will produce no increase in peak effect. Adverse effects of NSAIDs include gastrointestinal (GI) and renal toxicity. From the standpoint of morbidity and mortality, GI side effects constitute the most important toxicity that includes GI ulceration, perforation, and hemorrhage.[57-59] Serious GI toxicity may be seen without any warning sign and can be seen in 2-4% of the patients after one year of chronic use. The risk of NSAIDs gastropathy are increased in females, patients over the ago of 60, and those with a history of peptic ulcer disease or other morbidity. Concomitant use of NSAIDs and steroids may increase the risk of NSAIDs gastropathy up to four times. Ibuprofen in daily doses of 1,600 mg or less was associated with the lowest relative risk of severe GI toxicity. Aspirin and diclofenac are 1.6-1.8 times more likely, and ketoprofen is moreover 4 times likely to cause gastropathy with chronic use. Misoprostol, an FDA approved agent to reduce the risk of GI ulceration should be used with caution in childbearing age females due to its teratogenic potential.

NSAIDs can cause small asymptomatic aminotransferase elevation in 1-15% of patients taking NSAIDs chronically. Prior to starting chronic NSAIDs treatment aminotransferase should be checked as a baseline and periodically thereafter.

Renal toxicity may be seen in patients with reduced renal blood flow or systemic hypovolemia. In addition, NSAIDs can affect renal tubular function, causing edema, mild hypertension, and hyperkalemia.

Nonacetylated salicylates and choline magnesium trisalicylate in particular has the advantage of analgesic effect similar to aspirin although causing substantially less GI toxicity and little or no effect on platelets.

Acetaminophen, which is as potent as aspirin, is an analgesic and antipyretic but is much less effective as an anti-inflammatory agent and does not interfere with platelet function or cause any significant GI toxicity. It also does not cross-react in aspirin-sensitive asthma. Liver toxicity may be encountered with daily doses above 4 g, especially in patients that are fasting, alcoholics or patients with prior liver injury. Recently, FDA changed the labeling for the over-the-counter pain relievers adding a warning to highlight the potential for liver toxicity, particularly when using acetaminophen in high doses, when taking more than one product with acetaminophen, and when taken with moderate amount of alcohol.

Tramadol ■ Tramadol (Ultram), classified as opioid analgesic in some European countries is not a schedule II analgesic in the United States. Having some opioid-activity it also inhibits serotonin/norepinephrine reuptake. It is generally weaker that other opioids (10-fold less potent in μ receptor binding than codeine) and has a ceiling dose. In some European trials, it was shown to be safe and effective in a double-blind randomized placebo-controlled trial for the treatment of diabetic neuropathic pain.[60,61] The risk of abuse and dependence with tramadol has been found to be very low. It has been shown to produce synergistic analgesic response in preclinical studies at 1:8 mg-to-mg tramadol:acetaminophen ratio. Ultracet, a combination of tramadol 37.5 mg and acetaminophen 325 mg is now available in the United States. A long-acting tramadol has been approved in the United states recently and is now available for clinical use. Its onset of action is significantly longer than short-acting tramadol, so long-acting formulation should be taken regularly on a fixed schedule.

Tapentadol ■ The FDA just approved tapentadol hydrochloride, an immediate-release oral tablet for the relief of moderate to severe acute pain. It has a duel analgesic effect: opioid agonist and norepinephrine reuptake inhibitor. It is a synthetic drug that is available in doses of 50, 75, or 100 mg.

Opioid Analgesics

The opioid analgesics as a class consist of heterogeneous compounds whose pharmacologic effects are derived from their interaction with multiple CNS opiate receptors.[62] The morphine agonist drugs bind to discrete opiate receptors and produce analgesia. The opioid antagonists block and reverse the effects of opioid receptors. All clinically available opioids are mu-opioid agonists and only oxycodone has been suggested to be a kappa-opioid agonist activity as well. A number of opioid analgesics is available for clinical use and are listed in Table 69-6.

Codeine is considered to be a weak opioid and has a limited analgesic efficacy. It is used for the management of mild to moderate pain and has been included in step 2 of the analgesic ladder.[63] Codeine is metabolized to morphine that is its main active metabolite. It is about

Table 69-5 **Nonopioid Analgesics Commonly Used for Mild to Moderate Pain**

Name	Starting Oral Dose Range (mg)	Comments (Precautions)
Aspirin	650	Often used in combination with opioid analgesics (renal dysfunction; avoid during pregnancy, in hemostatic disorders, and in combination with steroids)
Choline magnesium trisalicylate (Trilisate)	1500	Does not affect platelet function
Acetaminophen (Tylenol)	650	Like aspirin but does not affect platelet function
Ibuprofen (Motrin, Advil)	200-400	Higher analgesic potential than aspirin
Diflunisal (Dolobid)	500-1000	Longer duration of action than ibuprofen; higher analgesic potential than aspirin
Naproxen (Naprosyn)	250-300	Like diflunisal
Ketorolac (Toradol)	10 (30 IM)	Not to exceed 5 days
Tramadol (Ultram)	50-200	Weak μ agonist and serotonergic and catecholamine reuptake inhibitor
Cox-2 inhibitors		
Celecoxib (Celebrex)	100-200	Contraindicated in sulfa-allergic patients

Table 69-6 ■ **Opioid Analgesics Commonly Used for Moderate to Severe Pain Narcotic Agonists**

	Parenteral (mg)	Oral (mg)	Conversion Factor (IV to PO)	Comments
Morphine	10	30	3	Standard of comparison for opioid analgesics; lower dose for aged patients and patients with impaired ventilation, bronchial asthma, increased intracranial pressure, liver failure, renal failure
Hydromorphone (Dilaudid)	1.5	7.5	5	Slightly shorter-acting
Methadone (Dolophine)	10	20	2	Good oral potency, long plasma half-life; like morphine, may accumulate with repetitive dosing, causing excessive sedation
Fentanyl	100μg = 4 mg morphine IV	–	–	Short half-life; transdermal and transmucosal preparations available
Meperidine (Demerol)	75	300	4	Not recommended in chronic cancer pain due to toxic metabolite, impaired renal function, or if receiving monamine oxidase inhibitors
Levorphanol (Levo-Dromoran)	2	4	2	Like methadone
Codeine	130	200	1.5	Often used in combination with non-opioid analgesics; biotransformed, part, to morphine
Oxycodone (Roxicodone, Tylox)	–	30	–	Also in combination with non-opioid analgesics, that limit dose escalation
Oxymorphone (Numorphan)	1	–	6 (rectal)	Like methadone; not available orally

6 times weaker than morphine. In single-dose studies of cancer, dental, and postoperative pain codeine 60 mg was found to be equianalgesic to aspirin 650 mg or acetaminophen 600-1000 mg. Approximately 15% of the population cannot convert codeine to morphine because of the lack of a specific enzyme and thus cannot gain pain relief. At the higher doses required to treat severe pain, codeine is poorly tolerated by patients because it produces significant nausea. When used in combination with acetaminophen (Tylenol #2, #3, and #4) the maximum daily dosing should not exceed the maximum acetaminophen dosing.

Oxycodone is included in both step 2 and step 3 of the analgesic ladder. It binds to both the mu- and kappa-opioid receptors.[64] Oxycodone is available in combination with acetaminophen (Percocet, Tylox) or alone in tablet form and liquid form. Oxycodone is 10 times more potent than codeine. Oxycodone 5 mg has similar analgesic effect to acetaminophen 500 mg. When used in combination with acetaminophen it offers enhanced analgesia, an "opioid-sparing" effect and improved side effect and safety profile.[65] Simultaneous use of other acetaminophen products or NSAIDs limits the maximum daily doses of the combination products.

Bioavailability of oxycodone is about 50%. Its potency compares with oral morphine, ratio being about 3:2.[66,67] Oxycodone is reported to cause fewer hallucinations, pruritis, and nausea compared with morphine.[68,69] While oxycodone accumulates in the patients with renal insufficiency, its only active metabolite oxymorphone does not. Oxycodone is available as 5, 10, and 30 mg immediate-release preparations, variety of doses when combined with acetaminophen, as well as extended release OxyContin.

Morphine remains the drug of choice for the management of patients with pain and cancer because of its place on the essential drug list of the WHO, its familiarity to physicians, and its wide oral use in the management of cancer pain.[10] Morphine, the prototypic drug, has an oral bioavailability that is about 35% and a plasma half-life of 2-3 h in a young patient with normal renal and liver function. With repeated administration, the pharmacokinetics of morphine and its metabolites, morphine-3-glucuronide (M-3-G, 55%) and morphine-6-glucuronide (M-6-G, 15%) usually remain linear, but may change significantly in elderly patients and in patients with renal or liver insufficiency.[70,71] Conflicting data have been reported on the role of M-3-G and the development of tolerance.[72] Some studies suggest that the accumulation of M-3-G may be associated with the side effects of CNS excitation (eg, myoclonus and delirium), whereas M-6-G accumulation may result in the depressive side effects (eg, drowsiness and respiratory depression).[73] Half-life of M-6-G, a potent opioid agonist, in an elderly patient or a patient with significant renal insufficiency may be up to a few days and cause sedation that outlives the normally expected analgesic and sedating effects of morphine.[71,72,74-76] As judged by single-dose studies, the relative potency of parenteral to oral morphine is 1:3, ie, 10 mg parenteral morphine produce analgesia equal to 30 mg of oral morphine.

Morphine is now available in a wide variety of preparations, including immediate-release tablets, oral solutions, controlled-release tablets (for 8, 12, or 24 h), buccal tablets, rectal suppositories, and parenteral forms (intravenous, subcutaneous, epidural, and intrathecal). Morphine delivered by a new delivery system, Avinza was shown to offer 24 h pain relief in an arthritis model, providing 10% of the dose as immediate release. Because of the preservative, fumaric acid, its daily dose should not exceed 1600 mg. It can be sprinkled on food, but should not be dissolved to avoid immediate release of the 24-hour morphine dose. Kadian is another 24-hour formulation of slow-release morphine that can be sprinkled on food and given via percutaneous gastrostomy tube as well.

Hydromorphone (Dilaudid) is a strong opioid (1.5 mg of hydromorphone intravenously is equipotent to 10 mg of intravenous morphine) and a useful alternative to morphine in the treatment of moderate to severe cancer pain. Although myoclonus has been described in the setting of continuous high-dose infusion, possibly due to accumulation of hydromorphone-3-glucuronide,[71] hydromorphone may be a suitable alternative to morphine in the setting of morphine toxicity. Given its water solubility, availability in a high-potency formulation (10 mg/mL), and 87% bioavailability, hydromorphone is the drug of choice for chronic subcutaneous administration. It is also available in a suppository form. It has less histamine-release effects compared to the other morphine cogeners and can be used in patients who develop histamine-induced headache or itch.

Fentanyl is a mu opioid with shortest half-life that together with the unique transdermal delivery system makes it an opioid of choice for patients with renal or liver insufficiency or those who need to bypass GI tract or are noncompliant due to forgetfulness or other cognitive problems. Transdermal fentanyl is commonly used for the long-term management of pain in patients with advanced cancer of head and neck, and other malignancies.[74-76] It is available for intravenous use, in a transdermal patch, and in an oral transmucosal preparation. Fentanyl is about 25 times more potent than morphine. Transdermal fentanyl patch can only be used in opioid-tolerant patients. After the patient is started on a fentanyl patch there is a 6-12 h delay in the onset of analgesia, and therefore, patients need to have their pain controlled by the immediate-release medication during this titration phase. With transdermal application of fentanyl the patch has to be changed every 72 h in the majority of patients, but about 15% of patients may experience end-of-dose failure reporting escalation of pain on day 3. Escalation of the dose or changing the fentanyl patch (Duragesic) every 48 h should then be considered. Steady state is generally achieved within 12-24 h following application of the patch.

Some studies have suggested that patients who receive transdermal fentanyl may be more satisfied with analgesia and side-effect profile when compared with those who receive sustained-release morphine.[74-76] Administration of fentanyl patch may not eliminate or even significantly decrease the need for PRN short-acting opioids in some patients.

Heat may increase the amount of fentanyl that reaches the blood and can cause life-threatening breathing problems and death. Patients should not use heat sources such as heating pads, electric blankets, saunas, or heated waterbeds or take hot baths or sunbathe while wearing a patch. A patient or caregiver should call the patient's doctor right away if the patient has a temperature higher than 102° while wearing a patch.

Oral transmucosal fentanyl citrate (OTFC) is a valuable option for the treatment of highly prevalent cancer-related breakthrough pain, a transient increase in pain over a well-controlled baseline pain.[77,78] Two formulations of OTFC are currently approved for use in the United States (Table 69-7).

Fentanyl Actiq is available in a wider range of dosages (200-1600 µg) and is indicated for the management of breakthrough pain in opioid-tolerant adults. From 25% to 50% of both preparations are absorbed transmucosally over a 15-minute period, and an additional 25% is absorbed via the GI tract over the following 90 min. Onset of relief may occur within 5 minutes.[78] In dose-titration trials, OTFC has been shown to be safe and effective in comparison with other agents used for breakthrough pain.[79,80] In multicenter dose-titration trials, the effective OTFC dose fentanyl was associated with fewer side effects than morphine.

Table 69-7 Oral Transmucosal Fentanyl Citrate

Current Actiq Dose (mcg)	Initial Fentora Dose (mcg)
200	100
400	100
600	200
800	200
1200	400
1600	400

Actiq should be stored in a safe place out of the reach of children. Accidental ingestion by a child is a medical emergency and can result in death. Actiq contains sugar. Cavities and tooth decay have occurred in patients taking Actiq. When taking Actiq, the patients should talk to their dentists about proper dental care.

Fentora is a potent fentanyl formulation that is used only for treatment of breakthrough pain in opioid-tolerant cancer patients. For this purpose the FDA defined opioid-tolerant patients as those who are taking at least 60 mg oral morphine a day, at least 25 mcg transdermal fentanyl per hour, at least 30 mg of oral oxycodone daily, at least 8 mg oral hydromorphone daily or an equianalgesic dose of another opioid for a week or longer. FDA recently emphasized that patients should NOT take more than two Fentora tablets per breakthrough pain episode and MUST wait at least 4 h before treating another breakthrough episode with Fentora. It should be titrated from 100 mcg per dose with incremental increases in dosing to as high as 800 mcg, depending on the toleration of side effects and the therapeutic relief. For most patients, Fentora will be dosed in a smaller mcg dosing level with allowance for one additional dosing after 30 min of the initial dose, if pain is not relieved. Fentora cannot be substituted for Actiq because Fentora delivers more fentanyl to the blood than Actiq; substituting Fentora for Actiq using the same dose can result in a fatal overdose.

Oxymorphone hydrochloride, which was previously only available by injection, has recently been approved for oral use. Opana is an immediate-release formulation for moderate to severe acute pain, and Opana ER is an extended release formulation of oxymorphone.

Levorphanol is a second-line drug with the potential drug accumulation associated with its long half-life (12-16 h). The d-isomer of levorphanol (dextrorphan) is relatively devoid of analgesic action but acts as an NMDA receptor antagonist that may offer additional value in pain management. Steady-state plasma concentrations should be achieved by the third day of dosing. Levorphanol is rapidly distributed (<1 h) and redistributed (1-2 h) following IV administration. Levorphanol is well absorbed after PO administration with peak plasma concentrations occurring approximately 1 h after dosing. Plasma concentrations of Levorphanol following chronic administration in patients with cancer can reach 2-5 times those following a single dose, depending on the patient's individual clearance of the drug.

Methadone is an old opioid that has been increasingly used in cancer pain management over the last few years. Advantages to the use of methadone in cancer pain include 48-96% bioavailability, lack of active metabolites, low cost, long half-life resulting in larger intervals between doses, and improved patient compliance. Methadone is a potent opioid with a variable half-life, ranging from a few hours to a few days. This leads to potential drug accumulation even if the patient continues to take the stable dose that was initially prescribed. This dose accumulation and resulting escalation of blood levels associated with increased analgesia and possible increasing side effects may be seen 1-2 days to 7 days after the initiation of methadone treatment. Sedation, confusion, and even death can occur when patients are started on an excessive dose of methadone that initially may be well tolerated. Concerns about safety of methadone have led to its limited use, especially in frail patients.[81,82] The original equianalgesic table was based on single-dose studies, which demonstrated morphine: methadone ratio as 1:1. The latest literature suggests starting with 10:1 ratio. That means that when switching from 10 mg morphine IV per hour to IV methadone, the initial parenteral dose methadone should be 1 mg IV/hour.[83-85] In addition, numerous reports in the literature suggest that the equianalgesic ratio may be significantly influenced by the previous opioid dose and the length of time the patients were receiving the previous opioid.[86-88] In rotating patients from morphine to methadone, Ripamonti and colleagues used a dose ratio of 4:1 for patients who received 30-90 mg of morphine daily, 6:1 for patients who received 90-300 mg daily, and 8:1 for patients who received 300 mg or more.[86] Bruera and colleagues demonstrated that the hydromorphone/methadone ratio is correlated with total opioid dose, and that in switching from hydromorphone to methadone, much lower doses than expected may provide satisfactory analgesia.[85] In patients receiving more than 330 mg of hydromorphone prior to the switch, the dose ratio was 1.6:1, whereas in patients receiving less than 330 mg of hydromorphone daily, the dose ratio was 0.95:1.[84]

After calculating a safe starting dose (conservative estimation of 10:1 IV morphine to IV methadone ratio should be used in an opioid-tolerant patient), the total daily dose of methadone should be given either continuously IV or in 3-4 divided doses IV or PO. Understanding that such calculation may be very conservative and result in undertretament of pain in the first 2-3 days, it is essential to have the PRN doses available liberally. The PRN dose should be half or equal to regular schedule dose. Some groups suggest that methadone should be administered at a fixed calculated dose, but patient-controlled intervals. Using the rescues liberally the patient self-titrates methadone to the effective dose over 2-3 days. After titrating methadone to the effective therapeutic dose, the new daily dose should be administered in 3-4 divided doses with PRN available for breakthrough pain. Some clinicians and patients prefer to have a short-acting rescue opioid such as hydromorphone as a rescue. During the titration period, PRN methadone is preferred if appropriate supervision (daily phone calls or inpatient monitoring) is available for 2-5 days after initiating methadone. Considering the long half-life and dose accumulation of methadone, if excellent analgesia occurs within 24 h and no PRN medication is needed, a 50% reduction of the total dose should be considered.

The safety of methadone has also been demonstrated in the presence of chronic liver and renal disease, common at the end of life.[89] Mercandante and colleagues recently reported that in comparing the use of methadone vs morphine in pain management of advanced cancer at home, those who received methadone required fewer dose escalations, supporting a definite role for methadone in the hands of an experienced clinician.[90]

Overall, methadone is recommended for use only by physicians experienced in methadone prescribing or having access to the expert who can guide them.

Meperidine is an opioid with unique properties. Meperidine has been recently shown to block Na+ channels with molecular pharmacologic features of a local anesthetic. Mostly preclinical findings support classification of meperidine as a local anesthetic, but with less overall potency than lidocaine. Repetitive dosing of meperidine in a patient with renal insufficiency can lead to accumulation of a toxic metabolite, normeperidine, resulting in CNS hyperexcitability. This adverse effect is characterized by subtle mood changes followed by tremors, multifocal myoclonus, and occasionally, seizures. This complication occurs more commonly in patients with renal disease but can occur following repeated administration in patients with normal renal function.[91] The Agency for Health Care Policy and Research recommends its use for no longer than 48 h and in doses that do not exceed 600 mg per day.

Opioid Agonist/Antagonists and Partial Agonists

Opioid agonist/antagonists have the main advantage of causing less respiratory depression and having less abuse potential. However, the clinical use of these agents in cancer pain management is limited by the undesirable side effects and by ceiling analgesic effects. Pentazocine is a kappa-opioid agonist and a weak mu-opioid antagonist or partial agonist. Its analgesic effect is mediated mostly by kappa-opioid receptors. Higher doses (60-90 mg) elicit dysphoric and psychotomimetic effects, as well as increased blood pressure and heart rate. When given to a patient who is tolerant to opioids pentazocine may precipitate withdrawal symptoms. Ceiling effect for analgesia and respiratory depression are observed above 50-100 mg of pentazocine. Nalbuphine and butorphanol are similar to pentazocine in agonist/antagonist opioid effects. Buprenorphine is a partial agonist at the mu-opioid receptors and an antagonist at the kappa and delta receptors.[92] Unlike full mu-opioid agonists, at higher doses, buprenorphine's physiological and subjective effects, including euphoria, reach a plateau. This ceiling may limit the abuse potential and may result in a wider safety margin. Buprenorphine is approved for the treatment of opioid addiction. Prolonged use of buprenorphine can result in physical dependence. However, withdrawal symptoms appear to be mild to moderate in intensity compared with those of full μ agonists.

Start With a Specific Drug

Choosing an analgesic regimen requires knowledge of the pharmacokinetic and pharmacodynamic properties of the opioid analgesics and adjuvant analgesic medications. Each physician should become familiar with several drugs in these groups and adapt them to the needs of his or her clinical practice. Cherny and colleagues have documented the strategies used by pain physicians for the selection of analgesic drugs and routes of administration.

A common approach is to start a patient on a nonopioid, followed by the use of codeine or oxycodone alone or in combination with the nonopioid. For further opioid, titration combination drugs (opioids with acetaminophen or NSAIDs) should be avoided. Short-acting opioids are usually used for opioid titration and as needed (PRN) for breakthrough pain. After an effective stable 24-hour opioid requirement is established a switch to a long-acting formulation given in 1-4 divided dose should be considered. Long-acting opioids allow patients to achieve more consistent blood levels, reduce pain recurrence, improve compliance, and reduce the iatrogenic dependence. Rescue medications equivalent to one-half of the standing 4-hourly dose should be made available to patients.[77]

Overall, opioid dose, route, and titration schedule should be tailored to the patient's medical needs, treatment goals, and side-effect profile. There is no minimum or maximum dose. The opioid dose needs to be titrated to maintain the patient's desired balance between pain relief and opioid-related side effects. Selection of the opioids should be based on the physician's familiarity with the particular opioid, patient's analgesic history, potential for the drug accumulation, side effects, and severity of pain. It is critical that patients presenting with severe pain are treated with a strong opioid immediately.

Opioid Rotations

If a patient is receiving opioids but experiences side effects even at subtherapeutic doses an opioid rotation should be considered. This process of opioid substitution or rotation is a common clinical practice based on the significant interindividual variability in analgesia and side-effect profile.[93] These variable responses may, in part, be explained by the presence of different opioid receptor subtypes, including the differences mediated by the specific single nucleotide polymorphisms (SNPs) at the mu-opioid receptor and other genes.[94-96] Selected SNPs have been associated with the following opioid responses:

- Increasing dosage requirements of morphine and fentanyl
- Altered efficacy to mu-opioid antagonists
- Altered hypothalamic–pituitary–adrenal axis activation
- Increased adverse effects to M-6-G

Pending further definitive studies opioid rotation for now remains an empiric intervention based on the experience of the clinician. In a prospective study, 80 of 100 patients referred to the MSKCC Pain Service required changes in either opioid or route of administration to obtain adequate analgesia with tolerable side effects. About 80% of patients required one opioid switch, 44% of patients required two switches, and 20% of patients required three or more switches.[97]

The main advantages of the opioid rotation are minimizing polypharmacy, reduction of side effects, and improving analgesia. Change in the route of administration may improve convenience, compliance, absorption thus improving analgesia. Cost reduction is another reason opioid rotation may be desired. Among disadvantages are variable and unpredictable outcomes and potential need for consecutive opioid rotations and possibility of eventual need for a number of adjuvant analgesics.

Choose the Starting Dose

During the opioid rotation it is most useful to start with the dose that is equivalent to one-half the equianalgesic dose of the previous drug that provided good analgesia. Dose reduction may not be needed if at the time of the rotation pain control was suboptimal. Anticipating the dose accumulation of methadone within the first few days of stable dose administration should be remembered and a conservative dose of 10% of the previous morphine equivalent should be used if close monitoring for sedation and other side effects is not possible.

Choose the Route of Administration

Oral Route ■ The oral route is convenient, most cost efficient, and should be preferred unless specific reasons to bypass the GI tract exist. In general, orally administered drugs have a slower onset of action and a longer duration of effect; drugs administered parenterally have a more rapid onset of action but a shorter duration of effect.

Oral opioids differ substantially in the degree to which they are inactivated as they are absorbed from the GI tract and passed through the liver into the systemic circulation. As indicated in Table 69-6, morphine and hydromorphone have parenteral/oral potency ratios of 1:3 and 1:5, respectively, and methadone and levorphanol are subject to less presystemic elimination, resulting in an intravenous/oral potency ratio of 1:1 or 1:2. Conservative dosing should be used if close monitoring is not possible.

Intranasal, Sublingual, Buccal, Rectal, and Transdermal Routes ■ The intranasal, sublingual, buccal, rectal, and transdermal routes of administration provide alternative approaches for patients who cannot take oral drugs. Intranasal butorphanol, a mixed agonist-antagonist, provides adequate analgesia for patients with acute postoperative pain but is not commonly used for chronic cancer pain management.

Both fentanyl and methadone are well absorbed sublingually, as demonstrated in a study of normal volunteers.[98] An oral transmucosal formulation of fentanyl (Actiq and Fentora) has been demonstrated to be efficacious in treating breakthrough pain in cancer patients.

Morphine is poorly absorbed sublingually but has been reported anecdotally to be effective.[99]

Oxymorphone, hydromorphone, and morphine are available as rectal suppositories and are effective in managing chronic cancer pain. Studies of sustained-release morphine rectal suppositories in normal volunteers reported no significant differences in morphine absorption between the oral and rectal methods except that rectal absorption was delayed.[100]

The transdermal fentanyl patch offers a unique route of opioid administration. The patch is applied topically, but provides systemic drug administration (see earlier section). In the setting of significant malabsorption or unpredictable drug absorption, GI and head and neck malignancy interfering with oral drug administration, as well as noncompliance resulting from compulsory drug use or patient's forgetting to take opioids on a schedule, this route may be especially desirable.

Intravenous Boluses and Infusions ■ Intravenous boluses allow rapid onset of action as compared with other routes of administration. Continuous infusions provide more stable analgesia without the peak and trough effects seen with repeated boluses. The time to peak effect correlates with the lipid solubility of the opioid and can range from 5 to 15 min for fentanyl and morphine to up to 40 min for methadone.[101] The common use of permanent central catheters to provide intravenous access for intravenous boluses, continuous infusions, and patients controlled analgesia (PCA) is discussed in the following sections. Specific guidelines for the use of continuous infusions have been developed and are summarized in Table 69-8.[102]

Intermittent or Continuous Subcutaneous Infusions ■ This approach is an alternative to the intravenous infusion.[103-105] The infraclavicular and anterior chest sites provide the greatest freedom of movement for patients. The infusion site is changed every 3-7 days, and a wide variety of opioid analgesics, including morphine, hydromorphone, levorphanol, oxymorphone, heroin, and fentanyl, have been used safely and effectively by this approach. Methadone use has been complicated by the development of cutaneous rashes and inflammatory lesions thought to be a hypersensitivity response.[86] Limited pharmacokinetic studies have demonstrated that the bioavailability of drug from subcutaneous sites at steady state varies from 78% to 100%.[106,107] Guidelines for the use of this approach have been well described in the literature.[106,107]

Epidural and Intrathecal Infusions ■ Although the vast majority of cancer patients receive adequate analgesia with oral, transdermal, or intravenous opioids, some patients may experience intolerable side effects and may receive significant relief from epidural and intrathecal infusions with favorable side-effect profile.[108,109] Data suggest that depending on the medical setting, up to 10% of cancer patients require this approach to provide adequate analgesia.[110,111] The combination of opioids, low dose local anesthetics, clonidine, and recently ziconotide has expanded the usefulness of this technique in patients with neuropathic and other cancer pain.[112]

The availability of patient-controlled devices to which the epidural catheter has allowed patients to self-titrate opioids during pain escalation and remain fully ambulatory.[113] The pharmacokinetics of epidural opioids suggest that a substantial amount of opioid (about 10 times the amount that would be there from a systemic injection) diffuses into cerebrospinal fluid from the epidural space. There is concurrent systemic uptake of the drug comparable to an intramuscular injection that is the highest in lipophilic drugs such as fentanyl. Therefore, the epidural route is associated with both cerebrospinal fluid as well as systemic uptake of the drug. In contrast, intrathecal administration is associated with significantly less systemic uptake of drug.[114,115] The advantage of both these routes of administration is that smaller doses of opioids can be used, and the undesirable central effects (eg, somnolence and respiratory depression) of the opioids can be mini-

Table 69-8 ■ **Guidelines for the Management of Continuous Intravenous Infusion Opioids**

1. CII should be indicated (bolus effect, nursing considerations, or rapid titration of dose).
2. Select an appropriate drug (consider the efficacy of current analgesic, prior-opioid exposure, and pharmacokinetic factors such as half-life).
3. Choose the infusion device. (Flow-calibrated infusion pump should be used.)
4. Convert the latest 24 h total daily opioid consumption to equianalgesic IV dose.
5. If the current drug is used, infuse this quantity over the next 24 h.
6. For CII with a drug different from the current one, convert the daily quantity of opioid into IV equivalent of the new drug, and infuse over the next 24 h (a 50% dose reduction may be needed if pain is well controlled and the patient is tolerant to the opioids).
7. Increase infusion rate until analgesia is achieved or intolerable side effects develop. (If close monitoring is available, repeat the bolus injection, and increase the infusion rate by up to 50% every 20-60 min if pain is severe. If close monitoring is not available, offer a "rescue dose" [a dose of a short half-life drug equivalent to the loading dose administered] every 2 h as needed, and increase the infusion rate after 24 h to amount received during the preceding 24 h period.)
8. If possible, control side effects with adjuvant drugs; if not effective, an opioid rotation should be considered.

mized. Epidural clonidine may be useful in cancer patients with severe pain who cannot be optimally managed on opiates, due to side effects.[116,117] In a randomized placebo-controlled trial in the setting of intractable cancer pain, 45% of patients received analgesia vs 21% in the placebo group.[118] Clonidine was especially useful in patients with neuropathic pain. Given its properties as an α-2-adrenergic agonist, blood pressure and heart rate must be continuously monitored.

Patient-Controlled Analgesia ■ This term has been used to describe the use of specifically designed infusion pumps that can deliver a continuous infusion with bolus doses given on demand by the intravenous, subcutaneous, or epidural routes. This method of opioid administration allows the patient to self-titrate and thus individualize the analgesic doses within the limits set by the clinician. Each pump can be programmed to the needs of the individual patient with a set "lockout time" to prevent patients from overdosing themselves. This approach is most useful for managing the patient with acute pain, including postoperative or pain crisis, as well as the patient with chronic cancer pain who is unable to tolerate drugs by the oral route.[102,119] Intravenous bolus doses of opioids provide the most rapid onset and shortest duration of analgesia. In patients requiring frequent repeated parenteral boluses to maintain analgesia, a continuous infusion via PCA often is a more practical approach. This approach can be successfully used in patients in the terminal stages of their illness when oral drug administration is limited. The wide variety of PCA pumps, from simple devices to sophisticated computerized systems, combined with the use of intravenous or subcutaneous administration has been a major advance in cancer pain management.[120]

Adjuvant Drugs

There is a series of adjuvant drugs that are used in patients with pain and cancer (Table 69-9).[103]

These drugs have been developed and approved for clinical indications other than analgesia, including nausea, vomiting, anxiety, mania, depression, and seizures. Moreover, there are specific adjuvant drugs for the treatment of neuropathic pain and bone pain. The choice of the drugs must be individualized using the simplest but most potent of combinations.

Table 69-9 ■ Number Needed to Treat (NNT) Measurement of Analgesics

Analgesic	NNT
Opioids	2.79
Tramadol	4.76
Gabapentin	4.39
Pregabalin	4.93
Amitriptyline	2.64
Capsaicin	3.26
Lidocaine (Lidoderm)	2.00

Abbreviation: NNT, Number needed to treat for one patient to report 50% reduction in symptoms.

Antidepressant Drugs ■ This class of drugs appears to be the most useful in the management of patients with neuropathic pain.[104] Their analgesic effects are thought to be mediated in part by serotonergic and noradrenergic activity in the CNS. Controlled studies in migraine, postherpetic neuralgia, and diabetic neuropathy have demonstrated their efficacy. They appear to be equally useful in controlling chronic burning pain, continuous dysesthesia, and lancinating or shock-like pain common in patients with peripheral nerve injury.

Amitriptyline is the most commonly used drug, but imipramine, desipramine, and paroxetine have also been reported to be effective.[105,121] For amitriptyline, the suggested dosing schedule is to start at 10-25 mg in a single dose at bedtime, with dosing increments of the same amount. Doses can be increased every 1-2 days, particularly when using 10-mg tablets. Compliance with the regimen as well as the establishment of a therapeutic level can be verified by measuring drug plasma levels.

Recently, duloxetine hydrochloride (Cymbalta) was approved for the management of the pain associated with diabetic peripheral neuropathy and postherpetic neuralgia. This is the first drug specifically approved for these indication. The safety and effectiveness of duloxetine were established in two randomized, controlled studies of approximately 1074 patients. Although the mechanism of action is unknown, patients treated with Cymbalta reported a greater decrease in pain compared to placebo. In these trials, 51% of patients treated with duloxetine reported at least a 30% sustained reduction in pain. In comparison, 31% of patients treated with placebo reported this magnitude of sustained pain reduction.

Four randomized controlled trials (RCTs), compared analgesia from antidepressants amitriptyline, nortriptyline, or desipramine to placebo in PHN. These trails showed significant benefit of tricyclic antidepressants. Number needed to treat (NNT), a number of patients needed to be treated for one patient to report 50% pain reduction was 2.64 (2.1-3.54).

Anticonvulsant Drugs ■ These drugs have been used in the management of pain since the 1960s. Their clinical use in chronic neuropathic pain is considered when the pain is lancinating or burning. Carbamazepine (Tegretal) and gabapentin (Neurontia) are anticonvulsant drugs that suppress spontaneous neuronal firing. In patients with cancer, carbamazepine has been used specifically in managing the acute shock-like neuralgic pain in the cranial or the cervical distribution caused by tumor infiltration or surgical injury. This drug has also been effective in patients with stump pain secondary to traumatic neuroma and patients with lumbosacral plexopathy reporting acute lancinating pain. Patients should commonly start at 100 mg at bedtime, slowly titrating up to 400-600 mg per day. Three placebo-controlled studies of carbamazepine in trigeminal neuralgia had a combined NNT for 50% pain relief of 2.5. A single placebo-controlled trial of gabapentin in postherpetic neuralgia had an NNT of 3.2. For diabetic neuropathy NNTs for effectiveness were as follows (one randomized controlled trial for each drug): carbamazepine 2.3, gabapentin 3.8, and phenytoin 2.1. The NNT for gabapentin based on the polled data was 4.39 (3.34-6.07). The pooled NNT for a 50% pain reduction with pregabalin was 4.93 (3.66-7.58).

Gabapentin is also effective in improving analgesia in patients with neuropathic cancer pain already treated with opioids. Its excellent side-effect profile, lack of hepatic metabolism, and lack of any known drug–drug contraindications make it a prime choice. Although small numbers of patients report bothersome gastrointestinal side effects and mental clouding, it is generally well tolerated up to 4800 mg per day. The dose should be reduced in patients with renal insufficiency.

Both clonazepam (Klonopin) and valproic acid (Depakote) have been reported to be effective in a series of anecdotal case reports and may be considered as alternative agents in patients who are unable to benefit from carbamazepine, gabapentin, or phenytoin. Lamotrigine, (Lamictal) a new antiseizure medication, has been recently used for pain. Although a recent trial showed no significant effect of lamotrigine on spontaneous and evoked pain in complete and incomplete spinal cord injury, it reduced spontaneous pain and evoked pain in the area of spontaneous pain. In a prospective survey, out of 20 patients with chronic, neuropathic pain not responding to interventional therapy who received lamotrigine, four were temporary responders and six patients obtained sustained pain relief. Five patients regained opioid responsiveness and the drug combination produced excellent pain relief for more than 5 months.[122]

Phenothiazine Drugs ■ Methotrimeprazine (Levoprome, Nozinan) has been shown to have effects equianalgesic to morphine in single-dose studies in patients with postoperative pain and chronic cancer pain. This drug is not currently available in the United States.

Haloperidol (Haldol) is the drug of choice in the management of patients with acute psychosis and delirium. Animal studies demonstrate that haloperidol potentiates morphine analgesia and has an independent analgesic effect. The doses of haloperidol in patients with acute delirium or acute psychotic reaction start with 0.5-1 mg orally at bedtime to 2-3 mg 3 times a day, depending on the patient's symptomatology and ability to tolerate the drug.[6,104] For belligerent patient intramuscular injections can be given.

Atypical Neuroleptics ■ Evidence-based review of the available studies on the potential effectiveness of the atypical neuroleptics for the treatment of pain reveals that 90% of the published reports indicate that the atypical neuroleptics did have an analgesic effect. The overall strength and consistency of this evidence is variable. There are, however, few double-blind, placebo-controlled studies, and many of the reports/studies have less than 50 patients. As such, this question requires further research.

Risperidon (Risperdal) may be useful for treatment of both hyper- and hypoactive delirium. It is associated with fewer parkinsonian side effects. The same is true for olanzapine, (zyprexa) an atypical neuroleptic that may be quite sedating and in elderly patients may be associated with worsening delirium. Its sedating properties may be of great value under certain circumstances. It also comes as a dissolvable tablet that may be an advantage in dysphagia or if a patient is too sedated or weak to be able to cooperate.

Antihistamine Drugs ■ Hydroxyzine has been shown to have analgesic effects when combined with morphine or meperidine in doses of 100 mg parenterally.[105] Hydroxyzine (Vistetil, Atavax) also has antiemetic and sedative properties, both of which can be desirable in patients with nausea, vomiting, and acute anxiety. Common practice is to use hydroxyzine at doses of 25 mg in combination with opioids to control these other effects. Most published data are derived from the anecdotal reports.

Corticosteroids ■ Corticosteroids are the most widely used general-purpose adjuvant analgesics. Analgesic effects of steroids consist in part of the anti-inflammatory effect. In cultured dorsal root ganglia corticosteroids were shown to reduce ectopic neural discharge that is thought to be the explanation of their effectiveness in neuropathic pain. They may ameliorate pain and produce beneficial effects on appetite, nausea, and mood. They provide analgesia from pain syndromes associated with raised intracranial pressure, acute spinal cord compression, superior vena cava syndrome, metastatic bone pain, neuropathic pain due to infiltration or compression by tumor, or hepatic capsular distension.[28] Systemic, intra-articular and epidural routes of administration are most common. Patients with advanced cancer who experience pain and other symptoms that may respond to steroids are usually given relatively small doses (dexamethasone, 1-2 mg twice daily). In patients with epidural spinal cord compression, high doses (dexamethasone, 24 or 100 mg IV, followed by a slow taper) can be used to manage an acute episode of severe pain.[30]

About 85% of patients receiving 100 mg of dexamethasone as a part of a radiotherapy protocol reported significant relief associated with marked reduction in analgesic requirements within 24 h of administration of this dose. Several studies demonstrate prolonged survival times and reduced opioid doses in terminal cancer patients receiving steroids. In patients with prostate cancer, 30 mg of prednisone on a regular basis improves patients' quality of life and reduces their pain symptomatology.[28,121] Pain resulting from tumor infiltration of the brachial and lumbosacral plexus is often improved by the use of steroids. Steroids also improve the headache and radicular pain commonly seen in leptomeningeal disease. Corticosteroids may be particularly helpful in the patient who is admitted to the hospital with far-advanced disease and diffuse pain in an acute painful crisis. We often use a large dose of steroids in this setting (10-24 mg of dexamethasone IV) to stabilize the patient and provide rapid symptom control.

Steroid psychosis can complicate steroid use, However, and can occur during dose escalation or withdrawal. Steroid-induced psychosis is treated with dose reduction and neuroleptics.

In peripheral nerve hyperalgesia, an open RCT showed some improvement in analgesia after a single epidural injection of 80 mg methylprednisolone and 10 mg bupivacaine in the acute phase of herpes foster for neuritic pain, but the effect did not last beyond 1 month.[123]

Neurostimulant Drugs ■ Dextroamphetamine has been demonstrated to provide additive analgesia in patients receiving morphine for postoperative pain.[124] In a controlled repeated-dose trial, oral methylphenidate (Ritalin) reversed opioid-induced sedation and provided supplemental analgesia in a population of patients with cancer pain.[125,126]

Modafinil (Provigil) is a wakefulness-promoting agent for oral administration similar in action to amphetamine and methylphenidate, although its pharmacologic profile is not identical to that of sympathomimetic amines. Unlike sympathomimetic agents, modafinil has minimal effects on cardiovascular and hemodynamic parameters. The effectiveness of Provigil in reducing the excessive sleepiness associated with narcolepsy using American Sleep Disorders Association criteria was established in two multicenter, placebo-controlled, two-dose (200 or 400 mg per day), double-blind studies of outpatients.

Topical and Systemic Local Anesthetics ■ Topical drugs, including lidocaine and benzocaine creams are useful in the management of painful cutaneous and mucosal lesions and as a premedication prior to skin puncture. Controlled studies have demonstrated the effectiveness of a eutectic mixture of 2.5% lidocaine and 2.5% prilocaine (EMLA) in reducing pain associated with venipuncture, lumbar puncture, and arterial puncture.[127] Viscous lidocaine is frequently used in the management of oropharyngeal ulceration.[128] A lidocaine patch (Lidoderm) is a delivery system delivering 5% lidocaine transcutaneously with minimal blood concentrations. It is approved for postherpetic neuralgia and effective for other somatic pains. It is applied for 12 h of every 24 h to avoid tachyphylaxis.

Lidocaine (Xylocame), bupivacaine (Marcome), and ropivacaine (Naropin) are the most commonly used parenteral local anesthetics for trigger-point injections, intercostals, brachial, epidural, and intrathecal infusions. Unfortunately, positive response to lidocaine infusion does not predict analgesia. Epidural bupivacaine offers good motor and sensory separation and lasts 2-3 times longer than lidocaine. That leads to its frequent use in the epidural and intrathecal infusions. Bupivacaine is quite cardiotoxic when given parenterally and caution is required in patients receiving both epidural bupiracaine and intravenous infusions simultaneously. Special marked tubing to deliver bupivacaine should be used to avoid administration errors.

Adjuvants for Bone Pain ■ Bisphosphonate drugs (pamidronate (Aredia), clodronate, zoledronate (tometa), and bandronate (Boniva) bind to bone hydroxyapatite, inhibiting osteoclast activity, and are highly effective in the management of painful a metastatic disease to the bone and in managing multiple myeloma. Some randomized double-blind studies have demonstrated their efficacy not only in relieving bone pain but also in reducing skeletal complications[129] and mortality.

Combined analysis of two multicenter, randomized, placebo-controlled studies of pamidronate disodium for the palliation of bone pain in men with metastatic prostate cancer failed to demonstrate a significant overall treatment effect.[130] In women with advanced breast cancer and clinically evident bone metastases, the use of bisphosphonates (oral or intravenous) in addition to hormone therapy or chemotherapy, when compared with placebo or no bisphosphonates, delayed any skeletal event and reduce the risk of developing one.[131]

Zoledronic acid (4 mg) has been compared to placebo in a randomized phase III trail involving 422 men with hormone-refractory prostate cancer metastatic to bone. Zoledronic acid demonstrated a significant advantage over placebo for median time to first skeletal related event.[131]

In January 2008, the FDA issued an alert about the possibility that patients on biphosphonates can develop severe musculoskeletal pain starting within days, months, or even years after initiating treatment. The FDA's concern is that the association between biphosphonates and severe musculoskeletal pain may be overlooked by health care professionals, delaying diagnosis, prolonging pain and/or impairment, and necessitating the use of analgesics.

Strontium-89 (^{89}Sr) among other radiopharmaceuticals, is an effective treatment of patients with chemotherapy-refractory prostate cancer but careful and prolonged monitoring of hematologic parameters after therapy is required. In a recent study of the 14 administered treatments, 8 (57%) resulted in improved pain control, with 2 patients being able to stop analgesia. The median duration of response was 56 days. There was significant and prolonged bone marrow toxicity, with six patients requiring red blood cell transfusion.[132] ^{89}Sr is effective and safe in bone pain palliation in breast cancer. In a recent study 25 patients with painful multifocal bone metastases from breast cancer received 148 MBq ^{89}Sr IV. The global response rate was 84%. The duration of pain relief ranged from 2 to 14 months (mean of 125 days). A moderate hematological toxicity resolved within 12 weeks after ^{89}Sr administration.[133]

Ketamine infusions has produced analgesia in cancer patients in doses much lower than those required for anesthesia (typically 0.1-1.5 mg/kg/h). A double-blind crossover study evaluating the effect of intrathecal ketamine on spinal morphine analgesia revealed that ketamine enhanced the analgesic effect and reduced the amount of morphine required.[134] Ketamine significantly reduced the pain intensity, and can improve morphine analgesia in difficult pain syndromes, such as neuropathic pain. The occurrence of central adverse effects should be taken into account. However, especially when using higher doses. Increasing number of good outcomes with oral, subcutaneous, and intravenous ketamine in cancer patients has been reported in noncontrolled studies.

These observations should be tested in studies of prolonged ketamine administration. Ketamine is usually considered when respiratory depression and extreme uncontrollable sedation pose risks for the opioid and sedating adjuvant analgesics.

It is recommended to start ketamine at a low dose of 0.02-0.05 mg/kg/h by continuous intravenous infusion and rapidly titrate up as needed, escalating the dose by up to 100% every 4-6 hours, depending on the pain intensity and side-effect profile. Cognitive side effects have occurred infrequently at these doses. However, at doses of 10-20 mg/h, 30-50% of patients are reported to develop drowsiness, nightmares, and hallucinations. Due to the limited quality of the published data, the role of ketamine is not yet established. To develop evidence-based guidelines for cancer patients, additional studies are needed.

Treatment of Side Effects

Depending upon the circumstance, a number of side effects associated with opioid analgesics can be characterized as desirable or undesirable. Sedation, confusion, nausea, vomiting, constipation, multifocal myoclonus, and respiratory depression are the most common side effects encountered in the clinical use of opioids. When evaluating for opioid-related side effects, clinician should attempt to establish whether the side effects are due to the opioid, other drugs, or the disease progression.

Sedation ■ This side effect is particularly bothersome for patients who are trying to maintain their normal daily work and social activities. Tolerance develops to this effect within several days. In patients who are excessively sedated but who are obtaining adequate analgesia, opioid dose reduction may be tried first. If opioid dose cannot be reduced without compromising analgesia the use of caffeine, modafinil, dextroamphetamine, or methylphenidate, as described previously, may counteract this effect (Table 69-10). Level 1 evidence now exists to support the use of the psychostimulants to treat opioid-induced sedation and fatigue.

Table 69-10 ■ **Algorithm for the Management of Persistent Opioid-Induced Sedation**

Eliminate nonessential psychoactive medications
If analgesia is satisfactory, reduce opioid dose by 25%
Consider addition of a psychostimulant
Consider:
Addition of a nonopioid or adjuvant drug
Opioid substitution
Use of an anesthetic or neurosurgical approach

Nausea and Vomiting ■ Nausea and vomiting can occur from the action of opioid analgesics on the medullary chemoreceptor trigger zone (CTZ) and direct effect on the gastrointestinal mortality. Opioids may delay gastric emptying by more than 10 h. The incidence of nausea and vomiting is markedly increased in ambulatory patients, suggesting that the opioid drugs also alter vestibular sensitivity. Opioid-induced nausea and vomiting appears to vary with the drug and the patient, so that some advantage may result from switching to an equianalgesic dose of another opioid. Alternatively, an antiemetic may be used at the initiation of the opioid. Commonly used drugs for control of nausea and vomiting associated with opioids include prokinetic agents prochlorperazine and metoclopramide. Scopolamine may be advantageous in a patient with mostly orthostatic nausea. Lorazepam may be particularly effective in anticipatory nausea, but can be quite sedating. Dexamethasone is a potent antinausea medication associated with significant side effects with long-term use. The 5-HT3 antagonists ondansetron, granisetron, and others are well tolerated, but quite expensive, which may decrease patient compliance, especially if they have to pay for the medications. Tolerance to this side effect generally develops within 2-3 days.

Constipation ■ Constipation is the most common adverse effect of the opioid analgesics. These drugs act at multiple sites in the gastrointestinal tract and spinal cord to produce a decrease in intestinal secretions and peristalsis, resulting in a dry stool and constipation. Tolerance to constipation develops slowly if at all making laxatives an absolutely necessary component of the opioid therapy. Provision for a regular bowel regimen including cathartics and stool softeners should be instituted. The use of an osmotic cathartic (lactulose) may be the next step. Whatever approach is taken, it should be used regularly and aggressively to prevent fecal impaction and bowel obstruction.

Multifocal Myoclonus ■ In chronic systemic administration of opioids, especially with rapid dose escalation, the corresponding opioid blood levels and metabolites may increase causing multifocal myoclonus. Multifocal myoclonus if untreated may degenerate into a grand mal seizure. Standard approach to this side effect is to switch the patient to an alternative opioid. If myoclonus is observed in a dying patient, the use of benzodiazepines or barbiturates to suppress the myoclonic jerks may be preferred.

Confusion and Hallucinations ■ In chronic systemic administration of opioids, especially with rapid dose escalation, the corresponding metabolites may increase steadily with increased doses and exceed the highest tolerated levels causing delirium. This occurs in 40-90% of patients at the end-of-life, and it is one of the most distressing symptoms for patients and their families (Table 69-10). Uncontrolled pain with delirium is usually managed by an "opioid rotation" to another opioid. Sequential therapeutic trials used to determine the most favorable drug has become a standard strategy in pain management. When switching opioids in the treatment of cancer pain, one should be aware that 80% of patients require one switch, 44% require two switches and 20% require three or more switches. Delirium should be viewed as a medical emergency, evaluated and treated urgently.

Respiratory Depression ■ Respiratory depression is potentially the most serious adverse effect. The morphine-like agonists act on brain stem respiratory centers to produce, as a function of dose, increasing respiratory depression to the point of apnea. In man, death from an overdose of a morphine-like agonist is nearly always due to respiratory arrest. Therapeutic doses of morphine may depress all phases of respiratory activity: rate, minute volume, and tidal exchange.

However, as carbon dioxide accumulates, it stimulates central chemoreceptors, resulting in a compensatory increase in respiratory rate, which masks the degree of respiratory depression. At equianalgesic doses, all the morphine-like agonists produce an equivalent degree of respiratory depression. Respiratory depression most commonly occurs in opiate-naive patients after acute administration of an opioid and is typically associated with other signs of CNS depression, including sedation and mental clouding.

Tolerance develops rapidly to this effect with repeated drug administration, allowing the opioid analgesics to be used in the management of chronic cancer pain without significant risk of respiratory depression. If respiratory depression does occur, it can be rapidly reversed by the administration of the specific opioid antagonist, naloxone. The use of naloxone should be based on the prior-opioid exposure of the patient. In patients chronically receiving opioids who develop respiratory depression, the standard naloxone dose, 0.4 mg/mL, should be diluted in 9 cc of saline and slowly titrated in the patient to reverse respiratory depression. This approach prevents the patient from experiencing excruciating pain with reversal of the analgesic effects of the current opioid while providing improved respiratory function. If effective, naloxone reverses sedation and respiratory depression within seconds. One should be aware that in a patient with CO_2 narcosis, naloxone may not reverse the opioid-induced respiratory depression even if it blocks the opioid receptors. Intubation if appropriate needs to be considered if the patient has high CO_2 and does not respond to naloxone. Patients with cancer receiving opioids chronically are very sensitive to naloxone's effects, and patients who have been taking drugs with a long half-life, such as methadone or levorphanol, or who have been taking a slow-release morphine preparation or using a transdermal patch will require a continuous infusion of naloxone to maintain a stable respiratory pattern.

The dose of naloxone for continuous infusion should be calculated from the initial dose used to reverse depression. Commonly, 1.2 mg of naloxone is diluted in 250 mL of saline and slowly titrated to the needs of the individual patient. Before administering naloxone to a comatose patient, an endotracheal tube should be placed to prevent aspiration, given the possibility of respiratory compromise, excessive salivation, and bronchial spasm.

Hypogonadism ■ Profound hypogonadism has been noted in patients receiving intrathecal opioids. It has been increasingly recognized that chronic opioid exposure can cause hypogonadism presenting with severe fatigue and decreased sexual drive. Survivors of cancer who chronically consumed opioids experienced symptomatic hypogonadism with significantly higher levels of depression, fatigue, and sexual dysfunction. With the increasing use of opioids among patients with cancer, monitoring, and if appropriate, supplementation of testosterone may be needed.

Psychological and Behavioral Approaches

Psychological management of cancer pain includes the use of psychotherapeutic, cognitive-behavioral, and psychopharmacologic interventions. The use of short-term supportive psychotherapy based on a crisis intervention model allows patients to receive emotional support, information, and skills and information to assist in adapting to a pain crisis.[6] Psychiatrists and psychologists trained in psycho-oncology can be pivotal in managing patients who have significant psychological morbidity associated with their cancer pain. Cognitive-behavioral techniques are helpful in promoting an increased sense of control, thus reducing the sense of hopelessness and helplessness, common to many cancer pain patients.[135,136] These techniques are most useful in three clinical situations: (1) in the management of patients with intermittent predictable pain (such as pain associated with procedures), (2) in the management of incident pain (eg, in the patient with pain on movement), and (3) in the management of chronic cancer pain. A series of cognitive-behavioral approaches used with cancer patients are listed in Table 69-11. The goal of such interventions is to enhance the sense of personal control of a patient in pain. Some techniques are primarily cognitive, focusing on perceptual, and thought processes, and others are predominantly behavioral, directed at developing modulation of behavior to help patients cope with pain and cancer. These approaches are used concurrently with analgesic drug therapy and anesthetic and neurosurgical approaches.

Anesthetic Approaches

Anesthetic approaches can be divided into six major types: (1) trigger-point injections, (2) peripheral nerve blocks, (3) autonomic nerve blocks, (4) epidural and intrathecal infusions, (5) surgical approaches, and (6) neurostimulatory approaches. The techniques for each of these procedures have been described in detail in standard textbooks.[111]

Short-acting and long-acting anesthetics are used for temporary and diagnostic nerve blocks whereas phenol, alcohol neurolysis, cryo- and radiofrequency lesioning are used for permanent blocks, although it is not uncommon that a permanent nerve block provides analgesia for about 2-3 months only. Destruction of neurons with hypertonic solution and ice crystal formation with cryotherapy is partially reversible by regeneration of the affected nerve. Alcohol causes a nonselective tissue destruction by dehydration

Table 69-11 ■ **Cognitive-Behavioral Techniques for Cancer Pain**

Preparatory information
Cognitive restructuring
Focusing
Controlled mental imagery
Distraction
Controlled attention
Mental, behavioral
Music therapy
Hypnosis
Biofeedback

and extraction of lipids and coagulating mucoproteins and lipoproteins.

Trigger-Point Injections

Patients with significant musculoskeletal pain often describe specific tender trigger-point areas and significant pain relief may be achieved when these trigger points are injected with saline, local anesthetic, or Botox.[137] Effective relief, however, is not diagnostic of musculoskeletal pain alone, and evaluation of the cause of pain is still necessary to rule out the specific etiology.

Peripheral Nerve Blocks

Peripheral nerve blocks can be used to localize the nerve distribution and for therapy. The usefulness of this technique is limited to areas of the body in which interruption of both motor and sensory function will not interfere with the patient's functional status. This approach is most commonly used in patients who have pain in the head (gasserian ganglion, glossopharyngeal, trigeminal nerve and its branches, occipital, and other blocks), extremities (interscalene, supraclavicular, infraclavicular and axillary brachial plexus blocks, musculocutaneous, ulnar, median and radial nerve blocks, sciatic, femoral, and other nerve blocks), and chest (intercostals, paraspinal blocks).[138-141] In intercostal and paraspinal nerve blocks multiple nerves usually must be blocked to provide adequate analgesia. The highest blood levels of local anesthetic are seen with multilevel intercostals nerves. Risk of bleeding, infection, and pneumothorax should be considered. Anesthesia dolorosa is a potentially devastating complication of a permanent nerve block when the patient develops painful anesthesia at the site of the block. Thus, neurolytic blocks are most suitable for patients with localized unilateral pain and a short-life expectancy.[142] This approach has very limited value in managing upper and lower limb pain associated with brachial and lumbosacral plexopathy because of the high risk of associated motor function loss. Epidural neurolysis, when neurolysis is performed via the epidural catheter carries a somewhat higher risk of spinal cord injury. Permanent nerve blocks and epidural neurolysis may be considered in the following instances: (1) exhaustion of the appropriate antitumor approaches (radiation, surgery), (2) clear clinical and radiologic definition of the cause of pain, (3) failure of pharmacological interventions to produce adequate analgesia without significant side effects, (4) a favorable response to a temporary block with a local anesthetic, and (5) magnetic resonance imaging performed before the procedure to rule out epidural tumor infiltration.

Neurosurgical Approaches

Laminectomies and vertebral body resection with reconstruction are usually used for pain associated with spinal cord compression or spine instability, usually caused by a pathological collapse. Vertebroplasty with intravertebral methyl methacrylate can be sufficient when cord compression does not exist (Table 69-12).[143,144] Neuroablative procedures are designed to interrupt pain pathways in either the peripheral or CNS. Risk of the loss of function resulting from such procedure is a major concern. Patients will rarely give up neurologic function for improvement in pain, particularly if the neurologic deficit may be associated with incontinence or leg weakness. Chemical *hypophysectomy,* reported to be effective especially in breast and prostate cancer patients, has become a rare procedure. *Dorsal rhizotomy* involves cutting the dorsal roots. It can be performed as an open surgical procedure following laminectomy or by a percutaneous radiofrequency technique through the intervertebral foramina under radiographic control.[188] *Cordotomy* can be performed as an open or percutaneous unilateral or bilateral surgical procedure (Fig. 69-2).[145] A unilateral cordotomy remains the neurosurgical treatment of choice for patients with refractory cancer pain, but neurosurgical procedures have become less frequent. The procedure is performed using radiographic visualization. Penetration of the cord by a fine electrode, usually in the C1-C2 interspace is monitored by electrical impedance. The ability to complete the procedure technically varies from 70% to 99% of attempts. This approach is particularly useful in patients with unilateral pain below the T1 region. Pain relief reports vary from 70% to 95% and may last from 3 weeks to 6 months.[146]

Table 69-12 ■ Neurosurgical Procedures for Cancer Pain

Antitumor procedures
Anterior vertebral body resection and reconstruction
Decompressive laminectomy
Ventricular shunts for headache due to increased intracranial pressure
Debulking of tumor in brachial and lumbosacral plexus
Analgesic procedures
Peripheral neurectomy
Cranial neurectomy (trigeminal, glossopharyngeal)
Dorsal rhizotomy
Dorsal root entry zone lesion
Cordotomy (unilateral or bilateral)
Chemical hypophysectomy
Neurostimulatory procedures
Transcutaneous electrical nerve stimulation (TENS)
Peripheral nerve or plexus stimulation
Dorsal column stimulation
Thalamic stimulation
Neuropharmacologic procedures
Epidural opioids, local anesthetic and clonidine infusions
Intrathecal opioids, local anesthetic and clonidine infusions
Intraventricular opioids

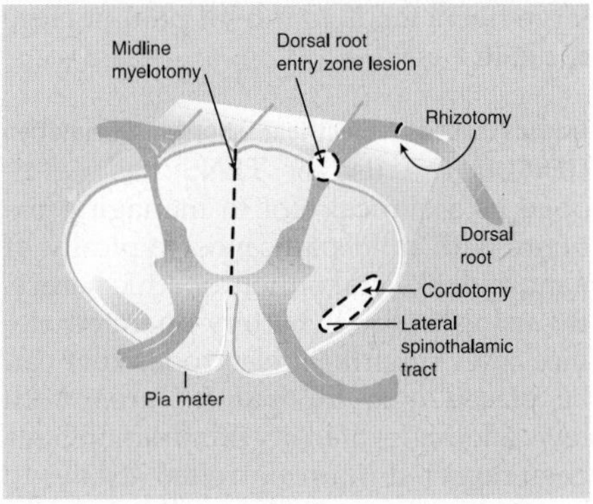

Figure 69-2 ■ Cross-section of the spinal cord showing sites of neuroablative procedures for pain control. *Source:* From Ref. 143.

Dorsal Root Entry Zone Lesion

This procedure was developed to manage predominantly neuropathic pain by producing a surgical lesion in the dorsal root entry zone. In a group of patients with Pancoast's tumor infiltration of the brachial plexus, Sindou and Lapras reported that 66% obtained pain relief.[193] In general, the practicality of dorsal root entry zone lesions for the management of cancer patients remains undefined.

Cingulotomy

Cingulotomy has recently received new attention in the treatment of some patients with cancer pain. The development of a stereotactic procedure using magnetic resonance imaging for guidance to place a radiofrequency lesion has led to new interest in this procedure. In a group of patients recently reported by Hassenbusch and colleagues, four patients with pain from widely metastatic diffuse bone disease and who were receiving opioid analgesics reported immediate pain relief with bilateral cingulate lesions.[194] The pain relief persisted in this group of patients until death in 2-6 weeks. This procedure has previously been used to treat patients with psychiatric illness.

Neurostimulatory Procedures

These procedures are based on the Gate Theory of Pain, which suggests that a neurophysiologic gating mechanism exists in the spinal cord, probably within the substantia gelatinosa. Stimulation of the small fibers tends to promote pain or open the gate whereas stimulation of large fibers tends to inhibit pain or close the gate.

Transcutaneous Electrical Nerve Stimulation (TENS) ■ The use of TENS has developed as a clinical tool in managing patients with mild pain, most typically of a musculoskeletal or neuropathic nature. By using a small battery-operated device with superficial electrodes that can be placed over the painful area, both low- and high-intensity stimulation have been reported in uncontrolled studies to be effective in controlling mild pain in a peripheral nerve distribution.

Peripheral Nerve Stimulation ■ Stimulation of peripheral nerves by implantation of electrodes was proposed on the basis of the concept of selectively activating large nerve fibers to suppress activity in small, presumably pain, fibers.[147] Experience to date suggests up to 30-50% incidence of relief, with a general falloff in efficacy within the first 2 years.

Dorsal Column Stimulation ■ As the large nerve fibers ascend in a compact bundle through the dorsal column, they are accessible to selective electrical stimulation. The dorsal column stimulating technique involves introducing an electrode into the epidural or intrathecal space and advancing it to the appropriate level overlying the dorsal columns. The main indication for placement of a dorsal column stimulator is intractable dysesthetic or neuropathic pain of the limbs or trunk, such as occurs in patients with radiation-induced brachial or lumbosacral plexopathy. This procedure is effective in 43-75% of patients and carries a low morbidity rate.[148,149] The trial is considered positive if more than 50% improvement is achieved. The most common complication is failure of the device itself, which occurs in approximately 10% of patients annually. Other complications include infections, cerebrospinal fluid (CSF) fistula, allergy or rejection response to the device material, and changes in stimulation overtime, which may be related to cellular changes around the electrode or shifts in its position.

Thalamic Stimulation ■ The stereotactic insertion of stimulating electrodes into the medial thalamus has been most commonly used to manage intractable pain characterized by a predominantly neuropathic component described as a steady, tingling, burning element of pain.[198,199] Complications with this procedure include infection in 2-15% of patients, electrode migration in 2-27%, and worsening neurologic dysfunction in 2-15%.

Intrathecal Pumps ■ Implantation of intrathecal pumps are the most common neurosurgical procedure today in cancer pain management. Patients with uncontrolled cancer pain and inability to tolerate higher oral opioids and who have a life expectancy of more than 6 months (3 months are paid for by some insurance companies) may be considered. Opioids, clonidine, and local anesthetics may be added to the intrathecal solution, a drug combination not available by intravenous route. Magnetic resonance imaging must be performed prior to the procedure to rule out epidural tumor infiltration that may increase the risk of bleeding into the epidural and intrathecal space. Before the implanted pump or permanent epidural catheter is placed it is important to perform an appropriate trial. An epidural catheter allows patient-controlled analgesia (ie, rescue [PRN] drug administration), in addition to the continued infusion not available by the intrathecal route. Drug combinations can be delivered epidurally as well. As a rule, the epidural dose is significantly smaller than the equianalgesic dose of the oral opioid. The dose reduction is even more pronounced when opioid is administered intrathecally. Surgical complications include perioperative bleeding that may lead to pocket hematoma as well as epidural and intrathecal hematomas with neurological injury. This and other complications are rare, but should be watched for.

Specific Autonomic Nerve Blocks

Celiac plexus block is commonly used for intolerable upper abdominal and upper back pain associated with localized pancreatic carcinoma. Outcome is generally worse when liver metastases or retroperitoneal lymphadenopathy is present. Patients usually continue to require opioids, but may need less dose or slower dose escalation for up to 2-3 months after the celiac plexus block. The major side effect of the procedure is transient hypotension and diarrhea. Patients must be well hydrated and monitored during the procedure and for 4-6 h afterward. Significant neurologic complications such as paraparesis and renal hemorrhage occur in less than 1% of patients if proper technique is used. The procedure should only be performed under radiologic guidance to avoid such complications. Splanchnic nerve block may provide relief of pain in patients who fail to obtain relief from celiac plexus block. In patients with cancer it may help to reduce opioid requirements and improve function.

Hypogastric and ganglion of Impar blocks are usually considered for treating intractable pelvic pain. In postsurgical/postradiation pelvic cancer pain results may be limited due to the disturbed anatomy.

Sedation in the Imminently Dying

Close adherence to established pain management guidelines produces effective and satisfactory analgesia in 70-100% of cancer patients. Ventafridda and colleagues reported that up to 50% of patients in his home-care palliative service had uncontrolled symptoms in the last days of life and required sedation for adequate control.[150] In those patients whose pain cannot be relieved without cognitive impairment, the use of sedation is an acceptable strategy when the intent is to relieve suffering. The United States Supreme Court has defined sedation as appropriate care of the dying, different from physician-assisted suicide.[151-153] In patients who are sedated for symptom control, such an approach should include an open discussion with the patient's family, a do-not-resuscitate order, the appropriate use of drugs for symptom control, and dose escalation only to manage clearly defined signs and symptoms. By invoking the principle of double effect, pain medication may be provided in doses that may risk respiratory depression to the point of death, if required for symptomatic relief. The primary intention must always be pain relief although the foreseen but unintended result may be sedation or death. Such practices are considered an important part of appropriate and compassionate care of the dying at cancer centers worldwide.[154,155]

Tolerance

Tolerance is a pharmacologic effect characterized by the fact that with repeated administration, increasing doses are necessary to provide the same effect.[130] Tolerance develops at different rates for the various opioid effects. Tolerance to respiratory depression, as discussed previously, develops rapidly in contrast to no or slow tolerance to the constipating effects. The first sign of analgesic tolerance is the patient's report that the duration of analgesic effect is reduced from its initial interval. The patient who reports the shorter duration of pain relief is often labeled as a clock-watcher, and that patient's report may be misinterpreted by health care professionals as an early sign of addiction. It is common for patients even with stable pain to increase their dose of opioid analgesic during the titration phase until they have reached steady state and are stabilized on a dose. This stabilized dose may be reached over a 2- to 4-week period. Dose escalation in cancer patient most often is a sign of disease progression and should prompt a thorough medical investigation. It is critical to remember that in patients with increasing pain, the degree of relief of pain and its analgesic effect are based on a log-dose relationship, and doubling the dose may therefore be necessary to provide adequate analgesia.

During opioid titration intolerable side effects occur before adequate analgesia is achieved. Switching to an alternative analgesic, using adjuvant drugs and employing a neurosurgical approach may be used in this instance.

Differentiate Physical Dependence From Psychological Dependence

Physical dependence is the term used to describe the phenomenon of withdrawal when an opioid is abruptly discontinued or when an opioid-mixed agonist-antagonist or antagonist (eg, naloxone) is administered. The severity of this withdrawal is a function of the dose and duration of prior-opioid administration. Prior exposure to an opioid agonist can greatly increase a patient's sensitivity to an antagonist.

Symptoms of opioid withdrawal include:

- Anxiety, irritability, insomnia,
- Sweating, increased salivation, tearing, rhinorrhea
- Hot flashes, chills
- Diarrhea, abdominal cramping, nausea, vomiting

To prevent acute withdrawal, patients receiving opioids should not be discontinued abruptly, but be tapered off their drug. Around 25% of the previous daily dose will usually prevent signs and symptoms of withdrawal in a majority of patients, but to minimize the withdrawal symptoms, downward titration by 25% every 1-3 days is commonly preferred.

In contrast to physical dependence, *psychological dependence* is a term used to describe a behavioral pattern of drug use characterized by continued craving for an opioid for effects other than pain relief. An overwhelming involvement with drug use and procurement as compulsive traits are the salient features of this type of dependence. Cancer patients chronically receiving opioids become physically but not psychologically dependent on their drugs. Patients' and physicians' fears of addiction are the major barrier to adequate cancer pain management.[156-158] Patients with poorly managed and/or undertreated pain may mimic the signs of psychological dependence, displaying a behavioral pattern known as *pseudoaddiction*.[159] The prevalence of true psychological dependence among cancer patients without history of addiction is extremely rare.

Addiction and Drug Abuse in Cancer Pain Patients

The American Academy of Pain Medicine, the American Pain Society, and the American Society of Addiction Medicine (2001) defined addiction as a primary, chronic, neurobiologic disease, with genetic, psychological, and environmental factors influencing its development and manifestations. It is characterized by behaviors that include one or more of the following: impaired control over drug use, compulsive use, use despite harm, and craving.

The WHO characterizes addiction as:

- Usage out of control
- Obsession with obtaining a supply
- Use causes personal and legal difficulties
- Use continues despite problems
- User denies taking the substance
- Quality of life is NOT improved

Known risk factors and prevalence of addiction/chemical coping in the general population correlate with similar rate, 10% (3-18%), of aberrant drug behavior in pain patients.[132,133,160,161]

The management of pain in cancer patients with history of chemical dependency requires a comprehensive assessment and requires a treatment approach directed both at pain and the associated problems. Loss of control over the use of opioids, preoccupation with obtaining opioids despite the presence of adequate analgesia and adverse consequences associated with opioid use are suggested by the consensus statement of the *Academy* and Societies mentioned previously (2001). Personal history of substance abuse, poor social support and substance abuse in the family and friends, and psychiatric history may influence the follow-up and clinical monitoring strategy that needs to be implemented. Psychiatric assessment, social worker assessment, and referral to a pain management group may be helpful for one time evaluation of support throughout the treatment period. It is hard to overestimate the importance of a team approach, consistent treatment plan, and exchange of information between providers participating in care for the cancer pain patient with substance abuse to insure good analgesia and safety. On the other hand, it is important to keep in mind that patients with a history of substance abuse are at high risk of under treatment of pain, both because of the clinician's caution in prescribing opioids at the doses they would be comfortable with in a patient without history of addiction, but also because many of the patients with history of substance abuse are opioid tolerant and need relatively high opioid-dose.

When starting opioid analgesics in a high-risk patient the clinician should monitor the patient to ensure that the opioids:

- Reduce pain levels
- Improve functionality ("uptime") and mood
- Improve activities of daily living
- May help to return to work
- May lead to reduced consumption of health care resources

After a high-risk patient is identified the following steps may be taken:

- Educate the patient and the family
- Monitor supportive environment
- Prevent unilateral dose escalation
- Rule out psychiatric comorbidity as uncontrolled anxiety, depression or psychosis

A clinician should be aware that a patient with a history of chemical dependency has increased stress during cancer treatment. A worsening of prognosis may precipitate a relapse.

Pseudoaddiction ■ Pseudoaddiction is behavior that is reminiscent of addiction, but is driven by undertreatment of pain and disappears with adequate analgesia. It is not uncommon for a patient with pseudoaddiction to exhibit anger and demanding behaviors, insisting on a specific drug or specific doses/route of administration.

Adequate analgesia in a patient with pseudoaddiction leads to the resolution of the aberrant behavior.

Urine drug testing in clinical practice is a consensual diagnostic test directed to the verification of the compliance with the medications prescribed and abstinence from illicit or nonprescribed substances. In order to perform the urine drug test, the clinician has to provide full explanation regarding the nature and purpose of testing to the patient and obtain at least verbal consent from the patient. The clinician ordering the test must be familiar with the reliability of the urine toxicology laboratory chosen. Codeine and heroin are metabolized to morphine and will test positive for morphine in urine. Generally, semisynthetic and synthetic opioids such as oxycodone and methadone are not detected unless chromatography/mass spectrometry is used. Hydromorphone is partially metabolized to morphine and may test positive for it. Most opioids will reliably test positive for the first 2 days after the last dose; cocaine metabolites test positive for 2-4 days, propoxyphene for 6-48 h, and cannabinoids for 5-28 days, depending on the frequency and the dose. If not familiar with the assays used in the institution the clinician may need to be in close contact with the laboratory to interpret the urine drug test results correctly. If used appropriately, such testing, especially in a high-risk patient, may help to set and enforce boundaries based on mutual trust and honesty.

In summary, most cancer patients presenting with pain have advanced disease and need opioids for analgesia. Concerns about addiction, lack of access, and other barriers should not interfere with the availability of opioids and other analgesics to the patient in need.

Selected References

The complete reference list can be found at www.CANCERMEDICINE8.com

1. Cherny NI, Portenoy RK. Practical management of cancer pain. In: Wall PD, Melzack R, eds. *Textbook of Pain*, 3rd ed. Edinburgh: Churchill Livingstone; 1994:1437–1468.
2. Elliott K, Foley KM. Neurologic pain syndromes in patients with cancer. In: Portenoy RK, ed. *Neurology Clinics. Pain: Mechanisms and Syndromes*, Vol. 7. Philadelphia: W.B. Saunders; 1989:333.
3. Agency for Health Care Policy and Research. Management of cancer pain: clinical practice guideline. Rockville (MD): U.S. Public Health Service Agency for Health Care Policy and Research; 1994. Publication No.: 94–0592.
4. Fishman B, Pasternak S, Wallenstein SL, et al. The Memorial pain assessment card: a valid instrument for the evaluation of cancer pain. *Cancer.* 1987;60:1151.
5. Graham C, Bond SS, Gerkocic MM, Cook MR. Use of McGill pain questionnaire in the assessment of cancer pain: replicability and consistency. *Pain.* 1980;8:377.
11. Grond S, Zech D, Diefenbach C, Bischoff A. Prevalence and pattern of symptoms in patients with cancer pain: a prospective evaluation of 1,635 cancer patients referred to a pain clinic. *J Pain Symptom Manage.* 1994;9:372–382.
12. Portenoy RK, Kornblith AB, Wong G, et al. Pain in ovarian cancer patients: prevalence, characteristics, and associated symptoms. *Cancer.* 1994;73:907–914.
13. Twycross RG, Fairfield S. Pain in far-advanced cancer. *Pain.* 1982;14:303.
14. Ferrell BR, Wisdon C, Wenzl C. Quality of life as an outcome variable in management of cancer pain. *Cancer.* 1989;63:2321.
15. Cleeland CS, Gonin R, Hatfield A, et al. Pain and its treatment in outpatients with metastatic cancer. *N Engl J Med.* 1994;330:592–596.
16. Cleeland CS. The impact of pain on patients with cancer. *Cancer.* 1984;54:263.
17. Levin D, Cleeland CS, Dar R. Public attitudes toward cancer pain. *Cancer.* 1985;56:2337.
18. Gonzales GR, Elliott KJ, Portenoy RK, Foley KM. The impact of a comprehensive evaluation in the management of pain. *Pain.* 1991;47:41–44.
19. The SUPPORT principal investigators. A controlled trial to improve care for seriously ill hospitalized patients: the study to understand prognosis and preferences for outcomes and risks of treatments. *JAMA.* 1995;274:1591–1598.
20. van den Beuken-van Everdingen MH, de Rijke JM, Kessels AG, Schouten HC, van Kleef M, Patijn J. Prevalence of pain in patients with cancer: a systematic review of the past 40 years. *Ann Oncol.* 2007;18:1437–1449.
40. Mayer EA, Gebhart GF. Basic and clinical aspects of visceral hyperalgesia. *Gastroenterology.* 1994;107:271–293.
41. Sengupta JN, X Su, Gebhart GF. Kappa, but not mu or delta, opioids attenuate responses to distention of afferent fibers innervating the rat colon. *Gastroenterology.* 1996;111:968–980.
42. Burton MB, Gebhart GF. Effects of kappa-opioid receptor agonists on responses to colorectal distension in rats with and without acute colonic inflammation. *J Phannacol Exp Ther.* 1998;285:707–715.
43. Foley KM, Portenoy RK. World Health Organization/International Association for the Study of Pain: joint initiative in cancer pain treatment. *J Pain Symptom Manage.* 1993;8:335–339.
44. Foley KM. Pain assessment and cancer pain. In: Doyle D, Hanks GW, MacDonald RN, eds. *Oxford Textbook of Palliative Medicine*, 2nd ed. New York Oxford University Press; 1998:310–330.
45. Portenoy RK, Lipton RB, Foley KM. Back pain in the cancer patient an algorithm for evaluation and management. *Neurology.* 1986;37:134.
46. DuPen SL, DuPenn AR, Polissar N, et al. Implementation of guidelines for cancer pain management results of a randomized controlled clinical trial. *J Clin Oncol.* 1999;17:361–370.
47. Jadad AR, Bowman GP. The WHO analgesic ladder for cancer pain management. Stepping up the quality of its evaluation. *JAMA.* 1996;274:1870–1873.
48. Ventafridda V, Tambourini M, Caraceni A, et al. A validation study of the WHO methods for cancer pain relief. *Cancer.* 1987;59:850–856.
49. Zech Detlev FJ, Grond S, Lynch J, et al. Validation of WHO guidelines for cancer pain relief: a 10-year prospective study. *Pain.* 1995;63:65–76.
50. Payne R. Issues pertinent to the revision of national guidelines, NCCN proceedings. *Oncology.* 1998;12:169–175.
75. Payne R, et al. Quality of life and cancer pain: satisfaction and side effects with transdermal fentanyl versus oral morphine. *J Clin Oncol.* 1998;16:1588–1593.
76. Ahmedzai S, Brooks D. The TTS-Fentanyl Cooperative Trial Group. Transdermal fentanyl versus sustained-release oral morphine in cancer pain: preference, efficacy, and quality of life. *J Pain Symptom Manage.* 1997;13:254–261.
77. Portenoy RK, Hagen NA. Breakthrough pain: definition, prevalence, and characteristics. *Pain.* 1990;41:273–281.
78. Farrar JT, Cleary J, Rauck R, et al. Oral transmucosal fentanyl citrate; randomized, double-blinded, placebo-controlled trial for treatment breakthrough pain in cancer patients. *J Natl Cancer Inst.* 1998;90:611–616.
79. Portenoy RK, et al. Oral transmucosal fentanyl citrate (OTFC) for the treatment of breakthrough pain in cancer patients, a controlled dose titration study. *Pain.* 1999;79:303–312.
80. Christie JM, et al. Dose-titration multicenter study of oral transmucosal fentanyl citrate for the treatment of breakthrough pain in cancer patients using transdermal fentanyl for persistent pain. *J Clin Oncol.* 1998;16:3238–3245.
81. Fainsinger RB, Schoeller T, Bruera E. Methadone in the management of cancer pain: a review. *Pain.* 1993;52:137–147.
82. Grochow L, Sheidler V, Grossman S, et al. Does intravenous methadone provide longer lasting analgesia than intravenous morphine? A randomized, double-blind study. *Pain.* 1989;38:141.
83. Crews JC, Sweeney NJ, Denson DD. Clinical efficacy of methadone in patients refractory to other mu-opioid receptor agonist analgesics for management of terminal cancer pain. Case presentations and discussion of incomplete cross-tolerance among opioid agonist analgesics. *Cancer.* 1993;72:2266–2272.
84. Lawlor PG, Turner KS, Hanson J, Bruera ED. Dose ratio between morphine and methadone in patients with cancer pain: a retrospective study. *Cancer.* March 15, 1998;82:1167–1173.
125. Bruera E, Watanabe S. Psychostimulants as adjuvant analgesics. *J Pain Symptom Manage.* 1994;9:412–415.
126. Dalal S, Melzack R. Potentiation of opioid analgesia by psychostimulant drugs: a review. *J Pain Symptom Manage.* 1998; 18:245–253.
127. Maunuksela EL, Korpela R. Double-blind evaluation of a lignocaine-prilocaine cream (EMLA) in children: effect on the pain associated with venous cannulation. *Br J Anaesth.* 1986;58:1242.
128. Camel SB, Blakeslee DB, Oswald SG, Barnes M. Treatment of radiation- and chemotherapy-induced stomatitis. *Otolaryngol Head Neck Surg.* 1990;102:326.
129. Berenson JR, Lipton A. Use of bisphosphinates in patients with metastatic bone disease. *Oncology.* 1998;12:1573–1580.
130. Foley KM. Changing concepts of tolerance to opioids: what the cancer patient has taught us. In: Chapman CR, Foley KM, eds. *Current and Emerging Issues in Cancer Pain: Research and Practice.* New York: Raven; 1993:331–349.
131. Lipton A, Small E, Saad F, et al. The new bisphosphonate, Zometa (zoledronic acid), decreases skeletal complications in both osteolytic and osteoblastic lesions: a comparison to pamidronate. *Cancer Invest.* 2002;20(Suppl 2):45–54.
132. Adams NJ, Plane MB, Fleming MF, et al. Opioids and the treatment of chronic pain in a primary care sample. *J Pain Symptom Manage.* 2001;22:791–796.
133. Fishbain DA. Report on the prevalence of drug/alcohol abuse and dependence in chronic pain patients (CPPs). *Subst Use Misuse.* 1996;31:945–946.
134. Yang C-Y, Wong O-S, Chang J-Y, Ho S-T. Intrathecal ketamine-reduced morphine requirements in patients with terminal cancer pain. *Can J Anaesth.* 1996;43: 379–383.
135. Fishman B. The treatment of suffering in patients with cancer pain: cognitive-behavioral approaches. In: Foley KM, Bonica JJ, Ventafridda V, eds. *Advances in Pain Research and Therapy.* Vol. 16. Second International Congress on Cancer Pain. New York: Raven; 1990:301.
165. Eisenberg E, Berkey CS, Carr DB, et al. Efficacy and safety of nonsteroidal antiinflammatory drugs for cancer pain: a meta-analysis. *J Clin Oncol.* 1994;12:2756–2765.
166. Donner B, Zenz M, Strumpf M, Raber M. Long-term treatment of cancer pain with transdermal fentanyl. *J Pain Symptom Manage.* 1998;15:168–175.
167. Halperin DL, Koren G, Attias D, et al. Topical skin anesthesia for venous, subcutaneous drug reservoir and lumbar punctures in children. *Pediatrics.* 1989;84:218.
168. Tumbull IM, Shulman R, Woodhurst WB. Thalamic stimulation
169. Acute Pain Management in Infants, Children, and Adolescents: Operative and Medical Procedures, in US Department of Health and Human Services. 1992. Agency for Health Care Policy and Research. Procedure. Rockville, MD.

70 Primary Neoplasms of the Central Nervous System in Adults

Craig Nolan, MD ▪ Lisa M. DeAngelis, MD

Introduction

Tumors of the central nervous system (CNS) are a heterogeneous group of both benign and malignant intracranial and intraspinal neoplasms. Intracranial tumors are classified into two groups: those that grow within the brain (intracerebral) and those that grow outside the brain but within the cranial vault (extracerebral). Similarly, intraspinal tumors are classified into two groups: those that arise within the spinal cord (intramedullary) and those that originate from outside the spinal cord (extramedullary). Historically, tumors of the CNS have been intractable to standard therapies of surgical resection, radiotherapy, and chemotherapy. However, over the past several decades, advances in diagnostic imaging, surgical techniques, and radiation oncology have improved survival and quality of life. Most important, we are acquiring a better understanding of the molecular events associated with the malignant phenotype of a brain tumor. This understanding has led to the development of several novel chemotherapeutic approaches to the treatment of brain tumors. Despite these recent advances, many adults with a malignant brain tumor rarely survive more than 1 year. A continued multidisciplinary clinical approach in combination with the efforts of the tumor biologist is needed to gain long-term disease control and, ultimately, a cure for malignant brain tumors.

Epidemiology

Most primary intracranial tumors are uncommon or rare illnesses. The overall annual incidence of brain tumors, both benign and malignant, in the United States is estimated at 14.80 cases per 100,000 person-years leading to an estimated 64,000 new cases diagnosed each year (Central Brain Tumor Registry of the United States Statistical Report [CBTRUS] 1998–2002).[1] More than 40% are gliomas, and two-thirds of these are high-grade tumors. The incidence of glial tumors is 6.42 per 100,000 person-years, with a higher incidence in males (7.67 per 100,000 person-years) than in females (5.35 per 100,000 person-years).[1] The American Cancer Society (ACS) estimated the number of new brain and nervous system tumors in 2008 to be 21,810 (11,780 males and 10,030 females), more than twice that of Hodgkin disease. Primary brain tumors are the second most common cancer in childhood after leukemia with an incidence of 4.0 per 100,000 person-years, and they are the second leading cause of cancer death in men aged 20–39 and the fifth in women of that age.[2,3]

Neuroepithelial tumors account for approximately 49% of CNS tumors (of which glioblastoma (GBM) comprises the majority at 23%), meningiomas account for 26%, sellar tumors 7%, CNS lymphomas 3%, and other brain tumor types 8%.[1] Both the incidence and histologic type of intracranial tumors differ by race, sex, age, and social class.[4] The overall incidence of brain tumors (especially gliomas) is greater in Whites than Blacks. However, meningiomas are more frequent in Blacks than Whites.[4] Pituitary adenomas are also more common in Blacks than Whites. Sex differences are apparent. The male to female ratio is 1.7 for oligodendrogliomas, 1.6 for astrocytomas, and 1.0 for malignant meningiomas. For benign meningiomas, the female to male ratio is 1.5 for intracranial meningiomas and 3.5 for spinal meningiomas. Lymphomas and germ cell tumors are more common in males. These data are from the National Cancer Institute's (NCI) SEER registry (Surveillance, Epidemiology, and End Results) and confirmed by the CBTRUS data.[5]

CNS tumors can occur at any age. Both the overall incidence and histological type vary by age. There is a small peak before age 10 and a steady rise from age 15. The average age of onset for all primary brain tumors is 54 years. The average age of onset of GBM and meningioma is 62 years, whereas for oligodendroglioma the mean age of onset is 16 years.[1] Low-grade gliomas, such as astrocytomas, are more common in the young, and high-grade tumors, such as GBM, are more common in the elderly. The CBTRUS data show that the highest incidence for all brain tumors occurs in the 75–84-year-old age group, with GBMs occurring most frequently in patients older than 65 years.

Reported brain tumor incidence also varies by geography. The most developed countries report higher rates of primary brain tumors than less-developed countries. Incidence rates are similar in the United States, Canada, Western Europe, and Australia. Rates in Scandinavia are slightly higher than those in the United States. The lowest incidences are seen in Japan, India, and Singapore.[4] Migrant populations usually have rates that are closer to those of natives of their adoptive country than those who remain in their country of origin, suggesting that environmental factors are important. The reported incidence of brain tumors also varies by social class.[4] In several studies, the incidence of brain tumors increased with social class, this being more evident in men than in women. The explanation of social class difference, if real, is unknown.

An increase in the incidence of and mortality from primary brain tumors in adults has been noted over the past several decades.[6–9] Certainly, some of these increases are the result of improved ascertainment owing to better diagnostic imaging, improved access to medical care, and the increasing age of the population. Important to the clinician is the change in the relative frequency of specific tumors. For example, primary CNS lymphomas (PCNSL) are increasing both in incidence and frequency when compared to other primary brain tumors in both the immunosuppressed and immunocompetent populations.[10] The increasing recognition of oligodendroglial features in a glioma has resulted in a reclassification of this tumor from an astrocytoma accounting for the rise in overall incidence of oligodendrogliomas; a change that is not necessarily accurate.[11]

The relative 2- and 5-year survival rates for patients with primary malignant brain tumors are 36.2% and 27.6%, respectively. Age and tumor histology are very significant prognostic factors. For instance, the 5-year relative survival rate for patients with pilocytic astrocytomas (a common childhood tumor) is 87.2%, compared to 3.2% in patients with GBMs.[12] Other prognostic factors include extent of disease, extent of resection, and tumor location.

Risk Factors

Risk factors that are significant for CNS tumorigenesis are elusive (Table 70-1). Definitive identification of risk factors for malignant brain tumors is problematic

Table 70-1 ■ Risk Factors for Primary Brain Tumors of Neuroepithelial, Meningeal, or Lymphocytic Origin

Definite risk factors

1. Ionizing radiation
2. Hereditary syndromes
3. Family history of brain tumors
4. Immunosuppression

Possible risk factors

1. Prior cancers
2. Infectious agents or immunologic response: viruses, *Toxoplasma gondii*
3. Head trauma
4. Epilepsy, seizures, or convulsions
5. Diet: nitrosamine/nitrosamide/nitrate/nitrite consumption
6. Tobacco smoke exposure (women)
7. Occupations and industries: synthetic rubber manufacturing, vinyl chloride, petroleum refining/production work, licensed pesticide applicators, agricultural work, and others
8. Left-handedness (fewer gliomas in left-handed persons)
9. Sociodemographic status (more low-grade tumors in affluent; more high-grade tumors in lower socioeconomic groups)

owing to the heterogeneity of primary brain tumors, differences in histological classifications, and various retrospective exposure surveys. Even in large population–based studies, the number of brain tumors is relatively small and statistically significant differences may not be reliably reproducible. Furthermore, most studies consider brain tumors as a group and do not stratify by histology which is important because there are undoubtedly different risk factors for different tumor types, eg, meningiomas compared to gliomas.

Although there have been a large number of studies examining the relationship between the environment and the occurrence of brain tumors, only two unequivocal risk factors have been identified: ionizing radiation and immune suppression.[4] The role of low- and high-dose therapeutic ionizing radiation as a significant risk factor for brain tumors has been confirmed in many studies. Irradiation for intracranial tumors, eg, medulloblastoma or extracranial head and neck cancers, including prophylactic irradiation for leukemia, increase the incidence of both gliomas and sarcomas seven-fold in those who survive more than 3 years. The cumulative relative risk of secondary brain tumors in patients treated with cranial irradiation for leukemia is 1.39 at 20 years; approximately two-thirds of the tumors are gliomas, and one-third are meningiomas.[13] High-grade gliomas have a median latency of 9.1 years from the cranial radiotherapy compared to 19 years for meningiomas. Some studies suggest that the concurrent use of antimetabolites during radiation therapy may increase the number of brain tumors.[14] Low-dose radiation such as that used to treat tinea capitis, a fungal infection of the scalp, and skin hemangiomas in children is associated with an increased risk of brain tumors.[15] A relative risk of 18, 10, and 3 have been observed for nerve sheath tumor, malignant meningioma, and glioma, respectively.

Acquired immune suppression, such as human immunodeficiency virus (HIV) infection, or the use of immunosuppressive drugs after organ transplantation, increases the incidence of PCNSL.[16] HIV infection may also increase the frequency of glioma and intracranial leiomyosarcomas.[17] Congenital immunosuppressive illnesses such as the Wiskott–Aldrich syndrome are also associated with an increased incidence of cerebral lymphomas. PCNSL in immunosuppressed patients is driven by pre-existing latent Epstein–Barr viral infection of B-lymphocytes. When a lymphoma occurs in an immunosuppressed patient, it is twice as likely to occur in the brain as elsewhere in the body.[18,19]

Other studies of environmental risk factors are less convincing than those of ionizing radiation and immunosuppression. Some investigators have shown that dietary exposure to N-nitrosourea compounds could be a risk factor.[20] Some evidence suggests that the consumption of cured meats that contain N-nitroso compounds, may not only predispose to brain tumors in the adult consumer but also in the children of mothers who consume them during pregnancy.[21] Some evidence suggests that vitamins and other antioxidants may protect against N-nitroso compounds.[22] Fruit and vegetable consumption may also decrease risk. Other studies have identified high protein diets and alcohol as risk factors.[4] The role, if any, of nutrition in either causing or protecting from brain tumors remains unknown.

Several studies have evaluated the risk of certain occupations and the development of brain tumors. Industries that have been reported to show an increased risk are pesticide and fertilization manufacturing, synthetic rubber production, vinyl chloride synthesis, and petrochemical industries.[4] Formaldehyde has been identified as a possible causal factor for brain tumor development. Increased risks of brain tumors were found in embalmers and pathologists.[23]

Additional research evaluating the association of brain tumors with head trauma, cigarette smoking, seizure history, maternal alcohol use, and infection has been inconclusive. Some reports find SV40 large T-antigen sequences at high frequency in gliomas and medulloblastomas.[24] One study suggests that prior varicella-zoster infection protects against glioma.[25]

Exposure to electromagnetic fields (EMF), especially through the use of cellular phones, has been of interest. Several studies have demonstrated no association between cellular phone use and brain tumors.[26–28] Diagnostic radiation therapy exposures from medical and dental radiographs do not appear to be significant risk factors in glioma formation, despite the increased risk associated with therapeutic irradiation.[29]

Molecular Genetics

The malignant transformation of a glial cell is a multistep process involving tumor-suppressor gene inactivation and oncogene activation and overexpression. There are also alterations in the regulation of the cell cycle, abnormalities in signal transduction pathways, glioma cell invasion, and angiogenesis. The location and nature of these molecular abnormalities are being identified in particular tumor types; GBM is the best studied tumor.

There is evidence that different molecular pathways may lead to the development of an identically appearing GBM. There appear to be at least two types of GBM: primary (de novo) and secondary (Table 70-2).[20] Although histologically indistinguishable, each has unique molecular alterations. Primary GBMs occur in patients in the sixth and seventh decades of life without a history of a previous low-grade glioma. Secondary

Table 70-2 ■ Pathways to Glioblastoma Formation

Activates signal transduction pathways	*EGFR* amplification (7p12)	Cells of Origin ↓	*PDGF, FGF2* overexpression	Activate signal transduction pathways
Disrupts $p14^{ARF}$ and $p16^{INK4A}$ pathways	*INK4A* loss (9q26)	Low-grade glioma ↓	*p53* mutation (17p13)	Disrupts $p14^{ARF}$ pathway, inhibits apoptosis and promotes genomic instability
Activates signal transduction pathways	*PTEN* loss (10q24)	Anaplastic glioma ↓	*CDK4* amplification (12q13) *RB* loss (13q13)	Disrupt $p16^{INK4A}$ pathway
		GBM (primary) ← direct from Cells of Origin; GBM (secondary)	*PTEN* loss (10q24)	Enhances AKT activity

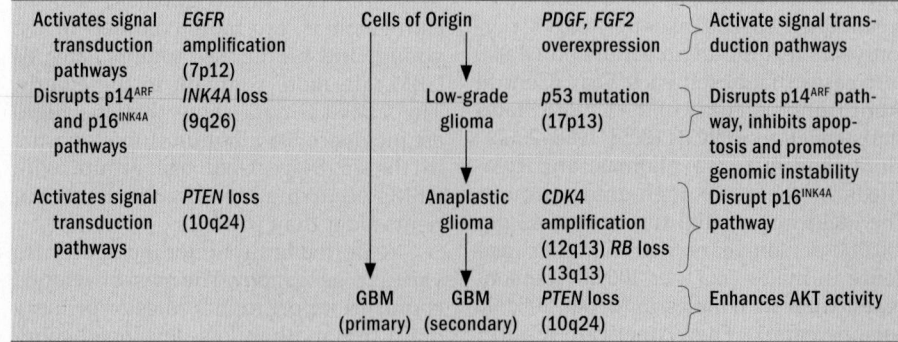

Source: From Ref. 296.

GBMs are found in patients in the fourth and fifth decades of life and arise from the transformation of a preexisting low-grade glioma. Amplification of the epidermal growth factor receptor (EGFR) occurs in primary GBMs but not secondary tumors. In the latter, mutations of the p53 gene are seen.[30] The EGFR gene has been localized to chromosome 7p11-p12 and plays a role in cell proliferation and transformation. It is the most frequently amplified oncogene in astrocytomas and has been reported to occur in 62% of anaplastic astrocytomas (AA) and GBMs.[30] Amplification of EGFR has not been shown to correlate with survival.

Another growth factor receptor important in the development of astrocytomas is platelet-derived growth factor receptor (PDGFR), also a member of the tyrosine kinase family of receptors (Table 70-3).[31–34] PDGFR occurs in two isoforms (alpha and beta). PDGFR-alpha overexpression is an early event in tumorigenesis and is present in most tumor grades.[35] PDGFR-beta is found in higher grade tumors. Protein kinase C (PKC) is another tyrosine kinase involved in signal transduction and is highly expressed in malignant gliomas.[36–38] There are several isoforms of PKC and nonselective inhibition of these isoforms, such as with high-dose tamoxifen, can inhibit tumor growth.[39–40]

Tumor suppressor genes produce proteins that inhibit cell growth or promote cell differentiation. Tumor suppressor genes important to brain tumors include p53, PTEN/MMAC, and CDKN2.[41] The p53 gene encodes a 53-kDa protein that modifies cellular function, including the cell cycle, DNA repair after radiation damage, genomic stability, and the induction of apoptosis. The p53 gene product prevents progression of the cell cycle beyond the G1/S checkpoint when damaged DNA is present. If the DNA can be repaired, the cell cycle proceeds; if not, p53 directs the cell to die (apoptosis). If p53 does not function normally, cells with abnormal DNA can reproduce uncontrollably causing a neoplasm. The most common alterations of the p53 gene are point mutations or deletions. Immunohistochemistry can detect p53 mutations in tumors, whereas lack of p53 immunoreactivity indicates the presence of the wild-type p53 gene.[42–44]

PTEN is a tumor suppressor gene located on chromosome 10q23. Functional PTEN suppresses proliferation and promotes apoptosis. PTEN mutations are common in high-grade gliomas and occur more frequently in GBM than in AA. PTEN also has prognostic significance in that PTEN mutations have been associated with decreased survival in both GBM and AA.[45–48]

In addition to oncogene amplification and tumor suppressor gene inactivation, malignant tumors acquire the ability to invade adjacent neural structures and form a new blood supply via angiogenesis. Glial tumors are extremely invasive neoplasms and typically extend beyond their macroscopic borders making local control of tumor growth nearly impossible. Glioma cells secrete matrix metalloproteases (MMPs) that break down adjacent neural tissues and allow tumor cells to invade.[49] There are ongoing clinical trials using MMP inhibitors in an attempt to reduce tumor invasion into normal brain tissue.[50] In addition to direct invasion, angiogenesis is also an important factor in CNS tumor growth. Angiogenesis leads to vascular hyperplasia, which is the pathological hallmark of a GBM. Vascular endothelial growth factor (VEGF) is the most important mitogen in angiogenesis in gliomas.[51–53] VEGF is not expressed in normal brain endothelium but is upregulated in the endothelium of tumor vessels. Overexpression of VEGF is found in gliomas, which are highly vascular and often hypoxic tumors. Hypoxia induces VEGF expression, and tumor cells that become hypoxic increase VEGF secretion in an attempt to survive. VEGF also increases vascular permeability and hence may also play a role in peritumoral edema seen in malignant gliomas. Several studies of angiogenesis inhibitors are currently on-going to treat malignant gliomas.

Table 70-3 **Molecular and Cytogenetic Abnormalities Associated With Common Primary Brain Tumors**

Tumor	Abnormalities	Prevalence (%)	Gene
Astrocytoma	17p loss or mutation	65	*p53*
	PDGFR overexpression	60	*PDGFR*
	22q (loss)		Unknown
	13q	25	*Rb*
Anaplastic astrocytoma	9p (loss)	50	*INKA-ARF*
	13p (loss)	25	*Rb*
	19q (loss)	50	Unknown
	11q (loss)		Unknown
	CDK4 amplification	10–20	*CDK4*
Glioblastoma	10q (loss)	80	*PTEN (MMAC1, TEP1)*[a]
	EGFR amplification, rearrangement	40	*EGFR*
	17p (loss)	30	*p53*
	9p (loss)	70	*INK4A*
	13q	40	*RB*
	CDK4 amplification	10–20	*CDK4*
	MDM2 amplification	10	*MDM2*
Oligodendroglioma	19q (loss)	50–80	Unknown
	1p (loss)	40–92	Unknown
	17p (loss)	10–15	*p53*
	7 (gain)		*EGFR*
Anaplastic oligodendroglioma	9p (loss)		*INK4-ARF*
	10q (loss)		*?PTET (MMAC1)*
	EGFR amplification		*EGFR*
	CDK4 amplification		*CDK4*
Medulloblastoma	9q (loss)	10–20	*ptcl*
	11p (loss)	30–45	Unknown
	17p (loss)	30–50	Unknown
Meningioma	1p (loss)		Unknown
	9q (loss)		Unknown
	10q (loss) (only malignant)		Unknown
	14q (loss)		Unknown
	17p (loss)		*p53*
	22q (loss)	60	*NF2*, other
Ependymoma	17p (loss)		Unknown
	22q (loss)	30	Unknown
Hemangioblastoma	3p (loss)	100	*VHL*

[a]Only 30% of 10q loss is attributed to *PTEN*.

Familial Tumor Syndromes of the CNS

Familial brain tumor syndromes are a heterogeneous group of disorders characterized by an association of brain tumors with systemic features primarily dermatologic. Some of these syndromes include neurofibromatosis types 1 and 2, tuberous sclerosis (TS), Sturge–Weber syndrome, Von Hippel–Lindau (VHL) disease, and Li–Fraumeni syndrome (Table 70-4).

Neurofibromatosis 1

Neurofibromatosis 1 (NF-1), also known as von Recklinghausen disease, is the

Table 70-4 ■ CNS Tumor Syndromes

Disorders	CNS Tumors	Tumors of Other Organs and Tissues	Skin Lesions	Genes	Chromosomes
Neurofibromatosis-1	Glioma, neurofibroma	Iris hamartoma, osseous lesions, pheochromocytoma, leukemia	Café au-lait spots, cutaneous axillary freckling, neurofibromas	*NF1*	17q11.2
Neurofibromatosis-2	Schwannoma, meningioma	Posterior lens opacities, retinal hamartoma	None	*NF2*	22q12.2
von Hippel–Lindau disease	Hemangioblastoma	Retinal hemangioblastoma, renal cell carcinoma, pheochromocytoma, visceral cysts, endolymphatic sac tumor	None	*VHL*	3p25–p26
Tuberous sclerosis	Astrocytoma	Cardiac rhabdomyoma, adenomatous polyps of the duodenum and small intestine, cysts of the lung and kidney, lymphangioleiomyomatosis, renal angiomyolipoma	Cutaneous angiofibroma ("adenoma sebaceum"), peau de chagrin, subungual fibromas	*TSC1, TSC2*	9q34
Li-Fraumeni syndrome	Gliomas (10%)	Breast carcinoma; bone and soft tissue sarcoma; adrenocortical, lung, and GI carcinoma; leukemia	None	*P53*	17p13.1
Cowden disease	Cerebellar mass (Lhermitte-Duclos disease)	Hamartomatous polyps of the eye, colon, and thyroid; breast carcinoma, thyroid cancer	Multiple trichilemmomas, fibromas	*PTEN*	10q22.3
Turcot A syndrome	Medulloblastoma	Colorectal polyps, colon carcinoma		*APC*	5q21–22
Turcot B syndrome	Glioma	Colon cancer, no polyps	Café au-lait spots	*MLH1* *PMS2*	3p21.3 7p22
Nevoid basal cell carcinoma syndrome (Gorlin syndrome)	Medulloblastoma (anaplastic)	Jaw cysts, ovarian fibromas, skeletal abnormalities	Multiple basal cell carcinomas, palmar and plantar pits	*PTCH*	9q22.3–31
Retinoblastoma	Pineal tumor	Retinal tumor, osteosarcomas and other tumors	None	*RBI*	13q14
Bloom syndrome	Medulloblastoma, meningioma	Characteristic face and voice, gonadal failure, diabetes, immunodeficiency	Sun sensitivity, patches of hyper-and hypopigmentation	*BLM*	15q26.1
Fanconi anemia	Astrocytoma, medulloblastoma	Anemia, skeletal malformations, enlarged cerebral ventricles, gastrointestinal malformations	Café au-lait spots, hyperpigmentation and hypopigmentation	*FANCA*	16q24.3
			Patches of hyperpigmentation	*MLM*	1p36
Familial melanoma	Astrocytoma	None		*CDKN2 A/p14 ARF*	9p21
Rhabdoid predisposition syndrome	PNET, choroid plexus carcinoma	Renal tumors, extrarenal malignant rhabdoid tumors	None	*HSNFA/INH1*	22q11
Multiple endocrine neoplasia (MEN-1 Carney complex)	Pituitary adenomas	Hyperparathyroidism, gastrinoma, insulinoma, thyroid/bronchial carcinoid	Facial angiofibroma, lipoma, collagenoma	*MEN1*	11q13
Ataxia-telangiectasia	Astrocytoma, medulloblastoma, cerebellar ataxia	Lymphomas, hypogonadism, radiation sensitivity, insulin resistance, premature aging, small stature	Telangiectasias	*ATM*	11q22–q23

Abbreviation: PNET, primitive neuroectodermal tumor.

most common hereditary disease predisposing to CNS cancer, with a prevalence of 1 in 4000.[54] The incidence is equal in men and women. It is an autosomal dominant disorder with 100% penetrance but is highly variable in its expressivity with both minimally and severely affected individuals within the same family. The NF-1 gene has been mapped to chromosome 17q11.2 and encodes a tumor suppressor, neurofibromin.[55]

The typical clinical features of NF-1 include neurofibromas, benign tumors appearing beneath the skin and along peripheral nerves; Lisch nodules, brown growths appearing on the surface of the iris; Café-au-lait spots, hyperpigmented flat patches of skin; axillary freckling and bony abnormalities. NF-1 patients are predisposed to other neoplasms, benign and malignant. These include malignant schwannomas, rhabdomyosarcomas, and GBMs. The predominant CNS tumors in NF-1 are optic pathway and brainstem gliomas. Optic pathway gliomas are usually pilocytic astrocytomas and brainstem gliomas are astrocytomas. The typical peripheral nerve tumor is the plexiform neurofibroma, which often involves the paraspinal and cranial nerves.

Neurofibromatosis 2

Neurofibromatosis 2 (NF-2), known as central neurofibromatosis, is an autosomal dominant disorder with a much lower prevalence than NF-1 and accounts for only 10% of all neurofibromatosis cases.[55] The NF-2 gene is a tumor suppressor gene located on chromosome 22q12.[57,58] The predominant CNS tumors in NF-2 are vestibular schwannomas, often bilateral, and meningiomas. Cutaneous manifestations are much less common in NF-2 than in NF-1.

Tuberous Sclerosis

Tuberous sclerosis (TS) formerly known as Bourneville disease is an autosomal dominant disorder and is the second most common neurocutaneous syndrome after NF-1.[58,59] There is a continuum of variable expressivity. TS has been mapped to two different loci: TS complex 1 located on chromosome 9q34 encodes the protein hamartin and TS complex 2 located on chromosome 16p13.3 encodes the protein tuberin.[60,61] The classic clinical triad of mental retardation, seizures, and facial angiofibromas occurs only in the most severe cases. Skin lesions are seen in 96% of patients.[62] These include angiofibromas, uncal fibromas, hypomelanotic skin patches known as "ash leaf spots," and dental pits. The hallmark CNS tumor is the subependymal giant cell astrocytoma. They are pathologically benign tumors and occur in 5% to 10% of TS patients.[63] Their location near the foramen of Monroe may cause death in TS patients from blockage of cerebrospinal fluid and subsequent obstructive hydrocephalus. Other CNS lesions include cortical tubers and subependymal glial nodules known as "candle gutterings." Although cortical tubers are also benign lesions, they may cause seizures.[64]

von Hippel–Lindau Disease

von Hippel–Lindau (VHL) disease is a tumor syndrome involving a variety of neoplasms in multiple organ systems including hemangioblastomas in the cerebellum, spinal cord, and retina and pheochromocytomas and renal cell carcinoma. Other less common lesions include pancreatic and renal cysts and endolymphatic sac tumors. The hemangioblastomas are associated with overexpression of VEGF.[65] VHL disease is an autosomal dominant disorder mapped to chromosome 3p25-p26.[66] It has a high penetrance but variable expressivity.

Li-Fraumeni Syndrome

Li-Fraumeni syndrome is a rare autosomal dominant disorder seen in children and young adults leading to multiple different tumors. It is caused by germ line mutations of p53.[67,68] However, some families do not have the p53 mutation and their genetic defect is unknown. Overall penetrance of the gene is about 50% by age 30 and 90% by age 60.[69] Common tumors seen are breast, osteosarcoma, and brain tumors, primarily AA and GBMs. Some develop medulloblastomas and supratentorial primitive neuroectodermal tumors.[70] Other less common tumors include soft tissue sarcomas, leukemia, and lung, adrenal, gastric, and colon cancers. Except for the generally younger age of patients with brain tumors with this syndrome and the slightly higher male/female ratio compared with sporadic tumors, the brain tumors in these patients do not differ clinically from their sporadic counterparts.

Histological Classification of CNS Tumors

WHO classifies tumors by their patterns of differentiation and presumed cell of origin (Table 70-5). Primary CNS tumors comprise approximately 70% of intracranial tumors, with the majority being neuroepithelial tumors (Table 70-5).[71] The cell of origin is the glial cell (usually astrocyte) that accounts for 90% of brain cells. The remainder arise from meningeal, pituitary, lymphocytic, or germ cells. Neurons constitute less than 10% of brain cells and are an uncommon source of CNS neoplasms.

Table 70-5 Partial WHO List of Common Tumors of Neuroepithelial Tissue

I. Astrocytic tumors
   1. Diffuse astrocytoma (fibrillary, protoplasmic, gemistocytic, mixed)
   2. Anaplastic astrocytoma
   3. Glioblastoma (giant cell, gliosarcoma variants)
   4. Pilocytic astrocytoma
   5. Pleomorphic xanthoastrocytoma
   6. Subependymal giant cell astrocytoma
II. Oligodendroglial tumors
   1. Oligodendroglioma
   2. Anaplastic oligodendroglioma
   3. Oligoastrocytoma
   4. Anaplastic oligoastrocytoma
III. Ependymal tumors
   1. Ependymoma (cellular, papillary, clear cell, tanycytic)
   2. Anaplastic (malignant) ependymoma
   3. Myxopapillary ependymoma
   4. Subependymoma
IV. Choroid plexus tumors
   1. Choroid plexus papilloma
   2. Choroid plexus carcinoma
V. Neuronal and mixed neuronal-glial tumors
   1. Gangliocytoma
   2. Ganglioglioma
   3. Anaplastic ganglioglioma
   4. Dysembryoplastic neuroepithelial tumor (DNET)
   5. Central neurocytoma
VI. Pineal tumors
   1. Pineocytoma
   2. Pineoblastoma
   3. Pineal parenchymal tumor of intermediate differentiation
VII. Embryonal tumors
   1. Medulloblastoma (desmoplastic, large cell, melanotic, medullomyoblastoma)
   2. CNS primitive neuroectodermal tumors (PNETs)
      a. Neuroblastoma
      b. Ganglioneuroblastoma
      c. Ependymoblastoma
      d. Medulloepithelioma

In general, children most frequently develop primitive neuroectodermal tumors, PNET, low-grade astrocytomas, and ependymomas. Seventy percent of these tumors are infratentorial and occur near the midline. In contrast to children, adults tend to present with supratentorial tumors that are off the midline and are higher grade astrocytic tumors. GBM, a WHO grade 4 tumor, is hypercellular with nuclear pleomorphism, mitotic figures, endothelial proliferation, and necrosis. Microvascular proliferation is indicative of this tumor type's ability to formulate its own blood supply for rapid growth and invasion. AAs, WHO grade 3 tumors, also have increased cellularity, nuclear atypia, and mitosis, but necrosis and microvascular proliferation are absent. WHO grade 2 astrocytomas typically comprise a fairly uniform group of astrocytes in a background of fibrillary matrix. There is significantly less nuclear atypia and cellular pleomorphism than in grade 3 and 4 tumors. Mitotic figures are rare, and there is an absence of vascular proliferation and necrosis.

Glial tumors can be very heterogeneous, and there can be different grades within a lesion and even different histologic features with astrocytic and oligodendroglial appearing regions within the same tumor. This can be very challenging diagnostically and highlights the need to get an adequate pathologic sample for examination. The highest grade found within the lesion determines the diagnosis and dictates treatment.

Grade 1 tumors, juvenile pilocytic astrocytomas (JPA), occur almost exclusively in children. They are characterized by low cellularity, Rosenthal fibers, they may develop cysts, and do not infiltrate surrounding tissue extensively. They may contain rare mitoses and hyperchromatic nuclei, although these are not features of malignancy in these tumors. In young children, they occur most commonly in the cerebellar hemispheres. After surgical resection, they have a 95% 5-year progression-free survival (PFS) rate.[72] The other low-grade glial tumors also tend to be discreet and less infiltrative. These include pleomorphic xanthoastrocytoma (PXA), ganglioglioma, neurocytoma, and dysembryoplastic neuroepithelial tumor (DNT). These tumors usually require an experienced neuropathologist to diagnose.

Oligodendrogliomas are characterized by a relatively uniform array of small round cells with artifactual perinuclear halos in a background of fine capillary ("chicken-wire") vasculature. They are typically described as having a "fried-egg" appearance. Occasionally, oligodendrogliomas have features of anaplasia, pleomorphism, and necrosis and are classified as grade 3 anaplastic oligodendrogliomas (AO). They tend to have a better clinical prognosis than their astrocytic counterparts. Some oligodendrogliomas have a molecular alteration characterized by loss of genetic material on chromosomes 1p and 19q.[73] Increased sensitivity to treatment has been reported in tumors with these deletions.

PNET are a group of neoplasms characterized by groups of undifferentiated small blue cells with Homer–Wright rosettes (cells arranged around a true lumen). They are usually fast growing tumors and tend to disseminate along

CSF pathways. They are most common in children and are often found in the cerebellum (medulloblastoma) and in the pineal gland (pinealoblastoma). Although these lesions are histologically identical, the medulloblastoma is more amenable to treatment and has a better outcome.

Ependymomas are neoplasms that arise from ependymal cells that line the ventricles and spinal canal. They can arise wherever ependymal cells are present and a particular predilection is the fourth ventricle. They are the most frequent neuroepithelial tumor of the spinal cord, accounting for more than 50% of spinal gliomas in both children and adults. They are histologically characterized by perivascular pseudorosettes (tumor cells arranged radially around blood vessels), and Homer–Wright rosettes. There are several histologic subtypes including clear cell, cellular, and papillary, but these different histologic features have no clinical importance. These tumors are usually low grade but can be aggressive and spread along CSF pathways.

Clinical Presentation

Patients with brain tumors may present with generalized, nonfocal signs and symptoms or with focal manifestations related to the specific location of the tumor in the brain. Factors that contribute to the presenting signs and symptoms include tumor location, size, growth rate, and secretions. Supratentorial tumors are more likely to present with seizure, whereas infratentorial tumors more commonly present with headache, nausea, and vomiting. Superficial cortical tumors are more likely to cause seizure only, whereas deeper tumors are more likely to cause personality and cognitive changes. Seizure is the presenting symptom in about 15% of patients with brain tumors but is seen in less than 5% of patients with an acute stroke—which is often considered in the differential diagnosis of patients with a primary brain tumor. Tumors in eloquent areas of the brain will result in more focal symptoms such as aphasia, hemiparesis, or sensory loss. Tumors in the brainstem typically present with cranial nerve deficits such as diplopia or facial weakness. Tumors of the cerebellum may cause ipsilateral ataxia, unsteady gait, and nystagmus.

The growth rate and size of the tumor is important in determining symptoms. Slowly growing tumors (such as low-grade astrocytomas) usually present with seizure without focal neurologic deficit, whereas fast growing tumors (GBM) often present with a focal neurologic deficit. Large tumors may cause generalized symptoms owing to mass effect or false localizing signs owing to CSF obstruction (hydrocephalus) or brain herniation. Generalized symptoms from local mass effect or edema include headache, nausea, emesis, and depressed level of consciousness. False localizing signs resulting from hydrocephalus or brain herniation include diplopia, ipsilateral hemiparesis, cortical blindness, tinnitus, and anosmia.

Some intracranial tumors can cause symptoms not just by their size and location, but also by their secretions. Pituitary tumors may secrete growth hormone associated with acromegaly or prolactin-causing galactorrhea and amenorrhea. Pineal region tumors have been reported to interfere with melatonin secretion causing insomnia and personality change. Some tumors secrete cytokines such as interleukin and tumor necrosis factor that alter brain neuropeptides, which may affect cognitive function and behavior.

Diagnostic Neuroimaging

Patients with signs and symptoms suggestive of an intracranial lesion should have a neuroimaging study. Magnetic resonance imaging (MRI) is the modality of choice for CNS tumors. MRI has changed the presenting symptoms of a brain tumor. In the past, physicians were hesitant to suggest invasive diagnostic tests, such as angiogram or pneumoencephalogram unless the patient had significant neurologic symptoms. With the use of MRI, brain tumors are often diagnosed in patients long before they develop symptoms of raised intracranial pressure.

MRI is superior to CT because MRI clearly visualizes the entire intracranial contents in three dimensions (3D). In CT, bone and teeth create artifacts that obscure lesions, particularly in the posterior fossa. With MRI, multiplanar images are available, which facilitate the diagnosis. In addition, patients are not exposed to radiation or iodinated contrast eliminating possible allergic reactions.

There are certain signal characteristics seen on MRI that distinguish a brain tumor. The increased water content of brain tumors and their surrounding edema create a hypointense (darker than normal brain) T1 image and a hyperintense (lighter than normal brain) T2 image. T1 and T2 refer to proton relaxation time. Disruption of the blood–brain barrier occurs in certain tumors. The contrast agent gadolinium leaks across the disrupted blood–brain barrier and enters the brain tumor's extracellular space, causing hyperintensity (enhancement) on T1 images. High-grade tumors such as GBM tend to disrupt the blood–brain barrier and have the characteristic appearance of a hypointense center surrounded by a hyperintense irregular rim of contrast enhancement (Fig. 70-1). In comparison, low-grade tumors have an intact blood–brain barrier and usually do not contrast enhance. Fluid-attenuated inversion recovery (FLAIR) sequences provide rapid distinction between normal brain and brain tumor or edema and provide the best tumor to background contrast ratios to delineate the full extent of the lesion. On FLAIR imaging, however, tumor cannot be differentiated from edema. Diffusion-weighted imaging (DWI) assesses the mobility of water molecules and may differentiate among ischemia, cytotoxic edema within a tumor, radiation-induced necrosis, and vasogenic edema. Perfusion images measure blood volume and vascularity and correlate with tumor grade and with ^{18}fluorodeoxyglucose (FDG) positron emission tomography (PET) studies.

There are some limitations to MRI. Many pathological processes appear hypointense on T1 images and hyperintense on T2 images. They include primary brain tumor, radiation necrosis, ischemic stroke, infection, inflammatory process, and demyelination. Contrast enhancement does not always correlate with tumor grade. An example is the JPA, a low-grade brain tumor with areas of dense contrast enhancement. Enhancement does not accurately determine the border of the tumor or the full extent of disease. This is confirmed on T2 and FLAIR images where diffuse hyperintensity is often seen beyond the margins of tumor enhancement and represent infiltrating disease as well

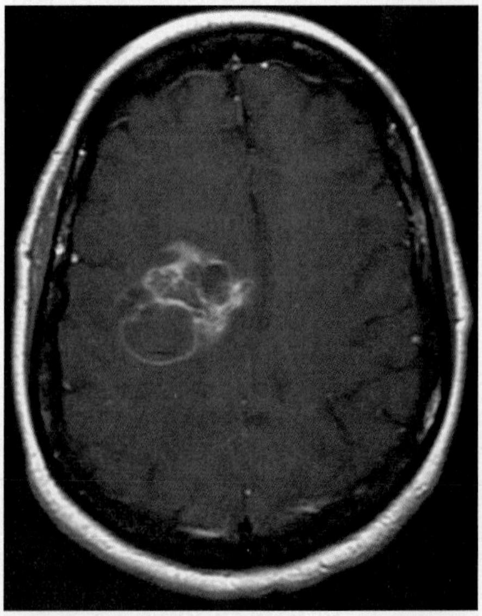

Figure 70-1 ■ Glioblastoma. This is a post-gadolinium T1-weighted MRI of a right posterior frontal glioblastoma. There is irregular contrast enhancement with focal areas of necrosis.

as perilesional edema. In addition, in patients treated for a brain tumor, it is often difficult to determine recurrence from posttreatment effect such as radiation injury with MRI. Despite these limitations, MRI remains the standard imaging technique for brain tumors.

Other Imaging Techniques

PET has several uses in the diagnosis of brain tumors. PET can help distinguish between recurrent tumor and radiation necrosis, may differentiate low-grade lesions from high-grade lesions, and may guide stereotactic biopsy to the site of active or high-grade tumor within an apparently low-grade lesion seen on MRI (Fig. 70-2).[74,75] PET is performed by injecting substances such as glucose, an amino acid such as methionine, or even a nucleotide labeled with a positron-emitting isotope such as O15, C11, N13, and F18. FDG is the most commonly used isotope for evaluating brain tumors.[76,77] The differential accumulation of this metabolite in brain tumor tissue compared with normal brain can provide information about tumor grade.[78] FDG imaging defines the metabolic rate of the area being examined. Hypermetabolism (increased FDG uptake) is common in high-grade tumors and hypometabolism (low FDG uptake) is common in low-grade tumors. FDG PET can distinguish radiation necrosis from recurrent tumor. Whereas both may appear similar on MRI, radiation necrosis is typically hypometabolic on PET in comparison to recurrent high-grade tumor, which is either isometabolic with normal brain or hypermetabolic on PET. Although these characteristics are usual, there are patients with radionecrosis that is hot on PET (presumably from macrophage infiltration) and high-grade tumors that are iso- or hypometabolic. FDG PET scans are often done on patients suspected of having a low-grade tumor prior to biopsy.[79] In a patient with a nonenhancing lesion on brain MRI and a PET scan that is completely hypometabolic who presents only with seizures well-controlled on medication, we may elect to follow with serial MRI scans and not biopsy the lesion. In contrast, if the same patient has an area of hypermetabolism on the FDG PET, biopsy should target that area to confirm a diagnosis of a high-grade tumor that would require treatment.

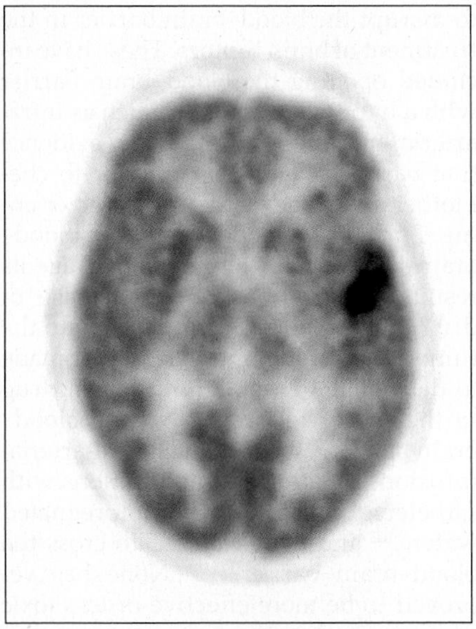

Figure 70-2 Low-grade glioma. This is an FDG PET image of a left temporal low-grade glioma showing an area of focal hypermetabolism that corresponded to a focal area of anaplasia.

Magnetic resonance spectroscopy (MRS) measures nuclear signals from metabolites of interest in brain tumors such as *N*-acetyl-aspartate (NAA), choline, lactate, and creatine. Choline levels are elevated when there is increased cell turnover. Lactate indicates anaerobic metabolism and is never seen in normal brain; it indicates hypoxic areas of tumor or radiation injury. Lipids may accumulate in areas of necrosis. The exact role of NAA is unknown but appears to be involved in lipid synthesis and is localized to neurons. The patterns of these chemicals may distinguish the grade and histologic type of glioma and also distinguish tumor from infection, demyelination, or radiation necrosis.[80] In general, necrotic areas of tumor and necrosis owing to radiation will have reduced levels of choline, lactate, and NAA. Active tumors will show an increase in choline and a reduction in NAA; lactate may be increased in hypoxic tumor areas and absent in necrotic areas. Demyelinating disorders are marked by normal or decreased NAA and increased choline. Brain abscesses show absent creatine, choline, and NAA but a large lactate peak. However, these patterns overlap and MRS rarely provides definitive information.

Functional MRI (fMRI) is an increasingly important technique that maps the functional organization of the brain, particularly the primary motor, sensory, and language cortices. The fMRI is based on the concept that increased neuronal activity results in increased cerebral blood flow (CBF). The resulting increased oxygen delivery exceeds the tissues' ability to extract the increased oxygen content. Therefore, there is an increase in oxyhemoglobin and a reciprocal decrease in deoxyhemoglobin.[81] This focal change in the oxyhemoglobin to deoxyhemoglobin ratio results in an increased signal on MRI. The fMRI is useful in presurgical planning and allows a surgeon to map eloquent cortex and then plan resection while preserving neurologic function; this facilitates maximal resection without neurologic deficit.

Principles of Therapy

The treatment of a primary brain tumor includes both definitive and supportive therapy. Definitive therapy encompasses surgery, radiation therapy, and chemotherapy. Supportive therapy considers management of tumor symptoms such as treatment of focal and general symptoms with corticosteroids, seizure control with antiepileptic medication, treatment of deep venous thrombosis with anticoagulants, and the provision of psychosocial support when needed.

Surgery

Surgery is the most important single modality in the treatment of brain tumors.[82,83] Benign or low-grade tumors are often cured by surgery. For tumors that cannot be cured, such as GBM, extent of surgical resection is a significant prognostic factor, and biopsy alone has inferior survival for GBM patients compared with more extensive resection. A retrospective analysis of three prospective RTOG randomized trials of 645 GBM patients revealed a statistically significant improvement in survival between GBM patients who had gross total resection (median 11.3 months) versus those who had biopsy only (median 6.6 months).[84] The goals of surgery are multifactorial: establish a tissue diagnosis, decompress the tumor mass, alleviate symptoms, and reduce steroid dose. The ultimate goal of surgery is gross total resection. Biopsy, in particular stereotactic needle biopsy performed under CT or MRI guidance, is indicated in the following circumstances: (1) a surgically inaccessible tumor such as those in the brainstem, basal ganglia, or thalamus; (2) multifocal tumors or gliomatosis cerebri; (3) PCNSL, a tumor better treated with chemotherapy than surgery; (4) in a patient with medical comorbidity resulting in a high surgical/anesthetic risk. Needle biopsies have several limitations. There is a limited tissue sample that can often compromise diagnosis, both with respect to tumor type and grade. There may also be a sample error because tissue from the edge of a lesion may be of low-grade histology and not represent deeper areas of higher grade tumor. There is also a greater risk of bleeding or hematoma with a needle biopsy compared with an open procedure where the surgeon can visualize and control bleeding.

When surgical cure is not possible, even removing large portions of an infiltrating tumor has several beneficial effects. Resection reduces the number of tumor cells that must subsequently be eliminated by radiotherapy (RT) and chemotherapy. RT and chemotherapy exert their effects by killing a percentage of tumor cells irrespective of tumor volume. These modalities are more likely to enhance survival when there is less tumor present. A reduced tumor volume also reduces areas of hypoxia, which increases radiosensitivity. Surgical resection reduces postoperative complications compared to biopsy. Removal of a substantial portion of tumor provides more intracranial space for any postoperative swelling and most patients improve following resection, whereas many deteriorate following biopsy alone. Preoperative fMRI (see earlier text) and awake intraoperative cortical mapping are techniques that facilitate tumor removal without neurologic injury.

Radiation Therapy

Radiotherapy is an effective adjuvant treatment for malignant glioma. For some tumors, such as germinomas, RT is curative. In prospective trials, RT gives better survival than surgery alone, or surgery plus chemotherapy. After surgical resection, RT is the single most effective treatment for malignant glioma. In the original Brain Tumor Study group of high-grade glioma, the median survival of patients treated by surgery alone was 14 weeks, whereas those receiving postoperative whole brain RT of 50–60 Gy was 36 weeks.[85] Improved RT techniques now allow for higher doses to the tumor while sparing normal brain. The goal of the modern radiation oncologist is to deliver radiation to the tumor in a precise manner, usually defined by the area of contrast enhancement on MRI scan with a margin of 2–3 cm, sparing surrounding normal brain tissue. Standard fractionated external beam radiation therapy involves delivering the optimum dose of 60 Gy in daily fractions of 1.8–2.0 Gy/day over 6 weeks.[86] Each fraction kills a similar proportion of tumor cells, resulting in a logarithmic decline in the number of surviving cells as the number of fractions increase. The biological basis for fractionation is that dividing a dose into fractions spares normal tissues because sublethal damage of normal cells is repaired between dose fractions, whereas tumor cells are not repaired. Late complications of RT in the nervous system are primarily influenced by the total dose and the dose per fraction. Acute toxicity is mostly related to the fraction size causing an exacerbation of edema; this can be prevented and ameliorated with corticosteroids.

The development of three dimensional conformational treatment (3D-CRT) planning permits the administration of a high dose of radiation to a 3D target volume while sparing the dose to surrounding tissues.[87] An advanced form of 3D-CRT is intensity modulated radiation therapy (IMRT). IMRT adds an additional refinement to dose modulation by conforming the dose to the shape of the target volume around adjacent critical structures.[88] Radiosurgery is another technique used to treat some brain tumors. Stereotactic radiosurgery (SRS) delivers highly focal external irradiation to a clearly defined small target, typically in a single dose.[89] SRS can be delivered by a gamma knife (cobalt 60 sources) or a linear accelerator with equivalent results. The radiation beam is directed using coordinates on a standard stereotactic head frame. Multiple radiation beams intersect at points known as isocenters within the skull after entering through numerous points or arcs distributed over the head. To maintain a steep dose gradient, the target volume must be small—less than 4 cm. Radiosurgery is primarily used to treat small lesions such as metastatic tumors, meningiomas, acoustic neuromas, and pituitary adenomas. It is rarely used in the treatment of malignant glioma because this infiltrative disease does not lend itself to focused RT.

Interstitial brachytherapy is the surgical implantation of radioactive isotopes into a tumor cavity at the time of resection.[90] The seeds remain in place until the desired dose is delivered. The seeds and catheters are then removed from the patient, or less commonly, low-dose seeds are left permanently. The most commonly used radiation source is iodine 125. Randomized controlled trials have failed to demonstrate any advantage of this form of therapy in patients with malignant gliomas over conventional radiation.[91,92] Neurologic complications from radionecrosis with brachytherapy are also significant.

Protons, neutrons, and heavy charged particles have also been used to treat CNS tumors.[93] Proton beams interact with nuclei of atoms rather than their electrons. Large doses of radiation are deposited in a targeted area sparing adjacent tissue. Because of this feature, protons and heavy charged particles such as helium ions have been used for radiosurgery to delivery fractionated radiation. Charged particle beams can be made to stop in front of critical structures, and in combination with oblique beams can be wrapped around a sensitive structure that could not withstand such high intensity exposure.[94] This technique is ideal for skull base tumors such as chordomas, meningiomas, and chondrosarcomas. It may also be used to treat tumors adjacent to the optic nerves, optic chiasm, and brainstem.

Radiosensitizers are chemical modifiers of the radiation response. Oxygen assists in the DNA damage caused by radiation. Hypoxia protects cells from radiation injury; the radiation dose must be increased by a factor of 3 to obtain the same effect in hypoxic cells as those that are oxygenated. The radioresistance of GBM may be due in part to the presence of hypoxic but viable tumor cells in necrotic areas. Some classes of radiosensitizers that have been studied in brain tumor patients include nitroimidazoles, halogenated pyrimidine analogs, and the herpes thymidine kinase gene, but none has resulted in clinical benefit.[95,96,97]

Chemotherapy

Chemotherapeutic drugs have traditionally not been successful in the treatment of most brain tumors.[98,99] Some exceptions include PCNSL, germinomas, and some oligodendrogliomas. The role of chemotherapy in the treatment of astrocytomas is limited with respect to extending survival compared with surgery and radiation alone. There are no adequate chemotherapeutic agents for acoustic neuromas, meningiomas, and pituitary adenomas.

There are several problems specific to the chemotherapy of brain tumors. These include the role of the blood–brain barrier, the paucity of lymphatics in the brain, the heterogeneity of gliomas, the intrinsic resistance of gliomas, and a low therapeutic/toxic ratio. Many chemotherapy agents cannot penetrate a tumor in the brain due to an intact blood–brain barrier. In tumors such as metastases and high-grade gliomas, there is disruption of the blood–brain barrier allowing variable penetration of water soluble chemotherapeutic agents to the tumor. However, in certain tumors such as low-grade gliomas, the blood–brain barrier is intact and water soluble chemotherapeutic agents cannot reach the disease. In high-grade gliomas, the blood–brain barrier is intact at the infiltrative margin of the tumor, where the cells are most viable. Many attempts have been made to disrupt the blood–brain barrier in the treatment of brain tumors. These have included opening the blood–brain barrier with a hyperosmolar agent such as intra-arterial mannitol.[100] There is no evidence that barrier opening is superior to chemotherapy alone without barrier opening. Furthermore, opening of the blood–brain barrier with hyperosmolar agents results in a proportionate increase of drug into the normal brain than into the tumor. Other attempts have been made to deliver higher concentrations of drug to the tumor to circumvent the blood–brain barrier. These include intra-arterial infusions,[101] intratumoral injections with catheters, implanting drug-impregnated wafers,[102] and drugs altered to cross the blood–brain barrier.[103,104] None has yet proved to be more effective or less toxic than conventional routes.

In addition to the obstacle of the blood–brain barrier, most brain tumors have intrinsic resistance to chemotherapeutic agents probably because of the heterogeneity of higher-grade gliomas.

Thus, most conventional agents are ineffective even if they achieve adequate concentrations in tumor tissue. When RT or chemotherapy does succeed in killing tumor cells, the deficiency of a lymphatic system in the brain prevents the easy removal of detritus caused by treatment. Necrotic tissue is not readily removed and serves as a nidus for edema and worsening neurologic function.

Standard Chemotherapeutic Agents ■ Standard chemotherapeutic agents used to treat brain tumors include both cytotoxic and cytostatic drugs. Cytotoxic drugs are agents that inhibit tumor growth by directly killing tumor cells. These agents rely upon tumor cells dividing more rapidly than normal cells to achieve a therapeutic index. In contrast, cytostatic agents impair tumor growth without causing cell death. Many cytotoxic drugs have their effect by inhibiting DNA synthesis. The alkylating agents such as carmustine (BCNU), temozolomide, lomustine (CCNU), procarbazine, carboplatin, and cisplatin cause alkyl groups to bind to DNA, producing DNA cross-links. Antimetabolites such as methotrexate and cytarabine are cell cycle specific and impair normal cell cycle activities. The vinca alkaloids such as vincristine and vinblastine impair cell division by interfering with microtubular formation.

Nitrosoureasn ■ Carmustine (BCNU) and lomustine (CCNU) are common alkylating agents that have been used to treat gliomas as single agents or in combination therapy.[105–107] They alkylate the O-6 position of guanine in DNA. Substantial evidence indicates that patients whose tumors express the repair enzyme methyl guanine 6-methyltransferase (MGMT) are more resistant to the chemotherapeutic effects of nitrosoureas.[108] Inhibitors of the enzyme are being used experimentally to increase tumor sensitivity to nitrosoureas and other chemotherapeutic agents, although they also enhance myelosuppression.[109] BCNU is given intravenously. CCNU has better oral bioavailability and is given in pill form. The primary toxicity for both BCNU and CCNU is myelosuppression. Fatigue, nausea, and emesis may also be seen. A less common, but serious toxicity, is pulmonary fibrosis.

Temozolomide, Procarbazine, and Dacarbazine ■ Temozolomide is an imidazotetrazine derivative of dacarbazine (DTIC). Its metabolite acts as an alkylating agent, methylating the O-6 position of guanine. It has been used to treat both high- and low-grade gliomas as adjuvant therapy and at recurrence.[110,111] Major toxicities include myelosuppression, constipation, fatigue, and nausea. It has excellent oral bioavailability. As a result of its relatively good efficacy and tolerability it has become the mainstay of glioma chemotherapy.

Procarbazine ■ Procarbazine has an active metabolite that is a nonspecific inhibitor of DNA and RNA synthesis. Major toxicities include myelosuppression, rash, nausea, and emesis. It also acts as a weak monoamine oxidase inhibitor; therefore, patients taking procarbazine need to avoid tyramine containing foods such as red wine, cheese, and fava beans. It can be given as a single agent or in combination with lomustine (CCNU) and vincristine (PCV chemotherapy). It has been shown to have activity against high-grade gliomas, and PCNSL.[112,113]

Platinum Compounds ■ Carboplatin and cisplatin are cell cycle nonspecific drugs that alkylate the N7 position on guanine.[114] Both are water soluble and excluded by an intact blood–brain barrier. These drugs are efficacious against germinomas and medulloblastomas and although widely used in the treatment of malignant gliomas, their role is not clearly established. Toxicities include myelosuppression, ototoxicity, nephrotoxicity, and neuropathy.

Vinca Alkaloids ■ Vincristine and vinblastine are vinca alkaloids that cause cell cycle arrest via interference with microtubule formation. They penetrate the blood–brain barrier poorly.[115] They do not have a clear role in the treatment of high-grade glioma. Vincristine is used as part of some chemotherapeutic regimens in the treatment of PCNSL. The primary toxicity is neuropathy.

Taxanes ■ Paclitaxel and docetaxel impair microtubule formation. They have been used as single agents for high-grade glioma and as radiosensitizers. They are water soluble and are given intravenously. Toxicities include myelosuppression, alopecia, and cardiac arrhythmia.

Antimetabolites ■ Methotrexate is an S–phase specific folic acid analogue that decreases the intracellular folate pool. It is given intrathecally or intravenously. Toxicities include myelosuppression, nephrotoxicity, mucositis, nausea, and emesis. It has been used mainly in the treatment of PCNSL and for leptomeningeal disease. Cytarabine is another antimetabolite with indications similar to methotrexate.

Cytostatic Agents ■ These agents have been assuming a larger role in the chemotherapy of brain tumors.[116] They have a selective mode of action and a good therapeutic index. These drugs include *cis*-retinoic acid, tamoxifen, thalidomide, and celecoxib. At high doses, *cis*-retinoic acid, a vitamin A analogue, makes high-grade gliomas assume a less-aggressive phenotype. It is used rarely as a single agent but often in combination with cytotoxic drugs. At high doses tamoxifen inhibits PKC and has some activity against glioma.[117] Celecoxib is a cyclooxygenase-2 (COX-2) inhibitor. Because COX-2 is overexpressed in glioma cells, celecoxib has been investigated as a potential chemotherapeutic agent for malignant glioma, but its efficacy remains uncertain.

Experimental Therapies

The relatively low efficacy of standard chemotherapeutic agents in the treatment of brain tumors has led to the development of experimental modalities particularly in the form of immunotherapy, gene therapy, angiogenesis inhibitors, and growth factor inhibitors that are discussed later.

Supportive Therapy

In addition to surgery, radiation, and chemotherapy, where the goal of treatment is to extend survival, various types of supportive therapy are also required to treat the neurologic symptoms of a brain tumor and improve the patient's quality of life. Supportive therapy includes the use of anticonvulsants for seizure management, corticosteroids for the control of symptoms associated with tumor edema, and anticoagulants in the treatment of deep venous thrombosis.

Seizures comprise one of the most common symptoms of patients with brain tumors. They usually occur as the presenting symptom or as a complication of surgery. All seizures from a brain tumor begin as a focal seizure even if the focal seizure is not observed clinically. The seizures may stay focal or generalize leading to loss of consciousness. Focal seizures usually resolve spontaneously and rarely cause permanent neurologic damage. Occasionally, repetitive seizures lead to status epilepticus. Patients with brain tumors who have had a seizure either at presentation or during the course of their treatment should be treated with an anticonvulsant. There is no evidence that anticonvulsant drugs prevent seizures in patients with brain tumors who have never had a seizure.[118]

Corticosteroids dramatically relieve the symptoms from edema caused by brain tumors, thus reducing intracranial pressure. Symptomatic improvement usually takes hours and patients may be symptom free within 24 to 48 hours. Corticosteroids are indicated in all patients with brain tumors who exhibit neurologic symptoms from the tumor. One exception is the patient with presumed PCNSL. In patients with lymphoma, corticosteroids may cause tumor necrosis owing to their lymphocytic effect, compromising a histologic diagnosis if the steroids are administered prior to biopsy.

The optimal dose of corticosteroid to be administered is not clear. The typical dose is 16 mg of dexamethasone per day. The drug is long-acting and there is no need to administer it more than twice a day. Once begun, the administration of a corticosteroid is continued until the patient's symptoms are relieved. The dose is then tapered to the lowest dose commensurate with good neurologic function. There is no upper limit to the dose of steroids used. If the recommended dose of 16 mg a day does not improve neurologic function, then higher doses may be effective. A dose of 100 mg a day for 48 hours may be needed to gain neurologic improvement in patients with marked elevation of intracranial pressure. For patients on steroids greater than 6 weeks, prophylactic treatment for *Pneumocystis carinii* infection is indicated.

Deep venous thrombosis (DVT) is a common complication of brain tumors and their therapy. Factors that contribute to their development include immobility, neurosurgery, the release of thromboplastins from the brain, and hypercoagulability related to cancer and chemotherapy. Most DVTs occur in proximity to the patient's surgery. The use of pneumatic compression boots perioperatively decreases the incidence of DVT.[119] The use of perioperative subcutaneous heparin is safe and effective in preventing DVT;[120] its use does not increase the risk of intratumoral hemorrhage.[121,122] Anticoagulants can be used to treat established thromboembolism in patients with brain tumors. They are safe and effective. Those with contraindications to anticoagulants can undergo placement of a vena cava filter.

Glioblastoma and Anaplastic Astrocytoma

Glioblastomas develop in approximately 5 per 100,000 individuals per year in North America, making them the most common brain tumor in adults.[123] Although GBMs account for only 1% of adult cancers, they account for 2% of cancer deaths. The mean age of patients with GBM is 54 years, compared with a mean age of 45 years for AA. Both GBMs and AAs are slightly more common in men than in women. GBMs are twice as common in Whites than in Blacks.[124] GBMs are more commonly located in the temporal lobes; AAs are more commonly found in the frontal lobe.[125] The median survival for AA ranges between 3 and 5 years.[125] The median survival for GBM ranges between 6 and 24 months.[125]

Prognostic Factors

Favorable prognostic factors include age younger than 50 years at diagnosis, a high Karnofsky performance score (KPS), and surgical resection versus biopsy alone.[126] A higher proliferation rate (M1B1) may predict a worse prognosis on patients with astrocytomas but does not predict survival in GBM.[127]

Pathology

The histopathology of both GBM and AA was discussed under "Histologic Classification of CNS Tumors." Both GBMs and AAs are very hypercellular and infiltrative. AAs tend to have a lower labeling index than GBMs. GBMs are pathologically distinguished from AAs by the presence of necrosis and/or vascular hyperplasia. There is a class of GBM referred to as giant cell glioblastoma. These tumors have the characteristic features of GBM but are also characterized by the presence of large multinucleated giant cells in a reticulin network; they arise de novo and are more common in younger patients. Gliosarcomas display the typical pathologic features of GBM in combination with densely packed spindle-shaped cells in herring bone patterns. Gliosarcomas have the same prognosis as GBM and are treated identically.

Neuroimaging

The appearance of a GBM and AA is very similar on MRI and most often indistinguishable. Both appear as contrast enhancing lesions exerting mass effect (Fig. 70-1). They both display heterogeneous signal intensities on T1 and T2 weighted images. Almost 95% of GBMs will enhance with gadolinium. This frequency of contrast enhancement is less in AAs. GBMs also have a greater tendency to spread along white matter tracts, in particular the corpus callosum, to cross to the contralateral cerebral hemisphere, giving the so-called butterfly appearance.

Surgical Diagnosis and Treatment

In patients with both GBM and AA, surgery establishes the diagnosis, alleviates neurologic symptoms, and prolongs survival. Gross total resection is the goal because most studies suggest that extensive surgery increases both duration and quality of survival. In a prospective multi-institutional series, the morbidity among 408 patients undergoing craniotomy for newly diagnosed malignant glioma was 24%; mortality was 1.5%. Fifty-three percent of patients improved neurologically after craniotomy, and only 8% were neurologically worse.[128] Biopsy offers no opportunity for neurologic improvement.

Radiation Therapy

After surgical resection, patients with GBM and AA are treated with RT and, usually, with chemotherapy.[129] The standard treatment schedule is external beam RT to a dose of 60 Gy administered in 1.8–2.0 Gy fractions 5 days per week for 6 weeks. Elderly patients (>70 years of age) treated with surgery and RT survive longer than those treated with surgery alone, but the prognosis still remains poor.[130] Some have suggested reducing the dose and duration of radiation therapy for patients over 70 years (45 Gy/25 fractions). Occasionally, shorter courses of hypofractionated RT (30 Gy/10 fractions) are used for older patients in poor condition to achieve rapid palliation; efficacy appears comparable to more protracted regimens.

Chemotherapy

Historically, chemotherapy has been administered to patients with malignant glioma after the completion of radiation therapy.[131] As per the most recent reports, cytotoxic chemotherapy is given concurrently with external beam radiotherapy and is typically continued in the adjuvant phase of treatment.

For newly diagnosed GBM, the current standard treatment following surgical resection is RT with concurrent daily temozolomide followed by at least six cycles of adjuvant temozolomide. A prospective randomized trial of 573 patients with newly diagnosed GBM showed that patients treated with RT plus continuous daily temozolomide (75 mg/m^2/day) followed by 6 months of adjuvant temozolomide (150–200 mg/m^2/day for 5 days of a 28-day cycle) had a median survival of 14.6 months compared with 12.1 months in patients treated with RT alone. Furthermore, the 2-year survival rate was 26.5% compared with 10.4%.[132] There was minimal toxicity in the combined RT/chemotherapy group. The significance of the DNA repair enzyme, MGMT, was also demonstrated. Hegi et al analyzed the methylation status of the MGMT promotor in approximately one-half of the subjects from the phase III study.[133] There was a distinct survival advantage for any patient whose promotor was methylated and therefore less active. Median survival of patients treated with RT plus temozolomide was 21.7 months for those with a methylated MGMT promotor and 15.3 months for those without (p = 0.007). Although patients whose tumors have a methylated promotor benefit the most from the addition of temozolomide chemotherapy, to date there is no established alternative therapeutic strategy for those with an unmethylated promoter. These studies included only those patients with GBM, but this approach has been widely adopted for patients with AA as well.

At recurrence, a variety of treatment options may be explored. Re-resection may debulk disease, improve neurologic function and confirm the presence of tumor recurrence and not radionecrosis. SRS is rarely indicated. Preliminary data from a randomized study suggest that survival is identical when bevacizumab is used with or without irinotecan in patients with recurrent GBM. Anti-angiogenic treatment may work in combination with cytotoxic agents. A recent study of recurrent GBM reports an unusually high radiographic response rate (60%) with the combination of bevacizumab, a recombinant monoclonal antibody targeting VEGF, with the cytotoxic drug irinotecan.[134] The investigators reported a 6- month PFS rate of 30% and a median survival of 9 months, which is superior to clinical trials of standard cytotoxic agents alone at recurrence.

The molecular profiling of malignant gliomas has led to the targeting of specific pathways in tumor growth. There are several ongoing trials for recurrent GBM looking at the role of EGFR inhibitors, mTOR inhibitors, PKC inhibitors, and interruptions in RAS signaling.[135] Gene therapy has not been a promising treatment of malignant glioma.[136] Glioma cells may be transduced in situ with the herpes simplex virus-thymidine kinase (HSV-TK) gene, thus making them susceptible to ganciclovir-mediated killing. In preclinical studies this approach was effective, but the promise was not confirmed in early clinical studies. Cytotoxic viral therapy may be another therapeutic approach. Reovirus, a virus that causes upper respiratory tract infections in healthy individuals, appears to be tumoricidal in glioma models.[137]

Immunotherapy has emerged as a novel treatment strategy for gliomas using processed tumor antigens, often from the patient's own tumor.[138] Immunotherapy using dendritic cells or a peptide vaccine is capable of producing an antiglioma response. Dendritic cell vaccinations may increase sensitivity of tumor cells to chemotherapy and improve survival. Data are very preliminary and further results are pending.[139,140]

Overall, the survival outcome for patients with recurrent malignant glioma is poor. Wong and colleagues reviewed the outcome of patients with recurrent malignant glioma treated in eight consecutive phase 2 chemotherapy trials.[141] Of the 225 cases with recurrent GBM, the median PFS was only 9 weeks, and for the 150 patients with recurrent AA, median PFS was 13 weeks. Overall, the median survival was 30 weeks for the entire cohort. A response to treatment predicted better PFS.

Low-Grade Gliomas and Oligodendrogliomas

Low-grade gliomas (LGG) include astrocytomas, oligodendrogliomas, and mixed oligoastrocytomas.[142] Less common low-grade tumors include central neurocytoma and ganglioglioma. A distinct LGG is the JPA found in children and young adults. It has the characteristic MRI appearance of a cyst with an enhancing nodule, typically seen in the cerebellum. However, pilocytic astrocytomas can occur in other locations as well including the optic nerve, thalamus, and hemispheres. Complete surgical resection is curative when feasible. There is a great histologic diversity to LGGs that makes generalizations about their treatment and prognosis difficult. In general, they are slow-growing tumors and may not require immediate therapeutic intervention. However, their major risk lies in their tendency to transform to a higher-grade glioma at which time their prognosis is dictated by the new histology.

LGGs constitute approximately 10% of all primary brain tumors.[142] The median age at diagnosis, excluding JPA, is 37 years, with a mean age ranging from 10 to 66 years. The male female ratio is 1.5:1. Patients with NF-1 and NF-2 are at an increased risk of these tumors, especially for low-grade astrocytomas of the optic pathway. LGGs may occur in many areas of the brain, in particular in the optic nerve, cerebellum, hypothalamus, brainstem, and cerebral hemispheres. Oligodendrogliomas have a tendency to arise in the white matter of the frontal (40%), parietal (30%), and temporal (20%) lobes of young adults. They represent 10% of all LGGs in adults and 5% of LGGs in children.

The most common presenting symptom of patients with LGG is seizure.[143–145] In most series, seizure is reported to be the initial symptom in 60–80% of patients. Headache is an uncommon presenting symptom, occurring only in 5% of patients at diagnosis. The majority of patients are neurologically well at presentation; 90% will have a KPS of 90–100 at diagnosis. The majority of seizures are focal rather than generalized, and the most common presenting sign is a sensory or motor deficit specific to the location of the lesion. The median duration from the onset of symptoms to the time of diagnosis is 6–17 months. Children with JPA often present with ataxia, headache, and nausea owing to the typical cerebellar location of these lesions.

A CT scan in an emergency department is typically the first diagnostic test done in a patient who presents with a seizure. The appearance of an LGG on CT is that of a hypodense lesion that is occasionally cystic.[146] Cerebral astrocytomas in adults are often solid, hypodense, and may be diffusely infiltrating. There is typically minimal mass effect. They may or may not enhance. Oligodendrogliomas appear as a hypodense or isodense lesion with variable enhancement. Oligodendrogliomas often have calcification reflecting the mineralization within their blood vessel walls. The appearance of an astrocytoma and oligodendroglioma on MRI is similar. Both are hypointense or isointense on T1WI and hyperintense on T2WI or FLAIR (Fig. 70-3). Contrast enhancement is variable. Signal voids may be seen on T2WI in areas of calcification in oligodendrogliomas.

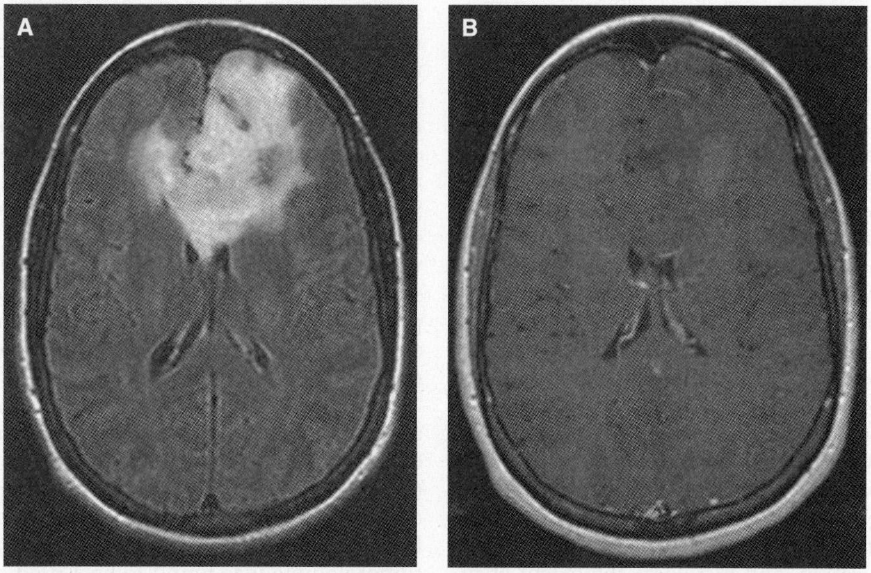

Figure 70-3 ■ Low-grade glioma. (**A**) FLAIR image demonstrating extensive infiltrative disease predominantly of the left frontal lobe extending across the anterior corpus callosum and involving the deep right frontal white matter. (**B**) Postcontrast images show no evidence of enhancement of this large large lesion.

Although patients with LGGs have a better prognosis when compared with patients with malignant gliomas, 50–75% will die from their disease.[147] The median survival of patients with LGGs has been reported to range between 5 and 10 years.[148] There is controversy over prognostic indicators in LGG. Histology plays an important role in survival. Survival increases with a greater ratio of oligodendrocytes: astrocytes within a tumor. The median survival for a low-grade oligodendroglioma is 9.8 years compared with 4.7 years for a low-grade astrocytoma.[149] Age is also important. Patients less than 40 years of age have a median survival of 10.8 years compared with 8.1 years in patients older than 40 years of age.[149] Some studies suggest that seizures preceding the diagnosis by 6 months or more are a good prognostic indicator.[150] Overall tumor volume and extent of surgical resection may play an important role in survival. Complete resection may improve survival and larger tumors may have a faster growth rate and tend to recur more frequently after surgical resection.

At present, the only agreed upon intervention in the management of LGGs is obtaining tissue for histologic diagnosis. There is no unanimous approach to the treatment of LGG because of the paucity of prospective randomized trials. Most treatment suggestions to date result from retrospective reviews of LGGs. Treatment options include observation, biopsy alone, surgical resection, radiation, chemotherapy, or some combination of the former. Factors that influence treatment selection are patient age at diagnosis, neurological deficit, tumor location, extent of surgical resection possible, and histology. Childhood JPA is the only exception to the treatment controversy in LGG. Complete surgical resection of JPA may be curative.

There is growing evidence to suggest that a greater extent of resection at diagnosis may be a favorable prognostic factor. Many series have shown that the reduction of tumor volume by surgery will lengthen the time to tumor progression. In a series by Berger et al, 15% of patients recurred with a median time to tumor progression of 50 months if the residual postoperative tumor volume was less than 10 cm^3 compared with 46% of patients with a median time to tumor progression of 30 months if the postoperative tumor volume was greater than 10 cm^3.[151] In a more recent review of 216 patients with LGG who underwent surgical resection, Smith et al demonstrated that after adjusting for age, KPS, tumor location, and histology, the extent of resection remained a significant factor in overall survival and PFS.[152] Predicted overall survival was diminished even with residual tumor volumes on the order of 10 cm^3. In addition, there was no association between extent of resection and postoperative neurologic deficit. These data strongly argue in favor of achieving a maximal resection in LGGs. Most series report 80% or greater 5-year survival rates in patients who undergo gross total resection based on review of immediate postoperative MRIs.[148]

The timing of surgical resection is also controversial. Some studies have shown no benefit of immediate surgery compared to observation with serial MRIs.[153] However, there are several potential risks of delaying surgery, including malignant transformation of the tumor, tumor growth that would make the lesion unresectable, and the surgical risk of treating a larger tumor in an older patient. Malignant transformation of a LGG is common. Many published series report that 13–86% of LGGs recur at a higher grade.[154,155] Factors leading to transformation are unknown. Some series suggest there is an inverse relationship between age at diagnosis and length of time to malignant transformation.[156] In some reports, low-grade glioma in patients ≥45 years of age behaved like a high-grade glioma.[157]

The utility and timing of RT in the treatment of LGG is also controversial. Most studies done before 1975 reported a beneficial role for radiation in the treatment of LGG.[158–162] However, these studies often failed to stratify based on histology, tumor location, and patient age. The EORTC conducted a prospective phase III trial in adults with supratentorial LGGs, randomizing them to observation only or to initial treatment with radiation alone.[163] The median PFS was 5.3 years in the treated group compared with 3.4 years in the observation arm ($p < 0.0001$). However, the overall survival rate was similar (median 7.4 and 7.2 years respectively). Two-thirds of patients in the observation arm eventually received radiation. Therefore, observation and deferral of radiation may be justified without compromising overall survival. Some studies suggest benefit to radiation in patients older than 50 years of age who have had biopsy alone.[164] Three-year survival rates were reported at 50% for patients who had postbiopsy radiation compared with 25% for patients who did not receive radiation after biopsy.

Two prospective randomized trials compared postbiopsy low-dose radiation (45–50 Gy) to a higher dose (59.4–64 Gy).[165,166] There was no difference in PFS or overall survival between low- and high-dose groups. However, tumor volume was found to be a predictor of outcome and the higher RT doses were associated with greater toxicity. Therefore, patients with well-controlled seizures who are neurologically intact can be followed and treatment deferred until there is clinical or radiographic progression. Patients with poorly controlled seizures or serious neurologic deficits, such as cognitive impairment, need immediate treatment. RT is effective but can probably be administered in lower doses with good efficacy, either when used immediately or later unless there is evidence that the lesion has transformed to a higher grade.

The role of chemotherapy in the treatment of LGGs is not well established. Historically, these tumors have been poorly responsive to cytotoxic chemotherapy. This lack of response may be owing to their low rate of cell growth and indolent nature, their genetic instability, and an intact blood–brain barrier. To date there are only two published randomized trials. The first is a trial of the Southwest Oncology Group where 66 patients with LGG were randomized to RT alone or to RT in combination with CCNU.[167] There was no difference in survival between the two arms. There is a more recent trial (RTOG 9802) where patients were stratified based on risk factors (age and extent of resection) into favorable and unfavorable patients.[168] Favorable patients were observed (group 1), and unfavorable patients were treated with RT+/- procarbazine, CCNU, and vincristine (PCV) (groups 2 and 3). The 5-year OS for groups 1, 2, and 3 was 93%, 62%, and 71%, respectively. The addition of PCV did not increase survival.

The response of malignant glioma to temozolomide has generated interest for its use in LGG. Several series have shown that temozolomide has activity in patients with LGGs who have had progression after radiation.[169–174] Among these patients, 47–67% had some tumor shrinkage (>25%) with a median PFS of 10–22 months. Several small studies have explored the use of temozolomide as the initial postsurgical therapy for LGGs.[175–177] Response rates, when minor responses are included, range from 31% to 61%, and median time to progression ranges from 31 months to 36 months. These encouraging results have led the EORTC to initiate a phase 3 trial randomizing patients with LGG to radiation or temozolomide; this study is ongoing.

Chemotherapy is effective in treating LGG but the best drug or combination of drugs, as well as the timing of therapy, is unknown. LGGs with 1p and 19q chromosomal deletions may respond better to chemotherapy.[178,179] These chromosomal changes indicate an oligodendroglial lineage. The unique chemosensitivity of oligodendrogliomas was first recognized in patients with (AO).[180,181] Oligodendrogliomas account for 5–20% of all primary brain tumors. They are predominantly a tumor of adults with a peak incidence between the fourth and sixth decades of life. They commonly occur in the frontal, parietal, and temporal lobes. They are more frequently low-grade than high-grade tumors.

Like all diffuse gliomas, AOs infiltrate brain tissue diffusely. Histologically, they are hypercellular. They may lose the characteristic morphology known as the "fried-egg" appearance seen in lower-grade oligodendrogliomas. Also, the "chicken wire" pattern of branching blood vessels may not be present in AOs. They exhibit typical features of anaplasia such as high cell density, mitotic figures, nuclear atypia, microvascular proliferation, and necrosis. There are no specific immunohistochemical markers for AO. Occasionally, neurocytomas, ependymomas, or pilocytic astrocytomas may resemble oligodendrogliomas. Some AOs have astrocytic features and may be GFAP positive. There are no definite criteria that define how much of an oligodendroglial component must be present in an astrocytoma before it is considered an oligoastrocytoma. Many studies require an arbitrary 25% oligodendroglial representation, but this is also subject to sampling error.[182] Deletion of the short arm of chromosome-1 (1p) and the long arm of chromosome 19 (19q) is a unique feature of oligodendroglial neoplasms.

Codeletion of 1p/19q occurs in 61–89% of AOs but only in 14–20% of mixed anaplastic oligoastrocytomas.[183,184] The 1p/19q LOH represents a balanced translocation. AOs usually have additional chromosomal deletions; in particular, loss of heterozygosity for 9p or deletion of the CDKN24 gene.[185,186]

On MRI or CT, most AOs are characterized by enhancement (Fig. 70-4A and B). The pattern of enhancement of 1p/19q codeleted tumors may be somewhat different: more patchy and homogeneous, in contrast to the ring-like enhancement with necrosis seen in GBMs and AOs without 1p/19q deletion.[187]

The presence or absence of combined loss of 1p/19q is the most important prognostic factor for oligodendroglial tumors.[188–190] Codeletion is associated with a more indolent behavior and a better response to chemotherapy and RT. The median overall survival in AO without 1p/19q loss is 2 to 3 years but greater than 6 to 7 years in patients with tumors with combined 1p and 19q loss.[191] One study showed that 100% of AO patients with 1p or combined 1p and 19q loss had an objective response to chemotherapy (24 of 24 and 22 of 22, respectively).[191] In contrast, only 25% and 31% of those patients whose tumors retained these alleles responded. The 5-year survival rate for patients with tumors with 1p/19q LOH is 95% as opposed to 25% for those whose tumor retained these alleles.

Randomized trials have shown that adjuvant radiation provides significant yet modest improvement in survival for patients with high-grade glioma.[192] No trial specifically addresses the role of radiation in AO alone, but the conventional dose is 60 Gy in 30–30 fractions based upon the studies of GBM and AA. Some trials have found benefit from postoperative RT in patients with AO. Others have found benefit from RT only in patients with neurologic deficit or in those who had a biopsy only. AOs with 1p/19q loss have a superior outcome after RT compared with those without 1p/19q loss. AOs have a more favorable response to chemotherapy than high-grade astrocytomas. Initial studies investigated PCV, with more recent studies focusing on the use of temozolomide. The reason for the favorable response of AO to chemotherapy is unknown. There are indications that MGMT is expressed less in AO and perhaps even more so in 1p/19q codeleted tumors than in astrocytomas.[193] MGMT promotor methylation occurs in 80–90% of codeleted AOs and in only 50% of GBMs.[194–196]

The unique chemosensitivity of AOs was first appreciated in recurrent disease. Approximately two-thirds of patients with recurrent AOs after RT had a response to PCV chemotherapy. The time to progression in these patients was 12–18 months;[198–200] the reported response rate of recurrent AO to temozolomide varies between 46% and 55%, with 12 month PFS between 40% and 50%.[196,200] No formal comparison between PCV and temozolomide is available.

There have been two large randomized trials of patients with AO at initial diagnosis.[201,202] Both examined the administration of RT +/- PCV chemotherapy; one trial used PCV in the neoadjuvant setting and the second used it following RT. Both trials demonstrated that chemotherapy significantly prolonged PFS but not OS. In both studies, patients who received RT alone usually received PCV at progression. Furthermore, patients with 1p/19q deleted tumors fared best. Therefore, these studies mainly examined the timing of chemotherapy that seemed to work as well when it was part of the initial regimen as when given at recurrence. However, PCV has high toxicity and has largely been replaced with temozolomide, which is much better tolerated.[201]

The chemosensitivity of AO has made upfront chemotherapy attractive. The rationale for initial chemotherapy is to defer radiation. A few small studies using temozolomide exist. One trial of upfront temozolomide therapy shows a short time to progression (8 months) in patients who did not have 1p loss, in contrast to patients with 1p loss who were free from progression at 24 months.[202] In a phase 2 trial of 69 patients who had newly diagnosed AO, an intensive PCV regimen was followed by high-dose thiotepa with autologous stem cell rescue, without RT.[203] The median PFS in the 39 patients who received the stem cell procedure was 78 months and the OS has not been reached. A second study is underway using temozolomide induction and busulfan and thiotepa for transplant with promising initial results. These data provide conflicting information regarding the optimal approach to patients with AO. The variety of options is reflected by the large range of treatment decisions made by experienced neuro-oncologists.[204]

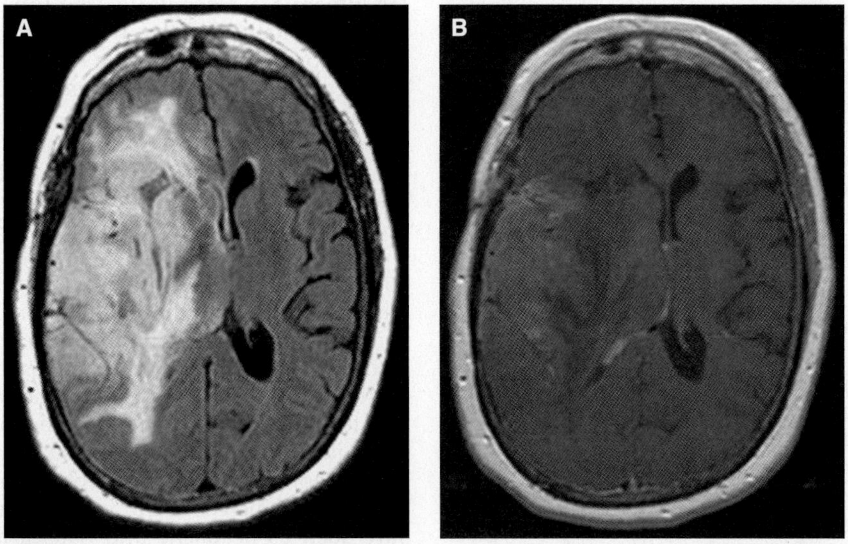

Figure 70-4 Anaplastic oligodendroglioma. (**A**) FLAIR image showing extensive tumor infiltrating the right hemisphere. (**B**) Patchy enhancement os seen throughout the tumor.

Ependymoma

Ependymomas account for approximately 5% of all intracranial tumors in adults and 10% in children; they are the most common intracranial tumor in children under the age of 5 years. There is a slight male predominance. Ependymomas have a bimodal incidence with a major peak at 5 years and a smaller peak at 35 years.

Pathology

Ependymomas are tumors comprising ependymal cells that tend to occur along the surfaces of the ventricles. They may also occur in the brain parenchyma adjacent to the ventricles or anywhere along the spinal canal. More than 60% of ependymomas occur in the posterior fossa and arise from the caudal floor of the fourth ventricle. Supratentorial ependymomas are typically parenchymal rather than intraventricular in location and most common in the frontal and parietal lobes. They can extend along the subarachnoid space and seed the CSF.

The WHO divides ependymomas into ependymomas (WHO grade II), anaplastic ependymomas (WHO grade III), subependymomas, and myxopapillary ependymomas (both WHO grade I). There are four histiologic variants of WHO grade II ependymomas: cellular, papillary, clear cell, and tanycytic, which do not carry any prognostic or therapeutic significance. In general, ependymomas comprise uniform cells in a collagenous background. They typically have infrequent mitoses and little necrosis. They may contain cysts, calcification, or hemorrhage. Pseudorosettes are the most common epithelial feature; they appear as eosinophilic zones surrounding a blood vessel. Anaplastic ependymomas have histologic features that resemble GBM. They have nuclear pleomorphism, a high mitotic rate, endothelial proliferation, and necrosis. They are more commonly found in the supratentorial compartment.

A number of genetic abnormalities have been reported in ependymomas, none characteristic.[205,206] The most common is loss of chromosome 22 reported to occur in 16–60% of tumors. Chromosome 22 loss is more common in spinal ependymomas. Other reported genetic associations are loss of chromosome 6q and the X chromosome as well as gains of 1q and 9q.

The overall prognosis for intracranial ependymomas is not favorable. Reported 5-year survival ranges from 40% to 80% and only 25% to 50% of patients have a 5-year PFS.[207–212] Young age (<5 years) is associated with a worse survival. Supratentorial ependymomas have a better prognosis than posterior fossa ependymomas. Furthermore, tumors that arise from the foramen of Luschka have a worse prognosis than tumors that arise from the center of the fourth ventricle. The most consistent factor associated with survival is extent of surgical resection. The correlation between pathologic grade and prognosis is unclear.[213,214] In many series, postoperative survival does not correlate with anaplastic pathology, although most reviews indicate that necrosis, a high mitotic rate, and endothelial proliferation are associated with a worse prognosis. Other poor prognostic indicators are up regulation of the erb-B2 receptor, low GFAP expression, and the presence of diploid DNA.

Clinical findings depend upon the tumor location. The symptoms caused by ependymomas most commonly arise from CSF obstruction but may also occur from either brainstem compression or focal cerebral involvement. Common symptoms of CSF obstruction are headache, nausea, and vomiting. Lower cranial nerve palsies are less common presenting signs. Supratentorial tumors may present with seizure or focal motor or sensory deficits. MR scan demonstrates a tumor that is heterogeneously hypo- and isointense on T1 and hyperintense on T2 and may or may not enhance. Calcification is present in 60% of infratentorial tumors and areas of necrosis and cysts are seen in 80% of tumors.

The initial treatment of ependymomas is surgical. A gross total resection will prolong survival but may not always be possible depending upon the location of the tumor. Most supratentorial ependymomas can undergo a gross total resection in comparison to posterior fossa tumors that often require removal of the inferior cerebellar vermis. This procedure may result in cerebellar mutism. Surgical resection should be followed by RT. The optimal dose is 45 Gy administered in 1.6–1.8 Gy fractions. The amount of tissue to be treated has been debated in the literature.[207] The need for entire neuraxis radiation has been challenged. Despite the fact that about 15% of ependymomas will seed the leptomeninges, they do so at recurrence, so that radiation is delivered to the tumor bed and not to the entire neuraxis unless CSF spread is documented at diagnosis on spine MRI and CSF cytology which should be done in all patients for staging. The literature also shows that patients treated with local radiation have preserved cognitive functioning compared with those treated with craniospinal radiation.

Like glial tumors, ependymomas are primarily chemoresistant tumors. There is no role for adjuvant chemotherapy in the treatment of ependymoma as it does not prolong survival. Chemotherapy may be considered at recurrence. Some investigators have reported response rates of up to 65% with platinum drugs. Some studies also suggest that temozolomide or etoposide may be effective.[215–218]

Primary Central Nervous System Lymphoma (PCNSL)

PCNSL is a high or intermediate grade non-Hodgkin lymphoma restricted to the brain, CSF, spinal cord, and eyes.[219,220] Previously known by a variety of names including microglioma, reticulum cell sarcoma, perivascular sarcoma, and lymphosarcoma, PCNSL represented about 1% of primary brain tumors. However, among immunocompetent individuals the incidence of this lymphoma has risen three-fold in the past two to three decades for no clear reason. It has an estimated incidence of 0.3/100,000/year. It has a higher incidence in the immunosuppressed patient, whether immunosuppression is congenital (Wiskott–Aldrich syndrome) or acquired (AIDS, organ transplant patients, or drug-induced). In this subpopulation, PCNSL is usually associated with the Epstein–Barr virus (EBV).[221,222,223,224,223–226]

PCNSL occurs in all age groups with a peak incidence in the sixth and seventh decades of life. Immunocompromised patients are younger, and the median age of onset among AIDS patients is 40 years. There is a slight male preponderance in immunocompetent patients; however, 90% of AIDS-related PCNSL occurs in men. Older age and poor performance have been associated with shorter survival.[225] PCNSL is a highly treatable disease; like all lymphomas, it is both chemosensitive and radiosensitive.

The majority of PCNSLs are diffuse large cell, or large cell immunoblastic lymphomas. Most exhibit a B-cell immunophenotype with less than 3% of T-cell origin.[226,227] The tumor cells have a characteristic perivascular growth pattern. They tend to grow in perivascular spaces and form concentric rings around vessel walls without invading the vascular lumen. Macroscopically, the tumors are white matter lesions, which may be solitary or multiple. Multiple lesions are more common in AIDS patients, and occur in 30–40% of sporadic cases. Unlike high-grade gliomas, PCNSL in immunocompetent patients lacks vascular proliferation and necrosis. However, necrosis is seen commonly in AIDS-related PCNSL.

PCNSL is a rapidly growing tumor, so symptoms are usually present for only a few weeks prior to diagnosis. The most common presenting symptoms are cognitive deficits or personality changes that can be attributed to the tumor's predilection for the frontal lobe and its tendency for multifocality. Lateralizing neurologic deficits appropriate to the involved area and signs of increased intracranial pressure such as headache and nausea are also common. PCNSL forms a parenchymal mass in more than 90% of patients, but it can involve all compartments of the nervous system including the spinal fluid, spinal cord, and eye. Leptomeningeal involvement is seen in about 40% of parenchymal PCNSL, but primarily leptomeningeal PCNSL is rare. Patients rarely have symptoms of leptomeningeal disease such as cranial neuropathies, lumbosacral radiculopathies, or communicating hydrocephalus. Therefore, clinicians cannot rely upon the clinical presentation to indicate the presence or absence of leptomeningeal spread of the tumor. All patients with PCNSL should undergo lumbar puncture for cytological evaluation.

Ocular involvement of PCNSL is common. It may be the initial manifestation of the disease, or occur at relapse. Patients who develop ocular lymphoma first have a 50–80% chance of developing cerebral lymphoma. The diagnosis of ocular lymphoma can be difficult because symptoms often mimic benign inflammatory conditions such as uveitis, chorioretinitis, and vitreitis. The most frequent symptoms are floaters and visual blurring. Diagnosis is made from slit lamp exam, ocular ultrasound, and often vitreal biopsy.

The radiographic appearance of PCNSL is similar on both CT and MRI. Prior to contrast administration, PCNSL is usually iso- or hyperdense on CT and isointense on T1 weighted MRI. After contrast administration the lesions enhance diffusely (Fig. 70-5). The lesion borders are indistinct, and the amount of edema is variable. Unlike high-grade gliomas in immunocompetent patients, there is no central necrosis. Radiographically, PCNSL often responds to corticosteroids and may transiently vanish from imaging studies.

PCNSL is a highly treatable disease. It is very chemo- and radiosensitive, similar to systemic non-Hodgkin lymphoma. Despite this sensitivity to treatment, PCNSL has a high recurrence rate with a 5-year survival of 25–50%.[228] Age at diagnosis and performance status are the most important prognostic factors in patients with PCNSL, regardless of treatment. Surgical resection does not contribute to survival, and the median survival is only 4 to 5 months with surgery alone. Owing to their oncolytic effect on malignant lymphocytes, steroids should be held prior to surgical biopsy so as not to interfere with the pathologic diagnosis.

Cranial RT (40–50 Gy) had been the cornerstone of treatment for PCNSL increasing survival rates to 12 to 14 months.[229] Although highly effective at producing a remission, tumor recurs after 1 year with RT, and the 5-year survival is only 3% to 4%. Severe neurotoxicity is also an important concern with WBRT.

Standard chemotherapy regimens for systemic lymphoma such as CHOP (cyclophosphamide, doxorubicin, vincristine, and prednisone) have not proven beneficial in the treatment of PCNSL.[230,231,232,,233,] The use of drugs that can penetrate the blood–brain barrier and achieve high concentrations in both the brain and CSF, such as high-dose methotrexate and cytarabine, are essential to treatment regimens for PCNSL. Methotrexate is the most effective and commonly used single drug for the treatment of PCNSL. High-dose methotrexate produces response rates of 60–90% when used as a single agent or in combination with other drugs. A wide range of high-dose methotrexate regimens are reported in the literature, and they can achieve a median overall survival of 30 to 60 months.[234–243] Cytarabine is the other agent commonly used that has good penetration into the CSF and the intraocular compartment. It is often used as consolidation therapy after radiation therapy or in combination regimens. Recently, rituximab has been investigated for its potential role in PCNSL.[244,245] It penetrates an intact blood–brain barrier poorly but does reach areas of bulky disease that enhance on MRI and can produce responses. It is now being combined with chemotherapy in a number of ongoing clinical trials.

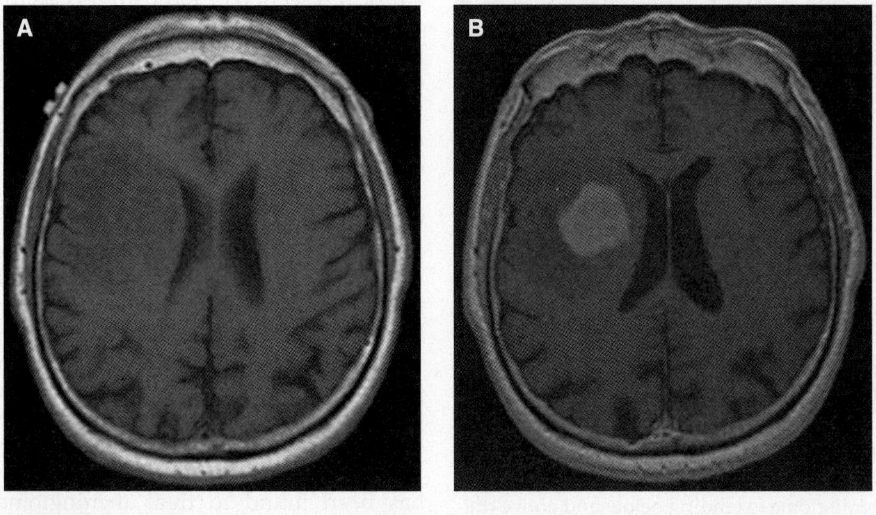

Figure 70-5 PCNSL. Pre-gadolinium (**A**) and postgadolinium (**B**) images of a right frontal diffusely enhancing PCNSL. Note the edema that surrounds the enhancing mass.

Meningioma

Meningiomas account for approximately 25% of intracranial tumors. They are extra-axial tumors and arise from arachnoidal cap cells rather than the dura itself. They are more common in woman than in men. Female preponderance is not seen in malignant meningiomas.[246] A greater incidence is seen among African Americans than other ethnic groups. Meningiomas typically occur during the fourth through sixth decades. Approximately 85% of meningiomas are supratentorial, and multiple meningiomas occur in 10% of sporadic cases.

Meningiomas have been associated with both radiation exposure and hormones. Ionizing radiation is the only established risk factor for meningioma.[247–250] Both low- and high-dose radiation have been associated with the development of meningiomas. These meningiomas are more often atypical or malignant and are often multifocal. Most meningiomas are estrogen receptor negative and progesterone receptor positive; however, there are no convincing data that sex hormones cause meningiomas.[251–253] The absence of progesterone receptors is associated with malignant tumors and a shorter time to recurrence after surgical resection.

Multiple cytogenetic changes have been noted in meningioma. The most consistent is the deletion of chromosome 22, which occurs in 50% of meningiomas and probably involves the NF-2 tumor suppressor gene.[253] Chromosomal changes are more frequent in atypical and malignant meningiomas. Other alterations include losses on chromosomes 1p, 3p, 6q, 9q, 10q, 14q, and 17p. Certain peptides, such as VEGF and EGFR, have growth effects upon meningiomas.[254,255]

The prognosis after treatment of meningiomas depends upon the histology of the tumor and the extent of resection.[256,257,258] Age at diagnosis and tumor size may also play a role. Younger patients fare better than the elderly. The recurrence rate for a completely resected typical meningioma is 20% at 5 years and 25% at 10 years. Tumors that are incompletely resected have about a 60% chance of recurrence without RT. McCarthy et al published a survey of more than 9000 patients with meningiomas treated in the United States and included in the

National Cancer Data Base.[259] The 5-year overall survival was 60%; 81% for patients <65 years and 56% for patients > 65 years. The estimated 5-year survival for benign tumors was 75% and 55% for malignant tumors. Population-based studies reported a 5-year survival rate near 90%.

Macroscopically, meningiomas are smooth, lobulated tumors that are well demarcated from adjacent brain and have broad dural attachments. Typically, meningiomas compress rather than invade adjacent brain. However, they may invade venous structures such as the superior sagittal sinus.

The histologic appearance of meningiomas varies with the type of meningioma. The three most common subtypes of meningiomas are meningothelial, transitional cell, and fibrous. There are some features common to all meningiomas including a lobular structure, calcification, and psammoma bodies. Most meningiomas react with epithelial membrane antigen (EMA) and vimentin. EMA immunoreactivity is less common in atypical and malignant tumors. Most histological subtypes do not have clinical significance; however, rhabdoid and clear cell meningiomas are frequently more aggressive tumors.

Atypical meningiomas have a higher mitotic index as well as increased cellularity, a high nucleus/cytoplasm ratio, prominent nucleoli, necrosis, and patternless growth. Typically at least three of these features must be seen to classify a meningioma as atypical. Brain invasion alone warrants the diagnosis of an atypical meningioma but is not sufficient to classify a meningioma as malignant. A malignant meningioma must have at least 20 mitoses per 10 high power fields or histology resembling carcinoma or sarcoma. Whereas only 1% of meningiomas metastasize, about one half of malignant meningiomas metastasize, usually to liver, bone, and lung.

Most meningiomas are very slow growing and may be asymptomatic; many are found incidentally on imaging done for other reasons. When meningiomas do produce clinical symptoms and signs, they typically do so by compression of brain structures, edema, or hydrocephalus. Although most meningiomas do not cause significant brain edema, secretory meningiomas may cause edema resulting in significant neurologic symptoms. Convexity meningiomas may cause seizure. Meningiomas in particular locations may have typical clinical syndromes. Olfactory groove meningiomas may cause anosmia and the Foster Kennedy syndrome (optic atrophy and scotomata in the ipsilateral eye and papilledema in the contralateral eye). Cavernous sinus meningiomas may cause diplopia, proptosis, and other oculomotor abnormalities.

CT and MRI readily diagnose meningiomas. On CT, meningiomas are hyperdense extraaxial masses (Fig. 70-6). Calcification is present in 25% of tumors. Because meningiomas are typically slow growing, bone erosion of the overlying skull may be seen. Meningiomas demonstrate dense uniform contrast enhancement. Atypical, malignant, and large meningiomas more commonly cause surrounding brain edema. On T1- and T2-weighted MRI images, most meningiomas have signal intensity similar to surrounding grey matter. A dural tail sign on contrast-enhanced images is characteristic. Some tumors may have flow voids indicating marked vascularity of the tumor. MRS shows well-defined peaks for choline, a low phosphocreatine/creatine ratio, and a decrease in NAA. An alanine peak is characteristic of meningiomas.

The first step in the management of a patient with a meningioma is to decide whether treatment is necessary. Many meningiomas may be followed for years if they do not exhibit growth or cause neurologic symptoms.[260] If seizures are the only symptom and are well controlled with medication, surgical resection may not be necessary. Other meningiomas are not resected because tumor removal may be dangerous. This is usually the case in larger lesions and those located at the skull base and cavernous sinus. These meningiomas may encase portions of the intracavernous carotid artery as well as multiple cranial nerves.

The treatment for most meningiomas is surgical resection.[26,262] In many instances, the tumor can be removed completely and a cure is achieved. Meningiomas with the best potential for complete removal are those located along the convexity. The main consideration in the removal of these tumors is the extent of involvement of the sagittal sinus; the anterior third of the sinus may be excised without serious neurologic sequelae. Preoperative embolization may be done to reduce the size and vascularity of the tumor, making resection easier. Even in those patients in whom a complete removal has been accomplished, approximately 15–20% of these tumors will recur and may require additional surgery or RT.

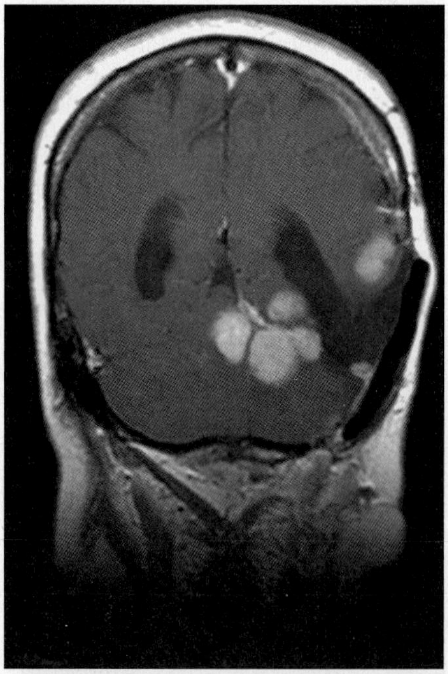

Figure 70-6 Meningioma. A coronal postgadolinium view of a multilobulated meningioma extending below and above the tentorium. There is a second lesion in the left occipito-parietal cortex.

RT is used in the treatment of meningiomas in inoperable tumors, in partially resected tumors in some patients, at recurrence, and in all resected tumors that are malignant. The role of RT in atypical meningiomas is unclear. In the past, meningiomas were reputed to be radioresistant tumors. However, more recent data suggest that RT can be effective. The low dose (30–40 Gy) used in older studies may have contributed to the poor results seen.[263,264] Doses in the range of 45–60 Gy are effective in patients with incomplete resection of tumor, improving 5-year recurrence free survival to that seen with complete surgical resection.[265–269] In addition, new 3D planning techniques and stereotactically guided conformational RT allow for reductions in the volume of normal tissue irradiated and less neurotoxicity.[270,271] The use of protons in the treatment of some meningiomas has also been of benefit in reducing toxicity and delaying recurrence.

Stereotactic RT is an important treatment option for atypical, malignant, and recurrent meningioma. Radiosurgery has also become the preferred treatment for small typical meningiomas less than 3 cm. In a retrospective comparison of 198 adult patients who underwent either surgical resection or radiosurgery as initial treatment of their meningioma, Pollack et al found that both modalities had equivalent tumor control.[271] Tumor control rates with stereotactic radiosurgery are higher than 90% in most series with complication rates less than 5%.

There is a small group of patients in whom, despite multiple surgical resections and RT, the meningioma recurs. In these patients, medical therapy with hormonal or chemotherapy agents may be considered when surgical and RT options are exhausted. The use of the progesterone antagonist, mifepristone, initially appeared effective, but this was not sustained with further testing.[275,276]

To date, no effective chemotherapy has been found to treat meningioma. There have been some attempts with anthracyclines, cisplatin, and irinotecan but without definite success.[272,273274.] There are several small series of patients with recurrent meningioma that report a response to hydroxyurea, but most patients do not appear to benefit,[275,276,277,278,279,280,281] Newton et al reported that 18/20 patients responded to hydroxyurea for a median of more than 3 years.[277] Minor hematologic toxicity was reported. Some meningiomas are characterized by marked angiogenesis and VEGF expression. There is in vitro evidence that interferon can inhibit growth of meningioma cells via inhibition of angiogenesis, and there are small patient series reporting a response of meningioma to interferon.[282–284] There are no large trials examining more potent anti-angiogenic agents.

Spinal Cord Tumors

Epidemiology and Etiology

Primary spinal cord tumors constitute approximately 10–15% of all CNS neoplasms, and they are grouped by location which is often dependent on their cell of origin. Spinal cord tumors fall into three major groups: intramedullary, intradural extramedullary, and extradural.

Intramedullary tumors typically are derived from glial or ependymal cells (astrocytomas and ependymomas) and are found throughout the spinal cord. They are rare, accounting for only 5–10% of all spinal cord tumors.[285,286] Intradural extramedullary tumors include nerve sheath tumors (neurofibromas and schwannomas) and meningiomas. These tumors account for approximately 55–65% of all spinal cord tumors.[287,288] The most common extradural tumor is a metastatic lesion from another primary. The leading primary sites of metastatic tumors to the spine in order of frequency are lung, breast, and prostate.[289] In general, intramedullary tumors are more common in children, and extramedullary tumors are more common in adults.

Clinical Presentation and Neuroimaging

Clinical symptoms of spinal cord tumors include back pain, motor and sensory disturbances, and bladder, bowel, and sexual dysfunction. Focal back pain at the tumor location is the most common presenting symptom. This pain is worse at night and in the supine position. Slowly growing tumors may cause little or no symptoms, whereas rapidly growing tumors may have significant neurologic symptoms and signs at initial presentation. Intramedullary tumors frequently do not present with pain but rather with signs of central cord dysfunction. These patients will often present with weakness, long tract signs, loss of pain and temperature sensation, and bowel, bladder, and sexual dysfunction. Intramedullary tumors are said to cause sacral sparing (intact sensation over the sacral region) because they arise from the central part of the cord, and the sacral fibers are located at the most peripheral portion of the spinal cord. However, this is an unreliable finding. Intradural extramedullary tumors typically present with radicular signs of pain, and motor and sensory disturbances. Extradural metastases present with focal back pain and commonly produce signs of spinal cord compression with paraparesis and sensory loss in the legs.

MRI is the mainstay of radiographic diagnosis for all spinal cord tumors. In many cases, MRI accurately predicts the histology of the tumor. Intramedullary astrocytomas and ependymomas typically result in parenchymal expansion of the spinal cord and are often associated with a cystic cavity or syrinx. Astrocytomas enhance heterogeneously and are often cystic. Ependymomas display more uniform enhancement and are less commonly cystic. Meningiomas commonly occur in the neural foramen and have a characteristic "dumbbell" appearance on MRI. Extradural metastatic tumors typically arise in the boney part of the vertebral column and compress or deform the spinal cord (Fig. 70-7). They often obliterate the surrounding subarachnoid space of the spinal cord.

Pathology

Primary tumors of the spinal cord or nerve roots are similar to intracranial tumors in cellular type. They may arise from glial cells giving rise to astrocytomas or ependymomas, or from Schwann cells of the nerve roots, or meningeal cells from the coverings of the spinal cord. Metastatic tumors have a histology similar to the primary tumor.

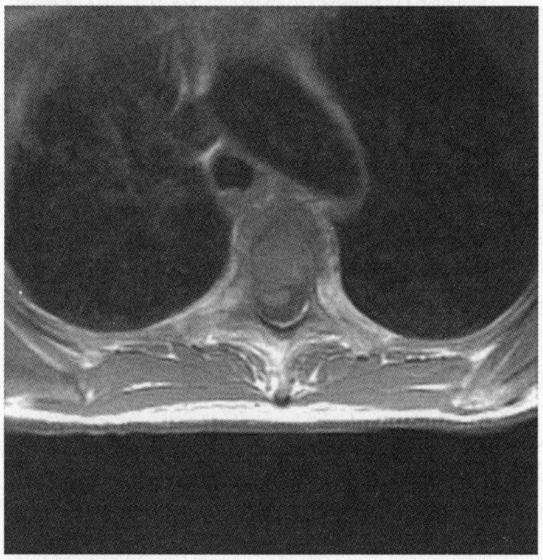

Figure 70-7 Epidural spinal cord compression from breast cancer. On this axial T1 weighted MRI one can appreciate the metastatic tumor extending from the vertebral body and compressing the spinal cord ventrally and predominantly on the right. This is extraaxial compression.

Treatment

The goals of surgery for spinal cord tumors are to establish a diagnosis and to relieve symptoms. Gross total resection is the goal for meningiomas, nerve sheath tumors, and ependymomas. Astrocytomas account for 90% of intramedullary tumors in adults. Unlike ependymomas, astrocytomas do not demonstrate a clear line of demarcation from tumor and normal spinal cord. Therefore, the risk of subtotal resection must be weighed against the risk of neurologic deficit. Five-year overall survival for spinal cord astrocytomas is 50–60%.[290–292] Extent of resection has not been shown to affect survival. Most of these tumors in adults are grades 1 and 2, with only about 10% being higher grade. Histologic grade is the most significant prognostic factor. Five-year survival for grade 1 tumors reaches 80%, whereas 5-year survival for grades 2 and 3 tumors is 15%.[292] For most diffuse spinal cord astrocytomas, only a biopsy is done for diagnosis.

Unlike spinal astrocytomas, spinal cord ependymomas can more commonly undergo gross total resection. The majority of these tumors are low-grade, well-circumscribed lesions. Cure, with preservation of neurologic function, can be achieved with complete resection of spinal meningiomas. Myxopapillary ependymomas are found exclusively at the filum terminale and are grade 1 lesions. They have a good prognosis and are associated with a 10-year survival rate of 90%.[293,294]

Reports in the literature regarding the effects of radiation dose, extent of the radiation field, and the type of radiation have been conflicting. A recent review of 183 patients with spinal cord glial tumors from six institutions compared the PFS and OS of 82 patients who received surgery alone with 101 patients who received surgery and postoperative radiation treatment.[295] As many as 120 patients had ependymomas, the remainder astrocytomas. The median total radiation dose was 49.5 Gy for ependymomas and 50 Gy for astrocytomas. In the ependymoma patients, there was no benefit from RT with respect to OS and PFS. In the astrocytoma patients, radiation did not affect OS. However, radiation did significantly reduce the risk of disease progression in patients with low to intermediate grade astrocytomas compared to patients who underwent surgery alone.

There is no clear role for adjuvant chemotherapy in the treatment of spinal cord intramedullary tumors. There are a few case reports of patients having transient responses to temozolomide, nitrosoureas, and platinum compounds.

Selected References

The complete reference list can be found at www.CANCERMEDICINE8.com

1. Central Brain Tumor Registry of the United States. Primary Brain Tumors in the United States Statistical Report, 1998–2002. Hinsdale, IL: CBTRUS (2005).
8. Werner MH, Phuphanich S, Lyman GH. The increasing incidence of malignant gliomas and primary central nervous system lymphoma in the elderly. Cancer 1995;76:1634–42.
13. Walter AW, Hancock ML, Pui CH, et al. Secondary brain tumors in children treated for acute lymphoblastic leukemia at St Jude Children's Research Hospital. J Clin Oncol 1998;16:3761–7.
27. Inskip PD, Tarone RE, Hatch EE, et al. Cellular-telephone use and brain tumors. N Engl J Med 2001;344:79–8.
28. Kan P, Simonsen SE, Lyon JL, Kestle JR. Cellular phone use and brain tumor: a meta-analysis. J Neuro-Oncol 2008;86:71–8.
29. Bondy ML, Wang LE, El-Zein R, et al. Gamma-radiation sensitivity and risk of glioma. *J Natl Cancer Inst* 2001:93:1553–7
73. Cairncross JG, Ueki K, Zlatescu MC, et al. Specific genetic predictors of chernotherapeutic response and survival in patients with anaplastic oligodendrogliomas. J Natl Cancer Inst 1998;90:1473-9.
84. Simpson JR, Horton J, Scott C, et al. Influence of location and extent of surgical resection on survival of patients with glioblastoma multiforme: results of three consecutive Radiation Therapy Oncology Group (RTOG) clinical trials. Int J Radiat Oncol Biol Phys 1993;26:239-44.
96. Lammering G, Valerie K, Lin PS, et al. Radiosensitization of malignant glioma cells through overexpression of dominant-negative epidermal growth factor receptor. Clin Cancer Res 2001;7:682-90.
99. DeAngelis LM. Medical progress: Brain tumors. N Engl J Med 2001;344:1 14-323.
102. Brem H, Piantadosi S, Burger PC, et al. Placebo-controlled trial of safety and efficacy of intraoperative controlled delivery by biodegradable polymers of chemotherapy for recurrent gliomas. The Polymer-brain Tumor Treatment Group. Lancet 1995;345:1008-12.
111. Yung WK, Albright RE, Olson J, et al. A phase II study of temozolomide vs. procarbazine in patients with glioblastoma multiforme at first relapse. Br J Cancer 2000;83:588-932.
118. Glantz M, Friedberg M, Cole B, et al. Double-blind, randomized, placebo-controlled trial of anticonvulsant prophylaxis in adults with newly diagnosed brain metastases. Proc ASCO 1994;13:176.
122. Constantini S, Kanner A, Friedman A, et al. Safety of perioperative minidose heparin in patients undergoing brain tumor surgery: a prospective, randomized, double-blind study. J Neurosurg 2001;94:918-21.
123. Wrensch M, Minn Y, Chew T, et al. Epidemiology of primary brain tumors: current concepts and review of the literature. Neuro-Oncol 2002;4:278-99.
126. Curran WJ Jr. Scott CB, Horton J, et al. Recursive partitioning analysis of prognostic factors in three Radiation Therapy Oncology Group malignant glioma trials. J Natl Cancer Inst 1993;85:704-10.
127. Moskowitz SI, Jin T, Prayson RA. Role of M1B1 in predicting survival in patients with glioblastomas. J Neurooncol 2006:76(2): 193-200.
128. Chang SM, Parney IF, McDermott M, et al. Perioperative complications and neurological outcomes, of first and second craniotomies among patients enrolled in the Glioma Outcome Project. J Neurosurg 2003;98:1175-81.
129. Laperriere NJ, Leung PM, McKenzie S, et al. Randomized study of brachytherapy in the initial management of patients with malignant astrocytoma. Int J Radiat Oncol Biol Phys 1998;41:1005-11.
132. Stupp R, Mason WP, Van den Bent MJ, et al. Radiotherapy plus concomitant and adjuvant temozolomide for glioblastoma. N Engl J Med 2005;352:987-96.
133. Hegi ME, Diserens AC, Gorlia T, et al. MGMT gene silencing and benefit from temozolomide in glioblastoma. N Engl J Med 2005;352:997-1003.
134 Vredenburgh JJ, Desjardins A, Herndon JE 2nd, et al. Bevacizumab plus irinotecan in recurren glioblastoma multiforme. J Clin Oncol 2007;25:4722-9.
135. Stupp R, Hegi ME, Gilbert MR, et al. Chemoradiotherapy in malignant glioma: standard of care and future directions. J Clin Oncol 2007;25:4127-36.
141. Wong ET, Hess KR, Gleason MJ, et al. Outcomes and prognostic factors in recurrent glioma patients enrolled onto phase II clinical trials. J Clin Oncol 1999; 17:2572-8.
142. Louis DN, Ohgaki H, Wiestler OD, Cavenee WK, editors. World Health Organization Classification of Tumours the Central Nervous System (4th Edition). Lyon; IARC Press, 2007.
146. Henson JW, Gaviani P, Gonzalez RG. MRIin the treatment of adult gliomas. Lancet Oncol 2005 ;6:167-75.
147. Gilbert MR, Lang FF. Management of patients with low grade gliomas. Neurol Clin 2007;25:1073-88.
155. van den Bent MJ, Afra D, de Witte O, EORTC Radiotherapy and Brain Tumor Groups and the UK Medical Research Council, et al. Long-term efficacy of early versus delayed radiotherapy for low-grade astrocytoma and oligodendroglioma in adults: the EORTC 22845 randomised trial, Lancet 2005;366:985-90.
165. Karim AB, Maat B, Hatlevoll R, et al. A randomized trial on dose-response in radiation therapy of low-grade cerebral glioma: European Organization for Research and Treatment of Cancer (EORTC) Study 22844. hit J Radiat Oncol Biol Phys 1996;36:549-56.
170. van den Bent MJ, Taphoorn MJ, Brandes AA, European Organization for Research and Treatment of Cancer Brain Tumor Group et al. Phase II study of first-line chemotherapy with temozolomide in recurrent oligodendroglial tumors: the European Organization for Research and Treatment of Cancer Brain Tumor Group Study 26971. J Clin Oncol 2003;21:2525-8.
176. Hoang-Xuan K, Capelle L, Kujas M, et al. .Temozolomide as initial treatment for adults with low-grade oligodendrogliomas or oligoastrocytomas and correlation with chromosome lp deletions. J Clin Oncol 2004;22:3133-3138.
177. Levin N, Lavon I, Zelikovitsh B, et al. Progressive low-grade oligodendrogliomas: response to temozolomide and correlation between genetic profile and O6-methylguanine DNA methyltransferase protein expression. Cancer 2006;106:1759-65.
187. Jenkinson MD, du Plessis DG, Smith TS, et al. Histological growth patterns and genotype in oligodendroglial tumours: correlation with MRI features. Brain 2006; 129:1884-1891.
189. Cairncross G, Berkey B, Shaw E, et al. Phase III trial of chemotherapy plus radiotherapy compared with radiotherapy alone for pure and mixed anaplastic oligodendroglioma: Intergroup Radiation Therapy Oncology Group Trial 9402. J Clin Oncol 2006;24:2707-14.
190. van den Bent MJ, Carpentier AF, Brandes AA, et al. Adjuvant procarbazine, lomustine, and vincristine improves progression-free survival but not overall survival in newly diagnosed anaplastic oligodendrogliomas and oligoastrocytomas: a randomized European Organisation for Research and Treatment of Cancer phase III trial. J Clin Onco1 2006;24:2715-22.
191. Jenkins RB, Blair H, Ballman KV, et al. A t(l;19)(qlO;plO) mediates the combined deletions of lp and 19q and predicts a better prognosis of patients with oligodendroglioma. Cancer Res 2006;66:9852-61
196. Brandes AA, Tosoni A, Cavallo G, et al. Correlations between O6-methylguanine DNA methyltransferase promoter methylation status, Ip and 19q deletions, and response to temozolomide in anaplastic and recurrent oligodendroglioma: a prospective GICNO study. J Clin Onco1 2006;24:4746-53.
201. Mohile NA, Forsyth P, Stewart D, et al. A phase II study of intensified chemotherapy alone as initial treatment for newly diagnosed anaplastic oligodendroglioma: an interim analysis. J Neurooncol 2008;89:187-93.
203. Abrey LE, Childs BH, Paleologos N, et al. High-dose chemotherapy with stem cell rescue as initial therapy for anaplastic oligodendroglioma: long-term follow-up. Neuro Oncol 2006;8:183-8.
204. Abrey LE, Louis DN. Paleologos N.et al. Treatment recommendations for anaplastic oligodendroglioma. Neuro Oncol 2007;9:314-8.
215. Gornet MK, Buckner JC, Marks RS, et al. Chemotherapy for advanced CNS ependymoma. J Neurooncol. 1999;45:61-67.
229. Henry JM, Heffner RR Jr, Dillard SH, et al. Primary malignant lymphomas of the central nervous system. Cancer 1974; 1293-1302,
239. Batchelor T, Carson K, O'Neill A, et al. Treatment of primary CNS lymphoma with methotrexate and deferred radiotherapy: a report of NABTT 96-07. J Clin Oncol. 2003;21:1044-1049.
270. Sajja R, Barnett GH3 Lee SY, et al. Intensity-modulated radiation therapy (JJVIRT) for newly diagnosed and recurrent intracranial meningiomas: preliminary results. Technol Cancer Res Treat , 2005;4:675-82.
278. Mason WP, Gentili F, Macdonald DR, et al. Stabilization of disease progression by hydroxyurea in patients with recurrent or unresectable meningioma. J Neurosurg 2002;97:341-6.

71 Brain Metastases

Lisa M. DeAngelis, MD

Metastasis is the most common tumor affecting the brain. Autopsy studies find intracranial metastases in approximately 25% and brain metastases in 15% of patients who die of cancer.[1] Between two-thirds and three-quarters of such patients had symptoms from the intracranial metastasis during life which approximates the 9.6% incidence of brain metastasis reported in a recent population-based study.[2,3] Thus, approximately 70,000 patients have symptomatic intracranial metastases annually, a number that far exceeds the 17,000 patients with malignant primary brain tumors. Most brain metastases present late during the course of what is usually a widely metastatic cancer. In a smaller percentage of patients (perhaps about 10% of patients with lung cancer), a brain metastasis may be the first evidence that the patient suffers from cancer; alternatively, a patient with cancer believed to be localized may have an asymptomatic brain metastasis found on a screening computed tomography (CT) or magnetic resonance imaging (MRI).[4] In recent years, with more effective systemic therapy, brain metastases are emerging as the only site of relapse in many patients with otherwise controlled cancer.[5-8] Because of the increasing incidence of brain metastasis as the sole site of relapse, prophylactic cranial radiation is often administered to those patients with small cell lung cancer who achieve a complete remission from initial chemotherapy and radiotherapy.[9,10] Recent data suggest there may be a subset of patients with nonsmall cell lung cancer who also benefit from prophylactic cranial irradiation.[10]

In adults, the most common sources of brain metastases are lung and breast carcinoma and melanoma (Table 71-1). However, any malignant neoplasm can metastasize to the brain and it is likely that one will see an increasing number of metastases from what are believed to be uncommon sites, for example, ovary,[6] endometrium,[7] or multiple myeloma.[11] In as many as 10% of patients with brain metastases, no primary tumor is found on initial search although immunocytochemical analysis of the brain metastasis may help identify the primary site.[12] On rare occasions, the primary tumor is not identifiable even at autopsy.

Brain metastases are only one of many neurologic complications of cancer. We discuss the others, both metastatic and nonmetastatic, in Chapter 123.

Pathophysiology of the Metastatic Process

To reach the brain, a systemic cancer must develop its own blood supply, invade local tissues, and enter the circulation either by invading venules or lymph channels that eventually reach the venous circulation (Fig. 71-1).[1,13] Because systemic tumors enter the venous circulation and, ultimately, the right side of the heart, the first capillary bed they encounter is in the lung. Accordingly, the majority of patients with brain metastases have either primary lung tumors or lung metastases at the time the brain lesions become symptomatic. To reach the arterial circulation, the tumor must either (1) grow in the lung and seed the pulmonary venous circulation[14]; (2) traverse the lung capillary bed to enter the left side of the heart; or (3) cross a patent foramen ovale to enter the left heart directly. Some have proposed that tumor reaches the brain via the vertebral venous system (Batson's plexus) to explain the absence of lung metastases.[15]

Two factors promote intracranial metastases: (1) In the resting state, the brain receives 15-20% of the body's blood flow, thus making it likely that circulating tumor cells will reach the brain. (2) Certain tumor cells find the brain a propitious place for arrest and growth. This is one of the reasons that the probability of brain metastasis varies among tumor types and that the site of a brain metastasis may vary depending on the histology of the primary tumor. For example, certain primary tumors such as those from the kidney and colon are more likely to metastasize to the cerebellum than are lung cancers or those arising elsewhere in the body.[16] Once in the intracranial cavity, the tumor must arrest within the capillary bed, cross the endothelium and vessel wall, grow within the organ, vascularize itself through the process of angiogenesis, and then grow large enough to cause symptoms. At each step in the metastatic process, the tumor cells may fail, so that probably only a minute fraction of cells that reach the circulation ever become metastases.[17]

Tumors may metastasize to virtually any portion of the intracranial cavity, but the overall distribution of brain metastasis is also determined by the size of the region and its vasculature. Thus, about 85% of brain metastases are found in the cerebral hemispheres, usually in the posterior portion of the hemispheres at the watershed between the middle and posterior cerebral arteries. There is also an over-representation in the anterior border zone between the anterior and middle cerebral arteries. Approximately 10-15% of metastases are found in the cerebellum, a number somewhat larger than might be expected on the basis of blood supply, and probably represents the predilection for some pelvic tumors to metastasize to the cerebellum. Only approximately 3% of metastases are found in the brainstem.

Table 71-1 **Source of Brain Metastases in 729 Patients With Cancer Lesions**

Primary Tumor	Total (%)	Single	Multiple
Lung cancer	288 (39)	137	151
Nonsmall cell	178	89	89
Small cell	110	48	62
Breast	121 (17)	59	62
Melanoma	80 (11)	39	41
Genitourinary	81 (11)	49	32
Renal cell	45	25	20
Bladder	14	9	5
Prostate	11	9	2
Testicular	11	6	5
Gynecologic	52 (7)	28	24
Uterine/vulvar	38	20	18
Ovarian	14	8	6
Gastrointestinal	45 (6)	30	15
Unknown	33 (5)	23	10
Miscellaneous	29 (4)	19	10
Total	729	384	345

Source: Adapted from Ref. 56.

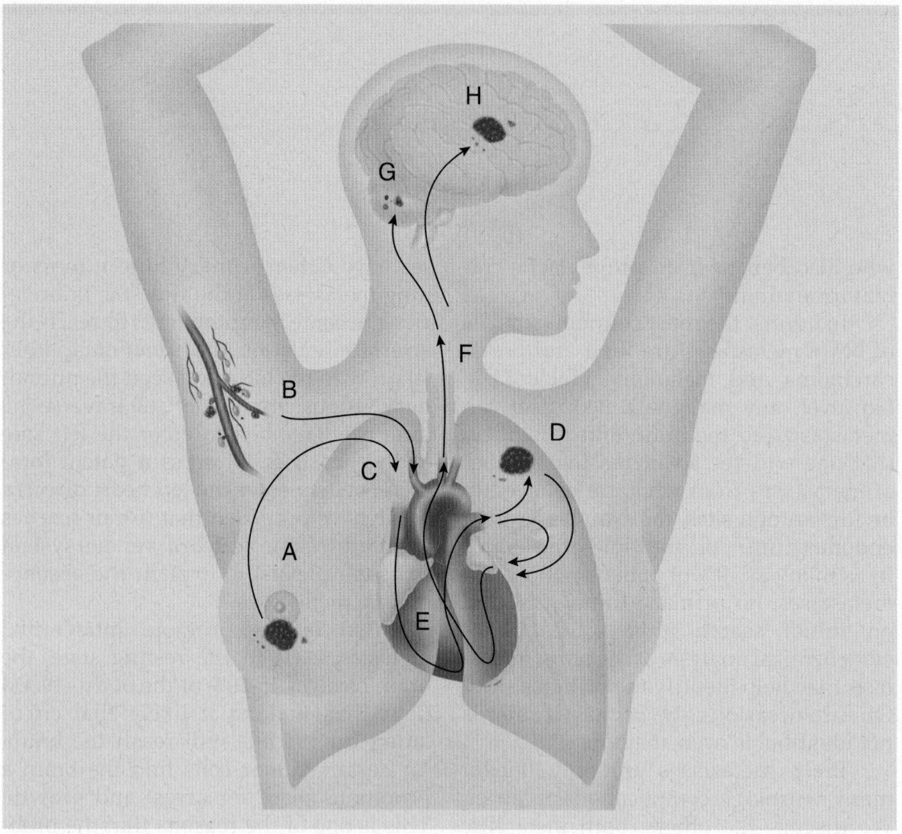

Figure 71-1 Pathophysiology of the metastatic process. Metastasis is a multistep process. In this illustration: **(A)** malignant neoplasm arises in an organ distant from the central nervous system and, as it grows, it develops its own vascular supply. **(B)** Clone(s) of malignant cells with metastatic potential enter blood or lymph channels and eventually reach the venous circulation. **(C)** The malignant cells enter the right heart with the venous circulation and either exit through the pulmonary artery to the lung **(D)**, or cross a patent foramen ovale **(D)**, to enter the systemic circulation. Most tumors that enter the lung either arrest in the pulmonary capillary bed, grow as pulmonary metastases and subsequently seed the pulmonary venous circulation, or, alternately, **(E)**, transverse the pulmonary vascular bed without arresting **(E)**, to enter the pulmonary venous circulation. Malignant clones in the pulmonary venous circulation then enter the left heart and exit into the systemic circulation **(F)**, along with those cells that may have crossed a patent foramen ovale **(F)**. Once in the systemic circulation, the likelihood of entering the cerebral circulation is high because, in the resting state, 15-20% of cardiac output supplies the central nervous system. Tumor cells entering the cerebral circulation must then arrest in brain capillaries or venules, cross the vessel wall, and grow within the brain **(G, H)**. *Source*: From Ref. 1.

In patients whose systemic tumor is otherwise controlled, the brain is often a site for isolated metastatic disease. Neither blood flow nor the nature of the central nervous system (CNS) microenvironment fully explains this phenomenon, but the blood–brain barrier may. In the first half of the twentieth century, when no treatment was available for acute leukemia, CNS involvement was rare because patients died from uncontrolled systemic leukemia. As chemotherapeutic agents became effective in controlling systemic disease, the incidence of CNS involvement began to rise to the point where it reached almost 50% in patients with acute lymphoblastic leukemia. The chemotherapeutic agents used to treat leukemia were largely water-soluble and did not cross the blood–brain barrier. The few leukemic cells that reached the CNS were protected from these drugs by the blood–brain barrier, and they could proliferate until they produced neurologic symptoms. "Prophylactic" treatment of the CNS by radiation therapy and/or intrathecal drugs decreased the incidence of CNS metastases from leukemia to under 10%.[18] However, once tumor is established in the brain, the blood–brain barrier is disrupted and the CNS becomes accessible to treatment with agents that do not normally cross it. Furthermore, some water-soluble systemic agents can penetrate an intact blood–brain barrier when given in high doses (eg, high-dose methotrexate).

The CNS as a sanctuary site of microscopic disease may apply to breast, small-cell lung, and perhaps other cancers.[8,19] When a chemosensitive tumor has relapsed in the CNS, it does not necessarily mean that the CNS disease is resistant to the chemotherapeutic agents that controlled the systemic tumor. The blood–brain barrier may have prevented those tumor cells from ever seeing a significant concentration of the drug, thus preserving the tumor cells' intrinsic chemosensitivity to that agent.[20]

Clinical Features

The symptoms and signs of brain metastases are related to the involved brain area (Table 71-2). Focal symptoms include weakness (hemiparesis), gait disturbances, visual field defects, and aphasia. Generalized symptoms usually relate to increased intracranial pressure and include headache, cognitive or behavioral abnormalities, nausea, and vomiting. Often, edema surrounding a brain metastasis increases brain volume, and thus intracranial pressure, much more than the tumor itself. Because brain edema responds to corticosteroids, the initial treatment of brain metastases with steroids (see below) often relieves both generalized and focal symptoms and signs. The tumor itself usually causes symptoms by compressing surrounding brain rather than destroying it. As a result, removing the tumor often returns the patient's neurologic state to normal.

Symptoms usually evolve over a few weeks; sometimes the symptoms begin acutely, corresponding to a hemorrhage into the metastasis or a seizure with a prolonged postictal state. Any intracranial metastatic tumor can hemorrhage, but certain primary tumors, such as melanoma, thyroid, renal, and choriocarcinoma, have a propensity to bleed. However, the most common source of a hemorrhagic brain metastasis is lung cancer because of its high frequency of CNS metastases. When multiple metastases are present, it is common to see simultaneous hemorrhage into many of the lesions; the mechanism for this is unclear. On occasion, focal seizures can cause neurologic signs that do not resolve. The tumor probably causes ischemia in the surrounding brain by stealing its blood supply, thus causing the seizure.

Table 71-2 **Signs and Symptoms of Brain Metastases at Presentation**

	% of Patients
Headache	24
Hemiparesis	20
Cognitive and behavioral disturbances	14
Seizures (focal or generalized)	12
Ataxia	7
Other	16
No symptoms	7

The only necessary diagnostic test is an MRI. Although the scan cannot unequivocally differentiate metastases from other lesions, certain abnormalities suggest metastases. Metastases are usually spherical and have more regular margins than primary tumors. They are usually found at gray–white matter junctions in watershed areas of the brain.[16,21] When small, they uniformly contrast enhance, and when larger, they may ring enhance. The tumor is usually surrounded by substantial edema. Very small metastases may appear as small dots of contrast enhancement with or without hyperintensity on the T2-weighted image; they usually lack surrounding edema. Fifty percent of patients have a single identifiable brain metastasis, 20% have two metastases, and 13% have three metastases. The remainder has more than three.[16]

A characteristic MRI in a patient with known cancer usually establishes the diagnosis. However, the diagnosis can be incorrect in approximately 10% of patients, and other diagnostic considerations include abscesses, primary brain tumors, demyelinating lesions, or inflammation.[22] If there is sufficient uncertainty about the diagnosis, biopsy may be necessary.

Treatment

The therapeutic approach to patients with brain metastases depends on the number and location of metastases, on the biology of the primary tumor, and on the extent of systemic disease. Treatment is divided into supportive and definitive measures (Table 71-3).

Table 71-3 ■ Treatment of Brain Metastases

Supportive
Corticosteroids (usual dose 8-16 mg dexamethasone daily)
Anticonvulsants (not for prophylaxis)
Antibiotics (prophylaxis for pneumocystis)
Anticoagulants (deep vein thrombosis)
Definitive
Surgery (1-3 metastases)
Whole-brain radiation therapy (multiple lesions, postoperative)
Stereotactic radiosurgery
Gamma knife
Linear accelerator
Single dose
Fractionated
Chemotherapy (chemosensitive primary)

Supportive Care

Corticosteroids ■ Supportive care may include corticosteroids, anticonvulsants, psychotropic drugs, antibiotics, and anticoagulants.[1] Corticosteroids are necessary only for symptomatic metastases, where they usually produce a dramatic response, and during the course of definitive treatment with surgery or radiation therapy (RT). Corticosteroids are not required for asymptomatic patients with small metastases unless RT or surgery is imminent. Because of their frequent side effects, the dose of corticosteroids should be tapered to the lowest level that controls neurologic symptoms. In patients expected to be on corticosteroids for more than 6 weeks, prophylactic antibiotics to prevent *Pneumocystis carinii infection* are indicated.

Anticonvulsants ■ Anticonvulsants have no prophylactic benefit and are used only if the patient has had a seizure.[23,24] Patients who require anticonvulsants should be placed on agents that do not enhance the hepatic microsomal system. Drugs such as phenytoin, phenobarbital, and carbamazepine increase p450 activity, which can reduce the serum level of many chemotherapeutic agents, thus compromising treatment of the underlying malignancy. Some of the newer anticonvulsants, such as topiramate, levetiracetam, or gabapentin are better choices.

Anticoagulants ■ Thromboembolic disease requiring treatment with anticoagulants is common in patients with cancer. Brain metastases are not a contraindication to the use of anticoagulants provided there is no intracranial hemorrhage. Anticoagulants are more effective than inferior vena cava filters in these patients and are safe provided that the anticoagulant is maintained in the therapeutic range.[25]

Definitive Treatment

Surgery ■ Two controlled trials clearly indicate that for patients with a single brain metastasis, surgical removal is superior to whole-brain radiation therapy, both in preventing brain relapse and in improving quality of life.[22,26] A third trial found no benefit, but many of the patients randomized to radiotherapy alone underwent resection at relapse.[27] In patients whose systemic disease is quiescent or controllable, surgical removal of a single brain metastasis substantially improves survival. Technological improvements in surgery, including functional magnetic resonance imaging (fMRI) preoperatively to locate eloquent areas of the brain, stereotactic surgical resection, intraoperative ultrasonography, intraoperative MRI, and cortical mapping, have helped assure complete resection with lower surgical morbidity and virtually no mortality.[28] Two-year survivals are 15-20%, depending on the primary tumor; 5-year survival rates are approximately 10%, and occasional "cures" are reported. Retrospective analysis supports the resection of two or even three metastases, with the outcome comparable to a surgically treated single brain metastasis.

A randomized controlled trial indicates that patients with a single resected metastasis who receive postoperative RT have fewer recurrences of cancer in the brain and are less likely to die of neurologic causes than are similar patients treated with surgery alone.[29] However, overall survival was comparable between the two groups because patients with controlled cerebral disease died of progressive systemic tumor. These data suggest that an appropriate patient with a single, surgically accessible brain metastasis should have that metastasis removed and receive postoperative whole-brain radiation therapy (WBRT). However, because of the toxicity of WBRT, particularly in the over 60 age group, many physicians do not use it in the immediate postoperative period, but reserve radiation until relapse, even though RT may be less effective once a tumor has recurred.

Radiation Therapy ■ The time-honored treatment of brain metastases has been WBRT, delivering 3000 cGy in 10 fractions. For patients with extensive systemic disease or multiple brain metastases, this remains the best option. Most patients have at least a transient response to radiation (Fig. 71-2); they symptomatically improve with steroids and RT, and are less likely to die of their neurologic disease than are patients who do not receive this treatment. However, survival is short, with a median of 4-6 months, because most patients die of uncontrolled systemic tumor. Even those patients who respond to RT and whose tumors are controlled are at risk for reseeding the brain from systemic tumor. In occasional patients, RT actually sterilizes the brain metastases and they do not recur. Because of late-delayed radiation toxicity in those patients whose systemic prognosis is more than a year, we recommend a dose of 4000-5000 cGy given in 180-200 cGy fractions. The lower dose per fraction is believed to diminish radiation toxicity but cognitive dysfunction may occur even with small fractions, especially if the patient has received chemotherapy.[30] Cognitive deficits from RT are more severe in children under 3 years of age and in adults over 60 years of age, and in those who receive extensive chemotherapy. Nevertheless, even young adults often complain of memory loss after WBRT.

Radiosurgery ■ Radiosurgery is increasingly employed instead of surgery for the treatment of single or even multiple brain metastases that are <3-4 cm in diameter.[1,31-33] Radiosurgery can be delivered either using the gamma knife or a linear accelerator, and can be given either as a single dose or can be fractionated. The treatment appears to be most effective against those tumors that are

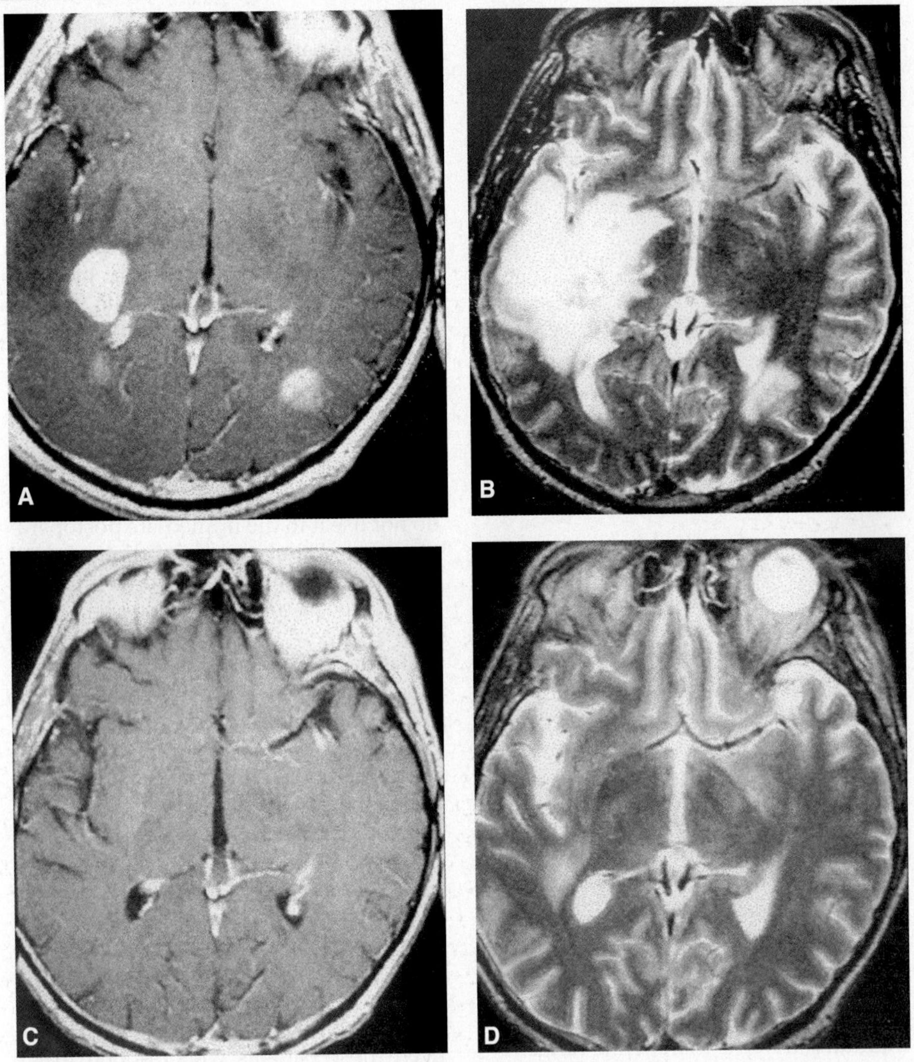

Figure 71-2 ■ Metastatic small cell lung cancer before and after radiation therapy. **(A)** The T1-weighted image before radiation shows two of the multiple contrast enhancing metastases; the larger is surrounded by hypointense brain edema. **(B)** The T2-weighted image before radiation shows hyperintense edema surrounding the relatively hypointense tumor. **(C and D)** MRI scans after radiation show an excellent response to radiation therapy.

relatively resistant to conventional external beam RT, such as melanoma[34] and renal cell carcinoma.[35] The reason is unclear, but the higher dose per fraction may eliminate otherwise resistant tumor cells. Most report approximately 80% tumor control with <10% complications. Tumor control is defined as disappearance, decrease in size, or no increase in size of the treated lesion. Postradiosurgery MRI may show a transient increase in tumor size because of radiation injury or tumor necrosis.[36] This can resolve over a few months and, therefore, an increase in lesion size a few weeks to months after stereotactic radiosurgery does not necessarily indicate tumor progression. Local control may be maintained over two years in 60% of patients, but with increasing survival, symptomatic recurrence becomes increasingly likely.[37] Radiosurgery has advantages over surgery in that it is relatively noninvasive, rarely requires hospitalization, and can often reach areas that are surgically inaccessible.[38] Radiosurgery has the disadvantage that it is not useful for tumors larger than 3-4 cm.

A recent randomized, prospective trial comparing WBRT and WBRT followed by a stereotactic radiosurgery boost in 331 patients with one to three newly diagnosed brain metastases, showed no survival advantage with the addition of radiosurgery.[39] Those with a single brain metastasis had longer survival when radiosurgery was added to WBRT (median 6.5 vs 4.9 months, $p = .0393$), but survival was not improved for those with multiple metastases. There was no significant difference between treatment groups in time to tumor progression or neurologic death rates.

A separate randomized controlled trial examined stereotactic radiosurgery with and without WBRT in patients with 1-4 brain metastases. Similar to the findings in the postoperative WBRT study, WBRT significantly reduced brain recurrence but had no effect on survival.[40] Furthermore, these authors demonstrated that improved cognitive function was associated with CNS disease control although WBRT may contribute to impaired neurocognitive function in some long-term survivors.[41]

There have been no randomized, prospective studies comparing neurosurgery and radiosurgery as treatment of solitary brain metastasis, and retrospective studies have shown conflicting results. One case-controlled, retrospective trial of the two modalities found that patients lived longer and did better with surgical resection.[42] This was partially attributed to the propensity for radiosurgery to cause brain necrosis that in itself is symptomatic and may require surgery for removal. A more recent retrospective study comparing surgical resection and stereotactic radiosurgery in patients with tumor size less than 35 mm and similar use of postprocedure WBRT (82% vs 96%, respectively) yielded similar survival rates during the first year after the procedure, but the neurosurgical patients survived longer during the second year; however, the difference in overall survival was not statistically significant ($p = .15$).[43] Recurrence rates were similar between the neurosurgical and radiosurgery groups (30% vs 29%), but there were significantly more local recurrences in the neurosurgical group compared with the radiosurgical group ($p = .02$). At this time, we use surgery to resect single lesions from accessible locations if they are >3-4 cm, associated with significant vasogenic edema or hemorrhage, or causing obstruction of CSF flow. Radiosurgery is an excellent option for smaller lesions or those in a surgically inaccessible location; we rarely treat more than three lesions in a patient, and usually do not administer WBRT concurrently.

Chemotherapy ■ Chemotherapy is increasingly being recognized as efficacious for brain metastases from chemosensitive systemic cancers. These include germ cell tumors, breast cancer, small-cell lung cancer, and some others.[44-46] Chemotherapy is often reserved for patients whose brain metastases have recurred after surgery or WBRT, but chemotherapy may also be considered in asymptomatic patients with brain metastases discovered on a screening MRI who are scheduled to receive chemotherapy for their systemic disease. This implies a primary cancer that is relatively sensitive to chemotherapeutic agents.

There are several reasons for administering chemotherapy before radiation: (1) It is useful to judge tumor response to chemotherapy before initiating radiation therapy. If the tumor is responsive, the chemotherapy can be continued even after radiation is given. (2) Radiation therapy decreases the blood supply to the tumor and thus may decrease the amount of chemotherapeutic agent that reaches the metastases. (3) Some evidence suggests that chemotherapy delivered before radiation is less neurotoxic than the converse because RT may open the blood–brain barrier and allow entry of potentially toxic agents that are given post-RT. The evidence is best for methotrexate but may apply to other drugs as well. Despite blood–brain barrier disruption, overall blood flow to the tumor is reduced so that drug delivery to the metastases is not necessarily enhanced by radiotherapy.

In addition to standard chemotherapeutic agents, small molecule inhibitors may be effective against brain metastases. This has been best described using erlotinib in non small-cell lung cancer and sunitinib for renal cancer.[47-49] Initial reports of lapatinib's efficacy against brain metastases from breast cancer failed to meet the expected response rate in a recent phase II trial.[50] Furthermore, some risk of intracerebral hemorrhage may be seen using these agents in patients with brain metastases.[51]

Prognosis ■ Untreated symptomatic brain metastases usually cause death within 1 or 2 months.[1] Patients treated with corticosteroids survive a little longer with a median of 1.3 months. Patients treated with whole-brain radiotherapy have a median survival of 4-6 months, and those treated by surgery followed by whole-brain radiation have a median survival of about 9 months. Patients with controlled systemic disease treated by surgery and radiation have a 10-15% 5-year survival and an occasional apparent cure. Prolonged survival can also be seen after radiosurgery.[52]

Prognostic factors include mental status, response to steroids, activity of the systemic tumor, and treatment modality. In one series, site of the primary tumor, age, and the number of brain metastases were prognostic factors, although with lesser importance than those indicated above. In patients with lung primaries, male sex was a significant factor. In patients with breast primaries, the interval between the primary tumor and the development of brain metastases was also significant, with a longer interval correlating with better survival. The RTOG performed a recursive partitioning analysis of prognostic factors in 1200 patients with brain metastases treated with WBRT on three RTOG trials.[53] They segregated patients into three classes based only on KPS, age, and the presence of extracranial metastases. Class 1 patients had a KPS ≥ 70, and were <65 years of age with a controlled primary and no extracranial metastasis; median survival was 7.1 months. Class 3 patients had a KPS < 70 and a median survival of 2.3 months. Class 2 included all other patients and had a median survival of 4.2 months. This classification scheme may apply to patients treated with surgery and radiosurgery.[54,55]

Approach ■ All patients with cancer and neurologic symptoms should undergo contrast-enhanced MRI. Asymptomatic patients at high risk for development of brain metastases (eg, lung cancer, melanoma) should be considered for screening of the brain for occult cerebral metastases. Screening is particularly important if the patient is to undergo a major surgical procedure for treatment of the primary tumor. If a single or, in some cases, two or three surgically accessible lesions are found in a patient with a good performance status and a reasonable systemic prognosis (at least 6-12 months), the lesion(s) should be removed surgically or radiosurgery considered if the lesions are sufficiently small. The decision concerning radiation after removal of a single metastasis should be made on an individual basis, depending on the surgeon's view of the success of tumor removal, the patient's general state, and the patient's age. Patients with one to three surgically inaccessible lesions smaller than 4 cm, particularly from radioresistant tumors such as melanoma and renal cell carcinoma, should be considered for radiosurgery. Symptomatic patients with multiple metastases or whose systemic prognosis is poor can be treated with palliative whole-brain radiation therapy. Patients with systemic disease about to undergo systemic chemotherapy, whose brain lesions are small and either asymptomatic or only mildly symptomatic, should be evaluated for their response to chemotherapy prior to radiation or surgery. If it is clinically possible, corticosteroids should be withheld unless they are part of the chemotherapy regimen. Patients who fail surgery and radiation should also be considered for chemotherapy.

Selected References

The complete reference list can be found at www.CANCERMEDICINE8.com

1. DeAngelis LM, Posner JB. *Neurologic complications of cancer*, 2nd ed. New York: Oxford University Press; 2008.
17. Nguyen DX, Massague J. Genetic determinants of cancer metastasis. *Nat Rev Genet.* 2007;8:341–352.
22. Patchell RA, Tibbs PA, Walsh JW. A randomized trial of surgery in the treatment of single metastases to the brain. *N Engl J Med.* 1990;322:494–500.
23. Forsyth PA, Weaver S, Fulton D, et al. Prophylactic anticonvulsants in patients with brain tumour. *Can J Neurol Sci.* 2003;30:106–112.
25. Schiff D, DeAngelis LM. Therapy of venous thromboembolism in patients with brain metastases. *Cancer.* 1994;73:493–498.
26. Vecht CJ, Haaxma-Reiche H, Noordijk EM, et al. Treatment of single brain metastasis: radiotherapy alone or combined with neurosurgery? *Ann Neurol.* 1993;33:583–590.
29. Patchell RA, Tibbs PA, Regine WF, et al. Postoperative radiotherapy in the treatment of single metastases to the brain: a randomized trial. *JAMA.* 1998;280:1485–1489.
30. Fonseca R, O'Neill BP, Foote RL, et al. Cerebral toxicity in patients treated for small-cell carcinoma of the lung. *Mayo Clin Proc.* 1999;74:461–465.
32. Flannery TW, Suntharalingam M, Regine WF, et al. Long-term survival in patients with synchronous, solitary brain metastasis from non-small-cell lung cancer treated with radiosurgery. *Int J Radiat Oncol Biol Phys.* 2008;72:19-23.
33. Omuro AM, Abrey LE. Brain metastases. *Curr Neurol Neurosci Rep.* 2004;4:205–210.
39. Andrews DW, Scott CB, Sperduto PW, et al. Whole brain radiation therapy with or without stereotactic radiosurgery boost for patients with one to three brain metastases: phase III results of the RTOG 9508 randomised trial. *Lancet.* 2004;363:1665–1672.
40. Aoyama H, Shirato H, Tago M, et al. Stereotactic radiosurgery plus whole-brain radiation therapy vs stereotactic radiosurgery alone for treatment of brain metastases: a randomized controlled trial. *JAMA.* 2006;296:2483–2491.
41. Aoyama H, Tago M, Kato N, et al. Neurocognitive function of patients with brain metastasis who received either whole brain radiotherapy plus stereotactic radiosurgery or radiosurgery alone. *Int J Radiat Oncol Biol Phys.* 2007;68:1388–1395.
43. O'Neill BP, Iturria NJ, Link MJ, et al. A comparison of surgical resection and stereotactic radiosurgery in the treatment of solitary brain metastases. *Int J Radiat Oncol Biol Phys.* 2003;55:1169–1176.
45. Ekenel M, Hormigo AM, Peak S, et al. Capecitabine therapy of central nervous system metastases from breast cancer. *J Neurooncol.* 2007;85:223227.
47. van Pawel J, Wagner H, Duell T, et al. Erlotinib in patients with previously irradiated, recurrent brain metastases from non-small cell lung cancer: two case reports. *Onkologie.* 2008;31:123–126.
49. Koutras AK, Krikelis D, Alexandrou N, et al. Brain metastasis in renal cell cancer responding to sunitinib. *Anticancer Res.* 2007;27:4255–4257.
52. Sheehan JP, Sun MH, Kondziolka D, et al. Radiosurgery for non-small cell lung carcinoma metastatic to the brain: long-term outcomes and prognostic factors influencing patient survival time and local tumor control. *J Neurosurg.* 2002;97:1276–1281.
53. Gaspar L, Scott C, Rotman M, et al. Recursive partitioning analysis (RPA) of prognostic factors in three Radiation Therapy Oncology Group (RTOG) brain metastases trials. *Int J Radiat Oncol Biol Phys.* 1997;37:745–751.
54. Regine WF, Rogozinska A, Kryscio, et al. Recursive partitioning analysis classifications I and II: applicability evaluated in a randomized trial of resected single brain metastases. *Am J Clin Oncol.* 2004;27:505–509.

72 Neoplasms of the Eye

Amy C. Schefler, MD ■ David H. Abramson, MD ■ Ira J. Dunkel, MD ■ Beryl McCormick, MD

Introduction

This chapter reviews benign and malignant ocular, orbital, and lid tumors in both children and adults. The most common of these are listed in Table 72-1.

Pediatric Ophthalmic Oncology: Ocular Diseases

Benign Disease

Benign pediatric ocular lesions are very rare. Choroidal nevi, which are present in more than 10% of the adult population, are rare before puberty and are never seen in the infant. Conjunctival and iris nevi are also extremely rare in prepubertal children. Iris nevi detected in children often represent Lisch nodules, a manifestation of neurofibromatosis type 1.

Benign retinal tumors are also rare. When found they are usually astrocytic hamartomas and are frequently part of the tuberous sclerosis syndrome. When viewed with indirect ophthalmoscopy, astrocytic hamartomas usually have a thin, transparent membrane overlying the retina and typically obscure retinal blood vessels. They may enlarge and calcify with time. They may be confused with myclinated nerve fibers which are white, follow the distribution of the nerve fiber layer, and obscure retinal vessels.

Hamartomas of the retinal pigment epithelium are rare in children. They are frequently near the optic disc and are pigmented, with distortion of retinal vessels and a slightly opaque appearance. They have no malignant potential.

Primary Malignant Disease (Retinoblastoma)

Introduction to Retinoblastoma ■ The most common primary ocular malignancy of childhood is retinoblastoma.[1] Retinoblastoma arises from an unidentified retinal progenitor cell. Although retinoblastoma is relatively rare, it has been the subject of great interest because of its well-studied genetic inheritance pattern and molecular biology.[2]

Retinoblastoma has a cumulative lifetime incidence rate of one in 18,000-30,000 live births worldwide. Surveys suggest a relatively constant occurrence in this century.[3] The incidence in the United States is relatively low, at 3.58 cases for each million children under the age of 15 years, and decreases with advancing age. The overall median age at diagnosis in the United States is 18 months, with the median age of diagnosis of bilateral cases occurring at 12 months and of unilateral cases at 24 months.[4] In rare instances, retinoblastoma is detected prenatally via ultrasound or during adulthood.[5-7]

Survival rates for retinoblastoma patients in the developed world have increased dramatically over the past century. The mortality of retinoblastoma was reported as 83% in 1897 in children who were treated with enucleation, and as 43% in all children in 1916.[8] In contrast, recent cancer registry reports in Europe and the United States have demonstrated 5-year survival rates of 90% and 98%, respectively.[9,10] The improved survival rate is due to earlier detection of the tumor and improved techniques for local tumor control. In contrast to developed countries, however, developing nations report dramatically low survival rates, as patients in these countries typically present with widespread metastatic disease.

There are no differences in incidence by sex, race, or right versus left eye.[11] Some data suggest geographic clustering, but convincing evidence is lacking. Retinoblastoma does appear to occur more commonly in poor patients worldwide.

Molecular Biology of Retinoblastoma ■ The traditional view of retinoblastoma genetics, widely held until recently, was that the disease occurs in two forms, germinal and nongerminal. Both forms occur as a result of loss or mutation of both alleles of the retinoblastoma gene (*rbl*). In nongerminal cases, both *rbl* alleles are inactivated somatically in a single developing retinal progenitor cell, whereas in germinal cases, the first mutation occurs in the germline and only the second mutation is somatic. Nongerminal retinoblastoma is always unilateral and unifocal, although the tumor may break apart resulting in hundreds of tiny intraocular seeds. More recent study over the past decade has indicated that nearly all retinoblastoma patients probably demonstrate a degree of mosaicism for the *rbl* mutation.[12] Furthermore, recent evidence suggests that genomic instability, microsatellite instability, defects of the DNA mismatch repair system, and alterations in DNA methylation and acetylation/deacetylation may also be necessary for the malignant transformation of retinoblastoma after the loss of pRB.[13-15]

The proposed retinoblastoma gene was localized to chromosome 13ql4 through deletion studies and linkage analysis.[16-18] A candidate gene was isolated from this locus in 1986 by Friend et al.[19] Further characterization of the gene revealed that it spans 180 kb and is composed of 27 exons. The gene encodes a 4.8 kb mRNA transcript which is expressed in all adult tissues. The 110 kD nuclear phosphoprotein (pRB) consists of 928 amino acids.

The protein is a regulator at the cell cycle checkpoint between G1 and entry into the S-phase (Fig. 72-1). The phosphorylation pattern of pRB varies during the cell cycle and the current model suggests

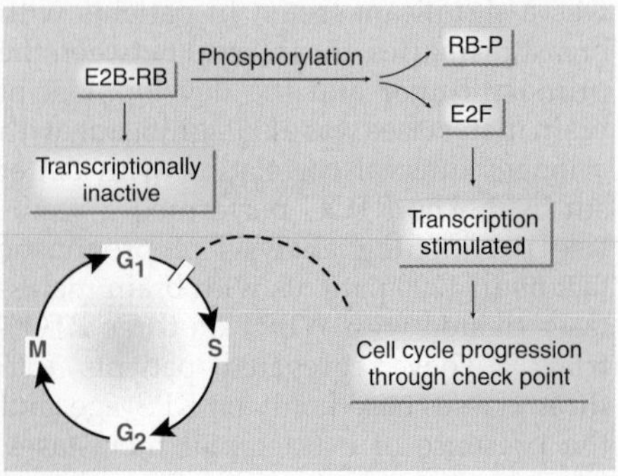

Figure 72-1 ■ Artistic rendition of molecular mechanism of retinoblastoma gene action.

Table 72-1 ■ **Most Common Ophthalmic Neoplasms, Benign and Malignant**

	Benign	Malignant	
		Primary	Secondary
Children			
Ocular	—	Retinoblastoma	Leukemia
Orbital	Capillary hemangioma	Rhabdomyosarcoma	Leukemia
Adult			
Ocular	Choroid nevus	Uveal melanoma	Metastasis (lung, breast)
Orbital	Cavernous hemangioma	Lymphoma	Sinus cancer
Lids	Chalazion	Basal cell carcinoma	Lymphoma

that the hypophosphorylated normal pRB binds transcriptional regulators that promote entry into the S-phase. This function of pRB is inactivated by phosphorylation or by viral oncoprotein binding of pRB. When phosphorylated, pRB dissociates from the transcription factor E2F, freeing E2F to bind to DNA and stimulate transcription of downstream genes that promote progression through the cell cycle. Loss of normal *rbl* function, as in the case of the tumors, allows for uncontrolled entry into the S-phase and more rapid cell division.[20]

Rbl was the first tumor suppressor gene to be identified. The tumor suppressive function of the *rbl* gene was confirmed in studies that demonstrated the loss of both alleles of the gene in tumor tissue specimens.[21] Later studies showed that a germinal *rbl* mutation was present in virtually all retinoblastoma kindreds and that inheritance of the mutant *rbl* allele predicted disease.[22,23] The tumor suppressive function of the gene has furthermore been demonstrated in transfection studies showing that the introduction of wild-type expression in pRB-defective cell lines partially reverses the malignant phenotype.[24]

Genetic Testing ■ Both population data gathered from families and our current understanding of the molecular mechanisms of inheritance of the disease have enabled us to predict the likelihood that new offspring in families affected by retinoblastoma will develop the disease (Table 72-2). Karyotypic studies, which analyze the morphology of entire chromosomes, are generally not useful for the clinical diagnosis of retinoblastoma because they can only identify deletions spanning 2-5 million base pairs and only 3-5% of retinoblastoma patients carry deletions this large.[25] Instead, more sophisticated indirect and direct techniques that detect smaller mutations are used.[26,27] At the present time, a single genetic test is unlikely to detect all germline RB gene mutations in patients with retinoblastoma because of the variety of types and locations of mutations that occur. However, adaptation of a routine clinical protocol including a series of complementary tests based on the observation that most mutations alter the protein size and disrupt the large pocket domain may be able to rapidly detect the majority of mutations.[25]

Presenting Signs and Symptoms of Retinoblastoma ■ The most common presenting signs and symptoms of retinoblastoma vary depending on the socioeconomic conditions in which the patient presents. In developing countries, children have often developed extraocular disease before they are diagnosed and frequently present with proptosis and an orbital mass (Fig. 72-2). These children are older at diagnosis (age 4-6 years) than patients in the United States and few survive. Many large retrospective studies over the past quarter-century have examined the most common presentations of retinoblastoma in large developed nations.[28-31] In the United States, the most common presenting sign (60% of cases) is leukocoria, a white pupillary reflex (Fig. 72-3). The reflex is caused either by the reflection of incoming light off the tumor or by the retinal detachment caused by the underlying tumor.

Presenting signs in the United States that occur less commonly include strabismus, (misalignment of the eyes), inflammatory signs (mimicking orbital cellulitis), anisocoria (different sized pupils), heterochromia (different colored irides), hyphema (blood in the anterior chamber), tumor hypopyon (tumor in the anterior chamber) and nystagmus. Two large retrospective studies on large populations of retinoblastoma patients have recently examined the patterns of detection of retinoblastoma in the United States. The vast majority of patients' disease was discovered by a family member (80%) rather than by a pediatrician (8%) or an ophthalmologist (10%).[29]

Diagnostic Testing ■ The differential diagnosis of retinoblastoma includes lesions that can simulate a solitary ocular tumor such as astrocytic hamartomas and toxocara canis and lesions that can cause a total

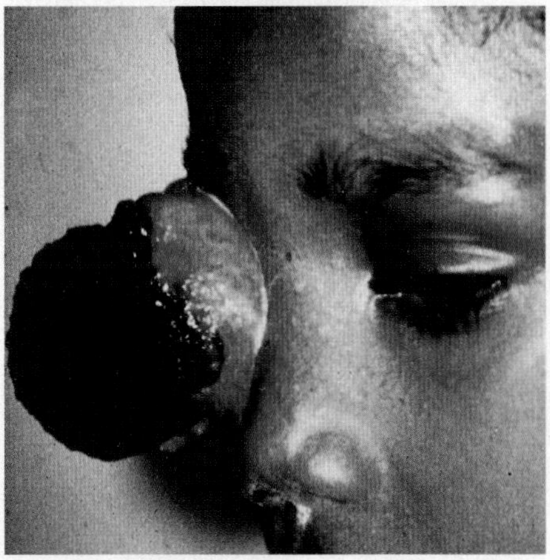

Figure 72-2 ■ Advanced orbital presentation of retinoblastoma. *Source:* Courtesy of A. Wachtel, M.D., Lima, Peru.

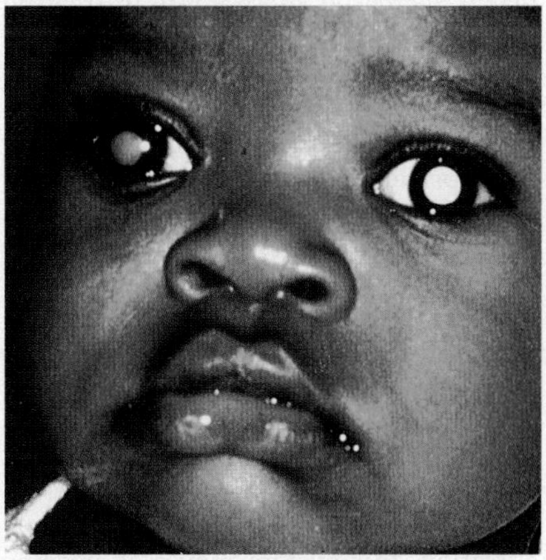

Figure 72-3 ■ Leukocoria (white pupillary reflex) caused by retinoblastoma. The tumor can be seen in the vitreous. There are seeds in the anterior chamber, anterior to the iris.

Table 72-2 ■ **Genetic Counseling for Retinoblastoma**

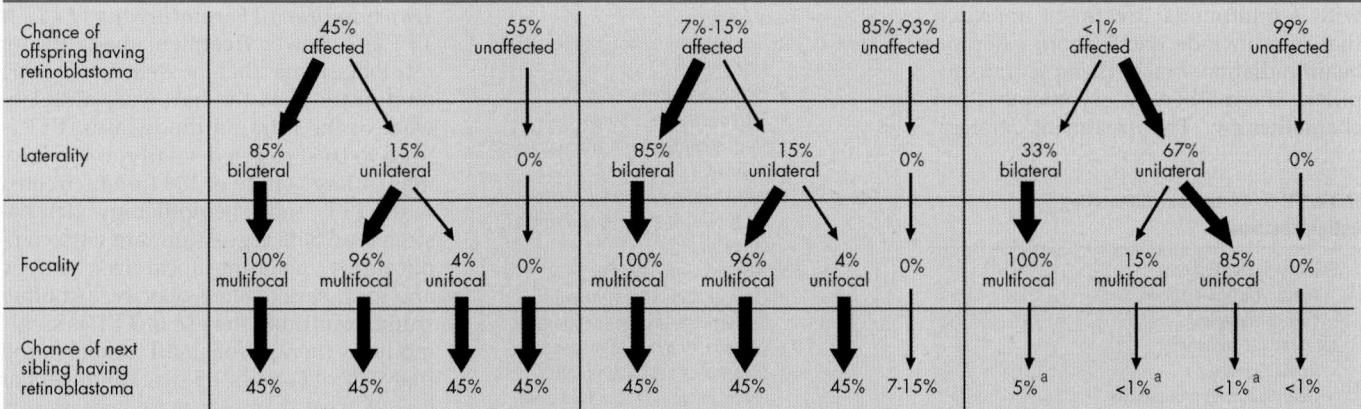

Chance of offspring having retinoblastoma	45% affected			55% unaffected	7%-15% affected			85%-93% unaffected	<1% affected			99% unaffected
Laterality	85% bilateral	15% unilateral		0%	85% bilateral	15% unilateral		0%	33% bilateral	67% unilateral		0%
Focality	100% multifocal	96% multifocal	4% unifocal	0%	100% multifocal	96% multifocal	4% unifocal	0%	100% multifocal	15% multifocal	85% unifocal	0%
Chance of next sibling having retinoblastoma	45%	45%	45%	45%	45%	45%	45%	7-15%	5%[a]	<1%[a]	<1%[a]	<1%

[a]If parent is a carrier, then 45%.

retinal detachment such as Coats disease, retinopathy of prematurity, and persistent hyperplastic primary vitreous (persistent fetal vasculature syndrome) (Table 72-3). Patients suspected of having retinoblastoma should undergo indirect ophthalmoscopy and fundus photography as well as ophthalmic ultrasonography. Ultrasonography is useful as it demonstrates masses with high reflectivity that block sound, causing characteristic shadowing behind the tumor. Needle biopsies are rarely performed for suspected retinoblastoma, as puncturing the eye can lead to tumor seeding with orbital invasion and even death from metastatic disease.

Staging of Intraocular Retinoblastoma ■ The Reese–Ellsworth classification scheme is the most commonly used classification system for describing intraocular tumors (Table 72-4A).[32] It is not a true staging scheme, for untreated patients do not progress from Group I to higher groups but it has served as an excellent ocular reference for comparison of different series and treatment schemes. A higher numeric classification signified that a tumor was more anterior and that there was a decreased success rate in treating the lesion with lateral port external-beam radiation. In recent years, its usefulness has been questioned by many ophthalmic oncologists who feel it is no longer appropriate given the current trend away from the use of external-beam radiation. A new classification system was recently developed and has been used clinically by several centers in a collaborative study (Table 72-4B).[33] It has also been shown to correlate with the response to treatment with the most common current approach to the treatment of intraocular disease, chemotherapy combined with focal therapy.[34] As with the Reese–Ellsworth classification, this system may also become antiquated as treatment trends inevitably change in the future.

Treatment of Intraocular Retinoblastoma ■ Survival rates in excess of 95% are currently achieved for most patients treated at major centers in developed countries with a multimodal treatment approach that may include enucleation, external-beam radiation, brachytherapy, transpupillary thermotherapy, cryotherapy, and chemotherapy. The treatment strategy for each patient depends on several factors: involvement of one or both eyes, heredity of the disease, age of the patient, tumor volume and localization, stage of disease (including Reese–Ellsworth classification), and presence of extraocular disease.[35]

Table 72-3 ■ **Lesions Simulating Retinoblastoma**

Solitary ocular tumor
Astrocytic hamartoma
Toxocara canis
Total retinal detachment
Coats disease
Retinopathy of prematurity
Persistent fetal vasculature (PFV)

Enucleation ■ Enucleation is surgical removal of the eye without resecting the lids or extraocular muscles. Patients considered for enucleation include those with advanced retinoblastoma in one or both eyes, active tumor in a blind eye, and painful glaucoma from tumor invasion. More than 99% of patients with unilateral retinoblastoma without microscopic or macroscopic extraocular disease are cured with this procedure.[36]

Table 72-4A ■ **Reese–Ellsworth Scheme for Intraocular Retinoblastoma**

Group I
a. Solitary tumor, less than 4 disc diameters in size, at or behind the equator
b. Multiple tumors, none over 4 disc diameters in size, all at or behind the equator
Group II
a. Solitary tumor, 4 to 10 disc diameters in size, at or behind the equator
b. Multiple tumors, 4 to 10 disc diameters in size, behind the equator
Group III
a. Any lesion anterior to the equator
b. Solitary tumors larger than 10 disc diameters behind the equator
Group IV
a. Multiple tumors, some larger than 10 disc diameters
b. Any lesion extending anteriorly to the ora serrata
Group V
a. Massive tumors involving over half the retina
b. Vitreous seeding

Table 72-4B ■ **New International Classification for Retinoblastoma**

Group A	Rb ≤ 3 mm in basal dimension or thickness
Group B	Rb > 3 mm or with one or more of the following: • Macular location (≤3 mm to foveola) • Juxtapapillary location (≤ 1.5 mm to optic nerve) • Additional subretinal fluid (≤3 mm from margin)
Group C	Retinoblastoma tumor with one of the following: • Subretinal seeds ≤ 3 mm • Vitreous seeds ≤ 3 mm • Both subretinal and vitreous seeds ≤ 3 mm
Group D	Retinoblastoma tumor with one of the following: • Subretinal seeds > 3 mm • Vitreous seeds > 3 mm • Both subretinal and vitreous seeds > 3 mm
Group E	Extensive retinoblastoma occupying > 50% of globe or any of the following: • Neovascular glaucoma • Opaque media from vitreous hemorrhage in anterior chamber, vitreous, or subretinal space • Invasion of postlaminar optic nerve, choroid (> 2 mm), sclera, orbit, or anterior chamber

External-Beam Radiation ■ External-beam radiation, once employed in many patients with intraocular retinoblastoma, has fallen out of favor in recent years due to its association with the development of second nonocular cancers in germinal retinoblastoma patients. Several studies have indicated that radiation given after patients reach one year of age does not increase the risk of second cancers, and thus some clinical centers believe that this treatment modality may be used with impunity after this milestone.[37,38] When radiation is given, it is often used as salvage therapy after focal therapies have failed. In cases of bilateral advanced intraocular disease, external-beam radiation can be used bilaterally. In these cases, one or both eyes may eventually require salvage enucleation.

Survival of children who undergo external-beam radiation in the United States is 85-100%, mirroring the excellent survival rates of children with this disease in general.[39-41] Overall local control in the radiated eye, defined as preservation of the eye (avoidance of enucleation), varies in different series from 58% to 95%. Rates of eye preservation are as high as 95% for Reese–Ellsworth Group I-III eyes, and an 83% 3-year eye preservation rate was observed in the most recent large series of Group IV and V eyes treated with a standard lateral beam approach.[42] A recent study of Reese–Ellsworth Group Vb eyes alone demonstrated a 81% 1-year ocular survival rate and a 53% 10-year ocular survival.[43] Location of the tumor determines the likelihood that it will respond to external-beam radiation; tumors in the posterior pole tend to have the best results with this treatment.

Transpupillary Thermotherapy (TTT) ■ TTT is a newer treatment modality for retinoblastoma that is delivered using modifications to the hardware and software of the infrared diode laser. TTT is used to treat selected small retinoblastomas. A large study of 108 tumors treated with TTT and chemotherapy demonstrated an 86% regression rate with complications including focal iris atrophy and focal paraxial lens opacity.[44] Another study examining the use of TTT as single modality therapy for small tumors found that 92% of tumors 1.5 disc diameters or less in base diameter were successfully cured with TTT alone.[45]

Cryotherapy ■ Cryotherapy is used as a primary treatment for small peripheral retinoblastomas or as secondary treatment for recurrent tumors treated previously with external-beam radiation. Rapid freezing (-90°C per minute) results in intracellular ice crystal formation, protein denaturation, pH changes, and finally cell membrane rupture. All studies examining the use of cryotherapy alone have demonstrated 90-100% cure rates in tumors that are less than 3 mm in diameter and less than 1 mm in thickness with minimal complications.[46-48]

Brachytherapy ■ Episcleral brachytherapy was pioneered in 1933 by the British ophthalmologist Henry Stallard.[49] Over the last few years, radioactive plaques have been used more commonly as primary therapy in the effort to avoid external-beam radiation therapy. Relative indications for radioactive plaques include tumors that are classified as Reese–Ellsworth Stage IVa or less and tumors that are between 4 and 10 disc diameters in size. Brachytherapy can also be used as a salvage technique in eyes that have failed other types of therapy including external-beam radiation, photocoagulation, or cryotherapy. ^{125}Iodine is currently the most commonly used isotope in brachytherapy for retinoblastoma. This isotope is advantageous because the radioactive seeds can be placed into a custom-built plaque designed to match the size of the lesion.

A tumor recurrence rate of 12% at one year post-treatment has been reported when plaques are used as primary treatment for retinoblastoma.[50] Radioactive plaques can also be successful when used as salvage therapy for eyes that have failed other treatment methods. Merchant et al. recently reported a 60% overall eye preservation rate (15/25 eyes) for salvage brachytherapy after primary chemotherapy or radiation therapy.[51] Shields et al. reported on 148 tumors treated with plaques after failure of other methods.[50] Tumor recurrence at one year was detected in 8% of tumors previously treated with chemotherapy and 25% of tumors previously treated with external-beam radiotherapy.

Systemic Chemotherapy ■ The indications for chemoreduction are not yet well-established. Most commonly this treatment is used for patients who have visual potential in eyes containing tumors which are too large to treat initially with focal methods. Chemoreduction is used to shrink these tumors so that focal treatments such as cryotherapy, thermotherapy, or radioactive plaques can be administered afterword.

Most studies of chemoreduction for retinoblastoma since 1996 have utilized vincristine, carboplatin, and an epipodophyllotoxin, either etoposide or teniposide.[52-70] The addition of cyclosporine as a P-glycoprotein inhibitor has also been suggested to decrease the ability of tumor cells to transport antineoplastic drugs from the intracellular space thereby allowing the cells to develop multi-drug resistance.[52,57] Choice of agents as well as number and frequency of cycles varies currently at different institutions.

The results of recent studies examining the efficacy of chemoreduction followed by focal therapies have been most promising for patients with Reese–Ellsworth Group 1-3 eyes. For these patients, many authors have demonstrated that enucleation can be successfully avoided almost 100% of the time. Results for patients with Reese–Ellsworth Groups 4 and 5 eyes have been more discouraging. In a meta-analysis of patients treated with chemoreduction, 37% of eyes avoided *both* external-beam radiation and enucleation. Forty-one percent of eyes required radiation but avoided enucleation, and 40% of eyes required enucleation (with or without prior radiation).[71]

Intra-arterial Chemotherapy ■ Clinicians in Japan were the first to postulate that another method of local drug delivery, intra-arterial infusions of chemotherapy, may increase penetration of the drug into small intraocular tumors and decrease systemic side effects.[72] In a study of 187 patients, melphalan infusions were performed using a catheter tip placed just distal to the orifice of the ophthalmic artery with temporary occlusion of the internal carotid artery during the infusion. Common side effects included bradycardia during injection, facial erythema, and mild eyelid edema. Local tumor control rates and eye preservation rates were not reported. Our group recently reported a novel technique in which the ophthalmic artery of ten patients with advanced retinoblastoma was selectively cannulated in order to perform a local injection of melphalan.[73] Twenty-seven cannulations were performed and dramatic regression of tumors, vitreous seeds, and subretinal seeds were seen in each case (Fig. 72-4A-C). No sepsis, anemia, neutropenia, fever, strokes, or death occurred. This technique may eventually replace enucleation as the primary approach for advanced intraocular disease if longer follow-up and larger patient cohorts demonstrate continued safety and success. We are currently investigating the use of other agents as well.

Treatment of Extraocular Retinoblastoma ■ In the most developed nations, extraocular disease occurs only in a small minority of patients. For more complete infor-

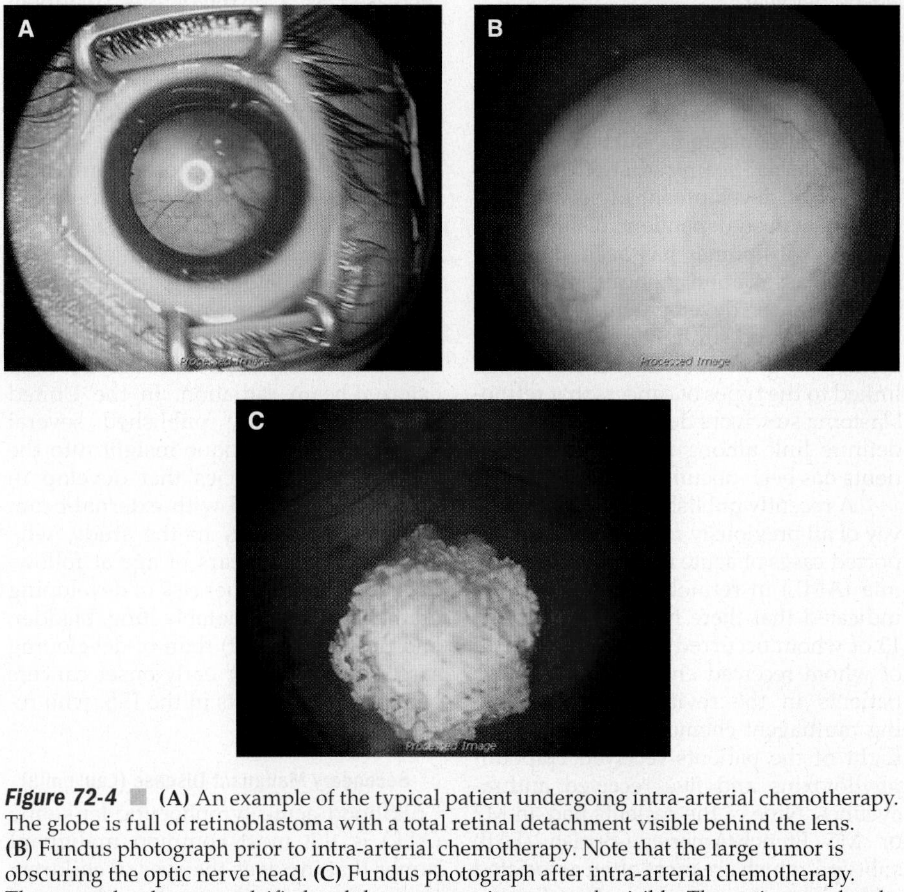

Figure 72-4 ■ **(A)** An example of the typical patient undergoing intra-arterial chemotherapy. The globe is full of retinoblastoma with a total retinal detachment visible behind the lens. **(B)** Fundus photograph prior to intra-arterial chemotherapy. Note that the large tumor is obscuring the optic nerve head. **(C)** Fundus photograph after intra-arterial chemotherapy. The tumor has become calcified and there are no vitreous seeds visible. The optic nerve head can now be visualized above the tumor. The retina is flat.

Table 72-5 ■ **Risk Factors for Second Nonocular Cancer Development in Retinoblastoma Survivors**

Factor	Strength of Association With Incidence of 2nd Cancers
Presence of germinal mutation in *rbl* gene	Definite causation (necessary risk factor)
Dose of external-beam radiation	Dose-dependent causation
External-beam radiation given at <1 year of age	Very likely association
Presence of lipomas	Definite association (noncausative)
Smoking	Definite association
Chemotherapy	Possible association
Sun exposure	Possible association
Growth hormone	Possible association

mation on the treatment of extraocular retinoblastoma, the reader is encouraged to consult more extensive sources.[74-90]

Second Malignancies ■ In 1949, it was first recognized that some retinoblastoma patients develop second nonocular neoplasms years after the successful treatment of the eye cancer.[91] Since then the incidence of additional nonocular cancers in survivors of retinoblastoma who carry the *rbl* mutation has been reviewed extensively.[37,38,92-98] Previous analyses have also shown that additional nonocular cancers are the leading cause of death in survivors of germinal retinoblastoma in the United States.[96] Of the survivors of germinal retinoblastoma, cumulative incidence reports of second malignancies vary, but most large studies with adequate long-term follow-up have reported yearly incidence rates of approximately 0.5-1% per year.[38,99]

Several clinical risk factors and treatment-related exposures have been shown to have an association with the development of second nonocular cancers in retinoblastoma survivors (Table 72-5). External-beam radiation increases the risk of development of second cancers in a dose-dependent fashion. The presence of lipomas has been shown to have an association (noncausative) with second cancer development.[92] Exposure to smoking and sunlight as well as treatment with growth hormone, have been linked to the types of cancers that retinoblastoma survivors develop, although no definite link among retinoblastoma patients has been documented.

A recently published worldwide survey of all previously reported and nonreported cases of acute myeloblastic leukemia (AML) in retinoblastoma survivors indicated that there have been 15 cases, 13 of whom occurred in children and 12 of whom received chemotherapy.[100] The patients in the review received varying multiagent chemotherapy regimens. Eight of the patients received epipodophyllotoxins and five received anthracyclines. Nine of the patients had an M2 or M5 French-American-British (FAB) subtype, which are most often associated with chemotherapy-induced malignancies. Ten of the patients died of AML. The overall incidence of secondary AML in this population appears low given the large cohort of retinoblastoma patients who have received etoposide worldwide over the last 10 years. The number of patients at risk is likely increasing since the continued upsurge in the use of chemotherapy for intraocular disease since the mid-1990s. The latency period of epipodophyllotoxin-induced malignancies in other patient populations is typically relatively short (6 years or less) and therefore a short follow-up interval does not explain the low incidence. Of note, the incidence of secondary AML in the oldest cohort of patients followed continuously in the United States (since 1914 in New York) who were historically treated with surgery and radiation is nearly zero. This observation suggests that although the current incidence of secondary AML in the chemotherapy era is low, it has increased as a result of this treatment approach. Only time and international collaboration will resolve this clinical question.

Second malignancies observed in retinoblastoma survivors in the U.S. include, in order from most common to least: osteogenic sarcomas of the skull and long bones, soft tissue sarcomas, pineoblastomas, cutaneous melanomas, brain tumors, Hodgkin's disease, lung cancer, breast cancer, salivary gland, and oral cancers. This reflects a cohort who historically received large doses of external-beam radiation. In the United Kingdom, a study published several years ago offers unique insight into the types of malignancies that develop in patients not treated with external-beam radiation.[101] Patients in the study, who were all over 25 years of age at follow-up, had a much higher risk of developing epithelial cancers (notably lung, bladder, and probably breast) than of developing sarcomas and other early-onset cancers compared to patients in the U.S. who received radiation.

Secondary Malignant Disease (Leukemia)

Childhood acute lymphocytic leukemia (ALL) is the most common malignant tumor that involves the eyes of children. Leukemia primarily involves the uveal tract: the iris, ciliary body, and/or choroid. It can also involve the retina, optic nerve, and orbit.

Leukemic iris infiltrates can appear as creamy clusters of cells floating on the surface of the iris. When iris infiltrates are present, they can manifest as heterochromia (different color irides), cells in the anterior chamber (tumor hypopyon mimicking idiopathic iritis), or bleeding in the anterior chamber (hyphema). Hyphema can be associated with glaucoma and a painful, photophobic, red, sensitive eye. In contrast to iris involvement, leukemic infiltration is virtually impossible to detect ophthalmoscopically in the ciliary body or choroid because ALL diffusely invades the choroidal blood vessels. This subtle thickening is often detectable only by B-scan ultrasound.[102] Leukemic infiltration in the choroid has been identified in 90% of eyes at autopsy after death from leukemia. Retinal involvement is rare.

Leukemic infiltration of the eye can presents in different time sequences in relation to the overall presentation of the disease. Most commonly, the infiltration presents simultaneously with the initial presentation of the leukemia. The majority of patients with ALL demonstrate ultrasonic ocular findings at presentation. When the leukemia is treated, the choroidal involvement usually disappears within days. Leukemic infiltration of the eye can also present as an isolated site of relapse following induction treatment and CNS radiation prophylaxis. In these children the CNS has often been treated with radiation but the eye has escaped treatment, functioning as a sanctuary site. Treatment of the eye alone in such cases may be justified. Finally, leukemic infiltration can present as a sign of CNS recurrence with or without evidence of a gross mass in the CNS. These patients frequently have leukemic cells near the posterior pole and in the vitreous. In these cases, the tumor cells enter the eye via the optic nerve which has been seeded directly from the CNS.[103] In these cases, treatment to the brain with chemotherapy or external-beam radiation is generally considered.

Pediatric Ophthalmic Oncology: Orbital Diseases

Benign Disease

Capillary Hemangiomas ■ Benign tumors of the orbit in children are frequently incidental problems detected on CT scan or observed because of lid or orbital asymmetry. Many require no treatment. The most common benign orbital tumor of childhood is the capillary hemangioma.[104] On CT, capillary hemangiomas are usually associated with congenitally enlarged orbits while rhabdomyosarcomas are not.

Treatment of these hemangiomas is difficult. The tumors respond to low dose radiation and we have used fractionated doses up to 800 cGy with success. There have also been several reports of treatment with recombinant interferon alpha.[105] Local injections of short and long-acting steroids are probably the treatment of choice when mandated by visual or overwhelming cosmetic reasons.

Dermoid Cysts ■ Dermoid cysts are benign and represent congenital ectodermal rests. Treatment is surgical, but utmost care must be taken because many have bilobed posterior orbital extensions that can extend intracranially.

Lymphangioma ■ Despite the fact that lymphatics do not exist in the orbit, benign lymphangiomas do.[106] These tumors are thought to be congenital and have no malignant potential, but in contrast to hemangiomas are rarely present at birth. They are most commonly seen at around age 6 with explosive proptosis caused by bleeding of the tumor into the cystic spaces referred to as *chocolate cysts*. Treatment is difficult. They do not respond to steroids or radiation. Surgery with electrocautery laser is the treatment of choice. Satisfactory cosmetic results are difficult to attain.

Malignant Disease

Rhabdomyosarcoma ■ The most common primary malignant orbital tumor of childhood is rhabdomyosarcoma. The average age at diagnosis is 6-10 years with equal incidence in both sexes and both orbits. Although the hallmark presentation of an orbital rhabdomyosarcoma is rapid, progressive, painless proptosis, patients can present with a less dramatic course with slow, progressive proptosis or with ptosis, strabismus, or a subconjunctival fleshy mass.[107] The diagnosis of rhabdomyosarcoma should be considered whenever rapid progressive proptosis occurs in the first 20 years of life. The most common location in the orbit is superonasal. CT or MRI scans can help define the extent of the tumor.

Urgent biopsy is mandatory. All attempts should be made to biopsy the lesion directly without going through the sinuses or skull because of the possibility of causing metastatic disease by tracking tumor cells along the biopsy path. The most common histologic type is an embryonal rhabdomyosarcoma. When rhabdomyosarcomas present in the inferior orbit they are usually histologically alveolar type. These malignancies do not originate from extraocular muscles but from undifferentiated pluripotential mesenchymal elements in the orbital soft issues.

External-beam radiation was first utilized in the mid-1960s and later combined with chemotherapy producing excellent local cures and better than 90% long term survival. The Intergroup Rhabdomyosarcoma studies in the 1980s demonstrated that the most effective combination for disease localized to the orbit was vincristine, actinomycin-D and radiation.[108] In giving radiation, the eye was not spared or shielded. Long-term follow-up demonstrated that after a median of 7 years, only 14% of such eyes were enucleated, but vision was impaired in 70% of them.[109] A more recent meta-analysis completed by four international collaborative groups found no significant difference in survival for those patients treated with chemotherapy alone versus chemotherapy plus radiation.[110]

Adult Ophthalmic Oncology: Ocular Diseases

Benign Disease

Benign tumors of the lid, conjunctiva, iris and choroid are common while those of the retina and cornea are rare. Benign tumors of the lens and vitreous do not occur. The most important benign tumors of the eye in adults are the choroidal nevi.

Choroidal Nevi ■ Choroidal nevi are never present at birth, but generally present around puberty. In the United States, 10-13% of the adult population have choroidal nevi. They are racially related; choroidal nevi in blacks are very rare.

Choroidal nevi are flat, pigmented benign lesions with edges that can be feathered and irregular or rounded (Fig. 72-5). They are usually slate-gray to light chocolate in color. Over time (months to years), there can be associated changes visible by ophthalmoscopy. Many demonstrate changes on their surface such as drusen or have associated findings such as subretinal fluid or neovascular membranes. They may also cause visual field defects. Since 10% of the adult population has choroidal nevi and there are only 1500 choroidal melanomas in the United States yearly, it is assumed that the chance of a choroidal nevus becoming a melanoma is less than one in a thousand. A number of studies have now demonstrated which nevi are more likely to undergo malignant transformation. The predictive factors are shown in Table 72-6.

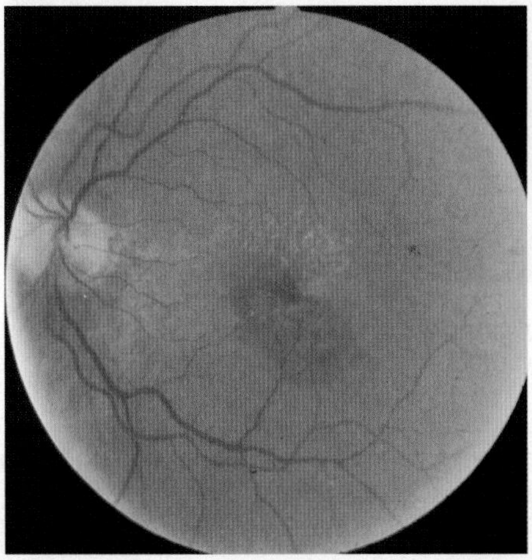

Figure 72-5 ■ Choroidal nevus located inferior to the macula. Note the yellow drusen indicating benign status.

Table 72-6 ■ **Predictive Factors: Nevus to Melanoma Transformation**

- *Size*: The greater the thickness of a choroidal nevus, the greater the chance of it becoming a melanoma. Of nevi 2.5 mm in thickness, approximately 1% per month become melanomas.
- *Location*: Nevi at the posterior portion of the eye more commonly become melanomas than those situated anteriorly.
- *Orange Pigment*: When choroidal nevi develop orange pigment on their surface, the chance of a melanoma developing greatly increases.
- *Serous Fluid*: Serous fluid in the form of an overlying retinal detachment can be seen with nevi, but such nevi more likely become melanomas.
- *Absence of Drusen*: Drusen are a strong indicator of chronicity and benignity and lesions with drusen rarely transform.
- *Hot Spots* on fluorescein angiography
- *Symptoms* (decreased vision or visual field defect)

A melanocytoma is a special type of choroidal nevus often observed in darker-skinned Caucasians of Mediterranean origin. Melanocytomas are brown-black lesions that most commonly originate from the optic nerve head, but can evolve from the choroid, ciliary body, or iris. The lesions may be several millimeters high, can grow slowly, and can affect the visual field or visual acuity. Pathologically, the lesion is a magnocellular nevus with jet black pigmentation. While the lesions are benign, rare cases of transformation to malignancy have been recorded although no deaths have been documented.

The differential diagnosis of a choroidal nevus includes: congenital hyperplasia of the retinal pigment epithelium (CHRPE), hamartomas of the retinal pigment epithelium, and hemorrhages within the retina, especially hemorrhages beneath the retinal pigment epithelium (most commonly associated with age-related macular degeneration). Ophthalmoscopic appearance as well as results of a fluorescein angiogram and ultrasonography are used to distinguish these lesions from each other.

Iris Nevi and Melanomas ■ Iris nevi are benign lesions of the iris that appear on slit lamp examination as pigmented flat areas. They are common, may be multiple, and occur more often in blue-eyed patients. Like choroidal nevi, iris nevi are rarely present at birth and present around puberty. Rarely, they can appear elevated and can grow and shed pigmented cells into the anterior chamber angle, clogging the trabecular meshwork and causing a severe secondary glaucoma that can blind the eye. These lesions have often been referred to as iris melanomas. Widespread metastases, however, are seen rarely if ever. Many clinicians have theorized that the reason for the less aggressive behavior observed in iris melanomas versus choroidal melanomas is simply the smaller size of these lesions. However, recent studies suggest that they are distinctly different from choroidal lesions in that a significant percentage demonstrate an activating mutation in exon 15 of the BRAF gene which is common in cutaneous melanoma, but almost never seen in choroidal lesions.[111] Management of iris melanoma is based on the presence or absence of glaucoma, and should not be guided by a need to prevent metastases. Melanomas that originate in the ciliary body and extend into the iris, however, often demonstrate very aggressive behavior and can metastasize.

Malignant Disease

Introduction to Choroidal Melanoma ■ Choroidal melanoma is the most common primary ocular malignant tumor in adults. There are about 1500 new cases per year of choroidal malignant melanoma in the United States. The average age at diagnosis is 55-65 years with men and women equally affected and no predilection for right versus left eye. In the United States, 99% of choroidal melanomas occur in Caucasians. The most common way in which the tumor is detected is on routine exam (41%).[112] Men more often present with symptoms and when there are symptoms the right eye is more often found to have the tumor. The most common symptom is a perceived deficit in the peripheral visual field followed by decreased vision. The lesion is not painful, unlike metastatic tumors to the eye in which pain is not unusual.

The visual field defect is characteristic. There is an absolute scotoma overlying the tumor associated with a surrounding relative field defect that does not obey the horizontal meridian (as most ocular defects do) and does not observe the vertical meridian (as many CNS defects do).[113]

Melanomas of the choroid originate in melanocytes that normally lie within the choroid. The choroid, the layer between the sclera and retina is a rich, high-flow syncytium of vascular lobules that not only supply blood to the photoreceptors (rods and cones) of the retina but also serve as a heat sink to dissipate heat energy liberated by absorbed visible light.

Whether all melanomas of the choroid originate from choroidal nevi is not known, but patients with flat, pigmented, untreated nevi followed for more than 20 years have developed melanomas arising from the previously dormant lesion. The cause of choroidal melanomas is unknown but predisposing medical conditions include: melanosis oculi (nevus of Ota), dysplastic nevus syndrome, pregnancy, and possibly HIV. Medications that have been shown to cause increased growth of the tumors include estrogen replacement therapy and levodopa. Occupational associations include agriculture and farming work and several industrial operations.[114] We have also seen an increased risk in World War II holocaust survivors.

Diagnosis of Choroidal Melanoma ■ The diagnosis of choroidal melanoma can usually be made on the basis of ophthalmoscopic examination alone. The lesions most often appear as elevated, dome-shaped masses that can rupture Bruch's membrane (Fig. 72-6). When Bruch's membrane is ruptured, the tumors are referred to as mushroom-shaped or collar-button because of their characteristic shape. The lesions can also be multilobed or flat and diffuse. Lesion color varies from patient to patient and from area to area within the tumor. As many as 40% of the tumors have no pigment clinically. When pigmented, the tumors are frequently a dusky gray to charcoal in color but occasionally they are deep brown.

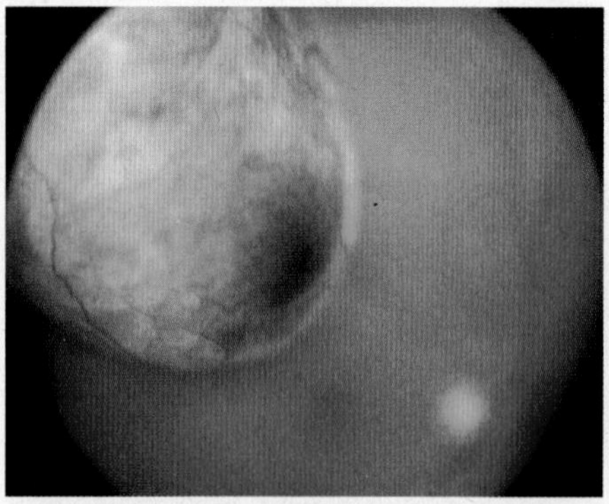

Figure 72-6 ■ Malignant melanoma of the choroid.

Ocular ultrasonography and sometimes fluorescein angiography can also aid in diagnosis. All choroidal melanomas have associated retinal detachments. In some cases it may be difficult to detect the detachments ophthalmoscopically while in others the retinal detachment may be so extensive that the melanoma is not seen clinically. Typically the B-scan ultrasound demonstrates an elevated solid tumor[115] and the A-scan demonstrates medium to low reflectivity.[116] With the use of rigorous and standardized ophthalmic and systemic examinations, a diagnostic accuracy of 99.7% was reached in the Collaborative Ocular Melanoma Study (COMS).[117] Since clinical accuracy is so high, needle biopsy is rarely needed.

Since there are no lymphatics in the eye or within the orbit, melanomas of the choroid metastasize through vascular channels. Approximately 68% of single site metastases occur within the liver.[118] The median survival has been reported as 6 months to 1 year[118,119]; however, Rietchel et al. have reported that there is a substantial subset of patients, 22%, who survive to 4 years postdiagnosis.[118]

Clinical and Pathologic Risk Factors ■ A number of clinical and pathological features have been shown to correlate with patient survival.[120] First, larger tumors, measured clinically using the height, and/or greatest base diameter to volume, are more likely to metastasize. Second, location of the melanoma affects prognosis. Patients with melanomas originating in the iris have the best outcome. Ciliary body melanomas have a threefold mortality compared with choroidal melanomas. Third, patients younger than 60 have better survival than those older than 60. Fourth, patients with extraocular extension have higher mortality rates than those who do not. Finally, many pathologic features (only available in cases where the eye has been removed) correlate with survival and are covered extensively elsewhere.[121] The best known of these is cell type. Epithelioid cells, which are larger and more pleomorphic, are more likely to be contained in large tumors, and carry a worse prognosis.

The COMS Group, which included 44 institutions across the United States, was a series of prospective, randomized clinical trials and other reports on the prognosis and treatment of small, me-

Table 72-7 ■ **Final Size Classifications of Choroidal Melanomas in the Collaborative Ocular Melanoma Studies (COMS)**

	Small Melanomas (mm)	Medium Melanomas	Large Melanomas
Apical height	1-2.5	2.5-10 mm AND	>10 mm OR
Largest basal diameter	5-16	<16 mm	Greater than 16 mm (when 2 mm or greater in height)

Table 72-8 **Results of the Collaborative Ocular Melanoma Study (COMS)**

	Small	Medium	Large
Reference	*Arch Ophthalmol.* December 1997; 115(12):1537-1544	*Arch Ophthalmol.* July 2001; 119(7):969-982	*Am J Ophthalmol.* June 1998; 125(6):779-796
Type of study	Nonrandomized, prospective follow-up	Prospective randomized clinical trial	Prospective randomized clinical trial
Number of patients in study	204	1317	1003
Size of melanomas included in study	Apical height: 1.0-2.5 mm Largest basal diameter: 5 mm	Apical height: 2.5-10.0 mm Largest basal diameter: 5-16 mm	Apical height: 10.0 mm or larger Largest basal diameter: 16 mm or larger
Objective of study	To describe time to tumor growth and determine baseline characteristics associated with growth of small tumors	^{125}I Brachytherapy vs enucleation for treatment of medium tumors	Pre-enucleation radiation vs enucleation alone for treatment of large tumors
Findings of study	21% grew by 2 years 31% grew by 5 years Characteristics associated with growth: initial tumor thickness and diameter, presence of orange pigment, absence of drusen, absence of retinal pigment epithelial changes	No clinically or statistically significant difference in survival rates between the 2 treatments for up to 12 years after treatment	No significant difference in survival rates between the 2 treatments Age and largest basal diameter of the tumor are the only factors that affect prognosis

dium, and large choroidal melanomas. The COMS size classification scheme is shown in Table 72-7 and the results of the studies are detailed in Table 72-8.

Genetic Analysis ■ In recent years, interest in analysis of chromosomal changes and gene expression patterns in choroidal melanoma has greatly increased. Several chromosomal abnormalities, including gain or loss of chromosomal material in chromosomes 3, 6, and 8, have been detected in primary uveal melanoma tissue and have been associated with metastasis.[122] Monosomy 3 in uveal melanoma is a statistically significant predictor of both relapse-free and overall survival.[123] Prescher et al. reported that while no patients with disomy 3 developed metastatic disease, 57% of patients with monosomy 3 developed metastases within 3 years.[123]

Gene expression microarray analysis has been performed examining 3075 genes in 25 enucleated eyes.[124] The authors identified 2 groups: class 1 (low-grade tumors) and class 2 (high-grade tumors). Class 2 tumors demonstrated downregulated gene clusters on chromosome 3 and upregulated clusters on chromosome 8q. These classifications strongly predicted metastatic death with a 95% Kaplan–Meier-based survival prediction at 92 months of 95% in class 1 and 31% in class 2. The classifications outperformed other clinical and pathologic prognostic indicators.

The number of clinical centers performing karyotyping, single nucleotide polymorphism (SNP) analysis, fluorescent in situ hybridization (FISH) analysis, and/or comparative genomic hybridization (CGH) on fine-needle aspiration and enucleation specimens has dramatically increased in the last few years. Some groups have also begun to perform FISH or microsatellite array on fine-needle aspiration biopsy specimens.[125,126] Biopsies have been attempted via pars plana and transscleral approaches. In recent series, sufficient tissue material for diagnosis was obtained for FISH in 98% of cases and for microsatellite assay in 86% of cases.[125,126] Because no effective treatment is available for metastatic uveal melanoma at this time, it is unclear what, if any, interventions or screening programs for metastases should be offered to patients whose lesions are shown to be high-risk for metastasis on biopsy. Nonetheless, as new treatments or prophylactic drugs for metastatic melanoma are developed and available for clinical trials, it will be important to identify which patients are appropriate for entry into such studies.[127,128]

Treatment and Prognosis of Small Melanomas ■ In the COMS, the definition of a small melanoma was a lesion that was 1-2.5 mm in thickness and 5-16 mm in largest basal diameter. This observational study demonstrated that, of choroidal melanomas initially managed by observation, 21% demonstrated growth to medium or large tumors by 2 years and 31% by 5 years.[129] However, there were no defined criteria or threshold for treatment and this group may have included patients whose lesions demonstrated no growth or high-risk features. Factors significantly associated with growth by statistical analysis in the study were greater initial tumor thickness and diameter, presence of orange pigment, absence of drusen, and absence of areas of retinal pigment epithelial changes adjacent to the tumor (Table 72-6).

Since the COMS brachytherapy trials were published, most ophthalmologists in the United States have continued to use the COMS tumor size guidelines in order to designate a tumor as medium and institute brachytherapy. Nonetheless, some investigators have raised the question of whether small melanomas should also be treated with brachytherapy. Although the COMS indicated that the long-term mortality rate for these patients is low (eight-year all-cause mortality of 14.9%),[130] it may be significant enough to justify the consideration of brachy therapy in these patients. There has been only one study examining the outcomes of patients with small melanomas initially observed, then treated with a standardized brachytherapy protocol after growth or new orange pigment was observed. Sobrin et al. reported a 3.9% (95% confidence interval, 0-11.2%) melanoma-specific five-year mortality rate.[131] The melanoma-specific five-year mortality rate for the tumors in the COMS small tumor study was 1%[130]; however, the calculation of this rate included a substantial number of patients whose suspected tumors did not grow and were never treated. A randomized, prospective trial of visual and survival outcomes in patients managed by observation versus prompt treatment is needed to answer this critical question.[131]

Treatment and Prognosis of Medium Melanomas ■ The COMS completed a prospective, randomized clinical trial enrolling 1317 patients with medium-sized melanomas in which patients were randomly assigned to enucleation or brachytherapy with ^{125}I plaques at a tumor dose of 10,000 cGy.[132] The study concluded mortality rates following brachytherapy (81% 5-year survival) did not differ from mortality rates following enucleation (82% 5-year survival) for up to 12 years after treatment. Given the findings of this study, patients with medium-sized melanomas are offered both enucleation and brachytherapy as potential treatment options. Brachytherapy with ^{125}I plaques is usually administered at doses of 7500-10,000 cGy to the tumor apex. The fractionation schemes vary markedly without an apparent effect on local control, metastasis or complications. Complications include radiation retinopathy and optic neuropathy.[133] As a result of these complications, 43% of patients have 20/200 vision or worse by 3 years of follow-up.[134]

Treatment and Prognosis of Large Melanomas

■ In the past, patients with large tumors were generally treated with enucleation, with or without preoperative radiation. The COMS prospective, randomized clinical trial for patients with large tumors found that there was no survival difference between patients treated with enucleation alone (5-year survival 57%) and patients treated with pre-enucleation radiation (5-year survival 62%).[135] The patients assigned to the pre-enucleation radiation group in this study were treated with 5 fractions of 200 cGy external-beam radiation and enucleation within 72 hours. Patients with large melanomas are now generally treated with enucleation alone.

Metastatic Disease

The most common malignant neoplasm in the eye or orbit, in children or adults, is metastatic carcinoma to the choroid. While there are only 350 cases of retinoblastoma and 1500 cases of choroidal melanoma yearly in the United States, it is estimated that 30,000-100,000 patients with cancer develop metastases to the eye each year.[136]

Most cancers metastasize to the uveal tract (iris, ciliary body, and choroid), with choroidal metastases occurring most frequently. Metastases to the lids, conjunctiva, optic nerve, orbit, extraocular muscles and orbital bones are also reported. Metastases to the retina are rare.

Choroidal metastases are usually amelanotic, multiple, bilateral, minimally elevated, and painful when situated around the optic nerve or invading the sclera. In contrast, ocular melanomas are typically pigmented, solitary, unilateral, significantly elevated, and painless. Metastatic tumors, like ocular melanomas, always have an associated serous detachment but the amount of detachment is proportionally greater with metastases. Ultrasonographically, most metastases have high reflectivity on ultrasound. Most ocular melanomas are detected on routine examinations, whereas ocular metastases are typically identified because of symptoms of decreased visual field and diminished visual acuity due to serous retinal detachments.

Metastasis to the eye most commonly occurs in adults aged 55-65, the same age distribution as that for ocular melanomas. Metastases originate most commonly from a primary lung cancer and second most commonly from a primary breast cancer. As many as 34% of patients who present with metastases to the choroid have no previously known history of a primary cancer.[137] Many other cancers metastasize to the eye, including G.I., prostate (though more commonly to orbital bones), thyroid, ovarian, and cutaneous melanoma. Virtually all cancers have been found to be capable of metastasizing to the eye.

The most striking feature of metastatic ocular lesions is their association with concurrent CNS metastases. While the true concordance of these two lesions is unknown, it has been our experience that more than 75% of cases of ocular metastasis have concurrent CNS disease, though frequently the CNS disease is initially undetectable with imaging. It has therefore been speculated that some ocular metastases do not arrive through blood borne routes but that CNS metastases may actually seed the choroid via the subarachnoid space as they do in childhood leukemia.

Treatment for ocular metastasis is considered when symptoms of diminished vision, pain, or diplopia are present. Treating the ocular lesion rarely has an impact on survival, except in carcinoid metastases, but may significantly alter the quality of life. Many ocular metastases respond to chemotherapy the way other systemic metastases respond. Chemotherapy and/or hormonal manipulation may cause rapid regression of the tumor and of subretinal fluid. External-beam radiation is also used to palliate symptoms from ocular metastases. Except for carcinoid and breast cancer, however, median survival in patients with metastatic choroidal lesions is just over 6 months.

Cancer-Associated Retinopathy (CAR)

Cancer-associated retinopathy (CAR) is a paraneoplastic disorder characterized by visual loss in patients with cancer. Patients report photopsias or entopic phenomenon as well as light sensitivity and night blindness. Examination reveals decreased visual acuity, decreased color vision, and scotomas.[138] A CAR antibody, a 23 kDa protein commonly found on blood testing, is known to be specific for a photoreceptor and bipolar cell-specific calcium binding protein. The underlying tumor is thought to express recoverin and stimulate this antibody response. The circulating antibodies then react with the retina resulting in photoreceptor degeneration. Although antibodies to recoverin account for the majority of cases, additional antibodies to 46, 45, 60, and 65 kDa proteins have been described.[138] Lung cancer, endometrial sarcoma, lymphoma and prostate cancer have been associated with the syndrome. Treatment is difficult. Steroids, plasmapharesis, intravenous immunoglobulin (IVIG), and treatment of the underlying tumor have been attempted. Although individual successes have been reported, most patients have little improvement and there is no clear consensus as to the best treatment.[139,140]

Ocular Lymphoid Tumors

Non-Hodgkin lymphomas can occasionally infiltrate the intraocular tissues and become clinically apparent even before identification of the systemic disease. Immunocompromised patients, especially those with viral illness such as those with HIV/AIDS, show an increased incidence of this disease.

Primary malignant lymphomas of the eye have historically been called *reticulum cell sarcoma* or *microgliomatosis,* and usually present with cells in the vitreous with associated retinal and optic nerve involvement. Diagnosis is made by vitrectomy or lumbar puncture. Treatment is accomplished with systemic steroids and external-beam radiation therapy of 2400 cGy to the affected eye and/or chemotherapy. These patients frequently have CNS disease but rarely have systemic disease. There is controversy about whether to treat the brain in those cases in which diagnostic lumbar puncture and MRI demonstrate no disease. Median survival is 3.5 years and is usually determined by the extent of brain involvement.

Uveal lymphoid infiltration is a rare disorder characterized by localized or diffuse infiltration of the uveal tract by lymphoid cells. Patients typically present with painless, progressive visual loss. Nodular amelanotic thickening of the choroid or exudative retinal detachment with secondary glaucoma can be present.[141] Biopsy confirmation should be targeted to the most accessible tissue. Management emphasizes globe conservation aimed at visual presentation and generally involves oral steroids and/or external-beam radiation. Prognosis for survival is excellent, and generally based on the degree of systemic involvement. Associated CNS involvement is rare.

Adult Ophthalmic Oncology: Orbital Diseases

Introduction to Orbital Tumors

Fortunately, malignant tumors of the orbit are unusual. Neoplasms account for approximately 20-25% of orbital disease and are most common in patients in their sixties or older. Biopsy is rarely needed for definitive diagnosis even in cases of metastatic disease to the orbit. Malignant primary cancers of the orbit that do require biopsy and surgical management include lacrimal gland tumors and orbital lymphoma.

All cases of suspected orbital tumor should undergo imaging, including ophthalmic ultrasound, CT scans with or without contrast, and/or MRI with or without contrast in order to define more clearly the location of the tumor.

Benign and Malignant Disease

Well-Delineated Orbital Masses ■ The most common benign orbital tumor of adults is the cavernous hemangioma. Patients have slowly progressive painless proptosis with a mass indenting the globe, showing striae in the retina and a flattened globe on imaging studies. Treatment is surgical, and complete removal is possible. Other well-circumscribed lesions include neurofibromas, schwannomas, hemangiopericytomas, meningioma, and gliomas.

A mucocele or mucopyocele is a cystic, encapsulated mass originating in a paranasal sinus (usually the frontal sinus) that follows repeated bouts of sinusitis often leading to recurrent orbital cellulitis. It is the most common cause of proptosis in children. The bony wall is not intact on imaging studies. Treatment involves antibiotics. Surgical drainage is necessary if antibiotics fail to achieve resolution of the pyomucocele or if optic nerve compression is present.

Diffuse Orbital Masses ■ Diffuse orbital masses usually require a biopsy and include orbital lymphoma, orbital cellulitis, fibrous histiocytoma (benign and malignant), neurofibromas, and sarcomas. Lymphoproliferative neoplasms account for greater than 20% of all orbital mass lesions. The incidence of non-Hodgkins lymphoma of all anatomic sites has been increasing at a rate of 3-4% per year and orbital lymphomas have been increasing at an even greater rate, although the factors responsible for this rise are poorly understood.[141] Historically, lymphoid tumors were classified as either active lymphoid hyperplasia or malignant lymphoma. More recently, it has been recognized that lymphoproliferative lesions represent a continuum and that ulimate behavior is difficult to predict. Currently, 70-90% of orbital lymphoproliferative lesions are designated as malignant lymphomas on the basis of molecular genetic studies and monoclonal cell surface markers.

The typical lymphoproliferative lesion presents as a gradually progressive painless mass. It can be located anteriorly in the orbit or beneath the conjunctiva. Orbital imaging reveals the characteristic molding of the tumor around normal structures, and bony erosion is rare except in high-grade lesions. Up to 50% of all lesions arise in the lacrimal fossa, and up to 17% of lesions occur bilaterally. For all lesions, early biopsy is recommended to establish a diagnosis and characterize the lesions to reflect distinct morphologic, immunologic, cytogenetic, and molecular properties under the Revised European American Lymphoma (REAL) classification.[142,143] This classification has been shown to predict differences in the clinical behavior of these lesions. The classification allocates adnexal lymphomas to one of five categories: marginal zone lymphoma (MALT), diffuse lymphoplasmacytoid/lymphoplasmacytic lymphoma, follicle center lymphoma, diffuse large B-cell lymphoma, and other rare lymphomas.

Management of adnexal lymphoma involves a metastatic work-up by an oncologist. Ocular disease is generally treated with 2000-3000 cGy of external-beam radiation therapy, which results in local control in virtually all cases and may prevent systemic spread. However, at least 50% of patients eventually have systemic lymphoma detected and treatment of systemic dissemination is based on the pathologic grade of the lesion and its characteristic degree of aggressiveness. Some indolent lymphomas are refractory to chemotherapy and are associated with long-term survival, whereas more aggressive lymphomas may be cured with aggressive chemotherapy and/or radiation.

Some studies suggest that patients with bilateral orbital involvement have a poorer prognosis. Conjunctival lesions have the lowest likelihood (20%) of developing systemic disease. Eyelid lymphomas have the highest likelihood (67%), with orbital lesions in between (35%).[144]

Lacrimal Gland Tumors

Lacrimal gland tumors can be easily identified with ophthalmic ultrasonography, but a more clear definition of tumor location, especially bony involvement, is best demonstrated with CT scans. When lacrimal gland masses are bilateral on orbital imaging, they generally represent lesions such as sarcoid, orbital pseudotumor, or lymphoma. Of those lacrimal gland masses not presenting with inflammatory signs, the majority represent lymphoproliferative disorders, as fully 50% of orbital lymphomas develop in the lacrimal fossa. Only a minority of lacrimal fossa lesions are primary epithelial neoplasms of the lacrimal gland. Biopsy is necessary in suspected cases to establish a pathologic diagnosis.

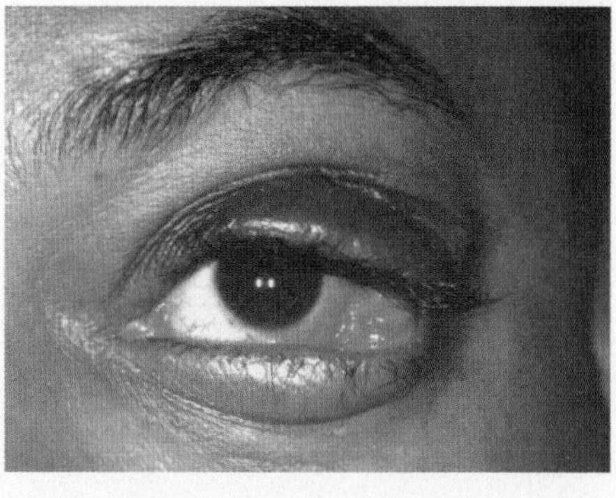

Figure 72-7 ■ Adenoid cystic carcinoma of the lacrimal gland in a patient who underwent 2 biopsies of the mass, both of which were equivocal. The patient developed metastases to the parotid gland and later died.

Approximately 50% of primary epithelial neoplasms of the lacrimal gland are benign mixed tumors (pleomorphic adenomas) and about 50% are carcinomas. Approximately half of the carcinomas are adenoid cystic tumors (Fig. 72-7), and the remainder include malignant mixed tumors, primary adenocarcinomas, mucoepidermoid carcinomas, and squamous carcinomas. Treatment for primary malignant lacrimal gland tumors includes excisional surgery and radiation therapy. Except for pleomorphic adenomas that undergo successful surgical removal without a preliminary biopsy (with resultant tumor capsule rupture, increasing risk of recurrence), the clinical course for most of these tumors is that of multiple painful recurrences with ultimate mortality from intracramal extension or systemic metastases, often occurring a decade or more after initial presentation.

Selected References

The complete reference list can be found at www.CANCERMEDICINE8.com

1. Abramson DH. Retinoblastoma. *Pediatr Emerg Casebook*. 1985;3:3–15.
3. Tamboli A, Podgor MJ, Horm JW. The incidence of retinoblastoma in the United States: 1974 through 1985. *Arch Ophthalmol*. 1990;108:128–132.
5. Salim A, Wiknjosastro GH, Danukusumo D, Barnas B, Zalud I. Fetal retinoblastoma. *J Ultrasound Med*. 1998;17:717–720.
7. Singh AD, Black SH, Shields CL, Shields JA. Prenatal diagnosis of retinoblastoma. *J Pediatr Ophthalmol Strabismus*. 2003;40:222–224.
9. Sant M, Capocaccia R, Badioni V. Survival for retinoblastoma in Europe. *Eur J Cancer*. 2001;37:730–735.
11. Abramson DH, Ellsworth RM, Grumbach N, Kitchin FD. Retinoblastoma: survival, age at detection and comparison 1914-1958, 1958-1983. *J Pediatr Ophthalmol Strabismus*. 1985;22:246–250.
12. Sippel KC, Fraioli RE, Smith GD, et al. Frequency of somatic and germ-line mosaicism in retinoblastoma: implications for genetic counseling. *Am J Hum Genet*. 1998;62:610–619.
13. Duesberg P. Chromosomal chaos and cancer. *Sci Am*. 2007;296:52–59.
14. Mastrangelo D, De Francesco S, Di Leonardo A, Lentini L, Hadjistilianou T. Retinoblastoma epidemiology: does the evidence matter? *Eur J Cancer*. 2007;43:1596–1603.
15. Dimaras H, Khetan V, Halliday W, et al. Loss of RBI induces non-proliferative retinoma; increasing genomic instability

correlates with progression to retinoblastoma. *Hum Mol Genet*. 2008.
21. Fung YK, Murphree AL, T'Ang A, Qian J, Hinrichs SH, Benedict WF. Structural evidence for the authenticity of the human retinoblastoma gene. *Science*. 1987;236:1657–1661.
22. Dunn JM, Phillips RA, Becker AJ, Gallie BL. Identification of germline and somatic mutations affecting the retinoblastoma gene. *Science*. 1988;241:1797–1800.
23. Dunn JM, Phillips RA, Zhu X, Becker A, Gallie BL. Mutations in the RBI gene and their effects on transcription. *Mol Cell Biol*. 1989;9:4596–4604.
24. Muncaster MM, Cohen BL, Phillips RA, Gallie BL. Failure of RBI to reverse the malignant phenotype of human tumor cell lines. *Cancer Res*. 1992;52:654–661.
25. Harbour JW. Overview of RB gene mutations in patients with retinoblastoma. Implications for clinical genetic screening. *Ophthalmology*. 1998;105:1442–1447.
36. Abramson DH, Ellsworth RM. The surgical management of retinoblastoma. *Ophthalmic Surg*. 1980;11:596–598.
37. Abramson DH, Frank CM. Second nonocular tumors in survivors of bilateral retinoblastoma: a possible age effect on radiation-related risk. *Ophthalmology*. 1998;105:573–579; discussion 9–80.
38. Moll AC, Imhof SM, Schouten-Van Meeteren AY, Kuik DJ, Hofman P, Boers M. Second primary tumors in hereditary retinoblastoma: a register-based study, 1945-1997: is there an age effect on radiation-related risk? *Ophthalmology*. 2001;108:1109–1114.
39. Blach LE, McCormick B, Abramson DH. External beam radiation therapy and retinoblastoma: long-term results in the comparison of two techniques. *Int J Radiat Oncol Biol Phys*.1996;35:45–51.
40. Zelter M, Damel A, Gonzalez G, Schwartz L. A prospective study on the treatment of retinoblastoma in 72 patients. *Cancer*. 1991;68:1685–1690.
52. Gallie BL, Budning A, DeBoer G, et al. Chemotherapy with focal therapy can cure intraocular retinoblastoma without radiotherapy. *Arch Ophthalmol*. 1996;114:1321–1328.
54. Murphree AL, Villablanca JG, Deegan WF, 3rd, et al. Chemotherapy plus local treatment in the management of intraocular retinoblastoma. *Arch Ophthalmol*. 1996;114:1348–1356.
56. Greenwald MJ, Strauss LC. Treatment of intraocular retinoblastoma with carboplatin and etoposide chemotherapy. *Ophthalmology*. 1996;103:1989–1997.
58. Shields CL, Shields JA, Needle M, et al. Combined chemoreduction and adjuvant treatment for intraocular retinoblastoma. *Ophthalmology*. 1997;104:2101–2111.
60. Friedman DL, Himelstein B, Shields CL, et al. Chemoreduction and local ophthalmic therapy for intraocular retinoblastoma. *J Clin Oncol*. 2000;18:12–17.
61. Beck MN, Balmer A, Dessing C, Pica A, Munier F. First-line chemotherapy with local treatment can prevent external-beam irradiation and enucleation in low-stage intraocular retinoblastoma. *J Clin Oncol*. 2000;18:2881–2887.
62. Vazquez E, Castellote A, Piqueras J, et al. Second malignancies in pediatric patients: imaging findings and differential diagnosis. *Radiographics*. 2003;23:1155–1172.
63. Wilson MW, Rodriguez-Galindo C, Haik BG, Moshfeghi DM. Merchant TE, Pratt CB. Multiagent chemotherapy as neoadjuvant treatment for multifocal intraocular retinoblastoma. *Ophthalmology*. 2001;108:2106–2114; discussion 14–15.
64. Shields CL, Honavar SG, Meadows AT, et al. Chemoreduction plus focal therapy for retinoblastoma: factors predictive of need for treatment with external beam radiotherapy or enucleation. *Am J Ophthalmol*. 2002;133:657–664.
65. Shields CL, Honavar SG, Shields JA, Demirci H, Meadows AT, Naduvilath TJ. Factors predictive of recurrence of retinal tumors, vitreous seeds, and subretinal seeds following chemoreduction for retinoblastoma. *Arch Ophthalmol*. 2002;120:460–464.
66. Brichard B, De Bruycker JJ, De Potter P, Neven B, Vermylen C, Cornu G. Combined chemotherapy and local treatment in the management of intraocular retinoblastoma. *Med Pediatr Oncol*. 2002;38:411–415.
67. Shields CL, Honavar SG, Meadows AT, Shields JA, Demirci H, Naduvilath TJ. Chemoreduction for unilateral retinoblastoma. *Arch Ophthalmol*. 2002;120:1653–1658.
68. Rodriguez-Galindo C, Wilson MW, Haik BG, et al. Treatment of intraocular retinoblastoma with vincristine and carboplatin. *J Clin Oncol*. 2003;21:2019–2025.
69. Balasubramanya R, Pushker N. Bajaj MS, Rani A, Ghose S, Arya LS. Visual outcome in macular retinoblastoma treated with primary chemotherapy. *Ophthalmologica*. 2003;217:417–421.
70. Sussman DA, Escalona-Benz E, Benz MS, et al. Comparison of retinoblastoma reduction for chemotherapy vs external beam radiotherapy. *Arch Ophthalmol*. 2003;121:979–984.
86. Saleh RA, Gross S, Cassano W, Gee A. Metastatic retinoblastoma successfully treated with immunomagnetic purged autologous bone marrow transplantation. *Cancer*. 1988;62:2301–2303.
87. Namouni F, Doz F, Tanguy ML, et al. High-dose chemotherapy with carboplatin, etoposide and cyclophosphamide followed by a haematopoietic stem cell rescue in patients with high- risk retinoblastoma: a SFOP and SFGM study. *Eur J Cancer*. 1997;33:2368–2375.
88. Schvartzman E, Chantada G, Fandino A, de Davila MT, Raslawski E, Manzitti J. Results of a stage-based protocol for the treatment of retinoblastoma. *J Clin Oncol*. 1996;14:1532–1536.
89. White L. Chemotherapy in retinoblastoma. *Am J Pediatr Hematol Oncol*. 1991;13:189–201.
90. Puccetti D. Treatment of extraocular retinoblastoma. In: Albert DM, Polans A, eds. *Ocular Oncology*. New York: Marcel Dekker, Inc.; 2003:489–498.
122. Sisley K, Rennie IG, Cottam DW, Potter AM, Potter CW, Rees RC. Cytogenetic findings in six posterior uveal melanomas: involvement of chromosomes 3, 6, and 8. *Genes Chromosomes Cancer*. 1990;2: 205–209.
124. Onken MD, Worley LA, Ehlers JP, Harbour JW. Gene expression profiling in uveal melanoma reveals two molecular classes and predicts metastatic death. *Cancer Res*. 2004;64:7205–7209.
126. Shields CL, Ganguly A, Materin M, et al. Chromosome 3 analysis of uveal melanoma using fine-needle aspiration biopsy at the time of plaque radiotherapy in 140 consecutive cases. *Arch Ophthalmol*. 2007;125:1017–1024.
128. Tsai T, O'Brien JM. The future promise and the current reality of genetic prognostication in patients with uveal melanoma. *Arch Ophthalmol*. 2008;126: 413–415.
130. Mortality in patients with small choroidal melanoma. COMS report no. 4. The Collaborative Ocular Melanoma Study Group. *Arch Ophthalmol*. 1997;115:886–893.
141. Orbit, eyelids, and lacrimal system. In: *Basic and Clinical Science Course*. San Francisco: American Academy of Ophthalmology Publishers; 2004:81–89.
142. Coupland SE, Krause L, Delecluse HJ, et al. Lymphoproliferative lesions of the ocular adnexa. Analysis of 112 cases. *Ophthalmology*. 1998;105:1430–1441.
143. Johnson TE, Tse DT, Byrne GE, Jr., et al. Ocular-adnexal lymphoid tumors: a clinicopathologic and molecular genetic study of 77 patients. *Ophthal Plast Reconstr Surg*. 1999;15:171–179.
144. Knowles DM, Jakobiec FA, McNally L, Burke JS. Lymphoid hyperplasia and malignant lymphoma occurring in the ocular adnexa (orbit, conjunctiva, and eyelids): a prospective multiparametric analysis of 108 cases during 1977 to 1987. *Hum Pathol*. 1990;21:959–973.

73 Neoplasms of the Endocrine Glands: Pituitary Neoplasms

Chirag D. Gandhi, MD ■ Kalmon D. Post, MD

Pituitary adenomas are epithelial tumors arising from the adenohypophysis that can manifest with neurological symptoms from local mass effect such as headaches, visual disturbances, increased intracranial pressure, and cranial nerve palsies, or as a variety of clinical entities depending on the hormones that they secrete. In rare cases (<1%) patients can also present with diabetes insipidus. Pituitary adenomas constitute 10-15% of intracranial tumors, although the incidence is as high as 24% in autopsy series. They are most common in the third and fourth decades of life and overall affect both sexes equally. There are, however, differences in frequency between the sexes for certain subtypes, such as Cushing disease, which is more frequent in women; prolactin (PRL)-secreting adenomas, which are more common in young women; and null-cell adenomas, oncocytomas, and gonadotropin-secreting adenomas, which are more common in men.

The classification of pituitary neoplasms has undergone a variety of modifications since its conception. Classically, they were separated based on the light microscopy characteristics of cell cytoplasm and were divided into acidophilic, basophilic, and chromophobic tumors. Acidophils were thought to produce excess amounts of growth hormone (GH) and were linked to acromegaly and gigantism; basophils were thought to secrete adrenocorticotrophic hormone (ACTH) and cause Cushing disease; and chromophobes were regarded as hormonally inactive. This system has only limited value since it does not take into consideration either hormone secretion or cellular derivation. It has been well established that both acidophilic and basophilic adenomas may secrete other hormones and that chromophobes can be hormonally active and may secrete GH, PRL, ACTH, thyroid-secreting hormone (TSH), follicle-stimulating hormone (FSH), luteinizing hormone (LH), or α-subunit.[1]

Adenomas are now classified based on the hormones they secrete.[2,3] Endocrinologically, they are considered either active or inactive and are classified as active only if the amount of hormone they secrete exceeds normal levels in the blood and is clinically evident. Inactive adenomas contain secretory and cellular components necessary for hormone production, but they are not associated with clinical and biochemical evidence of hormone excess. The reason is not well understood, but it is thought that "inactive" cells either produce undetectable levels of hormone or abnormal hormone that is not recognized by the antibody in radioimmunoassay, or that these cells have lost the ability to produce any hormone through some acquired genetic defect.[4] This functional classification is now being further modified to incorporate recent advances in molecular and immunohistochemical advances in pituitary research.

Recent investigations in pituitary tumorigenesis have shown that adenomas are monoclonal proliferations[5-7] and that neoplastic progression is related to oncogenes and to defects in tumor suppressor genes. The only initiating mutation that has been identified so far is in a subset of 10-40% of GH-secreting tumors that possess a constitutive activation of the cAMP pathway owing to a point mutation in the α-chain of the GTP binding protein, Gs. This results in elevated cAMP formation and subsequent GH hypersecretion and adenoma proliferation.[8] Although it has been theorized that adenomas with this gsp oncogene mutation are smaller and more sensitive to medical therapy, recent studies have failed to demonstrate any phenotypic differences in patients with and without the gsp mutation.[9] Extensive research has resulted in a multiplicity of other factors that influence pituitary tumor progression. Other oncogenes that have been linked to adenoma progression include cAMP-responsive nuclear transcription factor, CREB, which is also thought to be promoted by the overexpression of Gsα[9]; ras oncogene mutations that have been detected in aggressive prolactinomas[10]; and more recently, the pituitary tumor transforming gene, PTTG, which may be a new marker for invasiveness in secretory adenomas.[11] Tumor suppressor genes such as Rb, menin, TP53, p27, p16[12,13] as well as promoting factors such as hypothalamic neurohormones and locally produced growth factors and cytokines are also being studied to aid in the understanding of adenoma growth. Novel therapeutic target receptors are also being investigated. These include galectin-3 (Gal-3), found only in PRL and ACTH hormone-secreting tumor lines, as well as the nuclear receptor, peroxisome proliferator-activated receptor gamma (PPAR-γ), which has been isolated in a variety of adenoma lines.[14-16] The exact molecular mechanisms of pituitary adenoma proliferation are still incompletely understood, but once they are better defined, additional treatment options may be available.

Patients presenting with a suspected or known pituitary adenoma need to undergo a complete radiographic and endocrine assessment prior to the initiation of either medical or surgical therapy. Magnetic resonance imaging (MRI) is the modality of choice and should be requested with a localized pituitary protocol that includes thin cuts in the coronal and sagittal planes (Figs. 73-1A and 73-1B). MRI helps to depict tumor size, extension, and characteristics such as hemorrhagic and cystic changes (T2-weighted images). Gadolinium is also essential for increasing the diagnostic yield for microadenomas (<10 mm) and useful in delineating normal and abnormal tissue in macroadenomas (T1-weighted images pre- and post-gadolinium).[17] In general, a hypointense lesion on a noncontrast MRI that demonstrates less enhancement with gadolinium than normal pituitary tissue raises the suspicion of a pituitary adenoma. This is particularly important in parasellar invasive tumors. Based on radiographic imaging, Jules Hardy first classified pituitary adenomas based on their extent of intrasellar and extrasellar extension as well as their invasiveness (Fig. 73-2).[18] In addition to radiographic imaging, the patient's baseline endocrine panel should include serum GH, insulin-like growth factor (IGF-1), TSH, free T4, T3, PRL, ACTH, cortisol, LH, FSH, and testosterone. Following these tests, the determination of further medical or surgical treatments can be made.

With the exception of prolactinomas, which can be medically managed long term with dopamine agonists, and asymptomatic, endocrine-inactive tumors that can be followed with serial imaging, surgery is the preferred definitive treatment of pituitary adenomas. Based on innovative work by Cushing, Guiot, and Hardy the transsphenoidal approach is the preferred surgical technique for most adenomas.[19] The goals of surgery include the reduction of any mass effect created by the tumor, the cessation of endocrine hyperactivity, and the preservation or restoration of pituitary function. These goals can now be achieved quickly with minimal morbidity through the trans-

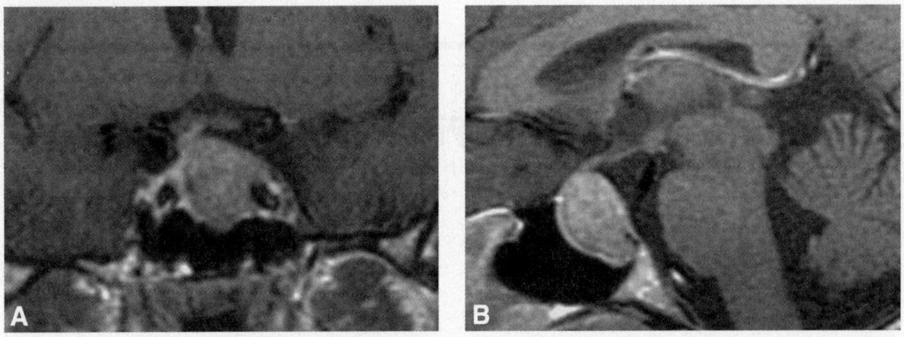

Figure 73-1 ■ A 38-year-old woman with an ACTH-secreting adenoma. (**A**) Coronal T1-weighted MRI with contrast demonstrates a hypointense macroadenoma within the sella that extends into the left cavernous sinus and encases part of the carotid artery. (**B**) Sagittal T1-weighted MRI with contrast demonstrates a hyperintense macroadenoma within the sella.

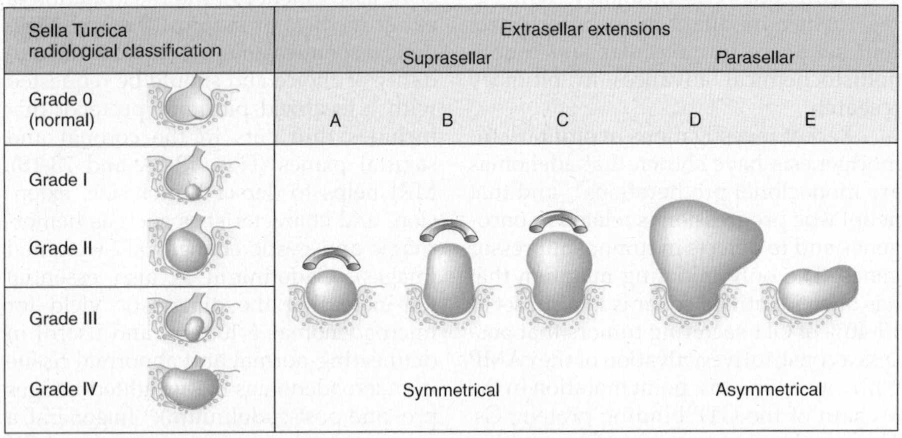

Figure 73-2 ■ Hardy's classification of pituitary adenomas. Grades 1 and 2 are enclosed within the sella. Grades 3 and 4 are invasive. Extrasellar classifications A, B, and C are increasing amounts of direct suprasellar adenomas. D is asymmetric extension, and E is lateral extension into the cavernous sinus. *Source*: Adapted from Ref. 18.

sphenoidal approach.[20] Postoperatively, based on the type of pituitary adenoma, hormone status, and the degree of extrasellar extension, decisions regarding adjuvant therapy can then be made.

Prolactin-Secreting Pituitary Adenomas

Prolactinomas are the most commonly diagnosed pituitary adenoma, representing approximately 30% of cases.[21] Rarely life threatening, they cause symptoms primarily as a result of hyperprolactinemia, which, in turn, results in alterations in reproductive and sexual function, but may also cause symptoms related to mass effect. This is the only pituitary tumor in which a reliably effective medical treatment is available, and that in most cases is the favored primary therapy (Fig. 73-3). Surgical treatment, however, provides similar results as in other endocrine-secreting adenomas and is applicable as the primary intervention for prolactinomas in certain cases.

Clinical Presentation

Although prolactinomas are distributed evenly between men and women at autopsy, women are 4 times more likely to become symptomatic than men. With very few exceptions, prolactinomas are slow growing and the clinical presentation differs in men and women. In women of reproductive age, the symptoms are typically oligomenorrhea or secondary amenorrhea, galactorrhea, and sterility followed by decreased libido, dry vaginal mucosa owing to a deficiency in estrogen, weight gain, and psychological symptoms such as depression and anxiety. Approximately 5% of women with primary amenorrhea and 25% of women with secondary amenorrhea (excluding pregnancy) have a prolactinoma.[22] When galactorrhea accompanies amenorrhea, the incidence increased to 70-80%.[23] In men and in postmenopausal women the tumors grow to much larger sizes and are only detected once they begin to produce mass effect resulting in headaches, visual disturbances (most commonly a bitemporal hemianopsia from chiasmal compression), hypopituitarism, ophthalmoplegia, and, rarely, hydrocephalus from obstruction of the foramen of Monro. Men may also experience a diminished libido, impotence, gynecomastia, and infertility from decreased androgen production.

There still exists significant debate on the exact mechanism of hypogonadism caused by hyperprolactinemia. The most likely explanation is that PRL, through dopamine inhibition, alters the hypothalamic release of gonadotropin-releasing hormone (GnRH), causing disruptions in the normal pulsatile secretion of LH.[24] Prolonged periods of hyperprolactinemia have also been linked to bone demineralization, which is the result of hypogonadism and not of the elevated PRL levels per se, as previously believed, since bone density is normal in eumenorrhic hyperprolactinemic women.[25]

Diagnosis

Besides prolactinomas, hyperprolactinemia can be associated with a variety of causes such as pregnancy, hypothyroidism, PRL-stimulating drugs (eg, phenothiazines, butyrophenones, metoclopramide), and renal failure that need to be considered in the differential diagnosis. In addition, physiological hyperprolactinemia can occur from psychological and physical stresses, such as exercise, surgery, and hypoglycemia, but the PRL

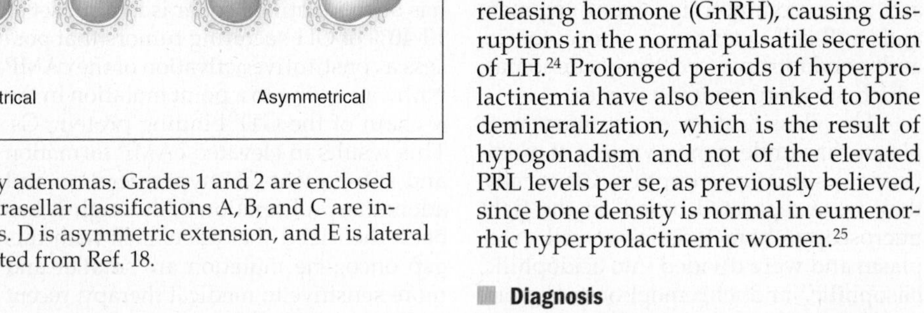

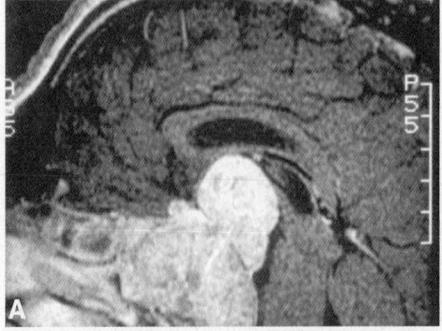

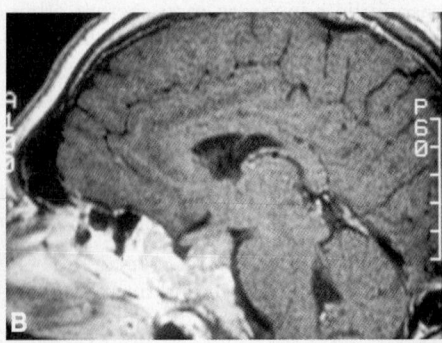

Figure 73-3 ■ A 52-year-old male with diminished libido and a macroprolactinoma. (**A**) Sagittal T1-weighted MRI with contrast demonstrates a large sellar/suprasellar adenoma with compression of the optic chiasm. (**B**) Sagittal T1-weighted with contrast demonstrates a significant reduction in tumor volume after treatment with bromocriptine.

level rarely exceeds 40 ng/mL in these cases.[26] A definitive diagnosis of prolactinoma is difficult and in most cases requires radiographic evidence in addition to elevated PRL levels. In men, a basal PRL value greater than 100 ng/mL is usually indicative of a prolactinoma. In women, levels over 200 ng/mL are also highly suggestive of prolactinomas and values 100-200 ng/mL are likely to be associated with PRL-secreting adenomas.[27,28] The greatest diagnostic uncertainty lies in women with PRO values from 50 ng/mL to 100 ng/mL, which is termed moderate hyperprolactinemia. In these cases, the elevated PRL could be from a PRL-secreting tumor, but could also be from "stalk effect" caused by a nonsecreting adenoma that interferes with the flow of prolactin-inhibitory factor (PRIF) from the hypothalamus. Although various endocrine stimulation tests to differentiate these two possibilities have been suggested, they have not proven to be reliable.[29]

Serum PRL levels are an index of secretory activity and have been found to be associated with the size of the prolactinoma, excluding any associated cystic or necrotic component. If the PRL is less than 200 ng/mL, 80% of tumors are microadenomas; if PRL is greater than 200 ng/mL, 20% are microadenomas. This relationship, however, does not hold true for giant prolactinomas (>4 cm). The PRL may be greater than 1,000 ng/mL, but falsely low serum PRL levels (25-150 ng/mL) have also been described despite the existence of giant or invasive prolactinomas; the phenomenon is know as the "hook effect."[30,31] Briefly, the hook effect occurs when during radioimmunoassay the antibody binding sites become saturated and the binding curve is no longer proportional to the PRL level. This can be resolved by performing serial dilutions.

Treatment

The treatment options available to a patient with a prolactinoma include observation, medical therapy, surgical therapy, and radiotherapy. The best treatment depends on tumor size, PRL level, clinical manifestations, tolerance of medical therapy, and the desire for fertility. Studies have demonstrated that the vast majority of microprolactinomas (<10 mm) do not increase in size.[28] Additionally, autopsy series have found the frequent occurrence of incidental microprolactinomas. Based on this, if patients have only mildly elevated PRL, normal pituitary function, no clinical symptoms, and no desire for pregnancy, observation with serial radiographic and endocrine evaluation is reasonable.

Lactotrophs are controlled by a negative dopaminergic effect from the hypothalamus, and therefore, dopamine agonists have become the standard medical therapy. Unlike long-term medical treatment of other endocrine-active pituitary disorders, dopamine agonists have been remarkably effective in both reducing the size of the tumor as well as normalizing serum PRL levels below the accepted remission level of 25 ng/mL. Bromocriptine was the first of these medications, but more recently, others such as cabergoline, quinagolide, lisuride, pergolide mesylate, and terguride are also used. Biomolecular studies have shown that dopamine agonists selectively activate type D2 dopamine receptors blocking the transcription of the PRL gene.[32] The shrinkage of PRL cells results in amyloid deposition in and fibrosis of the tumor.[33] Dopamine agonists have been shown to have a high response rate with reports of normalization of PRL in 70-80%, tumor shrinkage in 80-90%, and restoration of ovulation in 80-90%.[34] Based on these results, some would argue that medical treatment should be used in all patients except the 10% who have significant side effects.[35] In addition, an important recent study indicates that a majority of patients who respond to cabergoline with normalization of PRL levels and a reduction in tumor size may experience remission of hyperprolactinemia following discontinuation of the drug.[36] Although the follow-up period has been relatively short, this study suggests the potential for a curative treatment with medical therapy in a select group of patients.

Dopamine agonists do have some significant disadvantages that may temper their use in all patients. The effects are reversible, making the therapy lifelong in most cases, and thus requiring significant compliance. Additionally, there can be significant side effects including nausea, vomiting, postural hypotension, headaches, as well as depression and anxiety that can make long-term compliance even more difficult in some patients. In cases of pituitary apoplexy and in tumors with large cystic components, dopamine agonists are not effective in shrinkage. A group of bromocriptine-resistant prolactinomas with increased aggressiveness and increased incidence in males has also been recently described.[37] Two recent articles in the New England Journal of Medicine[38,39] reported risks for cardiac valve regurgitation in patients receiving long-acting dopamine agonists such as cabergoline. However, these were patients with Parkinson's disease who were receiving doses which were approximately seven times higher than the maximal dose used for treatment of prolactinomas.[40] Valvular disease has not been seen in this lower dose population.

The role of surgery in the treatment of prolactinomas has been under discussion. Some argue that surgery should be the initial treatment, with medical therapy as an adjunct only in cases without remission.[41] The rate of long-term remission varies significantly, depending on the size of the tumor and preoperative PRL levels. The most favorable results have been demonstrated in microadenomas with levels below 200 ng/mL with remission rates ranging from 50% to 84% in long-term follow-up.[34,41-43] The remission rate drops with macroadenomas and with PRL levels from 200 to 500 ng/mL, even though these tumors are amenable to surgical resection. Surgery has not been shown to be useful in giant adenomas and in tumors with PRL levels greater than 500 ng/mL, where the remission rate decreases to 0%. These lesions are better treated with medical therapy, possibly in conjunction with surgery and radiation. Overall, the lower the PRL level, the greater the chance of long-term cure.

Because of the successful long-term control of prolactinomas with medical and surgical options, conventional radiotherapy is generally not considered a primary mode of treatment. It is used in certain invasive tumors, but even that indication is under debate.[44] The use of stereotactic radiosurgery as either a primary treatment modality[45] or as an adjuvant therapy[46] is becoming increasingly common. In various recent studies, in addition to a decrease in the PRL level, the endocrine cure rates with radiosurgery have been approximately 30%.[47] These results, however, are confounded by variations in the number of patients who are on medical therapy at the time of radiosurgery, making a true assessment of efficacy unclear.

Recommendation

Based on the results discussed above, the recommendations for the optimum treatment of prolactinomas needs to be tailored to the tumor size, PRL level, and the patient's wishes. Medical therapy is the first option for almost all prolactinomas. Treatment with a dopamine agonist can be considered as the primary treatment with almost all microadenomas, including patients desiring pregnancy or those with primary amenorrhea.

Based on the most current literature, surgical removal with a high remission can be recommended for most macroadenomas with PRL less than 200 ng/mL. For tumors larger than 2 cm and PRL less than 500 ng/mL, patients should be first treated with a dopamine agonist to reduce the tumor volume and then undergo surgical resection. Any residual tumor can then be treated medically. For very large or invasive tumors or for tumors with PRL greater than 500 ng/mL, medical therapy should be the primary treatment modality.

The subgroup that needs specific discussion comprises patients who are pregnant and harbor prolactinomas. There is a small but serious risk related to the possible rapid expansion of the tumor. Complications occur primarily from macroprolactinomas that have suprasellar extension; they are much less frequent in cases of microprolactinomas.[48] If the patient becomes symptomatic, a dopamine-agonist can be administered. The data regarding the effects of continuous dopamine-agonist therapy on the fetus are limited, however, but suggest no ill effect. During pregnancy, surgery should be undertaken only if the tumor does not respond to medical treatment and if there are progressive neurological symptoms. Patients with macroadenomas who desire pregnancy should undergo a transsphenoidal resection prior to conception, or remain on bromocriptine during the pregnancy.

Growth Hormone-Secreting Pituitary Adenomas

GH secretion is under hypothalamic control through somatostatin and growth hormone releasing hormone (GHRH). Upon release, GH causes the production of IGF-1 from the liver, which, in turn, affects bone and tissue growth and also inhibits further release of GH and GHRH. These inhibitory feedback loops are ineffective in acromegaly, and GH release continues autonomously. The clinical manifestations of GH-secreting pituitary tumors have been found to correlate better with IGF-1 levels than with GH levels.

Clinical Presentation

These tumors account for about 30% of all endocrine-active pituitary tumors and most patients present in their third to fifth decade with macroadenomas with a long subclinical course ranging from 4 years to 10 years.[49] GH excess classically presents as acromegaly or gigantism, both marked by an insidious coarsening of features with frontal bossing and prognathism, macroglossia, and exaggerated acral growth. Patients are also found to develop organomegaly, hypertension, cardiomyopathy, congestive heart failure, restrictive lung disease, sleep apnea, and arthropathies. Additionally, a very high percentage of acromegalic patients have impaired glucose metabolism and diabetes mellitus. Common symptoms include fatigue, headaches, arthralgias, oily skin, hyperhidrosis, and in patients with a co-secreting PRL variant, amenorrhea, galactorrhea, and loss of libido. The slow, progressive symptoms are associated with mortalities as high as 50% by the age of 50 in untreated patients, 2-3 times that of the general population.[50]

Diagnosis

The diagnosis is usually apparent based only on the characteristic physical appearance and the frequent subclinical history. Elevated basal fasting GH levels greater than 2.5 ng/mL or, more accurately, an elevated IGF-1 is suggestive of acromegaly. IGF-1 levels must be corrected for age and sex. These values are more accurate than GH levels because they are more stable throughout the day. Dynamic testing is usually not useful in diagnosis and is usually reserved for monitoring therapeutic efficacy. The most common test is the oral glucose tolerance test (OGTT), which involves the tracking of serial GH levels after a 75- to 100-g oral glucose load. In normal patients, GH levels should suppress below 1 ng/mL. A lack of suppression is diagnostic for a GH-secreting tumor. Owing to the improved sensitivity and specificity of the GH assay, there have been questions about whether GH suppression criteria during an OGTT in patients with acromegaly should be modified for gender or age similar to those for IGF-1. A recent study of 92 patients with acromegaly, however, suggests that nadir levels of GH did not vary significantly based on either age or gender.[51]

Once the clinical and biochemical diagnosis is confirmed, an MRI determines the location and size of the tumor. If this fails to demonstrate a pituitary tumor, a possible ectopic GHRH source, occurring in about 1% of cases, should be sought in the chest or abdomen.

Treatment

Outcome measures for cure have been modified multiple times since the initial availability of a GH assay in the 1960s. Currently, the biochemical goals of therapy are to reduce basal GH levels to less than 2.5 ng/mL, to normalize IGF-1 levels, and to achieve a nadir GH level of less than 1 ng/mL with an OGTT[52] (Fig. 73-4). A complete cure should lead to recovery of normal pituitary function in most cases and a slow reversal of both cosmetic and physiological abnormalities.

Transsphenoidal surgery remains the primary treatment of these adenomas.[50] The advantages of surgery include a prompt decrease in GH levels, relief of mass effect, and a tissue diagnosis. At our institution, a 14-year review of 115 patients yielded a biochemical remission in 61% of cases with transsphenoidal surgery alone.[53] The rate was 88% for microadenomas and 53% for macroadenomas. Tumor size and preoperative GH levels were found to correlate negatively with surgical outcome. Immediate postoperative GH levels were found to correlate with long-term outcome. In cases where the postoperative GH level was less than 3 ng/mL, the chance of favorable long-term outcome was 89%. Postoperative radiotherapy was given to 32 patients and 31% of these cases are still in remission. An additional 3 patients are in remission with surgery, radiotherapy, and medical treatment. The overall

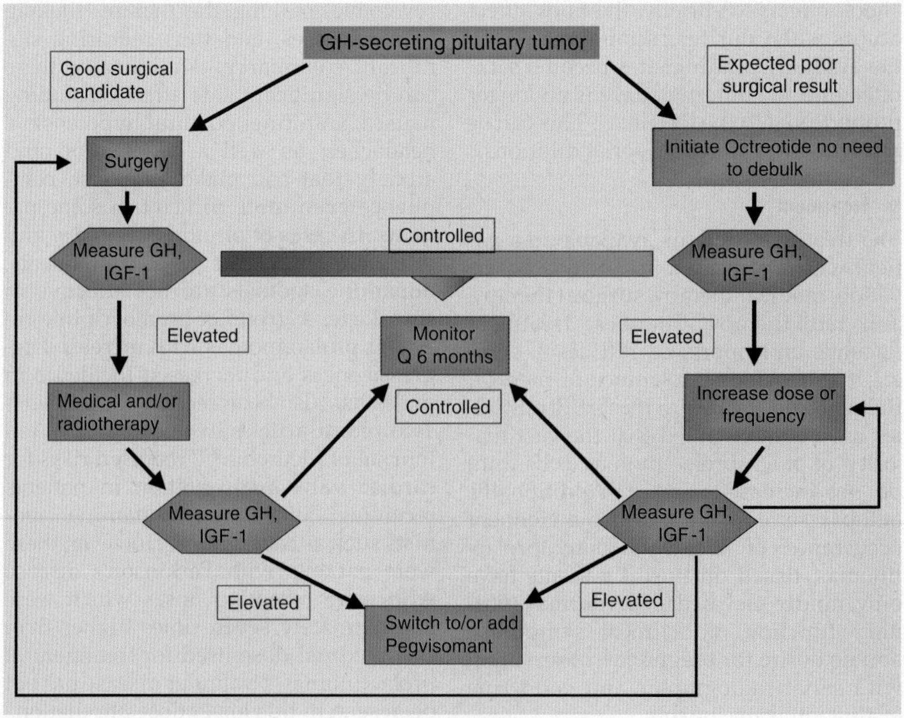

Figure 73-4 The algorithm for the management of acromegaly. Control is characterized by a glucose-suppressed GH less than 1 ng/mL, a normalized age and gender matched IGF-1. *Abbreviation*: DXRT, radiation therapy. *Source*: From Ref. 50.

complication rate was 6.9%, with no CSF leaks, meningitis, permanent diabetes insipidus, or new hypopituitarism. The recurrence rate was 5.4%. Other studies have reported similar results.[54,55]

Both radiotherapy and, more recently, radiosurgery have been used for the treatment of acromegaly. The use of conventional external radiation has been found to reduce GH levels to less than 5 ng/mL in 50-70% of cases, but these effects can take as long as a decade to occur.[56] Hypopituitarism has been found in 50% of patients 10 years after irradiation, with an increasing incidence annually thereafter.[57] Radiosurgery has demonstrated that normalization of GH levels can be achieved within 3-5 years.[58] A similar rate of hypopituitarism is likely to occur, however. Additionally, damage to the optic chiasm remains a concern, and a safety distance of 4 mm should be followed in the management of all types of pituitary adenomas. In general, radiosurgery continues to be an adjunctive therapy after failed transsphenoidal surgery. Remissions have been demonstrated in an additional 30-50% of patients within 2 years.[54,59,60] A recent review found that a significant problem in the interpretation of radiosurgical results was the inconsistent definition of "normal."[47] Endocrine cure rates in a variety of small studies were found to range from 0% to 96% and improvement in 0%-67%. Out of 20 studies reviewed, 6 did not cite their criteria for cure, and 11 of 14 other studies used different criteria to define cure. These results are further confounded by the inconsistent use of somatostatin analogs in patients undergoing radiosurgery. Current studies on the efficacy of radiosurgery also have limited long-term follow-up. Additional randomized studies are needed.

Medical management as the primary or adjuvant treatment of acromegaly remains a controversial topic. In patients who do not have visual loss, some neuroendocrinologists have advocated treatment with somatostatin analogs as the primary treatment.[61] Most practitioners, however, citing the significant morbidity associated with acromegaly, advocate surgical resection followed by adjuvant medical treatment or radiotherapy if needed. 3 classes of drugs are used to treat acromegaly: dopamine agonists, somatostatin analogs, and GH-receptor blockers. Dopamine agonists such as bromocriptine and cabergoline have been shown to provide symptomatic relief in some acromegalic patients. However, these medications rarely reduce the basal GH to less than 2.5 ng/mL and normalize IGF-1 in less than 30% of patients.[62] Their effectiveness is also limited by the side effects. Despite their limited efficacy as compared with other medical options, dopamine agonists remain popular because of their lower cost and ease of oral administration. Somatostatin analogs such as octreotide have been found to be more effective. Octreotide normalizes IGF-1 levels and reduces GH levels to less than 5 ng/mL in approximately 50% of patients.[63] The long-acting analogs such as lanreotide and octreotide LAR can reduce GH below 2.5 ng/mL in 70% of cases and normalize IGF-1 in 88% of patients.[64-66] The newest medication group is the GH-receptor antagonist pegvisomant, which does not act on the pituitary gland, but instead prevents dimerization of the GH-receptor, and thus inhibits the generation of IGF, the primary effector of GH action. A recent study demonstrated 97% of patients treated with pegvisomant had a reduction in their age-adjusted IGF-1 to normal levels.[67] Additional studies, however, have raised concerns about the elevation of liver transaminases and enlargement in tumor size in a small number of patients on this medication.[68] These side effects make interval MRI and liver function testing imperative in patients using this medication.

Medical treatment has been found to provide symptomatic relief of headaches and hyperhidrosis as well as to improve arthropathy and cardiac function. Recent studies have demonstrated that in patients whose glucose-suppressed GH levels and IGF-1 normalized, left-ventricular ejection fraction (LVEF) improved. In a majority of patients with uncontrolled acromegaly, LVEF deteriorated.[69,70] Although current medical therapies are well tolerated and demonstrate good efficacy, they are required lifelong, with recurrence once the medication is discontinued. The significant cost and problems with patient compliance long term continue to make medical treatments more useful as an adjuvant treatment after surgery and radiosurgery have been used.

Between 20% and 30% of GH-secreting adenomas co-secrete PRL. Women often report amenorrhea and galactorrhea, men may develop impotence, and both sexes may complain of loss of libido. Dopamine agonists have been found to be particularly effective in the treatment of acromegalic patients with mixed GH- and PRL-secreting tumors, but transsphenoidal surgery remains the primary treatment.[71]

ACTH-Secreting Adenomas

In Cushing disease, the largest subset of Cushing syndrome, hypersecretion of ACTH by the pituitary results in adrenal hyperplasia and hypercortisolism. Cushing's disease is considered by many to be the most challenging pituitary endocrinopathy to diagnose and treat. The problems in long-term cure arise from difficulties in detection of minute tumors, even with MRI. Furthermore, aggressive macroadenomas have a high rate of recurrence. The incidence is 9 times more frequent in women and usually occurs in the third and fourth decades.

Clinical Presentation

Only about 10-20% of ACTH-secreting adenomas are large enough to produce mass effect, resulting in visual field deficits, cranial nerve involvement, or hypopituitarism. Over 50% of tumors are less than 5 mm and first become evident because of the endocrine presentation. Patients with Cushing disease most commonly present with centripetal obesity, moon facies, buffalo hump, hirsutism, purple abdominal striae, and acne. The main signs include hypertension, osteopenia, proximal myopathy, diabetes mellitus, and significant psychiatric disorders. These clinical syndromes not only cause severe morbidity, but also a 5-year mortality rate of 50% among untreated patients.[72]

Diagnosis

The accurate diagnosis of Cushing disease is actually a 2-step process once a patient has suggestive clinical signs and symptoms. The first step is to determine that the hypercortisolism is actually the result of a pituitary adenoma and not the result of either an adrenal or another ectopic source. The second step is the accurate localization of the adenoma, which in many cases is not possible by static MRI alone. The algorithm for a complete diagnosis is nearly 100% accurate,[73] but each test alone carries a failure rate of 10-30%[74] (Table 73-1).

Hypercortisolism can be quickly verified by an elevation in the 24-hour urinary free cortisol and 17-OH corticosteroids. More recently, a midnight salivary cortisol level has been demonstrated to be a highly sensitive and specific method by which to diagnose hypercortisolism.[75] The diagnosis of Cushing disease may then be suggested with a low-dose dexamethasone suppression test that does not suppress serum cortisol to less than 10 μg/dL. Adrenal cortisol-producing adenomas can be ruled out if plasma ACTH is more than 5 ng/L.[76] After ACTH-dependent hypercortisolism has been established, the next step is the exclusion of an ectopic ACTH syndrome by a high-dose dexamethasone suppression test. In 95% of Cushing disease cases, the plasma cortisol levels are reduced to less than 50% of baseline, whereas in ectopic ACTH or adrenal tumors cortisol levels remain unchanged. Corticotropin-releasing hormone (CRH) stimulation is also advo-

Table 73-1 ■ Biochemical Evaluation for Cushing Syndrome

A. Screening for Cushing syndrome
1. Measurement of 24 h UFC in 2 or 3 collections. Test is unequivocal for hypercortisolism if the cortisol level is 4-fold that of normal in 2 of 3 screens. If equivocal, proceed to the low-dose DST. Salivary cortisol levels are also highly sensitive and specific.
2. Low-dose DST. 1 mg dexamethasone is administered at 11 pm and serum cortisol is drawn the following day at 8 am. A 2-day test is also commonly performed.
If < 5 μg/dL: Cushing syndrome is excluded
If 5-10 μg/dL: Indeterminate and retesting is necessary
If > 10 μg/dL: Cushing syndrome is probably present

B. Tests to distinguish primary Cushing disease from ectopic or adrenal tumors
1. Serum ACTH is low in adrenal tumors. Plasma ACTH (values > 10 pg/mL are suggestive of ACTH-dependent disease; values < 5 pg/mL are suggestive of ACTH-independent disease).
Abdominal CT can help identify a unilateral adrenal mass or bilateral adrenal enlargement in ACTH-dependent cases
2. High-dose DST. 8 mg of dexamethasone is administered at 11 pm and serum cortisol is drawn the following day at 8 am. A 2-day test is also commonly performed.
In 95% of cases of Cushing disease, plasma cortisol is suppressed by 50%
No suppression is seen with ectopic or adrenal sources
3. CRH stimulation test. Can be used after an equivocal high-dose DST.
Cushing disease responds to CRH with further increases in plasma cortisol levels
Ectopic and adrenal tumors do not respond to CRH
4. IPSS is reserved for persistent equivocal testing or in re-operations in which IPSS was not initially performed.
After CRH administration, an inferior petrosal sinus/plasma ACTH gradient > 3:1 is suggestive of Cushing disease and aids with lateralization

Abbreviations: DST, dexamethasone suppression test; UFC, urinary free cortisol; CRH, corticotrophin releasing hormone; IPSS, inferior petrosal sinus sampling.

cated in conjunction with the dexamethasone suppression test in order to increase sensitivity.[77] In patients where this testing is not compelling, inferior petrosal sinus sampling (IPSS) may be performed to confirm the pituitary etiology.

After the definitive diagnosis of Cushing disease has been established, the tumor must be localized before treatment can be initiated. If an MRI demonstrates a possible adenoma, treatment can then be initiated. The threshold for most MRI techniques is an adenoma 3 mm in diameter; however, 50% of ACTH-secreting tumors may thus be undetected. In this case IPSS and cavernous sinus sampling to measure the levels of ACTH after CRH stimulation should be performed. A gradient of 2:1 localizes the adenoma within the pituitary gland. The results may suggest laterality in the pituitary gland with this technique, but there is a 25-30% error rate in the localization.[78]

Treatment

Transsphenoidal surgical resection is the first option for treatment of Cushing disease. A review of the current surgical literature demonstrates that the remission rates range from 76% to 91%, and in microadenomas, from 84% to 94%.[79] Outcomes with the latter group were found to be dependent on the ability to visualize that adenoma on MRI.[80] The outcomes in macroadenomas appear to be dependent on the degree of invasiveness, with a reported 64% cure rate with surgery alone and 83% with adjuvant radiotherapy.[79] During the immediate postoperative period there is a rapid decline in both serum cortisol and ACTH levels, and patients must be monitored closely for symptoms of hypocortisolism (Addisonian crisis). Most patients require replacement therapy for up to 1 year as their own hypothalamic-pituitary axis recovers from the chronic overstimulation by ACTH. Various studies have attempted to assess the predictors of long-term cure.[81,82] Subnormal levels of cortisol and ACTH postoperatively are strong indicators for full remission, but even in these cases a 15-25% recurrence rate may occur over time.[16,83] In our experience, even normal cortisol and restoration of normal dexamethasone suppression do not necessarily indicate lasting remission. Because of this, long-term follow-up is essential in these patients.

Both radiotherapy and radiosurgery have been commonly used as adjuvant treatment of patients with recurrent or invasive tumors that are not cured by surgery alone. The cure rates of conventional radiotherapy have been reported to be as high as 90% at 5 years post-treatment. A large proportion of these patients began to experience hypopituitarism in later years, and 5% developed Nelson's syndrome.[84] Conventional radiation is not used as a primary modality because remission cannot be achieved for a long-period, and patients continue to suffer from the symptoms and morbidities of Cushing disease. As an alternative, radiosurgery has the advantage of having an effect on ACTH secretion much sooner than conventional radiation. Cure rates of 35-90% are reported, and much lower rates of hypopituitarism.[85,86] The reported rates of success, however, are confounded by inconsistent measures of "cure" and limited long-term follow-up. Radiosurgery as a primary treatment modality has limited outcome assessment.

For patients who fail surgical treatment or in whom surgery cannot be tolerated, the most common medical treatment is ketoconazole, which acts by blocking adrenal steroid synthesis. Occasionally, ketoconazole is also used for a few weeks preoperatively to control the severe manifestations of hypercortisolism. Cortisol and ACTH levels can return to normal in up to 90% of patients, but patients must be monitored closely for hepatotoxicity; the effects of ketoconazole stop immediately after discontinuation.[87] Other agents have also been employed, including aminoglutethimide, metyrapone, mitotane, and cyproheptadine. Recent studies are attempting to assess the role of dopamine agonists in the treatment of ACTH-secreting tumors. The administration of cabergoline therapy for 3 months was found to inhibit cortisol secretion in 60% of patients, with a normalization in 40% of patients.[88] This study also demonstrated dopamine receptor (D2) immunostaining in a majority of ACTH-secreting adenomas and requires further study. The PPAR-γ ligand rosiglitazone is also being studied as a possible new treatment option.[89]

Total adrenalectomy can also control hypercortisolism but requires lifelong dependence on exogenous glucocorticoid and mineral corticoid replacement. Additionally it can result in Nelson syndrome in 10-30% of patients and carries a generally unfavorable prognosis. Nelson's syndrome presents as hyperpigmentation from loss of cortisol inhibition and the stimulation of melanocytes by elevated ACTH. Most patients that present with Nelson syndrome harbor large, invasive pituitary adenomas that are very difficult to cure surgically and often require adjuvant radiotherapy and medical treatment. Studies have demonstrated variable effectiveness of neurosurgical treatment of Nelson's syndrome, ranging from 10% to 70%. These small series, however, have been plagued by lack of uniform definitions of "cure" and limited long-term follow-up.[90,91] More recently, a report on 13 patients with Nelson syndrome with a median follow-up of 17 years more convincingly demonstrated the efficacy of neurosurgical intervention.[92] Fortunately, the overall incidence has declined significantly since transsphenoidal surgery replaced bilateral adrenalectomy as the primary treatment of Cushing disease.

In the event of a noncure, a second surgical procedure with a more aggressive exploration of the pituitary gland for tumor is usually effective, since the most common cause of surgical failure is that the adenoma could not be found.[93] If IPSS was not performed prior to the first surgery, it should be before a second surgery. A complete hypophysectomy, even after initial failure, is rarely indicated; it is performed at our institution only for patients with a tenuous condition or in those who insist on it. In the event of surgical failure after a second surgery, medical therapy, radiation, or even bilateral adrenalectomy can be considered. Because of the significant rate of recurrence, even many years after surgery, patients in remission need to follow-up with interval endocrine evaluations.

Silent ACTH-Secreting Adenomas

A more recently described entity is that of silent ACTH-secreting adenomas in which immunohistochemical staining demonstrates reactivity for ACTH without any preoperative signs or symptoms of hypercortisolism. The exact incidence is unclear but has been reported to be between 6% and 43% in published studies.[94] In addition to the lack of any clinical findings of Cushing disease, there is also no evidence of hypercortisolism on laboratory testing. This is usually a surprise diagnosis, and the role of the pathologist in accurately determining the entity is critical for the immediate postoperative period as well as for long-term management. Studies have suggested that silent corticotrophic adenomas behave aggressively with a high rate of recurrence, as high as 37%.[95,96] This underscores the reason for long-term follow-up as well as the possibility of postoperative radiation. In addition, studies have also shown that in the immediate postoperative period, a subgroup of silent ACTH-secreting adenomas develop ACTH-cortisol axis dysfunction and require postoperative steroid replacement.[94]

Gonadotropin-Secreting and Nonsecreting Pituitary Adenomas

Approximately 1/3 of pituitary tumors are considered nonsecreting adenomas. They are generally associated with an older age population, with a peak in the fifth decade. Patients usually present with signs and symptoms of hypopituitarism, and commonly with associated visual field defects and other ophthalmologic problems. Despite their similar clinical presentation, endocrine-inactive tumors are a heterogeneous group of tumors. Ultrastructural studies have demonstrated that these tumors actually contain secretory granules and that a majority of them synthesize FSH, LH, and the α-subunit with a smaller subset producing other anterior pituitary hormones that do not show clinical manifestations.[97] However, no clear and consistent difference in treatment or prognosis has emerged among the various subtypes.

Clinical Presentation

Because endocrine-inactive tumors do not cause hypersecretion syndromes, they usually present with symptoms associated with mass effect. Patients usually complain of headaches, visual changes, and symptoms of pituitary insufficiency. In a majority of cases, the tumor is a macroadenoma at the time of diagnosis.

Diagnosis

Aside from undergoing a routine endocrine evaluation, patients with a suspected endocrine-inactive tumor should have determination of the FSH, LH, and glycoprotein α- and β-subunits. Elevated levels of FSH and LH may be suggestive of a gonadotropin-cell adenoma, especially in postmenopausal women. Secretion of uncombined α- or β-subunits has been recognized with increasing frequency in pituitary tumors, suggesting the existence of still unknown defects in the coupling process.[98] In some patients, the tumor mass may interfere with the normal dopamine-modulated suppression within the pituitary stalk and result in a mildly elevated PRL level.

Treatment

Surgery remains the primary treatment of patients with inactive adenomas. The goals are to relieve the mass effect, restore pituitary function, and to obtain a tissue diagnosis. As with other pituitary adenomas, the preferred approach is transsphenoidal, but cases with significant extension outside the sella may require a transcranial approach. The results of surgery for endocrine-inactive tumors are not as clearly described as for other adenomas because there are no clear criteria for cure. Studies have consistently demonstrated that 70-80% of patients experience significant improvement in visual function.[99] In addition, nearly 100% of patients report resolution of headaches,[100] and there is an improvement in pituitary function ranging from 15% to 57%, depending on the series and the criteria for hypopituitarism.[99]

Clinical improvement is not suggestive of complete tumor removal. Postoperative imaging a few months after surgery is required to assess the extent of tumor resection. Early imaging may not be as helpful or accurate because of confounding edema, postoperative hemorrhage, and hemostatic material. Studies report that residual tumor is identified in 66-86% of patients, but the rate of recurrence with gross resection is highly variable in the literature.[101,102]

Radiotherapy or radiosurgery is rarely used as the primary treatment of inactive adenomas, but rather as an adjuvant in patients found to have residual tumor postoperatively or significant suprasellar or cavernous sinus involvement preoperatively. Because of the significant risks of radiation therapy to the pituitary region, however, many practitioners advocate that residual tumors should be followed with serial imaging and radiated only if the tumors grow.[103,104] A recent study by Tanaka and colleagues focuses on the "natural history" of residual nonfunctioning adenoma by correlating tumor-volume doubling time, patient's age, and a proliferation index (MIB-1).[105] In 40 patients with a mean follow-up of 53 months, they found a significant difference in doubling time in patients below and above 61 years of age. Specifically, doubling time was much longer in older patients, suggesting that age should be taken into consideration when deciding on adjuvant treatment strategies.

A variety of studies have confirmed the limited efficacy of the medical management of non-secreting adenomas. In a recent evaluation of tumor volume in 9 nonfunctioning adenomas after 1 year of cabergoline treatment, expression of D2 dopamine receptors was found in 67% of cases.[106] Tumor shrinkage by MRI was observed in 56% of cases, but was truly notable in only 2 cases. Various other medical therapies, including bromocriptine, other dopamine-agonists, octreotide, and GnRH agonists and antagonists, have been tried without consistent shrinkage in tumor size and are seldom used.

TSH-Secreting Pituitary Adenomas

TSH-secreting adenomas are the least common of the pituitary tumors, representing only 1-2% of cases.[107]

Clinical Presentation

Patients can present with constitutional complaints consistent with long-standing thyroid dysfunction such as heat intolerance, diarrhea, weight-loss, fatigue, and exophthalmos, or complaints from the local mass effect such as headaches, visual changes, and symptoms of hypopituitarism. There is often a delay in diagnosis of these tumors because they are commonly misdiagnosed as Graves disease and are only detected when already large and invasive. They can be difficult to cure.[108]

Diagnosis

A large proportion of TSH-secreting tumors are associated with elevated levels of TSH, in spite of elevated free T3 and free T4. Additionally, documentation of an elevated α-subunit/TSH ratio increases the sensitivity of the biochemical diagnosis. Ultrasensitive immunometric TSH assays allow a distinction between patients with primary hyperthyroidism and those with central hyperthyroidism or resistance to thyroid hormone.

Treatment

Prior to any surgical intervention, the hyperthyroidism should be controlled in order to minimize the risk of cardiac arrhythmias that may occur intraoperatively or during induction of anesthesia. This is commonly done with a preoperative beta blocker. If the surgery is nonemergent, an antithyroid drug (propylthiouracil or methimazole) can also be added. Transsphenoidal surgery is the primary treatment, but is associated with cure rates of only about 35-62% with surgery alone and 55-81% in conjunction with medical treatment and radiotherapy.[109-111] The criteria for cure in TSH-secreting adenomas have not yet been well defined. External radiation is used if clinical remission is not obtained with surgery alone but not as a primary treatment modality.

Medical treatment of tumors with octreotide has been reported to be effective in 92% of TSH-secreting adenomas, with a normalization of TSH and tumor shrinkage in the vast majority.[112] Octreotide is often useful as an adjuvant therapy, but the long-term costs and problems of compliance preclude octreotide as the primary treatment in most cases. More recent reports have also shown that lanreotide, a long-acting analog, may have efficacy similar to that of octreotide.

Conclusion

Pituitary adenomas are a heterogeneous tumor population that require different management paradigms depending on the individual subtype. Transsphenoidal surgery remains the most common intervention in the treatment of these tumors. Adjuvant medical and radiation therapies continue to play a significant role in long-term control. In addition, recent advances in molecular biology, drug development, and improved radiosurgical outcomes hold significant promise for future treatment improvements.

Selected References

The complete reference list can be found at www.CANCERMEDICINE8.com

2. Landolt AM. Ultrastructure of human sella tumors. Correlations of clinical findings and morphology. *Acta Neurochir (Wien).* 1975;Suppl 22:1.
4. Kovacs K, Horvath E, Vidal S. Classification of pituitary adenomas. *J Neurooncol.* 2001;54:121.
6. Lloyd RV. Molecular pathology of pituitary adenomas. *J Neurooncol.* 2001;54:111.
8. Landis CA, Masters SB, Spada A, Pace AM, Bourne HR, Vallar L. GTPase inhibiting mutations activate the alpha chain of Gs and stimulate adenylyl cyclase in human pituitary tumours. *Nature.* 1989;340:692.
10. Cai WY, Alexander JM, Hedley-Whyte ET, et al. ras mutations in human prolactinomas and pituitary carcinomas. *J Clin Endocrinol Metab.* 1994;78:89.
13. Woloschak M, Roberts JL, Post KD. Loss of heterozygosity at the retinoblastoma locus in human pituitary tumors. *Cancer.* 1994;74:693.
16. Kreutzer J, Fahlbusch R. Diagnosis and treatment of pituitary tumors. *Curr Opin Neurol.* 2004;17:693.
20. Jane JA, Jr, Thapar K, Kaptain GJ, Maartens N, Laws ER, Jr. Pituitary surgery: transsphenoidal approach. *Neurosurgery.* 2002;51:435.
23. Liu JK, Couldwell WT. Contemporary management of prolactinomas. *Neurosurg Focus.* 2004;16:E2.
27. Randall RV, Scheithauer BW, Laws ER, Jr, Abbound CF, Ebersold MJ, Kao PC. Pituitary adenomas associated with hyperprolactinemia: a clinical and immunohistochemical study of 97 patients operated on transsphenoidally. *Mayo Clin Proc.* 1985;60:753.
29. Persani L, Beck-Peccoz P, Medri G, Conti A, Faglia G. Thyrotropin alpha- and beta-subunit responses to thyrotropin-releasing hormone and domperidone in normal subjects and in patients with microprolactinomas. *Neuroendocrinology.* 1991;53:411.
32. Maurer RA. Dopaminergic inhibition of prolactin synthesis and prolactin messenger RNA accumulation in cultured pituitary cells. *J Biol Chem.* 1980;255:8092.
36. Colao A, Di Sarno A, Cappabianca P, Di Somma C, Pivonello R, Lombardi G. Withdrawal of long-term cabergoline therapy for tumoral and nontumoral hyperprolactinemia. *N Engl J Med.* 2003;349:2023.
37. Delgrange E, Sassolas G, Perrin G, Jan M, Trouillas J. Clinical and histological correlations in prolactinomas, with special reference to bromocriptine resistance. *Acta Neurochir (Wien).* 2005;147:751.
38. Schade R, Andersohn F, Suissa S, Haverkamp W, Garbe E. Dopamine agonists and the risk of cardiac-valve regurgitation. *N Engl J Med.* 2007;356:29.
39. Zanettini R, Antonini A, Gatto G, Gentile R, Tesei S, Pezzoli G. Valvular heart disease and the use of dopamine agonists for Parkinson's disease. *N Engl J Med.* 2007;356:39.
40. Melmed S. Update in pituitary disease. *J Clin Endocrinol Metab.* 2008;93:331.
51. Freda PU, Landman RE, Sundeen RE, Post KD. Gender and age in the biochemical assessment of cure of acromegaly. *Pituitary.* 2001;4:163.
52. Giustina A, Barkan A, Casanueva FF, et al. Criteria for cure of acromegaly: a consensus statement. *J Clin Endocrinol Metab.* 2000;85:526.
53. Freda PU, Wardlaw SL, Post KD. Long-term endocrinological follow-up evaluation in 115 patients who underwent transsphenoidal surgery for acromegaly. *J Neurosurg.* 1998;89:353.
54. Laws ER, Vance ML, Thapar K. Pituitary surgery for the management of acromegaly. *Horm Res.* 2000;53(Suppl 3):71.
55. Trepp R, Stettler C, Zwahlen M, Seiler R, Diem P, Christ ER. Treatment outcomes and mortality of 94 patients with acromegaly. *Acta Neurochir (Wien).* 2005;147:243.
59. Kim SH, Huh R, Chang JW, Park YG, Chung SS. Gamma Knife radiosurgery for functioning pituitary adenomas. *Stereotact Funct Neurosurg.* 1999;72(Suppl 1):101.
60. Kim MS, Lee SI, Sim JH. Gamma Knife radiosurgery for functioning pituitary microadenoma. *Stereotact Funct Neurosurg.* 1999;72(Suppl 1):119.
65. Stewart PM, Kane KF, Stewart SE, Lancranjan I, Sheppard MC. Depot long-acting somatostatin analog (Sandostatin-LAR) is an effective treatment for acromegaly. *J Clin Endocrinol Metab.* 1995;80:3267.
66. Ayuk J, Stewart SE, Stewart PM, Sheppard MC. Long-term safety and efficacy of depot long-acting somatostatin analogs for the treatment of acromegaly. *J Clin Endocrinol Metab.* 2002;87:4142.
67. Stewart PM. Pegvisomant: an advance in clinical efficacy in acromegaly. *Eur J Endocrinol.* 2003;148(Suppl 2):S27.
68. van der Lely AJ, Hutson RK, Trainer PJ, et al. Long-term treatment of acromegaly with pegvisomant, a growth hormone receptor antagonist. *Lancet.* 2001;358:1754.
69. Colao A, Cuocolo A, Marzullo P, et al. Effects of 1-year treatment with octreotide on cardiac performance in patients with acromegaly. *J Clin Endocrinol Metab.* 1999;84:17.
74. Graham KE, Samuels MH, Nesbit GM, et al. Cavernous sinus sampling is highly accurate in distinguishing Cushing's disease from the ectopic adrenocorticotropin syndrome and in predicting intrapituitary tumor location. *J Clin Endocrinol Metab.* 1999;84:1602.
75. Trilck M, Flitsch J, Ludecke DK, Jung R, Petersenn S. Salivary cortisol measurement—a reliable method for the diagnosis of Cushing's syndrome. *Exp Clin Endocrinol Diabetes.* 2005;113:225.
76. Newell-Price J, Trainer P, Besser M, Grossman A. The diagnosis and differential diagnosis of Cushing's syndrome and pseudo-Cushing's states. *Endocr Rev.* 1998;19:647.
81. Chen JC, Amar AP, Choi S, Singer P, Couldwell WT, Weiss MH. Transsphenoidal microsurgical treatment of Cushing disease: postoperative assessment of surgical efficacy by application of an overnight low-dose dexamethasone suppression test. *J Neurosurg.* 2003;98:967.
82. Rollin GA, Ferreira NP, Junges M, Gross JL, Czepielewski MA. Dynamics of serum cortisol levels after transsphenoidal surgery in a cohort of patients with Cushing's disease. *J Clin Endocrinol Metab.* 2004;89:1131.
83. Bochicchio D, Losa M, Buchfelder M. Factors influencing the immediate and late outcome of Cushing's disease treated by transsphenoidal surgery: a retrospective study by the European Cushing's Disease Survey Group. *J Clin Endocrinol Metab.* 1995;80:3114.
90. Pereira MA, Halpern A, Salgado LR, et al. A study of patients with Nelson's syndrome. *Clin Endocrinol (Oxf).* 1998;49:533.
91. Wislawski J, Kasperlik-Zaluska AA, Jeske W, et al. Results of neurosurgical treatment by a transsphenoidal approach in 10 patients with Nelson's syndrome. *J Neurosurg.* 1985;62:68.
92. Kelly PA, Samandouras G, Grossman AB, Afshar F, Besser GM, Jenkins PJ. Neurosurgical treatment of Nelson's syndrome. *J Clin Endocrinol Metab.* 2002;87:5465.

74 Neoplasms of the Thyroid

Steven I. Sherman, MD

It was estimated that more than 37,000 individuals would be diagnosed in 2008 with carcinoma of the thyroid gland and that about 1600 patients would die as a consequence of complications of these diseases or their treatments.[1] Now the sixth most commonly diagnosed malignancy in women, the age-adjusted incidence of thyroid carcinoma has risen faster than that of any other cancer, and the age-adjusted mortality is also among the most rapidly increasing.[2] Histologically, 80% and 14%, respectively, are either papillary or follicular carcinomas, differentiated carcinomas that derive from the thyroid hormone producing follicular epithelial cells. Another 4% are medullary carcinoma, a neuroendocrine malignancy, and the remaining 2% are the highly aggressive anaplastic carcinoma. Rates of disease recurrence and cancer-specific mortality are increased in patients with metastases, especially those with extracervical spread. In the Surveillance, Epidemiology, and End Results (SEER) report of 15,700 patients, the overall 10-year age-and gender-corrected survival rates were 98% for papillary, 92% for follicular, 80% for medullary, and 13% for anaplastic carcinoma.[3] Older age at diagnosis and wider spread of disease are associated with a worse prognosis, independent of the type of cancer. Although differentiated carcinomas have a 2:1 female predominance, male gender confers a slightly worse prognosis.

Because of a lack of randomized comparative trials, decisions regarding the selection of treatments for these diseases are based largely on retrospective analyses and consensus recommendations.[4,5] Therapy routinely involves multiple modalities, including surgery and thyroid hormone, radioiodine (for differentiated tumors), and external radiation and chemotherapy for selected patients with advanced disease. However, the poor response to treatment for metastatic thyroid cancer has recently triggered development of newer therapies.

Diagnostic Evaluation of the Solitary Thyroid Nodule

The most common clinical presentation of a patient with thyroid carcinoma is with a solitary thyroid nodule, of which 5% are malignant (Table 74-1).[6] Whereas about 5% of individuals have a palpable nodule, ultrasonography reveals clinically unsuspected nodules in 20-70% of individuals without palpable lesions, and multiple nodules are frequent.[7] Sonographic criteria that increase the likelihood of malignancy include the presence of microcalcifications, hypoechogenicity, irregular infiltrative margins, and increased intranodular vascularity.[8] Incidentally detected thyroid nodules are also seen in 1-2% of Fluorodeoxyglucose-Positron Emission Tomography (FDG-PET) scans, for which the risk of malignancy up to 40%.[9] Thyroid ultrasound with cytologic examination of a fine needle aspirate (FNA) of solitary nodules at least 1 cm in size is the most appropriate diagnostic procedure; in the setting of multiple nodules, those with suspicious sonographic appearances (and if none are present, the largest) should be preferentially aspirated. Papillary, medullary, and anaplastic carcinomas can be readily diagnosed on the basis of cytologic criteria.[10] However, the distinction between follicular carcinoma and benign follicular adenoma requires histologic demonstration of either invasion through the tumor capsule or vascular invasion. Hence, follicular adenomas and carcinomas are grouped together cytologically as indeterminate or suspicious follicular neoplasms. Up to 25% of aspirations are inadequate or nondiagnostic, largely because of aspiration of cystic, hemorrhagic, or hypocellular colloid nodules. The false-positive and false-negative rates for nodules characterized as "malignant" and "benign," respectively, are less than 5%. For suspicious follicular lesions, the overall rate of carcinoma is approximately 20%, with higher rates associated with larger nodule size, older age, and male gender. Intraoperative frozen section evaluation adds little to the evaluation of follicular neoplasms, but may occasionally be helpful to confirm the diagnosis of cytologically suspected papillary carcinoma.[11] For nodules in which fine-needle aspiration yields inadequate diagnostic material, repeat aspiration, particularly with ultrasonography guidance, can augment the accuracy of the procedure.[12]

By radionuclide scanning, malignant thyroid lesions are usually hypofunctioning or "cold," but this finding is both nonspecific and nondiagnostic. In contrast, a "hot" hyperfunctioning nodule causing thyrotoxicosis is highly likely to be a benign follicular adenoma. Thus, only patients with a suppressed thyroid stimulating hormone (TSH) should undergo radioiodine scanning to determine the function of significant nodules, and FNA performed only for nonfunctioning lesions. Other imaging procedures, such as computed tomography (CT), magnetic resonance imaging (MRI), and PET have no role in the routine diagnostic evaluation of thyroid nodules.

Table 74-1 Differential Diagnosis of a Thyroid Nodule

Benign thyroid disease
Macrofollicular
Colloid adenoma
Adenomatoid hyperplasia
Microfollicular
Follicular adenoma
Hürthle cell adenoma
Toxic adenoma
Hashimoto thyroiditis
Graves disease
Infection
Tuberculosis
Fungal
Pneumocystis
Abscess
Thyroid cyst
Infiltrative and granulomatous disease
Malignant thyroid disease
Differentiated thyroid carcinoma
Papillary thyroid carcinoma
Follicular thyroid carcinoma
Medullary thyroid carcinoma
Anaplastic thyroid carcinoma
Primary thyroid lymphoma
Metastatic
Breast carcinoma
Renal cell carcinoma
Lung carcinoma
Melanoma
Colon carcinoma
Gastric carcinoma
Extrathyroidal disease
Parathyroid adenoma, cyst, or carcinoma
Esophageal diverticulum
Lipoma
Aberrant subclavian artery

Differentiated Thyroid Carcinoma

Pathogensis

The only well-established risk factor for differentiated thyroid cancer is radiation exposure, especially during infancy. Therapeutic irradiation for benign conditions, such as thymic and tonsillar enlargement, or for malignant diseases, such as Hodgkin lymphoma and before bone marrow transplantation, is associated with an excess relative risk for thyroid malignancy of 3-9 per Gy.[13] Exposure to internal sources of radiation after the Chernobyl nuclear accident led to marked increase in the incidence of papillary carcinoma, the highest risks seen in younger children.[14]

Differentiated carcinoma is a component of several inherited syndromes, including familial adenomatous polyposis, Gardner syndrome, Cowden disease, Turcot syndrome, and Carney complex. Familial nonmedullary carcinoma, described in families with at least two first-degree relatives with the disease, has been reported in 5% of all papillary carcinoma patients, and may portend a more-aggressive disease course.[15,16] Putative susceptibility loci have been identified on chromosomal regions 1p13.2-1q22, 2q21, 14q32 and 19p13.2.[17]

Follicular cell tumorigenesis may develop along several paths, many of which are also common in other solid tumors. For papillary carcinoma, an early initiating event is usually activation of intracellular signaling upstream from the mitogen-activated protein (MAP) kinase, including (1) the V600E mutation in the bioinformatic resources and application facility (BRAF) kinase, (2) one of several chromosomal rearrangements forming *RET/PTC* oncogenes, or (3) activated *RAS*.[18] *BRAF* mutations have been associated with more aggressive histologic variants, greater frequency of recurrence, and less radioiodine responsiveness.[19] Other factors that may contribute to progression of papillary carcinomas include overexpression of other intracellular kinases, deoxyribonucleic acid (DNA) hypermethylation and histone deacetylation leading to silencing of tumor-suppressor genes, and cell-cycle dysregulation.[20,21] In contrast, follicular carcinomas may rarely arise from benign adenomas as a result of transforming events. Mutations in *RAS*, which are also common in follicular adenomas, may lead to greater genomic instability, increased allelic loss, and more risk for transforming chromosomal rearrangements, such as t(2;3)(q13;p25) that fuses the DNA binding domain of a thyroid-specific transcription factor, PAX8, to peroxisome proliferator-activated receptor (PPAR)-gamma-1 in follicular carcinoma but not benign lesions.[22]

Pathologic Features

Papillary carcinomas are characterized by the presence of papillae consisting of a well-defined fibrovascular core surrounded by one or two layers of tumor cells (Fig. 74-1). Follicles and colloid are typically absent. Nuclei tend to be large, oval, and appear crowded and overlapping on microscopic sections. The nuclei contain hypodense powdery chromatin, cytoplasmic pseudoinclusions caused by a redundant nuclear membrane, and nuclear grooves.

Of the several histologic subtypes, the follicular variant accounts for approximately 10% of all papillary carcinomas. The cells are organized into follicles rather than papillae, but cytologically, they display the typical nuclear features of papillary carcinomas. Rates of recurrence and survival with the follicular variant are very similar to those of patients with common-type papillary carcinomas.[23] In contrast, the tall cell variant of papillary carcinoma is a more aggressive tumor, characterized by eosinophilic tumor cells that are twice as tall as they are wide. The primary tumors tend to be large, are often invasive, and frequently have both local and distant metastases at the time of diagnosis. The 5-year survival rate is 75-85%.[24]

Follicular carcinomas are distinguished from benign follicular lesions on the basis of invasiveness. These tumors are commonly encapsulated, and invasion can commonly be demonstrated in one or more foci along the capsule or across vascular endothelial walls. Semiquantitative assessment of the magnitude of invasion can separate follicular carcinomas into minimally invasive and widely invasive lesions; a minimally invasive follicular carcinoma has only scattered foci of capsular or vascular invasion. In contrast to papillary carcinomas, cytologic features do not reliably distinguish benign from malignant follicular lesions.

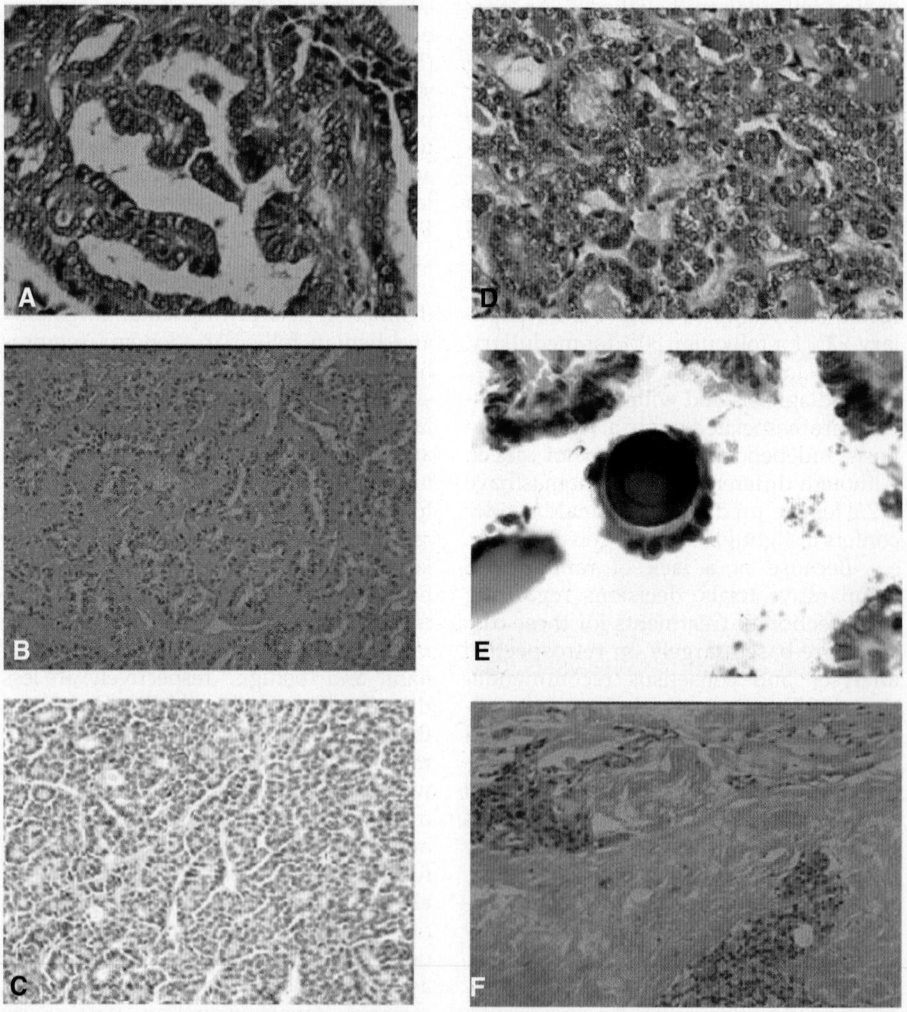

Figure 74-1 Pathologic features of differentiated thyroid carcinoma. (**A**) Papillary carcinoma, with characteristic fibrovascular papillary formation, crowded nuclei, and nuclear clearing. (**B**) Follicular variant of papillary carcinoma, with typical cells of papillary carcinoma in follicular formations. (**C**) Tall cell variant of papillary carcinoma, with cells at least twice as tall as they are wide and eosinophilic cytoplasm. (**D**) Psammoma body of papillary carcinoma. (**E**) Microfollicular neoplasm, with scant colloid. (**F**) Follicular carcinoma, demonstrating invasion across a thick capsule into neighboring thyroid.

Hürthle cell neoplasms are formed by cells containing numerous mitochondria, which impart a granular, eosinophilic appearance to their cytoplasm.[25] Most have a follicular architecture and are diagnosed as adenomas or carcinomas by the same criteria applied to other follicular neoplasms. A Hürthle-cell variant of papillary carcinoma is much less common and tends to be more aggressive than typical papillary carcinomas.

Insular carcinomas, characterized by small cells arranged in nests, are often placed in the intermediate category of poorly differentiated thyroid carcinomas. These tumors generally concentrate radioiodine and are therefore treated as differentiated cancers.

Clinicopathologic Staging

Although multiple clinicopathologic staging schemes exist for differentiated thyroid carcinoma, the sixth edition of the AJCC/UICC staging approach (Table 74-2) is generally recommended for use, but evidence for a superior value for predicting death caused by thyroid cancer has only been reported for the previous fifth edition.[26-28] Both versions classify patients with distant metastases but who are under the age of 45 years as being at "low risk" for death, one of several significant caveats to clinical use of these schemes. The importance of histologic features such as tumor size and extrathyroidal invasion underscore the need for pathologists to report these data uniformly on thyroidectomy specimens.[29]

Primary Surgical Management

Total thyroidectomy has been the initial surgical procedure for up to 90% of patients with differentiated thyroid carcinoma.[30] This choice is supported by these arguments: (1) foci of papillary carcinoma are commonly found in both thyroid lobes[31,32]; (2) contralateral recurrence occurs in 5-10% of patients who undergo unilateral surgery; and (3) the efficacy of therapy with radioiodine and the specificity of serum thyroglobulin levels as a tumor marker are maximized by resection of as much thyroid tissue as possible, In a retrospective analysis of the outcomes of 1685 low-risk patients, the 20-year recurrence rate after lobectomy was 22%, compared with 8% for patients treated with total thyroidectomy.[33] Other retrospective studies (although not all) reported similar results of reduced recurrence. Most recently, analysis of a multicenter prospective thyroid cancer registry database has demonstrated improved survival associated with total or near-total thyroidectomy in patients with stages II to IV disease (risk ratio for mortality compared with less than near-total thyroidectomy 0.64 for stage II, 0.79 for stages III and IV combined).[34] In contrast, the major argument put forth to support a unilateral procedure is the higher risk for complications following bilateral surgery, including hypoparathyroidism and recurrent laryngeal nerve paralysis that may not be justified by small differences in survival in low risk patients.[35,36]

In the absence of prospective trials, consensus panels have generally recommended that a near-total or total thyroidectomy should be performed by an experienced thyroid surgeon if the primary papillary carcinoma or Hürthle cell carcinoma is at least 1 cm in diameter, if there is extrathyroidal extension of tumor, or if there are metastases.[4,5] In selected patients whose papillary tumor is <1 cm in diameter and confined to one lobe of the gland, a unilateral lobectomy may be sufficient.[37] For patients with a cytologically suspicious follicular neoplasm, unilateral lobectomy and isthmusectomy should be performed; a complete thyroidectomy is done if there is a diagnosis of malignancy.

Although microscopic regional nodal metastasis of papillary carcinoma occurs in up to 80% of patients, only about 35% have cervical or mediastinal node metastasis grossly detectable at the time of surgery, most commonly found in lateral cervical compartments.[38] Unlike most other malignancies, the presence of lymph node metastasis is only a minor risk factor for mortality.[39] Whereas resection of clinically involved central compartment (level VI) nodes has been associated with improved survival and is commonly recommended, the potential benefit of prophylactic level VI neck dissection may only outweigh the potential surgical morbidity when performed by experienced thyroid surgeons.[40] Compartment-oriented modified radical lateral dissections should be performed if node involvement is identified.[41] Results suggesting that neck dissections at the time of initial thyroidectomy may decrease the incidence of regional recurrence support the practice of routine preoperative ultrasonography to evaluate regional lymphatics.[42,43] In the presence of invasion of aerodigestive tract structures, similar survival rates are achieved from either complete surgical resection or shave excision leaving only microscopic residual disease.[44] In the presence of frank cartilage destruction or intraluminal involvement of the aerodigestive tract structures, a shave excision cannot

Table 74-2 **TNM (Tumor, Node, Metastases): The AJCC (American Joint Committee on Cancer) Staging Scheme for Thyroid Carcinomas (Sixth Edition)**

T: Tumor status		
T1	<2 cm	
T2	2–4 cm	
T3	>4 cm or minimal extraglandular invasion	
T4	Extraglandular invasion	
T4a	Gross invasion	
T4b	Prevertebral, carotid, or mediastinal invasion	
Tx	Tumor status unknown	
N: Regional node status		
N0	No nodes involved	
N1a	Cervical level VI nodes positive	
N1b	Unilateral, contralateral or bilateral cervical levels II-V or mediastinal nodes positive	
Nx	Nodes status unknown	
M: Distant metastases		
M0	No distant metastases	
M1	Distant metastases	
Mx	Metastases status unknown	
Stage assignments		
	Differentiated carcinoma (<45 years)	Differentiated carcinoma (>45 years) or medullary carcinoma
Stage I	Any T, any N, M0	T1, N0 M0
Stage II	Any T, any N, M1	T2, N0, M0
Stage III		T3–4, N0, M0 Any T, N1a, M0
Stage IV		A: T4a, any N, M0 Any T, N1b, M0 B: T4b, any N, M0 C: Any T, any N, M1
Anaplastic carcinomas		
All are classified as stage IV		

be performed without leaving gross tumor behind, leading to a 50% death rate within 4 years. Surgery in patients with extensively invasive thyroid carcinoma should, therefore, aim to remove all gross tumors, attempting to retain as much airway, vocal, and digestive function as possible. However, only if the tumor is unresectable or the patient does not agree to a radical resection should gross tumor be left behind in the neck.[45]

Postoperative Adjuvant Therapy

Radioiodine

Adjuvant radioiodine therapy following primary surgery has two rationales: (1) to destroy any residual microscopic foci of disease within a thyroid bed remnant or in regional nodal metastases, and (2) to increase the specificity and negative predictive value of subsequent serum thyroglobulin measurements and 131I scanning for detection of recurrent or metastatic disease by eliminating residual normal tissue (referred to as "ablation"). Conflicting data have been reported from multiple retrospective studies of the efficacy of radioiodine. In a recent meta-analysis, only one of the seven included studies reported improved survival following adjuvant radioiodine and improved locoregional disease-free survival was observed in only three; conclusions were unchanged following a recent update of the analysis.[46,47] In a recent multicenter thyroid cancer registry, improved survival was associated with postoperative radioiodine use in stages II to IV disease patients after adjustment for extent of thyroidectomy, and in stage III to IV patients when also adjusted for thyroid hormone suppression therapy.[34] For patients with residual disease following optimal surgery, including extracervical metastases, radioiodine therapy is also recommended. In contrast, ablation may be withheld for patients with small solitary primary tumors without evidence of extrathyroidal invasion or metastasis, particularly if under age 45 at diagnosis.

The efficacy of radioiodine depends on patient preparation, tumor-specific characteristics, sites of disease, and administered radioiodine activity. Iodide uptake by thyroid tissue is stimulated by TSH and is suppressed by increased endogenous iodide stores. Following thyroidectomy, the patient's thyroid hormone levels must decline sufficiently to allow the TSH concentration to rise sufficiently. This period of hormone withdrawal typically lasts 4-5 weeks. To minimize the resulting symptoms of hypothyroidism, the shorter-acting hormone liothyronine (T3) is often administered at doses of up to 25 μg two times per day. Lower doses are administered to elderly patients and those with ischemic heart disease. Liothyronine is stopped at least 2 weeks prior to radioiodine dosing. An alternative to thyroid hormone withdrawal is the use of exogenous recombinant human thyrotropin alfa, which in a recent small randomized study limited to low risk patients appeared equivalent to thyroid hormone withdrawal for stimulating radioiodine uptake and successful ablation.[48] In one nonrandomized case series, short term recurrence rates were similar regardless of method of TSH stimulation.[49] Patients should avoid foods with high iodine content for 1-2 weeks prior to the scanning.[50] For similar reasons, radioiodine uptake can be iatrogenically suppressed for 1-3 months after administration of iodinated intravenous contrast for radiographic procedures. Urinary iodine content can be measured to confirm excessive iodine intake if suspected.

Whole body radioiodine scans for localization of uptake prior to ablation or therapy are frequently performed 24-72 h after administration of a diagnostic activity of 2-5 mCi of ^{131}I. Most patients demonstrate significant uptake of radioiodine within the thyroid bed following thyroidectomy, presumably from normal residual thyroid. Greater sensitivity for the detection of residual or metastatic tumor can be attained with the use of higher amounts of ^{131}I. But larger radioisotope activities can lead to "stunning," in which reduced uptake of the subsequent ablative or therapeutic dose occurs as a consequence of radiation delivered by the diagnostic dose.[51] Use of 123I, with a lower radiation dose to thyroid tissue, may prevent stunning of therapeutic uptake after a diagnostic scan without loss of diagnostic accuracy, whether endogenous hypothyroidism or exogenous recombinant human TSH is used to stimulate uptake.[52,53] However, the exact utility of scanning before therapy in the absence of known metastatic disease is undefined, and therefore scanning before ablation may be considered optional for patients who are apparently free from gross metastases.[5,54] An alternative approach is to use a low activity of ^{123}I to measure radioiodine uptake in the thyroid bed before treatment, without requiring greater activities necessary for imaging.

With postoperative radioiodine uptake in the thyroid bed, or if no pretherapy scanning or uptake has been performed, an empirically selected activity of ^{131}I is administered for adjuvant ablation, typically 30-100 mCi. In general, higher efficacy rates have been reported with larger administered activities. Assuming that the 24-h radioiodine uptake is less than 5%, this lower activity has a similar efficacy of successful ablation and could be considered for patients with disease entirely confined to the thyroid gland.[55] Nonetheless, there is scant information about long-term outcomes, and considerably more study is required before such low doses can be generally recommended.[56] Alternatively, quantitative dosimetry can be applied to estimate the radioiodine activity necessary to deliver an effective radiation dose to the tissue of at least 30,000 cGy, which may reduce the risk of excessive marrow radiation exposure especially in older patients.[57] When substantial yet unsuspected locoregional disease or excessive thyroid remnants are detected, strong consideration is given to additional surgery before radioiodine administration.

A post-treatment scan is performed several days after administration of the radioiodine dose, but the diagnostic utility of such scans immediately after treatments is maximal in patients whose thyroid bed activity was previously ablated.[58]

Thyroid Hormone

Patients require life long thyroid hormone administration to treat postsurgical hypothyroidism and to minimize TSH stimulation to tumor growth. With TSH-suppressive thyroid hormone therapy, both overall survival and disease-free survival may be improved two to threefold, particularly in Tumor, Node, Metastases (TNM) or National Thyroid Cancer Treatment Cooperative Study (NTCTCS) stages III and IV patients.[34,59] Lesser degrees of suppression may also improve overall survival in stage I and II patients.[34] However, potential morbidity from overly aggressive thyroid hormone suppression therapy includes acceleration of osteoporosis,[60] provocation of atrial fibrillation,[61] and possibly cardiac hypertrophy and dysfunction and impaired quality of life.[62] The clinician must balance the risk for disease recurrence or progression with the risk for thyrotoxic complications in determining the degree of TSH-suppressive therapy. At least during the initial years of follow-up, patients at lower risk for thyroid cancer morbidity and mortality should have their TSH levels maintained between 0.1 and 0.5 mU/L, whereas patients at higher risk should have TSH levels suppressed to less than 0.1 mU/L.[5] Patients who remain disease-free for 5-10 years may potentially have their degree of TSH suppression reduced by lowering their doses of thyroid hormone; other mitigating factors, such as concurrent cardiac disease, may also dictate a need for reduced hormone dosing.

External Beam Radiation

External beam radiotherapy (EBRT) may be an effective adjuvant therapy to prevent locoregional recurrence in older patients with locally invasive papillary carcinoma.[63] A review of 282 patients found that postoperative EBRT did not significantly affect the locoregional control or disease-specific survival rates. However, in a subgroup of 155 patients with papillary histology and microscopic residual disease (evidence of disease at or within 2 mm of the resection margin, or tumor that was shaved off cervical structures), EBRT produced a significant improvement in 10-year rates of locoregional control (93% vs. 78%) and disease-specific survival (100% vs. 95%).[64] Increased freedom from locoregional and distant relapse has been reported in patients older than age 40 years with extrathyroidal extension and lymph node involvement from papillary carcinoma, when treated with adjuvant EBRT in addition to total thyroidectomy, two courses of ^{131}I, and TSH suppression.[65] In neither study was a benefit of adjuvant EBRT demonstrated for patients with follicular carcinoma. Adjuvant EBRT is likely of little benefit to those younger than age 45 years, and esophageal and tracheal side effects may be poorly tolerated by the elderly patient (>65 years). Intensity modulated radiotherapy (IMRT) may be associated with reduced toxicity.[66] EBRT, 40-50 Gy to the thyroid bed, is recommended in the setting of gross extrathyroidal invasion with presumed microscopic residual disease, as well as following incomplete resection near aerodigestive structures.

Long-Term Follow-Up

Diagnostic Imaging and Serum Thyroglobulin Monitoring

The follow-up paradigm for differentiated thyroid carcinomas has undergone significant changes in the past several years, in part due to the improved utility of cervical ultrasound and serum thyroglobulin measurements. Whereas patients following initial radioiodine ablation previously underwent routine radioiodine scanning, this procedure is now being used more selectively.[67] Ultrasonography of the thyroid bed and cervical node compartments can accurately identify locoregional metastases and recurrence measuring several millimeters in diameter and facilitate confirmatory FNA of such lesions.[68,69] Sensitivity of FNA to detect recurrent disease can be enhanced by measurement of thyroglobulin in the needle washout.[70] Neither CT nor MRI is as sensitive for detecting such small lesions, although these techniques are more readily standardized and less operator-dependent. Routine chest radiographs are of limited sensitivity, and probably can be avoided in low risk patients.[71]

The synthesis and secretion of thyroglobulin (Tg) is a differentiated characteristic of thyroid follicular cells.[72] In the long-term follow-up of patients, measurement of the serum Tg concentration aids the detection of residual, recurrent, or metastatic disease, particularly given the rough correlation between tumor size and Tg level. After thyroid resection and ablation, serum Tg concentrations should approach the limits of assay detectability, but may take several years to decline to an undetectable nadir following primary therapy.[73,74] An important factor in the interpretation of Tg concentrations is the concurrent level of TSH, given the dependence on TSH for Tg production. The sensitivity for detection of residual cancer is enhanced by elevation of the serum TSH during thyroid hormone withdrawal or by the use of recombinant TSH (thyrotropin alfa).[75] The sensitivity of detecting disease by measurement of Tg following TSH stimulation is 85-95% but may be as low as 50% during TSH suppression or with dedifferentiated tumors.[76] The utility of stimulated Tg measurements in the absence of scanning combined with cervical ultrasound has the greatest accuracy in low risk patients, but radioiodine scanning remains valuable for follow-up in high risk patients.[77,78] Recently introduced Tg assays with functional sensitivities as low as 0.1 ng/mL may potentially obviate the need for TSH-stimulated testing, but the clinical significance of such minimally detectable levels remains uncertain, particularly if stable or declining during follow-up.[79]

In immunometric assays, reported Tg concentrations can be falsely lowered by autoantibodies that bind Tg and prevent antigen interaction with assay's antibodies.[80] For the 25% of the thyroid cancer population with anti-Tg autoantibodies, serum Tg levels must be interpreted with caution. The persistence of anti-Tg autoantibodies following thyroidectomy and radioiodine ablation may in itself indicate the presence of residual thyroid tissue and an increased risk for recurrence.[81]

Therapy of Metastatic Disease

Surgery

Function-preserving compartmental node dissection is preferred, if possible, for patients with nodes >1 cm in diameter, and may produce undetectable Tg levels in up to 40% of patients.[82,83] In the setting of disease invading aerodigestive structures, grossly complete surgical excision can improve survival, but may require more extensive procedures such as tracheal resection and anastomosis or pharyngectomy. Palliative procedures can be employed when curative resection is not feasible, and can include tracheal stents, tracheotomy, and laser ablation, in addition to partial excision. For extracervical metastases, surgical resection can lead to improved survival in selected patients. In one report, nearly 30% of patients who underwent complete resection of their skeletal, pulmonary or intraabdominal metastases remained disease free after an average follow-up of 8 years.[84] Among patients with one or more brain metastases, surgical removal significantly improved median survival from 4 to 22 months; radio surgery may yield similar outcomes.[85,86] Symptom palliation can also result from surgical treatment, particularly for lesions causing pain or spinal cord compression.

Radioiodine

^{131}I treatment of regional nodal metastases yields a complete response in 80% of patients when at least 8000-10,000 cGy is delivered, but can be suboptimal in patients with bulky disease.[87] Patients with residual postoperative disease in the thyroid bed or in the regional lymph nodes are treated with high activities of ^{131}I. Efficacy has been reported with 150 mCi as an average dose, either as a result of empiric therapy or as determined by dosimetry.

Patients treated for iodine-concentrating pulmonary metastases, which occur in approximately 5% of cases of differentiated cancer, have a 5-year survival rate of 60-80%, as compared with a 5-year survival rate of 30% for those whose tumors do not take up iodine.[88,89] Long term survival is highest in those patients with pulmonary metastases seen on ^{131}I scanning, but not seen on chest radiography or CT. Nevertheless, only a minority of patients with such micronodular disease has a complete remission, and even cumulative ^{131}I activities greater than 600 mCi are rarely effective.[89] Patients with macronodular pulmonary metastases seen on chest radiography but not detected by ^{131}I scanning have the worst prognosis, and only rarely respond to large doses of ^{131}I. Radioiodine activities of 150-175 mCi are recommended for empiric treatment of pulmonary metastases. Advocates of dosimetry suggest treatment of distant metastases with the maximum tolerable doses ie, that dose which delivers no more than 200 cGy to the red marrow and 80-120 mCi whole-body retention. Such activities may exceed 300-400 mCi, but are calculated to allow the greatest degree of tumor kill without dose-limiting toxicity.[90] ^{131}I treatment of skeletal metastases may yield complete resolution of disease in fewer than 10% of treated patients, and partial remission in only 35%.[91] Patients with follicular carcinoma may be more likely to respond (Fig. 74-2). Empiric doses of 200 mCi are generally suggested for distant metastases outside the lungs. Following surgical debulking, radioiodine therapy can also be administered to patients with iodine-concentrating intracerebral metastases.[85]

Acute and chronic complications of ^{131}I can limit the usefulness of this treatment. In the short-term, radiation thyroiditis, painless neck edema, sialoadenitis, and tumor hemorrhage or edema occur in 10-20% of patients, particularly when higher doses are given. Over the long-term, ^{131}I therapy may be associated with dose-related development of secondary neoplasms, such as colorectal carcinoma, salivary tumors, and acute leukemias. Excess absolute risks are 14.4 solid cancers and 0.8 leukemias per GBq of ^{131}I at 10,000 person-years of follow-up.[92] Cumulative ^{131}I activities above 500-600 mCi are associated with a significant increase in risk. Oligospermia and transient ovarian failure also occur, but subsequent infertility is rare, except after high doses.[93,94] Patients who receive repeated high radiation doses to the lung parenchyma from radioiodine treatment of diffuse pulmonary metastases rarely develop pulmonary fibrosis. In contrast, administration of even a single treatment with 150 mCi ^{131}I can result in chronic epiphora due to nasolacrimal duct obstruction that may require dacryocystorhinostomy.[95]

As production of Tg and incorporation of radioiodine represent distinct differentiated functions of follicular cells, metastatic disease can be suspected by the presence of a detectable serum Tg in the absence of radioiodine uptake. Such "false-negative" results occur in up to 15% of diagnostic radioiodine scans in patients with detectable Tg levels following thyroid ablation. Despite a high frequency of post-therapy scans demonstrating foci of radioiodine uptake combined with a subsequent decrease in the serum Tg level when ^{131}I is administered in this setting, there is no evidence that these endpoints are associated with improved patient outcomes.[73,96] Instead, diagnostic imaging should be performed to identify foci of disease that could be surgically resected or treated by other means (Fig. 74-3), such as cervical ultrasonography, CT, or MRI. FDG-PET imaging can be particularly useful in localizing disease in patients with Tg levels greater than 10 ng/mL and negative radioiodine imaging, with minimal increase in sensitivity following thyrotropin injection.[97] In the absence of surgically resectable disease, only patients with evidence of progressive metastases, rising Tg levels greater than 10 ng/mL, or who are at high risk for disease-related mortality might receive a therapeutic trial of ^{131}I before embarking on other systemic treatment modalities. However, for younger patients with stable or minimally elevated Tg levels and no radiographic evidence of disease, evidence of benefit is insufficient to warrant empiric radioiodine.

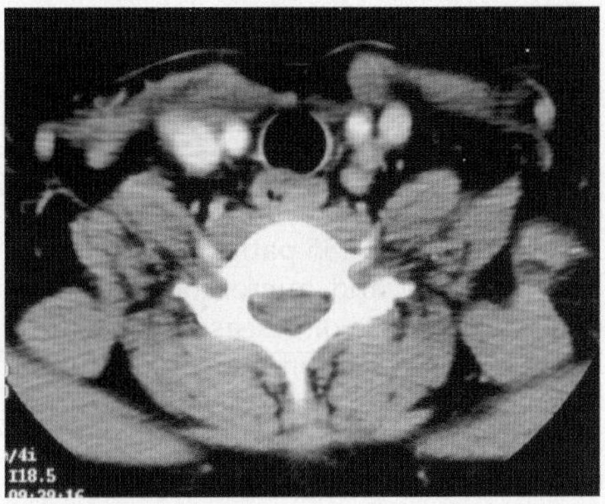

Figure 74-3 Contrast-enhanced CT of the neck in a patient with recurrent papillary thyroid carcinoma. Patient had previously undergone thyroidectomy and radioiodine ablation. Although a diagnostic radioiodine scan performed 1 week previously had shown no pathologic uptake, her serum TSH-stimulated thyroglobulin level was elevated, leading to the radiographic study. Following surgical resection of the two lymph nodes identified posterior to the left internal jugular vein and carotid artery, the serum thyroglobulin level became undetectable.

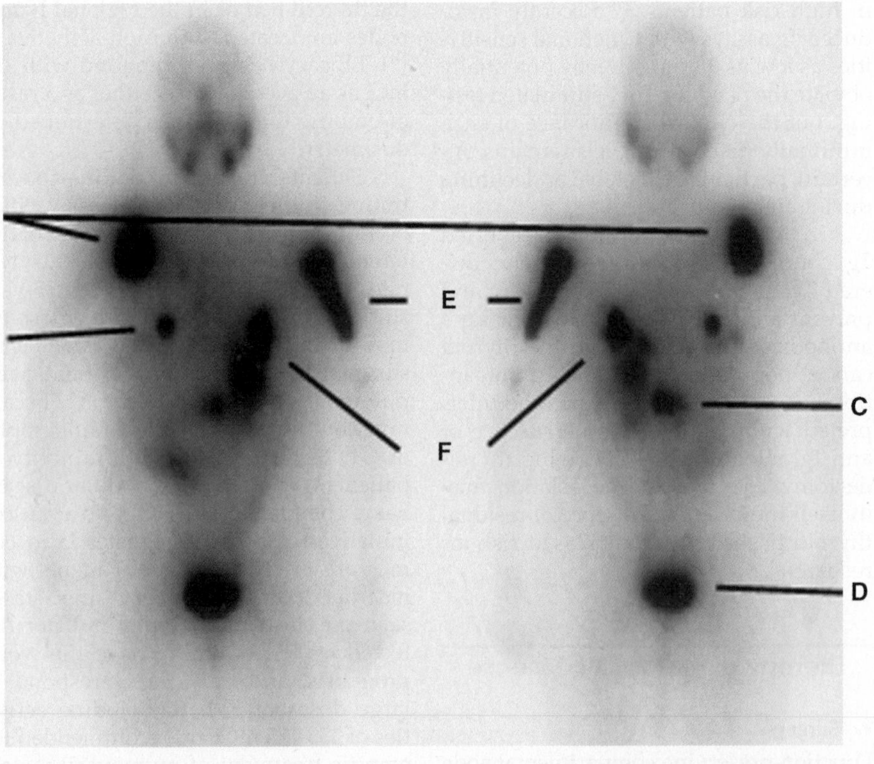

Figure 74-2 Anterior and posterior views of whole-body ^{131}I imaging in a patient with metastatic follicular thyroid carcinoma. Two years after a thyroidectomy and radioiodine ablation, the patient developed back and extremity pains. Following thyroid hormone withdrawal, a radioiodine scan was performed that revealed multiple skeletal and pulmonary metastases. External beam radiotherapy and multiple repeated doses of radioiodine led to resolution of her pain and stabilization of her disease. **(A)** Right shoulder metastasis. **(B)** Right lung metastasis. **(C)** Thoracic vertebra metastasis. **(D)** Radioiodine excreted in bladder. **(E)** Left humerus metastasis. **(F)** Left lung metastases superimposed on physiologic excretion into stomach.

External-Beam Radiation

Patients with unresectable gross locally invasive or metastatic disease in the neck may also benefit from the addition of EBRT, with 5-year local control and disease-specific survival rates of about 65%.[64] EBRT can also benefit patients with painful skeletal metastases. When surgical resection is not feasible, palliative radiation should be offered to patients with bone lesions that either cause pain or pose a risk for pathologic fracture. Radiation doses of 50 Gy in 25 fractions may be given for solitary lesions, but reduced doses should be administered for vertebral foci.

Chemotherapy

Until recently, little progress has been made since the original reports of transient partial responses to doxorubicin in approximately one-third of patients treated for distant metastases.[98] The recommended dose is 60-75 mg/m^2 every 3 weeks, and cumulative doses of up to 600 mg/m^2 can be administered in responsive patients. In one comparative trial, the combination of doxorubicin, 60 mg/m^2, and cisplatin, 40 mg/m^2, induced complete or partial response in 16%, whereas doxorubicin alone yielded a 31% response rate.[99] Toxicities, including pancytopenia and gastrointestinal side effects, are markedly more common and severe, however, during these combination therapies, without clear evidence of greater benefit.

Recently completed phase 2 trials demonstrate that anti-angiogenic therapies may produce partial response rates of up to 30% and stabilize another 40-50% of patients with progressive metastatic disease.[100-104] Clinical benefit lasting at least 24 weeks was observed in about half of patients. In studies of orally available antiangiogenic tyrosine kinase inhibitors (axitinib, motesanib diphosphate, and sorafenib), thyroid cancer patients experienced side effects similar to other solid tumor populations, including hypertension, diarrhea, fatigue, skin rashes and erythema, and weight loss. Multiple other agents are in clinical trials, targeting pathways involved in angiogenesis, cell cycle regulation, and tumor differentiation. For patients with clinically progressive metastatic disease who cannot enter clinical trials, therapy with sorafenib is appropriate as initial therapy.

Management of Differentiated Carcinoma in Special Populations

Thyroid carcinoma in children and adolescents is uncommon, and few large series have evaluated the long-term prognosis and appropriate therapy for young patients with these malignancies. A recent series described the extended follow-up of 112 young patients with differentiated thyroid carcinoma treated at the MD. Anderson Cancer Center.[105] One-fourth of the 99 living patients had developed recurrent disease, and 6 patients died of thyroid cancer at a mean of 26 years after initial diagnosis. One patient who had lung metastases at the time of diagnosis died of progressive pulmonary disease after 36 years. The other 5 patients developed lung and bone metastases and died after a 2- to 20-year disease-free interval. Three more patients died from complications of radiation therapy, one because of tracheal necrosis 26 years after diagnosis and two because of cervical sarcomas over 20 years after diagnosis. Two died from subsequent breast cancer. In another series of 61 young patients treated for thyroid cancer, the 20-year survival rate was 97%.[106] Two patients died of progressive metastatic thyroid cancer within 10 years of the initial operations. Three of the 10 patients who had lobectomy or subtotal thyroidectomy developed local recurrence in the residual thyroid gland, whereas none of the 51 patients who had total or near-total thyroidectomy developed a local recurrence, Given the high frequency of multifocal intrathyroidal disease, locoregional spread, and extracervical metastases, total thyroidectomy with nodal dissection and adjuvant radioiodine therapy should be offered to all young patients with differentiated carcinoma. Lifelong close surveillance is warranted because of the risk of late recurrences and disease progression. For the rare adolescent whose metastatic disease is radioiodine unresponsive, sorafenib may induce partial remission.[107]

Differentiated carcinoma is the second most common malignancy diagnosed in the prenatal and postpartum period, affecting 0.1% of all pregnancies.[108] There has been some concern that the hormonal factors associated with pregnancy might accelerate the progression of disease, but outcomes of pregnant women diagnosed with differentiated carcinoma do not differ from those of age-matched nonpregnant women.[109,110] In most cases, thyroidectomy can be performed in the second trimester when diagnosed early in pregnancy, whereas surgery can be deferred until the postpartum period for those found later; radioiodine, however, is only administered postpartum.

Medullary Thyroid Cancer

Medullary thyroid carcinoma (MTC) derives from the neuroendocrine parafollicular or C cells of the thyroid (Fig. 74-4). Sporadic MTC accounts for 80% of all cases of the disease, with the remainder of patients having inherited tumor syndromes, such as multiple endocrine neoplasia (MEN) type 2A, MEN2B, or familial medullary thyroid carcinoma (FMTC).[111,112] Because the C cells are predominantly located in the upper portion of each thyroid lobe, patients with sporadic disease typically present with upper pole nodules. Metastatic cervical adenopathy is noted in approximately 50% of patients at initial presentation, and symptoms of upper aerodigestive tract compression or invasion are reported in up to 15% of patients with sporadic disease. Symptoms from distant metastases in the lungs or bones may be elicited from 5% to 10% of patients. The ability of the tumor to oversecrete measurable quantities of calcitonin, occasionally along with other hormonally active peptides, such as adrenocorticotrophic hormone or calcitonin gene-related peptide, leads to unexplained diarrhea, symptoms of Cushing syndrome, or facial flushing in many patients with advanced disease. Rarely, MTC is suggested by the presence of dense calcifications seen on radiologic imaging of the anterior neck or sites of metastatic disease. The typical age of sporadic presentation is in the fifth or sixth decade, and there may be a slight female preponderance.

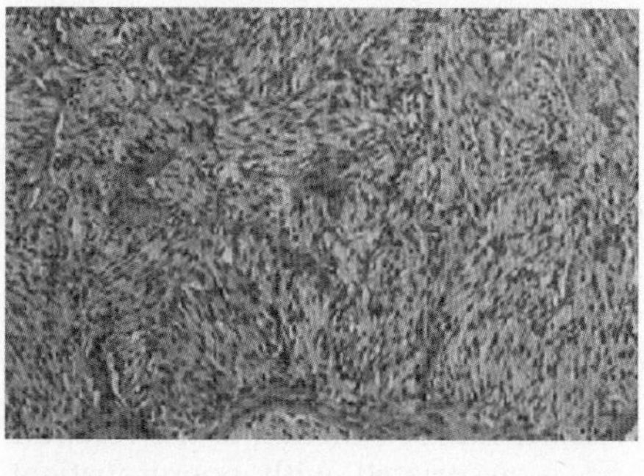

Figure 74-4 Medullary thyroid carcinoma, with nests of spindle-shaped cells. Such nests are often interspersed with clusters of round-to-oval cells, all immunostaining for calcitonin.

The diagnosis of sporadic MTC is usually suspected following FNA of a solitary nodule. Although routine measurement of the serum calcitonin concentration has been suggested as a cost-effective means of identifying MTC without an FNA, the enhanced sensitivity to detect microscopic MTC or C cell hyperplasia in the absence of familial disease is of uncertain clinical significance.[113] However, if the serum calcitonin level has been measured, an unstimulated level greater than 100 pg/mL is associated with a high likelihood of MTC.[114]

In known families with inherited MTC, prospective family screening identifies disease carriers long before clinical symptoms or signs are noted.[115] When compared with sporadic disease, the typical age of presentation for familial disease is the third decade, without gender preference; in MEN2A, signs or symptoms of hyperparathyroidism or pheochromocytoma uncommonly present before those of MTC, even in the absence of prospective screening. All familial forms of MTC are inherited in an autosomal dominant fashion. Mutations in *RET*, which codes for a cell membrane-associated tyrosine kinase receptor for glial cell line-derived neurotrophic factor, are found in about 95% of families with familial forms of MTC.[115] Mutations associated with MEN2A and

FMTC have been primarily identified in several codons of the cysteine-rich extra-cellular domains of exon 10, 11, 13, and 14 whereas MEN2B and some FMTC mutations are found within the intracellular exons 15 and 16 (Table 74-3).[116] Somatic mutations in exons 11, 13, and 16 have also been found in 40-50% of sporadic MTC tumors, particularly the codon 918 mutation that activates the tyrosine kinase function of the receptor and is associated with poorer patient prognosis.[117] Furthermore, approximately 6% of patients with clinically sporadic MTC carry a germ line mutation in *RET*, leading to identification of new families with multiple previously undiagnosed affected individuals.[118] Genetic counseling and testing for *RET* proto-oncogene mutations should be offered to all patients newly diagnosed with clinically apparent sporadic MTC, as well as for screening children and adults in known families with inherited forms of MTC.[115] On the basis of the relative frequency of mutations in certain exons, mutational analysis using direct DNA sequencing methodology should start with exon 11, followed sequentially by exons 10, 16, 13, 14, and 15.[116] In the patient with clinically sporadic MTC, the likelihood of a false negative *RET* germline test for familial disease is less than 1%; however, if the family history is suggestive for an autosomal inherited disorder, complete sequencing of *RET* can be considered, and the family should be screened clinically and biochemically for possible MTC.

The primary approach to staging of medullary carcinoma is the American Joint Committee on Cancer (AJCC) based TNM system.[26] In a multivariate analysis of prognostic factors, patients between 40 and 65 years of age at diagnosis had a 2-fold and over age 65 7-fold higher risk for death than those under age 40.[119] Patients with inherited disease appear to have a better prognosis, even after correcting for the early age of diagnosis in familial disease. Despite being typically diagnosed during childhood, patients with MEN2B are more likely than those with either MEN2A or FMTC to have locally aggressive disease.[119] Other factors that may be important for predicting a worse prognosis include the heterogeneity and paucity of calcitonin immunostaining of the tumor, rapidly rising serum carcinoembryonic antigen (CEA), and postoperative residual hypercalcitoninemia. Preoperative imaging studies should include neck ultrasound in all patients, and contrast-enhanced CT of the neck, chest, and liver when cervical metastases are present or either the calcitonin level is >400 pg/mL or CEA < 100 ng/mL.[120,121]

Initial Surgical Management

Unless MEN2 has been ruled out by germline *RET* testing, serum calcium and plasma free metanephrines should be measured to exclude coexistent hyperparathyroidism and pheochromocytoma, respectively. Total thyroidectomy is indicated in all patients with MTC, especially given the high frequency of bilateral disease in both sporadic and familial disease, and has been associated with improved survival.[122] Even in the absence of clinically detectable nodal metastases, central neck compartment dissection should be performed in all patients, and ipsilateral lateral neck and/or mediastinal dissections should be strongly considered when the primary tumor is >1 cm or when central compartment disease is present. Disfiguring radical node dissections do not improve prognosis and are not indicated. In the presence of grossly invasive disease, more extended procedures with resection of involved neck structures may be appropriate, but function-preserving approaches are preferred. Post-operative thyroid hormone therapy is indicated, but TSH suppression is not appropriate as C cells lack TSH receptors.

Table 74-3 Common *RET* Protooncogene Mutations in Hereditary Medullary Thyroid Carcinoma

Mutated Codon/Exon	Clinical Syndrome	Risk for Mortality (7th International MEN Workshop)[115]
609/10	FMTC; MEN2A with or without Hirschsprung disease	High risk
611/10	FMTC; MEN2A with or without Hirschsprung disease	High risk
618/10	FMTC; MEN2A with or without Hirschsprung disease	High risk
620/10	FMTC; MEN2A with or without Hirschsprung disease	High risk
630/11	FMTC; MEN2A	High risk
634/11	FMTC; MEN2A; MEN2A with or without cutaneous lichen amyloidosis	High risk
635/11	MEN2A	Not described
768/13	FMTC; MEN2A	Least high risk
790/13	FMTC; MEN2A	Least high risk
791/13	FMTC; MEN2A	Least high risk
804/14	MEN2B	Least high risk
883/15	FMTC	Highest risk
891/15	FMTC	Least high risk
912/16	MEN2B	High risk
918/16	MEN2B	Highest risk

Source: From Ref. 155.

Adjuvant Radiation Therapy

EBRT should be considered in patients after maximal surgical therapy and those who are considered at high risk for regional recurrence. After radiotherapy for microscopic residual disease, extra glandular invasion, or lymph node metastases, the locoregional relapse-free rate at 10 years was 86%, as compared with 52% for those patients who did not receive adjuvant therapy.[123] With conformal or intensity-modulated radiotherapy, 60 Gy administered in 30 fractions, local control is readily achieved with acceptable toxicity even in the setting of distant metastases.[124] As for differentiated carcinoma, EBRT can be given to palliate painful bone metastases.

Persistently Elevated Calcitonin

Three months postoperatively, serum concentrations of calcitonin and CEA should be measured, although nadir values may occasionally occur months later.[125,126] Most patients with palpable or macroscopic MTC who undergo attempted curative resection will have detectable serum calcitonin values postoperatively, indicative of residual disease. Those with values <150 pg/mL can be followed conservatively with neck ultrasound, but those with values >150 pg/mL should be re-evaluated for either residual resectable disease in the neck or the presence of distant metastases. A recent study reported 5 year survival rates of 100%, 92%, and 25% in patients with postoperative calcitonin levels that double in >24, 6-24, and <6 months, respectively; shorter doubling times of both CEA and calcitonin are also predictive of radiographic disease progression.[127,128]

Given the general failure of routine lymphadenectomy or excision of palpable tumor to normalize the serum calcitonin concentrations in most patients, attention has been directed toward detection and eradication of microscopic deposits of tumor. However, most case series report that undetectable postoperative calcitonin levels are seen in only a small proportion of patients, and clinical recurrence may yet occur.[129,130] Thus, only patients with overt disease in the neck and no distant metastases should undergo reoperative neck surgery.

Prophylactic Surgery for Gene Carriers

Given the identification of patients with malignant disease as early as age 6 years, prophylactic thyroidectomy by age 5 has been recommended for at-risk family members who are identified as carriers of a familial *RET* mutation. Of 50 *RET* mutation carriers, 88% had normal levels of plasma calcitonin when evaluated 5-10 years after prophylactic thyroidectomy.[131] Surveillance with calcitonin measurements and thyroid ultrasound and delayed surgery may be appropriate for children with the least virulent *RET* mutations in codons 768, 790, 791, 804, and 891, particularly if the family history is of less aggressive disease.[115]

Management of Distant Metastatic Disease

Systemic chemotherapy has been reported to yield response in up to 30% of patients with metastases of MTC involving liver, lung or bones. Most regimens in current use combine dacarbazine with other agents including vincristine, 5-fluorouracil, cyclophosphamide, or doxorubicin, without significant advantage of one combination compared with another.[132] More recently, therapies targeting key intracellular signaling cascades have demonstrated benefit in clinical trials and case series.[133] Vandetanib, a multikinase inhibitor targeting RET, VEGFR, and EGFR, induced partial responses in 10-20% of patients with metastatic inherited MTC, and prolonged stable disease with symptomatic improvement was reported in another 30% in two phase 2 trials; a randomized, placebo-controlled trial is underway.[134,135] Other multikinase inhibitors reported to produce significant responses and/or prolonged stabilization include sorafenib, sunitinib, XL184, and motesanib diphosphate.[136-141] For patients with clinically progressive or symptomatic metastatic disease who cannot enter clinical trials, therapy with sorafenib is appropriate as initial therapy.

Anaplastic Thyroid Carcinoma

Anaplastic thyroid carcinomas are aggressive undifferentiated tumors, with a disease-specific mortality approaching 100%.[142-144] Patients with anaplastic carcinoma are older than those with differentiated carcinomas, with a mean age at diagnosis of about 65 years. Fewer than 10% of patients are younger than 50 years, and 60-70% are women.[3] Approximately 50% of patients with anaplastic cancer have either a prior or coexistent differentiated carcinoma. Anaplastic carcinoma develops from more differentiated tumors as a result of one or more dedifferentiating steps, particularly loss of the p53 tumor-suppressor protein, amplification of phosphatidylinositol 3-kinase, and overexpression of receptors for various growth factors.[145-147] However, no specific precipitating events have been identified, and the mechanisms leading to anaplastic transformation of differentiated carcinomas are uncertain.

Patients with anaplastic carcinoma present with extensive local invasion, and distant metastases are found at initial disease presentation in 15-50% of patients.[142] The lungs and pleura are the most common sites of distant metastases, being seen in up to 90% of patients with distant disease. Approximately 5-15% of patients have bone metastases, 5% have brain metastases, and a few have metastases to the skin, liver, kidneys, pancreas, heart, and adrenal glands.

The diagnosis of anaplastic carcinoma is usually established by FNA or surgical biopsy. CT of the neck and mediastinum can accurately determine the extent of the thyroid tumor and identify tumor invasion of the great vessels and upper aerodigestive tract structures. Most pulmonary metastases are nodules that can be detected by routine chest radiography. Bone lesions are usually lytic.

Treatment and Prognosis

There is no effective therapy for anaplastic carcinoma, and the disease is uniformly fatal.[142] The median survival from diagnosis ranges from 3 to 7 months, and the 1- and 5-year survival rates are approximately 25% and 5%, respectively.[3] Death is attributable to upper airway obstruction and suffocation (often despite tracheostomy) in half the patients and to a combination of complications of local and distant disease and/or therapy in the remainder. Patients with disease confined to the neck at diagnosis have a mean survival of 8 months, as compared to 3 months if the disease has extended beyond the neck. Other variables that may predict worse prognosis include older age at diagnosis, male gender, and dyspnea as a presenting symptom.

Except for patients whose tumors are small and confined entirely to the thyroid, total thyroidectomy with complete tumor resection does not prolong survival.[143,148] EBRT, administered in conventional doses, also does not prolong survival.[144] Although up to 40% of patients may respond initially to radiation therapy, most have local recurrence. The introduction of hyperfractionated radiotherapy, combined with radiosensitizing doses of doxorubicin, may increase the local response rate to about 80%, with subsequent median survival of 1 year; distant metastases then become the leading cause of death. Similar improvement in local disease control has been reported with the combination of hyperfractionated radiotherapy and doxorubicin, followed by debulking surgery in responsive patients.[149] However, the addition of larger doses of other chemotherapeutic drugs has not been associated with improved control of distant disease or improved survival. Paclitaxel has been associated with short-term stabilization in a minority of patients, and may provide some palliative benefit.[150] Although one patient with a prolonged complete response was reported in a phase 1 study of the vascular disrupting agent combretastatin, a subsequent phase 2 study yielded no responses and a median survival of only 20 weeks.[151,152] Based on preclinical data suggesting enhanced activity in combination with cytotoxic chemotherapy, a randomized phase 3 trial of combretastatin combined with paclitaxel and carboplatin versus paclitaxel and carboplatin alone is ongoing.[153] Similarly, the thiazolidinedione derivative CS7017, combined with paclitaxel, is being evaluated in a phase 1/2 trial on the basis of promising findings in animal models of anaplastic carcinoma.[154]

Selected References

The complete reference list can be found at www.CANCERMEDICINE8.com

3. Gilliland FD, Hunt WC, Morris DM, et al. Prognostic factors for thyroid carcinoma: a population-based study of 15,698 cases from the Surveillance, Epidemiology and End Results (SEER) program 1973–1991. *Cancer*. 1997;79:564–573.
5. Cooper DS, Doherty GM, Haugen BR, et al. Management guidelines for patients with thyroid nodules and differentiated thyroid cancer. *Thyroid*. 2006;16:109–142.
7. Fish SA, Langer JE, Mandel SJ. Sonographic imaging of thyroid nodules and cervical lymph nodes. *Endocrinol Metab Clin North Am*. 2008;37:401–417.
8. Papini E, Guglielmi R, Bianchini A, et al. Risk of malignancy in nonpalpable thyroid nodules: predictive value of ultrasound and color-Doppler features. *J Clin Endocrinol Metab*. 2002;87:1941–1946.
10. Baloch ZW, LiVolsi VA, Asa SL, et al. Diagnostic terminology and morphologic criteria for cytologic diagnosis of thyroid lesions: a synopsis of the National Cancer Institute Thyroid Fine-Needle Aspiration State of the Science Conference. *Diagn Cytopathol*. 2008;36:425–437.
14. Ron E. Thyroid cancer incidence among people living in areas contaminated by radiation from the Chernobyl accident. *Health Phys*. 2007;93:502–511.
18. Nikiforova MN, Nikiforov YE. Molecular genetics of thyroid cancer: implications for diagnosis, treatment and prognosis. *Expert Rev Mol Diagn*. 2008;8:83–95.
19. Lupi C, Giannini R, Ugolini C, et al. Association of BRAF V600E mutation with poor clinicopathological outcomes in 500 consecutive cases of papillary thyroid carcinoma. *J Clin Endocrinol Metab*. 2007;92:4085–4090.
21. Kondo T, Asa SL, Ezzat S. Epigenetic dysregulation in thyroid neoplasia. *Endocrinol Metab Clin North Am*. 2008;37:389–400.

33. Hay ID, Grant CS, Bergstralh EJ, et al. Unilateral total lobectomy: is it sufficient surgical treatment for patients with AMES low-risk papillary thyroid carcinoma? *Surgery.* 1998;124:958–964; discussion 64–66.
34. Jonklaas J, Sarlis NJ, Litofsky D, et al. Outcomes of patients with differentiated thyroid carcinoma following initial therapy. *Thyroid.* 2006;16:1229–1242.
42. Kouvaraki MA, Shapiro SE, Fornage BD, et al. Role of preoperative ultrasonography in the surgical management of patients with thyroid cancer. *Surgery.* 2003;134:946–954.
46. Sawka AM, Brierley JD, Tsang RW, et al. An updated systematic review and commentary examining the effectiveness of radioactive iodine remnant ablation in well-differentiated thyroid cancer. *Endocrinol Metab Clin North Am.* 2008;37:457–480.
48. Pacini F, Ladenson PW, Schlumberger M, et al. Radioiodine ablation of thyroid remnants after preparation with recombinant human thyrotropin in differentiated thyroid carcinoma: results of an international, randomized, controlled study. *J Clin Endocrinol Metab.* 2006;91:926–932.
54. Cailleux AF, Baudin E, Travagli JP, et al. Is diagnostic iodine-131 scanning useful after total thyroid ablation for differentiated thyroid cancer? *J Clin Endocrinol Metab.* 2000;85:175–178.
61. Sawin CT, Geller A, Wolf PA, et al. Low serum thyrotropin concentrations as a risk factor for atrial fibrillation in older persons. *N Engl J Med.* 1994;331:1249–1252.
62. Biondi B, Cooper DS. The clinical significance of subclinical thyroid dysfunction. *Endocr Rev.* 2008;29:76–131.
65. Farahati J, Reiners C, Stuschke M, et al. Differentiated thyroid cancer. Impact of adjuvant external radiotherapy in patients with perithyroidal tumor infiltration (stage pT4). *Cancer.* 1996;77:172–180.
67. Torlontano M, Crocetti U, Augello G, et al. Comparative evaluation of recombinant human thyrotropin-stimulated thyroglobulin levels, 131I whole-body scintigraphy, and neck ultrasonography in the follow-up of patients with papillary thyroid microcarcinoma who have not undergone radioiodine therapy. *J Clin Endocrinol Metab.* 2006;91:60–63.
68. do Rosario PW, Fagundes TA, Maia FF, et al. Sonography in the diagnosis of cervical recurrence in patients with differentiated thyroid carcinoma. *J Ultrasound Med.* 2004;23:915–920.
76. Haugen BR, Pacini F, Reiners C, et al. A comparison of recombinant human thyrotropin and thyroid hormone withdrawal for the detection of thyroid remnant or cancer. *J Clin Endocrinol Metab.* 1999;84:3877–3885.
77. Pacini F, Molinaro E, Castagna MG, et al. Recombinant human thyrotropin-stimulated serum thyroglobulin combined with neck ultrasonography has the highest sensitivity in monitoring differentiated thyroid carcinoma. *J Clin Endocrinol Metab.* 2003;88:3668–3673.
85. Chiu AC, Delpassand ES, Sherman SI. Prognosis and treatment of brain metastases in thyroid carcinoma. *J Clin Endocrinol Metab.* 1997;82:3637–3642.
89. Durante C, Haddy N, Baudin E, et al. Long-term outcome of 444 patients with distant metastases from papillary and follicular thyroid carcinoma: benefits and limits of radioiodine therapy. *J Clin Endocrinol Metab.* 2006;91:2892–2899.
92. Rubino C, de Vathaire F, Dottorini ME, et al. Second primary malignancies in thyroid cancer patients. *Br J Cancer.* 2003;89:1638–1644.
97. Leboulleux S, Schroeder PR, Schlumberger M, et al. The role of PET in follow-up of patients treated for differentiated epithelial thyroid cancers. *Nat Clin Pract Endocrinol Metab.* 2007;3:112–121.
100. Ain KB, Lee C, Holbrook KM, et al. Phase II study of lenalidomide in distantly metastatic, rapidly progressive, and radioiodine-unresponsive thyroid carcinomas: preliminary results. *J Clin Oncol.* 2008;28:6027.
101. Sherman SI, Wirth LJ, Droz JP, et al. Motesanib diphosphate in progressive differentiated thyroid cancer. *N Engl J Med.* 2008;359:31–42.
102. Cohen EEW, Rosen LS, Vokes EE, et al. Axitinib (AG-013736) is an active treatment for all histological subtypes of advanced thyroid cancer: results from a phase II study. *J Clin Oncol.* published online June 9, 2008, 10.1200/JCO.2007.15.9566; 2008.
103. upta-Abramson V, Troxel AB, Nellore A, et al. Phase II trial of sorafenib in advanced thyroid cancer. *J Clin Oncol.* 2008.
105. Vassilopoulou-Sellin R, Goepfert H, Raney B, et al. Differentiated thyroid cancer in children and adolescents: clinical outcome and mortality after long-term follow-up. *Head Neck.* 1998;20:549–555.
109. Yasmeen S, Cress R, Romano PS, et al. Thyroid cancer in pregnancy. *Int J Gynaecol Obstet.* 2005;91:15–20.
113. Cheung K, Roman SA, Wang TS, et al. Calcitonin measurement in the evaluation of thyroid nodules in the United States: a cost-effectiveness and decision analysis. *J Clin Endocrinol Metab.* 2008;93:2173–2180.
115. Brandi ML, Gagel RF, Angeli A, et al. Guidelines for diagnosis and therapy of MEN type 1 and type 2. *J Clin Endocrinol Metab.* 2001;86:5658–5671.
116. Eng C, Clayton D, Schuffenecker I, et al. The relationship between specific RET proto-oncogene mutations and disease phenotype in multiple endocrine neoplasia type 2. International RET mutation consortium analysis. *JAMA.* 1996;276:1575–1579.
117. Elisei R, Cosci B, Romei C, et al. Prognostic significance of somatic RET oncogene mutations in sporadic medullary thyroid cancer: a 10-year follow-up study. *J Clin Endocrinol Metab.* 2008;93:682–687.
127. Barbet J, Campion L, Kraeber-Bodere F, et al. Prognostic impact of serum calcitonin and carcinoembryonic antigen doubling-times in patients with medullary thyroid carcinoma. *J Clin Endo Metab.* 2005;90:6077–6084.
129. Fialkowski E, Debenedetti M, Moley J. Long-term outcome of reoperations for medullary thyroid carcinoma. *World J Surg.* 2008;32:754–765.
131. Skinner MA, Moley JA, Dilley WG, et al. Prophylactic thyroidectomy in multiple endocrine neoplasia type 2A. *N Engl J Med.* 2005;353:1105–1113.
132. Ball DW. Medullary thyroid cancer: monitoring and therapy. *Endocrinol Metab Clin North Am.* 2007;36:823–837.
135. Wells SA, Jr., Gosnell JE, Gagel RF, et al. Vandetanib in metastatic hereditary medullary thyroid cancer: follow-up results of an open-label phase II trial. *J Clin Oncol.* 2007;25:6018.
137. Kelleher FC, McDermott R. Response to sunitinib in medullary thyroid cancer. *Ann Intern Med.* 2008;148:567.
140. Cohen EEW, Needles BM, Cullen KJ, et al. Phase 2 study of sunitinib in refractory thyroid cancer. *J Clin Oncol.* 2008;26:6025.
142. Neff RL, Farrar WB, Kloos RT, et al. Anaplastic thyroid cancer. *Endocrinol Metab Clin North Am.* 2008;37:525–538.
144. Kebebew E, Greenspan FS, Clark OH, et al. Anaplastic thyroid carcinoma. Treatment outcome and prognostic factors. *Cancer.* 2005;103:1330–1335.
149. Kim JH, Leeper RD. Treatment of locally advanced thyroid carcinoma with combination doxorubicin and radiation therapy. *Cancer.* 1987;60:2372–2375.
150. Ain KB, Egorin MJ, DeSimone PA. Treatment of anaplastic thyroid carcinoma with paclitaxel: phase 2 trial using ninety-six-hour infusion. *Thyroid.* 2000;10:587–594.
152. Cooney MM, Savvides P, Agarwala S, et al. Phase II study of combretastatin A4 phosphate (CA4P) in patients with advanced anaplastic thyroid carcinoma (ATC). *J Clin Oncol.* 2006;24:5580.

75 Neoplasms of the Adrenal Cortex

David E. Schteingart, MD

Adrenal cortical carcinomas (ACC) are rare, highly malignant tumors that account for only 0.2% of deaths due to cancer. Their incidence has been estimated at two per million people annually. About half of these tumors produce hormonal and metabolic syndromes that lead to their discovery. The other half are silent and are discovered with metastasis or when the primary tumor becomes large enough to produce abdominal symptoms.

Pathogenesis

The etiology of ACC remains unknown. Although ACC can occur at any age, most cases occur between ages 30 and 50 years.[1] Risk of developing the dise ase is increased in men who smoked more than 25 cigarettes daily (odds ratio 2:0; 95% confidence interval [CI] 1.0–4.4) and in women who used oral contraceptives, especially before age 25 (odds ratio 1:8; 95% CI 1.0–3.2).[2]

Clonality studies of adrenal cortical tumors, using X-chromosome inactivation analysis, indicate monoclonal expansion of a single cell as the origin of ACC. There are multiple chromosomal alterations in ACC. Chromosomal gains are observed in chromosomes 5, 12, and 19 and most losses occur in chromosomes 1p, 17p and 11.[3] Mutations in key genes involved in adrenal cortical cell proliferation may lead to tumor development.[4] Cases of adrenal cancer have been described in families with a hereditary cancer syndrome who exhibit mutations in tumor-suppressor genes. One such condition is the Li-Fraumeni syndrome, a rare autosomal-dominant syndrome caused by germ-line mutations in the TP53 tumor-suppressor gene and associated with high susceptibility to a variety of malignancies, including sarcoma, breast cancer, brain tumors, lung cancer, laryngeal carcinoma, leukemia, and ACC. However, adrenal cancer occurs infrequently in this syndrome. The deleterious genotype in these cases is expressed through several generations in both children and adults.[5,6] Studies on the genetics of these familial syndromes helped identify mutations in sporadic cases. Somatic mutations of the tumor suppressor gene TP53 are associated with 1/3 of ACC, with p53 protein nuclear accumulation and a worse prognosis. Studies of specific genes and pangenomic analysis show that the insulin-like growth factor II (IGF-II) gene is the most commonly expressed, being detected in 85% of cases of ACC.[7] Transcriptome studies have identified an IGF-II cluster of genes (containing mainly growth factors and growth factor receptor genes) significantly over expressed in ACC. Perturbation of the IGF-II locus appears to be a dominant event in ACC. In contrast, a cluster of steroidogenic genes (CYP11A, CYP11B, HSD3B1) is more frequently expressed in adenomas. Transcriptome analysis also suggest that the Wnt signaling pathway is activated in ACC. About a third of adrenal cortical tumors harbor somatic activating mutations of the β-catenin gene.[8] In the absence of the Wnt signal, β-catenin is captured within a destructive complex and eventually degraded. In contrast, activation of Wnt signaling allows β-catenin to accumulate and enter the nucleus where it activates genes that instruct the cell to proliferate and remain in an undifferentiated state. Using transcriptome profiling, a set of genes identified with Wnt dysregulation was identified in ACC.[7] Another potential mechanism of tumorogenesis involves upregulation of telomerase, a multi-subunit ribonucleoprotein complex that adds telomere repeats to the ends of linear chromosomes, a process critical for normal tissue progenitor cell function and cancer development.[9] Telomerase is found to be up-regulated in 90% human cancers where it serves to stabilize telomeres and allow unlimited cell division. In the presence of p53, senescence is activated as an anti-oncogenic mechanism. With the loss of p53 seen in adrenal cancer, telomere maintenance mechanisms are active and lead to tumor development. As proposed in other malignant solid tumors, activated adrenal cortical cancer stem cells may provide a mechanism for perpetuating progenitor cells that ultimately contribute to the persistent proliferation of mature cancer cells. Microarray analysis of adrenal tumors and normal adrenals has also shown upregulation of Jagged1 and Notch pathways in a majority of adrenal cortical carcinomas. These pathways could be important contributors to adrenal tumorigenesis and targets for pharmacological inhibition of cell proliferation.[10] *FOXM1*, a proliferation specific transcription factor of the Forkhead family, was also shown to be over expressed in malignant vs benign tumors or normal tissues. Thus, *FOXM1* may be a good marker for malignant adrenocortical tumors and may play a role in tumorigenesis.[11]

A variety of other genetic defects have been described in ACC but it is uncertain what role they play in the initiation and progression of the neoplastic process. As with the TP53 gene, allelic loss at the Rb gene locus on chromosome 13q has been described in ACC.[12] Other genetic markers examined have included the H19, and the p57kip2 genes. These genes have been mapped to chromosome 11p15.513 and appear to be important for fetal growth and development. The levels of expression of the H19 are very high in human fetal adrenal glands,[13] but they subsequently decrease by 50% in adults. The gene product for p57kip2, a member of the p21cip1 cyclin-dependent kinase family, appears to regulate cell proliferation, exit from the cell cycle, and maintenance of differentiated cells. Loss of activity of the p57kip2 gene product has been detected in virilizing adenomas and ACC[14] suggesting that this gene product plays a role in the normal maintenance of adrenal cortical differentiation and function. H19 and p57kip2 gene expression is adrenocorticotropic hormone (ACTH) dependent, and regulation of the p57kip2 gene appears to be related to the cyclic adenosine monophosphate (cAMP)-dependent protein kinase pathway. The gene product for p57kip2 is usually found to be high in most normal human tissues. A markedly reduced expression of the H19 gene has been found in both nonfunctioning and functioning ACC, especially in tumors that produce cortisol and aldosterone. Reduced expression of the p57 kip2 has been found in Beckwith-Wiedemann syndrome, a congenital overgrowth disorder characterized by high risk of development of childhood tumors, including ACC. In general, genetic changes increase as the tumor increases its malignancy grade.

Oncogenic virus infection as cause of ACC has been investigated. There are studies showing involvement of Human Cytomegalic Virus infection in functioning ACC. The virus can stimulate not only cell proliferation, but more importantly it can stimulate steroidogenic enzyme expression.[15]

Some of the genetic changes described are uncovered in the late stages

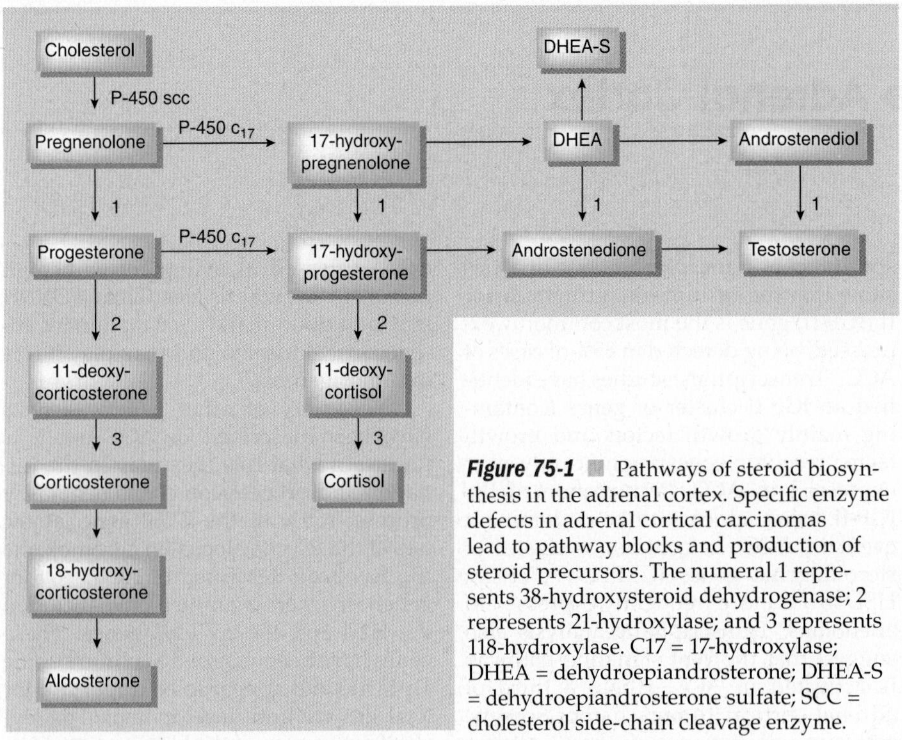

Figure 75-1 Pathways of steroid biosynthesis in the adrenal cortex. Specific enzyme defects in adrenal cortical carcinomas lead to pathway blocks and production of steroid precursors. The numeral 1 represents 38-hydroxysteroid dehydrogenase; 2 represents 21-hydroxylase; and 3 represents 118-hydroxylase. C17 = 17-hydroxylase; DHEA = dehydroepiandrosterone; DHEA-S = dehydroepiandrosterone sulfate; SCC = cholesterol side-chain cleavage enzyme.

of the disease, and it is likely that a better understanding of early events may lead to a more effective control of the process of tumorigenesis. The recent identification of specific genetic defects in adrenal cortical carcinomas are likely to be important in understanding the process of tumorigenesis as well as the diagnosis, prognosis and targeted therapy of adrenal cancer.

Diagnosis

Cushing syndrome is the most common clinical presentation in adult patients with adrenal cancer. Characteristically, these patients describe rapid development (3-6 months) of the clinical manifestations of cortisol excess, including weight gain, muscle weakness, easy bruising, irritability, and insomnia. In addition, commonly there are manifestations of androgen excess, including hirsutism, acne, and irregular menses or amenorrhea in women. Although virilization frequently accompanies Cushing syndrome, the predominant clinical manifestations may be those of androgen excess with only subtle evidence of hypercortisolism. The androgen excess may decrease the severity of the catabolic effect of hypercortisolemia such that skin and muscle atrophy may not be as readily apparent as in those patients with benign tumors. Patients with metastatic disease complain of anorexia and weight loss rather than weight gain. Adrenal cortical carcinomas causing Cushing syndrome are large, with an average weight of 800 g, but the clinical manifestations of hormone excess may lead to earlier diagnosis and the finding of smaller tumors.

Hormonal findings in patients with clinical manifestations of Cushing syndrome include high urinary-free cortisol, serum cortisol, dehydroepiandrosterone sulfate (DHEA-S) at baseline, and failure to suppress with a high (8 mg) dose of dexamethasone. ACTH levels are usually suppressed. The steroid profile in serum or urine can help distinguish between benign and malignant adrenal cortical tumors because of the presence of intermediary precursors in the steroid biosynthesis pathway or their metabolites in patients with malignant neoplasms (Fig. 75-1). Specifically, serum levels of progesterone, pregnenolone, 17-hydroxyprogesterone, 17-hydroxypregnenolone and dehydroepiandrosterone measured by gas chromatography/mass spectroscopy (GC/MS) are increased in ACC. Levels of 11-deoxycortisol are less specific a measurement because they are increased in both, benign and malignant tumors.

Sex hormone-producing carcinomas lead to virilization in women and feminization in men. Women with virilizing ACC present with marked androgen-type hirsutism, male-pattern baldness, deepening voice, breast atrophy, clitoral hypertrophy, decreased libido, and oligo- or amenorrhea. In contrast, manifestations of androgen excess are less noticeable in men. Prepubertal boys with androgen excess develop precocious puberty without concomitant testicular enlargement. Feminizing tumors in women cause breast tenderness and dysfunctional uterine bleeding. These tumors in men are associated with gynecomastia, breast tenderness, testicular atrophy, and decreased libido. Prepubertal girls with feminizing tumors experience early breast and uterine development and onset of menarche.

Patients with virilizing tumors demonstrate high serum levels of testosterone, androstenedione, and DHEA-S, whereas patients with feminizing tumors have high serum estradiol levels. Total testosterone levels in virilized women are >2 ng/mL (normal 0.3-0.6 ng/mL).

Aldosterone-producing ACC are extremely rare. Patients present with hypertension and hypokalemia, which are typical clinical manifestations of primary aldosteronism. Compared with patients with benign aldosterone-secreting adenomas, those with carcinoma have larger tumors, higher aldosterone levels, and more severe hypokalemia.[16,17] Evaluation should include measurement of serum electrolytes, aldosterone, and plasma renin levels. Findings include severe hypokalemia with potassium levels below 2.5 mEq/L, hypernatremia, and metabolic alkalosis. Serum aldosterone levels are high, and plasma renin levels are suppressed.

Silent ACC do not present with recognizable symptoms of excessive hormone production, are detected when they attain large size and cause local symptoms, or are detected incidentally in the course of investigation of unrelated abdominal complaints. A hormonal profile on patients with suspected silent adrenal tumors should also be obtained. Some of these tumors produce steroid biosynthesis pathway intermediates, such as progesterone and 11-deoxycortisol.[18] It is important to determine the level of these steroids prior to surgical resection of the tumor because they can be used as biochemical markers in the postoperative follow-up.

Differential Diagnosis

A major dilemma in the differential diagnosis of adrenal cancer arises with incidentally discovered adrenal masses found in 1-3% of patients undergoing abdominal scans by computed tomography (CT). Most of these masses are benign, and adrenal cortical adenomas are 60 times more common than primary carcinoma.[19] Malignant adrenal masses are frequently metastatic from extra-adrenal neoplasms. Age, ethnic background, and comorbidities should be considered when evaluating an incidentally discovered adrenal mass. These masses are uncommon under the age of 30, but their prevalence increases with age. Thus, an incidentally discovered adrenal mass in a young person is of greater concern and should be monitored more closely and for a longer period of time to rule out malignancy. Silent adrenal masses are more common among African Americans and patients with diabetes mellitus, obesity, and hypertension.

The size of the mass is an important consideration in determining if it is benign or malignant. Masses less than 3 cm in diameter are usually benign[20]; in contrast, the probability that the mass is malignant is generally increased when it measures more than 6 cm. The mean tumor size of ACC is 10 cm, and 95% are larger than 5 cm. The prevalence of carcinoma increases with the larger tumors: 2% in tumors <2 cm, 6% in tumors 4 to 6 cm, and 25% in tumors 6 cm. Since early resection of these tumors offers the best chance for cure or long-term survival, an accurate diagnosis of a small tumor is very important. Nonfunctioning small adrenal masses less than 3 cm in diameter usually remain stable for many years. Malignant masses, however, may be initially small but enlarge over time. In contrast, functioning adrenal tumors are associated with significant morbidity that depends on the metabolic effects of the hormones produced in excess. Fine needle aspiration (FNA) biopsies under CT guidance are occasionally performed in order to determine if a mass is of adrenal cortical origin and benign or malignant. One should not perform this procedure routinely unless there is a strong probability the adrenal lesion is metastatic and confirming this could determine the resectability of a non-adrenal primary malignancy. There is always the risk of breaching the tumor capsule and seeding neoplastic cells in adjacent sites. In addition, the amount of tissue extracted is seldom sufficient to establish a diagnosis. As described below, it is usually possible to determine the nature of an adrenal cortical lesion using appropriate imaging techniques.

Imaging Characterization

A variety of imaging procedures can be useful in the localization and evaluation of the benign or malignant character of an adrenal cortical neoplasm and the extent of disease.

Computed Tomography

Unenhanced and contrast-enhanced CT have been used to distinguish benign from malignant adrenal masses on the basis of their lipid content.[21,22] Lipid-rich masses are usually benign, while lipid-poor masses are frequently malignant. Enhancement is measured in Hounsfield units (H). Low-attenuation lesions have low H values. Using unenhanced CT, it was shown that adenomas have values less than +10 H, whereas nonadenomas have values greater than +18 H. These criteria give a sensitivity of 73% for distinguishing adenomas from nonadenomas and a specificity of 96%. CT images obtained 1 hour after the injection of contrast show an enhancement of 11 ± 13 H (<30) for adenomas and of 49 ± 8.3 H (>30) for nonadenomas, with a sensitivity of 95% and a specificity of 100%. Adenomas also exhibit a >60% washout within 15 min of contrast injection, whereas nonadenomas exhibit a greater retention of contrast. Malignant adrenal masses are generally larger than 5 cm, have an inhomogeneous pattern because of areas of necrosis within the tumor, and are frequently invasive of the upper pole of the adjoining kidney and of the inferior vena cava (Fig. 75-2). The CT procedure also helps determine the presence of involved lymph nodes and hepatic or pulmonary metastases. A definition of metastatic involvement is important in determining the stage of the disease and treatment goals.

Ultrasonography

Malignant lesions vary in echo texture and are heterogeneous in appearance, with focal or scattered echopenic or echogenic zones representing areas of tumor necrosis, hemorrhage, or calcification.[23,24]

Magnetic Resonance Imaging

Tumors appear as hypointense masses compared with the liver on T1-weighted images and hyperintense on T2-weighted images. Magnetic resonance imaging (MRI) also demonstrates displacement or invasion of adjacent organs as well as liver metastases. Superior blood vessel identification and the multiplanar capabilities of MRI make it the imaging modality of choice in evaluating the extent of disease and planning surgical excision.[25] The distinction between benign and malignant masses on the basis of the presence of lipid can also be determined by chemical shift MRI. Lipid-rich adenomas show a 34% change in relative signal intensity between in-phase and out-of-phase imaging, whereas non-adenomas do not change. This technique gives a specificity of 100% and a sensitivity of 81% in distinguishing these lesions.[26] However, there is no evidence suggesting that MRI is superior to CT in distinguishing between benign and malignant adrenal masses.

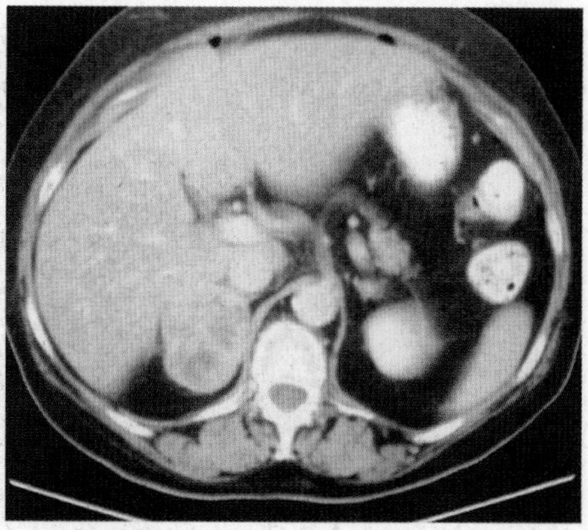

Figure 75-2 CT appearance of a right adrenal cortical carcinoma. The mass is inhomogeneous, secondary to areas of necrosis within the tumor.

Positron Emission Tomography Scanning

Positron emission tomography (PET) has been used to image various types of primary tumors and metastatic disease, taking advantage of the increased metabolic activity of neoplastic tissue. Most of these PET studies have used fluorodeoxyglucose (FDG) [^{18}F].[27] However, false negative findings were reported in 46% of patients in one series.[28] The limiting factor in detecting lesions with PET is their size. If lesions are smaller than 8 mm, they fall below the discrimination limit for this imaging procedure and are missed. The best use of FDG-PET is to determine if a lesion seen on CT is likely to be malignant. Malignant lesions exhibit increased metabolic activity and will appear as areas of increased radioligand uptake. A better imaging tracer for adrenal tumors may be [^{123}I] Iodometomidate.[29] This tracer is quite specific for adrenal tissue and although it may not distinguish benign from malignant tumors, the presence of uptake in extra-adrenal sites may indicate recurrence of disease or metastasis in patients who have undergone resection of an adrenocortical carcinoma. In spite of the clear usefulness of FDG-PET in the evaluation of adrenal cancer it is not yet standard of practice and its cost not routinely reimbursable.

Staging

Adrenal cortical carcinoma can be staged on the basis of the size of the primary tumor and extent of regional or distant tumor involvement, according to the 4 stage MacFarlane classification,[30] as modified by Sullivan.[31] In this older classification, patients in stage I have tumors that measure less than 5 cm in diameter and have no evidence of lymph node involvement or metastases; patients in stage II have tumors larger than 5 cm but are also free of lymph node involvement or metastases. Patients in stage III exhibit tumors of any size with local lymph node involvement or local tissue invasion. Patients in stage IV have distant metastases. The sites of tumor spread in stage IV are summarized in Table 75-1. The most frequent sites for metastases are the lung, liver, lymph nodes, and bone. Until 2004, no official tumor nodes and metastasis (TNM) classification was available for ACC, although one can be derived from the modified McFarlane classification (Table 75-2). The new Union Internationale Contre le Cancer (UICC) staging system published by the WHO in 2004 essentially endorsed the McFarlane classification.[32] The stage at which an adrenal cortical carcinoma is defined determines the prognosis.[31,33] Whereas 50% of patients in stage I, II, or III are alive 40 months after diagnosis, only 10% of patients in stage IV are alive at that time. However, the prognostic value of the established staging system has never been validated in a large series of patients. Using data from 455 patients with ACC in the German Registry, an attempt was made to analyze parameters used in the definition of stages for their respective predictive value for survival. Distant metastases were the strongest predictor with a hazard ratio (HR) of 6. In patients without distant metastases, the predictors were in the following order: tumor thrombus/invasion in the inferior vena cava or renal vein (HR 3.4), lymph node involvement (HR 2.4) and local adipose tissue infiltration (HR 2.0).[34] According to these observations, stage III could be subdivided into sub-categories with different prognostic implication.

Pathologic Diagnosis

Pathologic criteria, alone or in combination with histochemical biomarkers, genetic profiles and clinical features, can be used in the differential diagnosis of benign and malignant adrenal cortical tumors and in assessing their prognosis.[35]

Table 75-1 ■ Sites of Metastasis in Stage IV Adrenal Cortical Carcinoma

Organ	Percent
Lung	45
Liver	42
Lymph nodes	24
Bone	15
Pancreas	12
Spleen	6
Diaphragm	12
Miscellaneous (brain, peritoneum, skin, palate)	12

Table 75-2 ■ MacFarlane Classification of Adrenal Cortical Carcinoma Based on Size and Extent of Disease

Stage	Tumor Size	Lymphadenopathy	Invasion	Metastases	TNM
I	< 5cm	–	–	–	T1-N0-M0
II	< 5cm	–	–	–	T2-N0-M0
III	Any size	+	+	+	T1 or T2-N1-M0
IV	Any size	+	+	+	T1 or T2-N1-M1

Abbreviation: TNM, tumor-node-metastasis.

Adrenal adenomas are usually well encapsulated and homogeneous on cross section (Fig. 75-3A) and do not metastasize; in contrast, adrenal carcinomas are large, multilobulated tumors with areas of necrosis and evidence of capsular and vascular invasion (Fig. 75-3B).

Various systems of histologic diagnosis have been proposed, but the most commonly used system is the one described by Medeiros and Weiss.[36] Nine histologic findings have been described: (1) high nuclear grade, (2) mitotic grade greater than 5 mitoses/50 high-power fields (HPF), (3) atypical mitosis, (4) low percentage of clear cells, (5) diffuse architecture, (6) necrosis, (7) venous invasion, (8) sinusoidal invasion, and (9) capsular invasion. According to these criteria, a Weiss score (0-9) can be determined for each patient. Malignant tumors meet four or more of these histologic criteria. The three most commonly found are a mitotic rate greater than 5 mitoses/50 HPF, atypical mitosis, and venous invasion.

The mitotic rate is an important criterion not only for distinguishing malignant from benign tumors, but also for predicting the clinical virulence of adrenal cortical carcinomas. Patients with carcinomas having a high mitotic rate (>20 mitoses/10 HPF) have a shorter disease-free survival period than patients whose carcinomas have a low mitotic rate (<20 mitoses/10 HPF).

Most adrenal cortical carcinomas are large, but size alone either has no effect on survival time or has minimal effect. Depending on the degree of cell differentiation, adrenal cortical carcinomas have been classified as well-differentiated or anaplastic. Although well-differentiated carcinomas may have a less aggressive course than the anaplastic tumors, cell differentiation may not predict survival independently of the mitotic rate.

Attempts have been made to study adrenal cortical carcinomas by immunohistochemical analysis. Proliferation markers such as Ki67, are helpful to confirm malignancy, determine malignancy grade and predict tumor recurrence. The Ki67 labeling index ranges from 1% to 26%. Kaplan Meier analysis showed that a labeling index of >7% is significantly associated with shortened disease-free survival.[37] Other markers, such as D11, Melan-A and chromogranin A help define the adrenocortical origin of the tumor. In the future, identification of specific gene mutations by gene chip analysis in adrenal cortical carcinomas may be helpful in determining not only diagnosis, but also the malignant grade and prognosis of individual tumors. Using hierarchical clustering of data derived from genotyping adrenal cortical tumors, it is possible to separate a cluster of tumors with higher mitotic grade, greater proliferation markers, increased chromosomal instability and aneuploidy.[38] Tumors with nuclear β-catenin also have worse prognosis.

Carcinoma Management

Therapeutic interventions used to treat patients with adrenal cancer include sur-

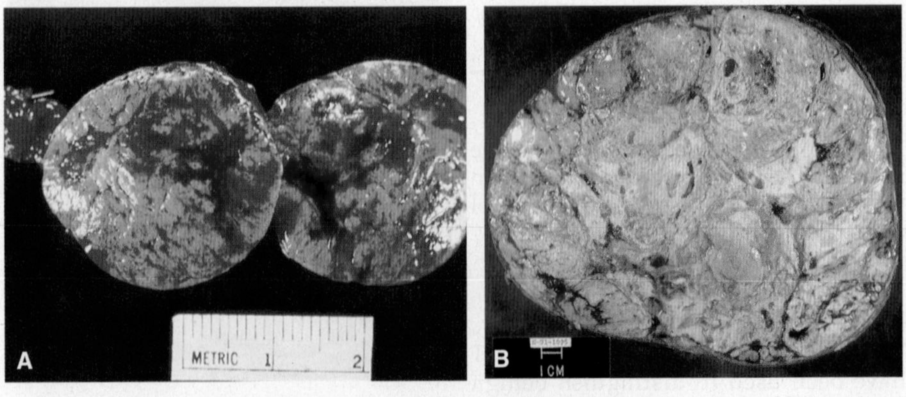

Figure 75-3 ■ Comparison of gross anatomical appearance of benign adrenal adenomas and malignant adrenal cortical carcinomas: (**A**) 2.5-cm benign adrenal adenoma causing Cushing syndrome. The tumor is well encapsulated and of homogeneous appearance. (**B**) 25-cm adrenal cortical carcinoma with lobulated appearance and areas of necrosis.

gery, radiation therapy, cytotoxic chemotherapy, and mitotane.[39]

Surgery

Patients with presumed stages I to III tumors will always be offered surgery. Surgical resection, even if incomplete, should be considered as the initial step in therapy. Because most adrenal carcinomas are large, the surgical approach should be either transabdominal or thoracoabdominal, with an incision of sufficient length to allow adequate exploration and resection of contiguous organs, if necessary, to remove gross tumor. For this reason, laparoscopic surgery is not recommended for the large tumors.[40] There are differences of opinion regarding the surgical approach for smaller tumors. Some reports suggest a higher risk of peritoneal carcinomatosis with laparoscopic surgery (89%) than with open adrenalectomy (15%),[41] while another report[42] suggests that laparoscopic adrenalectomy for malignancy can be performed in appropriately selected cases with equal oncologic outcome while providing advantages in patient morbidity. Ultimately, the outcome appears very dependent on the surgeon's skill and experience. The danger of breaching the tumor capsule with peritoneal spillage is a major risk with laparoscopic surgery. The open approach also facilitates lymph node dissection and regional exploration for tumor spread. A compromise in the surgical strategy for uncertain lesions can be initial laparoscopic approach with conversion to an open adrenalectomy if there is good evidence during the procedure the tumor is malignant. The surgical goal should be the resection of the entire tumor mass, whenever possible. Even if this is not possible because of local extension into other structures, tumor debulking should be carried out to the maximum degree possible. It is frequently necessary to remove the adjoining kidney en bloc with the tumor because of invasion of the upper pole with adrenal cancer. Multiorgan resection may be required in one third or more of patients. Following tumor removal at first operation, a definite staging should be assessed together with pathological assessment of the tumor including Weiss score, histochemical markers and genotyping. In case of complete resection, the recurrence risk should be assessed and adjuvant therapy should be considered. In case of residual tumor, further local radiofrequency ablation, local radiation therapy or general chemotherapy should be considered.

Surgical resection should be considered for relapses in highly selected patients with excellent performance status, symptomatic disease (ie, from hormone hypersecretion), limited loco-regional recurrence or isolated distant metastases if complete resection can be achieved. In cases of liver metastases, a partial lobectomy or segmentectomy, with resection of the involved portion of the liver, has led to long-term remission.[43] Adherence to or invasion of the wall of the inferior vena cava may require resection of that portion of the wall and a patch. Surgery for resection of local recurrences or metastases can often be limited by the location of lesions and by repeated recurrences. These aggressive efforts to excise all grossly visible tumors are justified because chemotherapy appears to be most effective when the tumor burden is minimal. Resection of metastases is also recommended when their number is limited and they are surgically accessible (lung, liver). Resection of these lesions should be considered, especially in patients who have had long disease-free intervals after resection of the primary tumor and have favorable tumor biology.[44]

Radio-Frequency Ablation (RFA) and Radiation Therapy

RFA of hepatic lesions and local recurrence has resulted in temporary control of metastatic disease but its utility and value remain to be proven. RFA can be considered in the treatment of lesions less than 6 cm in size that are not near indispensable tissues or large blood vessels. There are very little data in the medical literature documenting the efficacy of radiation therapy in ACC. In earlier reports, adrenal cortical carcinomas were reported to be resistant to radiation therapy.[45] However, limited data and anecdotal reports suggest that radiation therapy is likely as effective as in the majority of other solid tumors. As with other solid tumors, radiation therapy is recommended in the treatment of bone, brain, and other metastases, and for symptomatic local recurrences. The risk/benefit ratio of this treatment should be individually assessed. Radiation treatment of the adrenal bed can be administered to a patient with an incomplete local resection or after local recurrence. The latter should not replace surgery, especially in patients without evidence of residual disease, but could be used postoperatively as an adjunct to surgery. Another approach to radiotherapy is the use of selective radioligands with high affinity with adrenal cortical tissue. Preliminary studies using high dose [^{123}I] Iodometomidate in patients with metastatic ACC showed decreased size of metastatic lesions.[29]

Systemic Chemotherapy

Adjuvant Therapy ■ Adjuvant therapy should be offered to patients in stages I, II and III after apparently complete resection of the primary tumor. The main drug used for this purpose is mitotane but the benefit of this type of therapy remains controversial. Retrospective analysis of a large cohort of patients in stages I, II and III who had received adjuvant mitotane therapy following radical resection of the primary tumor showed that treatment with mitotane prolonged recurrence free survival.[46] Patients were treated with 3-4 gm/day and reached therapeutic levels (14 mcg/ml) after 3-6 months. Of the 23 patients studied, 35 patients showed relapse after 5-31+ months of follow-up. Prospective randomized clinical trials involving limited number of patients in single institutions failed to show a beneficial effect of mitotane in extending life expectancy. However, a multicenter, randomized clinical trial with larger number of patients still needs to be done in order to validate the benefit of this type of adjuvant therapy.[47] Because of the results reported with the most recent retrospective studies, adjuvant mitotane therapy is recommended for patients in stages I, II and III following complete resection of the primary tumor. Adjuvant radiation therapy following resection of the primary tumor has been investigated. Although it appears to prevent local recurrence, it does not prevent metastases and does not prolong life expectancy.

Systemic Chemotherapy for Advanced (Stage IV) Disease ■ The efficacy of first line chemotherapy is very limited with only temporary improvement. Chemotherapeutic protocols used as first line therapy include combinations of etoposide + doxorubicin + cisplatin + mitotane and streptozotocin + mitotane with complete or partial response rates of up to 50% of patients. For second-line therapy, agents are used that have not been used as first line. They include paclitaxel, 5-fluorouracil, vincristine sulfate and cyclophosphamide. However, these treatments have not been validated by large, well-controlled studies. The consensus from several series is that systemic chemotherapy is not very effective when given in stage IV; however, several factors contribute to the difficulty of comparing treatment outcomes. These include a relatively small number of patients per series, variability of treatment between and within series, lack of definition of the extent of disease at the time of treatment, and variable grades of malignancy. Some series include patients with low-grade malignancy as well as patients with high-grade malignancy. In addition, treatments are difficult to compare because there is a lack of a uniform definition of response, the duration of response is not always clearly stated, patients within a series frequently receive multiple drugs in variable sequence, and radiation therapy is sometimes combined with chemotherapy.[39,48]

Mitotane has been used in the treatment of patients with metastatic adrenal cortical carcinoma, either as monotherapy or in combination with other chemotherapeutic drugs, but there is no consensus regarding its efficacy.[49,50] Mitotane is an adrenalytic drug with selective action on the adrenal cortex. It belongs to the class of drugs that require transformation into active metabolites for therapeutic action. The active metabolites may covalently combine with specific targets in the cells responsive to the drug and/or induce oxygen activation, leading to toxicity. There is evidence that mitotane is transformed to an acyl chloride by a mitochondrial P-450–mediated hydroxylation and that the acyl chloride covalently combines with specific bionucleophiles within the adrenal cortical cell for the adrenolytic effect to take place. It is possible that adrenal tumors vary in their ability to affect metabolic transformation or initiate free-radical production, thereby expressing variable sensitivity to mitotane.[47] In a series of reports,[51] mitotane has been associated with partial or complete response in 33% of patients with adrenal cancer. Mitotane causes significant toxicity in therapeutically effective doses. The adverse effects of mitotane are dose dependent and usually intolerable when doses exceed 6 g daily, a dose that may be required to achieve therapeutic blood levels of 14-20 μg/mL.[52] Treatment begins with doses of 1 g twice daily, and the dose is gradually increased to tolerance. The drug is best administered with fat-containing foods, since its absorption and transport appear coupled to lipoproteins. Patients treated with mitotane should be monitored clinically by measuring urinary-free cortisol, serum electrolytes, serum cholesterol and liver enzymes. Mitotane increases the binding of cortisol to corticosteroid-binding globulin, and serum cortisol levels can be elevated even when the circulating free cortisol level is not.[53] Treatment with mitotane inhibits hormone production and eventually causes necrosis of the contralateral adrenal gland. Patients must receive cortisol replacement of 25-35 mg daily. Synthetic glucocorticoids, such as prednisone and dexamethasone, are less desirable because their metabolism may be enhanced by mitotane, making it difficult to determine the optimal replacement dose. In low doses (2-4 g daily), mitotane has less adrenalytic effects on the zona glomerulosa and is less likely to suppress aldosterone production. With larger doses, replacement with fluorocortisol may be necessary. Cholesterol levels may increase during treatment because mitotane is an HMG-CoA reductase activator. Treatment with statins reduces these levels.

Long-Term Treatment Outcome

Medical therapy for adrenal cortical carcinoma is of limited effectiveness;[54,55] however, there are a significant number of patients whose life expectancy has been extended with acceptable morbidity. Combined surgical and medical treatment appears to be more effective than medical treatment alone, especially for patients with localized or regional disease (stages I–III). In a comparison of 18 patients treated with mitotane alone and 15 treated with combined surgical resection and mitotane chemotherapy, those who underwent surgical treatment had a more favorable response, with 33% of patients surviving more than 5 years from the time of first recurrence.[44] A study of 49 patients with adrenal carcinoma concluded that surgical excision offered the best chance for prolonged survival. Forty-three percent of patients with a completely resected tumor were alive with no evidence of disease 7.3 years postoperatively.[56] Comparing various types of therapy in 110 patients with adrenal cortical carcinoma, it was noted that 56% of patients responded to surgery for localized and regional disease with a disease-free survival time of at least 2 years. In contrast, abdominal radiation therapy was effective in 15%, systemic chemotherapy in 9%, and mitotane therapy in 29%.[57]

In a review of 82 patients, it was noted that survival of patients with metastatic disease was poor and not improved by treatment with mitotane, cytotoxic chemotherapy, or radiation therapy.[58] In a series of 28 patients with stage IV disease, a combination of etoposide (100 mg/m² on days 5-7), doxorubicin (20 mg/m² on days 1 and 8), cisplatin (40 mg/m² on days 1 and 9), and mitotane (4 g/d) was given. Two patients had a complete response, and 13 had a partial response, for an overall response rate of 53.5%; stable disease was observed in 8 patients. Time to progression was 24.4 months.[59] In another series of 40 patients with adrenocortical carcinoma, a phase II trial was conducted with streptozocin and mitotane. Streptozocin was administered in doses of 1.0 g/d for 5 days, followed by 2 g once every 3 weeks; mitotane was given orally in doses of 1-4 g/d. Complete or partial response was obtained in 22 patients with measurable disease. Overall, 2-year survival was 70% and 5-year survival, 32.5%. Significant effect on the disease-free interval (p = .02) and on survival (p = .01) was noted in 17 adjuvantly treated cases, compared with patients without any therapy after complete resection.[60]

Thus, survival of patients with adrenal carcinoma with recurrent or metastatic disease is better for those who are able to receive surgical treatment rather than medical treatment alone. With surgical treatment, 50% of patients survive an average of 70 months, whereas less than 10% of patients are alive for this length of time with medical treatment alone. The surgical treatment involves not only resection of the primary tumor, but also repeated resection of metastases. A management algorithm for each stage of the disease is provided in Figure 75-4.

The prognosis of patients with adrenal cortical carcinoma is poor, but the

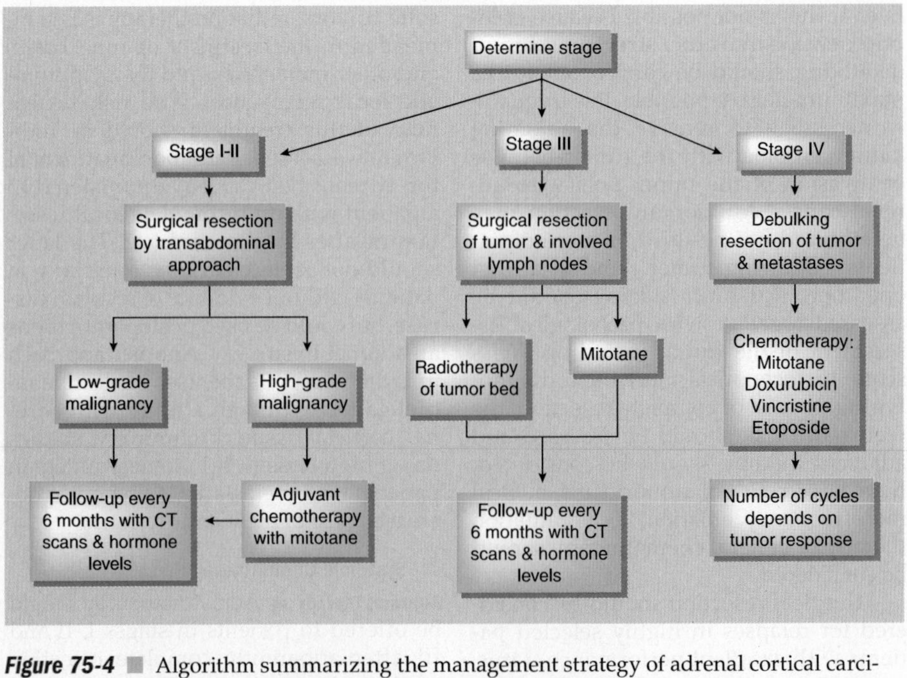

Figure 75-4 ■ Algorithm summarizing the management strategy of adrenal cortical carcinoma based on stage of the disease. Hormone measurements should be followed as tumor markers in patients with functioning adrenal cortical carcinoma.

life expectancy of patients in stages I, II, and III can be significantly extended by a combination of surgical resection and chemotherapy. There are individual cases in which curative resection has been possible and others in which metastatic lesions have regressed on chemotherapy. Early diagnosis is possible in patients with functioning neoplasms, in whom the metabolic manifestations of hormone excess can lead to the discovery of tumors in stages I and II. In contrast, the prognosis of patients in stage IV is poor.

Adrenal Function Inhibitors in Treatment

The metabolic changes associated with excessive hormonal production can cause significant morbidity and shortened life expectancy in patients with residual disease who do not respond to antitumor therapy. Inhibitors of adrenal function have been used to suppress steroid hormone production and improve the clinical manifestations of the disease. The most commonly used inhibitors are ketoconazole and aminoglutethimide.

Ketoconazole is an imidazole derivative that inhibits the synthesis of cortisol by inhibiting mitochondrial cytochrome P-450-dependent enzymes, such as cholesterol side-chain cleavage and 11 β-hydroxylase, in rat and mouse adrenal preparations. It is also an important inhibitor of gonadal and adrenal steroidogenesis in vivo when given in doses as low as 200-600 mg/d. Ketoconazole has been used to treat patients with Cushing syndrome and virilization caused by adrenal carcinoma.[61] Clinical improvement occurs frequently, but regression of metastatic disease is rare.[62] When patients are treated with ketoconazole, adrenal insufficiency is avoided by decreasing the dose sufficiently to maintain normal cortisol levels. The most frequent adverse reactions with ketoconazole are nausea and vomiting, abdominal pain, and pruritus in 1-3% of patients. Hepatotoxicity, primarily of the hepatocellular type, has been associated with its use.

Aminoglutethimide inhibits cholesterol side-chain cleavage and the conversion of cholesterol to pregnenolone in the adrenal cortex. As a consequence, the synthesis of cortisol, aldosterone, and androgens is suppressed. The drug has been used both in adults and children in doses of 500-2000 mg/d.[63] Cortisol levels fall gradually with regression of the clinical manifestations of Cushing syndrome[61] and eventually patients may need cortisol replacement. The effect of aminoglutethimide is promptly reversed by interruption of therapy. Aminoglutethimide causes gastrointestinal (anorexia, nausea, vomiting) and neurologic (lethargy, sedation, blurred vision) side effects and can cause hypothyroidism in 5% of patients. A skin rash is frequently observed during the first 10 days of treatment, but it usually subsides with continuation of treatment. Headaches have also been reported with the larger doses.

Another drug, mifepristone, is available as a glucocorticoid receptor antagonist and able to reverse the clinical manifestations of hypercortisolemia. It is given in doses of 600-900 mg daily. The drug is not FDA approved and is not commercially available but can be obtained from the manufacturer on a compassionate use basis.

Future Prospects

More effective therapy is needed for adrenal cortical carcinomas, and it is likely to come from a better understanding of tumor biology, including the oncogenic and tumorigenic processes that induce early mutations and drive progression with growth and dissemination of an established tumor. Future approaches to the treatment of adrenal cortical carcinoma are likely to be based on blocking or reversing the biologic mechanisms of tumorigenesis.

Molecular targeted therapy is promising but still experimental. Like many other proliferative pathways, those involved in adrenal tumorogenesis appear to involve signaling through receptor tyrosine kinases and their downstream signaling pathways. Tyrosine kinases that are upregulated include the IGF-I receptor as well as the Fibroblast Growth Factor receptor 1. There is no experience with tyrosine kinase inhibitors in adrenal cancer. IGF-II is highly expressed in ACC and preclinical studies with IGF antagonists have shown tumor suppressive activity. Early phase I and II clinical trials with IGF antagonists have shown promising responses. Antiangiogenic strategies have been tested in preclinical studies, but the response in clinical situations has not been validated.[62] Rosiglitazone, a thiazolidinedione insulin sensitizer has been shown to block cell proliferation and migration in a human, steroid-secreting adrenal cortical carcinoma cell line as well as to induce cell differentiation and apoptosis through activation of PPAR. This effect appears to be mediated through impairment of IGF-I in adrenal cancer cells. Rosiglitazone has not been studied as an anticancer drug in adrenal cortical carcinoma.

The difficulty in assessing the effectiveness of published treatment protocols stems from the fact that most series are limited in the number of patients studied. There is great variability in the drugs used, the stage and extent of the tumor, and the grade of malignancy. Because adrenal cancer is rare, collaborative, worldwide, multicenter controlled studies are necessary in order to reach consensus on the efficacy and safety of treatment protocols.[64] This type of international collaboration currently exists in the form of registries, tissue banks and multicenter clinical trials and offers the prospect of propelling the field forward within the next decade.

Selected References

The complete reference list can be found at www.CANCERMEDICINE8.com

1. Brennan MF. Adrenocortical carcinoma. *CA Cancer J Clin*. 1987;37:348–365.
16. Farge D, Chatellier G, Pagny JY, et al. Isolated clinical syndrome of primary aldosteronism in four patients with adrenocortical carcinoma. *Am J Med*. 1987;83:635–640.
17. Arteaga E, Biglieri EG, Kater CE, et al. Aldosterone-producing adrenocortical carcinoma. Preoperative recognition and course in three cases. *Ann Intern Med*. 1984;101:316–321.
18. Grondal S, Curstedt T. Steroid profile in serum: increased levels of sulphated pregnenolone and pregn-5-ene-3 beta, 20 alpha-diol in patients with adrenocortical carcinoma. *Acta Endocrinol*. 1991;124:381–385.
19. Copeland PM. The incidentally discovered adrenal masses. *Ann Surg*. 1984;199:116–122.
24. Hamper UM, Fishman EK, Hartman DS, et al. Primary adrenocortical carcinoma: sonographic evaluation with clinical and pathologic correlation in 26 patients. *Am J Roentgenol*. 1987;148:915–919.
30. MacFarlane DA. Cancer of the adrenal cortex: the natural history, prognosis and treatment in the study of the fifty-five cases. *Ann R Coll Surg Engl*. 1958;23:155–186.
31. Sullivan M. Adrenal cortical carcinoma. *Urology*. 1978;120:660–665.
33. Hogan T. A clinical and pathological study of adrenocortical carcinoma: therapeutic implications. *Cancer*. 1980;45:2880–2883.
35. Weiss LM. Comparative histologic study of 43 metastasizing and non-metastasizing adrenocortical tumors. *Am J Surg Pathol*. 1984;8:163–169.
43. Thompson NW. Adrenocortical carcinoma. In: Thompson NW, Vinik AI, eds. *Endocrine Surgery Update*. New York: Grune and Stratton; 1983:119–128.
45. Percarpio B, Knowlton AH. Radiation therapy of adrenal cortical carcinoma. *Acta Radiol Ther Phys Biol*. 1976;15:288–292.
49. Hogan TF, Citrin DL, Johnson BM, et al. o,p′-DDD (mitotane) therapy of adrenal cortical carcinoma: observations on drug dosage, toxicity and steroid replacement. *Cancer*. 1978;42:2177–2181.
63. Schteingart DE, Cash R, Conn JW. Aminoglutethimide and metastatic adrenal cancer: maintained reversal (six months) of Cushing's syndrome. *JAMA*. 1966;198:1007–1010.

76 Tumors of the Diffuse Neuroendocrine and Gastroenteropancreatic Endocrine System

Evan Vosburgh, MD

Introduction

The diffuse neuroendocrine system (DES) is represented by small numbers of cells spread through the body, and the fascinating collection of tumors that derive from these cells present a bewildering spectrum of epidemiologic, pathologic, biologic and clinical features. Clinical and scientific investigation of these rare tumors, which include inherited multiple endocrine neoplasia (eg, MEN-1, MEN-2), unique clinical syndromes secondary to secretion of specific peptides (eg, insulinomas, glucagonomas, VIPomas), and many patients with long survival, are challenging. The more common presentation of these sometimes clinically dramatic tumors is often characterized by nonspecific or absent symptoms and signs of small, difficult to detect tumors (<1 cm in size) that even when suspected may have already metastasized. The above features in part explain the long term cancer registry data showing 5-year survivals for tumors of the neuroendocrine system that have not improved in the past several decades, and that remain about 30–60%, leading many to argue stridently for the avoidance of the term "benign" for neuroendocrine tumors as a group.

However, detailed understanding of somatostatin receptor biology improved imaging for diagnosis and follow-up, and resulted in a major advance in control of symptoms through the use of somatostatin analogues. Other advances in biochemical markers and improved imaging techniques for diagnosis and localization, coupled with screening based on specific familial syndromes associated with defined gene mutations, now offer a small opportunity for screening and early detection as well as for curative surgical treatment of many of these rare tumors. Ongoing investigation of the biology of growth factor receptors, tyrosine kinases, and other signaling pathway inhibitors specific to neuroendocrine tumors, as well as empiric clinical trials of targeted therapies in early phase trials is beginning to yield therapeutic advances following decades of disappointing results with cytotoxic chemotherapy.

The discussion of tumors of the DES in this chapter will focus on the gastroenteropancreatic neuroendocrine tumors (GEP-NET), representing the majority of all tumors of the DES. Specific subgroups include the following:

- Carcinoid tumors, a group of well-differentiated GEP-NET, representing over one-half of all GEP-NET.
- Pancreatic neuroendocrine tumors (PNETs), the second highest incidence of GEP-NET, divided into non-secretary tumors and those with a variety of unique immunochemical and clinical features related to secretion of specific peptides (ie, insulinomas).
- Multiple endocrine neoplasia (MEN) syndromes 1, 2a, 2b, and familial medullary thyroid carcinoma (FMTC), which are well-characterized (familial) cancer syndromes involving multiple tissues where cells of the DES are found.
- Pheochromocytoma and parathyroid tumors, both sporadic and seen in association with MEN syndromes

The Diffuse Endocrine System

The diffuse endocrine system (DES) had its descriptive origins in early histology and cell biology that defined a population of normal chromium-avid epithelial cells widely scattered through the intestinal tract (enterochromaffin cells) and other organs (chromaffin or clear cells).[1–3] Pearse[4] proposed the APUD (amine precursor uptake and decarboxylation) system and with other investigatators expanded the description of the APUD/DES secretory products to include a list of over 100 bioactive peptides, monamines, and eicosanoids.[5] In the gut, these cells are scattered from stomach to rectum and represent less than 1% of the surrounding cell population.

The Neuroendocrine Cell

It was originally believed that all cells of the DES shared embryologic origin in the neural crest (neuroectoderm). However it is now clear that the gut enteroendocrine cells arise from gut endoderm,[6,7] and the four epithelial cell types of the gut, including enteroendocrine cells, are derived from a common pluripotential stem cell found in the intestinal crypts.[8] However, these cells of the gut DES share phenotypic and biochemical features with neural cells. Along with the large core dense vesicles (LCDV) of endocrine cells, the DES cells also contain synaptic-like microvesicles (SLMV) characteristic of the synaptic regions of neural cells. The complex and diverse biochemistry and control of secretion from LCDV and SLMV of the DES cells is discussed in detail by Weidenmann and colleagues.[9] Many of the molecules shared by neurons and neuroendocrine cells have been used to study neuroendocrine tumors, including the "general markers" of chromogranin A (CgA), synaptophysin, and neuron-specific enolase (NSE) and the "specific markers" found in subtypes of neuroendocrine tumors consisting of the peptide and amine hormones (see below).

A number of peptides originally isolated from gut endocrine tissues including gastrin, cholecystokinin, vasoactive intestinal polypeptide (VIP), and substance P (SP) occur in nerves. Peptides found primarily in nervous tissues have been identified in gut endocrine cells and include somatostatin (somatotropin release-inhibiting factors [SRIF]), encephalin, neurotensin, and thyrotropin-releasing hormone (TRH).[10,11,12] Unique to the GEP axis is the ability of the endocrine cell to secrete a variety of peptides and amines.

The Gastroenteropancreatic (GEP) Cells

Despite the unifying characteristics of this unique set of DES cells with shared endocrine and neural features, a closer look at the accumulated information on the general and specific histologic, morphologic, hormonal content, and tissue distribution characteristics defined a heterogeneous population of distinct cell types. Table 76-1 describes the 15 cell types found in the stomach, pancreas, and intestine of man as outlined by Solcia and colleagues[13] and updated by Rindi and colleagues.[14] Only a limited number of the 15 cell types have been associated with a specific endocrine tumor, and sev-

Table 76-1 ■ **Endocrine Cells of the Adult Gastroenteropancreatic System by Cell Type, Hormone Content, Vesicle Markers, and Location**

		Gastroenteropancreatic Vesicle Markers		Location						
Cell Type	**Hormone Content**	**LDCV**	**SLMV**	**Pan**	**C/F**	**A**	**D**	**J**	**I**	**LI**
P/D1	Ghrelin	CgA, VMAT2			+					
EC	5-HT	CgA, VMAT1	Syn		+	+	+	+	+	+
ECL	Histamine	CgA, VMAT2	Syn		+					
A	Glucagon	CgA > CgC VMAT2	Syn	+						
B	Insulin	CgA,VMAT2 NESP55	Syn	+						
CCK	Cholecystokinin						+	+		
D	Somatostatin	CgA	Syn	+	+	+	+	+		
G	Gastrin	CgA	Syn			+	+			
GIP	GIP/Xenin	CgA					+	+		
PP	PP	CgA, CgC VMAT2	Syn	+						
L	PYY/GLI	CgC > CgA	Syn					+	+	+
M	Motilin						+	+		
N	Neurotensin	CgA						+	+	
S	Secretin, 5-HT	CgA					+	+		

Abbreviations: 5-HT, 5-Hydroxyhistamine; a, antrum; c/f, corpus/fundus; CgA, chromogranin A; CgC, chromogranin C; d, duodenum; GLP-1, glucagon-like immunoreactants.; I, ileum; j, jejunum; LDCV, large dense core vesicle; li, large intestine; NESP55, neuroendocrine secretory protein 55; pan, pancreas; PP, pancreatic polypeptide; PYY, PP-like peptide; SLMV, synaptic-like microvesicle; Syn, synaptophysin; VMAT, vesicular monamine transporter.
Source: Modified from Ref. 14.

eral of the peptides identified in these cells have yet to be identified as being actively secreted by any endocrine tumor. The most important distinguishing feature of each cell type is the presence of a specific peptide or bioactive amine.

Neuroendocrine Markers

Neuroendocrine markers are utilized in the histologic and immunohistochemical categorization of neuroendocrine tumors, and to some degree as clinical markers for diagnosis and assessment of response and relapse. The markers are both general and specific, with general markers related to cellular compartments, such as vesicles or the cytosol, and specific markers being related to the individual hormones/amines synthesized and secreted by the various GEP-NET. These are described for some of the most important markers below.

Serotonin and Metabolites ■ The rate-limiting step in those GEP-NET that synthesize and secrete serotonin (eg, carcinoid tumors) is the conversion of tryptophan into 5-hydroxytryptophan (5-HTP), catalyzed by the enzyme tryptophan hydroxylase. 5-HTP is rapidly converted to 5-HT that is either stored in the neurosecretory granules or may be secreted directly into the vascular compartment where it is converted into the urinary metabolite 5-hydroxyindoleacetic acid (5-HIAA).[15] The quantification of 5-HIAA in a 24-h urine collection is s the best characterized and most frequently used clinical assay for diagnosis and follow-up for GEP-NETs that synthesize and secrete serotonin.[16]

Patients with neuroendocrine tumors of bronchopulmonary and gastric origin have relatively little 5-HIAA, but large amounts of 5-HTP, presumed due to low intracellular levels of dopa-decarboxylase that impairs the conversion of 5-HTP into 5-HT.[16]

Chromogranin A ■ Chromogranin A (CgA) is a member of the chromogranin family of glycoproteins that are stored along with numerous peptide hormones in the large dense core vesicles (LDCV) of endocrine and neuroendocrine cells,[17] and as such is actively secreted. It therefore can serve as an immunohistochemical marker at diagnosis, as well as a plasma marker. CgA is considered as a "general marker" of neuroendocrine differentiation along with synaptophysin, and the loss of CgA staining correlates with tumor evolution to an undifferentiated histology. Of the numerous endocrine markers shown to be elevated above normal concentrations in serum/plasma of neuroendocrine patients,[18] CgA has been generally accepted as the most useful marker in GEP-NET patients with a sensitivity above 90%.[19] The CgA level correlates with metastatic versus non-metastatic disease at presentation,[20] and can be used to follow patients for relapse following surgery.[21]

NESP-55 ■ Neuroendocrine secretory protein-55 (NESP-55) is a member of the chromogranin family, with a less widespread distribution in endocrine and neural tissue than chromogranin A. Srivastava and colleagues[22] studied 63 neuroendocrine tumors for a variety of neuroendocrine markers, and showed that NESP-55 staining was restricted to endocrine tumors of the pancreas and adrenal medulla, and proposed that this marker could be used to assign origin to metastatic neuroendocrine tumors.

Synaptophysin ■ Synaptophysin (p38) is a major neuronal protein concentrated in the membrane of small synaptic vesicles of nerve cells.[23] Weidenmann and colleagues[24] demonstrated the presence of synaptophysin in a wide range of normal neuroendocrine cells and neuroendocrine tumors. Buffa and colleagues[25] combined immunohistochemistry and ultrastructural studies on the normal and tumor tissues to localize the synaptophysin to a population of small, clear vesicles distinct from the peptide-containing (CgA-positive) secretory vesicles. The synaptophysin-positive vesicles are now commonly referred to as SLMV.

Neuron-Specific Enolase ■ Neuron-specific enolase (NSE) derives its name from the early observations that the enzyme was restricted to central neurons. It was later found in peripheral autonomic nerves and a number of endocrine cells. Bishop and colleagues[10] demonstrated NSE in all identifiable endocrine and nerve cells of the gastrointestinal (GI) tract and pancreas. NSE has replaced earlier histologic argentaffin stains as a cytosolic general marker of normal neuroendocrine cells and tumors.

VMAT1, 2 ■ The vesicular monamine transporter protein has two isoforms, *VMAT1* and *VMAT2*, which serve as amine transporters in the granule/vesicular membrane of a variety of cell types. They differ in cellular distribution, substrate specificity, and drug sensitivity.[26] *VMAT1* is expressed primarily in the enterochromaffin (EC) cells of the GI tract and the adrenal chromaffin cells. *VMAT2* is expressed in gastric enterochromaffin-like (ECL) cells, adrenal chromaffin cells, as well as various central and peripheral neurons (including enteric).[27] Rindi and colleagues[28] proposed *VMAT2* as an ECL cell and tumor marker. In a study of 211 GI tumors *VMAT1* was expressed primarily on ileal and appendicial carcinoids (EC cell-derived tumors) that synthesize serotonin, and *VMAT2* was expressed primarily on gastric carcinoids (also ECL cell-derived tumors) that synthesize histamine. There was little or no VMAT1 or VMAT2 expression in the peptide producing PNET and rectal carcinoids and nonendocrine tumors of the GI tract.[29]

Tumors of the DES

Coincident with the description of the normal cells of the DES, Siegfried Oberndorfer (see Modlin et al.[1]) in 1907 separated out a group of monotonous-appearing GI tumors labeled "karzinoide" (carcinoid), carcinoma-like, as distinct from the more aggressive adenocarcinomas.[30] Masson[31] then established the relationship between the normal EC cells of the gut and the cells of the tumor, establishing a relationship between the DES and carcinoid tumors. Carcinoids were soon reported in numerous locations, including the lung, bronchi, pancreas, and throughout the GI tract. The term carcinoid has, for almost 100 years, been generally applied to all tumors of the DES that share a similar histological appearance and that, to this day, are described as monotonous small cells with regular, well-rounded nuclei with insular, trabecular, glandular, undifferentiated, and mixed growth patterns.[32] With an increased understanding of the DES, more specifically the GEP cells, and the parallels between normal cell types and specific tumor types, the description and classification of "carcinoids" evolved and attempts have been made to further classify tumors into more biologically and clinically relevant groups.

Williams and Sadler[33] in 1963 proposed a classification based on embryologic division into tumors arising from the foregut, midgut, and hindgut. The foregut tumors were perhaps the most diverse group and included two distinct foregut carcinoid tumors: sporadic primary, and tumors secondary to achlorhydria. The skin manifestations of carcinoid syndrome for these tumors is referred to as atypical and tends to be of long duration with a purplish or violaceous rather than pink or red hue, and frequently results in telangiectasia and hypertrophy of the skin of the face and upper neck that may result in a "leonine" facies. It is not unusual for these tumors to metastasize to bone. The cells of origin include the Kulchitsky cells of the bronchus and the ECL cell of the stomach and upper GI tract.

Midgut carcinoid tumors were found in locations distal to the second portion of the duodenum, the jejunum, the ileum, and the ascending colon. The midgut carcinoids arise from EC cell and characteristically have high serotonin and low histamine content and often produce other vasoactive compounds, such as kinins, prostaglandins, and SP. The classic carcinoid syndrome (see below) of flushing and diarrhea with or without wheezing is most closely associated with the midgut tumors. These tumors may rarely produce ACTH and infrequently metastasize to bone.

Hindgut carcinoid tumors were located in the transverse colon, left colon, and rectum. These tumors are often silent (hormonal symptoms) in their presentation and more frequently metastasize to bone. Though clinically useful in characterizing patient groups, and still informally used today, the embryologic classification has been replaced by several WHO classifications described below.

WHO Classification

The first WHO classification solidified the use of term *carcinoid* by using it to refer to the majority of neuroendocrine tumors, except neuroendocrine tumors of the pancreas/thyroid, paragangliomas, small-cell lung carcinoma, and Merkel cell tumors of the skin. Incorporated into the revised classification were additional histologic characteristics, such as those described by Soga and Tazawa,[32] who described growth patterns such as acinar or trabecular. Kloppel and colleagues[34] attribute the failure of the initial WHO classification to the overuse by pathologists of the term carcinoid at a time when the clinical and biological characterization of these tumors was defined by distinct subtypes, and most clinicians were restricting the use of the term carcinoid to those neuroendocrine tumor patients who demonstrated the carcinoid syndrome.

The revised WHO classification published in 2000 by Solcia and colleagues[35] adapted the term *(neuro)endocrine* so as to avoid the varied historical definitions of carcinoid. The 2000 WHO classification introduced the term GEP-NET, and defined three broad groups (Table 76-2A) based on pathology. Table 76-2B details further refinements of clinically meaningful groups, using the three broad histologic groups and additional clinical features. The tumors were then defined in more detail within the categories of stomach, duodenum (and upper jejunum), appendix, ileum (and distal jejunum), colon-rectum, and pancreas, with criteria that included tumor size, differentiation, angioinvasion, proliferative activity, local organ invasion, metastases, hormonal secretion, and association with distinct clinical syndromes (ie, carcinoid syndrome) or diseases (ie, neurofibromatosis)—clearly incorporating more than was seen under the microscope.

There remains no broadly accepted histologic classification system for GEP-NET that provides prognostic information for the individual patient. A tumor grading system has been tentatively developed for pancreatic and gastric tumors.[36] The assignment of a histologic diagnosis of "carcinoid" remains common, with most using the term as equivalent to the WHO category of well-differentiated neuroendocrine tumor, with or without clinical evidence of the carcinoid syndrome. Numerous efforts are under way to characterize the phenotype by molecular and genetic techniques that will perhaps add more clinically relevant annotation to the often deceptive histology.

Somatostatin and Somatostatin Receptors

The biology of somatostatin and the somatostatin receptors (SSTRs) and their expression on GEP-NET have yielded information that remains central to the diagnosis and therapy of this group of tumors. Somatostatin analogues serve as one of the earlier examples of targeted cancer therapy and contributed greatly to improve the medical and surgical management and quality of life. Unfor-

Table 76-2 Classification of GEP-NET

A: Broad Histologic Categories

Group	WHO Nomenclature	Common Synonym
1a	Well-differentiated neuroendocrine tumor	Carcinoid
1b	Well-differentiated neuroendocrine carcinoma	Malignant carcinoid
2	Poorly differentiated neuroendocrine carcinoma	Same

B: Clinical and Pathologic Modifiers Used to Refine Prognosis

Clinicopathologic Features	Benign	Uncertain	Malignant
Tumor size (cm)	<2	>2	>2
Local spread	No	Yes	Yes
Vascular invasion	No	Yes	Yes
Nuclear atypia	No	Yes	Yes
Tissue invasion	No	No	Yes
Metastases	No	No	Yes

Source: Modified from Refs. 259 and 260.

tunately SSTR agonist and antagonists have yet to provide a biologically active target that results in significant tumor cell death. The development of radioconjugated somatostatin analogues as imaging agents provide valuable clinical data, and the further extension of these agents as peptide receptor radiotherapy (PRRT) with measurable responses in refractory patients is nearing clinical approval in the United States and Europe, following closely on the clinical efficacy demonstrated for radioconjugated antibodies for certain lymphomas.

Somatostatin and SSTR Biology

Somatostatin is a peptide that inhibits a wide variety of physiologic activities, the most relevant for the treatment of GEP-NET being the inhibition of hormone secretion. Somatostatin is found in the central nervous system, hypothalamic-pituitary system, GI tract, exocrine and endocrine pancreas, and immune effector cells. It exists as somatostatin-28 and somatostatin-14.[37] Somatostatin-14 (14 amino acids) is pictured in Figure 76-1 with octreotide and several of the somatostatin analogues currently in use or under clinical investigation. Somatostatin, octreotide, and other analogues bind at the plasma membrane with varying affinities to a family of receptor subtypes, referred to as SSTR 1–5 (Table 76-3). The five subtypes have been cloned, each with a unique chromosomal location, and partially characterized as members of a superfamily of G-protein–coupled receptors (GCPR).[38,39] SSTR isoforms share between 40% and 60% homology, but have different biological effects mediated through activation of these receptors by somatostatin (or analogues). The increased activation of tyrosine phosphatase occurs via SSTR1 and SSTR2, and activation of adenyl cyclase via SSTR5 can result in decreased cellular proliferation, and the activation of SSTR3 can increase apoptosis.[37,40,41]

The SSTR1–5 are found in varying distribution on normal tissues in the CNS, anterior pituitary, adrenal gland, and pancreas, where the islets express all five SSTR subtypes. GEP-NET and other neuroendocrine tumors, as well as tumors with neuroendocrine components arising from cells of the DES often express SSTR subtypes—often more than one subtype—in high densities.[42–45] The GEP-NET, particularly the midgut carcinoid and pancreatic islet-cell tumors, express multiple SSTR subtypes, the most common and highest density being SSTR2 in over 80% of cases, followed by SSTR5.[45–47] The expression of SSTR2 has been central to the development of somatostatin analogues as therapy to control secretory symptoms, for diagnostic and follow-up nuclear imaging, and for the emerging therapeutic option of peptide receptor radiotherapy (PRRT).

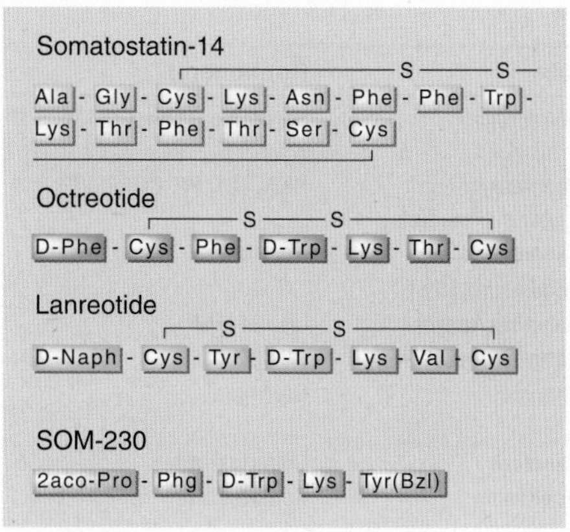

Figure 76-1 Somatostatin and analogue structures (including SOM 230).

Clinical Features of GEP-NET

Generally speaking, the GEP-NET are difficult to recognize at initial presentation. Pulmonary nodules, pancreatic masses, hepatic metastases, and gastric and rectal lesions at endoscopy often are thought to be more common malignancies prior to pathology reports being issued. The GEP-NET are all rare tumors and, as such, no simple screening program has been developed except in the even rarer familial syndromes. The early symptoms are often nonspecific (ie, abdominal pain and diarrhea), and even when more dramatic or classic secretory symptoms occur, the primary tumors are still often small and difficult to localize. All too often patients have long-standing symptoms and are diagnosed following the development of symptoms related to more advanced local or distant metastatic disease. However, once the diagnosis is considered, advancements in nonspecific (ie, CgA) and specific tumor markers (ie, 5-HIAA, gastrin) along with the imaging capabilities with radiolabeled somatostatin analogues, complemented by ultrasound, computed tomography (CT), magnetic resonance imaging (MRI), and positron emission tomography (PET) scanning, permit a strong presumptive or confirmed diagnosis to guide medical and surgical management. The variability in the location, secretory status, and biological behavior of these rare tumors has made clinical investigation difficult, resulting in few controlled trials. Despite the lack of comparative trials, consensus based on clinical evidence is available for guiding management of GEP-NET.[48,49] Many GEP-NET share common features of diagnosis, staging, and surgical and medical management, and by necessity are understood clinically through study of the more common ileal carcinoids and PNET.

Epidemiology

One of the challenges facing the classification systems over the past century for carcinoid and related neuroendocrine tumors is that the histology is not particularly informative and tends to be similar for benign and malignant biologic phenotypes. One distinction that has been maintained with some consistency over time has been the separation of classic carcinoid tumors from the pancreatic islet cell, or PNETs.

The two broad groups of tumors, carcinoid (WHO: well-differentiated neuroendocrine tumors), and PNET, are of approximately equal incidence and together comprise over 80% of all tumors of the DES. The carcinoid tumors represent more than 50% of neuroendocrine tumors in clinical practice. The most common site being in the small intestine (ileum) where they are often diagnosed following operative management of small bowel obstruction or bleeding or found incidentally during endoscopic procedures, and frequently only after local or distant metastases are present. The remaining neuroendocrine tumors in clinical practice are divided roughly as follows: 25% "nonfunctional" PNET, and 75% functional PNET consisting of 35% gastrinomas, 25% insulinomas, 10% VIPomas, 5% glucagonomas, and less than 3% neurotensinomas, somatostatinomas, and other rare ectopic hormone-secreting tumors.[50] Many of these "nonfunctional" tumors actually store and secrete pancreatic polypeptide (PP), a hormone, with no defined clinical effects. Other "nonfunctional" PNETs stain for specific peptides and amines but do not secrete amounts sufficient to cause a clinical syndrome. The use of the suffix "-oma" in gastrinoma, glucagonoma, insulinoma and VIPoma should be reserved for patients with elevated serum levels of the specific peptide and the associated clinical syndromes. Table 76-4 details the numerous clinical syndromes associated with GEP-NET.

Table 76-3 **Somatostatin Analogue Binding Affinities (IC_{50} [nM]) to SSTR**

	sstr1	sstr2	sstr3	sstr4	sstr5
Somatostatin 14	0.93 ± 0.12	0.15 ± 0.02	0.56 ± 0.17	1.5 ± 0.4	0.29 ± 0.04
Octreotide	280 ± 80	0.38 ± 0.08	7.1 ± 1.4	> 1000	6.3 ± 1.0
Lanreotide	180 ± 20	0.54 ± 0.08	14 ± 9	230 ± 40	17 ± 5

Abbreviation: SSTR, somatostatin receptor.
Source: From Ref. 261.

Table 76-4 ■ The Clinical Syndromes

Clinical Syndrome	Tumor Type	Site	Hormone(s)
Flushing/diarrhea/ wheezing	Carcinoid	Mid foregut	Serotonin, substance P
		Pancreas/foregut Adrenal medulla	NKA, TCT, PP, CGRP, VIP
Ulcer disease	Gastrinoma	Pancreas (85%), duodenum (15%)	Gastrin
Hypoglycemia	Insulinoma sarcomas	Pancreas/uterus	Insulin/TNF
	Hepatoma	Retroperitoneal liver	IGF/BP
Dermatitis/dementia Diabetes/DVT	Glucagonoma	Pancreas	Glucagon
Diabetes/steatorrhea	Somatostatinoma	Pancreas	Somatostatin
Cholelithiasis/ neurofibromatosis	Somatostatinoma	Duodenum	Somatostatin
Silent/liver mets	PPoma	Pancreas	PP
Acromegaly	GEP	Pancreas	GH (GHRH)
Cushing	GEP	Pancreas	ACTH/CRF
Hypercalcemia	VIPoma	Pancreas	VIP
	GEP	Pancreas	PTHrP
Pigmentation	GEP	Pancreas	MSH

Abbreviations: ACTH, adrenocorticotropic hormone (corticotrophin); BP, binding protein; CGRP, calcitonin gene, related peptide; CRF, corticotropin releasing factor; DVT, deep venous thrombosis; GEP, gastroenteropancreatic; GH, growth hormone, somatotropin; GHRH, growth hormone-releasing hormone; IGF, insulin-like growth factor; MSH, melanocyte stimulating hormone; NKA, neurokinin A; PP, pancreatic polypeptide; PTHrP, parathyroid hormone related peptide; TCT, thyrocalcitonin; TNF, tumor necrosis factor; VIP, vasoactive intestinal peptide.

In a comprehensive epidemiologic review of carcinoid tumors, Modlin and colleagues[51] report. based on SEER (Surveillance, Epidemiology, and End Results) program data, and patterned the analysis to provide continuity with prior reports based on data from the End Results Group (1950–1969) and the Third National Cancer Survey (TNCS) (1969–1971), permitting analysis of incidence data over a half century. The multidecade analysis of over 13,000 tumors shows, that this group of tumors, representing 0.49% of all malignancies, has increased in overall incidence for the past 30 years, with increases and decreases in specific sites. The GI tract is the site of over 65% of carcinoids, with an additional 25% occurring in the bronchopulmonary system (Fig. 76-2). Within the GI tract, the small bowel remains the most common site with a stable incidence over time, as opposed to the gastric and rectal carcinoids that have increased in recent decades. The changes in gastric and rectal incidence have been attributed to both changes in attribution within TNCS and SEER as well as the increased detection rate with the increasing use of upper and lower endoscopies. Over the same period, the incidence of carcinoids of the appendix decreased, perhaps reflecting the decrease in open abdominal procedures and bystander appendectomies.[52]

The reported overall incidence for carcinoids is about 2 cases per 100,000 (0.002%) in the United States,[51] and just under 1 case per 100,000 population (0.001%) in Scotland and England,[52] Italy,[53] and Japan.[54] These reported incidences are much lower than the reported incidence in autopsy series where Moertel and colleagues[56] from the Mayo Clinic reported carcinoids of the small bowel in 0.65% of unselected autopsies, and Berge and Linell[57] from Sweden reported a 1.2% incidence over a 12-year unselected series of autopsies. A similar large difference in incidence has been seen for PNET where the incidence of diagnosed PNET is about 0.04 per 100,000 and autopsy incidence exceeds 300 per 100,000.[57] It is not known how many of the large number of small bowel carcinoids and PNET found at autopsy would become clinically evident, or even how closely related in biology they are to symptomatic carcinoids. It is of interest that in series of 198 patients who received a gastric bypass operation for morbid obesity at a single center, there were three cases of incidental ileal carcinoids, for an incidence of about 1.5%.[58]

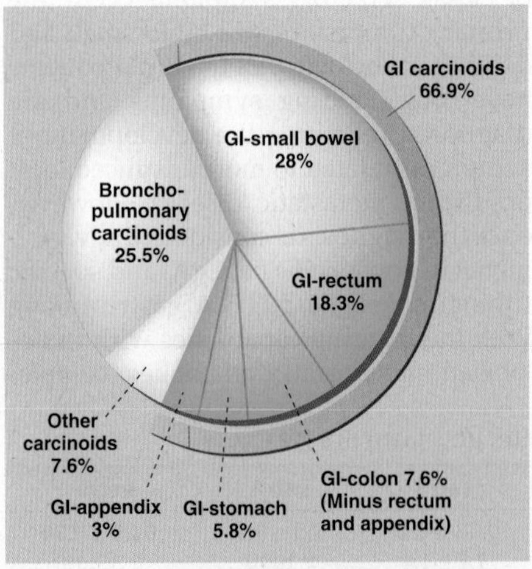

Figure 76-2 ■ Relative incidence of all carcinoid tumors and subgroup of gastrointestinal carcinoids. *Source*: From Ref. 51.

Imaging

The GEP-NET are a collection of rare tumors with varied presentations and clinical features. This fact limits the ability to conduct and publish large comparative studies. To date there are very few studies of GEP-NET that fit the criteria for evidence-based clinical decision making. Imaging of GEP-NET is no exception and has been addressed directly by the European Network of Neuroendocrine Tumors (ENET) in a Delphi process that sought to standardize guidelines for diagnostic imaging procedures in neuroendocrine tumors.[59] It was recognized at the outset that there were considerable center-to-center differences, reflecting the lack of controlled studies, but the process was able to yield five suggested diagnostic algorithms for different clinical presentations. A strong consensus emerged that somatostatin receptor scintigraphy (SRS) was central to the diagnosis of most cases of GEP-NET, and that CT and MRI provided further anatomical definition of SRS-documented disease and were more useful to follow tumor growth than SRS, and that the role of PET scans was still undetermined. Other authors support the opinion that since SRS is noninvasive and has high sensitivity for locating both primary and metastatic lesions (including bone), it should be used as the initial imaging modality in patients with confirmed and suspected GEP-NET, except those with insulinoma.[60–62]

Three-phase high resolution computerized tomography (CT) remains and MRI has emerged as useful procedures for the clinical staging and follow-up of GEP-NET because both provide a clear anatomical definition of tumors.[63] Both procedures can assess the extent of tumor spread to the mesentery and bowel wall as well as metastases to the lymph nodes and liver. The typical appearance of mesenteric invasion by carcinoid tumors on CT is a mesenteric mass with radiating linear densities representing thickened neurovascular bundles.[64] The advantage of CT is its ability to localize the tumors precisely in relation to the adjacent structure. GEP-NET that metastasize to the liver tend to be hypervascular and can appear isodense on CT scan following intravenous contrast. Therefore, suspected and confirmed liver metastases should be evaluated with CT scans before and after the administration of contrast.[64] MRI may be a very sensitive technique for the detection of liver metastases in some patients whose tumors are not seen well even on three-phase CT, and it may be more sensitive for the diagnosis of skeletal disease than CT. MRI needs further evaluation as a primary modality for the diagnosis and staging of carcinoid tumors because it can be done with less radiation exposure and without the oral contrast used with CT, which usually aggravates carcinoid diarrhea.[65]

Positron emission tomography (PET), increasingly used in oncology for diagnosis, staging and follow-up of certain tumors, has been found to be of limited use in neuroendocrine tumors. The low proliferative capacity of neuroendocrine tumors is thought to account for the low sensitivity of ^{18}FDG-PET for carcinoid and related tumors.[66] Recent data strongly supports a role of 11C-5-HTP-PET (taking advantage of the serotonin metabolism of NET) as an imaging technique that is more sensitive than both CT and SRS, detecting more lesions and smaller lesions that either CT or SRS alone.[67] ^{11}C-5HTP PET is currently limited by the requirement of a cyclotron at the imaging site given the several minute half-life of ^{11}C.

Scintigraphic Detection With Methyliodobenzylguanidine (MIBG) or Octreotide Scanning ■ The first report of ^{131}I-MIBG for the imaging of a carcinoid tumor was that of Fischer and colleagues in 1984, in which hepatic metastases that were seen as photopenic areas on a ^{99}mTc-phytate liver scan concentrated ^{131}I-MIBG.[68] Since this initial description, there have been a number of reports of successful imaging of carcinoid tumors using ^{131}I-MIBG.[69] The number of patients studied are far less than those reported for pheochromocytoma or neuroblastoma, however, overall sensitivity is calculated to be 55%. Because MIBG is taken up by a wide variety of neuroendocrine tumors, specificity depends on the certainty of the clinical and biochemical diagnosis and its use should be reserved for very select cases of GEP-NET where other imaging modalities are not informative.

Several somatostatin analogs (Fig. 76-1) have been developed that have preferential high affinity binding to SSTR2, SSTR5,[40,41] corresponding to the two SSTR expressed in 70–90% of GEP-NET.[45–47] The first octapeptide developed for clinical use, octreotide, was also the first analogue used in development for SRS. The first generation incorporated ^{123}I-tyr3-octreotide,[70] but was replaced by the currently most commonly used agent, ^{111}In-pentreotide ([^{111}Indium-DPTA] octreotide, OctreoScan).[71]

SRS with ^{111}In-DTPA octreotide was evaluated in a European multicenter trial in 350 patients with a histologically or biochemically proven neuroendocrine gastroenteropancreatic (GEP-NET) tumor.[72] Tumor sites were detected by conventional imaging methods in 88%, whereas SRS was positive in 80%. SRS was positive for most GEP-NET, yielding detection rates of glucagonomas (100%), VIPomas (88%), carcinoids (87%) and nonfunctioning islet cell tumors (82%). The low detection rate (46%) noted for insulinomas is related to the lower incidence of SSTR2 on insulinoma cells. Not only was SRS able to identify know sites of involvement, but it also revealed another 166 unsuspected lesions; 40% of these unsuspected lesions were later confirmed as true positive findings, leading to management changes in 40% of the 235 patients. This imaging technique is also valuable in identifying metastatic disease to extra-abdominal sites (Fig. 76-3).

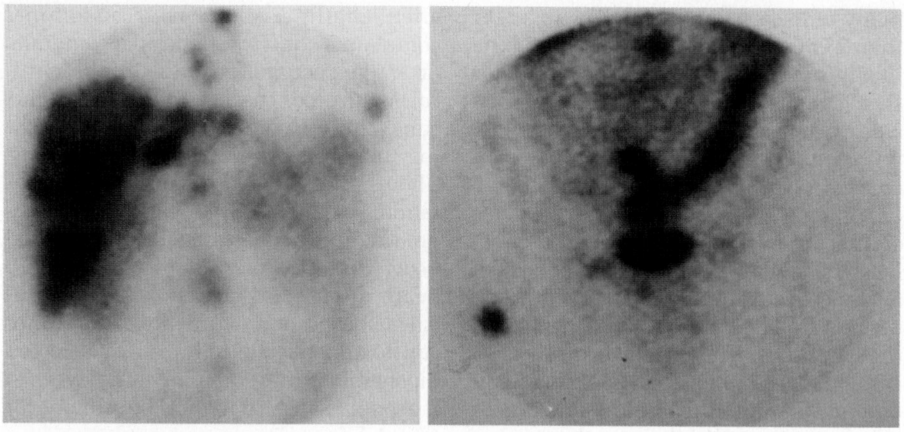

Figure 76-3 ■ Octreotide scan at 24 h showing liver and pelvic metastases in a patient with malignant carcinoid tumor.

Carcinoid Tumors

Carcinoid tumors, or well-differentiated endocrine tumors of the gastroenteropancreatic system, are the most commonly occurring gut endocrine tumors. The nonautopsy incidence is estimated to be approximately 1.5 cases per 100,000/year of the general population (ie, approximately 2500 cases/year in the United States). Nonetheless, they account for 13–34% of all tumors of the small bowel and 17–46% of all malignant tumors of the small bowel.[56,] Carcinoids have been reported as occurring in a multitude of less common locations, and other than the need to recognize that these very rare tumors are often misdiagnosed and managed,[73] most of the practical clinical literature on carcinoids addresses the more common sites of ileal, bronchus, gastric, appendix, and rectal.

Age Distribution ■ Carcinoid tumors have been reported from the first to the tenth decade. Modlin and colleagues[51,73] report the average age of all carcinoids in their analysis has increased from 59.9 years in the old SEER database, to 61.4 years in the more recent SEER database. The average age for carcinoids of the small intestine, common enough to generate reliable incidence data, shows an average age of 65.4 years, almost the same as the average age for noncarcinoid small intestinal tumors overall.

Natural History ■ Except for the small percentage of patients who present with undifferentiated neuroendocrine carcinomas,[74] the tumors at all sites are slow growing, often remain undiagnosed for many years, and sometimes are recognized only by symptoms related to metastatic spread to lymph nodes, liver, and, less often, bone.

Small Bowel GEP-NET ■ Small bowel GEP-NET (carcinoids) is frequently present with small bowel obstruction, abdominal pain, diarrhea, or GI bleeding.[53] Because tumors located in the distal small bowel in most cases have a low intramural profile (Fig. 76-4), it is not surprising that

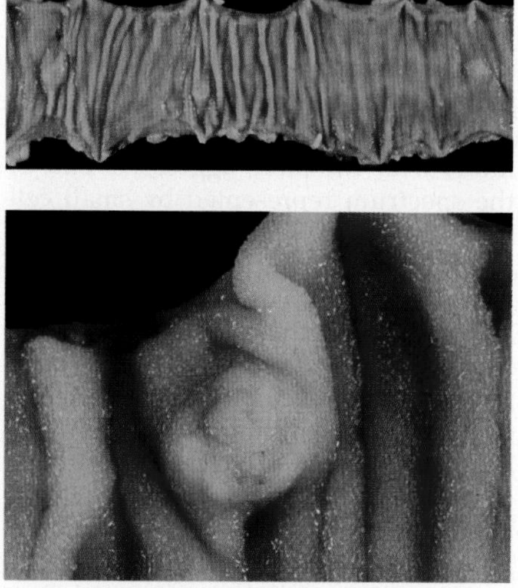

Figure 76-4 ■ Multiple carcinoids of the small bowel. Three small (<1 cm) intestinal carcinoids found in a young male on inspection of the terminal ileum at colonoscopy. *Source*: Courtesy of Ed Uthman, MD.

many of these tumors can grow to larger than 2 cm and remain undiagnosed. The likelihood of metastases relates to tumor size. The incidence of metastases associated with ileal GEP-NET is less than 15% with a tumor smaller than 1 cm, but increases to 95% with tumors larger than 2 cm. The ability of small tumors to cause significant local symptoms is in part related to the development of events such as ischemia, strangulation, and intussusception from the marked fibrotic reaction they produce. The causes of fibrosis of carcinoids remains poorly understood and of "paramount clinical and scientific importance" to their further understanding and treatment.[75] Small bowel GEP-NET account for upwards of 90% of patients with the carcinoid syndrome, described below.[76]

Gastric Carcinoids ■ Gastric carcinoids are divided into three distinct groups based on histology and clinical features.[77] The largest group comprises approximately 75% of tumors (type I) and involves an association between pernicious anemia, atrophic gastritis, chronic thyroiditis, and gastric carcinoid tumors. These tumors arise from the gastric ECL cell and usually are small and multiple and rarely metastasize. Development of these tumors is believed to be secondary to long-standing basal hypergastrinemia. The second largest group comprises approximately 20% of tumors (type 2), are not associated with hypergastrinemia, present as sporadic large solitary gastric carcinoids and tend to metastasize more frequently and have a worse prognosis. The third group comprise approximately 10% of tumors (type 3), small gastric carcinoids seen in association with MEN-1 and the Zollinger-Ellison syndrome (ZES).

Pulmonary (Tracheobronchial) Carcinoids ■ Pulmonary (tracheobronchial) carcinoids (well-differentiated neuroendocrine tumors) are the more indolent of the spectrum of pulmonary neuroendocrine tumors, with the more aggressive end of the spectrum represented by small cell lung carcinoma. These tumors comprise about 2% of all lung tumors, present on average in the fifth decade of life, and are associated with the carcinoid syndrome in fewer than 5% of cases. They have been responsible for ectopic hormone secretion leading to Cushing disease (ACTH) and acromegaly (GH). Overall, they have a favorable prognosis compared with other lung cancers and other carcinoids, with 5-year survivals of about 90%.[73,77,78]

Diagnosis

When not delivered as a surgical or endoscopic diagnosis, the confirmation of carcinoid tumors might be made only after lengthy evaluation of abdominal complaints or iron-deficiency anemia, or astute recognition of a unique clinical syndrome, the carcinoid syndrome, consisting of complaints such as flushing, diarrhea, wheezing, and myopathy. Though not often diagnosed at presentation, patients with longstanding carcinoid syndrome can develop right-sided heart disease, referred to as carcinoid heart disease (discussed below). Clinical suspicion of a neuroendocrine tumor can fortunately be followed by selected biochemical and imaging studies with reasonable sensitivity and specificity for GEP-NET.

No single measurement detects all cases of carcinoid syndrome, although the urine 5-HIAA appears to be the best screening procedure. The normal range for 5-HIAA secretion is 2–8 mg/24 h, and the quantification of serotonin and all its metabolites usually permits the detection of 84% of patients with carcinoid tumors.[79] False positives can occur with ingestion of serotonin rich foods, such as nuts, avocados, kiwi, pineapple, and bananas.[80] Chromogranin A has been found to be elevated in 100% of carcinoid syndrome patients, but is lacking in specificity of tumor location because it is elevated in PNET and other neuroendocrine tumors.[81] Other peptides involved include SP, neuropeptide K, and PP. In carcinoids of the GI tract, other peptides are less informative, with neurotensin elevated in 43%, SP in 32%, motilin in 14%, somatostatin in 5%, and VIP rarely.[16]

Carcinoid Syndrome

Carcinoid syndrome occurs in less than 10% of patients with carcinoid tumors. Ninety-one percent of cases only occur after metastatic spread to the liver.[82] Principal features include flushing, wheezing, diarrhea, abdominal pain, and after long-standing symptoms, endomyocardial fibrosis with tricuspid and pulmonary valve involvement, and very rarely, pellagra. Diarrhea is found in 83% of cases, flushing in 49%, dyspnea in 20%, and bronchospasm in 6%.[82] Serotonin and its metabolites are thought to be responsible for the majority of carcinoid syndrome symptoms, but other mediators, such as prostaglandins, SP, kallikrein, dopamine, and neuropeptide K, are thought to be involved.[16]

The diarrhea syndrome that occurs with carcinoid tumors usually is of a secretory nature, with diarrhea persisting during fasting or intravenous feeding. Flushing in carcinoid syndrome is of two varieties. First, with small intestinal and pancreatic tumors the flush usually is of a faint pink to red color and involves the face and upper trunk as far as the nipple line. The flush is initially provoked by alcohol and food containing tyramines (eg, blue cheese, chocolate, red sausage, and red wine). With time, the flush may occur spontaneously and without provocation. It usually is ephemeral, lasting only a few minutes, and may occur many times per day, but generally does not leave permanent discoloration. In contrast, in the second variety seen with bronchopulmonary and gastric tumors the flush is often more intense, of longer duration, purplish in hue, frequently followed by telangiectasia, and involves not only the upper trunk but may also affect the limbs. The limbs may become acrocyanotic, and the nose resembles that of rhinophyma. The skin of the face may thicken, with the appearance of a leonine facies resembling that seen in leprosy and acromegaly.[16]

Carcinoid Heart Disease

Carcinoid heart disease develops in half to two-thirds of patients with the carcinoid syndrome[83,84] and is characterized by predominantly right-sided valvular lesions described as plaques with proliferation of myofibroblasts and dense extracellular collagen and myxoid deposits.[85] The cardiac disease is a structural disease with thickening and retraction of the valves causing regurgitation (followed later by fusion of fibrous changes to cause stenosis), resulting in right-sided congestive heart failure as the most common cause of cardiac-related death.[86] Moller and colleagues[87] reported on over 100 patients followed with serial echocardiograms or referred for surgery based on initial echocardiograms. Peak 5-HIAA levels and prior chemotherapy were independent predictors of progression of carcinoid heart disease. Evidence for serotonin, and its metabolites, as the primary cause of valvular lesions includes proliferation in vitro of cardiac valve fibroblasts that could lead to connective tissue deposition seen on valves in carcinoid heart disease.[88] Indirect evidence includes the histologic similarities to the valvular lesions seen with the diet drugs fenfluramine-phentermine.[89] Studies to date suggest that control of serotonin (5-HIAA) levels after carcinoid heart disease has been established does not prevent progression of valvular disease.[87,90]

Prognosis

Arecent review of over 13,000 cases of carcinoid tumors[51] and over 50 years of data supports that there has been little change in overall survival, and in survival by site and extent of disease (localized, regional, and distant). The conclusion is supported by a lengthy literature showing the lack of success, despite extensive clinical trial efforts, in documenting a clear survival advantage with a long list of chemotherapies (single agent and combined), somatostatin analogues (without and with radionuclides), interferons, aggressive surgical approaches to metastatic lesions, and early trial results with some of the newer targeted agents. Though the general prognosis for neuroendocrine tumors is excellent compared with that of metastatic adenocarcinomas of the colon, stomach, and pancreas, Modlin and colleagues[51] emphasized that combining all tumors, there was documentation of metastatic disease at diagnosis in 12.9%, with an overall 5-year survival of 67.2%—concluding that these data support that carcinoids, and by extension GEP-NET in general, should not be thought of as generally benign tumors.

Pancreatic NET (PNET) (Islet-Cell Tumors)

Most of the noncarcinoid neuroendocrine tumors of the GEP do in fact occur in the pancreas, thus the common use of the classification of PNETs. As a group, they have histologic features that are largely similar to the GEP-NET labeled as carcinoids,[91] and despite efforts to subdivide based on growth patterns and granule ultrastructure, there is not yet a classification scheme that correlates with the type of hormone secreted that is responsible for clinical symptoms, nor a classification that predicts the likelihood of malignant spread for a given patient.[92] The annual incidence is approximately 10 cases per million population, with clinically evident tumors at an incidence of about 3.5–4.0 per million. As is often true with neuroendocrine tumors, the incidence at autopsy is much higher; in the case of PNET, the incidence has been reported as high as 10% when particular attention is taken to examine the pancreas in detail.[93] The PNET represent just under half of all neuroendocrine tumors, but represent only a small fraction, 1–2%, of all pancreatic tumors. The individual PNET are defined by the clinical syndromes associated with their specific secretory products (Table 76-4). Nonfunctioning (PPoma) and gastrinoma are the most common malignant PNET, and insulinoma is the most common benign PNET, followed in incidence by a list of rare and interesting tumors. The different PNET have unique biological features relevant to their presentations, diagnostic evaluations, and initial surgical and medical management. Unfortunately, once metastatic neither the surgical nor medical management is curative, but rather, offers palliation of significant symptoms. These therapies will be commented on for all PNET as a group.

Nonfunctioning PNET

Nonfunctioning PNET are defined by having no specific associated clinical syndrome, despite staining for one or several peptides and amines or even having quantifiable serum levels of certain neuroendocrine markers. Included in the nonfunctioning PNET are the PPomas. PP is evident on staining of upwards of 75% of these tumors and measured in the serum of the majority of patients. However, PP has not been found to lead to any identified clinical symptoms or signs. There is no evidence to suggest that the biological characteristics and clinical presentation of PPomas and nonfunctioning PNET without elevated PP are different entities. These tumors secrete, in addition to PP, markers that include chromogranin A, B, C, α-, and β-HCG subunits.[94]

Clinical Presentation and Diagnosis ■ Nonfunctional PNET and PPomas together account for about 15–30% of the PNET.[94] Because they have no associated secretory symptoms, they often present with bulky disease in patients in the fourth or fifth decade, with presenting complaints of abdominal pain in 36%, jaundice in 28%, and incidental finding at surgery in 16%.[95] For the same reason, there is a high reported incidence of metastases at diagnosis that ranges from 60% to 90%. PP is elevated in a variety of NET- and non-NET–related conditions, so cannot be used alone to make the diagnosis of a PPoma. Serum chromogranin A and B are elevated in close to 100% of nonfunctioning PNET.[81] Localization of nonfunctioning PNET is less important than other PNET, given the late presentation with obvious primary tumors. Once diagnosed, CT and MRI along with SRS are used to stage and follow metastatic disease.

Surgery ■ As for most GEP-NET, the treatment of choice and the only therapy that can achieve a cure is surgery. Given the late presentation and high percentage of patients with metastatic disease at presentation, surgical cure is not often possible for nonfunctional PNET/PPomas. However, procedures such as surgical debulking and relief of biliary obstruction can provide significant palliation.

Gastrinoma

The gastrinoma syndrome, first named the ZES, is based on a report of two patients with severe peptic ulcer disease and non-β islet-cell tumors of the pancreas,[96] with later identification of gastrin as the secreted hormone.[97] Gastrinoma patients are characterized by a severe ulcer diathesis and persistent basal gastric acid hypersecretion that is also thought responsible for the frequent symptom of diarrhea resulting from the direct effect of gastric acid on the intestinal mucosa, inactivation of lipase, and precipitation of bile salts. Gastrinomas account for about 25% of all PNET, are found primarily in the duodenum (70%) and pancreas (25%), and demonstrate malignant behavior in approximately 50% of cases. About 20% of gastrinoma patients are found to have MEN-1,[98] and their presentation and course differ from sporadic cases (see MEN-1 Syndrome). The incidence of malignant disease exceeds 50% at diagnosis, and increases over time even after surgical resection.[99,100]

Clinical Presentation and Diagnosis ■ The possibility of gastrinoma syndrome should be considered in patients with unexplained secretory diarrhea and patients with ulcer disease that is recurrent, refractory to therapy, or occurs in unusual locations. Before development of the radioimmunoassay, 80% of patients with gastrinoma presented with a severe ulcer diathesis, bleeding, intestinal obstruction, or perforation. Today, the diagnosis of gastrinoma can be made even before ulcers develop, based on diarrhea or mild duodenitis. A history of improvement in the diarrhea with administration of H2-receptor antagonists or proton pump inhibitors is strongly suggestive of the gastrinoma syndrome. Many patients currently present without any abdominal pain, and in fact, it is found that diarrhea is perhaps more common than ulcer-related pain and can be the only symptom in upwards of 20% of patients.[98]

The diagnosis requires the demonstration of an elevated fasting serum gastrin and elevated basal acid output. It must be noted that gastrin levels may also be elevated in disorders associated with gastric acid hypersecretion, and in those disorders that result in hypo- and achlorhydria. Infection with *Helicobacter pylori* can elevate both serum gastrin and the basal acid output. The *H. pylori* should be treated and tests repeated before considering a diagnosis of ZES. Elevated serum gastrin levels are associated with low basal acid output in patients on antisecretory therapy (ie, omeprazole), and can be seen in chronic gastritis, pernicious anemia, atrophic gastritis, and postvagotomy states.[101] The most sensitive and accurate test remains the secretin stimulation test for gastrin secretion. Secretin, 2 μ/kg, is given intravenously and blood samples for gastrin drawn at 2, 5, 10, 20, and 30 min. A rise of more than 100 pg/mL is strongly suggestive of ZES.[102]

Gibril and colleagues compared in a prospective study the sensitivity of SRS with that of CT, MRI, ultrasonography, and selective angiography in the detection of primary and metastatic gastrinomas.[103] The SRS scans proved the single most sensitive method for imaging either primary or metastatic liver lesions in patients with ZES.

Improvements in localization by imaging, including intraoperative and endoscopic ultrasound, along with more aggressive surgical techniques, have led to a larger percentage of gastrinomas being diagnosed when localized to the pancreatic head, duodenum, and peripancreatic lymph nodes.[104]

Histology of the primary tumor does not predict for malignancy. Weber and colleagues[100] showed that primary tumor size was the best predictor of malignancy, with liver lesions found in 4% of gastrinomas <1.0 cm, 28% of tumors >1.0 cm and <2.9 cm, and 61% of tumors 3.0 cm or larger. Duodenal gastrinomas have a lower percentage of malignant tumors (5%) compared with pancreatic gastrinomas (52%), but this might simply reflect that pancreatic tumors are generally larger than duodenal gastrinomas at diagnosis.[100]

Surgery ■ With the ability to control gastric acid hypersecretion over long periods, the quality of life and prognosis of ZES improved significantly, to the point where the long-term survival of patients with very slow growing gastrinomas are now determined largely by the eventual malignant behavior of the tumor.[97,104] Surgery has evolved from gastric resections to control ulcer disease to complex surgery using pre- and intraoperative imaging to localize and resect often small local and regional metastatic disease. The overall survival rate for gastrinomas, excluding patients with MEN-1, at 5 years is between 60% and 80%, and at 10 years is between 45% and 75%.[100,105,106] Norton and colleagues report that in a series of patients operated on with curative intent, the 10-year survival is 94%.[104] Fraker and colleagues report on a study of surgical versus medically managed patients and demonstrate a lower percentage of liver metastases developing in the surgical patients over long-term follow-up.[107]

Medical Therapy ■ Treatment of the gastrinoma syndrome has undergone significant changes since the first case was described in 1955.[96] Until the development of drugs to control excessive acid production, the purpose of operative intervention was to excise the acid-secreting stomach to avoid the excessive morbidity and mortality from massive hemorrhage or perforation. Successive generations of medical therapies including anticholinergics, histamine H2 receptor blockers, and the now more potent and widely used inhibitors of the H+-K+ adenosine triphosphatase/proton pump inhibitors (ie, omeprazole).[94,102,108] Though failure rates in controlling acid hypersecretion with various agents and in different studies over time have varied, failure rates with omeprazole are about 5%, with average omeprazole dosages of 20–80 mg/day.[108]

As with carcinoids, gastrinomas in general have a low response rate to single and multiagent chemotherapy. This includes the randomized trials by Moertel and colleagues that explored streptozotocin-based regimens, and the small-cell lung cancer regimen of cisplatin and etoposide.[109–111] The use of chemotherapy remains a decision individualized for each patient, and is generally reserved for patients with metastatic disease, in whom other measures to control symptoms from secretion of hormones and bulk disease have failed. Presence of metastatic disease alone might not require therapy in this slow-growing tumor; over half of liver lesions in gastrinomas show no or minimal growth over a mean follow-up period of 29 months.[112]

Fifteen gastrinoma patients treated with long-acting lanreotide included in a study by Shojamanesh and colleagues[113] demonstrated that only patients classified as slowly progressing before entry in the trial had a clinical or radiological response.

Insulinoma

Insulinomas were first described by Whipple in a 1938 report of 30 patients with pancreatic adenomas and hypoglycemia.[114] Insulinomas are the second most common functioning PNET, with an incidence of 0.8–0.9 cases per million. Overall, the incidence of metastatic disease, about 5–15%, is low compared with other PNET. The tumors are often well encapsulated, solitary nodules found evenly distributed throughout the pancreas.[115] The finding of multiple insulinomas should prompt testing for MEN-1, present in about 10% of patients.[116]

Clinical Presentation and Diagnosis ■ Almost all cases of insulinoma present with symptoms of hypoglycemia, with neuroglycopenic symptoms (visual complaints, altered consciousness, weakness) more common than adrenergic symptoms alone (sweating, tremulousness).[115] Diagnosis of suspected cases is made by a supervised fast, where over 90% of patients will develop a serum glucose of <50 mg/dL during a 48-h fast, and the corresponding serum insulin level at the time of hypoglycemia will equal or exceed 5 μU/mL.[117]

It is generally recommended that in the absence of documented metastases, all insulinomas be surgically removed, even in those with mild symptoms. With surgery, 80–90% of all insulinoma patients will be cured.[115] This is supported by the increasing role of endoscopic ultrasound (EUS), which has a reported sensitivity of 80%, including tumors less than 1 cm.[118] Intraoperative ultrasound (IOUS) can be used to avoid blind pancreatic resections when even EUS cannot localize a lesion. Perhaps the most sensitive test is selective intra-arterial injection of calcium with hepatic venous sampling, a technique with a reported sensitivity of 94% for insulinomas.[119,120]

Medical Therapy ■ Insulinoma patients frequently discover on their own, prior to diagnosis, that they can reduce hypoglycemic symptoms by eating small, frequent meals; this approach can be used effectively, short term, post-diagnosis. Diet is coupled with medical therapy, including diazoxide and octreotide. Diazoxide, which directly blocks release of insulin from the β-cell, is initiated at a dosage of 150–200 mg daily, and increased to a maximum of 600–800 mg daily.[121] Octreotide, in dosages from 50 μg to as high as 1500 μg daily of short-acting formulations, can control symptoms in as high as 60% of patients.[122] Little is known about the long-term control of insulinomas with medical therapy because most patients have surgery soon after diagnosis.

VIPoma

The VIPoma (vasoactive intestinal polypeptide) was first described by Verner and Morrison,[123] followed by a review of 55 patients with the syndrome.[124] The diagnostic terms also used include the Verner-Morrison syndrome, as well as the descriptive acronym WDHA syndrome (watery diarrhea, hypokalemia, and achlorhydria), or as proposed by Kvols,[16] the expanded WDHHA syndrome to account for the hypochlorhydria in most cases and the acidosis that results from bicarbonate wasting in some cases. The hormone VIP is thought to be largely responsible for the direct inhibition of gastric acid secretion, stimulation of intestinal secretion, and the resulting electrolyte abnormalities that account for the symptoms of a VIPoma. Unlike other PNET, there are distinct adult and pediatric subsets of patients. VIPoma are rarely seen in patients with an MEN syndrome.[116,125]

Clinical Presentation ■ The VIPomas are quite rare, accounting for only about 5% of the PNET. The mean age of diagnosis in adults is 50 years with a range of 32–81 years, distinct from the mean age of diagnosis in children of 2–4 years with a range from 10 months to 9 years.[126] In adults, 90% of the tumors are found in the pancreas, most often as solitary nodules. The tumor histology alone cannot distinguish VIPomas from other PNET;[121] however, immunohistochemical detection of tumor VIP is highly suggestive because it is found in very few other neuroendocrine tumors. In adults, upwards of 60% of cases present with or develop metastatic disease. In children, on the other hand, most VIP-secreting tumors are extrapancreatic and are neurogenic in origin, with the most common histology being ganglioneuroblastomas and ganglioneuromas.[127] The diagnosis requires the documentation of elevated plasma VIP concentrations and documentation of large volume secretory diarrhea.[128] The diarrhea generally exceeds 3 L/day and, importantly, does not decrease significantly with oral fasting. Surprisingly, some patients will go months and years prior to diagnosis, partly because the diarrhea is episodic at first and during quiet periods the VIP level may normalize. As the tumor size increases the diarrhea, cramping, and other symptoms become more persistent. The diarrhea could be confused with laxative abuse, other benign secretory diarrheas, and with the diarrhea syndrome caused by another PNET, a gastrinoma (Zollinger-Ellison syndrome). The distinguishing features of gastrinoma and VIPoma (WDHHA) diarrhea are shown in Table 76-5. The mean fasting plasma VIP levels in VIP patients = 900 pg/mL, far exceeding the normal levels of <170 pg/mL in most laboratories.[127,128]

Medical Therapy ■ In patients with a suspected VIPoma, the first therapeutic intervention is to correct the hypovolemia, hypokalemia, and acidosis if present. A variety of medications have been used to control the diarrhea but have largely been replaced with the somatostatin analogue octreotide. Octreotide controls symptoms in over 80% of patients, corresponding with a drop in the VIP plasma level.[122] The dosages required range from standard octreotide dose of 50 µg three (3) times a day to as high as 1200 µg/day. In patients refractory to even high doses, the addition of a corticosteroid is sometimes successful. Chemotherapy, as discussed below, has shown only occasional responders.

Surgery ■ Once symptoms are controlled and electrolytes corrected, imaging studies should be done to localize the VIPoma and evaluate for possible surgical resection for cure. Long and colleagues[127] reported that in 52 patients with pancreatic VIPomas, the average lesion was 9 cm in diameter, and thus readily visible by CT or ultrasound. Other studies have shown that some VIPomas require angiography with or without selective venous sampling for VIP levels.[129] The role of SRS, supported by the ENET consensus,[59] is to localize extra-pancreatic primary lesions and detect metastatic disease. Complete resections have resulted in long-term control of symptoms in 30–50% of adult patients.[121,126] If metastatic disease is present and not readily resectable, then medical therapy can be maximized prior to considering palliative surgery to help control symptoms.

Glucagonoma

Glucagonoma was first reported in 1966 by McGavran and colleagues, who called attention to a syndrome that included acquired diabetes and glucagon-producing tumors.[130] This rare tumor, estimated to account for 1% of GEP-NET, was later recognized to include a characteristic skin rash, necrolytic migratory erythema (NME).[131–133] The tumor occurs almost exclusively in adults over 40 years of age and is rarely associated with MEN-1.[125]

Clinical Presentation ■ The largest reported single-institution experience was from the Mayo Clinic, which reported on 21 patients seen between 1975 and 1991.[134] The main presenting features of the glucagonoma syndrome included weight loss (71%), the characteristic NME rash (67%), mild diabetes mellitus (38%), diarrhea (29%), and painful glossitis and angular stomatitis (29%). The NME rash can be insidious in onset and typically precedes the diagnosis of the glucagonoma by several years. It usually is widespread, but major sites of involvement are the perioral and perigenital regions along with the fingers, legs, and feet (Fig. 76-5).

The findings of diabetes, NME rash, weight loss, diarrhea, stomatitis, and glossitis is thought to be largely due to the direct effects of high circulating levels of glucagon and its known effects on glycogenolysis, gluconeogenesis, ketogenesis, lipolysis, insulin secretion, intestinal and pancreatic secretion, and intestinal motility. In addition, the amino acid depletion that results from excess glucagon causes, or at least worsens, the NME rash.[136] Another poorly explained feature of the glucagonoma syndrome is that patients have a significant risk of thromboembolic complications, particularly pulmonary embolism.

At diagnosis, the glucagonomas are almost all found as single lesions in the pancreas (tail > body), averaging 5–10 cm in size, and metastatic disease is already present in over 60% of patients, most often to the liver, as is generally true for all PNET.[121,137] The histology of glucagonomas is similar to other PNET, particularly in that many other PNET stain positive for glucagon. Therefore, the diagnosis requires documentation of increased plasma glucagon levels. Fasting glucagon levels in normal individuals rarely exceed 200 pg/mL. Disorders causing elevated plasma glucagon levels include diabetes mellitus, burn injury, acute trauma, bacteremia, cirrhosis, renal failure, and Cushing syndrome, and can result in fasting plasma glucagon levels as high as 500 pg/mL. Glucagonoma patients have levels >500 pg/mL in almost 100% of cases, and >1000 pg/mL in over 90% of cases.

If the diagnosis is made while the tumor is still localized, surgical resection

Table 76-5 ■ **Differentiation of Gastrinoma and WDHHA Syndrome**

Feature	Gastrinoma	WDHHA
Diarrhea	Acid	Alkaline (HCO_3 loss)
Gastric acid	Increased	Decreased
Gastric volume	Increased	Normal or decreased
Nasogastric suction	Diarrhea improves	Diarrhea unchanged
Motility	Increased[a]	Increased slightly[b]
Abdominal pain	Marked	Rare (initially)
Stool K^+ loss	Slight	Marked
Metabolic acidosis	No (alkalosis with gastric suction)	Yes
Lesion location	Primary pancreas (also liver, wall of stomach, and duodenum)	Primary pancreas
Mediator	Gastrin	VIP/other

[a]Motility enhanced secondary to gastric acid stimulation.
[b]Motility may be slightly increased secondary to direct effects of either intraarterial or intraluminal VIP.
Abbreviations: VIP, vasoactive intestinal peptide; WDHHA, watery diarrhea, hypokalemia, hypochlorhydria, and acidosis.

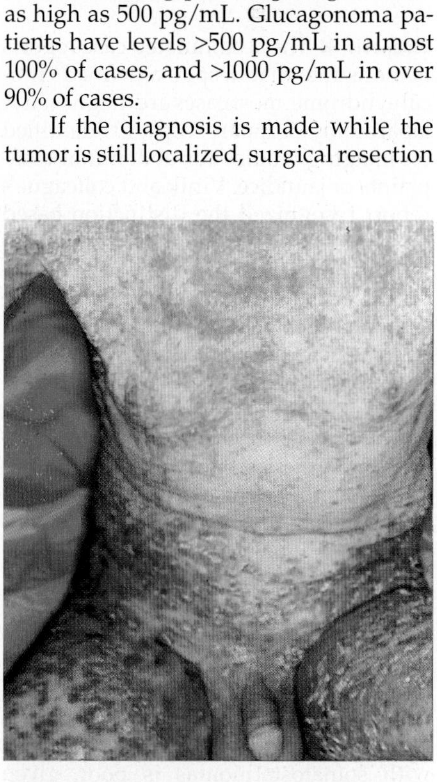

Figure 76-5 ■ Migratory necrolytic erythema of glucagonoma syndrome.

can be curative.[137,138] As in other islet-cell tumors, even when malignant these tumors tend to be extremely slow growing. Almost invariably, the NME rash resolves after successful removal of a glucagon producing tumor, even if the rash has been present for several years.[139] In addition, in those patients who do not undergo curative resection but are treated with chemotherapeutic agents, the NME rash and other skin manifestations improve as the glucagon levels decrease.[140]

Octreotide has been used to improve the preoperative condition of patients and to treat symptoms related to unresectable and metastatic disease. Both the NME rash and diarrhea, but generally not the glucose intolerance/diabetes, respond in over 50% of the patients, with complete disappearance of symptoms in about 30% of patients.[121,122]

Somatostatinoma

Somatostatinomas are rare PNET, with about 50 cases reported to date. The first cases were reported in 1977 by Ganda and colleagues[141] and Larsson and colleagues.[142]

Krejs and colleagues[143] reported a series of 8 cases in 1979, and Vinik and colleagues reported the largest review on 48 cases in 1986.[12] The rarity of this tumor and the advanced stage at presentation has not permitted the collection of much information on approaches to diagnosis, imaging, and treatment. Somatostatinomas are rarely seen in association with MEN-1,[125] but an association with MEN-2 and neurofibromatosis is suggested.[12,144]

Diagnosis ■ The accumulated case reports demonstrate that despite a defined clinical syndrome, most cases are diagnosed at laparotomy or laparoscopy, or identified on imaging studies for abdominal complaints or jaundice. Vinik and colleague's report recognized the distinction based on clinical presentations of somatostatinomas presenting in the pancreas, intestine, and extra-pancreatic sites.[145] The central clinical features of the somatostatinoma syndrome consist of diabetes, diarrhea, steatorrhea, gallbladder disease, hypochlorhydria, and weight loss. An elevated plasma level of somatostatin-like immunoreactivity (SLI), an immunoassay that reacts with several forms of somatostatin, is thought to be responsible for the majority of symptoms. The tumors tend to present as large masses, reflecting the high levels of somatostatin thought necessary to create symptoms. At diagnosis, 85% of the pancreatic and 50% of the intestinal primaries had evidence of metastatic spread.[146] Though the data are minimal, the outlook for those with somatostatinomas is poor, given the high incidence of malignant spread. Close to half of reported patients died within a year and others survived up to as long as 5 years.[145]

Growth Hormone Releasing Factor

First described in 1982 by Guillemin and colleagues,[147] growth hormone releasing factor (GRF)omas are perhaps the least common GEP-NET. The clinical features are due to excess plasma growth hormone and are indistinguishable from the acromegaly that results from pituitary tumors. GRFomas have presented with ZES or Cushing's diseases as well. The tumors are found in the pancreas, lung, and small intestine and are often greater than 6 cm at diagnosis. The histology is typical of other GEP-NET. The diagnosis should be expected in any patient with acromegaly and no pituitary adenoma, or acromegaly and an abdominal mass. Plasma GRF levels confirm the diagnosis.[148]

Therapy for GEP-NET

In general, carcinoids and other GEP-NET are slow growing, and symptoms are most often attributable to secretory products. Even patients with extensive metastatic disease can enjoy a normal quality of life as long as the endocrine syndrome is quiescent. For those patients whose tumors are not resectable at diagnosis or who later develop metastatic disease, given the general lack of curative therapies at this stage, the focus is on control of symptoms. The use of the long-acting somatostatin analogs and interferon to decrease secretion of vasoactive and other hormones, combined with bulk-reducing procedures primarily directed at hepatic lesions, the quality of life of GEP-NET patients can be maintained for extended periods of time.

Surgery ■ ***Primary*** ■ Prophylactic treatment with a somatostatin analogue (see below) should be considered before all surgical procedures, in even in suspected carcinoid patients. In general, surgical removal of the primary tumor is the treatment of choice for small and localized tumors as well as for the alleviation of any obstructive symptoms, but surgical cure of GEP-NET tumors is uncommon in the presence of intra-abdominal and hepatic metastases. Gastric and duodenal GEP-NET can, in select cases with tumors <1 cm, be excised endoscopically.[149] Carcinoids of the small bowel that appear localized should be resected en bloc with lymphadenectomy and removal of the mesentery.[150] Carcinoids of the appendix and rectum are both generally treated by appendectomy if <2 cm, and resection if >2 cm.[151] Localized low-grade neuroendocrine tumors of the tracheobronchial tree can be successfully treated in a high percentage of cases with segmental or wedge resections.[78]

Hepatic Ablation Therapies ■ A number of ablation therapies used in the management of metastatic disease to the liver have been applied to neuroendocrine tumors. Procedures include hepatic resection, hepatic artery embolization without and without chemotherapy, ethanol injections, and radiofrequency ablation.

Hepatic Resections ■ Que and colleagues recently performed a meta-analysis summarizing reports in the medical literature over 26 years.[152] Surgery may involve hemihepatectomy, trisegmentectomy, or wedge resection. The operative mortality after partial hepatectomy for carcinoid tumors in this series was 2.3%. More than 80% had improvement in symptoms related to hormone excess (ie, carcinoid syndrome) and the duration of response ranged from 4 to 120 months.

Radiofrequency Ablation ■ It is estimated that >90% of patients with hepatic metastases have lesions that are too large, too numerous, or diffuse disease that preclude resection. Radiofrequency ablation (RFA) has been used in these patients to reduce bulk of disease and control symptoms. The largest series to date of RFA in metastatic neuroendocrine tumors involving patients treated over a 10-yer period at a single institution demonstrated perioperative morbidity of <5%, a 90% partial and 72% complete relief of symptoms, and median duration of symptom control of approximately 1 year.[153]

Hepatic Artery Vaso-occlusive Therapy ■ Vaso-occlusive therapy to reduce bulk of hepatic lesions to decrease secretory syndromes and mass effects should be attempted after careful consideration given the high risk of complications in the immediate "postembolization" phase as well as longer-term complications and death. Overall, vascular-occlusion therapies have led to biochemical responses as high as 50%, and tumor reduction is as high as 40%, and generally of short duration.[154] Hepatic arterial occlusion combined with sequential chemotherapy has resulted in biochemical responses as high as 80%, with a median duration of 18 months or more.[155,156]

Hepatic Transplantation ■ A recent review of the first 103 liver transplants in Europe for NET tumors showed 5-year overall and disease-free survival of 46% and 24% respectively.[157] However, the restrictive transplant criteria, significant morbidity and mortality of the procedure, and the general lack of transplantable organs makes transplant a limited therapeutic option.

Though there are no direct comparative studies for different ablative approaches, a single institution retrospective analysis by Osborne and collegues[158] showed an overall survival advantage for surgical approaches over embolization.

Somatostatin Analogues

Somatostatin analogues have had a major impact on the flushing, diarrhea, and wheezing in most patients with metastatic carcinoid and the carcinoid syndrome. Most patients with secretory symptoms related to a GEP-NET are treated first with a somatostatin analog, most often octreotide, to control the symptoms of diarrhea and flushing.[145] Janson and colleagues[159] and Kvols and colleagues[160] have shown that patients with carcinoid and other neuroendocrine tumors with positive SRS scans all responded with improvement in symptoms to octreotide, whereas all patients with negative scans failed to respond. The marked symptomatic improvement with somatostatin analogues has precluded any clinical trial evaluation of these agents versus placebo or observation to determine if they have survival advantage in the treatment of newly diagnosed (symptomatic) patients. Also not proven, but clinically accepted, is the fact that the somatostatin analogues have simplified and reduced the risks of surgery, and perhaps allowed many more patients to benefit from more aggressive surgical approaches. As an example, Kvols and colleagues treated a patient, who soon after the induction of anesthesia had a fall in blood pressure that was unresponsive to intravenous fluid, calcium, norepinephrne, or epinephrine administration, and within 1 min of 100 µg of octreotide given intravenously, blood pressure rose, and the patient made an uneventful recovery.[161]

Of the currently available SST analogues used for treatment of GEP-NET, octreotide and a long-acting formulation (somatostatin-LAR) are available in the United States[162] All of the currently available analogues and their long-acting formulations bind with high affinity to SSTR2 and SSTR5 and have in vitro antisecretory and anti-proliferative activities, and there are reports that binding to SSTR3 occurs with higher doses and can induce apoptosis.[163,164] SOM 230, a somatostatin analogue with broad binding affinity to SSTR1–5, is currently in phase II development for GEP-NET.

Most of the clinical studies over the past three decades with somatostatin and its analogues have included patients with multiple histologies, generally GEP-NET patients diagnosed as carcinoid or pancreatic islet cell, and the vast majority had a defined secretory syndrome (most often carcinoid) or symptomatic bulky disease. As such, the response endpoints are varied and most often included symptomatic (SR), biochemical markers (BR), and radiological objective response (OR), and most reported on stabilization of tumor growth (SD) in groups of patients who were generally highly symptomatic with evidence of progressive tumor growth. Delaunoit and colleagues[165] reviewed the literature for three decades of use of somatostatin analogues in the treatment of GEP-NET. Most studies are single arm with relatively small numbers and a heterogeneous collection of patients. The conclusions that most authors concur with are that complete tumor responses are rare (2–5%), stabilization of disease can occur in as high as 40% of patients, biochemical responses are commonly in the 70–80% range, and symptomatic response is seen in most patients with front-line therapy. An analysis of over 60 published studies by Harris and Redfern[166] showed control of symptoms of diarrhea and flushing in over 80% of patients, and over 70% of those patients showed a decrease in 5-HIAA levels. As is unfortunately typical, octreotide responses were maintained for a median of only 4 months in 40% of patients, with the remainder of patients having sustained control of symptoms from 1 to as long as 2.5 years. The comparative studies of short- and long-acting agents demonstrated similar data, with no significant differences between the agents in terms of response, safety, and efficacy.[167,168] Many of the adverse effects of the agents are mild and resolve with continued use. The most notable adverse events seen with long-term use of somatostatin analogues relates to the effect on the biliary tree. Of patients treated longer than 18 months, 62% had dilatation, sludge, or stones in the gallbladder. Newly documented stones were documented in 24%; however, only 1% of patients required a cholecystectomy.[165]

High-Dose Somatostatin Analogues ■ Several authors have investigated high doses of both octreotide and lanreotide (not approved for GEP-NET in the US) based on preclinical data that suggested a dose-response relationship, and possible recruitment of the SSTR3 pathway has been implicated in apoptosis of neuroendocrine cells in vivo and in animal models.[41] Eriksson and colleagues[169] treated 19 patients with progressive GEP-NET at a lanreotide dosage of 12 mg/day, and Faiss and colleagues[170] treated 30 patients at a lanreotide dosage of 15 mg/day, and all types of responses seem comparable and not particularly better than other lanreotide studies. No systematic study of a dose-response relationship has yet been done for any of the somatostatin analogues.

Biologic Agents

Interferon ■ Oberg and colleagues pioneered the use of leukocyte interferon in carcinoid GEP-NET[171] and reviewed the early trials in 2000.[172] Most trials investigating interferon in GEP-NET have been conducted in patients who have been previously treated with a somatostatin analogue. In the majority of these cases, the addition of interferon resulted in symptomatic responses in a significant number of patients. Two studies from the Uppsala group[173,174] and a study by Frank and colleagues[175] demonstrated that a biochemical response could be achieved in 63–77% of patients, with over 50% reporting stable disease and a rare complete or partial response. These studies and others suggested that the combination of a somatostatin analogue and an interferon as front-line therapy might be more efficacious than either agent alone. One of the few multicenter, randomized, comparative trials done in the field of GEP-NET to date, however, showed that the objective responses were no higher with the combination as compared with either agent alone.[176] There was a higher symptomatic and biochemical response rate in the combination therapy group, but at the expense of increased toxicity. It remains unanswered whether the combination as front-line therapy, or sequential use of the agents, provides the greatest long-term benefit to the patient.

External Beam Radiotherapy

There are no data that support the routine use of radiation therapy for GEP-NET patients unless they have symptomatic bone metastases, spinal cord compression, bronchial obstruction, or some other symptomatic site of disease.

Peptide Receptor Radiotherapy

Despite the lack of demonstrated radiosensitivity, the targeting to over expressed SSTR provided by somatostatin analogues has led to the development of PRRT reagents for GEP-NET.[177] Currently no radiolabeled somatostatin analogues are approved for therapeutic indications, and they remain available only through clinical trials or for compassionate use in selected centers. Generally speaking, PRRT has been investigated in patients with inoperable primary cancers and those with metastases, and as such, patients have often been previously treated with and failed somatostatin analogues, chemotherapy, and possibly other agents. PRRT is a logical extension of diagnostic imaging with Octreoscan ([^{111}In-diethylenetriaminepentaacetic acid (DTPA)]octreotide) for tumor localization, whereby the localization documents the opportunity for selective delivery of a radiopharmaceutical at the site of SSTR2 expressing tumors. The initial trials were in fact performed with high doses of the Octreoscan imaging agent,[178,179] and though a biological response was seen in several patients, objective responses were few, and significant bone marrow and other toxicities occurred. The poor results were felt in large part due to the use of ^{111}Indium and its poor tissue penetration and the relatively low affinity of the agent for SSTR2 and other SSTRs.

Two other radiolabeled somatostatin analogues have undergone phase I and II clinical trial evaluation in GEP-NET. Five studies involved the compound [^{90}Y-DOTA, Tyr3] octreotide that substituted ^{90}yttrium for ^{111}Indium with a different coupling agent. Over 180 patients have been evaluated in long term follow-up after treatment, and the studies show overall response rates (CR + PR) ranging from about 10–30%, with about 50–60% of patients developing stable disease,[180] a significant improvement over the [^{111}In(DTPA)]octreotide results. There continued to be grade 3–4 hematologic toxicity in up to 20% of patients as well as several cases of renal and liver toxicity and a few cases of myelodysplasia. Renal toxicity in most of the recent studies has been decreased, even with higher cumulative radiation doses, through the use of amino acid infusions.[181] Another PRRT agent, [^{177}Lu-DOTA0, Tyr3] octreotate, incorporates the combined β- and γ-emitting radionuclide ^{177}Luthium, and the use of a modification of the octreotide molecule, octreotate, that has a marked increase in binding affinity to the SSTR2.[183] The most recent follow-up on patients with GEP-NET treated with [^{177}Lu-DOTA0, Tyr3] octreotate as PRRT shows less toxicity, with temporary bone marrow suppression, a single case of MDS with a history of prior alkylating agent exposure, and a case of progressive renal insufficiency. The responses included one CR (1%), 22 PRs (29%), and stable disease in 30 (40%), and median time to progression not having been reached at 25 months.[184] Clearly, though there were clinically significant responses seen with these agents in even refractory patients, there are numerous clinical questions yet to be addressed in clinical trials that await the approval and wider use of these agents.

Chemotherapy for GEP-NET

In malignant GEP-NET, chemotherapy has not been shown to be effective for most patients, and this approach should still be considered investigational. Numerous trials over several decades have been conducted with every class of chemotherapy given by numerous routes including hepatic artery infusion. This extends to some of the more recently introduced chemotherapeutic agents such as docetaxel.[185] Given the rarity of GEP-NET, and the variety of tumors within this group, many trials could be criticized as being small and including patients with poorly defined criteria, often heavily pretreated, where it may have been difficult to identify drugs with low but appreciable response rates. However, most studies were repeated at more than one institution or in cooperative groups, and still no drug has shown a more significant cytotoxic effect.

Several authors have reviewed the history of treatment of carcinoid, and other GEP-NET, with single-agent and multiagent chemotherapy.[16,186] The single agent most studied in carcinoid tumor is 5-fluorouracil, which accounted for observed response rates of 26% and 18% in single-institution and multi-institutional trials, respectively. Melia and colleagues[187] reported a high complication rate with little benefit when 5-fluorouracil was administered by intra-arterial, portal or peripheral intravenous routes. Other trials showing minimal or no response include single agents intravenous doxorubicin, 60 mg/m^2, every 3–4 weeks, and dactinomycin and dacarbazine in metastatic carcinoid tumor,[188,189] and rare objective responses to either cisplatin or etoposide, and no responses to carboplatinum. Activity was seen with pancreatic NET, but not carcinoid using streptozotocin.[16]

Initial experience with combination chemotherapy suggested that this modality might be effective against malignant carcinoid tumor. Early nonrandomized studies of combinations of cyclophosphamide plus methotrexate, streptozotocin plus 5-fluorouracil, or weekly streptozotocin plus doxorubicin reported response rates in excess of 50%; however, rigid criteria for response were not always employed and complete responses were not seen. Based on these observations, the Eastern Cooperative Oncology Group conducted a series of multi-institutional randomized trials of combinations that all contained streptozotocin, despite the low activity of this drug when used alone. In two studies of 170 evaluable patients, the response rates ranged from 23% to 33%. The most recent trial, a randomized control trial of 249 patients, streptozocin and fluorouracil were compared to fluorouracil and doxorubicin, and no significant difference was found.[190] In a prospective trial, the Southwest Oncology Group reported similar response rates of brief duration following a combination of 5-fluorouracil, cyclophosphamide, and streptozotocin with or without doxorubicin. Generally speaking, streptozocin is no longer recommended for carcinoid therapy, but is still utilized in pancreatic NET where the response rates appear somewhat greater.[191]

Thus, in the absence of randomized trials that contain a no-treatment arm, there is no persuasive evidence that single-agent or combination chemotherapy provides any significant impact on disease progression or on survival in patients with malignant carcinoid tumor. Chemotherapy is generally reserved to provide palliation of hormone excess and symptoms related to tumor bulk. There is a serious unmet medical need for effective systemic therapy for advanced GEP-NET.

Targeted Therapies ■ The association of some carcinoid and PNETs with inherited disorders including MEN1 and 2 (see below) as well as tuberous sclerosis, von Hippel-Lindau, and neurofibromatosis are contributing to an understanding of potential tumor suppressors relevant to these tumors. Early genetic studies of these tumors have demonstrated consistent deletions on chromosome 18 in carcinoids, and deletions of chromosome 11 (location of *MEN* gene) in islet cell and pancreatic NET. These changes as well as observations of VEGF, EGFR and other growth factor receptor pathways have provided justification of a series of clinical trials of targeted agents.[192]

Early phase trials have been completed for several novel targeted therapies. Minimal or no response was seen in phase II studies of the tyrosine kinases inhibitors imatinib[193] and gefitinib.[194] More encouraging are the responses seen in phase II trials of the broad tyrosine kinases inhibitor sunitinib[191] and the VEGF inhibitor bevacizuimab.[192] Additional trials, including combinations, of targeted therapies are currently planned and underway.

Adjuvant Therapy

Adjuvant therapy has been proposed for use following potentially curative resection of intestinal and pancreatic primaries to lower the risk of recurrence. However, the general lack of effective systemic therapies and the often long time interval (years) before recurrence presents formidable barriers to achievable clinical trial designs. Perhaps advances in histologic, and molecular characterization of tumors along with identification of more effective therapies will facilitate clinical studies of subsets of patients at high risk of recurrence. Clinical trial planning is underway to study anti-VEGF and other therapies as adjuvant treatment immediately following successful complete resection of limited hepatic metastatic disease where there is a high risk of recurrence in the first few years following surgery.

Parathyroid Carcinoma

Parathyroid carcinomas, unlike parathyroid hyperplasia and adenomas, are not related to MEN syndromes and as such are discussed separately.

Epidemiology and Etiology

In contrast to benign parathyroid tumors, which have been diagnosed increasingly since the introduction of automated multichannel analyzers in the 1970s, with an annual age-adjusted incidence of 28 per 100,000, parathyroid carcinomas remain rare. In collected cases of hyperparathyroidism, parathyroid carcinomas usually represent <1% of the cases. Only about 400 cases have been reported, and their etiology is unknown.[195]

Clinical Features

Parathyroid carcinomas are usually slow-growing tumors with a tendency to recur locally and metastasize late.[195] The great majority of them (95%) are functioning and produce a more severe picture of primary hyperparathyroidism compared with parathyroid adenomas or hyperplasia (Table 76-6). The major distinguishing features of malignant hyperparathyroidism are younger mean age of onset, presence of a palpable neck mass, and severe hypercalcemia, often >14 mg/dL.[196] Metastases occur late and are seen most often in the lung (40%), cervical nodes (30%), and the liver (10%).[195]

Laboratory Tests

Hypercalcemia, the hallmark of hyperparathyroidism, is usually severe in patients with parathyroid carcinoma. The serum calcium level is above 14 mg/dL in about two-thirds of the patients, compared with less than 10% of patients with benign hyperparathyroidism. By far the most important test to diagnose primary hyperparathyroidism is the serum level of immunoreactive PTH (iPTH). Rarely more than twice normal in benign hyperparathyroidism, the value of iPTH is markedly elevated often five or more times the upper limit of normal, in cases of functioning parathyroid carcinoma. Ectopic production of PTH is exceptional and has been documented in very few cases of non-parathyroid carcinomas, where the cause of hypercalcemia is frequently related to a distinct hormone named PTHrP (PTH related peptides).

Biopsy

Biopsy is not necessary in the majority of cases before definitive surgery for either benign or malignant parathyroid tumors and is in fact generally contraindicated based on documented cases of tumor seeding.[197]

Imaging Techniques

In benign hyperparathyroidism, first-time exploration of the neck by an experienced surgeon will successfully detect the tumor(s) in more than 90% of cases. Imaging techniques are most useful in cases of recurrent or persistent hyperparathyroidism after initial surgery. They are also useful before initial surgery whenever a carcinoma is suspected on clinical grounds, allowing evaluation of the local extent of the tumor.

Noninvasive Techniques

High resolution ultrasonography is an excellent noninvasive technique, although its overall results are operator-dependent.[16] In a prospective comparison based on 100 patients with benign parathyroid tumors before surgery, overall sensitivities were as follows: scintigraphy 73%, CT 68%, MRI 57%, sonography 55%, with respective specificities of 94%, 92%, 87%, and 95%.[198] For patients with parathyroid carcinoma, CT scanning appears most useful at this time since it has good sensitivity for detecting the primary tumor and allows evaluation of its local extent and metastases.

Treatment

Surgery is the major and only curative treatment of parathyroid carcinoma.[199] Despite the slow growth of these tumors, the surgery is best performed as early as possible before local and distant spread has occurred. The technique involves removal of the tumor en bloc, with all involved surrounding structures and without violating its capsule. Surgery is the recommended treatment of recurrent tumor as well, offering long-term control of hypercalcemia in the absence of a cure.[200] Parathyroid carcinomas are resistant to radiotherapy, although it can occasionally be useful for palliation of pain from bone metastasis. The experience with chemotherapy is limited to case reports.[201,202] The 5-year survival is about 50% (including 30% without recurrence) and the 10-year survival varies from 13% to 35%, with patients who survive many years despite repeated recurrences and metastasis.[197]

Table 76-6 Clinical Features of Primary Hyperparathyroidism Due to Parathyroid Carcinoma and Benign Tumors

	Cancer	Benign
Incidence	2–4%	96–98%
Female:male	1:1	3:1
Age (yrs)		
Mean	45	58
Range	12–84	17–83
Palpable neck mass	42%	Rare
Serum calcium		
Mean mg/dL (mmol/L)	15 (3.75)	11–12 (2.75–3.0)
>14 mg/dL (3.5 mmol/L)	64%	<10%
Renal disease	56%	20%
Lithiasis	49%	20%
Nephrocalcinosis	23%	Rare
Decreased function	51%	14%
Bone disease	63%	6%
Osteitis fibrosa cystica	36%	4%
Renal and bone disease	39%	Rare
Gastrointestinal disease		
Peptic ulcer	11%	8%
Pancreatitis	11%	Rare
Asymptomatic	3%	47%

MEN Syndromes

The MEN-1 and MEN-2 syndromes describe individuals and families with hyperplasia and/or tumors of multiple endocrine tissues. The MEN-1 and MEN-2 syndromes, however, differ in the type and how often certain endocrine tissues are involved, etiology, clinical presentation, preventive and therapeutic surgery, screening, and follow-up of affected individuals. The neuroendocrine tumors that occur within the MEN syndromes have both similarities and differences to the same tumors when they occur sporadically. Both MEN-1 and MEN-2 involve hyperparathyroidism secondary to hyperplasia or tumors. MEN-1 includes many of the PNET discussed earlier in this chapter. MEN-2 includes medullary carcinoma of the thyroid and pheochromocytoma, which have not been discussed, therefore, both MEN-related, other familial, and sporadic tumors will be discussed below. Pituitary adenoma, pheochromocytoma, and medullary thyroid carcinoma were each initially identified as independent pathological entities. The clustering of MEN syndromes was described later.

MEN-1 Syndrome

This syndrome was first referred to as Werner syndrome, after the person who published the observation of groups of individuals with multiple adenomas that appeared to be inherited in an autosomal dominant pattern.[203] In 1968 Steiner and colleagues characterized the collection of multiple endocrine tumors/hyperplasia into two groups referred to as "multiple endocrine adenomatosis [later changed to neoplasia] types 1 and 2."[204] A somewhat unpredictable cluster of neuroendocrine and nonendocrine tumors from a total of about 20 different histologies characterizes MEN-1 syndrome cases and families (Table 76-7). Though there is no "typical" grouping of neuroendocrine tumors for all MEN-1 syndrome families, data from many families show that the most common tumors are parathyroid, including hyperplasia (90%), enteropancreatic (70%), and anterior pituitary (25%).[205] A practical clinical guideline for diagnosis of an MEN-1 individual is to have two of the three principal tumors diagnosed, and a MEN-1 family would involve at least one case as defined above and at least one first-degree relative with at least one of the principal tumors types.

It is now recognized that about 80% of familial MEN-1 individuals and about 50% of sporadic MEN-1 individuals have a heterozygous germline mutation in the *MEN-1* gene.[206–209] A recent update of 1336 mutations have been characterized and they are spread across the coding region of the *MEN-1* gene, leading in large part to truncation mutants of MENIN that impair binding with the numerous proteins such as JUN-D, Smad3, and NF-KappaB, FANCD2, HDAC1 and others.[211] MENIN, the product of the *MEN-1* gene, acts as a tumor suppressor and has recently been shown to interact through the lysine-3-histone deactylase,[210] and the various mutations act as loss-of-function mutations. Despite the varied genotypes, no correlation of genotype to predictable clinical phenotype has been determined that could allow a more focused algorithm to justify preventive surgery and a more focused screening of affected family members with specific mutations.[211] This is despite the fact that the gene shows high penetration with over 90% of documented carriers having clinical or biochemical evidence of disease by age 50 years. Similar inactivating somatic mutations are also found to a varying degree in sporadic tumors of the same histology as found in MEN-1 syndromes. MEN-1 mutations remain the most common form of genetic predisposition to neuroendocrine tumors, including those associated with RET, TSC 1, TSC2, and VHL.[212] In general, the familial and somatic mutations differ clinically in that the familial cases have an earlier age of onset, affect multiple organs, and often develop multiple tumors within the same organ.[213] Despite these differences, diagnostic and therapeutic decisions often rely on data from studies of the more common non-MEN-1 patients.

MEN-1 and Parathyroid Lesions

Most patients first present with symptoms of hyperparathyroidism, asymptomatic hypercalcemia, or if in a known MEN-1 family undergoing screening, with biochemical or imaging evidence of parathyroid tumor(s). The average age of onset is 25-30 years old, and by age 50, nearly 100% of the MEN-1 patients will have evidence of HPT. The converse is not true, only 2-4% of cases of sporadic HPT investigated will be found to have mutations in the *MEN-1* gene,[214] and the average age of onset is 55-60 years old.

In adults first suspected of the MEN-1 syndrome because of manifestations of a PNET (eg, gastrinoma), hyperparathyroidism is often only diagnosed after obtaining serum calcium and parathyroid hormone levels, even though such patients may have had a decade-long history of renal stones.[16]

MEN-1 patients characteristically have multi-glandular nodular hyperplasia as the cause of their hyperparathyroidism. Often, the individual gland involvement is variable and is best described as asymmetrical hyperplasia, resulting in enlargement of only one or two glands, particularly in younger patients. This disease usually takes a slow but progressive course, and eventually all glands are involved.

Micro- or macroadenomas of the pituitary gland are commonly detected in MEN-1 patients when biochemical and imaging studies have been performed. Most tumors are functionally active and secrete prolactin. Less frequently, MEN-1 patients may develop tumors that secrete ACTH or growth hormone and present with Cushing syndrome or acromegaly. In the MEN-1 patient it is especially important to establish that the Cushing syndrome is pituitary dependent (Cushing disease) rather than caused by an adrenal adenoma or the ectopic secretion of ACTH or corticotropin-releasing factor (CRF) from islet-cell tumors or a bronchial carcinoid tumor.[16]

Table 76-7 ■ **MEN-1 Tumor Type Distribution and Estimated Penetrance (%) by Age 40 Years**

Endocrine Tumors (Common)	Endocrine Tumors (Less Common)	Nonendocrine Features
Parathyroid adenoma (90%)	Thymic carcinoid (2%)	Collagenomas (70%)
Gastrinoma (40%) PP (nonfunctioning) oma (20%)	Bronchial carcinoid (2%)	Facial angiofibromas (85%)
Prolactinoma (20%)	PNET (VIPoma, glucagonoma, etc) (2%)	Lipomas (30%)
Insulinoma (10%)	ACTH, GH (2%)	
ECL tumor (10%)	Pheochromocytoma (<1%)	
	TSH (rare)	

Note. Nonfunctioning adrenal tumors are found in as high as 25% of MEN-1 patients on full evaluation.
Source: From Ref. 203.

MEN-1 and Gastrinoma

Gastrinoma, a functioning islet-cell tumor secreting gastrin, is responsible for the ZES, the next most common tumor to follow HPT in MEN-1 patients. Prior to the introduction of potent proton pump inhibitors, ZES was responsible for multiple peptic ulcers and high morbidity and mortality.

Approximately 20% of gastrinomas are associated with the MEN-1 syndrome.[98] Gastrinomas diagnosed in association with the MEN-1 syndrome are quite different from those associated with sporadic gastrinomas. Tumors in the MEN-1 syndrome usually present at an earlier age and are multiple, often small or undetectable, and less frequently (7–12%) malignant. The role of surgery for gastrinoma in MEN-1 patients therefore remains poorly defined. Surgery with curative intent might include complete pancreaticoduodenectomy. Given the high biochemical recurrence postsurgery in MEN-1 patients, it is generally recommended to avoid surgery and manage medically, with periodic evaluations for radiological progression of tumors. When there is no evidence of metastatic disease and venous sampling demonstrates an anatomically localized source of gastrin, enucleation (pancreatic head) or resection (body or tail) may offer excellent palliation, but rarely a cure.[16] Based on the correlation between tumor size and risk of liver metastases, some advocate surgery for those MEN-1 patients with a tumor exceeding 2.0–2.5 cm.[104]

MEN-1 Medical and Surgical Management

The clinical features of patients with MEN-1 depend entirely upon the natural history of the individual tumors and endocrine hyperfunction. Most patients with MEN-1 pancreatic disease requiring surgical intervention present with a syndrome caused by hypersecretion of a specific hormone such as gastrin, insulin, VIP, or glucagon. Overall, patients with familial MEN-1 neoplasms have long survival, which is significantly better than that for patients with sporadic endocrine pancreatic tumors.[16]

The surgical treatment of the MEN-1 syndrome is dependent on the phenotypic expression in the individual patient. Because components of the syndrome may be metachronous, surgical procedures involving different endocrine organs may be required over a period of many years. Regardless of initial findings, MEN-1 patients must be followed for life for involvement of the pituitary gland, parathyroid glands, endocrine pancreas or duodenum, adrenal glands, thymus, and lungs (bronchial carcinoids).

A lack of predictable genotype-phenotype relationships does not permit preventive surgery and requires a broad sweep of follow-up tests for affected family members. Brandi and colleagues include one of several consensus positions on screening of suspected and confirmed MEN-1 mutation carriers that include both biochemical and imaging tests.[205] With improved medical management of hypercalcemia and peptic ulcers, more than 30% of MEN-1 patients can be managed successfully for years and now die at later ages of malignancies related to MEN-1.[215,216] The timing (childhood vs adult) and type of operation (total vs partial parathyroidectomy) for prevention of HPT remains controversial, balancing risk of recurrence with adverse effect of possible lifelong hypoparathyroidism.

MEN-2 Syndromes

The MEN-2 syndromes represent several distinct clusters of neuroendocrine tumors with strong association between specific gene mutations of the *RET* proto-oncogene and phenotype, permitting preventive surgery and focused follow-up and screening of patients and families for specific "at-risk" tumors. There have been between 500 and 1000 MEN-2 families reported worldwide, with the subtype *MEN-2b* representing about 80% of families.[216] MEN-2 has two distinct subtypes, MEN-2A and MEN-2B, and most would also include FMTC as a MEN-2 syndrome as well (Table 76-8). The syndromes were first recognized by clinical patterns of tumor involvement[204] and later shown to be caused by specific mutations in the *RET* oncogene. MEN-2A patients are characterized by medullary thyroid carcinoma in 95%, pheochromocytoma(s) in 50%, and hyperplasia/adenoma of the parathyroid glands in 15–30% of cases.[219] MEN-2B patients have medullary thyroid carcinoma in 100%, pheochromocytoma(s) in 50%, and varied reported incidences of mucosal neuromas and marfanoid body habitus.[218,219] Over 95% of the *RET* mutations in MEN-2A reported to date

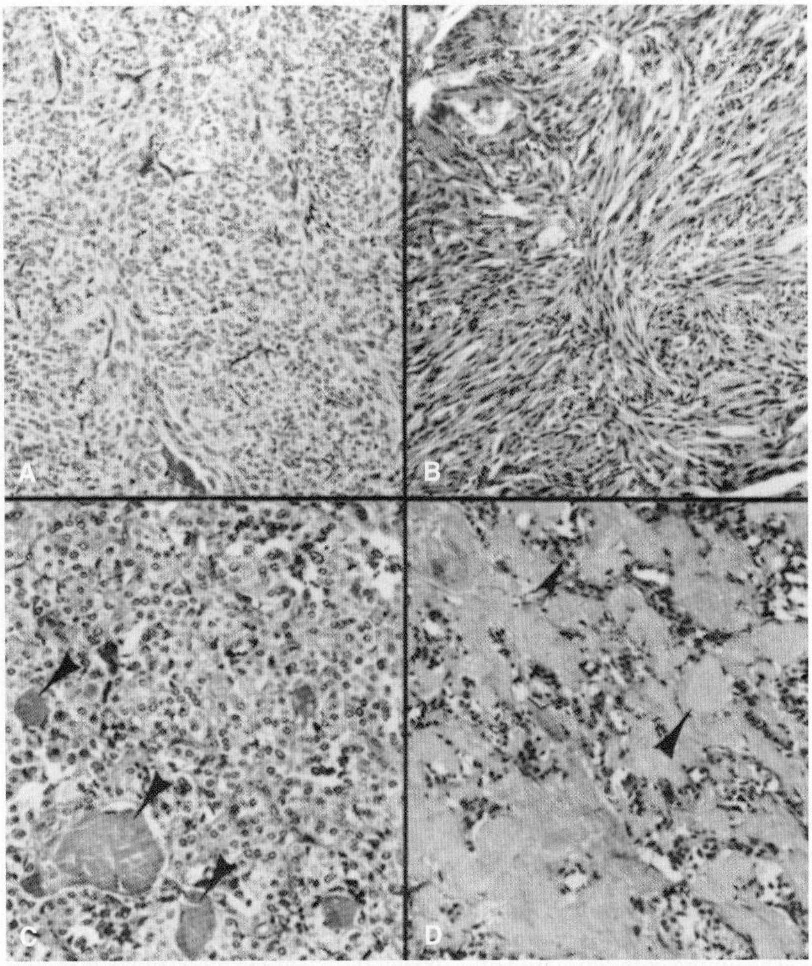

Figure 76-6 Histologic features of medullary thyroid cancer. **(A)** Nests of polygonal cells. **(B)** Spindle-shaped cells. **(C)** Amyloid deposits (*arrows*). **(D)** Large amount of fibrous stroma with sparse cells and amyloid nodules (*arrows*).

involve exons 10 and 11, corresponding to the cysteine-rich extracellular domain of the receptor.[220] About 90% of FMTC have identified RET mutations, including some overlap with mutations at specific codons seen in MEN-2A. Over 95% of MEN-2b cases have the same missense M918T mutation at codon 918 in exon 16, and a few cases are reported with A883F mutations in exon 15, both corresponding to the intracellular domain of the receptor.[221]

Medullary Thyroid Carcinoma

Medullary thyroid carcinomas are derived from the thyroid C-cells and are preceded and accompanied by pathologic findings of C-cell hyperplasia (Fig. 76-6). C-cell hyperplasia is also seen in 5% of the normal population, and therefore can confuse the screening and evaluation of MEN patients.[222]

MTC represents about 5–10% of new cases of thyroid cancers, or about 1000 cases per year in the United States. Of these, about 75% have no family history of MTC (sporadic MTC) and are generally diagnosed around the age of 50–60 years.[223] All MEN patients are at high risk of medullary thyroid carcinoma (Table 76-8). MEN-2A patients often present with MTC before pheochromocytoma or parathyroid disease. In known MEN-2A families, biochemical evidence of early MTC usually occurs between the ages of 5 and 25 years.[224] The MEN-2B patients have an earlier age of onset of cancers and a more aggressive phenotype of medullary thyroid carcinoma leading to a worse prognosis compared with MEN-2A patients.[225,226] Fortunately, some of these children are recognized prior to the diagnosis of MTC based on the marfanoid body habitus and mucosal neuromas.[227]

MTC and C-cell hyperplasia are suspected in the presence of elevated serum calcitonin levels, a sensitive and specific

Table 76-8 **Classification of MEN-2 Syndromes**

	MEN-2 Cases	MTC	Pheo	Parathyroid Hyperplasia/ Adenoma
MEN-2A	60–90%	95%	50%	20–30%
MEN-2B	5%	100%	50%	Uncommon
FMTC	5–35%	100%	0%	0%

Abbreviations: FMTC, familial medullary thyroid carcinoma; MTC, medullary thyroid carcinoma; Pheo, pheochromocytoma.
Source: From Refs. 216, 217, 239.

marker for both conditions. In patients at risk, confirmed MTC cases after treatment or MEN-2 family members, the more sensitive calcitonin stimulation test can be performed where calcitonin levels are drawn before and 5 min following a calcium infusion.[224] Both MTC and CCH can result in a positive calcitonin stimulation test, and not all cases of CCH will progress to MTC.[222,224] Patients not identified by early screening, about 30% of MTC patients, will present with a (painful) neck mass, and/or diarrhea associated with high calcitonin levels. Unfortunately most of these patients already have local or distant spread of their tumors.[223,228]

Treatment of MTC involves total thyroidectomy and lymph node dissection in almost all cases, with autotransplantation of parathyroid tissue if possible, followed by lifelong thyroid replacement. Of these patients, approximately 50% will develop recurrent disease,[229] so it is recommended that they be screened with a yearly calcitonin stimulation test. Recent data suggest that FDG-PET might be particularly sensitive in detection of MTC metastases.[230] Chemotherapy and radiation therapy have generally been found to result in few responses.[231] Prophylactic thyroidectomy (and autotransplant of parathyroid tissue) is accepted therapy for all patients with documented *RET* germline mutations. The timing of the surgery, still controversial, can in fact be guided by the specific *RET* codon affected.[205]

Familial Medullary Thyroid Carcinoma

The designation of FMTC, as opposed to MEN-2A, MEN-2B, and sporadic MTC, is defined as families with four or more cases of MTC in the absence of a diagnosis of pheochromocytoma or parathyroid hyperplasia/adenoma.[232] Of these cases, almost 90% will be found to have an identifiable *RET* mutation.[233] It is recommended that all FMTC cases undergo regular screening tests for pheochromocytoma, and parathyroid disease given that some families are later classified as MEN-2A or B.[239] The therapy for FMTC is the same as for MTC in association with MEN-2A, MEN-2B, though the clinical course and prognosis is more favorable for FMTC.[235]

Pheochromocytoma

Pheochromocytomas arise in the chromaffin cells of the adrenal medulla (Fig. 76-7). Paragangliomas arise from tissue of the sympathetic and parasympathetic nervous system. Paragangliomas of the sympathetic nervous system, often called extra-adrenal pheochromocytomas, are most often located in the retroperitoneum. Paragangliomas of the parasympathetic nervous system are

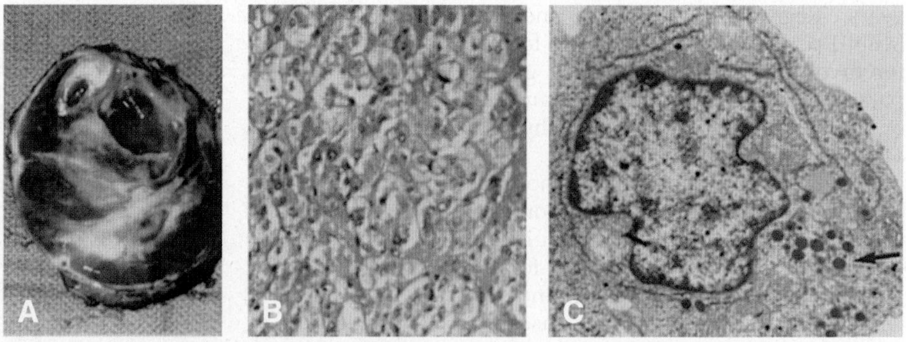

Figure 76-7 ■ Pheochromocytoma. **(A)** Gross appearance of a surgically removed hemisected extra-adrenal pheochromocytoma. **(B)** Histopathologic appearance of a pheochromocytoma showing typical cords of glandular cells separated by bands of stroma (H&E, ×25). **(C)** Ultrastructural appearance of a single pheochromocytoma cell showing dense neurosecretory granules (*arrow*) (×6000).

often located in the region of the aortic arch, neck, and base of skull (ie, carotid body paragangliomas).[236] Pheochromocytomas are rare. Mayo Clinic data estimate that approximately 800 cases of pheochromocytoma are diagnosed in the United States each year.[237] They are found in approximately 0.1–0.5% of hypertensive patients.[238]

Clinical Features and Diagnosis ■ Discussions of the diagnosis and management of pheochromocytoma often consider the "rough rule of tens": 10% of neoplasms occur in children, 10% of sporadic cases are bilateral, 10% are extra-adrenal, and 10% are malignant. Previously, this rule included that 10% of pheochromocytomas were familial, but recent updates [239,240] document that pheochromocytoma patients without personal or family history of associated endocrine neoplasia are in fact found to harbor mutations in over 25% of cases, and those germ-line mutations are found in one of the five susceptibility genes for this disease: VHL, *RET, NF-1, MEN-1*, and succinate dehydrogenase subunits D,B,C (*SDHD, SDHB, SDHC*). Overall, including familial and apparent sporadic tumors, about 30% of all pheochromocytoma cases are now thought to have an identifiable germ-line mutation, leaving over 60% as sporadic tumors. It is now recommended that genetic counseling and possible genetic testing, be considered for all patients diagnosed with pheochromocytoma, particularly those diagnosed under age 50 years with a family history or multifocal disease where the a priori risk of identifying a mutation clearly exceeds 10%.[241] The documentation of a germline mutation impacts on the medical management of both the patient and family.

Patients may present anywhere in the spectrum from normotensive and asymptomatic to a severe, life-threatening hypertensive crisis.[242] In clinically diagnosed patients, hypertension can be either sustained or episodic, and each occurs in approximately half of patients with pheochromocytoma. The most common symptoms are headache, sweating, and palpitation; each occurs in about 60% of patients.

The fundamental basis for the diagnosis of pheochromocytoma is a high index of clinical suspicion with confirmation by biochemical determinations for catecholamines or catecholamine metabolites in blood or urine. Plasma metanephrines are though to be the single best test for the diagnosis of pheochromocytoma. However, not all laboratories provide plasma metanephrine assays, and one can rely on the more widely available measurements of 24-h urinary excretion for catecholamines, metanephrines, or vanillylmandelic acid (VMA). In patients with borderline results, a clonidine suppression test can be performed.[243] CT scanning, as well as MRI, can visualize over 90% of adrenal pheochromocytomas in patients with biochemical evidence of a pheochromocytoma.[244,245] MIBG is a structural analogue of guanethidine and is taken up and stored in secretory granules of the chromaffin cells.[246] ^{131}I-MIBG scans have been shown to have a sensitivity of 87% and a specificity of 97%.[247,248] All patients should have an MIBG scan to confirm that the tumor seen on CT scan/MRI is a pheochromocytoma (Fig. 76-8). Because of the risk of catastrophic hemorrhage or hypertensive complications, fine-needle aspiration should not be attempted for cytologic diagnosis.

Surgical Management of Benign or Recurrent Resectable Disease ■ Nearly all benign pheochromocytomas can be cured by surgical resection. Because of its slow growth rate and accompanying significant morbidity, complete resection of local recurrence or limited metastases of malignant pheochromocytoma should be attempted. The value of debulking surgery for patients whose tumor cannot be completely resected is not established, but reports of

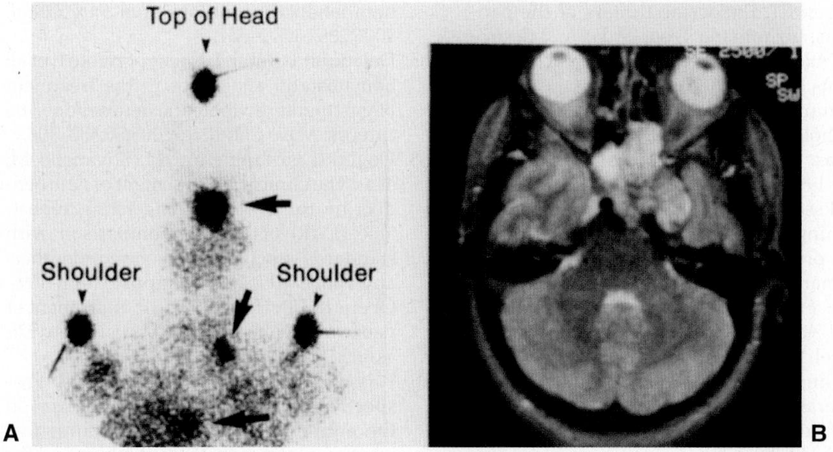

Figure 76-8 ■ Diagnostic imaging in metastatic pheochromocytoma. **(A)** Gamma camera image of the upper body of a patient 48 h following injection of ^{131}I-metaiodobenzylguanidine. Areas of abnormal isotope uptake are noted at the base of the brain, the cervical region, and the mid-thoracic spine (*arrows*). **(B)** T2-weighted magnetic resonance image of the same patient demonstrating a signal-intensive mass encroaching the circle of Willis, the left temporal lobe, and the left optic nerve.

successful control of symptoms following surgery have been reported.[249]

Medical Treatment of Recurrent or Metastatic Disease ■ It is estimated that only about 5–25% of all pheochromocytomas are malignant.[250] The diagnosis of malignant pheochromocytoma can be made only when the tumor is locally invasive and unresectable, recurs after primary extirpation, or is found to be metastatic. Although the natural history of the disease in each of these situations may be variable and somewhat unpredictable, advanced malignant pheochromocytoma is associated with a high morbidity and mortality. The limited data suggest a significant number of patients with disseminated disease may live for long periods without specific antineoplastic therapy.[251]

Targeted radiotherapy using high specific activity MIBG has been evaluated in several small studies, and overall it was found that the majority of patients with malignant pheochromocytoma do not take up and retain sufficient MIBG to deliver an effective radiation dose to the tumor. There is a symptomatic improvement in about 75% of patients, an objective tumor response in about 20%, with few complete responses, and recurrence of symptoms and progression of disease of most cases.[252]

The CVD (cyclophosphamide, vincristine, and dacarbazine) regimen that is effective in children with advanced neuroblastoma was adapted for use in malignant pheochromocytoma. In a study by Averbuch and colleagues[253] of 14 patients with advanced, progressive, and symptomatic pheochromocytoma, there were 57% complete and partial responses, 79% complete and partial biochemical responses, and median duration of responses of 21–22 months, respectively. Currently, CVD is considered the preferred treatment of symptomatic, disseminated pheochromocytoma.

MEN-2 and Pheochromocytoma ■ Pheochromocytomas in MEN-2 patients are diagnosed between the ages of 20 and 30 years (with MEN-2B patients generally being younger than MEN-2A patients), earlier than the sporadic pheochromocytomas diagnosed between 35 and 45 years old.[254] The earlier age of diagnosis is in part due to MEN-2 patients being screened based on earlier diagnosis of another endocrine tumor or a family history. About 25% of MEN-2A patients present with pheochromocytoma as their first tumor.[255,256] Up to 75% of patients are diagnosed concurrently with medullary thyroid carcinoma[254] MEN-2 patients with pheochromocytomas develop bilateral tumors and appear to have a lower incidence of malignant transformation than patients with sporadic tumors.[257] Given the low incidence of malignancy in MEN-2 patients, unilateral or bilateral subtotal resection with preservation of adrenocortical function can be considered in this population to avoid lifelong replacement therapy. The MEN-2A patients are often asymptomatic, but can develop hypertensive crises during surgery, such as for hyperparathyroidism or medullary thyroid carcinoma. Therefore, all patients with MEN-2 should be carefully screened for the presence of pheochromocytoma before any surgery or invasive procedure and, if present, treated with α-adrenergic blockade to control blood pressure.

Within MEN-2 families, the specific *RET* mutation at codon 634 is highly associated with the presence or eventual development of pheochromocytoma and should be considered in following these patients. Overall, the general recommendation is to screen all MEN-2 patients for pheochromocytoma on a yearly basis.[241]

Familial Isolated Pheochromocytoma ■ It has been well documented that sporadic pheochromocytoma (those without any personal or family history of MEN-2) have been associated with germline mutations in *VHL*, succinate dehydrogenase B (*SDHB*) and succinate dehydrogenase D (*SDHD*) and *RET*, now referred to as familial isolated pheochromocytomas (Table 76-9).

Between 0.1% and 6% of all NF-1 patients, and between 20% and 50% of hypertensive NF-1 patients, will develop pheochromocytoma. However, the diagnosis of NF-1 is often made on clinical grounds in childhood, long before the presentation of a pheochromocytoma in the third or fourth decade. The clinical features of NF-1–associated pheochromocytomas are similar to sporadic cases.[258]

Table 76-9 ■ **Germline Mutations Found in Selected Pheochromocytoma Patients Without Personal or Family History Suggestive of MEN-2 (Sporadic Cases)**

Gene	No. Patients Tested	No. Found to Have Mutation	Percent With Mutation
VHL	157	9	6
SDHD	37	3	8
SDHB	24	1	4
RET	137	1	<1
			Total 19

Source: From Ref. 260.

Selected References

The complete reference list can be found at www.CANCERMEDICINE8.com

1. For a definitive historical discussion on carcinoid tumors, the reader is encouraged to read: Modlin IM, Shapiro MD, Kidd M. Siegfried Oberndorfer: origins and perspectives of carcinoid tumors. *Human Pathol.* 2004;35:1440–1451.
14. Rindi G, Leiter AB, Kopin AS, et al. The "normal" endocrine cell of the gut—

changing concepts and new evidences. *Ann NY Acad Sci.* 2004;1014;1–12.
19. Oberg K. Biochemical diagnosis of neuroendocrine GEP tumor. *Yale J Biol Med.* 1997;70:501–508.
20. Nehar D, Lombard-Bohas C, Olivieri S, et al. Interest of Chromogranin A for the diagnosis and follow-up of endocrine tumors. *Clin Endocrinol.* (Oxford). 2004;60:644–652.
32. Soga J, Tazawa K. Pathology analysis of carcinoids: histologic reevaluation of 62 cases. *Cancer.* 1971;28:990–998.
34. Kloppel G, Perren A, Heitz PU. The gastroenteropancreatic neuroendocrine cell system and its tumors: the WHO classification. *Ann NY Acad Sci.* 2004;1014:13–27.
35. Solcia E, Kloppel G, Sobin LH, et al. *Histologic Typing of Endocrine Tumours.* 2nd ed. WHO International Classification of Tumours. Berlin: Springer-Verlag; 2000.
37. Patel Y. Somatostatin and its receptor family. *Front Neuroendrinol.* 1999;20:157–198.
40. Lamberts SW, van der Lely AJ, de Herder WW, et al. Octreotide. *N Engl J Med.* 1996;334:246–254.
45. Ruebi JC, Waser B, Schaer JC, Laissue JA. Somatostatin receptor sst1-sst5 expression in normal and neoplastic human tissues using receptor autoradiography with subtype—selective ligands. *Eur J Nuc Med.* 2001;28:836–846.
51. Modlin IM, Lye KD, Kidd M. A 5-decade analysis of 13,715 carcinoid tumors. *Cancer.* 2003;97:936–959.
55. Moertel CG, Sauer WG, Docherty MB, Baggenstoss AH. Life history of the carcinoid tumor of the small intestine. *Cancer.* 1961;14:291–293.
70. Krenning EP, Bakker WH, Breeman WA, et al. Localization of endocrine-related tumours with radio-iodinated analogue of somatostatin. *Lancet.* 1989;i:242–244.
73. Modlin IM, Shapiro MD, Kidd M. An analysis of rare carcinoid tumors: clarifying these clinical conundrums. *World J Surg.* 2005;29:92–101.
74. Kulke MH, Mayer RJ. Carcinoid tumors. *N Engl J Med.* 1999;340:858–868.
77. Modlin IM, Kidd M, Laitch I, etal. Current status of gastrointestinal carcinoids. *Gastroneterology.* 2005;128:1717–1751
82. Soga J, Yakuwa Y, Osaka M. Carcinoid syndrome: a statistical evaluation of 748 reported cases. *J Exp Clin Cancer Res.* 1999;18:133–141.
84. Anderson AS, Krauss D, Lang R. Cardiovascular complications of malignant carcinoid disease. *Am Heart J.* 1997;134: 693–702.
85. Simula DV, Edwards WD, Tazelaar HD, et al. Surgical pathology of carcinoid heart disease: a study of 139 values from 75 patients spanning over 20 years. *Mayo Clin Proc.* 2002;77:139–147.
91. Jensen RT. Endocrine tumors of the pancreas. In: Yamada T, ed. *Textbook of Gastroenterology.* New York, NY: Lippincott Williams & Wilkins; 2003.
93. Kimura W, Kuroda A, Morioka Y. Clinical pathology of endocrine tumors of the pancreas. Analysis of autopsy cases. *Dig Dis Sci.* 1991;36:933–942.
94. Eriksson B, Oberg K. PPomas and nonfunctioning endocrine pancreatic tumors: clinical presentation, diagnosis, and advances in management. In: Mignon M, Jensen RT, eds. *Endocrine Tumors of the Pancreas: Recent Advances in Research and Management.* Basel, Switzerland: S. Karger;1995:120.
96. Zollinger RM, Ellison EH. Primary peptic ulceration of the jejunum associated with islet cell tumors of the pancreas. *Ann Surg.* 1955;142:709–723.
98. Roy PK, Venzon DJ, Shojamansesh H, et al. Zollinger-Ellison syndrome. Clinical presentation in 261 patients. *Medicine.* (Baltimore) 2000;79:379–411.
108. Metz DC, Strader DB, Orbuch M, et al. Use of omeprazole in Zollinger-Ellison: a prospective nine-year study of efficacy and safety. *Alimnet Pharmacol Ther.* 1993;7:597–610.
113. Shojamanesh H, Gibril F, Louie A, et al. Prospective study of the antitumor efficacy of long-term octreotide treatment in patients with progressive metastatic gastrinoma. *Cancer.* 2002;94:331–343.
115. Grant CS. Insulinoma. *Surg Oncol Clin North Am.* 1998;7:819–844.
124. Verner JV, Morrison AB. Endocrine pancreatic disease with diarrhea: report of a case due to diffuse hyperplasia of non-beta islet tissue with a review of 54 additional cases. *Arch Intern Med.* 1974;133:492–499.
130. McGavran MH, Unger RH, Recant L, et al. A glucagonsecreting alpha-cell carcinoma of the pancreas. *N Engl J Med.* 1966;274:1408–1413.
141. Ganda PO, Weir GC, Soeldner JS, et al. Somatostatinoma: a somatostatin-containing tumor of the endocrine pancreas. *N Engl J Med.* 1977;296:963–967.
142. Larsson LI, Hirsch MA, Holst J, et al. Pancreatic somatostatinoma clinical features and physiologic implications. *Lancet.* 1977;1:666–668.
152. Que FG, Nagnorney DM, Batts KP, et al. Hepatic resection for metastatic neuroendocrine carcinomas. *Am J Surg.* 1995; 169:36–43.
153. Mazzaglai PJ, Berber E, Milas M, Siperstein AE. Laparoscopic radiofrequency ablation of neuroendocrine liver metastases: a 10-year experience evaluating predictors of survival. *Surgery.* 2007;142:10–19.
158. Osborne DA, Zervos EE, Strosberg J, et al. Improved outcome with cytoreductive versus embolization for symptomatic hepatic metastases of carcinoid and neuroendocrine tumors. *Ann Surg Oncol.* 2006;206;13:572–581.
165. Delaunoit T, Rubin J, Neczyporenko F, et al. Somatostatin analogues in the treatment of gastroenteropancreatic neuroendocrine tumors. *Mayo Clin Proc.* 2005;80:502–506.
168. Dogliotti L, Tampellini M, Stivanello M, et al. The clinical management of neuroendocrine tumors with long-acting repeatable (LAR) octreotide: comparison with standard subcutaneous octreotide therapy. *Ann Oncol.* 2001;12(suppl 2);S105–109.
172. Oberg K. Interferon in the management of neuroendocrine GEP tumors: a review. *Digestion.* 2000;62(suppl 1):92–97.
176. Faiss S, Pape UF, Bohmig M, et al. Prospective, randomized, multicenter trial on the antiproliferative effect of lanreotide, interferon alfa, and their combination for therapy of metastatic neuroendocrine gastroenteropancreatic tumors—the International Lanreotide and Interferon Alfa Study Group. *J Clin Oncol.* 2003;21:2689–2696.
184. Kwekkeboom DJ, Bakker WH, Kam BL, et al. Treatment with Lu-177 DOTA-Tyr3-octreotate in patients with neuroendocrine tumors: interim results. *Eur J Nucl Med Mol Imaging.* 2003;30:S231.
185. Kulke MH, Kim H, Stuart K, et al. A phase II study of docetaxel in patients with metastatic carcinoid tumors. *Cancer Invest.* 2004;22:353–359.
186. Schnirer II, Yao JC, Ajani JA. Carcinoid: a comprehensive review. *Acta Oncol.* 2003;42:672–692.
191. Kulke M. Gastrointestinal neuroendocrine tumors: a role for targeted therapies? *Endocrine Related Can.* 2007;14:207–219.
192. Yao JC. Molecular targeted therapy for carcinoid and islet-cell carcinoma. *Best Prac & Res Clin Endocrin & Metabolism.* 2007;21:163–172.
195. Shane E. Clinical review 122: parathyroid carcinoma. *J Clin Endocrinol Metab.* 2001;86:485–493.
206. Chandrasekharappa SC, Guru SC, Manickam P, et al. Positional cloning of the gene for multiple endocrine neoplasia-type 1. *Science.* 1997;276:404–407.
211. Lemos MC, Thakker RV. Multiple endocrine neoplasia type I (MEN1): analysis of 1336 mutations reported in the first decade following identification of the gene. *Human Mutation.* 2008;29:22–32.
217. Marini F, Falchetti A, Del Monte F, et al. Multiple endocrine neoplasia type 2. *Orphanet J of Rare Dis.* 2006;1:45–50.
238. Pacak K, Linehan WM, Eisenhofer G, et al. Recent advances in genetics, diagnosis, localization, and treatment of pheochromocytoma. *Ann Intern Med.* 2001;134:315–329.
250. Goldstein RE, O'Neil JA, Holcomb GW, et al. Clinical experience over 48 years with pheochromocytoma. *Ann Surg.* 1999;229:755–766.

77 Neoplasms of the Head and Neck

Michael E. Kupferman, MD ■ Erich M. Sturgis, MD, MPH ■ David L. Schwartz, MD ■ Adam Garden, MD ■ Merrill S. Kies, MD

Introduction

Approximately 48,000 new cases of head and neck cancer will be diagnosed in the United States and over 11,000 Americans will die from these malignancies in 2009.[1] Although head and neck cancer accounts for only 3% of all new cancer cases and only 2% of all cancer deaths in the United States annually, these malignancies as a group are the fifth most common malignancy among men worldwide.[2] Tobacco and alcohol are the primary etiologic agents in these cancers, pointing out that prevention (tobacco/alcohol control and cessation) should be the primary public health goal of the field.[3] However, a rising proportion of these cancers (particularly those found in the oropharynx) are likely attributable to oncogenic human papillomavirus (HPV)[4,5] and the impact of population-wide HPV vaccination will have on incidence rates has yet to be determined. Evidence also suggests that inherited factors and exposure to other environmental agents modulate risk and will help refine prevention strategies in the future.[6-9] Head and neck cancers have a much greater impact in certain parts of the world, especially where cigarette smoking and/or chewing of carcinogenic stimulants is more prevalent, and thus head and neck cancers are important causes of cancer mortality worldwide.[2,9] In addition, even in the developed world significant disparities in incidence and mortality remain for select populations, such as African Americans.[6] The more widespread adoption of multidisciplinary care likely underlies improvements in survival rates for some sites (nasopharynx and oropharynx)[7,8]; however, long-term survival rates are either stagnant or have worsened for other sites[10,11]

The survival advantages provided by the adoption of aggressive multidisciplinary care have been undermined by the significant percentage of patients with head and neck squamous cell carcinoma (HNSCC) who subsequently recur at distant sites, develop second primary malignancies, or succumb to comorbid conditions.[12] Despite marked advances in reconstructive surgery and rehabilitation, intensity-modulated radiotherapy (IMRT) and conservation approaches to certain malignancies, HNSCC patients continue to have significant functional deficits and detriments to their quality of life. These compelling problems highlight the importance of neoadjuvant chemotherapy, smoking cessation, chemoprevention, and speech/swallowing rehabilitation. Combined-modality approaches involving both chemotherapy and radiation are now standards of care for locally advanced disease and for organ preservation. Understanding the biology of head and neck cancer and developing molecular-targeted therapeutic agents have advanced substantially, and molecular-targeted chemoprevention also is advancing. These new therapeutic and preventive approaches appear to hold great promise for improving the control of head and neck cancer and its sequalae. This chapter reviews both the current status of and future investigative directions for the epidemiology, biology, chemoprevention, diagnosis, and therapy of head and neck cancer.

Descriptive Epidemiology

Incidence

In the United States, estimates for 2008 were for 22,900 new cases of oral cavity cancer, 12,410 new cases of pharyngeal cancer, and 12,250 new cases of laryngeal cancer. While the United States has benefited from tobacco control efforts with declining smoking prevalence beginning in the 1960s and subsequent declines in incidence rates for most head and neck cancer sites beginning in the 1980s, more recently cancers of the oropharynx appear to be increasing in incidence.[4-7] Approximately 1 in 2 oral cavity cancers occur in women, while only 1 in 4 pharyngeal and laryngeal cancers occur in women. Both oral cavity/pharyngeal and laryngeal cancer incidence rates in men have steadily declined over the last two decades to 15.5/100,000 and 6.0/100,000, respectively, in 2004 (age-adjusted to the US 2000 Standard). Over the last 15 years, women have enjoyed similar trends in both oral cavity/pharyngeal and laryngeal cancer incidence rates to 6.0/100,000 and 1.3/100,000, respectively, in 2004 (age-adjusted to the US 2000 Standard). Although blacks and whites have similar rates of oral cavity/pharyngeal cancer, black men have double the rate of laryngeal cancer of white men; and black women have a 40% higher rate of laryngeal cancer than that of white women. Hispanics have the lowest rates of oral cavity/pharyngeal cancer, and Asians have the lowest rates of laryngeal cancer.

The median age at diagnosis for HNSCC is approximately 60 years, but the incidence of these cancers in young adults (age <45 years) appears to be increasing.[13] This increase has not been apparent in blacks, and carcinomas of the tonsil, oral tongue, and base of tongue account for the majority of this increase in incidence.[6,13] It has been suggested that these increases are related to increasing numbers of oropharyngeal cancers associated with oncogenic HPV.[5] Recent analysis of the Surveillance, Epidemiology, and End Results (SEER) database demonstrates that the increasing incidence of oropharyngeal cancers is principally among white men presenting with oropharyngeal cancers between 39 and 60 years of age.[9,14]

Head and neck cancer is relatively common in many parts of the world and represents the most common malignancy afflicting men in some parts of the world. For example, in South Central Asia, home to one-fifth of the world's population, head and neck cancer accounted for approximately 155,400 new cases of cancer in 1990 (17% of all cancers and 25% of all cancers occurring in men.[2,9] Although the 80% of head and neck cancers in South Central Asia are oral cavity and pharyngeal (excluding nasopharyngeal) cancers, in other regions of the world, laryngeal cancers and nasopharyngeal cancers account for a much higher percentage of head and neck malignancies. For example, in the developed world, laryngeal cancer accounts for approximately one-third of head and neck cancers, and in Southern and Eastern Europe, approximately 40% of all head and neck cancers are laryngeal cancers)[2,14] In China, nasopharyngeal cancer accounts for 55% of all head and neck cancers, and in Southeast Asia, nasopharyngeal cancer accounts for 70% of all head and neck cancers and 5% of all cancers in men)[2,14].

Prevalence

Highlighting the impact of cancer survivorship, approximately 350,000 individuals were living in the United States with a history of head and neck cancer in November, 2007 (240,176 with a history of oral cavity/pharyngeal cancer and 93,096 with a history of laryngeal cancer).[6] As expected, the sex distribution of these prevalent cases reflects the sex of the incident cases. However, African Americans accounted for only 11.5% of the prevalent population of individuals with a history of laryngeal cancer and only 7.3% of the prevalent population of individuals with oral cavity/pharyngeal cancer. These small percentages of the prevalent populations of these cancers likely reflect the poorer overall survival of African Americans diagnosed with HNSCC. Over the past decade, African Americans have demonstrated survival rates approximately 20% worse than whites for oral cavity/pharyngeal cancer and 15% worse than whites for laryngeal cancer.[6]

As a group, head and neck cancers are the third most prevalent cancer worldwide after breast and colorectal cancers, accounting for 7% of the 22.4 million individuals diagnosed with distribution cancer in 2000, excluding nonmelanoma skin cancer.[2,15] Of the approximately 1.6 million individuals with a history of head and neck cancer in 2000, 707,100 had a diagnosis of oral cavity cancer, 458,100 had a diagnosis of laryngeal cancer, 248,800 had a diagnosis of oro/hypopharyngeal cancer, and 171,500 had a diagnosis of nasopharyngeal cancer.[2,15]

Survival Mortality

In 2008 in the United States, 5390 deaths will be attributed to oral cavity cancer, 2200 to pharyngeal cancer, and 3670 to laryngeal cancer. However, head and neck cancer accounts for less than 2% of all cancer deaths in the United States annually. Broader use of and improvements in multidisciplinary care likely underlie the significantly improved survival rates for nasopharyngeal, oropharyngeal and hypopharyngeal cancer patients and trends toward improved oral cavity cancer survival rates; however, laryngeal cancer survival rates appear to be worsening.[7,8,10,11] Mortality rates reflect not only the improvements in treatment/survival but also declining incidence attributable to tobacco control. Mortality rates (age-adjusted to the 2000 US Standard) for oral cavity/pharyngeal cancers have declined steadily over the past two decades and for laryngeal cancers for the past decade. Blacks have higher oral cavity/pharyngeal and laryngeal cancer mortality rates than whites. Hispanics have the lowest oral cavity/pharyngeal cancer death rates, while Asians have the lowest laryngeal cancer death rates.[6]

In 2002, head and neck cancer accounted for approximately 350,000 deaths worldwide, with 127,459 due to oral cavity cancers, 89,956 due to laryngeal cancers, 83,993 due to oro/hypopharyngeal cancers, and 50,332 due to nasopharyngeal cancers.[2] As with other cancer sites, mortality/incidence ratios for head and neck cancers are much higher in developing countries for both men and women as compared with the United States.[2,15] This likely reflects the better survival for these cancers seen in the United States; however, an opposite trend is seen for nasopharyngeal cancer.[2,15]

Risk Factors

Tobacco ■ In the late 1950s, a landmark case-control study by Dr Ernst Wynder established the link between tobacco use and oral cavity cancer.[16] This was followed a year later by a cohort study of over 180,000 men that demonstrated an increased risk of death from HNSCC in cigarette smokers as compared with men who never smoked.[17] These studies also demonstrated elevated risks for HNSCC death in cigar and pipe smokers. In 1964, the Advisory Committee to the Surgeon General on Smoking and Health published its report linking smoking to cancer based on many of Hill's classic criteria of disease causality.[18] Because of limitations of sample size and follow-up time, Doll and Hill's classic cohort study of over 40,000 British physicians showed only a borderline risk of HNSCC related to smoking.[19] However, their criteria linking HNSCC and tobacco smoking have been clearly demonstrated over the past 40 years in multiple independent studies.[3] Most importantly, the strength and consistency of the association between smoking and HNSCC have been demonstrated in numerous case-control and cohort studies with significant relative risks or odds ratios in the 3-fold to 12-fold range.[16,17,19-22] Furthermore, a dose-response effect is consistently shown in these studies between the duration and dose of smoking with increasing risk of HNSCC and between the time since quitting and the decreasing risk of HNSCC.[20-23] Other mucosal malignancies of the head and neck such as nasopharyngeal carcinoma (NPC) and sinonasal malignancies have a weaker association with tobacco smoking.[24] The specificity of the link between tobacco and HNSCC (and not the nonmucosal/unexposed head and neck malignancies), the coherence and analogy of the explanation of tobacco-induced HNSCC to lung carcinogenesis, and the biologic plausibility of the well-established tobacco-induced carcinogenesis model have all helped establish tobacco as the chief etiologic agent in HNSCC.

Although the risk of bronchogenic carcinoma appears to be less significant for cigar and pipe smokers than for cigarette smokers, these forms of tobacco use are also clearly associated with an increased risk of HNSCC.[16,23,25,26] The pooling of saliva containing carcinogens in gravity-dependent regions may account for the site distribution of HNSCC based on consumption patterns; in fact, it appears that in the US floor of mouth (FOM), laryngeal, and hypopharyngeal cancers are almost exclusively found in smokers.[27] Smokeless tobacco and related product users and pipe smokers often have a habitual position for the quid or pipe stem, and these products are also associated with cancer of the oral cavity.[28] In south central Asia where the use of such products is common, the gingivobuccal region is the most common site for HNSCC.[9,29]

Although smoking rates are declining in the developed world, smoking rates are rising in developing countries, home to four-fifths of the world's population. In the United States, smoking rates have declined since the Surgeon General's warning in 1964.[5,30] In 1965, 42.4% of the US adult population were current smokers, while in 2006 only 20.8% were current smokers.[31] Although the reduction in cigarette smoking has been much greater in men over the last three decades, the rate of current cigarette use remains higher in men (23.9%) than for women (18.05%), and 32.4% of Native Americans continue to smoke.[31] Worldwide, striking variations in head and neck cancer sites and incidence are seen among different regions, cultures, and demographic groups and are due, in large part, to differing patterns of tobacco and other substance abuse.[2,9,14,15] For instance, in South Central Asia "pano" (betel leaf, lime, catechu, and areca nut) is commonly chewed and is a strong risk factor independent of tobacco use for carcinoma of the oral cavity, one of the most common cancers in men and women in this region.[9,32]

Alcohol ■ Alcohol, too, is an important promoter of carcinogenesis and is a contributive factor in at least 75% of HNSCCs.[20,22,23] Furthermore, alcohol appears to have an effect on risk of HNSCC independent of tobacco smoking, but these effects are consistently significant only at the highest level of alcohol consumption.[16,20,22,33] Although studies attempting to correlate the type of alcoholic beverage with specific cancer risks have been conflicting, most investigators believe that ethanol itself is the main causative factor.[22,34] Nevertheless, it appears that the major clinical significance of alcohol consumption is that it potentiates the carcinogenic effect of tobacco at every level of tobacco use. However, this effect is most striking at the highest levels of exposure, and the magnitude of this effect is at least additive, but may be multiplicative, dependent on the subsite of HNSCC and the levels of exposure.[20,22]

Infectious Agents ■ Although it has been suggested that various infectious agents play a role in head and neck carcinogenesis, only Epstein-Barr virus (EBV) and HPV can be implicated as etiologic agents in head and neck carcinogenesis based on current scientific evidence. EBV appears to be associated with most NPCs, and HPV (most commonly type 16) is associated with approximately 50% of oropharyngeal carcinomas.[4,5] HPV may also play a role in the etiology of squamous cell carcinomas arising in the sinonasal tract.[35] Although herpes simplex viruses have been suggested as a risk factor for oral cavity cancer,[36] and *Helicobacter pylori* has been suggested as a risk factor for laryngeal cancer,[37] confirmation of these findings is lacking.[38,39]

While laboratory evidence supporting the role of HPV as a risk factor for HNSCC is somewhat circumstantial, HPV has been established as an etiologic agent in cervical cancer,[40] and over the last decade, several investigators have suggested that infection with HPV, especially the high-risk type HPV-16, is a risk factor for oropharyngeal carcinoma.[27,41-47] The chief oncoproteins of HPV-16 are encoded by the genes *E6* and *E7*. The E6 protein targets the tumor suppressor gene *TP53* for ubiquitination and degradation. In fact, degradation of *TP53* in HPV-positive cells is fully dependent on the presence of E6.[48] The E7 oncoprotein is involved in suppression of pRb function. Reduced pRb expression is common in HPV-positive tonsillar cancer.[49] In vitro experiments support the tumorigenicity of HPV-16 in human epithelial cells. Furthermore, numerous studies using methods such as polymerase chain reaction (PCR), Southern blotting, and in situ hybridization have detected HPV DNA in the tumor tissue and sera of oropharyngeal cancer patients.[27,42,44-46] Oropharyngeal tumors and tumors in nonsmokers are the most frequent HPV-positive head and neck malignancies.[27,42] Although oropharyngeal cancer patients presenting without the classic tobacco exposures more commonly have HPV-16-associated tumors,[27] it also possible that there may be synergistic interactions between the traditional oropharyngeal risk factors of tobacco and alcohol with HPV-16.[50] The circumstantial, mechanistic, and molecular epidemiologic evidence strongly supports the role of HPV-16 infection in oropharyngeal carcinogenesis. The potential effect of HPV-16 immunizations in the prevention of cervical carcinomas may help prevent oropharyngeal cancers as well.[5]

The epidemiologic link between EBV and nasopharyngeal cancer is quite strong.[51-56] NPC may be the best example of a virus-related epithelial carcinoma and has served as a model for the study of virus-induced carcinogenesis elsewhere in the body. The fundamental and early role of EBV in the pathogenesis of NPC is further supported by the identification of EBV DNA in premalignant nasopharyngeal lesions. Regardless of histopathologic subtype (World Health Organization [WHO] I to III), geographic or ethnic setting, sporadic or endemic pattern, and premalignant or malignant status, NPC is an EBV-associated malignancy. Although WHO types II and III are overwhelmingly positive for EBV, EBV is also associated with well-differentiated (WHO type-I) NPC.[55] Both serologic and mucosal swab evidence of EBV infection has been used to enhance the screening for NPC in endemic areas.[51,57] Evidence of EBV DNA in cervical lymph node metastases of unknown primary origin has been used to identify nasopharyngeal primaries.[52] More recently, the detection of EBV DNA in peripheral blood (both cellular and cell-free component) has demonstrated prognostic significance for predicting survival and distant metastases and may become a standard biomarker to follow these patients.[58-61]

Genetic Susceptibility ■ The predominant risk factor for HNSCC is a history of exposure to tobacco and alcohol, with a rising proportion of these cancers attributable to HPV16.[4,5] However, since only a fraction of smokers develop cancer, variations in genetic susceptibility may be equally important in the disease etiology. A genetic component to this disease is also supported by large family studies demonstrating a 3-fold to 8-fold increased risk of HNSCC in first-degree relatives of patients with HNSCC.[62-65] Furthermore, there is molecular epidemiologic evidence supporting the concept of genetic susceptibility in head and neck cancer patients.[66] Emerging data from case-control studies of several phenotypic and genotyping assays support the hypothesis that genetic susceptibility plays an important role in the etiology of HNSCC. According to this hypothesis, inherited differences in the efficiencies of carcinogen metabolizing systems, deoxyribonucleic acid (DNA) repair systems, and/or cell-cycle control/apoptosis systems influence one's risk of tobacco-induced cancers.[67,68] Identifying such at-risk individuals in the general population by use of these biomarker assays would have a profound impact on primary prevention, early detection, and secondary prevention strategies. Three recent high-impact publications of genome-wide association studies have identified the same lung cancer susceptibility locus in separate populations.[69-71] These studies will likely be followed in the near future by similar explorations of genome-wide HNSCC association studies and suggests that tailored prevention of tobacco-associated cancers may be a realistic goal.

Environmental Tobacco Smoke ■ Environmental tobacco smoke or secondhand smoking, first received mass attention when the Surgeon General advocated changes in smoking policies in public and work places because nonsmokers exposed to environmental tobacco smoke are at an increased risk for developing lung cancer and later when the United States Environmental Protection Agency classified environmental tobacco smoke as a human carcinogen.[72,73] A high-profile legal case in Australia later brought significant attention to the risk of HNSCC secondary to environmental tobacco smoke exposure. In May of 2001, the New South Wales Supreme Court found that a 62-year-old nonsmoker's HNSCC was significantly associated with long-term exposure to environmental tobacco smoke in her job as a bar attendant and imposed liability on her employer.[74] Two case-control studies supported the court's finding. In a study of 173 cases of HNSCC and 176 cancer-free controls, environmental tobacco smoke was associated with a more than twofold increased risk of HNSCC, and a dose-response relationship was also observed.[75] In a separate study of 44 nonsmokers with HNSCC and 132 cancer-free nonsmoker controls, environmental tobacco smoke was associated with a significantly increased risk of HNSCC, and this was particularly true for females and for those reporting exposure at work.[76]

Laryngopharyngeal Reflux ■ Observational and anecdotal studies have long suggested that gastroesophageal reflux may be associated with laryngeal cancer.[77,78] Furthermore, multiple studies have objectively documented a high prevalence of gastric reflux into the laryngopharynx in patients with laryngeal cancer via 24-hour pH probe monitoring.[79-82] Furthermore, a retrospective case-control study of 10,140 hospitalized patients and 12,061 outpatients with laryngeal and pharyngeal cancer and 40,561 hospitalized and 48,244 outpatient controls has been performed using US Department of Veterans Affairs databases.[83] The diagnosis of gastroesophageal reflux disease was associated with a significantly elevated risk of laryngeal cancer (OR = 2.4 [2.15-2.69] and OR = 2.3 [2.1-2.5] for hospitalized and outpatient groups, respectively) and of pharyngeal cancer (OR = 2.4 [1.9-3.0] and OR = 1.9 [1.7-2.2] for hospitalized and outpatient groups, respectively).

Furthermore, these risk estimates were adjusted for age, gender, ethnicity, smoking, and alcohol consumption. However, a large Swedish cohort study of 66,965 patients with discharge diagnoses of heartburn, hiatal hernia, or esophagitis with a follow-up of 376,622 person-years concluded that there was no evidence of a causal association between gastroesophageal reflux and either laryngeal or pharyngeal cancer.[84]

Marijuana ■ Marijuana smoke has a four times higher tar burden and a 50% higher concentration of benzopyrene and aromatic hydrocarbons than does tobacco smoke. Although anecdotal evidence has long suggested that marijuana is a risk factor for HNSCC, few reports have found direct evidence of marijuana as an etiologic factor for HNSCC because most users of marijuana are also exposed to tobacco and alcohol.[85,86] A recent case-control study including 173 HNSCC patients and 176 cancer-free controls demonstrated a cigarette-adjusted risk of HNSCC of over twofold associated with marijuana use, with evidence of a dose-response relationship.[87] Contrarily, a large retrospective cohort of 64,855 health maintenance organization (HMO) members found no association with tobacco-related cancers.[88] Problems of under reporting of marijuana use and limited sample size of heavy users limit conclusions regarding marijuana use and HNSCC risk.[89]

Diet ■ Epidemiologic evidence from traditional case-control study designs suggests that diets high in animal fats and low in fruits and vegetables may be risk factors for HNSCC.[90-94] Several studies have used case-control methodology to correlate salted fish consumption with NPC risk, and this risk may be due to the high content of nitrosamine compounds in preserved foods such as salted fish.[95,96] Some evidence suggests vitamin A and beta-carotene may be responsible for the protective effect of diets high in fruits and vegetables, and deficiencies of carotenoids appear to be a risk factor for HNSCC and lung cancers.[91] It is not known, however, which of the more than 500 carotenoids are protective, what chemical interactions may occur, or what protective role other micronutrients in carotenoid-rich foods may play. Others have found that total intake of vitamins C and E are also protective.[92,93] Moreover, diets are complex and difficult to assess and validate; in particular, there are often inaccuracies in translating foods into constituent nutrients. Further studies are needed to more precisely define the relationship between dietary intake and serum levels of the various carotenoid components. It may be impossible to determine which of the vast array of compounds is most beneficial, and controlling for other dietary variables and confounding risk factors has remained a difficult methodological problem. Further confounding this situation, smoking has been associated with reduced dietary intake and serum levels of carotenoids. Despite these many problems, prospective and retrospective nutritional (serum and dietary) epidemiologic studies have provided important clues to the development and prevention of these cancers.

Occupation/Air Pollution ■ Although occupational exposures probably play a minor role overall in the development of HNSCC, they are major risk factors for malignancies of the sinonasal region.[97-101] The most important exposures occur in the metalworking, refining, woodworking, and leather/textile industries.[97-100] Indoor air pollution is a significant problem in much of the developing world where indoor stoves using biomass or fossil fuels are the primary method of cooking and heating. Not only are these exposures likely risk factors for HNSCC, but they also contribute to the risk of paranasal sinus cancers and lung cancers, chronic pulmonary diseases, and childhood illnesses.[101-106] Although some evidence does not support asbestos as a risk factor for HNSCC, an expert committee of the National Academy of Sciences has concluded that there is sufficient evidence to consider asbestos as a significant independent risk factor for laryngeal cancer.[107,108]

Radiation ■ No significant association has been demonstrated between ionizing radiation and the development of HNSCC. However, squamous cell carcinomas of the lip, like skin cancers, are associated with ultraviolet radiation exposure. Furthermore, exposure to gamma radiation is associated with thyroid cancers, sarcomas of the head and neck, and salivary gland malignancies, including paranasal sinus cancers. Although therapeutic irradiation of head and neck malignancies does not appear to induce second primary squamous cell carcinomas of the aerodigestive tract, it is associated with an increased risk of sarcomas of the head and neck.[109] This is a particular concern for children who have received therapeutic irradiation. Furthermore, environmental, medical diagnostic, and therapeutic radiation exposure to the head and neck are all significantly associated with salivary gland malignancies.[110,111] These studies have found a significant dose-response relationship with risk increasing with dose, and mucoepidermoid carcinomas appear to be the most common radiation-induced salivary malignancy.[110,111] In the past, the uses of radium for watch dial painting and thorotrast contrast in sinonasal imaging were both associated with an increased risk of paranasal sinus malignancies; however, these materials are no longer employed. Occupational studies have suggested that indoor exposure to radon gas or volatile chemicals may also increase the risk for HNSCC.[101]

Ultimately, the public health goal is better prevention and early detection of these malignancies by reducing the use of tobacco and alcohol, preventive vaccination against HPV-16, discovering and avoiding other causative agents, and identifying the genetically susceptible. Unfortunately, HNSCC screening has not been effective, likely due to the rarity of the disease.[112] However, in parts of the world where HNSCC account for a major portion of the cancer burden, prevention and screening programs have been very effective where implemented.[9] It is clear that tobacco/alcohol control and cessation can reduce HNSCC mortality as well as limit the suffering from this disease, and it is likely that HPV-16 vaccination will ultimately prevent a major portion of these cancers that occur in nonsmokers.

Pathologic Assessment and Biology

Aside from stating that a particular tumor is SCC, additional information reported by the pathologist usually includes tumor grade or differentiation. Traditionally, tumor grading has been based on criteria developed over 50 years ago by Broder.[113,114] Unfortunately, differentiation grade has not been consistently accurate in reflecting the biologic aggressiveness of squamous carcinomas.[114] The difficulty in predicting the behavior of individual tumors is well recognized. Prognosis is influenced by many factors other than grade.[115,116]

These include tumor size; site; vascularity; lymphatic drainage; surface expression of epidermal growth factor receptor; host immune response; the patient's age, sex, nutritional, and performance status; and other as yet unrecognized variables.

The comprehensive histological evaluation of squamous cell carcinomas includes characteristics of tumor–host interactions; Jakobsson and colleagues pioneered their incorporation into the determination of tumor grade.[117] Characteristics considered include degree of keratinization, nuclear grade, mitotic rate, inflammatory response, vascular-stromal response, vascular invasion, and pattern of invasion. These characteristics have variably correlated with biologic behavior. Keratinization is the major determinant of Broder grade. Better-differentiated tumors that produce more keratin are thought to be less likely to metastasize. Nuclear grade assesses nuclear pleomorphism. Enlarged, hyperchromatic nuclei are associated with less-differentiated tumors. Nuclear grade accurately predicts the behavior of advanced laryngeal cancers.[118] Enlarged nuclear size and staining presumably reflect chromosomal abnormalities and increased DNA content. Numerous studies of DNA content have demonstrated high rates of aneuploidy in squamous cell cancers that range from 50% to 70%. Aneuploidy has been associated with poor prognosis[119,120] have also importantly shown that ploidy analysis of premalignant squamous lesions is critically important in predicting progression to malignancy as well as death from these cancers. Mitotic rate and labeling index have also been used to reflect proliferative activity, but large-scale studies of head and neck cancers have been lacking.

Features reflecting aggressive disease include lymphatic invasion, perineural invasion, lymph node metastases, and penetration of the tumor through the capsule of involved lymph nodes (extracapsular spread [ECS]). The presence of regional lymph node metastases is the most important determinant of prognosis in head and neck cancer and is associated with a 50% decrease in survival rates as compared with patients without regional metastases.

More recently, the histological pattern of invasion of these cancers was systematically studied. Tumors that invade with thin fingerlike projections or single disassociated cells behave more aggressively regardless of differentiation grade and tend to be associated with vascular and neural invasion.[117] The presence of ECS of tumor in the neck has been directly associated with high rates of distant metastases. These various histological features play an important role in therapeutic decision making.

A complete discussion of the molecular pathology underpinning SCC is beyond the scope of this chapter, and the reader is referred to some of the many reviews on this area.[120] Intense investigation is ongoing regarding the complex interplay of cellular and genetic alterations that contribute to carcinogenesis and the metastatic phenotype in HNSCC. The fundamental roles of p53, dysregulated receptor tyrosine kinase signaling, apoptotic resistance, angiogenesis, and chemotherapeutic resistance are under active study in numerous laboratories. These scientific studies should prove fruitful in the pursuit of novel diagnostics and effective therapies.

Anatomy

The term "cancer of the head and neck" refers to a diverse collection of neoplasms of varying histologies arising from the variety of anatomic sites that make up the upper aerodigestive tract (UADT).[119] This chapter, however, deals predominantly with SCC of the UADT as it accounts for approximately 90% of the malignancies of the upper aerodigestive tract.[121] The UADT consists of a complex mucosa-covered conduit for food and air that extends from the vermilion surface of the lips to the cervical esophagus. In common usage, this terminology has been applied primarily to those cancers arising from the mucosal surfaces of the lips, oral cavity, pharynx, larynx, and cervical esophagus. Included in this designation, however, are other important sites, such as the nose and paranasal sinuses, salivary glands (major and minor), thyroid and parathyroid, and skin (both melanoma and nonmelanoma skin cancers). Some cancers arising in this region are typically excluded from the generic designation of head and neck cancer. Examples are tumors of the central nervous system, ocular neoplasms, primary tumors of lymphatic origin, and neural and endocrine malignancies.

Because of the diversity of sites and tissues of origin, the biology of tumor growth, patterns of metastases, natural boundaries for tumor extension, and signs and symptoms of disease are quite varied. The anatomy of the region has also dictated that optimal evaluation, diagnosis, and treatment require specific multidisciplinary expertise, including neurosurgery, otolaryngology, head and neck surgery, oral and maxillofacial surgery, cosmetic and reconstructive disciplines, and specialists in radiology, pathology, radiation therapy, and chemotherapy. The clinical manifestations of disease are varied and have a significant impact on the cosmetic and functional integrity of the head and neck region. Although the anatomic structures are only millimeters apart, the low metastatic potential and high curability of vocal cord cancers stand in extreme contrast to the early dissemination and grim prognosis of stage-matched pyriform sinus cancers.[122-127] Clinical differences between cancers in different sites are not explained solely by anatomic factors, but also by major biologic differences. Regrettably, the relatively small number of head and neck cancer patients often requires grouping patients for trials. Associated morbidities of disease and treatment involve the special senses to varying degrees, notably speech, swallowing, smelling, breathing, and masticatory functions critically important for social interaction, a good quality of life, and ultimately, survival.

Oral Cavity

The oral cavity is defined as starting at the vermilion border of the lips and extends posteriorly to include the lips, buccal mucosa, anterior tongue, floor of the mouth, hard palate, and upper and lower gingiva. The tongue occupies a major portion of the oral cavity and is contiguous with the floor of the mouth. The gingival mucosa overlying the mandibular and maxillary alveolar ridges adheres to the underlying periosteum. The hard palate forms the roof of the oral cavity and consists of mucosa overlying the palatine portion of the maxilla extending from the superior alveolar ridge to the junction with the soft palate, which lies in the oropharynx. Although the delineation between oral cavity and oropharynx might seem artificial, the distinction is important because of varying natural history, individualized therapeutic approaches, and numerous functional considerations.

Pharynx

The pharynx is a musculomembranous tube suspended from the skull base to the level of the sixth cervical vertebra, supported by overlapping constrictor muscles (superior, middle, and inferior) and other muscles arising from the styloid process and skull base.

This musculomembranous conduit communicates with the oral cavity anteriorly, the nasopharynx superiorly, and the hypopharynx and larynx inferiorly. It is divided into four sites of clinical importance: the tonsillar area, which makes up the major portion of the lateral pharyngeal wall and blends with the tongue base, soft palate, and retromolar trigone; the tongue base; the soft palate; and the posterior pharyngeal wall. Innervation of the pharynx is via the pharyngeal plexus, with contributions from the glossopharyngeal (sensory) and vagus nerves (motor and sensory).

The hypopharynx is divided into three distinct regions: the pyriform sinuses; the posterior surface of the larynx (postcricoid area); and the inferior, posterior, and lateral pharyngeal walls. The pyriform sinuses are paired mucosal pouches wrapped around the larynx, which funnel food around the larynx and into the esophagus. They are bounded superiorly by the pharyngoepiglottic folds and inferiorly by the cricoid cartilage. The sinuses come together at the esophageal introitus and cervical esophagus at the level of C6.

Larynx

The larynx consists of a mucosally-covered cartilaginous framework (thyroid and cricoid cartilages) suspended from the hyoid bone above by the thyrohyoid membrane and attached below to the trachea. The opening to the larynx is continuous with the pharyngeal airway. Unlike the rest of the pharynx, the mucosa of the larynx consists largely of columnar, ciliated, respiratory-type epithelium. Stratified squamous epithelium is found on the upper posterior epiglottis, aryepiglottic folds, and true vocal folds. It is important to note that although they are lymphatics in the upper larynx, they are sparse in the true vocal folds, or glottis.

The larynx is divided into three anatomic regions: the supraglottic larynx, the glottic larynx, and the subglottic larynx. The supraglottic larynx includes the epiglottis, aryepiglottic folds, laryngeal surface of the arytenoids, false vocal cords, and ventricles. The glottic larynx is derived from the tracheobronchial anlage and consists of both true vocal cords and the mucosa of the anterior and posterior commissures. It extends from the lateral-most apex of the laryngeal ventricle to 1 cm below the free edge of the vocal folds toward the cricoid. It has few, if any lymphatics. The subglottic larynx consists of the region bounded by the glottis above and the inferior border of the cricoid cartilage. Lymphatic supply to the subglottic larynx is extensive and bilateral. The infraglottic lymphatics drain to the cervical nodes through the cricothyroid membrane, while supraglottic lymphatics drain through the thyrohyoid membrane.

Nose and Paranasal Sinuses

The term "nose and paranasal sinuses" refers to the region of the upper aerodigestive tract that starts at the vestibule of the nose anteriorly, is covered by squamous epithelium, and extends posteriorly to the posterior choana, where the nasopharynx begins. By definition, paranasal sinus malignancy does not include the nasopharynx unless by extension. It does include the paranasal sinuses, specifically, the maxillary, ethmoid, frontal, and sphenoid sinuses. Although the most common malignancy of the nose and paranasal sinuses is SCC, the nose and paranasal sinuses pose a particular set of problems that deserve separate consideration. As a result, the topic of nose and paranasal sinus malignancy is covered in a later section.

Neck

Anatomic considerations in the treatment of cancers of the head and neck must include a thorough understanding of the neural, vascular, and, especially, the lymphatic structures of the neck. Detailed anatomic studies have described the organization of the lymphatic drainage of the UADT. Specific regions of the head and neck and the tumors that arise there have lymphatic drainage that is consistent and predictable. There are 12 major groups of lymph nodes (six each bilaterally) in the head and neck (Fig. 77-1),[128] although only levels I to V play a major role in aerodigestive tract SCC of the head and neck (SCCHN) Primary and secondary echelons of lymph node drainage have been defined for each major region of the head and neck mucosa. A standard rule of thumb is that the lymphatic drainage for any particular region is predicted by the arterial supply of that region. The lip, cheek, and anterior gingiva drain to submandibular and submental lymph node groups. In addition, the cheek and upper lip also drain to inferior parotid and facial nodes, while the posterior gingiva and palate drain to the internal jugular chain and lateral retropharyngeal groups. Lymphatic drainage for the tongue drains to the internal jugular, subdigastric, omohyoid, submandibular, and submental nodal groups. Midline lesions often drain bilaterally. Although metastases to the lower neck nodes are infrequent from the oral cavity, generally the more anterior the tumor location in the tongue, the more likely it is that metastases also will spread to lower jugular nodes. The FOM drainage is similar to that of the tongue. The upper portion of the pharynx drains directly to the upper cervical lymph nodes along the internal jugular chain. The oropharynx and tonsil drain through the parapharyngeal space to the midjugular region, particularly to the jugulodigastric nodes. Retro and lateral pharyngeal nodes can also be involved. The regions of the hypopharynx and larynx drain primarily along the routes of their vascular supply to either the deep cervical nodes along the midjugular (upper pharynx, larynx) or the deep nodes along the lower jugular and paratracheal region (lower pharynx, larynx).

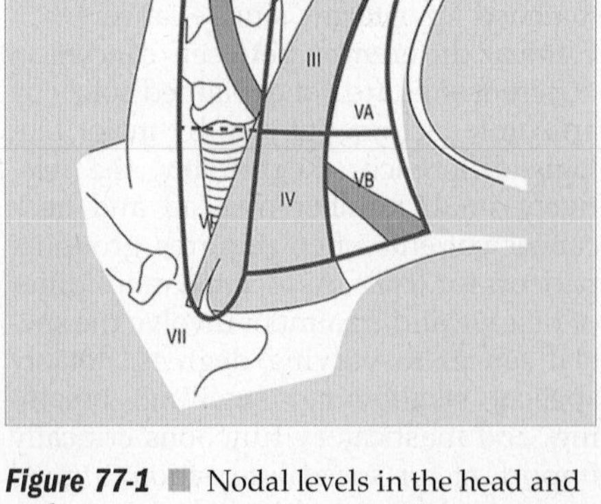

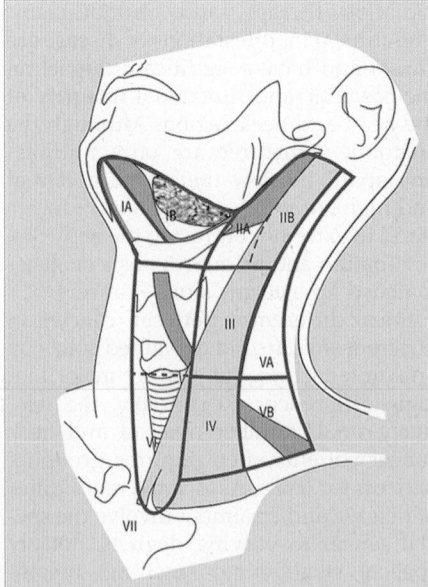

Figure 77-1 ■ Nodal levels in the head and neck.

For the purposes of local treatment, the various lymph node groups of the neck have been divided into levels. Level I includes the submental group of nodes (IA), located within the triangle bounded by the anterior belly of the digastric muscles and the hyoid bone, and the submandibular group (IB), bounded by both bellies of the digastric muscle and the body of the mandible. Level II nodes consist of the upper jugular lymph nodes located in proximity to the upper third of the internal jugular vein and extending from the skull base to the level of the bifurcation of the carotid artery. The anterior and posterior boundaries are the lateral border of the sternohyoid muscle and the posterior border of the sternocleidomastoid muscle, respectively. Level II is further divided into those lymph nodes located anteroinferior to the vertical plane of the spinal accessory nerve (IIA) and those lymph nodes posterosuperior to the nerve (IIB). Level III nodes include those nodes located adjacent to the middle third of the internal jugular vein from the carotid bifurcation to the plane marked by the omohyoid muscle's crossing over the jugular vein (the level of the cricoid cartilage). Anterior and posterior boundaries are the same as level II. Level IV nodes include the lower jugular group extending from omohyoid muscle above to the clavicle below. Level V nodes are those located in the posterior triangle in the region of the spinal accessory nerve and the transverse cervical artery. This level is bounded by the anterior border of the trapezius muscle, the posterior border of the sternocleidomastoid muscle, and the clavicle below. This level, too, is further divided into Va and Vb nodes, with Va nodes being those nodes located above the plane along the inferior edge of the cricoid and including the chain of nodes superior to the spinal accessory nerve posterior to the sternocleidomastoid muscle. Vb nodes are the nodes below the cricoid plane, inferior to the spinal accessory nerve and include the nodes along the transverse cervical artery and all of the supraclavicular fossa.

Diagnosis and Staging

The identification and appropriate management of malignant mucosal lesions in the head and neck are important aspects of patient care that have major impact on overall survival rates. Since stage (extent) of disease at the time of diagnosis is the most important prognostic factor in the treatment of HNSCC, the identification and early treatment of small cancers correlates with excellent survival. Most dysplastic lesions or in situ carcinomas of the oral mucosa occur as red (erythroplasia) or white (leukoplakia) patches that may be readily apparent on visual examination. In areas less easily visualized directly, such as the larynx and hypopharynx, early lesions cause such symptoms as chronic hoarseness and sore throat and, later, referred otalgia, or dysphagia. Such symptoms demand visualization of the larynx and hypopharynx usually by fiber-optic approaches.

Dysphagia, odynophagia, otalgia, hoarseness, mucosal irregularities and ulceration, pain, weight loss, and the presence of an unexplained neck mass are the most common presenting symptoms of invasive HNSCC. The predominant symptoms vary with the site: Chronic dysphagia or odynophagia (for 6 weeks or even less) demands thorough visualization of the oropharynx, hypopharynx, and esophagus; chronic hoarseness demands visualization of the larynx; chronic unilateral serous otitis media in an adult may be a result of cancer of the nasopharynx blocking the eustachian tube; and unilateral nasal polyps, nasal obstruction, or epistaxis is a common presenting sign of nasal cavity or paranasal sinus neoplasms. A firm or hard unilateral cervical mass represents malignancy until proven otherwise. In persons older than 20 years, such a mass represents neoplasm more than 80% of the time, and 60% of these neoplasms are due to metastatic spread from an UADT primary.

In patients presenting with a suspicious neck mass, a complete head and neck examination usually reveals the primary malignant tumor (Fig. 77-2). If it does not, a thorough search for occult primary cancers both above and below the clavicles is warranted. Technologic advances in fiber optics and in flexible and rigid endoscopes now provide excellent upper airway visualization and biopsy capabilities that can be performed routinely in the clinic setting.[129] Endoscopic evaluation should include the nasopharynx, oropharynx, hypopharynx, larynx, and upper esophagus. Endoscopic evaluation should be accompanied by chest radiography and axial imagining of the head and neck. If these fail to reveal a primary, then consideration should be given for esophagoscopy as well, since it is much more sensitive for mucosal lesions of the esophagus than is computerized tomography. Most commonly, occult primaries responsible for neck metastases occur in the nasopharynx, tongue base, tonsil, or hypopharynx. In the absence of an identifiable mass, directed biopsies of these sites are indicated during endoscopic evaluation, and, if present, bilateral tonsillectomies should be performed if a primary is not identified. Metastasis to a solitary left supraclavicular lymph node (Virchow's node) is occasionally seen with infraclavicular cancer, especially colon cancer. Generally, isolated metastatic supraclavicular masses (level IV) derive from breast, lung, or infradiaphragmatic neoplasms. Thyroid malignancies may also metastasize to this area.

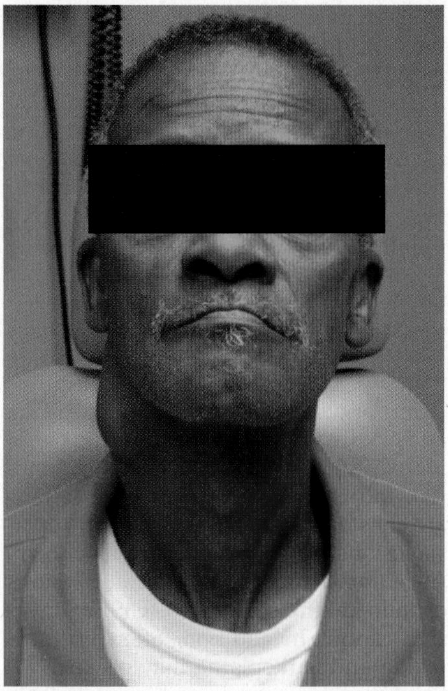

Figure 77-2 ■ Untreated N3 disease in a patient with HNSCC.

Three-dimensional imaging with computed tomography (CT) and magnetic resonance imaging (MRI) is frequently used to supplement the clinical evaluation and staging of the primary tumor and regional lymph nodes. Ultrasonography, when combined with fine-needle aspiration (FNA) technique, is an effective means for staging the neck, thyroid and salivary glands. FNA of neck lesions often aids in the diagnostic evaluation of head and neck malignancies. Open biopsies should be performed only after attempts by FNA are nondiagnostic. If an excisional biopsy is required because FNA is inconclusive or not feasible, then the surgeon and patient should be prepared for definitive neck dissection if the mass should prove to be metastatic squamous cell carcinoma. The potential ramifications of false-negative results on FNA are inherently obvious. Accuracy of the cytological interpretation of the aspirate is directly dependent on the skill and experience of the ultrasonographer and pathologist.

More recently, positron emission tomography (PET) imaging has shown promising results in head and neck cancer. Highly elevated primary tumor fluorodeoxyglucose standardized uptake values (FDG SUVs) may predict for more aggressive disease and inferior treatment outcomes.[130-132] FDG-PET can provide over 90% sensitivity and specificity for upfront staging of both primary and cervical neck nodal disease,[133] can localize occult local primary disease[134,135] or distant metastases[136] not elicited by anatomic imaging or physical exam. Combined FDG-PET/CT imaging may further improve neck staging accuracy results.[137-140] Incremental superiority of FDG-PET for regional staging of the neck relative to CT or MRI alone was confirmed by a recent meta-analysis of retrospective and prospective studies encompassing over 1200 FDG-PET imaging cases with confirmatory neck dissection pathology.[141] Analysis of this dataset revealed FDG-PET to be sensitive (79%, 95% CI: 72% to 85%) and specific (86%, 95% CI: 83% to 89%) for this indication. Recent prospective series in early-intermediate T-stage oral cavity and oropharyngeal cancer patients suggest that FDG-PET can potentially guide more appropriate management of clinically N0 patients when directly correlated with CT and sentinel node biopsy[142] or (less ideally) with CT/MRI findings.[143]

Considerable interest has recently focused on FDG-PET monitoring of disease response to radiotherapy or chemoradiotherapy. A number of groups have found that FDG-PET posttreatment restaging provides high negative predictive power;[144-147] accordingly, there is now growing acceptance of withholding consolidative neck dissection following radiotherapy in the absence of residual FDG-avid adenopathy,[148] although others argue that expert clinical interpretation of serial CT imaging could achieve similar results.[149,150] FDG-PET/CT may eventually prove useful for improving delineation of disease targets for advanced radiotherapy planning.[151] However, challenges for this remain, particularly for identification of validated thresholding techniques to precisely distinguish FDG-avid disease from bystander tissues.[152,153] At MD Anderson Cancer Center, we routinely use FDG-PET/CT to supplement anatomic imaging and clinical examination for radiotherapy planning; however, we do not use negative FDG-PET results to defer treatment of suspicious findings identified by exam or conventional staging techniques.

Staging criteria for cancers arising in the UADT, paranasal sinuses, and salivary glands have been developed by the American Joint Committee on Cancer (AJCC) (Table 77-1). The criteria undergo regular reevaluation and modification. The stage groupings used for head and neck cancer are based on T (primary tumor), N (regional node), and M (distant metastasis) designations. Because of variations in the growth, behavior, and prognosis of head

Table 77-1 ■ Clinical Tumor Stage and Groupings for Head and Neck Cancer

Stage 0	Tis	N0	M0
Stage I	T1	N0	M0
Stage II	T2	N0	M0
Stage III	T3	N0	M0
	T1	N1	M0
	T2	N1	M0
	T3	N1	M0
Stage IVA	T4a	N0, N1 or N2	M0
	Any T	N2	M0
Stage IVB	Any T	N3	M0
	T4b	Any N	M0
Stage IVC	Any T	Any N	M1

and neck cancers according to site of origin and extent, differences exist in the staging criteria for each anatomic site. Staging criteria for the primary lesion are site specific. However, except for tumors arising in the nasopharynx and those of the thyroid, there is uniformity in the nodal staging criteria and stage grouping (Table 77-2).

Careful documentation of tumor extent and accurate staging classification are also important for the comparison of the results of different treatment regimens. Accurate evaluation of the results of a given treatment or the efficacy of new treatment strategies requires comparisons among patient groups with tumors of similar extent and behavior. Restaging after treatment or for recurrent cancers must be clearly designated and separate from the primary staging of previously untreated cancers. Postsurgical, or pathologic, staging is important in the primary treatment of head and neck cancers because of the increasing use of postoperative radiation therapy and/or adjuvant chemotherapy for patients with locally aggressive tumors, ECS into the soft tissues of the neck close or positive margins, and perineural invasion.[154]

It should be noted, however, that as good as the widely accepted AJCC staging system is for head and neck cancer, it still falls short in that it too often fails to distinguish between deeply infiltrative tumors and those that are superficial or exophytic. Experience shows that this distinction is an important one and can have a significant impact on survival. Another factor that merits consideration in future revisions to the AJCC is HPV status for oropharyngeal cancers, which has striking prognostic value in this disease.[155]

Treatment

General Principles

After a histological diagnosis has been established and tumor extent determined, the selection of appropriate treatment of a specific cancer depends on a complex array of variables, including tumor site, prognosis, relative morbidity of various treatment options, patient performance and nutritional status, concomitant health problems, social and logistic factors, therapy anticipated for potential recurrences or second primaries, and patient preference. These variables are each considered with respect to the established effectiveness of various treatment regimens available.

The overall management goals in treating patients with head and neck cancer are to achieve the highest cure rates at the lowest cost in terms of functional and cosmetic morbidity. These goals include early diagnosis, effective rehabilitation, and appropriate palliation, when indicated. The achievement of these goals requires the close cooperation of an interdisciplinary team of practitioners representing surgery, radiation and medical oncology, chemotherapy, prosthodontics, dentistry, speech language pathology, social services, dietetics, physical and rehabilitative medicine, pathology, nursing, and often psychiatry.

Effective rehabilitation is an important part of the overall treatment of head and neck cancers. Modern advances in surgical reconstruction, microvascular free-tissue transfer, and prosthodontics have significantly improved posttreatment function.[156] Rehabilitation concerns must be addressed at initial treatment planning and carefully integrated with the various treatment modalities used. Pretreatment dental evaluations and speech and swallowing assessments should be routinely performed. Needed dental care and/or extractions should be planned prior to radiation to reduce the risks of dental-associated mucositis and osteoradionecrosis. The overall impact of treatment and rehabilitation on patients' quality of life is an important issue that may require specialized social or psychiatric support systems for the patient and family. Furthermore, attention must be paid to nutritional support, and early intervention with the placement of enteral access for gastrostomy feeding should be entertained in selected patients. Contemporary combined approaches of chemotherapy and radiotherapy place a long-term burden on the patient that must be compensated. Indeed, it is this close attention to nutrition and general supportive care that makes combined treatment regimens possible. Finally, the prolonged nature of treatment of advanced disease, which may extend over many months, requires consideration of the social and financial impact of treatment decisions on the patient, the family, and the patient's career.

Biopsies of primary tumors need not be excisional unless the biopsy procedure is sufficient for local control. Oncologic principles of surgical resection must not be compromised by ill-conceived reconstructive efforts or attempts at modifying the necessary resection in order to minimize functional or cosmetic morbidity. Gross residual cancer or positive surgical margins after tumor resection portend inevitably for treatment failure. Appropriate management must also include the use of precise modern techniques of conservative surgical resection (eg, partial laryngectomy and functional neck dissection) that, in selected patients, have cure rates similar to those of more radical techniques.[157]

Table 77-2 ■ Clinical Tumor Staging Characteristics for Regional Lymph Nodes and Distant Metastases

Regional lymph nodes	
Nx	Regional lymph nodes cannot be assessed
N0	No evidence of regional lymph node metastases
N1	Metastasis in single, ipsilateral regional lymph node <3 cm in greatest dimension
N2a	Metastasis in single, ipsilateral regional lymph node between 3 and 6 cm in greatest dimension
N2b	Metastasis in multiple ipsilateral regional lymph nodes, none >6 cm in greatest dimension
N2c	Metastasis in bilateral or contralateral regional lymph nodes, none >6 cm in greatest dimension
N3	Metastasis to regional lymph node >6 cm in greatest dimension
Distant metastases	
Mx	Presence of distant metastasis cannot be assessed
M0	No evidence of distant metastasis
M1	Distant metastases are present in one or more locations

Oral Premalignancy

Appropriate management of leukoplakia and erythroplakia lesions includes a high index of suspicion, particularly in high-risk individuals. Although both lesions are considered premalignant, erythroplasia lesions are of greater clinical concern, since approximately half of these lesions contain carcinoma in situ (CIS) or invasive cancer. In addition, often erythroplakia and leukoplakia may coexist.[158,159] Erythroplakia mandates biopsy to rule out invasive cancer. The management of erythroplakia and leukoplakia depends on the location, extent, and histology. The diffuse field effect and multifocal nature of the epithelial carcinogenic process support the need for effective prevention. Various molecular markers, including aneuploidy, loss of heterozygosity (LOH) and podoplanin expression portend for a high risk of transformation in dysplastic oral intraepithelial neoplasia (IEN).[160-162] White lesions can be confused with mucositis; lichen planus; local tissue irritation from mechanical, thermal, or chemical trauma; histoplasmosis; candidiasis; and other infectious processes. Topical supravital staining with toluidine blue of suspicious lesions can be helpful in identifying areas for biopsy and in screening high-risk populations. Toluidine blue staining was found to be associated with LOH in dysplastic, minimally dysplastic, or nondysplastic oral IEN, which suggests the potential of toluidine blue for identifying oral IEN with a molecularly marked high risk of cancer and perhaps for helping guide surgical margin widths.[163,164] Lesions that persist despite the removal of local irritating factors, or those that are associated with ulceration, vertical growth, induration, a recent change in size, or pain, should be sampled by biopsy and/or excised. Despite aggressive local therapy, complete surgical resection (as defined by the absence of dysplasia at the margins) does not prevent oral carcinoma development in cases of aneuploid dysplastic leukoplakia.[161] In these situations, a targeted chemoprevention with inhibitors of epidermal growth factor receptor (EGFR) and cyclooxygenase-2 have shown some promise.[161,165] Complete resection, however, can reduce the relatively low cancer rate associated with diploid dysplastic leukoplakia. Complete resection of oral IEN did not statistically significantly reduce the overall risk of cancer development, but did significantly reduce the cancer risk associated with high-risk lesions, as defined by LOH patterns[166] These findings reflect the critical importance of molecular confirmation of complete resection of oral IEN, in which the surgical margins are often narrow, nonexistent, or not assessed. Future research in this area should evaluate the roles of optimal surgical margin width and complete resection as confirmed by molecular analyses in reducing the cancer risk associated with molecularly defined high-risk oral IEN.

General Overview of Natural History and Treatment by Site

Oral Cavity

Both tumor and treatment significantly compromise speech and deglutition, particularly for those patients in whom cancer involves the tongue, the floor of the mouth, or the mandible. Furthermore, the diversity of potential sites of cancer development in the oral cavity and variations of lymphatic drainage and rates of node metastases lend added complexity to treatment planning.[167,168] Despite the fact that this region is readily amenable to visual examination and bimanual palpation, more than 50% of patients are diagnosed in advanced stages. The current T-staging of oral cavity primaries is presented in Table 77-3.

Lips ■ SCCs of the mucosal surface of the lips are the most common oral cavity cancers. An important distinction must be made between cancers of the skin surrounding the lips, which are considered cutaneous malignancies, and those that occur on the mucosa of the lips, which are classified as oral cancers. Over 90% occur on the lower lip, usually on the exposed vermilion border, midway between the midline and the oral commissure. Upper lip cancers are most commonly basal cell carcinomas.[169] Well-differentiated and verrucous cancers rarely metastasize. Poorly differentiated and spindle cell varieties tend to grow aggressively and metastasize commonly. Perineural infiltration of large nerves is indicative of aggressive disease and requires aggressive, often combined therapies.

Considerations in the treatment of lip cancers include: (1) oncological control of the disease, (2) a functional oral sphincter with oral competence and (3) acceptable cosmetic outcome.[170,171] These goals are achieved equally well with either primary radiation or surgery when the tumors are less than 2 cm in size or are very superficial. Larger lesions, however, are best treated with surgical resection and reconstruction, which allows for greater accuracy in evaluating the extent of tumor and nerve or lymphatic involvement.[172,173] Frequently, adjacent precancerous changes are present that can also be treated with surgery (lip shaving and advancement) to prevent recurrences or the development of second primary tumors.[174,175] For larger lesions, primary reconstruction with local, regional, and sometimes free-tissue flaps avoids defects that result from tissue loss with radiotherapy, provides for future reconstructive and treatment options, and decreases the very real risk of osteoradionecrosis of the mandible. Lesions demonstrating extensive infiltration, bone involvement, or lymphatic metastases should be managed with combined surgery and postoperative radiation.

Table 77-3 ■ **Primary Tumor Staging Characteristics for Oral Cavity Carcinoma**

Tx	Primary tumor cannot be assessed (as occurs after excisional biopsy)
T0	No evidence of primary (as in unknown primary tumors)
Tis	Carcinoma in situ
T1	Tumor is 2 cm or less in greatest dimension
T2	Tumor is between 2 and 4 cm in greatest dimension
T3	Tumor is >4 cm in greatest dimension
T4	A: Tumor invades adjacent structures (through cortical bone, maxillary sinus, skin, tongue musculature, deep tissue, nerves B: Tumor invades masticator space, pterygoid plates, skull base, carotid artery

Radiation therapy techniques for management of lip cancers include external irradiation, interstitial implants, and combinations of both. Local tumor control rates with irradiation exceed 80%,[176-178] with determinant survival at 5 years (including surgical salvage) in excess of 95%. Similar tumor control and survival rates are reported with primary surgical excision.[179] Regional metastasis decreases the survival rates to 36% to 55%.[176,180] The 5-year survival rates for patients with carcinomas of the upper lip are lower than for those with similar lower-lip lesions and range from 40% to 60%.[181,182] Involvement of both lips and the lateral commissure is uncommon. The prognosis for commissure lesions is not as good as for cancers of other areas of the lip. Cross reported a 5-year survival rate of 34% for patients with oral commissure carcinoma.[180]

Tongue ■ Tongue cancers account for over 25% of oral cavity SCCs and most commonly arise in the anterior two-thirds of the tongue on the lateral or ventral surface. SCCs on the dorsum of the tongue are less common. Infiltration of the underlying tongue musculature occurs early. The intrinsic tongue muscles are loosely arranged and endowed with a rich vascular and lymphatic supply, which may explain the high rate of regional metastases and ECS. Prognosis is directly related to the degree of infiltration and the presence of regional metastases and ECS. The biologic aggressiveness of T1 and T2 (<4 cm) tongue cancers is noteworthy and is reflected in higher rates of occult regional metastases than those of similarly staged lesions arising from other oral sites. Occult nodal metastases are present in 30% to 40% of early lesions.[183-186] Approximately 40% of patients have clinical evidence of node metastases at diagnosis.[187] Primary echelon node drainage is to the upper deep cervical lymphatics; however, involvement of middle and lower neck nodes (levels III and IV) is not uncommon. Bilateral nodal involvement can occur with cancers of the tip or the midline of the tongue. Locoregional recurrence in patients with tongue cancer accounts for 60% to 70% of cancer deaths.[188-190] Distant metastases account for 15% of deaths, and second primaries in the upper aerodigestive tract account for 20% to 40%. The management of carcinomas of the tongue has been significantly influenced by an increased appreciation of the aggressiveness of seemingly small but deeply infiltrative lesions, the high rate of occult lymph node metastases, and improvements in soft tissue and bony reconstruction. Although surgical excision alone has been the mainstay of treatment, combined surgery and adjuvant radiation therapy to include the primary site and regional nodes is commonly used for most advanced cancers (stages III and IV) and is being used increasingly for small stage II cancers that exhibit pathologic indicators of lymph node metastasis or perineural invasion (Fig. 77-3). Postoperative chemoradiotherapy is indicated for adverse pathologic findings of perineural invasion, extracapsular lymph node extension or close surgical margins.[191]

For stage I cancers, surgical excision is effective and expeditious, with excellent preservation of function. For stage II lesions that are infiltrative, hemiglossectomy or partial glossectomy achieves excellent tumor control rates and should be combined with dissection of neck nodes at risk (supraomohyoid dissections) to provide accurate information about staging and determine the need for adjuvant treatment, specifically, postoperative radiotherapy. While hemiglossectomy will result in some functional morbidity in terms of articulation and deglutition, surgery remains the mainstay of treatment in oral tongue malignancies. Free-tissue transfer reconstruction can significantly offset the morbidity of hemiglossectomy. Primary therapy with radiation doses of 65 Gy to 70 Gy can be administered via external megavoltage radiation but this paradigm has fallen out of favor for the primary treatment of oral cancer, due to high rates of osteoradionecrosis, fibrosis, and impaired function.

Extension of cancer to the floor of the mouth or the mandible may necessitate partial mandibulectomy or segmental mandibular resection. Modern reconstructive techniques with vascularized composite bone and soft tissue free flaps, titanium metal prostheses, and dental implants have improved the functional and cosmetic results of major mandibular resections. An elective neck dissection is recommended for lesions with greater than 4 mm of invasion owing to the risk of occult nodal disease. When tumors grossly involve bone, radiation therapy is less effective in these poorly vascularized tissues and requires high doses that are associated with osteoradionecrosis. After local failure of interstitial radiotherapy implants, complication rates for salvage surgical resections are extremely high and are associated with significant morbidity from fistulization, radionecrosis, and failure of primary reconstructive efforts. Although the surgical salvage of radiation failures is often successful in early lesions, success drops to less than 50% in advanced lesions.

For more advanced primary lesions (stages III and IV), surgery and postoperative external beam radiation are generally used, although primary chemoradiotherapy is under investigation at the University of Chicago.[192] No prospective controlled trials have proved the superiority of combined therapy over surgery alone for disease without nodal metastases, but retrospective studies indicate improved locoregional control rates.[193-197] These improvements have generally been offset, in part, by an increased frequency of distant metastases and second primaries. Surgical management generally consists of partial glossectomy and neck dissection, with the mandible being spared unless directly involved. In instances with limited periosteal invasion, coronal and other partial mandibular resections can be performed that spare mandibular continuity and maintain function. Where tumors extend to the midline or involve the tongue base, subtotal or total glossectomy may be necessary. Continued improvements in reconstructive techniques have improved the functional results of these aggressive resections. Provision for temporary tracheostomy and prolonged enteral nutrition should be made. Total glossectomy or sacrifice of both hypoglossal nerves frequently necessitates permanent feeding gastrostomy. Current experience indicates that total glossectomy can, in highly select patients, be accomplished without the need for laryngectomy although prolonged or even permanent parenteral feeding will likely be required.[198] Postoperative radiotherapy is generally administered within

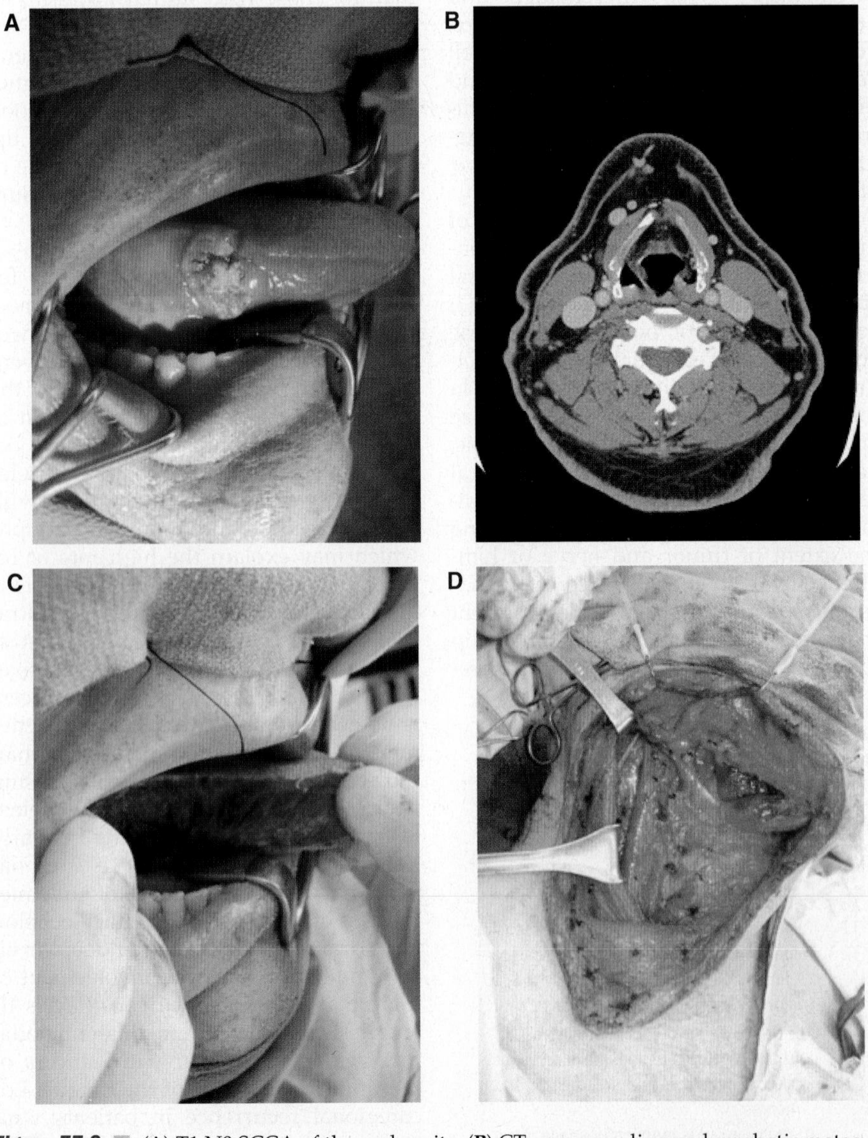

Figure 77-3 ■ (**A**) T1 N0 SCCA of the oral cavity. (**B**) CT scan revealing no lymphatic metastasis. (**C**) Hemiglossectomy resection. (**D**) Staging supraomohyoid neck dissection.

4-6 weeks of surgery. High-risk surgical margins or ECS can be treated to a high-dose or with concomitant chemoradiotherapy. For advanced oral cavity cancers, both ipsilateral and contralateral necks are irradiated, with the dosage determined by the extent of disease. Close surgical margins require high doses (70 Gy) because of the difficulty in eradicating even small amounts of tumor in the tongue after glossectomy.[199] Even with combined therapy, estimated 2-year disease-free and overall survival rates for advanced disease are about 50%.[200] The 5-year survival rates range from 50% to 70% for stages I and II to 15% to 30% for stages III and IV.[188]

The management of the neck is of particular interest in patients with tongue cancer because of the high rate of nodal metastases. For T2 or larger lesions, rates of occult metastases exceed 40%, and some form of neck treatment is generally indicated. When the primary tumor can be adequately excised via a transoral technique, unilateral or bilateral neck dissections should be performed based on the location of the primary disease. Concomitant chemoradiotherapy should be used postoperatively if surgical margins are involved or there is ECS. Radiation therapy alone should be considered when there is more than one metastatic lymph node.

Floor of Mouth (FOM) ■ FOM cancers occur with a frequency similar to that of tongue cancer. Early spread to adjacent areas (gingiva and periosteum of the mandible) is common. The periosteum of the mandible is a natural barrier to invasion. Fixation of the tongue is a sign of deep invasion. The tumor may extend to or through the mylohyoid muscle, which serves as a natural barrier to direct spread below the hyoid bone. Lymph node metastases at presentation are seen in approximately 40% of patients, and an additional 20% have occult lymphatic metastases.[184] The occult metastatic rate increases with the T stage of the primary: T2 tumors have a 40% and T3 tumors a 70% occult metastasis rate.

First-echelon nodes of lymphatic drainage include the submandibular and jugulodigastric lymph nodes (levels I and II). Submental node involvement is comparatively less frequent. Evaluation for early mandibular involvement is facilitated by palpation since fixation to the mandible indicates periosteal involvement and direct bone invasion is present in 50% to 60% of such tumors. This distinction is often aided with bone windows on computed tomography.

Small cancers (T1, T2) are generally treated effectively by wide resection. Lateral FOM tumors can often be resected transorally and the resection defect closed with the advancement of adjacent mucosa, skin grafts, or secondary intention. Sialodochoplasty of the severed submandibular duct can be performed for superficial lesions. Small cancers involving the mandible (T4) are best treated surgically because bone involvement compromises radiation efficacy. An elective selected neck dissection is performed for T1 tumors with more than 4 mm of invasion and for all T2-4 cancers. Bilateral neck dissections should be performed for anterior FOM lesions, as both necks are at risk for occult metastasis due to the nature of lymphatic drainage in this region. If nodal metastases are present, therapeutic neck dissection is indicated. Surgery remains the mainstay of treatment of early FOM malignancies, achieving excellent functional and curative results.

More advanced FOM cancers (T3, T4) are generally treated with resection combined with similar approaches to that described for oral tongue cancers in the prior section (Fig. 77-4). Again, mandibular continuity-sparing procedures with cortical resections can often be employed. In these instances, we have found fasciocutaneous flaps to offer excellent FOM and tongue reconstructive potential. Large mucosal and soft tissue surgical defects are typically reconstructed with free-tissue transfers, and contemporary management of mandibular defects entails bony reconstruction with either a fibula or scapula free flap.

Treatment results are influenced by the size of the primary tumor, presence of lymph node metastases, degree of mandibular involvement, and adequacy of resection. The 5-year survival rates for localized stage I and II FOM carcinomas range from 60% to 80%. Cancers that cross the midline or involve the tongue or the mandible are associated with 5-year survival rates of 50% to 60%.[201] Survival rates for more advanced lesions (stages III and IV) are less than 50%. Lymph node metastases decrease survival rates to approximately 25%.

The major advantage of combined treatment (radiation and surgery) in these patients is improved control of ipsilateral and contralateral neck disease. Because rates of occult nodal disease are high in advanced primary lesions, elective treatment of the neck with radiation or bilateral neck dissections is indicated. Recurrence in the untreated, clinically negative neck is the most frequent site of failure in patients treated only with surgery.[202] For patients with multiple nodal metastases, systemic therapy may be warranted due to the high risk of distant metastases to the lungs. Continuing surveillance for the development of a second primary in the head and neck, esophagus or lungs is advised.

The development of second primary cancers is a major cause of morbidity and death. Fu and colleagues reported that 55 of 153 (36%) patients developed second primaries, of whom 30 died of their second cancer.[203] Distant metastases occur in 10 to 15% of patients.[202,203]

Gingival and Buccal Mucosa ■ Gingival cancers occur most commonly (80%) in the lower gingiva, posterior to the bicuspids.[204] For both sites, trismus is an ominous sign indicating extension to the masseter or pterygoid muscles. Clinical staging criteria are similar to those for other oral sites. Overall, regional metastases occur in approximately 15% of gingival cancers.[205] Recently, occult nodal metastases have been documented in as high as 30% of buccal cancers and elective neck dissection recommended in all but the earliest of cancers.[206] Exophytic tumors tend to be papillary or verrucous in appearance and can be confused with benign hyperkeratosis.

Small, superficial gingival cancers can be effectively treated with surgical resection with excellent preservation of function.[207] Generally, the amount of bone resected for small lesions is minimal and resection can be accomplished transorally. Even larger lesions requiring partial maxillectomy or alveolectomy can

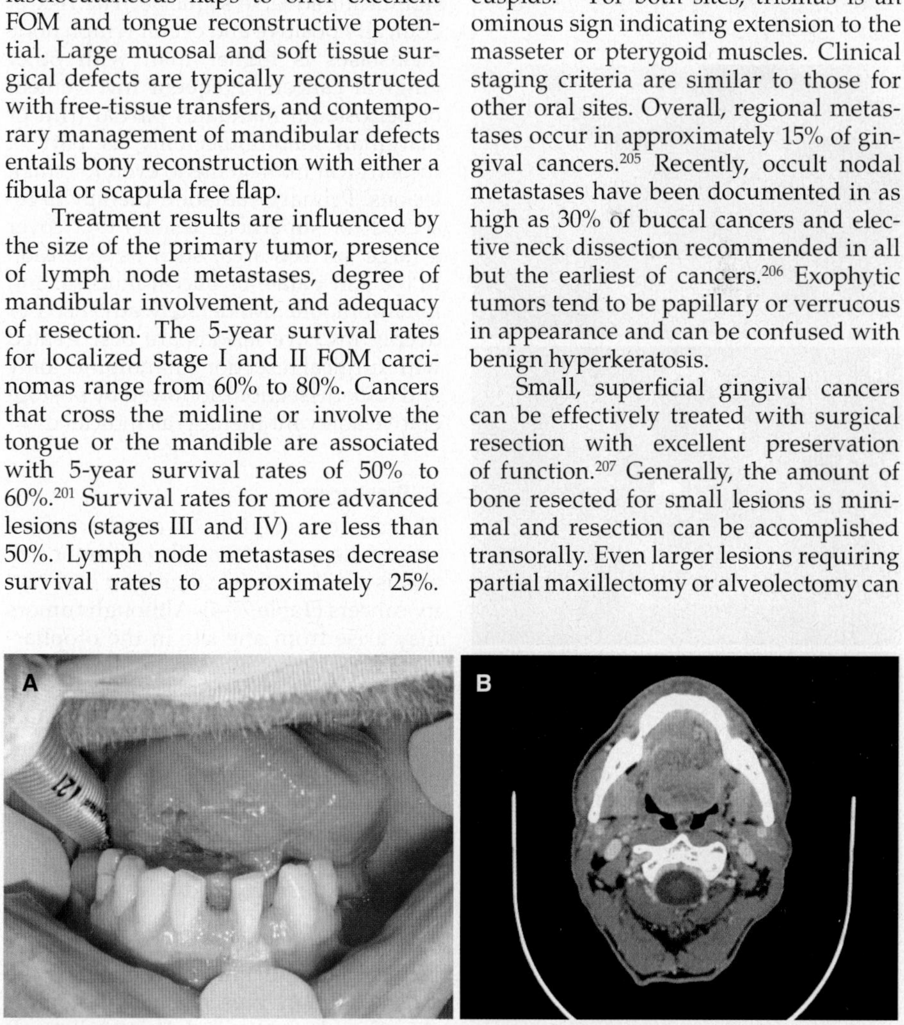

Figure 77-4 ■ (**A**) T3 N0 floor of mouth SCCA. (**B**) Deep infiltration of the intrinsic tongue musculature on axial imaging.

be resected without external incision. External beam irradiation is not as effective in local tumor control once gross bone involvement has occurred. The intermediate (T2 or larger) lesions are best handled surgically; the risk of osteoradionecrosis is thereby avoided. For larger lesions (T3 and T4), segmental mandibulectomy and/or maxillectomy is required, and adjuvant radiation is frequently recommended (Fig. 77-5). Elective neck dissection should be performed for advanced lesions of the mandibular gingival, as these lesions tend to have occult metastases. Limited data are available on the behavior of maxillary ridge and hard palate cancers, but these lesions can metastasize to the lateral neck nodes, and thus elective management of the neck is strongly encouraged, whether with neck dissection or neck irradiation.[208] Clinically positive neck nodes warrant neck dissection at the time of the resection of the primary tumor.

Overall survival rates for gingival and buccal cancers depend on tumor size, bone involvement, and node metastases. The 5-year survival rates for gingival lesions range from 78% for stage I to 15% for stage IV disease.[209] Surgical results are clearly superior to those of radiation when bone involvement is present. Survival rates (5-year) for stages I and II buccal carcinomas range from 65% to 75%. Determinant survival for stages III and IV disease varies from 20% to 30%.[27,46,205] For both gingival and buccal mucosal cancers, overall survival rates have improved over recent years as surgical management has replaced radiation therapy as the primary treatment.

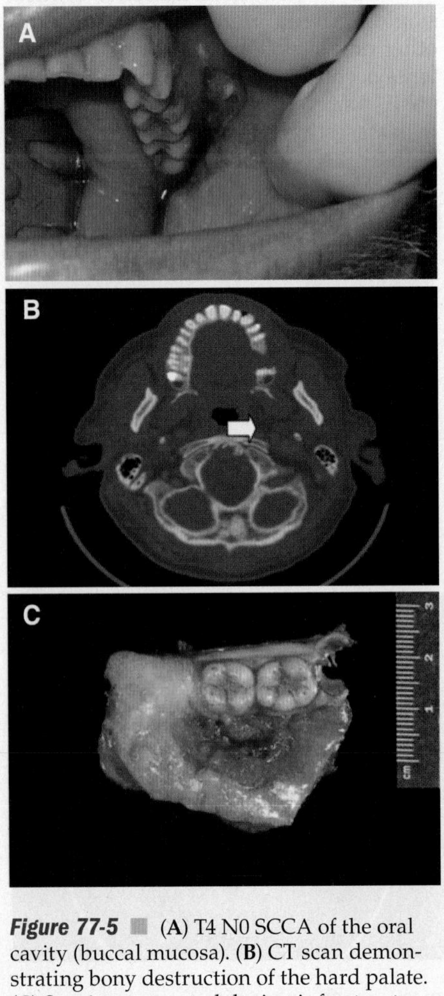

Figure 77-5 ■ (**A**) T4 N0 SCCA of the oral cavity (buccal mucosa). (**B**) CT scan demonstrating bony destruction of the hard palate. (**C**) Specimen resected during infrastructure maxillectomy.

Retromolar Trigone ■ Cancers arising in the retromolar trigone (the narrow band of mucosa that lies behind the mandibular molars and covers the ascending ramus of the mandible) are rarely confined to that gingiva, but often involve adjacent buccal mucosa, anterior tonsillar pillar, the floor of the mouth, and/or posterior gingiva. Thus, retromolar trigone cancers that involve the anterior tonsillar pillar have a tendency to behave more like oropharyngeal cancers than like oral cavity primaries. However, bony invasion is common and must be considered when determining the optimal treatment strategy. As mentioned earlier, primary irradiation to the mandible can lead to significant adverse sequelae. The risk of clinically positive and occult lymph node metastases is higher than with other gingival cancers. Frequent involvement of periosteum mandates partial (rim or marginal) mandibulectomy as part of the surgical management, even for small lesions. Primary radiation therapy is reserved for superficial lesions that cover a large surface area, such as extension to the soft palate or buccal mucosa, and remain mobile. Moderately advanced or deeply invasive lesions are best treated with surgical resection (mandibulectomy and neck dissection), followed by postoperative adjuvant therapy, as indicated.

■ Oropharynx

The clinical staging of oropharyngeal cancers depends primarily on tumor size and is similar to the staging of oral cavity cancers (Table 77-4). Although tumors may arise from any site in the oropharynx, they arise most commonly from the palatine arch, which includes the tonsillar fossa and base of the tongue. Traditionally patients with oropharyngeal cancer are in their sixth and seventh decade of life with a significant history of tobacco use. More patients are being seen at a younger age without typical tobacco exposures, and it is likely that the tumors in many such patients are associated with HPV-16.[27,46] Aside from a cervical mass of unknown etiology, the most common presenting symptom is chronic odynophagia (often unilateral) and referred otalgia. Change in voice, dysphagia, and trismus are late signs.

Table 77-4 ■ **Primary Tumor Staging Characteristics for Cancer of the Oropharynx**

Tx	Tumor cannot be assessed (as occurs with previous biopsy)
T0	There is no evidence of a primary (as occurs with an unknown primary tumor)
Tis	Carcinoma in situ
T1	Tumor is <2 cm in greatest dimension
T2	Tumor is between 2 and 4 cm in greatest dimension
T3	Tumor is >4 cm in greatest dimension
T4	A: Tumor invades adjacent structures (medial pterygoid, hard palate, mandible, deep muscles of tongue, larynx)
	B: Tumor invades lateral pterygoid, pterygoid plates, carial nerves, carotid artery (encasement), lateral nasopharynx, skull base

Regional lymphatic metastases occur frequently and are related to the depth of tumor invasion and tumor size. Upper cervical nodes are generally first involved, but lower nodes can become clinically involved with skipping of the upper first-echelon nodes. Bilateral lymphatic metastases can occur, particularly with cancers of the soft palate, tongue base, and midline pharyngeal wall. The retropharyngeal lymph nodes are also common sites of metastasis and warrant evaluation when planning treatment.

Tonsil ■ The treatment of early tonsillar neoplasms (stages I and II) is usually radiation therapy as a single modality. Transoral wide local excision of small, superficial lesions may be locally effective, but does not address the high potential of occult lymph node metastasis. While surgery and primary radiation offer comparable locoregional control for small tumors, patients will require postoperative radiotherapy.[210] Surgical management of advanced cancers require extensive resections of the pharyngeal wall or mandible,[209,211] with free-tissue transfer and postoperative radiotherapy. Patient function after intensive treatment is often poor, with a significant number dependant upon gastrostomy tube for nutrition and a tracheostomy for pulmonary toilet. Thus, a shift toward nonsurgical management with combined chemotherapy and radiotherapy approaches for tonsillar cancers has prevailed (Fig. 77-6).

Radiation for early tonsillar cancers offers the advantage of treating upper-echelon lymph nodes along with the primary tumor. Treatment is usually unilateral unless extension to the tongue base or midline soft palate is present, which warrants treatment of contralateral lymphatics.[212] Ipsilateral treatment portals allow sparing of the contralateral mucosa and salivary glands. Because much of the tumor may be medial to the mandible,

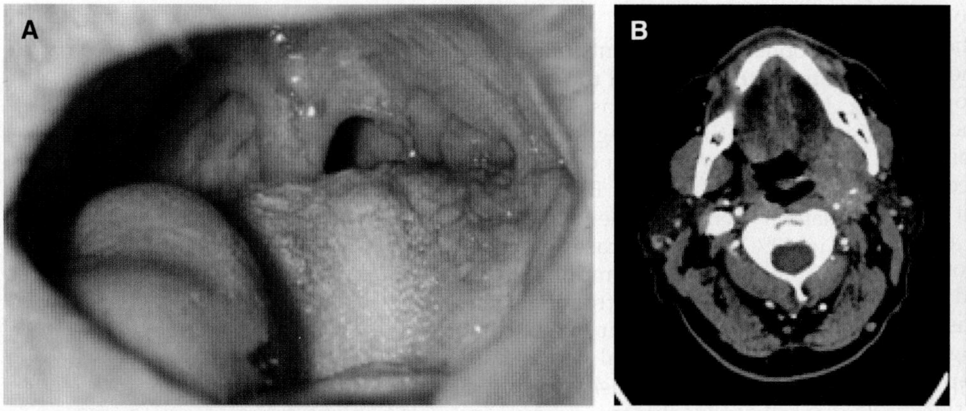

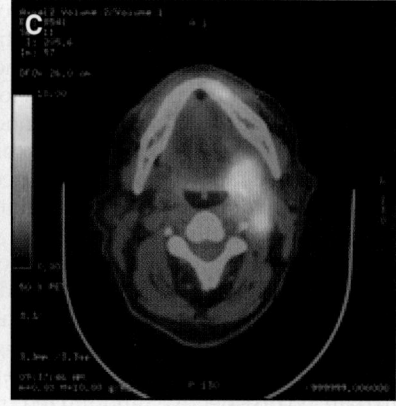

Figure 77-6 (**A**) T2 N2b SCCA of the oropharynx, clinically small lesion. (**B**) Deep infiltration into the parapharyngeal space is evident on CT scanning. (**C**) On PET-CT imaging, two distinct lesions are evident, the primary tumor and a posterior lymphatic metastasis.

deeper dose calculation with electron beam therapy is used, which can be combined with a small interstitial implant if invasion of adjacent tongue is present. Modern treatment techniques, such as intensity-modulated radiotherapy, permit conformal dose delivery which can reduce the potential morbidity of either unilateral or bilateral radiation treatment for tonsillar disease, particularly by reducing radiation-related xerostomia.[213] Initial institutional reports have indicated encouraging treatment outcomes with the use of IMRT in oropharyngeal cancer patients;[214-218] this is discussed in greater detail below in the section "Radiotherapy."

Radical radiotherapy to lymph nodes controls approximately 90% of limited nodal disease (N1) if the primary tumor is controlled, but nodal failure increases to more than 20% if failure occurs at the primary tumor site. Overall 5-year survival rates for patients with advanced primary tumors or regional metastases are generally less than 25% with single-modality therapy.[219-222] Combination of chemotherapy and radiotherapy has been shown to be effective in controlling locoregional disease in stage III and IV tonsillar cancers, and thus, surgery is frequently avoided. In addition, HPV status is highly predictive of patient outcomes in this disease. This is discussed further in the section "Chemotherapy and Radiation for Locally Advanced Disease" below. In general, surgery is rarely recommended for advanced tonsillar carcinoma unless the mandible is grossly invaded. When surgery is planned, postoperative concomitant therapy should be anticipated.

Tongue Base ■ Cancers of the base of the tongue pose a more difficult therapeutic problem than do tonsillar carcinomas. Most patients present with advanced disease due to the silent nature of these tumors, resulting in frequent regional metastases, greater treatment morbidity, and poor patient survival. Because of the functional deficits associated with gross total resection of even small tongue-base cancers, most tumors are treated with definitive radiation with or without chemotherapy, as described for tonsillar cancer above. Owing to the rich network of lymphatics present in the base of the tongue, 75% of patients will present with stage III or IV disease (Fig. 77-7). It is not uncommon for patients with small T1 or T2 tumors to develop multilevel, bilateral, or even contralateral metastases. Understaging of the primary tumor is common because these cancers tend to be diffusely infiltrative beyond their clinical appearance. This may account for similarities in local tumor control rates for both early and advanced lesions. Poor outcome is largely attributable to late diagnosis.[223]

The staging of tongue-base carcinomas is principally dependent on primary tumor size and the extent of regional metastases. Lymph node involvement is present in approximately 60% of patients with small (T1, T2) primaries.[224] Overall 5-year survival rates range from 11% to 45%.[225,226] The 5-year survival rates decrease from over 60% for N0 patients to less than 30% for N1 patients.[224-227] The results of radiation therapy alone as definitive treatment of small primary tumors (T1, T2) are better for exophytic than for deeply invasive tumors.[224] Radiation alone is generally reserved for those patients without clinical nodal metastases, but can be combined with planned neck dissection for patients with clinically positive nodes that persist after the completion of radiation-based approaches. The use of twice-daily, hyperfractionated radiotherapy or concomitant chemotherapy and radiotherapy appears to result in improved tumor control without many of the complications associated with implants for larger tumors.[228,229] Local recurrence is more frequent after radiation alone in most series,[224,225,230] and salvage rates for local failure is poor. The use of interstitial brachytherapy has fallen out of favor at most institutions in the United States, due to the high morbidity associated with their use. Surgical management of early superficial primary tongue-base tumors (T1) achieves results similar to those from radiation alone. In most cases, however, primary tumors are moderately advanced and require transcervical resection via mandibulotomy or lateral pharyngotomy approaches, combined with elective or therapeutic

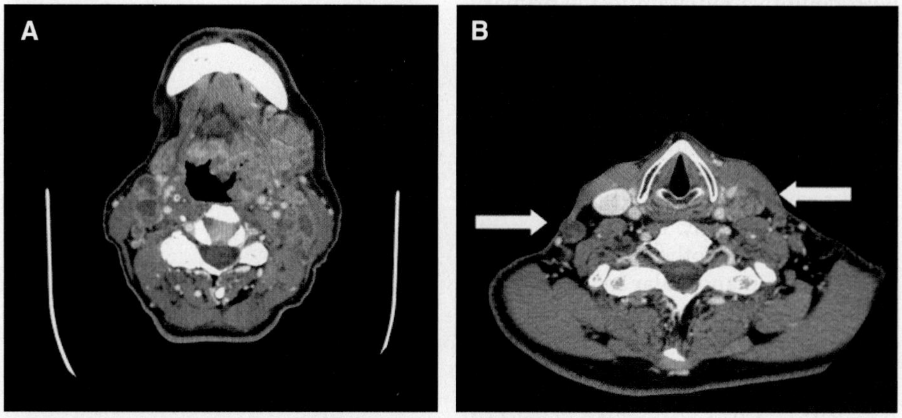

Figure 77-7 (**A**) Massive T4 N2c SCCA of the oropharynx (left base of tongue). (**B**) Multilevel bilateral nodal metastases present.

neck dissection. Advances in robotic surgery have prompted the application of this technology in the management of limited tongue-base cancers.[231] However, because of the high rates of nodal metastases, patients should receive postoperative radiotherapy to the neck. Local tumor control rates are superior to those with radiation alone,[224,225] but regional control is poor if clinically positive nodes are present. Elective neck dissection can serve an important role as a staging procedure, thereby providing a rationale for adjuvant radiation therapy. To date, no prospective randomized trial data are available that compare surgery alone with combined surgery with either preoperative or postoperative radiation. Survival rates are depressed for patients with T4 and advanced nodal disease.

Soft Palate and Pharyngeal Wall ■ Cancers of the soft palate and pharyngeal wall are less common than other oropharyngeal neoplasms. Many soft-palate cancers occur on the anterior surface of the palate and tend to be superficial. Posterior wall lesions tend to be superficial with less tumor bulk than similarly staged lesions elsewhere in the oropharynx. Advanced lesions with deep invasion have ready access to the prevertebral fascia, infratemporal fossa, and skull base and can be associated with extensive submucosal spread with clinical skip areas. Such patients often present with skull-base pain and neck stiffness.

Radiation-based approaches as curative treatment are preferred in most cases, even for T3 primary tumors.[232] Resection of most soft-palate lesions is associated with severe functional disability. The rates of occult regional metastases are difficult to determine because elective irradiation of bilateral nodal groups is included as part of primary treatment and must include the retropharyngeal lymphatics. Clinically positive lymph nodes at presentation occur in 30% of patients.[233] Small primary tumors with positive nodes can be effectively treated with definitive radiation to the primary tumor and neck. Neck dissections should be performed if disease in the neck persists at 6 to 8 weeks following the completion of external beam therapy. Extensive pharyngeal wall cancers or palate cancers with extension to the tonsil and those cases with advanced regional metastases are usually treated with combined chemoradiotherapy approaches unless gross mandibular involvement is noted. Overall 5-year survival rates for soft-palate and faucial pillar cancers are 60% to 70% and range from 80% to 90% for T1 and T2 lesions to 30% to 60% for stages III and IV lesions.[221] Locoregional recurrence is the most frequent cause of failure.[234]

Hypopharynx

The hypopharynx represents one of the most lethal sites for SCC of the head and neck. Lymph node metastases are clinically evident at time of diagnosis in 70% to 80% of patients[122,123,235] and are indicative of advanced disease. Bilateral and contralateral lymph node metastases occur in 10% to 20% of cases, particularly if tumors cross the midline of the hypopharynx. Primary tumor extension beyond the hypopharynx is common.[236,237] Hypopharyngeal cancers are characterized by a propensity to spread submucosally to involve the oropharynx or esophagus. Ulcerated deep infiltration and skip areas are anticipated. This leads to difficulties in adequately assessing the margins of the tumor and contributes to poor local tumor control, even with the addition of adjuvant radiation.[238] The majority (more than 75%) of hypopharyngeal cancers arise in the pyriform sinus, while 20% occur in the posterior pharyngeal wall (Fig. 77-8). Postcricoid cancers are rare (less than 5% of hypopharyngeal cancers). Pyriform cancers spread early to other contiguous structures, such as the larynx, postcricoid area, thyroid gland, and thyroid and cricoid cartilages. Most pyriform sinus cancers arise along the medial wall followed by the lateral wall of the sinus. The postcricoid mucosa is contiguous with the apex of the pyriform and tumor can spread circumferentially to involve the entire lower hypopharynx. Because of the locale of hypopharyngeal cancers and their growth patterns and proximity to the larynx, surgical management often entails total laryngopharyngectomy.[126] Extension to the esophagus will necessitate a cervical esophagectomy.

The staging of hypopharyngeal cancer is based on the subsite involved, the size of the tumor, the presence of vocal cord fixation, and the extent of lymph node metastases (Table 77-5). Distant metastases at the time of diagnosis are rare. Staging evaluation is critical for treatment planning and must include endoscopic evaluation to determine the extent including evaluation of adjacent structures and the presence of second primary tumors or skip areas.[239] Determination of the precise site of origin and inferior extent of a tumor can be difficult with large tumors or with those obstructing the esophageal inlet.

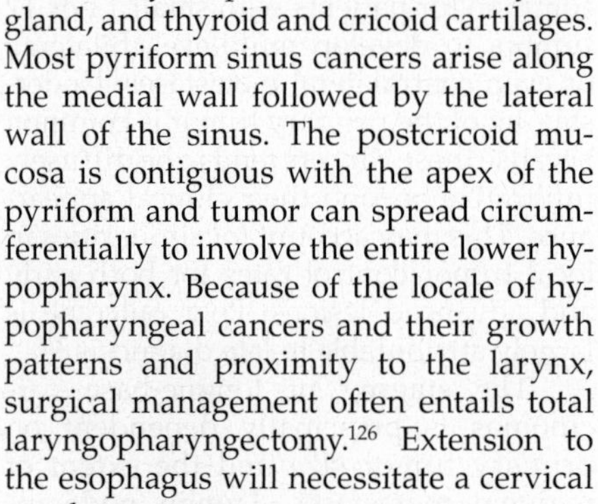

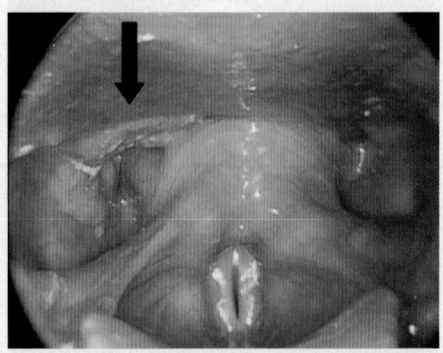

Figure 77-8 ■ T1 SCCA of the hypopharynx, involving the posterior pharyngeal wall and extending into the esophageal inlet.

Table 77-5 ■ **Primary Tumor Staging Characteristics for Cancer of the Hypopharynx**

Tx	Tumor cannot be assessed (as occurs with previous biopsy)
T0	There is no evidence of a primary (as occurs with an unknown primary tumor)
Tis	Carcinoma in situ
T1	Tumor limited to one subsite in the hypopharynx and <2 cm in greatest dimension
T2	Tumor involves more than one subsite in the hypopharynx or adjacent site, or measures between 2 and 4 cm in greatest dimension and without fixation of the hemilarynx
T3	Tumor measures >4 cm in greatest dimension or there is fixation of the hemilarynx
T4	A: Tumor invades adjacent structures (thyroid/cricoid cartilage, esophagus, thyroid gland, central compartment soft tissues B: Tumor invades prevertebral fascia, mediastinum or encases carotid artery

Because of the necessity to remove the larynx as part of the surgical treatment of most hypopharyngeal cancers, radiation therapy, for early T1 and T2 and in combination with chemotherapy for T3 disease has been investigated.[240] Retrospective analyses have consistently demonstrated that survival rates are lower and locoregional failure rates higher with radiation alone as compared with surgery or surgery and radiotherapy.[123,236-238,241,242]

Nevertheless, the functional implications of primary surgery for even the earliest of hypopharyngeal cancers have brought about the primary role of radiation-based approaches. However, for small (T1) cancers of the hypopharynx, and particularly for superficial posterior pharyngeal wall lesions, radiation therapy alone has been used effectively, with surgery reserved for salvage.[243,244] Radiation therapy offers the advantage of treating bilateral occult lymph node disease, including that of retropharyngeal nodes, which are frequently involved when cancer arises from the posterior pharyngeal wall.[237] Most patients, however, present with advanced primary tumors (T3 to T4) and positive lymph nodes. In such patients, local control rates with radiation alone decrease to 50% and salvage surgery is rarely successful. Thus, surgical management remains the mainstay of treatment of most advanced hypopharyngeal cancers. This is especially true when function is poor at diagnosis. Specifically, although there is emerging evidence that combinations of chemotherapy and radiotherapy are effective for controlling locoregional disease, one can expect that if a patient's speech and swallowing function are poor at diagnosis as evidenced by weight loss, cord fixation, dysphagia, and/or odynophagia, then function is likely to remain poor even if chemoradiotherapy eradicate disease. In such patients, we recommend surgery followed most commonly by radiotherapy. Resections may entail partial pharyngectomy, pharyngolaryngectomy, or total pharyngectomy combined with neck dissection and the associated difficulties in posttreatment function. Although free-flap reconstructions have improved results, there still remain the difficulties of lack of sensation and dysphagia.

Tumors arising in the lower hypopharynx or postcricoid mucosa often spread to involve the esophagus. Distal submucosal spread into the esophagus can be extensive and requires partial or total esophagectomy. Reconstruction with transposition of the stomach (gastric pull-up), jejunal free graft, or tubed fasciocutaneous free flap is currently recommended.[10,245-247] With improved locoregional control following the advent of total laryngopharyngectomy and postoperative radiation therapy, disease recurrence more commonly occurs in distant sites (ie, the lung). Treatment approaches with combined preoperative or postoperative radiation have dramatically improved the control of locoregional disease, but survival rates have not improved as substantially over those with surgery alone because of the increased rates of distant metastases. Postoperative radiation is currently preferred to preoperative radiation because of its lower local recurrence rates, fewer complications, and less difficulty in accurately assessing tumor margins.[123,238,241] The presence of lymph node metastases, extra-capsular lymph node involvement, and direct extension of the primary tumor into the soft tissues of the neck are adverse prognostic factors and are indications for postoperative chemoradiotherapy. Locoregional recurrence continues to account for the greatest number of deaths from disease.[127,248]

Overall 5-year survival rates range from 10% to 30% for posterior pharyngeal wall cancers[244,249-252] and from 20% to 40% for pyriform sinus cancers (Table 77-7).[122,123,127,237,241,242] Distant metastases are uncommon at the time of presentation, but may appear many years after primary therapy and seem to correlate with extent of regional lymph node involvement.[123,253] The rates of distant metastases range from 20% to 50%[123,127] and increase with the extent of lymph node disease.

Larynx

Because of the prominent role the larynx plays in communication, swallowing, respiration, protection of the lower airway, and, therefore, quality of life, the treatment of cancer of the larynx presents formidable dilemmas regarding functional consequences in addition to the intrinsic threat to life posed by these cancers. More so than with any other site of head and neck cancer, quality-of-life issues have been incorporated into treatment decisions and have echoed throughout the management strategy of the other head and neck sites.[254,255] Cancer of the glottic larynx is generally diagnosed at an earlier stage than are other head and neck sites, primarily owing to the early manifestation of symptoms, most commonly hoarseness. As a result, cure rates are generally higher than for other sites.

The larynx is divided into three subsites that form the basis for classifying laryngeal cancers. These separations exist because each site is associated with differences in patterns of local spread, risks of lymphatic metastasis, and control rates. These differences exist as a result of differences in embryologic development and vascular and lymphatic anatomy. The TNM staging for these subsites is listed in Table 77-6.

Considerable attention has been devoted to anatomic studies of the vascular and lymphatic compartments of the larynx.[256-258] These studies have defined natural anatomic barriers to cancer spread within the larynx and have contributed to the development of select surgical procedures for partial laryngeal resections of certain cancers.[259,260]

The true vocal cords present an effective boundary between supraglottic and subglottic lymphatic spread within the larynx. This anatomic barrier can be compromised by tumors involving the anterior or posterior commissures and with deeply invasive tumors that extend vertically across the true and false vocal cords (transglottic cancers). Normally, the inner perichondrium of the thyroid cartilage also presents an effective barrier to cancer spread. However, cancer involvement of the anterior commissure or transglottic extension is associated with invasion of the thyroid cartilage in 40% to 60% of cases.[259,261]

Early diagnosis is critical for achieving high survival rates and larynx preservation.[262] Most cancers that are diagnosed at an early stage of development arise in the glottic larynx. This is because minimal changes of the vibrating vocal cord from tumor growth result in changes in its vibrating characteristics and presents early as dysphonia or hoarseness. Supraglottic cancers are usually more advanced than glottic cancers at the time of diagnosis because they do not generally produce early symptoms of hoarseness. Rather, the earliest symptoms of a supraglottic cancer are usually sore throat, dysphagia, referred otalgia, or the development of a neck mass representing regional metastasis. Airway compromise may be an early symptom with subglottic cancer.

Modern clinical evaluation of laryngeal cancers includes fiber-optic laryngoscopy, direct laryngoscopy, CT, and MRI of the larynx and neck, as well as videostroboscopic analysis (Fig. 77-9). The radiological assessments are of value in assessing direct extension to the preepiglottic and paraglottic spaces of the larynx, detecting cartilage invasion and evaluating the soft tissues and lymph nodes of the neck. However, the precise evaluation of tumor extent still requires direct laryngoscopy under

Table 77-6 Primary Tumor Staging Characteristics for Carcinoma of the Larynx

Supraglottis	T1	Normal vocal cord motility and tumor limited to one laryngeal subsite
	T2	Tumor invades one adjacent site, normal vocal cord motility
	T3	Tumor limited to larynx with arytenoids fixation and/or extends to postcricoid area or preepiglottic tissues, limited thyroid cartilage involvement (inner cortex)
	T4	A: Tumor extends beyond thyroid cartilage and\or invades soft tissues of neck, thyroid, esophagus, tongue musculature, strap muscles or trachea
		B: Tumor invades prevertebral fascia, mediastinum or encases carotid artery
Glottis	T1	Tumor limited to one vocal cord (s) with normal motion
		T1a: Tumor limited to one cord
		T1b: Tumor involves both cords
	T2	Tumor extends to supraglottis or subglottis and/or with impaired vocal cord motility
	T3	Tumor limited to larynx but with vocal cord\arytenoid fixation, paraglottic space invasion, limited thyroid cartilage involvement (inner cortex)
	T4	A: Tumor extends beyond thyroid cartilage and\or invades soft tissues of neck, thyroid, esophagus, tongue musculature, strap muscles or trachea
		B: Tumor invades prevertebral fascia, mediastinum or encases carotid artery
Subglottis	T1	Tumor limited to subglottis
	T2	Tumor extends to glottis but with normal or impaired motion
	T3	Tumor limited to larynx but with vocal cord\arytenoid fixation
	T4	A: Tumor extends beyond thyroid cartilage and\or invades soft tissues of neck, thyroid, esophagus, tongue musculature, strap muscles or trachea
		B: Tumor invades prevertebral fascia, mediastinum or encases carotid artery

Table 77-7 **Primary Tumor Staging Characteristics for Carcinoma of Nasopharynx**

T1	Tumor confined to the soft tissues of the nasopharynx
T2	Tumor extends to the soft tissues of the oropharynx and/or nasal fossa
	T2a: Without parapharyngeal extension
	T2b: With parapharyngeal extension
T3	Tumor invades bony structures and/or paranasal sinuses
T4	Tumor exhibits intracranial extension and/or involvement of cranial nerves, infratemporal fossa, hypopharynx, or orbit

anesthesia. With large, obstructive tumors, this may require tracheostomy. In some patients, debulking the tumor mass at the time of direct laryngoscopy can obviate the need for tracheostomy and thereby reduce the potential risk of tumor seeding of the tracheostomy site. Even with precise clinical evaluation, inaccurate estimation of tumor extent (usually underestimation) occurs in 30% to 40% of cases.[263-265] Most often this involves failure to identify invasion of the laryngeal cartilage framework, although a fine-cut CT scan of the larynx performed as part of the staging process will detect these aggressive features.

Supraglottic primary tumors account for 25% to 50% of all laryngeal cancers.[263,264] A knowledge of the laryngeal compartments aids in understanding the spread and staging of supraglottic and glottic cancers. The staging of supraglottic cancers is based on the subsite or region of the supraglottis involved in the cancer. Subsites include the false vocal cords, arytenoids, lingual and laryngeal surfaces of the epiglottis, and aryepiglottic folds. The epiglottis itself is also subdivided into the region extending above the plane of the hyoid and that below the hyoid. Suprahyoid epiglottic tumors tend to have a better prognosis than infrahyoid cancers with the exception of those invading the aryepiglottic fold (marginal area) to involve the pyriform sinus. This, again, is due to the richer network of lymphatics in the infrahyoid portion of the epiglottis. Early cancers (T1 and T2) can involve one or more subsites but have normal vocal cord motion. Those cancers that cause fixation of the arytenoid or involve the postcricoid region, medial wall of the pyriform sinus, or preepiglottic space are staged T3. Those that extend beyond the larynx or invade thyroid cartilage are staged T4.

The staging of glottic carcinomas is also determined by functional and anatomic features. Cancers limited to the true vocal cords are T1 (T1a—one vocal cord involved; T1b—both vocal cords involved), and those with extension to an adjacent site or with impaired cord mobility are staged T2. Impaired vocal cord motion is also staged as T2 and is due to muscular invasion and some element of paraglottic disease spread. Whereas, as impaired motion is staged as T2, arytenoid fixation and vocal cord immobility upstages a lesion to a T3. Those tumors with cartilage involvement or extension outside the larynx are T4.

True subglottic cancers that are limited to the subglottic region (T1) or to the subglottis and true vocal cords (T2) are early cancers but, unfortunately, are diagnosed late because of a lack of symptoms. Fixation of the vocal cord (T3) and cartilage invasion or extension outside the larynx (T4) is associated with a worse prognosis. The nodal classification for staging is the same as for other HNSCC sites.

Although a great deal of controversy exists regarding the optimal treatment of approach for larynx cancer, at The University of Texas M. D. Anderson Cancer Center, curative radiotherapy is generally the treatment of choice for early-stage laryngeal lesions. For moderately advanced lesions one must consider the trade-offs between definitive radiotherapy with salvage surgery held in reserve versus definitive surgery or, more recently, combined chemotherapy and radiation therapy approaches. A number of factors, aside from stage, warrant consideration in determining the optimal treatment strategy for patients, including: age, medical comorbidities, laryngeal function and rehabilitative potential. Advanced T4 lesions are treated with surgery and postoperative radiotherapy.

Examination under anesthesia and biopsy make up the gold standard in the assessment of early lesions, combined with radiographic imaging for assessment of the paraglottic space and thyroid cartilage. Radiation therapy remains the management of choice for early glottic cancers. Nevertheless, in some instances, patients may choose conservation laryngeal surgery, including endoscopic laser excision of localized lesions, or partial laryngeal surgery. Both require frozen-section analysis of margins if the patient and tumor factors support such an approach. In addition, in many instances, conservation laryngeal surgical salvage is effective in those 10% to 20% of cases in which external beam therapy has been unsuccessful for stages I and II cancers.

The design of radiation treatment must be tailored to the individual patient, but some general comments can be made. Early-stage (T1-2, N0) glottic lesions are treated with conventional fields localized to the primary tumor; T1 tumors are typically treated once-daily to doses of approximately 6300 to 6600 cGy, while T2 tumors are treated more aggressively with twice-daily or concomitant-boost fractionation.[266] T2 tumors with bulky subglottic extension or with anterior involvement with potential extralaryngeal spread outside the thyroid cartilage are at higher risk for treatment failure, and can be considered for concurrent chemoradiotherapy. Supraglottic tumors have access to a richer lymphatic drainage than do tumors of the glottic larynx, and so radiation fields must be larger in order to treat cervical and retropharyngeal nodal basins at risk for metastatic disease. With conventional techniques, one treats the primary tumor volume and regions at risk of subclinical metastatic disease to 5000 cGy, and then reduces the field size to areas of gross disease and delivers an additional 2000 to 2400 cGy. The spinal cord is shielded at 4500 cGy, and megavoltage electron beams are used to treat the posterior cervical nodes to higher doses as required. Because of the V shape of the anterior neck, wedge-compensating filters are often required to ensure uniform radiation dose distributions. If the anterior supraclavicular fossa is at risk of micrometastatic disease, it is treated to 5000 cGy, using an anterior field suitably matched to the upper-neck fields. Conventional treatment fields for advanced supraglottic and glottic disease pass through the parotid glands and can cause posttreatment xerostomia. IMRT is an alternative to conventional treatment in such cases. IMRT can treat tumor and

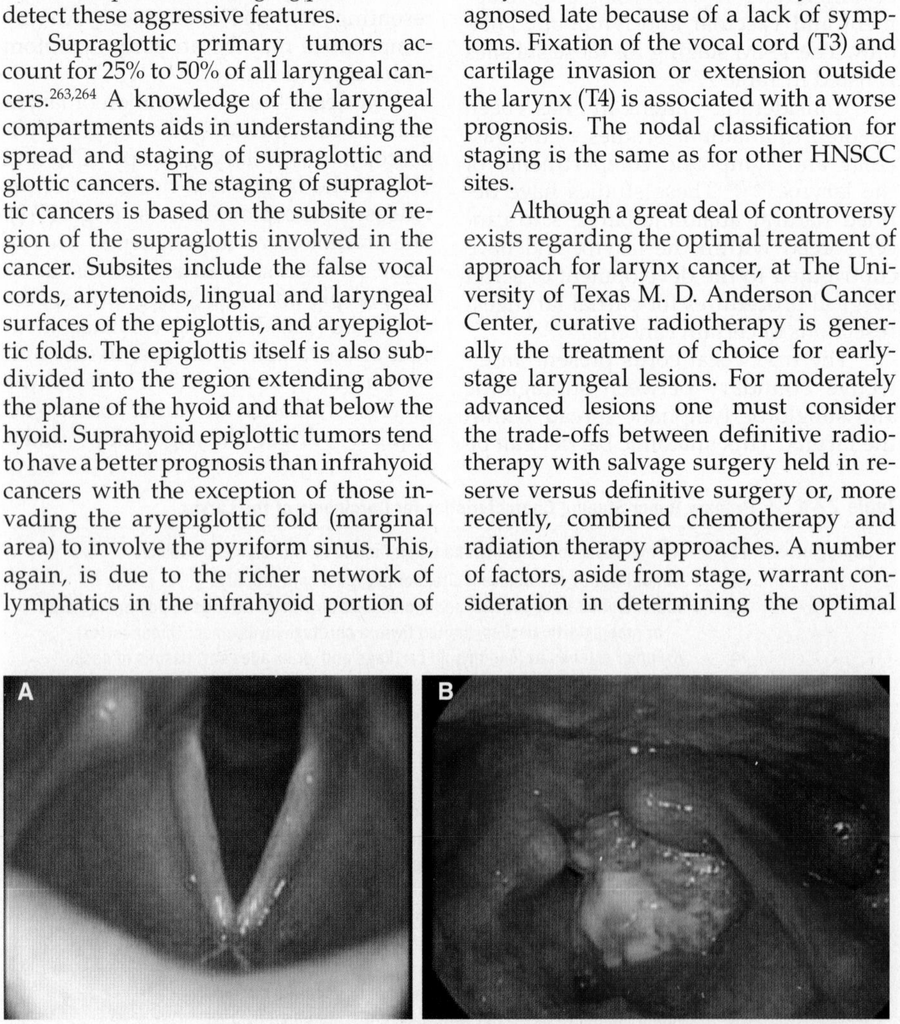

Figure 77-9 (**A**) Normal larynx. (**B**) T3 left glottic SCCA, with obliteration of the normal vocal cord anatomy. Extension onto the supraglottis and onto the arytenoid is evident.

nodal regions with conformal sparing of normal tissues, such as parotids and spinal cord. With IMRT, distinct volumetric targets are designed to encompass gross primary and nodal disease, immediately adjacent soft tissues and nodes, and at-risk draining nodal stations requiring prophylactic coverage. These targeted volumes are treated to specified doses comparable to those delivered with conventional techniques. Further details regarding IMRT are provided below in the section "Radiotherapy". As a final note, tumors originating from or involving the subglottic larynx can spread to the upper paratracheal nodes as well as to the nodes in the cervical chain; therefore, radiation fields for this disease must therefore include the upper mediastinum.[267]

The treatment of more advanced laryngeal cancers (T3 and T4) has historically included surgery with or without radiation therapy. Prospective randomized studies have shown convincingly that chemotherapy and radiation therapy (including surgical salvage) are equally effective in the long-term survival of patients with T3 laryngeal cancers as compared with surgery with or without radiation therapy. It is important to note that approximately 60% of patients may preserve their larynx, and thus quality of life has significantly improved.[240,268] Speech communication profiles are clearly better in the group of patients randomized to the larynx preservation arm, but there was no determination of swallowing function.[269] However, local control was poorer for patients with T4 lesions. Current standard of care argues that laryngeal preservation approaches or protocols be considered in treating such patients, with the corollary that patients with poor function at diagnosis will likely have poor laryngeal function after conservation treatment. Thus, a primary surgical approach should be strongly entertained for patients with significant aspiration based upon pretreatment swallowing studies. In addition, due to the toxicity of combined chemoradiotherapy regimens, those with pulmonary and cardiac comorbidities that may limit treatment intensity may be best managed with surgery and radiotherapy.

Many surgical procedures for laryngeal carcinoma involve the creation of a tracheal stoma. This area is sometimes at significant risk of tumor recurrence, which is most likely associated with paratracheal nodal metastases. For this reason, bilateral paratracheal dissections should be performed in T4 glottic cancers and radiation therapy provided postoperatively if metastases to this echelon of nodes are found pathologically. Once a stomal recurrence has developed, the prognosis is grave regardless of salvage treatment. Sisson and colleagues reported on a series of 28 patients with stomal recurrences treated with one or more surgical resections.[270] The 5-year survival was only 17%. Schneider and colleagues reported on patients with tracheal recurrences treated with radiotherapy; good palliation of local pain and/or bleeding was achieved, but the 2-year survival rate was only 6%.[271] If risk factors for stomal recurrence are present, then the tracheal stoma should be irradiated as part of the initial management.

Supraglottic Cancers ■ Important factors in selecting therapy for supraglottic cancers are tumor location, cord fixation and preepiglottic extension. Tumors limited to the suprahyoid epiglottis are amenable to radiation with fields that encompass neck regions at risk of lymphatic metastases. In addition, some proponents of limited surgical interventions recommend endoscopic laser excision separate from management of the neck. Tumors involving the aryepiglottic folds, pyriform sinuses, or infrahyoid epiglottis tend to be more aggressive, are deeply infiltrative, and frequently involve the preepiglottic space. Radiation alone is less effective than surgery, resulting in more frequent local recurrences that require surgical salvage. The addition of systemic concomitant chemotherapy will positively impact the outcomes of patients with these tumors. Persistent post-radiation edema of the supraglottic larynx is not uncommon and contributes to difficulty in detecting recurrence, which occurs in 40% to 50% of cases.[272-274] Supraglottic recurrences are difficult to detect at a stage when they are amenable to laryngeal conservation surgery. Most patients who recur will ultimately require a salvage total laryngectomy.

Preepiglottic extension of cancer carries a poor prognosis. However, such a situation can be managed effectively with horizontal supraglottic laryngectomy, which allows preservation of the voice. Indeed, even advanced tumors with extension of cancer to the vallecula and tongue base can often be treated by extended supraglottic laryngectomy with results equal to those of total laryngectomy. Very superficial tumors of the suprahyoid epiglottis can also be treated with simple epiglottectomy. Because supraglottic laryngectomy is associated with variable degrees of postoperative aspiration, adequate pulmonary status is a prerequisite for this surgery, as is intact mobility of the true vocal cords.

In any patient undergoing partial laryngectomy, preoperative consent should be obtained for total laryngectomy in case the surgical findings dictate that more extensive surgery is needed. Approximately 20% of patients require prolonged tracheostomy, and this is usually related to edema secondary to postoperative radiation. The rates of persistent swallowing difficulties are low however, and the need for completion laryngectomy for persistent aspiration ranges only from 0% to 5%.[275-277]

The frequency of neck node metastases is at least 20% with T2 or greater tumors. Treatment of the clinically negative neck may be accomplished with surgery or radiation. Surgical approaches should include removal of bilateral primary nodal groups at risk of occult disease (levels II, III, and IV).298-300 For T1 and T2 lesions, most authors demonstrate overall cure rates of 68% to 73%[278-280] with determinate 3-year survival rates of 80% to 85%[263,278,279] when elective neck dissection is included. Most recurrences occur in the neck, and this argues for prophylactic neck treatment.[281]

Radiation is also effective for early lesions. Local control rates for patients with supraglottic tumors treated with radiation alone range from 68% to 94%, and survival rates are 50% to 89%. The latter set of survival figures are comparable to those for planned surgery and adjuvant radiotherapy, which range from 46% to 90%. Although the figures are comparable for T1 and T2 lesions, there is a trend favoring the combined approach for larger lesions. Nonrandomized series from different institutions are not strictly comparable since unstated patient selection factors are generally involved. For example, the excellent local control results reported by Goepfert and colleagues for T3 and T4 lesions are for a selected set of tumors that were exophytic in nature.[282]

While acceptable local-regional control can be achieved for supraglottic cancers, survival rates are adversely impacted due to the development of second primary tumors or intercurrent disease. Cure rates range from 73% to 75% for radiotherapy[283-286] and increase to 80% to 85% with the addition of surgical salvage.[287-289] Most recurrences are local, and preservation of voice is successful in 65% to 70% of patients when salvage surgery is included.[287]

The treatment of more advanced supraglottic cancers (T3, T4) remains controversial, with laryngeal preservation remaining a focus of treatment (Fig. 77-10). Combined chemoradiotherapy is often curative, but toxicities remain significant. The addition of chemotherapy will not only enhance the therapeutic benefits of radiotherapy, but may also increase mucositis, odynophagia and long-term fibrosis and xerostomia. As described above, patients with T4 lesions are best managed with laryngectomy and radiotherapy, as cartilage and bone invasion are difficult to control with radiation with an acceptably high rate of disease recurrences. However, some experienced

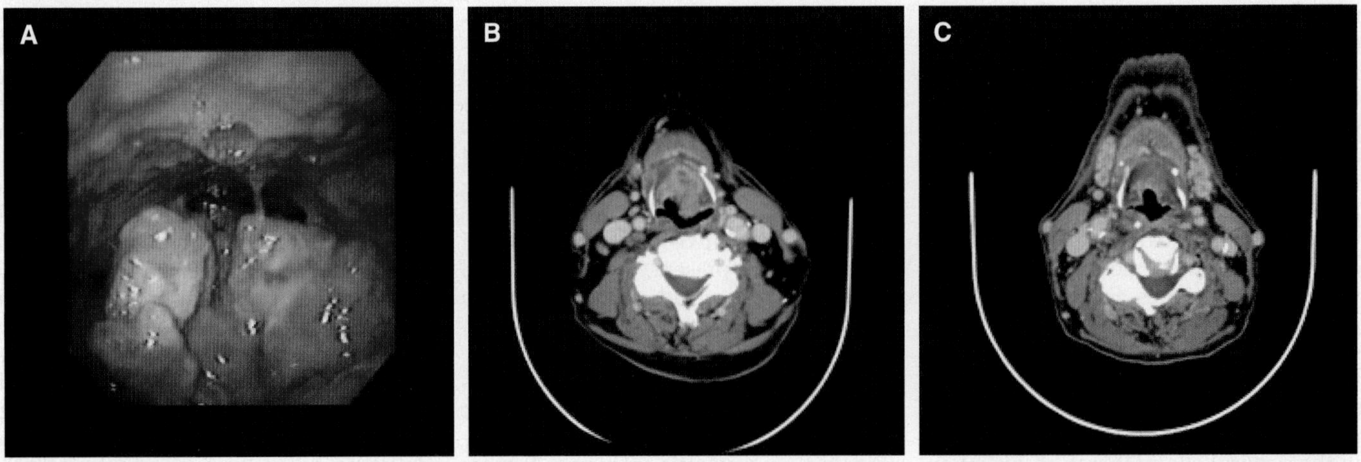

Figure 77-10 (A) T3 N0 SCCA of the supraglottis. Destruction of the epiglottis is evident. (B) Invasion of the pre-epiglottic space is seen on CT scan, prior to concomitant chemoradiotherapy. (C) Posttreatment imaging, demonstrating a complete response at the primary site.

centers have treated patients with minimal laryngeal framework invasion with combined chemoradiotherapy with high success. Further analysis of this selected patient cohort is necessary to determine the optimal treatment. One area of controversy surrounds the management of patients with bulky T3 lesions and poor pretreatment function. While a nonsurgical approach will allow the patient to preserve the larynx, the preexisting compromised functions portend for uncertain functional outcome after treatment. These patients ultimately may require long-term or permanent enteral nutrition and tracheostomy for significant aspiration, and may ultimately require a laryngectomy for pulmonary toilet. One novel approach that has been advocated is to utilize induction chemotherapy to assess both tumor and functional responses. Those with improvement of their function after one cycle of chemotherapy may tolerate concomitant chemoradiotherapy and avoid laryngectomy. Alternatively, those with minimal or no response would be best managed with surgery and postoperative radiotherapy.

Although the stigma of laryngectomy remains, contemporary postoperative laryngeal rehabilitation offers quite acceptable functional outcomes. The advent of tracheo-esophageal punctures (TEP), in conjunction with intense rehabilitation, has markedly improved the functional outcomes of laryngectomized patients. A laryngeal speech can be realized within 2 weeks after surgery. In the salvage surgical setting, TEP placement should be deferred for at least 3 months while the surgical site matures. Early TEP placement resulted in fistula formation and poor wound healing.

Planned neck dissections at the conclusion of treatment for N2 disease or greater is often performed. Approximately 50% of patients have clinically palpable lymph nodes at the time of diagnosis, and 20% to 25% have bilateral nodal involvement. In the clinically negative neck, elective neck dissection revealed metastases in 15% to 30% of patients, and thus bilateral elective neck irradiation is warranted. Failure to control disease in the neck is a major cause of mortality in supraglottic cancers. In most reports, radiation alone for the control of supraglottic cancers with N2 or N3 nodes is clearly inferior to combined therapy. Overall 5-year survival rates for supraglottic cancers range from 40% to 50%.[289,290] Local failures occur in approximately 10% of patients and regional failures in 15% to 20%. Rates of distant metastases range from 11% to 18%,[289,291,292] with rates approaching 30% in patients with stage IV disease.[293] Second primaries (20-25% of failures) are a major cause of death[289] and intercurrent illness accounts for up to 20% of deaths.[292-294]

Glottic and Subglottic Cancers The treatment of glottic cancer is greatly influenced by the secondary goal of voice preservation. Mobility of the vocal cords is a critical factor in selecting treatment. For small cancers (T1, T2) with mobile vocal cords, radiation therapy alone for cure achieves excellent local control rates (T1, 85-95%; T2, 65-75%) and overall survival rates similar to those for surgical resection.[295,296] Voice quality, although often impaired by radiation, is generally better than that following surgical resection.[297,298] Local recurrences after definitive radiation can often be salvaged by subsequent surgery. Tumor involvement of the anterior commissure or arytenoids has been associated with higher local recurrence rates for radiation alone, but this may have been related to understaging. As with supraglottic cancers, careful clinical tumor staging is necessary since underestimation of tumor extent is common. The "irradiate-and watch" treatment strategy is predicated on close follow-up in order to detect recurrences when they are still salvageable by surgery. Delay in the diagnosis of recurrent glottic cancers after radiation is more frequent than with supraglottic cancers[282] and may requires total laryngectomy for cure. A supracricoid laryngectomy is another primary or salvage treatment option of glottic carcinomas.

Survival figures in radiotherapy series are comparable to local control rates for surgery, reflecting the effectives of surgical salvage and the fact that few patients with early glottic cancer die of their disease. The 5-year survival rates for T1 lesions range from 85% to 95% with either primary surgery or radiation. Rates for T2 lesions are generally in the range of 75% to 85%, but these rates decrease by 10% to 15% (local control rates by 20-25%) when the mobility of the vocal cords is impaired[299] or when there is transglottic spread.[300] Lesions with impaired mobility owing to muscle invasion behave more like T3 cancers and have a poorer prognosis with radiotherapy alone.[295,301-304] Transglottic cancers and those with subglottic extension have higher rates of regional metastases and more often require total laryngectomy for cure (Fig. 77-11). In selected patients with these more advanced lesions, extended supraglottic laryngectomy or supracricoid partial laryngectomy may effectively salvage the patient and avoid a permanent stoma.[198,305] Voice quality is typically poor with these procedures, and permanent tracheostomy may be needed. In addition, these procedures are technically challenging and require a high level of training and experience dependent. However, with proper patient selection, these procedures can be well tolerated and effective.

Management of advanced T3 glottic cancers has historically consisted of total laryngectomy with or without postoperative radiation therapy. Although older series show suboptimal control rates (20-35%) and survival rates

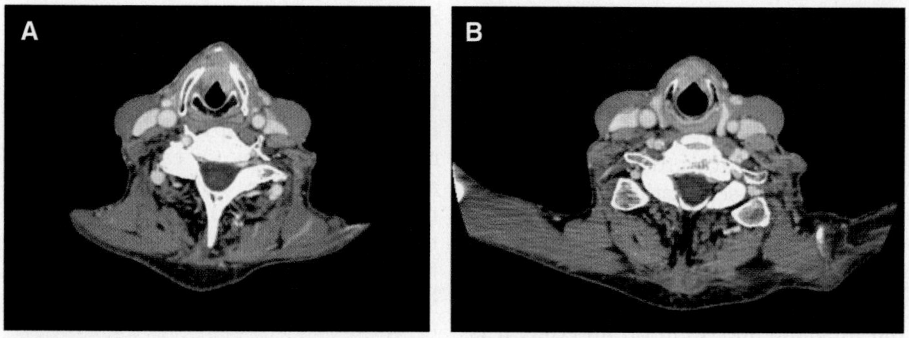

Figure 77-11 Small volume laryngeal SCCA with both glottic (**A**) and subglottic (**B**) involvement. The lesion is staged T4 due to the extensive cartilagenous invasion, with extension into the soft tissue of the neck.

(10-50%) for unselected sets of T3 and T4 tumors treated with radiation alone, it is now recognized that with proper selection, radiotherapy control rates for T3 lesions can approach 70-80%,[306] which is enhanced by the addition of systemic therapy with a platinum-based protocol. In patients without regional metastases, local tumor control rates with surgery alone are excellent. Significant increases in local control with the addition of radiation therapy have not been clearly demonstrated. However, in patients with regional metastases, overall prognosis is poor and recurrence in the neck is a major problem when surgery alone is used. Improved regional tumor control rates are achieved with the addition of adjuvant radiation therapy.[282] Because rates of occult regional metastases approach 30% in patients with advanced glottic (T3, T4) cancers, elective modified or selective node dissections for staging purposes are recommended when surgery is performed for primary disease. Demonstration of histologically positive nodal metastases has been used as an indication for postoperative radiation. Surgery alone is curative in 50% to 80% of patients without nodal metastases,[285,302,307-309] but this decreases to less than 40% if metastases are present.[302,310,311]

Considerable controversy surrounds the use of definitive radiation with surgical salvage in patients with advanced (T3N0, T4N0) but localized glottic cancers.[307,312,313] Overall survival rates range from 50% to 55%,[310,312,314] with larynx preservation in 60% to 70% of these patients.[300,310,312] High complication rates, however, have been reported with late surgical salvage of radiation failures, and may require the use of free-tissue transfer for reconstruction.[310] Postoperative fistulas may occur in 30-50% of patients, a source of significant morbidity. The resolution of this controversy will require carefully designed prospective studies that include assessments not only of survival, but also of voice and quality-of-life issues and complication rates.

Subsets of laryngeal cancers that warrant special consideration are those that involve both the glottic and supraglottic regions (transglottic). These cancers are usually advanced and are associated with a high incidence (30-50%) of regional metastases.[300,315] These tumors can be difficult to control with radiation alone, and may warrant the addition of chemotherapy in the treatment plan.

It was previously thought that distant metastases from laryngeal cancers were uncommon, accounting for less than 10% of failures. However, with improved locoregional control, the recognized incidence of distant metastasis is increasing. Distant spread is approximately four times more common with supraglottic than with glottic cancers.[125] Rates of distant metastases associated with glottic cancer have increased, however, with the use of combined therapy and have been reported in approximately 20% of patients with advanced disease.[316] Rates appear to be directly related to the extent of nodal disease, with reported rates as high as 40% to 50% of failures attributed to distant metastases in patients with N2 or N3 disease.

Subglottic carcinomas are a rare variant of squamous carcinomas of the larynx possessing a high risk for paratracheal metastases, local recurrence, and death from disease.[317-319] Surgery is the preferred therapy except in early superficial diseases of this site.[317-319]

Carcinoma In Situ (CIS) A special issue relates to the treatment of CIS of the vocal cords.[114,320] This disease often can be managed with vocal cord stripping, but if enough serial sections are examined, foci of invasive carcinoma are often found. For diffuse CIS of the glottis, radiation therapy has been advocated, due to significant risk of malignant transformation and the inability to clear this disease surgically. Very superficial cancers limited to the free edge of the vocal cord or CIS can be effectively treated by limited excision by conventional means or with laser excision, with excellent voice preservation.[316,321] More extensive disease requires cordectomy, vertical hemilaryngectomy, or supracricoid laryngectomy.[322] Numerous methods have been devised for reconstructing the vocal cords after conservation surgery, although, in fact, they are probably not necessary if proper patient selection is pursued. In general, voice results are inferior to those achieved with radiation therapy alone for early lesions. The patient with CIS, however, by inference has diffuse premalignant mucosal findings and certainly should be targeted for novel prevention strategies owing to the likelihood of later developing invasive disease.

Nonsurgical Treatment There has been an increasing focus on the use of chemotherapy in the management of laryngeal cancers of all stages. Laccourreye and others have published a series of articles that suggest that exclusive chemotherapy may be effective in select cases.[323,324] Randomized trials have demonstrated that the concomitant administration of chemotherapy and radiotherapy improves local-regional disease control and overall survival in patients with locally advanced squamous cell carcinomas of the head and neck (SCCHN). Induction chemotherapy with cisplatin and fluorouracil has long been recognized as highly active with clinical partial and complete responses observed in 80% to 90% of previously untreated patients.[325-327] It was postulated that a substantial response to initial treatment with chemotherapy would lead to an improvement of therapeutic efficacy for surgery or radiotherapy. This led to the Department of Veterans Affairs Laryngeal Cancer Study,[328] in which 332 patients with stage III or IV SCC of the larynx were randomized to receive either induction chemotherapy consisting of cisplatin and fluorouracil followed by radiotherapy or surgery and postoperative radiotherapy. Patients who experienced no tumor response to chemotherapy or those who had locally persistent or recurrent cancer underwent salvage laryngectomy. Two-year survival for both treatment groups was 68%, and 41% of patients randomly assigned to the experimental arm were alive with a functional larynx at 2 years. Thus, the efficacy of chemotherapy followed by radiotherapy (with surgical salvage) was similar to that of surgery followed by radiotherapy and established organ preservation as a realistic goal of nonsurgical treatment administered with curative intent. Lefebvre and colleagues[240] later reported the potential for effective sequential induction chemotherapy followed by radiotherapy in a European trial involving patients with cancers of the hypopharynx.

In the Veterans Affairs study,[328] there were observed trends in patterns of tumor relapse, with 20% of patients in the chemotherapy arm having locoregional recurrence versus 7% in the surgery arm. Distant disease recurrence was more likely in the surgical arm, affecting 17% of patients versus 11% in the chemotherapy/radiotherapy group. Salvage laryngectomy was required more often in patients with glottic cancer than in those with supraglottic primary sites (43% vs 31%), in patients with fixed vocal cords than in those with mobile vocal cords (41% vs 29%), and in patients with gross invasion of thyroid cartilage compared with patients without (41% vs 35%). Salvage laryngectomy was required in 56% of patients with T4 cancers compared with 29% of patients with smaller primary tumors ($p = .001$).

The Veterans Affairs Larynx study prompted further investigations of chemotherapy and radiotherapy in the treatment of intermediate-stage larynx cancer using the sequential administration of induction chemotherapy, consisting of cisplatin and fluorouracil, followed by radiotherapy as the control arm. This was compared with concomitant cisplatin and radiotherapy, and radiotherapy administered as a single treatment modality.[329,330] Patients with stage III and IV disease were eligible, T2/3, N0-3, M0. T1 and most T4 patients were not eligible. For all groups, totaling 547 patients, surgical salvage was reserved for those patients with persistent or locally recurrent disease. Survival did not seem to be affected by treatment assignment. At a median follow-up of 3.8 years, patients randomly assigned to concomitant cisplatin and radiotherapy achieved a higher rate of laryngeal preservation, 84% versus 72% in patients receiving sequential chemoradiotherapy ($p = .005$) or radiotherapy alone 67% ($p < .001$). At 2 years, 78% of patients on the concomitant chemoradiotherapy arm achieved locoreional control versus 61% of patients receiving sequential chemotherapy and then radiation and 56% of patients treated with radiotherapy alone. As expected, acute toxic effects of treatment were greatest in the patients who received radiotherapy with concomitant cisplatin.

These trials indicate that for patients with intermediate-stage SCC of the larynx, a combined treatment program with the objectives of tumor eradication and laryngeal preservation is appropriate. It is also important to recognize that patients with locally advanced destructive primary laryngeal cancers were not included in the multi-institutional trial. These patients may require total laryngectomy for optimal tumor control and to preserve swallow function.

Nasopharynx

Presentation and Staging ■ In the United States, NPC accounts for 2% of all HNSCC. Its unusual epidemiologic and natural history features include a remarkable tendency toward early regional and distant dissemination. NPC also is extremely sensitive to radiotherapy and cytotoxic chemotherapy.

In the adult, the nasopharynx is a chamber that is approximately cuboidal in shape and 4 cm on an edge. It is bounded anteriorly by the choana of the nasal cavity, superiorly by the clivus, and inferiorly by the soft palate. Its posterior wall is the mucosa that overlies the superior constrictor muscles of the pharynx and the C 1 and C2 vertebral bodies. The lateral walls contain the eustachian tube orifices. The epithelium of the superior lateral walls contains pseudostratified columnar cells and occasional goblet cells, while the inferior lateral and posterior walls are stratified squamous in nature. The region is richly endowed with lymphatics that drain to the retropharyngeal and deep cervical nodes.

Malignant neoplasms of the nasopharynx are primarily epithelial, with the presence of keratin associated with a poorer prognosis. The WHO recognizes three histopathologic types of NPC: type 1, differentiated SCC (of varying degrees); type 2, nonkeratinizing carcinoma; and type 3, undifferentiated lymphoepithelial carcinoma.[331] Mixed patterns are common.

About one-third of patients present with a neck mass without other complaints, and about 70% to 75% of patients have enlarged neck nodes at presentation. Other common complaints are epistaxis, nasal stuffiness, headache, and hearing loss (generally unilateral). The tumor can spread laterally and superiorly to cause bony destruction of the base of the skull. Frequently, there are cranial nerve findings, with the sixth nerve being most commonly involved.[332] There are two principal cranial nerve syndromes associated with NPC: (1) the retroparotidian syndrome, involving cranial nerves IX, X, XI, and XII; and (2) the petrosphenoidal syndrome, involving cranial nerves III, IV, V, and VI (and occasionally cranial nerve II via extension through the foramen lacerum into the middle cranial fossa). Evaluation of the nasopharynx should consist of direct visualization with a fiber-optic scope. An MRI scan is important in evaluating base-of-skull involvement and the possible presence of occult-involved lymph nodes.

The most recent revision of the AJCC/Union Internationale Contre le Cancer (UICC) staging system recognizes the uniqueness of NPC among other head and neck tumors. Both the criteria for T and N staging have been revised, as has the stage grouping. These are summarized in Table 77-7.

Treatment ■ Standard treatment of NPC is radiation therapy or concomitant chemoradiotherapy for early and locally advanced disease, respectively. Surgical resection even for early-stage disease is technically difficult because of the anatomic location of the primary tumor and frequent bilateral cervical and retropharyngeal node involvement. The role of the surgeon is limited to obtaining tissue for diagnosis, resecting residual adenopathy after definitive radiotherapy, and surgery for rare non-WHO histologies such as adenoid cystic carcinoma. Fortunately, most NPCs tend to be fairly radiosensitive, and even large lymph nodes often respond to moderate doses of radiotherapy.[333] Prior to initiating therapy, dental consultation is advised since it is necessary to irradiate the parotid glands bilaterally, and the resulting xerostomia predisposes to serious oral problems.

The initial radiation fields encompass the adjacent base of the skull as well as the nasopharynx itself. The fields are bilaterally directed and include the retropharyngeal drainage and the anterior and posterior cervical chains. A dose of 4500 cGy is given, using megavoltage photons, and then the fields are reduced to spare the spinal cord and an additional 500 cGy are given. Megavoltage electrons are used to bring the posterior cervical nodes to this same dose. The fields are then reduced in size and an additional 2000 to 2200 cGy are given to the nasopharyngeal primary. Regions of positive cervical adenopathy are also boosted with megavoltage photons and/or electrons to total doses of 6500 to 7500 cGy, depending on the original size of the node and its response to the first phase of therapy.[334] In selected patients, the boost dose to the nasopharynx itself can be given with an intracavitary implant.[335] Critical normal structures in the treatment region include the cervical cord, the brain-stem, the optic nerves, and orbital contents. Proper shielding and limiting the delivered dose to these structures are necessary to avoid untoward complications. An anterior supraclavicular field is generally matched to the initial large lateral fields, and approximately 5000 cGy are given to treat submicroscopic disease in this area.

More recently, IMRT has been utilized in an attempt to improve the therapeutic index of external beam radiotherapy for nasopharyngeal cancer. Increasing the conformality of radiation delivery is an attractive approach, given the many critical neural, vascular, and soft tissues surrounding this anatomic site. Several investigators have directly compared the dose delivery of IMRT to conventional techniques. Xia and colleagues demonstrated that IMRT can provide accelerated delivery of high-dose (68 Gy) to over 95% of nasopharyngeal disease while improving normal tissue sparing relative to conventional treatment.[336] Likewise, Hunt and colleagues demonstrated the feasibility of increasing delivered dose to gross nasopharyngeal disease with IMRT (77.3 Gy vs 67.9 Gy with the traditional plans).[337] MRT improved coverage of parapharyngeal regions, skull base, and medially-located nodal basins while reducing doses to all normal structures, including, mandible, temporal lobes, and parotid glands. Beyond technical improvements, early institutional data from Memorial Sloan-Kettering Cancer Center confirmed encouraging 91% local and 93% regional three-year disease-control rates in a 74 patient cohort treated with IMRT (with 69 receiving chemotherapy) and followed for a median of 35 months.[338] This group observed 100% local control for Stage T1/T2 disease, versus 83% local control for T3/T4 disease ($p = 0.01$). Likewise, Lee and colleagues[339] have reported on the UCSF experience using IMRT for nasopharyngeal cancer, which yielded a 97% locoregional recurrence-free survival rate in 67 patients, with a median follow-up time of 31 months. There was less toxicity than would have been expected using concomitant chemotherapy and conventional radiotherapy. These encouraging North American results have been echoed by series from two separate groups from Hong Kong, which demonstrated greater than 90% two or three-year disease control rates with IMRT in Asian patient populations presenting with advanced disease.[340,341] Treatment results are related to both stage and histopathology, but many series do not adequately document outcome as a function of these variables. Huang combines the above-listed T1, T2, and T3 stages into his T1/T2 categories.[342] For the clinically negative neck, he reports 5-year survival of 65%. For groups corresponding to T4N--N2 and T4N3, he found respective 5-year survivals of 41.3% and 23%. Vikram and colleagues noted a 5-year locoregional control rate for early T-stage N0 patients of 65%.[343] Scanlon and colleagues found a clear worsening of prognosis with increasing cervical adenopathy with 5-year survivals of 67%, 24%, and 14% when the patient had no clinical adenopathy, unilateral adenopathy, or bilateral adenopathy, respectively.[344] It is important to note that these series were treated prior to routine CT/MRI scanning, which would have the tendency to increase the clinical stage of the neck disease.

A clear correlation exists between the degree of cervical adenopathy and the subsequent development of distant metastases, with patients with bilateral adenopathy having a 5-year actuarial risk of approximately 80% of developing distant metastases. Common sites of distant metastases are the lung, bone, and liver. In selected cases, a failure at the primary site alone can be salvaged using a combination of external beam radiotherapy and an intracavitary implant.[345] However, the morbidity associated with this may be substantial. Long-term study has shown that brachytherapy with permanent radioactive gold grain interstitial implantation is an effective salvage treatment in persistent and recurrent NPC patients who have nasopharynx-confined disease.[346] Five-year local control rates were the best for patients with persistent disease (87.2%) versus those with a first recurrence (62.7%) or second recurrence (23.4%, $p = .0004$). Overall 5-year survival rates for these three patient groups were 79.1%, 53.6%, and 42.9%, respectively. Lesion size was not an independent prognostic factor for local control. Complications (including headache, palatal fistula, and mucosal radiation necrosis at site of gold grain implantation) of this brachytherapy approach occurred most often in patients with persistent disease (28.3% vs 18.9% and 16% in patients with first and second recurrence, respectively).

Although effective in early stages, standard radiotherapy (despite achieving high complete response rates) produces 5-year survival rates in stage III disease of only 10% to 45% and in stage IV disease of 0% to 30%.[347,348] Despite major differences between NPC and other HNSCC, many chemotherapy studies have included NPC patients, which confounds study results.

The efficacy and toxicity of systemic therapy is presently evaluated in trials that include NPC as a distant entity, and efforts are made to define patient cohorts according to the WHO classification. Including NPC with squamous cancers in studies of other head and neck sites will confound study outcomes in part because of the exquisite sensitivity of NPC to chemotherapy and radiation, but also because of the distinctive patient demographics and patterns of tumor recurrence in NPC.

Reports of phase 2 trials demonstrate single-agent activity for cisplatin, carboplatin, fluorouracil, bleomycin, methotrexate, anthracycline, vinca alkaloids, and taxanes.[349,350] Response rate ranges from 20% to 60%, with complete responses uncommon. More recent reports of cisplatin-based drug combinations describe tumor responses in 50% to 80% of patients clinically complete in 20% to 25% of these.[351-354] Moreover, Fandi and colleagues[355] have reported durable disease remissions in a cohort of patients followed over a period of years. Chan and colleagues[356] have recently reported that the combination of cetuximab, a chimeric monoclonal antibody directed against the EGFR, and carboplatin has activity (overall disease-control rate 60%) even in heavily previously treated NPC patients.

For patients with staging III and IV at diagnosis, chemoradiotherapy has become the standard of care. Concomitant chemotherapy and radiation appears to be the backbone of treatment. In 1995, Chan and colleagues[357] reported no difference in local tumor control or survival in a small study ($n = 77$) testing the value of chemotherapy with cisplatin/5-fluorouracil (5-FU) administered in a sandwich fashion as neoadjuvant and adjuvant treatment with radiotherapy. In the United States, an Intergroup Cooperative Study (IG0099) tested radiotherapy–alone arm versus an experimental arm consisting of concomitant cisplatin given on days 1, 22, and 43 during radiotherapy followed by three courses of adjuvant cisplatin and 5-FU chemotherapy.[358] A total of 147 evaluable patients with stages III and IV tumors were entered onto this study. Notably, approximately one-third of patients in this study were classified WHO 1, unlike most reports from the Pacific Rim in which greater than 95% of patients are WHO 2/3. At 3 years there was improved progression-free survival (69% vs 24%, $p = .001$), improved overall survival (76% vs 46%, $p = .005$), and reduced distant metastases (13% vs 35%, $p = .002$) for the experimental arm. The results of this trial changed the standard of care in the United States. These data were corroborated by another randomized phase 3 trial, which compared concurrent cisplatin (40 mg/m^2 weekly) and radiotherapy with radiotherapy alone in 350 patients with local and regionally advanced (Ho stage N2 and N3, or N1 with nodal disease ≥4 cm) NPC.[359] This study found that treatment with combined chemotherapy plus radiotherapy prolonged progression-free survival (hazard ratio (HR), 1.367; 95% CI, 0.93-2.0). The treatment effect had a notable covariate interaction with tumor stage, and subgroup analysis showed a significant difference in patients with Ho stage T3 disease in favor of the concomitant-therapy arm ($p = .0075$; HR, 2.328; 95% CI, 1.26-4.28). The time to first distant failure also was statistically prolonged in patients with T3 tumors of the concomitant-treatment arm versus T3 tumor patients of the radiotherapy-alone arm ($p = .016$). Treatment in the chemotherapy-plus radiation arm was well tolerated.[359] An updated report[360] concludes that overall survival benefits after chemoradiotherapy most clearly obtain in patients with T3/4 staging ($p = .013$). Lin and colleagues[361] conducted a prospective phase 3 trial with randomization to radiation therapy (RT) alone or RT with 2 cycles of concomitant cisplatin and fluorouracil administered during weeks 1 and 5 of RT. Overall survival again favored the combined treatment arm (Table 77-8).

Alternatively, strategies with induction chemotherapy have much appeal because of the high risk of systemic tumor dissemination in patients with NPC. However, a survival advantage for this approach has not been conclusively demonstrated. Chua and colleagues[362] have analyzed pooled data from two large phase 3 trials investigating the role of induction chemotherapy in NPC. In these trials, a total of 784 patients were randomized to receive 2 to 3 cycles of cisplatin-based combination drug therapy then radiotherapy or radiotherapy alone. The 5-year relapse-free survival was 50.9% and 42.7%, respectively (p = .014), and disease-specific survival was 63.5% and 58.1% (p = .029). Overall survival was not found to be significantly different between the arms (p = .092). Hui et al.[363] have recently reported favorable progression-free and overall survival results in a phase 2 study of induction cisplatin and docetaxel preceeding chemoradiotherapy. One can conclude that concomitant chemoradiotherapy is the treatment of choice for locally advanced NPC, much in accordance with the Intergroup 0099 trial. However, induction chemotherapy followed by radiotherapy is an option for patients who are not good candidates for concomitant treatment.

The report of Chan and colleagues[356] is notable as data are accumulating to show that the EGFR is a potential therapeutic target in NPC[364,365] and that high surface expression may correlate with poor outcome.[366] Thus, clinical studies of EGFR inhibitors are underway. Small molecule EGFR tyrosine kinase inhibitors are also under study and have demonstrated activity in SCC of other primary head and neck sites.[367] Surface expression of EGFR, phosphorylated EGFR, MAPK, and Akt are potential molecular markers that may be useful in the future to select patients for treatment with EGFR inhibitor treatment protocols. We anticipate that new molecular treatment regimens will be evaluated in clinical trials of promising induction systemic therapies followed by chemoradiotherapy. This approach uses the induction (neoadjuvant) format as a vehicle to test new drug compounds or regimens in treatment-naïve patients, while retaining active therapeutic programs administered with curative intent.

Nose and Paranasal Sinuses

As mentioned previously, the nose and the paranasal sinuses pose a unique set of problems that deserve separate consideration from SCC of the UADT. Although SCC is still the most common histology, it accounts for less than 50% of disease. The three most common malignant histologies of the paranasal sinuses are SCC, adenocarcinoma and adenoid cystic carcinoma, but a number of other histologies are prevalent in this region, including sinonasal undifferentiated carcinoma (SNUC), neuroendocrine carcinoma, and esthesioneuroblastoma (often referred to as olfactory neuroblastoma).

Cancer of the nose and paranasal sinuses is relatively rare (Table 77-9).When taken as a whole, these malignancies account for only 0.2% to 0.8% of cancers diagnosed annually, or approximately 3% of cancers of the UADT. The incidence is generally reported as 0.3 to 1 per 100,000 population.[368-370] These cancers tend to occur most commonly in the fifth decade of life, although they can occur at any age. Cancer of the nose and paranasal sinuses is rare in children except for some sarcomas, such as rhabdomyosarcoma.[371,372] Although there are numerous environmental factors associated with cancer of the nose and paranasal sinuses, as industry has modernized, these have become somewhat less important. There continues to be a relationship between these malignancies and tobacco exposure, however.[373]

Table 77-8 Selected Concomitant Chemoradiotherapy Trials in Locally Advanced NPC

Study	*n*	Treatment Arms	Outcomes
Al-Sarraf et al.[358]	78	cddp 100 mg/m² weeks 1,4,7-RT + adj cddp/fu	5-yr PFS 58% and OS 67% CM vs 29% 29% and 37% RT
	69	RT	(p < .001)
Lin et al.[361]	141	cddp 20 mg/m²/day +fu 400 mg/m²/day 96 h infusion weeks 1 + 5-RT	5-yr PFS 72% and OS 72% CM vs 53% and 54% RT
	143	RT	(p = .001 + .002)
Chan et al.[359,360]	174	cddp 40 mg/m² weekly-RT	5-yr PFS 60% and OS 70% CM vs 52% and 59% RT
	176	RT	(p = .06 + .05)
Hui et al.[363]	34	Doc 75 mg/m² +cddp 75 mg/m² x2	3-yr PFS 88% and OS 94% vs 60%
	31	→ CRT	(p = .12) and 68% (p = .01)
		CRT	

Abbreviations: cddp, cisplatin; CM, combined modality; doc, docetaxel; fu, fluorouracil; OS, overall survival; PFS, progression-free survival; RT, radiotherapy.

Table 77-9 Distribution of Malignant Tumors of Paranasal Sinuses

Location	Percentage
Maxillary sinuses	55-63
Nasal walls	27-35
Ethmoid sinuses	9-10
Frontal sinuses	2
Sphenoid sinuses	1

Neoplasms of the nose and paranasal sinuses do not present early. This is because these tumors tend to be asymptomatic and usually contained within either a sinus or the nasal cavity. It is not until the patient develops symptoms from nasal airway obstruction or acute sinusitis that the patient seeks medical attention.[368,373] Early symptoms usually include nasal airway obstruction, rhinorrhea, sinusitis, epistaxis, and, occasionally, dental problems such as dental pain, numbness, and loose teeth. Late symptoms include cranial nerve deficits, proptosis, facial pain and swelling, ulceration through the palate, and trismus, all of which are ominous signs (Fig. 77-12).

The diagnosis of nose and paranasal sinus cancers is made by having a high index of suspicion in a patient who presents with nasal airway obstruction and a nasal mass. Key to this is a thorough endoscopic or fiber-optic examination of the entire nasal cavity to rule out benign disease such as nasal polyposis or uncomplicated acute or chronic sinusitis. Biopsy is indicated when a mass is found. However, great care should be taken as these lesions can hemorrhage, especially neuroendocrine carcinoma and esthesioneuroblastoma, which have a propensity toward epistaxis. When taking a patient to the operating room for an endoscopic examination and biopsy, a frozen section should be obtained.[368] It is critical to consider minimizing exposure of uninvolved structures, therefore, biopsy only should be performed without Caldwell Luc procedures, septoplasty, or entry into uninvolved sinuses. Although it may be impossible to determine the exact histology of a particular lesion on frozen section, the pathologist is usually able to make a distinction between benign and malignant histology. This allows the surgeon to terminate the procedure if a more extensive resection is necessary in the management of an aggressive tumor.

When evaluating the patient with a sinonasal mass, imaging plays an important part in not only the diagnosis and staging of these lesions, but also the surgical planning. CT and MRI both play important roles in the evaluation of sinonasal neoplasms.[368,373] The combination of CT and MRI provides useful information for surgical planning,

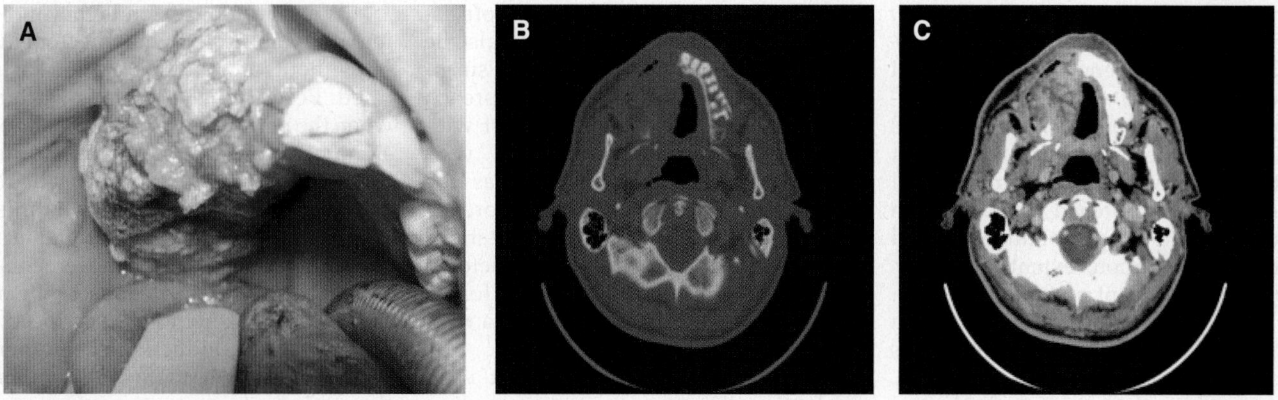

Figure 77-12 (A) T4 SCCA of the maxillary sinus, with extension into the oral cavity. (B) Bone windows on CT scan reveals complete replacement of the maxillary sinus with tumor and destruction of the pterygoid plates. (C) Soft tissue windows reveal extra-osseous extension into the midface.

especially with regard to skull-base involvement. Although CT provides more information regarding bony anatomy and helps with surgical planning, MRI is better at assessing perineural involvement and skull-base involvement and is better able to distinguish neoplasm from inspissated mucus.

The staging of cancer of the paranasal sinuses is made radiographically.[369,371,374] Because these malignancies rarely present as early stage, the accepted staging systems are not commonly used in clinical practice; however, for completeness, they are provided for the maxillary sinuses and for the ethmoid sinuses (Tables 77-10 and 77-11). Special note is made of "Ohngren's line," or the malignant plane. The plane is defined by an imaginary line drawn from the medial canthus to the ipsilateral angle of mandible and passes through the infraorbital foramen. Tumors above this line (suprastructure) are unfavorable, while those below (infrastructure) are considered favorable.

Table 77-10 **AJCC Staging for Malignant Primary Tumors of Maxillary Sinuses**

TNM	Staging Characteristics
Tx	Primary tumor cannot be assessed
T0	No evidence of primary tumor
Tis	Carcinoma in situ
T1	Tumor limited to antral mucosa and without invasion or erosion of bone
T2	Tumor casing bone erosion or destruction (except the posterior wall or orbit)
T3	Tumor invades any of the following: posterior wall of the maxillary sinus, subcutaneous tissues, skin of cheek, floor or medial wall of orbit, infratemporal fossa, pterygoid plates, ethmoid sinuses
T4	Tumor invades orbital contents and/or extends to orbital apex, cribriform plate, skull base, nasopharynx, sphenoid or frontal sinuses

Table 77-11 **Primary Tumor Staging Characteristics for Carcinoma of Ethmoid Sinuses**

TNM	Tumor Extent
T1	Tumor confined to the ethmoid sinuses
T2	Tumor extends to the nasal cavity
T3	Tumor extends to the anterior orbit and/or maxillary sinuses
T4	Tumor exhibits extension to the orbital apex, sphenoid or frontal sinuses, or intracranially and/or to external nose

Histology The histology of neoplasms of the nose and paranasal sinuses is varied and can be divided into benign and malignant disease.[368,371,375,376] The most common sinonasal tumor, by far, is benign allergic nasal polyposis. If this is excluded, then the relationship between benign and malignant disease is approximately one to one. The most frequent malignant histologies are listed in Table 77-12. After benign nasal polyposis, inverting papilloma accounts for the majority of noninflammatory pathologies. It is generally felt that inverting papillomas arise from the squamous, or Schneiderian, mucosa. Although inverting papillomas are benign, they can be very aggressive locally, causing destruction of vital structures, invasion of the orbit, diplopia, and significant deformities. Furthermore, these are associated with an approximately 15% incidence of malignancy. As a result of their aggressive nature and risk of malignancy, all inverting papillomas should be excised promptly and completely. Varied approaches exist for the resection of inverting papilloma. These approaches vary in terms of their cosmetic impact on the patient but also in their ability to access different areas of the sinonasal cavities. Although cosmesis is important, the surgeon must maintain complete excision of the inverting papilloma as his primary goal. Despite complete excision, these tumors can recur locally (9%) and degenerate into malignant disease. As sarcomas and salivary gland malignancies are covered in separate sections, this section will deal only with SCC, SNUC, neuroendocrine carcinoma, and esthesioneuroblastoma.

Table 77-12 **Most Frequent Histologies Found in Malignant Tumors of Nose and Paranasal Sinuses**

Squamous cell carcinoma
Sinonasal undifferentiated carcinoma (SNUC)
Neuroendocrine carcinoma
Melanoma
Adenocarcinoma
Salivary gland neoplasms
Sarcomas
Esthesioneuroblastoma (olfactory neuroblastoma)
Metastases

Treatment The treatment of neoplasms of the sinonasal cavity are varied and primarily determined by the histology.[374,377-380] Traditionally, surgery with postoperative radiotherapy has been advocated for many of these tumors, with some exception. Although very effective for smaller tumors of select histologies, this approach provides poor control in many instances. This is because these tumors usually present with advanced disease involving the orbit, skull base and soft tissues of the face. The shortcomings of traditional treatment have led to the incorporation of new approaches, including chemotherapy. Due to the poor outcomes associated with this disease, a role for chemotherapy is evolving. An induction based approach, with patients triaged to either concurrent chemoradiotherapy or surgery with postoperational radiation based upon the response to chemotherapy, is currently under investigation among patients with advanced tumors.

A complete discussion of the surgical management of paranasal sinus malignancies is beyond the scope of this chapter, but highlights of surgical considerations will be briefly presented. A distinction between the surgical approach and the type of resection must be made. Surgical approaches include (1) open transfacial; (2) midface degloving/sublabial; and (3) endoscopic. Surgical resections include: (1) medial maxillectomy; (2) infrastructure maxillectomy; (3) total maxillectomy with or without orbital exenteration; and (4) craniofacial resection. The approach and resection utilized should be personalized, based upon tumor location, extent, histology, cosmesis, and patient preference.

The open lateral rhinotomy incision lies along the side of the nose and extends from the medial canthus to the nasal ala, extending into the nasal vestibule and allows excellent visualization of the nasal cavity (Fig. 77-13). It provides excellent exposure for tumors of the lateral nasal wall and septum, which can be managed with medial maxillectomy and septectomy. The midface degloving approach avoids external incisions but offers limited lateral and superior exposure, and requires a thorough understanding of rhinoplasty techniques. Nasal deformity is a common postoperative complication.

For total maxillectomy, the lateral rhinotomy incision can be combined with lip-splitting and infraorbital extensions to provide greater access to the orbit, lateral maxilla, zygoma and masticator space. Cosmesis and ectropion are concerns, but this incision provides the necessary exposure to the lateral maxilla for performing extended resections. This incision can also incorporate an orbital exenteration when necessary. An alternative approach entails extending the lateral rhinotomy into the Lynch incision and may avoid postoperative ectropion without sacrificing surgical access.

The endoscopic approach is being increasingly used in the management of paranasal sinus cancers. This approach provides excellent visualization with angled telescopes, the ability to remove bone with high-speed drills and soft tissue with microdebriders, and can also be complemented by intraoperative surgical navigation. However, this approach requires a high degree of comfort with the technology and experience with endoscopic techniques, as well as the ability to convert to an open approach when necessary. Some of the limitations include: inability to repair large defects, access to the orbit, and the need for an experienced surgical assistant for a two-handed technique.

Medial maxillectomy is best used for benign disease or those diseases limited to the medial wall of the maxilla or lateral wall of the nasal cavity. It can be performed through a lateral rhinotomy, midface degloving or endoscopic approach. This is a very effective operation for inverting papilloma and requires no reconstruction. Meticulous closure of the lateral rhinotomy usually leads to a very favorable cosmetic result as well.

Maxillectomy includes removal of the antral walls of the maxillary sinus but leaves the orbital periosteum and the malar strut. It is indicated for T1 and T2 lesions of the maxillary antrum without erosion beyond the sinus. This operation can be tailored to a particular tumor in order to decrease postoperative morbidity. Specifically, when feasible, rather than making a straight midline incision through the palate, the palatal excision can be curved away from the premaxilla, thus saving the incisors and cuspids. This provides a better functional result postoperatively. In addition, the orbital floor can also be preserved if the tumor is located inferiorly. This prevents diplopia, enophthalmos, and helps to prevent contracture of the skin, and avoids ectropion. The reconstruction of this defect is usually limited to a split-thickness skin graft and prosthetic rehabilitation.

When tumor extends beyond the maxillary sinus, total maxillectomy with or without orbital exenteration is indicated. Resection of the eye is warranted when the periorbita is breached, although significant controversy surrounds the indications for exenteration, particularly .when only the orbital periosteum is involved. In instances when orbital fat and especially if extraocular movements are restricted because of muscle involvement, the eye should be sacrificed. Innovations with induction chemotherapy may eventually lead to preservation of the eye in certain situations. Once again, reconstruction is best accomplished through the use of a split-thickness skin graft and prosthesis. Occasionally, a free flap may be required for more extensive resections or to protect the osseous skull base, which frequently will be postoperatively managed by radiation therapy.

Finally, combined craniofacial resections are indicated when tumors extend to the skull base. Although many combined operations can be performed exclusively from below by an experienced head and neck surgeon, combination with neurosurgery allows approach of the tumor from above, and protects the brain from iatrogenic injury. In this situation, a pericranial flap is usually used to resurface the sinonasal roof and protect dura and intracranial contents. If significant facial or orbital resection is performed, a free flap will be needed to protect the cranial vault and provide midface soft tissue bulk. A role for robotic surgical approaches to the skull base is currently under investigation by a number of groups, but has not found widespread use to date.

The complications of these operations are varied and depend on the particular approach utilized. The most common problem is dysfunction of the

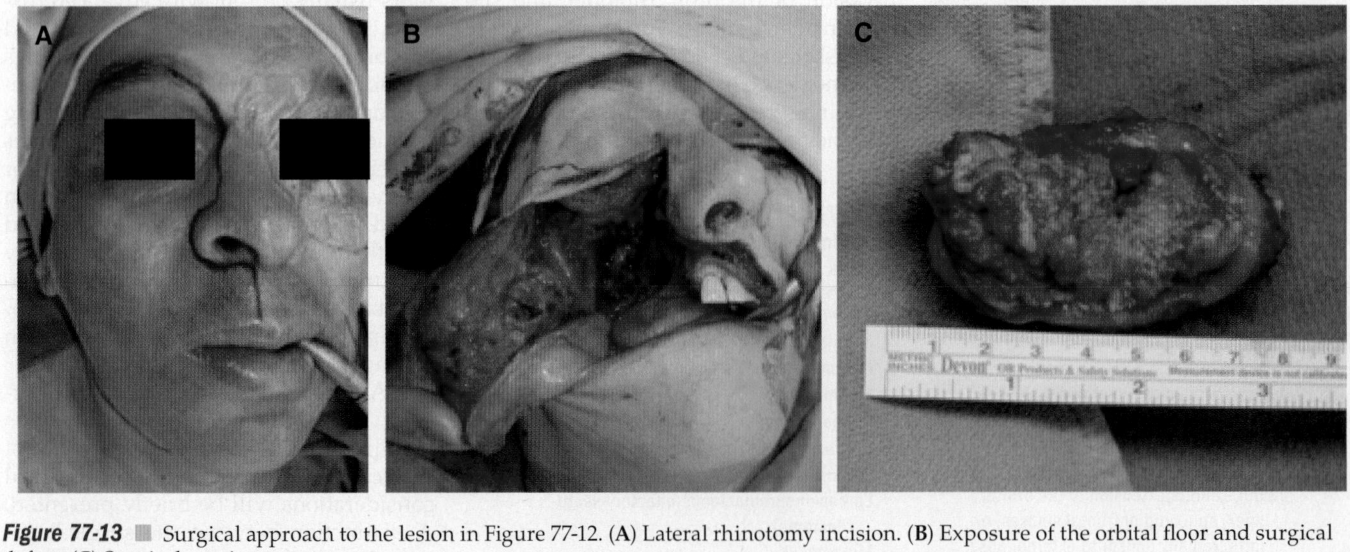

Figure 77-13 Surgical approach to the lesion in Figure 77-12. (**A**) Lateral rhinotomy incision. (**B**) Exposure of the orbital floor and surgical defect. (**C**) Surgical specimen.

lacrimal apparatus. This is especially important for patients who are likely to receive postoperative radiation therapy. Marsupialization of the lacrimal duct at the time of surgery can avoid lacrimal obstruction, but a formal dacryocystorhinostomy (DCR) may be performed when there is disruption of the lacrimal apparatus. In addition, as many as 20% of patients will have postoperative diplopia owing to loss of support from the bony floor. Despite tethering of the medial canthus along the nasal bones and supporting the eye medially, this problem persists. Early intervention by ophthalmology is beneficial. Reconstruction of the orbital floor with a free bone graft or titanium can be effective, but can pose problems with wound care and healing when postoperative radiation is administered. In addition, posttreatment surveillance can be difficult when the maxilla has been reconstructed. The indications for orbital reconstruction are not clear and deciding whom to reconstruct is the subject of current investigations. With combined craniofacial resections, pneumocephalus is a dreaded life-threatening complication. It has previously been felt that tracheostomy should be performed in all craniofacial patients to decrease the risk of pneumocephalus, but with meticulous closure of the pericranial flap and the use of free flaps as indicated, however, we have not found this to be the case. Rarely do we feel that tracheostomy is indicated for combined craniofacial resections. Pneumocephalus is also an indication of a persistent cerebrospinal fluid leak that can often lead to meningitis and death.

Radiotherapy plays a major role in the management of sinonasal malignancies. It is used both preoperatively and postoperatively and can be used in select cases as definitive therapy for small T1 and T2 lesions, especially those limited to the nasal vestibule and anterior nasal cavity.[381] In this situation, high locoregional control rates and good cosmetic outcome should be expected. With the increased use of radiotherapy in combination with surgery, ever-improving rates of locoregional control have been achieved. However, this has also lead to higher recognized rates of distant metastasis. Surgery with postoperative radiation therapy remains the standard of care for advanced sinonasal cavity tumors. As mentioned above, concomitant chemoradiotherapy can be utilized in selected patients. Patients with inoperable tumors or those who are not felt to be good surgical candidates, may be best treated with radiation therapy alone for local control and palliation.

Treatment-related sequelae from radiation to the paranasal sinuses and skull base are common. Acute complications include skin desquamation, nasal dryness, mucositis, xerophthalmia and fistula formation. Chronic side effects include nasal dryness, xerophthalmia, visual impairment, atrophic rhinitis, osteoradionecrosis and pituitary dysfunction. Dry eye can range from mild dryness alleviated with over-the-counter drops to significant keratitis, corneal ulceration, and even blindness. Enucleation may even be necessary for debilitating ophthalmoplegia. Although the retina, like most neural structures, is radioresistant, visual impairment can occur as a result of damage to the lens and/or microvasculature that supports both the retina and optic nerve. Frontal lobe necrosis is a devastating complication that may require neurosurgical intervention.

Although chemotherapy as a component of concomitant treatment with radiation[382-384] is covered more extensively in a separate section, some aspects of chemotherapy deserve special consideration and will be mentioned briefly here. Traditionally, chemotherapy has been used for sinonasal tumors in palliative situations or for patients with recurrent tumors. However, the use of induction chemotherapy in select patients with involvement of the eye has shown promising results in preserving the orbit.[385] Choi and colleagues reported results of concomitant chemoradiotherapy and investigators at the University of Chicago[378] have used induction chemotherapy with cisplatin and infusional 5-FU to achieve improved rates of locoregional control and preserve the eye.[385,386] Studies at various centers are currently ongoing to validate the use of this approach for advanced sinonasal malignancies. Some investigators have utilized intra-arterial chemotherapy followed by surgery and/or radiation therapy for advanced sinonasal malignancies.[387-390] Although these studies have shown some benefit with regard to locoregional control, the morbidity associated with intra-arterial therapy does not appear to justify this approach. For patients with unresectable skull-base neoplasms, concomitant chemoradiotherapy is a reasonable approach that may offer locoregional control in up to 50% of patients.[385] SNUC, neuroendocrine carcinoma and ENB represent a spectrum of tumors with neuroendocrine differentiation that can be difficult to distinguish histologically. Immunohistochemistry is often necessary to accurately diagnose these lesions, which may also be confused with sinonasal melanoma, rhabdomyosarcoma, PNET, or lymphoma. An experienced head and neck pathologist should be consulted prior to determining a treatment plan. Misdiagnosis is not infrequent, and can have a significant impact on patient management and outcome.

SNUC is a rare but lethal cancer typically presenting as advanced disease in elderly patients (Fig.). Traditional treatment has been surgery followed by postoperative radiation therapy, but this has provided poor long-term control. These tumors may be chemosensitive and a response to induction chemotherapy may identifty patients for concomitant chemoradiotherapy as definitive treatment.[387,391-393] Surgical salvage after nonsurgical therapy has a uniformly dismal prognosis, but in light of the poor locoregional control achieved with traditional surgery and postoperative radiation therapy, most agree that study of concomitant chemoradiotherapy is warranted.

Neuroendocrine carcinomas have also been traditionally treated with surgery and postoperative radiation therapy. However, the literature seems to suggest that they should be treated much like neuroendocrine carcinoma at other primary sites, such as small cell carcinoma of the lung.[394-396] Our treatment strategy has focused on the use of induction chemotherapy with cisplatin and etoposide. If patients achieve a complete response, they proceed directly to radiotherapy. For nonresponders and partial responders, surgery followed by radiation therapy is the treatment of choice. This has led to improvements in locoregional control rates, with decreased morbidity from surgery.

Finally, esthesioneuroblastoma, or olfactory neuroblastoma, is a rare neoplasm of the sinonasal cavity, emanating from the olfactory neurofilaments at the cribriform plate. Invasion of the anterior cranial fossa occurs early in the disease process, and eventually involves the brain parenchyma (Fig. 77-15).[371] Patients often present with nasal obstruction and epistaxis. Pathological misdiagnosis is common, and IHC is imperative to distinguish this tumor from other small rounds blue cell tumors. Treatment centers around surgical resection and postoperative radiotherapy Investigators from the University of Virginia reported on 34 consecutively treated patients and the use of preoperative radiation therapy and chemotherapy.[397] They found that patients who responded to induction regimens had decreased disease-specific mortality and had 5-year and 10-year survival rates of 81% and 55%, respectively. Finally, a recently published single-institution trial tested carboplatin, lomustine, and vincristine systemically (median 4 cycles) and/or regionally (median 17 cycles) every 2 months in 6 patients with metastatic esthesioneuroblastoma involving the central nervous system.[398] Our experience demonstrated effective locoregional control and overall survival with surgery and postoperative radiotherapy. Chemotherapy is reserved

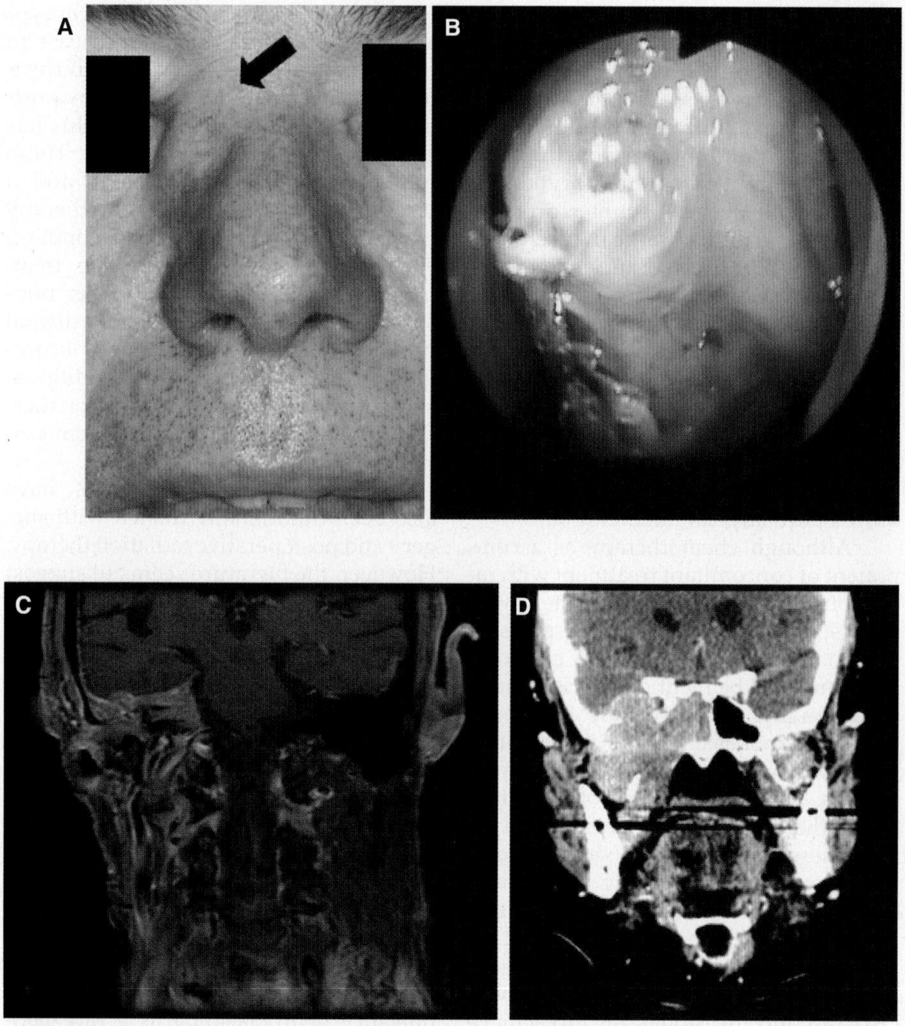

Figure 77-14 ■ (A) Sinonasal undifferentiated carcinoma with extension into the facial soft tissues. (B) Intranasal view of the lesion. (C) MRI demonstrating infratemporal fossa and epidural extension. (D) CT scan demonstrating bony destruction of the middle cranial fossa and extension into the pterygoid plates and sphenoid sinus.

for patients with extensive intracranial or orbital disease that would otherwise require an extensive resection. In the induction setting, chemotherapy may be studies as a cytoreductive approach, allowing complete surgical resection.[399]

Nonsquamous Histologies

Skin

A detailed discussion of nonmelanoma skin cancer of the head and neck is beyond the scope of this chapter, but key clinical issues will be briefly reviewed. The majority of these tumors are basal cell carcinomas (80%), with squamous cell carcinomas accounting for approximately 15% of these skin cancers. Although the skin of the head and neck accounts for less than 10% of the body's surface area, 70% to 80% of cutaneous malignancies occur in this region. As a result of greater sun exposure during occupational and recreational activities (with increased ultraviolet-B exposure), the incidence of skin cancer is increasing and the initial age at presentation is decreasing. About 3000 yearly deaths are attributable to nonmelanoma cutaneous malignancies, and morbidity occurs in a manyfold greater number of people, however, in terms of medical costs, cosmetic deformity, and loss of function. About 1,000,000 new nonmelanoma skin cancers are projected annually in the United States. Treatment is protracted because of the recurrent nature of the disease, the need for repeated reconstructive efforts, and the propensity of second primary skin cancers to occur. Most early lesions are successfully controlled on the first attempt with conservative local therapy.

However, advanced skin cancer of the head and neck is not controlled easily, and its frequently devastating physical consequences can have tremendous influence on a patient's psychological well-being. A recent study (n = 210 patients) was conducted to identify nonmelanoma (squamous cell) skin cancer patients at the greatest risk of disease-specific mortality.[400] The individual clinical-pathologic factors most highly associated with adverse disease-specific survival were invasion beyond subcutaneous tissues (p = .009), perineural invasion (p = .002), and lesion size (≥4 cm) (p = .0003). These patients are also at risk for the development of lymphatic and distant metastasis and may require multimodality therapies, including surgery, radiation and chemotherapy. The efficacy of targeted molecular agents for

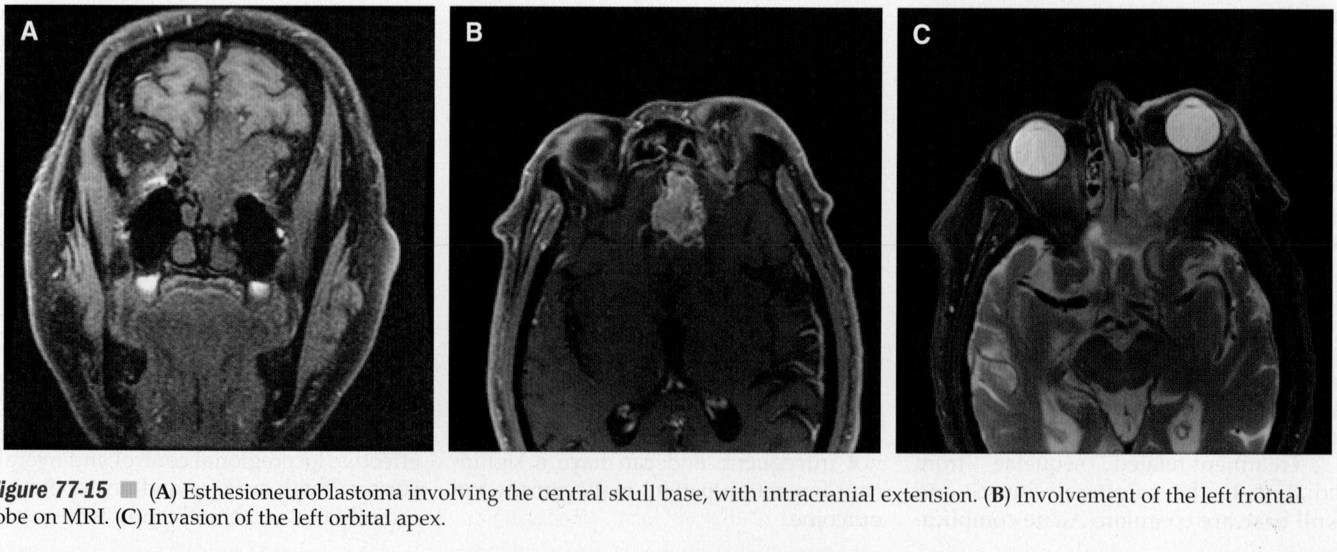

Figure 77-15 ■ (A) Esthesioneuroblastoma involving the central skull base, with intracranial extension. (B) Involvement of the left frontal lobe on MRI. (C) Invasion of the left orbital apex.

advanced and recurrent cancers is currently under investigation.

Salivary Glands

Anatomy Salivary gland tissue is ubiquitous in the submucosa of the upper gastrointestinal tract and is grouped into three major salivary glands: the parotid, the submaxillary (or submandibular), and the sublingual glands. The most common sites of tumors of minor salivary glands are the palate, the base of the tongue, and the buccal mucosa.[121,401,402]

The majority of salivary gland tumors arise in the parotid glands, and although nearly 80% of these are benign, these glands are the origin of the majority of malignant tumors. Tumors arising in the submandibular, sublingual, or minor salivary glands are more likely to be malignant.

The largest salivary glands are the parotids, which are located on the cheeks anterior to the external auditory canal and pinna. The gland wraps around the mandible, and as the facial nerve passes through the parotid, it divides it into superficial, or lateral, and deep lobes. About 80% of the gland lies lateral to the facial nerve, and 20% lies deep to this nerve, behind and medial to the mandible. The internal carotid artery, the internal jugular vein, the cervical sympathetic chain, and cranial nerves IX, X, and XI are in close proximity to the deep lobe of the parotid. The lymphatic drainage of parotid tumors is to intraparotid lymph nodes, external jugular chain, and the upper jugular lymph nodes (levels II and III). Additional lymphatic drainage is to adjacent levels, including the posterior triangle or level V. Depending on histology, many nodes may be involved. The presence of nerves within the parotid gland, especially the facial nerve and the auriculotemporal branch of the trigeminal, can be involved by tumors, especially adenoid cystic carcinoma and SCC, which may exhibit perineural extension. Any parotid mass warrants evaluation, and surgical excision is often the only solution since progression of even benign neoplasms may not only cause facial asymmetry, but also place the facial nerve at risk. Further, benign lesions may transform into high-grade malignancies over time, as in the case of carcinoma ex-pleomorphica.

The second largest glands are the submandibular glands, located in the triangle formed by the two bellies of the digastric muscle and the mandible. Malignant tumors in this location can spread to the lymph nodes in levels II, III, and IV, as well as grow along the nerves, preferentially the branches of the lingual nerve, the nerve to the mylohyoid, and occasionally the mandibular branch of the facial nerve. Seldom will growth occur along the hypoglossal nerve, in spite of the close proximity of the structure. About half of the tumors in the submandibular glands are benign.

The sublingual glands are the smallest of the major salivary glands and are formed of a conglomeration of glands located underneath the mucosa of the floor of the mouth and surrounding the excretory duct of the submandibular gland, Wharton's duct.

Diagnosis The clinical presentation of malignant salivary gland tumors is variable, depending on the site and histology. The presence of a facial nerve paralysis is uncommon but generally indicates a malignant lesion. Tumors of the deep lobe of the parotid are notorious for producing dysphagia and submucosal deformity of the soft palate. When major invasion of the parapharyngeal space occurs, involvement of cranial nerves IX, X, XI, and even XII can occur. The usual presentation of submandibular gland tumors is a painless swelling below the mandible, and such tumors need to be distinguished from the much more frequent bacterial sialoadenitis of this gland.

On physical examination, a palpable mass without superficial ulceration of either skin or mucosa is the most frequent finding. An important diagnostic procedure to be considered, provided that expert cytology opinion is available, is fine-needle aspiration. The objective of this cytological diagnosis is to rule out neoplasia or confirm the presence of malignancy. This procedure, especially in the parotid and submandibular gland, has gained increasing acceptance and should be considered whenever the information that can be obtained will have an impact on treatment or prognosis. The accurate typing of tumor is often less important and may be deferred to the definitive histological examination. This has to be applied judiciously in spite of the high accuracy reported by experts (ie, sensitivity, 94%; specificity, 97%; accuracy, 95%).[403]

Histopathology Benign lesions are the most frequent tumor of the parotid gland. The basic histological classification of malignant salivary tumors was developed by Foote and Frazzell (Table 77-13).[404] Over the years, this classification has been reviewed and expanded to include some less frequently found malignant tumors, and the present WHO classification is most often quoted.[402,405] Mucoepidermoid carcinomas constitute about 26%, 21%, and 10% of malignant salivary gland tumors of the palatal, parotid, and submandibular glands, respectively.[404] Mucoepidermoid carcinoma is the most frequent cancer of the parotid gland and is classified into high-grade, intermediate, and low-grade tumors (Fig. 77-16).[406,407] Well-differentiated, low-grade mucoepidermoid carcinoma is characterized by a slow growth rate, a low recurrence rate after complete surgical excision (about 15%), and rare incidence of metastasis. High-grade tumors are more aggressive, and the local recurrence rate after surgery alone approaches 60%.[404] Local recurrences and distant metastases may occur many years after treatment.[121,408] About 50% of patients with high-grade mucoepidermoid carcinomas present with regional metastases, and 30% develop metastases at distant sites.[406,409,410] Acinic cell carcinomas are usually well differentiated and account for approximately 13% of the cancers arising from the parotid glands. Lymph node metastases occur in about 15% of cases. Again, local recurrence and distant metastases may occur many years after treatment.[121,411] Adenoid cystic carcinomas, once called cylindromas, account for approximately 10% of parotid gland malignancies but 60% of malignant neoplasms of the submandibular or minor salivary glands.[404,412,413] Three subtypes have been identified that correlate to biological behavior: cribiriform type (least aggressive), tubular and solid (most aggressive). A remarkable feature of this neoplasm is its propensity to invade major nerves and spread along the endoneural and perineural sheaths. This has significant prognostic importance and must be taken into account when

Table 77-13 **Most Common Malignant Tumors of Salivary Glands**

Mucoepidermoid carcinoma (low, intermediate, or high grade)
Acinic cell carcinoma
Adenoid cystic carcinoma
Adenocarcinoma
Malignant mixed tumor (carcinoma-expleomorphic adenoma)
Squamous cell carcinoma

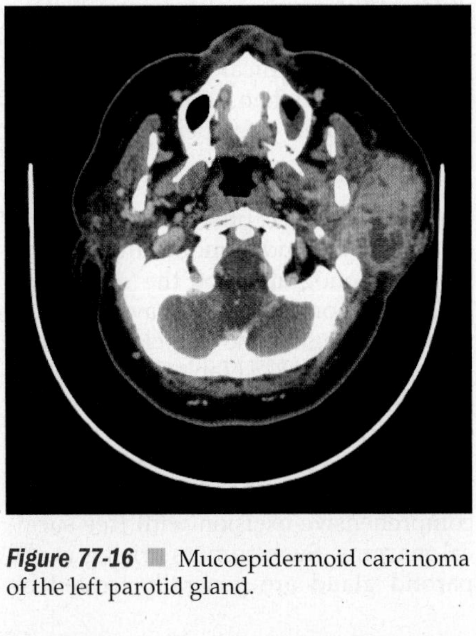

Figure 77-16 Mucoepidermoid carcinoma of the left parotid gland.

deciding treatment and, specifically, when considering postoperative radiotherapy. Although these tumors often follow an indolent course, as many as 40% of patients ultimately develop regional and distant metastases.[412,413]

Adenocarcinomas account for 10% of parotid gland cancers but are more common in the minor salivary glands.[414] The majority of them are high-grade tumors. About 36% of patients either present with or subsequently develop regional lymph node metastases; therefore, the regional lymph nodes need to be addressed in treatment strategies for high-grade adenocarcinomas.[415,416] Lung and bone are frequent sites of distant metastases.

Carcinoma ex-pleomorphica arises from preexisting benign pleomorphic adenoma. The risk of malignant transformation increases with time and age of the patient. Of adenomas of less than 5 years' duration, 1.6% can dedifferentiate, and 9.4% of adenomas present for more than 15 years can dedifferentiate.[417] True malignant mixed tumors are very rare, constituting only 2% to 5% of all malignant salivary gland tumors. These are typically aggressive tumors. The neck nodes are involved in 25% of patients.[121] One histology that deserves mention is salivary ductal carcinoma, which appears microscopically similar to breast carcinoma. The role of HER2 receptor expression in this disease has treatment implications-adding transtuzumab, the monoclonal antibody targeting HER2, may be beneficial in this disease. Primary SCC of the salivary gland is rare, accounting for less than 3% of parotid neoplasms. This lesion must be distinguished from metastatic SCC to the parotid lymph nodes from cutaneous malignancies or from other sites. SCC of the skin of the forehead, temple, or ear may metastasize to this region. Such primary sites must be excluded before the diagnosis of primary squamous carcinoma of the parotid can be made. Primary SCCs of the parotid gland may develop regional lymph node metastases in 50% of patients, a clinical feature that must be considered when patients are treated by surgery and postoperative radiation therapy.

Staging ■ The accepted staging system for salivary gland tumors can be found in the monographs of the AJCC and UICC. Both organizations have agreed to changes bringing the two classifications into agreement[405,418] (Table 77-14).

The treatment of benign and malignant salivary gland tumors is surgery. Early-stage (T1 or T2) and especially low-grade tumors should be treated with comprehensive excision with free surgical margins. Such tumors arising in the parotid gland are generally treated by

Table 77-14 ■ **Primary Tumor Staging Characteristics for Carcinoma of the Salivary Glands**

Stage	Tumor Characteristics
Tx	Primary tumor cannot be assessed
T0	No evidence of primary tumor
T1	Tumor limited to gland and <2 cm in greatest dimension
T2	Tumor limited to gland and between 2 and 4 cm in greatest dimension
T3	Tumor limited to gland and between 4 and 6 cm in greatest dimension
T4	Tumor limited to gland but >6 cm in greatest dimension

Subdivisions: Each of the above T-stages is divided into (a) local extension or (b) without local extension. Local extension is defined as clinical or macroscopic evidence of tumor invasion of bone, skin, soft tissues of the neck, or nerve.

parotidectomy with preservation of the facial nerve. Early-stage high-grade tumors of any histology are treated with surgical resection of the primary site, with an attempt to achieve free surgical margins. This often is not possible, and microscopic spread, especially of adenoid cystic carcinoma, may occur along tissue planes, submucosal spaces, and perineural pathways. The dissection of regional lymph nodes should be done judiciously; elective nodal dissection is seldom indicated except in high-grade malignancies, especially salivary duct carcinoma, mucoepidermoid carcinoma and SCC.[419] Salivary glands malignancies were thought to be resistant to conventional photon radiation, but over the years it has become established that postoperative irradiation is highly effective for eradicating subclinical disease.[413,416,420-424]

Incomplete removal, recurrences of benign tumors following prior surgical treatment, facial nerve involvement and aggressive tumor types are the primary indications for radiotherapy.[420,424] Postoperative radiotherapy also indicated for major and minor salivary gland cancers when either of the following exists: (1) the tumor is high grade or is metastatic SCC, regardless of surgical margins; (2) the surgical margins are close or microscopically positive (which also may include tumors arising in the deep lobe of the parotid gland), regardless of grade; (3) a resection has been performed for a recurrent cancer, regardless of the histology or margin status; (4) the tumor has invaded beyond the capsule of the gland into skin, bone, nerve, or glandular tissue; (5) regional lymph nodes contain metastatic cancer; or (6) if there is gross residual or unresectable disease.. In addition, preoperative radiotherapy prior to planned surgery may actually facilitate parotidectomy in advanced cases and allow preservation of the facial nerve. If the facial nerve is involved at presentation (as evidenced by nerve weakness) then surgery and postoperative radiotherapy is favored.

For T3 and T4 parotid cancer, unless the facial nerve is circumferentially encompassed by tumor or grossly enlarged by cancer, nerve-sparing surgery may be used followed by radiotherapy. Radiation therapy doses to the primary site and involved structures are in the range of 5500 to 65 Gy, depending on tumor type and postsurgical status. Generally, for low-grade mucoepidermoid carcinomas and acinic cell carcinomas, it is not necessary to treat the clinically uninvolved neck. For all other high-grade histologies, the neck nodal drainage is generally treated to doses in the range of 5000 cGy. In the case of adenoid cystic carcinomas, the radiation fields should include the anatomic course of named nerve trunks to the base of the skull.[413] Management of the facial nerve is one of the more controversial and complex issues surrounding the treatment of salivary gland cancers. Resection of the nerve results in profound cosmetic and functional deficits. Even resection of a single branch, particularly the frontal branch, can lead to significant morbidity. Thus, patients must be extensively counseled preoperatively regarding the intraoperative management of the nerve. Compromised function preoperatively portends for poor functional outcome, even with nerve grafting. When the normally-functioning facial nerve is found intraoperatively to be involved by cancer and cannot be preserved, resection and primary nerve grafting should be performed. Postoperative radiotherapy can be administered to nerve grafts, although the long-term functional outcomes remain suboptimal.

Prognosis ■ The results of treatment depend on both the histological type and the tumor site. In a series from The University of Texas M. D. Anderson Cancer Center, 5-year survival rates were 100% for patients with acinic cell carcinoma, 95% for patients with adenoid cystic carcinoma, 90% for patients with low-grade mucoepidermoid carcinoma, 80% for patients with high-grade mucoepidermoid carcinoma, 70% for patients with adenocarcinoma, and 59% for patients with malignant mixed tumors.[416,422] At the Princess Margaret Hospital, primary parotid disease was controlled by surgery alone in 24% of cases and by surgery and radiotherapy in 74% of cases.[421]

In the case of submandibular gland tumors, approximately half of treated patients are free of disease after 5 years, compared with a lesser number of patients with high-grade mucoepidermoid histology.[425] Minor salivary gland tumors, especially tumors in the paranasal sinuses, often present with advanced-stage disease. In the M. D. Anderson series, the 2-year local control rate was 47% in patients treated with surgery alone and 76% in patients treated with surgery and postoperative radiation therapy.[414] Results of minor salivary gland tumors are usually more favorable.[422,426-428] In selected instances for minor salivary gland tumors, radiotherapy alone might be an option, but local control is less favorable T-stage affects local control of disease, and the extent of disease is more important than the site itself.

Neutron Radiotherapy n For patients with large inoperable salivary gland tumors or for patients who are at high risk of local recurrence after an incomplete resection, fast-neutron radiotherapy is an alternative to standard radiotherapy. Fast neutrons have different radiobiological properties when compared with standard radiation, and in vivo data from Batterman and colleagues on the response of pulmonary metastases to fractionated radiotherapy show a relative biologic effectiveness (RBE) factor in the range of 8.0 for salivary gland tumors, compared with RBEs in the range of 3.0 to 3.5 for late effects in most normal tissues.[429] To put this in perspective, if one were to give a dose of 20 neutron-Gy to a parotid tumor, the biologic effect in terms of the mucosa and temporomandibular joint would be equivalent to 60 to 70 photon-Gy, but the biologic effect on the tumor would be equivalent to 160 photon-Gy—a theoretical therapeutic gain of a factor of 2.3 to 2.6.

The Radiation Therapy Oncology Group (RTOG) in the United States and the Medical Research Council (MRC) in England performed a phase 3 randomized clinical trial to compare fast-neutron radiotherapy versus conventional photon irradiation for inoperable salivary gland tumors. The fast-neutron group achieved significantly improved tumor clearance at both the primary site and in the regional lymph nodes. At the 2-year endpoint, the local/regional control rates were 67% for the neutron group compared with 17% for the photon group ($p < .005$), and survivals were 62% for the neutron group compared with 25% for the photon group ($p = .1$). Because of the significantly greater locoregional control rate achieved in the fast-neutron group, the study was closed early for ethical reasons. Ten-year data continued to show improved locoregional control on the neutron arm (56% vs 17%, $p = .009$) but no difference in overall survival because of deaths from distant metastases.[430] A summary of single-institution comparative data is consistent with the results of the randomized trial showing a local control rate of 67% for 309 patients treated with fast neutrons compared with 26% for 298 patients treated with conventional photon irradiation.[431]

Modern neutron treatment facilities allow for three-dimensional conformal approaches to treatment, and this has resulted in further improvement of outcome. Douglas and colleagues reviewed the University of Washington experience involving 148 patients with major salivary gland tumors (mixed histologies).[432] Local control was found to be a function of tumor size, with long-term control being achieved in 78% of patients with tumors smaller than 4 cm compared with 40% for patients with tumors larger than 4 cm. The probability of a patient developing distant metastases was found to be strongly dependent on lymph node status being 52% at 5 years for the node-positive group compared with 32% for the node-negative group. It was found that an initial surgical resection was beneficial in terms of reducing the amount of disease present at the time of neutron radiotherapy.

Another analysis by Douglas and colleagues focused strictly on patients with adenoid cystic histologies.[433] This series consisted of 151 patients with tumors arising in both major and minor salivary glands and who had gross tumor at the time of treatment. The overall 5-year local control rate was 59%, with a 5-year actuarial survival rate of 72%. In patients who had undergone an incomplete surgical resection and in whom there was no skull-base involvement by tumor, the local control rate was 80%.

Neutron radiotherapy has also been used to treat patients with multiply-recurrent pleomorphic adenomas. The initial treatment of choice for these benign tumors is surgery, with long-term local control rates being in the range of 95%. However, some patients experience multiple recurrences following surgical resection. These cases present a difficult management problem since further surgery may entail a higher than acceptable risk of damage to the facial nerve. In these situations, neutron radiotherapy offers an alternative form of treatment. The number of patients with multiply-recurrent pleomorphic adenomas treated with fast neutrons is small compared with the number of frankly malignant tumors that have been treated, but results appear quite encouraging. Douglas and colleagues reported on 16 patients who were treated with a median time at risk of 96 months.[434] The 15-year actuarial local control was 76% for patients with gross tumors and 100% for those with only positive minimal disease following their last surgical resection.

Systemic therapy for salivary cancer remains an investigational endeavor, with no standard regimen universally accepted. Discussed above, all agree that there should continue to be an emphasis on local therapy, most often surgical resection then postoperative radiotherapy dependent on the surgical pathology. Chemotherapy, as a component of primary management, is usually in the setting of a clinical trial.

Previous studies have demonstrated single-agent activity for methotrexate, doxorubicin, cisplatin, 5-FU, the vinca alkaloids, and, more recently, taxanes. Response rates are in the range of 15% to 20%. Combination therapy provides some increase in response but with no clear survival advantages. A regimen with cyclophosphamide, doxorubicin, and cisplatin (CAP) has produced responses in 40% to 50% of patients treated, with duration 4 to 6 months.[435] Responses are more often observed in patients with adenocarcinomas, and less likely adenoid cystic carcinoma. There has been relatively little demonstrated efficacy for newer targeted compounds and more work is needed.

A decision to proceed with systemic therapy should be considered with attention given to tumor histology, stage, time to disease progression after primary therapy, patient performance status, and the pace of disease progression. Efforts are also underway to identify molecular markers, which may enhance our ability to individualize therapy in determining an applicable treatment plan. Most head and neck oncologists tend to separate patients with adenoid cystic carcinoma from others in developing a treatment strategy. After diagnosis, surgical resection is performed if feasible, and for many patients consideration is given to postoperative radiotherapy. Chemotherapy may be reserved in primary management for patients with locally advanced and unresectable disease. More often, chemotherapy becomes a treatment option for patients with distant disease recurrence, and common sites of involvement are lung and bone. In this setting, an understanding of the number of metastatic sites, tumor bulk, and the timing of disease progression are important. As metastatic adenoid cystic carcinoma will often be indolent in its growth pattern, a short period of observation is typically indicated, particularly in debilitated or elderly patients. At times, there may be only slow growth over a period of years. However, if serial evaluations show more aggressive cancer, then it would be appropriate to consider an investigational trial or chemotherapy perhaps with a platin-based regimen. Partial response rates of 40% to 50% have been reported in selected patients for CAP and cisplatin-based therapy.[435-439] Airoldi and colleagues[440,441] have combined vinorelbine with cisplatin in a phase 2 experience with a mix of salivary tumor histologies. They observed moderate activity with occasional complete responses, some long-term survivors, and even activity (CR + PR, 44.4%) in adenoid cystic carcinoma.

In patients with high-grade mucoepidermoid carcinoma or salivary duct adenocarcinoma, traditional cisplatin-based chemotherapy combinations may be more routinely active. In this group of patients, the taxanes are observed to be active as single agents and are being tested in combination chemotherapy regimens.[442] Clinical and pathological data are accumulating, which indicate that the expression of biomarkers such as mutant p53 proteins, expression of vascular endothelial growth factor, and surface EGFR overexpression may predict or identify more aggressive tumor phenotypes, and may also represent potential therapeutic targets. Our group recently reported[443] an early experience with gefitinib, a small molecule, EGFR tyrosine kinase inhibitor, administered in a phase 2 protocol for patients with advanced salivary tumors. We are observing stabilization of disease in 30% to 40% of patients with adenoid cystic carcinoma. Glisson and colleagues have reported that HER/2-neu overexpression is common in salivary duct carcinomas (10 of 12 patients studied).[444] A high level of c-kit expression has also been identified in adenoid cystic carcinoma, but preliminary trials with imatinib mesylate have not demonstrated clinical benefit.[445]

In summary, the emerging molecular biomarker data may have important prognostic implications and hopefully will lead to more active systemic treatment strategies. The observation of HER2 positivity in salivary duct carcinoma may be the basis for systematic study of chemotherapy and trastuzumab in this uncommon group of patients. However, given the relative rarity of salivary cancers in general, formal trials may require collaboration among multiple, large tertiary centers or implementation through the cooperative oncology group mechanism.

Sarcomas of the Head and Neck

Overall, sarcomas are particularly rare neoplasms as they constitute only 1% of all cancer diagnosed in the United States and 1% of all head and neck primary cancers.[435,446] Furthermore, these tumors do not commonly manifest as primary malignancies in the head and neck region except in the pediatric population, in which as many as 35% of all sarcomas affect head and neck sites.[447] The most commonly encountered sarcomas of the head and neck region are osteogenic sarcoma, malignant fibrous histiocytoma, rhabdomyosarcoma, and angiosarcoma.

The rarity of sarcomas, as well as the multitude of histological subtypes, can make definitive diagnosis difficult, and an experienced pathologist is key to the initial evaluation. Appropriate pathologic characterization forms the basis for prognosis and subsequent treatment selection. The biology of a neoplasm and its propensity for locally aggressive growth and systemic dissemination are clearly reflected in its histology and grade. Size and location of the lesion, which have become more precisely delineated with improvements in radiographic modalities, also impart reliable prognostic information. All of these factors, along with the complexities of head and neck anatomy (especially regarding function and cosmesis), make optimal treatment difficult to determine in many cases.

Traditionally, surgery has formed the cornerstone of therapy for head and neck sarcomas. However, multimodality treatment of these tumors incorporating a multidisciplinary approach has yielded encouraging results. Data collected by ongoing cooperative studies such as the Intergroup Rhabdomyosarcoma Study Group (IRSG) have demonstrated improved outcomes for those patients treated with surgery along with other nonsurgical modalities. These protocols also serve as a model for the evolving roles of chemotherapy and radiation either as adjuvant treatments or even primary therapy in selected patients. As a result, many patients, particularly children, are now able to avoid surgery in functionally and cosmetically critical areas of the head and neck without compromising their survival. Detailed discussion of the management of these cancers may be found elsewhere in this textbook.

Metastasis

Metastatic lesions in the jaws may arise from distant sites. A comprehensive review of the English language literature was published in 1994 that culled 390 cases.[448] Of the 384 cases that were usable for analysis, there were 200 women and 184 men with an age range of 6 months to 88 years with a mean of 45.5 years. Eighty-one percent of these lesions were reported in the posterior mandible, with 13.6% in the maxilla (Fig. 77-17) and 5.4% occurring in both jaws. For all patients, in order of decreasing frequency, the sites were breast (21.8%), lung (12.6%), adrenal (8.7%), kidney (7.9%), bone (7.4%), colorectal (6.6%), and prostate (5.6%). For women the order was breast (42%), adrenal (8.5%), colorectal (8%), genitourinary (7.5%), and thyroid (6%), while for men it was lung (22.3%), prostate (12%), kidney (10.3%), bone (9.2%), and adrenal (9.2%). In the first decade of life the most common site was the adrenal and in the second decade it was bone. In older groups, breast predominated for women and prostate for men. Seventy percent of the tumors were epithelial. In about one-third of the cases, the first presentation of malignant disease was the metastatic lesion of the mandible. The most common complaints were swelling (57%), pain (39%), and parasthesia (23%). Radiographically, most of the lesions were radiolytic with ill-defined borders. Prostate was the most likely lesion to demonstrate a pattern of mixed lucency-opacity or predominant opacity. The presence of a metastatic lesion of the jaws indicated a grave prognosis, with the average time from diagnosis of metastasis to death being 7.3 months.[448]

Diagnosis is established by biopsy of the jaw lesion. However, a warning is in order. Prostate and renal cell carcinomas, constituting one-third of all the metastatic lesions in men, both may be associated with impaired hemostasis. Biopsy of either lesion may result in significant bleeding. The definitive treatment is that of the primary disease with expectation of a generally poor outcome.

Radiation Therapy

Radiotherapy plays an integral role in the treatment of most head and neck cancers. Used as the sole modality for the treatment of select early-stage disease (T1 and T2), it gives comparable results to a surgical resection, often with less morbidity. For tumors arising in the larynx, it may be preferred to surgery because it may maintain a function and vocal quality. For advanced-sized lesions, it is used as an adjuvant to surgery in order to improve locoregional control. When used as an adjuvant, it is important that there be good communication between the surgeon and the radiation oncologist in order to avoid inadvertent delays that can compromise outcome. For example, Vikram and colleagues[449] have noted that the rate of locoregional tumor recurrence was greater if there was more than a 6-week delay between surgery and the initiation of adjuvant radiotherapy. The adverse impact of a delay in beginning treatment has been confirmed by Mackillop and colleagues,[450] who found an approximate 10% lowering of local control in patients with advanced tonsillar carcinoma per month of delay in beginning radiotherapy. For advanced inoperable lesions and for tumors arising in certain sites, such as the nasopharynx, radiation therapy may be the only potentially curative modality. Its effectiveness has been increased by the concomitant use of chemotherapy and by using more optimal treatment fractionation schemas (discussed below).

Ionizing radiation (high-energy photons, electrons, neutrons, protons, and other charged particles) interacts with matter in subtle ways and should not be thought of as simply a form of cautery.[451] Tumors and normal tissues

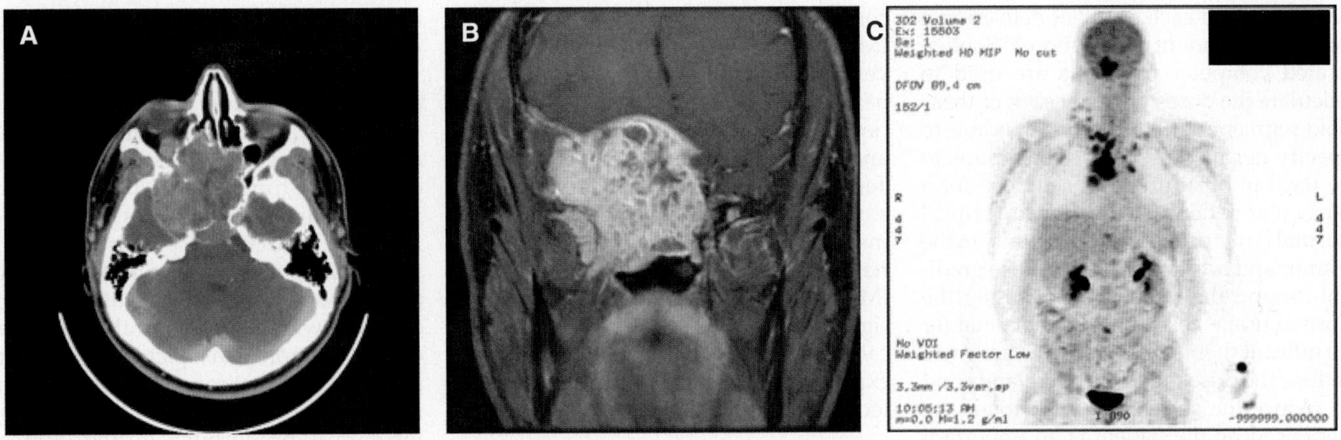

Figure 77-17 (A) Destructive central skull base metastasis from a non-small cell lung cancer (NSCLC). (**B**) MRI demonstrating compression of the temporal lobe. (**C**) PET-CT revealing large right lung NSCLC with numerous mediastinal metastases.

can vary dramatically in their ability to repair the cellular damage caused by ionizing radiation. This makes it possible to use treatments such as chemotherapy and hyperthermia to reduce the repair capability of tumors and to design fractionation schemes that effectively widen the therapeutic window between tumor control and normal tissue damage. HNSCC are generally characterized as being "moderately radiosensitive," meaning that fairly large amounts of radiation must be delivered in order to achieve a high probability of tumor control. Fortunately, the required doses are within the tolerance range of most tissues in the head and neck.

The effectiveness of a given dose of radiation depends on how it is given.[450] Over the past 30 years, various "standard" treatment regimens have evolved to treat head and neck cancer. In the United States, the traditional "curative" treatment regimen consists of giving 180 to 200 cGy once-a-day for 5 days a week to a total dose of 6500 to 7400 cGy; in England and Canada, higher daily doses of 220 to 250 cGy are given once a day for 5 days a week to a total dose of 5000 to 5500 cGy. These two schemas have evolved empirically, and a review of the literature seems to indicate that they provide comparable tumor control with the main debate relating to differences in complications. Various altered fractionation regimens have been compared with the standard regimens in clinical trials and some of these appear to be evolving into new "standards."

Radiation kills the stem cells in the basal layer of the skin and mucosa, and several weeks later, the cells in the more superficial protective layers are not adequately replaced when they are lost through normal physiologic processes. This denudes the epithelium, giving rise to a mucosal reaction that can greatly inhibit a patient's ability to swallow solids and liquids. This does not occur immediately but is progressive after several weeks of radiotherapy. The use of concomitant chemotherapy and/or altered fractionation treatment regimens can make this reaction occur sooner and be more severe. Patients must be monitored closely to ensure that they maintain adequate nutrition during therapy, and often a feeding tube is required. Placement of such a tube is preferable to giving the patient a break in therapy, which can lower the tumor control probability due to repopulation.[452-454] A similar reaction can occur in the skin in the treatment portals, giving rise to a severe sunburn-like reaction. Amifostine, a radioprotective agent, has been shown to reduce the incidence and severity of these side effects, but is itself associated with nausea as a side effect.[455,456] Thus far, it appears that this agent does not impart any radioprotective effect to patients with HNSCC.

Radiation to the head and neck area can cause significant changes in salivary gland function and taste perception.[457-459] The severity and duration of these changes are dose dependent. In the absence of amifostine, there is transient loss of saliva and taste after doses of 1000 to 1500 cGy; doses of 4000 to 5000 cGy cause permanent changes. A University of Michigan study showed substantial reduction in salivary output if the mean dose to the parotid glands was more than 24 Gy. Pilocarpine (Salagen) is effective in maximizing any residual salivary gland output.[460] Both the decrease in the amount of saliva and the changes in its chemical composition allow changes in the distribution of microorganisms inhabiting the mouth, which in turn can markedly increase the risk of dental caries.

Aggressive dental prophylaxis prior to beginning radiotherapy is mandatory in the dentulous patient because the incidence of osteoradionecrosis can be considerably reduced if the necessary repairs and/or extractions are done prior to treatment rather than in heavily irradiated tissues after treatment.[461] If extractions are necessary, a delay of 2 to 3 weeks between the extractions and the initiation of radiotherapy is necessary in order to allow for adequate healing. If extractions or other invasive procedures are required after high-dose radiotherapy, hyperbaric oxygen treatments are helpful in reducing the risk of osteoradionecrosis, particularly if the mandible is involved.[462,463]

Technologic Advances

Advances in radiotherapy have been tied to advances in technology. In the early days, low-energy orthovoltage devices and radium 226 sources were used to treat HNSCC. Then came megavoltage beams from linear accelerators and cobalt 60 units and brachytherapy isotopes such as cesium 137, iridium 192, and iodine 125 produced in nuclear reactors. Modern radiotherapy centers use sophisticated linear accelerators producing photon beams of different energies and megavoltage electron beams that can easily treat posterior neck lymph nodes without risk of spinal cord damage. Computer-controlled multileaf collimators facilitate custom blocking techniques to spare uninvolved normal tissues and sequential changes in field geometry as a patient progresses through treatment. CT and MRI are used to locate tumors, with many radiation oncology centers having dedicated scanners used exclusively for simulation and treatment planning. CT, MRI, and PET scans are fused to give the clinician a broader perspective in locating regions at risk of tumor. Noncoplanar field configurations, often using vertex presentations, are standard techniques.

Intensity-Modulated Radiotherapy (IMRT)

IMRT is the next step in the saga to improve dose localization. In this approach, many different treatment fields are used, with each field being divided into multiple segments, and each segment delivering a prescribed amount of radiation.[464] Sophisticated computer programs are used to calculate the doses given by each of these field segments, and the clinician is able to specify normal tissue dose constraints to be used in obtaining the "solution" for a particular patient. There often are critical normal structures in close proximity to the tumor, and achieving a sharp dose gradient around the target while limiting the normal tissue dose offers the potential for significant therapeutic gain. The ability to reduce the dose to the parotid glands and to reduce the subsequent xerostomia experienced by the patient is an important advantage of this technique.[42] Likewise, additional anatomic regions important for functional swallowing, such as larynx and pharyngeal constrictor muscles, are being identified for future IMRT dose sparing strategies to improve functional recovery following treatment.[465]

Why are these advances important clinically? The advantages of improved tumor imaging are obvious as there should be fewer "marginal misses" than in the past. Another advantage relates to being able to give higher radiation doses to the tumor in a safe manner. Other things being equal, higher doses of radiation lead to a higher tumor control probability. In the case of HNSCC, dose-response curves generally exhibit a steep region, wherein modest increases in radiation dose will give rise to significant improvement in outcome.[466-468] Initial institutional series suggest promising treatment outcomes in HNSCC patients with IMRT.[135] Taking oropharyngeal cancer as an example, De Arruda and colleagues from Memorial Sloan-Kettering Cancer Center reported results for 50 patients with oropharyngeal primaries (78% of whom had stage IV disease) treated with IMRT and followed for a median of 18 months.[215] Two-year estimates of local progression-free, regional progression-free, distant metastases-free, and overall survival were 98%, 88%, 84%, and 98%, respectively. Reported xerostomia severity decreased with time from the end of treatment, and among patients with at least 9 months of follow-up there was 67% grade 0-1 and 33% grade 2 toxicity. Garden and colleague reported our initial results from M.D. Anderson Cancer Center for patients with small volume T-stage oropharyngeal disease.[217] Fifty-one patients were included for analysis. Median follow-up was 45 months. The 2-year actuarial locoregional control, recurrence-free, and overall survival rates were 94%, 88%, and 94%, respectively. Additional series echo these encouraging locoregional disease-control rates for oropharyngeal disease,[214,216,218] but it is important to emphasize that these are early retrospective, single-institution findings; controlled randomized data comparing IMRT to conventional treatment are not yet available for oropharynx or other head and neck disease sites. The Radiation Therapy Oncology Group (RTOG) and the Groupe Oncologie Radiotherapie Tete et Coe (GORTEC) are prospectively studying IMRT for HNSCC in the multi-institutional setting, with results currently maturing. Given the complexity of IMRT treatment planning and delivery, rigorous quality assurance and technical support, as well as adequate clinician experience are critical to the ultimate effectiveness of IMRT.[469]

Curative Radiotherapy

HNSCC responds to radiation injury through a loss of reproductive capability, resulting in a clonogenic rather than an interphase death. Within the context of a given fractionation schema, the amount of cell killing is essentially an exponential function of this approach is to take advantage of the difference in the shapes of the cell survival curves between tumors and late-responding tissues in order to deliver a higher dose of radiation without increasing the late effects of treatment. A typical example for head and neck cancer would be to give 120 cGy per fraction (Fx) twice daily (bid) to a total dose of 8160 cGy.[470-472] The interval between fractions must be approximately 4.5 to 6 hours to allow for repair of damage to normal tissues.

Accelerated fractionation refers to using a fraction about the same size (or perhaps slightly smaller) as in conventional fractionation, multiple daily treatments, a shorter overall treatment time, and a total dose about the same as (or perhaps slightly less than) given in the conventional radiation schema. The basic idea with this approach is to overcome the effects of tumor repopulation by shortening the overall time. Theoretically, this should improve tumor control for the same radiation dose without increasing the overall late effects. Following Ang,[473] the various accelerated fractionation schemas can be classified into three categories: (1) a short, intensive course; (2) a split course; and (3) a concomitant-boost. The continuous hyperfractionated accelerated radiotherapy (CHART) regimen, [474] which consists of giving 150 cGy/Fx three times a day on 12 consecutive days to a total dose of 5400 cGy, is a prototype regimen in category A. The approach of Wang and colleagues [475,476] (160 cGy/Fx bid to a total dose of 6720 cGy with a 2-week break after 3840 cGy) is a prototype regimen in category B. The concomitant-boost approach of Ang and colleagues[473,476] (180 cGy/Fx qd to 5400 cGy, with an additional daily treatment of 150 cGy/Fx to the final target volume being delivered during the final 12 days of therapy) is a prototype regimen in category C.

Model calculations that show which of these approaches would be expected to produce the best results is critically dependent on the radiobiologic parameters of the tumor (eg, α/β, and the tumor proliferative properties [eg, TD and F1]).[451,477,478] In clinical practice, even tumors arising from the same anatomic site and having the same basic histology can exhibit a wide variation in these parameters. To simplify this picture, it is generally assumed that for a given level of tumor control, the required radiation dose for cure is proportional to the number of clonogenic cells in the tumor.[451,479-481] In the context of a once-a-day treatment regimen with daily doses in the range of 180 to 200 cGy, subclinical microscopic disease requires a dose of approximately 5000 cGy, a 1 cm tumor requires approximately 6500 cGy, and large T3 or T4 tumors require approximately 7000 to 7500 cGy.[479] Patients with head and neck tumors are generally treated with shrinking field techniques, wherein the various regions at risk receive doses commensurate with the amount of tumor they are thought to contain. In the past, doses greater than 7500 cGy required the use of interstitial radioactive implants to limit the doses received by adjacent normal tissues. Today, however, the use of IMRT and proton beam therapy also allows the clinician to achieve high tumor doses in a safe manner.[452,482] The summary by Laramore describes representative local control rates and survival data for patients with HNSCC treated with definitive radiotherapy delivered in a standard fractionation scheme.[483] Local control rates are excellent for the early-stage tumors, but there is an obvious need for improvement in regard to the more advanced lesions. Hence, altered fractionation approaches and the concomitant use of chemotherapy and radiotherapy are topics of current research interest.

Many factors affect the choice between radiotherapy and surgery as the primary definitive form of treatment. For early lesions of the larynx, the two modalities may yield equivalent locoregional control and survival, but radiation therapy is perceived to yield a better functional result, making it the treatment of choice. In certain cosmetically sensitive areas, such as the lip or in early lesions of the nose or eyelid, radiation therapy gives a better ultimate result even after reconstructive surgery. For tumors of the nasopharynx, a site that is surgically unapproachable, radiotherapy is the mainstay of treatment. Fortunately, nasopharyngeal tumors tend to be among the more sensitive of the HNSCCs. For early tumors of the tonsil and the base and lateral aspects of the tongue, the overall results between surgery and radiotherapy are approximately equivalent, and informed patient choice should guide the treatment management decision. Radiotherapy is also given following the diagnosis of SCC metastatic to cervical lymph nodes from an unknown primary head and neck site. The treatment fields encompass the probable sites of tumor origin (nasopharynx, tonsillar fossa, tongue base, and hypopharynx), with patient survivals at 2 to 3 years being in the range of 30% to 60%.[484,485]

Accelerated and Hyperfractionated Radiotherapy

An area of current interest in the treatment of head and neck cancer is to use "nonstandard" radiation treatment regimens to improve the therapeutic ratio between tumor control and normal tissue damage. Standard once-a-day treatment approaches developed empirically, and although they are convenient from the viewpoint of operating a radiation oncology department, there is no reason to think that they cannot be improved. There are currently two basic approaches that are being investigated in an attempt to find a more optimal radiation treatment fractionation schema.

Hyperfractionation refers to using smaller fraction sizes, multiple daily treatments, a higher total dose of radiation, and a total treatment time that is about the same duration as for conventional radiotherapy. The basic idea with this approach is to take advantage of the difference in the shapes of the cell survival curves between tumors and late-responding tissues in order to deliver a higher dose of radiation without increasing the late effects of treatment. In the absence of predictive assays that would allow the clinician to individualize the treatment of a given patient, large-scale clinical trials are necessary to compare one approach with another for the treatment of specific classes of tumors.

In the United States, early work using hyperfractionation to treat locally advanced head and neck cancer took place at the University of Florida.[427] Doses of up to 8011 cGy were given, using 120 cGy bid. Compared with historical controls, there was better locoregional control, a greater degree of acute mucositis, and equivalent late effects. The first large phase 3 trials took place outside the United States. Datta and colleagues [486] reported on 176 patients treated in India who were randomized to standard fractionation to 6600 cGy versus 120 cGy bid to 7920 Gy. At 2 years, locoregional control was 63% on the hyperfractionation arm versus 33% on the standard arm ($p < .001$). Pinto and colleagues [487] reported on 98 patients treated in Brazil who were randomized to either 6600 cGy via standard fractionation or 110 cGy bid to 7040 cGy. Their patients all had stages III and IV carcinomas of the oropharynx and so represented a reasonably homogeneous population. Locoregional control was 84% on the hyperfractionation arm versus 64% on the standard arm ($p = .02$). Horiot and colleagues[488] reported on a European Organization for Research and Treatment of Cancer (EORTC) study involving 356 patients with oropharyngeal tumors who were randomized to either 7000 cGy standard fractionation or 115 cGy bid to 8050 cGy. Locoregional control was 40% on the standard arm versus 59% on the hyperfractionation arm ($p = .02$). In all of these trials, the acute mucositis was more severe on the hyperfractionation arm, but the late effects were similar.

One of the most aggressive of the accelerated treatment regimens is the CHART approach. Doses of 150 cGy/Fx are given 3 times a day on 12 consecutive days to a total dose of 5400 cGy. An early analysis of a phase 1/2 study showed more severe early effects and four cases of radiation myelitis in patients whose spinal cords received 4500 to 4800 cGy.[474] This high incidence of myelitis cannot be satisfactorily explained on the basis of incomplete repair of nerve tissue between fractions. However, when the regimen was taken into a phase 3 trial, the cord dose was limited to 4000 cGy. The randomized trial showed no difference in locoregional control or survival but there were no additional cases of myelitis with this lower dose.[489]

In 1991 the Radiation Therapy Oncology Group (RTOG) began a randomized phase 3 trial testing four different radiation fractionation schemas for patients with inoperable squamous cell tumors of the head and neck.[472] Standard fractionation at 200 cGy/Fx to 7000 cGy was the control arm. Another arm was hyperfractionation radiotherapy at 120 cGy/Fx bid to a total dose of 8160 cGy, which was determined to be an unacceptable dose on a prior dose-searching study.[471] The remaining two arms were categories B and C variants of an accelerated fractionation schema. One of these arms was the split-course regimen of Wang and colleagues (described above), and the other was the concomitant-boost regimen of Ang and colleagues (also described above). The study closed in 1997 with 1073 patients being evaluable for analysis.[472]

Analysis of the three altered fractionation regimens was done in comparison with the standard fractionation arm. There was no improvement in locoregional control with the accelerate/split course, but there was a statistically significant benefit with the hyperfractionated ($p = .045$) and concomitant-boost ($p = .05$) regimens. There was also a trend toward improved disease-free survivals, which did not reach statistical significance. As might be expected, with death due to locoregional failure being only about 50% of the total deaths, all the arms were equivalent in terms of absolute survival. The incidence of grade 3 or greater (RTOG/EORTC scoring scheme) acute toxicity was worse on all three altered fractionation arms, with the differences being statistically significant. Only the concomitant-boost regimen had significantly worse late effects when compared with standard fractionation. However, this may be an artifact of the definition of "late effects" as those that are present 90 days or longer following treatment. The "acute effects" on the concomitant-boost arm persisted longer than on the other arms, and hence the difference in scoring. If a longer cutoff time is chosen, then the late effects spectra are the same on all four arms.

The Meta-analysis of Chemotherapy in Head and Neck Cancer (MACH-NC) Collaborative Group has recently conducted a study that asked the question as to whether there was any evidence that altered fractionation radiation schema could improve patient survival when compared with patients treated with standard fractionation schemas.[490] This analysis was based on individual patient data and included 6515 patients from 15 different trials. Overall, there was an absolute survival benefit of 3% at 5 years with altered fractionation schemas (39% vs 36%, $p = .04$). There was also a benefit to absolute local control (8%) and nodal control (3%). However, when the analysis was restricted to studies comparing hyperfractionation to standard fractionation (no trials utilizing an accelerated fractionation schema), the absolute improvement in survival was 9%. Hence, it would seem that an increase in total dose rather than a decrease in overall treatment time was a more effective approach.

Fraction size may be important in determining late effects. Jen and colleagues[491] have reported an increased risk of temporal lobe necrosis in patients with nasopharyngeal tumors who were treated with 160 cGy bid instead of 120 cGy bid. In both fractionation schemas, the time interval between same-day fractions was kept at 6 hours. In the 120 cGy fraction group, the total tumor dose was higher at 8000 cGy, while in the 160 cGy fraction group, the dose was in the range of 6840 to 7640 cGy. The portal configuration was the same in each group. None of the 70 patients treated with the 120 cGy fractions developed temporal lobe necrosis, whereas 3 of 11 (27%) of patients treated with 160 cGy fractions developed symptomatic temporal lobe necrosis. The estimated doses to the temporal lobes were, respectively, 6000 to 7440 cGy on the 120 cGy bid arm and 4480 to 6700 cGy on the 160 cGy bid arm.

Combined Surgery and Radiotherapy

Radiotherapy is often given as an adjuvant to surgery for moderately advanced but resectable tumors. For most head and neck sites, giving adjuvant radiotherapy improves local control for T3 or T4 primaries or in situations where there is pathologic involvement of cervical lymph nodes.

Radiotherapy can be given either preoperatively or postoperatively. The aims of preoperative radiotherapy are to sterilize microscopic disease outside the resection field and to shrink the tumor bulk, making surgery more tractable. Theoretically, preoperative radiotherapy should also reduce the risk of disseminating viable tumor cells at the time of surgery. Dosages of 5000 cGy over 5 to 5.5 weeks are generally given, with no significant wound healing problems occurring at this dosage.[492] Preoperative radiotherapy is rarely indicated today.

In the postoperative setting, the surgical procedure has disrupted the regional blood supply. Conventional wisdom suggests that higher doses of radiation are needed because of the increased likelihood of hypoxic tumor cells, which would be more radioresistant than their well-oxygenated counterparts. Generally, 5500 to 6000 cGy in 180 to 200 cGy fractions are given for microscopic residual disease. If the surgical margins are grossly positive or if there is a high likelihood of macroscopic residual disease, then higher doses are used. Peters and colleagues[493] have shown that at least 6300 cGy should be given if extracapsular nodal extension is found in the operative specimen. Postoperative radiotherapy has the advantage of being given only to those patients thought to be at significant risk of locoregional recurrence based on a review of the pathologic data. It has the additional advantage of not delaying the surgical procedure, which is the most important treatment modality for patients with advanced, operable tumors. Currently, extracapsular extensions and perineural invasion are indications for concomitant chemotherapy and radiation therapy or clinical protocols addressing these adverse pathologic findings.

Although it is generally felt that there is little use for a debulking surgical procedure unless one can achieve microscopic disease levels, there may be situations where a gross total resection followed by high-dose radiotherapy is preferable to treatment with radiotherapy alone. An analysis by the Head and Neck Intergroup (IG0034) showed that excluded patients with positive surgical margins had improved locoregional tumor control compared with matched cohorts from the RTOG databases of patients treated with radiotherapy alone.[494] At 4 years, respective locoregional control rates were 44% versus 24% ($p = .007$). However, there was no difference in survival. Since this was not a randomized study, the authors do not argue for changing traditional resectability criteria, but, rather, testing this concept in the context of a controlled clinical trial.

Locoregional disease relapse following surgery is particularly common in patients with positive surgical margins, extracapsular nodal disease, or multiple positive nodes. Based on retrospective analyses, [495,496] adjuvant radiation reduces the relative risk of relapse by approximately 50%. However, locoregional recurrence rates remain as high as 35-60% in this population,[497] prompting the addition of chemotherapy to postoperative radiation. Two landmark multi-institutional phase 3 trials demonstrated improved outcomes with this approach. In the first trial,[498] the EORTC randomized 334 subjects to 66 Gy with or without cisplatin 100 mg/m^2 × 3 cycles. Estimated three-year local control (85% vs 70%), disease free survival (60% vs 40%), and overall survival (65% vs 50%) were improved by the addition of cisplatin. Acute toxicity was exacerbated by chemotherapy, but severity of late effects purportedly remained equivalent. The RTOG conducted a complementary trial,[191] randomizing 459 patients to nearly identical treatment arms as the EORTC trial: 60-66 Gy with or without cisplatin 100 mg/m^2 × 3 cycles. Chemotherapy improved estimated two-year local control (82% vs 72%, $p = 0.01$) and disease-free survival (70% vs 60%, $p = 0.05$). As with the EORTC trial, this was at the cost of higher acute grade 3 or greater toxicity. The trials had different inclusion criteria, study populations, and follow-up intervals. However, joint reanalysis of both trials strongly suggested significant clinical benefit to combined adjuvant therapy for patients with either positive surgical margins or extracapsular nodal disease.[498]

Systemic Therapy

Chemotherapy and Radiation for Locally Advanced Disease

Induction Chemotherapy ■ Treatment with chemotherapy used in sequence before surgery or radiotherapy—known as induction or neoadjuvant chemotherapy—has potential advantages. It is feasible. Patients are not debilitated by surgery, radiotherapy or a combination of the approaches. Drug activity may be optimal because there has been no disruption of normal vascularity. Effective systemic therapy in this setting is likely to induce a favorable tumor response and clearly there is a reduction in the risk of distant disease recurrence.[192,328,329,499] The potential for induction chemotherapy to affect local disease control following surgery or radiotherapy is under study. Early studies demonstrated that cisplatin and infusional 5-FU (PF) is a highly active regimen[500]; a substantial response to chemotherapy predicts for tumor sensitivity to radiotherapy; and that there appeared not be a major adverse effect on surgical or radiotherapy morbidity.[499]

Discussed in part above, the VA Laryngeal Cancer Study Group[328] demonstrated the feasibility of induction PF followed by radiotherapy for patients with stage III/IV squamous cell carcinomas of the larynx. Patients were randomly assigned to receive standard therapy with laryngectomy and postoperative RT or 2-3 cycles of PF followed by radiotherapy. Surgery was reserved for salvage of patients with persistent or progressive disease. After 3 years follow-up, 66% of surviving patients in the induction therapy group had a preserved and functional larynx. Moreover, there ware no overall survival differences between the treatment arms. A subsequent study conducted by the EORTC in patients with squamous cancer of the hypopharyx compared induction PF followed by radiotherapy in responding patients to laryngopharyngectomy and radiation.[240] No survival differences were observed and 28% of the chemotherapy group survived with a functional larynx. The larynx preservation rate at 3 years was 42%. These studies demonstrated the potential for sequential chemotherapy and radiotherapy to be effective treatment strategies and that anatomic organ preservation is a reasonable therapeutic objective for many patients.

In follow-up to the VA study[329], the Head and Neck Intergroup conducted a prospective three-arm study with sequential PF and radiotherapy as the control arm compared to concomitant cisplatin and radiotherapy and radiotherapy administered as a single modality. Surgical salvage was implemented for patients with persistent or progressive tumor. For entry, patients had stage III/VI disease but T1 and advanced T4 lesions were not eligible. With no difference in overall survival, the concomitant arm produced superior local disease control resulting in larynx preservation in 88% versus 75% in patients receiving sequential chemotherapy and radiation and 70% in patients treated with radiation alone. Notably, patients with destructive T4 primary tumors were excluded.

A sequence of studies has focused on the addition of taxanes to the PF regimen, to advance the antitumor activity (Table 77-15). Hitt et al.[501] compared cisplatin and fluorouracil with a three-drug combination of paclitaxel, cisplatin and

Table 77-15 ■ **Selected Induction Taxane Trials**

Studies	Schema	Primary Objectives	Study Outcomes
Madrid[501]	R: PF / PPF → CT-RT	CR rate, in multisite, stage III/IV cancers (N-387)	14% CR ($p < .001$) 33% CR
Tax 323[502]	R: PF / TPF → RT	PFS, in stage III/ IV M0 multisite "unresectable" SCC (N-358)	PFS TPF:PF ($p = .007$) HR 0.72
Tax 324[503]	R: PF / TPF → RT+ cbdca	OS, in stage III/IV M0 multisite SCC (N-501)	45% 3-yr OS ($p = .006$) vs 62%

Abbreviations: cbdca, carboplatin; OS, overall survival; PF, cisplatin and 5-fluorouracil; PFS, progression-free survival, PPF, paclitaxel, cisplatin and fluorouracil; RT, radiotherapy
Sources: From Ref. 501–503.

a modified dose of fluorouracil (PCF). Responses were better in the experimental arm (33% CR vs 14%) with no overall increase in toxicity. More recent studies have generated much excitement. The EORTC studied 358 patients in a prospective trial [502] comparing induction PF versus docetaxel, cisplatin and fluorouracil (TPF). After induction chemotherapy for 4 cycles, all patients received radiotherapy as a single modality. With a median follow-up of 32 months, TPF produced superior tumor responses, a progression-free survival advantage with HR 0.72, and increased survival, HR 0.73. In the TAX 324 phase 3 trial [503] 501 patients were randomized to receive either induction chemotherapy with docetaxel (75 mg/m^2), cisplatin (100 mg/m^2) and fluorouracil (1000 mg/m^2/day CI x 4d) or the standard cisplatin and fluorouracil regimen. After 3 cycles, chemoradiotherapy with weekly carboplatin was administered. A fraction of patients underwent surgery for advanced nodal disease. A significance difference in disease-free and overall survival obtained, with 62% of patients receiving TPF alive at 36 months compared to 48% of the control group.

At this time there are ongoing randomized studies[192,499] designed to more precisely define the value of induction chemotherapy, in patients with locally advanced disease. After the induction treatment, patients proceed to chemoradiotherapy. Two such trials in North America are accruing patients and both are testing the TPF regimen. Survival is the primary endpoint. We anticipate that future phase 1 and 2 studies will explore novel systemic programs with integration of molecularly targeted components. We look forward to the day when individual patient characteristics, tumor site and stage, and tumor biologic markers will lead to personalized therapy based on validated selection factors.

Concomitant Chemotherapy and Radiation ■ A sequence of randomized trials[228,329,382,384,504-509] and meta-analysis[510] demonstrate that the concomitant administration of chemotherapy and radiation leads to improved local control and overall survival in patients with locally advanced squamous cell carcinomas, particularly of the oropharynx (Table 77-16). However, most reported trials include patients with invasive squamous cell carcinomas from a mix of primary sites. Scrutiny of these manuscripts is advised as the percentage of patients with oral cavity, pharyngeal, and laryngeal primary sites may vary in reports from different centers, and this may markedly affect study outcomes. Most often, patients with unknown primary head and neck cancers and nasopharyngeal cancers are reported separately. It should be emphasized that concomitant chemoradiotherapy is associated with marked, acute mucocutaneous toxicity requiring expert supportive medical care. Speech and swallow rehabilitation consultation is routinely needed. Gastrostomy feeding tubes are placed in a high percentage of patients. The risk of long-term complications such as osteonecrosis and oropharyngeal fibrosis are under study.

At The University of Texas MD Anderson Cancer Center, oral cavity primary tumors are most often approached surgically if there are no medical contraindications. As discussed in this chapter, cancers of the oral tongue, FOM, and buccal surface are amenable to surgical resection followed by reconstructive procedures. Depending upon tumor histology, size, pathologic margins, and the extent of nodal involvement, postoperative radiotherapy is administered. An older French study[511] tested weekly cisplatin and concomitant radiotherapy. Recent trials[191,498,512] have explored the potential value of postoperative chemoradiotherapy with cisplatin administered every 3 weeks in "high-risk" patients (Table 77-17). In a review of data from these American and European studies, it appears that patients with positive surgical margins

Table 77-16 ■ **Selected Randomized Trials Comparing Radiotherapy With Concomitant Chemoradiotherapy**

Authors	Year	No. of Patients	Chemotherapy	Radiation (GY)	Survival Benefit	Locoregional Control Benefit
Jeremic et al.[585]	1997	159	P	70	Yes	Yes
Al-Sarraf et al.[358b]	1998	147	P	70	Yes	Yes
Jeremic et al.[507]	2000	130	P	77	Yes	Yes
Adelstein et al.[504]	2003	295	P	70	Yes	Yes
Huguenin et al.[506]	2004	224	P	74[a]	No	Yes
Adelstein et al.[586]	1997	100	PF	66-72	Yes[c]	Yes
Wendt et al.[384]	1998	270	PFL	70.2[a] (split)	Yes	Yes
Brizel et al.[382]	1998	116	PF	70-75[a]	Yes	Yes
Calais et al.[228]	1999	226	CpF	70	Yes	Yes
Staar et al.[509]	2001	240	CpF	69.9[a]	Yes[d]	Yes[d]
Budach et al.[505]	2005	384	MF	70.6-77.6[a]	Yes	Yes
Bensadoun et al.[587]	2006	163	PF	75.6-80.4[a]	Yes	Yes

Abbreviations: Cp, carboplatin; F, fluorouracil; L, leucovorin; M, mitomycin; P, cisplatin.
[a]Altered fractionation radiation.
[b]Disease-free survival.
[c]Relapse-free survival.
[d]Oropharynx cancer subset.
Source: Modified after Ref. 195.

Table 77-17 Postoperative Radiotherapy After Definitive Surgical Resection for High-Risk SCCHN With or Without Cisplatin: Phase 3 Trials

Study	Eligibility	Treatment Arms	n	Outcomes
Bachaud et al.[511]	Stage III/IV and nodal ECS	RT (65-74 Gy, 1.7qd) vs RT + weekly cddp, 50 mg	44 39	LRC 77% CM vs 59% RT (p = .08); 5-yr OS 36% CM vs 13% RT (p< .01)
RTOG 9501[191]	Microsurgically involved surgical margins, ≥2 nodal metastases, or ECS	RT (60-66 Gy, 2 Gy qd vs RT + cddp (100 mg/m² dL, 22, 43)	231 228	2-yr LRC 82% CM vs 72% RT (p = .04)
EORTC [512]	pT3/4 or any N2/3, ≈ margins, ECS, perineural infiltration, or vascular tumor emboli	RT (54-66 Gy, 2Gy qd) vs RT + cddp (100 mg/m² dL, 22, 43)	167 167	5-yr LRC 82% CM vs 69% RT (p = .007); 5yr OS 53% CM vs 40% RT (p = .02)

Abbreviations: cddp, cisplatin; CM, combined modality treatment; ECS, extracapsular spread; LRC, locoregional control; OS, overall survival; RT, radiotherapy; SCCHN, squamous cell carcinoma of the oral cavity, pharynx, larynx.

or the presence of extra-capsular nodal involvement were most likely to benefit from "combined therapy" rather than with radiotherapy administered as a single modality.[512] Disease-free survival was significantly longer after chemoradiotherapy (HR for recurrent disease or death 0.78, p = .04), but not overall survival in the RTOG/Intergroup study,[191] while significant advantages for both local control and survival were observed by the EORTC[498] despite use of virtually the same chemoradiotherapy schedule. There were some differences in eligibility criteria. Daily fractionated radiotherapy was given with cisplatin, 100 mg/m², administered on days 1, 22, and 43 of the radiotherapy regimen. Notably, acute treatment-related grade 3/4 toxicity, particularly mucocutaneous effects, were greater after chemoradiotherapy relative to radiotherapy alone (77% vs 34%, p < .001[191] and 41% vs 21%, p = .001[498] respectively), although there were no clear differences in late adverse effects in either study.

As a generalization, the data indicate that concomitant chemotherapy and radiation reduce risk of local or regional tumor recurrence compared with radiotherapy as a single modality. Related to this, overall survival improves. This has also been a finding of the postoperative chemoradiotherapy trials discussed above. There has not been a widely perceived advantage for concomitant chemoradiotherapy with regard to distant disease control or reduction in risk of second primary tumors. However, some investigators have reported that concomitant chemoradiotherapy may have beneficial effects on local and distant disease control.[329,499,507]

With regard to toxicity, usually a brisk mucocutaneous reaction occurs with chemoradiation, necessitating the use of oral rinses for hygiene, analgesics, attention to fluid and calorie intake, and involvement of speech and swallowing rehabilitation specialists. Moreover, there is concern that long-term xerostomia, fibrosis, and related swallowing dysfunction may be more likely after concomitant chemoradiotherapy than radiation therapy administered alone. Brizel and others have reported the potential for amifostine, a radioprotector, to reduce acute and chronic xerostomia after radiotherapy.[513] Long-term functional data for most patients have not been routinely reported. In the recent Intergroup larynx trial [329] and the postoperative chemoradiotherapy trials,[191,498,512] there appeared not to be a high risk of chronic deleterious effects of combined therapy relative to control groups treated with radiotherapy.

In a very exciting recent trial, Bonner and colleagues[514] report a prospectively randomized multi-institutional trial in which previously untreated patients with locally advanced SCC of the oropharynx, hypopharynx, or larynx received definitive radiotherapy with or without cetuximab. As discussed below in the section "Novel Therapeutics," cetuximab is a chimeric human and murine monoclonal antibody directed against the EGFR and is under intense study for the treatment of SCCHN. In this phase 3 trial, 424 patients were entered and median duration of follow-up was 38 months. Notably, there was no increase in severe-grade radiation-related mucocutaneous toxicity. Moreover, median survival (28 months vs 54 months) and 3-year survival (44% vs 57%) favored the combined therapy arm with a significant advantage in locoregional tumor control. At this time, the Radiation Therapy Oncology Group is conducting a large prospective trial for patients with locally advanced SCCHN of the oropharynx, hypopharyx and larynx. Patients receive chemoradiotherapy with cisplatin and radiation, with or without cetuximab.

Thus, the current standard of care for patients with stage III and IV SCCHN, who are not candidates for surgery, is to be treated with concomitant chemoradiotherapy. Most centers agree that cisplatin administered with once-daily radiotherapy is a widely accepted approach. Alternative chemoradiation treatment plans, hyperfractionated radiotherapy with chemotherapy, other drug or multidrug regimens, and sequential chemoradiotherapy (induction or adjuvant drug treatment) should be further studied and may best be administered within the context of a clinical trial. Furthermore, the promising early results of the radiotherapy and cetuximab trial predict the integration of molecular therapy into multimodal treatment strategies.

Recurrent and Metastatic Disease: Cytotoxics

Activity of cytotoxic chemotherapy with single agents has been demonstrated in phase 2 trials, and expected response rates for multiple drugs are presented in Table 77-18. Treatment responses are generally more likely to be obtained in patients with ECOG performance status 0/1; in patients presenting with distant metastases or with tumor recurrence greater than 6 months from primary therapy; and in patients with sites of involvement such as lung not previously radiated.

Methotrexate has been a traditional choice of many oncologists for palliation of recurrent or metastatic SCCHN.[515-518] The standard dosage schedule is 40 mg/m²/week intravenously or intramuscularly, with dosage escalation to 60 mg/m²/week, until mild toxicity or a tumor response is achieved. This approach is relatively nontoxic, inexpensive, and convenient, features that are critical to palliative therapy.

Cisplatin is an important component of drug therapy for SCCHN and often is administered in an intermittent schedule (75-100 mg/m² every 3-4 weeks). The dose-response relationship for cisplatin in SCCHN has been studied by several groups but remains uncertain.[519] Driven by the activity and toxicities of cisplatin, analogue development has also been a focus of much activity. Carboplatin is a second-generation platinum complex

Table 77-18 Single-agent Activity in Recurrent Head and Neck Cancer

Agent	Approximate Response %
Methotrexate	25
Bleomycin	15
Cisplatin	25
Carboplatin	20
5-Fluorouracil	15
Paclitaxel	30
Docetaxel	30
Ifosfamide	20

with substantial activity and less toxicity than cisplatin. Bolus carboplatin has a pharmacokinetic profile similar to continuous-infusion cisplatin but with significantly less renal, otologic, neurologic, and gastrointestinal (nausea/vomiting) toxicity. Reversible myelosuppression (primarily thrombocytopenia) is the dose-limiting toxicity for carboplatin.

Older single-agent studies of carboplatin given monthly in bolus infusion or in fractionated schedules produced objective response rates of 20% to 30% in recurrent and metastatic SCCHN.[515] 5-FU has limited single-agent activity in SCCHN. It has been given in varying doses as an intravenous infusion or bolus daily (for 5 days), weekly, or every 3 to 4 weeks. The dose-limiting toxicities of bolus administration are mucositis, diarrhea, and cutaneous erythema. Schedule dependency of 5-FU treatment has received little study in SCCHN, although long-term continuous low-dose infusion (eg, over 6 weeks) may be effective palliation for recurrent disease. Continuous-infusion regimens were designed initially to reduce myelosuppression and seem to have enhanced activity. This agent has most commonly been used in combination with cisplatin, as discussed elsewhere in this chapter. Despite modest single-agent activity, preclinical studies indicating synergistic interaction with radiation and enhanced cytotoxicity with chemical modulators (eg, leucovorin) have led to much study of this agent in combination with other principles.

Phase 3 studies have directly compared cisplatin and methotrexate (randomized, two-arm design).[515] In one of these studies, Hong and colleagues[517] gave cisplatin at 50 mg/m^2 on days 1 and 8 every month versus methotrexate at 40 to 60 mg/m^2/week. Response rates were 28.6% and 23.5%, respectively. Taxanes have demonstrated single-agent activity. The taxanes constitute a distinctive class of established active agents in SCCHN.[519-521] Use of docetaxel has produced response rates ranging from 21% to 42% in phase 2 studies in patients who have not previously received palliative chemotherapy.[519,520]

Combination chemotherapy may produce responses in 30% to 40% of patients, but without significant survival advantages over single-agent therapy, which is usually in the range of 6 to 9 months (Table 77-19). For patients with disease not amenable to local therapy with curative intent, the goal of chemotherapy is to provide palliation with achievement of a tumor response. For some patients achieving substantial disease regression, this may lead to increased survival. In the appropriate context, combination chemotherapy with either PF or a platin/taxane combination

Table 77-19 **Selected Randomized Phase 3 Trials of Chemotherapy in Recurrent or Metastatic Squamous Cell Carcinoma of the Head and Neck**

Trial	No. of Patients	Regimen	Response Rate (%)	Survival (p Value)
Jacobs et al.[253]	79	cddp/fu	32	NS
	83	cddp	17	
	83	fu	13	
Forastiere et al.[588]	87	cddp/fu	32	NS
	86	cbdca/fu	21	
	88	mtx	10	
Clavel et al.[589]	127	cddp/mtx/bleo/vcr	34	NS
	116	cddp/fu	31	
	122	cddp	15	
Schrijvers et al.[590]	122	cddp/fu/ifnα-2b	47	NS
	122	cddp/fu	38	
Forastiere et al.[591]	101	cddp/pac (high dose)	35	NS
	98	cddp/pac (low dose)	36	
Gibson et al.[522]	104	cddp/fu	22	NS
	100	cddp/pac	28	
Vermorken et al.[592]	215	platin/fu	20	7.4 mos median
	219	platin/fu - cet	36	10.1 mos median p = .04

Abbreviations: bleo, bleomycin; cbdca, carboplatin; cddp, cisplatin; fu, fluorouracil; ifnα-2b, interferon alfa-2b; mtx, methotrexate; NS, not statistically significant; pac, paclitaxel; vcr, vincristine.
Source: Modified from Ref. 650.

has become the standard of care in good-performance patients with advanced or recurrent SCCHN. A report of the Eastern Cooperative Oncology Group is notable. Gibson and colleagues[522] conducted a prospective phase 3 trial comparing cisplatin and infusional fluorouracil with cisplatin and paclitaxel. Two hundred eighteen patients were entered. There was no difference in response rate (27% and 26%, respectively) or survival 8.7 months versus 8.1 months, respectively. Toxicity was similar.

In a major recent report, Vermorken and colleagues[523] have tested the addition of cetuximab to the platin-fluorouracil combination and have demonstrated in a prospective phase 3 study involving 442 patients, treated for recurrent or metastatic disease, a response advantage and improved median survival from 7.4 to 10.1 months. There was no unusual toxicity. This is the first report of improved survival after the addition of a targeted compound to cytotoxic chemotherapy.

It is concluded that survival for patients with recurrent or widely metastatic SCC of the head and neck remains poor. Approximately 30% of patients survive 1 year. The experience thus far has been that chemotherapy is much more active in previously untreated patients. There is a pressing need for continuing new drug development and more efficacious systemic strategies.

Novel Therapeutics ■ Invasive squamous cell cancers emerge after the accumulation of multiple genomic events in a multistep process.[524-528] There appear to be essential molecular alterations that are biologically significant, which confer a survival advantage for cancer cells and which constitute the process of carcinogenesis.[524] As we understand better the underlying cancer biology, potential therapeutic targets have been identified and have led to innovative treatment strategies.

Epidermal Growth Factor Receptor ■ EGFR is a transmembrane glycoprotein activation of which triggers a cascade of "downstream" intracellular signaling events important for regulation of epithelial cell growth.[527,529-534] Epidermal growth factor (EGF) and transforming growth factor- alpha (TGF-α) are ligands for the receptor. Ligand binding to the extracellular receptor domain prompts intracellular phosphorylation, which, in turn, leads ultimately to transcription of genes that participate in cell growth. Overexpression of EGFR or its principal ligand, TGF-α, has been observed in approximately 90% of SCCHN.[533] This increase in both TGF-α and EGFR forms an autocrine loop that results in increased EGFR signaling, which has been linked to cell proliferation, tumor progression, tumor angiogenesis, and increased cell survival.[535-539] Furthermore, surface EGFR and TGF-α expression appears to correlate inversely with overall survival following surgery and RT.[533,540,541] Preclinical studies have demonstrated promise for treatment strategies with monoclonal antibodies (eg, cetuximab) or tyrosine kinase inhibitors (eg, gefitinib) that target the EGFR, most often as a component of a combination regimen. Phase 3[542,543] and 3[514,523] trials in humans represent a relatively advanced area of new drug development.

Gefitinib and erlotinib are small molecules that inhibit phosphorylation of cytoplasmic tyrosine kinases of the EGFR. Both agents are administered orally and have been tested as single agents in recurrent or metastatic SCCHN.[192,544,545] Of interest, the Chicago group has observed tumor responses in 12% of patients treated with gefitinib, 500 mg daily[544] , but in a subsequent study the response rate diminished to 3% at the 250 mg dose[192] commonly used for patients with nonsmall-cell lung cancer. Moreover, reports of "gain-of-function" EGFR mutations have not surfaced in SCCHN in contrast to NSCLC, where abnormalities in the exon range 18 to 21 are strong predictors for a response to gefitinib. The oral tyrosine kinases may be administered per gastrostomy feeding tubes, a matter of consequence for many head and neck cancer patients. In these phase 2 studies, an association between development of skin rash and survival has also been observed.[192]

Cetuximab is a chimeric human/murine monoclonal antibody directed against the extracellular portion of EGFR. Shin and colleagues[546] have reported a phase 1 experience combining cetuximab and cisplatin, observing tumor responses in 6 of 9 evaluable patients with recurrent SCCHN. Moreover, tumor saturation was achieved at the generally well-tolerated loading dose of 400 mg/m^2 followed by weekly 250 mg/m^2 administrations. Binding of the monoclonal antibody competes with ligand activation and prevents receptor dimerization, with consequent abrogation of multiple downstream signals. In phase 2 trials, cetuximab was combined with cisplatin in treating patients refractory to platin-based chemotherapy,[542,547] continuing the administration of the platinating agent after adding cetuximab. Tumor responses were observed in 12% to 14% of patients, a striking result in this very poor prognostic group. Moreover, Vermorken and colleagues [543] have more recently reported responses in 13% of patients, similarly platin-refractory, with cetuximab administered as a single agent. In aggregate, these trials also demonstrated a relationship between skin rash and activity.

The Eastern Cooperative Oncology Group has completed a randomized placebo controlled trial testing cisplatin with or without cetuximab in recurrent or metastatic SCCHN as first-line therapy.[548] This trial enrolled 123 patients and demonstrated a 26% response rate in the treatment arm versus 10% in the control group (p = .029). However, the two cohorts did not differ with respect to the primary end point of progression-free survival (4.1 vs 3.4 months, p = .27) or a secondary end point of overall survival (9.2 vs 8 months, p = .18). More recently, Vermorken et al.[523] have demonstrated in a phase 3 trial that the addition of cetuximab to cisplatin or carboplatin and fluorouracil favorable affects tumor response rates and overall median survival, 7.4 month in the control arm increased to 10.1 months in the cetuximab group. Of great importance, Bonner and colleagues[514] have also recently reported preliminary results of a prospective randomized phase 3 trial of radiotherapy, administered with or without cetuximab. As discussed earlier, this study showed that local tumor control and overall survival was significantly improved in the combination therapy arm.

The association of skin toxicity with activity has been repeatedly observed[192,549] and needs further exploration. If indeed this relationship exists, it would imply a mechanistic etiology and, since skin rash occurs more frequently at higher doses, possibly a dose-response relationship for these compounds. Furthermore, this would support testing a strategy of escalating dose until rash or dose-limiting toxicities develop.

Angiogenesis ■ New blood vessel formation is a necessary process for tumor growth, and angiogenic molecules are potential therapeutic targets in SCCHN. Interleukin-8 (IL-8) is a major angiogenic factor associated with oral SCC cell lines[550] and is found in SCCHN tumor samples.[551] Vascular endothelial growth factor (VEGF) is a multifunctional cytokine and a potent stimulator of the growth of endothelial cells. VEGF activates receptor tyrosine kinases, which are located on the surface of endothelial cells, and is critical to the regulation of both normal and cancer-related blood vessel formation. Increased VEGF protein expression is seen in many cancers, including SCCHN, [552-554] and after radiotherapy and may play an important role in the induction of angiogenesis. Experimental evidence has demonstrated that tumor growth can be diminished by inhibiting neovascularization[524,550,555-560], making antiangiogenic therapy an attractive potential treatment strategy. Seiwert and Cohen present a useful review[561] of angiogenesis targeting in head and neck cancer indicating that available agents for testing include VEGF ligand targeted therapy with the fully humanized monoclonal antibody, bevacizumab; small molecule VEGFR2/KDR receptor inhibitors; small molecule VEGFR2 inhibitors such as sorafenib, sunitinib, and ZD 6474; integrin antagonists; enzymes that affect the extracellular matrix; and cytotoxics such as taxanes that may have direct endothelial cell toxicity.

There are reports of the combination of antiangiogenic compounds with chemotherapy and/or radiotherapy. Bevacizumab prevents VEGF binding to receptor tyrosine kinases (VEGFR1 and VEGFR2) with resultant inhibition of tumor cell growth. Kies et al.[562] has combined cetuximab and bevacizumab in an ongoing phase 2 trial with a preliminary analysis showing responses in 25% of patients with recurrent disease and no serious hemorrhagic complications. The University of Chicago group has combined bevacizumab with chemotherapy and radiation with promising response rates in the range of 90% to 100%, and no major observed increase in toxicity.[563] Much excitement has recently been generated by the experience with chemotherapy in adenocarcinoma of the lung. In a prospective, randomized study of 444 patients receiving conventional paclitaxel and carboplatin chemotherapy, with or without bevacizumab, there was a response and survival superiority for the experimental arm.[564] Vokes and colleagues[565] combined bevacizumab with gefitinib in a phase 1 trial in patients with advanced SCCHN and observed tumor responses in 14%, with little toxicity. A solitary patient had grade 4 hemorrhage, although this event was not clearly related to VEGF inhibition.

Intracellular Signaling ■ Newer, targeting compounds that inhibit signal transduction, influence cell cycle activity and apoptosis, regulate transcription, and affect extracellular matrix and angiogenesis are the subjects of intensive study.[524] Most of these compounds are in preclinical or early clinical development and not so far along as the EGFR inhibitors. Cyclin-dependant kinase (CDK) inhibitors are in phase 1 trials. CDK dependent phosphorylation crucial intermediates that regulates cell cycling. Cyclin D is commonly overexpressed in SCCHN and p16, which is a crucial induction inhibitor of CDK4, may be deleted or not transcribed in many tumors. Flavopiridol and another CDK inhibitor, CI-799, which is a structural analog of rapamycin, are under study. Src is activated in response to stimulation of receptor kinases and with EGFR may be vulnerable to targeted therapy. Insulin Growth Factor Receptor inhibition is under study. Alterations of the ras oncogene have been observed in SCCHN,[566] and more frequently in nonsmall-cell lung cancer. Related to this, farnesyl transferase inhibitors were developed to block ras recruitment to the cell membrane and subsequent signal transduction.[567] However, recent studies have raised speculation regarding the actual target.[568-570] In a phase 1b trial designed to test the value of the farnesyl transferase inhibitor SCH 66336 in SCCHN, Kies and colleagues[571] administered the drug for 2 weeks preoperatively to 29 patients. Inhibition of farnesylation was reported in all patients tested, despite the short duration of therapy. This phase 1 study demonstrates the potential for trials with induction systemic therapy as a vehicle wherein new drugs or combinations can be tested with regard to activity, toxicity, and the extent to which there is biochemical inhibition of a molecular target.

Tissue Hypoxia ■ Tissue hypoxia is associated with poor outcomes and resistance to treatment in SCCHN, prompting an intense search for agents specifically toxic to this cell population, particularly in combination with RT.[572-575] Mitomycin C is a bioreductive antibiotic with modest single-agent activity and is under study as a radiation sensitizer.[576] Haffty and colleagues[577] conducted a randomized trial of concomitant radiotherapy combined with mitomycin C or porfiromycin with 128 patients. Local tumor control (82% vs 65%) was superior in patients receiving mitomycin. Tirapazamine is a benzotriazine compound that requires reduction to its active free radical form in an hypoxic environment. This agent has demonstrated synergy in vitro with cisplatin.[578] A phase 2 study with tirapazamine, cisplatin, and radiation in selected patients demonstrated feasibility and activity, with 3-year locoregional control 84% in previously untreated patients with stage III or IV disease.[579] However, the addition of tirapazamine to concomitant cisplatin/RT did not add to treatment efficacy, in an early report of a phase 3 trial.[580] New targeting strategies are under investigation. HIF-1 is a key transcriptional factor for hypoxia associated genes and inhibitors are under development.[581]

Gene Therapy ■ Approaches utilizing adenovirus-mediated wild-type *TP53* gene transfer have generated excitement following the demonstration of tumor responses in some patients.[582] Khuri and colleagues[583] conducted a multicenter phase 2 trial combining ONYX-015, which is a selective replicating adenovirus, with cisplatin and 5-FU in treating patients with advanced SCCHN. A response rate of 52% was observed in 30 patients with fully evaluable tumors. In a subset analysis of patients with tumors injectable and not accessible for injection, there was observed a substantial difference with tumor responses observed more often after chemotherapy and ONYX-015 administration (p = .006). Ongoing trials with TP53 replacement strategies continue for patients with recurrent SCCHN accessible to injection and as a chemoprevention strategy. However, gene therapy remains highly investigational.

Chemoprevention ■ Adjuvant chemotherapy administered as a single modality to eradicate micrometastases following definitive local therapy has not been successful. A number of randomized trials have evaluated the impact of adjuvant multiagent chemotherapy with no clear survival impact.[515,521] However, concomitant chemoradiotherapy in the adjuvant setting has produced very promising results in phase 3 trials of "high-risk" patients (see the section "Chemotherapy and Radiation for Locally Advanced Disease" above).

It is critically important to develop effective chemopreventive agents for patients with definitively treated primary cancers of the head and neck because of the high risk of second primary tumors (SPTs), which develop at a rate of 3% to 4% per year during follow-up. There also is an intense research interest in distinguishing, largely through molecular assessments, between recurrences and SPTs [524], and chemoprevention has evolved, in part, from adjuvant therapy in this setting. A relatively small randomized controlled adjuvant trial of high-dose 13-cis-retinoic acid (13cRA) for 1 year in stage I-IV disease was neutral with respect to recurrences, but produced a significant reduction in SPTs.[555] This trial led to a NCI Intergroup trial of low-dose 13cRA for 3 years to prevent SPTs in over 1000 patients with definitively treated early-stage head and neck cancer. Although better tolerated than the high-dose 13cRA regimen, the low-dose trial had no effect on SPTs, recurrence, or survival.[584] This trial, however, did provide the first definitive proof that the survival rate in former smokers is significantly better than in current smokers, further supporting public health efforts in smoking cessation. Promising phase 2 data have suggested that a high-dose bioadjuvant regimen of 13cRA, interferon-alpha (IFN-α), and vitamin E can substantially reduce recurrence and SPTs associated with locally advanced head and neck cancer.[559] Based on these data, a phase 3 trial (coordinated by ECOG) has attempted to test this regimen for adjuvant therapy in locally advanced disease. These adjuvant/SPT prevention trials evolved largely out of a pioneering program of human chemoprevention involving the translational study of retinoids in oral IEN patients. Further discussion (including the relevant randomized controlled trials) is presented in Chapter 33, "Chemoprevention of Cancer."

New approaches, such as bioadjuvant therapy with 13cRA, IFN-α, and vitamin E, must be developed to prevent second primary tumors as well as recurrences. Definitively treated head and neck cancer patients also may benefit from molecular-targeted agent combinations especially if molecular markers indicate a high SPT risk. The ability to identify individuals at risk for invasive cancer is a focus of trials analyzing allelic imbalances in patients with oral premalignant lesions showing LOH of specific loci in chromosome 3p and/or 9p. At the MD Anderson Cancer Center eligible patients are randomized to receive erlotinib or placebo in the "Erlotinib Prevention of Oral Cancer Study" (EPOC). This project is designed to determine the potential efficacy and toxicity of a molecularly targeted agent applied to a selected and high risk patient population

Current Directions

Systemic therapy is now an integral part of SCCHN treatment. Many patients with locally advanced disease are treated with chemotherapy and radiation. The increasing appreciation of HPV as an etiologic and favorable prognostic factor can be expected to affect patient management and the design of clinical trials. Options for the treatment of recurrent disease now include re-irradiation, cytotoxic chemotherapy, and molecularly targeted therapy. We can expect intensive study of more specific targeting compounds aimed at enhancing efficacy and reducing toxicity. Combining targeting agents, as has been demonstrated with bevacizumab and gefitinib, is also anticipated. The recent report of a survival advantage for radiotherapy administered with cetuximab over radiotherapy as a single modality heralds the integration of targeted therapy as a component of primary treatment in SCCHN. It also appears that cetuximab adds to the efficacy of traditional cytotoxic chemotherapy when used in combination. Thus, these compounds appear to hold great promise for advancing our therapeutic armamentarium.

Selected References

The complete reference list can be found at www.CANCERMEDICINE8.com

1. Jemal A, Siegel R, Ward E, et al. Cancer statistics, 2009. *CA Cancer J Clin.* 2009; 59(4):225–249.
8. Chen AC, Schrag N, Hao Y, et al. Changes in treatment of advanced oropharyngeal cancer, 1985–2001. *Laryngoscope.* 2006;117:16–21.
17. Hammond EC, Horn D. Smoking and death rates: report on forty-four months of follow-up of 187,783 men. 2. Death rates by cause. *J Am Med Assoc.* 1958;166(11):1294–1308.
27. Dahlstrom KR, Adler-Storthz K, Etzel CJ, et al. Human papillomavirus type 16 infection and squamous cell carcinoma of the head and neck in never-smokers: a matched pair analysis. *Clin Cancer Res.* 2003;9(7):2620–2626.
32. Merchant A, Husain SS, Hosain M, et al. Paan without tobacco: an independent risk factor for oral cancer. *Int J Cancer.* 2000;86(1):128–131.
36. Maden C, Beckmann AM, Thomas DB, et al. Human papillomaviruses, herpes simplex viruses, and the risk of oral cancer in men. *Am J Epidemiol.* 1992;135(10):1093–1102.

44. McKaig RG, Baric RS, Olshan AF. Human papillomavirus and head and neck cancer: epidemiology and molecular biology. *Head neck*. 1998;20(3):250–265.
53. Henle W, Henle G, Ho HC, et al. Antibodies to Epstein-Barr virus in nasopharyngeal carcinoma, other head and neck neoplasms, and control groups. *J Natl Cancer Inst*. 1970;44(1):225–231.
59. Lin JC, Chen KY, Wang WY, et al. Detection of Epstein-Barr virus DNA the peripheral-blood cells of patients with nasopharyngeal carcinoma: relationship to distant metastasis and survival. *J Clin Oncol*. 2001;19(10):2607–2615.
60. Lin JC, Wang WY, Chen KY, et al. Quantification of plasma Epstein-Barr virus DNA in patients with advanced nasopharyngeal carcinoma. *N Engl J Med*. 2004; 350(24):2461–2470.
68. Neumann AS, Sturgis EM, Wei Q. Nucleotide excision repair as a marker for susceptibility to tobacco-related cancers: a review of molecular epidemiological studies. *Mol Carcinog*. 2005;42(2):65–92.
70. Hung RJ, McKay JD, Gaborieau V, et al. A susceptibility locus for lung cancer maps to nicotinic acetylcholine receptor subunit genes on 15q25. *Nature*. 2008; 452(7187):633–637.
81. Koufman JA. The otolaryngologic manifestations of gastroesophageal reflux disease (GERD): a clinical investigation of 225 patients using ambulatory 24-hour pH monitoring and an experimental investigation of the role of acid and pepsin in the development of laryngeal injury. *Laryngoscope*. 1991;101(4 Pt 2 Suppl 53):1–78.
83. El-Serag HB, Hepworth EJ, Lee P, Sonnenberg A. Gastroesophageal reflux disease is a risk factor for laryngeal and pharyngeal cancer. *Am J Gastroenterol*. 2001;96(7):2013–2018.
95. Farrow DC, Vaughan TL, Berwick M, et al. Diet and nasopharyngeal cancer in a low-risk population. *Int J Cancer*. 1998;78(6):675–679.
96. Ning JP, Yu MC, Wang QS, Henderson BE. Consumption of salted fish and other risk factors for nasopharyngeal carcinoma (NPC) in Tianjin, a low-risk region for NPC in the People's Republic of China. *J Natl Cancer Inst*. 1990;82(4):291–296.
98. Luce D, Gerin M, Morcet JF, Leclerc A. Sinonasal cancer and occupational exposure to textile dust. *Am J Ind Med*. 1997;32(3):205–210.
111. Saku T, Hayashi Y, Takahara O, et al. Salivary gland tumors among atomic bomb survivors, 1950–1987. *Cancer*. 1997;79(8):1465–1475.
115. Snow GB, Annyas AA, van Slooten EA, et al. Prognostic factors of neck node metastasis. *Clin Otolaryngol Allied Sci*. 1982;7(3):185–192.
118. Gregg CM, Beals TE, McClatchy KM, et al. DNA content and tumor response to induction chemotherapy in patients with advanced laryngeal squamous cell carcinoma. *Otolaryngol Head Neck Surg*. 1993;108(6):731–737.
137. Schoder H, Yeung HW, Gonen M, et al. Head and neck cancer: clinical usefulness and accuracy of PET/CT image fusion. *Radiology*. 2004;231(1):65–72.
141. Kyzas PA, Evangelou E, Denaxa-Kyza D, Ioannidis JP. 18F-fluorodeoxyglucose positron emission tomography to evaluate cervical node metastases in patients with head and neck squamous cell carcinoma: a meta-analysis. *J Natl Cancer Inst*. 2008;100(10):712–720.
145. Porceddu SV, Jarmolowski E, Hicks RJ, et al. Utility of positron emission tomography for the detection of disease in residual neck nodes after (chemo)radiotherapy in head and neck cancer. *Head neck*. 2005;27(3):175–181.
150. Tan A, Adelstein DJ, Rybicki LA, et al. Ability of positron emission tomography to detect residual neck node disease in patients with head and neck squamous cell carcinoma after definitive chemoradiotherapy. *Arch Otolaryngol Head Neck Surg*. 2007;133(5):435–440.
152. Ford EC, Kinahan PE, Hanlon L, et al. Tumor delineation using PET in head and neck cancers: threshold contouring and lesion volumes. *Med Phys*. 2006;33(11): 4280–4288.
156. Baker SR, Sullivan MJ. Osteocutaneous free scapular flap for one-stage mandibular reconstruction. *Arch Otolaryngol Head Neck Surg*. 1988;114(3):267–277.
160. Kawaguchie H, El-Naggar AK, Papadimitrakopoulou V, et al. Podoplanin: a novel marker for oral cancer risk in patients with oral premalignancy. *J Clin Oncol*. 2008;26(3):354–360.
176. Jorgensen K, Elbrond O, Andersen AP. Carcinoma of the lip. A series of 869 cases. *Acta Radiol Ther Phys Biol*. 1973;12(3): 177–190.
191. Cooper JS, Pajak TF, Forastiere AA, et al. Postoperative concurrent radiotherapy and chemotherapy for high-risk squamous-cell carcinoma of the head and neck. *N Engl J Med*. 2004;350(19):1937–1944.
197. Vikram B, Strong EW, Shah JP, Spiro R. Failure at the primary site following multimodality treatment in advanced head and neck cancer. *Head Neck Surg*. 1984;6(3):720–723.
201. Panje WR, Smith B, McCabe BF. Epidermoid carcinoma of the floor of the mouth: surgical therapy vs combined therapy vs radiation therapy. *Otolaryngol Head Neck Surg*. 1980;88(6):714–720.
202. Shaha AR, Spiro RH, Shah JP, Strong EW. Squamous carcinoma of the floor of the mouth. *Am J Surg*. 1984;148(4):455–459.
210. Laccourreye O, Hans S, Menard M, et al. Transoral lateral oropharyngectomy for squamous cell carcinoma of the tonsillar region: II. An analysis of the incidence, related variables, and consequences of local recurrence. Arch *Otolaryngol Head Neck Surg*. 2005;131(7):592–599.
219. Chung TS, Stefani S. Distant metastases of carcinoma of tonsillar region: a study of 475 patients. *J Surg Oncol*. 1980;14(1):5–9.
224. Weber RS, Gidley P, Morrison WH, et al. Treatment selection for carcinoma of the base of the tongue. *Am J Surg*. 1990;160(4): 415–419.
237. Pingree TF, Davis RK, Reichman O, Derrick L. Treatment of hypopharyngeal carcinoma: a 10-year review of 1,362 cases. *Laryngoscope*. 1987;97(8 Pt 1):901–904.
245. Harrison DF. Surgical management of hypopharyngeal cancer. Particular reference to the gastric "pull-up" operation. *Arch Otolaryngol*. 1979;105(3):149–152.
248. Jacobs C. Adjuvant chemotherapy for head and neck cancer. *J Clin Oncol*. 1989;7(7):823–826.
255. Mirimanoff RO, Wang CC, Doppke KP. Combined surgery and postoperative radiation therapy for advanced laryngeal and hypopharyngeal carcinomas. *Int J Radiat Oncol Biol Phys*. 1985;11(3):499–504.
257. Kirchner JA, Cornog JL, Jr., Holmes RE. Transglottic cancer. Its growth and spread within the larynx. *Arch Otolaryngol*. 1974;99(4):247–251.
265. Pillsbury HR, Kirchner JA. Clinical vs histopathologic staging in laryngeal cancer. *Arch Otolaryngol*. 1979;105(3):157–159.
269. Hillman RE, Walsh MJ, Wolf GT, et al. Functional outcomes following treatment for advanced laryngeal cancer. Part I—Voice preservation in advanced laryngeal cancer. Part II—Laryngectomy rehabilitation: the state of the art in the VA System. Research Speech-Language Pathologists. Department of Veterans Affairs Laryngeal Cancer Study Group. *Ann Otol Rhinol Laryngol Suppl*. 1998;172:1–27.
273. Wang CC. Megavoltage radiation therapy for supraglottic carcinoma. Results of treatment. *Radiology*. 1973;109(1): 183–186.
280. DeSanto LW, Lillie JC, Devine KD. Surgical salvage after radiation for laryngeal cancer. *Laryngoscope*. 1976;86(5):649–657.
312. Harwood AR, Bryce DP, Rider WD. Management of T3 glottic cancer. *Arch Otolaryngol*. 1980;106(11):697–699.
335. Wang CC, Busse J, Gitterman M. A simple afterloading applicator for intracavitary irradiation of carcinoma of the nasopharynx. *Radiology*. 1975;115(3):737–738.
339. Lee N, Xia P, Quivey JM, et al. Intensity-modulated radiotherapy in the treatment of nasopharyngeal carcinoma: an update of the UCSF experience. *Int J Radiat Oncol Biol Phys*. 2002;53(1):12–22.
343. Vikram B, Mishra UB, Strong EW, Manolatos S. Patterns of failure in carcinoma of the nasopharynx: I. Failure at the primary site. *Int J Radiat Oncol Biol Phys*. 1985;11(8):1455–1459.
356. Chan AT, Hsu MM, Goh BC, et al. Multicenter, phase II study of cetuximab in combination with carboplatin in patients with recurrent or metastatic nasopharyngeal carcinoma. *J Clin Oncol*. 2005;23(15):3568–3576.
371. Batsakis JG. The pathology of head and neck tumors: nasal cavity and paranasal sinuses, part 5. *Head Neck Surg*. 1980;2(5):410–419.
375. Batsakis JG, Regezi J, Solomon A, Rice D. The pathology of head and neck tumors: mucosal melanomas, part 12. *Head Neck Surg*. 1982;4:404–418.
376. Batsakis JG, Rice D, Solomon A. The pathology of head and neck tumors: squamous and mucous-gland carcinomas of the nasal cavity, paranasal sinuses, and larynx, part 6. *Head Neck Surg*. 1980;2: 497–508.
377. Jesse RH. Preoperative versus postoperative radiation in the treatment of squamous carcinoma of the paranasal sinuses. *Am J Surg*. 1965;110(4):552–556.
378. Lee MM, Vokes EE, Rosen A, et al. Multimodality therapy in advanced paranasal sinus carcinoma: superior long-term results. *Cancer J Sci Am*. 1999;5(4):219–223.
379. Nishino H, Miyata M, Morita M, et al. Combined therapy with conservative surgery, radiotherapy, and regional chemotherapy for maxillary sinus carcinoma. *Cancer*. 2000;89(9):1925–1932.

78 Cancer of the Lung

Charles Lu, MD ▪ Amir Onn, MD ▪ Ara A. Vaporciyan, MD ▪ Joe Y. Chang, MD, PhD ▪ Bonnie S. Glisson, MD ▪ Ritsuko Komaki, MD ▪ Ignacio I. Wistuba, MD ▪ Jack A. Roth, MD ▪ Roy S. Herbst, MD, PhD

Historical Note

From a practically nonexistent malignancy early in the twentieth century, lung cancer has become the most common cancer in the world and, in many countries, the most common cause of cancer-related death. The association between cigarette smoking and lung cancer is well established, and many of the molecular events in lung carcinogenesis have been identified. The long time period between initial exposure to tobacco carcinogens and the development of clinical lung cancer suggests that multiple steps are required for expression of the malignant phenotype, which is characterized by distinct tumor heterogeneity. Between 80% and 90% of all lung cancer cases are non-small cell lung cancer (NSCLC), and most of the others are small cell lung cancer (SCLC). In contrast to other common solid cancers, lung cancer has no well-established methods for early detection, and most cases are diagnosed at an advanced stage. Although there has been improvement in treatment options, including surgical techniques, chemotherapy, and radiation therapy, the overall 5-year survival rate for patients with lung cancer remains low, approximately 15%.[1] The landscape of lung cancer is beginning to change. In recent years, our understanding of the biology in different subsets of lung cancer has improved significantly, leading to the discovery of several potential molecular targets and the development of novel agents that inhibit their activity. These findings are already translating into improvements in patient survival and quality of life (QOL). Most dramatic has been the introduction of the epidermal growth factor receptor (EGFR) tyrosine kinase inhibitors (TKIs) gefitinib (Iressa, Astra-Zeneca) and erlotinib (Tarceva, Genentech). Monotherapy with these drugs may prolong survival and improve symptoms in subsets of lung cancer patients. Furthermore, gain-of-function somatic mutations of EGFR have been identified and correlated with response to EGFR inhibitors.[2] Advances have been noted in angiogenesis therapy, and bevacizumab (Avastin, Genentech), a monoclonal antibody to vascular endothelial growth factor (VEGF), has been found to prolong survival in patients with advanced disease when administered in combination with chemotherapy.[3] In addition to advances in molecular targeted therapy, newer and safer strategies for chemotherapy and radiation therapy are being implemented: Adjuvant platinum-based chemotherapy has been introduced for some patients undergoing surgery for early-stage disease,[4] newer chemotherapeutics such as pemetrexed (Alimta, Eli Lilly) have efficacies similar to those of older agents with fewer adverse events (AEs),[5] and newer regimens have shown beneficial efficacy and safety profiles in the elderly.[6] This review provides a current overview of the causes, diagnosis, and therapy of lung cancer.

Etiology and Epidemiology

Worldwide, lung cancer is the most common (1.35 million of 10.9 million new cases) and the deadliest form of cancer (1.18 million of 6.7 million cancer-related deaths).[7] The United States 2007 cancer statistics, published recently,[1] suggest that lung cancer is the second most common cancer for both men and women (15% and 15% of all cases, respectively), but, as in previous years for both sexes, it is the number one cause of cancer death (89,510 men, or 31% of all cancer-related deaths in men, and 70,880 in women, 26% of all cancer-related deaths in women). In fact, more people in the United States die of lung cancer than of the next three causes of cancer-related deaths combined, which are prostate cancer, breast cancer, and colorectal cancer.[1] In 1920, fewer than 1000 cases of lung cancer were reported, and it was regarded as a rare malignancy. Since the 1950s, however, lung cancer has been recognized as a major public health problem. The incidence of new cases rose first in men and reached a peak in the mid 1980s; a steady decline has been noted since then. The incidence in women increased until the late 1990s and has recently stabilized. These changes occurred in parallel to the widespread adoption of cigarette smoking by both sexes. The decline in lung cancer incidence and mortality among men has been explained by reduction in smoking rates.[8] Recent data indicate that the proportion of lung cancer patients with SCLC has decreased over the past 20 years, possibly due to declining smoking rates and the change to low-tar filtered cigarettes.[9]

Smoking and Lung Cancer

Tobacco is the world's single most avoidable cause of death. The World Health Organization (WHO) has calculated that the 5.6 trillion cigarettes smoked per year at the close of the twentieth century will cause nearly 10 million fatalities per year by 2030. Lung cancer is the most common tobacco-related cause of cancer mortality: One case occurs for every 3 million cigarettes smoked. As described by Proctor, cancers caused by tobacco were among the earliest discovered environmental cancers.[10] First reports on the association between tobacco use and cancer of the oral cavity and lip were published in Europe in the eighteenth and nineteenth centuries. More than 60 years ago, Muller in Germany was the first to recognize the positive association between cigarette smoking and lung cancer. Since then, multiple epidemiological studies have confirmed these observations and elaborated on the molecular mechanisms of smoking carcinogenesis, providing sufficient evidence to establish a strong causal association between cigarette smoking and cancer of the aerodigestive tract (lung, oral cavity, pharynx, larynx, nasal cavities, paranasal sinuses, nasopharynx, esophagus, stomach, liver, and pancreas), urinary bladder, kidney (renal cell carcinoma), and uterine cervix, as well as myeloid leukemia. Other forms of tobacco smoking, such as cigars, pipes, and bidis, also increase risk of cancer, including cancer of the lung and parts of the upper aerodigestive tract. A meta-analysis of over 50 studies on never-smokers showed a consistent and statistically significant association between exposure to environmental tobacco smoke and lung cancer risk.[10]

Smoking is currently responsible for one-third of all cancer deaths in many Western countries and is a rapidly growing cause of morbidity and mortality in many other countries. It has been estimated that every other smoker will be killed by tobacco.[11] To date, smoking accounts for about 85% to 90% of lung cancer deaths in both sexes. The rate at which lung cancer develops is strongly correlated with the duration of tobacco exposure. After 45, 30, and 15 years of cigarette smoking, the annual incidence rates of lung cancer are 0.5%, 0.1%, and under 0.01%, respectively. Thus, a 3-fold increase in the duration of tobacco use can increase the annual incidence of lung cancer by 50-fold. As smoking ceases, the annual risk remains roughly constant thereafter. For instance, after 30 years of smoking, the risk is approximately 0.1%, and if a smoker stops after 30 years, this annual rate will persist indefinitely. Thus, 15 years later, the annual risk is 0.1% instead of 0.5%, which it would have been if smoking had continued. About 80% of the risk is, therefore, avoided by stopping smoking.[12]

In contrast to the decline in smoking rates in men are worrisome reports of increases in cigarette smoking among youngsters, and especially on college campuses nationwide, where approximately 40% of students define themselves as active smokers. This is irrespective of the type of college or students' sex, ethnicity, or year in college.[13]

Passive Smoking

Smokers are not the only people at increased risk from exposure to tobacco smoke. "Passive smoking" from environmental tobacco smoke also increases the risk of lung cancer death. According to the Environmental Protection Agency (EPA), each year about 3000 nonsmoking adults die of lung cancer as a result of breathing the smoke of others' cigarettes. Analysis has shown that the sidestream smoke emitted from a smoldering cigarette between puffs contains virtually all carcinogenic compounds that have been identified in the mainstream smoke inhaled by smokers. Even though passive smokers are exposed to much lower concentrations of these carcinogens than active smokers, environmental tobacco smoke has become the only agent ever classified by the EPA as a human carcinogen for which an increased cancer risk has actually been observed at typical environmental levels of exposure.[14] The risk of dying of lung cancer is 30% higher for a nonsmoker living with a smoker than for those living in a totally tobacco-free household.[15]

Cigarette Smoke Composition

Dozens of compounds have been identified in cigarette smoke, both particles (solid phase) and gases (vapor phase). More than 60 of these agents have been shown to be carcinogenic in laboratory animals, and some of them are also carcinogenic in humans, including benzo[a]pyrene, a polycyclic aromatic hydrocarbon; aromatic amines; formaldehyde; benzene; and miscellaneous inorganic and organic compounds. Tobacco also contains specific carcinogens related to nicotine, such as 4-(N-methyl-N-nitrosamino)-1-(3-pyridyl)-1-butanone (NNK), a strong carcinogen in rodents.[16] Following 5 to 20 years of exposure to these agents, certain changes occur in airway epithelium as described in the next sections, leading in some cases to the development of cancer.[10]

Lung Cancer in Women

For most of the past 100 years, lung cancer has generally been thought of as a disease affecting primarily men. In the past several decades, however, the incidence of lung cancer has risen among women in the United States and most other parts of the world. Although incidence is still higher among men than women, the gap has narrowed and lung cancer has become the leading cause of cancer death among American women. The rise in rates of lung cancer among women has paralleled the increase in the prevalence of cigarette smoking. Just as in men, the majority (85–90%) of lung cancers among women are considered the result of smoking. There is accumulating evidence suggesting that the development of lung cancer is different in women than in men. For example, women smokers are more likely than men to develop adenocarcinoma of the lung, and women who have never smoked are more likely to develop lung cancer than men who have never smoked. Furthermore, the 5-year survival rate for women who have lung cancer is 15.6%, while it is 12.4% for men; women survive longer after surgical resection of early-stage lung cancer as well as after treatment of metastatic disease; female sex has been associated with longer survival in SCLC as well. Hormonal, genetic, and metabolic differences between the sexes are believed to account for these clinical differences. Indeed, estrogens were found to be involved in lung carcinogenesis, either by acting as estrogen receptor ligands and activating cellular proliferation pathways, or by metabolic activation to reactive intermediates that can produce DNA adducts and cause oxidative damage.[17,18]

Since smoking remains the primary cause of lung cancer, the differences in the clinical profile of the disease between the sexes have been attributed to different response to tobacco carcinogens. Indeed, in the 1990s, several case-control studies indicated that relative risks of lung cancer associated with specific amounts and duration of cigarette smoking may actually be higher among women than among men. Bain and colleagues recently performed a meta-analysis on prospective cohorts to examine this hypothesis and found that women do not appear to have a greater susceptibility to lung cancer than men, given equal smoking exposure.[17] These data were important because they arise from carefully conducted monitoring since 1986 of large cohorts of female nurses (>60,000) and male health professionals (>25,000). In total, approximately 1300 lung cancers were observed in current and former smokers in these cohorts, a sufficient number of cases for the kind of detailed analyses needed to control covariates such as age at start of smoking, age at quitting smoking, height, weight, and diet. The key finding was that the ratio of exposure-standardized lung cancer incidence rates for female current smokers to male current smokers was 1:1. The same ratio of 1:1 was also found for former smokers (95% confidence interval [CI] 0.95–1.31). In analyses by histologic type of lung cancer, the data confirmed previous findings that female smokers did have a significantly higher rate of adenocarcinoma than male smokers.[17] The equal rates of lung cancer mortality in younger U.S. men and women, corresponding to an era when smoking prevalence in the sexes was equal, also provide evidence against a major sex difference in susceptibility to smoking-induced lung cancer.[19] These data suggest that, although women are not more susceptible than men to smoking-induced lung cancer, the clinical characteristics of their disease differ from those of lung cancer in men.

Familial Predisposition

It is interesting that the vast majority of cigarette smokers, including heavy smokers, do not develop lung cancer. This suggests that cancer formation is dependent on an inherited predisposition or cofactors such as additional carcinogens. Studies that have compared risk factors of individuals with histologically confirmed lung cancer and of individuals with other smoking-related cancers found that having relatives with lung cancer did not increase the risk of developing lung cancer, but it did increase the risk of having cancer at some site.[20] This suggests a heritable variation in response to carcinogens. Respiratory diseases also predispose to development of lung cancer. Studies of families predisposed to lung cancer showed that the development of lung cancer in young individuals (aged ≤50 years) was compatible with Mendelian codominant inheritance or a rare autosomal gene.[21] This gene was involved to a lesser degree in individuals older than 50 years who developed lung cancer, suggesting that the cause of cancer in these noncarriers was long-term exposure to tobacco. Bailey-Wilson and colleagues recently studied the susceptibility genes for familial lung cancer and conducted a genome-wide linkage analysis of 52 extended pedigrees ascertained through probands with lung cancer who had several first-degree relatives with the same disease. The results localized a major susceptibility locus influencing lung cancer risk on chromosome 6q23–25.[22]

Table 78-1 **Documented Occupational Lung Carcinogens**

Substance	Occupational Exposures
Arsenic	Smelters, pesticide manufacturers
Asbestos	Miners, millers, insulators, railroad and shipyard workers
Chloromethylethers	Ion-exchange resin manufacturers
Chromium	Chromate and pigment manufacturers
Hydrocarbons	Coal-gas workers, roofers
Mustard gas	Poison-gas manufacturers
Nickel	Refiners
Radiation	Miners of uranium and other ores

Source: Adapted from Frank AL. Epidemiology of lung cancer. In: Roth JA, Ruchdeschel T, Weisenburger T, eds. *Thoracic Oncology*. Philadelphia: WB Saunders; 1989.

Table 78-2 **Major Genetic Aberrations in NSCLC and SCLC**

		NSCLC (%)	SCLC (%)
MYC	Amplifications	5-20	20-35
RAS	Mutations	15-20	<1
EGFR	Mutations	20	–
INK4a	LOH	70	50
p16INK4A	Mutations	20-50	< 5
p14ARF	Mutations	20	65
TP53	LOH	60	75-100
	Mutations	50	75
RB	LOH	30	70
	Mutations	15-30	90
FHIT	Mutations	40	80
TSG101	Mutations	–	90[a]
DMBT1	Mutations	40-50	100
LOH in various regions	*3p*	70-80	90-100
	4p	10-20	50
	4q	30	80
	8p	80-100	80-90
Promoter hypermethylation			
RASSFIA	30–40	90-100	
INK4a	*p16*	25-40	ND
	p14ARF	8	ND
RAR		40	70
TIMP-3		25	ND
CDH1		55	ND
DAPK		19	ND
GSTP1		1	ND
MGMT		20-40	ND

[a]Aberrant transcripts detected, but no point mutations.
Abbreviations: CDH1, E-cadherin; DAPK, death-associated protein kinase; DMBT1, deleted in malignant brain tumor; GSTP1, glutathione S transferase P1; LOH, loss of heterozygosity; MGMT, O6-methylguanine-DNA methyltransferase; ND, not determined; NSCLC, nonsmall-cell lung cancer; SCLC, small-cell lung cancer; TIMP-3, tissue inhibitors of metalloproteinase-3.
Source: Modified from Meuwissen R, Berns A. Genes Dev. 2005;19:643–664.

Other Environmental Causes

Lung cancer occurs in association with occupational and environmental exposures to carcinogenic agents other than tobacco smoke. Occupational agents classified as Group 1 carcinogens by the International Agency for Research on Cancer include inorganic arsenic, asbestos, bis(chloromethyl)ether, chromium (hexavalent), nickel and nickel compounds, polycyclic aromatic compounds, radon, and vinyl chloride. Group 2A of probable carcinogens include acrylonitrile, beryllium, cadmium, formaldehyde, acetaldehyde, synthetic fibers, silica, and welding fumes. Currently, occupational exposures have been estimated to account for 5% to 15% of all lung cancer cases worldwide (Table 78-1). In areas where shipbuilding was or is a major industry, asbestos exposure appears to be a clear etiologic agent, synergistically with cigarette smoking. Occupational risk for miners traditionally included development of pneumoconioses, chronic obstructive pulmonary disease (COPD), and lung cancer when exposed to radon, uranium, and others compounds. Radon is a gas that accumulates in basements, and indoor radon exposure has been reported to be an important cause of lung cancer in the general population.[23]

Molecular Pathogenesis

The rapidly developing technology of molecular biology has allowed the identification of multiple genes responsible for lung carcinogenesis. Interestingly, these genes are altered forms of genes normally present in eukaryotic cells. The plethora of genetic abnormalities and redundancy of altered pathways induced by tobacco and other carcinogens determines lung cancer heterogeneity, which is remarkable in comparison to that of other solid tumors. In this regard, it has to be remembered that individual tumors are characterized by specific genetic alternation(s) and that there is a gradual accumulation of abnormalities in a given tumor, from normal epithelium to invasive carcinoma. Table 78-2 lists genes that have been implicated in lung carcinogenesis. A detailed review of cancer biology may be found in other sections of this textbook.

Molecular Abnormalities in Premalignancy

Structural and genetic epithelial changes occur gradually, and invasive carcinoma develops 5 to 20 years after initial insult to the airways (Fig. 78-1). Loss of specific chromosomal regions on a single allele (loss of heterozygosity [LOH]) has been detected frequently in lung cancers and bronchial epithelia exposed to tobacco carcinogens. The regions of earliest and most frequent allelic loss are 3p21, 3p22–24, 3p25, and 9p21.[24] It is noteworthy that many of these changes are seen in histologically normal bronchial epithelium from smokers, but not nonsmokers.[25] However, these changes appear to become more frequent and extensive in terms of chromosome loss with advancing abnormality of premalignancy. In some cases, these molecular changes appear to be clonally independent. Methylated sequences of tumor suppressor gene promoters can be detected in tumors, smoking-damaged normal lung (preneoplastic changes), sputum, and blood. These represent attractive surrogate biomarkers for early detection and

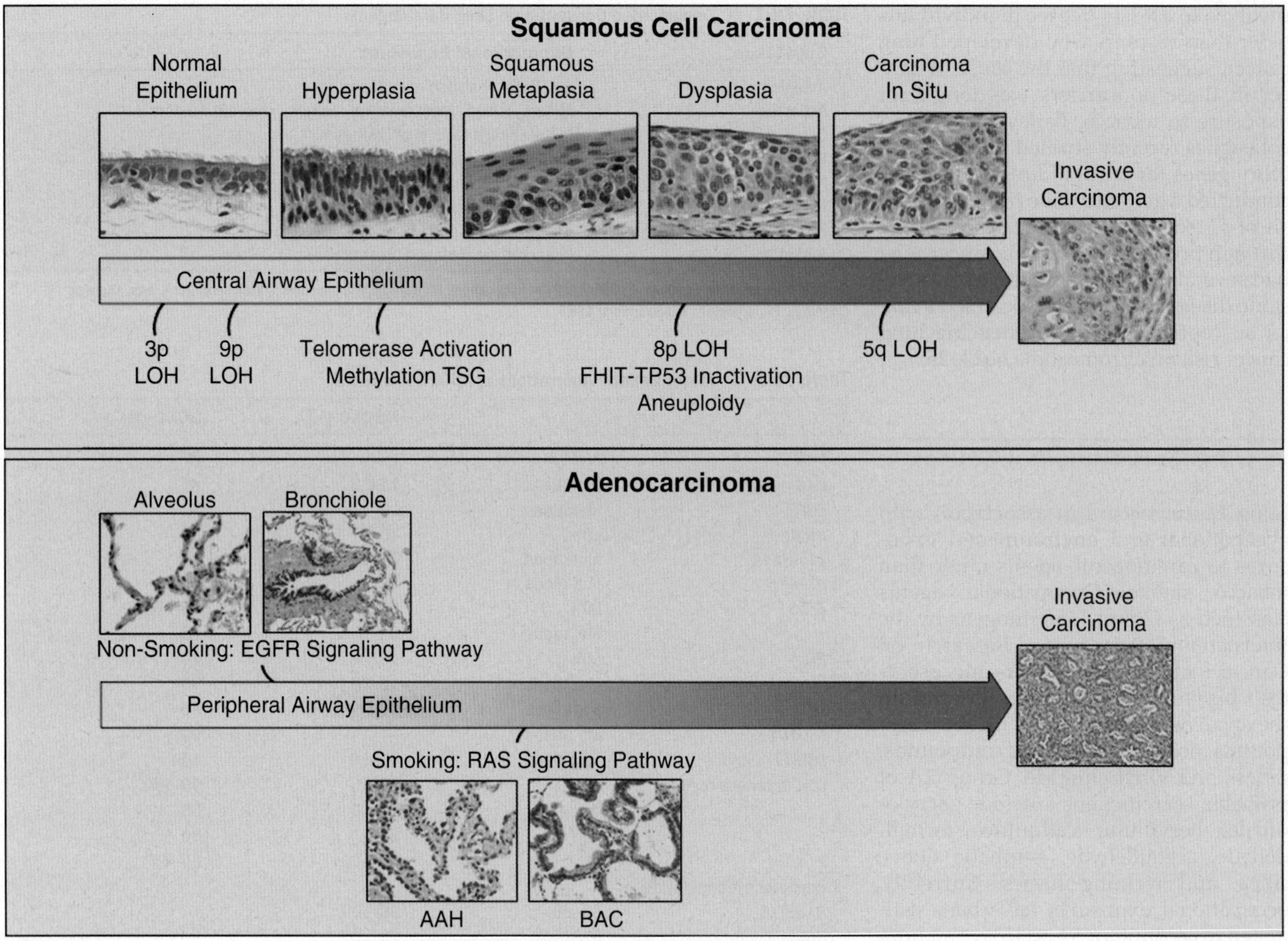

Figure 78-1 Summary of histopathologic and molecular changes involved in the pathogenesis of squamous cell carcinoma and adenocarcinomas of the lung. Some molecular changes commence at a histologically normal epithelium stage. Two molecular pathways, smoking- and non-smoking-related, have been identified in the pathogenesis of lung adenocarcinoma. For this tumor histology, the only known preneoplastic lesion is atypical adenomatous hyperplasia (AAH), which appears to be the precursor for the subset of lung adenocarcinomas with bronchioloalveolar carcinoma (BAC) features. Both pathways lead to the development of invasive adenocarcinoma. *Abbreviations*: LOH, loss of heterozygosity; TSG, tumor suppressor gene.

monitoring of chemoprevention, smoking cessation, and response to therapy.

Second Primary Cancers

Patients who have had a primary epithelial cancer of the upper aerodigestive tract (head and neck, esophagus, or lungs), have a 10% to 44% risk of developing a simultaneous or subsequent second primary cancer in the region or in distant organs, probably as a result of exposure to the same carcinogen. This effect is called "field cancerization." Many studies have implicated inactivation of TP53 in both primary and secondary lesions as a factor in this phenomenon. The incidence of second primary tumors is especially high following treatment of laryngeal carcinoma, and up to 25% of these cases develop lung cancer in the first 14 years of follow-up. The most common histologic type of lung cancer in these patients was squamous cell carcinoma, but nonsquamous tumors were noted and occurred more frequently in women.[26] For patients who survive resection of a NSCLC, the risk of developing a second lung cancer is approximately 1–2% per patient per year. For survivors of SCLC, the corresponding risk appears to be even higher, approximately 6% per patient per year.[27]

Pathology of Lung Cancer

From histopathologic and biologic perspectives, lung cancer is a complex neoplasm. The histologic classification is based on analysis of lung tumors by light microscopy with standard staining techniques, and guidelines were published by the World Health Organization (WHO) in 2004 (Table 78-3).[28] The most common histologic types of lung cancer are NSCLCs, which include squamous cell carcinoma, adenocarcinoma (including the noninvasive type of bronchioloalveolar carcinoma) and large cell carcinoma, and SCLCs.[28] Lung neoplasms are generally classified by the best-differentiated region of the tumor and graded by its most poorly differentiated portion.

Precursor Lesions

Lung cancers are believed to arise after the development of a series of progressive

Table 78-3 WHO Lung Cancer Classification

I. Epithelial tumors
A. Benign
1. Papillomas
2. Adenomas
B. Dysplasia/carcinoma in situ
C. Malignant
1. Squamous cell carcinoma
a. Spindle-cell variant
2. Small-cell carcinoma
a. Oat-cell carcinoma
b. Intermediate-cell type
c. Combined oat-cell carcinoma
3. Adenocarcinoma
a. Adenocarcinoma, mixed subtype
b. Acinar adenocarcinoma
c. Papillary adenocarcinoma
d. Bronchioloalveolar carcinoma: nonmucinous, mucinous, mixed nonmucinous and mucinous or indeterminate
e. Solid adenocarcinoma with mucin production
f. Fetal adenocarcinoma
g. Mucinous (colloid) adenocarcinoma
h. Mucinous cystadenocarcinoma
i. Signet-ring adenocarcinoma
j. Clear-cell adenocarcinoma
4. Large-cell carcinoma
a. Giant-cell carcinoma
b. Clear-cell carcinoma
5. Adenosquamous carcinoma
6. Carcinoid tumor
7. Bronchial gland carcinoma
8. Others
II. Soft tissue tumors
III. Mesothelial tumors
A. Benign
B. Malignant
IV. Miscellaneous tumors
A. Benign
B. Malignant
V. Secondary tumors
VI. Unclassified tumors
VII. Tumor-like lesions

Source: Adapted from Ref. 37.

pathological changes (preneoplastic or precursor lesions) in the respiratory mucosa. The recent 2004 WHO histological classification of preinvasive lesions of the lung lists three main morphologic forms[28]: (1) squamous dysplasia and carcinoma in situ (CIS); (2) atypical adenomatous hyperplasia (AHH); and (3) diffuse idiopathic pulmonary neuroendocrine cell hyperplasia (DIPNECH), which has been associated with the development of carcinoid tumors of the lung.[29] While the sequential preneoplastic changes have been defined for centrally arising squamous carcinomas, they have been poorly documented for large cell carcinomas, adenocarcinomas and SCLCs.[29,30]

Squamous Dysplasia

Mucosal changes in the large airways that may precede or accompany invasive squamous cell carcinoma include hyperplasia, squamous metaplasia, squamous dysplasia and CIS.[29,30] In hyperplasia, epithelial basal cells proliferate. Then, as a result of chronic exposure and repeated injury by inhaled agents, the columnar hyperplastic epithelium is replaced with stratified squamous epithelium. Dysplastic lesions may be categorized as mild, moderate, or severe; however, these lesions represent a continuum of cytologic and histologic atypical changes that may show some overlap between categories. Whereas mild dysplasia is characterized by minimal architectural and cytological disturbance, moderate dysplasia exhibits more cytological irregularity, which is even higher in severe dysplasia and is accompanied by considerable cellular polymorphism. When the dysplasia involves the full thickness of the epithelium, CIS is present. Invasion of the basement membrane and infiltration of malignant cells into the underlying stroma is the first sign of invasive cancer. Dysplastic lesions are often not detected by conventional white-light bronchoscopy or gross examination. However, the utilization of fluorescent bronchoscopy, such as lung-imaging fluorescent endoscopy (LIFE), greatly increases the sensitivity for detection of dysplastic lesions and CIS.[31] Little is known about the rate and risks of progression of squamous dysplasia to CIS and ultimately to invasive squamous cell carcinoma; however, it has been estimated that the duration of this process may be 5 to 20 years. Multiple molecular studies have helped to characterize a sequence of molecular events involved in the progression of dysplastic lesions.[32,33]

Atypical Adenomatous Hyperplasia (AAH)

It has been suggested that adenocarcinomas may be preceded by AAH in peripheral airway cells;[29,34] however, the respiratory structures and the specific epithelial cell types involved in the origin of most lung adenocarcinomas are unknown. AAH is a discrete parenchymal lesion arising in the alveoli close to terminal and respiratory bronchioles. Because of their size, AAH lesions are usually incidental histological findings, but they may be detected grossly, especially if they are 0.5 cm or larger. The increasing use of high resolution CT scans for screening purposes has led to an increasing awareness of this entity, as it remains one of the most important differential diagnoses of air filled peripheral lesions, often described radiographically as ground glass opacities. AHH maintains an alveolar structure lined by rounded, cuboidal or low columnar cells. The postulated progression of AAH to adenocarcinoma with bronchioloalveolar (BAC) features, apparent from the increasingly atypical morphology, is supported by morphometric, cytofluorometric, and molecular studies.[30,34] Distinction between highly atypical AAH and non-mucinous BAC is sometimes difficult. Somewhat arbitrarily, BAC is considered generally >10 mm in size, with more cellular atypia than their AAH counterparts. In addition, several molecular changes frequently present in lung adenocarcinomas are also present in AAH lesions, and they are further evidence that AAH may represent true preneoplastic lesions.[35]

Invasive Tumors

Adenocarcinoma

This tumor type accounts for nearly 40% of all lung cancers (Fig. 78-2A). According to the 2004 WHO classification, adenocarcinoma can be sub-classified into five major subtypes: acinar, papillary, solid with mucin production, bronchioloalveolar, and mixed adenocarcinomas.[28] Most adenocarcinomas are heterogeneous, consisting of two or more of the histological subtypes; thus, most (80%) adenocarcinomas fall into the mixed subtype.[36] When tumor cells grow in a purely lepidic fashion without evidence of invasion, they are regarded as BAC.[37] Well, moderate and poorly differentiated histologies are recognized among acinar and papillary tumors. While the BAC pattern is usually well differentiated, the solid adenocarcinoma pattern is, by definition, poorly differentiated. On histologic examination, these poorly differentiate tumors usually demonstrate mucus production as shown by mucicarmine or periodic acid-Schiff staining. Lung adenocarcinomas typically immunostain for thyroid transcription factor-1.

Adenocarcinomas usually originate within the periphery of the lung and may be single or multiple with a wide range in size. Adenocarcinoma may develop in a background of underlying fibrosis; however, adenocarcinoma of the lung arising in association with a focal scar is uncommon.[38] The current notion is that most of the scars associated with adenocarcinomas of the lung are caused by tumor growth.[39] While adenocarcinomas of the lung spread primarily by lymphatic and hematogenous routes, aerogeneous dissemination often occurs in BAC and is characterized by spread of tumor cells through the airways forming lesions separate from the main mass.[39]

Bronchioloalveolar Carcinoma (BAC)

BAC is defined as an adenocarcinoma of the lung, which grows in a lepidic fashion along the alveolar septae without invasion of stroma, blood vessels, or pleura (Fig. 78-2B).[39] Unfortunately, this strict definition of BAC as a true noninvasive

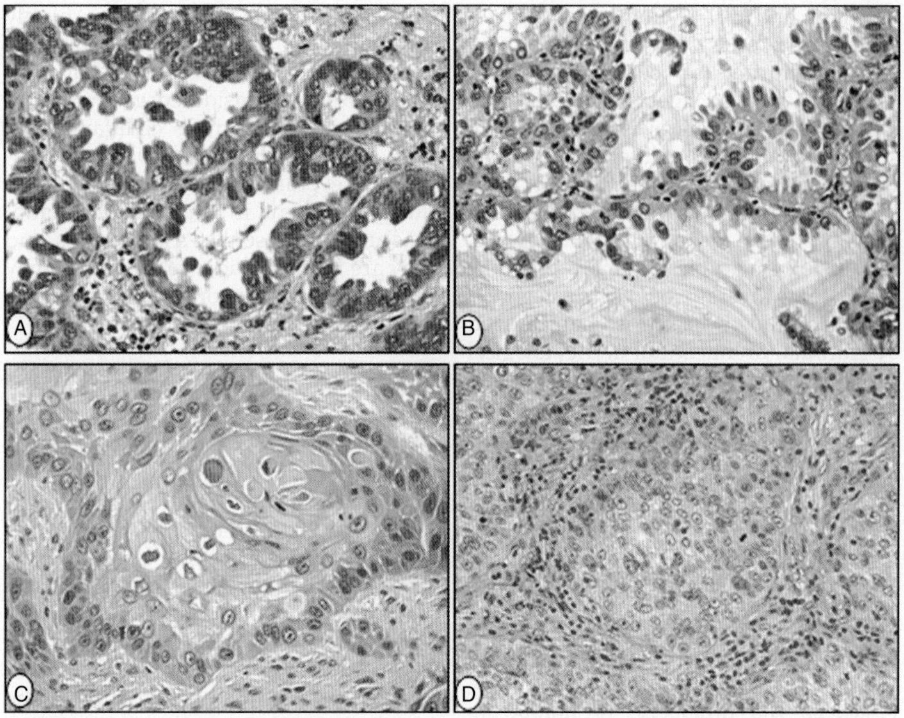

Figure 78-2 Histopathology characteristics of major forms of NSCLC: **(A)** adenocarcinomas, **(B)** adenocarcinoma with bronchioloalveolar pattern, **(C)** squamous cell carcinoma, and **(D)** large cell carcinoma of the lung.

tumor is not uniformly applied, with pathologists frequently labeling mixed tumors with varying degrees of lepidic growth as either BAC tumors or adenocarcinomas with BAC features. BAC has been sub-classified in three types: non-mucinous, mucinous, and mixed mucinous and non-mucinous. The non-mucinous BAC consists of varying mixtures of type 2 pneumocytes and Clara cells. Although a BAC-like pattern of spread is common at the edge of conventional adenocarcinomas, histologically pure BAC is uncommon, comprising only 3% of all lung cancers.[37] BAC and mixed subtype adenocarcinomas with a BAC component may present as different gross pathologic findings in the lung, including a solitary peripheral nodule, multiple nodules, and lobar consolidation.[37] When multiple nodules occur, they may be unilateral or bilateral. It has been shown that while patients with small peripheral lung adenocarcinomas with a pure BAC pattern and no invasion had 100% 5-year survivals, those with mixed BAC with invasive components and BAC with purely invasive growth patterns demonstrated 5-year survivals of 75% and 52%, respectively.[38]

Squamous Cell Carcinoma

This tumor type accounts for approximately 30% of all lung cancers. Intercellular bridges, squamous pearl formation and individual cell keratinization characterize squamous differentiation in this tumor type (Fig. 77–2C). While all these features are very apparent in well-differentiated squamous cell carcinomas, they are difficult to find in poorly differentiated tumors. The histologic subtypes described include basaloid, small cell, papillary and clear cell types.[28] Approximately 70% of squamous cell carcinomas of the lung present as central lung tumors.[40] The tumor may grow to a large size and central cavitation secondary to necrosis is a common gross finding.[41] Central squamous cell carcinomas may form intraluminal polypoid masses and may occlude the bronchial lumen. Similar to other lung cancer types, squamous cell carcinomas spread primarily by lymphatic and hematogenous routes. In addition, squamous cell carcinomas may directly invade mediastinal lymph nodes and other mediastinal structures by extending through peribronchial tissues.[40] Thus, locoregional recurrence after surgical resection is more common in squamous cell carcinomas than other cell types.[42] There are no squamous cells normally present in the respiratory mucosa, and they develop from metaplastic cells that usually arise as a result of tobacco exposure.

Adenosquamous Carcinoma

Adenosquamous carcinoma of the lung is characterized by the presence of squamous cell carcinoma and adenocarcinoma with each comprising at least 10% of the tumor.[43] They account for 1% to 2% of lung cancers and are usually located in the periphery of the lung and may contain a central scar. The routes of dissemination and metastasis are similar to the other NSCLCs.

Large Cell Carcinoma

Large cell carcinoma is an undifferentiated carcinoma that lacks the features of squamous cell carcinoma, adenocarcinoma, or SCLC.[44] Thus, it is a diagnosis of exclusion. They account for approximately 9% of all lung cancers, and they represent a spectrum of morphology, and most large cell carcinomas consist of large cells with abundant cytoplasm and large nuclei with prominent nucleoli (Fig. 78-2D).[41] They also include some specific variants, including large cell neuroendocrine carcinomas (LCNEC), lymphoepithelioma-like carcinomas, clear cell carcinomas, and large cell carcinomas with rhabdoid component.[44] LCNEC demonstrates neuroendocrine differentiation.[45] Lymphoepithelioma-like carcinoma is characterized by dense lymphocytic infiltration and the presence of EBV viral sequences.[46,47] Many poorly differentiated squamous cell carcinomas and adenocarcinomas may show a component of large cell carcinomas; however the tumors are classified according to their best-differentiated component. Most large cell carcinomas are usually large, peripheral masses.[44] The tumor usually invades the visceral pleura, chest wall, or adjacent structures. The pattern of spread of large cell carcinomas is similar to other NSCLCs.

Large Cell Neuroendocrine Carcinoma (LCNEC)

This tumor types is defined by the presence of large undifferentiated cells with prominent nucleoli, neuroendocrine pattern of growth, high mitotic rate and neuroendocrine differentiation demonstrated by immunohistochemistry (Fig. 77–3B).[45] They are usually peripheral, nodular masses, with necrosis. LCNEC is considered an aggressive malignancy with a prognosis similar to SCLC.[45] The term combined LCNEC is used for tumors associated with other better differentiated types of NSCLC, mostly adenocarcinomas.[44]

Sarcomatoid Carcinomas

Sarcomatoid carcinomas of the lung are a group of poorly differentiated NSCLCs that contain a component of sarcoma or sarcoma-like (spindle and/or giant cell) differentiation.[48] Currently, there are five variants identified: pleomorphic carcinoma, spindle cell carcinoma, giant cell carcinoma, carcinosarcoma, and pulmonary blastoma.[48,49] Sarcomatoid carcinomas are rare tumors (0.3–1.3%).[36,48] They can arise in the central or peripheral lung. Peripheral tumors are usually large masses, and they invade the chest wall.[50] Pleomorphic carcinoma is a poorly differ-

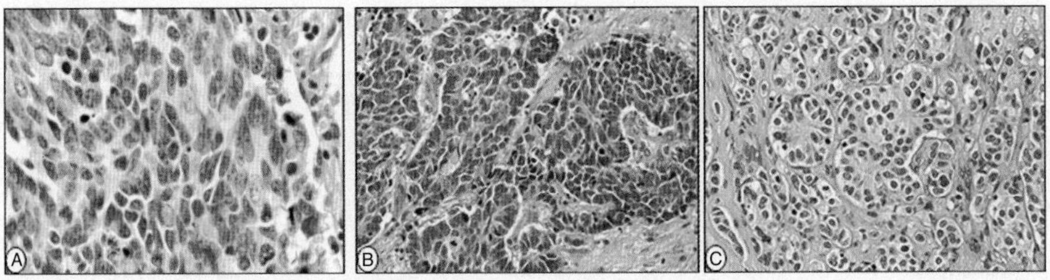

Figure 78-3 Lung tumors with neuroendocrine differentiations: **(A)** SCLC, **(B)** LCNEC, and **(C)** carcinoid

entiated type of NSCLC (squamous cell carcinoma, adenocarcinoma or large cell carcinoma) containing at least 10% spindle or giant cells.[48] Spindle cell carcinoma is a NSCLC consisting exclusively of spindle-shaped tumor cells, which resemble spindle cells found in sarcomas.[48] Giant cell carcinomas are composed entirely of highly pleomorphic and multinucleated giant cells.[48] Carcinosarcoma is defined as a tumor with a mixture of usual NSCLC and sarcomatous elements, such as malignant cartilage (chondrosarcoma), bone (osteosarcoma), and muscle (rhabdomyosarcoma).[48] Pulmonary blastoma is a mixed tumor containing a primitive epithelial component that may resemble well-differentiated fetal adenocarcinoma and a primitive mesenchymal stroma, with some sarcomatous components.[48] While most sarcomatoid carcinoma variants are exclusively composed of epithelial tumor cells, the sarcomatoid element present in carcinosarcoma and pulmonary blastoma are truly sarcomatous, and these subtypes represent mixed epithelial and mesenchymal malignancies.

Small Cell Lung Carcinoma (SCLC)

This tumor type accounts for approximately 15% of all lung cancers.[51] They characteristically consist of small epithelial tumor cells with finely granular chromatin and absent or inconspicuous nucleoli (Fig. 78-3A).[51] Necrosis is frequent and extensive and the mitotic count is high. Although there is not a precise upper limit for cell size to be defined as small cell, it has been suggested that the cells should measure approximately the diameter of two or three small mature lymphocytes.[52] While SCLC represents a light microscopic diagnosis, electron microscopy shows neuroendocrine granules in at least two-thirds of cases and immunohistochemistry for neuroendocrine markers (chromogranin and synaptophysin) is positive in most (~90%) cases.[52,53] Less than 10% of SCLCs demonstrate a mixture with NSCLC histologic types, usually adenocarcinoma, squamous cell carcinoma or large cell carcinoma, and they are termed combined SCLCs.[51]

Most SCLCs present as a perihilar mass. SCLCs are typically situated in a peribronchial location with infiltration of the bronchial submucosa and peribronchial tissue.[51] Extensive lymph node metastases are common.[54] The tumors are large masses with extensive necrosis. Diagnosis is usually made by bronchoscopy with bronchial and trans-bronchial lung biopsies and cytology, and it is highly unusual to encounter SCLC as a surgical specimen.[52] Approximately 5% of SCLCs present as peripheral small lesions.[51]

Carcinoid Tumors

Lung tumors with neuroendocrine morphology and differentiation include the low-grade typical carcinoid, intermediate-grade atypical carcinoid, high-grade LCNEC, and SCLC.[55] Carcinoid tumors are characterized by organoid growth pattern, uniform cytologic features, and immunohistochemical expression of neuroendocrine markers, such as chromogranin and synaptophysin (Fig. 78-3C).[56] Carcinoid tumors have been divided into two categories, typical and atypical types, based on their clinical behavior and pathologic features, with atypical crinoids having more malignant histologic and clinical features.[57] Typical and atypical crinoids are also referred to as low and intermediate grade neuroendocrine carcinomas, respectively. Histologically, typical carcinoids show fewer than 2 mitoses per 2 mm^2 field and lack necrosis, while atypical carcinoids show 2–10 mitosis per 2 mm^2 field and/or foci of necrosis.[56]

Typical carcinoids are uniformly distributed throughout the lungs, whereas atypical carcinoids are more commonly peripheral tumors.[58] Compared to typical carcinoids, atypical carcinoids have a larger tumor sizes, a higher rate of metastases, and their survival is significantly reduced.[58] At presentation, approximately 10–15% of typical and 40–50% of atypical carcinoids demonstrate regional lymph node metastases.[56]

Clinical Manifestations

Clinical Presentation

Some patients present with an asymptomatic lesion discovered incidentally on chest radiograph. The majority of lung cancers, however, are discovered because of the development of a new or worsening clinical symptom or sign. Although no set of signs or symptoms is pathognomonic for lung cancer, they may be divided into four categories: (1) those due to local tumor growth and intrathoracic spread, (2) those due to distant metastases, (3) nonspecific systemic symptoms, and (4) paraneoplastic syndromes.

Manifestations of Local Tumor Growth and Intrathoracic Spread

Signs and symptoms referable to the primary tumor vary depending on location and size of the tumor. Centrally located tumors produce cough, a localized wheeze, hemoptysis, and symptoms and signs of airway obstruction and postobstructive pneumonitis such as dyspnea, fever, and productive cough. Occasionally, large tumor masses, usually of squamous or large cell histologic type, cavitate and present as malignant lung abscesses. Peripheral tumors are more likely to be asymptomatic when they are small and confined within the lung; occasionally, cough and pleuritic chest pain may be evident.

Intrathoracic spread of lung cancer, either by direct extension or by lymphatic metastasis, is associated with a variety of sign and symptom complexes. The importance of these symptoms and signs is that they generally indicate that the patient is no longer a candidate for curative surgery. Mediastinal invasion may be manifested as vague, poorly localized chest pain in association with other findings of nerve entrapment, vascular obstruction, and/or compression or invasion of the esophagus. One of the most common neurologic disorders arising from mediastinal involvement is hoarseness owing to entrapment of the recurrent laryngeal nerve. Because of its longer intrathoracic course, the left recurrent laryngeal nerve is more likely to be the source of hoarseness than the right recurrent laryngeal nerve.[59] With recurrent laryngeal nerve paralysis, a patient may develop dysphagia for both solids and liquids, resulting in recurrent aspiration. Compression of the esophagus by the tumor also may lead to dysphagia. The formation of a tracheoesophageal or bronchoesophageal fistula, which occurs with a frequency of 0.16%, can be manifested by vigorous cough, especially on swallowing, and recurrent aspiration pneumonia.[60] Involvement of the phrenic nerve is associated with hiccups early, and later leads to paralysis and elevation of the hemidiaphragm with resulting dyspnea.

The principal vascular syndrome associated with the extension of lung cancer into the mediastinum is superior vena cava (SVC) syndrome, most commonly caused by invasion of the vein and extrinsic compression by the tumor, but also by intraluminal thrombosis.[61] Lung cancer accounts for 65% to 90% of all cases of SVC syndrome, and in approximately 85% of these cases the primary lung tumor is on the right, primarily in the right upper lobe or right mainstem bronchus. By cell type, SCLC predominates as the cause of SVC syndrome, followed by squamous cell carcinoma. Establishment of a histologic diagnosis is important before initiating treatment, because the SVC syndrome is no longer considered a radiotherapeutic emergency.

With apical tumors, the classic Pancoast syndrome (lower brachial plexopathy, Horner syndrome, and shoulder pain) may become manifest owing to local invasion of the lower brachial plexus (C8 and T1 nerve roots), satellite ganglion, and chest wall.[62] The tumor may cause symptoms through involvement of the first or second rib or vertebrae and other nerve roots. The radiographic signs are those of an asymmetric apical cap or an apical mass. Most superior sulcus tumors are squamous cell carcinomas, although they may be adenocarcinomas, or even in 1-2% of cases, SCLC, underscoring the importance of establishing a histologic diagnosis.

Approximately 15% of patients with lung cancer have pleural involvement at initial presentation, and 50% of patients with disseminated lung cancer develop pleural effusion during the course of their illness. A pleural effusion may be asymptomatic when small, but it is usually associated with dyspnea, cough, or chest pain.[63] A number of pathogenic mechanisms have been suggested, but the presence or absence of malignant cells in cytology specimens does not significantly influence survival outcome, although the presence of malignant cells in pleural washings at the time of pulmonary resection for lung cancer has been shown to have a negative impact survival.[64] Rarely, lung cancer can present as an ipsilateral spontaneous pneumothorax, generally attributed to erosion of the visceral pleura by a peripheral tumor, but underlying emphysema also may play a role.

Pericardial involvement arises from direct extension of the tumor or as a result of retrograde spread through mediastinal and epicardial lymphatics. Lung cancer is the single most frequent source of pericardial metastases.[65] In many cases, the process is not diagnosed before the patient's death. Clinical findings include cardiac dysrhythmias, enlargement of the cardiac silhouette on the chest radiograph, and, infrequently, signs and symptoms of cardiac tamponade (Table 78-4).

Table 78-4 ■ Clinical Manifestations Caused by Local Tumor Growth and Intrathoracic Spread at Presentation

	Frequency (%)	
Clinical Manifestation	**SCLC**	**NSCLC**
Cough	50-76	40
Dyspnea	34-40	30-40
Chest pain	35-36	25-40
Hemoptysis	15-23	15-35
Pneumonitis	21-25	13-24
Vocal cord paralysis	15	Uncommon
SVC syndrome	12	<10
Pleural effusion	10-15	15
Pancoast's syndrome	Rare	3
Pericardial effusion	Uncommon	Rare

Abbreviations: NSCLC, non-small cell lung cancer; SCLC, small cell lung cancer; SVC, superior vena cava.

Manifestations of Distant Metastases

Approximately 60% of SCLC and 30% to 40% of NSCLC patients present with stage IV metastatic disease. Although lung cancer can metastasize to virtually any organ site, the most common sites of hematogenous spread that are clinically apparent are the central nervous system (CNS), bones, liver, and adrenal glands. Many of these patients do not have symptoms that can be attributed to a specific distant site. Bone pain appears to be common, however, one-third of patients in one large series had "pain other than chest pain" at presentation, and the majority of those episodes were due to bony involvement. Symptoms related to liver involvement (right upper quadrant pain) are less common or nonspecific (nausea, weight loss, anemia). Involvement of the adrenal glands is often asymptomatic, and most adrenal metastases are discovered incidentally during staging evaluation or at autopsy. If symptomatic, it presents with unilateral pain in the flank, abdomen, or costovertebral angle. Much less commonly, signs or symptoms point to brain and CNS involvement. These can range from nonspecific headache or mental status change to focal or generalized seizures and localized weakness. Epidural and intramedullary spinal cord metastases may be the sole neurologic manifestations of lung cancer. Diffuse meningeal involvement is uncommon at the time of initial presentation, but it may be seen later in the course of the disease, particularly with SCLC. The lymphatic spread of lung cancer may manifest with cough and dyspnea, depending on the extent of parenchymal involvement.

Systemic, Nonspecific Signs, and Symptoms

As shown in Table 78-5, systemic, nonspecific signs and symptoms are common in both SCLC and NSCLC. The 30% rate of anorexia is probably underreported. Weight loss, which is usually but not always accompanied by anorexia, occurs in approximately one-half of the patients and generalized weakness in one-third. Fever and anemia occur less frequently, in fewer than 20% of the patients. Fever is generally not considered paraneoplastic in lung cancer patients; if present, it is usually associated with a documented infection (eg, postobstructive pneumonia) or with liver metastases.

Paraneoplastic Syndromes

Table 78-6 lists 21 paraneoplastic syndromes, which induce signs and symptoms away from the primary tumor or its metastasis. The major categories of paraneoplastic syndromes include endocrine, neurologic, cutaneous, and musculoskeletal, and cardiovascular and hematological manifestations.[66]

Endocrine Syndromes ■ ***Syndrome of Inappropriate Secretion of Antidiuretic Hormone*** **■** Excess secretion of arginine-vasopressin associated with hyponatremia are the hallmarks of the syndrome of inappropriate secretion of antidiuretic hormone (SIADH). The cardinal findings are hyponatremia with corresponding

Table 78-5 ■ Clinical Manifestation Caused by Systemic Effect at Presentation

	Frequency (%)	
Clinical Manifestation	**SCLC**	**NSCLC**
Anorexia	30	30
Weight loss (≥10 lb)	35-52	45-52
Fatigue	23-42	35
Fever	11-15	7-16
Anemia	11-15	16-20

Abbreviations: NSCLC, non-small cell lung cancer; SCLC, small cell lung cancer.

Table 78-6 ■ Major Paraneoplastic Manifestations of Lung Cancer

Syndrome	Clinical Frequency (%)	Comments
Endocrine		
Inappropriate ADH	5–10	Mainly SCLC
Atrial natriuretic factor	Mainly SCLC	–
Ectopic ACTH	3–7	Most commonly with SCLC
Hypercalcemia of malignancy	10	Most commonly with squamous cell types
Gynecomastia	6	More with large-cell type
Other hormones	–	No significant clinical manifestations
Neurologic		
Eaton-Lambert	6	Mainly SCLC
Subacute sensory neuropathy	Rare	Mainly SCLC
Subacute cerebellar degeneration	Rare	Mainly SCLC
Limbic encephalopathy	Rare	Mainly SCLC
Visual paraneoplastic syndrome	Rare	Mainly SCLC
Subacute necrotic myelopathy	Rare	Mainly SCLC
Cutaneous/musculoskeletal		
Hypertrophic pulmonary osteoarthropathy	<10	More with adenocarcinoma
Acanthosis nigricans	Rare	–
Tylosis	Rare	–
Dermatomyositis	Rare	–
Cardiovascular/hematologic		
Nonbacterial thrombotic endocarditis	Uncommon	More with adenocarcinoma
Migratory thrombophlebitis	Uncommon	More with adenocarcinoma
Hypercoagulable status	10–15	Renal
Glomerulonephritis	Rare	–
Nephrotic syndrome	Rare	–

Abbreviations: ACTH, adrenocorticotrophic hormone; ADH, antidiuretic hormone; SCLC, small cell lung cancer.

hypo-osmolality of the serum and extracellular fluid; continued renal excretion of sodium; absence of clinical evidence of fluid volume depletion; osmolality of the urine greater than that appropriate for the concomitant osmolality of the plasma, ie, urine less than maximally diluted; and normal function of kidneys, adrenals and thyroid glands. SIADH may be caused by a variety of malignant tumors, and SCLC is the most common (up to 15%, though only one-third of them are symptomatic). Water restriction is usually sufficient to control symptoms until systemic anticancer treatment is initiated, which typically leads to improvement or resolution of the hyponatremia. Saline infusion, furosemide, or demeclocycline is infrequently required. Other conditions associated with SIADH must be considered, such as CNS disorders, pulmonary infections, and positive pressure ventilation. Also, a large number of pharmaceutical agents have been shown to produce SIADH, including a number of cytotoxic drugs such as vincristine, vinblastine, cisplatin, cyclophosphamide, and melphalan. Malignant tumors that cause SIADH are primary brain tumors, hematologic malignancies, intrathoracic nonpulmonary cancers, skin tumors, gastrointestinal cancers, gynecological cancer, breast and prostate cancers, and sarcomas.

Syndrome of Ectopic Adrenocorticotropic Hormone ■ Hyperadrenocorticism in association with ectopic adrenocorticotropic hormone (ACTH) production (>200 pg/mL) is a frequently observed hormonal syndrome in lung cancer, particularly in SCLC. Serum ACTH levels are elevated in 30% to 72% of SCLC patients, and cortisol secretion is abnormally regulated in 51%, but only 3% to 7% of SCLC patients become symptomatic. Patients with ectopic ACTH syndrome generally fit the demographic characteristics of lung cancer patients and rarely exhibit the classic cushingoid features of centripetal obesity or moon facies. Severe weakness and weight loss are universal as are excessive mineralocorticoid effects such as edema (30–40%) and hypertension (30–60%). Hyperpigmentation occurs in 25% to 30% of patients. Distinctive laboratory features of ectopic ACTH syndrome include severe hypokalemic alkalosis (70–90% of patients have a serum potassium level <3.0 mEq/L), elevated urinary 17-hydroxycorticoid excretion, and high serum ACTH levels (>200 pg/mL in 65% of patients). The ectopic ACTH syndrome is best managed by effective treatment of the underlying disease, but hypokalemia and hypertension may require appropriate, immediate adjunctive management. Ectopic ACTH syndrome was found to be associated with frequent complications from chemotherapy and shortened survival in patients with SCLC.[67]

Other Hormone Production ■ Other hormones elevated in lung cancer, particularly in patients with SCLC, include calcitonin, growth hormone, prolactin, serotonin, insulin, gastrin, and melanocyte stimulating factors. In most cases, however, these laboratory abnormalities bear minimal clinical significance.

Hypercalcemia of Malignancy ■ It has long been known that cancer patients may have hypercalcemia even without demonstrable bone metastases. Hypercalcemia has been reported to occur in up to 20% to 30% of patients with cancer at some time during the course of their disease. This incidence may be falling owing to the wide use of bisphosphonates in patients with multiple myeloma or breast cancer, although data are lacking. Hypercalcemia leads to progressive mental impairment, including coma, as well as renal failure. These complications are particularly common terminal events among patients with cancer. The detection of hypercalcemia in a patient with cancer signifies a very poor prognosis; approximately 50% of such patients die within 30 days. A parathyroid hormone-related protein, which shares an N-terminal sequence with the parathyroid hormone but has a unique C-terminal portion, has been shown to be responsible for the majority of cases of hypercalcemia of malignancy. Squamous cell carcinoma is the lung cancer mostly associated with hypercalcemia, and SCLC is rarely involved. Hypercalcemia may be completely reversible with effective treatment of the underlying cancer, and bisphosphonates may be used as a specific therapeutic modality.[68]

Neurologic Syndromes ■ Neurologic syndromes associated with lung cancer may occur through autoimmune mechanisms, and they occur mainly in patients with SCLC. Symptoms may precede diagnosis of the cancer by many months or may be the first sign of tumor recurrence. Direct metastatic effects or metabolic or infectious processes must be excluded as contributors to the neurologic findings. The severity of neurologic symptoms is unrelated to tumor bulk, and a primary malignant lesion may be undetected before death, despite disabling symptoms. Most of these conditions are not specific for malignancy.

Eaton-Lambert Syndrome ■ A myasthenia gravis-like disorder that was originally linked to SCLC but was found in other cancers, this syndrome, characterized by proximal limb muscle weakness and fatigue, is caused by the formation of IgG antibodies directed at calcium channels present in both the tumor and the neuromuscular junction. A type 1 antineuronal nuclear autoantibody (ANNA-1, also known as "anti-Hu") has been identified as a marker of neurological autoimmunity that is highly associated with SCLC (97%) and other paraneoplastic neurologic disorders.[69]

Subacute Sensory Neuropathy ■ This is the most characteristic peripheral neuropathy associated with SCLC. Clinical symptoms characterized by progressive impairment of all sensory modalities, with areflexia and marked sensory ataxia followed by stabilization after a period of weeks, may precede the diagnosis of SCLC by several months. It may be accompanied by more widespread evidence of paraneoplastic encephalitis, with cerebellar brainstem dysfunction and dementia.

Cutaneous and Musculoskeletal Syndromes ■ Digital clubbing and hypertrophic pulmonary osteoarthropathy (HPO) are the other major paraneoplastic syndromes associated with lung cancer, most exclusively with NSCLC. Digital clubbing (ie, subungual soft tissue thickening, most commonly involving the fingernails) is more common than HPO, which often resembles rheumatoid arthritis. It is characterized by a symmetric polyarthritis (usually involving the ankles, wrists, and knees), proliferative periostitis of the long bones, and neurovascular changes of the hands and feet, often with little or no evidence of clubbing. Although these conditions are also reported in several disorders not related to cancer and in other tumors metastatic to the chest, lung cancer accounts for more than 80% of cases of HPO in adults.[70] Radionuclide bone scans typically demonstrate increased uptake at the distal ends of the affected long bones, and the results may be confirmed by evidence of new bone formation on plain films; the spine is spared. The onset of HPO is often acute, may precede the diagnosis of cancer by months, and is usually but not invariably associated with inoperability. The cause of HPO is unknown. A variety of underlying mechanisms have been suggested, including the release of platelet-derived growth factor by megakaryocytes or platelet clumps that bypass the pulmonary capillary network. The syndrome may resolve with response of the cancer to therapy. No effective form of treatment is recognized, including aspirin and nonsteroidal antiinflammatory agents.

Other cutaneous paraneoplastic syndromes include dermatomyositis, acanthosis nigricans, and tylosis or hyperkeratosis of the palms and soles. These conditions are rarely seen in patients with lung cancer.

Cardiovascular and Hematologic Manifestations ■ Arterial and, more commonly, venous thrombosis is a frequent complication of cancer and sometimes a harbinger of occult cancer. Moreover, the use of new and aggressive therapy for cancer increases the risk of thrombosis. The two most notable manifestations in lung cancer are nonbacterial thrombotic endocarditis (NBTE) and venous thromboembolism (VTE).

NBTE, also known as marantic endocarditis, has been described most commonly in conjunction with adenocarcinoma and BAC; at autopsy, the incidence of NBTE in each of these cancer subtypes was approximately 7%, and the mitral valve was typically involved. Clinically significant emboli to the CNS, kidneys, and coronary arteries have been found.[71]

Pulmonary embolism and deep venous thrombosis are the two manifestations of VTE. Approximately 20% of VTE in the general population is associated with cancer, and cancer increases the risk of VTE about fivefold. Therapy for cancer, including surgery, chemotherapy, hormonal therapy, growth factors, angiogenesis inhibitors, and central venous catheters, add to the risk of thrombosis. Migratory thrombophlebitis was reported in patients with adenocarcinomas from different origins, mostly gastrointestinal tract (eg, pancreas) and lung.

A hypercoagulable state is noted in 10% to 15% of lung cancer patients. Thrombocytosis (60% of patients), hyperfibrinogenemia (54% of solid tumor patients), and general activation of the clotting system result in thrombosis and occasionally bleeding in lung cancer patients.

Recommended definitive therapy for established VTE includes low-molecular-weight heparin (LMWH) for most patients, unfractionated heparin for patients with renal failure, thrombolysis in cases of massive pulmonary embolism, and inferior vena cava filters when anticoagulation therapy is contraindicated.[72] Most authorities recommend 6 months therapy for secondary prevention. Lee and colleagues suggested that long-term treatment or secondary prophylaxis of VTE in cancer patients should include at least 6 months of LMWH rather than warfarin. (Their data showed probabilities of recurrence of thromboembolism of 17% in the warfarin group and only 9% in the LMWH group at 6 months, without increasing the risk of bleeding).[73]

Miscellaneous Paraneoplastic Associations ■ Renal disorders, such as membranous glomerulonephritis and subsequent nephrotic syndrome, have been reported as paraneoplastic phenomena in patients with lung cancer. The onset frequently precedes the diagnosis of cancer and probably is related to glomerular deposition of circulating antigen–antibody complexes. It is a poor prognostic sign among patients with all types of carcinoma, with a median survival duration of only 12 months from the time of diagnosis of the syndrome and only 3 months from the time of tumor diagnosis. The glomerulonephritis may normalize with appropriate treatment.

Diagnostic and Staging Techniques

The methods used to establish a diagnosis of lung cancer depend on the individual clinical situation. In some cases, such as a patient who presents with an asymptomatic solitary pulmonary nodule, tissue diagnosis may not be established until the time of definitive surgical resection. However, since many clinicians prefer to establish a diagnosis prior to consideration of a surgical procedure, several modalities are used for this purpose. Least invasive is the collection of a sputum sample for cytologic studies. In any instance, the evaluation begins with a thorough history and physical examination. Because 50–75% of all patients present with metastatic disease, clues to clinical stage will often be evident on their evaluation. The cervical, supraclavicular, and scalene regions should be examined carefully for possible lymphadenopathy; the skin for cutaneous or subcutaneous nodules; the axillary regions for masses or adenopathy; the chest for signs of bronchial or vascular obstruction or pleural effusion; and the abdomen for hepatic enlargement. Neurologic signs or symptoms or bone pain warrant appropriate imaging evaluation to rule out distant metastases.

Accurate clinical staging includes a combination of noninvasive and invasive procedures. Noninvasive studies include sputum cytology and imaging studies; most commonly used are chest radiography, computed tomographic (CT) scanning, and positron emission tomographic ([PET]usually PET-CT) scanning. For mediastinal or spinal lesions magnetic resonance imaging (MRI) is considered. Invasive procedures include bronchoscopy, CT or ultrasound-guided fine needle aspiration (FNA) or biopsy, lymph node biopsy, and surgical (open) biopsy using mediastinoscopy or thoracoscopy. Patients who present with clinical or radiographic evidence of extensive disease usually require the least invasive procedure to establish both the diagnosis and disease stage. Cytologic or histologic confirmation through FNA or biopsy usually is sufficient to confirm suspicion of N3 or M1 disease. Thoracentesis or pericardiocentesis should be performed on associated effusions to assess possible T4 disease. Other patients with less extensive disease often present with subtle radiographic findings that require more invasive techniques for adequate staging, particularly when mediastinal lymph node involvement is suspected. It is of note that the level of evidence for these recommendations is low and relies mostly on usual practice and expert opinion.

Noninvasive Studies

Sputum Cytology ■ Cytologic evaluation of sputum, bronchial washings, bronchial brushings, and FNA specimens have high diagnostic yield, but the positive and negative predictive values of each and their accuracy of diagnosis certainly are dependent on sampling error, tissue preservation, processing quality, and observer experience. Sputum cytology is a simple test with a specificity rate of 99%. However, the sensitivity rate is approximately 70% for central tumors, and less than 50% for peripheral lesions. To increase the yield, three specimens are usually collected. In practice, more invasive measures to obtain a diagnosis are used in most cases.

Imaging ■ Lung cancer is generally first imaged by chest radiography. CT scan, PET scan, and occasionally MRI is used to stage a known or suspected lung cancer and monitor response to therapy. The radiographic morphology of lung cancer may be correlated with cell type, with the following generalizations[74]: (1) Adenocarcinoma usually presents as a solitary pulmonary nodule, and most malignant solitary pulmonary nodules are adenocarcinomas. (2) Large central masses are usually squamous cell carcinoma (an endobronchial lesion thus may result in postobstructive changes) or SCLC (may involve mediastinal and hilar lymph nodes, sometimes without an overt parenchymal lesion). (3) A large peripheral mass usually represents large-cell or squamous cell carcinoma. Peripheral squamous cell carcinomas are more prone to central necrosis and formation of a cavity than other histologic types. Lobulated lesions with central masses associated with necrosis and thicker walls than typical for lung abscesses characterize cavitary squamous cell carcinoma. Adenocarcinoma occasionally manifests as a large peripheral mass. (4) Airspace disease (termed "ground glass opacity") or multiple nodules may occur with BAC, and sometimes with adenocarcinoma. (5) A sclerotic pattern may be identified in adenocarcinomas, as well as areas of chronic scar in association with a long-standing interstitial fibrotic pattern (a finding termed "scar carcinoma").

Chest Radiography ■ Posterior-anterior and lateral chest radiographs remain the simplest method for identifying patients with lung cancer. It is widely available, has low cost, and low radiation dose, but most cases are identified at an advanced stage. A standard chest radiograph can detect a lesion as small as 3 mm in diameter; however, unsuspected nodules generally are not seen unless larger than 5 mm in diameter. Associated atelectasis, postobstructive pneumonitis, abscess, bronchiolitis, pleural reaction, rib erosion, pleural effusion, or bulky mediastinal lymphadenopathy may be identified on radiographs, raising suspicions of a primary lung malignancy.

Plain chest radiography may identify abnormal pulmonary nodules. There are no absolute criteria to confirm a benign lesion on the basis of its radiographic appearance, but stability of size for 2 years and the presence of specific patterns of calcification (multipunctate foci, a dense central nidus, a popcorn ball, or laminated "bull's eye" appearance) are considered indicators of benignancy. However, some tumors such as BAC and typical carcinoids occasionally appear to be stable for 2 or more years. Since the absence of appreciable growth over a 2-year period had a predictive value of only 65% for a benign lesion, the dictum that 2- year stability on plain-film radiography indicates a benign process should be used with caution.[75]

Computed Tomography ■ As a single comprehensive study, CT scan remains the most effective noninvasive technique for evaluating suspected or known lung cancer and the mediastinum, which may contain associated metastatic disease. However, the accuracy of CT scanning in identifying metastatic disease in mediastinal lymph nodes is highly variable and its sensitivity ranges from 51% to 95%. Such a wide range in accuracy is secondary to variations in the criteria for nodal abnormality, which are based on size and shape of a lymph node, CT scanner differences, and nonuniformity in nodal mapping. A lymph node size of 1 cm or more in shortest diameter has been generally accepted as the criterion of abnormal nodal enlargement. Approximately 8% to 15% of patients considered to have a negative CT scan for mediastinal nodal enlargement, with lymph nodes sized 1 cm or less, will ultimately be found to have mediastinal nodal involvement at the time of operation. Mediastinal lymph nodes that are more than 2 cm in diameter contain metastatic disease in over 90% of cases. Lymph nodes that are 1.5–2 cm in size contain disease in over 50% of cases. Lymph nodes that are 1 to 1.5 cm in size harbor metastatic disease in 15% to 30% of cases. The negative predictive accuracy of CT scan is 85% to 92% for mediastinal lymph node metastases. For these reasons, many centers are now using PET-CT imaging.

Magnetic Resonance Imaging ■ MRI is not used for the routine evaluation of patients with lung cancer, but it does have specific advantages over CT scan. Because of its heightened ability to discern neurologic and vascular structures, tumors that reside in close proximity to neurovascular structures may be more accurately assessed by MRI than by CT scan. MRI is most useful in evaluating patients with superior sulcus tumors.

Positron Emission Tomographic Scanning ■ Over the past several years, PET scanning with 2-[18F]fluoro-2-deoxy-D-glucose (FDG-PET) has been increasingly used in the diagnosis, staging, and monitoring therapy of lung cancer. This test identifies areas of increased glucose metabolism, which is a common trait in pulmonary tumors. Since commercial PET scanners provide nominal spatial resolution of 4.5–6.0 mm in the center of the axial field of view, even lesions that are less than 1 cm in diameter can be detected on the basis of an increased uptake of FDG. Although initially heralded as a reliable noninvasive method of identifying and staging pulmonary neoplasms, a number of limitations have become apparent. Many inflammatory processes such as abscesses and active granulomatous diseases, as well as hypoxic conditions such as those that exist after radiotherapy, may cause high FDG uptake and lead to false-positive results. Treatment-induced hypermetabolic inflammatory changes also may lead to difficulty differentiating between treatment effects and those of the residual tumor. False negative results have occurred primarily in tumors with low glucose metabolism (carcinoid and BAC) and in small tumors, owing to the limited spatial resolution of current PET scanners.[76]

Integrated PET-CT PET provides imprecise information on the exact location of focal abnormalities. Thus, even if the results of PET and CT scan are visually correlated, the precise location of lesions is sometimes difficult to determine. To overcome this limitation, integrated PET-CT was recently introduced.[77] Recent studies suggested that integrated PET-CT had improved the diagnostic accuracy of NSCLC. Tumor staging was significantly more accurate with integrated PET-CT than with CT scan alone ($p = .001$), PET alone ($p < .001$), or visual correlation of PET and CT scan ($p = .013$); node staging was also significantly more accurate with integrated PET-CT than with PET alone ($p = .013$).[77] This technology is currently being tested in many centers in the world.

Invasive Studies

Bronchoscopy ■ Fiberoptic bronchoscopy (FOB) is an essential and standard technique for the evaluation of patients with pulmonary neoplasms; it remains the most important procedure for determining the endobronchial extent of disease. FOB permits careful survey of the supraglottic, glottic, tracheal, and bronchial regions to the level of most subsegments. Tumor (T) status can be defined by measuring tumor proximity to the carina and various bronchi and by identifying unsuspected occult lesions that indicate multiplicity of disease. For lesions that are visible by endoscopy, an accurate histologic diagnosis can be achieved in over 90% of cases. For central lesions, cytologic studies via needle aspiration, washings, and brushings, coupled with biopsy, heightens the diagnostic yield to over 95%. Peripheral lesions not visible endoscopically may be approached by cytologic studies of brushings and bronchioloalveolar lavage (BAL), which yield a diagnosis in 50 to 60% of patients. Cytologic studies, coupled with transbronchial FNA (TBNA), greatly enhance diagnostic yield. The efficacy of bronchoscopy in establishing an accurate diagnosis depends on the location of the lesion, the histologic characteristics of the lesion, its accessibility via bronchoscopy, and the level of experience of the cytopathologist.

Fine-Needle Aspiration Biopsy (FNA) ■ ***Transthoracic Percutaneous FNA Biopsy (TPNA)*** ■ TPNA has significantly heightened the ability to diagnose intrathoracic pathologic processes. With CT or ultrasound guidance, tissue samples can be obtained from poorly accessible sites in the lung, mediastinum, abdomen, and retroperitoneum. The procedure is performed under local anesthesia using a small-gauge needle. Aspirated material is immediately processed with optimal procedural coordination. Many centers use an on-site cytopathologist for interpretation. Should the material be inadequate, a repeat aspiration can be performed. TPNA has been shown to be over 90% effective in establishing a final diagnosis. The false-positive rate is low (1%) and the false-negative rate ranges from 23% to 29%. Complications after TPNA include pneumothorax (20–28%), with 5 to 7% requiring chest tube insertion; transient hemoptysis (2–4%); and, rarely, air embolism. Implantation of tumor cells along the needle tract has been reported in isolated cases but is considered extremely rare.[78]

Transbronchial FNA Biopsy (TBNA) ■ TBNA was introduced by Wang and Terry using fiberoptic bronchoscopy.[79] It has been used most widely to sample endobronchial and peripheral lesions, and significantly improves the diagnostic yield when coupled with standard diagnostic measures (washings, brushings, and biopsies). TBNA is best performed in a suite that is equipped with fluoroscopy to enhance localization of the lesion. One of the most important applications of TBNA is the evaluation of mediastinal lymphadenopathy. The true sensitivity and specificity of TBNA appear to range from 14-50% and 96-100%, respectively. Thus, negative results require definitive operative confirmation, but the risk of a false positive finding appears to be quite low.[78]

Advances in Bronchoscopy ■ The development of linear echo-endoscopes has opened up new diagnostic possibilities for patients with lung cancer. Transoesophageal endoscopic ultrasound-guided FNA (EUS-FNA) and endobronchail ultrasound-guided transbronchail needle aspiration (EBUS-TBNA) are both minimally invasive diagnostic techniques that enable real-time controlled aspirations of mediastinal lymph nodes and centrally located lung tumors. Evolving reports using these technologies suggest that EBUS-FNA has higher sensitivity than TBNA and that EUS plus EBUS may allow near-complete minimally invasive mediastinal staging in patients with suspected lung cancer. These newer diagnostic technologies may serve as an alternative approach for mediastinal staging in patients with suspected lung cancer.[80]

Electromagnetic Navigation Diagnostic Bronchoscopy ■ Advances in technology have led to the recent development of a new type of real-time guidance for sampling of peripheral lung lesions. Electromagnetic registration and guidance combines virtual bronchoscopy, three-dimensional (3-D) CT images, and a steerable probe to aid in the biopsy of lung lesions. The yield and safety of this technology are being tested in several centers.[81]

Mediastinoscopy ■ Transcervical mediastinoscopy is the best method for invasive evaluation of the middle mediastinum to include the peritracheal and subcarinal lymph nodes. The indication remains preoperative mediastinal nodal assessment in patients with CT scan evidence of cross-sectional lymph node enlargement of more than 1 cm. In such patients who are proven to have lung cancer, the chance that these nodes contain metastasis is over 7%. If the nodes are enlarged to 1.5 to 2 cm or more, the risk of having metastatic involvement is over 30%. The accuracy of cervical mediastinoscopy ranges from 80% to 90%, and the false-negative rate ranges from 10% to 12%. The lymph node station most commonly missampled is the subcarinal region, which is difficult to access in some patients and challenging to biopsy completely in most patients. The subaortic and aortopulmonary window regions are inaccessible by standard cervical mediastinoscopy.[82] Extended cervical mediastinoscopy, a variation of standard mediastinoscopy, has been useful for staging lesions in the left upper lobe. The standard mediastinoscopy incision is used, with the plane of dissection extending anterior to the innominate artery and aorta, anterolaterally to the level of the aortopulmonary window. Direct tumor invasion into the mediastinum or nodal disease within the prevascular space and aortopulmonary window can be assessed with this technique. Accuracy rates are over 91%. "Anterior mediastinotomy," originally described by McNeil and Chamberlain, permits direct visual access to the anterior mediastinum through the second, third, or fourth anterior interspace, with or without removal of a short portion of the adjacent cartilage. For right-sided lesions, the procedure provides access to the proximal pulmonary artery and SVC. The procedure is used on the left side to evaluate disease in the subaortic and lateral aortic regions.

Thoracoscopy ■ Thoracoscopy and video-assisted thoracoscopy (VATS) are used in a broader range of applications, including resectional techniques. The VATS approach is used in many thoracic conditions, and its role continues to evolve regarding the evaluation and management of lung cancer. It is currently considered for the evaluation and treatment of pleural tumors and effusions and in the diagnosis of indeterminate pulmonary nodules, and has a complementary role to standard mediastinoscopy in the staging of mediastinal lymph nodes. It has also become an accepted approach for resection of peripheral early-stage lung cancer in many centers.[83]

Operative Staging

Operative staging provides the opportunity to verify histologically the extent of gross and microscopic disease. The surgeon is responsible for performing a complete nodal dissection or nodal sampling as an integral part of the thoracotomy. Lymph nodes are removed and labeled according to the location of the station on the regional station map (Fig. 78-4). Lymph node maps were introduced in the 1970s when nodal dissection was recognized as an important component of surgical staging. In 1983, the American Thoracic Society (ATS), using transverse section anatomy as defined by CT scan and viewed at thoracotomy, developed a regional lymph node staging map, which was further revised

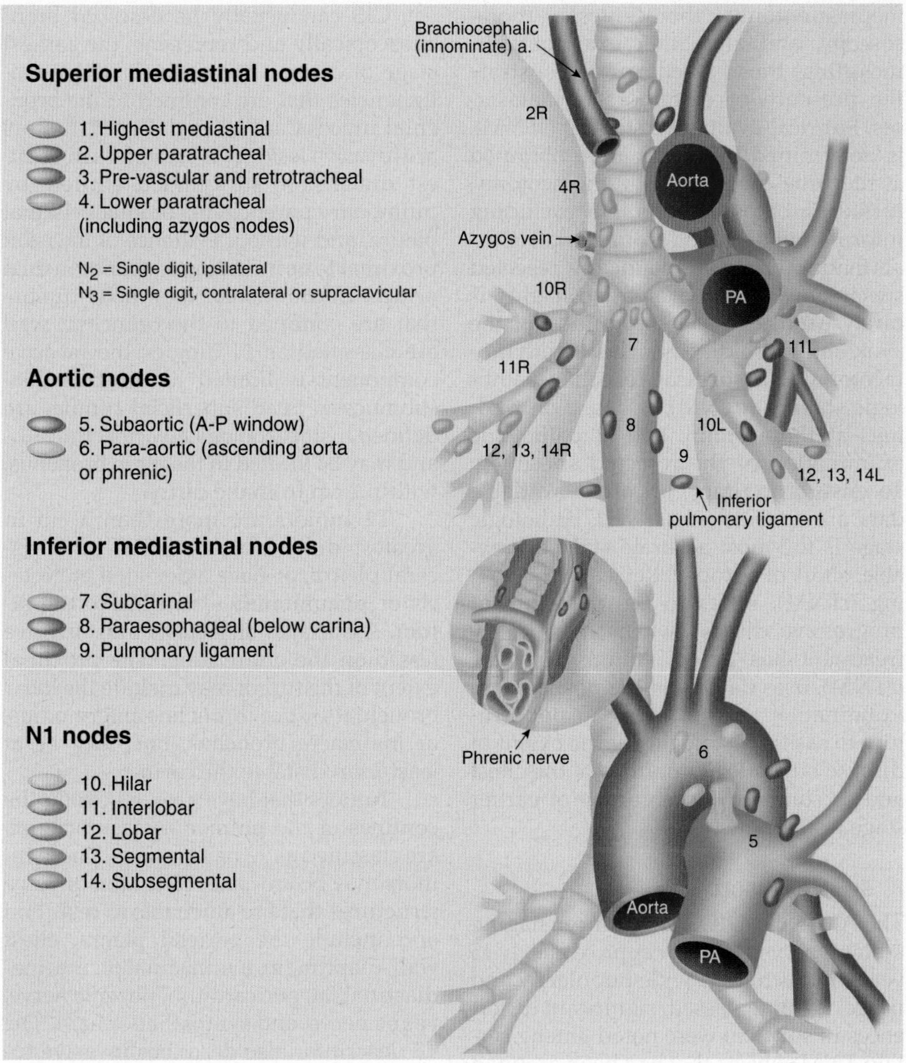

Figure 78-4 Regional lymph node stations for the staging of lung cancer. The location of the lymph nodes and assigned numbers are determined by the surgeon at the time of operation. *Source*: Adapted from Ref. 84.

by the Lung Cancer Study Group (LCSG). Another map, which is commonly used, was developed by Naruke, proposed by the Japan Lung Cancer Society (JLCS), and recommended by the American Joint Committee on Cancer (AJCC). The important difference between the two nodal maps is the location of station 10. In the ATS/LCSG map, station 10 represents mediastinal lymph nodes. In the AJCC/JLCS map, station 10 represents hilar lymph nodes. The current staging system places station 10 lymph nodes within the hilar nodes; therefore, they represent N1 nodes. The distinction between station 10 (N1 nodes) and station 4 (N2 nodes) is based on the position of the node relative to the visceral-to-mediastinal pleural reflection. Nodes covered by visceral pleura are level 10.[84] Within the mediastinum, a phantom midline exists to differentiate N2 and N3 nodes. Ipsilateral positive lymph nodes are N2 nodes, and contralateral positive lymph nodes are N3 nodes. If a lymph node straddles the midline and has its major component residing on one side, the nodal station is labeled according to the site of predominant location. Subcarinal nodes always bridge the midline but are classified as N2 nodes. If nodes within the subcarinal region obviously reside on the contralateral side, they should be labeled as N3 nodes. The surgeon ultimately is responsible for determining the boundary of the mediastinal and visceral pleura and for documenting the precise location of all lymph nodes prior to submitting them to the pathologist for examination.

Cancer Screening and Early Detection

Because symptoms of early-stage localized disease are insidious and nonspecific, they are frequently attributed to the effects of smoking. By the time the patient seeks medical attention, the disease is usually advanced so that complete surgical resection is possible in fewer than 30% of cases, and the overall 5-year survival rate is less than 15%. Clearly, screening and early detection of cancer at a more treatable stage is a desirable goal. Unfortunately, to date there have been no randomized controlled studies that have demonstrated a disease-specific mortality advantage attributable to screening methods of lung cancer.

In the 1970s, the National Cancer Institute (NCI) sponsored three separate randomized trials to assess the efficacy of lung cancer screening in male smokers (aged 45 years or older who smoked at least one pack per day).[85] By 1978, a total of 31,360 patients had been enrolled, and the results of a 5-year follow-up study were published in 1984. The Mayo Lung Project assessed the screening potential of routine chest radiographs versus symptom development, while the other two projects, the Johns Hopkins Lung Project and the Memorial Sloan-Kettering Lung Cancer Screening Program, evaluated the screening potential of routine sputum cytology with chest radiographs versus chest radiographs alone. Chest radiographs detected lung cancer at an earlier phase, improving resectability rates, whereas sputum cytology had no further impact. Final results of all three studies were unable to demonstrate a disease-specific mortality reduction, and for this reason there is no US policy on standardized screening for lung cancer.[86]

The introduction of low-radiation-dose spiral CT (LDCT) renewed interest in screening high-risk individuals for early lung cancer.[87] Initial data from separate centers suggested that LDCT improves detection of malignant disease by nearly 4- to 10-fold, but at the cost of a significantly high false-positive rate. These false-positive cases require further radiographic and/or invasive evaluation. Though LDCT is still an unproven technique, some medical establishments have been advocating its use for screening for lung cancer in the community at large.

The NCI-sponsored National Lung Screening Trial (NLST) is now conducting a randomized controlled trial to test whether LDCT scanning can reduce lung cancer mortality in asymptomatic individuals. Subjects are randomized to undergo screening with LDCT or chest x-ray. The NLST will enroll 50,000 high-risk heavy smokers (and former heavy smokers who quit within 15 years before randomization), aged 55 to 74 years. Participants will undergo an initial screening and two subsequent annual screenings and will be observed for a minimum of 4.5 years. The trial is powered to detect a modest but clinically relevant reduction of 20% in lung cancer mortality with LDCT screening. Randomization for the NLST began in September 2002 and was closed to further enrollment in 2004. Final analyses are expected in 2009.[88]

The Mayo Clinic recently presented its interim analysis of the NLST data. In a 5-year prospective study of LDCT in 1520 individuals at high risk of lung cancer, participants (who were aged 50 years or older and had smoked at least 20 pack-years) underwent five annual (one initial and four subsequent) CT scan examinations. Results suggested that CT allowed detection of early-stage lung cancers, and that the benign nodule detection rate was high. However, there was no significant difference in lung cancer mortality rates.[89]

Staging Systems

Staging is the determination of the extent of disease, with the intent of grouping patients with similar levels of disease for analytical, therapeutic, and prognostic purposes. The staging of lung cancer provides a scale of relative disease, which can be assigned to all patients with primary lung malignancies. Accurate staging of lung cancer is essential for defining operability, for selecting treatment regimens, for predicting survival, and for reporting comparable end results.

The staging system used in lung cancer has been based primarily on anatomic and morphologic criteria. The tumor-nodes-metastasis (TNM) system developed by Pierre Denoix in 1946 for staging of malignant tumors has remained the fundamental scheme for the classification of primary lung carcinoma. The TNM system has been used as the basis for the staging systems developed by both the AJCC and the International Union Against Cancer (UICC), and more recently for that developed by the International Staging System (ISS), which has replaced the earlier systems.

The accuracy of staging depends on available clinical information and relies on preoperative and subsequent evaluations at different times during the course of the disease: clinical-diagnostic staging (c), surgical-evaluative staging (s), postsurgical resection-pathologic staging (p), retreatment staging (r), and autopsy staging (a). These letters are used as a prefix to the TNM descriptors to identify the point during the course of the disease at which the stage was established (eg, cTNM for clinical-diagnostic staging). Clinical diagnostic staging (cTNM) is based on the anatomic extent of disease that can be determined by any diagnostic testing short of thoracotomy. Such an evaluation may include findings from the history, physical examination, routine and special radiography, bronchoscopy, esophagoscopy, mediastinoscopy, mediastinotomy, thoracentesis, thoracoscopy, and any other examinations, including those used to demonstrate the presence of extrathoracic metastases. Surgical-evaluative staging (sTNM), is determined by information obtained at the time of exploratory thoracotomy, including biopsy results, but excluding information obtained from complete examination of a therapeutically resected specimen. Surgical-evaluative staging is rarely used today in recognition of the avoidable morbidity associated with thoracotomy. Postsurgical resection-pathologic staging (pTNM), is based on findings at thoracotomy and at pathologic examination of the resected specimen. To ensure accuracy, all other available data are considered as well. Pathologic stage is the most accurate stage achievable, short of autopsy. Retreatment staging (rTNM), refers to the restaging of progressive disease when the primary treatment has failed. Autopsy staging (aTNM), uses data from the postmortem examination and provides an opportunity to assess histologically the extent of disease beyond the confines of the chest and to compare the accuracy of earlier stage evaluations.

Staging of NSCLC

The AJCC and UICC lung cancer staging systems served well for approximately 15 years and achieved wide popularity and usage. As time passed, significant differences in survival were noted among certain TNM subsets that had been grouped prospectively into the same clinical stage. To achieve uniformity in the descriptors of the TNM system and to heighten accuracy in predicting stage-specific survival, the AJCC and the UICC in 1985 together developed a single system that has become the primary system used internationally, the ISS. This system was revised in 1997 to allow greater specificity in identifying patient groups with similar prognoses and treatment options (Tables 78-7, 78-8, and 78-9).[90] Since its inception, the ISS has gained worldwide acceptance and remains the predominant system for the staging of lung cancer.

TNM Descriptors

The primary tumor descriptor T derives its classification on the basis of size, location, and extent of local invasion. T0 indicates no evidence of a primary tumor and is used primarily during retreatment staging. TX describes tumors that are identified cytologically by malignant cells in sputum samples or bronchial washings, but no specific site of origin can be recognized radiographically or bronchoscopically. TX also is used to describe tumors that cannot be adequately assessed during retreatment staging.

CIS can usually be assessed bronchoscopically and represents the earliest stage of disease. Accordingly, those malignancies that are confined to the bronchial mucosa are labeled Tis. T1 tumors are invasive lesions 3.0 cm or less in greatest dimension, surrounded entirely by pulmonary parenchyma or intact visceral pleura, and without evidence of invasion proximal to or including a lobar bronchial orifice. Uncommonly, superficial tumors that are confined to the bronchial wall are classified as T1 tumors; the invasive component is limited to the bronchial submucosa. Such superficial tumors are defined histopathologically, not clinically, and may be located in the main bronchus, within 2 cm from the carina.

T2 tumors are more than 3 cm in greatest dimension, or invade the visceral pleura, or have associated atelectasis or pneumonitis extending to the hilum. Associated atelectasis must involve less than the entire lung. The proximal extent of the tumor may include the lobar bronchial orifice, bronchus intermedius, or mainstem bronchus, but must be at least 2 cm distal to the carina.

Tumors that have grown beyond the confines of the pulmonary parenchyma are classified as T3 or T4 lesions. These tumors may be any size. T3 tumors involve structures that are amenable to resection and include the parietal pleura, chest wall, diaphragm, mediastinal pleura, mediastinal fat, pericardium, phrenic nerve, vagus nerve, and sympathetic chain. The T3 descriptor also describes invasive tumors that reside within 2 cm of the carina without involving the carina. Atelectasis of the entire lung is considered consistent with T3 status. T4 includes tumors that invade the structures of the deep mediastinum (including the heart, great vessels, trachea, esophagus, vertebral body, and carina), are associated with a pleural effusion containing malignant cells, or have a satellite tumor nodule(s) in the primary tumor lobe of the lung. The implication of a pleural effusion in conjunction with lung cancer is addressed later in the chapter.

Regional lymph node involvement is classified with the descriptor N. When no demonstrable metastases exist in regional lymph nodes, the N0 descriptor is given. Metastatic disease to the hilar lymph nodes is classified as N1 disease, and metastasis to the ipsilateral mediastinal lymph nodes or subcarinal lymph nodes is classified as N2 disease. The specific locations of involved hilar and mediastinal lymph nodes are important to staging and are discussed later. Metastatic disease located in lymph nodes in the contralateral mediastinum, contralateral hilum, or on either side outside the thorax (scalene or supraclavicular) is classified as N3 disease.

Table 78-7 TNM Descriptors

Primary Tumor (T)	
TX	Primary tumor cannot be assessed, or tumor proven by the presence of malignant cells in sputum or bronchial washings but not visualized by imaging or bronchoscopy
T0	No evidence of primary tumor
Tis	Carcinoma in situ
T1	Tumor ≤3 cm in greatest dimension, surrounded by lung or visceral pleura, without bronchoscopic evidence of invasion more proximal than the lobar bronchus[a] (ie, not in the main bronchus)
T2	Tumor with any of the following features of size or extent: >3 cm in greatest dimension Involves main bronchus, ≤2 cm distal to the carina Invades the visceral pleura Associated with atelectasis or obstructive pneumonitis that extends to the hilar region but does not involve the entire lung
T3	Tumor of any size that directly invades any of the following: chest wall (including superior sulcus tumors), diaphragm, mediastinal pleura, parietal pericardium; or tumor in the main bronchus, ≤2 cm distal to the carina but without involvement of the carina; or associated atelectasis or obstructive pneumonitis of the entire lung
T4	Tumor of any size that invades any of the following: mediastinum, heart, great vessels, trachea, esophagus, vertebral body, carina; or tumor with a malignant pleural or pericardial effusion,[b] or with satellite tumor nodule(s) within the ipsilateral primary-tumor lobe of the lung
Regional Lymph Nodes (N)	
NX	Regional lymph nodes cannot be assessed
N0	No regional lymph node metastasis
N1	Metastasis to ipsilateral peribronchial and/or ipsilateral hilar lymph nodes, and intrapulmonary nodes involved by direct extension of the primary tumor
N2	Metastasis to ipsilateral mediastinal and/or subcarinal lymph node(s)
N3	Metastasis to contralateral mediastinal, contralateral hilar, ipsilateral, or contralateral scalene, or supraclavicular lymph node(s)
Distant Metastasis (M)	
MX	Presence of distant metastasis cannot be assessed
M0	No distant metastasis
M1	Distant metastasis present[c]

[a] The uncommon superficial tumor of any size with its invasive component limited to the bronchial wall, which may extend proximal to the main bronchus, is also classified T1.

[b] Most pleural effusions associated with lung cancer are due to tumor. However, there are a few patients in whom multiple cytopathologic examinations of pleural fluid show no tumor. In these cases, the fluid is nonbloody and is not an exudate. When these elements and clinical judgment dictate that the effusion is not related to the tumor, the effusion should be excluded as a staging element, and the patient's disease should be staged T1, T2, or T3. Pericardial effusion is classified according to the same rules.

[c] Separate metastatic tumor nodule(s) in the ipsilateral nonprimary-tumor lobe(s) of the lung also are classified M1.

Table 78-8 Stage Grouping in Lung Cancer: TNM Subsets[a]

Stage	TNM Subset
v0	Carcinoma in situ
IA	T1 N0 M0
IB	T2 N0 M0
IIA	T1 N1 M0
IIB	T2 N1 M0
	T3 N0 M0
IIIA	T3 N1 M0
	T1 N2 M0
	T2 N2 M0
	T3 N2 M0
IIIB	T4 N0 M0
	T4 N1 M0
	T4 N2 M0
	T1 N3 M0
	T2 N3 M0
	T3 N3 M0
	T4 N3 M0
IV	Any T, Any N, M1

[a] Staging is not relevant for occult carcinoma, designated TX N0 M0.

Metastases to distant organs or lymph node sites beyond the N3 sites, or ipsilateral involvement in lobe(s) of the lung other than the site of the primary tumor, chest wall, or pleural nodules discontinuous from the primary tumor, are identified by the M1 descriptor.

Stage 0 includes CIS (Tis N0 M0). Stage I comprises T1 or T2 lesions without any lymph node metastases or distant metastases (stage IA, T1 N0; stage IB, T2 N0). Stage II includes T1 or T2 tumors with metastasis to the lymph nodes in the peribronchial or ipsilateral hilar region only, or locally more advanced tumors without any nodal involvement (stage IIA, T1 N1, stage IIB, T2 N1, T3 N0). Stage IIIA disease represents T3 with metastasis limited to the peribronchial or ipsilateral hilar nodes or any metastasis to ipsilateral mediastinal lymph nodes (T3 N1, T1 N2, T2 N2, T3 N2). Stage IIIB disease includes any tumor more extensive than T3, any tumor with supraclavicular or contralateral mediastinal lymph node involvement, or any tumor with a malignant pleural effusion but without evidence of distant metastasis (any T N3, T4, any N). Stage IV disease pertains to distant metastatic spread (any T, any N, M1).

Staging of NSCLC has been modified in recent years with the introduction of FDG-PET. This modality, and more so integrated PET-CT, may provide a combination of anatomical and functional assessment of the primary tumor and suspected areas of metastasis. Guidelines for their use in the preoperative setting are evolving gradually.[91]

Revisions to the AJCC Cancer Staging Manual are expected in 2009, and a proposal for the revision of the NSCLC TNM stage groupings were recently published by the International Association for the Study of Lung Cancer (IASLC) based on analyses of a large international database of over 67,000 NSCLC cases treated between 1990 and 2000.[92] The IASLC recommendations for revisions of the T stage descriptors included: Subclassifying T1 as T1a (≤2 cm) and T1b (>2 cm and ≤3 cm); subclassifying T2 as T2a (>3 cm and ≤5 cm, or T2 by other criteria and ≤5 cm) and T2b (>5 cm and ≤7 cm); Reclassifying T2 tumors >7 cm as T3; Reclassifying the subset of T4 tumors defined by additional nodules in the same primary lobe as T3; Reclassifying the subset of M1 disease defined by additional nodules in an ipsilateral but different lobe as T4. Recommendations for revisions of the M stage descriptors included: Reclassifying pleural dissemination, defined by malignant pleural effusions and/or pleural nodules, as M1a; subclassifying M1 disease defined by contralateral lung nodules as M1a and disease defined by distant metastases outside the lung/pleura as M1b. There were no recommended changes for the N stage descriptors. Revisions to the resulting TNM stage groupings included: Reclassifying T2a N1 M0 disease as stage IIA, T2b N0 M0 disease as stage IIA, and T4 N0-1 M0 disease as stage IIIA. It is expected that these proposed changes will be adopted, further enhancing the clinical relevance of the TNM staging system.

Staging of SCLC

When the TNM system was first developed for NSCLC in the 1960s, it was not prognostic when applied to a population of patients with SCLC. This was most likely explained by the very low incidence or stage I or II SCLC and the fact, that without chemotherapy, all patients with SCLC had very short survival. In a placebo-controlled trial of cyclophosphamide, The Veterans Administration Lung Group (VALG) developed a two-stage system for SCLC.[93] They separated patients into two groups, termed limited or extensive, based on whether or not their disease could be encompassed by a radiation port. The former group included those with malignant pleural effusion; the latter group all those with metastatic disease to distant sites. This classification was prognostic in patients on both arms of the trial, with median survival rates twice as long in limited stage patients.

Table 78-9 ■ **Lymph Node Map Definitions**

Nodal Station	Anatomic Landmarks
N2 nodes: All N2 nodes lie within the mediastinal pleural envelope	
1. Highest mediastinal nodes	Nodes lying above a horizontal line at the upper rim of the brachiocephalic (left innominate) vein where it ascends to the left, crossing in front of the trachea at its midline
2. Upper paratracheal nodes	Nodes lying above a horizontal line drawn tangential to the upper margin of the aortic arch and below the inferior boundary of No. 1 nodes
3. Prevascular and retrotracheal nodes	Prevascular and retrotracheal nodes may be designated 3A and 3P; midline nodes are considered to be ipsilateral
4. Lower paratracheal nodes	The lower paratracheal nodes on the right lie to the right of the midline of the trachea between a horizontal line drawn tangential to the upper margin of the aortic arch and a line extending across the right main bronchus at the upper margin of the upper lobe bronchus, and contained within the mediastinal pleural envelope; the lower paratracheal nodes on the left lie to the left of the midline of the trachea between a horizontal line drawn tangential to the upper margin of the aortic arch and a line extending across the left main bronchus at the level of the upper margin of the left upper lobe bronchus, medial to the ligamentum arteriosum and contained within the mediastinal pleural envelope. Researchers may wish to designate the lower paratracheal nodes as No. 4s (superior) and No. 4i (inferior) subsets for study purposes; the No. 4s nodes may be defined by a horizontal line extending across the trachea and drawn tangential to the cephalic border of the azygos vein; the No. 4i nodes may be defined by the lower boundary of No. 4s
5. Subaortic (aortopulmonary window)	Subaortic nodes are lateral to the ligamentum arteriosum or the aorta or left pulmonary artery and proximal to the first branch of the left pulmonary artery and lie within the mediastinal pleural envelope
6. Para-aortic nodes (ascending aorta or phrenic)	Nodes lying anterior and lateral to the ascending aorta and the aortic arch or the innominate artery, beneath a line tangential to the upper margin of the aortic arch
7. Subcarinal nodes	Nodes lying caudal to the carina of the trachea, but not associated with the lower lobe bronchi or arteries within the lung
8. Paraesophageal nodes (below carina)	Nodes lying adjacent to the wall of the esophagus and to the right or left of the midline, excluding subcarinal nodes
9. Pulmonary ligament nodes	Nodes lying within the pulmonary ligament, including those in the posterior wall and lower part of the inferior pulmonary vein
N1 nodes: All N1 nodes lie distal to the mediastinal pleural reflection and within the visceral pleura	
10. Hilar nodes	The proximal lobar nodes, distal to the mediastinal pleural reflection and the nodes adjacent to the bronchus intermedius on the right; radiographically, the hilar shadow may be created by enlargement of both hilar and interlobar nodes
11. Interlobar nodes	Nodes lying between the lobar bronchi
12. Lobar nodes	Nodes adjacent to the distal lobar bronchi
13. Segmental nodes	Nodes adjacent to the segmental bronchi
14. Subsegmental nodes	Nodes around the subsegmental bronchi

Through the past 20 years the "limited" classification has been refined to identify those who are candidates for curative-intent chemoradiation. This modification of the VALG definition requires that disease be encompassed in a tolerable radiation port and excludes patients with malignant pleural and pericardial effusions. Further, because large ports encompassing very advanced nodal disease are not feasible, patients with contralateral supraclavicular or contralateral hilar nodes are also excluded. The TNM system is applied in evaluating resectablity of the unusual patient with SCLC who presents with a T1-2 primary and appears clinically node-negative. This represents approximately 5% of SCLC.

As in NSCLC, the process of staging of SCLC is key to determining therapy and prognosis. The main goal of thorough staging is to identify patients who are candidates for curative intent chemoradiation. Patients who have clinically evident metastatic disease (extensive-stage) do not require thorough staging for all potential sites of spread. Because the major intent of staging is to determine therapy, the case can be made to image the brain in all patients since positive findings are an indication for eventual brain radiation. A critical part of the initial evaluation is determining the physiologic or functional status, the major prognostic indicator in SCLC, and a reflection of both short and long-term prognosis. Poor performance status in SCLC increases risk of early treatment-related death during initial chemotherapy.

A complete history and physical examination are fundamental and often can give clues to the extent of disease. Standard chest radiography with posterior-anterior and lateral views can assess the primary tumor and concurrent parenchymal disease. Mediastinal lymph node involvement often can be suggested by mediastinal widening. CT scan is important in further evaluating the primary tumor and local regional disease. It is critical to planning the ports for administration of radiation therapy in patients with limited stage. There are emerging data that FDG-PET imaging as an adjunct to CT optimizes radiation planning, although this practice is not yet standard.[94]

One of the most common sites of extrathoracic metastatic disease is the bone. Approximately 38% of patients who present with SCLC have bone metastases. For this reason, radionuclide bone scan is important. If bone scan reveals suspect regions that suggest metastatic disease, site-specific bone radiographs are recommended for confirmation. Bone scan is associated with some degree of error because it often highlights areas of benign disease such as osteoarthritis, compression fractures, and prior trauma. For this reason, bone scan alone should not be used for therapeutic decision making.

Bone marrow examination is indicated in the staging of patients with SCLC if unexplained cytopenias are documented. The bone marrow is involved with metastatic disease in 17% to 23% of patients. Bone marrow involvement is diagnosed by bone marrow aspiration and biopsy, which are complementary tests. The bone marrow is removed from the iliac crests, and bilateral biopsies increase the yield by approximately 10%. Fewer than 5% of patients present with bone marrow metastases as the only site of extrathoracic disease. Thus, it has been abandoned as a routine staging procedure.

Because the CNS is involved by disease in close to 20% of patients at the time of diagnosis, careful attention should be paid to the neurologic review of systems and examination. Metastases to the nervous system have been noted to occur in over 40% of patients over the entire course of the disease, and may occur at autopsy in up to 65% of patients.[95,96] CT scan of the brain documents occult metastases in 5% to 10% of patients. On the basis of its apparent higher sensitivity rate, MRI may improve the accuracy of staging and is used more frequently for that reason. Suspected spinal or leptomeningeal disease with carcinomatous meningitis can be confirmed by MRI coupled with cerebrospinal fluid cytologic studies.

Metastasis to the liver is present in 22% to 28% of patients with SCLC at diagnosis. Liver function tests and abnormal liver enzymes are not sensitive nor specific as a screening tool, although patients whose test results are within normal ranges rarely have associated hepatic metastasis. Abdominal CT scan is an important addition to staging to evaluate the liver as well as the adrenal glands, kidneys, spleen, pancreas and intra-abdominal lymph nodes.

Prognostic Factors in SCLC ■ The strongest clinical prognostic factors in patients with SCLC include extent of disease, performance status, sex, and age. Abnormalities in laboratory factors that have implications for prognosis include hemoglobin, white cell and platelet counts, and biochemical abnormalities such as lactate dehydrogenase, sodium, bicarbonate, and alkaline phosphatase levels.[97]

Like NSCLC staging, staging of SCLC has been modified in recent years with the introduction of FDG-PET. This modality, and more so the integrated PET-CT, may provide a combination of anatomical and functional assessment of the primary tumor and suspected areas of metastasis.[98] One small series in patients with SCLC showed that FDG-PET upstages 8% of patients otherwise deemed limited stage.[94]

Performance Status

In both NSCLC and SCLC, the patient's functional status or performance status (PS) is a key determinant of not only the patient's ability to undergo therapy, but also the patient's prognosis. PS is a general measure of a patient's physiologic status, taking into account the cancer and its associated effects along with other concurrent medical problems, such as cardiac or pulmonary disease. The PS is measured by two scales, the Zubrod and the Karnofsky.

Patients who are fully ambulatory and either asymptomatic (Zubrod PS 0) or mildly symptomatic but fully ambulatory (PS 1) usually tolerate therapy well. Patients who are symptomatic and spend up to 50% of the day in bed (PS 2) do not tolerate therapy as well, are at higher risk of complications of chemoradiotherapy, and usually are not surgical candidates. Patients with NSCLC who are symptomatic and in bed more than 50% of the day, but not bedridden (PS 3), and those patients who are bedridden (PS 4) usually are not candidates for chemotherapy. Introduction of measures to correct medical problems, such as infection, anemia, electrolyte imbalances, malnutrition, and cardiac dysfunction, may improve the PS to permit therapy. In the case of SCLC, PS 3–4 is not considered a strict contraindication to chemotherapy, though modification of doses, routine incorporation of growth factor support, and initial use of palliative thoracic radiation may be considered to reduce the risk of early treatment-related death in these patients.

In a study of more than 5000 NSCLC and SCLC patients entered into VALG protocols between 1968 and 1978, 77 prognostic factors were analyzed.[99] The most important prognostic factor was PS at the time of diagnosis. Extent of disease, weight loss greater than 10% in the previous 6 months, and the presence of any systemic symptoms were identified as other key prognostic factors. Analyses of other large patient cohorts have confirmed the prognostic significance of PS.[100,101]

General Guidelines for Lung Cancer Staging

Patients who present with a new lung lesion and no evidence of metastatic disease by history, physical examination, or chest radiography should undergo CT scanning of the chest, including the liver and adrenal glands. Sputum cytologic studies can provide a diagnosis in about 10% of patients; it is more sensitive in patients with central lesions. A diagnosis also can be obtained by FOB or FNA as already discussed. In some circumstances, when a clinical stage I malignancy is suspected, invasive diagnostic studies can be waived, and the patient can undergo resection for diagnosis and treatment. If a resection beyond a lobectomy is required or if the patient is a high surgical risk, it is best to attempt preoperative diagnosis of the lesion. If the patient requires pneumonectomy, a cancer diagnosis should be made before proceeding with the resection.

Asymptomatic patients who have no abnormal results on physical examination and who are potential surgical candidates with clinical stage I, stage II, or stage IIIA (N0 or N1) disease can undergo resection. Patients with chest CT scan evidence of metastatic disease, particularly N2 or N3 disease, should undergo invasive studies, which may include cervical mediastinoscopy. In some instances, FNA biopsy can be performed. For patients with potentially resectable stage III disease, the status of the mediastinal lymph nodes is the most important factor in determining therapy. If the lymph nodes are radiographically enlarged (>1 cm in cross-sectional diameter), histologic or cytologic evaluation is necessary prior to proceeding to thoracotomy. Evidence of improved outcome using neoadjuvant chemotherapy in this population has allowed some of these patients to come to resection. Randomized trials and institutional series have sought several different treatment strategies for potentially resectable stage IIIA (N2) disease: preoperative chemotherapy and/or radiation therapy, or chemotherapy and radiation therapy with no surgery. These studies are discussed in more detail later in this chapter. If N3 (stage IIIB) disease is discovered, nonoperative management is appropriate.

The invention of PET significantly changed lung cancer staging. The American College of Surgeons Oncology Group Z0050 studied the use of PET in staging potentially operable NSCLC. Results suggested that in patients with suspected or proven NSCLC considered resectable by standard staging procedures, PET can prevent nontherapeutic thoracotomy in a significant number of cases. The authors concluded that use of PET for mediastinal staging should not be relied on as a sole staging modality, and positive findings should be confirmed by mediastinoscopy. In addition, they suggested that metastatic disease, especially a single site, identified by PET, required further confirmatory evaluation.[102]

If a diagnosis of SCLC is made, a thorough search for metastatic disease should be undertaken, followed by appropriate treatment in the form of chemotherapy or chemoradiotherapy. In only a small minority of cases (5%), can a patient with SCLC be considered for surgical intervention; these are cases of very early stage disease, that is, disease confined only to the lung without evidence of nodal or metastatic disease.

If the history and physical examination are suggestive of metastatic disease, other noninvasive staging studies directed to the area of concern should be performed. In addition to a chest CT scan, these studies may include a PET scan, a CT scan or MRI of the brain, bone scan, and a CT scan of the abdomen if the CT scan of the chest did not include the liver and adrenal glands. FDG-PET is substituted for bone scan in many institutions. The bone scan remains the most sensitive imaging study to detect skeletal metastases, but the apparent false-positive rate is as high as 50%. Bone scan detects metastases in only 3% to 4% of asymptomatic patients, most of whom have other foci of metastases. Bone scanning in asymptomatic patients should generally be reserved for those patients with locally advanced (T3, T4, or N2) or stage IV disease. These scans can be helpful in identifying unsuspected sites of metastases. Should such areas be identified, they should be confirmed radiologically and, if need be, by histologic or cytologic studies.

Upper abdominal CT scan should not be routinely performed for patients with clinical stage I or stage II disease. Extrathoracic metastases are unusual under such circumstances. In one series of patients with potentially resectable disease, 12% had unsuspected hepatic involvement. In the same series, unsuspected adrenal metastases were identified in 8% of patients. In another consecutive series of 172 patients who underwent adrenal CT scanning, 12% had metastatic disease; more than one-half of those patients had no other identifiable site of disease, and metastatic disease was confirmed cytologically by FNA biopsy in all patients. Approximately 10% of all lung cancer patients have CNS metastases at the time of diagnosis. CNS metastases are most common in patients with SCLC. Occult brain metastases are present in approximately 3% to 6% of patients with NSCLC. CT scanning of the brain identified a 13% incidence of metastases in patients being evaluated for resection, although only 21% of these were unsuspected by virtue of unremarkable neurologic examination findings. Because of this low incidence of occult brain metastases, particularly in patients with early clinical stages of disease, routine CT scanning of the brain is not performed.

In patients with locally advanced (T3, T4, or N2) or stage IV disease, a CT scan of the brain and a bone scan are essential. These should be performed, even if extensive disease elsewhere has been confirmed, since the discovery of brain metastases alters the type of therapy. MRI is probably more sensitive than CT scans for identifying and diagnosing asymptomatic metastatic disease to the brain, but its role in routine staging remains to be defined.

Therapy for NSCLC

In patients with NSCLC, the most important prognostic factor is tumor stage, and this factor largely determines treatment.[103] Surgery is the standard mode of treatment of patients with stage I and II tumors and for some patients with stage III tumors; with preoperative or postoperative radiation therapy or chemotherapy (or both) added if the tumor invades the mediastinal lymph nodes. The use of combined-modality therapy in locally advanced stage III NSCLC is an area of intense investigation, as discussed later in this chapter. Patients with stage IV disease are treated with chemotherapy or palliative radiation therapy or with supportive therapy alone. Patients with histologically documented unresectable or inoperable NSCLC are evaluated first for definite therapy "for cure" with a combined chemoradiation therapy approach. If there are pressing symptomatic needs for palliation, such as complete obstruction of a major airway, hemoptysis, SVC obstruction, painful bony metastases in the weight-bearing areas, or symptomatic brain metastases, the initial treatment is radiotherapy with or without chemotherapy. If a patient has evidence of disseminated disease and there is no pressing need for radiotherapy, the approach includes consideration of systemic chemotherapy, or supportive therapy alone if the patient's general condition is not suitable for systemic chemotherapy. Each of the three main disciplines involved in the treatment of lung cancer—surgery, radiotherapy, and chemotherapy—is discussed individually. SCLC, whose treatment is radically different from that of NSCLC, is discussed as a separate section, albeit with similar organization.

Results by Stage

Stages IA and IB ■ The average 5-year survival rate for patients with stage I NSCLC is approximately 65% (range 55–90.5%). Within this group, several factors appear to influence survival: T status, tumor size independent of T status, and histology. The more favorable tumors are T1 squamous cell carcinoma and T1 BAC. Focal T1 N0 BAC has been reported to have a 5-year survival rate as high as 90.5%.[104] Significant prognostic factors that adversely affect survival include mucin production by the tumor and diffuse invasion.

Overall survival rates of all patients with T1 N0 disease have been reported to be 82% at 5 years and 74% at 10 years, while those for patients with T2 N0 disease are 68% at 5 years and 60% at 10 years.[105] In this series of 598 patients, the overall incidence of recurrence was 27% (local or regional 7%, systemic 20%). Second primary tumors developed in 206 patients (34%). Of these 206 tumors, 70 (34%) were second primary lung cancers, for an overall incidence of second primary lung cancers of 11.7% (70 of 598). These findings, confirmed by other investigators, prompted division of stage I into two groups, stage IA (TI N0) and IB (T2 N0).

The median survival period for all patients with T1 N0 NSCLC is approximately 8 years. The long-term prognosis for patients with T1 N0 NSCLC has been evaluated by the LCSG, which reported recurrence rates per eligible patient per year of 0.042 for patients with squamous tumors and 0.088 to 0.106 for patients with nonsquamous tumors within the first 5 years after surgery.[106] A later report suggested, however, that the rate of recurrence decreased (from 0.043 to 0.013), whereas the rate of new primary lung cancer increased (from 0.009 to 0.016), with no significant differences between the two histologic subgroups.[105]

Stages IIA and IIB ■ The average 5-year survival rate for patients with stage II disease is 41.2% (range 29–51%). Several studies have evaluated this group to identify tumor characteristics that affect survival. The LCSG reported significant survival differences between patients with squamous carcinoma and those with adenocarcinoma and between patients with a T1 lesion and those with a T2 lesion.[107] More specifically, patients with T1 squamous carcinoma had a 5-year survival rate of 75%, while those with T2 adenocarcinoma had a 5-year survival rate of 25%. Mountain, in 1986, reported 5-year survival rate in 317 patients: 54% for those with a T1 lesion and 40% for those with a T2 lesion. These persistent differences in survival based on T status led to division of stage II into IIA and IIB.

Patients whose tumor is staged T3 N0 because of chest wall invasion have a favorable 5-year survival rate, as high as 56%. Patients with T3 N2 disease, however, have a 5-year survival rate ranging from 16% to less than 5%. Survival rates are worse in those patients who have incomplete resections. The similarity of the outcomes for T3 N0 and T2 N1 disease supported its reclassification as stage IIB.[64,90]

Adjuvant or Neoadjuvant Chemotherapy ■ Supplementing surgery with chemotherapy has been tested by several studies with promising results.[4] Such an approach in selected patients may prolong survival with reasonable toxicity. This approach is becoming a standard of care in many cases in early-stage disease, and is discussed later in this chapter.

Stage IIIA ■ Approximately 25% to 40% of patients with NSCLC have stage III disease. Of these, approximately one-third present with potentially resectable disease, stage IIIA (T1–3 N2, T3 N1). The median survival duration for all patients with stage IIIA (clinical or surgical stage) disease is 12 months, and the 5-year survival rate is 9% to 15%. Within the stage IIIA subset, however, survival rates vary widely.[64,90]

Burt and colleagues conducted a review of T3 and T4 tumors that involve the mediastinum, but not the mediastinal lymph nodes. The overall 5-year survival rate was 19%, with median survival duration of 18 months. Factors that were found to affect survival were complete resectability and histologic type. The 5-year survival rate with complete resection was 30%, and the 5-year survival rate of patients with adenocarcinoma or large-cell carcinoma was 30%, while that of patients with squamous cell carcinoma was 14%.[108]

Patients with clinical (preoperative) N0 or N1 disease but pathologic (postresection) N2 disease survive longer than patients with clinical N2 disease, and 3- and 5-year survival rates of 47% and 34%, respectively, were reported for such patients.[109] Pearson and colleagues noted that patients with negative mediastinoscopy findings who were found to have N2 disease following resection had a 24% 5-year survival rate; the 5-year survival rate was only 9% for those who underwent resection after positive mediastinoscopy.[110] Patients with "completely resected" pathologic N2 disease have a median 5-year survival rate approaching 22%.

The role of combined-modality treatment remains somewhat unclear. Many trials that included combinations of surgery, radiation therapy, and chemotherapy have been conducted for patients with stage III disease. The various treatment regimens and results are discussed in later sections.

Stage IIIB ■ The median survival duration for stage IIIB patients is 8 months, and the 5-year survival rate is 5% or less.[64,90] The vast majority of these patients receive nonoperative therapy. There is, however, a select group of patients that can be considered for surgical resection: the rare patient with IIIB disease on the basis of a T4 tumor involving the carina and occasionally the SVC, aorta, or atrium. With increased but acceptable operative morbidity and mortality rates, extended resection and reconstruction techniques can be undertaken. After carinal resection, 3- and 5-year survival rates are directly related to nodal status, and range from 0% to 43%. Extended resections for selected patients with other T3/T4 tumors have been associated with 5-year survival rates that vary from 0% to 18.3%, depending on nodal status.

Stage IV ■ Stage IV disease is beyond the reach of surgical cure, with 5-year survival rate of less than 5%. Treatment of this disease is well outlined in the following sections. On rare occasions, patients with solitary brain metastasis and an otherwise resectable lesion can undergo resection of both tumors. In this select group, surgery seems to prolong life and improve quality of life better than nonsurgical treatment, although no prospective studies have been performed. The 5-year survival rate has been shown to range from 13% to 21%, with median survival duration of 14 months.

Surgical Treatment

Preoperative Assessment ■ For any patient being considered for pulmonary resection, specific risk factors play an important role in determining operability and the chances of perioperative complications. Factors that are known to be associated with increased perioperative morbidity and mortality are greater age, continued cigarette use, cardiac disease, restricted pulmonary function, and pneumonectomy. In association with these factors, PS is a key general indicator of physiologic function and, as such, is another factor determining risk. With the increasing use of adjuvant and induction therapy, concurrent systemic illnesses (renal or hepatic dysfunction, weight loss, anemia, leukopenia) and a diminished PS score associated with therapy can heighten a patient's intolerance to surgical intervention. Recent reviews of preoperative therapy for patients with stage III lung cancer have noted higher rates of complications than cited in historic reviews, although long-term survival appears to have been positively affected.[111] Several cooperative groups have evaluated the influence of PS on survival in large numbers of patients with inoperable lung cancer.[99] Each study found that a patient's initial PS had a definite impact, not only on prognosis, but also on the ability to tolerate aggressive therapy. A similar observation can be made in the evaluation of patients being considered for aggressive therapy in the form of surgical resection; those with a poor PS are at a higher risk than those with a good PS. Consideration of operability must include careful assessment of a patient's PS in addition to other key risk factors.

Cardiac Function ■ The most common untoward perioperative events are cardiopulmonary ones. For this reason, the cardiopulmonary system must be carefully evaluated and optimally prepared before operative intervention. If there is a history of cardiac or vascular disease or suggestive symptoms, a thorough investigation of the cardiovascular system beyond initial assessment is imperative. Following screening electrocardiography, which should be performed in all patients, further tests to detect cardiac dysfunction or coronary artery disease may be necessary. Stress testing, echocardiography, multigated acquisition (MUGA) scanning, dobutamine echocardiography, or stress/Persantine thallium scanning may give clues to a heightened risk of ischemic disease. Coronary angiography ultimately may be necessary. Au and colleagues reported a postpneumonectomy mortality rate of 21% in patients older than 70 years.[112] The mortality rate was significantly adversely affected if the patient had a history of ischemic heart disease ($p = .001$). Miller and colleagues found that routine thallium scanning identified over 10% of patients with significant asymptomatic coronary artery disease and made a difference in management in half these patients.[113] Their review underscores the importance of careful questioning for possible underlying cardiac pathology. For patients unable to undergo a standard exercise test, Persantine thallium testing is very useful for predicting patients at risk of developing a postoperative cardiac event following major general or vascular procedures (sensitivity 100%, specificity 43%).

If studies reveal significant coronary or valvular disease that should be operatively corrected, angioplasty, coronary artery bypass, or valve repair can be performed prior to or during pulmonary resection. A series of 45 patients who underwent pulmonary resection for lung cancer either at the time of cardiac surgery or within a median of 2 months following surgery revealed operative mortality rates of 6.7% or 0%, respectively.[114] Another study on 11 concomitant cardiac and pulmonary resections for lung cancer revealed no operative deaths. The disadvantage of concomitant surgery is the inability to perform an adequate lymph node dissection for staging.

Patients who have had a recent myocardial infarction (MI) are at a significantly increased perioperative risk of re-infarction or death. Steen and colleagues showed that performance of any operation requiring general anesthesia within 3 months after an MI results in a 27% incidence of re-infarction.[115] The risk dropped to 11% 3 to 6 months after infarction and to 5% thereafter. Wells and colleagues reported no re-infarction in 48 patients who required an operation within 3 months of an MI. Their excellent results may have been secondary to very aggressive perioperative cardiac monitoring and early initiation of medical management. The nature of the procedures and the selection criteria in this study are not well outlined, but the results do suggest that the risk in this group of patients can be reduced with aggressive perioperative measures.[116] The best time to perform a pulmonary resection following an MI is unclear. Certainly, the risk of the operation and possible re-infarction should be weighed against the possibility of growth and spread of the malignancy. Mathisen and Wain postpone resection to at least 4 to 6 weeks after the event.[117] Our approach agrees with that of Mathisen and Wain. If such management is not feasible, alternative treatment should be considered.

Pulmonary Function ■ Most patients with lung cancer have associated chronic lung disease because of many years of smoking. The degree of underlying parenchymal pathology and abnormal chest mechanics may be subtle or subjectively insignificant because of compensatory lifestyle changes. On the other hand, concurrent benign pulmonary disease may be severely, subjectively debilitating for unclear reasons and without objective proof. Various objective studies, noninvasive and invasive, can provide good information in the overall assessment of pulmonary function and can provide the surgeon with a good estimate of risk.

Because pulmonary resection reduces lung volume, precise measurements of pulmonary function and reserve are imperative. Predicted postoperative volumes, based on spirometry, are useful in estimating the amount of lung that can be removed. Spirometric studies measure overall lung capacity, reserve volumes, functional residual capacity, and forced expiratory volumes. These simple tests give a relatively crude but highly useful estimate of lung function and pulmonary mechanics. The presence and extent of underlying disease can be quickly determined, along with any response to therapy (eg, bronchodilators).

Patients with abnormal pulmonary function are known to have an associated increase in perioperative complications. Several spirometric parameters have been analyzed by various authors and are useful in identifying patients at increased risk (Fig. 77–5). No single parameter is used alone to select or exclude patients from surgery. The information is always considered collectively, along with other parameters noted below. Patients with limited pulmonary function in the noted risk categories generally are more susceptible to perioperative complications because of limited functional reserve to adapt to post-resection changes and underlying lung disease that is more susceptible to dysfunction caused by inflammation or infection. To optimize pulmonary function, patients are strongly encouraged to stop smoking 2 weeks in advance of surgery to reduce the amount of bronchorrhea and smoking-related bronchitis. Pulmonary physiotherapy is initiated with bronchodilators, incentive spirometry and coughing, appropriate antibiotics, and a walking program. Patients with poor pulmonary function test (PFT) results should have the tests repeated following this 1- to 2-week physiotherapy program. In some instances of severe bronchospasm, a short course of steroid therapy can be helpful.

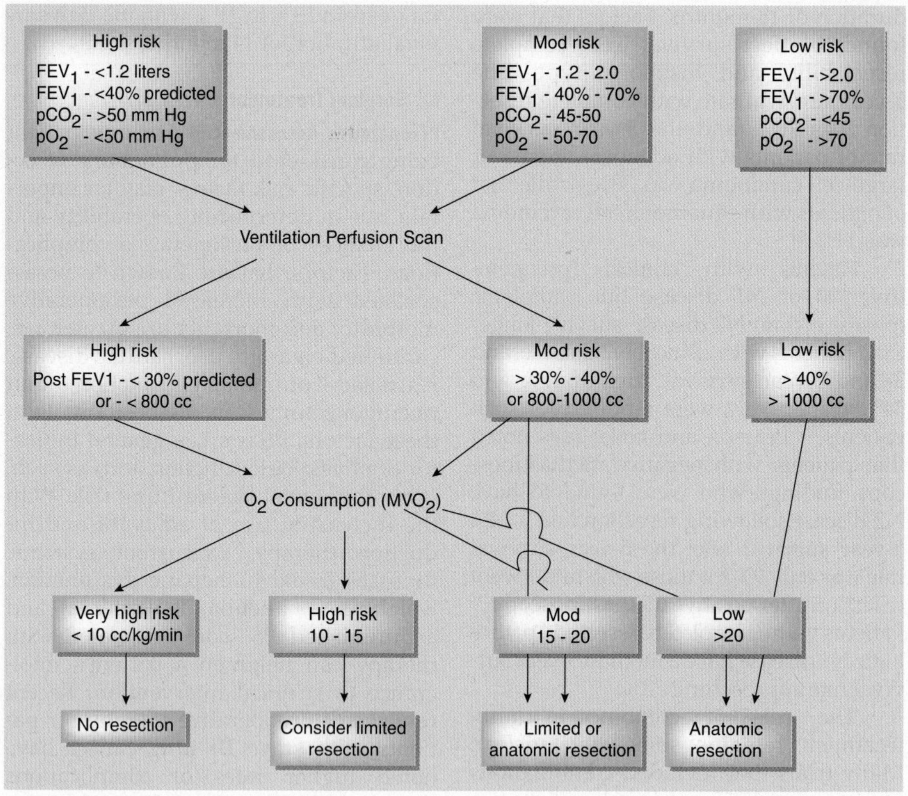

Figure 78-5 ■ Pulmonary risk based on spirometry results, arterial blood gases (ABG), and oxygen consumption studies (MVO2). *Abbreviations:* CXR, chest radiography; FEV, forced expiratory volume.

Arterial Blood Gases ■ Resting hypoxia or hypercapnia is a subtle indicator of chronic pulmonary disease that affects proper gas exchange. A variety of etiologies, both pulmonary and cardiac, can cause blood gas abnormalities. The most common cause in patients with lung cancer is ventilation/perfusion mismatch caused by chronic obstructive pulmonary disease. Areas of pneumonia, atelectasis, or arterial obstruction from a lung tumor only exacerbate a pre-existing mismatch. An arterial oxygen pressure (Po_2) less than 60 mm Hg and a resting partial pressure of carbon dioxide (Pco_2) over 50 mm Hg are indicators of high risk of perioperative complications. Whether because of the tumor, other underlying disease, or both, the presence of abnormal arterial blood gases indicates a problem that can be worsened by resection of an already limited resource of lung.

Xenon Scanning ■ Careful analysis of normally perfused and ventilated lung segments can be helpful in identifying those patients who can safely undergo resection. Split lung function studies using inhaled ^{133}Xenon and injected ^{99m}Tc-labeled macroaggregated albumin give percentages of the total ventilation and perfusion in each lung. The post-resection volumes can be calculated by multiplying the ventilation or perfusion percentage to the remaining lung.

Oxygen Consumption Study ■ The previously mentioned tests are performed primarily with the patient in a resting state without the benefit of exertional stresses. Measurement of a patient's capacity to exercise may, in fact, be a better predictor of candidacy for surgery. A good measure of exercise capacity is the maximal amount of oxygen that can be consumed during a given period of time. This oxygen consumption study (MVO_2) measures the end product of cardiac and pulmonary interaction in a real-time stress situation that appears to better simulate the physiologic demands of surgery. Several studies have shown the usefulness of MVO_2 in predicting increased risk of perioperative complications.[118] Patients with an MVO_2 higher than 20 mL/kg/min are at low risk of complications, whereas those with an MVO_2 less than 10 mL/kg/min are at a very high risk of complications. Those with values from 10 to 15 are at high risk but may be candidates for limited resection or possibly lobectomy, depending on spirometric results. Patients with values from 15 to 20 have a low to moderate risk and usually can tolerate major resection, including pneumonectomy.

Diffusing Capacity ■ Other parameters of underlying pulmonary disease include abnormal gas diffusion and exchange and an imbalance of ventilation and perfusion. The diffusing capacity for carbon monoxide (DLCO) estimates pulmonary capillary surface area and indirectly reflects pulmonary capillary hemoglobin content. DLCO also estimates alterations in alveolar microarchitecture, indicating the presence of emphysematous changes. Ferguson and colleagues showed the value of measuring DLCO and its usefulness in predicting postoperative pulmonary complications in patients who have underlying parenchymal changes despite having acceptable spirometry results.[119] In their group of patients, as the predicted DLCO percent worsened, the prevalence of pulmonary complications and mortality increased, particularly when the DLCO was less than 60%. In a more recent, updated study of diffusing capacity, Ferguson and colleagues showed a direct correlation between worsened diffusing capacity and postoperative complications and mortality. They concluded that the predicted postoperative diffusing capacity percentage is the strongest single predictor of risk of complications and mortality after lung resection. They found little relationship between the predicted postoperative diffusing capacity percentage and the predicted postoperative forced expiratory volume in 1 second and suggested that these two values be evaluated independently in estimating operative risk.[119] The usefulness of DLCO as a predictor of pulmonary complications has been confirmed by other investigators.

Assessment of Pulmonary Hypertension ■ In patients with chronic lung disease manifested by abnormal arterial blood gas values, reduced diffusing capacity, low values in oxygen consumption studies, or poor spirometric results underlying pulmonary hypertension may be present and often to some degree. Unrecognized pulmonary hypertension can contribute to pulmonary complications and mortality in patients undergoing resection, particularly in those undergoing pneumonectomy. Right ventricular work is already increased in patients with pulmonary hypertension. With resection, further work is imposed and can lead to hemodynamic compromise. Eventually, failure can ensue. The specific values of pulmonary pressures that place a patient at risk of resection are unclear. If marginal spirometry and poor oxygen consumption values coexist with abnormal indicators of right heart function and pulmonary vascular resistance, alternative therapy may need to be considered.

Surgical Technique ■ *Conduct of Anesthesia* ■ Pulmonary resections are conducted under general anesthesia. After placement of adequate intravenous access and appropriate monitoring devices, general anesthesia is induced, and the patient is intubated with a single-lumen endotracheal tube. Fiberoptic bronchoscopy is performed if it has not been performed previously by the operating surgeon. Bronchoscopy provides the opportunity to assess the airway, the extent of endobronchial disease, and other possible sites of unsuspected lesions. Following bronchoscopy, in most instances, a double-lumen endotracheal tube is placed to provide selective ventilation. In such a fashion, the operated lung can be deflated, facilitating access to the hilar structures without respiratory activity impeding visualization. In instances of complex resections for which bronchoplastic or vascular reconstruction is required, variations in the conduct of anesthesia may include cross-table ventilation, jet ventilation, or cardiopulmonary bypass. At the completion of the operation, the patient is awakened in the operating room and extubated, depending on the extent of the operation and the condition of the patient. Pain management is key to a smooth recovery. Some accepted modalities for adequate control of post-thoracotomy discomfort are continuous epidural analgesia and continuous intravenous analgesia delivered via a patient-controlled analgesia pump. These methods usually provide satisfactory relief from pain while permitting patients to cough, breathe deeply, and ambulate effectively. Supplemental nonsteroidal agents are used when breakthrough pain occurs. Other methods for pain relief are also used, such as intercostal nerve cryoablation, continuous delivery of local anesthetic agents, and intercostal nerve blocks.

Incisions ■ Several approaches to the chest cavity are used for resection of pulmonary tumors. The most frequently used incision is the posterolateral thoracotomy; it permits the best overall exposure to the pleural space. For this and most other thoracic incisions, the patient is placed in the lateral decubitus position with the table slightly flexed. A "lazy S"-shaped incision is made, passing under the tip of the scapula. The chest cavity is commonly entered through the fifth intercostal space. For resections that must include a portion of the chest wall, the incision is tailored accordingly; in particular, for superior sulcus tumors, the incision is carried posterosuperiorly with division of the trapezius muscle. At the completion of the operation, chest tubes are placed and brought out through separate incisions. Closure is accomplished by reapproximating the ribs and closing the chest wall musculature and subcutaneous tissue in individual layers.

The anterior thoracotomy is used primarily for noncomplex lesions located in the mid, lower, and anterior lung fields. The patient is placed in the supine position. The incision travels in a curvilinear fashion under the border of the pectoralis muscle, although in some instances, some fibers of the pectoralis are divided. In women, the incision is made in the inframammary fold and can be carried laterally or medially as needed. The disadvantage of the anterior thoracotomy is limited exposure of the superior and posterior mediastinum.

The axillary thoracotomy can be used for uncomplicated and straightforward pulmonary resections, primarily for an upper or middle lobectomy. A horizontal or transversed incision can be used to expose the underlying musculature with care to avoid the long thoracic nerve. The only muscle divided is the intercostal muscle, along with splitting of a few fibers of the serratus anterior. The chest cavity is entered through the fourth or fifth intercostal space. The advantages of this approach include better cosmesis, smaller incision length, and quicker opening and closure. Also, the recovery time may be shorter because relatively fewer muscles are divided. Two other types of muscle-sparing thoracotomy are also available: anterior and posterior. In anterior muscle-sparing thoracotomy, the skin incision is placed along the anterior portion of the posterolateral thoracotomy. The latissimus musculature is retracted posteriorly, and the serratus anterior musculature is retracted anteriorly to expose the rib cage. The posterior muscle-sparing thoracotomy is placed along the posterior portion of the posterolateral thoracotomy. The latissimus and underlying serratus are reflected anteriorly, while a small rim of exposed trapezius muscle is retracted posteriorly. The chest cavity is entered through the desired interspace, usually the fifth or sixth. The primary disadvantage of muscle-sparing thoracotomies is their inability to provide adequate access for the opening of an interspace higher than the fifth and a limited ability to spread the ribs for exposure that may be critical in more complex resections.

A median sternotomy or clamshell incision can be used for resections of tumors located in the upper lobes or in cases of bilateral disease when exploration of both thoracic cavities is desired. Sternotomy provides good access to both hemithoraces, facilitates anesthesia by keeping the patient in the supine position, and is a less painful incision than any thoracotomy. The disadvantages of sternotomy are that exposure of the lower lobes is poor, and resection of tumors in this location is difficult. Moreover, mediastinal lymph node dissections are not as complete as those performed through a thoracotomy. Access to the lower lobes is better through a clamshell incision, but this method of exposure is much more painful than a sternotomy.

Thoracoscopic resection (also called VATS) has gained significant attention over the past decade and especially in the past 3–5 years.[120] Multiple investigators have shown the ability to perform anatomic lobectomies and even pneumonectomies using a VATS approach without any rib spreading. Series of over a 1000 patients including all stages of disease have been reported and the outcomes, compared to modern historical controls, have been similar. There is mounting data that the postoperative recovery is greatly shortened compared to standard rib spreading techniques. Other advantages that have been documented include decreased postoperative air leaks, pneumonia, atrial fibrillation, length of stay and even mortality. These advantages have led some investigators to hypothesize that better tolerance of adjuvant chemotherapy will be seen following thoracoscopic lobectomy versus standard approaches. These claims have not been substantiated in a randomized trial, and it is likely that no such trial will be performed since enrollment in such a trial would be limited by patient preference. The penetration of VATS lobectomy into the standard of care for early stage lung cancer will likely parallel what was seen with the rise of minimally invasive cholecystectomy in the 1990s. No large scale randomized studies comparing open cholecystectomy to minimally invasive cholecystectomy were preformed but patient preference and a wealth of retrospective data provided the impetus for a change in the treatment of gallbladder disease. It is likely that a similar trend will be seen with VATS lobectomy.

Exploration of the Chest ■ After entry into the chest, the pleural cavity, lung, and mediastinum are evaluated thoroughly to assess resectability and possible metastatic disease. Parietal pleural implants are indicative of T4 disease, whereas implants extending beyond the parietal pleura into the chest wall or diaphragmatic implants represent metastatic disease. Both situations preclude resection. The presence of pleural fluid indicates the possibility of a malignant effusion, and intraoperative cytologic evaluation should be performed prior to any resection; a malignant effusion also indicates T4 disease and precludes resection. If no diagnosis has been achieved preoperatively, the lesion in question is assessed and biopsied, if this can be accomplished easily and safely. Often, a wedge excisional biopsy is done to completely remove a peripherally located tumor. If the lesion is located centrally, an FNA or Tru-cut biopsy can be performed. An anatomic resection may be necessary if the lesion cannot be safely or adequately biopsied or if tumor spillage can occur as a consequence of a biopsy. A pneumonectomy should not be performed, however, without a tissue diagnosis.

The presence of mediastinal lymphadenopathy does not preclude the potential for complete resection. In contrast to mediastinal lymph nodes that are found to contain metastatic disease prior to thoracotomy, microscopically positive mediastinal lymph nodes (N2) that are discovered at thoracotomy do not carry as poor a prognosis. Patients with clinical (preoperative) N0 or N1 disease but pathologic (postresection) N2 disease survive longer than patients with clinical N2 disease. Tumors that extend deeply into the pulmonary hilum or are densely fixed to the mediastinum or chest wall may require a more extended resection than anticipated. In most instances, resectability can be determined by preoperative noninvasive studies, exploratory thoracotomy revealing unresectable disease in only about 5% of patients. In such circumstances, where unexpected findings occur at thoracotomy, the surgeon decides the feasibility of an extended resection. The first priority remains the safety of the patient and whether an extended resection can be reasonably and completely performed on the basis of the studies that evaluated the patient's cardiac and pulmonary functions. If physiologic evidence indicates an acceptable risk, resectability is then determined, taking into account the factors that differentiate T3 and T4 tumors. The determinants of a T3 tumor usually do not prevent a safe and complete resection; a resection that accomplishes removal of the tumor with negative gross and microscopic margins provides the best opportunity for long-term survival. If the tumor is T4, the likelihood of complete resectability is low except in isolated circumstances in which advanced techniques can be used. These situations are discussed in the section "Extended Surgical Procedures."

Standard Surgical Procedures ■ Pneumonectomy, the total removal of the lung, is indicated for tumors that cannot be completely resected with a lesser procedure. Pneumonectomy is often indicated for central lesions that involve either the mainstem bronchus or the main pulmonary artery, tumors that are located in both the upper and lower lobes, and locally recurrent tumors. The procedure is most commonly performed through a posterolateral thoracotomy. The vascular structures are mobilized, ligated, and divided within either the thoracic or pericardial cavity (for central tumors). The main bronchus is mobilized to the level of the carina and stapled (or suture closed) no more than 0.5 cm from the carina. Following division of the bronchus and removal of the specimen, the mediastinal lymph nodes are dissected.

Usually, postoperative pleural drainage is unnecessary, unless fluid or blood drainage from the hemithorax needs to be monitored. Aggressive pulmonary toilet and pain control are mandatory to reduce the incidence of pulmonary complications.

Operative mortality and morbidity rates have improved over the past 25 years owing to improvement in perioperative monitoring, anesthetic techniques, postoperative care, and antibiotics. Mortality rates vary depending on the magnitude of the resection. The 30-day mortality rates for limited resection, lobectomy, and pneumonectomy are 1.4% to 3.8%, 1.8% to 3.8%, and 5% to 12%, respectively. Mortality rates for pneumonectomy as high as 21% to 43% have been reported when coupled with aggressive preoperative, concomitant chemotherapy, and radiation therapy. Complications from all causes occur in over one-fourth of all patients. Cardiopulmonary complications (pneumonia, acute respiratory distress syndrome, atelectasis, aspiration, atrial fibrillation, and myocardial infarction) are the most frequent morbidities associated with pulmonary resection and occur in approximately 20% to 30% of patients. Postoperative pneumonia is responsible for the majority of the postoperative deaths. Empyema occurs in approximately 2% of patients undergoing pneumonectomy. Mortality rates for pneumonectomy range from 6% to 12%. For older patients or those undergoing a right pneumonectomy, the mortality rate is higher and can approach 10.6% to as high as 37% for some high-risk patients who have undergone preoperative therapy.[121–124]

Lobectomy is the most common type of resection performed for lung cancer and accounts for approximately 65% to 75% of all resections at our institution. Such anatomic resections provide a method for removing the primary tumor, associated disease, and lymph node-bearing areas while leaving a significant amount of residual functional parenchyma. Cancer survival is equivalent for patients undergoing lobectomy or pneumonectomy for all stages of disease when a complete resection is performed. Lobectomy requires isolation, ligation, and division of the individual segmental arterial and venous branches supplying the lobe. Division of the fissure between the lobes is usually performed with a stapling device to reduce the air leak that occurs from incising the pulmonary parenchyma. The lobar bronchus is closed with a stapler or with sutures. For lesions that are located close to the lobar orifice, an adequate margin of resection often cannot be achieved. In such circumstances, a portion of the main bronchus must be included with the resection. This type of resection is termed a sleeve resection and is performed as a parenchyma-sparing procedure to avoid pneumonectomy (Fig. 78-6). It is most commonly performed for lesions located in the right upper lobe, but it may be used for tumors in the left upper lobe, left lower lobe, or bronchus intermedius. The procedure is performed to include a small segment of grossly normal bronchus (5 mm) to ensure an adequate margin. Once frozen section analysis confirms negative margins, the two ends of the bronchus are reapproximated with interrupted sutures, achieving an airtight seal. In selected patients, bronchial sleeve resection has proven to be a safe and effective method for pulmonary preservation, with cancer survival rates comparable with those following pneumonectomy.[125] The overall 5-year survival rate in patients with stage III disease who undergo sleeve lobectomy is 21%. A 5-year survival rate of 38% has been reported following sleeve resection of T3 lesions; the survival rate appears to be directly related to the extent of N2 nodal involvement. As for pneumonectomy, pulmonary complications are the most common event after lobectomy and are the primary cause of postoperative mortality. The overall procedural mortality rate, however, is only 1% to 3%. Sleeve resections also have low operative mortality but carry a 5% risk of anastomotic complications (leak or stricture).[126]

Limited resections include segmentectomy, wedge resection, and lumpectomy. Any segment of lung can be resected, but this form of limited resection requires a bit more tedious dissection through the lung parenchyma than standard lobectomy. A segmentectomy indicates that a distinct anatomic resection was performed. The pulmonary artery and segmental bronchus are individually isolated and divided. The segment is removed from the remaining lobe by stapled excision or blunt dissection, and the segmental pulmonary venous branches are divided as encountered. Wedge excision, in contrast, is performed without identifying the adjacent anatomic landmarks. It is a simple and quick procedure. A stapling device usually is used to remove the lesion, including a rim of grossly normal lung to provide a clear margin. Wedge resections can be used only for peripherally located lesions. Lesions that reside more deeply within the pulmonary tissue often are not amenable to wedge resection and may require precise local excision with laser or electrocautery assistance (lumpectomy). The pulmonary tissue is directly incised and the lesion is removed, with preservation of the surrounding lung. Postoperative air leaks usually are minimal.

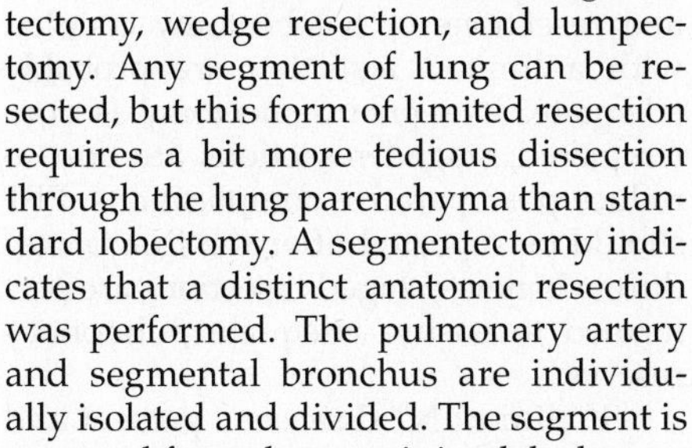

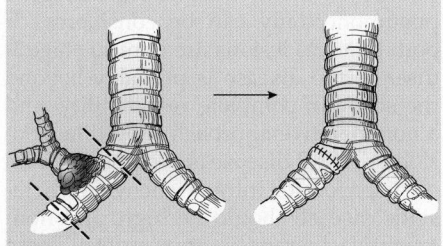

Figure 78-6 ■ A standard right upper lobectomy cannot be performed in this circumstance because residual tumor will remain in the bronchial stump. Rather than performing a pneumonectomy, a sleeve lobectomy is performed to ensure negative margins while still preserving the right middle and lower lobes.

Over the past 35 years, lobectomy has been regarded as the procedure of choice for the treatment of early-stage lung cancer. The LCSG completed a prospective phase 3 trial comparing limited resection (segmentectomy or wedge resection) with lobectomy for patients with small peripheral tumors staged intraoperatively as T1 N0 malignancies.[127] Patients were randomized to undergo standard lobectomy, segmentectomy, or wedge resection. Patients who underwent limited resection had a significantly higher rate of local recurrence. Survival tended to favor patients treated by lobectomy, particularly those with nonsquamous tumors, but the difference was not statistically significant. There was no significant difference in either morbidity or mortality among any of the procedures. The conclusions were that lobectomy should remain the standard procedure for patients with early-stage disease. Nakamura and colleagues recently performed a meta-analysis to compare survival after limited resection and after standard lobectomy for patients with stage I disease. They studied 14 articles, including the sole randomized controlled trial that was reported by the LCSG, and found that survival after limited resection for stage I lung cancer was comparable to that after lobectomy.[128] Most authorities, however, follow the LCSG guidelines and reserve limited procedures for patients with pulmonary function problems or other illnesses that preclude lobectomy.[129] These conclusions are being challenged in an era of earlier detection with high resolution computed tomography. A number of authors have reexamined the role of limited resections for very early (<1 cm) lesions. In addition, alternative treatment modalities such as radiofrequency ablation and radiosurgery are being examined as well. Additional studies to delineate the role of these treatments and the patients for whom they are suited still need to be done. Ad hoc use of these modalities should be discouraged and enrollment of the patient in a trial designed to evaluate these modalities should be encouraged.

Extended Surgical Procedures ■ Patients with tumors considered T3 N0 because of chest wall invasion who undergo chest wall resection have 5- year survival rates ranging from 26% to 60%. In patients with T3 N2 tumors, on the other hand, the 5-year survival rate is less than 5%, although Martini has reported a 5-year survival rate of 21% for patients with regional lymph node involvement. Other factors adversely influencing survival are incompleteness of resection and depth of invasion of the tumor into the chest wall. Overall 5-year survival rates for patients with surgically resected T3 tumors have ranged from 12% to 40%.[130]

Tumors involving the carina are considered T4 lesions. Most lesions involving the carina are not amenable to surgical resection (Fig. 78-7). There are, however, several indications for resection: (1) tumors restricted to the carina, such as rare cases of primary lung cancer arising on the carina, and less common neoplasms such as adenoid cystic carcinoma or mucoepidermoid carcinoma; (2) tumors of the mediastinal trachea that extend to involve the origin of the main bronchus or carina; (3) primary carcinoma of the lung extending proximally to involve the origin of the main bronchus and carina on either the right or left side, which may, in very rare instances, be managed by carinal resection or sleeve pneumonectomy; and (4) rare cases of benign disease involving the carina with local destruction. These are indications that have been defined by Pearson.[131]

Operative mortality rates for carinal resection and sleeve pneumonectomy are significantly higher than for traditional pulmonary resections and have been reported to range from 10% to 30%. In selected patients with tumors confined to the carina or tracheobronchial angle, sleeve pneumonectomy can achieve a complete resection; however, the significant 30-day mortality risk of 8% to 20.9%

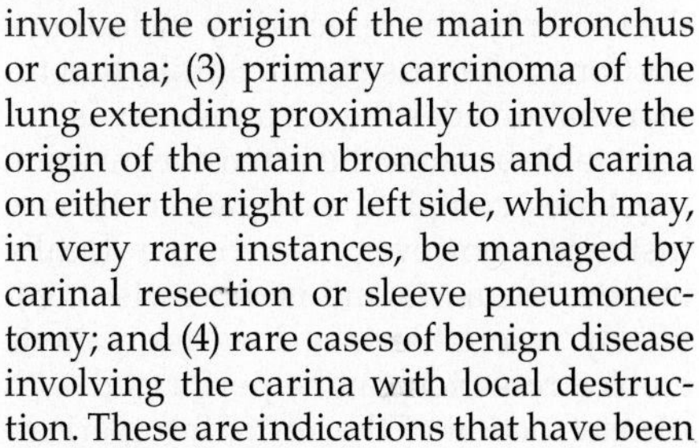

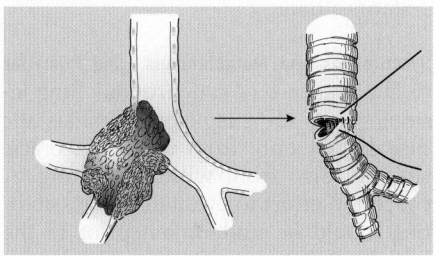

Figure 78-7 ■ A sleeve pneumonectomy. The tracheal carina is resected with a small segment of distal trachea and an anastomosis is made with the proximal left main stem bronchus.

indicates that caution must be used in recommending such a procedure. Five-year survival rates for these procedures have been reported as high as 23% to 35%. Survival after resection of T4 tumors that involve the carina is directly related to the extent of nodal disease; 3-year survival rates are 43% for N1 disease, 34% for disease involving only the subcarinal node, and 0% when the upper mediastinal nodes are involved.[132,133]

Tumors that involve the vena cava, aorta, main pulmonary artery, or left atrium are considered T4 tumors. If the vena cava becomes directly involved by the primary pulmonary neoplasm, the effect is compression or wall invasion. Compression or obstruction of the vena cava is manifested by distal venous engorgement, which most frequently compromises the SVC, causing SVC syndrome. Although the more common cause of SVC syndrome is compression from metastatic disease in lymph nodes in the superior mediastinum, direct tumor compression can cause the same process. In most instances, such tumors represent extensive disease and carry a poor prognosis. Treatment is usually nonsurgical, although in a few cases of localized disease with vena cava involvement, the tumor can be resected by including a portion of the vessel wall. Similarly, a tumor that invades the aorta usually is unresectable because the extensive invasion precludes complete extirpation. In rare instances, however, if a tumor locally invades the aorta and is otherwise completely resectable in a low-risk patient, en bloc resection can be performed with reconstruction of the aorta. Intrapericardial extension of the tumor not uncommonly involves the left atrium, precluding resection. In some instances of local invasion of the left atrium, a complete resection can be accomplished without hemodynamic compromise. Tsuchiya and colleagues reported a 5-year survival rate of 22% after resection of the left atrium to achieve a complete resection.[134] Such reports suggest the feasibility of aggressive approaches for selected T4 tumors, and for this reason patients should not be denied a surgical evaluation based on their T status alone.

Synchronous and Metachronous Lung Primaries

■ The presence of synchronous lung lesions raises the suspicion of metastatic disease not only from an extrathoracic site, but also from within the lung. A concerted effort to evaluate all possibilities should be undertaken prior to the initiation of any treatment. The histology is particularly important. If adenocarcinoma is found in the lung, numerous potential extrathoracic sites of origin can exist. A complete examination that includes a thorough evaluation of the gastrointestinal tract, breast, and reproductive system is imperative. If the lung lesion is squamous carcinoma, a systematic inspection of the upper aerodigestive tract and rectum should be performed. This includes panendoscopy (nasopharyngoscopy, laryngoscopy, bronchoscopy, and esophagoscopy), with biopsies of any suspicious lesions. Only after an exhaustive search has been undertaken to rule out nonpulmonary sources should lung primaries be considered. If the lesions are present within the same lobe, these lesions probably originated from the same source. The larger of the two should be considered the primary, while the other represents a satellite lesion, an intraparenchymal metastasis. Satellite lesions are discussed in the next section.

Synchronous primary lung cancers occur in 0.26% to 1.7% of all patients with lung cancer.[135] Practical pathologic and clinical criteria have been proposed as guidelines to distinguish primary and metastatic tumors.[136–138] Probable or definite synchronous lung cancers are physically separate and located in a different segment, lobe, or lung, with no regions of common lymphatic involvement. They have a different histologic type or are proven to arise from different endobronchial lesions by bronchoscopy or from separate foci of CIS at pathologic examination. Patients with unilateral tumors and hilar or mediastinal lymph node metastases are not considered to have synchronous tumors. When synchronous tumors are confirmed as individual primaries, they should be staged separately and independently according to standard TNM definitions. The patient's overall tumor stage should be determined by the higher-staged lesion.

Survival rates after complete resection of synchronous lung cancers are worse than for isolated lesions of similar stage. The overall 5-year survival rate for all patients with synchronous lesions ranges from 0% to 44%, and the median survival duration ranges from 11 to 43 months; patients with no hilar or mediastinal node metastases generally survive longer.[136,139]

Metachronous (asynchronous) lesions are distinct tumors that arise in separate anatomic sites and are of different histologic types; they may be of the same histologic type if there was previous complete resection of the initial primary lung cancer without stump involvement, the tumors originated in separate lobes or lungs, there is no cancer in the common lymphatics or extrapulmonary disease at the time of diagnosis, and the site of origin of the second primary can be identified (or, if the original site is unknown, there is an interval of at least 2–3 years between the two tumors).[137] As the number of patients successfully treated for lung cancer increases, the incidence of second primaries will also increase. Multiple lung cancers occur in 10% to 25% of patients who survive longer than 3 years.[140] Patients in whom the multiple lesions are metachronous survive significantly longer (10-year survival rates from time of diagnosis of the original tumor reported as 42%) than those in whom the multiple lesions are synchronous. Survival is strongly influenced by the interval to recurrence and the stage of the second primary. The time interval between the development of asynchronous primary lesions may exceed 10 years.

The treatment of these lesions should follow the same pattern of evaluation that has been previously discussed. The only difference pertains to evaluation of the mediastinum. If the chest CT scan does not demonstrate adenopathy and bilateral lesions exist, it has been our practice to perform mediastinoscopy to rule out occult N2 disease prior to performing pulmonary resection. The method for resection depends on the location of the disease and the degree of concomitant pulmonary disease. If both lesions are clinical stage I disease and the patient has normal PFT results, either sternotomy with bilateral resection or staged thoracotomies can be performed. Because lobectomy provides the best opportunity for local control and possible cure, lobectomies are most desirable; such procedures are best performed in a staged fashion. If pulmonary function is limited or sternotomy is performed, limited resections or a lobectomy coupled with a limited resection are probably adequate. If a pneumonectomy is contemplated, staged resections are best to reduce postoperative complications. PFT should be repeated after the first procedure whenever staged resections are performed to ensure adequate pulmonary reserve.

If clinical N1 disease is present and the lesions are unilateral, intraparenchymal metastases are probably present, indicative of higher-stage (stage IV) disease. In the absence of N2 disease, a pneumonectomy can be considered. If both bilateral lesions are clinical stage II disease, the disease is probably beyond the scope of complete resectability, and a nonoperative approach should be considered. If N2 disease is present, the level of suspicion for intraparenchymal metastatic disease should be high, and nonoperative therapy is appropriate. These situations also pertain to metachronous lesions.

Survival rates after treatment of synchronous or metachronous primary lung lesions are better than those for metastatic or locally recurrent disease. Locally recurrent disease has been reported to develop at a median time interval of 13 months and to have a 4-year survival rate of 5% to 23%.[140]

Satellite Lesions Satellite lesions are separate foci of tumor that coexist with the lung primary tumor in the same lobe and represent intraparenchymal metastases. Mountain and colleagues and Deslauriers and colleagues have noted the implications of satellite lesions in their series of patients.[141,142] In the series of Deslauriers and colleagues, patients with a stage I, stage II, or stage III lesion who had an associated satellite tumor had 5-year survival rates of only 32%, 12.5%, and 5.6%, respectively, rates that are clearly worse than expected for early stages of disease. Accordingly, Mountain has recommended that tumors with associated satellite lesions be considered T4 tumors.

Surgery for N2 Disease The frequency of mediastinal lymph node involvement in patients with resectable NSCLC ranges from 22% to 33%.[143] Approximately 33% of patients with stage IIIA disease (based on N2 nodal metastases) present with a single positive node, whereas the remainder present with multiple nodes involved at a single station or at multiple stations. Patients with multiple-station involvement have a significantly worse prognosis than patients with single-node involvement.[144] In patients with metastases involving a single station, a significant survival difference has not been demonstrated between those with subcarinal metastases and those with metastases to other stations.

In patients with multiple-station metastases, the significance of subcarinal involvement is uncertain. The significance of metastases to the highest mediastinal lymph node and the definition of an incomplete resection based on N2 lymph node metastases are unclear.[145] The overall survival rate for patients with completely resected N2 disease is approximately 22%.

Patients with intranodal disease have a significant survival advantage over patients with extranodal extension.[146] Lymph nodes that extend beyond the confines of the nodal capsule have an increased propensity to involve adjacent tissue, reducing the chances of a complete resection. Such gross perinodal spread confers the possibility of microscopic residual disease, which may account for increased local recurrence rates and carry a worse prognosis.[147]

Positive Margins (Bronchial and Parenchymal) At the time of resection, the bronchial margin should be assessed by frozen section to ensure a complete resection. If the margin contains evidence of disease, all reasonable attempts to achieve a negative margin should be undertaken. It can be surmised that the risks of residual disease evolving into gross and potentially metastatic disease are higher in the face of an incomplete resection on the basis of a positive bronchial margin. But several studies have shown that reasonable survival rates can be achieved in the face of a positive bronchial margin. When microscopic disease or CIS exists within the mucosa, 5-year survival rate can approach 24%.[148] Shields and colleagues also showed a reasonable survival rate in patients with carcinoma in the bronchial mucosa.[149] In this cohort of patients, however, survival was poor when disease was present outside of the bronchial mucosa or within the peribronchial lymphatics, a finding similar to those of other studies.[148,150]

The role of radiotherapy in patients with positive margins of resection is unclear. Definitive studies that address this issue are difficult to perform. No current evidence indicates that radiation therapy improves rates of survival or local recurrence. Despite this fact, and on the basis of success with radiation therapy in the treatment of gross disease (locally advanced and stage IV), it is assumed that radiation will reduce the increased risk of local recurrence implied by a positive margin. At our institution, the standard of care remains radiation therapy if gross or microscopic disease remains after resection.

Surgery for Metastatic Disease Approximately 25% to 30% of all patients who present with NSCLC have stage IV disease (any T, any N, M1). These patients are usually treated with systemic therapy or palliative radiotherapy; their 5-year survival rate is generally less than 5%.[64] There is one subset of patients who can be considered for surgical intervention: those with resectable lung carcinoma and a resectable solitary brain metastasis. In this select group, surgery seems to prolong life and improve quality of life more effectively than nonsurgical treatment. The 5-year survival rate for the patients who undergo surgery has been shown to range from 13% to 30%, and the median survival duration ranges from 14 to 27 months. It has been suggested that adrenal metastases can be resected in patients with lung cancer, but the benefit, other than local control, is unclear. For lack of evidence to the contrary, conventional therapy for metastatic disease should not typically include the option of surgery except in highly selected cases.[151,152]

Management of Malignant Pleural Effusions Many patients either present with malignant pleural effusion or develop an effusion during or after therapy. Symptomatic effusions should be palliated with the greatest expediency to allow a rapid return of the patient's quality of life. Standard therapy has been thoracoscopy with talc pleuradage or tube thoracostomy with some form of chemical or talc pleurodesis. Both require hospitalization and either a general anesthetic or prolonged placement of an uncomfortable tube thoracostomy. A recent alternative is placement of a chronic indwelling catheter that can be drained by the patient at home and achieves prompt resolution of symptoms and eventual pleural symphysis. This system has the same success rate as tube thoracoscopy when the end point for evaluation is symptomatic relief. Its ease of insertion, minimal patient discomfort, rapid return to an ambulatory status, and reduced cost in this usually preterminal condition makes this system a very attractive option.[153]

Surgery for High-Risk Patients Many patients with potentially resectable disease are excluded from surgery because of severe cardiac or pulmonary limitations. Such high-risk patients are categorized by specific objective criteria. Usual pulmonary measures of high risk include the following: (1) preoperative forced expiratory volume in one second (FEV_1) less than 40% of predicted, (2) predicted post-resection FEV_1 less than 33% of predicted as determined by radioisotopic ventilation–perfusion studies, and (3) resting hypercarbia on arterial blood gas analysis ($Pco_2 > 45$). Cardiac criteria of high risk include (1) MI 3 to 6 months before the anticipated surgery, (2) evidence of class III angina, (3) hemodynamically significant valvular heart disease, (4) atrial fibrillation, (5) age over 75 years, (6) a history of cerebrovascular accident or transient ischemic attack, and (7) an echocardiogram with an ejection fraction of less than 50%. The introduction of improved methods to assess cardiopulmonary function has helped to better assess a patient's candidacy for surgery. The increased operative mortality associated with surgery for these patients can erode the oncologic survival advantage usually achieved with surgery. For most of these patients, radiotherapy carries considerably less risk and achieves similar rates of cure. Highly selected patients with these risk factors can sometimes still be offered surgery. Some examples include resection of a right upper lobe tumor in patients with severe bullous emphysema confined to the upper lobes or correction of cardiac disease immediately before or during pulmonary resection. A surgical evaluation, therefore, should not be denied solely because of cardiac or pulmonary limitations.

Radiotherapy

Radiation therapy for lung cancer has changed rapidly in recent years. Our ability to define target volumes and avoid normal structures has been aided by advancements in CT technology and in FDG-PET scanning. It is now possible, moreover, to measure and account for individual variations in respiratory tumor motion. Treatment-planning algorithms can account for tissue heterogeneity, which can improve dose distributions to target volumes. 3-D-conformal radiotherapy is routinely achieved by using International Commission on Radiation Units and Measurements (ICRU) definitions of volumes and doses. Intensity-modulated radiotherapy (IMRT) is being implemented and proton therapy is becoming a reality. We also look forward to the rational integration of new biologic therapies into standard treatment.

More than 60% of lung cancer patients will receive radiotherapy at some point in their disease, 45% for initial treatment and 17% for palliation.[154] This means that over 100,000 Americans with lung cancer are irradiated yearly. Therefore, it is critical that we aggressively implement the optimal treatment. Experienced teams are required to manage the care of these patients optimally, particularly when combined-modality therapy is used; outcomes are demonstrably better when patients are treated by experienced personnel.[155,156]

Radiation Treatment Techniques and Volumes for Lung Cancer ■ The ICRU has defined several important volumes for the modern treatment of lung cancer, which are described in the following paragraphs:

Gross Tumor Volume (GTV) ■ GTV is defined as visible tumor by any imaging modality. FDG-PET scanning is quite important for radiation treatment planning.[157] It can reduce interobserver differences in GTV contouring,[158] and it can help to categorize suspect mediastinal/hilar lymph adenopathy as either benign or malignant; higher standard uptake values (SUVs) are predictive of metastatic disease. It can also help to identify tumors within an atelectatic lobe, and thereby decrease the amount of normal lung irradiated. Finally, because FDG-PET scans detect distant metastases in about 30% of NSCLC patients (particularly those with otherwise advanced disease), it can help significantly with patient triage.[159]

Clinical Target Volume (CTV) ■ CTV is defined as the volume that is likely to contain gross and microscopic disease. A radiographic–histopathologic comparison of lung tumor size was recently completed.[160] This study demonstrated that to include the tumor within the CTV with 95% accuracy requires GTV to CTV expansions of 6 mm for squamous cancers and 8 mm for adenocarcinomas. Expansions for other histologic types have not been determined, but a conservative approach would be to use 8 mm. Appropriate CTV for the mediastinum has not been rigorously determined. We empirically use 8-mm expansions around involved nodes (either gross involvement or FDG-PET positivity).

Planning Target Volume (PTV) ■ PTV is defined as CTV with a margin to account for daily setup error and target motion. PTV is designed to take setup uncertainty and motion into account. Setup uncertainty is likely both technique dependent and institution dependent and should be measured individually for each technique.

Accounting for respiratory-dependent tumor motion is similarly challenging and can be approached in several ways. It is clear, however, that two-dimensional (2-D) measurement of tumor motion, such as might be done by fluoroscopy, is inadequate. Such motion is unpredictable and is independent of tumor size, location, and PFT results.[161] Thus, tumor motion is best assessed individually for each patient. Recent 4-D CT imaging showed that approximately 40% of lung cancers move more than 5 mm and 10% of lung cancers move more than 10 mm during the respiration. For patients with tumors moving less than 5 mm, simple expansion along the axis of motion is adequate. However, for patients with tumors moving more than 5 mm, particularly more than 10 mm, the treatment machine can be gated with respiration or the patient can use an assisted breath-hold technique or, possibly, an internal target volume (ITV)-based approach can be used. A commercially available system can be used to gate the linac.[162] This technique uses an externally placed fiducial that is tracked as the patient breathes. The beam can be triggered at a chosen point in the respiratory cycle, typically end-expiration because this is the longest and most reproducible portion of the respiratory cycle. This requires that patients be able to breathe slowly in a regular pattern. Active breathing control and deep inspiration breath hold are two techniques that have been pioneered to help patients hold their breaths at reproducible points in the respiratory cycle.[163,164] The radiation beam is then initiated. These two techniques limit patient respiratory excursion to fixed volumes. They limit diaphragm excursion to about 5 mm instead of 10 to 15 mm.[165] These techniques require very cooperative patients who are able to hold their breath for at least 15 sec. Unfortunately, patients with poor pulmonary function (who would most benefit from reduction in irradiated lung volumes) are the patients least able to comply with breath-holding techniques. Thus, it is not clear which is the best method to temporally immobilize lung tumors.

Internal Target Volume (ITV) ■ ITV is an expansion of CTV in which target motion is explicitly measured and taken into account as defined by ICRU62. Using new technologies such as multislice detectors and faster imaging reconstruction, it is now possible to image patients during real-time breathing and assess organ motion using 4-D CT.[166] To determine the ITV from the 4-D CT images, the tumor volume outlined on expiratory phase of the 4-D images is registered on other phases of the images to create a union of target contours enclosing all possible positions of the target. The same principle can be applied to the images acquired with inspiration and expiration breath holds. Attention should be paid to irregular breathing and variation of breathing patterns over the course of the treatment, and the effects of such on the ITV margin. Even with 4-D CT, the freebreathing ITV is only a snapshot and a single stochastic sampling of the patient breathing during the 4-D CT acquisitions. Thus, the true ITV margin should be enlarged on the basis of the uncertainty of patient's breathing during the treatment course.

A more interesting and challenging application for 4-D CT images is 4-D treatment planning in which the actual dose distributions for free-breathing treatment can be calculated. In this process, the dose distributions are calculated for each phase of the breathing cycle and then added together by deformation registration. Such composite dose distribution and DVHs demonstrate the actual dose that the patient is receiving from the treatment if he/she breathes the same way as the 4-D CT images are representing.[167]

Intensity Modulated Radiation Therapy (IMRT) and Proton Radiotherapy ■ IMRT offers the benefit of dose escalation without causing greater toxic effects to surrounding normal tissue for patients with prostate or head and neck cancer.[168] However, the application of IMRT to lung cancer has been delayed due to concerns that IMRT may deliver low yet damaging doses to a larger volume of normal lung tissue. Moreover, the possible movement of a tumor because of respiration introduces another level of complexity to both the IMRT dosimetry and the technique used.

We investigated dosimetric improvement with respect to target dose, tumor conformity, and normal tissue sparing, comparing IMRT with 3-D CT for early and locally advanced NSCLC.[169,170] We found that IMRT may be more suitable than 3-D CT treatment planning for cases of advanced stage disease with a larger GTV and thus a greater volume of normal lung involvement. Using IMRT, the median absolute reduction in the percentage of lung volume irradiated above 10 and 20 Gy were 7% and 10%, respectively. This corresponded with decreases of more than 2 Gy in the mean total lung dose and 10% in the risk of radiation pneumonitis. The volumes of the heart and esophagus irradiated above 40 to 50 Gy and normal thoracic tissue irradiated above 10 to 40 Gy were reduced using the IMRT plans. In contradiction of the common belief, the integral dose delivered to the patient was also reduced with IMRT in certain cases. There was a marginal increase in the spinal cord maximum dose and lung volume above 5 Gy in the IMRT plans in half of cases, which could have been caused by the significant increase of monitor units and thus leakage dose in IMRT for the sliding window delivery technique used in these studies.

Although IMRT may be effective in reducing normal tissue toxicity and improving tumor coverage, its high-dose gradient and conformity require a high level of precision in dose delivery and tumor localization. In the meantime, the complexity introduced by tumor motion must be recognized when using IMRT. Unlike 3-D conformal radiotherapy (3-D CRT), IMRT treats only a portion of the target volume at a particular time. There is a great deal of concern as whether target motion and collimator motion during IMRT delivery will have significant interplay effect, thus degrading the planned dose distributions. For IMRT to be feasible and more effective in treating NSCLC, motion reduction techniques should be explored further, such as breath holding and tumor tracking. Our preliminary clinical data indicated that IMRT may reduce toxic effects in normal tissue in selected cases, particularly for tumor moves less than 5 mm, and allow further dose escalation.[171] We have recently developed IMRT guidelines for NSCLC using image-guided radiotherapy.[172]

The proton is a charged particle that, compared to the photon, possesses a well-defined range of penetration determined by both the beam's energy and the density of the tissue through which it passes. As the proton beam penetrates the body, the particles slow down and deposit the dose sharply near the end of its range, a phenomenon known as the Bragg peak. By modulating the Bragg peak across the target volume, proton beams can deliver a full, localized, uniform dose of energy to the treatment site while sparing the surrounding normal tissues. The physics of the proton beam is ideal for treatments where organ preservation is paramount, such as lung cancer. The preliminary clinical data from Shioyama and colleagues and Bush and colleagues using escalated/accelerated proton radiotherapy showed promising clinical results comparable to those of surgical resection in stage IA cases.[173,174] Again, the accuracy of target delineation and tumor motion consideration are critical for both proton and photon treatment. Proton treatment is more sensitive to anatomical motion, position uncertainties, and tissue inhomogeneity.[172]

In our preclinical study, we found that proton radiotherapy significantly reduced dose to normal lungs, esophagus, spinal cord, and heart in both stage I and stage III NSCLC even with dose escalation (87.5 Gy for stage I, 74 Gy for stage III) compared with standard dose of photon radiotherapy (66 Gy for stage I and 63 Gy for stage III) using either 3-D or IMRT.[175] The improvement was more dramatic in stage I disease and the contralateral lung. Our preliminary clinical data indicated that proton therapy may reduce acute side effects even with higher proton doses in lung cancer patients treated with concurrent chemoradiotherapy. Long-term follow up is needed. Further improvement of proton planning, particularly for complicated stage III cases, can be achieved by adding wedges, coordination between beam arrangement, and/or intensity modulated proton therapy.

We also designed and evaluated several image-guided radiotherapies to study the impact of respiratory motion on dose distributions for 3-D CRT, IMRT, and proton radiotherapy and to assess the potential benefits of accounting for respiratory motion with gating or breath hold.[176] We found that tumor motion has a significant effect on radiation dose distribution. This motion should be considered for both photon and proton radiotherapy. ITV or gated radiotherapy can significantly reduce target missing owing to tumor motion. Compared with photon 3-D CRT and IMRT with gated or non-gated radiotherapy, proton radiotherapy (gated or free-breathing with ITV approach) significantly improves normal tissue sparing, especially at low dose levels.[172] Our data showed that it is possible to have escalated/accelerated proton radiotherapy without significantly increasing toxic effects to normal tissue. This approach may translate to better local control and survival rates for patients with stage I NSCLC. At MD Anderson Cancer Center, we are going to conduct phase 2 clinical trials using imaging-guided proton radiotherapy for stage I and stage III NSCLC. PET/CT studies will be used in all patients for both stage and treatment planning. We plan to deliver a total dose of 87.5 CGE (cobalt gray equivalent): 2.5 CGE per fraction for stage I disease and 74 CGE with concurrent chemotherapy followed by adjuvant chemotherapy for stage III disease. A 4-D CT study will be required to account for tumor motion, and to assist in deciding on a treatment delivery technique (free-breath, breath-hold, or gated treatment).

In summary, IMRT and proton treatments represent the most recent technological developments in radiation oncology. These new treatment modalities have the potential to reduce the toxic effects to normal tissue compared with 3-D CRT. However, high-dose conformity and dose sculpting from the IMRT and proton treatments require a greater degree of precision in treatment delivery and careful management of organ motion. Image-guided targeting, and patient positioning will possibly become the standard of practice for future IMRT and proton treatments. The clinical significance of possible increased exposure of low-dose (<10 Gy) to the chest by IMRT is unknown. IMRT should be used only in selective cases, and target volume motion and low-dose exposure to the lung should be minimized. Proton holds a great potential for sparing normal tissues and may allow further radiation dose escalation/acceleration without significantly increasing normal tissue toxicities.

Primary Radiation Therapy for Stage I and II NSCLC ■ Patients who have surgically resectable NSCLC but are medically inoperable because of their lung function, cardiac function, bleeding tendency, or other comorbid conditions, or patients who refuse surgery, may be considered for conventional fractionated radiotherapy (60–70 Gy with 2 Gy/fraction). Observation only is a poor choice for patients with stage I NSCLC, as most will die of their cancer. Primary radiotherapy for early-stage NSCLC is considered reasonable for such patients, with reported 5-year survival rates ranging from 10% to 30% with conventional fractionated radiotherapy.[177,178] Several studies have reported a benefit to dose escalation suggesting a dose-response relationship in both survival and local control in these patients.[178–181] Since early-stage NSCLC is not inherently a systemic disease from diagnosis, and since local control is poor after conventional radiotherapy, research measures aimed at improving survival should put significant emphasis on improving local tumor obliteration.

It should be kept in mind that lung cancer in such patients is always staged clinically, which makes comparison with surgically treated patients difficult. Several surgical series demonstrate a 24% to 37% upstaging of cT1-T2 N0 disease, which partially explains the poorer results seen in clinically staged irradiated patients.[127] Small early-stage NSCLC is uncommon in radiation oncology clinics. As we develop better screening tools for early-stage NSCLC, however, the number of patients with small but medically inoperable tumors will increase.[87]

At MD Anderson Cancer Center, between 1978 and 2003, 200 patients with clinical stage I disease were treated with curative intent by primary radiotherapy. Among them, 85 patients were treated with 3-DCRT. 3-DCRT was associated with improved survival (36% at 5 years) and local-regional control (70% at 5 years) compared with 2-D radiotherapy (10%, 34% respectively at 5 years, $p < .001$). On multivariate analysis, male gender, age >70-year-old, weight loss >5%, and tumor size >4 cm were associated with decreased survival. The most important prognostic factor documented in the literature is usually tumor size. Doseretz and colleagues. reported that rates of distant metastasis were correlated to the size of the primary tumor.[179] The incidence of metastasis in 3 years was 8% in tumors smaller than 3 cm, 27% in tumors measuring 3 to 5 cm, and 50% in tumors larger than 5 cm. They reported that the local control rates at 3 years were 77% for 4 cm lesions and 48% for those larger than 4 cm.

Stereotactic Body Radiation Therapy in Early-Stage NSCLC ■ The development of 3-D CRT and stereotactic body radiation therapy (SBRT) have allowed precise targeting and delivery of radiotherapy. SBRT for lung cancer utilizes elements of 3-D CRT and also incorporates a variety of systems for taking tumor motion into consideration and decreasing setup uncertainty using image-guided radiotherapy techniques. These systems allow reduction of treatment volumes facilitating hypofractionation with markedly increased daily doses (>10 Gy) and a significantly reduced overall treatment time. The combination of multiple beam angles to achieve sharp dose gradients, high precision localization, and a high dose per fraction in extracranial locations is referred to as SBRT. This approach delivers a high biological effective dose (BED) to the target while minimizing toxic effects to normal tissue; which may translate into improved local control and survival rates.

Dr. Onishi and colleagues reported on the use of SBRT in stage I NSCLC in Japan,[182] retrospectively evaluating results from a Japanese multi-institutional study. Patients with stage I NSCLC ($n = 245$; median age 76 years; T1 N0 M0, $n = 155$; T2 N0 M0, $n = 90$) were treated with hypofractionated high-dose SBRT in 13 institutions. Stereotactic 3-D treatment was performed using noncoplanar dynamic arcs or multiple static ports. A total dose of 18 to 75 Gy at the isocenter was administered in 1 to 22 fractions. The median calculated BED was 108 Gy (range 57–180 Gy). During follow-up (median, 24 months; range 7–78 months), pulmonary complications of National Cancer Institute Common Toxicity Criteria grade 2 or higher were observed in only 6 patients (2.4%). Local progression occurred in 33 patients (14.5%), and the local recurrence rates were 8.1% for BED = 100 Gy and 26.4% for BED < 100 Gy ($p < .05$). The 3-year overall survival rates of medically operable patients were 88.4% for BED = 100 Gy and 69.4% for < 100 Gy ($p < .05$). Their data showed that hypofractionated high-dose SBRT with BED < 150 Gy was feasible and beneficial for curative treatment of patients with stage I NSCLC. For all treatment methods and schedules, local control and survival rates were better with BED = 100 Gy than with BED < 100 Gy. Survival rates in selected patients (medically operable, BED = 100 Gy) were excellent and were potentially comparable to those of surgery.

In our institution, we have treated more than 220 patients using imaging-guided SBRT (4-D CT simulation and daily CT on rail for tumor localization and setup accuracy) at doses of 50 Gy delivered in 4 fractions (daily treatment for 4 days). Based on preliminary analysis, the local control rate at the primary site is higher than 95%, and toxicity is minimal even for centrally located lesions.[183] Long-term follow-up is needed to confirm these data.

The Radiation Therapy Oncology Group (RTOG) recently completed patient enrollment for phase 2 clinical trials to analyze the efficacy of SBRT in peripheral stage I NSCLC with 60 Gy in 3 fractions delivered over 2 weeks. Preliminary data appear promising. An international randomized study to compare SBRT with surgery in stage I NSCLC has been planned by our group and will start to enroll patients in 2008.[184] SBRT may become the future standard radiotherapy for peripheral inoperable stage I NSCLC and its role in operable stage I NSCLC is under study.

Postoperative Radiotherapy ■ Postoperative radiotherapy (PORT) is currently contraindicated in patients with stage I completely resected disease on the basis of the PORT meta-analysis.[185] Data for stage II and higher-stage disease neither support nor refute the use of PORT (because the hazard ratio error bars include 1.0), although it clearly improves regional control.

The use of PORT for stage II and III NSCLC was first tested in a controlled trial by the LCSG, which randomized 210 patients to receive either 50 Gy in 25 fractions or no treatment.[186] Local recurrence rate was significantly reduced (3% vs 41%), but there was no effect on overall survival or disease-free survival because of the high rate of distant failure. However, recent data from subgroup analyses of a phase 3 randomized study examining surgical resection with/without adjuvant chemotherapy (ANITA Trial) indicated that PORT may improve overall survival in patients with N2 disease.

In patients with resectable or marginally resectable NSCLC, 5-year survival rates and collective results of surgery alone for stage III (N2) ranged from 14% to 30%. Many patients who have clinical N0 disease (even when it is staged by mediastinoscopy) are found to have occult mediastinal lymph node metastases. Approximately 15% of patients with resected T1 tumors have N2 disease, and 40% to 45% of patients with T2-T3 tumors will have N2 disease. Patients with incomplete resection, including positive margins, multiple levels of lymph node involvement, extracapsular extension, and N2 disease, usually have poor local control, and PORT is usually indicated.

Preoperative Chemotherapy and Chemoradiotherapy ■ If N2 disease is bulky and the potential for complete resection is questionable, patients can be treated by neoadjuvant chemotherapy followed by surgery. At MD Anderson, 60 patients were randomized to undergo chemotherapy and surgery or surgery alone. Twenty-eight patients received three cycles of cyclophosphamide, etoposide, and cisplatin and then underwent surgery, and they were compared with 32 patients treated with surgery alone.[187] The median survival durations were 64 months versus 11 months, favoring neoadjuvant chemotherapy. The 2-year survival rate was 56% in the neoadjuvant group and 15% in the surgery-only group ($p = .008$). In this study, the patients who had positive margins, multiple levels of positive lymph nodes, or extracapsular extension received PORT between 50 and 60 Gy, and only two patients developed local recurrences. Rosell and colleagues from Barcelona randomized 60 patients treated with or without mitomycin C, ifosfamide, and cisplatin as neoadjuvant chemotherapy.[188] Thirty patients received neoadjuvant chemotherapy followed by surgery, and the other half underwent surgery alone; the median survival duration was 26 months in the neoadjuvant group and 8 months in the surgery only group. The 2-year survival rates were 29% among the patients who received neoadjuvant chemotherapy and 0% among the patients who received surgery alone ($p = .001$), although both groups had PORT of 50 Gy in 5 weeks.

Increasing numbers of patients with stage III disease are now undergoing induction chemotherapy, followed by surgery, on the basis of the work of Rosell and colleagues and Roth and colleagues.[187,188] To study the issue of surgical resection after induction chemoradiation, the Southwest Oncology Group (SWOG) conducted a phase 2 trial of concurrent induction chemotherapy, cisplatin, and etoposide, with thoracic radiation therapy in 74 patients with biopsy proven stage IIIA (N2) NSCLC. Study results suggested that this approach may improve patient survival with reasonable toxicity.[189] On the basis of the results from this study, the NCI had launched a phase 3 multicenter trial (RTOG [chair], SWOG, National Cancer Institute of Canada Clinical Trials Group [NCIC CTG], Eastern Cooperative Oncology Group [ECOG], Cancer and Leukemia Group B [CALGB], North Central Cancer Treatment Group [NCCTG]) for patients with biopsy-proven N2 disease and potentially resectable NSCLC (NCI Protocol INT 139). Patients were stratified by PS and T status and were randomized to receive induction chemoradiotherapy followed by surgery or chemotherapy with definitive radiotherapy as follows: following randomization, all patients received cisplatin (50 mg/m^2 IV days 1, 8, 29, 36), etoposide (50 mg/m^2 IV days 1–5, 29–33), and thoracic radiotherapy (45 Gy, 1.8 Gy/day, begin day 1) for 5 weeks. Patients in arm 1 who had no local progression or distant metastases at restaging underwent resection approximately 3 to 5 weeks after completion of course 2. Patients in arm 2 without local progression or distant metastases at restaging underwent full-course radiotherapy to 61 Gy. All patients received an additional two courses of chemotherapy. Initial results showed better PFS rate in the trimodality arm. Follow-up data, including survival data, were presented in 2005 by Albain and colleagues.[190] The study was closed in November 2001 after accrual of 484 patients. At the time the data were presented, all patients had follow-up of more than 2.5 years. Study results confirmed significantly greater PFS for arm 1. Survival curves were superimposed through year 2 and then separated. By year 5, an absolute survival benefit of 7% favored the surgery arm (OR 0.63 [0.36, 1.10], p = .10). Subgroup analysis revealed better survival for patients who underwent a lobectomy (p = .002). However, trimodality therapy was not optimal when a pneumonectomy was required owing to the high mortality risk. Finally, N0 status at surgery significantly predicted a higher 5-year survival rate. The authors suggested that surgical resection after chemoradiation can be considered for fit patients if lobectomy is feasible.

Radiation Therapy for Unresectable Stage III NSCLC ■ For patients with unresectable stage III NSCLC, conventional radiotherapy alone resulted in a median survival time of 10 months and a 5-year survival rate of 5%. To improve the outcome of treatment, chemotherapy was added to radiotherapy. Chemotherapy and radiotherapy can be delivered sequentially or concurrently. The most well-known trial, reported by the CALGB, compared standard radiotherapy to 60 Gy to sequential cisplatin and vinblastine chemotherapy for two cycles followed by radiotherapy to 60 Gy. Median survival times and 5-year survival rates were superior for the chemoradiotherapy arm (13.8 months vs 9.7 months, 19% vs 7%, respectively).[191]

These results led the RTOG to conduct a three-arm trial (RTOG 88-08) comparing standard radiotherapy, sequential chemoradiotherapy (CALGB regimen), and 69.6-Gy hyperfractionated radiotherapy. Sequential chemoradiotherapy was statistically superior to standard and hyperfractionated radiotherapy.

Schaake-Koning et al.[192] compared radiotherapy alone with radiotherapy plus daily cisplatin or weekly cisplatin. There was no difference in distant failure rates between the groups with or without cisplatin. However, the survival rate in the radiotherapy-plus-cisplatin group was 54% at 1 year, 26% at 2 years, and 16% at 3 years, compared with 46%, 13%, and 2% in the radiotherapy-alone group (p = 0.009). Therefore, this study showed that a gain in local tumor control seems to have translated into increased survival time.

Furuse and colleagues compared patients receiving two cycles of mitomycin, vindesine, and cisplatin given every 28 days concurrent with split-course radiotherapy (total dose of 56 Gy) with patients receiving two cycles of mitomycin, vindesine, and cisplatin followed by continuous radiotherapy (total dose of 56 Gy). The concurrent treatment yielded an improved 5-year survival rate compared with the sequential treatment.[193] A subsequent report demonstrated that the difference in survival was attributed to better intrathoracic tumor control in the patients receiving concurrent treatment.

The RTOG (RTOG 9410) conducted a three-arm randomized trial to analyze whether the concurrent delivery of cisplatin-based chemotherapy with thoracic radiation treatment (TRT) improves survival compared with the sequential delivery of these therapies for patients with locally advanced, unresected stage II-III NSCLC.[194] The sequential therapy consisted of cisplatin (P, 100 mg/m^2) and vinblastine (5 mg/m^2) followed by 60 Gy of radiation. The concurrent treatment used the same chemotherapy with 60 Gy of radiation beginning on day 1 of chemotherapy (CON-QD RT). The third treatment was concurrent P (50 mg/m^2) and oral etoposide (50 mg) with 69.6 Gy of radiation in 1.2-Gy BID fractions beginning on day 1 (CON-BID RT). With minimum and median follow-up times of 4.0 and 6.0 years, the median survival times and 4-year survival rates were 14.6 months and 12% for patients receiving sequential treatment, 17.1 months and 21% for patients receiving CON-QD RT, and 15.2 months and 17% for patients receiving CON-BID RT. The CON-QD RT group had better survival times and rates than the sequential group (p = 0.046). RTOG9410 demonstrated that the concurrent delivery of cisplatin-based chemotherapy with TRT conferred a greater long-term survival benefit than did the sequential delivery of these therapies. The locoregional failure rates were 50% for patients receiving sequential treatment, 43% for patients receiving CON-QD RT, and 34% for patients receiving CON-BID RT. The rate of acute toxic effects were higher in the CON-BID RT group (68% grade 3 and above) than in the CON-QD RT group (48% grade 3 and above). There was no significant difference in late toxic effects and survival between these two groups. However, the rate of radiotherapy in-field failure was lower in the CON-BID RT group than in the CON-QD RT group. The higher rate of toxic effects in the CON-BID RT group may explain its lack of a survival benefit. In RTOG 9410, radiotherapy was based on 2-D planning, which is usually associated with higher toxic effect rates.

A third trial comparing concurrent with sequential chemoradiotherapy reported in 2001 and updated in 2005 also explored the use of consolidation chemotherapy.[195] In this phase 3 trial from France, 205 patients were assigned to receive two cycles of cisplatin plus vinorelbine followed by 66 Gy of radiation or cisplatin/etoposide and concurrent radiation to 66 Gy followed by two cycles of consolidation chemotherapy with cisplatin and vinorelbine. Local control rates were improved with the concurrent regimen (40% vs 24%), and the median survival times and 4-year survival rates were numerically superior (but not statistically superior) in the concurrent arm of the trial (16.3 vs 14.5 months and 21% vs 14%, respectively). However, the incidence of grade 3 esophagitis was significantly higher in the concurrent arm (32% vs 3%), and the toxic effects-related death rates were high in both arms (9.5% in the concurrent arm and 5.6% in the sequential arm).

These three phase 3 trials consistently demonstrated longer survival times for patients receiving concurrent chemoradiotherapy, and this difference was significant in 2 of the 3 trials. On the basis of these results, concurrent chemoradiotherapy has been the standard of care since 2001. It is important to note that toxic effects are significantly more common with concurrent chemoradiotherapy than with sequential chemoradiotherapy.

In RTOG 9410, the locoregional failure rate after concurrent chemoradiotherapy was still around 34% to 43%. To improve the local control rate, three groups (RTOG, NCCTG, and the University of North Carolina) have separately performed radiation dose-escalation trials for patients with inoperable stage III NSCLC and reported results supporting the safety of 74 Gy. University of North Carolina conducted a phase 1/2 dose-escalation clinical trial using high-dose 3DCRT (60–74 Gy) for inoperable stage IIIA/IIIB NSCLC with induction chemotherapy followed by concurrent chemoradiotherapy.[196] They reported a 3-year survival rate of 36% and a 13% locoregional relapse rate as the only site of failure. For patients who finished radiotherapy, the 3-year survival rate was 45%.

Because of the promising local control, good survival data, and acceptable toxic effects obtained using 3DCRT to doses of 74 Gy with concurrent chemotherapy, RTOG has initiated a phase 3 study to compare conventional dose (60 Gy) with escalated dose (74 Gy) radiotherapy concurrently with weekly paclitaxel and carboplatin in patients with stage IIIA/B NSCLC. The primary end point is overall survival. IGRT is strongly recommended and IMRT is allowed if tumor motion has been taken into consideration. Consolidation chemotherapy is required.

Special Considerations Superior Vena Caval Obstruction ■ Superior vena caval obstruction (SVCO), also known as SVC syndrome, is a not an uncommon finding in patients with lung cancer and requires prompt recognition and treatment. Approximately 65% to 97% of all cases of SVC syndrome occur secondary to malignancy. Three to five percent of patients with cancer of the lung present with edema of the face, neck, or arms and a prominent venous pattern in the chest wall, indicative of SVCO. Usually, the lung tumors are right-sided lesions. 10-15% of patients with right-side malignancies may develop a component of SVCO. Commonly, they have associated shortness of breath, dyspnea, and headache, but rarely is glottic occlusion, laryngeal swelling, airway compromise, or cerebral venous hypertension a problem. Contrary to earlier thinking, SVCO is very rarely an oncologic emergency because few, if any, patients have died of the syndrome. Symptoms usually occur gradually, with accompanying venous collateralization manifested through cutaneous venous engorgement in the upper extremity, neck, and torso. Sometimes, symptoms can occur rather acutely from thrombosis of the major veins. Often the presenting symptoms are compounded by tracheal compression, recurrent nerve paralysis, and airway compromise. Even in such circumstances, treatment should not be initiated without a diagnosis, which usually can be obtained through cytologic or histologic testing. It is usually possible to obtain sputum, bronchial brushings or biopsies, or percutaneous aspirates that will establish the diagnosis. If SCLC is found, standard small cell treatment protocols are initiated, that is, systemic chemotherapy followed by thoracic irradiation or concurrent chemoradiotherapy. NSCLC causing SVCO is an indication for rapid thoracic irradiation. Large daily doses of 3.5 to 4.0 Gy are delivered for 3 or 4 days; the daily dose is then reduced to 1.8 or 2.0 Gy, and treatment is continued to the usual total doses. Over 80% of patients so treated are relieved of the obstruction. Surgical intervention is rarely indicated, except for highly selected patients with severe symptoms, complete occlusion of the SVC, refractory symptoms after radiotherapy with or without chemotherapy, and thrombosis of venous collaterals. Bypass procedures reroute the venous blood flow of the upper compartment to the right atrium. Other surgical options are en bloc removal of the SVC or stent insertion. The prognosis is slightly worse for patients with SVCO than for patients who do not develop this syndrome because of the volume and extent of the tumor and lower PS. A recent review tested the evidence on the efficacy of different modalities in the treatment of SVCO in lung cancer. The authors suggested that chemotherapy and radiotherapy are effective in relieving SVCO in a proportion of patients, while stent insertion appears to provide relief in a higher proportion and more rapidly. The optimal timing of stent insertion (whether at diagnosis or following failure of other modalities) is currently uncertain. The effectiveness of steroids in SVCO remains uncertain.[197]

Superior Sulcus Tumors ■ Superior sulcus tumors (SST) represent an uncommon presentation of lung cancer, accounting for approximately 3% of all lung cancers. SST with associated Pancoast syndrome, Horner syndrome, pain in the C8-T1 distribution, and atrophy of the intrinsic muscles of the hand (usually extrinsic involvement of the brachial plexus) represent a unique subset of these tumors. Irrespective of vertebral body or vascular invasion, tumors with Pancoast syndrome (true "Pancoast tumors") carry a poor prognosis and should be classified as T4 lesions. The T3 descriptor is appropriate when the rib, intercostal muscle, sympathetic chain, stellate ganglion, or lowest cord of the brachial plexus is involved. Other poor prognostic findings include N2–3 status, the use of wedge resection instead of lobectomy with en bloc chest wall resection, and incomplete resection. The majority of tumors are of non-small cell histologic types, but occasionally SCLC occurs. The diagnosis can usually be established by FNA. SCLCs are treated with nonoperative therapy by standard small-cell protocols, whereas NSCLCs are usually treated with combined-modality therapy. Magnetic resonance angiography can be helpful in determining the extent of tumor. In many cases, SST can be completely resected, including the lowest chord of the brachial plexus, the sacrifice of which causes minimal neurologic compromise. Tumors that invade the vertebral body, subclavian vessels, or deep aspects of the brachial plexus present difficult surgical problems that may be ameliorated by induction chemotherapy. In some circumstances of limited invasion, however, the subclavian artery can be resected and reconstructed. When the tumor is adherent to the vertebral body, a portion can be removed with an en bloc resection, or the entire vertebral body can be removed and reconstructed.

For patients who have potentially resectable lesions, the best timing for radiotherapy is unknown. Certainly, radiation therapy can diminish the size of the tumor and perhaps improve resectability, particularly in patients who have improvement in their pain during the course of their preoperative radiation therapy. Radiation has its greatest effect when a full and uninterrupted dose can be delivered in the range of 60 to 65 Gy. When radiation therapy is given preoperatively, the usual dosage range is from 30 to 45 Gy. Higher preoperative radiation doses generally increase the perioperative complication rate, although a 5-year survival rate over 60% with full-dose preoperative therapy over 55 Gy, with conventional fractionation of 175 to 200 Gy/day vs high-dose fractionation of 275 to 300 Gy/day, has been reported in association with minimal perioperative morbidity. It should be kept in mind that split-course techniques generally have been found to be inferior to continuous course irradiation. A retrospective analysis at the Massachusetts General Hospital suggested that induction chemoradiation was superior to radiation alone prior to resection, although the radiation dose was 12 Gy higher in the combined group.[198] A prospective phase 2 intergroup study demonstrated that induction chemoradiation followed by surgery can result in significant complete pathologic responses and very good survival, especially for patients with T2 N0 disease.[199]

At our institution, we feel that the best care for patients with a potentially resectable tumor is immediate thoracotomy followed by PORT. In a retrospective analysis of patients with an SST who received definitive care at MD Anderson between January 1977 and December 1987, 85 patients were identified.[200] The male-to-female ratio was 2.7 to 1, and the ages ranged from 35 to 80 (median, 59) years. Karnofsky PS was 80 or higher in 70 of the patients (82%). Thirty patients (35%) had 5% or more loss of body weight. All had histologic or cytologic confirmation of carcinoma: 25% were squamous cell, 2% SCLC, 54% adenocarcinoma, 6% large-cell carcinoma, and 12% unclassified. After complete evaluation, 43 patients were classified as having clinical stage IIIA disease, and 42 as having stage IIIB. One patient with stage IIIA disease underwent surgery; 13, surgery plus radiation therapy; 2, surgery plus radiation therapy plus chemotherapy; 17, radiation therapy plus chemotherapy; and 4, chemotherapy alone. Surgery was a component of therapy more frequently in stage IIIA disease than in stage IIIB disease ($p \leq .05$), and systemic treatment was used significantly more often in stage IIIB disease ($p = .0042$). The one patient treated with surgery alone lived 2 years. Twenty-three percent (7 of 31) of patients who had radiotherapy alone and none of the 4 patients who had chemotherapy alone lived 2 years. Of the 25 patients who underwent surgery as part of their treatment, 13 (52%) lived over 2 years, while 13 of the 60 (22%) patients who did not undergo surgery lived over 2 years. Of the patients who received radiation therapy as part of their treatment, 31% lived 2 years, and of those who received chemotherapy, 18% lived 2 years. Fifty-two patients (61%) had local control of the tumor; their survival duration was significantly longer ($p = .01$) than those who had local failure. In patients with unresectable tumors, total dose of radiotherapy was important ($p = .01$) in achieving local control; patients treated with less than 65 Gy had a 38% local control rate, while those treated with more than 65 Gy achieved a 69% local control rate. Ten of 11 patients treated with neutron beam therapy had good local control. Split-course radiotherapy was disadvantageous. High PS, weight loss of less than 5%, and no involvement of the vertebral bodies were significant factors ($p = .01$) in prolonging survival. The conclusions of the study were that surgical resection should be used whenever possible for SST. Patients with unresectable disease should receive high-dose photon or neutron radiotherapy, if available.[200] There is a high likelihood of close or positive surgical margins for SST; we have generally preferred induction chemotherapy followed by postoperative radiation to 50 Gy if surgical margins are adequate, 60 Gy for microscopically positive margins, and at least 66 Gy for grossly positive margins (all delivered at 2 Gy per day). Others have used preoperative radiation followed by intraoperative brachytherapy in SST. There is no established role for chemotherapy alone for these tumors.

The overall 5-year survival rate for patients with resected SST ranges from 28% to 56%. The presence of nodal disease significantly shortens survival. For patients who receive radiotherapy alone, the 5-year survival rate ranges from 1.6 to 23%.[201]

In summary, combinations of surgery and radiotherapy have been the hallmark of treatment of SST. Aggressive surgery with lobectomy and en bloc chest wall resection and lymphadenectomy is still essential. However, the use of neoadjuvant chemotherapy followed by surgery and radiotherapy has the potential to improve outcome as it has for other stage III NSCLC.

Brachytherapy ■ Endotracheal or endobronchial lesions may cause shortness of breath, postobstructive pneumonitis, and hemoptysis. Endobronchial brachytherapy has been used to achieve high radiation doses to these relatively accessible tumors, either as a component of potentially curative therapy or, more commonly, in the palliative setting after external radiotherapy has failed. High-dose-rate brachytherapy has been shown to accomplish rapid alleviation of symptoms and improve functional status without causing esophagitis, pneumonitis, or the bone marrow suppression seen with external irradiation. High dose-rate brachytherapy is ideal for patients who need either short-term palliation or quick resolution of symptoms before they undergo definitive treatment. Doses of 35 to 42 Gy in 7 Gy weekly fractions have been delivered to such tumors using high-dose-rate brachytherapy remote afterloading techniques.

Between 1988 and 1993, 81 patients with lung cancer underwent endobronchial brachytherapy at MD Anderson.[202] Presenting symptoms were shortness of breath in 65 patients (notably 16 did not have any dyspnea), cough in 53, hemoptysis in 22, wheezing in 31, and chest pain in 11. Squamous cell carcinoma was detected in 46% of cases. Eleven percent (9 of 81) of the patients had endobronchial treatment 3 times at 2-week intervals, and 67% (54 of 81) had treatment twice with 2-week intervals. Ninety-three percent of the patients received 1500 cGy calculated at a distance of 0.6 cm from the center of sources for mainstem lesions, and the rest of the patients had the same dose calculated at a distance of 0.75 cm from the center of the sources for tracheal lesions. Twenty-six patients (32%) showed improvement, and 25 patients had moderate improvement. Seventeen patients had minimal improvement, and 11 patients showed no change. Five patients became slightly worse and two became much worse after the endobronchial brachytherapy. Thus, 85% achieved some response, including 32% who had an excellent response. The median duration of responses was 4.5 months. Median survival duration was 5 months for all patients, ranging from 0.5 to 43 months. There was no significant difference between groups on the basis of histology, although SCLC patients appeared to have less symptom relief, probably because they were more likely to have extrinsic causes of bronchial obstruction.

Chemotherapy

Single Agents ■ The clinical development of chemotherapeutic agents has traditionally been in the setting of stage IV disease. Customarily, drug activity has been reported with respect to response rate, and of the many drugs tested in lung cancer in the early 1980s, six have been found to have predictable and reproducible antitumor activity with response rates in excess of 15%: cisplatin, ifosfamide, mitomycin C, etoposide, vindesine, and vinblastine. Variability in dose and schedule relate to response rates observed, and interpretation of early trial data were further complicated by the heterogeneity of the patient populations tested.

More recently, a new generation of compounds has been demonstrated to possess significant activity against NSCLC. These include topoisomerase I inhibitors, taxanes, and active analogues of previously established chemotherapeutic compounds (ie, gemcitabine, vinorelbine). When these agents are used in combination with other active agents such as the platinum compounds, response rates have exceeded 50%. Of the taxanes, docetaxel has had response rates of approximately 30% in multiple trials, and paclitaxel has demonstrated response rates in excess of 20%. Gemcitabine (deoxy-fluorocytidine) is a fluoridated derivative of cytosine arabinoside with single-agent response rates greater than 20%. Myelosuppression is not a dose-limiting toxicity, and therefore this agent has become quite useful when administered in combination with others. Vinorelbine is an active synthetic vinca alkaloid with less neurotoxicity than vinblastine. Pemetrexed is a newer multitargeted antifolate, also with demonstrated activity in NSCLC. Response rates in the range of 20% have been observed.[5,203,204]

Combination Chemotherapy ■ Because single agents have modest activity, combination chemotherapy regimens have developed with the majority including a platinum compound. In summary, these drug combinations consistently produce objective tumor response in 20% to 40% of patients with advanced NSCLC and a median survival duration of 6 to 8 months in most randomized trials. A complete tumor response is quite uncommon, however, and no single regimen has emerged as the standard treatment approach. The ECOG conducted a randomized phase 3 study to determine if one of four platinum-based combinations had superior efficacy in patients with advanced NSCLC.[204] This trial involved 1207 patients randomly assigned to receive the control combination of cisplatin and paclitaxel or cisplatin and gemcitabine, cisplatin and docetaxel, or carboplatin and paclitaxel. The results of this modern trial are notable, because the overall response rate was only 19%, and the median survival duration was 7.9 months. The 1-year survival rate was 33%, and the 2-year survival rate 11%. Neither response rate nor survival duration differed significantly among the treatment arms. Patients with an ECOG PS of 2 had a lower rate of survival than those with a PS of 0 or 1. None of these regimens emerged as superior. Since the carboplatin and paclitaxel treatment arm was associated with less toxicity overall, particularly with respect to febrile neutropenia and nausea, it was adopted by many oncologists in the United States. Several studies have compared cisplatin-based two-drug combination regimens with single agents, and on balance, combination regimens appear to fare better, prolonging survival. Cisplatin and vindesine or vinorelbine prolonged survival over the comparator arms, vinorelbine or vindesine alone. However, other investigators could not confirm these results. Similarly, randomized trials have failed to demonstrate a survival advantage for the combination of cisplatin and etoposide over cisplatin or etoposide given as single agents. Nonetheless, more recent trials have shown that combinations with cisplatin appear to yield consistently higher response rates than cisplatin alone. This improvement is modest but still has translated into a survival advantage, at least for combinations with vinorelbine and gemcitabine. In aggregate, these studies indicate that two-drug regimens are significantly more active in the treatment of NSCLC than cisplatin given alone.[203,204]

Chemotherapy for Advanced NSCLC

Chemotherapy vs Best Supportive Care

A series of trials has demonstrated that treatment with chemotherapy yields superior results to purely supportive care (symptom relief) in patients with advanced NSCLC. The results of earlier studies with long-term alkylating agents were disappointing, but most recent trials using platinum-based combinations have resulted in superior survival for patients receiving active treatment.[205,206] On balance, benefits are modest, with median survival ranging from 20 to 30 weeks versus 10 to 17 weeks. The variability of results is due to differences among studies with small numbers of patients, variable access to care, and a lack of standardization of "best supportive care." An estimate of the relative benefit of 27% reduction in the probability of death in the year following diagnosis with cisplatin-based chemotherapy compared with best supportive care alone emerged from a meta-analysis using individual patient data from cisplatin-based trials.[207] For 778 patients, the pooled hazard ratio was 0.73 (95% CI 0.63–0.85, p = .0007). Median survival for treated patients was 5.5 months, while that for patients who received supportive care was 4.0 (p = .001). This approach was consistent in elderly patients as well. In an Italian study, single-agent chemotherapy with vinorelbine prolonged the survival of patients 70 years or older over purely supportive care (p = .03).[208] In this trial, median survival duration increased from 21 to 28 weeks. A Canadian multicenter trial has been comprehensively analyzed.[209] In this study, best supportive care, including radiation therapy, was compared with two chemotherapy regimens: vindesine and cisplatin or cyclophosphamide, doxorubicin, and cisplatin. The vindesine/cisplatin regimen was associated with significantly longer survival than supportive care (p = .01). A cost-effectiveness analysis concluded that there was no disadvantage to chemotherapy. Indeed, the major cost for each of the treatment arms was hospitalization and not the use of chemotherapy. Moreover, chemotherapy may provide important symptom control in a substantial number of patients, such as decreased cough, dyspnea, pain, and hemoptysis.

First-Line Therapy for Advanced NSCLC ■ Although existing data clearly indicate that chemotherapy is warranted in appropriately selected patients with advanced NSCLC, an optimal chemotherapy regimen has not been identified. Until the mid 1990s, cisplatin combinations, most often with a vinca alkaloid or etoposide, were commonly used. More recently, drug regimens with a platinum, either cisplatin or carboplatin, and a second newer drug with known activity are more widely used. That second agent could be a taxane, vinorelbine, gemcitabine, or a camptothecin. Choosing one regimen from among many has been a difficult task, however, since there is no clearly documented survival advantage for one drug program over the others. At times, subtle differences in eligibility criteria (eg, inclusion of patients with stage III tumors or those with poor PS) make it difficult to directly relate the results among trials. Nonetheless, there is a trend indicating that regimens containing platinum with a taxane or gemcitabine probably produce higher response rates and also better survival outcome in some series.

There have been a number of studies of paclitaxel in combination with cisplatin or carboplatin, and other agents. In a three-arm randomized ECOG trial (ECOG 5592), 560 eligible, previously untreated patients were randomized to receive a combination of cisplatin plus etoposide or paclitaxel, either low-dose (135 mg/m^2 over 24 h) or high-dose (250 mg/m^2 over 24 h with growth factor) paclitaxel in.[210] The response rates for the low-dose and high-dose paclitaxel arms were 26.5% and 32.1%, respectively, significantly better than the cisplatin/etoposide arm. There was also an improvement in overall survival, but it reached statistical significance only when the two paclitaxel arms were combined into a single group and compared with the third arm. In a European trial of similar design, cisplatin plus paclitaxel led to improved response rate and quality of life parameters, but there was no overall survival difference compared with a standard regimen of cisplatin and teniposide.[211]

In a recent survey, paclitaxel plus carboplatin was found to be the most widely favored option for first-line chemotherapy in all stages of NSCLC among U.S. medical oncologists.[212] This relates to ease of administration on an outpatient basis, manageable toxicity profiles compared with cisplatin-containing regimens, and promising phase 2 trial results. SWOG investigators reached similar conclusions. Although several regimens seemed to provide comparable palliation in advanced NSCLC, they favored a paclitaxel plus carboplatin regimen for future studies because of its favorable toxicity profile and better tolerability and compliance.[213] A recent randomized phase 3 study compared the efficacy and safety of weekly paclitaxel in combination with carboplatin administered every 4 weeks to the standard regimen of paclitaxel and carboplatin administered every 3 weeks. Results suggest that all efficacy parameters were similar between the two treatment arms. The authors concluded that the favorable nonhematologic toxicity profile of the weakly paclitaxel arm makes it an alternative treatment option in this setting.[214]

Like vinorelbine and paclitaxel, gemcitabine is approved by the U.S. Food and Drug Administration (FDA) for NSCLC. A series of successful phase 2 trials of cisplatin plus gemcitabine led to pivotal phase 3 studies.[215–217] The Hoosier Oncology Group compared gemcitabine plus cisplatin with cisplatin alone and showed that the association yielded a modest improvement in median and 1-year survival rates.[217] On the other hand, the Spanish and Italian trials that compared gemcitabine plus cisplatin with another regimen of cisplatin plus etoposide or mitomycin plus ifosfamide plus cisplatin, respectively, failed to demonstrate survival benefit, although there were significant improvements in overall response rates with the gemcitabine plus cisplatin regimens.[215,216] A phase 3 trial of cisplatin and docetaxel versus gemcitabine and docetaxel enrolled 441 subjects.[218] There were no significant differences in overall response rates or median survival durations. The interpretation of the authors was that both drug combinations had comparable activity.

The TAX 326 study group performed a large multicenter, multinational study of two docetaxel/platinum regimens for NSCLC.[219] In a 1218-subject, three-arm trial comparing docetaxel and cisplatin, docetaxel and carboplatin, and vinorelbine and cisplatin (VC), median survival duration was longest for the docetaxel and cisplatin arm, 11.3 months, with a 1-year survival rate of 46% (vs 41% for VC) and a 2-year survival rate of 21% (vs 14% for VC) ($p = .03$). A Japanese phase 3 trial compared docetaxel and cisplatin with vindesine and cisplatin in 311 patients.[215] Docetaxel/cisplatin produced a significantly higher response rate than vindesine/cisplatin, 37.1% versus 21.2% ($p < .01$), and the duration of response trended longer (13.1 vs 9.3 weeks).[220]

In 2006 The U.S. FDA approved the use of bevacizumab in combination with carboplatin and paclitaxel for the initial treatment of patients with unresectable, locally advanced, recurrent or metastatic, non-squamous, NSCLC. This approval was based on an improvement in survival time when bevacizumab was added to a standard chemotherapy regimen. In 2007 bevacizumab was approved in Europe for the first-line treatment of patients with advanced NSCLC, in combination with any platinum-based chemotherapy regimen. This new paradigm is discussed in more detail in the "Molecular Targeted Therapy" section.

Certainly, quality of life concerns should enter the treatment decision-making process, and this area is now receiving increasing scrutiny. With respect to ideal duration of chemotherapy, there are probably no clear guidelines because the nature of treatment itself is rapidly changing. ASCO has recommended that not more than six cycles of currently accepted chemotherapy regimens be administered to individual patients. This issue was examined in a prospective phase 3 trial comparing a defined duration of therapy with carboplatin/paclitaxel versus continuous treatment in advanced NSCLC.[221] Despite differences in the median number of treatment cycles delivered, there were no significant differences in response rates or survival among the 236 randomized patients. A general consensus is that most conventional chemotherapy regimens should be given for a finite number of cycles and that continuing a maintenance approach is not beneficial. After four to six cycles, chronic treatment-related toxic effects may outweigh benefits.

Second-Line Chemotherapy for Advanced NSCLC ■ With the gradual increase in the efficacy of systemic therapy, a growing number of patients who develop progressive or recurrent disease following first-line treatment are appropriate candidates for consideration of second-line therapy. The role of docetaxel has been established in this setting. In a pivotal phase 3 trial, 373 subjects were randomized to receive docetaxel (100 or 75 mg/m^2) or a control regimen of vinorelbine or ifosfamide at the choice of the investigators as second-line therapy.[222] Response rates in the docetaxel arms were 10.8% and 6.7%, respectively (0.8% response with vinorelbine or ifosfamide), but patients who received docetaxel achieved a longer time to tumor progression and a superior 1-year survival rate at the 75 mg/m^2 dose (32%). Previous exposure to paclitaxel did not decrease the likelihood of response to docetaxel, nor did it appear to have an impact on survival. Treatment appeared to be well tolerated. The researchers concluded that the 75 mg/m^2 every-3-week schedule offers meaningful benefit to patients with advanced disease. A second phase 3 multicenter international study enrolled 204 subjects who had progressed on or after at least one cisplatin-containing chemotherapy regimen and randomly assigned them to receive either docetaxel or best supportive care. The initial dose of docetaxel was 100 mg/m^2, but it was reduced to 75 mg/m^2 because of toxicity. The overall response rate was only 6%. However, time to progression and survival duration were significantly longer for docetaxel-treated patients. Median survival duration was 7.5 months for patients who received 75 mg/m^2 and 4.6 months for patients who received supportive care ($p = .01$). A striking finding was that the 1-year survival rate for patients who received docetaxel at 75 mg/m^2 was 37%, while it was 12% for patients in the best supportive care arm ($p = .003$). Quality of life analyses also have provided evidence favoring treatment with docetaxel in selected patients.[223]

Pemetrexed (Alimta) is a multitargeted antifolate drug that targets the enzymes thymidylate synthase, dihydrofolate reductase, and glycinamide ribonucleotide formyl transferase. The phase 3 trial of pemetrexed in NSCLC was a survival comparison between pemetrexed and docetaxel in relapsed NSCLC.[5] In this noninferiority study, both pemetrexed and docetaxel were given on day 1 of a 21-day cycle. Patients in both arms were premedicated with dexamethasone. Patients in the pemetrexed arm also received folate and B_{12} supplementation. Response rates were 9.1% and 8.8%, and median survival times were 8.3 and 7.9 months in the pemetrexed and docetaxel arms, respectively. The docetaxel arm had higher incidences of grade 3 and 4 neutropenia (40% vs 5%), neutropenic fever (13% vs 2%), and neuropathy (8% vs 3%) than the pemetrexed arm. Thus, pemetrexed produced similar results and was better tolerated than docetaxel in the treatment of patients with pretreated NSCLC, leading to the FDA approval of pemetrexed for relapsed NSCLC.

Despite these advances in treatment, improvements in the survival of patients with NSCLC in recent years have been modest. For patients with advanced disease with good enough PS to tolerate and thus receive third- or fourth-line chemotherapy, a retrospective analysis reported the median overall survival from the start of the last treatment as 4 months.[224]

Combined-Modality Treatment of NSCLC ■ *Advances in Neoadjuvant/Adjuvant Chemotherapy* ■ Despite undergoing resection, the vast majority of lung cancer patients experience recurrent and/or metastatic disease; two-thirds of these recurrences and metastases occur systemically and one-third locally. Therefore, supplementing surgery with chemotherapy is a rational treatment strategy.[4] Considerable effort has been directed toward improving therapeutic outcomes (except for the prognostically favorable T1 N0 M0 cancers) with the administration of systemic chemotherapy and/or radiotherapy in conjunction with surgery. Results from older chemotherapy trials have been disappointing, and in some cases were associated with shorter survival in the subjects receiving chemotherapy compared to those receiving no treatment. Nevertheless there remains much interest in improving systemic treatment strategies, since many patients eventually develop distant metastatic disease.

Neoadjuvant Chemotherapy ■ SWOG recently conducted a phase 3 North American trial (S9900) comparing primary surgery alone with induction chemotherapy (paclitaxel/carboplatin [PC]) followed by surgery. Preliminary data from this multicenter Intergroup trial were presented at the 2005 ASCO annual meeting.[225] Patients with clinical stage T2 N0, T1–2 N1, or T3 N0–1 NSCLC were randomized to receive preoperative PC for three cycles or surgery alone. The trial closed early following publication of positive data on adjuvant treatment from other studies. Although not statistically significant, there were trends in progression-free and overall survival which favored preoperative PC. A recent European study randomized 519 patients with stage I-III NSCLC to surgery alone or three cycles of platinum-based chemotherapy followed by surgery. This study did not find differences in the overall survival between the two arms.[226] A French Phase 3 trial randomized patients with stage IB-IIIA disease to receive preoperative mitomycin, ifosfamide, and cisplatin, in addition to postoperative chemotherapy for responding patients, or surgery alone. Although not statistically significant, improved overall survival was observed with chemotherapy, and subset analysis demonstrated that subjects with N0 and N1 disease had significantly better survival with chemotherapy.[227]

Adjuvant Chemotherapy ■ The LCSG and the Ludwig Lung Cancer Study Group of Europe have conducted a series of trials investigating the potential benefit of adjuvant chemotherapy in patients with completely resected early-stage lung cancer. The LCSG compared four cycles of cyclophosphamide, doxorubicin, and cisplatin (CAP) with no further treatment in 269 patients.[228] After a mean follow-up duration of 6.4 years, no benefits in disease-free or overall survival rates were apparent. However, compliance was poor, because only 80% of patients randomized to receive chemotherapy actually did so, and only 53% of patients completed all four planned treatment cycles. Another study yielded more encouraging results in 110 patients with T1–3 NSCLC (90% of whom had T1–2 N0 staged tumors).[229] Fifty-four patients were randomized to receive six cycles of CAP and 54 to receive no further therapy. Although time to recurrence and overall survival duration were significantly better in the chemotherapy-treated patients, an imbalance in randomization resulted in the assignment of twice as many patients who had undergone pneumonectomy to the control group. After adjustment for this imbalance, results were less impressive.

A more definitive recent trial was conducted by the ECOG.[230] This prospective randomized study was designed to determine whether combination chemotherapy with cisplatin/etoposide and thoracic radiotherapy was superior to thoracic radiotherapy alone for patients with completely resected stage II or IIIA NSCLC. A total of four chemotherapy cycles were administered, the first two given concomitantly with radiotherapy. Radiation was given in a daily fractionation sequence to a total dose of 50.4 Gy and was identical in the two treatment arms. The median duration of follow-up was 44 months for 488 patients entered. Although the combined postoperative treatment was generally well tolerated, there was no decrease in the risk of intrathoracic recurrence for the experimental arm, nor was there evidence of a survival difference between the treatment arms.

A meta-analysis in 1995 compared surgery alone with surgery followed by cisplatin-based chemotherapy. This study included eight trials and 1394 patients, and showed a 13% reduction in the risk of death, suggesting that adjuvant chemotherapy afforded an absolute benefit of 5% at 5 years ($p = .08$). This was not affected by patient sex, PS, or age, or by tumor histologic subtype.[231] The International Adjuvant Lung Trial study included 1867 patients who underwent randomization to receive either three or four cycles of adjuvant cisplatin-based chemotherapy or to undergo observation. The investigators concluded that cisplatin-based adjuvant chemotherapy prolonged survival among patients with completely resected NSCLC.[232] Three studies on adjuvant chemotherapy were presented at the ASCO 2004 annual meeting: two moderate-sized studies showed a significant survival benefit: 15% at 5 years for the NCIC JBR10 study,[233] and 12% at 4 years for the CALGB 9633 study.[234] Furthermore, a Japanese meta-analysis of 2003 patients randomized in six trials of uracil-tegafur showed a 5% benefit at 7 years,[235] confirming the results of the Japanese Lung Cancer Research Group study.[236] Current ASCO guidelines indicate that adjuvant cisplatin-based chemotherapy is recommended for routine use in patients with stages IIA, IIB, and IIIA disease. Those recommendations include selected patients older than 65 years old. Although there has been a statistically significant overall survival benefit seen in several randomized clinical trials (RCTs) enrolling a range of people with completely resected NSCLC, results of subset analyses for patient populations with stage IB disease were not significant, and adjuvant chemotherapy in stage IB disease is not currently recommended for routine use. To date, very few patients with stage IA NSCLC have been enrolled onto RCTs of adjuvant therapy, and adjuvant chemotherapy is not recommended for this stage group.[237]

Unresectable Stage III NSCLC ■ Thoracic irradiation has been the standard therapy for patients with inoperable IIIA/IIIB NSCLC in the United States for many years. Although chest radiotherapy improves cancer-related symptoms and reduces the frequency of local tumor regrowth, the outcomes with chest radiotherapy alone were poor, with a median survival of approximately 10 months and a 5-year survival rate of less than 5%. Efforts to improve these results have included altered radiation dose-fractionation schedules and combined chemoradiation approaches. These trials are discussed in the section "Radiotherapy" above.

Chemotherapy in the Elderly ■ Approximately one-third of all patients with NSCLC are aged 70 years or older, and, although these patients are likely to have an increased risk of comorbid conditions and impaired organ function, most studies have suggested that age alone should not be a factor in the decision to treat patients with chemotherapy. Retrospective studies of patients treated for advanced NSCLC found no major differences between patients older than and younger than 65 years of age,[238] and an analysis of age as a risk factor in chemotherapy trials found that the response, toxicity, and survival rates of elderly patients were similar to those of younger patients.[239]

Two phase 3 randomized studies of chemotherapy in the elderly have been reported.[240,241] The ELVIS (Elderly Lung Cancer Vinorelbine Italian Study) group performed a multicenter, randomized trial of single-agent vinorelbine as a first-line agent in elderly patients with advanced NSCLC. Results demonstrated that the addition of vinorelbine to best supportive care significantly prolonged survival in this group of patients.[240] Median survival for best supportive care plus vinorelbine was 28 weeks, while it was 21 weeks for best supportive care alone. This benefit was achieved at the cost of some drug related toxicity, reflected in lower scores on quality-of-life subscales that were directly related to drug toxicity (eg, nausea and constipation). Patients who received vinorelbine scored better than control patients on overall health status and quality-of-life, however, and suffered less from the lung cancer symptoms of shortness of breath, cough, and hemoptysis. Recently, the Multicenter Italian Lung cancer in the Elderly Study (MILES) randomized elderly patients with advanced NSCLC to receive vinorelbine, gemcitabine, or vinorelbine plus gemcitabine. Results demonstrated that the combination of gemcitabine plus vinorelbine does not improve survival or quality of life compared with single-agent chemotherapy with vinorelbine or gemcitabine in this patient population. The combination treatment was more toxic than the agents administered alone.[241]

The recommendations of an international expert panel were presented recently.[6] The panel recommended a comprehensive geriatric assessment to better define prognosis and predict tolerance to treatment. They suggested that randomized phase 3 trials with adequate power are warranted to address unanswered questions regarding the efficacy and tolerability of platinum-based chemotherapy. The panel also reviewed the role of biologic therapy in this age group and suggested that, on the basis of present data, target-based agents as first-line treatment of elderly NSCLC patients are not yet recommended. They concluded that single-agent chemotherapy with a third-generation drug (vinorelbine, gemcitabine, a taxane) should be the recommended option for nonselected elderly patients with advanced NSCLC. Platinum-based chemotherapy is a viable option for fit patients with adequate organ function. Best supportive care remains important, in addition to chemotherapy or as the exclusive option for patients who are unsuitable for more aggressive treatment.[6] Novel therapeutics are extensively studied in this population, as discussed in the next section.

Molecular Targeted Therapy ■ Advances in our understanding of cancer biology have led to the discovery of a number of potential molecular targets and the development of novel agents that, unlike conventional cytotoxic agents, specifically target tumor cells or their blood vessels. This approach has been termed "molecular targeted therapy." Most advanced in clinical research for NSCLC-targeted therapies are epidermal growth factor receptor (EGFR) and vascular endothelial growth factor (VEGF) inhibitors. Indeed, the first targeted therapies for NSCLC were gefitinib (Iressa, AstraZeneca) and erlotinib (Tarceva, Genentech), EGFR tyrosine kinase inhibitors (TKI) that have been approved as monotherapy for advanced NSCLC. The rationale for EGFR inhibition as a target for cancer therapy was proposed nearly 25 years ago, when it was discovered that EGFR was frequently overexpressed in human tumors, and in many cases was associated with poor outcome.[242] Several strategies have been developed to target the EGF family of receptors. These include monoclonal antibodies, which either bind the ligand or compete with the ligand for the extracellular domain of the receptor; inhibitors of receptor dimerization; small-molecule inhibitors of the intracellular tyrosine kinase domain; antisense oligonucleotides; and inhibitors of the EGFR downstream signaling network.

Inhibitors of EGFR ■ Gefitinib and erlotinib are small molecules that reversibly target EGFR tyrosine kinase. Two randomized phase 2 multicenter trials of gefitinib were conducted in over 400 patients.[243,244] These studies showed that monotherapy with gefitinib induces radiographic response in 12% to 18% and improves symptoms in 40% to 43% of NSCLC patients with advanced disease who experienced chemotherapy failure at a dose of 250 mg/day. On the basis of these data, gefitinib received approval in Japan and South Korea in July 2002 as second-line chemotherapy for advanced NSCLC, and in May 2003 in the United States as third-line monotherapy treatment of advanced disease. However, the results of the gefitinib phase 3 trial were negative. In multicenter study 709, Iressa Survival Evaluation in Lung Cancer (ISEL), 1692 patients were randomized to receive gefitinib 250 mg/day or placebo. This study demonstrated a difference between gefitinib and placebo in terms of survival, although this did not reach statistical significance in the overall population. In preplanned subgroup analyses, however, gefitinib therapy was associated with significantly increased survival in never-smokers and those of Asian ethnicity.[245]

Erlotinib was investigated in a phase 2 trial in 56 patients with advanced NSCLC whose disease had failed to respond to platinum-based chemotherapy. Unlike the gefitinib studies, patients were included only if their tumors overexpressed EGFR (> 10% positive cells). In this study, erlotinib was given continuously at a fixed dosage of 150 mg/day, which produced an acneiform rash in 78% of patients. Twelve percent of patients responded to erlotinib, and 39% of patients had prolonged stable disease during the treatment. The results of the erlotinib phase 3 trial were positive: In a randomized, placebo-controlled trial (NCIC BR.21) involving 731 patients, single-agent erlotinib was shown to prolong survival in NSCLC patients after first- or second-line chemotherapy. Overall response to erlotinib was 9%, and the overall survival durations were 6.7 months for erlotinib and 4.7 months for placebo (p = .001).[246] On the basis of this study, the first randomized trial to confirm that an EGFR TKI prolongs survival after first- or second-line chemotherapy, erlotinib received approval by the FDA in 2004.

The reasons for the differences between BR21 and ISEL results are not clear. Possible explanations for the discrepancy are that erlotinib was given at a dose closer to its maximal tolerated dose than gefitinib; that the study populations were not comparable (ISEL was almost twice as large), including a higher rate of refractory disease in ISEL; and that these drugs are different after all. The negative ISEL data resulted in a label change for gefitinib in NSCLC patients in the United States and other countries, and withdrawal from marketing authorization application in the European Union.

Since gefitinib and erlotinib do not induce myelosuppression, it seemed reasonable to test them in combination with chemotherapy. However, results of four large phase 3 results were negative. Two large, randomized, placebo-controlled, phase 3 trials were conducted with gefitinib (Iressa NSCLC Trial Assessing Combination Treatment (INTACT) trials 1 (gemcitabine and cisplatin) and 2 (paclitaxel and carboplatin)).[247,248] Patients were randomly assigned to receive placebo, gefitinib 250 mg/day, or gefitinib 500 mg/day in addition to chemotherapy. Patients continued with gefitinib or placebo until disease progression. Results showed that gefitinib did not add therapeutic benefits over chemotherapy alone. In two large, randomized similarly designed trials of chemotherapy with or without erlotinib, erlotinib was given concomitantly with a combination of carboplatin and paclitaxel (the TRIBUTE study; n = 1059) or a combination of cisplatin and gemcitabine (TALENT; n = 1172).[249,250] Selection of patients for these trials was not based on biologic features. Like the gefitinib phase 3 trials, these studies showed that erlotinib offered no survival benefit or improvement in response rate over chemotherapy alone. Several ongoing studies are examining the efficacy and safety of gefitinib or erlotinib with chemotherapy in subsets of NSCLC patients.

Monoclonal antibodies that target EGFR, such as cetuximab, are also being tested in clinical trials. Cetuximab has demonstrated significant activity in colorectal and head and neck cancer patients. In a large ongoing phase 3 trial in NSCLC patients whose tumors express EGFR, subjects are randomized to receive chemotherapy (cisplatin and vinorelbine) with or without cetuximab.[251] The feasibility of combining chemoradiotherapy and cetuximab has been demonstrated in a phase 2 study in patients with unresectable stage III disease.[252] It remains possible that in the near future monoclonal antibodies against EGFR will become another molecular targeted agent available for patients with NSCLC.

Prediction of EGFR TKI Response ■ Better understanding of the biology of the EGFR system in lung cancer has been the focus of intense research in the past few years. Retrospective analyses of gefitinib or erlotinib study data revealed several clinical predictors of response. They repeatedly showed that responses were more frequent among patients who had never smoked, women, patients with adenocarcinomas, and patients of East Asian ethnicity.[2] Two groups from Boston in two pivotal studies examined gain-of-function somatic mutations of EGFR in exons 18–21 and correlated them with response to EGFR inhibitors. Lynch and colleagues[253] and Paez and colleagues[254] found increased sensitivity to gefitinib in patients with these EGFR mutations, and that patients who did not express a mutation had a low probability of responding.

The group from Memorial Sloan Kettering Cancer Center extended these data and showed that similar EGFR mutations are also associated with responses to erlotinib.[2] These findings are supported by a report of correlation between these clinical predictors of response and EGFR mutation status.[255] Compiling these data reveals that EGFR mutations are identified in 80% of responders to EGFR small molecule TKIs, whereas mutations in K-ras (exon 2) are associated with lack of sensitivity to either erlotinib or gefitinib.[2] The role of EGFR or K-ras mutation status in prediction of response to EGFR inhibitors in general, and EGFR TKI in particular, are being studied in prospective studies. For example, Cappuzzo and colleagues conducted a phase 2 trial of gefitinib in patients who never smoked or had increased EGFR gene copy number or activation of Akt.[256] An interim analysis suggested that gefitinib was active and well tolerated and that EGFR FISH analysis was an accurate predictor of response to therapy. Further prospective studies will be required to determine the most reliable, validated biomarkers of response to EGFR TKI therapy.

Angiogenesis Inhibitors in Lung Cancer ■ VEGF, which is an endothelial cell survival factor, is essential for tumor angiogenesis. One approach to the modulation of VEGF-mediated angiogenesis is to use antibodies against the VEGF protein itself or VEGFR. Bevacizumab (Avastin, Genentech) is a recombinant humanized monoclonal antibody to VEGF that acts synergistically with chemotherapy. It was approved for use in the United States and Europe for first-line treatment of metastatic carcinoma of the colon or rectum.

In a phase 1 trial, bevacizumab reduced serum VEGF concentrations to undetectable levels when administered at dosages of at least 3 mg/kg/week and showed no pharmacologic interactions when studied in combination with a variety of chemotherapeutic agents. In a phase 2 study, patients with stage IIIB/IV NSCLC were randomly assigned to undergo standard therapy with carboplatin and paclitaxel alone or with 7.5 mg/kg or 15 mg/kg of bevacizumab.[257] Subjects in the control group (chemotherapy only) who experienced disease progression were allowed to enter the high-dose bevacizumab arm. Response rates were higher (40.0% vs 21.9%) and time to progression (7.0 vs 3.9 months) and median survival (17.7 vs 11.6 months) were longer in the high-dose arm than in the low-dose arm. An unusual and unexpected toxic effect was the development of life-threatening hemoptysis in six patients, which resulted in four fatalities. This event did not appear to be dose dependent, since all but one of these six cases occurred in the low-dose bevacizumab arm. Bleeding arose from centrally located tumors close to major blood vessels and cavitation or necrosis had occurred in most cases. This adverse event has not been noted in studies of other tumor types.

Because multivariate analysis identified squamous cell histology as a risk factor, the phase 2/3 NSCLC study comparing bevacizumab (15 mg/kg) plus carboplatin and paclitaxel with carboplatin and paclitaxel alone included only patients whose tumors were of nonsquamous histologic type. This trial, ECOG study 4599, recruited 878 patients.[3] Chemotherapy was administered every 3 weeks for six cycles, and bevacizumab was administered every 3 weeks until disease progression or toxic effects were intolerable. In addition to histology of squamous cell carcinoma, other exclusion criteria were presence of brain metastases or clinically significant hemoptysis. Median survival was prolonged (12.3 vs 10.3 months) in the group assigned to chemotherapy plus bevacizumab, as compared with the chemotherapy-alone group (hazard ratio for death, 0.79; $p = .003$). The median progression-free survival in the two groups were 6.2 and 4.5 months, respectively (hazard ratio for disease progression, 0.66; $p < .001$), with corresponding response rates of 35% and 15% ($p < .001$). Rates of clinically significant bleeding were 4.4% and 0.7%, respectively ($p < .001$). There were 15 treatment-related deaths in the chemotherapy plus bevacizumab arm, including 5 from pulmonary hemorrhage. The researchers concluded that in these selected NSCLC patients, the addition of bevacizumab to chemotherapy has a significant survival benefit, with risk of increased treatment-related deaths. Based on these results, bevacizumab with platinum-based chemotherapy is indicated for selected NSCLC patients in the US and Europe.

Combination of Treatment Strategies ■ Different combinations of conventional therapy (chemotherapy or radiation therapy) or combinations of targeted therapy are being explored, and some examples are discussed in this section. As already discussed, the mainstay for cancer therapy is still chemotherapy. Concurrent administration of gefitinib or erlotinib with chemotherapy did not improve results of chemotherapy alone.[238–241] Several studies are looking at potential explanations for this phenomenon and studying whether the sequence of administration of these combinations is clinically relevant. Another approach is the combination of growth factor receptor TKI and monoclonal antibodies to improve signaling inhibition. Preliminary preclinical data are encouraging.[249,250]

As alternatives, drugs are now being developed to block several signaling pathways. Vandetanib (ZD6474, Zactima, Astra-Zeneca) is a TKI of VEGFR and EGFR currently being tested in the clinic.[258] It has been suggested that, besides complementing chemotherapy regimens, targeted agents could enhance the therapeutic efficacy of radiation therapy. The combination of different EGFR and VEGFR blockers to improve target inhibition was examined with bevacizumab and erlotinib in 40 patients with stage IIIB/IV or recurrent NSCLC of nonsquamous cell histology.[259] Treatment with bevacizumab (15 mg/kg IV every 21 days) plus erlotinib (150 mg/day orally) resulted in eight partial responses (20%, CI 7.6–32.4%) and 26 patients with stable disease (65%, CI 50.2–79.8%). The median survival of 34 patients treated in the phase 2 part of the study was 12.6 months, and 52% of patients were alive at 1 year. No pharmacokinetic interactions were observed between the two agents, and the most common adverse events were mild to moderate rash, diarrhea, and proteinuria. These encouraging data support further evaluation of VEGF/EGF inhibition for the treatment of advanced NSCLC, and a randomized study is currently ongoing.[258] Some of these drugs are listed in Table 78-10.

Summary of the MD Anderson guidelines for diagnosis and therapy of NSCLC are presented in Fig. 78-8.

Molecular Prognostic Markers

The identification of validated molecular markers that can reliably identify patients with different clinical outcomes would have significant impact on patient care. For patients who have undergone complete surgical resection of NSCLC, the ability to stratify this population into groups with either a high or low risk of cancer recurrence would facilitate decisions regarding the use of adjuvant therapy. Many groups have focused on identifying molecular prognostic factors in patients with early-stage NSCLC because of the availability of surgical tumor specimens.[260–263] In a case-control study of stage I NSCLC patients who recurred within 40 months of resection, promoter methylation of four genes (*p16*, *CDH13*, *RASSF1A*, and *APC*) was associated with early disease recurrence.[260] The development of gene expression microarray technology recently has allowed investigators to employ a genomics approach to identify gene expression profiles associated with clinical outcome. Based on gene-expression profiles in 89 patients with early-stage NSCLC, investigators developed a gene-expression model with

Table 78-10 **Molecular Targeted Therapy for Lung Cancer**

Agent	Activity	Comment
Gefitinib, erlotinib	EGFR TKI	Approved as monotherapy third line in advanced NSCLC
Erbitux, panitumumab, EMD732000	Monoclonal antibodies to EGFR	
Bevacizumab	Monoclonal antibody to VEGFR	Approved for first line colon cancer with chemotherapy
ZD6474, AEE788	VEGFR and EGFR TKI	
BAY43-9006 (Sorafenib)	Raf-1, VEGFR, and PDGFR-β TKI	
PTK787	VEGFR TKI	
SU11248	VEGFR, PDGFR, c-Kit, and CSF-1 TKI	

Abbreviations: CSF-1, colony-stimulating factor-1; EGFR, epidermal growth factor receptor; NSCLC, nonsmall-cell lung cancer; PDGFR, platelet-derived growth factor receptor; TKI, tyrosine kinase inhibitor; VEGFR, vascular endothelial growth factor receptor

a predictive accuracy of 72% and 79% for NSCLC recurrence when applied to two separate validation cohorts.[263] Another group employed a similar approach to identify five genes (*DUSP6*, *MMD*, *STAT1*, *ERBB3*, and *LCK*) associated with recurrence and survival from 125 NSCLC patients who had undergone surgical resection.[261] The resulting five-gene signature, when tested on two validation cohorts, similarly predicted relapse-free and overall survival.

Molecular Predictive Markers

Oncologists still lack the necessary tools to personalize lung cancer therapy due to the absence of validated predictive molecular markers. If one could identify which patients are more likely to respond to specific agents, strategies could be devised which maximize efficacy and minimize unnecessary drug toxicity. Distinguishing a prognostic from a predictive molecular marker can be tedious, however, requiring prospective randomized trials with appropriate control arms. A recent analysis of a placebo-controlled, randomized trial of the EGFR tyrosine kinase inhibitor erlotinib in advanced NSCLC patients investigated molecular (EGFR protein expression, *EGFR* gene copy number, and *EGFR* mutation status) and clinical predictors of outcome.[264] Interestingly, survival was significantly improved with erlotinib in subjects with EGFR protein expression and with polysomy or amplification of *EGFR*, but not in a smaller group of patients with *EGFR* mutations. Analysis of a large randomized trial of adjuvant chemotherapy in patients with completely resected NSCLC indicates that lack of protein expression of the DNA-repair enzyme excision repair cross-complementation group 1 (ERCC1) is a predictive marker of benefit from adjuvant cisplatin-based therapy.[265] It is anticipated that ongoing and future studies incorporating high-throughput genomic and proteomic technologies will accelerate the development of clinically useful predictive molecular profiles, which will allow better individualization of NSCLC therapy.

Therapy for SCLC

SCLC differs from NSCLC in its rapid growth rate, propensity for early systemic spread, and short natural history. Of the patients whose disease is managed without resection of the primary tumor, very few have no evidence of tumor dissemination beyond the thorax at autopsy. A series published in 1973 showed that of patients who underwent an attempt at curative resection and died within 30 days from postoperative complications, 63% had distant metastases at postmortem examination.[266] Ninety percent of these patients had metastases to mediastinal lymph nodes. These aggressive clinical features are reflected in the short overall survival of these patients. Before effective systemic treatment became available, the median survival was 12 weeks for those with limited-stage disease and 5 weeks for those with extensive-stage disease. Patients rarely survived longer than 35 weeks. It is important to recognize, however, that staging procedures were primitive in that era. Thus, with more accurate staging, both groups would likely have better outcomes.

Locoregional therapy, with either surgery or radiation, prolonged survival only slightly, primarily for patients with what was then defined as limited-stage disease. An overwhelming majority of patients did not benefit. Only 20% survived for a year, and 5-year survival was rare. In a landmark trial conducted by the Medical Research Council in England in the 1960s, patients who were considered candidates for surgical resection by the standards of the time were randomized to undergo thoracotomy or definitive irradiation of the primary tumor and regional lymphatics. Radiation therapy resulted in slightly better mean survival duration (6.5 vs 10 months, $p = .04$); 1-, 2-, and 5-year survival rates were 22%, 10%, and 4%, respectively, for radiotherapy and 21%, 4%, and 1%, respectively, for surgery. Notably, the one 5-year survivor in the surgery arm was ultimately unable to undergo surgery and was given radiation therapy instead. This and other experiences led to the abandonment of surgery as a primary modality of treatment of SCLC, with the possible exception of patients with node negative solitary pulmonary nodules. Moreover, chest radiotherapy as a sole treatment would also soon be superseded.

In 1969, Green and colleagues reported the results of a placebo-controlled randomized trial evaluating single-agent alkylating agents in the treatment of lung cancer. Three courses of intravenous cyclophosphamide nearly tripled the median survival duration (from 6 to 17 weeks) in patients with extensive-stage and doubled that of limited-stage patients (from 12 to 24 weeks). Subsequent trials in the 1970s documented survival impact from the use of chemotherapy as an adjunct to radiation, compared to radiation alone, despite the use of suboptimal chemotherapy. Combination chemotherapy was developed in that same decade with improved complete response rates and survival duration relative to single agents. With the general acceptance of SCLC as a systemic disorder and recognition of the superiority of multimodal regimens over local therapy alone, chemotherapy became the cornerstone of SCLC management.[267]

Surgical Treatment

Although it has been established that surgical resection does not customarily play a role in the treatment of SCLC, there are still some clinical settings in which surgery may be of potential benefit. The most accepted role for surgery is in the case of peripheral SCLC. Although two-thirds of patients have extensive disease at the time of presentation, there is a small subset, fewer than 5% of patients with SCLC, who present with the tumor confined to the lung, with or without N1 lymph node metastases. These patients commonly present with a solitary pulmonary nodule on an incidental chest radiograph. Overall 5-year survival rate for patients who have undergone surgery followed by adjuvant chemotherapy has been shown to range from 28% to 60% for patients with stage I disease and 20% to 35% for patients with T1 N1 disease.[268] Isolated reports have described 5-year survival rates as high as 70% to 80% for selected groups of patients with very limited stage disease. The great disparity between the

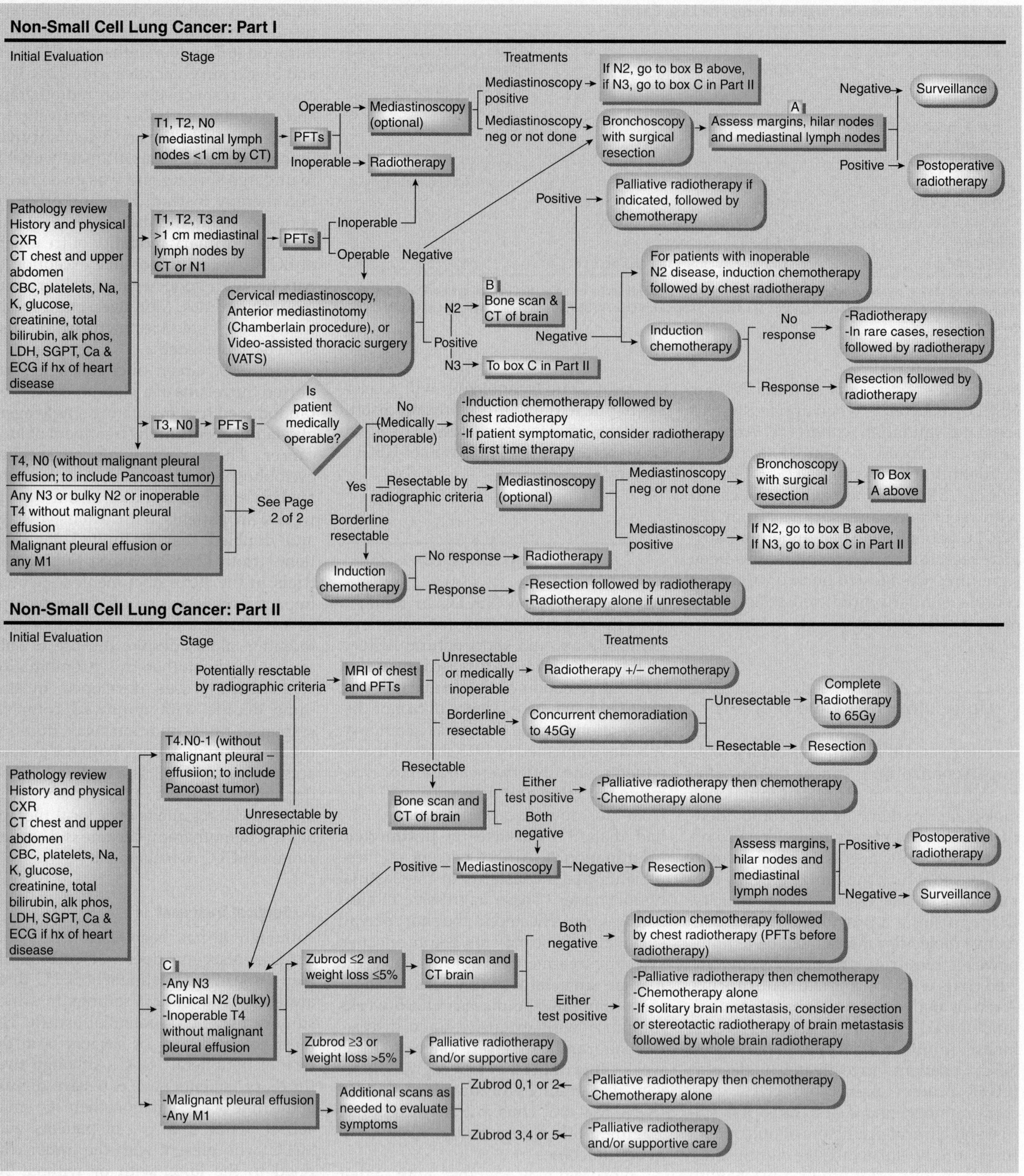

Figure 78-8 Management of non-small cell lung cancer.

survival rates of these patients and the survival rates of the more common central SCLC has led to several hypotheses. Some investigators believe that these tumors represent a variant of SCLC with altered biology; however, others believe that these tumors are inaccurately diagnosed and may in fact be well or moderately-differentiated neuroendocrine carcinomas (typical or atypical carcinoids).[269]

Most patients with peripheral SCLC have the diagnosis made at the time of thoracotomy. A select few, however, have the diagnosis established preoperatively with FNA. The rare but established presentation of SCLC as a peripheral lesion, along with the fact that NSCLC and carcinoids can be misdiagnosed as SCLC on FNA, should prompt the clinician to continue to consider the patient for surgical treatment rather than refer immediately for chemotherapy. In light of this preoperative diagnosis, staging should be even more thorough than usual to reflect the high incidence of occult mediastinal and systemic metastasis associated with SCLC. Thorough radiographic staging, as well as mediastinoscopy, are employed prior to consideration of surgery. The presence of mediastinal involvement would obviate the role of surgery, but the presence of hilar adenopathy on radiographic staging is not an absolute contraindication to surgery. These patients may still undergo exploration as a means of establishing the presence of disease within the hilar nodes and, in good candidates, resection can still be offered if a complete resection is possible. All patients with surgically treated SCLC, regardless of whether the diagnosis was established before, during, or after resection, should receive postoperative chemotherapy. In trials reported by the Veterans Administration Surgical Adjuvant Group, patients who received postoperative chemotherapy did better than those who did not. When the timing of chemotherapy was examined, there appeared to be no advantage to giving chemotherapy preoperatively.[267]

Radiotherapy

Surgical local control is applicable to a very small subset of patients with SCLC. The remainder requires some form of local control as part of their treatment, and radiotherapy fulfills this role. Two meta-analyses employing different methods confirmed the value of thoracic irradiation to decrease local recurrence and prolong survival. The first study, based on results from 11 trials, showed an absolute increase in overall survival rate of 5.4% at 2 years.[270] The second study collected data on 2140 patients from 13 randomized trials comparing chemotherapy alone with chemotherapy plus thoracic irradiation and found an improvement in absolute survival rate of 5.4%, from 15% to 20.4%, at 3 years.[271] Of note, the trials included in these meta-analyses were not recent studies, and none of them employed cisplatin and etoposide, the current standard chemotherapy regimen. In addition, these trials included both sequential and concurrent chemoradiotherapy.

Timing of Thoracic Radiotherapy Relative to Chemotherapy ■ Although the optimal schedule of chemoradiotherapy for LD SCLC continues to evolve, the current data from randomized trials, including recent meta-analyses, favor concurrent chemoradiotherapy and the administration of radiotherapy earlier in the course of treatment.[272–274] One of the first influential studies was performed by the National Cancer Institute of Canada Clinical Trials Group, which randomized 308 subjects to receive concurrent chemoradiotherapy with the radiotherapy beginning either with the second or the sixth chemotherapy cycle. The chemotherapy regimen was cyclophosphamide, doxorubicin, and vincristine (CAV) alternating with etoposide and cisplatin (EP), for a total of six cycles of chemotherapy. Progression free and overall survival were significantly improved in the early radiotherapy arm.[275]

A subsequent trial by the Japan Clinical Oncology Group (JCOG 9104) randomized 231 patients with LD SCLC to either sequential chemoradiotherapy (four cycles of EP followed by thoracic radiotherapy) or concurrent chemoradiotherapy (four cycles of EP with radiotherapy beginning with cycle 1).[276] Radiotherapy in both arms was given at 1.5 Gy bid × 30 fractions in 3 weeks. Although median survival rates were improved in the concurrent arm (27.2 vs 19.7 months), the difference did not achieve statistical significance (p = 0.09). However, 2-year (54 vs 35%) and 5-year (24 vs 18%) survival rates and a HR for death of 0.7 (p = .02) clearly support early concurrent chemoradiation as opposed to sequential chemotherapy and radiation. A recent systematic overview analyzed all phase 3 chemoradiotherapy trials that administered platinum and etoposide with chest radiotherapy.[277] The most important predictor of improved survival was a short time interval between the first day of chemotherapy and the last day of radiotherapy, supporting the early administration of concurrent chemoradiation for LD SCLC.

Fractionation of Thoracic Radiotherapy With Concurrent Chemotherapy ■ Because SCLC is radiosensitive, without a shoulder in the radiation dose-response curve, and has a rapid doubling time, the use of multiple reduced-dose fractions in theory may increase efficacy. This approach is also hypothesized to protect normal tissues from late effects, especially those with a shoulder in their dose response.[278] Several phase 2 trials of hyperfractionated and accelerated chemoradiation in LD SCLC patients yielded encouraging 2-year survival outcomes compared to historical controls with conventionally fractionated radiation.[279,280] Standard daily fractionation (1.8 Gy per fraction × 25 fractions in 5 weeks) and accelerated fractionation (1.5 Gy twice daily × 30 fractions in 3 weeks) were compared in a pivotal intergroup phase 3 trial (INT-0096) of 417 patients with LD SCLC.[281] Patients received a total dose of 45 Gy of thoracic radiation, given in the first 5 weeks of chemotherapy in control patients and, more intensely, in the first 3 weeks on the experimental arm. Concurrent chemotherapy consisted of cisplatin 60 mg/m^2 IV on day 1 and etoposide 120 mg/m^2 IV on days 1–3 for four cycles. No dose reductions were permitted in the first two cycles of therapy. The accelerated radiation was associated with prolonged median (23 vs 19 months) and 5-year (26 vs 16%) survival compared with concurrent once-daily radiotherapy (p = .04). The only significant difference in toxicity between the arms was in grade 3 esophagitis, which was significantly more frequent with twice-daily thoracic radiotherapy (27% vs 11%, $p < .001$).

Another phase 3 trial compared twice-daily split-course radiotherapy with once-daily radiotherapy, although there were significant differences in trial design compared to INT-0096.[282] Patients received three cycles of induction EP, and those without progressive disease were then randomized. In contrast to INT-0096, the twice daily radiotherapy was interrupted by a 2.5 week break, resulting in the same intensity of radiation on both the hyperfractionated and daily radiation arms. There were no differences in progression free and overall survival between the two treatment arms.

Notably the thoracic radiation schemas and the 5-year survival rates on the experimental arms of INT-0096 and JCOG 9104 are essentially identical. Further, the 26% and 24% 5-year survival rates, respectively, represent the best long-term outcome for LD SCLC yet reported in large phase 3 trials. Despite these favorable results, this approach has not been widely adopted in the community, possibly because of the difficulty of scheduling and the increased rate of esophagitis.[283]

Total Tolerable Dose ■ Radiation dose to the thorax is another controversial area.[284] The NCIC developed an important study to show dose response in the thorax.[285] A dose response was clearly demonstrated by the results: thoracic PFS was prolonged by giving 37.5 Gy in 15 fractions over 3 weeks rather than 25 Gy in 10 fractions over 2 weeks as consolidation after completion of induction chemotherapy. Arriagada and colleagues published a report of 173 patients with limited-stage SCLC treated in three consecutive trials at the Institute Gustave-Roussy, France. The total dose of thoracic radiotherapy ranged from 45 to 65 Gy, administered by split courses interdigitating with chemotherapy. Dose of radiotherapy did not significantly impact local control or survival.[286] Strategies were considered that might increase the local control rate for concurrent chemotherapy and radiation therapy without increasing the esophageal toxicity rate to unacceptable levels. One strategy considered was to increase the total dose by administering daily thoracic radiation therapy at higher levels. Considering the value demonstrated by accelerated fractionation even to a total dose of just 45 Gy in 3 weeks, there was concern that a greater overall duration of thoracic radiation therapy might be disadvantageous.

Accelerated fractionation via concomitant boost is associated with improved locoregional control in patients with head and neck cancer compared to conventional daily fractionation.[287] This strategy uses once-daily irradiation through approximately 4–5 weeks of treatment and then twice daily irradiation in approximately the last 2 weeks of treatment, delivering one daily fraction to the large field and one fraction to boost the dose to the small field. Thus, it is termed concomitant boost. Taking a lead from its success in head and neck cancer, the RTOG evaluated a similar strategy in SCLC.

In a phase 1 trial (RTOG 97-12) concomitant boost radiation was administered concurrent with the first two cycles of EP.[288] The dose was escalated from 50.4 to 64.8 Gy over 5 weeks. Daily radiation dose was 1.8 Gy to the large field followed by dose escalation to the boost fields to minimize esophagitis.The maximum tolerated dose (MTD) was 61.2 Gy over 5 weeks, which was subsequently tested in a phase II trial (RTOG 0239). TRT was administered to large fields to a dose of 28.8 Gy at 1.8 Gy per fraction, 5 days per week for 16 fractions followed by twice-daily treatment (large field in AM, the boost field in PM), then off-cord boost twice-daily for the last 9 days, all at 1.8 Gy per fraction for a total dose of 61.2 Gy in 34 fraction over 5 weeks. Preliminary results indicate that that the toxicity profile of this approach is acceptable, though survival data are not yet reported.[289]

Theorizing that daily radiation to a dose greater than 45 Gy might be as efficacious as 45 Gy given bid in 3 weeks, the CALGB compared the MTDs of once-daily and twice-daily radiotherapy in LD SCLC patients.[290] Radiotherapy was started with the fourth cycle of chemotherapy, and the recommended phase 2 dose in the once-daily arm was 70 Gy. Not surprisingly the MTD of the accelerated therapy was 45 Gy. A subsequent phase 2 trial (CALGB 39808) demonstrated that 70 Gy in daily fractions was feasible with carboplatin and etoposide after induction chemotherapy with paclitaxel and topotecan.[291] The median survival of 22.4 months reflects the best outcome reported for conventional daily fractionation in LD SCLC. The rate of grade 3–4 esophagitis was 21%, compared to 17% in RTOG 0239, and estimated in a much larger number of patients, 32% in INT-0096.

Given the reduced esophageal toxicity and predicted maintained efficacy of the radiation regimens in CALGB 39808 and RTOG 0239, a pivotal Intergroup trial will compare those two experimental arms with a control arm of 45 Gy administered twice-daily, all with early concurrent EP (cycle 1).

Prophylactic Cranial Irradiation (PCI) in SCLC

Symptomatic brain metastases are detected in approximately 10% of SCLC patients at initial presentation, and an additional 10% may have occult metastases on MRI or CT imaging, with the likelihood of new brain metastases developing increasing with lengthening survival.[292] In the absence of specific therapy to the CNS, the actuarial cumulative probability reached 80% at 28 months of follow-up when the cases of CNS metastasis found at autopsy were included and 58% at 24 months when only clinical brain metastases were counted. At postmortem examination, much higher incidences were reported, ranging up to 65%. With the hope that the CNS would be the only site of residual disease, PCI was incorporated as an initial part of treatment of SCLC in the early 1970s.[267]

Since the early 1980s, PCI has been recommended for complete responders on the basis of the findings from a retrospective study from the NCI. Between 1977 and 1995, 11 prospective randomized trials of PCI were published. Although all but two trials reported a significant reduction in the incidence of brain metastasis, none demonstrated an improvement in survival with PCI. Four trials have addressed the issue of PCI in complete responders. All four studies failed to demonstrate any survival benefit of PCI, even among the complete responders, despite significant reduction in the frequency of brain metastases. This lack of survival benefit was attributed to the fact that in most patients the disease progresses at other sites, which is the predominant factor influencing survival. In a most definitive large randomized study of 300 SCLC patients who achieved CR following various chemotherapy regimens, PCI (24 Gy given in eight fractions over 12 days) significantly reduced the rate of brain metastasis as the isolated first site of relapse (45% vs 19% at 2 years, $p < .01$, and overall brain relapse rate at 2 years 67% vs 40%, $p < .01$). The 2-year survival rate of 29% in the PCI group was not significantly different from that of the control group, who did not receive PCI (21.5%, $p = .14$).[96]

Although these trials failed to demonstrate any survival benefit of PCI, a meta-analysis concluded that PCI prolongs both overall survival and disease-free survival among SCLC patients in complete remission.[293] This analysis was based on individual data from 987 patients, 85% with LD, who were enrolled in seven randomized trials to evaluate the role of PCI in complete remission. The relative risk of death in the treatment group, compared with the control group, was 0.84 (95% CI 0.73–0.97; $p = .01$), which corresponds to a 5.4% increase in the rate of survival at 3 years (15.3% in the control group vs 20.7% in the PCI group). PCI has not been routinely applied, even to patients who achieved CR to thoracic radiotherapy and chemotherapy, because of concern for neurological toxic effects, which were attributed to the PCI, and lack of associated benefit to overall survival. When more fractionated radiotherapy was given to patients with a CR and the radiotherapy was separated temporally from chemotherapy, there was reduction in the incidence of intracranial metastasis without severe neurotoxicity.

When patients with limited-stage SCLC were evaluated before and after PCI by an expert neuropsychologist applying detailed neuropsychological testing, 83% (25 of 30 patients) were found to have minor cognitive dysfunction prior to PCI, and no significant differences were found in the comparison of pretreatment and post-treatment neuropsychological results.[294] A subsequent analysis of a larger cohort of limited stage patients who received PCI did not demonstrate any consistent decline in cognitive function following PCI. These data indicate that concerns over PCI-associated neurotoxicity should not deter patients from receiving PCI.[295]

The meta-analysis revealed that PCI improved not only overall survival rate, but also disease-free survival rate by 8.8%, from 13.5% to 22.3% ($p = .001$), and reduced cranial recurrence rate by 25.3%, from 58.6% to 33.3% ($p < .001$). There was a trend to reduction of brain metastasis in the subset of PCI patients who received at least 36 Gy in 12 fractions rather than lower doses of PCI.[267] A decision-analytic model examining quality-adjusted life expectancy (QALE) in a cohort of SCLC patients concluded that current data supported the use of PCI in patients with limited SCLC who achieved a complete response to therapy.[296] A recent randomized trial for patients with extensive small-cell lung cancer who achieved a response to chemotherapy has shown that PCI reduced the incidence of symptomatic brain metastases and prolonged disease-free and overall survival. PCI increased median survival from 5.4 to 6.7 months ($p = .003$), and 1-year survival rates were 27.1 % in the PCI group compared to 13.3% in the control group ($p = .003$).[297] This difference in survival in the PCI patients may be attributed in part to increased treatment for extra-CNS progression in that group (68 vs 45%) and a low rate of brain radiation for patients with brain recurrence on the control arm (59%).

Chemotherapy

In its initial presentation, SCLC is quite sensitive to a variety of cytotoxins in the following drug classes: alkylators, anthracyclines, camptothecin derivatives, epipodophyllotoxins, platinating agents, vinca alkaloids, and taxanes. While the nitrogen mustard derivatives, methotrexate, vinorelbine, and gemcitabine do have activity, they are less active than other drugs and not commonly utilized. Drugs considered active are associated with single agent response rates generally greater that 30%.

The combination of etoposide and cisplatin (EP), first studied as a salvage regimen in the 1980s, has over the past 25 years become the standard of care for initial therapy of both LD and ED patients. Randomized trials have generally shown equivalent efficacy for EP and other more toxic regimens in patients with ED; thus it is the standard based on higher therapeutic index.[298] In patients with LD, in combination with concurrent thoracic radiation, it was associated with survival impact when compared to cyclophosphamide, epirubicin and vincristine.[299] This may in part relate to the ability to deliver full doses of EP in this setting without prohibitive midline, lung parenchymal, and bone marrow toxicity, that is observed with anthracycline-alkylator regimens.

The general response rates and survival outcomes observed in clinical trials by disease stage are shown in Table 78-11. Current outcomes in community practice, relative to those of 30 years ago, from the Surveillance, Epidemiologic, and End Results (SEER) program of the National Cancer Institute have shown only modest improvement. For ED SCLC, 2-year survival increased from 1.5% in 1973% to 4.6% in 2000, while In LD SCLC, 5-year survival increased from 4.9% in 1973 to 10% in 1998.[9]

Despite evidence from summaries of randomized trials in both LD and ED SCLC that progress was being achieved when data from the early 1980s were compared to the nineties, there is little argument that therapeutic outcomes have plateaued over the past approximately 15–20 years.[300,301] Further, improved supportive care likely contributes to better outcomes in the modern era.

Combination Chemotherapy ■ In general, older randomized studies demonstrated predictable advantages of combination programs compared to single agent therapy or sequential use of multiple single agents. On the basis of a large number of combination chemotherapy trials, which reported much higher response rates and better survival outcomes than single-agent trials, combination chemotherapy became accepted as standard in the early 1980s. More recent trials have compared single agent etoposide to combination regimens in the elderly, frail population. These were all positive for survival impact with combination therapy.[302,303]

As discussed above, after decades of study, the standard regimen for initial therapy in North America is EP. A minimum of four courses of EP is recommended based on a Southeastern Cancer Study Group phase 3 trial which randomized patients to receive either four courses of EP, six courses of cyclophosphamide, doxorubicin, and vincristine (CAV), or alternating EP and CAV.[298] Many strategies based on modifications of chemotherapy have been investigated in an effort to improve on EP, and with few exceptions these have not been successful in improving survival. The strategies which have been investigated are reviewed below and include alternating therapy, primarily with CAV, dose-dense therapy with growth factor support, high-dose therapy with marrow or stem cell rescue, prolonged chemotherapy, and addition of other cytotoxins to the EP base.

Data from the Japanese Clinical Oncology Group (JCOG) trial 9511 provided a notable exception to the above-summarized negative studies. In this randomized phase 3 trial, patients with ED were treated with either EP or irinotecan and cisplatin (IP).[304] Patients in the IP arm had improved median and long-term survival, compared to patients on etoposide (median survival 12.8 vs 9.4 months, $p = 0.002$, 2-year survival 20 vs 5%). The experimental arm in this study consisted of cisplatin and irinotecan given at 4-week cycles, with cisplatin 60 mg/m^2 on day 1 and irinotecan 60 mg/m^2 on days 1, 8, and 15. A slight modification of this schedule was used in a subsequent trial in North America which attempted to confirm these findings.[305] However, this trial, in a predominantly Caucasian population, demonstrated no benefit for patients on the IP arm. Toxicities were different with more diarrhea due to irinotecan, and more myelosuppression on the EP arm. The results of a third similar trial from the SWOG 0124 are awaited. This study replicated the dose and schedule of IP from JCOG 9511 and completed accrual in late 2006. Interestingly, comparison of pharmacogenomic analysis in JCOG 9511 and SWOG 0124 patients has been presented in abstract form. These data suggest that polymorphisms in genes involved in irinotecan metabolism may explain toxicity differences between the Japanese and American patients. Another topoisomerase I inhibitor, topotecan, has also been substituted for etoposide in a doublet with cisplatin and the two arms compared in a large, randomized phase 3 trial. This study also failed to show benefit for topotecan, with similar outcomes for both arms.[306]

Carboplatin substitution for cisplatin in combination with etoposide has been studied in two randomized trials. The first of these was a large trial with 350 patients which documented improved outcome in LD patients, but not ED, for the cisplatin arm (median survival 14 vs 12 months).[307] The second trial included 143 LD and ED patients and found no detriment in survival for patients treated with carboplatin with either stage of disease (median survival ED: 10.4 months, LD: 14.1 months).[308] Further, carboplatin was substantially less toxic as regards neutropenic infection, emesis, and neurotoxicity. Current practice standards hold that carboplatin with etoposide is reasonable therapy for patients with ED, and based on favorable toxicity profile, is preferred in those with poor performance status and/or significant co-morbidities. EP is preferred for the therapy of LD patients treated with curative intent.

Dose Response, Dose Escalation/Intensity ■ In preclinical studies, dose escalation has been an important strategy for overcoming drug resistance, yielding higher response and complete remission rates and increasing curability. Having been recognized as one of the most chemosensitive common solid tumors of adulthood, there was rationale that dose escalation and/or dose dense therapy would improve survival in SCLC.

Dose Escalation ■ Although two randomized trials of high-dose compared to low-dose cyclophosphamide, methotrexate, and lomustine (CMC) were positive for survival impact on the high-dose arms in the 1970s, the results of multiple randomized trials in the 1980s and 1990s have generally been negative as regards survival benefit.[309,310] Most relevant in the modern era is a trial of standard-dose and high-dose EP in which administration of 67% higher doses of EP over the first 6 weeks of therapy were compared.[311] Despite 68% higher actual doses delivered and 46% higher dose-rate intensity, there was no benefit in terms of CR rate (23% vs 22%, $p = .44$) or median survival duration (10.7 vs 11.4 months, $p = .68$). There was predictably increased myelosuppression with high-dose EP.

One positive trial randomized 105 patients with LD SCLC to receive a 33% higher dose of cyclophosphamide and a 25% higher dose of cisplatin in only the first of six cycles of treatment with

Table 78-11 ■ **Postoperative Adjuvant Chemotherapy in Early-Stage Lung Cancer**

Study	Pts	Stage IB	% Chemo	↑5 Yr %	HR	95% CI	p Value
JBR.10(227)	482	45	VbPac	15	0.70	0.52–0.92	.012
CALGB(228)	344	100	PacCb	12–4 yr	0.62	0.41–0.95	.028

Abbreviations: Cb, carboplatin; CI, confidence interval; HR, hazard ratio; Pac, paclitaxel; Pts, patients; Vb, vinorelbine.

cyclophosphamide, cisplatin, doxorubicin, and etoposide. Patients receiving the higher doses of the two drugs survived significantly longer, with 2- and 5-year survival of 42% versus 20% and 26% versus 8%, respectively ($p = .03$).[312,313] Thoracic radiation was administered alternating with chemotherapy after cycles 2, 3, and 4. It should be noted that the survival in the "high-dose" arm of this trial is essentially identical to what was obtained with standard dose EP and early accelerated hyperfractionated radiation in INT-0096 (#283). It is possible that benefits of higher doses are of greater magnitude in patients with limited-stage SCLC; however, these data in particular do not seem relevant in the context of modern chemoradiation regimens.

Using time, as opposed to dose, as the variable, Steward et al randomized 300 patients (both LD and ED) to receive vincristine, ifosfamide, etoposide, and cisplatin in a 3 week, as opposed to 4 week, cycle.[314] There were no substantial differences in toxicity between the arms, suggesting that the 3 week regimen could be considered "standard." Survival at 2 years was 33% versus 18%, favoring the 3-week cycle. A second randomization in the study to receive granulocyte-macrophage colony stimulating factor not did not influence efficacy or toxicity.

Dose Escalation With Marrow or Peripheral Blood Stem Cell Support ■ To obtain greater tumor cell kill, several investigators have studied myeloablative doses of chemotherapy, with either autologous bone marrow or peripheral blood stem cell support, often in a protected environment. Reasoning that only patients with smaller tumor burden would benefit from the intensive treatment approach, Carmustine, at standard dose or ablative dose with marrow rescue.[315] Though the efficacy outcomes in the subset of 32 patients with LD suggested impact from high dose therapy, they did not achieve statistical significance (19 vs 14 months). Further, the high incidence of isolated locoregional recurrence in the absence of thoracic radiation (11/16, 69%) lessens the relevance of this approach today, with similar and superior outcomes with modern chemoradiation regimens.

Another small trial randomized 83 patients (79 with LD) to six cycles of standard ifosfamide, etoposide, and carboplatin (ICE) or two courses of epirubicin and paclitaxel followed by stem cell harvest and three courses of high-dose ICE.[316] There was a progression-free (15 vs 11.1 months) and a median (30.3 vs 18.5 months, $p = .001$), survival benefit for patients on the high-dose arm. Given the quantitative difference in benefit for time to progression, as opposed to overall survival, the impact of the induction chemotherapy is called into question.

Similarly, increasing dose density by reducing the cycle interval and supporting with granulocyte or granulocyte-macrophage colony stimulating factors (G-CSF, GM-CSF) has not generally been successful. An exception to this is noted in a randomized trial from the United Kingdom. Recently Thatcher et al randomized 403 patients (152 with LD, 44 with ED) to doxorubicin, cyclophosphamide, and etoposide (ACE) every 3 weeks as compared to every 2 weeks in the intensive arm with G-CSF support.[317] Although the median survival for the two arms was not substantially different, the 1-year (47 vs 39%) and 2-year (13 vs 8%) survival rates favored intensified ACE ($p = .04$) It is notable, however, that 2-year survival for the intensified patients with LD was only 20%, clearly inferior to what is obtained with modern chemoradiation and EP. This same group had previously published a randomized trial with G-CSF supported, intensified vincristine, ifosfamide, carboplatin, and etoposide in 65 patients (60 with LD).[318] Although 2-year survival favored the intensified arm (32 vs 15%), this result is again an inferior outcome for LD patients.

Overall, there have been no convincing data supporting the benefit of intensification of therapy with marrow or stem cell support or dose-dense therapy in SCLC. A recent review documents the absence of consistent survival benefit for these approaches.[319] There are currently no data justifying chemotherapy as a routine initial treatment in doses that cause more than moderately severe myelotoxicity.

Alternating and Sequential Chemotherapy ■ Goldie and Coldman have provided a mathematical model of the spontaneous development of drug-resistant clones at a mutation rate proportional to the number of actively dividing tumor cells.[320] This model predicts that multiple active agents should be given at full doses to maximize the chance of eradication of the entire tumor cell population; because of overlapping myelosuppressive toxic effects, however, all possible drugs cannot be given simultaneously. More feasibly, the alternate or administration of two equally effective, partially noncross-resistant combination regimens was tested in a series of trials in the 1980s.

Three trials compared CAV with CAV alternating with EP, regimens which are at best minimally non-cross resistant. In an early Canadian trial, the alternating schedule of CAV/EP prolonged the overall survival in patients with extensive-stage SCLC compared with six cycles of CAV (9.6 vs 8.0 months, $p = .03$).[321] However, the survival difference did not reach statistical significance when patients with only locoregional disease were excluded from the analysis. Also, because EP alone was not tested in this trial, the possibility could not be eliminated that the superiority of the alternating regimen was due to the better treatment regimen rather than the alternating schedule. Two subsequent studies compared treatment with CAV and EP alone and alternating the two regimens. The Japanese trial showed significant improvement in the overall survival of patients who received the CAV/EP alternating regimen.[322] The median survival duration of that group was 11.8 months, while that of the CAV or PE induction groups was 9.9 months. This survival benefit was seen only in patients with limited-stage SCLC; the median survival duration of the CAV/PE arm was 16.8 months, significantly superior to that of the CAV arm (12.4 months, $p = .014$) or the PE arm (11.7 months, $p = .023$). For the patients with extensive-stage SCLC, there was no difference in overall survival among the three treatment arms. Similar results were obtained for extensive-stage SCLC by the Southeastern Cancer Study Group (SECSG) showing that four cycles of EP resulted in identical response/survival benefit as six cycles of CAV or three cycles of alternating therapy.[298]

For patients with limited-stage SCLC, SWOG investigators conducted a large randomized trial comparing induction with the alternating CAV/PE regimen to that with CAVE. There was no difference in median survival duration between the two arms (16.5 vs 15.1 months, $p = .58$).[323] Canadian investigators failed to show an advantage of the alternating CAV/EP strategy in patients with limited-stage SCLC when it was compared with sequential treatment with CAV (three times) followed by EP (three times).[324] German investigators also failed to show the advantage of the alternating chemotherapy treatment strategy over sequential treatment with ifosfamide/etoposide followed by CAV.[325]

Overall the data from these studies suggests impact from E or EP exposure in patients with LD, as opposed to alternating therapy per se. This is supported by an SECSG trial for LD in which two courses of EP following six cycles of CAV prolonged median survival by nearly 7 months compared to CAV alone.[326] The advantage of EP as a base regimen in LD has been confirmed more recently in a randomized trial with cyclophosphamide, epirubicin, and vincristine.[299] As regards the Goldie-Coldman hypothesis, however, it is important to note that none of the trials discussed above studied regimens that were noncross-resistant in any significant percentage of patients.

Duration of Induction Chemotherapy ■ Generally randomized trials have not shown survival impact from prolonged administration of chemotherapy beyond

4–6 cycles, though improvement in time to progression has been observed.

The value of three courses of oral etoposide following four cycles of ifosfamide/EP was studied in 233 patients with ED.[327] Significant benefit was limited to improved progression-free (8.2 vs 6.5 months) and trends to improved 1-year (51 vs 40%) and median (12.2 vs 11.2 months) survival in patients receiving oral etoposide. Four courses of topotecan given after four courses of EP in a similar randomized study showed modest improvement in time to progression (3.6 vs 2.3 months), but no benefit for median survival (8.9 vs 9.3 months) in topotecan-treated patients.[328]

Based on the SECSG trial four cycles of EP for induction is accepted as a minimum standard of care, though many trials continue to include options for up to six cycles.[298] Second line chemotherapy should be offered at the time of recurrence.

Three and four drug regimens randomized studies have not generally shown significant survival impact from the addition of ifosfamide or paclitaxel to an EP base.[329,330] Toxicity, however, has consistently been increased with triplet therapy. Comparison of EP to the four drug regimen EP + cyclophosphamide and epirubicin did demonstrate improved median (10.5 vs 9.3 months) and 1-year (40 vs 29%) survival rates.[331] However, severe myelosuppressive toxicity, such as febrile neutropenia (70 vs 18%), was problematic on the experimental arm with a 9% treatment-related mortality. Similar efficacy and toxicity data with the four drug regimen of EP + ifosfamide and vincristine administered every 4 weeks, compared to EP or cyclophosphamide, epirubicin, etoposide given every 3 weeks, have reinforced EP as a standard of care.[332]

Management of the Elderly ■ Currently representing more than one-third of patients with SCLC, the proportion of those who are elderly (age >70 years) will continue to increase in the future as our population ages. Although the heterogeneity in this group is substantial, there is general agreement that they represent a population at higher risk for treatment-related morbidity and mortality based on the high frequency of co-morbidities, lower functional status, and reduced organ, especially bone marrow, reserve. Although randomized trials are few in number, reducing the intensity of therapy in this group by using single agents or low dose chemotherapy has been associated with inferior efficacy and shortened survival, and it is not recommended.[302,303] Multiple phase 2 trials of etoposide and carboplatin in this population have revealed good tolerance and reasonable efficacy.[333,334] In a recent randomized trial, full dose EP was safely given to elderly patients with G-CSF support and resulted in efficacy similar to outcomes in younger patients.[335] In this trial 95 patients, 46% with ED, older than 70 with ECOG PS 0–2 were randomized to EP at standard (E, 100 mg/m^2 IV days 1–3; P, 40 mg/m^2 IV days 1–2) or attenuated dose (E, 60 mg/m^2 IV days 1–3, P 25 mg/m^2 IV days 1–2). Patients on full dose EP also received lenograstim 5 mg/kg sc days 5–12. Overall response rates (55 vs 39%), median (41 vs 31 weeks) and 1-year (39 vs 18%) survival rates all favored the full dose arm. Further, both regimens were well-tolerated with only one treatment related death (full-dose arm).

As regards management of the elderly patient with LD, analysis of patients >70 years on INT-0096 has been reported by Yuen et al.[336] The elderly had an increased death rate in the first 6 months after randomization, with a 10% treatment-related death rate compared to the 1% rate in those <70 years. Severe myelosuppressive toxicity was greater in the elderly with 78%, compared to 90% of younger patients receiving the planned four courses of EP. Other toxicities were similar. Both median (21.6 vs 14.4 months) and 5-year (22 vs 16%) survival rates were worse in the elderly, reflecting, at least in part, the increased death rate during treatment and early in follow-up. These data suggest that the elderly with LD and retained performance status benefit from standard chemoradiation. However, this group should be carefully selected with respect to performance status and deserve greater use of supportive care measures. The lowest effective doses of EP or E-carboplatin should be given. Consideration of prophylaxis with G-CSF upon completion of chemoradiation is recommended.

Special Clinical Situations SVC Syndrome ■ For patients with SVC syndrome, acute airway obstruction, or CNS metastases, radiotherapy is a powerful local treatment modality and is widely used. However, as experience accumulated with chemotherapy, it became apparent that chemotherapy provides rapid palliation of SVC syndrome in most SCLC patients and is begun more feasibly on an urgent basis. Therefore, chemotherapy alone is appropriate for the initial treatment of SVC syndrome, especially if other pressing extrathoracic disease exists. Similarly, combination chemotherapy alone is also appropriate for airway obstruction at initial presentation.

Brain Metastases ■ Formerly, systemic chemotherapy was believed to play a limited role in the treatment of brain metastases because of the widely held view of the brain as a pharmacologic sanctuary. In the 1980s, several groups observed in prospective trials that systemic chemotherapy alone, without brain irradiation, could induce objective regression of brain lesions. These results clearly indicate that once contrast-enhancing metastases are evident with MRI or CT, the blood–brain barrier is not intact and response rates to chemotherapy are similar in the brain and in extra-CNS sites.[337,338] As has been the case with SVC syndrome in SCLC, first-line therapy with cranial irradiation may not be necessary, even though this has not been addressed in a randomized trial setting. Ultimate irradiation of the brain is indicated, however, given an increase in complete response rates with its addition. For patients with intracranial relapse, the available data indicate that the efficacy of second-line chemotherapy is generally much less than in previously untreated patients and initial whole brain radiation is standard. Conversely, patients with recurrent brain metastases after previous cranial irradiation should not be denied a trial of systemic chemotherapy.

Second-Line Therapy for SCLC ■ The prognosis is poor for patients who receive second-line therapy after relapse with median survival generally in the range of 4–6 months. Response to additional therapy and survival from the time of relapse is influenced by response to initial chemotherapy and the progression-free interval following its completion. Giaccone et al were the first to observe this in a trial with teniposide reported in 1988.[339] In this study none of seven patients who had not responded to initial treatment responded to teniposide. Of 16 whose progression-free interval was ≤ 2.6 months, only 2 (12%) responded to teniposide. This can be contrasted with the 42% response rate (10/24) in those with response to initial chemotherapy and 53% response rate (9/17) with more prolonged progression-free interval. Although the numbers are small in each one of the subgroups, these observations were confirmed in multiple trials that followed in the 1990s. Disease that relapses less than 2–3 months after first-line therapy is commonly termed refractory, and rates of response in this setting are lower than disease that relapses later, which is usually termed sensitive.

Although there is no generally accepted standard regimen for relapse, topotecan is the most extensively studied agent, and it is the only drug with an FDA indication for treatment of sensitive relapse SCLC. This indication derived from a trial which compared topotecan, 1.5 mg/m^2 days 1–5, to CAV in patients who had responded to initial chemotherapy and relapsed ≥60 days after its completion.[340] The response rates were 24.3% in 107 topotecan-treated patients and 18.3% in 104 patients treated with CAV (p = .285). There was no difference in median time to progression (13.3 vs 12.3 weeks, p = .552) or median survival duration (25.0 vs 24.7 weeks, p = .795) between the two groups. Symptoms improved to a greater degree in the topotecan group than in the CAV group for four of eight categories evaluated, including dyspnea, anorexia, hoarseness, and fatigue, as well as interference with daily activity (p = .043). Grade 4 neutropenia occurred in 38% of topotecan courses and 51% of CAV courses (p < .001). Grade 4 thrombocytopenia and grade 3 or 4 anemia occurred more frequently with topotecan, occurring in 10% and 18% of topotecan courses and 1% and 7% of CAV courses, respectively (p < .001 for both). Subsequent randomized phase 2 and 3 trials compared oral topotecan (2.3 mg/m^2) to the intravenous formulation and identified similar efficacy outcomes with the more convenient oral form. Toxicity is altered somewhat with the oral form producing less neutropenia but more diarrhea than the intravenous drug.[306,341]

Oral topotecan has been compared to best supportive care in a recent trial which documented the survival impact of second-line chemotherapy on SCLC. Patients with both refractory and sensitive relapse who were not candidates for standard intravenous therapy were randomized to best supportive care versus oral topotecan (n = 141).[342] Although response rates to topotecan were low at 7%, 44% of treated patients attained stable disease, and had improved symptom control and maintenance of quality of life. The impact of topotecan on progression and survival was seen equally in patients with refractory or sensitive relapse. Median survival was 26 weeks versus 14 weeks for topotecan and control patients, respectively (p = 0.0104). Survival at 6 months was also favorably impacted by treatment, 49% versus 26%. The evidence for impact from chemotherapy in this setting was persuasive and should influence our use of chemotherapy in this setting both in and outside of clinical investigation.

Other choices for management of recurrent SCLC include use of the initial induction regimen, especially if progression-free survival after discontinuation of induction is prolonged, typically 6 months or longer. Irinotecan, while not studied nearly as extensively as topotecan in recurrent patients, appears to have similar benefits.[343] Limited evaluation of taxanes and anthracyclines, either alone or in combination with other drugs, also suggest low level activity in recurrent disease.[344] Palliative radiation to chest, brain, and bone is also effective and used commonly in drug-resistant and recurrent SCLC.

Targeted Therapy ■ Patients with SCLC are yet to benefit from enhanced knowledge of the abnormal biology that is associated with its development and progression. Numerous leads have been investigated in phase 2 and 3 trials; the vast majority of these have not been promising.[345] Approaches combining molecularly targeted therapies with standard chemotherapy seem most promising as single-agent evaluation of biologics has proven very ineffective thus far. Examples of active areas of clinical research with this design include agents which target processes such as angiogenesis and apoptosis, and signal transduction pathways such as m-TOR and the insulin-like growth factor axis. Given the plateau in survival for patients with SCLC over the past 20 years, there is much hope that this new paradigm will lead us to more effective therapy.

Conclusion and Future Prospects

Elimination of tobacco consumption is certainly the most effective way to reduce lung cancer incidence. However, this goal remains elusive because of continuing social and economic pressures. In addition, lung cancer also occurs in people who have never smoked. Lung cancer will continue to be a significant public health burden well into the twenty-first century. Thus, early detection and new therapeutic options are needed to improve the dismal rate of survival for lung cancer patients. Progress in defining the molecular events involved in the genesis of lung cancer cells has been rapid over the past 15 years, and the potential benefits from this progress for patients may be substantial. The use of molecular profiles to identify persons at high risk of developing lung cancer may enable cost-effective implementation of prevention and early detection programs. For example, low activity of the DNA repair enzyme 8-oxoguanine DNA N-glycosylase has been associated with increased risk of developing lung cancer.[346]

The mainstay of cancer therapy is still surgery, radiotherapy, and chemotherapy, and recent years have shown improvement in patient outcome by their combination and optimization. (Fig. 78-9). A large effort has been dedicated to further impact lung cancer outcome by adding biological therapy. Such an approach utilizes alteration of oncogene expression with recombinant gene constructs to allow reversal of the transformed phenotype. In addition, a wealth of biologically active agents that interfere with signal transduction events in the development and progression of lung cancer are now being explored. Rather than targeting the actual genetic errors, these treatments correct or interfere with the sequelae of those genetic changes. For example, genetic mutations that lead to increased expression or activity of a growth factor receptor could be targeted, either by blocking the receptor itself or by interfering with its downstream signal transduction pathways. The first drugs of this kind are the EGFR TKIs recently approved for management of lung cancer. In parallel, monoclonal antibodies to VEGF are combined with conventional chemotherapy to improve survival of patients with lung cancer, colorectal cancer, breast cancer, and renal cell carcinoma

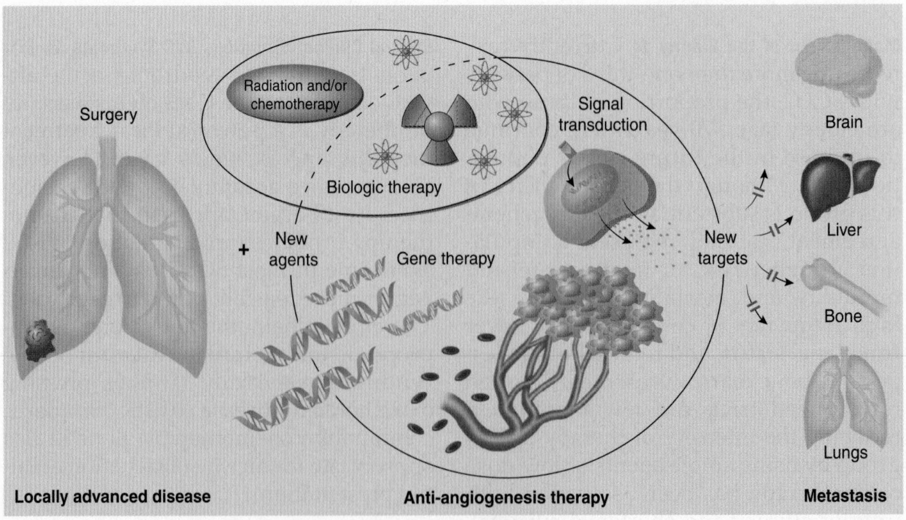

Figure 78-9 ■ Most patients with non-small cell lung cancer die from metastatic disease. Treatment in the locally advanced setting will likely require chemotherapy or radiation therapy in combination with biologic therapy to enhance its effectiveness and prevent metastatic spread of tumor.

among others. The reader is encouraged to follow the literature closely (eg, by using MEDLINE searches) and to keep up to date on current protocols (eg, by following the protocol lists via the Physician's Data Query at the NCI Web page: http://cancernet.nci.nih.gov/cancertopics).

In summary, lung cancer therapy efforts in recent years have focused on cancer prevention, early detection and multimodality therapy. Improvements in systemic therapy (chemotherapy and molecular targeted therapy) will certainly have an impact on all stages of disease. Since lung cancer is a heterogeneous disease, it will also be essential to identify and better understand specific molecular targets, and select patients for therapy according to their tumor's biological profile. It is hoped that advances in translational proteomic and genomic research will be the key to identifying reliable, validated predictive biomarkers. Progress in these areas will hopefully lead to better control of this disease while minimizing treatment-related side effects.

Selected References

The complete reference list can be found at www.CANCERMEDICINE8.com

3. Sandler A, Gray R, Perry MC, et al. Paclitaxel-carboplatin alone or with bevacizumab for non-small-cell lung cancer. *N Engl J Med.* 2006;355(24):2542–2550.
5. Hanna N, Shepherd FA, Fossella FV, et al. Randomized phase III trial of pemetrexed versus docetaxel in patients with non-small-cell lung cancer previously treated with chemotherapy. *J Clin Oncol.* 2004;22(9):1589–1597.
17. Bain C, Feskanich D, Speizer FE, et al. Lung cancer rates in men and women with comparable histories of smoking. *J Natl Cancer Inst.* 2004;96(11):826–834.
27. Johnson BE. Second lung cancers in patients after treatment for an initial lung cancer. *J Natl Cancer Inst.* 1998;90(18):1335–1345.
32. Wistuba, II, Mao L, Gazdar AF. Smoking molecular damage in bronchial epithelium. *Oncogene.* 2002;21(48):7298–7306.
76. Vansteenkiste J, Fischer BM, Dooms C, Mortensen J. Positron-emission tomography in prognostic and therapeutic assessment of lung cancer: systematic review. *Lancet Oncol.* 2004;5(9):531–540.
87. Henschke CI, Yankelevitz DF. CT screening for lung cancer: update 2007. *Oncologist.* 2008;13(1):65–78.
92. Goldstraw P, Crowley J, Chansky K, et al. The IASLC Lung Cancer Staging Project: proposals for the revision of the TNM stage groupings in the forthcoming (seventh) edition of the TNM classification of malignant tumours. *J Thorac Oncol.* 2007;2(8):706–714.
122. Harpole DH, Jr., DeCamp MM, Jr., Daley J, et al. Prognostic models of thirty-day mortality and morbidity after major pulmonary resection. *J Thorac Cardiovasc Surg.* 1999;117(5):969–979.
127. Ginsberg RJ. A randomized comparative trial of lobectomy versus limited resection for patients with T1 N0 non-small cell lung cancer. *Lung Cancer.* 1991;7:83–88.
184. Chang JY, Roth JA. Stereotactic body radiation therapy for stage I non-small cell lung cancer. *Thorac Surg Clin.* 2007;17(2):251–259.
185. Postoperative radiotherapy in non-small-cell lung cancer: systematic review and meta-analysis of individual patient data from nine randomised controlled trials. PORT Meta-analysis Trialists Group. *Lancet.* 1998;352(9124):257–263.
186. Effects of postoperative mediastinal radiation on completely resected stage II and stage III epidermoid cancer of the lung. The Lung Cancer Study Group. *N Engl J Med.* 1986;315(22):1377–1381.
191. Dillman RO, Seagren SL, Propert KJ, et al. A randomized trial of induction chemotherapy plus high-dose radiation versus radiation alone in stage III non-small-cell lung cancer. *N Engl J Med.* 1990;323(14):940–945.
193. Furuse K, Fukuoka M, Kawahara M, et al. Phase III study of concurrent versus sequential thoracic radiotherapy in combination with mitomycin, vindesine, and cisplatin in unresectable stage III non-small-cell lung cancer. *J Clin Oncol.* 1999;17(9):2692–2699.
204. Schiller JH, Harrington D, Belani CP, et al. Comparison of four chemotherapy regimens for advanced non-small-cell lung cancer. *N Engl J Med.* 2002;346(2):92–98.
208. Shidelli C, Perrone F, Ralls C. Effects of vinorelbine on quality of life and survival of elderly patients with advanced non-small-cell lung cancer. The Elderly Lung Cancer Vinorelbine Italian Study Group. *J Natl Cancer Inst.* 1999;91(1):66–72.
219. Fossella F, Pereira JR, von Pawel J, et al. Randomized, multinational, phase III study of docetaxel plus platinum combinations versus vinorelbine plus cisplatin for advanced non-small-cell lung cancer: the TAX 326 study group. *J Clin Oncol.* 2003;21(16):3016–3024.
222. Fossella FV, DeVore R, Kerr RN, et al. Randomized phase III trial of docetaxel versus vinorelbine or ifosfamide in patients with advanced non-small-cell lung cancer previously treated with platinum-containing chemotherapy regimens. The TAX 320 Non-Small Cell Lung Cancer Study Group. *J Clin Oncol.* 2000;18(12):2354–2362.
223. Shepherd FA, Dancey J, Ramlau R, et al. Prospective randomized trial of docetaxel versus best supportive care in patients with non-small-cell lung cancer previously treated with platinum-based chemotherapy. *J Clin Oncol.* 2000;18(10):2095–2103.
227. Depierre A, Milleron B, Moro-Sibilot D, et al. Preoperative chemotherapy followed by surgery compared with primary surgery in resectable stage I (Except T1N0), II, and IIIa non-small-cell lung cancer. *J Clin Oncol.* 2002;20(1):247–253.
230. Keller SM, Adak S, Wagner H, et al. A randomized trial of postoperative adjuvant therapy in patients with completely resected stage II or IIIA non-small-cell lung cancer. Eastern Cooperative Oncology Group. *N Engl J Med.* 2000;343(17):1217–1222.
231. Stewart LA and Pignon JP Chemotherapy in non-small cell lung cancer: a meta-analysis using updated data on individual patients from 52 randomised clinical trials. Non-small Cell Lung Cancer Collaborative Group. *BMJ.* 1995;311(7010):899–909.
232. Arriagada R, Bergman B, Dunant A, Le Chevalier T, Pignon JP, Vansteenkiste J. Cisplatin-based adjuvant chemotherapy in patients with completely resected non-small-cell lung cancer. *N Engl J Med.* 2004;350(4):351–360.
233. Winton T, Livingston R, Johnson D, et al. Vinorelbine plus cisplatin vs observation in resected non-small-cell lung cancer. *N Engl J Med.* 2005;352(25):2589–2597.
244. Kris MG, Natale RB, Herbst RS, et al. Efficacy of gefitinib, an inhibitor of the epidermal growth factor receptor tyrosine kinase, in symptomatic patients with non-small cell lung cancer: a randomized trial. *JAMA.* 2003;290(16):2149–2158.
246. Shepherd FA, Rodrigues Pereira J, Ciuleanu T, et al. Erlotinib in previously treated non-small-cell lung cancer. *N Engl J Med.* 2005;353(2):123–132.
253. Lynch TJ, Bell DW, Sordella R, et al. Activating mutations in the epidermal growth factor receptor underlying responsiveness of non-small-cell lung cancer to gefitinib. *N Engl J Med.* 2004;350(21):2129–2139.
259. Herbst RS, Johnson DH, Mininberg E, et al. Phase I/II trial evaluating the anti-vascular endothelial growth factor monoclonal antibody bevacizumab in combination with the her-1/epidermal growth factor receptor tyrosine kinase inhibitor erlotinib for patients with recurrent non-small-cell lung cancer. *J Clin Oncol.* 2005;23(11):2544–2555.
272. De Ruysscher D, Pijls-Johannesma M, Vansteenkiste J, Kester A, Rutten I, Lambin P. Systematic review and meta-analysis of randomised, controlled trials of the timing of chest radiotherapy in patients with limited-stage, small-cell lung cancer. *Ann Oncol.* 2006;17(4):543–552.
281. Turrisi AT, 3rd, Kim K, Blum R, et al. Twice-daily compared with once-daily thoracic radiotherapy in limited small-cell lung cancer treated concurrently with cisplatin and etoposide. *N Engl J Med.* 1999;340(4):265–271.
284. Cox JD. Dose-response in small cell carcinoma. *Int J Radiat Oncol Biol Phys.* 1988;14(2):393–394.
293. Auperin A, Arriagada R, Pignon JP, et al. Prophylactic cranial irradiation for patients with small-cell lung cancer in complete remission. Prophylactic Cranial Irradiation Overview Collaborative Group. *N Engl J Med.* 1999;341(7):476–484.
297. Slotman B, Faivre-Finn C, Kramer G, et al. Prophylactic cranial irradiation in extensive small-cell lung cancer. *N Engl J Med.* 2007;357(7):664–672.
305. Hanna N, Bunn PA, Jr., Langer C, et al. Randomized phase III trial comparing irinotecan/cisplatin with etoposide/cisplatin in patients with previously untreated extensive-stage disease small-cell lung cancer. *J Clin Oncol.* 2006;24(13):2038–2043.
340. von Pawel J, Schiller JH, Shepherd FA, et al. Topotecan versus cyclophosphamide, doxorubicin, and vincristine for the treatment of recurrent small-cell lung cancer. *J Clin Oncol.* 1999;17(2):658–667.

79 Malignant Mesothelioma

Harvey I. Pass, MD ■ Michele Carbone, MD, PhD ■ Hedy Lee Kindler, MD

Historical Perspective

In a seminal report, Wagner[1] and colleagues reported asbestos as the etiologic agent in 32 of 33 cases of malignant pleural mesothelioma, largely by environmental exposure in the "Asbestos Hills" of Cape Province in South Africa. This singular relationship, confirmed in many other countries, including the United States,[2] established the disease as a distinct entity.

Incidence and Epidemiology

The incidence of mesothelioma has been underestimated in mortality statistics.[3] Presently, pleural mesotheliomas are responsible for approximately 15,000-20,000 deaths annually worldwide. Cases are clustered in areas of asbestos product plants and shipbuilding facilities, not only in the United States, but also in other industrialized countries, such as England.[4,5] The male to female ratio is approximately 4:1, and 80% arise from the pleura.[6] In autopsy studies, the frequency of malignant mesothelioma varies from 0.02% to 0.7%, with a rate of 0.2% in the largest series.[7] In most hospital series, the pleura is more often involved than the peritoneum, with a predominance of the right side over the left (60:40).[8] In some epidemiologic studies monitoring cohorts of asbestos workers, however, the peritoneal form is more common than the pleural. The mean age of patients is approximately 60 years,[9] but the disease can occur at any age, including in childhood.[10,11]

Etiology

Mesotheliomas are not only connected to asbestos exposure, but also may be related to previous Simian Virus 40 (SV40) infection and quite possibly to genetic predisposition.

Beginning 15 years after onset of exposure, approximately 6-10% of asbestos workers older than age 35 years will die of mesothelioma.[12] It is estimated that from 1940 through 1979, approximately 27.5 million workers were occupationally exposed to asbestos in the United States, with a calculated annual death rate from mesothelioma of approximately 2000 in 1980 up to 3000 in the late 1990s.[13] Insulation, construction, shipyard industries, and automobile brakes are among the many sources of occupational exposure.[14] Although asbestos exposure and cigarette smoking act synergistically to produce lung cancer, smoking is not a factor for mesothelioma, although an association between cigarettes using "micronite" filters has been postulated.[15] Exposure can also occur by household contamination of women and children, usually through the work clothes of an asbestos' worker.

Genomic and molecular analyses have elucidated multiple cytogenetic and molecular abnormalities that contribute to the development of MPM. It is commonly believed that asbestos inhalation leads to deposition of fibers deep in the lung parenchyma and eventual migration and implantation of fibers in the pleural lining. Repeated episodes of inflammation and healing, oxygen free radical production from inflammatory cells and the iron moiety within asbestos,[16] and direct damage to DNA by the fibers are generally accepted pathogenic features of asbestos exposure . Karyotype and comparative genomic hybridization (CGH) analyses of primary MPM tumors and cell lines detected frequent deletions, duplications, and translocations with genomic losses more common than gains.[17] Deletions within chromosomes 1p, 3p, 4p, 4q, 6q, 9p, 13q, 14q, and 22q are common and notable for the loss of the tumor suppressor genes *p16/CDKN2A*, p53, and NF2 located within these loci.[18] Testa and colleagues demonstrated that heterozygous *Nf2* (+/-) mice exposed to asbestos exhibited frequent homozygous deletions of the *Cdkn2a/Arf* and *Cdkn2b* loci and activation of *Akt* with rapid development of MPM, suggesting that these molecular events may be critical to tumorigenesis.[19,20] In addition, the Wilms' tumor gene (WT1), which encodes a transcription factor that represses the transcription of a number of growth factors and proto-oncogenes, is often mutated in both MPM primary tumors and cell lines.[21] Loss of tumor suppressor gene activity may be a key to the transformation into malignant mesothelioma.

Interestingly, the dose-dependent cytotoxicity of asbestos is not lethal to the asbestos-sensitive mesothelial cells. In fact, a recent paper has illustrated the critical role of tumor necrosis factor alpha (TNF-α) and NF-κ signaling in the survival of damaged mesothelial cells.[22] The inflammatory response to asbestos deposition in the pleura is mediated by macrophages and mesothelial cells, with both cell types secreting TNF-α, and the mesothelial cell expressing TNF-α receptor (TNF-R1), in an autocrine and paracrine interaction. TNF-α then stimulates the NF-κ pathway, which regulates pro-survival cellular mechanisms and may allow asbestos-induced, DNA damaged cells, to divide rather than undergo apoptosis. This response imparts a survival advantage that permits the asbestos-injured cells to transform and progress into malignant mesothelioma.

Other cytokines and growth factors produced by malignant mesothelial cells are associated with asbestos carcinogenesis. Platelet derived growth factor-A chain and, C-sis, an oncogene *that* encodes for the platelet derived growth factor beta chain (PDGF-β), are overexpressed in cell lines derived from primary and metastatic MPM whereas C-sis expression is virtually nonexistent in normal mesothelial cells.[23,24] In addition, transforming growth factor beta (TGF-β) is a growth-regulatory and immunomodulatory cytokine expressed in high levels in MMP cell lines. TGF-β may play a role in PDGF receptor expression in MMP. Pleural fluid from MPM patients also shows increased levels of IL-6 and IL-8, both important cytokines involved in angiogenesis.[25]

Asbestos also causes direct activation of cell-signaling pathways (Fig. 79-1). Crocidolite fibers can stimulate autophosphorylation of the epidermal growth factor receptor (EGFR), which activates extracellular regulated kinase 1 and 2 (ERK1 and ERK2). ERK1/2 activation in turn increases activator protein (AP)-1 activity with subsequent increased mitosis of the mesothelial cells.[26,27] Recent work by Jablons and colleagues have implicated the Wnt pathway in the development of MPM and have recently shown that promoter hypermethylation of Wif-1 results in constitutive activation of Wnt signaling, suggesting a mechanism for the inhibition of apoptosis in abnormal mesothelial cells.[28] SV40 is a DNA virus that deserves mention with regard to the development of malignant mesothelioma. This virus is found in rhesus monkeys and in humans and is thought to have been transferred from one to the other via contaminated polio vaccines,

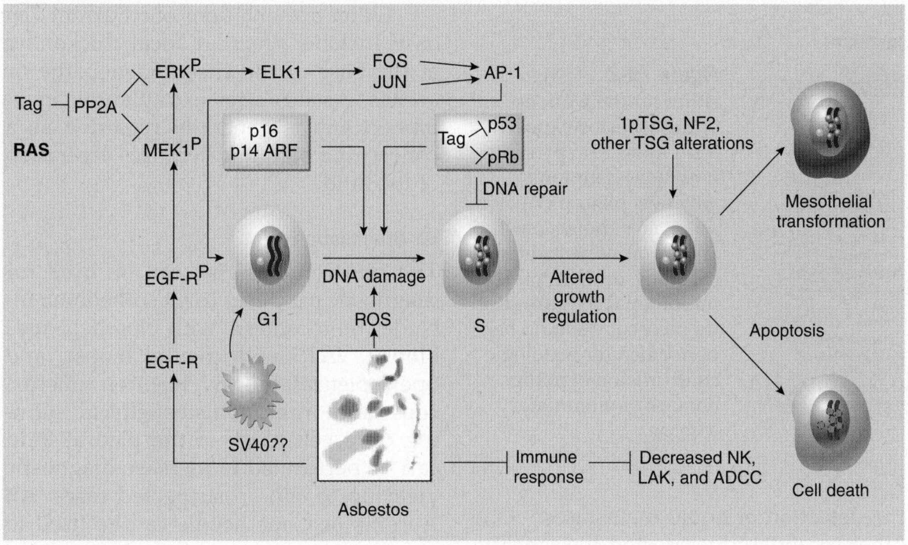

Figure 79-1 Mesothelioma pathogenesis, with known and hypothesized mechanisms possibly linking asbestos and nonasbestos mechanisms of transformation. Increased levels of activator protein 1 (AP-1) stimulate cell division. AP-1 is upregulated through a pathway that involves phosphorylation of the EGF receptor (EGF-R phosphorylated to EGF-RP), activation of ras, and eventual phosphorylation of MEK1 kinase and the extracellular regulated kinases (ERK). Through activation of intermediary kinases including Elk1, and transcription factors such as fos and jun, AP-1 stimulates cell division. Crocidolite asbestos can start this cascade of events since it induces both DNA mutations and phosphorylation of EGF-R. Asbestos can also induce DNA alterations such as p16 loss, and abnormalities of p14 ARF through the production of reactive oxygen species (ROS) that are generated by alveolar macrophages which phagocytize asbestos fibers. Moreover, asbestos is known to have profound effects on the immune system by decreasing natural killer cell (NK) and lymphokine activated killer cell (LAK) number and activity, as well as interfering with antibody dependent cell-medicated cytotoxicity (ADCC). Tag of SV40 could have profound effects in concert with the asbestos including (1) inhibition of phosphatase 2A (PP2A) leading to unregulated AP-1 production, (2) direct DNA damage and (3) binding of p53 and the protein of the retinoblastoma gene (pRB), thus inhibiting cell cycle check points, as well as potential repair of the mutated cells. The mutated cells could then become immortalized through other abnormalities of tumor suppressor genes (TSG), including the neurofibromatosis 2 gene (NF-2), and escape immune surveillance due to the immunomodulatory effects of asbestos. An asbestos body surrounded by alveolar macrophages is depicted in the inset. The green circle represents SV40 DNA that has not integrated into the chromosomes of the mesothelial cell.

which were administered worldwide between 1953 and 1963.[29-31] SV40 causes mesothelioma in hamsters within 6 months, but can also be found in human mesothelioma specimens. As most malignancies are multifactorial SV40 alone is not the sole causative agent, but along with asbestos SV40 can be considered a cocarcinogen.[32]

Other causative agents include radiation as has been observed in young adults who have received RT for Wilms tumor or for mediastinal lymphoma.[33]

Genetic Predisposition to Mesothelioma

Various other fibers, such as zeolites (erionite type) from volcanic rocks, have been incriminated in Turkey, and a few deposits have been found in Oregon in the United States. The potential of zeolites to produce mesotheliomas has been confirmed experimentally after intraperitoneal injection.[34] After inhalation, the mesothelioma yield from zeolites exceeds that of any other fiber. In certain villages in Cappadocia, a region in Central Anatolia, Turkey, 50% or more of deaths are caused by malignant mesothelioma. Closer observation revealed that mesotheliomas only occurred in certain homes and not in others (homes in these areas are inhabited by multiple generations and passed down), even though all homes contained similar amounts of erionite according to recent mineralogical analysis. Pedigree analyses of families who lived in homes where mesotheliomas occurred showed that these mesotheliomas appeared to be inherited in an autosomal-dominant pattern.[35,36] About 50% of descendents of affected parents developed mesotheliomas. When members of unaffected families married into affected families, 50% of their descendents also developed mesotheliomas. Whether genetics alone or in conjunction with erionite are responsible for these mesotheliomas remains unknown, but clearly, genetics is a key factor, since mesotheliomas do not develop in nonaffected families regardless of environmental exposure.

Diagnosis of the Patient With Possible Mesothelioma Histology (Fig. 79-2)

There are three different types of mesothelioma. The epithelial type, the fibrous morphology type, also called sarcomatoid type, and a combination called biphasic or mixed type. The majority of mesotheliomas (50%) are of the epithelial type, 10% are sarcomatoid, and the remaining mesotheliomas are mixed. Immunohistochemical markers are necessary to help distinguish between metastatic carcinomas and mesothelioma. These markers include positive pankeratin, keratin 5/6, calretinin, and WT-1. Negative markers include CEA, CD15, Ber-EP4, Moc-31, TTF-1, and B72.3. Such markers are important as mesothelioma may be difficult to distinguish from other malignancies, ie, biphasic mesotheliomas from carcinosarcomas or fibrous mesothelioma from metastatic pleural sarcomas.[37]

Symptoms and Signs

The onset of mesothelioma is associated with chest pain, dyspnea, or cough. Progressive invasion of the chest wall often leads to intractable pain. Pleural effusion is present initially in up to 95% of cases. Often the fluid is viscous due to high content of hyaluronic acid. Later, tumor growth usually results in complete obliteration of the pleural space and encasement of the lung. Late symptoms of bulky mesotheliomas include mediastinal invasion with dysphagia, phrenic nerve paralysis, pericardial effusion, and superior vena cava syndrome.[38] Peritoneal mesothelioma is characterized by ascites and intestinal compromise leading to cachexia.

Laboratory Evaluation

There are several lab abnormalities associated with mesothelioma. Of these the presence of thrombocytosis with platelet counts greater than 400,000 is probably the most common. Others include hypergammaglobulinemia, eosinophilia, anemia of chronic disease, elevated homocysteine levels, folic acid deficiency, and Vit B12 and Vit B6 deficiency.[38]

Tumor Markers

The two basic tumor markers for this disease are osteopontin (OPN) and mesothelin (SMRP). Osteopontin is a glycoprotein biomarker that is expressed by certain cancers, including lung, breast, colorectal, gastric, ovarian, and melanoma. Osteopontin is also involved in cell signaling pathways that are associated with asbestos induced carcinogenesis. A recent study compared OPN levels in patients with mesothelioma with OPN

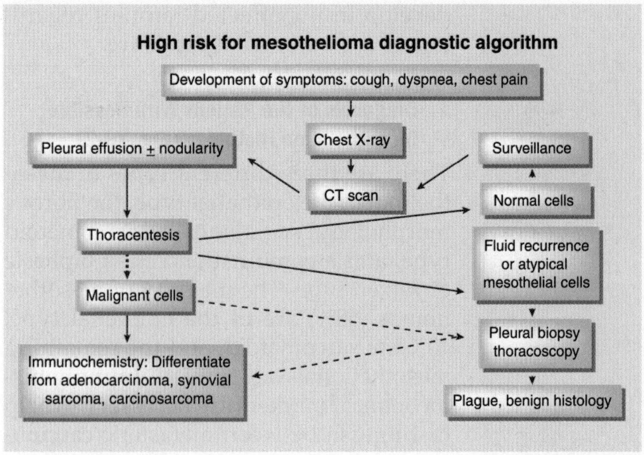

Figure 79-2 Algorithm for the work up of the asbestos-exposed individual who presents with new symptoms. Any new pleural effusion must have thoracentesis and immunohistochemical analyses. If atypical mesothelial cells are seen, thoracoscopy should be performed for histologic confirmation of malignancy or inflammatory disease.

levels in patients with asbestos related diseases that were not malignant. This study showed that OPN can be used to separate those patients that had asbestos exposure with mesothelioma from those who had asbestos exposure without malignancy.[39]

SMRP or mesothelin, originally described by Pastan,[40] is also a glycoprotein and is found in mesothelioma, ovarian cancer, and pancreatic cancer. Robinson and colleagues demonstrated in 48 patients that SMRP is a serum biomarker with 83% sensitivity and 95% specificity.[41,42] In an even more recent study by Pass et al SMRP was shown to be a promising marker for malignant pleural mesothelioma in blood and pleural fluid. Serum SMRP levels were higher in MPM patients when compared to lung cancer patients, as were the SMRP levels in pleural fluid when compared to benign pleural fluid or other non-MPM pleural effusions.[43]

Imaging Modalities

Imaging is very important for the diagnosis, staging, and clinical management of patients with mesothelioma. The imaging techniques used include: CXR, CT scan, MR, and PET/CT. Chest X-ray can show a pleural effusion, pleural thickening, nodularity, pleural masses, contraction, and fixation of the chest as well as mediastinal shift toward the volume loss.

CT is the current primary modality for diagnosis, staging, and response assessment.[44] MR may be of additional benefit to detect diaphragm invasion or involvement of the endothoracic fascia. An isolated area of chest wall involvement might potentially be better evaluated with MR.

With PET/CT the primary tumor is FDG avid and this modality has been shown to improve the localization of regions that have higher uptake and also the accuracy of staging. In addition it has the ability to detect distant extrathoracic metastases. Flores et al reported a sensitivity of 19% for T staging and 11% for the detection of nodal metastases.[45] One other recent study reported the sensitivity, specificity, positive predictive value, negative predictive value, and accuracy of PET/CT for N2 disease to be 38%, 78%, 60%, 58%, and 59%, respectively. The corresponding percentages for T4 status were 67%, 93%, 86%, 82%, and 83%, respectively.[46] PET/CT improves the overall staging of patients with mesothelioma and thus may potentially improve selection of patients for surgical resection.

PET may be useful in determining the extent of distant metastatic disease, but had a sensitivity of only 11% in detecting metastatic lymph node disease.[47] However, the same study found that a high SUV correlated with N2 disease at the time of resection. More recently, research from the same institution showed that an SUV value 10 greater correlated with a significantly shorter survival time and a 3.3 times greater risk of dying compared to SUV levels below 10.[48] This suggests that PET results may help to stratify patients for different treatments according to their metabolic activity. Integrated CT-PET imaging combines the anatomic data from CT with the functional data of PET and may be able to increase the diagnostic accuracy and staging of MPM patients. In a study of 29 MPM patients, integrated CT-PET correctly assigned the overall stage in 72% of cases, showed increased sensitivity for T4 disease, 67% vs 19% for PET alone, identified 7 patients with extrathoracic disease missed by conventional radiographic studies, and identified 12 patients that would have been precluded from surgical resection based on conventional studies.[49]

RECIST criteria using CT scan have been applied in order to evaluate response to therapy in mesothelioma.[50] A complete response means that there is no evidence of tumor, whereas a partial response requires a 30% reduction for at least 4 weeks. A 20% increase in total tumor measurement or the appearance of a new lesion would be consistent with disease progression.

Other presentations of recurrent disease include irregular focal thickening at the base of the chest, adenopathy or ascites. Ascites after extrapleural pneumonectomy is generally regarded as a concerning sign and requires aspiration of the fluid.

Diagnostic Tools

The interventions that can be used for diagnostic purposes in mesothelioma include: thoracentesis with closed pleural biopsy, VATS with pleural biopsy, and open pleural biopsy. Electron microscopy and immunohistochemical staining on a cell block of the pleural fluid can be performed to increase diagnostic yield up to 84% in suspected cases. An Abrams or Cope needle can be used to aid in diagnosis as well. Video assisted thoracoscopy is useful in the group of patients with large or recurrent effusions.[51] A recent study confirmed the utility of this technique among patients undergoing surgery for mesothelioma, but also pointed out the difficulty in obtaining correct histologic diagnosis.[52] Information about parietal, visceral, and diaphragmatic pleural involvement can be obtained as well as this might have prognostic value for survival.[53] Open pleural biopsy is required when there is no free pleural space.

Natural History and Prognostic Indicators

Most patients with mesothelioma, whether treated or not, die from the local complications of the disease. Enlarging tumor bulk causes respiratory failure, chest wall pain, and dysphagia from esophageal compression. Performance status remains the most important predictor of survival. Data from CALGB clinical trials revealed that survival for treated mesothelioma is 7 months for those patients with a performance status of 1 to 2 but 13-14 months for those with a 0 (no impairment) status.[54] Other than performance status nonepithelial histology, male gender, hemoglobin levels, platelet counts, LDH, and white blood cell counts are all prognostic indicators.[55] In a more recent study from a large tertiary referral center factors such as tumor histology, pathologic stage, gender, asbestos exposure, smoking, symptoms, laterality, and clinical stage were all considered.[56] PET CT also has been examined with regard to its prognostic value. In fact low SUV and epithelial histology have better prognosis than high SUV and nonepithelial histology. Higher SUV tumors had a higher risk of death than lower SUV tumors.[57]

Staging

Historically, staging for MPM used nonstandardized criteria that resulted in substantial differences in the reported rates of survival and treatment efficacy. In response, the International Mesothelioma Interest Group (IMIG) published their guidelines for the staging of MPM that more accurately documented the progression of disease and the importance of nodal involvement[58] (Table 79-1). The American Joint Commission on Cancer (AJCC) has adopted these guidelines and the current TNM staging system used is generally accepted. Staging is essential for operative planning. Patients with stage I to stage III disease are candidates for surgical cytoreduction. In an effort to stratify patients for survival, CALGB and EORTC studies found that performance status is the best predictor of survival, while age, histologic subtype, and gender are other important prognostic factors.[59,60] Most patients will succumb to their disease due to respiratory failure or pneumonia. Metastatic disease to the peritoneum and contralateral lung are the most common sites, although distant metastases, which commonly remain asymptomatic, are found in 33-49% of patients.[61] Molecular analysis using DNA microarray technology has developed a 4-gene expression ratio that accurately predicted outcomes independent of histologic subtype.[62] A new 27-gene chip array predicted time to progression with 95% accuracy and data from another group showed that expression of Aurora kinases A and B correlated with a more aggressive phenotype.[63,64] However, none of the microarray data has been validated by other investigators to date.

Table 79-1 IMIG Staging System for Pleural Mesothelioma

T1	
T1a	Tumor limited to the ipsilateral parietal ± mediastinal ± diaphragmatic pleura, no involvement of the visceral pleura
T1b	Tumor involving the ipsilateral parietal ± mediastinal ± diaphragmatic pleura, tumor also involving the visceral pleura
T2	Tumor involving each of the ipsilateral pleural surfaces (parietal, mediastinal, diaphragmatic, and visceral pleura) with at least one of the following features: • Involvement of diaphragmatic muscle • Extension of tumor from visceral pleura into the underlying pulmonary parenchyma
T3	Describes locally advanced but potentially resectable tumor Tumor involving all of the ipsilateral pleural surfaces (parietal, mediastinal, diaphragmatic, and visceral pleura) with at least one of the following features: • Involvement of the endothoracic fascia • Extension into the mediastinal fat • Solitary, completely resectable focus of tumor extending into the soft tissues of the chest wall • Nontransmural involvement of the pericardium
T4	Describes locally advanced technically unresectable tumor Tumor involving all the ipsilateral pleural surfaces (parietal, mediastinal, diaphragmatic, and visceral pleura) with at least one of the following features: • Diffuse extension or multifocal masses of tumor in the chest wall, with or without associated rib destruction • Direct transdiaphragmatic extension of tumor to the peritoneum • Direct extension of tumor to the contralateral pleura • Direct extension of tumor to mediastinal organs • Direct extension of tumor into the spine • Tumor extending through to the internal surface of the pericardium with or without a pericardial effusion; or tumor involving the myocardium
N-Lymph nodes	
NX	Regional lymph nodes cannot be assessed
N0	No regional lymph node metastases
N1	Metastases in the ipsilateral bronchopulmonar or hilar lymph nodes
N2	Metastases in the subcarinal or the ipsilateral mediastinal lymph nodes including the ipsilateral internal mammary nodes
N3	Metastases in the contralateral mediastinal, contralateral internal mammary, ipsilateral, or contralateral supraclavicular lymph nodes
M-Metastases	
MX	Presence of distant metastases cannot be assessed
M0	No distant metastasis
M1	Distant metastasis present
Stage I	
Ia	T1aN0 M0
Ib	T1bN0 M0
Stage II	T2 N0 M0
Stage III	Any T3 M0
	Any N1 M0
	Any N2 M0
Stage IV	Any T4
	Any N3
	Any M1

Abbreviations: T, primary tumor; T1, limited to ipsilateral pleura only (parietal pleura, visceral pleura); T2, superficial local invasion (diaphragm, endothoracic fascia, ipsilateral lung, fissures); T3, deep local invasion (chest wall beyond endothoracic fascia); T4, extensive direct invasion (opposite pleura, peritoneum, retroperitoneum); N, lymph nodes; N0, no positive lymph node; N1, positive ipsilateral hilar nodes; N2, positive mediastinal nodes; N3, positive contralateral hilar nodes; M, metastases; M0, no metastases; M1, metastases; blood-borne or lymphatic.

Source: Adapted Refs.[19,230]

Treatment Options (Table 79-2)

The treatment options for mesothelioma depend on several parameters, including performance status, medical comorbidities, pulmonary function, stage, and age of the patient as well other factors. Surgical options are considered as long as the bulk of the disease can be removed without leaving gross disease behind. If this cannot be accomplished, then supportive measures for palliation can be used.

Supportive Measures

The techniques that can be used for the palliation of this disease are directed toward the management of the pleural effusion and chest pain. The options for managing the pleural fluid include thoracentesis, talc pleurodesis, pleuroperitoneal shunting, and finally placement of a tunneled indwelling pleural catheter (PleurX catheter, Denver Biomedical). Talc pleurodesis can be performed either through a chest tube or via thoracoscopy. The success rate with the use of talc pleurodesis is estimated to be approximately 90%. Loculated effusions or trapped lung can be treated with a PleurX catheter.[65] A potential downside related to the use of indwelling pleural catheters is catheter tract metastases, but this can be treated with external beam radiotherapy without catheter removal. Chest pain is manageable with narcotic analgesia and referral to a pain management team. If this treatment is not adequate, radiation can be used with a 60% response rate, but often not a durable response.[66]

Surgical Options

The surgical treatment options for mesothelioma include those already mentioned for palliation as well as extrapleural pneumonectomy and pleurectomy decortication. Appropriate preoperative evaluation of pulmonary and cardiac status is absolutely essential. Pulmonary function, arterial blood gases, ventilation perfusion scanning as well as echocardiography and stress testing are all routinely performed. Determination of clinical stage can be performed with a CT scan as well as PET CT. All patients with IMIG stages I-IV may be considered for surgical therapy, but the role of surgery in stages III and IV may be only palliative for pleural effusion

Table 79-2 **Treatment Options for Mesothelioma**

Supportive care	
Effusion control	Talc pleurodesis
	Vats assisted
	Slurry
	Pleurex catheter
	Repeated thoracenteses
Pain control	Narcotics
	Permanent epidural catheter
	Localized radiation
Surgery	Pleurectomy with decortication
	Extrapleural pneumonectomy
Chemotherapy[a]	Pemetrexed (Alimta) and cisplatin[a]
	Gemcitabine and cisplatin[a]
	Vinorelbine (Navelbine)
	Phase I/II trials with targeted agents
Multimodality therapy	Induction chemotherapy, surgery, and postoperative radiotherapy[b]
	Surgery and postoperative radiotherapy
	Surgery and postoperative chemotherapy
	Surgery and novel cytotoxic/targeted agents[b]
Novel intrapleural therapies	Hyperthermic chemoperfusion[b]
	Photodynamic therapy[b]
	Gene therapy[b]
Novel radiation techniques at selected centers	Intensity-modulated radiation therapy

[a]Most commonly used in recent phase II/III trials.
[b]Under investigation.

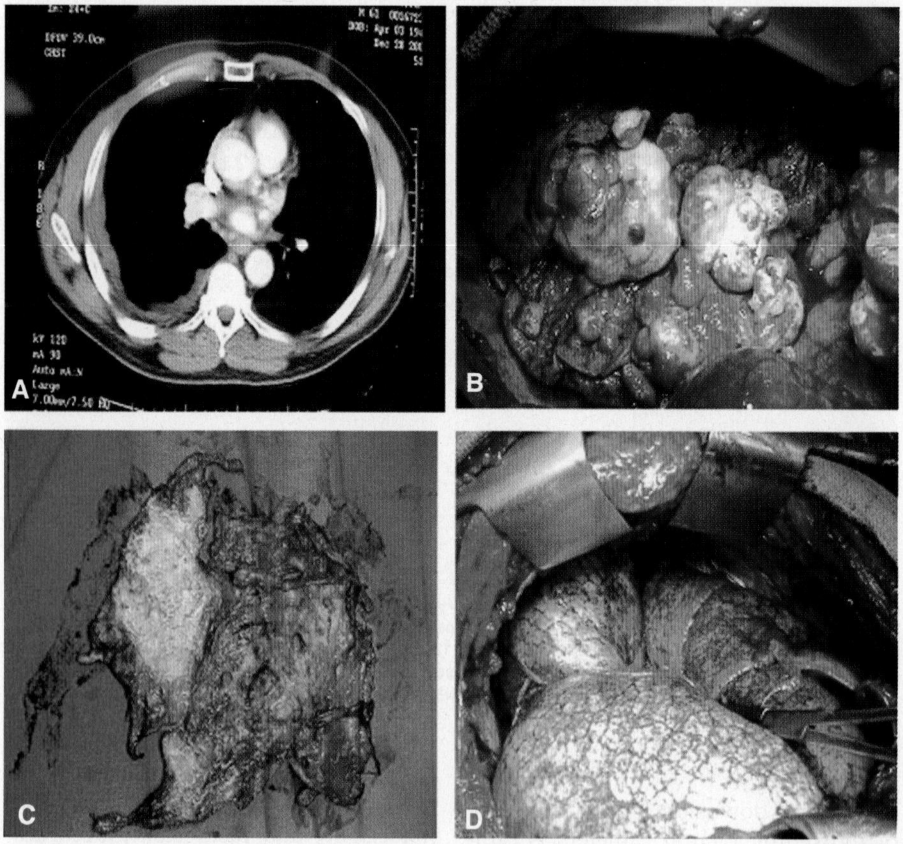

Figure 79-3 Pleurectomy for mesothelioma: (**A**) typical computer tomogram reveals thickened pleura; (**B**) operative view reveals disease primarily on the parietal pleura; (**C**) operative specimen; (**D**) completion of satisfactory cytoreduction with sparing and decortication of the lung.

management depending upon the performance status of the patient. Evaluation of lymph node status can be performed for suspicious PET CTs and can be done with mediastinoscopy if the nodes are believed to be accessible through this means.[67] A recent study suggests that this might not be adequate since the extent of nodal involvement may actually be below the subcarinal level.[68] In those cases of lower lymph nodes that are suspicious, EUS–FNA can be performed for more accurate assessment of the lower mediastinal lymph nodes.[69]

Whether to offer mesothelioma surgery to patients with nodal involvement remains controversial. Many studies have revealed that mesothelioma patients with nodal disease found at surgery do poorly. Most recently, pleurectomy with positive nodes had a median survival of 16 months, while extrapleural pneumonectomy (EPP) gave 15 months.[70] The question of whether EPP should be performed at all is currently being addressed in the Mesothelioma and Radical Surgery trial. In this trial induction chemotherapy is given followed by EPP and radiotherapy. The control arm comprises patients with mesothelioma randomized to nonsurgical treatment.[71]

Pleurectomy (Fig. 79-3)

Pleurectomy for mesothelioma can be performed with less mortality than that associated with EPP, and in a recent review was in the 1.5-2.0% range. Death was from respiratory failure and hemorrhage. Pleurectomy is mostly performed through a thoracotomy incision, but in some cases can be performed with VATS, as described by Nakas et al.[72]

Extrapleural Pneumonectomy (Fig. 79-4)

Radical resection of both the visceral and parietal pleura, lung, pericardium, and diaphragm can be performed for the treatment of malignant mesothelioma with reasonable mortality rates. Traditionally this operation has been performed through a posterolateral thoracotomy, but it also can be performed through a sternotomy, particularly for right sided tumors.[73] Complications are common with this operation, the most frequent being cardiac arrhythmia in up to 20-40% of patients as described in Sugarbaker's most recent report.[74] In a more recent study by Schipper et al[75] complications in their group of patients were divided into major and minor. Major complications included empyema, respiratory failure, and bronchopleural fistulae among others. Minor complications included in this series were blood transfusions and arrhythmia. Overall mortality was 6.3%, comparable to that described by Rusch and colleagues at 6-8%.[76] Sugarbaker et al reported their mortality at a benchmark low percentage of 3.4%. Death is usually from myocardial infarction and presumed pulmonary emboli. Overall survival ranges from 9.3 to 17 months. These results are consistent with most series in the United States, such as those by Pass et al,[77] Rusch et al,[78] Sugarbaker et al,[79] and Flores et al.[80]

Pleurectomy or EPP

The operation of choice, especially for early pleural mesothelioma, has yet to be defined. There is no doubt that EPP

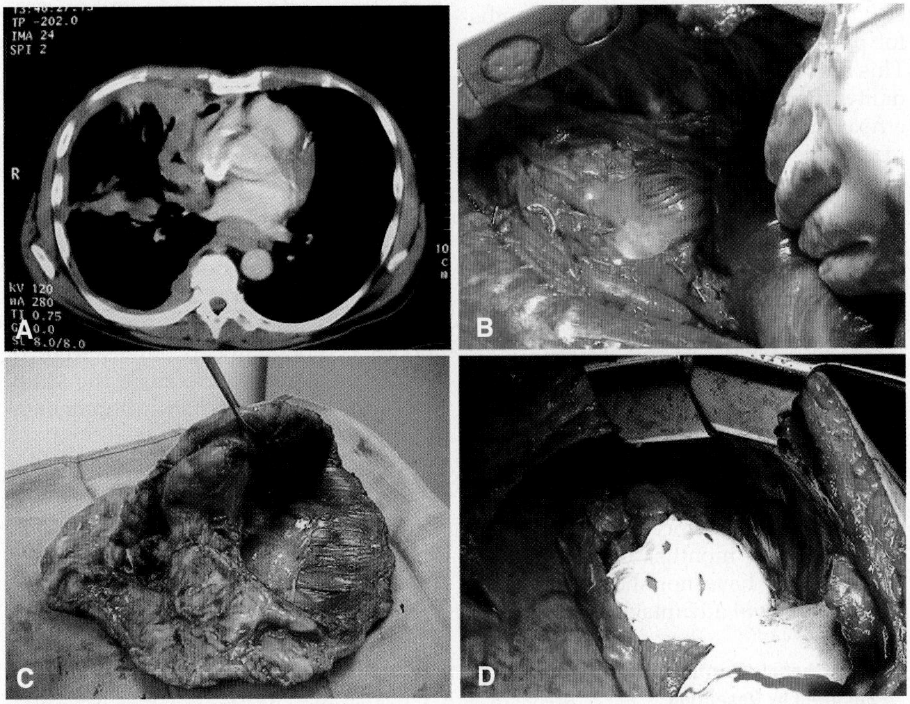

Figure 79-4 Extrapleural pneumonectomy for mesothelioma: (**A**) Computer tomography reveals thickened pleura, pericardium and disease in the fissures. (**B**) Intraoperative view after the resection with hand on the liver. Stapled bronchial stump, right atrium, and extent of pericardiotomy is seen. (**C**) Operative specimen reveals diaphragmatic resection to the right and thickened pleura encasing the lung. (**D**) Reconstruction of the diaphragm and pericardium with Gore-Tex patches.

is a more extensive dissection and may serve to remove more bulk disease than a pleurectomy, chiefly in the diaphragmatic and visceral pleural surfaces. Some surgeons, however, will include diaphragmatic resection and pericardial resection with their pleurectomies to accomplish removal of "all gross disease." For EPP, when performed in patients with bulky disease, it is almost a necessity to include pericardiotomy, with or without resection, since this maneuver aids in the exposure of the vessels and allows intrapericardial control to prevent a surgical catastrophe. There are no real guidelines preoperatively that one can use to assure the patient which operation will be necessary to accomplish tumor removal. The presence of irregular, bulky disease on the CT scan that infiltrates into the fissures probably dictates the necessity for EPP; a large effusion with minimal bulk disease may call for pleurectomy decortication. Moreover, the philosophy of the surgeon regarding the operation may impact on his choice, for some surgeons reserve EPP for those patients with bulky disease that prevents simple pleurectomy, whereas others feel that the greatest chance for complete gross excision will be via EPP performed in the patient with minimal disease. This important factor—preoperative quantitative bulk of disease—may not only influence the choice or resection, but may also be an important preoperative prognostic factor in any patient with mesothelioma.[81]

Recently, a large combination series from the Memorial Sloan Kettering Cancer Center, the National Cancer Institute, and the Karmanos Caner Institute, reviewed the results of surgery for pleural mesothelioma. From 1990 to 2006, 663 consecutive patients underwent surgical resection. Median age was 65 years (26-93 range), including 538 men and 125 women. Operative mortality was 7% for EPP (n = 27/385) and 4% for pleurectomy/decortication (P/D) (n = 13/278). Kaplan–Meier analysis demonstrated significant differences for AJCC stages I-IV ($p < .001$), epithelioid vs nonepithelioid histology ($p < .001$), and EPP vs P/D ($p < .001$). Stratified analysis revealed that there was no statistical difference in median survival for stage I and II patients having P/D (n = 98; 23 months) vs EPP (n = 96; 19 months, p = .07). However, a trend toward improved survival was observed in stage I and stage IV disease with P/D and in stage II disease with EPP. A Cox proportional hazards analysis demonstrated a HR of 1.2 for EPP (p = .04) controlling for stage (HR =1.9, $p < .001$) and histology (HR =1.5, $p < .001$).[82] These provocative data demonstrate that the choice of operation for mesothelioma is not limited to EPP in early stage disease.

Radiation Therapy

Recently the use of radiation therapy for the treatment of malignant mesothelioma has been discussed more in terms of multimodality therapy or for palliation. The use of radiation as curative treatment for MPM is technically challenging because of all the organs that have to be included in the radiation field. There is obvious concern for the normal surrounding tissue and the potential toxicity. There have been several documented studies on the use of high-dose radiotherapy as primary treatment for mesothelioma. The most recent is from Holsti et al who reported 2 and 5 year survivals of 21% and 9%, respectively, in 57 patients.[83]

Concurrent Chemotherapy and Radiation

The very poor results that were obtained with use of radiation therapy alone for mesothelioma led to the idea of using chemotherapy and radiation together. Several published series by Alberts et al,[84] Ruffie et al,[85] Linden et al,[86] and Herscher et al[87] investigated the use of combined modality chemoradiation therapy.

Surgery Followed by Radiation

In a recent retrospective review performed at Memorial Sloan Kettering, 123 patients who underwent pleurectomy decortication (P/D) received ipsilateral hemithoracic radiotherapy with a mean dose of 42.5 Gy postoperatively. The 2-year survival was 23%, and the study pointed out that residual disease could not be eradicated with external radiation with or without brachytherapy.[88] There is a high locoregional failure rate associated with this technique, and because of this a more aggressive approach with EPP and radiation was reviewed by Stevens et al.[89] In this study the 3-year survival ranged from 20% to 55% with EPP and RT. Local failure rates were 6% for intensity modulated RT and 30% for 3D conformal radiation. Chan et al have described a novel radiation therapy technique combining electrons with intensity-modulated photons after surgery in six patients after EPP and five after P/D. This study showed that IMRT is a viable treatment option for mesothelioma patients. The addition of electrons helped normal tissue sparing.[90] More recently a study by Rice et al reviewed the use of IMRT after EPP with good local control and median survival of 10.2 months.[912] As one might expect, distant metastases are the problem with this approach and occurred in up to 54% of patients.

Multimodality Therapy

After the demonstration of systemic failure with surgical options followed by radiation, the next possible schema was the addition of chemotherapy in the setting of multimodality therapy. In the past this included the combination of debulking surgery with intrapleural chemotherapy and postoperative chemotherapy. Rusch et al[92,93] used intrapleural cisplatin and cytarabine after surgical debulking followed by systemic chemotherapy. The median survival of these patients was 17 months, and failures with this technique were local. Zellos et al[94] reported their standard approach with EPP followed by postop radiation and chemotherapy. Paclitaxel and carboplatin were used concurrently with 40.5 Gy of radiation. Median survival was also 17 months.

Induction Chemotherapy Followed by Surgery and Radiation ■ Recently, several studies have reported encouraging results using induction chemotherapy. Weder et al showed in a small pilot study that neoadjuvant chemotherapy with cisplatin and gemcitabine followed by EPP and postoperative radiation could produce a median survival of 23 months. 1-year and 2-year survival rates were 79% and 37%, respectively.[95] Flores et al in another small study found that early stage MPM patients successfully completing a course of neoadjuvant chemotherapy with cisplatin and gemcitabine, followed by EPP and 54 Gy of radiotherapy, had a median survival of 33.5 months.[96] A more recent Swiss, multicenter phase II trial of induction therapy followed by EPP and radiation, that included 61 patients, reported a 23-month median survival in those patients who underwent EPP. These data suggest that induction therapy may prolong survival compared with upfront surgery. Postoperative morbidity was 62% and mortality was 3.2%, which is comparable to the Brigham experience.[97] A large industry sponsored North American Trial investigated neoadjuvant pemetrexed plus cisplatin, followed by extrapleural pneumonectomy (EPP) and hemithoracic radiation (RT) in stage I-III malignant pleural mesothelioma (MPM). Patients received pemetrexed 500 mg/m^2 plus cisplatin 75 mg/m^2 for 4 cycles. Patients without disease progression underwent EPP followed by RT (54 Gy). The primary endpoint was pathologic complete response (pCR) rate. 77 patients received chemotherapy. All 4 cycles were administered to 83% of patients. The radiological response rate was 32.5% (95% CI: 22.2, 44.1), and 3 pCRs were observed (5.3% of EPP). A total of 57 patients proceeded to EPP, which was completed in 54 patients, and 40 patients completed radiation. Median survival in the overall population was 16.8 months (95% CI: 13.6, 23.2, censorship: 33.8%). Patients completing all therapy had a median survival of 29.1 months and a 2-year survival rate of 61.2%. Radiological response of CR or PR was associated with a median survival of 26.0 months compared with 13.9 months for patients with an SD or PD (p = .05). This multicenter trial showed that trimodality therapy with neoadjuvant pemetrexed plus cisplatin is feasible with a reasonable long-term survival rate, particularly for patients who completed all therapy. Radiological response but not gender, histology, disease stage, or nodal status was associated with improved survival (JCO in press, 2009)

Intrapleural Photodynamic Therapy

Pass et al[98,99] conducted a series of phase I through phase III trials randomizing patients to surgery with intraoperative photodynamic therapy (PDT) vs surgery without PDT and demonstrated that there was no difference in survival.(14.4 months vs 14.1 months). Other phase II trials of PDT have not shown any convincing survival advantage.

Hyperthermic Perfusion of the Pleura Followed by Resection

Sugarbaker et al described the use of hyperthermic cisplatin to perfuse the pleura and the abdomen after pleurectomy and decortication in a phase I/II trial. Overall survival was 10.5 months except for the group receiving surgery, which had an overall survival of 22 months.[100] Data regarding this technique after EPP are forthcoming.

Chemotherapy for Mesothelioma

Historically, anthracyclines, platinum agents, and antimetabolites have been used as single agents against MPM with response rates ranging from 10% to 20% and median survival times less than one year. Meta-analysis has determined that, cisplatin is the most active single agent.[101] More recent studies of combination chemotherapies, particularly with a platinum Compound have yielded modestly superior response rates and median survival times. Chemotherapy for MPM can also improve symptoms such as pain and dyspnea.[102]

The current benchmark regimens for mesothelioma contain platinum and an antifolate. Pemetrexed, an antifolate that targets thymidylate synthase, dihydrofolate reductase, and glycinamide ribonucleotide formyltransferase, is currently the only FDA approved agent for MPM.[103] A landmark phase III trial randomized 456 chemotherapy-naive patients to cisplatin plus either pemetrexed or placebo. The combination yielded a significantly higher response rate (41% vs 17%; $P < .001$), median survival (12.1 vs 9.3 months; p = .020), and time to progression (5.7 vs 3.9 months, p = .001) than single-agent cisplatin. Combination treatment also produced a significant improvement in pulmonary function, quality of life, and symptoms including dyspnea and pain. Vitamin supplementation with dietary doses of folate and vitamin B12 resulted in improved response rates and survival, and reduced the incidence of severe toxicity.[104]

A smaller European phase III trial randomized 250 MPM patients to cisplatin with or without the antifolate raltitrexed. Once again, combination therapy yielded higher response rates (23.6% vs 13.6%) and an improved median overall survival (11.4 months vs 8.8 months), though the p values were of borderline significance, since the study was underpowered. Vitamin supplementation was not used in this trial.[105]

The substitution of carboplatin for cisplatin achieves similar results, with potentially less toxicity, which is important in a disease in which the majority of patients are elderly. In a 102 patient phase II study, the combination of pemetrexed plus carboplatin yielded a 19% response rate, a median time to progression of 6.5 months, and a median overall survival of 12.7 months.[106]

Gemcitabine has limited single-agent activity against MPM, but the combination of gemcitabine plus cisplatin is quite active, yielding response rates ranging from 12% to 48%.[107-110] These differences in response rates are most likely a result of heterogeneity in patient selection and inconsistency in response assessment between trials. Other gemcitabine doublets with activity in MPM include gemcitabine plus carboplatin, (26% response rate, 15.1 month median overall survival),[111] and gemcitabine plus oxaliplatin (40% response rate, 13 month median overall survival).[112] Gemcitabine plus pemetrexed is only modestly more active than either agent alone, at the expense of greater toxicity.[113]

At 24%, vinorelbine has one of the highest response rates of any single-agent in this disease,[114] while in the second-line setting, a response rate of 16% and a median survival of 9.6 has recently been reported.[115] As with other combinations, the addition of cisplatin appears to increase response rates and survival, to 30% and 16.8 months, respectively.[116] The phase III MS01 trial suggests that vinorelbine may also improve survival in MPM. Four hundred and nine newly-diagnosed MPM patients were randomized to active symptom control (ASC) with or without chemotherapy (vinorelbine or mitomycin-vinblastine-cisplatin (MVP)). Pooled survival data for the two chemotherapy arms achieved only borderline significance in favor of chemotherapy (7.6 vs 8.5 months, p = .32) but when this was analyzed by the type of chemotherapy given, ASC and MVP resulted in similar survival (7.6 and 7.8 months, respectively), while vinorelbine-treated patients survived a median of 9.4 months (HR 0.81, p = .11).[117]

Biologic Therapies

Ribonuclease inhibitors, such as ranpirnase, are a novel biologic approach to MPM treatment. Cytotoxic ribonucleases specifically target tumor cell tRNA resulting in inhibition of protein synthesis and cell cycle arrest at the G1 phase. A phase III trial comparing single-agent ranpirnase to doxorubicin that enrolled 154 MPM patients resulted in better overall and 2-year survival in a subset of low-risk patients treated with ranpirnase.[118] An international phase III trial comparing doxorubicin to combination doxorubicin plus ranpirnase is ongoing.

Targeted Therapies

Epidermal growth factor receptor (EGFR), vascular endothelial growth factor (VEGF), and platelet derived growth factor (PDGF) are important growth factors involved in MPM pathogenesis. Numerous studies of agents that target these pathways have been relatively disappointing. Despite promising preclinical data phase II trials of the EGFR tyrosine kinase inhibitors erlotinib and gefitinib have shown no efficacy.[119,120] Imatinib an inhibitor of the tyrosine kinase activity of the platelet derived growth factor, is also inactive.[121] A randomized multicenter, double-blind placebo-controlled phase II trial of gemcitabine plus cisplatin with either the anti-VEGF monoclonal antibody bevacizumab or placebo, concluded that the addition of bevacizumab did not affect progression-free or median overall survival.[122] Similarly, phase II studies of the VEGF inhibitors SU5416, vatalanib, thalidomide, and sorafenib have demonstrated only modest single agent activity, comparable to other single-agents in this disease.[123] Despite the relative lack of activity of these tyrosine kinase inhibitors, other pathways are currently being examined, including src, which is frequently expressed and activated in mesothelioma. Dasatinib, a potent inhibitor of src family kinases, which inhibits migration and invasion of mesothelioma in preclinical models[124] *is currently* being evaluated in a phase II CALGB study in previously treated patients.

Suberoylanilide hydroxamic acid (SAHA, voyinostat), an oral histone deacetylase inhibitor has preclinical activity in mesothelioma. Two partial responses in 13 MPM patients were observed in the phase I trial of SAHA, and all patients with stable or responding disease experienced symptomatic improvement.[125] These data led to an ongoing double-blind, placebo-controlled, randomized phase III trial in 660 previously treated MPM patients. Overall survival is the primary endpoint.

The proteasome inhibitor bortezomib inhibits constitutive activation of NFkB and enhances the cytotoxicity of cisplatin and pemetrexed in preclinical mesothelioma models.[126,127] Two European trials are currently testing bortezomib as a single-agent and in combination with cisplatin.

Three drugs that target mesothelin are currently in phase I and II trials. SSIP is a recombinant immunotoxin. MORAb-009 is a chimeric humanized monoclonal antibody and CRS-207 is an attenuated listeria vector that encodes human mesothelin. SSIP and MORAb-009 have completed phase I evaluation and are being tested with pemetrexed plus cisplatin.[37,38,128]

Conclusion

Mesothelioma remains a very difficult malignancy to treat with poor survival overall. Several new approaches with regard to better staging may help select out the patients who are more appropriately treated with surgery. Multimodality therapy appears to be the most acceptable current approach for treatment. Several new drugs and immune therapies might alter the course of this disease, but overall it remains a challenge to all of those who continue to treat this entity.

Selected References

The complete reference list can be found at www.CANCERMEDICINE8.com

1. Wagner JC, SLEGGS CA, Marchand P. Diffuse pleural mesothelioma and asbestos exposure in the North Western Cape Province. *Br J Ind Med.* October 1960;17:260–271.
15. Cugell DW, Kamp DW. Asbestos and the pleura: a review. *Chest.* March 2004;125(3):1103–1117.
16. Xu A, Zhou H, Yu DZ, Hei TK. Mechanisms of the genotoxicity of crocidolite asbestos in mammalian cells: implication from mutation patterns induced by reactive oxygen species. *Environ Health Perspect.* October 2002;110(10):1003–1008.
18. Ivanov SV, Miller J, Lucito R, et al. Genomic events associated with progression of pleural malignant mesothelioma. *Int J Cancer.* February 1, 2009;124(3):589–599.
20. Altomare DA, You H, Xiao GH, et al. Human and mouse mesotheliomas exhibit elevated AKT/PKB activity, which can be targeted pharmacologically to inhibit tumor cell growth. *Oncogene.* September 8, 2005;24(40):6080–6089.
22. Yang H, Bocchetta M, Kroczynska B, et al. TNF-alpha inhibits asbestos-induced cytotoxicity via a NF-kappaB-dependent pathway, a possible mechanism for asbestos-induced oncogenesis. *Proc Natl Acad Sci USA.* July 5, 2006;103(27):10397–10402.
29. Pershouse MA, Heivly S, Girtsman T. The role of SV40 in malignant mesothelioma and other human malignancies. *Inhal Toxicol.* November 2006;18(12):995–1000.
30. Pass HI, Bocchetta M, Carbone M. Evidence of an important role for SV40 in mesothelioma. *Thorac Surg Clin.* November 2004;14(4):489–495.
32. Kroczynska B, Cutrone R, Bocchetta M, et al. Crocidolite asbestos and SV40 are cocarcinogens in human mesothelial cells and in causing mesothelioma in hamsters. *Proc Natl Acad Sci USA.* September 19, 2006;103(38):14128–14133.
35. Carbone M, Emri S, Dogan AU, et al. A mesothelioma epidemic in Cappadocia: scientific developments and unexpected social outcomes. *Nat Rev Cancer.* February 2007;7(2):147–154.
38. Kaufman AJ, Pass HI. Current concepts in malignant pleural mesothelioma. *Expert Rev Anticancer Ther.* February 2008;8(2):293–303.
39. Pass HI, Lott D, Lonardo F, et al. Asbestos exposure, pleural mesothelioma, and serum osteopontin levels. *N Engl J Med.* October 13, 2005;353(15):1564–1573.
42. Robinson BW, Creaney J, Lake R, et al. Mesothelin-family proteins and diagnosis of mesothelioma. *Lancet.* November 15, 2003;362(9396):1612–1616.
43. Pass HI, Wali A, Tang N, et al. Soluble mesothelin-related peptide level elevation in mesothelioma serum and pleural effusions. *Ann Thorac Surg.* January 2008;85(1):265–272.
45. Flores RM. The role of PET in the surgical management of malignant pleural mesothelioma. *Lung Cancer.* July 2005;49 (Suppl 1):S27–S32.
51. Carbone M, Albelda SM, Broaddus VC, et al. Eighth international mesothelioma interest group. *Oncogene.* October 25, 2007;26(49):6959–6967.
56. Flores RM, Zakowski M, Venkatraman E, et al. Prognostic factors in the treatment of malignant pleural mesothelioma at a large tertiary referral center. *J Thorac Oncol.* October 2007;2(10):957–965.
58. Rusch VW. A proposed new international TNM staging system for malignant pleural mesothelioma. From the International Mesothelioma Interest Group. *Chest.* October 1995;108(4):1122–1128.
62. Gordon GJ, Rockwell GN, Godfrey PA, et al. Validation of genomics-based prognostic tests in malignant pleural mesothelioma. *Clin Cancer Res.* June 15, 2005;11(12):4406–4414.
63. Pass HI, Liu Z, Wali A, et al. Gene expression profiles predict survival and progression of pleural mesothelioma. *Clin Cancer Res.* February 1, 2004;10(3):849–859.
64. Lopez-Rios F, Chuai S, Flores R, et al. Global gene expression profiling of pleural mesotheliomas: overexpression of aurora kinases and P16/CDKN2A deletion as prognostic factors and critical evaluation of microarray-based prognostic prediction. *Cancer Res.* March 15, 2006;66(6):2970–2979.
68. Edwards JG, Stewart DJ, Martin-Ucar A, Muller S, Richards C, Waller DA. The pattern of lymph node involvement influences outcome after extrapleural pneumonectomy for malignant mesothelioma. *J Thorac Cardiovasc Surg.* May 2006;131(5):981–987.
71. Treasure T, Utley M. Mesothelioma: benefit from surgical resection is question-

able. *J Thorac Oncol*. October 2007;2(10): 885–886.
74. Sugarbaker DJ, Jaklitsch MT, Bueno R, et al. Prevention, early detection, and management of complications after 328 consecutive extrapleural pneumonectomies. *J Thorac Cardiovasc Surg*. July 2004;128(1):138–146.
77. Pass HI, Kranda K, Temeck BK, Feuerstein I, Steinberg SM. Surgically debulked malignant pleural mesothelioma: results and prognostic factors. *Ann Surg Oncol*. April 1997;4(3):215–222.
78. Rusch VW, Venkatraman ES. Important prognostic factors in patients with malignant pleural mesothelioma, managed surgically. *Ann Thorac Surg*. November 1999;68(5):1799–1804.
80. Flores RM, Pass HI, Seshan VE, et al. Extrapleural pneumonectomy versus pleurectomy/decortication in the surgical management of malignant pleural mesothelioma: results in 663 patients. *J Thorac Cardiovasc Surg*. March 2008;135(3):620–626.
90. Stevens CW, Forster KM, Smythe WR, Rice D. Radiotherapy for mesothelioma. *Hematol Oncol Clin North Am*. December 2005;19(6):1099–1115, vii.
93. Rusch V, Saltz L, Venkatraman E, et al. A phase II trial of pleurectomy/decortication followed by intrapleural and systemic chemotherapy for malignant pleural mesothelioma. *J Clin Oncol*. June 1994;12(6):1156–1163.
97. Flores RM. Induction chemotherapy, extrapleural pneumonectomy, and radiotherapy in the treatment of malignant pleural mesothelioma: the Memorial Sloan-Kettering experience. *Lung Cancer*. July 2005;49(Suppl 1):S71–S74.
99. Pass HI, Temeck BK, Kranda K, et al. Phase III randomized trial of surgery with or without intraoperative photodynamic therapy and postoperative immunochemotherapy for malignant pleural mesothelioma. *Ann Surg Oncol*. December 1997;4(8):628–633.
102. Berghmans T, Paesmans M, Lalami Y, et al. Activity of chemotherapy and immunotherapy on malignant mesothelioma: a systematic review of the literature with meta-analysis. *Lung Cancer*. November 2002;38(2):111–121.
106. Van Meerbeeck JP, Manegold C, Gaafar R, et al. A randomized phase III study of cisplatin with or without raltitrexed in patients (pts) with malignant pleural mesothelioma (MPM): an intergroup study of the EORTC Lung Cancer Group and NCIC. *Proc Am Soc Clin Oncol*. 22[14S]. 2004. Ref Type: Abstract.
107. Ceresoli GL, Castagneto B, Zucali PA, et al. Pemetrexed plus carboplatin in elderly patients with malignant pleural mesothelioma: combined analysis of two phase II trials. *Br J Cancer*. July 8, 2008;99(1):51–56.
109. Nowak AK, Byrne MJ, Williamson R, et al. A multicentre phase II study of cisplatin and gemcitabine for malignant mesothelioma. *Br J Cancer*. August 27, 2002;87(5):491–496.
115. Steele JP, Shamash J, Evans MT, Gower NH, Tischkowitz MD, Rudd RM. Phase II study of vinorelbine in patients with malignant pleural mesothelioma. *J Clin Oncol*. December 1, 2000;18(23):3912–3917.
120. Garland LL, Rankin C, Gandara DR, et al. Phase II study of erlotinib in patients with malignant pleural mesothelioma: a Southwest Oncology Group Study. *J Clin Oncol*. June 10, 2007;25(17):2406–2413.
125. Tsao AS, He D, Saigal B, et al. Inhibition of c-Src expression and activation in malignant pleural mesothelioma tissues leads to apoptosis, cell cycle arrest, and decreased migration and invasion. *Mol Cancer Ther*. July 2007;6(7):1962–1972.
127. Sartore-Bianchi A, Gasparri F, Galvani A, et al. Bortezomib inhibits nuclear factor-kappaB dependent survival and has potent in vivo activity in mesothelioma. *Clin Cancer Res*. October 1, 2007;13(19):5942–5951.
129. Hassan R, Ho M. Mesothelin targeted cancer immunotherapy. *Eur J Cancer*. January 2008;44(1):46–53.

80 Thymomas and Thymic Tumors

A. Philippe Chahinian, MD ■ Alberto M. Marchevsky, MD

The thymus can be the site of a large variety of neoplasms of epithelial, lymphoid, and other origin that account for less than 1% of all tumors (Table 80-1). The majority of thymic neoplasms in adult patients are thymomas, malignant lymphomas, germ cell tumors, and less often, thymic carcinomas or neuroendocrine carcinomas.[1] The majority of thymic neoplasms arising in children and young adults are malignant lymphomas and germ cell tumors.

History

Givel published a detailed historical review of the thymus gland and thymomas.[2] The first description of a thymic tumor is credited to Sir Astley Paston Cooper, a surgeon from London, in 1832. In 1849, the British microscopist Arthur Hill Hassall described the corpuscles unique to the thymus. The first association between myasthenia gravis (MG) and thymoma was discovered in 1899 by the German neurologist Hermann Oppenheim. The first thymectomy for MG was performed in 1911 by Ernst Ferdinand Sauerbruch in Zurich, Switzerland. The thymus showed hyperplasia but no tumor, and myasthenia improved markedly after surgery. Alfred Blalock at Vanderbilt University in Nashville, Tennessee, pioneered the surgical technique of total thymectomy in 1936 (case published in 1939) and advocated it for the treatment of MG.

Table 80-1 ■ Primary Thymic Neoplasms

Thymic epithelial tumors
Thymomas
Thymic carcinomas
Germ cell tumors
Seminoma
Embryonal carcinoma
Yolk sac tumor
Choriocarcinoma
Teratoma
Mixed germ cell tumor
Germ cell tumor with somatic-type malignancy
Germ cell tumor with associated hematologic malignancy
Mediastinal lymphomas
Primary mediastinal B-cell lymphoma
Thymic extranodal marginal zone B-cell lymphoma of mucosa Associated lymphoid tissue (MALT)
T-cell lymphoma
Hodgkin lymphoma
Histiocytic and dendritic cell tumors
Myeloid sarcoma
Mesenchymal tumors
Thymolipoma
Solitary fibrous tumor
Sarcoma

Etiology and Epidemiology

There are no known etiologic factors for thymomas, although a few cases have developed following radiation therapy to the chest. For example, among 23 patients with thymoma, two had received radiation therapy for an enlarged thymus during childhood, 17 and 28 years prior to the diagnosis of a thymic neoplasm.[3] Epstein-Barr virus (EBV) has been associated with thymic lymphoepithelioma, a rare variant of thymic carcinoma that is usually more frequent in young patients.[4] A few patients with the multiple endocrine neoplasm type I syndrome (MEN I) have had associated thymomas or neuroendocrine carcinomas of thymic origin.[5-8]

Thymomas have an incidence of approximately 1-5 million population/year and present with an equal incidence in men and women.[9,10] They can develop in a wide age range with a peak incidence in the fourth and fifth decades of life. Thymomas are unusual neoplasms in children and tend to have a more aggressive clinical course than in adults.[11-13]

Anatomic Pathogenesis

Embryology and Anatomy

The thymus is embryologically derived from the endodermal epithelium of the third pharyngeal pouches (which also give rise to the lower pair of parathyroid glands) and, less constantly, the fourth ones as well.[1] The right and left thymic anlagen migrate downward into the anterosuperior mediastinum, joining together without complete fusion to form a bilobate organ.[1] Although most thymic tumors are located in the anterosuperior mediastinum, variations in migration account for the findings of gross or microscopic thymic tissue anywhere between the hyoid bone superiorly and the diaphragm inferiorly.[14] Wide exposure of the mediastinum and even the neck is therefore necessary if surgical removal of the entire thymus is indicated, as in patients with thymoma or those with MG (with or without associated thymoma). The absolute weight of the thymus reaches its peak in the pubertal years (mean 34 ± 15 g between age 10 and 15 years) and then gradually decreases, although this age-related involution normally is never complete.[1]

Histologically, the normal thymus shows distinctive lobules with a sharp demarcation between the cortex, rich in lymphocytes, and the medulla, rich in epithelial cells and characteristic Hassall's corpuscles, formed by concentric layers of mature epithelial cells.

The thymus plays a critical role in the maturation of bone marrow-derived lymphocytes into T cells and, as such, in cell-mediated immunity. It has a rich blood supply but no afferent lymphatics. Efferent lymphatics apparently originate from perivascular spaces and drain into the mediastinal and lower cervical nodes.[1]

Pathology of Thymic Epithelial Neoplasms

Pathology of Thymomas

Thymomas appear grossly as single or multiple encapsulated neoplasms that range in size from microscopic lesions to large tumors replacing the entire anterior mediastinum and compressing the adjacent intrathoracic structures.[15-20] Grossly, most thymomas are well encapsulated (Fig. 80-1) but some thymomas can be locally invasive extending into mediastinal soft tissues, superior vena cava and other vascular structures, lymph nodes, pleura, pericardium, trachea, and/or other intrathoracic structures adjacent to the thymus (Fig. 80-2). The incidence of transcapsular invasion varies considerably in different cohorts of thymomas from 9.2% to 59.2%. On section thymomas exhibit a distinctive fibrous capsule and multiple fibrous septa that divide the lesion into a characteristic lobulated appearance (Fig. 80-3). Thymomas can undergo degenerative changes with cystic degeneration. Rarely, thymomas present as a mediastinal cyst that needs to be distinguished from a thymic and other intrathoracic cysts by the presence of focal solid areas in the cyst wall.[21-23]

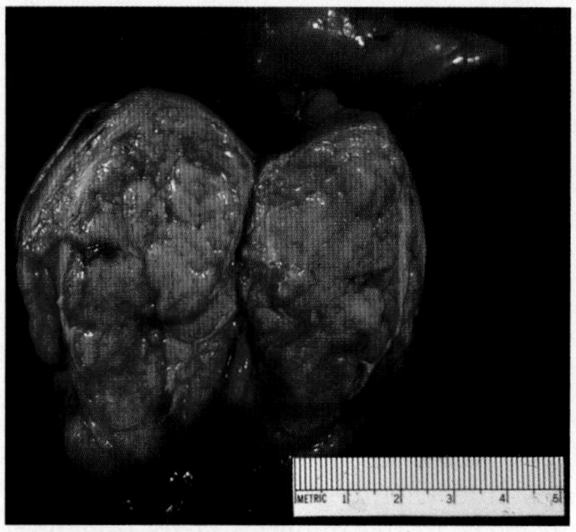

Figure 80-1 ■ Gross photograph of thymoma showing an encapsulated tumor with a gray, soft surface exhibiting characteristic fibrous septa.

Microscopically, thymomas are composed of epithelial cells that can have elongated or polygonal shaped nuclei admixed with a variable number of mature lymphocytes.[24,25] The epithelial and lymphoid cells of thymomas are usually arranged in solid sheets divided by fibrous septa in a somewhat lobulated appearance that can be observed grossly and at low power microscopy in most thymomas (Fig. 80-3).[18,19,26] Other histologic features of thymomas include, in order of frequency, perivascular spaces (56%) (Fig. 80-4), collections of foamy macrophages (27%), pseudorosette formations of epithelial cells (20%), gland-like structures (20%), Hassall's corpuscles (16%), areas of cystic degeneration that can result in cystic thymomas (16%), lymphoid follicles with germinal centers (8%), and a variable number of hemorrhagic, necrotic, and/or calcified areas.

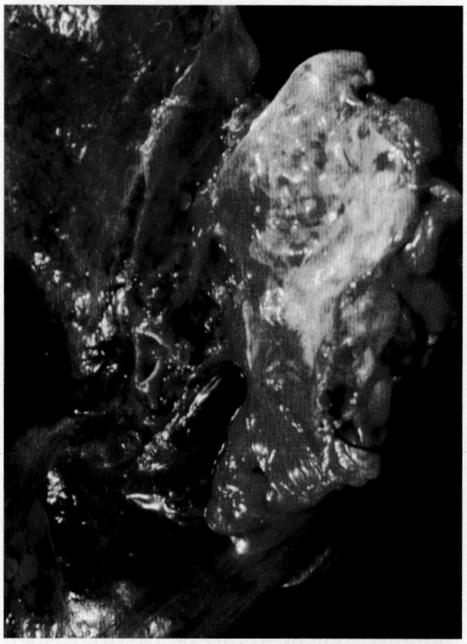

Figure 80-2 ■ Gross photograph of invasive thymoma showing invasion of mediastinal soft tissues and bronchial wall.

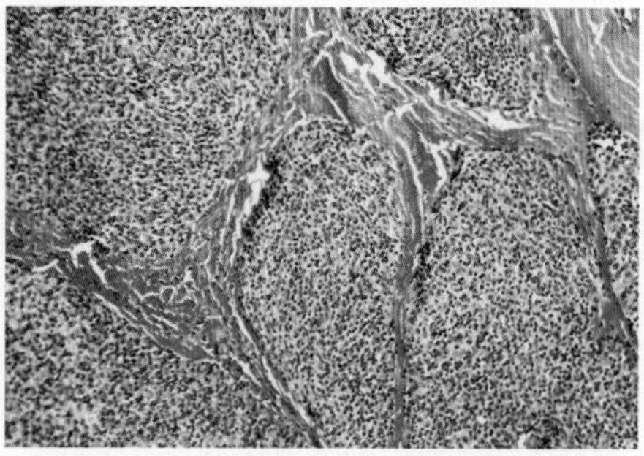

Figure 80-3 ■ Photomicrograph of thymoma showing the characteristic lobulations of the lesion. The epithelial and lymphoid cells are separated by thin fibrous septa (H&E; x40).

Occasionally, scattered macrophages among the lymphocytic component can mimic a "starry sky" appearance, not to be confused with Burkitt's lymphoma. Myoid cells, so designated because their cytoplasm contains cross-striations identical to those of skeletal muscle fibers, have also been identified in rare cases. Mitoses and necrosis are unusual in thymomas and should raise the suspicion of a thymic carcinoma.[27]

World Health Organization Classification of Thymomas

Different classification schema have been proposed for the categorization of thymic epithelial neoplasms.[20,26-31] The most widely used classification scheme of these tumors has been proposed by the World Health Organization (WHO) in 1999 and has been modified in 2004 (Table 80-2).[32-35] The WHO classification, which was initially designed as a translation tool to compare other classification schema, uses the unusual approach of distinguishing various histologic types of thymomas using the letters A through C combined with the numbers 1 through 3 for thymomas B.[30] Thymic carcinomas are classified as thymoma C in the 1999 version of the WHO classification of thymic epithelial neoplasms and as thymic carcinomas in the more recent 2004 version.[27] In the past, it has been controversial whether thymomas should be further subdivided into benign and malignant lesions based on the absence or presence of capsular invasion (Fig 80-5). The concept that encapsulated thymomas are benign neoplasms is no longer accepted after reports of metastases in patients with such lesions.[36] Currently all thymomas are considered as low-grade malignant lesions with variable potential to recur and/or metastasize that is highest in thymomas C. Thymic carcinomas are malignant neoplasms with a considerably more aggressive clinical behavior than thymomas, akin to carcinomas arising in the lung and other locations.[15,27,37-39]

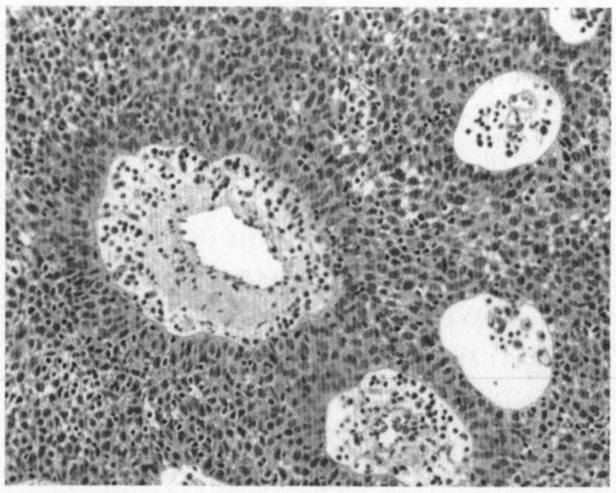

Figure 80-4 ■ Photomicrograph of thymoma at higher power showing the tumor cells arranged around blood vessels, in a characteristic perivascular growth pattern. The tumor cells are polygonal, with minimal cytologic atypia. They are admixed with small mature lymphocytes (H&E; x100).

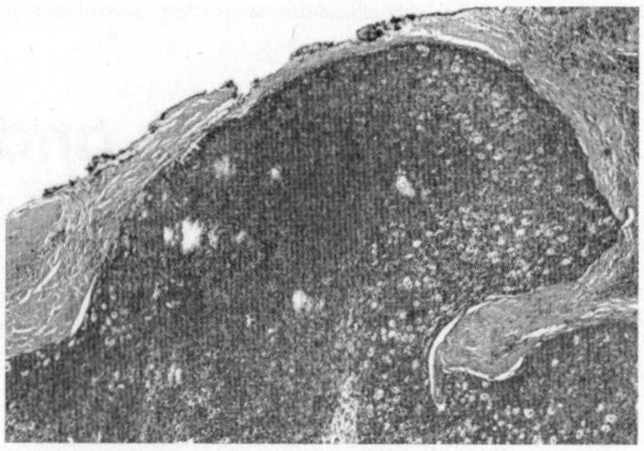

Figure 80-5 ■ Photomicrograph of a thymoma showing invasion of the capsule (H&E; x40).

The WHO classification system designates the lesions composed predominantly of spindle epithelial cells as thymoma A (Fig. 80-6 and Fig. 80-7).[19,20,35,40] Patients with thymoma A have a lower incidence of myasthenia gravis than those with other thymoma histologic types and a greater incidence of aplastic anemia. Tumors composed of polygonal epithelial cells are designated as thymoma B while neoplasms containing variable proportions of both spindle and polygonal epithelial cells are classified as thymoma AB. Thymoma B is further subclassified into B1, B2, and B3 lesions. B1 thymomas are composed of inconspicuous polygonal epithelial cells admixed with a large number of mature lymphocytes. These lesions have been designated in the past as lymphocyte-predominant thymomas because of the sparsity of visible epithelial cells in histologic sections stained with hematoxylin and eosin (H&E) and can be particularly difficult to distinguish from lymphomas without the aid of immunostains. B2 thymomas are composed of polygonal cells that are more conspicuous than those seen in B1 lesions and frequently exhibit slight nuclear variability and focally prominent nucleoli (Fig 80.8). B3 thymomas, classified in other schema as "atypical thymoma" are composed of polygonal or spindled epithelial cells that exhibit moderate variability in

Table 80-2 **World Health Organization Classification of Thymomas**

Type A (Spindle cell; medullary)
Type AB (Mixed)
Type B1 (Lymphocyte-rich, lymphocytic; predominantly cortical; organoid)
Type B2 (Cortical)
Type B3 (Epithelial; atypical; squamoid; Well differentiated carcinoma)
Micronodular Thymoma
Metaplastic Thymoma
Microscopic Thymoma
Sclerosing Thymoma

cell size and shape (anisocytosis), focal nuclear hyperchromasia and cytologic atypia. B3 thymomas characteristically have fewer lymphocytes than seen in B1 and B2 lesions and can be difficult to distinguish from low-grade thymic carcinomas. The terminology "well-differentiated thymic carcinoma" has been used inconsistently in the literature.

Thymomas are frequently heterogenous neoplasms and can exhibit different WHO "types" on different sections taken from the same lesion.[31]

Immunohistochemistry and Other Ancillary Techniques The epithelial cells of thymomas exhibit cytoplasmic immunoreactivity to keratin AE1/AE3, a feature that is generally very helpful to confirm the diagnosis of thymoma on needle biopsies and other pathologic materials (Fig. 80-9).[18,26,41] A variety of other epitopes have been shown in the different WHO histologic types of thymomas, such as laminin, collagen IV, metallothionein, PE-53, cytokeratins such as CAM 5.2, CK7, CK14 and CK18, CD57, and others.[9,17,18,42-44] However, they have limited diagnostic value and are not helpful to stratify thymomas into various WHO types or to estimate prognosis. CD5 is an immunohistochemical marker that is usually negative in thymomas other than thymoma C. However, a more recent study showed that only approximately 20% of thymic carcinomas exhibited CD5 immunoreactivity.[18] Antibodies to Foxnl and CD205 are two novel markers of thymic epithelial cells that may be useful to distinguish different thymomas and thymic carcinoma.[43] For example, Foxnl nuclear immunoreactivity has been reported as positive in all thymomas AB and B, all but one thymoma A, focally in 76% of thymic carcinomas, and 13% of cutaneous squamous cell carcinomas. This marker is negative in squamous cell carcinomas of other origins. CD205 cytoplasmic immunoreactivity has been reported as positive in all thymomas B and AB, 89% of thymoma A, and 59% of thymic carcinomas.[43] It is less specific for thymic differentiation than Foxnl and can be expressed in 27% of head and neck squamous cells carcinomas, few lung tumors, and other neoplasms.

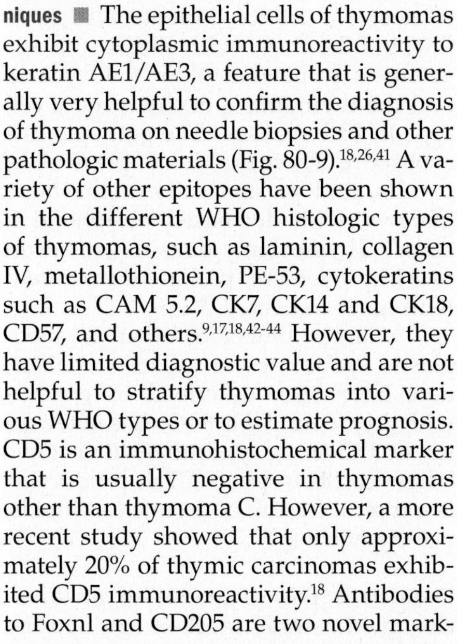

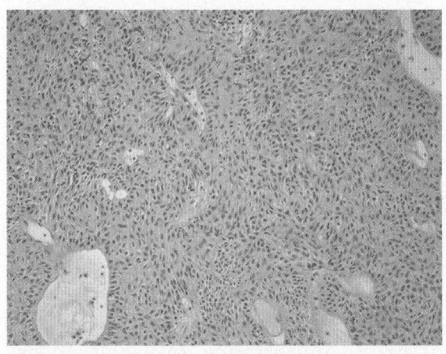

Figure 80-6 Photomicrograph of spindle cell thymoma (thymoma A). The tumor cells have elongated nuclei. Note the paucity of mature lymphocytes (H&E; x100).

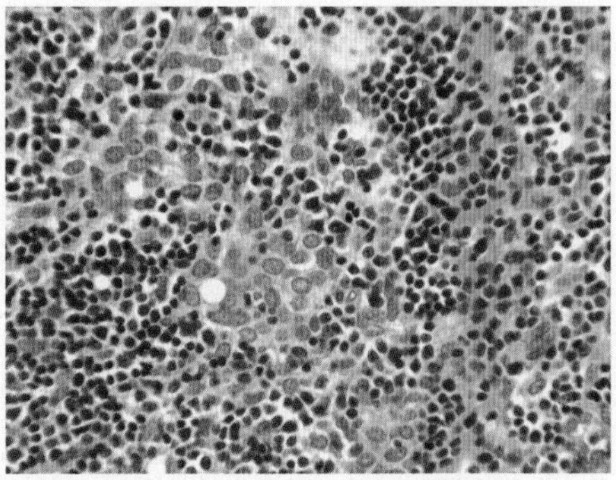

Figure 80-7 Photomicrograph of thymoma A showing small polygonal epithelial cells with round nuclei, lack of visible nucleoli and scanty cytoplasm. They are admixed with numerous lymphocytes (H&E; x200).

Electron microscopy is seldom used for the routine diagnosis of thymomas.[45,46] The tumor cells reveal ultrastructural features that are characteristic for epithelial differentiation such as desmosomes, tonofilaments, elongated cell processes, and a lack of dense core granules. The malignant epithelial cells form an irregular mesh with multiple communicating spaces and channels containing mature lymphomas and resembling the normal ultrastructural features and microenvironment of the thymus gland. Few studies have addressed the genetic changes of thymomas.[47-49] The most common genetic abnormality was loss of heterozygosity in the region of chromosome 6q23.3-25,3, which occurred in 45.8% of 26 thymomas.[50] Alterations of tp53 were found in 2 of 17 cases of benign thymomas vs 11 of 18 cases of malignant thymomas and 7 of 9 cases of thymic carcinomas.[51] In another study, tp53 protein expression was seen in only 1 of 17 thymomas vs 14 of 19 cases of thymic carcinomas.[52] An inverse correlation between tp53 and bcl-2 protein expression has been described in thymomas.[53]

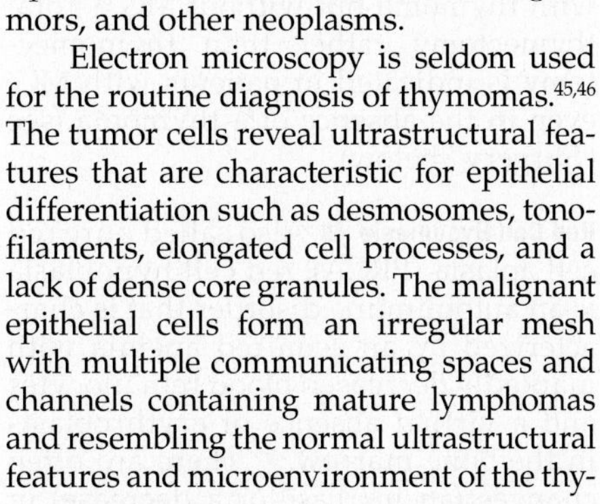

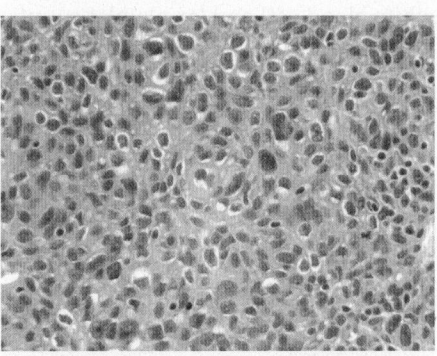

Figure 80-8 Photomicrograph of thymoma B3 (so-called atypical thymoma). The tumor cells exhibit considerable variation in size and shape, hyperchromasia and somewhat irregular nuclear membranes. There are relatively few lymphocytes in the background (H&E; x200).

Histologic Prognostic Features in Thymomas Thymomas A (spindle cell thymomas) have been considered as benign lesions in the past, but this concept is not supported by descriptions of patients with these lesions that develop recurrences and/or progression of their disease.[9,54] Marino et al and Muller-Hermelink et al have postulated that the classification of thymomas into cortical, medullary, and mixed differentiation lesions reflective of the anatomy of the normal thymus may have prognostic significance.[55,56] In their view, patients with medullary and mixed thymomas usually show a lower incidence of local invasiveness and recurrences and better survival rates than patient with cortical thymomas, even in the presence of capsular invasion. Patients with medullary and mixed thymomas also have a lower incidence of myasthenia gravis than those with cortical thymomas. However, the inter-observer reproducibility and prognostic value the Marino and Muller-Hermelink classification of thymomas have been controversial and this schema is not routinely used for the classification of thymomas in most U.S. hospitals.[40]

The prognostic value of nuclear deoxyribonucleic acid (DNA) content

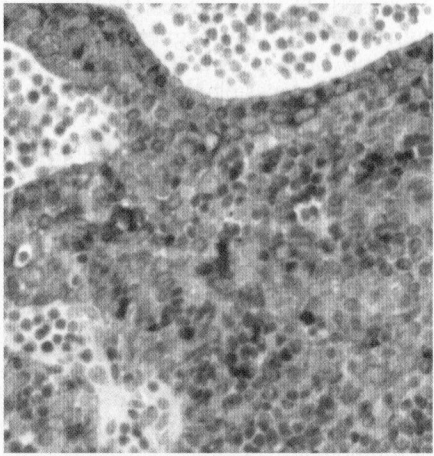

Figure 80-9 The epithelial cells of thymomas exhibit cytoplasmic immunoreactivity when stained for keratin AE1/AE2 (Immunostain; x200).

measured by flow cytometry is also controversial.[57] Although the percentage of cells in the S phase does not appear to have any prognostic significance, other studies have found that aneuploidy correlates with poorer survival.[57] For example in one study the 5-year survival rate was 91% for 11 patients with diploid thymomas and only 23% for 12 patients with aneuploid thymomas.[58]

Clinical Features of Thymomas

Most tumor-related symptoms are vague (cough, dyspnea, chest pain) or secondary to local and regional mediastinal spread (pleural effusion, superior vena cava syndrome, or pericardial effusion) and, therefore, often indicate invasiveness. Occasionally, thymomas may present as diffuse pleural tumors and simulate malignant mesothelioma.[59] About half of thymomas occur in asymptomatic persons and are discovered fortuitously on a chest radiograph, which shows a retrosternal mass in the anterosuperior mediastinum forming a bulge in the cardiovascular silhouette. The tumor may be best seen on oblique and lateral views. Computed tomography (CT) is invaluable for detecting small thymomas and assessing possible invasion of surrounding structures, such as the mediastinum, pleura, and pericardium. It can show calcifications in or at the periphery of the tumor in approximately 20% of cases,[60] although they bear no relation to invasiveness. The presence of a fat plane all around the tumor is a good sign of noninvasiveness, but, conversely, fibrous adherence to surrounding structures may simulate invasion.[61] CT can also help differentiate thymomas from vascular structures and tumors, such as aneurysms, particularly when intravenous contrast is used.[61] Thymomas show increased T1- and T2-weighted image signal intensity by magnetic resonance imaging, but the role of that technique in detecting possible capsular and vascular invasion, compared with CT, needs further study.[61] The use of positron emission tomography with 18-fluorodeoxyglucose to distinguish malignant from benign mediastinal tumors has been evaluated.[62] Thymic carcinomas and invasive thymomas show high uptake, whereas noninvasive thymomas show low uptake. It should be emphasized, however, that surgical exploration and pathologic evaluation remain the most reliable means to assess the invasiveness of thymomas.

Associated Paraneoplastic Syndromes

A remarkable number of paraneoplastic syndromes are associated with thymomas. They are mostly related to autoimmune mechanisms and are dominated by three characteristic entities (Table 80-3).

Myasthenia Gravis ■ Myasthenia gravis (MG) occurs in approximately 33-50% of patients with thymoma, and approximately 10% of patients who have MG have a thymoma.[1,63] Such patients are usually older than those with MG without thymoma, although the clinical signs of MG are similar in both groups. Few features distinguish the histologic appearance of thymomas in patients with MG; predominantly spindle cell thymomas are rare in this group, and the surrounding thymic tissue reveals the presence of lymphoid follicles with germinal centers in approximately 50% of the cases (vs only 5-8% of cases involving thymomas without MG).[1] MG is an autoimmune disorder that is characterized by the presence of antibodies to the acetylcholine receptors of the neuromuscular junction. Such serum antibodies are found in 90% of patients with generalized MG.[61] The triggering mechanisms are unknown. Myoid cells in the normal thymus raise the possibility of in situ sensitization.[64] Serum striational antibodies directed against elements of the sarcomere, such as titin, are found in 80% of patients with MG and thymoma and in 25% of patients with thymoma but without MG.[61] Total thymectomy rather than thymomectomy is indicated in patients with MG, even in the absence of a thymoma (see "Surgery" below).

Red Call Hypoplasia ■ Also called pure red cell aplasia (PRCA), red cell hypoplasia is an autoimmune disorder that is characterized by an acquired anemia with markedly decreased blood reticulocytes and a virtual absence of erythroblasts in the bone marrow.[1,65] There are often changes (an increase or a decrease) in white blood cell and/or platelet counts. PRCA is seen in approximately 5% of patients with thymoma, but 50% of patients with PRCA have a thymoma, which is of the spindle cell type in two-thirds of these patients.[1] PRCA generally occurs in patients older than 40 years of age who have thymoma, and the incidence of local invasion is not different from other thymomas. The bone marrow is usually quite cellular, and erythropoietin levels are typically high.[65] An immunoglobulin (Ig)G inhibitor of erythroblastic growth has been described in the serum of some patients.[65] Thymectomy produces remission of the anemia in approximately 30% of cases.[65] Corticosteroids and immunosuppressive agents are also effective. Recently, a prolonged complete remission (with tumor regression) was described in one case with the combination of octreotide and prednisone.[66]

Table 80-3 ■ **Thymomas: Associated Disorders**

Myasthenia gravis	Lymphomas
Red cell aplasia	Kaposi sarcoma
Hypogammaglobulinemia	Eaton-Lambert syndrome
Collagen diseases	Nephrotic syndrome
Sjögren's syndrome	Endocrine disorders
Pemphigus	
Cancer (nonthymic)	
Leukemias	

Source: Adapted from Ref. 101.

Hypogammaglobulinomia ■ First reported by Good in 1954,[67] this acquired syndrome results in extreme susceptibility to recurrent, and often serious, infections.[68] It occurs in approximately 5-10% of patients with thymoma, and a thymoma is found in 10% of patients with acquired hypogammaglobulinemia.[1,60] There is a decrease in all major Igs, particularly IgG and IgA, and decreased eosinophils in the blood and bone marrow. A combined deficit in cell-mediated immunity can also be seen. Almost a third of patients also have PRCA. Like those with PRCA, the age group is somewhat older (>40 years), and the thymoma is of the spindle cell type in 75% of cases.[1] The pathogenesis is obscure. There is a lack of pre-B cells, B cells, and plasma cells in the bone marrow, with decreased peripheral B cells.[68] Thymectomy does not result in any improvement; palliative treatment with Igs is indicated.[68]

A large number of other paraneoplastic syndromes or associated disorders have been described in patients with thymoma (Table 80-3). It is noteworthy that Cushing syndrome with ectopic adrenocorticotropin (ACTH) production is a typical feature of thymic carcinoids, not thymomas.[1,69]

Diagnosis ■ The diagnosis of an anterior mediastinal mass is guided by the clinical suspicion of its etiology. Invasive incisional biopsy techniques, with mediastinoscopy or mediastinotomy for thymoma, carry the risk of violating the tumor capsule and disseminating tumor cells.[70] Otherwise, percutaneous fine-needle aspiration or core biopsy under fluoroscopic or CT guidance is generally considered safe and effective. Combined with special stains and electron microscopy, if necessary, it has a sensitivity of 80% and specificity greater than 90%.[60] It is of prime importance, however, to establish a firm pathologic diagnosis in view of the many other tumor types that may require specific therapies, as discussed below.

Other Thymic Tumors

Thymic Carcinomas

Thymic Carcinomas are epithelial tumors comprising approximately 0.06% of thymic neoplasms and composed of epithelial cells that exhibit cytologic features characteristic of malignancy, such as considerable pleomorphism, hyperchromasia, prominent nucleoli, increased mitotic activity and/or necrosis.[27,37,71] The terms "carcinoma" and "thymoma" have been used inconsistently in the literature and both neoplasms are currently considered as malignant, although patients with thymic carcinoma have a considerably more guarded prognosis. Thymic carcinomas are unusual, and for example, only 16 cases have been seen at the Mayo Clinic in 75 years.[27] Approximately 300 cases including multiple histologic types have been reported in the literature. Squamous cell carcinomas are probably the most frequent variant of these neoplasms and other forms of thymic carcinomas such as mucoepidermoid carcinoma, clear cell carcinoma, adenocarcinoma and others have been reported as case reports or small series. Lymphoepithelioma of the thymus is a particularly interesting variant of thymic carcinoma frequently associated with the Epstein–Barr virus (EBV) expression and exhibits similar histopathologic features to those seen in the head and neck area.[72,73] One of us (APC) reported, in 1985, the first case of such a thymic carcinoma associated with EBV.[4,74] That 19-year-old male patient had a serologic profile similar to that of patients with EBV-associated pharyngeal carcinoma, with elevated antibody titers to the viral capsid antigen (VCA) (IgG and IgA anti-VCA), to the diffuse components of the early antigen (IgG anti-D), and to EBV nuclear antigen. Moreover, hybridization techniques detected an average of 49 EBV genomes per tumor cell. Another such case was reported in 1988 in a 30-year-old woman.[75] The embryologic origin of the thymus from the primitive pharynx further reinforces a possible unified theory about the pathogenesis of lymphoepithelioma-like carcinomas of the pharynx and the thymus.[4] Since then, other investigators have demonstrated the presence of EBV genomes in cases of lymphoepithelioma-like thymic carcinoma, but the role of EBV in other thymic tumors (thymomas and other types of thymic carcinomas) is not established.[76-78] Carcinoma with t(15;19) translocation is a recently described aggressive variant of thymic carcinomas that affects children and young adults.[79]

The prognosis of patients with thymic carcinomas is worse than the outcome of patients with thymoma. The overall 5-year survival rate of 60 cases of thymic carcinoma was 33.3%.[80] Patients with a low-grade histology did much better than those with a high-grade histology.

Thymic Carcinoid and Neuroendocrine Tumors

Carcinoid tumors can arise in the thymus and were distinguished from thymomas in 1972.[1,69] They are currently classified by WHO as thymic neuroendocrine carcinomas because they are more aggressive than their counterparts in the lung and other organs. Indeed extrathoracic metastases are present in 30-40% of cases of primary thymic carcinoid tumor at diagnosis. The association with Cushing syndrome with ectopic ACTH production in a patient with a thymic tumor should raise this possibility because it occurs in 30% of patients with thymic carcinoid tumor but not in patients with thymoma.[1,69] Other paraneoplastic syndromes, such as osteoarthropathy and Eaton-Lambert syndrome, and an association with multiple endocrine neoplasia (type I or II) have been described.[69] Carcinoid syndrome has not been reported. Thymic neuroendocrine carcinomas are subclassified into well-differentiated lesions, including typical carcinoid and atypical carcinoid and poorly differentiated neuroendocrine carcinomas including large cell neuroendocrine carcinoma and small cell carcinoma, neuroendocrine type. All these lesions exhibit histopathologic features at low-power microscopy characteristic of neuroendocrine differentiation, including the formation of cellular nests, trabeculae and pseudorosettes. The tumor cells vary according to the cell type. Carcinoid tumors are composed of round to elongated nuclei with "salt-and-pepper" nuclear chromatin, variable hyperchromasia and minimal pleomorphism. Typical carcinoid tumors usually lack mitosis and necrosis while atypical carcinoid tumors exhibit low mitotic activity and focal areas of necrosis. Large cell neuroendocrine carcinoma of the thymus are composed of large, pleomorphic, hyperchromatic cells that can exhibit focally prominent nucleoli.[84] Small cell carcinomas of the thymus are composed of small hyperchromatic cells with nuclear molding and inconspicuous nucleoli.[85] Both variants of high-grade thymic neuroendocrine carcinomas exhibit frequent mitosis, usually higher than 10 mitosis in 10 high power fields and extensive areas of necrosis.[86] The tumor cells of all variants of thymic neuroendocrine carcinoma exhibit cytoplasmic immunoreactivity to chromogranin and synaptophysin and dense core neuroendocrine granules under electron microscopy. Immunostains for Ki-67 can be used to estimate the proliferative fraction of these lesions.

Thymic Lymphomas

Lymphomas are, with thymomas, the most common tumors of the thymus. Although the thymus is a T-cell organ, the most frequent lymphomas of the thymus in adult patients are Hodgkin lymphoma and B-cell lymphomas.[87-91] Primary Hodgkin lymphoma of the thymus tends to be limited to the gland and is, as a rule, of the nodular sclerosis type.[69,92-94] It is frequently associated with cystic change in the adjacent thymic tissue. B-cell lymphomas of the mediastinum frequently involve the thymus and lymph nodes and frequently exhibit histologic features that are unusual for B-cell lesions in other locations, such as sclerosis with compartmentalization of the tumor cells, clear cell features, and focal formation of cellular nests simulating an epithelial malignancy.[89,91,92] They tend to follow an aggressive clinical course. Lymphomas involving the thymus and mediastinal lymph nodes in children include Burkitt's lymphoma, and lymphoblastic lymphoma, a lesion of T-cell origin. It is of prime importance to differentiate a lymphoma from a thymoma in view of the different therapeutic approaches. Special stains and electron microscopy may be necessary in difficult cases.

Germ Cell Tumors of the Thymus

The thymus is a classic site of extragonadal primary germ cell tumors. This may be explained by the proximity of the urogenital ridge to the primitive pharynx in the embryo.[1,69] The most common ones are seminomas (sometimes difficult to differentiate from thymoma) and teratomas (mature or immature).[95,96] Almost every type of germ cell tumor, however, has been reported in the thymus, either in a pure or mixed form, including embryonal carcinomas, yolk sac tumors, teratocarcinomas, and choriocarcinomas.[95] Most of these tumors occur in men in their twenties or thirties, although mature teratomas occur with equal frequency in males and females.[69] Testicular examination (by palpation and sonography) fails to reveal a tumor, confirming an extragonadal origin. It is of prime importance to recognize germ cell tumors of the thymus and to distinguish them from thymomas because of the therapeutic implications. A liberal practice of obtaining serum markers, including alpha-fetoprotein and human chorionic gonadotropin, may help identify a germ cell tumor in patients otherwise diagnosed as having undifferentiated carcinoma of the mediastinum.[97,98] Tissue staining for such markers should also be performed and can be positive even when serum levels are normal. Germ cell tumors are highly responsive to radiotherapy (RT) (seminomas) or chemotherapy, although the overall results and long-term survival are usually inferior to those of corresponding testicular primary tumors.

Other Thymic Tumors

Other thymic tumors include thymolipomas, which may become quite large, thymic cysts, metastases to the thymus and other neoplasms listed in Table 80-1.

Staging of Thymomas

Stage and completeness of excision have been shown to be the most reliable prognostic features for patients with thymomas. The modified Masaoka staging system is generally used.[99] It divides the lesions into stages I-IV (Table 80-4). A recent meta-analysis has shown that patients with thymomas in stage I and II have similar prognosis, ranging from 84% to 100% 10-year survival rates.[36,71] Patients with stage III and IV have a higher incidence of local recurrence, pleural invasion and/or distant metastases with 10-year survival rates of 30-50%. Metastases in thymomas patients are usually intrathoracic (pleura, pericardium) and may represent direct implants from the primary lesion. Extrathoracic and embolic metastases were so rare that only 12 cases were collected from the literature in 1971.[100] In more recent series, however, extrathoracic metastases to the bone, liver, lymph nodes, and other organs were seen in up to 45% of patients, probably as a result of referral selection, a longer survival, or better imaging techniques.[100]

Differential Diagnosis of Anterosuperior Mediastinal Tumors

Although thymic neoplasms are by far the most common tumors of the anterosuperior mediastinum in adult patients, other mass lesions in that location include thyroid or parathyroid tumors, lymphomas, Castleman disease, mediastinal germ cell tumors, aneurysms, myxomas, lipomas, solitary fibrous tumor, paragangliomas, thymic and bronchogenic cysts and rarely sarcomas.[46,101] Lymphomas can be difficult to distinguish from thymomas on needle biopsies, particularly from B1 lesions. Thymoma A can be difficult to distinguish from solitary fibrous tumor, hemangiopericytoma and other mesenchymal lesions composed of spindle cells. Thymoma C can be difficult to distinguish from primary thymic carcinomas and metastases. Carcinomas usually exhibit greater nuclear atypia, mitoses and necrosis, histologic features that are usually absent or present only focally in thymoma C.

Table 80-4 ■ **Staging of Thymomas**

Stage	Extent of Disease	No. of Cases	Read: Survival (%)	
			5 Years	10 Years
I	Totally encapsulated	37	96	67
II	Microscopic or macroscopic capsular invasion into surrounding fat or mediastinal pleura	13	86	60
III	Invasion of surrounding organs (pericardium, lung, great vessels)	32	70	58
IV	(A) Pleural or pericardial implants (B) Embolic metastasis	11	50	0

Source: Adapted from Ref. 99.

Therapy

Surgery

Because there are no reliable histologic criteria for the malignant nature of thymomas, all such tumors should be considered potentially malignant. Total thymectomy (rather than thymomectomy) is the procedure of choice, even for stage I encapsulated tumors.[60,102] It is also the procedure indicated for patients with MG, with or without thymoma. The usual approach is by median sternotomy, although additional thoracic or cervical incisions may be necessary, and some surgeons advocate maximal thymectomy with exploration of all of the possible areas in which ectopic thymic tissue might be found.[14] There is a need for the surgeon to carefully explore the mediastinum for evidence of local invasion, which is the most reliable indication of malignancy and the most important prognostic factor. The tumor capsule should not be breached. Systematic microscopic examination is necessary to search for capsular invasion and to distinguish it from simple adhesions. Following total thymectomy, the recurrence rate is usually low (about 2%) for stage I encapsulated thymomas.[1] Recently, video thoracoscopic approaches were performed for well-encapsulated small thymomas, 49 but the long-term results are unknown.[103]

In patients with thymoma and MG, remission of MG occurs in approximately 10-30% following thymectomy, often after a delay of up to 2 years or more, compared with a remission rate of approximately 40-80% after thymectomy for MG without a thymoma.[1,60,102,104,105] An additional fraction of patients show improvement of MG. Early thymectomy (within 1 year) after onset of MG is associated with a higher percentage of less invasive thymomas.[106] Recurrence, and even first occurrence, of MG after apparent total thymectomy has been observed and could be related to tumor regrowth or persistent ectopic thymic tissue.[60] In the past, MG was a poor prognostic sign in patients with thymoma. Most recent surgical series, however, do not show a significant difference in survival for patients with thymoma, with or without MG.[99,102,107,108] Such a change is attributed to better surgical and anesthesia techniques, which have largely prevented postoperative deaths from MG.

Local invasion is seen in approximately 30-40% of thymomas at surgery,[99,107,108] but the slow-growing nature of the tumor and the rarity of distant metastases justify attempts at radical surgery. Identification of the phrenic, recurrent laryngeal, and vagus nerves is of major importance.[14] Extended resections—including one lung, one phrenic nerve, pericardium, or even resection and repair of great vessels, such as the innominate vein or superior vena cava—have been performed. They should be undertaken only if they lead to complete tumor resection. Radiotherapy is indicated in cases of invasive thymoma. With modern techniques of peri- and postsurgical care, surgical mortality is low (0-5%), even in patients with MG.[99,104,108]

In four large series with a total of 744 patients, the 5- and 10-year survival rates were 75-85% and 63-80%, respectively, for patients with noninvasive encapsulated thymomas.[99,107,108] Survival figures for patients with invasive thymomas were 50-67% at 5 years and 30-53% at 10 years. Whereas invasiveness is the major prognostic factor in patients with thymoma, most series also report a better prognosis for spindle cell thymomas and those with a higher ratio of lymphocytes to epithelial cells.[99,107,108] Local recurrences and/or metastases (often intrathoracic) may also be amenable to surgical resection.

Radiotherapy

Thymomas are radiosensitive, and the efficacy of radiotherapy (RT) has been emphasized in many reports. Following surgical biopsy, or partial excision, survival of more than 10 years after RT has been seen.[100] Most authors do not believe that it is only the lymphocytic component rather than the epithelial one that is sensitive to RT.[100]

The role of RT is best discussed according to stage. For stage I disease following total surgical resection, postoperative RT is not indicated in view of the very low relapse rates. For stages II and III disease, the use of postoperative RT is recommended even after total surgical resection.[60,99,102,107,109] In a review of the literature, as well as their own experience, Curran and colleagues reported a 28% intrathoracic relapse rate after complete surgical resection without RT, as opposed to 5% when postoperative RT was given.[110] The latter figure may be unusual, however, because others have reported no such differences in favor of RT after complete surgical resection.[3] The systematic use of RT after complete resection has been recently questioned particularly for stage II patients, but the small number of cases and the retrospective nature of the collected data as well selection of patients do not allow a definitive conclusion in the absence of prospective randomized trials. The irradiated volume should include the mediastinum with adjacent areas and probably the supraclavicular areas, which are possible sites of relapse.[100] The total dose is usually about 45 Gy, with appropriate protection of the spinal cord, although doses of 50 Gy and higher have been given.[100,110] Radiation pneumonitis, mediastinitis, pericarditis, coronary artery fibrosis, hypothyroidism as well as secondary cancers are potential complications.

RT is also given to patients with residual disease, following biopsy only or incomplete surgical resection for stage III disease. In 20 such cases, Curran and colleagues observed 4 mediastinal recurrences and 5 others outside the mediastinum, whereas no local relapse was seen when RT was given after total surgical resection for stage II or III disease.[110] Partial tumor debulking by surgery prior to RT in patients with stage III or IV disease does not appear to be beneficial.[111] The 5-year survival rate for such patients was 45% overall, including 61% for stage III and 23% for stage IV disease after RT. Collaboration between the surgeon and the radiotherapist is essential to delineate areas of tumor involvement by radiopaque clips and to plan the treatment.

Chemotherapy

Thymomas are relatively chemosensitive. As experience with chemotherapy is increasing, good response rates and sometimes dramatic tumor regressions have been observed.[112]

Single Agents for Thymomas The rarity of thymomas precludes knowledge of the efficacy of many agents.[100,113] The two most commonly used and most active known single agents are cisplatin and corticosteroid therapy (Table 80-5).[100,114-125] In the literature, of 28 patients treated with cisplatin at various doses (up to 130 mg/m²), there were three complete and six partial responses, for a response rate of 32%. A rather low dose of cisplatin (50 mg/m² every 3 weeks) was used in 21 of these patients as part of an Eastern Cooperative Oncology Group trial.[121] Only two partial responses were seen, raising the possibility of a dose-response relationship. The occurrence of complete responses and the long duration of some responses (over 20 months) further indicate that cisplatin is an effective agent. Corticosteroid therapy, either as ACTH or glucocorticoids, is effective in inducing tumor regression in patients with invasive or metastatic thymoma. The thymolytic effects of these drugs, especially for cortical lymphocytes, have been reported even in relatively corticosteroid-resistant species, such as humans.[100] The relative role of this lympholytic effect vs a direct oncolytic effect on the neoplastic epithelial cells of thymomas remains to be determined. It is of note, however, that glucocorticoid receptors have been found in the cytosol of human thymoma cells,[126] including those with a pure epithelial histology,[127] suggesting a possible direct antineoplastic effect. In 13 reported patients, there were 2 complete and 9 partial responses or improvement from steroid therapy (Table 80-5). Some of these responses were long-lived (23-36 months) or could be reinduced by resumption of higher daily doses after relapse.[128]

The efficacy of other single agents is largely anecdotal. Ifosfamide, at a dose of 1.5 g/m² daily for 5 days every 3 weeks with mesna, has been evaluated in 13 patients, with 5 complete responses (38%) with a median duration of response of 66+ months and 1 partial response.[129] Doxorubicin has produced regressions of short duration in two of three patients. The taxanes have not been evaluated.

Since thymomas express somatostatin receptors, as shown by radiolabeled octreotide scan, a trial of octreotide at a dose of 0.5 mg subcutaneously three times daily was undertaken by the Eastern Cooperative Oncology Group.[125] Patients were evaluated at 2 months, and those who responded continued on octreotide alone for a maximum of 1 year, whereas those who progressed were given prednisone 0.6 mg/kg orally per day in addition to octreotide for a maximum of 1 year. Of 32 evaluable patients with thymoma, there were 2 complete (6%) and 10 partial (31%) objective responses. Of these, 4 partial responses (12.5%) were observed on octreotide alone. None of an additional 6 patients (5 thymic carcinomas and 1 thymic carcinoid) responded. The overall 1- and 2-year survival rates were 86.6% and 75.7%, respectively.

Combination Chemotherapy of Thymomas Various regimens of combination chemotherapy have been reported in small numbers of patients.[100,113] The overall cumulative response rate for cisplatin-containing regimens is 68%, with 22% complete responses (Table 80-6)[100,130-143] which is not much different from regimens without cisplatin (65% response with 35% complete responses) (Table 80-7).[144-151] In the absence of prospective randomized trials, there is no basis to recommend one regimen over another.

These results are highly encouraging because many patients experienced prolonged responses. Patients with thymoma and severe MG that is resistant to conventional medical therapy can

Table 80-5 **Single Agents in Thymoma**

Agent (Ref.)	Patients (*n*)	CR	PR	Response Duration (Months)	Survival (Months)
Cisplatin (118-124)	1	1	-	13	-
	1	1	-	10+	-
	1	-	1	4	13
	1	-	1	1	-
	1	1	-	20+	-
	1	1[a]	-	24	24+
	1	-	1	1	-
	21	0	2	-	-
Steroids[b] (126-128)	12	2	8	-	-
	1	-	1	23	-
Ifosfamide (129)	13	5	1	66+	-
Maytansine (1)	4	0	2	1.5, 4.5	-
Doxorubicin (146,153)	3	0	2	-	-
Vincristine (146,153)	2	0	0	-	-
Chlorambucil (146,153)	2	0	0	-	-
Nitrogen mustard (146,153)	1	0	0	-	-
Octreotide	32	0	4	-	-
+ Prednisone (125)	21	2	6	-	-

[a]With radiotherapy.
[b]Adrenocorticotropin or corticosteroids.
Abbreviations: CR, complete responses; PR, partial response.

Table 80-6 ■ Combination Chemotherapy With Cisplatin in Thymoma

Regimen (Ref.)	Patients (n)	Response Type	Duration (Months)
BAPP (100,134)	9a	1 CR, 5 PR[a]	6–37+
CAP (114,135,137)	1	1 CR	12+
	29	3 CR, 12 PR	Med. 11.8
	23	5 CR, 11 PR	
CAP ± prednisone (115,138)	6a	2 CR, 3 PR	4–49+
	13	3 CR, 8 PR	
	22	3 CR, 14 PR	
AP (139-141)	1	1 PR	6
	1	1 PR	3
	2	2 CR	4+, 12+
EP (142)	16	5 CR, 4 PR	Med. 41
PVB (143)	5	2 CR	48+, 72+
		2 PR	3, 9
ADOC (144)	32	15 CR, 14 PR	Med. 11
VIP (145)	28	9 PR	Med. 11.9
Total	188	42 CR (22%), 87 PR (46%)	

[a]Includes one patient with thymic carcinoma.

Abbreviations: ADOC, Adriamycin (doxorubicin), cisplatin, Oncovin (vincristine), and cyclophosphamide; AP, Adriamycin (doxorubicin) and cisplatin; BAPP, bleomycin, Adriamycin (doxorubicin), cisplatin, and prednisone; CAP, cyclophosphamide, Adriamycin (doxorubicin), and cisplatin; CR, complete response; EP, etoposide and cisplatin; PR, partial response; PVB, cisplatin, vinblastine, and bleomycin; VIP, etoposide, ifosfamide, and cisplatin.

Table 80-7 ■ Combination Chemotherapy Without Cisplatin in Thymoma

Regimon (Ref.)	Patients (n)	Response Type	Duration (Months)
MVPV (146)	2	2 PR	0.8, 3
ACVB (146)	1	1 PR	2
COPP (147)	5	4 PR[a]	
DC (149)	1	1 CR	13
VCC ± prednisons (150)	9	4 CR	31–62
		1 PR	2
CAV (148)	4[b]	1 CR	12+
		3 PR	4–9
CHOP (151)	1	1 CR	12
CHOP ± bleomycin (161)	13	5 CR	
COP ± procarbazine (161)	6	3 CR, 1 PR	
PCb (162)	1	1 PR	
Total	43	15 CR (35%), 13 PR (30%)	

Abbreviations: ACVB, Adriamycin (doxorubicin); CAV, cyclophosphamide, Adriamycin (doxorubicin), and vincristine; CCNU, vincristine and bleomycin; CHOP, cyclophosphamide, doxorubicin, vincristine, prednisone; COP, cyclophosphamide, Oncovin (vincristins), and prednisone; COPP, cyclophosphamide, Oncovin (vincristine), prednisone, and procarbazine; CR, complete response; DC, doxorubicin and cyclophosphamide; MVPV, nitrogen mustard, vincristina, procarbazine, and vinblastine; PCb, paclitaxel and carbhoplatin; PR, partial responses; VCC, vincristine, cyclophosphamide, and CCNU.

[a]Two patients in CR for 33 and 34 months after radiotherapy was added.

[b]A fifth patient without a measurable tumor had complete remission of myasthenia gravis following chemotherapy.

sometimes benefit dramatically from chemotherapy for the relief of myasthenia symptoms. Some patients requiring ventilatory support have been weaned from the respirator just a few days after receiving chemotherapy.[148]

Chemotherapy has also been combined with RT in patients with thymoma.[152] This approach has been effective in patients with stage III disease using cyclophosphamide, Adriamycin (doxorubicin), and cisplatin (CAP). In one trial with 23 patients, the response rate was 69.6% and the median survival was 93 months.[114] In another trial, chemotherapy with CAP plus prednisone was followed by surgery and radiotherapy, leading to a 73% disease-free survival at 7 years.[115] Such studies emphasize the importance of combined-modality therapy in patients with advanced thymomas.

The effectiveness of chemotherapy in thymoma may lead to its preoperative use in patients with large or extensively invasive thymomas.[100] The management of such patients requires a combined-modality approach with chemotherapy, surgery, and RT in the most appropriate sequence, according to the individual case. In patients with unresectable thymoma, treatment with RT, chemotherapy, or both can induce tumor regression and allow surgical resection of residual disease, if any. By using this approach, complete tumor eradication was achieved in 5 of 8 patients in one study[116] and in 11 of 16 patients in another study.[117] Thus, the treatment was successful in two-thirds of the patients. This was confirmed more recently in 22 patients with Masaoka stage III or IV thymoma treated with induction Chemotherapy (modified CAP regimen plus prednisone), with a 77% response rate (14% complete response) followed by complete surgical resection in 76% of patients. This was followed by RT and chemotherapy. The overall survival at 5 years was 95%, with 77% progression-free survival.[136] Hence, excellent long-term results are within reach, and it seems justified to add invasive thymoma to the list of neoplasms that are curable even at an advanced stage.[112]

Chemotherapy of Thymic Carcinomas ■ The results of chemotherapy for thymic carcinomas are much less favorable.[153] The efficacy of single agents is virtually unknown. Cisplatin combinations, including cisplatin, etoposide, and bleomycin or cisplatin, etoposide, and ifosfamide, have been evaluated in very small numbers of patients, with response rates of 20-60%.[153,154] Single case reports have shown good results with various regimens, including combinations of bleomycin, doxorubicin, cisplatin, and prednisone,[4] or of bleomycin, vinblastine and cisplatin, or of 5-fluorouracil, methotrexate with cisplatin or doxorubicin and cisplatin, as well as irinotecan alone.[153]

Targeted Therapies ■ Recently, genetic studies have revealed that KIT (CD117), a tyrosine kinase receptor, is frequently overexpressed in thymic carcinomas (86% positivity), whereas it is absent in thymomas or normal thymus.[155] Of interest is the fact that a patient with a poorly differentiated epidermoid thymic carcinoma harboring mutations of KIT similar to those seen in gastrointestinal stromal tumors (in-frame deletion in exon 11) experienced a response to imatinib (400 mg/day) for about 6 months.[156] A personal patient of one of us (APC) also with a poorly differentiated squamous thymic carcinoma positive for C-KIT by immunohistochemistry and heavily pretreated with chemotherapy failed to respond to imatinib, however. Dasatinib has been reported to induce a partial resolution in a patient with B2 type thymoma who also had lymphoid blast crisis of chronic myeloid leukemia, the latter being previously treated with imatinib.[157] Thymomas often express epidermal growth factor receptor, but mutations are rare.[158] Three patients with thymoma have been reported to respond to cetuximab.[159,160] The activity of targeted agents deserve future trials in this disease.

Selected References

The complete reference list can be found at www.CANCERMEDICINE8.com

1. Rosai J, Levine GD. Tumors of the thymus. In: *Atlas of Tumor Pathology*. 2nd Series. Fascicle 13. Washington DC: Armed Forces Institute of Pathology; 1976.
2. Givel JC. Historical review. In: Givel JC, Merlini M, Clarke DB, Dusmet M, editors. *Surgery of the Thymus. Pathology, Associated*

Disorders and Surgical Technique. Berlin: Springer-Verlag; 1990:1.
4. Leyvraz S, Henle H, Chahinian AP, et al. Association of Epstein-Barr virus with thymic carcinoma. *N Engl J Med.* 1985;312:1296.
12. Dhall G, Ginsburg HB, Bodenstein L, et al. Thymoma in children: report of two cases and review of literature. *J Pediatr Hematol Oncol.* 2004;26:681.
14. Jaretzki A III, Wolff M. "Maximal" thymectomy for myasthenia gravis. Surgical anatomy and operative technique. *J Thorac Cardiovasc Surg.* 1988;96:711.
18. Suster S. Diagnosis of thymoma. *J Clin Pathol.* 2006;59:1238.
20. Suster S, Moran CA. Histologic classification of thymoma: the World Health Organization and beyond. *Hematol Oncol Clin North Am.* 2008;22:381.
24. Marchevsky A. The mediastinum. *Pathology (Phila).* 1996;3:339.
25. Marchevsky AM, McKenna RJ, Jr., Gupta R. Thymic epithelial neoplasms: a review of current concepts using an evidence-based pathology approach. *Hematol Oncol Clin North Am.* 2008;22:543.
27. Moran CA, Suster S. Thymic carcinoma: current concepts and histologic features. *Hematol Oncol Clin North Am.* 2008;22: 393.
30. Marchevsky AM, Gupta R, McKenna RJ, et al. Evidence-based pathology and the pathologic evaluation of thymomas: the World Health Organization classification can be simplified into only 3 categories other than thymic carcinoma. *Cancer.* 2008;112:2780.
32. Chalabreysse L, Roy P, Cordier JF, et al. Correlation of the WHO schema for the classification of thymic epithelial neoplasms with prognosis: a retrospective study of 90 tumors. *Am J Surg Pathol.* 2002;26:1605.
37. Rieker RJ, Muley T, Klein C, et al. An institutional study on thymomas and thymic carcinomas: experience in 77 patients. *Thorac Cardiovasc Surg.* 2008;56:143.
39. Yano M, Sasaki H, Yokoyama T, et al. Thymic carcinoma: 30 cases at a single institution. *J Thorac Oncol.* 2008;3:265.
42. Azad NS, Ahmad Z, Ahsan A, et al. Thymoma: a clinicopathologic association of world health organization histologic subtype and invasive behaviour. *J Coll Physicians Surg Pak.* 2007;17:658.
55. Marino M, Muller-Hermelink HK. Thymoma and thymic carcinoma. Relation of thymoma epithelial cells to the cortical and medullary differentiation of thymus. *Virchows Arch A Pathol Anat Histopathol.* 1985;407:119.
56. Muller-Hermelink HK, Marino M, et al. Immunohistological evidences of cortical and medullary differentiation in thymoma. *Virchows Arch A Pathol Anat Histopathol.* 1985;408:143.
64. Drachman DB. Myasthenia gravis. *N Engl J Med.* 1994;330:1797.
67. Good RA. Agammaglobulinemia: a provocative experiment of nature. *Bull Univ Minn Hosp.* 1954;26:1.
69. Wick MR, Rosai J. Neuroendocrine, germ cell, and nonepithelial tumors. In: Givel JC, Merlini M, Clarke DB, Dusmet M, eds. *Surgery of the Thymus. Pathology, Associated Disorders and Surgical Technique.* Berlin: Springer-Verlag; 1990:109.
71. Marchevsky AM, McKenna RJ, Jr., Gupta R. Thymic epithelial neoplasms: a review of current concepts using an evidence-based pathology approach. *Hematol Oncol Clin North Am.* 2008;22:543.
74. Rosai J. Lymphoepithelioma-like thymic carcinoma: another tumor related to Epstein-Barr virus [editorial]. *N Engl J Med.* 1985;312:1320.
80. Suster S, Rosai J. Thymic carcinoma. A clinicopathologic study of 60 cases. *Cancer.* 1991;67:1025.
83. Moran CA, Suster S. Neuroendocrine carcinomas (carcinoid tumor) of the thymus. A clinicopathologic analysis of 80 cases. *Am J Clin Pathol.* 2000;114:100.
85. Rosai J, Levine G, Weber WR, Higa E. Carcinoid tumors and oat cell carcinomas of the thymus. *Pathol Annu.* 1976;11:201.
92. Davis RE, Dorfman RF, Warnke RA. Primary large-cell lymphoma of the thymus: a diffuse B-cell neoplasm presenting as primary mediastinal lymphoma. *Hum Pathol.* 1990;21:1262.
96. Moran CA, Suster S. Germ-cell tumors of the mediastinum. *Adv Anat Pathol.* 1998;5:1.
97. Fox EM, Woods RL, Tattersall MHN, McGovern VJ. Undifferentiated carcinoma in young men: the atypical teratoma syndrome. *Lancet.* 1979;1:1316.
98. Richardson RL, Schoumacher RA, Fer MF, et al. The unrecognized extragonadal germ cell cancer syndrome. *Ann Intern Med.* 1981;94:181.
99. Masaoka A, Monden Y, Nakahara K, Tanioka T. Follow-up study of thymomas with special reference to their clinical stages. *Cancer.* 1981;48:2485.
100. Chahinian AP, Bhardwaj S, Meyer RJ, et al. Treatment of invasive or metastatic thymoma. Report of eleven cases. *Cancer.* 1981;47:1752.
101. Marchevsky A, Kaneko M. *Surgical Pathology of the Mediastinum.* New York: Raven Press; 1988.
104. Jaretzki A III, Penn AS, Younger DS, et al. "Maximal" thymectomy for myasthenia gravis. Results. *J Thorac Cardiovasc Surg.* 1988;95:747.
105. Papatestas AE, Albert LI, Osserman KE, et al. Studies in myasthenia gravis: effects of thymectomy. Results on 185 patients with nonthymomatous and thymomatous myasthenia gravis 1941-1969. *Am J Med.* 1971;50:465.
107. Verley JM, Hollmann KH. Thymoma. A comparative study of clinical stages, histologic features and survival in 200 cases. *Cancer.* 1985;55:1074.
108. Maggi G, Giaccone G, Donadio M, et al. Thymomas. A review of 169 cases, with particular reference to results of surgical treatment. *Cancer.* 1986;58:765.
110. Curran WJ, Kornstein MJ, Broks JJ, Turrisi AT III. Invasive thymoma: the role of mediastinal irradiation following complete or incomplete surgical resection. *J Clin Oncol.* 1988;6:1722.
112. Holland JF. Karnofsky Memorial Lecture. Breaking the cure barrier. *J Clin Oncol.* 1983;1:75.
113. Bhardwaj S, Chahinian, AP. Chemotherapy for invasive thymomas. In: Givel JC, Merlini M, Clarke DB, Dusmet M, eds. *Surgery of the Thymus. Pathology, Associated Disorders, and Surgical Technique.* Berlin: Springer-Verlag; 1990:293.
114. Loehrer PJ, Chen M, Kim K, et al. Cisplatin, doxorubicin, and cyclophosphamide plus thoracic radiation therapy for limited-stage unresectable thymoma. An Intergroup trial. *J Clin Oncol.* 1997;15:3093.
115. Shin DM, Walsh GL, Komaki R, et al. A multidisciplinary approach to therapy for unresectable malignant thymoma. *Ann Intern Med.* 1998;129:100.
116. Kirschner PA. Reoperation for thymoma. Report of 23 cases. *Ann Thorac Surg.* 1990;49:550.
125. Loehrer PJ, Wang W, Johnson DH, Ettinger DS. Octreotide alone or with prednisone in patients with advanced thymoma and thymic carcinoma. An Eastern Cooperative Oncology Group phase II trial. *J Clin Oncol.* 2004;22:293.
129. Highley MS, Underhill CR, Parnis FX, et al. Treatment of invasive thymoma with single-agent ifosfamide. *J Clin Oncol.* 1999;17:2737.
130. Giaccone G, Ardizzoni A, Kirkpatrick A, et al. Cisplatin and etoposide combination chemotherapy for locally advanced or metastatic thymoma. A phase II study of the European Organization for Research and Treatment of Cancer Lung Cancer Cooperative Group. *J Clin Oncol.* 1996;14:814.
134. Chahinian AP, Holland, JF, Bhardwaj S. Chemotherapy for malignant thymoma. *Ann Intern Med.* 1983;99:5.
137. Loehrer PJ, Kim K, Aisner SC, et al. Cisplatin plus doxorubicin plus cyclophosphamide in metastatic or recurrent thymoma. Final results on an Intergroup trial. *J Clin Oncol.* 1994;12:1164.
142. Giaccone G, Ardizzoni A, Kirkpatrick A, et al. Cisplatin and etoposide combination chemotherapy for locally advanced or metastatic thymoma. A phase II study of the European Organization for Research and Treatment of Cancer Lung Cancer Cooperative Group. *J Clin Oncol.* 1996;14:814.
145. Loehrer PJ, Jiroutek M, Aisner S, et al. Combined etoposide, ifosfamide and cisplatin in the treatment of patients with advanced thymoma and thymic carcinoma. An Intergroup trial. *Cancer.* 2001;91:2010.
153. Chahinian AP. Chemotherapy of thymomas and thymic carcinomas. *Chest Surg Clin N Am.* 2001;11:447.

81 Tumors of the Heart and Great Vessels

Sai-Ching Jim Yeung, MD, PhD ■ Carmen Escalante, MD ■
Sarina van der Zee, MD ■ A. Philippe Chahinian, MD ■ Valentin Fuster, MD, PhD

Introduction

Primary cardiac tumors are rare, with a prevalence of less than 0.5% in autopsy series,[1-3] and three quarters of all primary cardiac tumors are benign (Table 81-1).[4,5] Pediatric tumors, most commonly hamartomas, are associated with genetic syndromes in many cases. In adults, most benign tumors are myxomas, fibroelastomas and lipomas; surgical resection is often curative. The majority of malignant primary cardiac tumors are sarcomas and lymphomas, which carry a poor prognosis despite treatment.[6] Metastases to the heart are significantly more common than primary tumors in adults.[7] While most primary tumors arise from the endocardium, followed by the myocardium and then the pericardium,[8] the latter is the most common site for metastases.[9]

Clinical Features

The clinical features of cardiac tumors frequently reflect the cardiac structure affected and the friability of the tumor rather than its histology,[9] The predominant site of common cardiac tumors is shown in the Figure 81-1.

Tumors of the endocardial surface may present with valvular dysfunction or intracavitary obstruction. Right atrial tumors can lead to tricuspid valve obstruction and symptoms of right heart failure, while left atrial tumors may present with dyspnea and orthopnea as a consequence of mitral valve obstruction. Obstruction of the coronary ostia may lead to angina. Rarely, complete cavitary obstruction may lead to sudden death, Myocardial invasion may present as arrhythmia, systolic dysfunction, or diastolic dysfunction. Pericardial involvement can present as pleuritic chest pain or cardiac tamponade. Friable tumors, such as some myxomas and papillary fibroelastomas, may present with evidence of cerebral, pulmonary, visceral or peripheral emboli. Systemic manifestations, frequently seen in myxomas as well as malignant cardiac tumors, include fever, weight loss, myalgias, arthralgias, fatigue and weakness.

Patients with cardiac tumors may present with the symptoms described above, or masses may be discovered incidentally on imaging studies, particularly when small. Physical examination may disclose a murmur, either systolic or diastolic, that varies with body position if the tumor is mobile. The characteristic "tumor plop" of a mobile tumor such as a myxoma is heard in diastole following the second heart sound and is thought to be due to the tension on the tumor stalk as the mass prolapses from atrium to ventricle or to the tumor striking the myocardium.[10] The tumor plop may be mistaken for a third heart sound or mitral opening snap. The electrocardiogram may show nonspecific ST-T abnormalities, atrial or ventricular arrhythmias, bundle branch block, or low voltage QRS complexes in the case of pericardial effusion. Chest x-ray findings include cardiomegaly and tumor calcification. Laboratory abnormalities include anemia (possibly hemolytic) or erythrocytosis, leukocytosis, thrombocytopenia,

Table 81-1 ■ **Type and Frequency of Primary Tumors of the Heart and Pericardium in Two Series From the Armed Forces Institute of Pathology**

Type	1976–1993 Series		Pre-1977 Series	
	n	%	*n*	%
Benign tumors				
Myxoma	114	27.9	130	29.3
Papillary fibroelastoma	31	7.6	42	9.5
Rhabdomyoma	20	4.9	36	8.1
Lipoma	2	0.5	45	10.1
Fibroma	20	4.9	17	3.8
Hemangioma	17	4.2	15	3.4
Atrioventricular nodal tumor	10	2.4	12	2.7
Teratoma	4	1.0	14	3.2
Lipomatous hypertrophy, atrial septum	12	2.9	0	0.0
Granular cell tumor	4	1.0	3	0.7
Lymphangioma	2	0.5	2	0.5
Benign fibrous tumor	3	0.7	0	0.0
Neurofibroma	0	0.0	3	0.7
Histiocytoid cardiomyopathy	2	0.5	0	0.0
Inflammatory pseudotumor	2	0.5	0	0.0
Myocytic hamartoma	2	0.5	0	0.0
Paraganglioma	2	0.5	0	0.0
Epithelioid hemangioendothelioma	1	0.2	0	0.0
Total	248	60.6	319	71.8
Malignant tumors				
Angiosarcoma	37	9.0	39	8.8
Unclassified sarcoma	35	8.6	0	0.0
Rhabdomyosarcoma	6	1.5	26	5.9
Mesothelioma	8	2.0	19	4.3
Fibrosarcoma	9	2.2	14	3.2
Osteosarcoma	13	3.2	5	1.1
Malignant fibrous histiocytoma	16	3.9	0	0.0
Lymphoma	7	1.7	7	1.6
Leiomyosarcoma	12	2.9	1	0.2
Myxosarcoma	8	2.0	0	0.0
Synovial sarcoma	5	1.2	1	0.2
Malignant teratoma	0	0.0	4	0.9
Neurogenic sarcoma	0	0.0	4	0.9
Thymoma[a]	0	0.0	4	0.9
Liposarcoma	2	0.5	1	0.2
Malignant schwannoma	2	0.5	0	0.0
Yolk sac tumor	1	0.2	0	0.0
Total	161	39.4	125	28.2
Total tumors	409		444	

[a]From thymic rests in the parietal pericardium.
Source: Adapted from Refs. 4 and 5. Cysts are excluded.

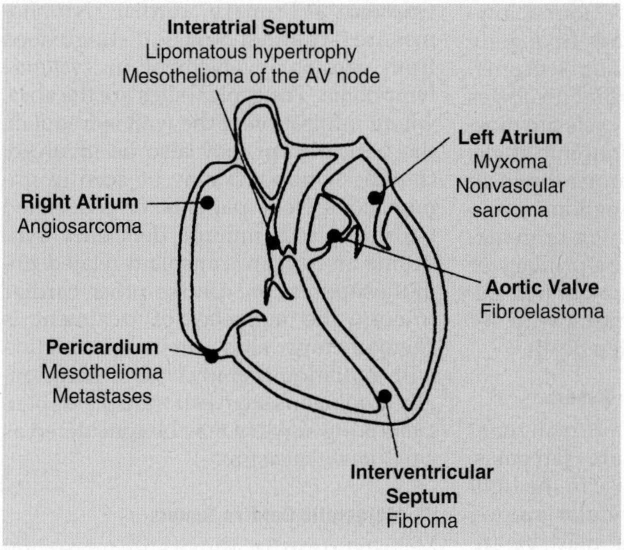

Figure 81-1 ■ Predominant sites of common cardiac tumors.

increased serum immunoglobulin levels, and elevated acute-phase reactants such as erythrocyte sedimentation rate and C-reactive protein.[10]

Diagnosis

Two-dimensional echocardiography provides excellent spatial and temporal resolution of cardiac masses and is the initial imaging modality that should be pursued. However, while transthoracic echocardiography (TTE) is useful as a screening method, transesophageal echocardiography (TEE) allows for better tumor characterization and assessment of intra- and extracardiac invasion.[11] Three-dimensional echocardiography can help define complex tumor geometry but is still investigational.[12] Magnetic resonance imaging (MRI) and computed tomography (CT) can be gated to the ECG and offer additional information in the evaluation of cardiac tumors, including dynamic visualization of tumor motion.[13,14] MRI provides the highest degree of soft tissue contrast of any imaging modality and provides outstanding tumor localization, tissue characterization, visualization of the entire mediastinium, and flexibility in the selection of imaging planes (Fig. 81-2).[15,16] In addition, tailored imaging sequences allow more specific characterization of particular tumors.[16] Although the spatial resolution of CT is greater than MRI, but less than echocardiography, the soft tissue characterization of CT is inferior to MRI and thus, CT can be considered an intermediate modality appropriate in select patients.[9,13] Cardiac angiography, once a mainstay in the diagnosis of cardiac tumors, has fallen out of use for that purpose given the risk of embolization during the procedure. However, imaging of the coronary arteries remains appropriate prior to cardiac surgery in older patients to evaluate the need for a concomitant coronary bypass procedure.

The differential diagnosis for a cardiac mass discovered on imaging includes thrombus and vegetation.[17,18] Thrombi are usually seen in the context of heart disease including arrhythmia, cardiomyopathy, or myocardial infarction, or in patients with thrombophilia. A prominent Eustachian valve or Chiari network may present as a right atrial mass.[19]

Cardiac Tumors

Benign Primary Cardiac Tumors

Myxomas ■ Histologically, these soft gelatinous tumors are thought to arise from the subendocardial mesenchyme and contain polygonal to stellate myxoma cells ("lepidic cells"), often around vascular channels in an eosinophilic matrix, with various areas of hemorrhage.[5] The cells are positive for factor VIII and can also express neuron-specific enolase and S-100 protein.[10] The majority of myxomas arise in the left atrium and are usually attached to the fossa ovalis. In a meta-analysis of 32 reports encompassing 1029 patients, 83% of myxomas were found to occur in the left atrium.[20] The remainder are found in the right atrium, or rarely, either ventricle or multiple sites. They often present as mobile masses attached by a stalk to the endocardial surface.[21] The mean age is 50 years at presentation, and more women are affected than men.[20,22] The classic clinical presentation includes a triad of constitutional symptoms, valvular obstruction, and embolization. Embolic phenomena, seen in 30-40% of patients, are more likely when the tumor surface is irregular (polypoid or myxoid) rather than smooth.[9] Surgery is generally recommended at the time of diagnosis due to embolic risk, and involves en bloc resection along with margins of normal tissue as well as the fossa ovalis. Recurrence is rare, but long-term follow-up is necessary.[23]

Although most myxomas are sporadic, familial syndromes have been described. The Carney complex is a multiple endocrine neoplasia syndrome that includes cardiac, endocrine, neural and cutaneous tumors in addition to skin and mucosal pigmentation.[24,25] The diagnostic criteria are shown in Table 81-2.[26] Two disease manifestations and one genetic criterion are necessary for the diagnosis. Familial myxomas are inherited in an autosomal dominant fashion. Mutations in *PRKAR1A*, the gene for which is located on chromosome 17q22-24 and encodes a regulatory subunit of cyclic-AMP dependent protein kinase A, have been identified in approximately one half of affected patients.[27-30] A variant associated with

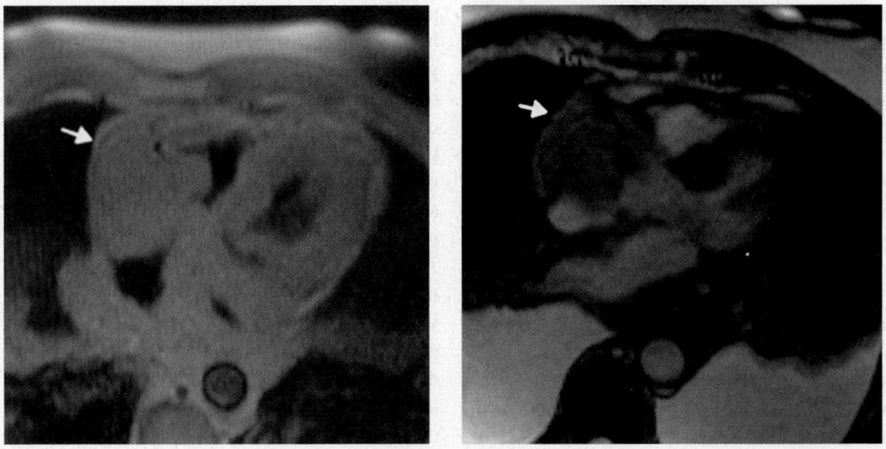

Figure 81-2 ■ Cardiac MRI of a 69-year-old man with lymphoma demonstrating a large homogeneous mass (*arrows*) occupying most of the right atrium and extending into the right ventricle and posterior mediastinum. The image on the left is a dark-blood image in the four-chamber view obtained using T2-weighted half-Fourier acquisition single-shot turbo spin echo. The image on the right is a bright-blood image in the four-chamber view obtained using steady-state free precession; note the large bilateral pleural effusions.

Table 81-2 Diagnostic Criteria for the Carney Complex

Disease manifestations
Spotty skin pigmentation, distribution typically involving conjunctiva, lips, canthi, vaginal or penile mucosa
Cutaneous or mucosal myxoma
Cardiac myxoma
Breast myxomatosis (or suggestive magnetic resonance findings)
Primary pigmented nodular adrenocortical disease or Liddle's test with paradoxical positive response of urinary glucocorticosteroids to administration of dexamethasone
Acromegaly from growth hormone–producing adenoma
Large cell calcifying Sertoli cell tumor or characteristic calcification on testicular ultrasonography
Thyroid carcinoma or multiple ultrasonographically demonstrated nodules in a young patient
Psammomatous melanotic schwannoma
Multiple blue nevi
Multiple ductal adenomas of the breast
Osteochondromyxoma
Supplemental criteria
First-degree relative with the Carney complex
Inactivating mutation of the *PRKAR1A* gene

Source: Adapted from Ref. 26 with permission from The Endocrine Society, Copyright 2001.

distal arthrogryposis has been linked to a missense mutation in the myosin heavy-chain gene on 17p12-p13.1.[31] Familial myxomas present at a younger age, are more likely to be multiple, and are more likely to recur after resection than sporadic myxomas.[32] Identification of first-degree relatives facilitates the identification of myxomas at risk for embolization.

Fibroelastomas ■ Fibroelastomas are sometimes compared to sea anemone,[33] as they are composed of papillary fronds similar to normal chordae tendinae. They usually arise from the valvular endocardium, most commonly the aortic valve, and occur over a wide range of ages.[34,35] Fibroelastomas may be asymptomatic or may present with transient ischemic attack, stroke, heart failure, angina, myocardial infarction, or sudden death.[36] As the risk of embolization is high, patients with large, mobile masses, symptoms, or who are undergoing cardiac surgery for other reasons should be considered for surgical resection.[37-39]

Other Benign Tumors ■ Rhabdomyomas occur almost exclusively in children and are described below. Lipomatous septal hypertrophy is an exaggeration of the normal accumulation of fat within the atrial septum and is typically visualized as a right atrial mass.[40] The role of surgery is controversial as the finding is often incidental, but may be considered in cases of vena cava obstruction, atrial arrhythmia, and congestive heart failure.[9,40] Lipomas and hemangiomas may be found anywhere in the heart. Fibromas frequently arise in the interventricular septum.[41] Hamartomas of mature cardiac myocytes are very rare.[21] Pericardial cysts are most common in the right costophrenic angle, and bronchogenic cysts can be found in the myocardium.[5] Paragangliomas and mesotheliomas may be benign or malignant. Mesotheliomas may be primary or metastatic to the pericardium, or may occur in the AV node, presenting with AV block, arrhythmia, or sudden death.[42]

Malignant Primary Cardiac Tumors

Sarcomas ■ The majority of malignant primary cardiac tumors are sarcomas. Angiosarcomas usually arise in the right atrium near the atrioventricular groove, although other chambers may be involved, and are associated with areas of hemorrhage, pericardial invasion and effusion. The peak age for angiosarcomas is between 20 and 50 years, with a two- to threefold male predominance.[5] The presentation may include including palpitations, dyspnea, and chest pain (pleuritic and/or pericardial), or signs and symptoms related to congestive heart failure or thromboembolism.[3] The relationship between cardiac angiosarcoma and Kaposi's sarcoma, in which cardiac involvement has been described, requires further investigation.[43] Endomyocardial-based sarcomas, often with smooth muscle or myofibroblastic differentiation, are usually located in the left atrium and consist of multiple subtypes, including undifferentiated pleomorphic sarcoma, osteosarcoma, leiomyosarcoma, fibrosarcoma, and myxofibrosarcoma.

Prognosis of cardiac sarcomas is poor, with a mean survival of 16.5 months after diagnosis,[6] as many patients have metastases at the time of presentation.[44] Complete surgical resection of cardiac angiosarcomas, as in other cardiac malignancies, is usually impossible. Orthotopic heart transplantation, at times combined with bilateral lung transplantation, has been described in a few small series and case reports. Although, in most cases, heart transplantation followed by chemotherapy does not affect the long-term outcome,[45] selected patients may have good outcomes with transplantation.[46,47] A survey of the 173 heart transplant centers in the United States and Canada, with a 76% reply rate, revealed only 24 cases of transplantation for primary cardiac malignancy, and an accompanying literature review revealed 104 published cases. One-year survival was 54% in the survey and 32% in the review, although at least five patients survived more than 4 years.[48] A novel surgical approach in recurrent atrial malignancies is atrial homograft transplantation using donor atria from a tissue bank.[49]

Lymphomas ■ Primary cardiac lymphomas are rare and should be distinguished from cardiac involvement in systemic lymphoma. The typical sites are the atria, where infiltration of the wall is frequent; the pericardium may also be involved. Cardiac lymphoma may be seen in immunocompetent patients or associated with acquired immune deficiency syndrome and organ transplant-related immunosuppression. Unlike other cardiac tumors, the mainstay of treatment is chemotherapy, alone or in combination with radiation therapy,[6,50] and occasionally autologous stem cell transplantation. Debulking surgery may be considered as a palliative measure.

Metastatic Cardiac Tumors

Metastatic cardiac tumors are more common than primary tumors. In one series of 133 resected cardiac tumors, 14% were metastases.[5] Mechanisms of metastasis include direct extension, hematogenous spread, lymphatic spread and cavoatrial or pulmonary vein extension.[7] Malignancies likely to metastasize to the heart are shown in Table 81-3.[21] According to statistics from 6240 autopsies of cancer patients from two large series, the frequency of heart metastases was, in decreasing order, melanoma (46%), malignant germ cell tumor (38%), leukemia (33%), lung carcinoma (17%), lymphoma (17%), sarcoma (15%), esophageal carcinoma (13%), renal carcinoma (11%), and breast carcinoma (10%).[21] Almost any cancer, however, can metastasize to the heart. We found a high frequency of cardiac metastasis and/or invasion in patients with malignant pleural mesothelioma.[51] In 19 autopsies, cardiac invasion was found in 14 (74%), with more than half involving the pericardium and more than one-quarter the myocardium.[52] Treatment is generally palliative. Palliative resection may be considered in selected instances.

Pediatric Tumors

In contrast to adults, metastases to the heart are rarely observed in the pediatric population. Many cardiac neoplasms in

Table 81-3 Tumors Likely to Metastasize to the Heart

Melanoma
Malignant germ cell tumor
Leukemia and lymphoma
Breast carcinoma
Lung carcinoma
Hepatocellular carcinoma
Renal cell carcinoma
Sarcoma
Esophageal and gastric carcinoma
Mesothelioma (may be primary to pericardium or metastatic)

children occur in the context of familial syndromes (see section on the Carney Complex, above). The majority are hamartomas. Rhabdomyomas account for the majority of pediatric cardiac tumors[53] and are associated with tuberous sclerosis, an autosomal dominant disorder characterized by benign neoplasms of the heart, kidneys, brain, lungs and skin.[5] They occur most commonly in the ventricles and, in the context of familial syndromes, often regress spontaneously; surgical resection is usually necessary only if outflow tract obstruction is present.[54-56] Cardiac fibromas, also frequently found in the ventricle, occur in a minority of patients with Gorlin syndrome, another autosomal dominant disorder presenting with multiple neoplasms, including basal cell carcinomas and medulloblastomas as well as odontogenic keratocysts and skeletal abnormalities.[57,58] Neurofibromas are found in patients with von Recklinghausen's disease.[21]

Tumors of the Great Vessels

Primary tumors involving the aorta, pulmonary artery, and vena cavae are rare, appearing in the literature mainly as case reports or in small retrospective case series.[59-61] Risk factors for the development of tumors of the great vessels remain poorly defined. Prior radiation exposure has been postulated as a possible causative factor.[62] Plastic polymers, such as Dacron, have been linked to aortic tumors in animal studies; nonetheless, aortic tumors arising around a Dacron graft in humans, although reported, are extremely rare.[63] Tumors of the great vessels typically present with thromboembolic events or an obstructive syndrome.[59] TEE and MRI are useful in differentiating tumors of the great vessels from intraluminal thrombus, mediastinal lymphadenopathy, or adjacent lung tumors.[61]

Benign tumors of the aorta include endothelial papillary fibroelastomas arising in the aortic sinuses, which may present with intermittent prolapse into a coronary artery or with emboli to the heart or brain.[64] Intra-aortic myxomas have also been described, presenting with recurrent arterial emboli.[60]

Malignant tumors of the aorta and pulmonary artery are often aggressive, poorly differentiated sarcomas arising from intimal cells and showing myofibroblastic differentiation ("intimal type"). Rarely, malignant tumors of the great vessels are identified as angiosarcomas, leiomyosarcomas, hemangioendotheliomas, schwannomas, and fibrous histiocytomas.[59,65-67] Sarcomas of the inferior vena cava tend to be well-differentiated leiomyosarcomas. Whereas sarcomas of the aorta present at a mean age of 62 years, sarcomas of the pulmonary artery present at a mean age of 41 years. In a review of 60 cases, the median age was 52 years, with a male-to-female ratio of 1:2[68] and a median duration of symptoms of 10 months. The clinical picture was suggestive of pulmonary embolism, with dyspnea (70%), chest pain (48%), cough (34%), hemoptysis (30%), and syncope (25%). Metastases to lung (67%) and lymph node (20%) were common. Although patients tend to present with advanced disease and prognosis is poor, a minority respond to resection and chemotherapy.[69]

The cornerstone of therapy for the tumors of the great vessels is complete surgical excision.[70] The use of various grafts has been advocated,[71] along with postoperative radiation and chemotherapy, often with an anthracycline-based regimen.[59,65] A combination of etoposide, vincristine, ifosfamide, and doxorubicin may regress pulmonary metastases.[71] Although mean survival for patients with tumors of the great vessels is only 10 months, patients with sarcoma of the pulmonary artery may have a better prognosis compared with sarcoma of the aorta (23 vs 5 months).[59,71,72] Prolonged survival is extremely rare but has been reported.[73] For patients with unresectable disease, endovascular stent grafting may improve quality of life.[74]

Selected References

The complete reference list can be found at www.CANCERMEDICINE8.com

1. Heath D. Pathology of cardiac tumors. *Am J Cardiol.* 1968;21(3):315–327.
2. Reynen K. Frequency of primary tumors of the heart. *Am J Cardiol.* 1996;77(1):107.
3. Travis WD, B.E., Mueller-Hermelink HK, Harris CC (Editors). *World Heath Organization Classification of Tumors.* Lyon: France; 2004.
4. Perchinsky MJ, Lichtenstein SV, Tyers GF. Primary cardiac tumors: forty years' experience with 71 patients. *Cancer.* 1997;79(9):1809–1815.
5. McAllister JHA, Fenoglis JJ. *Tumors of the cardiovascular system. In: Atlas of tumor pathology. 2nd Series. Fascicle 15.*Washington, DC: Armed Forces Institute of Pathology; 1978.
6. Donsbeck AV, et al. Primary cardiac sarcomas: an immunohistochemical and grading study with long-term follow-up of 24 cases. *Histopathology.* 1999;34(4): 295–304.
7. Bussani R, et al. Cardiac metastases. *J Clin Pathol.* 2007;60(1):27–34.
8. Lam KY, Dickens P, Chan AC. Tumors of the heart. A 20-year experience with a review of 12,485 consecutive autopsies. *Arch Pathol Lab Med.* 1993;117(10):1027–1031.
9. Burke A, Jeudy J, Jr., Virmani R. Cardiac tumours: an update. *Heart.* 2008;94(1): 117–123.
10. Allard MF, T.J., Wilson JE, McManus BM. *Atlas of Heart Diseases, Volume III,* ed. B. E. 1995, St Louis: Mosby; 1995:15.1-6.5.
11. Geibel A, et al. Diagnosis, localization and evaluation of malignancy of heart and mediastinal tumors by conventional and transesophageal echocardiography. *Acta Cardiol.* 1996;51(5):395–408.
12. Lokhandwala J, et al. Three-dimensional echocardiography of intracardiac masses. *Echocardiography.* 2004;21(2):159–163.
13. Araoz PA, et al. CT and MR imaging of primary cardiac malignancies. *Radiographics.* 1999;19(6):1421–1434.
14. Feuchtner G, et al. Images in cardiovascular medicine. Prolapsing atrial myxoma: dynamic visualization with multislice computed tomography. *Circulation.* 2004;109(12):e165–e166.
15. Kaminaga T, Takeshita T, Kimura I. Role of magnetic resonance imaging for evaluation of tumors in the cardiac region. *Eur Radiol.* 2003;13(Suppl 4):L1–L10.
16. Grizzard JD, Ang GB. Magnetic resonance imaging of pericardial disease and cardiac masses. *Cardiol Clin.* 2007;25(1):111–140, vi.
17. Zee-Cheng CS, et al. Giant vegetation due to Staphylococcus aureus endocarditis simulating left atrial myxoma. *Am Heart J.* 1986;111(2):414–417.
18. Auriti A, et al. Giant vegetation of the mitral valve simulating primary cardiac tumor. *Echocardiography.* 2004;21(2):183–185.
19. Alam M, Sun I, Smith S. Transesophageal echocardiographic evaluation of right atrial mass lesions. *J Am Soc Echocardiogr.* 1991;4(4):331–337.
20. Kuon E, et al. The challenge presented by right atrial myxoma. *Herz.* 2004; 29(7):702–709.
21. Burke A, Virmani R. *Tumors of the Heart and Great Vessels.* Atlas of Tumor Pathology, Series 3, Fascicle 16, ed. A.F.I.o. Pathology. 1996, Washington (DC).
22. Burke AP, T.H., Gomez-Roman JJ, et al. Benign tumors of pluripotent mesenchyme, in Pathology and genetics of tumours of the lung, pleura, thymus and heart. In: B.E. Travis WD, Mueller-Hermelink HK, Harris CC, editors, Editor. 2004, IARC Press: Lyon, France.
23. Attum AA, et al. Malignant clinical behavior of cardiac myxomas and "myxoid imitators." *Ann Thorac Surg.* 1987;44(2):217–222.
24. Carney JA, et al. The complex of myxomas, spotty pigmentation, and endocrine overactivity. *Medicine (Baltimore).* 1985;64(4):270–283.
25. McCarthy PM, et al. The significance of multiple, recurrent, and "complex" cardiac myxomas. *J Thorac Cardiovasc Surg.* 1986;91(3):389–396.
26. Stratakis CA, Kirschner LS, Carney JA. Clinical and molecular features of the Carney complex: diagnostic criteria and recommendations for patient evaluation. *J Clin Endocrinol Metab.* 2001;86(9):4041–4046.
28. Stratakis CA. Mutations of the gene encoding the protein kinase A type I-alpha regulatory subunit (PRKAR1A) in patients with the "complex of spotty skin pigmentation, myxomas, endocrine overactivity,

and schwannomas" (Carney complex). *Ann N Y Acad Sci*. 2002;968:3–21.
29. Bourdeau I, et al. 17q22-24 chromosomal losses and alterations of protein kinase a subunit expression and activity in adrenocorticotropin-independent macronodular adrenal hyperplasia. *J Clin Endocrinol Metab*. 2006;91(9):3626–3632.
30. Carney JA. The complex of myxomas, spotty pigmentation, and endocrine overactivity. *Arch Intern Med*. 1987;147(3):418–419.
31. Veugelers M, et al. Mutation of perinatal myosin heavy chain associated with a Carney complex variant. *N Engl J Med*. 2004;351(5):460–469.
32. Carney JA. Differences between nonfamilial and familial cardiac myxoma. *Am J Surg Pathol*. 1985;9(1):53–55.
33. McAllister HA, Jr., Hall RJ, Cooley DA. Tumors of the heart and pericardium. *Curr Probl Cardiol*. 1999;24(2):57–116.
34. Gowda RM, et al. Cardiac papillary fibroelastoma: a comprehensive analysis of 725 cases. *Am Heart J*. 2003;146(3):404–410.
44. Ogle GD, Bell DR. Angiosarcoma of the heart. *Aust N Z J Med*. 1987;17(1):74–76.
45. Uberfuhr P, et al. Heart transplantation: an approach to treating primary cardiac sarcoma? *J Heart Lung Transplant*. 2002;21(10):1135–1139.
46. Grandmougin D, et al. Total orthotopic heart transplantation for primary cardiac rhabdomyosarcoma: factors influencing long-term survival. *Ann Thorac Surg*. 2001;71(5):1438–1441.
47. Aravot DJ, et al. Primary cardiac tumours–is there a place for cardiac transplantation? *Eur J Cardiothorac Surg*. 1989;3(6):521–524.
48. Rodriguez-Cruz E, Cintron-Maldonado RM, Forbes TJ. Treatment of primary cardiac malignancies with orthotopic heart transplantation. *Bol Asoc Med P R*. 2000;92(4–8):65–71.
49. Stoica SC, et al. Atrial transplantation for recurrent cardiac sarcoma. *J Heart Lung Transplant*. 2001;20(11):1220–1223.
50. Percy RF, et al. Prolonged survival in a patient with primary angiosarcoma of the heart. *Am Heart J*. 1987;113(5):1228–1230.
51. Chahinian AP, et al. Diffuse malignant mesothelioma. Prospective evaluation of 69 patients. *Ann Intern Med*. 1982;96(6 Pt 1): 746–755.
52. Wadler S, et al. Cardiac abnormalities in patients with diffuse malignant pleural mesothelioma. *Cancer*. 1986;58(12):2744–2750.
56. Bosi G, et al. The natural history of cardiac rhabdomyoma with and without tuberous sclerosis. *Acta Paediatr*. 1996;85(8): 928–931.
69. Mayer F, et al. Primary malignant sarcomas of the heart and great vessels in adult patients–a single-center experience. *Oncologist*. 2007;12(9):1134–1142.
70. Park BJ, et al. Surgical management of thoracic malignancies invading the heart or great vessels. *Ann Thorac Surg*. 2004;78(3):1024–1030.
71. Zerkowski HR, et al. Primary sarcoma of pulmonary artery and valve: multimodality treatment by chemotherapy and homograft replacement. *J Thorac Cardiovasc Surg*. 1996;112(4):1122–1124.
73. Mattoo A, et al. Pulmonary artery sarcoma: a case report of surgical cure and 5-year follow-up. *Chest*. 2002;122(2):745–747.
74. Totaro M, et al. Cardiac angiosarcoma arising from pulmonary artery: endovascular treatment. *Ann Thorac Surg*. 2004; 78(4):1468–1470.

82 Primary Germ Cell Tumors of the Thorax

John D. Hainsworth, MD ■ F. Anthony Greco, MD

The biology and clinical characteristics of mediastinal germ cell tumors have been defined during the last 30 years. These neoplasms, although rare, are of particular interest because they usually affect young males and because curative therapy is now available for many patients. The clinical and pathologic characteristics of benign and malignant germ cell tumors and of poorly differentiated carcinoma of the mediastinum are presented, with special attention focused on the treatment of these neoplasms.

Benign Teratomas of the Mediastinum

Although benign teratomas of the mediastinum (mature cystic teratomas or dermoid tumors) account for only 3-12% of mediastinal tumors, they comprise 60-70% of all mediastinal germ cell tumors.[1,2] These tumors have been described in patients with ages ranging from 7 months to 65 years; however, most occur in young adults, with an approximately equal incidence in males and females.[2,3] No predisposing conditions or associated abnormalities have been recognized in patients developing these tumors.

Benign mediastinal teratomas have a histologic appearance identical to that of benign teratomas arising in the more common ovarian location. These tumors are usually well encapsulated and are composed either of a single large cystic cavity or of several smaller intercommunicating cystic spaces. On histologic examination, mature tissue from ectodermal, mesodermal, and endodermal germ cell layers is typically present. Mature tissue that recapitulates the histology of any human organ can be found in these tumors. However, the ectodermal component (ie, skin, sebaceous tissue, neural tissue) is usually predominant.[3]

Approximately 95% of benign teratomas arise in the anterior mediastinum; the remainder arise in the posterior mediastinum.[2,3] These tumors are slow growing, and in recent years, 50-60% of patients have been asymptomatic at the time of diagnosis by routine chest radiography.[3] When symptoms are present, dyspnea, and substernal chest pain are the most common. Cough productive of hair or sebum is pathognomonic of a benign mediastinal tumor. However, this distinctive symptom is extremely rare and occurs late in the natural history of this condition following tumor rupture into the tracheobronchial tree. Superior vena cava syndrome is also rare and is a late manifestation. Most patients with benign mediastinal teratomas appear to be healthy, and physical examination contributes little to the diagnosis. Likewise, laboratory evaluation is usually normal. Serum levels of human chorionic gonadotropin (HCG) and alpha-fetoprotein are always normal in patients with benign teratoma.

The chest radiograph typically reveals a well-circumscribed anterior mediastinal mass that often protrudes into one of the lung fields. These tumors are usually large at the time of diagnosis; in one large series, the median size was $10 \times 8.5 \times 5.4$ cm^3. Occasionally, chest radiography identifies teeth within the tumor, a pathognomonic finding. Calcification is present in up to 25% of tumors, occurring in fragments of bone, in the tumor wall, or in other areas throughout the tumor, in addition to its occasional occurrence in teeth.

Surgical excision is the treatment of choice for benign teratoma of the mediastinum. Median sternotomy is usually the best surgical approach, although successful resection can also be accomplished by thoracotomy. Surgical removal is sometimes difficult because of the large size of the tumor and the involvement of other structures such as the pericardium, lung, great vessels, thymus, chest wall, hilar structures, and diaphragm, in decreasing order of frequency. Some 10-15% of patients require additional procedures (eg, lobectomy, pericardiectomy) for complete tumor resection. Benign teratomas are resistant to radiation and cytotoxic drugs, and these modalities have no role in their treatment.

Tumor recurrence is rare following complete surgical resection.[2-4] Prolonged survival has also been reported in patients who underwent only subtotal resection, owing to the involvement of vital mediastinal structures. The operative mortality rate in recent years has been very low.

Malignant Germ Cell Tumors

Etiology

Malignant mediastinal germ cell tumors of various histologies were first described as a clinical entity approximately 50 years ago.[5,6] Mediastinal and other extragonadal germ cell tumors were initially thought to represent isolated metastases from an inapparent gonadal primary site. However, there is now abundant clinical evidence to substantiate the extragonadal origin of these tumors.[1,7] Extragonadal germ cell tumors, particularly those arising in mediastinal and pineal sites, represent a malignant transformation of germinal elements distributed to these sites and can occur in the absence of a primary focus in the gonad. Some investigators suggest that this distribution arises as a consequence of abnormal migration of germ cells during embryogenesis.[6,8] Others hypothesize a widespread distribution of germ cells to multiple sites during normal embryogenesis, with these cells conveying genetic information or providing regulatory functions at somatic sites.[9]

Epidemiology

Malignant germ cell tumors of the mediastinum are uncommon, representing only 3-10% of tumors originating in the mediastinum.[10] They are much less common than germ cell tumors arising in the testes and account for only 1-5% of all germ cell neoplasms.[11] These figures, most of which are derived from retrospective series reported between 1950 and 1975, may underestimate the true occurrence of mediastinal germ cell tumors. The histology of these tumors may be similar to other poorly differentiated mediastinal tumors, including malignant thymoma and high-grade non-Hodgkin's lymphoma. Some patients with poorly differentiated neoplasm or poorly differentiated carcinoma of the mediastinum have the i(12p) chromosomal abnormality frequently present in germ cell tumors.[12] Other patients with poorly differentiated carcinoma of the mediastinum have clinical characteristics and treatment responses typical of patients with extragonadal germ cell tumors.[13] Although there is no doubt that mediastinal germ cell tumors are uncommon, increasing familiarity with the tumors by both clinicians and pathologists will probably result in their increased recognition.

The great majority of mediastinal malignant germ cell tumors occur in patients between 20 and 35 years of age. For unknown reasons, most are found in males. In the rare occurrences reported in females, mediastinal malignant germ cell tumors appeared to be histologically and biologically identical to those occurring in males. The relative rarity of extragonadal germ cell tumors in women parallels the lower incidence of female gonadal germ cell tumors compared with their incidence in males. Although the incidence of primary testis tumors is low among racial minorities in the United States, the occurrence of extragonadal germ cell tumors is somewhat more common (7% vs 16% of cases, respectively).[14,15]

Patients with nonseminomatous extragonadal germ cell tumors have a subsequent increased risk of developing testicular cancer, strengthening the concept of a precursor abnormality (the so-called "testicular intraepithelial neoplasm") in the germ cells of these patients.[16]

Histopathology

Mediastinal germ cell tumors appear to be histologically identical to germ cell tumors arising in the testis and contain the same range of histologic subtypes. However, the frequency of yolk sac tumor and taratocarcinoma is higher in mediastinal germ cell tumors, while embryonal carcinoma is less common. In a review of 229 malignant mediastinal germ cell tumors seen between 1960 and 1994 at the Armed Forces Institute of Pathology, pure seminoma was the most common histology, accounting for 52% of cases.[17] Nonseminomatous histologies included teratocarcinoma (20%), yolk sac tumor (17%), choriocarcinoma (3.4%), embryonal carcinoma (2.6%), and mixed nonseminomatous tumors (5.2%).

Clinical Characteristics

Unlike benign germ cell tumors of the mediastinum, malignant mediastinal tumors are usually symptomatic at the time of diagnosis. Most mediastinal malignant tumors are large and cause symptoms by compressing or invading adjacent structures, including the lungs, pleura, pericardium, and chest wall. Pure seminomas are somewhat slower growing and have less potential for early metastasis than do tumors with nonseminomatous elements. Pure seminomas and tumors with nonseminomatous elements are therefore discussed separately, although substantial overlap exists in their clinical characteristics.

Seminoma ■ Seminomas grow relatively slowly and can become very large before causing symptoms. Tumors 20-30 cm in diameter can exist with minimal symptomatology. Approximately 20-30% of seminomas are detected by routine chest radiography while still asymptomatic.[18] The most common initial symptom is a sensation of pressure or dull retrosternal chest pain. Additional symptoms include exertional dyspnea, cough, dysphagia, and hoarseness. Superior vena cava syndrome develops in approximately 10% of patients. Systemic symptoms related to metastatic lesions are uncommon.

At the time of diagnosis, only 30-40% of patients with mediastinal seminoma have localized disease; the remainder have one or more sites of distant metastases.[19] The regional lymph nodes (cervical, upper abdominal) are the most common metastatic sites; lung and bone are the most common visceral sites.[20] The retroperitoneum is an uncommon site of metastasis in patients with mediastinal seminoma.[1,19,20]

Pure seminoma appears radiographically as a large, noncalcified anterior mediastinal mass that can compress or deviate the trachea or bronchiif of sufficient size. A computed tomographic (CT) scan of the chest typically shows a large homogeneous anterior mediastinal mass that obliterates the fat planes surrounding mediastinal vascular structures.[21] The radiographic findings are not specific enough to allow the distinction of mediastinal seminoma from other mediastinal tumors.

Elevated serum levels of HCG are detected in up to 40% of mediastinal seminomas.[20] However, most of these are low-level elevations (2-10 ng/mL); levels of HCG exceeding 100 ng/mL are unusual and suggest the presence of nonseminomatous elements. The serum alpha-fetoprotein level is always normal in pure mediastinal seminoma, and any elevation of this tumor marker indicates the presence of nonseminomatous elements. Serum lactic dehydrogenase is elevated in the majority of patients with mediastinal seminoma.[19,20]

Nonseminomatous Germ Cell Tumor ■ Few patients with these rapidly growing neoplasms are asymptomatic at diagnosis. Symptoms caused by compression or invasion of local mediastinal structures are identical to those seen in patients with mediastinal seminoma. However, presenting symptoms caused by metastatic lesions are much more common because 85-95% of these patients have at least one metastatic site at the time of diagnosis.[22-24] Common metastatic sites include the lungs, pleura, lymph nodes (particularly supraclavicular and retroperitoneal), and liver. Less frequent sites of involvement include the bone, brain, and kidney. High levels of HCG sometimes are associated with gynecomastia. Neoplasms with elements of choriocarcinoma have a marked hemorrhagic tendency; these patients may have catastrophic events related to uncontrolled hemorrhage at a metastatic site (eg, massive hemoptysis, intracranial hemorrhage).[25] Constitutional symptoms, including weight loss, weakness, and fever, are more common in these patients than in those with pure seminoma.

Chest radiographic features of mediastinal nonseminomatous germ cell tumors are similar to those seen in mediastinal seminomas. The CT scan frequently shows an inhomogeneous mass, with multiple areas of hemorrhage and necrosis, differing from the usually homogeneous appearance of mediastinal seminoma.[21]

The serum tumor markers HCG and alphafetoprotein are usually abnormal in patients with mediastinal nonseminomatous germ cell tumors. Alpha-fetoprotein is most frequently abnormal and is elevated either alone or in conjunction with HCG in 80-90% of patients, whereas elevation of HCG occurs in only 30-35% of patients.[26,27] This pattern of marker elevation differs slightly from that seen in testicular cancer, in which elevations of HCG and alpha-fetoprotein occur with nearly equal frequency and are seen in 50-70% of patients with metastatic tumor. As in mediastinal seminoma, elevation of serum lactic dehydrogenase is frequent, occurring in 80-90% of patients.[23]

Syndromes Associated With Mediastinal Nonseminomatous Germ Cell Tumors

Klinefelter Syndrome

Klinefelter syndrome is a relatively common chromosomal abnormality characterized by hypogonadism, azoospermia, and elevated gonadotropin levels in association with a 47,XXY karyotype. Men with this syndrome have increased incidence of several types of cancer.[28] The association of Klinefelter syndrome and mediastinal nonseminomatous germ cell tumors is now well recognized.[29,30] Four of 22 consecutive patients (18%) treated at Indiana University for primary mediastinal germ cell tumors had karyotypic confirmation of Klinefelter syndrome, and an additional patient had clinical features.[31] The average age of patients with Klinefelter syndrome who develop extragonadal germ cell tumors is approximately 18 years, 10 years younger than the median age of those developing this tumor in the absence of Klinefelter syndrome. Testicular germ cell neoplasms have rarely been reported in association with Klinefelter syndrome; therefore, the association with mediastinal germ cell tumor seems specific.

The explanation for this association is unknown, but it seems reasonable to assume that the chromosomal abnormality plays some role. Increasing evidence indicates that many individuals who develop germ cell tumors have underlying germ cell defects. Many patients with extragonadal germ cell tumors have histories of infertility, and testicular biopsy in these patients shows various abnormalities, including decreased spermatogenesis, peritubular fibrosis, and interstitial edema.[32] In addition, patients who are successfully treated for extragonadal germ cell tumors have a markedly increased risk of developing a subsequent testicular germ cell tumor.[16] These data suggest that either a congenital or an acquired germ cell defect contributes not only to defective spermatogenesis but also to the development of extragonadal germ cell tumors.

Hematologic Neoplasia

A unique association between mediastinal nonseminomatous germ cell tumors and a variety of hematologic neoplasms is now well described.[33-39] Hematologic neoplasms have included acute myeloid leukemia, acute nonlymphocytic leukemia, acute lymphocytic leukemia, erythroleukemia, acute megakaryocytic leukemia, myelodysplastic syndrome, and malignant histiocytosis. In a series of 635 patients with extragonadal germ cell tumors, 17 patients developed hematologic malignancies at a median of 6 months after the extragonadal germ cell tumor was diagnosed.[39] All hematologic neoplasms developed in the 287 patients with mediastinal nonseminomatous germ cell tumors, for a 2% incidence in this group. Median survival was only 5 months after the hematologic disorder was diagnosed, and no patient survived for more than 2 years.

Recent evidence indicates that the hematologic neoplasms in this setting are not treatment related but rather arise from clones of malignant lymphoblasts or myeloblasts contained within the mediastinal germ cell tumor. Foci of malignant lymphoblasts have been recognized histologically in several mediastinal germ cell tumors.[35,36] More importantly, several patients have had an identical chromosomal abnormality (an isochromosome of the short arm of chromosome 12) in the neoplastic cells from the mediastinal germ cell tumor and the hematologic neoplasm, providing strong evidence of a common origin.[36-38] However, the specific association of leukemias and other hematologic neoplasms with mediastinal nonseminomatous germ cell tumors, rather than with all germ cell tumors, remains unexplained.

In addition to hematologic neoplasia, several cases of idiopathic thrombocytopenia in association with mediastinal nonseminomatous germ cell tumors have been reported.[40,41] These patients had normal numbers of megakaryocytes in the bone marrow; however, immune destruction of platelets could not be demonstrated. Prednisone and splenectomy were unsuccessful in increasing the platelet count; persistent thrombocytopenia caused significant morbidity in all patients and made treatment extremely difficult. At present, the cause of this syndrome is unknown.

Pretreatment Evaluation and Staging

The diagnosis of a mediastinal germ cell tumor should be considered in all young males with a mediastinal mass. In addition to physical examination and routine laboratory studies, initial evaluation should include CT of the chest and abdomen and determination of serum levels of HCG and alpha-fetoprotein. Any symptoms suggestive of distant metastases should be appropriately evaluated with radiologic studies.

In patients with suspected mediastinal germ cell tumor, a histologic diagnosis should be made using the least invasive approach because rapid initiation of definitive systemic therapy is important. Because these neoplasms are poorly differentiated, specimens obtained by fine-needle aspiration biopsy are sometimes insufficient for a definitive diagnosis. In such patients, surgical biopsy via median sternotomy or limited thoracotomy is indicated. Attempts at complete surgical resection of these mediastinal neoplasms are not indicated because curative results with other treatment modalities are superior.

Treatment of Seminoma

Pure mediastinal seminomas are curable in the large majority of patients, even when metastatic at the time of diagnosis. These tumors are highly sensitive to radiation therapy and to combination chemotherapy, and the selection of treatment therefore depends on the disease stage and the size of the mediastinal tumor.

Highly effective systemic combination chemotherapy now offers the best option for curative treatment for most patients with mediastinal seminoma. When used in advanced testicular seminoma, intensive cisplatin-based regimens are at least as active as they are against nonseminomatous germ cell tumors. Table 82-1 summarizes the experience with modern cisplatin-based combination regimens in the treatment of pure mediastinal seminoma.[19,22,24,42-48] Even with bulky local tumors and frequent metastatic disease, all recent series have shown cure rates of >80% with initial cisplatin-based chemotherapy. In a large, retrospective analysis of 51 patients treated at 10 centers between 1975 and 1996, 93% of patients treated with cisplatin-based first-line chemotherapy achieved complete remission, with subsequent relapses in only 14%.[48] Therefore, cisplatin-based chemotherapy, using regimens effective in advanced testicular cancer, should be the treatment of choice for all patients with mediastinal seminoma who have bulky (>6 cm) masses or evidence of metastatic disease.

Radiation therapy is also a potentially curative treatment for mediastinal seminoma.[4,19,49,50] Approximately 60% of patients with localized tumors are cured with radiotherapy; the relapse rate is correlated with tumor size. In patients with localized tumors <6 cm in diameter, the cure rate is high with radiation therapy or chemotherapy, and choice of treatment should be individualized. For young patients without contraindications, curative treatment with chemotherapy avoids potential long-term consequences of mediastinal irradiation (eg. coronary artery disease, valvular disease, constrictive pericarditis, second cancers).[51,52] Patients who are poor candidates for chemotherapy should have mediastinal radiation therapy (35-50 Gy). Patients who relapse after radiation therapy have a high salvage rate with chemotherapy[22,42]; in these patients bleomycin-containing regimens should be avoided to minimize the risk of pulmonary toxicity.

Patients with bulky seminoma at any site frequently have residual radiographic abnormalities on CT scan after chemotherapy. In most patients, these masses represent dense scirrhous reactions rather than viable seminoma or benign teratoma.[48,53,54] Residual seminoma is more frequent when residual lesions are >3 cm in diameter.[54] However, because of dense fibrosis following chemotherapy, surgical exploration and resection of the residual mediastinal mass are technically difficult and are associated with frequent morbidity and mortality. PET scanning is useful in differentiating residual seminoma from necrotic or fibrotic masses in patients with residual CT abnormalities following chemotherapy.[55] In one series, tumor status in all 19 patients with residual lesions >3 cm and in 95% of patients with lesions ≤3 cm was correctly predicted by PET. Therefore, PET scanning should be performed approximately 8 weeks after completion of chemotherapy in patients with residual CT abnormalities. Patients with normal PET scans should be followed without further treatment, whereas those with abnormal PET scans should undergo surgical resection. Patients who do not have surgical exploration should

Table 82-1 ■ Mediastinal Seminoma: Treatment With Cisplatin-Based Combination Chemotherapy

Study, Year	No. of Patients	Received Previous Radiotherapy	Treatment Regimen	No. of Complete Responses (%)	No. of Long-Term Disease-Free Survivors (Mo)
Hainsworth et al, 1982[22]	4	3	PVB	3 (75)	3 (> 24)
Jain et al, 1984[19]	11	0	VAB-6, 8, PVB 1, DDP/CTX 2	10 (91)	10 (19 + –46)
Logothetis et al, 1985[24]	4	Unspecified	DDP/CTX 3, CISCA 21	4 (100)	4 (unspecified)
Loehrer et al, 1987[42]	9	7	PVB ± A or BEP	8 (89)	7 (unspecified)
Bukowski et al, 1993[43]	8	0	PVB/EBAP	5 (63)	4 (>24)
Delgado et al, 1993[44]	6	0	VAP-6, PVB, BEP	5 (83)	5 (5-103)
Goss et al, 1994[45]	8	0	BEP 6, BEP + RT 1, VAB-6 1	8 (100)	8 (4-132)
Mencel et al, 1994[46]	19	0	VAP-6, EP	19 (100)	18 (>24)
Gerl et al, 1996[47]	4	1	VIP, EIP	4 (100)	4 (>24)
Bokemeyer et al, 2001[48]	51	0	Cisplatin based	NA	45 (88%)
Total	124			66 (90%)	108 (87%)

Abbreviations: A, Adriamycin (doxorubicin); BEP, bleomycin 30 U weekly, etoposide 100 mg/m² intravenously (IV) × 5 days, cisplatin 20 mg/m² IV × 5 days, cycles repeated q 3 weeks; CISCA, multidrug regimen developed at The University of Texas M. D. Anderson Cancer Center; CISCA2, multidrug regimen developed at M.D. Anderson; CTX, cyclophosphamide; DDP, cisplatin; EBAP, etoposide, bleomycin, cisplatin; EIP, etoposide, ifosfamide, cisplatin; EP, etoposide, cisplatin; NA, not available; PVB (Einhorn regimen), cisplatin 20 mg/m² IV × 5 days, vinblastine 0.15 mg/kg D 1,2, bleomycin 30 U weekly, cycles repeated of 3 weeks VAB-6, multidrug regimen developed at Memorial Sloan-Kettering Cancer Center; VIP, vinblastine, ifosfamide, cisplatin.

have serial CT scans performed every 3 months during the first year following treatment, with biopsy of any enlarging mass on chest CT.

In summary, most patients with mediastinal seminoma can be cured with therapy, and all patients should be approached with this intent. For most patients, initial cisplatin-based chemotherapy is the treatment of choice. Optimal chemotherapy includes four courses of bleomycin, etoposide, and cisplatin, as is recommended for poor-prognosis testicular germ cell tumors.[56] Patients with mediastinal masses <6 cm in diameter (usually asymptomatic) have the option of radiation therapy as primary therapy, with cisplatin-based chemotherapy available for those who relapse.

Treatment of Nonseminomatous Tumors

Prior to the development of effective cisplatin based chemotherapy, no effective therapy was available for nonseminomatous mediastinal germ cell tumors.[57] Local treatment modalities were ineffective because of the high percentage of patients with metastatic disease and the relative radioresistance of these tumors.

The use of intensive cisplatin-based chemotherapy developed for the treatment of advanced nonseminomatous testicular neoplasms has improved the previously dismal outlook in patients with mediastinal nonseminomatous germ cell tumors. Although overall cure rates remain lower than those achieved in the treatment of testicular cancer, a compilation of results from reported series containing 10 or more patients and using optimal chemotherapy indicates a 41% long-term survival rate (Table 82-2).[22-24,26,27,43,44,47,58-61] The large bulk of most mediastinal germ cell tumors at the time of diagnosis contributes to these relatively poor results. Comparable long-term survival rates of 40-50% have been reported when testicular germ cell tumors with far advanced, bulky metastases are treated with similar cisplatin-based regimens.[62] However, it is now recognized that inherent biologic differences between mediastinal and testicular germ cell tumors also play a role in determining the relatively low cure rate.[63]

At present, treatment for all histologic subtypes of mediastinal nonseminomatous germ cell tumor should follow the same guidelines. Early reports of an unfavorable outcome for patients with pure endodermal sinus tumors have not been confirmed when modern cisplatin-based chemotherapy is used.[64] Pure mediastinal choriocorcinoma probably has a worse prognosis [22]; however, there is currently no rationale for treating these patients differently from other patients with nonseminomatous mediastinal germ cell tumors.

The treatment for mediastinal nonseminomatous germ cell tumors should follow guidelines for poor-prognosis testicular cancer. Initial treatment with four courses of bleomycin, etoposide, and cisplatin is considered standard therapy.[56] As in the treatment of testicular cancer, administration of chemotherapy at full doses and on schedule is important in obtaining optimal results. Following the completion of therapy, patients should

Table 82-2 ■ Results of Initial Treatment With Cisplatin-Based Combination Chemotherapy in Nonseminomatous Mediastinal Germ Cell Tumors

Study, Year	No. of Evaluable Patients	Chemotherapy Regimen	No. of Complete Responders (%)	No. of Long-Term (>24 Mo) Disease-Free Survivors (%)
Funes et al, 1981[56]	13	PVB	6 (46)	5 (38)
Hainsworth et al, 1982[22]	12	PVB ± A	7 (58)	7 (58)
Logothetis et al, 1985[24]	11	CISCA II CISCA/VBIV	NA	4 (36)
Israel et al, 1985[23]	11[a]	VAB-6	NA	4 (36)
Kay et al, 1987[57]	11	PVB, BEP	7 (64)	5 (45)
Nichols et al, 1990[26]	31	PVB ± A, BEP	18 (58)	13 (42)
Bukowski et al, 1993[43]	16	PVB/EBAP	9 (56)	9 (56)
Delgado et al, 1993[44]	40	VAB-6, PVB, BEP	15 (38)	14 (35)
Gerl et al, 1996[47]	12	PVB, BEP, ECBC	8 (67)	6 (50)
Hidalgo et al, 1997[58]	27	Cisplatin based	11 (41)	8 (30)
Fizazi et al, 1998[59]	29	VAP-6, PveVB, PVB, BEP	19 (60)	10 (34)
Ganjoo et al, 2000[27]	75	Cisplatin based	49 (65)	36 (48)
Total	288		49 (56)	121 (42)

Abbreviations: A, Adriamycin (doxorubicin); BEP, bleomycin 30 units weekly, etoposide 100 mg/m² intravenously (IV) × 5 days, cisplatin 20 mg/m² IV × 5 days, cycles repeated every 3 weeks; CISCA II, CISCA/VBIV, multidrug regimens developed at The University of Texas M. D. Anderson Cancer Center; EBAP, etoposide, bleomycin, Adriamycin (doxorubicin), cisplatin; ECBC, etoposide, cisplatin, bleomycin, cyclophosphamide; NA, not available; PVB, cisplatin 20 mg/m² IV × 5 days, vinblastine 0.15 mg/kg days 1 and 2, bleomycin 30 U weekly; PveVB, cisplatin, etoposide, vinblastine, bleomycin; VAB-6, multidrug regimen developed at Memorial Sloan-Kettering Cancer Center.

[a]Includes patients with retroperitoneal tumors.

be restaged with repeat serum tumor markers and CT scans of the chest and abdomen.

Subsequent management is determined by the response to initial chemotherapy (Fig. 82-1). Patients with normal CT scans and tumor marker levels should receive no further therapy. Approximately 20% of these patients subsequently relapse, with almost all relapses occurring during the first 2 years after completion of therapy. Standard follow-up of these patients includes monthly physical examination, chest radiography, and serum tumor marker determinations during the first year and similar evaluations every 2 months during the second year following therapy.

The large majority of patients have residual radiographic abnormalities in the mediastinum after completion of chemotherapy.[27] In these patients, surgical resection of residual masses should be performed if technically feasible. Persistent elevation of serum tumor markers is not a contraindication to surgical resection in this setting because salvage chemotherapy regimens for patients with persistent carcinoma are usually ineffective.[65,66] Pathologic findings in resected specimens have varied widely in different reported series, probably based on differences in patient selection criteria. Residual germ cell carcinoma is found in a substantial proportion of patients (25-66%).[67-69] A small percentage of patients have residual cancer of various non-germ cell histologies (eg, sarcoma, adenocarcinoma, neuroendocrine carcinoma).[69] The remainder of patients have either benign teratoma, necrosis, or fibrosis without active carcinoma. Patients with a large component of teratocarcinoma in the original biopsy are more likely to have residual benign teratoma.

Surgical resection of all residual radiographic abnormalities is curative for a substantial proportion of patients. Patients with no viable tumor remaining (ie, necrotic tumor, fibrosis, and/or benign teratoma only) have the same low risk of subsequent relapse as do patients achieving complete remission with chemotherapy alone.[67,69] Resection of benign teratoma is therapeutic because these can undergo slow local growth or subsequent malignant degeneration when left in place. Patients with resection of residual germ cell carcinoma have a high risk of future relapse; however, surgical resection is curative in 20-30%.[68,69] In these patients, two additional courses of chemotherapy postoperatively may reduce the recurrence rate. Most patients with residual non-germ cell histologies do poorly even with complete resection, although occasional long-term survivors have been reported.[69] Further systemic treatment after resection in these patients has been ineffective.

The prognosis is very poor for patients in whom complete surgical resection is not feasible, as well as in those who relapse after surgical resection. Standard second-line cisplatin-based

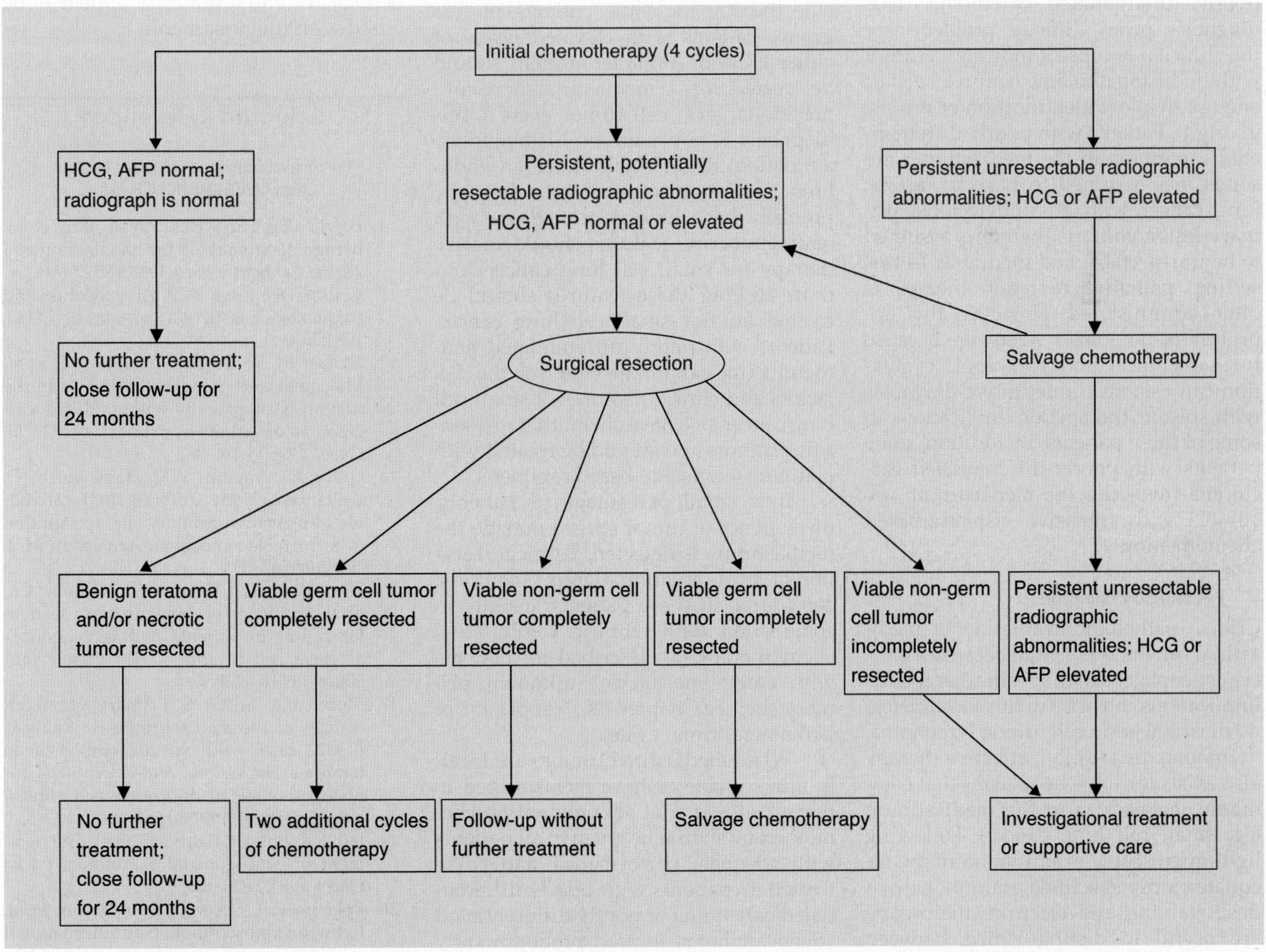

Figure 82-1 Management of mediastinal nonseminomatous germ cell tumors after completion of first-line chemotherapy. *Abbreviations:* AFP, alpha-fetoprotein; HCG, human chorionic gonadotropin. *Salvage regimens used in advanced testicular germ cell tumors are less effective for mediastinal tumors.

regimens and high-dose chemotherapy regimens are curative in 20-50% of patients with recurrent testicular cancer but are effective in only 11% of patients with mediastinal nonseminomatous germ cell tumors.[65,66] High-dose chemotherapy as salvage treatment is also unsuccessful in these patients, in contrast to the favorable results in patients with relapsed nonseminomatous testicular germ cell tumors.[70] The combination of paclitaxel/ifosfamide/cisplatin has improved the salvage therapy of patients with relapsed testicular germ cell tumors, but has not been evaluated in patients with mediastinal germ cell tumors.[71] Treatment with this regimen or inclusion in a clinical trial evaluating novel therapy are reasonable choices for salvage therapy in this difficult group.

Poorly Differentiated Carcinoma of the Mediastinum

Occasionally, the biopsy diagnosis in a patient with a mediastinal tumor is poorly differentiated carcinoma. This diagnosis poses difficult problems for the clinician because it indicates a tumor with no histopathologic features specific enough to allow identification of the site of origin. Patients with poorly differentiated carcinoma in the mediastinum are sometimes assumed to have metastatic lung cancer with an undetectable primary lesion and are, therefore, assumed to be unresectable and incurable. In this setting, palliative radiation therapy is often administered. However, this approach is no longer adequate because further clinical and pathologic evaluation can establish a definitive diagnosis with specific therapeutic implications in some of these patients. In addition, some patients with poorly differentiated carcinoma involving the mediastinum are curable with intensive cisplatin-based chemotherapy.[13,72]

Pathologic Evaluation

Critical pathologic evaluation of mediastinal tumors is essential because a variety of neoplasms with specific therapeutic implications can arise in this location (eg, mediastinal germ cell tumor, lymphoma, thymoma). In addition, effective therapy also exists for some neoplasms that commonly metastasize to the mediastinum (eg, small cell lung cancer). Following light microscopic examination of an adequate biopsy specimen, immunoperoxidase staining and electron microscopy are useful in distinguishing between the various neoplasms occurring in the mediastinum. By using these methods, lymphoma and neuroendocrine tumors (including small cell lung cancer) can be reliably identified, and appropriate therapeutic approaches can be defined. Molecular genetic analysis should also be considered in young men, because identification of an i(12p) chromosomal abnormality is diagnostic of a germ cell tumor.[12]

Diagnostic Evaluation and Staging Workup

All patients should have CT scans of the chest and abdomen, as well as measurement of serum levels of HCG and alpha-fetoprotein. PET scanning is also effective in identifying a primary site in a minority of patients, and is now routinely included in the diagnostic evaluation of patients with carcinoma of unknown primary site.[73] Fiber-optic bronchoscopy should be performed if other studies are nondiagnostic. Small cell lung cancer should be suspected when neuroendocrine features are found in patients with a history of cigarette smoking.

Treatment

The diagnostic evaluation defines specific therapy for some patients in this group. Patients with elevated levels of either HCG or alpha-fetoprotein should be treated for a mediastinal nonseminomatous germ cell tumor even if this diagnosis is not made by histologic examination. Patients who have an endobronchial lesion found at bronchoscopy probably have lung cancer, those with neuroendocrine features should receive therapy for small cell lung cancer, and those lacking these features should be treated for non-small cell lung cancer. Patients with poorly differentiated neuroendocrine carcinoma who lack the risk factors and clinical features of small cell lung cancer also have chemotherapy-sensitive tumors and should be treated with platinum/etoposide-based regimens.[74,75]

In a small percentage of patients, no evidence of tumor spread outside the mediastinum is detected. Surgical resection or local radiation therapy should be considered in these patients, usually in conjunction with empiric combination chemotherapy (as described for patients with carcinoma of an unknown primary site; see Chapter 120: Neoplasms of Unknown Primary Site).

When mediastinal tumors are locally unresectable or have metastasized to distant sites, a trial of combination chemotherapy should be given to all patients with adequate performance status. We treated 43 patients with poorly differentiated carcinoma or poorly differentiated adenocarcinoma located predominantly in the mediastinum.[72] These patients represented 19% of our entire group of patients with poorly differentiated carcinoma of an unknown primary site. The median age was 38 years; 32 patients had other metastatic sites in addition to the mediastinum. Only 5 of 43 patients (12%) had elevated serum levels of HCG or alpha-fetoprotein. All patients received cisplatin-based chemotherapy; 13 patients (30%) had a complete response, and 7 patients (16%) are long-term disease-free survivors. A review of the light microscopic features in these patients failed to reveal any previously unsuspected germ cell tumors or lymphomas.

In summary, patients with mediastinal tumors initially diagnosed as poorly differentiated carcinoma are a heterogeneous group. Some of these patients actually have well-defined tumor types that can be identified with additional pathologic or clinical evaluation. Patients in whom a specific tumor is identified should be treated according to standard guidelines for that tumor type. A trial of platinum-based chemotherapy should be given to patients in whom no well-defined tumor type is recognized. Some of these patients have highly responsive neoplasms, and a minority appear to be cured with this treatment.

Selected References

The complete reference list can be found at www.CANCERMEDICINE8.com

3. Lewis BD, Hurt RD, Payne WS, et al. Benign teratomas of the mediastinum. *J Thorac Cardiovasc Surg.* 1983;86:727–731.
11. Collins DH, Pugh RCB. Classification and frequency of testicular tumors. *Br J Urol.* 1984;36:1–11.
12. Motzer RJ, Rodriguez E, Reuter VE, et al. Molecular and cytogenetic studies in the diagnosis of patients with mid-line carcinomas of unknown primary site. *J Clin Oncol.* 1995;13:274–282.
13. Greco FA, Vaughn WK, Hainsworth JD. Advanced poorly differentiated carcinoma of unknown primary site: recognition of a treatable syndrome. *Ann Intern Med.* 1986;104:547–553.
16. Hartmann JT, Fossa SD, Nichols CR, et al. Incidence of metachronous testicular cancer in patients with extra-gonadal germ cell tumors. *J Natl Cancer Inst.* 2001;93:1733–1738.
17. Moran CA, Suster S. Primary germ cell tumors of the mediastinum—I. Analysis of 322 cases with special emphasis on teratomatous lesions and a proposal for histopathologic classification and clinical staging. *Cancer.* 1997;80:681–690.
19. Jain KK, Bosl GJ, Bains MS, et al. The treatment of extra-gonadal seminoma. *J Clin Oncol.* 1984;2:820–827.
20. Bokemeyer C, Droz JP, Horwich A, et al. Extragonadal seminoma: an international multicenter analysis of prognostic factors and long term treatment outcome. *Cancer.* 2001;91:1394–1401.

22. Hainsworth JD, Einhorn LH, Williams SD, et al. Advanced extragonadal germ cell tumors. Successful treatment with combination chemotherapy. *Ann Intern Med.* 1982;97:7–11.
23. Israel A, Bosl GJ, Golbey RB, et al. The results of chemotherapy for extragonadal germ cell tumors in the cisplatin era: the Memorial Sloan-Kettering Cancer Center experience (1975 to 1982). *J Clin Oncol.* 1985;3:1073–1078.
26. Nichols CR, Saxman S, Williams SD, et al. Primary mediastinal nonseminomatous germ cell tumors—a modern single institution experience. *Cancer.* 1990;65:1641–1646.
27. Ganjoo KN, Rieger KM, Kesler KA, et al. Results of modern therapy for patients with mediastinal nonseminomatous germ cell tumors. *Cancer.* 2000;88:1051–1056.
31. Nichols CR, Heerema NA, Palmer C, et al. Klinefelter's syndrome associated with mediastinal germ cell neoplasms. *J Clin Oncol.* 1987;5:1290–1294.
34. Nichols CR, Roth BJ, Heerema N, et al. Hematologic neoplasia associated with primary mediastinal germ cell tumors. *N Engl J Med.* 1990;322:1425–1429.
39. Hartmann JT, Nichols CR, Droz JP, et al. Hematologic disorders associated with primary mediastinal nonseminomatous germ cell tumors. *J Natl Cancer Inst.* 2000;92:54–61.
46. Mencel PJ, Motzer RJ, Mazumdar M, et al. Advanced seminoma: treatment results, survival, and prognostic factors in 142 patients. *J Clin Oncol.* 1994;12:120–126.
48. Bokemeyer C, Droz JP, Horwich A, et al. Extragonadal seminoma: an international multicenter analysis of prognostic factors and long-term treatment outcome. *Cancer.* 2001;91:1394–1401.
51. Majewski W, Majewski S, Maciejewski A, et al. Adverse effects after radiotherapy for early stage (I, IIa, IIb) seminoma. *Radiother Oncol.* 2005;76:257–264.
53. Schultz SM, Einhorn LH, Conces DJ, et al. Management of postchemotherapy residual mass in patients with advanced seminoma: Indiana University experience. *J Clin Oncol.* 1989;7:1497–1503.
54. Puc HS, Heelan R, Mazumdar M, et al. Management of residual mass in advanced seminoma: results and recommendations from the Memorial Sloan-Kettering Cancer Center. *J Clin Oncol.* 1996;14:454–460.
55. DeSantis M, Becherer A, Bokemeyer C, et al. 2-18Fluorodeoxy-D-glucose positron emission tomography is a reliable predictor for viable tumor in postchemotherapy seminoma: an update of the prospective multicentre SEMPET trial. *J Clin Oncol.* 2004;22:1034–1039.
61. Fizazi K, Culine S, Droz JP, et al. Primary mediastinal nonseminomatous germ cell tumors: results of modern therapy including cisplatin-based chemotherapy. *J Clin Oncol.* 1998;16:725–732.
67. Kesler KA, Rieger KM, Ganjoo KN, et al. Primary mediastinal nonseminomatous germ cell tumors: the influence of postchemotherapy pathology on long-term survival after surgery. *J Thorac Cardiovasc Surg.* 1999;118:692–699.
68. Vuky J, Bains M, Bacik J, et al. Role of postchemotherapy adjunctive surgery in the management of patients with nonseminoma arising from the mediastinum. *J Clin Oncol.* 2001;19:682–688.
69. Schneider BP, Kesler KA, Brooks JA, et al. Outcome of patients with residual germ cell or non-germ cell malignancy after resection of primary mediastinal nonseminomatous germ cell cancer. *J Clin Oncol.* 2004;22:1195–1200.
72. Hainsworth JD, Johnson DH, Greco FA. Cisplatin-based combination chemotherapy in the treatment of poorly differentiated carcinoma and poorly differentiated adenocarcinoma of unknown primary site: results of a twelve-year experience at a single institution. *J Clin Oncol.* 1992;10:912–922.
73. Seve P, Billotey C, Broussole C, et al. The role of 2-deoxy-2-[F-18] fluoro-D-glucose positron emission tomography in disseminated carcinoma of unknown primary site. *Cancer.* 2007;109:292–299.
74. Hainsworth JD, Johnson DH, Greco FA. Poorly differentiated neuroendocrine carcinoma of unknown primary site: a newly recognized clinicopathologic entity. *Ann Intern Med.* 1988;109:364–371.
75. Hainsworth JD, Spigel DR, Litchy S, Greco FA. Phase II trial of paclitaxel, carboplatin, and etoposide in advanced poorly differentiated neuroendocrine carcinoma: a Minnie Pearl Cancer Research Network study. *J Clin Oncol.* 2006;29:3548–3554.

83 Neoplasms of the Esophagus

Stephen G. Swisher, MD ■ David C. Rice, MD ■ Jaffer A. Ajani, MD ■ Ritsuko K. Komaki, MD ■ Mark K. Ferguson, MD

Neoplasms of the esophagus and gastroesophageal junction are among the most challenging oncologic problems. Management of this disease is plagued by nihilism because of high rates of mortality. Early mortality is common because the majority of the cancers are in an advanced stage at the time of diagnosis and because current therapies are relatively ineffective once the tumor has reached an advanced stage. Esophageal cancer was recognized as early as the twelfth century, and pathologic descriptions were produced in the sixteenth and seventeenth centuries.[1] Initial attempts to treat the tumor included resection of a cervical esophageal cancer in 1877 and an intrathoracic cancer in 1913.[2,3] Surgical resection became the mainstay of therapy beginning in the 1940s. Radiotherapy was initially used in the 1920s, but it was not until the development of megavoltage techniques in the 1950s that this modality was used with any frequency. Active chemotherapeutic agents were first identified in the 1960s and have been increasingly incorporated into the treatment of advanced tumors.

Anatomy and Histology

The esophagus is a muscular organ that extends from the cricopharyngeus muscle at its cephalad margin to the esophagogastric junction (EGJ). It is divided into regions on the basis of both anatomy and the proclivity for certain neoplasms to develop in specific regions (Fig. 83-1). The cervical esophagus extends from the cricopharyngeus muscle to the thoracic inlet (15–18 cm from incisors). The upper third of the thoracic esophagus extends from the thoracic inlet to the tracheal bifurcation, just below the level of the aortic arch (18–24 cm). The middle thoracic esophagus extends from the tracheal bifurcation to a point midway between the carina and the EGJ (24–32 cm). The lower thoracic esophagus extends from this midway point to the EGJ (32–40 cm). Tumors of the EGJ and gastric cardia are often included in discussions of esophageal cancer because of their pathophysiologic similarities to adenocarcinomas of the distal esophagus.[4] Classifications of EGJ tumors have developed that define the different types of tumors according to the epicenter of the mass (ie, type I, >1 cm above EGJ; type II, 1 cm above to 2 cm below EGJ; type III, >2–5 cm below EGJ).[5]

The muscle tissues of the esophagus are arranged in an outer longitudinal layer and an inner circular layer. The proximal one-third to one-half of the muscularis propria is derived from the bronchial arches, making it principally skeletal (striated) muscle and giving it the potential to develop rhabdomyosarcomas (Table 83-1). The remainder of the esophageal musculature comprises smooth muscle, as does the rest of the foregut, in which leiomyomas or leiomyosarcomas may occur. Fibrous, fatty, and connective tissues interspersed in the wall of the esophagus may also give rise to sarcomas.

The esophagus is lined over most of its length with squamous epithelium, which can give rise to squamous cell carcinoma and is the most common neoplasm of the esophagus in most of the world. These cancers occur most often in the cervical esophagus and in the upper and middle thoracic esophagus. Carcinosarcomas and spindle cell carcinomas, which are subtypes of squamous cell cancer, infrequently occur in these regions. The distal 2–3 cm of the esophagus and the cardia are lined by columnar epithelium, in which adenocarcinomas may occur.[5] The development of intestinal metaplasia, known as Barrett esophagus, more proximally because of gastroesophageal reflux and other factors allows the development of adenocarcinomas in the middle and upper thoracic esophagus in isolated instances. Other cellular elements in the mucosa, submucosal glands, and muscularis propria may give rise to unusual neoplasms, such as small cell cancer, malignant melanoma, granular cell tumors, mucoepidermoid carcinoma, and adenoid cystic carcinoma.[6,7] The histologic types of benign and malignant tumors of the esophagus are shown in Table 83-1.

Etiology

In most of the world, dietary and nutritional factors are the most common etiologic agents and are associated with the development of predominantly squamous cell carcinomas. Among the most frequently cited carcinogens are nitrosamines, which have been found to be in high concentrations in foods in endemic areas of esophageal cancer in northern China.[8] Contamination of food

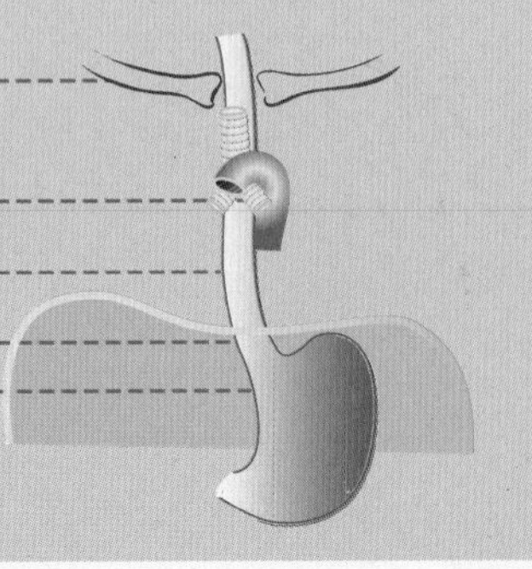

	Squamous carcinoma	Adeno-carcinoma	Total
Cervical	5%	0%	5%
Upper thoracic	15%	1%	16%
Middle thoracic	9%	2%	11%
Lower thoracic	2%	28%	30%
Cardia	0%	38%	38%
	31%	69%	100%

Figure 83-1 ■ The distribution of malignant neoplasms of the esophagus according to cell type and site of occurrence.

Table 83-1 ■ **Neoplasms of the Esophagus**

Epithelial
- Squamous cell carcinoma
  - Spindle cell carcinoma
  - Carcinosarcoma
- Adenocarcinoma
- Adenosquamous carcinoma
- Mucoepidermoid carcinoma
- Adenoid cystic carcinoma
- Small cell carcinoma

Nonepithelial
- Leiomyoma
- Leiomyosarcoma
- Malignant melanoma
- Rhabdomyoma
- Rhabdomyosarcoma
- Granular cell tumors
- Malignant lymphoma

by fungi that reduce nitrate to nitrite may further aggravate this situation. Mechanical factors that have been cited include drinking beverages at excessively high temperatures and consumption of foods containing silica or other substances, such as crushed seeds, that directly irritate the esophagus.[8,9] Deficiencies of folic acid, vitamins A and C, and riboflavin, molybdenum, and selenium also have been implicated in the development of esophageal neoplasms.[10-12]

In the western hemisphere, social factors figure more prominently in the development of esophageal cancer. Heavy alcohol consumption increases the risk of cancer 10 to 25 times, depending on the concentration of alcohol in the beverage.[13] Cigarette smoking has been linked to the development of both squamous cell cancers and adenocarcinomas.[14] The combined exposure to low levels of tobacco and alcohol increases the risk of esophageal cancer by a factor of 10 to 20, whereas the synergistic effect of exposure to high levels of both alcohol and tobacco increases the risk by a factor of over 100.[15] Chronic esophageal injury due to gastroesophageal reflux has also been shown to be a risk factor for the development of adenocarcinoma, with severe, longstanding reflux symptoms increasing the risk of cancer by a factor of 40.[16] Chronic gastroesophageal reflux is believed to be etiologically related to the development of Barrett esophagus, which occurs primarily in white males and is associated with a 40-fold increase in the risk of adenocarcinoma of the esophagus.[17] A relationship between reflux and the development of squamous cell cancers has also been suggested in patients who consume a diet high in linoleic acid.[18] The lifetime risk of squamous cell cancer of the esophagus is 5–10% in patients with esophageal achalasia, a 15-fold increase in incidence that is likely due to chronic irritation from retained food.[19-21]

Race and gender are associated with varying incidences of cancer of the esophagus in the western hemisphere. Men are more commonly affected than are women, blacks develop squamous cell cancers more often than do whites, and white males develop adenocarcinomas more often than do females or individuals of other race groups.[22] However, none of these increased frequencies has yet been linked to genetic factors, and most have been explained by variations in socioeconomic status and the attendant social habits described earlier. The single proven genetic abnormality that is associated with a 25% lifetime incidence of squamous cell cancer of the esophagus is tylosis A, the late-onset, familial form of palmar and plantar hyperkeratosis.[23] A number of genetic alterations are associated with neoplasms of the esophagus, including allelic losses at chromosomes 3p, 5q, 9p, 9q, 13q, 17p, 17q, and 18q. Abnormalities of TP53, Rb, cyclin D1 and c-myc have also been associated with esophageal cancer development.[24]

Infectious agents, including human papillomavirus (HPV), have been implicated in the development of neoplasms of the esophagus. Transforming proteins from high-risk HPV subtypes 16, 18 cause loss of function of the tumor suppressor genes TP53 and Rb, resulting in abnormal proliferative states.[25] HPV has been documented in up to 50% of patients with squamous cell cancers of the esophagus and appears to be more common in areas in which esophageal cancer is endemic.[26] These findings have not been universally reproducible, however.[27]

Epidemiology

The most common neoplasm worldwide is squamous cell carcinoma; in the United States and Europe, adenocarcinoma now predominates (Fig. 83-2). The incidence of esophageal cancer varies more worldwide than any other cancer. In the United States, the incidence of esophageal cancer is approximately 7 cases per 100,000 people, whereas in high-risk areas in China, Iran, and Russia, it can be more than 100 per 100,000. In rural Linxian, China, esophageal cancer is the leading cause of death.[28,29] These geographical variations imply a strong role for local environmental carcinogens in esophageal carcinogenesis. The long-term survival rate for patients with esophageal cancer, regardless of histology, is less than 10%, which is due, in large part, to the advanced stage at which these cancers are detected. The age-adjusted mortality rate from esophageal cancer in the United States is 4.4 per 100,000 population per year, a figure that increased by 22% between 1973 and 1999.[30] These data translate to an estimated incidence of 13,900 new cases and about 13,000 deaths from esophageal cancer in 2003 (excluding tumors of the EGJ).[31]

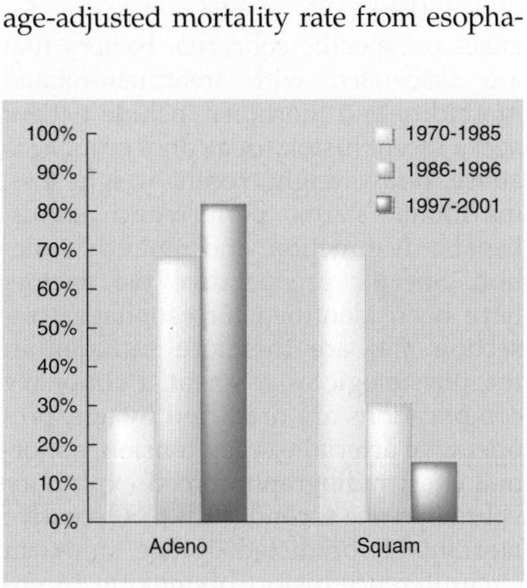

Figure 83-2 ■ The proportion of adenocarcinoma and distal esophageal tumors has increased over time. *Abbreviations:* Adeno, adenocarcinoma; squam, squamous cell carcinoma. *Source:* From Ref. 79.

Besides geographical differences, there are other important differences that have been described in the Western hemisphere. Esophageal carcinoma is more common in men than women regardless of the histologic subtype, and squamous cell cancers tend to occur more frequently in blacks than in whites. In addition, there has been a striking increase in the incidence of adenocarcinoma in the United States and Europe, whereas squamous cell carcinoma has remained stable.[32] Adenocarcinoma of the distal esophagus and cardia have risen by more than 350% among white males since the mid-1970s, increasing at a more rapid rate than any other solid tumor (Fig. 83-2).[22,33-37] The reasons for these dramatic changes in the Western hemisphere are not clear but may include increased Barrett esophagus, gastroesophageal reflux, obesity, and over-the-counter medications as well as changing smoking and alcohol use.[16] In other areas of the world (outside Europe and North America), squamous cell carcinoma of the esophagus predominates and adenocarcinoma has not increased.

Patients usually present because of complaints of dysphagia, which requires either the involvement of the entire circumference of the esophagus by the neoplasm or the growth of a large, polypoid obstructing mass. Dysphagia first develops in response to dense solid foods and progresses to result in difficulties with soft foods and then liquids. Accompanying vomiting and regurgitation are common. Symptoms of heartburn or gastroesophageal reflux (40%) are often associated and occur more frequently in patients with adenocarcinoma.[38] The most common symptom in the absence of dysphagia is pain (25% of cases).[38] It may be related to swallowing (odynophagia) or local extension of the tumor into adjacent structures such as the vertebral bodies, pleura, or mediastinum. In some instances, it may be due to bony metastases from systemic spread. Weight loss is noted in more than 70% of patients and is due to the inability to swallow or to systemic manifestations of the disease.[38] Patients with weight loss have a significantly worse prognosis in many series.[39,40]

The location of the tumor depends in large part on histology. Adenocarcinoma is located predominantly in the lower esophagus, whereas squamous cell carcinoma predominates in the cervical, upper, and middle esophagus (Figs. 83-1 and 83-2). Unfortunately, because of the distensible nature of the esophagus, these symptoms often do not occur until the tumors are quite large and no longer localized to the esophagus.

In contrast to patients who present because of symptoms of dysphagia, a smaller subset of earlier stage adenocarcinoma patients are increasingly being identified in North America and Europe with endoscopic abnormalities noted during endoscopic surveillance for gastroesophageal reflux symptoms or Barrett esophagus. These patients tend to present with smaller, earlier stage tumors that are more likely to be localized and amenable to treatment. In addition, in some areas of China where squamous cell cancer is endemic, routine cytologic screening is performed, and if results are diagnostic or suspicious, follow-up endoscopy is performed. These mass screening efforts have led to early diagnosis in many areas of China, with 5-year survivals of more than 90%.[29] The low incidence of esophageal cancer in most areas of the world, however, makes this type of mass screening impractical and cost ineffective from a public health standpoint.

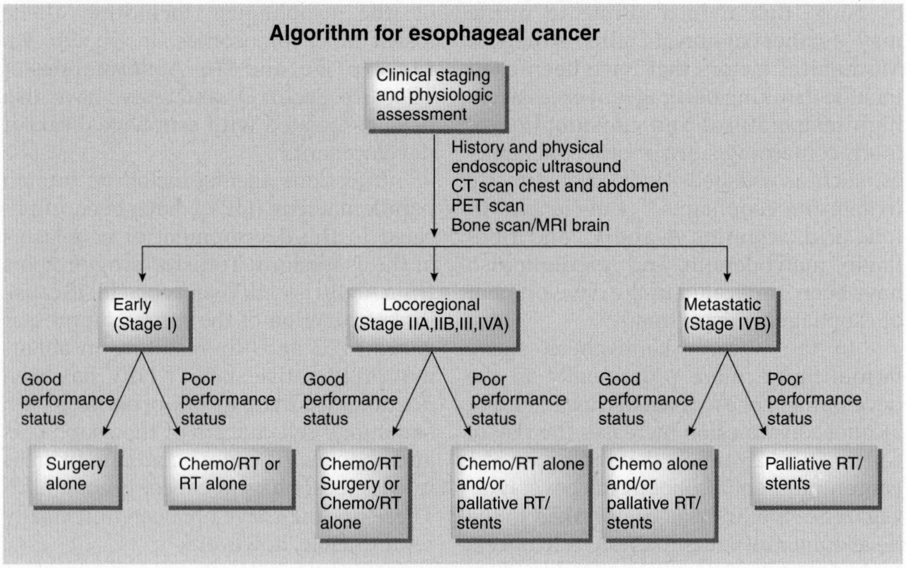

Figure 83-3 Current treatment recommendations for esophageal cancer based on performance status and clinical stage at the University of Texas M.D. Anderson Cancer Center. *Abbreviations:* Chemo, chemotherapy; CT, computed tomography; MRI, magnetic resonance imaging; PET, positron emission tomography; RT, radiotherapy.

Treatment Overview

Patients who present with suspected esophageal cancer, either because of the above-mentioned symptoms or mass screening efforts, initially require pathologic confirmation of malignancy (see "Diagnosis" below). Once the pathologic diagnosis has been obtained, patients are assessed for therapy by determining the clinical stage (see "Staging Evaluation") of the tumor and the physiologic status of the patient (see "Pretreatment Assessment"). With this information, an informed decision about treatment can be made that optimizes the chance to cure or palliate the disease while minimizing the treatment-related morbidity (see "Therapy") (Fig. 83-3).

Diagnosis

Symptomatic patients or patients in whom an esophageal mass is diagnosed by screening require endoscopy to enable biopsy for histologic examination and/or brushing for cytologic examination. The overall accuracy of histologic diagnosis of esophageal cancer using flexible endoscopy with biopsy is about 80%.[41,42] Endoscopically directed cytologic brushings have a diagnostic accuracy in excess of 90%. Combining these techniques yields an overall diagnostic accuracy of 98%.[41] If flexible endoscopic diagnostic techniques fail, rigid endoscopy with biopsy, which has a diagnostic accuracy close to 100%, should be considered.[42] In selected patients who have symptoms or findings on physical examination suggestive of metastatic disease, biopsy of the suspected metastatic site provides both a tissue diagnosis and a confirmation of stage.

Pretreatment Assessment

In addition to a careful history and physical examination, the overall assessment of a patient with esophageal cancer focuses on specific concerns. Factors that are associated with treatment-related morbidity and mortality include patient age, a recent history of alcohol or tobacco abuse, body weight, recent weight loss, nutritional status, performance status, hepatic dysfunction, and renal dysfunction. Specific preoperative risk factors have been identified for esophageal resection and are therefore included in the physiologic assessment. Pulmonary complications are predicted by age, preoperative arterial oxygen tension, abnormal chest radiograph, forced expiratory volume in one second (FEV_1).[43] Operative mortality is predicted by age, mid-arm circumference, history of smoking, incentive spirometry, performance status, and the frequency with which the operation is performed in an institution.[43,44] Any symptoms of cardiac disease necessitate careful evaluation with electrocardiography (ECG), echocardiography, stress tests, and coronary arteriography as indicated. Patients with significant coronary artery disease are at increased risk of morbidity and mortality and cardiac intervention may be warranted prior to treatment of the esophageal neoplasm. These physiologic assessments allow patients to be classified as good or poor performance status, which then allows the aggressiveness of treatment to be tailored to their specific risks (Fig. 83-3).

Staging Evaluation

Assessment of stage permits medical practitioners to discuss the status of individual patients with accuracy, allows informed recommendations about therapy, and gives patients and their families necessary information about prognosis. The typical assessment for most patients often includes upper gastrointestinal endoscopy, contrast radiography of the esophagus, computed tomography (CT) of the chest and abdomen, endoscopic ultrasonography (EUS) and positron emission tomography (PET). Other examinations are selected on the basis of specific findings in individual patients, such as neurologic symptoms (magnetic resonance imaging [MRI] of brain), musculoskeletal symptoms (bone scan), or supraclavicular nodes (neck ultrasonography and biopsy). Staging techniques allow patients to be accurately placed into groups in which risk can be assessed as well as the optimum type of therapy.

Presentation

Contrast Radiography of the Esophagus

A contrast study of the esophagus is often the initial diagnostic examination obtained in patients with dysphagia. It allows confirmation of mucosal irregularity and serves as guide for subsequent endoscopy. It also allows evaluation of the esophagus and stomach distal to the area of stenosis, which cannot also be assessed by endoscopy with tight strictures.

Endoscopy ■ Upper gastrointestinal endoscopy allows a pathologic diagnosis to be obtained in the majority of patients. The gross appearance of the tumor can be categorized as advanced or superficial, and the extent of the tumor can be accurately determined. Additional unsuspected malignancies that may be present in up to 20% of patients with squamous cell cancer may also be identified. Endoscopy also permits assessment of the mobility of a tumor, indicating whether it is fixed within the mediastinum.

Endoscopic Ultrasonography ■ EUS improves the staging accuracy of primary tumors and regional and some nonregional lymph nodes. It has become a essential tool to help identify patients with early-stage carcinoma who do not need multimodality treatment (Fig. 83-3). EUS depicts the normal esophagus as five alternating hyperechoic and hypoechoic layers representing the mucosa and lamina propria, muscularis mucosa, submucosa, muscularis propria, and adventitia. Depth of tumor invasion is determined by assessing the level to which the tumor extends. EUS is also useful for assessing whether there is involvement of the aorta, but airway invasion is not accurately determined because of interference of the ultrasound signal with the intratracheal air column. The accuracy of EUS determination of primary tumor stage is related to the pathologic tumor stage, being more accurate for more advanced stages of disease, with an overall accuracy of about 80%.[45-47] EUS is substantially less accurate in staging primary tumors after chemoradiotherapy is administered, primarily because of overstaging. The technique is not able to distinguish between treatment-induced fibrosis and residual tumor, leading to a mean overall accuracy in this setting of 45%.[48]

In assessing lymph nodes with EUS, three criteria are used: size, border characteristics, and internal architecture. Lymph nodes that are enlarged, have a well-defined external border, and are characterized by relatively uniform, hypoechoic internal architecture are more likely to be malignant. Using these criteria, the overall accuracy of lymph node staging by EUS is about 75%.[46,49] After chemoradiotherapy, the accuracy of EUS for staging lymph nodes decreases to just over 50%.[48] Development of fine needle aspiration techniques have allowed pathologic confirmation of enlarged lymph nodes in both regional and nonregional sites.[47-50]

CT of the Chest and Abdomen ■ CT has become a standard technique for esophageal cancer staging since its inception in the late 1970s because it has allowed better identification of patients with metastatic (M1b) and locally invasive tumors (T4). CT is not very accurate for determining the depth of the primary tumor (T) status, but it is helpful in identifying patients who might have direct invasion of local structures, such as the aorta or major airways, either of which precludes surgical intervention.[45] Aortic invasion is suspected when more than 25% of the aortic circumference is effaced by an esophageal cancer.

CT does not accurately determine lymph node (N) status since normal lymph nodes often vary in size according to their location in the mediastinum and abdomen, and a single size limit for nodes is not possible to establish. In addition, lymph nodes involved by metastatic spread are often not enlarged.[51-54] The sensitivity for CT detection of involved lymph nodes is therefore poor (30-60%), and the overall accuracy of nodal detection by CT is less than 60%.[55-57]

CT is most useful for detecting distant often unsuspected metastatic (M) disease. The most common sites for metastatic spread, aside from nonregional lymph nodes, are (in decreasing order of frequency) the liver, lung, peritoneum, adrenal gland, bone, and kidney. CT of the thorax and abdomen evaluates almost all these regions. Accuracy of the CT detection of liver metastases is in excess of 90%.[51,56,58,59]

Bronchoscopy ■ Bronchoscopy should be performed for all patients who are candidates for surgical therapy and whose tumors are adjacent to the trachea or mainstem bronchi. This permits direct assessment of tumor invasion into the airway lumen or submucosa.

Magnetic Resonance Imaging ■ As a method for routine staging of esophageal neoplasms, MRI offers no advantages compared with CT and is therefore seldom used since it is a more difficult and expensive test to obtain. Both techniques have similar specificities, sensitivities, and overall accuracy for determining resectability with regard to direct invasion of the aorta and airway.[52,53,56] Neither test provides much useful information about regional or metastatic lymph nodes, and MRI offers no improvements over CT in evaluating the liver for metastatic disease. Whether advances in MRI technology will offer improved staging capabilities remains to be seen.

Positron Emission Tomography ■ PET scanning to detect involved lymph nodes and sites of metastatic disease through increased metabolism with 18F-fluorodeoxyglucose was introduced as an investigational staging technique for esophageal cancer in the mid-1990s. PET is most useful in helping identify patients with unsuspected metastatic disease. Given the possibility of false positive results from inflammation, biopsies are still required to definitively confirm metastatic disease in PET positive patients. The PET scan often serves as a guide to help identify suspected areas of metastatic disease for confirmatory biopsy. Another potential role for PET may be in determining response to chemotherapy and radiation therapy although false positives induced by chemotherapy and radiation-induced inflammation remain a problem.[60-62] PET may also have a role in identifying recurrent esophageal cancer by allowing targeting of unsuspected areas of increased metabolic activity.[63]

Bone Scintigraphy ■ Bone scans have been used for decades for staging patients with esophageal neoplasms, although their utility is unproven. In patients without bone pain or other evidence for metastatic disease, the likelihood of identifying skeletal metastases is less than 5%.[64]

Neck Ultrasonography ■ Cervical and supraclavicular lymph nodes are affected by metastatic spread in up to 30% of patients with neoplasms of the thoracic esophagus, and most are not detectable on physical examination. The use of routine ultrasound examination of the neck in patients without palpable lymph nodes yields unsuspected nodal metastases in over 10% of patients.[65] The overall accuracy of cervical and supraclavicular nodal assessment with ultrasonography is about 90%.[66,67] The addition of routine needle aspiration under ultrasound guidance for cytology may improve the yield of this potentially valuable technique.[67] At the present time, however, this is not a commonly used screening technique.

Minimally Invasive Surgical Staging ■ Laparoscopy has been used since the early 1980s, and thoracoscopy has been used since the early 1990s in an effort to improve staging of esophageal neoplasms. Both are used in some centers prior to preresectional therapy. The need for general anesthesia and a separate invasive procedure has limited the popularity of this staging procedure.

Biologic Staging ■ A variety of biologic markers have been investigated for their utility in estimating prognosis in patients with esophageal neoplasms. These include growth factors (epidermal growth factor [EGF], transforming growth factor [TGF]-β, platelet-derived growth factor [PDGF]), oncogenes (*c-myc, int-2, hst-1, cyclin D, EGFR, HER-2/neu, h-ras*), tumor suppressor genes (*Rb,TP53, p73, APC, MCC, p27*), the cell adhesion molecule E-cadherin, the oncodevelopmental marker CEA, and deoxyribonucleic acid (DNA) content and ploidy.[68-70] To date, none of these techniques have become generally accepted staging techniques except in isolated referral centers.

TNM (Tumor, Node, Metastasis) Staging System ■ These pretreatment staging evaluations allow patients to be clinically staged by a cTNM staging system that can help determine the optimum therapy (Fig. 83-3). The current staging system for esophageal cancer includes epithelial tumors of the cervical, thoracic, and intraabdominal esophagus, as well as of the EGJ (Table 83-2).[71] Tumors are staged according to clinical findings from noninvasive tests and pathologic findings resulting from any invasive staging procedures. It is useful to specify lymph node locations during biopsy and resection because their location determines whether they are considered regional nodes or nonregional metastatic nodal disease (Fig. 83-4). The prognosis of patients with esophageal cancer is determined by the depth of penetration of the primary tumor (transmural vs nontransmural), whether there is lymph node involvement, the relative number of lymph nodes involved, and whether distant metastases are present.[71-81,87-92] The long-term survival in patients with esophageal neoplasms correlates well with the pathologic stage (Fig. 83-5).[72,78] The ability of the clinical cTNM staging system to accurately predict the pTNM status has improved with time as the use of endoscopic ultrasound, CT of the chest and abdomen, and PET scan has increased.[79]

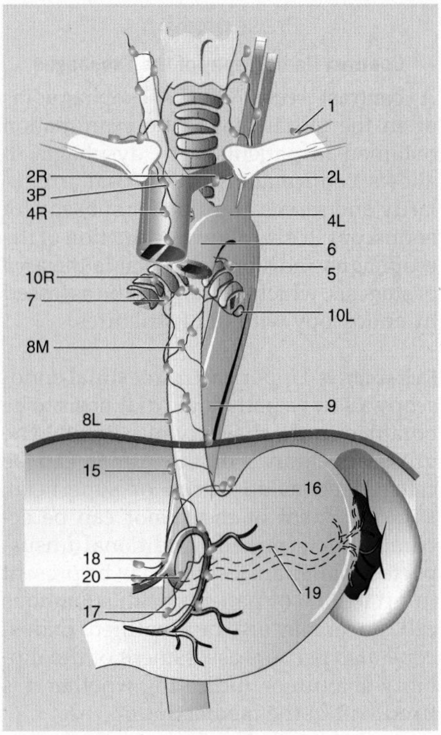

Figure 83-4 ■ Lymph node staging map for neoplasms of the esophagus. *Source*: From Ferguson, MK. Carcinoma of the esophagus and cardia. *Surgery of the Alimentary Tract*. 5th ed, vol. 1: *The Esophagus*, Elsevier.

Table 83-2 ■ **TNM Staging System for Esophageal Neoplasms**

Primary tumor (T)			
TX		Primary tumor cannot be assessed	
TO		No evidence of primary tumor	
Tis		Carcinoma in situ	
T1		Tumor invades lamina propria or submucosa	
T2		Tumor invades muscularis propria	
T3		Tumor invades adventitia	
T4		Tumor invades adjacent structures	
Regional lymph nodes (N)			
NX		Regional lymph nodes cannot be assessed	
NO		No regional lymph node metastases	
N1		Regional lymph node metastasis	
Distant metastasis (M)			
MX		Distant metastasis cannot be assessed	
MO		No distant metastasis	
M1		Distant metastasis	
		Tumors of the lower thoracic esophagus	
		M1a	Metastasis in celiac lymph nodes
		M1b	Other distant metastasis
		Tumors of the midthoracic esophagus	
		M1a	Not applicable
		M1b	Nonregional lymph nodes and/or other distant metastasis
		Tumors of the upper thoracic esophagus	
		M1a	Metastasis in cervical nodes
		M1b	Other distant metastasis
Stage grouping			
Stage 0	Tis NO	MO	
Stage 1	T1	NO	MO
Stage IIA	T2	NO	MO
	T3	NO	MO
Stage IIB	T1	N1	MO
	T2	N1	MO
Stage III	T3	N1	MO
	T4	Any N	MO
Stage IV	Any T	Any N	M1
Stage IVA	Any T	Any N	M1a
Stage IVB	Any T	Any N	M1b

Regional lymph nodes: Cervical esophageal tumor: scalene, internal jugular, upper cervical, periesophageal, supraclavicular, cervical not otherwise specified. *Intrathoracic esophageal tumor:* Tracheobronchial, superior mediastinal, peritracheal, carinal, hilar, periesophageal, perigastric, paracardial, mediastinal not otherwise specified.
Source: From Ref. 71.

Therapy

Standard curative treatment options for esophageal cancer include surgical resection, external beam radiotherapy, chemotherapy, or combinations of two or three of these options. The selection of appropriate therapy is often challenging because few comparisons of these options have been performed in prospective, randomized fashion. In addition, these trials have often been performed over a long time period with an inadequate number of patients during which significant changes in histology and types of treatment have occurred (ie, different radiation equipment, dosages and fields, and different surgical techniques and chemotherapy agents). Clinical staging techniques have also evolved over time, leading to stage migration and poor correlation with pathologic stage, especially from studies prior to CT scan, endoscopic ultrasound and PET.[79] These problems make comparisons between different trials or treatment arms difficult. Treatment strategies have therefore evolved over time based on regional experiences and biases. In an effort, to guide current treatment strategies, we have included an esophageal treatment algorithm that incorporates different treatment strategies based on the physiologic status and clinical stage of the patient (Fig. 83-3). This algorithm reflects the treatment

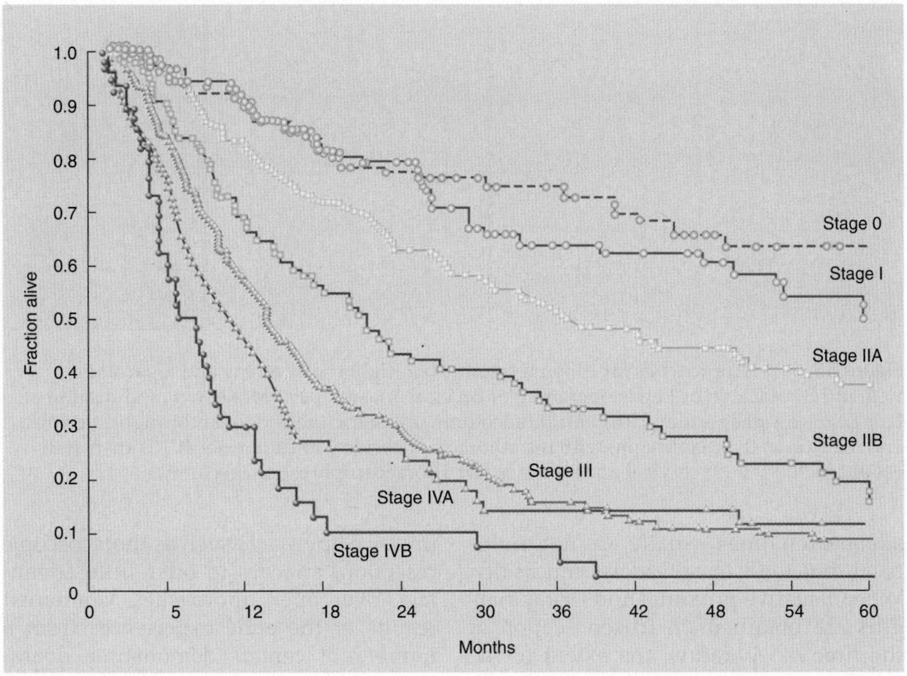

Figure 83-5 Long-term outcome according to pathologic stage of resected esophageal cancers at the University of Texas M.D. Anderson Cancer Center from 1970 to 2000 ($N = 917$).

biases of the authors and is meant only to give some guidance in an otherwise confusing therapeutic arena.

In esophageal cancer, local control of the disease, as well as cure, are the primary objectives of therapy because of the debilitating effects of dysphagia caused by progressive tumor growth and esophageal obstruction. Early-stage cancers (stage 0, I) traditionally have been treated by resection in good performance patients and by radiotherapy with or without radiation sensitizing chemotherapy in patients who cannot tolerate surgery. Recently newer noninvasive modes of treatment include endoscopic mucosal resection and other ablative therapies. Most patients, however, present with locoregionally advanced esophageal cancer because of the long period of asymptomatic tumor growth. These patients (stage II, III, and IVa) then to have poor outcome when treated with a single modality such as surgery or radiation therapy because of the development of metastatic and locoregional recurrences. Attempts have therefore focused on treating these patients with multimodality approaches combining locoregional (surgery/radiation) therapies with systemic (chemotherapy) treatments. Although controversial, many oncologists in North America currently recommend treating these patients with definitive chemoradiation alone or preoperative chemoradiation and surgery. The data to unequivocally support these approaches are lacking as demonstrated in the often conflicting randomized trial results (Table 83-3) and some centers have argued that more aggressive en bloc resection and 3-field lymphadenectomies are also important. Surgery and chemotherapy are often avoided in poor performance status locoregionally advanced patients because of treatment-related morbidity. In these patients, locoregional palliation can often be achieved with palliative stents and/or radiation. For patients who are initially recognized to be in advanced (metastatic) stages of disease, chemotherapy with or without palliative radiotherapy has been the mainstay of treatment. The development of endoesophageal stents has provided additional locoregional palliation and has limited the need for palliative surgical bypass even in patients with tracheoesophageal fistulas (Fig. 83-3).

Surgery

Resection is the mainstay of treatment of neoplasms of the esophagus. It is the best single modality for managing patients with early-stage cancers. Surgery is an integral element in multimodality therapy for regionally advanced cancers because patients who undergo preoperative

Table 83-3 **Results of Randomized Trials of Definitive Chemoradiotherapy for Locoregionally Advanced Esophageal Cancer**

Author	Year	Treatment	Tech.	Hist.	Pts.	Median Survival	*p* Value
Chemo/RT vs RT alone							
Roussel et al[120]	1989	Methotrexate + 56 Gy	C~RT	S	77	9 mo	NS
		56 Gy			73	8 mo	
Araujo et al[116]	1991	5-FU, bleomycin, mito + 50 Gy	C/RT	S	28	18 mo	NS
		50 Gy			31	16 mo	
Hatlevoll et al[121]	1992	Cisplatin, bleomycin + 53 Gy	C~RT	S	46	6 mo	NS
		53 Gy			51	6 mo	
Slabber et al[122]	1998	Cisplatin, 5-FU + 40 Gy	C/RT	S	34	6 mo	NS
		40 Gy			36	5 mo	
Smith et al[117]	1998	Mitomycin, 5-FU + 40 Gy	C/RT	S > A	60	15 mo	.04
		40 Gy			59	9 mo	
Cooper et al[119]	1999	Cisplatin, 5-FU + 50 Gy	C/RT	S > A	61	13 mo	.01
		64 Gy			62	9 mo	
Chemo/RT (high dose) vs chemo/RT (low dose)							
Minsky et al[114]	2002	Cisplatin, 5-FU + 50 Gy	C/RT	S > A	10	18 mo	NS
		Cisplatin, 5-FU + 64y	C/RT		9	13 mo	
Chemo/RT/surgery vs chemo/RT alone							
Stahl et al[148]	2005	Cis, 5-FU, Etop.~Cis, Etop.+ 40 Gy ~ Surgery	C~C/RT~S	S	86	16.4 mo	NS
		Cis, 5-FU, Etop.~Cis, Etop.+ 65 Gy	C~C/RT		86	14.9 mo	
Bedenne et al[149]	2007	Cis, 5-FU,+ 46 Gy ~ Surgery	C/RT~S	S > A	129	17.7 mo	NS
		Cis, 5-FU, 66 Gy	CRT		130	19.3 mo	
Chemo/RT (5-FU) vs chemo/RT (no 5-FU)							
Ajani et al[168]	2008	Cis, 5-FU, Paclitaxel ~ 5-FU, Paclitaxel + 50.4 Gy	C~RT	S > A	41	28.2 mo	NS
		Cis + Paclitaxel ~ Cis + Paclitaxel + 50.4 Gy	C~RT		43	14.9 mo	

(neoadjuvant) therapy have a 75% incidence of residual local disease amenable to resection, although this remains controversial since some oncologists argue that surgery should be reserved only for patients who relapse with locoregional disease. Improvements in endoesophageal stenting have allowed patients with metastatic or poor performance locoregionally advanced disease to be palliated in with nonsurgical approaches.

Approaches to Resection ■ Surgical approaches to resection include a transthoracic operation, mobilization of the esophagus via a transhiatal route, and thoracoscopic/laparoscopic resection (Table 83-4; Fig. 83-6).

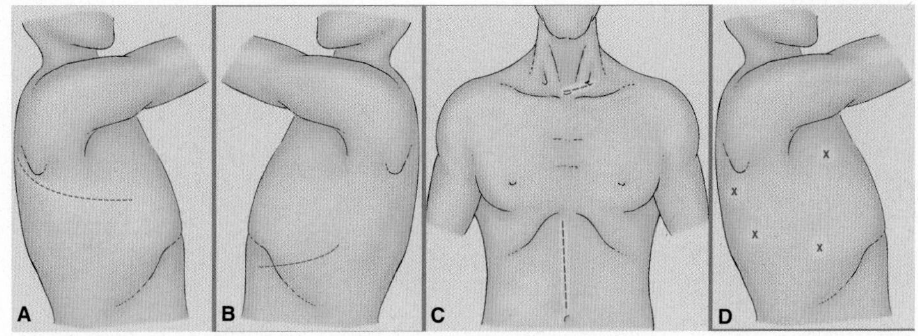

Figure 83-6 ■ Approaches for esophagectomy. **(A)** Right thoracotomy and laparotomy with intrathoracic (Ivor Lewis operation) or cervical anastomosis (McKeown modification of Ivor Lewis esophagectomy). **(B)** Left thoracotomy, accessing the abdomen through a peripheral incision in the diaphragm, with intrathoracic or cervical anastomosis. **(C)** Transhiatal esophagectomy with cervical anastomosis. **(D)** Thoracoscopic esophagectomy.

Open transthoracic approaches provide the ability to perform a more complete dissection of the primary tumor and lymph nodes than is possible using a transhiatal approach. The transhiatal approach allows the operation to be done more quickly with fewer incisions and potentially less trauma. This latter concept has been expanded with the use of thoracoscopic/laparoscopic techniques, which were introduced in the mid-1990s as a means to perform a thorough esophageal and nodal dissection while theoretically limiting operative morbidity and the duration of postoperative hospital stay.

The selection of an operative approach is dependent, in part, on tumor location and histology. Squamous cell cancers are most often located in the middle and upper thoracic esophagus, a location to which a transhiatal approach is often contraindicated except in the most experienced hands. In contrast, adenocarcinomas, which most often arise in the distal esophagus or cardia, are easily amenable to open transthoracic and transhiatal approaches. Squamous cell cancers are multifocal in nearly 20% of patients, and near-total esophagectomy is recommended to minimize the risk of performing an incomplete resection.[80,81] This usually necessitates a cervical anastomosis for reconstruction. In contrast, adenocarcinomas usually are not multifocal, but tend to spread submucosally. When negative proximal and distal margins are obtained on frozen section at the time of operation, the extent of the esophageal resection is theoretically satisfactory. Recently the performance of esophagectomy using minimally invasive techniques has been described.[82,83] The procedure begins with thoracoscopic mobilization of the thoracic esophagus, followed by laparoscopic creation of the gastric conduit. The specimen is delivered through a cervical incision and the gastric conduit anastomosed to the cervical esophagus. A complete mediastinal and celiac axis lymph node dissection is usually performed without difficulty. The largest series reported to date included 222 patients and documented a very low mortality rate of 1.4% and a major morbidity rate of 32%.[84] Although there have been no prospective comparisons between minimally invasive esophagectomy and open esophagectomy, in a retrospective review, Nguyen and colleagues[85] reported that patients who had minimally invasive esophagectomy had shorter operative times, less blood loss, fewer transfusions, and shortened intensive care unit and hospital courses than patients who underwent open procedures. Recently Horgan and colleagues[86] have described robotic-assisted, minimally invasive esophagectomy. The chief advantage of the surgical robot appears to be enhanced visualization and ability to dissect the thoracic esophagus via a transhiatal approach, which obviates thoracoscopic mobilization.

Table 83-4 ■ **Operative Approaches to Resection for Esophageal Cancer**

Transthoracic
• Ivor Lewis (laparotomy, right thoracotomy, high intrathoracic anastomosis)
• McKeown modification of Ivor Lewis (cervical anastomosis)
• Left thoracotomy with intrathoracic anastomosis
• Left thoracotomy with cervical anastomosis
• Thoracoabdominal incision
Transhiatal
Minimally invasive
• Thoracoscopically assisted
• Laparoscopically assisted
• Thoracoscopic/laparoscopic

It is difficult to demonstrate an advantage of any technique over the other. Results from 44 published reports of transthoracic or transhiatal esophagectomy for cancer demonstrate a higher incidence of anastomotic complications in the latter group, but otherwise no important differences in operative morbidity or mortality and similar 5-year survival rates.[88-93] Similarly, the use of a minimally invasive approach, such as thoracoscopic resection, appears to offer little advantage over open approaches. Combined results of the early experiences from a number of centers demonstrate operative morbidity and mortality, as well as postoperative duration of hospital stay, to be similar to results for open procedures.[93-101] Currently, the choice of the approach to esophageal resection depends largely on the training, experience, and personal preference of the surgeon.

Effects of Preoperative Therapy ■ The use of preoperative therapy before surgery has the potential of increasing perioperative morbidity and mortality. One prospective randomized study reported that septic complications, respiratory complications, and operative mortality were higher in patients who underwent preoperative chemotherapy compared with surgery alone.[102] However, several other studies assessing neoadjuvant chemotherapy or chemoradiotherapy have shown no important differences in postoperative complications or operative mortality.[39,103-107] The complexity of esophageal surgery mandates that the procedure be performed at a high-volume referral center to minimize operative morbidity and mortality.[44] Medicare data suggest that high-volume centers can perform esophageal resections with a mortality of 3%, whereas less experienced centers have a mortality of 19%.[44] This morbidity and mortality may be even further increased when preoperative therapy is used. At less experienced centers, the morbidity and mortality of the procedure may be greater than the potential benefit, especially when considering the low likelihood of cure in locoregionally advanced patients.

Surgery for Cervical Esophageal Cancer ■ Neoplasms of the cervical esophagus pose special problems with regard to surgical therapy. To obtain adequate surgical margins in tumors that extend to the cricopharyngeus muscle or invade the proximal trachea, it is necessary to include a laryngectomy as part of the resection, which adds substantial long-term morbidity to what is often a palliative procedure. As a result, a higher percentage of patients with cervical esophageal cancer are treated nonsurgically than is the case for patients with cancers in other locations. Resection provides good palliation for dysphagia but does not appear to substantially influence long-term survival and the morbidity has led most people to recommend chemoradiation in this subset of patients.[108-111]

Reconstruction After Esophagectomy ■ Reestablishing alimentary tract continuity after esophageal resection in a manner that permits ingestion of a normal diet is an important component of surgery for esophageal cancer. Options for reconstruction include using the stomach as a substitute or interposing a segment of colon or jejunum between the proximal esophageal remnant and the stomach (or duodenum after total gastrectomy). The use of the stomach for reconstruction is by far the most common technique because the stomach has the most reliable blood supply among any of the reconstructive options and because only a single anastomosis is required, compared with the three anastomoses necessary for bowel interposition. Cervical anastomoses are favored by some surgeons because they decrease the incidence of acid reflux into the esophageal remnant and because anastomotic leaks are usually easily managed by simple cervical drainage. The disadvantages of cervical anastomoses are a higher incidence of recurrent laryngeal nerve injury and more frequent anastomotic leaks. Whether the additional tumor-free proximal margin provided by a cervical anastomosis offers a survival advantage has not been proven.[112] Use of the posterior mediastinum (esophageal bed) for reconstruction optimizes emptying of the reconstructive organ but may predispose to tumor infiltration if a complete resection is not performed.[113]

Radiation Therapy

Radiotherapy has been used for decades in the management of neoplasms of the esophagus and as with surgery targets the locoregional tumor rather than the systemic disease. The primary roles of radiotherapy, as with surgery, are as a potentially curative single modality for localized disease and as a palliative therapy for advanced tumors. Results of both uses have been disappointing because of a lack of complete response of the primary tumor and the development of radiation-induced strictures that limit its palliative benefits. More recently, the use of radiation has expanded to include an important adjuvant role in multimodality therapy to further improve the locoregional control obtained with surgery alone.

Treatment is planned to uniformly irradiate gross tumor and margins suspected of harboring microscopic disease, while minimizing injury to adjacent normal tissues, such as the lung, heart, and spinal cord. Regional nodal basins are usually included, typically cervical and supraclavicular nodes for cervical cancers, supraclavicular and subcarinal lymph nodes for upper thoracic cancers, and celiac axis nodes for lower thoracic and cardiac cancers. Initial treatment is to opposed, anterior-posterior and posterior-anterior fields using high energy (6–24 MV) photons. In patients receiving potentially curative high-dose therapy, the final treatments are delivered at an oblique angle to minimize the total dose to the spinal cord. Daily treatments of 1.8–2 Gy to a total of 60–70 Gy were formerly used for curative intent, although this has been modified since recent trials have demonstrated equal efficacy and less toxicity with the lower dose (50.4 Gy).[114] Palliative doses tend to be even lower to further reduce this morbidity (30–40 Gy).

Radiation as Single Modality Therapy ■ The use of radiation therapy as a single modality for esophageal cancer is sometimes indicated as a potentially curative therapy in patients who are unable to tolerate (or who refuse) resection or combined definitive chemoradiotherapy. Radiation therapy alone achieves 5-year survival rates of 0–20% in patients without distant metastatic disease, with the majority of survival rates being less than 10%. Although low, these survival rates may be biased by patient selection since good performance status patients are usually treated with surgery while radiation is often reserved for the poor performance status group. Treatment of unresectable but localized esophageal cancer with radiotherapy yields results similar to those reported for potentially resectable cancers, with survival rates at 5 years of less than 10%.[115-122] One small randomized study has demonstrated increased survival with surgery alone versus radiation therapy alone, although the authors focused more on endpoints of quality of life.[123]

Radiotherapy as an Adjuvant to Resection ■ In an effort to obtain better local control of disease, radiotherapy has been used both preoperatively and postoperatively as an adjunct to resection (Table 83-5).[124-128] The interval between completion of radiotherapy and resection is typically 3–5 weeks (1 week/10 Gy), which is felt to minimize perioperative complications from bleeding and radiation-induced fibrosis. In the proper setting, postoperative complication and mortality rates are not increased by the administration of preoperative radiotherapy, although this may be contingent on performing the surgical procedure in a high-volume center.[44] Most randomized, controlled studies have not demonstrated a survival advantage compared with surgery alone although these studies were often performed with outdated radiation therapy techniques.[124-128] Meta-analysis of the combined data from all randomized studies that have been published do not demonstrate improved survival with preoperative radiotherapy.[129]

The use of radiotherapy postoperatively enables the administration of higher radiation doses than are feasible

Table 83-5 ■ **Results of Randomized Trials of Pre- and Postoperative Radiotherapy for Locoregionally Advanced Esophageal Cancer**

Authors	Year	Treatment	Histology	Patients (No.)	5-Year Survival	*p* Value
Preoperative RT vs surgery alone						
Launois et al[124]	1981	Surgery alone	S	57	11.5%	NS
		Surgery + 40 Gy		67	7.5%	
Gignoux et al[125]	1988	Surgery alone	S	106	10%	NS
		Surgery + 33 Gy		102	9%	
Wang et al[126]	1989	Surgery alone	S	102	30%	NS
		Surgery + 40 Gy		104	35%	
Arnott et al[130]	1992	Surgery alone	S	86	17%	NS
		Surgery + 20 Gy		90	9%	
Nygaard et al[128]	1992	Surgery alone	S	41	4%	.08
		Surgery + 35 Gy		48	18%	
Postoperative RT vs surgery alone						
FUASR[133]	1991	Surgery alone	S	119	18%	NS
		Surgery + 45–55 Gy		102	20%	
Fok et al[131]	1993	Surgery alone	S	65	11% (4yr)	NS
		Surgery + 49–52.5 Gy		65	11% (4yr)	
Ziernan[132]	1995	Surgery alone	S	35	20% (3yr)	NS
		Surgery + 56 Gy		33	23% (3yr)	

with preoperative radiotherapy although this treatment has been associated with increases in the incidence of anastomotic strictures and prolonged recovery from surgery, adversely affecting the quality of life.[130-132] There is also some evidence that median survival is worse in patients who undergo postoperative radiotherapy, compared with resection only, as a result of an earlier appearance of distant metastatic disease and because of irradiation-induced deaths, although selection bias may also play a role.[131] Postoperative irradiation appears to decrease the local recurrence rate but overall has no proven influence on long-term survival.

Intraluminal brachytherapy has been added in some centers to curative or palliative external beam radiotherapy in an effort to improve local control of disease. Doses of 10–20 Gy are administered after completion of external beam treatment in one or more fractions using Iridium-192. In patients with potentially curable disease, the addition of intraluminal brachytherapy appears to enhance locoregional control, compared with external beam radiotherapy alone, but is associated with a higher incidence of radiation-induced esophageal strictures.[133-135] Reducing the dose per fraction of intraluminal brachytherapy may in the future limit the incidence and severity of these local complications.[136] The use of brachytherapy in patients with unresectable or recurrent esophageal cancer is still under investigation but may provide better symptomatic relief than other modalities, such as gastric bypass surgery, chemotherapy, laser therapy, and stenting.[137-139]

Chemotherapy and Combination Therapy

Most patients with carcinoma of the esophagus have advanced disease at the time of diagnosis, and long-term survival is dismal even in operable patients. These factors have led to the investigation of systemic chemotherapy in an effort to improve both local and distant control of disease and to prolong survival. Chemotherapy has an emerging role in the treatment of esophageal cancer, either as neoadjuvant or postoperative adjuvant therapy or as part of concomitant chemoradiotherapy.

Single-Agent Chemotherapy ■ A number of agents have been investigated as sole therapy for esophageal cancer, including cisplatin, irinotecan, bleomycin, mitomycin, 5-fluorouracil (5-FU), paclitaxel, methotrexate, vinorelbine, mitoguazone, vindesine, doxorubicin, and etoposide. phase 2 trials have demonstrated responses of 15–30% for these agents, with cisplatin, mitomycin, 5-FU, paclitaxel, and vindesine being the most active.[140] The responses have been short lived and have not led to any meaningful prolongation of survival.

Multiagent Chemotherapy ■ The observation that single-agent chemotherapy provided modest and short-lived responses has led to the investigation of multidrug therapy for esophageal cancer. The drug combinations, which usually have been cisplatin based, have been evaluated as sole therapy for patients with recurrent or metastatic disease and as preoperative therapy for patients with regionally advanced disease. Responses are better than with single-agent therapy, averaging about 50%, and have become the mainstay of therapy for patients with metastatic esophageal cancer (Fig. 83-3).

In locoregionally advanced esophageal cancer, combination chemotherapy has been investigated in combination with radiation or surgery to try to reduce the high rate of systemic relapse noted when surgery or radiation therapy alone is used. Attempts to use chemotherapy with surgery have included preoperative and postoperative strategies usually with cisplatin-based multiagent regimens. The randomized trials with preoperative chemotherapy usually consist of two or three chemotherapy cycles followed by resection. Some studies have also added postoperative chemotherapy to the regimen. There is no apparent difference in response to chemotherapy based on histology. There is no clear increase in perioperative complications noted with preoperative chemotherapy when the surgery is performed at an experienced center. As Table 83-6 demonstrates, recent randomized trials have demonstrated a survival benefit with preoperative chemotherapy especially when larger number of patients are randomized.[40,104,107,108,129,141-144] The reasons for the failure of the majority of trials may be due in part to the small numbers of patient in each study. Meta-analyses have suggested with larger number of patients that there is a significant benefit to preoperative chemotherapy especially in patients with adenocarcinoma.[145]

Table 83-6 ■ **Results of Randomized Trials of Pre- or Postoperative Chemotherapy for Locoregionally Advanced Esophageal Cancer**

Author (Ref.)	Year	Treatment	Histology	Patients (No.)	Resectability	Op. Mort.	Median Survival (Mo)	*p* Value
Preoperative chemotherapy								
Roth et al[40]	1988	Cisplatin, bleomycin, vindesine + surgery	S > A	19	–	10%	9	NS
		Surgery alone		20	–	0%	9	
Nygaard et al[128]	1992	Cisplatin, bleomycin + surgery	S	50	58%		10	NS
		Surgery alone		41	69%	13%	7	
Schlag et al[103]	1992	Cisplatin, 5-FU + surgery	S	21	69%	–	6	NS
		Surgery Alone		24	79%	–	8	
Maipang et al[141]	1994	Cisplatin, bleomycin, vinblastine + surgery	S	24	–	–	17	NS
		Surgery alone		22	–	–	17	
Ancona et al[142]	1995	Cisplatin, 5-FU + Surgery	S	35	78%	7%	–	NS
		Surgery alone		43	86%	5%	–	
Law et al[106]	1997	Cisplatin, 5-FU + surgery	S	73	95%	9%	13	NS
		Surgery Alone		74	89%	8%	17	
Kelsen et al[107]	1998	Cisplatin, 5-FU + surgery	A > S	213	76%	7%	15	NS
		Surgery alone		227	89%	6%	16	
Clarke et al[144]	2002	Cisplatin, 5-FU + surgery	A > S	400	78%	10%	17	<.05
		Surgery alone		402	70%	10%	13	
Cunningham et al[169]	2006	Epirubicin, cisplatin, 5-FU + surgery	A	250	69%	6%	23	<.01
		Surgery alone	25% GEJ					
			75% Gastric	253	66%	6%	20	
Postoperative chemotherapy								
Ando et al[129]	1997	Cisplatin, vindesine + surgery	S	105	–	–	58	NS
		Surgery alone		100	–	–	47	

Abbreviations: A, adenocarcinoma; NS, not significant; S, squamous cell; 5-FU, 5-fluorouracil.

Table 83-7 Results of Randomized Trials of Preoperative Chemoradiotherapy for Locoregionally Advanced Esophageal Cancer

Author (Ref)	Year	Treatment	Histology	Patients (No.)	Technique	Op. Mort.	Medial Survival (Mo)	*p* Value
LePrise et al[146]	1994	Cisplatin, 5-FU + 20 Gy + surgery	S	41	Sequential	9%	10	NS
		Surgery alone		45		7%	10	
Walsh et al[150]	1996	Cisplatin, 5-FU + 40 Gy + surgery	A	58	Concurrent	12%	17	.01
		Surgery alone		55		3%	12	
Bosset et al[151]	1997	Cisplatin + 37 Gy + surgery	S	143	Concurrent	12%	19	NS
		Surgery alone		139		4%	19	
Urba et al[152]	2001	Cisplatin, 5-FU + 45 Gy + surgery	A	50	Concurrent	4%	18	.15
		Surgery alone		50		2%	17	
Burmeister et al [153]	2005	Cisplatin, 5-FU + 35 Gy + surgery	A,S	128	Concurrent	5%	22	NS
		Surgery alone		128		5%	19	
Tepper et al[170]	2008	Cisplatin, 5-FU + 50.4 Gy + surgery	A > S	30	Concurrent	0%	54	.002
		Surgery alone		26		4%	22	

Abbreviations: A, adenocarcinoma; NS, not significant; S, squamous cell; 5-FU, 5-fluorouracil.

Postoperative chemotherapy (cisplatin, 5-FU) for patients after esophagectomy has not demonstrated to date a survival advantage compared with surgery alone and has been associated with increased treatment-related complications (Table 83-7).[146] Even in meta-analyses there has not been a clear benefit demonstrated with postoperative chemotherapy.[147]

Definitive chemoradiotherapy with selective surgery has also been evaluated as a strategy to improve survival in locoregionally advanced esophageal cancer. These studies have used both sequential and concurrent treatment strategies. The concurrent use of chemotherapy and radiotherapy is theoretically appealing because, in addition to the systemic effects of chemotherapy, certain agents behave as radiosensitizers. Randomized studies with a concurrent strategy demonstrate an advantage to combined treatment versus radiation therapy alone (Table 83-4).[115,117,118,120-123,148] Definitive chemoradiotherapy strategies with surgery used only as salvage appear most effective in squamous cell carcinoma and less effective in adenocarcinoma where long-term survival is lower.[108] Two trials have been performed in Europe randomizing squamous cell carcinoma patients to definitive chemoradiation or preoperative chemoradiotherapy and surgery.[148,149] These studies demonstrated similar survivals between groups and suggest that definitive chemoradiation may be an acceptable strategy for squamous cell carcinoma of the upper and middle esophagus. The optimum dose for definitive chemoradiotherapy is currently 50.4 Gy as suggested by a randomized trial in which increased doses of radiation were associated with increased treatment-related mortality without a survival advantage.[114]

Preoperative chemoradiotherapy has also been investigated in locoregionally advanced esophageal cancer as a strategy in an attempt to reduce both the high locoregional and systemic relapse rate noted with surgery alone or preoperative chemotherapy and surgery. The theoretical advantages to preoperative as opposed to postoperative chemoradiation therapy include (1) the ability to control subclinical systemic metastases prior to the immune suppression that results from surgery; (2) downstaging locoregional disease to increase the likelihood of a complete resection at surgery; and (3) the ability to administer full doses of chemoradiation that would not be possible to administer postoperatively because of perioperative debility. As Table 83-7 demonstrates, the results are not consistent, although sequential chemoradiation does not appear to be beneficial.[146,148,150-153] There have been several trials that have been encouraging for concurrent preoperative chemoradiation in locoregionally advanced esophageal cancer especially in adenocarcinoma, but statistical significance has not been achieved in all trials. Meta-analyses with larger numbers of patients have suggested that preoperative chemoradiation and preoperative chemotherapy have survival advantages compared with other strategies, although these studies are limited by different preclinical staging techniques and heterogenous patient populations (Fig. 83-7).[145] A survival benefit for combined therapy is evident in most studies in patients who are found to have a complete pathologic response in the surgical specimen and have provided strong incentives to continue the investigations of this strategy. In addition, since surgery alone or radiation therapy alone has such poor outcomes, many oncologists currently use definitive chemoradiotherapy alone or preoperative chemoradiation and surgery for nonmetastatic, locoregionally advanced esophageal cancer (Fig. 83-3). Two randomized trials from Europe have been reported comparing defini-

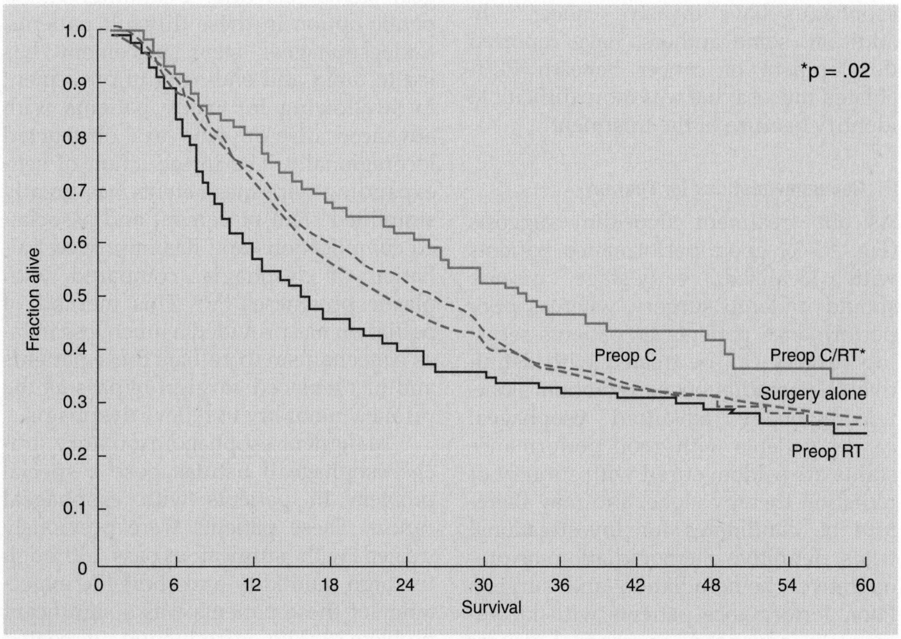

Figure 83-7 Improved long-term survival noted in patients undergoing preoperative chemoradiation (Preop C/RT) prior to surgery (surg) at the University of Texas M.D. Anderson Cancer Center (*n* = 879). *Source*: From Ref. 79.

tive chemoradiation versus preoperative chemoradiation and surgery in squamous cell carcinoma.[148,149] Preliminary results demonstrated improved locoregional control with surgery but no survival advantages. Although operative mortality was higher than expected these trials suggest definitive chemoradiation may be an acceptable strategy in squamous cell carcinoma of the upper and middle esophagus especially in institutions where trimodality treatment-related mortality is high.[148,149]

Photodynamic Therapy

Photodynamic therapy (PDT) has been investigated in the treatment of patients with carcinoma in situ or superficial cancers who are unable to tolerate or who refuse surgical resection. PDT is performed by first systemically administering a photosensitive compound, and after its uptake in tumor, strong areas of concern are endoscopically treated with low-level laser light to activate the compound, causing selective cell death through release of toxic oxygen metabolites. The complete response rate of 75–80% endures for several years, suggesting that some patients may be cured with this therapy although long-term follow-up is still required.[154-157] PDT also is being investigated as one of several techniques, including laser photocoagulation, argon beam cautery, and electrocautery, for ablating Barrett mucosa as a means of preventing the development of adenocarcinoma, although some authors have expressed concern for this approach since current staging techniques are relatively inaccurate, and up to 50% of patients who undergo resection for high-grade dysplasia in Barrett esophagus have invasive cancer.[158] In addition, some authors, have reported development of cancer beneath PDT-ablated mucosa that was more difficult to identify because of the treatment.

Recommendations for Therapy

As our treatment algorithm suggests (Fig. 83-3), good performance patients with localized, early-stage disease should undergo surgery, whereas poor performance patients or patients refusing surgery can be treated with definitive chemoradiation or radiation alone. Locoregionally advanced esophageal cancer patients with good performance status are seldom cured with surgery or radiation therapy alone, and may therefore be candidates for investigational trials, definitive chemoradiation, or preoperative chemoradiation and surgery. Poor performance patients with locoregionally advanced esophageal cancer should be treated with chemoradiation or palliative radiation therapy and/or stents. Metastatic esophageal cancer patients who are good performance status may be offered chemotherapy alone with the addition of palliative radiation and/or stents for locoregional control. Chemotherapy should not be used if the patients have a poor performance status since the focus should be on palliation.

Palliative Therapy of Esophageal Obstruction

In patients with advanced esophageal cancer not amenable to potentially curative therapy, a primary goal of treatment is relief of dysphagia.[159] This can be accomplished with palliative resection, but high operative morbidity and mortality rates as well as the prolonged period of recovery that is necessary preclude meaningful palliation and most oncologists currently recommend nonsurgical means for palliation. External beam radiotherapy, as an isolated modality or in combination with chemotherapy, is noninvasive but requires considerable time to complete and results in strictures in up to 30% of patients. Intraluminal brachytherapy is another option that is considered in some centers.[160,161] Photocoagulative laser therapy is another option that is usually performed with an Nd:YAG laser, with an initial improvement in dysphagia in 85% of patients and a mean duration of response of less than 1 month. PDT offers a similar initial efficacy but provides a more enduring response, although skin photosensitivity is an undesirable side effect.[162]

The development of endoesophageal stents has offered another therapeutic option in these difficult patients. Endoesophageal stent placement has led to rapid and enduring improvement in swallowing for many patients with advanced disease who are obstructed locoregionally. The introduction of self-expanding wire mesh stents has greatly simplified stent placement and associated complications and has improved palliation of dysphagia, compared with plastic prostheses.[163,164] This method of palliation has provided a much less invasive mechanism to palliate these patients and has replaced surgical bypass as the primary modality to relieve dysphagia.

Malignant esophagorespiratory (tracheoesophageal) fistulas pose a special problem in patients with esophageal cancer. These patients were previously treated with surgical bypass although the high morbidity and short life expectancy of these patients was a significant problem.[165] The introduction of coated wire mesh stents offers a better option for the treatment of such fistulas because they palliate dysphagia while occluding the fistula without requiring an extensive surgical procedure in an often debilitated and poor performance status patient.[166,167]

Selected References

The complete reference list can be found at www.CANCERMEDICINE8.com

3. Torek F. The first successful case of resection of the thoracic portion of the esophagus for carcinoma. *Surg Gynecol Obstet.* 1913;16:614–617.
5. Siewert JR. Adenocarcinoma of the esophagogastric junction: classification, pathology and extent of resection. *Dis Esophagus.* 1996;9:173–182.
14. Yu MC, Garabrant DH, Peters JM, et al. Tobacco, alcohol, diet, occupation, and carcinoma of the esophagus. *Cancer Res.* 1988;48:3843–3848.
24. Montesano R, Hollstein M, Hainaut P. Genetic alterations in esophageal cancer and their relevance to etiology and pathogenesis: a review. *Int J Cancer.* 1996;69:225–235.
35. Powell J, McConkey CC. Increasing incidence of adenocarcinoma of the gastric cardia and adjacent sites. *Br J Cancer.* 1990;62:440–443.
38. Swisher SG, Hunt KK, Holmes EC, et al. Changes in the surgical management of esophageal cancer from 1970-1993. *Am J Surg.* 1995;169:609–614.
40. Roth JA, Pass HI, Flanagan MM, et al. Randomized clinical trial of preoperative and postoperative adjuvant chemotherapy with cisplatin, vindesine, and bleomycin for carcinoma of the esophagus. *J Thorac Cardiovasc Surg.* 1988;96:242–248.
44. Swisher SG, DeFord L, Merriman KW, et al. Effect of operative volume on morbidity, mortality and hospital use after esophagectomy for cancer. *J Thorac Cardiovasc Surg.* 2000;119:1126–1134.
46. Beseth BD, Bedrod R, Isacoff WH, et al. Endoscopic ultrasound does not accurately assess pathologic stage of esophageal cancer after neoadjuvant chemoradiotherapy. *Am Surg.* 2002;66:827–831.
49. Rice TW, Boyce GA, Sivak MV. Esophageal ultrasound and the preoperative staging of carcinoma of the esophagus. *J Thorac Cardiovasc Surg.* 1991;101:536–544.
57. Krasna MJ, Reed CE, Jaklitsch MT, et al. Thoracoscopic staging of esophageal cancer: a prospective, multiinstitutional trial. *Ann Thorac Surg.* 1995;60:1337–1340.
63. Flamen P, Lerut A, Van Cutsem E, et al. The utility of positron emission tomography for the diagnosis and staging of recurrent esophageal cancer. *J Thorac Cardiovasc Surg.* 2000;120:1085–1092.
71. American Joint Committee on Cancer. *AJCC Cancer Staging Manual.* 5th ed. Philadelphia: Lippincott, Williams and Wilkins; 1997:65–69.
76. Nigro JJ, DeMeester SR, Hagen JA, et al. Node status in transmural esophageal adenocarcinoma and outcome after en bloc esophagectomy. *J Thorac Cardiovasc Surg.* 1999;117:960–908.
79. Hofstetter W, Swisher SG, Correa AM, et al. Treatment outcomes of resected esophageal cancer. *Ann Surg.* 2002;236:376–385.

84. Luketich JD, Alvelo-Rivera M, Buenaventura PO, et al. Minimally invasive esophagectomy: outcomes in 222 patients. *Ann Surg.* 2003;486–496.
88. Hulscher JBF, van Sandik JW, De Boer AGEM, et al. Extended transthoracic resection compared with limited transhiatal resection for adenocarcinoma of the esophagus. *New Engl J Med.* 2002;347:1662–1669.
91. Putnam JB Jr, Suell DM, McMurtry MJ, et al. Comparison of three techniques of esophagectomy within a residency training program. *Ann Thorac Surg.* 1994;57:319–325.
96. Akaishi T, Kaneda I, Higuchi N, et al. Thoracoscopic en bloc total esophagectomy with radical mediastinal lymphadenectomy. *J Thorac Cardiovasc Surg.* 1996;112:1533–1540.
102. Lerut T, Coosemans W, De Leyn P, et al. Reflections on three field lymphadenectomy in carcinoma of the esophagus and esophagogastric junction. *Hepato-Gastroenterol.* 1999;46:717–725.
103. Schlag PM, Chirirgische Arbeitsgemeinschaft fuer Onkologie der Deutschen Gesellschaft fuer Chirurgie Study Group. Randomized trial of preoperative chemotherapy for squamous cell cancer of the esophagus. *Arch Surg.* 1992;127:1446–1450.
104. Walsh TN, Noonan N, Hollywood D, et al. A comparison of multimodal therapy and surgery for esophageal adenocarcinoma. *N Engl J Med.* 1996;335:462–467.
105. Bosset J-F, Gignoux M, Triboulet J-P, et al. Chemoradiotherapy followed by surgery compared with surgery alone in squamous cell cancer of the esophagus. *N Engl J Med.* 1997;337:161–167.
106. Law S, Fok M, Chow S, et al. Preoperative chemotherapy versus surgical therapy alone for squamous cell carcinoma of the esophagus: a prospective randomized trial. *J Thorac Cardiovasc Surg.* 1997;114:210–217.
107. Kelsen DP, Ginsberg R, Pajak TF, et al. Chemotherapy followed by surgery compared with surgery alone for localized esophageal cancer. *N Engl J Med.* 1998;339:1979–1984.
108. Chakkaphak S, Krishnasamy S, Walker SJ, et al. Treatment of carcinoma of the proximal esophagus. *Surg Gynecol Obstet.* 1989;168:307–310.
114. Minsky BD, Paj ak TF, Ginsberg RJ, et al. INT 0123 (Radiation Therapy Oncology Group 94-05) phase III trial of combined-modality therapy for esophageal cancer: high-dose versus standard-dose radiation therapy. *J Clin Oncol.* 2002;20:1167–1174.
116. Arauj o CMM, Souhami L, Gil RA, et al. A randomized trial comparing radiation therapy versus concomitant radiation therapy and chemotherapy in carcinoma of the thoracic esophagus. *Cancer.* 1991;67:2258–2261.
119. Cooper JS, Guo MD, Herskovic A, et al. Chemoradiotherapy of locally advanced esophageal cancer. *JAMA.* 1999;281: 1623–1627.
124. Launois B, Delarue D, Campion JP, Kerbaol M. Preoperative radiotherapy for carcinoma of the esophagus. *Surg Gynecol Obstet.* 1981;153:690–692.
125. Gignoux M, Roussel A, Paillot B, et al. The value of pre-operative radiotherapy in esophageal cancer: results of a study by the EORTC. *Recent Rep Cancer Res.* 1988;110:1–13.
127. Arnott SJ, Duncan W, Kerr GR, et al. Low dose preoperative radiotherapy for carcinoma of the oesophagus: results of a randomized clinical trial. *Radiother Oncol.* 1992;24:108–113.
128. Nygaard K, Hagen S, Hansen HS, et al. Preoperative radiotherapy prolongs survival in operable esophageal carcinoma: a randomized, multicenter study of pre-operative radiotherapy and chemotherapy. The Second Scandinavian Trial in Esophageal Cancer. *World J Surg.* 1992;16:1104–1110.
129. Ando N, Iizuka T, Kakegawa T, et al. A randomized trial of surgery with and without chemotherapy for localized squamous carcinoma of the thoracic esophagus: the Japan Clinical Oncology Group study. *J Thorac Cardiovasc Surg.* 1997;114:205–209.
130. Arnott SJ, Duncan W, Gignoux M, et al. Preoperative radiotherapy in esophageal carcinoma: a meta-analysis using individual patients data (Oesophageal Cancer Collaborative Group). *Int J Radiat Oncol Biol Phys.* 1998;41:579–583.
131. Fok M, Sham JST, Shoy D, et al. Postoperative radiotherapy for carcinoma of the esophagus: a prospective, randomized controlled study. *Surgery.* 1993;113:138–147.
144. Medical Research Council Oesophageal Cancer Working Party. Surgical resection with or without preoperative chemotherapy in oesophageal cancer: a randomised controlled trial. *Lancet.* 2002;359:1727–1733.
145. Gebski V, Burmeister B, Smithers BM, Foo K, Zalcberg J, Simes J, for the Australasian Gastro-Intestinal Trials Group. Survival benefits from neoadjuvant chemoradiotherapy or chemotherapy in oesophageal carcinoma: a meta-analysis. *Lancet Oncol.* 2007;8:226–234.
146. Le Prise E, Etienne PL, Meunier B, et al. A randomized study of chemotherapy, radiation therapy, and surgery versus surgery for localized squamous cell carcinoma of the esophagus. *Cancer.* 1994;73:1779–1784.
148. Stahl M, Stuschke M, Lehmann N, et al. Chemoradiation with and without surgery in patients with locally advanced squamous cell carcinoma of the esophagus. *J Clin Oncol.* 2005;23:2310–2317.
149. Bedenne L, Michel P, Olivier B, et al. Chemoradiation followed by surgery compared with chemoradiation alone in squamous cancer of the esophagus: FFCD 9102. *J Clin Oncol.* 2007;25:1160–1168.
150. Walsh TN, Noonan N, Hollywood D, et al. A comparison of multimodal therapy and surgery for esophageal adenocarcinoma. *N Engl J Med.* 1996;335:462–467.
151. Bosset J-F, Gignoux M, Triboulet J-P, et al. Chemoradiotherapy followed by surgery compared with surgery alone in squamous-cell cancer of the esophagus. *N Engl J Med.* 1997;337:161–167.
152. Urba S, Orringer M, Turrisi A, et al. Randomized preoperative locoregional chemoradiation versus surgery alone in patients with resectable esophageal cancer. *J Clin Oncol.* 2001;19:305–313.
153. Burmeister BH, Smithers BM, Fitzgerald L, et al. Surgery alone versus chemoradiotherapy followed by surgery for resectable cancer of the esophagus: a randomized controlled phase III trial. *Lancet Oncol.* 2005;6:659–668.
157. Overholt BF, Panjehpour M, Haydek JM. Photodynamic therapy for Barrett's esophagus: follow-up in 100 patients. *Gastrointest Endosc.* 1999;49:1–7.
166. Raijman I, Lynch P. Coated expandable esophageal stents in the treatment of digestive-respiratory fistulas. *Am J Gastroenterol.* 1997;92:2188–2191.
168. Ajani JA, Winter K, Komaki R, et al. Phase II randomized trial of two nonoperative regimens of induction chemotherapy followed by chemoradiation in patients with localized carcinoma of the esophagus: RTOG 0113. *J Clin Oncol.* 2008;26:4551–4556.
169. Cunningham D, Allum WH, Stenning SP, et al. Perioperative chemotherapy versus surgery alone for resectable gastroesophageal cancer. *New Engl J Med.* 2006;355:11–20.
170. Tepper J, Krasna MJ, Niedzwiecki D, et al. Phase III trial of trimodality therapy with cisplatin fluorouracil, radiotherapy, and surgery compared with surgery alone for esophageal cancer; CALGB 9781. *J Clin Oncol.* 2008;26:1086–1092.

84 Carcinoma of the Stomach

James C. Yao, MD ■ Christopher H. Crane, MD ■ Takeshi Sano, MD ■ Paul F. Mansfield, MD

Epidemiology

The incidence of gastric cancer is declining worldwide, but nowhere more so than as in the United States where it has dropped precipitously since the 1930s, when it was the leading cause of cancer deaths of men in the United States. That decline followed by 20-30 years the widespread availability of refrigeration—proposed to account for much of the phenomenon.[1] In 2005, the age-adjusted incidence of gastric cancer in the United States was 7.2 per 100,000 population (Fig. 84-1) and represents an average annual change of −1.6% since 1975.[2]

The decline in the incidence of gastric cancer is really a decline in the incidence of distal lesions. The presenting anatomic location of primary lesions underwent a massive shift from noncardial sites to cardial sites. Since 1976, the incidence of proximal cardial and gastroesophageal (GE) junction adenocarcinoma in the United States and Europe has in fact increased.[3] This rise in incidence suggests a common pathogenesis distinct from that of distal gastric lesions; one that is unclear.

In the United States, it is estimated that 21,500 people developed gastric cancer and 10,880 died from the disease in 2008.[4] The risk of developing gastric cancer varies by gender and race. In 2005, the incidence among men and women were 10.4 and 4.8 per 100,000, respectively.[2] In the United States, by race (Fig. 84-1) and ethnicity, white had the lowest incidence. Black, Asian/Pacific Islander, and Hispanics were 2.0, 2.2, and 1.9 times as likely as whites to develop gastric cancer.[2]

Despite a worldwide decline in gastric cancer incidence, with an estimated 934,000 new cases in 2002 gastric cancer remains the second most common cause of cancer related death.[5] Gastric cancer is particularly common in China (accounting for 42% cases worldwide), South America, Eastern Europe, and Japan and Korea, where it is the most common malignancy.[5]

The age-adjusted death rate has been on the decline in the United States over the last 30 years and was 3.8 per 100,000 in 2005.[2] However, this is mostly due to declining incidence; survival in patients with diagnosed gastric cancer remains poor. Only modest improvements in survival have been observed. According to the Surveillance, Epidemiology, and End Results (SEER) registry, the 5-year survival rate gastric cancer (all stages) increased from 16.3% between 1975 and 1979 to 23% in 2000.[2] It should be noted that these data predates the publication of major trials of multimodality therapy with positive results and widespread acceptance.

Etiology

Mucosal changes brought about by a variety of environmental insults can eventually lead to atrophic gastritis. Chronic atrophic gastritis and the resulting intestinal metaplasia appear to be precursor conditions for intestinal-type gastric cancer.[6] Host-related, environmental, and infectious causes have been implicated in the etiology of gastric cancer.

A variety of host-related factors have been associated with gastric cancer. For example, low serum ferritin levels[7] and pernicious anemia have been associated with an increased risk of this disease. Furthermore, whereas medically treated peptic ulcer disease does not appear to be associated with an increased risk of gastric cancer, patients who have undergone distal gastrectomy for benign peptic

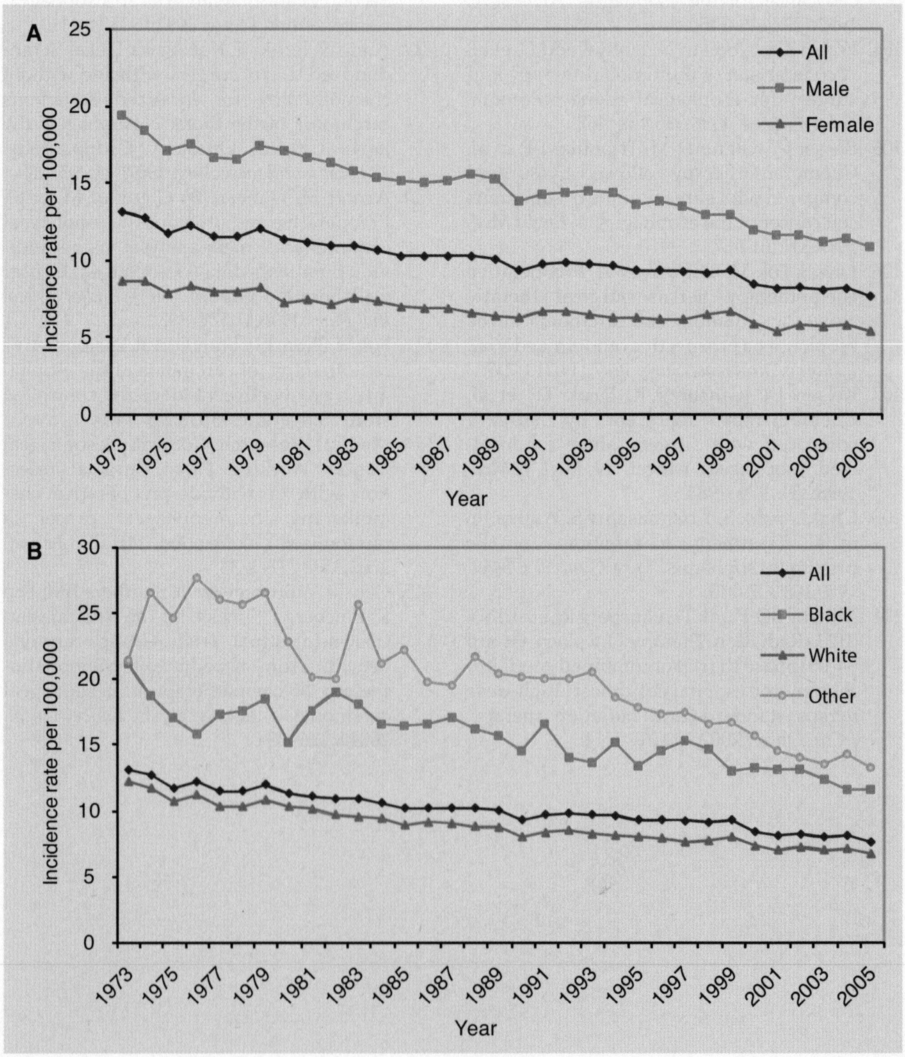

Figure 84-1 ■ SEER data from 1973 to 2005 showing time changes in the incidence of gastric cancer (per 100,000 people) by (**A**) gender, and (**B**) race. *Source*: National Cancer Institute, DCCPS, Surveillance Research Program, Cancer Statistics Branch; released April 2008 based on the November 2007 submission.

ulcer disease have been reported to have as much as a fivefold increase in risk albeit many years out from the procedure.[8]

Clear evidence shows a heritable risk of gastric cancer in a small number of patients, as discussed below. Familial predisposition has been reported[9] and appears to be independent of environmental factors.[10] This predisposition has also been examined in controlling for dietary risk in patients with hereditary nonpolyposis colorectal cancer (HNPCC) and familial adenomatous polyposis (FAP). Patients with HNPCC have an increased risk of gastric cancer, whereas those with FAP do not appear to have an increased risk of it.[11]

The most compelling evidence for an environmental cause of intestinal-type gastric cancer comes from studying migrants. Japanese, South American, and Eastern European migrants to the United States have a decreased risk of gastric cancer after two to three generations in a lower risk environment and diet.[12,13] Dietary and environmental factors, particularly early in life, appear to influence the risk.[12] The widespread availability of refrigeration has paralleled the reduction in the incidence of intestinal-type gastric carcinoma.[14] Use of refrigeration may have reduced dietary exposure to various carcinogens, such as nitrates and nitrites, and by reducing bacterial and fungal contamination of food. Investigators seeking to correlate nitrate concentrations in drinking water with stomach or esophageal cancer incidence found no such relationship.[15] Another possibility is that increased use of refrigeration led to a reduction in the consumption of smoked, cured, and salted foods. The correlation of these dietary factors with gastric carcinoma rates in epidemiological studies led to the performance of prospective studies, which found no association with gastric cancer. It should be noted, however, that the lag time for these effects is measured in decades. Increased consumption of fresh fruit is associated with decreased incidence of gastric cancer,[16] but it does not appear to be related to plasma levels of vitamin C.[17] A diverse diet, especially with regard to fruits and vegetables, has been reported to be protective.[1] A modest increase in risk has been reported with increased consumption of meat,[18] and a positive correlation between gastric cancer risk and increased meat-cooking time has been reported in retrospective studies of food intake and for food preparation preference.[19] Other environmental factors, such as smoking[16] and industrial dust exposure,[20] may be associated with gastric cancer. A causative role for alcohol has not been established.[21-23]

Infectious factors in gastric cancer, such as *Helicobacter pylori* infection, have been reported in epidemiological studies,[24] and infection rates have been reported to be high in endemic areas.[25] Prospective serological studies have shown that patients with *H. pylori* infection have a threefold to fivefold increase in risk of noncardial lesions only.[26] Recent evidence identified a specific strain of this species, cagA-positive *H. pylori*, and infection early in life as risk factors for gastric cancer.[27] A reduction in the risk of this disease with treatment of *H. pylori* infection has not been demonstrated, but such treatment has been approved by the Japanese health insurance system. In addition, gastric cancer screening has been determined to be substantially more cost-effective in endemic areas.[28] The correlation between *H. pylori* and gastric lymphoma (discussed in lymphoma chapter) must also be considered. A cohort study looking at stored serum suggested that chronic Epstein-Barr virus infection may play an etiological role in a subset of patients.[29] There are undoubtedly additional environmental factors that have not yet been identified.

Over the past decade, a trend of increasing incidence of proximal gastric cancer has been reported by a number of American investigators.[3,30] A similar change in the pattern of gastric cancer localization has been observed in Europe and Asia (Table 84-1).[31-33] In a report of the National Cancer Data Base, of the patients with gastric cancer classified proximal to distal in orientation, approximately 50% had localization in the gastric cardia or fundus.[34] The cause of this increase in the incidence of proximal gastric cancer is under investigation.

Proximal gastric cancer has a different pattern of clinical and biological behavior from that of distal gastric cancer. Specifically, several investigators have reported a worse prognosis for patients who have proximal gastric cancer than for those whose cancer is located in the mid or distal portion of the stomach.[32,34] In addition, the incidence of proximal gastric cancer is higher in white patients than in patients of other ethnicities.[3] Furthermore, obesity may play a role in its pathogenesis. Two case-controlled studies conducted in the United States and one conducted in Sweden found an association between a high body mass index and adenocarcinoma of the gastric cardia.[26,35] Our recent analysis of 1339 consecutive cases of gastric and GE junction cancer at the University of Texas MD Anderson Cancer Center showed that proximal localization was strikingly more frequent in non-Hispanic white men, while non-Hispanic white women had a pattern of gastric cancer localization similar to other ethnic-racial groups.[36]

GE junction cancers are classified at the discretion of the treating physician. There are no distinct morphological features that separate esophageal, GE junction, and gastric cancers. However, when investigators compared distal Barrett's associated esophageal, GE junction, and gastric cardial cancers by using comparative genomic hybridization, they found that loss of 14q31-32.1 was distinctly more common in patients with Barrett's esophageal cancer.[37] This loss was uncommon in patients with gastric cardial cancer and occurred with intermediate frequency in patients with GE junction cancer, implying that the latter is a mixture of cancers arising from the distal esophagus and gastric cardia.

Histology

Adenocarcinoma is the dominant histology in gastric cancer and accounts for 87% of cases in the SEER registry diagnosed between 2001 and 2005. The Lauren and WHO classifications are the

Table 84-1 Gastric Cancer Localization in Selected Countries

Tumor Location	United States[34]		Germany[236]		The Netherlands[129]		Japan[33]		Korea[32]
	Reported	Adjusted[a]	Reported	Adjusted[a]	Reported	Adjusted[a]	Reported	Adjusted[a]	Reported
	n = 33,085		*n* = 1750		*n* =711		*n* = 668		*n* = 10,783
Proximal	31%	45%	28%	30%	10%	10%	18%	21%	13%
Mid	5%	7%	37%	39%	28%	28%	33%	37%	87%[§]
Distal	25%	36%	25%	26%	54%	55%	38%	43%	
Diffuse	8%	12%	5%	5%	7%	7%	[c]	[c]	[d]
Unknown[b]	30%		5%		<1%		11%[c]		[d]

[a]Excludes cases in which the primary tumor location is unknown or cannot be classified in a proximal to distal orientation (greater curve, lesser curve).
[b]Primary tumor location is unknown or cannot be classified in a proximal to distal orientation.
[c]Author classified diffuse cases with unknown.
[d]Author only reported location as proximal versus distal two thirds.

two major classification systems used for the histology of gastric adenocarcinoma. The Lauren's system simply classifies cancer as intestinal or diffuse.[38] This system does recognize that there are cases in which the histology is mixed, with components of both intestinal and diffuse disease. The simplicity of this system has resulted in widespread use of it.

Intestinal-type gastric cancer is also call epidemic-type gastric cancer. It features a retained glandular structure and cellular polarity. Grossly, it usually has a sharp margin. It arises from the gastric mucosa and is associated with chronic gastritis, gastric atrophy, and intestinal metaplasia. *H. pylori* and environmental factors likely play a major role in its pathogenesis.

The diffuse-type histology is associated with an invasive growth pattern. Scattered clusters of uniform-sized malignant cells frequently infiltrate the submucosa. However, it has little glandular formation. Mucin production is common. Studies of gastrectomy specimens obtained from patients without clinical disease have shown early diffuse-type gastric cancer arising below normal-appearing epithelium.[39] Tumor cells in this type appear to arise from the superficial layer of the lamina propria.

An infiltrative growth pattern in diffuse-type gastric cancer often results in the absence of a mass. Endoscopically, the cancer may be difficult to identify without the presence of an ulceration or mass. Malignant cells can infiltrate well beyond the apparent tumor margin. In advanced cases this leads to linitis plastica with a leather-bottle-like stomach.

WHO Classification

The WHO scheme classifies gastric cancer into more detailed groups than the Lauren classification does. Specifically, the papillary and tubular groups correspond with the intestinal type of gastric cancer in the Lauren's classification, whereas the mucinous and signet-ring cell histologies correspond with the diffuse type. The undifferentiated type may lack features that further identify its origin. Mixed histologies with multiple components are common. Although it classifies gastric cancer into more groups than the Lauren's system does, the WHO classification is not uniformly used in Western countries.

Clinical Manifestations

The symptoms of gastric cancer are often nonspecific, leading to diagnosis at an advanced stage. This is caused in large part by the fact that both the stomach and abdominal cavity are large and distensible. Early symptoms, such as vague discomfort as well as, episodic nausea, vomiting, and anorexia, are common in patients without cancer. So, they initially are often not of concern to patients or physicians unless they persist or progress over a period of time. Outside of Japan, early detection of gastric cancer is not attempted. In the United States, it is not uncommon for patients to undergo several months of therapy for peptic ulcer disease prior to a diagnosis of gastric cancer.

Table 84-2 Symptoms at Diagnosis by Gastric Cancer Localization

Symptom	Proximal (n = 553)	Nonproximal (n = 689)	p Value
Abdominal pain	276 (50%)	447 (65%)	<.001
Weight loss	222 (40%)	277 (40%)	NS
Dysphagia	210 (38%)	83 (12%)	<.001
Nausea/vomiting	88 (16%)	182 (26%)	<.001
Early satiety	73 (13%)	132 (19%)	.005
Bleeding	89 (16%)	116 (17%)	NS

Abbreviation: NS, not singnification.

The most common symptoms of gastric cancer at diagnosis are abdominal pain (50-65%) and weight loss (40%). Although anemia is also a frequent finding, among patients with gastric cancer, overt upper gastrointestinal bleeding is much less common. Our analyses of more than 1000 cases of gastric cancer at MD Anderson Cancer Center have shown that symptoms vary according to the location of the primary lesion (Table 84-2). Dysphagia occurs predominantly in patients with proximal cancer localization, whereas nausea and vomiting are more common in patients with nonproximal cancer. Early satiety can be especially prominent in patients with linitis plastica.

Physical examination findings are late events that indicate advanced, unresectable disease. A palpable epigastric mass indicates a large locally advanced tumor. Jaundice usually indicates hepatic metastasis or metastatic lymphadenopathy in the portal region. Peritoneal metastases into the pelvis can occur as Blumer shelf nodules. Krukenberg tumors of the ovaries can occur in the absence of peritoneal disease. A periumbilical mass can arise from lymph node metastasis or, more commonly, from peritoneal metastasis. One more site of palpable lymphadenopathy is in the left supraclavicular area, ie, Virchow's node. Other, less common dermatological findings include acanthosis nigricans and multiple seborrheic keratoses.

Pattern of Spread

Gastric cancer can spread in several ways. Adjacent organs, such as the liver, diaphragm, pancreas, spleen, and colon (or its mesentery), are frequently involved by direct extension. It can also spread through the lymphatic system to distant nodes. Hematogenously, the liver is frequently involved. Finally, as the cancer penetrates the gastric wall, peritoneal metastases frequently occur. End-organ failure because of liver and or peritoneal metastases is a frequent cause of death.

Japanese investigators noted that the histology and patient's age may affect the pattern of spread of gastric cancer. In their autopsy study of 173 cases of gastric cancer, investigators found diffuse histology to be associated with peritoneal metastasis and intestinal histology to be associated with hepatic metastasis.[40] They also found peritoneal metastasis to be more common in younger patients. In a separate surgical study, researchers analyzed case records of 216 patients who had synchronous peritoneal or hepatic metastasis,[41] finding poorly differentiated histology associated with the former and well to moderately differentiated histology the later.

On a molecular level, expression of vascular endothelial growth factor (VEGF) and its receptor KDR has been associated with liver metastasis.[42,43] The role of VEGF in angiogenesis is compatible with the presumed hematogenous route of dissemination of gastric cancer to the liver. Expression of VEGF-C, which can cause neogenesis of lymphatic vessels, is associated with lymph node metastasis.[44,45] In addition, dysregulation of cellular adhesion is likely central to peritoneal metastasis. CD44H has been linked with increased gastric cancer cell adhesion to mesothelial cells and increased peritoneal metastasis in animal models.[46] C-met amplification has also been linked with peritoneal metastasis.[47,48] Further translational research of the molecular biology of metastasis may improve our ability to predict sites of failure and refine therapeutic strategies.

Molecular Biology of Gastric Cancer

Molecular markers in gastric cancer and their clinicopathological correlations are presented in Table 84-3.

Table 84-3 Molecular Markers With Clinicopathological Correlations

Marker	Involvement	Dominant Histology	Clinical Correlation
Epigenetic			
Hypermethylation	Common	Both	
MSI	31-39%	Intestinal	Conflicting for survival, favorable or no difference
Tumor suppressor			
p53	47-74%	Both (intestinal early event, diffuse late event)	Correlates with stage in diffuse-type cancer
APC	8-34%	Intestinal	–
MCC	24-33%	Diffuse	–
DCC	12-49%	Intestinal	–
FHIT	49-67%	–	Correlates with stage, conflicting for survival
Adhesion			
E-cadherin	54-83%	Diffuse	–
α-catenin	83-92%	Diffuse	–
γ-catenin	91-100%	Diffuse	–
β-catenin	–	Intestinal (GSK3β region)	Poor survival
CD44	31-72%	CD44v6-intestinal	CD44v6 in intestinal-type cancer correlates with inferior survival
Tyrosine kinases			
EGFR	35-81%	Both	Correlates with stage, conflicting for survival.
HER2/neu	10-38%	Intestinal	Poor survival
PDGF α	42-45%	Both	Correlates with stage and poor survival
c-Met	34-71%	Diffuse	Correlates with stage and peritoneal metastasis
Angiogenesis			
VEGF	–	Intestinal	Correlates with hepatic metastasis
bFGF	–	Intestinal	Increased recurrence

Hereditary Gastric Cancer

Familial clustering has been noted to occur in approximately 1% of gastric cancer cases. Known germline mutations account for only a small portion of these cases. The search for other candidate genes is ongoing. The understanding of genetic abnormalities underlying hereditary gastric cancer offers not only the opportunity for prevention and surveillance for affected individuals but also clues regarding the molecular pathology and development of sporadic gastric cancer.

Hereditary Diffuse Gastric Cancer Syndrome ■ Germline mutations of the E-cadherin gene (*CDH1*) in families with a history of gastric cancer was first reported in three Maori kindreds in 1998.[49] Since then, multiple families with a history of gastric cancer and mutations of this gene have been identified, establishing the hereditary diffuse gastric cancer syndrome. However, detectable E-cadherin mutation accounts for only a small percentage of families with a history of diffuse gastric cancer. Most detected germline mutations of the E-cadherin gene have resulted in truncated E-cadherin protein.

The E-cadherin gene is involved in cellular adhesion. Defects in this gene have been linked with diffuse-type gastric cancer and lobular breast cancer.[50] Histologically, most cancers in this syndrome have a poorly-differentiated, infiltrative, and signet-ring cell histology, though a mixed histology with an intestinal component has also been reported.[50]

Affected individuals inherit one copy of the defective E-cadherin gene. Somatic mutation, deletion, or promoter methylation inactivates the other copy. The cancer appears with an autosomal dominant pattern with high penetrance. Moreover, when prophylactic gastrectomy is performed, multifocal early gastric cancers are nearly always found in the resected specimen.[39] Genetic counseling is recommended in suspected cases, taking into consideration the degree of penetrance and age of onset of known cases of gastric cancer in the family, and the paucity of log term outcomes data for prophylactic gastrectomy.

FAP ■ Germline mutations of the *APC* gene result in FAP. This disorder is inherited in an autosomal dominant pattern with high penetrance. Polyps in such cases frequently undergo malignant transformation. Although the colon is the most common site of polyp formation, gastric polyps occur in 27-70% of affected individuals.[51,52] Whereas fundic gastric polyps are usually thought to be hamartomas, foveolar dysplasia and invasive adenocarcinoma have been described by a number of investigators.[51,52]

HNPCC ■ HNPCC is a genetic disorder characterized by germline mutations in a group of mismatch repair genes, including *hMSH2, hMLH1, hMSH6, hPMS1*, and *hPMS2*. Defects in these genes result in genomic instability characterized by microsatellite instability (MSI). Although colorectal and endometrial cancers are the most common manifestations of HNPCC, gastric carcinoma has also been observed. An analysis of the Korean Hereditary Tumor Registry showed a 3.2-fold increase in the relative risk of gastric cancer in families carrying the HNPCC mutation.[53] However, germline mutation of one of the mismatch repair genes accounts for only a small percentage of gastric cancers with MSI.

Li-Fraumeni Syndrome ■ Li-Fraumeni syndrome is characterized by multiple primary malignancies.and caused by mutations in the p53 tumor suppressor gene. Although gastric cancer has been observed as part of Li-Fraumeni syndrome, it does not significantly contribute to the overall number of cases of familial gastric cancer.[54]

Epigenetic Changes

Hypermethylation ■ Methylation of CpG islands in the CpG promoter region regulates the expression of various genes. Aberrant methylation of normally unmethylated promoters is now recognized as an alternative pathway for inactivation of various tumor suppressor and tumor-related genes. Promoter methylation of the *E-cadherin, hMLH1*, and *p16* genes has been observed. Hypermethylation may be involved in the early carcinogenesis of both intestinal- and diffuse-type gastric cancer.

A defect in the mismatch repair gene, *hMLH1*, has been linked with MSI. Several investigators have examined the relationship between hypermethylation of the *hMLH1* gene promoter and MSI. In one study, investigators found hypermethylation of the *hMLH1* promoter in 17 of 18 MSI-positive gastric cancer cases.[55] Furthermore, they observed hypermethylation in the surrounding nonneoplastic tissue in 71% of the cases. Other investigators searching for mutations and hypermethylation of the *hMHL1* gene in patients with MSI-positive gastric cancer[56] found biallelic *hMLH1* promoter hypermethylation in all of the cases, but no mutations in the *hMLH1* gene.

Besides germline mutations, hypermethylation of the E-cadherin promoter is commonly observed as an alternative pathway of *CDH1* gene inactivation.[57,58] Aberrant hypermethylation of other genes has also been detected in patients with gastric cancer. These genes include *DCC, p16, O6-methylguanine-DNA methyltransferase*, and *RUNX3*.[59-61] Epigenetic changes resulting from CpG island hypermethylation may lead to development of the replication error (RER) phenotype, silencing of tumor suppressor genes, and altered cellular adhesion because of silencing of E-cadherin. These early changes may lead to further accumulation of mutations and progression of cancer.

MSI ■ Microsatellites are monotonous tandem repeats found throughout the human genome. Germline mutations in DNA repair genes, *hMSH2, hMLH1, hMSH6, hPMS1,* and *hPMS2* lead to MSI and the hereditary HNPCC phenotype. Altered lengths of microsatellite markers are the hallmark of the RER phenotype and have been described in a number of human malignancies, including gastric cancer.

Sporadic gastric cancers may be classified as microsatellite stable, MSI low, or MSI high. The frequency of MSI (high and low) in gastric cancer has been reported to range from 31% to 39%.[62,63] MSI is likely to occur early in gastric carcinogenesis in patients with the RER phenotype, leading to inactivation of other tumor suppressor genes. Studies have found MSI in areas of intestinal metaplasia, dysplasia, and gastric adenoma in patients with gastric cancer.[64] Likewise, several presumed downstream mutations have been associated with MSI. Specifically, mutations in the transforming growth factor-β2 gene have been observed in a large percentage of gastric tumors with MSI.[65]

Several investigator have reported that MSI is associated with an intestinal histology.[62,64] Likewise, MSI has been associated with distal gastric cancer.[64] At this time, whether the MSI status affects outcome in patients with gastric cancer is not clear.

Tumor Suppressor Genes

p53 ■ *p53*, which is located on chromosome 17q, is a key tumor suppressor gene. Germline mutations of *p53* lead to multiple malignancies at a high frequency. *p53* regulates cell replication and apoptosis. Wild-type *p53* is usually not detected with the use of immunohistochemical techniques. However, mutants are more stable than wild-type *p53*, accumulate in the nucleus, and lead to so-called *p53* overexpression, which commonly occurs in gastric cancer. Studied according to loss of heterozygosity (LOH), allelic deletions involving the *p53* locus have been detected in up to 64% of gastric cancer cases.[66] Furthermore, studies have shown other *p53* abnormalities to be involved in 47-74% of gastric cancer cases.[66,67]

There are distinct differences in the pattern of *p53* involvement in the two major types of gastric cancer. Some have found mutation of *p53* to be an early event in the development of intestinal-type gastric cancer not correlated with stage progression.[67,68] With the use of immunohistochemical techniques, mutation of this gene has been detected in 46-50% of cases of early intestinal-type gastric cancer. *p53* abnormalities have also been detected in areas of high-grade dysplasia but not metaplasia.[68] In diffuse-type gastric cancer, mutation of *p53* is less common, as it has been found in only 10-20% of cases of early-stage disease.[67,68] However, *p53* abnormality is associated with stage progression in diffuse-type gastric cancer being detected in only 17% of cases of T1 diffuse-type gastric cancer but 50% of cases of T2 or higher disease.[67]

APC* and *MCC ■ Both the *APC* and *MCC* genes are located on chromosome 5q21. Deletion and somatic mutation of the *APC* gene have been described in 8-34% of gastric cancer cases.[66,67] Several investigators have reported that mutation of *APC* is more common in well and moderately differentiated cases of intestinal-type gastric cancer though differences may vary by histology.[67]

LOH of *MCC* locus has been described in two studies. In one, LOH was observed in 33% of the cases without regard to histology.[66] In the other, LOH was present in only 24% of the undifferentiated cases and none of the differentiated cases.[69] The effect of *APC* and *MCC* mutations on clinical outcome remains poorly understood.

DCC ■ The *DCC* gene, which is located on chromosome 18q21, was initially found to correlate with colon cancer progression and metastasis. It has become clear that this gene is also frequently involved in gastric cancer. Methods of *DCC* inactivation include allelic deletion as well as promoter hypermethylation.[67,70] Overall, studies have found loss of *DCC* expression in 12-49% of gastric cancer cases.[67,70,71] Two of these studies found *DCC* involvement to be significantly more common in advanced intestinal-type gastric cancer.[67,71] Furthermore, Wu et al.[67] examined LOH at the *DCC* locus in gastric cancer; separating cases by histology and stage, they found LOH in none of the T1 cases, 4% of the advanced diffuse-type cases, and 32% of the advanced intestinal-type cases.

RUNX3 ■ *Runx3* is a recently discovered putative tumor suppressor gene involved in gastric carcinogenesis. This gene is normally expressed in gastric epithelia. In experimental animal models, *Runx3* knockout mice have been shown to exhibit gastric epithelial hyperplasia with suppression of apoptosis.[61] Examination of human gastric cancer cell line and tissue has uncovered frequent silencing of *Runx3* expression by hypermethylation and mutations. Further investigations into the role of *Runx3* in gastric carcinogenesis are under way.

Cellular Adhesion

Loss of normal cellular adhesion is an important feature of human cancer development. Specifically, metastasis is characterized by loss of adhesion that allows cancer cells to invade and leave the site of origin and subsequently adhere to other sites, such as lymph nodes, the liver, and the peritoneum. Diffuse-type gastric cancer is characterized by aberrant cellular adhesion with a pattern of infiltrative growth by a small cluster of or sometimes single tumor cells. In conjunction with catenins, the cadherins play a critical role in cell adhesion and polarity.[72] Up to 90% of gastric cancer cases have an abnormality in at least one component of the cadherin-catenin complex.[73]

E-Cadherin ■ E-cadherin, which is encoded by the *CDH1* gene, is the major cadherin in epithelial cells. A defect in E-cadherin is recognized as an important feature of diffuse-type gastric cancer. Immunohistochemical analyses have found abnormal E-cadherin staining in more than half of cases of sporadic diffuse-type gastric cancer.[73,74]

Using polymerase chain reaction and LOH analyses, investigators found mutations of the E-cadherin gene in approximately 50% of diffuse gastric cancer cases.[75] Others found E-cadherin mutations in 14% of cases of mixed-type gastric cancer.[76] In contrast, they detected only silent mutations in cases of intestinal-type gastric cancer. Promoter hypermethylation is an alternative pathway of inactivation for E-cadherin.[57,58] Overall, E-cadherin promoter hypermethylation was observed in about half of cases of gastric cancer, however, it was observed in 83% of cases with the diffuse histology.

Catenins ■ When interacting with the cytoplasmic domain of E-cadherin, the α-, β-, and γ-catenin complexes bind the intracellular domain of E-cadherin to the actin filaments to maintain cellular adhesion. Similar to that of E-cadherin, abnormal expression of α- and γ-catenin is associated with diffuse-type gastric cancer.[74] Immunohistochemical studies have shown abnormal expression of α- and γ-catenin in 84-92% and 91-100% of diffuse-type gastric cancer cases, respectively.[73,74]

β-Catenin also interacts with the product of the *APC* gene. While the expression of β-catenin did not correlate with histology in some studies,[73,77] one group of investigators reported that mutations in GSK3b correlated with intestinal histology.[78] In addition, reduction in the membranous expression of β-catenin is associated with poor survival.[73,77]

CD44 ■ *CD44* is a transmembrane glycoprotein involved in cellular adhesion. It has several splice variants that may modulate invasion and metastasis. Silencing of *CD44* by promoter hypermethylation has been reported in human gastric carcinoma cell lines.[79] In animal models, transforming growth factor-β1, has been shown to increase expression of the CD44H isoform in diffuse-type gastric cancer, allowing for increased adhesion to mesothelial cells and increased potential for peritoneal metastasis.[46]

The reported frequency of *CD44* expression in human gastric cancer specimens varies widely, ranging from 31% to 72%, likely reflecting differences within study populations.[80] The intensity of *CD44* expression has been found to correlate with the depth of invasion.[80] Specifically, in patients with stage II or IIIa gastric cancer, *CD44* expression correlated with an inferior 5-year survival rate (43% vs 63%; $p = .002$).

Multiple investigators have examined the significance of the *CD44v6* isoform in gastric cancer observing an association with intestinal histology.[81] Immunohistochemical techniques demonstrate that *CD44v6* is positive in 67-92% of cases with intestinal histology and 17-48% of cases with diffuse histology. Investigators have also reported that *CD44v6* expression is associated with increased depth of invasion, nodal involvement, and metastasis.[81] Among patients with intestinal-type gastric cancer, *CD44v6* has also been reported to predict poorer survival.[81] Though, multivariate survival analysis of this isoform has not been performed, the observation about survival was confirmed by other investigators.

Tyrosine Kinases

Epidermal Growth Factor Receptor (EGFR) (c-erbB-1) ■ EGFR is a transmembrane receptor tyrosine kinase that has been implicated in the pathophysiology of a number of malignancies. It has been reported to be expressed in 35-81% of cases of gastric cancer.[82,83] Gene amplification has been detected in 9% of gastric cancer cases.[47] There does not appear to be any association of EGFR with any particular histology.[82]

EGFR has been associated with increased depth of invasion in resected gastric cancer specimens. Similarly, some investigators have reported inferior survival rates in EGFR-positive cases.[47] However, this was not confirmed by other studies. With the recent development of antibodies and small molecule inhibitors, interest in combining chemotherapy with EGFR inhibition has increased.

***HER2/neu* (c-erbB-2)** ■ *HER2/neu* is an oncogene that belongs to the erbB family of membrane receptor tyrosine kinases. It is located on chromosome 17q21 and produces a 185-kDa transmembrane glycoprotein. It forms homodimers and heterodimers with other members of the erbB family, resulting in tyrosine phosphorylation. Amplification of *HER2/neu* has been identified in patients with gastric cancer. Using immunohistochemical, Southern blot, and fluorescence in situ hybridization analysis, investigator reported *HER2/neu* overexpression in 10-38% of gastric cancer cases with some differences based on subtypes.[67,82,83] When grouped by Lauren's histology, *HER2/neu* is more common in cases of intestinal-type gastric cancer (14-49%) than in cases of diffuse-type disease (0-19%).[67,82] When grouped by primary tumor location, *HER2/neu* overexpression was not found in proximal gastric cancer cases, but it was found in 10% of distal gastric cancer cases.

Several investigators have examined the effect of *HER2/neu* status on clinical outcome. When compared with patients with *HER2/neu*-negative tumors, those with *HER2/neu*-positive tumors had a more advanced stage and higher histological grade.[82] In three studies, the median survival duration in patients with *HER2/neu*-positive gastric cancer was half of that in patients with *HER2/neu*-negative disease.[82]

c-Met ■ *c-Met* is the receptor for hepatocyte growth factor. Overexpression of *c-Met* has been reported in 34-71% of gastric cancer cases.[48,67,84] c-Met overexpression is associated with the diffuse histology, an advanced stage, and an infiltrative growth pattern.[48,67,84] Investigators have described an increased tendency toward peritoneal metastasis in patients with *c-Met* amplification.[48]

Angiogenesis

Angiogenesis appears essential for the growth of solid tumors. Tumor angiogenesis is governed by a number of proangiogenic and antiangiogenic factors. Recent advances have led to improved understanding of the mechanism of tumor angiogenesis and development of antiangiogenic therapy. Increased angiogenesis in tumor specimens portends an unfavorable prognosis in patients with gastric cancer.[42] VEGF and basic fibroblast growth factor (bFGF) are major regulators of angiogenesis, have prognostic value, and are targets for antiangiogenic therapy in patients with gastric cancer.

VEGF ■ Studies of resected gastric cancer specimens have shown that the level of *VEGF*-A (VEGF) expression correlates with the tumor microvessel density.[42,43] Increased expression of *VEGF* has been linked with increased rates of invasion, metastasis, and disease recurrence.[42] *VEGF*-C expression is involved in the neogenesis of lymphatic vessels. In particular, studies of gastric cancer have linked *VEGF*-C expression with increased rates of lymph node metastasis.[45] Furthermore, circulating *VEGF* levels in the blood may predict outcome in patients undergoing surgical resection of gastric cancer.[85]

VEGF expression and tumor vascularity have also been linked with the histology and patterns of metastasis of gastric cancer. In one study, expression of VEGF and its receptor KDR was observed more frequently in intestinal-type gastric cancer than in diffuse-type disease.[42] Furthermore, primary tumors in patients with synchronous hepatic metastases showed higher vessel counts and *VEGF* expression levels than did tumors in patients with synchronous peritoneal metastases. Similarly, *VEGF* expression has been linked with hepatic relapse of gastric cancer following resection.[43]

bFGF ■ *bFGF* can be detected in the blood of gastric cancer patients and both it and its receptors are expressed in gastric tumors.[42,86] *bFGF* expression is stronger in intestinal-type cases than in diffuse-type cases.[42] In one small study, *bFGF* expression was associated with an increased rate of cancer recurrence after surgery.[86] No significant differences in microvessel density or sites of metastasis were associated with *bFGF* expression in the study by Takahashi et al.[42]

Transcription Factors

Evidently, gastric cancer cells express multiple growth factors and growth factor receptors. This results in potentially redundant signal transduction pathways. Sp1 is a transcription factor for many genes that regulates multiple aspects of tumor-cell survival, growth, and angiogenesis. Abnormal expression of Sp1 in cases of human gastric cancer has recently been reported.[87] On the molecular level, the degree of VEGF expression correlated highly with Sp1 expression. Clinically, higher Sp1 expression was associated with higher disease stages and nodal involvement. Furthermore, in multivariate analyses, Sp1 expression was superior to VEGF expression as a predictor of outcome after gastrectomy.[87]

Mammalian Target of Rapamycin

Mammalian target of rapamycin (mTOR) is a highly conserved serine/threonine kinase that regulates cell growth and metabolism in response to environmental factors. It also mediates signaling transduction downstream of key receptor tyrosine kinases, such as insulin-like growth factor (IGF) receptor, VEGFR, and EGFR. Activation and phosphorylation of tyrosine kinases leads to activation of phosphatidylinositol 3-kinase, which in turn activates the serine/threonine kinase Akt. While mutations in mTOR have not been detected in cancer, dysregulation of the pathway is common.

Phosphorylated mTOR has been reported to be present in approximate 62% of gastric cancers and appears to correlate with depth of invasion.[88] In-vivo studies in human gastric cancer zenograft models showed that mTOR inhibition was associated with inhibition of tumor growth and reduced angiogenesis.[88,89]

Pathological and Clinical Staging

The most widely used staging system for gastric cancer is the American Joint Committee on Cancer (AJCC)/Union Internationale Contre le Cancer (UICC) system, which follows a standardized evaluation of the primary tumor (T), regional lymph nodes (N), and distant metastatic disease (M).[90] Table 84-4 shows the current system as revised in 2004. Figure 84-2 shows the correlation between disease stage and survival and underscores the extremely poor overall survival of gastric cancer in the United States from a large review of the National Cancer Data Base by Huyndahl et al.[34] The T stage is categorized according to four levels based on the depth of penetration of the wall of the stomach. T1 tumors are the most superficial, with involvement only as deep as the submucosa. This group is further separated in the Japanese system, and its main importance is in evaluating which tumors are amenable to endoscopic mucosal resection. T2 tumors invade into the muscularis propria, whereas T3 tumors invade through the serosa. In the only significant change from the prior staging system of 1997, T2 tumors are classified as T2a (invasion of the muscularis propria) or T2b (invasion into the subserosa) tumors, but this does not change the stage groupings. The extent of serosal involvement is also assessed in the Japanese system and has some correlation with the risk of failure in the peritoneal cavity. Finally, T4 tumors directly invade adjacent organs.

The AJCC staging system reflects the importance of the number of lymph nodes retrieved resected and evaluated in a specimen. The greater the number of nodes evaluated, the more accurate the staging. However, it is imperative that at least 15 lymph nodes be examined. Nodal staging is divided into four groups:

- N0: no positive nodes;
- N1: 1-6 positive lymph nodes with tumor;
- N2: 7-15 positive lymph nodes with tumor; and
- N3: more than positive 15 lymph nodes with tumor.

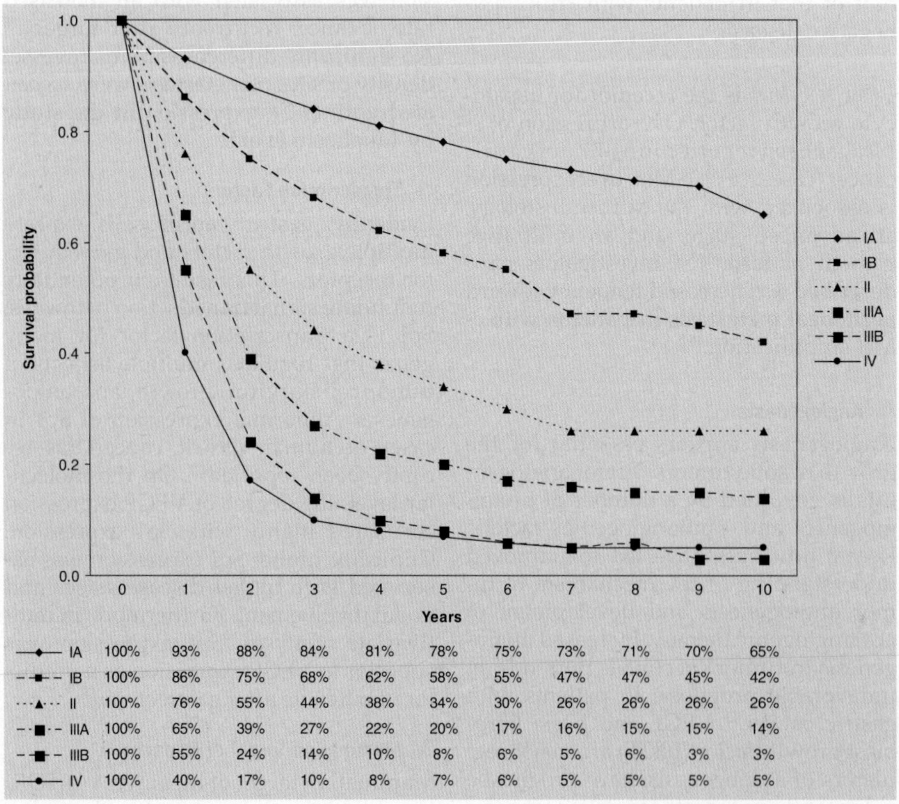

	0	1	2	3	4	5	6	7	8	9	10
IA	100%	93%	88%	84%	81%	78%	75%	73%	71%	70%	65%
IB	100%	86%	75%	68%	62%	58%	55%	47%	47%	45%	42%
II	100%	76%	55%	44%	38%	34%	30%	26%	26%	26%	26%
IIIA	100%	65%	39%	27%	22%	20%	17%	16%	15%	15%	14%
IIIB	100%	55%	24%	14%	10%	8%	6%	5%	6%	3%	3%
IV	100%	40%	17%	10%	8%	7%	6%	5%	5%	5%	5%

Figure 84-2 One-year through 10-year survival rates of patients with gastric cancer after gastrectomy. *Source*: Adapted from Ref. 34.

Table 84-4 **AJCC Stage Grouping for Gastric Cancer**

	Nodal Stage			
T Stage	N0	N1	N2	N3
T1	Ia	Ib	II	IV
T2a/b	Ib	II	IIIa	IV
T3	II	IIIa	IIIb	IV
T4	IIIa	IIIb	IV	IV

Of note is that all patients with N3 disease are classified as having stage IV disease.

The well-described Japanese system that the previous AJCC/UICC system was based on defined nodal stage by anatomic location and proximity to the primary tumor. A detailed description of this system is found in the surgical section below.

There are several aspects of appropriate clinical staging of gastric cancer that should be performed in a stepwise fashion. These steps are physical examination, laboratory studies, computed tomography (CT), endoscopic ultrasound (EUS), and laparoscopy. The role of positron emission tomography for gastric cancer is still evolving; we have seen mixed results of this test, though there is some evidence that is can be used to evaluate response to therapy. Physical examination should be directed toward detecting evidence of muscle wasting (particularly around the temples) and spread of the cancer. Palpation for adenopathy in the supraclavicular fossa (Virchow node), periumbilical area (Sister Mary Joseph node), and the left axilla (Irish node) is essential.[91] The abdomen is palpated for any masses and examined ascites. In addition, a digital rectal exam is performed to assess any masses or a Blummer shelf. Laboratory studies, which include a complete blood count; electrolytes, blood urea nitrogen, and creatinine; and liver function tests (lactate dehydrogenase, alkaline phosphatase, at least one transaminase, and bilirubin). Evaluation of tumor markers such as CEA, CA19-9 and CA125 may be considered. CT scanning of the abdomen and pelvis (and the chest for proximal lesions) is performed to detect evidence of the primary tumor (linitis plastica often will have a distinctive appearance, although one must be sure not to it confuse it for a stomach that has not distended for other reasons), liver metastases, ascites, peritoneal nodules, and nodal metastases beyond the area or areas of resection. EUS is reasonably accurate in assessing the T stage of a tumor, but is very operator dependent. It has an accuracy rate slightly better than 50% in evaluating nodal status. The ability to perform needle biopsy analysis of a node endoscopically can be helpful, however, full nodal status can only be determined accurately by pathological assessment of a resected specimen. We believe that EUS should be considered for two purposes: (1) full staging and evaluation of patients entering neoadjuvant therapy trials and (2) assessment of early-stage lesions that might be amenable to endoscopic mucosal resection. With a neoadjuvant therapy approach EUS may provide a baseline for treatment, it cannot differentiate between tumor and scar tissue and hence should not be used to evaluate response.[92]

Laparoscopy is essential for complete staging of all cases of gastric cancer with the exception of those with a sonographically detected T1 lesion with a moderately differentiated or well-differentiated histology. Laparoscopy for gastric cancer was first described in 1984; since then, multiple studies have demonstrated the benefits of performing laparoscopy in conjunction with other staging modalities for otherwise potentially resectable gastric cancer. Laparoscopy results in upstaging in one fifth to one fourth of patients, primarily through detection of peritoneal metastases not seen on CT scans.[92-94] The detection rate of liver metastases not seen on high-quality CT scans by laparoscopy should be less than 5%.[93] An other benefit of laparoscopy is that a feeding jejunostomy tube can be placed with minimal morbidity at the time of staging for nutritional support during neoadjuvant therapy. If ascites is identified, a feeding jejunostomy tube should generally not be placed. In addition, Burke et al.[94] demonstrated the cost-effectiveness of laparoscopy.

Therapy for Locoregional Disease

Endoscopic Mucosal Resection

Because gastrectomy can have significant complications and long-term sequelae and many patients with very early-stage gastric cancer can expect to have close to a normal life expectancy, better methods of managing these patients have been sought. In Japan, where nearly half of the patients early-stage gastric cancer (owing to significant screening efforts), surgeons have explored the use of endoscopic removal of very early-stage cancers, which have little likelihood of nodal involvement. The polyp removal techniques for patients with colon cancer formed the rationale behind this approach. Fortunately, the wall of the stomach is significantly thicker than that of the colon, allowing for safer excision of mucosa with a reduced chance of perforation. Overall, the incidence of nodal positivity with T1 tumors is approximately 10%. However, in this overall favorable prognosis group, numerous features of the primary tumor can delineate patients who have an extremely low likelihood of having nodal metastases and therefore are good candidates for endoscopic resection. The first of these features is a tumor confined to the mucosa versus a tumor that invades the submucosa, where the incidence of nodal positivity increases from 1% to 3% to roughly 15%.[95] Patients with a Borrmann classification of the primary tumor (types 1-5), the presence of poorly differentiated or signet-ring cell tumors, evidence of lymphatic invasion, a large tumor size (>2 cm), and female gender are far more likely to harbor nodal disease than those without these features.[96] Hence, patients whose tumor is well differentiated, has a superficial appearance (Japanese classification type 0-I, IIa, IIb, IIc), and is T1 tumor as determined EUS have a very low chance of nodal disease.

In Japan, with its aggressive screening programs, endoscopic resection has gained widespread acceptance for tumors with a low histological grade.[97] With this technique, the specimen is carefully analyzed; if penetration into the submucosa is identified, the patient then undergoes gastrectomy. Although Japanese treatment guidelines established strict criteria for application of this technique, some endoscopists in high volume centers have proposed expanded criteria based on their large database.[98] They are now removing large, even ulcerated lesions using a special technique called endoscopic submucosal dissection (ESD). It should be noted that, even in this aggressive procedure, careful histological evaluation of the resected specimen and confirmation of T1 (mucosa) disease is essential. Long-term survival data are awaited. The major problem with this approach in the United States is a lack of patients who are legitimate candidates for endoscopic mucosal resection. Hence, very few endoscopists develop the requisite skills and experience for performing this technique. An alternative for patients with early-stage tumors with favorable prognostic features is a laparoscopic wedge excision. This procedure was first described in 1994; since then, several authors have expanded laparoscopic surgery to include formal total gastrectomy.[99,100] Limited procedures can be considered when the risk of nodal metastasis is low; however, their precise role in the comprehensive management of gastric cancer is still evolving. The application of laparoscopic gastrectomy is increasing. While its role evolves, the adequacy of nodal dissection will remain an important issue.[101]

Surgical Considerations

Several factors must be considered when contemplating surgical resection, including organ system function (pulmonary, cardiac, hepatic, and renal) and general performance status. Some patients are so frail or debilitated that surgical resection cannot reasonably be considered. Patients with evidence of cirrhosis have an increased risk of surgical morbidity/mortality, although there have been a few reports of small numbers of patients with even Child class C cirrhosis who have undergone resection. In a study by Isozaki et al.,[102] the mortality rate was 10% in cirrhotic patients who underwent gastrectomy and 16% in patients who underwent a D2 dissection, which is significant in a nation where the operative mortality rate for gastrectomy is routinely 1% or 2%.

The indications for resection of gastric cancer must be carefully considered whether it is for potential cure or as a palliative intervention. When considering palliative resection, one must be very explicit as to the degree of the patient's symptoms. Whereas a patient with a true obstruction likely needs operative palliation, the ability of most patient's (≥80%) to eat will improve with the use of chemotherapy.[103] Therefore, obstruction is a relative indication rather than an absolute one. Patients with significant bleeding obviously should at least be considered for palliative resection. One must have these considerations in mind prior to taking a patient to the operating room, as intraoperative findings may change the intent of the planned operation. One should be aware that the surgical mortality rate can be quite high with palliative resection.[104] Palliative bypass also carries a very high mortality rate and frequently fails to achieve the desired benefit.[104,105] Palliative care in such patients is discussed more thoroughly near the end of this chapter.

One must consider factors such as the type of operation to be performed, method of reconstruction, and any previous procedures a patient may have undergone when planning the surgical management of gastric cancer. While still unusual, increasingly in the United States, patients are being seen who have had prior surgery for reflux or obesity, which further complicates surgical planning. Patients who have a dilated stomach because of outlet obstruction (and so are likely candidates for a subtotal gastrectomy) generally should be brought into the hospital 2-3 days prior to a planned resection for nasogastric (NG) tube suctioning to decompress the stomach.[106] This maneuver as well as leaving a relatively small gastric pouch will minimize the possibility of postoperative delayed gastric emptying. Patients who do not have an obstruction generally undergo a bowel-prep the day prior to surgery, which can almost always be accomplished on an outpatient basis.

Surgical Controversies

The major surgical issues that have been studied, with varying degrees of success, include the (1) extent of luminal resection, (2) extent of lymph node dissection, (3) role of splenectomy, and (4) method of reconstruction. The choice of operation for gastric cancer depends on the tumor location, histological type, and disease stage. Gastrectomy is the most widely used approach for the treatment of invasive gastric cancer and offers the greatest likelihood of long-term survival. The choices for gastric resection include segmental resection and distal subtotal, total, and proximal subtotal gastrectomy. The type of both gastric resection and nodal dissection may be limited or quite extensive depending on the surgeon's level of experience and biases, the location of the tumor, and the pathological features of the tumor.

Extent of Luminal Resection ■ Prospective and randomized studies have revealed no survival advantage of performing a total gastrectomy for tumors of the distal stomach as opposed to distal subtotal gastrectomy when all of the disease can be removed with adequate margins.[107,108] In particular, Gouzi et al.[108] conducted a prospective randomized trial of total versus subtotal gastrectomy in 169 patients with adenocarcinoma of the gastric antrum who underwent resection with curative intent. The postoperative mortality rate was 1.3% for total gastrectomy and 3.2% for subtotal gastrectomy. The complication and 5-year survival rates in the two groups did not differ significantly. The Italian Gastrointestinal Tumor Study Group conducted a similar prospective randomized trial and found 5-year survival rates of 65% and 62% in the subtotal and total gastrectomy group, respectively.[107] In most series, the quality of life after a subtotal gastrectomy is superior to that after a total gastrectomy; therefore, subtotal gastrectomy should be performed when an adequate margin can be obtained while maintaining a reasonably sized gastric remnant.[109,110] Likewise, one should always be mindful of maintaining an adequate blood supply to the remaining stomach. After radical lymphadenectomy along the lesser curvature, the remaining stomach receives blood supply only from the branches of the splenic artery (short gastric vessels and posterior gastric artery). For this reason, subtotal gastrectomy with splenectomy may result in stump necrosis and should be avoided.

Tumors of the proximal stomach and GE junction require significant consideration for resection and reconstruction. They are often classified according to the Siewert classification.[111,112]

- Type I: adenocarcinoma of the distal esophagus, which usually arises in Barrett esophagus and may infiltrate the GE junction from above;
- Type II: true carcinoma of the cardia arising immediately at the GE junction within 1 cm above and 2 cm below the junction; and
- Type III: subcardial gastric carcinoma infiltrating the junction and distal esophagus from below.

In patients with an advanced tumor involving the GE junction, the site of origin of the tumor may be unclear. Patients with type I tumors should virtually never be considered for a purely transabdominal approach. They are best considered for either a gastric pull-up to the neck (with the stomach, jejunum, or colon) or an Ivor-Lewis procedure. The section on cancer of the esophagus contains a description of and considerations for this procedure.

Type II and III tumors can be treated with either a total gastrectomy or a proximal subtotal gastrectomy (transabdominally, as an Ivor-Lewis procedure, or through a left thoracoabdominal incision, though the later approach recently met with disfavor) depending on the local extent of the tumor.[113,114] For lesions that do not invade a significant portion of the esophagus, a total gastrectomy may be the more appropriate operation. The two main reasons for this are that (1) reflux esophagitis is extremely rare after a Roux-en-Y reconstruction as opposed to the roughly one third of patients who will have significant reflux after proximal subtotal resection,[109,115,116] and (2) proximal subtotal gastrectomy may fail to fully remove the lymph nodes along the entire lesser curvature, which is the most common site of nodal metastasis. However, not all authors agree that total gastrectomy offers fewer quality-of-life problems than proximal subtotal gastrectomy does, and they therefore champion the latter approach.[114]

For patients whose gastric cancer is associated with Barrett esophagus, the appropriate operation usually requires removal of more of the esophagus than can be safely done trans-abdominally. The relative merits of the Ivor-Lewis procedure versus a gastric pull-up to the neck are beyond the scope of this chapter, although the morbidity of an anastomotic leak in the chest is clearly far greater than that of one in the neck, even though the risk of a leak is greater with the pull-up procedure. For poorly differentiated tumors, the general recommendation is to resect a wider margin. Some surgeons have advocated the use of total esophago-gastrectomy with colonic interposition for advanced tumors of the GE junction.[117] This operation, as may be expected, can carry a significant morbidity and mortality risk and therefore should be considered under only the most extenuating circumstances. Considerations may include previous surgery (for obesity or reflux) or other conditions rendering the stomach unsuitable for reconstruction. In some circumstances, the jejunum can be brought up as high the carina (without the need for a vascular anastomosis) or neck with supercharging from the carotid and jugular vessels. With advances in microvascular techniques, the later approach is gaining increasing favor, and is preferable to colonic interposition, in high volume centers for such cases.

Two high volume centers in the Netherlands compared transhiatal and transthoracic approaches to the mid-to-distal esophageal and cardia adenocarcinoma in a randomized controlled study and found a better 5-year survival by extended transthoracic esophago-gastrectomy than limited transhiatal resection in Siewert type I but not type II and III tumors.[118] A Japanese cooperative group studied the role of left thoracoabdominal approach to Siewert type II/III tumors in a randomized study, found no survival benefit of this extended surgery over transabdominal approach and increased morbidity, recommending this approach be avoided.[119] These studies suggest that Siewert type II/III tumors should be treated as a gastric cancer with abdominal approach while type I tumors should be treated as an esophageal carcinoma with transthoracic resection.

Nodal Dissection ■ The extent of lymph node dissection remains the most controversial concern in the surgical management of gastric cancer. The surgeons in Japan, among those in other countries, have for years advocated the use of radical lymph node dissection. This often includes removal of periaortic lymph nodes. Over the past decade or so, several investigators have attempted to better define how radical a dissection should be performed and for what extent of disease through both randomized trials, which are discussed below, and more careful evaluation of the likelihood of a tumor to spread to specific nodal areas.[120,121] The Japanese Gastric Cancer Association defined the extent of lymph node dissection using the designation "D" based on their large survival data.[122] Roughly speaking, a D1 dissection includes just the perigastric lymph nodes. A classic D2 dissection also includes nodes along the hepatic, left gastric, celiac, and splenic arteries as well as those in the splenic hilum. A D3 dissection includes nodes along the porta hepatis and in the retropancreatic and periaortic regions.

To more accurately evaluate surgical specimens, the Japanese Research

Society for Gastric Cancer created a classification system that divides the draining lymph node basins into 16 stations consisting of 6 perigastric stations and 10 stations along the adjacent major vessels, in the splenic hilum, behind the pancreas, and along the aorta. What is actually present in these nodal stations was elucidated in a study by Wagner et al.,[123] who carefully dissected cadavers and assessed each nodal station. They found tremendous variation in the number of nodes recovered from each station and that the lesser curvature was the only area to have nodes recovered in every patient. Similarly, it is important to know that the number of nodes recovered is affected not only by natural variation among patients and the surgical technique used but also by the rigor with which the pathologist examines the specimen. Dissecting and sending these specimens separately may increase the total yield of nodes recovered simply by heightening the awareness of the pathologist regarding the task at hand. Use of a fat-clearing technique can double the number of nodes recovered, which can then clearly alter the pathological assessment.[124] The impact of a lack of staging information was perhaps best demonstrated in the National Cancer Data Base study in 1985 by Lawrence et al.,[125] which found that more than half of the patients did not have a stage determination. By 1991, the number of patients without staging decreased, but nearly one out of every four patients still did not have a stage designation.

Retrospective studies from Japan have suggested that extended lymphadenectomy can improve survival, particularly in patients with stage II or III tumors, and can do so with a perioperative mortality rate of 1%.[126] In comparison, the German Gastric Cancer Study Group conducted a prospective nonrandomized study of node dissections.[127] In this study, most of the patients were designated to undergo a D2 dissection. However, a significant number of patients were designated to undergo a D1 dissection primarily based on the number of nodes recovered. In this study, a radical dissection was defined as one containing 27 or more nodes in the specimen. When comparing patients who underwent R0 (potentially curative) resections and examination of at least 15 nodes, patients with stage II or IIIA disease had a significant survival advantage. Clearly, based on the percentage of patients with each stage of disease, stage migration may be at least partially responsible for the perceived benefits of D2 dissection.

Five prospective randomized trials have examined the extent of lymph node dissection in patients with gastric cancer. One of these trials, which was performed by Dent et al.,[128] randomized patients to undergo a D1 or D2 dissection. The authors evaluated more than 400 patients but found only 43 who were intraoperative candidates for the study. They found no difference in survival, yet the operative time, blood loss, and hospital stay were all greater in the D2 dissection group. The operative mortality rate was similar in the two groups.

Two large prospective randomized trials of D1 versus D2 dissection in Western patients were completed and reported.[129-131] In the Dutch trial surgeons who served as reference surgeons for the study were trained in the technique of radical lymph node dissection by a highly experienced senior Japanese surgeon. The surgical quality control in this study was carefully scrutinized. More than 1000 patients were entered into this study, 711 of whom underwent an R0 resection, thus making them eligible for evaluation. The operative morbidity and mortality rates were both significantly greater in the D2 group than in the D1 group (43% and 10%, respectively, vs 25% and 4%, respectively; $p < .01$). This trial failed to show a benefit of extended lymph node dissection with a follow-up duration of more than 10 years. However, a careful review of the data from this study revealed that the increase in the mortality rate was associated with either male patients undergoing D2 dissection or patients undergoing splenectomy and distal pancreatectomy for complete nodal dissection. Patients who underwent a D2 dissection with preservation of the spleen/tail of the pancreas had a risk of operative mortality quite similar to that of patients who underwent a D1 dissection with preservation of the spleen. The rate of recurrence was lower in patients who underwent a D2 dissection than in those who underwent a D1 dissection at 5 years (37% vs 43%). In the final report at this trial subset analysis showed that patients with N2 disease fared better with a D2 dissection than did those with a D1 dissection. The design of this Dutch trial was based on the assumption that lymph node dissection would increase the survival rate from 20% to 32%. Unexpectedly, 40% of the patients were found to have early-stage gastric cancer. In addition, the investigators may have overestimated the potential benefit of extended lymph node dissection. The anticipated benefit of extended lymph node dissection may be determined by multiplying the frequency of lymph node metastasis at certain sites by the survival rate of patients with known metastases at these sites. In such a study, Sasako et al.[121] found that the incidence of splenic hilar lymph node metastasis was roughly 10% and that the survival rate was 10% in patients with metastasis-positive nodes in that site Therefore, the potential increase in survival rate with removal of these nodes is only 1%. In patients with metastasis-positive lymph nodes along the common hepatic, celiac, and left gastric sites, these numbers are higher. Specifically, the overall increase in survival rate with extended lymph node dissection may be 5-8%, which is less than the additional increase in mortality seen with the use of splenectomy and distal pancreatectomy to achieve D2 dissection in both this trial and one performed by the Medical Research Council (MRC).

The MRC trial randomized 200 patients per arm (out of 737 registered patients) to undergo D1 or D2 dissection.[131] Thirty-two surgeons participated in this study, which took 7 years to complete. Distal pancreatectomy and splenectomy were liberally applied to achieve D2 dissection. The operative mortality rate was 13% in the D2 group and 7% in the D1 group. The researchers found no survival advantage for the more aggressive procedure. Similar to the Dutch trial described above, this study found that the increase in morbidity and mortality rate associated with D2 dissection was almost entirely attributable to the use of splenectomy and distal pancreatectomy. Japanese physicians have routinely used splenectomy to achieve complete nodal dissection and have not discerned any increased morbidity with this procedure. A large cooperative group prospective randomized trial in Japan is currently addressing this issue.[132]

More aggressive para-aortic dissection was evaluated in a Japanese randomized controlled trial. In JCOG-9501, patients with T2 or greater tumors, cancer negative peritoneal cytology, and an R0 resection, were intraoperatively randomly assigned to D2 lymphadenectomy or D2 lymphadenectomy plus para-aortic nodal dissection.[133] A total of 523 patients were entered into this study. The overall operative mortality rate was 0.8% in each arm of the study. Forty percent of the patients underwent a total gastrectomy with splenectomy. In the final survival analysis at 5 years after the close of accrual, the overall survival curves of the two groups completely overlapped (5-year survival rates 69.2% and 70.3%). The investigators concluded that prophylactic para-aortic lymphadenectomy should not be performed for curable non-early gastric cancers.[133]

Only surgeons who have performed aggressive lymph node dissection with extremely low operative morbidity and mortality rates should consider it. One study in the United States reported an operative mortality rate of 1.8% for gastrectomy with aggressive lymph node dissection.[134] This should be compared with data from the American College of Surgeons showing the mortality rate for gastrectomy ranges from 8% to 9% in the United States.[135]

The American College of Surgeons has also conducted large studies of patterns of care for gastric cancer across the United States.[136,137] Data from these studies have demonstrated the need for careful evaluation of resected specimens for proper staging. In one of these studies, lymph nodes in the resected specimen were not reported in one third of the patients. A similar finding was seen in the Intergroup 0116 trial of adjuvant therapy, in which nodes in the resected specimen were not reported in more than half of the patients.[138] This is likely the product of a less aggressive operation and a less aggressive evaluation on the part of pathologists.

Linitis plastica, an extremely virulent form of gastric cancer, is considered incurable by many clinicians, and some feel that patients with it should never undergo gastrectomy.[139] At best, the 5-year survival rates in patients with this disease are in the single digits. One approach to patients with linitis plastica is to evaluate with staging laparoscopy and the patient still has potentially resectable disease, treat with neoadjuvant therapy to further select out patients with the most aggressive disease who will never benefit from a gastrectomy. Only those patients who remain free of distant disease are then considered for resection. Similarly, if a patient with linitis plastica has a positive margin, careful consideration should be paid to how far to chase the margin with error on the side of caution if tissues appear grossly normal.

Multivisceral Resections

One of the concerns raised by the results of the Dutch and MRC trials described above is the role of multivisceral resections in the treatment of gastric cancer. In those studies, the mortality rate clearly increased to roughly 15% with the application of distal pancreatectomy and splenectomy. This prompted a reassessment of such aggressive surgery in Western patients. Piso et al.[140] reviewed 33 patients who underwent gastrectomy with pancreatectomy (total, distal, or head) and evaluated operative morbidity and mortality. The overall operative mortality rate was 9%, which is remarkable considering that 9 patients (27%) underwent a palliative resection in the face of known peritoneal or liver metastases. In patients who underwent an R0 resection, the median survival duration was 17 months. The authors also found that only 39% of patients had pathological confirmation of direct invasion of the pancreas. A group from Memorial Sloan-Kettering Cancer Center reported on this issue with the use of their prospective database.[141,142] They found of more than 800 patients who underwent an R0 resection over a 15-year period, roughly one third of the patients underwent resection of an additional organ. Most importantly, the operative mortality rate was only 4%, which was similar to that reported in the Dutch and MRC trials for limited dissection but far lower than that for D2 dissection with adjacent organ resection. Interestingly, the likelihood of actual adjacent organ invasion was very low (14%) in the final pathological examination. The 5-year survival rate in these patients was 32%, lower than the rate of 50% in patients who did not need a multivisceral resection to achieve an R0 resection. These data clearly support the appropriate application of multivisceral resection of gastric cancer when required to achieve an R0 resection at centers where the operative mortality rate can be kept low.

Resection Techniques

There are many different ways to perform a gastrectomy. This section describes the approach to subtotal and total gastrectomy most commonly used at MD Anderson Cancer Center. Once a patient is taken to the operating room for a gastrectomy, he or she is placed in the supine position. If the patient has a T2 tumor or greater and has not undergone staging laparoscopy, the procedure is performed at this juncture (if a truly palliative resection is not to be considered). A midline incision is made from the xiphoid to the umbilicus. Some surgeons use a bilateral subcostal incision; however, we have found that a midline incision provides ample visualization of the upper abdomen and is less painful. Next, the left lateral segment of the liver is mobilized, and the falciform ligament is divided and ligated near the umbilicus and can be used as a pedicled flap to reinforce either the duodenal stump or the esophagojejunostomy. A self-retaining retractor system is then placed and exploration is again performed to confirm the presence or absence of metastatic disease. The omentum is then dissected off the transverse colon. Some surgeons prefer to perform an omental bursectomy (resection of the anterior leaf off of the transverse mesocolon and the peritoneum off of the pancreas) at this time. The rationale for this is resection of microscopic peritoneal metastases, which may be present at this location. This is difficult to justify, however, as a subtotal gastrectomy leaves a portion of the lesser sac regardless of the type of resection performed, and there is no evidence that total gastrectomy (which would be required to remove the entire omental bursa) is a better oncological procedure than subtotal gastrectomy, as noted above. Moreover, the belief that removal of microscopic carcinomatosis in and of itself would confer any survival advantage may be overly optimistic. Depending on the blood supply and viability, the infracolic omentum may be left in place or completely removed.

Next, the patient is placed in a slight reverse Trendelenburg's position. The spleen is brought down into the operative site with moist packs placed behind it to minimize the risk of injury to the spleen and improve visualization. With this technique and careful dissection of the left gastroepiploic vessels (and short gastric vessels for a total gastrectomy), the risk of iatrogenic splenectomy should be only about 1%. With the stomach and omentum reflected in a cephalad direction, dissection is performed in the left side of the abdomen with identification and ligation of the left gastroepiploic vessels. The omentum is then divided over to the greater curvature of the stomach for a subtotal gastrectomy and continues in a cephalad direction, dividing the short gastric vessels for a total gastrectomy. Once the left side of the stomach is fully mobilized, the packs behind the spleen may be removed. Dissection of the omentum continues to the right and, at a point near the hepatic flexure dissection, is carried up to the duodenum. The right gastroepiploic vein is then identified entering into the middle colic vein and divided. A packet of lymph nodes is adjacent to the right gastroepiploic artery as it arises off the gastroduodenal artery; these nodes are dissected up with the specimen, and the artery is ligated. The right gastric vessels are then divided near the hepatic artery, and the duodenum is mobilized. With the duodenum elevated, the fatty attachments along the inferior border are ligated with 3-0 silk. Electrocautery should not be used here, as these vessels are fragile and tend to bleed. The duodenum is then transected, typically with a stapler. The gastrohepatic ligament is divided with the use of electrocautery, employing great care to detect an accessory or replaced left hepatic artery, which can almost always be taken with impunity. However, if the artery is extremely large, a test clamping should be performed.

Dissection is carried over to the esophagus with incision of the peritoneum along the right crux of the diaphragm. The stomach is retracted in a cephalad direction, and dissection is performed across the superior border of the pancreas, reflecting the nodal bearing tissue in a cephalad direction. Next, the left gastric vein is identified, ligated, and divided. This vein may be located either in front of or behind the hepatic artery and may be quite fragile (Fig. 84-3). The dissection continues toward the gastroduodenal artery. The nodal bearing tissue is reflected in a cephalad direction across the hepatic artery. Dissection continues out of the splenic artery to the posterior gastric artery, arising from the splenic artery and providing blood supply to the upper posterior medial wall of the stomach. The left gastric artery is then identified at its origin, ligated, and divided, and the nodal bearing tissue around the celiac axis is dissected back to the crux of the diaphragm. On the left side of the abdomen, the tissue anterior to the adrenal gland is a reasonable plane to work through. The dissection then returns to the right side of the esophagus. In a subtotal gastrectomy, the nodal bearing tissue along the right cardia is dissected off of the GE junction and upper stomach and swept in a caudal direction. All of the right cardial nodes are resected, even in a subtotal gastrectomy. At this point, for a subtotal gastrectomy, a point at least 5 cm proximal to the upper border of the tumor is then selected, and the stomach is transected, usually with a stapler. For a subtotal gastrectomy, the resection is complete at this point, with blood supply coming from the preserved short gastric vessels. For a total gastrectomy, all of the short gastric vessels would have been divided previously; thus, the esophagus is divided with the appropriate margin. If greater exposure of the esophagus is needed, the diaphragm hiatus should be opened; ligation and division of the left phrenic vein usually provides ample exposure of much of the distal esophagus. Stay sutures with 2-0 silk are placed full thickness in the esophagus prior to transection. It is important to remember to perform frozen section analysis of the resection margins prior to reconstruction.

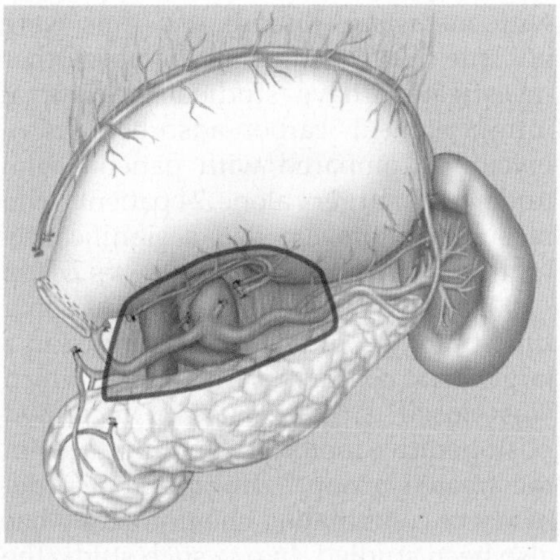

Figure 84-3 Critical area of D2 dissection (spleen-preserving method).

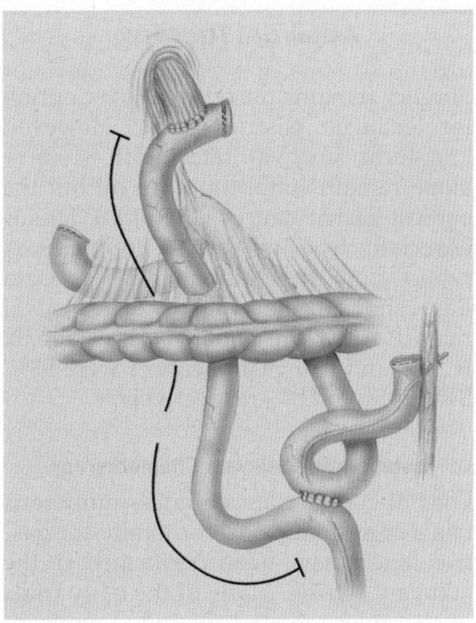

Figure 84-4 Reconstruction after total gastrectomy with a 45-cm Roux limb and defunctionalized short segment for jejunostomy tube placement.

Reconstruction

Many different methods of reconstruction can be used. For total gastrectomy, the options include the standard Roux-en-Y operation (Fig. 84-4), pouch construction, and jejunal interposition (with or without a pouch). Although each of these approaches has its advocates, and numerous small trials have been conducted, there is not a consensus regarding the best method, with various studies supporting each approach.[115,143-151] These studies have looked at both the nutritional implications of and quality-of-life considerations for various reconstruction methods and the benefits of pouch construction versus standard Roux-en-Y reconstruction, with results both for and against pouch reconstruction.[146,151] One type of reconstruction that does make physiological sense is jejunal interposition of a 45-cm segment of the small bowel between the esophagus and duodenum. Studies of this technique have not been conclusive.[150] The biggest downside of this type of reconstruction is that three anastomoses are performed in series (esophagojejunostomy, duodenojejunostomy, and jejunojejunostomy). However, patients who undergo jejunal interposition tend to lose less body weight and have a lower incidence of cholelithiasis with food passing through the duodenum. This type of reconstruction should at least be considered for patients who otherwise appear to be likely to have significant nutritional problems, such as those who have undergone a bowel resection, or in patients undergoing prophylactic gastrectomy. The most common reconstruction method that we perform for subtotal or total gastrectomy is the Roux-en-Y operation.

Reconstruction options for subtotal gastrectomy include Billroth I gastroduodenostomy, loop reconstruction (Billroth II), jejunal interposition, and Roux-en-Y reconstruction. Loop reconstruction (or Roux-en-Y reconstruction) can be performed either at the staple line by removing the staple line and creating an anastomosis from the end of stomach to the side of the small bowel or on the posterior surface of the stomach (Fig. 84-5). If sewn, this is typically performed as a two-layer anastomosis with an inner layer of a running 3-0 absorbable monofilament suture and an outer layer of 3-0 silk Lembert sutures. We most frequently perform Roux-en-Y reconstruction by dividing the small bowel roughly 25 cm distal to the ligament of Treitz (or at the site of a previously placed feeding tube used with neoadjuvant therapy). A vascularized limb of the small bowel is then brought, in a retrocolic fashion up to the posterior wall of the stomach. This is aligned in a manner to create a stapled side-to-side anastomosis with the tip of the small bowel directed toward the left shoulder. For either anastomosis, one should make sure that the anastomosis is at least 6 cm in length to provide optimal emptying of the gastric remnant.[152] One should also make sure that the gastric remnant left in place is not too large, so as to avoid delayed gastric emptying. Roux-en-Y reconstruction prevents the difficult problem of bile reflux, which can occur with Billroth II reconstruction, particularly if the entire lesser curvature has been cleared. The enteroenterostomy is created roughly 45 cm downstream

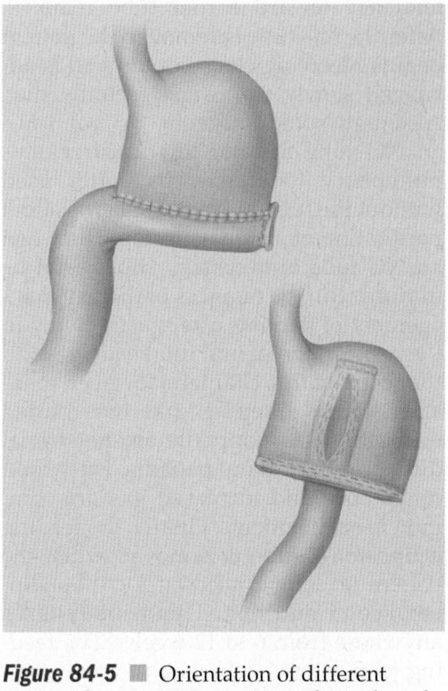

Figure 84-5 Orientation of different options for gastrojejunostomy after subtotal gastrectomy.

from the gastrojejunostomy. This is done in a side-to-side fashion with a short defunctionalized side limb through which a feeding jejunostomy tube can be placed.

Reconstruction after total gastrectomy can be a bit more elaborate than after subtotal gastrectomy (although it need not be). The most common reconstruction method for total gastrectomy is the Roux-en-Y operation. This is usually done in an end-of-esophagus to side-of-jejunum fashion. This anastomosis can be performed by either using a circular or linear stapler technique or sewing in either two or one layers, the latter of which is our preferred approach (a single layer with interrupted 3-0 silk sutures). The principal reason for using the sewing technique is the lower rate of anastomotic stricture when compared with stapling. In general, there appears to be no substantial difference in the leak rate between sewn and stapled anastomoses. One should also note that even surgeons who routinely staple an anastomosis sew the anastomosis in roughly 10% of the cases.

The NG tube is passed across the anastomosis and used to test the anastomosis with air under water prior to completion of the procedure. The falciform ligament, if it is long enough, can be wrapped around the esophagojejunostomy to bolster the anastomosis. Postoperatively, we do not routinely perform a contrast study, but if the patient has unexplained tachycardia or fever or is slow to regain intestinal function, we do perform a barium swallow, or CT scan. Typically, the NG tube is removed when there is evidence of bowel function and low output from the NG tube. Otherwise, the tube is usually left in for 5-7 days, though there is an increasing tendency toward earlier tube removal. After the NG tube is removed the patient begins receiving clear liquids and is advanced slowly to postgastrectomy diet. Although some surgeons do not leave an NG tube in after total gastrectomy, pulmonary toilet may be better used without the tube in place, concerns about perforation of a fresh anastomosis when an NG tube is necessary should not be minimized. The nuances of dietary management of patients after gastrectomy in the resumption of oral intake are beyond the scope of this chapter. However, management of dumping and overcoming transient loss of appetite are not trivial difficulties for many patients. Fatty food intolerance and increased gas are common in such patients. Finally, the feeding jejunostomy tube is removed when the patient no longer needs it for the maintenance of nutrition. This usually takes anywhere from 6 to 12 weeks. The feeding jejunostomy tube is an excellent insurance policy when a leak develops and prolonged oral intake must be avoided.

Adjuvant Therapy

Surgery remains the only curative option for localized gastric cancer. However, long-term survival rates with surgery alone remain suboptimal for all but the earliest gastric cancer (T1N0M0). This is especially true in Western countries. A report from the National Cancer Data Base showed that the 5-year survival rates in American patients with stage Ib, II, IIIa, and IIIb gastric cancer were 58%, 34%, 20%, and 8%, respectively.[34]

Postoperative Adjuvant Chemotherapy

Over the past four decades, numerous trials of systemic chemotherapy for gastric cancer have been performed in the adjuvant setting. Many of the early trials were underpowered, included improper control groups, or used suboptimal methodologies. These limitations along with heterogeneous inclusion criteria rendered much of their results unreproducible.[153] Meta-analyses of these trials were fraught with difficulties and could not recommend a particular regimen. Nevertheless, two large analyses were performed with conflicting results.[154,155] Each analysis recommended treatment for subgroups such as patients with node-positive disease and Asian patients. Selected trials reporting benefits are described below.

Most of the chemotherapy agents considered to be active against advanced gastric cancer have reported response rates of 15-20% when administered alone. Consequently, to determine the expected survival benefit, random-assignment trials involving hundreds to thousands of patients would be needed. In particular, the activity of single-agent mitomycin in the adjuvant setting was first reported by Japanese investigators in 1977.[153] They summarized four trials of adjuvant mitomycin. One of these trials showed an improved 5-year survival rate in treated patients when compared with control patients. A subsequent small trial from Spain also reported a survival advantage for patients who received mitomycin when compared with surgery-alone controls.[153] However, the improved survival rate seen in two of these five trials with single-agent mitomycin must be balanced with the first trial's lack of reproducibility and the second trial's small number of subjects. The numerous trials using mitomycin-containing regimens that demonstrated no survival benefit must also be considered.[153]

Using an anthracycline-based regimen, investigators randomly assigned patients to undergo surgery followed by treatment with epirubicin, 5-fluorouracil (5-FU), and folinic acid or surgery alone; they observed an improved 3-year survival rate in the treated group.[153] However, this was a small trial, with only 55 patients receiving treatment. Confirmation is needed.

Prolonged continuous administration of an oral 5-FU prodrug has been attractive to a number of investigators. In one trial, 85 patients were randomly assigned to receive treatment with mitomycin alone every 6 weeks for four cycles or at the same dosage with daily tegafur for 36 consecutive days each cycle. The 5-year survival rate was significantly higher in the group that received mitomycin and tegafur.[153] However, the small number of patients, long accrual time (11 years), and lack of a surgery alone control group make these results questionable.

In a more recent Japanese study, investigators from the ACT-GC group randomly assigned 1059 patients with stage II or III gastric cancer who had an R0 gastrectomy with D2 or higher lymphadenectomy to surgery alone or postoperative S-1.[156] Improved relapse-free survival and overall survival were observed in the S-1 treated group. The 3-year relapse-free survival rates were 72.2% in the S-1 treated group and 59.6% in the surgery-alone group ($p < .01$). Similarly, the 3-year overall survival rates were 80.1% in the S-1 treated group and 70.1% in the surgery alone group ($p < .01$). However, it should be noted that the safety profile of S-1 differs between Western and Asian patients and that S-1 is currently not available in United States.

Intraperitoneal Therapy

The peritoneal cavity is a frequent site of relapse of gastric cancer. Intraperitoneal administration of chemotherapeutic agents may result in improved delivery to microscopic residual disease. Several trials have examined the feasibility of such an approach. Two trials compared surgery alone with surgery followed by intraperitoneal delivery of cisplatin.[153] No survival differences were observed. However, both trials included patients with metastatic disease and thus were not true trials of adjuvant therapy. Other investigators have studied the use of intraperitoneal carbon-adsorbed mitomycin.[153] Compared with patients who underwent surgery alone, 24 patients who received mitomycin had a significantly higher 2-year survival rate (69% vs 27%; $p < .005$). However, the advantage of using this strategy could not be confirmed in a larger trial conducted in Austria, which was closed early because of increased postoperative morbidity and mortality in the treated group.[153] Intraperitoneal delivery of combination chemotherapy has also been studied. In one such study, the investigators randomly assigned 248 patients to undergo surgery alone or with intraperitoneal mitomycin and 5-FU but found no significant difference in overall survival between the two groups.[153]

Continuous hyperthermic peritoneal perfusion was designed to favorably alter the distribution and kinetics of agents used in intraperitoneal chemotherapy.[153] A number of randomized trials of adjuvant continuous hyperthermic peritoneal perfusion have been performed in Japan. As part of a phase 1 study of intraperitoneal hyperthermic perfusion at our institution, 12 patients with gastric cancer were treated with this approach.[153] Survival durations were significantly longer for patients who underwent perfusion when compared with a nonrandomized group of patients with stage IV disease who were candidates for perfusion during the same period but received systemic chemotherapy. Unfortunately, two operative deaths (17%) occurred, and all of the patients eventually died of their disease.

Postoperative Adjuvant Immunotherapy

Immunotherapy has been explored in the postoperative setting in hopes of decreasing relapse and improving survival in patients with gastric cancer. However, few immunotherapy trials have had a no-treatment control arm. One of these was a three-arm randomized study that compared surgery followed by observation only, surgery followed by chemotherapy with 5-FU and methyl CCNU, and surgery followed by chemotherapy with 5-FU and methyl CCNU plus levamisole.[157] The overall survival rate at 5 years was 50% in all three groups.

The nonspecific immune stimulant OK-432 (Picibanil) has also been studied in randomized trials. In one such trial, patients were randomly assigned to undergo surgery alone; surgery followed by chemotherapy with mitomycin, 5-FU, and cytarabine; or surgery followed by the same chemotherapy regimen plus OK-432.[158] After a median follow-up duration of 5 years, the investigators found no significant difference in overall survival among the three groups. In addition, Korean investigators studied OK-432 in two randomized trials.[159] In one of the trials, 64 patients underwent surgery alone, and 74 patients underwent surgery followed by chemotherapy with mitomycin, 5-FU, cytosine arabinoside, and OK-432. The 5-year survival rate was higher in the treated group (45% vs 23%; $p < .05$). In the other trial, 159 patients received mitomycin, 5-FU, and OK-432; 77 patients received only mitomycin and 5-FU; and 94 patients underwent surgery alone. The 5-year survival rate was 45%, 30%, and 24%, respectively. The results of these trials are encouraging but must be confirmed in larger trials.

Chemoradiation for Incompletely Resected Disease

Several early trials evaluated the role of chemoradiation in patients with incompletely resected gastric cancer. Specifically, a randomized trial conducted at Mayo Clinic administered radiation at 35-40 Gy both with and without a bolus of 5-FU for 3 days for a variety of unresected tumors.[160] The investigators analyzed a small group of patients with gastric cancer and found the patients who received concurrent 5-FU to have a superior 5-year survival when compared with those who received radiation alone (12% vs 0%), providing evidence of the efficacy of this chemoradiation regimen, which has been used for three decades. A subsequent randomized trial conducted by the Gastrointestinal Tumor Study Group evaluated chemotherapy alone with 5-FU and methyl CCNU compared with chemoradiation (split course: 5000 cGy with a bolus of 5-FU given at the start of each course of radiotherapy) in patients with incompletely resected gastric cancer.[161] The trial was stopped early because of six treatment-related deaths and six disease-related deaths within the first 6 months of therapy in the combined-modality arm. In spite of this, the investigators found a statistically significant survival benefit in the combined-modality arm at 5 years (survival rate, 20% vs 6%; $p < .01$). In this study, the gastrointestinal and hematological toxic effects were not managed optimally. Modern supportive care, including jejunostomy tube feeding and cytokine support could have enhanced the difference in survival in favor of the combined-modality arm. To confirm these results, investigators designed a second trial with similar entry criteria comparing 5-FU, methyl CCNU, and doxorubicin alone with the same regimen followed by chemoradiation (4320 cGy with a bolus of 5-FU) starting on day 57.[162] Unfortunately, this trial was hampered by poor accrual and compliance (of 59 patients, 11 did not receive the prescribed dose of radiation, and 7 did not undergo radiotherapy), which may explain why it showed no difference in survival.

Others have investigated postoperative radiotherapy alone for gastric cancer. For example, the British Stomach Cancer Group conducted a phase 3 trial that stratified 436 patients by age, symptom duration, and disease stage and randomized them to undergo surgery alone, surgery followed by 5-FU, doxorubicin, and mitomycin (FAM) chemotherapy alone, or surgery followed by radiotherapy (45 Gy in 25 fractions with or without a 5.4-Gy boost) alone.[163,164] In spite of the fact that one third of the patients had residual disease, 18% had positive margins, and one third received 40 Gy of radiation or less, the researchers found a locoregional control advantage in the radiotherapy arm (90% vs 73% for surgery alone and 81% for surgery followed by chemotherapy; $p < .01$). The cause-specific and overall survival rates were not statistically different. Even though it did not include a chemoradiation arm, the failure of this study to show a survival impact has influenced the direction of subsequent investigations.

Evidence of the importance of 5-FU administration was demonstrated in a randomized study conducted by the European Organisation for Research and Treatment of Cancer (EORTC),[165] which showed a survival advantage in patients who underwent chemoradiation when compared with those who received radiation alone (to 55.5 Gy). All patients with gross disease who had no progressive disease received 5-FU concurrently and for 18 months after chemoradiation. Subsequent studies have shown that chemoradiation can be curative in a small percentage of patients with unresectable or partially resected gastric cancer.[160]

Postoperative Adjuvant Chemoradiation

Postoperative adjuvant 5-FU-based chemoradiation for gastric cancer was reported 25 years ago when a randomized trial was conducted with patients with completely resected gastric cancer who underwent observation or postoperative chemoradiation (37.5 Gy with a bolus of 5-FU at 15 mg/kg for 3 days).[166] By design, the investigators obtained the patients' informed consent after randomization and did not stratify the patients for known prognostic factors. Ten of 39 patients with favorable prognostic factors refused to undergo adjuvant therapy after randomization. The locoregional control, overall survival, and relapse-free survival rates were all higher in the adjuvant therapy arm than in the controls. Strikingly, the overall survival rate was highest in patients who refused treatment after randomization. Upon analysis by intent to treat, survival was higher in the group that received postoperative chemoradiation, but the difference was not statistically different (20% vs 12%).

Although they provided some evidence of the benefit of chemoradiation in patients with gastric cancer, the studies described above did not provide definitive conclusions because of small patient numbers, inclusion of patients with gross residual disease, use of nonstandardized surgery, administration of suboptimal doses of 5-FU or radiation, or inadequate supportive care. Subsequently, investigators designed an Intergroup trial (INT 0116) in an attempt to minimize these shortcomings.[138] Eligible patients had stage IB-IV gastric cancer that had been treated with curative resection, but the majority of the 556 evaluable patients had positive lymph nodes (85%) or T3/T4 lesions (68%). Patients were randomly assigned to undergo postoperative chemoradiation (45 Gy with a bolus of 5-FU) or observation after complete surgical resection. At 3 years, patients in the treatment arm had a 9% absolute (22% relative) survival advantage (50% vs 41%; p = .0005) at the cost of significant gastrointestinal (33% [grade 3/4]) and hematological (54% [grade 3/4]) toxic effects. Although CT scanning was not required during follow-up, they reported that the rate of local failure was significantly reduced (19% vs 29%). Additional improvement in local control could improve outcome further. The importance of the radiotherapy technique is illustrated by the fact that technical radiotherapy errors had to be corrected with a centralized quality assurance effort in 35% of the cases. Concerns have been raised about the extent of surgery performed in this trial. Specifically, although D2 resection was recommended, only 10% of the patients underwent this procedure, and 54% underwent less than a D1 resection. Because study enrollment and randomization were performed after surgery, this information is probably a reflection of the pattern of surgical practice and pathologic assessment in the United States rather than protocol noncompliance. Interestingly, the extent of nodal dissection did not correlate with disease-free or overall survival (p = .80) This trial established postoperative adjuvant 5-FU-based chemoradiation as the standard of care for resected gastric cancer in the United States. Table 84-5 shows the treatment regimen used in this trial. Several single-institution studies and SEER analyses have also reported an advantage with postoperative radiotherapy with or without concurrent chemotherapy. It has been argued that chemoradiation may not have a benefit if a D2 dissection is performed. However, in a large retrospective analysis from Korea, the median duration of overall survival was noted to be significantly longer among patients who received 5-FU-based chemoradiation after D2 dissection than among patients who underwent D2 dissection alone (95 vs 63 months, p = .02).[167] These results are, however, subject to potential selection bias.

Intraoperative Radiotherapy

A randomized study from Japan showed a survival advantage with intraoperative radiotherapy (IORT) for stage II-IV gastric cancer but not for stage I gastric cancer with the use of doses ranging from 28 to 35 Gy.[168] Although it suffered from methodological flaws, this study demonstrated the proof of principle for the role of IORT for gastric cancer and for cancer in general. A smaller study showed a significant local control advantage with IORT.[169]

Irradiation Technique and Supportive Care

A comprehensive consensus report of important treatment-planning issues in gastric cancer has been reviewed elsewhere[170] and is summarized below. When planning treatment of gastric cancer all available imaging (CT and barium swallow), endoscopic, pathological, and operative findings should be reviewed prior to simulation. Patients should undergo simulation on an empty stomach (nothing by mouth for 3 h) and receive treatment in the morning before eating to minimize stomach distention. An oral contrast agent should be given 15-30 min prior to simulation, and treatment devices used for arm elevation should be employed. Patients can undergo treatment with either opposed anterior and posterior portals or a multiple-field technique with or without three-dimensional treatment planning. The use of four or more radiation fields has been reported to significantly decrease the rate of grade 4 or 5 toxicity when compared with the use of two fields.[171] However, lateral fields are not always advisable for patients with an intact stomach, because the gastric fundus frequently extends too far posteriorly. In such instances, the kidneys and spinal cord cannot be shielded without shielding the target. CT-based treatment planning with dose-volume histograms is helpful in objectively evaluating various technical treatment options in individual patients. For instance, with the use of three-dimensional planning, beam arrangements can be optimized so that the radiation dose delivered to the kidneys and liver is minimized. Using slight right anterior oblique and left posterior oblique beams facilitates coverage of the porta hepatis while avoiding irradiation of the right kidney. Customized blocking should be used to shield the critical structures in the field, including the small bowel, liver, spinal cord, and kidneys.

There is no uniform agreement about which lymph node groups should be treated, but treatment volumes should be tailored to the location of each individual tumor. There are detailed data regarding the risk of nodal involvement from lymphadenectomy series,[172] which can guide physicians. Depending on the location of the primary tumor in the stomach, perigastric, gastroepiploic, celiac, porta hepatis, subpyloric, gastroduodenal, splenic-suprapancreatic, and retropancreaticoduodenal nodes can be at risk for metastatic spread. The gastric remnant, the perigastric nodes, and the branches of the celiac axis should be treated in all cases. In addition, a 5-cm esophageal mucosal margin and the paraesophageal nodes should be included in the cephalad treatment volume for lesions involving the cardia or GE junction. However, including the duodenal mucosa and periduodenal nodes in the treatment volume for these proximal lesions is not necessary. For distal lesions at or near the gastroduodenal junction, the entire C-loop should be covered to ensure a 5-cm margin of the duodenal mucosa, and the suprapancreaticoduodenal nodes should be treated. In a very small minority of cases it is necessary to use intensity modulated radiation therapy (IMRT) to adequately spare organs at risk such as the liver and kidneys. IMRT may also be helpful in lesions of the gastric cardia to spare the lungs, heart, and liver adequately.

The importance of aggressive supportive care administered by a multidisciplinary care team cannot be overemphasized and was illustrated by the experience of the Gastrointestinal Tumor Study Group,[161] as discussed above. Malnutrition can lead to treatment-related death. When performing radiotherapy for gastric cancer, the routine use of prophylactic antiemetics and jejunostomy tube feeding vastly im-

Table 84-5 Selected Adjuvant Therapy Options

Postoperative chemotherapy and chemoradiation (INT0116 study)
Chemotherapy (one 28-day cycle)
5-FU 425 mg/m²/day IV on days 1-5
Folinic acid 20 mg/m²/day IV on days 1-5
Chemoradiation (5 weeks)
5-FU 400 mg/m²/day IV on days 1-4 and on the last 3 days of radiotherapy
Folinic acid 20 mg/m²/day IV on days 1-4 and on the last 3 days of radiotherapy
External-beam radiation, 45 Gy at 1.8 Gy/day 5 days per week
1-month recovery period
Chemotherapy (two 28-day cycles)
5-FU 425 mg/m²/day IV on days 1-5
Folinic acid 20 mg/m²/day IV on days 1-5
Perioperative chemotherapy (MAGIC study)
Chemotherapy ECF (three 21-day cycle)
Epirubicin 50 mg/m² IV on day 1
Cisplatin 60 mg/m² IV on day 1
5-FU 200 mg/m²/day CIV infusion on days 1-21
Surgery
3-6 week rest period prior to surgery
6-12 week rest period after surgery
Chemotherapy ECF (three 21-day cycle)
Epirubicin 50 mg/m² IV on day 1
Cisplatin 60 mg/m² IV on day 1
5-FU 200 mg/m²/day CIV infusion on days 1-21

Abbreviations: IV, intravenously; CIV, continuous intravenous infusion.

proves treatment tolerance. Nutritionists should monitor patients' calorie intake and weight, provide them with calorie goals, and serve as a resource for other nutrition-related issues.

Preoperative Chemotherapy

Despite recent advances in curative gastrectomy followed by postoperative chemoradiation, 5-year survival rates remain below 50% after this procedure.[138] Several potential advantages make preoperative therapy an attractive target of investigation. For example, early initiation of systemic therapy may eliminate micrometastases. Likewise, the ability to assess tumor response may enable early termination of ineffective therapy. Furthermore, preoperative therapy can downstage the primary tumor and may improve the R0 resection rate. In patients with occult chemo-resistant metastases that manifest during treatment, nontherapeutic gastrectomy may be avoided. Preoperative therapy also adds prognostic information. An analysis of 83 patients on preoperative chemotherapy protocols at MD Anderson showed that response to preoperative chemotherapy was the single most important predictor of survival.[173] However, these findings must be balanced with the potential risk of delaying definitive local therapy. Treatment-resistant clones may develop during therapy, and the performance status may decrease, potentially increasing surgical risk, though at MD Anderson, this has not translated into increased mortality.

Accurate clinical staging of gastric cancer is essential in preoperative clinical trials. Because of the potential for down-staging, pretreatment endoscopic sonography and laparoscopy are needed for all enrolled patients for comparison with control groups. A number of chemotherapeutic regimens have been studied in small trials. The patient-selection and treatment plans in these trials were heterogeneous, making the results difficult to compare. However, they show that preoperative therapy is feasible and can downstage tumors.

The recently reported Medical Research Council Adjuvant Gastric Infusional Chemotherapy (MAGIC) trial has changed the landscape of treatment options for patients with locally advanced gastric cancer.[174] This randomized phase 3 trial compared surgery alone to surgery with 3 cycles of both preoperative and postoperative epirubicin, cisplatin and fluorouracil (ECF) chemotherapy (Table 84-5). Among 503 patients accrued to this trial, ECF chemotherapy toxicity was manageable and the rates of postoperative morbidity and mortality were similar in the surgery-alone and ECF groups. The resected tumors were smaller (3 cm vs 5 cm, $p < .001$) and had less advanced T (T1/T2, 51.7% vs 36.8%, $p = .002$) and N (N0/N1, 84.4% vs 70.5%, $p = .01$) stages than the ECF group. With a median follow-up of 4 years, patients in the ECF group had significantly better 5-year overall survival (36% vs 23%, $p = .009$) and progression-free survival (HR = 0.66; 95% CI 0.53-0.81; $p < .001$) rates. This trial clearly establishes this treatment regimen as a viable option for patients seen prior to gastrectomy. It is important to realize only 42% of patients completed the prescribed protocol. No information on patterns of failure is available, pathologic complete response did not occur with preoperative chemotherapy alone. Since endoscopic ultrasonography was not routinely performed, the tumor size reduction data is based on endoscopic measurement of the maximal tumor diameter and the T and N stage down-staging data are based on the assumption of a random distribution of T and N stage at diagnosis since CT scans could not provide accurate staging detail.

The United Kingdom National Cancer Research Institute Upper Gastrointestinal Clinical Studies Group ST03 trial (otherwise known as MAGIC-B) addresses this concern by prospectively evaluating T and N stage by endoscopic ultrasonography. The follow-up trial, MAGIC-B randomizes resectable gastric cancer patients to perioperative chemotherapy with epirubicin, cisplatin, and capecitabine with or without the anti-VEGF antibody bevacizumab.

Preoperative Chemoradiation

Combined-modality chemoradiation in the preoperative setting allows for treatment with the target organ in place. When compared with postoperative radiotherapy, this may result in reduced radiotoxicity in the intestines, and adjacent organs. When using the strategy, feeding gastrostomy tubes should be avoided, as they rarely function well during irradiation and increase the risk of subsequent surgery. In comparison, routine placement of feeding jejunostomy tubes (outside of the radiation field) enhances tolerance and decreases the need for parental support and hospital admission.

Preoperative radiotherapy both with and without chemotherapy has been reported to improve outcome in prospective randomized trials.[175-177] These trials, which were conducted in Russia, showed increased resectability and survival without increased morbidity with the use of suboptimal radiation doses without concurrent chemotherapy. Similarly, in a pilot study conducted at MD Anderson, 24 patients received 45 Gy of external-beam radiation at 1.8 Gy per day 5 days per week concurrent with continuous-infusion 5-FU at 300 mg/m^2 per day on days when irradiation was performed.[178] Surgery was carried out 4-6 weeks after completion of the chemoradiation in 19 (79%) of these patients. IORT (10 Gy) was given at resection. A complete pathological response was observed in 2 (8%) patients.

The use of induction chemotherapy followed by chemoradiation is currently under investigation. In a small multi-institutional study, patients received two courses of 5-FU, folinic acid, and cisplatin followed by 5-FU-potentiated radiotherapy (45 Gy). Twenty-eight patients underwent surgical resection without experiencing excessive complications. Of the treated patients 30% had a pathologically confirmed complete remission.[179] Investigators are at present studying induction chemotherapy followed by chemoradiation and surgery with the incorporation of newer chemotherapeutic agents in phase 2 trials. The many theoretical advantages of this preoperative strategy for resectable gastric cancer will have to be proven in large random-assignment trials.

Approaches to Adjuvant Therapy

Recent results from three well-powered multicentered studies have demonstrated significant survival benefits for adjuvant therapy compared to surgery alone using three differing approaches. Regardless of patient population, tumor localization, and extent of lymph node dissection, surgery alone is no longer adequate for patients with more than early gastric cancer and otherwise fit to undergo therapy. A direct comparison across studies is not advisable due to differences in study design, patient population, proportion of patients with node positive disease, and extent of node dissection. It is, however, interesting to note that the magnitude of reported survival benefit compared to surgery alone were similar among these studies. The hazard ratios for treated groups compared to surgery alone control groups in the INT0116 study, the MAGIC study, and the ACTS-GC study were 0.74 (95% CI 0.60-0.92), 0.75 (95% CI 0.60-0.93), and 0.68 (95% CI 0.52-0.87) respectively.

We therefore advise a practical approach for recommending adjuvant therapy. Patients with apparent early disease (stage IA by EUS), or patients having indication for upfront surgery (such as those with acute bleed) should have surgery and proceed with postoperative chemotherapy and chemoradiation as in the INT0116 study if found to have stage IB-IV disease on final pathology. Patients with borderline resectable disease or GE junction tumor requiring an esophagogastrectomy with thoracic or neck anastomosis should be considered for preoperative chemotherapy as in the MAGIC study or be enrolled into clinical trials. Finally, for Asian patients located where S-1 is available, postoperative chemotherapy with S-1 should be considered.

Systemic Therapy for Advanced Disease

In patients with unresectable gastric cancer at the time of their diagnosis or with metastatic disease that occurs after primary therapy, the cancer is incurable; thus, therapy is palliative. Despite numerous randomized trials, the survival rates in such patients remain poor. Poor performance status or multiple sites of metastases are associated with significantly worse outcomes. An analysis of the SEER 9 registry showed only modest improvements in overall survival in patients with metastatic disease over the past three decades.[2] The median survival duration in unselected patients diagnosed with metastatic gastric cancer in 2004 was less than 5 months.[180] The median survival durations reported in clinical trials have ranged from 7 to 10 months. Considering this dismal prognosis, several investigators have examined systemic chemotherapy to see whether it has a role for advanced gastric cancer. Four small random-assignment trials assessed the impact of palliative chemotherapy on survival duration and quality of life.[181-184] All four trials reported superior survival durations in patients receiving treatment when compared with those who received best supportive care (Table 84-6). Those who received best supportive care had median survival durations ranging from 3 to 5 months, whereas those who received chemotherapy had median survival durations ranging from 8 to 12 months. Improvements in symptoms and quality of life were also apparent in the chemotherapy group. These findings are consistent with the fact that gastric cancer is a somewhat chemosensitive disease. Side effects of chemotherapy must be balanced against the potential benefits of it and symptoms associated with unchecked cancer growth. Palliative chemotherapy should be considered for most patients with an adequate performance status and nutritional support.

One difficult and controversial area is therapy for nonevaluable disease in asymptomatic patients (such as those with low-volume abdominal carcinomatosis). Although some advocate the immediate use of chemotherapy, others advise observation. The rationale for performing observation lies in the fact that only 30-40% of patients will have an objective response to any particular chemotherapeutic regimen. Delaying treatment until the appearance of early symptoms or evaluable disease may spare patients from experiencing unnecessary toxic effects and preserve their quality of life. These patients should be closely observed with a medical history, physical examination, and CT scans, if necessary. Treatment may be initiated when evaluable disease is established or symptoms appear, though if obstructive symptoms occur (due to peritoneal disease) systemic therapy may not be able to be initiated.

Table 84-6 ■ **Trials of Palliative Chemotherapy Versus Best Supportive Care**

Regimen	No. of Patients	Median Survival	*p* Value	Reference
FAMTX versus	30	9.0 months	.001	182
BSC	10	3.0 months		
FEMTX versus	17	12.0 months	.001	183
BSC	19	3.0 months		
ELF versus	18	7.5 months	Not stated	184
BSC	19	4.0 months		
ELF or LF versus	31	8.0 months	.120	181
BSC	30	5.0 months		

Abbreviations: BSC, best supportive care; FEMTX, 5-FU, epirubicin, methotrexate.

Table 84-7 ■ **Selected Data From Phase 2 Trials of Single-Agent Chemotherapy for Advanced Gastric Cancer**

Reference	Agent	No. of Patients	Response Rate (%)	95% CI (%)
237	5-FU	51	20	9-30
238	UFT	188	28	22-34
239	S-1	51	49	36-62
240		51	44	30-59
241	Pemetrexed	27	22	6-38
237	Mitomycin	211	30	24-36
242	Doxorubicin	188	23	17-29
243		93	13	6-19
244		34	21	7-35
245	Epirubicin	24	17	2-32
246		39	8	0-16
247	Etoposide	26	19	3-35
248		14	21	0-42
249	Irinotecan	66	23	13-34
237	Cisplatin	115	20	13-27
250	Paclitaxel	30	17	6-35
251		23	5	0-21
252	Docetaxe	33	24	9-39
253		41	17	8-30
254		59	24	14-37

Abbreviations: S-1, tegafur plus 5-chloro-2,4-dihydropyrimidine; UFT, uracil plus tegafur.

■ Chemotherapy

Single Agents ■ Numerous commercially available chemotherapeutic agents have been used in single-agent therapy for gastric cancer. With the exception of S-1, which has a reported response rate of 40-50%, the response rate for agents to be considered active in single-agent therapy for gastric cancer is about 20% (Table 84-7).

Combination Chemotherapy ■ A number of combination chemotherapy programs have been developed based on agents with known single agent activity in gastric cancer. Key randomized trials are summarized in Table 84-8, and selected combination regimens are listed in Table 84-9.

In gastric cancer, promising response rates in phase 2 studies have not always translated into improved overall survival. For example, a North Central Cancer Therapy Group trial comparing 5-FU alone, 5-FU plus doxorubicin, and FAM showed an increasing response rate with the addition of more agents (18%, 27%, and 38%, respectively).[185] However, the median survival duration in all three groups was identical. A similar trial comparing 5-FU alone with 5-FU plus mitomycin also showed no difference in overall survival.[186] Finally, the Japan Clinical Oncology Group Study compared 5-FU alone with 5-FU and cisplatin or with uracil plus tegafur and mitomycin failed to show survival benefits of the combination therapy despite improved response rates in the 5-FU and cisplatin group.[187] Selection of the chemotherapy regimens in clinical practice should be based on the results of phase 3 trials.

To increase the activity of 5-FU-based regimens, investigators combined 5-FU, doxorubicin, and methotrexate (FAMTX).[188] They found that the response rate to FAMTX was 58% and that the complete remission rate was 12%. However, the treatment-related mortality rate was high (3%). The EORTC carried

Table 84-8 **Selected Randomized Trials of Chemotherapy for Advanced Gastric Cancer**

Reference	Treatment Group	No. of Patients	Response Rate (%)	Median Overall Survival (months)	*p* Value (Survival)
185	5-FU	51	18	7.0	NS
	5-FU + doxorubicin	49	27	7.0	
	FAM	51	38	7.0	
186	5-FU	123	16	6.0	NS
	5-FU+	127	19	5.0	
187	5-FU	105	11	7.0	NS
	5-FU + cisplatin	105	34	7.0	
	UFT + mitomycin C	70	9	6.0	
189	FAM	103	9	7.0	.004
	FAMTX	105	45	10.5	
255	5-FU + cisplatin	103	51	9.0	NS
	FAM	98	25	7.0	
	5-FU	94	26	7.0	
191	EAP	30	20	6.0	NS
	FAMTX	30	33	7.0	
192	FAM	52	15	6.0	NS
	PELF	85	43	8.0	
194	ECF	111	46	9.0	.0005
	FAMTX	108	21	6.0	
197	5-FU + cisplatin	81	20	7.0	NS
	ELF	79	9	7.0	
	FAMTX	85	12	7.0	
206	5-FU + cisplatin		25	8.6	.02
	DCF		37	9.2	
210	S-1	150	54	13.0	.04
	S-1 + cisplatin	148	31	11.0	
207	ECF	263	41	9.9	.02
	ECX	250	46	9.9	(EOX vs ECF
	EOF	245	42	9.3	comparison)
	EOX	244	48	11.2	
208	5-FU + cisplatin	108	25	TTP: 3.8	NS
	5-FU + oxaliplatin	112	34	TTP: 5.7	
209	5-FU + cisplatin	156	29	9.3	NS
	Capecitabine + cisplatin	160	41	10.5	

Abbreviations: NS, not significant; UFT, uracil and tegafur.

Table 84-9 **Selected Combination Chemotherapeutic Regimens for Advanced Gastric Cancer**

5-FU, cisplatin (28-day cycle)
5-FU 750 mg/m²/day CIV infusion on days 1-5
Cisplatin 20 mg/m²/day IV on days 1-5
5-FU, cisplatin, docetaxel (21 to 28-day cycle)
5-FU 750 mg/m²/day CIV infusion on days 1-5
Cisplatin 75 mg/m²/day IV on day 1 only
Docetaxel 75 mg/m² IV on day 1 only
ECF (21-day cycle)
Epirubicin 50 mg/m² IV on day 1
Cisplatin 60 mg/m² IV on day 1
5-FU 200 mg/m²/day CIV infusion on days 1-21
EOX (21-day cycle)
Epirubicin 50 mg/m² IV on day 1
Oxaliplatin 130 mg/m² IV on day 1
Capecitabine 625 mg/² twice daily (1250 mg/m² per day) on days 1-21
EOF (21-day cycle)
Epirubicin 50 mg/m² IV on day 1
Oxaliplatin 130 mg/m² IV on day 1
5-FU 200 mg/m²/day CIV infusion on days 1-21
ECX (21-day cycle)
Epirubicin 50 mg/m² IV on day 1
Cisplatin 60 mg/m² IV on day 1
Capecitabine 625 mg/m² twice daily (1250 mg/m² per day) on days 1-21
Irinotecan plus cisplatin (42-day cycle [alternative 21-day cycle])
Irinotecan 50-65 mg/m² IV on days 1, 8, 15, and 22 [days 1 and 8])
Cisplatin 25-30 mg/m² IV on days 1, 8, 15, and 22 [days 1 and 8])
S-1[a] plus cisplatin (Japanese regimen based on SPIRITS trial; 35-day cycle)
S-1 40-60 mg twice daily (80-120 mg/day) on days 1-21
BSA < 1.25 m²: 40 mg
BSA 1.25-1.5 m²: 50 mg
BSA > 1.5 m²: 60 mg
Cisplatin 60 mg/m² IV on day 8
S-1[a] plus cisplatin (Regimen used in the global phase 3 study; 28-day cycle)
S-1 25 mg/m² twice daily (50 mg/m2/day) on days 1-21
Cisplatin 75 mg/m² IV on day 1

Abbreviations: CIV, continuous intravenous; IV, intravenously.
[a]Toxicity of S-1 differ between Asian and Western patients. S-1 at present is not approved by the FDA in the United States.

out a multicenter random-assignment trial comparing FAM and FAMTX.[189] The response rate in the FAMTX group was significantly higher than that in the FAM group (45% vs 9%; $p < .0001$). In addition, the median survival duration was longer in the FAMTX group (10.5 months vs 7.0 months).

To explore the possible synergy between etoposide and cisplatin, a phase 2 trial examining the combination of etoposide, doxorubicin, and cisplatin (EAP) for advanced gastric cancer was performed.[190] In 67 evaluable patients, the response rate was 64% (95% CI 52-76%), and the complete remission rate was 21%; the median survival duration was 8.9 months. However three subsequent phase 2 trials of EAP found excessive treatment-related mortality.

Furthermore, a randomized phase 2 trial compared EAP and FAMTX.[191] The trial was stopped early, however, because of excessive toxic effects and treatment-related deaths (4 of 30 patients [13%]) in the EAP group. The response rate was 33% in the FAMTX group and 20% in the EAP group, with overlapping confidence intervals between the two groups. The median survival rates in the two groups were also similar (6 months in the EAP group, 7 months in the FAMTX group).

Italian investigators compared the combination of cisplatin, epirubicin, leucovorin, and 5-FU (PELF) with FAM.[192] In this random-assignment trial, 85 patients received PELF, and 52 patients received FAM. Patients in the PELF arm had a higher response rate than patients in the FAM arm did (43% vs 15%; $p = .001$). In a follow-up trial, 200 patients were randomly assigned to receive PLEF or FAMTX.[193] The investigators noted an improved response rate for PELF (39% vs 22%; $p = .009$). However, the differences in the 1- and 2-year survival rate were not statistically significant.

Investigators have also compared ECF with FAMTX. In one phase 3 trial, 274 patients received treatment.[194] The response rate in the ECF group was 46% (95% CI 37-55%), whereas that in the FAMTX group was 21% (95% CI 13-28%). Moreover, the median survival duration was longer in the ECF arm (9 months vs 6 months; $p = .0005$).

Etoposide, leucovorin, and 5-FU (ELF) were combined in an effort to develop an active, less toxic chemotherapy regimen. Etoposide and 5-FU are both active against gastric cancer and do not have any cumulative organ toxicity.[195] Myelosuppression was the only major toxic effect, with 16% of the patients experiencing grade 3 leukopenia and 4% having grade 4 leukopenia. The same ELF regimen given every 3 weeks was studied at MD Anderson with granulocyte-macrophage colony-stimulating factor support.[196] Of 29 previously untreated patients, a partial response was observed in 13% of those who were assessable.

To compare these active regimens, the EORTC conducted a three-arm randomized trial of FAMTX, ELF, and 5-FU plus cisplatin. A total of 399 patients were enrolled. In a recent update of this study, the response rate in 245 patients with measurable disease was 12% for FAMTX, 9% for ELF, and 20% for 5-FU plus cisplatin.[197] The median survival duration was 7 months in all three groups.

To investigate the role of newer agents in combination chemotherapy programs, three phase 2 trials examined the combination of irinotecan and cisplatin. In particular, in a phase 1/2 study using a 4-week cycle, the maximum tolerated dose of irinotecan was 80 mg/m^2 on days 1 and 15 when the cisplatin dose was fixed at 80 mg/m^2 on day 1.[198]Similarly, the response rate was 42% (95% CI 22-61%). The recommended phase 2 dose of irinotecan was 70 mg/m^2. In a similar study, 44 Japanese patients received irinotecan at 70 mg/m^2 every 4 weeks on days 1 and 15 and cisplatin at 80 mg/m^2 on day 1.[199] The response rate was 48% (95% CI 33-63%). One complete remission was reported, and the median survival duration was 9 months. At MD Anderson, these two drugs were evaluated on a weekly schedule.[200,201] Cisplatin was given at 30 mg/m^2 per week, and irinotecan was given at 50-65 mg/m^2 per week (50 mg/m^2 per week for previously treated patients and 65 mg/m^2 per week for previously untreated patients) on days 1, 8, 15, and 22 of a 42-day cycle. The response rate was 58% in previously untreated patients and 31% in previously treated patients.

Building on the 5-FU and cisplatin regimen, Korean investigators tested the combination of 5-FU, cisplatin, and paclitaxel in a phase 2 trial.[202] Of the 41 patients who received treatment, 51% (95% CI 37-66%) had an objective response. The median survival duration was 6 months.

Docetaxel-based chemotherapy regimens have also been extensively studied in patients with gastric cancer. Several investigators conducted phase II trials with the combination of docetaxel and cisplatin. They administered 75-85 mg/m^2 docetaxel and 75 mg/m^2 cisplatin on day 1 of a 21-day cycle.[203-205] The response rates ranged from 33% to 56%, and the median survival durations ranged from 9 to 10 months.

A random-assignment phase 3 trial compared the combination of docetaxel, cisplatin, and 5-FU (DCF) with 5-FU plus cisplatin in study that involved 445 patients.[206] Use of DCF resulted in a superior response rate (37% vs 25%; p = .01), time-to-progression (median, 5.6 months vs 3.4 months; p < .01), and overall survival (median 9.2 months vs 8.6 months; p = .02). However, the DCF regimen resulted in substantial treatment-related toxic effects. Specifically, 82% of the patients had grade 3/4 neutropenia, and 69% of the patients had at least one grade 3/4 treatment related adverse event.

Built on earlier success with the ECF regimen, a recent phase 3 study (REAL-2) investigated the role capecitabine and oxaliplatin in GE cancer using a two-by-two design.[207] The study randomly assigned 1002 patients to treatment with either ECF or epirubicin and cisplatin plus capecitabine (ECX) or treatment with either epirubicin and oxaliplatin plus fluorouracil (EOF) or epirubicin and oxaliplatin plus capecitabine (EOX).[207] Approximately 65% of patients had carcinoma of stomach or GE junction, and 88% had adenocarcinoma histology. Response rates and median overall survival were 41% and 9.9 months for ECF, 46% and 9.9 months for ECX, 42% and 9.3 months for EOF, and 48% and 11.2 months for EOX. Investigators concluded noninferiority of capecitabine compared to 5-FU and of oxaliplatin compared to cisplatin.

These findings of noninferiority were confirmed in two phase 3 studies investigating the role of capecitabine or oxaliplatin in gastric cancer. In one study, 220 patients were randomly assigned to treatment with infusional 5-FU and leucovorin plus either cisplatin (FLP) or oxaliplatin (FLO).[208] While the response rates were higher in the FLO arm (34% vs 25%; p < .01), compared to FLP, differences in time to progression were not statistically significant (HR 0.8; 95% CI, 0.58-1.09). A second contemporaneous phase 3 study compared cisplatin plus capecitabine (XP) and cisplatin plus 5-FU (FP).[209] Three-hundred-sixteen patients were randomly assigned to XP or FP. Response rate was higher in the XP group (41% vs 29%; p = .03). There were, however, no significant differences in PFS (HR 0.8; 95% CI 0.63-1.03) or OS (HR 0.85; 95% CI 0.64-1.13).

Recently, Japanese investigators tested the combination of S-1, and cisplatin in a phase 3 study (SPIRITS).[210] In this study 305 patients were randomly assigned to treatment with S-1 or S-1 plus cisplatin. Response rate (54% vs 31%), PFS (median, 6 months vs 4 months; p < .01), and OS (median, 13 months vs 11 months; p = .04) were superior in the combination arm. However, it is known that the toxicity profile of S-1 differs between Asian and Western patients due to differences in PK. In fact, a global phase 3 study, which enrolled over a thousand patients, compared S-1 or 5-FU plus cisplatin,using a lower dose S-1 and different schedule. Unfortunately, the study failed to achieve its primary endpoint of superior overall survival (Taiho press release, July 18, 2008).

Molecularly Targeted Agents

Despite the incorporation of newer agents, the median survival of patients with advanced gastric cancer remains less than 1 year with cytotoxic chemotherapy. Clearly, development of novel therapeutic strategies beyond traditional cytotoxic chemotherapy is needed.

As in solid tumors, angiogenesis has been shown to be an important part of gastric cancer progression. Recently, bevacizumab was studied in a phase 2 trial in advanced gastric cancer, showing promising results in combination with irinotecan and cisplatin.[211] Among 34 patients with measurable disease, investigators observed a response rate of 65%. Overall survival was 12.3 months. However, 6% of patients experienced gastric perforation or near perforation, and 25% of patients experienced grade 3/4 thromboembolic complications.

Strategies targeting EGFR have also gained considerable interest. The Southwest Oncology Group conducted a stratified phase 2 study of erlotinib in GE junction and gastric carcinoma.[212] Investigators reported a 9% response rate among 43 patients with GE junction carcinoma. No responses were observed in the gastric group. Several ongoing studies are investigating the addition of EGFR inhibitors to cytotoxic chemotherapy. In one completed study that enrolled 38 patients with EGFR positive tumors, cetuximab was combined with 5-FU, folinic acid and irinotecan (FOLFIRI).[213] Response rate was 44%. Median time to progression was promising at 8 months.

Results from early studies in gastric cancer incorporating targeted agents are mixed. Larger randomized studies are needed to define the role of these and newer agents in gastric cancer.

Approaches to Systemic Therapy

While the incorporation of novel agents targeting VEGF and EGFR appears promising in these single arm phase 2 studies, random assignment phase 3 studies are needed to define the role of these agents in the management of advanced gastric cancer. In general, three drug combinations can be considered for patients with good performance status (Table 84-9). Doublet or single-agent chemotherapy should be considered for patients with suboptimal performance status who desire systemic therapy. Enrollment of eligible patients on clinical trials should be strongly encouraged.

Symptom Management

The issue of palliation is critical for gastric cancer patients. This section explores the factors involved in deciding how to best provide palliation and which methods are best for achieving those ends. Given the relatively high percentage of patients who present with incurable disease, the issues of quality of life and palliation are particularly germane. Unlike in Japan, where 50% of patients present with early-stage gastric cancer only 10% or less of patients do so in the United States.[136] In fact, 40-50% of patients are found to have distant metastatic disease upon completion of the initial staging.[93,94] Inconsistencies, discrepancies, and misunderstandings regarding the level of symptoms, when palliation is required, and what conditions can be palliated further cloud this issue. Furthermore, some surgeons take a nihilistic approach, classifying all patients with locally advanced tumors in the palliative rather than the potentially curative category despite an R0 resection, making evaluations of survival difficult, at best.

Patients with gastric cancer may present with symptoms including bleeding, obstruction, pain, early satiety, and weight loss. A review by Miner et al.[214] examined 307 patients with gastric cancer who underwent a noncurative resection entered in a single institution's prospective database. Roughly half of the patients had what they termed a truly palliative resection, most commonly for bleeding (20%), obstruction (43%), or pain (29%), and only 2% of the procedures were performed emergently, which could have been a reflection of the tertiary-care nature of the institution. As might be expected, patients in the palliative group had much poorer survival than did those in the nonpalliative group, which contained many patients who had positive margin resections. Age was also a significant risk factor, with older patients having worse survival. Kahlke et al.[215] found similar results in their review of 169 patients with incurable gastric cancer who underwent surgery. They classified symptoms as major (significant bleeding, confirmed obstruction, or perforation) or minor (all others). They also determined whether patients underwent a resection or simply an exploratory procedure. They found that major symptoms portended poorer survival but, interestingly, that the type of surgical procedure had no bearing on survival.

In a large review, the American College of Surgeons surveyed more than 18,000 patients with gastric cancer, demonstrating that most patients do not need immediate surgical palliation.[136] Relatively few patients present with complete obstruction, however, early satiety and dysphagia are fairly common. Similarly, patients with gastric cancer do not usually present with massive bleeding; however, many patients are anemic. These differences at presentation permit a broader range of treatment options and allow the amount of time necessary for a complete staging work-up for most patients. Surgery clearly provides the best chance for long-term survival and should be performed for any patient without distant disease unless extenuating circumstances preclude it. However, surgery is not necessarily the best way to obviate symptoms caused by gastric cancer in patients with metastasis as noted above. When making decisions about surgical palliation, physicians must keep in mind the expected life span of patients with metastatic disease. Among patients with carcinomatosis, the median survival duration is only about 5 months, and 1-year survivors are relatively unusual.[93] Patients with hepatic metastases survive only slightly longer, with a median survival of about 6-8 months. Furthermore, in our experience, patients with distant nodal disease have a median survival of 8-12 months. Patients with ascites may survive for only 2 months or less, as may those with lymphangitic spread to the lungs or leptomeningeal disease, both of which are quite rare and usually quickly fatal. Bone marrow metastases also carry a dismal prognosis. Hence to properly evaluate palliative interventions for gastric cancer, one must understand the disease as well as the morbidity of and time to recovery from the planned treatment. The typical presenting symptoms of gastric cancer and options for alleviating them are described below.

Pain

Pain is clearly the most subjective symptom a patient with gastric cancer may have. Patients' pain ranges from no pain at all to pain requiring massive quantities of narcotics. Pain may be caused by invasion of the celiac plexus, intestinal obstruction, or bone metastases. Obstruction can further confound the problem of pain management. In the absence of obstruction, long-acting oral narcotics can be used easily. However, if obstruction is present, other methods must be employed. Until recently, the need for intravenous pain management often required patients to spend their last days in the hospital receiving intravenous medication. However, the development of transdermal fentanyl patches as well as fentanyl lollipops and sublingual morphine and anxiolytics, as well as the expansion of home health services have allowed patients to remain at home and relatively free from pain at the end of life.

Although celiac axis block has been employed somewhat frequently for pancreatic cancer, it is used far less often for gastric cancer. Nevertheless, this technique should be considered for patients with severe intractable pain. Pain may also be caused by raw gastric mucosa; in such patients, sucralfate slurry frequently improves the pain. Ablative surgery is rarely indicated purely for the management of pain in these patients.

Several studies have examined pain as an aspect of quality of life. These studies have demonstrated an improvement in quality of life with the use of chemotherapy. For example, Glimelius et al.[181] performed a prospective randomized trial of 5-FU and leucovorin (plus etoposide in younger patients or those with a good performance status) versus best supportive care alone (control). They assessed the quality of life in 61 patients by using the EORTC-QLQ-C30 instrument. A statistically significantly greater percentage of patients in the chemotherapy-plus-supportive care arm had an improvement in or prolongation of a high quality of life when compared with the control arm (45% vs 20%; $p < .05$). These results were found with a minimum follow-up duration of 4 months and evaluation by the patients. The physician assessment resulted in a higher perception of improvement in the chemotherapy-plus-supportive care arm (55%; $p < .01$) but mirrored the patient evaluation in the control arm. In addition, the quality-adjusted duration of survival and time to progression were significantly greater in the treatment arm (5 months vs 2 months; $p = .03$), whereas the difference in overall survival was not significant. In an earlier study, the same group found that among patients with the common gastrointestinal cancers (gastric, pancreatic, and colon), those with gastric cancer were the only group to experience a benefit in terms of survival when receiving palliative chemotherapy versus supportive care alone (10 months vs 4 months; $p < .02$).[181] They also found that whereas the average cost of all medical care was about 50% higher in the chemotherapy group, the cost per day was equivalent in the two groups and so supported the use of chemotherapy in these patients.

Bone metastasis is relatively unusual with gastric cancer, occurring in only about 1-2% of patients. However, it does appear to be more common in patients with diffuse-type disease and in younger patients. In our experience, approximately 10% of patients with linitis plastica will experience bone metastasis. Bone pain may be best treated with external-beam radiation as described in a study by Yoshikawa and Kitaoka.[216] They evaluated 23 patients with bone metastases seen over a 10-year period. They found that radiotherapy but not chemotherapy alleviated their pain but that patients survived only a few months after the discovery of bone metastases. Metastases rarely develop in weight-bearing bones; when this does happen, it may require orthopedic intervention. Life expectancy is so short in most of these patients that such intervention is not necessary, but it must be considered carefully.

Bleeding

Given the broad spectrum of severity of bleeding, there are perhaps more treatment options for it than for any other symptom of gastric cancer. Massive bleeding may be treated with arterial embolization or endoscopy; however, resection is often required to control the hemorrhage. Only in cases of widely metastatic disease should one consider avoiding intervention for bleeding. Telling a patient with newly diagnosed gastric cancer and his or her family about this is very difficult, but in some instances, it is the right thing to do. Embolization is a temporizing procedure, and as such, it may be used to buy time to complete work-up or discuss resuscitation status. Endoscopy can also temporarily control bleeding with the use of either a heater probe or an argon coagulator. For patients who are experiencing slow oozing and need a transfusion every 1-2 weeks, endoscopy may be successful. Chemotherapy may be risky for patients who are losing blood at such a rate. However, once it is given, it will often further slow blood loss in patients who were losing blood at a slow rate. But the risk of this is that the patient may have a major bleeding event while his or her blood counts are low. Savides et al.[217] evaluated 42 patients with malignancy and blood loss. In half of these patients, the loss was acute and severe. Patients underwent a combination of cautery and injection of epinephrine. One third of the patients had a recurrence of bleeding, and just over 40% needed an operation. Even with these interventions, the 1-year survival rate was only 11%. In addition, Loftus et al.[218] reported on 15 patients with major upper gastrointestinal bleeding from malignancy that was treated endoscopically. Eleven of these patients had gastric cancer. The patients underwent epinephrine injections and heater probe or laser coagulation. The bleeding initially stopped in 10 patients. However, 8 of the 10 had a recurrence of bleeding, and one third of the patients had major complications. Two patients died of treatment-related causes.

We have found chemoradiation to be very effective in controlling blood loss in patients who are slowly losing blood. Roughly 80% of patients will no longer need transfusions after undergoing chemoradiation. We have preferred to use a radiosensitizing dose of 5-FU at 300 mg/m^2 per day administered by continuous infusion while using external-beam radiation to a dose of 45 Gy over 5 weeks. Several series have indicated that 50-75% of patients experience improvement of bleeding, gastric outlet obstruction, and pain with this method.[219,220]

As described above, physicians must decide whether patients who are bleeding massively are surgical candidates and then either take them to the operating room or simply make comfortable and allow them to die. Endoscopic and embolization maneuvers can occasionally allow for the necessary time to have these often difficult discussions.

Obstruction/Dysphagia/Early Satiety

The occurrence of proximal gastrointestinal tract obstruction in patients with gastric cancer is highly dependent on the location of the primary tumor. However, given the high incidence of peritoneal metastases in these patients, small bowel and colonic obstructions occur relatively frequently with advanced disease. Aranha et al.[221] reviewed 73 patients with small bowel obstruction secondary to metastatic carcinoma, some of whom some had gastric cancer. They found relatively high operative morbidity and mortality rates in these patients. The mortality rate dropped over time, but even in the most recent period, it exceeded 10%. In general, patients with small bowel obstruction secondary to metastatic gastric cancer have survival durations that range from a few weeks to months.

Dysphagia is typically graded on a scale of 0-4, with 0 being no dysphagia, 1 being dysphagia to solid foods, 2 being dysphagia to soft foods, 3 being dysphagia to liquids, and 4 being complete obstruction. Tumors in the body of the stomach are rarely obstructive unless they are of the linitis plastica variety, in which case it is more of a functional obstruction as opposed to a mechanical one. Cardial tumors may be obstructive in a manner very similar to esophageal tumors, whereas prepyloric tumors may be obstructive in a manner more like pancreatic cancer. Many of the evaluations of treatment options for obstruction by proximal tumors mix patients with these tumors with patients with esophageal tumors. In many instances, the differences are irrelevant. The treatment options for obstruction include laser recanalization, stenting, radiotherapy, bypass, drainage tubes, and resection. Studies have evaluated interventions ranging from supportive care only to aggressive resection. In the face of metastatic disease, however, resection should be applied very cautiously. In the absence of large prospective randomized trials, when evaluating all of the studies that discuss resection for palliation, caution should be exercised considering the inherent bias of not attempting resection in patients with very advanced disease and then attempting to compare patients who have undergone resection with these patients. If a patient's disease is so advanced that the physician will not consider resection, it should not be surprising if the patient fares poorly as seen in the report by Miner et al.[214]

The technology of expandable stents, such as the Wall stent, has grown dramatically over the past few years. In a systematic review, Dormann et al.[222] reviewed 136 publications reporting the use of self-expanding metal stents for gastroduodenal malignancies in 32 case series. They found that in 606 patients, stent placement was successful in 97% of the patients, and that the placement was technically successful in 87% of them. They found no procedure-related mortality and a relatively low number of complications. However, in 18% of the cases, the stent became occluded secondary to tumor ingrowth. Further, Fiori et al.[223] conducted a small (18 patients) prospective randomized trial comparing bypass and stenting. They found no difference in morbidity, mortality, emptying, or clinical outcome with these two procedures, suggesting that stenting is an effective alternative to bypass in patients with gastric cancer.

Endoscopic ablative techniques have also been used to relieve dysphagia. The rate of improvement with these techniques is most often rapid, usually requiring only one treatment, and complication rates are relatively low. Success rates are typically high (about 90%), but durability is a potential concern. Carter et al.[224] treated malignant dysphagia in 141 patients with an Nd:YAG laser system and found that 92% of the patients had an improvement in swallowing, with 6% suffering a perforation and 3% having a fistula. Mason et al.[225] reported a similar rate of initial improvement of symptoms in 189 patients. However, after 6 months, almost 90% of the patients had died. Most of these patients appeared to have had an improvement in their measured quality of life early after treatment. However, as patients near death, their quality of life deteriorates rapidly.[226] In yet another study, Heindorff et al.[227] used argon-beam electrocoagulation in 83 patients. More than half of the patients were able to eat normal food after one treatment, whereas 16% of the patients were never able to eat normal food again. They repeated the treatment every 4 weeks as needed. The investigators found seven perforations and were able to manage all but one of them conservatively.

Sargeant et al.[228] conducted a prospective randomized trial of the addition of external-beam radiation to laser ablation for the palliation of dysphagia. They randomized 67 patients to receive 30 Gy in 10 fractions or no radiation and then observed them. While there was no difference in the immediate improvement of symptoms, the radiotherapy decreased the need for subsequent ablations, doubling the time between treatments. This did not come without a price, however, as several of the irradiated patients needed dilatation, which resulted in fistulae and perforations in a few cases. Spencer et al.[229] had a similar intent with the use of brachytherapy in 19 patients. They administered 10 Gy after laser ablation and then observed the patients. One third of the patients needed no further therapy, and those who did need further ablation did not need a repeat of the procedure for a median of 11 weeks; the median survival duration was about 8 months. In addition, Highley et al.[230] prospectively evaluated the use of post-treatment systemic chemotherapy (cisplatin, epirubicin, and 5-FU) in 34 patients with malignant dysphagia treated with laser ablation. Almost 60% of the patients had a response to the chemotherapy with a significant improvement in dysphagia and decrease in the need for additional laser ablation.

Lo et al.[231] examined the use of gastrojejunostomy in 51 patients with gastric cancer and reported an operative mortality rate of 22% and an operative morbidity rate of 55%. The median survival duration was only 14 weeks (two of which were spent recuperating in the hospital), and more than 20% of the patients suffered delayed gastric emptying. In this manner, nearly 50% of the patients (those with delayed gastric emptying plus operative mortality) did not benefit from the procedure. Nevertheless, the authors concluded that gastrojejunostomy was a satisfactory palliative intervention. Kikuchi et al.[105] also examined the use of gastrojejunostomy in 52 patients with antral obstruction, finding a median survival duration of only 5 months and a median palliation duration of less than 3 months. They concluded that justification of this approach is difficult for patients with antral obstruction.

One of the most difficult problems in evaluating the role of resection in palliation is determining the true intent of the operation. Although many surgeons may consider a procedure to be palliative based on their pessimism as noted in the report by Miner et al.,[214] the reality may be far different. One telling example of this concern is the report by Ekbom and Gleysteen,[232] who reviewed 144 patients with gastric cancer, 55 of whom appeared to have undergone palliative resection, and 20 of whom underwent bypass procedures (the remainder underwent potentially curative resections). Both the survival and symptom relief duration were markedly better in the resection group than in the bypass group. However, determining whether these are truly comparable groups is difficult. The finding of long survival duration in patients ostensibly receiving palliative treatment often raises questions as to the intent of the operation as documentation is often poor. In comparison, Ouchi et al.[233] evaluated 95 patients who had undergone 64 resections, 15 bypasses, and 16 explorations alone—in the palliative setting. Ninety-three of the patients had stage IV disease. In many of these patients, the stage was based on the presence of disease in sites other than the peritoneum, as the disease was staged as P = 0 or 1 (no visible peritoneal disease or only peritoneal disease adjacent to the stomach) in 62 patients and P = 2 or 3 (few scattered metastases to the distant peritoneum or numerous metastases throughout the peritoneum) in 33 patients. Overall, the 3-month hospitalization-free survival rate was 70%. In patients with P2 or P3 disease, the median survival was 7 months, which, not surprisingly was less than that in the group with little or no peritoneal disease. Patients who underwent a total gastrectomy with P2 or P3 disease had a median survival of less than 6 months, whereas those who underwent a distal resection had a median survival of about 8 months; there were no 2-year survivors in the total gastrectomy group. The authors concluded that there was no benefit of either total gastrectomy or bypass in patients with any peritoneal disease away from the stomach.

One of the more aggressive approaches for proximal gastric tumors was reported by Saidi et al.[117] In 70 patients, 49 of whom had stage IV disease, they performed a total gastrectomy with mucosectomy of the esophagus and colonic interposition through the deepithelialized esophagus. The operative mortality rate was 10%, and 58 patients had a median survival duration of 17 months. The authors suggested that this provided distinct palliation, although this is debatable. As described above with the median survival duration of 17 months, one cannot be sure of the likely potential curative aspect in many such patients.

For patients at an advanced age, some authors have suggested that the benefits of potentially curative resection diminish to the point that all such maneuvers are to be considered palliative. Specifically, Ishigami et al.[234] found that one out of every four patients with gastric cancer over the age of 85 years was an unfit candidate for surgery and that those who did undergo surgery had significantly more complications. We take a very selective approach to such patients and consider resection based on a patient's physiologic condition. Matsushita et al.[235] concluded in a study of 24 patients over the age of 80 years that age alone should not be a reason to avoid the use of potentially curative procedures.

Dysphagia/obstruction is one of the biggest problem in patients with gastric cancer and has the widest array of management options. Unfortunately, each option has its benefits and risks such that in the absence of an institutional protocol, one must strongly consider patient comfort and compliance concerns as well as the expertise within his or her institution before determining the best treatment approach.

Nutrition

Roughly half of all patients with gastric cancer have experienced weight loss by the time of presentation. For many patients, maintaining a proper diet is simply a matter of changing to more nutritious foods. Others may need to change to a completely liquid diet with nutritional supplements. The remaining patients are not able to maintain adequate caloric intact regardless of dietary manipulations. As part of our complete staging of gastric cancer, we routinely perform laparoscopy. In this setting, using a T-fastener kit, we place a feeding jejunostomy tube (except in the face of ascites) either for nutritional support during planned therapy (preoperative or definitive) or for supportive care. Patients who so desire can have the tube removed after several weeks if they have chosen to simply let their disease take its course, although few actually do so. There are numerous supplements available, so patients may have to experiment to find which ones they tolerate best. We structure feedings so that they take place at night to help facilitate as normal a lifestyle as possible. The use of total parenteral nutrition for patients with metastatic gastric cancer is very difficult to justify with the rare exception of a patient who would otherwise be a candidate for aggressive systemic therapy.

One must understand their patients well and communicate the pros and cons of the various options for palliative care to them in a coherent fashion. There is no best approach to palliation with gastric cancer. However, understanding what can and should be palliated will help physicians go a long way toward determining the best method of palliation. We generally encourage consideration of protocol-based chemotherapeutic options for patients with metastatic disease who are able to tolerate it. For patients with slow blood loss, we generally use chemoradiation to effectively control the bleeding. Patients with metastatic disease remain the most difficult group of patients with gastric cancer to care for.

Conclusions

Fortunately, the incidence of gastric cancer is decreasing around the world. However, with this decrease, the patterns regarding more aggressive variants of the disease are changing. Despite some progress in all areas of the management of gastric cancer (surgery, chemotherapy, and radiotherapy), most patients in the United States diagnosed with gastric cancer will die of it. The ability to define who will have this disease will allow us to develop screening and preventive measures.

As we enter the age of molecular targeted therapy, agents targeting the VEGF and EGFR systems are entering phase 2 trials in gastric cancer. Improvements in our understanding of molecular biology and molecular classification of gastric cancer may lead to the rational development of novel therapeutic strategies for gastric cancer.

Selected References

The complete reference list can be found at www.CANCERMEDICINE8.com

2. Ries LAG, Melbert D, Krapcho M, et al. SEER Cancer Statistics Review, 1975-2005. Bethesda, MD: National Cancer Institute; 2008.
12. Correa P, Cuello C, Duque E, et al. Gastric cancer in Colombia. III. Natural history of precursor lesions. J Natl Cancer Inst. 1976;57:1027–1035.
17. Webb PM, Bates CJ, Palli D, et al. Gastric cancer, gastritis and plasma vitamin C: results from an international correlation and cross-sectional study. The Eurogast Study Group. Int J Cancer. 1997;73:684–689.
26. Chow WH, Blot WJ, Vaughan TL, et al. Body mass index and risk of adenocarcinomas of the esophagus and gastric cardia. J Natl Cancer Inst. 1998;90:150–155.
35. Lagergren J, Bergstrom R, Nyren O. Association between body mass and adenocarcinoma of the esophagus and gastric cardia. Ann Intern Med. 1999;130: 883–890.
49. Guilford P, Hopkins J, Harraway J, et al. E-cadherin germline mutations in familial gastric cancer. Nature. 1998;392: 402–405.
55. Endoh Y, Tamura G, Ajioka Y, et al. Frequent hypermethylation of the hMLH1 gene promoter in differentiated-type tumors of the stomach with the gastric foveolar phenotype. Am J Pathol. 2000;157:717–22.
61. Li QL, Ito K, Sakakura C, et al. Causal relationship between the loss of RUNX3 expression and gastric cancer. Cell. 2002;109:113–124.
65. Myeroff LL, Parsons R, Kim SJ, et al. A transforming growth factor beta receptor type II gene mutation common in colon and gastric but rare in endometrial cancers with microsatellite instability. Cancer Res. 1995;55:5545–5547.
68. Brito MJ, Williams GT, Thompson H, et al. Expression of p53 in early (T1) gastric carcinoma and precancerous adjacent mucosa. Gut. 1994;35:1697–1700.
87. Yao JC, Wang L, Wei D, et al. Association between expression of transcription factor Sp1 and increased vascular endothelial growth factor expression, advanced stage, and poor survival in patients with resected gastric cancer. Clin Cancer Res. 2004;10:4109–4117.
93. Lowy AM, Mansfield PF, Leach SD, et al. Laparoscopic staging for gastric cancer. Surgery. 1996;119:611–614.
94. Burke EC, Karpeh MS, Conlon KC, et al. Laparoscopy in the management of gastric adenocarcinoma. Ann Surg. 1997;225:262–267.
98. Gotoda T. Endoscopic resection of early gastric cancer. Gastric Cancer. 2007;10:1–11.
101. Miura S, Kodera Y, Fujiwara M, et al. Laparoscopy-assisted distal gastrectomy with systemic lymph node dissection: a critical reappraisal from the viewpoint of lymph node retrieval. J Am Coll Surg. 2004;198:933–938.
103. Ajani JA, Ota DM, Jessup JM, et al. Resectable gastric carcinoma. An evaluation of preoperative and postoperative chemotherapy. Cancer. 1991;68:1501–1506.
107. Bozzetti F, Marubini E, Bonfanti G, et al. Subtotal versus total gastrectomy for gastric cancer. Five year survival rates in a multicenter randomized Italian trial. Ann Surg. 1999;230:170–178.
113. Harrison LE, Karpeh MS, Brennan MF. Total gastrectomy is not necessary for proximal gastric cancer. Surgery. 1998;123:127–130.
114. Shiraishi N, Adachi Y, Kitano S, et al. Clinical outcome of proximal versus total gastrectomy for proximal gastric cancer. World J Surg. 2002;26:1150–1154.
118. Omloo JM, Lagarde SM, Hulscher JB, et al. Extended transthoracic resection compared with limited transhiatal resection for adenocarcinoma of the mid/distal esophagus: five-year survival of a randomized clinical trial. Ann Surg. 2007;246:992–1000.
119. Sasako M, Sano T, Yamamoto S, et al. Left thoracoabdominal approach versus abdominal-transhiatal approach for gastric cancer of the cardia or subcardia: a randomised controlled trial. Lancet Oncol. 2006;7:644–651.
121. Sasako M, McCulloch P, Kinoshita T, et al. New method to evaluate the therapeutic value of lymph node dissection for gastric cancer. Br J Surg. 1995;82:346–351.
128. Dent DM, Madden MV, Price SK. Randomized comparison of R1 and R2 gastrectomy for gastric carcinoma. Br J Surg. 1988;75:110–112.
130. Hartgrink HH, van de Velde CJ, Putter H, et al. Extended lymph node dissection for gastric cancer: who may benefit? Final results of the randomized Dutch gastric cancer group trial. J Clin Oncol. 2004;22:2069–2077.
131. Cuschieri A, Weeden S, Fielding J, et al. Patient survival after D1 and D2 resections for gastric cancer: long-term results of the MRC randomized surgical trial. Br J Cancer. 1999;1522–1530
133. Sasako M, Sano T, Yamamoto S, et al. D2 lymphadenectomy alone or with para-aortic nodal dissection for gastric cancer. N Engl J Med. 2008;359:453–462.
138. Macdonald JS, Smalley SR, Benedetti J, et al. Chemoradiotherapy after surgery compared with surgery alone for adenocarcinoma of the stomach or gastroesophageal junction. N Engl J Med. 2001;345:725–730.
142. Martin RC, Jaques DP, Brennan MF, et al. Extended local resection for advanced gastric cancer: increased survival versus increased morbidity. Ann Surg. 2002;236:159–165.
149. Mochiki E, Kamimura H, Haga N, et al. The technique of laparoscopically assisted total gastrectomy with jejunal interposition for early gastric cancer. Surg Endosc. 2002;16:540–544.
151. Svedlund J, Sullivan M, Liedman B, et al. Quality of life after gastrectomy for gastric carcinoma: controlled study of reconstructive procedures. World J Surg. 1997;21:422–433.
156. Sakuramoto S, Sasako M, Yamaguchi T, et al. Adjuvant chemotherapy for gastric cancer with S-1, an oral fluoropyrimidine. N Engl J Med. 2007;357:1810–1820.
157. The Italian Gastrointestinal Tumor Study Group. Adjuvant treatments following curative resection for gastric cancer. Br J Surg. 1988;75:1100–1104.
162. The Gastrointestinal Tumor Study Group. The concept of locally advanced gastric cancer. Effect of treatment on outcome. Cancer. 1990;66:2324–2330.
164. Allum WH, Hallissey MT, Ward LC, et al. A controlled, prospective, randomised trial of adjuvant chemotherapy or radiotherapy in resectable gastric cancer: interim report. British Stomach Cancer Group. Br J Cancer. 1989;60:739–744.
169. Sindelar WF, Kinsella TJ, Tepper JE, et al. Randomized trial of intraoperative radiotherapy in carcinoma of the stomach. Am J Surg. 1993;165:178–186; discussion 186–187.
173. Lowy AM, Mansfield PF, Leach SD, et al. Response to neoadjuvant chemotherapy best predicts survival after curative resection of gastric cancer. Ann Surg. 1999;229:303–308.
174. Cunningham D, Allum WH, Stenning SP, et al. Perioperative chemotherapy versus surgery alone for resectable gastroesophageal cancer. N Engl J Med. 2006;355:11–20.
178. Lowy AM, Feig BW, Janjan N, et al. A pilot study of preoperative chemoradiotherapy for resectable gastric cancer. Ann Surg Oncol. 2001;8:519–524.
187. Ohtsu A, Shimada Y, Shirao K, et al. Randomized phase III trial of fluorouracil alone versus fluorouracil plus cisplatin versus uracil and tegafur plus mitomycin in patients with unresectable, advanced gastric cancer: The Japan Clinical Oncology Group Study (JCOG9205). Am J Clin Oncol. 2003;21:54–59.
194. Waters JS, Norman A, Cunningham D, et al. Long-term survival after epirubicin, cisplatin and fluorouracil for gastric cancer: results of a randomized trial. Br J Cancer. 1999;80:269–272.
206. Van Cutsem E, Moiseyenko VM, Tjulandin S, et al. Phase III study of docetaxel and cisplatin plus fluorouracil compared with cisplatin and fluorouracil as first-line therapy for advanced gastric cancer: a report of the V325 Study Group. J Clin Oncol. 2006;24:4991–4997.
207. Cunningham D, Starling N, Rao S, et al. Capecitabine and oxaliplatin for advanced esophagogastric cancer. N Engl J Med. 2008;358:36–46.
208. Al-Batran S, Hartmann J, Probst S, et al. A randomized phase III trial in patients with advanced adenocarcinoma of the stomach receiving first-line chemotherapy with fluorouracil, leucovorin and oxaliplatin (FLO) versus fluorouracil, leucovorin and cisplatin (FLP). J Clin Oncol. 2006;24:182S.

85 Treatment of Liver Metastases

Nancy E. Kemeny, MD ■ Michael D'Angelica, MD

The liver is a frequent site for metastases from other sites. For cancers that occur in the gastrointestinal (GI) tract, the course of metastatic disease to the liver is easily explained, since the venous drainage of most GI organs takes place via the portal vein, which passes through the liver. It is not surprising, therefore, that for tumors such as colorectal cancer, the liver is the most common and, frequently, the only site of metastatic disease. Extraabdominal tumors, such as bronchogenic carcinoma, breast cancer, and malignant melanoma, often spread hematogenously to the liver. In an autopsy series of 10,736 extrahepatic primary tumors, liver metastases with or without metastases to other organs were present in 41% (Table 85-1).[1] Therefore, it is clear that metastatic disease to the liver represents a significant oncologic problem.

Although it is recognized that liver metastases play a major role in the morbidity and mortality associated with many cancers, until recently, the approach to hepatic metastasis has been nihilistic. However, in the last few decades, therapies have been developed for hepatic metastases that offer not only effective palliation, but also cure in selected cases. Improved imaging modalities such as ultrasonography, computed tomography (CT), magnetic resonance imaging (MRI), and positron emission tomography (PET) have allowed early detection of metastases that allows for effective therapy. Improvements in surgical and anesthetic techniques now permit hepatic resection with a perioperative mortality of <4%, making potentially curative resections acceptable from the standpoint of risk. In addition, development of other techniques, such as regional chemotherapy and ablation, offer effective palliative options when curative resections are impossible. In this chapter, we discuss the different modalities used to eradicate hepatic metastases, and we summarize the clinical data supporting the various treatment modalities for liver metastases.

Table 85-1 ■ **Common Primary Site for Cancer Metastatic to the Liver**

	Metastatic Site		Metastatic Cases with Liver Involvement %
	Liver Only	Liver ± Other	
Lung	602	593	50
Breast	328	643	66
Colon/rectum	145	383	73
Stomach	123	158	56
Pancreas	32	148	79
Uterus	264	200	43
Ovary	154	177	53
Skin	118	160	58

Imaging Techniques

Imaging modalities have become indispensable in the treatment of the patient with liver metastases. Early, accurate detection of liver metastases permits discovery of tumors at a curable stage, assists in choosing among the alternative therapies, facilitates preoperative planning, and enhances response monitoring in cases when a nonsurgical approach is most reasonable. Modalities that are currently useful are listed below.

Computed Tomography

Computed tomography is one of the most useful tests for detecting liver metastases. A narrow window setting and a lower width (100–150 HU) are the most useful, since these settings increase contrasts between the normal liver parenchyma and abnormal areas. Noncontrast CT is helpful in identifying hypervascular metastases (especially carcinoid, islet cell tumors, and renal cell carcinomas) and in visualizing calcifications or hemorrhage. Dynamic CT (where there is a rapid intravenous infusion of contrast) is better for detecting tumors that are hypovascular, such as colorectal carcinomas. One problem with this modality is that lesions may not be distinguishable from liver parenchyma during the equilibrium phase of the contrast injection (when the intravascular and interstitial concentrations equilibrate).[2] However, high quality, thin cuts with precise timing of contrast can characterize liver tumors at multiple phases of contrast flow through the liver. Such scans, referred to as triphasic CT, can identify and characterize the majority of liver tumors, and are used to create angiograms of the hepatic vasculature. Triphasic CT provides extraordinary anatomic detail of the liver in multiple dimensions. CT portography (contrast given via a superior mesenteric vein injection) delivers contrast to the normal parenchyma via the portal vein. Since colorectal metastases are largely nourished by the hepatic artery and derive little blood supply from the portal vein, they appear as filling defects surrounded by liver parenchyma, which is contrast-enhanced because most parenchymal blood supply comes from the portal vein.[2]

Magnetic Resonance Imaging

T1-weighted spin echo images generally show metastases as low-intensity lesions, whereas T2-weighted images of metastases are areas of high signal intensity (Fig. 85-1). At all field strengths, T2-weighted sequences are generally superior for the detection and characterization of liver masses. Benign cysts and hemangiomas are generally homogeneous and have a bright appearance (termed a "light bulb" sign), whereas metastatic lesions are more heterogeneous and not as bright. On MRI, hemangiomas can be confused with highly vascular tumors and with cysts; however, if dynamic gadolinium injections are given, hemangiomas can be more accurately diagnosed, since they will demonstrate peripheral nodular enhancement. MRI is also useful to distinguish fatty infiltration from metastases (Fig. 85-1).[3] Demonstration of extrahepatic pathology by MRI is inferior to CT. The value of MRI is to characterize hepatic masses of unclear etiology such as cysts, hemangiomas, and other benign masses from metastases in a patient with multiple lesions.

Ultrasonography

Transcutaneous and Intraoperative ■ Transcutaneous ultrasonic evaluation of the liver for metastases represents the least invasive and least expensive of the diagnostic modalities. Its usefulness depends primarily on the expertise and diligence of the operator. In addition, since overlying air may obscure ultrasonic imaging of

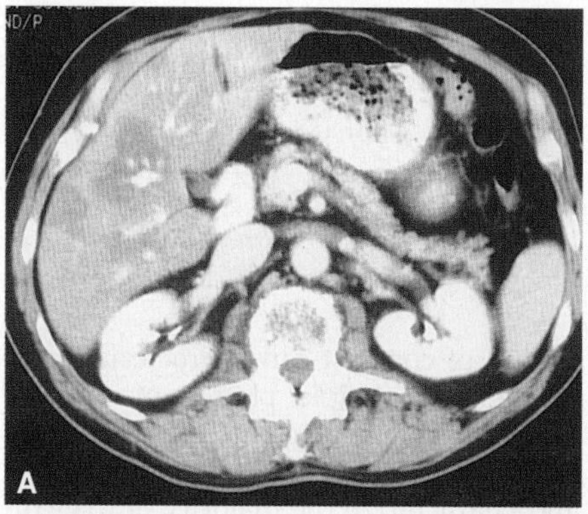

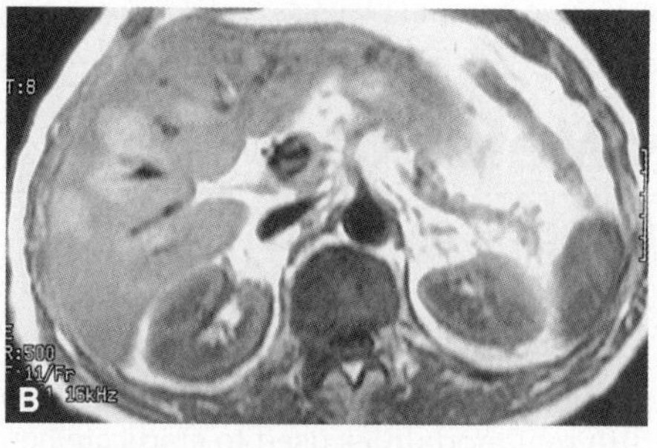

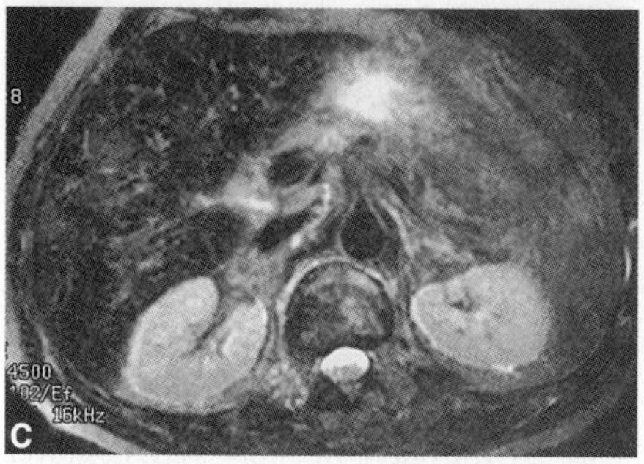

Figure 85-1 ■ **(A)** A CT scan of abdomen showing lesions that were read as metastatic disease. On closer inspection, vessels are seen coursing through the lesions, suggesting fatty infiltrations. **(B)** A T1-weighted spin echo MRI (TR 500, TE111) in which the brightness of the lesions is hyperintense relative to liver, which is a clue that they are fatty infiltrated. **(C)** A T2-weighted fast-spin echo (TR 4500, TE 102) with fat saturation. Areas that were bright are now suppressed, indicating fatty liver with vessels coursing through it.

the liver, overlying bowel and lung tissue may obscure imaging of lesions, particularly at the dome of the liver. Nevertheless, in expert hands, this modality may be as accurate as CT or MRI in determining the number and size of lesions, as well as their relationship to major vessels.[3]

Intraoperative ultrasound (IOUS) is equally operator-dependent, but has become indispensable in the surgical treatment of liver tumors. This modality is now used to detect small and deep hepatic lesions that are not palpable. In studies of patients with colorectal cancer who underwent colon resection, lesions missed on surgical palpation were detected by IOUS (14 in 1 study and 7 in the other).[3] With improved preoperative imaging, the yield of IOUS has decreased and rarely finds patients to be unresectable.[4,5] Contrast-enhanced ultrasound has been developed, can be used intraoperatively, and is currently being evaluated.

Positron Emission Tomography (PET)

It has long been noted that colon cancer cells use glucose at a higher rate than normal tissues. PET exploits this characteristic of tumor cells in order to image tumor sites. When a positron emitting glucose analogue 2-[18F]-fluoro-2-deoxyglucose (18F-FDG) is administered to patients with colorectal cancer, the radiolabeled glucose analogue is transported into tumor cells by the same cell-surface hexose transporters that transport glucose and it undergoes phosphorylation to FDG-6--phosphate. 18F-FDG6-phosphate is not subject to further metabolism in most tumor cells, and therefore is selectively retained.[6,7] Imaging by positron detectors allows whole-body staging for cancer.

Four early studies sought to determine the utility of this modality in the preoperative assessment of patients with liver metastases.[8–11] These preliminary studies suggested that 18F-FDG-PET may detect additional occult disease in up to one-third of patients with metastatic colorectal cancer. Three definitive studies have since further defined the role of FDG-PET in this patient population. In a study examining long-term outcome of patients with hepatic colorectal metastases who were assessed by FDG-PET prior to liver resection, higher resectability, lower recurrence rates, and improved long-term survival were associated with use of FDG-PET.[12] This study suggests that improved patient selection using this imaging modality may enhance ultimate patient outcomes. As would be expected, the yield of the FDG-PET is related to the risk of occult disease. A recent study has suggested that a clinical risk score that has been developed for stratification of risk of recurrence can be used to predict yield of FDG-PET scanning.[13] Finally, a study has also shown that although FDG-PET is quite useful in detecting extrahepatic metastases, its utility in detection of small intrahepatic metastases is questionable. This study correlated pathologically assessed liver tumors to preoperative PET scanning, and found that subcentimeter tumors in the liver are only detected 20% of the time.[14] In patients undergoing preoperative chemotherapeutic treatments, the record is even worse: Only 5% of subcentimeter lesions were detected. From these recent data, a few conclusions about FDG-PET can be drawn. It is a useful test in the preoperative staging of patients with metastatic colorectal cancer. Patients with synchronous liver metastases or with high clinical risk scores[15] are particularly good candidates for scanning. However, FDG-PET should not be used as the sole test in the follow-up of patients after hepatic resection when liver is the site of recurrence.

Liver Resection

Liver metastases are common with colorectal cancer, and most liver resections are performed for cancers that originate in the colon or rectum. Resection is pursued because the liver is often the only site of metastases, alternative treatments are rarely curative, and surgical excision can be performed safely and is potentially curative. Of the 150,000 patients presenting each year in the United States with colorectal cancer, over 50,000 will be found to have hepatic metastases during the course of their disease.[16–18] If untreated, patients with hepatic colorectal metastases can expect a median survival of 5 to 10 months, with <0.5% surviving 5 years.[16,19–24] Systemic chemotherapy, although now associated with median survivals approaching 2 years, rarely results in 5-year survival.[25–32]

On the basis of the hypothesis that metastatic disease may be limited to the liver, and encouraged by autopsy findings that one-third of patients dying of colorectal cancer have the liver as the only site of metastatic disease, surgeons have resected hepatic metastases in an attempt to cure disease that is clinically confined to the liver. A number of retrospective studies on resection of metastatic colorectal cancer to the liver provide evidence that major liver resection can be performed safely and provide prolonged disease-free survival and cure (Table 85-2). Some retrospective studies have documented that patients with resectable metastases who do not undergo resection rarely survive >5 years, whereas those who are resected have a potential for 5-year and even 10-year survival.[33] The reported complication rate in most studies was approximately 20% (Table 85-3). Most complications are pulmonary, with symptomatic pleural effusions occurring in 5–10% of patients,[34,35] pneumonia in 5–22%,[36,37] and pulmonary embolism in 1%.[38,39] Hepatic insufficiency occurs in 3–8% of all major resections,[36–38,40] bile leak and biliary fistula in approximately 4% of all patients,[36–38] and perihepatic abscess in 2–10%.[34,36,38,39] Significant hemorrhage is rare (1–3%), but can be a major cause of

Table 85-2 Results of Hepatic Resection for Metastatic Colorectal Cancer

	Operative Mortality		Survival (%)			
Study	***n***	**%**	**1 Yr**	**3 Yr**	**5 Yr**	**10 Yr**
Foster[42]	78	5	–	–	22	–
Thompson[42]	22	11	80	37	31	–
Adson[41]	141	2	82	40	25	–
Fortner[39]	75	7	89	57	35	–
Butler[44]	62	10	–	50	34	21
Iwatsuki[54]	60	0	95	53	45	–
Hughes[45]	607	–	–	–	33	–
Nordlinger[34]	80	5	5	41	25	16
Cobourn[46]	56	0	–	–	25	–
Schlag[36]	122	4	85	40	30	–
Doci[37]	100	5	–	–	30	–
Younes[47]	133	–	91	–	–	–
Scheele[58]	219	6	–	–	39	21
Rosen[48]	280	4	84	47	25	–
Gayowski[68]	204	0	91	45	34	–
Scheele[58]	469	4	–	45	38	23
Fong[59]	577	3	88	59	38	–
Nordlinger[60]	1568	2	88	44	28	–
Rees[61]	150	1	94	–	37	–
Jamison[62]	280	4	84	46	27	20
Fong[15]	1001	3	89	57	37	22
Choti[49]	226	1	93	57	40	26
Fernandez[51]	100	1	86	66	58	–
Pawlik[50]	557	–	97	74	58	–
Wei[52]	423	1.6	93	–	47	28

Table 85-3 Complications of Liver Resection (%)

	Scheele[33]	**Schlag[36]**	**Doci[37]**	**Fortner[39]**	**Nordlinger[34]**
Total number	219	122	100	75	80
Liver-related complications					
Hemorrhage	7(3)	–	3	1(1)	1(1)
Bile fistula	8(4)	5(4)	4	–	–
Perihepatic abscess	4(2)	11(9)	5	5(7)	2(3)
Liver failure	17(8)	–	3	3(4)	1(1)
Renal failure	3(1)	–	1	–	–
Portal vein thrombosis	–	–	–	1(1)	–
Infections					
Wound	–	7(6)	–	1(1)	–
Sepsis	–	3(2)	2	–	4(5)
General complications					
Gastrointestinal bleeding	–	M	–	–	1(1)
Deep vein thrombosis	2(1)	M	–	1(1)	–
Pulmonary embolism	4(2)	M	–	1(1)	1(1)
Cardiac/MI	2(1)	6(5)	1	1(1)	1(1)
Pneumonia	0(0)	10(8)	22	3(4)	–
Pleural effusion	–	M	–	6(8)	3(4)

Abbreviation: MI, myocarcinoid infarction.

perioperative mortality. However, the high incidence of complications does not always translate into mortality or prolonged hospital stays. Even for resections of up to 80% of the liver, the mortality associated with elective liver resection for colorectal metastases is <5% and 1% in the most recent series (Table 85-2).[34,36–39,41–52] The reported median hospital stay in centers experienced with liver surgery was typically 1 to 2 weeks, but many centers have decreased hospital stay to <1 week. In a recent series of 1001 consecutive resections from Memorial Sloan-Kettering Cancer Center (MSKCC), including 237 trisegmentectomies, the mortality rate was 3%, the median hospital stay was 9 days, and intensive care unit (ICU) admission was required for only 4% of patients.[40] In a more recent publication from MSKCC on patients undergoing resection of bilobar metastases (over 80% lobar resection or more), the 90-day mortality has dropped from 6% in 1994 to 1% in 2003.[53]

Long-term results after resection of hepatic colorectal metastases clearly indicate the potentially curative nature of such treatment, and justify the risks and costs involved. Representative studies on long-term outcome after liver resection for metastatic colorectal cancer are summarized in Table 85-2.[15,37,45,47,49–52,54–62] The 3-year survival is above 40%, and the 5-year survival is between 25% and 58%. There has been a clear improvement in survival, with many modern series now demonstrating 5-year survivals >50% and median survivals over 4 years. In series with longer follow-up, the 10-year survival is reported to be 20%.[34,38,44] While most reported survival statistics are predicted without complete long-term follow-up, a recent study demonstrated that with 10-year actual follow-up, at least 17% of patients are truly cured of disease with a liver resection.[63] The results of surgery are therefore far superior to supportive care or chemotherapy, in that the modality is associated with long-term survival and is potentially curative. Surgical resection must therefore be regarded as the standard of care for resectable colorectal metastases.

Many of the published studies attempted to identify prognostic factors for poor outcome in order to refine patient selection criteria. Although differences exist between studies, the most consistent predictors of poor outcome have been stage of the primary (node-positive), shorter disease-free interval from the time of the primary presentation, size of the largest metastasis, carcinoembryonic antigen (CEA) level, multiple tumors, positive resection margins, and bilobar location of tumors.[15,17,34,36,37,39,41–48,54,58,59,61,62,64–69] Interestingly, the presence of any one of these factors does not preclude the possibility of long-term survival. A few factors, however, are associated with nearly universal recurrence, and these include ≥4 liver metastases, the presence of extrahepatic disease, and a positive margin.[70,71] In our recent MSKCC analysis of 10-year survivors from hepatic resection, the only factor that precluded cure was the presence of a positive hepatic resection margin.Contraindications to hepatectomy have been difficult to define aside from the technical inability to resect all disease. Traditionally, the presence of 4 or more metastases, close margins, and extrahepatic disease were felt to contraindicate hepatic resection, since publications from the 1980s showed these factors to be associated with poor survival. These data came from an era of poor imaging and staging as well as from an era of ineffective chemotherapy. We now know that resection of ≥4 tumors or close margins can still result in 5-year survival in approximately one-third of patients, despite high recurrence rates.

Until recently, the presence of extrahepatic disease has been an absolute contraindication to hepatic resection. This has been challenged, and in the era of effective chemotherapy, selected patients with limited extrahepatic disease are being considered for resection.[73] With the development of effective chemotherapy for metastatic colorectal cancer as well as improvements in the technique of hepatic resection, the indications for hepatectomy are expanding; just how far these indications will expand still requires definition.

With the increasing role of surgery in the treatment of hepatic metastases, there is a growing need for a simple prognostic scoring system to permit selection of patients for liver resection. In addition, such a scoring system would be important for stratification of patients in clinical trials. In a recent MSKCC analysis of 1001 consecutive liver resections, several preoperative factors were found to be most influential for poor outcome. They include: (1) liver tumors >5 cm; (2) disease-free interval between colon and liver disease <12 months; (3) number of liver tumors >1; (4) lymph node-positive primary; and (5) preoperative CEA level >200 ng/mL. However, presence of any one of these characteristics was still associated with a 5-year survival of 24% to 34%, and therefore none can be considered complete contraindications to resection. Now the clinical risk score based on these five criteria guides patient selection and stratification. Assigning 1 point to each of these factors predictive of poor prognosis, the clinical risk score consists of the sum. A score of ≤2 places a patient in a good prognostic group for whom resection is ideal and associated with 5-year survival of nearly 50%. For scores of 3, 4, or 5, outcome is less favorable, and patients should be considered for novel trials of adjuvant therapy. Interestingly, despite lower survival rates, long-term survival is still seen in these patients with high clinical-srisk scores.[72] This clinical risk score is also now being used to help with preoperative assessment. A high clinical risk score has been associated with sufficient yield to justify both FDG-PET scanning[13] and laparoscopy[74] in the preoperative staging of patients with hepatic colorectal metastases.

Gastrointestinal low-grade neuroendocrine tumors metastatic to the liver are the second most common tumors seen by hepatic surgeons for consideration of resection. Neuroendocrine tumors present different issues than those seen in colorectal carcinoma. First, they can be indolent, with long periods of disease stability even in the absence of treatment, and second, many are associated with hormonal production that can be crippling to patients. Therefore, the role of resection is to potentially prolong survival and to attempt to provide durable symptom control. All the clinical data addressing the role of resection in this disease are retrospective and fraught with selection bias, in that the patients who undergo resection are those who tend to have indolent disease and less tumor burden. Nonetheless, the largest series of resection for neuroendocrine liver metastases showed a 5-year survival ranging from 50% to 75% and symptom control in over 90% of patients. Approximately 60% of patients experience recurrence of symptoms at 5 years. Resection of at least 90% of gross disease appears to be an important issue in symptom control. Recurrence after resection, however, is common, occurring in at least 85% of patients.

Other ablative techniques that can be useful in controlling symptoms and treating tumor include chemoembolization, radioembolization, and radio frequency ablation (RFA). Published experience with these techniques is relatively small, but the main benefit of these techniques is that they are minimally invasive. Comparisons between ablative techniques and surgery usually suggest that surgery results in better outcome; however, selection bias makes retrospective comparisons between these techniques difficult.

A number of diseases can present with limited hepatic metastases amenable to resection, and in the literature tend to be labeled "noncolorectal, nonneuroendocrine" (NCNN) metastases. Experience with liver resection for these other metastases is limited, and every report is plagued with small numbers, extreme selection bias, as well as tremendous variety in tumor histology. Nevertheless, initial studies show that in well selected patients, long-term survival is feasible with over one-third of patients surviving over 5 years. In addition, it was found that longer disease-free interval, complete resection, and tumor type were associated with improved survival. The best outcomes were seen in patients with genitourinary tumors such as testicular, adrenal, renal, and gynecologic cancers.[77] In an updated series from MSKCC analyzing hepatic resection for NCNN metastases (excluding sarcoma), 141 patients were studied. Overall median survival was 42 months, with a 57% 3-year survival. There were 24 5-year survivors with 49 still at risk. Multivariate analysis revealed negative margins, reproductive tract histology, and a disease-free interval >2 years to be associated with improved survival. The best survival was seen in gynecologic, testicular, breast, renal, and adrenocortical tumors, while the worst outcomes were seen in patients with melanoma and GI (other than colorectal) cancers.[78] A multi-institutional study from France has recently analyzed outcomes in 1452 patients who underwent hepatic resection for NCNN metastases. Five-year survival was 36% (median 35 months). However, 5-year relapse-free survival was only 14% (median 11 months). Factors associated with improved outcome in this study included age <60 years, tumor type (squamous histology and ocular melanoma fared the worst), longer disease-free interval, lack of extrahepatic disease, response to chemotherapy, and clear margins.[79]

A study from MSKCC specifically studied liver resection for metastatic sarcoma. Of 4270 patients with primary sarcoma and 331 with liver metastases, only 56 underwent hepatectomy, which underlines the extreme selection bias. Five-year survival after hepatectomy was 30% (median 39 months), which was better than those being treated without resection. Recurrence occurred in nearly all patients. A disease-free interval >2 years was independently associated with an improved outcome.[80] This report was published before the discovery of imatinib and its utility in the treatment of GI stromal tumors (GIST). GIST is now commonly referred for cytoreductive procedures including hepatectomy because of the high response rates with imatinib, although the exact role of metastasectomy in GIST remains to be defined.

Adjuvant Chemotherapy After Liver Resection

Nearly two-thirds of patients selected for liver resection of metastatic colorectal cancer will have a recurrence due to microscopic residual disease undetected at the time of the original liver resection. This provides a rationale for adjuvant chemotherapy.

Adjuvant Systemic Chemotherapy

Few trials have evaluated the role of adjuvant systemic therapy after liver resection. O'Connell and colleagues treated 26 patients with 5-fluorouracil (5-FU) and semustine after liver resection, and compared them to 26 patients with closely matched prognostic factors treated with liver resection alone. There was no significant survival advantage in the adjuvant chemotherapy group.[81] Portier and colleagues randomized 173 patients to IV 5-FU or no chemotherapy after liver resection, and demonstrated a 5-year survival of 50% and 40%, respectively ($p = .15$).[82] A similar trial by Langer and colleagues reported a 4-year survival of 57% and 47%, respectively, with a median survival of 53 months and 43 months, respectively ($p = .39$).[83]

At present, patients who have not received chemotherapy are usually offered adjuvant oxaliplatin (Oxa), 5-FU, and leucovorin (LV), based on an adjuvant chemotherapy trial after primary colon resection.[84] For patients who have had prior chemotherapy, the use of adjuvant systemic therapy has not been studied, but because second-line therapy has less activity in the metastatic setting, it would be reasonable to consider alternate therapies to adjuvant systemic therapy alone.

Adjuvant Hepatic Arterial Infusion (HAI)

A number of trials have evaluated the use of adjuvant HAI chemotherapy after liver resection. Regional adjuvant treatment was pursued because in many series the most common site for tumor recurrence after resection was the residual liver.[17,18,34,85]

Five randomized trials examined the role of adjuvant HAI after liver resection. The MSKCC trial[86] was a large, single-institutional study in which 156 patients were randomized to systemic 5-FU and leucovorin (LV) systemic therapy (SYS) or HAI floxuridine (FUDR) plus dexamethasone with systemic 5-FU and LV (HAI+SYS).[86] The primary endpoint was 2-year survival. The 2 treatment groups were stratified by the number of metastases and the type of treatment received prior to the study. Approximately 20% of each group had >4 liver metastases. Baseline characteristics were well matched, including poor prognostic variables (positive hepatic resection margins, synchronous disease), the number receiving large resections (trisegmentectomy or lobectomy), the number with Dukes' C or rectal primaries, and the number of patients with abnormal expression of p53 or high thymidylate synthetase.

Two-year survival was significantly greater for the HAI+SYS group (86% and 72% for the HAI+SYS and SYS groups, respectively; p = 0.03). The endpoint of the study was accomplished.[86] When first publicized, the 2-year hepatic disease-free survival was significantly longer in the HAI group but progression-free survival was not. Now with a median follow-up of 10 years, median overall disease-free survival is 31 months for HAI+SYS and 17 months for the SYS-alone group (p < .02). Ten-year survival is 41% for HAI+SYS and 27% for SYS-alone. (Fig. 85-2). Median survival is 68.4 months and 58.8 months for the HAI+SYS versus SYS-alone groups, respectively. Updated median hepatic-free survival has not been reached for the HAI+SYS group, and is 32.5 months for the SYS-alone group (p < .001). Hepatic toxicity was higher in the HAI+SYS group, with increased bilirubin in 11%, and 5 patients requiring biliary stents. If patients are divided into good-risk and bad-risk categories, the 10-year survival is still high for patients who received HAI (Fig. 85-3).

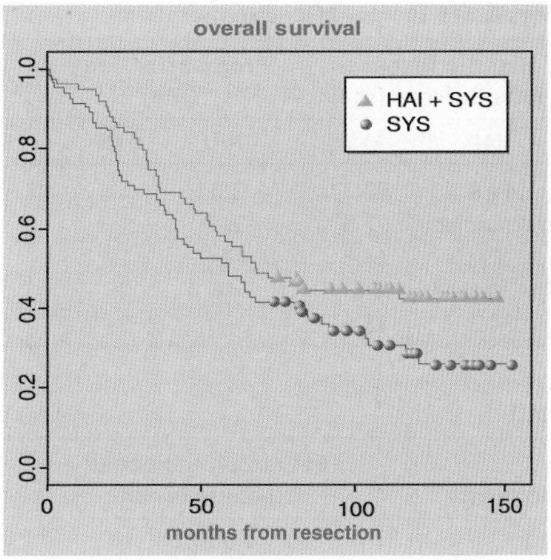

Figure 85-2 Kaplan–Meier estimates of overall survival in the groups assigned to either HAI + systemic chemotherapy or systemic chemotherapy alone. The estimated median survival was 68.4 months in the combined-therapy group (29 of the 74 patients died) and 58.8 months in the monotherapy group (38 of 82 patients died).

Another trial conducted by the Eastern Cooperative Oncology Group (ECOG) randomized patients to observation alone versus a combination of hepatic arterial FUDR and systemic infusional 5-FU.[87] The study was powered to detect a difference in disease-free survival: 109 patients were randomized, and randomization was done prior to surgery. Twenty-nine patients, although randomized, were not in the study because of extrahepatic disease or unresectable disease. If the patients who actually entered the study are considered, of the 45 patients in the control group, 77.8% recurred—53% in the liver. In the 30 patients in the HAI group, 53% had recurrence and only 26% had liver recurrence. The 4-year recurrence-free survival was improved—46% versus 22%, in the HAI and control groups, respectively (p= .04). The endpoint was recurrence-free survival, which was accomplished. Five-year survival for the patients who actually were in the study was 59% HAI+SYS versus 40% of those in the control group. Median survival was 63.7 months for the HAI+SYS group and 49.4 months for the control group (p = .60) (Table 85-4).

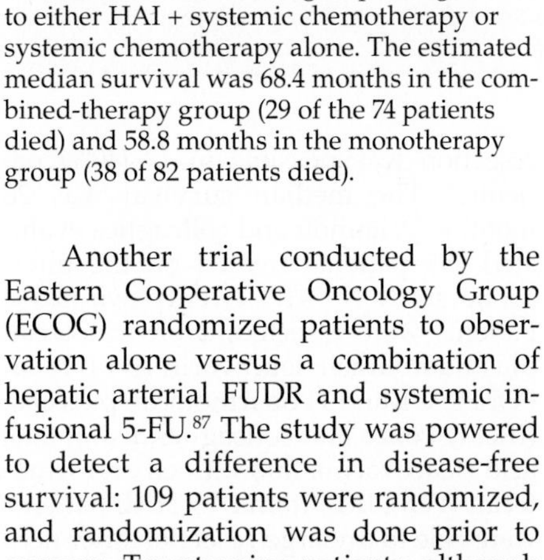

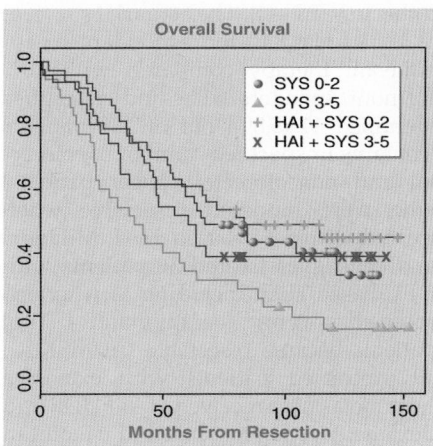

Figure 85-3 Kaplan–Meier estimates of overall survival in the groups assigned to either HAI + systemic chemotherapy or systemic chemotherapy alone with stratification based on the preoperative clinical risk score. Using the clinical risk score for predicting recurrence after hepatic resection defined by Fong et al.[13] outcomes were significantly better with combined therapy compared to monotherapy in patients with higher clinical risk scores (3 to 5).

A German Cooperative Group performed a randomized trial after hepatic resection of adjuvant HAI of FU and LV versus control.[88] Patients were stratified according to number of liver metastases (1–2 vs 3–6) and the site of the primary tumor (colon and upper rectum vs mid or lower rectum). Despite initial randomization, 21% in the HAI arm did not receive the assigned treatment for various reasons including anatomic variants, extrahepatic disease at the time of surgery, technical complications with port placement, and patient refusal after randomization. By the end of the trial, 77% of patients randomized to the HAI+SYS arm had received this treatment and only 30% finished therapy. At 18-month interim analysis, 33% of patients receiving adjuvant therapy and 37% of patients treated with resection alone had relapsed, and no survival advantage was seen. When the outcomes were analyzed to look at treated patients, median survival was 44.8 months in the treated group (n = 87) versus 39.7 months in the control group (n = 114), respectively. Median time to liver progression doubled in the group receiving HAI: 20 months versus 12.6 months for the control group. The study used arterial ports rather than pumps (allowing for more clot formation) and used FU, which has less hepatic extraction than FUDR. Another troubling point is that at the time of reporting, only 38% of patients were followed for at least 2 years.

In a study from Greece, 143 patients were randomized after liver resection to: (A) Mitomycin, FU, LV, and IL-2 given via port into the hepatic artery and intravenously, or (B) the same drugs given intravenously only. The survival at 2-years was 92% versus 75% and at 5 years 73% versus 60% for groups A and B, respectively. Median survival was 79 months versus 66 months, and 5-year survival was 40% and 34% for groups A and B, respectively (p = .04). Three patients in A and two patients in B required biliary stents. Median survival with no hepatic involvement was 79 and 44.5 months for A and B, respectively (p = .0003).[89] Two smaller studies also demonstrated an improvement in survival with HAI therapy.[90,91]

Table 85-4 Randomized Trials of Adjuvant (HAI) versus SYS Therapy After Liver Resection

	No. of Patients	Median Survival (Mo)		Hepatic Disease-Free Survival (Mo)		Progression-Free (Mo)	
		HAI	SYS	HAI	SYS	HAI	SYS
Lorenz M[88]	226	44.8	39.7	44.8	23.3	20	12
Kemeny N[86]	156	68.4	58.8	Not reached	32.5	31.3	17.2
Lygidakis NJ[89]	122	76	66	79	44.5	45.5	19
Kemeny M[87]	75	65	50	Not reached	20	46	25
Kusunoki M[90]	58	60	30	34.2	18.4	–	–

Table 85-5 Drugs for Hepatic Arterial Infusion (HAI)

Drug	Half-life (min)	Estimated Increased Exposure by HAI
Fluorouracil (FU)	10	5-10-Fold
5-Fluoro-2-deoxyuridine (FUDR)	<10	100-400-Fold
Bischloroethylnitrosourea (BCNU)	<5	6-7-Fold
Mitomycin-C	<10	6-8-Fold
Cisplatin	20-30	4-7-Fold
Adriamycin (doxorubicin hydrochloride)	60	2-Fold

Source: From Ref. 120.

These studies clearly show a significant increase in disease-free survival (Table 85-5). There is also an increase in median survival in some studies, although most were not powered to show a significant increase in survival. One study was powered for 2-year survival, and did show an increase in survival with HAI. A small study using HAI plus systemic Oxalydation (Oxa) 5Fu and LV had a 4-year survival of 88%.[92] We presently believe that in institutions that have experience with HAI treatment for patients undergoing liver resection for colorectal metastases, adjuvant treatment should consist of HAI therapy. The question of whether the new systemic agents can complement regional therapy or replace it is subject to ongoing investigation.

Neoadjuvant Chemotherapy

The fact that some patients with unresectable tumors were rendered resectable with systemic chemotherapy prompted further investigation of neoadjuvant chemotherapy.[93,94] In a retrospective trial by Bismuth and colleagues, 330 patients who were considered unresectable because of large lesions, multiple nodules, poor location, or extrahepatic disease, were treated with chronomodulated Oxa/5-FU/LV, and 53 (16%) patients proceeded to liver resection. The 5-year survival following liver resection was 40%. Adam and colleagues updated these results, identifying 701 patients with unresectable liver metastases treated with neoadjuvant chemotherapy, 95 (13.6%) of whom underwent a potentially curative resection.[95] The 5-year survival rate for the resected patients was 34%.

Subsequent trials confirmed the ability of neoadjuvant chemotherapy to render patients resectable. Alberts and colleagues reported a 60% response rate in 42 patients using Oxa (FOLFOX)-4; resection was possible in 17 (40%) patients.[96] The median survival was 26 months. Delaunoit and colleagues evaluated 795 patients treated on the intergroup study N9741.[97] Twenty-two (3.3%) patients were resected, 2 on irinotecan plus fluorouracil/leucovorin (IFL), 11 on FOLFOX-4, and 11 on irinotecan plus Oxa (IROX). Pozzo and colleagues, using folic acid (leucovorin), fluorouracil and irinotecan (FOLFIRI), found 13 of 40 patients were able to undergo resection after neoadjuvant therapy.

Some of the neoadjuvant HAI chemotherapy trials have used HAI alone. Clavien and colleagues, using HAI FUDR and LV, induced resectability in 6 (26%) out of 23 previously treated patients (including 20 previously treated with camptothecin [CPT]-11). The actuarial survival at 3 years was 84% for responders to neoadjuvant therapy compared with 40% for nonresponders. Elias and colleagues identified 14 (5.8%) out of 239 patients (contains unspecified number of colorectal and noncolorectal cancer patients) who were rendered resectable when treated with 5-FU-based HAI. Milandri and colleagues treated 36 patients with 5-FU-based HAI (including 13 who also received systemic therapy), and 4 (11%) patients became resectable. At MSKCC, 49 pretreated patients with extensive liver metastases received HAI FUDR and dexamethasone plus Oxa and irinotecan systemic chemotherapy. The response rate was 92%, and although the majority of patients had previous chemotherapy before entry into this trial (many already progressing on systemic therapy), surgical resection of liver metastases was then possible in 47%.[102,103]

Neoadjuvant therapy has certain advantages. Some studies suggest that progression of disease on systemic therapy leads to worse survival rates. Adam and colleagues demonstrated a 5-year survival of 30% in patients who underwent liver resection after a response to chemotherapy and 8% if there was progression on chemotherapy.[104] A recent review of 120 patients with synchronous disease found no difference in survival in patients who progressed or who had response prior to liver resection, but 40% of these patients were treated with HAI therapy after liver resection.[105] However certain chemotherapies can lead to liver toxicity. In a report of preoperative therapy with Oxa, 40% of patients developed perisinusoidal and veno-occlusive fibrosis.[106]

Systemic Chemotherapy

Some tumors are more responsive to chemotherapy. Responses of liver metastases to systemic chemotherapy vary and usually reflect the responsiveness of the primary tumor. Most studies of systemic therapy do not differentiate between patients who have only liver metastases and those with generalized metastatic disease. Combination chemotherapy has substantially improved the response rates in breast cancer, but liver metastases still have a lower response rate than do soft tissue or pulmonary metastases. In a Southwest Oncology Group study of 262 patients, those with disease sites other than the liver had a 71% response rate (110 of 154) versus a 47% (41 of 88) response rate for patients with liver metastases only ($p < .001$).[107]

For patients with gastric carcinoma, with fluorouracil, epirubicin, glutathione, and filgrastim, the response rate was 62% for all metastatic sites, whereas the response rate for those with hepatic metastases was 55% versus 77% for lymph nodes.[108]

In patients with colorectal cancer, the liver is the most common site of dissemination, with up to 70% of patients developing liver metastases during the course of their disease.[30,32,109–113] The overall response with older regimens was low, as was the response rate in the liver.[25,26,30,31,114,115] Recently, however, a number of new agents have become available for the treatment of colorectal cancer. Studies with irinotecan combined with 5-FU and LV have increased response rates and survival over 5-FU/LV alone.[116] The addition of Oxa to 5-FU/LV has further improved response rate and survival.[117] In a randomized trial comparing Oxa/5-FU/LV (FOLFOX) to irinotecan/5-FU/LV (IFL), there was an increase in response rate (45% vs 35%) and survival (19.5 vs 15 months) for the FOLFOX group versus the IFL group, respectively.[118] Using an anti-VEGF monoclonal antibody, bevacizumab, with IFL versus IFL alone, there was a statistically significant improvement in response rate and survival as well (Table 85-6).[119] None of these new trials separated the response rate for patients with liver metastases from the entire group.

For primary liver cancers, a number of trials are using gemcitabine either alone or in combination for biliary cancers including cholangiocarcinoma, producing response rates generally around 30%.[120-122] However, chemotherapy still produces a low response in hepatocellular cancers.

Table 85-7 Second-Line IV Chemotherapy for Metastatic Colorectal Cancer

Study	Regimen	Response (%)	Survival (Mo)
Systemic			
Rothenberg[255]	CPT-11	11	9.9
Rothenberg[256]	FOLFOX-4	10	9.8**
Cunningham[257]	C225/CPT-11	23	8.6**
Saltz[258]	C225	9	6.4
HAI			
Kemeny[153]	FUDR/Dex/LV	52	13.5
Kemeny[154]	FUDR/Mito-C	70	19
Kemeny[166]	FUDR/Dex+Sys CPT-11	74	20
Kemeny[102]	FUDR/Dex+Sys Oxal+CPT-11	90	28

Table 85-8 Hepatic Arterial Infusion (HAI) for Breast Cancer

Investigator	No. of Patients	Drugs	Partial Response (%)	Median Survival (Mo)
Fraschini[168]	34	Cisplatin + Vinblastine	33	11
Estape[169]	16	VP-16-Cytoxan	50	16
Fraschini[170]	25	Vinblastine	52	11[a]
Fraschini[171]	26	Cisplatin	19	11
Maral[172]	15	Mitomycin-C + FUDR	53	18[b]
Arai[173]	56	FU + Doxo + Mitomycin	81	12.5
Tada[174]	45	Doxorubicin + Mitomycin-C	37	7.5

[a]Mean survival only for responders.
[b]Some patients in study also had colon cancer.

Second-Line Therapy for Colorectal Cancer

The use of second-line therapy for colorectal cancer is now possible because of the new agents. However, with the majority of new agents, the response rate to second-line therapy ranges from 9% to 22%. In small studies using HAI therapy, alone or combined with systemic chemotherapy, second-line therapy produced response rates of 52% to 90% and a median survival of 13–28 months (Table 85-7).

Hepatic Arterial Chemotherapy

The rationale for hepatic arterial chemotherapy is based on both anatomic and pharmacologic factors. Liver metastases are perfused almost exclusively by the hepatic artery (once lesions are >3 cm in diameter), although normal liver hepatocytes derive their blood supply mostly from the portal vein.[123] In addition, certain drugs are largely extracted by the liver during the first pass through the arterial circulation, which results in high local concentrations of the drug with minimal systemic toxicity. Ensminger and colleagues[124] demonstrated that 94–99% of FUDR is extracted by the liver during the first pass, compared with 19–55% of FU. The pharmacologic advantage of various chemotherapeutic agents for HAI is summarized in Table 85-8.[124] Drugs with high total body clearance and short plasma half-life are more useful for hepatic infusion. If a drug is not rapidly cleared, recirculation through the systemic circulation diminishes the advantage of hepatic arterial delivery.[125,126] Newer drugs such as irinotecan have not exhibited increased activity when delivered by HAI.[127]

The liver is often the first and only site of metastatic disease. The theory of the stepwise pattern of metastatic progression proposes that hematogenous spread occurs first via the portal vein to the liver, then from the liver to the lungs, then to other organs.[128,129] If this theory is valid, aggressive treatment of metastases confined to the liver (resection and/or hepatic infusion) may yield prolonged survival for some patients.

Regional hepatic arterial therapy can be delivered using either a hepatic arterial port or a percutaneously placed intra-arterial catheter connected to an external or a totally implantable pump. Early studies with percutaneously placed hepatic artery catheters produced high response rates, but clotting of the catheters and of the hepatic artery, duodenal ulcers, and bleeding from around the catheters[130] led physicians to abandon this method. The development of a totally implantable pump allowed long-term hepatic artery infusion with good patency of the catheter and the hepatic artery, and a low incidence of infection.[131] One study compared three groups: (1) surgical placement of a hepatic artery catheter, (2) percutaneous placement of the catheter, and (3) surgical placement of a reservoir. The reported ability to administer chemotherapy was highest for the reservoir group—115 days versus 31 and 25 days for groups 1 and 2, respectively.[132] A number of trials using the implantable pump produced high response rates with good survival rates.[133-140]

Currently, 10 randomized studies are comparing hepatic arterial chemotherapy with systemic chemotherapy (Table 85-9). In a study at MSKCC, all patients underwent exploratory laparotomy to exclude those with extrahepatic disease. Patients were stratified by percent of liver involvement and baseline lactate dehydrogenase (LDH) values. Both groups received a 14-day continuous infusion of FUDR, but the dose was lower in the systemic group, since the higher dose could not be tolerated as systemic infusion. The response rate was 52% for HAI, and 20% for systemic therapy ($p = .001$). Crossover from systemic therapy to hepatic infusion was permitted. The median survivals for the HAI and systemic groups as randomized were 17 and 12 months, respectively ($p = .424$). The pa-

Table 85-6 Select Randomized Trials of First-Line Chemotherapy for Metastatic Colorectal Cancer

Study	Regimen	% Response	Survival (Mo)	p-Value
Doulliard[254]	5-FU/LV/Irinotecan	41	17.4	<.05
	5-FU/LV(LV5FU2/AIO)	23	14.1	
Saltz[116]	5-FU/LV/Irinotecan	39	14.8	<.05
	5-FU/LV(bolus)	21	12.8	
DeGramont[117]	5-FU/LV/Oxa	51	16.2	<.05
	5-FU/LV	22	14.7	NS
Goldberg[118]	FOLFOX-4	38	18.6	<.05
	IFL bolus	29	14.1	
	Irinotecan/Oxa	29	16.5	
Hurwitz[119]	IFL+Avastin	44.8	20.3	.004
	IFL	34.8	15.6	≤.001

Table 85-9 **Randomized Trials of HAI for Unresectable Liver Metastases**

Study Group, Date (Ref.)	Arms	*n*	No. (%) Receiving Assigned Therapy	X-over	Responses (CR+PR)	Median TTP (mo)	Median TTHP (mo)	Median Survival (mo)
MSKCC, 1987 (129)	HAI FUDR	48	45 (94)	Yes	50%[a]	9[a]	NR	17
	IV FUDR	51	48 (94)		20%	5	NR	12
NCI, 1987 (131)	HAI FUDR	32	21 (66)	No	62%[a]	NR	NR	17
	IV FUDR	32	29 (92)		17%	–	NR	12
NCOG, 1989	HAI FUDR	67	50 (75)	Yes	42%[a]	NR	13*	16.5
	IV FUDR	76	65 (86)		10%	NR	6.5	15.8
City of Hope, 1990	HAI FUDR	31	31 (100)	Yes	55%[a]	8.8	NR	13.8
	IV FU	10	10 (100)		20%	7.5	NR	11.6
NCCTG, 1990 (132)	HAI FUDR	39	33 (85)	No	48%	6.0	15.7[a]	12.6
	IV FU/LV	35	36 (103)		12%	5.0	6.0	10.5
French, 1992 (133)	HAI FUDR	81	70 (87)	No	44%[a]	NR	14.5[a]	15*
	IV FU	82	41 (50)		9%	NR	5.5	11
English, 1994 (134)	HAI FUDR	51	49 (96)	No	NR	NR	NR	13.5[a]
	IV FU	49	10 (20)		NR	NR	NR	7.5
German, 2000 (137)	HAI FUDR	54	37 (69)	Yes	43%[a]	5.9	NR	12.7
	HAI FU/LV	57	40 (70)		45%[a]	9.2	NR	18.7
	IV FU/LV	57	52 (91)		20%	6.6	NR	17.6
MRC/EORTC 2003 (138)	HAI FU/LV	145	95 (66)	No	22%	7.7	NR	14.7
	IV FU/LV	145	126 (87)		19%	6.7	NR	14.8
CALGB, 2003 (L)	HAI FUDR	68	59 (87)	No	48%[a]	5.3	9.8[a]	24
	IV FU/LV	67	58 (87)		25%	6.8	7.3	20

[a]Statistically significant difference ($p < .05$) compared with control group.

Abbreviations: BSC, best supportive care; CR, complete response; FU, 5-fluorouracil; FUDR, floxuridine; HAI, hepatic arterial infusion; IV, intravenous; LV, leucovorin; *n*, number of patients enrolled; NR, not reported; OS, overall survival; PR, partial response; TTHP, time to hepatic progression; TTP, time to progression; X-over, crossover to HAI arm.

tients who did cross over had a median survival of 18 months compared with 8 months for those who did not cross over to HAI ($p = .04$).[133]

A similar randomized study conducted by the Northern California Oncology Group also used FUDR infusions in both groups.[134] Forty-two percent responded to HAI and 10% to systemic therapy ($p < .001$). The median time to progression was 401 and 201 days for the HAI and systemic groups, respectively ($p < .009$), although median survivals were 503 and 484 days, respectively. Eventually 43% of patients on systemic therapy received HAI, which may have obscured survival differences. For the group that crossed over, the median survival was twice as long as for the group that never received HAI. Another flaw in the study was that patients with metastases to hepatic lymph nodes were also included.

At the National Cancer Institute, 64 patients were randomized to HAI or systemic FUDR. The response rates were 62% and 17%, respectively ($p < .003$).[135] In the subset of patients without extrahepatic disease, the 2-year survival was 47% in the HAI group versus 13% in the systemic group ($p < .03$).

In another small study conducted by the Mayo Clinic, HAI FUDR was compared to systemic bolus FU for 5 days in 69 patients.[136] Objective tumor response was observed in 48% and 21% ($p = .02$), and time to hepatic progression was 15.7 and 6 months, respectively ($p = .001$). Despite the increase in response rate and time to hepatic progression, survival was similar in the 2 groups (12.6 and 10.5 months, respectively). However, this survival information is difficult to interpret because 48% of the HAI group was either not adequately treated or had extrahepatic disease.

In a large French trial, patients were randomized to HAI FUDR versus systemic bolus FU.[137] The response rates were 49% and 14%, median time to hepatic progression was 15 and 6 months, and median survival was 14 and 10 months for the HAI and systemic therapy groups, respectively. The 2-year survival was 22% for HAI and 10% for the systemic group ($p = .02$). One criticism of this trial is that some patients in the systemic therapy group received chemotherapy late, since only symptomatic patients were treated in the systemic group. A British study was designed in a similar manner (only symptomatic patients were treated in the systemic group).[138] The HAI group had a significantly longer survival. Patients in the HAI group had significantly longer normal performance status than the patients in the systemic therapy group.

A German cooperative group randomized 168 patients to (1) HAI FUDR, (2) HAI FU/LV, or (3) systemic FU/LV.[141] The median time to progression was 5.9, 9.2, and 6.6 months; and median survival times were 12.7, 18.7, and 17.6 months, respectively. In this study, the median survival was better for HAI-FU/LV. Tumor response rates were 43.2%, 45%, and 19.7%; and development of extrahepatic disease was 40.5%, 12.5%, and 18.3%, respectively. Toxicity data indicate that FU/LV therapy was much more toxic than FUDR. The incidence of stomatitis was 8%, 75%, and 64.6%, and of diarrhea was 0%, 11%, and 11% for HAI FUDR, HAI FU/LV and IV FU/LV, respectively. A port instead of a pump was used, and dosing for FUDR was different than in the American studies in that FUDR was reduced from 0.2 to 0.15 mg/kg/day after 3 cycles rather than adjusting for patient toxicity. It should be pointed out that although an intention-to-treat analysis was used, only 68.5% randomized to HAI FUDR were treated, but all were included in the survival analysis.

The Medical Research Council/European Organization for the Research and Treatment of Cancer (MRC/EORTC)[142] conducted a randomized trial of IV versus HAI FU/LV in 290 patients. Median and 2-year survival rates were 13.4 months and 23% in the IV arm versus 14.7 months and 20% in the HAI arm. However, 37% of patients allocated to the HAI arm did not receive the treatment, and 29% had to stop treatment, so approximately 50% of patients in the HAI group did not receive treatment or had inadequate treatment and are included in the survival analysis. No breakdown of the treated patients was given.

The Cancer and Leukemia Group B (CALGB) trial differs from others in that it includes the use of dexamethasone and LV in the HAI arm versus 5-FU+LV in the systemic arm, with no crossover. The endpoint was survival, which was 24.4 months and 20 months in the HAI and systemic groups, respectively ($p = .0034$). The time to hepatic progression was better in the HAI arm (9.8 months vs 7.3 months, $p = .034$), but the time to extrahepatic progression was better in the systemic arm (7.7 months vs 14.8 months,

$p < .029$) for the HAI and systemic groups, respectively. Quality of life was improved at 3 and 6 months in the HAI group.[143]

Toxicity of Hepatic Arterial FUDR Infusion

The most common problems with HAI are hepatic toxicity and ulceration of the stomach and duodenum. Myelosuppression, nausea, vomiting, and diarrhea do not occur with HAI or FUDR. If diarrhea does occur, shunting to the bowel should be suspected.[144] Clinically, biliary toxicity is manifested as elevations of aspartate transaminase (AST), alkaline phosphatase, and bilirubin. In the early stages of toxicity, hepatic enzyme elevations will return to normal when the drug is withdrawn and the patient is given a rest period, although in more advanced cases, it does not resolve. The bile ducts derive their blood supply almost exclusively from the hepatic artery[145] and thus are undoubtedly perfused with high doses of chemotherapy.

In patients who develop jaundice, an endoscopic retrograde cholangiopancreatogram (ERCP) may demonstrate lesions resembling idiopathic sclerosing cholangitis in 5% to 29% of patients treated by experienced clinicians.[139] Because the ducts are sclerotic and non-dilated, sonograms usually do not show dilation. The strictures may be focal and present at the hepatic duct bifurcation; therefore, drainage procedures either by ERCP or by transhepatic cholangiogram may be helpful. Duct obstruction from metastases should first be excluded by a liver CT.

Close monitoring of liver function tests is necessary to avoid biliary complications. If the serum bilirubin becomes ≥3 mg/dL, no further treatment should be given until the bilirubin returns to normal, and then with a 75% reduction in dose to prevent the development of sclerosing cholangitis.

Ulcer disease results from inadvertent perfusion of the stomach and duodenum with drug via the small collateral branches from the hepatic artery. This can be prevented by careful dissection of these collaterals at the time of pump placement.[140] In a large series reviewing 544 patients who received pumps, other toxicities included dislodgement of the catheter (3%), occlusion of catheter (2%), extrahepatic perfusion (3%), and pump infection (2.5%).[146]

Decreasing Hepatic Toxicity of HAI ■ Three approaches have been tried in the attempt to decrease hepatic toxicity: (1) HAI dexamethasone (D), (2) circadian modification, and (3) HAI- FU alternating with FUDR. The hepatic toxicity induced by HAI of FUDR may be related to portal triad inflammation, which could lead to ischemia of the bile ducts. Hepatic arterial administration of dexamethasone may decrease inflammation and thereby decrease biliary toxicity. In patients with established hepatobiliary toxicity from HAI, dexamethasone promotes resolution of liver function abnormalities. A randomized study of FUDR+D versus FUDR alone showed a trend toward decreased bilirubin elevation in patients receiving FUDR+D compared with the group receiving FUDR alone (9% vs 30%, $p = .07$).[147] The response rate with FUDR+D was 71% versus 40% for FUDR alone ($p = .03$). Survival was also 23 and 15 months, respectively. The use of circadian modification of HAI FUDR is another way to decrease hepatic toxicity. In a University of Minnesota nonrandomized study comparing constant (flat) infusion versus circadian-modified (CM) hepatic arterial FUDR, the patients with CM infusion tolerated almost twice the daily dose of FUDR, with a decrease in hepatic toxicity compared with patients receiving flat infusions.[148]

The third approach is to decrease toxicity by alternating drugs such as HAI FUDR with hepatic arterial (HA) FU. Weekly HA bolus of FU does not cause hepatobiliary toxicity; however, it frequently produces treatment-limiting systemic toxicity or arteritis. Stagg and colleagues used alternating HAI followed by HA bolus FU via the pump side port.[149] The response rate was 51%, and median survival was 22.4 months. In contrast to the experience with single-agent HAI FUDR, no patient has had treatment terminated because of drug toxicity. Using an infusion of FU and mitomycin-C, Metzger and colleagues found that median survival was 18 months, with a partial response rate of 57%.[150] Sclerosing cholangitis did not occur, but mucositis and leukopenia did. Catheter complications led to premature termination of treatment in one-third of the patients. Although the dose of FUDR fits into an implanted pump, FU requires an external pump for infusion or bolus weekly side port injections. Van Riel and colleagues, employing a MediPort to administer FU infusion 1000 mg/m^2 for 5 days, reported a 34% response rate in 145 patients with a 14.3-month median survival. Arterial thrombosis was seen in 48% and catheter dislocation in 22%.[151] With a higher dose of FU (2200 mg/m^2 over 24 h weekly with LV), objective responses were seen in 28 out of 50 (56%) patients, with a median survival of 23 months.[152]

Increasing Response Rate to HAI ■ The addition of LV and mitomycin-C to FUDR have increased response rates but also produced biliary sclerosis. In previously treated patients, FUDR+LV and D produced a 50% response rate, and mitomycin side port injection added to HAI FUDR+D produced a 70% response rate.[153,154] Both trials, however, increased biliary sclerosis. 5-FU, LV, and interferon with degradable starch microspheres via an HAI catheter produced a response rate of 70% and a median survival of 24 months in 95 patients. The major toxicity was diarrhea in 58%; there were problems with catheter occlusion in 46%.[155]

Another approach is to use new agents via the HAI route. Van Riel and colleagues treated 25 patients with a 5-day continuous infusion of HAI irinotecan every 3 weeks.[156] In 22 assessable patients, 14% had a partial response and 40% had stable disease, with a median survival was 8.1 months. There was lack of hepatic extraction of the drug despite the increased conversion of irinotecan to its active metabolite SN38.[157] Fiorentini treated 12 patients with HAI irinotecan and reported a 33% response rate. Similarly Vogl and colleagues noted a partial response of 33% in 9 patients.[158]

A number of trials have evaluated HAI/Oxa combinations. Kern and colleagues demonstrated an objective response rate of 59% using HAI/Oxa and 5-FU and folinic acid.[159] Ducreux and colleagues used a similar regimen in a phase II study, and achieved an objective response rate of 79% (with 3 of 14 patients undergoing complete resection of their metastases after response to therapy) and a 6-month survival of 86%.[160] Other trials have recorded response rates of 13% to 69% for HAI Oxa combined with other chemotherapies given via the IV route.[161–164] Using HAI with concurrent systemic chemotherapy has increased response rates in small phase II trials. Two trials used HAI chemotherapy plus systemic irinotecan. Zelek and colleagues gave HAI pirarubicin plus systemic irinotecan/5FU/LV to 31 patients, and reported a response rate of 48% with a median survival of 20.5 months.[165] At MSKCC, HAI FUDR and systemic irinotecan in 35 previously treated patients produced a partial response rate of 74% — the median survival was 20 months.[166] Further work with Oxa/irinotecan produced a 90% response rate in previously treated patients. Table 85-7 outlines treatment with systemic or HAI ± systemic therapies in second line therapy.

Hepatic Arterial Infusion

Conclusions ■ In 7 randomized trials, the response rate was higher with HAI compared with systemic therapy. The time to hepatic progression was significantly longer in the HAI groups versus the systemic groups. The randomized pump studies do not clearly evaluate the issue of survival because crossover was allowed; patients with positive portal nodes were included; and the number of patients entered was small.

A meta-analysis[167] of HAI FUDR versus systemic FU or FUDR showed a significant increase in response rate (41% vs 14%) and a significant increase in survival (16 months vs 12 months) for HAI and systemic therapy, respectively. The use of HAI therapy after progression on systemic therapy looks promising compared with second-line systemic therapy after progression on first-line treatment (Table 85-7). The use of HAI for other tumor types has not been studied as extensively. Some of the breast studies with HAI are shown in Table 85-8 and for biliary cancers in Table 85-10.[168-174] Most of these studies were conducted in patients whose tumors were failing to respond to systemic therapy, yet response rates of ≥50% were seen in 5 of the 8 studies in breast cancer. For uveal melanoma, the response with HAI fotemustine (40%) was higher than that obtained with other modalities.

Cryoablation

It is well known that the freeze/thaw process can bring about cellular destruction. Surgeons have long tried to harness the destructive capacity of the freezing process to treat liver tumors, and over the last 2 decades, advances in the design of cryosurgical instruments and mass marketing of the instruments have generated enthusiasm for this modality in the treatment of liver tumors. Traditionally, cryoablation has been performed with an open operation, which is the optimal way to execute this technique because it allows for mobilization of the liver, utilization of intraoperative ultrasound, and accurate staging of disease. The downside of open cryoablation is the large incision involved and the possibility of associated morbidity. Cryoablation can also be performed laparoscopically[175] or percutaneously,[176] but experience with these techniques is limited.

Cryoablation is particularly attractive for treatment of HCC because of the frequent association of HCC with cirrhosis. Hepatic resection in cirrhosis has a high-risk of complications, including liver failure; cryoablation allows preservation of liver parenchyma and function in the setting of cirrhosis. The attractiveness of cryoablation in the setting of compromised hepatic function encouraged extensive investigations, which resulted in data supporting the use of this modality for HCC.[177,178]

For metastatic tumors within the liver, however, a role for this modality is less well defined. Most series of cryoablation in liver metastases have focused on metastatic colorectal cancer but with limited numbers and limited follow-up, making conclusions about efficacy and comparison with other treatment modalities almost impossible. Since cryoablation has never proved to be curative, it should not be used in lieu of resection unless medical circumstances or the condition of the liver preclude safe resection.

Cryotherapy has limitations in terms of the size and numbers of lesions that can be treated. Most surgeons would not cryoablate more than 5 or 6 lesions, and the responsiveness of any tumor over 5 cm is probably limited (Although many series on cryoablation claim that it is only performed in "unresectable patients," any lesion that is can be ablated can also likely be resected by an experienced hepatic surgeon.). Ravikumar and colleagues reported that 18 of 24 patients with colorectal carcinoma were rendered disease-free by cryosurgery. Of these 18 patients, 39% were alive and free of disease at the time of publication.[179] In 18 patients treated by Onik and colleagues, 14 were not adequately treated and recurred; 4 (22%) had a complete response.[180] Morris and Ross reported less encouraging results.[181] In their report, 75% of the 67 patients treated with cryosurgery alone experienced relapse of preoperative CEA levels within 6 months.[182]

The most commonly identified prognostic factors involving this technique are size of metastases, volume of liver replaced, pretreatment CEA, absence of extrahepatic disease, complete ablation, and normalization of CEA after treatment. Reports from more recent series show 4-year and 5-year actuarial survival ranging from 22% to 36%; and 5-year survivors have been reported.[175,183,184] Complete response in treated tumors ranges from 60% to 90%, with most recurrences occurring at distant intrahepatic sites with or without synchronous extrahepatic metastases. This finding underscores the need for adjuvant therapy. Cryotherapy, like any local therapy for liver metastases, should be followed by additional chemotherapy, and regional HAI chemotherapy has been particularly promising.[166]

Survival after hepatic resection for metastatic colorectal cancer (5 year, 25–58%) yields better results than cryoablation, but the patient population is not easily comparable. Nonetheless, resection, when possible, is the standard of care; and the utility of cryoablation is primarily in patients who cannot undergo resection or who have parenchymal liver disease that precludes resection. Another application of cryotherapy is to enhance margins in resections that come unexpectedly close to tumors. This strategy has yielded favorable local tumor control.[185] With the expanding indications for resection of metastases, cryoablation has been used to treat deep tumors contralateral to a resection in otherwise unresectable patients. This approach has had some early success, and is another indication for cryotherapy.[186]

Although less morbid than resection, cryoablation can potentially result in morbidity and mortality. In the largest series, morbidity ranged from 10% to 40%, and mortality ranged from 0% to 8%. In a review of 869 patients reported in 20 different series, the overall mortality was 1.6%.[187] The most common complications included generalized hypothermia, hemorrhage, biliary fistulae, bile collections, and cryoshock. Although rare, cryoshock is of particular concern as it involves multiorgan failure, renal failure, and disseminated intravascular coagulation.[177,179,180,188,189]

Cryosurgical methods should be used only by surgeons familiar with liver anatomy and resection, since adequate mobilization of the liver and appreciation of the location of the major intrahepatic blood vessels and bile ducts are essential for safety. Furthermore, the possibility of resection as an alternative should be evaluated by experienced hepatic surgeons.

Radiofrequency Ablation

Radiofrequency ablation (RFA) is a method that uses heat to kill tumor cells.[190] Radiofrequency electrodes (which look like a long needle), direct electrical energy from radiofrequency generators to ablate tumors. Such RF electrodes can be guided into position by sonographic, CT, or MRI guidance; and ablation monitored by similar imaging modalities. RFA can be performed at open laparotomy by laparoscopic surgery, or percutaneously.

The major advantage of RFA over cryoablation is the lower cost of the equip-

Table 85-10 Biliary Tract Carcinoma: Hepatic Arterial Infusion (HAI) Trials

Study	No. of Patients	HAI Therapy	% Response	Median Survival (Mo)
Warren[259]	15	Doxorubicin	60	NR
Smith[260]	11	5-FU/ mitomycin-C	64	12.5
Makela[261]	27	Mitomycin-C	48	14
Cantore[262]	26	Epirubicin/cisplatin systemic 5-FU IVCI	40	13.2

ment, less time involved, and the possibility of performing such ablations percutaneously. The small size of the electrodes permits RFA without laparotomy. The major obstacle to this ablative technique is the limited size of the lesions that can be ablated. As heat is generated within the tumor, charring of tissues occurs, decreasing the conduction of heat. Patients with 1 to 3 lesions located in the periphery of the liver that are <3 cm are good candidates for RFA. Research is also being undertaken to increase the size of the areas that can be ablated. Improvements in technology, such as use of higher-power generators, saline-cooled-tip electrodes,[191] and larger arrays may soon allow ablation of lesions up to 5 cm (7 cm zones of ablation). It is important that lesions are not adjacent to bowel, kidney, gallbladder, or diaphragm. Follow-up images may be difficult to interpret, since the defect in the liver is larger with hypoattenuation after ablation. Any residual enhancement or increase in size or irregularity should raise a concern for recurrence.

Studies with relatively long follow-up are beginning to emerge,[192,193] indicating that ablations are safe and may offer durable treatment. In the largest of these studies, Livrhaghi and colleagues reported on a 41-center study with 2320 patients (1610 with HCC and 501 with metastatic colorectal cancer).[194] In total, 3554 lesions were treated. There were 6 deaths (0.3%) and 50 major complications (2.2%). In a recent comprehensive review, Decadt summarized the known literature published in the English language.[195] Local recurrence rates after RFA were reported as 1.5% to 28%, with the typical rate approximately 10%.

Recurrence is clearly related to tumor size and technique. Surgical ablations are associated with better tumor control than percutaneous ablation, but have a longer recovery time.[191] Elias et al used RFA for recurrences after liver resection to increase his local cure rate and decrease the need for resection.[196] Livraghi evaluated RFA in a series of 88 patients who had resectable metastases from colon cancer. He and his colleagues found they could get a complete ablation in 53 patients, thus 98% were spared surgical resection, either because they remained tumor free (44%) or developed additional metastases (56%).[197] For those using RFA, factors that increase survival include tumor size <3 and lower baseline CEA[198] There was a median survival of 38, 34, and 21 months for lesions <3 cm, 3–5 cm, and >5 cm, respectively (p = .03).[197] In an MD Anderson series of 348 patients, 190 had resection alone, 101 patients had RRA plus resection, and 57 had RFA alone. Recurrences were seen in 52%, 64%, and 84% of patients, respectively.[199] However, this is not a true comparison since RFA may have been preformed when resection was not possible. Pawlik reported a 25% 5-year survival in 124 patients with liver metastases from colon cancer using RFA, and resection in patients where resection alone was not possible.[200] RFA can also be used for other malignancies such as breast, with good results.[201] Livraghi reported on 24 breast cancer patients whose liver lesions were treated with RFA; 10 are still alive and free of disease with a median follow-up of 10 months.[202] In 240 patients with HCC and 44 patients with liver metastases treated with RFA, patients with liver metastases had a higher extrahepatic recurrence (p = .019) and shorter disease-free survival (p = .007).[203] In neuroendocrine tumors, RFA can relieve symptoms in 95% of patients.[204]

Radio frequency ablation is most useful for patients with hepatocellular cancer who also have cirrhosis. Curley and associates[205] presented a series of 110 patients with cirrhosis who received RFA for hepatocellular cancer, with no recurrences occurring in 50%. Curley reported on 110 HCC patients whose local recurrence was 3.6%, recurrence in liver 45%.[206] Toxicities from RFA have been outlined in a review of 312 patients (226 had percutaneous procedures).[207] The most frequent toxicities included liver abscesses (7), portal vein thrombosis (3), pleural effusion (5), colon perforation (1), and renal insufficiency (1).[207]

Compared with other ablative techniques, RFA is simpler to perform than cryotherapy. However, it is easier to assess areas of ablation during cryoablation, where the generated ice ball appears unequivocally as a homogeneous, hypoechoic lesion on ultrasound. Cryoablation allows ablation of larger lesions and has a longer track record.

As instrumentation improves to allow ablation of larger tumors and experience with these instruments increases, the indication for RFA will undoubtedly expand. These 2 ablative techniques will likely remain complementary techniques in the treatment of patients with metastatic colorectal cancer located predominantly within the liver.[208]

The most proven uses of ablative techniques for hepatic colorectal metastases are in combination with resection for patients with bilateral metastases.[184] Other indications include ablation after previous liver resection when a re-resection is not technically possible, or as primary local therapy when the patient with small tumors is medically unfit for surgery or unwilling to have surgery. Many ongoing studies are attempting to define the optimal chemotherapy to be administered after such ablative therapies.

The combination of RFA and HAI may be useful. In a small study of 50 patients, 32% remained tumor free at a 20-month median follow-up, with 10% recurrences at site and new liver metastases in 30%.[209] Martin treated 21 patients with RFA and HAI FUDR. With a follow-up of 24 months, the median survival is 30 months.

The most intriguing line of investigation related to ablative therapies is currently attempting to define the role of such therapies in patients with liver-predominant colorectal metastases. As most patients with liver metastases die of the liver disease, ablative therapies have become safe and effective at local control. Many patients have only limited extrahepatic disease that may be controllable by systemic therapies; investigators are attempting to determine if ablative therapies can add to effective systemic therapies in improving patient outcome. Currently a multicenter trial is randomizing patients with predominant liver metastases to systemic therapy versus combined liver tumor ablation with systemic therapy. Progression was documented in 65% of those receiving RFA and FOLFOX versus 86% in those receiving chemotherapy alone.[210] RFA may have a role during liver resection when one side is resected and small disease exists on the other side that cannot be resected. In patients who have undergone a resection and develop a small recurrence, percutaneous or laparoscopic RFA can be preformed if the lesion can be reached easily and is not close to large vessels. The presence of blood vessels near the tumors causes conduction of thermal energy away from the tumor and spares killing the tumor near the blood vessel.[195] The Europian Organisation for Research and Treatment of Cancer (EORTC) and additional studies of RFA in combination with other modalities will address the question of whether this RFA adds to other modalities.

Embolization

Normal liver parenchyma derives its nutrient blood supply from two sources: the hepatic artery and the portal vein. Of the two, the portal vein provides the majority of nourishment for a normal liver, and the hepatic artery can usually be ligated or occluded with little effect on liver function. Hepatic metastases, however, derive their blood supply from the hepatic artery. Interruption of the hepatic artery may preferentially injure liver tumors, while preserving liver function. The earliest attempts at arterial interruption involved surgical ligation of the hepatic artery. Although such ligations often produce necrosis and shrinkage of tumor, usually only a transient effect is achieved because of collateral vessels rapidly develop. Hepatic arterial ligation has therefore been largely abandoned in favor of transcutaneous embolization.[211] Embolization of oils, gelatin, plastic, collagen, or glass particles (Table 85-11) can interrupt arterial blood flow to tumors and has the advantage of being nonsurgical. Lipiodol is an ionized oil contrast medium that also can be used. It is taken up preferentially by hepatocellular carcinoma cells and retained for a long time after injection into the hepatic artery. Because of its selective uptake and retention, its main function is to act as a delivery system.[212] Moreover, such embolizations can be repeated to occlude collateral vessels that develop. Such therapy has become standard treatment for unresectable primary HCC. For metastatic cancers, however, the benefits are less clear, except in the case of metastatic neuroendocrine tumors.

A number of studies have been performed examining the utility of embolization for metastatic colorectal cancers to the liver. In a study randomizing 61 individuals with hepatic colorectal metastases to embolization, intraoperative embolization and hepatic artery ligation, or no treatment, median survivals were 9, 13, and 10 months, respectively.[213] In another study that examined 67 patients who were randomized to hepatic artery ligation alone or in conjunction with portal vein infusion of FU, there was only 1 response.[214] The median survival in both groups was 12 months. These studies suggest that arterial interruption is ineffective for colorectal cancer, not surprising, because hepatic metastases from colorectal cancer are not particularly vascular. For highly vascular tumors, such as metastatic neuroendocrine tumors, however, hepatic artery embolization (HAE) has a definite role to play.[215] Ajani and colleagues studied HAE in 22 patients with islet cell carcinoma, using polyvinyl alcohol particles (Ivalon) and gelatin sponge particles (Gelfoam). The median survival in this study was 33 months from initiation of embolization (range 1–72 months). Prospective studies have shown a decrease in tumor progression with transarterial embolization/transarterial chemoembolization (TAE/TACE) versus untreated controls.[216] In one study, patients had a partial response associated with subjective improvement and a decrease in hormone levels. Other studies corroborate these results,[215–219] and show HAE to be effective in symptomatic relief and in reducing circulating levels of secreted hormones. Some rare tumors such as ocular melanoma and GI stromal tumors with liver metastases have increased response rates with chemoembolization.[213,220]

Though embolization is relatively safe in patients without associated cirrhosis, many complications have been described. Common systemic symptoms include nausea, vomiting, fever, pain, and changes in liver function tests. Problems less commonly encountered but more ominous include (1) liver necrosis, (2) acute cholecystitis, (3) ischemic necrosis of the bowel by embolization of one of the vessels to the intestinal tract, (4) pancreatic infarction and pancreatitis by embolization of one of the pancreatic vessels, and (5) dyspnea by embolization of the lungs.[215–219] Rapid cell death may also result in tumor lysis syndrome, with symptomatic hyperuricemia leading to uric acid nephropathy and oliguria.

It is clear that morbidity and mortality are related to pre-embolization liver function status and amounts of tumor embolized. Patients with cirrhosis, portal vein occlusion, and biliary tract obstruction are usually excluded. When a large tumor burden is present, staged embolizations should be performed. Vigorous hydration and prophylactic allopurinol may also be indicated. In carcinoid tumors, HAE may cause a life-threatening carcinoid crisis with the rapid release of hormones from the tumor cells. Somatostatin analogues may be given, either prior to the procedure or if a carcinoid crisis occurs.

Chemoembolization

Chemoembolization is an extension of traditional percutaneous embolization techniques. With chemoembolization, investigators embolize tumors with Gelfoam or Ivalon particles soaked with chemotherapeutic agents. The theoretical advantage is that such embolizations will not only provide vascular occlusion but will produce sustained therapeutic levels of chemotherapy in the tumor areas. Generalized ischemia would reduce the ability of the cell to protect itself from the toxicity of chemotherapy. In human hepatoma and colon carcinoma cell cultures, hypoxia increased uptake of daunomycin.[220] Despite the widespread usage of such chemoembolization, few randomized studies have demonstrated that the theoretical advantage of adding chemotherapy to embolization translates into a clinical advantage. Llovet randomized 112 patients to (1) chemoembolization with doxorubicin and lipiodol; (2) embolization (Gelfoam particles only); and (3) symptomatic treatment. The 1-year, 2-year, and 3-year survival rates were 82%, 63%, and 29% for chemoembolization and 75%, 50%, and 29% for embolization.[221] Chemoembolization was associated with a reduced incidence of subsequent portal vein invasion.[222] Lin and colleagues,[223] Llovet et al.,[221] and Ikeda and colleagues[224] found no advantage in adding chemotherapy to embolization. Both the first and second studies show an advantage of embolization versus no treatment. The Groupe D'Etude de Traitment du Carcinome Hepatocellulaire randomized 96 patients to chemoembolization with lipiodol versus no treatment and found no increase in survival, although the treatment reduced tumor growth.[225] Llovet's review of the literature suggested chemoembolization does improve survival over control.[226] A meta-analysis found no difference of transarterial chemoembolization versus embolization in patients with HCC.[227] A few other meta-analyses have looked at chemoembolization or embolization in patients with HCC (Table 85-12).[228,229] In patients with hepatitis B a prospective study of TACE versus hepatic resection in HCC demonstrated a significant increase in survival with resection in the Cancer of the Liver-Italian Program (CLIP) 0 patients but no difference in resection versus TACE in the CLIP 1–2 subgroups.[230] Chemoembolization for liver metastases from colon cancer is less effective. Stagg and colleagues reviewed patients receiving chemoembolization: 19 of 84 (23%) patients with hepatoma responded versus 3 of 38 (9%) patients with colorectal cancer.[231] Other trials using chemoembolization are listed in Table 85-13. Although responses are high in some studies, most report median survivals of 7 to 8 months.

Another form of chemoembolization involves enclosing chemotherapeu-

Table 85-11 Chemoembolization for Hepatocellular Carcinoma (HCC)

	No. of Patients	Response (%)	1-Year Survival (%)
Pelletier[260]	37	24	51
Bruix[261]	40	55	70
Lo[262]	40	27	57
Ikeda[263]	20	70	75
Kawai[264]	208	-	69
Okamura[265]	58	19	86

Table 85-12 Agents Used for Embolization

Agents	Particle Size (μm)
Ivalon-polyvinyl alcohol foam	150–500
Collagen-angiostat	20–250
Gelfoam-gelatin sponge particles	1–2
Spherex-degradable starch micro	45

tic agents in a microsphere. Degradable starch microspheres injected intra-arterially are trapped in an extracapillary network formed in liver metastases.[232,233] The drug dissolved in the microsphere suspension will be retained in the blood vessels of the target organ as long as the blood flow is blocked, and then will gradually release the chemotherapeutic agents, resulting in a longer duration of tumor exposure to the drug. Use of such drug-containing microspheres is considered experimental, and should be performed within the confines of formal prospective investigations.

Radiation Therapy

External beam radiation, although effective in the treatment of primary tumors such as colorectal cancer, has not been widely used in treating liver metastases because of the low tolerance of normal hepatic parenchyma to radiation. Whole liver radiation with doses of >3500 cGy is associated with a significant likelihood of radiation hepatitis and liver failure.[234] External beam radiation effective palliates symptoms in approximately 60% of patients. Recently, 3 different strategies have increased the applicability of external beam radiation to treatment of liver metastases: (1) 3-dimensional (3-D) conformal radiation treatment planning,[235] (2) the delivery of radioisotopes, and (3) simultaneous administration of radiosensitizing chemotherapeutic agents. Lawrence and colleagues delivered smaller doses of radiation to the normal liver and larger doses to the tumor by conformal 3-D treatment planning.[236] Lawrence and colleagues produced a 48% response rate in previously treated patients. In 18 patients with colorectal cancer who had localized hepatic metastases, the median survival was 22 months. From their group, this technique of conformal RT and HAI of FUDR in 128 patients with intrahepatic malignancies produced a median survival of 15.8 months.[226] Response and survival for cholangiocarcinoma, colorectal, and HCC were 26%, 13.3 months; 59%, 17.2 months; and 40%, 15.2 months, respectively. Using 3-D conformal radiation to treat 37 patients with hepatocellular cancer who had failed or were not suited for embolization, Liu obtained a 64% response rate with a 2-year survival of 40%.[237] Other strategies for radioablation of liver tumors have attempted to selectively target tumors while minimizing radiation doses to normal parenchyma.

The main strategies that are being explored for specific radioablation of tumors are antibody-directed radioablation, radioembolization, and intraoperative interstitial irradiation using afterloading catheters. In antibody-directed radioablation, a radioisotope such as yttrium-90 or Re is attached to an antibody specific for the tumor, such as antibodies to CEA. It is hoped that injection of such radiolabeled antibodies will concentrate therapeutic radionuclides at the tumor sites.[238] Such an approach is still experimental, but has reached the stage of clinical trials for colorectal metastases. Results in the near future should define the utility of radioimmunotherapy.

Attempts have been made at radioembolization in order to deliver the therapeutic radionuclide physically to the liver tumor. Instillation of glass microspheres containing yttrium-90 into the hepatic artery is one approach. This isotope is a beta emitter with a half-life of 64 h and a mean energy of disintegration of 0.937. It has a mean tissue penetrance of 2.5 mm and maximum penetrance of 10 mm.[239] With these characteristics, yttrium-90 is well suited for localized internal radiation therapy. Gray and colleagues reported embolization of 10 patients with hepatic colorectal metastases in 1989.[240] The radiation doses ranged between 755 and 2500 MBq, and resulted in significant decreases in circulating CEA. No long-term results were reported. Herba and colleagues reported on yttrium-90 embolization of 12 metastatic colorectal cancers, 1 carcinoid and 1 islet cell tumor.[241] At 7-month follow-up, 10 patients had stable disease and 4 had progression. Andrews and colleagues reported on yttrium-90 embolization of 17 patients with colorectal metastases and 6 with metastatic neuroendocrine tumors.[242] Although doses of up to 12,500 cGy were relatively well tolerated, partial response was noted in only 5 patients.[242] In a small study, 21 patients with colorectal cancer were randomized to microspheres containing yttrium-90 plus 5FU/LV or 5FU/LV alone. The median survival was 29 and 13 months, respectively.[243] Using yttrium[90] microspheres with escalating doses of Oxa, Sharma et al found that the maximum tolerated dose (MTD) was 60 mg/m^2 for the first 3 cycles.[244] The progression-free survival (PFS) was 9.3 months and hepatic PFS was 12.3 months in 20 patients.[244] Sato et al reported on 137 patients who were chemotherapy refractory—43% responded to yttrium[90] microspheres injected inta-arterially[245] (51 patients had colon primaries, 19 had neuroendocrine primaries). Attempts have also been made to treat metastatic colorectal cancer by embolization with ^{131}I-labeled lipiodol, but with little success.[246] The reason that response rates for radioembolization of metastatic tumors are far less than those reported for treatment of primary HCC is that most metastatic tumors—except for neuroendocrine primaries—are far less vascular than HCC. Comparative trials of radioembolization to other treatment modalities need to be performed.

Percutaneous Ethanol Injection

Direct injection of absolute alcohol into a tumor produces tumor necrosis and death. The first attempts to use this modality to treat hepatic tumors were performed in Japan in 1983.[247] Under ultrasound guidance, up to 30 cc of ethanol

Table 85-13 Chemoembolization for Colon Cancer

Investigator	No. of Patients	Agent	Partial Response %	Median Survival (mo)
Daniels[263]	55	Collagen	34	–
		Cisplatin		
		Doxorubicin		
		Mitomycin-C		
Stuart[264]	20	FU	59	7
		Mitomycin-C		
		Ethiodized oil		
		Gelatin		
Tellez[265]	30	Angiostat	62	8
		Cisplatin		
		Adriamycin		
		Mitomycin-C		
Link[266]	17	Lipiodol	0	7
		Adriamycin		
Lang[267]	46	Lipiodol	17	–
		Doxorubicin	–	
Martinelli[268]	13	Polyvinyl	24	–
		Alcohol		
		FU and Interferon	–	
Stagg[269]	12	Gelfoam	0	–
		Doxorubicin		
		Mitomycin-C		
		Cisplatin		

can be injected percutaneously with the aim of ablating the tumor. The injections can also be guided by CT. In a report from Italy on 26 patients with metastatic disease, those with lesions of 2 cm had responses in 13 of 15 lesions; those with lesions of 2–3 cm had responses in 4 of 5 lesions, but in lesions of 4 cm, there were 0 of 6 responses.[248] Because of the relation of effectiveness to tumor size, most physicians performing percutaneous ethanol injection therapy (PEIT) will only treat <4 lesions, each being <4 cm in diameter. PEIT is most frequently used for treatment of primary hepatocellular carcinoma,[248–250] since the multifocal nature of the disease and the common association with cirrhosis often make resection of even small amounts of liver prohibitively dangerous. For metastatic disease to the liver, PEIT has been less helpful. Most cases of liver metastases are not associated with cirrhosis, so up to 80% of the liver can be resected with relatively low mortality. Most cases suitable for alcohol injection, therefore, are resectable. In addition, colorectal metastases, unlike hepatomas, are very hard tumors, making instillation of alcohol difficult. It is not surprising that the reported experience of alcohol injection for metastatic disease to the liver is modest, and no trial comparing PEIT with more accepted therapy has been published. In the largest study to date, Giovannini and Seitz gave alcohol injections to 40 patients who had metastatic disease to the liver.[251] These included 32 cases of colorectal cancer, 9 metastatic mammary cancers, 5 carcinoid tumors, 4 undifferentiated tumors, 3 uterine cancers, 1 esophageal cancer, and 1 bronchogenic carcinoma. No major complication was associated with such treatment. For patients with colorectal metastases, the median survival was 28 months, but there were no 4-year survivors. Amin and colleagues compared PEIT.[252] to interstitial photocoagulation. and had a median survival of 6.5 months with the alcohol treatments.

Alcohol injection is a rather safe procedure. However, the simplicity and effectiveness of RFA make it a much more attractive method of local tumor destruction for small tumors, although cryoablation remains the ablative treatment of choice for large tumors. Some advocate the use of PEIT and RFA or embolization together.[253]

Summary

Metastatic cancer is frequently found in the liver. For colorectal metastases in the liver, resection may be curative and should be considered standard therapy, if the liver is the only site of disease and resection is possible. For other metastatic tumors to the liver, the role of surgical resection remains to be defined. Even when resection cannot be performed with curative intent, cryoablation, intra-arterial chemotherapy, arterial embolization, conformal radiation and radioembolization are modalities that may provide effective palliation. The relative merits of each method of therapy in the various tumor types remains to be determined by ongoing and future clinical trials.

Selected References

The complete reference list can be found at www.CANCERMEDICINE8.com

1. Pickren JW, Tsukada Y, Lane W. Liver metastases: analysis of autopsy data. In: Weiss E, Gilbert H, eds. *Metastases*. Boston: GK Medical Publishers; 1982:2.
4. Jarnagin WR, Bach AM, Winston CB, et al. What is the yield of intraoperative ultrasonography during partial hepatectomy for malignant disease? *J Am Coll Surg*. 2001;192:577–583.
11. Fong Y, Saldinger PF, Akhurst T, et al. Utility of 18F-FDG positron emission tomography scanning on selection of patients for resection of hepatic colorectal metastases. *Am J Surg*. 1999;178:282–287.
15. Fong Y, Fortner J, Sun RL, Brennan MF, Blumgart LH. Clinical score for predicting recurrence after hepatic resection for metastatic colorectal cancer: analysis of 1001 consecutive cases. *Ann Surg*. 1999;230:309–318; discussion 18–21.
28. Kemeny N, Cohen A, Bertino JR, Sigurdson ER, Botet J, Oderman P. Continuous intrahepatic infusion of floxuridine and leucovorin through an implantable pump for the treatment of hepatic metastases from colorectal carcinoma. *Cancer*. 1990;65:2446–2450.
33. Scheele J, Stang R, Altendorf-Hofmann A. Hepatic metastases from colorectal carcinoma: impact of surgical resection on the natural history. *Br J Surg*. 1990;77:1241–1246.
45. Hughes KS, Simon R, Songhorabodi S, et al. Resection of the liver for colorectal carcinoma metastases: a multi-institutional study of patterns of recurrence. *Surgery*. 1986;100:278–284.
49. Choti MA, Sitzmann JV, Tiburi MF, et al. Trends in long-term survival following liver resection for hepatic colorectal metastases. *Ann Surg*. 2002;235:759–766.
58. Scheele J, Stang R, Altendorf-Hofmann A, Paul M. Resection of colorectal liver metastases. *World J Surg*. 1995;19:59–71.
63. Tomlinson JS, Jarnagin WR, DeMatteo RP, et al. Actual 10-year survival after resection of colorectal liver metastases defines cure. *J Clin Oncol*. 2007;25:4575–4580.
69. Nordlinger B, Vaillant J, Guigiet M, et al. A scoring system to select candidates for resection of colorectal liver metastases based on 1568 cases. *SSO Abstract Book*. 1996;17:11.
70. Are C, Gonen M, Zazzali K, et al. The impact of margins on outcome after hepatic resection for colorectal metastasis. *Ann Surg*. 2007;246:295–300.
71. Kornprat P, Jarnagin WR, Gonen M, et al. Outcome after hepatectomy for multiple (four or more) colorectal metastases in the era of effective chemotherapy. *Ann Surg Oncol*. 2007;14:1151–1160.
73. Elias D, Liberale G, Vernerey D, et al. Hepatic and extrahepatic colorectal metastases: when resectable, their localization does not matter, but their total number has a prognostic effect. *Ann Surg Oncol*. 2005;12:900–909.
77. Harrison L, Brennan M, Newman E, et al. Hepatic resection for noncolorectal, nonneuroendocrine metastases: a 15-year experience with 96 patients. *Surgery*. 1997;121:625.
79. Adam R, Chiche L, Aloia T, et al. Hepatic resection for noncolorectal nonendocrine liver metastases: analysis of 1,452 patients and development of a prognostic model. *Ann Surg*. 2006;244:524–535.
86. Kemeny N, Huang Y, Cohen AM, et al. Hepatic arterial infusion of chemotherapy after resection of hepatic metastases from colorectal cancer. *N Engl J Med*. 1999;341:2039–2048.
87. Kemeny MM, Adak S, Gray B, et al. Combined-modality treatment for resectable metastatic colorectal carcinoma to the liver: Surgical resection of hepatic metastases in combination with continuous infusion of chemotherapy—an intergroup study. *J Clin Oncol*. 2002;20:1499–1505.
88. Lorenz M, Muller H-H, Schramm H, et al. Randomized trial of surgery versus surgery followed by adjuvant hepatic arterial infusion with 5-fluorouracil and folinic acid for liver metastases of colorectal cancer. German Cooperative on Liver Metastases (Arbeitsgruppe Lebermetastasen). *Ann Surg*. 1998;228:756–762.
92. Kemeny N, Tong W, Gonen M, et al. Phase I study of weekly oxaliplatin plus irinotecan in previously treated patients with metastatic colorectal cancer. *Ann Oncol*. 2002;13(9):1490–1496.
96. Alberts SR, Horvath WL, Sternfeld WC, et al. Oxaliplatin, fluorouracil, and leucovorin for patients with unresectable liver-only metastases from colorectal cancer: a North Central Cancer Treatment Group phase II study. *J Clin Oncol*. 2005;23(36):9243–9249.
99. Clavien PA, Selzner N, Morse M, Selzner M, Paulson E. Downstaging of hepatocellular carcinoma and liver metastases from colorectal cancer by selective intra-arterial chemotherapy. *Surgery*. 2002;131:433–442.
102. Kemeny N, Fong Y, Jarnagin W, et al. Phase I trial of systemic oxaliplatin combination chemotherapy with hepatic arterial infusion in patients with unresectable liver metastases from colorectal cancer. *J Clin Oncol*. 2005;23:4888–4896.
103. Kemeny N, Huitzil M, Capanu M, et al. Conversion to resectability using hepatic artery infusion plus systemic chemotherapy for the treatment of unresectable liver metastases from colorectal carcinoma. Accepted in *J Clin Oncol*. 2009.
104. Adam R, Pascal G, Castaing D, et al. Tumor progression while on chemotherapy: a contraindication to liver resection for multiple colorectal metastases? *Ann Surg*. 2004;240:1052–1061; discussion 61–64.
105. Gallagher DJ, Zheng J, Capanu M, et al. Response to neoadjuvant chemotherapy does not predict overall survival for

patients with synchronous colorectal hepatic metastases. *Ann Surg.* 2009.

123. Breedis C, Young C. The blood supply of neoplasms in the liver. *Am J Pathol.* 1954;30:969.
133. Kemeny N, Daly J, Reichman B, Geller N, Botet J, Oderman P. Intrahepatic or systemic infusion of fluorodeoxyuridine in patients with liver metastases from colorectal carcinoma. A randomized trial. *Ann Intern Med.* 1987;107:459–465.
134. Hohn D, Stagg R, Friedman M, et al. A randomized trial of continuous intravenous versus hepatic intra-arterial floxuridine in patients with colorectal cancer metastatic to the liver: The Northern California Oncology Group Trial. *J Clin Oncol.* 1989;7:1646–1654.
137. Rougier P, Laplanche A, Huguier M, et al. Hepatic arterial infusion of floxuridine in patients with liver metastases from colorectal carcinoma: long-term results of a prospective randomized trial. *J Clin Oncol.* 1992;10:1112–1118.
138. Allen-Mersh T, Earlam S, Fordy C, Abrams K, Houghton J. Quality of life and survival with continuous hepatic artery floxuridine infusion for colorectal liver metastases. *Lancet.* 1994;344:1255–1260.
142. Kerr DJ, McArdle CS, Ledermann J, et al. Intrahepatic arterial versus intravenous fluorouracil and folinic acid for colorectal cancer liver metastases: a multicentre randomised trial. *Lancet.* 2003;361:368–373.
146. Allen P, Nissan A, Picon A, et al. Technical complications and durability of hepatic artery infusion pumps for unresectable colorectal liver metastases: an institutional experience of 544 consecutive cases. *J Am Coll Surg.* 2005.
171. Fraschini G, Fleishman G, Yap H-Y, et al. Percutaneous hepatic arterial infusion of cisplatin for metastatic breast cancer. *Cancer Treat Rep.* 1987;71:313–315.
173. Arai Y, Sone Y, Inaba Y, Ariyoshi Y, Kido C. Hepatic arterial infusion chemotherapy for liver metastases from breast cancer. *Cancer Chemother Pharmacol.* 1994;33(S): 142–144.
181. Morris D, Ross W. Australian experience of cryoablation of liver tumors: metastases. *Surg Oncol Clin NA.* 1996;5:391–397.
185. Gruenberger T, Jourdan JL, Zhao J, King J, Morris DL. Reduction in recurrence risk for involved or inadequate margins with edge cryotherapy after liver resection for colorectal metastases. *Arch Surg.* 2001;136:1154–1157.
191. Lencioni R, Goletti O, Armillotta N, et al. Radio frequency thermal ablation of liver metastases with a cooled-tip electrode needle: results of a pilot clinical trial. *Eur Radiol.* 1998;8:1205–1211.
194. Livraghi T, Solbiati L, Meloni MF, Gazelle GS, Halpern EF, Goldberg SN. Treatment of focal liver tumors with percutaneous radio-frequency ablation: complications encountered in a multicenter study. *Radiology.* 2003;226:441–451.
195. Decadt B, Siriwardena AK. Radio frequency ablation of liver tumours: systematic review. *Lancet Oncol.* 2004;5:550–560.
200. Pawlik TM, Izzo F, Cohen DS, Morris JS, Curley SA. Combined resection and radio frequency ablation for advanced hepatic malignancies: results in 172 patients. *Ann Surg Oncol.* 2003;10:1059–1069.
208. Bilchik AJ, Wood TF, Allegra D, et al. Cryosurgical ablation and radio frequency ablation for unresectable hepatic malignant neoplasms: a proposed algorithm. *Arch Surg.* 2000;135:657–662; discussion 62–64.
217. Carrasco C, Charnsanparej C, Ajani J, et al. The carcinoid syndrome: palliation by hepatic artery embolization. *AJR.* 1986;147:149–154.
221. Llovet JM, Real MI, Montana X, et al. Arterial embolisation or chemoembolisation versus symptomatic treatment in patients with unresectable hepatocellular carcinoma: a randomised controlled trial. *Lancet.* 2002;359:1734–1739.
226. Llovet JM, Bruix J. Systematic review of randomized trials for unresectable hepatocellular carcinoma: chemoembolization improves survival. *Hepatology.* 2003;37:429–442.
228. Reidy DL, Schwartz JD. Therapy for unresectable hepatocellular carcinoma: review of the randomized clinical trials-I: hepatic arterial embolization and embolization-based therapies in unresectable hepatocellular carcinoma. *Anticancer Drugs.* 2004;15:427–437.
236. Lawrence TS, Ten Haken RK, Kessler ML, et al. The use of 3-D dose volume analysis to predict radiation hepatitis. *Int J Radiat Oncol Biol Phys.* 1992;23:781–788.
240. Gray BN, Burton MA, Kelleher DK, Anderson J, Klemp P. Selective internal radiation (SIR) therapy for treatment of liver metastases: measurement of response rate. *J Surg Oncol.* 1989;42:192–196.
260 Smith GW, Bukowski RM, Hewlett JS, et al. Hepatic artery infusion of 5-fluorouracil and mitomycin C in cholangiocarcinoma and gallbladder carcinoma. *Cancer.* 1984;54:1513–1516.
261 Makela JT, Kairaluoma MI. Superselective intra-arterial chemotherapy with mitomycin for gallbladder cancer. *Br J Surg.* 1993;80:912–915.

86 Primary Neoplasms of the Liver

Max W. Sung, MD ■ Swan N. Thung, MD

The liver, next to lymph nodes, is the most frequent site of metastases from malignant tumors outside the liver. This is particularly true for the gastrointestinal cancers, with their direct venous drainage via the portal vein to the rich sinusoidal vascular network in the liver. These metastatic tumors are termed secondary hepatic neoplasms. Tumors can also arise directly from cells within the liver, and are termed primary hepatic neoplasms. Hepatocellular carcinoma (HCC), which arises from hepatocytes, constitutes 70–85% of primary hepatic neoplasms, while cholangiocarcinoma (intrahepatic bile duct cancer), which arises from cholangiocytes (epithelial cells lining bile ducts), constitutes 10–15% of primary hepatic neoplasms. The remaining 5% are uncommon tumors such as primary hepatic angiosarcoma, epithelioid hemangioendothelioma or hemangiopericytoma (arising from vascular lining cells), or primary hepatic lymphoma (arising from immune cells in the liver). This chapter will discuss separately HCC, cholangiocarcinoma, and the other less common primary liver cancers.

Hepatocellular Carcinoma

Epidemiology

Worldwide, primary liver cancer is the third leading cause of cancer deaths, and is the fifth and eighth most common new cancer in men and women, respectively. It is responsible for 680,000 deaths and 711,000 new cases per year (as estimated for 2007).[1]

The incidence of HCC is remarkable for its large geographical variation, from high incidence areas per 100,000 such as Mongolia (99), Korea (49), African Congo (32), Japan (29), to low incidence areas such as Northern Europe (3), Australia and New Zealand (4), and North America (4).[2] Of new cases 84% occur in developing countries, with 55% in China alone. This geographical variation is largely due to the geographical variations in risk factors, such as chronic hepatits B (HBV) and C (HCV) infections, alcohol abuse, and aflatoxin exposure.

Global trends in HCC incidence have recently shown an increase in low incidence areas (Europe, America) and a decrease in high incidence areas (China, India, Singapore), with the exception of Japan, a high incidence region where an increase in HCC has been noted.[3,4] These trends most likely reflect recent changes in the control of risk factors in the various regions.

The higher incidence of HCC in men compared to women has been shown across geographic regions, with generally higher male to female ratios in high incidence regions (3.7) compared to low incidence areas (2.0).[5] The incidence of HCC increases with increasing age, although the age at which this trend starts varies from region to region, depending on the mode of viral transmission and the risk factors involved. For instance, the age threshold is younger when the predominant risk factor is vertical transmission of HBV (Southeast Asia, Africa), and older with HCV acquired during adulthood (United States, Japan).[6]

Risk Factors

The most common risk factor for HCC is cirrhosis, which is present in 80–90% of HCC cases.[7,8] It is hypothesized that chronic hepatic necroinflammation from a variety of etiologies leads to cirrhosis and HCC due to increased hepatocyte regeneration and hyperplasia predisposing to mutations and malignant transformation. The time from chronic liver disease to cirrhosis and HCC may vary from an average of two decades in HBV and HCV infection, to only a few years for nonalcoholic steatohepatitis (NASH) and hereditary hemochromatosis.[9] One-fifth of HCC occurs in the absence of cirrhosis, and in these cases, a direct mutagenic effect from genetic events such as HBV DNA integration into host chromosomes and specific genetic mutations arising from aflatoxin exposure has been reported.

HBV and HCV ■ It has been estimated that 75–80% of HCC is associated with chronic infections with HBV (50–55%) or HCV (25–30%)[10]. Depending on the geographical region, the association with HBV and HCV varies from 60–20% in Asia and Africa to 20–60% in Japan, Europe, and North America.

For HBV, a direct mutagenic effect has been postulated, due to integration of HBV DNA in the host genome adjacent to cellular oncogenes or to the transactivating effect of the HBx protein on cellular gene expression.[11–13] The finding that 20% of HBV-related HCC occurs in the absence of cirrhosis suggests a direct effect of the virus. In contrast, HCV-related HCC virtually always occurs in the presence of cirrhosis or severe fibrosis, and may reflect the lack a direct mutagenic effect from genomic integration, which does not occur with HCV, an RNA virus.[14–16]

Transmission of HBV is via parenteral exposure such as during obstetric delivery (vertical transmission), blood transfusions, sexual intercourse, intravenous drug abuse, and close physical contact, particularly with infants and small children, who are at much higher risk (90%) for developing viral persistence following acute infection.[17,18] Transmission of HCV is also via parenteral exposure but primarily through blood transfusions and intravenous drug abuse.[19,20] The 5-year cumulative risk for developing HCC from HBV is 10% (North America and Europe) to 15% (Asia), and for HCV, 17% (North America and Europe) to 30% (Japan).

The development of effective blood donor screening for HBV in 1980 and HCV in 1990 has reduced the incidence of transfusion-associated viral hepatitis from 33% of hepatitis cases to 0.3% in the United States.[21] The development of effective HBV vaccines (>90%) for pre-exposure prophylaxis and in combination with hepatitis B immune globulin for post-exposure prophylaxis has dramatically reduced the incidence of HBV infection.[22,23] In Taiwan, the incidence of HCC in children following the institution of universal HBV vaccination has decreased from 0.70 per 100K to 0.35 per 100K.[24] The incidence of HCV has also decreased following blood donor screening in 1990, but because of the 20-year lag time from acute infection to cirrhosis and HCC, the impact of the decrease in HCV will not be seen until after the year 2015. In the meantime, it is expected that the incidence of HCV-related HCC will continue to increase. An effective vaccine against HCV has yet to be developed because of the high mutation rate of the virus. For patients with established chronic HBV or HCV infection, prior treatment with alpha interferon has been associated with reduced incidence of HCC (International Interferon-alpha Hepatocellular Carcinoma Study Group).[25–27] A reduction of serum HBV DNA titers over time, either spontaneously or through long-term treatment with nucleoside/nucleotide analogs, has been shown to be associated with a lower cumulative risk for developing HCC.[28] Long-term treatment with low-dose interferon for HCV, however, has not been shown to reduce HCC incidence (US HALT-C study).[29,30] These studies indicate that primary prevention of acute viral infection as well as the effective treatment of chronic infection may reduce the incidence of HCC in the near future.

Alcohol ■ Oral ingestion of alcohol produces a spectrum of liver impairment, from fat accumulation and acute necroinflammation to cirrhosis. HCC generally does not develop in the absence of cirrhosis, and risk is increased with concurrent HBV or HCV infection.[16] The 5-year cumulative risk for HCC in alcoholic cirrhosis is 8%. Cessation of alcohol intake may reduce the risk of progression to cirrhosis, and may accelerate the growth of established HCC.

Aflatoxins ■ Aflatoxins are potent hepatocarcinogens produced by fungi and are contaminants in stored grains. When controlled for HBV infection, HCC incidence in Africa varied 5-fold and is correlated with the extent of aflatoxin exposure in the diet.[31] A consistent genetic mutation in codon 249 of the tumor suppressor p53 gene (GC to TA transversion) has been identified and positively correlated with aflatoxin exposure in a meta-analysis of 49 studies.[32,33] Aflatoxins are synergistic with chronic HBV infection towards the development of HCC. Primary prevention measures include improving grain storage to avoid moldy contamination, and tighter regulation of aflatoxin content in foods prepared from stored grains. Secondary prevention measures take into account the metabolic pathways of aflatoxin (metabolic activation to carcinogenic intermediates and detoxification of these intermediates by conjugation). For instance, Oltipraz in clinical trials has been shown to inhibit metabolic activation and enhance detoxification, with corresponding decrease in affatoxin conjugates in the urine.[34] Alternatively, chlorophyllin can reduce bioavailability of dietary aflatoxin by forming complexes with aflatoxin and inhibiting their absorption.

Obesity and Diabetes ■ With the increasing prevalence of obesity and diabetes mellitus in developed countries, the association with HCC has raised public health concerns. In epidemiologic studies, the relative risk of HCC for obesity has been shown to increase to 4.52 for men and to 1.69 for women.[36] For diabetes, the risk of HCC was increased 4-fold and 2.1-fold in a Danish study for men and women, respectively.[37] Of obese individuals, 90% have fatty livers, ranging from nonalcoholic fatty liver disease (NAFLD) to NASH.[38] Progression to cirrhosis occurs in 8–26%, after which there is an increased risk for malignant transformation to HCC.[39,40] Pathogenetic mechanisms include lipid peroxidation and free radical oxidative stress as tumor initiation and promotion steps, chronic activation of inhibitor kinase kappa beta leading to inflammation, and hepatic fibrosis due to hyperinsulinemia and hyperglycemia.[41] Primary prevention of obesity includes the promotion of healthy dietary habits. There has been however no evidence that HCC incidence can be reduced with secondary prevention measures such as weight loss and medical interventions.[42] Of concern is the development of portal inflammation and fibrosis in morbidly obese individuals who underwent rapid weight loss of more than 1.6 kg per week.[43]

Hemochromatosis ■ Hemochromatosis is an autosomal recessive disorder with a prevalence rate of 2–5 per 1,000 in the Caucasian population. In this inherited disorder, mutations have been documented in the HFE gene on chromosome 6 (C282Y and H63D), the HFE-2 gene on chromosome 1, and the HFE-3 gene on chromosome 7. The increased absorption of dietary iron and accumulation in tissues such as the skin, heart, and liver leads to heart failure and cirrhosis, primarily in C282Y homozygotes and C282Y/H63D compound heterozygotes.[44] The 5-year cumulative risk for HCC in hemochromatosis-associated cirrhosis (21%), even higher than for HCV cirrhosis in Europe and North America.[20] Primary prevention includes the screening of first-degree relatives of hemochromatosis patients for C282Y and H63D mutations; homozygotes should be checked for elevation in serum ferritin and transferrin saturation. Treatment with therapeutic phlebotomy or iron chelation therapy prior to onset of cirrhosis may be effective in preventing the development of cirrhosis and HCC in these patients.

Alpha-1-Antitrypsin Deficiency ■ Alpha-1-antitrypsin is an autosomal recessive disorder with mutations in the serine protease inhibitor gene, alpha-1-antitrypsin.[45] The disorder, which has codominant expression for each allele, causes impaired transport of the inhibitor protein from hepatocytes, leading to accumulation in the liver and decreased circulating serum concentrations of the protein. Clinically, patients with alpha-1-antitrypsin deficiency develop emphysema (even in the absence of smoking), hepatic necroinflammation, cirrhosis, and HCC.[46] There is currently no evidence that medical treatment, which enhances secretion of the inhibitor protein and increases intrahepatic degradation, is clinically effective. For patients with decompensated cirrhosis, liver transplantation is effective in correcting the underlying metabolic disorder.

Hormonal Factors

The higher incidence of HCC reported in males when compared to females suggest the influence of hormonal factors on hepatocarcinogenesis. Long-term use of oral contraceptives for women or anabolic steroids has been associated with the development of HCC.[47] The exact pathogenetic mechanisms are not known, but it is known that normal hepatocytes express estrogen, progesterone, and androgen receptors, and that a subgroup of HCC in males expresses variant forms of the estrogen receptor, which do not bind to antiestrogens.[48] Hypothyroidism has been reported to be associated with a 2.1-fold excess risk of HCC compared to controls, but this effect was noted only in women.[49] The pathogenetic mechanism for this association is not understood.

Pathology (Fig. 86-1A and 86-1B)

The malignant transformation of hepatocytes to HCC is a multistep process associated with genetic mutations, allelic losses, epigenetic alterations, and perturbation of molecular cellular pathways. The phenotypic expression of these changes can be manifested by precursor lesions, which accompany HCC spatially and temporally and are termed dysplastic nodules.[50,51] These nodules are distinct

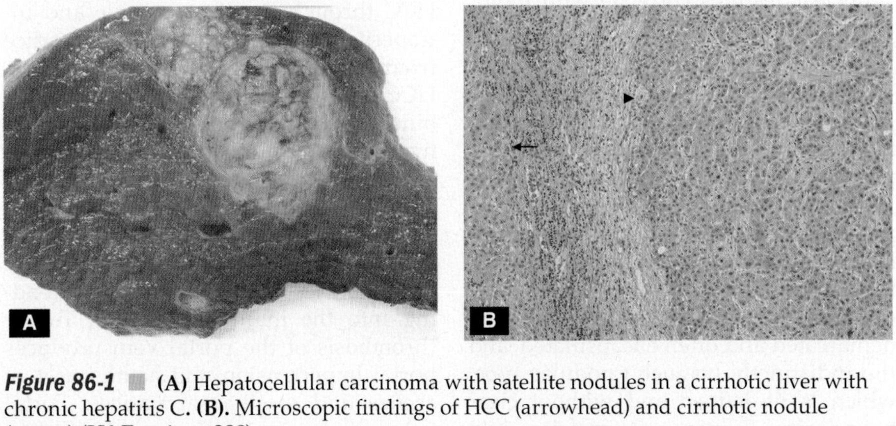

Figure 86-1 ■ **(A)** Hepatocellular carcinoma with satellite nodules in a cirrhotic liver with chronic hepatitis C. **(B).** Microscopic findings of HCC (arrowhead) and cirrhotic nodule (arrow) (H&E stain, ×200).

from the benign regenerative nodules associated with cirrhosis by virtue of their high proliferative index and clonality. The International Working Party of the World Congress of Gastroenterology classified dysplastic nodules, which are distinctly nodular lesions greater than 5 mm in diameter into low-grade dysplastic nodule (LGDN) and high-grade dysplastic nodules (HGDN).[52] LGDNs show only mild dysplasia and have no link to neoplasia. In contrast, HGDNs are characterized by higher cell density (small cell change) than the surrounding tissue, exhibit nodule-in-nodule formation, and closely resemble well-differentiated HCCs both on radiologic and pathologic examination.[53] Distinguishing HGDNs from early HCCs is an unresolved challenge. A panel of 3 immunohistochemical markers of malignant transformation: heat shock protein 70, glutamine synthetase, and glypican 3 has been used to separate HCCs from HGDNs.[54] Molecular data based on quantitative gene expression profiles of 3 genes, LYVE1, E-cadherin, and survivin allow a reliable diagnosis of early HCC.[55]

While genetic profiling of HCC most likely will allow more effective and targeted therapy for patients with HCC, gross and microscopic characteristics of HCC have been widely used to correlate with the natural history of the disease and with prognosis.

1. Tumors that grossly are classified as spreading, infiltrative, or diffuse would be more rapidly progressive and would have a worse prognosis than those that are solitary, although this has never been proven.
2. "Encapsulated" HCCs, which almost always arise in cirrhotic livers, tend to be solitary and slow growing; and pedunculated HCCs, due to their resectability, have a relatively good prognosis.[56]
3. The different microscopic variants of HCC, such as pseudoglandular or spindle cell features, do not seem to have any clinical significance.
4. The degree of tumor differentiation and Edmonson and Steiner grading of nuclear features correlate with tumor growth rate and survival.[50,51]

Early HCC

Advances in diagnostic imaging modalities and the establishment of screening protocols in populations at high risk for HCC have made detection of early HCC possible. Early HCC is grossly a small HCC of up to around 2 cm in diameter. It is classified into 2 types: small HCC of distinctly nodular type, which is well demarcated and often encapsulated, and the indistinctly (vaguely) nodular type, which is ill-defined and without clear boundaries. Tumor cell invasion into the portal vein and minute intrahepatic metastases adjacent to the tumor are observed in distinctly nodular small HCCs, but not the distinctly nodular small HCCs.[57,58]

Progenitor Cell HCC

Hepatic progenitor cell marker CK19 is expressed during embryonic and fetal life.[59,60] Expression of this oncofetal antigen in a number of HCC suggests that transformation of progenitor cells in the liver can give rise to the cancer.[61] Transformation of liver progenitor cells may result in HCC, cholangiocarcinoma, mixed forms of HCC and cholangiocarcinoma, or cholangiolocellular carcinoma.[62–65] Furthermore, several studies have correlated CK19 expression in HCC with worse prognosis, faster recurrence after surgical treatment, and distant metastases.[66,67] Combined or mixed hepatocellular-cholangiocarcinoma accounts for approximately 1–2% of HCCs. The clinical behavior of these tumors is similar to HCC.[68]

Vascular Invasion in HCC

Vascular invasion, usually classified as gross or microscopic, has been identified as a risk factor for tumor recurrence following hepatic resection.[69,70] Microvascular invasion represents a wide spectrum, between no invasion and gross vascular invasion, however. Histological features of microvascular invasion that include invasion of a vessel with a muscular wall and invasion of vessels more than 1cm from the tumor border do have adverse prognostic significance.

Clinical Presentation and Natural History

Dysplastic nodules and early HCC are generally asymptomatic and are usually incidental findings on radiographic studies or detected as a result of screening procedures. Early HCC may remain indolent or slow growing for up to 1 year before seeming to undergo more rapid tumor progression. Symptoms may include upper abdominal pain from distention of the liver capsule, acute pain with vascular collapse from rupture of HCC through the liver capsule and intraperitoneal hemorrhage, and jaundice from biliary tract obstruction by tumor. HCC may also present with hyperbilirubinemia without biliary obstruction or hypercalcemia without bone metastases as a paraneoplastic syndrome.

HCC, in its early stages, generally progresses stepwise, with increase in tumor size, followed by invasion directly into branches of the portal vein, extending into the main portal vein. Tumor thrombosis of the portal vein produces portal hypertension and acute onset of ascites and esophageal varices. Portal vein invasion is usually accompanied by a rapid increase in serum AFP despite no changes in the size of the primary tumor in the liver. The tumor can also invade directly into branches of the hepatic veins or into the intrahepatic inferior vena cava, then propagating as a tumor thrombu to the superior vena cava and into the right atrium. Invasion into the hepatic artery is much less common.

Dissemination of HCC occurs in later stages, and is primarily via the blood stream to the lungs, bones, and brain. These metastatic lesions are typically hypervascular like the primary tumor and predispose to bleeding (hemoptysis and intracranial hemorrhage). Metastatic involvement of the bones may be solitary or multiple and can produce isolated symptomatology such as cranial or peripheral nerve compression.

Multiple tumors in the liver may arise from multiple primary tumors in a cirrhotic liver, particularly with chronic HCV infection, or may represent hepatic metastases from tumor thrombosis of the portal from the primary tumor and hematogenous dissemination back to the liver. The distinction between multifocal HCC and intrahepatic metastases is important since the former tend to respond better to regional therapeutic approaches and liver transplantation.

Malignant ascites and peritoneal carcinomatosis are rare in HCC and are generally associated with prior tumor rupture with intraperitoneal hemorrhage, or contamination of the peritoneum during percutaneous needle biopsy or hepatic resection.

The prognosis for patients with HCC is dismal. Overall survival varies from several weeks to 1 year depending on extent of tumor involvement and other prognostic factors.

Diagnosis

The American Association for the Study of Liver Diseases (AASLD) has previously issued its guidelines for the diagnosis of HCC.[71] These guidelines suggest that, for patients with cirrhosis, a liver mass detected on a radiographic study does not need biopsy confirmation for the diagnosis of HCC: the liver lesion must however be at least 2 cm in diameter, and exhibit typical vascular patterns on dynamic imaging with CT scan, contrast ultrasound, or MRI (enhancement during arterial phase with washout during portal venous phase). For lesions between 1cm and 2 cm in diameter, 2 dynamic imaging studies with typical enhancement characteristics of HCC are required. Lesions less than 1 cm in diameter should be followed with ultrasound every 3–6 months. These guidelines are supported by the high incidence of regenerative nodules in cirrhotic livers that remain stable for many years, but can undergo malignant transformation to HCC with a shift in vascular supply from the portal vein to the hepatic artery and an increase in size. Hence, HCC can be isodense on single-phase contrast CT scan, but detectable with triple phase or dual phase dynamic contrast CT, where the scans are performed serially without contrast, during the arterial phase and during the portal venous phase. Percutaneous biopsy of a liver lesion in a cirrhotic patient has an increased risk for hemorrhage, seeding of the needle track with malignant cells, and false negative results due to inaccurate radiographic localization particularly with small lesions.

Serum AFP, a normal glycoprotein produced by the fetal liver and yolk sac, may become elevated with the development of HCC. AFP is particularly indicative if the level is higher than 500 mcg/L (normal range 10–20 mcg/L).[72] Up to 20% of HCC are not associated with a high serum AFP, however, and moderate elevations of AFP can be found in other conditions such as active hepatic inflammation from any etiology (virus, drugs, autoimmune), fetal abnormalities such as spina bifida in a pregnant patient, and other cancers such as germ cell and gastric cancers. A consistent rising serum AFP in a patient with chronic liver disease without active hepatic inflammation (normal liver function tests) is suspicious for HCC and radiographic investigation should be initiated. The use of serum AFP has also been found to enhance the sensitivity of non-contrast ultrasound, from 71% to 29%, in the screening of high-risk individuals for early HCC.[73]

For the detection of metastatic disease from HCC, CT scans with contrast of the head, chest, abdomen, and pelvis and radionuclide bone scans are standard tests. Dynamic contrast is not generally necessary, but if used, can demonstrate the same type of arterial enhancement in the metastatic lesions as in the primary tumor. PET scanning with 19F-Flurodency glucose has not been found to be consistently reliable to warrant routine testing in HCC staging. Malignant portal venous involvement is generally detected as a filling defect in the portal vein on dynamic imaging or duplex Doppler ultrasound examination.

Staging

Due to the close association of HCC with cirrhosis, the prognosis of individual cases depends both on the extent of malignant involvement and the severity of cirrhosis. Most of the staging systems for HCC prognosis incorporate both elements of tumor extent and severity of cirrhosis, and differ by the elements chosen for each system. TNM parameters for T include size, multifocality, bilaterality, gross vascular involvement, and distant metastases, but do not include cirrhosis parameters.[74]

Cirrhosis parameters as used in the Child-Pugh scoring system to predict prognosis of patients with cirrhosis are incorporated in most staging systems including the CLIP (Cancer of the Liver Italian Program score), JIS (Japan Integrated Staging score), CUPI (Chinese University Prognostic Index), and French Prognostic Classification.[75–77] The BCLC (Barcelona Clinic Liver Cancer) system includes, in addition, a treatment algorithm based on staging.[78] There is currently no consensus as to the most predictive staging system worldwide.

The Child-Pugh scoring system for cirrhosis assigns points to serum bilirubin, serum albumin, prothrombin time, ascites, and encephalopathy, the sum of which places patients into A, B, and C categories.[79] The 1-year survival of non-HCC patients with Child-Pugh A, B, and C has been reviewed and was 67%, 37%, and 18%. The CLIP scoring system, which assigns a maximum of 6 points to Child-Pugh status, tumor extent, serum AFP, and macrovascular invasion, has been reviewed for prognostic prediction in HCC patients. The 1-year survival of HCC patients according to CLIP score was reported as 92% (0), 80% (1), 52% (2), 37% (3), 4% (4), 0% (5), and 0% (6). CLIP is widely used in clinical trials of HCC.

BCLC stages HCC patients as very early, early, intermediate, advanced, and terminal, based on Child-Pugh status, performance status, tumor size, multifocality, and presence of portal vein invasion. BCLC also offers a treatment algorithm based on staging. Patients with very early or early stages are amenable to curative treatment modalities including resection, orthotopic liver transplantation (OLT), percutaneous ethanol injection, or radiofrequency thermo-ablation, while patients with intermediate stage are amenable to treatment with chemoembolization. For advanced stage patients, recommended treatment includes sorafenib or enrollment in clinical trials of investigative agents. Terminal stage patients are generally not considered eligible for sorafenib treatment or clinical trials, and are best treated for symptom control.

There will most likely be modifications to existing classification schemes as well as newer staging systems for both prognosis and treatment of HCC as more is known regarding the natural history and response to treatment of the different subgroups of HCC patients.

Treatment

The stepwise progression of HCC, from tumor(s) only in the liver to portal venous involvement and distant metastases, allows for treatment approaches suitable for each stage of the disease. The safety of these treatment modalities depends on the severity of chronic liver disease or cirrhosis as well as other comorbid medical conditions.

Surgical Resection ■ For HCC limited to the liver, surgical resection with curative intent provides superior long-term survival when compared to non-surgical treatment modalities. However, only 10-15% of patients with newly diagnosed HCC are suitable candidates for surgical resection: tumors must be confined to a single lobe amenable to an anatomic resection, there must be no portal venous involvement, and the uninvolved liver must have adequate function and reserve to sustain a hepatic resection without post-operative liver failure. When these conditions are met, post-operative mortality can be reduced to 0.8%, and 5-year survival can be as high as 78%.[80,81]

The assessment of adequate hepatic reserve depends on the extent of planned hepatic resection and the volume of liver remaining post-resection. The post-resection liver volume can be increased by pre-operative portal venous embolization of the lobe planned for resection, which results in hypertrophy of the unembolized lobe.[82] In addition, the uninvolved liver should be functioning well, as evidenced by Child-Pugh status A, normal serum bilirubin, and, optionally, absence of portal hypertension as measured by wedged hepatic venous pressure gradient, and clearance of indocyanine green at 15 minutes.

Poor prognostic factors following hepatic resection include tumor size (>5 cm), vascular invasion, resection margins of less than 0.5 cm, pre-operative serum AFP greater than 10,000 ng/mL, absence of a tumor capsule and poorly differentiated histology. Tumor recurrence is unfortunately high: 50-60% at 3 years and 70-100% at 5 years post-resection. There is no evidence to support the use of adjuvant chemotherapy or transarterial chemoembolization.[83] However, adjuvant transarterial radioembolization using 1–131 lipiodol has been in shown in a randomized controlled trial to result in a significant increase in disease-free survival and overall survival at 5 years: 62% and 67%, respectively, in the treated group compared to 36% and 38% in the control group.[84]

Orthotopic Liver Transplantation ■ OLT is theoretically an ideal treatment modality for patients with HCC since it can remove both the tumors as well as the chronically diseased liver, thereby eliminating the potential complications of end stage liver disease as well as the source for subsequent HCC. The disadvantages are the complications of drugs administered post-OLT to prevent allograft rejection, which can induce diabetes and chronic renal insufficiency, as well as increase the risks for the development of other cancers such as Kaposi's sarcoma and post-transplant lymphoproliferative disease. For patients with HCC in the absence of cirrhosis, hepatic resection produces no differences in survival at 3 and 4 years when compared to OLT, and without the added complications of chronic immunosuppression. For patients with HCC in the presence of cirrhosis, however, survival outcomes are superior for OLT compared to hepatic resection.[85]

OLT series in the past have shown that overall survival is the same at 5 and 10 years for patients transplanted for the treatment of HCC are comparable to patients transplanted for non-malignant reasons. This is seen for patients with HCC of 5 cm or less; patients with larger tumors or associated with vascular invasion, however, have tumor recurrence within 1 year and poor survival outcomes. These outcomes reported for early HCC prompted the organization that allocates donor organs in the United States (United Network for Organ Sharing-UNOS) to adopt guidelines to expedite OLT for patients with Stage II HCC (American Liver Tumor Study Group), defined as single tumor between 2cm and 5 cm, or 2 or 3 tumors none greater than 3 cm. These guidelines are also called the Milan criteria.[86] Retrospective studies of HCC patients who have undergone OLT have been conducted to see if the Milan criteria can be expanded and still retain the survival benefits of OLT. For patients who exceeded the Milan criteria who had 4 nodules, with the largest nodule measuring 4 cm., 5 year survival was 53.6% compared to 73.3% for patients who met Milan criteria.[87] These data suggest that transplant criteria can be expanded beyond the Milan criteria. Other countries which perform OLT may not follow the restrictions of the Milan criteria and may have shorter waiting times, while some countries have cultural obstacles to organ donation and limited OLT services.

Local-Regional Treatment Modalities for HCC ■ For HCC patients who are not candidates for hepatic resection, the liver tumors may be ablated by a variety of methods.

Percutaneous Ethanol Intra Tumora Ablation (PEIT) ■ Ethanol mediates destruction of tissues on direct contact and has been used to inject directly into small liver tumors. The procedure is generally performed by percutaneous injection of small aliquots of 95% ethanol directly into the tumors in separate injections twice a week for 4–12 sessions. The procedure is relatively low-invasive and low-cost, but requires operator expertise to inject into all parts of the tumors. Tumors smaller than 5 cm in diameter are effectively treated by PEIT, although the local recurrence rates are high for tumors larger than 3 cm. 3- and 5-year survival rates for solitary tumors less than 5 cm treated with PEIT are 79% and 47%, respectively. Larger tumors can be treated in a single session with a large volume of ethanol during laparoscopy under general anesthesia.

Cryoablation ■ Liquid nitrogen at-70°C is effective in mediating destruction of tumor tissues. The liquid nitrogen is circulated via a probe placed with the tip in the center of a liver tumor. The tumor is allowed to freeze (monitored by concurrent ultrasound monitoring) to beyond the margins, then allowed to thaw. Generally, at least two freeze-thaw cycles are required to completely ablate the tumor. The procedure can be performed under general anesthesia via laparoscopy or laparotomy, or percutaneously under ultrasound visualization.

Radiofrequency Thermoablation (RFA) ■ Heat above 60°C generated by high frequency alternating current can be used to directly destroy tumors. The heat is delivered by percutaneous or laparoscopic placement of a probe directly into the liver tumor under ultrasound guidance. The probe contains of small tines containing electrodes, which can be extended within the tumor to 2–4 cm, thereby allowing heat to be generated throughout the tumor, and permitting effective treatment of tumors up to 5 cm in diameter. 5-year survival of 63% has been reported following RFA of tumors not greater than 2 cm. Small randomized trials have shown that tumors not greater than 5 cm treated with either RFA or hepatic resection had similar overall and disease-free survival at 3 and 4 years.

Transarterial Chemoembolization (TACE) ■ The liver as an organ is unique in having a dual blood supply from the hepatic artery and the portal vein, meeting in the hepatic sinusoids, and draining out of the liver via the hepatic veins. HCC is supplied primarily by the hepatic artery while the liver parenchyma is supplied primarily by the portal vein. Delivery of chemotherapy as well as embolic particulates will therefore target HCC while sparing the normal liver. Hepatic arterial delivery of chemotherapeutic agents therefore has a pharmacokinetic advantage over systemic delivery; the undiluted drug is delivered directly to the hepatic tumor, and if metabolized by the liver, exits the liver with a lower drug concentration, there by reducing adverse effects to organs supplied by the systemic circulation. The addition of embolic particles reduces blood flow and enhances the pharmacokinetic advantage of hepatic arterially delivered chemotherapy, while the embolization reduces oxygen and nutrient supply resulting in anoxic damage to the tumor.

Transarterial chemoembolization is generally performed by catheterization of the femoral artery and threading the catheter via the aorta to the hepatic artery. A hepatic angiogram is then performed to assess patency of the portal vein with centrifugal flow, absence of arteriovenous or arterioportal shunting, and to demonstrate a hypervascular tumor blush indicating hepatic arterial supply to the tumor. The dose and type of chemotherapy drugs for TACE have not been well defined, but generally single agent doxorubicin or triple drug combination of doxorubicin, mitomycin, and cisplatin have been used. These drugs are extracted to varying extents by the liver and hence derive pharmacokinetic advantage from hepatic arterial delivery. The chemotherapy agents are generally mixed with either lipiodol, which can enhance delivery of the drug to the tumor, or with embolizing agents to benefit from the reduced blood flow and prolonged exposure of the tumor to the chemotherapeutic agents. It is not clear if lipiodol confers additional activity to the TACE procedure, or which embolizing agent is optimal. Generally, smaller size embolizing particles (<100 um) provides more ischemic embolizing effects than larger size particles. Degradable embolizing particles are preferable to agents that produce permanent obstruction in order to facilitate repeated TACE treatments. Examples of embolizing agents used for TACE include gel foam, microfibrillar collagen, embospheres, and DC beads (Polymeric Polyvinyl alcohol spherules). DC beads are unique in that they can be loaded with doxorubicin which is then slowly released from the beads following embolization in the tumor vessels. A number of controlled trials have been reported for TACE versus supportive care, some with negative and others with positive results. 2 meta-analyses of these trials have been reported which showed statistically significant improvement in 2-year survival when compared to supportive care or suboptimal therapy.[88,89] Overall survival ranges from 57% (1 year) and 26% (3 years) in one series to 82% (1 year) and 63% (2 years) in another series.[90] Adverse effects of TACE include transient hepatic dysfunction, occasional myelosuppression, and hepatic failure, particularly in patients with elevated bilirubin or hepatic encephalopathy pre-TACE.

Systemic Treatment Initial reports in 1975 of the activity of single agent doxorubicin administered intravenously at a dose of 75 mg/m^2 in HCC (3/13 compete responses, 11/13 response rate, median survival 8 months) was unfortunately not repeated in subsequent trials of doxorubicin, where median survival averaged 3 months.[91] A small randomized trial of doxorubicin 60 mg/m^2 versus supportive care in 106 patients showed a median survival of 10.6 versus 7.5 weeks for the control group (p <0.036).[92] The response rate was 3%, and treatment-related mortality occurred in 25%, underlying the inclusion of patients with severe hepatic dysfunction in the trial. The combination of cisplatin, interferon-alpha, doxorubicin, and 5-fluorouracil (PIAF) produced 26% response rates with a median survival of 9 months in a phase 2 trial, but randomized phase 3 trial of PIAF versus doxorubicin showed no superiority in response rates or survival benefit (median survival 8.7 vs 6.8 months, NS).[93] Following promising results in single-arm trials, nolatrexed was evaluated in a large phase 3 randomized controlled trial in HCC with doxorubicin as the control treatment with 445 patients. Nolatrexed showed minimal activity for the treatment of HCC; median survival was 22.3 weeks for nolatrexed and 32.3 weeks for doxorubicin, (HR = 0.753).[94] Response rate was 1.4% for nolatrexed and 4.0% for doxorubicin.

Following promising results in a phase 2 trial in HCC,[95] sorafenib, a multi-targeted tyrosine kinase inhibitor was shown in a large randomized placebo-controlled phase 3 trial in patients with HCC and Child-Pugh status to have a survival advantage at the prespecified second interim analysis.[96] The trial enrolled 602 patients; median survival was 10.7 months in the sorafenib group compared to 5.9 months in the placebo group (HR = 0.69, p = 0.00058). There were, however, no complete responses; partial responses by RECIST criteria were noted in 2.3% in the sorafenib group compared to 0.7% in the placebo group. These trials provided the basis for FDA approval of sorafenib for the treatment of patients with unresectable HCC in November 2007. A similar phase 3 trial for unresectable HCC in Asian patients showed the same survival benefit when compared to placebo.[97] Adverse effects included diarrhea, hand-foot syndrome, rash, cardiac ischemia, and hypertension. It should be noted that the phase 2 trial of sorafenib included Child-Pugh status A and B patients, and elevations in serum bilirubin were seen in 40% of Child-Pugh B patients compared to 18% of Child-Pugh A patients. Treatment of HCC patients with Child-Pugh status B with sorafenib should therefore be approached with great caution.

Other targeted therapies have been evaluated in phase 2 trials, including the EGFR inhibitor erlotinib (median survival 13.0 months),[98] the anti-EGFR monoclonal antibody cetuximab (median survival 9.6 months),[99] and the anti-VEGF monoclonal antibody bevacizumab (median survival 12.4 months).[100] A phase 2 trial of erlotinib in combination with bevadizumab showed response rates of 21% and a median survival of 19 months.[101] Survival advantage of doxorubicin plus sorafenib compared to doxorubicin plus placebo (median survival 6.9 vs 2.4 months) has been referred in a randomized double-blind phase 2 trial.[102] This survival benefit could have been due to the effect of sorafenib. A phase 3 trial in HCC is currently in progress to evaluate if doxorubin plus sorafenib confers a survival advantage to sorafenib alone.

Cholangiocarcinoma

Cholangiocarcinomas, commonly called intrahepatic bile duct cancers, arise from cholangiocytes which are epithelial cells lining intrahepatic bile ducts and ductules. These tumors are distinct from extrahepatic bile duct and gallbladder cancers, which arise from epithelial lining of the extrahepatic biliary system.

Cholangiocarcinomas are responsible for 10–15% of primary liver cancer, while HCC accounts for 70–85%.

Epidemiology

As with HCC, there is a large geographical variation in the incidence of cholangiocarcinoma worldwide, ranging from 96 per 100,000 in men in Thailand to 0.85 per 100,000 in men in North America.[6] This variation is most likely due to the geographical variation in risk factors associated with the development of cholangiocarcinomas. In the United States, the incidence has been rising, from 0.32 per 100,000 (1975–1979) to 0.85 (1995–1999), a 165% increase.[103] The incidence of cholangiocarcinoma in men is higher than in women, possibly because one of the major risk factors, primary sclerosing cholangitis, is seen predominantly in men.

Risk Factors

The major pathogenetic mechanism for the development of cholangiocarcinoma is chronic inflammation of the bile ducts, which results in generation of reactive oxygen species, local production of cytokines such as interleukin 6 and hepatocyte growth factor, and increase in cholangiocyte proliferation and cell turnover. The 3 main conditions associated with chronic bile duct inflammation are:

1. Primary sclerosing cholangitis, which confers a lifetime risk for developing cholangiocarcinoma of 8–20%.[103] One-third of patients who develop cholangiocarcinoma do so within 2 years of the diagnosis of primary sclerosing cholangitis.
2. Parasitic infestations such as Opisthorcis viverrini in Thailand and Chlonorchis sinensis in Korea.[104,105] Opisthorcis viverrini is a flatworm which lives in the bile ducts, and lays eggs, which are excreted in feces. The lifecycle continues when the eggs, which are ingested by snails, hatch cercariae and penetrate fish, which are then are eaten by humans. Two-thirds of cholangiocarcinoma cases worldwide can be attributed to Opisthorcis viverrini infestations, and Thailand has the highest incidence rates of cholangiocarcinoma in the world.
3. Hepatolithiasis, a condition common in Asia but rare in Europe and North America. Hepatolithiasis induces a cycle of bile stasis, bacterial infection, leading to stenosis, bile duct obstruction, and chronic inflammation.[106]
4. Congenital choledochal cysts, which result in bile duct dilatation, bile stasis, reflux of pancreatic enzymes, and chronic bile duct inflammation. The risk for developing cholangiocarcinoma is 15% after the second decade.[107]

Like HCC, cholangiocarcinoma has been associated with chronic viral hepatitis and cirrhosis. In a Danish study of patients with cirrhosis, there is a 10-fold increased risk for cholangiocarcinoma after follow-up for 6 years.[108] In a prospective Japanese study in patients with HCV-related cirrhosis, 2.3% developed cholangiocarcinoma.[109] Hepatitis C virus seropositivity has been detected in up to 36% of patients.[110] The notion that hepatitis C core antigen is present in proliferating bile ductules in patients with HCV infection and could be associated with the development of cholangiocarcinoma was suggested by Yamamoto et al.[111] Furthermore, the portal inflammation might enhance the development of dysplastic or hyperplastic changes in the biliary lining. Some patients with cholangiocarcinoma associated with HCV infection had been given the diagnosis of HCC or combined HCC-cholangiocarcinoma. while the risk of developing cholangiocarcinoma in primary sclerosing cholangitis is not associated with the presence of liver cirrhosis,[92,93] the peripheral type is one of the characteristics of cholangiocarcinoma that develops in HCV-related cirrhosis. For patients who received Thorotrast as a radiographic contrast in the 1940s and 1950s, the estimated risk for cholangiocarcinoma is 300 times that of the general population.

Natural History

Unlike extrahepatic bile duct cancers, intrahepatic cholangiocarcinomas may not present with obstructive jaundice and hence the diagnosis may not be made until the cancer has become advanced. The diagnosis is made with the finding of hepatic mass or focal bile duct dilatations on ultrasound, CT or MRI scans, or endoscopic retrograde cholangiography. A rising serum CA19–9 in patients with primary sclerosing cholangitis may indicate the development of cholangiocarcinoma in the inflamed bile ducts. Histological confirmation can be made by brush cytology of bile duct strictures during ERCP, or by fine needle biopsy of suspicious areas along the bile ducts.The prognosis of cholangiocarcinoma is poor with 5-year survival of less than 5%.[112] The most common appearance of cholangiocarcinoma is moderately differentiated adenocarcinoma within a desmoplastic stroma (Figure 86-2A and 86-2B). Perineural invasion is often seen. Other variants of cholangiocarcinoma include papillary adenocarcinoma, signet ring carcinoma, squamous cell or mucoepidermoid carcinoma, and lymphoepithelioma-like form. Interestingly dysplasia and p53 mutation in the biliary epithelia may precede cholangiocarcinoma in patients in primary sclerosing cholangitis.[113]

Treatment

Surgical resection with complete excision of the tumor with negative margins, including partial hepatectomy if needed, can result in 5-year survival rates of 50%.[114] Patients are considered resectable if there is no evidence of liver, nodal, or peritoneal metastasis on CT and laparoscopy/laparotomy, and if the extent of malignant involvement of the biliary system does not preclude a curative resection. There is no evidence that adjuvant chemotherapy or chemoradiation is of benefit in patients with negative margins and nodes following resection. For patients with microscopic residual disease, adjuvant radiation therapy including intraoperative and post-operative external beam radiotherapy has produced statistically significant survival benefit compared to surgery alone (39.2% vs 13.5% 5-year survival).[115]

OLT for the treatment of cholangiocarcinoma has been reported with 5-year survival rates of 23%, with a median time to recurrence of 9 months.[116] OLT in combination with neoadjuvant chemoradiation, however, has 1-, 3-, 5-year survival rates of 92%, 82%, 82% compared to 82%, 48, 21% with resection alone.[117]

For patients with unresectable cholangiocarcinoma, systemic chemotherapy has made some progress in the past decade. Single agent chemotherapy with capecitabine or gemcitabine has produced response rates of 6% and 30%, and median survival of 8.1 and 9.5 months, respectively.[118,119] Combination chemotherapy with gemcitabine and capecitabine has a response rate of 31% with a median survival of 14 months,[120] while gemcitabine-oxaliplatin combinations produced a response rate of 36% with a median survival of 15.4 months.[121]

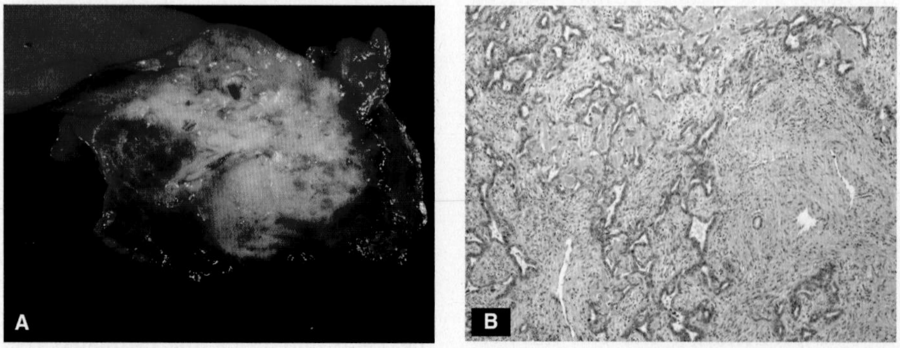

Figure 86-2 (A) Cholangiocarcinoma in a noncirrhotic liver. (B) Microscopic picture showing glandular formation within desmoplastic stroma (H&E, ×200).

Cholangiolocellular Carcinoma

Cholangiolocellular carcinoma (CLC) is a very rare liver cancer, accounting for 1% of primary liver cancers. CLC is thought to originate from the hepatic progenitor cells that are located in the bile ductules (cholangioles) and/or canals of Hering.[122,123] CLC is characterized by small cords resembling cholangioles or bile ductules in desmoplastic stroma (Fig. 86-3). Tumor cells are monotonous, cuboidal, and smaller in size than normal hepatocytes, with scanty eosinophilic cytoplasm. The nuclei are round and contain distinct nucleoli. Tumor cells show very mild atypia and resemble non-malignant cholangioles; the diagnosis of malignancy maybe difficult on needle biopsy specimen. Hepatocytes and bile ductular cells share the same hepatic stem/progenitor cells.[124] It is not surprising, therefore, that small focal areas of HCC-like and cholangiocarcinoma -like cells may be present. The biological behavior of CLC remains obscure, but reports seem to suggest that CLCs have aggressive behavior.[122]

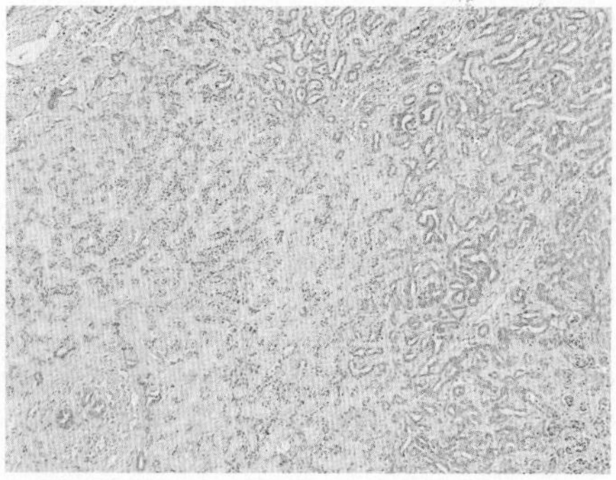

Figure 86-3 Microscopic picture of cholangiolocellular carcinoma showing bile ductule-like tumor cells within desmoplastic stroma (H&E, ×100).

Primary Hepatic Angiosarcoma

Primary hepatic angiosarcoma is also very rare, accounting for 2% of primary liver tumors. Derived from the malignant transformation of hepatic endothelial cells, hepatic angiosarcomas are notable for their association with environmental carcinogens such as thorotrast (contrast agent used in radiographic studies in the 1940s and 1950s), vinyl chloride (used in the plastics industry), arsenicals (prolonged use of Fowler's solution and agricultural interludes [Paris gum]), and androgenic-anabolic steroids. In most cases, there is no associated cirrhosis and no clear etiologic factor can be identified.[125,126] The disease is usually advanced at the time of diagnosis, with diffusely infiltrative disease or multifocal tumors in the liver.[127] Liver biopsy can show only massive necrosis of the liver, and patients are often referred for OLT. Prognosis is poor for this tumor, even with liver transplantation. The effectiveness of chemotherapy, including regimens known to be effective for soft tissue sarcomas, has not been well documented for hepatic angiosarcoma.

Epithelioid Hemangioendothelioma of the Liver

Epithelioid hemangioendothelioma (EHE) of the liver is, like hepatic angiosarcoma, derived from vascular endothelial cells and is a very rare primary cancer of the liver. The prognosis for EHE is better than for hepatic angiosarcoma, but can be very variable, ranging from aggressive variants to indolent cases lasting up to 28 years.[128] These tumors are usually multiple and are positive for one or more endothelial markers (Factor VIII-Ag, CD34, or CD31). Tumor cellularity is a better prognostic indicator than mitotic rate, which can be low even in aggressive variants. EHE has been treated with OLT with 54% of patients in 1 series alive at 4.5–18 years, even in cases with extrahepatic metastases at time of transplantation.[129] Anti-angiogenesis inhibitors such as thalidomide are potential therapeutic agents for these tumors of vascular origin.[130] Epithelioid hemangiopericytoma (EHP) of the liver is another rare malignant liver tumor, derived from pericytes of the vascular system, and shares with EHE a variable prognosis. Like hepatic angiosarcoma, EHP has been associated with exposure to vinyl chloride in plastics workers.[108]

Selected References

The complete reference list can be found at www.CANCERMEDICINE8.com

1. Garcia A, Jemal A, Ward EM, et al. *Global Cancer Facts & Figures 2007.* Atlanta, GA: American Cancer Society; 2007.
2. Bosch FX, Ribes J, Diaz M, Cleries R. Primary liver cancer; worldwide incidence and trends. *Gastroenterol.* 2004;127: S5–S16.
3. Kiyosawa K, Umemura T, Ichigo T, et al. Hepatocellular carcinma: recent trends in Japan. *Gastroenterology.* 2004;127:S17–S26.
10. Bosch FX, Ribes J, Borras J. Epidemiology of primary liver cancer. *Semin Liver Dis.* 1999;19:271–285.
11. Moroy T, Marchio A, Etiemble J, et al. Rearrangement and enhanced expression of c-myc in hepatocellular carcinoma of hepatitis virus infected woodchucks. *Nature.* 1986;324:276–279.
12. Wang J, Chenivesse X, Henglein B, Brechot C. Hepatitis B virus integration in a cyclin A gene in a hepatocellular carcinoma. *Nature.* 1990;343:555–557.
13. Andrisani OM, Barnabas S. The transcriptional function of the hepatitis B virus X protein and its role in hepatocarcinogenesis. *Int J Oncol.* 1999;15:373–379.
14. Colombo M. The role of hepatitis C virus in hepatocellular carcinoma. Recent results. *Cancer Res.* 1998;154:337–344.
19. Alter MJ. Epidemiology of hepatitis C in the West. *Semin Liver Dis.* 1995;15:5–14.
20. McMahon JM, Pouget ER, Tortu S. Individual and work-level risle factors for hepatrlis C Intection among heterosexual drug.
21. Alter HJ, Houghton M. Clinical Medical Research Award. Hepatitis C virus and eliminating post-transfusion hepatitis. *Nat Med.* 2000;6:1082–1086.
38. Neuschwanter-Tetri BA, Caldwell SH. Nonalcoholic steatohepatohepatitis: summary of an AASLD Single Topic Conference. *Hepatology.* 2003;37:1202–1219.
39. Powell EE, Cooksley WG, Hanson R, et al. The natural history of nonalcoholic steatohepatitis: a follow-up study of forty two patients for up to 21 years. *Hepatology.* 1990;41:372.
40. Bugianesi E, Leone N, Vanni E, Marchesini G. Expanding the natural history of nonalcoholic steatohepatitis: from cryptogenic cirrhosis to hepatocellular carcinoma. *Gastroenterology.* 2002;123:134.
41. Edmison J, McCullough AJ. Pathogenesis of non-alcoholic steatohepatitis: human data. *Clin Liver Dis.* 2007;11:75–104.
42. Kadayifci A, Merriman RB, Bass NM. Medical treatment of non-alcoholic steatohepatitis. *Clin Liver Dis.* 2007;11:119–140.
43. Andersen T, Gluud C, Franzman MB, et al. Hepatic effects of dietary weight loss in morbidy obese subjects. *J Hepatology.* 1991;12:224–229.
44. Edwards CQ, Griffen LM, Goldgar D, et al. Prevalence of hemochromatosis among 11.065 presmaly healthy blood donors. *N Engl J Med.* 1988;318:1355.
45. Stoller J, Aboussouan. Alpha 1-antitrypsin deficiency. *Lancet.* 2005;365:2225–2236.
46. Eriksson S, Carlson J, Velez R. Risk of cirrhosis and primary liver cancer in alpha 1-antitrypsin deficiency. *N Engl J Med.* 1986;314:736–739.
47. Giannitrapani L, Soresi M, La Spada E, Cervello M, D'Allessandro N, Montalto G. Sex hormones and liver cancer. *Ann N Y Acad Sci.* 2006;1089:228–236.
48. Villa E, Colantoni A, Grottola A, et al. Variant estrogen receptors and their role in liver diseae. *Mol Cell Endocrinol.* 2002;193:65–69.
84. Kau WY, Lai EC, Leug TW, Yu SC. Adjuvant intra-arterial iodine-131-labelled lipiodol for resectable hepatocellular carcinoma: a prospective randomized trial—update on 5-year and 10-year survival. *Ann Surg.* 2008;247:43.
85. Iwatsuki S, Starzl TE, Sheahan DG, et al. hepatic resection versus transplantation for hepatocellular carcinoma. *Ann Surg.* 1991;214:221.
88. Llovet J, Bruix J. Systematic review of randomized trials for unresectable hepatocellular carcinoma. Chemoembolization improves survival. *Hepatology.* 2003;37:429.
89. Marelli L, Sigliano R, Triantis C, et al. Transarterial therapy for hepatocellular carcinoma: which technique is more effective? A systematic review of cohort and randomized studies. *Cardiovasc Interent Radiol.* 2007;30:6.
92. Lai CL, Lok AS, Wu PC, Chan GC, Lin HJ. Doxorubicin versus no antitumor therapy in inoperable hepatocelular carcinoma. A prospective randomized trial. *Cancer.* 1988;62:479–483.
93. Yeo W, Mok TS, Zee B, et al. A randomized phase III study of doxorubicin versus cisplatin/interferon α-2b/doxorubicin/fluorouracil (PIAF) combination chemotherapy for unresectable hepatocellular carcinoma. *J Natl Cancer Inst.* 2005;97:1532–1538.
96. Llovet JM, Ricci S, et al. Sorafenib in advanced hepatocellular carcinoma. *N Engl J Med.* 2008;359:378–390.
97. Cheng A, Chan Z, Mazzaferre et al. Efficacy and safety of sorafenib in patients in the Asia-Pacific region with advanced hepatocellular carcinoma: a phase III randomised, double-blind placebo-controlled trial. *Lancet Oncol.* 2008;10:25–34.
100. Thomas MB, Morris JS, Chadhs R, et al; Phase II Arial of the combination of bevacizumab and erlotinib in patients who have advanced hepatocellular carcinoma. J Clin Oncol. 2009,27:843–850.
101. Thomas MB, et al. the combination of bevacizumab and erlotinib shows significant biological activity in patients with advanced hepatocellular carcinoma. *J Clin Oncol.* 2007;25:4567.
104. Haswell-Elkins MR, Mairiang E, Mairiang P, et al. Cross-sectional study of Opisthorchis viverrini infection and cholangiocarcinma in communities within a high-risk area in Northeast Thailand. *Int J Cancer.* 1994;59:505–509.
105. Lim, MK, Ju YH, Granceschi S, et al. Chlonorchis sinensis infection and increasing risk of cholangiocarcinoma in the Republic of Korea. *Am J Trop Med Hyg.* 2006;75:93.
108. Sorensen HT, Friis S, Olsen JH, et al. Risk of liver and other types of cancer in patients with cirrhosis: a nationwide cohort study in Denmark. *Hepatology.* 1998;28:921–925.
109. Kobayashi M, Ikeda K, Saitoh S, et al. Incidence of primary cholangiocellular carcinoma of the liver in Japanese patients with hepatitis C virus-related cirrhosis. *Cancer.* 2000;88:2471–2477.
112. Broome U, Olsson R, Loof L, et al. Natural history and prognostic factors in 305 Swedish patients with primary sclerosing cholangitis. *Gut.* 1996;38:610–615.
113. Batheja N, Suriawinata A, Saxena R, et al. Expression of p53 and PCNA in cholangiocarcinoma and primary sclerosing cholangitis. *Modern Pathol.* 2000;13: 1265–1268.
116. Meyer CG, Penn I, James L. Liver transplantation for cholangiocarcinoma: results in 20 patients. *Transplantation.* 2000;69:1633–1637.
117. De Vreede I, Steers JL, Burch PA, et al. Prolonged disease-free survival after orthotopic liver transplantation plus adjuvant chemoirradiation for cholangiocarcinoma. *Liver Transpl.* 2000;6:309–316.
119. Kubicka S, Rudolph KL, Tietze MK, et al. Phase II study of systemic gemcitabine chemotherapy for advanced unresectable hepatobiliary carcinomas. *Hepatogastrenterology.* 2001;48:783–789.
120. Knox JJ, Hedley D, Oza A, et al. Combining gemcitabine and capecitabine in patients with advanced biliary cancer; a phase II trial. *J Clin Oncol.* 2005;23:2332–2338.
123. Steiner PE, Higginson J. Cholangiolocellular carcinoma of the liver. *Cancer.* 1959;12:753–759.
124. Roskams T. Liver stem cells and their implication in hepatocellular and cholangiocarcinoma. *Oncogene.* 2006;25:3818–3822.
127. Nuetow PC, Buck J, Ros PR, et al. Malignant vascular tumors of the liver: radiographic pathpogic correlation. *Radio Graphics.* 1994;14:153.
128. Makhlouf HR, Ishak KG, Goodman D. Epithelioid hemangioendothelioma of the liver: a clinicopathologic study of 137 cases. *Cancer.* 1999;85:562–582.

87 Gallbladder and Bile Duct Cancer

Ahmed O. Kaseb, MD ▪ Melanie B. Thomas, MD, MS ▪ Steven A. Curley, MD, FACS

Gallbladder Cancer

Adenocarcinoma of the gallbladder is the sixth most common digestive-system malignancy in the United States. In Western countries such as the United States, where there is a low incidence of hepatocellular carcinoma (HCC), gallbladder cancer is relatively more common. The American Cancer Society estimates that about 9520 new cases of gallbladder cancer and bile duct cancer (excluding bile ducts within the liver) would be diagnosed in 2008 in the United States. About 3340 people would die of these cancers in 2008. Of these new cases and deaths, about half are due to gallbladder cancer.[1] Between 1980 and 1995, mortality rates from gallbladder cancer decreased in the United States, Canada, Australia, and the United Kingdom, while increasing in Japan, Italy, Spain, and Chile.[2] Unlike HCC and cholangiocarcinoma, gallbladder carcinoma has a higher incidence in females than males.[2] The preponderance of this cancer in females is even greater in patients <40 years old, with a female-to-male ratio of 20:1.[3]

Gallbladder carcinoma is more common in Southwest Native American than in the general American populace. Incidence rates for U.S. white males, U.S. black males, and Native American males in New Mexico are 0.4, 0.6, and 3.8 cases per 100,000 per year, respectively. The corresponding rates for females are 1.0, 0.8, and 10.3.[2] Gallbladder carcinoma has been found in 6% of Southwest Native American is undergoing biliary tract surgery.[4] Gallbladder carcinoma is the second most common gastrointestinal malignancy in this population, and the youngest reported case of gallbladder carcinoma occurred in an 11-year-old Navajo girl.[5]

Other human populations also have an increased incidence of gallbladder cancer. In Chile, the incidence of gallbladder cancer is rising, and gallbladder cancer is the number one cause of cancer mortality in Chilean women.[6] The geographic and population-based variations in the incidence of gallbladder cancer suggest that environmental risk factors, including carcinogens, infectious agents like *Salmonella typhi* and *Helicobacter pylori*, and diet have a role in gallbladder tumorigenesis.

Causative Factors

There are no apparent associations between gallbladder carcinoma and hepatitis B or C virus infection, cirrhosis, or mycotoxin exposure. Similarly, chemical hepatocarcinogens have not been clearly demonstrated to increase the risk of developing gallbladder carcinoma. However, there are suggestions that workers exposed to carcinogenic substances, such as methylcholanthrene and nitrosamines, have a higher incidence and earlier onset of gallbladder carcinoma when compared with control populations.[7] There is a significant association between gallstones and gallbladder carcinoma, with gallstones present in 74-92% of patients with gallbladder carcinoma.[8-9] The risk of developing gallbladder carcinoma increases directly with increasing gallstone size.[10] Patients with gallstones 2.0-2.9 cm in diameter have a 2.4 times higher relative risk of developing gallbladder carcinoma, whereas patients with gallstones greater than 3.0 cm in diameter have a 10.1 times higher risk. Patients with longstanding chronic cholecystitis can develop calcification of the gallbladder wall, also known as porcelain gallbladder. It is possible that chronic inflammation and/or infection of the gallbladder increases the risk of developing gallbladder carcinoma because 22% of patients with calcified gallbladders have gallbladder carcinoma.[11] Furthermore, pathogenic bacteria are cultured from the gallbladders of patients with gallbladder cancer at a significantly greater frequency than from patients with simple cholelithiasis.[12] Cholelithiasis and cholecystitis are more common in females, which may in part explain the higher incidence of gallbladder carcinoma in females.[13]

Patients with these premalignant lesions may progress to invasive gallbladder carcinoma. Epithelial dysplasia, atypical hyperplasia, and carcinoma in situ have been identified in the gallbladder mucosa of 83%, 13.5%, and 3.5%, respectively, of patients undergoing cholecystectomy for cholelithiasis or cholecystitis.[14] Areas of mucosal dysplasia can be observed in >90% of patients with invasive gallbladder carcinoma.[15] There is also evidence that adenomatous polyps arising from the gallbladder mucosa are premalignant lesions. A review of 1605 cholecystectomies reported 11 benign adenomas, 7 adenomas with areas of malignant transformation, and 79 invasive gallbladder carcinomas.[16] There appears to be an increased expression of epithelial growth factors and protooncogene, particularly ras, in the progression from chronic cholecystitis to dysplasia and then to invasive carcinoma.[17] In patients with anomalous pancreaticobiliary ductal union, a condition known to be associated with an increased risk of developing gallbladder cancer, chronic inflammation results in hyperplasia of the gallbladder epithelium.[18] K-*ras* mutations were noted in some of these patients with high-grade dysplasia, suggesting that mutations in this protooncogene may be an early event in gallbladder mucosal proliferation leading to carcinogenesis. Studies performed in patients with invasive gallbladder carcinoma have demonstrated that the majority have abnormal or mutated tumor suppressor (*p53* and *p16*), cell cycle regulation (cyclin E), and apoptosis regulation (Bcl-2) genes, as well as increased expression of angiogenesis factors (VEGF).[19,20]

Pathology

The gross appearance of gallbladder carcinoma varies, depending on the stage of the disease and extent of spread. Early-stage lesions that have not infiltrated through all layers of the gallbladder wall may be indistinguishable from chronic cholecystitis. Occasionally, a sessile or pedunculated tumor is present and suggests the diagnosis of a gallbladder carcinoma.[21] More advanced gallbladder carcinomas are grossly evident by infiltration into the liver or contiguous organs, such as the duodenum or stomach.[22]

Microscopically, >90% of gallbladder carcinomas are adenocarcinomas, with the remaining cases being adenosquamous, squamous, and anaplastic carcinomas, and, rarely, carcinoid tumors or embryonal rhabdomyosarcoma.[8,21] Carcinoma in situ is an early lesion, with the malignant cells involving only the mucosal layer of the gallbladder wall. Gallbladder adenocarcinomas generally have a predominant papillary or tubular arrangement of cells.[21] Papillary adenocarcinoma is characterized by an extended stroma covered by columnar cells. The tubular formations of tubular adenocarcinoma may be lined by tall columnar cells or by cuboidal epithelium. Mucin production and signet ring cells can be identified frequently in gallbladder adenocarcinomas.[21] More poorly differentiated carcinomas have solid sheets or nests of small, scattered cells infiltrating into the stroma and destroying the normal gallbladder wall architecture. Vascular, lymphatic, and perineural invasion by the carcinoma can be demonstrated frequently.

Advanced locoregional disease usually is present at the time of diagnosis of gallbladder carcinoma. Only 10% of patients with this disease have cancer confined to the gallbladder wall.[8] Direct extension of the carcinoma into the gallbladder fossa of the liver is present in 69-83% of patients.[22-24] Direct invasion of the liver usually indicates the presence of other regional disease because fewer than 12% of patients with liver involvement have no other sites of regional disease. Direct invasion of the extrahepatic biliary tract occurs in 57% of cases; the duodenum, stomach, or transverse colon is involved in 40%; and the pancreas is involved in 23%. The hepatic artery or portal vein is encased by tumor in 15% of patients. Regional lymph node metastases in the cystic, choledochal, or pancreaticoduodenal lymphatic drainage basins are present in 42-70% of patients.[22] More distant lymph node metastases occur along the aorta or inferior vena cava in approximately 25% of cases. Importantly, lymph node metastases can occur in the absence of liver or other contiguous organ involvement by the gallbladder carcinoma.

The pattern of lymph node metastases from gallbladder carcinoma is predictable on the basis of anatomic studies that have identified three pathways of lymphatic drainage of the gallbladder (Fig. 87-1).[25] The main pathway is the cholecysto-retropancreatic pathway, with lymphatic vessels on the anterior and posterior surfaces of the gallbladder that converge at a large retroportal lymph node. This principal retroportal lymph node communicates with the choledochal and pancreaticoduodenal lymph nodes. The cholecysto-celiac pathway consists of lymphatics from the anterior and posterior walls of the gallbladder that run to the left in front of the portal vein and then communicate with groups of pancreaticoduodenal lymph nodes or aorticocaval lymph nodes lying near the left renal vein. The final pattern of spread of gallbladder carcinoma is related to vascular invasion. Noncontiguous liver, pulmonary, and bone metastases have been found in 66%, 24%, and 12% of gallbladder carcinoma patients, respectively.[22]

The staging systems used for gallbladder carcinoma are based on the pathologic characteristics of local invasion by the tumor and lymph node

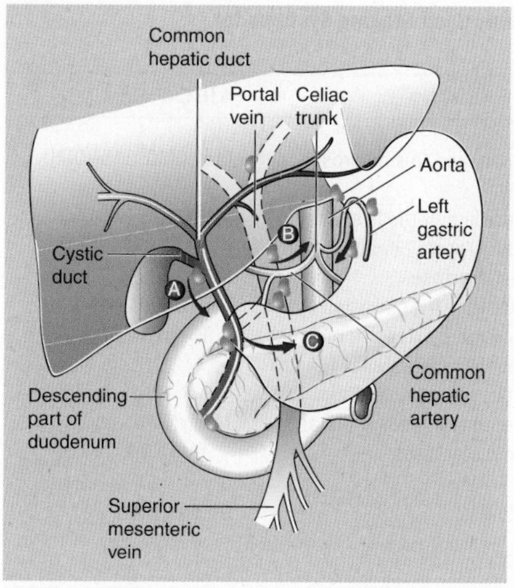

Figure 87-1 ■ Patterns of lymphatic drainage from the gallbladder. **(A)** The main pathway of lymphatic drainage, and thus, lymph node metastasis from gallbladder cancer is to the cholecysto-retropancreatic nodes. This pathway drains from the gallbladder to nodes along the cystic duct and common bile duct and then to nodes posterior to the duodenum and pancreatic head. **(B)** The cholecysto-celiac pathway courses from the gallbladder through the gastrohepatic ligament to celiac nodes. **(C)** The third lymphatic drainage route is the cholecysto-mesenteric pathway, coursing from the gallbladder posterior to the pancreas to aortocaval lymph nodes.

metastases. Before the American Joint Cancer Committee (AJCC) developed a tumor-node metastasis (TNM) staging schema for gallbladder carcinoma, the Nevin and colleagues staging system was used frequently.[26] Studies of gallbladder carcinoma performed in Japan generally apply the staging system of the Japanese Society of Biliary Surgery.[27] Most recent studies stage patients according to the TNM criteria. Carcinoma in situ corresponds to a T1aN0M0 tumor in the AJCC staging system. The characteristics of these three staging systems are outlined in Table 87-1.

Clinical Presentation

The most common symptoms and signs in patients with gallbladder carcinoma are nonspecific. Right upper quadrant abdominal pain, which may or may not be exacerbated by eating a fatty meal, is the predominant presenting complaint in 75-97% of patients.[2,8,28] Right upper quadrant abdominal tenderness is present in a slightly smaller percentage of patients. These symptoms and signs usually are ascribed to cholelithiasis or cholecystitis. Nausea, vomiting, and anorexia are present in 40-64% of patients; clinically evident jaundice is present in 45%; and weight loss of greater than 10% of normal body weight is noted in 37-77%.

Although 45% of patients obviously are jaundiced at presentation, 70% of patients present with a serum bilirubin elevated at least two times greater than normal.[28] Serum alkaline phosphatase levels are elevated in two-thirds of patients with gallbladder carcinoma. Alanine aminotransferase and aspartate aminotransferase levels are elevated in one-third of patients and are consistent with advanced hepatic invasion and metastases. In these patients with TNM stage III or IV disease, the serum CEA level is elevated in >80% of patients.[28] The incidence of elevated serum CEA levels in early-stage disease is not known.

Diagnostic Studies

Before ultrasonography and CT became widely available, the preoperative diagnosis rate for gallbladder carcinoma was only 8.6-16.3%.[2] Ultrasonography is the primary imaging study for symptomatic patients with presumed cholelithiasis or choledocholithiasis. High-resolution ultrasonography is able to detect early and locally advanced gallbladder carcinoma.[29] An early tumor as small as 5 mm can be recognized as a polypoid mass projecting into the gallbladder lumen or as a focal thickening of the gallbladder wall.[30] In patients with locally advanced gallbladder carcinoma, ultrasonography can demonstrate extrahepatic and intrahepatic bile duct obstruction, porta hepatis lymphadenopathy, direct hepatic extension of tumor, and hepatic metastases. Preoperative ultrasonography may suggest the correct diagnosis in up to 75% of patients with gallbladder carcinoma.[30,31] However, ultrasonography does not accurately detect celiac or paraortic lymphadenopathy or peritoneal dissemination of tumor.[32] Blood flow studies with color Doppler ultrasonography are also useful because gallbladder cancers have high-velocity arterial flow in 90% of cases, while benign lesions have minimal flow.[33] Recent advances in endoscopic ultrasonography, including the use of contrast-enhancing agents, may improve the diagnostic accuracy in assessing the T stage of the gallbladder cancer.[34]

CT scans are performed less frequently in patients with presumed benign biliary tract disease. However, if gallbladder carcinoma is suspected, CT findings can predict correctly the diagnosis in 88-95% of patients.[35,36] The CT characteristics of gallbladder carcinoma include diffuse or focal gallbladder wall thickness of greater than 0.5 mm in 95% of patients, gallbladder wall contrast enhancement in 95%, intraluminal mass in 90%, direct liver invasion by tumor in 85% (Fig. 87-2), regional lymphadenopathy in 65%, concomitant cholelithiasis in 52%, dilated intrahepatic or extrahepatic bile ducts in 50%, noncontiguous liver

Table 87-1 **Comparison of the Three Most Commonly Used Staging Systems for Gallbladder Carcinoma**

Stage	Nevin	JSBS	AJCC-TNM
I	Cancer confined to the mucosa	Cancer confined to subserosal layers	T1aN0M0, T1bN0M0
II	Cancer involves the mucosa and muscularis	Direct invasion of the liver and/or bile duct, porta hepatis lymph node metastases	T2N0M0
III	Cancer extends through the serosa (all three layers of the gallbladder wall involved)	More extensive liver invasion by cancer, more extensive regional lymph node metastases (gastrohepatic, retropancreatic)	T1N1M0, T2N1M0, T3AnyNM0
IV	Tumor through all three layers of the gallbladder wall with cystic lymph node metastasis	Liver, peritoneal, and/or distant organ metastases	T4AnyNM0, any TAnyNM1
V	Tumor invades the liver by direct extension and/or metastasis to any distant organ	No stage V	No stage V

Abbreviations: AJCC, American Joint Committee on Cancer; JSBS, Japanese Society of Biliary Surgery; T, primary tumor; Tx, primary tumor cannot be assessed; T1, tumor invades mucosa or muscle layer; T1a, tumor invades mucosa; T1b, tumor invades muscle; T2, tumor invades perimuscular connective tissue, no extension beyond serosa or into liver; T3, tumor invades beyond serosa or into one adjacent organ or both (extension <2 cm into liver); T4, tumor extends >2 cm into liver and/or into two or more adjacent organs (stomach, duodenum, colon, pancreas, omentum, extrahepatic bile ducts); N, regional lymph nodes; Nx, regional lymph nodes cannot be assessed; N0, no regional lymph node metastasis; N1, regional lymph node metastasis; N1a, metastasis in cystic duct, pericholedochal, and/or gastrohepatic lymph nodes; N1b, metastasis in peripancreatic, periduodenal, periportal, celiac, and/or superior mesenteric artery lymph nodes; M, distant metastasis; Mx, presence of distant metastasis cannot be assessed; M0, no distant metastasis; M1, distant metastasis.

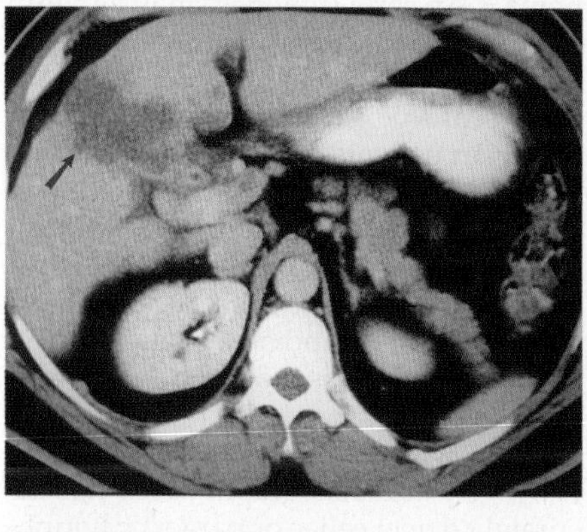

Figure 87-2 High-resolution, helical CT scan in a patient with gallbladder carcinoma. Direct tumor invasion into the hepatic parenchyma is evident.

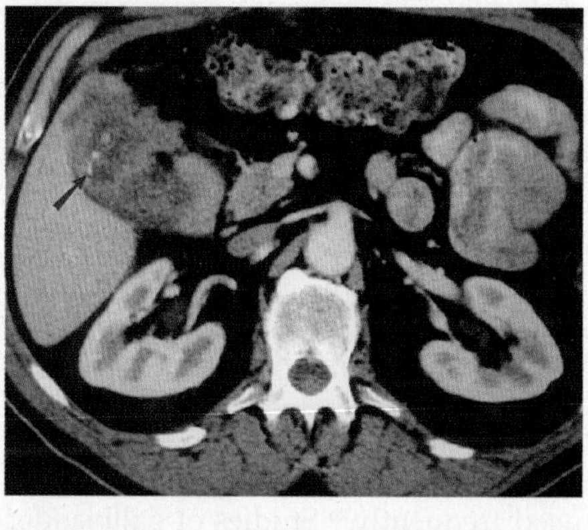

Figure 87-3 A high-resolution, helical CT scan in another patient with gallbladder cancer. A locally invasive tumor is again noted with areas of calcification (*arrow*) noted in the thickened gallbladder wall.

metastases in 12%, invasion of contiguous gastrointestinal tract organs in 8%, and intraluminal gallbladder gas in 4%.[35] CT can also demonstrate calcification of the gallbladder wall (Fig. 87-3).

Treatment

Resection The curative resection rates for gallbladder carcinoma range from 10% to 30%.[37] The majority of patients are not candidates for curative resection because of extensive locoregional disease, noncontiguous liver metastases, and/or distant metastases. Although it is clear that long-term survival can be achieved in some patients with resectable lesions, the extent of resection remains a controversial issue.

Simple cholecystectomy is an adequate therapy for gallbladder carcinoma confined to the mucosa (T1aN0M0). The 5-year survival rate for patients undergoing simple cholecystectomy for disease confined to the mucosa ranges from 57% to 100%.[38,39] There is not universal agreement on simple cholecystectomy as the sole therapy for patients with T1aN0M0 tumors; some authors recommend that extended cholecystectomy (cholecystectomy, wedge resection of the gallbladder fossa including a 3-5 cm margin of normal liver, and a cystic, pericholedochal, gastrohepatic, pancreaticoduodenal, and paraortic lymphadenectomy) be performed to treat patients with these very early-stage lesions.[40,41]

These authors recommend that all gallbladders be opened at the time of cholecystectomy for frozen section evaluation of any suspicious areas in the mucosa. If an unsuspected gallbladder carcinoma is diagnosed by frozen section biopsy or if a T1aN0M0 gallbladder carcinoma is diagnosed on final pathology, these authors advocate that an extended cholecystectomy be performed. The bias for this aggressive surgical treatment of T1aN0M0 gallbladder carcinoma is based on the small number of cases of regional lymph node recurrence in patients treated with simple cholecystectomy alone. No rationale is provided for the liver resection because the small number of patients who did fail after simple cholecystectomy developed metastases in the pericholedochal or cystic lymph nodes and not in the liver. Furthermore, the incidence of subsequent lymph node metastases in T1aN0M0 patients was <10% in the small groups of 32 and 36 patients, respectively.[40,41] The incidence of lymph node metastases in 201 patients with gallbladder carcinoma confined to the mucosa was only 2.5% in a study of patients who underwent cholecystectomy and regional lymphadenectomy.[38] The mortality rate for extended resection ranges from 2% to 5%, and major postoperative morbidity occurs in 13-40%.[38,39,42] Therefore, the morbidity and mortality associated with extended cholecystectomy is excessive compared with the potential survival benefit that would occur in <5% of patients with T1aN0M0 lesions.

There is a rationale for performing extended cholecystectomy in patients with T1b tumors or AJCC-TNM stage II and III gallbladder carcinomas (Fig. 87-4). In 165 patients with T1b gallbladder carcinomas, there was a 15.6% incidence of regional lymph node metastasis.[38] Of 867 patients with a T2 primary lesion, 56.1% had regional lymph node metastases.[38] The 453 patients with T3 tumors had a 74.4% incidence of regional lymph node metastases. The 5-year survival rate following extended cholecystectomy for AJCC stage II and III gallbladder carcinoma ranges from 7.5% to 71%.[38,39,42,43] Regional lymph node metastases and/or direct tumor invasion of the hepatic parenchyma are indicators of poor prognosis, with significant reductions in 5-year overall survival rates associated with these pathologic findings.[44,45] Microscopically positive liver resection margins also have a negative impact on survival because these patients had a median survival of 8.9 months compared with 67.2 months for patients with tumor-free margins.[44] Preoperative helical CT scans and intraoperative ultrasonography are used to assess the extent of direct invasion into the hepatic parenchyma, which assists with decision making regarding the extent of liver resection necessary to clear all disease. If adequate tumor-negative resection margins are attained, the radicality of liver resection does not affect survival, as attested by similar long-term survival rates following right lobectomy, extended right lobectomy, right trisegmentectomy, and central bisegmentectomy for gallbladder cancer.[38,39,46-48] T1b patients are classified as stage I in the AJCC system, but, arguably, with a 15.6% incidence of regional lymph node metastases, long-term survival benefit may occur in a significant number of these patients who undergo an extended cholecystectomy (Fig. 87-4).

All authors do not perform an en bloc resection of the extrahepatic bile duct as part of an extended cholecystectomy. Because gallbladder carcinoma is found to invade the extrahepatic bile duct in 57% of cases, with almost all cases occurring in patients with T3 or T4 tumors, an en bloc resection of the proper hepatic and common bile ducts with Roux-en-Y hepaticojejunostomy should be included in an extended cholecystectomy of transmurally invasive tumors. This includes those individuals in whom a clinically unsuspected gallbladder carcinoma is diagnosed pathologically following a simple cholecystectomy with a positive margin at the cystic duct. Gallbladder cancer involving the cystic duct and gallbladder neck frequently grows along the proper hepatic and right bile ducts, necessitating a right or extended right hepatic lobectomy and excision of the extrahepatic ducts to remove all disease.[49]

Extremely radical operations have been proposed for patients with extensive T3N1M0 or T4N01M0 tumors. This includes hepatopancreatic duodenectomy and abdominal organ cluster transplantation for locally advanced gallbladder carcinoma.[38,50,51] The operative mortality rate for these radical procedures is at least 15%, with a greater than 90% incidence of major morbidity. Resection of the portal vein and/or hepatic artery with vascular reconstruction frequently is necessary to resect completely all gross malignant disease. The largest report of patients undergoing hepatopancreatic duodenectomy for gallbladder carcinoma is 150 cases from Japan, with a 5-year survival rate of 14%.[38] The patients who did not die from intraoperative or postoperative complications all succumbed to recurrent and/or metastatic carcinoma.

It is estimated that 80,000 laparoscopic cholecystectomies are performed each year in the United States. On average, gallbladder carcinoma is diagnosed in 2% of patients undergoing cholecystectomy for presumed benign biliary tract disease. Thus, approximately 1600 patients who annually undergo laparoscopic cholecystectomy could suffer inadvertent dissemination of gallbladder carcinoma.[52-55] However, the potential laparoscopic dissemination of tumor cells may not significantly alter the natural history of gallbladder cancer in most patients. A review of our experience at the University of Texas MD Anderson Cancer Center with diagnostic and therapeutic laparoscopy in patients with gastrointestinal malignancies indicated that port site recurrence is a harbinger of widespread metastasis in >95% of patients; thus, it is rarely an isolated site of recurrent malignant disease.[56] Furthermore, a report drawn from the National Cancer Data Base between 1989 and 1995 revealed no change in incidence or survival from gallbladder cancer during the time laparoscopic cholecystectomy supplanted open cholecystectomy as the procedure of choice for gallbladder disease presumed benign.[57] Nonetheless, because of the large number of cholecystectomies being performed laparoscopically and the small but measurable risk of dissemination of tumor cells, it has been recommended that (1) unless the surgeon feels capable of performing a definitive

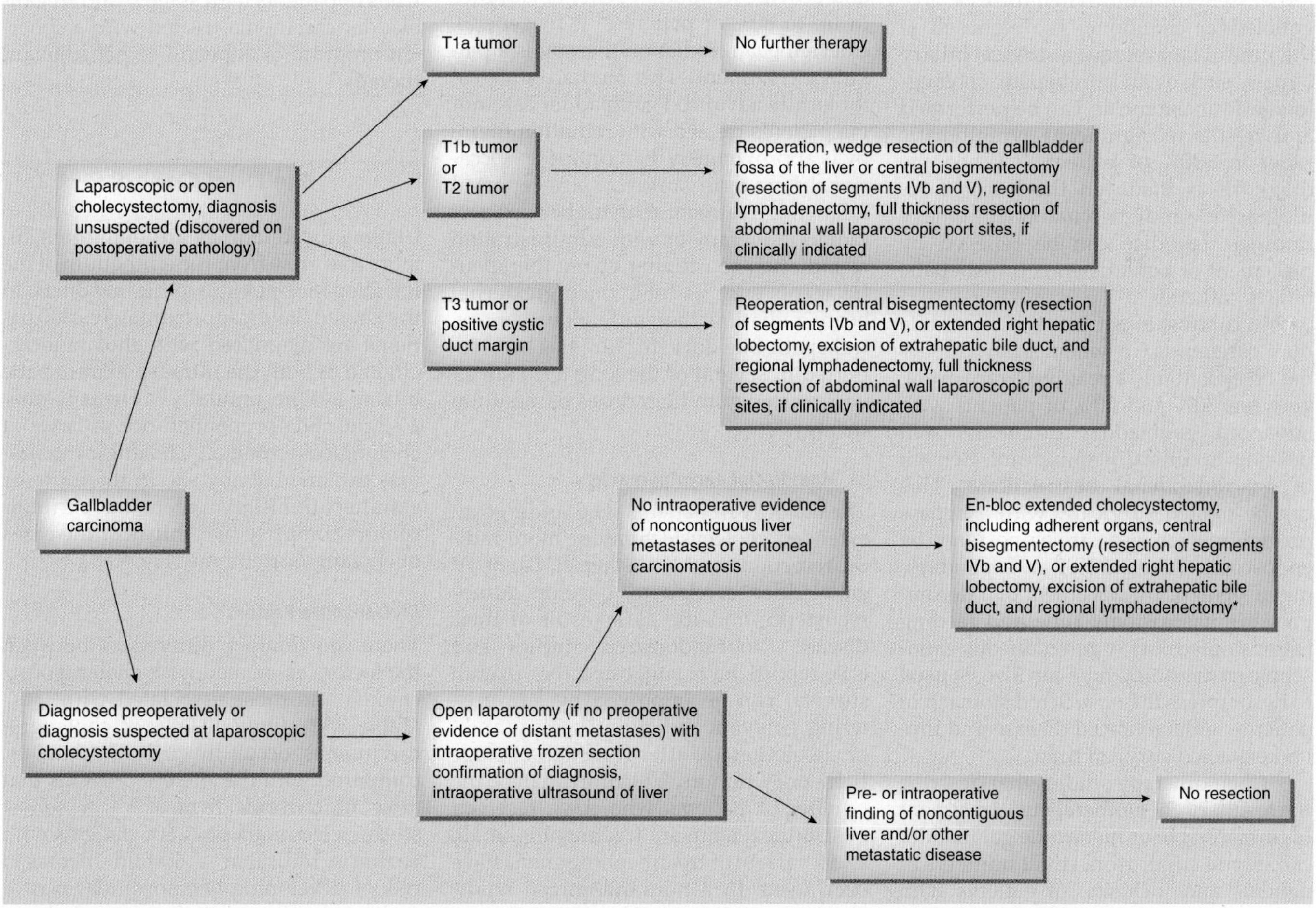

Figure 87-4 Algorithm to guide surgical decision making for patients with gallbladder cancer. *Regional lymphadenectomy includes complete dissection and removal of the cystic, pericholedochal, pancreaticoduodenal, gastrohepatic, and paraortic lymph nodes.

extended cholecystectomy for gallbladder carcinoma, patients in whom gallbladder carcinoma is suspected preoperatively by clinical or radiologic criteria should be referred without laparoscopy, laparotomy, or percutaneous biopsy, and (2) if gallbladder carcinoma is suspected on visual inspection during an attempted laparoscopic cholecystectomy, either an open definitive operation should be performed or the operation should be terminated without biopsy and the patient referred for appropriate surgical therapy.[52] Patients who underwent laparoscopic cholecystectomy and were then found on pathologic analysis to have gallbladder cancer should still be considered for aggressive surgical treatment because long-term disease-free survival will result in a subset of these patients.[58]

Palliation ■ The majority of patients with gallbladder carcinoma are diagnosed at an advanced, unresectable stage of disease. As in patients with hilar bile duct cancer, relief of symptomatic jaundice is a consideration. Patients with unresectable gallbladder carcinoma frequently have extensive involvement of the extrahepatic bile duct and may have bulky porta hepatis lymphadenopathy, which makes endoscopic placement of an internal stent difficult. When unresectable gallbladder carcinoma is diagnosed at the time of laparotomy, a surgical biliary bypass, such as an intrahepatic cholangioenteric anastomosis, can be performed and results in significant symptomatic relief in >90% of patients.[59] When the diagnosis is made on the basis of radiographic and percutaneous biopsy findings, jaundice can be relieved by placement of percutaneous transhepatic biliary catheters.

In contrast to patients with hilar bile duct carcinoma, in whom gastroduodenal obstruction is a relatively rare event, between 30% and 50% of patients with advanced gallbladder carcinoma will develop a clinically significant element of gastroduodenal obstruction.[60] This can be treated surgically with a bypass procedure such as gastrojejunostomy, by endoscopic placement of an expandable metal stent, or by placement of a decompressing gastrostomy tube and feeding jejunostomy tube. A percutaneous endoscopic gastrostomy tube can also be used to decompress the obstructed stomach in patients with advanced disease and limited expected survival time.

Chemotherapy studies that describe the results of chemotherapeutic treatment of unresectable or metastatic gallbladder carcinoma suffer from small numbers of patients and inclusion of patients with hilar bile duct carcinoma. A study of 53 patients with gallbladder carcinoma who received systemic chemotherapy with 5-fluorouracil (5-FU) or 5-FU plus other chemotherapeutic agents showed objective antitumor responses in 12% or less of the patients in each treatment arm.[61] Fluoropyrimidines combined with doxorubicin administered systemically have produced objective response rates of 30-40%.[62,63] Gemcitabine as a single agent may produce similar response rates, but these responses are rarely durable for more than 3-6 months.[64] Complete remission is rare and in most studies, median survival is 11 months or less. However, the literature regarding treatment results with specific regimens is limited because most series are small, and many reports consist of a mix of bile duct cancers, gallbladder cancer, and either pancreatic or hepatocellular cancer. More details of recent clinical trials are explained in cholangiocarcinoma section.

Radiation Therapy ■ Analysis of the patterns of failure after resection of gallbladder carcinoma revealed that local recurrence was the first and, in a significant number of cases, the only site of failure in more than one-half of patients.[65] External beam radiation therapy to a total dose of 45 Gy can produce radiographic evidence of tumor reduction in 20-70% of these tumors and provide temporary relief of jaundice in up to 80% of patients.[66-68] In general, external beam radiation therapy is a palliative treatment. The median survival for locally advanced gallbladder carcinoma patients treated with radiation therapy is approximately 10 months.[65-68] Occasional long-term survivors are reported following treatment with higher doses of radiation therapy or with administration of radiation-sensitizing chemotherapeutic agents such as 5-FU during external beam radiation therapy.[65] However, extrahepatic bile duct stricture has been reported in several of the long-term survivors treated with high doses of radiation therapy.[69]

Multidisciplinary Approaches

The majority of patients who undergo an extended cholecystectomy or more radical resection for AJCC stage II, III, or IV gallbladder carcinoma develop tumor recurrence and die as a result of their disease. Nonrandomized studies and case reports have suggested that overall survival can be improved by administering adjuvant radiation therapy and/or chemotherapy after resection of stage II, III, or IV tumors.[70,71] Unfortunately, the number of patients who have received postsurgical adjuvant treatment is small, and a variety of treatment regimens have been used. In a nonrandomized study, 9 patients with stage IV gallbladder carcinoma were treated with complete surgical resection alone, while 17 patients were treated with complete resection combined with 20-30 Gy of intraoperative radiation therapy.[72] Ten of these 17 patients also received 36.4 Gy of postoperative external beam radiation therapy. The surgical procedures performed in both groups of patients included extended cholecystectomy and a variety of more radical procedures, including hepatopancreatic duodenectomy. There were no 3-year survivors among the nine patients treated with resection alone, but there was a 3-year survivorship of 10.1% in the 17 patients treated with resection and radiation therapy. There is a single report of 18 patients treated with preoperative chemoradiation therapy (4500 cGy, 180 cGy/fraction, 5 days/week, continuous intravenous infusion of 5-FU 350 $mg/m^2/day$ on days 1 to 5 and 21 to 25) prior to a planned resection of known gallbladder cancer.[73] Thirteen of the 18 patients underwent resection; one patient refused operation, one patient did not complete preoperative chemoradiation, one patient had disease progression after chemoradiation, and two patients had unresectable disease found at laparotomy. The actuarial 5-year survival rate in the 13 resected patients was 57%. Unfortunately, there are no randomized trials of patients with stage II and III gallbladder carcinoma treated with a coherent program of adjuvant or neoadjuvant therapy.

Bile Duct Cancer

Cholangiocarcinomas are malignant tumors that arise from the epithelium of the intrahepatic or extrahepatic bile ducts. In the United States, approximately 3000 patients are diagnosed with cholangiocarcinoma of both the intra- or extrahepatic biliary system annually.[74] There is only a slight male preponderance of cases of cholangiocarcinoma. Cholangiocarcinomas can arise at any site in the intra- or extrahepatic biliary system, but perihilar tumors comprise two-thirds of the cases of cholangiocarcinoma (Fig. 87-5).[75]

Causative Factors

There are distinct differences between the factors associated with cholangiocarcinoma and those associated with HCC (Table 87-2). Only 10-20% of cholangiocarcinomas occur in cirrhotic patients, compared with the 70-90% of HCCs that arise in cirrhotic livers.[74,76,77] A cohort study in Denmark of 11,605 patients with cirrhosis indicated a 60-fold increased risk of developing hepatocellular cancer and a 10-fold increased risk of cholangiocarcinoma.[77] Frequently, the cirrhosis

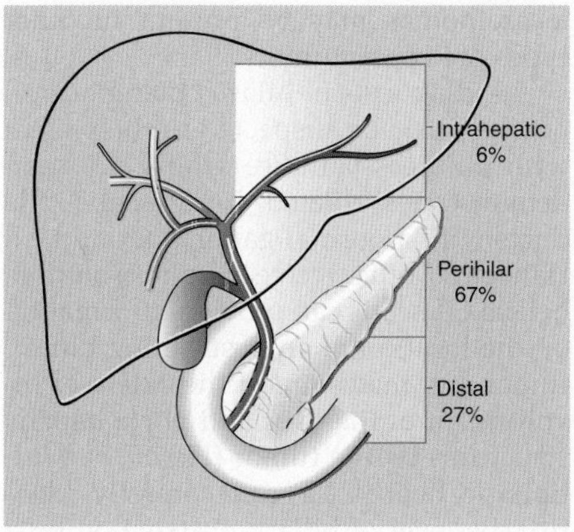

Figure 87-5 The distribution of 294 cholangiocarcinomas into intrahepatic, perihilar, and distal subgroups. *Source*: From Ref. 75.

associated with cholangiocarcinomas is a subacute secondary biliary type that results from the neoplastic obstruction of the bile ducts, indicating that, in some cases, cirrhosis in cholangiocarcinoma patients is the result of the tumor rather than its cause.

Cholangiocarcinoma is more prevalent in Southeast Asia than in other parts of the world. The higher incidence in this geographic region is related to parasitic infection with the liver flukes *Opisthorchis sinensis* and *Opisthorchis viverrini*.[78,79] Liver flukes induce hyperplasia, fibrosis, and adenomatous proliferation of human biliary epithelium and are associated with hepatolithiasis. The fluke infestation suggests a direct etiologic role in the subsequent development of cholangiocarcinoma, but this relationship is not established unequivocally.

Several disorders that can produce chronic inflammation of the bile ducts have been associated with an increased risk of developing cholangiocarcinoma. These include polycystic liver disease, choledochal cysts, congenital dilation of the intrahepatic bile ducts (Caroli syndrome), sclerosing cholangitis (occasionally in association with inflammatory bowel disease), hepatolithiasis, and cholelithiasis.[80-85] Hepatolithiasis is not a common disorder, and only 5-7% of patients with documented hepatic stones develop cholangiocarcinoma.[84,85] The reported incidence of cholangiocarcinoma developing in areas of congenital cystic dilation of the bile duct, including choledochal cysts and Caroli disease, ranges from 3% to 30%.[86,87] Patients with primary sclerosing cholangitis are also at increased risk to develop cholangiocarcinoma, with incidence rates ranging from 9% to 40%.[88,89] Patients with ulcerative colitis may also develop sclerosing cholangitis, but cholangiocarcinoma occurs in only 0.4-1.4% of individuals with ulcerative colitis.[88] In patients with sclerosing cholangitis, whether associated with ulcerative colitis or not, radiologic distinction between sclerosing cholangitis and cholangiocarcinoma is often impossible. One study showed that the serum tumor marker CA19-9 had an 89% sensitivity and 86% specificity in diagnosing cholangiocarcinoma in patients with sclerosing cholangitis.[90] Combining serum CA19-9 levels with serum CEA levels may further increase the diagnostic accuracy to detect cholangiocarcinoma in patients with sclerosing cholangitis.[91]

Patients who underwent diagnostic radiography with intravenous injection of Thorotrast (thorium dioxide) are at high risk of developing HCC, angiosarcoma, and cholangiocarcinoma.[92] Cholangiocarcinoma is the most frequent hepatic neoplasm reported in patients who have received Thorotrast. Exposure to several drugs or carcinogens has also been linked to an increased risk to develop cholangiocarcinoma (Table 87-2). Because cholangiocarcinoma is a relatively rare neoplasm, it has been difficult to prove its pathogenesis related to any of these factors, but it is clear that chronic inflammation of the biliary tree by any cause is associated with an increased risk of developing cholangiocarcinoma.

Chronic inflammation of the biliary system or exposure to genotoxic agents concentrated in bile may produce damage to the DNA of biliary epithelial cells, leading to the development of cholangiocarcinoma. Mutations in the p53 tumor suppressor gene and in the K-ras protooncogene have been identified in cholangiocarcinoma patients.[93,94] There may be geographic and population-based differences in the mutation rates of these two genes in cholangiocarcinoma, but alterations in p53 and K-ras are observed in significant proportions of patients with any of the identified factors (Table 87-2) that increase risk to develop cholangiocarcinoma. Overexpression of c-erbB-2, a protooncogene that encodes a transmembrane protein that is highly homologous to epidermal growth factor receptor (EGFR), has been confirmed in human cholangiocarcinoma cells and in benign proliferative biliary epithelium from patients with hepatolithiasis, primary sclerosing cholangitis, and liver fluke infestation.[95] Alterations in *c-erbB-2* expression may occur early in the chronic inflammation-induced proliferation of biliary epithelium leading to malignant transformation. Chronic inflammation may also produce the overexpression of the *Bcl-2* protooncogene observed in cholangiocarcinomas, which may promote tumorigenesis by inhibiting normal apoptotic processes.[96]

Table 87-2 **Factors Associated With Increased Risk to Develop Cholangiocarcinoma vs Hepatocellular Carcinoma**

Cholangio carcinoma	Hepatocellular Carcinoma
Liver fluke infection	Cirrhosis
Ophisthorchis sinensis	Chronic hepatitis B virus infection
Opisthorchis viverrini	Chronic hepatitis C virus infection
Congenital/chronic cystic dilation	Aflatoxin B1 ingestion of the bile ducts
Choledochal cyst	Chronic ethanol ingestion
Caroli disease	Primary biliary cirrhosis
Hepatolithiasis	Hemochromatosis
Primary sclerosing cholangitis	α-1-Antitrypsin deficiency
Ulcerative colitis	Glycogen storage disease
Thorotrast exposure	Hypercitrullinemia
Cholelithiasis	Porphyrias
Asbestos	Hereditary tyrosinemia
Dioxin (Agent Orange)	Wilson disease
Polychlorinated diphenyls	Hepatotoxin exposure
Nitrosamines	Thorotrast
Isoniazid	Polyvinyl chloride
Methyldopa	Carbon tetrachloride

Clinical Presentation

The clinical features of cholangiocarcinoma are nonspecific and depend on the location of the tumor. The usual clinical presentation of patients with hilar cholangiocarcinoma is painless jaundice. Patients may also report concomitant onset of fatigue, pruritus, fever, vague abdominal pain, and anorexia. The serum liver function tests in patients with hilar cholangiocarcinoma commonly demonstrate obstructive jaundice, with alkaline phosphatase and total bilirubin levels elevated in greater than 90% of patients.[74] Cholangiocarcinomas that arise in peripheral bile ducts within the hepatic parenchyma usually reach a large size before becoming clinically evident. Patients with these large peripheral hepatic tumors usually present with hepatomegaly and an upper abdominal mass, abdominal and back pain, and weight loss.[74] Jaundice and ascites are late and usually preterminal sequelae in patients with large intrahepatic cholangiocarcinomas. Jaundice associated with a large hepatic cholangiocarcinoma is caused by a combination of extension of the tumor to the bifurcation of the left and right hepatic ducts, and by compression of contralateral bile ducts by the expanding tumor.

Serum alkaline phosphatase levels are elevated in >90% of patients with cholangiocarcinoma.[75] Serum bilirubin also is elevated in the majority of cholangiocarcinoma patients, particularly in those with a tumor arising in the central portion of the liver or the extrahepatic hilar bile ducts.[97] In contrast to HCC, serum α-fetoprotein levels are abnormal in fewer than 5% of cholangiocarcinoma patients.[75] There is an increase in serum CEA levels in 40-60% of cholangiocarcinoma patients.[75,98] Another tumor marker, CA19-9, is elevated in >80% of patients with cholangiocarcinoma.[98]

Pathology

Cholangiocarcinomas originating in the periphery of the hepatic parenchyma usually are solitary and large, but satellite nodules occasionally are present.[99] Gross tumor invasion of the large portal or hepatic veins occurs much less frequently than in HCC. The gross and microscopic appearance of intrahepatic cholangiocarcinomas may have prognostic significance because tumors with periductal infiltration have a higher incidence of lymph node and intrahepatic metastasis.[100] Metastases to the regional lymph nodes, lungs, and peritoneal cavity are more common in cholangiocarcinoma than in HCC. When the tumor causes longstanding biliary obstruction, the liver may show secondary biliary cirrhosis.

Microscopically, cholangiocarcinoma is characterized by low cuboidal cells that resemble the normal biliary epithelium. Varying degrees of pleomorphism, atypia, mitotic activity, hyperchromatic nuclei, and prominent nucleoli are noted from area to area in the same tumor. Rarely, a clear cell variant of cholangiocarcinoma occurs, which must be distinguished from clear cell renal carcinoma with liver metastasis.[101] Cholangiocarcinomas are mucin-secreting adenocarcinomas, and intracellular and intraluminal mucin often can be demonstrated. The presence of mucin is useful in differentiating cholangiocarcinoma from HCC. The absence of bile production by cholangiocarcinoma can also be useful in distinguishing this tumor from a HCC. Immunohistochemical staining that is positive for epithelial membrane antigen and tissue polypeptide antigen may be useful in confirming a diagnosis of cholangiocarcinoma.[102,103] Immunohistochemical staining for cytokeratin subtypes can be helpful in differentiating cholangiocarcinoma from metastatic colorectal carcinoma.[104] Cholangiocarcinomas are usually locally invasive, which spread along nerves or in subepithelial layers of the bile ducts.

Diagnostic Studies

Peripheral intrahepatic cholangiocarcinoma is often difficult to distinguish pathologically and radiographically from a deposit of metastatic adenocarcinoma within the liver. Although transabdominal ultrasonography can detect an intrahepatic malignant tumor greater than 2 cm in diameter, ultrasound findings do not differ between cholangiocarcinomas, liver metastases from extrahepatic adenocarcinomas, and multinodular HCC.[105] CT demonstrates a rounded, low attenuation mass with irregular or lobulated margins (Fig. 87-6). Satellite lesions may be evident, particularly when using helical CT during the optimal period of hepatic contrast enhancement. Calcification within the tumor is present in 25% of cases, and a central scar is observed in 30%.[106] MRI shows a nonencapsulated mass with irregular margins that is hypointense compared with the normal liver on T1-weighted and hyperintense on T2-weighted images. The peripheral rim of the tumor usually enhances following MRI contrast administration. A hyperintense central scar is best seen on T2-weighted images, but the CT and MRI characteristics of intrahepatic cholangiocarcinomas may be present in other types of hepatic tumors.[106]

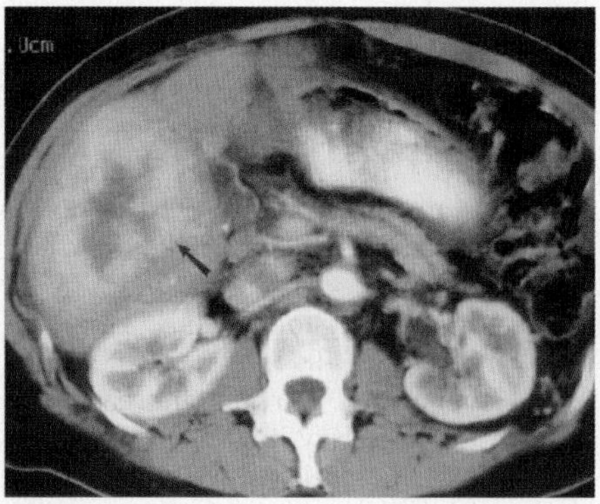

Figure 87-6 ■ High-resolution, helical CT scan during the arterial contrast phase in a patient with an intrahepatic cholangiocarcinoma. The periphery of the tumor (*arrow*) has irregular margins and enhances with contrast. A relatively hypovascular area of scar and tumor necrosis is evident in the center of the tumor.

A diagnosis of hilar cholangiocarcinoma should be suspected in the patient with painless jaundice whose CT scan demonstrates dilated intrahepatic bile ducts with a normal gallbladder and extrahepatic biliary tree. High-resolution, helical CT scans can provide information on the location of an obstructing biliary tumor and may suggest the extent of involvement of the liver and porta hepatis structures by the tumor (Fig. 87-7). Multiphasic helical CT can correctly identify the level of biliary obstruction by a hilar cholangiocarcinoma in 63-90% of patients.[107,108] Preoperative helical CT is also useful in demonstrating lobar or segmental liver atrophy caused by bile duct obstruction or portal vein occlusion (Fig. 87-8).[108] However, helical CT is not accurate in assessing the resectability of hilar cholangiocarcinomas because of limited resolution in evaluating intraductal tumor spread and significant false-positive and false-negative rates in demonstrating portal vein or hepatic artery involvement by tumor.[107,108]

Like the CT scan, ultrasonography can demonstrate a nondilated gallbladder and common bile duct associated with dilated intrahepatic ducts. In addition, as grayscale ultrasonography has improved, the diagnosis of cholangiocarcinoma is supported by finding a hilar bile duct mass in 65-90% of patients.[109] Ultrasonography and CT scan may be used to demonstrate the presence of intrahepatic tumor due to direct extension or noncontiguous metastases and enlarged periportal lymph nodes, suggesting nodal metastases.[110] Even intraoperative ultrasonography is suboptimal for detecting intraductal spread by hilar cholangiocarcinoma, cor-

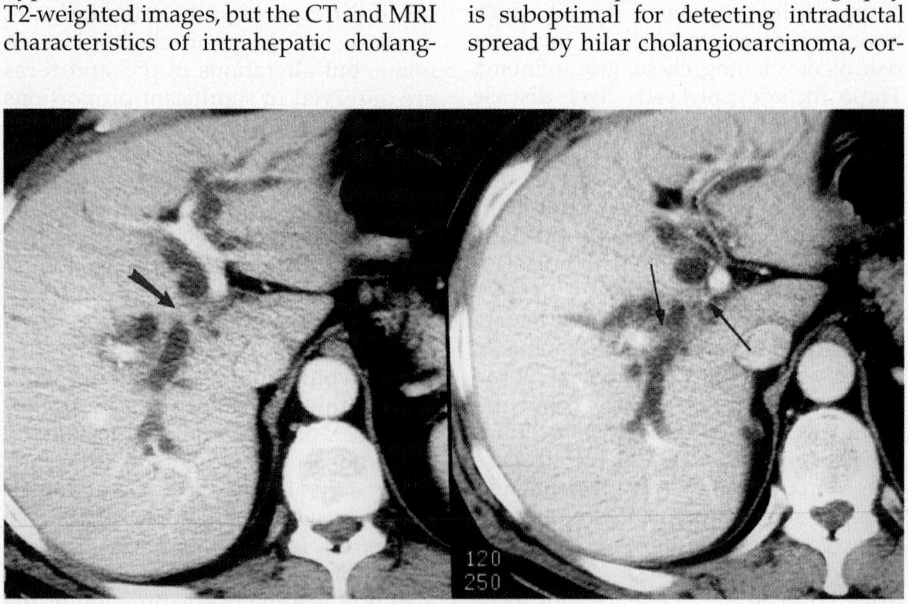

A B

Figure 87-7 ■ High-resolution, helical CT scan in another patient presenting with obstructive jaundice. The tumor mass **A**, (*large arrow*) producing marked intrahepatic biliary duct dilatation is evident. Areas of tumor invasion of the portal vein **B**, (*small arrows*) suggested on the CT scan were confirmed at the time of operation to be tumor invasion of the portal vein.

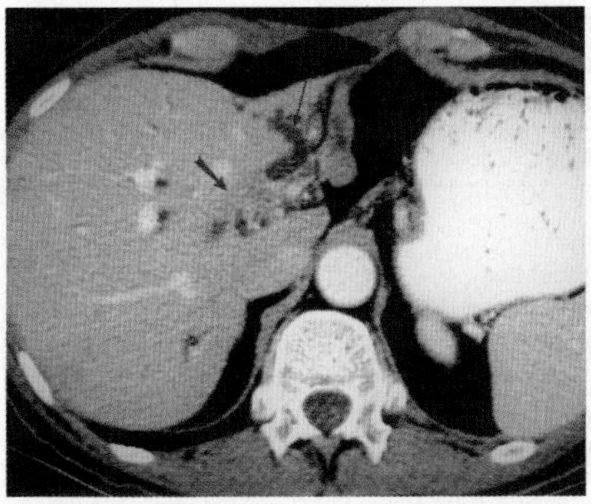

Figure 87-8 ■ High-resolution, helical CT scan in a patient presenting with several months of increasing pruritus followed by the development of clinically evident jaundice. The relatively hypodense hilar cholangiocarcinoma (*large arrow*) is evident. Marked atrophy of the left hepatic lobe is noted with dilated intrahepatic bile ducts (*small arrow*), but little remaining hepatic parenchyma is evident.

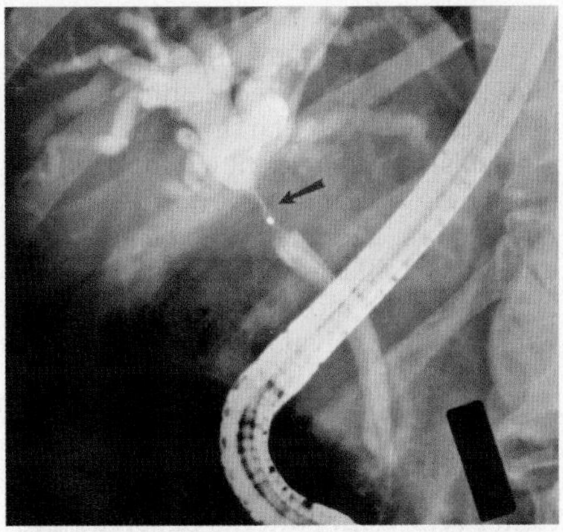

Figure 87-9 ■ Endoscopic retrograde cholangiopancreatography showing a focal stricture of the proper hepatic bile duct (*arrow*) with marked dilatation of the intrahepatic bile ducts. This hilar cholangiocarcinoma was completely resected with Roux-en-Y hepaticojejunostomy reconstruction of biliary-enteric continuity.

rectly demonstrating the extent of tumor spread away from the primary biliary tumor in only 18% of cases.[111] Intraoperative ultrasonography can be used to screen for noncontiguous liver metastases from the primary biliary cancer and can accurately detect direct tumor invasion of the portal vein and hepatic artery in 83.3% and 60% of cases, respectively.[111]

Similar to the intrahepatic variety, hilar cholangiocarcinoma usually shows hypointensity on T1- and hyperintensity on T2-weighted MRI. Dilated intrahepatic bile ducts are evident in patients with obstructing tumors, and lobar atrophy is seen in cases of portal venous occlusion. Fast low-angle shot (FLASH) MR with contrast-enhanced coronal imaging has been used to demonstrate intraluminal extension of tumor and to distinguish between blood vessels and bile ducts.[112] Magnetic resonance cholangiopancreatography (MRCP) and MR virtual endoscopy can demonstrate hilar bile duct obstruction by tumor with dilated intrahepatic ducts.[112,113] The advantages of MRCP over direct cholangiography include noninvasiveness and possible visualization of isolated bile ducts.

Cholangiography definitively demonstrates a lesion obstructing the left and right hepatic ducts at the hilar confluence (Fig. 87-9), and percutaneous transhepatic cholangiography (PTC) and endoscopic retrograde cholangiopancreatography (ERCP) are both useful in assessing patients with extrahepatic biliary obstruction. A prospective, randomized comparison of PTC and ERCP in patients with jaundice concluded that the two techniques had similar diagnostic accuracy.[114] PTC was 100% accurate in demonstrating obstruction at the confluence of the left and right hepatic ducts, while ERCP had an accuracy of 92% in demonstrating these lesions. ERCP has the additional benefit of providing a pancreatogram. A normal pancreatogram helps to exclude a small carcinoma of the head of the pancreas as a cause of biliary obstruction. Cytologic specimens can be obtained at the time of PTC and ERCP. The presence of malignant cells in bile or bile duct brushings is confirmed in approximately 50% of patients undergoing PTC or ERCP.[109,114–116]

Drainage of the obstructed biliary tree with partial or complete relief of jaundice and associated symptoms can be achieved with PTC. Improvements in catheter technology led to the development of endoprostheses that can be placed across the malignant obstruction into the duodenum to allow internal drainage.[117] It must be emphasized that providing symptomatic relief for patients by decompressing the biliary tract should not be the primary reason to place these catheters. Prospective, randomized studies have failed to demonstrate a benefit in terms of a decrease in hospital morbidity or mortality by preoperative decompression of biliary obstruction.[118] However, the catheters are useful in identifying and dissecting the hepatic duct bifurcation at the time of operation and aid in the reconstruction of the biliary tract following extirpation of the tumor.[119,120]

Positron emission tomography (PET) is being evaluated as a diagnostic tool in patients with all types of malignant tumors. PET assesses in vivo metabolism of positron-emitting radiolabeled tracers like [^{18}F] fluoro-2-deoxy-D-glucose (18FFDG), a glucose analog that accumulates in various malignant tumors because of their high glucose metabolic rates. FDG-PET does not provide anatomic detail to assess resectability of hilar cholangiocarcinomas or intrahepatic malignancies, but it may prove useful in detecting distant metastatic disease that would preclude a curative resection. In patients with primary sclerosing cholangitis, FDG-PET studies may be able to detect small hilar and intrahepatic cholangiocarcinomas and thus may be useful in therapeutic and transplant decision making in these patients.[126] PET has recently been used to aid in the diagnosis and staging of patients with bile duct cancer.[122] PET scan images correctly detected the primary cholangiocarcinoma in 24 of 26 patients (sensitivity 92.3%) and was true negative in eight patients with benign bile duct disease (adenoma, sclerosing cholangitis, Caroli disease). Distant metastatic disease was diagnosed correctly in 7 of 10 patients with histologically proven metastases, but regional lymph node metastases were identified in only 2 of 15 patients (13.3%).

The role of laparoscopy as part of the diagnostic and staging evaluation of patients with hilar cholangiocarcinoma is being evaluated at our institution. Several patients with seemingly resectable tumors have avoided an exploratory laparotomy when peritoneal tumor implants were found with laparoscopy. In addition, patients at high risk of developing peritoneal carcinomatosis may be identified by positive cytologic specimens obtained from laparoscopic washings. Finally, laparoscopic ultrasonography can be used to exclude the presence of noncontiguous liver metastases or extensive hilar tumor infiltration in patients with extrahepatic bile duct cancers.[123]

Treatment of Intrahepatic Cholangiocarcinomas

Intrahepatic cholangiocarcinomas may be detected in 30-45% of patients before they metastasize or cause jaundice.[124,125] These patients should be considered for operation because long-term survival has been reported in a proportion of the patients undergoing curative liver resection for intrahepatic cholangiocarcinoma.[76,125-127] A study of 19 patients who underwent resection of intrahepatic cholangiocarcinoma demonstrated that patients with no porta hepatis lymph node metastases had a 3-year survival rate of 64% compared with 0% for patients with nodal metastases.[126] A larger cohort of 32 patients who underwent resection of intrahepatic cholangiocarcinomas confirmed the negative prognostic impact of regional lymph node metastases and large size (>5-cm diameter) of the primary tumor.[127] The 5-year overall survival rates reported for patients who underwent a margin-negative liver resection for intrahepatic cholangiocarcinoma range from 20% to 48%, with regional lymph node metastases, presence of satellite tumor nodules, portal vein invasion by tumor, and large tumors identified as a poor-prognosis indicator.[125-127] Large size of the primary tumor is a poor-prognosis indicator because of the increased frequency of vascular and lymphatic invasion by the tumor as well as growth along neighboring bile duct walls.[128]

Hilar Bile Duct Cholangiocarcinoma

In 1890, Fardel first described a primary malignancy of the extrahepatic biliary tract. A report in 1957 described three patients with small adenocarcinomas involving the confluence of the left and right hepatic ducts.[129] Such primary cholangiocarcinomas arising at the bifurcation of the extrahepatic biliary tree are known commonly as Klatskin tumors, following his report in 1965 of a larger series of patients with these lesions.[130]

Prognostic Factors

In contrast to reports, the most important factor affecting prognosis is the resectability of the tumor. Patients who undergo curative resection (margin-negative) have 3-year survival rates from 40% to 87% and 5-year survival rates between 10% and 73%.[59,131] The wide range of survival rates is explained by variations in the incidence of factors that portend a poor prognosis in the various series. Significant determinants of improved prognosis in patients undergoing curative resection include well-differentiated tumors, absence of lymph node metastases, absence of direct tumor extension into the liver, papillary histology (versus nodular or sclerotic), serum bilirubin at presentation of <9 mg/dL, and a near-normal or normal performance status. Palliative resection, surgical bypass procedures, and various types of intubation and drainage procedures are associated with 3-year survival rates of 0-4%.[131] Hilar cholangiocarcinomas have a poorer prognosis than do carcinomas arising in the middle or distal thirds of the extrahepatic bile duct, which is related directly to the presentation of hilar tumors at a more locally advanced stage with bilobar liver involvement by tumor and resultant lower rates of curative resection.[132] However, like hilar cholangiocarcinoma, the presence of regional lymph node metastases reduces the 5-year overall survival rate following resection of middle or distal third bile duct cancer to 21% compared with the 65% survival rate in patients with node-negative disease.

Pathologic features of the bile duct cancer are predictors of outcome after resection. Prognosis is affected adversely if the tumor infiltrates the serosa of the bile duct, invades directly into the liver, demonstrates vascular invasion, or has metastasized to regional lymph nodes. Histologic type and grade are also important factors. Patients with the relatively unusual papillary bile duct adenocarcinoma have the most favorable prognosis, with 3-year survival rates up to 75%.[131,133] Patients with the more common nodular or sclerotic types of hilar cholangiocarcinoma have 3-year survival rates of <30%. A pathologic study that correlated gross tumor type with patterns of spread provides evidence that may explain the observed differences in survival outcomes. Papillary and superficial nodular tumors spread predominantly by mucosal extension, rarely invading the deeper layers of the bile duct wall or lymphatic channels, whereas nodular infiltrating or diffuse infiltrating tumors spread by direct or lymphatic extension in the submucosa.[134] The distance of mucosal or submucosal spread away from the gross tumor can be as great as 30 mm, but there were no local or anastomotic recurrences if at least a 5-mm tumor-free margin was attained. Patients with well- or moderately differentiated carcinomas have a 3-year survival rate of up to 51%, whereas no patient with a poorly differentiated carcinoma survived longer than 2 years.[135]

Treatment

Resection of a hilar cholangiocarcinoma affords the patient the best chance for significant survival; however, 5-year survival rates after resection of hilar cancers are 40% in the most hopeful reports and 10% or less in other accounts. Long-term survival rates after resection of middle or distal common bile duct cholangiocarcinomas, the latter requiring pancreaticoduodenectomy, are generally higher compared with hilar tumors.[75] This is most likely related to higher rates of margin-negative resection with middle or distal extrahepatic bile duct tumors and the absence of direct tumor extension into the liver.

The patterns of failure after curative extrahepatic bile duct resection for hilar cholangiocarcinoma have been described in a few series of patients (Table 87-3).[135] Locoregional tumor recurrence developed in a high percentage of patients, with failure in the liver (62%), tumor bed (42%), and regional lymph nodes (20%). The caudate lobe is the most frequent site of liver recurrence. Regional lymph nodes include porta hepatis, retroduodenal, and perigastric node groups along the gastrohepatic ligament. Distant metastasis develops in the majority of patients who exhibit a locoregional recurrence; however, it was the site of first failure in only 24%.

Table 87-3 Sites of Tumor Recurrence After Curative Resection of Proximal Hilar Cholangiocarcinomas

Site	Frequency (%)
Liver	62
Tumor bed	42
Regional lymph nodes	20
Peritoneum	16
Lungs	71
Bone	31
Skin	7

Detailed anatomic studies have offered an explanation for the high incidence of liver and local recurrence following resection of a hilar cholangiocarcinoma. In a series of 25 patients undergoing surgery for hilar cholangiocarcinoma, direct invasion of hepatic parenchyma at the hilum was noted in 12 patients (46.2%), with 11 patients (42.3%) also having carcinoma extending into the bile ducts draining the caudate lobe or directly invading the caudate lobe parenchyma.[136] A study of 106 adult human cadavers showed that 97.2% had bile ducts draining the caudate lobe that entered directly into the main left hepatic duct, right hepatic duct, or both. These caudate lobe bile ducts frequently enter the main left or right hepatic ducts within 1 cm of the proper hepatic duct. Thus, a carcinoma arising at the confluence of the right and left hepatic ducts need not be large to extend into the bile ducts draining the caudate lobe.

Because cholangiocarcinoma is known to spread along the wall of the bile ducts and because the caudate lobe and hepatic hilum are frequent sites of tumor recurrence following extrahepatic duct resection, a number of authors now recommend more aggressive resections to include the caudate lobe and hepatic hilar parenchyma.[137-140] An understanding of the Bismuth-Corlette classification of hilar cholangiocarcinoma is useful in planning the extent and site of liver resection (Fig. 87-10).[141] The median survival associated with a more radical surgical approach has varied from 10 to 37 months, with 5-year survival rates of 20-44% and 10-year survival rates as high as 14%.[137-140] Although aggressive surgical resection of hilar cholangiocarcinomas, including hepatic resection, provides the best chance for long-term survival, these operative procedures are associated with significant risk. The operative mortality rate in modern series ranges from 5% to 12%, with postoperative liver failure following an extensive liver resection being the most common cause of death.[137-140] Surgical complications are reported in 25% to 45% of the surviving patients. Infectious complications are the most common postoperative problem, and

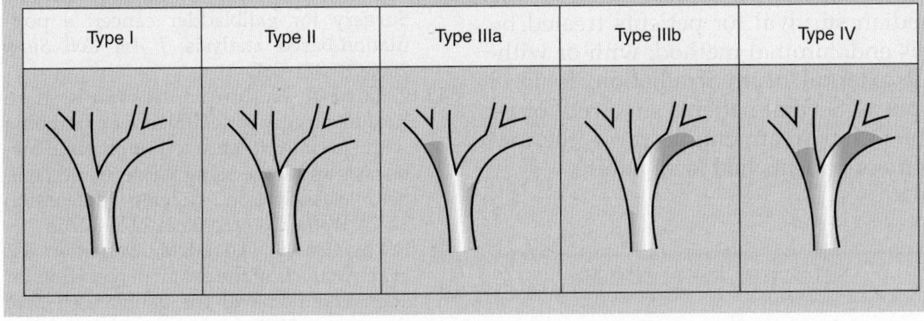

Figure 87-10 Bismuth-Corlette classification of hilar cholangiocarcinoma. Types 1 and 2 can be resected with excision of the extrahepatic bile duct with or without the hilar plate and caudate lobe. Types 3A and 3B can be resected with the addition of an en bloc right or left hepatic lobectomy, respectively. Type 4 is, by definition, unresectable. *Source*: From Ref. 141.

preoperative placement of biliary stents with resultant contamination of the obstructed biliary tree increases the incidence of infection.[142]

We recently reviewed our experience in patients with extrahepatic cholangiocarcinoma treated at the University of Texas MD Anderson Cancer Center.[143] Of 91 patients evaluated between 1983 and 1996, 51 (56%) presented with unresectable disease and 40 (44%) underwent resection. The median survival for the resected patients was 22.2 months versus 10.7 months in patients with unresectable disease ($p < .0001$). Nine patients, 5 with hilar and 4 with distal common duct cholangiocarcinoma, were treated with preoperative chemoradiation therapy (continuous intravenous infusion of 5-fluorouracil at 300 mg/m^2/day combined with external beam irradiation). Three of these nine patients had a pathologic complete response to chemoradiation treatment; the remaining six patients had varying degrees of histologic response to treatment. The rate of margin-negative resection was 100% for the preoperative chemoradiation group compared with 54% for the group not receiving preoperative treatment ($p < .01$). The patients treated with preoperative chemoradiation had no operative or postoperative complications related to treatment. Thus, it appears that neoadjuvant chemoradiation for extrahepatic bile duct cancer can be performed safely, produces significant antitumor response, and may improve the ability to achieve tumor-free resection margins.

Liver Transplantation Total hepatectomy with immediate orthotopic liver transplantation (OLT) has been described in patients with hilar cholangiocarcinoma.[144-149] The 90-day mortality from hemorrhage, sepsis, and graft rejection was 23.1%. Of the patients who survived <3 months following transplantation, the median survival was 11 months in the series prior to 1992 but has improved to 23 months in the recent series. In the older series of patients, the 5-year survival rate was 5.0%. In patients who died 3 months after transplantation, death was due to tumor recurrence in 85.4%. The 5-year survival rate following OLT for extrahepatic cholangiocarcinoma in current studies is 25%, and in the highly selected subset of patients with stage I or II disease, 5-year survival is 73%. Nonetheless, because of the poor results in most reports, many transplantation centers no longer perform liver transplantations in patients with hilar cholangiocarcinoma. Liver transplantation for hilar cholangiocarcinoma should probably be considered only as part of a prospective protocol evaluating multimodality treatment.

Palliation In general, curative surgical resection is possible in <30% of patients with hilar cholangiocarcinoma.[59,131,132] In patients deemed unresectable on the basis of the findings of diagnostic studies, laparotomy can be avoided by placing percutaneous external drains or endoscopically placed endoprostheses.[150,151] Conventional 10- or 12-French polyethylene endoprostheses have a high rate of occlusion and cholangitis.[152] However, new expandable metal wall stents appear to have improved long-term patency rates and may be used to deliver palliative high-dose rate endoluminal brachytherapy.[153,154] When unresectability is determined at the time of laparotomy, a decision must be made on a surgical bypass versus an operative intubation to provide drainage of the obstructed biliary tree. It is clear that techniques for surgical bypass, operative intubation, and percutaneous external drainage are equivalent in partial or complete relief of jaundice in 70-100% of patients.[59] Seemingly, the only potential advantage to the patient who undergoes surgical bypass instead of operative intubation is the absence of an external drainage catheter in the former group. The advantage of not having an external biliary drainage catheter or an internal endoscope is considering the quality-of-life issues related to chemotherapeutic toxicity; systemic chemotherapy has not demonstrated a distinct advantage in patients with hilar cholangiocarcinoma.

Radiotherapy Radiotherapy for bile duct cancer is even more confusing because of the various types, doses, routes of administration, and association with resected and unresected tumors, all in small numbers of patients. Internal radiation with 16 169Ir wires or seeds may have a palliative role in improving the patency of obstructed bile ducts; however, the number and frequency of episodes of cholangitis were not reduced, so the overall benefit is uncertain.[155] Internal radiation has been associated with prolongation of survival to an average of 16 months, and occasionally patients with unresectable disease survived >5 years.[156-158] Although the use of external beam radiotherapy alone to treat patients with unresectable hilar cholangiocarcinoma has not provided significant differences in overall patient survival, rare long-term survivals have been reported.[159] Intraoperative radiotherapy also has been evaluated in association with resectable and unresectable tumors.[160,161] Again, there is a suggestion of a slight prolongation of survival in patients with unresectable tumors, but the most interesting use of intraoperative radiotherapy may be as an immediate surgical adjuvant in the resected high-risk tumor bed.

Chemotherapy Given the high percentage of unresectable hilar cholangiocarcinomas, various chemotherapeutic regimens and radiotherapeutic regimens have been used in the hope of providing improved palliation and prolongation of survival. One trial suggested a benefit for chemotherapy over best supportive care alone. The study randomly assigned 90 patients with advanced pancreatic or biliary cancer ($N = 37$) to 5-FU-based systemic chemotherapy versus best supportive care alone and reported a median survival of 6 versus 2.5 months, respectively.[162] In general, no single drug or combination has consistently increased median survival beyond the expected 6-8 months. The most active agents are gemcitabine, capecitabine, 5-FU, and oxaliplatin.

A 1988 review of systemic chemotherapy for bile duct cancer noted that 97 patients had been treated with nine different treatment programs.[163] Mitomycin-C, doxorubicin, and 5-fluorouracil are the agents that have shown the greatest activity against cholangiocarcinoma. The collective partial response rate in the 97 patients was 29%, with no complete responses. The median survival of these patients receiving systemic chemotherapy ranged between 6 and 11 months. One study of 5-FU interferon alpha 2b

(IFN-a2b) given to 35 patients with biliary tract cancer reported 34% partial response (11 of 32 patients) and a median time to progression of 9.5 months, and a median survival of 12 months.[164] Response rates with gemcitabine alone range from 13% to 60%, with a median survival of <8 months in general.[165] In another study of 75 patients (45 cholangiocarcinoma, 3 ampulla of Vater, and 27 gallbladder), gemcitabine plus capecitabine combination was well tolerated.[166] The study reported response rate of 29%, median progression-free and overall survival rates were 6.2 and 12.7 months, respectively. In another study of gemcitabine and oxaliplatin (GEMOX) combination, those who had a good performance status of 0-2, bilirubin <2.5× normal and received GEMOX as first-line chemotherapy (N = 33) had a response rate of 33%, a median progression-free survival of 5.7 months, and a median survival of 15.4 months.[167] A more recent pooled analysis of 104 trials of different chemotherapy regimens in advanced biliary cancer concluded that the gemcitabine/cisplatin combination offered the highest rates of objective response and of tumor control (objective response plus stable disease) compared to either gemcitabine-free or cisplatin-free regimens.[168] However, this did not translate into significant benefit in terms of either time to tumor progression or median overall survival. More recently, several investigators studies targeted agents in biliary tract cancers. One study of 42 patients suggested benefit from anti-EGFR by the oral tyrosine kinase inhibitor erlotinib.[169] There were 3 partial responses and 7 patients remained progression-free at 6 months.

Interventional Radiology and Internal Radiotherapy ■ With no significant increase in survival and coniary drainage tubes, a combination of external beam plus endoluminal boost irradiation is an attractive treatment program. The favored treatment sequence is to start with external beam irradiation to obtain tumor regression, which provides a better dose distribution from the endoluminal boost irradiation to treat any residual tumor. The use of endoluminal ^{169}Ir alone for palliative treatment of patients with unresectable hilar bile duct cancers has been reported.[170] Endoluminal doses ranged from 15 to 35 Gy when combined with external beam irradiation (usually 45-50 Gy), or when endoluminal doses of up to 60 Gy were used alone. The dose reference point may vary from 0.5 to 1.0 cm from the central catheter. The total nominal doses of external beam plus endoluminal boost irradiation are between 60 and 70 Gy to the tumor, and although this range exceeds the liver and small intestine tolerance, the highest doses are confined to a small volume of tissue. The median survival for patients treated by this endoluminal method, with or without external beam irradiation, is 15-18 months. Several patients survived for >4 years after treatment; however, the majority of patients had local failure.

Selected References

The complete reference list can be found at www.CANCERMEDICINE8.com

2. Lazcano-Ponce E, Miguel JF, Munoz N, et al. Epidemiology and Molecular pathology of gall bladder cancer. *CA Cancer J Clin.* 2001;51:349–364.
4. Nelson BD, Porvaznik J, Benfield JR. Gallbladder disease in Southwestern American Indians. *Arch Surg.* 1971;103:41–43.
7. Mancuso TF, Brennan MJ. Epidemiological considerations of cancer of the gallbladder, bile ducts and salivary glands in the rubber industry. *J Occup Med.* 1970;12:333–341.
9. Khan ZR, Neugut AI, Ahsan H, Chabot JA. Risk factors for biliary tract cancers. *Am J Gastroenterol.* 1999;94:149–152.
12. Csendes A, Becerra M, Burdiles P, et al. Bacteriological studies of bile from the gallbladder in patients with carcinoma of the gallbladder, cholelithiasis, common bile duct stones and no gallstones disease. *Eur J Surg.* 1994;160:363–367.
14. Albores-Saavedra J, Alcantra-Vazquez A, Cruz-Ortiz H, Herrera-Goepfert R. The precursor lesions of invasive gallbladder carcinoma. Hyperplasia, atypical hyperplasia and carcinoma in situ. *Cancer.* 1980;45:919–927.
17. Yukawa M, Fujimori T, Hirayama D, et al. Expression of oncogene products and growth factors in early gallbladder cancer, advanced gallbladder cancer, and chronic cholecystitis. *Hum Pathol.* 1993;24:37–40.
20. Quan ZW, Wu K, Wang J, et al. Association of p53, p16, and vascular endothelial growth factor protein expressions with the prognosis and metastasis of gallbladder cancer. *J Am Coll Surg.* 2001;193:380–383.
22. Fahim RB, McDonald JR, Richards JC, Ferris DO. Carcinoma of the gallbladder. A study of its modes of spread. *Ann Surg.* 1962;156:114–122.
25. Ito M, Mishima Y, Sato T. An anatomical study of the lymphatic drainage of the gallbladder. *Surg Radiol Anat.* 1991;13:89–104.
28. Perpetuo MD, Valdivieso M, Heilbrun LK, et al. Natural history study of gallbladder cancer. A review of 36 years experience at MD Anderson Hospital and Tumor Institute. *Cancer.* 1978;42:330–335.
31. Dalla Palma L, Rizzatto G, Pozzi-Mucelli RS, Bazzocchi M. Grey-scale ultrasonography in the evaluation of carcinoma of the gall bladder. *Br J Radiol.* 1980;53:662–667.
34. Hirooka Y, Naitoh Y, Goto H, et al. Contrast-enhanced endoscopic ultrasonography in gallbladder diseases. *Gastrointest Endosc.* 1998;48:406–410.
37. Kohya N, Miyasaki K. Hepatectomy of segment 4a and 5 combined with extra-hepatic bile duct resection for T2 and T3 gallbladder carcinoma. *J Surg Oncol.* 2008 1;97:498–502.
40. Coburn NG, Cleary SP, Tan JC, Law CH. Surgery for gallbladder cancer: a population-based analysis. *J Am Coll Surg.* 2008;207:371–382.
43. Chijiiwa K, Noshiro H, Nakano K, et al. Role of surgery for gallbladder carcinoma with special reference to lymph node metastasis and stage using Western and Japanese classification systems [discussion 1277]. *World J Surg.* 2000;24:1271–1276.
46. D'Angelica N, Dalal KM, Dematteo RP, et al. Analysis of the extent of resection for adenocarcinoma of the gallbladder. *Ann Surg Oncol.* 2008.
49. Yamaguchi K, Chijiiwa K, Shimizu S, et al. Anatomical limit of extended cholecystectomy for gallbladder carcinoma involving the neck of the gallbladder. *Int Surg.* 1998;83:21–23.
52. Fong Y, Brennan MF, Turnbull A, et al. Gallbladder cancer discovered during laparoscopic surgery. Potential for iatrogenic tumor dissemination. *Arch Surg.* 1993;128:1054–1056.
55. Contini S, Dalla Valle R, Zinicola R. Unexpected gallbladder cancer after laparoscopic cholecystectomy: an emerging problem? Reflections on four cases. *Surg Endosc.* 1999;13:264–267.
58. Fong Y, Hefernan N, Blumgart LH. Gallbladder carcinoma discovered during laparoscopic cholecystectomy. Aggressive reresection is beneficial. *Cancer.* 1998;83:423–427.
61. Falkson G, MacIntyre JM, Moertel CG. Eastern Cooperative Oncology Group experience with chemotherapy for inoperable gallbladder and bile duct cancer. *Cancer.* 1984;54:965–969.
65. Buskirk SJ, Gunderson LL, Adson MA, et al. Analysis of failure following curative irradiation of gallbladder and extrahepatic bile duct carcinoma. *Int J Radiat Oncol Biol Phys.* 1984;10:2013–2023.
68. Kopelson G, Harisiadis L, Tretter P, Chang CH. The role of radiation therapy in cancer of the extra-hepatic biliary system. An analysis of thirteen patients and a review of the literature of the effectiveness of surgery, chemotherapy and radiotherapy. *Int J Radiat Oncol Biol Phys.* 1977;2:883–894.
71. Athlin LE, Domellof LK, Bergman FO. Advanced gallbladder carcinoma. A case report and review of the literature. *Eur J Surg Oncol.* 1987;13:449–453.
74. Thuluvath PJ, Rai R, Venbrux AC, Yeo CJ. Cholangiocarcinoma. A review. *Gastroenterologist.* 1997;5:306–315.
77. Sorensen HT, Friis S, Olsen JH, et al. Risk of liver and other types of cancer in patients with cirrhosis: a nationwide cohort study in Denmark. *Hepatology.* 1998;28:921–925.
79. Kurathong S, Lerdverasirikul P, Wongpaitoon V, et al. *Opisthorchis viverrini* infection and cholangiocarcinoma. A prospective, case-controlled study. *Gastroenterology.* 1985;89:151–156.
81. Voyles CR, Smadja C, Shands WC, Blumgart LH. Carcinoma in choledochal cysts. Age-related incidence. *Arch Surg.* 1983;118:986–988.
83. Wee A, Ludwig J, Coffey RJ Jr, et al. Hepatobiliary carcinoma associated with primary sclerosing cholangitis and chronic ulcerative colitis. *Hum Pathol.* 1985;16:719–726.
86. Robertson JF, Raine PA. Choledochal cyst. A 33-year review. *Br J Surg.* 1988;75:799–801.

89. Kaya M, de Groen PC, Angulo P, et al. Treatment of cholangiocarcinoma complicating primary sclerosing cholangitis. The Mayo Clinic experience. *Am J Gastroenterol.* 2001;96:1164–1169.
92. Ito Y, Kojiro M, Nakashima T, Mori T. Pathomorphologic characteristics of 102 cases of thorotrast-related hepatocellular carcinoma, cholangiocarcinoma, and hepatic angiosarcoma. *Cancer.* 1988;62:1153–1162.
95. Terada T, Ashida K, Endo K, et al. c-erbB-2 protein is expressed in hepatolithiasis and cholangiocarcinoma. *Histopathology.* 1998;33:325–331.
98. Jalanko H, Kuusela P, Roberts P, et al. Comparison of a new tumour marker, CA 19-9, with alpha-fetoprotein and carcinoembryonic antigen in patients with upper gastrointestinal diseases. *J Clin Pathol.* 1984;37:218–222.
101. Yamamoto M, Takasaki K, Yoshikawa T, et al. Does gross appearance indicate prognosis in intrahepatic cholangiocarcinoma? *J Surg Oncol Suppl.* 1998;69:162–167.
103. Pastolero GC, Wakabayashi T, Oka T, Mori S. Tissue polypeptide antigenÑa marker antigen differentiating cholangiolar tumors from other hepatic tumors. *Am J Clin Pathol.* 1987;87:168–173.
105. Colli A, Cocciolo M, Mumoli N, et al. Peripheral intrahepatic cholangiocarcinoma. Ultrasound findings and differential diagnosis from hepatocellular carcinoma. *Eur J Ultrasound.* 1998;7:93–99.
108. Han JK, Choi BI, Kim TK, et al. Hilar cholangiocarcinoma. Thin-section spiral CT findings with cholangiographic correlation. *Radiographics.* 1997;17:1475–1485.
111. Kusano T, Shimabukuro M, Tamai O, et al. The use of intra-operative ultrasonography for detecting tumor extension in bile duct carcinoma. *Int Surg.* 1997;82: 44–48.
113. Neri E, Boraschi P, Braccini G, et al. MR virtual endoscopy of the pancreaticobiliary tract. *Magn Reson Imaging.* 1999;17:59–67.
116. Tanaka M, Ogawa Y, Matsumoto S, Nakayama F. The role of endoscopic retrograde cholangiopancreatography in preoperative assessment of bile duct cancer. *World J Surg.* 1988;12:27–32.
119. Cameron JL, Broe P, Zuidema GD. Proximal bile duct tumors. Surgical management with silastic transhepatic biliary stents. *Ann Surg.* 1982;196:412–419.
122. Kluge R, Schmidt F, Caca K, et al. Positron emission tomography with [(18)F] fluoro-2-deoxy-D-glucose for diagnosis and staging of bile duct cancer. *Hepatology.* 2001;33:1029–1035.
125. Lieser MJ, Barry MK, Rowland C, et al. Surgical management of intrahepatic cholangiocarcinoma. A 31-year experience. *J Hepatobiliary Pancreat Surg.* 1998;5:41–47.
127. Pichlmayr R, Lamesch P, Weimann A, et al. Surgical treatment of cholangiocellular carcinoma. *World J Surg.* 1995;19:83–88.
130. Klatskin G. Adenocarcinoma of the hepatic duct at its bifurcation within the porta hepatis. *Am J Med.* 1965;38:241–248.
132. Burke EC, Jarnagin WR, Hochwald SN, et al. Hilar cholangiocarcinoma. Patterns of spread, the importance of hepatic resection for curative operation, and a presurgical clinical staging system. *Ann Surg.* 1998;228:385–394.
134. Ouchi K, Suzuki M, Hashimoto L, Sato T. Histologic findings and prognostic factors in carcinoma of the upper bile duct. *Am J Surg.* 1989;157:552–526.
138. Bengmark S, Ekberg H, Evander A, et al. Major liver resection for hilar cholangiocarcinoma. *Ann Surg.* 1988;207:120–125.

88 Neoplasms of the Exocrine Pancreas

Robert A. Wolff, MD ■ Christopher H. Crane, MD ■ Donghui Li, PhD ■ Douglas B. Evans, MD

Introduction

Pancreatic cancer is the fourth leading cause of cancer-related death for both men and women (following lung, colon, and breast cancer) and now accounts for 6% of all cancer-related deaths. In 2008, adenocarcinoma of the exocrine pancreas led to 34,290 deaths in the United States and worldwide, it is estimated to cause over 200,000 deaths annually.[1,2] Pancreatic cancer is not often discovered while it is still localized and surgically resectable, the only chance for cure. Rather, exocrine pancreatic cancer is characterized by early spread to regional lymph nodes and vascular dissemination with occult liver, or lung metastases frequently present at the time of diagnosis, even when findings from imaging studies are normal. Late diagnosis, coupled with its aggressive biologic behavior, make the incidence rates of pancreatic cancer virtually the same as its mortality rates.

Prognosis is highly dependent on the extent of disease and the patient's performance status at diagnosis. Clinical staging categorizes tumors as resectable (stage I or II), locally advanced (stage III), or metastatic (stage IV). Importantly, there is now emerging recognition of a subset of tumors best classified as borderline resectable.[3] With the exception of borderline resectable disease, the American Joint Commission on Cancer (AJCC) Cancer Staging Manual has been appropriately modified to reflect the emphasis on stage-specific treatment planning, which recognizes that most patients are not surgically staged.[4]

Patients who undergo upfront surgical resection for localized, nonmetastatic adenocarcinoma of the pancreatic head have a long-term survival rate of approximately 20% and a median survival ranging between 16 and 23 months.[5-8] Results from recent clinical trials support the delivery of adjuvant therapy after surgery with curative intent, but these strategies have not led to significant improvements in long-term survival for the past 20 years.[9] Alternative approaches to resectable disease include neoadjuvant therapy and delivery of novel therapeutics, which are now being investigated.

Patients with locally advanced pancreatic cancer have a median survival of 10-12 months and while chemoradiation remains a standard option, the role and timing of chemoradiation is now being reexamined.[10-12] Presentation with metastatic disease carries a dismal prognosis. Without active therapy, median overall survival is only 3-4 months, and with treatment, survival is typically improved by only a few months.[13-15] Thus far, the integration of molecular agents into therapy has not had meaningful impact on survival when delivered to unselected patients, prompting an interest in a more personalized approach to therapy.[16-18]

In this chapter, we will review the current literature relevant to the epidemiology, molecular and cellular biology, diagnosis and treatment of pancreatic cancer. The diagnostic algorithms emphasize the use of state-of-the-art imaging to include dynamic-phase computed tomography (CT) and endoscopic ultrasound (EUS) and in select cases, laparoscopy, to identify those patients most apt to gain from surgical intervention. Selection mechanisms, which identify patients who may benefit from aggressive combined modality therapy, will also be examined. Clinical trials, which involve novel treatments based on the known molecular mechanisms involved in tumorigenesis, will also be discussed.

Epidemiology

The risk of pancreatic cancer is low in the first three to four decades of life but increases sharply after age 50 years. Most patients are diagnosed between the ages of 60 and 80 years.[19] Historically, pancreatic cancer was more common in men than women, but now the incidence is about the same for both sexes, probably as a result of the increased use of tobacco by women.[19]

Pancreatic cancer incidence and mortality statistics are similar throughout the world. Incidence rates are highest in industrialized societies and western countries. In Europe, rates are highest in the Nordic countries.[19] In the United States, rates are relatively high among native Hawaiians and Korean Americans. The highest rates are observed in African Americans, considerably higher than for native Africans, suggesting an environmental influence. The reasons for slight regional and ethnic differences in the incidence of pancreatic cancer are unknown, but may be due to a trend toward a decline in tobacco use in certain groups and regions.[20] Unfortunately, these broad epidemiologic categories do little to identify specific individuals at high risk of pancreatic cancer.

Etiologic Factors

Diabetes Mellitus

An association between diabetes mellitus and pancreatic cancer has been known for decades, but the precise relationship has yet to be defined, and not all studies have supported such a link.[21] Diabetes mellitus has been implicated both as an early manifestation of pancreatic cancer and as a predisposing factor.[22-28] Two meta-analyses published 10 years apart have both reported that pancreatic cancer occurred with increased frequency in patients with longstanding diabetes (diagnosed at least 5 years prior to the diagnosis of pancreatic cancer or death due to pancreatic cancer).[29,30] The authors from these studies have therefore concluded that longstanding diabetes mellitus is an independent risk factor for pancreatic cancer.

While longstanding diabetes mellitus appears to be a risk factor for pancreatic cancer, a number of studies suggest new-onset diabetes may be a manifestation of it.[31,32] Ductal adenocarcinoma can induce peripheral insulin resistance.[33] In addition, a putative cancer-associated diabetogenic factor has been isolated from conditioned medium of pancreatic cancer cell lines and patient serum.[34] The expression of a diabetogenic factor is also supported by clinical observations showing diabetes can resolve after surgical resection of the primary tumor.[35] Some experts have gone on to suggest that evaluation of new-onset diabetes could lead to earlier diagnoses of pancreatic cancer, particularly if linked to an as yet undefined biomarker, which can distinguish benign diabetes mellitus from diabetes associated with an underlying pancreatic cancer.[36,37]

Hyperinsulinemia, Obesity, and the Metabolic Syndrome

Recent cohort studies have also shown that abnormal glucose metabolism may be associated with an increased risk of pancreatic cancer.[38,39] High insulin concentrations in the microenvironment of the pancreatic duct cell may contribute to malignant transformation[40,41] and hyperglycemia in the local tumor environment may promote perineural invasion often seen with pancreatic cancer.[42]

Of note, impaired glucose tolerance, insulin resistance, and secondary hyperinsulinism are associated with obesity and inactivity. Positive associations between obesity and pancreatic cancer risk have been reported in several large prospective studies.[43-48] A recent meta-analysis of 21 independent prospective studies involving 3,495,981 individuals and 8062 pancreatic cancer patients showed that the relative risk of pancreatic cancer per 5 kg/m^2 increase in body mass index was 1.16 (95% CI: 1.06-1.17) in men, and 1.10 (95% CI: 1.02-1.19) in women.[49] It has been estimated that obesity-associated pancreatic cancer accounts for ¼ of the cases in the US population.[43]

Further support for a link between obesity, insulin resistance, and pancreatic cancer comes from emerging recognition of the metabolic syndrome. While definitions vary, this syndrome is characterized by type 2 diabetes mellitus, truncal obesity, hypertension and dyslipidemia, which together increase the risk of cardiovascular disease.[50] More recent epidemiologic data have suggested the metabolic syndrome as a risk factor for pancreatic cancer.[51] Given the dramatic rise in the prevalence of the metabolic syndrome over the last several years, the epidemiology of pancreatic cancer may begin to shift. Moreover, since the metabolic syndrome has been associated with ongoing inflammation, the mechanisms driving pancreatic carcinogenesis may have similarities to other inflammatory conditions associated with an increased risk of cancer. Of note, fatty infiltration of the pancreas may lead to steatopancreatitis, suggesting a potential link between obesity, nonalcoholic fatty pancreatic disease, nonalcoholic steatopancreatitis, and pancreatic cancer.[52]

Pancreatitis

Although an association between pancreatitis and an increased risk of pancreatic cancer has long been suspected, the magnitude of the risk remains uncertain. Older clinical studies suggested that chronic forms of pancreatitis were most closely associated with the development of pancreatic cancer.[53,54] A later retrospective cohort study of 2015 patients from six countries also demonstrated an increased risk of pancreatic cancer in patients with chronic pancreatitis, with the cumulative incidence of pancreatic cancer increasing with longer follow-up.[55] In contrast were the findings of Karlson and colleagues,[56] who identified 230 patients with pancreatic cancer among 29,530 patients in the Swedish national registry discharged 1 year or more after a hospital admission for pancreatitis. Although they found that, the standardized incidence ratio (observed/expected) for the development of pancreatic cancer was increased in patients with pancreatitis (2.8; 95% confidence interval [CI], 2.5-3.2), after 10 years or more, the excess risk declined and of borderline significance. The authors concluded that the data did not support a causal association between pancreatitis and pancreatic cancer and suggested that alcohol consumption and smoking were contributing factors, which led to the increased cancer risk. Nevertheless, inflammation has been implicated in many other malignancies, and therefore, a causal relationship between pancreatitis and pancreatic cancer remains plausible.[57-59] Preclinical studies support the role of inflammation as a necessary component of malignant transformation. For example, in adult mice with K-ras mutations, induction of low-grade chronic pancreatitis was necessary to develop premalignant precursor lesions or invasive ductal adenocarcinoma.[60]

The incidence of pancreatic adenocarcinoma is also increased in patients with hereditary pancreatitis or tropical pancreatitis. Hereditary pancreatitis has an autosomal dominant pattern of transmission with 80% penetrance.[61] Symptoms usually arise by age 40 years, but can occur before age 5 years. To examine the possibility of a connection between hereditary pancreatitis and pancreatic cancer, Lowenfels and colleagues obtained data about 246 patients with hereditary pancreatitis.[62] The estimated cumulative risk of pancreatic cancer developing by age 70 was approximately 40%. In addition, molecular data strongly suggests that mutations in the cationic trypsinogen gene play an important role in hereditary and possibly acquired forms of pancreatitis, increasing the risk of pancreatic cancer.[63]

Inherited Cancer Syndromes

Selected inherited cancer syndromes are also associated with an increased risk of pancreatic cancer.[64] One of these is hereditary breast-ovarian cancer syndrome, which is associated with mutations in BRCA1 or BRCA2. BRCA2 is a tumor suppressor gene on chromosome 13q12 and its protein product is involved in the repair of DNA strand breaks. Germline mutations in the BRCA2 gene have been found in 10% of patients with familial pancreatic cancer and in 7% of patients thought to have sporadic pancreatic cancer.[65-67] Germline BRCA2 mutations represent the most common inherited predisposition to pancreatic cancer and are associated with an up to a 10-fold greater risk of pancreatic cancer than in the general population.[68] Another inherited cancer syndrome associated with pancreatic cancer is the Peutz-Jeghers syndrome, an autosomal dominant trait caused by mutations in the LKB1/STK11 tumor suppressor gene on chromosome 19p13. This syndrome is characterized by the presence of hamartomatous gastrointestinal polyps and mucocutaneous pigmentation and is associated with an increased risk of several gastrointestinal cancers.[69] Although patients with Peutz-Jeghers syndrome are at significant risk of pancreatic cancer, the exact magnitude of the risk is unclear. Of note, biallelic inactivation of the LKB1/STK11 gene was also found in 4% of patients with resected sporadic pancreatic cancers.[70] The familial atypical multiple-mole melanoma (FAMMM) syndrome is a rare autosomal dominant disorder with incomplete penetrance caused by germline mutations in the p16 tumor suppressor gene on chromosome 9p21 and causes the development of multiple nevi, including malignant melanoma. FAMMM-pancreatic carcinoma (FAMMM-PC) is the new term for the form of FAMMM associated with pancreatic cancer.[71] Both early-onset and late-onset pancreatic cancer have been seen in affected families. Hereditary nonpolyposis colon cancer (HNPCC) is an autosomal dominant condition caused by germline mutations in mismatch repair genes resulting in an increased risk of both colorectal cancer and other cancers, including cancer of the breast, endometrium, ovary, and pancreas.[72]

Familial pancreatic cancer kindreds have also been identified that are not affected by any defined inherited cancer syndrome or familial pancreatitis. At-risk patients for familial pancreatic cancer include those with a minimum of two first-degree relatives with pancreatic cancer.[73] In a study of a family with familial pancreatic cancer, the susceptibility locus for autosomal dominant pancreatic cancer was located on chromosome 4q32-34.[74] However, this finding has not been confirmed by other investigators.[75]

Infectious Diseases

Older data suggested an association between Helicobacter pylori (H. pylori) and pancreatic cancer.[76,77] H. pylori may cause subclinical pancreatitis or increased gastrin levels, with resultant trophic effects on the pancreas. In addition, given that the gastric carriage of H. pylori is a known risk factor for peptic ulcer formation and gastric cancer, it may explain the association between gastric resection and pancreatic cancer.[78] At variance with this observation is a recent necropsy-based, case-control study performed in Sweden, that found no relationship between the development of pancreatic cancer and a remote history of gastric resection.[79]

Hepatitis B may also be a risk factor for pancreatic cancer. In a recent study involving 476 patients with pathologically confirmed adenocarcinoma of the pancreas and 879 age-matched, sex-matched, and race-matched healthy controls, a possible association between past exposure to hepatitis B virus and pancreatic cancer was discovered.[80] The proximity of the liver to the pancreas and the fact that the liver and pancreas share common blood vessels and ducts may make the pancreas a potential target organ for hepatitis viruses. In fact, hepatitis B surface antigen (HBsAg), a marker for chronic HBV infection, was detected in pure pancreatic juice and pure bile juice[81] and there was evidence of HBV replication in pancreatic cells and concurrent damage to exocrine and endocrine epithelial cells with an inflammatory response.[82,83] The possibility that viral hepatitis can lead to pancreatic damage is further supported by findings of elevated pancreatic enzyme levels in a substantial percentage of patients with acute and chronic HBV and HCV infection.[84]

Environmental Factors

Tobacco

The risk factor most firmly associated with pancreatic cancer is cigarette smoking.[85-88] In animals, pancreatic malignancies can be induced through the long-term administration of tobacco-specific N-nitrosamines or the parenteral administration of other N-nitroso compounds.[89,90] These carcinogens are metabolized to electrophiles that readily react with DNA, leading to miscoding and activation of oncogenes. Numerous US and European case-control and cohort studies have shown an increased risk of pancreatic cancer in smokers; indeed, it is currently estimated that approximately 25% of cases of pancreatic cancer are due to cigarette smoking.[91] Studies have also shown that the risk of pancreatic cancer increases as the amount and duration of smoking increase and that long-term smoking cessation (>10 years) reduces the risk by approximately 30% relative to the risk in current smokers.[87,91] The detection of carcinogen-DNA adducts in human pancreas tissues and tobacco-specific compounds in pancreatic juice further confirm the link between cigarette smoking and pancreatic cancer.[92-94] Recent molecular epidemiological studies have also shown that individual variability in carcinogen metabolism and DNA repair may partially determine the susceptibility to smoking-related pancreatic cancer.[95-98] This may facilitate strategies to identify high-risk individuals for primary prevention of pancreatic cancer.

Whether the use of smokeless tobacco products increases the risk of pancreatic cancer remains controversial.[99] Some studies do suggest an increase in risk,[100] but others have found no definite association between smokeless tobacco use and pancreatic cancer.[101,102]

Diet

Various dietary factors have also been implicated in the development of pancreatic cancer. Generally, high intakes of fat or meat increase the risk; whereas high intakes of fruits and vegetables reduce the risk.[103-106] Recent studies suggest that the method of meat preparation and subsequent intake of food mutagens may contribute to the development of pancreatic cancer.[107-109] Cooking meat at high temperature, (deep-fried, grilled, or barbequed), produces potential carcinogens such as heterocyclic amines and polycyclic aromatic hydrocarbons.

The associations of dietary carbohydrates, refined sugars, and glycemic index or load with pancreatic cancer have been investigated in many studies but the results are inconsistent.[110-118] The glycemic index represents the postprandial glucose response of individual food items compared with a reference food; refined grains, such as white bread or white rice, produce a larger increase in postprandial glucose levels than whole grain foods. A high dietary glycemic index or load could increase the risk of pancreatic cancer due to the adverse effect of a high postprandial glucose level and resulting insulin demands. The inconsistent results on the associations of dietary glycemic index and risk of pancreatic cancer could be related to study design issues, such as small sample size, inadequate control for diabetes and other confounders, or incomplete exposure information.

Decreased pancreatic cancer rates have been associated with the high consumption of vegetables, citrus fruits, fiber, and vitamin C.[103] The protective effects of these food items may have been mediated through folate as indicated by findings from a study of male smokers showing that dietary folate intake and serum folate levels were inversely associated with the risk of pancreatic cancer.[119] However, the association of folate intake and risk of pancreatic cancer was not observed in other studies.[120,121]

Although heavy alcohol consumption is an established risk factor for pancreatitis and type 2 diabetes mellitus, a clear association between alcohol consumption and pancreatic cancer has not been firmly established. Even though most studies have failed to demonstrate a positive association of alcohol and pancreatic cancer, some studies have shown a significant increased risk associated with total ethanol intake more than 30 grams per day.[122-124]

Occupational Exposures

The role of occupational or industrial factors in pancreatic cancer has been investigated extensively. Increased risk of pancreatic cancer has been associated with exposures to some chemicals (eg, organochlorines, chlorinated hydrocarbons, and formaldehyde), or some specific occupations (eg, stone miners, cement workers, gardeners, and textile workers). However, the statistical power of most of these studies is quite low and firm conclusions about occupational exposures and pancreatic cancer risk cannot be drawn.[19]

In summary, cigarette smoking and obesity may each be responsible for as many as 25% of the cases of pancreatic cancer implying that half of pancreatic cancer cases may be preventable.[41,44] Conversely, the proportion of pancreatic cancer cases attributable to known inherited pancreatic cancer syndromes is small. However, these high-risk individuals are the focus of intense research into the pathophysiology of pancreatic tumorigenesis and potential prevention strategies. The management of such individuals remains extremely controversial; options range from close observation to aggressive surgical intervention with a variety of approaches in evolution.[125-128]

Pathology

Histopathology

The normal architecture of the pancreas is typical of the architecture of a secretory gland. A background of acinar cells accounts for approximately 80% of the cell number and volume of the gland and clusters of islet cells account for 1-2%. Single-layered, cuboidal ductal cells comprise 10-15%, and the remainder is a sparse interlacing network of blood vessels, lymphatics, nerves, and stroma. In carcinoma, this architecture is markedly altered. Almost all malignant neoplasms of pancreatic origin (95%) arise from the exocrine portion of the gland and have light microscopic features consistent with those of adenocarcinomas.[129] The predominant histologic feature is a dense collagenous stroma with atrophic acini, remarkably preserved islet cell clusters, and a slight-to-moderate increase in the number of ducts, both normal- and malignant-appearing. The diagnosis of ductal adenocarcinoma rests on the identification of mitoses, nuclear and cellular pleomorphism, discontinuity of ductal epithelium, and evidence of perineural, vascular, or lymphatic invasion.[129]

Table 88-1 Histologic Classification of Tumors of the Exocrine Pancreas

Malignant
Carcinoma in situ (PanIn III; pancreatic intraepithelial neoplasia)
Ductal adenocarcinoma[a]
Intraductal papillary mucinous carcinoma (invasive IPMN)
Mucinous cystadenocarcinoma
Acinar cell carcinoma
Pancreatoblastoma
Premalignant
Intraductal papillary-mucinous neoplasm (noninvasive IPMN)[b]
Mucinous cystadenoma
Uncertain malignant potential
Solid pseudopapillary tumor
Benign
Serous cystadenoma[c]

[a]Variants include adenosquamous carcinoma, mucinous adenocarcinoma, signet ring cell carcinoma, and undifferentiated carcinoma (spindle cell, giant cell, and small cell types).
[b]Previous names include intraductal mucin-hypersecreting neoplasm, duct ectatic mucinous cystadenoma or carcinoma, and mucinous ductal ectasia.
[c]May exhibit uncontrolled local tumor growth, causing the designation "benign" to be questioned.

Tumors arising from the islets of Langerhans (endocrine) cells of the pancreas are much less common, and primary nonepithelial tumors of the pancreas (eg, lymphomas or sarcomas) are extremely rare. A current view of the histologic classification of exocrine pancreatic neoplasms is presented in Table 88-1.

Molecular Pathology

Studies of archival human pancreatic tumor tissue and human pancreatic cancer cell lines have identified several characteristic genetic abnormalities associated with pancreatic cancer. In particular, specific point mutations have been found at codon 12 of the K-ras oncogene, located on chromosome 12p13, in 75-90% of pancreatic adenocarcinoma specimens.[130,131] Mutations in the K-ras oncogene are thought to be an early event in the transformation of normal duct epithelium,[132] and preliminary data suggest that K-ras may be the site of action of environmental carcinogens such as cigarette smoke or organochlorine compounds.[133,134] The detection of mutant K-ras in body fluids and biopsy specimens is also currently being explored as a technique for the early diagnosis of pancreatic cancer in selected patients.[135-137] The RAS oncoprotein is an important signal-transduction mediator for receptor protein tyrosine kinases.[138] Transforming mutations of RAS are resistant to the GTPase-activating function of GTPase-activating proteins and result in a constitutively active RAS protein, unregulated cellular proliferation signals, and susceptibility to transformation. All RAS proteins are produced in the cytoplasm as biologically inactive precursor molecules and must undergo posttranslational modification in order to localize to the membrane, which is necessary for full biologic activity. The enzyme farnesylprotein transferase catalyzes the first of a series of steps necessary for the translocation of the RAS protein to the cell membrane and therefore, inhibitors of farnesylprotein transferase were developed and studied in patients with pancreatic cancer. Unfortunately, clinical results have been disappointing.[139]

In the progression model of pancreatic cancer proposed by Hruban and colleagues,[132] inactivation of the p16 tumor suppressor gene is thought to occur after mutation of K-ras. The p16 protein, whose gene is located on chromosome 9p21, belongs to a class of cyclin-dependent kinase (Cdk)-inhibitory proteins (including p21/WAF1/Cip1) and inhibits the cyclin D1/Cdk-4 complex that normally acts to phosphorylate the retinoblastoma (Rb) protein. Phosphorylation of Rb results in the release of transcription factors that promote the transcription of genes necessary for progression through the G1 phase of the cell cycle. Therefore, inactivation of p16 leads to hyperphosphorylated Rb that, in turn, leads to unregulated cell growth. Abrogation of the Rb/p16 pathway can also result from inactivation of the RB1 gene or the overexpression of cyclin D1 or Cdk-4. In approximately 95% of pancreatic carcinomas, the Rb/p16 pathway is inactivated when the p16 gene is inactivated as the result of homozygous deletion, the loss of one allele combined with an intragenic mutation in the other, or hypermethylation of the promotor of the p16 gene.[140] Germline mutations in the p16 tumor suppressor gene are associated with the newly described FAMM-PC syndrome discussed previously.

Loss of the TP53, DPC4, and possibly BRCA2 tumor suppressor genes are thought to occur late in the development of pancreatic cancer.[132] The TP53 gene is the most commonly mutated gene in human cancer. This tumor suppressor gene, located on chromosome 17p13, regulates progression through the cell cycle and induction of cell death. Following DNA damage, TP53 protein levels increase because of posttranslational changes in protein stability. These increased TP53 protein levels lead to the transcriptional activation of p21wAF1/CIP1, which inhibits cyclin-dependent kinase activity and prevents cell-cycle progression from the G1 phase to the S phase.[141] In addition to its effect on the cell cycle, TP53 also modulates apoptosis in response to DNA damage through the transcriptional activation of additional genes.[142] Approximately 50-75% of pancreatic adenocarcinomas show loss of TP53 function.[143,144]

The SMAD4/DPC4 tumor suppressor gene on chromosome 18q21 is an important component of the transforming growth factor-β signaling pathway that normally downregulates the growth of epithelial cells, stimulates differentiation, and promotes apoptosis.[145,146] Loss of this important growth regulatory pathway contributes to unregulated cell growth. The DPC4 gene is inactivated in approximately 55% of human pancreatic tumors through homozygous deletion or the loss of one allele coupled with an intragenic mutation in the second allele.[147] Clinically, loss of SMAD4 expression appears to be associated with poor prognosis in patients with resected pancreatic adenocarcinoma since the presence of SMAD4 expression in the tumor was associated with a median survival advantage of 5 months.[148] The ability to restore (and possibly overexpress) DPC4 function in human pancreatic cancer cells remains an active area of investigation because of its obvious therapeutic implications.[149]

Recently, Jones et al performed a comprehensive genetic analysis of 20,661 protein-coding genes in 24 pancreatic cancers.[150] More than 1000 mutated genes were detected in these analyses. Although the number of mutations varied from tumor to tumor, the altered genes affected a core set of 12 cellular signaling pathways and regulatory processes, including apoptosis, regulation of G1/S phase transition, hedgehog signaling, K-ras signaling, TGF-β signaling, and Wnt/Notch signaling, c-Jun N-terminal kinase signaling, regulation of invasion, DNA damage control, homophilic cell adhesion, small GTPase–dependent signaling (other than K-ras), and integrin signaling. The authors pointed out that pancreatic cancer is different from certain forms of leukemia, in which tumorigenesis appears to be driven by a single, targetable oncogene. Pancreatic cancers result from genetic alterations of a large number of genes that function through a relatively small number of pathways and processes. Thus, the best hope for therapeutic development may lie in the discovery of agents that target the physiologic effects of the altered pathways and processes rather than their individual gene components. An increased understanding of these molecular alterations may lead to new treatment strategies. Although advances in genomic and proteomic technology are revealing new and exciting targets for therapy, they also are demonstrating the complex nature of tumorigenesis and metastasis.[132,144,151,152]

Tumor Biology

The cellular events leading to pancreatic tumorigenesis, invasion, and metastasis continue to be elucidated. Pancreatic carcinogenesis likely results from cellular injury, DNA damage, and epigenetic changes caused by environmental exposure to tobacco smoke, carcinogens in foods, or other ingested material. Persons with compromised metabolic pathways designed to detoxify carcinogens may therefore be at increased risk for DNA damage and epigenetic alterations. These genetic and epigenetic perturbations, amplified by inherited or acquired defects in DNA repair pathways, ultimately result in oncogene activation and tumor suppressor gene inactivation as detailed previously. Such events eventually give rise to groups of genetically mutated, phenotypically normal-appearing cells with a proliferative advantage over their normal cellular counterparts. Subsequent malignant transformation may be further promoted by a microenvironment of inflammation precipitated by the presence of infectious agents, pancreatitis, or steatopancreatitis, with hyperglycemia, hyperinsulinemia, or both accelerating tumorigenesis. Once an invasive phenotype is established, tumor cells are capable of recruiting or reprogramming other stromal elements to provide an environment conducive to tumor cell survival, migration, invasion, and metastatic spread. Pancreatic cancer cells have a propensity for perineural and lymphovascular invasion, which may facilitate local recurrence along arterial structures and spread to locoregional nodes. This alone can be lethal with autopsy series showing that about 20% of patients who succumb to pancreatic cancer do so only with locoregional disease.[153] Tumor cells can also readily metastasize to more distant sites to include the liver, lung, and peritoneal cavity, and ultimately can result in death.

Cell of Origin in Pancreatic Cancer: The Acinar Cell

For years, pancreatic ductal epithelial cells were thought to explain the origins of pancreatic cancer. More recently, however, several groups have shown compelling evidence for acinar or centroacinar cells as the early progenitors of pancreatic cancer.[60,154,155] Acinar cells can transdifferentiate into duct-like epithelia, passing through a nestin-positive intermediate, which is dependent on Notch signaling pathways.[156] These duct-like epithelial cells are metaplastic with the potential to develop premalignant precursors. The ability of acinar cells to transdifferentiate appears to be dependent on a variety of signals to include RAS, matrix metalloproteinase 7, and Notch. In the future, screening and prevention strategies pancreatic cancer may focus on identification of cellular injury within the acinar cell population and the use of specific therapies to reverse or minimize it.

The Stem Cell Model of Pancreatic Cancer

Over the last several years, the stem cell model of malignancy has emerged from in vitro and in vivo observations demonstrating that no more than 1-2% of the cells comprising a tumor have self-replicating and tumorigenic potential. In this model, malignant stem cells give rise to more differentiated progeny, which represent the bulk of any given tumor mass. In a variety of malignancies, relatively small numbers of cancer stem cells have been identified by their expression of specific cell surface markers. Cancer stem cells have been characterized by their potential for self-renewal, the presence of aberrant developmental signaling pathways, such as sonic hedgehog, and signaling cascades that are integral for tumor metastasis.[157] Moreover, these malignant stem cells are notable for resistance to standard chemotherapy and radiation. Simeone and colleagues have begun to characterize pancreatic cancer stem cells from primary human pancreatic cancer specimens grown in immunocompromised mice. They have identified a very small subset of cells (0.2-0.8%), which are positive for the cell surface markers CD44, CD24, and epithelial specific antigen (ESA).[158] As few as 100 of these highly tumorigenic cells injected into mice can generate tumors are histologically identical to the human tumors from which they are derived. From a clinical standpoint, the identification of cancer stem cells within human pancreatic cancers has important implications for treatment since these cells are likely responsible for the development of cancer metastases and recurrence after clinical remission. Future strategies for improved pancreatic cancer control and eradication will likely require a two-pronged approach: debulking tumors using the known weaponry of systemic cytotoxic therapy, molecular therapy, limited-field radiotherapy, and in some cases surgery, combined with a yet undefined treatment to eradicate the cancer stem cell population.

The Tumor Microenvironment and the Role of Pancreatic Stellate Cells

Pancreatic cancer cells are notorious for creating a permissive environment within the host for local tumor growth, invasion, and metastasis. Although the prerequisite cellular events remain poorly defined, there is growing appreciation for the role of the tumor microenvironment as critical to cancer cell survival, metastasis, shelter from immune surveillance, and resistance to conventional anticancer therapies. Thus far, clinical efforts to impact the tumor microenvironement using matrix metalloproteinase inhibitors (to prevent basement membrane degradation and invasion) and antiangiogenic agents have been disappointing,[17,159,160] but new research may provide other opportunities for exploitation of the tumor-host interface. For example, stromal fibroblasts (also known as pancreatic stellate cells) have been recently shown to promote tumor cell growth, migration, invasion, and metastases.[161] Theoretically, targeting the interaction between these stromal elements and the cancer cells, perhaps in combination with other cytotoxic therapy, may provide another clinically meaningful treatment approach in the future.

Clinical Manifestations of Pancreatic Cancer

Virtually all patients with periampullary neoplasms and approximately 50% of patients with pancreatic cancer have jaundice at diagnosis as the result of extrahepatic biliary obstruction. Tumors arising in the ampulla of Vater or within the intrapancreatic portion of the common bile duct cause biliary obstruction early in the disease course and, therefore, may be associated with a better prognosis. Small tumors of the pancreatic head strategically located near the intrapancreatic portion of the bile duct also may obstruct the bile duct and cause the patient to seek medical attention while the tumor is still localized and potentially resectable. In contrast, adenocarcinomas arising in the pancreas that do not obstruct the intrapancreatic portion of the bile duct are often not diagnosed until they become locally advanced or have metastasized. In the absence of extrahepatic biliary obstruction, few pancreatic cancer patients present with potentially resectable disease.

If jaundice is not present, presenting complaints are often nonspecific, as are the clinical signs on physical examination. The pain typical of locally advanced pancreatic cancer is a dull, fairly constant pain of visceral origin localized to the middle and upper back; the pain is due to tumor invasion of the celiac and mesenteric plexus. Some patients have vague, intermittent epigastric pain; its etiology is less clear. Fatigue, weight loss, anorexia and early satiety are common even in the absence of mechanical gastric outlet obstruction. Pancreatic exocrine insufficiency, when present, is due to obstruction of the pancreatic duct and commonly results in malabsorption, steatorrhea, and mild changes in stool frequency. Recognition of pancreatic insufficiency is important since it is easily addressed with supplemental pancreatic enzymes. Moreover, in this setting, weight loss should not be assumed a manifestation of locally advanced or metastatic disease. Symptomatic diarrhea attributable to lack of pancreatic enzymes entering into the intestinal lumen is uncommon. However, patients with high-grade biliary obstruction often report loose stools; this usually resolves with restoration of bile flow into the gastrointestinal tract. As previously discussed, hyperglycemia is a common finding at the time of presentation and it may develop during the course of disease.

Diagnostic Evaluation

With the increasing subspecialisation of medicine, the diagnostic workup of patients ultimately found to have pancreatic cancer can be fragmented and inefficient. Surgeons or subspecialty oncologists may be asked to evaluate a patient at any point in the diagnostic process to include evaluation of abdominal pain, suspicion of pancreatic cancer, or biopsy-confirmed malignancy with or without complete staging evaluation. Important clinical information, having direct implications for therapy, can be obtained from a thorough history and physical examination. Some of this information cannot be obtained from imaging studies and includes assessment of performance status, cardiopulmonary function, the presence or absence of left supraclavicular or periumbilical adenopathy, or evidence for venous thromboembolism. With this in mind, a general outline of appropriate diagnostic and staging studies can be reviewed.

Imaging

Biliary obstruction is usually evaluated with abdominal ultrasonography (US) to confirm the mechanical nature of the obstruction and to determine whether the site of obstruction originates from the intrahepatic or extrahepatic portion of the biliary tree. When extrahepatic biliary obstruction is evident, further work-up can proceed directly with a combination of CT and endoscopic retrograde cholangiopancreatography (ERCP). In the setting of localized disease, EUS may provide additional staging information and this combined with fine needle aspiration (FNA), is our preferred method for tissue confirmation of malignancy. For patients presenting with abdominal pain or back pain, the diagnostic work-up is often less directed, but eventually leads to a suspicion of pancreatic cancer. Figure 88-1 for the diagnostic schema for patients with suspected pancreatic cancer, which emphasizes the importance of high-quality CT.

High-quality CT can identify most pancreatic tumors and accurately define the relationship of the tumor to the celiac axis and superior mesenteric vessels.[162] The development of multislice or multidetector CT (MDCT) allows imaging of the entire pancreas during the bolus phase of contrast enhancement. In addition, scan data can be processed to display images in three-dimensional and multiplanar formats.[163] MDCT performed with contrast enhancement and a thin-section technique can accurately assess the relationship of the low-density tumor to the celiac axis, hepatic artery, SMA, and superior mesenteric–portal vein (SMPV) confluence. At least two phases of contrast-enhanced helical scanning are required. The first (arterial) phase is performed from the diaphragm through the horizontal portion of the duodenum in order to define the relationship of the tumor to the adjacent arteries and to determine the presence or absence of aberrant arterial anatomy. When IV contrast is properly injected and timed, acquired images optimize the difference in density between the pancreas and tumor. The second (venous) phase is performed to define the relationship of the tumor to the surrounding venous structures (SMV, portal vein, and splenic vein) and to uncover metastases in the liver and remainder of the abdomen.

For treatment planning, it is of critical importance to use standardized, objective radiologic criteria for preoperative tumor staging. The CT findings defining a potentially resectable pancreatic cancer (AJCC stages I or II) are: (1) the absence of extrapancreatic disease, (2) a patent SMPV confluence (assuming it is technically

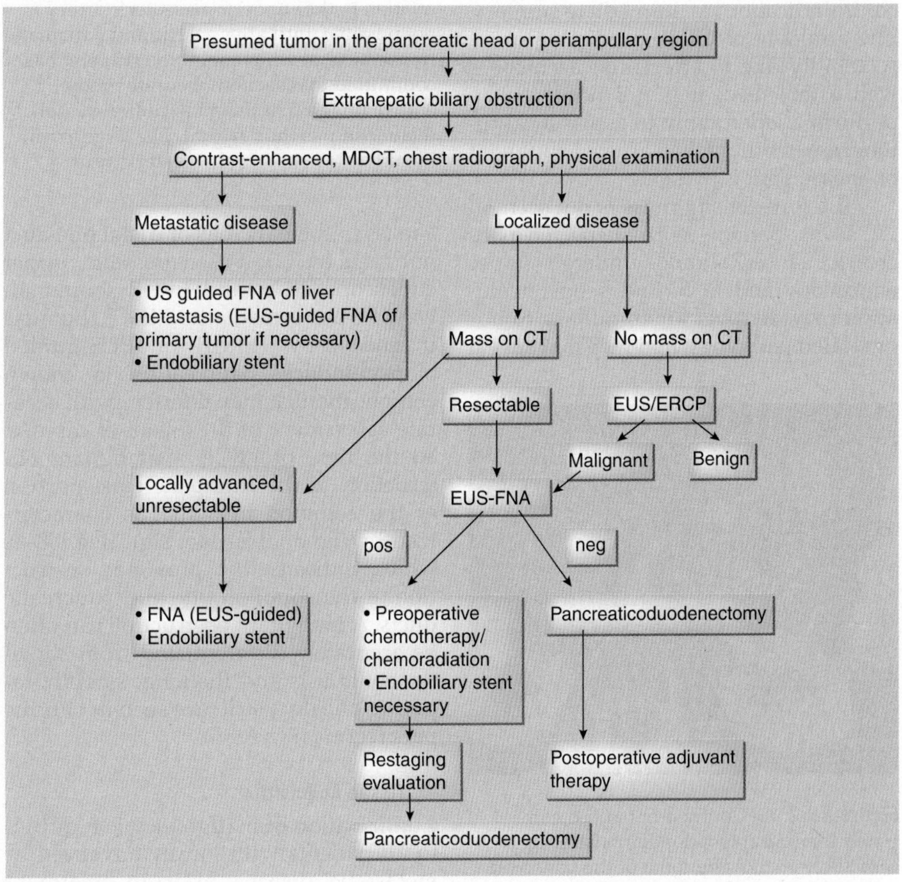

Figure 88-1 Management algorithm employed at our institution for patients with suspected or biopsy-proven adenocarcinoma of the pancreatic head. Accurate radiographic imaging allows patients to be staged as having resectable, locally advanced, or metastatic disease. In patients with locally advanced or metastatic disease, biopsy confirmation of malignancy is mandatory prior to the initiation of specific anticancer therapy. Similarly, before the initiation of neoadjuvant therapy cytologic confirmation of malignancy is required. The development of endoscopic ultrasound (EUS)-guided fine-needle aspiration (FNA) has greatly simplified tissue acquisition for patients with localized, nonmetastatic pancreatic cancer. In patients without cytologic evidence of malignancy (negative biopsy) in whom clinical and radiographic evidence support the diagnosis of a pancreatic or periampullary cancer, we proceed directly to pancreaticoduodenectomy (followed by postoperative adjuvant therapy if indicated). Laparoscopy should be considered prior to opening the abdomen in patients with potentially resectable disease; however, we rarely perform laparoscopy as a separate staging procedure. *Abbrevations:* CT, computed tomography; ERCP, endoscopic retrograde cholangiopancreatography.

possible to resect isolated involvement of the SMV or SMPV confluence and perform a suitable venous reconstruction), and (3) no direct tumor extension to the celiac axis or SMA (Fig. 88-2). A patient is deemed to have locally advanced, unresectable disease (AJCC stage III) when CT images demonstrate tumor extension to the SMA or celiac axis for greater than 180° of the circumference of the vessel (now referred to encasement) or occlusion of the SMPV confluence (Fig. 88-3). Limited arterial abutment (tumor–vessel interface of 180° or less) is now referred to as borderline resectable and patients with this extent of disease may be amenable to an initial nonoperative multimodality treatment approach followed by eventual surgery.[164] In general however, tumor extension to the celiac axis, common hepatic artery, or SMA (abutment or encasement) should be considered a contraindication to immediate surgery. The accuracy of CT in predicting unresectability due to arterial encasement is well established; it is not necessary to perform a laparotomy to assess local tumor resectability when arterial abutment or encasement is present.

If a low-density mass is not seen on CT scans, patients with suspected pancreatic cancer should undergo upper endoscopy and EUS. Endoscopic evaluation may discover an ampullary tumor or related pathology, and EUS may reveal a mass in the pancreas or distal bile duct not seen on CT. When possible, upper endoscopy, EUS, and ERCP should always be performed after MDCT, because if endoscopy (ERCP or EUS-guided biopsy)-induces pancreatitis, (a known complication), it may interfere with accurate assessment of the extent of disease. At the time of ERCP, a malignant obstruction of the intrapancreatic portion of the common bile duct is characterized by the double-duct sign (Fig. 88-4), which indicates the proximal obstruction of the common bile and pancreatic ducts. A malignant obstruction can often be accurately differentiated from choledocholithiasis and the long, smooth, tapering bile duct stricture seen in chronic pancreatitis (Fig. 88-5).

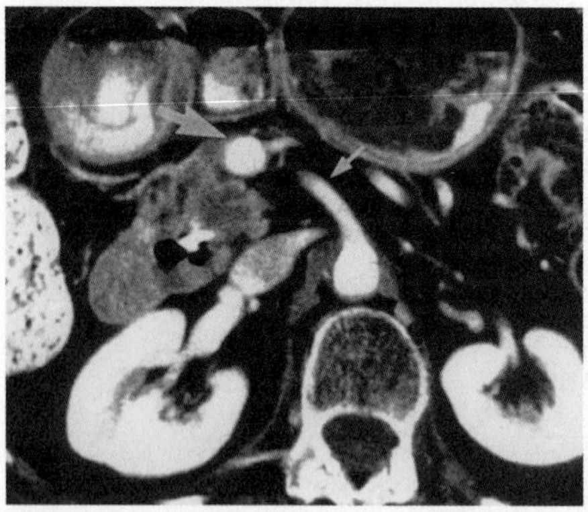

Figure 88-2 ■ Contrast-enhanced computed tomorgraphy scan demonstrating a resectable adenocarcinoma of the pancreatic head. The low-density tumor is easily seen in the pancreatic head. Note the absence of tumor extension to the superior mesenteric artery (*small arrow*); there is a normal fat plane between the low-density tumor and the superior mesenteric artery. However, the tumor (area of low density) does extend to the superior mesenteric vein just inferior to the tip of the large arrow. This patient may require venous resection and reconstruction at the time of pancreaticoduodenectomy. This subtle finding would not be apparent on a lesser quality scan. The intrapancreatic portion of the common bile duct contains a stent that was endoscopically placed for biliary drainage.

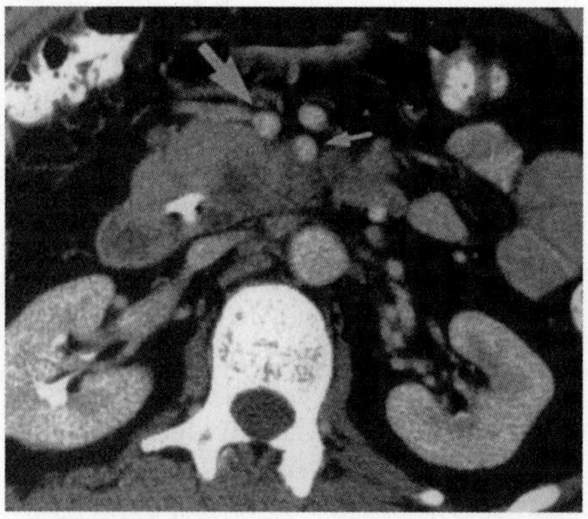

Figure 88-3 ■ Contrast-enhanced computed tomography scan demonstrating an unresectable adenocarcinoma of the pancreatic head and uncinate process. The low-density tumor is inseparable from the posterior wall of the superior mesenteric artery (*small arrow*). Direct intraoperative assessment of the extent of retroperitoneal tumor growth in relation to the superior mesenteric artery is not possible until after gastric and pancreatic transection, at which point the surgeon has committed to resection; accurate preoperative imaging of this vital tumor–vessel relationship is thus critical. The large arrow identifies the superior mesenteric vein.

Tissue Acquisition

Confirmation of malignancy is required in all patients with locally advanced or metastatic disease prior to treatment with systemic therapy or radiotherapy. For patients with radiographic evidence of metastatic disease, biopsies (usually of the metastatic site) can be obtained percutaneously either with US-guidance or CT-guidance. For patients with localized disease, which may be amenable to surgical resection upfront or after a period of neoadjuvant therapy, we prefer EUS-guided biopsy to minimize the risk of tumor seeding. Furthermore, EUS-guided biopsy is probably better than percutaneous CT-guided biopsy for tumors, which are smaller, or difficult to access using CT-guidance.[165] EUS-guided FNA of the pancreas is notable for its accuracy and safety.[166] When FNA material is examined by an experienced cytopathologist, false-positive results should be rare; however, false-negative biopsies do occur, especially when small tumors are involved. Therefore, negative results from EUS-guided FNA should not be considered definite proof that a malignancy does not exist, and repeat EUS-guided FNA may improve diagnostic accuracy in those patients with suspected malignancy.[167]

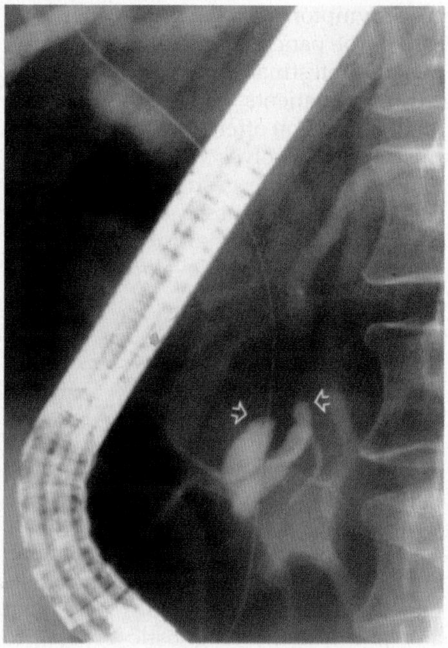

Figure 88-4 ■ Endoscopic retrograde cholangiopancreatography demonstrating the classic double-duct sign seen with adenocarcinoma of the pancreatic head. The open arrows identify the common bile and pancreatic ducts, which are obstructed by the pancreatic cancer.

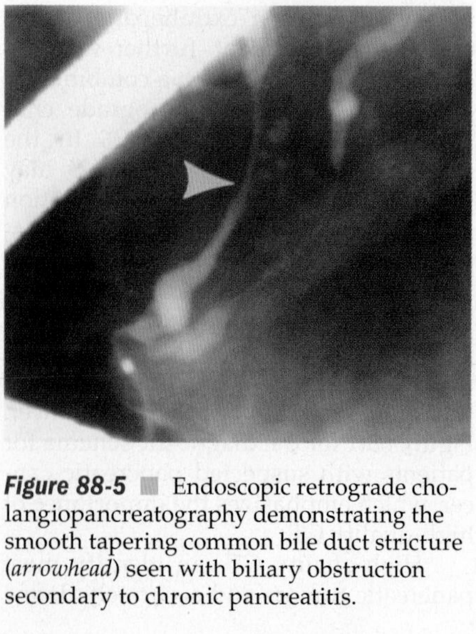

Figure 88-5 ■ Endoscopic retrograde cholangiopancreatography demonstrating the smooth tapering common bile duct stricture (*arrowhead*) seen with biliary obstruction secondary to chronic pancreatitis.

Importantly, in a patient who presents with extrahepatic biliary obstruction, a malignant-appearing stricture of the intrapancreatic portion of the common bile duct, and no history of recurrent pancreatitis or alcohol abuse, the absence of a mass on CT or EUS images should not be grounds for ruling out a carcinoma of the pancreas or bile duct. Instead, the results of EUS, with or without FNA, should be considered in the context of the clinical picture and as a complement to CT and ERCP findings. As discussed above, high-quality CT imaging should be performed before an FNA is attempted because of the risk of biopsy-induced pancreatitis, which may distort the pancreatic and peripancreatic anatomy. Further, FNA biopsy should only be performed if a mass is visualized; blind biopsy of the pancreas is inappropriate.

Laparoscopic Staging

the past, laparoscopy has been performed in patients who have radiologic evidence of localized pancreatic cancer to detect extrapancreatic tumor not seen on CT scans, thereby limiting laparotomy to those patients who truly have localized disease.[168] However, with the availability of high-quality contrast-enhanced CT, which can better identify metastatic disease,[169] the role of laparoscopy in staging under a separate anesthesia induction appears to be decreasing.[170] More recent studies have suggested that CT occult extrapancreatic disease is found in only 4-13% of patients with tumors otherwise deemed resectable.[171] Of note, the yield of staging laparoscopy may be improved with preoperative measurement of serum carbohydrate antigen (CA) 19-9 and acquisition of preoperative CA 19-9 levels is recommended as part of the staging work-up.[172,173] If the suspicion of extrapancreatic disease is high, or the patient is a marginal surgical candidate based on comorbidities, it may be appropriate to perform staging laparoscopy as a stand-alone procedure. In general, however, we typically perform laparoscopy at the time of anesthesia for planned laparotomy in patients with presumed localized, resectable pancreatic cancer; laparoscopy can be performed quickly and in an occasional patient obviate the need to undergo a nontherapeutic laparotomy. Importantly, the rapidly expanding body of literature on laparoscopic staging has drawn attention to the need to avoid nontherapeutic laparotomy and there is now consensus that primary tumor resectability should be assessed prior to laparotomy.

Biliary Drainage

The practice of placing endobiliary stents prior to surgery or other treatment modalities in patients with malignant distal bile duct obstruction has become increasingly common for a number of reasons. First, the point of patient entry into the health care system is often the gastroenterologist, internist, or family practitioner, none of whom has subspecialty expertise in the treatment of pancreatic cancer. These physicians may not have a contemporary understanding of the rapidly expanding stage-specific treatment options for patients with pancreatic cancer. In such situations, placement of a plastic biliary stent is a common way of relieving symptomatic (pruritus, anorexia, etc) jaundice. Second, for patients with potentially resectable disease, surgery is often delayed until referral to a high-volume center can be arranged. Third, because most patients with pancreatic cancer have extrapancreatic metastatic disease (even if not apparent on imaging studies), there has been a greater emphasis on multidisciplinary treatment, including the delivery of chemotherapy or chemoradiation prior to surgery, which requires normal hepatic function.

For patients considered to have locally advanced or metastatic pancreatic cancer based on the findings from noninvasive imaging studies or laparoscopy, the debate over the merits of surgical bypass versus endoscopic stenting has ended owing to the advent of expandable metal stents. An endobiliary self-expandable metal stent has superior long-term patency compared with plastic stents.[174,175] However, certain groups of patients with symptomatic distal bile duct obstruction should not undergo endobiliary metal stent placement. Patients who present a diagnostic dilemma, such as those without an obvious mass in the head of the pancreas or with a history of pancreatitis, should have a plastic stent placed at the first endoscopic intervention in order to permit easy stent removal and additional diagnostic studies as needed. Though covered metal stents can also be removed endoscopically,[176] they should not be used to provide temporary biliary decompression in a patient without a tissue diagnosis of malignancy. Those patients who require endobiliary decompression for only a few weeks prior to surgery, such as those who require detailed medical evaluation to optimize their preparation for major surgery, may receive a plastic or metal (if the diagnosis is established) stent. There may also be a role for plastic stent placement in those patients with such a significant burden of metastatic disease that survival beyond 2 months in unlikely. However, insertion of a metal stent is acceptable in this subset of patients since survival duration (and the time to plastic stent occlusion) is variable.

In patients who are brought to the operating room for a planned pancreaticoduodenectomy, but are found to have locally advanced or extrapancreatic metastatic disease, we recommend removal of the endobiliary stent and surgical biliary bypass to avoid any possibility of future stent occlusion. If an expandable metal stent is already in place and the biliary bypass looks to be more difficult than usual, operative biliary bypass may be deferred. Such situations may include, for example, tumor extension into the porta hepatus or occlusion of the superior mesenteric or portal vein resulting in cavernous transformation of the portal vein and extensive dilated collateral veins anterior to the bile duct. When operative biliary bypass is performed, the bile duct is preferred for biliary decompression rather than the gallbladder, and the gallbladder should never be used for biliary decompression in the setting of acute or chronic gallbladder disease, cephalad tumor extension, or prolonged stent placement prior to surgery. A further consideration is that hypertrophy and fibrosis of the wall of the bile duct may make the cystic duct–common bile duct junction unsuitable for biliary decompression in patients with a previous endoscopic stent. Therefore, we prefer biliary bypass as a Roux-en-Y choledochojejunostomy or hepaticojejunostomy. The gallbladder is removed and the common bile duct transected. The endoscopic stent, if present, is removed, the distal bile duct is closed, and an end-to-side choledochojejunostomy is created with a single layer of interrupted monofilament sutures.

Treatment of Localized, Potentially Resectable Disease

Surgical Considerations

The accurate preoperative assessment of resectability (local and distant disease) is the most critical aspect of the diagnostic and staging work-up in patients with pancreatic cancer. Quality survival time will be greatly improved by avoiding nontherapeutic laparotomy in patients with unresectable pancreatic cancer. Indeed, laparotomy for those who undergo surgical exploration and are found to have unresectable disease is associated with a risk of perioperative morbidity, a hospital stay of at least 1 week, and a median survival after surgery of only 7-10 months.[177] If the primary tumor cannot be resected completely (gross complete resection), surgery for pancreatic cancer (pancreaticoduodenectomy) offers no survival advantage. Patients who undergo a gross incomplete resection have an expected median survival of less than 1 year, which is no different from the survival duration seen in patients with locally advanced, unresectable (stage III) disease who are treated with chemotherapy and irradiation without surgery.[178] In addition, even microscopically positive surgical margins may have a negative impact on overall survival (in the absence of multimodality therapy), and when planning upfront surgery, the ability to obtain a margin-negative resection should be viewed as an important contribution to the goal of achieving long-term survival.[179] Therefore, in contrast to the situation in selected patients with gastric or colorectal cancer, there are no data supporting palliative (incomplete or grossly positive margins) resection for adenocarcinoma of the pancreas.

Owing to recent advances in operative technique, anesthesia, and critical care, the 30-day in-hospital mortality rate is 2% or less in patients who undergo pancreaticoduodenectomy performed by experienced surgeons.[180-182] Data from a study conducted by Birkmeyer and colleagues have also demonstrated that higher hospital volume is associated with lower surgery-related mortality.[183] Furthermore, subsequent analysis has also shown that patients who undergo cancer surgery at high-volume hospitals are also less likely to experience late mortality.[184]

Importantly, when upfront surgery is contemplated for a patient with potentially resectable disease, it should be linked to the patient's potential to recover adequately from surgery in order to receive postoperative therapy. Such an assessment should occur preoperatively. A number of randomized trials and analysis of large data sets support the delivery of adjuvant therapy after surgery. Surgery alone as an intervention for resectable pancreatic cancer may have little or no survival advantage over what can be achieved with nonsurgical therapy.[185,186]

Pancreaticoduodenectomy ■ Standard surgical procedure for neoplasms of the pancreatic head and periampullary region is pancreaticoduodenectomy, which involves removal of the pancreatic head, duodenum, gallbladder, and bile duct with or without the gastric antrum. The current technique of pancreaticoduodenectomy has evolved from the procedure first described by Whipple and colleagues in 1935.[187] Their two-stage pancreaticoduodenectomy consisted of biliary diversion and gastrojejunostomy during one operation, followed by resection of the duodenum and pancreatic head after the patient recovered from the earlier procedure (usually about 3 weeks later). By 1941, the world experience totaled 41 cases, with a perioperative mortality rate of 30%.[188] Before 1940, the pancreatic remnant was not reanastomosed to the small bowel, and the high mortality rate was largely because of the development of a pancreatic fistula from the oversewn pancreatic remnant. In 1941, Whipple modified his reconstruction to include a pancreaticojejunostomy, with the entire procedure done in one operation.[188]

As stated above, prior to opening the abdomen, laparoscopy is performed and the abdomen carefully explored to exclude extrapancreatic metastatic disease. Sites of suspected liver or peritoneal metastatic lesions are biopsied, and the material submitted for frozen-section histologic analysis. Primary tumor resection should not be done when biopsy-proven liver or peritoneal metastases are found. Our recommended technique for pancreaticoduodenectomy utilizes a midline or bilateral subcostal incision. In patients who have resectable disease, there is no indication for routine intraoperative pancreatic biopsy. Whether to perform lymph node biopsy for frozen-section analysis remains controversial. Although positive lymph nodes are a prognostic factor (along with poorly differentiated histology, microscopically positive resection margins, etc) that predicts decreased survival,[180,189] microscopic metastases are found in regional lymph nodes on permanent-section pathologic evaluation in 60-90% of patients who undergo pancreaticoduodenectomy. Further, recent data have documented 5-year survival in up to 20% of node-positive patients who were treated with combined modality therapy.[190] In a good-risk patient with localized, resectable pancreatic cancer, lymph node metastases are not an absolute contraindication to pancreaticoduodenectomy when it is part of a combined-modality treatment approach.[191] Therefore, random lymph node sampling for frozen-section analysis at the time of pancreaticoduodenectomy is not recommended. However, in some circumstances, when a patient is considered high-risk because of medical comorbid conditions or when there are oncologic concerns (such as a very high CA19-9 level) or suspicious adenopathy is present, a positive regional lymph node may be viewed as a contraindication to pancreaticoduodenectomy.

At the time of surgical exploration for a pancreatic head cancer, a Kocher maneuver is traditionally the first maneuver performed so that the tumor's relationship to the SMA can be determined. In this maneuver, by mobilizing the pancreatic head and duodenum from their retroperitoneal attachments, the surgeon attempts to palpate a plane of normal tissue between the firm tumor and the posterior pulsation of the SMA. The relationship of the tumor to the right lateral wall of the SMA is the most critical aspect of the pretreatment staging evaluation. Importantly, this critical tumor–vessel relationship should be accurately evaluated by MDCT before the patient is taken to the operating room. In the case of larger tumors, tumors with significant peritumoral fibrosis, or at reoperation (following a previous unsuccessful attempt at pancreaticoduodenectomy), it is often impossible to accurately determine by palpation the relationship of the primary tumor to the SMA (after mobilization of the duodenum). The second maneuver traditionally performed to assess resectability is to develop a plane of dissection between the anterior surface of the SMPV confluence and the posterior surface of the pancreatic neck to exclude tumor involvement of the SMV or SMPV confluence. Such tumor involvement precludes resection, in the opinion of most surgeons. However, the rationale for performing this maneuver early in the operation is also unclear because tumors of the pancreatic head or uncinate process are prone to invade the lateral or posterior wall of the SMPV confluence, but rarely involve the anterior wall. The relationship of a pancreatic head tumor to the lateral and posterior walls of the SMPV confluence (and the SMA) can be directly seen only after gastric and pancreatic transection, at which point the surgeon has already committed to resection. Again, preoperative imaging using high-quality, contrast-enhanced MDCT can alert the surgeon to the possible need for venous resection and reconstruction.[182]

The technique of pancreaticoduodenectomy currently used in the United States incorporates selected aspects of the traditional Whipple procedure and emphasizes the importance of removing all soft tissue to the right of the SMA. The surgical resection is divided into six clearly defined steps (Fig. 88-6); the most oncologically important and difficult part of the operation is step six, during which the pancreas is divided and the specimen is removed from the SMPV confluence and the right lateral border of the SMA.[191] After traction sutures are placed on the superior and inferior borders of the pancreas, the pancreas is transected with electrocautery at the level of the portal vein. If tumor adheres to the portal vein or SMV, the pancreas can be divided more distally in preparation for segmental venous resection. The small venous tributaries to the uncinate process and pancreatic head are then ligated and divided so that the specimen can be separated from the SMPV. Only after full medial mobilization of the SMPV is it possible to identify the SMA.[192] The pancreatic head and all soft tissue to the right of the SMA are then removed by direct ligation of the inferior pancreaticoduodenal artery or arteries. Failure to fully mobilize the SMPV confluence risks injury to the SMA and

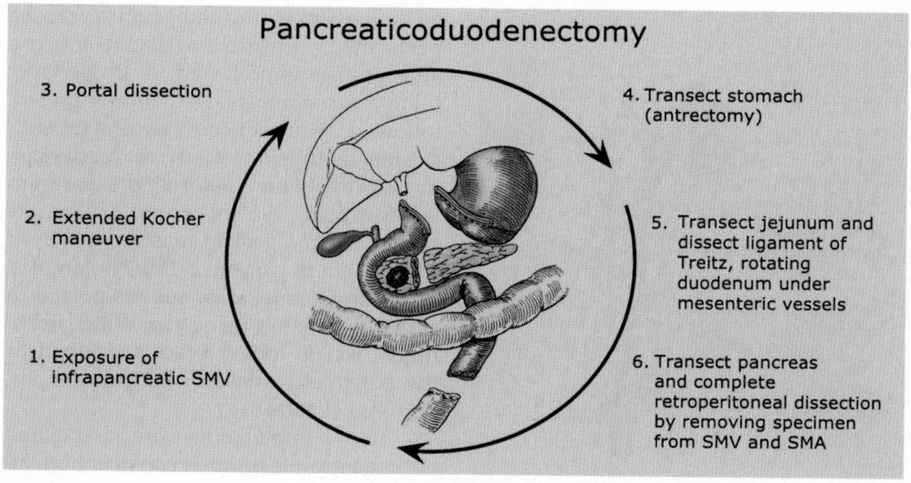

Figure 88-6 ■ Six surgical steps of pancreaticoduodenectomy.

usually results in a positive resection margin because of incomplete removal of the uncinate process and the mesenteric soft tissue adjacent to the SMA.[193] Furthermore, if the SMPV confluence is not completely mobilized, one cannot expose the SMA, which is necessary for the inferior pancreaticoduodenal arteries to be directly ligated. Mass ligation of this vessel (or vessels) with surrounding mesenteric soft tissue is the major cause of postoperative retroperitoneal hemorrhage, as this vessel can retract from a poorly placed tie or ligature.

The high incidence of local recurrence after standard pancreaticoduodenectomy requires particular attention to the SMA margin. The SMA margin (also referred to as the retroperitoneal or mesenteric margin) is the soft tissue margin along the right lateral border of the proximal SMA (Fig. 88-7).[4] It is critical that this margin be identified for the pathologist and assessed histologically; the residual disease status (termed "R" factor) cannot be determined if the retroperitoneal margin is not assessed histologically.[193,194] Perineural invasion involving the mesenteric plexus at the SMA origin and tumor cell infiltration of lymphatic vessels and connective tissue may extend microscopically beyond the confines of the palpable tumor.[182,193] During step six of pancreaticoduodenectomy, therefore, the SMPV confluence must be fully mobilized and the SMA exposed so that the specimen can be completely and safely dissected from the right lateral aspect of the proximal SMA.

Vascular Resection ■ Segmental resection of the SMPV confluence is necessary when the tumor cannot be separated from the lateral wall of the SMV or portal vein.[182,191] However, such isolated venous resection should be performed only in patients whose tumors adhere to the SMV or SMPV confluence but who have no evidence of tumor extension to the SMA or celiac axis. Invasion of the SMV or portal vein is not associated with histopathologic variables (positive lymph nodes) that suggest a poor prognosis, and patient survival after pancreaticoduodenectomy is not affected by the need for venous resection.[182] Because the need for venous resection is unexpected in many patients and is discovered only after gastric and pancreatic transection, when nonresectional procedures are no longer an option, surgeons who perform pancreaticoduodenectomies should be familiar with the anatomy of the mesenteric venous system and standard vascular techniques for resection and reconstruction of the SMPV confluence.[192]

The standard technique for segmental venous resection involves transection of the splenic vein.[195,196] Division of the splenic vein allows complete exposure of the SMA medial to the SMV and provides increased SMV and portal vein length (since they are no longer tethered by the splenic vein) for a primary venous anastomosis following segmental vein resection. However, preservation of the splenic vein–portal vein junction is preferred whenever possible (Fig. 88-8).[182,197] The splenic vein can only be preserved, however, when tumor invasion of the SMV or portal vein does not involve the splenic vein confluence. Preserving the splenic vein–SMPV confluence significantly limits mobilization of the portal vein and prevents primary anastomosis of the SMV (following segmental SMV resection) unless segmental resection is limited to less than 2 cm; therefore, an interposition graft is required in most patients who undergo SMV resection with splenic vein preservation. The internal jugular vein is our preferred conduit for interposition grafting.[197] Preserving the splenic vein adds significant complexity to venous resection because it prevents

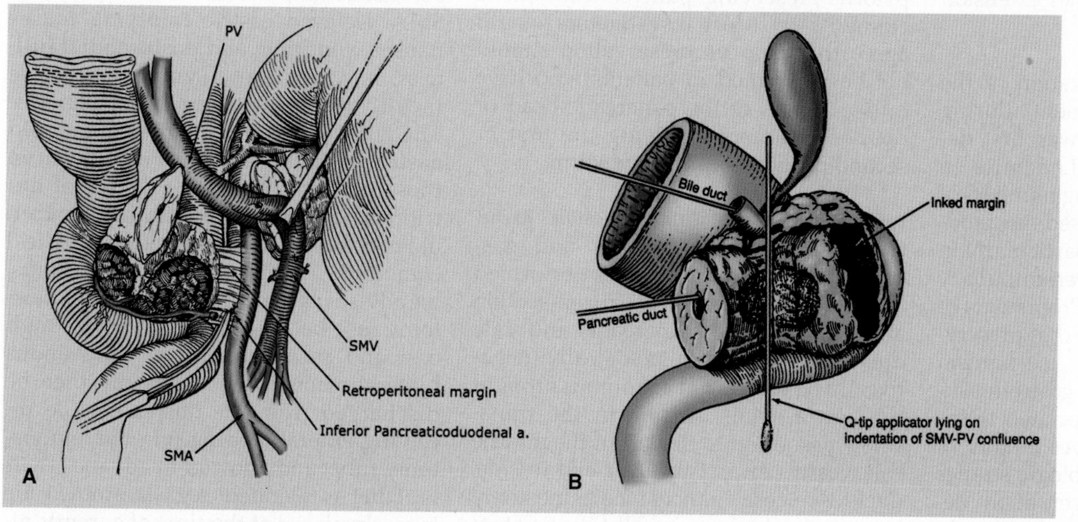

Figure 88-7 ■ Illustration of the retroperitoneal margin as defined at the time of tumor resection (**A**). Medial retraction of the superior mesenteric vein (SMV) and superior mesenteric–portal vein confluence facilitates dissection of the soft tissues adjacent to the lateral wall of the proximal superior mesenteric artery (SMA); this site represents the retroperitoneal margin. Complete permanent-section analysis of the pancreaticoduodenectomy specimen requires that it be oriented for the pathologist to enable accurate assessment of the retroperitoneal margin of excision and other standard pathologic variables. The retroperitoneal margin must be identified and inked with the pathologist (**B**); it cannot be assessed retrospectively. As shown here, a probe is in both the pancreatic duct and the bile duct, and a Q-tip applicator lies on the indentation of the SMPV confluence. One can then ink (for final pathologic assessment) the soft-tissue margin adjacent to the proximal SMA; this represents the retroperitoneal (or mesenteric) margin of excision.

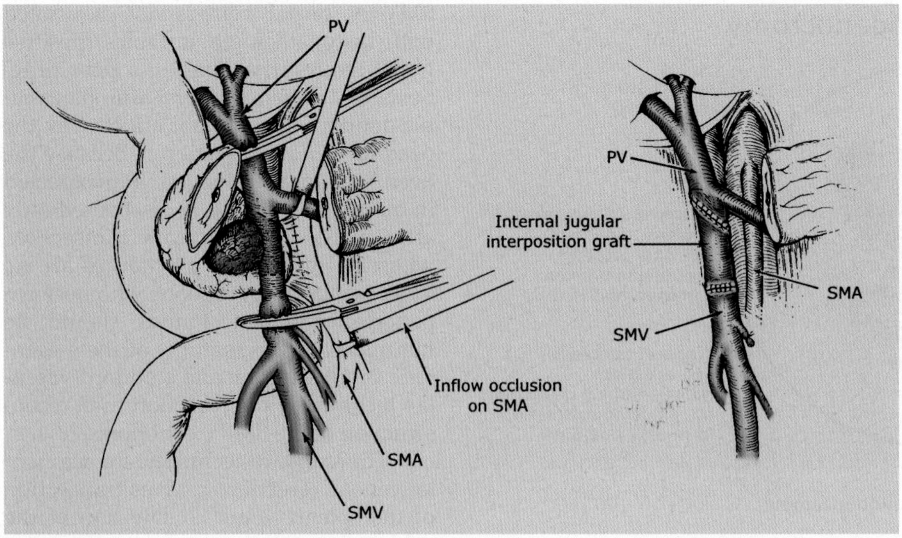

Figure 88-8 ■ Illustration of resection of the superior mesenteric vein (SMV) with splenic vein preservation. The intact splenic vein tethers the portal vein (PV), making a primary anastomosis impossible in most cases. Our preferred method of reconstruction of the SMV is to use an internal jugular vein interposition graft. With the splenic vein intact, exposure is inadequate to separate the specimen from the lateral aspect of the proximal superior mesenteric artery (SMA). Therefore, the graft can be placed prior to specimen removal, thereby allowing medial retraction of the reconstructed superior mesenteric–portal vein confluence, or after separation of the specimen from the SMA posteriorly. Segmental resection of the SMV with splenic vein preservation adds significant complexity to this operation.

direct access to the most proximal 3-4 cm of the SMA (medial to the SMV).

It is important to emphasize the distinction between regional pancreatectomy and pancreaticoduodenectomy with segmental resection of the SMV or SMPV confluence.[198] Venous resection is not an attempt to improve en-bloc lymphatic and soft tissue clearance, as is performed in regional pancreatectomy. Larger local-regional resections (to the left of the SMA and celiac axis) in poorly selected patients with advanced disease are unlikely to affect survival.[199] Venous resection should be performed only in patients whose tumors adhere to the SMV or SMPV confluence but no evidence of tumor extension to the SMA or celiac axis.

Pylorus Preservation ■ Preservation of the antropyloroduodenal segment during pancreaticoduodenectomy was first described by Traverso and Longmire in 1978.[200] Since then, increasing numbers of pancreatic surgeons have used this modification of the procedure, particularly in patients who have small periampullary lesions or benign disease. Proponents of pylorus preservation argue that preserving the antropyloric pump mechanism improves long-term upper gastrointestinal tract function, has associated nutritional benefits, and improves quality of life.[201,202] In addition, physiologic studies suggest that pylorus preservation decreases intestinal transit time, lessens diarrhea (steatorrhea), normalizes glucose metabolism, and improves postoperative weight gain.[203,204] Detractors of pylorus-preserving pancreaticoduodenectomy counter that the reported improvements in gastrointestinal tract function and nutrition are small, if any, and come at the expense of an increased risk of delayed gastric emptying in the early postoperative period.[205,206] Recently, modifications of the pylorus-preserving surgical approach with mechanical intraoperative dilation of the pylorus or preservation of the left gastric vein have both been suggested as a means of limiting delayed gastric emptying.[207,208]

In summary, currently available findings from randomized trials suggest no difference in perioperative factors or patient outcome between standard and pylorus-preserving pancreaticoduodene ctomy.[206,209,210] Most investigators would agree that pylorus preservation should not be performed in patients who have bulky tumors of the pancreatic head or duodenal tumors involving the first or second portions of the duodenum.

Pancreatic, Biliary, and Gastrointestinal Reconstruction ■ Pancreatic, biliary and gastrointestinal reconstruction is performed after confirmation by frozen-section analysis that the pancreatic and bile duct margins are histologically negative.[191] The transected jejunum is brought through a small incision in the transverse mesocolon to the left of the middle colic vessels, and a two-layer, end-to-side, duct-to-mucosa pancreaticojejunostomy is performed over a small Silastic stent (if the pancreatic duct is not dilated). If the pancreatic duct is not suitable for a duct-to-mucosa anastomosis, a two-layer anastomosis that invaginates the cut end of the pancreas into the jejunum can be performed. However, a duct-to-mucosa anastomosis is preferred. A single-layer biliary anastomosis is then completed, followed by an anticolic, two-layer, end-to-side gastrojejunostomy or duodenojejunostomy (when pylorus preservation is performed). We are careful to separate the biliary and gastric anastomoses by at least 50 cm to prevent reflux cholangitis. A feeding jejunostomy tube is placed in selected patients using the Witzel technique; we no longer place a drain near the pancreatic anastomosis prior to abdominal closure.

Two complications are associated with gastrointestinal reconstruction after pancreaticoduodenectomy: leak at the pancreaticojejunostomy and delayed gastric emptying. Leaks from the biliary and gastric anastomoses should be rare, however, and were more prevalent in connection with early gastrointestinal reconstruction techniques that involved simple closure of the pancreatic stump. Once the high rate of pancreatic fistula formation was recognized, surgeons quickly switched to implanting the pancreatic remnant into the jejunum.[211] An alternative is to implant the pancreatic remnant into the posterior wall of the stomach.[212] Regardless of the technique used, the results seem to depend on the experience of the surgeon: the incidence of complications decreases with greater experience.

Delayed gastric emptying is common after standard pancreaticoduodenectomy and may occur more frequently with pylorus preservation.[205,213] In the absence of an intra-abdominal infection (pancreatic anastomotic leak), delayed gastric emptying is largely related to denervation of the upper gastrointestinal tract during resection of the pancreatic head and attached soft tissues and nerves to the right of the SMA. Delayed gastric emptying causes nausea, vomiting, and postprandial fullness; however, these symptoms resolve in 4-12 weeks in virtually all patients. The nutritional consequences of delayed gastric emptying are most significant in those patients with some degree of nutritional depletion preoperatively and in older patients with significant medical comorbid conditions. In such patients, we advise placement of a feeding jejunostomy tube because of the otherwise high cost and inconvenience of intravenous hyperalimentation. Patients can then be discharged from the hospital while receiving enteral feeding (via the jejunostomy tube) and allowed to advance their oral diet as tolerated. A gastrostomy tube is rarely placed at the time of surgery, although in selected patients it effectively avoids prolonged nasogastric tube placement due to temporary gastric emptying dysfunction.

Table 88-2 TNM Staging System

Definitions			
Primary Tumor (T)			
TX	Primary tumor cannot be assessed		
T0	No evidence of primary tumor		
Tis	In situ carcinoma		
T1	Tumor limited to pancreas and 2 cm or less in greatest dimension		
T2	Tumor limited to pancreas and more than 2 cm in greatest dimension		
T3	Tumor extends beyond the pancreas but without involvement of the celiac axis or the superior mesenteric artery		
T4	Tumor involves the celiac axis or the superior mesenteric artery (unresectable primary tumor)		
Regional Lymph Nodes (N)			
NX	Regional lymph nodes cannot be assessed		
N0	No regional lymph node metastasis		
N1	Regional lymph node metastasis		
Distant Metastasis (M)			
MX	Distant metastasis cannot be assessed		
M0	No distant metastasis		
M1	Distant metastasis		
Stage Grouping			
Stage 0	Tis	N0	M0
Stage IA	T1	N0	M0
Stage IB	T2	N0	M0
Stage IIA	T3	N0	M0
Stage IIB	T1-3	N1	M0
Stage III	T4	N0/1	M0
Stage IV	T1-4	N0/1	M1

Source: Adapted from Exocrine pancreas. Greene FL, Page DL, Fleming ID, et al., editors. *AJCC Cancer Staging Manual*, 6th Edition. New York: Springer; 2002:157-164.

Pathologic (Surgical) Staging

The staging system of the AJCC and International Union Against Cancer is given in Table 88-2.[4] The modifications to the TNM staging system in the sixth edition allow the accurate staging of patients even if they do not undergo pancreatic resection. The T4 (and stage III) designation is reserved for locally advanced unresectable primary tumors in the absence of distant metastases.

When the pancreaticoduodenectomy specimen is evaluated pathologically, the surgeon and pathologist should first evaluate frozen sections of the common bile duct transection margin and the pancreatic transection margin. The SMA margin (the soft tissue margin directly adjacent to the proximal 3-4 cm of the SMA) (Fig. 88-7) is then evaluated on permanent sections by inking the margin and sectioning the tumor perpendicular to the margin.[193] The pathologist must evaluate the SMA margin at the time of tumor resection because it is not possible to identify later. Reresection is performed in the event of a positive bile duct or pancreatic transection margin; however, this is not possible in the retroperitoneum/SMA mesentetry, where the aorta and the origin of the SMA limit the extent of surgical resection. The R status of resection cannot be determined if the SMA margin is not assessed histologically. Most importantly, the surgeon and pathologist should classify this margin after integrating the operative findings and the histologic assessment of this margin. All pancreatic resections should be classified according to the R status: R0, no gross or microscopic residual disease; R1, microscopic residual disease (microscopically positive surgical margins with no gross residual disease); and R2, grossly evident residual disease. The pathologist cannot usually differentiate an R1 (microscopically positive) from an R2 (grossly positive) SMA margin. The R designation should appear in the final operative note or other highly visible aspect of the medical record and should be consistent with the pathology report. For example, if the surgeon states that gross tumor was encountered when completing the retroperitoneal dissection, a positive histologic margin should be deemed an R2 resection in the operative report (dictation). If a complete gross resection was performed, the final R designation cannot be determined until the pathologic assessment of the SMA margin; a positive margin would imply an R1 resection, which should then appear in the medical record. The operative report should routinely be finalized until the status of the SMA margin is determined histologically. The difficulty in differentiating R1 from R2 resections has significant implications for the conduct of clinical trials examining the potential survival benefits of subsequent nonsurgical therapies.

The final pathologic evaluation of the permanent sections should include a description of the tumor histology and differentiation, gross and microscopic evaluation of the tissue of origin (pancreas, bile duct, ampulla of Vater, or duodenum), and a measurement of the maximum transverse tumor diameter, involved lymph nodes and total lymph nodes examined, and the presence or absence of perineural, lymphatic, and vascular invasion. If segmental venous resection has been performed, the area of presumed tumor invasion of the vein wall is serially sectioned and examined to discriminate benign fibrous attachment from direct tumor invasion. If the patient received preoperative chemoradiation therapy, the grade of the treatment effect is assessed using the grading schema developed by Cleary and reported by Evans and colleagues.[214] The Japanese staging system involves an extremely detailed analysis of margins and lymph node groups and is not practical for widespread application.[215] As multimodality treatment strategies for pancreatic cancer become more commonly used, standardized pathologic assessment of tumor specimens will become even more important.

Prognostic Factors

Prognostic factors in patients with localized, potentially resectable pancreatic cancer are used to guide treatment recommendations, especially in older patients whose medical comorbid conditions may increase the risks associated with major pancreatic surgery. However, unlike the approach taken with solid tumors, pathologic prognostic variables do not guide the use of adjuvant therapy because, despite a potentially curative pancreaticoduodenectomy, disease recurs in at least 80% of patients. Therefore, in general, adjuvant therapy (as discussed in the next section) is administered to all patients with exocrine pancreatic cancer regardless of the pathologic findings in resected specimens.[216] The prognostic factor of greatest significance for survival, one that is available to the clinician prior to surgery and the pathologic assessment of the resected specimen, is the preoperative radiographic assessment of local tumor extension, because it predicts the eventual resection margin status.[5,178] The margin of greatest importance is the SMA (retroperitoneal or mesenteric) margin along the right lateral border of the SMA as discussed above in detail. In centers using strict radiographic criteria for resectability, approximately 20% of patients who undergo a grossly complete resection for pancreatic adenocarcinoma will be found to have a microscopically positive SMA margin (R1 resection).[193,217] However, reports from other university centers suggest that R1 resections occur quite frequently (37-50% of resections) and are independent predictors of poor surivival.[180,218-221] In contrast, other publications have shown no clear difference between the survival of patients undergoing an R0 resection and those undergoing an R1 resection.[193,222,223] This may be related to the overall quality of the surgical resection, technique used for margin analysis, use of adjuvant therapy, treatment sequencing and patient selection; clearly many variables will affect the endpoints of survival and local disease control. It has been suggested that strict criteria for surgical margin assessment have not been broadly applied and greatly underestimate the frequency of R1 resections, possibly misclassifying some as R0 resections.[194] The impact of a truly microscopically positive-margin (in the setting of a grossly complete resection) treated with multimodality therapy has not been evaluated outside of experiences of single institutions.[193] An occasional patient will have microscopic extension of tumor cells along the pancreatic duct (positive pancreatic transection margin), but the clinical significance of this is uncertain. Importantly, dysplastic cells secondary to tumor-induced pancreatitis are frequently found at the pancreatic transection margin and should not be cause for further pancreatic resection (in the absence of histologic evidence of invasive adenocarcinoma).

Another clinical parameter, which appears to have prognostic significance is the serum CA 19-9 level. A number of studies have shown that elevated serum levels of CA 19-9 drawn preoperatively and/or postoperatively have prognostic significance.[224-226] Whether elevated CA 19-9 levels obtained preoperatively should alter planned management (to defer surgery until neoadjuvant therapy has been delivered) has not been prospectively studied. As discussed previously, elevated preoperative CA 19-9 levels increase the yield with staging laparoscopy and in the setting of an otherwise apparently resectable pancreatic cancer, a preoperative serum CA 19-9 level above 100-150 U/mL should prompt further staging.[172,173]

Investigators have examined pathologic factors of the resected tumor in an effort to establish reliable prognostic variables associated with decreased survival.[180,227] Metastatic disease in regional lymph nodes, poorly differentiated histology, and increased size of primary tumors have been associated with decreased survival duration. For example, in a study conducted by Yeo and colleagues,[228] 45 patients with pancreatic adenocarcinoma who underwent complete resection with both negative resection margins and negative regional lymph nodes had a median survival of 32 months and a 5-year survival of 40%. However, in an analysis of 12 5-year survivors (following complete resection) done by Conlon and colleagues,[229] 4 had poorly differentiated histology, 5 had metastatic disease in regional lymph nodes, 9 had histologic evidence of extrapancreatic soft tissue extension of the tumor, and 10 patients had histologic evidence of perineural invasion.[229] In a recent report of actual 5-year survivors from our group at the University of Texas, MD Anderson Cancer Center (UTMDACC), 36% were node-positive, and 20% of all node-positive patients survived 5 years.[190]

In an otherwise good-risk patient with localized, potentially resectable pancreatic cancer (as shown by objective CT criteria that have already been reviewed), the lymph node status, degree of differentiation of the primary tumor, and other histologic (or molecular) prognostic variables are of modest clinical relevance. Regardless of these findings, we would treat such a patient with multimodality therapy that includes chemotherapy, surgery, and possibly chemoradiation therapy as part of a protocol-based treatment program. However, in elderly patients with comorbid conditions that may increase their risk from pancreaticoduodenectomy, knowledge of poorly differentiated histology and the positive status of regional lymph nodes (information that can now be obtained at major referral centers through the use of EUS-FNA) may be cause to recommend systemic therapy or chemoradiation therapy rather than proceeding directly to major pancreatic surgery.

Lastly, intraoperative variables, such as the perioperative blood loss, the number of red blood cell transfusions, and operative time have also been examined.[5,228] An increase in perioperative blood loss and the need for blood transfusion were both associated with a decrease in survival duration. However, increased tumor size would logically be associated with a more difficult operation, resulting in greater blood loss and the high likelihood of incomplete resection.

Postoperative (Adjuvant) Therapy

Adjuvant therapy for patients with resected pancreatic cancer has been in evolution since the first report of its benefit was published in 1985 by the Gastrointestinal Tumor Study Group (GITSG).[230] In that prospective randomized study of adjuvant chemoradiation (500 mg/m^2/day of 5-fluorocil (5-FU) for 6 days and 40 Gy of radiation) followed by weekly bolus 5-FU (500 mg/m^2/week for 2 years) versus observation alone after pancreaticoduodenectomy, a survival advantage was seen for multimodality therapy (20 months vs 11 months with resection alone, $p = 0.035$). Given the striking difference in survival, the study was closed before it reached its planned accrual of 100 patients. To support their original observation, the investigators submitted a subsequent report on the survival of an additional 30 patients undergoing curative resection who received the experimental arm of the protocol without randomization; they had virtually the same survival as that previously reported.[231] Since those publications, several other prospective randomized trials have been conducted and published (Table 88-3).[6-8,232] Taken together, these studies have led to some confusion regarding the overall merits of adjuvant therapy and the relative contributions of chemotherapy and radiation as components of adjuvant therapy. Nevertheless, careful review of Table 88-3, combined with other available data regarding adjuvant therapy provides for some conclusions.[9]

First, of the three trials that randomized patients to active therapy or to observation after surgery, all demonstrate improved survival compared with surgery alone ranging from 2 to 10 months. The GITSG trial and EORTC 40891 showed improvement in survival using 5-FU-based chemoradiation, while the CONKO-001 trial showed improvement with the delivery of systemic gemcitabine. It should be noted that in the EORTC trial, although the survival advantage for those patients who randomized to

Table 88-3 **Selected Ongoing Randomized Trials for Patients With Locally Advanced Pancreatic Cancer**

Study	Design	Arms
ECOG 1200	Randomized phase 2	Gem 500 mg/m^2 + Cisplatin + 5-FU *followed by* PVI 5-FU + XRT 50.4 Gy + 5.5 weeks Gem 500 mg/m^2 weekly × 5 + XRT 50.4 Gy over 5.5 weeks
ECOG/RTOG 4201	Randomized phase 3	Gem 1 gm/m^2 weekly × 3 (max 7 cycles) XRT 50.4 Gy over 5.5 weeks + Gem 600 mg/m^2 *followed by* Gem 1 g/m^2 weekly × 3 (max 5 cycles)
RTOG PA 0411	Phase 2	XRT 50.4 Gy over 5.5 weeks + Cape 825 mg/m^2 (PO bid Mon – Fri) + Bev 5 mg/kg every 2 weeks *followed by* Gem 1 g/m^2 weekly × 3 (max 3 cycles) + Bev 5 mg/kg every 2 weeks

Abbreviations: Bev, bevacizumab; bid, twice daily; Cape, capecitabine; ECOG, Eastern Cooperative Oncology Group; 5-FU, 5-fluorouracil; Gem, gemcitabine; OS, overall survival; PO, orally; PVI, protracted venous infusion; QOL, quality of life; RFS, relapse-free survival; RR, response rate; RTOG, Radiation Therapy Oncology Group; XRT, radiotherapy.

chemoradiation was clinically significant (17.6 months vs 12.1 months), it was not statistically significantly different from the survival of patients randomized to observation alone ($p = 0.09$). Based on the relatively small number of patients with pancreatic cancer enrolled on the study (114), critics have argued the EORTC 40891 is an underpowered positive study[233] and one group has used an alternative statistical analysis to support this position.[234] Conversely, after longer term follow-up, the EORTC investigators have stood by their original conclusion that adjuvant chemoradiation offers no survival advantage over surgery alone.[235] More recently, using gemcitabine monotherapy as the experimental arm, the results from CONKO-001 have also support the use of adjuvant therapy after surgery. Although the median survival advantage was quite modest for patients randomized to gemcitabine (22.8 months vs 20.2 months, $p = 0.005$), the 3-year and 5-year survival rates show the clear superiority of treatment with gemcitabine over observation (26% vs 18% and 20% vs 9%, respectively).

Second, the observed deleterious effects of chemoradiation as adjuvant therapy reported in the European Study Group for Pancreatic Cancer (ESPAC)-1 trial have not been reported elsewhere. This study was conducted by 83 participating physicians in 61 hospital centers between 1994 and 2000. ESPAC-1 enrolled 541 patients following resection for adenocarcinoma of the pancreas. The trial used a four-arm, 2 × 2 factorial design to compare (1) adjuvant chemoradiation (40 Gy in a split course and 5-FU), (2) adjuvant chemotherapy (5-FU and folinic acid), (3) chemoradiation therapy followed by chemotherapy, and (4) observation alone following pancreaticoduodenectomy for pancreatic and periampullary carcinomas. Two-hundred eighty-five patients (53%) were entered into the randomized 2 × 2 factorial design. The median survival durations for the 285 patients randomized in the 2 × 2 factorial design were 16.9 months (observation), 13.9 months (chemoradiotherapy), 21.6 months (chemotherapy), and 19.9 months (chemoradiation plus chemotherapy). This analysis did not have the statistical power to compare these median survivals directly. However, the median survival among the 147 patients randomized to receive chemotherapy (alone or with chemoradiotherapy) was 20.1 months versus 15.5 months among the 142 patients who did not receive chemotherapy (hazard ratio for death, 0.71; 95% CI, 0.55-0.92; $p = .009$). The median survival among the 145 patients randomized to receive chemoradiotherapy (alone or with chemotherapy) was 15.9 months versus 17.9 months in the patients not assigned to receive chemoradiation (hazard ratio for death, 1.28; 95% CI 0.99-1.66; $p = .05$). Of the 145 patients randomized to receive chemoradiation, only 90 (62%) received the assigned 40 Gy of EBRT and the survival duration of those who did and did not receive intended therapy was not reported. No other available data has demonstrated 5-FU-based chemoradiation as harmful to patients who have undergone surgery with curative intent including two large retrospective analyses reported separately from the Johns Hopkins Hospital (JHH) and the Mayo Clinic.[236,237] Furthermore, analysis of large U.S. databases has also suggested a benefit with the delivery of adjuvant chemoradiation after pancreatic cancer surgery compared with surgery alone (29 months vs 12.5 months, $p = 0.0003$).[186]

Third, the CONKO-001 results, taken together with the results from Radiation Therapy Oncology Group (RTOG) 97-04 study imply that systemic gemcitabine is superior to surgery alone, and probably superior to infusional 5-FU. Fourth, Table 88-3 demonstrates that in the interval from 1985 to 2008, no significant improvements in survival have been made for patients with resected pancreatic cancer.[9] Lastly, no matter what adjuvant strategy is employed, local failure rates are alarmingly high (26-60%) despite enrollment of a small proportion of patients having an R1 resection.

At present, the results from CONKO 001 represent the best evidence for the delivery of adjuvant therapy with single-agent gemcitabine to patients who have undergone a potentially curative resection for pancreatic cancer. This regimen is straightforward, and is capable of delivery in the community setting with acceptable toxicity. Importantly, though, the patients enrolled in CONKO 001, represented a fairly select group, having adequately recovered from surgery (with a recommendation to begin therapy within 42 days of surgery), and to have postoperative serum CEA and CA 19-9 levels no more than 2.5 times the upper limit of normal for each participating center. The benefit of adjuvant gemcitabine for patients with slow recovery from surgery, or with significant postoperative elevations of serum tumor markers, has not been clearly defined.

In the future, clinical trials of adjuvant therapy should demonstrate more disciplined methodology than has been employed previously.[9] This should include the application of strict radiographic criteria to assess resectability of the primary tumor using MDCT or high-quality MR imaging, standardized surgical techniques, and appropriate guidelines to ensure adequate assessments surgical margins.[4] Furthermore, given the experience from a number of published preoperative studies, it can be conservatively estimated that 15-20% of patients undergoing upfront surgical resection will develop radiographic evidence of metastatic disease within the usual postoperative recovery period (6-12 weeks).[214,238-241] Therefore, prior to the initiation of adjuvant therapy, restaging studies with CT or MR, (and possibly the acquisition of a postoperative CA 19-9 level),[224,226] should be mandated to identify those patients with rapid onset of metastatic disease or otherwise unfavorable prognosis.

Ongoing Adjuvant Therapy Trials

Current phase 3 trials of adjuvant therapy are continuing to test gemcitabine in the adjuvant setting. The ESPAC investigators, having dismissed radiotherapy as a component of adjuvant therapy, have been enrolling patients on ESPAC-3, a multicentered trial with planned accrual of 900 patients. ESPAC-3 randomizes patients having undergone curative resection of pancreatic cancer and adequate recovery, to receive gemcitabine (1000 mg/m^2 over 30 min, weekly × 3, every 28 days) for 6 months, or bolus 5-FU and leucovorin (as administered in ESPAC-1) for 6 months.[8]

Meanwhile, the EORTC continues to investigate the role of adjuvant chemoradiation in EORTC 40013. This is a phase 2 or 3 trial of gemcitabine followed by gemcitabine-based chemoradiation versus 6 months of systemic gemcitabine alone. Currently, there is limited experience with adjuvant gemcitabine-based chemoradiation following pancreaticoduodenectomy. In a phase 2 trial conducted by Blackstock and his colleagues, gemcitabine-based chemoradiation was delivered to 46 patients who had undergone potentially curative pancreatic cancer resection.[242] Gemcitabine was given twice weeky at a dose of 40 mg/m^2 concurrently with radiation to a total dose of 50.4 Gγ given over 5.5 weeks. While toxicities were acceptable, median survival was only 18 months, no better than that reported using 5-FU based chemoradiation.

Other Approaches to Adjuvant Therapy

Despite results using radiation as a component of adjuvant therapy in European studies, 5-FU-based chemoradiation remains a cornerstone of recently completed phase 2 adjuvant therapy trials in the US Investigators from Virginia Mason Medical Center previously designed and reported their results using an intense course of chemoradiation, which consists of external-beam radiation therapy (EBRT) at a dose of 45-54 Gy (25 fractions over 5 weeks) and three-drug chemotherapy: continuous infusion 5-FU (200 mg/m^2 daily, days 1-35), weekly intravenous bolus cisplatin (30 mg/m^2 daily, days 1,8,15,22,29), and subcutaneus alpha, interferon (IFNα) (3 × 10^6 units, days 1-35). Chemoradiation is followed by further infusional 5-FU (200 mg/m^2 daily, weeks 9-14 and 17-22). This regimen was delivered to 43 patients after pancreaticoduodenectomy performed between 1995 and 2002; with a mean follow-up time of 31.9 months, median survival had not yet been reached.[243] The American College of Surgeons Oncology Group subsequently conducted a phase 2 trial (Z5031) in an attempt to confirm these favorable results; reported in abstract form only, the median survival of 89 study patients was 27 months.[244] This is consistent with results from Washington University where a modification of the Virginia Mason regimen was used with lower doses of 5-FU (175 mg/m^2) and cisplatin (25 mg/m^2) and IFNα given only 3 times weekly. In addition, two cycles of postchemoradiation gemcitabine was delivered rather than infusional 5-FU. This modified regimen was administered to 53 resected patients at Washington University and resulted in a median survival of 25 months.[245] Although all three trials of the Virginia Mason regimen have led to median survivals, which are favorable compared with historical controls, this therapy can be toxic and cannot be endorsed as a standard approach to adjuvant therapy off protocol or in centers with limited experience in its delivery.

Another novel approach to adjuvant therapy is being studied at JHH with a focus on the potential benefits of tumor vaccination after conventional surgery and 5-FU-based chemoradiation. Investigators there have developed an allogeneic pancreatic tumor cell vaccine genetically manipulated to express granulocyte-macrophage colony stimulating factor (GM-CSF), to enhance T-cell responsiveness. In a pilot study of 14 patients undergoing pancreaticoduodenctomy for pancreatic cancer, allogeneic pancreatic tumor cells engineered to secrete GM-CSF, were injected subcutaneously at various doses 8 weeks after surgery. Chemoradiation was subsequently delivered, and for those patients without relapse at completion, further vaccinations were delivered monthly for up to 3 additional months. Of note, three patients receiving the highest number of allogeneic tumor cells (greater than 10 × 10^7) had increased delayed hypersensitivy responses and were reported to have the best survival.[246] A phase 2 trial using vaccination as a component of adjuvant therapy has been completed with 60 patients enrolled; 30% of these had a R1 resection. Preliminary results of this trial have been reported with an observed median survival of 26 months.[247] While these results are encouraging, larger randomized phase 2 or 3 trials will be required to support the incorporation of immunotherapy into standard adjuvant therapy.

Preoperative (Neoadjuvant) Therapy

There are many practical and theoretical advantages to preoperative treatment of patients with localized pancreatic cancer. Most compelling is the ability to provide immediate systemic therapy for a disease that is systemic at diagnosis in virtually all patients. A second more practical advantage is improved patient selection for pancreatic surgery—an operation associated with significant patient morbidity even when performed in experienced hands. This improved patient selection arises because patients with rapidly progressive systemic disease are identified as part of the restaging evaluation performed following neoadjuvant treatment (prior to planned surgery). In prospective trials, approximately 25% of patients who receive preoperative treatment do not undergo successful resection of their primary tumor as a consequence of disease progression or evolution of clinically significant medical comorbidity.[216] These patients are spared the morbidity and prolonged recovery sometimes associated with pancreaticoduodenectomy. In a series of trials performed at UTMDACC, patients who demonstrated disease progression after preoperative chemoradiation had a median survival of only 7 months.[189,239,240] In addition, the high frequency of positive-margin resections with upfront surgery supports the concern that the retroperitoneal margin of excision, even when negative, may be only a few millimeters, making surgery alone inadequate local therapy for most patients. Thus, many institutions have begun to investigate the role of chemotherapy and/or chemoradiation given preoperatively, and this overall strategy is becoming more common in the off-protocol setting.

Since 1988, five prospective preoperative trials have been completed at our institution.[214,239,240,248,249] These trials have had identical eligibility criteria using a CT-based definition of resectable disease (as previously described), a uniform surgical technique for the performance of pancreaticoduodenectomy, and a standardized system for pathologic evaluation of surgical specimens, including resection margins. This has maximized the number of variables held constant, while varying only the chemoradiation regimens. All eligible patients were required to have biopsy-proven adenocarcinoma of the pancreatic head. In our initial preoperative study reported in 1992, 28 patients received a course of infusional 5-FU (300 mg/m^2/day) in combination with standard-fractionation external beam radiation therapy (EBRT; 50.4 Gy; 180 cGy/fraction for 28 fractions over 5.5 weeks).[214] The gastrointestinal toxic effects (nausea, vomiting, and dehydration) were severe enough to require hospital admission in a third of patients. Preoperative (postchemoradiation) restaging radiographic evaluation 4-5 weeks after completing preoperative therapy disclosed evidence of metastatic disease in 25% of patients. Another 15% had intraoperative evidence of metastatic disease at laparotomy for an overall resectability rate of 60%. Median survival for the patients who underwent pancreaticoduodenectomy with curative intent was 18 months. The degree of tumor cell kill was graded using a standardized scoring system, and 40% of the resected specimens had a pathologic partial response to therapy (>50% of the tumor cells were nonviable). Although the results from this initial trial of preoperative therapy appeared equivalent to those seen with postoperative therapy, the toxicity and hospitalization rate was discouraging. These findings led to a change in the delivery of EBRT in all subsequent preoperative trials performed at UTMDACC.

A rapid-fractionation program of EBRT was developed and delivered with 18-MeV photons using a four-field technique to a total dose of 30 Gy (3 Gy/fraction, 10 fractions over 2 weeks). This was designed to avoid the gastrointestinal toxicity associated with standard-fractionation chemoradiation delivered over 5.5 weeks, while maintaining the excellent local tumor control achieved with multimodality therapy.[239] Three sequential preoperative chemoradiation trials have evaluated three different radiosenzitizers (continuous infusion 5-FU, paclitaxel, and gemcitabine), all given as single agents, with our rapid-fractionation EBRT.[239,240,248] Again, restaging with contrast-enhanced CT and chest radiography was performed 4-5 weeks after the completion of chemoradiation, in preparation for pancreaticoduodenectomy. In our first study of rapid-fractionation EBRT with infusional 5-FU, 35 patients were enrolled, 27 were taken to surgery, and 20 (57%) underwent successful pancreaticoduodenectomy.[239] Local tumor control and patient survival were equal to the results with standard-fractionation (5.5 weeks) chemoradiation. Of note, only 2 (10%) of the 20 patients who underwent pancreaticoduodenectomy developed local-regional recurrence, and the median survival for all 20 resected patients was 25 months. Prior to the advent of gemcitabine, paclitaxel was investigated as a preoperative radiosensitizer in a group of patients with resectable pancreatic cancer.[240] Paclitaxel did not provide an advantage over 5-FU-based chemoradiation in terms of resection rate, local treatment effect, or overall survival.

Based on the superiority of gemcitabine over 5-FU in the setting of advanced disease, an interest in gemcitabine-based chemoradiation emerged and a phase 1 study of gemcitabine in combination with rapid-fractionation EBRT was performed in patients with locally advanced disease.[250] This regimen used our rapid-fractionation EBRT with 7 weekly infusions of gemcitabine. The maximum tolerated dose (MTD) of gemcitabine using this treatment schedule was 350 mg/m^2/week, roughly one-third the standard weekly dose. The dose-limiting toxic effects included fatigue, anorexia, nausea, vomiting, and dehydration; febrile neutropenia occurred in only one patient. Objective tumor regression was observed in 24% of patients, and one patient had a dramatic radiographic response, resulting in eventual surgical resection; the tumor was resected with negative surgical margins and histologically, 95% of the tumor specimen was nonviable. These results were sufficiently encouraging to proceed with a study of gemcitabine-based preoperative chemoradiation (GemXRT) in a group of patients with potentially resectable disease. A total of 86 patients were enrolled in this clinical trial.[248] Toxicities were similar to those observed in the initial phase 1 trial. Despite a longer elapsed time from enrollment to surgery (pancreaticoduodenectomy) compared with previous trials with 5-FU and EBRT (11-12 weeks rather than 7-9 weeks), 74% of patients underwent successful pancreaticoduodenectomy (compared with 60% with 5-FU–based chemoradiation). A pathologic partial response (>50% of tumor cells nonviable) was seen in over half of the surgical specimens, and there was one pathologic complete response. Overall, median survival for all 86 patients was 23 months with an actual 5-year survival of 27%. Median survival was 34 months for the 64 patients who completed all therapy to include surgical resection in the form of pancreaticoduodenectomy, and 7 months for the 22 patients who did not undergo pancreatic resection (due to disease progression or evolving medical co-morbidities). The actual 5-year survival for those who did and did not complete all therapy was 36% and 0% respectively. Neoadjuvant GemXRT was able to accurately distinguish patients who would benefit from surgery from patients with initially radiographically occult metastatic disease, which became apparent after preoperative therapy. For these latter patients, a large operation would simply add morbidity with no clinical benefit. Using preoperative GemXRT, major sites of disease recurrence were distant (liver, peritoneum, lung). Therefore, in our subsequent neoadjuvant trial, we delivered additional systemic therapy prior to chemoradiation and planned surgery. Published as a companion manuscript in the same issue of the *Journal of Clinical Oncology*, preoperative gemcitabine (750 mg/m^2) and cisplatin (30 mg/m^2) was given every 2 weeks for 4 doses followed by chemoradiation consisting of 4 weekly infusions of gemcitabine (400 mg/m^2) combined with radiation therapy (30 Gy in 10 fractions over 2 weeks) delivered 5 days per week (Gem-Cis-ART).[249] Patients underwent restaging 4-6 weeks after completion of chemoradiation and, in the absence of disease progression, were taken to surgery. The study enrolled 90 patients and 79 (88%) completed chemo-chemoradiation. Sixty-two (78%) of 79 patients were taken to surgery and 52 (66%) of 79 underwent pancreaticoduodenectomy. Median survival for the 79 patients who completed Gem-Cis-XRT was 19 months, with a median survival of 31 months for the 52 patients who received all therapy to include surgery and 10.5 months for the 27 patients who did not undergo surgical resection of their primary tumor due to disease progression ($p < .001$). The results observed with Gem-Cis-XRT were not superior to those observed with Gem-XRT. The median survival for the 52 patients who underwent surgery after Gem-Cis-XRT was 31 months; less, although not statistically different, than the 34 month median survival observed for the 64 patients who underwent surgery following Gem-XRT ($p = 0.41$). There was insufficient power to detect differences in survival based upon the sizes of the two study populations and it remains unclear if there were other confounding variables unique to such complicated treatment sequencing in patients with pancreatic cancer. However, there was a statistically significant increase in the number of patients with node-positive disease in the Gem-Cis-XRT trial compared to Gem-XRT, which was most likely due to a greater number of node-positive patients at study entry; the treatment effect in the primary tumor was identical in both trials suggesting a similar "downstaging" of node positive disease. Nevertheless, the results from these two preoperative gemcitabine-based chemoradiation trials are sufficiently compelling to justify broader investigation of neoadjuvant treatment for localized stage I/II pancreatic cancer to include the incorporation of molecular targeted therapies in addition to chemotherapy and radiation in the preoperative setting. Further, the very favorable survival data from this experience opens the door for consideration of a surgery-last treatment approach in patients with resectable pancreatic cancer even in an off-protocol setting. Clearly, if there is any concern over local tumor resectability, as in the case of borderline resectable tumors (discussed further below) surgery should only be considered after induction therapy.[251]

Unfortunately, many reports of neoadjuvant therapy for pancreatic cancer have included heterogeneous patient populations, enrolling patients with locally advanced or marginally resectable pancreatic cancer. Few investigators report clear anatomic definitions of locally advanced disease, and many studies incorporate intraoperative assessment of the extent of local tumor growth, data, which are subjective and not reproducible. In general, patients with locally advanced pancreatic cancer should not be included in studies of preoperative therapy because their inclusion confounds reports of overall resection rates, the frequency of R0 and R1 resections, and complicates comparisons to other studies. Therein lies the importance of using accurate and reproducible anatomic definitions for resectability, based on high-quality CT imaging.

Challenges associated with the delivery of neoadjuvant therapy include the need for a pretreatment pancreatic biopsy and the frequent need for intermediate-term palliation of jaundice using endoscopically placed biliary stents.[166,181,252] In addition, these stents can occlude during preoperative treatment leading to biliary stent-related morbidity. The insertion of coated metal stents in patients about to receive preoperative therapy is now routine since stent occlusion is more common when the preoperative interval exceeds 2-3 months.

Radiotherapy Technique and Dose in Localized Disease

When radiotherapy is delivered postoperative setting, the standard dose of radiotherapy in the postoperative setting is typically 50.4 Gy in 28 fractions. Field reductions are often made after 45 Gy. The boost volume should include the superior mesenteric vessels the tumor bed, and the celiac axis. In the neoadjuvant setting, standard-fractionation EBRT to 50.4 Gy has also been used. As discussed above, delivery of 30 Gy in 10 fractions has been successful in the neoadjuvant settting. Standard preoperative or postoperative adjuvant radiotherapy is typically directed to the regional lymphatics as well as the tumor bed with concurrent 5-FU or capecitabine. When concurrent gemcitabine is used as the radiosensitizer, smaller more localized fields are recommended to either the intact gross tumor (or the tumor bed in the postoperative setting). It is important to avoid the duodenul mucosa or jejunal reconstruction as much as possible. The benefits of chemoradiation either delivered preoperatively or postoperatively probably result from the treatment of the SMA margin. Although there may not be universal agreement about the size and shape of standard radiation fields, the superior mesenteric artery origin and the celiac axis must be covered with adequate margins. CT planning is recommended to target these structures and to contour the fields for organs at risk to include the kidneys, liver, and spinal cord. A three- or four-field technique using anterior, posterior, and opposed lateral fields allows optimal sparing of these critical tissues. Omitting the posterior field in a three field plan is often preferred if a large amount of the right kidney is in the anterior and posterior fields.

For tumors located in the pancreatic head, the anterior and posterior fields typically cover the T11-L3 vertebral bodies, being mindful that the visceral anatomy is quite variable in relation to the bony anatomy. The porta hepatis should be identified on CT and included in all fields. Inferiorly, the goal is to cover the tumor and duodenal bed with a 2 cm margin. The right border of the anterior and posterior fields and the anterior extent of the lateral fields are defined by the preoperative location of the duodenum. The left border of the anterior and posterior fields is placed 2 cm to the left of the vertebral body edge, as long as there is adequate coverage of the preoperative tumor volume. This usually means that the upper right border of the anterior and posterior fields is located 4-5 cm to the right of the vertebral body edge, and the anterior aspect of the lateral field is 5-6 cm from the anterior vertebral body edge. Blocking is placed over the inferior pole of the right kidney in the anterior and posterior fields, bisecting the vertebral bodies in the lateral fields. Corner blocks are typically placed in the anterior aspect of the lateral fields as well. For lesions of the pancreatic body and tail, similar principles are applied to field location, except that the splenic hilum is covered while the porta hepatis and duodenal bed are not; the right field border is typically located 2 cm from the right vertebral body edge.

Approach to the Patient With Potentially Resectable Disease

Clinical decisions regarding patients with potentially resectable disease should be made in the context of evidence-based principles of cancer care. First, surgery should only be performed in patients whose tumors appear to be resectable (ie, with a high-probability of R0 resection) based on MDCT and who have a good performance status (ECOG 0-1). Second, pancreaticoduodenectomy should be performed as part of a multimodality treatment program that includes preoperative or postoperative chemotherapy with or without EBRT. If upfront surgery is being considered, it should be linked to a reasonable probability that the patient will be capable of receiving postoperative therapy. Importantly, published perioperative mortality rates support the referral of patients with potentially resectable disease to centers that frequently perform major pancreatic resections for cancer.[183,253] Third, current and future treatment programs for patients with resectable pancreatic cancer should emphasize the use of systemic therapy (currently consisting of gemcitabine or gemcitabine-based combinations, 5-FU, or targeted agents). Since 80% of patients who appear to have resectable disease also have regional lymph node or distant organ metastases at the time of diagnosis, approaches that emphasize local therapies are misguided. Fourth, because of the modest survival rates seen with previously published treatment programs, the enrollment of all patients into clinical trials of new combinations of surgery, chemotherapy, chemoradiation, and newly developed systemic agents is strongly encouraged.

For patients who undergo upfront surgery, adjuvant therapy should be considered for all those with adequate recovery from surgery and no postoperative radiographic evidence of metastatic disease. Off-protocol, therapy should include the delivery of standard doses of gemcitabine either as a single modality for 6 cycles,[7] or given before and after 5-FU-based chemoradiation.[6] The role of radiation in the setting of an R1 resection remains controversial. Some have supported the delivery of postoperative chemoradiation to patients undergoing R1 resections based on nonrandomized retrospective studies.[193,236,237] Others have argued against the delivery of adjuvant radiation after R1 resection and have advise the delivery of chemotherapy only in this situation.[223] This can be resolved by the conduct of a randomized clinical trial, which limits enrollment to patients who have undergone an R1 resection.

In general, preoperative therapy should be delivered in the context of a clinical trial. At present, for those patients who receive have preoperative therapy with subsequent surgical resection, the role of postoperative chemoradiation or chemotherapy has not been clearly defined.

Management of Borderline Resectable Pancreatic Cancer

With the advent of MDCT, tumors that are neither clearly resectable, nor clearly unresectable have become increasingly recognized. These tumors are now being described as borderline resectable and have emerged as a distinct clinical entity in pancreatic cancer. While definitions vary, borderline resectable tumors can be broadly defined as tumors, which abut but do not encase critical arterial structures such as the SMA, hepatic artery, or celiac axis, or tumors with varying degrees of involvement of the SMV, portal vein, and superior mesenteric–portal venous confluence.[3,254] As such, a borderline resectable tumor puts the patient at high risk for a margin-positive resection (R1 or R2) and argues for an initial nonoperative approach. This is supported by several lines of evidence. First, reports from around the world suggest that upfront margin-positive resections are independent predictors of poor survival.[180,218-221] Although other reports have not demonstrated a statistically significant survival disadvantage in those patients undergoing an R1 resection,[222,223] some of these analyses have not adhered to strict pathologic criteria to define R status.[194] Second, in patients with potentially resectable disease, neoadjuvant chemoradiation leads to low R1 resection rates,[240,248,249] or reduces the risk of an R1 resection compared with upfront surgery.[255] Third, older single-institution studies have demonstrated the potential of preoperative chemoradiation therapy to occasionally convert locally unresectable pancreatic cancer to resectable disease.[256-258] For example, in a study conducted at the New England Deaconess Hospital, 16 patients who had locally advanced, unresectable pancreatic cancer were treated with 45 Gy of EBRT and infusional 5-FU to enhance resectability; two (13%) of the patients were able to undergo subsequent resection.[256] Likewise, investigators from Duke University and the University of California, Los Angeles have reported that between 8% and 10% of patients with locally advanced pancreatic cancer can be treated with chemoradiation and ultimately undergo complete resection.[257,258] Tumor-downstaging has also been reported from the early experiences, which combined gemcitabine with EBRT for locally advanced pancreatic cancer.[250,259] Finally, when preoperative regimens that include radiation are delivered to patients more strictly defined as having borderline resectable disease, subsequent surgical resection can occur with higher frequency. Mehta and colleagues have reported on the Stanford University experience using preoperative infusional 5-FU and radiation in patients with marginally resectable disease.[260] Fifteen patients received chemoradiation, and of these, 9 (60%) ultimately underwent surgical resection with negative margins. Two patients were reported to have complete pathological responses.[260] Further support for preoperative chemoradiation comes from our experience showing that approximately 40% of patients with borderline resectable disease can ultimately undergo surgical resection, with a median overall survival for the subset undergoing surgical resection equal to 40 months. Moreover, an R0 resection was achieved in 94% of resected patients.[251]

Given these lines of evidence, upfront surgery should be discouraged in patients with borderline resectable disease, since positive surgical margins would be expected to occur quite frequently. Rather, preoperative chemotherapy or chemoradiation should be considered since sufficient tumor destruction, particularly at the tumor's periphery, could render a tumor resectable with curative intent (ie, negative surgical margins). Given the frequency of systemic relapse after surgery for pancreatic cancer, serious concerns about borderline resectable tumors may be unfounded. However, recent data from both adjuvant and neoadjuvant trials suggest that gemcitabine is somewhat better than 5-FU for improving survival[6,248,249] and imply that as systemic therapy improves further (albeit slowly), complete surgical resection will become increasingly relevant for long-term survival. Thus, strategies that improve the chance of achieving a R0 resection for patients with borderline resectable disease should take precedence over upfront resection, which by definition is high-risk for R1. In the future, adherence to strict radiographic definitions of resectable, borderline resectable, and locally advanced disease, will allow for the design of specific protocols for each of these distinct entities. As will be discussed below, the incorporation of biologic agents into preoperative programs for borderline resectable tumors is predicted to be an area of future interest.

Treatment of Locally Advanced Disease

Chemoradiation Versus Radiation Alone or Chemotherapy Alone

Chemoradiation therapy has been part of the foundation of therapy for locally advanced disease and has previously been shown to prolong survival compared with radiation alone and chemotherapy alone. In GITSG studies of 5-FU-based chemoradiation therapy in patients with locally advanced pancreatic adenocarcinoma,[12,261] patients were randomly assigned to receive 40 Gy of radiation plus 5-FU, 60 Gy plus 5-FU, or 60 Gy without chemotherapy. Radiation therapy was delivered as a split course, with 20 Gy given over 2 weeks followed by a 2-week rest. 5-FU was delivered IV at a bolus dosage of 500 mg/m^2/day for the first 3 days of each 20-Gy cycle and iven weekly (500 mg/m^2) following the completion of chemoradiation therapy. The median survival was 10 months in each of the chemoradiation therapy groups and only 6 months for the group that received 60 Gy without 5-FU. In subsequent GITSG studies, neither doxorubicin (Adriamycin)[262] used as a radiation potentiator nor multidrug chemotherapy (streptozocin, mitomycin, and 5-FU [SMF]) alone or continued after chemoradiation therapy[263] was found to be superior to 5-FU-based chemoradiation therapy. Additional chemotherapy after 5-FU-based chemoradiation therapy increased the toxicity without an apparent therapeutic benefit.

In contrast to the results from the GITSG study demonstrating better survival with 5-FU-based chemoradiation therapy than with SMF chemotherapy alone, an ECOG study suggested no benefit to chemoradiation therapy over 5-FU alone.[264] The study randomly assigned patients with locally advanced or incompletely resected pancreatic adenocarcinoma to receive chemoradiation therapy (40 Gy and 5-FU at 600 mg/m^2/day for 3 days) or 5-FU alone (600 mg/m^2/week). The chemoradiation therapy group received weekly bolus administration of 5-FU following chemoradiation therapy until disease progression. Similar to the GITSG studies, all patients were surgically staged and entered in the study within 6 weeks of surgery. Patients with incomplete resections and patients with limited peritoneal involvement were also allowed to participate. The median survival was 8.3 months in the group that received chemoradiation therapy and 8.2 months in the group that received 5-FU alone. Of note, as discussed later in the section on metastatic disease, it was evident in the GITSG studies and in the ECOG trial that patients with locally advanced, unresectable pancreatic cancer who are not fully ambulatory secondary to ongoing symptoms, did not benefit from anticancer therapy.

The introduction of gemcitabine and the recognition of benefit in patients with advanced disease stimulated the design of trials that compared gemcitabine to modern chemoradiation. A recently presented randomized trial from the French foundation Francophone de Cancérologie Digestive and Société Française de Radiothérapie Oncologique (FFCD-SFRO) was a randomized trial that has compared chemotherapy to chemoradiation in patients with locally advanced pancreas cancer.[11] Patients were treated with gemcitabine alone in one arm or radiation (total dose 60 Gy) with concurrent 5-FU and cisplatin, followed by gemcitabine in the second arm. The median overall survival in the gemcitabine alone arm was unusually high: 14.3 months. These results are not consistent with the reported median survivals for patients with locally advanced pancreatic cancer patients treated with gemcitabine-based chemotherapy alone in contemporaneous randomized trials. For example, in ECOG 6201, a trial which compared three gemcitabine-based systemic treatments without radiation for patients with advanced pancreatic cancer, the median survival of patients with locally advanced disease was 9.1 months.[265] Similarly, in a trial of gemcitabine-based chemotherapy alone (Cancer and Leukemia Group B [CALGB] 308303), patients with locally advanced disease had a median survival of 9.9 months.[17]

Conversely, the FFCD-SFRO study also reported unusually poor survival (8.4 months) among the patients treated with 5-FU/cisplatin chemoradiation followed by gemcitabine; this is significantly lower than results typically reported using 5-FU based chemoradiation: 10-12 months. Of further concern was high rate of the acute toxicity observed in the chemoradiation arm; this led to poor compliance with the regimen and probably contributed to the poor outcome for the cohort. Factors that likely contributed to the poor tolerance were the inclusion of cisplatin as a radiosensitizer, the use of a high dose of radiation (60 Gy) and the inclusion of regional nodal fields in the radiation portal.

In the United States, the only recent trial to compare chemotherapy to chemoradiation has been ECOG 4201. This trial compared gemcitabine-based chemoradiation (gemcitabine given at 600 mg/m^2 weekly with radiation to regional nodal volumes to a dose of 50.4 Gy in 28 fractions) followed by weekly gemcitabine (1000 mg/m^2 weekly, 3 of 4 weeks) with standard treatment using gemcitabine alone. Although it closed prematurely after accruing only 74 of a planned 316 patients, a statistically significant median survival benefit was seen in the arm that received chemoradiation compared to the arm that received chemotherapy alone, 11.0 versus 9.2 months, ($p = 0.034$ two-sided, stratified Log rank). This benefit came at the cost of increased gastrointestinal toxicity (grade 3 or greater gastrointestinal toxicity 38% vs 14% $p = 0.03$ and fatigue, 32% vs 6%).[266] Thus, the addition of radiation to standard chemotherapy resulted in a modest prolongation of median survival at the cost of a modest increase in toxicity that remained manageable.

Chemotherapy Alone Versus Chemoradiation: An Important Controversy?

The reality of current pancreas cancer treatment today is that both chemotherapy and chemoradiation have significant limitations. Both modalities should be rationally used in individual patients to maximize survival and minimize morbidity. Patients probably benefit modestly in different ways from both systemic therapy and chemoradiation; these approaches are complementary and should both be considered in all patients with locally advanced disease. Selection of patients that are most appropriate for chemoradiation is probably best accomplished with an initial strategy of gemcitabine-based chemotherapy for 2-4 months in patients without significant local symptoms, followed by consolidation with chemoradiation in patients who do not have rapidly progressive distant disease.[267,268] Serial measurements of CA 19-9 can be obtained and may serve as an indicator of response. Chemoradiation directed to the gross tumor can then be used when there is local progression, symptomatic progression, if the CA 19-9 level begins to plateau or rise, or the chemotherapy becomes poorly tolerated. Such a strategy has been employed at UTMDACC, and a recent analysis indicates improved median survival among patients treated with chemotherapy followed by chemoradiation compared to those treated with chemoradation initially (11.9 months vs 8.5 months, $p < 0.001$).[10] This likely reflects the value of patient selection by delivering chemotherapy first. This approach can help identify those patients who rapidly develop distant disease and spare them chemoradiation, which is unlikely to be of benefit.[10]

Gemcitabine-Based Chemoradiation Trials ■ The introduction of gemcitabine was a modest step forward in the treatment of pancreatic cancer. Its value as a systemic agent in pancreatic cancer and discovery of its potent radiosensitizing properties,[269] stimulated the study of combinations of gemcitabine with EBRT for patients with localized pancreatic cancer.[250,270-273] Several strategies have been investigated, including seven weekly injections of gemcitabine with rapid-fractionation EBRT (30 Gy) discussed previously, twice weekly gemcitabine with 50.4 Gy of EBRT, weekly gemcitabine with 50.4 Gy of EBRT, and full dose weekly gemcitabine with escalating doses of radiation. Most of these studies suggested gastrointestinal toxicity as a dose-limiting factor, but hematologic toxicity has also been observed. Now, there is no standard approach for combining gemcitabine and radiation, but several variables appear to be important in predicting the MTD. These include variations in the size of the radiation portal, the total radiation dose, possibly the dose of radiation per fraction, and whether gemcitabine is administered once or twice weekly.[274]

Three multi-institutional studies have been completed evaluating gemcitabine-based chemoradiation. In a small study performed in Taiwan, 34 patients with locally advanced pancreatic cancer were randomized to receive 5-FU-based chemoradiation (500 mg/m^2 daily for 3 days, every 14 days with radiation to a total dose of 50.4-61.2 Gy) or gemcitabine and radiation (600 mg/m^2 weekly with equivalent doses of radiation).[275] The objective response rate to gemcitabine and radiation was 50% and only 13% for 5-FU chemoradiation. In addition, median survival was substantially better using gemcitabine compared with 5-FU (14.5 months vs 6.7 months, $p = .027$). The efficacy results must be interpreted with caution because of the limited accrual (34 patients), the poor results in the control group and therapy that was poorly tolerated in both arms. A phase 2 study conducted in patients with locally advanced pancreatic cancer by the Cancer and Leukemia Group B evaluated gemcitabine given at 40 mg/m2 twice weekly. In that study, there were 35% and 50% grade 3 or 4 gastrointestinal and hematologic toxicities, respectively, and the median survival was only 8.5 months.[276] Both of these studies used regional nodal fields that likely contributed to the significant gastrointestinal toxicity. In contrast, the approach developed at the University of Michigan delivers the manufacturer's recommended dose of gemcitabine (1 g/m^2) with a slightly lower radiotherapy dose (36 Gy in 15 fractions over 3 weeks), with conformal radiation fields encompassing the gross tumor volume alone. At that institution, the irradiation of a smaller volume of normal tissue was reported to be well tolerated.[271] Investigators have since embarked on a multi-institutional phase 2 study evaluating the same regimen. Results indicate that approximately 25% of patients experience grade 3 nausea and grade 3 vomiting each occurred in about 10% of the 41 enrolled patients.[277]

Several points about gemcitabine-based chemoradiation are worth emphasizing. First, all chemoradiation regimens studied in patients with locally advanced disease, including gemcitabine-containing regimens, have significant efficacy limitations. Similar to its value as a systemic agent,[13] gemcitabine is probably only modestly better than 5-FU when it is used with radiotherapy, but early experience suggest it is somewhat more toxic.[278] Second, the degree of gastrointestinal toxicity reported in the three multi-institutional studies using gemcitabine calls into question whether the combination of gemcitabine and radiotherapy will be tolerated well enough for future studies to build on these experiences. Finally, compared with radiotherapy fields that target the gross tumor only, elective regional nodal irradiation leads to more gastrointestinal toxicity. Since currently available chemoradiation regimens cannot fully control the primary tumor, irradiation of microscopic regional nodal metastases probably does not improve the outcome of patients with locally advanced pancreatic cancer, regardless of the concurrent chemotherapeutic agent used. Certainly, if gemcitabine is used in combination with irradiation on esophageal, gastric, or duodenal mucosa, the volume of mucosa being treated should be minimized or there will be a significant risk of severe acute toxicity. Given the significant acute toxicity and limited efficacy reported using various combinations of gemcitabine and radiotherapy, gemcitabine-based chemoradiation is unlikely to be widely embraced in clinical practice for patients with locally advanced disease.

Novel Approaches to Chemoradiation ■ ***Molecular Agents as Radiosensitizers*** Oncology has entered an era of molecular therapy, and just as molecular agents have been combined with cytotoxic chemotherapy, the delivery of targeted agents as radiosensitizers is showing some promise.[279] In pancreatic cancer, integrating molecular agents into chemoradiation regimens requires that the cytotoxic chemotherapy backbone has predictable and acceptable toxicity. In that context, capecitabine has emerged as an attractive agent to combine with radiation in advanced pancreatic cancer. Capecitabine is an orally administered agent reported to have clinical benefit response and objective tumor response similar to that of gemcitabine in advanced pancreatic cancer.[280] Moreover, in colorectal cancer, capecitabine shows similar efficacy to intravenously administered 5-FU with a more favorable toxicity profile.[281,282] Last, capecitabine has also been shown to have a favorable toxicity profile when combined with EBRT for a number of GI tumors including pancreatic cancer.[283] In contrast to gemcitabine and EBRT, the favorable acute toxicity profile of capecitabine makes it an attractive chemoradiation platform upon which to integrate biologic agents.

As described elsewhere in this text, bevacizumab (a monoclonal antibody directed against vascular endothelial growth factor [VEGF]), and cetuximab (a monoclonal antibody against epidermal growth factor receptor [EGFR]), have changed the standard of care for patients with a variety of advanced solid tumors when combined with cytotoxic drugs. In pancreatic cancer, when erlotinib (an oral EGFR inhibitor), is delivered with gemcitabine, it provides more benefit to patients with pancreatic cancer compared with treatment with gemcitabine alone.[16] Importantly, these molecular therapies may play important roles as radiosensitizers and presently, bevacizumab's radiosensitizing properties are now being investigated in the clinic.[284,285] The precise mechanism of radiosensitization has not been defined, but possibilities include enhanced lethality of the endothelial cell,[286] the tumor cell,[287] or the improvement in vascular physiology leading to a reduction in tumor hypoxia.[288] In a recently completed phase 1 dose escalation study conducted at UTMDACC, capecitabine and bevacizumab were administered in combination with radiation (50.4 Gy) to 47 patients with locally advanced pancreatic cancer.[285] The study demonstrated that bevacizumab is generally safe when combined with chemoradiation in patients with locally advanced pancreatic cancer. The acute toxicity was minimal and easily managed with dose adjustments of capecitabine, without interruption or attenuation of either the bevacizumab or the radiation dose. Of note, although there was a 43% incidence of grade 2 gastrointestinal toxicity and a 21% incidence of grade 2 hand-and-foot syndrome, decreasing the dose of oral capecitabine was sufficient to avoid grade 3 toxicity in the majority of patients. In addition, limiting radiotherapy fields to the gross tumor volume alone probably contributed further to the small incidence of grade 3 acute toxicity and in general, bevacizumab did not appear to enhance acute toxicity. However, tumors with invasion of the duodenum appeared to be at higher risk of bleeding or perforation. Overall, the tumors in 9 of 46 evaluable patients (20%) had an objective partial response to initial therapy. This included 6 of 12 tumors treated at a dose of 5 mg/kg of bevacizumab.[285] The RTOG has now completed a phase 2 trial to evaluate capecitabine-based chemoradiation with bevacizumab (RTOG PA04-11), followed by systemic therapy with concurrent gemcitabine and bevacizumab. Patients with tumor invasion of the duodenum have been specifically excluded because of the risk of duodenal hemorrhage, and bleeding with in the radiation field was not a significant problem.

Similarly, EGFR inhibitors hold promise as radiosensitizers,[279] although none of the currently available inhibitors (gefitinib, erlotinib, or cetuximab) have been evaluated in multi-institutional trials in combination with radiation for pancreatic cancer. A phase 1 trial has evaluated gemcitabine-based chemoradiation (gemcitabine dosed at 40 mg/m^2 twice weekly) in combination with erlotinib.[289] The maximal tolerated dose of erlotinib was 100 mg daily; the combination led to an objective response rate of 35% and a reported median survival of 18.7 months among the 17 patients who completed the therapy (a total of 21 patients enrolled). A phase 2 study our institution is currently evaluating gemcitabine, oxaliplatin, and cetuximab, followed by capecitabine, radiation therapy (50.4 Gy), and cetuximab, followed by gemcitabine and cetuximab until progression. Trials that combine cetuximab or erlotinib with bevacizumab and EBRT for the treatment of pancreatic cancer are anticipated in the near future. Of note, although neither VEGF or EGFR inhibitors have been proven to improve outcomes for patients with advanced pancreatic cancer when combined with chemotherapy,[17,18] this should not discourage investigation of VEGF or EGFR inhibitors as radiosensitizers since these agents may have important modulating effects on the tumor cells or the tumor microenvironment when delivered with radiation.

Another novel approach to radiosensitization involves tumor necrosis factor-alpha (TNFα. In preclinical models, TNFα enhances radiation effects in esophageal cancer.[290] However, when TNFα is administered systemically, significant toxicity has been observed, limiting its use as a radiosensitizer. TNFerade is a replication deficient adenovector that expresses human TNFα under control of the radiation-inducible Egr-1 promoter. TNFerade has been directly injected into tumors with subsequent treatment with EBRT in a phase 1 study involving 36 patients with advanced solid tumors.[291] Six patients had pancreatic cancer; and three of the five pancreatic cancer patients evaluable for response had objective tumor response. TNFerade is now being studied in a randomized phase 2 or 3 trial comparing TNFerade plus standard of care chemoradiation with chemoradiation alone in patients with locally advanced pancreatic cancer.[292]

Stereotactic Radiation Body Therapy (SBRT) for Pancreatic Cancer?

Stereotactic body radiotherapy (SBRT) is capable of precisely delivering high doses of radiation to small tumor volumes. Critical components of this strategy include accurate and reproducible imaging, the integration of organ motion (commonly due to respiration) into treatment, meticulous patient immobilization, and careful patient selection. The CyberKnife is an innovative approach that incorporates real-time tracking of implanted fiducials to potentially address organ motion into real-time therapy. Patient selection is critical in the application of this technology. For primary or metastatic tumors of the lung or liver, this approach is particularly appealing because these tumors move with respiration and the ablation of a small volume of surrounding normal liver or lung tissue to the tumor usually does not result in a significant clinical consequence. However, if a radiosensitive structure such as the duodenum, small bowel, or stomach is inseparable from a radioresistant target, such as a pancreatic neoplasm, real-time motion tracking may minimize the volume of tissues that are treated, but the duodenum cannot be completely avoided. In fact, the duodenum is usually the critical normal tissue dictating technique and dose of radiation therapy. The feasibility of SBRT as a pancreatic cancer treatment has been investigated in a phase 1 dose escalation trial of a single fraction of radiation therapy in patients with locally advanced pancreatic cancer at Stanford University.[293] The authors commented from that trial that the "...duodenum is in close proximity to the majority of the pancreatic tumors treated, and it was impossible to avoid treating this structure to a relatively high dose." and recommended a dose of 25Gy.[293] In an attempt to improve on the median survival of 8.0 months at the 25Gy dose level, the same investigators then conducted a phase 2 trial using 45Gy of intensity-modulated radiation therapy with concurrent 5-FU followed by a stereotactic boost of 25Gy. This strategy did appear to be effective. The trial enrolled 19 patients, 16 of whom actually completed the therapy; median survival for these 16 patients was only 6.3 months.[294] The Stanford group has recently investigated treatment with gemcitabine before and after a single 25Gy fraction of SBRT.[295] Although median survival was more encouraging (11.4 months), late GI toxicity was significant with five patients having grade 2 duodenal ulceration, 1 patient having a grade 3 duodenal stricture, and one patient experiencing a grade 4 duodenal perforation. Given the lack of any convincing prospective evidence for improved outcome, at present, there is no role for the use of SBRT outside the setting of a clinical trial in pancreatic cancer patients.

Radiotherapy Technique for Patients With Locally Advanced Disease

Patients with locally advanced tumors probably do not benefit from regional lymph node irradiation; radiotherapy fields should therefore be confined to the gross tumor. This strategy reduces the gastrointestinal toxicity of chemoradiation. Thus, it is important to identify the pancreatic tumor correctly. On contrast-enhanced CT, pancreatic tumors are typically hypodense compared with the surrounding pancreatic parenchyma. When there is doubt about the location of the primary tumor, CT images should be reviewed with an experienced radiologist. Administration of an oral contrast agent at the time of simulation illuminates the duodenal "c-loop." Endobiliary biliary stents can also be visualized, which facilitates identifying the common bile duct.

The pancreas and duodenum move a median of 1 cm with respiratory excursion.[296] If the gross tumor alone is to be treated, respiratory motion must be either controlled or accounted for in radiotherapy planning. This is commonly accomplished by simply adding an additional margin to the planned radiation fields in the cranial and caudal directions. However, because axial tumor motion is negligible, an additional margin for motion in the axial directions is not necessary. Radiation treatment that is gated to the respiratory cycle (respiratory gating)[297] is a necessary component of radiation dose escalation studies that seek to deliver > 60 Gy to the primary tumor while sparing the duodenum. Thus, radiation fields designed to spare the duodenum that are tightly confined to the primary tumor without correction for organ motion could lead to under-dosing of the tumor target, or "marginal miss." A four-field technique is recommended with equally weighted anterior, posterior, and opposed lateral fields. A 2 cm block margin is used in the radial directions, and a 3 cm margin is used in the cranial and caudal directions.

Tumors of the Pancreatic Body and Tail

Because adenocarcinomas of the pancreatic body and tail do not obstruct the intrapancreatic portion of the common bile duct, early diagnosis is rare, and most patients have locally advanced or metastatic disease at the time of diagnosis. The celiac axis or SMA is encased in most patients, except for the anecdotal patient who presents with upper gastrointestinal hemorrhage resulting from sinistral hypertension due to splenic vein occlusion by a small tumor. In the rare patient who appears to have resectable disease on CT scans (no arterial encasement and no extrapancreatic disease), laparoscopy prior to laparotomy is a logical initial step because this frequently reveals peritoneal metastases.[171,298] Accurate preoperative imaging and a selective approach to surgical therapy will avoid surgery-related morbidity and mortality in patients who do not have potentially resectable disease.

The scant data on surgical resection confirm the short survival and poor prognosis in this subgroup of patients.[299,300] As a general rule, patients with adenocarcinomas of the body and tail should undergo staging laparoscopy. If there is no evidence for metastatic disease, we strongly recommend delivery of neoadjuvant chemotherapy or chemoradiation. Distal subtotal pancreatectomy is then considered in the rare patient who shows no evidence of disease progression on restaging radiographic studies after neoadjuvant therapy and who has a performance status acceptable for major abdominal surgery. In all other patients, enrollment in phase 2 investigational trials should be considered.

Approach to Locally Advanced Pancreatic Cancer

Prior to initiation of therapy, a careful appraisal of a patient's symptoms and overall functional status (before and after symptoms of pancreatic cancer developed) should be completed. In general, for patients with good PS and adequate pain control, we favor induction chemotherapy over initial chemoradiation to select those patients with more favorable tumor biology, who may ultimately benefit from subsequent delivery of chemoradiation.[10,267,268] Under these circumstances, staging laparoscopy offers no distinct advantage over delivery of chemotherapy. For those patients with marginal or poor PS, supportive measures to include adequate biliary drainage, stabilization of pain, and control of other symptoms (fatigue, nausea, vomiting, diarrhea, or constipation) should be instituted ahead of anticancer therapy. In patients who appear to have locally advanced pancreatic cancer, but having a clinical picture suggestive of metastatic disease, staging laparoscopy may be useful to avoid the toxicity and futility of chemoradiation at any point in the patient's treatment.

It should be noted that chemoradiation has been touted for its potential palliative benefits in locally advanced disease, and in a prospective phase 1 trial of capecitabine-based chemoradiation, pain and other symptoms were improved after completion of therapy.[301] However, the overall clinical benefits associated with chemoradiation has not been rigorously studied. In one retrospective review of 25 patients with locally advanced disease, Fisher and colleagues observed a clinical benefit in only 24% of patients undergoing chemoradiation, suggesting that the benefit may actually be equivalent to that observed with gemcitabine.[13,302]

It remains unclear if patients who have received chemoradiation should be treated immediately with further systemic therapy or followed expectantly for clinical and/or radiographic evidence of progressive disease. Progressive disease may take the form of local tumor progression with increasing pain, gastric outlet obstruction, or recurrent biliary obstruction; distant metastatic disease with liver or lung metastases; or peritoneal carcinomatosis.

Whenever possible, patients with locally advanced disease having a good performance status should be treated in the context of a clinical trial. This may involve a predefined course of chemotherapy followed by chemoradiation, or alternatively a program of chemoradiation with a targeted agent, followed by further systemic therapy.

Outside of a clinical trial, systemic therapy with gemcitabine may improve both pain control and performance status,[13] and avoids the gastrointestinal toxicity associated with chemoradiation. For those patients with stable or responding disease after a few months of systemic therapy, chemoradiation can then be considered to maximize local-regional tumor control. This treatment sequence has the advantage of avoiding the toxicity of chemoradiation in those patients who show evidence progressive disease following systemic therapy.

Management of Gastric Outlet Obstruction

Patients with symptomatic gastric outlet obstruction and a reasonable performance status require gastric bypass, which can be performed by laparotomy or laparoscopy. However, the performance of prophylactic gastric bypass at the time of laparotomy in patients found to have unresectable disease remains controversial. Those in favor of prophylactic gastrojejunostomy state that it can be performed safely, is not associated with postoperative delayed gastric emptying, and will prevent subsequent gastric outlet obstruction in 10-20% of patients.[303,304] Those who do not recommend prophylactic gastric bypass believe that concomitant gastrojejunostomy (at the time of therapeutic biliary bypass) significantly increases operative morbidity; that the incidence of subsequent gastric outlet obstruction in patients who receive only a biliary bypass is much less than 10%; and that if clinically evident gastric outlet obstruction does occur, it is usually a manifestation of end-stage disease.[305-308] Lillemoe and colleagues[309] reported the results of a prospective randomized trial of prophylactic gastrojejunostomy in patients with adenocarcinoma of the pancreatic head and periampullary region. Patients found to have unresectable disease (and not to have intraoperative evidence of impending gastric outlet obstruction, in which case the patients were excluded from analysis) at the time of laparotomy were randomized to undergo either a prophylactic gastrojejunostomy or no further surgery. Subsequent gastric outlet obstruction developed in 8 (19%) of the 43 patients who did not undergo a gastric bypass and in none of the 44 patients who underwent a gastrojejunostomy. Postoperative delayed gastric emptying (2% of patients) and mean hospital stay (8 days) were not different between groups. Further, there were no perioperative deaths, and the mean survival duration was 8.3 months in both groups. The authors therefore concluded that a retrocolic gastrojejunostomy should be performed routinely when a patient with pancreatic or periampullary cancer is found at laparotomy to have unresectable disease.

The opposite conclusion was reached by Espat and colleagues[308] from Memorial Sloan-Kettering Cancer Center, who reported the longitudinal follow-up findings in 155 patients who were found to have unsuspected locally advanced or metastatic disease at the time of staging laparoscopy for presumed localized pancreatic cancer. They found a low incidence of gastric outlet obstruction in patients with advanced pancreatic cancer. Only two patients underwent elective gastric bypass (one was performed laparoscopically). At a median follow-up of 6 months (by which time 81% of patients had died of disease), only 3 (2%) of the 155 patients had undergone a subsequent open palliative surgical procedure, including a gastrojejunostomy for symptomatic gastric outlet obstruction in 2 of these patients. One additional patient required a percutaneous gastrostomy tube to relieve poor gastric emptying during the terminal phase of his disease. The median survival was 6.2 months for those with metastatic disease and 7.8 months for those with locally advanced disease, suggesting that these patients did not have high-volume metastatic disease at the time of laparoscopy. Raikar and colleagues[310] also reported a low incidence of subsequent gastric outlet obstruction in patients with unresectable pancreatic cancer who underwent endoscopic biliary decompression. In that study, only 1 (3%) of 34 patients treated with endoscopic biliary decompression required surgical bypass for gastric outlet obstruction. These two nonrandomized studies therefore do not support the routine practice of prophylactic gastric bypass.

In general, we do not recommend prophylactic surgery in patients with pancreatic cancer. However, if a patient is found to have unresectable disease during a planned pancreaticoduodenectomy, a gastrojejunostomy may be considered when clinical symptoms or anatomic findings suggest impending obstruction. In all other patients with good PS and newly discovered locally advanced or limited metastatic disease at the time of surgery, creation of a retrocolic gastrojejunostomy is justified.[309]

Treatment of Metastatic Disease

Progress in the treatment of metastatic pancreatic cancer has lagged behind that of other gastrointestinal malignancies. Pancreatic cancer is resistant to conventional cytotoxic agents, and more recently has proven to be insensitive to an array of molecular targeted agents. In addition, many patients present with decreased functional status, an independent predictor of poor survival; treating such patients with cytotoxic therapy may actually be counterproductive. Furthermore, even when patients present with good performance status, in the absence of meaningful tumor stabilization or regression, most will experience clinical decline, making the delivery of subsequent anticancer therapy more difficult, and usually, less effective. Not surprisingly therefore, despite significant efforts to alter the natural history of metastatic disease using gemcitabine, cytotoxic gemcitabine doublets, nongemcitabine containing regimens, and novel therapeutics, clinically meaningful improvements in survival have not been observed since gemcitabine's introduction in the mid-1990s. However, sluggish progress cannot be blamed merely on aggressive cancer biology and ineffective therapies, but may also be attributed to suboptimal clinical trial design, poor patient selection, and in the emerging era of molecular therapy, a general lack of predictive biomarkers. These impediments are now being recognized, and with a better understanding of the genetic and molecular perturbations driving tumor growth and metastases, there is an emerging perception within the pancreatic cancer community that more advances that are significant are soon possible. A brief historical perspective and a review of modern trials of systemic will aid the reader in this regard.

Early Trials of Chemotherapy in Pancreatic Cancer: The 1950s-1980s

After its synthesis in the 1950s, 5-FU, usually administered as a bolus injection, became the most widely used drug for the treatment of advanced pancreatic cancer and early experience suggested respectable antitumor activity. In a review of trials dating back to the 1960s and 1970s, the overall response rate to bolus 5-FU was estimated to be 28%.[311] However, these initial studies used unreliable methods to assess response including physical examination, ultrasonagraphy, and liver-spleen scintillography, likely overestimating the single-agent activity of bolus 5-FU.[312-314]

Nevertheless, since single-agent 5-FU was initially considered active in advanced pancreatic cancer, 5-FU combinations were subsequently investigated. The Southwest Oncology Group (SWOG) performed a randomized phase 2 trial comparing newer single agents (methylglyoxal-bis-guanylhydrazone [MGBG], dihydroxyanthracenedione [DHAD], and aziridinylbenzoquinone [AZQ]) to a combination of 5-FU, doxorubicin, mitomycin C, and streptozocin (FAM-S).[315] There were no significant differences in survival among patients randomized to the various single agents or to FAM-S. Other trials evaluated combinations of 5-FU, doxorubicin, and mitomycin C (FAM), 5-FU streptozotocin, mitomycin C, (SMF), and the Mallinson regimen, (consisting of induction therapy with 5-FU, cyclophosphamide, methotrexate, and vincristine followed by maintenance treatment with 5-FU and mitomycin C). Initial results using these 3 regimens in phase 2 trials were encouraging and appeared superior to historical results obtained with single-agent 5-FU,[316-318] but in larger randomized trials, none of them demonstrated any significant survival advantage over any other combination.[319-321]

Modern Cross-Sectional Imaging Confirms Chemoresistance: 1980s-1990s

Once modern cross-sectional CT and MR imaging became more widely available in the 1980s and early 1990s, a growing appreciation for the chemoresistance of pancreatic cancer emerged. In addition to completion of a number of phase 2 and phase 3 trials of 5-FU-based combinations (which proved disappointing), this period was marked by investigation of a wide array of cytotoxic drugs to assess their single-agent activity. These included studies of iproplatin, trimetrexate, edatrexate, fazarabine, AZQ, MGBG, amonafide, topotecan, and ZD1694 (Tomudex).[322] While some of these drugs appeared modestly effective in small phase 2 trials, none was reproducibly active and no clear winner emerged.

Despite a complete lack of progress in systemic therapy at the time, some important observations were made, which still have implications for the conduct of clinical trials and the selection of patients for appropriate therapy. First, it became apparent that prognosis was dependent on stage at presentation, with patients generally characterized as having potentially resectable disease, locally advanced, unresectable disease, or disseminated disease. In 1985, Kalser and his colleagues reported on the survival of 393 patients having resected, locally advanced, or metastatic pancreatic cancer, all of whom enrolled in protocols conducted by the Gastrointestinal Tumor Study Group.[323] There were striking differences in survival observed among these three groups of patients, with resected patients having a median survival of 73 weeks, and those with disseminated disease surviving only 10 weeks. Those with locally advanced disease had intermediate median survival approaching 35 weeks. Second, it was recognized that assessing objective response to therapy, particularly for the primary tumor, was a challenge. Ductal adenocarcinoma within the pancreas often leads to intense desmoplastic changes surrounding small clusters of malignant ductal epithelium.[324] Recent investigations suggests this is caused by the microenvironement, specifically pancreatic stellate cells and proliferating fibroblasts, which produce fibrotic changes leading to a protective and supportive environment for the malignant epithelium.[325] These primary tumors are generally resistant to chemotherapy and radiation, but even when meaningful tumor destruction occurs, it may not be reflected on subsequent imaging studies. In addition, radiographic changes caused by peritumoral inflammation and pancreatitis may resolve during therapy, without any real change in the viability of the malignant epithelium, confounding the significance of an apparently smaller pancreatic mass.[326] Third, performance status was appreciated as a significant predictor of survival and patients with poor functional status have very poor survival.[323,327] Recent studies have confirmed this finding and have further suggested that more aggressive therapies may only benefit the subset of patients with good performance status (discussed later).[328]

The Emergence of Gemcitabine as Standard Therapy

Gemcitabine (2-fluoro, 2-deoxycytidine) a deoxycytidine analog, was developed in the early 1990s and had advantages over other deoxycytidine analogs such as cytarabine, with improved lipophilic properties and less myelosuppression.[329] During the past decade, it has emerged as the standard cytotoxic drug for the treatment of advanced pancreatic cancer.[13,330,331] Two of the initial phase 2 trials of gemcitabine were reported in 1994 and 1996. Between these two studies, a total of 72 evaluable patients were treated with response rates ranging from 6% to 11%.[330,331] Importantly, symptomatic improvement was observed among the patients enrolled in these trials. These observations led to the registration trial for gemcitabine with clinical benefit, not survival, as the primary end point.[13] Chemonaive patients with advanced pancreatic cancer were randomized to receive weekly gemcitabine versus bolus weekly 5-FU. Patients treated with gemcitabine had a higher response rate (5.4% vs 0%), improved median survival (5.65 vs 4.41 months, $p = 0.0025$) and a better 1-year survival rate (18% vs 2%) compared with patients treated with bolus 5-FU.[13] Most importantly, gemcitabine was found to have more clinically meaningful effects on disease-related symptoms compared with bolus 5-FU (24% vs 4% respectively). These clinical benefits were also documented in patients treated with gemcitabine after disease progression while receiving 5-FU.[332] The clinical benefit and modest survival advantage produced by gemcitabine compared with bolus 5-FU, led to its approval by the US Food and Drug Administration and its acceptance as first-line therapy for patients with advanced pancreatic adenocarcinoma. Since that time, few drugs given as single agents have been directly compared with gemcitabine, and to date, none has been established as superior. These include the matrix metalloproteinase inhibitors marimastat and BAY 12-9566, and the camptothecin, exatecan mesylate.[159,333,334] Thus, in virtually all recent large prospective randomized trials of frontline chemotherapy for advanced pancreatic cancer, treatment with gemcitabine monotherapy has been the control arm.

Importantly, although studies have firmly established the lack of efficacy of bolus 5-FU,[13,335] there is evidence that infusional delivery of 5-FU and oral capectabine have some activity in pancreatic cancer.[280,336] Given the toxicity profiles of these drugs, which are relevant to patients with advanced pancreatic cancer, a randomized trial comparing gemcitabine to infusional 5-FU or capecitabine would be welcomed.

Chemotherapy Is Better Than Best Supportive Care

Even though the benefits of cytotoxic therapy in patients with advanced pancreatic cancer are fairly small, a recent analysis supports the delivery of chemotherapy over best supportive care.[337] In a series of meta-analyses, Sultana and colleagues evaluated the possible survival advantages of chemotherapy in patients with locally advanced or metastatic pancreatic cancer. Several comparisons were examined: chemotherapy versus best supportive care; 5-FU versus 5-FU-based combinations; gemcitabine versus FU; and gemcitabine versus gemcitabine-based combination therapy. Of the 113 relevant trials reviewed, 51 trials involving 9970 patients met the inclusion criteria with particular attention to overall survival as a major endpoint. The results showed that chemotherapy improved survival compared with best supportive care (HR = 0.64; 95% CI, 0.42-0.98). As previously reported in primary data, 5-FU-based combination chemotherapy did not result in better overall survival compared with 5-FU alone (HR = 0.94; 95% CI, 0.82-1.08). Unfortunately, there was insufficient power to detect significant survival differences between patients receiving gemcitabine and those receiving 5-FU. Of note however, the authors also analyzed several trials, which compared treatment with gemcitabine monotherapy against gemcitabine-based combinations to determine if there was any difference in overall survival. The findings of this analysis will be discussed in the section below.

Fixed-Dose Rate Gemcitabine: An Effort to Improve Gemcitabine Therapy

Gemcitabine is a pro-drug, which requires intracellular phosphorlyation for cytotoxic activity either as an inhibitor of ribonucleotide reductase, or by incorporation into an elongating chain of DNA. During early clinical trials of gemcitabine, the rate of gemcitabine phosphorylation was noted to be subject to saturation kinetics.[338] Further studies demonstrated that the rate of intracellular gemcitabine triphosphate accumulation and peak intracellular concentrations were highest at a dose rate of 350 mg/m^2 per 30 min (~10 mg/m^2/min).[338] These pharmacokinetic findings suggested that increasing the infusion time for gemcitabine while holding the dose rate constant would increase the intracellular levels of phosphorylated species of gemcitabine and thus improve antitumor efficacy.

To test this hypothesis, a randomized phase 2 trial was conducted in patients with metastatic pancreatic cancer.[339] Patients were randomized to receive either FDR gemcitabine (infused at 10 mg/m^2/min) or gemcitabine given using the standard 30-min bolus technique. FDR gemcitabine (1500 mg/m^2 over 150 min) led to a similar objective response rate compared with gemcitabine at 2300 mg/m^2 given over 30 min, but patients treated with FDR gemcitabine had a trend toward improved survival compared with those patients who received gemcitabine delivered over 30 min (8.0 months vs 5.0 months, respectively, $p = 0.13$). This provocative result has led to further investigation of FDR gemcitabine. In a phase 2 trial conducted by Louvet et al, FDR gemcitabine (1000 mg/m^2 IV over 100 min) given on day 1, was followed by oxaliplatin (100 mg/m^2 over 120 min) on day 2 (GemOx).[340] The response rate to this combination was 30.6%, much higher than those previously reported for gemcitabine alone and median survival for the group was 9.2 months; this is also better than historical data using gemcitabine. A subsequent prospective randomized trial found that GemOx improved progression free survival (PFS) compared with gemcitabine monotherapy given at 1000 mg/m^2 over 30 min in patients with advanced pancreatic cancer.[15] Whether the higher response rate seen with GexOx was attributable to the addition of oxaliplatin, or to the delivery of FDR gemcitabine was the subject of a subsequent Eastern Cooperative Oncology Group (ECOG) trial E6201.[265] E6201 enrolled 832 patients with advanced pancreatic cancer and randomized them to receive standard infusion gemcitabine, FDR gemcitabine, or GemOx as previously described by Louvet. Preliminary results showed a slight improvement in response rates for both FDR gemcitabine and GemOx (9-10%) compared with gemcitabine alone (5%), but there was no significant difference between FDR gemcitabine and GemOx in terms of overall survival.

The results from E6201 suggest that the benefit of GemOx may be explained by the improved efficacy of FDR gemcitabine rather than the addition of oxaliplatin. However, as discussed below, PS may be an important factor in predicting response to more aggressive gemcitabine-based cytotoxic combinations, to include GemOx. Currently, results from the randomized phase 2 trial of FDR gemcitabine given near MTD, and ECOG 6201 both demonstrate the modest superiority of FDR gemcitabine over gemcitabine given as a 30 min bolus and is proof of principle that optimal delivery of minimally effective therapies provides some clinical benefit. Later in the chapter, a rationale for investigation of FDR gemcitabine given at lower doses will be discussed.

Gemcitabine-Based Cytotoxic Combinations: Benefit Limited to Good PS Patients?

Given the consistent, albeit modest single-agent activity of gemcitabine, gemcitabine-based combinations have been investigated over several years. In most phase 2 trials, gemcitabine was combined with one other cytotoxic agent such as docetaxel, capecitabine, oxaliplatin, 5-FU, cisplatin, UFT, irinotecan, premetrexed, and epirubicin.[340-350] Generally, response rates to these gemcitabine doublets have been higher than those typically reported for gemcitabine alone and median overall survival better than those historically reported for gemcitabine. Unfortunately, just as 5-FU based combinations have not led to improved overall survivals compared with 5-FU alone in large phase 3 trials, neither have gemcitabine-based regimens compared with gemcitabine alone (Table 88-4).[351-356] For most tested combination regimens, overall survival has been somewhat improved compared with gemcitabine monotherapy. The reasons for this are not entirely clear, but may be explained in part by low response rates (no matter what the therapy), patient crossover from gemcitabine monotherapy to a gemcitabine doublet, or patient selection. As note above, in the study conducted by Louvet, which randomized patients to gemcitabine or gemcitabine and oxaliplatin (GemOx) (progression-free survival PFS) was improved using combination therapy (5.8 months for GemOx, 3.7 months for gemcitabine, p = 0.04).[15] Unfortunately, no statistically significant overall survival advantage was observed among the patients randomized to GemOx. The authors reported that some of the patients who were randomized to receive gemcitabine were subsequently treated with doublet therapy that involved GemOx or gemcitabine and cisplatin. Such cross over might obscure the potential survival benefit of any gemcitabine doublet. In addition, inappropriate patient selection may further explain the disappointing results with gemcitabine doublets based on the enrollment of patients with poor PS. These issues have spurred two recent meta-analyses of trials comparing gemcitabine monotherapy to gemcitabine-based combinations. In the report by Sultana previously described, survival was improved using gemcitabine combination chemotherapy compared with gemcitabine alone (HR = 0.91; 95% CI, 0.85-0.97). A separate meta-analysis was performed by Heinemann and colleagues and also showed a survival advantage for patients treated with gemcitabine + "X" when X represented either oxaliplatin or cisplatin (HR for death = 0.85 [95% CI: 0.76-0.96], p = 0.010), or 5-FU (HR = 0.90 [95% CI: 0.81-0.99], p = 0.030). No survival benefit was seen when X was premetrexed, exatecan, or irinotecan. Importantly, the results reported by Heinemann suggested that only patients with good PS (defined as a Karnovsky PS ≥ 80%) derived benefit from gemcitabine-based combination therapy (HR = 0.76; 95% CI: 0.67-0.87; p < 0.0001) whereas patients with KPS < 80% appeared to do slightly worse with combination therapy compared with the delivery of gemcitabine alone (HR = 1.08; 95% CI: 0.90-1.29, p = 0.40). While cytotoxic gemcitabine-doublet therapy cannot be broadly endorsed as standard, these two meta-analyses do provide support for the use of gemcitabine doublets (particularly gemcitabine-platinum combinations). Furthermore, doublet therapy should probably be limited to centers with experience using these combinations, and only administered to patients with good PS.

Table 88-4 Selected Phase 3 Trials of Gemcitabine vs Gemcitabine Doublets for Patients With Advanced Pancreatic Cancer

Author, Year	No. of Patients	Median Survival (Months)		p-Value
		Gem-Monotherapy	Gem-Doublet	
Berlin, 2002[234] (Gem ± 5-FU)	322	5.4	6.7	.09
Colucci et al., 2002[307] (Gem ± CDDP)	107	4.6	7.0	.43
Louvet, 2004[308] (Gem ± Oxaliplatin)	313	7.1	9.0	.13
O'Reilly, 2004[278] (Gem ± Exatecan)	349	6.2	6.7	.52
Herrmann, 2005[309] (Gem ± Capecitabine)	319	7.3	8.4	.314
Moore, 2005[310] (Gem ± Erlotinib)	569	5.91	6.37	.011

Abbreviation: Gem, gemcitabine.

Molecular Agents: Disappointment Even Before the 21st Century

Some readers might be surprised to learn that investigations of targeted therapy actually began over 20 years ago with the delivery of hormonal agents, which were thought to have biologic relevance in pancreatic cancer. Preclinical studies performed both in vitro and in vivo demonstrated the presence of sex hormone receptors and gut hormone receptors on tumor cells. Unfortunately, subsequent clinical trials, which investigated the efficacy of tamoxifen, flutamide, and the somatostatin analog, octreotide, have all been negative.[357-360] Although these drugs were tested prior to the development of gemcitabine, there is no ongoing effort to retest these drugs in combination with it.

Attempts to improve pancreatic cancer therapy using modern molecular therapeutics have been equally disappointing. Although molecular agents have changed the face of cancer therapy in other gastrointestinal tumors to include hepatocellular carcinoma[361] and advanced colorectal cancer,[362] minimal improvements have been observed in pancreatic cancer. Table 88-5 shows the results of one randomized phase 2 and several large phase 3 trials comparing the efficacy of gemcitabine, or a gemcitabine combination to the same regimen with the addition of a targeted agent.[16-18,139,160,363,364]

These trials have investigated a wide variety of molecular agents to include tipifarnib, a farnesyl transferase inhibitor designed to prevent localization of the RAS oncoprotein to the cell membrane, thereby abrogating its function, marimastat, a matrix metalloproteinase inhibitor intended to prevent tumor cell invasion, metastasis, and angiogenesis, erlotinib and cetuximab, both EGFR inhibitors, and bevacizumab, an antiangiogenic agent. With the exception of erlotinib, which leads to a small incremental improvement in median overall survival when added to gemcitabine, compared to treatment with gemcitabine alone (hazard ratio for death 0.82 [95% CI 0.69-0.099, p = 0.038]), none of the other molecular agents have led to an improvement in survival. Nevertheless, results from these large trials can be informative, and provide insights for the design and conduct of the next generation of clinical studies using molecular agents in pancreatic cancer.

First, in none of the trials summarized in Table 88-5, was there any requirement for the target to be relevant as a criterion for enrollment. The enrolled patients therefore represented unselected groups in terms of tumor or host characteristics, which might predict responsiveness to

Table 88-5 **Summary of Completed Randomized Trials of Gemcitabine Alone (or With Placebo) vs Gemcitabine With a Targeted Agent in the Treatment of Advanced Pancreatic Cancer**

Principal Investigator Year Gemcitabine ± Targeted Agent	No. of Patients	Objective Response Rate	Median Survival (Days)	% 1-Year Survival	*p*-Value (Median Survival Comparison)
Van Cutsem, 2004[319]					
Gem + placebo	347	8%	182	24%	
vs					
Gem + tipifarnib	341	6%	193	27%	.75
Bramhall, 2002[331]					
Gem + placebo	119	11%	164	18%	
vs					
Gem + marimastat	120	11%	165.5	17%	.95
Moore, 2005[310]					
Gem	284	8.0%	177	17%	
vs					
Gem + erolotinib	285	8.6%	191	24%	.025

Abbreviation: Gem, gemcitabine.

the study drug. At the time these studies were conducted, this was defensible since no predictive biomarkers were established to predict response to any given agent. As an example, in SWOG S0205 reported by Philip and colleagues, gemcitabine monotherapy was compared to gemcitabine plus cetuximab in patients with advanced pancreatic cancer. The trial demonstrated no statistically significant improvement in PFS or overall survival with the addition of cetuximab (6.4 months for gemcitabine/cetuximab vs 5.9 months for gemcitabine alone, $p = 0.14$).[18] At the time, tumor tissue was required for entry to assay the presence or absence of EGFR overexpression, a parameter, which has not been predictive of response to cetuximab in other studies. Given the recent data in colorectal cancer showing that patients with tumors containing a wild-type K-ras oncogene, have a greater chance of benefit with cetuximab compared with patients having mutant K-ras tumors,[365] the availability of sufficient tumor tissue for K-ras mutational testing should now be a minimal prerequisite for enrollment in a trial studying an EGFR inhibitor. (Some investigators might insist on the presence of wild-type K-ras within the tumor as necessary for enrollment in a trial of an EGFR inhibitor.)[366] In the future, selecting patients with specific host-specific, or tumor-specific characteristics will be critically important for meaningful progress in the clinic.

Second, with the exception of the study conducted by Cascinu and colleagues, the summarized trials were all large phase 3 trials, which taken together, enrolled over 3400 patients. In general, these trials were launched based on single-arm phase 2 data, which demonstrated some improvement in survival compared with historical controls treated with gemcitabine alone. For example, cetuximab was considered worthy of further investigation in SWOG after a phase 2 trial of standard dose gemcitabine with cetuximab in 41 patients with advanced pancreatic cancer showed an objective response rate 12.2%, an overall median survival of 7.1 months, and a 1-year survival rate of 31.7%.[367] Likewise, bevacizumab was studied by the CALGB based on results from a single-arm phase 2 trial of standard dose gemcitabine (1000 mg/m^2 over 30 min, days 1, 8, and 15 every 28 days) combined with bevacizumab (10 mg/kg days 1 and 15 every 28 days), demonstrated a response rate of 21% and a median survival of 8.8 months among of group of 52 patients, all of whom had metastatic disease.[368] In the near future, a decision to commit large numbers of patients and resources to randomized phase 3 trials based on results from small single-arm exploratory trials may be ill advised.

Third, CALGB 80303, which compared gemcitabine plus placebo to gemcitabine plus bevacizumab, recapitulated findings from the 1980s; performance status is an important predictor of survival. In that trial, patients were stratified based on ECOG PS (0, 1, or 2), with reported median survival times of 8.0, 4.8, and 2.8 months respectively; this was irrespective of assigned therapy. This suggests that patients with advanced pancreatic cancer having ECOG PS ≤ 2 may not benefit from cytotoxic therapy and calls for investigation of a noncytotoxic molecular drug or drugs as an alternative to treatment with cytotoxic drugs.

Finally, in the majority of trials summarized in Table 88-5, enrolled patients were allowed to have either locally advanced, or metastatic disease. As previously discussed, the prognosis associated with these two stages is distinctly different and when the patient population is heterogeneous either in terms of PS, or stage, comparing outcomes between treatment arms can be difficult, and comparing results across studies even more so.

The Future of Systemic Therapy: Not Just Targeted Therapy, Personalized Therapy

Only one conclusion can be drawn from all available evidence regarding the efficacy of systemic therapy in pancreatic cancer: it barely works, and thus far, has depended on the delivery of cytotoxic drugs. Over the next several years, while continued development and investigation of molecular agents is welcomed, a reexamination of the optimal and tailored delivery of conventional cytotoxics is essential. This is particularly true since recent studies suggest a renewed interest in cytotoxic drugs for pancreatic cancer. Most importantly however, an emphasis on personalized cancer therapeutics designed to optimize efficacy and minimize toxicity is far more important than continued empiric delivery of any drugs in various combinations.

Gemcitabine: Is it a Molecular Agent?

To date, oncologists have been trained in 2 potentially conflicting paradigms: use conventional cytotoxic drugs at MTD but deliver molecular agents at biologically relevant doses. These paradigms require realignment, with particular attention to cytotoxic drug dosing. Continued delivery of cytotoxics dosed at, or close to MTD may be counterproductive, leading to toxic effects, which overwhelm any improvement in efficacy. Since future studies are likely to combine cytotoxic drugs with molecular agents, rational dosing of the cytotoxic backbone is essential. In this context, gemcitabine and other conventional cytotoxic drugs need to be revisited.

As discussed previously in the chapter, gemcitabine is a pro-drug, which requires phosphorylation for antitumor activity within the tumor cell. This agent is generally considered an antimetabolite, which inhibits ribonucleotide reductase thereby depleting intracellular pools of trinucleotides (GTP, TTP, CTP, and ATP) necessary for DNA synthesis. Gemcitabine triphosphate can also incorporate into an elongating chain of DNA, leading to premature DNA chain termination.[369] It can therefore be argued that gemcitabine is a targeted agent, inhibiting ribonucleotide reductase and DNA synthesis. Currently, a standard regimen of gemcitabine consists of 1000 mg/m^2 given over 30 min, on days 1, 8, and 15 of a 28 day cycle. However, results from a variety of sources suggest that gemcitabine can be effective, and likely better tolerated, at far lower than standard doses.

When gemcitabine was initially studied in phase 1, objective responses were observed in two patients: one patient with colorectal cancer responded to a dose of 180 mg/m^2 and another patient with nonsmall cell lung cancer had an objective response at a dose of 525 mg/m^2.[370] In this study, gemcitabine was infused over 30 min in all patients and at doses higher than 350 mg/m^2, no further increases in intracellular concentrations of gemcitabine triphosphate were observed in mononuclear cells obtained from participating patients. The investigators therefore suggested that intracellular accumulation of the gemcitabine nucleotide was saturated at higher doses of gemcitabine infused over 30 min. They further concluded that the MTD of gemcitabine should be 790 mg/m^2.[370] Other support for administration of lower doses of gemcitabine comes from a study in Japan which attempted to determine the individualized maximal repeatable dose (iMRD) of gemcitabine in a group of 18 patients with metastatic pancreatic cancer.[371] The iMRD ranged from 300 to 700 mg/m^2 and these doses (30-70% of standard dose) led to objective responses in 16% of patients and an overall median survival of 9.5 months; both endpoints are impressive in a cohort comprised of patients with metastatic disease. Last is the data from the our trial of preoperative GemXRT in patients with potentially resectable pancreatic cancer.[248] In this study, gemcitabine was given at a dose of 400 mg/m^2 over 30 min weekly for 7 weeks. The overall survival for all 86 patients was 23 months even though 25% of patients did not undergo surgery with curative intent. Among the 64 patients who did undergo resection, median survival was 34 months; superior to reports from other large trials of neoadjuvant or adjuvant therapy. Of interest, gemcitabine at 400 mg/m^2 was infused over 30 min (13 $mg/m^2/min$) approximating FDR gemcitabine.[338] Of further note, the total cumulative dose of gemcitabine given to the patients in our preoperative trail (2800 mg/m^2) is less than 20% of the total cumulative dose of gemcitabine delivered to patients in the CONKO 001 trial (18,000 mg/m^2), which proved the benefit of adjuvant gemcitabine.[7] Taken together, these studies suggest gemcitabine at 1000 mg/m^2 infused over 30 minutes lacks pharmacologic rationale, and is not an optimal dose for efficacy, or toxicity. Delivery of lower doses of FDR gemcitabine is therefore an important research question; broad support from within the pancreatic cancer community of researchers will be required to support such clinical trials.

Other Cytotoxic Agents for Personalized Pancreatic Cancer Therapy

Over the last several years, germline mutations in BRCA1, and especially BRCA2, have been shown to increase the risk of pancreatic cancer.[68] These genes play important roles in DNA repair mechanisms and preclinical studies have shown that tumors with BRCA2-like mutations are quite susceptible to the DNA damaging effects of ionizing radiation, mitomycin C and platinum analogs.[372,373] Although germline mutations in BRCA2 are relatively rare in pancreatic cancer, they may account for up to 6% of pancreatic cancer cases observed in high-risk families.[374] Furthermore, some experts have suggested that perturbations in BRCA-dependent DNA repair pathways may be clinically relevant in sporadic pancreatic cancers.[375] Thus, delivery of therapies with the potential to lead to DNA double strand breaks, such as mitomycin C, platinum analogs, or ionizing radiation may have relevance to patients with tumors associated with "BRCAness."[375,376] Initial efforts in personalized cancer therapy for pancreatic cancer might therefore investigate the efficacy of agents such as mitomycin C or platinum agents in patients with documented or suspected mutations in BRCA2. In addition to the study of cytotoxics agents for tumors associated with aberrations in BRCA -DNA repair pathways, testing novel molecular agents such as poly (ADP) ribose polymerase (PARP) inhibitors, which foster synthetic lethality in these tumors has also been proposed.[376]

Similarly, although the frequency of microsatellite instability (MSI)-high tumors in pancreatic cancer remain relatively low (13%),[377] delivery of a camptothecin analog to patients with MSI-high tumors warrants further research.[378] Of note, as shown previously in Table 88-4, the combination of gemcitabine with irinotecan proved no better than gemcitabine alone for the treatment of advanced pancreatic cancer, and unless biologically relevant selection mechanisms are used to enroll patients into research trials, empiric drug combinations will likely result in continued failure.[354]

Another cytotoxic agent with potential as a personalized cancer therapeutic is nanoparticle, albumin-bound (nab)-paclitaxel. Previous data in breast cancer suggests that nab-paclitaxel may be especially useful in tumor microenvironments that overexpress secreted protein acidic and rich in cysteine (SPARC).[379] In pancreatic cancer, SPARC overexpression in stromal cells rather than in tumor cells has been associated with poor prognosis in patients with resected pancreatic cancer.[380] This prompted a phase 1 study of gemcitabine with nab-paclitaxel for the treatment of advanced pancreatic cancer. In a preliminary report released by von Hoff and colleagues, the combination led to an objective response in 9 of 16 evaluable patients (56%).[381] While entry into the trial did not require SPARC overexpression, this biomarker should be assessed in future trials as a potential predictor of response to nab-paclitaxel.

Another taxane with potential use as a targeted cytotoxic agent is Endotag-1.[382] Endotag-1 is paclitaxel bound to cationic liposomes, which theoretically target tumor associated endothelial cells. In a completed 4-arm randomized phase 2 trial, the combination of Endotag-1 combined with gemcitabine improved overall survival compared with treatment using gemcitabine alone. Of note, survival appeared to correlate to treatment with higher doses of Endotag.[383]

Novel Molecular Agents for Pancreatic Cancer Therapy

Other drugs worth brief mention in the expanding arena of molecular targeted agents for pancreatic cancer include axitinib, an oral receptor tyrosine kinase inhibitor of VEGF receptor and insulin-like growth factor-1 (IGF-1) receptor inhibitors. Axitinib is an oral tyrosine kinase inhibitor of the platelet-derived growth factor receptor (PDGF-R), VEGF receptors 1, 2, and 3, and colony stimulating factor-1 receptor. It has demonstrated antitumor activity in renal cell, thyroid, lung, and pancreatic cancer.[384] Axitinib has been tested in a randomized phase 2 trial, which compared axitinib plus gemcitabine to gemcitabine alone in patients with advanced pancreatic cancer.[385] The combination led to an increase in median overall survival compared with treatment with gemcitabine alone (6.9 months vs 5.4 months, respectively), which prompted further study of this combination in a larger phase 3 trial.[385] Unfortunately, a recent press release from the sponsor reported that a preliminary analysis showed that axitinib plus gemcitabine did not improve survival compared with treatment using gemcitabine alone.

Given the role of insulin and insulin-like growth factor-1 in the progression of pancreatic cancer, significant interest in the IGF-1 signaling pathway as a potential target in pancreatic cancer has emerged.[386] A number of small molecule inhibitors and monoclonal antibodies to the IGF-1 receptor are being developed and now entering phase 1 clinical testing; clinical results are not as yet available.[387] Importantly, clinical development of these agents may require development of specific biomarkers to determine the importance of the IGF-1 signaling pathway in an individual patient's pancreatic cancer to select those patients who may benefit from IGF-1 receptor blockade.

Future Clinical Trials in Pancreatic Cancer

The last decade has led to pessimism about the integration of any new drugs into pancreatic cancer therapy, and failures of the past should inform future efforts. For the time being, smaller randomized phase 2 trials may more quickly determine those drugs or drug combinations worthy of larger investments of money and patients in confirmatory phase 3 trials. In addition, clinical trials, which assess the presence of specific molecular tumor characteristics as a requirement for enrollment, will probably be more fruitful than trials that enroll unselected patients. Lastly, inclusion criteria which limit enrollment to those patients with good PS and a specific stage of disease (resected, locally advanced, or metastatic) will allow for cleaner comparisons between various trials.

Approach to the Patient With Metastatic Disease

Metastatic pancreatic cancer is characterized by anorexia, cachexia, and pain. Jaundice may result from the primary tumor or intrahepatic metastases. Local tumor progression can lead to worsening pain, gastric outlet obstruction, or gastroparesis, and patients with peritoneal carcinomatosis may suffer from intractable ascites, intestinal dysmotility, or mechanical obstruction. Constipation is also very common. Patients are also at risk of venous thromboembolism, but the risk is not clearly higher than that associated with other gastrointestinal tumors.[388] Palliation must always be the primary goal and is facilitated by a multidisciplinary team. Symptomatic relief of biliary obstruction and pain should be addressed before initiation of systemic therapy. For most patients, adequate pain control can be obtained with the use of long- or short-acting narcotics, without excessive sedation.[389] However, if pain is not well controlled with oral or transdermal narcotics or if these agents are poorly tolerated, patients should be evaluated for celiac plexus or splanchnic plexus ablation. Whether EUS-guided neurolytic blocks are superior to fluoroscopic-guided blocks, or CT-guided blocks remains an open question, but EUS-guided neurolysis was shown to be superior to CT-guided blockade in patients with chronic pancreatitis.[390]

Given the poor prognosis for patients with metastatic disease, biliary obstruction should be relieved with nonsurgical means. On occasion, percutaneous biliary drainage may be required to relieve an extrahepatic biliary obstruction. The use of duodenal stents in patients with mechanical gastric outlet obstruction and poor prognosis is becoming more widely accepted.[391] For patients with intractable symptomatic ascites, paracentesis is generally perceived as most efficacious,[392] but it is not an intervention with durable benefits. Diuretics may be of some utility, but often lead to intravascular volume contraction with minimal effect on abdominal girth and, therefore, are rarely effective. Shunting procedures for ascites should be reserved for selected patients, but specific indications can not be easily defined and each case must be reviewed on an individual basis.[393]

Systemic therapy for metastatic disease should be actively discouraged in patients with poor performance status (ECOG > 2) or significant metastatic tumor burden. End-of-life discussions and planning are appropriate at the time of diagnosis in patients with metastatic disease. However, if a patient has an adequate performance status, a trial of gemcitabine as first-line therapy is reasonable. The addition of a platinum analog or other cytotoxic drugs should be reserved for those patients who have a Karnovsky PS ≥ 80%. At present, for patients being considered for treatment with gemcitabine monotherapy, the addition of erlotinib is reasonable; the anticipated benefits of this drug should not be overstated.[16]

If gemcitabine is recommended, it is usually delivered on a day 1, 8, 15 schedule, repeated every 28 days. Restaging studies should usually be performed every 2 cycles and should include CT of the abdomen and pelvis. Chest CT imaging is indicated when lung metastases are present. For patients advised to continue treatment beyond 2 cycles, restaging studies should be performed every 8-12 weeks.

Whenever possible, patients with good performance status should be encouraged to enroll in a clinical trial. Patients whose disease progresses during treatment in a clinical trial that does not include gemcitabine may be considered for gemcitabine-based therapy, since some clinical benefit from gemcitabine has been observed for such patients.[332] Recent data suggest that patients who fail gemcitabine may derive some benefit from treatment with a fluoropyrimidine in combination with oxaliplatin although second-line therapy should probably be limited to those patients who are maintaining adequate PS in the face of disease progression.[394,395] Supportive care is always a reasonable alternative to continued anticancer therapy.

In summary, clinically meaningful advances in the treatment of metastatic pancreatic cancer have developed quite slowly. However, with a greater understanding of the underlying genetic and molecular abnormalities involved in pancreatic carcinogenesis, rational chemotherapy, radiation therapy, molecular therapy, in conjunction with other supportive methods are expected to alter the natural course of this disease in the near future. Continued efforts to enroll patients with advanced pancreatic cancer into well-designed clinical trials should remain a high priority for oncologists across all disciplines.

Selected References

The complete reference list can be found at www.CANCERMEDICINE8.com

1. Jemal A, Siegel R, Ward E, et al. Cancer statistics, 2008. *CA Cancer J Clin.* 2008;58:71–96.
3. Varadhachary GR, Tamm EP, Abbruzzese JL, et al. Borderline resectable pancreatic cancer: definitions, management, and role of preoperative therapy. *Ann Surg Oncol.* 2006;13:1035–1046.
4. Exocrine pancreas. In: Greene FL, Page DL, Fleming ID, et al., editors. *AJCC Cancer Staging Manual*, 6th ed. New York: Springer; 2002:157–162.
6. Regine WF, Winter KA, Abrams RA, et al. Fluorouracil vs gemcitabine chemotherapy before and after fluorouracil-based chemoradiation following resection of pancreatic adenocarcinoma: a randomized controlled trial. *JAMA.* 2008;299:1019–1026.
7. Neuhaus P, Reiss H, Post S, et al. CONKO 001: final results of the randomized, prospective, multicenter phase III trial of adjuvant chemotherapy with gemcitabine versus observation in patients with resected pancreatic cancer. *J Clin Oncol.* 2008;26:LBA 4504. www.asco.org/ASCO/Abstracts+%26+Virtual+Meeting/Abstracts?&vmview=abst_detail_view&confID=55&abstractID=34749
8. Neoptolemos JP, Stocken DD, Friess H, et al. A randomized trial of chemoradiotherapy and chemotherapy after resection of pancreatic cancer. *N Engl J Med.* 2004;350:1200–1210.
11. Chauffert B, Mornex F, Bonnetain F, et al. Phase III trial comparing intensive induction chemoradiotherapy (60 Gy, infusional 5-FU and intermittent cisplatin) followed by maintenance gemcitabine with gemcitabine alone for locally advanced unresectable pancreatic cancer. Definitive results of the 2000-01 FFCD/SFRO study. *Ann Oncol.* 2008;19:1592–1599.
12. Moertel CG, Frytak S, Hahn RG, et al. Therapy of locally unresectable pancreatic carcinoma: a randomized comparison of high dose (6000 rads) radiation alone, moderate dose radiation (4000 rads + 5-fluorouracil), and high dose radiation + 5-fluorouracil: the Gastrointestinal Tumor Study Group. *Cancer.* 1981;48:1705–1710.
13. Burris HA, 3rd, Moore MJ, Andersen J, et al. Improvements in survival and clinical benefit with gemcitabine as first-line therapy for patients with advanced pancreas cancer: a randomized trial. *J Clin Oncol.* 1997;15:2403–2413.
15. Louvet C, Labianca R, Hammel P, et al. Gemcitabine in combination with oxaliplatin compared with gemcitabine alone in locally advanced or metastatic pancreatic cancer: results of a GERCOR and GISCAD phase III trial. *J Clin Oncol.* 2005;23:3509–3516.
16. Moore MJ, Goldstein D, Hamm J, et al. Erlotinib plus gemcitabine compared with gemcitabine alone in patients with advanced pancreatic cancer: a phase III trial of the National Cancer Institute of Canada Clinical Trials Group. *J Clin Oncol.* 2007;25:1960–1966.
17. Kindler HL, Niedzwiecki D, Hollis D, et al. A double-blind, placebo-controlled, randomized phase III trial of gemcit-

abine plus bevacizumab versus gemcitabine plus placebo in patients with advanced pancreatic cancer: a preliminary analysis of Cancer and Leukemia Group B 80303. *J Clin Oncol.* 2007;25:4508. www.asco.org/ASCO/Abstracts+%26+Virtual+Meeting/Abstracts?&vmview=abst_detail_view&confID=47&abstractID=32921

18. Philip PA, Benedetti J, Fenoglio-Preiser C, et al. Phase III Study Comparing Gemcitabine plus Cetuximab versus Gemcitabine in Patients with Locally Advanced or Metastatic Pancreatic Adenocarcinoma: Southwest Oncology Group Protocol S0205. *J Clin Oncol.* 2007;25: LBA4509. www.asco.org/ASCO/Abstracts+%26+Virtual+Meeting/Abstracts?&vmview=abst_detail_view&confID=47&abstractID=32920
30. Huxley R, Ansary-Moghaddam A, Berrington de Gonzalez A, et al. Type-II diabetes and pancreatic cancer: a meta-analysis of 36 studies. *Br J Cancer.* 2005;92:2076–2083.
51. Russo A, Autelitano M, Bisanti L. Metabolic syndrome and cancer risk. *Eur J Cancer.* 2008;44:293–297.
57. Coussens LM, Werb Z. Inflammation and cancer. *Nature.* 2002;420:860–867.
60. Guerra C, Schuhmacher AJ, Canamero M, et al. Chronic pancreatitis is essential for induction of pancreatic ductal adenocarcinoma by K-Ras oncogenes in adult mice. *Cancer Cell.* 2007;11:291–302.
64. Foulkes WD. Inherited susceptibility to common cancers. *N Engl J Med.* 2008;59:2143–2153.
127. Canto MI, Goggins M, Hruban RH, et al. Screening for early pancreatic neoplasia in high-risk individuals: a prospective controlled study. *Clin Gastroenterol Hepatol.* 2006;4:766–781.
130. Almoguera C, Shibata D, Forrester K, et al. Most human carcinomas of the exocrine pancreas contain mutant c-K-ras genes. *Cell.* 1988;53:549–554.
132. Hruban RH, Goggins M, Parsons J, Kern SE. Progression model for pancreatic cancer. *Clin Cancer Res.* 2000;6:2969–2972.
139. Van Cutsem E, van de Velde H, Karasek P, et al. Phase III trial of gemcitabine plus tipifarnib compared with gemcitabine plus placebo in advanced pancreatic cancer. *J Clin Oncol.* 2004;22:1430–1438.
150. Jones S, Zhang X, Parsons DW, et al. Core signaling pathways in human pancreatic cancers revealed by global genomic analyses. *Science.* 2008;321:1801–1806.
158. Li C, Heidt DG, Dalerba P, et al. Identification of pancreatic cancer stem cells. *Cancer Res.* 2007;67:1030–1037.
160. Bramhall SR, Schulz J, Nemunaitis J, et al. A double-blind placebo-controlled, randomised study comparing gemcitabine and marimastat with gemcitabine and placebo as first line therapy in patients with advanced pancreatic cancer. *Br J Cancer.* 2002;87:161–167.
164. Katz MH, Pisters PW, Evans DB, et al. Borderline resectable pancreatic cancer: the importance of this emerging stage of disease. *J Am Coll Surg.* 2008;206: 833–846.
179. Howard TJ, Krug JE, Yu J, et al. A margin-negative R0 resection accomplished with minimal postoperative complications is the surgeon's contribution to long-term survival in pancreatic cancer. *J Gastrointest Surg.* 2006;10:1338–1345.
180. Winter JM, Cameron JL, Campbell KA, et al. 1423 pancreaticoduodenectomies for pancreatic cancer: a single-institution experience. *J Gastrointest Surg.* 2006;10: 1199–1210.
182. Tseng JF, Raut CP, Lee JE, et al. Pancreaticoduodenectomy with vascular resection: margin status and survival duration. *J Gastrointest Surg.* 2004;8:935–949.
183. Birkmeyer JD, Siewers AE, Finlayson EV, et al. Hospital volume and surgical mortality in the United States. *N Engl J Med.* 2002;346:1128–1137.
191. Evans DB, Lee JE, Tamm EP, Pisters PWT. Pancreaticoduodenectomy (Whipple Operation) and total pancreatectomy for cancer. In: Fisher JF, editor. *Mastery of Surgery,* 5th ed. Philadelphia: Lippincott, Williams and Williams; 2007:1299–1317.
193. Raut CP, Tseng JF, Sun CC, et al. Impact of resection status on pattern of failure and survival after pancreaticoduodenectomy for pancreatic adenocarcinoma. *Ann Surg.* 2007;246:52–60.
212. Yeo CJ, Cameron JL, Maher MM, et al. A prospective randomized trial of pancreaticogastrostomy versus pancreaticojejunostomy after pancreaticoduodenectomy. *Ann Surg.* 1995;222:580–588.
214. Evans DB, Rich TA, Byrd DR, et al. Preoperative chemoradiation and pancreaticoduodenectomy for adenocarcinoma of the pancreas. *Arch Surg.* 1992;127:1335–1339.
224. Ferrone CR, Finkelstein DM, Thayer SP, et al. Perioperative CA19-9 levels can predict stage and survival in patients with resectable pancreatic adenocarcinoma. *J Clin Oncol.* 2006;24:2897–2902.
226. Berger AC, Garcia M, Jr., Hoffman JP, et al. Postresection CA 19-9 predicts overall survival in patients with pancreatic cancer treated with adjuvant chemoradiation: a prospective validation by RTOG 9704. *J Clin Oncol.* 2008;26:5918–5922.
230. Kalser MH, Ellenberg SS. Pancreatic cancer. Adjuvant combined radiation and chemotherapy following curative resection. *Arch Surg.* 1985;120:899–903.
232. Klinkenbijl JH, Jeekel J, Sahmoud T, et al. Adjuvant radiotherapy and 5-fluorouracil after curative resection of cancer of the pancreas and periampullary region: phase III trial of the EORTC gastrointestinal tract cancer cooperative group. *Ann Surg.* 1999;230:776–782.
243. Picozzi VJ, Kozarek RA, Traverso LW. Interferon-based adjuvant chemoradiation therapy after pancreaticoduodenectomy for pancreatic adenocarcinoma. *Am J Surg.* 2003;185:476–480.
246. Jaffee EM, Hruban RH, Biedrzycki B, et al. Novel allogeneic granulocyte-macrophage colony-stimulating factor-secreting tumor vaccine for pancreatic cancer: a phase I trial of safety and immune activation. *J Clin Oncol.* 2001;19:145–156.
248. Evans DB, Varadhachary GR, Crane CH, et al. Preoperative gemcitabine-based chemoradiation for patients with resectable adenocarcinoma of the pancreatic head. *J Clin Oncol.* 2008;26:3496–3502.
249. Varadhachary GR, Wolff RA, Crane CH, et al. Preoperative gemcitabine and cisplatin followed by gemcitabine-based chemoradiation for resectable adenocarcinoma of the pancreatic head. *J Clin Oncol.* 2008;26:3487–3495.
251. Katz MHG, Pisters PWT, Evans DB, et al. Borderline resectable pancreatic cancer: the importance of this emerging stage of disease. *J Am Coll Surg.* 2008;206:833–846.
285. Crane CH, Ellis LM, Abbruzzese JL, et al. Phase I trial evaluating the safety of bevacizumab with concurrent radiotherapy and capecitabine in locally advanced pancreatic cancer. *J Clin Oncol.* 2006;24:1145–1151.
291. Senzer N, Mani S, Rosemurgy A, et al. TNFerade biologic, an adenovector with a radiation-inducible promoter, carrying the human tumor necrosis factor alpha gene: a phase I study in patients with solid tumors. *J Clin Oncol.* 2004;22:592–601.
311. Carter SK, Comis RL. The integration of chemotherapy into a combined modality approach for cancer treatment. VI. Pancreatic adenocarcinoma. *Cancer Treat Rev.* 1975;2:193–214.
327. Ishii H, Okada S, Nose H, et al. Prognostic factors in patients with advanced pancreatic cancer treated with systemic chemotherapy. *Pancreas.* 1996;12:267–271.
370. Abbruzzese JL, Grunewald R, Weeks EA, et al. A phase I clinical, plasma, and cellular pharmacology study of gemcitabine. *J Clin Oncol.* 1991;9:491–498.
387. Hewish M, Chau I, Cunningham D. Insulin-like growth factor 1 receptor targeted therapeutics: novel compounds and novel treatment strategies for cancer medicine. *Recent Patents Anticancer Drug Discov.* 2009;4:54–72.

89 Neoplasms of the Small Intestine, Vermiform Appendix, and Peritoneum, and Carcinoma of the Colon and Rectum

James C. Padussis, MD ▪ Georgia M. Beasley, MD ▪ Nicole S. McMahon, BS ▪ Douglas S. Tyler, MD ▪ Kirk A. Ludwig, MD

Tumors of the Small Intestine

The small intestine represents 75% of the total length of the gastrointestinal (GI) tract and comprises 90% of its mucosal surface area, yet rarely does this region develop malignant tumors.[1] Recent figures show that less than 3% of all alimentary tract tumors and 0.4% of all malignancies arise in the small bowel.[2] Five thousand three hundred new small bowel malignancies were predicted for 2004 with an estimated 4 stomach tumors and 28 colorectal tumors for every tumor found in the small bowel.

Several mechanisms have been postulated to explain the low incidence of neoplastic transformation within the small intestine. The most important of these are the rapid transit of content through the small bowel, which provides a shorter exposure of its mucosa to carcinogens, increased lymphoid tissue in the small intestine with a high level of immunoglobulin A expression, and a lower bacterial load in the small bowel that results in a decreased conversion of bile acids into potential carcinogens by anaerobic microorganisms.[3,4] In addition, the liquid contents of the small bowel may cause less mucosal irritation than the more solid contents of the large intestine, and there is the presence in the small intestine of mucosal detoxifying enzymes such as benzopyrene hydroxylase.[5]

Although 75% of small bowel tumors found at autopsy are benign, most of the symptomatic lesions and tumors discovered during surgery are malignant. Adenocarcinomas comprise 30% to 50% of small bowel malignant tumors, followed by carcinoids (25-30%), lymphomas (15-20%), and, to a lesser extent, sarcomas. Leiomyomas account for 25% of all benign tumors, while others include adenomas and lipomas, and rarer neoplasms such as fibromas, fibromyxomas, neurofibromas, ganglioneuromas, hemangiomas, and lymphangiomas.[6]

Certain conditions are associated with an increased incidence of particular types of small bowel tumors. Familial adenomatous polyposis is known to be a powerful risk factor for adenocarcinoma, with small bowel cancer being the most common cancer after colon cancer itself.[7] The relative risk (RR) of small bowel carcinoma in these patients has been described as being greater than 100.[8] Other hereditary syndromes associated with small bowel tumors include Peutz–Jeghers (PJ) syndrome (increased incidence of hamartomatous polyps in the jejunum and ileum), Gardner syndrome (adenoma and adenocarcinoma), and von Recklinghausen disease (paraganglioma). Small bowel inflammatory disorders are associated with increased malignancy, including, most notably, Crohn's disease, which may increase the risk of small bowel adenocarcinoma by greater than 100.[9] Other disorders associated with increased risk of malignancy are celiac disease (lymphoma and adenocarcinoma) and immunoproliferative disease (diffuse intestinal lymphoma and immunoproliferative small intestinal disease).[5]

Clinical Presentation

Many small bowel tumors are asymptomatic until late in their course because of their relatively slow growth and the ease with which the liquid contents of the small bowel can pass even a partially obstructing lesion. Half of small bowel cancers are found only at autopsy. The remainder are usually found as a result of the symptoms of partial obstruction: nausea and vomiting if the lesion is proximal, as well as crampy abdominal pain, or other nonspecific findings such as weight loss. Hemorrhage is frequently found in those tumors that penetrate beyond the submucosa, but almost always is occult, presenting as microcytic anemia or stool that is positive on guaiac testing. Certain small bowel tumors have more specific presenting symptoms, such as jaundice (ampullary carcinoma) and fever, diarrhea, and weight loss (lymphoma). Endocrine tumors of the gut, the most common of which are carcinoid tumors, may present with their own set of classic symptoms, such as flushing, diarrhea, cyanosis, and intermittent respiratory distress. Only a small proportion of patients with carcinoid tumors have these symptoms, the vast majority being asymptomatic or having symptoms secondary to mass lesion effects.

Eventually, malignant tumors cause enough symptoms for the ensuing medical work-up to reveal the tumor. Unfortunately, some time may pass between the first symptom and diagnosis.[10] In one series, almost one-third of the patients had symptoms for 5 years or more prior to definitive diagnosis.[11] A more recent study demonstrated a mean duration of symptoms of 7 months prior to diagnosis. Many patients eventually diagnosed with small bowel tumors present as an emergency with either bowel obstruction or perforation.

Diagnostic Imaging

Radiographic studies often aid in the diagnosis of these lesions, especially in advanced disease. However, such studies, on many occasions, are not useful for early diagnosis of curable malignancy. Plain films of the abdomen are unlikely to be of use, except to demonstrate the presence of obstruction or perhaps displacement of the bowel by a mass. The small bowel follow-through, although noninvasive and relatively inexpensive, is often insensitive. A more sensitive procedure is the double-contrast modality of enteroclysis, which involves placing a nasogastric tube into the descending duodenum and infusing barium and methylcellulose under pressure. This technique enables better visualization of the intestinal lumen and mucosal surface, and has a 90% sensitivity for small bowel tumors versus only 33% with small bowel follow-through.[12] Computed tomographic (CT) scanning with oral contrast has led to nearly 100% recognition of small bowel tumors in some series, although it has limited ability to differentiate among tumor types.[13] This modality appears to be most useful for preoperative staging and metastatic evaluation.[14] In one series, the sensitivity for CT in determining T (tumor) stage was 57%, compared with 61% and 42% for colon and gastric cancer, respectively.[15-17] Angiography and nuclear scanning may be useful in the case of a bleeding tumor or a suspected hemangioma. Endoscopic ultrasonography (EUS) is used to detect and stage small bowel tumors and allows real-time interventional diagnostic procedures, mainly in the periampullary region. EUS has been shown to be superior to CT and magnetic resonance imaging (MRI) in predicting vascular invasion and overall assessment of T stage of ampullary neoplasms.[18,19]

In the past decade, small bowel endoscopy has become increasingly useful as a diagnostic tool. There are three main types of small bowel endoscopy: push enteroscopy, intraoperative or laparoscopically assisted enteroscopy, and, most recently, double-balloon enteroscopy. Push enteroscopy involves an intestinal intubation of a 220- to 250-cm instrument, usually with fluoroscopic assistance, and can be used to examine the jejunum for mean lengths of 120 cm beyond the ligament of Treitz.[20] During intraoperative endoscopy, the surgeon manually manipulates through the small bowel wall with either a push endoscope (anterograde) or a colonoscope (retrograde) to examine the entire small bowel. The surgeon can mark the lesions of interest, usually by suture, and resect at the completion of the enteroscopy. This invasive diagnostic and therapeutic technique is useful in cases of multiple lesions, such as in PJ syndrome and when other modalities have failed in diagnosis. The recent addition of laparoscopically-assisted enteroscopy provides a less invasive technique than interoperative enteroscopy, but still requires general anesthesia and both a surgeon and endoscopist.[21] In double-balloon enteroscopy, an endoscope and a soft flexible overtube, each of which has an inflatable balloon attached to its distal end, are employed together. The two tubes are advanced over one another repeatedly using alternating inflation of the balloons to hold position, allowing deep advancement into the small intestine. The entire small intestine can be examined using this method with less discomfort than experienced with the push method.[22] After receiving the Federal Drug Administration (FDA) approval in 2001, a small, swallowable imaging capsule was introduced by Swain and colleagues that is propelled by peristalsis through the intestinal tract and transmits data to a receiver that captures video images.[23] The clinical indications for the use of capsule endoscopy are becoming clearer in light of recent studies. One such study evaluating 52 patients found that capsule endoscopy was more effective in detecting small tumors in the small intestine than traditional modalities.[23] However, in this study, two jejunal tumors were missed as a result of poor bowel preparation. Though capsule endoscopy is a promising technique, several shortcomings still exist, including lack of forward and backward movement to examine an area of interest, inability to use instruments to carry out biopsy or treatment, reliance on a good bowel prep and inadequate image resolution.[23-25] The main indication for capsule endoscopy remains occult gastrointestinal bleeding (OGIB).

Treatment

The treatment of small bowel tumors is generally surgical, with simple resection for benign lesions and an aggressive approach for malignant lesions. Overall, the survival for adenocarcinomas, carcinoids, lymphomas, and sarcomas was better in 328 cases from a population-based registry than that for all other organs, except the breast, colon, prostate, and uterus.[26] In most cases, the surgical resection must include wide margins, resection of lymph nodes, and removal of the supporting mesentery. In rare cases, radiation or chemotherapy may precede surgery. Duodenal tumors may require pancreatico-duodenectomy if malignant, whereas tumors of the terminal ileum may require right hemicolectomy to ensure complete resection and adequate margins.

Malignant Neoplasms of the Small Bowel

Adenocarcinomas ■ Adenocarcinomas are the most common malignant tumors in the small bowel, accounting for approximately 30% to 50% of all malignant small bowel tumors.[27,28] They most commonly arise in the seventh decade of life and are seen slightly more often in men than in women.[29] While primary tumors arise most often in the duodenum (48-52%) and jejunum (23-25%) and less commonly in the ileum (13-16%), the reason for this distribution is unclear.[30,31] Some have postulated that the richness of immunoglobulin A (IgA)-secreting cells in the ileum accounts for its relative sparing from adenocarcinoma by neutralizing luminal carcinogens.[4] Others have noted that the abundance of the enzyme benzopyrene hydroxylase may play a protective role by detoxifying potential carcinogens.[32]

The histogenesis of small bowel adenocarcinoma most likely follows the adenoma-carcinoma sequence described initially for large bowel cancer.[33] As a result, the single most important risk factor for small bowel adenocarcinoma is preexisting adenoma, either single or multiple, as associated with multiple polyposis syndromes.[34] Small bowel adenocarcinomas have also been associated with alcohol (but not tobacco), nontropical sprue, regional enteritis, celiac disease, and urinary diversion procedures such as ileal conduit.[35-39]

Despite the well-known correlation of colonic cancer with ulcerative colitis, much less evidence exists to indict Crohn's disease as a cause of adenocarcinoma of the small bowel.[40] The few reports that are available show a slightly increased risk of tumors associated with Crohn's disease to occur in the terminal ileum and in other sites where Crohn's disease is active.[41-43] The age at diagnosis is usually 10 years younger for the Crohn's patients than for the population at large. As with ulcerative colitis (UC) and tumors of the colon, the diagnosis of Crohn's disease precedes small bowel tumors by about 10 years. Several risk factors have been identified in patients with Crohn's disease who develop adenocarcinoma of the small bowel: duration of Crohn's disease, male gender, fistulization, presence of strictures, and surgical creation of blind excluded loops of intestines.[44,45]

Celiac sprue, while well-known to predispose to intestinal lymphoma, is also associated with adenocarcinoma of the small bowel.[37] The numbers cited in case reports are few, but the presence of disease in otherwise noncharacteristic locations seems to lend credence to the theory that gluten-mediated jejunoileitis is also an independent risk factor for the development of adenocarcinoma of the small bowel as well as lymphomas.[28,37] Adenocarcinoma of the small intestine, often aggressive, can affect children and is usually associated with degeneration of a PJ hamartoma.[34]

The genetic mechanisms involved in the carcinogenesis of the small bowel remain unknown, most likely because of the small number of cases. Blaker and colleagues from Germany showed that although small intestinal carcinomas reveal complex genetic changes, a significant number of tumors share karyotypic instability and losses of chromosome 18q21-q22. 18q deletions often target the SMAD4 gene and disrupt tumor suppression through TGFβ-signaling.[46] Svrcek and colleagues, using tissue microarray analysis, determined that inactivation of the SMAD4/DPC4 gene is involved in small intestinal adenocarcinoma tumorigenesis and that over expression of TP53 and abnormal expression of β-catenin are two common events in small intestinal adenocarcinoma.[47]

Symptoms of adenocarcinoma of the small bowel range from obstructive symptoms, such as vomiting and jaundice for those with duodenal tumors, to indistinct abdominal pain, weight loss, and anemia for more distal lesions. The most common complaint is abdominal pain in 30% to 70% of patients. Weight loss is also common, occurring in more than 50% of patients. Obstruction is found in 40% to 70% of patients prior to presentation. In the collected Mayo series, 71% of patients had either overt or clinical evidence of blood loss.[48] Adenocarcinomas, especially duodenal tumors, usually become symptomatic earlier than other small bowel tumors, allowing for earlier diagnosis and intervention. Despite this, 30% to 35% of small bowel adenocarcinomas are metastatic at the time of diagnosis.[30,31] Metastasis can occur via lymphatics, by a hematogenous route (liver, lungs, and bone most commonly), or by direct extension through the serosal surfaces and into the peritoneal cavity. Because of the insidious nature of adenocarcinomas, they tend to present late with either lymph node involvement or distant metastases. One hypothesis for early metastasis is that, unlike large-bowel mucosa, small bowel mucosa contains lymphatics that course through the villi, extending near the luminal surface, allowing invasion of the mucosal tumor into the lymphatics.

In a recent study conducted by the American College of Surgeons on 5000 small bowel adenocarcinomas, the overall 5-year disease-free survival (DFS) was 30.5%.[49] The median survival in this series was 19.7 months. Staging of adenocarcinomas of the small bowel is carried out by the tumor, node, metastases (TNM) classification system. The primary treatment of adenocarcinomas is wide surgical resection, with removal of lymph nodes and the vascular pedicle. Margins of 5 cm are considered acceptable. Recent reports indicate that even this treatment does not yield good survival rates for node-positive patients. In a recent study examining 217 patients with small bowel adenocarcinoma followed over a 10-year period at MD Anderson Cancer Center, patients with stage IV disease had a shorter 5-year overall survival (OS) than those with I-III disease (5% vs 36%).[31] The 5-year survival was significantly shorter if the positive lymph node ratio (number of positive lymph nodes/number of total lymph nodes) was greater than 75% versus less than 75% (12% vs 51%). In patients with involvement of the proximal duodenum, pancreatoduodenectomy may be necessary. In those with disease in the terminal ileum, a right hemicolectomy is indicated. In those with jejunal involvement, wide resection is recommended.

All attempts should be made to resect the primary lesion to prevent mucosal bleeding. For patients deemed unresectable at the time of laparotomy, some have advocated the use of intraoperative radiation therapy.[50-52] The lack of clinical trials makes this therapy difficult to recommend in a setting other than specialized centers. External beam radiation may be helpful to palliate symptoms, but again, there is a lack of published experience with this treatment. Chemotherapy usually incorporates 5-fluorouracil (5-FU) and nitrosoureas. In some settings, these agents have led to tumor regression and increased lengths of survival.[52]

Carcinoid Tumors ■ Carcinoid tumors represent approximately 25% to 30% of malignant tumors of the small bowel. They were first described by Lubarsch over 100 years ago.[51,53] Obendorfer used the term "karzinoide" in 1907,[54] but the exact nature of the tumor was not determined until 1928 when Masson described its origin as the chromaffin cell.[55] The most recent population-based review of carcinoid tumors comes from the epidemiologic study by Maggard and colleagues, who analyzed 11,427 cases of carcinoid tumors.[56] The most frequent sites for carcinoids were the GI tract (54.5%) and the bronchopulmonary system (30.1%). Within the GI tract, most occurred in the small bowel (44.7%), rectum (19.6%), and appendix (16.7%). In contradistinction to adenocarcinoma, the carcinoid tends to arise in the distal small intestine rather than in more proximal sites. In the series reported by Moertel, all surgically confirmed, 3% were in the duodenum, 5% in the jejunum, 32% in the proximal ileum, and 60% in the distal ileum.[57] The median age at discovery is 60.9 years, and females constitute 54.2% of patients.[56]

A unique feature of carcinoid tumors is their ability to produce a variety of protein and peptide products, the most characteristic of which is serotonin. Systemic serotonin is thought to cause most of the symptoms of the carcinoid syndrome, including diarrhea, flushing, wheezing, and right-sided heart disease. Carcinoid syndrome is seen in 5% to 7% of patients with large tumor burdens and metastatic disease.[58,59] It is believed that the metastatic component is necessary to ensure drainage of the compounds involved in the syndrome into the systemic circulation and to provide an adequate tumor mass to produce large amounts of peptidergic products.

Carcinoid tumors are traditionally classified according to their embryonic site of origin and their usual histologic type.[60] In 1963, Williams and Sandler reported that those discovered in the foregut (bronchi, stomach, pancreas, biliary tract, and parts one and two of the duodenum) tended to have a histologic pattern of trabeculae and were occasionally associated with the carcinoid syndrome. Those arising from the midgut, the most common site, had a histologic pattern of nests and invading cords and were most commonly associated with the carcinoid syndrome. Finally, those found in the hindgut (descending colon and rectum) had a mixed histologic picture, but were infrequently involved with the carcinoid syndrome.[60]

The clinical manifestations of carcinoid are often vague or absent and the definitive diagnosis is often not made prior to surgery. In a series of 145 patients with gastrointestinal carcinoid tumors, only 12 had a proper diagnosis before surgery and those 12 had definite symptoms of carcinoid syndrome.[57,61] Most often, patients are operated on for signs of bowel obstruction, not by the tumor itself, but by a desmoplastic reaction that leads to shrinking of the mesentery as a result of fibrosis and kinking of the bowel.[58,62] Standard imaging techniques such as CT, ultrasonography, and even enteroclysis rarely identify the primary tumor, making preoperative diagnosis of small bowel carcinoid very difficult.[59,63] A useful diagnostic tool, if a carcinoid tumor is suspected, is the measurement of carcinoid products and their metabolites including serotonin and 5-HIAA. A diagnosis of carcinoid syndrome is confirmed if the 24-hour urine 5-HIAA level is more than 10 mg.[60,64] In one study involving primarily patients with metastatic disease, elevated 5-HIAA excretion predicted the presence of carcinoid tumor with a sensitivity of 73% and a specificity of 100%.[61,65] Scintigraphy with radiolabeled octreotide has been successfully used to localize undetected primary and metastatic lesions.[66] Two large European studies show carcinoid lesion detection with a sensitivity of 89% by using this diagnostic tool.[67]

The metastatic potential of a carcinoid tumor correlates closely with its size. In the Moertel series, there were no metastases in tumors less than 0.5 cm in diameter, 15% in tumors 0.5 to 0.9 cm in diameter, 72% in tumors 1.0 to 1.9 cm in diameter, and 95% metastases in tumors larger than 2 cm.[57] However, small bowel carcinoids may still metastasize when less than 1 cm. Recent evidence based on 5-HIAA levels, suggests that most cases of metastatic carcinoid of unknown primary probably arise from small ileal tumors. Extent of disease, which mainly comprises either lymph node (regional) or liver (metastatic) involvement, is a definite predictor of outcome. In Maggard's analysis of 11,427 carcinoids, 5-year survival for localized, regional, and distant disease of the small intestine was 70.4%, 64.1%, and 32.4%, respectively.[68] Given these statistics, outside of duodenal and rectal carcinoids, discussed below, and appendiceal carcinoids, discussed later in the chapter, there is no place for limited resection of intestinal carcinoids. Even with small tumors, an extended resection with relevant lymph node drainage is required. This is the only approach that allows definitive histopathologic staging, resection of occult lymph node metastasis, and prevention of local complications caused by a desmoplastic resection.[60] Careful intraoperative examination is mandatory, because most series report that 30% of these tumors are multicentric.[48] Another reason for meticulous exploration is that associated neoplasms occur with small intestinal carcinoids in 16.6% of cases.[68] In the case of advanced disease, there may be some benefit to debulking procedures, but this remains controversial, because the absolute size of the tumor does not correspond well with the degree of symptoms.[48,69,70] Some authors recommend aggressive treatment even in patients with widely metastatic disease, including resection of all intraabdominal tumor deposits, segmental liver resection as needed, and hepatic arterial embolization. Cholecystectomy also has been performed to prevent gallbladder necrosis during hepatic embolization. Although it has not been proven whether this aggressive surgical approach increases survival, it has yielded biochemical remission in up to 25% of patients and regression of hepatic metastases for long periods.[68,71] In the MD Anderson experience of 81 patients with carcinoid disease metastatic to the liver who underwent hepatic artery embolization or chemoembolization, 67% experienced a partial response with a mean duration of response of 17 months. Overall, 63% of patients had reduction in their tumor-related symptoms and the OS time was 31 months.[72]

Duodenal and rectal carcinoid tumors are similar in that they are relatively rare and may be amenable to endoscopic or local resection. Primary duodenal carcinoids account for only 2.6% of carcinoid tumors in the United States, although they are increasingly recognized with the more widespread use of upper GI endoscopy.[73] Because of the rarity of this disease, management recommendations for duodenal carcinoids have been extrapolated from the experience with midgut and hindgut carcinoids. A recent study by Mullen and colleagues however demonstrated successful margin negative endoscopic resection in six patients with tumors less than 1.5 cm.[73] Interestingly, this study found lymph node metastases to be present in 54% of patients with duodenal carcinoid, including two patients with tumors smaller than 1 cm and limited to the submucosa. The impact of lymph node metastasis in duodenal carcinoids is uncertain, however, in that no patient developed distant metastases or carcinoid syndrome in this series. Similarly, rectal carcinoids are uncommon tumors, representing 1.8% of malignant anorectal neoplasms.[74] Rectal carcinoids less than 1 cm are adequately treated by wide local excision alone or even by endoscopic resection if less than 0.5 cm. Tumors between 1 and 2 cm should be locally resected by a wide, local, full-thickness excision with abdominoperineal resection (APR) or low anterior resection (LAR) recommended for tumors that invade the muscularis propria. Even though major oncologic operations were once recommended for rectal carcinoids greater than 2 cm, it is now appreciated that the risk of distant metastasis is so high that radical surgery should not be considered if the tumor can be removed by wide local excision. Every attempt should be made for sphincter preservation in patients with carcinoids of the rectum of greater than 2 cm because of the high likelihood of distant failure and the marginal benefit obtained from radical local therapy.[74]

Medical therapy in the form of somatostatin analogues is effective in relieving symptoms of the carcinoid syndrome, though demonstrated tumor regression is rare. Octreotide is an eight amino acid, long-acting somatostatin analogue that binds to receptor subtypes 2, 3, and 5 and has been widely used for both detection and treatment of carcinoid tumors.[75] In one study, octreotide was delivered subcutaneously at a dosage of 150 μg three times a day, showing improved symptoms in 88% of patients and decreased urinary 5-HIAA in 72% of patients.[76]

Prognosis of patients with carcinoid disease varies according to several factors. Size of the primary tumor is an important predictor of metastasis and survival. Carcinoid tumors greater than 2 cm in diameter portend a worse prognosis than those less than 2 cm.[77] This is most likely a result of the propensity to metastasize and not increased biologic aggressiveness of these larger tumors. In the Maggard series, increased tumor size was associated with a greater likelihood of lymph node involvement.[56] In the carcinoid series at Duke University, a direct correlation was found between size of the primary tumor and extent of disease at presentation.[78] In addition, after controlling for stage of disease, region of origin of primary tumor predicted prognosis in this series of patients. In patients with distant metastases at presentation, those with midgut tumors had markedly better prognosis than did patients with foregut or hindgut tumors. The reasons for the relative indolence of metastatic midgut tumors are unclear.

Composite tumors, those that display characteristics of both carcinoid tumors and adenocarcinomas, are well described in the appendix but are less well-known in the small intestine. These tumors are relatively rare, with most reports to date encompassing only one or two cases. They are aggressive tumors with a metastatic potential similar to that of adenocarcinoma and should be treated as adenocarcinomas. Lymphatic metastasis appeared histologically to be adenocarcinoma in two cases and carcinoid in one; thus, it seems that these tumors may arise from cells with pluripotential patterns of differentiation.[79]

Gastrointestinal Stromal Tumors ■ Gastrointestinal stromal tumors (GIST) is the current nomenclature for a diverse group of benign or malignant GI neoplasms derived from embryonic mesoderm that may have smooth muscle (smooth muscle GIST), neural differentiation (gastrointestinal autonomic nerve tumor), characteristics of both (mixed GIST), or may appear as undifferentiated spindle cell lesions (GIST not otherwise specified). Malignant GISTs constitute 15% to 20% of the malignant tumors found in the small bowel.[80] GISTs most often classified, until recently, as leiomyomas and leiomyosarcomas, are now known to represent a discrete neoplastic entity. The cellular origin of GIST is proposed to be the interstitial cell of Cajal, an intestinal pacemaker cell.[81] GISTs are characterized by mutations in the protooncogene C-kit that lead to constitutive activation of its glycoprotein product KIT and the subsequent tyrosine kinase activity.[82] More than 90% of GISTs express KIT and biochemical evidence of KIT can be found in almost all GISTs.[83] In the majority of these cases, this activation is linked to a somatic mutation KIT, usually involving exon 9 or 11.[82]

Most GISTs present as an abdominal mass causing bowel obstruction evidenced as nausea, vomiting and abdominal pain, or as GI bleeding. GISTs usually grow rapidly, with masses 5 cm in diameter or greater being common.[84] This rapid rate of growth explains the propensity for GI blood loss, because these tumors may outgrow their blood supply, become necrotic, and ulcerate. Blood loss is usually chronic, with laboratory studies revealing a microcytic anemia.[80,84] Fistulas and abscesses are also caused by tumor necrosis. GISTs usually occur in patients older than age of 50 years, with similar rates of occurrence in both genders.[85] These tumors tend to spread by local extension, growing into the mesentery, surrounding serosal surfaces, or omentum. Vascular metastases are common, but lymphatic spread is unusual. GISTs are usually easy to detect with radiologic examination because of their large size, with CT scanning providing an excellent diagnostic test.

As with other tumors of the small bowel, the primary treatment of GIST is surgical resection with wide margins. Because lymph node involvement is not common, extensive lymphadenectomy appears to provide no added survival benefit. One study analyzing 200 cases of GIST over a 16-year period found that in patients with primary disease who underwent complete resection of gross disease, the 5-year actuarial survival rate was 54%.[86] Survival was predicted by tumor size but not microscopic margins of resection. In a study reviewing 50 cases of GIST specific to the small intestine, Crosby and colleagues identified subgroups with significantly longer OS in univariable analysis were those with localized or locally advanced disease (stage I) and those who underwent complete gross resection.[87] Even with complete surgical resection, the majority of tumors will recur, often involving the liver and peritoneal surface. In the largest series of GIST recurrences, the group from Memorial Sloan-Kettering Cancer Center retrospectively analyzed 69 such patients.[86] Local recurrence was seen in 76% of patients, of which half had synchronous liver lesions. Surgical resection for recurrent disease was completed in one-third of cases with median survival of 15 months. Neither complete nor partial resection resulted in significantly improved survival, although the subgroup of patients with isolated, resectable hepatic lesions showed a trend toward longer survival.

With the high recurrence rate after surgery, effective adjuvant therapy is needed. GIST tumors are resistant to standard chemotherapy and irradiation, with no current role for treatment with these modalities.[88] Because GISTs express a mutated C-*kit* tyrosine kinase, the tyrosine kinase inhibitor imatinib mesylate has shown promise in early clinical trials. There have been two American College of Surgeons Oncology Group (ACOSOG) trials looking at the role of adjuvant imatinib mesylate after resection for those patients at intermediate or high risk of recurrence. ACOSOG Z9000 was the first phase II trial studying the efficacy of adjuvant imatinib following complete resection of GIST at high risk of recurrence.[89] Patients underwent complete gross resection of a KIT-expressing primary GIST that was at high risk of recurrence (tumor size greater than 10 cm, tumor rupture, or less than 5 peritoneal metastases). Following resection, patients received oral imatinib 400 mg/day for 1 year. At a median follow-up of 4 years, the 1- 2- and 3-year OS rates were 99%, 97%, and 97%, respectively. The 1, 2, and 3-year recurrence free survival rates were 94%, 73%, and 61%, respectively. These results compared favorably with historical controls for both recurrence free survival and OS. ACOSOG Z79001 was a follow-up phase III trial in which patients were randomized to 1 year of oral imatinib or placebo following resection.[90] This study showed that while imatinib was well tolerated and increased recurrence free survival, OS was not increased compared to placebo. In addition, there is an ongoing Radiation Therapy Oncology Group (RTOG) trial looking at the role of imatinib mesylate in the neoadjuvant setting.[91] Neoadjuvant imatinib mesylate holds much promise because it can lead to marked shrinkage in tumor size, which can frequently be predicted within 2 to 4 weeks of initiating therapy using positron emission tomography (PET) scans. Whether it will allow surgeons to do smaller operations or will improve survival remains to be determined, but appears most applicable to GIST tumors near the gastroesophageal junction, ampulla and in the rectum.

In the metastatic setting, there is much clearer evidence of the effectiveness of imatinib mesylate. In an early report by Joensuu and colleagues, the promise of selectively inhibiting the constitutive activity of mutated KIT in GIST with imatinib mesylate as an effective therapeutic strategy was realized.[92] In this study, a 50-year-old patient with metastatic GIST who had undergone resection of multiple recurrent tumors, as well as chemotherapy, continued to have progressive, unresectable disease. After a 2-week trial of imatinib mesylate, MRI showed a 41% decrease in tumor size; at 14 months there was a greater than 80% decrease. In a European Organization for Research and Treatment of Cancer (EORTC) phase I study, the highest feasible dosage of imatinib was 400 mg twice a day.[93] The dose-limiting side effects at higher doses included severe nausea, vomiting, edema, and rash. A phase II study of 147 patients randomized to receive either 400 mg or 600 mg of imatinib mesylate daily demonstrated a sustained objective response in more than 50% of the patients with advanced unresectable or metastatic GIST with no significant differences in toxic effects or response between the two doses.[94] These favorable results led to rapid development of randomized multicenter phase III trials in the United States and Europe. The EORTC's phase III trial randomized 946 patients to 400 mg of imatinib either once or twice a day and found that if response induction is the only aim of treatment, a daily dose of 400 mg, given for 4 to 6 months, is sufficient. However, in patients with widespread metastatic disease, the prolonged progression-free survival (PFS) achieved with 400 mg twice a day, would be a more ideal dosage.[95] The US Phase III Sarcoma Group Study S0033 had a similar design and compared the same two daily doses.[96] The major difference in the two studies was that the primary endpoint of the S0033 was OS whereas the EORTC's was PFS. In the 746-patient S0033 study there was no significant difference in PFS at 2 years between the 400 mg and 800 mg dosages (50% vs 53%).[96] Additional tyrosine kinase inhibitors are currently available including sunitinib. These are useful in patients that progress on imatinib or do not tolerate it. Molecular studies suggest that imatinib is most effective in patients with exon 11 C-kit tyrosine kinase mutations and sunitinib may be more effective in patients with exon 9 mutations.

Lymphoma ■ Lymphoma accounts for 15% to 20% of all malignant small bowel tumors.[97] The stomach is the most common site of GI lymphoma (>60%), followed by an equal distribution between the large and small intestines.[98] There is a slight male predominance of approximately 1.5:1, and the median age is lower than that of persons with other small bowel tumors (49 years in one large series).[99,100]

Lymphomas are the most frequent malignant neoplasms in transplant recipients, appearing on average 20 months after the initiation of cyclosporine.[101] Prognosis is better than for other forms of intestinal lymphomas with two-thirds cured with resection, radiotherapy, acyclovir, and reduction of immunosupression.[102,103]

Small bowel lymphomas also occur in AIDS. Virtually all lesions are B-lymphocyte in origin. Peri-cecal lymphoma may perforate and simulate acute appendicitis. The prognosis is poor but is dominated by the HIV-related disease such that life expectancy for these patients is not significantly inferior to similar patients without lymphoma.[102]

The clinical presentation of GI lymphoma includes abdominal pain, nausea, vomiting, fatigue, weight loss, and GI bleeding, which may be occult. Perforation may occur in some patients, causing an acute abdomen.[85] Systemic signs of lymphoma, such as lymphadenopathy and fever, may also be present. Radiographic studies, such as a CT scan with oral contrast are of value in making the diagnosis.[85] A mass with bulky adenopathy is highly suggestive of abdominal lymphoma.[104]

Multiple staging systems have been proposed for GI lymphomas, including the Ann Arbor, Musshoff, and newly revised European-American classification system. Each of these major staging systems recognizes four major stages of small bowel lymphoma: stage I for local disease, stage II for regional involvement, and stages III and IV for advanced disease with metastasis. The overall prognosis of the more advanced stages is fair, with a 5-year survival of only 25% to 30%.[104] In a retrospective analysis of 32 cases of primary small bowel lymphoma treated with either radical surgery (for stages I and II) plus chemotherapy versus chemotherapy alone (for stages III and IV), the overall 5-year survival was 59%, while the relapse-free survival rate among the complete responders was 72%.[105] These results suggest aggressive multimodal therapy may be beneficial.

Resection of small bowel lymphoma is important for local control but rarely eradicates the disease. Disease is often advanced so that fewer than 30% of intestinal tumors are amenable to primary curative resection.[105] Adjuvant therapy is an essential part of the treatment. The surgical resection should always be attempted for localized disease and should involve removal of the bowel segments, with wide margins, and the involved mesenteric lymph nodes, if possible. Margins need to be completely clear of tumor since lymphomas may spread for long distances in the submucosal plane. Adjuvant chemotherapy in patients after potential curative resection is advocated.[106,107] In patients with unresectable lymphoma, radiation therapy and chemotherapy are recommended.[108]

Small bowel lymphoma is particularly common in the Middle East, especially in southern Iran. This Mediterranean lymphoma is found in children and young adults.[109,110] Patients tend to be from lower socioeconomic groups with a background of malnutrition. The tumor progenitor cell is believed to be the perifollicular B cell, which produces IgA. The tumor releases an excess of alpha heavy chains, which are detectable in the serum.[111] Combination chemotherapy is useful in unresectable disease, although an optimal regimen has not been defined.[112] This lymphoma behaves differently from other small bowel lymphomas and appears to have a worse prognosis.

Metastatic Neoplams ■ Metastatic neoplasm involvement of the small bowel is more frequent than primary small intestinal neoplasia. Primary tumors of the colon, ovary, uterus, and stomach involve the small bowel, most often by direct invasion or peritoneal spread. Primaries from the breast, lung, and melanoma metastasize to the small intestine hematogenously.[112] Within the GI tract, the small bowel is the most frequent site of metastasis of melanoma, most likely because of its rich blood supply. In one recent series of metastatic melanoma of the intestinal tract, the metastases were the presenting sign that lead to diagnosis of melanoma in 50% of the cases.[113] A retrospective study of 103 cases of malignant melanoma performed by the Armed Forces Institute of Pathology stated that small bowel involvement by melanoma, even in the absence of a known primary, is usually metastatic.[114] Prolonged survival after resection of small bowel melanoma is poor, but aggressive resection in cases without a known primary site may improve quality of life.[115]

Tumors of the Appendix

Malignancies of the appendix are rare, making up less than 4% of all intestinal neoplasms.[116] Among 71,000 appendectomy specimens taken over a 40-year period, Collins found 958 malignant tumors, with an overall incidence of 1.35%.[117] In their series of 8699 appendectomies in a 23-year period at a single institution, Schmutzer and colleagues reported a total of 101 tumors, of which 60 were malignant, for an incidence of 1.2% overall and 0.7% for malignant tumors.[118]

In 1943, Uihlein and McDonald classified appendiceal malignancies into three categories on the basis of morphology: carcinoid tumors, malignant mucoceles, and adenocarcinomas of the colonic type.[119] Although many authors consider the malignant mucocele and adenocarcinoma to be histologically identical and argue that they should be regarded as the same process, others have described significant differences in their clinical features. As a result, despite their microscopic similarity, the natural histories of the two tumors are distinct enough that most consider them different disease processes.[120] In the series by Collins, carcinoids made up 51% of the malignant tumors found, mucoceles accounted for 32%, and 6% were adenocarcinomas.[117] The remainder consisted of a large number of rare tumors, including sarcomas. In addition, Warkel and colleagues described a complex appendiceal tumor distinct clinically and pathologically from carcinoids and adenocarcinomas, but sharing features of both.[121] For this lesion, the term adenocarcinoid is used.

Carcinoids

Carcinoids are the most common appendiceal tumor, comprising 32% to 77% of appendiceal neoplasms.[122,123] In 1975, Godwin reported a series of 2837 carcinoid cases identified by the End Results Group (ERG; 1950-1969) and the Third National Cancer Survey (TNCS; 1969-1971) programs of the National Cancer Institute (NCI) between the years 1950 and 1971.[124] This survey reported that the majority of carcinoids were in the appendix (ERG: 43.9%; TNCS: 35.5%). Modlin and Sandor updated this classic study in 1997 by adding to the existing database 5468 cases collected from 1973 to 1991 through the Surveillance, Epidemiology, and End Results (SEER) program.[68] This study reported a decrease in appendiceal carcinoids from 43.9% (ERG) to 7.6% (SEER) over a 20-year time period. The authors warned that this information should be evaluated cautiously because the ERG file contains both benign and malignant appendiceal carcinoids, whereas the first 14-year period of the SEER program does not. Another explanation offered was the decreased surgical commitment to appendectomy in the past 2 decades.

The SEER study also revealed a sex predominance for appendiceal carcinoids, with tumors from females comprising 68% of the cases. Similarly, Roggo and colleagues retrospectively analyzed 41 cases of appendiceal carcinomas and reported that 80.5% of the cases occurred in females.[125] This female predominance may reflect the increased number of pelvic procedures performed in women, leading to more incidental findings, including carcinoids of the appendix. Appendiceal carcinoids mostly present at an early age, averaging 32 to 42 years in the literature.[68,125]

Moertel and colleagues, in their evaluation of 150 appendiceal carcinoids over a period of 51 years, noted that 4.7% of the cases metastasized but none of the tumors less than 2 cm exhibited metastatic spread.[126] In general, metastases in appendiceal carcinoids less than 2 cm in diameter are uncommon. Because large carcinoid tumors of the appendix are rare, the overall rate of metastasis in most series is in the range of 1.3 to 4.7%.[127,128] Nonlocalized appendiceal lesions, which in Modlin's ERG registry comprised only 5% of all appendiceal carcinoids, increased significantly to 35.4% in the SEER file. It is unclear whether this increase is due to an elevated awareness of the biology of the lesion and greater sampling of lymph nodes and surrounding tissue, or reflects the inclusion of autopsy data in the SEER group.[68]

The majority of carcinoid tumors of the appendix may be treated with a simple appendectomy.[129] At laparotomy, these tumors appear as small yellow nodules, usually in the distal third of the appendix. Histologically, the cells are small, uniform, and contain a central nucleus with few mitoses. Almost all carcinoids show invasion of the muscular layer of the wall of the appendix and involvement of lymphatic vessels adjacent to the tumor is essentially universal.[129] This being said, few patients have regional or distant dissemination of disease. Malignant carcinoid syndrome is rarely associated with appendiceal carcinoids with only six cases reported, all of which had distant metastases.[68] In view of these observations, the standard recommendation is that tumors less than 2 cm require only an appendectomy as adequate treatment, while those greater than 2 cm require a hemicolectomy. However, because metastases have been found even with primary tumors of 1.5 to 2 cm in diameter, some authors recommend that patients in this group undergo right hemicolectomy. Although hemicolectomy has been advocated for these larger tumors, no prospective studies establish whether aggressive surgery is associated with a better prognosis. Some authors suggest hemicolectomy if mesoappendiceal involvement is found. Given the frequency of invasion of the mesoappendix by carcinoid (16%), mesoappendiceal involvement alone does not warrant right hemicolectomy.[68] In a review of the Danish Cancer Registry, Svendson and Bulow found 10 cases of appendiceal carcinoid tumors involving the mesoappendix. Eight of the 10 cases were associated with primary tumors less than 1 cm and were treated with appendectomy without recurrence.[130]

Three series have described experiences with carcinoids of the appendix in the pediatric population. The youngest patient reported was 3 years old. In the most recent of the series, the largest tumor found was 1.2 cm. In 65% of pediatric patients, there was invasion of the muscularis or of the muscularis and serosal layers, which compares with 77% to 90% in other series. In all cases, the tumor was less than 2 cm in diameter, and only appendectomy was performed. There have been no recurrences.[128,130-132] It appears that appendectomy alone is sufficient treatment in children if the initial lesion is less than 2 cm in diameter.

Because most carcinoids are found at the tip of the organ and are small, it has been estimated that only 10% result in acute appendicitis.[133] Distal location was found in 82% of patients in the series reported by Collins[117] and in 71% of patients by Moertel and colleagues.[122] In these series, of appendiceal tumors discovered during appendectomy for appendicitis, only 30% were apparently involved in causing the appendicitis because of obstruction of the appendiceal lumen.[117,122,126]

In Modlin's review of 8305 carcinoids, the 85.9% 5-year survival for appendiceal carcinoids exceeded that of carcinoids in any other location.[68] This good prognosis is confirmed in reports throughout the literature.[134,135] The reasons for this excellent survival rate may include the anatomic site of the lesion, incidental early discovery, and simple surgical management in the majority of cases.

Mucocele

An appendiceal mucocele is any one of a number of lesions that is characterized by dilation of the appendiceal lumen, alteration of the mucosal lining, hypersecretion of mucus, and occasional extension outside of the appendix.[136] The underlying pathology may be a hyperplastic polyp; a benign neoplasm, such as cystadenoma; or a malignant tumor, such as cystadenocarcinoma. In the original classification system proposed by Uihlein and McDonald, mucoceles make up one of the three major types of appendiceal malignancies. The authors admit the rigid division between malignant mucoceles and adenocarcinoma is not universally accepted.[119] Many authors support the use of a system based on histologic findings, rather than on the presence of a cystic lesion.[136] In this system, mucoceles of the appendix are classified into simple (obstructive) and mucoceles with proliferative epithelial changes. Benign neoplastic proliferative changes may be localized, as in adenoma of colonic type, or diffuse, as in mucinous adenoma or mucinous cystadenoma. Malignant proliferative groups may be classified as colonic type adenocarcinoma, mucinous cystadenocarcinoma, and mixed carcinoid-adenocarcinoma.[137] The preneoplastic potential of hyperplastic epithelium and the premalignant nature of adenomatous epithelium are seen by the coexistence of hyperplastic, adenomatous, and carcinomatous epithelium all in the same lesion.[137] A consequence of mucoceles of the appendix (cystadenomas and cystadenocarcinomas) is pseudomyxoma peritonei. This lesion, characterized by large quantities of mucus-like material in the peritoneal cavity, is considered to represent dissemination of mucinous cystadenocarcinoma within the peritoneal cavity (see the section on Pseudomyxoma Peritonei).[138]

Though the diagnosis of appendiceal mucocele is usually an incidental finding at celiotomy, mucinous cystadenomas and cystadenocarcinomas are among the few appendiceal tumors that may be diagnosed preoperatively.[129] Computed tomography strongly suggests a mucinous tumor if a mass is present in the right lower quadrant with near water density. Ultrasound shows a diagnostic variable sonographic echogenicity because of the combination of mucin with more anechoic fluid. Although both imaging techniques may be helpful in diagnosing a mucocele, other cystic lesions of the peritoneal cavity, such as ovarian cysts, duplication cysts, mesenteric and omental cysts, or an abscess, may have a similar appearance.[139]

Treatment is surgical resection, with the extent of resection dependent on the underlying histology. In the case of hyperplastic polyps or cystadenoma, a simple appendectomy is considered curative. In the series reported by Higa and colleagues, 36 of the 46 patients with mucinous cystadenomas were treated with appendectomy alone with no recurrence.[136] In patients with mucinous cystadenocarcinoma, a substantial number will present with extensive abdominal metastases or pseudomyxoma peritonei. Treatment of the primary lesion includes a formal right hemicolectomy with removal of draining lymph nodes.[140] Stephenson and Brief reviewed 53 appendiceal mucinous cystadenocarcinomas treated by either simple appendectomy or right hemicolectomy. At 10 years, survival was 65% among patients treated with hemicolectomy, in contrast to a 37% rate among patients who had received an appendectomy alone.[141] Surgical debulking of metastatic deposits and evacuation of mucus collections are also recommended.

Pseudomyxoma Peritonei

Pseudomyxoma peritonei (PMP) is a unique condition characterized by diffuse collections of gelatinous material in the abdomen and pelvis and mucinous implants on the peritoneal surfaces. The term PMP was originally applied to intraperitoneal mucinous spread originating from a cystadenoma of the appendix. As the tumor grows and occludes the lumen, mucus accumulates and the appendix ruptures. The peritoneum is then seeded with mucus-producing cells, which continue to proliferate and produce mucus.[142] Over the years, the term PMP has begun to be used more generally by clinicians to signify not only intraperitoneal mucinous dissemination from rupture of a benign cystadenoma, but also peritoneal dissemination of mucus-producing adenocarcinomas of the appendix, large and small bowel, as well as lung, breast, pancreas, stomach, bile ducts, gallbladder, and fallopian tubes/ovary.[143,144] PMP is more common in females, and is found unexpectedly in approximately 2 of 10,000 laparotomies.[143] The most common presenting symptom in both men and women is increasing abdominal girth; in men the second most common symptom is an inguinal hernia, while for women it is an ovarian mass palpated at the time of a routine pelvic examination.[142]

The radiographic appearance of PMP is characteristic. On CT scan, the mucinous material is similar in density to fat, and appears heterogeneous. Scalloping of the liver, spleen, and mesentery is found, and calcifications are common. The undersurface of the diaphragm may be greatly thickened by large cystic masses of mucinous tumor. A striking early finding is the characteristic peripheral location of tumor within the abdomen and pelvis and relative sparing and central displacement of the small bowel and mesentery.[142]

Standard treatment for PMP is repeated surgical debulking for symptomatic disease.[143] This treatment is not curative, but aims to resect gross disease to limit the buildup of mucus and its pressure effect. Disease recurrence requires repeated and progressively more difficult surgery due to adhesions and fibrosis. Cytoreduction and intraperitoneal chemotherapy is a more aggressive approach that includes radical surgical removal of all intraadbdominal and pelvic disease and the administration of intraperitoneal heated chemotherapy. It has been adopted by some clinicians, aiming fur cure. Drug penetration is enhanced by heating the perfusate containing chemotherapy, an approach termed intraperitoneal hyperthermic chemotherapy (IPHC).[145-148] This approach is best suited to patients with minimal residual disease (deposits smaller than 2 to 2.5 mm) after surgical cytoreduction. It is unlikely that even a heated solution of chemotherapy could penetrate large tumor deposits.

Sugarbaker and colleagues have written the most extensively about treatment of peritoneal surface malignancy with aggressive surgical debulking and IPHC.[148] His group uses four clinical assessments to select patients who are most likely to benefit from combined treatment. First, histopathologic assessment in which noninvasive malignancies such as true PMP or cystic mesothelioma are more likely to be made visibly disease-free through a peritonectomy procedure, and are less likely than other invasive histologies to have spread to regional nodes, liver, or other systemic sites. Second, preoperative contrast-enhanced CT of the chest, abdomen, and pelvis to exclude not only liver or other systemic metastases, but also to determine if small bowel obstruction or tumor nodules greater than 5 cm are present, which portends a poor prognosis. Two other clinical indices, the peritoneal cancer index (PCI, a quantitative indicator of prognosis derived from the size and distribution of nodules on the peritoneal surface), and the completeness of cytoreduction score (the size of persisting tumor nodules after maximal cytoreduction), are derived intraoperatively. A 2001 report by Sugarbaker and colleagues included 108 patients with PMP treated over a 10-year period (1983-1993) with surgical debulking and intraoperative intraperitoneal heated mitomycin followed by intraperitoneal 5-FU during postoperative days 1 to 6, and three subsequent courses of adjuvant intravenous mitomycin and intraperitoneal 5-FU.[149] Of the 65 patients with true PMP, 5-year survival was 75% and 10-year survival was 68%. Those with carcinomatosis had a poorer outcome with 5- and 10-year survival rates of 26% and 9% respectively. It should be noted that the favorable results achieved by international experts in the field may not be replicated in routine clinical practice.

Aggressive cytoreduction and IPHC has been tried for secondary peritoneal carcinomatosis in several centers throughout the world, although only one prospective controlled trial has been completed.[150] This Dutch trial randomly assigned 105 patients with peritoneal carcinomatosis from appendiceal (n = 18) or colorectal (n = 87) cancer without evidence of other metastases to surgical debulking (aiming to achieve deposits less than 2.5 mm) with IPHC versus systemic chemotherapy without debulking. Only palliative surgery was permitted in the control patients, and they received 5-FU and leucovorin given weekly until progression. In the experimental group, after debulking, the abdominal cavity was perfused for 90 minutes with isotonic dialysis fluid containing mitomycin and heated to 41°C. Systemic chemotherapy similar to the control arm was started 6 weeks after cytoreduction and IPHC. At 8-year follow-up, the median PFS was 7.7 months in the control arm and 12.6 months in the cytoreduction arm. The median disease-specific survival was 12.6 month in the control arm and 22.2 months in the cytoreduction arm. The 5-year survival was 45% for those patients in whom an R1 resection (no evidence of gross disease) was achieved, which compared favorable with the 20% 5-year survival for the entire group.

Adenocarcinoma

Primary adenocarcinoma of the appendix is a rare neoplasm, with fewer than 300 total cases described worldwide.[151] The primary adenocarcinoma is a colorectal-type tumor that develops from an adenoma.[136] The mean age of presentation is 50 years and a male predominance is noted of anywhere from 4:1 to 2.8:1.[151-153] The clinical presentation in the majority of patients in the literature is acute appendicitis or an abdominal mass, though the diagnosis is rarely made preoperatively. Perforation may complicate the clinical picture, occurring in up to 40% of cases, but perforation alone has little effect on OS.[154]

Histologically, primary adenocarcinoma is distinguished from an adenoma by invasion of the wall of the appendix by the neoplastic tissue. Lymph node metastases are noted in 25% of cases at presentation.[155] Adenocarcinoma of the appendix has a metastatic potential between that of appendiceal carcinoid and colonic adenocarcinoma, with metastases developing in 20% of patients, often to the ovary.[156] The degree of metastatic involvement varies with the histologic grade; about 30% of the well-differentiated tumors are found to have metastasized, whereas nearly 70% of the poorly differentiated tumors are metastatic at the time of laparotomy.[151,152] The overall 5-year survival rate is 55% and varies with Dukes stage (A 100%, B 67%, C 50%, D 6%).[157]

The extent of tumor invasion is the most important factor when determining treatment of appendiceal adenocarcinoma. Because these tumors behave in a fashion similar to that of colonic adenocarcinomas, they must also be treated with the same aggressive surgical approach. For any lesion with invasion beyond the mucosa, right hemicolectomy with resection of draining lymph nodes is advocated.[158] In the presence of such invasion, the 5-year survival after right hemicolectomy is 60% compared with 20% after appendectomy alone.[157] For lesions truly confined to the mucosa, though there are strong advocates for both hemicolectomy and appendectomy, but the consensus is that such a lesion may be treated by appendectomy alone. Any suggestion that the tumor has extended beyond the mucosa is indication for a right hemicolectomy.[159] In one series, a second primary tumor at a distant site (colon, cervix, breast, prostate, esophagus, stomach, ovary, or bladder) was found in 11% of patients,[152] and in the series reported by Chang and Attiyeh, 32% had second tumors. This suggests some genetic role, mutation, loss of a tumor-suppressor gene, or a defect in immunosurveillance.[151]

A rare lesion of the appendix, intermediate between adenocarcinoma and carcinoid, is the adenocarcinoid. This lesion arises from the base of glands and spares the luminal mucosa; it is composed of slender tuboglandular structures, nests of goblet cells, or a mixture of both.[160] The tumor represents, at most, only 5% of all appendiceal neoplasms.[161] Despite their small size when found at celiotomy, adenocarcinoids behave quite energetically, with a propensity to metastasize to the ovaries. They should be treated aggressively with right hemicolectomy, which is considered curative if the margins are clear and there are no involved lymph nodes.

Carcinoma of the Colon and Rectum

Epidemiology

Colorectal cancer (CRC) continues to be an important health issue both globally and in the United States. It is the third most common malignant tumor and the fourth most common cause of cancer death in the world.[162] While prevalent in many countries, CRC is more common in developed nations. In the United States alone, it is estimated that 24,260 men and 25,700 women will die of CRC in 2008. In addition in the United States, CRC has the third highest incidence in both sexes with an estimated 77,250 new cases in men and 71,560 new cases in women in 2008.[163] It is thought that dietary and lifestyle habits, in conjunction with genetic factors, account for the increased incidence in developed countries. Research shows that individuals who migrate from regions where CRC is less common to regions of high incidence will inherit the risk of the host country.[164]

There are disparities in CRC incidence and mortality among races and ethnic groups. African Americans have the highest rates of both incidence and mortality when compared to the White, Asian American, American Indian, and Hispanic populations.[163] The reasons for the disparities are not entirely known, however it has been postulated that differences in access to high-quality regular screening, timely diagnosis and treatment, dietary and lifestyle factors, and socioeconomic status could play a role.[163,165]

Despite the high prevalence of CRC in the United States, both the incidence and overall mortality from CRC has been declining over the past few years. For both males and females, CRC incidence rates have decreased at a rate of approximately 2.3% between the years 1998 and 2004.[163] In addition, mortality has been declining for both sexes at a rate of 1.7% between 2002 and 2004.[163] This decline in mortality has been present, but less dramatic for the African-American population at 0.3%.[165] Studies have shown that increased screening and detection can reduce the chance of developing or dying from CRC by 10-75%, depending on which screening tests are used and how often they are performed.[166] This increased screening could also be a reason for the shift in anatomic distribution of CRC from rectum and left-sided cancers to more right-sided cancers. Data from the National Cancer Database from the years 1988 and 1993 show an increase from 51% to 55% of all CRC to be proximal to the splenic flexure.[167] Multiple studies have confirmed a higher rate of proximal colon cancer rates compared to distal colon or rectal carcinoma rates, both in the United States and globally.[167-170]

Risk Factors

Age and Racial Background ■ Age is a known risk factor for CRC. The vast majority of cases of CRC occur in people over age 50, with incidence continuing to increase thereafter.[166] The SEER statistics from the NCI between the years 2001 and 2005 report 18 cases of CRC per 100,000 for individuals under 65 and 273 cases per 100,000 for individuals 65 and older (NCI 2005). As discussed, African-American individuals have a higher incidence and mortality rate of CRC compared to other racial and ethnic populations.[165-167]

Personal or Family History ■ Patients with a personal history of adenomatous polyps or previous CRC have an increased risk of developing colon cancer in the future. Size, number, and histology of polyps are important prognostic factors, with size >1 cm, villous or tubulovillous histology, and multiple polyps conferring a greater risk for CRC.[171] Patients with an isolated tubular adenoma of <1 cm do not appear to be at an increased risk of developing CRC.[171] In patients with previous CRC, the incidence of metachronous CRC is 6% and the incidence of metachronous adenomas is 25%.[172]

Family history of CRC in a first degree relative increases the risk of developing CRC two- to threefold, while cancer in a second-degree relative increases the risk of CRC by 25-50% above average.[173,174] In addition, risk increases if there are more than one first-degree relative with colon cancer or if they are diagnosed before age 55. It is thought that having a first-degree relative with colon cancer gives a patient the same risk at age 40 that the general population has at age 50 for developing CRC.[175] Family history of colonic adenoma also increases the risk of colorectal cancer, especially if the adenoma is diagnosed early. A large or histologically advanced adenoma confers the same risk as a positive family history of CRC.[176]

Inflammatory Bowel Disease ■ UC and Crohn's disease are well-known risk factors for colorectal carcinoma. For UC, the extent of disease and the duration of disease are the primary prognostic factors. Patients with pancolitis have a 5-fold to 15-fold increased risk of developing CRC compared to a threefold increased risk with colitis limited to the left side.[177] In addition, the risk for any patient with UC increases the longer the disease is present. The risk increases from 2-8% to 18% for patients with UC at 10, 20, and 30 years after diagnosis, respectively.[178] Similar characteristics and incidence of CRC have been reported in Crohn's disease.[179,180] In Crohn's disease, long standing duration of disease and the presence of fistulas in communication with the colon are risk factors for developing CRC.[181]

Diet and Lifestyle ■ There are numerous diet and lifestyle factors that have been shown to be correlated with an increased risk of CRC. Westernized dietary habits, including an increased consumption of red meat and fat with a decreased consumption of fruits and vegetables, is associated with colorectal cancer. In terms of fruits and vegetables, there is conflicting evidence about their protective benefit, but the general consensus is that while increased consumption does not provide a protective benefit, a very low consumption does increase risk of developing CRC.[182-184] The typical Western diet also contains high levels of fats and processed red meat. A high-fat diet containing mixed lipids and saturated fat has been shown to promote colon carcinogenesis.[185] Also, high consumption of red and processed meats is associated with an increased risk of developing distal colon cancer.[186] In addition, the Cancer Prevention Study II Nutrition Cohort study found that prolonged intake of red and processed meat was associated with an increased risk of distal colon cancer, while intake of poultry and fish was protective.[187]

Obesity has also been shown to be correlated with an increased risk of CRC in both men and women.[188] A meta-analysis of 31 studies found a relative risk for CRC of 1.19, comparing obese (BMI $\geq$ 30 kg/m^2) with normal weight (BMI < 25 kg/m^2) people and 1.45 comparing those with the highest to the lowest level of central obesity.[189] In addition, physical activity is correlated with a decreased risk of CRC. One study in women found women exercising greater than 4 h/week had a 40% lower risk of colon cancer than those exercising less than 1 h/week. Similarly, a meta-analysis of 19 cohort studies found that physical activity was protective against colon cancer, but not rectal cancer.[190]

Diabetes Mellitus and Hyperinsulinemia ■ There is increasing evidence that diabetes mellitus and/or insulin resistance are risk factors for colorectal cancer. A meta-analysis of 15 studies found the estimated risk of CRC in diabetics was 30% higher than nondiabetics (RR 1.30, 95% CI 1.20-1.40).[191] A possible explanation is the hyperinsulinemia associated with diabetes or even chronic insulin treatment for diabetes.[192] Insulin is a growth factor for colonic mucosal cells and increased plasma concentrations of insulin-like growth factor (IGF)-1 have found to increase the risk for CRC while IGF-binding protein-3 was found to be correlated with a decreased risk.[193]

Alcohol and Tobacco ■ Heavy alcohol consumption, defined as greater than 30 g/d (or 2+ drinks per day), is correlated with a moderately increased risk of CRC (RR 1.07-1.41). The association becomes weaker with lower alcohol intake and is irrespective of the type of alcoholic beverage consumed.[194,195] The association between smoking and CRC is not as straightforward. Most evidence has found that cigarette smoking may have a greater impact on CRC risk in patients with certain polymorphisms. For example, two different polymorphisms in CYP1A1, a gene involved in the activation and metabolism of hydrocarbons in tobacco, confer a greater risk for CRC in cigarette smokers.[196]

Genetics

Colorectal tumorigenesis is most certainly a disease of the genes, with accumulation of genetic alterations and progressive waves of clonal expansion of cells that have a growth advantage over their progenitors. Three major categories of genes have been implicated in the development of colorectal cancer, namely oncogenes such as K-*ras*, tumor-suppressor genes such as adenomatous polyposis coli (*APC*), deleted in colorectal carcinoma (*DCC*), *p53*, and mutated in colon cancer (*MCC*), and the mismatch repair genes *hMSH2, hMLH1, hPMS*, and *hPMS2*.

CRC develops from a multistep gene mutation sequence termed loss of heterozygosity (LOH) that can be observed in inherited and sporadic colorectal cancer. Fearon and Vogelstein first postulated in 1990 that at least five genes had to be mutated in order to progress in the adenoma to carcinoma sequence.[197] Further studies showed that at least seven genetic alterations take place before the development of cancer. Important genes in the LOH model include *APC*, K-*ras*, *DCC*, and *p53*. An entirely different pathway of cancer development is initiated by defects within the mismatch repair genes. In this case, replication errors increase, leading to microsatellite instability and malfunction of the gene. This pathway is referred to as replication error (RER) and occurs in 20% of all colorectal tumors.[198] Thus, there are multiple environmental factors that may act on a genetic predisposition or acquired defects, resulting in colorectal malignancy.

***APC* Gene** ■ The *APC* gene is located on the long arm of chromosome 5 (5q). It is mutated in familial adenomatous polyposis and Gardner syndrome and in most cases of Turcot syndrome. A mutated *APC* gene is found in the majority of colorectal tumors, being detectable in 63% of adenoma and carcinoma but not in the surrounding tissues, indicating that this is a somatic mutation. Because *APC* is a tumor suppressor gene, inactivation of the second allele must occur for the cell to lose the tumor-suppressing activity of the *APC* gene. There is considerable evidence that *APC* mutations occur early and may be the first event in sporadic colorectal mutagenesis. The function of the *APC* protein is incompletely understood, but felt to be important in adhesion and communication between cells as well as in anchoring the cytoskeleton.

***DCC* Gene** ■ The *DCC* gene is located on the long arm of chromosome 18 (18q). The gene product is involved in cell-cell adhesion and cell-matrix interactions, which may be important in preventing tumor growth, invasion, and metastasis. In sporadic colorectal cancer, *DCC* seems to play a critical role in the ability of a tumor to metastasize and as such is being considered for a prognostic marker regarding the metastatic status.

***p53* Gene** ■ The *p53* gene is so named because the gene product migrates in a gel as a 53-kDa protein. It is located on the short arm of chromosome 17 (17p). p53 seems to be the most important determinant of malignancy during colorectal tumorigenesis. *p53* is considered a transcription factor because of its ability to activate expression of genes. As a tetramer, *p53* binds sequences of DNA in the promoter region of other genes to enhance their transcription.[199] Most genes activated by *p53* are thought to be involved in the inhibition of growth. Therefore, inactivation of P53 function allows unregulated cell growth. Mutations of *p53* can be found in more than half of all human cancers, making it a component in biochemical pathways central to human carcinogenesis.[200]

K-*ras* Proto-oncogene ■ K-*ras* is an oncogene, which acts in a classic dominant fashion and is located on the short arm of chromosome 12 (12p). The K-*ras* protein interacts with putative effector molecules, conveying a growth response. The signal transduction process is perturbed with a mutant K-*ras* protein leading to tumor formation. In sporadic colorectal tumors, K-*ras* mutations have been found in 47% of carcinomas and in 50% of large adenomas.[201]

Mismatch Repair Gene ■ Mismatch repair genes are needed for cells to repair DNA replication errors and spontaneous base repair loss. The four DNA mismatch repair genes found in humans are *hMSH2* (chromosome 2p), hMSH6 (chromosome 2p), *hMLH1* (chromosome 3p), *hPMS1* (chromosome 2q), and *hPMS2* (chromosome 7p). They are regarded to contribute to hereditary nonpolyposis syndrome in various percentages.[202]

Inherited Syndromes ■ Even though the vast majority of cases of CRC are sporadic rather than familial, inherited susceptibility results in a dramatic increase in risk of developing CRC. The genetic syndromes are inherited in an autosomal dominant fashion and are associated with a very high risk of developing CRC.

Familial adenomatous polyposis (FAP) is characterized by numerous colonic adenomas which appear during childhood. This autosomal dominant syndrome has penetrance approaching 100% with the onset of symptoms and diagnosis generally around age 15 years.[203] If left untreated, FAP will invariably become CRC with a mean age of diagnosis and death of 39 and 42 years, respectively.[204] An attenuated form of APC (AAPC) is a milder phenotypic variant of FAP with a similar risk for developing colorectal cancer. AAPC is characterized by fewer adenomatous polyps and an older average age of diagnosis (usually in the early 50s). Both of these inherited syndromes are caused by different germ line mutations in the same *APC* gene, which is located on chromosome 5.[205]

Hereditary nonpolyposis colorectal cancer (HNPCC) is another autosomal dominant inherited syndrome which accounts for 1-5% of all colorectal carcinomas. Also known as Lynch syndrome, this disease is characterized by an early age of onset (some patients can present in their 20s while the mean age of diagnosis is 48 years), right-sided predominance, multiple synchronous or metachronous colonic tumors, and extracolonic manifestations. The extracolonic neoplasms can include endometrial cancer, renal pelvis and ureter cancer, small bowel cancer and skin lesions including sebaceous adenomas, keratoacanthomas, and sebaceous carcinoma.[206] As described above, HNPCC is caused by a mutation in one of the mismatch repair genes. MSH6 mutations are associated with a later age of diagnosis of CRC and a higher predominance of endometrial cancer.[207]

MYH-associated polyposis (MAP) is a recently described autosomal recessive polyposis syndrome associated with a somewhat attenuated phenotype compared to other familial polyposis syndromes.[208] Mutations in *MYH*, a base excision repair gene, are associated with an increased risk of multiple adenomas or polyposis coli.[209] In patients where no *APC* gene mutation is found, especially in those patients with 10-15 or more adenomas, work-up for an *MYH* gene mutation is indicated for diagnosis.[209,210] In addition, those patients with both heterozygous and homozygous mutations are at high risk for synchronous gastrointestinal cancers with 24% colorectal cancer.

PJ is an inherited hamartomatous polyposis syndrome that predisposes to colorectal cancer. The two major manifestations of PJ are pigmented mucocutaneous lesions and multiple colonic polyps which have the ability to undergo malignant transformation. PJ is associated with an increased risk of both GI and non-GI malignancies including ovarian, breast, pancreatic, uterine, Sertoli cell, and cervical neoplasms.[211-213] Juvenile polyposis (JP) is another inherited hamartomatous polyposis syndrome that can predispose to colorectal cancer. Patients with JP are also at increased risk for gastric, duodenal, and pancreatic cancers.[214,215]

Polymorphisms ■ Numerous genetic polymorphisms (normal variations in genes) have been found to be associated with developing CRC. Changes in genes such as carcinogen metabolism genes, methylation genes, and tumor-suppressor genes can lead to either an increase or decrease in cancer risk. Cytochrome P450 genes, Glutathione-S transferase genes,

N-acetyltransferase genes, and tumor suppressor genes have all been implicated in colorectal cancer. Cytochrome P450A1 (CYP1A1) is a phase I enzyme which acts on carcinogens found in tobacco smoke.[216] Polymorphisms such as A-->G at Ile462Val, exon 7 in the gene for CYP1A1 puts patients at an increased risk for developing CRC.[217] As mentioned above, patients who smoke cigarettes are especially at risk when they carry a polymorphism in this gene.

Glutathione-*S*-transferases are phase II enzymes responsible for the detoxification of mutagenic electrophiles, including polyaromatic hydrocarbons.[216] Glutathione-*S*-transferase Mu (GSTM1) and Theta (GSTT1) have both been discussed in relationship to colorectal cancer. In addition, *N*-acetyltransferases are phase II enzymes involved in detoxifyin arylamines, which are found in cooked meat.[216] Both GSTT1 and NAT2 rapid acetylator phenotype have been identified as causing an increased risk for CRC.[218]

The most common tumor repressor gene associated with CRC is the *APC* gene. A polymorphism at I1307K, found predominantly in the Ashkenazi Jewish population, confers a twofold increase in CRC risk.[219] Another polymorphism in the *APC* gene, I1317Q, also increases the risk of colorectal cancer.[220]

Some polymorphisms have been shown to be protective against CRC. Patients who eat a low fat diet and who are homozygous for a variant APC gene at codon 1822 have a reduced risk of colon cancer compared to those patients who are wild-type and eat a high-fat diet.[221] In addition, variations in a methylation gene for methylenetetrahydrofolate reductase (MTHFR), has been shown to influence CRC risk. Patients who carry the MTHFR 677TT genotype have a reduced risk of colorectal cancer.[222]

Presentation, Screening and Surveillance

Signs and Symptoms ■ The presentation of large-bowel malignancy generally falls into three categories: insidious onset of chronic symptoms, acute onset of intestinal obstruction, or acute perforation. The most common presentation is that of an insidious onset of chronic symptoms (77-92%), followed by obstruction (6-16%) and perforation with local or diffuse peritonitis (2-7%).[223-225]

Bleeding is the most common symptom of colorectal malignancy.[226] Unfortunately, patient and physician alike often attribute the bleeding to hemorrhoids. The error in this thinking was highlighted in a study in which 20% of patients over 40 years of age with rectal bleeding had colorectal neoplasia; 6% had colorectal adenocarcinoma and 14% had polyps. Bleeding may be occult or it may be seen as stool that is black, maroon or bright red depending on the location of the malignancy. Occult bleeding may present with iron-deficiency anemia and associated fatigue.

Change in bowel habits is the second most common complaint, with patients noting either diarrhea or constipation.[226] Constipation is more often associated with left-sided lesions because the diameter of the colon is smaller and the stool is more formed than on the right side. Patients may report a gradual change in the caliber of the stool or may have diarrhea if the narrowing has progressed sufficiently to cause obstruction. Carcinomas of the right side of the colon do not typically present with changes in bowel habits, but large amounts of mucus generated by a tumor may cause diarrhea, and large right-sided lesions or lesions involving the ileocecal valve may cause obstruction.

Abdominal pain is as common a presentation as change in bowel habits.[227] Left-sided obstructing lesions may present with cramping abdominal pain, associated with nausea and vomiting, and relieved with bowel movements. Right-sided malignancies may result in vague pain that is difficult to localize. Rectal lesions may present with tenesmus, but pelvic pain is generally associated with advanced disease after the tumor has involved the sacral or sciatic nerves. Less common symptoms include weight loss, malaise, fever, abdominal mass, and symptoms of urinary tract involvement (frequency, pneumaturia, and fecaluria). Bacteremia with *Streptococcus bovis* is highly suggestive of colorectal malignancy.[228,229]

Acute onset of intestinal obstruction was the presenting feature of 15% of 23,500 patients reported in 26 series. The symptoms of bowel obstruction, reviewed earlier, may be noted.[230] Physical exam is often unrevealing because the abdomen is distended, and masses, primary or metastatic, are not palpable. Tympany, ascites, and distention may be all that is noted on abdominal exam. Rectal exam will only rarely reveal an obstructing tumor. Colorectal malignancy should always be considered when patients present with large-bowel obstruction. The history, physical exam, and plain films of the abdomen may suggest the diagnosis. It may be confirmed with contrast enema, rigid or flexible endoscopy, or CT scans of the abdomen and pelvis.

Perforation is the third general class of presentation of colorectal malignancy. It may result in localized or generalized peritonitis or, if walled off, it may present with obstruction or fistula to an adjacent structures such as the bladder. Concurrent obstruction and perforation occurs in 12-19% of patients with obstruction.[231,232] When the perforation occurs proximal to the obstructing lesion, as with perforation of a dilated cecum proximal to an obstructing sigmoid carcinoma, the patients present with diffuse peritonitis and sepsis. Emergent surgical intervention after adequate fluid resuscitation is clearly indicated. However, in the case of perforation at the tumor, possibly secondary to tumor necrosis, the more indolent course may lead to confusion of the perforated tumor with inflammation associated with appendicitis, diverticulitis, or Crohn's disease.

Screening and Surveillance

Cancer screening refers to the testing of a population of apparently asymptomatic individuals to determine the risk of developing colorectal cancer. Surveillance refers to the ongoing monitoring of individuals who have an increased risk for the development of the disease. For colorectal cancer, surveillance is reserved for patients with inflammatory bowel disease, family cancer syndromes and those with a previous history of CRC or colorectal adenomas. Various screening and surveillance modalities are available to detect colorectal cancers and adenomatous polyps. Current screening and surveillance recommendations are listed below (Table 89-1).

Fecal Occult Blood Testing (FOBT) ■ Testing the stool for fecal occult blood was one the first tests used in CRC screening. The advantage of fecal occult testing includes availability, convenience, and low cost. Limitations include low sensitivity, low specificity, low compliance and inability to detect adenomas. Sensitivity is affected by slide storage, ascorbic acid, lesions not bleeding at the time of testing, and degradation of hemoglobin by colonic bacteria. Specificity is adversely affected by exogenous peroxidase activity by red meat and uncooked vegetables, and medications that may induce bleeding from noncolonic sources such as aspirin and other nonsteroidal anti-inflammatory drugs. In five large controlled studies including more than 300,000 patients, an increased detection of CRC in earlier stages was demonstrated,[233,234] and showed a significant reduction in mortality between 15% and 43%.[233-237] While office-based FOBT after digital rectal exam is not recommended as a stand-alone screening method, when the test is performed annually after the age of 50 on three consecutive stool samples, malignancy is detected at an earlier stage than if no screening is performed; making it a good option for those who refuse more invasive options.[238]

Table 89-1 US Multisociety Task Force on Colorectal Cancer (CRC): Screening Recommendations

Risk Category	Screening and Surveillance Recommendations
Asymptomatic: Average-risk, age 50 or greater	Flexible sigmoidoscopy or DCBE every 5 years or colonoscopy every 10 years starting at age 50
First-degree relative with CRC or adenomatous polyps at age 60 or greater, or two second-degree relatives affected with CRC	Colonoscopy every 10 years starting at age 40
First-degree relative with CRC or adenomatous polyps at age younger than 60 or two or more first-degree relative with CRC	Colonoscopy every 5 years starting at age 40 or 10 years younger than earliest family diagnosis
Gene carrier or at risk for familial adenomatous polyposis	Flexible sigmoidoscopy every year beginning at age 10-12
Gene carrier or at risk for hereditary nonpolyposis colorectal cancer	Colonoscopy every 1-2 years beginning at age 20-25 or 10 years younger than earliest family diagnosis

Flexible Sigmoidoscopy ■ Both rigid and flexible sigmoidoscopies are inexpensive, require no conscious sedation, are relatively safe (1-2 perforations per 10,000), and afford direct visualization and biopsy of polyps and cancers.[239] The advantage of the flexible sigmoidoscope over the rigid is that the 60-cm flexible scope allows the clinician to reach the descending colon and even the splenic flexure. The disadvantage of sigmoidoscopy is that the entire colon is not visualized with either procedure and lesions may be missed in the proximal bowel. Current American Cancer Society (ACS) screening recommendations are for sigmoidoscopy every 5 years with subsequent full colonoscopy if adenomatous disease is found.

Barium Enema ■ Barium enema combined with sigmoidoscopy allows for visualization of the entire colon and rectum. Single-contrast barium enema is significantly less sensitive and specific than double-contrast barium enema (DCBE) and should not be used as a screening tool for colorectal malignancy. DCBE has a sensitivity of 50% to 80% for polyps less than 1 cm, 70% to 90% for polyps greater than 1 cm, and 55% to 85% for stage I and II carcinomas.[240-242] When combined with sigmoidoscopy, the sensitivity reaches 98% and 99% for carcinomas and adenomas respectively.[243] Perforation as a result of DCBE has been reported at a rate of 1 per 25,000 studies.[244] Current ACS screening recommendations are for a barium enema every 5 years with subsequent colonoscopy if test results are positive.

Colonoscopy ■ Examination of the entire colon by colonoscopy is the gold standard CRC screening method. When performed by trained endoscopists, colonoscopy with polypectomy is a safe procedure with a perforation incidence of 0.1%, hemorrhage incidence of 0.3% and a mortality of 0.01% to 0.03%. The cecum is visualized in up to 98.6% of patients and a DCBE may be performed when the cecum is not reached.[245-250] Studies have shown that detecting and removing polyps reduces the incidence of colorectal malignancy, that detecting earlier lesions decreases disease-related mortality, and that fewer carcinomas develop in patients who have colonoscopy and polypectomy.[251,252] Colonoscopy is better than DCBE in detecting lesions <1 cm.[242] Furthermore, a tissue diagnosis or therapeutic intervention may be made at the time of initial evaluation. Colonoscopy also compares favorable with sigmoidoscopy because the entire colon may be directly visualized. In one study, a prevalence of 24% of new adenomas was found when 226 patients underwent colonoscopy within 1 year of flexible sigmoidoscopy. Advanced lesions proximal to the descending colon were found in 6% of these patients.[253] Current ACS screening recommendations are for a colonoscopy every 10 years.

CT Colonography ■ CT colonography (virtual colonoscopy) is an emerging technique for the diagnosis of colonic polyps in the screening population, that uses 3-dimensional reconstruction of the air distended colon. At the National Naval Medical Center, in 1223 average-risk adults who subsequently underwent conventional colonoscopy, virtual colonoscopy was as good or better at detecting relevant lesions.[254] However, it may be less accurate in surveillance populations, and subsequent multi-institutional studies have failed to confirm the excellent results from this series. The major limitations include uncertain accuracy, need for full bowel preparation, and follow-up colonoscopy for tissue diagnosis of radiographic abnormalities. Because virtual colonoscopy is considerably time and labor intensive from the standpoint of the radiologist, active investigations into methods of automating the evaluation process are ongoing. Current ACS screening recommendations are for a virtual colonoscopy every 5 years with subsequent colonoscopy if lesion found.

Preoperative Work-up and Staging

The general physical examination remains a cornerstone in assessing a patient preoperatively to determine the extent of local disease, disclosing distant metastases, and appraising the general operative risk. Special interest should be pain weight loss, pallor as a sign of anemia, and signs of portal hypertension. In addition, a complete workup-should include routine lab work, colonoscopy, chest x-ray, CT of the abdomen and pelvis, and transrectal ultrasound (TRUS) for those with rectal cancer.

Routine Laboratory Work ■ A complete blood count (CBC) may reveal the presence of anemia. Liver function tests (LFTs) may be abnormal in the case of liver metastases. Carcinoembryonic antigen (CEA) levels should be obtained as a baseline against which further values may be compared. Metastatic disease to the liver is often accompanied with very high levels of CEA, and levels surpassing 10 to 20 ng/mL are associated with increased chances of treatment failure for both node-negative and node-positive patients.[255]

Colonoscopy ■ Colonoscopy remains the single most important investigation in the evaluation of colonic diseases. It allows assessment of tumor size, but not depth of invasion, as well as localization in the colon. Further histology from the tumor can be obtained, synchronous tumors are detected, and synchronous polyps may be removed. Synchronous carcinomas occur in 2% to 7% of patients and synchronous polyps 29.7% of the time.[256] It has been suggested that preoperative colonoscopy alters the operative procedure in 30% of patients.[257]

Radiologic Evaluation ■ A chest x-ray rules out pulmonary lesions and serves as a rough guideline for cardiac as well as pulmonary status. The use of CT of the abdomen and pelvis in the preoperative evaluation of patients with colon cancer is controversial. It is our practice to obtain a CT in order to detect involvement of contiguous organs, para-aortic lymph nodes and the liver. Abnormal LFT's are present in only 15% of patients with liver metastases and may be elevated without liver metastases in up to 40%.[258] Therefore, we do not believe LFT's are a useful screening tool for determining the need for obtaining a CT scan. Transcutaneous abdominal ultrasound can be used in select patient to identify liver metastases, ascites, and gross adenopathy.

PET and now PET-CT, has emerged as a potentially important imaging modality for colorectal cancer. Using the glucose analog, fluorodeoxyglucose, metabolically active tissues are visualized. The standardized uptake value can provide a semiquantitative determination to help discriminate benign from malignant disease. Although potentially useful in recurrent cancer, it has not been helpful in the primary evaluation of patients with colon cancer due to false positive and high costs.

Transrectal ultrasound has become an invaluable component of preoperative assessment in rectal cancer patients. The layers of the rectal wall can be identified and the depth of penetration determined. Sensitivity ranges from 55% to 100% and specificity from 24% to 100% in different studies. The status of lymph nodes also can be predicted in 73% to 85%.[259] The depth of invasion and lymph node status is especially important if local excision is considered.

Staging ■ Staging systems are important for predicting outcomes, selecting patients for various therapies, and comparing therapies for like patients across institutions. For a tumor to be considered as an invasive cancer and staged, it must penetrate through the muscularis mucosa. Malignant cells superficial to this layer are thought to lack metastatic potential because of a paucity of lymphatic's and are considered carcinoma in situ. In 1932, Dukes proposed a classification based on the degree of direct extension along with the presence or absence of regional lymphatic metastases for the staging of rectal cancer, see table below. The TNM classification was proposed by the American College of Surgeons' Commission on Cancer to incorporate findings at laparotomy, see table below. The stages of the TNM system roughly correlate to the stages with Dukes' classification (Table 89-2).

Classification of histological grade, cell type, lymphatic, venous or perineural invasion, tumor ploidy, CEA level, presence of bowel perforation, and distal and tangential margins allow for further subclassification of the tumors and improved prognostication. The American Joint Committee on Cancer (AJCC) has settled on two grading classifications, low grade (well and moderately differentiated) and high grade (poorly and undifferentiated). DNA ploidy assessment is the measurement of the quantum amount of DNA in cells. Diploidy is correlated with good prognosis while aneuploidy is correlated with poor prognosis. Bowel perforation and elevated preoperative CEA are associated with poorer prognosis.

Although there are conflicting data on the relative power of various markers, in particular p53 expression and K-ras mutation, there is no evidence that any of these parameters singly or in combination replace or add significantly to the power of the conventional staging system.[260] Similarly, a variety of immunohistochemistry stains have been used in the recent years, but none appear clinically important.

Surgical Management of Colorectal Cancer

Management of Carcinoma in a Polyp ■ With the implementation of colonoscopic screening, colon cancers are being detected at earlier stages, including those that appear to be confined to or arise from an adenomatous polyp. These "malignant polyps," have their invasion limited to the submucosa. Their propensity for lymph node metastasis appears to be related to a number of histopathologic features including grade, presence of perineural/perivascular invasion, and overall gross morphology, sessile versus pedunculated.

The Haggitt classification system is used to define the depth of involvement of carcinoma into a polyp (Table 89-3). The risk of lymph node metastasis in Haggitt level 1, 2, and 3 lesions is less than 1%, and these lesions can usually be managed with complete endoscopic excision and India ink tattooing of the polypectomy site.[261] In these cases, careful colonoscopic surveillance of the polypectomy site is recommended. However, lymphovascular invasion, poor differentiation, or cancer close to the polypectomy resection margin (less than 2 mm) is usually an indication for a colectomy because of the increased risk of lymph node metastasis. In those scenarios, it is essential that the family be informed of the potential for not detecting cancer at all in the bowel wall or mesenteric lymph nodes of the resected specimen. Haggit level 4 lesions however, have an increased incidence of lymph node metastasis (12-25%) and should be managed with a colectomy.[261] In general, sessile polyps of the colon containing cancer should be managed with a colectomy as they are by definition Haggit level 4.

Most polyps throughout the colon can be removed through the colonoscope using the snare polypectomy technique. The polyp is visualized through the colonoscope, the snare wire is looped around the polyp and gently tightened while the electric current is applied. Whenever possible the polyp is retrieved for histology. When performed by trained endoscopists, colonoscopy with polypectomy is a safe procedure, with a perforation incidence of 0.3% to 1% and a hemorrhage incidence of 0.7% to 2.5%.[262]

Standard Resection Margins and Techniques ■ ***Bowel Preparation*** ■ Despite recent evidence challenging the benefit of mechanical bowel preparation, it remains a cornerstone in modern colorectal surgery. Mechanical cleansing may be accomplished by the use of vigorous laxatives along with repeated enemas until clearing. Until recently, an oral lavage with a polyethylene glycol hypertonic electrolyte solution such as GoLYTELY was used extensively. More recently, oral phospho-soda preparations have become increasingly popular but their use can be associated with fluid and electrolyte abnormalities.

Antibiotic Administration ■ Although there is no question that the preoperative antibiotic administration is beneficial in elective and emergency colorectal surgery,

Table 89-2 ■ **AJCC TNM Staging System for Colorectal Cancer**

TX	Primary tumor cannot be assessed
T0	No evidence of primary tumor
Tis	Carcinoma in situ
T1	Tumor invades into submucosa
T2	Tumor invades into muscularis propria
T3	Tumor invades through muscularis propria
T4a	Tumor perforates visceral peritoneum
T4b	Tumor directly invades other structures
NX	Regional lymph nodes cannot be assessed
N0	No regional lymph nodes
N1	1-3 lymph nodes
N2	4 or more lymph nodes
N3	Regional lymph nodes along with a named vascular trunk
MX	Presence of distant metastasis cannot be assessed
M0	No distant metastases
M1	Distant metastases

Stage	Depth	Nodal Status	Distant Metastasis
Stage 0	Tis	N0	M0
Stage I	T1, T2	N0	M0
Stage IIA	T3	N0	M0
Stage IIB	T4	N0	M0
Stage IIIA	T1-T2	N1	M0
Stage IIIB	T3-T4	N1	M0
Stage IIIC	Any T	N2	M0
Stage IV	Any T	Any N	M1

Dukes Staging System

Dukes	Tumor	Node Status	Distant Disease
A	Tis, T1, T2, T3	N0	M0
B	T4	N0	M0
C1	T1, T2, T3	Any N (except N0)	M0
C2	T4	Any N (except N0)	M0
D	Any T	Any N	M1

Table 89-3 ■ **Haggitt Classification of Malignant Polyps**

Haggit Level	Characteristics
0	Carcinoma in situ
1	Carcinoma invading into submucosa but limited to head of polyp
2	Carcinoma invading level of neck of polyp
3	Carcinoma invading stalk
4	Carcinoma invading submucosa below the stalk (above the muscularis propria)

the route of administration and antibiotic combination remains a matter of debate. Most surgeons start antibiotic prophylaxis at the day of operation using a combination to cover gram-positive, gram-negative, aerobic and anaerobic bacteria. Whether the antibiotic is given orally after bowel prep, such as erythromycin and neomycin, or intravenously, such as a second-generation cephalosporin, does not appear to matter so long as the antibiotic is administered before skin incision.

Right-Sided Colon Cancers ■ Cancers of the right colon account for up to 30% of primary colorectal cancers.[263] Patients with adenocarcinoma involving the cecum or ascending colon who do not have HNPCC or other synchronous lesions should be treated with a right hemicolectomy (Fig. 89-1A). The ileocolic, right colic (which is a branch of the ileocolic artery in over 85% of the cases and often not a separate artery of the SMA), and right branch of the middle colic arteries and veins should be ligated near their origin to assure an adequate lymphadenectomy. Approximately 5 to 10 cm of distal small intestine should be resected in continuity with the right colon to assure adequate blood supply at the stapled edge of the small intestine.

Transverse Colon Cancers ■ Transverse colon cancers are relatively uncommon, accounting for only 10% of colorectal primaries.[263] Lesions of the proximal and mid-transverse colon are usually best managed with an extended right hemicolectomy involving ligation of the ileocolic, right colic, and middle colic vessels (Fig. 89-1B). The ascending colon, hepatic flexure, transverse colon, and splenic flexures are removed with anastomosis of the ileum to the descending colon. It is advisable to avoid an anastomosis between the hepatic and splenic flexure because of concerns over adequacy of blood supply and tension at the anastomosis as the ascending and descending colon tend to migrate to and land in their anatomic position within the lateral gutters.

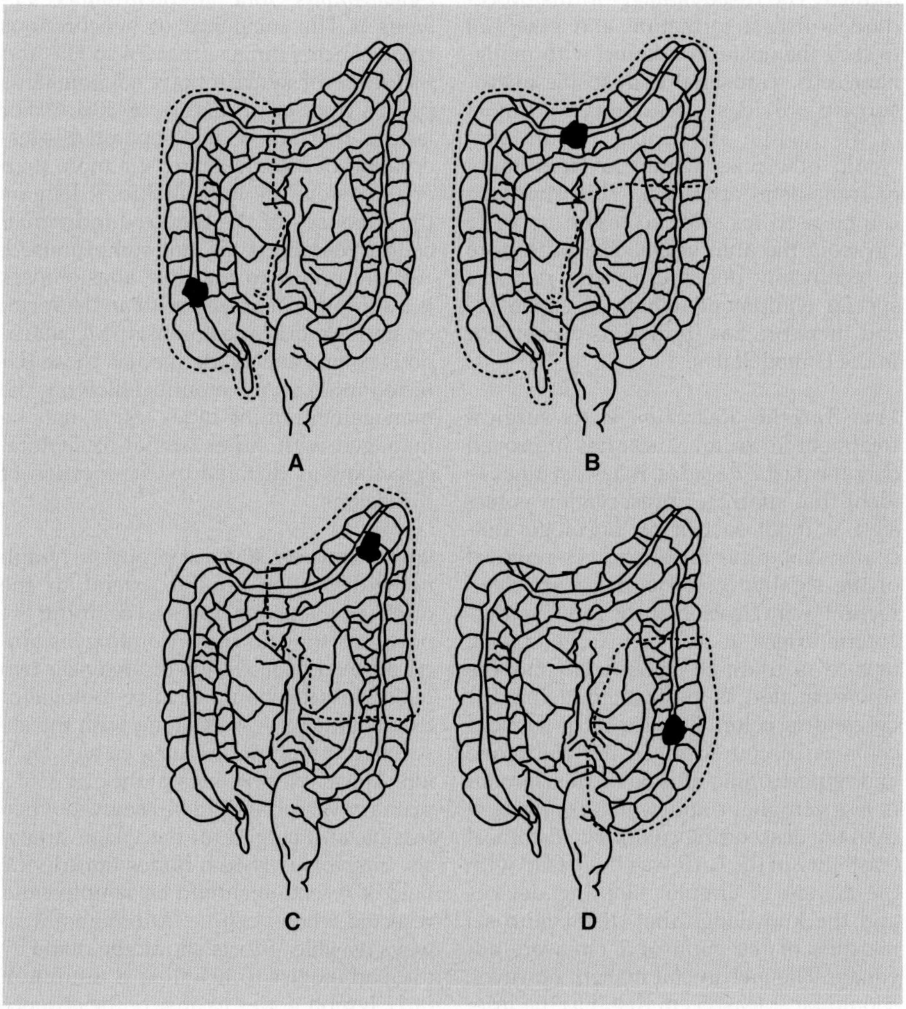

Figure 89-1 ■ Extent of resection for colon carcinoma: (**A**) Cecal or ascending colon cancer; (**B**) transverse colon cancer; (**C**) splenic flexure colon cancer; (**D**) sigmoid colon cancer. *Abbreviations*: ICA, ileocolic artery; IMA, inferior mesenteric artery; LCA, left colic artery; MCA, middle colic artery; RCA, right colic artery; SA, sigmoidal arteries; SHA, superior hemorrhoidal (rectal) artery.

Left Sided Colon Cancers ■ Lesions of the splenic flexure and descending colon are also uncommon, accounting for 15% of colorectal primaries.[263] Splenic flexure cancers may be managed with an extended right or left hemicolectomy (Fig. 89-1C). Cancers in the descending colon may be managed with a left hemicolectomy involving division of the left colic artery, preservation of the left branch of the middle colic artery, and anastomosis of the distal transverse colon to the distal sigmoid colon following a full splenic flexure mobilization. Alternatively, a left hemicolectomy may be performed with ligation of the inferior mesenteric vessels and an anastomosis between the transverse colon and the upper rectum.

Sigmoid Colon Cancers ■ Tumors of the sigmoid colon are common, accounting for 25% of colorectal primaries.[263] These tumors are usually removed by means of an anterior sigmoid colectomy, which usually involves division of the inferior mesenteric artery either above or below the left colic artery and the superior rectal arteries within the upper mesorectum with anastomosis of the descending colon to the upper rectum (Fig. 89-1D). Large, bulky sigmoid cancers located above the peritoneal reflection but at the level of the pelvic inlet present a unique challenge as their posterolateral borders abut the ureters, hypogastric nerves, and iliac vessels. Proper preoperative planning based on optimal imaging and consideration of ureteral stent placement is essential. In selected cases, preoperative chemoradiation has proven beneficial by virtue of tumor bulk reduction facilitating negative margins of resection while preserving important posterolateral structures.

Subtotal Colectomy ■ This resection involves the removal of the entire colon to the rectum with an ileorectal anastomosis. This procedure is indicated for multiple synchronous colonic tumors that are not confined to a single anatomical distribution, for selected patients with FAP with minimal rectal involvement (discussed below), or for selected patients with HNPCC and colon cancer. Although an excellent quality of life can be achieved after ileorectostomy, frequent loose bowel movements are common. Patients should be counseled regarding a bowel regimen and perianal care.

Total Proctocolectomy ■ The surgical treatment of FAP depends on the age of the patient, and the polyp density in the rectum. Surgical options include proctocolectomy with Brooke ileostomy, total abdominal colectomy with ileorectal anastomosis (IRA), or restorative proctocolectomy with ileal-pouch anal anastomosis (IPAA). Proctocolectomy with continent ileostomy is rarely performed today. Total abdominal colectomy with ileorectal anastomosis has a low complication rate, provides good functional results, and is a viable option for patients with fewer than 20 adenomas in the rectum. These patients must be observed with 6-month proctoscopic examinations to remove polyps and detect signs of cancer. If rectal polyps become too numerous completion proctectomy with Brooke ileostomy or IPAA, when technically possible, is warranted. The Cleveland Clinic has recently evaluated their registry of patients with FAP who were treated with IRA or IPAA. Prior to the use of IPAA for patients with high rectal polyp burdens, the risk of cancer in the retained rectum was 12.9% at a median follow-up of over 17 years.[264] Because of the use of IPAA for patients with large rectal polyp burdens and the selected use of IRA for those with small rectal polyp burdens, no patient has developed rectal cancer in the remaining rectum at a median follow-up of 5 years. Restorative proctocolectomy with IPAA has the advantage of removing all or nearly all large intestine mucosa at risk of cancer, while preserving transanal defecation. Complication rates are low when the procedure is done in large centers, but morbidity includes incontinence, multiple loose stools, impotence, retrograde ejaculation, dyspareunia, and pouchitis. Approximately 7% of patients have to be converted to permanent ileostomy due to complications from the procedure.[264]

Rectal Cancers ■ The surgical approach to rectal tumors depends upon depth of invasion and distance from the anal verge. The four categories include transanal approaches, transsacral approaches, LAR with total mesorectal excision (TME) and APR.

Local Excision ■ Local treatment alone as definitive therapy of rectal cancer was first applied to patients with severe comorbidities unable to tolerate radical surgery. Currently, conservative sphincter-saving local approaches are being more widely considered. Early studies of local excision have shown up to a 97% local control rate and 80% DFS for properly selected individuals.[265] Local treatment is best applied to T1 rectal cancers within 10 cm of the anal verge, tumors less than 3 cm in diameter involving less than one-fourth of the circumference of the rectal wall, highly mobile exophytic tumors, and tumors of low histologic grade. The decision to use local excision alone or to employ adjuvant therapy after local excision is based on the pathological characteristics of the primary cancer and the potential for micrometastases in draining lymph nodes. T1 lesions have positive lymph nodes in up to 18% of cases, whereas the rate for T2 ad T3 lesions is up to 38% and 70%, respectively. T2 tumors treated with local resection alone can have recurrence rates of 15% to 44%.[265] It is therefore our practice to treat T1 lesions with poor prognostic features and all T2 tumors with radical surgery. If local excision is performed, adjuvant therapy and close surveillance should be part of the treatment plan.

Local excision of distal rectal cancers can be accomplished by transanal excision, posterior proctectomy (Kraske procedure), or transanal endoscopic microsurgery. Transanal excision is the most straightforward approach and involves using the perirectal fat as the deep plane of dissection to achieve adequate circumferential margins of 1 cm. The Kraske procedure can be used for tumors in the middle and upper rectum and is more suitable for larger rectal lesions than transanal excision. In this procedure, a perineal incision is made just above the anus, the coccyx is removed, fascia divided and a proctectomy performed. The disadvantage of this procedure is fistula formation and potential to seed the posterior wound with malignant cells. Transanal endoscopic microsurgery provides accessibility to tumors of the middle and upper rectum that would otherwise require a laparotomy or transsacral approach. This approach can be used for selected lesion up to 15 cm from the anal verge. The procedure is technically demanding and requires special equipment, which is expensive and therefore has limited its acceptance in the United States.

Low Anterior Resection ■ As surgical treatment for rectal cancer has improved over the past 2 decades, it has become evident that sphincter preservation is feasible without sacrificing oncologic outcomes. The procedure involves removal of the sigmoid colon and the involved rectum, with ligation of the inferior mesenteric artery at its origin. The splenic flexure is routinely mobilized and the reconstruction is performed using the descending colon. The use of the sigmoid colon is discouraged, as the thickened and hypertrophic muscle of the sigmoid is less compliant and well vascularized than the descending colon. The technical feasibility of the LAR was increased with the advent of circular stapling devices and the knowledge that distal mucosal margins of resection of 2 cm were adequate. The mesorectal margin however, should be at least 5 cm distal to the inferior aspect of the tumor or to the end of the mesorectum at the pelvic floor. The technique of TME, which involves sharp excision and extirpation of the mesorectum by dissecting outside the investing fascia of the mesorectum, optimizes the oncologic operation by not only removing draining lymph nodes, but also maximizing lateral resection margins around the tumor. The effort at sphincter preservation was further enhanced by the results of the National Surgical Adjuvant Breast and Bowel Project (NSABP) R-03 trial which showed that neoadjuvant therapy was effective in converting probable APRs into sphincter-preserving operations.[266]

Abdominal Perineal Resection ■ For those patients who have cancers that overlap or abut the sphincter or who are incontinent of stool preoperatively, a combined approach of transabdominal and transperineal dissection is performed to remove the rectal specimen en bloc. Once the rectal specimen is removed via the perineal opening, the perineum is sutured closed and a permanent colostomy is created. The pelvis may be covered with omentum to keep small bowel out if radiation is contemplated.

Synchronous and Metachronous Lesions ■ The incidence of synchronous colon cancers ranges from 2% to 11% and incidence of synchronous adenomatous polyps may be in excess of 30%.[263] For lesions that are widely separated, preservation of colonic length via more than one anastomosis is desirable as long as the adequacy of the required individual cancer resections are not compromised. An alternative to multiple anastomoses is a subtotal colectomy with an ileorectal or ileosigmoid anastomosis. Metachronous colon cancers, defined as those detected more than 6 months following the management of the index lesion, may be managed with either partial or subtotal colectomy as dictated by the location of the lesions.

Lymphadenectomy ■ An appropriate lymph node dissection should extend to the origin of the primary vessel draining the portion of the colon incorporating the cancer. Resection of a lesion located near two major vessels should involve removal of the two major vessels along with the associated lymph nodes in an en bloc fashion. Apical lymph nodes, at the origin of a primary vessel, should be removed when feasible and tagged for pathologic analysis. Suspicious lymph nodes outside the field of resection should be sampled and resected when positive. Although not always feasible, efforts should be made by the pathologist to examine a minimum of 12 lymph nodes to ensure the absence of lymph node metastasis.[267,268] Although several series have demonstrated that sentinel node mapping and biopsy is feasible in patients with colon cancer, its true clinical utility in the management of patients with colon cancer awaits further investigation.[269]

Laparoscopic Colectomy ■ Laparoscopic resection of the colon was first described in 1990.[270] The proposed benefits to laparoscopic colectomy include a shorter recovery time and less narcotic use than the traditional open procedure. The technique of a laparoscopically-assisted colon resection consists of an intracorporal approach to explore the abdomen and mobilize the colon. The bowel is then exteriorized through a small incision for extracorporal resection and anastomosis. There was some initial concern regarding the ability to achieve an adequate oncologic resection and concern about the frequency of port-site recurrences using the laparoscopic technique for colon cancer.[271] However, the results of four large randomized trials, three of which have long-term follow-up, have provided solid evidence demonstrating laparoscopic colectomy in patients with colon cancer to be an accepted alternative to open colectomy.[272-275]

Three prospective randomized trials, Barcelona, Clinical Outcomes of Surgical Therapy Study Group (COST), and Conventional versus Laparoscopic-Assisted Surgery in Colorectal Cancer (CLASICC) have reported long-term follow-up data on the equivalence of laparoscopic colectomy to open colectomy for colon cancer.[272-274,276,277] Only short-term results are as yet available from the Colon Cancer Laparoscopic or Open Resection (COLOR) trial.[275] The first long-term cancer data from the single-center Barcelona study showed cancer-related survival was significantly higher in the laparscopically-assisted group than in the open surgery group.[272] This was accounted for by the significant improvement in cancer-related survival observed in patients with stage III colon cancer while there were no differences in patients with stage I or II disease. However, the COST and CLASICC trials showed no such differences between the two groups.[273,274] In a recent follow-up report of the COST trial, 5-year OS, 5-year DFS, recurrence rates, and sites of first recurrence were similar between groups.[276] Similarly, in a recent follow-up report from the CLASICC trial (which also included patients who underwent laparoscopically-assisted excision of rectal cancer), there were no differences at 3 years in OS, DFS, or local recurrence between the laparoscopic-assisted surgery group and the conventionally treated (open) group.[277] While no long-term data is yet available from the COLOR trial, patient benefits including earlier recovery of bowel function, need for fewer analgesics, and shorter hospital stay were reported in the laparoscopic cohort.[275] In all four studies, hospital stay was shorter while operating time for laparoscopically-assisted colectomy was longer.[272-275] The length of ileus was significantly less with laparoscopic colectomy in both the CLASICC and COST trials while the COST trial also observed significantly less time of use of oral analgesics with laprascopic colectomy.[273,274] While these short-term patient benefits have been observed, it is unclear if long-term patient benefits exist. In the CLASICC trial, no significant difference in the quality of life at 3 years for all scales was observed between the two groups.[277] In a meta-analysis of the four trials which included over 1500 patients, 3-year DFS and OS after laparoscopically assisted or open resection were similar, and disease-free OS rates for stages I, II, and III evaluated separately did not differ between the two treatments.[278] Laparoscopic-assisted colectomy when performed by experienced surgeons has proven to be an equivalent oncologic operation compared to open colectomy for patients with colon cancer.[279] Future directions in the study of the laparoscopic technique include maturation of more long-term data, appropriate patient selection for laparoscopic versus open procedures, and evaluating the cost-effectiveness of the laparoscopic technique. The rates of conversion to an open procedure from the COLOR, COST, and CLASICC trial were 17%, 21%, and 29% respectively.[273-275] Patients in the CLASICC trial treated with a converted procedure had higher complication rates making the selection of appropriate patients for laparoscopic surgery important.[274] The cost-effectiveness of the laparoscopic technique given the longer operating time and the advanced surgical training required also requires further evaluation.

The investigational experience with laparoscopic rectal cancer resection is not as complete as the data for laparoscopic colectomy. Surgical resection is an extremely important treatment modality for rectal cancer. The standard for middle and low rectal cancers is precise TME as described by Heald.[280] TME and adequacy of resection margins are associated with low recurrence and optimal survival.[281] Laparoscopic resection of rectal cancer must be able to achieve the same oncologic outcomes. The laparoscopic technique for rectal cancer involves transection of the distal bowel and mesorectum intracorporally and the division of the remaining mesentary and proximal bowel done extracorporally. An intracorporal end-to-end anastamosis is performed by positioning the anvil of the stapler in the descending colon and inserting the circular stapler through the rectum.[282,283] For low rectal cancers requiring laparoscopically-assisted APR, the mobilized rectum with mesorectum is retrieved through the perineal incision in the traditional fashion and the perineal wound is closed primarily.[283] Currently, laparoscopically-assisted resection of rectal cancer has not been definitely proven to be as oncologically effective as open surgery although currently available data strongly favors such a conclusion.

Several single-center case series of laparoscopically-assisted resection of rectal cancer have reported on the safety and feasibility of using the laparoscopic approach.[283-286] There have been two prospective randomized trials comparing laparoscopic and open techniques for resection of rectosigmoid cancer including the subset of patients in the CLASICC trial.[274,277,287] An initial observation in the CLASICC trial was a nonsignificant difference in the circumferential resection margin (CRM) positivity in patients undergoing laparascopically assisted anterior resection compared to those undergoing standard open LAR, a difference not seen in the APR laparoscopic procedure group. However, in a follow-up report, the higher positivity of CRM did not translate into an increased incidence of local recurrence.[277] This finding may have been a result of small numbers of patients and needs further investigation. Other results from this trial were discussed above in the laparoscopic colectomy section. In the other randomized trial which did not include any laparoscopically-assisted APR's (thereby only included sigmoid and upper rectal cancers), the were no significant differences in the probabilities of 5-year survival, 5-year DFS, or tumor recurrence.[287] Postoperative recovery was significantly better for the laparoscopic group while the operative time was significantly longer and the cost higher in the laparoscopic group.[287] Two meta-analyses have also been performed.[288,289] Aziz et al. analyzed a total of over 2000 patients and found no significant differences in the proportion of patients with positive radial margins or the number of lymph nodes harvested when considering the laparoscopic rectal cancer surgery, open rectal cancer, laparoscopic APR, and open APR groups.[288] Time to stomal function, first bowel movement, and length of hospital stay were significantly reduced after laparoscopic surgery. In the set of patients undergoing laparoscopically-assisted APR, a reduced rate of postoperative wound infection was observed.[288] In the other meta-analysis, short-term outcomes reported included a significantly lower morbidity but longer operating times in the laparoscopically resected group.[289] In addition, there was no difference in wound healing, leakage rates, or positive margins between the two groups.[289] Thus, increasing evidence supports the equality of laparscopically-assisted resection of rectal cancer to traditional open surgery.

In order to establish that laparoscopically-assisted resection of rectal cancer is not inferior to open resection, more long-term data on cancer recurrence and survival are needed. Furthermore, similar issues of cost-effectiveness of appropriate patient selection also apply to laparoscopic resection of rectal cancer as conversion rates from the two randomized trials were reported to be 23% and 34%. The laparoscopic procedure also requires longer operating time and advanced technical skill.[277,278] In order to further address concerns about the use of laparoscopically-assisted resection of rectal cancer, the American College of Surgery Oncology Group has developed a prospective, randomized phase II trial to determine if laparoscopic surgery is a technically and oncologically safe approach to the resection of rectal cancer.[290] Results of this trial will hopefully provide a more definitive evaluation of the technique and more clearly elucidate the role of laparoscopic surgery for rectal cancer.

Perforated Colon Cancers ■ Patients with perforated colon cancers often present with peritonitis. In this setting, the goals of surgical management are to remove the diseased segment of colon and prevent ongoing peritoneal contamination. Following resection and thorough irrigation of the peritoneal cavity, options for subsequent management include proximal diversion with creation of a mucous fistula/Hartmann pouch or primary anastomosis with proximal diversion via loop ileostomy. Perforated colon cancer is associated with a high rate of local recurrence and low rate of OS.[291]

Obstructing Colon Cancers ■ Cancer is the most common cause of large-bowel obstruction.[292] Obstructing right and transverse colon cancers are generally managed with a right hemicolectomy and primary anastomosis. Left sided colon cancers can be managed with either a single a single operation or a two-stage procedure.[292] The options for single-stage management include segmental resection or subtotal colectomy with ileorectal anastomosis. Subtotal colectomy is attractive because it removes the remaining of the potentially compromised colon, but it is a more extensive operation and may be associated with five to six bowel movements per day. On-table lavage has been used in the setting of segmental resection for obstruction, but postoperative complication rates remain a concern. A two-stage procedure involves first, resection of the primary tumor with proximal diversion and creation of a mucous fistula or Hartmann's pouch. The second stage, performed at a later time, involves reanastomosis of the colon. An alternative two-stage approach in select patients with an obstructing left colon lesion is resection with primary anastomosis and proximal fecal diversion with a loop ileostomy.[292]

Colonic stenting has recently been established as an option for patients with malignant colon obstruction.[293,294] Although it does not represent a long-term solution to the malignant colonic obstruction, stenting is useful in those whose prognosis is limited by the presence of metastatic disease or comorbidities. Stenting has also been used to allow transient relief of obstruction and bowel preparation with or without colonoscopic evaluation of the proximal colon before planned resection.[293,294]

Synchronous Distant Metastases ■ The liver is the most common site for colon cancer metastasis and approximately 17% of patients will present with synchronous liver metastasis.[263] Concomitant resection of colon and liver lesions may be undertaken safely in selected patients. Alternatively, management of liver metastasis may be dealt with at a subsequent operation. Systemic chemotherapy is also an essential component of therapy in these patients and will be discussed below.

Surveillance Following Resection ■ The goal of postoperative surveillance following resection of colon adenocarcinoma is identification of asymptomatic recurrences or new primaries that will allow for subsequent early treatment and lead to an improvement in survival. An expert panel assembled by the American Society of Clinical Oncology (ASCO) examined the evidence of supporting the role of various screening tests following resection of CRC (Table 89-4).[295] Interestingly, CBC, LFTs, FOBT and CT scanning were not considered essential components of surveillance. With these guidelines in mind, surveillance should be individualized depending on factors unique to a given case, including comorbidities and patient anxiety.

Local Recurrence ■ Local recurrence following resection of colonic adenocarcinoma occurs in approximately 4% of cases with the highest rates in advanced-stage tumors.[296] Although these patients generally have a poor survival, surgical resection of locoregional recurrence can result in long-term survival in up to 15% of patients.[296] Best results are obtained in patients with isolated small recurrences (less than 5 cm) that can be resected with negative margins.

***Table 89-4* ■ ASCO Guidelines for Colorectal Cancer Surveillance Following Resection**

Test	Recommendation
History and physical	Every 3-6 months for 3 year; then annually
Serum CEA	Every 2-3 months in stage II and III patients for at least 2 years
Colonoscopy	Every 3-5 years
Chest x-ray	Consider if rising CEA
Computed tomography	Consider if rising CEA

Adjuvant Therapy for Colorectal Cancer

5-Fluorouracil-Based Regimens ■ The antifolate 5-FU has been the cornerstone of chemotherapy for CRC since the 1960's. A metabolite of 5-FU, fluorodeoxyuridine monophosphate (FdUMP), inhibits thymidylate synthase (TS) and thus interferes with DNA synthesis.[297] 5-FU is also incorporated into RNA, which disrupts protein synthesis.[297] Studies however, did not show a survival advantage for adjuvant 5-FU until it was combined with a biomodulator. Leucovorin (folinic acid), levamisole (an antihelminthic agent), and methotrexate were all explored as modulators of 5-FU.[298-302] Leucovorin (LV) has been accepted as the standard biomodulator and increases cytotoxicity by stabilizing the FdUMP/TS complex and increasing the intracellular pool of reduced folate.

Multiple prospective trials have shown the clinical benefit of postoperative 5-FU in combination with either leucovorin or levamisole.[298-,299,301,302] The National Surgical Adjuvant Breast and Bowel Project C-03 trial showed that 6 months of 5-FU and LV each given weekly at 500 mg/m^2 for 6 of 8 weeks (Roswell Park Regimen) were superior to combination therapy with methyl 1-[2-chloroethyl-3-(4methyl-cyclohexyl)] (CCNU), vincristine, and 5-FU.[302] The incremental increases in DFS from 64% to 73% and in OS from 77% to 84% were proportionally similar to other randomized trials with 5-FU and LV.[302]

There are numerous 5-FU dosing schedules. In the adjuvant setting, these include bolus daily for 5 days every 4 weeks, the so-called Mayo Clinic regimen; weekly for 6 of every 8 weeks, or Roswell park regimen; and infusional schedules. Unlike the metastatic setting, continuous infusion 5-FU (CIFU) has not shown superiority over bolus-type adjuvant regimens. There was no difference in DFS or OS, but there was a suggestion that it may have an improved toxicity profile.[303,304]

The convenience of oral therapy and the prospect of avoiding long-term intravenous access complications, such as thrombosis and infection, have stimulated development of oral fluoropyrimidines. Capecitabine is a fluoropyrimidine carbamate that is converted to 5-FU in a three-step enzymatic cascade. Preclinical studies had shown that capecitabine exhibits selectivity for neoplastic cells because the final enzymatic conversion involves thymidine phosphorylase, which is preferentially expressed in tumor as opposed to normal tissues.[305,306] Twice-daily oral administration simulates continuous infusion of 5-FU without the costs and inconvenience of a pump.

The X-ACT trial showed that capecitabine was at least equivalent to bolus 5-FU in the adjuvant setting.[305] This noninferiority trial randomized 1987 patients with resected stage III colon cancer to 6 months of adjuvant capecitabine 1250 mg/m^2 twice daily for 2 weeks of a 3-week schedule or to bolus 5-FU 425 mg/m^2 and LV 20 mg/m^2 daily days 1 through 5 of a 28-day cycle (Mayo Regimen). The 3-year DFS was 64.2% in the capecitabine arm compared with 60.6% in the bolus 5-FU arm. With a hazard ratio of 0.87% and a $p < .001$, this study met its primary endpoint of equivalent DFS. The side effect profiles are slightly different, with capecitabine having an increased risk for hand-foot syndrome but markedly improved reductions in neutropenia and stomatitis seen in the bolus regimen.[305] It remains unknown whether capecitabine is equivalent to infusional regimens of 5-FU when added to oxaliplatin and bevacizumab, pending the results of the AVANT trial.

Oxaliplatin-Based Regimens ■ Oxaliplatin is a third-generation platinum compound that crosslinks DNA and induces apoptosis. Oxaliplatin has properties that are distinct from other platinum compounds such as cisplatin and carboplatin. The preclinical models showed both activity in cisplastin-resistant CRC cell lines and synergism when combined with 5-FU.[307] Oxaliplatin causes little nephrotoxicity, ototoxicity, and alopecia, but shares bone marrow suppressive properties and has its own sensory neuropathy that is typically reversible, cumulative, and exacerbated by exposure to cold.[307-310]

Oxaliplatin was quickly moved to the adjuvant setting after initial studies showed its efficacy in the metastatic setting. The MOSAIC trial randomized 2246 stage II (node-negative) and stage III patients to receive either oxaliplatin, folinic acid and 5-FU (FOLFOX-4) combination or infusional 5-FU/LV.[307,309,310] The infusional 5-FU was given every 2 weeks on a 28-day cycle as LV 200 mg/m^2 over 2 h followed by bolus 5-FU 400 mg/m^2, and then a 22-hour infusion of 5-FU at 600 mg/m^2 on days 1 and 2. FOLFOX-4 included the same regimen of 5-FU/LV with addition of oxaliplatin at 85 mg/m^2 over 2 h every 2 weeks of a 28-day cycle.[307] The probability of being free of disease was 78.2% in the FOLFOX-4 arm compared with 72.9% in the infusional 5-FU/LV arm. Subgroup analysis revealed that stage III patients derived more benefit as evidenced by DFS (72% receiving FOLFOX-4 vs 65% receiving 5-FU/LV, $p = .0002$) than stage II patients (87% receiving FOLFOX-4 vs 84% receiving 5-FU/LV, $p =$ ns). Oxaliplatin regimens are still restricted by its dose-limiting toxicity of neuropathy, which seriously affected 12% of patients during the trial but the percentage of patients affected dropped to 0.5% after 18 months.[307,309] Although follow-up has not been long enough to see a statistically significant improvement in OS, a recent update showed persistent improvement in DFS.[309] Moreover, 3-year DFS has been shown to be well correlated with OS across multiple colorectal trials.[307,309]

The benefit of oxaliplatin does not appear to be dependent on the schedule of 5-FU/LV. NSABP C-07 randomized 2407 patients with stage II/III colon cancer to bolus weekly 5-FU/LV (Roswell Park Regimen) or to FLOX (the same 5-FU/LV regimen with biweekly oxaliplatin).[308] The improvement in the hazard ratios and DFS was similar to that seen in the MOSAIC trial. The probability of being alive and free of disease at 3 years was 76.5% in the oxaliplatin arm compared with 71.6% in the control arm.[308] Although the efficacy of FLOX looked similar to the infusional 5-FU used in the MOSAIC trial, it does appear to be slightly more toxic, with increased diarrhea and dehydration.

Irinotecan-Based Regimens ■ Irinotecan is a camptothecin derivative that inhibits topoisomerase I by stabilizing DNA breaks that arise in DNA uncoiling for transcription and replication.[311] Two randomized controlled trials showed improved survival in patients receiving irinotecan along with 5-FU/LV, compared with 5-FU/LV alone, as first-line therapy in metastatic disease.[312,313] Despite the proven benefit in advanced disease, preliminary results from three large trials do not support the use of irinotecan in the adjuvant setting. CALGB C89803 compared a bolus version of irinotecan with 5-FU/LV (IFL) with 5-FU/LV alone and found an increase in grade III-IV toxicities (neutropenia, neutropenic fever, and death on treatment) without an improvement in DFS.[314] PETACC-3 and Accord02/FFCD9802 compared the addition of irinotecan with infusional 5-FU and also found increased toxicities in the experimental arm with no improvement in DFS in patients with stage III cancer.[315] On the basis of these trials, irinotecan-based regimens cannot be recommended in the adjuvant setting.[314,315]

Irinotecan is hydrolyzed in the liver to its active metabolite, SN-38, which in turn is glucoronidated to an inactive form by uridine diphosphate glucoronosyltransferase isoform 1A1 (UGT1A1).[311] The adverse events associated with irinotecan, including diarrhea, bone marrow suppression, and nausea or vomiting, have been shown in retrospective studies to correlate with polymorphisms of UGT1A1.[311] A diagnostic test has been approved by the FDA, and several current trials include adjustment of irinotecan dosages on the basis of genetic profiles (pharmacogenomics) of these metabolic enzymes.[311]

Biologic Agents ■ The two most recent FDA-approved therapies in metastatic colon cancer are "targeted," "biologic" agents rather than standard cytotoxic drugs. Both agents are monoclonal antibodies. Bevacizumab targets the vascular endothelial growth factor (VEGF) pathway and cetuximab is directed against the epidermal growth factor receptor (EGFR) pathway.

Bevacizumab is a humanized recombinant monoclonal antibody directed against VEGF. By binding ligand and preventing signaling of the VEGF receptor, bevacizumab is thought to interfere with the recruitment and growth of tumor-feeding blood vessels. Two phase-III trials have shown an improvement in both DFS and OS after the addition of bevacizumab to 5-FU based regimens combined with either oxaliplatin or irinotecan in the metastatic setting.[316,317] Side effects seen in these trials thought to be due to the addition of bevacizumab included reversible hypertension and proteinuria, as well as rare serious, but not statistically significant, side effects including gastrointestinal perforation, wound dehiscence, bleeding and clotting.[316,317] NSABP C-08 and MOSAIC-2 are two prospectively randomized trials designed to determine whether bevacizumab improves survival over FOLFOX-4 in the adjuvant setting.

Cetuximab is a monoclonal antibody directed against EGFR, which is involved with multiple growth signaling pathways. Cetuximab received FDA approval for treatment of irinotecan-resistant metastatic disease in 2004. In irinotecan-refractory disease, a 22% response rate was reached in patients treated with cetuximab/irinotecan compared with an 11% response rate with cetuximab as a single agent in a randomized phase II trial.[318] The side effects of cetuximab are relative mild, with an acneiform rash over the face, chest, and back occurring in most patients.[318] Allergic reactions also occur as cetuximab, unlike bevacizumab, is not fully humanized.[318] The US Intergroup N0147 trial is comparing FOLFOX-4 with and without cetuximab in the adjuvant setting for stage III colon cancer.

Summary Recommendations ■ The magnitude of benefit from adjuvant therapy appears to be proportional to the risk of relapse on the basis of pathologic stage. For stage III (node-positive) patients, the evidence supports the use of adjuvant chemotherapy for 6 months following resection.[319,320] FOLFOX-4 has the most convincing efficacy data but is associated with increased toxicities compared with 5-FU/LV alone. Capecitabine is a reasonable alternative to intravenous 5-FU/LV. Irinotecan-based regimens cannot be recommended in the adjuvant setting while the use of bevacizumab and cetuximab await further data. For stage II (node-negative) patients, the absolute benefit appears to be real but much smaller. The current trials were not powered to see a difference in this subgroup, so the role of adjuvant treatment for stage II patients is controversial.[319,320] Following the NCCN practice guidelines, FOLFOX-4 or 5-FU is often considered if the pathology displays high-risk features such as poor differentiation, lymphatic or vascular invasion, bowel obstruction, inadequate staging (<12 lymph nodes removed), perforation, or direct extension into other organs.[320] For stage II patients with no high-risk features, observation or enrollment in a clinical trial is recommended.[320]

The evidence also suggests that the elderly receive the same benefit from adjuvant chemotherapy as do younger patients.[321,322] A pooled analysis of three randomized clinical trials suggested that efficacy of adjuvant 5-FU-based chemotherapy was maintained in the elderly (defined as 70 years of age and older), and that toxicity was similar to younger patients except for an increase in leucopenia in one study.[322]

Neoadjuvant and Adjuvant Therapy for Rectal Cancer

As in colon cancer, surgical resection remains the cornerstone of the curative approach. However, unlike colon cancer, there is significant tendency for local failure after potentially curative resection. Improvements in the initial surgical procedure by performing a TME have reduced but not eliminated the risk of local recurrence. Salvage surgical procedures are technically difficult, often unsuccessful and fraught with morbidity. Therefore the major difference in the adjuvant treatment paradigm for rectal as compared with colon cancer is the addition of radiation therapy to reduce the risk of local failure.

Adjuvant Chemotherapy and Radiation ■ Studies in the 1980s and 1990s solidified the superiority of postoperative chemoradiation over surgery alone and surgery followed by radiation without chemotherapy. Chemoradiation reduced the risk of local failure, distant failure, and the risk of death.[323-325] In these studies, chemoradiation involved the use of seumustine (methyl-CCNU) in addition to 5-FU. Semustine carries a small but real risk of acute myeloid leukemia and is not longer used in adjuvant regimens for rectal cancer.[326] The North American intergroup trial confirmed the lack of additional benefit of semustine in addition to 5-FU and has established the role of continuous infusion 5-FU with radiation.[327] Comparing continuous infusion 5-FU (225 mg/m^2 per day for 5 weeks) to bolus 5-FU (500 mg/m^2 days 1-3 and days 36-39) at 4 years, the time to relapse was improved from 53% to 63%, and survival was improved from 60% to 70%. Unlike colon cancer, biomodulation with leucovorin or levamisole has not increased the efficacy of 5-FU in rectal cancer. Intergroup study 0144 completed accrual in 2000 and is designed to determine whether continued systemic therapy with infusional 5-FU improves survival over just using it during radiation.[327] In general, adjuvant therapy is recommended for any tumor that is T3 or greater in size or is node positive.

Neoadjuvant Chemotherapy and Radiation ■ The neoadjuvant approach is particularly attractive in rectal cancer because downstaging may increase ease and rates of respectability, allow potential sphincter preservation, and increase compliance by avoiding long postoperative recoveries. The Swedish Rectal Cancer Trial was the first to show that a short-term regimen of high-dose preoperative radiotherapy decreased the rate of local recurrence and improved survival compared with surgery alone.[328] The German phase III EORTC 22921 study was the first study to complete accrual in comparing neoadjuvant therapy with combined 5-FU/radiation to postoperative adjuvant 5-FU/radiation.[329] Patients with tumor extending through the muscle wall (T3) or with positive nodes (N1) were randomized to preoperative or postoperative chemoradiation. In both arms, the radiation (5040 GY in 28 fractions) was combined with 5-FU (1000 mg/m^2 over 120 h during the first and fifth week). All patients received additional systemic 5-FU for 4 months. The study failed to see an improvement in OS, but preoperative therapy was associated with an improved rate of local control (6% failure at 5 years compared to 13%), reduced acute and chronic toxicity, increased compliance, and an increased rate of sphincter preservation in patients with low-ling tumors.[329] Interestingly, posttreatment pathology results proved to be highly prognostic with patients who showed marked regression or negative nodes having improved DFS.[329]

The relative benefit of preoperative short course high-dose radiotherapy (Swedish approach) compared to conventional preoperative radiotherapy has not been studied. However, preoperative short course high-dose radiotherapy was directly compared to concomitant chemoradiotherapy using conventional radiotherapy and bolus 5-FU with leucovorin during weeks 1 and 5 in a Polish randomized trial involving 316 patients with T3-4 rectal cancer.[330] In an early report, the pathological complete remission rate was significantly higher in the chemoradiotherapy group (16% vs 1%), and there were fewer cases of radial margin positivity (4% vs 13%), but the rate of sphincter preservation in both groups was comparable (58% and 61%, respectively).[330] Local failure and survival rates were not reported. The Swedish approach has been adopted by many European oncologists but has not been widely accepted in the United States principally because of concerns for late treatment-related morbidity (such as anastomotic leak), and the desire to integrate concurrent chemotherapy with radiation.

Summary Recommendations ■ Although no survival benefit was achieved with preoperative compared with postoperative chemoradiotherapy, it is suggested that preoperative chemoradiotherapy is the preferred treatment for patients with locally advanced rectal cancer, given that it is associated with a superior overall compliance rate, an improved rate of local control, reduced toxicity, improved function and an increased rate of sphincter preservation in patients with low-lying tumors.[320] Although no trial has demonstrated conclusively that additional postoperative adjuvant 5-FU-based chemotherapy improves outcomes in patients who have undergone neoadjuvant chemoradiotherapy, guidelines from the National Comprehensive Cancer Network recommend that all such patients receive 5-FU-containing chemotherapy even if they have a pathologic complete remission to neoadjuvant therapy.[320]

Chemotherapy for Hepatic Metastasis

Conversion Therapy ■ Selected patients with initially unresectable liver metastases may become eligible for resection if the response to chemotherapy is sufficient. This approach has been termed "conversion therapy" to distinguish it from "neoadjuvant therapy" which applies to preoperative chemotherapy given to patients who present upfront with apparently resectable disease. The key parameter for selecting the specific regimen in this scenario is not survival or improved quality of life, but instead, response rate. Between 12% and 33% of patients with isolated but initially unresectable CRC liver metastases have a sufficient downstaging response to permit a subsequent complete resection.[331-335] Five-year survival rates average 30% to 35%, results that are substantially better than expected using chemotherapy alone. In the largest prospective study, 95 (14%) of 701 patients with initially unresectable CRC liver metastases were able to undergo resection after induction chemotherapy with chronomodulated 5-FU/LV and either oxaliplatin or irinotecan.[332] Patients with large or critically located lesions were most likely to become candidates for resection, and were also most likely to survive 5 years (60% and 49%, respectively) compared to those with multinodular disease or extrahepatic metastases (34% and 18%, respectively). Even if patients are refractory to initial chemotherapy, the addition of cetuximab to the regimen may increase the number of patients potentially eligible for resection.[336] Chemotherapy alone is not curative in this setting with the majority of radiographic completely responding lesions containing viable tumor. Thus, even in the setting of a complete clinical response, resection is still needed.

Neoadjuvant Therapy for Hepatic Metastasis ■ For patients with initially resectable liver metastases, the question of whether perioperative chemotherapy improves survival was addressed in an EORTC trial in which 364 patients with up to four metastases without prior exposure to oxaliplatin were randomly assigned to liver resection with or without FOLFOX-4 chemotherapy.[337] Six cycles of chemotherapy were administered prior to surgery, and six cycles were administered postoperatively. Sixty-seven of the 182 patients assigned to chemotherapy had an objective response, while 11 progressed, eight of whom were no longer considered resectable. Overall, 83% of patients were successfully resected, similar to the number who were successfully resected in the surgery alone group, 84%. The postoperative complication rate however was significantly higher in the chemotherapy group (25% vs 16%). Patients receiving perioperative chemotherapy had higher rates of hepatic failure, biliary fistulas and intraabdominal infection. Postoperative mortality rate was not higher than with surgery alone. Furthermore, there are an increasing number of reports of steatosis, vascular injury, and nodular regenerative hyperplasia in the livers of patients treated with preoperative irinotecan or oxaliplatin-containing chemotherapy regimens.[332, 338-340]

Adjuvant Therapy After Hepatic Resection ■ Adjuvant chemotherapy is commonly recommended following resection of hepatic colorectal metastasis despite the lack of data to support its use. There are many unknowns, including the timing of resection, optimal drug combination, schedule and duration of therapy. Because the presence of hepatic metastasis confers stage IV disease, either FOLFOX-4 or folinic acid, 5-FU and irinotecan (FOLFIRI) for 4 to 6 months is often used.[333] A targeted biologic agent may be considered despite the lack of data supporting use in stage II/III disease. Because of the risk of wound complications and other issues, it is recommended that bevacizumab be discontinued 8 weeks before or after major surgical procedures.[341]

Summary Recommendations ■ There are no widely accepted guidelines for determining which patients with CRC liver metastases should undergo immediate surgery and when neoadjuvant chemotherapy is indicated. However, the increasing reports of liver injury following neoadjuvant chemotherapy has prompted most physicians to recommend initial surgery for low risk (medically fit with four or fewer lesions), potentially resectable patients, followed by adjuvant chemotherapy.[342] On the other hand, neoadjuvant chemotherapy is reasonable for those who are higher risk or have borderline resectable or unresectable liver metastases. However, the duration should be limited, radiographic response assessment performed frequently, and surgery undertaken as soon as the metastases become clearly resectable.

Metastatic Colorectal Cancer

The last 5 to 10 years have seen unprecedented advances in the treatment of metastatic colorectal cancer. In the era when 5-FU was the sole active agent, OS was approximately 11 to 12 months. In the modern era, the average median survival duration has doubled with patients routinely living longer than 2 years. This increase has been mainly driven by the availability of new active agents. There are now five different classes of drugs with significant antitumor activity including the fluoropyrimidines, irinotecan, oxaliplatin, cetuximab and bevacizumab. For most patients, the goal of treatment will be palliative and not curative, with the treatment goals being to prolong OS and maintain quality of life (QOL) for as long as possible. For the vast majority of patients with noncurable metastatic CRC, rationally designed doublet combinations, such as FOLFOX (folinic acid, 5-FU, oxaliplatin) or FOLFIRI (folinic acid, 5-FU, irinotecan) should be considered the standard chemotherapy backbone for first-line palliative therapy. These regimens have well-documented activity and a tolerable toxicity profile.

FOLFOX ■ The first large size, randomized phase III trial comparing 5-FU and leucovorin versus FOLFOX-4 included 420 patients.[310] Patients received exactly the same regimen of a 2-hour infusion of 200 mg/m^2 of leucovorin followed by a bolus of 400 mg/m^2 and a 22-hour infusion of 600 mg/m^2 of 5-FU. All drugs were repeated for 2 consecutive days every 2 weeks. Half of the patients were assigned to receive 85 mg/m^2 of oxaliplatin as a 2-hour infusion on day 1 only.[310] Patients allocated to receive FOLFOX-4 had significantly longer PFS (median 9.0 vs 6.2 months; p = .0003) and better response rate (50.7% vs 22.3%; p = .0001) when compared with the control arm. However, although a trend could be seen, the improvement in OS did not reach significance (median, 16.2 vs 14.7 months, p = .12).[310] The lack of survival benefit in this European trial delayed FOLFOX acceptance in the United States. Shortly after, the NCCTG and the American intergroup conducted the N9741, a phase III trial with three arms.[343] The control arm received IFL regimen, and oxaliplatin was included in the two experimental arms. It was combined at 85 mg/m^2 with 200 mg/m^2 of irinotecan in the irinotecan and oxaliplatin (IROX) regimen, or with 5-FU and leucovorin, following the FOLFOX-4 regimen described above.[343] The final results showed a median time to progression of 8.7 months, response rate of 45% and median survival time of 19.5 months for those patients assigned to FOLFOX-4. These results were significantly superior to those observed for IFL (6.9 months, 31% and 15.0 months, respectively) or for IROX (6.5 months, 35%, and 1.4 months, respectively).[343] FOLFOX-4 was generally well tolerated but it was associated with a significantly higher rate of sensory neuropathy as described above.

Capcetabine, an orally active fluoropyrimidine, allows for the attractiveness of oral dosing, and the potential for eliminating the need for a central venous catheter and ambulatory infusion pump. At least five randomized phase III trials have directly compared XELOX (capcetabine, oxaliplatin) versus FOLFOX for first-line or second-line chemotherapy in metastatic CRC.[344-348] None showed that XELOX was inferior to FOLFOX-type regimens in terms of response rate, PFS, or OS. However, in nearly all cases, the PFS and OS curves for XELOX trailed beneath the curves for FOLFOX. In no case was this effect statistically significant or clinically meaningful. Thus, the available evidence supports the view that XELOX can be considered as a noninferior substitute for FOLFOX in palliative therapy.

FOLFIRI ■ The effectiveness of irinotecan was initially demonstrated in a randomized phase III trial conducted to evaluate irinotecan with or without standard bolus 5-FU and leucovorin versus a standard regimen of bolus 5-FU and leucovorin.[313] The combination regimen became known as the IFL regimen and included 5-FU 500 mg/m^2, leucovorin 20 mg/m^2, and irinotecan 125 mg/m^2 given weekly for 4 weeks every 6 weeks. Irinotecan alone was given at 125 mg/m^2 weekly for 4 weeks every 6 weeks, and the 5-FU/LV was given using the standard Mayo Regimen as described above.[313] The three drug regimen was superior to either 5-FU and leucovorin or to irinotecan alone, and the latter produced similar results as the 5-FU/LV regimen. In a comparison of IFL and the Mayo regimens, the median PFS improved from 4.3 months to 7.0 months, and the median OS improved from 12.6 months to 14.8 months.[313] FOLFIRI is a variation of IFL using infusional 5-FU, leucovorin, and irinotecan. There are several variations of FOLFIRI, but one of the favored regimens combines 180 mg/m^2 of irinotecan given on day 1 weekly, 400 mg/m^2 bolus leucovorin weekly, 400 mg/m^2 bolus 5-FU weekly followed by a 46 h infusion of 2400 mg/m^2 of 5-FU. The entire cycle is repeated every 14 days. A European trial compared the use of FOLFIRI versus FOLFOX as a first-line therapy for metastatic colorectal cancer.[349] Although it has been criticized for its relatively small size, this trial was important because it showed similar response rates and median survivals for FOLFOX and FOLFIRI.

While XELOX may be regarded as a valid substitute for FOLFOX, the situation is different for combinations of capecitabine with irinotecan (XELIRI) as an alternative to FOLFIRI. Capecitabine and irinotecan have partially overlapping toxicity profiles, particularly with regard to diarrhea. The potential for greater toxicity reduces the therapeutic advantage of an irinotecan/capecitabine combination and makes the selection of appropriate doses and schedules for this combination difficult.[350]

Bevacizumab ■ CRC was the first malignancy for which clear evidence for efficacy of an anti-VEGF strategy was obtained in randomized trials. In a pivotal early trial, the addition of bevacizumab to the bolus IFL regimen significantly improved response rates from 35% to 45%; PFS was extended from 7.1 months to 10.4 months, and more importantly, the OS improved from 15.6 to 20.3 months.[316] The adverse events in this trial were similar among the treatment with some notable exceptions. Patients receiving bevacizumab had an 11% incidence of grade 3 hypertension, and a 1.5% incidence of bowel perforations. No patients in the IFL arm presented with such problems.[316] The ECOG 3200 trial compared the use of FOLFOX to combination therapy of bevacizumab and FOLFOX.[317] The median survival for combination therapy was 12.5 months versus 10.7 months for FOLFOX alone. This confirmed that bevacizumab does significantly add potency to oxaliplatin-based regimens. Since 2004, the majority of patients with metastatic CRC have received bevacizumab as a component of first-line therapy regardless of the specific regimen chosen for chemotherapy backbone (FOLFOX, XELOX, FOLFIRI).

Cetuximab ■ The benefit of cetuximab added to first-line or second-line irinotecan-containing therapy has been addressed in the CRYSTAL trial and CALGB 80203.[351,352] In the CRYSTAL trial, 1198 previously untreated patients were randomly assigned to FOLFIRI with or without cetuximab.[351] Although the addition of cetuximab significantly improved PFS, the incremental gain was only 0.9 months. The addition of cetuximab also improved the response rate, but only by 8%.[351] The phase II CALGB 80203 trial, which randomly assigned 283 patients to FOLFOX or FOLFIRI with or without cetuximab as first-line therapy provides confirmatory data supporting the results of the CRYSTAL trial.[352] In a preliminary report, there was a clear demonstration of increased response rate with cetuximab in conjunction with both FOLFOX and FOLFIRI, while the impact on PFS was inconclusive.[352] Furthermore, a retrospective analysis of the CRYSTAL trial investigating the role of KRAS mutation status on PFS and response rate showed that in the KRAS wild-type population, the 1 year PFS rate for those who received cetuximab and FOLFIRI was 43% versus 25% for those who received FOLFIRI alone and the risk of progression was decreased by 32% in the combination treatment arm.[353] In the KRAS mutant population, however, there was no difference in PFS between the two arms. In summary, there is no convincing evidence to establish cetuximab as a component of front-line therapy in unselected patients.[353] The incremental gain in PFS in the CRYSTAL trial is not convincing enough to change current practice in view of the much larger gain in PFS obtained when bevacizumab is added to a first-line regimen. In view of the emerging data on K-ras mutation status effect on the effectiveness of cetuximab, it is hoped that future molecular advances will permit identification of those patients who are most likely to benefit from cetuximab.

Summary Recommendations ■ Initial combination therapy is preferred for patients with nonoperable metastatic CRC, in whom the palliative treatment strategy should aim to maximize the number of patients exposed to all active agents. This is best achieved by using well-established combination doublets (ie, FOLFOX, XELOX, or FOLFIRI) as the chemotherapy backbone, which would then only require one additional step to have all three active agents included in the treatment algorithm for second-line therapy (eg, FOLFOX followed by FOLFIRI, or FOLFIRI followed by FOLFOX). Bevacizumab should be considered a component of first-line therapy regardless of which regimen is chosen while data supporting the use of cetuximab in nonselected patients is lacking.

Selected References

The complete reference list can be found at www.CANCERMEDICINE8.com

5. Gill S, Mihas A. Small intestine neoplasms. *J Clin Gastroenterol*. 2001;33(4):267–282.
11. O'Riordan B, Vilor M, Herrera L. Small bowel tumors. An overview. *Dig Dis Sci*. 1996;14:245–257.
19. Cannon M, Carpenter S, Elta G, et al. EUS compared with CT, MRI, and angiography and the influence of biliary stenting on staging accuracy of ampullary neoplasms. *Gastrointest Endosc*. 1999;50:27–33.
21. Ingrosso M, Prete F, Pisani A, et al. Laparoscopically assisted total enteroscopy: a new approach to small intestinal diseases. *Gastrointest Endosc*. 1999;49:651–653.
22. Yamamoto H, Kita H, Sunada K, et al. Clinical outcomes of double-balloon endoscopy for the diagnosis and treatment of small intestinal diseases. *Clin Gastroenterol H*. 2004;2:1010–1016.
23. Mankanwal S, Ismail M. Capsule endoscopy: a review. *South Med J*. 2008;101: 407–414.
26. DiSario J, Burt R, Vargas H, McWhorter W. Small bowel cancer. Epidemiological and clinical characteristics from a population-based registry. *Am J Gastroenterol*. 1994;89:699–701.
29. Neugut A, Marvin M, Rella V, et al. An overview of adenocarcinoma of the small intestine. *Oncology*. 1997;11:529–536.
49. Howe J, Karnell L, Menck HR, et al. The American College of Surgeons Commission on Cancer and the American Cancer Society. Adenocarcinoma of the small bowel. Review of the National Cancer Data Base, 1985–1995. *Cancer*. 1999;86: 2693–2706.
56. Maggard M, O'Connell J, Ko C. Updated population-based review of carcinoid tumors. *Ann Surgery*. 2004;240:117–122.
61. Thompson G, van Heerden J, Martin J, et al. Carcinoid tumors of the gastrointestinal tract. Presentation, management, and prognosis. *Surgery*. 1998;98:1054–1063.
74. Kwaan M, Goldberg J, Bleday R. Rectal carcinoid tumors. *Arch Surg*. 2008;143: 471–475.
82. Rubin B, Singer S, Tsao C, et al. KIT activation is a ubiquitous feature of gastrointestinal stromal tumors. *Cancer Res*. 2001; 61:8118–8121.
89. DeMatteo R, Antonescu C, Chadaram V, et al. Adjuvant imatinib mesylate in patients with primary high risk gastrointestinal

stromal tumor (GIST) following complete resection: Safety results from the U.S. Intergroup Phase II trial ACOSOG Z9000. *J Clin Oncol.* 2005;23:9009.
97. Crump M, Gospodarowicz M, Shepard F. Lymphoma of the gastrointestinal tract. *Semin Oncol.* 1999;26:324–327.
114. Blecker D, Abraham S, Furth EE, et al. Melanoma in the gastrointestinal tract. *Gastrointestinology.* 1999;94:3427–3433.
126. Moertel C, Wieland L, Nagorney D, Dockerty M. Carcinoid tumor of the appendix. Treatment and prognosis. *N Engl J Med.* 1987;317:1699–1701.
129. Lyss A. Appendiceal malignancies. *Semin Oncol.* 1988;15:129–137.
148. Sugarbaker P. Managing the peritoneal surface component of gastrointestinal cancer. Patterns of dissemination and treatment options. *Oncology.* 2005;18:51–62.
150. Verwaal V, Bruin S, Boot H, et al. Eight-year follow-up of randomized trial: cytoreduction and hyperthermic intraperitoneal chemotherapy versus systemic chemotherapy in patients with peritoneal carcinomatosis of colorectal cancer. *Ann Surg Oncol.* 2008;15:2436–2432.
156. Rutledge R, Alexander J. Primary appendiceal malignancies. Rare but important. *Surgery.* 1992;11:244–250.
178. Eaden J, Abrams K, Mayberry J. The risk of colorectal cancer in ulcerative colitis: a meta-analysis. *Gut.* 2001;48:526–535.
188. Moghaddam A, Woodward M, Huxley R. Obesity and risk of colorectal cancer: a meta-analysis of 31 studies with 70,000 events. *Cancer Epidemiol Biomarkers Prev.* 2007;16:2533–2547.
202. Lynch H, Smyrk T. Hereditary non-polyposis colorectal cancer (Lynch syndrome). An updated review. *Cancer (Phila).* 1996;78:1149–1167.
203. Campbell WJ, Spence RA, Parks TG. Familial adenomatous polyposis. *Br J Surg.* 1994;81:1722–1733.
205. Burt R, DiSario J, Cannon-Albright L. Genetics of colon cancer: impact of inheritance on colon cancer risk. *Annu Rev Med.* 1995;46:371–379.
209. Sieber O, Lipton L, Crabtree M, et al. Multiple colorectal adenomas, classic adenomatous polyposis, and germ-line mutations in MYH. *N Engl J Med.* 2003;348:791–799.
251. Winawer S, Zauber A, Ho M, et al. Prevention of colorectal cancer by colonscopic polypectomy. The National Polyp Study Workgroup. *N Engl J Med.* 1993;329:1977–1981.
254. Pickhardt P, Choi J, Hwang I, et al. Computed tomographic virtual colonoscopy to screen for colorectal neoplasia in asymptomatic adults. *N Engl J Med.* 2003;349:2191–2200.
261. Nivatvongs S. Surgical management of malignant colorectal polyps. *Surg Clin North Am.* 2002;82:959–964.
272. Lacy A, Garcia-Valdecasas J, Delgado S, et al. Laparoscopy-assisted colectomy versus open colectomy for treatment of nonmetastatic colon cancer: a randomised trial. *Lancet.* 2002;359:2224–2229.
273. Nelson H, Sargent D, Wieand H, et al, for The Clinical Outcomes of Surgical Therapy Study Group. A comparison of laparoscopically assisted and open colectomy for colon cancer. *N Engl J Med.* 2004; 350:2050–2059.
274. Guillou P, Quirke P, Thorpe H, et al. Short-term endpoints of conventional versus laparoscopic-assisted surgery in patients with colorectal cancer (MRC CLASICC trial): multicenter, randomized controlled trial. *Lancet.* 2005;365:1718–1726.
275. Veldkamp R, Kuhry E, Hop W, et al. Laparoscopic surgery versus open surgery for colon cancer: short-term outcomes of a randomized trial. *Lancet Oncol.* 2005;6:477–484.
276. Fleshman J, Sargent D, Green E, et al. Laparoscopic colectomy for cancer is not inferior to open surgery based on 5-year data from the COST study group trial. *Ann Surg.* 2007;246:655–662.
277. Jayne D, Guillou P, Thorpe H, et al. Randomized trial of laparoscopic-assisted resection of colorectal carcinoma: 3-year results of the UK MRC CLASICC Trial Group. *J Clin Oncol.* 2007;25:3061–3068.
280. Heald R. Total mesorectal excision is optimal surgery for rectal cancer: a Scandinavian consensus. *Br J Surg.* 1995;82:1297–1299.
281. Arbman G, Nilsson E, Hallbook O. Local recurrence following total mesorectal excision for rectal cancer. *Br J Surg.* 1996;83:375–379.
294. Dionigi G, Villa F, Rovera F, et al. Colonic stenting for malignant disease: review of literature. *Surg Oncol.* 2007;16:S153–S155.
305. Twelves C, Wong A, Nowacki M, et al. Capecitabine as adjuvant treatment for stage III colon cancer. *N Engl J Med.* 2005; 352:2696–2704.
307. Andre T, Boni C, Mounedji-Boudiaf L, et al. Oxaliplatin, fluorouracil, and leucovorin as adjuvant treatment for colon cancer. *N Engl J Med.* 2004;350:2343–2348.
309. deGramont A, Boni C, Navarro M, et al. Oxaliplatin/5FU/LV in the adjuvant treatment of stage II and stage III colon cancer: efficacy results with a medical follow-up of 4 years. *J Clin Oncol.* 2005;23:3501–3507.
316. Hurwitz H, Fehrenbacher L, Novotny W, et al. Bevacizumab plus irinotecan, fluorouracil, and leucovorin for metastatic colorectal cancer. *N Engl J Med.* 2004; 350:2335–2344.
329. Sauer R, Becker H, Hohenberer W, et al. German Rectal Cancer Study Group: Preoperative versus postoperative chemoradiotherapy for rectal cancer. *N Engl J Med.* 2004;351:1731–1740.
334. Alberts SR, Horvath WL, Sternfeld WC, et al. Oxaliplatin, fluorouracil, and leucovorin for patients with unresectable liver-only metastases from colorectal cancer: a North Central Cancer Treatment Group phase II study. *J Clin Oncol.* 2005;23: 9243–9249.
338. Fernandez F, Ritter J, Goodwin J, et al. Effect of steatohepatitis associated with irinotecan or oxaliplatin pretreatment on resectability of hepatic colorectal metastases. *J Am Coll Surg.* 2005;200:845–853.
341. Ellis LM, Curley SA, Grothey A, et al. Surgical resection after downsizing of colorectal liver metastasis in the era of bevacizumab. *J Clin Oncol.* 2005;23:4853–4855.
342. Bilchik A, Poston G, Curley A, et al. Neoadjuvant chemotherapy for metastatic colon cancer: a cautionary note. *J Clin Oncol.* 2005;23:9073–9078.
351. Venook, A, Niedzwicki D, Hollis D, et al. Phase III study of irinotecan/5FU/LV (FOLFIRI) or oxaliplatin/5FU/LV (FOLFOX)±cetuximab for patients with untreated metastatic adenocarcinoma of the colon or rectum: CALGB 80203 preliminary results. *J Clin Oncol.* 2006;24:148s.
352. Van Cutsem E, Nowacki M, Lang I, et al. Randomized phase III study of irintoecan and 5-FU/FA with or without cetuximab in the first-line treatment of patients with metastatic colorectal cancer: the CRYSTAL trial. *J Clin Oncol.* 2007; 225:164s.

90 Neoplasms of the Anus

Bruce D. Minsky, MD ■ José G. Guillem, MD

Although an uncommon tumor, the incidence of anal cancer has increased over the last few decades.[1] This increase may be due to sexual transmission of HPV virus as well as the impact of HIV. Combined modality therapy (CMT) involving pelvic radiation and concurrent chemotherapy (5-FU combined with either mitomycin-c or cisplatin) has resulted in 5-year survival rates of approximately 80% while maintaining sphincter preservation for most patients. Surgery is reserved for selected patients with T1M0 disease who can undergo resection with acceptable functional outcomes or an abdominoperineal resection (APR) for salvage following CMT.

Gross Anatomy

There are three regions where anal cancers occur; the perianal skin or anal margin, the anal canal, and the lower rectum. The anal canal is 3-4 cm long and extends from the anal verge to the pelvic floor.[2] Cancers of the anal canal and the anal margin have different natural histories. The literature is confusing because of the various definitions of the anal canal and the anal margin. For example, some define the distal limit of the anal canal as the dentate line and all tumors below this as anal margin cancers,[3,4] others consider the distal extent of the anal canal as the anal verge,[5,6] while another definition of anal margin tumors are those tumors that arise within 5 cm of the anal verge.[7]

The incidence of anal margin and anal canal cancers is dependent on the anatomical boundaries. When the anal verge is defined as the distal margin of the anal canal, 15% of tumors arise from the anal margin, but this number increases to 30% when the dentate line is used as the distal limit. To clarify this issue, the American Joint Committee on Cancer (AJCC) and the Union Internationale Contra le Cancer (UICC) formed a consensus that the anal canal extends from the anorectal ring (dentate line) to the anal verge.[8,9] These two organizations agree that anal margin tumors behave in a similar fashion to skin cancers and therefore are classified and treated as skin tumors.

There is an extensive lymphatic system with many connections. The three main pathways include (1) superiorly from the rectum along the superior hemorrhoidal vessels to the inferior mesenteric lymph nodes, (2) from the upper anal canal and superior to the dentate line along the inferior and middle hemorrhoid vessels to the hypogastric lymph nodes, and (3) inferior from the anal margin and anal canal to the superficial inguinal lymph nodes.

Epidemiology

In the United States, cancers of the anal region account for 1-2% of all large bowel cancers and 4% of all anorectal carcinomas. In 2007, a total of 4650 cases of cancers of the anal region were reported in the United States, including 1900 men and 2750 women.[1] It is estimated that there will be 690 deaths per year.

Etiology

HPV Infection

Squamous cell carcinoma is closely correlated with HPV, most commonly types 16 and 18. In a population-based case control study from Scandinavia of 417 patients with anal canal cancers, a variety of behavioral factors such as sexual activity and venereal infection, tobacco consumption, and anal inflammatory lesions were examined.[10] A positive correlation was found both by univariate and multivariate analyses for the number of sexual partners and the risk of anal cancer. An association between venereal infection in both men and women was also noted.

Anal intraepithelial neoplasia (AIN) is rare in heterosexual men, while the incidence is 5-30% in HIV-negative homosexual males. These changes are rare among HIV-negative women. AIN is linked to HPV and is common in homosexual and immunosuppressed patients, especially those with HIV+.[11,12] In a report from Surawicz and colleagues of 90 homosexual men with an abnormal examination of the anal canal, 89% had HPV-associated changes.[13]

HIV (Human Immunodeficiency Virus)

There is a clear association between HIV and anal canal cancer. Cross-referencing US databases for AIDS with those for cancer, the relative risk of anal cancer in homosexual men at the time of or after AIDS diagnosis was 84.1.[14] The relative risk of anal cancer for up to five years before AIDS diagnosis was 13.9. In a series of 3595 patients undergoing a solid organ transplant the incidence of anal cancer was 0.11%.[15]

Anal canal carcinoma and AIN are associated with condylomata.[12] HPV-16 infection has a strong association with high-grade AIN and a risk of anogenital malignancy. However, HPV infection alone may be insufficient for malignant transformation, as many patients with HPV-positive cytology do not develop either AIN or anal cancer.[16]

Molecular Factors

Overexpression of p53 protein has been studied in patients receiving CMT. In an analysis involving approximately 20% of patients entered on both arms of the RTOG protocol 87-04 there was a trend toward adverse outcome (decreased local control and survival) in patients over expressing p53.[17] In one study of 55 patients, MIB-1 murine monoclonal antibody measuring KI 67 failed to predict outcome for patients treated with radiation with or without chemotherapy.[18] Patel et al proposed that activation of AKT, possibly through the PI3K-AKT pathway, is a component of the development of squamous cell cancers.[19]

Other Factors

The relationship between anal cancer and fistulas is conflicting. In one study, 41% of anal canal carcinomas were preceded by benign anorectal disease for at least 5 years.[20] However, two studies reveal only a temporal relationship but no evidence of causation.[21,22] In a separate study, homosexual males with a history of anal fissure or fistula had an elevated risk of anorectal squamous cell carcinoma (RR, 9.1).[23] Overall, the incidence of anal canal cancers in patients with Crohn's disease is low.[24] Immunosuppressed renal transplant patients have a 100-fold increase in anogenital tumors compared with the general population.[25]

Pathology

A variety of histologic cell types may occur in the anal area.[26] The majority of these (75-80%) are squamous cell carcinomas[27] and 15% are adenocarcinomas. In addition to the more common types seen in Table 90-1, other rare histologic entities can arise, such as small cell carcinomas[28] and lymphoma. Melanomas constitute 1-2% of all anal cancers.[29]

Squamous tumors may arise from the entire length of the anal canal as well as from the anal margin. Basaloid carcinomas, which are a variant of squamous carcinoma are commonly referred to as cloacogenic carcinomas. Adenocarcinomas arise from the glands at the dentate line. Small cell carcinomas are of neuroendocrine origin and are rare.

Tumors of the anal margin include squamous carcinoma, basal cell carcinoma, Bowen's disease, Paget's disease, verrucous carcinoma, and Kaposi's sarcoma. Malignant melanomas may arise from either location, but more commonly from below the dentate line.

Squamous cell tumors are divided into those with and without keratinization[30] and nonkeratinizing tumors are further subdivided into basosquamous, basaloid, and cloacogenic carcinomas. With the exception of melanoma and sarcoma, most clinicians conclude that prognosis is more dependent on stage rather than histology and treat all histologic varieties the same.[31,32] In contrast, using a multivariate analysis, Das and associates from the MD Anderson reported a higher distant metastasis rate for patients with basaloid histologies.[33]

Studies of flow cytometric analysis are conflicting and have reported both high-proliferative index but near-diploid peaks[34] as well as an aneuploid pattern.[35] In a multivariate analysis by Shepard et al, the depth of penetration, inguinal node involvement, and DNA ploidy were of independent prognostic significance.[36]

Natural History

The most common route of spread is by local extension proximally to involve other organs in the pelvis. Hematogenous spread occurs more often from tumors that arise at or above the dentate line.[37] This pattern of spread allows tumor cells into the portal system resulting in liver and lung metastases in 5-8% of patients[37] and bone in 2%.[38] Distant metastases occur with equal frequency independent of the histologic cell type involved. Distant metastases are rarely seen with anal margin tumors.

Lymphatic spread is common and involves the inguinal, pelvic, and mesenteric nodes. Inguinal lymph nodes are positive in 15-63% of cases.[39,40] The incidence of synchronous positive inguinal nodes is 15%.[37,41] In a series of 96 patients, metachronous positive inguinal nodes appeared in 25% with a median time to presentation of 12 months. Pelvic nodes are less commonly involved and mesenteric nodes are more likely to be involved if the tumors are proximal (50%) than distal (14%).[42] Positive mesenteric nodes in anal margin tumors are rare.

Historic surgical series report survivals of 0-20% following lymph node dissection with synchronous positive nodes.[43,44] Modern CMT has substantially improved this. Patients who undergo lymph node dissection for metachronous lesions have more favorable survivals with rates as high as 83%.[43,45] The majority of these recurrences occur by 2 years but may present as late as 8 years.[42]

Table 90-1 Histologic Types of Anal Cancer

Type	%
Squamous cell	63
Transitional (cloacogenic)	23
Adenocarcinoma	7
Basal cell	2
Melanoma	2
Paget's disease	2

Source: Modified from Ref. 138.

Diagnosis

The initial and most common symptom is bleeding, which occurs in over 50% of patients. Other common symptoms include pain, tenesmus, pruritus, change in bowel habits, abnormal discharge, and less commonly, inguinal lymphadenopathy.[42,46,47] Most of these symptoms are associated with benign conditions of the anus including fissure, fistula-in-ano, hemorrhoids, anal pruritus, and anal condyloma. Benign perianal conditions may coexist in 60% of anal margin tumors and in 6% of anal canal tumors.[48]

The most common physical finding is an intraluminal mass, which can be misdiagnosed as a hemorrhoid.[38,39] Endoscopically, the tumors may appear as flat or slightly raised lesions, as raised lesions with indurated borders, or as polypoid lesions. The use of transrectal ultrasound allows for the determination of depth of penetration and involvement of adjacent organs.[49]

An incisional biopsy is recommended for diagnosis. Excisional biopsies should be limited to small superficial lesions. Clinically palpable inguinal lymphadenopathy should be aspirated for cytological examination. A formal inguinal lymph node dissection is not recommended due to the associated morbidity, failure to have an impact on outcome, and the high-control rates with CMT. In a report by Garcia and associates of 46 HIV+ patients, anal brush cytology was more sensitive and specific for external compared with internal lesions.[50] High-resolution anoscopy is helpful in detecting both high-grade intraepithelial as well as invasive lesions in HIV+[51] and HIV-patients.[52]

Although a metastatic work up is commonly negative it includes computed tomography of the abdomen and pelvis to evaluate the primary tumor and to exclude liver metastases. A chest x-ray or chest computed tomography (CT) is required. In a series of 41 patients, positron emission tomography (PET) detected 91% of nonexcised primaries compared with 59% with CT alone.[53] In addition, 17% of inguinal nodes negative by CT and physical exam were positive by PET. However, PET, like sentinel node mapping[54] may be helpful but is not yet part of the standard work up. At the present time there are no reliable serum tumor markers.

Staging

A common staging system was developed by the American Joint Commission on Cancer (AJCC) and the Union Internationale Contre le Cancer (UICC) in 1997. This staging system accounts for the fact that anal canal carcinoma is primarily treated by chemoradiation (CMT) and abdominoperineal resection (APR) is reserved for treatment failure. The TNM classification is clinical. The primary tumor is assessed for size and for invasion of local structures such as the vagina, urethra, or bladder. The 6th edition of the AJCC staging system is seen in Table 90-2.[55] Compared with the 5th edition there are additional descriptors but they do not affect the stage grouping.

Prognostic Factors

As with most gastrointestinal cancers, the most important prognostic factors in anal cancer are T and N stage. In patients treated with radiation with or without chemotherapy, the most striking difference in results is seen when comparing T1-2 primary cancers (≤5 cm) vs T3-4 primary cancers (>5 cm). The local failure rates with T3-4 primary cancers are approximately 50% following CMT. When a complete response is achieved the local failure rate is 25%.

Peiffert et al reported an increase in local failure with T stage (T1: 11%, T2: 24%, T3: 45%, and T4: 43%) and a corre-

Table 90-2 **AJCC TNM Staging System for Anal Canal Cancer (6th Edition)**

Primary tumor (T)			
TX	Primary tumor cannot be assessed		
T_0	No evidence of primary tumor		
T_{is}	Carcinoma in situ		
T_1	Tumor ≤ 2 cm in maximum diameter		
T_2	Tumor > 2 cm but ≤ 5 cm in maximum diameter		
T_3	Tumor > 5 cm in maximum diameter		
T_4	Tumor of any size which invades an adjacent structure(s). (Involvement of the sphincter muscle(s) alone is not classified as T_4		
Regional lymph nodes (N)			
N_x	Regional lymph nodes cannot be assessed		
N_0	No regional lymph node metastasis		
N_1	Perirectal Lymph node metastasis		
N_2	Unilateral internal iliac and/or inguinal node metastasis		
N_3	Perirectal and inguinal node, and/or bilateral internal iliac and/or inguinal node metastasis		
Distant metastasis (M)			
M_x	Distant metastasis cannot be assessed		
M_0	No distant metastasis		
M_1	Distant metastasis		
Stage Groupings			
Stage			
0	T_{is}	N_0	M_0
I	T_1	N_0	M_0
II	T_{2-3}	N_0	M_0
IIIA	T_4	N_0	M_0
	T_{1-3}	N_1	M_0
IIIB	T_4	N_1	M_0
	T_{1-4}	N_{2-3}	M_0
IV	T_{1-4}	N_{0-3}	M_1

Note: Anal margin cancers are classified as skin cancers.

Additional Descriptors: Although they do not impact the stage grouping, additional prefixes are used which indicate the need for additional analysis:

Suffix	**Reason**
m	The presence of multiple primary tumors in a single site and is recorded in parenthesis: pT(m)NM.
y	When classification is performed during or following initial radiation and/or chemotherapy and is based on the amount of tumor present at the time of the examination, and not an estimate of tumor prior to therapy: ycTNM or ypTNM.
r	Indicates recurrent tumor: rTNM.
a	Indicates the stage at autopsy: aTNM.

Lymphatic Vessel Invasion (L)	
Lx	Cannot be assessed
LO	No lymphatic vessel invasion
L1	Lymphatic vessel invasion present

Venous Invasion (V)	
Vx	Cannot be assessed
VO	No venous Invasion
V1	Microscopic venous Invasion present
V2	Macroscopic venous invasion present

sponding decrease in 5-year survival (T1: 94%, T2: 79%, T3: 53%, and T4: 19%).[56] A similar decrease in 5-year colostomy free survival with T1-2 tumors vs T3-4 tumors was reported by Gerard and colleagues (T1: 83% and T2: 89% vs T3: 50% and T4: 54%).[57]

In contrast to T stage, the impact of positive lymph nodes is less clear. Unlike rectal cancer, inguinal lymph nodes in anal cancer are considered nodal (N) metastasis rather than distant (M) metastasis and patients should be treated in a potentially curative fashion. Cummings et al reported that patients with negative nodes who received CMT had a higher 5-year cause specific survival compared with those with positive nodes (81% vs 57%).[58]

The RTOG 87-04 trial (Table 90-3, reported a higher colostomy rate (which is an indirect measurement of local failure) in N1 vs NO patients (28% vs 13%).[59] In node negative and possibly node positive patients, the addition of mitomycin-C decreased the overall colostomy rates. The EORTC randomized trial (Table 90-3) of 45 Gy ± 5-FU/mitomycin-C also reported that patients with positive nodes experienced significantly higher local failure ($p = 0.035$) and lower survival ($p = 0.038$) rates compared to those with negative nodes.[60]

Allal et al reported that, by multivariate analysis, the only variable for which there was a possible impact was overall treatment time ($p = 0.09$).[61] In the EORTC randomized trial, multivariate analysis identified that positive nodes, skin ulceration, and male gender were independent negative prognostic factors for local control and survival.[60] Goldman and coworkers also found that women had a more favorable outcome than men.[62] The multivariate analysis of 167 patients by Das et al revealed that higher T and N stage correlated with increased local failure, N stage and basaloid histology was associated with distant failure, and N stage and HIV+ predicted for lower survival.[33] Other authors have reported that T stage, radiation dose, and percent hemoglobin were significant. In the Intergroup RTOG 98-11 trial (Table 90-3), multivariate analysis revealed that male gender ($p = 0.04$), clinically N+ ($p < 0.0001$), and tumor size > 5 cm (0.005) were independent prognostic factors for disease free survival.[63]

The histologic cell type for squamous cancers of the anal canal (squamous versus cloacogenic) has not been found to be of major prognostic significance. In some series cloacogenic carcinomas have been considered to have a slightly better prognosis[31,64] however, in 243 patients with resectable anal canal tumors, Papillon and Montbarbon reported a worse prognosis for patients with nonkeratinizing and basaloid carcinoma than for patients with keratinizing lesions.[65] Small cell carcinomas of the anus are rare and, similar to extrapulmonary small cell cancers in other parts of the body, appear to have a worse prognosis and a high incidence of metastatic disease.[28,66] Location has modest prognostic importance with anal margin tumors having a better outcome than those in the anal canal.

Three studies have examined DNA content (diploid vs nondiploid). Two found no prognostic impact of this factor[35,36] while in one multivariate analysis of 184 patients,[66] DNA ploidy was an independent prognostic factor for survival. In a separate study,[35] grade was a significant prognostic factor, with low-grade tumors resulting in a 5-year survival of 75% compared with only 24% for high-grade tumors. Data from the Princess Margaret Hospital suggest that the DT-diaphorase mutation is not a strong determinant of treatment outcome in patients who fail CMT.[67]

Tanum and Holm reported p53 expression in 34% of patients with anal carcinoma.[68] Pretreatment biopsies from 80 patients treated on the CMT arm of the intergroup RTOG 87-04 randomized trial were examined by immunohistochemistry for p53 expression.[69] For the total group, p53 protein was overexpressed in 47% of tumors. By multivariate analysis the 4-year local disease free survival was significantly decreased in those patients whose tumors overexpressed p53 (64% vs 88%, $p = 0.027$). However, significant differences were not seen in overall disease free or overall survival.

In a retrospective analysis from the Princess Margaret Hospital, p53 was measured by immunohistochemistry in

Table 90-3 ■ **Randomized Trials of Combined Modality Therapy for Anal Cancer**

Trial	No.	Initial treatment	Assessment/ Treatment of Residual		Arm	%CR	% With Colostomy	–% Local Crude	Control–Actuarial	%CFS	Survival—Overall	% Grade 4+ Early	Toxicity Late
Intergroup[59]	291 Pts	45 Gy EBRT pelvis	Residual	Boost	RT/5-FU	85	22	–	–	59	70 (4-yr)	7	
RTOG 8704	47% T3	5-FU: 1000/mg² × 96 h	Positive[a]	9 Gy +5-FU			*			*		*	
ECOG 1289	17% LN+	weeks 1 + 5		CDDP	RT/5-FU/MMC	92	9			71	75 (4-yr)	23	
			Negative	Observe									
		–vs–											
		45 Gy pelvis											
		5-FU: 1000 mg/m² × 96 h, wks 1+5											
		MMC: 10 mg/m², bolus day 1											
UKCCR[74]	585 Pts	45 Gy EBRT pelvis	≥50% CR[a]	15-20 Gy EBRT	RT	–	–	41	39 (3-yr)	–	58 (4-yr)	39	38
	51% T3			or brachytherapy				*	*			*	
	20% LN+				RT/5-FU/	–	–	64	61 (3-yr)	–	65 (4-r)	48	42
		–vs–	<50% CR	Salvage surgery	MMC								
		45 Gy EBRT pelvis											
		5-FU: 750-1000 mg/m² × 96-120 h, weeks 1+5											
		MMC: 12 mg/m², bolus day 1											
EORTC[60]	110 Pts	45 Gy EBRT pelvis	PR/CR[a]	15-20 Gy EBRT	RT	54	–	55	50 (5-yr)	40 (5-yr)	52 (5-yr)		
	85% T3			or brachytherapy				*	*	*			
	48% LN+	–vs–			RT/5-FU/	80	–	73	68 (5-yr)	72 (5-yr)	57 (5-yr)	↑ ulceration	
			<PR	Salvage surgery	MMC								
		45 Gy EBRT pelvis weeks 1+5											
		5-FU: 750 mg/m² × 120 h											
		MMC: 15 mg/m², bolus day 1											
Intergroup[63]	598 Pts	45 Gy EBRT pelvis	Positive[b]	10-14 Gy	5-FU/CDDP		20	26		48			
RTOG 98-11	28% T3	5-FU: 1000 /mg² × 96 h		5-FU/CDDP									
ECOG 1289	26% LN+	CDDP 95 mg/m² × 1		or MMC	5-FU/MMC	92	10	33		56			
		weeks 1,5,9,13	Negative	Observe	MMC								
		–vs–											
		45 Gy pelvis											
		5-FU: 1000 mg/m² × 96 h, wks 1+5											
		MMC: 10 mg/m², bolus day 1											

Abbreviations: CFS, Colostomy free survival; MMC, Mitomycin-C, CDDP, cisplatin, LN+, lymph node positive, CR, complete response, EBRT, external beam radiation therapy

*Statistically significant ($p \leq 0.05$)

[a]Biopsy at 6 weeks

[b]Biopsy at 8 weeks. The UKCCR trial includes 23% anal margin cancers.

49 patients who received CMT.[70] The incidence of p53 expression was 82%. By univariate analysis, p53 expression ≥5% was a poor prognostic factor for 5-year survival (78% vs 90%) compared with <5%. It was an independent poor prognostic factor for disease free survival ($p = 0.01$).

Treatment for Primary Disease

General Principles

Local Excision ■ Local excision has been used in selected patients with tumors that are <2 cm, well-differentiated, or tumors found incidentally at the time of hemorrhoidectomy. Of 188 patients with anal canal carcinoma treated at the Mayo Clinic, a subset of 19 were treated with local excision.[28] For the 12 patients with tumors confined to the epithelium and subepithelial connective tissues, 11 had tumors < 2 cm and 1 patient had two lesions. The survival was 100%. One of 12 patients recurred, and this patient was without evidence of disease 5 years after salvage APR. Patients with tumors penetrating into muscle who refused a colostomy had a higher recurrence rate. These patients often can be salvaged with an APR or CMT.

In summary, local excision alone is reasonable for those cancers found incidentally following hemorrhoidectomy and T1 tumors, which can be excised while maintaining sphincter continence. They require close follow-up and local recurrences can subsequently be treated with CMT.

Brachytherapy ■ In contrast with treatment programs in North America where patients receive CMT, patients treated in selected European centers receive external beam radiation therapy alone, with or without brachytherapy. The nonrandomized data suggest that the results of radiation therapy alone are comparable to CMT however, the radiation related toxicity is higher.[71] Brachytherapy techniques commonly involve afterloading ^{192}Ir. A frequent treatment approach is external beam for the first 45 Gy followed by an additional 15-20 Gy with a perineal boost or brachytherapy.

Ortholan and associates treated 66 patients with T1/TIS tumors with brachytherapy with or without small field external beam radiation.[72] With a median follow-up of 50 months there were only six local failures of which four occurred outside of the radiation field.

Abdominoperineal Resection ■ APR is reserved for salvage in patients who have failed radiation or in patients who have received prior pelvic radiation therapy. The results will be discussed later.

Combined Modality Therapy ■ The conventional treatment for anal canal cancer was APR until the late 1970s. This standard was challenged by Nigro et al in his initial report of three patients with squamous cell cancer of the anal canal who, following preoperative treatment with 30 Gy plus concurrent 5-FU and mitomycin-C, were found to have a pathologic complete response at the time of surgery.[73]

Since that time, many single-arm phase II studies have indicated that initial CMT yields a 80-90% complete response rate with APR reserved for salvage. Even in patients with large (≥5 cm) primary cancers, although the complete response rates are lower (50-75%), the majority of patients may be spared a colostomy and have an excellent overall survival.

Chemotherapy ■ Results of two prospective randomized trials (Table 90-3) from Europe of CMT vs radiation alone (EORTC[60] and UKCCCR[74]) support the use of CMT. In the UKCCCR trial, although the improvement in 4-year survival with CMT did not reach statistical significance (65% vs 58%) there was a significant improvement in 3-year actuarial local control (61% vs 29%).[74] In the EORTC trial, CMT resulted in a higher complete response rate (80% vs 54%), and a significantly higher 5-year actuarial local control rate (68% vs 50%) and colostomy free survival rate (72% vs 40%) but no significant difference in survival (57% vs 52%).[60] Although neither trial revealed a significant overall survival advantage, given the improvement in local control and colostomy free survival, they helped to establish CMT as the standard of care.

Results and Controversies

In the North America, CMT has been well established and randomized trials have focused on defining the ideal regimen. The role of mitomycin-C as a necessary component of CMT was confirmed by the Intergroup trial RTOG 87-04.[59] Patients were randomized to 45 Gy plus continuous infusion 5-FU with or without mitomycin-C. At 6 weeks following the completion of treatment patients with less than a complete response had an additional 9 Gy to the primary tumor plus concurrent 5-FU/cisplatin as salvage therapy. If there was still less than a complete response 6 weeks after the completion of this salvage therapy an APR was performed. Patients who received mitomycin-C had a higher complete response rate (92% vs 85%) and a significantly lower colostomy rate (9% vs 22%) and a corresponding significant increase in colostomy free survival (71% vs 59%) (Table 90-3). There was little difference in overall 4-year survival (75% vs 70%). Early grade 4+ toxicity was significantly increased in the mitomycin-C arm (23% vs 7%). Although overall survival was not significantly increased given the advantage in colostomy free survival, mitomycin-C is considered a necessary component of CMT.

The CMT arm using radiation/5-FU/mitomycin-C from RTOG 87-04 is the most common treatment approach. Patients received continuous course pelvic radiation to a total dose of 45 Gy (30.6 Gy whole pelvis followed by 14.4 Gy true pelvis) and two cycles (weeks 1 and 5) of concurrent continuous infusion 5-FU (1000 mg/m^2 days 1-4) and bolus Mitomycin-C (10 mg/m^2 bolus day 1). It is interesting to note that in the retrospective analysis of 167 patients reported by Das et al, 5 of the 5 pelvic recurrences occurred at the bottom of the SI joints. This is the superior border of the true pelvic field which begins at 30.6 Gy.[33]

Mitomycin-C vs Cisplatin ■ For patients who receive mitomycin-C based regimens, rates of complete response are 84% (81-87%), local control is 73% (64-86%), and 5-year survival rate is 77% (66-92%). For patients with T1-2 disease the complete response rates are >90% with ultimate local control rates following surgical salvage of 80-90%. In patients with T3-4 disease approximately 50% of patients will require a salvage APR. If they achieve a complete response following the completion of CMT then only 25% will require a salvage APR.

Although the results of 5-FU, mitomycin-C and concurrent 45 Gy are impressive there is room for improvement, especially in patients with T3-4 disease. A variety of treatment approaches have been tested. These include the use of 5-FU and cisplatin (as induction therapy and/or concurrently with radiation) and intensifying the radiation dose beyond 45 Gy using external beam or brachytherapy. The combination of 5-FU plus cisplatin is an attractive regimen: (1) patients who have failed 5-FU/mitomycin-C still respond to 5-FU/cisplatin and (2) cisplatin is a radiation sensitizer.

The Intergroup randomized trial RTOG 98-11 was developed to compare conventional CMT with 5-FU/mitomycin-c vs induction 5-FU/cisplatin chemotherapy followed by CMT with 5-FU/cisplatin (Table 90-3).[63] A total of 682 patients with stages T2-4 squamous (86%), basaloid, or cloacogenic carcinoma of the anal canal were randomized. Patients were stratified by gender, clinical node status, and tumor size and the primary endpoint was disease free survival. Overall, 27% had tumors > 5 cm, 35% had T3-4 tumors and 26% were clinically node positive.

Treatment details by arm were as follows. Conventional CMT arm: 5-FU

(1000 mg/m^2 days 1-4 and 29-32) plus mitomycin (10 mg/m^2 days 1 and 29) and radiation (45-59 Gy). Induction arm: 5-FU (1000 mg/m^2 days 1-4, 29-32, 57-60, and 85-88) plus cisplatin (75 mg/m^2 on days 1, 29, 57, and 85) and radiation (45-59 Gy beginning day 57).

Radiation doses and techniques were the same for both arms. The whole pelvis received 30.6 Gy (1.8 Gy/fx) followed by a 14.4 Gy cone down to the true pelvis. For NO patients the inguinal nodes were excluded after 36 Gy. For patients with T3-4 and/or N+ disease or for those T2 lesions with residual disease after 45 Gy a second cone down of 10-14 Gy to the gross disease or nodal disease was performed.

Palpable inguinal nodes were biopsied prior to treatment and a full thickness biopsy was optional 8 weeks following completion of CMT if any palpable residual abnormality was present in the inguinal node region. Local regional failure was defined as the present of disease in the radiation field at the 8 week follow-up.

With a median follow-up of 2.5 years, there was no significant benefit in 5-year disease free survival (60% vs 54%), 5-year survival(75% vs 70%), local-regional failure (25% vs 33%), and distant metastasis (15% vs 19%) rates in the mitomycin-C arm compared with the cisplatin arm.

The cumulative rate of colostomy was significantly improved in the mitomycin-C arm (10% vs 19%, p = 0.02). Although the overall acute grade 3+ toxicity was similar (87% vs 83%) the acute grade 3+ hematological toxicity was significantly higher in the mitomycin-C arm (61% vs 42%, $p < 0.001$).

In summary, compared with mitomycin-C based conventional CMT, induction 5-FU/cisplatin followed by CMT with 5-FU/cisplatin not only did not improve disease free survival but increased the colostomy rate. Conventional CMT with concurrent 5-FU/mitomycin-C remains the standard of care and is recommended in the NCCN guidelines.[75]

The ongoing ACT II UKCCR trial is a 4-arm trial comparing cisplatin vs mitomycin-C based CMT (50.4 Gy) with a secondary randomization to maintenance 5-FU/cisplatin vs observation. Preliminary results revent that patients who received mitomycin c significantly comparal with cisplatin had similar complate responde rates (94% vs 95%) and a higher grade 3+ hematologic toxicity note (25% vs 13%). Maintenance chenotherapy did not improve RFS or 3 year survival.[139] New CMT approaches including the use of cytotoxic agents such as capecitabine and oxaliplatin[76] are being investigated.

Dose Intensification ■ Conventional External Beam. In an attempt to improve local control and survival two parallel pilot trials of radiation dose intensification were performed. In both trials, patients received 36 Gy to the pelvis (30.6 whole pelvis plus 5.4 Gy to the true pelvis) and following a 2 week break, received an additional 23.4 Gy to the primary tumor with a 2-3 cm margin for a total dose of 59.4 Gy. The main differences between the two trials was the type of chemotherapy. The RTOG 9208 trial[77] used 5-FU and mitomycin-C whereas the ECOG 4292 trial(2297} used 5-FU and cisplatin.

The RTOG 9208 trial reported similar results to the standard regimen of 45 Gy plus 5-FU/mitomycin-C used in RTOG 87-04 except for a higher 2-year colostomy rate (30% vs 7%). Likewise, the ECOG 4292 trial did not reveal a benefit compared with conventional treatment.[78] The RTOG 98-11 trial allowed a boost of 10-14 Gy however, a dose response analysis has not been presented.[63]

Brachytherapy

Brachytherapy is an ideal method by which to deliver conformal radiation while sparing the surrounding normal structures. In most series, patients received 30-55 Gy of pelvic radiation with or without chemotherapy followed by a 15-25 Gy boost with Ir^{192} afterloading catheters. Most use low dose rate however some investigators have advocated high-dose rate.[79-81]

Combining the series, the mean results include a complete response rate of 83% (73-91%), local control rates of 81% (73-89%), and a 5-year survival rate of 70% (60-84%). The primary concern is anal necrosis and reports vary from 2% to as high as 76%[80] with an average of 5-15%.

Intensity Modulated Radiation Therapy (IMRT)

IMRT is being actively investigated as a method to deliver pelvic radiation therapy with lower acute and long term toxicity.[82,83] By identification of the dose limiting tissues surrounding the primary tumor and pelvic nodes and using multiple radiation fields to avoid them, IMRT may allow for dose escalation with less toxicity. Salama and associates treated 53 patients with IMRT based CMT.[84] Patients received 45 Gy whole pelvis followed by a boost to a median of 51.5 Gy. Acute grade 3 toxicities were 15% GI and 28% skin. Acute grade 4 toxicities included 30% leucopenia and 34% neutropenia. With a median follow-up of 15 months, freedom from failure included local (84%) and distant (93%) and survivals were colostomy free: 84% and overall: 93%. IMRT is being prospectively evaluated by the RTOG (RTOG 0529).

Radiation Therapy Alone ■ External Beam. Patients who receive radiation alone have an average local control rate of 74% (61-100%), and a 5-year survival rate of 63% (50-94%). Although the series of 18 patients from the Mayo Clinic had the highest survival and local control rate, they also had an increased complication rate requiring surgery (17%).[85] Overall, the results are comparable to patients who receive CMT with 45 Gy plus 5-FU and mitomycin-C. However, the average incidence of complications requiring surgery is 10% (range: 3-17%) which likely reflects the high-radiation doses that must be delivered to the primary site to control this disease when radiation therapy is the sole treatment modality.

Brachytherapy ± External Beam

The largest experience is from the Centre Leon Berard where 221 patients were treated over a 15-year period with external radiation therapy (Cobalt-60) to a dose of 35 Gy, followed 2 months later by an additional 15-20 Gy with an 192lr implant.[65] The serious complication rate was 3%, 5-year disease-free survival was 65%, and the locoregional control rate was 79%.

In summary, radiation therapy alone with either external beam or combined with brachytherapy may yield comparable local control and survival rates to CMT. However, since it is associated with an increase in anal necrosis even in experienced hands, it should be used with caution.

Is Biopsy Necessary at 6 Weeks?

There is considerable controversy as to the need for the first biopsy at 6 weeks following initial treatment. Data from the Princess Margaret Hospital suggest that squamous cell cancers regress slowly and continue to decrease in size for 3-12 months after the completion of CMT.[58] Based on these data, an increasing number of investigators advocate a more conservative approach and do not recommend a post-treatment biopsy. In the RTOG 87-04 trial, of the 25 patients with biopsy residual disease after 45 Gy and 5-FU/mitomycin-C who then received salvage therapy with 9 Gy plus 5-FU/cisplatin, 55% achieved a complete response 6 weeks later (a total of 12 weeks following the completion of the initial 45 Gy).[59] It is unclear if the complete response was a result of the "salvage" therapy or was due to an additional 6 weeks of tumor regression following initial therapy.

At many institutions, if there is residual disease at the 6 week post-treatment evaluation patients do not receive the 1 week of "salvage" therapy. The patients are examined every 6 weeks and providing the tumor continues to decrease in size, no salvage therapy is performed. However, if there is progression of disease or no response at 6 weeks following initial therapy, APR is necessary. In addition to careful physical exam, anal ultrasound may be helpful in following the tumor. In the Intergroup phase III anal canal cancer protocol RTOG 98-11, biopsy at 6 weeks following the initial 45 Gy was optional.

Treatment of the HIV-Positive Patient

In general, HIV+ patients have received lower doses of radiation and chemotherapy due to a concern that standard therapy may not be tolerated.[14] With a better understanding of the immunological deficiencies seen in HIV-positive patients, more recent reports have recommended therapy based on clinical and immunological parameters such as a history of prior opportunistic infections and CD4 counts.[86-88] The limited experience suggests that in patients with a CD4 count >200 µL who do not have signs or symptoms of other HIV-related diseases, aggressive CMT is appropriate. However, they need to be followed carefully and frequent modifications during therapy are likely to be necessary. For those patients with a CD4 count < 200µL or who have signs or symptoms of other HIV-related diseases, attenuated doses of radiation and/or chemotherapy are recommended. In one report there was no difference in acute or late toxicities based on CD4 counts.[86] It should be emphasized that most series include fewer than 20 patients and given the heterogeneity of the patients and treatments it is difficult to draw firm conclusions.

Toxicity of Treatment

As seen with other cancer therapies, pelvic radiation is associated with acute and long term toxicity. Large field sizes, a short overall treatment time, large fraction sizes (>2.0 Gy/day), low energy megavoltage radiation (Cobalt-60), doses of >50.4 Gy when there is small bowel in the field, the use of an AP/PA technique, treatment of only one field/day, the use of a direct perineal boost field, and the lack of computerized dosimetry all contribute to an increased incidence of radiation complications. Critical normal tissues that need to be considered in the treatment of anal canal cancer include bone marrow, rectum, small bowel, bladder, and skin. The acute toxicity is due to a combination of chemotherapy and radiation therapy. These include leukopenia, thrombocytopenia, proctitis, diarrhea, cystitis, and perineal erythema. Almost all patients will experience grade 3+ toxicity during the third week of CMT and require a 3-7 day treatment break. It must be emphasized that even when pelvic radiation is delivered with appropriate doses and techniques, approximately 1% will develop long term grade 3+ toxicity.

Although a number of reports demonstrate that radiation therapy can affect sphincter function and functional results in rectal cancer they are not directly applicable to anal cancer since patients do not undergo pelvic surgery.[89] There are limited reports of functional outcome in the anal cancer literature. One series reports that full function was maintained in 93% of patients[90] and a second series which used anorectal manometry reported complete continence in 56%.[91] Another reported good to excellent function in 93% of patients with a minimum of 1 year follow-up.[92]

Treatment of Anal Margin Cancer

Anal margin cancers are considered skin cancers. In brief, a reasonable approach is to recommend a local excision for smaller tumors (≤4 cm), which are not in direct contact with the anal verge. If the patient would require an APR due to anatomic constraints, or if a local excision would compromise sphincter function, or if the tumor is >4 cm and/or node positive, then nonoperative treatment is an appropriate alternative. Based on the randomized trial from the UKCCCR (which included 23% of patients with anal margin cancers) CMT is recommended. In a report from Erlangen, 5-year colostomy free (69%) and overall survival (54%) rates of anal margin tumors treated with CMT were lower than anal canal tumors. However, this may have been due to the higher T stages.[93]

Follow-Up After Treatment

Patients treated for anal cancer need to be followed carefully since those with local failure are amenable to salvage APR and can achieve long-term survival. Patients should be examined by physical exam and anoscopy every 6 weeks until a complete response is achieved then every 3 months for a total of 2 years. Follow-up examinations can then be decreased to every 6 months for the next 3 years and then yearly after 5-years. When failure of CMT occurs, 95% of the time it occurs within 3 years.[94]

The usefulness of computed tomography of the abdomen and pelvis or FDG-PET for follow-up is unclear. Christensen and colleagues reported that sensitivity for detecting recurrences was 1.0 for 3-D ultrasound combined with physical exam vs 0.86 for 3-D ultrasound alone vs 0.57 for 2-D ultrasound.[95] Since the most common site of failure is at the primary tumor site, there is no substitute for physical exam.

Management of Patients With Inguinal Node Involvement

When examining the impact of positive lymph nodes on local control and survival, it is important to identify the site of nodal disease as well as to differentiate synchronous versus metachronous nodal disease. Unfortunately, most series do not separate N1 vs N2 vs N3 disease. However, there are data examining synchronous vs metachronous nodal disease.

There are conflicting reports as to the prognosis of patients with synchronous nodal disease who are treated with CMT. Compared with node negative patients, Allal et al report a higher rate of local failure (N1-3: 36% vs N0:19%),[96] and the Intergroup RTOG 87-04 trial reported a higher colostomy rate (N1: 28% vs NO: 13%).[56] Although Cummings and associates reported a local failure rate of only 13% in node positive patients, 5-year cause specific survival was lower (N1-3: 57% vs NO: 81%).[58] By multivariate analysis, the EORTC randomized trial reported that positive nodes were an independent negative prognostic factor for local failure and survival.[60]

In contrast, in the CMT plus brachytherapy series from Gerard et al, patients with N1 vs N0 disease had similar 5-year disease specific and overall survival rates.[57] Likewise, complete response rates in the primary tumor are not affected by the presence of nodal disease. Doci and associates report similar rates in patients receiving cisplatin based therapy (N1-3: 92% vs NO: 100%)[97] and in a separate series of patients receiving mitomycin-C based therapy, all eight patients with N1-3 disease achieved a complete response.[98] Overall, external beam radiation alone[2,99-101] can control positive nodes in 65% of patients, and CMT[2,59,60,74] can achieve nodal control in approximately 90%.

The current treatment recommendations for patients with suspicious positive inguinal nodes include needle aspiration or at the most limited surgical sampling for confirmation of cancer followed by CMT with a boost of 45-50.4 Gy to the involved groin. Although inguinal node dissection should not be performed as part of the initial therapy it may be done for isolated inguinal recurrence in carefully selected patients since the morbidity from such an approach is significant.

The development of unilateral metachronous inguinal lymph nodes is not associated with such an ominous prognosis. After therapeutic groin dissection, the 5- to 7-year survival rates exceed 50% in two series,[41] but there were no long term survivors in a small series reported from the Mayo Clinic.[7] Current strategies in patients with metachronous isolated inguinal node metastases after CMT include a formal groin dissection followed by chemotherapy. The use of radiation in this setting depends on prior dose and fields.

Residual or Recurrent Cancer

Anal Margin

Locally recurrent anal margin cancers are more successfully controlled by local excision than are recurrences of anal canal cancer.[102,103] A series of recurrent tumors included 16 of 48 patients who, following a local excision, recurred locally (11), in the inguinal nodes (4), or both (1).[104] There were no visceral failures. The median time to recurrence was 26 months. Ten of the patients with local recurrences underwent repeat local excision, and only one required an APR. Nine of these patients survived more than 5 years. All four patients with inguinal node recurrences had inguinal lymphadenectomies, and two were long-term survivors. Although there is little reported experience with radiation therapy or CMT for patients with local recurrence after a local excision, it is a reasonable option for those who would otherwise require an APR.

Anal Canal

Following primary treatment of anal canal tumors with CMT, patients need to be evaluated for response to therapy. This is usually done 6 weeks after the completion of therapy, but Nigro[105] recommended waiting for 8 weeks and Cummings for at least 8-12 weeks.[58] If the tumor stops responding or begins to increase in size then a biopsy is recommended and if positive, the standard treatment is salvage APR.

A retrospective, nonrandomized study of patients from the V.A. Hospitals suggested that salvage surgery was superior to chemotherapy either with or without radiation therapy (53% vs19%, respectively).[106] Depending on the series, 5-year survival of local/regional failures of CMT range from 39-69%.[94,107-111] The variation in results are likely due to the small, retrospective nature of the series. The incidence of perineal wound sepsis/breakdown ranges from 42% to 70%.

In the RTOG 87-04 trial, biopsy was performed on most patients after their initial therapy.[59] For those with positive biopsies, salvage chemotherapy using cisplatin and 5-FU and concurrent 9 Gy was given. Of the 27 patients who received this "salvage" regimen, 24 underwent biopsy following its completion. Of these, 12 (50%) had a negative biopsy, and 5 of these had no further surgery after a minimum of 3 years follow-up. This indicates that at least some patients can have sphincter-sparing treatment despite failure to achieve a complete remission with first-line therapy. In the RTOG 98-11 trial, the full thickness biopsy at 8 weeks was optional.[63]

The literature is confusing regarding the outcomes of persistent vs recurrent disease. The more recent series from Ghouti[109] and Mullen[108] report not difference in the outcome of persistent vs recurrent disease.

Treatment of Metastatic Disease

Given the low incidence of anal cancer and the high success of CMT, the number of patients who develop metastatic disease is small. Single agent trials of doxorubicin (adriamycin) and of cisplatin resulting in limited responses have been reported by several investigators.[112,113] Combination chemotherapy with cisplatin and 5-FU has a response rate of approximately 50% using both systemic and regional (hepatic-arterial) routes.[114-116] Retreatment with 5-FU/mitomycin-c is an alternative. There is limited experience with newer agents such as irinotecan and cetuximab.[117]

Other Histologies

Melanoma

Anorectal melanomas are relatively rare, accounting for less than 1% of all anal canal tumors. The presenting stage, defined by the tumor thickness and nodal status, is the primary determinant of survival. Distant metastasis are common.[118-123]

Clinical Presentation and Pathologic Features ■ Anorectal melanomas are slightly more common in women, and the median age at presentation is in the sixth decade. Bleeding is the most common presenting symptom and is often attributed to hemorrhoids. Others include pain, tenesmus, pruritus, change in bowel habits, and weight loss. An initial error in diagnosis has been reported in up to 80% of patients who subsequently were diagnosed with anorectal melanoma.[118] A mass felt on rectal exam or seen extruding from the anus is common and it may appear pigmented in only one third of patients. Inguinal lymph nodes are frequently positive. The primary tumor may arise from the skin of the anal verge, the mucocutaneous junction, the transitional epithelium of the anal canal, or the rectal mucosa but is seldom found more than 5 cm from the dentate line. The pathologic characteristics of anorectal melanomas are the same as for cutaneous melanomas.

Patterns of Spread ■ Anorectal melanomas usually spread locally by direct extension proximal in the submucosal plane of the rectum, but they seldom invade bladder, vagina, sacrum, or prostate. Superior regional spread occurs via the lymphatic channels to the mesenteric system or laterally to the inguinal system. Synchronous inguinal nodes are present in 20% of patients and mesenteric nodes are involved in up to 65% undergoing radical surgery.[124] Hematogenous spread is found in up to 29% of patients at diagnosis[123,124] and overall in up to 69%.[125] Common sites of distant metastasis include the lungs, liver, and bone.

Treatment and Outcome ■ The traditional surgical approach was APR with pelvic lymph node dissection and bilateral groin dissection.[126] Since most patients with inguinal metastases died of disease, groin dissection is no longer performed.[126,127] Because of the high systemic failure rate, several authors have questioned the role of radical surgery and have advocated wide local excision.[118]

In the early reports from Memorial Sloan-Kettering,[128] the only long-term survivors were patients who had undergone an APR with or without lymphadenectomy. Similar results were found at the Mayo Clinic.[127] Despite a better local control rate with APR, most series have not shown a clear survival advantage for patients who have had an APR compared with patients having wide local excision.[118,119,124,129,130]

Several factors have been analyzed to determine their effect on outcome. Age and race are the only factors that have consistently been shown not to correlate with overall survival. Size was not an important factor in the results from Quan et al[126] but had a direct impact on survival in the study by Goldman and colleagues.[131]

A retrospective analysis of the SEER database of 126 patients treated from 1973 to 2001 with a variety of therapies was reported by Podnos et al[132] The 5-year survival based on disease status at presentation included local (32%), local/regional (17%) and distant (0%).

The inability to show a survival benefit for APR compared with wide local excision can be attributed to the small numbers of patients involved in the studies, selection bias, and the lack of randomized data. Any relative advantage of adjuvant immunotherapies, chemotherapy, and radiation therapy is similarly obscured and difficult to interpret. A histologic margin of at least 3 mm should be obtained if local excision is to be used. In view of possible higher local control rates, APR is still a reasonable option.[119-122,125,131]

Adenocarcinoma

Primary adenocarcinoma of the anal canal arising from the anal glands is rare. Most adenocarcinomas in the canal represent rectal cancer with distal spread. In general they should be treated like adenocarcinomas of the rectum. If T3 and or N+ then preoperative CMT followed by surgery and 4 months of postoperative adjuvant therapy is appropriate. However, the radiation fields should include the inguinal nodes. In a series of 13 patients, Beal and associates recommended the combination of CMT and APR and reported a 2-year actuarial survival of 62%.[133] Adenosquamous cancers of the anus are also rare and have a poor prognosis.[134] Given the squamous component, it is reasonable to treat these patients with combined 5-FU/mitomycin-C and concurrent radiation therapy with APR for salvage.

Sarcoma

Few cases of leiomyosarcoma of the anus have been reported. The optimal treatment for this neoplasm is not known. The standard surgical approach is APR. Using a technique well established for management for sarcomas of the extremities, one approach is local excision and Iridium-192 brachytherapy in an attempt to preserve the anal sphincter.[135-137] This technique may be an alternative to APR in selected patients.

Others

Bowen's disease, Paget's disease and Kaposi's sarcoma are commonly treated with surgery. Is settings where this could compromise sphincter function there are rare reports of treatment with CMT.

Selected References

The complete reference list can be found at www.CANCERMEDICINE8.com

1. Jemal A, Siegel R, Ward E, et al. Cancer statistics, 2007. *CA Cancer J Clin.* 2007;57:43–66.
8. American Joint Committee on Cancer. Anal canal. In: Fleming ID, Cooper JS, Henson DE, et al. *AJCC Cancer Staging Manual.* Philadelphia: Lippincott-Raven; 1997:91–96.
9. Anal canal. In: Sobin LH, Wittekind Ch. *TNM Classification of Malignant Tumors.* New York: Wiley-Liss; 1997:70–73.
11. Shepherd NA. Anal intraepithelial neoplasia and other neoplastic precursor lesions of the anal canal and perianal region. *Gastroenterol Clin North Am.* 2007;36:969–987.
12. Abramowitz L, Benabderrahmane D, Ravuad P, et al. Anal squamous intraepithelial lesions and condyloma in HIV-infected heterosexual men, homosexual men and women: prevalence and associated factors. *AIDS.* 2007;21:1457–1465.
17. Bonin SR, Pajak TJ, Russell AH, et al. Overexpression of p53 protein and outcome of patients with chemoradiation for carcinoma of the anal canal: a report of the randomized trial RTOG 87-04. Radiation Therapy Oncology Group. *Cancer.* 1999;85:1226–1233.
19. Patel H, Polanco-Echeverry G, Segditsas S, et al. Activation of AKT and nuclear accumulation of wild type TP53 and MDM2 in anal squamous cell carcinoma. *Int J Cancer.* 2007;15:2668–2673.
22. Lin AY, Gridley G, Tucker M. Benign anal lesions and cancer. *N Engl J Med.* 1995;332:190.
33. Das P, Bhatia S, Eng C, et al. Predictors and patterns of recurrence after definitive chemoradiation for anal cancer. *Int J Radiat Oncol Biol Phys.* 2007;68:794–800.
50. Garcia FU, Haber MM, Butcher J, et al. Increased sensitivity of anal cytology in evaluation of internal compared with external lesions. *Acta Cytol.* 2007;51:893–899.
51. Nahas CS, Lin O, Weiser MR, et al. Prevalence of perianal intraepithelial neoplasia in HIV-infected patients referred for high-resolution anoscopy. *Dis Colon Rectum.* 2006;49:1581–1586.
52. Pineda CE, Berry JM, Jay N, et al. High resolution anoscopy in the planned staged treatment of anal squamous intraepithelial lesions in HIV-negative patients. *J Gastrointest Surg.* 2007;11:1410–1415.
53. Cotter SE, Grigsby PW, Siegel B, et al. FDG-PET/CT in the evaluation of anal carcinoma. *Int J Radiat Oncol Biol Phys.* 2006;65:720–725.
54. Damin DC, Rosito MA, Schwartsmann G. Sentinel lymph node in carcinoma of the anal canal: a review. *Eur J Surg Oncol.* 2006;32:247–252.
56. Peiffert D, Bey P, Pernot M, et al. Conservative management by irradiation of epidermoid cancers of the anal canal: prognostic factors of tumor control and complications. *Int J Radiat Oncol Biol Phys.* 1997;37:313–324.
57. Gerard JP, Ayzac L, Hun D, et al. Treatment of anal canal carcinoma with high dose radiation therapy and concomitant fluorouracil-cisplatinum. Long term results in 95 patients. *Radiother Oncol.* 1998;46:249–256.
58. Cummings BJ, Keane TJ, O'Sullivan B, et al. Epidermoid anal cancer; treatment by radiation alone or by radiation and 5-fluorouracil with and without mitomycin-C. *Int J Radiat Oncol Biol Phys.* 1991;21:1115–1125.
59. Flam M, John M, Pajak T, et al. Role of mitomycin in combination with fluorouracil and radiotherapy, and salvage chemoradiation in the definitive nonsurgical treatment of epidermoid carcinoma of the anal canal: results of a phase III randomized intergroup study. *J Clin Oncol.* 1996;14:2537–2539.
60. Bartelink H, Roelofsen F, Eschwege F, et al. Concomitant radiotherapy and chemotherapy is superior to radiotherapy alone in the treatment of locally advanced anal cancer: results of a phase III randomized trial of the European Organization for Research and Treatment of Cancer radiotherapy and gastrointestinal cooperative groups. *J Clin Oncol.* 1997;15:2040–2049.
61. Weber DC, Kurtz JM, Allal AS. The impact of gap duration on local control in anal canal carcinoma treated by split-course radiotherapy and concomitant chemotherapy. *Int J Radiat Oncol Biol Phys.* 2001;50:675–680.
63. Ajani JA, Winter KA, Gunderson LL, Pedersen J, Benson III AB, Thomson CR et al et al. Fluorouracil, mitomycin, and radiotherapy vs Fluorouracil, cisplatin and radiotherapy in carcinoma of the anal canal. A randomized controlled trial. JAMA 2008;299:1914–21.
65. Papillon J, Montbarbon JF. Epidermoid carcinoma of the anal canal. *Dis Colon Rectum.* 1987;30:324–333.
69. Bonin SR, Qian C, Russell AH, et al. Overexpression of p53 protein is associated with decreased local disease-free survival in patients treated with chemoradiation for anal canal cancer: a report of RTOG 87-04. *Int J Radiat Oncol Biol Phys.* 1996;36:210–217.
74. UKCCCR Anal Cancer Trial Working Party. Epidermoid anal cancer: results from the UKCCCR randomised trial of radiotherapy alone versus radiotherapy, 5-fluorouracil, and mitomycin. *Lancet.* 1997;348:1049–1054.
75. Engstrom PF, Benson III, AB, Chen YJ, et al. Anal canal cancer: clinical practice guidelines in oncology. *J Natl Comp Cancer Network.* 2005;3:510–515.
77. John M, Pajak T, Flam M, et al. Dose escalation in chemoradiation for anal cancer: preliminary results of RTOG 92-08. *Cancer J Sci Am.* 1996;2:205–211.
78. Martenson JA, Lipsitz SR, Wagner H, et al. Initial results of a phase II trial of high dose radiation therapy, 5-fluorouracil, and cisplatin for patients with anal cancer (E4292): an Eastern Cooperative Oncology Group study. *Int J Radiat Oncol Biol Phys.* 1996;35:745–749.
79. Gerard JP, Mauro F, Thomas L, et al. Treatment of squamous cell anal canal carcinoma with pulsed dose rate brachytherapy. Feasibility study of a French cooperative group. *Radiother Oncol.* 1999;51:129–131.
81. RBruna A, Gastelblum P, Thomas L, et al. Treatment of squamous cell anal canal carcinoma (SCACC) with pulsed dose rate brachytherapy: a retrospective study. *Radiother Oncol.* 2006;79:75–79.
82. Meyer J, Czito B, Yin FF, et al. Advanced radiation therapy technologies in the treatment of rectal and anal cancer: intensity-modulated photon therapy and proton therapy. *Clin Colorec Cancer.* 2007;6:348–356.
84. Salama JK, Mell LK, Schomas DA, et al. Concurrent chemotherapy and Intensity-modulated radiation therapy for anal cancer patients: a multicenter experience. *J Clin Oncol.* 2007;25:4581–4586.

85. Martenson JA, Gunderson LL. External radiation therapy without chemotherapy in the management of anal cancer. *Cancer*. 1993;71:1736–1740.
86. Edelman S, Johnstone PAS. Combined modality therapy for HIV-infected patients with squamous cell carcinoma of the anus: outcomes and toxicities. *Int J Radiat Oncol Biol Phys*. 2006;66:206–211.
88. Wexler A, Berson AM, Goldstone SE, et al. Invasive anal squamous-cell carcinoma in the HIV-positive patient: outcome in the era of highly active antiretroviral therapy. *Dis Colon Rectum*. 2008; 51:73–81.
91. Vordermark D, Sailer M, Flentje M, et al. Continence and anorectal manometry after curative-intent radiation therapy for anal carcinoma. *Int J Radiat Oncol Biol Phys*. 1999;45s:340.
93. Grabenbauer GG, Kessler H, Matzel KE, et al. Tumor site predicts outcome after radiochemotherapy in squamous cell carcinoma of the anal region: long-term results of 101 patients. *Dis Colon Rectum*. 2005;48:1742–1751.
94. Renehan AG, Saunders MP, Schofield PF, et al. Patterns of local disease failure and outcome after salvage surgery in patients with anal cancer. *Br J Surg*. 2005;92:605–614.
96. Allal AS, Mermillod B, Roth AD, et al. The impact of treatment factors on local control in T2-T3 anal carcinomas treated by radiotherapy with or without chemotherapy. *Cancer*. 1997;79:2329–2335.
99. Schlienger M, Krzisch C, Pene F, et al. Epidermoid carcinoma of the anal canal treatment results and prognostic variables in a series of 242 cases. *Int J Radiat Oncol Biol Phys*. 1989;17:1141–1151.
100. Papillon J. Rectal and anal cancers. In: Papillon J, ed. *Rectal and Anal Cancers*. New York: Springer-Verlag; 1982:1–130.
102. Mendenhall WM, Zlotecki RA, Vauthey JN, et al. Squamous cell carcinoma of the anal margin treated with radiotherapy. *Surg Oncol*. 1996;5:29–34.
106. Longo WE, Vernava AM, Wade TP, et al. Recurrent squamous cell carcinoma of the anal canal. Predictors of initial treatment failure and results of salvage therapy. *Ann Surg*. 1994;220:40–49.
107. Schiller DE, Cummings BJ, Rai S, et al. Outcomes for salvage surgery for squamous cell carcinoma of the anal canal. *Ann Surg Oncol*. 2007;14:2780–2789.
108. Mullen JT, Rodriguez-Bigas MA, Chang GJ, et al. Results of surgical salvage after failed chemoradiation therapy for epidermoid carcinoma of the anal canal. *Ann Surg Oncol*. 2007;14:478–483.
110. Akbari RP, Paty PB, Guillem JG, et al. Oncologic outcomes of salvage surgery for epidermoid carcinoma of the anus initially managed with combined modality therapy. *Dis Colon Rectum*. 2004;47:1136–1144.
124. Brady MS, Kavolius JP, Quan SHQ. Anorectal melanoma: a 64-year experience at Memorial Sloan-Kettering Cancer Center. *Dis Colon Rectum*. 1995;38:146–153.
132. Podnos YD, Tsai NC, Smith D, et al. Factors affecting survival in patients with anal melanoma. *Am Surg*. 2006;72:917–920.
133. Beal KP, Wong D, Guillem JG, et al. Primary adenocarcinoma of the anus treated with combined modality therapy. *Dis Colon Rectum*. 2003;46:1320–1324.
137. Grann A, Paty PB, GuillemJG, et al. Sphincter preservation of leiomyosarcoma of the rectum and anus with local excision and brachytherapy. *Dis Colon Rectum*. 1999;42:1296–1299.
139. James R, Wan S, Glynne-Jones R, Sebag-Montefiore D, Kadalayil L, Northover J, Cunningham D, Meadows H, and Leadermann J. A randomized trial of chemoradiation using mitomycin or cisplatin, with or without maintencance cisplatin/5-FU in squamous cell carcinoma of the anus (ACT II). Proc ASCO 2000;27,797s.

91 Renal Cell Carcinoma

Brian I. Rini, MD ▪ Daniel Y.C. Heng, MD ▪ Ming Zhou, MD, PhD ▪ Andrew Novick, MD ▪ Derek Raghavan, MD, PhD, FACP, FRACP

Introduction

The incidence of renal cell carcinoma (RCC) is estimated at approximately 36,000 cases with 13,000 deaths in the United States annually.[1] The reported incidence of RCC has increased over time, largely but not entirely due, to an increase in the number of asymptomatic tumors incidentally detected with abdominal imaging obtained for other indications.[2,3]

Many advances in RCC have been made in recent years. Novel approaches to treating localized renal masses that emphasize less invasive and nephron-sparing approaches have been developed. Further, the biology underlying RCC has been elucidated, and agents targeting relevant biologic pathways have demonstrated robust clinical effect in the metastatic setting. This chapter will detail these advances and summarize the epidemiology, pathology, staging and treatment of RCC.

Epidemiology

RCC commonly presents in the sixth or seventh decade of life and develops in men twice as frequently as in women. A meta-analysis of 24 studies demonstrated that tobacco exposure is an established risk factor for RCC with a relative risk of approximately 2-3 fold.[4] Obesity is also a risk factor although specific dietary associations are not well-defined. Compared with men in the lowest three eighths of a cohort for body mass index (BMI), men in the middle three eighths had a 30-60% greater risk of renal-cell cancer, and men in the highest two eighths had nearly double the risk (P for trend, <0.001).[5] Hypertension, but not likely anti-hypertensive medicine, is associated with RCC development.[6] Acquired polycystic disease also predisposes to the development of RCC. A small percentage of patients (2-3%) will have one of several autosomal dominant syndromes which predispose patients to various RCC histologic subtypes which are detailed subsequently. One Australian study suggested that analgesic abuse is associated with RCC, although more commonly this association is found for cancer of the renal pelvis (see Chapter 92).

Clinical Presentation

In contemporary series, more than 50% of RCC patients present without initial symptoms as a result of abdominal CT scans or ultrasounds performed for an unrelated indication.[7-10] This has changed over the years as evidenced by the fact that in the 1970s, 10% of RCCs were discovered incidentally compared to 60% in 1998.[3,11]

The most common local symptoms of RCC include hematuria, flank pain and a palpable mass, although this classic triad is currently observed infrequently. Other local presentations include left scrotal varicoceles that may be observed in up to 11% of men because of obstruction of the gonadal vein by tumor in the left renal vein to which it directly empties. Venous involvement can also cause lower extremity edema, ascites, hepatic dysfunction and pulmonary emboli. Pain or dysfunction of specific organs may be the presenting feature of the patient with metastatic disease.

Systemic symptoms of paraneoplastic syndromes may also be an initial manifestation of RCC. Hypercalcemia is the most common paraneoplastic syndrome in RCC manifesting in 13-20% of patients. This is mediated by tumor production of parathyroid hormone (PTH) or PTH-related peptide. Patients who have bone metastases may have hypercalcemia as well, but the mechanism is due to direct bone release of calcium as opposed to a paraneoplastic process. Polycythemia occurs in 1-8% of cases and is postulated to be mediated by elevated erythropoietin levels. Stauffer syndrome is hepatic dysfunction in the setting of RCC without liver metastases. Endocrine abnormalities including elevated human chorionic gonadotropin (HCG) and adrenocorticotropic hormone (ACTH) have also been reported. Other systemic manifestations include constitutional symptoms such as fever, weight loss and fatigue.

Pathology

The WHO classification of renal neoplasms published in 2004 categorized malignant parenchymal renal cell neoplasms into three main and several other rare subtypes.[12] The most common RCC histology is the conventional clear cell subtype accounting for 75-80% of all RCCs. The remaining subtypes including papillary (10-15%), chromophobe (5-10%), medullary (<1%) and collecting duct carcinoma (<1%) (Fig. 91-1). Recently, several new entities, including RCC associated with Xp11.2/TFE3 translocation and mucinous tubular and spindle cell carcinoma, have also been described. Metanephric adenoma, oncocytoma, and papillary adenoma are benign tumors. Sarcomatoid differentiation is not a distinct histologic subtype, but rather represents a transformation to a higher grade malignancy that can occur across subtypes and is associated with a poor outcome.[13]

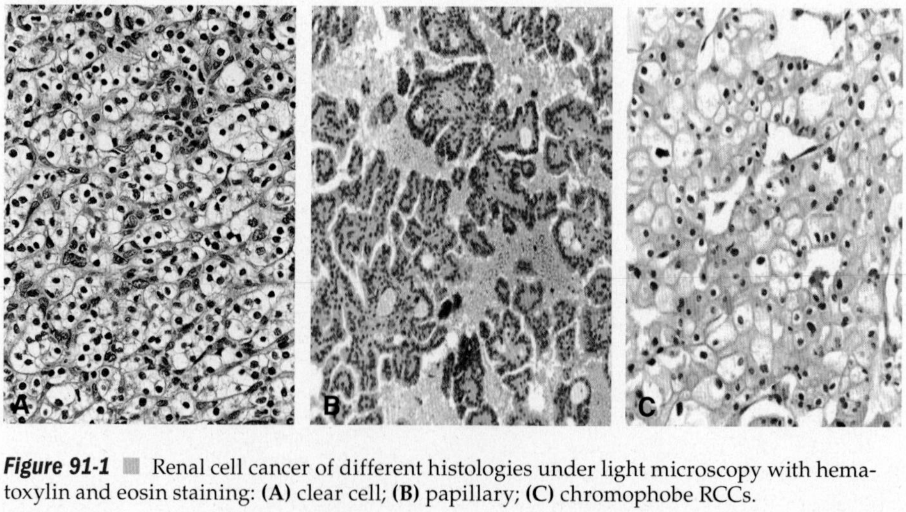

Figure 91-1 Renal cell cancer of different histologies under light microscopy with hematoxylin and eosin staining: **(A)** clear cell; **(B)** papillary; **(C)** chromophobe RCCs.

Conventional clear cell RCC arises from the proximal convoluted tubule and has clear cytoplasm on routine microscopic sections. The most common genetic alteration in clear cell RCC is a highly specific abnormality involving silencing of chromosome 3p (the von hippel-Lindau [*VHL*] gene) that occurs in approximately 35-50% of sporadic cases.[12] In addition, inactivation of the gene transcription by promoter hypermethylation is seen in 20% of the cases. Non-inherited clear cell RCC tends to present with larger, unilateral tumors. The inherited VHL syndrome (1/36,000 births) is a highly penetrant autosomal dominant disorder in which patients inherit a *VHL* gene defect on chromosome 3p25 and develop clear cell RCC and/or a constellation of cysts and tumors in the central nervous system and abdominal viscera.[14] Central nervous system lesions include retinal hemangioblastomas, endolymphatic sac tumors and craniospinal hemangioblastomas. The visceral lesions in these patients include clear cell RCCs, pheochromocytomas, pancreatic neuroendocrine tumors, epididymal cystadenomas and broad ligament cystadenomas.

Papillary RCC arises from the distal convoluted tubule and this is composed of tubulopapillary structures with hemosiderin deposition and foamy histiocytes within the fibrovascular cores. This is subdivided into type 1 and type 2 papillary RCC based on the morphology of the tumor cells lining the papillary structures.[12] Papillary carcinomas do not have *VHL* gene inactivation, but have trisomy of chromosomes 7, 17 and loss of Y chromosome as the most frequent genetic alterations. Other changes include chromosomal gain involving 3q, 8, 12, 16, and 20. Papillary tumors tend to have a multifocal nature and may present with bilateral kidney involvement. Two hereditary syndromes predispose to development of papillary RCC. Hereditary papillary renal carcinoma (HRPC) is characterized by c-Met proto-oncogene activation (chromosome 7q31-34) and the development of type 1 papillary RCC. Hereditary leiomyomatosis renal cell carcinoma (HLRCC) involves abnormalities of the fumarate hydratase gene (chromosome 1q42-43) and development of type 2 papillary RCC, leiomyomas of skin and uterine leiomyomas and leiomyosarcomas.[15]

Chromophobe RCC arises from the intercalated cells of the kidney and is characterized by large solid sheets of cells with pale or eosinophilic cytoplasm, a thick and distinct cell membrane and pleomorphic nuclei with an irregular nuclear membrane and perinuclear clearing.[12] The most frequent genetic alterations are a combination of loss of heterozygosity in chromosomes 1, 2, 6, 10, 13, 17, 21 and hypodiploidy. Patients with chromophobe histology tend to present with early stage disease with <5% of patients presenting with metastases.[16,17] Patients with Birt-Hogg-Dube (BHD) syndrome have a high proportion of RCCs with chromophobe-predominant histology. They possess loss of function mutations in the BHD gene on chromosome 17p, have prominent cutaneous manifestations (fibrofolliculomas) and are predisposed to pneumothoraces from rupture of pulmonary cysts.[18]

Prognostic Features

Grade

In patients with localized RCC, nuclear Fuhrman grade and tumor-node-metastasis (TNM) stage are consistently the most important prognostic factors.[19] The Fuhrman grading system scores the nuclear grade of RCCs on a scale of 1 (least aggressive) to 4 (most aggressive) based on nuclear and nucleolar size, shape and content.[20] Higher nuclear grade is associated with a worse 5-year overall survival. 5-year cancer-specific survival rates for localized grade 1, grade 2, and grade 3 or 4 tumors after nephrectomy are 89%, 65% and 46%, respectively.[19] A recent study demonstrated that Fuhrman grading is not useful for chromophobe RCC.[21]

Staging

In a patient with a suspected RCC, staging investigations including a CT of the chest (or CXR) and CT of the abdomen and pelvis are required to define the extent of the disease. The most common sites of metastases include the lungs, abdominal and mediastinal lymph nodes, liver and bone. Unless a patient has symptoms suggestive of bone or brain metastases, initial bone scans and CT scans of the head tend to be low yield. Whether baseline bone scans are indicated remains controversial, although, for purposes of consistency, they are often included in the protocols of clinical treatment trials.

The 2002 American Joint Committee on Cancer (AJCC) staging system is detailed in Table 91-1.[22] Patients with stage I disease have tumor confined within the kidney capsule. Stage II involves invasion through the renal capsule but within Gerota fascia. Stage III indicates regional lymph node, ipsilateral renal vein or inferior vena cava involvement. Stage IV disease requires distant metastases or involvement of adjacent organs other than the ipsilateral adrenal gland. This staging system reflects data that demonstrate poorer prognostic outcomes for patients with tumor extension through Gerota's fascia, venous involvement and lymph node metastases.

Treatment of Localized RCC

A number of treatment options exist for small (<4 cm) renal masses (Table 91-2). These include surgical excision, radiofrequency ablation (RFA) or cryotherapy (collectively called thermal ablation) or active surveillance with delayed intervention in very select populations. Surgical resection remains the cornerstone of the treatment of localized stage I and II RCC and usually obviates the need for a renal biopsy. Partial nephrectomy is preferred whenever feasible, especially in a patient with limited renal function, bilateral tumors and/or a patient with a solitary kidney. Although laparoscopic partial nephrectomy is less invasive, the technical skill required is high. In addition, the risk of hemorrhage is higher and increased operative times may lead to suboptimal intraoperative kidney perfusion. Therefore, more complex cases are best managed with an open surgical approach.

Table 91-1 AJCC (2002) Staging of Renal Cell Carcinoma

Tumor (T)	Node (N)	Metastases (M)	Stage
T0: No primary tumor			
T1: <7 cm limited to kidney			Stage I: T1 N0 M0
T1a: <4 cm			
T1b: 4-7 cm			
T2: >7 cm limited to kidney	N0: No nodes involved		Stage II: T2 N0 M0
T3: Involvement of major veins, adrenal gland and/or perinephric tissues but within Gerota fascia	N1: Involvement of single regional lymph node	M0: No distant metastases	Stage III: T3 N0 M0 Any N1 M0
T3a: Adrenal or perinephric tissue			
T3b: Renal vein or IVC			
T3c: IVC above diaphragm or involving IVC wall			
T4: Tumor invades beyond gerota fascia	N2: Involvement of more than one regional lymph node	M1: Distant metastases	Stage IV: T4 N0 M0 Any N2 Any M1

Table 91-2 ■ **Strategies in the Management of Small Renal Masses**

Modality	Advantages	Limitations
Radical nephrectomy	Established oncologic efficacy Technique in common community use	Increased risk of chronic kidney disease
Partial nephrectomy	Oncologic efficacy similar to radical nephrectomy for T1 tumors Preserves renal function	Small risk of postoperative hemorrhage or urinary leak Technically demanding
Thermal ablation	Minimally invasive Repeat ablation possible Better preservation of renal function compared to partial nephrectomy	Long-term oncologic efficacy not established Increased local tumor recurrenceDifficult to adequately treat tumors >3.5 cm diameter
Active surveillance	Most series have substantial selection bias and limited follow-up Average growth rates / risk of metastasis relatively low	Long-term oncologic outcomes not established Morbidity of intervention avoided in most patients, deferred in others

The preferred treatment of large tumors (>7 cm) and locally advanced tumors is a radical nephrectomy, either with a laparoscopic or open procedure. This involves ligation of the renal vasculature, excision of the kidney, Gerota fascia, and the ipsilateral adrenal grand. Laparoscopic radical nephrectomy is currently widely performed and has decreased postoperative pain to allow for shorter hospitalization and quicker recovery.

Thermal ablative options such as cryoablation and RFA are newer modalities. In RFA, electrodes are inserted directly into the tumor to deliver a high-frequency alternating current that causes ionic agitation and frictional heating that induces necrosis. In cryoablation, cryoprobes are inserted percutaneously and an ice ball formed at the tip of the probe within the tumor freezes surrounding tissue and induces necrosis. However, both of these procedures do not have rigorous long-term outcome data and there are reports that the risk of local recurrence is much higher in these procedures compared to traditional surgical excision.[23] Randomized controlled trials comparing these noninvasive approaches to traditional surgical treatment are not available. Thus, these procedures are usually limited to patients with smaller tumors (<4 cm) desiring an option other than surgery or who are not candidates for invasive operations.[24]

Lastly, a recent meta-analysis of patients with small renal masses that were initially observed demonstrated an average growth rate of only 0.28 cm per year, and only 1% of tumors metastasized.[25] This study is limited by short follow-up and an appropriately biased patient population with advanced age and comorbidities that made surgery less desirable. Thus, there may be a role for careful observation in this select group of patients.

Stage III disease involves the adrenal gland, perinephric tissues, lymph nodes and/or invasion of the renal vein or inferior vena cava. The procedure of choice for these individuals is an open radical nephrectomy for curative intent. Lymph node dissection should be carried out in patients with evidence of enlarged lymph nodes. In patients with no suspected nodal metastases, a routine extended lymph node dissection is controversial.

Metastatic Disease

Prognostic Factors

The most widely used prognostic factors for metastatic renal cell carcinoma were developed in the era where patients with metastatic RCC were treated primarily with immunotherapy. The Memorial Sloan-Kettering Cancer Center (MSKCC) criteria were developed via multivariable analysis in patients being treated for metastatic RCC with initial interferon (IFN) alpha based therapy (Table 91-3).[26] A clinical scoring system was developed and then validated by the bootstrap method and validated independently at the Cleveland Clinic.[27] These criteria classify patients into favorable, intermediate, and poor prognosis categories based on the number of adverse risk features present. The median progression free survival (PFS) for each of these categories was 8.3, 5.1, 2.5 months, respectively. The median overall survival for each prognostic category was 30, 14, and 5 months, respectively (log rank $p < 0.00001$).

Table 91-3 ■ **Memorial Sloan-Kettering Cancer Center (MSKCC) Prognostic Criteria for Metastatic RCC**

Adverse Prognostic Factors
Karnofsky performance status <80%
Diagnosis to treatment interval <1 year
Hemoglobin < lower limit of normal
Serum corrected calcium >10 g/dL
LDH > 1.5x upper limit of normal
Risk Categories and Clinical Outcome
0 prognostic factors (good risk): PFS: 8.3 m OS: 30 m
1-2 prognostic factors (intermediate risk): PFS: 5.1 m OS: 14 m
3-5 prognostic factors (poor risk): PFS: 2.5 m OS: 5 m

Abbreviations: OS, overall survival; PFS, progression-free survival.

New prognostic factors are being developed for contemporary patients being treated with targeted therapy described below.[28] The Cleveland Clinic adverse prognostic factors include the time from diagnosis to treatment 0, baseline platelet count :300 K/μL, baseline neutrophil count of :4.5 K/μL, and baseline corrected calcium of 10 mg/dL. Further prospective investigation will be required to further refine these criteria.

Levels of vascular endothelial growth factor (VEGF) expression have become a considerable subject of research due to potential biomarker capabilities. In retrospective series, serum VEGF is significantly increased in patients with RCC compared with controls (median 343.4 pg/mL vs 103.8 pg/ml; $p = 0.0001$).[29] In the placebo arm of a randomized trial of patients previously treated with immunotherapy, high levels of VEGF were associated with inferior survival. Patients with VEGF levels of less than or equal to 131 pg/mL had a median overall survival of 3.3 months while those with greater than 131 pg/mL had a median overall survival of 2.7 months ($p < 0.01$).[30] VEGF levels are thus prognostic of outcome in RCC, but have not yet proven predictive for response to VEGF-targeted therapy

Surgery in Patients With Metastatic Disease

Radical nephrectomy is also indicated in many patients with metastatic RCC (mRCC). Two phase 3 studies randomized patients to radical nephrectomy or not, followed by IFN in all patients. In a combined analysis of these trials, median survival was 7.8 months in patients treated with interferon-alpha alone versus 13.6 months for patients who underwent cytoreductive nephrectomy initially.[31-33] A greater survival advantage was observed in patients with better performance status. The cytoreductive paradigm remains predominant even though data in support of it are primarily empiric and has not been tested specifically in combination with the newer targeted agents described below. The observation of primary tumor responses with targeted agents may alter this paradigm in the future.

While cytoreductive nephrectomy appears to benefit many patients with metastatic RCC, it is not curative and should not be performed indiscriminate-

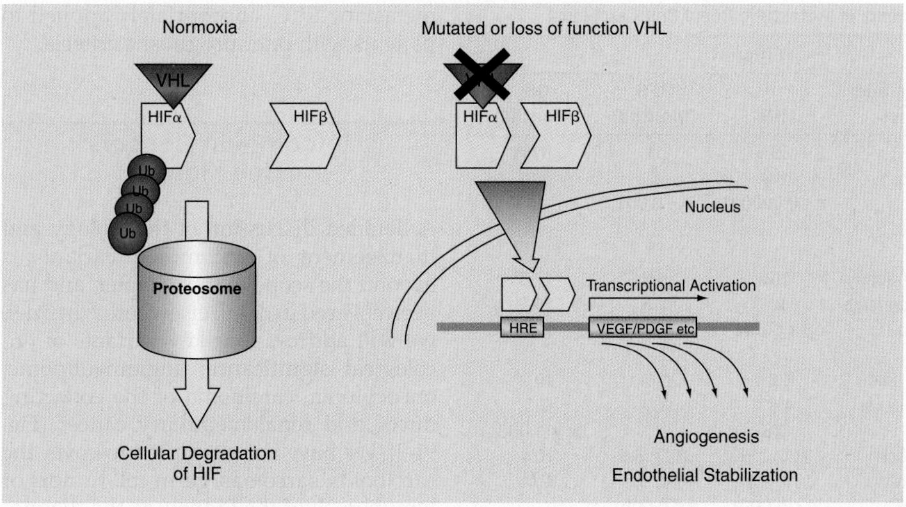

Figure 91-2 Normal function of VHL in the normoxic state compared to the aberrant VHL state/hypoxia. Under normal conditions, VHL binds to HIFα and polyubiquinates it to mark it for destruction in the cellular proteosome. In conditions of hypoxia or when VHL function is lost, HIFα binds HIFβ and then translocates into the nucleus to activate HIF responsive elements (HRE). This results in transcriptional activation of genes important in angiogenesis and endothelial stabilization such as VEGF and PDGF.

ly. Patients who are most likely to benefit from cytoreduction include those with: (1) substantial tumor burden (eg, :75%) in the involved kidney; (2) good performance status; and (3) no central nervous system or liver metastases (with rare exceptions).[34] Other considerations pertain to surgical resectability, particularly the potential for morbidity if there is proximity to vital structures, encasement of the renal hilum or other complicating factors.

Patients with disseminated RCC with solitary metastases may be considered for metastasectomy, although they represent a minority (2-3%) of cases. Favorable prognostic factors include a long interval between initial diagnosis and development of metastases, which reflects an indolent course and reinforces the likelihood that the metastasis is truly solitary. In addition, a complete resection of metastatic disease to render the patient to have no evidence of disease; eg, a solitary lung nodule must be feasible.[35] Patients with favorable features can anticipate up to a 30% 5-year survival with metastasectomy, and thus surgical resection of metastases should be considered in highly selected RCC patients.

Systemic Therapy for Metastatic Disease

Immunotherapy

As early trials employing chemotherapy did not produce any significant benefit,[36,37] immunotherapy had long been the standard of care for the treatment of metastatic RCC in an attempt to harness the innate immune response of RCC tumors. Interferon alpha has produced response rates of 10-15% with modest prolongation of overall survival versus inactive controls.[38] A pooled analysis investigating the use of high-dose interleukin-2 (IL-2) revealed an overall response rate of 14%, with 5% complete responses.[39] The majority of patients that achieved a complete response had durable disease remission. It is to be noted that there were significant side effects including capillary leak syndrome, which necessitated intensive blood pressure monitoring and the occasional requirement for vasopressors. Phase 3 trials of high-dose IL-2 failed to demonstrate significant benefits for the cohort versus alternative, low-dose cytokine regimens.[40,41] Thus, immunotherapy remains relevant in metastatic RCC due to the small percentage of patients who may dramatically benefit with a complete response, although attempts to identify and isolate the responding group have been uniformly unsuccessful. High-dose IL-2 is noteworthy for a small but real percentage of durable complete remissions, although it is only able to be applied to a highly selected minority of the RCC population at large. The occasional patient with very extensive disease, including the involvement of lung, bone and/or liver, may sustain a remission measured in years.

Targeted Therapy

New treatment approaches were developed through a better understanding of the biology and genetics of RCC. As noted previously, most clear cell RCCs demonstrate an abnormality of the *VHLs* gene (Fig. 91-2). When inactivated via mutation or methylation, the *VHL* gene product cannot regulate the degradation of a transcription factor called hypoxia inducible factor (HIF) alpha. HIF-alpha accumulates and leads to the transcription of a number of hypoxia-regulated genes including vascular endothelial growth factor (VEGF) and platelet-derived growth factor (PDGF). These growth factors bind to their respective tyrosine kinase receptors to promote angiogenesis and tumor growth.[14] These intricate pathways have become targets for drugs that have now revolutionized the scope of treatment for metastatic RCC (Table 91-4).

VEGF Ligand-Directed Therapy

Bevacizumab is a recombinant monoclonal neutralizing antibody that binds and neutralizes circulating VEGF. The activity of this agent in RCC was initially identified by small randomized trials.[42,43] A subsequent phase 3 clinical trial randomized nephrectomized patients with clear cell mRCC to the combination of IFN (3 times per week at a dose of 9 million international units (MIU) for up to 1 year) plus bevacizumab (10 mg/kg IV every 2 weeks) or IFN with placebo until disease progression.[44] The addition of bevacizumab to IFN significantly increased PFS (10.2 vs. 5.4 months) (HR 0.63; $p < 0.0001$) and objective tumor response rate (31% vs. 13%; $p < 0.0001$). A CALGB phase 3 trial of similar design confirmed a PFS benefit (8.5 vs. 5.2 months, $p < 0.0001$) and ORR benefit (25% vs. 13%, $p < 0.0001$) to bevacizumab plus IFN.[45] Common toxicities included hypertension and proteinuria with rare but serious toxicity including bowel perforation, arterial ischemic events and bleeding. It is unknown whether or not bevacizumab must be given in combination with interferon as there was no bevacizumab monotherapy arm in the phase 3 trials. Nevertheless, it is important in the armamentarium of treatments for RCC.

Receptor tyrosine kinases (RTKs) play an integral role in the signaling cascade of VEGF and PDGF.[46] RTKs have an extracellular domain that binds their respective ligand. There is a transmembrane region spanning the membrane into the cytoplasm and an intracellular domain that holds the tyrosine kinase responsible for downstream signaling. Upon ligand binding, the RTKs dimerize or multimerize to induce a conformational change that allows ATP binding resulting in autophosphorylation and transphosphorylation. These phosphorylated tyrosine domains are then able to activate downstream signal transduction through phosphorylation of various proteins.

Sunitinib is an oral multikinase inhibitor that blocks VEGFR-1, 2, and 3, PDGFR-B and related RTKs.[47] Initial phase 2 trials of sunitinib in metastatic RCC (a total of 169 patients who had failed prior

Table 91-4 Selected Clinical Trials of Targeted Agents in Metastatic Renal Cell Carcinoma

Agent	Mechanism	Population and Trial Arms	Efficacy RR	PFS (Months)	OS (Months)
Sunitinib[51]	Tyrosine kinase inhibitor of VEGF and related receptors	First-line sunitinib vs. IFN	39% 8% $p < 0.000001$	11 5 $p < 0.001$	N/A N/A
Sorafenib[54]	Tyrosine kinase inhibitor of VEGF and related receptors	Treatment-refractory, 2nd-line sorafenib vs. placebo	10% 2% $p < 0.001$	5.5 2.8 $p < 0.01$	17.8 15.2 $p = 0.14630$
Temsirolimus[56]	mTOR inhibitor	Poor risk first-line temsirolimus vs. IFN	8.6% 4.8% NS	N/A N/A	10.9 7.3 $p < 0.008$
Bevacizumab[44,45*]	VEGF ligand-binding antibody	First-line bevacizumab+ IFN vs. placebo+ IFN	31%, 25% 13%, 13% $p < 0.0001$	10.2, 8.5 5.4, 5.2 $p < 0.0001$	N/A N/A

*The results of two phase 3 bevacizumab trials are shown.
Abbreviations: IFN, interferon, N/A, not available or data not yet mature, NS, not statistically significant, *p* values for PFS are based on hazard ratios.

cytokine-based therapy) demonstrated an investigator-assessed objective response rate of 45%, a median duration of response of 11.9 months and a median progression-free survival (PFS) of 8.4 months.[48-50] The pivotal phase 3 randomized controlled trial[51] that enrolled 750 patients compared first-line sunitinib with interferon and demonstrated a statistically significant advantage in objective response rate (39% vs. 8%; $p < 0.000001$) and PFS (11 vs. 5 months) with a hazard ratio of 0.42 ($p < 0.001$). Of note, most patients enrolled (94%) had favorable or intermediate risk Memorial Sloan-Kettering Cancer Center (MSKCC) prognostic criteria.[52] Common toxicity included fatigue, hand-foot syndrome, diarrhea, mucositis and hypertension. This agent has become a standard of care for the first-line treatment of metastatic RCC.

Sorafenib was initially investigated for its ability to inhibit *Raf* thereby affecting the mitogen activated protein kinase (MAPK) signaling pathway responsible for downstream proliferation responses. However, it subsequently became clear that there was activity against VEGFR-2, VEGFR-3, PDGFB, Flt-3, and c-kit.[53] The Treatment Approaches in Renal Cancer Global Evaluation Trial (TARGET) was the largest study of previously-treated metastatic clear cell RCC, and enrolled 903 patients randomized to oral sorafenib 400 mg twice daily versus placebo.[54] All patients enrolled had favorable or intermediate risk MSKCC prognostic criteria. There was a clear median PFS benefit (5.5 vs. 2.8 months) in the sorafenib group. Objective response rate was minimal (10% investigator assessed), although over 70% of patients had some degree of tumor burden reduction. Based on these data, sorafenib has been FDA approved and become a standard of care for second-line treatment of mRCC after immunotherapy failure. However, in a randomized phase II trial of first-line sorafenib versus IFN, a PFS benefit could not be demonstrated.[55] Thus, sorafenib has assumed largely a second-line or later role in the treatment of metastatic RCC.

mTOR Inhibition

The "mammalian target of rapamycin" (mTOR) kinase is regulated by Akt and PI3 Kinase which are both downstream of VEGFR. mTOR is a component of intracellular pathways that promote tumor growth and proliferation and is a mediator of the hypoxic response. Temsirolimus is an FDA-approved mTOR inhibitor that binds to FKBP-12 to create a complex that directly inhibits mTOR. A phase 3 trial[56] included 626 previously untreated patients with poor prognostic criteria and randomized them to temsirolimus 25 mg IV weekly, interferon alpha 18 MU 3 times/week or temsirolimus 15 mg IV weekly + IFN 6 MU 3 times/week. Patients were required to have three or more of the following adverse risk features: Karnofsky performance status <80%, lactate dehydrogenase >1.5 times laboratory upper limit of normal, hemoglobin < laboratory lower limit of normal, serum calcium corrected for albumin >10 mg/dL, time from first diagnosis of RCC to start of therapy of <1 year and three or more metastatic sites. It is to be noted that 19% of patients included in this trial had non-clear cell histology. Temsirolimus monotherapy demonstrated an overall survival advantage compared to interferon alpha (10.9 vs. 7.3 months, log rank $p < 0.008$). The objective response rates were 8.6% for temsirolimus, and 4.8% for interferon which was not statistically significant. Temsirolimus has become a first-line standard of care for patients with metastatic RCC, appropriately applied to patients with poor prognostic criteria.

Uncommon Cancers of the Kidney

A detailed discussion of the biology and management of uncommon variants is beyond the scope of this chapter, and has been covered in detail elsewhere.[57] In brief, we will address four key variants of oncological significance: angiomyolipoma, oncocytoma, carcinoma of the collecting ducts, and renal medullary cancer (Fig. 91-3). We have not attempted to cover the carcinoids, sarcomas, germ cell tumors or lymphomas of the kidney, as the diagnosis and management are not unique to this organ site. Adult Wilms tumor is beyond the scope of this overview and has been discussed in detail elsewhere.[57]

Angiomyolipoma

Renal angiomyolipoma (AML) is a benign mesenchymal neoplasm, representing about 1% of resected renal tumors, which is most important in posing a diagnostic dilemma (vis-à-vis RCC).[57] It can present sporadically (80%) or in association with tuberous sclerosis, and in the latter situation, the tumors tend to be larger, present earlier, and to be associated more often with hemorrhage and multicentricity.[58] The higher prevalence in females, rapid growth in pregnancy and presence of estrogen and progesterone receptors suggest a possible linkage to sex hormone production. AML often has loss of heterozygosity of one of the genes that causes tuberous sclerosis, tuberous sclerosis 1 (TSC1) on chromosome 9q34 or TSC2 on chromosome 16p13. Once viewed as very uncommon, the widespread use of CT and MRI scanning has indicated that it is a relatively common, asymptomatic entity.

Pathologically this is usually a moderate to large sized, yellow-gray mass lesion, well demarcated from the kidney. AML can be solitary or multiple, can cause a mass effect (rather than infiltration), and is composed of thick walled blood vessels, adipocytes and smooth muscle cells. Immunohistochemically, this tumor is characterized by coexpression of smooth muscle and melanocyte markers, a range of non-specific proteins, but usually no epithelial markers.[59] Occasional lymph node involvement is thought to represent multicentric involvement, rather than true metastasis. The vast majority of the published literature suggests that these tumors rarely are aggressive, and more than 90% of AML less than 1-2 cm in diameter show no growth over 5 years.[57] This indolent neoplasm contrasts with the more dangerous vari-

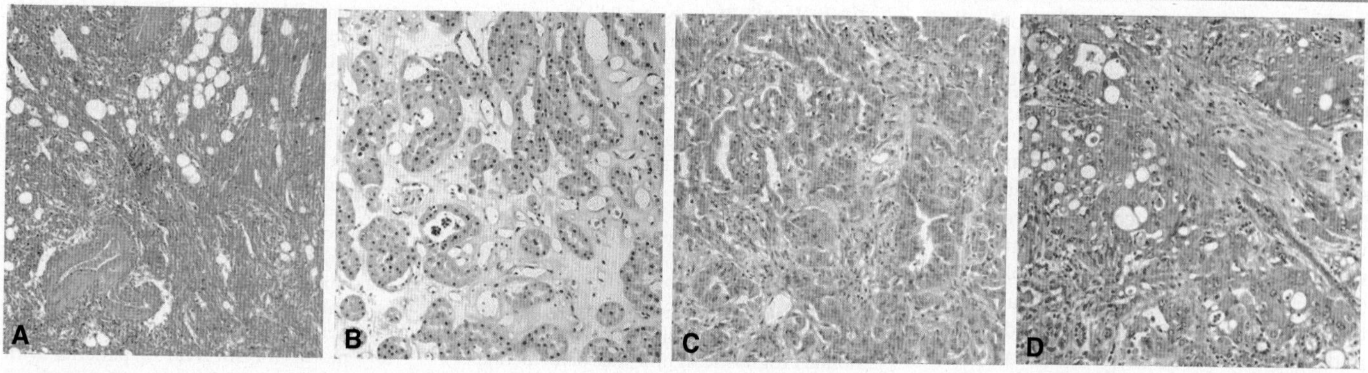

Figure 91-3 Uncommon cancers of the kidney. **(A)** Angiomyolipoma characteristically is composed of 3 elements: thick-walled blood vessels, adipocytes and smooth muscle cells. **(B)** Oncocytomas are uniform with abundant granular and eosinophilic cytoplasm embedded in a loose and myxoid stroma. **(C)** Collecting duct RCC consists of high-grade tumor cells forming complex and angulated tubules or tubulopapillary structures embedded in a remarkably desmoplastic stroma. **(D)** Renal medullary carcinoma comprises of high-grade tumor cells with desmoplastic stroma arranged in irregular nests with microcystic formation.

ant, epithelioid angiomyolipoma, which is potentially malignant, more heavily associated with tuberous sclerosis, with an even gender distribution and a somewhat younger age of onset.

The clinical presentation can be remarkably similar to that of RCC, either without symptoms or with classical features, such as pain, hematuria and a palpable mass. When the diagnosis is made on radiological imaging, the presence of intratumoral fat is the key, although this is not pathognomonic of this diagnosis. It should be remembered that RCC is sometimes associated with tuberous sclerosis.

AML is classically a slow growing tumor. The optimal approach to management is somewhat controversial, although there is general consensus that a diagnosis should be made, and that intervention may be required for tumors that are symptomatic or growing, for those tumors that are large at presentation, or where there is uncertainty whether this is AML or RCC. Treatment options include nephrectomy (complete or partial) or angiographic embolization. Nephron-sparing surgery is preferred. In our experience at the Cleveland Clinic, 27 patients with AML underwent partial nephrectomy, 21 of whom had a solitary kidney or impaired contralateral kidney; none required dialysis post-operatively, and none recurred at median follow up of 39 months.[58] Angiographic embolization is a relatively common alternative to surgical treatment, as is associated with complications in about 10% of cases, including abscess, hemorrhage, more generalized infection and pleural effusion.[58] There is no defined role for radiotherapy or chemotherapy in the management of these tumors.

Renal Oncocytoma

Renal oncocytomas are benign neoplasms that arise from the intercalated cells of the collecting duct and account for 3-5% of renal tumors in most large series.[60] They may be difficult to distinguish histologically from chromophobe RCC and clear cell RCC with eosinophilic cells. They are usually diagnosed incidentally although patients may occasionally present with flank pain, hematuria or a palpable mass. Most oncocytomas are confined within the renal parenchyma and are well circumscribed while capsular invasion or metastasis is rare.[57]

Pathologically, they are characterized by large uniform well-differentiated cells with abundant granular and eosinophilic cytoplasm embedded in a loose and myxoid stroma. The distinct perinuclear clearing seen in chromophobe RCC is absent in oncocytomas and examination using Hale's colloidal iron staining is mostly negative in oncocytomas but diffusely positive in chromophobe RCC.[57] Oncocytomas exhibit chromosomal alterations that generally fall into one of three groups: some have a deletion of chromosome 1 and X/Y, some have a balanced translocation involving 11q13, and others contain sporadic or no chromosomal alterations.[61]

The standard treatment of an oncocytoma is a curative partial nephrectomy. Patients who opt for a more conservative non-surgical approach should be closely monitored and should have surgical extirpation if there is rapid growth or evidence of concomitant RCC. Although renal oncocytomas are benign, their coexistence with RCC is not uncommon and can be seen in 10-32% of patients. Often, the inability of imaging and biopsy to reliably diagnose oncocytoma leads most patients to be treated surgically.[57]

Collecting Duct Carcinoma

Collecting duct carcinoma (CDC) represents less than 1% of kidney cancer.[57] It was originally thought to derive from distal tubular epithelium, but more recently has been show to arise in the collecting ducts. CDC, which is usually found in the renal medulla, ranges in size from small to greater than 10 cm and often has an irregular margin with evidence of local infiltration. Often surrounded by desmoplastic stroma, CDC has a variable tubular-papillary pattern of growth, with high grade nuclei and high mitotic activity. Mucin and sarcomatoid changes may be seen. There is no classical immunohistochemical appearance.

CDC is an aggressive tumor, often presenting at advanced stage. Common features include hematuria, flank pain or abdominal pain, and there are frequently metastases at first presentation, including lung, liver, bone, adrenals or lymph nodes. There is a 2:1 male predominance, with a broad age range of presentation. The appearance on CT scan is not specific, and consists mainly of a centrally arising infiltrative lesion without much contrast enhancement.

The diagnosis of CDC is usually made at surgery, which remains the definitive treatment for localized disease. However, this is one of the aggressive variants of renal cancer, and thus is often associated with early metastasis.[57,62] There is little evidence that immunotherapy has any significant utility, and thus most reports of treatment of metastatic disease have involved the use of systemic chemotherapy, mostly predicated on cisplatin-containing regimens.[57,62] Unfortunately remissions are relatively infrequent and of short duration. It has recently been suggested that the combination of cisplatin and gemcitabine has sustained activity,[63] although it is possible that the two cases treated in this report represented mis-diagnosed transitional cell cancer of the upper tract. Interestingly, these two case reports related to tumors occurring in adolescents.

Renal Medullary Carcinoma

This unusual tumor, located predominantly in the renal medulla, is frequently associated with hemoglobinopathies, such as sickle cell disease or trait.[57,64] It is thought to arise from the distal collecting duct. Similarly to CDC, it has an infiltrative pattern of growth. Histologically there are several variants, mostly characterized by hemorrhage, infiltration and necrosis, sometimes with areas of poorly differentiated cells, arrayed in sheets. The immunohistochemical appearances, similar to CDC, are not specific, although there appears to be a consistent reaction with markers of epithelial differentiation, such as antibodies to anti-cytokeratin (CAM 5.2) or epithetical membrane antigen (EMA).[64] There is no well-defined pattern of molecular or genetic features.

Like CDC, these tumors are often aggressive, found in a predominantly male population, and in particular in younger patients. Common presenting symptoms include hematuria, weight loss and abdominal or flank pain. Metastases are frequently present initially. Many of the case reports have been identified in African Americans with sickle cell trait or disease.

Surgical resection is the treatment of choice, when feasible, but as noted above, most patients present with metastatic disease. There is no defined optimal treatment for systemic spread. Immunotherapy seems to be relatively ineffective. There have been isolated case reports of the use of cytotoxic agents, including cisplatin based chemotherapy,[57,65] sometimes augmented with gemcitabine. It is unclear whether tyrosine kinase inhibition or other targeted therapies will have a definitive role. The quality of these data is predominantly disappointing, focused mostly on isolated case reports.

Conclusion

Renal cell carcinoma incidence is increasing worldwide. Surgery remains a mainstay of treatment for localized tumors and is part of multimodality therapy in the metastatic setting. An enhanced understanding of the biology of RCC has led to the clinical development of a number of targeted therapies that have substantially altered the therapeutic landscape. Future investigative endeavors include further refinement of the approach to the small renal mass, a better understanding of the biology of response and resistance to targeted therapy and clinical testing of combinations and sequences of targeted therapy in metastatic RCC.

Selected References

The complete reference list can be found at www.CANCERMEDICINE8.com

2. Chow WH, Devesa SS, Warren JL, Fraumeni JF, Jr. Rising incidence of renal cell cancer in the united states. *JAMA.* 1999;281:1628-1631.
3. Pantuck AJ, Zisman A, Belldegrun AS. The changing natural history of renal cell carcinoma. *J Urol.* 2001;166:1611-1623.
4. Hunt JD, van der Hel OL, McMillan GP, Boffetta P, Brennan P. Renal cell carcinoma in relation to cigarette smoking: meta-analysis of 24 studies. *Int J Cancer.* 2005;114:101-108.
5. Chow WH, Gridley G, Fraumeni JF, Jr, Jarvholm B. Obesity, hypertension, and the risk of kidney cancer in men. *N Engl J Med.* 2000;343:1305-1311.
7. Tsui KH, Shvarts O, Smith RB, Figlin R, de Kernion JB, Belldegrun A. Renal cell carcinoma: Prognostic significance of incidentally detected tumors. *J Urol.* 2000;163:426-430.
9. Mevorach RA, Segal AJ, Tersegno ME, Frank IN. Renal cell carcinoma: Incidental diagnosis and natural history: review of 235 cases. *Urology.* 1992;39:519-522.
10. Lee CT, Katz J, Fearn PA, Russo P. Mode of presentation of renal cell carcinoma provides prognostic information. *Urol Oncol.* 2002;7:135-140.
11. Nguyen MM, Gill IS, Ellison LM. The evolving presentation of renal carcinoma in the united states: trends from the surveillance, epidemiology, and end results program. *J Urol.* 2006;176:2397-2400; discussion 2400.
12. Pathology and genetics of tumours of the urinary system and male genital organs. In: Eble JN, Sauter G, Epstein JI, Sesterhenn IA, eds. Lyon, IARC Press; 2004.
13. Kwak C, Park YH, Jeong CW, et al. Sarcomatoid differentiation as a prognostic factor for immunotherapy in metastatic renal cell carcinoma. *J Surg Oncol.* 2007;95:317-323.
14. Cohen HT, McGovern FJ. Renal-cell carcinoma. *N Engl J Med.* 2005;353:2477-2490.
15. Delahunt B, Eble JN. Papillary renal cell carcinoma: a clinicopathologic and immunohistochemical study of 105 tumors. *Mod Pathol.* 1997;10:537-544.
16. Cheville JC, Lohse CM, Zincke H, Weaver AL, Blute ML. Comparisons of outcome and prognostic features among histologic subtypes of renal cell carcinoma. *Am J Surg Pathol.* 2003;27:612-624.
17. Patard JJ, Leray E, Rioux-Leclercq N, et al. Prognostic value of histologic subtypes in renal cell carcinoma: a multicenter experience. *J Clin Oncol.* 2005;23:2763-2771.
18. Pavlovich CP, Walther MM, Eyler RA, et al. Renal tumors in the birt-hogg-dube syndrome. *Am J Surg Pathol.* 2002;26:1542-1552.
19. Tsui KH, Shvarts O, Smith RB, Figlin RA, deKernion JB, Belldegrun A. Prognostic indicators for renal cell carcinoma: a multivariate analysis of 643 patients using the revised 1997 TNM staging criteria. *J Urol.* 2000;163:1090-1095; quiz 1295.
20. Fuhrman SA, Lasky LC, Limas C. Prognostic significance of morphologic parameters in renal cell carcinoma. *Am J Surg Pathol.* 1982;6:655-663.
22. Greene FL. *American Joint Committee on Cancer Cancer Staging Manual,* 6th Edition. New York: Springer-Verlag; 2002.
23. Kunkle DA, Egleston BL, Uzzo RG. Excise, ablate or observe: the small renal mass dilemma-a meta-analysis and review. *J Urol.* 2008;179:1227-1233; discussion 1233-1234.
24. Kaouk JH, Aron M, Rewcastle JC, Gill IS. Cryotherapy: clinical end points and their experimental foundations. *Urology.* 2006;68:38-44.
25. Chawla SN, Crispen PL, Hanlon AL, Greenberg RE, Chen DY, Uzzo RG. The natural history of observed enhancing renal masses: meta-analysis and review of the world literature. *J Urol.* 2006;175:425-431.
26. Motzer RJ, Bacik J, Mariani T, Russo P, Mazumdar M, Reuter V. Treatment outcome and survival associated with metastatic renal cell carcinoma of non-clear-cell histology. *J Clin Oncol.* 2002;20:2376-2381.
27. Mekhail TM, Abou-Jawde RM, Boumerhi G, et al. Validation and extension of the memorial sloan-kettering prognostic factors model for survival in patients with previously untreated metastatic renal cell carcinoma. *J Clin Oncol.* 2005;23:832-841.
28. Choueiri TK, Garcia JA, Elson P, et al. Clinical factors associated with outcome in patients with metastatic clear-cell renal cell carcinoma treated with vascular endothelial growth factor-targeted therapy. *Cancer.* 2007;110:543-550.
29. Jacobsen J, Rasmuson T, Grankvist K, Ljungberg B. Vascular endothelial growth factor as prognostic factor in renal cell carcinoma. *J Urol.* 2000;163:343-347.
30. Bukowski RM, Eisen T, Szczylik C, et al. Final results of the randomized phase III trial of sorafenib in advanced renal cell carcinoma: survival and biomarker analysis. *J Clin Oncol.* 2007;25:5023.
31. Flanigan RC, Salmon SE, Blumenstein BA, et al. Nephrectomy followed by interferon alfa-2b compared with interferon alfa-2b alone for metastatic renal-cell cancer. *N Engl J Med.* 2001;345:1655-1659.
32. Mickisch GH, Garin A, van Poppel H, de Prijck L, Sylvester R, European Organisation for Research and Treatment of Cancer (EORTC) Genitourinary Group. Radical nephrectomy plus interferon-alfa-based immunotherapy compared with interferon alfa alone in metastatic renal-cell carcinoma: a randomised trial. *Lancet.* 2001;358:966-970.
33. Flanigan RC, Mickisch G, Sylvester R, Tangen C, Van Poppel H, Crawford ED. Cytoreductive nephrectomy in patients with metastatic renal cancer: a combined analysis. *J Urol.* 2004;171:1071-1076.
34. Rini BI, Campbell SC. The evolving role of surgery for advanced renal cell carcinoma in the era of molecular targeted therapy. *J Urol.* 2007;177:1978-1984.
35. Pfannschmidt J, Hoffmann H, Muley T, Krysa S, Trainer C, Dienemann H. Prognostic factors for survival after pulmonary resection of metastatic renal cell carcinoma. *Ann Thorac Surg.* 2002;74:1653-1657.
36. Motzer RJ, Russo P. Systemic therapy for renal cell carcinoma. *J Urol.* 2000;163:408-417.
37. Yagoda A, Petrylak D, Thompson S. Cytotoxic chemotherapy for advanced renal cell carcinoma. *Urol Clin North Am.* 1993;20:303-321.
38. Coppin C, Porzsolt F, Awa A, Kumpf J, Coldman A, Wilt T. Immunotherapy for advanced renal cell cancer. *Cochrane Database Syst Rev.* 2005;(1):CD001425.
42. Yang JC, Haworth L, Sherry RM, et al. A randomized trial of bevacizumab, an anti-vascular endothelial growth factor antibody, for metastatic renal cancer. *N Engl J Med.* 2003;349:427-434.
43. Bukowski RM, Kabbinavar FF, Figlin RA, et al. Randomized phase II study of erlotinib combined with bevacizumab compared

with bevacizumab alone in metastatic renal cell cancer. *J Clin Oncol*. 2007;25:4536-4541.

44. Escudier B, Pluzanska A, Koralewski P, et al. Bevacizumab plus interferon alfa-2a for treatment of metastatic renal cell carcinoma: a randomised, double-blind phase III trial. *Lancet*. 2007;370:2103-2111.
48. Motzer RJ, Michaelson MD, Redman BG, et al. Activity of SU11248, a multitargeted inhibitor of vascular endothelial growth factor receptor and platelet-derived growth factor receptor, in patients with metastatic renal cell carcinoma. *J Clin Oncol*. 2006;24:16-24.
49. Motzer RJ, Michaelson MD, Rosenberg J, et al. Sunitinib efficacy against advanced renal cell carcinoma. *J Urol*. 2007;178:1883-1887.
51. Motzer RJ, Hutson TE, Tomczak P, et al. Sunitinib versus interferon alfa in metastatic renal-cell carcinoma. *N Engl J Med*. 2007;356:115-124.
52. Motzer RJ, Bacik J, Murphy BA, Russo P, Mazumdar M. Interferon-alfa as a comparative treatment for clinical trials of new therapies against advanced renal cell carcinoma. *J Clin Oncol*. 2002;20:289-296.
53. Ahmad T, Eisen T. Kinase inhibition with BAY 43-9006 in renal cell carcinoma. *Clin Cancer Res*. 2004;10:6388S-6392S.
54. Escudier B, Eisen T, Stadler WM, et al. Sorafenib in advanced clear-cell renal-cell carcinoma. N Engl J Med. 2007;356:125-134.
55. Szcylik C, Demkow T, Staehler M, et al. Randomized phase II trial of first-line treatment with sorafenib versus interferon in patients with advanced renal cell carcinoma: final results. *J Clin Oncol*. 2007;25:5025.
56. Hudes G, Carducci M, Tomczak P, et al. Temsirolimus, interferon alfa, or both for advanced renal-cell carcinoma. *N Engl J Med*. 2007;356:2271-2281.
57. Kalmadi SR, Zhou M, Novick A, Bukowski RM. Uncommon tumors of the kidney. In: Raghavan D, Brecher ML, Johnson DH, Meropol NJ, Moots PL, Rose PG, eds. *Textbook of Uncommon Cancer*, 3rd ed. Chichester, London: Wiley; 2006:1-17.
58. Fazeli-Matin S, Novick AC. Nephron-sparing surgery for renal angiomyolipoma. *Urology*. 1998;52:577-583.
59. Nelson CP, Sanda MG. Contemporary diagnosis and management of renal angiomyolipoma. *J Urol*. 2002;168:1315-1325.
61. Chao DH, Zisman A, Pantuck AJ, Freedland SJ, Said JW, Belldegrun AS. Changing concepts in the management of renal oncocytoma. *Urology*. 2002;59:635-642.
62. Dimopoulos MA, Logothetis CJ, Markowitz A, Sella A, Amato R, Ro J. Collecting duct carcinoma of the kidney. *Br J Urol*. 1993;71:388-391.
63. Peyromaure M, Thiounn N, Scotte F, Vieillefond A, Debre B, Oudard S. Collecting duct carcinoma of the kidney: a clinicopathological study of 9 cases. *J Urol*. 2003;170:1138-1140.
64. Swartz MA, Karth J, Schneider DT, et al. Renal medullary carcinoma: clinical, pathologic, immunohistochemical, and genetic analysis with pathogenetic implications. *Urology*. 2002;60:1083-1089.
65. Strouse JJ, Spevack M, Mack AK, et al. Significantresponsestocisplatin-basedchemotherapy in renal medullary carcinoma. *Pediatr Blood Cancer*. 2005;44:407-411.

92 Tumors of the Renal Pelvis and Ureter

Ali-Reza Golshayan, MD ■ Inderbir Gill, MD, MCh ■ Cristina Magi-Galluzzi, MD, PhD ■ Derek Raghavan, MD, PhD

Introduction

Tumors of the ureter and the renal pelvis are uncommon. They most frequently arise from the urothelium, and account for about 5% of urothelial malignancies. Approximately 3000 cases are diagnosed annually in the United States.[1] The incidence of these malignancies has increased over the past 20 years,[2] presumably because of changes in smoking, analgesic abuse and industrial exposure. Tumors of the renal pelvis are more common than ureteral cancers (2-4 times); most ureteral cancers occur in the distal ureter.[3] These tumors may occur synchronously or metachronously since the urothelium lines the entire urinary tract. Synchronous bilateral upper urinary tract cancers are very rare. In addition, these patients are at higher risk for bladder cancer both at diagnosis and in the future.[4] Although urothelial malignancies share many characteristics with carcinomas of the urinary bladder, many important differences distinguish these tumors which influence diagnosis, treatment and prognosis.

Epidemiology

Upper urinary tract tumors preferentially affect the elderly, especially in the fifth to eighth decades. The peak age of incidence is reported to be 60-65 years.[2,5] These tumors are two to three times more common in men than in women, although women have a 50% higher risk of death from this disease. They are twice as common in Caucasians as in African Americans.[6]

Etiology

Most tumors of the renal pelvis and ureter may be associated with environmental exposures in the workplace such as dyes, petrochemicals and plastics.[7] These tumors may occur up to 15 years after initial exposure. In the 1950s and 1960s, the ingestion of phenacetin-containing analgesics by factory workers was linked to the development of urothelial malignancy.[8] Analgesic abuse continues to be a significant factor to the present day.[9] Cigarette smoking has been associated with seven times increase in the risk of ureteral or renal pelvis cancer, and worldwide is likely the most common etiologic factor in this disease.[10]

Other etiologic factors that have been reported include hypertension, coffee consumption, industrial exposure, human papilloma virus exposure and chronic laxative use.[7,11-14] However, there has been no consistent cancer risk associated with food intake, vitamin use or body mass index.[15] In the Balkan regions, up to 50% of renal tumors are cancers of the renal pelvis because of an endemic familial interstitial nephropathy. Affected families have a 100-200 times increased risk of upper urinary tract cancers.[16] The risk of urothelial carcinomas is increased tenfold in those families with hereditary non-polyposis colon cancer.[17] These patients are more often younger and female.

Pathobiology

The urothelial lining represents a continuous epithelial layer from the renal calyces to the distal ureter, and is very similar to that of the bladder except for a less thick muscular layer. Urothelial carcinomas (UC) (also known as transitional cell carcinomas or [TCC]) account for the majority of upper urinary tract tumors (>90%), since they derive from the urothelium (Fig. 92-1). Urothelial carcinomas may be papillary or sessile. Papillary UCs account for 85% of the tumors of the renal pelvis and ureter. Grossly the lesions are soft, translucent, and occur most often in the lower portion of the ureters. Larger tumors have a tendency to have associated necrosis and hemorrhage. Invasion through and beyond the thinner muscular layer (subepithelial connective tissue) is more likely than in bladder cancer. UCs may also have associated urothelial carcinoma in situ (CIS), which may be difficult to identify and can present as a white plaque or a red patch.[18]

Squamous cell carcinomas (Fig. 92-2) account for approximately 8% of renal pelvis tumors. They have been associated with calculi, chronic bacterial infection, exposure to cyclophosphamide and hydronephrosis.[19,20] They have been reported to have a poorer prognosis than UCs as they tend to be more invasive at diagnosis.[21] Adenocarcinomas (Fig. 92-3) are rare, and may be associated with a poor prognosis. They tend to be raised, indurated lesions with a glistening surface, and have been associated with outflow obstruction.[20] Other even less common histologies include neuroendocrine carcinomas, sarcomas and plasmacytomas.

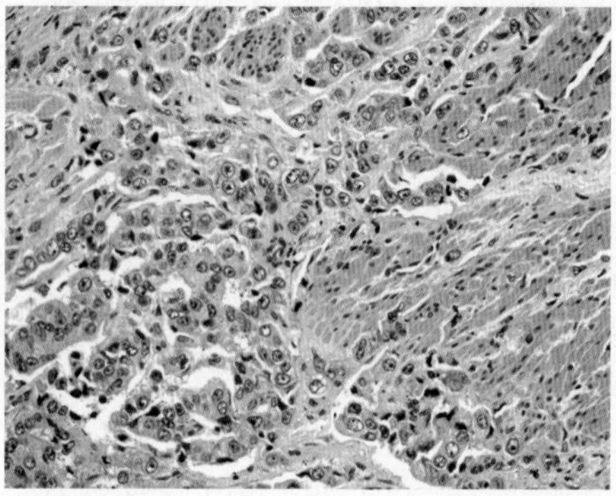

Figure 92-1 ■ Invasive urothelial carcinoma.

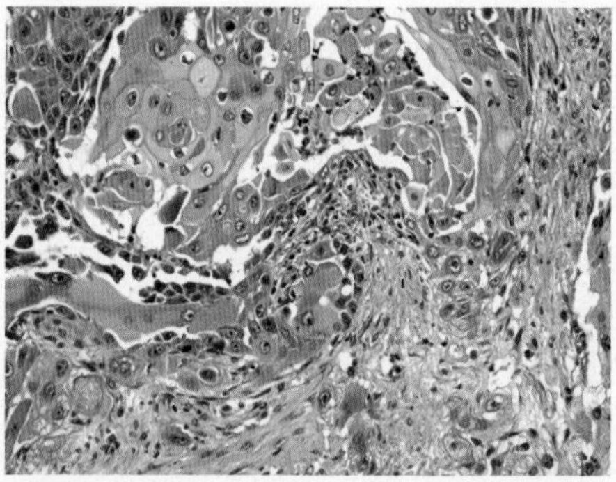

Figure 92-2 ■ Squamous cell carcinoma.

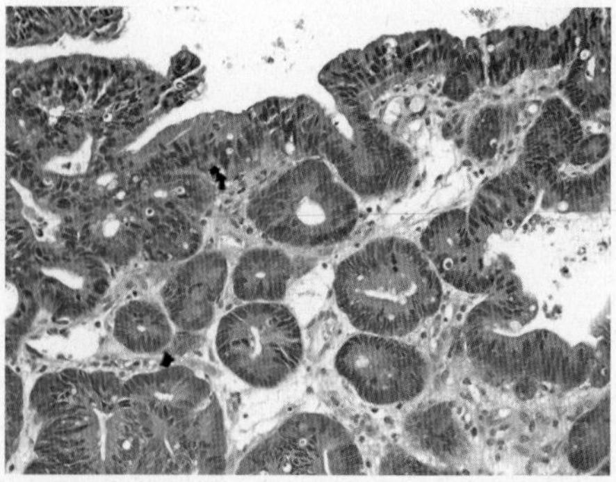

Figure 92-3 ■ Adenocarcinoma-colonic type.

Since the urothelium lines the entire urinary tract, tumors at multiple locations in the urothelium are common. This is especially true in patients with larger lesions and with urothelial CIS. This may be due to genetic changes along the entire urothelial surface from exposure to carcinogens. However, such multifocal carcinomas are most often monoclonal, suggesting a single focus of tumor which can spread via intraluminal seeding or intraepithelial migration. It is probable that both hypotheses play a role in this malignancy. A significant proportion of patients (20-50%) with tumors of the upper urinary tract will subsequently develop bladder urothelial carcinomas.[4]

Cytogenetics and Molecular Biology

Most of the available data have suggested that the karyotypic profiles of upper tract UCs are similar to those of bladder UC. The genetic changes associated with tumors of the upper urinary tract seem to be associated with the presence of the retinoblastoma gene, p53 and alterations on chromosome 9. Alterations of chromosome 9 seem to occur early and may be a factor in the development of papillary UC.[22] Renal pelvis UCs may be related to loss of heterozygosity on chromosomes 5q, 1p, 14q, and 8p. Trisomy 7 may be a poor prognostic factor in patients with this malignancy.[23] Trisomy 20 may be associated with an increased incidence of recurrence within the bladder.[24]

Field Defect: Association With Cancers of the Bladder

Similar factors responsible for cancers of the renal pelvis and ureter are known to contribute to bladder cancer. Therefore, one would expect these two malignancies to coincide as a function of a common field defect occurring throughout the urothelium. The incidence of involvement of the upper tract at time of radical cystectomy for bladder TCC has been estimated between 8% and 18%.[25] The relative risk for upper tract tumors after bladder cancer has been demonstrated as high as 64-75% at 2 years.[26] Up to 2-4% of patients with bladder cancer may develop upper urinary tract cancer.[27,28] Risk factors for the subsequent development of upper tract carcinomas include high grade, high stage, multifocal tumors, ureteral reflux, and presence of recurrent carcinomas.[29,30]

Conversely, the incidence of subsequent bladder cancer after prior upper tract urothelial carcinoma ranges from 20% to 50%.[4,31] Tumors of the bladder have been reported to present at a median interval of 14 months after complete resection of upper tract TCC.[32] These tumors are often multifocal. The risk of subsequent bladder cancer may be increased in those patients with chronic kidney disease and upper tract tumors treated by radical surgery.[33] A retrospective analysis has suggested that this risk of developing subsequent bladder cancer is associated with high tumor grade, and ureteral as opposed to renal pelvis location of primary tumor.[34] Therefore, individuals who have been treated with definitive therapy for upper urinary tract cancer should undergo close surveillance for primary tumors arising in the bladder. A common practice is to perform cystoscopy and cytology every three months for the first 2 years, every 6 months for the next 2 years, and then annually thereafter.

Presentation and Investigation

Clinical Presentation

Upper urinary tract tumors most often present with hematuria (70-95%), which may be gross or microscopic.[5,35] Flank pain is less common (8-40%), and may present as a result of ureteral obstruction from the tumor itself or due to a blood clot. Other symptoms reported include bladder irritation, constitutional symptoms or paraneoplastic syndromes (although the latter should raise suspicion that the tumor is actually a renal cell carcinoma).

As many as 10% of patients may be asymptomatic, at diagnosis. The physical examination is normally unremarkable, although an abdominal mass or tenderness may be elicited. The diagnosis of cancer of the upper urinary tract is often delayed as compared to bladder tumors, perhaps due to the relative difficulty in detecting admixed blood from the upper tract in the urine, the paucity of symptoms, the problems of imaging small lesions and the absence of adjacent structures whose structure or function will be damaged early by tumor extension.

Occasionally, the presentation will reflect the pattern of metastases, with common sites of involvement including lungs, liver, bone and lymph nodes, with less common metastases to brain, skin and other viscera.

Cytology

Urine cytology is often employed in the evaluation of hematuria, and necessary to exclude concurrent bladder lesions. It is a specific tool that is useful in the diagnosis of upper tract tumors. However, the sensitivity of cytology in the detection of UC of the upper tract can vary, with reported sensitivities up to 80% for high grade tumors and as low as 10-40% for low grade tumors.[36,37] Therefore, negative urine cytology does not rule out a malignancy. An experienced cytopathologist is critical for cytologic interpretation.

Selective ureteral urine sampling for cytologic analysis performed during endoscopy may improve sensitivity.[38] The nuclear characteristics may suggest the grade of tumor, but these findings do not correlate with the histologic grade or invasiveness. Urinary flow cytometry to evaluate abnormal DNA ploidy may be more accurate than cytology. It is an automated screening tool that requires a catheterized urine specimen. It may be useful in identifying patients at higher risk of a poorer prognosis, but the role of this technology in this malignancy is currently unclear.[39]

Radiologic Studies

Imaging the upper urinary tract often involves excretory urography. The historical standard of the intravenous pyelogram (IVP) provided a detailed picture of the entire renal collecting system and ureter. However, this has increasingly given way to CT urography, which can offer improved visualization of the collecting system, as well as the opportunity to evaluate for direct extension or nodal involvement. CT urography has been reported to have a sensitivity of up to 100%, a specificity of 60% and a negative predictive value of 100%.[40]

A solitary filling defect is seen in 50-75% of cases.[41] However, multiple filling defects, uteropelvic junction obstruction with hydronephrosis, infundibular stenosis, unilateral nonvisualization of the collecting system or splaying of the calices may also be seen. Calcification may be present in up to 70% of cases. Thickening of the wall of the ureter or adjacent involvement may be seen. In addition, CT scanning can stage the tumor, with assessment of lymph nodes, contralateral kidney, liver and other potential sites of metastases. MRI urography may be utilized for patients unable to tolerate iodinated contrast. In those patients with renal dysfunction or intravenous contrast intolerance, the method of retrograde pyleography can be used for imaging. In addition, retrograde pyleography should be employed if IVP or CT urography fails to show the entire urothelial surface.

Renal arteriography is not often employed in the evaluation of upper tract tumors. However, it may be useful in defining the nature of the filling defect, and in defining the vascular anatomy of a large or ill-defined tumor prior to surgical intervention. Renal arteriography may assist in differentiating these tumors from renal adenocarcinomas. Ultrasonography can distinguish renal pelvic tumors from renal calculi, but not from blood clots. The use of this procedure is relatively limited in this malignancy. Prior to any surgical intervention, it is recommended to perform isotope renal scanning to estimate the function of the remaining kidney.

Endoscopy

Endoscopic examination of the tissue by means of cystoscopy and ureteroscopy is the gold standard for diagnosis of upper urinary tract tumors. It allows for direct visualization and for a biopsy to be performed on any suspicious lesions. Although direct visualization alone can predict carcinoma in over 70% of cases, biopsy has been demonstrated to confirm diagnosis in approximately 90% of cases.[38,42,43] The procedure is safe and well tolerated in expert hands, with a complication rate of less than 7%. Deep biopsies should be avoided because of the thin walls of the ureter and renal pelvis, and to prevent tumor spillage into the peritoneum. The contra-lateral ureter is usually avoided to prevent inadvertent tumor seeding.

The correlation between endoscopic biopsy and pathologic stage has been evaluated in several studies. Biopsy grade has been demonstrated to predict accurately surgical grade in 78-90% of cases.[43,44] However, biopsy can understage the final pathology in up to 45% of cases.[44] Therefore, biopsies can not be recommended as the sole method for tumor staging.

Staging

Tumors of the upper urinary tract can spread by means of direct extension or disseminate via the vascular or lymphatic systems. Lymph nodes are often involved earlier, although metastases may occur in almost any organ. Clinical staging is based on the combination of radiographic studies, ureteroscopy and biopsy. However, due to the anatomy involved, the most accurate staging requires pathologic analysis of the surgically excised specimen.

The current American Joint Committee on Cancer (AJCC), tumor, nodes, metastases (TNM) staging for tumors of the ureter and renal pelvis is shown in Table 92-1. This system is pathologically based, and depends on the determination of the extent of invasion by the primary tumor as well evaluation of regional lymph nodes. Any lymph node invasion is categorized as stage IV disease.

The grade of urothelial carcinoma of the upper tract has generally been found to correlate with stage.[45] Superficial tumors are generally low-grade, whereas the majority of infiltrative tumors are high-grade. The prognosis is worse for patients with high-grade tumors than for those with low-grade tumors. High-grade tumors are more likely to be associated with urothelial CIS. The majority (55-75%) of ureteral tumors are low-grade and low-stage, and in the MD Anderson Cancer Center experience, these are the two most powerful prognostic determinants in multivariate analysis.[46]

Table 92-1 The AJCC TNM Classification of Cancers of the Ureter and Renal Pelvis

Primary Tumor (T)			
TX	Primary tumor cannot be assessed		
T0	No evidence of primary tumor		
Ta	Papillary noninvasive carcinoma		
Tis	Carcinoma in situ (CIS)		
T1	Tumor invades subepithelial connective tissue		
T2	Tumor invades the muscularis		
T3	*(For renal pelvis only)* Tumor invades beyond muscularis into peripelvic fat or the renal parenchyma		
T3	*(For ureter only)* Tumor invades beyond muscularis into periureteric fat		
T4	Tumor invades adjacent organs or through the kidney into the perinephric fat		
Regional Lymph Nodes (N)			
NX	Regional lymph node cannot be assessed		
N0	No regional lymph node metastasis		
N1	Metastasis in a single lymph node, 2 cm or less in greatest dimension		
N2	Metastasis in a single lymph node, more than 2 cm but not more than 5 cm in greatest dimension; or multiple lymph nodes, none more than 5 cm in greatest dimension		
N3	Metastasis in a lymph node more than 5 cm in greatest dimension		
Distant Metastasis (M)			
MX	Distant metastasis cannot be assessed		
M0	No distant metastasis		
M1	Distant metastasis		
Histologic Grade (G)			
GX	Grade can not be assessed		
G1	Well differentiated		
G2	Moderately differentiated		
G3-4	Poorly differentiated / undifferentiated		
Stage Grouping			
Stage 0a	Ta	N0	M0
Stage 0is	Tis	N0	M0
Stage I	T1	N0	M0
Stage II	T2	N0	M0
Stage III	T3	N0	M0
Stage IV	T4	N0	M0
	Any T	N1-3	M0
	Any T	Any N	M1

Source: From Ref. 89.

Prognosis

Following surgical resection, the 5-year overall survival rate is approximately 40%. Tumor stage and grade are reported as the most important prognostic factors for disease recurrence after surgical resection.[46-48] Low-grade, low-stage tumors are commonly associated with improved survival. If tumors are superficial and confined to the renal pelvis or ureter, they are potentially curable in more than 90% of patients. The 5 year survival rates for Ta tumors are >80%; but only 15-30% for T3 tumors. Overall 5-year survival is related to tumor stage: Ta, 95%; localized, 89%; regional, 63%; metastatic, 17%.[2] Unfortunately, up to 19% of patients may present with metastatic disease. The 5 year survival rates for patients with low-grade tumors is 94-100%, compared to 25-35% for those with high-grade tumors.[49]

Other prognostic factors are presented in Table 92-2. CIS of the upper urinary tract has been associated with a less favorable prognosis and an increased risk of future invasive urothelial carcinoma. In a retrospective multicenter study, 126 patients with UC of the renal pelvis and ureter were followed postoperatively for a median of 39 months.[50] Multivariate analysis demonstrated three independent prognostic factors for overall survival: pathologic T classification, presence of residual tumor following surgery, and location of tumor (renal pelvis vs. ureter +/- renal pelvis, with ureteral tumors being less favorable). No difference in survival was found between patients with solid vs papillary tumors.[48] Multifocal lesions appear to have a worse outcome than unifocal lesions at time of diagnosis.[46,51]

In a multicenter analysis of 269 patients over 16 years who underwent nephroureterectomy, multivariate anal-

Table 92-2 **Prognostic Factors in Cancers of the Ureter and Renal Pelvis**

Tumor features	Stage[2,47,48]
	Grade[47,48]
	Carcinoma in situ
	Ureter vs renal pelvis location[50]
	Lymphovascular invasion[53,54]
	Multifocal lesions[51]
	Synchronous muscle-invasive bladder UC[52]
Molecular markers	p53[90]
	Loss of heterozygosity 9p21[91]
	Aneuploidy[56]
	c-met[55]
	EGFR[57]
	p27[92]

ysis indicated that pathologic stage of the tumor and lymph nodes, history of prior bladder UC, tumor multifocality within the upper urinary tract and synchronous muscle-invasive bladder UC were independent predictors of cancer specific survival.[52] Of these, the factor associated with the worst disease-specific survival was synchronous muscle-invasive bladder UC.

The presence of lymphovascular invasion has been suggested as a prognostic factor for recurrence-free and disease specific survival.[53,54] Over-expression of the c-met oncogene may predispose to vascular invasion and more aggressive clinical behavior.[55]

Aneuploid DNA pattern on flow cytometry has been reported to have an unfavorable prognosis,[56] although other reports have disputed these findings.[51] Expression of epidermal growth factor receptor (EGFR) has been associated with high tumor stage, high tumor grade, and with metaplastic or glandular differentiation. High EGFR expression has been associated with the occurrence of metastatic disease.[57]

Surgery

Radical Nephroureterectomy

The standard treatment for localized upper tract urothelial carcinoma is radical nephroureterectomy.[2] This entails the complete removal of the kidney, with its surrounding fat and Gerota's fascia, removal of the affected ureter, as well as the en bloc resection of a bladder cuff. Up to 20-40% of patients present with recurrent tumors in cases when the entire ureter is not removed,[58] although it is clear that nephroureterectomy is no panacea, and that cure is elusive in patients with high-grade, high-stage tumors.[46] We believe that an ipsilateral lymph node dissection or sampling should be performed. This provides prognostic information, although any therapeutic benefit is a matter of debate.

Segmental lymph node excision has not been shown to improve the efficacy of surgery in high grade or high stage tumors, possibly because the overall results are so poor in these patients, and the fact that most of these patients will develop early metastases. In addition, lymph node involvement is uncommon in low-stage disease. If tumor invades the renal vein or inferior vena cava, thrombus extraction or partial vein dissection may be required.

Postoperatively patients should receive regular surveillance for disease recurrence. These include endoscopy of the contra-lateral ureter and bladder, CT scans or other appropriate imaging of the chest, abdomen and pelvis, as well as a focused history and physical examinations. The controversial role of adjunctive chemotherapy is discussed below.

Laparoscopic Radical Nephroureterectomy

In many urological applications, laparoscopy has allowed for decreased procedural morbidity compared to its open surgical counterpart, while conferring purportedly equivalent oncological clearance from a technical stand-point. Radical treatment of upper tract TCC ttraditionally has required open radical nephroureterectomy which usually involves two large, muscle-cutting, abdominal incisions. Laparoscopic radical nephroureterectomy (LNUx) is now considered to be a viable alternative to open surgery at many centers worldwide. Long-term oncological outcomes after LNUx are sparse in the literature: however, a few recent reports of intermediate-term outcomes have documented results comparable to open radical nephroureterectomy, although case selection bias may have influenced the results to some extent.[59,60]

We recently reported intermediate-term outcomes following LNUx for upper tract TCC.[61] Between December 1997 and August 2005, 100 patients underwent LNUx for upper tract TCC at the Cleveland Clinic Glickman Urological Institute. The median age of the patients at surgery was 73 years. The final pathological stage was pTis/pTa in 28%, pT1 in 31%, pT2 in 13%, pT3 in 24%, and pT4 in 4% of patients. High-grade lesions were present in 58% of patients, multifocal disease in 23%, and lymphovascular invasion in 9%. Positive surgical margins occurred in seven patients (7%). The median follow-up was 7 years (range, 2–10 years). At 2, 5, and 7 years, overall survival was 81%, 59%, and 50%, cancer-specific survival was 91%, 77%, and 72%, and recurrence-free survival was 66%, 50%, and 36%, respectively. Five-year cancer-specific survival by stage was: pTis/Ta 80%, pT1 70%, pT2 68%, pT3 60%, and pT4 0%. On univariate analysis, non organ-confined disease (p = 0.01) and lymphovascular invasion (p = 0.04) affected cancer-specific survival; on multivariate analysis only non organ-confined disease was a significant factor (p = 0.04). Concomitant bladder tumor at diagnosis was associated with a poor recurrence-free survival in both univariate (p = 0.02) and multivariate analysis (p = 0.01). These data suggest that our outcomes for LNUx may be comparable to open surgery with respect to tumor control. Given the recognized perioperative and morbity advantages of LNUx vis-à-vis open surgery, the acceptable long-term oncologic outcomes documented in this study provide additional rationale for LNUx to become the preferred treatment for upper tract TCC for organ-confined disease,[61] although true confirmation will require validation by a well-structured randomized clinical trial.

Nephron-Sparing Options

Nephron-sparing surgery has been advocated for certain settings such as: bilateral disease, solitary kidney, impaired renal function or significant comorbid medical conditions. These techniques include partial nephrectomy, partial ureterectomy, partial resection of renal pelvis and percutaneous resection of renal pelvic tumor. However, more recently, expanded indications for such procedures have been suggested. Advocates of such conservative surgery point to the high morbidity and mortality associated with radical surgery and to the poor prognosis of advanced lesions irrespective of the surgical procedure utilized. However, in the current clinical environment there is little difference in the perioperative morbidity and mortality between conservative and radical surgery.

When examining the literature on the subject, it should be emphasized that the results of both conservative and radical surgery reflect nonrandomized clinical trials, and that the patient populations are often quite different across trials. Studies of conservative management often involve highly selected patients. Generally the duration of follow-up for survival and disease recurrence in these studies have been shorter compared to those of radical nephroureterectomy. If conservative surgical management is contemplated, the potential risk for tumor recurrence anywhere in the urothelium, as well outside the renal pelvis, must be considered. This has been reported in the setting of residual ureteral stump, as well as in the disease of bladder cancer. Therefore, such patients require frequent surveillance. The decision to proceed with conservative surgery must be made on an individualized basis. Ureteral UC, which is superficial, low-grade and without any proximal disease, may be considered for segmental excision, ureteral implantation and regional lymphadenectomy. Selected patients with unifocal, low-grade, low-stage renal pelvic tumors may also be considered for conservative management, provided that ureteroscopy demonstrates minimal local extension and no skip lesions.

Endoscopic treatment may be appropriate in carefully selected patients, although its precise role is still being defined. The goal of this technique is to control the malignancy, and at the same time preserve renal function and ureteral integrity. These procedures involve resecting or ablating the tumor, and then fulgurating the tumor base, often with a laser. When performed by experienced surgical teams and in carefully selected cases, they have been shown to be effective and safe. Serious complications including ureteral perforation and ureteral stricture are uncommon.

It has been suggested that patients with low-grade tumors may be treated primarily by endoscopic means.[38,62,63] Tumors of the renal pelvis and calyceal system have been more difficult to resect using this method than those of the ureter, perhaps because of the convoluted anatomy, tumor multicentricity, or potential association with CIS. The small size of the instruments limits the volume of tumor that can be resected. Retrospective series have reported recurrence rates of 30-65%, and disease-free survival rates of 35-86%.[38,64,65] However, other reports have suggested a high recurrence rate in these patients in spite of initial good endoscopic local control.[63,66] Subsequent nephroureterectomy may be required in up to 20% of cases.[67]

Percutaneous management is another option considered primarily for patients with larger volume tumors when complete resection is the primary goal. Tumor visualization is improved compared to the endoscopic approach. However, this technique involves violation of urothelial integrity and therefore has been associated the risk of tumor spillage into the perirenal space and rare cases of port site recurrence.[68,69] Local recurrence has been observed in 23-35% of patients.[70-72] Tumor grade has been demonstrated to be a strong predictor of outcome in these patients.[73,74] Individuals with high-grade tumors are predisposed to disease recurrence and progression, and should be strongly considered for nephroureterectomy if they are surgical candidates.

Segmental ureterectomy may be performed for localized upper tract tumors. Noninvasive low-grade tumors of the proximal or middle ureter that are too large for endoscopic treatment may be treated by this method. In addition, this technique may be used for noninvasive high-grade or invasive tumors in patients who require nephron sparing surgery due to impaired renal function. Five year survival for stage T1 tumors has reported at 65%, and 50% for stage 2 tumors.[75] However, the risk of recurrence may be as high as 50%,[58] and therefore rigorous surveillance is required.

Radiotherapy

The role of radiotherapy in the management of upper urinary tract tumors has not been well defined. There is limited published information regarding the use of current techniques of radiation as definitive therapy or as neoadjuvant therapy in these patients. Adjuvant radiation therapy has been examined, but the published data do not really support a very useful role. The rarity of these tumors has precluded the application of large or randomized clinical studies. The available studies are presented in Table 92-3.

While the routine use of adjuvant therapy cannot be recommended, postoperative radiation may diminish the likelihood of local recurrence, but often without any significant impact on overall survival or the development of distant metastases.[50,76,77] It may be of benefit in select cases with high tumor stage, high tumor grade, and close surgical margins or with lymph node metastases. In a multivariate analysis, overall survival was found to be dependent on stage and age at diagnosis, with the use of adjuvant radiotherapy being of borderline significance ($p = 0.07$).[76] However, it is important to note that the number of patients in this study was quite small, and the results may have been influenced by case selection bias.

Chemotherapy

Intravesical and Intraureteral Therapy

The efficacy of intravesical therapy in the treatment of superficial urothelial carcinoma of the bladder led investigators to use these agents in upper urinary tract tumors. The most common approach has been to instill cytotoxic agents via a urinary catheter, and then to position the patient to ensure passive retrograde flow to the ureters via gravity. Alternatively, there have been reports of transcutaneous insertion of flexible catheters into the ureters, followed by infusion of agents. Anecdotal data suggest that tumor regression occurs in response to topical delivery of chemotherapy or immunotherapy, although the precision of the published information is not optimal.

When endoscopic resection is used as the sole primary therapy, the adjuvant use of topical therapy has been advocated to prevent or delay local recurrence. The use of bacillus calmette-guerin (BCG), mitomycin C, thiotepa and 5-fluorouracil as adjuvant therapy after endoscopic treatment have all been reported. Keeley and Bagley reported on 19 patients with urothelial carcinoma of the upper tract who underwent endoscopic treatment with laser and subsequently received with adjuvant intravesical mitomycin C.[78] Patients were chosen to receive adjuvant therapy if they had gross residual tumor, multifocal disease, high tumor grade or rapid recurrence of previous disease. Complete responses were seen in 35%, partial responses in 27%, and no

Table 92-3 **Adjuvant Radiotherapy After Surgery for Upper Urinary Tract Carcinomas**

	n	Radiation Dose (Median Gy)	Median Follow-up (Months)	Local Regional Failure	5-Year Overall Survival
Brookland et al. (1985)[77]	23[a]	50	40	9% vs 45%[f]	27% vs 17%[f]
Cozad et al. (1992)[93]	26[a]	50	13.5	11% vs 53%[f]	44% vs 24%[f]
Maulard-Durdux et al. (1996)[94]	26[b]	45	45	19%	49%
Catton et al. (1996)[95]	86[c]	35	111	34%	43%
Hall et al. (1998)[96]	74[a]	40	21	20% vs 6%[f] (Stage 3)	45% vs 40%[f] (Stage 3)
Ozsahin et al. (1999)[50]	126[d]	50	39	38% vs 65%[f]	21% vs 33%[f]
Czito et al. (2004)[86]	31[e]	46.9	31	45% vs 22%[g]	27% vs 67%[g]

[a]All patients ≥ Stage III; [b]63% ≥ Stage III; [c]73% ≥ Stage III; [d]65% ≥ Stage III; [e]81% ≥ Stage III. [f]radiotherapy vs. no radiotherapy, [g]radiotherapy vs. chemotherapy + chemoradiotherapy.

response was seen in 38% of patients. After a mean follow-up interval of 30 months, no patient had any systemic recurrence of disease. However, 50% had subsequent bladder tumors, all grade pTa.

In addition to intravesical administration, agents have been delivered via nephrostomy tube after percutaneous treatment. However, all of our current data are limited to retrospective series (Table 92-4), follow-up has been relatively short, and other reports have suggested an inferior outcome using this method. The outcomes may also have been influenced by the compromised clinical status of the patient population. The true efficacy of this approach has been difficult to assess to date. In general terms, in the context of recurrent superficial UC of the upper tracts, we do use topical therapy when feasible, to avoid additional aggressive surgery, focusing predominantly on BCG. This reflects the duration of remissions from the available anecdotal literature (Table 92-4) and our own experience.

Table 92-4 Reported Series of Adjuvant Topical Therapy for Cancers of the Ureter and Renal Pelvis

	Treatment	*N*	Recurrence Rate (%)	Median Follow-up (Months)
Sharpe et al. (1993)[97]	BCG	11	27	36
Eastham et al. (1993)[98]	Mitomycin-C	7	28.5	-
Bellman et al. (1994)[99]	BCG	16	12.5	-
Vasavada et al. (1995)[100]	BCG	8	12.5	22
Jarrett et al. (1995)[68]	BCG	30	33	55
Keeley et al. (1997)[78]	Mitomycin-C	19	50	30
Patel et al. (1998)[101]	BCG	12	15	15
Clark et al. (1999)[71]	BCG	17	35	20.5
Nonomura et al. (2000)[102]	BCG	11	22	20
See et al. (2000)[103]	Adriamycin	12	50	12
Okubo et al. (2001)[104]	BCG	11	36	49
Irie et al. (2002)[105]	BCG	9	11	36
Thalman et al. (2002)[106]	BCG	37	49	42
Hayashida et al. (2004)[107]	BCG	10	50	51

Systemic Adjuvant Therapy

Although there is extensive experience regarding the efficacy of systemic chemotherapy in urothelial malignancies as a whole, the benefit of adjuvant systemic chemotherapy in patients with completely resected ureteral and renal pelvic tumors is unproven at present. Compared to bladder cancers, tumors of the upper urinary tract are often associated with renal insufficiency, which can affect the toxicity profile of chemotherapeutic agents and portend for patients with a poorer performance status, less able to tolerate full doses of chemotherapy. However, there is evidence to suggest that upper tract tumors can respond to chemotherapy.[79-81] In our study comparing cisplatin vs the combination methotrexate, vinblastine, doxorubicin (Adriamycin) and cisplatin (MVAC) regimen for metastatic UC, we were able to show comparable response rates and survival for patients with upper and lower tract tumors.[81]

Based on retrospective studies, some investigators have proposed possible benefit from adjuvant chemotherapy,[82-85] although these studies do not constitute level 1 evidence. Bamias and colleagues reported on 36 patients with carcinoma of the upper urinary tract with T stage ≥ 3 or lymph node involvement treated with carboplatin and paclitaxel for four cycles after radical nephroureterectomy.[83] After a median follow-up of 40.6 months, 5 year disease free survival and overall survival were 40.2% and 52% respectively. No patients with grade 2 tumors relapsed, while the relapse rate for grade 3 tumors was 60%. In a more recent report, 32 patients with Stage pT2 or worse disease were treated with cisplatin-based chemotherapy.[84] Of those, 38% had disease recurrence over a median of 8.5 months. In comparison, 11 purportedly similar patients did not receive any adjuvant treatment, and 64% relapsed. However, another retrospective study, reported by a team of Korean investigators, investigated the use of adjuvant MVAC for patients with lymph node negative, pathologic stage T3 disease.[85] At 40 months of follow-up, 5/16 (31%) who received adjuvant therapy and 4/11 (38%) without added treatment had disease recurrence suggesting no obvious benefit for adjuvant therapy in this patient population. Again it is emphasized that case selection bias could have influenced this outcome.

Czito and colleagues examined the use of adjuvant radiotherapy ($n = 22$) compared to adjuvant methotrexate, cisplatin and vinblastine chemotherapy followed by concurrent radiation and cisplatin ($n = 9$).[86] Concurrent chemoradiotherapy was reported to improve disease-specific and overall survival in this small retrospective study. Although these results are interesting, and may have been over-interpreted, the reality is that there is little strong published evidence to clarify this situation, and well-powered, prospective randomized trials are required to provide concrete evidence of benefit for adjuvant chemotherapy.

Systemic Therapy for Advanced Disease

Although surgery is the treatment of choice in this disease, 50% of these patients will suffer from disease recurrence. The prognosis of these patients is poor. There are limited data available as to the best course of therapy because of the rarity of these tumors. Urothelial cancers are known to be responsive to cisplatin-based chemotherapy regimens.[81,87,88] As noted above, we have previously suggested that metastatic tumors from the renal pelvis and ureter are at least as responsive to MVAC chemotherapy as bladder UCs,[87] and our data and other series have shown response rates of 40-70%, depending on sites of involvement, with median survival figures in the range of 12-20 months. As the toxicity of the MVAC regimen is substantial, novel compounds have been assessed by our team and others, leading to the evolution of the doublet of gemcitabine and cisplatin as the basic component for novel compound development.[88] In current practice, patients with metastatic tumors of the upper urinary tract are usually treated with the protocols established for urothelial tumors arising from the bladder (as discussed in more detail in Chapter 93). Alternatively, these patients can be appropriately offered treatment on a clinical trial.

There are provocative preliminary data to suggest that targeted therapies, such as sunitinib, may have activity against UC, but specific information relating to upper tract tumors has not yet been published. This issue is discussed in more detail in Chapter 93 on bladder cancer.

Summary

Tumors of the upper urinary tracts are functionally and morphologically quite similar to those arising in the urinary bladder. The natural history is influenced by the reduced investment of surrounding tissues and the frequent association of such tumors with renal tract dysfunction and multifocality. As a result, the natural history outcome seems inferior to that established for lower tract tumors, although it is clear that surgical approaches can offer cure, especially for well differentiated and organ confined tumors. These tumors exhibit a similar responsiveness to chemotherapy as for other urothelial cancers, although data to support this are less clearly defined than for bladder cancer.

Selected References

The complete reference list can be found at www.CANCERMEDICINE8.com

1. Jemal A, Tiwari RC, Murray T, et al. Cancer statistics, 2004. *CA Cancer J Clin.* 2004;54:8–29.
2. Munoz JJ, Ellison LM. Upper tract urothelial neoplasms: incidence and survival during the last 2 decades. *J Urol.* 2000;164:1523–1525.
3. Anderstrom C, Johansson SL, Pettersson S, et al. Carcinoma of the ureter: a clinicopathologic study of 49 cases. *J Urol.* 1989;142:280–283.
5. Guinan P, Vogelzang NJ, Randazzo R, et al. Renal pelvic cancer: a review of 611 patients treated in Illinois 1975-1985. Cancer Incidence and End Results Committee. *Urology.* 1992;40:393–399.
8. Johansson S, Angervall L, Bengtsson U, et al. Uroepithelial tumors of the renal pelvis associated with abuse of phenacetin-containing analgesics. *Cancer.* 1974;33:743–753.
14. Ross RK, Paganini-Hill A, Landolph J, et al. Analgesics, cigarette smoking, and other risk factors for cancer of the renal pelvis and ureter. *Cancer Res.* 1989;49:1045–1048.
18. Melamed MR, Reuter VE. Pathology and staging of urothelial tumors of the kidney and ureter. *Urol Clin North Am.* 1993;20:333–347.
22. Fadl-Elmula I, Gorunova L, Mandahl N, et al. Cytogenetic analysis of upper urinary tract transitional cell carcinomas. *Cancer Genet Cytogenet.* 1999;115:123–127.
23. Dal Cin P, Roskams T, Van Poppel H, et al. Cytogenetic investigation of transitional cell carcinomas of the upper urinary tract. *Cancer Genet Cytogenet.* 1999;114:117–120.
25. Schumacher MC, Scholz M, Weise ES, et al. Is there an indication for frozen section examination of the ureteral margins during cystectomy for transitional cell carcinoma of the bladder? *J Urol.* 2006;176:2409–2413; discussion 2413.
26. Rabbani F, Perrotti M, Russo P, et al. Upper-tract tumors after an initial diagnosis of bladder cancer: argument for long-term surveillance. *J Clin Oncol.* 2001;19:94–100.
27. Oldbring J, Glifberg I, Mikulowski P, et al. Carcinoma of the renal pelvis and ureter following bladder carcinoma: frequency, risk factors and clinicopathological findings. *J Urol.* 1989;141:1311–1313.
28. Solsona E, Iborra I, Ricos JV, et al. Upper urinary tract involvement in patients with bladder carcinoma in situ (Tis): its impact on management. *Urology.* 1997;49:347–352.
31. Raman JD, Ng CK, Boorjian SA, et al. Bladder cancer after managing upper urinary tract transitional cell carcinoma: predictive factors and pathology. *BJU Int.* 2005;96:1031–1035.
37. Konety BR, Getzenberg RH. Urine based markers of urological malignancy. *J Urol.* 2001;165:600–611.
38. Blute ML, Segura JW, Patterson DE, et al. Impact of endourology on diagnosis and management of upper urinary tract urothelial cancer. *J Urol.* 1989;141:1298–1301.
40. Caoili EM, Cohan RH, Korobkin M, et al. Urinary tract abnormalities: initial experience with multi-detector row CT urography. *Radiology.* 2002;222:353–360.
41. Murphy DM, Zincke H, Furlow WL. Management of high grade transitional cell cancer of the upper urinary tract. *J Urol.* 1981;125:25–29.
42. El-Hakim A, Weiss GH, Lee BR, et al. Correlation of ureteroscopic appearance with histologic grade of upper tract transitional cell carcinoma. *Urology.* 2004;63: 647–650; discussion 650.
43. Keeley FX, Kulp DA, Bibbo M, et al. Diagnostic accuracy of ureteroscopic biopsy in upper tract transitional cell carcinoma. *J Urol.* 1997;157:33–37.
46. Brown GA, Busby JE, Wood CG, et al. Nephroureterectomy for treating upper urinary tact transitional cell carcinoma: time to change the treatment paradigm? *BJU Int.* 2006;98:1176–1180.
47. Huben RP, Mounzer AM, Murphy GP. Tumor grade and stage as prognostic variables in upper tract urothelial tumors. *Cancer.* 1988;62:2016–2020.
48. Heney NM, Nocks BN, Daly JJ, et al. Prognostic factors in carcinoma of the ureter. *J Urol.* 1981;125:632–636.
49. Lee SH, Lin JS, Tzai TS, et al. Prognostic factors of primary transitional cell carcinoma of the upper urinary tract. *Eur Urol.* 1996;29:266–270; discussion 271.
50. Ozsahin M, Zouhair A, Villa S, et al. Prognostic factors in urothelial renal pelvis and ureter tumours: a multicentre Rare Cancer Network study. *Eur J Cancer.* 1999;35:738–743.
52. Novara G, De Marco V, Gottardo F, et al. Independent predictors of cancer-specific survival in transitional cell carcinoma of the upper urinary tract: multi-institutional dataset from 3 European centers. *Cancer.* 2007;110:1715–1722.
55. Comperat E, Roupret M, Chartier-Kastler E, et al. Prognostic value of MET, RON and histoprognostic factors for urothelial carcinoma in the upper urinary tract. *J Urol.* 2008.
56. Blute ML, Tsushima K, Farrow GM, et al. Transitional cell carcinoma of the renal pelvis: nuclear deoxyribonucleic acid ploidy studied by flow cytometry. *J Urol.* 1988;140:944–949.
57. Leibl S, Zigeuner R, Hutterer G, et al. EGFR expression in urothelial carcinoma of the upper urinary tract is associated with disease progression and metaplastic morphology. *APMIS.* 2008;116:27–32.
59. Chung SD, Chueh SC, Lai MK, et al. Long-term outcome of hand-assisted laparoscopic radical nephroureterectomy for upper-tract urothelial carcinoma: comparison with open surgery. *J Endourol.* 2007;21:595–599.
60. Gill IS, Sung GT, Hobart MG, et al. Laparoscopic radical nephroureterectomy for upper tract transitional cell carcinoma: the Cleveland Clinic experience. *J Urol.* 2000;164:1513–1522.
61. Berger A, Haber G-P, Kamoi K, et al. Laparoscopic Radical Nephroureterectomy for Upper Tract TCC: oncologic outcomes at 7 years. *J Urol (In press).* 2008.
64. Elliott DS, Blute ML, Patterson DE, et al. Long-term follow-up of endoscopically treated upper urinary tract transitional cell carcinoma. *Urology.* 1996;47:819–825.
65. Chen GL, Bagley DH. Ureteroscopic management of upper tract transitional cell carcinoma in patients with normal contralateral kidneys. *J Urol.* 2000;164:1173–1176.
69. Huang A, Low RK, deVere White R. Nephrostomy tract tumor seeding following percutaneous manipulation of a ureteral carcinoma. *J Urol.* 1995;153:1041–1042.
70. Patel A, Soonawalla P, Shepherd SF, et al. Long-term outcome after percutaneous treatment of transitional cell carcinoma of the renal pelvis. *J Urol.* 1996;155:868–874.
76. Cozad SC, Smalley SR, Austenfeld M, et al. Transitional cell carcinoma of the renal pelvis or ureter: patterns of failure. *Urology.* 1995;46:796–800.
81. Loehrer PJ, Sr, Einhorn LH, Elson PJ, et al. A randomized comparison of cisplatin alone or in combination with methotrexate, vinblastine, and doxorubicin in patients with metastatic urothelial carcinoma: a cooperative group study. *J Clin Oncol.* 1992;10:1066–1073.
82. Michael M, Tannock IF, Czaykowski PM, et al. Adjuvant chemotherapy for high-risk urothelial transitional cell carcinoma: the Princess Margaret Hospital experience. *Br J Urol.* 1998;82:366–372.
83. Bamias A, Deliveliotis C, Fountzilas G, et al. Adjuvant chemotherapy with paclitaxel and carboplatin in patients with advanced carcinoma of the upper urinary tract: a study by the Hellenic Cooperative Oncology Group. *J Clin Oncol.* 2004;22:2150–2154.
85. Lee SE, Byun SS, Park YH, et al. Adjuvant chemotherapy in the management of pT-3N0M0 transitional cell carcinoma of the upper urinary tract. *Urol Int.* 2006;77:22–26.
86. Czito B, Zietman A, Kaufman D, et al. Adjuvant radiotherapy with and without concurrent chemotherapy for locally advanced transitional cell carcinoma of the renal pelvis and ureter. *J Urol.* 2004;172:1271–1275.
87. Sternberg CN, Yagoda A, Scher HI, et al. Methotrexate, vinblastine, doxorubicin, and cisplatin for advanced transitional cell carcinoma of the urothelium. Efficacy and patterns of response and relapse. *Cancer.* 1989;64:2448–2458.
88. Kaufman D, Raghavan D, Carducci M, et al. Phase II trial of gemcitabine plus cisplatin in patients with metastatic urothelial cancer. *J Clin Oncol.* 2000;18:1921–1927.
90. Keeley FX, Jr, Bibbo M, McCue PA, et al. Use of p53 in the diagnosis of upper-tract transitional cell carcinoma. *Urology.* 1997;49:181–186.
91. Amira N, Rivet J, Soliman H, et al. Microsatellite instability in urothelial carcinoma of the upper urinary tract. *J Urol.* 2003;170:1151–1154.
92. Kamai T, Takagi K, Asami H, et al. Prognostic significance of p27Kip1 and Ki-67 expression in carcinoma of the renal pelvis and ureter. *BJU Int.* 2000;86:14–19.
93. Cozad SC, Smalley SR, Austenfeld M, et al. Adjuvant radiotherapy in high stage transitional cell carcinoma of the renal pelvis and ureter. *Int J Radiat Oncol Biol Phys.* 1992;24:743–7453.
100. Vasavada SP, Streem SB, Novick AC. Definitive tumor resection and percutaneous bacille Calmette-Guerin for management of renal pelvic transitional cell carcinoma in solitary kidneys. *Urology.* 1995;45:381–386.
106. Thalmann GN, Markwalder R, Walter B, et al. Long-term experience with bacillus Calmette-Guerin therapy of upper urinary tract transitional cell carcinoma in patients not eligible for surgery. *J Urol.* 2002;168:1381–1385.
107. Hayashida Y, Nomata K, Noguchi M, et al. Long-term effects of bacille Calmette-Guerin perfusion therapy for treatment of transitional cell carcinoma in situ of upper urinary tract. *Urology.* 2004;63:1084–1088.

93 Bladder Cancer

Derek Raghavan, MD, PhD, FACP, FRACP ■ John P. Stein, MD‡ ■
Richard Cote, MD, FRCPath ■ J. Stephen Jones, MD, FACS

Introduction and Epidemiology

Bladder cancer is one of the most common malignancies in Western society, with an annual incidence of about 16 cases/100,000 males per year and 5 cases/100,000 females.[1,2] In the United States, this translates into about 67,000 new cases per year, with approximately 13,000 deaths per year. This is one of the malignancies for which the incidence and mortality figures have not changed greatly in the past 50 years, although it is possible that the incidence figures in males are beginning to plateau, reflecting the reduction in cigarette smoking. This is predominantly a disease of older aged males, with a median age at presentation of 60-65 years. There are geographical variations in incidence with increased rates in the Great Lakes region of the United States, in the littoral basin of the Middle East, and in regions with an increased incidence of schistosomiasis (most often squamous carcinoma). It occurs more often in Caucasians than in Asian or African American populations.[2]

The etiology is well-defined, with the most common association being cigarette smoking, and other factors including exposure to dyes and industrial reagents, motor exhaust, reduced intake of fluids (controversial), and analgesic (phenacetin) abuse.[1,2] Other associations include prior treatment with cyclophosphamide and other oxazophosphorine cytotoxics, high fat diet, chronic urinary infection, paraplegia, and prior pelvic irradiation.

Pathobiology and Molecular Determinants

Bladder cancer consists predominantly of urothelial carcinoma (UC), formerly known as transitional cell cancer. This type of cancer can occur anywhere along the urothelial tract, and may be multifocal in origin. About 90% of incident cases are UC, with about 5-10% being squamous cell carcinoma, 4-5% being adenocarcinoma, and the remainder consisting of rare cancers, such as small cell anaplastic cancer, sarcoma, melanoma or lymphoma. Occasionally other tumors metastasize to the bladder.

It is increasingly believed that bladder cancer arises from cancer stem cells,[3,4] and that the cancer stem cells have the ability to differentiate along different pathways. Thus it is not surprising that intermixed histological patterns will be found, although mostly UC predominates in such situations. Similarly, metastases will occasionally exhibit different histological patterns from the tumors of origin. These tumors are associated with a field defect of the urinary mucosa, probably due to antecedent carcinogenic stimuli, and thus can occur at multiple sites and with synchronous or metachronous presentations.

Urothelial carcinoma presents as either noninvasive or invasive disease. Within the noninvasive subset of tumors, two distinct histological subtypes are known, papillary vs flat carcinoma in situ (CIS). Noninvasive papillary carcinoma is the single most common presentation for bladder cancer, comprising more than 60% of incident cases. Noninvasive papillary carcinoma can be classified according to grade of disease, ranging from tumors generally considered benign (papilloma) to high-grade tumors with a high risk of developing invasion (grades 3 and 4) (Fig. 93-1). Several grading schemes have been introduced.[5] Grading systems are generally restricted to papillary neoplasms, as CIS is high-grade by definition, and virtually all invasive tumors are high-grade as well. Lower differentiation (high-grade) correlates with increased stage and reduced survival. Currently, generally used grading schemes include the Bergkvist system[6] and WHO/ISUP.[7] For invasive tumors, stage is the most important classical prognostic determinant, with the AJCC classification the most widely used.[8]

The predominant histologic type of urothelial cancer, formerly termed transitional cell cancer, may show a well organized pattern that is characteristic of grade 1 disease, with a high level of differentiation, reflecting the papil-

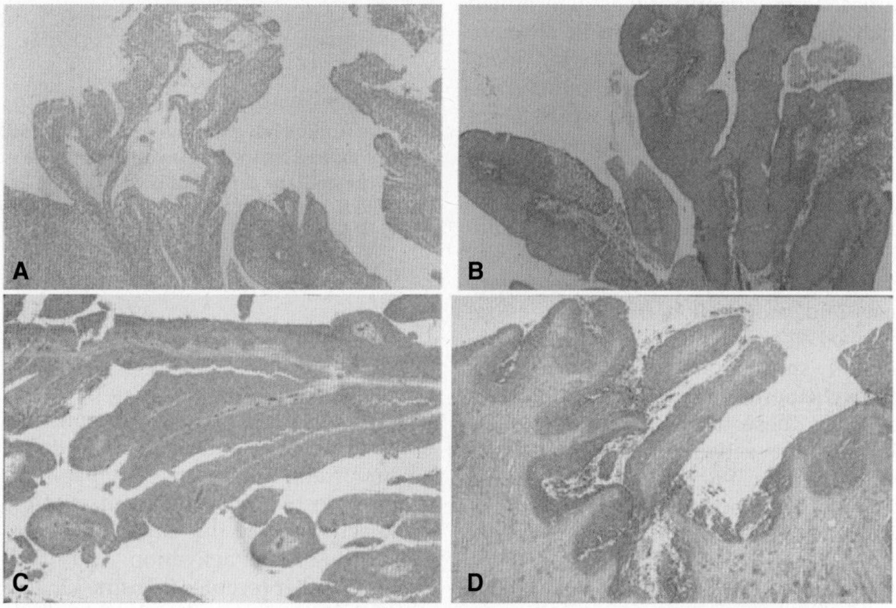

Figure 93-1 ■ Noninvasive papillary tumors of the urinary bladder. **(A)** Papillomas of the bladder have delicate fibrovascular cores, a relatively uniform urothelial lining with a pronounced umbrella cell layer, and orderly cells with nonpleomorphic nuclei. **(B)** Grade 1 papillary carcinomas are papillary neoplasms of low malignant potential, with essentially normal-appearing urothelium but greater thickness of cell layers and density. **(C)** Grade 2 papillary carcinomas are low-grade tumors with less delicate fibrovascular cores, multiple cell layers, loss of cellular polarity, and mild-to-moderate nuclear pleomorphism. **(D)** Grade 3 and 4 papillary carcinomas are high-grade tumors with thick fibrovascular cores, moderate-to-marked nuclear pleomorphism, and frequent mitoses. *Source:* From Ref. 5.

‡Deceased.

lary structure. A fibrovascular stalk is often seen. In grade 2 tumors, there is a higher nuclear to cytoplasmic ratio, and prominent nucleoli. Grade 3 disease is characterized by poorly differentiated or undifferentiated tissues that are increasingly disorganized and manifest a high mitotic index. The latest WHO nomenclature combines tumor differentiation into only low and high grades, based on the finding that tumor behavior is more accurately reflected in a dichotomized system than via a continuum of grades 1-3. However, acceptance of this innovation has been slow and not yet universal.

In the past, papillary tumors have been either classified as noninvasive or "superficial." Often, superficial included both noninvasive tumors and superficially invasive tumors (T1). It is becoming increasingly clear that this is an inappropriate designation, as the presence of any invasion announces the biological potential of the tumor, and should be distinguished from noninvasive disease.

Because the different morphologic subtypes of bladder cancer (in particular, papillary noninvasive tumors vs flat CIS) have been recognized for many years to have vastly different biologic behavior, these subtypes became the focus of molecular analysis.[9] The earliest cytogenetic studies in bladder cancer demonstrated alterations in chromosoms 9, 11, and 17, with allelic loss and loss of heterozygosity being the most common defects noted. This reflected the possible presence of tumor suppressor genes in these areas.[9] Subsequently, it was determined that the areas of alteration in chromosome 9 included the *INK4A/p16* locus and are commonly observed in noninvasive papillary carcinomas, while losses in chromosome 17p were commonly seen in flat CIS. On the basis of consistent and frequent genetic defects in bladder tumors, it has become clear that there are at least two distinct molecular pathways involved in bladder cancer tumorigenesis and progression (Fig. 93-2), as reviewed elsewhere.[9] Papillary tumors frequently show alterations in chromosome 9, particularly at the INK4a/p16 locus. Further, these tumors frequently show constitutive activation of the receptor tyrosine kinase-Ras pathway, exhibiting activating mutations in the HRAS and fibroblast growth factor receptor 3 (FGFR 3) genes. In contrast, flat CIS and invasive tumors frequently show alterations in the p53 gene and protein (TP53) and in the retinoblastoma(RB) gene. In fact, p53 gene mutations are among the most frequent alterations seen in invasive bladder cancers.[10]

An increasingly detailed understanding of the molecular mechanisms involved in UC tumorigenesis, progression and response to therapy has evolved.

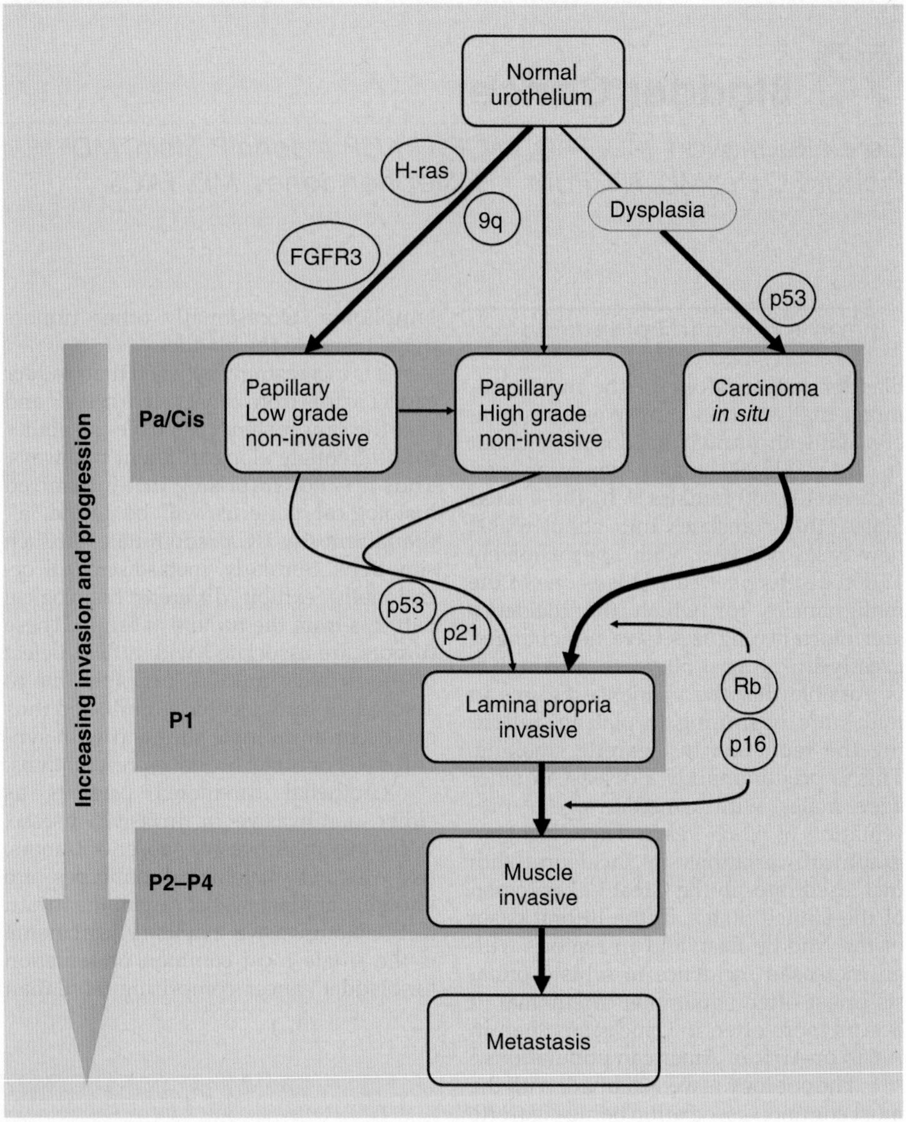

Figure 93-2 ■ Proposed model for urothelial tumorigenesis and progression. Superficial and invasive tumors have unique molecular profiles and arise from distinct pathways. The locations of molecules indicate events that pose a risk for progression of a particular phenotype. The rare papillary carcinomas that invade are more likely to have genetic alterations at crucial loci. The thickness of arrows represents the relative frequency of occurrence.
Source: From Ref. 9.

These findings are already beginning to have an impact on the way in which UC is evaluated and treated.

The RAS-MAPK signal transduction pathway has been demonstrated to be important in noninvasive papillary tumors. Most noninvasive papillary UC's show activation of this pathway, generally through the activation of FGFR3. However, other receptor tyrosine kinases are also known to be involved, such as epidermal growth factor receptor (EGFR) and Her2-neu, as reviewed previously.[9]

Cell cycle regulation has clearly been shown to be a critical pathway in flat CIS and invasive UC. A central molecule in this pathway is the p53 tumor suppressor protein, encoded by the *p53* gene. The p53 protein inhibits cell cycle progression at the G1-S transition, and mediates its control through transcriptional activation of p21 (WAF1/CIP1). Mutations in the *p53* gene constitute a central event in UC and many other cancers, and generally lead to alterations in p53 protein expression (over-expression).[10] Other molecules exerting cell cycle control have also been shown to be altered in UC, including p21 and the RB protein.[9] Further, it has been demonstrated that the accumulation of alterations in this pathway appears to be more important than any single alteration.[11] Patients showing alterations in two or three out of the three determinants (p53, p21, RB) had much poorer outcomes than patients with tumors showing alterations in none or only one of these determinants (Fig. 93-3).

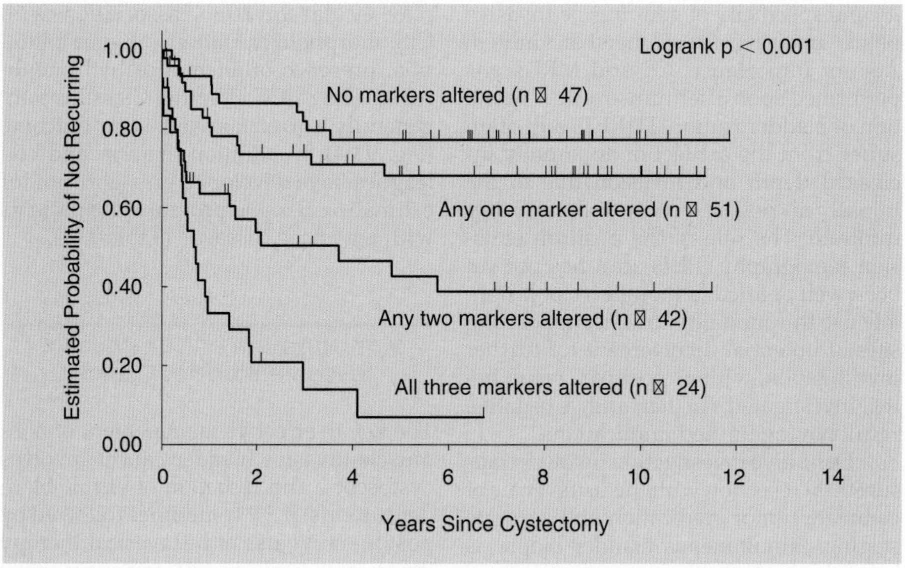

Figure 93-3 Probability of recurrence-free survival in 164 bladder cancer patients, who underwent radical cystectomy, based on alterations in p53, p21, and/or RB expression. The combined analysis shows an increased risk of recurrence with increasing number of deregulated molecules (logrank $p < .001$). *Source:* From Ref. 11.

Tumor angiogenesis is an important pathway in UC as well as other tumors. The first studies in UC examined angiogenesis as measured by microvessel density.[12] Angiogenesis involves a highly complex interaction between endothelial cell growth, migration and invasion. A large number of important and interrelated pathways control tumor angiogenesis. For example, thrombospondin has been demonstrated to be a key regulatory molecule in angiogenesis including a role in UC, and p53 has been shown to play a role in the regulation of thrombospondin expression.[13,14]

It is increasingly recognized that epigenetic alterations play an important role in UC. DNA methylation is the best described of the epigenetic events and involves the methylation of cytosine at CpG dinucleotides.[15] DNA methylation at promoter regions is believed to affect gene transcription and produce in many cases gene silencing, and is a frequent event in human cancer. Genes known to be affected by methylation in UC include RASSF1A, DAPK, and INK4A.[9]

Multiplex genome-wide expression analysis has become increasingly important in the analysis of UC and other cancers.[16] Sophisticated tools that allow for genome-wide expression analysis are being developed and used in the analysis of UC and other tumors. As molecular profiles emerge, they will not only provide a better understanding of progression and prognosis, but will also identify new therapeutic targets as well.

With increasing understanding of specific molecular alterations and their affect on UC progression, the development of therapies targeted to these alterations has begun in earnest. Some of the molecular alterations have been shown to affect response to conventional chemotherapy, with perhaps the most well-established example being *p53* alterations potentially promoting response to cisplatin-based therapies,[17] an observation that remains somewhat controversial,[18] and which will be rationalized when the results of a recent SWOG randomized trial are analyzed. In fact, therapies against targets mentioned above, along with many others, are being developed.[9,19] It is clear that the ability to target multiple pathways altered in UC will be a key to the success of individualized therapy for patients with bladder cancer.

Clinical Presentation

The presentation of bladder cancer usually reflects the extent of disease, with somewhat different patterns associated with non-muscle-invasive tumor, invasive disease, metastases, and the nonmetastatic manifestations of malignancy.[20,21] Patients with noninvasive tumors may present with asymptomatic hematuria (diagnosed on urinalysis), visible hematuria, and irritative patterns like frequency, dysuria, burning or nocturia. In patients with a prior history of non-muscle-invasive bladder cancer and prior transurethral resections, irritative bladder symptoms may be more prominent. Invasive tumors have a similar pattern of presentation, although more advanced tumors may be associated with pelvic pain, slowing of urinary stream, dyspareunia, and occasionally pneumaturia or fecal incontinence. Occasionally tumors involving the trigone will cause obstruction of ureters, with concomitant flank pain.

The presenting features of metastatic disease usually reflect the site(s) of involvement.[20,21] Common sites include distant lymph nodes, lung, liver and bone, and less commonly brain, skin, other viscera. In the present era of aggressive imaging, many metastases will first be detected upon routine follow-up scans. Pulmonary involvement will classically be associated with cough and dyspnea, and occasionally with hemoptysis or chest pain. Liver involvement may present with right upper quadrant pain or shoulder tip pain, and occasionally disruption of function, most commonly manifested by jaundice. Osseous metastases are often associated with bone pain, and less commonly with pathologic fracture, with common sites of involvement including spine, ribs, pelvis and skull. Brain metastases may be suggested by the development of headache, confusion or other motor features. A CT or MRI brain scan will usually reveal the problem, although rarely a spinal tap will be required to diagnose carcinomatous meningitis in a patient with a normal scan (especially in a patient who has received extensive prior chemotherapy for metastatic disease). Skin metastases are uncommon, but usually are manifest by an infiltrative pattern or isolated cutaneous or subcutaneous nodules.

The nonmetastatic manifestations of malignancy consist predominantly of serological syndromes, although occasional patients with present with the thrombo-embolic syndromes classically associated with advanced adenocarcinomas of the gastrointestinal (GI) tract. Bladder cancer is occasionally associated with the production of granulocyte-macrophage colony stimulating factors or other cytokines, and a greatly elevated white blood cell count may reflect this phenomenon, rather than underlying infection. Tumors with squamous differentiation may sometimes be associated with hypercalcemia, due to excess production of immunoreactive parathyroid hormone (PTH)-like substance. In general, these syndromes should be taken in context, and generally do not require specific management unless causing clinical syndromes—eg, severe hypercalcemia, significant thrombotic episodes.

Investigation and Staging

The specifics of the presentation will usually govern the nature of the investigations.[22] Presentation with hematuria or other urinary symptoms will usually lead to urinalysis and assessment of possible infection or urinary calculi. The absence of these conditions or the presence of sterile pyuria is usually grounds for assessing urinary cytology and/or progressing to cystoscopic examination. In some clinical practices, to improve upon the sensitivity of urine cytology, and to reduce the need for periodic cystoscopy in the follow-up of patients with non-muscle-invasive bladder cancer, novel biomarker dipstick assays have been developed, based on soluble bladder tumor antigens or cell-based markers (NMP22, BTA-TRAK, BLCA-4, Immunocyt). Molecular analysis (Urovysion) allows detection of aneuploidy reflecting changes in chromosomes 3, 7, and 17, which are associated with high-grade tumors, and loss of the 9p21 site that is characteristic of low-grade disease. Case-control and cohort studies have suggested that several of these markers may have higher sensitivity than urine cytology, and some have been approved by the FDA for use in combination with cystoscopy for the diagnosis of recurrence.[23] Their utility in initial diagnosis is more variable, with scanty data to support their use in this setting. As urinary cytology is said to be more than 98% specific, a positive reading mandates further investigation; however, negative findings are less helpful.

There is no specific serological work-up for bladder cancer. Routine hematological and biochemical testing may reveal chronic anemia of chronic disease or from blood loss, renal dysfunction (from obstruction or the underlying cause of the cancer), and occasionally evidence of metastases, such as raised alkaline phosphatase or liver function tests. No serological tumor markers have been shown to be specific to bladder cancer, although occasional elevation of carcinoembryonic antigen, human chorionic gonadotrophin, CA 19-9 or CA125 will be seen, the latter particularly in the presence of elements of adenocarcinoma.

Imaging of the urinary tract may be carried out before or after cystoscopy.[20,21] A relatively standard approach is to obtain an excretory urogram to delineate the anatomy of the urinary tract, including the presence of tumors of the bladder and upper tracts or hydronephrosis. CT urography is more commonly used in the current era, based on its ability to evaluate the renal parenchyma in addition to the urothelium, and it is performed more rapidly than excretory urography. MRI imaging may also be helpful to define the local anatomy and the extent of an invasive tumor, while also providing staging information about lymph node and distant sites of involvement. However, it should be emphasized that the sensitivity and specificity of non-muscle-invasive pelvic imaging are somewhat limited. Also of importance, CT and MRI scans performed soon after transurethral resection of bladder tumor (TURBT) will often suffer from the artifact of apparently increased depth and invasion due to the impact of post-resection inflammatory infiltrate. The role of the positron emission tomography (PET) scan has not yet been well defined, although we occasionally use this modality to assist in defining sites of potential involvement for further investigation, with a "positive" result being investigated further and a negative result having limited implications.

Definitive investigation involves transurethral resection with the usual goals of complete tumor eradication and accurate staging. Simultaneous bladder biopsy is helpful in only 10% of cases, and is typically reserved for the setting of a positive urinary cytology in the absence of adequate explanation. Bimanual examination at the time of transurethral resection (TUR) allows assessment of tumor stage and the presence of extravesical disease. In the setting of high-grade cancer, it is important to determine the existence of detrusor muscle invasion. Unless cystectomy is planned, repeat TUR within 6-8 weeks shows upstaging in 30% of patients with muscle identified in the original specimen, and 60% of patients in whom no muscle was present initially. Repeat TUR is also associated with improved response to intravesical chemotherapy.

Prognosis

The prognosis of bladder cancer largely reflects several of the factors already discussed, including stage and grade of the tumor, multifocality, presence of lymphovascular invasion, association with CIS, morphology, pattern of gene mutation, presence of anemia or hydronephrosis. The AJCC Staging Classification[8] generally correlates well with outcome (Fig. 93-4). In addition, Bajorin and colleagues have developed an algorithm for estimating risk and prognosis for patients with advanced disease[24] (Table 93-1).

Management of Non-muscle-Invasive Bladder Cancer

The key to effective management of non-muscle-invasive bladder cancer involves cystoscopy and resection of visible bladder tumor(s),[20,25,26] sometimes followed by postoperative use of intravesical therapy (immunological or cytotoxic reagents) to reduce the risk of recurrence.[27,28] As bladder cancer is associated with a field defect, multiple random biopsies of apparently normal urothelium should be performed to identify occult CIS if urine cytology is positive or in the presence of high-grade disease when bladder conservation is contemplated. Usually endoscopic resection is repeated within 4 weeks of the initial resection in patients with high-grade disease and/or T1 tumors, as up to 50% will have evidence of invasive bladder cancer into muscularis propria on re-biopsy.

The grade and stage of the tumor will dictate subsequent management. Patients with non-muscle-invasive, low-grade papillary bladder cancer are at low risk of progression to invasive disease, although the risk of recurrence may be as high as 70-80%. Patients at increased risk for recurrence on the basis of tumor size, multifocal tumors, or prior recurrent tumors are often given adjuvant intravesical therapy (usually weekly instillations

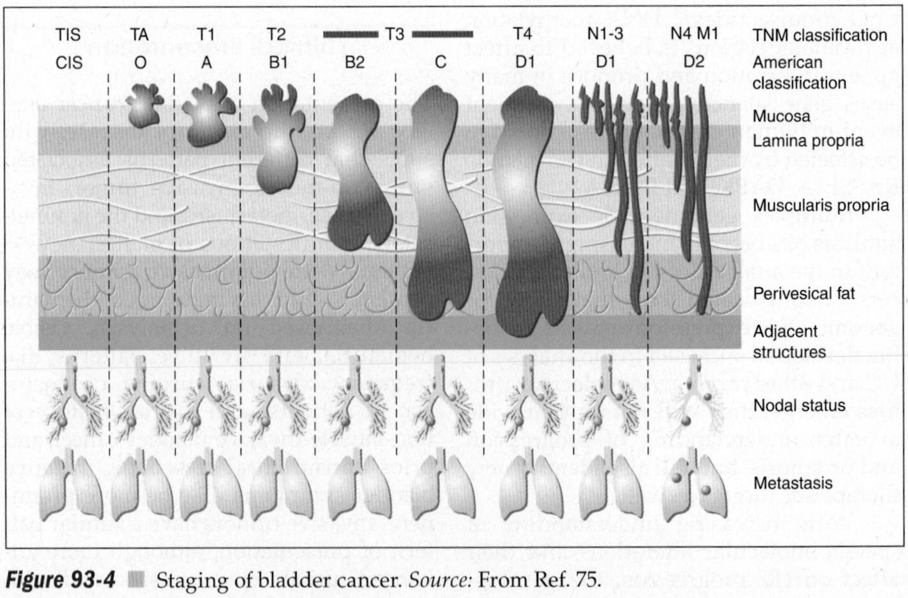

Figure 93-4 ■ Staging of bladder cancer. *Source:* From Ref. 75.

Table 93-1 **Risk Factors in Metastatic Bladder Cancer**

Variable	Statistical Significance (*p*)	Risk Ratio
3 Variables:		
Visceral metastases (yes/no)	.0001	1.99
Karnofsky P.S. (</≥80%)	.0001	2.05
Hemoglobin (normal/abnormal)	.0103	1.41
2 Variables:		
Visceral metastases (yes/no)	.0001	2.10
Karnofsky P.S. (</≥ 80%)	.0001	2.20

Source: Adapted from Ref. 24.

for 6-8 weeks) following resection, mostly with bacillus Calmette Guerin (BCG), which reduces the risk of recurrence by up to around 40%.[28] The mechanism of action of BCG is based on local immunological stimulation, perhaps with alteration of suppressor-helper T cell ratios. Effectively, such treatment allows the bladder to "reject" implantation and recurrence of bladder cancer.

Randomized trials suggest that BCG is superior to other intravesical agents at preventing tumor progression, and an initial bladder preservation strategy involving intravesical BCG is associated with long-term outcomes similar to early cystectomy for low-grade tumors.[25] Maintenance BCG is associated with a reduction in tumor recurrence and reduced requirement for cystectomy, compared to a single 6-week induction regimen. The optimal schedule of BCG administration has not been defined, and similarly the optimal commercial preparations and the ideal duration of administration remain controversial.

The side effects of all the intravesical agents in common use include irritative symptoms and hematuria. BCG may also cause a flu-like syndrome and, because it is an attenuated mycobacterium, it can produce local, regional and systemic TB-like infections. Granulomatous infections can occur at extravesical sites, including the prostate, epididymis, testes, kidney, liver and lungs. BCG sepsis is the most serious complication, and can be life-threatening. Systemic involvement ("BCG-osis") should usually be treated with triple-antituberculous therapy for 6 months.

In some centers, cytotoxic chemotherapy, with agents such as mitomycin C[28] or gemcitabine,[29] is preferred because of purportedly reduced toxicity, although it is not yet certain that this true, although a current SWOG trial should clarify this issue. For patients who refuse cystectomy for relapsed non-muscle-invasive disease, several lines of immunological or cytotoxic intravesical therapy may be feasible, and may delay recurrence and progression. In the past, thiotepa was often used as an intravesical agent, but fell into disfavor because of the risks of absorption (as it is a small molecule) with concomitant systemic toxicity, including myelosuppression and iatrogenic leukemia. Doxorubicin is also used occasionally, but randomized trials have suggested a lower efficacy than mitomycin C.

After completion of treatment, patients should be monitored closely with periodic cystoscopy and selective urine cytology and/or tumor marker evaluation at 3-6 month intervals to detect recurrence early. Patients with high-risk non-muscle-invasive bladder cancer (high-grade Ta, T1 or CIS) have at least a 50% risk of developing invasive bladder cancer and a 35% risk of dying from bladder cancer. Moreover, those with persistent or recurrent high-grade disease after one or two courses of intravesical therapy will develop muscle invasion and progression in 80% of cases. Thus we advocate timely radical cystectomy with urinary diversion for relapsed high-risk disease, particularly for patients with long life expectancy.[30,31] Cure rates approach 90% in this setting, and when cystectomy is delayed, true invasive disease develops and is associated with diminished survival.

Management of Invasive Bladder Cancer

Definitive Surgery

In the past 20 years, radical cystectomy with bilateral pelvic lymphadenectomy has increasingly been viewed as the standard treatment for clinically localized invasivebladdercancer.[20,31] Thistraditionally requires the en bloc removal of the anterior pelvic organs, which include the bladder, prostate, and seminal vesicles in men and the bladder, urethra, uterus, ovaries, and vaginal cuff plus anterior vaginal wall in women.[31] A urinary diversion is formed by the connection of the ureters to detubularized intestinal reservoir. Although the previous conventional approach was to drain the reservoir into a bag attached to a stoma in the skin, continent reservoirs, such as the Indiana pouch and orthotopic neobladder, are now standard approaches because they offer improved continence without the need for an external collecting bag. This, in turn, improves lifestyle and self-image, and thus may improve acceptance of extirpative therapy. Many of the "continent" reservoirs are emptied by intermittent self-catheterization, whereas the orthotopic neobladder involves creation of an intestinal reservoir which is attached to the urethra and enables the patient to void normally without self-catheterization.

Radical cystectomy, without adjuvant therapy, is curative in up to 60-70% of patients with invasive T2 bladder cancer,[20,31-33] depending on stage and other prognostic factors. The 5-year overall survival rates in large series of patients with T2-T3 disease range from *40-65%*. Relapse rates relate to stage, grade, presence of lymphovascular invasion, and expression of molecular prognosticators, and increase with the extent of disease. Radical cystectomy alone has been reported to be curative in 20-40% of patients with regional metastasis to pelvic lymph nodes, and the outcome is influenced by the primary tumor stage, number of involved lymph nodes, and the presence of extranodal extension.[20,31,32] It has been suggested that extended template node dissection, including presacral and common iliac nodes, may improve outcomes for patients with larger number of nodes and extranodal extension, and that removal of nodes in packages may improve outcomes.[31-33] However, this may reflect the case selection bias, surgical skill or support and salvage techniques available in centers of excellence.

Advances in Instrumentation

Laparoscopic radical cystectomy, with or without robotic assistance, has been reported in modest series from centers experienced in laparoscopic surgery, including our own.[34-36] The cystectomy and lymph node dissection are commonly performed laparoscopically and the urinary diversion is carried out through a midline incision smaller than is usual for conventional surgery. The potential advantages include reduced blood loss, less postoperative pain and shorter convalescence. The drawbacks include technical difficulty and possible limitations in oncological efficiency due to less clear observation of nodes and pelvic structures for evidence of tumor involvement. In addition, the available data have been derived from nonrandomized series, carried out by technically superb surgeons, and are characterized by careful case selection and relatively short follow-up.

Another innovation has been the use of prostate-sparing cystectomy, with the intent of ameliorating the extent of mutilation and late effects, although this has not yet been validated by randomized trials.[37] This concept faces the challenge that up to 50% of men undergoing cystectomy will be found to have direct urothelial cancer invasion into the prostatic urethra, ducts, or stroma, or previously unrecognized prostatic adenocarcinoma. Although we recognize the potential utility of novel technologies, and are exploring these at the Cleveland Clinic, we emphasize that caution must be exercised to ensure that cure rates are not negatively impacted by the innovations.

Role of Radiotherapy

For patients with invasive, clinically nonmetastatic bladder cancer who are not surgical candidates, either by their choice, technical considerations, or because of significant co-morbid conditions, radiation is the treatment of choice.[38-40] To date, there have been no well-designed, randomized studies comparing radiation with surgery in patients with similar characteristics. Favorable prognostic features for use of radiotherapy include small, localized, T2 tumors, absence of hydronephrosis, normal renal function and absence of anemia.[1,38-41]

A relatively standard radiotherapy approach is to deliver more than 65-70 Gy over 6-7 weeks, with the major component of dosage focused on the tumor and immediately surrounding areas, as defined by CT scanning in the prone position. In the present era, it is less common for radiotherapy to be delivered in isolation than for it to be administered in combination with systemic chemotherapy, largely based on the studies of the RTOG and the randomized trial conducted by the National Cancer Institute of Canada[42] in the 1980s and 1990s. These studies have shown significantly improved local control from chemoradiation, although a statistically significant survival benefit has been elusive.

Toxicities of radiation include cutaneous inflammation, proctitis that is occasionally complicated by bleeding and obstruction, cystitis or bladder fibrosis, impotence, incontinence, and development of secondary malignancies in the region surrounding the radiation field. Of importance, much of the documentation of severe pelvic side effects antedated the use of modern equipment, planning techniques, fractionation and field sizes.

Several innovations in radiation planning and treatment have been introduced in recent years, including Calypso and similar devices for tracking physiological movement of the tumor tissue and adjusting the radiation beam, and particle therapy, such as proton beam, with more focused beams and potentially less normal tissue toxicity. To date, no definitive, controlled studies on their application in bladder cancer management have been reported.

Combined Modality Strategies

Our first attempts to study systemic chemotherapy added to definitive local modalities (radiotherapy, transurethral resection of tumor, or cystectomy) were published more than 25 years ago,[43] and were based on the rationale that chemotherapy might reduce the extent of local tumor while controlling occult metastases. In the case of radiotherapy as definitive local treatment, it was hypothesized that some cytotoxic agents (5-fluorouracil, cisplatin, doxorubicin, paclitaxel, gemcitabine) might sensitize the tissues to an increased radiation effect. Nonrandomized trials of concurrent chemotherapy and radiation have, in fact, suggested that a higher rate of bladder preservation is possible with this approach, compared historically with radiation alone.[42-48] This has been confirmed by one randomized trial.[42] However, when chemoradiation fails, with local progression or relapse, salvage surgery becomes extremely difficult because of the formation of dense adhesions.

Neoadjuvant (Preemptive) Chemotherapy ■ We have known for quarter of a century that neoadjuvant or preemptive systemic chemotherapy can shrink primary bladder cancers, and result in downstaging, sometimes achieving a complete clinical and pathological remission.[43] Although the early randomized trials of neoadjuvant systemic chemotherapy, followed by definitive radiotherapy or cystectomy, showed no significant survival benefit from the combined modality approaches, these mostly tested single agent regimens which did not really have a major impact on survival in bladder cancer. However, the introduction of multidrug chemotherapy regimens, such as the methatrexate, vinblastine, doxorubicin, and cisplatin (MVAC) and cisplatin, methotrexate, and vinblastin (CMV) regimens, adapted from use in metastatic disease, into neoadjuvant protocols yielded survival benefit, as indicated by several randomized clinical trials and a meta-analysis (Table 93-2).[44-49] Of importance, when we designed the International Intergroup Trial more than 20 years ago, in which neoadjuvant CMV was assessed prior to definitive local treatment (either radiotherapy or surgery), it was believed that a minimum survival benefit of 10% should be achieved for the trial to achieve its goals. Thus with a smaller survival benefit, it was reported as a negative study.[45] The use of CMV chemotherapy in an RTOG trial of CMV plus chemo-radiation vs chemo-radiation alone did not show any difference in survival, perhaps because the chemo-radiation in both arms vitiated the difference.[50] Nonetheless, meta-analysis of several randomized trials confirmed that the overall trend is in favor of combined modality therapy and overall is statistically significant.[49]

Thus the consensus is now that neoadjuvant MVAC chemotherapy affords an absolute survival benefit of 8%, with an increase in median survival of up to 3 years, when added to radical cystectomy. A statistically significant survival benefit has not been proven when the primary treatment is radiotherapy. Despite these data for neoadjuvant MVAC plus cystectomy, a recent national survey of patterns of practice has indicated that relatively few urologists practice in a fashion consistent with these data, suggesting that change has come slowly in this area of clinical work.[51] What is not yet clear is whether an equivalent result can be achieved by the completion of radical cystectomy, with tailored use of subsequent adjuvant chemotherapy for selected patients with deeply invasive disease or adverse prognostic factors, such as lymphovascular invasion or nodal involvement.

To date, no multidrug cytotoxic regimen has been shown to be superior, or even equivalent to the MVAC or CMV regimens for neoadjuvant chemotherapy. However, the newer gentle regimens, such as gemcitabine-cisplatin or gemcitabine-carboplatin are increasingly being used for neoadjuvant therapy. This may be reasonable for the older or frail patients, but may lead to a greater risk of death from cancer for the more robust patient without intercurrent medical disorders. Ideally a randomized clinical trial would be needed to resolve this issue.

Table 93-2 ■ **Results of Clinical Randomized Trials of Neoadjuvant Chemotherapy for Invasive Bladder Cancer, Stages T1–T4**

Series	Neoadjuvant Regimen	Definitive Therapy	Median Survival With/Without Neoadjuvant Therapy (Months)	Actuarial Long-Term Survival With/Without Neoadjuvant Therapy
Shipley	CMV	RT/C	36/36	48%/49% at 5 yr
MRC-EORTC	CMV	RT/cystectomy	44/37.5	55%/50% at 3 yr
Intergroup	MVDC	Cystectomy	72/45	55%/45% at 6 yr
Nordic 1 trial	DC	Cystectomy	Not reached/72	59%/51% at 5 yr

Abbreviations: C, cisplatin; D, doxorubicin; M, methotrexate; Cy, Cyclophosphamide; V, vinblastine; MRC-EORTC, Medical Research Council/European Organization for Research and Treatment of Cancer; RT, radiotherapy.

Adjuvant Chemotherapy ■ Chemotherapy administered after radical cystectomy for patients with T3-T4 tumors and/or lymph node involvement may improve disease-free survival.[52-54] However, in the trials reported to date, most of which have been flawed by poor design and inadequate sample size, a statistically significant improvement in total survival has not been demonstrated. These flaws have been addressed in a large international randomized trial that has been in progress for several years, and which has suffered from poor accrual, leading to premature closure, and it seems unlikely that level 1 evidence on this issue will ever be available.

Although meta-analysis can sometimes help to resolve the failure of small trials to resolve an issue, the study published by the Cochrane group was heavily flawed.[55] It grouped a heterogeneous set of small trials that were either poorly designed, poorly executed, or which did not actually compare adjuvant chemotherapy with chemotherapy at relapse, and thus added nothing useful to the published literature, and actually confused the issue. Understanding the significant limitations of historical controls and poorly executed randomized trials, our group has concluded that it is possible that there is a survival benefit from adjuvant chemotherapy, and it is unlikely that there would be a survival deficit, and thus offers this approach to carefully selected patients with high-risk disease, otherwise healthy. That said, we would certainly support a well-designed randomized trial of adjuvant therapy if one were available.

Chemoradiation ■ As noted previously, the role of radiotherapy as a sole modality of treatment has diminished in the past 25 years, especially in North America. It is clear that the combination of chemotherapy plus radiotherapy, with either neoadjuvant or concurrent administration of cytotoxics, yields greater local control than radiotherapy alone, and thus potentially facilitates an improved chance of organ preservation. This is particularly useful in a patient with a T2 tumor who has not undergone multiple transurethral bladder tumor resections (which tend to increase the chance of a contracted, irritative bladder in the setting of chemoradiation). The approach popularized at Massachusetts General Hospital requires endoscopic assessment after 4000 cGy, with conversion to cystectomy for patients who have not shown a significant level of tumor cytoreduction.

There is a considerable body of literature from North America, the United Kingdom and Europe that supports the utility of chemoradiation for improving local control, based on phase I-II trials, as reviewed in detail elsewhere.[1,56] However, only one randomized trial has proven that improved local control occurs,[42] and there are no randomized trials that demonstrate a statistically significant improvement in overall survival. That said, Shipley and the investigators of RTOG have taken the philosophical view, in the design of their trials, that chemoradiation improves local control of the primary tumor, leaving it to systemic therapies to control the occult micrometastases that may be present at initial diagnosis.

Metastatic Bladder Cancer

Chemotherapy is the first-line treatment of choice for patients with metastatic bladder cancer. The single agent activity of 5-fluoruracil, methotrexate, the vinca alkaloids, doxorubicin and cisplatin was demonstrated between the 1960s and early 1980s. In 1985, Alan Yagoda and his team demonstrated that the combination of methotrexate, vinblastine, doxorubicin (Adriamycin) and cisplatin, the MVAC regimen produced objective responses in more than 60% of cases, with a median survival of 1 year.[57] In an International Intergroup study carried out by investigators in the United States, Canada, and Australia, we proved the utility of the MVAC regimen in a randomized trial against single agent cisplatin, and confirmed that the benefit persisted with a median follow-up beyond 6 years.[58] Others confirmed the superiority of MVAC to the combination of cyclophosphamide, doxorubicin and cisplatin.[59] The major limitation of the MVAC regimen was substantial toxicity, including *grade* 3-4 GI effects, stomatitis and myelosuppression, as well as occasional cases of renal dysfunction and cardiotoxicity.[58,59] Attempts were made to improve the regimen, and Sternberg et al demonstrated, in a randomized trial, that a dose-intense variant of MVAC yielded higher response rates and reduced toxicity compared to the original regimen,[60] but without achieving a major increment in median survival. However, at 5 years, the number of surviving patients was greater than for standard-dose MVAC, but did not reach statistical significance. Our late follow-up study of the comparison between cisplatin and the standard-dose MVAC regimen, which confirmed the benefit of the combination, showed that most patients in each arm had died of progressive cancer.[58] This opened the way for renewed investigation, of novel agents and strategies.

Single agent response rates of around 20-30% have been reported for paclitaxel, gemcitabine, docetaxel, ifosfamide, and pemetrexed. The combination of these agents with other standard or investigational drugs has resulted in response rates of 50-80%, sometimes with less toxicity than the conventional-combination MVAC regimen, but median survival figures have remained in the range of 12-20 months, and cure rates for patients with visceral metastases have not exceeded 10-15%.[61-66] After initial studies with the combination of gemcitabine and cisplatin revealed apparently equivalent response rates and substantially less toxicity than the MVAC regimen,[61] a randomized trial comparing gemcitabine-cisplatin vs MVAC confirmed these observations and showed that survival was similar.[66] As a consequence, an international consortium (International Intergroup) accepted gemcitabine-cisplatin as a new standard, and moved to compare gemcitabine-cisplatin with gemcitabine-cisplatin-paclitaxel for patients with previously untreated metastatic UCs. Although this study was modeled on a Spanish phase II trial,[65] with recruitment goals based on that trial, the Spanish data did not translate when applied by the International Intergroup, and analysis revealed the study to be underpowered to reveal a significant survival difference.[67] The investigators reported that this trial showed a slightly higher response rate from the triplet, but no clinically relevant or statistically significant difference in outcome, and thus concluded that there was no real clinical benefit from the addition of paclitaxel to the doublet of gemcitabine and cisplatin. Several other doublets and triplets have been assessed in phase I-II trials, but none has emerged as a major advance.

An important caveat in interpreting modern clinical trial data is that stage migration has occurred in the management of advanced bladder cancer, largely due to the increased use of aggressive post-surgical imaging via CT, MRI, and PET scans, and there has been increased use of systemic chemotherapy to treat patients with small volume, asymptomatic metastases. For example, at Memorial Sloan-Kettering Cancer Center, the initial experience with the MVAC regimen in 1985 produced a median survival of about 12 months whereas trial data from that institution in 1997 showed a median survival of 18 months with a variant of MVAC that has a relatively minor dose escalation. This should be borne in mind when considering the utility of novel combinations, such as the ITP regimen (ifosfamide, paclitaxel, and cisplatin), which also yields a median survival of about 18 months. Before novel regimens can be accepted into routine clinical practice, their safety and efficacy should be defined in randomized trials against accepted current standards. Irrespective of stage migration, it is quite clear that there has only been very modest progress in the development of novel cytotoxic agents for bladder cancer since the introduction of gemcitabine, both with respect to primary and salvage therapy for metastatic disease. The majority of patients with metastases still die of progressive tumor.

Because cytotoxic chemotherapy regimens have not improved the cure rate dramatically, alternative approaches are being investigated. In the past decade, we have focused on novel compounds that target the genes and proteins that control cellular growth, differentiation and apoptosis. Clinical trials are currently assessing the efficacy of agents that modulate the function of EGFR and other tyrosine kinase inhibitors. These agents are being tested both as monotherapy and in combination with chemotherapy. The ability to identify expression of the *HER-2/neu* oncogene, EGFR, and other molecular predictors of response to treatment may allow tailoring of more specific therapeutic strategies. For example, Hussain et al have assessed the utility of herceptin, in combination with a regimen of carboplatin, gemcitabine and paclitaxel, against bladder cancers expressing the *HER 2/neu* gene, and showed a response rate of 70%; however, the median survival of 14 months did not suggest that this was a major advance.[68]

Investigators at Memorial Sloan-Kettering Cancer Center have reported preliminary data indicating that the tyrosine kinase inhibitor, sunitinib (see Chapter 91: Renal Cell Carcinoma) can cause partial remissions in heavily pretreated bladder cancer, and that these remissions may be sustained for many months.[69] By contrast, others have reported lack of activity of sorafenib, another tyrosine kinase inhibitor, against bladder cancer.[70]

Another approach that is being investigated anew is the use of surgery to consolidate remissions achieved from chemotherapy.[71] This approach was pioneered in bladder cancer by Alan Yagoda 20 years ago. The rationale for this is based on the high relapse rate observed at responding sites of disease and is supported by the 33% incidence of viable cancer found within resected specimens after complete clinical response. Five year survival rates, as high as 30-40%, have been reported in patients following complete resection of metastatic sites after cisplatin-based chemotherapy, but it should be noted that these represent very heavily selected cases, dominated by single metastases.

Uncommon Histologic Variants

A detailed discussion of the management of adenocarcinoma, squamous carcinoma, small cell carcinoma and sarcoma of the bladder is beyond the scope of this brief review, and has been detailed elsewhere.[72-74] However, certain principles of management can be noted. All of the uncommon variants tend to be more resistant to chemotherapy than are the pure UCs, and thus a greater emphasis is placed on surgical resection or definitive radiotherapy when possible. Where unusual histologic patterns are noted, it is also important to exclude the diagnosis of second primary cancer.

The prognosis of metastatic tumors of nontransitional type reflects the sites of involvement, growth characteristics, and bulk of disease. As the yield from chemotherapy is less impressive than for urothelial cancer,[58] it is important to consider context (age, anticipated active life expectancy, intercurrent disease, sites of metastases) when planning the approach to chemotherapy.

As a general rule, squamous carcinomas are sensitive to combinations that include a platinum complex, paclitaxel, and gemcitabine, and occasional responses have been reported after treatment with methotrexate, bleomycin and the oxazophorines, such as ifosfamide. We have previously shown that the MVAC regimen is not especially useful for squamous carcinoma of the bladder.[58] Patterns of practice vary—at the MD Anderson Cancer Center, a combination of gemcitabine, ifosfamide and cisplatin is used; at the Cleveland Clinic, we commonly use a combination of paclitaxel, gemcitabine and cisplatin, and have seen long-term survivors treated for soft tissue advanced disease. Adenocarcinomas tend to respond transiently to regimens used for cancers of the GI tract, such as combinations involving oxaliplatin, irinotecan, and fluoropyrimidines, such as 5-fluorouracil or capecitabine, although there is a real paucity of well-structured phase II or phase III clinical trial data.

Investigators at the MD Anderson Cancer Center have reported a substantial experience with small cell anaplastic cancer of the bladder, revealing anticancer efficacy but few cures.[74] The regimens with utility resemble those used for small cell cancers of the lung, and generally involve combinations that include a platinum complex, etoposide, doxorubicin, a taxane, and an oxazophorine. However, there is a general consensus that these tumors are more resistant to chemotherapy than are bronchogenic small cell tumors, and there is thus a greater emphasis on the role of surgical extirpation in the control of the primary tumor. In addition, there is good level-2 evidence that chemotherapy adds to the survival impact of surgical resection.

Summary

There has been significant progress in the management of bladder cancer in the past 20 years, with refinement of our understanding of the underlying biology, relevance of gene expression and stem cell function, molecular prognostication, and improvement in the nature of surgery, reduction in toxicity of surgery, and rationalization of the role of chemotherapy for advanced disease. There is also a place for bladder conservation via radiotherapy or chemoradiation. Despite progress, many patients with metastatic disease die of their disease, and this has led to the search for new systemic therapies, including novel cytotoxics and the assessment of targeted therapies.

Selected References

The complete reference list can be found at www.CANCERMEDICINE8.com

1. Raghavan D, Shipley WU, Garnick MB, Richie JP, Russell PJ. Biology and management of bladder cancer. *N Engl J Med.* 1990;322:1129–1138.
2. Fleshner N, Kondylis F. Demographics and epidemiology of urothelial cancer of the urinary bladder. In: Droller M, ed. *American Cancer Society Atlas of Clinical Oncology: Urothelial Tumors*. London, Hamilton: BC Decker; 2004:1–16.
3. Brown JL, Russell PJ, Philips J, Wotherspoon J, Raghavan D. Clonal analysis of a bladder cancer cell line: an experimental model of tumor heterogeneity. *Brit J Cancer.* 1990;61:369–376.
5. Cote RJ, Soni R A, Amin MB. Bladder and urethra. In: Weidner N, Cote RJ, Suster S, Weiss L, eds. *Modern Surgical Pathology.* 1st ed. Philadelphia: Harcourt Health Sciences; 2003:1106.
8 Greene FL, Page DL, Fleming ID, et al, eds. Urinary bladder. In: *AJCC Cancer Staging Manual.* 6th ed. New York: Springer-Verlag, 2002:367–374.
9. Mitra AP, Datar RH, Cote RJ. Molecular pathways in invasive bladder cancer: new insights into mechanisms, progression, and target identification. *J Clin Oncol.* 2006;24:5552–5564.
11. Chatterjee SJ, Datar R, Youssefzadeh D, et al. Combined effects of p53, p21, and pRb expression in the progression of bladder transitional cell carcinoma. *J Clin Oncol.* 2004;22:1007–1013.
14. Grossfeld GD, Ginsberg DA, Stein JP, et al. Thrombospondin-1 expression in bladder cancer: association with p53 alterations, tumor angiogenesis and tumor progression. *J Natl Cancer Inst.* 1997;89:219–227.

18. Siu LL, Banerjee D, Khurana RJ, et al. The prognostic role of p53, metallothionein, P-glycoprotein, and MIB-1 in muscle-invasive urothelial transitional cell carcinoma. *Clin Cancer Res.* 1998;4:559–565.
19. Raghavan D. Molecular targeting and pharmacogenomics in the management of advanced bladder cancer. *Cancer.* 2003;97 (8 suppl):2083–2089.
21. Lagenstroer P, See W. Clinical pathogenesis and staging of urothelial bladder cancer. In: Droller MJ, ed. *American Cancer Society Atlas of Clinical Oncology: Urothelial Tumors.* London, Hamilton: BC Decker; 2004:58–72.
22. Jacques AET, Reznek RH. Radiological investigations in genitourinary cancer. In: Nargund VH, Raghavan D, Sandler HM, eds. *Urological Oncology.* 2008: 61–106.
24. Bajorin DF, Dodd PM, Mazumdar M, et al. Long-term survival in metastatic transitional-cell carcinoma prognostic factors predicting outcome of therapy. *J Clin Oncol.* 1999;17:3173–3181.
25. Cookson MS, Herr HW, Zhang ZF, et al. The treated natural history of high risk superficial bladder cancer: 15-year outcome. *J Urol.* 1997;158:62–67.
28. Huncharek M, Geschwind JF, Witherspoon B, et al. Intravesical chemotherapy prophylaxis in primary superficial bladder cancer: a meta-analysis of 3703 patients from 11 randomized trials. *J Clin Epidemiol.* 2000;53:676–680.
29. Dalbagni G, Russo P, Bochner B, et al. Phase II trial of intravesical gemcitabine in bacille-Calmette-Guerin-refractory transitional cell carcinoma of the bladder. *J Clin Oncol.* 2006;24:2729–2734.
30. Herr HW, Sogani PC. Does early cystectomy improve the survival of patients with high risk superficial bladder tumors? *J Urol.* 2001;166:1296–1299.
31. Stein JP, Lieskovsky G, Cote R, et al. Radical cystectomy in the treatment of invasive bladder cancer: long-term results in 1054 patients. *J Clin Oncol.* 2001;19:666–675.
32. Hautmann RE, Gschwend JE, dePetriconi RC, et al. Cystectomy for transitional cell carcinoma of the bladder: results of a surgery only series in the neobladder era. *J Urol.* 2006;176:486–492.
36. Haber GP, Gill IS. Laparoscopic radical cystectomy for cancer: oncological outcomes at up to 5 years. *BJU Int.* 2007;100:137–142.
38. Gospodarowicz MK, Hawkins NV, Rawlings GA, et al. Radical radiotherapy for muscle invasive transitional cell carcinoma of the bladder: failure analysis. *J Urol.* 1989;142:1448–1454.
39. Mameghan H, Fisher RJ, Watt WH, et al. The management of invasive transitional cell carcinoma of the bladder: results of definitive and preoperative radiation therapy in 390 patients treated at the Prince of Wales Hospital, Sydney, Australia. *Cancer.* 1992;69:2771–2774.
40. Borgaonkar S, Jain A, Bollina P, et al. Radical radiotherapy and salvage cystectomy as the primary management of transitional cell carcinoma of the bladder. Results following the introduction of a CT planning technique. *Clin Oncol.* 2002;14:141–147.
41. Chung PW, Bristow RB, Milosevic MF, et al. Long-term outcome of radiation-based conservation therapy for invasive bladder cancer. *Urol Oncol.* 2007;25:303–309.
42. Coppin C, Gospodarowicz M, James K, et al. Improved local control of invasive bladder cancer by concurrent cisplatin and preoperative or definitive radiation. The National Cancer Institute of Canada Clinical Trials Group. *J Clin Oncol.* 1996;14:2901–2907.
43. Raghavan D, Pearson B, Duval P, et al. Initial intravenous cis-platinum therapy: improved management for invasive high-risk bladder cancer? *J Urol.* 1985;133:399–402.
44. Grossman HB, Natale RB, Tangen CM, et al. Neoadjuvant chemotherapy plus cystectomy compared with cystectomy alone for locally advanced bladder cancer. *N Engl J Med.* 2003;349:859.
45. Neoadjuvant cisplatin, methotrexate, and vinblastine chemotherapy for muscle-invasive bladder cancer: a randomised controlled trial. International Collaboration of Trialists. *Lancet.* 1999;354:533.
49. Advanced bladder cancer meta-analysis collaboration: neo-adjuvant chemotherapy in invasive bladder cancer: a systematic review and meta-analysis. *Lancet.* 2003;361:1927–1934.
50. Shipley WU, Winter KA, Kaufman DS, et al. Phase III trial of neoadjuvant chemotherapy in patients with invasive bladder cancer treated with selective bladder preservation by combined radiation therapy and chemotherapy: initial results of Radiation Therapy Oncology Group 89-03. *J Clin Oncol.* 1998;16:3576.
52. Skinner DG, Daniels JR, Russell CA, et al. The role of adjuvant chemotherapy following cystectomy for invasive bladder cancer: a prospective comparative trial. *J Urol.* 1991;145:459–464.
53. Freiha F, Reese J, Torti FM. A randomized trial of radical cystectomy plus cisplatin, vinblastine and methotrexate chemotherapy for muscle invasive bladder cancer. *J Urol.* 1996;155:495.
54. Stockle M, Meyenburg W, Wellek S, et al. Advanced bladder cancer (stages pT3b, pT4a, pN1 and pN2): improved survival after radical cystectomy and 3 adjuvant cycles of chemotherapy: results of a controlled prospective study. *J Urol.* 1992;148:302.
56. Choueiri TK, Raghavan D. Chemotherapy for muscle invasive bladder cancer treated with radiotherapy—persisting uncertainties. *Nature Clin Pract Oncol.* 2008;5:444–454.
57. Sternberg CN, Yagoda A, Scher HI, et al. M-VAC (methotrexate, vinblastine, doxorubicin and cisplatin) for advanced transitional cell carcinoma of the urothelium. *J Urol.* 1988;139:461.
58. Saxman SB, Propert K, Einhorn LH, et al. Long-term follow up of phase III intergroup study of cisplatin alone or in combination with methotrexate, vinblastine, and doxorubicin in patients with metastatic urothelial carcinoma: a cooperative group study. *J Clin Oncol.* 1997;15:2564.
65. Bellmunt J, Guillem V, Paz-Arez L, et al. Phase I-II study of paclitaxel, cisplatin, and gemcitabine in advanced transitional-cell carcinoma of the urothelium. Spanish Oncology Genitourinary Group. *J Clin Oncol.* 2000;18:3247–3255.
66. Von der Maase H, Hansen SW, Roberts JT, et al. Gemcitabine and cisplatin versus methotrexate, vinblastine, doxorubicin, and cisplatin in advanced or metastatic bladder cancer: results of a large, randomized, multinational, multicenter phase III study. *J Clin Oncol.* 2000;17:3068.
72. Sternberg CN, Swanson DA. Non-transitional cell bladder cancer. In: Raghavan D, Scher HI, Leibel SA, Lange PH, eds. *Principles and Practice of Genitourinary Oncology.* Philadelphia: Lippincott-Raven; 1997:315–330.
73. Siefker-Radtke AO, Czerniak BA, Dinney CP, Millikan RE. Uncommon cancer of the bladder. In: Raghavan D, Brecher ML, Johnson DH, Meropol NJ, Moots PL, Rose PG, eds. *Textbook of Uncommon Cancer.* San Francisco, Chichester: Wiley; 2006:18–26.

94 Neoplasms of the Prostate

Christopher J. Logothetis, MD ▪ Jeri Kim, MD ▪ John Davis, MD ▪ Deborah Kuban, MD ▪ Paul Mathew, MD ▪ Ana Aparicio, MD

Introduction

Cancer of the prostate is the most commonly diagnosed non–skin neoplasm and the second leading cause of cancer-related mortality in men in the United States. Considerable advances have been made in the last decade in screening, diagnosis, and therapy options, particularly for early disease, but controversies about the diagnosis and management of prostate cancer, especially in the areas of screening and choice of therapy, continue to evolve. Although there are fewer controversies about prognosis in more advanced disease states, therapy options remain inadequate.

The clinical application of improved biopsy schemes and imaging methods and the continued widespread use of prostate-specific antigen (PSA) have resulted in increased detection of prostate cancer.

The evolving use of the serum PSA concentration and its change over time has not been paralleled by studies that test the relevance of those findings. The subsequent conflicting recommendations have resulted in confusion, exposing patients and physicians to the risks of delayed intervention or the choice of a more cautious approach, resulting in excessive adverse effects. It is hoped that replacement of the current morphologic and anatomic classification of prostate cancer with one based on its biology will address this challenge, although this has yet to be achieved. Novel approaches to elucidate prostate carcinogenesis and progression are providing realistic hope that reclassification of the disease is achievable.

Salient features that distinguish prostate cancer from other malignancies and that frame the dilemmas surrounding it are its striking age-dependent incidence, with progressively increasing frequency with increasing age; the variable lethality of morphologically identified cancers; the central role of androgen signaling; and the preponderance of bone-forming metastases on its lethal progression. The important advances made in each of these areas will, in the near future, modify the approaches currently used to prognosticate, treat, and prevent prostate cancer.

Biology of Prostate Cancer

Normal Anatomic and Histologic Features of the Prostate

The prostate gland sits in the pelvis, surrounded by the rectum posteriorly and the bladder superiorly, and it is anchored to the bladder pelvic floor; the urethra communicates between the bladder and the prostate into the penis (Fig. 94-1). The prostate is composed of stromal, ductal, and luminal epithelial cells and is organized around branching ducts and individual glands lined with secretory epithelial cells and basal cells.[1] The secretory epithelial cell is the major cell type in the gland. These androgen-regulated cells produce PSA and prostatic acid phosphatase (PAP). The central role of androgen signaling in prostate cancer biology likely accounts for the utility of PSA and PAP in determining disease status clinically. The vast majority of prostate cancers have cells that share properties with the secretory epithelial cells. Unlike the epithelial cells, the basal cell layer is not directly controlled by androgen signaling. Investigators have suggested that the basal cell population contains the prostate stem cells from which the epithelial cells develop. If correct, this view has obvious implications for the prevention and treatment of all stages of prostate cancer.

Neuroendocrine cells are also present within both the gland and the stroma, and they are thought to contribute to normal prostate function in a paracrine fashion.[2] The role of these cells has not been fully defined in terms of physiology or cancer biology. However, there is increasing appreciation that neuroendocrine pathways implicated in prostate carcinogenesis contribute to normal prostate development and function as well as to progression to the lethal phenotype.

The view that the prostate has a lobar pattern has been challenged. McNeal and colleagues[3] conducted detailed studies of the normal and pathologic anatomy of the prostate and introduced the concept of anatomic zones rather than lobes to describe the gland. There are four major zones within the normal prostate: peripheral, central, transition (constituting 70%, 20%, and 5% of the glandular tissue, respectively), and anterior fibromuscular stroma (Fig. 94-2). The peripheral zone, which extends posterolaterally around the gland from the apex to the base, is the most common site for the development of prostate carcinomas. The central zone surrounds the ejaculatory duct apparatus and makes up the majority of the prostatic base. The transition zone constitutes two small lobules that abut the prostatic urethra and is the region where benign

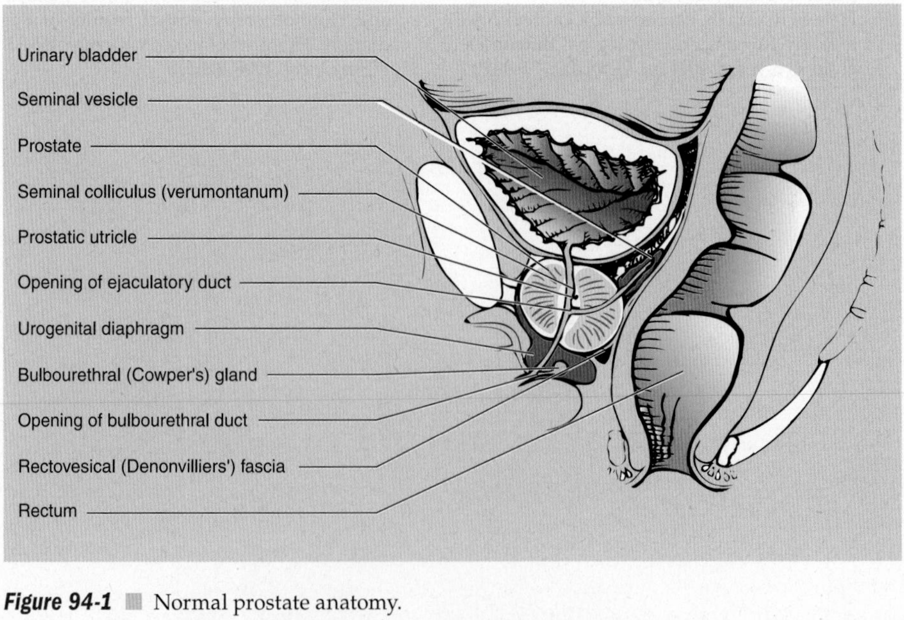

Figure 94-1 ▪ Normal prostate anatomy.

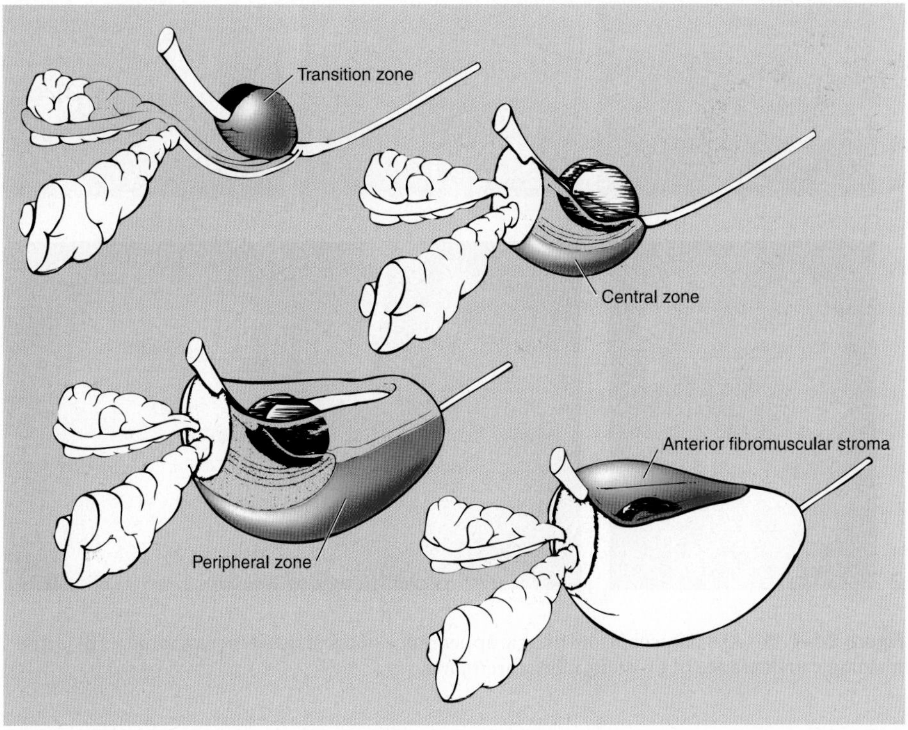

Figure 94-2 Zonal anatomy of the prostate: the three glandular zones of the prostate and the anterior fibromuscular stroma.

prostatic hypertrophy (BPH) primarily originates. Suggestions have been made that carcinomas that originate from the transition zone have lower malignant potential, but other study results have suggested that there is no difference in outcome compared with those originating in the peripheral zone, when controlled for grade and stage.[4,5]

Surrounding the gland is stroma, which includes fibroblasts, smooth muscle, nerves, and lymphatic tissue. The roles of stromal-epithelial interactions in prostate physiology and cancer development are being elucidated. Recent insights suggest that these interactions are critical in normal function, and increasing evidence implicates them in prostate carcinogenesis as well. The Stromal-epithelial interactions may exert both tumor-promoting and carrinogenesis- and progression- inbibitory effects. Furthermore, the stromal-epitthelial–interacting pathways implicated in the development of the tumor microenvironment in prostate cancer progression may be those that are shared by the prostate and bone in their normal development and function.[6]

A common misconception is that there is a distinct anatomic barrier surrounding the prostate—the prostate capsule; however, a true anatomic capsule does not exist. Instead, the smooth muscle of the prostatic stroma gradually extends into fibrous tissue that then ends in loose connective and adipose tissue. Of particular relevance is the absence of any semblance of a capsule at the gland's apex and anteriorly. This understanding of anatomic detail allows clinicians to determine the adequacy of prostate surgery by accurately defining the surgical margin with increasing confidence. It also allows the surgical delineation of disease as "organ confined" or "specimen confined." Organ confined implies that the cancer has not extended beyond the confines of the prostate, whereas specimen confined implies that the excision is adequate and no tumor extends beyond the cut margins. The distinction between these two terms is clinically relevant and important because they are used to determine the adequacy of surgery and the use of postoperative radiation therapy in selected patients.

A final anatomic note about the prostate is that Walsh and Donker[7] described the presence of two neurovascular bundles that pass adjacent to the gland posterolaterally. Acknowledgment of the role that these neurovascular bundles play in normal erectile function and defining their presence outside of the Denonvilliers fascia allowed Walsh to develop a "nerve-sparing" radical retropubic prostatectomy procedure that improves the odds of preserving potency.[8]

The last decade has seen the application of molecular profiles to the anatomy of the prostate. Further investigation into the molecular and cellular characterization of prostate cancer, integrated with anatomic and morphologic features of the gland, promises to refine prognostication, which may be used to guide selection of therapy and predict the effectiveness of specific local therapies—radiation, surgery, or both.

Premalignant Prostatic Lesions

Paradigms that are used to explain the progression of other solid tumors may not apply to prostate cancer.[9] Extensive information about the genetic and epigenetic phenomena associated with prostate cancer progression has been developed recently but has yet to pass the threshold of clinical utility to be truly useful. Most clinicians accept that premalignant lesions existing in the prostate may precede the development of cancer by many years. But given the lack of knowledge about the nature or rate of their progression, the morphologic identification of premalignant lesions on biopsy specimens achieves little more than providing the rationale for close monitoring of patients.

Morphologically heterogeneous lesions are included under the single term prostatic intraepithelial neoplasia (PIN) (Fig. 94-3).[10] PIN is defined as the presence of cytologically atypical or dysplastic epithelial cells within architecturally benign–appearing glands and acini. Three different grades have been described: 1 (mild), 2 (moderate), and 3 (severe). Grades 2 and 3 PIN are often combined as "high grade." PIN is presumed to be a premalignant lesion because it is commonly present adjacent to prostate adenocarcinomas.[11] The finding of PIN implies the existence of cancer in sites not sampled on biopsy or an increased risk of

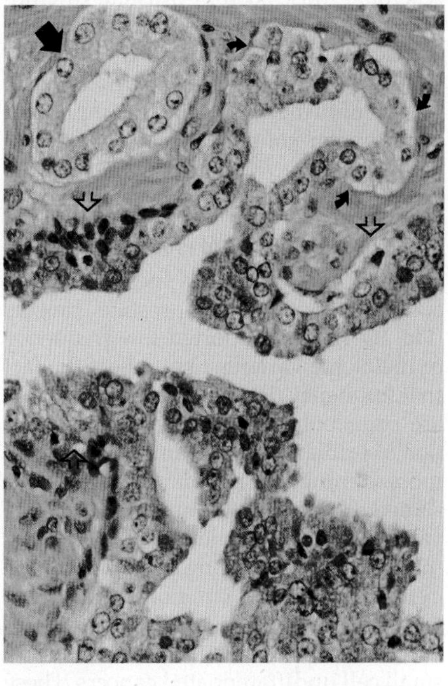

Figure 94-3 Photomicrograph of high-grade prostatic intraepithelial neoplasm (PIN) with basal cell layer (*open arrows*) with budding microacinus lacking basal cells (*curved solid arrows*). A microacinus of invasive Gleason pattern 3 adenocarcinoma is seen in the adjacent stroma (*straight solid arrow*). Hematoxylin and eosin ×160. (Courtesy of Thomas M. Wheeler, MD.)

developing a morphologic cancer at some later point. As noted above, the degree of risk and time to progression have not been determined with confidence.

Prospective studies have been small but have reinforced the hypothesis that PIN is the morphologic manifestation of a precursor lesion to morphologic prostate cancer. The data have suggested that the presence of high-grade PIN predicts the subsequent development of cancer, perhaps through a multistep carcinogenesis process. However, close clinical follow-up remains the standard of care after diagnosis of high-grade PIN alone.

Another lesion that may represent a premalignant change is atypical adenomatous hyperplasia (AAH), although existing data on this are scantier than they are for PIN. The characteristic appearance with AAH is the fulfillment of the architectural criteria for malignancy, with disruption of the basal cell layer, mainly in the transition zone, but without the cytologic changes diagnostic of cancer.[12] Some authors have suggested that a prostatic lesion composed of focal areas of epithelial atrophy associated with chronic inflammation (called proliferative inflammatory atrophy, or PIA) is a precursor of PIN and eventually prostate cancer.[13] Evidence for this hypothesis includes the observation that PIA often occurs adjacent to areas of PIN and prostate cancer[14] and that somatic genetic abnormalities seen in PIA often resemble those seen in prostate carcinoma.[15] Of particular relevance is that PIA implicates inflammation in the progression of prostate cancer.[16] If this hypothesis is confirmed and causally implicated with greater confidence in prostate cancer progression, that finding may lead to more effective prevention strategies.

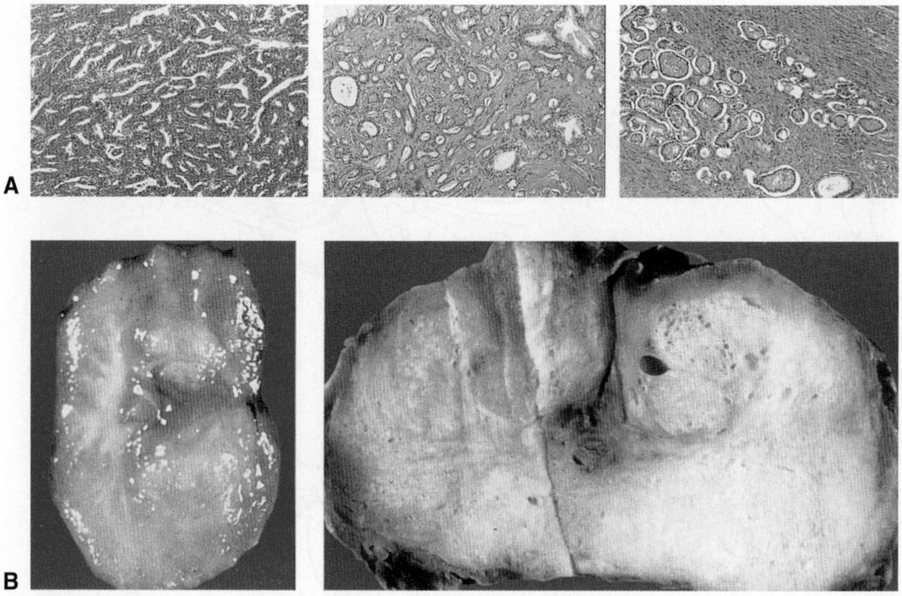

Figure 94-4 (A) Microscopic histologic appearance of prostate adenocarcinoma. (B) Gross histologic appearance of prostate adenocarcinoma.

Histologic Features of Prostate Cancer

Cancers that arise in the epithelium account for >95% of prostate cancers (Fig. 94-4).[17] The reported low frequency of histologic variants may reflect the fact that frequency determinations of variants are principally derived by the examination of primary cancers, among which the more common forms may be overrepresented. However, less common histologic varieties have been described, including mucinous or signet ring tumors; adenoid cystic carcinomas; carcinoid; large prostatic duct carcinomas (including the endometrial type); adenocarcinomas; and small cell undifferentiated cancers. These unusual subtypes are reported to occur in low frequencies. Because the histologic variants often present with advanced disease clinically, they are not subjected to surgery as often as the more common forms of prostate cancer. In addition, they occasionally manifest only in metastases during progression, thus in sites not often sampled. As a consequence, we may be underestimating their frequency because of their manifestation. This fact may be particularly important when attempting to estimate the true frequency of small cell carcinomas of the prostate, which have been reported with increasing frequency.[18] Nonetheless, it is important to recognize these unusual variants of prostate cancer because although standard hormonal therapies may be less effective in their treatment, they may be more responsive to chemotherapy than the more common type.[15,19]

Tumors with a neuroendocrine appearance (ie, carcinoid and small cell undifferentiated types) may arise from Kulchitsky cells, which are found in the basal regions of the prostatic epithelium.[2] Small cell carcinomas of the prostate share histologic and clinical features with other extrapulmonary small cell carcinomas. These cancers have been described as a histologic continuum, perhaps in some instances reflecting progression of acinar adenocarcinomas.[20] Thus, these "neuroendocrine" cancers of the prostate are likely to be a mechanistically and clinically heterogeneous grouping. Of importance is that they predict a specific pattern of anatomic progression: nonosseous visceral spread with lytic bone metastases and the probability of responsiveness to chemotherapy.

Transitional cell carcinomas involving the substance of the prostate may also be mistaken for prostate adenocarcinoma. It may be difficult to distinguish a transitional cell carcinoma arising in the transitional epithelium of the distal static products from a tumor arising in the bladder epithelium and spreading into the contiguous prostatic ducts.

Study findings have confirmed the primary prognostic importance of the degree of histologic differentiation of prostate adenocarcinoma. The degree of this differentiation is typically determined by patterns of gland formation and, less importantly, by cytologic detail. The most widely accepted grading scheme for adenocarcinoma of the prostate is that developed by Gleason (Fig. 94-5).[21] Gleason created a system for classifying prostate tumors based on two levels of scoring that recognize the heterogeneous nature of prostate carcinomas. The primary pattern of differentiation is assigned a

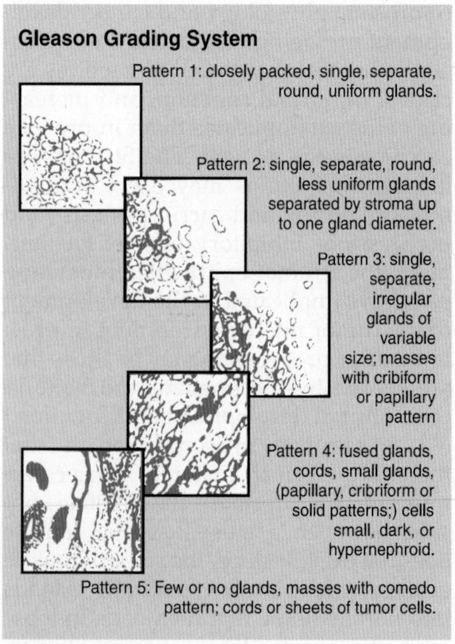

Gleason Grading System
Pattern 1: closely packed, single, separate, round, uniform glands.
Pattern 2: single, separate, round, less uniform glands separated by stroma up to one gland diameter.
Pattern 3: single, separate, irregular glands of variable size; masses with cribiform or papillary pattern
Pattern 4: fused glands, cords, small glands, (papillary, cribriform or solid patterns;) cells small, dark, or hypernephroid.
Pattern 5: Few or no glands, masses with comedo pattern; cords or sheets of tumor cells.

Figure 94-5 Histologic grading scheme for adenocarcinomas of the prostate. *Source*: Adapted from Ref. 69.

Gleason grade of 1 to 5 according to the dominant morphologic features of the specimen and its departure from normal appearance; the next most common pattern is also assigned a grade. This results in a two-digit score; for example, 3 + 4 = 7. The Gleason system has been criticized for inadequately recognizing the proportion of the tumor that is composed of the secondary pattern as well as for lacking adequate distinction between good and poor prognoses in patients whose cancers have Gleason scores of 5 to 7 (most patients). However, the reproducibility and reliability of Gleason grading between pathologists have consistently been shown to be excellent. Gleason's original work demonstrated a clear association between a higher score and a higher mortality rate, which others have since confirmed.[22] Many other predictors of the clinical behavior of prostate cancer have been explored, but the Gleason score still remains the most broadly applicable and prognostically useful histologic grading system.

Molecular Pathogenesis

Unlike the case of breast cancers, in which clinically relevant subsets of cancer have been identified on the basis of molecular profiles, the morphologic characterization of prostate cancer remains the standard.[23] Prostate cancer cells harbor a large number of somatic mutations, and in advanced disease, additional alterations accumulate. Alterations that affect the development and progression of prostate cancer include those in the hormonal and growth factor milieu, in hormonal and growth factor receptors, in intracellular signaling pathways, and in cell cycle regulation and apoptosis. The recent identification of chromosome 8q24 as a susceptibility locus supports the hypothesis that a significant portion of prostate cancers have genetic origins.

The hormonal and growth factor milieu to which the prostate is exposed has been consistently associated with the pathogenesis of cancer. In population-based studies, two hormones have been implicated: testosterone and insulin-like growth factor I (IGF-I). The association between testosterone and prostate cancer progression is well known. Several lines of evidence also suggest that IGF may be important in prostate cancer growth. First, several prostate cancer cell lines and prostate xenograft models express both IGFs I and II and their receptors.[24,25] Second, Chan and colleagues[26] reported on the relationship between plasma IGF-I concentration and prostate cancer, citing a relative risk of 4.3 for men in the highest quartile, compared with men in the lowest quartile. Moreover, a higher incidence of prostate cancer has been noted in patients who had relatively high IGF-I concentrations in plasma samples that had been obtained 5 years prior to the cancer diagnosis,[27] supporting the concept that IGF-I may be important early in the development of prostate cancer. Although this observation has yet to be confirmed, it does implicate IGF-I signaling in prostate cancer progression. It is likely that growth-factor and other stromal-epithelial interacting pathways cooperate in prostate cancer progression. Thus, a simple model centered on a single pathway is unlikely to lead to the understanding of human prostate cancer. Other growth factors—including epidermal growth factor, vascular endothelial growth factor (VEGF), platelet-derived growth factor (PDGF), and transforming growth factor beta (TGF-β)—may also be dysregulated in the development of prostate cancer (Table 94-1).[28]

The central role of androgen signaling in an endocrine fashion has dominated the understanding of the pathway in prostate cancer. It is clear that androgens are a major mediator of progression, though their role in prostate cancer susceptibility remains poorly understood. In fact, several hormonal receptors are altered in prostate cancer cells. Perhaps the best example is alterations in the androgen receptor (AR). In early cancer, AR mutations are relatively uncommon,[29] but germline variation (CAG repeats) in the *AR* gene has been shown to be a predictor of cancer aggressiveness[30] and may play a role in the frequency and aggressiveness of prostate cancer in African Americans.[31] It is interesting that AR mutations are more commonly seen in androgen-independent (castrate-resistant) prostate cancer,[29,32] arguing that the AR gene remains central in the growth and survival of prostate cancer even after the need for the ligand (androgens) has been mitigated. Several theoretical frameworks have been proposed for the development of androgen independence, most of which still postulate a cancer cell that depends on a functional *AR* but one that is amplified, oversensitive, promiscuous, or activated by up-regulated coactivators or down-regulated by corepressors.[33] For example, in LNCaP prostate cancer cells, an *AR* mutation, T877A, which is a substitution of alanine for threonine at position 877, results in an AR that is activated by other steroid hormones and by the androgen antagonist flutamide.[34] This *AR* mutation could help explain the "anti-androgen withdrawal syndrome." However, *AR* mutations occur too infrequently to account for the eventual evolution of most metastatic prostate cancers to a castrate-resistant state.

Table 94-1 Growth Factors Implicated in Prostate Cancer

Transforming growth factor beta
Fibroblast growth factor
Epidermal growth factor
Insulin-like growth factor
Platelet-derived growth factor
Vascular endothelial growth factor
Neurotensin
Endothelins
Colony-stimulating factors

Recent observations support the view that "intracrine" production of androgens acting in both autocrine and paracrine fashion are implicated in the progression of prostate cancer. Several lines of evidence support the concept that CYP17 lyase is implicated in remodeling the prostate cancer tumor microenvironment: androgens in the microenvironment are at a higher concentration than they are in the serum, CYP17 expression occurs in stage-dependent cancer progression, and tumor regression occurs clinically in castrate-resistant cancers. These data support the hypothesis that androgen signaling can be considered a stromal-epithelial interacting pathway. Difficulty in measuring the concentration of androgens in the local microenvironment continue to plague this concept and, although it is appealing, it remains unproven.

True androgen independence is likely to arise from alternative stromal-epithelial interacting or other signaling pathways. Several bone- and prostate-development pathways have been noted to be involved in prostate cancer progression and to be associated with higher grade cancers.[35] This attractive hypothesis could account for the bone-homing and bone-forming phenotype of prostate cancer and for its resistance to therapy in an organ-specific manner.

Molecules that alter intracellular signaling pathways also may be important in the pathogenesis and progression of prostate cancer to a castrate-resistant state. The clearest example to date is the tumor suppressor gene *PTEN*. This gene encodes for a phosphatase that is important in modulating the signal generated by activated growth factor receptors. Somatic mutations in *PTEN* occur at high frequency in prostate carcinoma cells, suggesting this as a frequent target for inactivation. One study documented a 60% rate of *PTEN* mutations; most of these were found in cell lines from metastatic disease, although mutations were also seen in primary cancers.[36] In fact, another group demonstrated higher rates of *PTEN* loss or mutation in tumors of advanced stage and grade.[37] Another pathway that may be inappropriately activated in prostate cancer is the hedgehog pathway. Normal hedgehog signaling is important in early development and patterning of the prostate epithelium. Recent work by Karhadkar and colleagues[38] demonstrated that activation of the hedgehog pathway distinguishes prostate cancer from normal prostate cells and, further, metastatic prostate cancer from localized cancer. Moreover, they demonstrated that hedgehog pathway inhibition results in PC3 xenograft regression. Both the PTEN and hedgehog pathways are therefore attractive targets for drug development.

Finally, alterations in molecules that regulate the cell cycle and apoptosis offer promising avenues for further investigation. TP53, p27, p21, and Rb have been studied, and the results have provided variable levels of evidence that they participate in the pathogenesis of prostate cancer.[39] Of particular relevance is that each of these molecules has been reported by some investigators to serve as prognosticators. The utility of these molecules as independent prognosticators or as part of a signature has yet to be prospectively validated. Signatures that predict disease recurrence after surgery have yet to find a role in the clinic.[40]

Early Detection of Prostate Cancer

Early detection of prostate cancer, when it remains confined to the prostate, brings patients and their physicians face to face with the controversial question of how localized disease may best be managed, that is, how patients can avoid overtreatment and preserve quality of life while simultaneously escaping from life-threatening disease.

Prostate cancer screening and early detection themselves are controversial because for every 18 cases detected, only 3 will result in death. The cost of radical prostatectomy, which removes the threat of disease if there is no metastasis, may be the imposition of impotence and urinary incontinence, which severely affect quality of life. To determine whether screening for prostate cancer and three other cancers reduces mortality, the National Cancer Institute's Division of Cancer Prevention undertook the randomized, controlled Prostate, Lung, Colorectal, and Ovarian Cancer Screening Trial (PLCO) at 10 sites in 1993. It is still under way. Participants undergo annual screening examinations for 13 years and follow-up for 8 years. The PLCO trial, consisting of 38,000 men 55-74 years old at their enrollment in the screening arm, tests them annually with a blood test for PSA level and a digital rectal examination (DRE) to detect palpable prostatic abnormalities. Investigators have reported that adherence to screening regimens is adversely affected by having false-positive results on previous prostate screens and other tests, by being African American, or by having less than a high school education.[41]

Also launched in the 1990s was the European Randomized Study on Screening for Prostate Cancer (ERSPC), which is also testing whether screening saves lives. Its findings are expected to be issued between 2009 and 2010.[42,43] In the United States, the American Cancer Society recommends annual prostate cancer screening (PSA blood test and DRE) for all men ages 50 and older who have a 10-year life expectancy,[44] but the U.S. Preventive Services Task Force and experts elsewhere, including the World Health Organization and the Council of the European Union, are waiting for the results of the PLCO and ERSPC studies to prove that prostate cancer screening reduces mortality before recommending it as general public health policy.[43,45,46]

Identifying Early Disease Using PSA and PSAV

Strategies to manage the diagnosis of localized prostate cancer include watchful waiting, radical prostatectomy, and radiotherapy. The PSA velocity (PSAV), one measure used in monitoring patients with localized disease, has been scrutinized as a tool for use in the diagnosis and prediction of outcomes. It is calculated using the log slope of at least three PSA values calculated over at least 2 years with no less than 6 months between measures.[47] Conceived as a way to capture the variability of prostate cancer or its progression, PSAV measures are used preoperatively and postoperatively. Researchers sometimes rely on measures taken closer together, consider fewer than three measures, and reduce the longitudinal period to less than 2 years. PSAV measures may have a role in watchful-waiting protocols in identifying patients whose cases require repeated biopsies.[47]

Prostate cancer screening can be oversimplified into an algorithm in which all patients with a certain threshold of PSA (eg, 2.5 or 4.0 ng/mL) or abnormal DRE findings are referred to a urologist for evaluation and possible biopsy. However, patients' overall interests are better served if a more comprehensive evaluation takes place that considers whether they are at increased risk of having prostate cancer because of ethnicity (eg, African Americans are at increased risk), age, and/or family history and whether a prostate cancer diagnosis would be likely to affect their overall survival because of a younger age and fewer competing comorbid conditions. A comprehensive PSA history may be beneficial for calculating PSAV, and the complexed PSA test may be useful as a front-line screening tool because it has slightly better specificity than total PSA in the total PSA range of 2.5-4.0 ng/mL.[48]

The PSA blood test has been described as a test that "neither excludes benign disease nor wholly predicts meaningful malignancies."[47] Ian Thompson, principal investigator of the Prostate Cancer Prevention Trial (PCPT), and his colleagues studied 8575 men from the study's placebo group to estimate the receiver operating characteristic (ROC) curve for PSA and concluded that no absolute cutoff value had the high degree of sensitivity and specificity simultaneously required for identification of a risk-free value.[49] Instead, they endorsed viewing all PSA values as a continuum of risk for prostate cancer.[49]

Single measures of PSA performed on blood samples taken decades before a patient's diagnosis have been statistically associated with levels of risk and have garnered great attention because of their apparent simplicity and efficiency and their ability to stratify patients for screening, but their reliability awaits verification.[50,51] These studies relied on blood samples drawn from 21,277 men in Sweden from 1974 to 1986 and on Sweden's cancer registry. From among these samples, prostate cancer diagnoses and blood samples were ascertained for 462, who were matched to controls. The median PSA level was about 0.6 ng/mL in the low-risk group. These investigators' most recent work bases prediction of cancer risk on a single PSA test before age 40.[51]

More widely investigated have been measures of PSAV, a calculation of rising PSA level that was introduced in the early 1990s as a marker of prostate cancer development, a means to reduce unnecessary biopsies, and a way to improve the specificity of PSA testing. However, current standards that shorten the minimum longitudinal monitoring period for calculating PSAV and push ever lower the levels of PSAV considered worrisome (now 3.5 ng/mL/year in men with a PSA <4 ng/mL in one algorithm) actually increase the likelihood of biopsy.[52-55] Cautious investigators[54] argue that to use PSAV to monitor men with a PSA <4 ng/mL, it is necessary to have evidence that such measures ensure that enough cases will be detected within the "window of curability" to make them worthwhile and that the financial and emotional costs of overdiagnosis will not undermine other advances. They also point out that relying on findings about PSAV in undiagnosed cases, which have been largely lacking, would be very different from relying on posttreatment PSAV findings and applying them to the detection setting. They and others have said that prospective studies are needed.[54,56]

An early study on the PSAV was one of men enrolled in a geriatrics trial. Carter et al.[52] concluded that in men with PSA values <4 ng/mL, a PSAV <0.75 µg/mL/year indicated absence of prostate cancer, and a PSAV ≥0.75 μg/mL/year indicated its presence. In work published 15 years later, Krejcarek et al.[57] reported that in the undiagnosed patients they studied who had PSAV values <1.0 ng/mL/year, only 6% of those younger than 70 years with cT1c disease had high-grade cancer; however, they found that a median PSAV value of 2.71 ng/mL/year, age, and clinical T stage were significantly related to high-risk disease (Gleason score 4+3). Because these subjects had undergone radiotherapy, the findings are not generalizable to patients treated with other therapeutic modalities. The study by Krejcarek et al. was a retrospective evaluation in 358 men to identify those at higher risk so they could improve outcomes by adding androgen-suppression therapy to radiotherapy and by improving the selection of radiotherapy fields.

A prospective trial conducted at the Royal Marsden Hospital and reported in 2008 studied 237 patients enrolled in an active surveillance trial who had a median PSA level of 6.5 ng/mL at the outset and a median pretreatment PSAV of 0.44 ng/mL/year.[58] The investigators determined that PSA density was a statistically significant independent determinant of PSAV in untreated patients: Those with a PSA density measure >0.185 ng/mL had a median PSAV of 0.92 ng/mL/year, and those with a PSA density measure <0.185 ng/mL had a median PSAV of 0.35 ng/mL/year. Because PSA density is a measure available at the outset of diagnosis and does not require longitudinal data collection, it will be a more efficient marker than PSAV is if others confirm this finding.

Staging of Prostate Cancer

Staging of cancer, which is integral to the treatment decisions that follow, comprises initial clinical staging based on findings from physical examination of the patient and diagnostic tests, and pathologic staging based on findings at surgery and on subsequent pathologic study of the removed prostate gland and other tissue. Less definitive than pathologic staging, clinical staging relies on palpation of the prostate, imaging studies, which for patients at low and intermediate risk are sometimes omitted, and needle biopsy results. Physicians can combine the clinical staging with two other significant prognostic factors, the Gleason score and the preoperative PSA value, to classify the case according to the D'Amico system, as low, intermediate, or high risk.[59] This system was first described in 1998 in the report of a retrospective study in which D'Amico et al. evaluated 1872 men with prostate cancer who had been treated with radical prostatectomy, external-beam radiotherapy, or radioactive implant with or without neoadjuvant androgen-deprivation therapy. In that study, clinical staging was based on DRE findings alone (American Joint Committee on Cancer tumor stage[60]). The researchers found that with that system, men who had been classified as being at low or intermediate risk had outcomes that were not statistically significantly different from others within their class. Most of this reliability is probably attributable to the Gleason score and the PSA level.

In the staging of prostate cancer, physicians rely on the TNM (tumor, node, metastasis) system of the American Joint Committee on Cancer to classify cases[60] (Table 94-2). It reports the extent of the tumor (T), the presence or absence of disease in the regional lymph nodes (N), and the extent of metastasis (M). In a second step of the staging process, the Gleason score is combined with the TNM classification, and cases are identified as stage I, II, III, or

Table 94-2 **TNM Clinical and Pathologic Staging of Prostate Cancer**

Clinical Stage		Pathologic Stage	
Primary Tumor			
TX	Primary tumor cannot be assessed		
T0	No evidence of primary tumor		
T1	Clinically inapparent tumor neither palpable nor visible by imaging		
T1a	Tumor incidental histologic finding in 5% or less of tissue resected		
T1b	Tumor incidental histologic finding in more than 5% of tissue resected		
T1c	Tumor identified by needle biopsy (e.g., because of elevated PSA)		
T2	Tumor confined within prostate[a]	pT2[b]	Organ confined
T2a	Tumor involves one half of one lobe or less	pT2a	Unilateral, involving one half of one lobe or less
T2b	Tumor involves more than one half of one lobe but not both lobes	pT2b	Unilateral, involving more than one half of one lobe but not both lobes
T2c	Tumor involves both lobes	pT2c	Bilateral disease
T3	Tumor extends through the prostate capsule[c]	pT3	Extraprostatic extension
T3a	Extracapsular extension (unilateral or bilateral	pT3a	Extraprostatic extension[d]
T3b	Tumor invades seminal vesicle(s)	pT3b	Seminal vesicle invasion
T4	Tumor is fixed or invades adjacent structures other than seminal vesicles: bladder neck, external sphincter, rectum, levator muscles, and/or pelvic wall	pT4	Invasion of bladder, rectum
Regional Lymph Nodes			
NX	Regional lymph nodes were not assessed	pNX	Regional nodes not sampled
N0	No regional lymph node metastasis	pN0	No positive regional nodes
N1	Metastasis in regional lymph node(s)	pN1	Metastasis in regional nodes
Distant Metastasis[e]			
MX	Distant metastasis cannot be assessed (not evaluated by any modality)		
M0	No distant metastasis		
M1	Distant metastasis		
M1a	Nonregional lymph nodes		
M1b	Bone(s)		
M1c	Other site(s) with or without bone disease		

[a] Tumor found in one or both lobes by needle biopsy, but not palpable or reliably visible by imaging, is classified as T1c.
[b] There is no pathologic T1 classification.
[c] Invasion into the prostatic apex or into (but not beyond) the prostatic capsule is classified not as T3 but as T2.
[d] Positive surgical margin should be indicated by an R1 descriptor (residual microscopic disease).
[e] When more than one site of metastasis is present, the most advanced category (pM1c) is used.
Source: Adapted from the AJCC Cancer Staging Manual (2002).

Table 94-3 ■ Prostate Cancer Stages

Stage	TNM Classification and Gleason Score
I	T1a, N0, M0, Gleason score 1
II	T1a, N0, M0, Gleason score 2, 3–4
	T1, T1b–T2, N0, M0, any Gleason score
III	T3, N0, M0, any Gleason score
IV	T4, N0, M0, any Gleason score
	Any T, N1, M0, any Gleason score
	Any T, any N, M1, any Gleason score

Source: Data from American Joint Committee on Cancer (2002).

IV, progressively representing advances in the extent of disease[60] (Table 94-3).

Prostate cancer is the most commonly diagnosed cancer in U.S. men, with the exception of skin cancers and in situ cancers.[61] About 3/4 of U.S. men report having been screened at least once, and early prostate cancer, because it has no symptoms, is often diagnosed in outpatient settings. Distinguishing between high- and low-risk localized prostate cancer, maximizing disease control and survival, and avoiding overtreatment, especially in men likely to die of comorbidities, are challenges physicians who treat these men face daily.[62]

The American Urological Association has characterized localized disease into three risk categories[63] (Table 94-4). Low-risk disease is generally characterized by a PSA value ≤ 10 ng/mL, a Gleason score ≤ 6, a lack of symptoms, and absence of both disease in the lymph nodes and metastases (ie, clinical stage T1c or T2). Disease is nonpalpable on DRE, but evidence of tumor may be detected by a transurethral resection of the prostate (TURP) performed because of what was thought to be benign prostatic hypertrophy (BPH) or by needle biopsy prompted by a high PSA level. PSA values >10 ng/mL but ≤20 ng/mL and/or a Gleason score of 7 (3+4 or 4+3) are associated with intermediate risk. PSA values >20 ng/mL and/or Gleason scores of 8-10 indicate high-risk cases.

Validated pretreatment nomograms that combine PSA, Gleason score, and clinical stage have been developed to give estimates of pathologic stage, which may be valuable to clinicians planning treatment.[64-67] In a 2007 update of the Partin tables, Markarov et al.[67] analyzed 5730 men who had undergone prostatectomy between 2000 and 2005 at Johns Hopkins Hospital and confirmed that, as these researchers had previously shown, clinical stage contributes significantly to the prediction, as do PSA level and Gleason score, and that cumulatively they are better predictors than any one alone. No patient's disease was clinically staged higher than T2c, and at prostatectomy, almost 75% had disease confined to the prostate. None of the 123 of 164 patients with a clinical Gleason score ≥ 8 who had a workup was found to have metastatic disease. In their series, as in others, the proportion of men presenting with organ-confined disease has been increasing: 54% in 1993,[64] 48% in 1997,[65] 64% in 2001,[66] and 73% in 2007 (year of publication).[67] New in this series was the absence of Gleason scores of 2 to 4, reflecting pathologists' belief that such scores represent sampling error.[68] Among patients with higher clinical stage, the authors reported a trend toward more accurate staging in their 2007 report over that in 2001 and perhaps indicating a broader need for surgery in those patients with higher clinical stage and Gleason scores.

Kattan[69] pointed out that Makarov et al.[67] did not report whether the data improved on the predictive accuracy of the former versions and that they did not incorporate in the statistical model such predictors as year the surgery was performed; Kattan suggested improving the tables by including metastatic workup or high-grade cancer as predictors.[69] The developers of the nomogram(s) themselves have questioned how changes in diagnostic workup or neoadjuvant therapy might affect the usefulness of the nomogram(s).[66] A more general problem with using the Partin tables is determining how applicable they are to general practice, inasmuch as they are based on care in an academic setting.[70]

Following up on previous work to improve the accuracy of identifying cases of low-volume low-grade disease,[71,72] researchers at The University of Texas M. D. Anderson Cancer Center have refined a nomogram specifically for identifying men for active surveillance.[73] This nomogram includes age, PSA density, and tumor length in a biopsy core. The low number of factors, the ease in ascertaining their values with only laboratory tests and extended biopsy, and their nonsubjective nature combined with an area under the curve (AUC) measure indicating good discriminatory power (ie, 0.727) make this nomogram attractive. The authors admitted that they cannot explain why their analysis indicates that older age would reduce the probability of low-volume, low-grade cancer and that younger men, with values appropriately low in the other categories, would be good candidates for surveillance. Nonetheless, their work offers for validation a new, practical tool for identifying these low-risk men.

Including a molecular marker as a predictor is another way investigators have attempted to improve a nomogram's accuracy. PCA3, a prostate-specific noncoding mRNA, is readily detected in urine when prostate cancer is present because it is overexpressed 60- to 100-fold 90% of the time.[74] Deras et al. undertook a prospective, multisite study of 570 men immediately before they underwent prostate biopsy and found PCA3 to be reliably sensitive and specific across PSA values <4 and >10 ng/mL and across various values of prostate volume and number of prior biopsies. Overall, PCA3 sensitivity was 54% (95% CI, 0.49-0.59) and specificity was 74% (95% CI, 0.71-0.77).[74]

Another marker with higher sensitivity and specificity values is now being intensively studied. EPCA-2, which had 92% specificity (95% CI, 0.85-0.96) in healthy men with BPH and 94% sensitivity (95% CI, 0.93-0.99) in men with prostate cancer, was reported in 2007.[75] Investigators tested serum samples from 330 individuals. PSA had a corresponding specificity of 65% (95% CI, 0.55-0.75). Relying on a cutoff point of 30 ng/mL, investigators reported that EPCA-2 detected 39 of 40 men with non–organ-confined disease and 36 of 40 men with organ-confined disease. Tests were also negative in men who were healthy (PSA < 2.5 ng/mL) but positive in men with prostate cancer whose PSA levels were <2.5 ng/mL.

Table 94-4 ■ Risk Stratification for Localized Prostate Cancer

Risk Level	PSA Level		Gleason Score		Clinical Stage
Low	≤10 ng/mL	*and*	≤6	*and*	T1c or T2a
Intermediate	>10-20 ng/mL	*or*	7	*or*	T2b *but not qualifying for high risk*
High	>20 ng/mL	*or*	8-10	*or*	T2c

Source: Adapted from the American Urological Association.

Therapy Options and Applications

Active Surveillance ■ In the pre-PSA era, "watchful waiting" implied an alternative to active treatment and described a period when patients were monitored but not treated until the disease progressed and/or symptoms developed. With the advent of PSA testing, a paradigm shift occurred, in which we now diagnose considerably more early prostate cancers, including those destined to remain clinically insignificant. New strategies are needed for managing select cases of low-risk prostate cancer without imposing immediate therapy. Such an approach has been called different terms, including "watchful observation with selective delayed intervention"[76] and "active surveillance."[77] This new strategy is to forego immediate treatment but closely follow patients with low-risk prostate cancer, pursuing early detection of tumor progression when the disease is still curable, and initiating definitive therapy appropriately. For this strategy to fulfill its promise, two clinical tools are mandatory: a method of identifying a priori patients harboring small low-grade, indolent tumors and a surveillance strategy that reliably detects tumor progression when the disease is still curable. Data supporting conservative management of cases with clinically localized prostate cancer can be gleaned from population-based studies[78,79] and a meta-analysis.[80] These pre–PSA era studies had a preponderance of older patients and patients with clinically evident cancers; therefore, their results cannot be directly extrapolated to the PSA-screened population. Other problems included the way patients had been diagnosed—many had not undergone a full workup for metastasis and, for many, diagnosis was based on fine-needle biopsy results[79]—and the fact that the researchers did not centralize pathology review.[78] Despite their limitations, these observational studies showed that men with low-grade prostate cancer have a protracted course of indolent disease and a very small risk of disease-specific death, even after 20 years of follow-up.[81]

In contrast, the risk of death from disease progression is higher for men with Gleason scores of 7-10. Watchful waiting and prostatectomy were compared prospectively in an important study by Swedish investigators who followed up their initial report with further analyses 3 years later.[82,83] The researchers studied 695 men with T0d, T1b, T1c, or T2 disease who were randomly assigned to undergo radical prostatectomy (n = 347) or watchful waiting (n = 348). Two-thirds had palpable tumors, but fewer than half in each group—43.8% of those undergoing prostatectomy and 39.7% of those assigned to watchful waiting—had symptoms. Statistically significant differences were found at a 10-year end point between those who underwent prostatectomy and those who who were not treated until local progression occurred (19.2% vs 44.3%; $P < .001$), distant metastasis developed (15.2% vs 25.4%; $P = .004$), and disease-specific mortality occurred (9.5% vs 14.9%; $P = .01$). These researchers urged physicians and patients to consider in treatment decisions the adverse effect on quality of life that prostatectomy and hormone treatment imposes. Whether these findings would be replicable in a U.S. study population is unknown because prostate cancer is typically diagnosed earlier here than it is in Sweden.[84] Inasmuch as the Prostate Cancer Intervention versus Observation Trial (PIVOT) pursues the same question with U.S. men, researchers are looking to that trial for resolution.[84] Two prospective cohort studies have examined the feasibility of active surveillance, or expectant management. Carter et al.[85] studied 81 men believed to have T1c low-volume prostate cancer for a median of 23 months (range 12-58 months). Their median age was 65 years (range 52-73 years). At baseline, all men had a PSA density ≤ 0.15 ng/mL/cm^3 and a Gleason score of <7. Free PSA in the men was a median of 17% (range 4.3-37%). Every 6 months, subjects underwent PSA measurement (both free and total) and DRE. Every 12 months, patients underwent transrectal ultrasound–directed biopsy, including evaluation of at least 12 cores. After at least 1 year in the study, 56 (69%) of the men were free of progression and still on surveillance. The other 25 men (31%) met the criteria of progression, which were adverse findings on prostate needle biopsy, including a Gleason score ≥ 7, any Gleason pattern of 4 or 5, more than two cores with cancer involvement, or 50% cancer involvement in any core. Their median time to disease progression was 14 months (range 12-52 months). The researchers found that in men who experienced progression by their definition, the PSA density was statistically significantly higher and the free PSA value statistically significantly lower than those values in men who did not experience progression.

In a larger phase II study, Klotz[86] reported findings on 299 men who at baseline had prostate cancer of grade T2b or lower, a PSA of <15 ng/mL, and a Gleason score ≤ 7. All subjects were older than 70 years. Surveillance included PSA measures, serial bone scans, and transrectal sonography (every 6 months for first 2 years and then annually thereafter), and biopsy within 1.5 or 2 years of entering the trial. Criteria for progression were that patients demonstrate PSA, clinical, and histologic disease progression. PSA progression was defined as having a PSA doubling time of <2 years (measured at least three times during a minimum of 6 months), a final PSA of >8 ng/mL, and a regression analysis of ln (PSA) on time $P < .05$. Clinical progression was defined as one of the following: doubling of the product of the maximum perpendicular diameters of the primary lesion (measured digitally); TURP necessitated by local progression; ureteral obstruction; or clinical or radiologic evidence of distant metastasis. Histologic progression was defined as a Gleason score ≥ 8 at subsequent biopsy. At 55 months, 60% remained on surveillance; at 96 months, disease-specific survival was 99% and overall survival was 85%. Thirty-five percent had a PSA doubling time of >10 years (median doubling time 7.0 years). Reasons for abandoning surveillance included patient preference (16%), rapid biochemical progression (12%), clinical progression (8%), and histologic progression (4%).

These two studies demonstrated the feasibility of active surveillance, given proper patient selection and careful follow-up, and the possibility of individualizing therapy.

Multisite clinical trials are seeking answers to satisfy the growing interest in watchful waiting. The investigators of a randomized phase III study, called Active Surveillance Therapy Against Radical Treatment in Patients Diagnosed with Favorable Risk Prostate Cancer, or START, are currently recruiting subjects to participate in this trial of watchful waiting or expectant management.[87] The primary aim of START is to compare the prostate cancer–specific mortality rate of those with low-risk disease who are carefully monitored with that of those who undergo treatment with radical prostatectomy or radiation. Evaluation of PSA doubling time is a secondary aim in evaluating outcomes.

Other trials include PIVOT[88] and ProtecT (Prostate Testing for Cancer and Treatment).[87] In PIVOT, investigators at 36 sites will compare intervention (radical prostatectomy) with expectant management and measure all-cause mortality as the primary end point in patients with localized prostate cancer.[89] PIVOT is increasing the generalizability of its findings by enrolling African Americans as one-third of its subjects and by requiring more than three-quarters of its total enrollees to have tumors detected by PSA testing.[87] Results are expected in 2010. Investigators of ProtecT, begun in 2001, expect to enroll more than 1500 men in the United Kingdom and to randomize them to treatment with conformal radiotherapy, prostatectomy, or active surveillance. START, like ProtecT, will compare active surveillance with active therapies. START investigators expect to enroll 2130 men in North America and the United Kingdom and to use three interventions—brachytherapy, external-beam radiotherapy, and surgery.[87] These and other trials should offer investigators more information about localized disease detected through PSA screening, helping physicians and patients understand the risks and benefits better and collaborate better in decision making.

Curative Therapy—An Anatomic Discussion of the Challenges of Disease Control and Minimizing Side Effects

The patient with early disease has the option to pursue one of a number of definitive therapeutic options, each with its own variations in technique. Fundamentally, the options are a radical prostatectomy or dose-escalated radiation therapy. Both treatment categories aim to treat the entire gland by surgical removal or radiation-based destruction. Alternative treatments have also emerged, such as cryotherapy and high-intensity focused ultrasound, that treat all or a portion of the gland. All treatments are associated with a risk of treatment recurrence and varying degrees of quality-of-life side effects specific to prostate cancer treatments: erectile dysfunction, urinary incontinence, urinary irritation and/or obstruction, and bowel dysfunction. The desire to diminish side effects and treatment recurrences has left the field with numerous updates in technique, entirely new technologies, and numerous comparisons. For each question involving treatment efficacy and side effects, the patient and practitioner want to know both the average results expected and any contributing features that help predict whether an individual patient will experience the favorable or unfavorable end of the range of results. In addition, studies have shed light on whether a particular procedure is reproducible across the range of treatment centers.[90-92] Most patients diagnosed today are very much aware of the potential for side effects and the concept that a practitioner's experience may affect outcomes.

The selection of patients for treatment is often derived by considering the slow natural history of prostate cancer and the life expectancy of the aging man. The most commonly accepted recommendation is that a patient may benefit from treatment if he has 10 or more years of life expectancy. However, this estimation may be a moving target because death from cardiac disease is declining with better treatments. Men should not be denied treatment on the basis of age alone,[93] but the study by Albertsen et al.[79] demonstrated significantly reduced prostate cancer–related death when the disease was diagnosed at age 70 and higher, especially for men with Gleason scores <7.

Radical Prostatectomy—A Model for the Treatment Dilemmas Concerning Therapy for Early Prostate Cancer

The challenges of treating early prostate cancer can be illustrated by an anatomic tour of a radical prostatectomy operation and by using the steps of the operation to highlight what the surgeon and radiotherapist must consider in achieving cancer control with minimal side effects. Refer to Figure 94-6 as we narrate our way through the intricate anatomy surrounding the prostate gland.

The radical prostatectomy operation involves complete removal of the prostate gland, seminal vesicles, and distal vas deferens. Conceptually, the prostate gland can be thought of as a conical structure with open ends—the bladder neck and the urethra. The sides of the cone have a capsular structure (although not a true histologic capsule) and are sur-

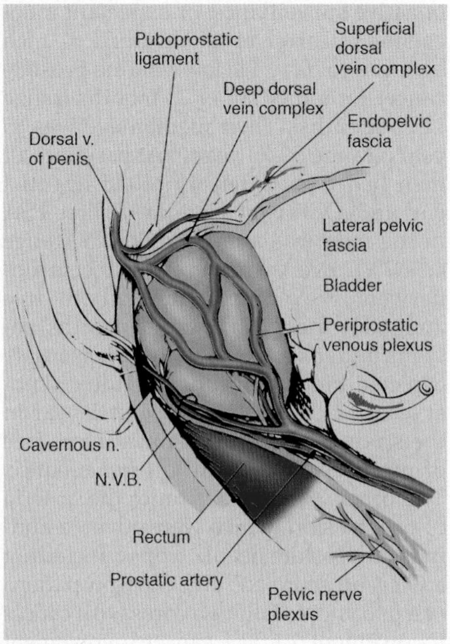

Figure 94-6 Surgical anatomy of the prostate in relationship to the deep dorsal vein complex, neurovascular bundle (NVB), and other surrounding periprostatic structures (lateral view).

rounded by endopelvic fascia laterally and by Denonvilliers fascia posteriorly. At its apex, the prostate is surrounded by the rhabdosphincter muscle and the dorsal vein complex, which is narrow over the urethra and then spreads into an apron-like structure as it traverses over the mid prostate, base of the prostate, and then over the bladder. Regardless of approach and technique, the removal of the prostate requires an intimate understanding of the intricate anatomic structures to be encountered, and a set of allowed surgical motions can be defined.

Access to the Prostate

The prostate gland is among the more difficult structures to access for surgery. It is covered anteriorly by the pubic arch, distally by the dorsal vein complex and rhabdoshpincter, inferiorly by the rectum, inferolaterally by the nerve bundles, and superiorly by the bladder. The prostate can be exposed with a lower midline abdominal incision from the pubic bone to the umbilicus, and the exposure progresses through extraperitoneal spaces. Alternative approaches include mini-laparotomy, laparoscopic access via 5 or 6 ports in the lower abdomen (extraperitoneal or transperitoneal), and perineal access. The mini-laparotomy incision is generally 8-10 cm rather than the 15-20 cm long needed for the standard laparotomy. Visualization of the prostate is similar in the two open abdominal approaches, but in the mini-laparotomy, the surgeon will rely more on instrument dissection than on manual dissection. The laparoscopic approach has become increasingly popular with the availability of robotic surgical systems to increase the laparoscopic surgeon's dexterity with instruments, with seven degrees of motion and three-dimensional camera view.

The choice of surgical approach depends on both the surgeon's training and the patient's characteristics. The retropubic approach has been taught in most residency programs worldwide; it provides access to the prostate and lymph nodes and entails a familiar transabdominal orientation. The perineal approach may be associated with less pain, and the scar is certainly less visible. There may be an advantage to this procedure in the circumstances of morbid obesity. However, the lymph nodes are not accessible, and this approach may be difficult for larger prostates, eg, those >60 g. The laparoscopic approach requires a steep learning curve of more than 100 cases, whereas the robot-assisted laparoscopic approach requires fewer.[94-96] Differences in postoperative pain and hospital discharge are not reliably seen between open retropubic and laparoscopic approaches[97,98] but may be decreased with the perineal approach.[99] Both perineal and laparoscopic approaches are associated with less bleeding, but in expert hands the transfusion rates are probably not significantly different.[100] Results from nonrandomized comparisons show increased transfusion rates in retropubic prostatectomy if the rates for this group are more than 10-15%.[101]

Moving forward with this discussion, we will discuss only the open retropubic and laparoscopic (both manual and robot-assisted types) operations. However, it is worth noting that although historic discussions on the perineal operation suggest that the outcomes may increase positive margin rates, decrease potency rates, and cause de novo rectal incontinence,[102] several high-volume centers have published very competitive outcomes,[99,103] and there is arguably a cost savings relative to the use of robotic approaches.[104,105]

Alternative treatments must also consider access to the prostate in their application. Brachytherapy is a form of whole-gland radiation treatment in which radioactively labeled seeds are inserted into the prostate by transperineal access using transrectal ultrasound for guidance. In cases of BPH, the anterior portion of the prostate may extend around the pubic bone's arch, creating a form of interference to needle placement. Thus, in the application of brachytherapy and cryotherapy (another transperineal-access ablative therapy), the prostate must be of a certain size (generally <60 g) and shape to allow for access. In contrast, modern external beam radiation treatments can handle a broader range of prostate sizes and shapes. The intensity-modulated radiation therapy (IMRT) technique, for example, uses multiple beams from different angles to boost the dose to the prostate while limiting the extraprostatic dose.

Exposure and Dissection of the Apex

The anterior and lateral surfaces of the prostate are covered by endopelvic fascia. This fascia can be cut sharply or by using cautery, with care to avoid or ligate varying networks of veins that course along the prostate and often penetrate the apex at 11 and 1 o'clock. The pubovesicle ligaments are cut by most surgeons to allow distal ligation of the dorsal vein complex. Mistakes in this region can cause significant blood loss in the open operation, although less so in the laparoscopic and/or robotic approaches because of the positive pressure of the CO_2 pneumoperitoneum.

The rhabdosphincter surrounds the urethra distally, and the apex of the prostate has no capsule-like structure. Therefore, there is tremendous potential for mistakes in this region, and this may be the step of the operation that improves the most with experience. In essence, the surgeon must control the dorsal vein complex with proximal and distal sutures and then make a tangential cut that is as close to the apex as possible to avoid damaging the rhabdosphincter complex yet avoid a positive apical margin. Numerous technique descriptions are available and cannot be fully catalogued, but the objectives of cancer control (ie, negative surgical margins) and urinary control are strongly influenced by this step.

Alternatives to surgery must also completely treat the apical region while avoiding side effects. Dose-escalated external beam and brachytherapy will inevitably reach both the apex and surrounding rhabdosphincter. However, because those structures are not specifically disrupted, stress incontinence results significantly less often than with surgery. Cryotherapy techniques include temperature monitors at the sphincter to avoid freezing outside of the apex.

Exposure and Dissection of the Bladder Neck

Dissection of the bladder neck is by comparison much easier than that of the apex in the open operation. The Foley catheter can be used as a guide, and electrocautery can be used safely. Care must be taken to preserve the posterior plate of the bladder neck and divide it away from the ureteral orifices. The bladder neck-sparing technique has been reported as possibly beneficial in avoiding urinary continence but is possibly associated with an increased incidence of positive margins.[106] A non–bladder neck-sparing plane can be reconstructed with sutures to match the urethral size for the anastomosis.

Alternatives to surgery must completely treat the base of the prostate while avoiding damage to the bladder. In conventional-dose radiation to the pelvis, the surrounding dose to the bladder and rectum was always a dose-limiting factor. Dose-escalation techniques, however, whether IMRT, proton therapy, or brachytherapy, effectively increase the dose to the prostate while holding down the dose to the bladder. Nevertheless, some of the dose does affect the bladder, accounting for the differing distribution of urinary side effects, including irritation, frequency, and hematuria.

Exposure and Dissection of the Seminal Vesicles

The seminal vesicles present their own surgical challenges. These structures lie immediately posterior to the bladder, with their tips coursing laterally. The vesicles are surrounded by several small arterial branches that must be controlled with clips or sutures. If uncontrolled, these branches may cause significant postoperative bleeding, which may require a second surgery. However, electrocautery must be avoided if possible because the tips of the vesicles lie immediately medial to the neurovascular bundles. Some researchers have reported the concept of leaving the tips intact to avoid nerve damage.[107] Laparoscopic surgeons may address this challenge by dissecting the seminal vesicles posterior to the bladder through the pouch of Douglas. For the radiotherapist, the seminal vesicles cannot be adequately treated by implant therapy but can be targeted by external technique. MRI with an endorectal coil can be used to stage the seminal vesicles for deciding whether to include them in the treatment plan—the tradeoff being increased bladder toxicity.

Neurovascular Bundle Dissection

The technique for neurovascular bundle dissections is usually retrograde (apex to base) for open surgery and anterograde (base to apex) for laparoscopic surgery. For the retrograde approach, the dorsal vein and urethral division steps are completed and the plane posterior to the Denonvilliers fascia is developed with blunt finger dissection. The bundles on each side can then be palpated. Visually, the neurovascular bundles blend well into the sides of the prostate through a series of lateral fascial layers. A triangle of fascia exists, with its borders being the prostatic fascia medially, the endopelvic fascia laterally, and the Denonvilliers fascia posteriorly. Regardless of the technique, the nerve bundle must be released at two junctions: the anterolateral junction of the prostatic fascia and levator fascia and the medial posterior junction of the Denonvilliers fascia.

During the course of neurovascular bundle dissection, the use of electrocautery must be avoided or the thermal transmission may produce irreparable nerve damage. The portion of the bundle from middle to apex has mostly parallel vessels and a few perforating veins that can be controlled with clips or just transected and left to clot. In contrast, the portion of the bundles near the base gives off perforating arteries to the prostate that must be controlled with clips to avoid hemorrhage. Alternative coagulation devices have been described that produce less thermal discharge, but the nerve bundles are very sensitive to heat, and an athermal technique is preferable. Two different planes of nerve-sparing dissection have been described: intrafascial and interfascial. Surgeons must use judgment in this area because although the closer margin obtained from the intrafascial approach may improve postoperative potency, it moves the inked margin of the resection closer to the prostate gland.[108]

Surgeons may choose to sacrifice the nerve bundles depending on the estimated risk of extraprostatic extension, as determined from pretreatment parameters such as PSA, clinical stage, biopsy Gleason score, number of biopsies with cancer, and volume of cancer on biopsies, and possibly by imaging with sonography or endorectal coil MRI. Nomograms may assist with arriving at this estimate,[67,109,110] but the surgeon's intuition and experience always play a role that is difficult to measure. In general, most patients prefer to have a nerve-sparing operation as long as cancer control can be maintained.

The proximity of the nerve bundle and the prostate capsule also relates to radiotherapy planning. With brachytherapy, the dose delivered can be quite high within the peripheral zone of the prostate but will steeply drop off outside the gland. As a result, intermediate- to high-risk disease may not be adequately treated when there is higher risk of microscopic extraprostatic extension. Many centers will recommend either radiotherapy, as the dose planning can be driven outside of the capsule, or a combination of brachytherapy and radiotherapy. Cryotherapists can also customize treatment in this region by either driving the ice ball extraprostatically if there is a concern or, if no cancer is present on a given side, they can warm the neurovascular bundle region and thus protect it from the ice ball.

Urethral Division

The urethra must be divided close to the prostate apex, essentially right near the verumontanum. The surrounding rhabdosphincter should be preserved, and excessive trauma from urethral dilators and catheters should be avoided.

Anastomosis

Both running and interrupted suture lines have been described, the latter more popular and feasible with the laparoscopic approaches. The objectives are to approximate the bladder to the urethra so that the anastomosis is watertight and the mucosal surfaces are in contact. Excessively large urethral bites that may shorten the functional urethral length should be avoided. Anastomoses that leak or separate may lead to a higher rate of scarring and contracture.[111]

Outcomes of Treatment for Early Disease

Cancer Control

Most modern studies use PSA recurrence-free survival as an end point because the data can be collected in a 5- to 10-year time frame rather than the 15- to 20-year time frame needed for longer end points such as disease-specific and overall survival rates. However, as the AUA guidelines[63] stress, PSA recurrence is inconsistently defined and does not directly correlate with longer survival. The most commonly used definition of PSA failure for surgery is a PSA level >0.2 ng/mL and, for radiation, the updated American Society for Therapeutic Radiology and Oncology (ASTRO) recommendation is PSA nadir plus 2 ng/mL.[112] Definitions of risk stratification also vary in different studies. The AUA guidelines recommend the D'Amico criteria and the options for each[59]:

- Low risk: PSA ≤ 10 ng/mL, a Gleason score ≤ 6, and clinical stage cT1c-cT2a.
- Intermediate risk: PSA >10-20 ng/mL or a Gleason score ≤ 7 or clinical stage T2b.
- High risk: PSA >20 ng/mL or a Gleason score ≤ 8-10 or clinical stage T2c.

According to these risk groupings, the expected cancer control outcomes of brachytherapy, external-beam radiotherapy, and radical prostatectomy in terms of PSA recurrence–free survival are seen in Figure 94-7.[63] For each modality, the 5-year range of outcomes are low risk, 75-95%; intermediate risk, 70-90%; and high risk, 30-80%. At 10 years, the ranges are low risk, 60-90%; intermediate risk, 40-80%; and high risk, 20-60%. On the basis of the limitations of lack of standardized reporting, different definitions of failure, and lack of head-to-head randomized controlled trials, the AUA panel stated that there are insufficient data to conclude that one treatment is superior to another. For patients choosing radiation therapy, the panel cited two randomized controlled clinical trials showing that higher-dose radiation may decrease the risk of a PSA recurrence.[113,114]

The topic of neoadjuvant and/or adjuvant androgen deprivation was also addressed by the AUA panel. Randomized clinical trials of neoadjuvant androgen deprivation plus radical prostatectomy showed no benefit in terms of PSA recurrence-free survival.[115,116] However, for intermediate-risk patients treated with radiotherapy, one trial showed that neoadjuvant and concurrent androgen deprivation for 6 months may prolong survival after radiotherapy.[117] For high-risk patients treated with radiotherapy,

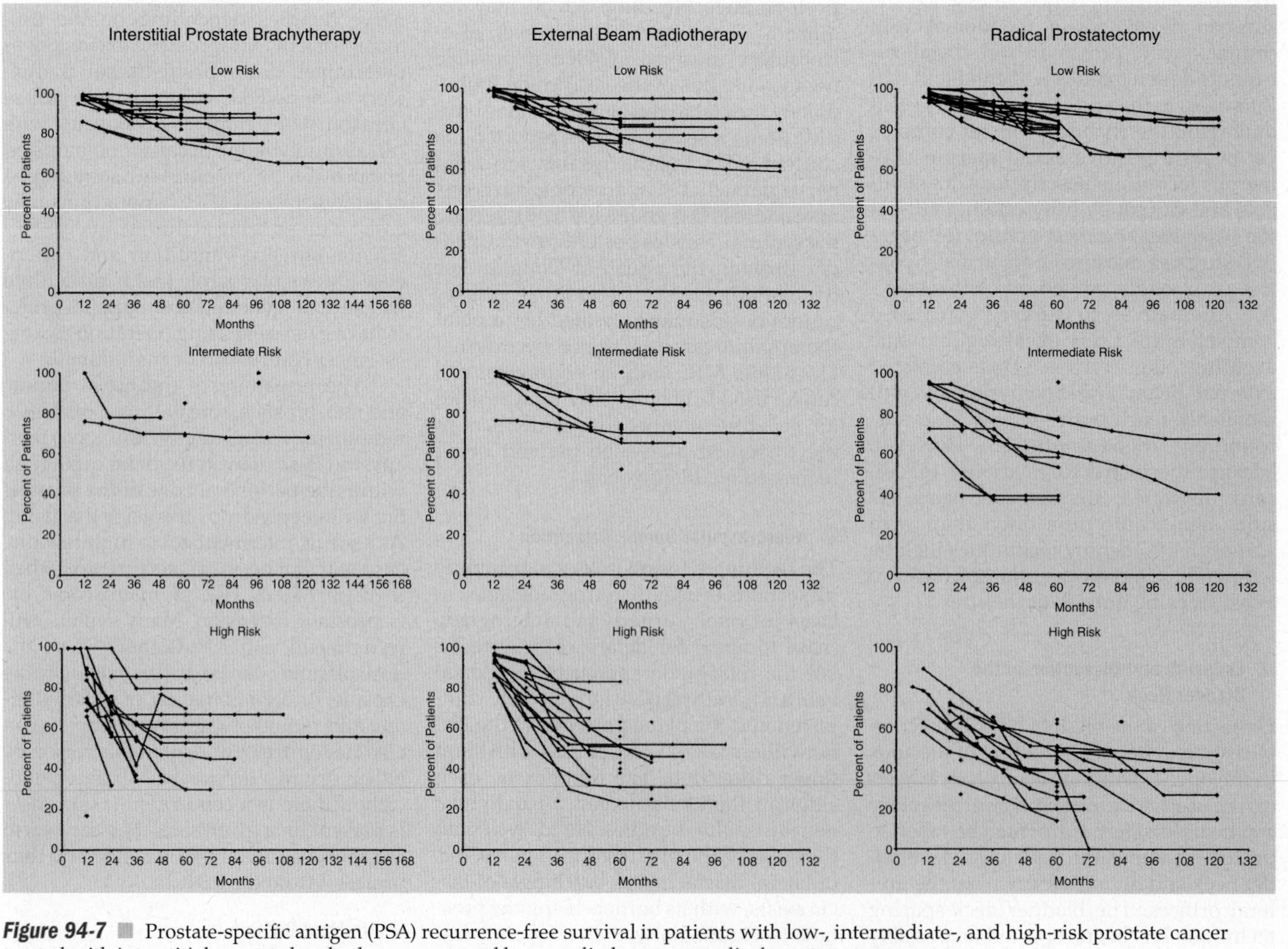

Figure 94-7 ■ Prostate-specific antigen (PSA) recurrence-free survival in patients with low-, intermediate-, and high-risk prostate cancer treated with interstitial prostate brachytherapy, external beam radiotherapy, or radical prostatectomy.

trials demonstrated a survival benefit for a longer duration of adjuvant androgen deprivation,[118] in the 2- to 3-year range. However, it is noteworthy that the radiotherapy used in these trials was conventional and not dose escalated.

In summary, the AUA guidelines list active surveillance, brachytherapy, radiotherapy, and radical prostatectomy as treatment options for low-, intermediate-, and high-risk disease. For radiotherapy, randomized controlled trials are cited regarding dosages and androgen deprivation use. For the high-risk patient, it is noted that recurrence rates are high and that patients should consider "clinical trials examining new forms of therapy, including combination therapies, with the goal of improved outcomes." It is also worth noting that the AUA panel concluded that first-line hormonal therapy is "seldom indicated in the patients with localized prostate cancer."[119]

The European Association of Urology has also issued a guidelines statement on prostate cancer, in which it cites many of the same randomized clinical trials regarding watchful waiting, surgery, and radiotherapy.[120] Additional recommendations based on lower levels of evidence are also cited. Some selected recommendations regarding early disease follow:

- Brachytherapy "may be proposed to patients cT1-T2a, Gleason score <7 (or 3+4), PSA ≤ 10 ng/mL, prostate volume ≤ 50 mL, without a previous TURP and with a good IPSS [International Prostate Symptom Score] (level of evidence: 2b)."
- Cryotherapy "has evolved from an investigational therapy to a possible alternative treatment method for CaP [prostate cancer] in patients unfit for surgery or in those with a life expectancy <10 years (grade C recommendation)."
- "All other minimally invasive treatment options, such as HIFU [high-intensity focused ultrasound], RITA [radiofrequency interstitial tumor ablation], microwaves, and electrosurgery, are still experimental or investigational. For all of these procedures, a longer follow-up is mandatory to assess their true role in the management of CaP (grade C recommendation)."

Another large-scale effort to summarize the state of the literature was prepared for the Agency for Healthcare Research and Quality and published in the *Annals of Internal Medicine*.[121] Again, the researchers met with difficulties because of variations in reporting and definitions, and only three randomized controlled trials compared the effectiveness between primary treatments (none with patients "primarily detected with PSA testing") so, essentially stated, no conclusions could be drawn.

Complications of Treatment

General ■ As a general statement, radical prostatectomy results in more urinary incontinence than radiotherapy or active surveillance do.[121] Brachytherapy and radiotherapy are associated with more bladder irritation and/or hematuria side effects and less incontinence. Radiotherapy has the higher risk of bowel urgency. All treatments have sexual side effects: although the pattern with radical prostatectomy is one of early loss with gradual improvement, the pattern with brachytherapy or radiotherapy is one of more gradual and delayed loss of function. Younger age and better preexisting function will predict better outcomes from all treatments.

However, there are numerous sources of bias and variability in comparisons, and there is no evidence that any one therapy "has a more significant cumulative overall risk of complications."[119] Although patients often request a single statistic, such as an incontinence rate or potency rate, it is accepted that more accurate quality-of-life research will result from the use of (a) validated instruments that ask multiple questions and offer a range of potential answers, (b) an instrument that is administered by someone other than the treating practitioner, (c) a prospective longitudinal design, including a pretreatment baseline measurement, and (d) an instrument that maintains response rates at >70% throughout the study period. The recent multicenter study by Ferrer et al.[122] evaluated the three standard treatments (radical prostatectomy, brachytherapy, and radiotherapy) with such an ideal method (except for treatment randomization). In the absence of comparisons of side effects in randomized controlled trials, various categories of studies can assist with our understanding of side effects: (a) results from multicenter community or academic series (ie, voluntary reporting of what goes on in the community), (b) single-surgeon high-volume series (ie, idealistic results), and (c) Medicare- or claims-based studies (ie, involuntary outcomes reporting).

Multicenter Studies ■ Penson et al.[123] reported the results from the Prostate Cancer Outcomes Study, which is a community-based cohort study conducted at six centers where men underwent radical prostatectomy in 1994 and 1995. In this study, the only relevant predictive information was that the men underwent a radical prostatectomy in the community, ie, no description of technique or quality analysis of the surgeon and/or surgery was given. Among the 1288 patients studied, frequent urinary leakage occurred in 3% at baseline, in 19% at 6 months, in 13% at 1 year, in 9% at 2 years, and in 11% at 5 years. At 5 years, the urinary control level was described as having total control in 35%; occasional leakage in 51%; frequent leakage in 11%; and no control in 3%.

Additional data were presented regarding pad use, irritative symptoms, and bother. Urinary bother started as no problem in 87% at baseline; at 5 years, 45% reported no problem, 42% reported a slight problem, and 13% reported a moderate to great problem. The percentages of patients who reported experiencing erections sufficient for intercourse were 81% at baseline, 9% at 6 months, 17% at 1 year, 22% at 2 years, and 28% at 5 years. Although urinary function and bother scores improved between 2 and 5 years, the percentages of men with no sexual activity were 15% at baseline, 44% at 1 year, and 46% at 5 years. Bilateral nerve sparing predicted a better return of erections at 5 years: 40% for bilateral compared with 23% for unilateral and 23% for non–nerve sparing. Age was also a predictor: In the most favorable group, 61% of men 39-54 years old reported erections.

Sanda et al.[124] reported on a multi-institutional cohort from nine university-affiliated centers, with surgery completed with open, laparoscopic, and robotic-assisted techniques. In theory, this group of surgeons has a high volume, but again, specific technique was not reported. Using the 100-point Expanded Prostate Cancer Index Composite (EPIC) scale, patients who underwent radical prostatectomy had a baseline score for urinary continence of just 90; the score dropped to 50 at 2 months, improved to 70 at 6 months, and plateaued at 80 at 12-24 months.

However, as the results from these two large studies demonstrate, the literature contains varying definitions of incontinence. Sexual function was adversely affected by both radical prostatectomy and radiotherapy. Among patients who underwent radical prostatectomy, potency was better preserved with nerve-sparing techniques. Among patients who underwent radiotherapy, however, potency was better preserved in patients treated with monotherapy than in those given a combination with hormonal therapy (even after a short duration of 6 months). Bowel function was most affected by radiotherapy and brachytherapy even after 1 year—9% with distress related to bowel function.

The AUA guideline panel review[63,119] reported a range of 3-74% for urinary incontinence and suggested that there are insufficient data to provide an overall assessment of urinary outcomes. Those AUA guidelines also provide a large-scale review of published results of erectile dysfunction after radical prostatectomy without details of surgical technique and experience. Rates of erectile dysfunction after 1 year are as high as 90%, and nerve-sparing techniques are helpful.

Expert Series ■ The nerve-sparing operation was initially described by Walsh et al. in the early 1980s,[125] and it became increasingly popular and oncologically safe after the introduction of PSA screening. As one can imagine, patient demand for Walsh's services and the services of other surgeons dedicated full time to this operation became quite high. Walsh et al. published a validated quality-of-life survey study that demonstrated the return of urinary control at 1 year in 93% of patients and a potency rate of 86% at 18 months.[126] A high-volume robot-assisted prostatectomy series also demonstrated excellent results: 1032 of 1110 patients (93%) wore one or no pads per day at 1 year, and potency was reported in 79.2%.[127] Although other studies have looked closely at factors affecting urinary control or potency rates, a recent trend has been to estimate the odds of achieving the "trifecta" of desired outcomes: cancer control, urinary control, and potency. The group from Memorial Sloan-Kettering Cancer Center has published the concept as a nomogram.[128]

Expert comparisons have extended across technique choices. Touijer et al.[129] performed a single-institution study involving two high-volume surgeons, one of whom performed laparoscopic and the other, open surgeries. There was an unexpected finding of better return of continence (defined as patient reports of no leakage or not requiring a pad) in the open-surgery group: at 12 months, 75% vs 48%. Descriptions of the surgical techniques were cited, but the true difference that affected outcomes was not described. Those authors suspected the result was due to the apical dissection in the laparoscopic approach and stated that further prospective analysis is needed.

Thus, a clear need in outcomes research in early disease is to better link technique to outcome. An example is seen in the study by Masterson et al.[130] which demonstrated that a specific technical improvement in nerve sparing can be described and the results measured. In the standard technique, the apex is dissected starting with the dorsal vein complex, cutting the urethra, and then bluntly mobilizing the posterior plane before releasing the posterolateral neurovascular bundles. In the modified technique, the sequence starts with dissection of the entire neurovascular bundle off the lateral aspect of the prostate from apex to seminal vesicle before the urethra is cut and posterior dissection performed. This avoids excessive traction applied to the neurovascular bundles. The 6-month recovery of erections improved from 40% with the standard technique to 67% with the modification. Such analogies can be seen in the literature on brachytherapy, in which the D90 analysis of the implant quality is a significant predictor of long-term biochemical disease–free interval.[131]

Variations in Outcomes and Medicare Databases ■ In multicenter studies and expert series, researchers voluntarily submit their own results and therefore have the ability to decide whether to participate. In the case of other studies, accessible data are used without such a decision to participate from each physician. Even among expert surgeons, complications vary.[132] The Medicare database and the Surveillance Epidemiology and End Results (SEER) registries are common sources for data from studies such as these. The advantages of these studies include their large numbers of patients and the opportunity they offer for studying a more average community cohort of patients. Their limitations include sampling only patients over age 65 and that their data end points are designed for billing purposes more than for research and can be incomplete in their assessment of the outcomes.

Quality-of-life data seen in such databases appear quite different from those in expert series. Benoit et al.[133] found urethral stricture in 19.5%, urinary incontinence in 21.7%, and erectile dysfunction in 21.5%. Begg et al.[134] looked at morbidity after radical prostatectomy in the SEER–Medicare linked database and found significant trends in the association between surgeon volume and complications and between hospital volume and complications. Recently, Hu et al.[135] analyzed a Medicare sample of patients who underwent minimally invasive radical prostatectomy versus open radical prostatectomy. The trends demonstrated fewer perioperative complications and shorter hospital stay for those who had a minimally invasive radical prostatectomy, although they had higher rates of salvage therapy and anastomotic strictures. However, the unfavorable outcomes with the minimally invasive radical prostatectomy procedure decreased significantly with increasing surgeon volume.

PSAV as a Predictor After Diagnosis ■ Researchers have also relied on PSAV to predict disease progression, relapse, and outcomes. In a retrospective study of 102 men who underwent radical prostatectomy,[136] researchers found a statistically significant association between a PSAV of 2 ng/mL/year in the year before diagnosis and tumor volume, which was 2.55 cm^3 in men with biochemical recurrence and 0.94 cm^3 in men who were disease free 5 years postsurgery ($P < .05$). The median PSAV in the men who experienced relapse was almost twice that of men who did not (1.98 ng/mL/year vs 1.05 ng/mL/year). Although these results help identify those at high risk, they may also help physicians identify patients whose tumors are more likely eradicable.

The results of two studies published in 2005 revealed associations between PSAV and outcomes. D'Amico et al.[137] studied PSAV in the year before diagnosis in 1095 men with localized prostate cancer to identify those most at risk of death from prostate cancer. They determined that a PSAV of >2.0 ng/mL/year was related to a statistically significantly shorter time to death from prostate cancer ($P < .001$) and to death from any cause ($P = .01$); those outcomes were also influenced by PSA level, tumor stage, and Gleason score at diagnosis. Factors that predicted time to death from prostate cancer were a clinical tumor stage of T2; a Gleason score of 8, 9, or 10; and an increasing PSA level at diagnosis.

In an even larger study with a follow-up of more than 7 years, Sengupta and colleagues[138] also found a significant association between increased risk of death from prostate cancer and both preoperative PSAV and PSA doubling time. In 2290 men who underwent radical prostatectomy, 460 with a PSAV of >3.4 ng/mL/year had a greater than sixfold increase in risk of prostate cancer death (hazard ratio [HR] 6.54; 95% CI 3.51-12.91) compared with those with lower PSAV values. In addition, the 506 men whose PSA doubling time was <18 months had a similar increased risk (HR 6.22; 95% CI 3.33-11.61) compared with those with lower PSA doubling times. The authors said that their findings that PSAV is a better predictor than PSA doubling time of biochemical progression while PSA doubling time is a better predictor than PSAV of clinical progression and death conform to the notion that prostate cancer growth follows an exponential rather than linear model.[138]

In a study in a group of 379 men with prostate cancer who experienced biochemical recurrence after radical prostatectomy, Freedland and colleagues found that PSA doubling time along with pathologic Gleason score and time from surgery to recurrence were statistically significant risk factors for prostate cancer–specific mortality[139]; in a separate study in a cohort with a PSA doubling time of <15 months, the same investigators found that 90% of deaths could be attributed to prostate cancer.[140] In studies of PSAV and PSA doubling time, those same investigators found no relationship between those variables and adverse pathologic findings or biochemical recurrence after radical prostatectomy.[141]

Furthermore, though African American men are at higher risk for prostate cancer than men of other races, researchers found no relationship between PSAV or PSA doubling time and race among whites, blacks, Hispanics, and Asians. As might be predicted, no relationship was found between PSAV and prostate volume.[136]

Prostate Cancer Chemoprevention: Large Trials

The PCPT (Prostate Cancer Prevention Trial) involved 18,882 men randomized to treatment with finasteride (a 5α-reductase inhibitor) or placebo.[142] PCPT ended more than a year earlier than planned because its Data Safety and Monitoring Committee determined that the trial had met its primary objective. Prostate cancer prevalence during the 7-year treatment period was 24.8% lower in the men taking finasteride than in men taking placebo (95% CI 18.6-30.6; $P < .001$). This good news was tempered, however, by the finding that tumors detected in those taking finasteride were 1.67 times more likely to be of a higher grade (Gleason score 7-10) than were those in subjects taking placebo (37.0% of graded tumors vs 22.2%; $P < .001$).

Newer studies of the PCPT data have reassured physicians that finasteride's ability to reduce cancer is clinically significant, explained why the initial results found high-grade disease more frequently in the finasteride arm, and endorsed its use. Taken together, the new results ease the concern that finasteride caused the rate of aggressive cancers to rise in the treated group and encourage physicians to offer finasteride to more men.[143]

According to other reevaluations of the PCPT data, a continuum of risk began at a PSA of even <4.0 ng/mL,[144] and new pathologic studies were undertaken of the PCPT prostate biopsy specimens on which data were available (finasteride, 519 patients; placebo, 716 patients) after results were initially reported to determine whether these tumors were clinically insignificant.[145] Results confirmed that the risk of clinically significant tumors rises with increasing PSA value and that of insignificant tumors falls (Table 94-5); nonetheless, 62% of cancers in men with Gleason scores ≤ 6 were deemed clinically significant, as were 75% of all cancers detected.[145]

In another reevaluation of the PCPT findings, Pinsky et al.[146] used a statistical model to tackle the problem of determining misclassification rates among the pathology findings in each arm and identifying a "true" relative risk for high-grade disease. They determined that misclassification from low- to high-grade disease from specimens at biopsy to those at radical prostatectomy is a function of the true ratio of low- to high-grade disease and misclassification rates. Although the results were not statistically significant in comparison with those for the placebo arm, the true rate of high-grade disease was lower in the finasteride arm (RR 0.84; 95% CI 0.68-1.05); also in the finasteride arm, the true rate of low-grade disease was both lower and significant (RR 0.61; 95% CI 0.51-0.71) compared with that in the placebo arm. The authors explained this paradox of similarly upgraded rates in both arms despite the finasteride group's having less misclassification as being the result of finasteride's decreasing the ratio of true low-grade to high-grade disease.

In response to evidence reported after the initial analysis of the PCPT[144,147] and to understand the effect of uncovered biases affecting that analysis, Redman and her colleagues[148] undertook a reanalysis, including evaluable patients omitted from the final analysis, estimating the true prevalence of cancer grade using the highest standard (radical prostatectomy), and studying the sensitivity of biopsy for prostate cancer. These reanalyses included one for selection bias and another that included grading information on radical prostatectomy in 500 cancer-diagnosed participants. Both produced greater risk-reduction estimates than the original study analysis had and attributed to finasteride no increased risk of high-grade cancer. In the first of those reanalyses, risk reduction was increased to 30% (RR 0.70; 95% CI 0.64-0.76; $P < .0001$), and prostate cancer rates were 21.1% in the placebo group (4.2% high-grade disease) and 14.7% (4.8% high-grade disease) in the finasteride group, with the 14% increase in high-grade disease nonsignificant (RR 1.14; 95% CI 0.96-1.35; $P = .12$). In the second reanalysis by Redman, risk reduction was increased to 27% (RR 0.73; 95% CI 0.56-0.96; $P = .02$), and risk of high-grade disease was lower in the finasteride group (placebo 8.2%; finasteride 6.0%). A third reanalysis found that biopsy sensitivity could significantly affect risk ratio estimates. The authors' conclusion was that men had no reason to worry about increased risk of high-grade cancer when they are treated with finasteride.[148]

Table 94-5 PSA and Identification of Significant and Insignificant Tumors

Tumor Type for which at Risk	PSA Value (ng/mL) 0–1.0	1.1–2.5	2.6–4.0	4.1–10.0
Significant tumors	15.6%	37.9%	49.1%	52.4%
Insignificant tumors	51.7%	33.7%	17.8%	11.7%

Source: Data from Ref. 147.

Earlier reevaluations of the PCPT data helped to explain how detection bias introduced by finasteride increased the sensitivity of PSA level for the end points of prostate cancer and high-grade disease (Gleason score 7-10) and how finasteride increased the sensitivity of the DRE (finasteride 21.3%; placebo 16.7%; $P = .015$).[144,147] Detection of high-grade disease by DRE was also found to be more sensitive than the PSA, but the difference was not statistically significant.[147]

Before these new analyses were published, principal investigator of the PCPT Ian Thompson and colleagues had answered in part the question their own research had posed when they demonstrated that finasteride's ability to increase the sensitivity of the PSA for prostate cancer and high-grade prostate cancer introduced detection bias for these end points.[144] When their end-of-study biopsy findings failed to demonstrate the increased detection of high-grade tumors in the finasteride arm that had been shown in the for-cause biopsies prompted by high PSA values or abnormal DRE findings, the researchers had a reason to suspect that finasteride might not have caused the changes. Thus, Thompson et al.[144] used AUC studies to demonstrate that the AUC for finasteride was significantly greater than that for placebo for cancer detection overall and for high-grade disease, whether the Gleason score was ≥ 7 or ≥ 8.

Thompson and colleagues[144] performed another analysis of PSA in the PCPT data, estimating the receiver operating characteristic (ROC) curve for PSA, and found that there was no cut point for PSA with both high sensitivity and specificity for monitoring healthy men for prostate cancer; rather, there was a continuum of prostate cancer risk at all PSA levels. The ROC curve was better for high-grade than for overall prostate cancer risk, but as subsequent analysis showed, there is a substantial risk of biopsy-detected prostate cancer and high-grade disease in men with PSA levels <4 ng/mL, which is generally thought to be in the normal range. Although PSA values <4 ng/mL are related to prostate cancer risk, it is not clear how this information should be applied to clinical decision-making. These data illustrate (a) the need for improved biomarkers of risk and prognosis of prostate cancer and (b) the value of biopsy-proven negative controls for assessing prostate cancer risk, biology, and prevention.

The most important National Cancer Institute (NCI)–supported chemopreventive initiative ongoing is the randomized, placebo-controlled trial called Selenium and Vitamin E Cancer Prevention Trial (SELECT), which is evaluating the effects of selenium and vitamin E, separately and combined, against those of placebo in preventing prostate cancer.[149] The serial collection of biospecimens from all SELECT study participants will enable the construction of risk models to help determine which men are most likely to develop prostate cancer and to help identify those most likely to benefit from selenium and vitamin E chemopreventive therapy.

Specimens from the other landmark NCI initiative for prostate cancer prevention, the PCPT, were recently released, making them available to researchers whether they are supported by NCI grants or not.[150]

Putative chemopreventive agents other than finasteride that have been studied or are in development include celecoxib, sulindac, toremifene, selenium, vitamin E, soy isoflavones, lycopene, and doxercalciferol. Currently under way are molecular epidemiologic studies of diet and prostate cancer risk as well as basic research into the carcinogenicity of specific diet-derived compounds such as heterocyclic amines. Statins have also been of interest. In 2003, the NCI's Division of Cancer Prevention awarded $42 million to fund a consortium made up of six programs headed by experienced cancer prevention principal investigators at six major institutions. Members were charged with becoming national leaders in prevention research and in initiating trials on agents of interest, including some of the agents named above.

Algorithm for Therapy: Future Directions

Future studies will affect therapy most dramatically if they address limitations reported in current reviews of the literature. These studies must (a) use a randomized design, including an untreated control group, (b) use standard definitions of cancer control and quality-of-life outcomes, (c) link specific techniques to outcome, and (d) demonstrate that a specific technique can be reproduced by multiple practitioners and produce an effect that is similar across settings in the same way that prescribing a drug produces similar effects across patient groups in different settings. After scientific standards are met, the study design should incorporate measures that will make progress possible by resolving questions, both large and small, posed by other work or by producing data that eliminate potential explanations that could undercut conclusions.

Using current knowledge, investigators can outline an algorithm for patients with localized disease as follows: make a determination about treatment, follow an evidence-based guideline or enroll the patient in a clinical trial if treatment is the option of choice, and incorporate molecular signatures to address tumor heterogeneity. First, patients and their physicians must cooperatively decide whether to pursue treatment. As described earlier, expectant management, also called watchful waiting or active surveillance, permits patients with localized disease to forgo treatment, and national organizations, including the National Comprehensive Cancer Network, have created guidelines for management[95]; however, in some active surveillance studies, as many as to 75% of men electing expectant management have been found to pursue therapy within 5 years, most because of rising PSA values.[151] Advances in better identification of low-risk cases with refined arrays of prognostic factors, including molecular markers, and closer surveillance may change that trend.

Critical to efforts in the future to spare patients with localized disease the side effects of unnecessary definitive therapy will be better tools for differentiating aggressive from indolent disease. Such tools, some of which are in development, may take the form of nomograms such as those described earlier, of a combination of one or more molecular markers added to PSA values, of genetic variants, or of discriminating molecular signatures.[152-154] With these combinations, we may be inspecting findings not for one specific value but for patterns of values within each collection of factors, and we may be able to obtain this information not only preoperatively but also before biopsy. Furthermore, predictions achieved this way may encompass not only therapeutic response but also natural disease progression.[153]

Locally Advanced Disease

Clinical Presentation

Locally advanced prostate cancer is heralded by disease extension outside the prostate capsule (T3a) or into the seminal vesicles (T3b). The tumor may grow laterally into the pelvic sidewall, centrally into the urethra, superiorly into the bladder neck and trigone, interiorly into the base of the penis, or posteriorly into the rectum. Although patients may be relatively asymptomatic when they are first seen, complaints are related to the direction of spread.

Common symptoms can be similar to those seen with BPH and vesicle outlet obstruction, such as urinary urgency, frequency, and hesitancy, nocturia, dysuria, and decreased stream. Invasion of the bladder or urethra can produce hematuria, and ureteral obstruction can lead to renal impairment. Hematospermia can be seen as well. Although Denonvilliers fascia is usually an effective barrier to tumor spread, rectal invasion produces symptoms similar to those seen in primary rectal cancer, such as hematochezia, constipation and obstruction, reduced stool caliber, and pelvic pain. Tumor extension inferiorly into the urogenital diaphragm or corporal bodies may result in perineal pain, priapism, or impotence.

In addition to DRE, the use of pelvic CT scanning or MRI, transrectal ultrasonography, cystoscopy, and rectosigmoidoscopy can help to better define the extent of disease and the adjacent organs involved. The PSA level is usually high in these patients, sometimes markedly so, although very high tumor grade, anaplastic tumors, and ductal variants may produce little PSA and, in these cases, the PSA level is disproportionate to the amount of disease present. In PSA-producing tumors, the PSAV is an important consideration because it is a measure of the growth rate and aggressiveness of the disease. A PSAV >2 ng/mL/year before treatment (prostatectomy or radiation) has been shown to relate to a higher rate of cancer-specific death.[155] A rapid PSA doubling time can also be an early indication of metastatic disease. Laboratory work related to the local extent of the tumor may show a low red blood cell count secondary to chronic bleeding or elevated blood urea nitrogen and creatinine values secondary to ureteral obstruction and renal impairment.

To assess potential disease outside the pelvis, abdominal CT or MRI, bone scanning, and chest x-ray are also indicated.

Therapy Options and Applications

According to the results of a patient care evaluation completed by the American College of Surgeons in 1990, the most common treatment for locally advanced prostate cancer at that time was radiation or hormone therapy. Combination treatment was used in just 12% of patients.[156] Poor outcomes and subsequent reports of superior results achieved with combined radiation and androgen deprivation therapy[157-160] led to a planned multimodality approach as the mainstay of treatment for these patients. Although surgery may be used selectively for locally advanced disease, it is usually combined with postoperative adjuvant radiation or with chemohormonal therapy or molecular targeting agents in a clinical trial.

Radiation and Hormone Therapy

Because radiation alone does not successfully eradicate the bulky local disease burden in patients with locally advanced disease (<50% chance) and this modality does not address the significant risk for metastasis in these patients, combined radiation and androgen deprivation has become the standard of care. The results of four randomized clinical trials—RTOG 85-31, EORTC 22863, RTOG 86-10, and RTOG 92-02—provide compelling supportive evidence for the use of combined therapy.[157-162] Patients with locally advanced tumors comprised the study group in the RTOG (Radiation Therapy Oncology Group) trials, and the EORTC (European Organization for Research on the Treatment of Cancer) trial patients had either T3 or T4 tumors or high-grade disease. The radiation dose in all of these trials was low by today's standards, 65-70 Gy. In all of those trials, the main drug was a luteinizing hormone–releasing hormone (LHRH) agonist. Results have been reported at 10 years posttreatment for the RTOG trials and at 5 years for the EORTC study.

In RTOG 85-31, hormone therapy was given indefinitely beginning after radiation, and in the EORTC trial, it was given concomitantly with radiation and then continued for 3 years. The results from both of these trials revealed a significant benefit in biochemical and clinical end points (local recurrence, distant metastasis, and disease-free survival) as well as in disease-specific and overall survival rates for the patients who received radiation and hormone therapy, as compared with those who received radiation alone.[157,158] In RTOG 85-31, subset analysis showed that this advantage was largely driven by patients with Gleason scores of 7 or higher.[157]

RTOG 86-10 compared the effects of 4 months of hormone therapy, started 2 months before radiation, to with those of radiation therapy alone. Patients benefited more from the combined radiation and hormone therapy in the end points of biochemical failure, distant metastasis, and disease-free and disease-specific survival.[159,161] The latest report revealed that just 4 months of adjuvant androgen-deprivation therapy had a profound effect on disease-specific survival[161]: ⅓ of the patients treated with radiation alone died as a result of prostate cancer within 9 years, whereas it took an additional 9 years for the same number of patients to die of their disease when hormone therapy had been added. However, there still was no significant difference in the overall survival rate.

RTOG 92-02 compared 4 months of hormonal therapy plus radiation (as in the combined treatment arm in RTOG 86-10) with radiation plus 28 months of hormone therapy (hormone therapy for 2 months before and 2 months during radiation followed by 24 more months). Similar to the results from the other studies, there was a between-group difference in all end points except overall survival, for which only patients with Gleason scores of 8-10 benefited from the longer duration of hormone therapy.[160,162]

These study results taken in conglomerate suggest that a longer duration of hormone therapy in conjunction with radiation better addresses not only local disease but also distant dissemination in patients who have a significant local tumor burden, especially in patients with high Gleason scores.

A study by D'Amico et al. included a mixture of patients at intermediate and high risk (T1b-T2b or low risk with T3 by endorectal MRI, PSA 10-40 ng/mL, or Gleason score 7-10). Patients were randomized to receive 70 Gy to the prostate and seminal vesicles alone or 70 Gy combined with 6 months of total androgen blockade starting 2 months before radiation treatment began. This study also showed an advantage in prostate cancer–specific mortality in patients receiving the combination therapy: 2% vs 8% at 8 years after treatment. Additionally, overall survival was 74% vs 61% in favor of the group treated with combination therapy.[163] Of note, however, is that although the survival benefit was of even greater magnitude in patients who had no or minimal cormorbidity (90% vs 64%), there was no benefit in patients with moderate or severe comorbidity. In the group with moderate or severe comorbidity, the survival rate was higher than it was in the group treated with radiation alone, although the difference was not statistically significant. D'Amico and colleagues suggested that hormone therapy increases the risk of myocardial infarction in this cohort.[164]

In another randomized trial in men with locally advanced (T2b-T4) disease, that of the Trans-Tasman Radiation Oncology Group (96.01), the addition of 6 months of total androgen blockade begun 5 months before radiation to a dose of 66 Gy significantly reduced biochemical, local, and distant failure and improved prostate cancer–specific survival.[165] The benefit of adding hormone therapy appeared to increase as the PSA and Gleason score became indicative of higher-risk disease. Although the current trend is to try to decrease the use of hormone therapy or at least limit its duration, because of the recent reports of cardiac morbidity, metabolic syndrome, and bone density effects,[164,166] the ideal duration of hormone therapy has yet to be determined on the basis of a maximal therapeutic ratio.[166]

Another EORTC trial, 22961, was designed to prove the non-inferiority of 6 months of hormone therapy and radiation compared with 3 years of hormone therapy and radiation in men with locally advanced prostate cancer (T2c-T4) and those with T1c-T2b N1-2 disease. The trial closed early after accrual of 990 patients, however, because an interim analysis showed the futility of trying to prove this hypothesis. Five-year PSA and clinical progression–free survival as well as overall survival rates were all lower in the patients who received 6 months of hormone therapy: 78% vs 59%, 82% vs 69%, and 85% vs 81%, respectively.[167] Thus, we must remain cautious in changing therapeutic recommendations without sufficient evidence. Of note, however, is the fact that current standard radiation doses are higher than those used previously, and this has been shown to both decrease local failure and subsequently affect distant metastasis.[168,169]

Radiation and Chemotherapy ■ Because the results of combined hormone therapy and radiation leave ample room for improvement, combinations with chemotherapy are being tested in clinical trials. In RTOG 99-02, patients with high-risk disease were randomized to treatment with radiation plus 2 years of androgen ablation or to treatment with the same combination followed by treatment with paclitaxel, estramustine, and etoposide for four cycles beginning 8 weeks after radiation.[170] Although this study was closed prematurely because of excessive thromboembolic toxicity, nearly 400 of the planned 1440 patients were accrued between 2000 and 2004. Future analysis may give some indication as to the efficacy of these agents delivered adjuvantly with radiation.[170] A follow-up study, RTOG 05-21, is underway; it has the same design as RTOG 99-02 but uses docetaxel and prednisone for six cycles after radiation as the adjuvant agents.

The investigators of small single-institution trials have reported using 5-fluorouracil[171] and docetaxel[172] as single agents concomitantly with radiation and estramustine and vinblastine in combination either concomitantly[173] or neoadjuvantly[174] with radiation. In these single-institution studies, the reported toxicity was greater than that which would be expected with radiation alone but was within the acceptable range. Unfortunately, the tumor control rates did not appear to be significantly affected in these trials.

Radical Prostatectomy

Although prostatectomy has been used to treat patients with locally advanced prostate cancer, the reported studies are usually qualified by including patients with less-extensive, resectable disease and lower-grade tumors than have been included in radiation trials. With prostatectomy, PSA disease–free outcome has been in the 50-60% range 5-10 years after treatment, and 60-80% of patients have required adjuvant and/or salvage radiation or hormone ablative therapy postoperatively.[175-178] Unlike the combined approach with radiation, the use of short-course androgen deprivation has not resulted in significant improvement in PSA disease–free progression when combined neoadjuvantly with prostatectomy.[179,180]

To date, surgery has not yielded results superior to those obtained with radiation plus hormonal therapy. A randomized trial comparing 8 weeks of treatment with diethylstilbestrol (DES) and either radiation or radical prostatectomy in patients with T2b-T3 tumors showed similar results with regard to biochemical, clinical progression–free, and cause-specific survival.[181] The dose of radiation used was only in the 60- to 70-Gy range, and the treatment-related morbidity was treatment specific, as might be expected.

Although several phase II studies have proven that various chemotherapeutic agents and hormonal therapy can be combined neoadjuvantly with surgery with an acceptable level of toxicity, a significant decrease in cancer progression or improvement in survival has yet to be seen.[182-184] The recently opened CALGB (Cancer and Leukemia Group B) 90203 trial randomizes patients to receive either six cycles of neoadjuvant docetaxel plus prednisone and androgen deprivation followed by radical prostatectomy or radical prostatectomy alone.

A series of studies conducted at M. D. Anderson Cancer Center expanded the concept of local control with surgery to more advanced disease states as part of an integrated treatment strategy for patients with more advanced cancers. Although the patients did not meet accepted criteria for prostatectomy, they were at risk for pelvic and urinary-outlet obstructive symptoms. No attempt has been made to date to establish the efficacy of this approach in large patient groups. A benefit of this approach is that it has provided relevant human prostate cancer to generate or test new hypotheses. The preoperative platform adds to the evidence that sonic hedgehog signaling is a therapy target for prostate cancer and can be therapeutically modulated in vivo.[185] These findings have prompted the further study of agents that inhibit sonic hedgehog signaling in the therapy of prostate cancer. In addition, we suggest that stromal-epithelial interacting pathways implicated in prostate cancer progression within the primary tumor are also those central to its progression in bone.[186] The clinical reasoning used to integrate surgery in patients with locally advanced cancers has been extended to patients with castrate-resistant progression, primarily in the case of prostates with "oligometastatic" cancer.[187] Taken together, these clinical observations establish feasibility.

Postprostatectomy Radiation ■ The results of three randomized trials have now shown similar benefit for adjuvant radiation after prostatectomy for the indications of extracapsular extension, seminal vesicle involvement, and positive surgical margins, the latter being the most significant predictor of the benefit of radiation.[188-190] All three of these studies demonstrated a benefit of approximately 20 percentage points in PSA disease–free survival 4-5 years after radiation, and in the Southwest Oncology Group (SWOG) trial report, Thompson and colleagues noted a benefit of this magnitude at 10 years posttreatment as well.[189] In all of these trials, the PSA failure rate decreased by half with adjuvant radiation, compared with surgery alone. The EORTC trial also showed a decrease in clinical failure.[188] At the latest update, with a median follow-up of 11.5 years, the SWOG trial has now shown a statistically significant difference in metastasis-free survival, which was the primary study end point.[191] At 15 years after treatment, 54% of the men treated with adjuvant radiation had developed metastatic disease or died, compared with 62% treated with prostatectomy alone; this is a hazard reduction of 25% in favor of the use of adjuvant radiation. Significant improvement in overall survival in the irradiated group was also seen.[191]

As the radiation dose is increased, targeting is improved, and candidates for prostatectomy are chosen more carefully by using newer imaging techniques to rule out metastatic disease, it is likely that the benefit of adjuvant radiation will only increase in the future.

Castrate-Resistant Locally Advanced Disease

Bulky tumor located within the prostate is especially problematic in patients with castrate-resistant disease. In these men, hormonal therapy will not debulk the tumor to achieve the desired response with radiation. In patients with metastatic disease, radiation alone can serve the purpose of relieving symptoms such as hematuria or recurrent urinary obstruction. In patients with greater expected longevity, chemotherapy may be used as a debulking agent prior to or in conjunction with radiation, although the duration and degree of response has not been well documented. Alternatively, prostatec¼tomy may be feasible and will provide symptomatic relief in these patients.[192]

Algorithm for Therapy: Future Directions

To apply the most appropriate treatment strategy, it is critical that physicians use diagnostic imaging, pathology review, PSA kinetics, and tumor markers to their fullest extent in assessing the tumor and individualizing therapy. The current emphasis is on exploring combined therapies that will not only eradicate local disease but will prevent or treat distant micrometastases as well. Trials using molecular targeting agents such as tyrosine kinase inhibitors and antiangiogenic agents in combination with radiation or prostatectomy are currently under way. The doses and toxic effects of these agents must be explored, along with their molecular effects in tissue. Ideally, in the future, molecular markers will enable more precise individualized therapy, predicting tumor growth and dissemination patterns (locoregional versus distant) so that treatment can be designed to effect the best response. The molecular targets of new agents and their effects on tissue—both tumor and stroma—must be defined in detail so that therapy can be matched to the tumor's molecular characteristics. It is in this manner that an individualized, multidisciplinary approach will provide the best strategies for both local and distant disease control as we move forward.

Metastatic Prostate Cancer

Among the leading causes of cancer-related deaths worldwide, metastases from adenocarcinoma of the prostate possess a highly conserved clinical phenotype, characterized by osteoblastic bone metastases. Although morbidity and mortality from advanced disease correlate with the volume of bone metastases, notable phenotypic variants observed in approximately 10% of patients include lymph node–dominant metastases, visceral-dominant (liver or lung) metastases, and locally advanced manifestations without bone metastases. Outgrowth of neuroendocrine or small cell carcinoma is a particular phenomenon associated with prostate cancer at the initial visit or, more commonly, after lengthy periods of hormonal therapy.

At the time of diagnosis of prostate cancer, overt radiologic evidence of metastatic disease varies from 10% to 15% of men from populations among which screening for the disease is commonplace to ≥70% of men from unscreened populations. After therapy directed toward localized disease, the earliest presentation of *micrometastatic disease* is most commonly a rising PSA serum level. Given that approximately ⅓ of patients treated for localized prostate cancer will experience treatment failure, it has been estimated that nearly 70,000 men are diagnosed yearly with the *rising PSA disease state* and the prevalence in the United States may be as high as 1 million.[193]

Biochemical recurrence of prostate cancer may be defined variably after surgery,[194] ie, time to PSA ≥0.2 ng/mL with the confirmatory value of >0.2 ng/mL, or radiation therapy,[195] ie, time to PSA nadir + 2 ng/mL. Such working definitions can assist in annotating and harmonizing reportable outcomes from therapy. It is important to recognize that a rise in PSA is not an absolute indicator of malignancy, an absolute indication for therapy, or fully predictive of disease progression or disease-specific mortality. The reasons for this are (a) benign explanations for PSA rise include incomplete prostatectomy or PSA bounces after radiation therapy, (b) the disease is capable of exceptional indolence, (c) early therapy has no established efficacy in improving overall survival or quality of life, and (d) comorbidities are common in aging men (the median age at diagnosis of the rising PSA disease state is 70 years), and alternative causes of death are incrementally dominant among lower-risk rising PSA disease states.

The *long natural history* of the disease after radical prostatectomy for localized adenocarcinoma of the prostate has been described as a median time to metastases of 8 years and a median life expectancy of 13 years.[196] The investigators of one randomized study of radical prostatectomy versus watchful waiting in 695 men reported a 19% cumulative incidence of metastases at 12 years in men with clinically localized disease who had undergone surgery at the time of diagnosis, compared with a 26% incidence of metastases in men who had undergone watchful waiting, without an observable plateau.[197] Outposts of disseminated and competent tumor cells persist for very long periods in suitable microenvironmental niches such as within the bone marrow. These clones are thought to remain clinically undetectable in dormant nonproliferative states or in balanced proliferative-apoptotic states before undergoing angiogenic switching to emerge as clinically detectable metastases.[198]

Using PSA doubling time, time to biochemical failure from surgery, and the histologic Gleason grade, for instance, different metastasis-free and overall survival outcomes can be estimated. For example, men with high-grade disease (Gleason score 8-10) and evidence of biochemical failure within 2 years of surgery have a 70% probability of developing metastases in 5 years,[196] and those with PSA doubling times of <3 months have a probability of prostate cancer–specific mortality of nearly 50% within 5 years.[199] In contrast, men with very long PSA doubling times (≥15 months) have prostate cancer–specific mortality rates of no greater than 10% at 10 years.[199] In younger patients, such as those with projected life expectancies of 15 years or longer, the predictive values of such PSA kinetics are less certain, and continued monitoring remains necessary.

Because the median age at diagnosis of men who have the rising PSA disease state is in their eighth decade, the integration of biomarkers of the lethal phenotype of the disease with the effects of aging and medical comorbidity into predictive models of life expectancy remains a significant challenge.[200,201] Biomarkers that can link the heterogeneous phenotype of metastatic disease to specific therapeutic strategies are required.

Diagnosis

A diagnosis of metastatic prostate cancer may be suspected with the emergence of symptoms or signs of the disease or with a rapidly rising and/or markedly elevated PSA concentration.

Symptoms and Signs of Metastatic Disease

The emergence of bone pain is perhaps the most common symptom of metastatic prostate cancer. Correctly diagnosing the cause of the pain is critical. A change in the character, location, and severity of preexisting "arthritis" pain, for example, should arouse suspicion. Malignant bone pain is usually unremitting and worsens over time. Base-of-skull syndromes can manifest as occipital pain or cranial nerve palsy; the sixth and twelfth nerves are frequently affected. Mental neuropathy presents as chin numbness related to unilateral or bilateral mandibular infiltration and compression of the vulnerable inferior alveolar nerve. A concomitant finding of exquisite sternal tenderness caused by replacement of the bone marrow with high-volume disease is reminiscent of acute leukemia. Referred pain from malignant nerve-root impingements can mimic benign disease; for example, L2 pain can be mistaken for degenerative disease of the hip, and lower thoracic root impingement, as an acute abdomen. The Lhermitte sign may signal spinal cord impingement. Back pain can result from bulky retroperitoneal adenopathy rather than from spinal metastases. On bone scans, benign disease such as vertebral compression fractures from osteoporosis, severe degenerative disease, and Paget's disease of the bone can mimic malignant progression.

The emergence of cough, shortness of breath, and interstitial perihilar infiltrates on chest x-ray suggests lymphangitic spread of disease; infection caused by *Pneumocystis carinii* is rare in men with prostate cancer, even those with long-term steroid exposure. Lung metastases are rarely the sole manifestation of distant disease; lung nodules and pleural effusions are other pulmonary manifestations. High-volume lung metastases, although unusual, should raise the suspicion of concomitant brain metastases. Liver metastases usually remain asymptomatic. High-volume liver metastases, lytic bone disease, and brain metastases can imply the presence of neuroendocrine or small cell carcinoma.

Local progression in the intact or irradiated prostate may be the dominant manifestation of advancing disease, and DRE is a surprisingly neglected diagnostic tool. Late emergence of irritative or obstructive urinary symptoms after radiation, rectal urgency, a change in stool caliber, or perineal pain suggests failure of local control and invasion of local structures. Lymphedema results from infiltration of regional lymphatics and can be particularly debilitating. Invasion of the base of the bladder can result in obstruction of the bladder outlet or ureter (with resultant hydronephrosis and renal failure), hematuria, and recurrent infections. Penile and scrotal metastases are less common.

Radiologic Studies ■ Radiologic studies that are most useful for staging metastatic disease include radionuclide bone scanning and CT of the abdomen and pelvis. A chest x-ray can identify less common pulmonary manifestations, and CT of the chest is occasionally useful to further characterize small pulmonary nodules, the presence of mediastinal lymphadenopathy, or lymphangitic disease. CT-guided needle biopsies are occasionally required to diagnose indeterminate lesions, but sampling errors and false negatives such as with small bone lesions remain a problem; follow-up is usually required to properly resolve the diagnostic question. MRI is useful for defining the presence of metastatic disease in bony lesions that are indeterminate on bone scans or plain x-rays, screening for suspected spinal cord compression or brain metastases, and evaluating the extent of infiltrative locally advanced disease in the pelvis. Positron-emission tomography and indium-labeled capromab penditide (ProstaScint, Cytogen Corporation, Princeton, NJ) imaging require further development with respect to sensitivity and specificity for metastatic disease and cannot be routinely recommended at this time.

Pathologic Studies ■ Pathologic studies to confirm a diagnosis of metastatic disease may include immunohistochemical testing for PSA and PAP expression; for example, PSA expression may be lost

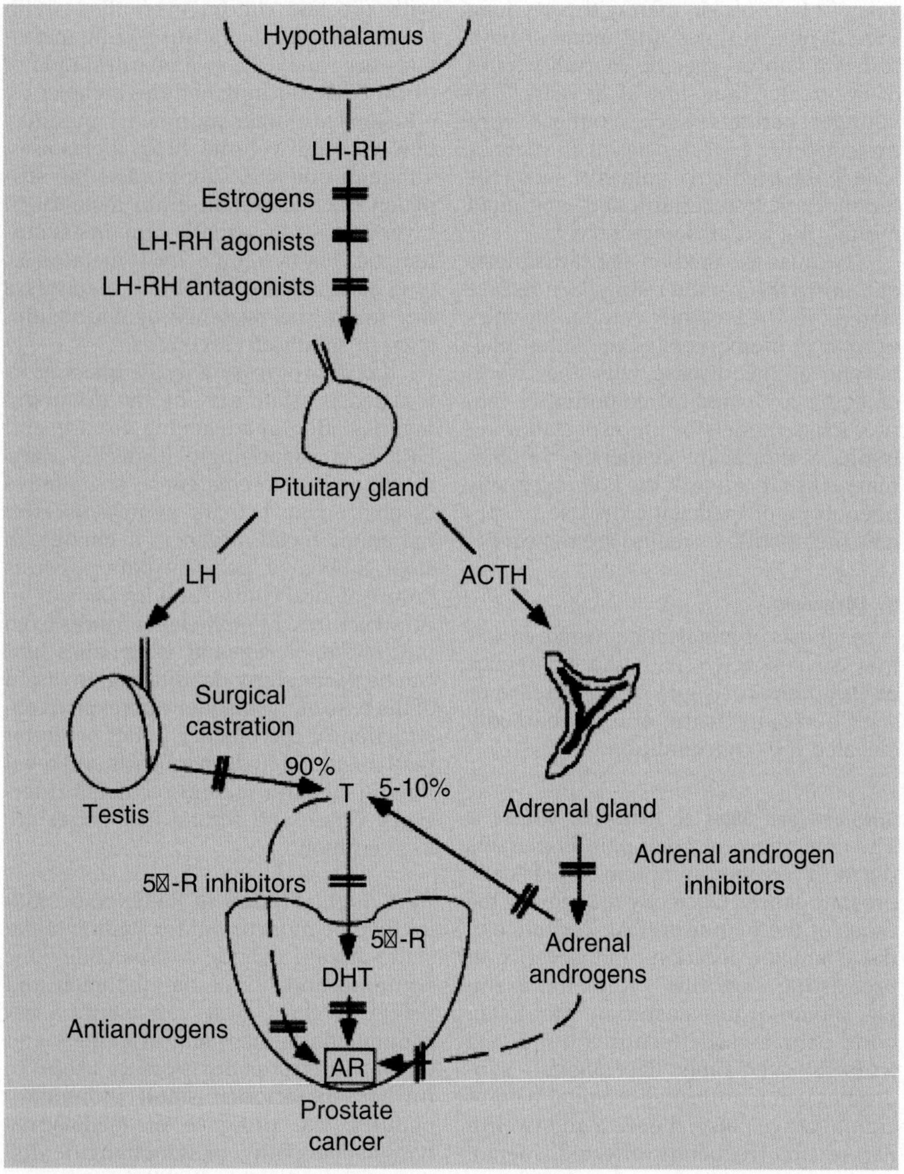

Figure 94-8 ■ Hormonal axis and therapeutic agents in prostate cancer. *Abbreviations*: LHRH, luteinizing hormone–releasing hormone; LH, luteinizing hormone; ACTH, adrenocorticotropin; AR, androgen receptor; DHT, dihydrotestosterone; 5α-R, 5-alpha-reductase. *Source*: From Ref. 203.

with androgen-deprivation therapy. In the future, molecular evidence of characteristic fusion genes may help resolve indeterminate cases. Men who have a markedly elevated serum PSA concentration (eg, >100 ng/mL) and a typical metastatic phenotype such as osteoblastic bone metastases at diagnosis rarely require a biopsy to confirm the presence of metastatic disease.

Currently Used Therapies

Hormonal Therapy ■ Since the discovery of the hormonal biology of prostate cancer,[202] hormonal therapy has been the mainstay in the control of advanced disease. Current therapies are directed toward lowering the concentrations of circulating androgens by surgical or medical castration therapy or by pharmacologic blockade of the binding of androgens to their receptor in target tissue[203] (Fig. 94-8). A combination of surgical and medical castration and androgen-receptor blockade, referred to as combined androgen blockade, may yield additional benefits[204] in subsets of patients still to be defined. Data supporting the integration of 5α-reductase inhibitors, which inhibit the conversion of testosterone to dihydrotestosterone, with combined androgen blockade, referred to as triple androgen blockade, are similarly limited. More effective antagonism of the androgen receptor such as with an avidly binding antagonist lacking partial agonist activity (eg, MDV3100) or more selective and potent inhibitors of androgen synthesis (eg, abiraterone acetate) are examples of novel hormonal approaches currently being investigated in phase I-III clinical trials.

In men with the rising PSA disease state, there is no evidence that the early application of hormonal therapy—before the emergence of metastases—improves overall survival or quality of life. The demonstration of improved survival with the integration of hormonal therapy and radiation therapy for high-risk localized disease[205,206] likely relates to improved local control and a decrease in a late wave of metastases from the primary[207] tumor rather than to the control of micrometastatic disease. In contrast, in a small study of immediate adjuvant versus deferred hormonal therapy for node-positive disease after radical prostatectomy, poorer than expected outcomes with hormonal therapy in the deferred-therapy arm[208] suggested that as in the antecedent Medical Research Council trial of immediate versus deferred hormonal therapy in metastatic disease,[209] late application of hormonal therapy results in inferior outcomes in some studies. There is a critical dearth of high-quality studies examining the role of hormonal therapy in the high-risk postoperative adjuvant setting or the rising PSA disease state in the overall survival and quality-of-life end points.

Complications of hormonal therapy[210] include hot flashes, weight gain, diminished libido and energy level, insomnia, mood and intellectual impairment, osteoporosis, sarcopenia, and acceleration of the metabolic syndrome or cardiovascular disease. Some part of these complications attributed to hormonal therapy, such as neurocognitive effects, may also relate to aging and the debilitating effects of advanced disease.[211] Monotherapy with nonsteroidal antiandrogens (eg, high-dose bicalutamide) may yield survival outcomes equivalent to those produced by medical castration in low-risk disease[212] but with lesser effects on bone mass, muscle strength, and libido.[213] Intermittent castration therapy with LHRH agonists reduces the cost and morbidity of therapy with no known adverse (or beneficial) effects in terms of duration of disease control; mature results from several randomized phase III trials are awaited.[214]

In men with either the rising PSA disease state or metastatic disease, the decline in PSA with castration therapy yields a nadir value that may be prognostically useful.[215,216] A nadir PSA >4 ng/mL in men with metastatic disease after 7 months of hormonal therapy was associated with a median overall survival of 13 months in contrast to a median survival of 75 months with a nadir PSA of ≤0.2 ng/mL.[216] (Fig. 94-9) These data suggest that a lethal phenotype can be identified in this manner for early intervention with experimental strategies.

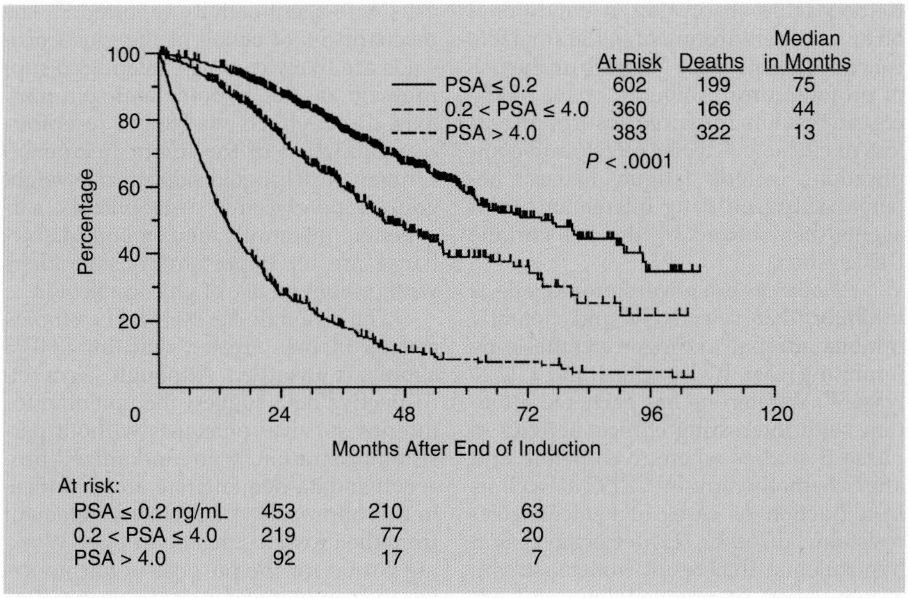

Figure 94-9 ■ Absolute PSA nadir after 7 months of hormonal therapy and median survival outcomes: PSA nadir > 4.0 ng/mL identifies a group with dire prognosis for early experimental therapeutics. *Source*: From Ref. 216.

To date, randomized studies in newly diagnosed metastatic disease have not identified a survival or quality-of-life benefit for early versus deferred introduction of chemotherapy combined with hormonal therapy.[217] Thus, the use of chemohormonal therapy in this setting remains experimental.

Nonhormonal Therapy ■ No convincing evidence supports the value of chemotherapy in treating hormone-naïve prostate cancer. A range of nonhormonal therapeutic agents, including vaccines, immunomodulators, angiogenesis and signal-transduction inhibitors, and differentiation agents have been legitimately studied in the rising PSA disease state and in asymptomatic metastatic disease. These settings have particular trial design challenges, including the lack of validated early surrogate end points for survival. To date, there is no evidence that a nonhormonal therapy has a major influence on the natural history of the disease.

Castrate-Resistant Disease

Durations of hormonal control vary from 6 years in men without metastases[217] to 18 months in men with metastatic disease.[218] When evidence of progressive disease emerges in the context of low serum concentrations of testosterone, by consensus <50 ng/dL,[219] the term *castrate-resistant prostate cancer* (CRPC) may be preferable to "hormone-refractory" or "androgen-independent" prostate cancer.[220] These tumors are often responsive to alternative hormonal therapeutic agents and hence are not strictly hormone refractory. Because persistent signaling via a "supersensitive" androgen receptor may occur despite the serum levels of testosterone after castration, they are often not truly androgen independent, either.

Prognosis

Few study reports have described the prognosis for men with CRPC defined by a rising PSA concentration alone. Observations from the placebo arm of a randomized controlled trial of zoledronic acid (201 men with castrate levels of serum testosterone, rising PSA values, and no evidence of bone metastases) demonstrated the potentially lengthy time to development of bone metastases, particularly in men with low PSA values and long PSA doubling times.[221] Overall, the risk of bone metastases in this cohort was 33% at 2 years, and the median bone metastasis–free interval was 30 months. More than 50% of the men with PSA doubling times of <6 months developed bone metastases within 18 months, whereas only 40% of those with PSA doubling times of >18 months had developed bone metastases within 3 years.

Although the median overall survival time in asymptomatic CRPC without metastases is 4 years, the prognosis of men with metastatic CRPC varies between symptomatic[222,223] and asymptomatic[224] disease and ranges from 9 to 23 months, respectively. Several predictive nomograms incorporate a range of easily determined clinical and biochemical parameters to predict 12- and 24-month overall survival rates.[225-227] A model that incorporated PSA doubling time, time to PSA progression after initiation of castration therapy, and presence of metastatic disease at the time of CRPC transition defined three prognostic groups to predict clinical progression or event-free survival (EFS)[227]: a low-risk group defined solely by a PSA doubling time of >10 months (median EFS 96 months); an intermediate-risk group with a PSA doubling time of <10 months and a time to PSA progression of >13 months (median EFS 33 months); and a high-risk group defined by a PSA doubling time of ≤10 months, the presence of metastatic disease at progression from androgen-dependent prostate cancer to CRPC transition, and a time to PSA progression of ≤13 months (median EFS 6 months).

Given these evident variations in the natural history of CRPC, there is clearly a need for reliable prognostic models both for routine clinical practice and for accrual stratification and reporting in clinical trials. Interpretations of differences in survival outcomes in clinical trials must take into account the potential effect of such variations, which may be incompletely accounted for by strategies of randomization and prognostic stratification.

Management of CRPC ■ A key principle in the management of CRPC is to balance the limitations of benefit of therapies and the variable threat of the disease. Current therapies can serve to control the disease by improving symptoms, reducing specific morbidity, and improving quality of life as well as overall survival time. CRPC occurs in an older population of men, with a median age of >72 years. The burden of androgen-deprivation syndrome, medical comorbidities, and attendant polypharmacy influences therapeutic choices.

Secondary Hormonal Therapy ■ Responses to secondary hormonal therapies are explained by the incompletely defined endocrine mechanisms that drive the progression of CRPC via the persistently expressed androgen receptor or androgen receptor–bypass pathways. No existing data formally quantify the quality-of-life or overall-survival benefit of second-line hormonal therapy compared with observation.

In general, the median duration of progression-free survival for an unselected population treated with secondary hormonal therapy is <6 months.[228,229] Although prognostic variables that define the frequency and duration of response among the various secondary hormonal therapies have not been determined, responses can be rewardingly prolonged for men with indolent profiles of castrate-resistant progression in particular. In contrast, men with short durations of primary hormonal control and with suboptimal PSA nadir response and rapid PSA doubling times are less likely to experience a prolonged response to secondary hormonal therapies. On a practical level, the choice of a secondary hormonal therapy in CRPC is influenced by details of prior hormonal therapy, comorbidity, and the risk of drug interactions.

A small but significant fraction of men with progressive CRPC given concurrent antiandrogen therapy will experience a 50% drop in PSA and objective regression of disease with *antiandrogen withdrawal* alone; this phenomenon has been described across the broad spectrum of steroidal and nonsteroidal antiandrogen agents. Estimates of the frequency and duration of the antiandrogen withdrawal response (AAWR) have varied, but the single largest prospective study of nonsteroidal antiandrogen agent (bicalutamide, flutamide, or nilutamide) withdrawal (n = 132) demonstrated a PSA decline by half in 11%, an objective response in 2%, and a median time to PSA progression of 6 months.[230] The mechanism of the AAWR is unknown as yet, although partial agonist activity of antiandrogens or androgen receptor mutations that confer agonist activity to antiandrogens have been posited to explain this phenomenon. Mutations of the androgen receptor were found in 10% of bone metastases, and these did not correlate with the AAWR.[231] Withdrawal responses have also been described with steroidal antiandrogens, including the progestins and glucocorticoids. These data suggest that the AAWR observation has yet to be fully elucidated and may be more complex than initially anticipated.

The probability of response to *deferred nonsteroidal antiandrogen therapy* in men receiving LHRH-agonist monotherapy has been linked to adverse PSA kinetics. Interestingly, progression of CRPC during therapy with one antiandrogen does not preclude a sequential response to another agent, although responses to sequential antiandrogen therapies appear to be linked to the probability of response to the first intervention.

High doses of the azole antifungal agent *ketoconazole* (400 mg 3 times daily) may function to enhance the effects of castration by ablating synthesis of adrenal androgens, themselves weak ligands of the androgen receptor but also a source of testosterone. Ketoconazole may also have direct cytotoxic effects on prostate cancer cells. Glucocorticoid replacement (eg, with 5 mg of prednisone 2 times daily or 30-40 mg of hydrocortisone daily) is required because iatrogenic adrenal insufficiency results from the use of ketoconazole. Ketoconazole also has detectable efficacy with low doses (200 mg 3 times daily), at which level glucocorticoid replacement is usually unnecessary. Ketoconazole absorption is conditional on an acidic environment in the stomach; concomitant atrophic gastritis or the use of proton-pump inhibitors or H2 blockers can result in impaired absorption and loss of efficacy. Adverse effects and complications include fatigue, nausea, hepatotoxicity, and drug interactions with agents metabolized by the cytochrome P450 system.

Abiraterone is a novel steroidogenesis inhibitor that selectively and potently inhibits adrenal androgen synthesis by inhibiting 17-α hydroxylase and C17,20 lyase.[232] Abiraterone has garnered attention, with interesting clinical activity in phase II studies when given before and after chemotherapy in CRPC as well as in a fraction of cases of ketoconazole-resistant disease. Hypertension and hypokalemia that result from upstream accumulation of pregnenolone and adrenocorticotropic hormone can be suppressed with prednisone supplementation. An ongoing large phase III trial compares abiraterone with prednisone, which has weak single-agent activity in CRPC, and excludes patients who have had prior ketoconazole exposure.

Estrogens have long been known to possess activity in prostate cancer, due at least in part to their castration effects. In the control of advanced disease, DES has demonstrated efficacy equal to that of LHRH agonist therapy, but DES has come into disrepute because of its well-documented thrombotic and cardiac complications, particularly with daily doses >3 mg. The efficacy of oral DES in lower doses, ranging from 1 to 3 mg daily,[233,234] as a single agent has been described without clear evidence of a dose-response relationship. The mechanism of action of DES has not been fully established, and correlations of response with tissue markers, such as estrogen receptor status, have not been made. Thrombotic complications of DES persist even with low doses; concomitant therapy with low-dose warfarin and enteric-coated aspirin or low–molecular weight heparin may offer prophylactic benefit. DES-related gynecomastia can be particularly troublesome, and prophylactic breast irradiation is recommended prior to initiation of therapy.

Progestins, including medroxyprogesterone and megestrol acetate, are rarely used because their efficacy appears to be minimal and their toxic effects include weight gain and thrombotic risks. Another progestin, cyproterone acetate, is not approved for use within the United States.

Glucocorticoids as single agents have modest activity in CRPC. The different glucocorticoids have not been compared directly, but dexamethasone in low doses (0.75 mg twice daily) has among the highest single-agent activity reported.[235] The mechanisms of action of the glucocorticoids are likely complex, relating to suppression of the hypothalamic-pituitary axis, direct effects via steroid receptors, or modulation of the tumor microenvironment. Cushingoid side effects, weight gain, hyperglycemia, osteoporosis, sarcopenia, insomnia, and mood disturbance are all important considerations with prolonged use of glucocorticoids.

The rationale for *continued castration therapy* in men treated with an LHRH agonist is unsettled. Although select retrospective data suggest the potential for inferior survival outcomes without persistent castration,[236] no randomized prospective data demonstrate an advantage to this approach. A consensus statement from the Prostate-Specific Antigen Working Group for the purpose of harmonizing the conduct of clinical trials in CRPC recommended maintenance of a castrate level of testosterone of <50 ng/dL.[219] The value of *orchiectomy* in men receiving LHRH agonist therapy is similarly unknown but is likely to be negligible or of short duration.

Serum testosterone levels of >50 ng/dL in men treated with optimal doses of LHRH agonist therapy or after orchiectomy are usually associated with low levels of free serum testosterone. Sex hormone–binding globulin elevations may yield spuriously elevated total testosterone concentrations; low doses of dexamethasone are usually effective in further suppressing such testosterone levels. However, rare instances of acquired LHRH-agonist resistance have been described, likely related to immunologic mechanisms; these cases emphasize the need for periodic monitoring of serum testosterone concentration.

In contrast to these considerations, PSA decreases and objective responses to *testosterone therapy* in prostate cancer have been described, a further reminder that a deeper understanding of the steroid-regulated biology of prostate cancer is necessary.[237]

Nonhormonal Therapy ■ As is the case with hormone-naïve metastatic disease, various nonhormonal therapeutic agents are being evaluated in clinical trials for use in asymptomatic or lower-risk CRPC in lieu of secondary hormonal therapy or chemotherapy. Experimental therapeutic agents in lower-risk settings are justified given the demonstrably limited benefits of standard chemotherapy.

Chemotherapy ■ Although there has been long-standing nihilism with regard to the role of chemotherapy in CRPC,[238] in the last few years, the results of two large phase III trials have demonstrated *overall-survival*[239,240] and *quality-of-life*[240]

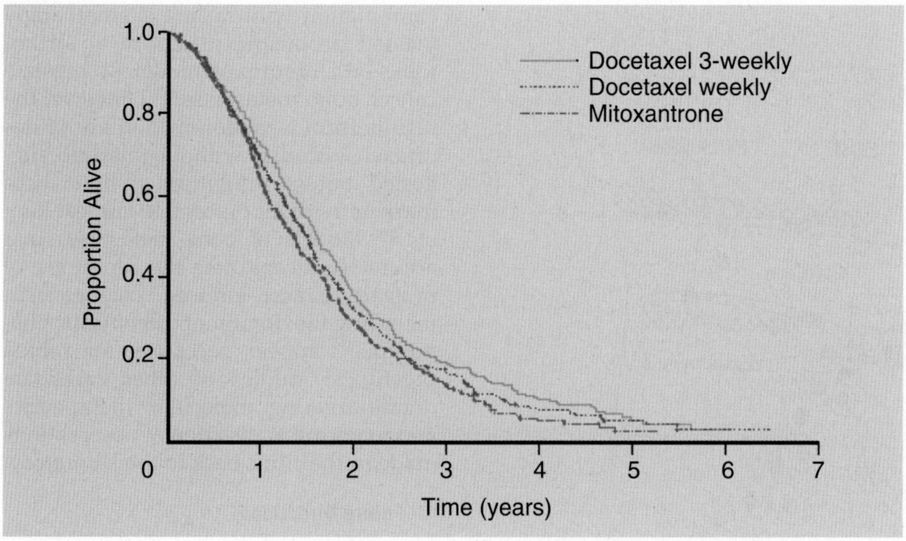

Figure 94-10 Updated results from TAX 327. Survival benefits are modest with docetaxel chemotherapy: median survival remains under 2 years, and an understanding of biologic subsets that benefit from therapy is required. *Source*: From Ref. 270.

advantages with docetaxel-based therapy compared with mitoxantrone plus prednisone (MP) therapy.

MP therapy with 12 mg/m^2 of mitoxantrone at 3-week intervals and and 5 mg of prednisone given twice daily was approved for use in the United States by the Food and Drug Association on the basis of greater pain relief with that regimen than with that achieved using prednisone monotherapy in symptomatic CRPC; however, no survival advantage for MP therapy was demonstrated in these studies.[222,223] In another study, the SWOG used treatment with 60 mg/m^2 of docetaxel given every 21 days plus 280 mg of estramustine given three times daily for 5 consecutive days and compared that regimen with treatment with MP; the results demonstrated an increase in progression-free survival from 3 to 6 months and an improvement in median survival by 2 months with the MP regimen.[239] In addition, the toxic effects attributed to estramustine were clinically significant, and the patients' quality of life was not improved.

In the multinational TAX 327 trial, a regimen of 10 mg of prednisone daily plus 30 mg/m^2 of docetaxel given weekly for 5 of 6 weeks and a regimen of 10 mg of prednisone daily plus 75 mg/m^2 of docetaxel given every 3 weeks were compared with a regimen of 10 mg of prednisone daily plus 12 mg of mitoxantrone given every 3 weeks.[240] A statistically significant improvement in median survival time similar to that in the SWOG trial (ie, 2 months) was described for the every-3--week schedule of docetaxel compared with the MP regimen[241] (Fig. 94-10). Similar improvement in PSA decline rates, pain response, and global quality of life were reported for the two dosing schedules of docetaxel compared with those resulting from the MP regimen; in contrast, objective responses were infrequent and no different in the three groups. Progression-free survival outcomes for the individual arms were not described.

The results from these studies prompted the U.S. Food and Drug Administration to approve a regimen of daily prednisone plus 75 mg/m^2 of docetaxel given every 3 weeks for the treatment of CRPC. These findings have also provided the necessary impetus for the further development of systemic therapeutic agents for CRPC to affect patients' overall survival time and quality of life.

When should patients with CRPC be offered chemotherapy? The optimum timing of initiation of chemotherapy in men with CRPC is still undetermined. Given its relative ease of administration and cost, secondary hormonal therapy is a reasonable choice for use in asymptomatic or minimally symptomatic patients, those with low burdens of metastatic disease, and those with rising PSA concentrations with adverse kinetics. Observation alone is reasonable for men with indolent PSA kinetics and/or no evidence of metastatic disease. In men with symptomatic CRPC, though, docetaxel chemotherapy is preferable to existing secondary hormonal therapeutic agents, given the data demonstrating the survival and quality-of-life benefits of docetaxel. When a single site of disease is dominant and symptomatic in a threatened area such as the spinal column or weight-bearing bone, the use of palliative radiation therapy is reasonable to secure this area before the initiation of chemotherapy. Asymptomatic patients with widespread disease should also be considered for docetaxel-based chemotherapy.

The *optimal duration* of chemotherapy in CRPC is also undetermined. Continued treatment to two cycles beyond the best response followed by observation is reasonable and commonly used because cumulative fatigue is common with docetaxel-based therapy. Intermittent chemotherapy with a view toward retaining control and providing interrupted therapy for quality-of-life purposes has been described,[242] but the drug holidays become progressively shorter as drug resistance invariably emerges. In addition, the role of maintenance chemotherapy in patients with a stable response is uncertain, and its use must be balanced against emergent toxicity.

The *limits of benefit* of chemotherapy are clear with docetaxel and with all other cytotoxic agents reported to date. Improvements in survival are tangible, but although they are comparable to those obtained in breast cancer, they remain modest. Another limitation is that therapeutic agents can be expensive and toxic, and the disease is still incurable, with few long-term survivors beyond 5 years.

Second-line therapy, used after treatment with docetaxel fails, has not been standardized, and for such patients, participation in a clinical trial should be strongly considered.[243] MP therapy has been considered the de facto standard after docetaxel fails, but the results observed to date have been discouraging, with 50% PSA decreases of only approximately 10%. The results with the use of the epothilones have been similarly discouraging, with taxane resistance. Combination mitoxantrone-epothilone studies are under way, but alternative strategies in the second-line setting are needed. When assessing therapeutic options for a patient whose disease is taxane resistant, unexplored secondary hormonal maneuvers should be considered.

Consistent with the data that the *microtubule* is an important target in CRPC, *paclitaxel* has also demonstrated significant activity when given weekly as a single agent as well as in several estramustine-containing combinations.[244-246] Cross-resistance between docetaxel and paclitaxel may be incomplete, but formal crossover studies have not been done. Similarly, other antitubule agents such as vinblastine, navelbine, and the epothilones have been studied, but the data thus far do not suggest major incremental advantages with their use. Oral cyclophosphamide given in chronic schedules has demonstrable activity in CRPC and is an alkylator-based approach, distinct from the approaches with the taxanes and anthracyclines described to date.[247,248] Etoposide[249] and carboplatin[250] have also been integrated into combination regimens in CRPC. It is highly unlikely that

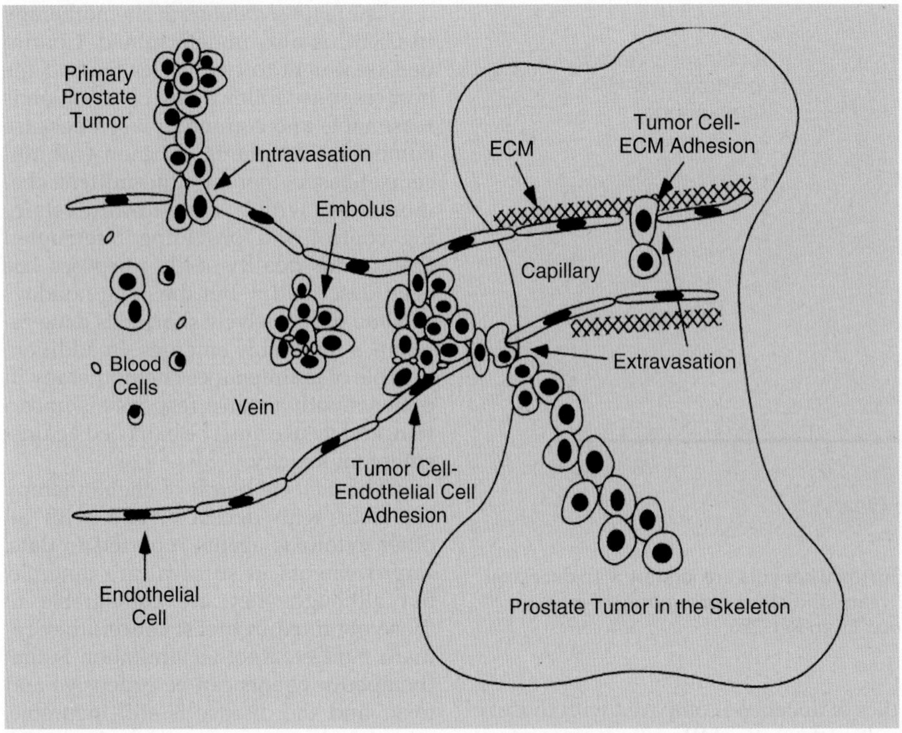

Figure 94-11 ■ The multistage process of metastases: the pathophysiology of early events in the metastatic cascade, undetected dormant micrometastatic disease, and proliferative disease in the bone microenvironment are likely regulated by distinctive events with differing implications for therapy. *Source*: From Ref. 251.

any of these agents will be formally studied for benefit in the future.

The Importance of Bone ■ The specific epithelial-stromal interactions that define the typical metastatic phenotype of prostate cancer are of critical interest. A mechanistic definition of the pathways to bone metastases, including epithelial-stromal interactions[251] (Fig. 94-11) may yield a therapeutic approach that can successfully modulate the natural history of the disease. Given that the dominant morbidity and mortality from the disease can be traced to bone metastases, an organ-targeting strategy has long been of interest to the field. The hallmark pathologic feature of advanced disease in bone is desmoplastic infiltration by carcinoma cells with robust proliferation of osteoblasts, voluminous woven bone, and scattered osteoclasts. There is intense research interest in modeling the early events of disease progression, including understanding the components and determinant physiologic characteristics of a putative metastatic niche in bone.

The principles of selective uptake in bone and prolonged retention of radiopharmaceutical agents at sites of increased bone mineral turnover guided initial studies of bone targeting in advanced prostate cancer. The natural affinity of the *radioisotope* strontium chloride Sr 89 (half-life 50 days) for bone, on the basis of its strong homology with calcium, and the phosphonate-coupled samarium Sm 153 (halflife 1.9 days) permit delivery of medium-energy β emitters to the tumor–bone matrix interface.[252] These agents offer a palliative option,[253] and observations of a survival benefit in CRPC with consolidative radioisotope therapy after the initial response to chemotherapy[254] have sparked further interest in an organ-directed approach.

Evidence of increased markers of bone resorption in cases of CRPC with bone metastases has justified the study of osteoclast-inhibitory bisphosphonates.[255] A large randomized phase III trial evaluating zoledronic acid in men with CRPC receiving concomitant chemotherapy demonstrated a reduction in bone pain and "skeletal-related events" with the use of this highly potent bisphosphonate.[256] The RANK (receptor activator of nuclear factor κB) ligand antibody denosumab has demonstrated promising activity in reducing bone lysis markers in men with progressive CRPC treated with zoledronic acid. Randomized phase III studies comparing zoledronic acid and denosumab in CRPC are in progress.

Several lines of evidence implicate the platelet-derived growth factor receptor (PDGFR) in the progression of disease in bone. Preclinical studies with the PDGFR inhibitor imatinib mesylate in combination with taxane chemotherapy yielded promising results in an orthotopic lytic-dominant model of prostate cancer bone metastases.[257] However, the results from a randomized study of docetaxel with and without imatinib suggested potent inhibition of bone lysis markers without detectable clinical benefit.[258] Models of bone metastases that accurately recapitulate the repertoire of prostate cancer–induced osteogenesis, including the dominant osteoblastic phenotype,[259] appear necessary for robust preclinical studies of other candidate organ-targeting molecular therapeutics and to permit translation of observations made in the clinic back to the laboratory.

Future Directions

The substantial limits of the efficacy of contemporary cytotoxic or available bone-targeting therapies in CRPC are known or predictable. It is highly unlikely that novel combinations, doses, or schedules of these agents will meaningfully transform the outcome of prostate cancer in patients. A deeper understanding of the molecular pathways involved in disease progression is now the necessary basis for reassessing our perspectives about the disease and for advancing the exploration of novel therapeutic approaches. In this regard, novel strategies need to exploit the unique biology of the malignant epithelial cell—its angiogenic, inflammatory, and immunologic microenvironment—and the physical and chemical components of the inorganic matrix that determine survival and progression of disease.

Current perspectives targeting the epithelial cell are centered on the *androgen receptor–dependent and -independent pathways of disease progression.*[260] Evidence that tissue androgens exist and androgen receptor signaling occurs despite medical castration[261] has justified continued androgen receptor targeting in castrate-resistant disease.[262] Androgen receptor inactivation, whether by reducing or eliminating ligand synthesis, blocking the ligand–receptor interaction, enhancing degradation of the receptor, inhibiting androgen receptor nuclear translocation, or interfering with the interaction between the androgen receptor and androgen-response elements,[248] may spare putative AR-negative stem cells that perpetuate the disease.[260] Autopsy series have demonstrated the heterogeneity of AR expression with 40% of metastatic sites expressing <10% AR by immunohistochemistry.[263] The frequent inactivation of the PTEN tumor suppressor in high-grade disease with activation of the *PI3-kinase/Akt signaling and downstream cell survival and proliferation pathways* is currently a dominant theme in the framework of defining the lethal molecular phenotype.[264] Therapeutic agents targeting the AR and PI3-kinase/Akt signaling pathways are currently in trials. A high frequency of *novel gene fusions* in primary prostate cancer specimens was reported in 2005.[265] A 5' untranslated region of a TMPRSS2 gene is fused to a 3' ETS-1 family member in most specimens studied to date. These and other novel fusion genes have thus far been found only in malignant epithelial cells across all Gleason grades. The fusions appear nonrandom and are largely exclusive within each individual tumor across all tumor foci. The 5' TMPRSS2 region contains an androgen-responsive promoter element, which also suggests that this gene fusion is a central biologic event in the progression of the disease. However, even if this were proven, because genomic events downstream and independent of the fusion gene or genes may drive later-stage disease, and these fusion genes are transcription factors that have hitherto been difficult to target, important therapeutic obstacles may exist.

An emerging understanding of shared and unique determinants of *vascular biology* of tumors has led to studies targeting the vasculature of CRPC. The addition of the vascular endothelial growth factor (VEGF) antibody bevacizumab to docetaxel in CRPC is under study in a phase III trial. Preclinical observation of *bone-specific* modifications of tumor vascular endothelial PDGFR activation[257] led to studies of PDGFR inhibitors in combination with chemotherapy in CRPC with bone metastases.[258] Thalidomide possesses antiangiogenic activity, and the results of a randomized phase II trial of docetaxel with thalidomide have suggested the potential for improved response and survival outcomes.[266] Although inhibitors of VEGF, PDGF, and epidermal growth-factor receptor signaling have not demonstrated notable single-agent activity to date, combined VEGF and PDGF receptor inhibition with sunitinib has demonstrated modest single-agent activity. It has been surmised that perhaps <10% of the molecular determinants of neoplastic angiogenesis have been discovered to date. Novel discovery platforms such as in vivo injection, recovery, and characterization of phage-bound peptide sequences binding to tissue-specific endothelial "vascular addresses"[267] may lead to novel antivascular therapeutic agents.

The broad scope of *immunotherapeutic* strategies in CRPC includes efforts to integrate the innate and adaptive immune response using vaccine strategies and immune adjuvant. The use of agents that can block negative regulatory components of the physiologic immune response, tumor-associated angiogenesis, may modulate the host response to the therapeutic benefit of patients. Although current vaccine approaches have not yielded major antitumor activity in phase II settings, the results of phase III trials with survival end points are awaited.[268]

The specific role of *stromal* components of the disease remains poorly understood. Experimental evidence suggesting that targeting osteoclasts with potent bisphosphonates such as zoledronic acid[255] or PDGFR inhibitors[258] has not changed the natural history of the advanced disease prototype. However, a large randomized adjuvant trial of zoledronic acid in high-risk localized disease is in progress, and the clinical results may revise these perspectives. RANK-ligand inactivation with denosumab or Src inactivation with dasatinib may further enhance osteoclast targeting. Because osteoblasts may play a major role supporting progression in bone[269] and fibroblast growth factor inhibition has demonstrated promise in an osteoblastic model of the disease,[259] clinical trials with fibroblast growth factor inhibitors are planned.

Similarly, the precise role of the inorganic matrix and how *tumor-matrix interactions*, such as those mediated by integrins, selectins, and cadherins, determine survival of malignant epithelial cells and disease progression, particularly in bone, remain incompletely understood. These are also under study as therapy targets.

Summary Perspectives

We have barely scratched the surface of understanding the biology of CRPC and its metastatic behavior. Important advances in the field await in turn the advance of foundational insights and informative preclinical models. Patients' participation in clinical trials is vital for assessing this biology with experimental agents and achieving incremental progress with novel therapeutic agents. *The heterogeneity of virtually all known therapeutic targets* indicates that assessing biologic subsets with disproportionate benefit to specific interventions and understanding subsequent emergent resistance remains a preeminent challenge in experimental design. Acquisition of informative biomarkers is difficult, given the unique distribution of heterogeneous disease to bone; the phenotype of circulating tumor cells may vary substantially from those embedded in a metastatic environment under distinctive paracrine influences. Eliminating or controlling micrometastatic disease may require different strategies from those used in controlling clinical metastases.

Palliative Care

At no time in the management of CRPC is a focus on symptom control inappropriate. The selective and strategic use of external-beam *radiation therapy* for palliation of bone pain, spinal cord compression, and prevention of fracture is critical in the management of CRPC. Early in the course of CRPC, external-beam radiation or radioisotope therapy must be used sparingly, however, because bone marrow reserve critical for support of systemic therapy may be significantly compromised. *Palliative surgery* on the spine or long bones to prevent or manage pathologic fractures is less commonly required in CRPC than in breast cancer or myeloma. Surgical extirpation of progressive symptomatic localized CRPC can prevent the grievous burden of pelvic floor invasion. The services of a *palliative care specialist* skilled in analgesic pharmacy and the management of a range of symptoms of advanced disease such as anorexia, nausea, constipation, depression, weight loss, insomnia, and delirium can be very valuable. The rediscovery of methadone as an effective and inexpensive opioid with a well-defined safety margin has been influential on patterns of care, and it is the rare patient for whom indwelling devices such as epidural pumps are necessary for maintaining effective analgesia. Finally, facilitation of end-of-life discussions and transition to hospice care at the appropriate time is of major benefit for patients and their families.

Histologic Variants

Markers

The WHO Histological Classification of Tumors of the Prostate[270] lists more than 30 histologic variants of tumors besides acinar adenocarcinoma that can affect the prostate (Table 94-6). This section describes the three most common of those variants.

Ductal Adenocarcinomas ■ Of the epithelial tumor variants, the most common are the ductal adenocarcinomas, originally described by Melicow and Pachter[271] as endometrial carcinoma of the prostatic utricle. Once thought to arise from the verumontanum, a müllerian duct remnant, their prostatic origin has been firmly established, but the more recent controversy is centered on whether they truly represent a separate category of prostatic adenocarcinomas with a distinct biology, as opposed to a "mere morphological variant of prostatic adenocarcinoma."[273,274] Ductal adenocarcinomas of the prostate have been reported to constitute 0.13%[275] to 6.3%[276] of all prostate carcinomas. They are characterized by duct-like structures lined by single layer or pseudostratified tall columnar cells with abundant eosinophilic to amphophilic cytoplasm

Table 94-6 ■ **WHO Histologic Classification of Tumors of the Prostate**

Tumor Class	Tumor Type	Tumor Subtype
Epithelial	Glandular neoplasms	Adenocarcinoma (acinar)
		Atrophic
		Pseudohyperplastic
		Foamy
		Colloid
		Signet ring
		Oncocytic
		Lymphoepithelioma-like
		Carcinoma with spindle cell differentiation (carcinosarcoma, sarcomatoid carcinoma)
		Prostatic intraepithelial neoplasia (PIN)
		Prostatic intraepithelial neoplasia, grade III (PIN III)
		Ductal adenocarcinoma
		Cribriform
		Papillary
		Solid
	Urothelial tumors	Urothelial carcinoma
	Squamous tumors	Adenosquamous carcinoma
		Squamous cell carcinoma
	Basal cell tumors	Basal cell adenoma
		Basal cell carcinoma
Neuroendocrine tumors		Endocrine differentiation within adenocarcinoma
		Carcinoid tumor
		Small-cell carcinoma
		Paraganglioma
		Neuroblastoma
Prostatic stromal tumors		Stromal tumor of uncertain malignant potential
		Stromal sarcoma
Mesenchymal tumors		Leiomyosarcoma
		Rhabdomyosarcoma
		Chondrosarcoma
		Angiosarcoma
		Malignant fibrous histiocytoma
		Malignant peripheral nerve sheath tumor
		Hemangioma
		Chondroma
		Leiomyoma
		Granular cell tumor
		Hemangiopericytoma
		Solitary fibrous tumor

Source: Adapted from Ref. 273.

displaying a papillary, cribiform, solid, or glandular architecture.[274] Up to 20% present as pure ductal adenocarcinomas, but most cases are mixed with elements of acinar adenocarcinomas.[276-278] Ductal adenocarcinomas do not express any specific markers that differentiate them from acinar adenocarcinomas. They are strongly positive for PSA and PAP and often express alpha-methylacyl coenzyme A racemase (AMACR) and occasionally carcinoembryonic antigen (CEA).[279-281] Approximately 30% of these tumors demonstrate residual basal cells, as demonstrated by positive staining for high molecular–weight cytokeratin (HMWCK or 34betaE12) and p63.[281]

Sarcomatoid Carcinomas ■ Carcinomas of the prostate with spindle cell differentiation, also known as carcinosarcomas or sarcomatoid carcinomas, are rare tumors (with only approximately 100 cases described in the literature[282]) that are characterized by the presence of both malignant high-grade epithelial and mesenchymal components. The epithelial component consists most commonly of acinar adenocarcinoma but may consist of ductal adenocarcinoma or contain elements of small cell or squamous cell carcinoma.[283-285] In approximately two-thirds of the cases, the mesenchymal component is a nonspecific malignant spindle-cell proliferation, but in one-third, it displays specific mesenchymal elements such as those of osteosarcoma, chondrosarcoma, or rhabdomyosarcoma.[284] The adenocarcinoma components are positive for keratin, and the sarcomatoid elements are positive for vimentin. The adenocarcinoma components are also positive for PSA in approximately 75% of the cases.[283]

Neuroendocrine Tumors ■ Of the nonepithelial variants of prostate cancers, neuroendocrine tumors are the most frequently encountered. The WHO classification includes focal neuroendocrine differentiation, carcinoid tumors, and small cell neuroendocrine carcinoma under this name.[270] Focal neuroendocrine differentiation, when defined as immunohistochemical staining for neurosecretory products such as chromogranin A, serotonin, or synaptophysin, is encountered to some extent in almost all cases of acinar adenocarcinoma[286] and appears to increase during treatment with androgen deprivation.[287,288]

Small Cell Carcinomas ■ Only 0.5-2% of clinical prostate tumor specimens contain small cell carcinomas, but 12-20% of cases in autopsy series have revealed small cell carcinoma in the context of acinar adenocarcinoma.[289-291] Between 42% and 75% of the clinical cases are preceded by a diagnosis of acinar adenocarcinoma, and mixed elements of high-grade acinar adenocarcinoma are present in 33-74% of the cases.[292-296]

Small cell carcinomas of the prostate are characterized by small round to spindle-shaped malignant cells displaying scanty cytoplasm, with hyperchromatic nuclei, coarse (salt-and-pepper) chromatin, nuclear molding, and absent or inconspicuous nucleoli. These cells are arranged in sheets with frequent necrosis and a high mitotic rate.[297] Most but not all small cell carcinomas stain positively for cytokeratin AE1/AE3 and CAM 5.2 (with a characteristic cytoplasmic dot-like pattern), as well as for neuroendocrine markers such as synaptophysin, chromogranin A, neuron-specific enolase, bombesin, and CD56.[294,296-299] They are also often positive for TTF-1 and P504S, occasionally positive for CEA, but rarely positive for PSA, PAP, or AR.[297,300]

Clinical Presentations

Ductal Adenocarcinomas

Ductal adenocarcinomas commonly manifest with symptoms of urinary obstruction and/or hematuria. Cystoscopic examination frequently reveals infiltration of the prostatic urethra and occasional polypoid or villous intraurethral projections arising at or near the verumontanum.[276,279] These tumors are typically high volume and locally advanced at diagnosis, with a 55-93% incidence of extraprostatic extension and a 20-47% incidence of positive margins reported in radical prostatectomy series.[277,278] In most instances, PSA levels are relatively high in patients with advanced disease,[277,301] although some cases manifest with serum PSA levels that are low relative to the tumor burden: in one series of 23 patients with metastatic disease, three patients (13%) had values <4 ng/mL.[302] Most prostatic ductal adenocarcinomas metastasize to bone and lymph nodes, as acinar adenocarcinomas do, but they have also been found to metastasize to unusual sites such as the penis, testis, and visceral organs.[302,303]

Sarcomatoid Carcinomas ■ Sarcomatoid carcinomas of the prostate typically manifest as large prostatic masses with local invasion, resulting in pelvic or perineal pain, lower abdominal mass, and symptoms of urinary obstruction with low serum PSA levels.[283,285,304] In more than half the cases, the diagnosis is preceded by a history of acinar adenocarcinoma treated with androgen deprivation or radiation therapy, with the time between the original diagnosis of acinar adenocarcinoma and the diagnosis of sarcomatoid carcinoma ranging from 2 months to 16 years.[283,284,305,306] Both the carcinomatous and sarcomatous elements can metastasize, and metastatic disease is often present at the time of diagnosis, with the most common sites of non–lymph node metastases being lung, bone, and brain.[283]

Small Cell Carcinomas

Most patients with primary small cell carcinomas have advanced-stage disease at their first visit, with large primary masses leading to lower urinary tract symptoms, bladder outlet obstruction, pelvic pain, ureteral obstruction, and/or hematuria.[292,295] Metastases are present in 75% of patients at the time of diagnosis of small cell carcinoma.[295] When preceded by a diagnosis of acinar adenocarcinoma of the prostate, the time between that original diagnosis and the diagnosis of small cell carcinoma can range between 1.5 months and 10 years.[292-295] Metastases are most often located in pelvic lymph nodes, liver, lungs, and bones,[292,295] although bony metastases are often osteolytic instead of osteoblastic, as would be typical for acinar adenocarcinoma.[294,299] Metastases to uncommon sites, such as the epididymis,[298] subcutaneous tissue,[293] pericardium,[299] or omentum,[292] have been described. Brain metastases occur in up to 20% of patients during the course of the disease, so MRI of the brain or contrast-enhanced CT should be performed as part of the staging workup.[294,295] Serum PSA and PAP levels are often within normal ranges, but serum CEA and lactic acid dehydrogenase levels have been found to be higher than normal in 53-65% and 39-76% of patients, respectively.[293,294] Elevated levels of circulating bombesin, calcitonin, adrenocorticotropic hormone, and somatostatin have also been observed.[294] As is the case for small cell carcinomas of the lung, a number of paraneoplastic syndromes have been described in association with small cell carcinomas of the prostate, including hypercalcemia,[298] elevated adrenocorticotropic hormone,[307] syndrome of inappropriate antidiuretic hormone,[299] myasthenic syndrome,[292] and hyperglucagonemia.[308]

Therapy Options and Applications

Ductal Adenocarcinomas ■ The natural history of ductal adenocarcinomas is debated. Some series describe cases with indolent courses and prolonged survival,[272,301,303,309] whereas others describe cases with aggressive courses and relatively low 5-year survival rates.[276-279] Some authors have proposed that the pure ductal adenocarcinomas have a more indolent behavior and the prognosis of the more common mixed ductal adenocarcinomas is dictated by the acinar component, which is frequently high grade.[301] Much like acinar adenocarcinomas, most ductal adenocarcinomas are sensitive to both radiation and hormone-deprivation therapies.[275] No published data support the use of chemotherapeutic treatments in this disease other than standard regimens for acinar adenocarcinomas.

Sarcomatoid Carcinomas ■ The prognosis of prostatic sarcomatoid carcinomas is poor, regardless of the histologic type of the sarcomatous elements.[283,284,304] In a 21-patient series with a median follow-up of 10 months (range 1-107 months), 18 patients died of their tumor within the follow-up period,[283] and in a more recent 32-patient series, the actuarial risk of death at 1 year was estimated at 20%.[284] Androgen-deprivation therapy is usually administered to target the malignant epithelial component, and the use of chemotherapy drugs typically administered for the treatment of sarcomas, such as ifosfamide and doxorubicin, has been reported.[285,304] However, among the nine patients given chemotherapy containing docetaxel, estramustine, carboplatinum, or cisplatinum in the series of Hansel et al.,[283] three died within 1 year of the diagnosis, and in five the cancer was unresponsive to chemotherapy. Given the morbidity caused by the local invasion of the primary tumors, palliative surgery (which often will need to involve anterior exenterations with urinary diversion) with or without adjuvant radiation may be appropriate. It is noteworthy that the only long-term survivor described by Dundore et al.[282] was treated by pelvic exenteration and resection of lung metastases. Two other patients in their series, who survived 89 and 107 months, were treated with intratumoral iodine 125 (^{125}I) before dying of carcinosarcoma.

Small Cell Carcinomas ■ Although chemotherapeutic agents are active in the treatment of small cell carcinomas of the prostate, the prognosis remains poor, with reported median survival times ranging from 5 to 17.5 months.[292-294,299] In a recent 83-patient retrospective series, patients with nonmetastatic disease at their initial visit appeared to do slightly better (median disease-specific survival 17.1 months vs 12.5 months in patients with metastatic disease at the initial visit), although only 20% of the patients with nonmetastatic disease received local therapy in addition to systemic therapy.[295] Since these are radiosensitive tumors[310] and at least one patient was apparently cured by surgical excision,[311] it is clear that the role of local therapies deserves further investigation in this patient population. In a 21-patient series described by Amato et al.,[292] four of eight patients responded to a combination of vincristine, doxorubicin, and cyclophosphamide. In a 38-patient phase II study of doxorubicin, etoposide, and cisplatin in patients with histologically proven small cell carcinoma of the prostate (either pure or mixed with adenocarcinoma), the response rate in patients with measurable disease was 61%, and 84% of symptomatic patients experienced pain reduction.[294] However, there were no complete responses, and the median time to progression and median overall survival were short, at 5.8 months and 10.5 months, respectively. It was concluded that the addition of doxorubicin to the standard etoposide–cisplatin regimen increased the toxic effects without any apparent increase in efficacy. It is also noteworthy that none of 13 patients subjected to anti-androgen withdrawal in this study responded to that maneuver.[294] It should be noted that even though small cell carcinomas do not appear to respond to androgen-deprivation therapies, a large proportion of cases have shown coexisting components of acinar adenocarcinoma, so it is recommended that hormonal therapy accompany chemotherapy in the treatment of this disease.[293,299]

Algorithm for Therapy: Future Directions

The main question about these histologic variants is whether they represent true biologic variants with different responses to standard treatments for prostate acinar adenocarcinomas that would require different therapeutic approaches. It seems clear that small cell carcinomas do represent a distinct biologic entity, and the questions that follow are: What makes it different, and what drives the progression of this disease so that specific therapies can be developed for this entity?

For all three variants, the role of local therapies remains to be determined, and in the case of small cell carcinoma, it is reasonable to ask whether prophylactic brain irradiation should be offered to patients whose systemic disease is otherwise controlled.

Selected References

The complete reference list can be found at www.CANCERMEDICINE8.com

1. McNeal JE. Normal histology of the prostate. *Am J Surg Pathol*. 1988;12:619–633.
6. Logothetis CJ, Navone NM, Lin SH. Understanding the biology of bone metastases: key to the effective treatment of prostate cancer. *Clin Cancer Res*. 2008;14(6):1599–1602.
8. Walsh PC. Anatomic radical prostatectomy: evolution of the surgical technique. *J Urol*. 1998;160(6 pt 2):2418–2424.
13. De Marzo AM, Marchi VL, Epstein JI, Nelson WG. Proliferative inflammatory atrophy of the prostate: implications for prostatic carcinogenesis. *Am J Pathol*. 1999;155:1985–1992.
17. Bostwick DG. The pathology of early prostate cancer. *CA Cancer J Clin*. 1989;39:376–393.
18. Papandreou CN, Daliani DD, Thall PF, et al. Results of a phase II study with doxorubicin, etoposide, and cisplatin in patients with fully characterized small-cell carcinoma of the prostate. *J Clin Oncol*. July 15, 2002;20(14):3072–3080.
21. Gleason DF. Classification of prostatic carcinomas. *Cancer Chemother Rep*. 1966;50:125–128.
26. Chan JM, Stampfer MJ, Giovannucci E, et al. Plasma insulin-like growth factor-I and prostate cancer risk: a prospective study. *Science*. 1998;279:563–566.
28. Ware JL. Growth factors and their receptors as determinants in the proliferation and metastasis of human prostate cancer. *Cancer Metastasis Rev*. 1993;12(3–4):287–301.
32. Taplin ME, Bubley GJ, Shuster TD, et al. Mutation of the androgen-receptor gene in metastatic androgen-independent prostate cancer. *N Engl J Med*. 1995;332:1393–1398.
40. Partin AW, Kattan MW, Subong EN, et al. Combination of prostate-specific antigen, clinical stage, and Gleason score to predict pathological stage of localized prostate cancer. A multi-institutional update. *JAMA*. 1997;277(18):1445–1451.
42. Schroder FH, Denis LJ, Roobol M, et al. The story of the European Randomized Study of Screening for Prostate Cancer. *BJU Int*. 2003;92(Suppl 2):1–13.
49. Thompson IM, Ankerst DP, Chi C, et al. Operating characteristics of prostate-specific antigen in men with an initial PSA level of 3.0 ng/ml or lower. *JAMA*. 2005;294(1):66–70.
51. Lilja H, Cronin AM, Scardino PT, Dahlin A, Bajartel A, Berglund G. A single PSA predicts prostate cancer up to 30 years subsequently, even in men below age 40. *J Urol*. 2008;179(206):abstract 589. Presented 18 May 2008 at the American Urological Association's Annual Meeting in Orlando, Florida.
54. Etzioni RD, Ankerst DP, Weiss NS, Inoue LY, Thompson IM. Is prostate-specific antigen velocity useful in early detection of prostate cancer? A critical appraisal of the evidence. *J Natl Cancer Inst*. 2007;99(20):1510–1515.
59. D'Amico AV, Whittington R, Malkowicz SB, et al. Biochemical outcome after radical prostatectomy, external beam radiation therapy, or interstitial radiation therapy for clinically localized prostate cancer. *JAMA*. 1998;280(11):969–974.
63. American Urological Association. *Guideline for the Management of Clinically Localized Prostate Cancer: 2007 Update*. Linthicum, MD: American Urological Association Education and Research, Inc.; 2007.
68. Epstein JI. Gleason score 2-4 adenocarcinoma of the prostate on needle biopsy: a diagnosis that should not be made. *Am J Surg Pathol*. 2000;24(4):477–478.
71. Ochiai A, Troncoso P, Chen ME, Lloreta J, Babaian RJ. The relationship between tumor volume and the number of positive cores in men undergoing multisite extended biopsy: implication for expectant management. *J Urol*. 2005;174(6):2164–2168.
77. Parker C. Active surveillance: an individualized approach to early prostate cancer. *BJU Int*. 2003;92:2–3.
78. Johansson JE, Holmberg L, Johansson S, Bergstrom R, Adami HO. Fifteen-year survival in prostate cancer: a prospective, population-based study in Sweden. *JAMA*. 1997;277:467–471.
79. Albertsen PC, Hanley JA, Gleason DF, Barry MJ. Competing risk analysis of men aged 55 to 74 years at diagnosis managed conservatively for clinically localized prostate cancer. *JAMA*. 1998;280:975–980.
86. Klotz L. Active surveillance with selective delayed intervention: using natural history to guide treatment in good risk prostate cancer. *J Urol*. 2004;172:S48–S51.
97. Wood DP, Schulte R, Dunn RL, et al. Short-term health outcome differences between robotic and conventional radical prostatectomy. *Urology*. 2007;70(5):945–949.
106. Marcovich R, Wojno KJ, Wei JT, Rubin MA, Montie JE, Sanda MG. Bladder neck-sparing modification of radical prostatectomy adversely affects surgical margins in pathologic T3a prostate cancer. *Urology*. 2000;55(6):904–908.
112. Roach M III, Hanks G, Thames H Jr, et al. Defining biochemical failure following radiotherapy with or without hormonal therapy in men with clinically localized prostate cancer: recommendations of the RTOG-ASTRO Phoenix Consensus Conference. *Int J Radiat Oncol Biol Phys*. 2006;65:965–974.
113. Pollack A, Zagars GK, Starkschall G, et al. Prostate cancer radiation dose response: results of the M. D. Anderson phase III randomized trial. *Int J Radiat Oncol Biol Phys*. 2002;53:1097.
118. Bolla M, Collette L, Blank L, et al. Long-term results with immediate androgen suppression and external irradiation in patients with locally advanced prostate cancer (an EORTC study): a phase III randomised trial. *Lancet*. 2002;360:103.
119. Thompson I, Thrasher JB, Aus G, et al. Guidelines for the management of clinically localized prostate cancer: 2007 update. *J Urol*. 2007;177(6):2106–2131.
137. D'Amico AV, Chen MH, Roehl KA, Catalona WJ. Preoperative PSA velocity and the risk of death from prostate cancer after radical prostatectomy. *N Engl J Med*. 2004;351(2):125–135.
144. Thompson IM, Chi C, Ankerst DP, et al. Effect of finasteride on the sensitivity of PSA for detecting prostate cancer. *J Natl Cancer Inst*. 2006;98(16):1128–1133.
145. Lucia MS, Darke A, Goodman PJ, et al. Pathologic characteristics of cancers detected in the Prostate Cancer Prevention Trial: implications for prostate cancer detection and chemoprevention. *Cancer Prev Res*.
154. U.S. National Institutes of Health. *Finasteride in Treating Patients Undergoing Surgery for Stage II Prostate Cancer*. J Kim, principal investigator. Bethesda, MD: U.S. National Institutes of Health, 2008. Available at: http://clinicaltrials.gov/ct2/show/NCT00438464.
158. Bolla M, Collette L, Blank L, et al. Long-term results with immediate androgen suppression and external irradiation in patients with locally advanced prostate cancer (an EORTC study): phase III randomized trial. *Lancet*. 2002;360:103–106.
161. Roach III M, Bae K, Speight J, et al. Short-term neoadjuvant androgen deprivation therapy and external-beam radiotherapy for locally advanced prostate cancer: long-term results of RTOG 8610. *J Clin Oncol*. 2008;26:585–591.
168. Kuban D, Tucker S, Dong L, et al. Long-term results of the M. D. Anderson randomized dose-escalation trial for prostate cancer. *Int J Radiat Oncol Biol Phys*. 2008;70:67–74.
179. Aus G, Abrahamson P, Ahlgren G, et al. Three-month neoadjuvant hormonal therapy before radical prostatectomy: a 7-year follow-up of a randomized controlled trial. *BJU Int*. 2002;90:561–566.
180. Gleave M, Goldenberg S, Chin J, et al. Canadian Uro-Oncoloy Group. Randomized comparative study of 3 versus 8-month neoadjuvant hormonal therapy before radical prostatectomy: biochemical and pathological effects. *J Urol*. 2001;166:500–506.
182. Pettaway C, Pisters L, Troncoso P, et al. Neoadjuvant chemotherapy and hormonal therapy followed by radical prostatectomy: feasibility and preliminary results. *J Clin Oncol*. 2000;18:1050–1057.
189. Thompson I, Tangen C, Paradelo J, et al. Adjuvant radiotherapy for pathologically advanced prostate cancer: a randomized clinical trial. *JAMA*. 2006;296(19):2329–2335.
196. Pound CR, Partin AW, Eisenberger MA, et al. Natural history of progression after PSA elevation following radical prostatectomy. *JAMA*. 1999;281:1591–1597.
205. Pilepich MV, Winter K, Lawton CA, et al. Androgen suppression adjuvant to definitive radiotherapy in prostate carcinoma—long-term results of Phase III RTOG 85-31. *Int J Radiat Oncol Biol Phys*. 2005;61:1285–1290.
206. Bolla M, Collette L, Blank L, et al. Long-term results with immediate androgen suppression and external radiation in patients with locally advanced prostate cancer (an EORTC study): a phase III randomized trial. *Lancet*. 2002;360:103–108.
209. The Medical Research Council Prostate Cancer Working Party Investigators Group. Immediate versus deferred treatment for advanced prostatic cancer—initial results of the Medical Council Research Trial. *Br J Urol*. 1997;79:235–246.
217. Millikan RE, Wen S, Pagliaro LC, et al. Phase III trial of androgen ablation with or without 3 cycles of systemic chemotherapy for advanced prostate cancer. *J Clin Oncol*. 2008 (in press).
223. Tannock IF, Osoba D, Stockler MR, et al. Chemotherapy with mitoxantrone plus prednisone or prednisone alone for symptomatic hormone-resistant prostate cancer: a Canadian randomized trial with palliative endpoints. *J Clin Oncol*. 1996;14:1756–1764.
226. Halabi S, Small EJ, Kantoff PW, et al. Prognostic model for predicting survival in men with hormone-refractory metastatic prostate cancer. *J Clin Oncol*. 2003;21:1232–1237.
255. Smith MR. Osteoclast targeted therapy for prostate cancer: bisphosphonates and beyond. *Urol Oncol*. 2008;26:420–425.

95 Tumors of the Penis and Urethra

Raymond S. Lance, MD ■ Donald F. Lynch Jr, MD

Cancer of the penis is an unusual disease in the United States and Europe, but is a major health problem in parts of South America, Africa, and Asia. The incidence of primary, malignant penile cancer in the United States using the Surveillance, Epidemiology, and End Results (SEER) database from 1973 to 2002 was 0.69 per 100,000.[1] The incidence decreased significantly over time from 0.84 per 100,000 in 1973-1982 to 0.69 per 100,000 in 1982-1992 to 0.58 per 100,000 in 1993-2002. White Hispanics had the highest incidence (1.01/100,000) followed by Alaska Natives and American Indians (0.77/100,000) and Blacks (0.62/100,000).[1] In 2008 an estimated 1250 new cases will be diagnosed with 290 deaths from primary penile cancer.[2] Approximately 95% of primary penile cancers are squamous cell carcinomas (SCCs). Other cancers involving the penis are epidemic Kaposi's sarcoma (KS), verrucous carcinoma, and transitional cell carcinoma.[3]

Urethral cancer is quite rare. A SEER database review found primary urethral carcinoma was identified in 1,075 men and 540 women, with an annual age-adjusted incidence rate of 4.3 per million and 1.5 per million, respectively. The annual incidence rate increased with age to a peak of 32 per million men and 9.5 per million women in the 75- to 84-year age group. The rate was 5.0 per million and 2.5 per million for African Americans and whites, respectively. The histologic types were transitional cell carcinoma in 888 patients (55%), SCC in 348 (21.5%), and adenocarcinoma in 265 (16.4%).[4]

Cancer of the Penis

Histopathology

Over 95% of penile cancers are SCCs (Fig. 95-1). Verrucous carcinoma, known alternatively as giant condyloma or Buschke–Lowenstein tumor, is a variant of squamous carcinoma which does not metastasize, but which spreads aggressively by local extension and destroys surrounding tissues (Fig. 95-2). Epidemic KS, associated with acquired immunodeficiency syndrome (AIDS), is being increasingly encountered (Fig. 95-3). Some 20% of male patients with AIDS may be expected to manifest a penile lesion in the course of the disease.[3] Melanoma, sarcoma, and basal cell carcinoma involve the penis infrequently but have been reported.

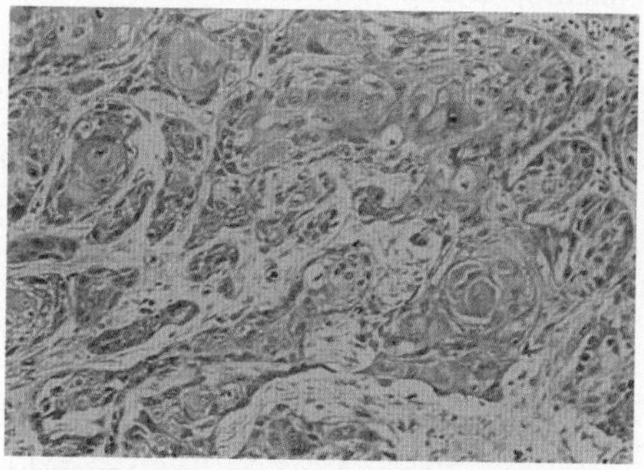

Figure 95-1 ■ Microscopic: Squamous cell carcinoma, moderately well differentiated, with characteristic keratin pearl formation.

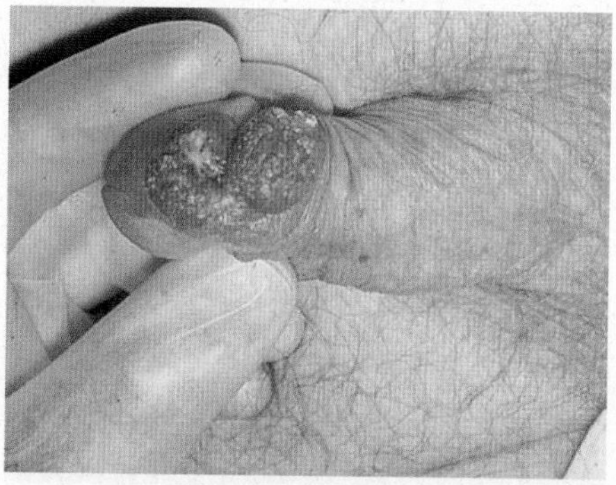

Figure 95-2 ■ Verrucous carcinoma (Buschke–Löwenstein tumor).

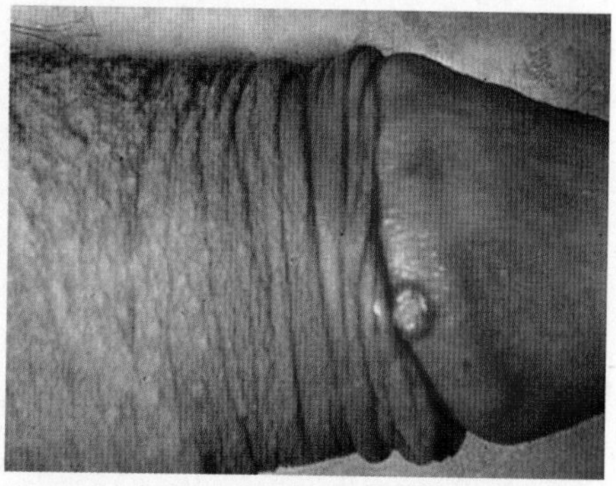

Figure 95-3 ■ Lesion of epidemic (AIDS-related) Kaposi sarcoma involving glans. *Source:* Courtesy of V. Marcial.

Bowen's disease is intraepithelial squamous CIS and is so called when it involves the base of the penis and the scrotum. When it involves the glans penis or prepuce, it is known as Erythroplasia of Queyrat. These lesions have the potential to develop into invasive squamous carcinoma.

Paget's disease of the penis is quite rare, but may develop primarily or as the result of an underlying adenocarcinoma of the urethra or periurethral glands. Balanitis xerotica obliterans, leukoplakia, and penile cutaneous horn may occasionally develop into squamous carcinoma. Bowenoid papulosis, a reddish, raised lesion resembling Erythroplasia of Queyrat but with a benign course may be difficult to distinguish from more problematic lesions. Biopsy is required to establish a diagnosis.

Epidemiology and Etiology

In countries where infant circumcision is common, such as Israel and the United States, the incidence of squamous carcinoma of the penis is low. Circumcision later in life does not seem to confer protection.[5] It has been thought that chronic exposure to smegma, a substance secreted by Tyson's glands in the prepuce, might be one mechanism promoting the development of squamous penile cancers. In the uncircumcized penis, proper hygiene may be made more difficult by phimosis, perpetuating chronic inflammation of the glans, and preputial tissues. In more developed countries with improved socioeconomic conditions, the incidence of penile cancer has fallen and the stage at presentation has also decreased, suggesting that a combination of improved education coupled with more attentive hygiene has reduced the incidence and severity of the disease.[6]

An association between cervical cancer in women whose spouses have penile cancer has been observed, and there is evidence to suggest that patients infected with human papillomavirus (HPV) types 16, 18, 31, and 33 may have a predisposition to develop squamous carcinoma in both the penis and the cervix.[7,8] Uncircumcized men are three times more likely to harbor HPV than uncircumcized men and female partners of uncircumcized men are much less likely to develop cervical cancer.[9]

Men may develop condyloma accuminata from this infection, may be totally asymptomatic carriers, or may harbor intraurethral lesions—unknown to the patient—which may shed the virus and expose a sexual partner. Balanitis xerotica obliterans (BXO) also known as lichen sclerosis et atrophicus (LS) is a premalignant lesion of the penis known to be associated with intact foreskin and HPV 16 infection and has been reported to increase the risk of subsequent SCC of the penis.[10] On examination LS is often associated with urethral meatal stenosis and has a well marginated white appearance. In 2001 Powell et al performed a retrospective review of 20 cases of penile SCC for histological evidence of LS. Overall, BXO histology associated with SCC was seen in 10 cases (50%) and some cases of BXO diagnosis preceded SCC by 10 years.[11]

Several large studies have shown that smoking is associated with an increased incidence of squamous carcinoma of the penis. Recent studies linking smoking to high-grade lesions of the cervix and vulva suggest an association between HPV, smoking, and cancer, which may also pertain in squamous carcinoma of the penis.[9,12]

Carcinoma-In-Situ (CIS)

Erythroplasia of Queyrat (Fig. 95-4) is characterized by a shiny, erythematous maculopapular patch, which is slightly raised, velvety in appearance, and typically involves the glans penis or prepuce. Bowen's disease appears scaly and red, is clearly demarcated, and often involves the scrotum and base of the penis. Histologically these lesions demonstrate dyskeratosis, vaculolization, and large nuclei with numerous atypical mitotic figures. The full thickness of the epithelium is involved. Clinically, Erythroplasia of Queyrat and Bowen's disease are the same disease, with a 10-20% association with progression to squamous carcinoma of the penis.[13]

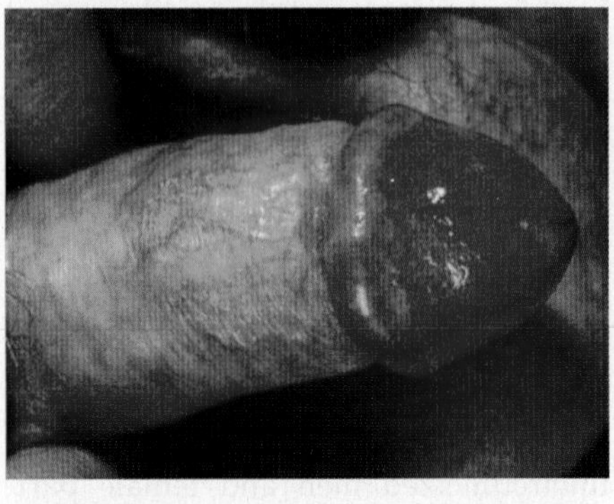

Figure 95-4 Large lesion of glans. Classic presentation.

Invasive Squamous Cell Carcinoma

Early invasive tumors may be small and largely unremarkable, sometimes resembling small abrasions or callused thickenings of penile skin. The initial lesion of squamous carcinoma most commonly presents on the glans or prepuce. It varies from a small, velvety, reddened, raised maculopapule to an ulcer, hyperkeratotic area, or exophytic papillary tumor (Fig. 95-5). Biopsy is required to make the diagnosis, and should include contiguous normal skin for comparison.

More advanced lesions may be exophytic or ulcerated (Fig. 95-6), and very advanced cancers may completely destroy the penile shaft. Metastases to the inguinal lymph nodes may produce large ulcerations in the groins late in the course of the disease. Well-differentiated tumors tend to metastasize infrequently, while more poorly differentiated tumors have a high propensity for early metastasis. Several studies have confirmed that higher tumor grade increases the likelihood of inguinal nodal metastases.[14-16]

Verrucous Carcinoma

Verrucous carcinoma, or Buschke–Lowenstein tumor of the penis, comprises about 5% of all penile cancers and represents a special variant of squamous carcinoma. It is well differentiated and does not metastasize, but spreads aggressively by local extension and may destroy penile tissues entirely if left untreated. These lesions are often associated with HPV types 6 and 11.[17,18]

Other Malignancies

Rarely transitional cell carcinomas of the bladder or urethra may extend to the glans and prepuce. Basal cell carcinoma, melanoma, and primary sarcomas are quite rare.[3] KS, usually the epidemic or AIDS-associated variety, is becoming an increasingly common problem. Local symptomatic management is recommended, although with large tumors surgical intervention may be required. KS is now categorized as (a) classic KS,

Figure 95-5 Verrucous carcinoma (Buschke-Lowenstein tumor).

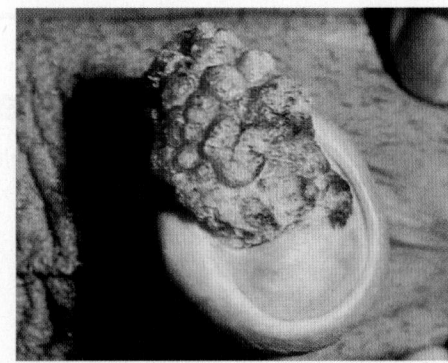

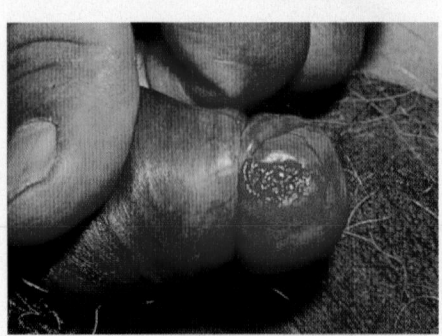

Figure 95-6 Large, papillary lesion of glans. *Source:* Courtesy of J. Vaeth.

which occurs in men without immunodeficiency and is generally indolent; (b) immunosuppressive treatment-related KS occurring in men on immunosuppressive treatment following organ transplantation or autoimmune treatment; (c) African KS, which occurs in younger men is some times aggressive but may be more indolent; and (d) epidemic or HIV-related KS which occurs in men with AIDS.[3] Infiltration of the penile structures with lymphoma or leukemia usually presents as priapism. A thorough search for systemic disease is always indicated. Treatment is with systemic chemotherapy.

Natural History and Course

Squamous carcinoma of the penis usually presents as a sore or ulcer of the glans, coronal sulcus, or prepuce. SCC is localized to the glans penis in approximately 34% of cases, to the prepuce in 15% and involves the body of penis alone in 3% of cases.[1] In the uncircumcised male, induration or swelling of the distal penis suggests tumor. Biopsy of the lesion following dorsal slit or circumcision confirms the diagnosis. Patients with penile cancer notoriously delay seeking care for suspicious lesions. In several large series up to 50% of such men delayed onset of care for more than one year. Biopsy prior to any radical surgery is mandatory. Confirmation of the disease is critical especially given the psychological impact of losing all or part of the phallus.

Erythroplasia of Queyrat, verrucous carcinoma, and various hyperkeratotic lesions including LS may evolve into squamous carcinoma or may coexist with it. Prompt treatment of these lesions is indicated.

Invasive squamous carcinoma of the penis follows a predictable pattern of metastasis. Lesions of the glans, coronal sulcus, prepuce, and distal shaft spread to the deep inguinal nodes, while lesions of the proximal shaft and base of the penis spread to the more lateral and superficial inguinal nodes. Subsequent spread to the external iliac, obturator, and iliac chains follows. Although "skip" metastases to the pelvic nodes have been reported, reevaluation of old reports and more recent series suggest that pelvic metastases in the absence of inguinal metastases probably do not occur.[19] Metastases to distant sites are infrequent and occur late in the course of the disease. Left untreated penile cancer progresses causing the deaths of the majority of those untreated within 2 years.[20]

Because primary lesions may be infected or chronically inflamed, secondary inflammation of the inguinal nodes is often present which may be impossible to distinguish from metastatic disease. Careful reexamination of the inguinal nodes following a 4- to 6-week course of broad-spectrum antibiotic therapy may help to differentiate inflammation from cancer.

Tumor Staging

Once the diagnosis of squamous carcinoma is established, complete staging is undertaken. Careful palpation of the inguinal nodes is carried out. Additional staging studies should include chest x-ray, computerized tomography (CT) of the pelvis and inguinal regions, and possibly magnetic resonance scanning (MRI). Where patients are obese or where the groins have been subjected to prior surgery, CT or MRI may be superior to palpation in detecting suspicious nodal enlargement. CT and MRI have supplanted lymphangiography as a staging procedure. MRI provides good discrimination of penile structures and may identify corpora cavernosal or spongiosal invasion. MRI of the penis for this purpose is enhanced by pharacological injection of prostaglandin El.[21] Currently PET scans have limited utility in staging penile cancer. Recently, MRI using lymphotrophic nanoparticles has been advocated. Ferumoxtran-10 is made of superparamagnetic iron oxide particles with iron oxide core measurements of 4.3-6.0 nm with whole particle size of 30-50 nm. Metastatic nodes show a sparing of nanoparticle uptake. Tabatabaei et al performed MR lymphangiography on seven men with penile cancer correlated with complete inguinal lymphadenectomy and documented a sensitivity and specificity of 100% and 97% respectively.[22] The role of MR lymphangiography remains investigational but holds great promise in staging penile cancer.

The American Joint Committee on Cancer (AJCC) Tumor, Nodes, Metastases (TNM) system of 2002 is the accepted staging system for penile cancer (Table 95-1).[23] The older Jackson system which is clinically based is no longer used, but is frequently encountered in the older literature (Table 95-2).

Table 95-1 AJCC (2002) Staging of Penile Cancer

Tumor (T)	
Tx	Primary tumor cannot be assessed
T0	No evidence of cancer
Tis	CIS
Ta	Noninvasive verrucous carcinoma
T1	Tumor invades subepithelial connective tissue
T2	Tumor invades corpus spongiosum or cavernosum
T3	Tumor invades urethra or prostate
T4	Tumor invades other adjacent structures
Nodes (N)	
Nx	Regional lymph nodes cannot be assessed
N0	No regional node metastasis
N1	Metastasis to a single, superficial inguinal lymph node
N2	Metastasis in multiple or bilateral superficial inguinal lymph nodes
N3	Metastasis in deep inguinal or pelvic lymph nodes, unilateral or bilateral
Metastasis (M)	
Mx	Presence of distant metastasis cannot be assessed
M0	No distant metastasis
M1	Distant metastasis

Source: From Ref. 17.

Surgical Treatment

Treatment of penile cancer is based on the extent of the primary tumor and its tumor grade, established by biopsy of the lesion. Antibiotic therapy is begun prior to biopsy and continued through surgical therapy and for 4-6 weeks afterwards. Once the tissue diagnosis is confirmed, small superficial tumors may be successfully treated with local surgical excision, topical chemotherapy, LASER surgery, Mohs' micrographic surgery, or superficial radiation therapy.[24-27]

Larger tumors with invasion may sometimes be managed with organ-sparing surgery or radiotherapy, but deeply invasive cancers, particularly those that deform the glans or involve the shaft structures, may not be amenable to conservative measures.

Lesions which involve the distal shaft or glans are usually managed by partial penectomy, providing that a 2-cm margin can be achieved while leaving enough penile length to allow the patient to void while standing and to engage in intercourse. More advanced lesions or tumors which involve the base of the penis are best managed by total penectomy with creation of a perineal urethrostomy.[3,28] More extensive lesions or those involving the base and bulbar urethral portion of the penis may require cystoprostatectomy or occasionally anterior or total pelvic exenteration, with urinary diversion.

Table 95-2 Jackson Staging System for Penile Cancer

I	Tumor confined to glans or prepuce
II	Invasion into shaft or corpora; no nodal or distant metastasis
III	Tumor confined to penis; operable inguinal nodal metastasis
IV	Tumor involves adjacent structures; inoperable inguinal nodes and/or distant metastasis

Source: From Ref. 16.

Management of the Regional Lymph Nodes

Inguinal or pelvic lymph nodes metastasis remains one of the most important factors predicting survival in men with SCC of the penis. Proper management of the inguinal and pelvic lymph nodes in patients with squamous carcinoma of the penis has been one of the most challenging and controversial aspects of penile cancer treatment. Lymphatic drainage of the penile shaft and base is to the superficial inguinal lymph nodes. Drainage from the glans, prepuce, and distal shaft is to the deep inguinal nodes. There is crossover of the lymphatic channels at the base of the penis so that a lesion on one side of the penis may metastasize to the contralateral inguinal nodes. The deep inguinal nodes drain to the external iliac and obturator chains and subsequently to the common iliac nodes and the retroperitoneal nodes surrounding the aorta and inferior vena cava.

Several clinical studies have shown that in patients with inguinal metastases, a meticulous inguinal node dissection will be curative in 40-60% of cases.[24,29,30] However, the traditional node dissection carries with it a high likelihood of morbidity—flap necrosis, wound infection, chronic lymphangitis, lymphocoele, and chronic lower limb edema. A modified, somewhat less extensive dissection has been adopted by most surgeons, which has reduced some of the unpleasant sequelae of groin dissection.[31] Nonetheless, an inguinal node dissection is not undertaken lightly, and the indications for a groin dissection in patients with no palpable inguinal nodes are not clear. Inguinal lymph nodes are palpable in 50-82% of patients at initial diagnosis.[32,33] In approximately 50% of these cases cancer is found on lymph node dissection. Lymphadenectomy is indicated if palpable nodes remain after 4-6 weeks of antibiotic therapy. While some 25% of patients with impalpable nodes have metastatic disease and must undergo a node dissection, others with no metastases may undergo needless surgery. Determining which patients should have inguinal lymphadenectomy and which may be followed expectantly continues to be a major challenge in the management of this disease. Those patients with metastases to the groins who do not undergo appropriate node dissection will usually die of their disease within 3 years.

Clinical staging of the inguinal nodes is highly inaccurate. Several studies have demonstrated that microscopic metastases may be present in impalpable nodes, while palpably enlarged nodes are benign half of the time.[27,34-36] Staging techniques using lymphangiography with aspiration of the nodes have proven to be unsatisfactory. As such, the sentinal node biopsy has emerged to decrease the morbidity of full bilateral inguinal lymph node dissections. The sentinel node is defined as the lymph node that receives lymphatic drainage directly from the primary tumor. The sentinel node biopsy, proposed by Cabanas and associates, while initially encouraging, has also proven to be unreliable and remains investigational.[19,37,38]

Tumor Grade

Recent studies have confirmed the importance of tumor grade as well as stage in assessing the risk of nodal metastases, and have helped clarify when node dissection should be performed. Patients with grade I tumors that are limited to the skin and superficial tissues of the penis are unlikely to have tumor metastasis to inguinal nodes. Patients with grade II or grade III lesions with any degree of invasion of the deeper penile structures have been shown to be at significant risk of groin metastases.[14-16] For many years patients with clinically negative inguinal nodes were followed expectantly and subjected to inguinal node dissection only if palpable node metastases developed, contemporary investigators recommend early surgery if high-grade tumor (grade II or III) and more than superficial invasion is documented on biopsy. At our institution, we treat patients with 4- to 6-weeks of broad-spectrum antibiotic therapy and then perform a modified bilateral inguinal node dissection on any patient with palpably enlarged inguinal nodes, and on patients with impalpable nodes who demonstrate invasion into the penile shaft or show grade II or grade III histopathology on their biopsy.

Pelvic Lymphadenectomy

Patients found to have inguinal node metastases should undergo pelvic lymphadenectomy on the affected side. This can be done extraperitoneally via a midline incision or through a modified Gibson or groin incision. At our institution, pelvic lymphadenectomy is done at the same time inguinal node dissection is performed, although at some centers the procedure is staged several weeks later.[3] Patients found to have fewer than three pelvic nodes, with all nodes below the bifurcation of the internal and external iliac vessels, often will fare well. Metastases above the bifurcation have been almost uniformly lethal.[39,40]

Radiotherapy (RT)

Primary RT of penile cancer is used more widely in Europe than in the United States, but may be appropriate in small superficial lesions or in selected larger lesions when organ preservation is the goal or when patients refuse surgery.[41-44] In more advanced lesions, however, tissue preservation may not be feasible. Concurrent chemotherapy usually bleomycin may enhance the effectiveness of RT.[45]

RT can be delivered either as external beam administered with peredex or wax block delivery, or as brachytherapy, with a mold or with Iridium^{192} wires. Irridium^{192} or Cesium^{137} may be used to boost dosages in bulky or extremely cornified tumors. Normally doses of 30-50 Gy given over 3-5 weeks are used. Boosts to 65-70 Gy utilizing various brachytherapy techniques may follow if clinically indicated. RT is often the treatment of choice in symptomatic lesions resulting from epidemic (AIDS-related) KS.[46] RT may be used as primary therapy in a select group of men presenting with localized penile cancer. This group is small but includes: young men with small superficial noninvasive lesions located on the distal penis, and those who refuse to have surgery as initial treatment. Additionally, RT is used for men with inoperable cancers.

Acute radiation reactions—edema and tissue inflammation, with concomitant skin irritation, tenderness, and dysuria—are common accompaniments of both external radiation and brachytherapy. Such symptoms usually subside promptly once therapy is completed. Long-term effects of treatment may include telangiectasia, hyperpigmentation, diminished sensation, scarring, and atrophy of the treated tissues. Fibrotic change and fistulization may occur in large lesions where significant tissue damage has occurred prior to radiotherapy. Late recurrences in radiated sites may occur up to a decade following definitive treatment, affirming that close follow-up is essential.[42]

Because of the rarity of penile cancer no randomized trials exist comparing RT to surgery. Ozsahin et al examined the impact of radiation therapy both primary and adjunctive in the treatment of clinically localized penile cancer in 60 men.[47] Locoregional relapse occurred in 13% treated with surgery compared to 56% treated with definitive primary radiation therapy. Of the RT failures, 73% were salvaged with surgery. The 5- and 10-year probability of survival with an intact penis in this series was 43% and 26%, respectively.

RT of clinically negative groins as a prophylactic measure is controversial as is adjuvant radiation to the groins following inguinal surgery. While some studies have suggested benefit from such treatment, others show no improvement when compared with patients treated with surgery alone.[48,49] RT to bulky unresectable lymph node metastases is rarely effective except as a palliative measure usually in concert with systemic chemotherapy.

Chemotherapy

Chemotherapy is used in treating penile cancer as an adjuvant to definitive surgical or radiation therapy or as a radiosensitizer. Experience with various treatment protocols is limited by the relative rarity of the disease. Multidrug combination chemotherapy programs have shown promise at several institutions. Pizzocaro and Piva of the Milan National Tumor Institute have used combination chemotherapy with vincristine, bleomycin, and methotrexate (VBM) and have been successful at rendering patients with fixed nodal metastases resectable.[50] Dexeus and associates from MD Anderson Cancer Center have used cisplatin-based chemotherapy as adjuvant therapy following surgery.[51] Leite et al from the Netherlands reported on the use of neoadjuvant chemotherapy in 20 men with inoperable tumors, and found that 12 (60%) were rendered operable including 8 (40%) who were long-term survivors.[52] In this series, the majority received bleomycin cisplatin and methotrexate. Similarly, a multi-institutional Southwest Oncology Group trial using methotrexate, cisplatin, and bleomycin to treat advanced, unresectable inguinal metastatic disease demonstrated a 32.5% response rate, although toxicity was high.[53] Several combination chemotherapy protocols which have shown effectiveness in treating squamous carcinoma of other sites such as, anus, esophagus, head and neck, remain to be tested in squamous carcinoma of the penis. Multi-institutional, multinational trials will be required to enroll sufficient numbers of patients to provide meaningful data.

Prognosis

Left untreated, squamous carcinoma of the penis is invariably lethal, killing most of those afflicted within 3 years.

Outcome is directly related to the extent of the disease at diagnosis and the presence or absence of inguinal metastases.[6,35,36,39]

Relative survival for localized tumor was 80%, with survival rates of 52% for regional (nodal) disease and 18% for distant disease. Horenblas and associates reported 93% 5-year survival when nodes were negative versus 50% in patients with clinically positive nodes.[49] Srinivas and associates reported a crude 5-year survival rate of 28% in patients with proven inguinal metastases. Patients with minimal nodal disease (N1,N2) had 50-80% 5-year survival rates, while those with N3/N4 disease had a much graver outcome, with only 4-12% survivals. Patients with negative groins had a 74% 5-year survival.[39,40] The outcome of patients with pelvic metastases has been very poor.

Conclusions

Squamous carcinoma of the penis is a preventable disease, and, in fact, incidence has fallen over the past two decades with improved socioeconomic conditions, attention to hygiene, and access to health care. Better understanding of the importance of tumor histology and a more aggressive approach to inguinal disease may provide further improvements in survival. Refinements in surgical and radiotherapeutic techniques have further improved outcome and quality of life. Early recognition of tumor lesions has allowed for effective but less extensive treatment and improvements in organ-sparing procedures.

Further research into combined modality therapies using chemotherapy in conjunction with surgery, radiation therapy, or both will likely further improve treatment results. Improved understanding of the role of possible causative agents (HPVs and HHVs) should improve both treatment and prevention.

Carcinoma of the Urethra

Female Urethral Carcinoma

The female urethra is largely contained within the anterior vaginal wall. In the adult it is 2-4 cm in length. Distally it is lined with stratified squamous epithelium changing to stratified or pseudostratified columnar epithelium more proximally. At the bladder neck, the mucosa is transitional cell epithelium.

The histopathology of female urethral cancer depends upon the tissue of origin. Squamous carcinoma is the most common, comprising about 50% of all tumors. Transitional cell carcinoma and adenocarcinoma are next most common and occur with roughly equal frequency. Unlike penile cancers, tumor grade does not appear to influence either propensity for metastasis or prognosis. Female urethral cancers occur more often in Caucasian women than in blacks.[54] Mixed tumors, undifferentiated carcinomas, melanoma, cloacogenic carcinoma, and clear cell adenocarcinoma have also been reported.[55,56]

Urethral cancers spread first by local extension and later metastasize via lymphatic channels and later hematogenously. The lymphatic drainage of the distal urethra and labia is to the superficial and deep inguinal nodes. The proximal urethra drains to the nodes of the iliac, obturator, presacral, and para-aortic lymphatic chains. Palpably abnormal lymph nodes are present in 20-50% of patients at presentation and almost always represent metastatic cancer. Metastases to distant sites such as liver, lung, brain, and bone—occur late and are more common with adenocarcinomas.[56-58]

Staging ■ The AJCC/UICC TNM staging system (2002) for urethral carcinoma is shown in Table 95-3.[59] One system is now used for both male and female patients. Older literature commonly refers to tumors as involving the distal third of the urethra as "anterior" or "distal" lesions, while those involving the proximal two thirds are described as "posterior" or "proximal" tumors.[54,55] These designations are useful in predicting the clinical behavior of urethral cancers and are still often used. Roughly half of tumors involve the entire length of urethra at diagnosis.

A rare variation of urethral cancer is carcinoma arising in a urethral diverticulum. These tumors are usually squamous carcinomas although adenocarcinoma has been reported and are usually located in the distal two thirds of the urethra.[60] They have been reported more frequently in black women than in Caucasians and likely arise from remnants of wolffian or mullerian ducts or ectopic cloacal epithelium.[61,62]

Surgical Management ■ In the female, most tumors present with bleeding or distal urethral mass. Distal urethral or anterior lesions usually present early and are diagnosed while at low stage. These tumors have been successfully managed with local excision, transurethral resection, partial urethrectomy, and fulguration or ablation with either neodymium: YAG or CO2 LASER techniques.[63-65] In rare instances, higher stage local lesions may be managed with total urethrectomy and preservation of the bladder with interposition of a catheterizable segment or with the Mitrofanoff procedure.

More proximal lesions present later and at higher stage than distal lesions. Progressive obstructive symptoms are the hallmark of proximal or "posterior" urethral lesions. For superficial tumors, transurethral resection or LASER surgery may be appropriate.[66-68] Advanced or extensive lesions, and those which involve the bladder or vagina, may necessitate cystectomy or anterior exenteration with urinary diversion.[54] Local recurrence in such high stage disease occurs frequently.

In advanced disease, metastases to the lymph nodes are present in 50% of

Table 95-3 ■ **AJCC (2002) Staging System for Male and Female Carcinoma of the Urethra**

Primary Tumor (T)	
TX	Primary tumor cannot be assessed
T0	No evidence of primary tumor
Ta	Noninvasive papillary, polypoid, or verrucous carcinoma
Tis	CIS
T1	Tumor invades subepithelial connective tissue
T2	Tumor invades any of the following: corpus spongiosum, prostate, periurethral muscle
T3	Tumor invades any of the following: corpus cavernosum, beyond prostate capsule, anterior vagina, bladder neck
T4	Tumor invades other adjacent organs
Regional Lymph Nodes (N)	
NX	Regional lymph nodes cannot be assessed
N0	No regional lymph node metastasis
N1	Metastasis in a single lymph node, 2 cm or less in greatest dimension
N2	Metastasis in a single lymph node more than 2 cm in greatest dimension, or in multiple nodes
Distant Metastasis (M)	
MX	Distant metastasis cannot be assessed
M0	No distant metastasis
M1	Distant metastasis

Source: From Ref. 47.

cases. Inguinal node dissection should be performed in the presence of palpably enlarged nodes, and pelvic node dissection should be performed when proximal involvement of the urethra is identified. There does not appear to be any therapeutic advantage to prophylactic node dissection when the inguinal nodes are not enlarged.

Radiation Therapy ■ Radiation therapy, administered as both external beam radiation and brachytherapy, has been used for definitive treatment of both localized and advanced tumors. It has also been used to downsize tumors before definitive surgical intervention. Results have been mixed, with 5-year survivals averaging about 35% in advanced disease.[54,61,66] Side effects and complications, including edema, fistulae, and damage to the bowel are commonplace.

Chemotherapy and Combined Therapy ■ The rarity of these tumors has precluded much meaningful clinical research in chemotherapeutic treatment, or in chemotherapy combined with radiation or surgery. Combination chemotherapy in conjunction with radiation and surgery has produced promising outcomes in squamous carcinomas of the head and neck, anus, and penis, and may be expected to demonstrate similar benefit in squamous cancers of the urethra.[65,67] However, multinational, multi-institutional trials will be required to provide clinical data to assess the efficacy of any such treatment regimens.

Prognosis ■ Long-term survival is related to the stage of the tumor at the time of diagnosis and appears to be independent of tumor histology or grade. Bracken and associates, in one of the few large series, report an overall 5-year survival of 32% in 81 patients.[54] Patients having tumors less than 2 cm in diameter did significantly better than those with tumors larger than 5 cm in diameter. Patients having tumors of the anterior or distal urethra have better survival than those with more proximal lesions, apparently because their tumors present earlier in their clinical course. Patients having tumors involving the entire urethra fare the worst, with only an 11% 5-year survival. Tumor recurrence rates of 66-100% have been noted.

Male Urethral Carcinoma

The male urethra averages some 18 cm in length, and is subdivided into the penile urethra, the membranous urethra, and the prostatic urethra. Beginning distally, the penile urethra is comprised of the meatus and fossa navicularis which is lined with stratified squamous epithelium. The pendulous urethra extends from the proximal fossa navicularis to the suspensory ligament of the penis, where it then becomes the bulbar urethra between the ligament and the urogenital membrane. These areas are lined with stratified or pseudo stratified columnar epithelium as is the short (1.5 cm) membranous urethra. This contains the external sphincter which is comprised of striated muscle fibers. The prostatic urethra passes through the prostate and is lined with transitional cell epithelium.

From 50% to 75% of male urethral cancers arise in the bulbar urethra. The remainder occurs predominantly in the fossa navicularis. Some 90% of male tumors demonstrate SCC histology.[57,58,68] Often there is an association with stricture of the urethra (Fig. 95-7). Infrequently, transitional cell carcinoma or undifferentiated tumor may predominate at the bladder neck or within the prostatic urethra. Poorly differentiated transitional cell cancers may show some squamous characteristics. Rarely adenocarcinoma may arise in the glands of Littre or the prostatic utricle. Metastases from distant tumor sites to the penis also occur infrequently.

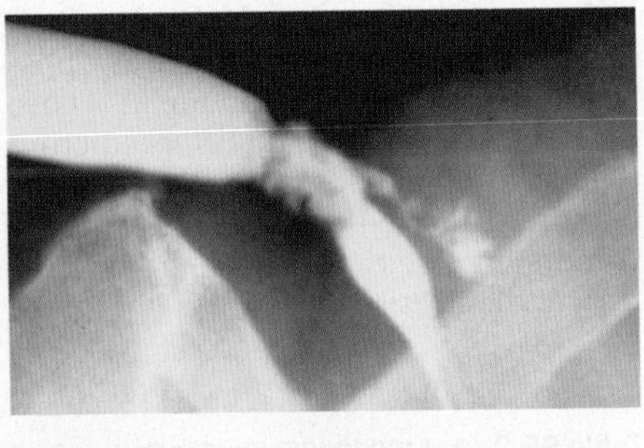

Figure 95-7 ■ Retrograde urethrogram demonstrating squamous carcinoma of bulbous urethra associated with a stricture.

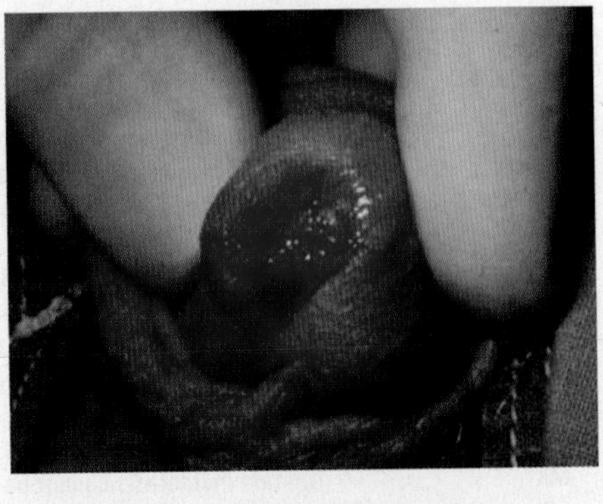

Figure 95-8 ■ Early pedunculated squamous cell carcinoma of the fossa navicularis/urethral meatus.

Obstructive symptoms are common in more proximal lesions, while urethral bleeding and palpation of a mass herald more distal lesions (Fig. 95-8). In general, the more proximal a tumor, and the later in its development, the higher its stage at diagnosis will be.

A special case exists in the urethral segment which is retained following cystectomy. These tumors are almost exclusively transitional cell carcinomas. Monitoring of the urethra in this situation and management of these tumors is discussed elsewhere.[69,70] When the urethra is excised, either in conjunction with cystectomy or as a secondary procedure, the entire urethra, including the fossa navicularis, must be excised.

Lymphatic drainage of the distal male urethra is similar to that of penile tumors. Tumors of the fossa and pendulous urethra drain to the superficial inguinal lymph nodes, while tumors of the bulbar, membranous, and prostatic urethral segments drain to the iliac, obturator, and presacral node groups. There may be crossover at the prepubic lymphatic plexus.

Staging ■ The AJCC/UICC Staging System for urethral carcinoma (2002) is shown in Table 95-3.[59] Special provision is now made for the staging of transitional cell carcinoma of the prostatic urethra and ducts. The terminology of distal or "anterior" tumors—those distal to the suspensory ligament—and proximal or "posterior" tumors—involving the bulbar, membranous, and prostatic segments—may be encountered.

Surgical Management ■ Low-grade, low-stage tumors of the urethra may lend themselves to transurethral resection or LASER fulguration, but such lesions are rare. Excisional biopsy may be feasible, and biopsy prior to LASER fulguration is essential to assess histopathology and tumor depth.

Selected lesions of the distal urethra may lend themselves to partial penectomy. Tumors must not involve the corpus spongiosum or the corpora cavernosa, and must be amenable to a 2-cm margin. More advanced or more proximal lesions may require a total penectomy with creation of a perineal urethrostomy. Proximal cancers may necessitate an anterior exenteration with radical cystoprostatourethrectomy and urinary diversion.[71]

Inguinal and pelvic lymphadenopathy portend metastatic disease. Careful serial palpation of the groins as well as interval pelvic CT evaluations are essential following curative treatment in the follow-up of a urethral cancer. Inguinal node dissection should be performed in the presence of clinically positive groin nodes. This has been curative in many cases. In several small series, 5-year survival rates ranged from 12% to 66% following inguinal node dissection.[72,73] Pelvic node dissection has also proven curative in an occasional case and is worthwhile, although the prognosis in pelvic nodal disease is much poorer than with inguinal node dissection.[72] In the absence of inguinal adenopathy, inguinal lymphadenectomy is probably not warranted.

Radiation, Chemotherapy, Combined Therapy Experience with these modalities is limited, although some success in treating superficial, low-grade lesions with external beam radiotherapy in both males and females has been achieved.[66,67] Brachytherapy implants and molds have also been used.[41,67] Successful management of urethral cancer with partial urethrectomy and combination chemotherapy has also been reported.[74]

The infrequency with which these tumors are encountered has made it impossible to amass much experience with chemotherapy, but it might be anticipated that combination chemotherapy with drugs similar to those used in squamous carcinoma of other sites or with transitional cell carcinoma of the bladder and penis may be similarly effective in urethral lesions of similar pathology. Again, the use of these treatment modalities as well as the employment of combined therapy programs will require large, international, multi-institutional studies to acquire data sufficient for meaningful interpretation.

Summary

Cancers of both the male and the female urethra are quite rare, but the disease may be devastating if not recognized and treated as early as possible. Early surgical or radiotherapeutic intervention may cure these tumors. Advanced disease, at least for the present, carries a grim prognosis. Reliably effective programs of surgery or radiotherapy combined with chemotherapy have not yet been developed, although such programs—based on experience with tumors of similar histopathology in other systems—have the potential for improving outcome. With further refinements in treatment and with increased availability of modern diagnostic techniques, combination chemotherapy, and worldwide communications and data transmission, there is hope that multinational, multi-institutional programs of treatment may provide effective therapy for those suffering from these cancers while expanding our effectiveness in managing them.

Selected References

The complete reference list can be found at www.CANCERMEDICINE8.com

1. Barnholtz-Sloan JS, Maldonado JL, Pow-sang J, Guiliano AR. Incidence trends in primary malignant penile cancer. *Urol Oncol*. 2007;25:361–367.
2. American Cancer Society. *Cancer Facts & Figures 2008*. Atlanta: American Cancer Society; 2008.
3. Pettaway CA, Lynch DF, Davis JW. Tumors of the penis. In: *Campbell-Walsh Urology,* 9th ed. Philadelphia: Saunders Elsevier; 2007:959–992.
9. Daling JR, Madeleine MM, Johnson LG, et al. Penile cancer: importance of circumcision, human papillomavirus and smoking in *in situ* and invasive disease. *Int J Cancer*. 2005;116:606–615.
10. Pugliese JM, Morey AF, Petersen AC. Lichen Sclerosus: review of the literature and current recommendations for management. *J Urol*. 2007;178:2268–2276.
11. Powell J, Robson A, Cranston D, Wojnarowska F, Turner R. High incidence of lichen sclerosus in patients with squamous cell carcinoma of the penis. *Br J Dermatol*. 2001;148:185–189.
12. Tsen HF, Morgenstern H, Mack T, et al. Risk factors for penile cancer: results of population-based case-control study in Los Angeles County (United States). *Cancer Causes Control*. 2001;12:267–277.
16. Theodorescu D, Russo P, Zhang ZF. Outcomes of initial surveillance of invasive squamous cell carcinoma of the penis and negative nodes. *J Urol*. 1996;155: 1626–1631.
17. Sherman RN, Fung HK, Flynn KJ. Verrucous carcinoma (Buschke–Lowenstein tumor). *Int J Dermatol*. 1991;30: 730–733.
18. Boshart M, zur Hausen H. Human papillomavirus (HPV) in Buschke–Lowenstein tumors: physical state of the DNA and identification of a tandem duplication in the non-coding region of a HPV-6 subtype. *J Virol*. 1986;58:963.
19. Fowler JE. Sentinel node biopsy for staging of penile cancer. *Urology*. 1984;23:352.
20. Misra S, Chaturvedi A, Misra NC. Penile carcinoma: a challenge for the developing world. *Lancet Oncol*. 2004;5:240–247.
21. Scardino E, Villa G, Bonomo G, et al. Magnetic resonance imaging combined with artificial erection for local staging of penile cancer. *Urology*. 2004;63: 1158–1162.
22. Tabatabaei, S, Harisinghani M, McDougal WS. Regional lymph node staging using lymphotrophic nanoparticle enhanced magnetic resonance imaging with ferumoxtran-10 in patients with penile cancer. *J Urol*. 2005;174:923–927.
23. Greene FL, Page DL, Fleming ID, et al., eds. Penis. In: *AJCC Cancer Staging Manual*. American Joint Committee on Cancer, 6th ed. New York: Springer; 2002.
24. Ekstrom T, Edsmyr F. Cancer of the penis: a clinical study of 229 cases. *Acta Chir Scand*. 1958;115:25.
25. Hanash KA, Furlow WL, Utz DC, Harrison EG Jr. Carcinoma of the penis: a clinicopathologic study. *J Urol*. 1970;104: 291.
26. Mohs FE, Snow SN, Messing EM, Kuglitsch MG. Microscopically controlled surgery in the treatment of carcinoma of the penis. *J Urol*. 1985;133:961–966.
27. Blastein LM, Finklestein LH. Laser surgery for treatment of squamous cell carcinoma of the penis. *J Am Osteopathic Assoc*. 1990;90:338.
28. deKernion JB, Tynbery P, Persky L, Fegen JP. Carcinoma of the penis. *Cancer*. 1973;32:1256.
29. D'Ancona CA, de Lucena RG, Querne FA, et al. Long-term followup of penile carcinoma treated with penectomy and bilateral modified inguinal lymphadenectomy. *J Urol*. 2004;174:498–501.
30. Bevan-Thomas R, Slayton JW, Pettaway CA. Contemporary morbidity from lymphadenectomy for penile squamous cell carcinoma: the MD Anderson experience. *J Urol*. 2002;167:1638–1642.
31. Catalona WJ. Modified inguinal lymphadenectomy for carcinoma of the penis with preservation of saphenous veins: technique and preliminary results. *J Urol*. 1988;140:306.
32. Ravi R. Morbidity following groin dissection for penile carcinoma. *Br J Urol*. 1993;72:941–945.
33. Ornellas AA, Kinchin EW, Nobrega BLB, et al. Surgical treatment of invasive squamous cell carcinoma of the penis: Brazilian National Cancer Institute long-term experience. *J Surg Oncol*. 2008;97: 487–495.
35. Stancik I, Holtl W. Penile cancer: review of the recent literature. *Curr Opin Urol*. 2003;13:467–472.
36. Ornellas AA, Correia AL, Marota A, Seixas ALC. Surgical treatment of invasive squamous cell carcinoma of the penis: retrospective analysis of 350 cases. *J Urol*. 1994;151:1244–1247.
37. Cabanas RM. An approach for the treatment of penile carcinoma. *Cancer*. 1977;39:456.
38. Perinetti EP, Crane DB, Catalona WJ. Unreliability of sentinel node biopsy for staging penile cancer. *J Urol*. 1980; 124:352.
39. Srinivas V, Morse MJ, Herr HW, Sogani PC, Whitmore WF Jr. Penile cancer: Relation of extent of nodal metastasis to survival. *J Urol*. 1987;137:880.
40. Lynch DF. Commentary on: Srinivas SV. Relation of extent of nodal metastasis to Survival. *Semin Urol Oncol*. 1997;15: 136–139.
41. Gerbaulet A, Lambin P. Radiation therapy of cancer of the penis. *Urol Clin North Am*. 1992;19:325–332.
45. Culkin DJ, Beer TM. Advanced penile carcinoma. *J Urol*. 2003;170:359–365.
51. Dexeus FH, Logothetis CJ, Sella A, et al. Combination chemotherapy with methotrexate, bleomycin, and cisplatin for advanced squamous cell carcinoma of the male genital tract. *J Urol*. 1991;146:1284–1287.

52. Leijte JAP, Kerst JM, Bais E, et al. Neoadjuvant chemotherapy in advanced penile carcinoma. *Eur Urol*. 2007;52:488–494.
53. Haas GP, Blumenstein BA, Gaggiano RG, et al. Cisplatin, methotrexate, and bleomycin for the treatment of carcinoma of the penis: a Southwest Oncology Group study. *J Urol*. 1999;161:1823–1825.
54. Mostofi FK, Davis CJ Jr, Sesterhenn IA. Carcinoma of the male and female urethra. *Urol Clin North Am*. 1992;19:347–358.
55. Bracken RB, Johnson DE, Miller LS, et al. Primary carcinoma of the female urethra. *J Urol*. 1976;116:188–192.
56. Chu AM. Female urethral carcinoma. *Radiology*. 1973;107:627–630.
57. Narayan P, Konety B. Surgical treatment of female urethral carcinoma. *Urol Clin North Am*. 1992;19:373–382.
58. Eng TY, Naguib M, Galang T, Fuller CD. Retrospective study of the treatment of urethral cancer. *Am J Clin Oncol*. 2003;26:558–562.
59. Greene FL, Page DL, Fleming ID, et al, eds. Urethra. In: *AJCC Cancer Staging Manual*. American Joint Committee on Cancer, 6th ed. New York: Springer; 2002.
60. Davis R, Peterson AC, Lance R. Clear cell adenocarcinoma in a female urethral diverticulum. *Urology*. 2003;61:644.
61. Tines SC, Bigongiari LR, Weigel JW. Carcinoma in diverticulum of female urethra. *AJR*. 1982;138:582.
62. Tesluk H. Primary adenocarcinoma of the female urethra. *Urology*. 1981;17:197.
63. Staeler C, Chaussy C, Jocham D, et al. The use of neodymium: YAG lasers in urology: indication, technique, and critical assessment. *J Urol*. 1985;134:1155–1160.
64. Schaeffer AJ. Use of the CO2 laser in urology. *Urol Clin North Am*. 1986;13:393404.
65. Dimarco DS, Dimarco CS, Zincke H, Webb MJ, Slezak JM. Surgical treatment for local control of female urethral carcinoma. *Urol Oncol*. 2004;22:404–409.
66. Weghaupt K, Gerstner GJ, Kucera H. Radiation therapy for primary carcinoma of the female urethra: a survey of over 25 years. *Gynecol Oncol*. 1984;17:58.
67. Dalbagni G, Donat SM, Eschwege P, Herr HW, Zelefsky MJ. Results of high dose rate brachytherapy, anterior pelvic exenteration, and external beam radiotherapy for carcinoma of the female urethra. *Int J Urol*. 2001;166:1759–1761.
69. Schellhammer PF, Whitmore WJ Jr. Transitional cell carcinoma of the urethra in men having cystectomy for bladder cancer. *J Urol*. 1976;115:56.
70. Varol C, Thalmann GN, Burkhard FC, Studer UE. Treatment of urethral recurrence following radical cystectomy and ileal bladder substitution. *J Urol*. 2004;172:937–942.
74. Franke HJ, Froehner M, Wirth MP. The treatment of primary urethral carcinoma—the dilemmas of a rare condition: experience with partial urethrectomy and adjuvant chemotherapy. *Onkologie*. 2001;24:48–52.

96 Testis Cancer

Christian Kollmannsberger, MD ■ Siamak Daneshmand, MD ■ Eric K. Hansen, MD ■
Christopher L. Corless, MD, PhD ■ Bruce J. Roth, MD ■ Craig R. Nichols, MD

Cancer of the testis is a relatively uncommon disease, accounting for approximately 1% of all cancers in males. However, it is an important disease in the field of oncology, as it represents a highly curable neoplasm, and the incidence of which is focused on young patients at their peak of productivity. Curative treatment of disseminated nonseminomatous germ cell tumors often combines surgery and chemotherapy. The goal of initial therapy is never palliation nor prolongation of survival, but cure.[1]

Epidemiology

Incidence

An age-related incidence curve of testicular cancer reveals a bimodal distribution. The major peak occurs between ages 15 and 35 years, owing almost exclusively to tumors of germ cell origin, which account for approximately 95% of all testicular cancer. Embryonal carcinoma represents the predominant histopathologic diagnosis up to the age of 35 years, after which seminoma is more common up to the age of 75 years. From 2001 to 2005, the median age at diagnosis for cancer of the testis was 34 years of age. Approximately 5.8% were diagnosed under age 20; 46.3% between 20 and 34; 29.2% between 35 and 44; 13.3% between 45 and 54; 3.3% between 55 and 64; 1.2% between 65 and 74; 0.6% between 75 and 84; and 0.2% 85+ years of age.[2]

The incidence of testicular cancer varies markedly based on geographic distribution. The incidence is highest in northern Europe and North America and lowest in Asia and Africa. There is also a striking influence of race, with the incidence among black and Hispanic males worldwide far less than that for their white counterparts.[3,4] In the US, estimates of the incidence ratio between white and African-American patients ranges from 4 to 5:1. Testicular cancer appears to be increasing among young white males in the Scandinavian countries, the United Kingdom, and the United States.[5] Standardized incidence rates increased annually 2-5%, with marginal differences between seminomas and nonseminomas. In the US, the annual percentage change from 1989 to 2005 was 0.8%. The trend may be attenuating in some countries, such as Denmark, and there appears to be large geographic differences in the changing incidences. It is estimated that 8090 cases of testicular cancer were diagnosed in the United States in 2008, with approximately 380 persons dying of the disease.[6]

Risk Factors

Cryptorchidism is the major identifiable risk factor associated with the development of testicular cancer, with a risk ratio variably reported between 2.5 and 14 in case-control studies.[7] The location of the maldescended testicle appears to be an important cofactor in the subsequent development of cancer, because those patients with intra-abdominal retention have a fourfold higher incidence of malignancy than those with the testicle etained in the inguinal canal. For a number of reasons, it seems unlikely that maldescent, in and of itself, represents the initiating event in the development of germ cell tumors: Only 10% of testicular tumors are associated with cryptorchidism, whereas 10-20% of the malignancies in patients with cryptorchidism occur in the contralateral, normally descended testicle; prepubertal orchiopexy fails to prevent the subsequent development of malignancy in the undescended testicle; and first-degree male relatives of patients with testicular cancer exhibit an increased incidence of cryptorchidism, hydroceles, and inguinal hernias, as well as testicular cancer.[8,9] These data suggest that some genetic predisposition and/or in utero environmental event may result in several genitourinary developmental abnormalities, including maldescent and germ cell neoplasia. Interestingly, an increase in the frequency of cryptorchidism has been observed and appears to parallel the timing and magnitude of the increase in incidence of testicular cancer. Brothers of men with testicular germ cell tumors (TGCTs) have an 8-fold to 10-fold risk of developing TGCT, whereas the relative risk to fathers and sons is approximately fourfold. This familial relative risk is much higher than that for most other types of cancer. A genome-wide linkage search yielded evidence for a testicular cancer susceptibility gene on chromosome Xq27 that may also predispose to undescended testes.[10]

TGCTs occur at increased frequency in men with human immunodeficiency virus (HIV). One multicenter study addresses the characteristics of these tumors. Thirty-five patients with HIV-related germ cell tumors (GCTs) were identified. The median age at germ cell tumor diagnosis was 34 years (range, 27-64 years). The median CD4 cell count was 315/mm^3 (range, 90-960/mm^3) at this time. The histologic classification was seminoma in 26 patients (74%) and nonseminomatous germ cell tumor in 9 patients (26%). Twenty-one patients (60%) had stage I disease and 14 patients had metastatic disease. Overall, six patients relapsed, three died from germ cell tumor, and seven died from HIV disease, resulting in a 2-year overall survival rate of 81%. HIV-related seminoma occurred more frequently than in the age-matched and sex-matched HIV-negative population, with a relative risk of 5.4 (95% confidence interval [CI] = 3.35-8.10); however, nonseminomatous germ cell tumor did not occur more frequently, and there was no change in the incidence of germ cell tumor since the introduction of highly active antiretroviral therapy. The conclusions of the authors were that testicular seminoma occurs significantly more frequently in HIV-positive men than in the matched control population. Patients with HIV-related GCTs present and should be treated in a similar manner to those in the HIV-negative population. Most of the mortality relates to HIV infection.[11]

An additional predisposition is the association of mediastinal nonseminomatous germ cell tumors with Klinefelter's syndrome. Approximately 10% of all patients with mediastinal nonseminoma have Klinefelter's syndrome, and there does not appear to be an increased incidence in patients with testicular or retroperitoneal primary tumors.[12]

An association of dysplastic nevus syndrome and testicular cancer has been observed.[13] A twofold higher incidence of multiple atypical nevi, and the attendant risk of melanoma, has been noted.

Patients with a history of unilateral testicular cancer are at risk of developing cancer in the other testicle. In a large Danish series, 2.7% of 2338 patients developed a contralateral testicular tumor during the period of follow-up.[14-16] Investigators at the Royal Marsden Hospital reported a similar rate of 2.75% for developing contralateral tumors among 760 men in an interval as long as 15 years.[17]

In the United States, the largest series is reported from Memorial Sloan-Kettering. Between 1950 and 2001, 3984 patients with testicular cancer were treated for germ cell tumor. A total of 58 patients with bilateral TGCTs were identified. Median follow-up was 60 months. Ten of the 58 patients (17%) had synchronous tumors, while the other 48 (83%) had metachronous tumors. Overall, seminoma was the most common histology of the synchronous and metachronous tumors. Most patients in the synchronous and metachronous tumor groups presented with low-stage disease. Of the 58 patients, 52 (89%) had no evidence of disease, and 6 (11%) were dead of disease at the last follow-up. Treatment of the second tumor appeared to be influenced by therapy for the first tumor in 16.7% of cases.[18]

Although risk estimates for synchronous and metachronous contralateral testicular cancers vary widely, many clinicians recommend routine biopsy of the contralateral testis for patients diagnosed with unilateral testicular cancer. Fossa and colleagues evaluated the risk of contralateral testicular cancer and survival in a large population-based cohort of men diagnosed with testicular cancer before age 55 years using Surveillance, Epidemiology and End Results (SEER) data. From 29,515 testicular cancer cases reported to the SEER Program of the National Cancer Institute (NCI), from 1973 through 2001, estimates of prevalence of synchronous contralateral testicular cancer, the observed-to-expected ratio (O/E), 15-year cumulative risk of metachronous contralateral testicular cancer, and the 10-year overall survival rate of both synchronous and metachronous contralateral testicular cancer were made. A total of 175 men presented with synchronous contralateral testicular cancer; 287 men developed metachronous contralateral testicular cancer (O/E = 12.4 [95% CI = 11.0-13.9%]; 15-year cumulative risk = 1.9% [95% CI = 1.7-2.1%]). In the multivariable analysis, only nonseminomatous histology of the first testicular cancer was associated with a statistically significantly decreased risk of metachronous contralateral testicular cancer (hazard ratio [HR] = 0.60; 95% CI = 0.46-0.79%; $p < .001$). Increasing age at first testicular cancer diagnosis was associated with decreasing risk of nonseminomatous metachronous contralateral testicular cancer (odds ratio = 0.90; 95% CI = 0.86-0.94%). The 10-year overall survival rate after metachronous contralateral testicular cancer diagnosis was 93% (95% CI = 88-96%), and that after synchronous contralateral testicular cancer was 85% (95% CI = 78-90%). The low cumulative risk of metachronous contralateral testicular cancer and favorable overall survival of patients diagnosed with metachronous contralateral testicular cancer is in accordance with the current US approach of not performing a biopsy on the contralateral testis.

These observations underscore the importance of continued long-term follow-up of patients with TGCTs.

Pathology

Origin and Molecular Genetics

Testicular tumors fall into several broad groups, as listed in Table 96-1. Classification of the germ cell tumors has historically been based on morphology, but recent molecular studies have yielded a more ontological scheme consisting of five distinct subtypes that differ in their proposed cell of origin.[19] According to this scheme, teratomas and yolk sac tumors arising in neonates and young children derive from primordial germ cells or very early gonocytes distributed along the gonadal ridge or in the testis/ovary. These tumors retain most of the genomic imprinting from both parental genomes. The teratomas remain diploid, while the yolk sac tumors show gains of chromosomes 1q, 12p13-14, and 20q, and losses of 1p, 4, and 6q.[19]

Spermatocytic seminoma is a second, distinct subtype of germ cell tumor thought to derive from postpubertal spermatogonia/spermatocytes. Accordingly, these tumors have a paternal pattern of genomic imprinting and show variable ploidy, sometimes with a gain of chromosome.[10]

Two of the other five proposed subtypes of germ cell tumor do not occur in the testis. Dermoid cysts of the ovary, which are thought to arise from oogonia/oocytes, are diploid/tetraploid and show maternal genomic imprinting. Hydatidiform mole (gestational trophoblastic disease) is a placental-derived neoplasm that contains a purely paternal genome as a result of fertilization of an empty ovum.

The fifth subtype of germ cell tumor consists of seminoma and the nonseminomatous germ cell tumor (NSGCT) patterns that, together, account for 95% of primary testicular neoplasms (Table 96-1). Variants of this germ cell tumor subtype also occur in the ovary (dysgerminoma), anterior mediastinum, and midline brain (germinoma). It is suggested that seminoma and NSGCT are derived from gonocytes that have lost their genomic imprinting as a result of being later in their development than those that give rise to infantile teratomas and yolk sac tumors. More-over, these gonocytes are polypoid (triploid or tetraploid), probably because of meiotic arrest. Depending on exactly when this arrest occurs during fetal development, the affected cells may be distributed to one or both testes, accounting for the bilateral germ cell tumors observed in 2-3% of patients.

Seminomas and NSGCT share a common precursor lesion called intratubular germ cell neoplasia, unclassified (ITGCNU). Growing in situ within seminiferous tubules, ITGCNU cells express markers shared with embryonic

Table 96-1 Primary Tumors of the Testis

Type	Relative Frequency	Genotype/Comments
Germ cell tumors		
Infants and children	~1% of all testis tumors	
Yolk sac tumor	65–80% of pre-pubertal	Aneuploid
Teratoma	20–35% of pre-pubertal	Diploid; mature elements; benign
Adolescents and adults	95% of all testis tumors	
ITGCNU	>90% of post-pubertal	Aneuploid (near triploid)
Seminoma	~45% of post-pubertal	Aneuploid (near triploid); iso12p
Nonseminomatous (NSGCT)	~55% of post-pubertal	Aneuploid (near triploid); iso12p
Embryonal carcinoma	~75% of NSGCT	
Yolk sac tumor	~50% of NSGCT	
Teratoma	~50% of NSGCT	Malignant (even mature elements)
Choriocarcinoma	~10% of NSGCT	
Adults (usually >50 yr)		
Spermatocytic seminoma	<1% of post-pubertal	Variable ploidy; gain of chromosome 9
Spermatocytic seminoma with sarcoma	Very rare	
Sex-cord stromal tumors		
Leydig cell tumor	~3% of all testis tumors	7–10% metastasis (post-pubertal)
Sertoli cell tumor	<1% of all testis tumors	
Granulosa cell tumor		
Adult type	Very rare	
Juvenile type	Uncommon	Infants <6 months
Mixed/indeterminate	Rare	
Mixed germ cell/sex-cord stromal tumors		
Gonadoblastoma	Very rare	

Table 96-2 ■ Markers of Testicular Germ Cell Tumors

Morphologic Subtype	Serum	Immunohistochemistry	FISH
ITGNCU		PLAP, KIT, OCT3/4	
Seminoma	HCG (low)	PLAP, KIT, OCT3/4	Excess 12p
Embryonal carcinoma	HCG (low)	CD30, OCT3/4, PLAP	Excess 12p
Yolk sac tumor	AFP	AFP, PLAP	Excess 12p
Choriocarcinoma	HCG (high)	HCG	Excess 12p
Teratoma			Excess 12p

Abbreviations: AFP, α-fetoprotein; FISH, fluorescence in situ hybridization; HCG, human choriogonadotropin; PLAP, placental/germ cell alkaline phosphatase.

stem cells, including the transcription factors OCT3/4 and NANOG.[20,21] These factors are essential to the development of embryonic stem cells in mice, but are not expressed in normal spermatogonia in mice or humans. Their presence in ITGCNU supports the theory that a pluripotent gonocyte is the cell of origin for both seminoma and NSGCT. In addition, OCT3/4 serves as a highly specific immunohistochemical marker in the diagnosis of extra-TGCTs (Table 96-2).[20,22]

Progression of ITGCNU to an invasive germ cell tumor is accompanied by a number of common events.[23] One is the acquisition of excess genetic material from the short arm of chromosome 12. In 80% of cases, this is accomplished through loss of 12q and reduplication of 12p (isochromosome 12p), while in the remaining 20%, the additional 12p sequences are distributed among other derivative chromosomes. Interestingly, the embryonic stem cell gene *NANOG* is on 12p. Fluorescence in situ hybridization (FISH) for 12p has already come into clinical use on paraffin sections as a diagnostic marker for germ cell tumors of all types and also for nongerm cell derivatives thereof.

Additional events associated with malignant progression of ITGCNU include loss of expression of the homeobox gene *NKX3.1*,[24] loss of the tumor suppressor PTEN,[25] and decreased expression of the cell cycle regulator p21.[26] Mutations of *TP53* are rare in postpubertal germ cell tumors, but the effects of this important tumor suppressor may be mitigated by *MDM2* overexpression,[26] or downregulation of *LATS2* by micro-RNAs mi-R372 and mi-R373. A genetic screen implicates miRNA-372 and miRNA-373 as oncogenes in TGCTs.[27]

Although seminoma and NSGCT share a common origin, they are clinicopathologically distinct cancers. Little is known of what determines their differences, but one interesting observation is that oncogenic mutations in KIT (a receptor tyrosine kinase) are found in 25% of seminomas and are essentially absent in NSGCT. These mutations may occur very early in seminoma tumorigenesis, as they are present in ITGCNU[28] and they have also been identified in dysgerminoma/germinoma of the ovary, mediastinum, and brain. Based on studies in mice, *KIT* gene function is essential to the development of primordial germ cells and to normal spermatogenesis; therefore, constitutive activation of this kinase may favor the seminoma pathway. It has also been suggested that *KIT* mutations are more common in patients who develop bilateral disease, but this remains controversial. Unfortunately, KIT kinase inhibitors such as imatinib are not likely to be of benefit to seminoma patients harboring *KIT*-mutant tumors, because most of the published mutations are inherently resistant to the drugs available.

Seminoma

Approximately 45% of all postpubertal TGCTs are pure seminoma ("classic" seminoma). The incidence is increased in cryptorchid testes, where it accounts for more than 60% of neoplasms. On gross examination, such tumors are generally homogeneous and well demarcated. Distinct lobulation may be apparent, with the nodules separated by dense fibrous bands. Areas of necrosis and hemorrhage may also be observed but are usually discrete. Microscopically, there is a monotonous distribution of uniform, rounded cells with large, centralized nuclei and nucleoli. The cytoplasm may be either clear or granular and will frequently stain positively for glycogen, lipid, and/or placental/germ cell alkaline phosphatase (PLAP). Stromal elements are equally characteristic, with an infiltrate rich in T-lymphocytes and containing occasional granulomas (Fig. 96-1). These features may predominate histologically and mimic granulomatous orchitis.

Seminoma presents most commonly in the fourth and fifth decades, usually as an enlarging, painless testicular mass. Approximately 70% of patients present with stage I disease (confined to testis), 20% with stage II (enlarged retroperitoneal lymph nodes), and only rarely with disease above the diaphragm. Lymphatic spread is to the para-aortic (PA) lymph nodes, then to the mediastinal or supraclavicular lymph nodes. Hematogenous dissemination to the lung, liver, bone, or adrenal is a late occurrence. Seminomas contain syncytiotrophoblastic giant cells that stain positively for human chorionic gonadotropin (HCG). Low-level HCG elevation is seen in 5–10% of patients with pure seminoma and likely reflects syncytiotrophoblastic elements present within the tumor (Table 96-2). Seminoma does not secrete α-fetoprotein.

Nonseminomatous Germ Cell Tumors

The most common postpubertal germ cell tumors of the testis are composed of one or more elements that are collectively known as "nonseminomatous." Four morphologic patterns are recognized among this group, as detailed below. In the great majority of cases, these patterns are intermixed in varying proportions, often subtly merging from one to the next. Areas of seminoma may be included (termed "mixed germ cell tumors" by some authors), but the prognosis is determined by the presence of the other elements and is less favorable, overall, than for pure seminomas.

Embryonal Carcinoma ■ Embryonal carcinoma is present in up to 90% of NSGCT cases. Macroscopically, it forms a soft, fleshy, inhomogeneous mass with areas of necrosis and hemorrhage. Direct invasion of the spermatic cord, epididymis, and tunica albuginea is not uncommon.

The microscopic appearance is extremely variable and may include papillary, solid, tubular, and glandular patterns, frequently interrupted by geographic necrosis (Fig. 96-2). Large polygonal cells with indistinct cytoplasmic borders (unlike seminoma) are the rule, with pale granular cytoplasm, large nuclei,

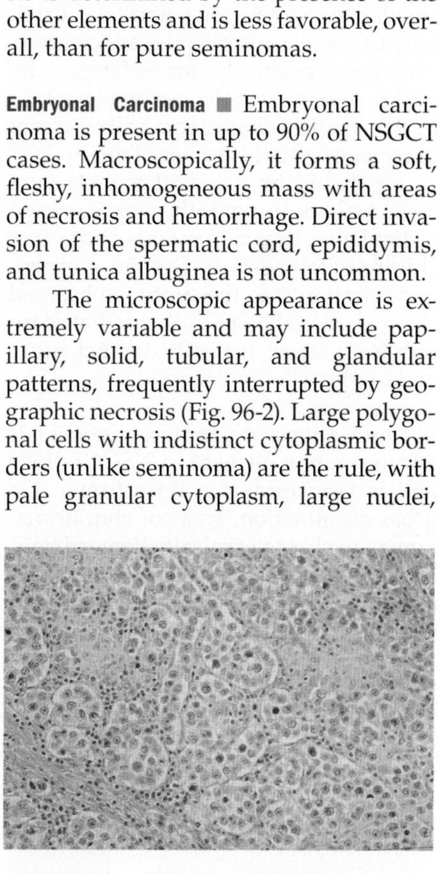

Figure 96-1 ■ Small nests of seminoma are separated by a lymphoid infiltrate and a focal granulomatous reaction.

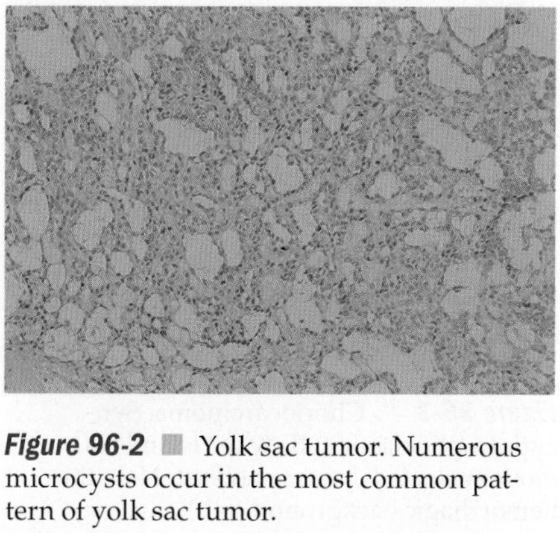

Figure 96-2 ■ Yolk sac tumor. Numerous microcysts occur in the most common pattern of yolk sac tumor.

and one or more centrally placed nucleoli. Mitotic figures and multinucleated cells are common. Clinically, these are aggressive tumors with lymph node metastases present in two-thirds of patients.

Yolk Sac Tumor ■ Yolk sac tumor, formerly called endodermal sinus tumor, is present in approximately half of NSGCT cases, but is rare in pure form in the postpubertal patient.[29] The most readily recognized pattern consists of a cluster of tumor cells surrounding a small central blood vessel, a structure referred to as a Schiller-Duval body (Fig. 96-3). The morphologic spectrum is quite broad, however, including microcystic (lacelike), micropapillary, solid, and hepatoid patterns. The tumor cell nuclei are somewhat smaller than those of embryonal carcinoma. Cytoplasmic globules are common and stain positively for α-fetoprotein, which accounts for the serum elevations in this marker characteristically present in patients with this tumor (Table 96-2).

It should be noted that in its pure form, yolk sac tumor is the most common testicular neoplasm in infants and young children (Table 96-1). Despite morphologic similarity to the subtype observed in postpubertal NSGCT, the pediatric tumor is an oncogenetically distinct entity and carries a better prognosis.

Choriocarcinoma ■ Choriocarcinoma is an uncommon element in NSGCT (15%) and is very rare as a pure tumor. On gross examination, areas of choriocarcinoma are characteristically hemorrhagic. Microscopically, the diagnosis requires a combination of cytotrophoblasts and syncytiotrophoblasts (Fig. 96-4). Stroma is sparse, but tends to be highly vascular. Choriocarcinoma of the testis represents the most aggressive subtype of NSGCT, often presenting with large-volume visceral metastases and/or brain metastases. Extreme elevations of serum HCG levels are characteristic.

Teratoma ■ Teratoma is defined as a tumor that contains elements of all three germ layers (endoderm, mesoderm, and ectoderm), present with varying degrees of differentiation. Teratomatous elements are recognized in approximately half of NSGCT cases, but are not usually pure. Macroscopically, teratomas tend to be large and have multiloculated cysts containing serosanguineous fluid as well as cartilaginous solid areas. Microscopically, all manner of tissue elements may be present, including cysts with squamous, respiratory or intestinal-type linings, mature cartilage, muscle, and fibroblastic stroma (Fig. 96-5). Areas that are less well differentiated ("immature teratoma") are often intermixed (Fig. 96-6). Regardless of the degree of differentiation, all teratomas in the postpubertal setting are regarded as malignant. In post-chemotherapy specimens (typically from retroperitoneal lymph node dissection) teratoma is the most common residual element. The presence of nonteratomatous NSGCT may be an indication for additional therapy.

A pure form of mature teratoma is common among pediatric patients under the age of four years. Although morphologically similar to mature areas of teratoma within NSGCT, these lesions arise through a different pathway and are essentially benign[30] (Table 96-1). Rarely, a nonteratomatous element is identified and may give rise to metastases.

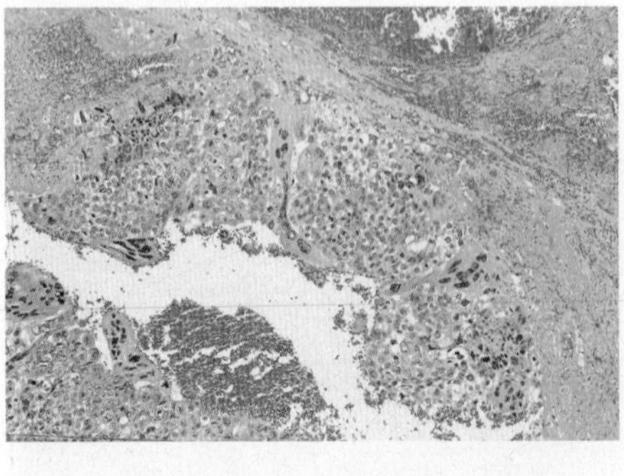

Figure 96-3 ■ Choriocarcinoma. Syncytiotrophoblastic cells "cap" islands of mononucleated cytotrophoblast. Note the hemorrhagic background.

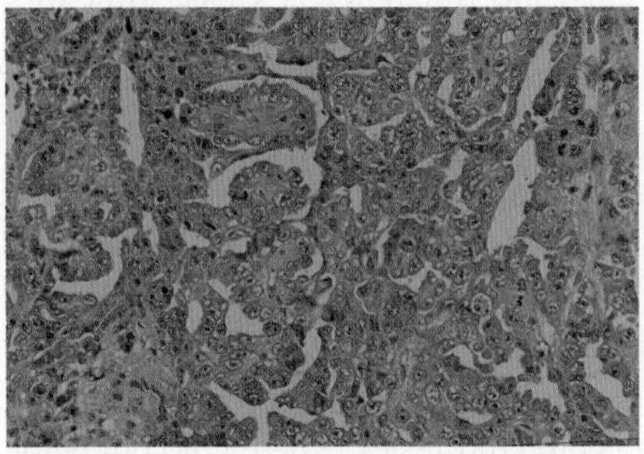

Figure 96-4 ■ Embryonal carcinoma. Irregularly shaped glands and papillae are lined by pleomorphic cells with vesicular, crowded nuclei and poorly defined cytoplasmic membranes.

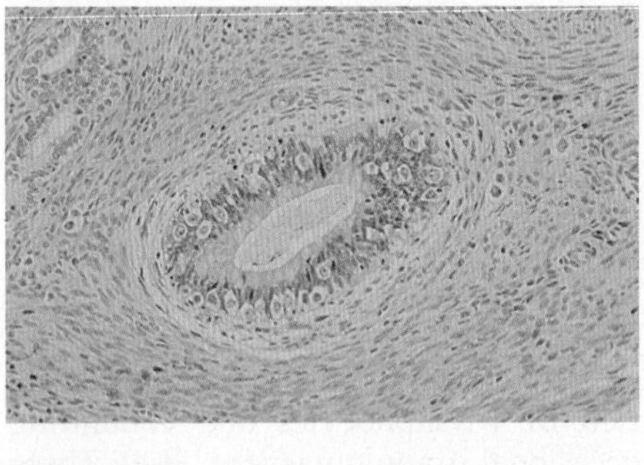

Figure 96-5 ■ Mature teratoma. There are mature-appearing small glands, a portion of a pilosebaceous unit, and bundles of smooth muscle.

Nongerm Cell Cancers Arising From Germ Cell Tumors

Given the pluripotent nature of the gonocytes from which seminomas and NSGCT are thought to arise, it is perhaps not surprising that in advanced cases of postpubertal testicular cancer, a nongerm cell element may emerge and become the dominant pattern. Among these are cancers morphologically resembling embryonal rhabdomyosarcoma, adenosquamous carcinoma, leiomyosarcoma, Wilms' tumor, glioblastoma multiforme, and primitive neuroectodermal tumor (PNET), all of which are associated with resistance to chemotherapy.[31] Myelodysplasia and leukemia may also evolve from NSGCT.[32]

Spermatocytic Seminoma

Spermatocytic seminoma accounts for only 1-2% of TGCTs. On gross examination, it has a grayish appearance and tends to be softer than classic seminoma. Microscopically, these tumors tend to form tubular clusters and are composed of round cells of highly variable size that bear resemblance to the cellular stages of normal spermatogenesis (Fig. 96-7). In contrast to classic seminoma, stromal lymphocytic infiltration is not a feature of spermatocytic seminoma. This tumor tends to occur over the age of 50, with a median age of 65 years. The prognosis following surgery is excellent, as there are only anecdotal reports of metastases.

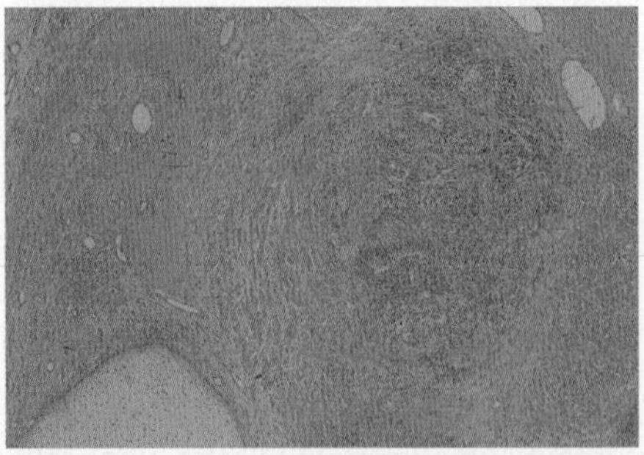

Figure 96-6 ■ Immature teratoma. An island of immature neuroepithelium is present adjacent to a nodule of hyaline cartilage.

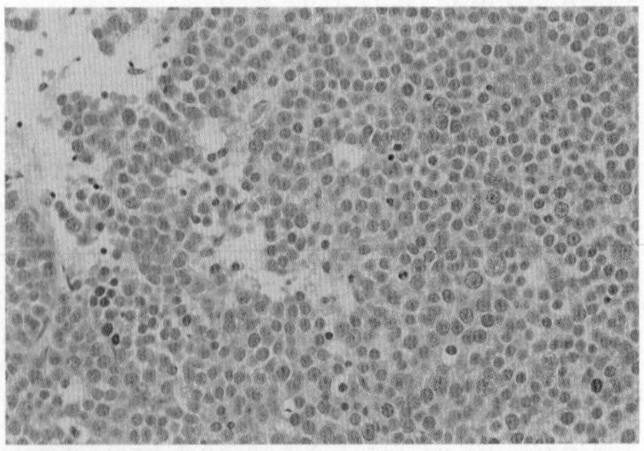

Figure 96-7 ■ Spermatocytic seminoma. There is a diffuse sheet-like arrangement of neoplastic cells that vary in size.

Sex Cord-Stromal Tumors

Tumors arising from stromal tissue account for only 4% of all adult testicular tumors, but represent almost 20% of childhood testicular tumors. These tumors are thought to arise from primitive gonadal mesenchyme and are subcategorized as Leydig cell tumor, Sertoli cell tumor, gonadoblastoma, granulosa cell tumor and mixed/indeterminate types (Table 96-1).

Leydig Cell Tumor ■ Leydig cell tumor represents about 3% of all testicular tumors, and although they may be seen in children, the median age of appearance is 60 years. Histologically, they are typified by cells with abundant oncocytic cytoplasm and round, regular nuclei. Clinical symptoms are usually related to the production of both androgens and estrogens by tumor cells, leading to precocious puberty in a child and gynecomastia in the adult. Approximately 10% of Leydig cell tumors metastasize, but this occurs only in the postpubertal patient. In patients with distant metastatic disease, treatment with radiation therapy or standard chemotherapeutic agents has generally been ineffective. Retroperitoneal lymph node dissection (RPLND) is an important staging procedure for these tumors. The therapeutic role of RPLND in low-volume metastatic retroperitoneal disease is unclear, but waiting to resect higher-volume tumor is ineffective. A prophylactic RPLND should, therefore, be considered in patients with clinical stage I tumors.

Sertoli Cell Tumor ■ Sertoli cell tumor shows no age predilection, presenting as a testicular mass that may be accompanied by gynecomastia or impotence secondary to tumor estrogen production. Microscopically, these lesions are composed of rounded cells with distinct cytoplasmic borders growing in cords and sheets in a fibrous background. As with other stromal tumors, therapy is primarily directed at resection of the primary lesion, with a staging work-up to include abdominal computed tomography (CT) scan and chest radiography. It is controversial as to whether an RPLND should be performed with clinical stage I disease. Large primary tumors with frequent mitoses or necrosis may prompt an RPLND. Unlike Leydig cell tumors, Sertoli cell tumors can respond to platinum combination chemotherapy.

Clinical Presentation

Most patients with testicular cancer seek medical attention because of the development of a swollen testis. Accompanying symptoms include a sensation of heaviness or aching in the affected gonad. Severe pain is quite rare, unless there is associated epididymitis or bleeding in the tumor. On occasion, because testicular cancer is commonly associated with low sperm counts, patients may present during the course of an infertility work-up.

Approximately 25% of patients with disseminated disease present with symptoms arising from metastatic disease.[33] Severe back pain from metastasis to the retroperitoneum is the most frequent symptom from metastatic disease of the testis and is the presenting symptom in patients with primary retroperitoneal germ cell tumors. Pulmonary complaints, such as shortness of breath, chest pain, or hemoptysis, are usually manifestations of far-advanced lung metastases. Primary mediastinal germ cell tumors are an exception, in that these tumors (if malignant) present with symptoms of mediastinal compression with pain, dysphagia, shortness of breath, and superior vena cava syndrome. Benign teratomas of the mediastinum produce few symptoms and are commonly discovered on routine chest film obtained for minor chest complaints. Other rare primary sites usually present with symptoms of local mass effect, for example, pineal, sacral presentations.

Diagnosis

Understanding the diagnosis and staging of TGCTs depends on understanding the anatomy of the vascular and lymphatic drainage of the testis as well as the likely sites of metastatic spread of the disease. The spermatic cord contains the lymphatic and vascular supply of the testis. The lymphatic and vascular supply diverges medially when the spermatic vessels cross ventral to the ureter. The landing zones for the lymphatic drainage of the right testis is the interaortocaval nodes below the renal vasculature and the ipsilateral distribution of nodes, especially the paracaval and preaortic nodes. The primary landing zone for a left-sided primary tumor includes in the PA nodes below the left renal vessels and the PA and preaortic nodes. Ipsilateral common iliac nodes are uncommonly involved unless large-volume disease is present.

Unusual patterns of disease can be seen (or created) in patients who have had prior pelvic surgeries including herniorrhaphy, abdominal orchiopexy, or scrotal violations.[34] It is important to emphasize here that the proper and only diagnostic procedure in this setting should be a radical inguinal orchiectomy. Transscrotal procedures can disrupt predictable patterns of lymphatic metastases and should not be done.

The evaluation for testicular cancer begins with a careful history and physical examination. The examination of the testis is performed by grasping the gonad between the thumb and first two fingers and carefully palpating the testis, epididymis, and cord. Tumors of the testis can present with a discrete nodular density or as diffuse infiltration of the entire testis (particularly seminoma and lymphoma). The other testis serves as a useful reference standard to make comparisons. If a testicular mass is suspected, transscrotal ultrasonography should be performed. The presence of a hypoechoic mass represents a testicular neoplasm, and a radical inguinal orchiectomy is required to make a definitive pathologic diagnosis, as well as to ensure local control of a primary testicular cancer.

Extragonadal germ cell tumors (EGCTs) arising within the retroperitoneum or mediastinum require specialized management. A diagnosis may be made on the basis of significantly elevated tumor marker levels in a patient with a mass in the anterior mediastinum or retroperitoneum. If there is no marker elevation, tissue confirmation is required. For mediastinal germ cell tumors, an anterior median sternotomy is favored for diagnosis. Because chemotherapy is the primary modality of treatment, attempts at debulking or total removal of mediastinal germ cell tumors as initial management are inappropriate. Primary retroperitoneal germ cell tumors may be associated with an occult testicular primary. Such patients should have a thorough evaluation of the gonads, including the use of testicular ultrasonography. If a previously unsuspected testicular tumor is found, orchiectomy can serve as the diagnostic procedure. Otherwise, fine-needle aspiration of the abdominal mass or exploratory laparotomy is required to provide tissue for diagnosis. In addition, an i(12p) chromosomal abnormality is diagnostic for germ cell tumor in a patient who presents with undifferentiated cancer.

A transscrotal biopsy should never be performed as this could seed the scrotal contents and, with disruption of regional lymphatics, lead to inguinal lymph node metastasis. Management of patients who have had a scrotal violation depends on the procedure performed and the anticipated treatment of the malignancy. If, at the time of scrotal orchiectomy, the surgeon identified the tumor and removed the testis in toto, then the only additional procedure that need be accomplished is removal of the inguinal portion of the spermatic cord. This can be done at the time of the retroperitoneal lymphadenectomy or through a separate inguinal incision. If a testicular biopsy was performed, management of the hemiscrotum depends on the primary treatment modality. Patients who are receiving primary chemotherapy do not need hemiscrotectomy. Inguinal lymphadenectomy is reserved for patients with palpable inguinal lymphadenopathy. For patients with early-stage seminoma who have had a scrotal violation, approximately 5-10% will experience local failure. Extending the field to include the groin and scrotum diminishes these prospects, but is associated with increased infertility. Such patients should be managed on a case-by-case basis, dependent on the desire to have a family and compliance with follow-up.

Tumor Markers

Serum HCG and α-fetoprotein represent the quintessential serum markers in oncology. They have significant value in the diagnosis, prognosis, and management of patients with germ cell tumors. α-Fetoprotein is a glycoprotein normally produced by the fetal yolk sac and is derived from the yolk sac or embryonal carcinoma elements of germ cell cancers. Elevated levels of α-fetoprotein are not seen in normal adults. The half-life of this protein in the serum is approximately 5 days. HCG is a smaller glycoprotein that is normally produced by trophoblastic tissues. In germ cell cancers, syncytiotrophoblastic components elaborate HCG. The protein comprises an alpha subunit and a beta subunit, each of which is antigenically distinct. The serum half-life of the entire protein is 18-30 h.

Serum HCG and/or α-fetoprotein are elevated in 85% of patients with disseminated nonseminomatous germ cell tumors. α-Fetoprotein alone is elevated in 40% of patients, and HCG alone is elevated in 50-60% of patients with disseminated nonseminomatous testicular cancer. Elevated lactic acid dehydrogenase (LDH) is a less specific marker and is mainly a correlate of disease bulk. Mediastinal nonseminomatous germ cell tumors more commonly have elevation of αfetoprotein (80%), because of frequent presence of yolk sac tumor, as compared with HCG (40%).

Pure seminoma is most frequently associated with normal α-fetoprotein and HCG, but approximately 10% of all cases, and up to 30% of patients with advanced disease, may have low-level elevation of HCG (usually < 100 mIU/mL).[35] Any elevation of α-fetoprotein in patients with seminoma must be viewed as evidence of nonseminomatous disease, and management should proceed as such.

α-Fetoprotein and HCG should be determined before and after orchiectomy, but the absence of marker elevation should not influence the decision to undertake the procedure. Likewise, normalization of serum markers after orchiectomy does not ensure that all disease has been removed, although persistence of marker elevation implies residual disease.

The rate of disappearance of elevated tumor markers is very useful in determining response to chemotherapy. HCG is the most useful in this regard; the most clinically helpful guideline is that a 10-fold decrease in the HCG level over a 3 week period is consistent with potentially curative chemotherapy. Less steep declines of HCG levels may correlate with the emergence of drug-resistant disease. Likewise, the reappearance of marker elevation often predates the radiographic appearance of recurrent disease and, as such, is an invaluable method of detecting early relapse.

Although the presence of tumor markers and their accurate determination serve as a luxury in the management of patients with germ cell cancer, the presence of these markers also can lead to errors in clinical management if not interpreted with caution. First, HCG determination can be nonspecific, and there is some cross-reactivity in the radioimmunoassay with luteinizing hormone. Also, HCG can be falsely elevated in patients who use marijuana. Low levels of HCG elevation, consequently, are difficult to interpret. A conservative approach to this dilemma is to repeat the HCG determination to ensure that the elevation is not a laboratory error. If the level is still high, the patient should be queried regarding drug usage. Testosterone should be given in a dose of 300 mg intramuscularly to ensure that a hypogonadal state with resultant high levels of luteinizing hormone is not interfering with the determination of HCG. If the level remains increased, restaging procedures and investigation of sanctuary sites (brain and contralateral testis) are in order.

A retrospective review by Zon and colleagues at Indiana University evaluated management problems in patients with very high HCG levels.[36] Forty-one patients with an HCG greater than 50,000 mIU/mL were included. All patients received cisplatin-based chemotherapy. Two of these 41 patients had normal HCG levels at the time of the fourth course of chemotherapy. Eight additional patients had normalized the HCG within 1 month of completion of the fourth course of therapy. Of these ten patients, seven remain continuously free of disease, and three are currently disease-free with salvage therapy. Thirty-one patients still had an abnormal HCG more than 1 month after completing the fourth course of primary chemotherapy. Fifteen of these patients are continuously disease-free, despite no further treatment. This review highlights a subset of patients with very high HCG levels who do not have a consistent predictable decline of HCG with treatment. Absolute dependence on predicted patterns of decline in these patients would have resulted in overtreatment or inappropriate initiation of salvage therapy. Our strategy has been to wait for a rising serum HCG before considering salvage therapy. False-positive elevation of α-fetoprotein is quite rare. Differential considerations include laboratory error, other tumor types (such as hepatocellular carcinoma), and liver inflammation from cirrhosis or hepatitis. An occasional patient may have baseline elevation of α-fetoprotein (usually < 100 ng/mL) that remains static over time and does not reflect active disease.[37]

Staging

Germ cell tumors are typically categorized as stage I, referring to tumors confined to the testis; stage II, indicating metastatic disease to the nodes of the periaortic or vena caval zone without pulmonary or visceral involvement; and stage III, which denotes metastasis above the diaphragm or involving other viscera. The American Joint Committee on Cancer (AJCC) has refined the classification system and included the important aspect of elevated tumor markers into the classification system. This TNM (tumornodes-metastasis)-based system adds important local prognostic parameters, such as vascular invasion; more regional nodal information, including size; and visceral versus nonvisceral metastasis and markers levels. This AJCC and World Health Organization (WHO) classification is the international standard (Table 96-4).[38]

Standard procedures to establish clinical stage include physical examination, abdominal and chest CT scans, and serum levels of α-fetoprotein, βHCG, and LDH. Brain imaging and bone scans should be performed only when clinically indicated. The role of positron emission tomography (PET) remains investigational in the initial staging of patients with germ cell tumors. However, in one series, PET imaging had a positive predictive value of 96% and negative predictive value of 90% when evaluating residual masses following chemotherapy.[39] PET scan will not reliably detect teratoma or microscopic carcinoma. PET scan has been investigated in patients with residual masses after chemotherapy for seminoma, and the persistence of PET avidity is associated with risk of recurrence.[40]

Table 96-4 ■ **AJCC Staging**

TNM Clinical Classification	
T:	*Primary tumor:* The extent of the primary tumor is classified after radical orchiectomy (see pT). If no radical orchiectomy has been performed, TX is used.
N:	*Regional lymph nodes*
NX	Regional lymph nodes cannot be assessed
N0	No regional lymph node metastasis
N1	Metastasis with a lymph node mass ≤2 cm in greatest dimension or multiple lymph nodes, not >2 cm in greatest dimension
N2	Metastasis with a lymph node mass >2 cm but not >5 cm in greatest dimension, or multiple lymph nodes, any one mass >2 cm but not >5 cm in greatest dimension
N3	Metastasis with a lymph node mass >5 cm in greatest dimension
M:	*Distant metastasis*
MX	Distant metastasis cannot be assessed
M0	No distant metastasis
M1	Distant metastasis
M1a	Nonregional lymph node or pulmonary metastasis
M1b	Distant metastasis other than to nonregional lymph node and lungs
pTNM Pathologic Classification	
pT:	*Primary tumor*
pTX	Primary tumor cannot be assessed (if no radical orchiectomy has been performed TX is used)
pT0	No evidence of primary tumor (eg, histologic scar in testis)
pTis	Intratubular germ cell neoplasia (carcinoma in situ)
pT1	Tumor limited to testis and epididymis without vascular/lymphatic invasion, tumor may invade tunica albuginea, but not tunica vaginalis
pT2	Tumor limited to testis and epididymis with vascular/lymphatic invasion, or tumor extending through tunica albuginea with involvement of tunica vaginalis
pT3	Tumor invades spermatic cord with or without vascular/lymphatic invasion
pT4	Tumor invades scrotum with or without vascular/lymphatic invasion
pN:	*Regional lymph nodes*
pNX	Regional lymph nodes cannot be assessed
pN0	No regional lymph node metastasis
pN1	Metastasis with a lymph node mass ≤2cm in greatest dimension and ≤5 positive nodes, none >2 cm in greatest dimension
pN2	Metastasis with a lymph node mass >2 cm but not >5 cm in greatest dimension; or >5 nodes positive, non >5 cm; or evidence of extranodal extension of tumor
pN3	Metastasis with a lymph node mass >5 cm in greatest dimension
pM:	*Distant metastasis*
	The pM category corresponds to the M category
S:	*Serum tumor markers*
SX	Serum marker studies not available or not performed
S0	Serum marker study levels within normal limits LDH HCG α-fetoprotein
S1	<1.5.N and <5000 and 1000
S2	1.5-10.N or 5000-50,000 or 1000-10,000
S3	>10.N or >50,000 or >10,000

N, the upper limit of normal for the lactate dehydrogenase assay.

Therapy

Carcinoma in Situ

Carcinoma in situ (CIS) or tubular intraepithelial neoplasia (TIN) is a true premalignant condition leading to both seminomatous and nonseminomatous invasive germ cell tumors in up to 50% of untreated cases (Figs. 96-8 and 96-9).[41] Management is controversial. Evaluated approaches for management include close observation, low-dose radiotherapy, and total orchiectomy. Observation after diagnosis of TIN offers the best chance of retained fertility, but requires a compliant patient and risks the possible requirement for more intensive treatment of invasive disease. Low-dose radiotherapy (18-20 Gy in 1.5-2.0 Gy fractions) will eradicate the TIN with high probability at the cost of decreased or eliminated fertility. These dose levels will not, however, usually affect potency, as Leydig cell function is preserved.[41,42] Total orchiectomy will obviously eliminate TIN

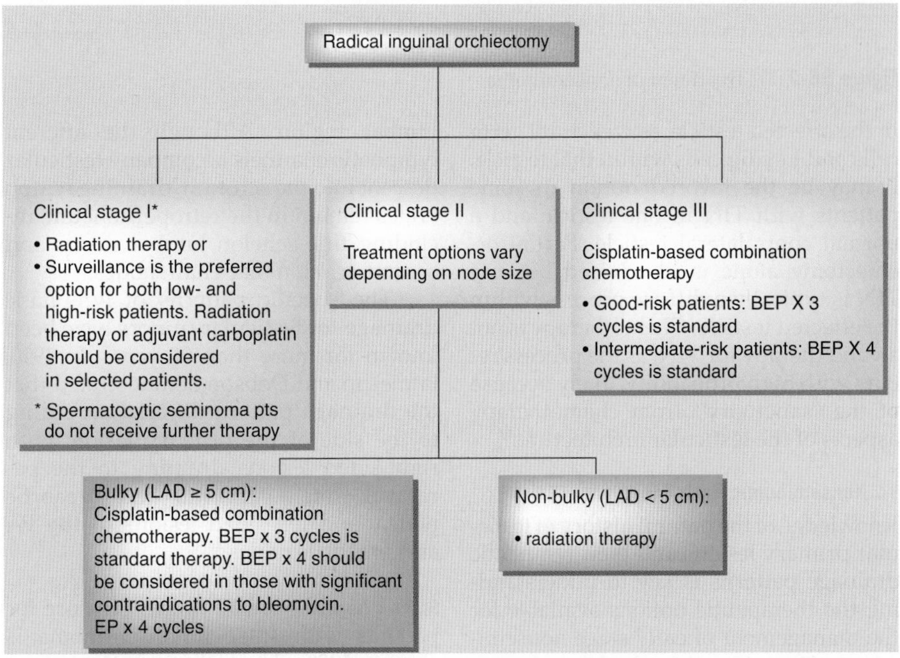

Figure 96-8 ■ Treatment of seminoma.

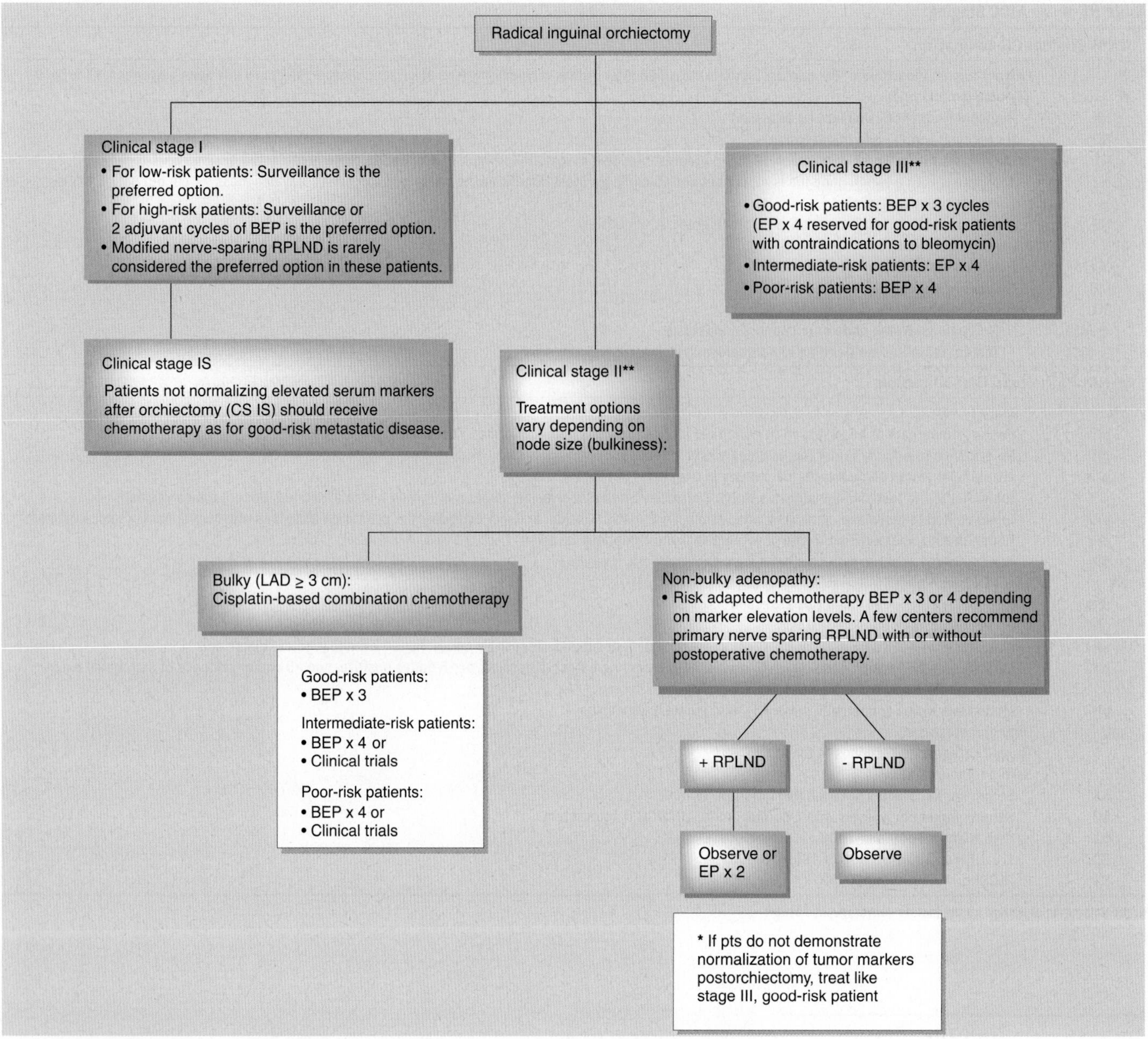

Figure 96-9 ■ Treatment of nonseminoma.

in the effected testicle, as well as all germ cells and Leydig cells within that testicle. It may be the favored option in some patients with TIN in one testicle and a normal contralateral testicle. Partial orchiectomy alone is ill advised because TIN is typically a diffuse process within the effected testicle. Chemotherapy is not a valid therapy for TIN, as the process recurs with high probability, likely because of the "sanctuary" from chemotherapy aspects of the testicular architecture.[43]

Nonseminoma: Early Stage

Knowledge of the natural history of testicular primary lesions and their lymphatic drainage patterns is key to understanding the therapeutic options available for the management of early-stage nonseminoma. Testicular lymphatics arise in proximity to the embryonic origin of the testicle, in the genital ridge in the high lumbar region. Although the afferent lymphatic channels accompany testicular descent into the scrotum, draining lymph nodes remain in the retroperitoneum, including first-echelon lumbar nodes and second-echelon iliac chain nodes.

The specific patterns of lymphatic drainage for testicular tumors have been known for more than 90 years. In 1910, Jamieson and Dobson demonstrated that the drainage pattern differed according to the side of the primary lesion, with right-sided lesions draining to the paracaval, interaortocaval, and preaortic nodes, and left-sided lesions to the PA and preaortic nodes.[44]

Stage I Nonseminoma ■ Today, the cure for patients with stage I nonseminoma is close to 100%. Three therapeutic options exist, primary RPLND, adjuvant chemotherapy and active surveillance, all of which result in a similarly excellent outcome. Attention has therefore been focused on the reduction in the toxicity of curative therapy. The accurate diagnosis of clinical stage I disease is critical to the consideration of less interventional therapy. Following inguinal orchiectomy and the diagnosis of nonseminoma, serum levels of βHCG and α-fetoprotein must return to normal (if elevated before orchiectomy), and abdominal CT, chest radiography, and/or chest CT must all be negative for metastatic disease before a patient can be labeled as having clinical stage I disease. In this clinical setting, approximately 30% of patients will suffer a relapse if no other therapy is administered, with the retroperitoneum remaining as the area at highest risk. Approximately 8-10% of patients will develop metastases outside of the retroperitoneum, mostly in the lungs.[45]

Prognostic factors have been identified to select a group of patients at higher risk of disease recurrence with clinical stage I disease. Freedman and colleagues developed a mathematical model on the basis of the four identified prognostic factors in the Medical Research Council (MRC) study in the United Kingdom and were able to identify a subset of patients with a 58% relapse rate at 2 years.[46] These four factors included invasion of testicular veins, invasion of testicular lymphatics, absence of yolk sac elements, and presence of undifferentiated tumor. pathologic T-stage higher than 1, the presence of components of embryonal carcinoma, and percent of the primary tumor occupied by teratoma, have also been described.[46-48] The importance of vascular invasion as the most dominating independent risk factor has been emphasised repeatedly in subsequent studies. Clinically, the presence of vascular invasion in the primary tumor specimen discriminates the "high-risk" patients with a risk of relapse of approximately 50% from the "low risk" patients without lymphovascular invasion and an approximately 15-20% risk of relapse. The other factors do not appear to add significantly to the prognostic value of lymphovascular invasion alone.

There is an ongoing controversy regarding the optimal management of patients with clinical stage I nonseminoma. All three options, RPLND, adjuvant chemotherapy and active surveillance are discussed below.

Retroperitoneal Lymph Node Dissection

Based on a predictable lymphatic pattern of spread of testicular tumors, RPLND emerged as a treatment option for testicular cancer as early as 1907.[49-51] In the United States, primary RPLND became the conventional approach for patients with clinical stage I nonseminomatous germ cell tumors, although this is currently being challenged. In Europe and Canada, consensus guidelines do not currently advocate primary RPLND in early-stage disease.[52,53] Nevertheless, RPLND does provide the most accurate method of detecting retroperitoneal nodal disease, which account for more than 90% of the first site of metastatic spread. RPLND alone can be curative in 50-80% of clinical stage I disease who are found to have limited nodal disease upon surgery (pN1). Those who have more than five metastatic lymph nodes, diseased nodes measuring more than 2 cm or any extra-nodal extension (pN2-3) are virtually all cured following two cycles of adjuvant chemotherapy.[54] Primary RPLND also has the advantage of removing retroperitoneal teratoma which is chemo-resistant, virtually eliminating the risk of late relapse of teratoma.[55] However even in pure teratomas, only 20% of patients will harbor occult retroperitoneal lymph node metastases at the time of diagnosis.[56] Relapses in the retroperitoneum are exceedingly rare in patients who undergo RPLND by experienced surgeons. The overall relapse rate for patients with disease limited to the testicle is approximately 10%, with the great majority of relapses occurring in the lungs, since the surgical procedure has effectively removed the retroperitoneum as a significant site of relapse.

A number of surgical techniques have been described to expose and resect retroperitoneal lymph nodes. Radical lymphadenectomy via a thoraco-abdominal (extra-peritoneal) approach was described in 1950,[57] and popularized by Skinner in the 1980s[58] while reports of pure abdominal (anterior) approaches dominated the 1970s,[59,60] with each approach having intrinsic advantages. The thoraco-abdominal approach allows excellent exposure on the ipsilateral side including suprahilar areas, however is associated with significantly higher morbidity including pain and chest complications albeit lower rates of small bowel obstruction owing to the extra-peritoneal approach.[58] In an effort to reduce morbidity Donohue and colleagues described the midline anterior approach and since the incidence of suprahilar metastases in clinical stage I disease was shown to be rare, the technique evolved to include only infrahilar RPLND.[61] The thoraco-abdominal incision is rarely used today for clinical stage I dissections, and has largely been replaced by the anterior midline approach. It is also possible to stay extra pleural and extra-peritoneal via a midline incision extended to the costochondral margin.

In experienced hands, the classic, bilateral RPLND is associated with minimal perioperative morbidity and virtually no mortality.[62] A major side effect of this approach, however, is the loss of antegrade ejaculation, with resultant need for assisted reproductive technology for fertility in over 90% of patients. An improved understanding of the nerves and pathways responsible for seminal emission and ejaculation along with meticulous anatomic studies of the distribution of right-sided and left-sided tumors led to further modification of the surgical "templates" for RPLND.[63,64] Several nerve-sparing modifications of the classic node dissection have now been described in an attempt to minimize ejaculatory dysfunction while maintaining the staging and/or therapeutic benefit of the procedure.[65-67] Any template used must adhere to strict principles of thoroughly resecting all interaortocaval lymph nodes and ipsilateral lymph nodes from the level of the renal hilum down to the bifurcation of the ipsilateral common iliac artery. Dissection is minimized on the contralateral side particularly below the level of the inferior mesenteric artery (IMA). In order to minimize retroperitoneal recurrence, some authors however advocate bilateral infrahilar dissections only sparing the contralateral nodes below the IMA.[68] Modified template nerve-sparing RPLND is now considered standard of care for patients undergoing surgery for clinical stage I disease. Meticulous preservation of the postganglionic sympathetic fibers arising from the sympathetic chain and the hypogastric plexus result in uniformly high rates of preservation of ejaculatory function (96-100%) while maintaining more than 99% cure rate.[59,66,69] Hospitalization times now average 4-5 days in experienced centers in the United States with rare ICU admissions postoperatively.

In an effort to further reduce the morbidity of surgery, laparoscopic techniques for RPLND have been used. More than 34 reports have been published to date detailing the results of more than 800 patients treated by laparoscopic RPLND.[70] Although operating room times are longer, long-term follow-up in over 550 patients has shown no difference in relapse rates compared with traditional open RPLND. However, the vast majority (>90%) of the patients with positive nodes have received adjuvant chemotherapy raising the question of the true efficacy of this approach. Laparoscopic RPLND is a technically challenging procedure that should only be undertaken by expert minimally invasive surgeons who are adept in retroperitoneal dissection. The same principles of modified templates and nerve-sparing approaches should apply to any laparoscopic approach.

Radiotherapy

Although previously utilized in stage I nonseminoma, radiotherapy is no longer used based on both the overwhelming success of combination chemotherapy, the safety of active surveillance as well as the limited efficacy of radiotherapy in nonseminomas.

Adjuvant Chemotherapy ■ The definition of a high-risk group by vascular invasion, the efficacy and safety of chemotherapy for good-risk metastatic disease and the near-perfect results of two cycles of chemotherapy in the setting of fully resected stage II disease have prompted investigators to consider the use of primary chemotherapy in high-risk stage I disease.

Based on data from stage II trials suggesting that 2 cycles of BEP may be sufficient adjuvant treatment, the MRC designed a prospective study offering 2 cycles of bleomycin, etoposide, and cisplatin (BEP) chemotherapy to patients with high-risk stage 1 NSGCTT.[71] The aim of the study was to evaluate the efficacy and long-term toxicity of adjuvant chemotherapy. One hundred and fourteen patients were treated and followed up for a median of 4 years. The 2-year recurrence-free survival was 98%. The 95% confidence interval excluded a true recurrence rate of more than 5%. Of the two patients who recurred, one was found to have adenocarcinoma of the rete testis rather than a germ cell tumour following histological review. Long-term toxicity was assessed by pretreatment and posttreatment analysis of renal function, lung function, semen analysis, and audiometry. No major, clinically significant changes were observed, although the median follow-up of 4 years is too short to conclusively assess long-term toxicity. Adjuvant chemotherapy with 2 cycles of BEP achieves a near-universal cure in patients with stage I disease with relapse rates in various studies ranging from 0% to 2%.

Two cycles of adjuvant BEP were subsequently adopted as the standard approach to patients with vascular invasion for the European Consensus Guidelines whereas patients with low risk disease are candidates for active surveillance.[72]

Recent data suggest that 1 cycle of BEP may result in similar outcome, although this needs further confirmation and follow-up.[73]

Active Surveillance ■ The main rationale for active surveillance is that systemic chemotherapy is highly effective and thus, patients who are cured by orchiectomy alone can be spared the treatment-related toxicity of a primary RPLND or adjuvant chemotherapy.

An early large prospective study of surveillance included 373 patients with a median follow-up of 5 years.[74] The recurrence rate was 27% and of these 80% recurred within the first year. Overall cure rate for the entire cohort of patients exceeded 98%. Vascular invasion was confirmed as the most important prognostic factor. The University of Toronto group recently presented 305 non risk-adapted patients on a prospective surveillance protocol.[75] With a recurrence rate of 25% and only two deaths (cancer-specific survival 97%) on long-term follow-up this series of surveillance underlines the efficacy of the approach. These data are consistent with other surveillance studies and the survival figures compare favorably with the best series for RPLND as well as adjuvant chemotherapy.

There are now reports of more than 3000 patients worldwide with clinical stage I disease who have had no other therapy administered following orchiectomy with relapse rates and survival remarkably similar between trials, regardless of the size of the study or country of origin.[76] Almost all patients on active surveillance relapse within 2 years after diagnosis with IGCCCG good prognosis disease.[74,77] Only 2-3% of relapses occur beyond 2 years. Thus careful surveillance plus chemotherapy at the earliest sign of recurrence is an effective management approach to patients with stage 1 NSGCTT. Active surveillance has been adopted as the standard of care for patients with low-risk disease by the European and for both low-risk and high-risk by the Canadian Consensus Guidelines.[72]

Based on a randomized prospective trial a sufficient follow-up schedule for vascular invasion negative patients consists of tumor markers and clinical examination every 2 months for the first 2 years and every 4-6 months for years 3-5. Chest X-rays are done every 4 months for the first 2 years and then every 6 months thereafter until year 5.[78] CT scans are performed at 3, 12, 24, and 56 months. Various surveillance schedules with closer follow-up and more frequent imaging exist for high-risk patients.

Management Preferences in Stage 1 NSGCTT ■ With the development of effective adjuvant chemotherapy, nerve-sparing RPLND and active surveillance, patients with stage 1 NSGCTT, especially those at high-risk of recurrence, now have a choice of management options. All options, when carried out meticulously, result in the same excellent survival prospects but with different shortcomings.

Arguments for retaining primary surgery are that, when done in one of the few high-volume centers in the US or elsewhere, results are excellent, infertility and complication rates are very low and such an approach, when performed in an experienced center, essentially eliminates the abdomen as a source of relapse making abdominal imaging unnecessary in follow-up. However, even in excellent centers, preoperative evaluations routinely fail to reliably identify the seventy percent of patients who are pathological stage I thus subjecting the majority of patients to major surgery without therapeutic benefit. In addition, 25-35% of patients will require additional 2 cycles of BEP due to extensive retroperitoneal disease. Most importantly, while reducing the risk of a retroperitoneal recurrence to 1-2%, RPLND does not eliminate the risk of recurrence outside the retroperitoneum (8-10%), The results of community level primary surgical management of stage I nonseminoma have not only demonstrated a numerically greater relapse rate as compared to adjuvant chemotherapy, but also a increased number of patients experiencing both scrotal and abdominal relapses strongly suggesting that primary RPLNDs performed by less experienced urologists result in inadequate cancer operations.[73]

Adjuvant chemotherapy, in particular for high-risk disease is considered the standard of care in many countries. While the recurrence rate is decreased to 2-4%, adjuvant chemotherapy will also result in overtreatment in at least 50% of patients.[76] All of these patients will experience hair loss, a significant disruption from work, school, and life, exposure to significant neutropenia with the rare risk of fatal complications, risk of vascular complications, rare acute chemotherapy reactions, at least temporary effects on fertility and the anxiety and fears that all patients receiving chemotherapy face. The potential long-term complications of one to two cycles of chemotherapy, although thought to be little, are currently unknown. With adjuvant chemotherapy, a low-level of recurrences still happens and most recurrences are seen in the abdomen. Thus, patients treated with adjuvant chemotherapy are not fully spared the fear of relapse or the inconvenience of ongoing imaging.

Concerns regarding the lack of compliance always serve as an argument against surveillance, in particular in high-risk CSI nonseminoma. Little research has been done to address the issue of compliance and its potential impact on overall outcome of CSI nonseminoma patients.[76] Reported compliance with surveillance visits range from poor to adequate however there is no evidence that the level of compliance across varying geographies materially impacts survival.[76,79,80] Survival rates consistently approach 100% even in series with reported "unsatisfactory" compliance. Educating patients about the risk of recurrence, the importance of reporting suspicious symptoms and the importance of adherence to recommended testing guidelines is crucial and that emphasizing that later identification of disease might well lead to more complicated and complex therapies is fully warranted. Concerns about the undissected retroperitoneum leading to a significant number of late refractory cancer or late recurrence of teratoma have not been realized in this and other studies.[76,79,81,82]

On surveillance, only patients who relapse will receive treatment. Treatment of these patients will be slightly longer than adjuvant BEP X 2 (6 vs 9 weeks).[83] In our opinion, there is only a small difference in toxicity between two and three courses of chemotherapy. However, there is a major difference between no chemotherapy and two courses. Active surveillance completely spares 70-75% of patients the burden of any active treatment and thus, minimizes treatment-related morbidity for the entire patient population.

In summary, patients with stage 1 NSGCTT can be successfully managed either by a policy of surveillance with chemotherapy in the event of recurrence, or by treatment with 2 cycles of adjuvant chemotherapy. Primary RPLND is no longer recommended as the standard approach. The importance of offering clear information about different treatment options to patients is key to the successful management of these patients.

Clinical Stage II

The presence of tumor marker positive disease and/or large-volume abdominal disease (>2 cm on abdominal CT, stage IIB) should be treated with primary chemotherapy. Standard treatment are 3 cycles of BEP according to the recommendations for IGCCCG good prognosis disease.[83] Only in case of significant contraindication to Bleomycin, 4 cycles of etoposide and cisplatin (EP) can be considered.[84] The majority of patients with stage IIA/B will achieve a clinical complete remission with resolution of all lymph node metastases and normalization of tumor markers. (80-90% in stage IIA and 65-85% in stage IIB).[83,84] Only patients with persistent retroperitoneal residual disease on the post-chemotherapy CT scan should undergo a post-chemotherapy RPLND. The relapse rate with this strategy is 4-9% for stage IIA and 11-15% for stage IIB.[85-87] Tumor marker negative stage IIA (lymph nodes ≤ 2 cm) represent a particular problem. Some of these patients will have benign lymph node enlargement, some of them, however, will have teratoma, pure embryonal carcinoma, or mixed tumors. There is currently no diagnostic tool to determine the nature of these masses reliably, including PET scanning. Management options include primary RPLND or a surveillance period with repeat imaging after 6-8 weeks. If the lesions shrink no further therapy is required, whereas for stable or even growing lesions, most centers would consider either primary chemotherapy, with a few selected centers considering primary RPLND.

Seminoma Early Stage

Orchiectomy and postoperative radiation therapy constituted the standard of care for early-stage seminoma patients during most of the twentieth century.[88-90] A properly performed radical orchiectomy by an inguinal approach is highly effective therapy for controlling disease at the primary tumor site. Occult or gross PA lymphatic tumor deposits can be eradicated with high probability after low doses of radiation therapy (20-25 Gy), owing to the extreme radiosensitivity of seminoma. More recently, trials have investigated surveillance in stage I seminoma. With a large majority of patients experiencing prolonged disease-free survival in early-stage seminoma, long-term quality of life end points will assume increasing significance in evaluating management options.

Stage I Seminoma: Primary and Adjuvant Therapy ■ Stage I disease comprises 85% of all seminoma cases diagnosed.[91] Stage I disease is where the most experience has been gained and the most evolution in treatment has occurred. Surveillance studies have demonstrated that a proper orchiectomy is curative approximately 80-85% of the time. Chemotherapy and/or radiation can be given as salvage therapy or as prophylaxis adjuvantly. Regardless of the elected management method, disease-specific survival at 5 years is over 99%.[92-95] The treatment of relapsed treatment-naïve disease appears to be as curable as it is at first presentation.

Four major series, the Princess Margaret Hospital, Danish Testicular Cancer Study Group, Royal Marsden Hospital, and Royal London Hospital, have demonstrated that surveillance is a viable option for treatment.[92-94,96-99] Their combined experience was pooled in an attempt to better identify candidates for treatment or surveillance.[93] In the entire group of 638 patients, 6 patients (0.9%) died of disease or complications of treatment of relapse. The overall 5-year and 10-year relapse-free rates were 82.3% and 78.7%, respectively. The majority (68.6%) of relapses occurred within 2 years, but still 7% of recurrences occur after 6 years. In an analysis of potential prognostic factors, the two most important were tumor size and rete testis invasion. Patients with tumors greater than 4 cm in diameter were twice as likely to relapse as those with smaller tumors. The rete testis is a communicating network of seminal channels traversing the mediastinum (or hilum) of the testis. Rete testis invasion was seen in 37% of the reported cases and defined as extension of the tumor into the testicular mediastinum without necessarily involving the tubular lumens. For patients with both factors of large tumor size and rete testis invasion, the rates of recurrence were as high as 33%. Although for patients without these factors, the recurrence rates were as low as 13%.

The schedule for surveillance testing is in flux and in general the previous intense schedules are being reversed downward. Many centers concentrate observations into the highest period of risk and use progressively less CT scans in follow up. Many schedules in seminoma are recommending a 3-2-1 with 3 abdominal/pelvic CTs the first year, 2 the second, and 1 the third with no CTs thereafter. Thus, although surveillance is a very attractive option, the frequency of follow-up imaging and tests cannot be reduced in any given patient. Therefore, patients who elect surveillance need to be compliant and reliable.

Patients with stage I seminoma have been successfully treated with orchiectomy and adjuvant radiation for over 60 years with overall survival rates now above 99%. Adjuvant PA radiation results in a 3-4% rate of relapse with most of those being salvageable with additional radiation and/or chemotherapy. Analogous to the movement for no initial therapy (surveillance) is a simultaneous drive to reduce the toxicity of initial adjuvant therapy by reducing radiation dose and volume treated.

Radiation dose has been gradually reduced to 20-25.5 Gy in 1.5-2 Gy fractions in current practice. The MRC TE18/ European Organization for the Research and Treatment of Cancer (EORTC) 30942 trial addressed whether the radiation dose could be safely lowered from 30 to 20 Gy.[100] Most patients received only radiation to the PA nodes and they were randomized to 30 Gy in 15 fractions versus 20 Gy in 10 fractions. The 0.7% absolute difference in relapse rates was statistically insignificant, and the lower dose was associated with less lethargy and inability to carry out normal work at 1 month.

Similarly, radiotherapy volume has been reduced. A previous MRC trial tested whether an ipsilateral pelvic lymph node field was a necessary in addition to the PA node field.[101] Ipsilateral pelvic lymph node irradiation did not significantly improve the 96% relapse-free survival at 3 years obtained with PA node field only radiation. However, four of nine of the patients who had been treated with PA node radiation had pelvic node involvement as a component of their relapse. Thus, the patients who receive PA node radiation alone must still be followed routinely with CT scans of the pelvis. Current practice is to treat the PA nodes from the top of T11 or T12 to the bottom of L5. Ipsilateral pelvic lymph node irradiation is still recommended, however, for patients who have had prior pelvic or inguinal surgery as this can disrupt normal lymphatic flow. But because of the less morbidity and better quality of life, PA node radiation alone is sufficient for patients with an undisturbed testicular lymphatic drainage.

Postorchiectomy Chemotherapy ■ Based on pilot studies of adjuvant carboplatin in patients with stage I seminoma and results of carboplatin-based treatment in disseminated seminoma, a large randomized trial was conducted by the EORTC/ MRC in which patients with well-staged clinical stage I seminoma were randomly allocated to standard prophylactic radiation therapy (primarily PA radiation at 20-30 Gy) or treatment with single-course, single-agent, carboplatin (AUC 7).[102,103] This trial was designed as a noninferiority trial powered to exclude an absolute increase in relapse at 2 years of 3%. In a 1:2 randomization scheme, 560 patients were assigned to single-agent carboplatin and 885 were assigned to standard radiation therapy. With median 4-year follow-up, the 3-year relapse-free survival rate was 95.9% for radiation compared with 94.8% for carboplatin, which was statistically insignificant ($p = 0.31$). There was a substantial difference in the pattern of relapse; however, with the majority of relapses on the carboplatin arm occurring in the abdomen, and almost all of the recurrences in the radiation arm occurring outside the radiation portal. Patients treated with carboplatin were less lethargic and less likely to take time off work than those given radiotherapy, but there was slightly less thrombocytopenia and neutropenia with radiotherapy. There were fewer new second primary TGCTs with carboplatin (two patients) versus radiotherapy (ten patients). The authors' conclusions were that single-agent carboplatin was a safe and effective adjuvant treatment of clinical stage I seminoma, but follow-up longer than 4 years is necessary. Criticisms of the study were that the pattern of abdominal relapse with the carboplatin-treated patients may necessitate abdominal imaging in follow-up and that short follow-up may underestimate the true incidence of relapse. This trial was updated in the plenary session at the 2008 American Society of Clinical Oncology Meeting.[103] With median 6.5 year follow-up, there remains no significant difference in 5-year relapse-free survival between carboplatin (95%) and radiotherapy (96%). Again, the rate of new second primary germ cell tumors was lower with carboplatin (2 patients) versus radiotherapy (15 patients).

Consensus guidelines have been developed in Europe and in Canada reflecting the collected work of experienced radiation oncologists, medical oncologists and urologists. The European consensus statement favors surveillance for all patients independent of the individual risk for relapse. Only if surveillance is not applicable, the equally effective alternatives are adjuvant radiation (20 Gy in 2 Gy fractions to PA field) or adjuvant carboplatin (one cycle, AUC 7). A risk-adapted strategy with selection of adjuvant treatment according to individual risk is currently being investigated and is still experimental.[258] The United States, to date, does not have a consensus statement on management of early-stage seminoma.

Stage II Seminoma ■ Several different staging systems have defined stage II seminoma, depending on how the distinctions are made for nodal size. Regardless of the specific staging system used, the potential for supradiaphragmatic involvement increases with the size of the subdiaphragmatic disease. At most centers, the arbitrary cutoff for systemic chemotherapy is 5 cm, while patients with nodal masses < 5 cm can be treated with radiation alone. Unlike with stage I, surveillance is not an option, and the expected 5-year relapse-free survival drops to 89-95% for patients treated with radiation alone.[104-106] The overall survival still remains around 97-99% because of the effectiveness of salvage therapy. For patients with stage II seminoma, the standard radiation field incorporates the PA and ipsilateral pelvic lymph nodes because of the possibility of retrograde lymphatic flow. Generally, this field is treated to 20-25.5 Gy in 1.5-2 Gy fractions, followed by a radiation boost to the enlarged node(s) to 30-36 Gy. The treatment of stage II seminoma with radiation has also evolved to less toxic treatment. Historically for a patient with stage II seminoma, radiation was delivered to the PA nodes, pelvic lymph nodes, and prophylactically to the mediastinum. This practice, although effective at limiting supradiaphragmatic failures, became associated with late cardiac morbidity. Chemotherapy is now favored for patients who are at significant risk of supradiaphragmatic involvement.

There is also an increasing experience with chemotherapy as primary management of small to moderate volume stage II seminoma.[107] A Spanish collaborative study has been recently reported, 72 patients were entered onto the study at 26 participating centers. Eighteen patients had stage IIA disease, and 54 patients had stage IIB disease. Eighty-three percent of patients achieved complete response, and 17% achieved partial response with residual mass. After a median follow-up time of 71.5 months, six patients with stage IIB disease experienced relapse, and one of these patients died as a result of seminoma. Three patients experienced nonseminoma-related deaths (two died from a further esophageal carcinoma, and one died from an upper digestive hemorrhage). The estimated 5-year progression-free survival rates for patients with stage IIA or IIB disease were 100% and 87% (95% CI, 77.5-97%), respectively. Five-year progression-free and overall survival rates for the whole group were 90% (95% CI, 82-98%) and 95% (95% CI, 89-100%), respectively mild to moderate emesis, stomatitis, and diarrhea were the most common nonhematologic effects. Such experiences strongly suggest that primary chemotherapy may be an effective alternative to abdominal radiation.

Therapy for Disseminated Disease

Chemotherapy: Precisplatin

A broad spectrum of chemotherapeutic agents were tested from 1952 to 1972 in disseminated germ cell tumors, and many were found to have some degree of activity in chemotherapy-naïve patients. In the early 1960s, the vinca alkaloids were tested. Vinblastine, as a single-agent, was able to induce complete remissions in 4 of 30 treated patients.[105] Although these were of short duration, they provided investigators with a rational component of subsequent combination regimens.

Several antitumor antibiotics were also found to have single-agent activity, including actinomycin D. Bleomycin was reported in 1970 to have significant activity, including the ability to induce complete remissions.[108,109]

An early combination regimen reported by Li and colleagues in 1960, which contained methotrexate, actinomycin D, and chlorambucil, remained popular throughout the rest of the decade.[110] Li reported an objective response rate of 52%, with more than half of those being complete responses. More importantly, they represented the first durable remissions, with 5 patients alive at 9-39 months after treatment at the time of the report.

A further advance in the development of effective chemotherapy for metastatic disease occurred when vinblastine and bleomycin were used in combination, as reported by Samuels and colleagues at the University of Texas M. D. Anderson Cancer Center.[111] This regimen resulted in 65% of patients achieving a complete remission, including some durable responses.

The most important event in the development of curative therapy for disseminated disease was the 1965 report by Rosenberg and colleagues of the antibacterial effect of platinum coordination compounds.[112] One of these compounds, cis-diamminedichloroplatinum (II) (cisplatin), was found also to have significant antitumor activity. Preclinical studies revealed testicular atrophy as a side effect in the dog model, prompting some investigators to predict activity for this compound against human testicular malignancies in the clinical setting. Cisplatin was soon reported to be the single most active agent against TGCTs, with response rates of 70% and complete remission rates of 50%.[110] Thirty years later, it remains the most active drug in germ cell tumors.

Indiana University Studies

In 1974, investigators at Indiana University began studies using vinblastine (PVB) in patients with disseminated testicular cancer. The initial study remains a landmark study in modern oncology.[113] This study incorporated principles of combination chemotherapy, as well as the concept of surgically resecting residual disease after the completion of chemotherapy. Induction chemotherapy was brief (three to four courses), and maintenance chemotherapy was given for 2 years after induction therapy. Thirty-three of 47 patients (70%) obtained a complete remission with chemotherapy. Of the remaining 14 patients, 5 obtained a complete remission with resection of residual disease after the completion of chemotherapy. Six of the patients attaining remission relapsed.

The initial study proved that PVB was remarkably effective, and yet there was substantial toxicity. The next study was designed to compare the original PVB program with a similar regimen with a lower dose of vinblastine (0.3 mg/kg vs 0.4 mg/kg).[114] Seventy-eight patients were entered into this study, with 70% of all patients remaining continuously free of disease with equivalent results with the different vinblastine dosages. As expected, however, the reduction in the vinblastine dose was associated with fewer episodes of sepsis and granulocytopenic fever. Thus, on the basis of equivalent therapeutic results with lesser toxicity, the lower dose of vinblastine, along with cisplatin and bleomycin, became the standard regimen for PVB.

Confirmation of the results of these trials at Indiana University was obtained in a large EORTC trial of chemotherapy for disseminated testicular cancer.[115] This trial tested the contribution of high-dose vinblastine (0.4 mg/kg) versus lower-dose vinblastine (0.3 mg/kg) and the value of maintenance vinblastine. The trial of 214 patients failed to demonstrate any advantage for patients assigned to high-dose vinblastine therapy or for those assigned to maintenance vinblastine.

A third-generation study was begun at Indiana University in 1978 in conjunction with the Southeastern Cancer Study Group (SECSG).[116] The previous studies had used maintenance therapy with monthly vinblastine for 2 years after the completion of induction therapy. This trial tested the contribution of maintenance chemotherapy. In this study, patients with disseminated testicular cancer were given four courses of induction chemotherapy with PVB. Patients obtaining a complete remission with chemotherapy, or after resection of teratoma, were randomized to receive maintenance vinblastine or no further therapy. This study failed to demonstrate an advantage for those patients randomized to the maintenance therapy arm, with a relapse rate of 12% for those receiving treatment versus 7% for patients receiving induction therapy only.

In the next study, Indiana University, in conjunction with the SECSG, designed a randomized trial comparing cisplatin plus bleomycin and either PVBs or etoposide (BEP).[117] Two hundred sixty-one patients with disseminated germ cell cancer were entered, and 244 were evaluable for response. Of these, 123 were randomly allocated to receive BEP, and 83% achieved a disease-free status. One hundred twenty-one patients were assigned to receive PVB, and 74% attained a disease-free status. In the combined subgroups of patients with minimal or moderate disease by the Indiana classification system, 90% achieved a disease-free status, with no difference between the two treatment arms. Whereas PVB and BEP gave equally good therapeutic results, there was a marked difference in neuromuscular toxicity, with the PVB patients experiencing significantly more paresthesias, myalgias, and abdominal cramping. Because BEP had substantially less neuromuscular toxicity with equal or superior therapeutic results, cisplatin, etoposide, and bleomycin became and remains a standard regimen.

Prognostic Classifications

An international consortium collected clinical data on patients receiving platinum-based therapy for metastatic germ cell tumor to develop a new prognostic model for disseminated disease.[118] Data on 5202 patients with nonseminomatous germ cell tumor and 660 patients with seminoma were analyzed. Independent predictors of outcome in univariate analysis were mediastinal primary site for nonseminomatous tumors, degree of α-fetoprotein, HCG, and LDH elevation, and the presence of nonpulmonary visceral metastasis. Using these factors, prognostic categories were derived. Good-risk patients with nonseminomatous disease were those with testicular or retroperitoneal primary, favorable markers, and no nonpulmonary visceral metastases (anticipated progression-free survival 90%). Poor prognosis included those patients with mediastinal primary nonseminoma, patients with nonpulmonary visceral metastases, or those with unfavorable elevation of tumor markers (anticipated progression-free survival 40%). An intermediate group had an anticipated progression-free survival rate of 75%. For seminoma, only good-risk and intermediate-risk groups were identified, with good and intermediate risks being discriminated by the absence or presence of nonpulmonary visceral metastases (Table 96-4). This classification should be the standard classification system for comparing results of clinical studies done at various institutions.

Table 96-4 International Germ Cell Consensus Classification

Good Prognosis:
Nonseminoma testis or retroperitoneal primary and no nonpulmonary visceral metastases and α-fetoprotein <1000 ng/mL, βHCG <5000 IU/L and LDH <1.5 upper limit of normal
Seminoma of any primary site and no nonpulmonary visceral metastases and normal α-fetoprotein, any βHCG, any LDH
Intermediate Prognosis:
Nonseminoma testis or retroperitoneal primary and no nonpulmonary visceral metastases and αfetoprotein >1000 ng/mL and <10,000 ng/mL or βHCG >5000 IU/L and <50,000 IU/L or LDH >1.5 normal and <10 normal
Seminoma of any primary site and nonpulmonary visceral metastases and normal α-fetoprotein, any βHCG, any LDH
Poor Prognosis:
Nonseminoma with mediastinal primary, nonpulmonary visceral metastases or α-fetoprotein >10,000 ng/mL or βHCG >50,000 IU/L or LDH >10 upper limit of normal

Abbreviations: LDH, lactate dehydrogenase; βHCG, β human chorionic gonadotropin.

Treatment of Good-Risk Disseminated Germ Cell Tumors

Patients with good-risk disease constitute approximately 56% of patients presenting with disseminated disease. The International Germ Cell Consensus Classification (IGCCC) for good-risk disease suggests that more than 90% of patients in this category enjoy long-term disease-free survival.

In the mid-1980s, several clinical trials were designed specifically for this group of patients. Because virtually all these patients achieve complete remission with standard chemotherapy, the trials addressed the possibility of reducing the amount of chemotherapy administered (thus decreasing acute and chronic toxicity), while maintaining the excellent cure rate. Several approaches to this reduction in therapy have been employed, including a shortening of the duration of therapy, use of chemotherapeutic agents with less single-agent toxicity, and a reduction in the number of agents used.

The SECSG performed a trial in which patients with good-risk disease were randomized to receive either three or four courses of BEP.[119] There was no difference in the percent of patients achieving complete remission with either arm, and 92% of patients on both arms were disease-free with a median follow-up of 19 months. On the basis of the results of this study, three courses of BEP (cisplatin 20 mg/m^2 plus etoposide 100 mg/m^2 intravenously [IV] days 1-5, repeated every 3 weeks, with bleomycin 30 units IV weekly) is standard therapy at Indiana University for patients with good-risk disease.

The Eastern Cooperative Oncology Group (ECOG) completed a trial randomizing patients with minimal or moderate disease to receive three courses of either BEP or EP alone in an attempt to eliminate the inconvenience (and possible pulmonary toxicity) of weekly bleomycin.[120] However, patients receiving bleomycin had superior survival. The EORTC has conducted a trial comparing four cycles of EP with or without bleomycin in patients with good-risk nonseminomatous germ cell tumor.[121] Complete remission rate (95% vs 89%) favored the bleomycin-containing arm, but relapse rates were similar. A trial at the Memorial Sloan-Kettering Cancer Center randomized good-risk patients to receive VP-16 (etoposide), combined with either cisplatin for four cycles (standard arm) or the platinum analog carboplatin.[122] In addition, the MRC/EORTC compared etoposide and bleomycin with either cisplatin or carboplatin in good-risk patients.[123,124] The advantages of carboplatin in this setting are its relative lack of nephrotoxicity and neurotoxicity and the ability to administer this compound on an outpatient basis without aggressive prehydration. Inferior survival was seen in the patients receiving carboplatin in these trials. Toner and colleagues reported inferior survival with four cycles of a dose-reduced version of BEP in comparison with standard BEP for three cycles.[125] In summary, analysis of all these trials attempting to further reduce toxicity by the elimination of bleomycin or the substitution of carboplatin for cisplatin has shown therapeutic inferiority for the experimental arm.

A final attempt to eliminate bleomycin from chemotherapy for good-risk regimens comes from the French collaborative study conducted by Culine and colleagues.[126] The trial enrolled 257 patients who were randomly allocated to standard therapy with three cycles of BEP or four cycles of EP (both regimens used 5-day schedules with 500 mg/m^2 of etoposide per cycle). At the time of trial initiation, an older prognostic classification was used. The trial was underpowered for survival analysis, but using the original prognostic classification system and when patients were reclassified by the IGCCCC system, there were more unfavorable outcomes and more deaths in the EP $\times$ 4 arm. A definitive trial would require a very large patient population to prove equivalence of the two regimens. Toxicity was not substantially different between the two arms with the exception of more skin and neurologic toxicity in the BEP arm and more neutropenia and thrombocytopenia in the EP arm. There were no therapy-related deaths in either arm and no difference in pulmonary toxicity. The authors concluded that BEP $\times$ 3 at standard "American" doses of cisplatin 20 mg/m^2 daily $\times$ 5, etoposide 100 mg/m^2 daily $\times$ 5 and bleomycin 30 units day 1, 8, and 15 represented standard therapy for good-risk disseminated germ cell tumors. They also concluded that further testing of this concept was not likely to be fruitful and that there was very little chance that EP $\times$ 4 could ever be proven a superior regimen. Such conclusions are reflected in both the European and Canadian consensus statements which endorse BEP $\times$ 3 as the standard regimen for IGCCC good-risk disseminated disease. We are unaware of any large ongoing trials in good risk disease addressing this issue.

Further reductions in the amount of therapy given are unlikely to reduce toxicity significantly, but certainly have the potential to reduce the cure rate in this stage of disease. Alternative schedules of BEP have also been reported. De Wit and colleagues report the results of a study from the EORTC and the MRC in which patients received either three cycles of BEP with etoposide given as 100 mg/m^2 days 1-5 or 165 mg/m^2 days 1-3, cisplatin given as either 20 mg/m^2 days 1-5 or 50 mg/m^2 on days 1 and 2 only, and weekly bleomycin. There was some mild increase in ototoxicity and gastrointestinal side effects with the three day schedule and long-term quality of life parameters and late toxicities are not available. These two versions of the BEP regimen yielded no significant difference in 2-year overall survival, with a 98% cure rate in patients with HCG < 1000.[127]

In conclusion, for patients with good-risk disseminated disease, BEP for three cycles is standard therapy. Carboplatin should not be substituted for cisplatin, and EP alone for 3 cycles should also not be used. EP alone for four cycles should only be used in the rare circumstances in which the good-risk patient has a significant contraindication to bleomycin.

Treatment of Patients With "Poor-Risk" Disseminated Disease

Patients with disseminated testicular cancer who present with poor prognostic features remain a therapeutic challenge. One approach for the initial treatment of these poor-risk patients is the exploration of chemotherapy dose intensification.

Preclinical models, as well as dose-intensity analysis of clinical trials, suggest a steep dose-response relationship for cisplatin. This relationship has been tested in the design of several clinical trials of intensive cisplatin therapy in patients with poor-prognosis germ cell cancer. Ozols and colleagues at the NCI reported the results of a randomized trial of aggressive, high-dose cisplatin therapy versus PVB in poor-risk testicular cancer patients.[128] In this trial, there was a 2:1 randomization of 52 poor-risk patients to receive an aggressive arm with cisplatin, 40 mg/m^2 (double the standard-dose) on days 1-5 with vinblastine, bleomycin, and etoposide in standard doses versus classic PVB with cisplatin given at 20 mg/m^2 on days 1-5. Of the patients receiving the aggressive arm, 88% had a complete response, as compared with 67% of the patients receiving PVB. The PVB arm had a high incidence of relapse, with 41% of the patients having disease recurrence, as compared with 17% of the patients receiving high-dose cisplatin, bleomycin, and VP-16 (PVeBV). Overall, 68% of the group randomized to the aggressive treatment remained disease-free, as compared with only 33% of the patients receiving standard therapy. Unfortunately, accompanying this apparent improvement in outcome was a substantial increase in toxicity. There was significantly more myelosuppression and hearing loss in the patients receiving the high-dose cisplatin therapy. Whether the apparent superiority of the high-dose regimen in this trial was attributable to the high-dose cisplatin, the inclusion of etoposide, or other factors, was not clear from the study design.

Rigid testing of the impact of high-dose cisplatin therapy in disseminated germ cell cancer was accomplished in a trial of the SECSG and the Southwest Oncology Group (SWOG) in advanced germ cell cancer.[129] This trial enrolled only patients with advanced disease by the Indiana classification system. Patients were assigned at random to receive standard doses of etoposide and bleomycin and either standard-dose cisplatin (20 mg/m^2 daily for 5 days) or high-dose cisplatin (40 mg/m^2 daily for 5 days). Between 1984 and 1989, 159 patients with advanced disseminated germ cell cancer were enrolled. Of these, 153 were evaluable for toxicity and response. Among 76 patients assigned to high-dose therapy, 52 (68%) became disease-free with chemotherapy alone or subsequent surgery. Among 77 patients on the standard-dose arm, 56 (73%) became disease-free with chemotherapy alone or surgical resection of residual disease. Overall, 74% of the patients receiving the high-dose cisplatin are alive, and 63% are continuously free of disease, as compared with 74% alive and 61% continuously free of disease on the standard-dose arm. In addition, the high-dose arm was associated with significantly more ototoxicity, neurotoxicity, gastrointestinal toxicity, and myelosuppression. In contrast to the NCI study, this large randomized trial found no therapeutic benefit of dose esçalation of cisplatin beyond standard doses.

In a follow-up to the SECSG trial of cisplatin dose-intensity, the ECOG conducted a trial testing the substitution of ifosfamide for bleomycin.[129] From 1987 to 1992, 304 patients with advanced-stage disseminated germ cell cancer by the Indiana classification system were entered into this trial, which randomized patients to either four standard courses of BEP or to four courses of VIP with etoposide (75 mg/m^2 daily for 5 days), ifosfamide (1.2 g/m^2 daily for 5 days), and cisplatin (20 mg/m^2 daily for 5 days). Two hundred ninety patients were fully evaluable for toxicity and 286 were evaluable for response. The rates for complete remission (VIP 37%, BEP 31%), favorable response (VIP 63%, BEP 60%), failure-free at 2 years (VIP 64%, VIP 60%), and 2-year survival (VIP 74%, BEP 71%) were not statistically different between the two treatments. Grade 3 or greater toxicity, primarily hematologic, was significantly greater on the VIP arm ($p < .0001$). There were five therapy-related deaths on each arm. This analysis failed to demonstrate benefit for the experimental arm, VIP, relative to standard therapy with BEP, as a treatment of poor-risk germ cell tumor.

A similar trial evaluating the role of ifosfamide in poor-risk patients with germ cell tumor was reported by the EORTC and MRC.[130] In this trial, patients were randomized to BEP/EP or intensively scheduled bleomycin, vincristine, and cisplatin followed by VIP-B. There were no differences in time to progression or overall survival. Grade 3 or 4 myelosuppression and weight loss were more pronounced in the bleomycin, Oncovin (vincristine), and prednisone (BOP)/VIP-B arm. The authors concluded that the intensive BOP/VIP-B therapy was more toxic, but without therapeutic advantage in treatment of poor-risk germ cell tumors.

High-Dose Chemotherapy as Primary Treatment of Poor-Risk Disease

Investigators in Hanover and at other institutions in Germany have attempted to intensify therapy for poor-risk patients by incorporating growth factors and peripheral blood progenitor cell support to give high-dose, repetitive chemotherapy cycles. In the most recent update of this phase 1/2 trial, patients with poor-risk disseminated germ cell tumors were given repetitive cycles of cisplatin 25-30 mg/m^2 on days 1-5, etoposide 100-250 mg/m^2 on days 1-5, and ifosfamide 2 g/m^2 on days 1-5 every 22 days for four cycles.[131] At the highest dose levels, support with growth factors and peripheral blood progenitor cells was required. With these supportive care techniques, this high-dose therapy was tolerated with no dose-limiting myelosuppression, mucositis, renal toxicity, or neurotoxicity. Three of the 32 patients at the highest dose levels died of causes related to therapy. Of the 23 evaluable for response, 20 (87%) attained disease-free status, and 3 patients relapsed.

A randomized trial of 115 patients from the Institut Gustave Roussey has been reported, wherein poor-risk patients were randomized to receive conventional therapy with cisplatin, vinblastine, etoposide, and bleomycin versus similar therapy followed by a single cycle of high-dose cisplatin, etoposide, and cyclophosphamide.[132] Unfortunately, this trial failed to demonstrate any advantage for the high-dose arm.

A large-scale trial has been conducted for poor-risk patients as defined by the International Staging System that compared two courses of standard therapy (BEP) followed by two cycles of very high-dose carboplatin, etoposide, and cyclophosphamide versus BEP × 4. The trial was conducted jointly by the Memorial Sloan-Kettering Cancer Center, the SWOG, ECOG, and the Cancer and Leukemia Group B (CALGB), and accrual finished in 2003.[133] Two hundred nineteen patients were randomly assigned to standard BEP × 4 ($n = 108$) or BEP × 2 followed by two high-dose cycles of carboplatin, etoposide and cyclophosphamide with stem cell rescue with each high-dose cycle. There were 10 deaths on treatment (6 on high dose arm and four on standard BEP) Toxicity particularly hematologic toxicity was more severe on the high dose arm. The one year durable complete remission rate was 52% on the high-dose arm and 48% on the standard BEP arm ($p = 0.53$). The authors conclude that there was no significant difference in outcome between the two arms and that standard-dose BEP remains the standard of therapy for intermediate and poor risk disseminated germ cell tumors.

A European trial comparing high-dose VIP to standard therapy in poor-risk germ cell tumors is also reported. This trial is based on the promising phase 1/2 trial reported by Schmoll and colleagues.[134] Between July 1993 and November 1999, 221 patients with either Indiana "advanced disease" ($n = 39$) or IGCCCG "poor-prognosis" criteria ($n = 182$) received one cycle of VIP followed by three to four sequential cycles of high-dose VIP chemotherapy plus stem cell support every 3 weeks, at six consecutive dose levels. After 4-year median follow-up, progression-free survival and disease-specific survival rates in the poor-prognosis subgroup were 69% and 79% at 2 years and 68% and 73% at 5 years, with 76% for gonadal/retroperitoneal versus 67% for mediastinal primaries. Severe toxicity included treatment-related death (4%), treatment-related acute myeloid leukemia (1%), long-term impaired renal function (3%), chronic renal failure (1%), and persistent grade 2-3 neuropathy (5%).

Additional investigations are underway in intermediate and poor-risk disease in Europe. EORTC is comparing BEP versus paclitaxel/BEP in intermediate-risk patients. In England investigators are comparing a platinating agent intense schedule plus vincristine to standard BEP as well as two-weekly versus three weekly BEP(Christian JCO 21 2003) . There have been previous negative randomized trials of such dose-dense, platinating agent intense regimens with an increase in toxicity in the intense arms without corresponding therapeutic benefit.[135]

Post-Chemotherapy Surgery

Introduction

Surgical resection of residual masses following chemotherapy for disseminated disease is a vital component of the multimodality treatment of testis cancer. Depending on the stage at diagnosis, 20-50% of patients who undergo induction chemotherapy for metastatic germ cell cancer have significant residual retroperitoneal disease requiring resection for complete cure. The presence of large residual masses around vital structures and the resultant severe desmoplastic reaction following chemotherapy often makes surgery in this setting exceptionally challenging. These operations should ideally be performed by experienced surgeons in high-volume centers.

Indications for Post-Chemotherapy RPLND (PC-RPLND)

Post-chemotherapy surgery should be considered only if serum tumor markers have normalized or reached a plateau. Typically PC-RPLND is indicated if there is radiographic evidence of residual disease post-chemotherapy, although the indications are different for seminomas than nonseminomas. Patients who have normalized their markers and have complete resolution of retroperitoneal adenopathy are considered at low risk of relapse and generally do not require surgery.[136] Some authors however advocate PC-RPLND in all cases of nonseminoma due to the increased presence of teratoma and viable germ cell tumor even in patients with complete radiographic and serologic response.[137] PC-RPLND should be performed 4-6 weeks following the last round of chemotherapy in order to allow patients to recover their counts. Imaging must include CT scan of the chest, abdomen and pelvis which should be performed reasonably close to time of surgery in order to ascertain persistence of residual disease in the retroperitoneum.

Nonseminoma ■ Although most authors advocate resection of "residual" masses following chemotherapy for NSGCT, there is no consensus on nodal size criteria. It is often difficult to measure the exact size of residual nodal tissue following chemotherapy, since nodes are often matted together in the retroperitoneum. The definition of a "normal" CT scan following chemotherapy for testis cancer varies, therefore it is imperative that treating physicians and surgeons carefully review the pre and posttreatment imaging.[138] Investigators have reported that up to one-third of small retroperitoneal post-chemotherapy masses measuring ≤2 cm in diameter contain residual teratoma or germ cell tumor.[139] There are currently no reliable imaging techniques or prediction models to accurately identify patients who have residual teratoma or viable GCT post induction chemotherapy.[140] The utility of 18-fluoro-deoxyglucose positron emission tomography (FDG-PET) scan is limited in the decision-making analysis of post-chemotherapy residual masses in NSGCT since it cannot distinguish fibrosis from teratoma. Although a positive PET scan is highly suggestive of residual viable tumor, false negative rates of up to 40% have been reported in a prospective trial.[141] Most experts agree that PC-RPLND is indicated when there are residual radiographically detectable lesions following first-line chemotherapy. Patients with teratoma present in the orchiectomy specimen are at increased risk of residual teratoma, and should be considered for PC-RPLND when there is any residual mass present post-chemotherapy.[139] Patients who have an increased serum AFP, teratoma in the primary tumor, and a post-chemotherapy cystic mass in the retroperitoneum may also be candidates for PC-RPLND rather than salvage chemotherapy. Beck et al. confirmed that cystic teratomas contain variably elevated levels of HCG and AFP and postulated that a leak into the bloodstream could explain the elevated tumor markers in this situation.[142] Teratomas can rarely invade the vena cava and present with a tumor thrombus and this should not be mistaken for a deep venous thrombosis.[143]

Seminoma ■ Following induction cisplatin-based chemotherapy, the presence of distinct residual masses is uncommon. CT scans often reveal a sheet like distribution of tissue around the IVC and/or aorta that resolves over a prolonged period.[144] Viable cancer is present in approximately 20% patients with residual masses >3 cm and almost no patients with residual masses <3 cm.[145] Since there is no concern about residual teratoma in pure seminomas, routine PC-RPLND for residual disease post-chemotherapy will result in overtreatment in approximately 80% of patients. PC-RPLND in this setting is one of the most challenging surgical scenarios that urologists encounter and rates of adjunctive surgery and complications tend to be higher.[146] In an effort to reduce the morbidity of surgery, a number of investigators have evaluated the role of FDG-PET in determining the presence of viable cancer. In a multicenter study ("SEMPET" trial), 56 PET scans were evaluated in 51 patients with CT-documented residual masses measuring 1-11 cm after adequate chemotherapy for bulky seminoma. All 19 cases with residual lesions >3 cm, and 35 of the 37 cases with residual lesions ≤3 cm were correctly predicted by PET scan. The sensitivity, specificity and positive predictive values of PET in determining residual viable disease was 80%, 100% and 100% respectively).[147] Not all studies have confirmed the reliability of PET and a number of false positives have been documented.[148,149] Nevertheless, PET scans may be the best noninvasive test to predict the presence of viable residual tumor in patients with post-chemotherapy residual masses. Resection of post-chemotherapy masses in seminoma remains controversial, and management should be individualized. Further management of patients with positive PET scans may include surveillance, biopsy, resection or radiation.

Extent of Surgery

PC-RPLND is a technically demanding operation requiring expertise in retroperitoneal surgery, vascular techniques, and detailed understanding of abdominal and retroperitoneal anatomy. The boundaries of surgical resection have been the topic of discussion since the first description of the procedure, and controversy regarding templates still exists. Although modified, nerve-sparing templates may be appropriate for lower stage disease, several investigators have demonstrated the presence of tumor outside these templates in advanced disease. In 113 patients with initial bulky retroperitoneal tumors, Wood et al. found that if the residual mass was removed accompanied by a modified retroperitoneal lymph node dissection nine patients (8%) would have tumor left in the retroperitoneum. Herr examined the outcomes of limited versus full bilateral PC-RPLND in 62 patients based on frozen section analysis of the resected mass. In patients with necrosis on frozen-section (37 patients), a limited dissection was performed and for those with teratoma or viable cancer, a full bilateral template was utilized. After a median follow-up of 6 years, there was 1 relapse of teratoma seen in the retroperitoneum in the group who underwent a limited dissection. The concordance between frozen-section and final pathology was 89%.[150] In a study of 50 PC-RPLND specimens, Ehrlich et al. found that all low-volume left side primary tumors followed a predictable pattern of spread to a modified left-sided template, whereas right-sided primaries had about a 20% crossover rate. Importantly after a mean follow-up of 53 months, there were no in-field recurrences noted.[151] Carver et al. at Memorial Sloan-Kettering reviewed their experience with 532 patients who underwent PC-RPLND for metastatic NSGCT and found that 7-32% patients had evidence of extra-template retroperitoneal disease, depending on the boundaries of the modified template. Interestingly 2/24 (8%) patients with residual masses less than 1 cm had extra-template metastases.[152] On the basis of these data, it appears that the most prudent approach would be a full bilateral dissection in the post-chemotherapy setting, although a limited template can be considered in low-volume left-sided primaries.

The surgical approach should be adapted to the size and location of the mass. Most masses can be accessed via a midline approach whereas larger masses and those requiring suprahilar dissections are best approached through a thoraco-abdominal incision or a midline incision extended to the costochondral junction. Thoraco-abdominal approaches afford the possibility of surgical resection of ipsilateral lung lesions. It should be noted that adjunctive surgery is required in about 20% of patients undergoing PC-RPLND. The most common adjunctive procedure includes a left nephrectomy and occasionally en bloc vena caval and/or aortic resection with graft placement is required.[153] Although simultaneous PC-RPLND and thoracic resections are feasible, more complex mediastinal masses are probably best approached in a staged manner in order to reduce complications rates. Findings of fibrosis in the retroperitoneal specimen should not preclude thoracic resections since up to 20% of patients can have teratoma or viable cancer in the chest.[154]

Complication rates following PC-RPLND performed at high-volume centers are higher than for primary RPLND ranging from 7% to 30% with a mortality rate of about 1%.[155,156] The most significant source of morbidity in this post-chemotherapy group is pulmonary toxicity related to prior bleomycin. Retrograde ejaculation remains a significant morbidity although patients with smaller masses are candidates for nerve-sparing approaches with about an 80% probability of preservation of ejaculatory function.[157,158]

Pathology

The histopathologic findings in post-chemotherapy surgical specimens determine the need for further treatment and surveillance protocol. In recent series, the incidence of persistent cancer is decreasing most likely due to optimized chemotherapy regimens and better selection of patients for surgery. Pathologic findings in patients with advanced NSGCT after induction therapy are approximately necrosis in 40-50%, teratoma in 35-40% and viable carcinoma in 10-15% of specimens.[159] Following salvage chemotherapy, the finding of viable carcinoma increases to about 50%.[160] Patients with viable disease resected at post-chemotherapy surgery are generally recommended to receive two postoperative cycles of cisplatin-based therapy, with two-thirds remaining disease-free in the long term.[129] Patients with completely resected very low-volume disease may also be observed. However, patients with unresectable disease, partial resection, or elevated tumor markers should be considered for full salvage chemotherapy.

"Desperation" RPLND

Patients with elevated or rising tumor markers who have undergone induction chemotherapy, failed salvage chemotherapy and have resectable retroperitoneal disease may be candidates for the so-called "desperation PC-RPLND." These patients often have chemotherapy resistant disease and surgery may afford the only chance for cure. PC-RPLND in this setting is technically arduous, often involving removal of adjacent organs and/or great vessels and is usually associated with significantly lower survival rates. Despite elevated markers, up to 50% of patients will harbor mature teratoma or necrosis/fibrosis in the surgical specimen.[161] In patients with viable germ cell cancers in the resected specimen, up to one-third will have long-term disease-free survival.[162] Incomplete resection portends a poor prognosis and patients should be carefully selected for extensive surgical procedures.

Chemotherapy of Seminoma

Modern chemotherapy series involving patients with bulky stage II or stage III disseminated seminoma report cure rates of more than 90%.[62] When compared with earlier studies of radiotherapy in this setting where cure rates ranged from 20% to 60%, cisplatin-based chemotherapy is clearly the treatment of choice in this clinical presentation. The role of single-agent carboplatin in patients with advanced seminoma has also been explored, but standard initial therapy remains cisplatin combinations.

Patients with disseminated seminoma and nonpulmonary visceral involvement do less well and are classified as intermediate risk.[122] Good-risk patients usually receive BEP × 3 and intermediate-risk patients receive BEP × 4.

An additional area of controversy is the management of patients with residual radiographic abnormalities after completion of cisplatin-based combination chemotherapy. Motzer and colleagues report results of 41 patients with bulky stage II, stage III, or stage IV disease treated with cisplatin-based combination chemotherapy.[163] At the completion of therapy, 23 patients had significant residual radiographic abnormalities, including 14 patients with masses ≥ 3 cm in size. Of these 23 patients, 19 underwent surgical exploration, and 5 were found to have significant findings other than fibrosis (4 viable seminoma and 1 teratoma). The authors recommend biopsy of residual radiographic abnormalities after chemotherapy for seminoma if the residual disease measures ≥ 3 cm.

At Indiana University and other centers, a different policy has been adopted. Surgery in this setting is extremely difficult because the surgeon commonly encounters a dense desmoplastic reaction. Also, these patients are older, sometimes have had abdominal radiotherapy as well as chemotherapy, and, as in several series, are prone to operative mortalities.[163] A review of seminoma from Indiana reports only a 10% incidence of relapse in the setting of residual radiographic disease greater than 3 cm post-chemotherapy.[164] There was no evidence in this series that risk of recurrence was related to the diameter of the residual mass. At Indiana University, close observation is the recommended approach in this setting. PET scans may be a useful predictor of viable tumor in post-chemotherapy residuals of patients with pure seminoma greater than 3 cm.[165]

However, there have been recent reports of significant rates of false-positive PET in this setting. A widely endorsed, conservative policy in this setting is to base evaluations and subsequent therapy on size and biopsy findings. Patients who have less than 3 cm residual mass after systemic chemotherapy are simply observed. Patients with 3 cm or greater residual masses are submitted to PET scanning. PET negative masses are observed without intervention. Patients with large PET positive masses undergo surgical biopsy or resection and subsequent approaches are defined by pathological findings.

In the past, radiation therapy for post-chemotherapy residual masses had been considered; however, very few of these masses contain seminoma. Furthermore, the curability with radiation is questionable if chemotherapy does not cure the patient. In addition, the risk of long-term complications, including leukemia, is increased when both chemotherapy and radiation are employed. Therefore, radiation for residual masses should not be performed.[40]

Salvage Chemotherapy

Despite the dramatic successes of chemotherapy in disseminated germ cell tumors, 20-30% of all such patients will fail to achieve durable complete remission with first-line therapy.[166] These individuals, as well as those who relapse from complete remission, are candidates for salvage chemotherapy. Because of the decreased efficacy and increased toxicity of second-line chemotherapy, this represents an important decision in the treatment of such patients and requires the expertise of individuals well versed in the intricacies of careful assessment of patients with germ cell tumors and of therapeutic options for this stage of testicular cancer.

Patient Selection ■ There are several clinical situations that may mimic persistent, progressive, or recurrent disease. One such situation involves the appearance of nodular lesions on the chest radiograph or chest CT scan at the end of chemotherapy or soon after completion of such therapy.[1] These nodules can represent bleomycin-induced pulmonary injury and are characteristically located in a subpleural region. This possibility should be considered in a patient who is otherwise responding serologically or radiographically and has new abnormalities in the lungs in separate sites from the original disease.

Another clinical situation frequently mistaken for progressive disease is the syndrome of growing teratoma.[167] Radiographically enlarging metastatic lesions during chemotherapy concurrently with normal or normalizing serologic markers often represent teratoma. Appropriate management of such a patient is surgical resection of residual radiographic abnormalities rather than administration of salvage chemotherapy. The causes of misinterpretation of tumor markers are detailed earlier in this chapter in the section "Tumor Markers" under the section "Clinical Presentation."

In general, a conservative policy is to reserve the initiation of salvage therapy until there is a clear demonstration of rising markers on serial determinations. The vagaries of interpretation of low-level marker elevation makes such a policy necessary to ensure that patients are not treated with intensive salvage chemotherapy on the basis of a false-positive marker elevation.

The possibility of occult central nervous system (CNS) metastasis should be considered in the setting of systemic sustained remission and elevation of serum tumor markers. In this situation, CT scans or magnetic resonance imaging (MRI) of the brain should be performed, along with evaluations for a testicular sanctuary site. The CNS evaluation should proceed even in the absence of clinical signs or symptoms if the only evidence of progressive disease is a rising marker.

The other important sanctuary site from chemotherapy in germ cell cancer is the testis. In most settings, the primary in the testis has been removed in the initial diagnostic process. However, in some patients presenting with advanced disease, chemotherapy is initiated without a tissue diagnosis. In such cases, the testis must be removed at the completion of chemotherapy, even if the primary tumor is no longer evident. The possibility of a metachronous contralateral testicular primary should also be entertained.

Prognostic Factors in the Salvage Situation

The importance of clinical prognostic factors in the second-line situation, similar to the first-line situation, has been increasingly recognized over the past years.[168,169] There is a great variability with regard to outcomes between the different conventional and high-dose regimens reported to date caused by the heterogeneity of the examined patient population. However, a universally accepted classification such as the IGCCCG for untreated patients has not yet been developed. Patients with gonadal primary tumor sites, cisplatin sensitive disease and relapse after complete response to first-line therapy are more likely to achieve a favorable treatment outcome with conventional-dose salvage therapy than patients with cisplatin-refractory disease, an incomplete response to first-line therapy or a mediastinal primary tumor site.[170] Other studies have also identified time to relapse,[171-173] serum markers at relapse[168,173,174] and histology, with seminoma being favorable[175] as prognostic factors.[170] These factors vary greatly in published salvage series, rendering comparison between regimens impracticable. Einhorn et al.[176] recently reported refractory disease, advanced initial tumor stage and the timing of high-dose chemotherapy (third or subsequent chemotherapy) as adverse prognostic factors. These risk factors discriminated a good, intermediate and poor-prognosis group with a long-term survival of approximately 80%, 60%, and 40% respectively.

Standard Salvage Therapy

Patients relapsing after cisplatin-based first-line chemotherapy have a less favorable-prognosis than patients at initial diagnosis, primarily because of the paucity of active single agents in patients refractory to cisplatin. During the three decades since the introduction of cisplatin, only a few new agents including etoposide (VP-16), ifosfamide, paclitaxel, gemcitabine and oxaliplatin have demonstrated activity in platinum-refractory patients. The rate of patients responding favorably to conventional salvage chemotherapy is approximately 50% and thus substantially lower than after first-line treatment. Long-term remissions are only achieved in 20-30% of patients.

The salvage chemotherapy regimen that serves as a basis for comparison is the regimen of vinblastine, ifosfamide, and cisplatin (VeIP) reported at Indiana University.[177] One hundred thirty-five patients who had not progressed during cisplatin-based therapy received VeIP as initial salvage chemotherapy. Toxicity of the regimen in this pretreated population was significant, with 71% developing granulocytopenic fever. Transfusions of platelets (27%) and red blood cells (49%) were common. Renal insufficiency (serum creatinine > 4 mg%) was observed in 7% of patients. Three patients died of causes related to treatment. Despite the formidable toxicity, the therapeutic results were gratifying. Fifty-six patients (45%) achieved a disease-free status with either chemotherapy alone (34 patients, 25%), or by resection of teratoma (15 patients, 12%), or of viable carcinoma (7 patients, 6%). Thirty-two (24%) of these patients are continuously disease-free, and 42 (32%) are currently disease-free (minimum follow-up, 5 years). Among the patients with extragonadal primaries, only 6 of 31 attained disease-free status, and only 1 is continuously disease-free. These results have been confirmed by other investigators.[178]

Investigators from Memorial Sloan-Kettering Cancer Center have evaluated a regimen consisting of paclitaxel plus ifosfamide plus cisplatin (TIP) as second-line therapy for patients with favorable prognostic features, but relapsed testicular cancers.[179] In that study 23 of 30 patients (77%) achieved a complete response to chemotherapy alone, and an additional patient achieved a durable partial remission with normal markers. Only two patients relapsed and treatment was generally well tolerated. This study underscores the importance of patient selection to favorable responses with standard salvage chemotherapy. With subsequent studies confirming these results, TIP has evolved into a widely used standard conventional-dose salvage regimen.[180,181]

Separate information suggests that recurrent seminoma may be uniquely sensitive to salvage chemotherapy. Miller and colleagues at Indiana University reported the results of VeIP in patients with seminoma recurring after primary cisplatin/ etoposide-based treatment.[182] Of these 23 patients, 19 (83%) achieved disease-free status, and 13 (56%) are continuously free of disease.

High-Dose Chemotherapy as Initial Salvage Therapy

High-dose chemotherapy has been studied as initial salvage chemotherapy. One of the first reports of such an approach is from Barnett and colleagues at the British Columbia Cancer Agency.[183] They reported the results of 18 patients with recurrent or persistent germ cell cancer after cisplatin-based primary therapy who were given conventional induction chemotherapy with cisplatin, etoposide, vincristine, and bleomycin on a weekly schedule or vinblastine, ifosfamide, cisplatin combinations. At the completion of conventional salvage chemotherapy, consolidation with high-dose chemotherapy was given with autologous bone marrow support. Patients received high-dose carboplatin, etoposide, and either cyclophosphamide or ifosfamide. There were 2 toxic deaths, it was too early to evaluate 2 patients, and 8 of 14 patients remained free of progression of germ cell cancer.

Siegert and colleagues in Germany reported the results of high-dose carboplatin, etoposide, and ifosfamide in the treatment of recurrent testicular cancer.[184] Patients received two induction courses of conventional-dose cisplatin, etoposide, and ifosfamide prior to receiving escalated therapy. Seventy-four patients received treatment with conventional therapy, followed by carboplatin 1500-2000 mg/m^2, etoposide 1200-2400 mg/m^2, and ifosfamide 0-10 g/m^2. Two patients (3%) died of causes related to treatment. Responses included 21 patients (28%) with complete remission with chemotherapy alone or with adjunctive surgery and 14 (19%) patients with marker-negative partial remission. Twenty-five of these patients (34%) maintained their response from 31 to 261 months.

The only randomized trial published to date looking at the concept of a single consolidating high-dose chemotherapy cycle after conventional induction chemotherapy was conducted in patients with favorable prognostic criteria. The vast majority of patients included into this study had primary gonadal or retroperitoneal germ cell tumors and all patients had previously achieved a complete or partial remission from platinum combination chemotherapy as first-line treatment. Patients were randomized to either 4 cycles of VIP or VeIP or 3 cycles of VIP followed by one high-dose cycle consisting of carboplatin, etoposide and cyclophosphamide. The 1-year event-free survival and 3-year survival rates (35% vs 42% in favor of high-dose chemotherapy) were essentially identical, although disappointingly low in particular for the high-dose arm.[185]

With the development of peripheral stem cell transplantation, sequential high-dose chemotherapy utilizing 2 or 3 high-dose chemotherapy cycles became feasible. Motzer et al.[186] reported a 41% long-term disease-free rate in 37 patients with cisplatin-resistant disease and unfavorable prognostic criteria after two cycles of conventional TIP chemotherapy followed by three cycles of high-dose carboplatin and etoposide.

At Indiana University, 184 patients have been treated with salvage tandem high-dose chemotherapy since 1989. One hundred and seventy patients received two consecutive courses of high-dose carboplatin and etoposide and 110 of the 184 patients underwent 1-2 cycles of cytoreductive conventional chemotherapy with vinblastin, cisplatin and ifosfamide prior to high-dose chemotherapy. All patients underwent aggressive resection of residual masses after chemotherapy whenever technically feasible. Overall, the long-term disease-free rate was 63%. Eighteen of 40 patients with progressive metastatic disease and tumors that were refractory to platinum remained disease-free after a median of 49 months confirming that high-dose chemotherapy is able to overcome cisplatin resistance in a substantial number of patients.

Sequential high-dose chemotherapy consisting of one cycle of VIP followed by three consecutive cycles of high-dose carboplatin and etoposide was compared with three cycles of VIP chemotherapy followed by a single high-dose cycle of carboplatin, etoposide and cyclophosphamide.[187] Known prognostic factors were well distributed between the two arms. No difference in survival probabilities between single high-dose and sequential high-dose chemotherapy arm was observed. The trial was underpowered to answer the question of whether one of the two high-dose regimens should be used as salvage treatment in any particular patient population. However, morbidity and mortality of sequential high-dose chemotherapy with a 2-drug regimen was lower compared to the single 3-drug regimen and 10% of patients with cisplatin-refractory disease achieved long-term survival.

In summary, high-dose chemotherapy yields excellent results in patients with relapsed germ cell cancer and carries an acceptable morbidity and low mortality in these young and fit patients. While the optimal regimen remains to be determined, sequential high-dose regimen with 1 or 2 conventional chemotherapy cycles followed by 2 or 3 high-dose cycles of carboplatin/etoposide, respectively, is the strategy of choice. While high-dose chemotherapy is an established treatment option for patients with unfavorable prognostic criteria, its role in patients with favorable prognostic criteria remains controversial. However, given the low morbidity and mortality, as well as the excellent results, high-dose chemotherapy serves as an alternative to conventional salvage therapy in this setting. Due to the complexity of the disease and therapeutic situation as well as the necessity of close multidisciplinary cooperation between medical oncologists, urologists and radiation oncologists, all relapsed patients should be referred to a specialized center.

Treatment of Multiply Recurrent Germ Cell Cancer

High-Dose Chemotherapy for Multiply Recurrent Germ Cell Cancer

Investigations into the use of high-dose carboplatin (CBCDA) and etoposide (VP-16) with autologous bone marrow support began at Indiana University in 1986. Initial investigations were on patients who were heavily pretreated and for whom no other curative therapeutic options existed.

The initial phase 1/2 dose escalation study examined the use of two courses of high-dose CBDCA and VP-16 in patients with germ cell tumors refractory to cisplatin (defined as progression after or within 4 weeks of the last cisplatin dose) or recurrent after primary therapy with cisplatin-based therapy and a salvage therapy with an ifosfamide-cisplatin combination.[188] Thirty-three patients were entered into the trial. Overall, seven (21%) of the patients died as a consequence of treatment. Deaths were primarily caused by infection, although one patient died of veno-occlusive disease of the liver. Of note, this was a very heavily pretreated patient population with more than half the patients having received three or more prior chemotherapy regimens, and 67% of patients were cisplatin-refractory. Eight patients obtained a complete remission and six had a partial remission, for an overall response rate of 44% (95% CI, 27-63%). Of the eight patients attaining complete remission, three are long-term disease-free survivors, and a fourth patient died at 22 months, free of germ cell cancer, from a therapy-related acute myeloid leukemia.[189] An overview of the experience at Indiana University with 49 patients with multiply relapsed and refractory germ cell cancer treated with double autologous transplantation demonstrated a 45% long-term disease-free survival after a median of 46 months follow-up.

Other Investigations

Other investigators have reported similar results using high-dose chemotherapy in patients with multiply relapsed testicular cancer. Taken as a whole, several conclusions can be drawn. First, high-dose chemotherapy can cure 15-20% of patients experiencing multiple cisplatin-fractory/relapses of germ cell cancer and should be the treatment of choice after failure of ≥2 conventional regimens. Second, therapy-related mortality in this heavily treated patient population is now <5%. Third, there is no standard high-dose salvage regimen. Last, in all these studies, patients with mediastinal nonseminomatous primary tumors fared particularly poorly and represent a group of patients who do not benefit from high-dose chemotherapy.

Salvage ("Desperation") Surgery

Some patients in the salvage setting are best approached with salvage surgery rather than chemotherapy. This is especially true for late relapsers or patients with relapsed disease confined to a single anatomic site. Indiana University has performed a retrospective review of all patients who were felt to have chemotherapy-refractory disease and were submitted to surgery for attempts at curative resection.[190] All patients had serologic or other evidence of progressive cancer. A total of 48 patients were reviewed, the majority of whom underwent isolated retroperitoneal lymphadenectomy (33 patients). Of these patients, 38 (79%) were rendered free of gross disease by surgery, and 29 (60%) attained a serologic remission. Ten patients (21%) remain continuously free of disease with follow-up ranging from 31 to 89 months. Clinical benefit was obtained only in that group of completely resected patients with a solitary site of disease at the time of surgery. Patients with multiple sites of metastasis, although resectable, were not cured. Albers et al. also reported a high long-term disease-free rate after salvage surgery for patients with persistently elevated tumor markers.[191] In carefully selected patients with chemotherapy-incurable disease, salvage surgery does offer a significant prospect of long-term disease-free survival. Such decisions about surgeries should be made at centers with significant experience in germ cell tumor management. In general, selection to attempt desperation surgery include slowly increasing tumor markers after an initial complete response to either first-line or second-line chemotherapy, radiographic respectable residual disease in 1 or 2 sites, and increasing markers with resectable disease after exhausting all chemotherapy options.[192]

New Agents

The development of new active compounds offers the best hope of truly changing the prospect for cure in recurrent or resistant germ cell tumors, as well as better therapy for patients presenting with poor-risk features. Several drugs have demonstrated single-agent activity, including oxaliplatin,[193] paclitaxel, and gemcitabine. A phase 2 study from ECOG evaluated the combination of paclitaxel and gemcitabine in 30 patients with refractory germ cell tumors.[194] The overall response rate was 21.4%, including three patients with complete remission CRs. Two patients remain continuously disease-free for 15+ and 25+ months. Oxaliplatin plus gemcitabine has been investigated in three studies with response rates of 16%, 32%, and 46%.[195-197] All of these studies have reported long-term survivors, in particular when chemotherapy was followed by resection of residual lesions. Targeted agents are currently explored within clinical studies.

Special Situations

Late Relapse

Of patients with disseminated testicular cancer who relapse after achieving a complete remission, most will suffer a recurrence within the first year following therapy, and the overwhelming majority within 2 years. A late relapse in this disease is generally accepted to be one that appears after a disease-free interval of more than 24 months. Late relapses following complete remission occur in 2-3% of cases, with recurrences as late as 32 years following complete remission. Those patients who have had recurrences with isolated mature teratoma in general have done well following excision, whereas those with marker positive carcinoma seem to have two phenotypes. One group have tended to recur with large-volume disease and have had less favorable responses to additional chemotherapy and/or surgery. Whereas there is a separate group particularly those who are chemotherapy-naïve who respond to chemotherapy and are seemingly cured easily with standard approaches.

At Indiana University, 81 patients were analyzed retrospectively who had recurrence of germ cell tumor after 2 or more years of being disease-free.[198] Sixty percent of these patients had recurrences after >5 years (maximum was 32 years). Serum marker elevation was seen, with 56% of patients having an elevated α-fetoprotein and 27% of patients an elevated HCG. Fifteen patients (19%) had a recurrence of teratoma, eight are continuously free of disease, and four patients are currently free of disease after further surgery (271-1021 months). Seven patients experienced recurrence with sarcomatous elements (with or without teratoma); four are currently disease-free. Fifty-nine patients had germ cell carcinoma as their initial late recurrence. Only 10 of these patients (17%) are continuously disease-free (101-781 months). Nine other patients are currently disease-free. Aggressive surgery was required in almost all these patients. Overall, 65 patients received cisplatin-based chemotherapy, and 17 (26%) achieved a disease-free status with chemotherapy with or without adjunctive surgery. Twelve of the 17 have relapsed. Only two patients treated with chemotherapy alone are continuously free of disease (neither of these patients had received previous chemotherapy). A second series at Indiana University of 77 additional patients demonstrate similar findings.[199]

Sharp and colleagues at Memorial Sloan-Kettering reviewed 75 patients who were seen from 1990 to 2004 for management of late relapse of germ cell tumor. In this modern series, the median time to late relapse was 6.9 years (range, 2.1-37.7 years). Overall, 56 patients (75%) had recurrence in the retroperitoneum. The 5-year cancer-specific survival was 60% (95% CI, 46-71%). Patients who underwent complete surgical resection at time of late relapse ($n = 45$) had a 5-year cancer specific survival of 79% versus 36% for patients without complete resection ($n = 30$; $P < .0001$). The 5-year cancer-specific survival for chemotherapy-naive patients was significantly greater than patients with a prior history of chemotherapy as part of their initial management (5-year cancer-specific survival, 93% vs 49%, respectively). As this was a series of patients referred at the time of late relapse, it is unknown how representative these results are for the late relapsing population as a whole. None the less, these and other data suggest that such patients can obtain long remissions or cures after late relapse. Patients who are chemotherapy naïve often are rendered disease-free with standard approaches including cisplatin-based chemotherapy coupled with post-chemotherapy surgery. A consistent feature of such studies is that patients who have late presentations with atypical yolk sac findings, elevated AFP and prior chemotherapy are best served by aggressive primary surgery for those with regional confined disease.

Although the appearance of late relapses is relatively rare (1-3% beyond 2 years), these data support current recommendations for continued lifetime follow-up. We recommend follow-up every 6 months for 2-5 years and then annually. The most appropriate schedule for imaging is unknown.

Long-Term Toxicity of Chemotherapy

Since the mid-1970s, the majority of testicular cancer patients with disseminated disease have been cured with combination chemotherapy with or without adjunctive surgery or radiation. Late complications of curative therapy have been seen in other malignancies, most notably Hodgkin's disease (eg, sterility, therapy-related second malignancies). Concerns about similar late effects of cisplatin-based therapy have been raised, and information is now available on a significant number of patients with follow-up of more than 10 years.

Nephrotoxicity

The acute effects of cisplatin on both renal glomerular and tubular functions are well documented, with decreases in both glomerular filtration rate (GFR) and effective renal plasma flow (ERPF) accompanied by magnesium wasting and elevated levels of 02-microglobulin, indicative of proximal tubule dysfunction. Most investigators have reported that the acute decreases in GFR and ERPF do not deteriorate further during the months to years following completion of chemotherapy; however, long-term subclinical impairment is frequently found.[200-202]

Vascular Toxicity

Raynaud's phenomenon is the most common vascular toxicity seen in patients following chemotherapy for testicular cancer. Although anecdotally reported after therapy with single-agent bleomycin, it is much more common following combination therapy. Vogelzang and colleagues reported a 21% incidence of this phenomenon in patients treated with vinblastine plus bleomycin, as compared with 41% when cisplatin was added to these two drugs.[203] Studies employing provocative testing suggest that even asymptomatic individuals may exhibit an exaggerated vasospastic response to cold stimuli.[203] The onset of the phenomenon tends to be delayed, with a median time to appearance of symptoms of 10 months.

Symptoms persist indefinitely, with 49% of patients in one series reporting continued symptoms at a median of 8.5 years from completion of therapy. The vasospasm has, in general, been refractory to therapy, although some success has been reported with the calcium channel blocker nifedipine.[204] The replacement of vinblastine by VP-16 in combination therapy with cisplatin and bleomycin has not reduced the incidence of Raynaud's phenomenon.[205]

The relationship of cisplatin-based chemotherapy to large-vessel ischemic events is less clear. There are case reports of myocardial ischemia and infarction, as well as cerebrovascular accidents, following vinblastine administration as a single-agent or combined with bleomycin. Several anecdotal reports of major cardiovascular events in young men receiving chemotherapy for testicular cancer suggested a causal association between chemotherapeutic treatments and these events.[118,206,207] Weijl and colleagues identified patients with liver metastases or those receiving high-dose corticosteroids to be at high-risk of developing thromboembolic complications.[208] To evaluate the risk of acute vascular events in patients receiving cisplatin-based chemotherapy for testicular cancer, questionnaires to assess cardiovascular toxicity were distributed to all participants in the Testicular Cancer Intergroup Study, and toxicity reviews from the chemotherapy flow sheets were conducted.[208] Patients with pathologic stage I testicular cancer were registered in the study and observed after retroperitoneal lymphadenectomy. Patients with pathologic stage II disease were randomized to receiving two postoperative courses of adjuvant cisplatin-based chemotherapy or observation. Any patient who experienced a recurrence after observation or adjuvant therapy was given four cycles of cisplatin-based chemotherapy.

A review of toxicity of treatment in those patients receiving adjuvant chemotherapy (n = 97) or chemotherapy for recurrent disease (n = 83) revealed no cases of acute cardiovascular toxicity. When the median follow-up after study enrollment was 5.1 years, 459 questionnaires were mailed, and 270 were returned. The percentage of returns was equal among the observed, adjuvant, and recurrent groups (59%, 54%, and 64%, respectively). There was a significant increase in the incidence of extremity paresthesias in the two groups receiving chemotherapy. Fatal myocardial infarction was reported in two patients in the observation group, and one nonfatal infarct was reported in the adjuvant treatment group. No patient in any group reported stroke. Three patients in the observation group and one patient in the recurrent group experienced a thromboembolic event.

Other population-based studies however do highlight a substantial increase in risk in cardiovascular disease particularly in patients who have received high cumulative doses of cisplatin. Fossa and colleagues identified 38,907 patients, who were 1-year survivors of testicular cancer within 14 population-based cancer registries in North America and Europe from 1943 through.[209] They used data from these registries to calculate standardized mortality ratios (SMRs) for noncancer deaths and to evaluate associations between histology, age at testicular cancer diagnosis, calendar year of diagnosis, and initial treatment and the risk of noncancer mortality. A total of 2942 deaths from all noncancer causes were reported after a median follow-up of 10 years, exceeding the expected number of deaths from all noncancer causes in the general population by 6% (SMR = 1.06, 95% CI = 1.02-1.10); the noncancer standardized mortality ratios did not differ statistically significantly between patients diagnosed before and after 1975, when cisplatin-based chemotherapy came into widespread use. Compared with the general population, testicular cancer survivors had higher mortality from infections (SMR = 1.28, 95% CI = 1.12-1.47) and from digestive diseases (SMR = 1.44, 95% CI = 1.26-1.64). Mortality from all circulatory diseases was statistically significantly elevated in men diagnosed with testicular cancer before age 35 years (1.23, 95% CI = 1.09-1.39) but not in men diagnosed at older ages (SMR = 0.94; 95% CI = 0.89-1.00). Men treated with chemotherapy (with or without radiotherapy) in 1975 or later had higher mortality from all noncancer causes (SMR = 1.34, 95% CI = 1.15-1.55), all circulatory diseases (SMR = 1.58, 95% CI = 1.25-2.01), all infections (SMR = 2.48, 95% CI = 1.70-3.50), and all respiratory diseases (SMR = 2.53, 95% CI = 1.26-4.53). Testicular cancer patients who were younger than 35 years at diagnosis and were treated with radiotherapy alone in 1975 or later had higher mortality from all circulatory diseases (SMR = 1.70, 95% CI = 1.21-2.31) compared with the general population.

In, longer follow-up of these patients, hypertension, glucose intolerance, unfavorable lipid profiles, and vascular events often arise.[210] The development of metabolic syndrome is well described in association with testicular cancer and cisplatin-based chemotherapy.[211]

Haugnes and colleagues examined this question in a Nordic national follow-up study (1998-2002). Patients >60 years were excluded in the present study, leaving 1135 patients eligible. The patients were divided in four treatment groups: surgery (n = 225); radiotherapy (n = 446) and two chemotherapy groups: cumulative cisplatin dose 850 mg (n = 376) and cisplatin dose >850 mg (n = 88). A control group consisted of 1150 men from the Tromsø Population Study. Metabolic syndrome was defined according to a modified National Cholesterol Education Program definition. Both chemotherapy groups had increased odds for metabolic syndrome compared with the surgery group, highest for the Cis >850 group [odds ratio (OR) 2.8, 95% CI 1.6-4.7]. Also, the Cis >850 group had increased odds (OR 2.1, 95% CI 1.3-3.4) for metabolic syndrome compared with the control group. The association between metabolic syndrome and the Cis >850 group was strengthened after adjusting for testosterone, smoking, physical activity, education and family status.

Patients with testicular cancer should be followed indefinitely. They need good medical management with weight reduction, smoking cessation, lipid profile monitoring, and appropriate blood pressure management. Patients and their treating physicians should remain cognizant of a persisting unfavorable cardiovascular risk profile in long-term survivors.[212,213]

Neurotoxicity

The peripheral neuropathy and ototoxicity observed in treated testicular cancer patients are attributable primarily to cisplatin, with a somewhat lesser contribution in older studies by vinblastine. The peripheral effects became manifest clinically as a distal sensory neuropathy, with paresthesias and dysesthesias, disturbances of position and vibratory sensation, and relative sparing of motor units.[214] Subjectively, these symptoms may be present for prolonged periods, with 43% of patients in one study reporting persistent symptoms 6-12 years after completion of therapy.[215] Objective studies confirm in 1984 the irreversibility of the neuropathy and suggest that the dorsal root ganglion represents the primary target of cisplatin-induced damage.

The ototoxicity associated with cisplatin administration is represented primarily by high frequency hearing loss and is related to the cumulative dose of cisplatin.[216,217] Other risk factors for the development of ototoxicity include a serum creatinine level higher than 1.5 mg/dL, increased age, and preexisting hearing impairment.

Second Malignancies

Although second primary cancers are a leading cause of death among men with testicular cancer, few studies have quantified risks among long-term survivors.[218] Travis and colleagues collaborated to review 14 population-based tumor registries in Europe and North America (1943-2001) and identified 40 576 patients, who were 1-year survivors of testicular cancer and ascertained data on any new incident solid tumors among these patients. A total of 2285 second solid cancers were reported in the cohort. The relative risk and excess annual risk decreased with increasing age at testicular cancer diagnosis ($P < .001$); the excess annual risk increased with attained age ($P < .001$) but the excess relative risk decreased. Among 10-year survivors diagnosed with testicular cancer at age 35 years, the risk of developing a second solid tumor was increased (RR = 1.9, 95% CI = 1.8-2.1). Risk remained statistically significantly elevated for 35 years (RR = 1.7, 95% CI = 1.5-2.0; $P < .001$). Cancers of the lung (RR = 1.5, 95% CI = 1.2-1.7), colon (RR = 2.0, 95% CI = 1.7-2.5), bladder (RR = 2.7, 95% CI = 2.2-3.1), pancreas (RR = 3.6, 95% CI = 2.8-4.6), and stomach (RR = 4.0, 95% CI = 3.2-4.8) accounted for almost 60% of the total excess. Overall patterns were similar for seminoma and nonseminoma patients, with lower risks observed for nonseminoma patients treated after 1975. Statistically significantly increased risks of solid cancers were observed among patients treated with radiotherapy alone (RR = 2.0, 95% CI = 1.9-2.2), chemotherapy alone (RR = 1.8, 95% CI = 1.3-2.5), and both (RR = 2.9, 95% CI = 1.9-4.2). For patients diagnosed with seminomas or nonseminomatous tumors at age 35 years, cumulative risks of solid cancer 40 years later (ie, to age 75 years) were 36% and 31%, respectively, compared with 23% for the general population.

Case reports and clinical alerts suggest that treatment with high-dose etoposide can result in the development of a unique secondary leukemia. To estimate the risk of developing leukemia in the more common clinical setting of patients receiving conventional doses of etoposide along with cisplatin and bleomycin, Nichols and colleagues reviewed records of patients with germ cell cancer entering clinical protocols using etoposide at Indiana University.[189] Between 1982 and 1991, 538 patients entered serial clinical trials, with planned etoposide doses from 1500 to 2000 mg/m^2 in combination with cisplatin plus either ifosfamide or bleomycin. Of these, 348 patients received an etoposide combination as initial chemotherapy, and 190 patients received etoposide as part of salvage treatment. In all, 315 patients are alive, and 337 patients have been followed up beyond 2 years. The median follow-up for patients still alive is 4.9 years. Two patients (0.37%) developed leukemia. One patient developed acute undifferentiated leukemia with a t(4:11)(q21:q23) cytogenetic abnormality 2.3 years after starting etoposide-based therapy, and one patient developed acute myelomonoblastic leukemia with normal chromosome studies 2 years after beginning chemotherapy. During this period, a number of patients were seen outside clinical trials, and we are aware of several hematologic abnormalities in this group, including one patient with acute monoblastic leukemia with a t(11:19)(q13:p13) abnormality. Secondary leukemia after treatment with chemotherapy including conventional-dose etoposide does occur. However, this low incidence of secondary leukemia does not alter the risk-benefit ratio of etoposide-based chemotherapy for germ cell cancer.

Fertility

Modern treatments cure most testicular cancer patients, so an important goal is to minimize toxicity. Fertility and sexual functioning have been evaluated in cross-sectional studies of long-term survivors of testicular cancer. In total, 680 patients treated between 1982 and 1992 completed the EORTC Qly-C-30 (qc30) questionnaire, the associated testicular cancer-specific module and a general health and fertility questionnaire. Patients were subdivided according to treatment received: orchidectomy either alone (surveillance [S] n = 169), with chemotherapy (C, n = 272), radiotherapy (R, n = 158), or both chemotherapy and radiotherapy (C/RT n = 81). In the surveillance group, 6% of patients had an elevated LH, 41% an elevated FSH and 11% a low (<10 nmolL^{-1}) testosterone. Hormonal function deteriorated with additional treatment, but the effect in general was small. Low testosterone was more common in the C/RT group (37% $P = 0.006$), FSH abnormalities were more common after chemotherapy (C 49%, C/RT 71% both $P < 0.005$) and LH abnormalities after radiotherapy (11%, $P < 0.01$) and chemotherapy (10%, $P < 0.001$). Baseline hormone data were available for 367 patients. After treatment, compared to baseline, patients receiving chemotherapy had significantly greater elevations of FSH (median rise of 6 (IQR 3-9.25) iu L^{-1} compared to 3 (IQR 1-5) iu L^{-1} for S; $P < 0.001$) and a fall (compared to a rise in the surveillance group) in median testosterone levels (-2 [IQR -8.0 to -1.5] vs 1.0 [IQR -4.0 to 4.0] $P < 0.001$). Patients with low testosterone (but not elevated FSH) had lower quality of life scores related to sexual functioning on the testicular cancer-specific module and lower physical, social and role functioning on the EORTC Qly C-30 (qc 30) questionnaire. Patients with a low testosterone also had higher body mass index and blood pressure. Treatment was associated with reduction in sexual activity and patients receiving chemotherapy had more concerns about fathering children. In total, 207 (30%) patients reported attempting conception of whom 159 (77%) were successful and a further 10 patients were successful after infertility treatment with an overall success rate of 82%. There was a lower overall success rate after chemotherapy (C 71%; CRT 67% compared to S 85% ($P = 0.028$)). Elevated FSH levels were associated with reduced fertility (normal FSH 91% vs elevated 68% $P < 0.001$).

In summary, gonadal dysfunction is common in patients with a history of testicular cancer even when managed by orchidectomy alone. Treatment with chemotherapy in particular can result in additional impairment. Gonadal dysfunction reduces quality of life and has an adverse effect on patient health. Most patients retain their fertility, but the risk of infertility is likely to be increased by chemotherapy. Screening for gonadal dysfunction should be considered in the follow-up of testicular cancer survivors.

Before the effects of therapy on fertility are examined, it must be recognized that up to 80% of testicular cancer patients will be oligospermic at diagnosis, prior to the initiation of any therapy.[221] Although the etiology of this oligospermia is not fully understood, several mechanisms have been proposed, including an autoimmune process or a primary endocrine dysfunction resulting in impaired spermatogenesis.[222,223]

The chemotherapy administered for testicular cancer has acute effects on both spermatogenesis and Leydig cell function; most patients remain azoospermic with elevated serum gonadotropins for the first 12 months following therapy. These toxic effects are reversible in a significant number of patients, however, as approximately 50% will see a return of both spermatogenesis and Leydig cell function during the second year after completion of therapy.[224,225] Several factors decrease the likelihood of the return of spermatogenesis, including age over 30 years, treatment duration of more than 6 months, and prior abdominal radiotherapy.[226,227] In the Indiana University experience, at least one-third of patients treated with chemotherapy alone have been able to father children without congenital anomalies, confirming previous data. Bohlen and colleagues reported that two cycles of adjuvant cisplatin-based chemotherapy given to patients with high-risk stage I germ cell tumors does not adversely affect fertility or sexual activity.[228] Lampe and colleagues, in an analysis of 170 patients, report that the probability of spermatogenesis increased after orchiectomy and cisplatin-based chemotherapy to 48% by 2 years and to 80% by 5 years.[229]

Pulmonary Toxicity

Bleomycin is solely responsible for the pulmonary toxicity observed in chemotherapy-treated testicular cancer patients. Pulmonary fibrosis develops in approximately 5% of individuals and can be fatal.[230] This toxicity is directly related to cumulative dose, with a significant increase above 450 units. The earliest physical finding of bleomycin-induced pulmonary injury is an inspiratory lag and should prompt immediate discontinuation of the drug. Subsequent signs and symptoms include bibasilar rales, nonproductive cough, and exertional dyspnea. Laboratory abnormalities include decreases in DLCO and late changes, including hypoxia and hypercapnia. Radiographic abnormalities include the appearance of subpleural-based nodules, visible on the chest radiograph or chest CT scan.

The risk of developing symptomatic bleomycin-induced lung disease increases with age > 70 years, prior or concomitant chest radiotherapy,[109,231] decreased renal function,[232] and high concentrations of inspired oxygen. Because the mortality for this condition approaches 50% and therapeutic interventions, such as corticosteroids, are ineffective, early diagnosis of asymptomatic patients and subsequent discontinuation of the drug are particularly important. The incidence of clinically significant bleomycin toxicity is negligible, however, with three cycles of BEP.

Response to chemotherapy may be determined by certain enzymes such as bleomycin hydrolase. Investigators from the Netherlands determined bleomycin hydrolase genotype in 304 patients treated with bleomycin containing chemotherapy. SNP A1450G was associated with a significant effect on TC survival. The (G/G) genotype was associated with a decreased survival compared to the wild type (A/A) or heterozygous variant (A/G).

Conclusion ■ The homozygous variant G/G of *BLMH* gene SNP A1450G is associated with reduced survival and higher prevalence of early relapses in TC patients treated with bleomycin-containing chemotherapy. This association is hypothesis generating and may eventually be of value for risk classification and selection for alternative treatment strategies in patients with disseminated TC.

Long-Term Toxicity of Radiation Therapy

Toxicity of Radiation

Acute ■ Acute radiation toxicity is dependent on what anatomical organs are irradiated, the radiation dose, and the volume. Two MRC trials have prospectively recorded the acute toxicity of radiation and demonstrate specifically how volume and dose contribute to toxicity. MRC TE10 trial randomized patients to PA only or PA with an ipsilateral pelvic field (dogleg [DL]).[101] The acute toxicity of nausea/vomiting was similar but slightly higher in the DL arm. As expected the DL field would not include much more small bowel than the PA area (p = .08). Nevertheless, both groups experienced nausea requiring medication in 25-30% of patients treated. For leukopenia where the DL treats much more bone marrow, the rates of mild leucopenia were almost twice as high when compared with the PA field alone. Nineteen percent experienced clinically detectable leucopenia for the PA arm versus 42% for the ipsilateral pelvic field arm (p < .0001). In addition, diarrhea was reported in only 7% of the PA arm only, but 14% in the ipsilateral pelvic field arm (p = .013).

In the MRC TE18 trial comparing 30 Gy with 20 Gy, patients were asked to complete a daily symptom diary in addition to their physician-recorded symptoms.[100] The patients who received 20 Gy tended to have less significant nausea than the patients who received the higher dose (p = .06). Leukopenia was also less (p = .02). Significantly more patients receiving 30 Gy reported moderate or severe lethargy (20% vs 5%) and an inability to carry out their normal work (46% vs 28%). But by 12 weeks, the two groups were similar. The lower doses and smaller fields in these trials reduced the acute toxicity without compromising treatment, and may lower the chronic and late sequelae of radiation.

At the time of presentation, approximately 50% of patients with seminoma have some degree of impairment in spermatogenesis with lower than average fertility.[232] Consequently, before adjuvant radiation, appropriate counseling, baseline fertility testing, and semen cryopreservation should be considered in patients considering having children in the future. Exposure of the remaining testis to internal radiation scatter from adjuvant radiotherapy to the PA or PA and ipsilateral pelvic nodes after orchiectomy may further impair fertility. The degree of fertility impairment is dose dependent, and available data suggest that temporary azoospermia may occur at dose levels as low as 40-50 cGy (0.4-0.5 Gy).[233-234] Permanent sterility occurs after 2-3.5 Gy. For a patient who is concerned about fertility, the radiation dose can easily be lowered to below the threshold where permanent spermatogenesis is affected. The difference in testicular dose depending on the treated field is illustrated by the MRC TE10 trial comparing the DL and PA field with the PA field alone. The median time to the first "normal" posttreatment sperm count was 13 months for PA patients and 20 months for DL patients, despite the fact that scrotal shielding was used in 63% of the DL patients and only 3% of the PA patients.[101] Testicular shielding with a clam shell reduces the dose to the testes by approximately 3-10 fold. For patients treated with PA and DL or PA radiation fields with gonadal shielding, the average testicular dose per fraction is 1.48 and 0.65 cGy, respectively.[235] Therefore, for men treated with testicular shielding, the cumulative testicular dose is approximately 0.5-2% of the prescription dose, and the majority of men will recover to their baseline sperm concentrations.[101,233,235] Hormonal changes require much higher doses and are not detectable based on testosterone. Subtle Leydig cell dysfunction, as measured by serum FSH and LH concentrations may occur, which are also dose and field dependent. Temporary mild elevation of FSH and LH (in the normal range) may occur with resolution to normal by 3 years with PA and DL fields, while minimal increase in FSH but not LH may occur after PA field only radiotherapy.[236]

Chronic ■ The avoidance of chronic toxicity or permanent late effects has raised the profile of surveillance as a preferred treatment option for many young patients with seminoma. Because radiation for seminoma historically incorporated a mediastinal field, cardiac toxicity developed in many patients. Zagars reviewed the M. D. Anderson experience of all 477 men with stage I or II testicular seminoma treated between 1951 and 1999.[237] After a median follow-up of 13.3 years, the cardiac-specific standardized mortality ratio was 1.61, while the cancer-specific standardized mortality ratio was 1.91. Both toxicities were only evident after 15 years of follow-up. Fifteen years may represent the latency period for chronic toxicity to develop, but it may also demonstrate that radiation treatment doses and fields prior to 1990 are much more toxic relative to more modern practices.

The risk of second malignancies for patients treated with historical methods around the advent of platinum-based chemotherapy was quantified in a large international population-based cancer registry study.[216] More than 40,000 survivors of testicular cancer were identified, having been diagnosed from as early as 1943 up to 2001. The risk of developing a second solid tumor among 10-year survivors was almost twice that of the general population with a relative risk (RR) of 1.9. Overall patterns were similar for seminoma and nonseminoma patients, with lower risks observed for nonseminoma patients treated after 1975. Significantly increased risks of solid cancers were observed among patients treated with radiotherapy alone (RR = 2.0, 95% CI = 1.9-2.2), chemotherapy alone (RR = 1.8, 95% CI = 1.3-2.5), and both (RR = 2.9, 95% CI = 1.9-4.2). For patients given radiotherapy alone, risks were 1.1, 1.5, and 2.0 in the follow-up periods of 1-4, 5-9, and 10 or more years. Relative risks tended to be highest among patients treated with radiation alone in typical infradiaphragmatic sites: stomach (RR = 4.1), pancreas (RR = 3.8), kidney (RR = 2.8), bladder (RR = 2.7), colon (RR = 1.9), and rectum (RR = 1.8). However, there was also increased risk of second malignancy in supradiaphragmatic sites as well, likely related to the supradiaphragmatic radiotherapy fields frequently applied in the past. The cumulative risk of solid cancer at age 75 for men diagnosed at age 35 was 36% for seminoma and 31% for nonseminomatous tumors compared with 23% for the general population. Although these results are instructive, they are difficult to extrapolate to current practice which uses smaller radiotherapy fields and lower doses. Nonetheless, these results reinforce our primary goals of maintaining high cure rates, while reducing the long-term impact of our therapies.

Sanctuary Sites and CNS Metastases

It is quite uncommon for patients to present with CNS metastasis as an initial manifestation of metastatic testicular cancer.[52,53] The rarity of this presentation makes CNS prophylaxis inappropriate for any subset of patients with advanced germ cell cancer. In patients with advanced hematogenous metastases or large-volume choriocarcinoma, however, clinical suspicion should be heightened and careful investigation of even minor CNS symptoms is warranted.

Patients with CNS involvement, either as a part of the initial presentation or as a manifestation of relapse, should be approached with curative intent. All patients require systemic therapy. Resection should be considered for superficial solitary metastasis. Patients with multiple brain metastases or CNS disease accompanying other advanced systemic involvement should receive whole-brain radiotherapy (30-50 Gy in 3-6 weeks at <2 Gy per fraction) along with appropriate systemic chemotherapy.[52,53,239,240] Patients relapsing with a solitary CNS metastasis without involvement of other sites undergo resection followed by CNS radiotherapy and two postoperative courses of "adjuvant" cisplatin-based chemotherapy.

The other important sanctuary site from chemotherapy in germ cell cancer is the testis. In most settings, the testicular primary was removed in the initial diagnostic process. However, in some patients presenting with advanced disease, chemotherapy is initiated without a tissue diagnosis. In such cases, the testis must be removed at the completion of chemotherapy even if the primary tumor is no longer evident. An intact primary can occasionally lead to some confusion and some difficulty interpreting marker elevations during and after chemotherapy. If there is an intact primary, one must consider this as a possibility as a source of persistent or increasing marker elevation during and after treatment.

The possibility of a metachronous contralateral testis primary must, at times, be entertained. In the setting of complete radiographic remission of systemic disease and a persistent or new elevation of serum tumor markers, the remaining testicle should be carefully examined and testicular ultrasonography be performed to rule out an occult primary in the remaining testis. For patients with a metachronous contralateral testis, organ-sparing surgery is now a viable option to preserve fertility.[241]

Extragonadal Germ Cell Tumors (EGCTs)

Germ cell tumors arise predominantly from within the testis, but an important subset of germ cell tumors are extragonadal in origin. Overall, approximately 5-10% of all germ cell cancers arise in nongonadal sites, particularly in the mediastinum and retroperitoneum. Beyond these sites EGCTs have been described in the pineal region, sacrococcygeal region and rarely also in the prostate, vagina, orbita, liver and gastrointestinal tract.

The initial theory regarding the genesis of these tumors was that they represented metastasis from an occult gonadal primary. Luna and colleagues reported the results of autopsy findings in 20 patients with extragonadal mediastinal germ cell tumors and found only one case of a testicular primary and one patient with a testicular scar.[244] Both these cases were associated with clinically occult lower retroperitoneal involvement. Primary retroperitoneal germ cell tumors are more commonly associated with an occult testicular primary site, especially when the tumor is not midline in origin.

There is now general acceptance that EGCTs represent malignant transformation of germinal elements distributed to these sites without a testicular focus. Some investigators suggest that this distribution is a consequence of abnormal cell migration during embryogenesis, while others have suggested that there is widespread distribution of germ cells to the liver, thymus, bone marrow, and brain, and that these cells provide important regulatory functions at these sites or convey important genetic hematologic or immunologic information.

In adults, the mediastinum is the most common extragonadal site for the development of germ cell tumors.[245,246] The most frequent symptoms at initial presentation include dyspnea (25%), chest pain (23%) and cough (17%) followed by fever (13%), weight loss (11%), vena cava occlusion syndrome and fatigue/weakness (6%).[247] The most common tumor in this site is mature teratoma.[248] This diagnosis can be suggested by the presence of a large circumscribed anterior mediastinal mass with normal serum HCG and α-fetoprotein. Management of mature teratoma is surgical, and there is no role for chemotherapy or radiotherapy. Although these tumors histologically are benign, removal is often difficult. The tumors are commonly adherent to adjacent structures, such as the pericardium, lung, and great vessels. Nonetheless, in this era of modern thoracic surgery, excellent outcome is the rule.[249] In a series from the Mayo Clinic, 64 of 69 patients were long-term survivors. Four of the remaining patients died as the result of surgical complications.

The principles of management of extragonadal nonseminomatous germ cell tumors parallel those of testicular germ cell cancer. The diagnosis should be considered in any young person with a poorly differentiated cancer arising in midline structures. Serum tumor markers should be obtained and, if the clinical condition is stable, a biopsy also should be obtained. In most settings, heroic efforts at surgical debulking should not be considered part of primary management. Cisplatin-based chemotherapy should be given as with testicular germ cell cancer. However, cure rates for nonseminomatous germ cell tumors of mediastinal origin are significantly inferior compared with those of testicular origin. An international analysis of 635 patients with EGCTs demonstrated an almost 90% change of cure with pure seminoma irrespective of the primary site, but only 45% survival at 5 years for patients with mediastinal nonseminomatous tumors.[247] High-dose chemotherapy with autologous stem cell support is not recommended outside of clinical trials.

Patients with residual radiographic abnormalities after completing chemotherapy for nonseminomatous EGCTs should be considered for surgical extirpation of residual disease whenever feasible even if elevated tumor markers have normalized. Vuky and colleagues report the surgical results of 32 patients with nonseminoma germ cell tumors arising from the mediastinum who underwent adjunctive surgery following chemotherapy.[250] Viable tumor was discovered in 66% of patients and teratoma in 22%.

Several important biologic associations with mediastinal nonseminomatous germ cell tumors have been described. There is a very high frequency of Klinefelter syndrome in patients with mediastinal nonseminomatous germ cell tumors. Two large series report an association in up to 20% of patients with Klinefelter syndrome.[12,251]

Approximately 10% of patients with mediastinal nonseminomatous germ cell tumors develop associated malignant hematologic dyscrasias. Between 1976 and 1989, of the 40 patients with mediastinal nonseminomatous germ cell tumors at Indiana University, six developed a hematologic malignancy.[32] In addition, 11 other patients were referred to Indiana University or case material was forwarded for evaluation of this association. Of this group of patients, six developed acute megakaryoblastic leukemia, five had acute nonlymphocytic leukemia (not M-7), two developed a virulent myelodysplastic syndrome, two were found to have extramedullary megakaryocytic myelosis, and two presented with massively elevated platelet counts and cytogenetic abnormalities or excess blasts in the marrow. The median time to the development of the hematologic abnormalities was 6 months, with five of the patients having simultaneous presentations of the two disorders. Thirty-three similar patients have been reported in the literature. The median interval between the two diagnoses in this review was 5 months, with 13 cases presenting simultaneously. A retrospective review of 287 patients with nonseminomatous mediastinal germ cell tumors revealed 17 patients with hematologic disorders with a median time of onset occurring 6 months after the diagnosis of germ cell tumor and a median survival of only 5 months after the diagnosis of the hematologic disorder.[252]

Careful clinical and cytogenetic analyses of these cases suggest that these tumors do not arise as a consequence of therapy for germ cell tumors, but represent a unique and biologically important association between these disorders. Similar cases are not found among those patients with testicular or retroperitoneal germ cell cancer treated with identical chemotherapy. Most compelling, however, is the finding of the most common karyotypic abnormality of germ cell cancer, isochromosome 12p, in a mediastinal germ cell tumor and in the leukemic blasts of one of these patients.[253] This implies that the mediastinal germ cell tumor and the hematologic malignancy arose from a common progenitor cell.

Patients with EGCTs, particularly those with retroperitoneal or nonseminomatous tumors, but also those with primary mediastinal EGCTs, are at an increased risk of metachronous testicular cancer.[254] The cumulative risk of developing a metachronous testicular cancer 10 years after a diagnosis of EGCT was approximately 14% for patients with retroperitoneal or nonseminomatous EGCTs.

Associations of mediastinal nonseminomatous germ cell tumors with other nonhematologic, nongerm cell tumors is unproven. Ulbright and colleagues found 269 cases of teratoma-containing material, including 209 testicular, 28 retroperitoneal, and 32 mediastinal primary sites in a review of germ cell tumor specimens seen at Indiana University from 1974 to 1982, Ulbright and colleagues found 269 cases of teratoma-containing material, including 209 testicular, 28 retroperitoneal, and 32 mediastinal primary sites.[255] Among this group of patients, 11 were identified who demonstrated malignant nongerm cell elements, including such variants as embryonal rhabdomyosarcoma, adenosquamous carcinoma, leiomyosarcoma, Wilms' tumor, and glioblastoma multiforme. They were identified prior to the initiation of therapy in 10 of the 11 cases. In patients with multiple samples available, histologic progression was often identified, moving from atypical features to overt nongerm cell elements. The authors suggested that these malignant nongerm cell elements are derived from the teratomatous elements within the tumor. Of particular interest, 3 of the 11 cases were patients with mediastinal primaries (27%), whereas mediastinal primaries made up only 12% of cases reviewed. In contrast, no association between nonhematologic, nongerm cell tumors and EGCTs was found in the largest series of EGCTs to date.[256]

Unrecognized Germ Cell Tumor Syndrome

On occasion, a patient will present with a clinical picture compatible with an EGCT, but without corroborating serologic or histopathologic evidence of a germ cell tumor. Work done at Vanderbilt University by Greco and colleagues suggests that such patients should undergo a very thorough histopathologic evaluation and, in some cases, receive empiric cisplatin-based chemotherapy.[257] The clinical features of the "unrecognized germ cell tumor syndrome" include patients younger than 50 years of age; tumor primarily involving the midline (mediastinum or retroperitoneum), lungs (in the form of multiple pulmonary nodules), or lymph nodes; an elevated βHCG or α-fetoprotein; or clinical evidence of rapid tumor growth. Seventy-one prospectively identified patients fitting this description were classified as having poorly differentiated carcinoma or poorly differentiated adenocarcinoma, and one or more of the above clinical features. Results of serologic investigation in this patient population revealed normal α-fetoprotein and HCG in 51 of these patients. Thirteen patients had elevation of one marker, and five had elevation of both markers. Light microscopy revealed poorly differentiated carcinoma in 48 patients (68%), poorly differentiated adenocarcinoma in 18 patients (25%), and poorly differentiated large cell carcinoma in five patients (7%). Electron microscopy resulted in a change in the histologic diagnosis in 17 (52%) of the 33 patients with poorly differentiated carcinoma undergoing this procedure, with neuroendocrine tumors being the most frequent new diagnosis. Sixty-eight of the patients were given some form of therapy, with 62 patients receiving cisplatin-based treatment. In this group, 15 patients (23%) had complete responses, and 18 patients (29%) had partial responses. Patients obtaining a response were generally young, male, and had midline involvement of the retroperitoneum, mediastinum, or cervical lymph nodes. All 15 had the light microscopic diagnosis of poorly differentiated carcinoma. A series of 41 patients with poorly differentiated carcinoma of unknown primary were evaluated by Motzer and colleagues at Memorial Sloan-Kettering Cancer Center.[258] Thirty percent of these patients were found to have tumors containing i(12p), increased copies of 12p, or a deletion of the long arm of chromosome 12. Seventy-five percent of patients demonstrating chromosomal structural abnormalities responded to cisplatin-based chemotherapy versus only an 18% response rate in patients for whom no diagnosis could be made.

These results suggest that poorly differentiated carcinomas of unknown primary are responsive to chemotherapy and may even be chemotherapy curable. A subset of these patients probably represents histologically and serologically atypical germ cell cancers. As such, patients with metastatic poorly differentiated carcinoma should be investigated to identify a primary site. Serum HCG and α-fetoprotein should be measured. Patients with a dominant pulmonary or mediastinal mass should have fiberoptic bronchoscopy. Thorough investigations with light microscopy, immunoperoxidase staining, and cytogenetics should be carried out to further characterize the tumor. Patients should receive a trial of cisplatin and etoposide-based chemotherapy.

Selected References

The complete reference list can be found at www.CANCERMEDICINE8.com

6. Jemal A, Thomas A, Murray T, Thun M. Cancer statistics, 2002. *CA Cancer J Clin.* 2002;52:23–47.
13. Raghavan D, Zalcberg JR, Grygiel JJ, et al. Multiple atypical nevi: a cutaneous marker of germ cell tumors. *J Clin Oncol.* 1994;12:2284–2287.
17. Sokal M, Peckham MJ, Hendry WF. Bilateral germ cell tumours of the testis. *Br J Urol.* 1980;52:158–162.
20. Jones TD, Ulbright TM, Eble JN, et al. OCT4 Staining in testicular tumors: a sensitive and specific marker for seminoma and embryonal carcinoma. *Am J Surg Path.* 2004;28:935–940.
22. Cheng L. Establishing a germ cell origin for metastatic tumors using OCT4 immunohistochemistry. *Cancer.* 2004;101:2006–2010.
30. Brosman S. Testicular tumors in prepubertal children. *Urology.* 1979;13:581–588.
36. Zon RT, Nichols C, Einhorn LH. Management strategies and outcomes of germ cell tumor patients with very high human chorionic gonadotropin levels. *J Clin Oncol.* 1998;16:1294–1297.
41. Dieckmann KP, Skakkebaek NE. Carcinoma in situ of the testis: review of biological and clinical features. *Int J Cancer.* 1999;83:815–822.
47. Hoskin P, Dilly S, Easton D, Horwich A, Hendry W, Peckham MJ. Prognostic factors in stage I nonseminomatous germ-cell testicular tumors managed by orchiectomy and surveillance: implications for adjuvant chemotherapy. *J Clin Oncol.* 1986;4:1031–1036.
53. Krege S, Beyer J, Souchon R, et al. European consensus conference on diagnosis and treatment of germ cell cancer: a report of the second meeting of the European Germ Cell Cancer Consensus Group (EGCCCG): part II. *Eur Urol.* 2008;53:497–513.
59. Donohue JP. Retroperitoneal lymphadenectomy: the anterior approach including bilateral suprarenal-hilar dissection. *Urol Clin North Am.* 1977;4:509–521.
67. Richie JP. Clinical stage 1 testicular cancer: the role of modified retroperitoneal lymphadenectomy. *J Urol.* 1990;144:1160–1163.
72. Krege S, Beyer J, Souchon R, et al. European consensus conference on diagnosis and treatment of germ cell cancer: a report of the second meeting of the European Germ Cell Cancer Consensus group (EGCCCG): part I. *Eur Urol.* 2008;53:478–496.
76. Groll RJ, Warde P, Jewett MA. A comprehensive systematic review of testicular germ cell tumor surveillance. *Crit Rev Oncol Hematol.* 2007;64:182–197.
79. Colls BM, Harvey VJ, Skelton L, et al. Late results of surveillance of clinical stage I nonseminoma germ cell testicular tumours: 17 years' experience in a national study in New Zealand. *BJU Int.* 1999;83:76–82.
83. Mead G, Group ftIGCCC. International Germ Cell Consensus Classification: a prognostic factor-based staging system for metastatic germ cell cancers. International Germ Cell Cancer Collaborative Group. *J Clin Oncol.* 1997;15:594–603.
88. Boden G, Gibb R. Radiotherapy and testicular neoplasms. *Lancet.* 1951;2:1195–1196.
94. Schmoll H-J, Souchon G, Bokemeyer C. European consensus on diagnosis and treatment of germ cell cancer: a report of the European Germ Cell Cancer Consensus Group (EGCCCG). *Ann Oncol.* 2004;15:1377–1399.
98. von der Maase H, Specht L, Jackobsen GK, et al. Surveillance following orchidectomy for stage I seminoma of the testis [comment]. *Eur J Cancer.* 1993;29A:1923–1924.
103. Oliver RT, Mead GM, et all. Radiotherapy versus carboplatin for stage I seminoma: updated analysis of the MRC/EORTC randomized trial (ISRTN27163214). *J Clin Oncol.* 2008;26:May 20 suppl:abstr 1.
108. Warwick OH, Alison RE, Darte JM. Clinical experience with vinblastine sulfate. *Can Med Assoc J.* 1961;85:579–583.
114. Einhorn L, Donahue J. Cis-diamminedichloroplatinum, vinblastine, and bleomycin combination chemotherapy in disseminated testicular cancer. *Ann Intern Med.* 1977;87:293–298.
117. Einhorn L, et al. The role of maintenance therapy in disseminated testicular cancer. *N Engl J Med.* 1981;305:727–731.
120. Einhorn LH, Williams SD, Loehrer PJ, et al. Evaluation of optimal duration of chemotherapy in favorable-prognosis disseminated germ cell tumors: a Southeastern Cancer Study Group protocol. *J Clin Oncol.* 1989;7:387–391.
124. Horwich A, Sleijfer DT, Fossa SD, et al. Randomized trial of bleomycin, etoposide, and cisplatin compared with bleomycin, etoposide, and carboplatin in good-prognosis metastatic nonseminomatous germ cell cancer: a Multi-institutional Medical Research Council/ European Organization for Research and Treatment of Cancer Trial. *J Clin Oncol.* 1997;15:1844–1852.
128. Ozols RF, Ihde DC, Linehan WM, et al. A randomized trial of standard chemotherapy v a high-dose chemotherapy regimen in the treatment of poor prognosis nonseminomatous germ-cell tumors. *J Clin Oncol.* 1988;6:1031–1040.
131. Kaye SB, Mead GM, Fossa S, et al. Intensive induction-sequential chemotherapy with BOP/VIP-B compared with treatment with BEP/EP for poor-prognosis metastatic nonseminomatous germ cell tumor: a Randomized Medical Research Council/ European Organization for Research and Treatment of Cancer study. *J Clin Oncol.* 1998;16:692–701.
135. Culine S, Kramar, A, et al. Randomized trial comparing bleomycin/etoposide/ cisplatin with alternating cisplatin/cyclophosphamide/doxorubicin and vinblastine/bleomycin regimens of chemotherapy for patients with intermediate- and poor-risk metastatic nonseminomatous germ cell tumors: Genito-Urinary Group of the French Federation of Cancer Centers Trial T93MP. *J Clin Oncol.* 2008;16:421–427.
137. Sheinfeld J. Risks of the uncontrolled retroperitoneum. *Ann Surg Oncol.* 2003;10: 100–101.
140. Vergouwe Y, Steyerberg EW, Foster RS, et al. Validation of a prediction model and its predictors for the histology of residual masses in nonseminomatous testicular cancer. *J Urol.* 2001;165:84–88; discussion 88.
143. Moore CJ, Daneshmand S, Kondagunta GV, et al. Management of difficult germ-cell tumors. *Oncology (Williston Park).* 2006;20:1565–1570, 1575; discussion 1575–1576.
148. Ganjoo KN, Chan RJ, Sharma M, et al. Positron emission tomography scans in the evaluation of postchemotherapy residual masses in patients with seminoma. *J Clin Oncol.* 1999;17:3457–3460.
152. Carver BS, Shayegan B, Eggener S, et al. Incidence of metastatic nonseminomatous germ cell tumor outside the boundaries of a modified postchemotherapy retroperitoneal lymph node dissection. *J Clin Oncol.* 2007;25:4365–4369.
156. Baniel J, Sella A. Complications of retroperitoneal lymph node dissection in testicular cancer: primary and post-chemotherapy. *Semin Surg Oncol.* 1999;17:263–267.
161. Beck SD, Foster RS, Bihrle R, et al. Post chemotherapy RPLND in patients with elevated markers: current concepts and clinical outcome. *Urol Clin North Am.* 2007;34:219–225; abstract ix–x.
164. Friedman EL, Garnick MB, Stomper PC, et al. Therapeutic guidelines and results in advanced seminoma. *J Clin Oncol.* 1985;3:1325–1332.
169. Nichols CR. Treatment of recurrent germ cell tumors. *Semin Surg Oncol.* 1999;17:268–274.
173. Fossa SD, Stenning SP, et al. Prognostic factors in patients progressing after cisplatin-based chemotherapy for malignant non-seminomatous germ cell tumours. *Br J Cancer.* 1999;80(9):1392–1399.
180. Kondagunta GV, Bacik J, et al. Etoposide and cisplatin chemotherapy for metastatic good-risk germ cell tumors. *J Clin Oncol.* 2005;23(36):9290–9294.
187. Lorch A, Kollmannsberger C, et al. Single versus sequential high-dose chemotherapy in patients with relapsed or refractory germ cell tumors: a prospective randomized multicenter trial of the German Testicular Cancer Study Group. *J Clin Oncol.* 2007;12(19):2778–2784.
193. Kollmannsberger C, Beyer J, et al. Combination chemotherapy with gemcitabine plus oxaliplatin in patients with intensively pretreated or refractory germ cell cancer: a study of the German Testicular Cancer Study Group. *J Clin Oncol.* 2004;22(1):108–114.
199. Meijer S, Mulder NH, Sleijfer DT, et al. Influence of combination chemotherapy with cis-diamminedichloroplatinum on renal function: long-term effects. *Oncology.* 1983;40:170–173.
204. Cantwell BMJ, Mannix KA, Roberts JT, et al. Thromboembolic events during combination chemotherapy for germ cell malignancy. *Lancet.* 1988;2:1086–1087.
209. Haugnes HS, Aass N, et al. Components of the metabolic syndrome in long-term survivors of testicular cancer. *Ann Oncol.* 2007;18(2):241–248.
215. Reddel RR, Kefford RF, Grant JM, et al. Ototoxicity in patients receiving cisplatin: importance of dose and method of drug administration. *Cancer Treat Rep.* 1982;66:19–23.
221. Morrish DW, Venner PM, Siy O, et al. Mechanisms of endocrine dysfunction in patients with testicular cancer. *J Natl Cancer Inst.* 1990;82:412–418.
226. Bohlen D, Burkhard FC, Mills R, et al. Fertility and sexual function after orchiectomy and two cycles of chemotherapy for stage I high-risk nonseminomatous germ cell cancer. *J Urol.* 2001;165:141–144.

97 Neoplasms of the Vulva and Vagina

Jacob H. Rotmensch, MD

Cancer of the Vulva

Incidence and Epidemiology

Vulvar cancer accounts for about 4% of cancers in the female reproductive organs and 0.6% of all cancers in women. It is the fourth most frequent gynecologic cancer.[1,2] The American Cancer Society estimates that in 2008, about 3460 cancers of the vulva will be diagnosed in the United States and about 870 women will die of this cancer.

Most vulvar carcinomas occur in older women, with more than 50% of the patients being 60-79 years of age. Invasive vulvar carcinomas are being seen with increasing frequency in younger patients, however, with 15% of vulvar cancers arising in women under the age of 40 years (Fig. 97-1).[3] This increased frequency in younger patients may be attributed to an increase in the number of sexual partners or venereal viral infections within the population.

Several epidemiologic studies suggest a sexually transmitted origin for carcinoma of the vulva. Condyloma acuminatum associated with human papillomavirus (HPV) has been noted in many patients with premalignant and malignant vulvar disease. It has been estimated that in the United States, over 1 million women each year develop perineal warts and that as many as 10% are infected with HPV.[4] Currently, HPV types 6 and 11 are most frequently found in benign vulvar warts, and HPV types 16, 18, 31, 33, and 45 are more frequently associated with intraepithelial neoplasia or invasive carcinoma.[4-6] HPV can be found in approximately 50% of vulvar carcinomas; the tumors are often multifocal and associated with vulvar dysplasias. HPV-negative tumors are often found in older women.[7,8]

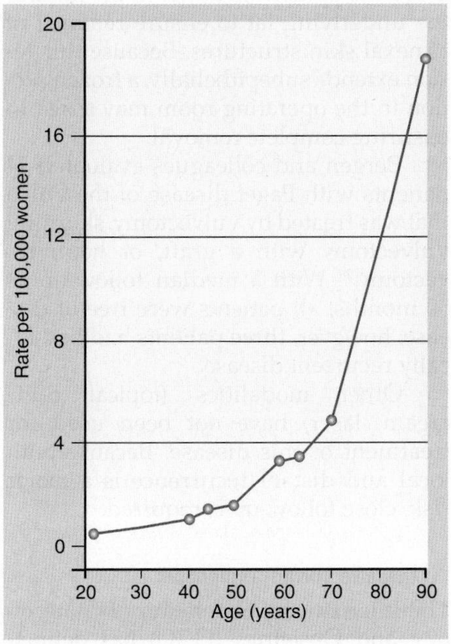

Figure 97-1 Age incidence curve for cancer of the vulva in white women in the United States. *Source:* From Menczer J, Voliovitch Y, Modan B, et al. Some epidemiologic aspects of carcinoma of the vulva in Israel. *Am J Obstet Gynecol.* 1982;143:893.

Although epidemiologic evidence strongly suggests a viral cause, other associations have been implied as well. Factors such as granulomatous diseases of the vulva, diabetes, hypertension, and obesity also have been associated with vulvar carcinoma, but perhaps this is because of the usually advanced age of patients. A case-control study by Mabuchi and colleagues found that domestic servants, or those working in laundry or cleaning plants, have an increased risk of vulvar carcinoma, thus suggesting an environmental component.[9]

The association of carcinoma in situ (CIS) with invasive carcinoma of the vulva indicates a continuum from preinvasive to invasive carcinoma. The progression of vulvar intraepithelial neoplasia to invasive carcinoma has been estimated to be on the order of 6%.[10,11] Progression, however, may differ between younger and older patients. Some authors suggest that the multifocal CIS of women in their thirties or forties may not be as likely to progress as that seen in older women.[12-14]

Vulvar Atypias

There has been a lack of uniformity in defining vulvar atypias. There are minimal data to support vulvar dystrophies being a cause of cancer. The International Society for the Study of Vulvar Disease has provided a standard nomenclature for these lesions, and this has been adopted by the International Society for Gynecologic Pathology (Table 97-1).[15] In 1985, the nomenclature was replaced by the terms CIS or vulvar intraepithelial neoplasia (VIN). In addition, the nonpremalignant squamous changes previously termed hyperplastic dystrophy are now considered under the classification of squamous hyperplasia.

Table 97-1 Classification of Vulvar Atypias

Pre-1985 classification:
Hyperplastic dystrophy
Without atypia
With atypia (mild, moderate, severe)
Lichen sclerosus
Mixed dystrophy
Without atypia
With atypia
Current classification:
Intraepithelial atypias
Mild dysplasia (VIN I)
Moderate dysplasia (VIN II)
Severe dysplasia—CIS (VIN III)
Lichen sclerosus
Miscellaneous

Abbreviations: CIS, carcinoma in situ; VIN, vulvar intraepithelial neoplasia.

Vulvar atypias can present with a variety of symptoms. The most common is irritation or itching; however, 20% of patients are asymptomatic.[16] Grossly, the lesions can be flat, raised (maculopapular), or verrucous. In color, they may be brown (hyperpigmented), red (erythroplastic), white, or discolored.

White lesions can appear to have a whitish, thickened keratin layer (leukoplakia) or a diffuse, white, brittle, paperlike appearance (lichen sclerosus) (Fig. 97-2). Areas of squamous hyperplasia (hyperplastic dystrophy) and dysplasia

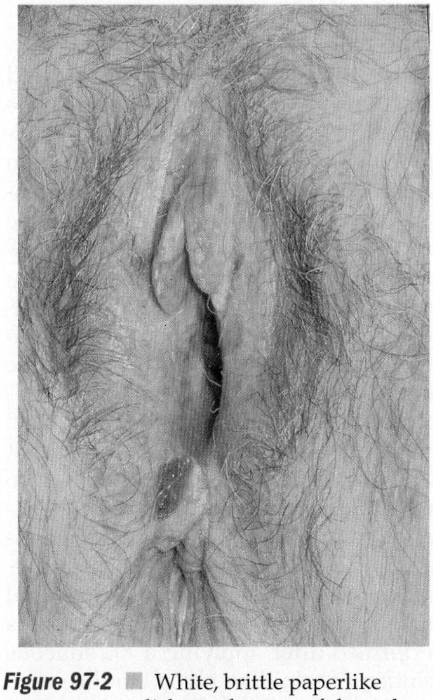

Figure 97-2 White, brittle paperlike appearance or lichen sclerosus of the vulva.

can also have a white appearance. Unlike lichen sclerosus, however, the tissue often is thickened, and the process tends to be focal or multifocal rather than diffuse.[15] It is important to biopsy lichen sclerosis since there may be an underlying vulvar carcinoma.[17,18]

Microscopically, atypical changes in the vulvar epithelium consistent with preinvasive lesions usually are marked by loss of maturation of the squamous epithelium. There is increased mitotic activity and an increase in the nuclear cytoplasmic ratio. Mild dysplasia (VIN I) is diagnosed if changes involve the lower third of the epithelium. If there is moderate dysplasia (VIN II), then half to two-thirds of the epithelium is affected. If there is severe dysplasia (VIN III), then two-thirds of the epithelium is affected. For CIS (also classified as VIN III) of the vulva, the full thickness of the epithelium usually is abnormal.

There is suggestion that there are two distinct causes of vulvar dysplasia of vulvar cancer. The first type is seen in younger patients and is related to HPV infection and smoking. This type presents itself as a "warty" dysplasia. The more common type is in elderly patients and is unrelated to smoking or HPV. This group is more related to lichen sclerosis adjacent to the tumor. Approximately 20% of vulvar cancer has been reported to have vulvar dysplasia.

It often is difficult to distinguish between benign squamous hyperplasia and intraepithelial neoplasia. Crum and colleagues suggested that nuclear size may be helpful in diagnosis because intraepithelial neoplasia of the vulva almost always contains nuclei that are fourfold or greater in size compared with benign condyloma or nonneoplastic epithelium.[19,20]

The best method of establishing a diagnosis is a high index of suspicion and early biopsy. Several methods also can be used to help assess these lesions. Cytology, colposcopy, and toluidine blue O can be used cautiously before biopsy. In general, however, cytologic evaluation of the vulva has not been helpful as a screening examination because the vulvar skin often is thickened and keratinized. Colposcopic examination of the vulva is difficult because unlike cervical lesions, the changes are difficult to recognize. Therefore, colposcopic examination is not used for routine vulvar examination; rather, it is primarily employed for patients who are being evaluated or followed for vulvar atypia or intraepithelial malignancies. The toluidine blue O test is nonspecific and stains nuclei in the superficial part of the epithelium. Colposcopy is performed after applying a 1% aqueous solution of toluidine blue O to the vulva for 1 minute and decolorizing the tissue with 1% acetic acid. Areas that retain the stain are biopsied. A positive test, however, does not always indicate a premalignant condition because 20% of benign areas on the vulva stain positively.[20]

To obtain the entire thickness of the skin for a definitive diagnosis, a biopsy of the vulva usually is done with a Keyes dermal punch. Occasionally, a larger biopsy is needed, in which case, a larger field can be locally anesthetized with lidocaine and a small scalpel or cervical biopsy punch used to obtain a specimen.[21]

Once the correct diagnosis has been established by biopsy, appropriate therapy can be undertaken. For lichen sclerosus, 2% topical testosterone propionate in petrolatum, used twice daily, is an effective preparation to overcome the epithelial atrophy. The medication should be given continuously or the atrophy returns. Side effects such as clitoral hypertrophy and increased hair growth can occur.

Local measures, for example, wearing cotton underclothes and avoiding strong soaps and detergents, often are used to diminish irritation. Topical fluorinated corticosteroids applied twice daily for 1-2 weeks are helpful in controlling pruritus, but prolonged use of these steroid preparations can lead to vulvar atrophy or contracture. If long-term therapy is needed, a nonfluorinated compound such as 1% hydrocortisone is used. Some patients with lichen sclerosus have severe contracture in the area of the posterior fourchette. Treating these areas surgically with plastic repair of the fourchette has been suggested.[22,23]

VIN can be treated by a variety of methods, and many authors have reported successful control of the disease by wide local excision.[8,22] Buscema and colleagues reported that 68% of 62 patients had no evidence of recurrence when treated by wide excision.[10] Adequate margins must be obtained with wide excision; however, this often may be difficult because of the multifocal nature of the disease. Friedrich and colleagues reported a 50% risk of recurrence if the margins were involved with neoplasia.[14]

Other modalities also have been reported in the treatment of VIN. Carbon dioxide laser vaporization and photodynamic therapy[24] of the vulva to a depth of 3 mm has been used, and current evidence indicates that laser therapy is as effective as surgical excision for the control of this disease. Before lasering the vulva, however, it is necessary to ascertain by histologic confirmation that invasive disease does not exist. Leuchter and colleagues treated 142 patients with CIS of the vulva.[25] Of those treated by laser, 17% had a recurrence, a result that is similar to that in lesions treated by local excision.

5-Fluorouracil (5-FU) cream has been used successfully to treat CIS of the vulva, and application of this has been reported to be successful in 75% of cases. With continuous application, however, this treatment causes edema and pain.

Paget Disease

Paget disease is a rare intraepithelial disorder of the vulvar skin that is seen in postmenopausal women.[26-28] Unlike VIN, the intraepithelial neoplastic cells are glandular rather than squamous. The lesion primarily occurs in whites of an average age of 65 years. Grossly, it appears as a reddish, eczematoid lesion. Microscopically, this type of lesion is characterized by large pale cells that often occur in nests and infiltrate the epithelium. Once the diagnosis is made, it is important to rule out the presence of an underlying cancer. Invasive vulvar Paget disease occur in approximately 10% of Paget disease.[18] If the anal area is involved, one needs to consider an anal carcinoma. A review by Lee and colleagues reported a total of 75 cases of Paget disease of the vulva: 16 (22%) of the patients had underlying invasive carcinoma of the adnexal structures and 7 (9%) had adnexal CIS.[27]

Paget disease of the vulva often spreads in an occult fashion, with margins extending beyond the normal appearance of the lesion.[28] If there is no evidence of an underlying malignant neoplasm, a wide local excision or total vulvectomy usually is performed.[29] If a wide local excision is performed, a slightly deeper excision is needed to remove the epidermis down to the level of the underlying fat to ensure removal of adnexal skin structures. Because this lesion extends subepithelially, a frozen section in the operating room may assist in ensuring complete removal.

Bergen and colleagues evaluated 14 patients with Paget disease of the vulva that was treated by vulvectomy, skinning vulvectomy with a graft, or hemivulvectomy.[29] With a median follow-up of 50 months, all patients were free of disease; however, three patients had had locally recurrent disease.

Other modalities (topical 5-FU cream, laser) have not been used for treatment of this disease. Because both local and distant recurrence is a major risk, close follow-up is required.

Invasive Vulvar Carcinomas

The International Federation of Gynecology and Obstetrics (FIGO) has defined four clinical stages of vulvar carcinoma.[30] In addition, many centers use the tumor, node, metastasis (TNM) classification. In 1988, the FIGO staging was modified to reflect lymph node status and the location of the tumor (Table 97-2). In this classification,

Table 97-2 **TNM Classification and Staging of Vulvar Carcinoma**

TNM Classification	
T	Primary tumor
Tis	Preinvasive carcinoma (CIS)
T1	Tumor confined to the vulva and/or perineum; 2 cm or less in diameter
T2	Tumor confined to the vulva and/or perineum; more than 2 cm in diameter
T3	Tumor of any size with adjacent spread to the urethra, vagina, or anus
T4	Tumor of any size infiltrating the bladder mucosa, the rectal mucosa, or both, including the upper part of the urethral mucosa, or fixed to the anus
N	Regional lymph nodes
N0	No nodes palpable
N1	Unilateral regional lymph node metastases
N2	Bilateral regional lymph node metastases
M	Distant metastases
M0	No clinical metastases
M1	Distant metastases (including pelvic lymph node metastases)

FIGO Staging (1988)		
0	Tis	CIS Intraepithelial carcinoma
I	T1N0M0	Tumor confined to the vulva and/or perineum; 2 cm or less in greatest dimension. No nodal metastasis.
II	T2N0	Tumor confined to the vulva and/or perineum; more than 2 cm in greatest dimension. No nodal metastasis.
III	T3N0M0 T1N1M0 T2N1M0 T3N1M0	Tumor of any size with (1) adjacent spread to the lower urethra and/or the vagina and/or the anus and/or (2) unilateral regional lymph node metastasis
IVA	T1N2M0 T2N2M0 T3N2M0 T4, any N, M0	Tumor invades any of the following: upper urethra, bladder mucosa, rectal mucosa, pelvic bone, and/or bilateral regional node metastasis.
IVB	Any T, any N, M1	Any distant metastasis including pelvic lymph nodes

Abbreviations: FIGO, International Federation of Gynecology and Obstetrics; TNM, tumor, node, metastasis.
Source: Adapted from Ref. 30.

a tumor that is located on the perineum is no longer considered to be stage III. In 1995, FIGO instituted a subclassification of stage I into IA and IB, based on whether there is stromal invasion greater than 1 mm. Clinical assessment of groin nodes is inaccurate in about 25% of cases. The error of clinical staging is about 18% of stage I compared to surgical staging.[31]

Vulvar cancer can spread by direct extension, lymphatic embolization or hematogenous dissemination. Metastasis to the femoral nodes without inguinal node involvement has been reported, but is uncommon. The direct lymphatic pathways from the clitoris to the pelvic nodes have been described but are not of clinical significance. The overall incidence of lymph node metastasis is approximately 30%. Pelvic node metastasis is uncommon with an overall frequency of 9%. Approximately 20% of patients with positive groin nodes have positive pelvic nodes.[32,33]

Squamous Cell Carcinoma ■ Squamous cell carcinomas comprise approximately 90% of primary vulvar malignancies. Grossly, these carcinomas usually appear as ulcerated or polyploid masses on the vulva. Biopsy reveals the characteristic histologic appearance: the tumor appears in nests and cords of squamous cells infiltrating the stroma, often with islands of keratin. On physical examination there is usually an ulcerated lesion or wart-like lesion. Recently, there has been an increased incidence of warty carcinoma accounting for 20% of all cases.

Different clinical results have been reported with this definition. Spread to regional lymph nodes has varied from 0% to 10% in tumors with less than a 5 mm depth of invasion.[34-39] For example, Hoffman and colleagues reported no nodal metastases in 43 patients whose tumor invaded less than 2 mm.[37] Lesions that were at risk of spreading to inguinal nodes included tumors with confluent tongues rather than those with individual tongues merely extending into the stroma. Hacker and colleagues, however, reported that six of seven patients with invasion of less than 3 mm had regional node involvement.[36]

The risk of nodal involvement may be decreased when CIS is present in the lesion. Rowley and colleagues noted that only 1 of 35 cases with adjacent CIS had nodal metastases.[38] By contrast, 5 of 27 had positive lymph nodes when superficial stage I lesions penetrating 2.1-5.0 mm did not have adjacent CIS.

Stage IA ■ For stage IA lesions, therapy may be less extensive than with invasive vulvar carcinoma. Different treatments have been reported, including wide local excision with or without ipsilateral node dissection, simple vulvectomy without node dissection, and radical vulvectomy without node dissection.[39-41] In younger patients, especially those with tumors located at a distance from the clitoris, an operation that spares the clitoris should be considered. DiSaia and colleagues recommended an operative procedure in which the superficial inguinal lymph nodes are removed and sent for frozen section.[40] If positive nodes are found, bilateral complete groin dissection and complete radical vulvectomy are performed; if the nodes are negative, wide local excision of the primary cancer is performed.

Iversen and colleagues reported an alternative approach, recommending a hemivulvectomy with ipsilateral groin dissection for lesions involving the labia.[41] For medial lesions, they suggest conventional radical vulvectomy with bilateral groin dissection. Boyce and colleagues recommended that conservative therapy can be used with minimal risk.[42] This recommendation appears to be advisable if invasion is greater than 1 mm and the tumor diameter is greater than 2 cm.

The pattern of spread for this carcinoma relates to the intricate lymphatic drainage of the vulva (Fig. 97-3).[5] Tumors located in the middle of either labium initially drain to the ipsilateral inguinal femoral nodes, whereas midline perineal tumors can spread either to the left or right side. Using technetium-99m colloid, Iversen and Aas showed that when radioactivity was injected to one side of the vulva, 98% of it localized in the ipsilateral nodes and less than 2% in the contralateral nodes.[33] Tumors along the midline in the clitoral or urethral areas may spread to either groin. From the inguinal-femoral nodes, lymphatic spread continues to the deep pelvic iliac and obturator nodes. Although there has been concern in the past that tumors in the clitoral-urethral area could spread directly to the deep pelvic nodes, current evidence indicates that this is rare.

There is no uniformly accepted definition regarding microinvasive carcinoma of the vulva, and this may result from confusion in measuring the depth of invasion. Microinvasion has been defined by some as a small lesion of the vulva less than 2 cm in diameter and invading less than 3 mm.[34] The International Society for the Study of Vulvar Diseases has recommended that the term microinvasive be dropped and that stage IA be used for tumors less than 2 cm in diameter and invading less than 1 mm from the epidermal-stromal junction, the basement membrane.

To identify patients who can be treated more conservatively, investigators have used intraoperative lymphatic mapping and sentinel node identification for squamous cell carcinoma. Investiga-

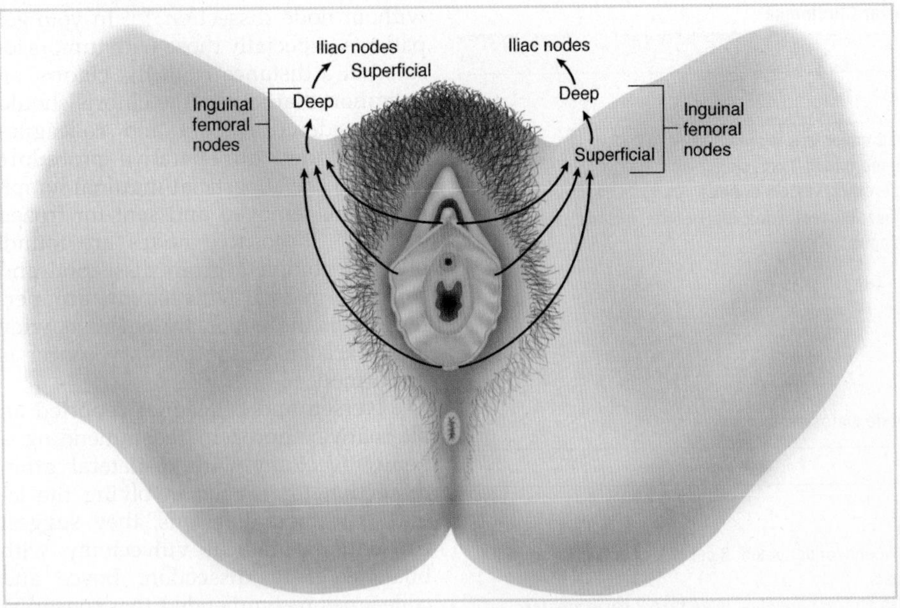

Figure 97-3 ■ Lymphatic drainage of the vulva.

tors have improved the rate of identification of the sentinel node by combining blue dye with radiolocalization.[43,44] Patients whose tumor invades the stroma less than 1 mm are at low risk of nodal involvement. In these cases, inguinal femoral lymphadectomy may not be indicated.

The feasibility of intraoperative lymphatic mapping with vulvar cancer has been demonstrated in 21 patients. In this series, the sentinel node was found in a variety of locations at the femoral vessels and at the medial border of Scarpa fascia. In no patients were the nonsentinel nodes positive if the sentinel nodes were negative.[44-46] False negative sentinel nodes have been reported with low incidence.[47-49]

Stages I, II, and III Invasive Carcinoma ■ The prognosis of a patient with vulvar carcinoma relates to the stage of disease (Fig. 97-4) and to the nodal status.[50] The presence of carcinoma in the regional lymph nodes correlates with the size and thickness of the primary lesion, the degree of tumor differentiation, and the involvement of vascular spaces by the tumor (Table 97-3). In 272 women with invasive vulvar carcinoma reported by the Gynecologic Oncology Group (GOG), regional nodes were involved in 8.9% of stage I, 25.3% of stage II, and 31.1% of stage III lesions.[51,52] If a lesion was less than 1 mm thick, there was a 3.1% incidence of positive nodes. With larger lesions, 4 mm or greater in thickness, 31% of nodes were positive. Hacker and colleagues reported an actuarial 5-year survival rate of 96% in those with negative nodes Survival decreased to 94% with one positive node, 80% with two positive

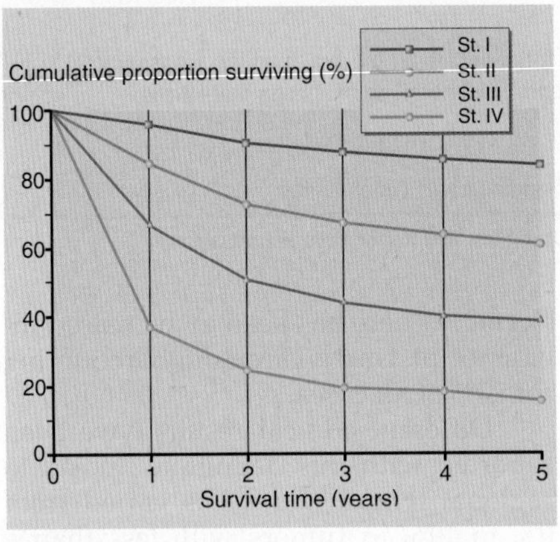

Figure 97-4 ■ Survival of patients with carcinoma of the vulva. *Source*: Adapted from the 20th Report on End Results of Therapy of Gynecologic Malignancies. Stockholm: International Federation of Gynecology and Obstetrics; 1988.

nodes, and 12% with three or more nodes involved by tumor.[53]

Not only is the number of nodes important, but there also appears to be a correlation with the size of the metastases. Hoffman and colleagues noted that 14 of 15 patients with inguinal lymph node metastases measuring less than 36 mm survived free of disease for 5 years compared with 12 of 29 patients whose tumor metastases measured greater than 100 mm.[54] No additional treatment is advised if only one lymph node in the groin in microscopically positive. The grade of tumor related to the percentage of positive nodes in the GOG study. Patients with stage 1 lesions did not have positive nodes, yet in patients with stage 4 lesions, 47.7% of nodes were positive. Vascular space involvement also was prognostic because 72% with vascular invasion showed tumor in regional nodes compared with 34% of those without vascular invasion. Nodal involvement also correlated with the location of the primary lesion.[55] Lesions on the labia are associated with 7.4% positive nodes, whereas clitoral lesions have a higher incidence of positive nodes (27.4%).[56] Boyce and colleagues reported that six tumors under 1 cm in diameter had no metastases to regional nodes but that the fraction of tumors with positive nodes rose to 55% for 29 cases with lesions over 4 cm.[42]

Therapy for stages I and II and early stage III vulvar carcinoma is accomplished with radical vulvectomy and bilateral inguinal femoral node dissection.[57] In the past, en bloc of radical vulvectomy and bilateral dissection of the groin and pelvic nodes was standard treatment. Over the last 20 years, there has been modification of this surgical approach. Since often the disease occurs in younger women with small tumors and concern of morbidity associated with en bloc resection. The deep pelvic nodes are rarely removed unless the inguinal nodes are involved. Most oncologists now remove only the inguinal and femoral nodes at the time of operation and treat the deep pelvic nodes with external radiation if superficial nodes are involved with tumor.

A wide variety of management options of the primary lesion have been proposed. Management of patients with small lesions should be individualized. Since the early 1980s, radical local excision has been advocated in patients with small tumors. The literature indicates that the incidence of local invasive recurrence is similar with local excision and more radical approaches. Radical local excision is most appropriate for unilat-

Table 97-3 ■ **Prognostic Factors of Stage, Grade, and Tumor Thickness Associated With Positive Regional Nodes**

Stage	Positive Nodes (%)	Grade	Positive Nodes (%)	Tumor Thickness (mm)	Positive Nodes (%)
I	8.9	1	0	<1	3.1
II	25.3	2	8.0	2	8.9
III	31.1	3	24.6	3	18.6
IV	62.5	4	47.7	>4	31.0

Source: Adapted from Sedlis A, Homesly H, Bundy BN, et al. Positive groin lymph nodes in superficial squamous vulvar cancer. *Am J Obstet Gynecol*. 1987;156:1159.

eral, isolated lesions. In a unilateral lesion less than 1 cm from the midline, radical wide local excision with possible postoperative radiation has been used. This approach has been used for risk factors such as large tumor sites, positive capillary-lymphatic space invasion, or surgical margins that are less than 8 mm. For midline lesions, standard management has varied from use of surgery as primary treatment to use of radiation with possible chemotherapy.

Different surgical approaches to invasive vulvar carcinoma have been evaluated. Classically, an en bloc dissection has been performed. Radical vulvectomy and groin dissection have been carried out through a single suprapubic incision that extends between the left and right anterior iliac spines (Fig. 97-5). This operation removed the entire vulva, including the clitoris, subcutaneous tissue, and inguinal femoral nodes. If the lesion involved the distal urethra, this has often been removed without the loss of urinary continence. In this procedure, the major complication has been wound breakdown and infection (occurring in 50% of the patients). Recently, modifications have been introduced to decrease the incidence of wound breakdown. These modifications include performing the inguinal femoral node dissection through separate inguinal incisions and then completing the radical vulvectomy. Tumor recurrences rarely occur in the skin bridge when separate groin incisions are used.[52,58]

Less mutilating procedures also have been reported in stage I disease. Rowley and colleagues reported using wide local excision and superficial inguinal node dissection in 20 patients with stage I lesions invading to a depth of less than 5 mm.[38] The superficial and contralateral inguinal femoral nodes were removed only if the superficial nodes contained tumor. This approach seems to be reasonable if a unilateral lesion is present; however, with a midline lesion, bilateral inguinal node dissection seems to be appropriate. In a recent update of a series of 50 patients initially reported by DiSaia and colleagues, only 1 patient died because of recurrent carcinoma treated with the latter conservative approach.[40] Six patients had only recurrent CIS or minimally invasive carcinoma. Modifying the approach for these early-stage lesions appears to be effective and is associated with less morbidity than the standard radical vulvectomy. If the nodes are free from tumor in stages I and II carcinomas of the vulva, no further therapy is required. If the nodes (especially the femoral nodes) are involved, pelvic irradiation is required. From a randomized study, Homesley and colleagues reported an improved survival rate in 118 patients with positive lymph nodes who received 4500-5000 cGy of radiation (Fig. 97-6).[51]

Advanced Vulvar Tumor ■ Large tumors of the vulva encroaching on the anorectal area and the urethra require more extensive treatment than a radical vulvectomy. In addition to a radical vulvectomy, it is usually necessary to perform a diversion of the urinary or fecal stream. Large defects may require skin grafts such as gracilis myocutaneous grafts. If the nodes are negative, a 5-year survival rate of 50% has been reported.[59,60]

However, newer approaches that involve a combination of preoperative radiation and surgery have been reported in treating these lesions. External radiation using newer techniques such as intensity modulated radiotherapy (IMRT) often is given to reduce the size of the tumor before surgical removal by radical vulvectomy, with or without regional lymph node dissection. Approximately 4000-4500 cGy is delivered to the pelvis and inguinal nodes, the operation being performed 5 weeks after the completion of radiation. This approach may obviate a urinary or fecal diversion. Boronow and colleagues reported a 5-year survival rate of 80% in 26 patients with primary carcinoma of the vagina and vulva who were treated with this technique.[61,62] Rotmensch and colleagues recently reported 16 patients with advanced vulvar lesions who were treated with preoperative radiation to the vulva and achieved an overall 5-year survival rate of 45%.[63] Recurrences were more likely if the resection margins were within 1 cm of the tumor. Complications have included stenosis of the introitus and urethra as well as rectovaginal fistula.

Recently, an approach has been to not only administer preoperative radiation for advanced lesions but also to add chemotherapy. Commonly, agents such as 5-FU, cisplatin, and mitomycin C have been used, producing up to 46% reduction in tumor with chemoradiation. The most common toxicities were acute cutaneous and wound complications.[64] Investigators have suggested that radiation-sensitive chemotherapeutic drugs, such as cis-platinum, may enhance the response to radiation. The Gynecologic Oncology Group (GOG) has attempted to expedite this; however, the study was terminated owing to a lack of sufficient patients. Because the vulvar skin is prone to radiation dermatitis, fibrosis, and ulceration, radiation as the sole therapy has been less than desirable. If the patient is inoperable because of medical conditions; however, radiation can be used as the primary treatment of a vulvar carcinoma.[65]

Recurrent Vulvar Cancer ■ Recurrences may be local or distant. More than 80% of recurrences occur in the first 2 years after therapy. The risk of recurrence of vulva carcinoma increases as the stage of disease increases. In an analysis of 224 patients with vulvar carcinoma, Podratz and colleagues reported a recurrence rate of 14% in stage I and 71% in stage IV disease.[66] Local recurrences were the most common. Local recurrences often occur in the skin bridge remaining after a radical vulvectomy.[67] Different modalities have been used to treat local recurrences. Both radiation therapy and resection of local vulvar recurrence provide effective control and a 5-year survival rate of approximately 50%. The combination of chemotherapy and radiation therapy has been used to treat recurrent disease and some large primary vulvar carcinomas. Thomas and colleagues reported the use of 5-FU (1 g/m^2) as a continuous intravenous infusion for 4-5 days every 4 weeks during radiation.[68] This combined approach was the sole treatment in nine patients, and six patients had a complete remission. Disseminated disease requires chemotherapy, but, unfortunately, no chemotherapy has been successful in this situation.

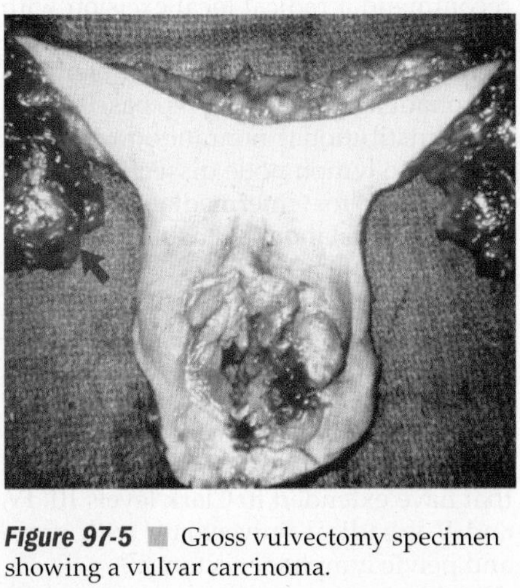

Figure 97-5 ■ Gross vulvectomy specimen showing a vulvar carcinoma.

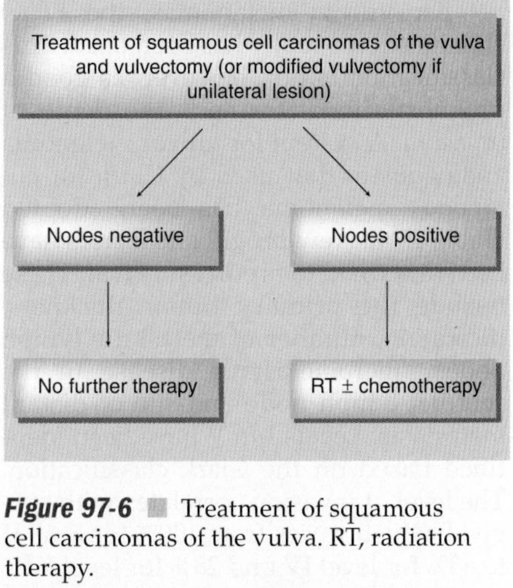

Figure 97-6 ■ Treatment of squamous cell carcinomas of the vulva. RT, radiation therapy.

Recurrence of vulvar cancer correlates with the number of positive groin nodes. Patients with less than three nodes have a lower risk of recurrence. Local vulvar recurrences can be further excised. Three patterns of local recurrences have been described. There is the primary tumor site recurrence, distal recurrence from the primary tumor, and recurrence in the skin incision. Local recurrence at a distant site (66.7% 3-year survival) has a better prognosis than recurrence at the primary tumor site (15.4% 3-year survival rate). Radiation therapy in combination with chemotherapy has been used to treat recurrences. The most active agents have been cisplatin, taxol, mitomycin, and 5-fluorouracil. However, response rates and duration of response has been low.

Bartholin Gland Carcinoma ■ Primary carcinoma of Bartholin gland accounts for 5% of all vulvar cancers, and over 200 cases have been reported;[69] approximately 50% of those tumors are nonepidermoid in nature. Bartholin gland carcinomas can be squamous if they originate near the orifice of the duct or papillary if they arise from the transitional epithelium of the duct, or they can be adenocarcinomas if they arise from the gland itself. An enlargement of Bartholin gland in a postmenopausal female should raise the suspicion of malignancy. These tumors are treated similarly to primary squamous cell carcinomas of the vulva, by radical vulvectomy and bilateral inguinal femoral lymphadenectomy. The overall 5-year survival rate of approximately 70% is below that reported for all carcinomas of the vulva and probably relates to a delay in diagnosis. A Bartholian gland carcinoma of the vulva is classified if the tumor is in the correct anatomic position, deeply located in the labium majora, the underlying skin is intact, and there is some normal gland present.

The adenoid cystic variety of Bartholin gland carcinoma invades locally and rarely metastasizes. It is slow growing with a tendency to recur locally and invade the perincular tissue. It usually requires only wide local excision for adequate therapy. Rosenberg and colleagues reported five cases of adenocystic carcinoma of Bartholin's gland, with four patients alive and free of disease 28-57 months after treatment.[70]

Basal Cell Carcinoma ■ Basal cell carcinoma is rarely encountered in the female genital tract. Such lesions are usually locally invasive, nonmetastatic tumors that are commonly found on the labium majus. Metastasis to the regional lymph nodes is uncommon. Therapy consists of wide local excision of the lesion. If the surgical margins are free of tumor, the disease is cured.

Verrucous Carcinoma ■ Verrucous carcinoma of the vulva is a variant of epidermoid carcinoma. Clinically, it appears as large, condylomatous lesions. They are locally aggressive, nonmetastatic, fungating tumors that gradually increase in size, pushing into rather than invading the underlying structures. Histologically, they consist of mature squamous cells with extensive keratinization. To establish the diagnosis, adequate biopsy is important because biopsy of a large verrucous carcinoma often can lead to an incorrect diagnosis of condyloma acuminatum.

These tumors tend to grow slowly and invade locally, rarely spreading to regional lymph nodes. In 24 cases of verrucous carcinoma, Japaze and colleagues found no lymph node metastases.[71] Depending on the size and location of the tumor, a wide local excision or simple vulvectomy is effective therapy; radical vulvectomy with inguinal node dissection or radiation therapy is not indicated as treatment for this entity. Radiation therapy is ineffective and can even worsen the prognosis, causing malignant changes within the tumor. The 17 cases treated surgically by Japaze and colleagues had an excellent 5-year survival rate of 94%. Close long-term follow-up is needed because disease can recur locally, especially if the tumor is large. If concurrent squamous cell carcinoma is found within the verrucous carcinoma, local excision is an inadequate therapy.[72]

Melanoma ■ Melanoma is the most frequent nonsquamous cell malignancy of the vulva and comprises approximately 5% of primary carcinomas of the vulva. Approximately 400 cases of melanoma of the vulva have been reported, with an overall 5-year survival rate of approximately 33%, irrespective of the therapeutic modality used. Patients with malignant melanoma of the vulva vary widely in age, ranging from 10 to 96 years, with an average age of approximately 60 years. These lesions most often affect the labia minora or the clitoris.[73]

For vulvar melanomas, the FIGO classification usually has been used. This classification is not, however, as good a prognostic indicator as is the depth of invasion. A system for vulvar melanoma analogous to that used by Clark for cutaneous melanoma has been adopted (Table 97-4). New prognostic factors have been described to predict survival. These include the primary tumor thickness, ulceration, number of metastatic lymph nodes, micrometastatic disease in the sentinel lymph node and site of distant metastasis. Levels I to V have been identified based on the Clark classification. The level of invasion correlates with survival, which varies from 100% for level II to 83% for level IV and 28% for level V.[74]

Table 97-4 ■ **Classification of Melanomas of the Vulva**

Clark Level	
I	Intraepithelial
II	Extension to papillary dermes
III	Filling the dermal papillae
IV	Invasive of collagen in reticular dermis
V	Extension into subcutaneous fat
Breslow Depth of Invasion	
I	<0.75 mm from skin surface
II	0.76-1.4 mm from skin surface
III	>1.5 mm from skin surface

Two varieties of melanoma have been described: nodular and superficial spreading melanoma.[75] The superficial spreading melanoma is more common and has a better prognosis, with a 5-year survival rate of 71%. Nodular melanoma has a worse prognosis, and this directly relates to its potential for vertical growth. The 5-year survival rate for nodular melanoma, which is more invasive, is only 38%.

The thickness of the tumor also may be useful in evaluating this lesion. Breslow reported a classification using depth of invasion as measured from the skin surface.[76] In his classification, Breslow reported the overall prognosis as excellent and the spread to regional nodes as unlikely for melanomas with a thickness of less than 0.76 mm, measured from the surface to the deepest point of penetration.

Wide local excision has been recommended for Clark level I and II disease when no palpable regional nodes are present.[77] In a report of 36 melanoma cases, Rose and colleagues noted that wide excision was as effective as radical vulvectomy.[78] Prognosis was better for younger patients, presumably because most had superficial spreading rather than nodular melanomas.

A reasonable approach is to excise a melanoma with a 2 cm margin and without node dissection for cases that are less than 2 mm thick. However, others would recommend a radical local excision with 1-2 cm margins from the primary lesions and an ipsilateral inguinofemoral lymphadenectomy. This is based on a multi-institutional nonrandomized trial of elective lymph node dissection versus obstruction for intermediate thickness cutaneous melanoma. This study showed elective lymph node dissection had a significantly better 5-year survival rate than observation for melanomas 1-4 mm.

An excision with a 2-3 cm margin combined with node dissection could be performed for more advanced melanomas. An alternative approach for lesions that have extended to Clark levels III, IV, and V is radical vulvectomy with groin and pelvic lymphadenectomy.[79]

It has been reported that melanoma of the vulva can metastasize to pelvic nodes, bypassing the inguinal femoral nodes, but current evidence indicates that pelvic node involvement does not occur without prior inguinal node involvement. A further therapeutic consideration is that patients with melanoma whose pelvic nodes are involved with tumor usually do not survive their disease.

Long-term results generally are not available for large series of melanomas. Most series of malignant melanoma report an overall survival rate of approximately 50%.[80] For lesions that correspond to Clark level I or II (lesions 0.76 mm thick) and are treated by wide local excision, the 5-year survival rate is in the vicinity of 100%. Prognosis becomes poorer with melanomas more than 3 mm thick. If the regional nodes are negative, the survival rate is approximately 60%; if the regional nodes are involved with tumor, survival is only 30%.

The role of chemotherapy for distant metastasis has not been well established. Regressions, but not cures, have been reported with various multiagent cytotoxic programs, including chemotherapy and/or immunotherapy.

Sarcoma ■ Sarcomas of the vulva are rare. Leiomyosarcomas appear to be the most frequently encountered sarcomas in this group of patients,[81] and surgical removal by wide local excision is the recommended initial treatment of choice. The 5-year survival rate is reported to be approximately 100%. Locally recurrent lesions are similarly treated. Chemotherapeutic considerations are the same as for those sarcomas in other sites of the female genital tract.[82]

Cancer of the Vagina

Primary vaginal cancers are rare, constituting less than 2% of all gynecologic malignancies.[1,83-85] Carcinoma of the vagina is defined as a primary carcinoma arising in the vagina and not involving the external os of the cervix superiorly or the vulva inferiorly. The majority of vaginal tumors are secondary to metastasis from other sites. Approximately 30% of primary vaginal cancers have in situ or invasive cervical cancers previously treated.

Vaginal cancer is rare and accounts for only about 3% of cancers of the female reproductive system. It is estimated about 2000 cases of vaginal cancer will be diagnosed in the United States and 800 women will die of this cancer.

The most common symptom of vaginal carcinoma is abnormal painless bleeding or discharge. With advanced tumors, pain or urinary frequency occasionally occurs, especially in cases of anterior wall tumors. Constipation or tenesmus has been seen with tumors involving the posterior vaginal wall. These tumors usually are diagnosed by direct biopsy of the tumor mass, and abnormal cytologic findings often will lead to diagnosis of a vaginal cancer.

The staging criteria for vaginal carcinomas according to the FIGO are given in Table 97-5.

Premalignant Vaginal Disease

Premalignant disease of the vagina is generally detected on cytologic screening. Once an abnormal cytology is obtained, a biopsy directed by colposcopic examination is required to verify the severity of the changes. Because vaginal intraepithelial neoplasia is often multifocal, it is necessary to inspect the entire vaginal canal.[86]

Most lesions occur at the vaginal apex. Audet-Lapointe and colleagues noted that 61 of 66 cases of vaginal intraepithelial neoplasia occurred in the upper third of the vagina.[87] These lesions usually can be excised locally. Other modalities often are preferred, however, because of the multifocal nature of this disease or the necessity of excising large areas, requiring skin grafting.[88]

Nonsurgical approaches for treating these lesions include laser ablation and 5-FU cream for widespread multifocal disease. Carbon dioxide laser frequently has been used and, if carried to a depth of 2-4 mm, allows for vaporization of abnormal tissue. Preliminary results reported by Petrilli and colleagues with this modality have shown a success rate of approximately 90%.[89] Radiation currently is not recommended for the treatment of noninvasive disease because of the proximity of the bladder and rectum and the availability of newer modalities.

Another approach to treating vaginal intraepithelial neoplasia is the use of 5% 5-FU cream for approximately 7 days, repeated every 3-4 weeks if the vaginal intraepithelial neoplasia persists. Hyperkeratotic lesions appear to be less sensitive to treatment because of their thickness and parakeratosis. Krebs reported on the use of 5% 5-FU daily for 10 days and noted that 17 of 20 patients with vaginal condylomas responded to this therapy.[90] Petrilli and colleagues and Ballon and colleagues reported success rates of 80-90% for vaginal intraepithelial neoplasia after multiple cycles of therapy.[89,91]

Table 97-5 **FIGO Staging Classification for Vaginal Carcinoma**

Stage	
0	CIS
I	Carcinoma limited to vaginal wall
II	Carcinoma involves subvaginal tissue but Has not extended to pelvic wall
III	Carcinoma extends to pelvic wall
IV	Carcinoma extends beyond true pelvis or involves mucosa of bladder or rectum

Abbreviation: CIS, FIGO, International Federation of Gynecology and Obstetrics.

Invasive Carcinomas of the Vagina

Squamous cell carcinomas of the vagina may appear grossly as either ulcerated or fungating tumors or they may be exophytic and protrude through the vaginal canal. They are the most common vaginal malignancy and account for 90% of primary vaginal cancers. The disease occurs primarily in women over 50 years of age. Most squamous cell carcinomas occur in the upper third of the vagina. In examining the patient, it is important to visualize the entire vagina because lesions on the posterior wall can be concealed by the speculum.[92] Microscopically, these tumors have the classic findings of invasive squamous cell carcinoma. They have pleomorphic squamous cells with occasional keratin pearls.

The location of the tumor determines the areas of lymphatic spread (Fig. 97-7).[93] The lymphatics of the middle and upper vagina communicate superiorly with the lymphatics of the cervix and drain into the pelvic nodes of the obturator, internal, and external iliac chains. The lymphatics of the distal third of the vagina drain to the inguinal and pelvic nodes, with a pattern of drainage similar to that of the vulva. The posterior wall lymphatics drain to the rectal lymphatic system. Positive inguinal nodes are present in 31.6% of disease in the lower vagina. The treatment for vaginal cancer is individualized.

Depending on the location, both radiation including high dose rate brachytherapy, and surgery have been used effectively in treating these lesions (Table 97-6). Treatment is often individualized, depending on the size, stage, and location of the tumor.[91,94]

If the tumor is less than 2 cm thick, some investigators advocate using only local radiation.[95,96] If the carcinoma is less than 0.5 cm thick, intracavitary irradiation with a vaginal cylinder to deliver 8000 cGy to the mucosa will give over 90% tumor control.[97] Spirtos and colleagues studied 23 stage I patients and noted only two local recurrences, and both of these had tumor doses of less than 7500 cGy.[98] For larger lesions, external radiation is used, with a concomitant reduction in the local vaginal component

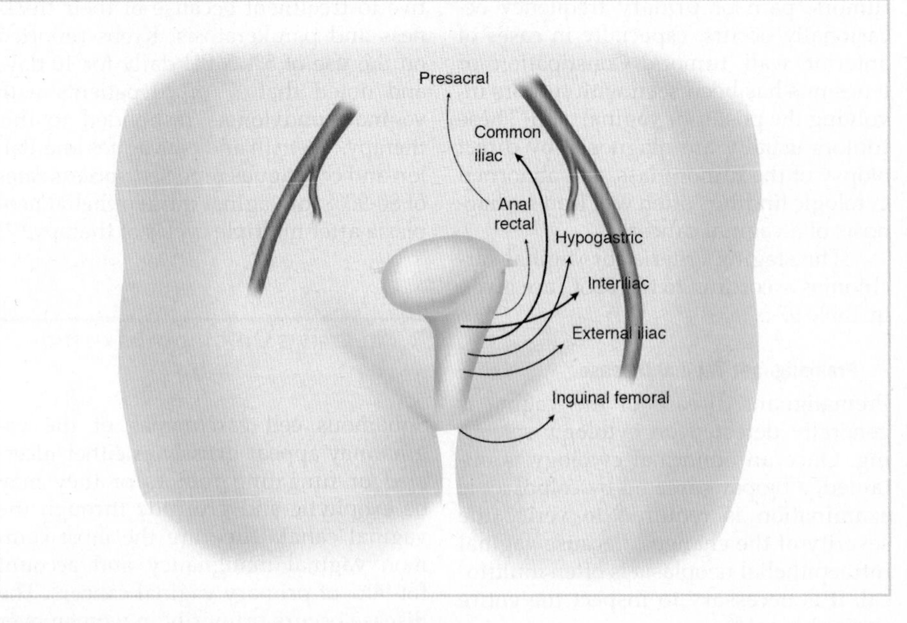

Figure 97-7 Lymphatic drainage of the vagina.

Table 97-6 **Treatment Scheme for Vaginal Carcinoma**

Stage	External Therapy (cGy)	Implant (Interstitial) cGy
I		
Σ, small tumors (<2 cm)	–	6000-7000
Σ, all others	Whole pelvis (4000)	3000-4000 cGy
II	Whole pelvis (4000-5000)	3000-4000 cGy
III	Whole pelvis (5000)	2000
IV	Whole pelvis (5000; an additional 1000–2000 through reduced field if implant not possible)	2000 (if possible)

1 cGy = 1 rad.
Source: Adapted from Nori Ref. 97.

of primary tumor treatment.[99] Implants, however, often cannot be used in patients with larger stage III or IV carcinomas. If such is the case, only external beam radiation is used, and a central boost is given after an initial whole-pelvis dose of 5000 cGy radiation.[100]

Small tumors located in the upper third of the vagina often can be excised.[101,102] In patients with these, a radical hysterectomy, partial vaginectomy, or pelvic lymphadenectomy usually is effective. Surgery has been preferred in younger patients.

If distant metastasis occurs, effective cis-platinum based chemotherapy for recurrent squamous cell carcinoma of the vagina has not been developed.[103] For squamous cell carcinoma, a variety of regimens using multiagent chemotherapy similar to those for cervical carcinoma have been employed.

The overall survival rate for patients with primary carcinoma of the vagina has been reported as approximately 45% and is related to the stage of the disease (Table 97-7). Even in patients with early stage I disease, the 5-year survival is only 70%.

Clear Cell Adenocarcinoma of the Vagina

Clear cell adenocarcinomas have been seen more frequently in young women since 1970 because of the association with intrauterine exposure to diethylstilbestrol.[104,105] Three predominant histologic patterns are found with clear cell carcinoma; they have been described as tubulocystic, solid, and papillary patterns.[106,107] Most clear cell carcinomas of the vagina are polypoid or nodular, with a reddish color.

Clear cell carcinomas can spread locally and by the lymphatic and hematogenous routes. Metastases to regional pelvic nodes have been found in approximately one-sixth of stage I cases. Spread to regional pelvic nodes becomes more frequent in higher-stage tumors.

Table 97-7 **Stage and Survival of Squamous Cell Carcinoma of the Vagina**

Stage	Survival Rate (%)
I	71
II	47
III	25
IV	8
Overall	45

Source: Adapted from Benedet JL, Murphy KS, Fairey RN, et al. Primary invasive carcinoma of the vagina. *Obstet Gynecol.* 1983;62:715.

Clear cell adenocarcinomas are staged as other carcinomas of the vagina are by the FIGO. Some 80% have been diagnosed as stage I or II.

Several prognostic factors have been identified. Older patients (ie, >19 years of age) have a more favorable prognosis than younger patients.[108] This difference has been associated with the presence of a more favorable tubulocystic pattern of clear cell adenocarcinoma, which is the most frequent histologic pattern found in older patients. In addition, smaller tumor diameter and superficial depth of invasion correlate with improved patient survival. Survival also depends on the stage of the disease. In 547 patients treated for clear cell adenocarcinoma of the vagina, the 5-year survival rate for those in stages I, II, III, and IV has been 93%, 83%, 37%, and 0%, respectively (Table 97-8).[108]

Because of the young age of these patients, surgery often is the primary therapy. For stage I and early stage II disease (Fig. 97-8), radical hysterectomy, partial or complete vaginectomy, pelvic lymphadenectomy, and replacement of the vagina with a split-thickness skin graft have been the approaches most frequently used.[109]

In patients with small stage I tumors of the vagina, efforts have been made to preserve fertility. The tumor has been excised with retroperitoneal lymph node dissection, followed by local radiation. Senekjian and colleagues reported that the survival rate of patients with small vaginal tumors treated with such an approach compares favorably with that of patients treated with conventional therapy.[109] In their series, eight pregnancies were reported in five patients who were treated locally.

Larger tumors have been treated with whole-pelvis radiation in addition to intracavitary implant. For tumors greater than 2 cm, whole-pelvis radiation of 4000-5000 cGy has been given, with an additional implant of 3000-4000 cGy.[110] In a few instances, exenterative surgery has been performed for larger tumors; how-

Table 97-8 **Survival at 5 and 10 Years for 547 Patients With Clear Cell Adenocarcinoma of the Vagina and Cervix**

	Survival (%)	
Stage	5 Years	10 Years
I	93	87
IIA	80	66
IIB	58	49
II (vagina)	83	67
III	37	12
IV	0	0

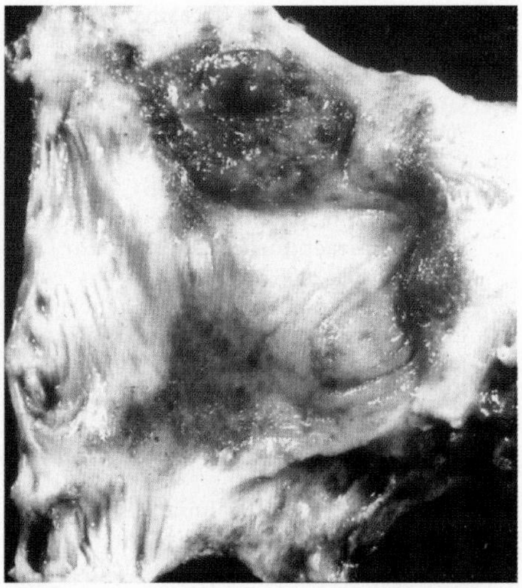

Figure 97-8 Clear cell adenocarcinoma of the anterior wall, with vaginal adenosis on the posterior wall at the edge of the tumor.

ever, this procedure usually has been applied to central recurrences following primary radiation therapy.[111]

If there is a recurrence, therapy consists of additional radical surgery, often requiring exenteration or extensive radiation localized to the pelvis. Systemic chemotherapy has been used in cases of metastatic disease. Cisplatin (75-100 mg/m^2) with a continuous infusion of 5-FU (1 g/m^2 for 3-5 days every 3-4 weeks) is currently recommended. However, no single agent or combination of chemotherapeutic agents has emerged as the most effective.[112] Prolonged follow-up is necessary because recurrences, especially in the lungs and supraclavicular areas, have been reported as long as 19 years after primary therapy.

Vaginal Melanomas

Malignant melanomas of the vagina are rare; they constitute less than 1% of all melanomas occurring in females. The age distribution of the neoplasm has ranged from 26 to 98 years,[58] with a median age of 70 years. Most patients are postmenopausal and present with vaginal bleeding, discharge, or a mass. Tumors may vary from 0.5 to 7.5 cm in diameter, with approximately 30% being 2 cm or less in diameter. Most of these tumors develop in the distal third of the vagina, commonly on the anterior wall. Primary vaginal melanomas presumably arise from vaginal melanocytes that are present in approximately 3% of normal females. Histologically, this neoplasm is similar to other melanomas found elsewhere and tends to be deeply invasive in the vagina.

The prognosis is worse than that of vulvar melanomas. Chung and colleagues reported a 5-year survival rate of only 21% in a series of 19 patients.[113] Reid and colleagues reported a 5-year survival rate of 17.4% in 15 cases, but the prognosis was improved for those tumors that were small and less than 3 cm in diameter.[114] More recently, Borazjani and colleagues reported improved survival for cases in which there were fewer than six mitoses/10 high-power fields.[115] The best prognostic factor is the size of the lesion.

Optimal treatment has not been established. Treatment usually consists of radical surgery or wide excision of the vagina and dissection of the regional lymph nodes, depending on the location of the lesion. Recently a more conservative approach has been used for wide local excision followed by pelvic radiation. Because of the poor prognosis, adjunctive radiation and chemotherapy have been used as local recurrences, and distant metastases with this disease are common.

Rare Vaginal Tumors in Young Females

Endodermal sinus tumor is a rare germ cell malignancy that is usually found in the ovary.[116] This tumor secretes alphafetoprotein, which often is a useful tumor marker for monitoring patients with this neoplasm. It is usually found in infants and children, and approximately 20 cases have been reported as occurring in the vaginas of infants who were under 2 years of age.[117,118] Patients generally present with complaints of bleeding or spotting from the vagina. On physical examination, there is a friable red to pinkish-white polypoid tumor. This tumor is aggressive, and most patients have died. Therapy has involved surgery, radiation, and chemotherapy. Young and Scully reported six patients who were disease free from 2 to 9 years after local therapy with operation, irradiation, or both, followed by systemic chemotherapy with vincristine, actinomycin D, and cyclophosphamide (VAC).[119] Copeland and colleagues reported similar results using the combination of chemotherapy and excision,[120] and Collins and colleagues recently noted the regression of tumor with chemotherapy alone.[121,122] In this report, a 5-month-old patient had regression of the tumor after VAC therapy.

Another rare tumor found in the vaginas of young females is sarcoma botryoides, or embryonal rhabdomyosarcoma.[123] This tumor is usually found in children less than 8 years of age. As with endodermal sinus tumor, the most common symptom has been vaginal bleeding. In 58 cases reviewed by Hilgers, the average age at onset of symptoms was 38.3 months.[56] This tumor resembles clusters of grapes and forms multiple polypoid masses that are believed to begin in the sub-epithelial layers of the vagina and to rapidly expand, filling the vagina. Histologically, these tumors are identified by the presence of rhabdomyoblasts that may contain cross-striations. Because of infiltration of the tumor under the vaginal epithelium, there is often a distinct subepithelial zone, called the cambium layer. The 5-year survival rate of these tumors in the past has ranged from 10% to 35%, and exenterative procedures have often been used.[124] Hilgers reviewed the literature on pelvic exenterations in 21 cases of embryonal rhabdomyosarcoma and found that this form of therapy was ineffective in curing these patients.[44] Effective control with less radical surgery has been achieved using multimodal treatment consisting of multiagent chemotherapy, VAC, combined with operation or radiation.

Hayes and colleagues recently reported 21 patients with vaginal rhabdomyosarcoma who received chemotherapy.[125] In their series, 7 relapsed, with 5 of these 7 having had residual disease following incomplete resection. In 17 of 21 patients who received chemotherapy before surgery, a subsequent delayed excision could be performed. Data regarding the long-term survival of a large number of patients are not available, but such a combined approach appears to result in effective therapy with less mutilating surgery.

A rare, benign, fibroepithelial vaginal polyp that resembles sarcoma botryoides can be found in the vaginas of infants or pregnant women.[75,126,127] Although large atypical cells are present microscopically, epithelial infiltration, a cambium layer, and strap cells are absent. Grossly, these polyps do not resemble the grape-like appearance of sarcoma botryoides. These hormonally stimulated hyperplastic lesions are called pseudosarcoma botryoides, and treatment by local excision is effective.

Selected References

The complete reference list can be found at www.CANCERMEDICINE8.com

4. Sutton GP, Stehman FB, Ehrlich CE, Roman A. Human papilloma virus deoxyribonucleic acid in lesions of the female genital tract: evidence for types 6/11 in squamous carcinoma of the vulva. *Obstet Gynecol*. 1987;70:564.
8. Stroup, AM. Demographic, clinical, and treatment trends among women diagnosed with vulvar cancer in the United States. *Gynecol Oncol*. 2008;108:577–583.
10. Buscema J, Woodruff JD, Parmley TH, Genadry R. Carcinoma in situ of the vulva. *Obstet Gynecol*. 1980;55:225.
14. Fredrich EF, Wilkinson EJ, Fu YS. Carcinoma in situ of the vulva: a continu-

ing challenge. *Am J Obstet Gynecol.* 1980; 136:830.

17. Raspollini MR, Asirelli G, Taddei GL. Analysis of lymphocytic infiltrate does not help in prediction of vulvar squamous cell carcinoma arising in a background of lichen sclerosus. *Int J Gynaecol Obstet.* 2008;100:190–191.
19. Crum PC, Liskow A, Petras P, et al. Vulvar intraepithelial neoplasia (severe atypia and carcinoma in situ). *Cancer.* 1984;54:1429.
21. Mulvany NJ, Allen DG. Differentiated intraepithelial neoplasia of the vulva. *Int J Gynecol Pathol.* 2008;27:125–135.
25. Leuchter RS, Hacker NF, Voet RL, et al. Primary carcinoma of the Bartholin gland: a report of 14 cases and review of the literature. *Obstet Gynecol.* 1982;60:361.
27. Lee SC, Roth LM, Ehrlich C, Hall JA. Extramammary Paget's disease of the vulva—a clinicopathologic study of 13 cases. *Cancer.* 1977;39:2540.
29. Bergen S, DiSaia PJ, Liao SY, Berman ML. Conservative management of extramammary Paget's disease of the vulva. *Gynecol Oncol.* 1989;33:151.
30. Creasman WT. New gynecologic cancer staging. *Obstet Gynecol.* 1990;75:287.
31. Zambo K, Szabo Z, Schmidt E, Koppan M, Repasy I, Bodis J. Is the clinical staging system a good choice in the staging of vulvar malignancies? *Eur J Nucl Med Mol Imaging.* 2007;35:1155–1165.
33. Iversen T, Aas M. Lymph drainage from the vulva. *Gynecol Oncol.* 1983;16:179.
34. Chu J, Tamimi HK, Ek M, Figge DC. Stage I vulvar cancer criteria for microinvasion. *Obstet Gynecol.* 1982;59:716.
36. Hacker NF, Nieburg RK, Berek JS, et al. Superficially invasive vulvar cancer with nodal metastases. *Gynecol Oncol.* 1983;15:65.
37. Hoffman JS, Kumar NB, Morley GW. Microinvasive squamous cell carcinoma of the vulva: a search for definition. *Obstet Gynecol.* 1983;61:615.
40. DiSaia PJ, Creasman WT, Rich WM. An alternate approach to early cancer of the vulva. *Am J Obstet Gynecol.* 1979;133:825.
43. Levenback C, Burke TW, Morris M, et al. Potential applications of intraoperative lymphatic mapping in vulvar cancer. *Gynecol Oncol.* 1995;59:216-220.
45. Iversen T, Tretli S. Intraepithelial and invasive squamous cell neoplasia of the vulva: trends in incidence, recurrence, and survival rate in Norway. *Obstet Gynecol.* 1998;91:969–972.
48. Hauspy J, Covens A, Beiner M, et al. Reply to sentinel lymph node in vulvar cancer. *Cancer.* 2008;112:1869–1870.
49. Moore RG, Robinson K, Brown AK, et al. Isolated sentinel lymph node dissection with conservative management in patients with squamous cell carcinoma of the vulva: a prospective trail. *Gynecol Oncol.* 2008;109:65–70.
51. Homesley HD, Bundy BN, Sedlis A, Adcock L. A randomized study of radiation therapy versus pelvic node resection for patients with invasive squamous cell carcinoma of the vulva having positive groin nodes. Gynecologic Oncology Study Group. *Obstet Gynecol.* 1986;68:733.
53. Hacker NF, Berek JS, Lagasse LD, et al. Management of regional lymph nodes and their prognostic influence in vulvar cancer. *Obstet Gynecol.* 1983;61:408.
54. Hoffman JS, Kumar NB, Morley GW. Prognostic significance of groin lymph node metastases of squamous carcinoma of the vulva. *Obstet Gynecol.* 1985;66:402.
57. Le T, Elsugi R, Hopkins L, Faught W, Fung-Kee-Fung M. The definition of optimal inguinal femoral nodal dissection in the management of vulva squamous cell carcinoma. *Ann Surg Oncol.* 2007;14: 2128–2132.
59. Weikel W, Schmidt M, Steiner E, Knapstein PG, Koelbl H. Reconstructive plastic surgery in the treatment of vulvar carcinomas. *Eur J Obstet Gynecol Reprod Biol.* 2008;136:102–109.
61. Boronow RC. Combined therapy as an alternative to exenteration of locally advanced vulvar vaginal cancer. *Cancer.* 1982;49:1085.
63. Rotmensch J, Rubin SJ, Sutton HG, et al. Preoperative radiotherapy followed by radical vulvectomy with inguinal lymphadenectomy for advanced vulvar cancer. *Gynecol Oncol.* 1990;36:181.
64. Moore DH, Thomas GM, Montana GS, et al. Preoperative chemoradiation for advanced vulvar cancer: a phase II study of the Gynecologic Oncology Group. *Int J Radiat Oncol Biol Phys.* 1998;42:1317–1323.
66. Podratz KC, Symmonds RE, Taylor WF. Carcinoma of the vulva and vagina. In: Coppelson M, ed. *Gynecologic Oncology.* New York: Churchill Livingstone; 1981;85-89.
69. Leuchter RS, Hacker NF, Voet RL, et al. Primary carcinoma of the Bartholin gland: a report of 14 cases and review of the literature. *Obstet Gynecol.* 1982;60:361.
76. Breslow A. Thickness, cross-sectional areas, and depth of invasion in the prognosis of cutaneous melanoma. *Ann Surg.* 1970;172:908.
79. Sugiyama VE, Chan JK, Shin JY, Berek JS, Osann K, Kapp DS. Vulvar melanoma: a multivariable analysis of 644 patients. *Obstet Gynecol.* 2008;110:296–301.
85. Beller U, Benedet JL, Creasman WT, et al. Carcinoma of the vagina. FIGO 6th Annual Report on the Results of Treatment in Gynecological Cancer. *Int J Gynaecol Obstet.* 2006;95:S29–S42.
86. Gonzalez Bosquet E, Torres A, Busquets M, Esteva C, Munoz-Almagro C, Lailla JM. Prognostic factors for the development of vaginal intraepithelial neoplasia. *Eur J Gynaecol Oncol.* 2008;29:43–45.
87. Audet-Lapointe P, Body G, Vauclair R, et al. Vaginal intraepithelial neoplasia. *Gynecol Oncol.* 1990;36:232.
90. Krebs HB. Treatment of vaginal condylomata acuminata by weekly topical application of 5-fluorouracil. *Obstet Gynecol.* 1987;70:68.
92. Gupta N, Mittal S, Dalmia S, Misra R. A rare case of primary invasive carcinoma of vagina associated with irreducible third degree uterovaginal prolapse. *Arch Gynecol Obstet.* 2007;276:563–564.
94. Beriwal S, Heron DE, Mogus R, Edwards RP, Kelley JL, Sukumvanich P. High dose rate brachytherapy (HDRB) for primary or recurrent cancer in the vagina. *Radiat Onc.* 2008;3:7.
95. Andersen ES. Primary carcinoma of the vagina: a study of 29 cases. *Gynecol Oncol.* 1989;33:317.
96. Otton GR, Nicklin JL, Dickie GJ, et al. Early-stage vaginal carcinoma—an analysis of 70 patients. *Int J Gynecol Cancer.* 2004;14:304–310.
98. Spirtos NM, Doshi BP, Kapp DS, Teng N. Radiation therapy for primary squamous cell carcinoma of the vagina: Stanford University experience. *Gynecol Oncol.* 1989;35:20.
102. Basaran A, Ayhan A. Cancer of the vagina treated with wide local excision and modified Martius (labial) flap interposition. *Gynecol Oncol.* 2008;108:455–456.
103. Samant R, Lau B, EC le T, Tam T. Primary vaginal cancer treated with concurrent chemoradiation using Cis-platinum. *Int J Radiat Oncol Biol Phys.* 2007;69:746–750.
113. Chung AF, Casey MJ, Flannery JT, et al. Malignant melanoma of the vagina: report of 19 cases. *Obstet Gynecol.* 1980;55:720.
117. Allyn DL, Silverberg SG, Salzberg AM. Endodermal sinus tumor of the vagina: report of a case with 7-year survival and literature review of so-called "mesonephromas." *Cancer.* 1971;27:1231.
123. Copeland LJ, Gershenson DM, Saul PB, et al. Sarcoma botryoides of the female genital tract. *Obstet Gynecol.* 1985;66:262.
127. Miettinen M, Wahlstrom T, Vesterinen E, Saksela E. Vaginal polyps with pseudosarcomatous features: a clinicopathologic study of seven cases. *Cancer.* 1983;51:1148.

98 Neoplasms of the Cervix

Anuja Jhingran, MD

Epidemiology

Incidence and Mortality

Cervical cancer is the second most common cancer among women worldwide, with an estimated 493,000 new cases and 274,000 deaths in the year 2002.[1] The incidence of cervical cancer in developing countries remains nearly twice that in developed countries, with the highest rates observed in Africa and Central and South America (29 per 100,000 per year) and the lowest in Oceania and North America (7.5 per 100,000 per year).[2] In developed countries, cervical cancer accounts for only 3.6% of all new cancers.[1] In the United States, it is estimated that there will be 11,070 new cases of cervical cancer in 2008, with 3, 870 related deaths,[3] making this neoplasm the third leading cause of cancer-related deaths in women between 20 and 39 years of age.[2] Cervical cancer is more frequently seen in the Hispanic population (13.8% of all cases of cervical cancer) followed by the African-American population (11.4%), Pacific Islanders/Asian (8.0%), whites (8.5%), and American Indians (6.6%).[3]

In the last 40 years, primarily because of the introduction of screening with the Pap smear, the incidence and mortality rates for cervical cancer have declined in most developed countries.[4] In the United States, incidence rates have declined nearly by 70% during this period. Rates of invasive cancer per 100,000 females have declined from 10.2 in 1998 to 8.5 in 2002.[5] In developing countries, however, cervical cancer continues to be a significant health problem due to suboptimal screening programs and a lack of therapy for precancerous conditions.

There are no reliable data on the prevalence and incidence of precancerous cervical lesions. In the United States, the National Cancer Institute estimates that each year approximately 300,000 women are found to have premalignant cervical lesions, whereas the American Cancer Society reported that in 2001, an estimated 65,000 women were found to have carcinoma in situ (CIS) of the cervix. From the SEER data, the overall incidence of squamous cell CIS among whites is 41.4 per 100,000 woman-years from 1991 to 1995.[6]

Risk factors for Cervical Neoplasia

Human Papillomavirus and Other Sexually Transmitted Agents ■ Epidemiologic evidence has long suggested a sexually transmitted etiology for cervical neoplasia. Supporting this hypothesis, several measures of sexual behavior (including multiple sexual partners, early age at first sexual intercourse, and sexual habits of male partners) have consistently been associated with an increased risk of cervical neoplasia.[7] Over the years, several sexually transmitted infectious agents have been the focus of research, including herpes simplex virus type 2 (HSV-2), *Chlamydia trachomatis*, *Trichomonas vaginis*, Cytomegalovirus, *Neisseria gonorrhoeae*, and *Treponema pallidum*.[8] In the mid-1970s, the hypothesis of a causal relationship between human papillomavirus (HPV) and cervical neoplasia was first proposed.[9] Since then, a large body of experimental, clinical, and epidemiologic research has accumulated supporting an etiologic role for some types of HPV.[10]

Of the more than 78 types of HPV that have been described, in excess of 35 types are associated with anogenital disease, and 30 or more are associated with cancer.[11] In an international study, HPV DNA was detected in 93% (range 75-100%) of cancer specimens collected in 22 countries and analyzed by the polymerase chain reaction (PCR) technique.[12] Similarly, HPV DNA has been detected by PCR in up to 94% of women with preinvasive lesions (cervical intraepithelial neoplasia [CIN]) and in up to 46% of women with cytologically normal tissue.[10,13]

HPV types classified as intermediate and high-risk have been identified in about 77% of high-grade squamous intraepithelial lesions (HGSILs) (CIN 2 and 3) and in 84% of invasive lesions.[14] In the series studied by Bosch and colleagues, HPV types 16, 18, 31, and 45 were detected in approximately 80% of the cases.[12] HPV 16 is by far the most prevalent HPV type in women with cervical neoplasia, present in up to 50% of HGSILs and invasive lesions, and it is the most common HPV type identified in cytologically normal women.[14-16]

The association between cervical neoplasia and HPV is independent of study population, study design, and HPV detection method.[10] Higher risk has been associated with specific HPV types (16, 18, 31, 33, 35, and 45), increasing viral load, and concurrent infection with multiple HPV types.[17,18] An increased risk of high-grade CIN ranging from 16-fold to 122-fold has been reported among women whose test results were positive for HPV of any type.[18] The percentage of cases of CIN attributed to HPV has been estimated to range from 60% to 92%.[13] In addition, adjustment for HPV status appears to account for most of the associations between cervical neoplasia and number of sexual partners and other characteristics of sexual behavior.[13,17,18]

Although a strong and consistent association between HPV and cervical neoplasia has been clearly established, the discrepancy between HPV prevalence and the incidence of cervical neoplasia suggests that other cofactors are necessary for the development and progression of the disease. The role of sexual and reproductive history, smoking habits, and hormonal and dietary factors, as well as their interaction with HPV, has been assessed in recent studies. Future research will need to assess the effect of recent changes in these factors on the occurrence of cervical cancer.[7]

Numerous studies have addressed the association between HIV and cervical neoplasia.[8] The Centers for Disease Control and Prevention added invasive cervical cancer to the list of conditions related to AIDS) in 1993.[16] HIV-positive women have been reported to have higher rates of cervical abnormalities, larger lesions, higher-grade histology, and higher recurrence rates than HIV-negative women. In addition, HIV-positive women have been reported to have higher HPV prevalence and HPV persistence rates than HIV-negative women. A meta-analysis by Mandelblatt and colleagues concluded that HIV is a cofactor in the association between HPV and cervical neoplasia, and this association seems to vary with the level of immune function.[19] Results from Ruche and colleagues in Africa support the theory of interaction between HIV-1 and HPV.[20] Although the biologic mechanism for this interaction is not as well understood; it could be explained by the effect of HIV infection on the immune system or by the existence of a molecular interaction between HIV and HPV.

Herpes simplex virus (HSV) was the focus of intensive study during the 1960s and 1970s. Serologic studies showed a higher prevalence of HSV-2 antibodies among women with cervical neoplasia than among controls. Two potential mechanisms of action have been suggested: a "hit-and-run" effect and a synergistic effect between HSV-2 and HPV.[21]

A statistically significant interaction between HSV-2 and HPV 16/18 was detected by Hildesheim and colleagues and Baldauf and colleagues; however, several recent studies continue to provide evidence against such an interaction.[19,22] An association between the presence of antibodies for *C. trachomatis* and cervical neoplasia that persists after controlling for HPV status and other potential factors has been reported.[23,24] However, others have failed to show an association with *Chlamydia trachomatis* using antibody determinations or other measures of exposure, including a self-reported history of *C. trachomatis* infection, culture[23-25] and PCR detection of *C. trachomatis*.[25]

Cytomegalovirus has been suspected as a risk factor for cervical neoplasia in previous studies. Higher levels of antibodies to cytomegalovirus have been reported among women with cervical neoplasia than among controls; however, some other studies have failed to identify an increased risk of cervical neoplasia associated with cytomegalovirus infection. The evidence remains conflicting, and the role of cytomegalovirus as an etiologic factor or cofactor is unclear.[22-25] Inconclusive evidence for other genital infectious agents, including Trichomonas vaginalis, Epstein-Barr virus, hepatitis B virus, hepatitis *C virus, N. gonorrhoeae, Gardnerella vaginalis*, and *T. pallidum*, has been reported.[8]

Other Molecular Markers ■ Other specific genetic abnormalities may also play an important role in carcinogenesis and the aggressiveness of cervical tumors, although, to date, the role of most of these genetic abnormalities in cervical cancer do not appear as important as the role of HPV. The c-*myc* oncogene is expressed in almost all differentiated cell types. It acts as a heterodimer with MAX (a related protein), binds DNA in a sequence-specific way, and acts as a transcriptional activator for genes critical in the regulation of cell growth.[26] The c-*myc* gene also plays a role in apoptosis; by binding MAX, it interacts with TP53, BAX, and BCLX. It induces apoptosis in cells deprived of growth factors.[27] Amplification of c-myc is the predominant route of activation in cervical cancer. Most studies report a 32-34% incidence of c-*myc* activation in cervical cancers. Amplication has been related to tumor size and nodal status as well as a risk factor for relapse.[28] The ras family of genes is also frequently mutated in cancers. Mutations have been reported in the *K-ras* and *H-ras* genes in cervical cancer at a rate of only 10-15%.[29] One report found that increased ras p21 expression correlated with risk of lymph node metastasis.[30]

In addition to overexpression of myc and mutation of ras, amplification or over expression of several different growth factor receptors has been implicated in cervical carcinogenesis. Overexpression of the epidermal growth factor receptor (EGFR) is usually related to amplification of the gene, and overexpression seems to confer a growth advantage to cells. EGFR is expressed not only in a large proportion of cervical carcinomas, but also in normal and premalignant epithelia. Investigators have found a strong correlation between the expression of EGFR and HER2/neu. The prognostic role of EGF-R in cervical carcinoma remains controversial, although two studies found EGFR prognostic for overall survival and disease-specific survival in patients with invasive cervical cancer.[31,32]

The apoptosis inhibitor Bcl2 prevents apoptosis. Overexpression of this gene leads to extension of the cancer cell's survival. Two studies have shown that Bcl2 is overexpressed in 61-63% of all cervical cancer and correlates inversely with overall survival,[33,34] whereas other studies have found no correlation with survival.[35]

Angiogenesis is critical for the progression of most cancers. Hockel and colleagues have reported an association between tumor hypoxia and progression of cervical cancer, and this would seem to correlate with the angiogenic potential of the tumor. However, attempts to correlate progression with actual vessel counts or angiogenic factors have proven more difficult. One angiogenic factor, VEGF, has recently been associated with cervical cancer,[36,37] but the precise role that angiogenic factors play in the development and progression of cervical cancer requires further elucidation.

Sexual Behavior ■ Although previous studies report a strong and consistent association between cervical neoplasia and some characteristics of sexual behavior of women and their male sexual partners, a weaker association has been found in more recent studies in which HPV infection has been taken into account.[17,38] The decrease in the magnitude of these associations after controlling for HPV status supports the notion that characteristics of sexual behavior may be only a proxy measurement for infection with HPV and other infectious agents that may be causally related to cervical neoplasia.

In most studies of preinvasive disease, the effect of the number of sexual partners is substantially reduced after adjustment for HPV, but in studies of invasive lesions, the association with the number of sexual partners remained statistically significant or at the border of significance.[17,39] Interestingly, no association is observed between number of sexual partners and cervical neoplasia among HPV-positive women, whereas a positive association remains among HPV-negative women.[17,40] Misclassification of HPV status, the effect of unmeasured cofactors, or a different etiology for the disease among HPV-negative women could explain the latter finding.

The association between early age at first sexual intercourse and increased risk has been less consistent. After controlling for HPV and other risk factors, a statistically significant association between age at first sexual intercourse and cervical neoplasia has remained in some studies, but in others, no association has been observed.[17,18,41] The association between cervical neoplasia and early age at sexual intercourse may indicate a period of higher susceptibility of the cervical tissue, a higher likelihood of exposure, or a longer period of exposure to carcinogenic factors. Whatever the mechanism underlying the association, establishing age at first sexual intercourse as an independent effect is difficult because of its high correlation with number of sexual partners.

An association between factors related to male sexual partners and an increased risk of cervical neoplasia has also been suggested.[42] High rates of cervical cancer in developing countries in which women are traditionally monogamous or have few sexual partners might be explained by the fact that males have large numbers of sexual partners and frequent contact with prostitutes. Penile HPV DNA prevalence is higher in husbands of women with cervical neoplasia than in husbands of women without cervical neoplasia.[13] Among men, the prevalence of HPV has been associated with the number of sexual partners and sexual contact with prostitutes.[43] In addition, higher HPV prevalence has been reported among males in geographic areas with higher rates of cervical cancer incidence than among males in geographic areas with lower rates, which supports a possible contribution of male partners to cervical carcinogenesis in their female sex partners.[43] Male circumcision has been associated with a reduced risk of penile HPV infection and, in the case of men with a history of multiple sexual partners, a reduced risk of cervical cancer in their current female partners.[44]

Reproductive Factors ■ No consistent relationships have been established between cervical neoplasia and menstrual or reproductive characteristics, including age at menarche or menopause, parity, number of spontaneous or induced abortions, age at first pregnancy, first live birth, or last birth, and number of vaginal deliveries or Cesarean sections. An association between higher parity and higher number of live births and increased risk of cervical neoplasia has been reported in six case-control studies after controlling for HPV status.[17,18,39,40]

There is also a strong association between invasive cervical cancer and early age at first birth reported by Bosch and colleagues,[45] coupled with the absence of an association with parity. A 70% increase in the risk of high-grade dysplasia (CIN 2 and 3) has been found among women with one or more vaginal deliveries. Becker and colleagues[46] found that an association also persisted after adjustment for ethnicity, HPV status, and other sexual and reproductive characteristics. Although there is no clear biologic mechanism to support this association, repeated trauma to the cervix during childbirth has been suggested as an etiologic factor.

Smoking Habits ■ Several epidemiologic studies have provided evidence supporting an association between cigarette smoking and cervical neoplasia. Most studies have shown a twofold increased risk among smokers and a dose-response relationship with duration and intensity of smoking.[47,48] Results from most recent studies controlling for HPV status have been inconsistent. Some support an independent effect of smoking, whereas others do not.[17,18,49] Although a possible interaction between HPV and smoking has been proposed, few studies have examined this joint effect.[21] Results from these studies have also been inconsistent.[39,50,51] In addition to the epidemiologic research; several studies have provided biologic plausibility for this association. High levels of nicotine, cotinine and tobacco-specific N-nitrosamines have been detected in the cervical mucus of active and passive smokers. DNA damage has been found in cervical tissue and exfoliated cells of women smokers. The local cell-mediated immune response is impaired in smokers. Furthermore, reduction of cervical lesion size has been documented among women participating in smoking cessation intervention.[52] In summary; although the mechanism of smoking-induced carcinogenesis in cervical tissue is not fully understood, current biologic, epidemiologic, and clinical studies suggest that cigarette smoking may be a risk factor for cervical neoplasia.

Oral Contraceptives ■ The role of oral contraceptives in the development of cervical neoplasia remains unclear, despite evidence in support of a biologic mechanism. Early studies showed a weak but statistically significant association, particularly for long-term users.[53] Interpretation of the results, however, is confounded by the correlation between oral contraceptive use, sexual behavior, and patterns of screening for cervical neoplasia; potential surveillance bias and selection of comparison groups; and lack of control for HPV in earlier studies.[53] Results from epidemiologic studies in which control for HPV status has been attained are conflicting.[17,18,39,41] Most of these studies failed to show an association between cervical neoplasia and different measures of oral contraceptive exposure.[17,18,39] An interaction between oral contraceptive use and HPV infection has been suggested; however, epidemiologic evidence of interaction is conflicting.[39] The analysis of an interaction effect is based on a very small number of cases, and results need to be interpreted with caution.

Dietary Factors ■ Several lines of evidence suggest that some nutrients may have a protective effect against cervical neoplasia, particularly vitamin A, carotenoids, vitamin C, vitamin E, and folic acid. The hypothesis that there is an inverse association between vitamin A intake and cervical neoplasia is based on the relationship between vitamin A and other epithelial tumors, mainly squamous cell carcinomas. Vitamin A is capable of reversing metaplastic changes in bronchial epithelium, providing a biologic basis for the association with cervical neoplasia.[54] Vitamin C plays a role in the maintenance of the normal epithelium and the protection of the normal epithelium against carcinogens. Folic acid functions as a coenzyme in the metabolism of single-carbon compounds, such as nucleic acid synthesis and amino acid metabolism.[54] It has been hypothesized that a subclinical folate deficiency may act as a cofactor in the integration of the HPV genome into host DNA.[55]

Despite these findings, epidemiologic studies on the association between vitamin A, carotenoids, vitamin C, and folic acid and cervical neoplasia have provided conflicting results.[7,56] Different methods of nutrient measurement, variation in selection of case and comparison groups, and differences in control for confounding factors make the comparison of these studies difficult. In addition, the correlation between nutrients makes the interpretation of the results a difficult task. In some studies in which control of confounding factors has been better, findings regarding an association between dietary or serum/plasma levels of nutrients and cervical neoplasia remain inconclusive.[50,57] An interaction between red blood cell folate levels and HPV 16–positive status, cigarette smoking, and parity has been suggested.[55] This interaction is consistent with current knowledge on the role of folate in carcinogenesis.

Risk Factors for Cervical Adenocarcinoma ■ Adenocarcinoma of the cervix accounts for more than 20% of all cervical cancers. However, in most developing countries the incidence is increasing, particularly among younger women. Between the early 1970s and mid-1980s, the incidence of adenocarcinoma more than doubled among women under 35 years of age.[58] Several investigators have reported a correlation between cervical adenocarcinoma and prolonged oral contraceptive use, but confounding issues need to be studied.[59] Alternatively, the increased incidence of cervical adenocarcinoma may be related to changes in the prevalence of HPV infection or to increased reporting of this histology.[60,61]

Summary

Cervical neoplasia continues to be a major health problem worldwide. Higher incidence and mortality rates are observed in developing countries. Among more developed countries, a significant decline in incidence and mortality has been observed in the last 50 years, which has been attributed to the introduction of screening programs. Current epidemiologic data support a strong role for HPV infection in the etiology of cervical neoplasia. This association satisfies all criteria for causality in epidemiologic research: strength, consistency, and specificity of the association; dose-response and temporal relationship; and biologic plausibility.[13] HPV infection appears to explain many of the established risk factors for cervical neoplasia, including sexual behavior and cigarette smoking. Nonetheless, the high prevalence of HPV infection in young healthy women compared with the low incidence of cervical neoplasia and the low progression rate of untreated CIN lesions support the existence of other cofactors in cervical carcinogenesis.[62] Future epidemiologic studies will need to further assess the role of these cofactors and their interaction with HPV. In addition, the role of viral factors such as HPV persistence and HPV variants in the progression of cervical neoplasia as well as of the determinant factors of HPV persistence will require further evaluation.[63] Similarly, the impact of recent trends in such environmental factors as smoking, exogenous hormones, and dietary factors deserves further attention.[7]

Histologic Classification of Epithelial Tumors

The histologic classification of epithelial tumors of the uterine cervix by the World Health Organization (WHO) separates them into three main groups: squamous cell carcinomas, adenocarcinomas, and other epithelial tumors (Table 98-1).[64,65]

Squamous Cell Carcinoma

The majority of cervical carcinomas are squamous cell carcinomas, which are

Table 98-1 **Modification of the WHO Histologic Classification of Epithelial Tumors of the Uterine Cervix**

- Squamous cell carcinoma
  - Microinvasive squamous cell carcinoma
  - Invasive squamous cell carcinoma
  - Verrucous carcinoma
  - Warty (condylomatous) carcinoma
  - Papillary squamous cell (transitional) carcinoma
  - Lymphoepithelioma-like carcinoma
- Adenocarcinoma
  - Mucinous adenocarcinoma
    - Endocervical type
    - Intestinal type
    - Signet-ring type
  - Endometrioid adenocarcinoma
  - Endometrioid adenocarcinoma with squamous metaplasia
  - Clear cell adenocarcinoma
  - Minimal-deviation adenocarcinoma
    - Endocervical type (adenoma malignum)
    - Endometrioid type
  - Serous adenocarcinoma
  - Mesonephric carcinoma
  - Well-differentiated villoglandular adenocarcinoma
- Other epithelial tumors
  - Adenosquamous carcinoma
  - Glassy cell carcinoma
  - Mucoepidermoid carcinoma
  - Adenoid cystic carcinoma
  - Adenoid basal carcinoma
  - Carcinoid-like tumor
  - Small cell carcinoma
  - Undifferentiated carcinoma

Source: Reproduced with permission from Carcinoma and other tumors of the cervix. In: *Blausteine's Pathology of the Female Genital Tract*, 4th ed.

classified as either large cell nonkeratinizing or large cell keratinizing. Nonkeratinizing carcinoma is characterized by squamous cells with somewhat hyperchromatic nuclei and a moderate amount of cytoplasm growing in discrete nests separated by stroma (Fig. 98-1). In the center of some of the nests, the squamous cells appear to differentiate and degenerate. Keratinizing carcinoma is characterized by cells with very hyperchromatic nuclei and densely eosinophilic cytoplasm growing in irregular invasive nests. Many of these nests have central "pearls" that contain abundant keratin. The average age of patients with squamous cell carcinoma is 51.4 years. Selected variants of squamous cell carcinoma are described in the following paragraphs.

Verrucous Carcinoma ■ Verrucous carcinomas are exophytic with frond like papillae and macroscopically resemble condylomas. They rarely metastasize, but local invasion can be extensive. Death usually occurs because of ureteral obstruction, infection, or hemorrhage. Histologically, the epithelium lacks cytologic atypia and

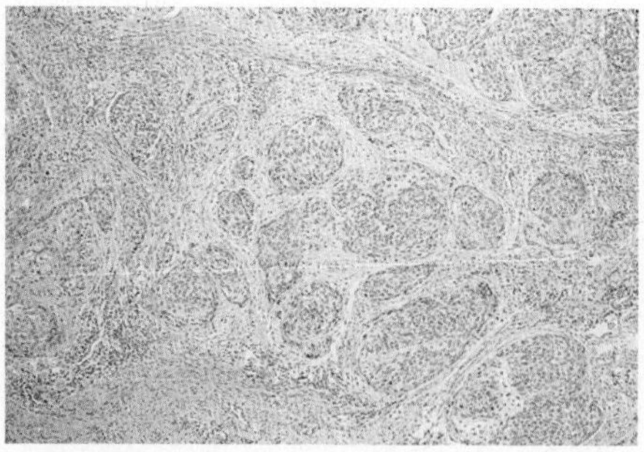

Figure 98-1 ■ Squamous cell carcinoma, nonkeratinizing.

mitotic activity, and the epithelial papillae lack a central fibroconnective tissue core. Mitotic activity may be evident in cells at the base of the tumor, and invasive nests of epithelium are observed along with well-circumscribed nests with a clearly visible or defined tumor-stroma interface. The inflammatory reaction at the epithelial stromal junction is marked.

This tumor rarely goes to the nodes, therefore, for early-stage disease, the treatment of choice is a type II modified radical hysterectomy without lymphadenectomy.

Papillary Squamous Cell Carcinoma ■ Papillary squamous cell carcinomas of the uterine cervix with transitional or squamous differentiation often resemble transitional cell carcinomas of the urinary tract (Fig. 98-2). Tumors with transitional cell differentiation have been described in every site in the female genital tract. Immunochemical tests identifying cytokeratin polypeptides cytokeratin 7 and cytokeratin 20 are useful in differentiating primary genital tract transitional cell carcinoma from urinary tract transitional tumors.[66] Urinary tract transitional cell carcinomas have a cytokeratin profile strongly positive for cytokeratin 20, whereas primary genital tract transitional cell carcinomas stain positive for cytokeratin 7. Invasive papillary transitional cell carcinomas of the uterine cervix are potentially aggressive carcinomas. It is important to distinguish these carcinomas from benign squamous papillomas and condyloma acuminata.[67] Biopsy material must include the underlying stroma to permit identification of invasion.

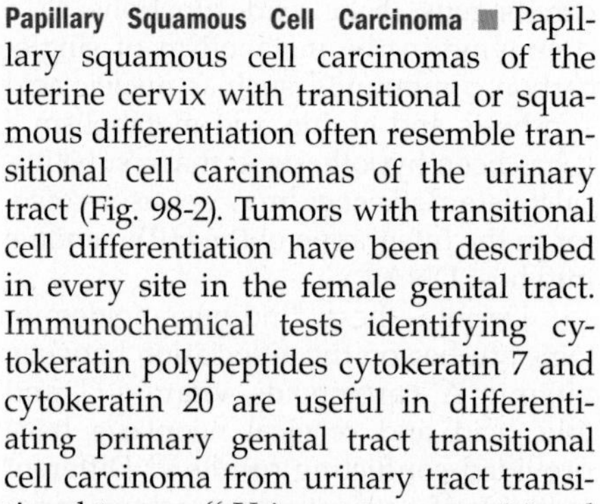

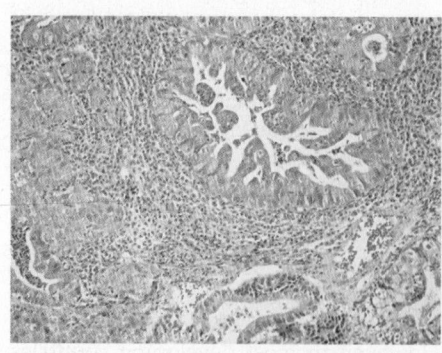

Figure 98-2 ■ Papillary squamous cell (transitional) carcinoma.

Lymphoepithelioma-Like Carcinoma ■ Lymphoepithelioma-like carcinomas are histologically similar to lymphoepitheliomas arising in the nasopharynx and salivary glands (Fig. 98-3). These carcinomas are usually well circumscribed and composed of undifferentiated cells. The cells are surrounded by inflammatory infiltrates composed of lymphocytes, plasma cells, and eosinophils.[68] Hasumi and colleagues reported 39 cases from the Cancer Institute Hospital in Tokyo. Their patients, 72% of whom were younger than 50 years of age, were treated with radical hysterectomy and pelvic lymphadenectomy. Two patients had positive lymph nodes. At the time of the report, 38 of the 39 patients were alive. The single death occurred 5 months after surgery and was due to serum hepatitis.

Adenocarcinoma

Adenocarcinomas represent 20-25% of cervical carcinomas today, whereas from 1950 to 1960 they represented only 5%.[69] This change in prevalence is a worldwide phenomenon.[70] The mean age at diagnosis for patients with invasive adenocarcinoma is between 47 and 53 years. Selected variants of adenocarcinoma are described in the following paragraphs.

Mucinous Adenocarcinoma ■ Mucinous adenocarcinoma is the most common type of cervical adenocarcinoma.[71] In the WHO classification, the first type of mucinous adenocarcinoma is composed of cells that resemble the columnar cells of the normal endocervical mucosa and is referred to as the endocervical type (Fig. 98-4). The second type is termed the intestinal type because it is composed of cells similar to those present in adenocarcinomas of the large intestine. A third type is composed of signet-ring cells and designated the signet-ring type. Frequently, mucinous adenocarcinomas are a mixture of these cell types.

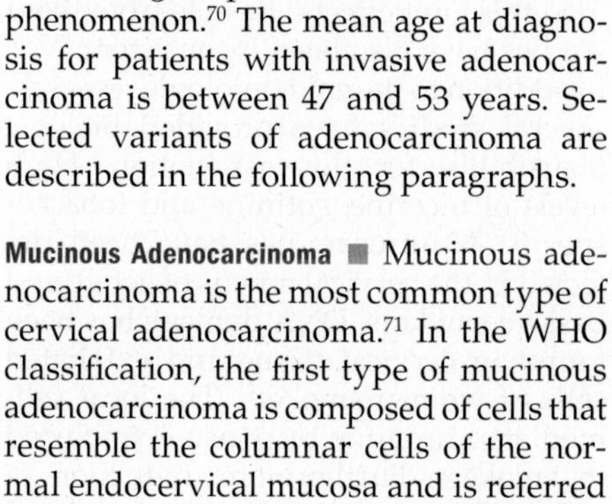

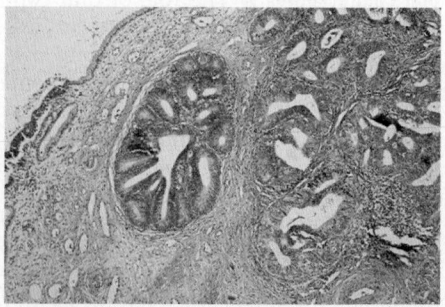

Figure 98-3 ■ Lymphoepithelioma-like carcinoma.

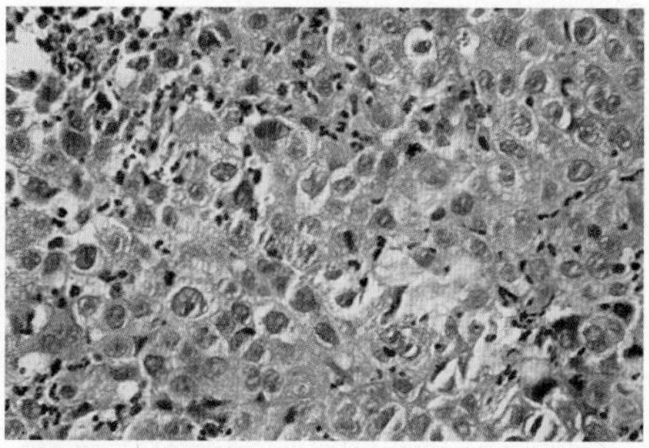

Figure 98-4 ■ Mucinous adenocarcinoma, endocervical type.

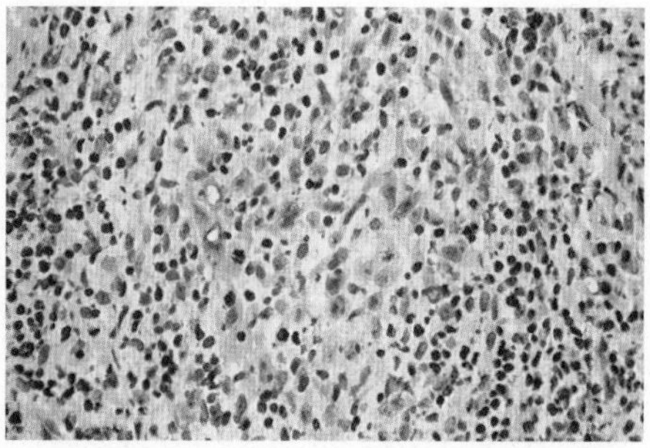

Figure 98-6 ■ Mucinous adenocarcinoma, endocervical type (adenoma malignum).

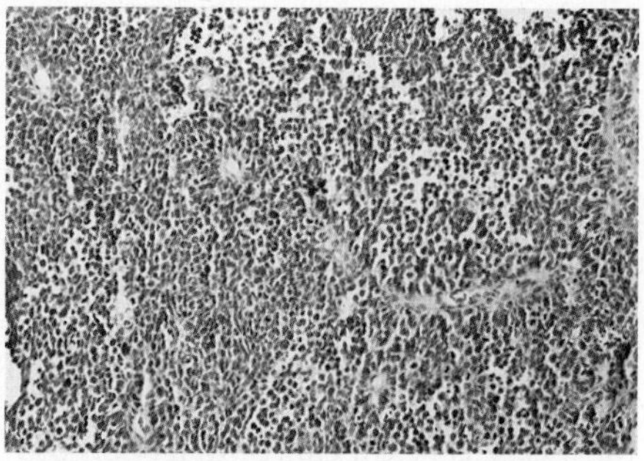

Figure 98-8 ■ Small cell carcinoma.

Endometrioid Adenocarcinoma ■ Endometrioid adenocarcinoma is the second most common type of primary endocervical tumor, accounting for 30% of all primary endocervical tumors. Endometrioid adenocarcinomas resemble typical endometrioid adenocarcinoma arising from the endometrial cavity (Fig. 98-5). Identification of the site of origin (ie, whether the primary tumor is in the endocervix or endometrium) may be difficult, but proper identification is important as the site or origin significantly influences therapy.

Adenoma Malignum ■ It is difficult to distinguish cytologically between adenoma malignum and normal endocervical glands (Fig. 98-6). Thus adenoma malignum is also referred to as minimal-deviation adenocarcinoma. A distinguishing feature of adenoma malignum is a bizarre and irregular glandular branching pattern. These irregular glands invade deeply into the stroma, and diagnosis requires a large tissue specimen (ie, one obtained with a cone biopsy). Diagnosis is frequently made on the basis of the hysterectomy specimen. Adenoma malignum is an extremely rare type of cancer and is sometimes associated with Peutz-Jegher syndrome.[72] The survival rate is poor if the well-differentiated pattern leads to undertreatment.

Other Epithelial Tumors

Adenosquamous Carcinoma ■ Adenosquamous carcinomas are defined as tumors that contain an admixture of histologically malignant squamous and glandular cells.[73] Adenosquamous carcinomas account for 5-25% of the cervical carcinomas in some series.[74,75] These carcinomas are similar in their clinical presentation, epidemiology, and pattern of spread to squamous cell carcinomas and adenocarcinomas. The poorly differentiated form of adenosquamous carcinoma has been referred to as glassy cell carcinoma. These carcinomas are made up of large uniform polygonal cells with a finely granular cytoplasm of the ground-glass type, hence the term "glassy cells" (Fig. 98-7). Similar to other undifferentiated tumors, glassy cell carcinomas spread early and are aggressive.[76] The mucoepidermoid carcinoma, also placed in this category, contain large cell nonkeratinizing or focally keratinizing squamous carcinoma, which stains positive for mucin but lacks recognizable glands. The mucinous component includes goblet or signet-ring-type cells localized in a nest of squamous cells. These carcinomas represent 20% of the carcinomas in some series if mucin is measured.

Small Cell Neuroendocrine Carcinoma ■ Small cell carcinomas, well defined in the WHO classification of cervical tumors, contain small anaplastic cells with scant cytoplasm (Fig. 98-8). These highly aggressive cancers diffusely infiltrate the cervical stroma.[77] Staining reveals neuroendocrine markers in most cases. Women with small cell carcinoma are likely to be 10 years younger than those with squamous cell carcinoma. Small-cell carcinomas tend to behave very aggressively and are frequently associated with widespread metastasis to multiple sites, including bone, liver, skin, and brain. These tumors should not be confused with small squamous cell carcinomas, which are associated with a better prognosis. Usually, there will be some areas showing squamous or glandular differentiation in the nonkeratinizing squamous cell carcinoma with small cells. Efforts to treat these cancers with approaches typically used for small cell carcinomas of the lung have had mixed results. Small cell carcinomas are different and more aggressive than nonkeratinizing squamous carcinoma with small cells.[78]

Non-small Cell Neuroendocrine Carcinoma ■ Nonsmall cell neuroendocrine carcinomas of the cervix have been reported, but they are not listed in the current WHO classification of cervical tumors.[79] The tumors contain intermediate to large cells, high-grade nuclei, and eosinophilic cytoplasmic granules of the type seen in neuroendocrine cells. A trabecular pattern is frequently evident, with or without glandular differentiation (Fig. 98-9). Tumors are usually immunoreactive for chromogranin. Reported survival rates for patients with these aggressive carcinomas are similar to those for patients with small cell carcinoma.

Terminology for cervical neuroendocrine tumors is confusing, and many pathologists are recommending application of the classification system used for the more common pulmonary neuroendocrine tumors (ie, typical carcinoid tumor, atypical carcinoid tumor, large cell neuroendocrine carcinoma, and small [oat] cell carcinoma).[80]

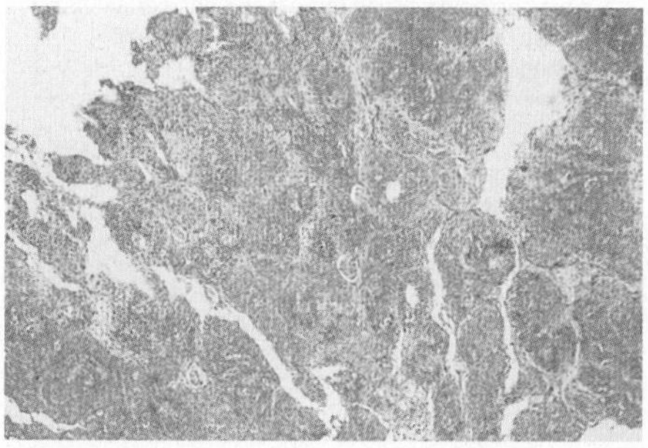

Figure 98-5 ■ Endometrioid adenocarcinoma.

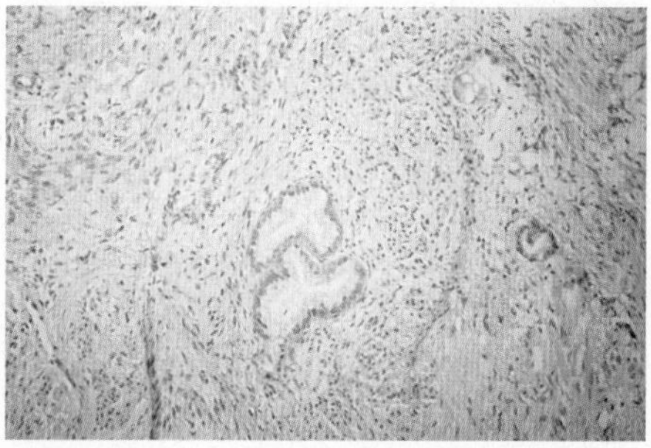

Figure 98-7 ■ Glassy cell carcinoma.

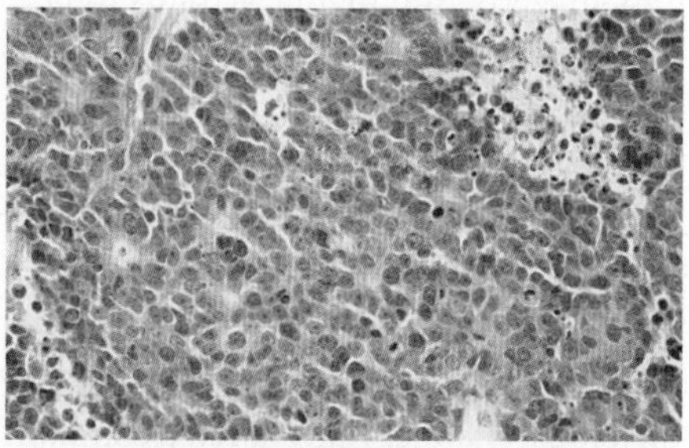

Figure 98-9 ■ Non-small cell neuroendocrine carcinoma.

Natural History of Carcinomas of the Uterine Cervix

Cullen described CIS, a precursor lesion for invasive cervical carcinoma, at the turn of the twentieth century. Broder reintroduced the term in the 1930s, and a relationship between CIS and invasive cervical carcinoma was described by a number of investigators. During the 1930s, cervical cancer detection programs based on cytologic screening to detect precursor lesions were being created. The identification of a spectrum of precursor lesions followed, and terminology was defined in the 1940s and 1950s. Reagan and Harmonic introduced the term dysplasia to refer to the spectrum of cervical abnormalities that featured cells whose abnormalities were fewer or less severe than those found in CIS.[81] Dysplastic cells resembled cells of the basal layer but had nuclear atypia and other cytoplasmic and nuclear abnormalities. The degree of dysplasia was classified on the basis of the relative thickness of the process in relationship to the thickness of the epithelium. By definition, in dysplasia, atypical cells did not occupy the full thickness of the epithelium, nor did they penetrate the basement membrane.[82] Mild or moderate dysplasia was thought to have a lower potential than severe dysplasia for progression to invasive carcinoma. The term "carcinoma in situ" (CIS) was reserved for atypical cells involving the full thickness of the epithelium. This division of noninvasive cervical lesions into two groups, dysplasia and CIS, was confusing. Clinicians considered dysplasia to be a potentially reversible lesion, whereas they thought of CIS as potentially dangerous and treated it with hysterectomy. Among pathologists, variability in distinguishing severe dysplasia from CIS was common, making a precise definition that had clinical application a necessity.

DNA ploidy studies had demonstrated a similarity between severe dysplasia and CIS. Both entities were found to consist of monoclonal proliferations of abnormal squamous epithelial cells with an aneuploid nuclear DNA content. These findings suggested that dysplasia and invasive carcinoma actually represented different points along the same disease spectrum. Richart introduced the term cervical intraepithelial neoplasia in the late 1960s.[83] The CIN terminology assumed that all types of lesions, from precursor lesions to invasive squamous cell carcinoma, represented a single disease process. Furthermore, because the CIN terminology represented a spectrum of histologic changes that shared a common etiology, its use fit nicely into a clinical treatment plan. When these lesions were diagnosed and adequately treated or destroyed, invasive carcinoma could be prevented.

The 1988 Bethesda System for Reporting Cervical/Vaginal Cytological Diagnoses and its most recent revision classifies precursor lesions as squamous intraepithelial lesions (SILs).[83] Generally, low-grade SILs (LGSILs) have cellular changes that are associated with a heterogeneous group of HPV types and are equivalent to mild dysplasia (CIN I). These lesions are usually diploid or polyploid. HGSILs are usually associated with intermediate-risk (31, 33, 35, 51, 58) or high-risk (16, 18, 56) HPV types. This category includes moderate dysplasia (CIN II), severe dysplasia (CIN III), and CIS. The high-grade lesions are typically aneuploid and are more likely to progress to invasive carcinoma, which makes the HGSILs the most important clinically. A significant percentage of these lesions will progress to invasive cancer if followed long term.[84] LGSILs usually behave in the opposite manner. One-half will regress spontaneously, and only 16% will progress to HGSILs.[85] Pathologists use a variety of terms for these precursor lesions. The written pathology report may use the new Bethesda system for both histologic and cytologic diagnoses, or it may use the new terminology only for the cytologic diagnosis. The older terminology for the histologic diagnosis remains popular. Mild dysplasia is CIN I, moderate dysplasia is CIN II, and severe dysplasia is CIN III or CIS.

The precursors of invasive adenocarcinoma of the cervix were recognized in the 1950s.[86] The best-defined precursor, if one exists, is adenocarcinoma in situ, which occurs infrequently in comparison with HGSILs. A large proportion of adenocarcinomas in situ occur in conjunction with SILs.[87] Adenocarcinoma in situ is associated with HPV DNA, mostly HPV 18, in contrast with SILs, which are associated with HPV 16. Adenocarcinoma in situ is less likely to be detected by Pap smear than SILs.[87] In the majority of cases, adenocarcinoma in situ involves the transformation zone and is unifocal.[88] The transition between normal glands and adenocarcinoma in situ is sharp. The cell type is usually endocervical and consists of atypical columnar glands.[89] Other types of adenocarcinoma in situ may contain colonic-type epithelium and endometrioid or clear cells.[90] The diagnosis of adenocarcinoma in situ is sometimes difficult and may pose a challenge to the experienced pathologist. Tissue specimens that are intact and properly oriented on arrival to the laboratory, of adequate size, and accompanied by the appropriate clinical history are extremely helpful in obtaining the correct diagnosis.

Diagnosis and Treatment of Precancerous Lesions

The most recent guidelines for screening for cervical cancer are listed in Figure 98-10. CIN is an increasingly common finding among sexually active young women. Since the introduction of the Bethesda system, the proportion of Pap smears identified as having low-grade cytologic abnormalities, minimal or ambiguous cytologic changes classified as atypical squamous cells of undetermined significance (ASCUS), or LGSILs has increased.[91] Approximately 50 million Pap smears are done yearly in the United States, and 5-10% of these smears are reported as having low-grade cytologic abnormalities. Although near consensus exists regarding the evaluation and management of HGSILs and carcinoma detected on Pap smears, controversy continues regarding appropriate management of ASCUS and low-grade abnormalities.[92] Issues include the risk of progression of the disease, the anxiety caused to the patient, the risk of overtreating patients with minor disease, and, more recently, the financial implications of prompt intervention and treatment.[93]

As more studies of women with mildly atypical Pap smears were published, data showed that 5-20% of women presenting with a single mildly atypical Pap smear were at risk of HGSILs or other more severe lesions.[94] In addition, it has recently been estimated that more than one-third of the HGSIL cases in a routine screening population are proceeded by a cytologic diagnosis of ASCUS.[95] This has led some clinicians to suggest that it is safer and more expeditious to perform colposcopy in women with a

- Screening should begin approximately three years after a woman begins having vaginal intercourse, but no later than 21 years of age.
- Screening should be done every year with regular pap tests or every two years using liquid-based tests.
- At or after age 30, women who have had three normal test results in a row may be screened every 2-3 years. However, doctors may suggest a woman be screened more if she has certain risk factors, such as HIV infection or a weakened immune system.
- Women 70 and older who have had three or more consecutive pap tests in the last 10 years may choose to stop cervical cancer screening.
- Screening after a total hysterectomy (with removal of the cervix) is not necessary unless the surgery was done as a treatment for cervical cancer.

Figure 98-10 Screening guidelines for the early detection of cervical cancer.

finding of ASCUS.[96] However, given the relatively high frequency of low-grade cytologic abnormalities in the absence of significant disease and the high financial and emotional cost of colposcopy, some have argued that these women should be evaluated by repeat cytology rather than colposcopy. The American College of Obstetricians and Gynecologists and a National Cancer Institute (NCI) consensus panel have acknowledged that managing a single mildly atypical Pap smear by repeating the test is an acceptable practice.[92,97]

The main goal in managing ASCUS and low-grade cytologic abnormalities is to identify those women at higher risk of HGSILs, primarily women more than 25 years old who cannot be relied on to return for long-term follow-up, who are suspected of having or known to have a history of abnormal cytologic findings or treatment of cervical neoplasia, who may be promiscuous, and who have no history of adequate screening.[98] Currently, two strategies are recommended for managing these lesions: The physician may repeat the Pap smear and perform a colposcopic evaluation, or, for patients with an ASCUS cytologic diagnosis or LGSILs without clinical evidence of cervical disease and without risk factors, the physician may repeat the Pap smear without performing colposcopy (Fig. 98-11).[92,98]

Management of Low-Grade Cytologic Abnormalities

Previously, low-grade cytologic abnormalities were usually considered benign and attributed to an underlying infection.[99] The common practice was to disregard the cytologic findings and repeat the Pap smear the following year.[99] In the 1970s, it was suggested that a more aggressive approach to mildly atypical Pap smear findings might be warranted. Stafl and Mattingly reported that approximately 25% of women with a colposcopic diagnosis of HGSILs (CIN II, III, and CIS) had been referred with an initial diagnosis of a mildly atypical Pap smear.[100] Similarly, Figge and colleagues reported that 15% of women with invasive cervical cancer had initially been referred because of a mildly atypical Pap smear.[101] Following these reports, most clinicians started treating any underlying vulvovaginal infection with antibiotics and repeating the smear several months later. If the smear result regressed to normal, the patient was scheduled for an annual Pap smear screening, whereas patients whose smears remained abnormal were referred for colposcopic evaluation, and Pap test every 4-6 months for 2 years. After three consecutive negative smears in the 2-year follow-up period, patients can be monitored using a routine cervical cancer screening protocol. For patients with clinical suspicion of cancer or persistent abnormal Pap smears during the 2-year follow-up, colposcopic evaluation is recommended. Depending on reliability for follow-up and the risk factor profile, women with persistent LGSILs can be treated with such ablative therapies as cryotherapy or loop electrosurgical excision procedure (LEEP). Patients undergoing treatment of LGSILs should be monitored every 4-6 months for up to 2 years by cytologic examination and colposcopic and histologic examination if required (Fig. 98-12).

In view of the costs, both emotional and economic, associated with evaluating women with low-grade cytologic abnormalities, considerable interest has arisen in developing novel cost-effective triage strategies for these patients. HPV DNA testing, automated cytology screening and cervicography are being evaluated as adjunct methods in the assessment and triage of patients with low-grade cytologic abnormalities. Most research has focused on the assessment of HPV testing.

In 1996, the NCI initiated a large multi-institutional study to establish the optimal management of mildly abnormal Pap smears With ASCUS or LGSIL.[102,103] Early available data reveal that a very high percentage of women (82.9%) with an LGSIL diagnosis from a Pap smear are positive for HPV DNA by the Hybrid Capture assay (Digene Diagnostics). As a result, it looks as though the potential for HPV testing to direct decisions about the clinical management of women with LGSIL is limited. On the other hand, testing for high-risk HPV DNA might be helpful in women with ASCUS. Preliminary analysis shows that the Hybrid Capture II assay has greater sensitivity in the detection of severe dysplasia or more severe lesions than a single additional cytologic test indicating ASCUS or a more advanced lesion. However, the specificity of

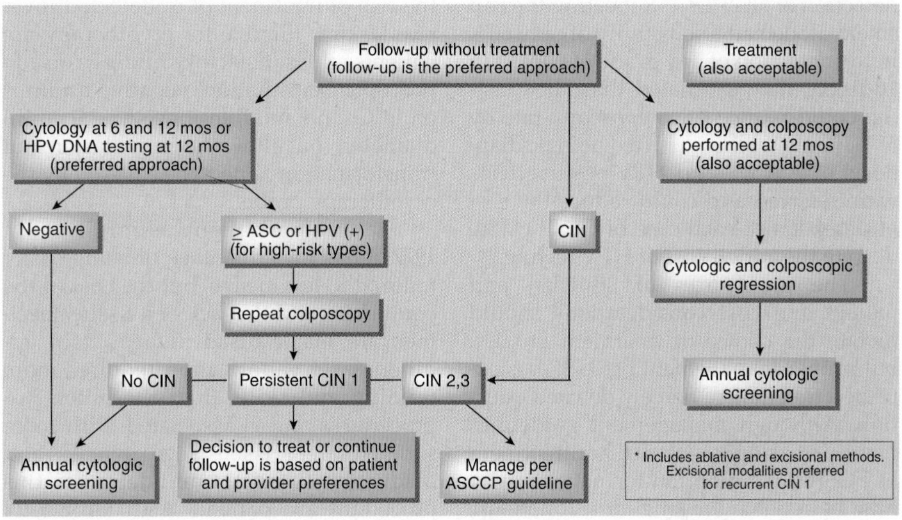

Figure 98-11 Management of women with biopsy-confirmed cervical intraepithelial neoplasia-grade 1 (CIN 1) and satisfactory colposcopy.

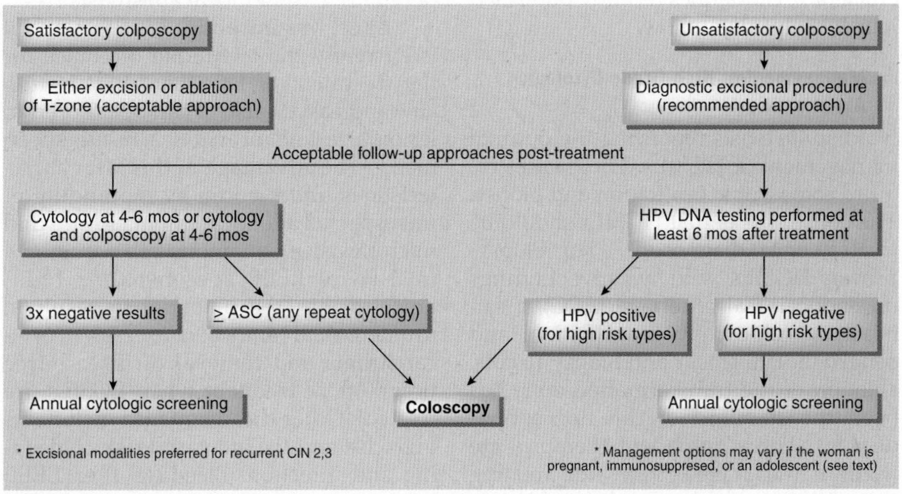

Figure 98-12 Management of women with biopsy-confirmed cervical intraepithelial neoplasia grades 2 and 3 (CIN 2.3).

the Hybrid Capture II assay was similar to that of repeat cytology. Future analyses and longer follow-up will hopefully help us determine the exact role of HPV testing in screening for cervical neoplasia.

Several researchers have assessed the value of HPV DNA testing as a specific and economical alternative for triage of low-grade cytologic abnormalities and as an adjunct to cervical cytology in primary screening.[104-107] With second-generation HPV DNA detection methods, including PCR based methods and the Hybrid Capture HPV DNA assay, both of which have a higher sensitivity and detect a broader range of HPV types with high oncogenic risk than earlier methods, results have been more consistent, supporting the role of HPV typing in the triage of patients with low-grade cytologic abnormalities and as an adjunct to cytology in primary screening.[104-107] Cox and colleagues reported that HPV testing had a sensitivity of 86% in the detection of CIN (any grade) and of 93% in the detection of HGSILs.[104] Repeating the Pap smear alone had a sensitivity of only 60% in the detection of any grade of CIN.[104] In addition, they estimated that HPV testing could reduce the colposcopy rate by 58% if only women with a cytologic diagnosis of ASCUS and HPV-positive tests were referred and could reduce the cost of detection of each case of CIN by 38% despite the added cost of HPV testing.[108]

The preferences of clinician and patient and cost considerations should dictate the choice of treatment of CIN, but proper management of LGSILs is expected to remain a fiercely debated question. Although management guidelines have increasingly included nontreatment of LGSILs as an option for patients who may be reliable for long-term follow-up, concerns over legal responsibility for progressive lesions continue to drive intensive follow-up protocols, particularly in the United States, that may not be cost-efficient.[109] Guidelines recently published may be helpful to follow.

Management of High-Grade Cytologic Abnormalities

No dispute exists regarding the optimal management of HGSILs. These cases require colposcopic evaluation and biopsy. The consensus is that HGSILs should be treated once diagnosed.[110] For biopsy-proven HGSILs with negative findings on endocervical curettage (ECC), a satisfactory colposcopy examination, and congruent Pap smear and biopsy results, ablation of the transformation zone has been the standard of care for several decades. Three outpatient therapies are used in the United States for treating these lesions: cryotherapy, laser ablation, and LEEP. For patients with unsatisfactory colposcopic examination findings, a Pap smear result more severe than the biopsy findings, presence of an adenomatous component, suspicion of invasive cancer, or positive findings on ECC, a cone biopsy is indicated. Cone biopsies (talked about later in the chapter) remove tissue to a depth of 20-30 mm and up to 30 mm in diameter, including the transformation zone.

The three outpatient therapies of cryotherapy, laser vaporization, and LEEP have been the focus of controversy. Safety, efficacy, and cost issues have dominated the debate. Cryotherapy, introduced in 1972, was the first outpatient treatment of CIN and remains a dependable treatment because of its reliability, low complication rate, ease of use, and low cost.[111] Another advantage of cryotherapy is that leaving a large dead viral HPV load within disrupted cells may improve the immune response to the causative agent of CIN. Major disadvantages include lack of ability to tailor treatment to the size of the lesion, lack of a tissue specimen, and the risk of treatment of undetected invasive lesions. Eligible for cryotherapy are patients with satisfactory findings on colposcopic examination, negative findings on ECC, and small lesions (2.5-3.0 cm in diameter) that allow the entire lesion and transformation zone to be covered by the cryotherapy probe.

Laser vaporization was introduced in 1977. It has the advantage of being easily tailored to lesion size, but the cost of the equipment and the lack of a tissue specimen are major disadvantages.[111] In addition, laser vaporization requires more training and skills than the other two procedures and is associated with more serious safety issues (eye injuries and inadvertent burns). Candidates for this procedure are patients with large CIN lesions, young women with suspicious or invasive lesions or adenocarcinoma in situ in whom preservation of fertility is desired, and patients unwilling to undergo LEEP under local anesthesia.

LEEP was introduced in 1989, and it is currently the technique of choice for the treatment of HGSILs. LEEP is reliable and easy to use. It can be tailored to lesion size and provides a tissue specimen.[111] The advantage of this last characteristic is underscored by the finding of unsuspected adenocarcinoma in situ and microinvasive squamous cell carcinoma in 2-4% of LEEP specimens.[98,111] LEEP, however, has the potential to result in unintentional removal of excessive cervical stroma and removal of disease-free tissue (more frequent when LGSILs are treated). Other disadvantages include its high cost and the increased risk of bleeding and infection. Bleeding after LEEP has been reported in 2-7% of cases.[111] The high rates of overtreatment observed with LEEP have been related to misdiagnosis of abnormality and multiple punch biopsies of small lesions prior to treatment.[98] The use of LEEP in see-and-treat protocols has been shown to improve patient compliance with treatment when patient selection is adequate. This strategy has been suggested as having the greatest potential benefit for populations with poor treatment compliance.[98]

No statistically significant differences in success rates (based on recurrence and persistence) between cryotherapy and laser vaporization have been reported, but variability in these rates from study to study is striking. In nonrandomized clinical studies, reported success rates range from 86% to 91% for cryotherapy and 89-97% for laser vaporization.[112] Similar success rates have been reported for LEEP (range, 84-95%). All these studies have shown an association between persistent or recurrent disease and high histologic grade, disease affecting endocervical gland crypts, and size of lesion. The only randomized controlled trial comparing the efficacy of all three treatment options reported no statistically significant difference in varying failure rates: cryotherapy, 24%; laser vaporization, 17%; and LEEP, 16%.[111] Similarly, no statistically significant differences in complication rates were observed between groups. Only lesion size was statistically associated with persistent disease, but risk of recurrence was associated with age more than 30 years, positivity for HPV 16 or 18, and previous treatment of CIN. Cold cone biopsy increases the risk of second-trimester abortions, preterm labor, and having infants of low birth weight. The amount of tissue removed by laser, cryotherapy, and LEEP is small, so these techniques have no adverse effect on pregnancy. Electro coagulation diathermy also has no adverse effect on pregnancy.

New Concepts in Diagnosis and Prevention

Fluorescence Spectroscopy The University of Texas MD Anderson Cancer Center and the University of Texas Optics Division have developed fluorescence spectroscopy, a very promising new technique. Fluorescence spectroscopy is completely noninvasive and involves the application of white light at different wavelengths to the surface of the cervix. It is a near real-time measurement that is fully automated and does not require the expertise needed for colposcopy. The higher the grade of the dysplasia, the more the absorption, the less the emitted fluorescence, and, therefore, the lower the signal from the tissue.[113] Preliminary data and cost analysis of this technique show that fluorescence spectroscopy of the cervix has a higher sensitivity than the Pap smear test and a higher specificity than colposcopy in differentiating squamous epithelial lesions from normal cervix and in differentiating LGSIL from HGSIL. Patients with an abnormal optical spectrum can be further evaluated with colposcopy, potentially on the same office visit.

Chemopreventative Management ■ One of the more exciting research areas in therapy for CIN is the use of chemopreventative agents. These therapies involve ingestion of an agent that reverses precancerous changes, returning the tissue to normal. Laboratory data have shown that retinoids can induce apoptosis in dysplastic cervical cells, suggesting that these compounds may be active in cell-cycle control.[114] Women with HGSIL and colposcopically evident lesions are the target population for chemoprevention studies because they have a higher risk of persistent disease or progression to cancer. α-Difluoromethylornithine and retinoids (vitamin A derivatives) are two drugs currently receiving attention in the United States and China.[115,116]

Vaccine Development ■ Papillomaviruses are epitheliotropic agents that induce benign papillomas of the skin and mucous membranes. In contrast to hepatitis B virus (HBV), there are more than 100 HPV genotypes (types). A subset of HPV types that are almost always transmitted sexually is the main cause of human cervical cancer. Infection with these HPV types is a strong risk factor for cervical cancer, and HPV DNA from one or more of these types is found in virtually all cervical tumors.[117,118] The virus encodes oncoproteins that appear to be required both for the induction and the maintenance of the cancer.

Because papillomaviruses contain oncogenes, and a prophylactic vaccine would be directed toward healthy young individuals, efforts to develop a prophylactic vaccine have emphasized a subunit approach, analogous to that used for HBV vaccine. Indeed, constitutive high-level expression of the L1 major structural viral protein, even in nonmammalian cells, leads to its efficient self-assembly into virus like particles (VLPs) that resemble authentic viral capsids structurally and antigenically. Preparative amounts of VLPs can be synthesized in insect cells or yeast. Such VLPs are suitable immunogens that, as is true of authentic virions, possess the immunodominant conformational epitopes capable of raising high titers of neutralizing antibodies.

Two vaccines have been developed: Ardasil, a quadrivalent vaccine targeting HPV 6, 11, 16, and 18, and Cervarix, a bivalent vaccine which targets HPV 16 and 18.[119] These vaccines are now licensed in more than 55 countries worldwide and are expected to be an enormous asset to cervical cancer prevention efforts. The FUTURE (Female United to Unilaterally Reduce Endo/Ectocervical Disease) II study group performed a randomized, double-blind, placebo-controlled trial in order to evaluate a quadrivalent vaccine (Gardasil) against HPV types 6, 11, 16, and 18 for the prevention of high-grade cervical lesions associated with HPV 16 and 18. Twelve thousand, one hundred and sixty seven women between the ages of 15 and 26 years were randomized to receive three doses of either HPV vaccine or placebo, administered on day 1, and at month 2 and month 6. Primary endpoint of this study was cervical intraepithelial neoplasia (CIN) grade 2 or 3, adenocarcinoma in situ or cervical cancer related to HPV 16 or 18. The subjects were followed up for an average of 3 years after the first dose of the vaccine and the efficacy of the vaccine in preventing the primary endpoint was 98% in the per-protocol susceptible population and 44% in an intention-to-treat population of all women who had undergone randomization (those with or without previous infection). Speculation that vaccines against HPV 16 and 18 will result in an increase in infections with other high-risk viruses was not seen in this population. The study concluded that the quadrivalent vaccine was highly effective in preventing HPV 16 and 18-related high-risk cervical lesions, and that widespread immunization of girls may result in a substantial decrease in cervical cancer resulting from infection with HPV 16 and 18.[119]

The interim analysis of the randomized double-blind controlled trial of the Papilloma Trial against Cancer In young Adults (PATRICIA) looking at the efficacy of prophylactic administration of bivalent vaccine against infection with HPV 16 and 18 was published in June 2007.[120] This vaccine has also shown evidence of cross-protection against HPV 45 and 31. In the study, 18, 644 women aged 15-25 years were randomized to receive either HPV 16/18 vaccine or hepatitis A vaccine at 0, 1, and 6 months. The primary endpoint of this trial was the efficacy of the vaccine against CIN 2+ lesions associated with HPV 16 or 18 and to assess in women who were seronegative and DNA negative for the corresponding vaccine type at baseline. The interim analysis for efficacy triggered when at least 23 cases of CIN 2+, with HPV 16 or 18 DNA in the lesion were detected in the total vaccinated cohort. The mean follow-up for women in the primary analysis for efficacy at the time of the interim analysis was 14.8 months, and 2 cases of CIN 2+ associated with HPV 16 or 18 DNA were seen in the vaccine group, and 21 were recorded in the control group. This gave the vaccine an efficacy of 90.4% and there were no significant safety profile differences between the study groups.[120]

HPV vaccines, as mentioned earlier, are currently licensed in 55 countries worldwide, and presently recommended for all 11-12-years old girls, though vaccination can be started as early as 9 years, and women between the age of 13 and 26 should also be vaccinated if they are not yet sexually active. Recent data from the United States suggest that HPV vaccination and biennial cervical screening from the age of 24 years will reduce the annual total Papanicolaou (PAP) test volume by 43% and result in the reduction in the workload at sexually transmitted disease clinics.[121] The Morkov model of incorporation of the HPV vaccination into a UK national cervical screening program predicts a 76% reduction in cervical cancer deaths and 66% reduction in high-grade lesions.[121] However, there are problems in world widespread distribution of the vaccinations including price of the vaccine, accessibility of the vaccines in countries due to lack of immunization infrastructure and opposition by conservative groups to the vaccination of young girls against what is perceived to be an sexually transmitted disease.[122]

Diagnosis and Treatment of Invasive Lesions Patterns of Spread

During the transition from in situ to invasive carcinoma, tumor cells penetrate the epithelial basement membrane and enter the underlying cervical stroma. Once the cervical stroma is invaded, the lymphatics and blood vessels are accessible, and dissemination beyond the cervix is possible.

The cervical, vaginal, and uterine lymphatic channels coalesce to form major drainage pathways. The major lymphatic trunks are the uteroovarian (infundibulopelvic), parametrial, and presacral, which drain into the paracervical, obturator, hypogastric, external iliac, common iliac, inferior gluteal, presacral, and lower aortic lymph nodes. A series studying the incidence and distribution pattern of retroperitoneal lymph node metastases in 208 patients with stages 1B, IIA, and IIB cervical carcinomas who underwent radical hysterectomy and systemic pelvic node dissection reported that 53 patients (25%) had node metastasis.[123] The obturator lymph nodes were the most frequently involved, with a rate of 19% (39 of 208), and the authors proposed them as sentinel nodes for cervical cancers. In fact, finding negative obturator nodes may be an indication that the pelvic lymph node dissection can be limited.

Lymph node status and the size and extent of the primary tumor are the most important prognostic factors in patients with cervical cancers. Among patients with early disease, the 5-year survival rate is only 60% in patients with three or more positive nodes and only 25-30% in patients with positive para-aortic nodes. Cervical cancers of similar size may have very different metastatic potentials, depending on their intrinsic aggressiveness and histologic cell type. Cervical carcinomas also invade directly. As the cancer grows, disease may extend to the lateral pelvic walls, into the bladder or rectum, or into the vagina.

The incidence of lymph node metastasis at diagnosis for each of the squamous cell carcinoma stages designated by the International Federation of Gynecology and Obstetrics (FIGO) has been well defined by surgical series.[124-126] Pelvic node involvement occurs in 10-25% of stage I carcinomas, 25-30% of stage II carcinomas, and 30-45% of stage III and IV carcinomas. Stage I carcinomas are more likely to metastasize to nodes once they reach 3 cm.[127,128] Because most patients with large bulky adenocarcinomas are treated with radiation therapy, the incidence of positive nodes by tumor size is not as well defined for adenocarcinoma as it is for squamous cell carcinoma. The incidence of positive nodes for poorly differentiated squamous cell carcinoma and for poorly differentiated adenocarcinoma is higher than that for the better differentiated carcinomas.

Carcinoma of the cervix spreads in an orderly manner. Nodes adjacent to the cervix are usually the first to be involved, and "skip" metastases are uncommon. Patients with positive para-aortic nodes usually have positive pelvic nodes. The incidence of positive para-aortic nodes in 978 patients with stage IB and IIA carcinoma whose aortic nodes were sampled prior to radical hysterectomy was 4.7% and 8.4%, respectively. The incidence of positive nodes in patients with adenocarcinomas is probably equal to that in patients with squamous cell-carcinomas when cancer size, histologic differentiation, and extent of tumor or FIGO stage are similar. Many large series report poorer survival rates for patients with adenocarcinomas than for patients with squamous cell carcinomas, especially those who have bulky lesions.[129,130] Small cell carcinoma and some of the carcinomas classified as other epithelial tumors are particularly aggressive. Carcinomas of the cervix, regardless of histology and size of the primary tumor, may contain highly malignant clones of cells that can prove unpredictable and spread extensively.

Clinical Symptoms

The clinical symptoms of carcinoma of the cervix are vaginal bleeding, discharge, and pain. The growth pattern of the carcinoma plays a role in the development of symptoms. Exophytic carcinomas bleed earlier in a sexually active patient (because of contact) than lesions that expand the cervix. Lesions that expand the endocervix in a barrel-shaped configuration may leave the squamous epithelium of the exocervix intact until the lesions exceed 5 or 6 cm in transverse diameter; therefore, carcinomas with this growth pattern may be silent and grow large before the patient bleeds. Cytologic findings may be negative unless the endocervix is sampled with a brush device. Ulcerative lesions that destroy the exocervix bleed early, and necrosis and infection induced by the cancer's outgrowing its blood supply result in a foul-smelling vaginal discharge.

Severe pelvic pain experienced during the pelvic examination may indicate salpingitis. Tubal infections require management before radiation therapy. Patients with an adnexal mass need surgical treatment before radiation therapy is started.

Paracervical extension of a carcinoma may remain silent until fixation to the pelvic wall occurs. Fixation with or without nodal involvement may obstruct a ureter. Ureteral encroachment is usually a silent process. Patients may present with bilateral ureteral obstruction with impending renal failure and report no history of urinary system complaints. Direct invasion of branches of the sciatic nerve roots causes back pain, and encroachment on the pelvic wall veins and lymphatics causes edema of a lower extremity. The triad of back pain, leg edema, and a nonfunctioning kidney is evidence of an advanced carcinoma with extensive pelvic wall involvement.

The anatomic position of the bladder, so closely adjacent to the cervix, favors contiguous spread from the cervix to the bladder. Urinary frequency and urgency are early manifestations of such spread; patients with advanced disease may present with hematuria or incontinence, suggesting direct extension of tumor to the bladder. Cystoscopy and biopsy should confirm the cause of hematuria or incontinence.

In contrast, posterior extension to the rectum and disruption of the rectal mucosa is an unusual pattern of disease spread in untreated patients. The deep cul-de-sac provides anatomic separation of the rectum and cervix. In patients who present with rectal mucosal involvement, there is usually extensive involvement of the posterior vaginal wall with direct extension to the rectum. For staging and treatment planning, cystoscopy and sigmoidoscopy are essential.

Metastatic carcinoma in para-aortic nodes may extend through the node capsule and directly invade the vertebrae and adjacent nerve roots. Back pain owing to involvement of the lumbar vertebrae and psoas muscles may be a manifestation of massive nodal disease; however, hematogenous spread to the lumbar vertebrae and involvement of the psoas muscle without significant nodal disease may occur.

Diagnosis

The diagnosis of cervical carcinoma is made by pathologic examination of a tissue specimen. A biopsy sample taken from the periphery of a tumor is more likely to contain morphologically intact neoplastic cells that are best able to represent the tumor pathologically. A biopsy specimen taken from the center of a tumor mass may include necrotic tumor debris; the result of hypoxia induced by the tumor's outgrowing its blood supply. Therefore, to rely on these dead and distorted cells is to compromise the accuracy of the histologic interpretation.

The endocervix should be curetted if no lesion is visible or if the cervix is enlarged, nodular, or hard. Older patients with adenocarcinoma require an endometrial biopsy. It may be difficult to distinguish an endocervical primary tumor from an endometrial primary tumor involving the lower uterine segment.

Patients with an abnormal Pap smear and no visible lesion require colposcopy and biopsy. The tissue specimen may be a simple colposcopy-directed biopsy specimen, an endocervical specimen obtained with a curette, or a conization specimen.

It is the current recommendation of FIGO to classify as stage IA any invasive cancer that can be identified only with a microscope. All gross lesions, even with superficial invasion, are at least stage IB cancers. Lesions with invasion of the stroma up to 3 mm in depth and no greater than 7 mm in width are classified as stage IA1. Lesions with invasion of stroma greater than 3 mm and no greater than 5 mm in depth and no wider than 7 mm are classified as stage IA2. For a lesion to be classified as IA2, the depth of invasion should not be more than 5 mm, measured from the base of the epithelium, either squamous or glandular, from which it originates. Vascular space involvement, either venous or lymphatic, should not alter staging.

Many clinicians prefer to use the term microinvasion and use criteria recommended by the Society of Gynecologic Oncologists instead of using the FIGO staging system. Microinvasion is invasion limited to 3 mm in depth, is measured from the base of the squamous or glandular epithelium of origin, and does not encompass lymphatic or vascular space involvement. A simple punch biopsy is inadequate for making the diagnosis of microinvasion: A conization specimen, containing the entire neoplastic process, is necessary. Additional tissue is required from patients with positive cone margins because an occult, frankly invasive carcinoma may lie adjacent to a positive margin.

Evaluation and Staging

Successful therapy planning requires detailed evaluation of the patient's general medical condition and the size and extent of the carcinoma. Medical illness must be stabilized and anemia must be corrected before treatment commences. Patients with anemia, which has been extensively studied, have a higher local relapse rate than patients with a normal hemoglobin (Table 98-2).[131,132] The patient's surgical history is important, and operative notes may describe the status of the abdominal organs as well as report abdominal and pelvic operations. Diagnoses of importance to therapy planning include ulcerative bowel disease, diverticulitis, and pelvic inflammatory disease. Such inflammatory conditions induce adhesions and fix loops of the intestines to each other, to adjacent organs, and to peritoneal surfaces.

Patients with small stage I carcinomas should undergo chest radiography, intravenous pyelography, a complete blood count, urinalysis, and blood chemistry analysis before treatment. Patients with advanced carcinomas require cystoscopy and proctoscopy. It is important to apply the FIGO rules for clinical staging (Table 98-3).[133] It is clearly stated in the FIGO guidelines that for staging purposes, the following examinations are permitted: cystoscopy, inspection, colposcopy, ECC, hysteroscopy, proctoscopy, intravenous pyelography, chest radiography, and skeletal radiography.[134] Findings from such examinations as lymphangiography, laparotomy, laparoscopy, computed tomography (CT), magnetic resonance imaging (MRI), and other examinations unnamed by FIGO should not be the basis for changing the clinical stage, despite the fact that such examinations or procedures can provide valuable information for planning therapy. The tumor-nodes-metastasis (TNM) staging categories have also been accepted by FIGO.[135] Lymph node status is not addressed in the FIGO staging system for carcinoma of the cervix, but three radiologic imaging techniques are available to evaluate lymph node status: CT, MRI, and fluorodeoxyglucose-positron emisssion tomography (FDG-PET) detect abnormal lymph nodes more lymphangiography.

The best radiologic imaging technique for detecting lymph node metastases is unclear. CT and MRI are good in identifying enlarged nodes; however, the accuracy of these techniques in the detection of positive nodes is compromised by their failure to detect small metastases, and many enlarged nodes are due not to metastases but to inflammation associated with advanced disease. The accuracy of MRI in the detection of lymph node metastases (72-93%) is similar to that of CT; however, when compared with surgical findings, MRI is superior to CT, clinical examination, and sonography in the evaluation of tumor location, tumor size, depth of stromal invasion, vaginal extension, and parametrial extension of cervical cancer.[136-139] Furthermore, studies suggest that MRI is a cost-effective method of evaluating cervical cancers.[139] Figure 98-13 shows an MRI of a patient with a cervical tumor.

PET is a new and rapidly expanding modality in oncologic imaging (Fig. 98-14). In a study of 101 patients with carcinoma of the cervix, Grigsby and colleagues reported that CT demonstrated enlarged pelvic lymph nodes in 20% and enlarged para-aortic lymph nodes in 7%, while PET demonstrated abnormal FDG uptake in pelvic lymph nodes in 67%, abnormal FDG uptake in para-aortic lymph nodes in 21%, and abnormal FDG uptake in supraclavicular lymph nodes in 8%.[140] The 2-year progression-free survival rate (PFS), based solely on para-aortic lymph node status, was 64% in CT-normal and PET-normal patients, 18% in CT-normal and PET-abnormal patients, and 14% in CT-abnormal and PET-abnormal patients. The authors

Table 98-2 Relapse Rates for Patients With Stage IIB or III Cervical Cancer

Hemoglobin (gm/dL)	Patients (No.)	Relapse Rate (%)		
		Local	Distant	Total
< 10	29	46	18	49
10–11.9	319	29	24	47
12–13.9	578	20	16	33
≥ 14	129	20	18	33

Relapse rates for patients with stage IIB or III cancer of the cervix according to average hemoglobin level during radiation therapy. *p* Values: $p = .002$ (local), $p = .1$ (distant), $p = .0007$ (total).
Source: From Ref. 131.

Table 98-3 Modified FIGO Staging

Stage	Description
0	CIS, intraepithelial carcinoma. Cases of stage 0 should not be included in any therapeutic statistics for invasive carcinoma.
I	The carcinoma is strictly confined to the cervix (extension to the corpus should be disre garded).
IA	Invasive cancer identified only microscopically. All gross lesions, even with superficial invasion, are stage IB cancers. Invasion is limited to measured stromal invasion with a maximum depth of 5 mm and a width no greater than 7 mm.
IA1	Measured invasion of stroma ≤ 3 mm in depth and ≤ 7 mm in width
IA2	Measured invasion of stroma > 3 mm and ≤ 5 mm in depth and ≤ 7 mm in width
IB	Clinical lesions confined to the cervix or preclinical lesions larger than stage IA
IB1	Clinical lesions ≤ 4 cm
IB2	Clinical lesions > 4 cm
II	The carcinoma extends beyond the cervix but has not extended onto the pelvic wall. Involves the vagina but does not extend as far as the lower third of the vagina
IIA	No obvious parametrial involvement
IIB	Obvious parametrial involvement
III	The carcinoma has extended onto the pelvic wall. On rectal examination, there is no cancer-free space between the tumor and the pelvic wall. The tumor involves the lower third of the vagina. All cases with hydronephrosis or a nonfunctioning kidney should be included unless they are known to result from another cause.
IIIA	No extension onto the pelvic wall but involvement of the lower third of the vagina
IIIB	Extension onto the pelvic wall or hydronephrosis or nonfunctioning kidney
IV	The carcinoma has extended beyond the true pelvis or has clinically involved the mucosa of the bladder or rectum.
IVA	Spread to adjacent organs
IVB	Spread to distant organs

Abbreviation: FIGO, International Federation of Gynecology and Obstetrics.
Source: From Ref. 133.

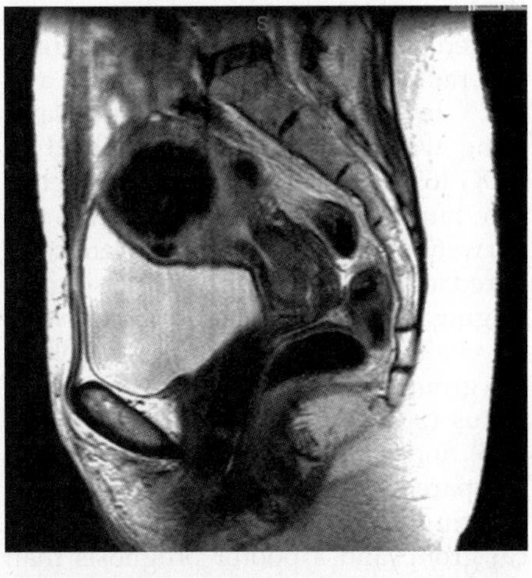

Figure 98-13 Magnetic resonance image of a patient with cervical tumor.

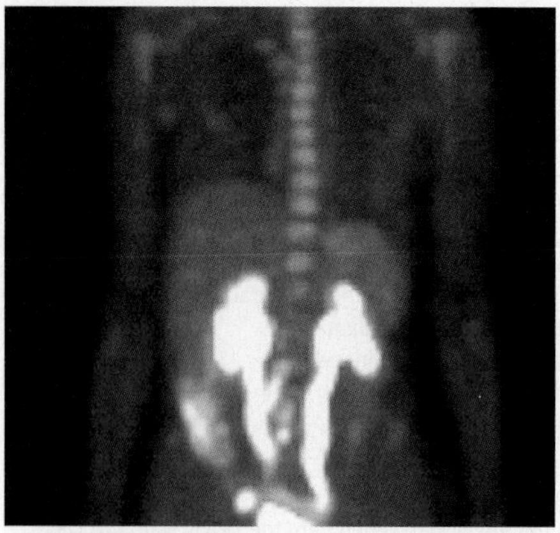

Figure 98-14 Positron emission tomography scan of a patient with cervical tumor showing positive nodes.

concluded that often than CT and that the findings on PET are a better predictor of survival than those on CT in patients with carcinoma of the cervix. Further studies are needed to confirm these results.

In some patients, surgical examination of the lymph nodes is warranted. The risk of occult para-aortic metastases is highest in patients with grossly involved pelvic nodes, and these patients may be the best candidates for operative exploration. These patients also may benefit from removal of the grossly enlarged nodes, which may be difficult to control with radiation alone.[141] When lymph node metastases are sought surgically, the extraperitoneal approach is currently the preferred technique.[142] It is preferred because high complication rates resulted from using a transperitoneal approach followed by radiation therapy.[143] Lymph node exploration and dissection may also be performed using a laparoscopic approach, which is associated with a shorter postoperative recovery time and probably less late radiation morbidity than open transperitoneal staging.[144] A recent retrospective review from the Gynecology Oncology Group (GOG) looked at three trials that are closed where patients with cervical carcinoma were treated with concurrent chemotherapy and radiation therapy: GOG 85, 120, and 165.[145] In GOG 85 and 120 surgical sampling was mandatory and optional in GOG 165, and this included 680 patients. Five hundred and fifty five patients underwent surgical staging and were compared to 130 patients who had no surgical staging prior to treatment, just radiological evaluation. Patients in the radiological group only had better performance status ($p < .01$), less advance stage ($p = 0.23$) and smaller tumor size ($p = .004$) compared to the surgical group, however in a multivariant analysis, the radiological group and a poorer prognosis than the surgery group (for disease progression, HR was 1.35 and for death it was 1.46). The authors conclude that surgical exclusion compared with radiographic exclusion of positive para-aortic nodes in patients with cervical cancer who received chemoradiation had a significant prognositic impact especially in Stage III disease.[145] Intraoperative lymphatic mapping may someday improve the accuracy of surgical staging of cervical cancer, and the GOG is currently opening a trial evaluating this approach.[146]

Prognostic Factors

FIGO stage correlates with survival and control of pelvic disease in patients with cervical cancer; however, prognosis is also influenced by other factors, including tumor characteristics and patient characteristics that are not included in the FIGO staging system.

Tumor Size and Local Extent Tumor size is one of the most important predictors of local recurrence and death in patients with cervical cancer treated with surgery or radiation therapy (Fig. 98-15). The FIGO staging classification for stage I disease was recently modified to include tumor diameter (ie, ≤4 cm, stage IB1; >4 cm, stage IB2).[147] For patients with more advanced disease, other estimates of tumor bulk that correlate with prognosis include presence of medial versus lateral parametrial involvement in FIGO stage IIB disease and unilateral versus bilateral pelvic wall involvement in FIGO stage IIIB disease.[148,149]

In patients who have had a radical hysterectomy, histologic evidence of extracervical spread (≥10 mm) and deep stromal invasion (>70% invasion) are associated with a poorer prognosis, as is parametrial extension, which is associated with higher rates of lymph node involvement, local recurrence, and death from cancer.[126,150-152] Uterine body involvement is associated with an increased rate of distant metastases in patients treated with radiation or surgery.[153]

Lymph Node Involvement Lymph node metastasis is another important prognostic factor for survival that is not part of the FIGO staging system. In several surgical series, after a radical hysterectomy, patients with positive pelvic lymph nodes had a 35-40% lower 5-year survival rate than patients with negative nodes.[124,126] However, recent studies suggest that postoperative chemoradiation improves these results.[154] Several authors have reported a correlation between size of the largest node involved or higher number of nodes involved and decreased survival rates. Patients with positive para-aortic nodes have a survival rate that is about half that of patients with similar-stage disease and negative para-aortic nodes.[124,126,151,155,156] With extended-field radiation therapy, patients with early-stage disease and positive para-aortic nodes have a cure rate of approximately 40-50%.

There is a strong correlation between positive lymph nodes in patients with cervical neoplasms and positive lymph-vascular space invasion (LVSI) in the tumor specimen. However, LVSI may be an independent predictor of prognosis, as a number of large series of patients treated with radical hysterectomy have demonstrated.[150,151,157,158] Roman and colleagues reported a correlation between the percentage of histopathologic sections containing LVSI and the incidence of lymph node metastasis.[159] In patients with adenocarcinoma of the cervix, there is a strong correlation between LVSI and outcome.[160,161]

Histologic Type There is controversy regarding whether adenocarcinomas of the cervix are associated with outcome similar to that seen with squamous carcinomas of the cervix. In several retrospective studies, investigators found that patients with adenocarcinomas of the cervix had outcome similar to that of patients with squamous carcinoma of the cervix treated with radiation therapy.[162,163] However, other investigators have come to an opposite conclusion. Among patients treated surgically, they found that patients with adenocarcinoma had unusually high relapse rates

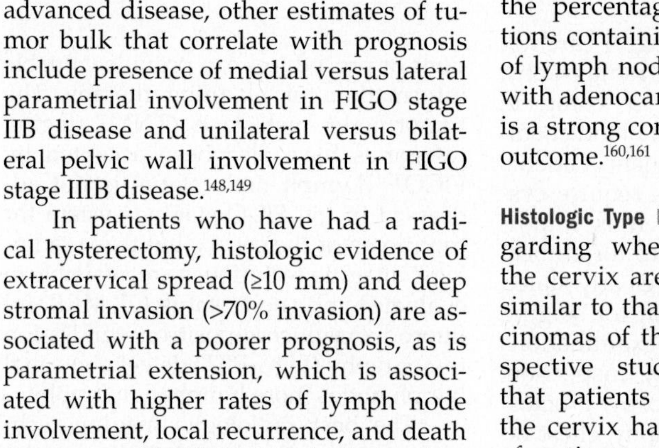

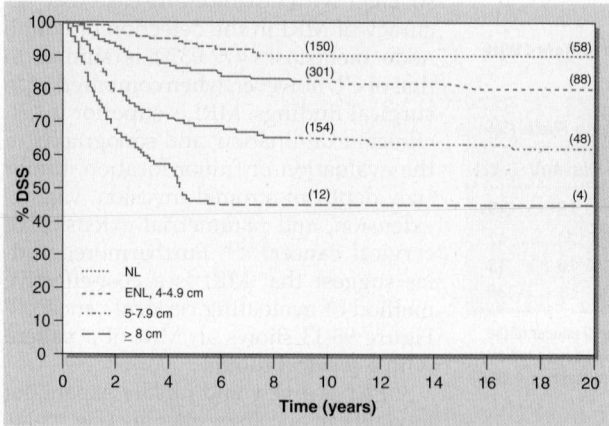

Figure 98-15 Disease-specific survival (DSS) is indicated for patients grouped according to size of cervix (NL, cervix of normal size; ENL, enlarged cervix, 4–4.9 cm). *Source*: From Ref. 131.

compared with the rates in patients with squamous cell carcinoma, and among patients treated with surgery or irradiation, they found that patients with adenocarcinoma had poorer survival rates than the rates seen in patients with squamous cell carcinoma.[164-166] Eifel and colleagues, in an analysis of 1767 patients treated with radiation for FIGO stage IB disease, reported that patients with adenocarcinoma had a significantly higher risk of recurrence and death from disease.[164] This finding was independent of age, tumor size, and tumor morphology. There was no difference in the rate of pelvic recurrence between patients with bulky adenocarcinoma (≥4 cm) and patients with squamous cell carcinoma; however, the rate of distant metastasis was almost twice as high in patients with adenocarcinoma as in patients with squamous cell carcinoma. Although the prognostic significance of histologic grade for squamous carcinomas has been disputed, there is a clear correlation between the degree of differentiation and the clinical behavior of adenocarcinomas.[161,167,168]

Other Tumor Factors ■ Baseline pretreatment serum squamous cell carcinoma antigen (SCCAg) level correlates well with stage of disease: 30-40% of stage I patients, 60-70% of stage II patients, and 80-90% of stage III and IV patients have elevated values.[169,170] The only exception to this trend is patients with bulky stage IB2 disease, in whom levels are more consistent with advanced-stage disease, suggesting that SCCAg level correlates with tumor bulk.[171] Pretreatment SCCAg levels have also been shown to correlate with tumor histology, grade, type of tumor (ie, exophytic vs infiltrative), microscopic depth of invasion, and risk of lymph node metastases in patients with early-stage disease.[172] The most important property of the pretreatment SCCAg level, however, is its ability to predict clinical outcome. Several authors have reported significantly lower survival rates in patients with very elevated values compared with patients with normal baseline levels, independent of stage.[172-175] Duk and colleagues reported a 5-year survival rate of 70% in stage IB patients with elevated pretreatment SCCAg levels, compared with 96% in patients with normal values.[175] SCCAg testing also provides a marker for monitoring the course of disease and response to treatment in patients with cervical cancer. Correlations of tumor response and SCCAg values have ranged from 72% to 95%.[176] For the detection of tumor recurrence, serial SCCAg testing has been proven to be more specific than sensitive, with specificities ranging from 90% to 100% and sensitivities ranging from 60% to 90%.[177] Monitoring of tumor response using SCCAg needs further investigation, especially studies designed to determine how often SCCAg measurement should be done, the level of SCCAg that is significant, which patients would benefit from this monitoring and the cost-effectiveness of using SCCAg as a tool for monitoring patients after treatment.[178]

Several authors have reported a correlation between HPV subtype and prognosis.[179-181] In two studies of patients with histologically negative lymph nodes, investigators reported higher rates of disease recurrence when findings on PCR assay of the lymph nodes were strongly positive for HPV DNA.[182,183]

Other molecular markers that have recently been evaluated for predictive power in cervical carcinoma are epidermal growth factor receptor and cyclooxygenase-2. Several studies have reported that overexpression of epidermal growth factor receptor in cervical carcinomas correlates with clinical predictors of poor prognosis such as large tumor size and lymph node involvement; however, this association is controversial, and study populations have generally been too small and heterogeneous to permit establishment of an independent association between epidermal growth factor receptor and prognosis. A preliminary study in patients with cervical cancer suggested that cyclooxygenase-2 overexpression was also correlated with poor prognosis, but, because of the small sample size, the study was not able to establish independent predictive value of this molecular marker.[184]

Other biologic features that have been investigated for their predictive power, with variable results, include inflammatory response in cervical stroma, peritoneal cytology, tumor vascularity and DNA ploidy or S-phase fraction.[185,186]

Patient Factors ■ Several investigators have reported correlations between low hemoglobin level before or during treatment and poor prognosis.[148,187]

It has been speculated that the poor prognosis of anemic patients is caused in part by hypoxia-induced radiation resistance. The strongest evidence that this may be true comes from a randomized study of 1978 patients at Princess Margaret Hospital. In one group, patients' hemoglobin levels were maintained, through the use of transfusions, at least 12 gm%; in the other group, hemoglobin levels were allowed to drop to as little as 10 gm%. The locoregional recurrence rate was significantly higher for the 25 anemic patients in the control arm than it was for the patients who received transfusions.[131] A recent retrospective study from Canada also found that hemoglobin levels of at least 12 gm% during radiation therapy were a significant predictor of successful radiation therapy and disease-free survival.[187] Subsequent studies investigating various techniques aimed at overcoming the theoretical radiobiological consequences of intratumoral hypoxia (use of hypoxic cell sensitizers, hyperbaric oxygen breathing, and neutron therapy) have not been successful. The GOG has recently started a study evaluating the effects of hemoglobin on prognosis. Accrual is slow at present, but if the trial is completed, it may help clarify the relationship between anemia and prognosis in patients with cervical carcinoma.

Other patient-related factors that have been shown to correlate with prognosis include age, platelet count, socioeconomic status, and smoking.[128,188-190] Kucera and colleagues reported that smokers with cervical cancer had a poorer 5-year survival rate than nonsmokers, and this relationship was statistically significant in patients with stage III disease (5-year survival rate 20.3% vs 33.9%, $p < .01$).[191] A recent study by Eifel and colleagues found that smokers had a significantly higher rate of grade 3 or 4 gastrointestinal complications than did nonsmokers in a group of patients with cervical carcinoma treated with definitive radiation therapy.[192]

Surgical Treatment Options

Cervical Conization and LEEP ■ Cervical conization is a procedure that removes or destroys the transformation zone and can be diagnostic, therapeutic, or both. A conization specimen is conical, as the name implies, and its size varies according to the area in question. The cone is shallow when an exocervical lesion is removed. The cone is deeper when the endocervix is being investigated. Patients requiring conization usually have one of the following: normal colposcopy findings and an abnormal Pap smear or positive ECC specimens; abnormal colposcopy findings in the form of failure to visualize the entire squamocolumnar junction or failure to define the extent of the lesion; microinvasive carcinoma in a biopsy specimen; adenocarcinoma in situ in a biopsy or ECC specimen; or a lack of correlation between cytologic (Pap smear), colposcopic, and histologic interpretations.

Cone biopsy is designed to completely remove the squamocolumnar junction and the lower portion of the endocervical canal in women with very small cervical cancers. The surgical specimen should include the entire lesion, as this permits measurement of both depth of invasion and extent of lateral spread.

Another surgical technique that can be used for conization is LEEP. In LEEP, a thin wire loop electrode is used to excise the lesion in patients with HGSIL. LEEP is an outpatient procedure. Although destructive techniques (such as laser ablation and cryotherapy) can provide effective treatment of suspicious lesions; the preferred technique is one that provides an appropriate histologic specimen, such as cervical cold knife conization (CKC) LEEP, or laser conization. Recently, Linares and colleagues compared CKC, laser conization, and LEEP and found that LEEP was associated with fewer complications and a shorter operating time then the other two procedures.[193] The only drawback of the LEEP procedure was a slightly shorter cone depth and a slightly higher risk of lesion recurrence.[193]

Patient Selection ■ Conization as sole treatment of early cervical cancers is a relatively recent concept. For women who have very limited risk of lymph node spread and who have a strong desire to maintain fertility, conization may be an option.[194,195] MD Anderson Cancer Center recommends that conization be considered only for patients with squamous cell lesions that invade less than 3 mm, have no LVSI, and have uninvolved resection margins.[196] There is very little information on which to base a recommendation regarding the use of conization as therapy for women with nonsquamous cervical cancer.[197]

Complications of CKC include hemorrhage, pelvic cellulitis, cervical stenosis, and incompetent cervix.[198] In addition, because this procedure requires general anesthesia, there is the additional burden of possible complications and cost of anesthesia.

Complications of LEEP are similar to but not the same as those of CKC: Infection, bleeding, burns to the vagina, cervical stenosis, cervical incompetence, and recurrence of dysplasia. With LEEP, however, stenosis is rare (occurring in 1% of patients) and is seen primarily in nulliparous, perimenopausal, or postmenopausal patients. Cervical incompetence is usually only a complication of multiple procedures. The other advantage of LEEP is that it does not require general anesthesia. As mentioned above, when three conization techniques (CKC, laser conization, and LEEP) were compared, LEEP was associated with fewer complication as well as decreased operative time.[193]

Radical Trachelectomy ■ Recently, for early-stage disease, several groups have tried to preserve the uterus and child-bearing capability by treating patients with a radical vaginal trachelectomy. This technique involves a laparoscopic pelvic lymphadenectomy followed by vaginal resection of the cervix, the upper 1-2 cm of the vaginal cuff, and the medial portions of the cardinal and uterosacral ligaments. The cervix is transected at the lower uterine segment, and a prophylactic cerclage is placed at the time of surgery. Several investigators recommend that this procedure be limited to patients with a tumor not exceeding 2 cm.[199,200]

Extrafascial Hysterectomy ■ Characterizing the extrafascial hysterectomy are the following: (1) the uterine vessels are skeletonized (to lessen the need to slide the tip of the clamp off the cervix) and are clamped and cut to allow the ligated vessels to fall away from the cervix, (2) the pubovesicocervical fascia is not separated from the cervix and is excised with the specimen, (3) the plane. for bladder separation from the cervix is created with sharp dissection because blunt dissection is more often associated with accidental entry into the bladder, and (4) the uterosacral ligaments are transected separately near their insertion into the cervix. This frees the uterus and cervix posteriorly and gains mobility for the specimen. This facilitates amputation of the vagina in front of the cervix, securing at least a 1 cm vaginal cuff. The extrafascial technique permits removal of the intact uterine fundus and cervix, leaving the parametrial soft tissues or a portion of the upper vagina. Extrafascial hysterectomy can be accomplished through an abdominal incision, transvaginally, or by using a combination of laparoscopic and transvaginal techniques.

Simple extrafascial hysterectomy is the standard definitive treatment option for women with stage IA1 cervical cancers and is sometimes performed following radiation therapy for bulky endocervical carcinomas. For patients with stage IA2 disease, there is some controversy regarding the most appropriate surgical procedure. These patients have 3-5% incidence of lymph node metastases and a higher rate of vaginal recurrence than patients with IA1 disease. So, although some data suggest that these IA2 lesions can be effectively resected with extrafascial hysterectomy, many American gynecologic oncologists limit this operation to women with IA1 tumors.[201,202] There is uniform consensus that conization-only therapy should not be offered to women with stage IA2 disease.

Radical Hysterectomy ■ Radical hysterectomy involves the en bloc removal of the uterus, cervix, parametrial tissues, and upper vagina. In the early twentieth century, Wertheim of Vienna described the radical hysterectomy for the treatment of cervical cancer. In the 1940s, Meigs of the United States championed the procedure, to which he added a pelvic lymphadenectomy. Today, radical hysterectomy with pelvic lymphadenectomy is the standard treatment in the management of stage IA2-IIA Tumors.

The type II (modified radical) hysterectomy is a less extensive version of the type III (radical) hysterectomy. The primary indication for type II hysterectomy is early invasive carcinoma, tumors less than 2 cm diameter. The type II operation ensures an adequate paracervical specimen and a vaginal cuff of 2-3 cm. In the type II operation, the medial half of the parametrium and upper one-third of the vagina are included in the surgical specimen. This is accomplished by exposing the ureters and taking the medial half of the cardinal and uterosacral ligaments instead of taking these ligaments where they attach to the pelvic wall and pelvic floor. The posterior approach is the surgeon's choice. The incidence of bladder and ureteral complications is lower with the type II operation than with a type III procedure. The type II hysterectomy can be performed with a modified or complete pelvic lymphadenectomy.

The type III (radical) hysterectomy is the classic Wertheim-Meigs radical hysterectomy. This operation is reserved for patients with stage IB and selected stage IIA carcinomas. The vaginal extension for stage IIA patients should be limited to no more than 1 cm. The parametrium, cardinal, and uterosacral ligaments are severed at the pelvic wall, and half of the vagina is removed. The uterine vessels are taken at their origin from the internal iliac vessels. The ureters are taken out of their tunnel and reflected laterally. This dissection of the distal ureters sacrifices the blood supply from the uterine and superior vesicle arteries. Reflection of the ureters clears the way for applying instruments across the parametrium along the pelvic wall. Complete removal of the cardinal ligaments and the rectal pillars and uterosacral ligaments at their base results in a greater risk of bladder atony, and loss of the distal-ureter blood supply results in a greater risk of fistulae. This operation produces an excellent cure rate in properly selected patients. In young patients, the ovaries are spared.

Intraoperative and immediate postoperative complications of radical hysterectomy include blood loss (average, 0.8 L), ureterovaginal fistula (occurring in 1-2% of patients), vesicovaginal fistula (<1%), pulmonary embolus (1-2%), small bowel obstruction (1-2%), and postoperative fever secondary to deep vein thrombosis, pulmonary infection, pelvic cellulitis, urinary tract infection, or wound infection (25-50%).[203] Subacute complications include lymphocyst formation and lower-extremity edema, the risk of which is related to the extent of the node dissection. Lymphocysts may obstruct a ureter, but hydronephrosis usually improves with drainage of the lymphocyst.[204] The risk of complications may be increased in patients who undergo preoperative or postoperative irradiation.

Although most patients have transient decreased bladder sensation after radical hysterectomy, with appropriate management severe long-term bladder complications are infrequent. However, chronic bladder hypotonia or atony occurs in approximately 3-5% of patients despite careful postoperative bladder drainage.[205] Bladder atony probably results from damage to the bladder's innervation and may be related to the extent of the parametrial and paravaginal dissection.[206] Radical hysterectomy may be complicated by stress incontinence, but reported incidences vary widely and may be influenced by the addition of postoperative radiation therapy.[207] Patients may also experience constipation and, rarely, chronic obstipation after radical hysterectomy.

Criteria for selecting patients who are appropriate candidates for radical hysterectomy include factors affecting the patient's suitability for major surgery as well as tumor characteristics, including tumor volume and lymphatic involvement. Patient factors play a very important role in the selection of primary radical surgery versus primary radiation therapy in patients with early-stage disease. The ability to preserve ovarian function as well as a more pliable vagina is important to young women facing this decision. Just as important, for women with significant medical problems, including obesity, primary radiation therapy may be the better treatment option.

In patients with early-stage (IA-IB1) disease, tumor characteristics play a very important role in treatment selection. Patients with high-risk factors may benefit from up-front definitive radiation therapy plus possible chemotherapy. Multiple studies have found that morbidity increases in patients who receive both radical surgery and radiation therapy.[208] High-risk tumor characteristics include large tumor size, which is associated with lymph node spread, increased chance of recurrence, and decreased survival rates. Eifel and colleagues found that disease-specific survival decreased significantly in patients with stage IB carcinoma if the tumor diameter was greater than 5 cm (88% vs 69%, $p < .0001$).[209] Other high-risk factors include lymph node metastases, parametrial involvement, and positive surgical margins.

Outcomes After Surgical Treatment

Reported 5-year survival rates for women with stage IB cervical cancer treated with radical hysterectomy and pelvic lymphadenectomy are approximately 80-90% (Table 98-4).[124-126,208,210-217] Patients with positive surgical margins or positive lymph nodes are at the highest risk of recurrence and poor outcome. Delgado and colleagues, in a large prospective study, reported 3-year disease-specific survival rates of 85.6% in patients with negative nodes and 50-74% in patients with positive nodes.[126] In the group with positive nodes, increasing number of positive nodes and involvement of common iliac nodes correlated with decreased survival. A recent randomized study showed that postoperative chemoradiation improved survival in patients with positive lymph nodes, positive surgical margins, or tumor present in the endometrium.[154]

Table 98-4 5-Year Survival Rates for Stage IB-IIA Cervical Cancer Patients After Radical Hysterectomy and Bilateral Pelvic Lymphadenectomy

First Aauthor (Ref.)	Stage	Year	*n*	Survival (%)
Morley (303)	IB	1976	156	87.2
Sall (215)	IB-IIA	1979	219	90.0
Kenter (213)	IB-IIA	1989	213	87.3
Lee (212)	IB-IIA	1989	343	87.2
Ayhan (124)	IB-IIA	1991	270	80.7
Hopkins (165)	IB	1991	213	92.5
Alvarez (208)	IB	1991	401	85
Burghardt (304)	IB	1992	443	83
Averette (123)	IIB-IIA	1993	726	90.1
Landoni (201)	IB–IIA	1997	172	83

Abbreviation: *N*, No. of patients.

Radiation Therapy

The management of invasive carcinoma of the cervix with primary radiation therapy involves a combination of external beam radiation therapy (EBRT) plus either low-dose rate (LDR) or high-dose rate (HDR) intracavitary irradiation. The goal of treatment is to balance these two elements in a way that optimizes the ratio of tumor control to treatment complications. The required dose varies according to the tumor burden in the cervix, paracervical sites, and regional nodes. Factors that influence the tolerable dose of radiation include the patient's vaginal and uterine anatomy, the degree of tumor-related tissue destruction and infection, and patient characteristics (eg, body habitus, comorbid illnesses, and smoking habits).

Treatment Options EBRT

EBRT is used as initial treatment in patients with bulky tumors. The usual plan is to give 40-45 Gy to the whole pelvis. This gives a homogeneous distribution to the central mass plus the regional lymph nodes. Such treatment reduces the primary tumor and any regional lymph nodes harboring disease, and it destroys microscopic foci in lymph-vascular spaces adjacent to the tumor. The shrinkage of the primary tumor allows better dose distribution from intracavitary irradiation.

High-energy photons (15-18 MV) are usually preferred for pelvic treatment because they spare superficial tissues that are unlikely to be involved with tumor. Simulation films, as well as CT, MRI, PET scan, and lymphangiography, guide the radiation oncologist in selecting boundaries for the portals. Typical radiation therapy fields are shown in Figure 98-16. A standard course of 40-45 Gy whole-pelvis EBRT plus two 48-h or equivalent intracavitary irradiation systems usually delivers at least 85 Gy to point A (a reference location 2 cm lateral and 2 cm superior to the cervical os) and 50-56 Gy to the lateral pelvic wall structures. Patients with grossly positive pelvic nodes within the 40- to 45-Gy field require a boost with a small field (Figs. 98-16 and 98-17).[218] The dose to the boost area is 8-10 Gy. The total dose to the positive nodes, including a 1-2 cm margin, is 60-62 Gy, which includes the contributions from two brachytherapy intracavitary systems. Intensity-modulated radiation therapy(IMRT)may be used to boost the dose to large pelvic nodes (up to approximately 70 Gy) in a very tightly defined volume.

There has been a recent interest in using IMRT in the treatment of cervical carcinoma. Unlike standard treatment, IMRT allows one to dose paint tissues in the area of treatment, ie, allowing higher doses to tumor while giving less dose to normal tissues especially small bowel (Fig. 98-17). Mundt et al. have published reports showing a decrease in both acute[219] and chronic[220] bowel toxicities in patients with endometrial or cervical carcinoma treated postoperatively to the pelvis with IMRT compared to standard treatment. However, the highly conformal dose distributions achieved by IMRT also increases the room of error. In particular, great attention needs to be given to internal organs motion (especially bladder and rectum) as well as tumor regression, and therefore at this time IMRT still is considered investigation

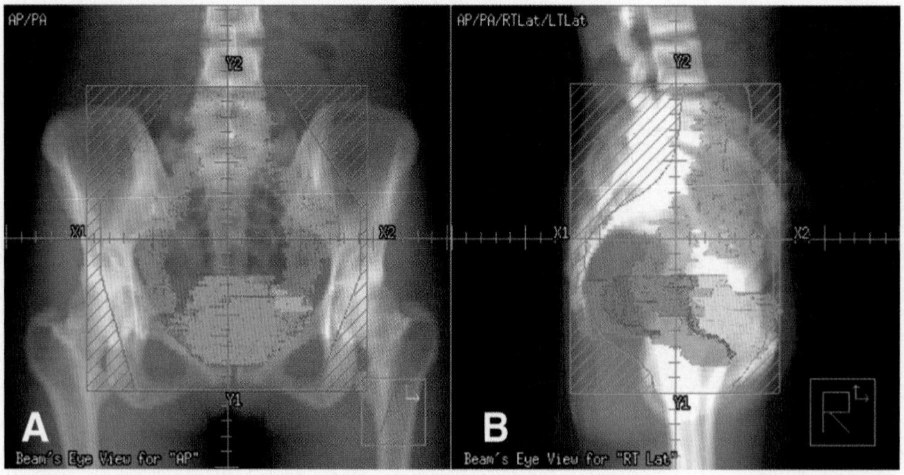

Figure 98-16 ■ Typical radiation fields for a patient with cervical cancer. (**A**) Anterior field; (**B**) lateral field.

therapy especially in the field of intact cervix.

Intracavitary Radiation Therapy (ICRT) ■ The importance of ICRT for cervical cancer should not be underestimated, because, although external beam radiation therapy plays a critical role in sterilizing pelvic wall disease and improving tumor geometry, too much reliance on external beam irradiation will compromise the chance for central disease control and increase the risk of complications.

Brachytherapy is usually delivered using afterloading applicators that are placed in the uterine cavity and vagina. Ideal placement of the intrauterine tandem and vaginal ovoids produces a pear-shaped radiation distribution, delivering a high radiation dose to the cervix and paracervical tissues and a reduced dose to the rectum and bladder. Several systems have been used throughout the world to determine dose rates and doses for cervical cancer. In the United States, the paracentral doses are most frequently expressed at a single point, point A, which is defined above. Point A bears no consistent relationship with the tumor or target volume but lies approximately at the crossing of the ureter and uterine artery. Other systems of dose specifications include the International Commission on Radiation Units and Measurements (ICRU) reference points based on ICRU Report 38 (1985) and the mg-h system. Whichever system of dose specification is used, emphasis should always be placed on optimizing the relationship between the intracavitary applicators and the cervical tumor and other pelvic tissues. Source, strength, and position should be carefully chosen to provide optimal tumor coverage with exceeding safe doses to normal tissue. In patients with bulky central disease, an effort should always be made to deliver at least 85 Gy (using low-dose rate brachytherapy) to point A. If the intracavitary placement has been optimized, this can usually be accomplished by not exceeding a dose of 70-75 Gy to the bladder reference point or 60-65 to the rectal reference point, doses that are usually associated with acceptably low risks of major complications. In addition, the dose delivered to the surface of the lateral wall of the apical vagina should not exceed 120-140 Gy.

In the past, clinicians regarded the radiobiological advantages of LDR intracavitary treatment (usually delivery of 40-60 cGy/h to point A) as a major factor contributing to the success of cervical cancer treatment. These low-dose rates permit repair of sublethal cellular injury, preferentially sparing normal tissues and optimizing the therapeutic ratio. During the past two decades, computer technology has made it possible to deliver brachytherapy at very high-dose rates (<100 cGy/min) using a high-activity cobalt 60 or iridium 192 source and remote afterloading. HDR therapy is slowly replacing conventional LDR therapy, primarily because of radiation safety. HDR intracavitary therapy is now being used for radical treatment of cervical cancer by a number of groups, including several in Japan, Canada, and Europe and, more recently, in the United States. Clinicians have found this approach attractive because it does not require that patients be hospitalized and may be more convenient for the patient and the physician.

Multiple randomized and nonrandomized studies have suggested that survival rates and complications rates with high-dose rate treatment are similar to those with traditional low-dose rate treatment. At least two studies from the United States have shown similar results with high-dose rate and low-dose rate therapy in early-stage disease; however, in stage IIIB disease, the survival rate was lower with high-dose rate than with low-dose-rate therapy.[221,222]

HDR brachytherapy is gaining increasing acceptance in the community and is considered standard therapy for patients with an intact cervix, and in 2000,[223] the American Brachytherapy Society suggested guidelines for the use of HDR brachytherapy for carcinoma of the cervix. The group emphasized the importance of factors that were already considered critical to successful LDR treatment—optimized applicator position, balanced use of external beam therapy and brachytherapy, compact overall treatment duration, and delivery of an adequate dose to tumor while respecting normal tissue tolerance limits.

Image-based brachytherapy is becoming increasingly common, particularly in Europe. Institutions are using MRI-based treatment-planning to plan their doses to tumor as well as doses to avoid structures such as the bladder and rectum; however large prospective studies and careful analysis will be needed prior to this becoming standard of care.

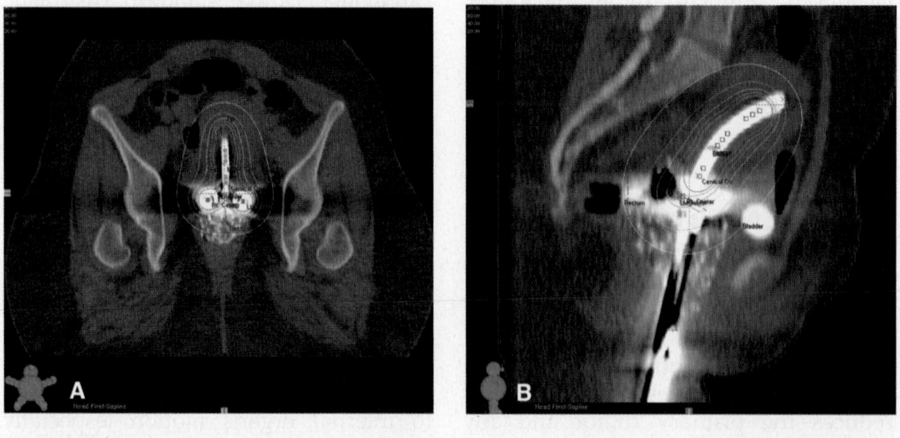

Figure 98-17 ■ Dose distribution of a typical intracavitary system; it is important to note how quickly the dose falls off the further one gets from the system. (**A**) Anterior view; (**B**) lateral view.

Interstitial Brachytherapy ■ Several groups have advocated the use of interstitial perinealtemplate brachytherapy in patients with poor anatomy or parametrial or pelvic sidewall disease. These implants are usually placed transperineally, with placement guided by a Lucite template that encourages parallel placement of hollow needles that penetrate the cervix and paracervical spaces and are usually loaded with iridium 192. Advocates state that the advantages of this method are the ease of inserting implants in patients whose uterus is difficult to probe, the ability to place sources directly into the parametrium, and the relatively homogeneous dose. Recent updates report poor survival rates and higher rates of major complications for patients with stage IIB and IIIB disease.[224,225] Outside of an investigational setting, interstitial treatment of primary cervical cancers should probably be limited to patients who cannot accommodate intrauterine brachytherapy and patients with distal vaginal disease that requires a boost with interstitial brachytherapy.

Patient Selection

For patients with IB1 tumors, the choice between surgery and radiation therapy is based primarily on patient preference, anesthetic and surgical risks, physician preference, and understanding of the nature and incidence of complications of radiation therapy and hysterectomy. In general, surgery is often chosen for younger patients in the hope of preserving ovarian function and hopefully reducing vaginal shortening, while radiation therapy is often selected for older postmenopausal women to avoid the morbidity of a major surgical procedure. Patients with stage IB2 disease can be treated with either surgery followed by radiation therapy or definitive radiation therapy. The biases are so large that the GOG could not complete a trial randomizing patients with stage IB2 disease between surgery followed by chemoradiation therapy and definitive radiation therapy. Radiation therapy is the primary local therapy for most patients with stage IIB-IVA disease.

Outcomes

Stage IB-IIA Disease ■ Radical radiation therapy achieves excellent survival and pelvic disease control rates in patients with stage IB-IIA cervical cancer. Eifel and colleagues reported 5-year disease-specific survival rates of 90%, 86%, and 67% in patients with stage IB tumors with cervical diameters of less than 4, 4-4.9 and greater than 5 cm, respectively.[209] The 5-year survival rates of patients with stage IIA disease range from 70% to 85% and, like survival rates in patients with stage IB disease, are strongly correlated with tumor size.[149,226,227] Recent studies suggest that results for patients with bulky tumors may be improved further by concurrent administration of chemotherapy.[228,229]

Table 98-5 ■ **Pelvic Disease Control and Survival Rates**[a]

FIGO Stage	Patients (*n*)	Control Rate (%)	Survival Rate (%)
I	229	93	89
IIA	315	88	85
IIB	314	80	62
IIIA	266	63	62
IIIB	216	57	50
IV	43	18	20

[a]Pelvic disease control rates and survival rates of 1383 patients with carcinoma of the intact uterine cervix treated with irradiation alone, according to the Fletcher guidelines: a French cooperative study.
Source: From Ref. 305.

Stage IIB-IVA Disease ■ Five-year survival rates of 65-75%, 35-50%, and 15-20% have been reported in patients who received radiation therapy alone for stage IIB, IIIB, and IV tumors, respectively (Table 98-5).[148,149,227,230] The addition of cisplatin-containing regimens may further improve local control and survival.[229,231,232]

Complications

Acute Side Effects ■ Acute side effects of pelvic irradiation include symptoms related to the bowel, bladder, rectum, and vagina. Most patients experience mild fatigue and mild to moderate diarrhea that usually is controllable with antidiarrheal medication and dietary modifications. Less frequently, patients may complain of bladder or urethral irritation. These symptoms may be treated with Pyridium or antispasmodics after urinalysis and urine culture have ruled out a urinary tract infection. Patients treated with extended-field radiation may have nausea, gastric irritation, and mild depression of peripheral blood cell counts. Acute symptoms may be increased in patients receiving concurrent chemotherapy. Unless the ovaries have been transposed, all premenopausal patients who receive pelvic radiotherapy experience ovarian failure by the completion of treatment.

Fatal or life-threatening complications of intracavitary radiation therapy are rare. Among 4042 patients who received 7662 LDR intracavitary treatments at MD Anderson between 1960 and 1992, there were 11 (0.3%) documented or suspected thromboembolic events resulting in four deaths (0.1%).[233] All four deaths were in patients who had extensive pelvic wall disease that may have obstructed flow in the pelvic vessels. Today, patients receive low-dose heparin during intracavitary radiation therapy to reduce the risk of thromboembolism. Uterine perforation, fever, vaginal laceration, and the usual risk of anesthesia are other less serious complications associated with intracavitary radiation therapy.

Problems After Therapy ■ For patients with cervical cancer, overall estimates of the risk of major complications of radiation therapy usually range between 5% and 15%.[234,235] The risk of experiencing a late complication is greatest within the first 3 years after treatment; however, major complications have been reported as late as 30 years or more after treatment. Lanciano and colleagues reported an overall actuarial rate of major complications of 14% at 5 years in a 1992 review of 1558 patients with cervical cancer treated in more than 100 facilities randomly selected for survey in the 1972 and 1978 Patterns of Care studies.[235] Eifel and colleagues reported an overall actuarial risk of major complications of 14.4% at 20 years in 1700 patients treated with radiation therapy for stage IB cervical cancer between 1960 and 1989.[234] At 5 years, the incidence was approximately 9.3%. Most complications occurring after radiation involve the rectum, bladder, or small bowel. During the first 3 years after treatment, rectal complications are most common and include bleeding, stricture, ulceration and fistula. In a study by Eifel and colleagues, the risk of major rectosigmoid complications was 2.3% at 5 years.[234] The average onset of major urinary tract complications tend to be somewhat later than that of intestinal complication, with an actuarial risk of hematuria requiring transfusion of 2.6% at 5 years.[234] The overall risk of developing a gastrointestinal or urinary tract fistula was 1.7% at 5 years with an increased risk of patients who underwent adjuvant hysterectomy or pretreatment transperitoneal lymphadenectomy.

The risk of small bowel obstruction is strongly correlated with a number of patient characteristics and treatment factors. Several studies have demonstrated a three- to fourfold increase in risk for patients who had transperitoneal lymphadenectomy before radiation.[234,235] However, there appears to be little added risk if the operation is performed with a retroperitoneal approach.[142] The risk of small bowel obstruction is also greater for patients who are very thin, have history of pelvic infection, or who smoke. A recent study from MD Anderson revealed a six fold increase in the risk of small bowel complications for patients who smoked more than one pack of cigarettes per day (12% vs 2% for nonsmokers).[192]

Patients who are treated with radiation for cervical cancer tend to have varying degrees of atrophy, telangiectasia, or scarring of the upper third of the vagina. Bruner and colleagues reported an average reduction in vaginal length of approximately 1 cm during the first 2 years after treatment.[236] However, more severe shortening can occur. Changes may be greater in patients with very extensive tumors and in patients who are elderly, sexually inactive, or hypoestrogenic.[234,236] Regular intercourse and use of vaginal dilators may help prevent vaginal shortening.

There are presently no prospective trials that have evaluated the role of chemotherapy and radiation therapy on quality of life of patients that survive their disease. In one retrospective cohort, severe (grade 3-4) late toxicities in the rectum, bladder, small intestine, and subcutaneous tissue were 12.3% and 1.1%, 11.2%, and 1.2%, 9.2% and 0.2% and 23.1% and 1.2%, respectively. Vaginal adhesion were seen in 29.6% of patients and vaginal stenosis in 33.9% of patients.[237] However, how these results effect patients and their quality of life is unknown and underscore the need for prospective quality of life studies on patients being treated with combination chemotherapy and radiation.

Current Practice by Disease Stage

CIS and Stage IA1 Disease

Treatment of HGSILs is rapidly changing. LEEP is one effective therapy for HGSILs. Other techniques such as cryosurgery and laser ablation have also proven effective. Regardless of the technique used, HGSILs should be entirely visible by colposcopy, the entire transformation zone should be visualized, and the ECC specimen should be negative. Conization with a knife is preferred when the ECC specimen is positive. All margins must be clear of intraepithelial lesions.

Stage IA1 (microinvasive) squamous cell carcinomas that invade the stroma less than 3 mm and have no LVSI are usually not visible to the unaided eye, and cytology is abnormal. The diagnosis requires cone biopsy, which yields a specimen adequate for diagnostic purposes. Conization alone is also potentially a low-risk therapy for patients who wish to retain fertility and who have invasion less than 3 mm in depth with no LVSI. It is important to remember that the margins of a cone specimen must be negative. When the conization specimen has a positive margin, a second tissue specimen must be obtained because foci of frankly invasive carcinoma may lie adjacent to the positive margin. Patients should be informed that the conservative approach carries a small risk. There is very little current information on which to base a recommendation regarding the use of conization as therapy for women with nonsquamous cervical cancers.[197] Patients who elect conization therapy must be willing to be monitored closely for the development of residual or recurrent cervical neoplasia.

The most conventional treatment of stage IA1 disease is a type 1 (simple extrafascial) hysterectomy. If the patient is young, the ovaries are left in place. Patients can also be treated with radiation therapy alone, usually consisting of intracavitary therapy alone. The 10-year disease control rate with radiation therapy alone is 95-100%.[238]

Stage IA2 Disease

Small lesions that invade 3-5 mm have an average risk of lymph node metastasis of about 5%. The standard treatment of patients with this stage of disease is type II (modified radical) hysterectomy and pelvic node dissection. However, if a patient wishes to preserve fertility, vaginal or abdominal radical trachelectomy is a viable option. In a review of 72 cases of stage IA,[239] IB, and IIA cervical cancer, with mean follow-up of 60 months, the recurrence-free survival was 95%. The recommendation from this study and others is that radical trachelectomy is a safe option for patients with tumor size less than 2 cm. This same group reported their rate of pregnancy after the procedure,[240] and there were a total of 50 pregnancies that occurred in 31 women. The majority (66%) had only one pregnancy, 19% had two pregnancies, and 16% had three pregnancies or more. A total of 36 pregnancies reached the third trimester, of which three (8%) ended prematurely. Based on their experience, they feel that the obstetrical results following radical trachelectomy are very encouraging and larger trials are needed.

If surgery is contraindicated, these patients can be treated with radiation alone, usually with pelvic radiation therapy plus brachytherapy. However, in special situations, brachytherapy alone may be sufficient in controlling disease. Hamberger and colleagues reported that all patients with stage IA disease and 96% of patients (89 of 93) with small stage IB disease (<1 cervical quadrant involved) were disease free 5 years after treatment using intracavitary irradiation alone.[241]

Stage IB1 and Small Stage IIA Disease

Treatment of invasive carcinoma or carcinoma of FIGO stage IB or greater is determined on the basis of tumor size and the presence or absence of lymph node metastases (Fig. 98-5).

Stage IB1 tumors, which are less than 4 cm in size, are considered small; however, they are associated with a significant risk of microscopic paracervical extension or lymph node metastasis. In a prospective study in patients treated with radical hysterectomy who had clinically estimated maximum tumor diameter less than 3 cm, the GOG reported that 16% of the patients (42 of 261) had lymph node metastases.[242] Landoni and colleagues found a 25% incidence of positive nodes (28 of 114 patients) in patients treated with radical hysterectomy for stage IB-IIA tumors that measured 4 cm or less on initial clinical examination.[208] Therefore, for patients with stage IB1 or small IIA (<4 cm diameter) disease, the treatment is either type III (radical) hysterectomy plus bilateral pelvic lymphadenectomy or radical radiation therapy. The goal of both of these treatment options is to destroy malignant cells in the cervix, paracervical tissues, and regional lymph nodes.

Overall survival rates for patients with stage IB1 or small IIA disease treated with either surgery or radiation therapy are usually in the range of 80-90%, suggesting that the two treatments are equally effective. However, only one prospective randomized trial has compared the two treatments directly.[208] In this study, patients with IB or IIA disease were randomized to receive either radical hysterectomy or radical radiation therapy. In the surgery arm, patients who had parametrial involvement, positive margins, deep stromal invasion, or positive nodes in the surgical specimen received postoperative pelvic radiation therapy. There were no significant differences in the rates of relapse or survival between the two arms, but the overall rate of grade 2 and 3 complications was greater for patients treated with hysterectomy. The dose of radiation therapy received by patients in the radiation therapy arms (76 Gy at point A) was low by conventional standards.

For patients with stage IB1 squamous carcinomas, the choice of treatment is based primarily on patient preference, anesthetic and surgical risks, physician preference, and an understanding of the nature and incidence of complications with radiation therapy and hysterectomy. For patients with similar tumors, the overall rate of major complications is similar with surgery and radiation therapy, although urinary tract complications tend to be more frequent after surgical treatment, and bowel complications are more common after radiation therapy. Surgical treatment tends to be preferred for young women with small tumors because it permits preservation of ovarian function and may cause less vaginal shortening. Radiation therapy is often selected for older, postmenopausal women to avoid the morbidity of a major surgical procedure.

The role of pelvic radiation therapy after radical hysterectomy is still being defined. The GOG, in a prospective trial, randomized patients with intermediate-risk of recurrence after radical hysterectomy for stage IB carcinoma to pelvic irradiation or no further treatment.[243] Patients were eligible if they had at least two of the following risk factors: greater than one-third stromal invasion, LVSI, or clinical tumor diameter of at least 4 cm. Patients with positive pelvic nodes were excluded. The authors reported a 47% reduction in the risk of recurrence when postoperative pelvic irradiation was given (15% vs 28%, $p = .008$). In this preliminary analysis, follow-up was too immature for a significance level to be assigned to the overall survival comparison, but there were 18 deaths (13%) in the radiation therapy arm versus 30 deaths (21%) in the no-further-therapy arm. An update of this study was recently published in 2006. In the update, radiation therapy continued to statistically reduce the risk of recurrence and the risk of progression or death from disease, however, there was not a statistical difference in overall survival between the two groups ($p = .074$).[244] The conclusions by the authors are that pelvic radiotherapy after radical surgery significantly reduces the risk of recurrence and prolongs PFS in women with stage IB cervical cancer, particularly in patients with adenocarcinoma or adenosquamous histologies.[244] The Southwest Oncology Group reported the results of a randomized trial of patients treated with radical hysterectomy followed by radiation therapy versus radiation therapy plus cisplatin-based chemotherapy. To be eligible, patients had to have pelvic lymph node metastases, parametrial involvement, or involved surgical margins. The authors found that patients who received radiation therapy plus chemotherapy had a significant improvement in survival compared with the survival of patients treated with radiation alone.[154]

Most practitioners agree that patients who have more than one positive lymph node, parametrial involvement, or positive margins require postoperative radiation therapy; however, the risk of late side effects is much higher with combined therapy (surgery plus radiation therapy) than with radiation therapy alone. A National Institutes of Health panel in 1996 concluded that "to minimize morbidity, primary therapy should avoid the routine use of both radical surgery and radiation therapy." However, if radiation therapy needs to be given after surgery, IMRT may help minimize the dose to small bowel and, therefore, hopefully reduce late complication (Fig. 98-18). Therefore, if a patient's initial work-up suggests that there is a high likelihood of parametrial invasion, deep stromal invasion, or lymph node metastases, strong consideration should be given to treating the patient with radiation therapy alone or with chemoradiation in select cases.

Stage IB2 Disease

Patients with tumors greater than 4 cm in diameter whose para-aortic lymph nodes are found to be free of disease have excellent survival rates when treated with whole-pelvis EBRT plus brachytherapy. However, these tumors appear on clinical examination to be technically resectable, and the ideal management of these tumors is a subject of considerable controversy. The approach to these tumors differs widely between centers, and the biases are so large that the GOG closed a trial early owing to a lack of accrual that compared surgery plus chemoradiation versus chemoradiation alone.

Although radiation therapy is effective for many patients with stage IB2 disease, central disease recurrences occur in at least 8-10% of patients with bulky endocervical cancers.[209,226,227] The literature contains numerous reports on the use of an adjunctive hysterectomy for patients with bulky endocervical carcinomas treated with primary radiation therapy. In 1991, Mendenhall and colleagues reported on the outcome of patients treated at the University of Florida before or after clinicians began to add adjuvant hysterectomy to the treatment of bulky (>6 cm) endocervical tumors.[245] They found no difference in pelvic disease control or survival rates with the two treatment policies, but they reported higher complication rates for patients who underwent adjuvant hysterectomy (18% vs 6%, $p = .027$). The GOG completed a trial in 1990 that compared using radiation alone versus radiation plus extrafascial hysterectomy in patients with stage IB cancers measuring 4 cm or more in diameter. In a 1997 abstract about this trial, Keys and colleagues reported no difference in overall survival rates between the two arms, but the final report of this trial has not yet been published.[246] At MD Anderson, at this time, extrafascial hysterectomy is used only if the optimal brachytherapy dose cannot be obtained because of multiple large fibroids in the uterus.

Several investigators recommend treating these tumors with initial surgery followed by postoperative radiation therapy or chemoradiation depending on the pathology findings. In a randomized trial by Landoni and colleagues, patients with stage IB2 tumors were randomized to initial surgery versus definitive radiation therapy.[208] In this trial, 84% of the patients treated with initial surgery required postoperative radiation therapy, which contributed to a higher complication rate in that arm. The overall survival rates were similar for patients treated with initial surgery or radiation, but the patients in the radiation arm received more protracted, lower-dose treatments than those recommended by most current experts in the field. A study recently published by Peters and colleagues suggested that chemoradiation should be considered standard therapy for patients with stage IB2 disease following initial surgery.[154]

Recently, several trials have been initiated to study the role of induction chemotherapy before surgical exploration in patients with bulky lesions who would otherwise be poor candidates for radical hysterectomy. In one trial, 205 patients with stage IB cervical cancer underwent surgery with or without an initial course of chemotherapy (cisplatin, vincristine, and bleomycin); all patients also received postoperative radiation therapy.[247] The authors reported that tumors treated with chemotherapy were more often resectable and that the 5-year survival rate of patients who had received neoadjuvant chemotherapy was better (81% vs 66%, $p < .05$). The GOG has recently closed a study also looking at neoadjuvant chemotherapy prior

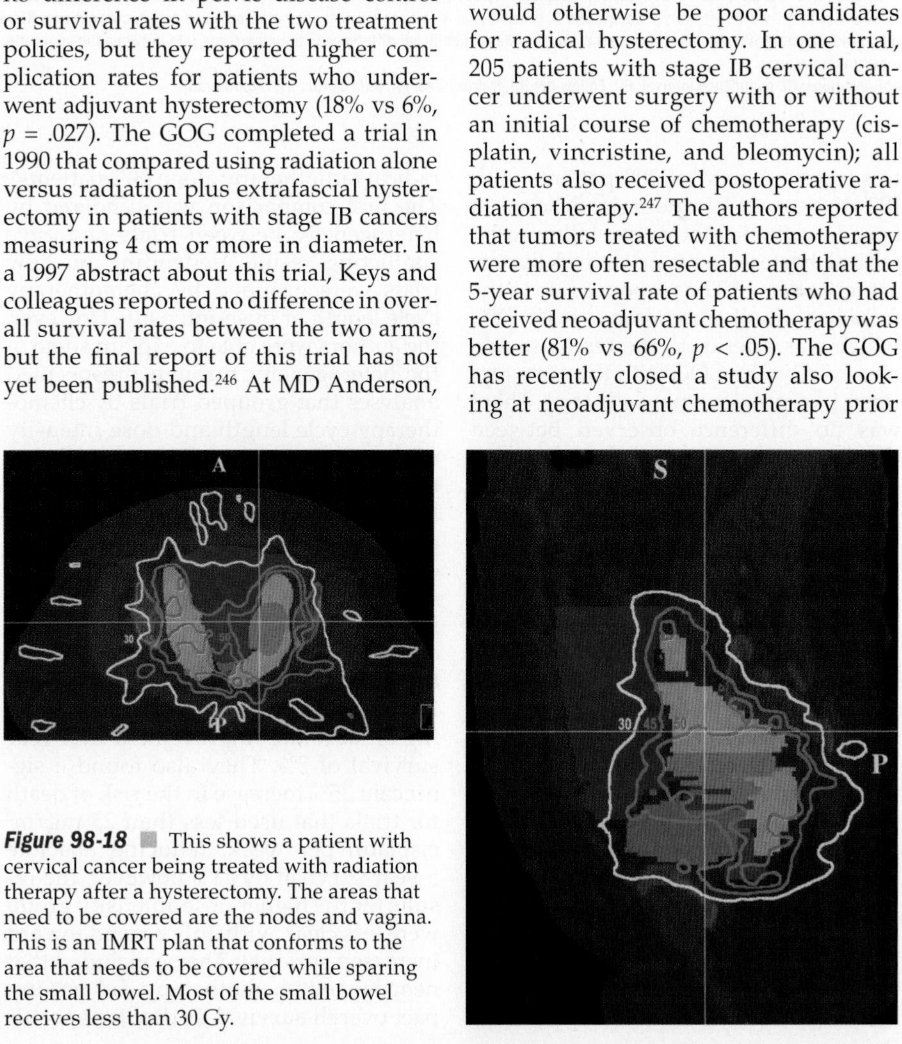

Figure 98-18 This shows a patient with cervical cancer being treated with radiation therapy after a hysterectomy. The areas that need to be covered are the nodes and vagina. This is an IMRT plan that conforms to the area that needs to be covered while sparing the small bowel. Most of the small bowel receives less than 30 Gy.

Table 98-6 **Prospective Randomized Trials: Role of Concurrent Radiotherapy and Cisplatin-Containing Chemotherapy[a]**

First Author (Ref.)	Eligibility	Patients (No.)	CT: Investigational Arm	CT: Control Arm	Relative Risk of Recurrence (90% CI)	*p* Values
Rose (229)	FIGO IIB-IVA	526	Cisplatin 40 mg/m²/wk (up to 6 cycles)	HU 3 g/m² (2×/wk)	0.57 (0.42-0.78)	<.001
			Cisplatin 50 mg/m²; 5-FU 4 g/m²/96 h; HU 2 g/m² (2×/wk) (2 cycles)	HU 3 g/m² (2×/wk)	0.55 (0.40-0.75)	<.001
Morris (227)	FIGO IB-IIA (≥5 cm); IIB-IVA or pelvic nodes involved	403	Cisplatin 75 mg/m²; 5-FU 4 g/m²/96 h (3 cycles)	None[a]	0.48 (0.35-0.66)	<.001
Keys (226)	FIGO IB (≥4 cm)	369	Cisplatin 40 mg/m²/wk (up to 6 cycles)	None[b]	0.51 (0.34-0.75)	.001
Whitney (230)	FIGO IIB-IVA	368	Cisplatin 50 mg/m²; 5-FU 4 g/m²/96 h (2 cycles)	HU 3 g/m² (2×/wk)	0.79 (0.62-0.99)	.03
Peters (152)	FIGO I-IIA after radical hysterectomy with nodes, margins, or parametrium positive	268	Cisplatin 50 mg/m²; 5-FU 4 g/m²/96 h (2 cycles)	None	0.50 (0.29-0.84)	.01
Pearcey (248)	FIGO IB-IIA (≥5 cm), IIB-IVA or pelvic nodes involved	259	Cisplatin 40 mg/m²/wk (up to 6 cycles)	None	0.91 (0.62-1.35)[c]	.43
Wong (250)	FIGO IB-IIA (>4 cm), IIB-III	220	Epirubicin 60 mg/m², then 90 mg/m² q4 wks for 5 more cycles[d]	None	~0.65	.02
Thomas (312)	FIGO IB-IIA	234	5-FU 4 g/m² over 96 h ×2	None	NS	
Lorvidhaya (251)[e]	FIGO IB-IVA	926	Mitomycin-C 10 mg/m² day 1 and 29 Oral 5-FU 300 mg/day days 1-14 and 29-42	None	0.001	

Results from prospective randomized trials that investigate the role of concurrent radiotherapy and cisplatin-containing chemotherapy for patients with locoregionally advanced cervical cancer.
[a]Patients in control arm had prophylactic para-aortic irradiation.
[b]All patients had extrafascial hysterectomy after radiotherapy.
[c]Survival.
[d]Chemotherapy was begun on day 1 and continued every 4 weeks throughout and after radiation therapy.
[e]This study had four arms: arm 1, conventional radiation therapy (RT); arm 2, conventional RT with adjuvant chemotherapy consisting of 5-FU orally at 200 mg/day given for 3 courses of 4 weeks, with a 2-week rest every 6 weeks; arm 3, conventional RT with concurrent chemotherapy; and arm 4, conventional RT with concurrent and adjuvant chemotherapy. The addition of adjuvant therapy did not affect recurrence, but here was a significant difference in the recurrence rate between the conventional RT and the conventional RT plus concurrent chemotherapy arms.
Abbreviations: CI, confidence interval; FU, Follow-up; HU, hydroxyurea; PA, para-aortic; RT, radiotherapy.

to surgery. A total of 288 patients with IB2 disease were randomized between neoadjuvant chemotherapy followed by radical hysterectomy or radical hysterectomy alone.[248] The response rate to the neoadjuvant chemotherapy was 52%, which was inferior to the response rate observed by the GOG with the same regimen in a previous phase II trial. There was no difference observed between the two arms in the rate of surgery performed (79% chemo + surgery vs 78% surgery), in the surgical-pathological findings and specifically in progressive free-survival (56% chemo + surgery vs 54% surgery) and overall survival (63% chemo + surgery vs 61% surgery) at 5 years. These results have led the GOG to recommend that neoadjuvant chemotherapy prior to surgery be avoided in any future trials.[248] A recent meta-analysis[249] collected individual patient data from 21 randomized trials of neoadjuvant chemotherapy in locally advanced cervical cancer. This analysis included data from comparison of the benefits of neoadjuvant chemotherapy followed by radical radiotherapy versus radical radiotherapy alone (2074), and for comparison of neoadjuvant chemotherapy followed by surgery (±radiotherapy) versus radical radiotherapy alone (872 patients). The first comparison was hindered by heterogeneity between trials and gave conflicting results depending on how trials were grouped by chemotherapy cycle length or dose-intensity. However, the authors were able to explain some of the heterogeneity through prespecified analyses that grouped trials by chemotherapy cycle length and dose-intensity of the cisplatin used. They found that the group of trials using cycles lasting longer than 14 days showed a significant 25% increase in the relative risk of death with neoadjuvant chemotherapy, representing an absolute 8% reduction in 5-year survival compared to shorter chemotherapy cycle lengths, where there was a significant 17% decrease in the relative risk of death, representing an absolute improvement in 5-year survival of 7%. They also found a significant 35% increase in the risk of death for trials that used less than 25 mg/m² cisplatin per week, reducing absolute 5-year survival by 11% however, the results for the higher dose-intensity group were less clear, with only a trend toward increased survival. They concluded that neoadjuvant chemotherapy did not impact overall survival or disease-specific survival to radiation therapy alone.[250] The second comparison showed that patients treated with neoadjuvant chemotherapy had a highly significant 35% reduction in the risk of death ($p = .0004$) that translated into a 14% absolute increase in 5-year overall survival. Unfortunately, this meta-analysis only included trials prior to 1999, when radiotherapy alone was still the standard treatment. Furthermore, it included two trials where all the patients received postoperative radiation therapy, two trials where at least 30% received radiation therapy and 50% of the patients came from the Italian trial where there was poor radiation therapy and prolonged treatment.[251] Ultimately, however, this approach may need to be compared with optimized chemoradiation to determine the most effective, least toxic therapy for these patients. The EORTC (European Organisation for Research and Treatment of Cancer) is currently running a trial addressing this specific question. Patients with IB2 cancers are being randomized to neoadjuvant chemotherapy followed by radiation or current chemotherapy and radiation. Another trial presently underway at Tata Memorial Hospital is randomizing approximately

700 patients with IB2 and IIB disease to weekly cisplatin and radiation therapy or three cycles of carboplatin and taxol followed by surgery. Hopefully these two large trials will help to resolve the role of neoadjuvant chemotherapy.

Two prospective randomized trials[228,229] indicate that patients who are treated with radiation for bulky central disease benefit from concurrent administration of cisplatin-containing chemotherapy. A third study suggests that patients who require postoperative radiotherapy because of findings of lymph node metastasis or involved surgical margins also benefit from concurrent chemoradiation.[252] These studies are discussed in more detail in the section "Concurrent Chemoradiation," later in this chapter. Patients who have stage IB1 cancers without evidence of regional involvement have excellent pelvic control rates (approximately 97% at 5 years) with radiotherapy alone and probably do not require chemotherapy when they are treated with primary radiotherapy.[209,227]

Stage IIB-IVA Disease

Radiation therapy is the primary local treatment of most patients with locoregionally advanced (stages IIIB-IVA) cervical carcinoma. The success of treatment depends on a careful balance between EBRT and brachytherapy that optimizes the dose to tumor and normal tissues and on the overall duration of treatment. Five-year survival rates of 65-75%, 35-50%, and 15-20% are reported for patients treated with radiation therapy alone for stage IIB, IIIB, and IV tumors, respectively.[148,149,230] In the French Cooperative Group study of 1875 patients treated with radiation therapy according to Fletcher guidelines, Barillot and colleagues reported 5-year survival rates of 70%, 45%, and 10% for patients with stage IIB, IIIB, and IVA tumors, respectively (Table 98-7).[149]

Local and distant disease recurrences continue to be a problem for patients with locally advanced disease. Neoadjuvant chemotherapy has produced excellent tumor responses; however, randomized trials have failed to demonstrate improvements in survival. In fact, in two trials, the survival rates were actually poorer when neoadjuvant chemotherapy was added to radiation therapy. Other approaches that have been used to try to improve outcome in these patients, including neutrons, hyperbaric oxygen, and hypoxic cell sensitizers, have also produced disappointing results.

Table 98-7 5-Year Survival Rates After Pelvic Exenteration: A Review of the Literature

Source	Patients (n)	5-Year Survival (%)
Bricker[306]	153	34.6
Symmonds[271]	198	32.0
Rutledge[269]	448	41.0
Ketcham[307]	162	38.0
Orr[270]	104	45.3
Morley[308]	100	61
Shingleton[309]	143	50
Magrina[310]	133	41

Concurrent Chemoradiation

In 1999, five prospective randomized trials involving patients with locoregionally advanced cervical cancer,[228,229,231,232,252] provided compelling evidence that the addition of concurrent cisplatin-containing chemotherapy to standard radiotherapy reduces the risk of disease recurrence by as much as 50%, and thereby improves the rates of pelvic disease control and survival (Table 98-8).

In two studies,[231,232] the GOG randomly assigned patients with stages IIB-IVA disease to receive either hydroxyurea or cisplatin-containing chemotherapy during external beam irradiation. All three of the cisplatin-containing regimens in these trials produced local control and survival rates superior to those for the control (hydroxyurea and radiation). In a third study,[228] patients with stage IB tumors measuring at least 4 cm in diameter were randomly assigned to receive radiation alone or radiation plus weekly cisplatin before an extrafascial hysterectomy. Patients who received cisplatin were more likely to have a complete histologic response and were more likely to be disease free at the time of preliminary analysis. A fourth study,[252] sponsored by the Southwest Oncology Group and the GOG, included patients who were treated with radical hysterectomy and were found to have pelvic lymph node metastases, positive margins, or parametrial involvement. Patients were randomly assigned to receive postoperative pelvic irradiation, alone or combined with cisplatin and fluorouracil (5-FU). In a preliminary analysis, patients who received chemotherapy in this study also had a better disease-free survival rate. An update of this trial found continued improvement of survival of chemotherapy and radiation therapy compared to radiation therapy alone at 5 years, however the benefit of the chemotherapy to the radiation therapy in a univariate analysis was less significant in tumors size <2 cm and patients with only one node positive.[253] The absolute improvement in 5-year survival for adjuvant chemotherapy in patients with tumors ≤2 cm was only 5% (77% vs 82%), while for those with tumors > 2 cm it was 19% (58% vs 77%). Similarly, the absolute 5-year survival benefit was less evident among patients with one nodal metastasis (79% vs 83%) than when at least two nodes were positive (55% vs 75%).[253]

Table 98-8 Single-Agent Chemotherapy for Cervical Cancer

Agent	Response (%)
Alkylating agents	
Cyclophosphamide	38/251 (15)
Chlorambucil	11/44 (25)
Melphalan	4/20 (20)
Ifosfamide	35/157 (22)
Mitolactol	16/55 (29)
Heavy metal complexes	
Cisplatin	190/815 (23)
Carboplatin	27/175 (15)
Antitumor antibiotics	
Doxorubicin	45/266 (17)
Bleomycin	19/176 (11)
Mitomycin	5/23 (22)
Antimetabolites	
Fluorouracil	29/142 (20)
Methotrexate	17/96 (18)
Hydroxyurea	0/14 (0)
Plant alkaloids	
Vincristine	10/55 (18)
Vinblastine	2/20 (10)
Etoposide	0/31 (0)
Miscellaneous agents	
Altretamine	12/64 (19)
Irinotecan (CPT-11)	36/192 (19)
Paclitaxel	14/74 (19)
Docetaxel	1/13 (8)
Topotecan	8/43 (19)
Hexamethylmelamine	12/64 (19)
Razoxane	5/28 (18)

Source: Data from Refs. 313–317.

During the same interval, the Radiation Therapy Oncology Group (RTOG)[229] conducted a trial in which radiotherapy alone was compared with pelvic irradiation (including prophylactic para-aortic irradiation) plus concurrent cisplatin and 5-FU. This study demonstrated a significant improvement in outcome for patients with stages III or IV disease as well as for patients with stages IB2 or II cervical cancer with concurrent chemotherapy. There was no significant difference in the incidence of late treatment-related complications.[229] An update of this trial, with a median follow-up period of 6.6 years for the surviving patients,[228] reported that the overall survival rate for patients treated with chemotherapy and radiation therapy compared to radiation therapy was still significantly better (67% vs 41% at 8 years, $p = < .0001$) and the conclusions by the authors was that chemotherapy with radiation therapy significantly improved the survival rate of women with locally advanced cervical cancer without increasing the rate of late treatment-related side effects.[254] Only one large randomized trial has failed to demonstrate a significant advantage from concurrent cisplatin-based chemotherapy in cervical cancer patients. This trial was published by Pearcey and colleagues in 2002.[255] The authors suggest that difference in technique could explain the difference between their results and the results of the five earlier trials, although the survival rate in their control arm indicated that the margin for improvement was smaller than that in the earlier trials. This trial was also the smallest of the six trials.

Taken together, the randomized trials provide strong evidence that the addition of concurrent cisplatin-containing chemotherapy to pelvic radiotherapy benefits selected patients with locally advanced cervical cancer. It remains to be resolved whether or not 5-FU plays a significant role. The combination of cisplatin plus FU was tested in four of the trials (RTOG 90-01, GOG 85, GOG 120, and Southwest Oncology Group [SWOG] 8797). In GOG 120, the frequency of grade 3 and 4 leukopenia was significantly higher in the arm with cisplatin/5FU and hydroxyurea compared to the arm with cisplatin and hydroxyurea alone, with equal effectiveness. Therefore, it was felt that cisplatin alone was equally effective as cisplatin-5FU and less toxic, although there has been no adequately powered direct randomized comparison of these two regimens without hydroxyurea.

A meta-analysis of 18 trials[256] with concurrent chemotherapy and radiation (4580 patients) in patients with cervical cancer concluded that concomitant chemotherapy and radiotherapy improved overall and PFS and reduced local and distant recurrence in selected patients with cervical cancer. Concomitant chemotherapy and radiation therapy produced a 12% absolute increase in survival with greater evidence of benefit in the trials using platinum-based chemotherapy than in those with nonplatinum-based chemotherapy.[245] More recently, a systematic review and meta-analysis based on individual patient data (IPD)[250] has documented a 7% absolute improvement in 5-year survival. The benefits were similar in the trials using platinum and nonplatinum chemoradiotherapy.[250] In this analysis, there is a suggestion that the magnitude of benefit with chemoradiotherapy varies according to stage, but not to other patients characteristics, suggesting a greater benefit in patients with early-stage disease compared to stage III and IV disease.[250] Currently in India, there is a large trial in progress comparing weekly cisplatin-based chemoradiotherapy with radiotherapy alone in women with FIGO stage IIIB cervical cancer. This trial will include a total of 850 patients and should provide a clear indication of the effect of cisplatin-based chemoradiotherapy in advanced cervical cancer. In the future, clinicians will be challenged to determine how these favorable results can be generalized to patients with cervical cancer who may not have been included in the prospective trials because of severe medical or social problems and to the developing nations where invasive cervical cancer is epidemic and where more patients present with locally advanced disease.

These studies raise other interesting questions that will undoubtedly be the subjects of future studies. Although North American studies have emphasized cisplatin-containing regimens, investigators in Southeast Asia have reported improved outcome when radiation was combined with epirubicin[257] or mitomycin and 5-FU.[258] Other drugs that are being studied for their radiosensitizing effects in patients with advanced disease are paclitaxel,[259] carboplatin,[260] nedaplatin,[261] topotecan,[262] and multiple biologic response modifiers. Another large study from Thailand, randomized 469 patients with locally advanced cervical cancer between concurrent weekly carboplatin and radiation therapy versus Tegafur-Uracil (an oral 5-FU agent), weekly carboplatin and radiation therapy. No difference was found between these two arms, concluding that weekly carboplatin with radiation therapy was effective in tumor control with acceptable toxicity and survival outcome.[263] Other ongoing randomized trials are investigating ways to enhance the benefits of standard weekly cisplatin-based chemotherapy. The GOG is presently conducting a phase III trial with platinum and tirapazamine in an attempt to sensitize hypoxic cells. They are also evaluating the addition of the ani-EGFR antibody C225 (Cetixumab) to cisplatin in patients with locally advanced cervical cancer, including patients with positive para-aortic nodes. The RTOG has completed a phase II trial looking at celebrex with a combination weekly cisplatin and radiation therapy and found no advantage with this regime[264] and presently are running a phase II trial evaluating avastin with weekly cisplatin and radiation therapy.

Metastatic Disease

Metastatic cancer in the para-aortic lymph nodes can be confirmed with fine-needle aspiration, laparoscopy, or extraperitoneal laparotomy. Laparoscopy and laparotomy, using the extraperitoneal approach, allows the removal of positive nodes and sampling of other para-aortic nodes, which may enhance control with radiation therapy and help design the treatment field.

The superior boundary of the extended EBRT portal provides a margin of 3 cm above the most cephalad of the positive nodes. The superior boundary limit is the T12 vertebra. Currently, patients with positive pelvic nodes or low common iliac nodes may have the field extended to the L1–L2 interspace.

Patients with para-aortic lymph node involvement can be treated effectively with extended-field irradiation. Five-year survival rates range from 25% to 50%.[265-267] The value of prophylactic extended-field irradiation was tested in two randomized trials. The RTOG studied 367 patients with stages 1B and IIA cancers greater than 4 cm in diameter or stage IIB disease in a randomized study. These patients received standard pelvic irradiation or extended-field radiation therapy prior to brachytherapy.[268] Patients treated with extended-field radiation therapy (45 Gy up to L1-L2) had a better absolute survival rate than did those treated with standard pelvic irradiation (67% vs 55% at 5 years), but there was no significant difference in the disease-free survival rates. Para-aortic recurrences were not analyzed separately, and there was no standard method of assessing initial node status.[81]

Another trial from the European Organisation for Research and Treatment of Cancer involved a similar randomization of patients between pelvic irradiation and extended-field irradiation (45 Gy up to L1-T12).[269] Twelve centers entered 441 patients. Two hundred and twenty eight patients underwent irradiation of the pelvis, and 213 underwent irradiation of the pelvis and para-aortic nodes. There was no statistically significant difference between the two treatment arms in terms of local control, overall distant metastases, and survival. The subset that received pelvic irradiation alone, which controlled the pelvic disease, had a higher incidence of subsequent para-aortic and distant disease. The incidence of enteric complications in this study was high, and the authors concluded that routine para-aortic irradiation for all high-risk patients with cervical carcinoma are of limited value.

The role of concurrent chemotherapy with extended-field irradiation has been evaluated in several phase II studies. Although side effects are greater when treatment fields are enlarged, combined therapy may be tolerable if careful consideration is given to the chemotherapy regimen, volume of tissue irradiated, and other factors that might increase the risk of serious toxicity. The RTOG studied the efficacy of twice-daily external irradiation to the pelvis and para-aortic field with concurrent chemotherapy consisting of cisplatin and fluorouracil. They concluded that this regimen had an unacceptably high rate (17%, 5 of 29) of grade 4 late side effects, and survival estimates were no better than with standard-fractionation irradiation without chemotherapy.[270] The GOG did a study combining once-daily extended-field irradiation with cisplatin and fluorouracil. Their treatment was better tolerated than that of the RTOG; however, their treatment time was more protracted, toxicity was still significant (18.6% grades 3-4 gastrointestinal toxicity, and 7 of 86 patients with late rectal toxicity), and there were numerous protocol deviations. However, the authors concluded that extended-field irradiation can be given safely with concurrent chemotherapy.[271] Malfetano and colleagues reported results of a combination of extended-field irradiation with weekly cisplatin (1 mg/kg, not to exceed 60 mg) in patients with negative para-aortic nodes.[272] The dose used in their regimen was similar to the 40 mg/m^2 used in the GOG with pelvic radiation and appeared to be well tolerated. The RTOG is evaluating extended-field radiation therapy and weekly cisplatin with or without amifostine therapy. In 26 patients treated with extended-field radiation therapy and weekly cisplatin, 81% experienced grades 3-4 acute nonhematologic toxicity and 40% grades 3-4 late toxicity. Eight patients underwent surgery for complications.[273] Results of treatment with amifostine has not yet been reported. In conclusion, it is tempting to extrapolate from the results achieved with combinations of pelvic radiation and chemotherapy; however, patients need to be informed that the cost-benefit ratio of concurrent chemotherapy and extended-field irradiation has not been formally tested.

Unsuspected Invasive Cancer Discovered After Simple Hysterectomy

Sometimes the pathologist discovers unsuspected invasive cervical carcinoma in the tissue specimen in patients who undergo hysterectomy for what is presumed to be a benign pelvic condition. Many factors can lead to such an event.[274] A false-negative Pap smear provides little opportunity for the gynecologist to avoid such events; however, the following oversights are avoidable: failure to evaluate an abnormal Pap smear, failure to perform a conization when indicated, and proceeding with a hysterectomy when there is a positive cone margin.

Patients with unsuspected invasive cervical carcinoma detected after simple hysterectomy have been classified in five groups according to the amount of disease and presentation: (1) microinvasive cancer, (2) tumor confined to the cervix with negative surgical margins, (3) positive surgical margins but no gross residual tumor, (4) gross residual tumor by clinical examination documented by biopsy, and (5) patients referred for treatment more than 6 months after hysterectomy (usually for recurrent disease).[275] The therapy plan is based on the amount of residual disease. Patients with minimal invasion and no residual disease require at most brachytherapy to the vaginal apex; patients with gross disease at the specimen margin require full-intensity therapy. Patients with minimal or no known gross residual disease (groups 1-3) have excellent 5-year survival rates (59-79%), whereas rates for patients with gross residual disease (groups 4 and 5) are poorer (in the range of only 41%).[276] The value of chemoradiation is unproven in this setting; however, in patients with gross disease, it is probably reasonable to add chemotherapy because of the relatively high local recurrence rates after radiation therapy alone.

Recurrent Disease

Prognostic Factors ■ Various clinicopathologic features have been associated with adverse outcomes in patients with recurrent cervical carcinoma in the pelvis; however, the relatively small numbers of patients and the heterogeneity of clinical and treatment parameters in most series preclude detailed statistical analysis of these factors. Two clinical factors commonly correlated with the probability of the success of salvage therapy are the location (central vs side wall involvement) and the size of the recurrent pelvic tumor.[277] The presence of nodal disease in conjunction with pelvic relapse portends a dismal outcome; other unfavorable clinical variables include nonsquamous histologies (particularly adenocarcinomas) and a higher FIGO stage at the time of diagnosis of the primary tumor.[278] Controversial factors include the interval between primary therapy and relapse and symptomatic versus asymptomatic pelvic failures.[212,278,279]

Radical Hysterectomy ■ In rare, carefully selected patients initially treated with primary radiation therapy, radical hysterectomy for salvage may be a feasible alternative to exenterative surgery. Coleman and colleagues reported 50 patients who underwent radical hysterectomy for persistent or recurrent disease after definitive radiation therapy.[280] The 5-year and 10-year survival rates were 72% and 60%, respectively. Severe complications were noted in 64% of patients, and 42% of patients had permanent complications. The authors concluded that radical hysterectomy was an alternative to exenteration in patients with small, centrally recurrent cervical cancer, but that it should be used only in carefully selected patients.[280]

Pelvic Exenteration ■ Pelvic exenteration is a potentially curative procedure for patients who, following radiation therapy, have a central pelvic recurrence or a new primary tumor in the irradiated field.[281-283] Advances in surgical technique, anesthesia, and postoperative care have decreased intraoperative and postoperative complications, and thus have greatly reduced operative mortality.[274,282,283] Advances in ostomy appliances and care have given patients the opportunity to live a nearly normal life and to be able to meet their personal needs and responsibilities after surgery. The type of exenteration is determined by the anatomical site of the cancer (Fig. 98-19).

Anterior Exenteration ■ Anterior exenteration encompasses the removal of the uterus, adnexa, bladder, urethra, and vagina. Patients selected for this operation have cancers that are sufficiently anterior to allow clearance of the rectum and do not extend to involve the vaginal apex or the posterior vaginal wall. Vaginal reconstruction is performed as indicated.

Posterior Exenteration ■ In posterior exenteration, the uterus, adnexa, anus, rectosigmoid colon, levator muscles, and vagina are removed. Many gynecologic oncologists leave a portion of the anterior vaginal wall to support the urethra, and this can lessen postoperative urinary incontinence. This procedure is performed in patients with lesions confined to the posterior vaginal wall and rectovaginal septum.

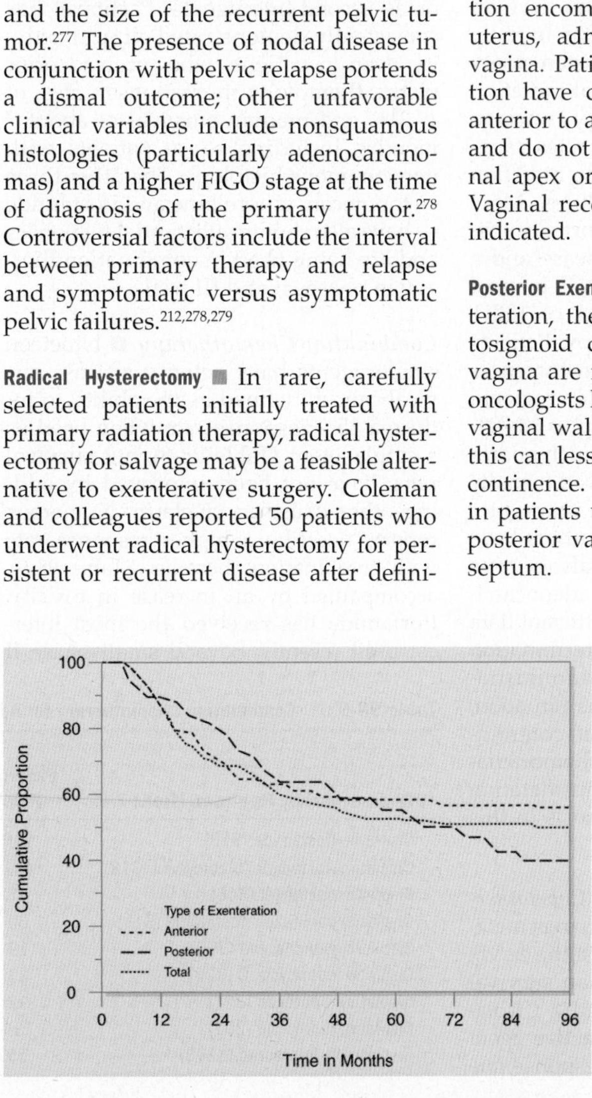

Figure 98-19 ■ Survival curves are shown to compare the three types of exenterations performed in an MD Anderson series (1955–1984). Although the curves are similar, it should be noted that posterior exenteration is performed more frequently than the other procedures for vulvar and anorectal cancer and is associated with more local cancer recurrences. *Source:* From Ref. 281.

Total Pelvic Exenteration ■ In total pelvic exenteration, the uterus, adnexa, bladder and urethra, vagina, rectosigmoid colon, levatores, and anus are all removed. Patients treated with this procedure usually have lesions that are central or involve the upper half of the vagina. Contiguous extension to the base of the bladder and rectovaginal septum leaves no opportunity to perform a less extensive operation. Vaginal reconstruction is performed for functional purposes and to aid in the reconstruction of the pelvic floor. An omental pedicled graft is required to aid in reconstruction of the pelvic floor, and this technique for bringing in a new blood supply has been a major factor in reducing postoperative complications.[284] In both anterior and total pelvic exenteration, a continent urinary conduit can be constructed.

Total pelvic exenteration is widely used, and 5-year survival rates of 40-50% can be expected (Table 98-7). At MD Anderson, a total of 448 exenterations were done from 1955 to 1984 and reported by Rutledge.[281] The 5-year survival rates for patients treated with exenteration are shown in Figure 98-19.

Radiation Therapy ■ Patients who have an isolated pelvic recurrence after initially being treated with a radical hysterectomy should be treated with radical radiation therapy. A literature review by Lanciano found disease-free survival rates ranging from 20% to 50% following radiation therapy for locoregional failures. More favorable outcomes were reported in patients with small-volume disease and a central pelvic relapse location.[277] In most patients, treatment consisted of EBRT with or without brachytherapy. Patients who have isolated central recurrences without pelvic wall fixation or regional metastasis can be cured in up to 60-70% of cases.[279] The prognosis is much poorer when the pelvic wall is involved (usually 10-20% of patients survive 5 years after radiation therapy). Several authors have reported significantly lower salvage rates in patients with recurrent adenocarcinoma of the cervix.[279,285] Insufficient data are available to permit determination of the benefit of concurrent administration of chemotherapy in this situation; however, in patients without contraindications to chemotherapy, chemoradiation may be a reasonable consideration given the overall poor prognosis in this population.[278,285,286]

Chemotherapy ■ *Single-Agent Chemotherapy* ■ Using chemotherapy to treat metastatic or recurrent carcinoma of the cervix is relatively ineffective. Median survival ranges between 4 and 8 months. Cisplatin is regarded as the most active agent in cancer of the cervix. The response rate is 17-21%.[287,288] Doses used range from 50 to 100 mg/m^2. Bonomi and colleagues276 compared 50-100 mg/m^2 and noted that the higher dose was associated with a better partial response rate (31% vs 21%) and a slightly better complete response rate (13% vs 10%). Response duration, PFS, and survival measures failed to improve with the higher dose.[288] Carboplatin given at 340-400 mg/m^2 every 28 days to 175 patients induced a complete response in 10 (5.7%).[289] The total response rate for carboplatin from a number of studies is 19%.

Ifosfamide has been studied as a single-agent in patients with recurrent cervical cancer in at least five phase II trials.[290-294] Response rates ranged between 33% and 50% in three studies that were conducted in patients who had received no previous chemotherapy.[292-295] However, the response rates were much lower in two phase II trials that included patients who had received prior systemic chemotherapy, with only three partial responses (8%) seen in 36 patients.[290,291]

The most active single agents include cisplatin, paclitaxel, topotecan, vinorelbine, and ifosfamide. These can be considered alone in patients who are not candidates for combination therapy or as second-line agents. Paclitaxel has consistently demonstrated clinical activity, even in patients who received prior platin therapy with response rates of 17-31% and median survival of about 7 months, including those patients with nonsquamous histology. The other three — topotecan, vinorelbine and ifosfamide — have also shown substantial responses and are being used in combination therapy in phases II and III trials.

Combination Chemotherapy ■ Nineteen single agents have activity against cervical cancer, defined as the ability to induce a 15% response rate when used as a single-agent (Table 98-8), but survival rates have not been improved by adding other drugs to cisplatin. Numerous reports describe a higher response rate with combination therapies (Table 98-9), accompanied by an increase in toxicity. Ifosfamide has received the most interest until recently. Several small phase II studies evaluated treatment with combinations of ifosfamide and either cisplatin or carboplatin in patients who had not received radiotherapy. Response rates for these combinations ranged between 50% and 62%.[296-299] A number of investigators have combined bleomycin with ifosfamide and a platinum compound. Three studies that included patients who had not received radiotherapy reported response rates of 65-100%.[300-302] Reports of treatment with these drugs in previously irradiated patients have yielded mixed but generally lower response rates of between 13% and 72%.[301-304]

Combinations of cisplatin and continuous infusion 5-FU,[305-307] cisplatin and paclitaxel,[308,309] cisplatin and vinorelbine,[310] and cisplatin and gemcitabine[311,312] also produce high response in previously untreated patients. The combination of carboplatin and liposomal doxorubicin has shown modest activity in this clinical setting.[313] Again, response rates decrease significantly if patients have had previous irradiation.[306,312,314]

A recent GOG randomized phase III trial reported that combining topotecan with cisplatin had a better response rate than cisplatin alone.[303] The response rate was 13% in the cisplatin arm and 27% in the combination arm. There was also an improvement in median survival by 3 months as well as a slight improvement in quality of life as determined by the functional assesment of cancer therapy-cervical (FACT-CX). They found the previous radio sensitizing chemotherapy and interval from diagnosis predicted for response. Response was more frequent in non-irradiated sites (70% vs 23%). This has led the GOG to their new prospective trial for primary stage IVB or recurrent/persistent carcinoma of the cervix. In this trial patients were randomized between four arms: arm 1, paclitaxel and cisplatin; arm 2, vinorelbine and cisplatin; arm 3, gemcitabine and cisplatin; and arm 4, topotecan and cisplatin. This study has recently been completed, but the results have not been published.

A number of barriers have impeded drug evaluations in patients with cervical cancer. Most patients have had high-dose

Table 98-9 ■ **Combination Chemotherapy for Advanced or Recurrent Cervical Cancer**

Chemotherapy Regimen (Ref.)	Patients (No.)	Previous Radiation Therapy (%)	Response (%)
Cisplatin/ifosfamide (318)	146	90	32
Cisplatin/ifosfamide/bleomycin (318)	141	87	31.2
Cisplatin/paclitaxel (246)	41	90	46.3
Cisplatin/paclitaxel/ifosfamide (319)	60	75	46
Cisplatin/gemcitabine (300)	19	53	41
Cisplatin/mitomycin-C (320)	33	96	42
Cisplatin/topotecan (321)	32	94	28
Cisplatin/topotecan (291)	294	47	27
Cisplatin/5-fluorouracil (293)	55	90	22

EBRT to the pelvis and lower vertebrae. The dose range of 40-55 Gy destroys the stem cell population of the bone marrow included within the treatment field. Because myelosuppression is the dose-limiting toxic effect of most drugs used for this disease, the reduced bone marrow reserve limits the amount of drug that can be given. In addition, patients with advanced carcinoma frequently have renal impairment because of ureteral obstruction and loss of a kidney. Marginal renal function prompts dose reductions for drugs requiring renal clearance. Cervical cancer often recurs in irradiated areas that are fibrotic and poorly vascularized. Such hostile environments repress drug deliverability. Tumor regression is difficult to measure by both physical examination and imaging techniques. Cellular mechanisms for chemotherapy and radiation therapy resistance need to be defined in patients with cervical cancer. Despite these obstacles, single-agent and combination chemotherapies have induced complete responses in patients with biopsy-proven carcinomas and hopefully combination chemotherapy will be better. However, the more recent randomized trials that compared platinum-doublets with single-agent cisplatin note a decline in the response rate seen for cisplatin that appears to parallel the number of patients who were treated with cisplatin-based chemoradiation for initial therapy of their cervix cancer and may reflect cisplatin-resistance in patients who relapse shortly after primary treatment with chemoradiation. We may need to develop new doublets that do not contain cisplatin to be used for patients who relapse within 12 months of having received platin-based chemoradiation. There should be a role for targeted biological agents, and presently many phase I and II trials are underway investigating these agents separately or in combination with chemotherapy. GOG has three phase II trials, GOG0076-DD with cetuximab plus cisplatin, GOG 0227-C with bevacizumab and GOG 0227-D with erlotinib.

Summary

In patients with recurrent cervical cancer, it is important first to determine if the patient is a candidate for definitive surgery or radiation therapy. Five-year survival rates range from 20% to 50% if one of these therapies can be administered. Systemic chemotherapy can be used for treatment of both recurrent and metastatic disease, but careful attention should be paid to balancing benefit and toxicity. Further research is needed to determine the impact of chemotherapy on quality of life and the sensitivity to chemotherapy of patients who received prior chemotherapy as part of chemoradiation therapy as well as the importance of biological agents.

Selected References

The complete reference list can be found at www.CANCERMEDICINE8.com

4. Coleman MP, Esteve J, Damiecki P, et al., editors. Trends in cancer incidence and mortality. *IARC Sci Publ*. 1993;121:1–86.
7. Brinton LA. Epidemiology of cervical cancer—overview. In: Munoz FB, Bosch FX, Shah KV, Meheus A, editors. *The Epidemiology of Human Papillomavirus and Cervical Cancer*. Oxford (UK): Oxford University Press; 1992:3–23.
12. Bosch FX, Manos MM, Munoz N, et al. Prevalence of human papillomavirus in cervical cancer: a worldwide perspective. International biological study on cervical cancer (IBSCC) study group [comments]. *J Natl Cancer Inst*. 1995;87:796–802.
13. Munoz N, Bosch FX. Cervical cancer and papillomavirus: epidemiological evidence and perspective for prevention. *Salud Publica Mex*. 1997;39:274–282.
62. Southern SA, Herrington CS. Molecular events in uterine cervical cancer. *Sex Transm Infect*. 1998;74:101–109.
102. The Atypical Squamous Cells of Undetermined Significance/Low-Grade Squamous Intraepithelial Lesions Triage Study (ALTS) Group. Human papillomavirus testing for triage of women with cytologic evidence of low-grade squamous intraepithelial lesions: baseline data from a randomized trial. *J Natl Cancer Inst*. 2000;92:397–402.
103. Solomon D, Schiffman M, Tarone R. Comparison of three management strategies for patients with atypical squamous cells of undetermined significance: baseline results from a randomized trial. *J Natl Cancer Inst*. 2001;93:293–299.
104. Cox JT, Lorincz AT, Schiffman MH, et al. Human papillomavirus testing by hybrid capture appears to be useful in triaging women with a cytologic diagnosis of atypical squamous cells of undetermined significance. *Am J Obstet Gynecol*. 1995;172:946–954.
108. Cox TJ. Evaluating the role of HPV testing for women with equivocal Papanicolaou test findings [editorial]. *JAMA*. 1999;281:1645–1647.
109. Cullen AP, Reid R, Campion M, et al. Analysis of the physical state of different human papillomavirus DNA's in intraepithelial and invasive cervical neoplasm. *J Virol*. 1999;65:606–612.
111. Mitchell MF, Tortolero-Luna G, Cook E, et al. A randomized clinical trial of cryotherapy, laser vaporization, and loop electrosurgical excision for treatment of squamous intraepithelial lesions of the cervix. *Obstet Gynecol*. 1998;92:737–744.
120. The HPV PATRICIA Study Group. Efficacy of a prophylactic adjuvanted bivalent L1 virus-like-particle vaccine against infection with human papillomavirus types 16 and 18 in young women: an interim analysis of a phase III double-blind, randomized controlled trial. *Lancet*. 2007;369:2161–2170.
122. Rogers LJ, Eva LJ, and Luesley DM. Vaccines against cervical cancer. *Curr Opin Oncol*. 2008;20:570–574.
127. Piver MS, Chung WS. Prognostic significance of cervical lesion size and pelvic node metastases in cervical carcinoma. *Obstet Gynecol*. 1975;46:507–510.
128. Mitchell PA, Waggoner S, Rotmensch J, et al. Cervical cancer in the elderly treated with radiation therapy. *Gynecol Oncol*. 1998;71:291–298.
140. Grigsby PW, Siegel BA, Dehdashti F. Lymph node staging by positron emission tomography in patients with carcinoma of the cervix. *J Clin Oncol*. 2001;19:3745–3749.
199. Lohe KJ, Burghardt E, Hillemanns HG, et al. Early squamous cell carcinoma of the uterine cervix. II. Clinical results of a cooperative study in the management of 419 patients with early stromal invasion and microcarcinoma. *Gynecol Oncol*. 1978;6:31–50.
208. Sasaki H, Yoshida T, Noda K, et al. Urethral pressure profiles following radical hysterectomy. *Obstet Gynecol*. 1982;59:101–104.
228. Keys HM, Bundy BN, Stehman FB, et al. Cisplatin, radiation, and adjuvant hysterectomy for bulky stage IB cervical carcinoma. *N Engl J Med*. 1999;340:1154–1161.
229. Morris M, Eifel PJ, Lu J, et al. Pelvic radiation with concurrent chemotherapy compared with pelvic and paraaortic radiation for high-risk cervical cancer. *N Engl J Med*. 1999;340:1137–1143.
231. Rose PG, Bundy BN, Watkins J, et al. Concurrent cisplatinbased chemotherapy and radiotherapy for locally advanced cervical cancer. *N Engl J Med*. 1999;340:1144–1153.
232. Whitney CW, Sause W, Bundy BN, et al. A randomized comparison of fluorouracil plus cisplatin versus hydroxyurea as an adjunct to radiation therapy in stages IIB–IVA carcinoma of the cervix with negative paraaortic lymph nodes: a Gynecologic Oncology Group and Southwest Oncology Group study. *J Clin Oncol*. 1999;17:1339–1348.
239. Plante M, Renaud MC, Francois H, et al. Vaginal radical trachelectomy: an oncologically safe fertility-preserving surgery. An updated series of 72 cases and review of the literature. *Gynecol Oncol*. 2004;94:614–623.
240. Plante M, Renaud MC, Hoskins IA, et al. Vaginal radical trachelectomy: a valuable fertility-preserving option in the management of early-stage cervical cancer. A series of 50 pregnancies and review of the literature. *Gynecol Oncol*. 2005;98:3–10.
242. Delgado G, Bundy BN, Fowler WC, et al. A prospective surgical pathological study of stage I squamous carcinoma of the cervix: a Gynecologic Oncology Group study. *Gynecol Oncol*. 1989;36:314–320.
243. Sedlis A, Bundy BN, Rotman MZ, et al. A randomized trial of pelvic radiation therapy versus No further therapy in selected patients with stage IB carcinoma of the cervix after radical hysterectomy and pelvic lymphadenectomy: a Gynecologic Oncology Group study. *Gynecol Oncol*. 1999;73:177–183.
244. Rotman M, Sedlis A, Piedmonte MR, et al. A Phase III randomized trial of postoperative pelvic irradiation in stage IB cervical carcinoma with poor prognostic features: follow-up of a Gynecologic Oncology Group Study. *Int J Radiat Oncol Biol Phys*. 2006;65:169–176.

245. Mendenhall WM, McCarty PJ, Morgan LS, et al. Stage IBIIA-B carcinoma of the intact uterine cervix greater than or equal to 6 cm in diameter: Is adjuvant extrafascial hysterectomy beneficial? *Int J Radiat Oncol Biol Phys*. 1991;21:899–904.
247. Sardi JE, Giaroli A, Sananes C, et al. Long-term follow-up of the first randomized trial using neoadjuvant chemotherapy in stage Ib squamous carcinoma of the cervix: the final results. *Gynecol Oncol*. 1997;67:61–69.
248. Eddy G, Bundy B, Creasman W, et al. Treatment of "bulky" stage IB cervical cancer with or without neoadjuvant vincristine and cisplatin prior to radical hysterectomy and pelvic/para-aortic lymphadenectomy: a phase III trial of the gynecologic oncology group. *Gynecol Oncol*. 2007; 106:362–369.
249. Neoadjuvant Chemotherapy for Cervical Cancer Meta-Analysis Collaboration. Neoadjuvant chemotherapy locally advanced cervical cancer: a systematic review and meta-analysis of individual patient data from 21 randomised trials. *Eur J Cancer*. 2003;39:2470–2486.
250. Tierney JF, Vale C, Symonds P. Concomitant and neoadjuvant chemotherapy for cervical cancer. *Clin Oncol*. 2008;20:401–416.
252. Peters WA 3rd, Liu PY, Barrett RJ 2nd, et al. Concurrent chemotherapy and pelvic radiation therapy compared with pelvic radiation therapy alone as adjuvant therapy after radical surgery in high-risk early-stage cancer of the cervix. *J Clin Oncol*. 2000;18:1606–1613.
253. Monk BJ, Wang J, Im S, et al. Rethinking the use of radiation and chemotherapy after radical hysterectomy: a clinical-pathologic analysis of a Gynecologic Oncology Group/Southwest Oncology Group/Radiation Therapy Oncology Group Trial. *Gyencol Oncol*. 2005;96:721–728.
254. Eifel PJ, Winter K, Morris M, et al. Pelvic irradiation with concurrent chemotherapy versus pelvic and para-aortic irradiation for high-risk cervical cancer: an update of radiation therapy oncology group trial (RTOG) 90-01. *J Clin Oncol*. 2004;22:872–880.
255. Pearcey R, Brundage M, Drouin P, et al. Phase III trial comparing radical radiotherapy with and without cisplatin chemotherapy in patients with advanced squamous cell cancer of the cervix. *J Clin Oncol*. 2002;20:966–972.
256. Green JA, Kirwan JM, Tierney JF, et al. Survival and recurrence after concomitant chemotherapy and radiotherapy for cancer of the uterine cervix: a systematic review and meta-analysis. *Lancet*. 2001;358:781–786.
257. Wong LC, Ngan HY, Cheung AN, et al. Chemoradiation and adjuvant chemotherapy in cervical cancer. *J Clin Oncol*. 1999;17:2055–2060.
258. Lorvidhaya V, Chitapanarux I, Sangruchi S, et al. Concurrent mitomycin C, 5-fluorouracil, and radiotherapy in the treatment of locally advanced carcinoma of the cervix: a randomized trial. *Int J Radiat Oncol Biol Phys*. 2003;55:1226–1232.
263. Veerasarn V, Lorvidhaya V, Kamnerdsupaphon P, et al. A randomized phase III trial of concurrent chemoradiotherapy in locally advanced cervical cancer: preliminary results. *Gynecol Oncol*. 2007;104:15–23.
269. Haie C, Pejovic MH, Gerbaulet A, et al. Is prophylactic para-aortic irradiation worthwhile in the treatment of advanced cervical carcinoma? Results of a controlled clinical trial of the EORTC radiotherapy group. *Radiother Oncol*. 1988;11:101–112.
270. Grigsby PW, Heydon K, Mutch DG, et al. Long-term follow-up of RTOG 92-10: cervical cancer with positive para-aortic lymph nodes. *Int J Radiat Oncol Biol Phys*. 2001;51:982–987.
271. Varia MA, Bundy BN, Deppe G, et al. Cervical carcinoma metastatic to para-aortic nodes: extended field radiation therapy with concomitant 5-fluorouracil and cisplatin chemotherapy: a Gynecologic Oncology Group study. *Int J Radiat Oncol Biol Phys*. 1998;42:1015–1023.
273. Small W, Winter K, Levenback C, et al. Extended-field irradiation and intracavitary brachytherapy combined with cisplatin chemotherapy for cervical cancer with positive para-aortic or high common iliac lymph nodes: results of ARM 1 pf RTOG 0116. *Int J Radiat Oncol Biol Phys*. 2007;68:1081–1087.
277. Lanciano R. Radiotherapy for the treatment of locally recurrent cervical cancer. *J Natl Cancer Inst Monogr*. 1996;21:113–115.
281. Rutledge FN. Pelvic exenteration: an update of the U. T. M. D. Anderson Hospital experience and review of the literature. In: Rutledge FN, Freedman RS, Gershenson DM, editors. *Gynecologic Cancer: Diagnosis and Treatment Strategies*. Austin (TX): University of Texas Press; 1987:7.
301. Kumar L, Bhargava V. Chemotherapy in recurrent and advanced cervical cancer. *Gynecol Oncol*. 1991;40:107–111.
302. Murad AM, Triginelli SA, Ribalta JCL. Phase II trial of bleomycin, ifosfamide, and carboplatin in metastatic cervical cancer. *J Clin Oncol*. 1994;12:55–59.
303. Long HJ 3rd, Bundy BN, Grendys EC Jr, et al. Randomized phase III trial of cisplatin (P) vs cisplatin plus topotecan (T) vs MVAC in stage IVB, recurrent or persistent carcinoma of the uterine cervix: a Gynecologic Oncology Group study [abstract 9]. *Gynecol Oncol*. 2004;92:397.
304. Tay SK, Lai FM, Soh LT, et al. Combined chemotherapy using cisplatin ifosfamide and bleomycin (PIB) in the treatment of advanced and recurrent cervical carcinoma. *Aust N Z J Obstet Gynecol*. 1993;32:263–266.

99 Endometrial Cancer

Jamal Rahaman, MD ■ Carmel J. Cohen, MD

It has been predicted that 39,080 new cases of uterine corpus cancer (the vast majority of which are endometrial cancer) will occur in the United States in 2007 and that the disease will result in 7400 deaths.[1] In 1991, the number of deaths from endometrial cancer in the United States began to exceed the number attributable to cervical cancer.[1,2] After declining between the mid-1980s and 1990s, the incidence rates for endometrial cancer increased by about 0.6% per year from 1988 to 1999. Norway, Czechoslovakia, and other northern European countries also reported significant increases in the incidence of endometrial cancer. Table 99-1 shows international survival figures as published in the Annual Report on the Results of Treatment in Gynecologic Cancer.[2]

Although the incidence of endometrial carcinoma is lower among black women than among white women, the mortality rates are higher in the former group of patients.[1,3] In their review of the National Cancer Data Base, Hicks and colleagues observed that black women were diagnosed with less favorable histologies, more advanced stages of disease, and poorly differentiated tumors than were white women.[3] Black women were less frequently treated surgically, and the surgically treated patients with advanced-stage disease received adjuvant radiotherapy (RT) less often and chemotherapy more often than did white patients. Most significantly, 5-year survival was poorer for black women, even for those with stage I disease who were treated surgically.[1,3]

Table 99-1 **Carcinoma of the Corpus Uteri**[a]

Volume	Year	No. of Patients	5-Year Survival (%)
16	1962-1968	14,506	63.0
17	1969-1972	10,720	65.4
18	1973-1975	11,501	66.6
19	1976-1978	13,581	67.7
20	1979-1981	14,906	65.1
21	1982-1986	19,402	69.7
22	1987-1989	13,040	72.7
23	1990-1992	7350	73.4
24	1993-1995	6260	76.5
25	1996-1998	7496	77.6
26	1999-2001	8110	80.0
Total		12,6872	

[a]Review of the 5-year survival rate reported in volumes 16 to 26 of the *Annual Report on the Results of Treatment in Gynecologic Cancer.*[2]

Risk Factors

The list of conditions thought to increase the risk of endometrial cancer has included body size, obesity, diabetes, nulliparity, a history of colon and/or breast carcinoma, syndromes of ovulation failure, syndromes of increased endogenous estrogen exposure, and exposure to exogenous estrogen. Nulliparity, compared with multiparity of five or more births, menopause after age 53 years, and 50 pounds of excess weight are all important risk factors that can increase a woman's probability for endometrial cancer by 5 to 10 times compared with patients without these risk factors. Increased risk from obesity relates to higher levels of estrogen synthesized by peripheral aromatization of precursors by the aromatase in fat. Diabetes in patients with a BMI <31.9 is not an independent risk for endometrial cancer.[4] Pathologic conditions that predispose to endometrial cancer often relate to increased levels of endogenous estrogen or exogenous estrogen supplementation.[5] Gusberg and Kardon reviewed the endometrial histology from 115 patients with estrogen-producing granulosa-theca ovarian tumors and found that 21% developed endometrial carcinoma and 43% had precancerous hyperplasia.[5] Others have not found the same incidence of adenocarcinoma, but have identified a high incidence of atypical hyperplasias.[6,7] Patients with polycystic ovary syndrome usually do not ovulate and thus are exposed to continuous estrogen production. When endometrial carcinoma occurs in women younger than 45 years of age, it is usually in patients with polycystic ovary syndrome[8,9] and is most frequently surrounded by atypical hyperplasia histologically. Finally, patients who are treated for ovarian dysgenesis and oophorectomy with unopposed estrogen replacement have developed endometrial carcinoma in the residual uterus.[10]

Unopposed use of exogenous estrogen can also predispose to endometrial cancer. In 1975, Smith and colleagues, in a retrospective case-control study of 317 women with endometrial carcinoma, noted a 4.5-fold relative risk among those women who had been treated with unopposed estrogen.[11] In 1993, mindful of the defects of the earlier studies, Brinton and Hoover, representing the Endometrial Cancer Collaborative Group, completed a hospital-based case-control study analyzing 300 menopausal women with new diagnoses of endometrial carcinoma and 207 matched-population controls.[12] These investigators identified a relative risk of 3.0 for all users of estrogen replacement, although the risks were higher for recent use, thin habitus, or cigarette smoking. No clear dose relationship was observed, but women who used low-dose estrogen preparations exclusively were found to be at lowest risk, although when low-dose use continued beyond 5 years, this advantage was lost. Although only 4% of the women used progestogens simultaneously with estrogen, there seemed to be a partial protective effect, but the risk was not eliminated. Some investigators have described an immediate decline in risk after cessation of estrogen use,[13] but Brinton and Hoover's study confirms the observation made by others that the excess risk can persist beyond 5 years after discontinuation of estrogen replacement, especially when there has been long-term exposure.[12]

The Centers for Disease Control and Prevention reported that oral contraceptive use for at least 12 months diminished the risk of endometrial cancer by 50% compared with the risk for women who had never used oral contraception. Nulliparous women seemed to benefit most, and the protection lasted for a decade following the discontinuation of oral contraceptive use.[14] Brinton and Hoover's study observed that previous oral contraceptive use did not protect women from increased relative risk of endometrial cancer when they employed unopposed estrogen in postmenopausal hormone replacement therapy, suggesting that the role of the progestogen in the combination oral contraceptive pills is essential in protecting against endometrial carcinoma.[12]

For more than 20 years, tamoxifen has been used to treat breast cancer, following the observation that it causes regression of metastatic tumor, diminishes the incidence of cancer in the contralateral breast, delays time to recurrence, and improves survival in subsets of patients. Several competitive inhibitors of steroid hormone receptors have been developed. These drugs are currently used for treatment of a variety of endocrine-related disorders and as selective tools allowing the dissection of the receptor transduction pathway. Most inhibitors bind competitively to the receptor and induce a conformational change in the ligand binding domain of the steroid hormone receptor. This altered conformation of the receptor promotes the dissociation of the receptor heat shock protein (HSP) complex, allowing the receptor to interact with deoxyribonucleic acid (DNA), but does not allow a productive association of the receptor and the transcriptional apparatus. Our understanding of the mechanism of action of anti-estrogens is the most evolved. Estrogen receptor (ER) contains two distinct transactivation domains: transactivation function 1 (TAF1) at the amino terminus of the receptor and TAF2, contained within the hormone-binding domain. In the presence of estrogen, these domains cooperate to produce a productive association of ER with the transcription apparatus. Tamoxifen is thought to function by disrupting TAF 1 or TAF2 cooperativity by inhibiting TAF2 transcriptional activity.[15] Clinically, tamoxifen diminishes serum cholesterol, increases sex hormone–binding globulin,[16] preserves bone density in the lumbar spine,[17] thickens the vaginal epithelium in some patients,[18] and is associated with the enlargement of uterine fibroids, the growth of endometrial polyps, and the development of endometrial neoplastic change. These are all estrogen-like functions. Paradoxically, the same drug is associated with the production of vaginal atrophy, the onset of vasomotor symptoms, and the development of clinical dyspareunia. These are features of estrogen deprivation.

The action of tamoxifen may be organ specific, just as it is known to be species specific in its association with hepatic neoplasia in laboratory animals. When immortalized breast cancer and endometrial cancer cell lines were implanted in athymic mice, both cancers grew well in the same animal. When tamoxifen treatment was given, the breast cancers were inhibited and the endometrial cancers continued to grow.[19] Several investigators have described an increase in the incidence of endometrial cancers among patients with breast cancer who were treated with tamoxifen.[20–22] Killackey and colleagues were the first to report endometrial carcinoma occurring in three breast cancer patients receiving anti-estrogens.[22] The strongest initial data implicating tamoxifen use in the subsequent development of endometrial carcinoma were reported by Fornander and colleagues, who reviewed the frequency of new primary cancers in the Swedish Cancer Registry for a group of 1846 postmenopausal women with early breast cancer.[20] There was a 6.4-fold increase in the relative risk of endometrial cancer in the 931 tamoxifen treated patients compared with controls. The dose of tamoxifen in this study was 40 mg/day. At doses of 20 mg/day, several investigators with small series have not observed an increased incidence of endometrial cancer. The National Surgical Adjuvant Breast and Bowel Project (NSABP) described observations on 3863 patients prospectively studied.[21] In the B-14 protocol, 2843 patients with node-negative, ER-positive breast cancer received either tamoxifen (20 mg/day) or placebo. An additional 1020 patients taking tamoxifen were registered in this project. The average time in the study was 8 years for the randomized patients and 5 years for the registered patients. Originally, 25 endometrial cancers were reported, but on review, 1 was found to be a sarcoma, and 2 of the cancers developed in women originally assigned to the placebo group, who were ultimately treated with tamoxifen before the discovery of their endometrial cancers. None of the patients who did not receive tamoxifen developed endometrial cancer. This is surprising because the relative risk for endometrial cancer in breast cancer patients is 1.4. The relative risk calculated for the tamoxifen-treated group compared with the placebo group was 7.5, with an annual hazard rate of 0.2 per 1000 for the placebo group and 1.6 per 1000 for the randomized tamoxifen-treated group. The distribution of pathologies among the 24 adenocarcinomas was the same as that reported in the National Cancer Institute's Surveillance, Epidemiology, and End Results (SEER) Program data for the years 1983 to 1987.

More recently, in the Breast Cancer Prevention Trial (P-1) of the NSABP, 13,388 women were randomly assigned to receive placebo (6707) or 20 mg/day of tamoxifen (6681) for 5 years.[23] Tamoxifen reduced the risk of invasive breast cancer by 49% and of noninvasive breast cancer by 50%. The rate of endometrial carcinoma was increased in the tamoxifen group (risk ratio 2.53); this increase occurred primarily in postmenopausal women aged 50 years or older. All endometrial carcinomas in the tamoxifen group were stage I, and no endometrial cancer deaths have occurred in this group.

In one report of 15 patients who developed endometrial cancer while exposed to tamoxifen, two-thirds of the patients had histologically virulent tumors. The patients with these tumors were significantly older than the general endometrial cancer patient population, however, and fell into an age group in which sarcomas and nonendometrioid carcinomas are likely to occur more frequently.[24] In several other series of similar size, the distribution of pathology among such patients was no different from that observed in endometrial cancer patients who have not been exposed to tamoxifen.[25] Similarly, Barakat and colleagues, in a retrospective review of 73 patients with a history of breast cancer who subsequently developed endometrial carcinoma, found no significant difference in stage, grade, or histologic subtype.[26]

More recently, studies have focused on the surveillance of breast cancer patients using tamoxifen. Runowicz and colleagues, in a summary analysis of the transvaginal ultrasound and endometrial biopsy data from NSABP (P-1), observed that ultrasonography had a sensitivity of 27% and a specificity of 70%.[27] Of 13 significant biopsies, only 1 showed invasive cancer; the other 12 revealed simple hyperplasia without atypia (9 patients) or complex hyperplasia without atypia (3 patients). The authors did not recommend the substitution of ultrasonography for endometrial biopsy for the assessment of endometrial hyperplasia or carcinoma in this group of patients. A similar prospective longitudinal study in Canada on 304 women with breast cancer receiving tamoxifen found that routine surveillance with ultrasonography was not useful in asymptomatic patients.[28] In another study, Barakat and colleagues evaluated 159 tamoxifen-treated patients by serial office endometrial biopsies obtained at the start of tamoxifen therapy and at 6-month intervals for 2 years, followed by three additional annual biopsies.[29] Although the procedure was feasible, significant pathology requiring hysterectomy was observed in only three patients, and the authors concluded that the utility of routine endometrial biopsy for screening in tamoxifen-treated women is limited. None of these studies provide strong support for screening with ultrasonography or endometrial biopsy in women who receive tamoxifen. Prompt evaluation of any vaginal bleeding is, however, mandatory. Clinicians should be not be reluctant to obtain endometrial biopsies or vaginal ultrasound in patients with multiple risk factors.

Although a large cohort of women with endometrial carcinoma is noted to have one or more risk factors, the background of hormonal aberration stemming from inappropriate estrogen exposure, either endogenous or exogenous, with all of the attendant typical phenotypes, accounts for no more than 30% of endometrial cancer patients. Historically, this figure was thought to be much higher, and conventional wisdom suggested that women of high parity, lean phenotype, and an unremarkable family history who had not had estrogen replacement therapy and had little intercurrent disease were relatively immune to endometrial cancer. Unfortunately, this is not the case, and many centers are reporting increasing numbers of patients with endometrial cancer who have no recognized risk factors. Such women frequently have more virulent disease (type II) histologically, with implied diminished survival, than do traditional endometrial cancer patients.[30,31]

Pathology

Endometrial Hyperplasia

When Gusberg and colleagues introduced the term "adenomatous hyperplasia" to describe the pattern of hyperplastic glands noted in association with, and often prior to, the development of endometrial adenocarcinoma, they included all of the variants of precursor histology. These ranged from a mild arrangement of densely crowded glands with eosinophilic cytoplasm through the spectrum of more disordered arrangements, with intraluminal tufting, and an increase in mitosis, pseudopalisading, and bizarre nuclei.[32] Hertig and Sommers similarly studied pre-invasive changes in the endometrium and described three intensities of abnormality, which they called "adenomatous hyperplasia," "atypical hyperplasia," and "carcinoma in situ."[33] Clinicians were confused because Hertig and Sommers' adenomatous hyperplasia implied a small risk of subsequent transition to cancer, whereas Gusberg and colleagues' adenomatous hyperplasia carried a 15% to 30% risk over time if it were not reversed by therapy.

Kurman and colleagues followed 170 patients with endometrial hyperplasia for a minimum of 1 year; the mean follow-up time was 13.4 years.[34] They established criteria for distinguishing lesions on the basis of architectural abnormalities and cytologic abnormalities. Only 1.6% of patients without cytologic atypia progressed to cancer compared with 23% of those with atypical cytology. Architectural abnormalities were not prognostically important. Table 99-2 presents the details of Kurman and colleagues' classification and observations. Their classification of simple or complex hyperplasia, with or without atypia, is now accepted for describing these lesions.

Endometrioid Adenocarcinoma

Endometrioid adenocarcinoma is the most common of the endometrial cancer histologies. It is characterized by the disappearance of stroma between abnormal glands that have infoldings of their linings into the lumens, disordered nuclear chromatin distribution, nuclear enlargement, and a variable degree of mitosis, necrosis, and hemorrhage. This classic variety accounts for 80% to 95% of the adenocarcinomas.

Adenosquamous Carcinoma

Adenosquamous cancer has malignant elements from both its squamous component and its adenomatous component. It usually accounts for 7% or less of the adenocarcinomas of the endometrium. However, in 1974, Reagan described a rising incidence of this entity in the University Hospitals of Cleveland, with adenosquamous cancer making up 20% of the endometrial cancers; these patients had a very poor prognosis.[35] Apparently, this change in the ratio of histologies has not been universal in the United States. The staging convention, now published in the 25th volume of the annual report, requires grading of this tumor on the basis of its glandular component and not its squamous component.[2] Although data are still maturing, it is suggested that when this convention is followed, adenosquamous cancer will not behave differently from endometrioid adenocarcinomas of the same stage and grade.

Uterine Papillary Serous Carcinoma

Described by Hendrickson and colleagues in 1982, uterine papillary serous carcinoma (UPSC) comprises 5% to 10% of stage I endometrial carcinomas and is characterized by an expansive papillary architecture with a fibrovascular matrix, marked cytologic atypia, bizarre nuclei, and widespread nuclear pleomorphism (Fig. 99-1).[36] The features are suggestive of papillary serous cystadenocarcinoma of the ovary. The lesion is highly virulent, usually found with deep myometrial penetration at the time of diagnosis, often extrauterine in location in patients with clinical early-stage disease, and almost always incurable when the disease has spread beyond the uterus. In one series, observations on 15 patients with UPSC were compared with 76 adenocarcinomas and 26 adenocarcinomas with papillary features, all treated in the same institution.[37] At 3 years, 75% of the adenocarcinoma group were alive without disease. For the adenocarcinomas with papillary features, the progression-free interval (PFI) was 33 months, and for the UPSC group, it was 9 months. In a study of recurrent disease, Lee and Belinson identified 28 recurrences in a series of 227 patients with clinical stage I endometrial carcinoma.[38] Of the 28 patients, 7 had no invasion of the endometrium at the time of diagnosis. Five of these 7 patients had histologic characteristics of UPSC, and all died of the disease.

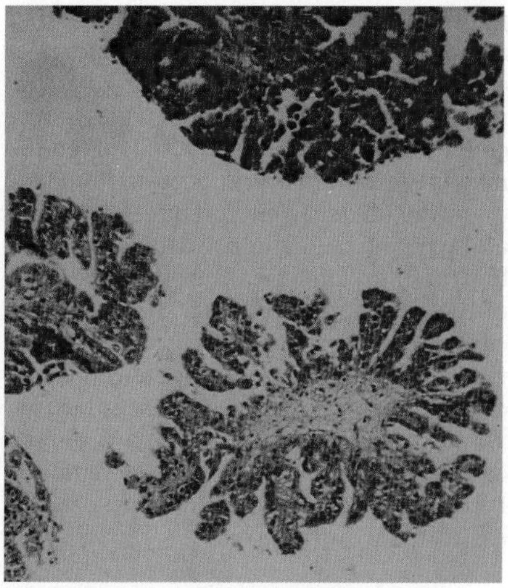

Figure 99-1 Uterine papillary serous carcinoma. Broad stalks supporting papillary fronds, appearing like papillary ovarian carcinoma. *Source*: Courtesy of Diane Deligdisch, MD, Mount Sinai School of Medicine. A correlation of the Federation Internationale de Gynecologie d'Obstetrique (FIGO), Unio Internationale Contre Cancrum (UICC), and American Joint Committee on Cancer (AJCC) nomenclatures.

Endometrial Papillary Adenocarcinoma

Endometrial papillary adenocarcinomas must be distinguished from UPSC because of their different behavior. They are characterized histologically as being usually well-differentiated endometrioid adenocarcinomas composed of very slender papillations, orderly neoplastic epithelial cells, few mitoses, and less cellular disorder than UPSC. The distinction between these two groups has been carefully detailed by Chen and colleagues.[39] The endometrial carcinomas with papillary features behave identically to the endometrioid adenocarcinomas.

Clear Cell Carcinoma

Kurman and Scully described clear cell cancers in detail.[40] Histologically,

Table 99-2 **Comparison of Follow-Up of 170 Patients With Simple and Complex Hyperplasia and Simple and Complex Atypical Hyperplasia**

	No. of Patients	Regressed *n* (%)	Persisted *n* (%)	Progressed to Carcinoma *n* (%)
Simple hyperplasia	93	74 (80)	18 (19)	1 (1)
Complex hyperplasia	29	23 (80)	5 (17)	1 (3)
Simple atypical hyperplasia	13	9 (69)	3 (23)	1 (8)
Complex atypical hyperplasia	35	20 (57)	5 (14)	10 (29)

Source: Adapted from Ref. 34.

although there are a variety of patterns, a presentation of polygonal or flattened cells with clear cytoplasm accounts for more than half of the cells. This group constitutes approximately 6% of endometrial carcinomas and occurs more frequently in older women. The 5-year overall survival rate is approximately 40%,[41] but this may be a result of the older age of the patients and the fact that clear cell carcinomas are generally found in patients with higher stages of cancer. Clear cells often appear in histologic mixtures when tumors are assigned to a different category on the basis of the prevalent cell type, and their presence usually confers a diminished prognosis.

Diagnosis

The median age for patients with adenocarcinoma of the endometrium is 61 years, with the largest number of women developing their cancers during the sixth decade. Only 5% develop adenocarcinomas before the age of 40 years, and these are usually women with the abnormal syndromes previously discussed. Eighty percent of patients have experienced menopause, and only 20% are diagnosed before they stop menstruating. Irregular or postmenopausal bleeding is the presenting symptom in at least 75% of patients, and at the time of diagnosis, 75% of patients have disease confined to the uterus. Thus, it is obvious that irregular bleeding is a critical symptom, and by explaining it histologically, one has an opportunity to identify endometrial cancer when it is highly curable by relatively uncomplicated therapy.

The traditional technique for diagnosis has been fractional dilation and curettage of the uterus, with careful sampling of both the endometrial cavity and the endocervical canal. Once a procedure for the hospital operating room, this is now performed as an office procedure with greater than 95% accuracy.[42,43] There will always be patients who require general anesthesia in a hospital setting, however, either because of very low pain threshold, cervical stenosis, or other intercurrent ailments.

Hysteroscopy, either by direct observation or with video-camera amplification, allows direct assessment of the topography of the endometrial cavity with the possibility for more selective sampling and the assurance of not missing any occult lesions. Many reserve this procedure as an accompaniment to formal dilation and curettage under anesthesia. However, caution should be exercised because hysteroscopic dissemination of malignant cells has been described in the literature.[44]

Noninvasive radiographic imaging techniques, such as magnetic resonance; imaging (MRI)[45] and ultrasonography,[46] are not cost-effective for screening. For diagnosis and documenting recurrence; however, imaging techniques (MRI, computed tomography [CT] scan, positron emission tomography [PET] scan and ultrasound) can achieve an accuracy rate above 80%.[47]

Staging

Historically, endometrial cancer staging was a clinical exercise, based on physical examination, noninvasive radiographic testing, and measurement of the depth of the uterine cavity. One can see from Table 99-3 that clinical staging for those with a large uterus very likely would be inaccurate and would lead to understaging, and possibly undertreating, a significant proportion of the stage I cancers. When tumor grade was identified as an important prognostic feature, many therapists argued for a staging system that would permit consideration of the histologic prognostic variables because a biopsy or curettage was required even to make the diagnosis. In 1971, tumor grade was officially incorporated into the staging system. During this same era, the Gynecologic Oncology Group (GOG) inaugurated a pilot study to perform staging laparotomy in the course of initial surgical treatment of patients with clinical stage I endometrial carcinoma.[48] This study noted that 16 of 140 patients evaluated had cancer in their lymph nodes, despite the fact that they had early-stage disease by preoperative clinical evaluation. In a subsequent expansion of this pilot study, it was noted that 9.6% of 843 patients in clinical stage I had lymph node metastasis.[49] In addition, extensive surgical staging detects extrauterine disease in 23.2% of patients with apparent preoperative clinical stage I disease.[50] These observations strengthened the impetus for more precise staging, and in 1988, the International Federation of Gynecology and Obstetrics (FIGO) introduced the requirement for surgical staging of patients with endometrial carcinoma.

Tables 99-4 and 99-5 present the latest modifications of the surgical staging system, which were promulgated in 1994 and 1995. This system requires the performance of total abdominal hysterectomy (TAH), bilateral salpingo-oophorectomy (BSO), washings for cytologic examination, lymph node sampling from the pelvic and para-aortic lymph nodes for those patients whose histology and depth of myometrial penetration (determined during the operation) are other than well-differentiated tumors with minimal myometrial penetration, and biopsies of any

Table 99-3 Definitions of the Clinical Stages in Carcinoma of the Corpus Uteri[a]

Stage 0	Atypical endometrial hyperplasia, carcinoma in situ Histologic findings are suspicious of malignancy Cases of stage 0 should not be included in any therapeutic statistics
Stage I	The carcinoma is confined to the corpus
Stage IA	The length of the uterine cavity is 8 cm or less
Stage IB	The length of the uterine cavity is more than 8 cm
Stage II	The carcinoma has involved the corpus and the cervix, but has not extended outside the uterus

[a]Correlation of the Federation Internationale de Gynecologie d'Obstetrique (FIGO), Unio Internationale Contre Cancrum (UICC), and American Joint Committee on Cancer (AJCC) nomenclatures.

Table 99-4 Staging for Corpus Uteri Carcinoma

FIGO Stage[a]	
I	Tumor confined to corpus uteri
IA	Tumor limited to endometrium
IB	Tumor invades up to or less than one-half of the myometrium
IC	Tumor invades to more than one half of the myometrium
II	Tumor invades cervix, but does not extend beyond uterus
IIA	Endocervical glandular involvement only
IIB	Cervical stromal invasion
III	Local and/or regional spread as specified in T3a, T3b, N1, and FIGO IIIA, IIIB, and IIIC below
IIIA	Tumor involves serosa and/or adnexa (direct extension or metastasis) and/or cancer cells in ascites or peritoneal washings
IIIB	Vaginal involvement (direct extension or metastasis)
IIIC	Metastasis to the pelvic and/or para-aortic lymph nodes
IVA	Tumor invades bladder mucosa and/or bowel mucosa
IVB	Distant metastasis excluding metastasis to vagina, pelvic serosa, or adnexa; including metastasis to intraabdominal lymph nodes other than para-aortic and/or inguinal lymph nodes

[a]Each staging category is subdivided into histologic grade 1, 2, or 3.

Table 99-5 Histopathology: Degree of Differentiation

G1	5% or less of a nonsquamous or nonmorular solid growth pattern
G2	6% to 50% of a nonsquamous or nonmorular solid growth pattern
G3	More than 50% of a nonsquamous or nonmorular solid growth pattern

suspicious areas. Employing the updated FIGO staging system, a recent report described disease-free survival as 90% for stage I, 83% for stage II, and 43% for stage III.[51] When surgical staging is completed, it becomes the strongest predictor of survival. Univariate analysis reveals that the 5-year survival rate for patients in surgical stage IA is 93.8%; in stage IB, 95.4%; and in stage IC, 75%.[52]

The adoption of a surgical staging system initially created controversy regarding what constitutes an adequate staging procedure, which patients should be surgically staged, and whether extensive staging or lymphadenectomy has therapeutic value.[50] While many investigators prefer complete surgical staging for all patients with endometrial cancer, recent data suggest that this is particularly appropriate for all intermediate and high-risk patients unless there is contraindication to such extensive surgery.[53]

Prognostic Factors

In a GOG study, 1180 patients with clinical stage I or II endometrial carcinomas were studied by surgical-pathologic staging.[54] Of this group, 895 patients were evaluable for all of the parameters derived from surgical staging, as well as for follow-up from postoperative treatment to recurrence, with documentation of recurrence site. From this experience and the other previously cited interim GOG reports of surgical staging outcome, one can appreciate those factors that are predictive of extrauterine spread of disease at the time of initial diagnosis and those factors that correlate with ultimate survival.

Surgical stage and age are highly significant prognostic features that maintain their significance in each of the analyses performed in the various reports.

Histologic Type

Whereas 80% to 95% of endometrial cancers are classic endometrioid adenocarcinomas, the remainder constitute a series of histologic types with a more unfavorable prognosis. These include serous papillary adenocarcinoma and clear cell, undifferentiated, and squamous cancers. These cell types confer an unfavorable prognosis, independent of other known prognostic factors.[55]

Tumor Grade

Within classic endometrioid adenocarcinomas, tumor grade is highly significant as an independent prognostic factor. In addition, numerous studies have demonstrated that, in general, there is a greater tendency for the less differentiated tumors to be associated with other poor prognostic factors, including deep myometrial penetration, vascular space invasion, and increasing stage.[54,56,57] Recently, Salvesen and colleagues showed that morphometric nuclear grade was a stronger prognostic factor than subjective histologic grade.[58] Further studies are needed to confirm the significance of these findings.

Myometrial Invasion

The depth of myometrial penetration is a very important independent prognostic factor for outcome in stage I disease. Deeper penetration is associated with higher probabilities of tumor recurrence and death.[54,56,59] Although increasing depth of invasion correlates with increasing grade of tumor, depth appears to be a more significant prognostic factor and predicts for the presence of extrauterine disease as detected at surgical staging procedures.[49] Regardless of grade, however, only 1% of patients with disease confined to the endometrium have extrauterine disease compared with patients with deep muscle invasion, for which the incidence of pelvic node invasion rises to 17% and para-aortic nodal involvement rises to 25%.[49] DiSaia and colleagues found that patients with only endometrial involvement had an 8% recurrence rate compared with 12% if there was superficial or intermediate myometrial invasion versus 46% if there was involvement of the outer third of the myometrium.[59]

Both relative and absolute measures of the degree of myometrial invasion have been used. Although it is clear from a number of studies that involvement of the uterine serosa is an extremely bad prognostic sign,[60] some difficulties arise in attempting to compare reports with absolute distances from the serosa versus those with relative degrees of penetration into muscle because the thickness of the myometrium varies from patient to patient. The current FIGO staging classification requires uterine thickness to be measured as less than or greater than invasion of 50% of the myometrial thickness.

Capillary-Lymphatic Space Invasion

Vascular space invasion is a significant risk factor for recurrence, but it is not as important as the grade and depth of myometrial penetration. Approximately 15% of endometrial adenocarcinomas invade capillary-like spaces.[49,61] There is a significantly increased probability of pelvic and para-aortic lymph node invasion when this happens. Where the capillary-like spaces are involved, pelvic and para-aortic lymph nodes are also involved in 27% and 19% of cases, respectively, representing about a fivefold increase over those without such involvement.[49]

Positive Peritoneal Cytology

The presence of positive peritoneal cytology in washings is associated with an increased risk of relapse.[54] Approximately 15% of patients have positive peritoneal cytology,[54] and this is often related to other poor prognostic factors, such as high grade or deep myometrial penetration. Thus, it is not surprising that it is also associated with an increased risk of metastases to pelvic and para-aortic lymph nodes. Opinions and data in the literature conflict with respect to interpreting the independent prognostic significance of peritoneal cytology. Approximately 5% of patients with positive peritoneal cytology have no evidence of extrauterine disease,[49] but approximately one-third of patients with extrauterine disease do have positive cytology.

Unfortunately, no study has correlated the sites of relapse with the presence or absence of positive peritoneal cytology. That positive cytology, independent of other negative prognostic features, conferred a worse prognosis would be more convincing if one could associate an increased risk of peritoneal and upper abdominal relapse in patients with positive cytology compared with those without. Three large series suggest that positive peritoneal cytology may be a poor independent prognostic factor,[62–64] but several small series and one review reported that there are no outcome differences between those with positive peritoneal cytology and those without.[65–67]

Race

Liu and colleagues reviewed the treatment patterns, risk factors, and survival of 219 patients treated surgically for endometrial cancer between 1990 and 1993.[68] In this study, black women, when compared with white women, had a higher incidence of unfavorable histology (38% vs 12%), advanced-stage disease (51% vs 19%), poor differentiation (49% vs 18%), and poor survival. There was no difference between the onset of bleeding and hysterectomy in the two groups. Even when corrected for hormone use, these differences persisted. From this study, it may be concluded that black women face a poorer prognosis for survival from endometrial cancer than do their white counterparts.

Hormone Receptor Status

The presence of cytoplasmic ER- and progesterone receptor (PR)-binding proteins has been quantitatively associated with better histologic differentiation,[69] favorable histologic subtype, and response to therapy.[70–72]

Ligand binding to ER and PR was higher in well-differentiated lesions and was significantly lower in grade 3 lesions and the nonendometrioid carcinomas.[72] Alterations in receptor expression, receptor assembly and activation, response element recognition, and/or receptor degradation are among the possible explanations for loss of hormone binding. In addition, recent evidence suggests that promoter site hypermethylation might account in part for the loss of ER.[73] Likewise, differential expression of the PR-alpha (PRA) and PR-beta (PRB) have been reported.[74] PRA appears to down-regulate ER action and PRB is the primary activator of the progesterone responsive gene, and the loss of either would theoretically result in an unopposed estrogen effect. Clinically, reduced levels of ligand interaction with the ER, PR, or both in endometrial cancer samples significantly ($p < .01$) correlate with recurrence and death from disease.[71,72]

Tumor Ploidy and Kinetics

Although tumor ploidy in endometrial cancer has been widely studied, the results are conflicting. Approximately 65% of these cancers are determined to be diploid by flow cytometry. In general, diploid patterns occur in the better differentiated tumors. In one study, flow cytometry measurements of ribonucleic acid, S-phase fraction, DNA index, and proliferative index were conducted on the tissues from 140 specimens.[75] Only in 19% of patients was advanced disease predicted on the basis of clinical evaluation. However, 40% of patients with advanced disease were found to be aneuploid, 69% had a high S-phase fraction, and 69% had a proliferative index greater than 14%.[75]

The nuclear Ki-67 antigen, which is expressed in all stages of the cell cycle except G0, may be detected by immunohistochemistry to estimate the proliferative activity in tumors. Salvesen and colleagues observed that Ki-67 expression was significantly higher among patients with FIGO stage III or IV disease, clear cell or serous papillary histology types, and poor histologic grade.[76] Ki-67 expression was significantly related to survival.

Refinements of this approach may hold great promise for prognostic assessment.

Oncogene Activation and Loss of Tumor Suppressor Function

The molecular events involved in the pathogenesis of endometrial carcinoma are poorly defined; however, several aspects of the molecular pathology of this disease were recently elucidated. Mutations in the TP53 tumor suppressor gene leading to overexpression of mutant TP53 protein are the most common molecular alterations described in human cancers to date.[77] Between 4% and 49% of endometrioid carcinomas,[77–88] and between 71.4% and 100% of serous carcinomas[81,83,86,89–91] overexpress TP53 protein. Of note, TP53 protein overexpression has been demonstrated in 10% to 15% of early-stage disease[77,90,92] and in 40% to 50% of advanced-stage disease;[77,80] but does not occur in endometrial hyperplasia.[77,83,84] This suggests that TP53 mutation may be a late event in the histogenesis of endometrial carcinoma[77,83,84] or that acquisition of a TP53 mutation leads to the development of a virulent endometrial cancer that does not pass through a phase of hyperplasia, as postulated by Berchuck and colleagues.[93] Several studies demonstrated a positive association between TP53 overexpression and high nuclear grade[79,81,94–96] and FIGO stage,[94] although these have not been universal findings.[88,94,96] In addition, overexpression of TP53 is independently associated with poor survival.[80,81,97] For example, Kohler and colleagues observed a median survival of 6.1 years in patients whose tumors did not overexpress TP53 in comparison with a median survival of 1.4 years in patients whose tumors overexpressed TP53.[80]

The ras family of G proteins (N, H, K-*ras*) plays a critical role in the regulation of cellular proliferation.[93] The most frequent site of mutation of the K-*ras* oncogene in endometrial carcinoma is codon 12. K-*ras* mutations have been identified in both complex atypical hyperplasia[98] and invasive carcinoma. However, there does not appear to be a significant relationship between K-*ras* mutation and survival in endometrial cancer.[99–102]

The *HER2/neu* gene encodes for a tyrosine kinase receptor that forms heterodimers with HER3 or HER4 and is then activated following binding of the ligand heregulin.[103] Several studies suggest that this oncogene product is overexpressed in 10% to 15% of endometrial cancers.[103–108] Hetzel and colleagues, in an immunohistochemical analysis of 247 patients with endometrial cancer, observed strong staining in 37 patients (15%), mild staining in 144 (58%), and no staining in 66 (27%) patients.[105] The 5-year progression-free survival (PFS) rate was 56% for the strong staining, 83% for the mild staining, and 95% for the nonstaining groups. Strong overexpression was associated with a poor (51%) overall survival. Likewise, Lukes and colleagues found high expression in 12% of patients.[104] Overexpression was more common in stage III and IV patients (24%) than in stage I or II patients (6%) and was associated with poor PFS in univariate analysis. However, in multivariate analysis, *HER2/neu* was found to be an independent variable only if DNA ploidy was excluded from the statistical model.

Phosphate and tensin homolog deleted on chromosome 10 (*PTEN*) is a candidate tumor suppressor gene that has been isolated from the 10q23–24 region, possesses growth inhibitory functions, and appears to be differentially expressed in endometrial cancers.[78,109] In fact, the frequency of *PTEN* mutations described by several investigators is several-fold higher than that described for any other gene mutated in endometrial cancers, including K-*ras* and *TP53*, making *PTEN* mutation the most common defined genetic alteration identified to date in endometrial cancers.[109,110] *PTEN* mutations are infrequent in nonendometrioid endometrial cancers but appear to be relatively common in the endometrioid subtype and are associated with early-stage, nonmetastatic disease and more favorable survival.[110] In addition, although *PTEN* mutations were not detected in normal endometrium, Mutter and colleagues identified mutations in 55% of precursor lesions and 87% of endometrioid carcinomas.[109] These observations suggest that *PTEN* mutations may play an early role in carcinogenesis, at least in type I endometrioid endometrial carcinomas.

The *FMS* oncogene encodes a tyrosine kinase that serves as a receptor for macrophage-colony stimulating factor (M-CSF). Expression of *FMS* in endometrial cancers correlates with advanced stage, high grade, and deep myometrial invasion.[111] Expression of *C-MYC* has been observed in normal endometrium and endometriosis, with higher expression in the proliferative relative to secretory phase. Several studies suggest that *C-MYC* is amplified in a fraction of endometrial carcinomas.[106]

Microsatellite instability is one of the major mechanisms of cancer susceptibility and has been identified in 17% to 43% of endometrial carcinomas.[78,89,112,113] Microsatellite instability was initially noted in colorectal patients with hereditary nonpolyposis colorectal cancer (HNPCC). Risinger and colleagues observed microsatellite instability in 17% of sporadic endometrial carcinomas and in 75% of those associated with HNPCC.[112] Of note, the sporadic endometrial carcinomas displaying microsatellite instability were all stage I adenocarcinomas with diploid or near-diploid DNA content, indicating that these tumors are from clinical type I patients.[103,112]

In a case-control study by Prasad and colleagues, tamoxifen and non–tamoxifen-associated endometrial carcinomas arising in women with breast cancer demonstrated genetic alterations (*PTEN*, K-*ras*, *TP53*, *CTNNB1*, and microsatellite instability) similar to those of sporadic endometrial carcinomas.[114]

Deligdisch and Holinka classified endometrial carcinoma into type I, which is associated with unopposed estrogen, good differentiation, endometrioid histology, early stage, and favorable prognosis, and type II, which is associated with older age, poor differentiation, nonendometrioid histology, advanced stage, and an unfavorable prognosis.[30,31] The studies discussed above suggest that this clinical classification can be expanded to include molecular features associated with type I and type II endometrial carcinomas. Table 99-6 illustrates these molecular features.

Treatment of Primary Disease

Surgery

The initial surgical staging procedure, outlined earlier (Table 99-4), is the standard therapeutic procedure as well. When there is disease outside the uterus and in the retroperitoneal nodes, there is no reason to believe that aggressive cytoreductive efforts might not help in presenting a reduced tumor burden during adjunctive therapy, despite the absence of a clinical trial suggesting efficacy.

There are occasions when, at the time of staging laparotomy, cervical or parametrial invasion is detected and a radical (Wertheim) hysterectomy with pelvic and aortic lymphadenectomy is performed to achieve clearance of all disease. However, the addition of tailored external beam radiation therapy (RT) following surgery has largely eliminated the routine performance of such procedures.

Surgery for recurrent disease is generally confined to those patients who have symptoms of intestinal or urinary tract obstruction, isolated regional recurrence, or isolated lung metastases that have not responded to cytotoxic or hormonal therapy. For such patients, surgery may be useful to correct functional deficits or to excise isolated recurrences or resistant metastatic deposits.

The first reports of surgical staging of endometrial carcinoma with the use of laparoscopy assisted vaginal hysterectomy and laparoscopic lymphadenectomy were in 1992.[115,116] Since then, several reports have included laparoscopic bilateral para-aortic lymph node dissections.[117] However, there is only one randomized clinical trial of appropriate design that compares laparoscopic management of endometrial carcinoma with traditional surgical therapy. The GOG conducted a prospective phase III study comparing laparoscopy assisted surgical staging with traditional total abdominal hysterectomy and staging. In addition to assessing variables such as completeness of surgical staging, complications, operating room time, and hospital stay, this study also evaluated expanded outcome variables, including patient-reported measures of quality of life. To date the data is available only in abstract form. Single-institution retrospective data have demonstrated that laparoscopic lymphadenectomy and vaginal or laparoscopic hysterectomy with BSO provided 5-year survival and recurrence rates similar to those of the traditional abdominal approach.[118–120] Recently, robotic assisted laparoscopic surgery has been increasingly applied, although the additional costs, operating time and availability of the expensive equipment necessary remain barriers to general application. Moreover the precise role for robotic surgery is yet to be defined.[121] Figure 99-2 presents an algorithm for the surgical management of endometrial carcinoma.

Radiation Therapy

Although surgery, where possible, constitutes the definitive primary treatment for most patients with endometrial carcinoma, it is clear that RT is also an effective modality in its management.

Table 99-6 ■ Clinical and Molecular Features of Endometrial Carcinoma

Features	Type I	Type II
Clinical[31]		
Risk factors	Unopposed estrogen	Age
Race	White > black	White = black
Degree of differentiation	Well differentiated	Poorly differentiated
Histology	Endometrioid	Nonendometrioid
Stage	I/II	III/IV
Prognosis	Favorable	Unfavorable
Molecular[93]		
Ploidy	Diploid	Aneuploid
K-*ras* overexpression	Yes	Yes
HER2/neu overexpression	No	Yes
TP53 overexpression	No	Yes
PTEN mutations	Yes	No
Microsatellite instability	Yes	No

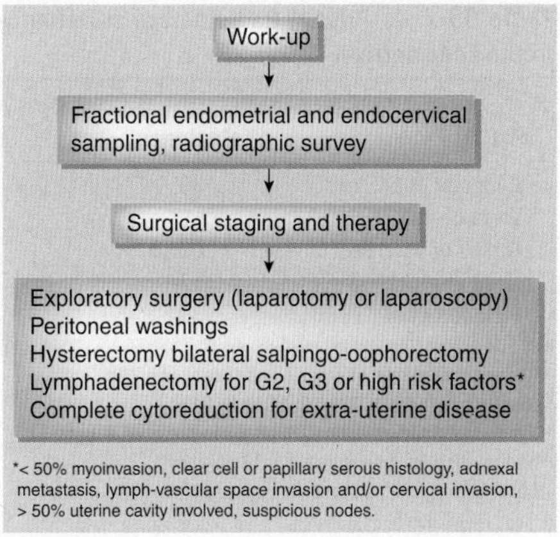

Figure 99-2 ■ Surgical management of endometrial carcinoma.

Definitive Irradiation for Inoperable Patients ■ Modern surgical techniques and improved postoperative care have diminished the number of patients considered inoperable. Nevertheless, because endometrial cancer is frequently a disease of the aged (over 65 years of age), who are often obese and sometimes diabetic, with other co-morbidities, surgery is not always possible. Table 99-7 shows five relatively large series in which patients received pelvic RT as their definitive management without initial surgery.[122–127]

The proportion surviving depends on tumor grade, just as for patients treated surgically; those with grade 1 tumors have better survival rates than do those with grade 3.[122] Significant numbers of patients die of causes unrelated to their primary carcinoma. In the case-control series (2 controls per case matched for age, stage, and grade) from Yale University, more deaths from intercurrent disease occurred within the inoperable stage I group than with the operable group (28 of 32 vs 3 of 15; $p < .0001$). Inoperable patients had a significantly shorter overall survival and more deaths owing to intercurrent disease than operable patients ($p < .0001$). However, inoperable patients who did not die from co-morbidities had a median 5-year survival rate that approached that of operable patients.[126]

Some patients with small uteri may be cured by intracavitary radiation only, but, usually, definitive management consists of both external beam and intracavitary irradiation because of more favorable radiation dosimetry. Complication rates are acceptable (usually less than 10%). After definitive irradiation, the pattern of failure, in contrast to that following surgery, consists mainly of central failure in the uterus. This observation is important for developing treatment strategies for patients with stage II disease. Removal of the uterus at some point in treatment provides better overall central

Table 99-7 **Primary Radiotherapy as Definitive Management of Inoperable Clinical Stage I Cancer of the Endometrium**

Study	Patients	Complication (%)	3-Year DFS (%)	5-Year DFS (%)	5-Year Survival
Abayomi et al., 1982[124]	39	15	[a]	–	–
Varia et al., 1987[122]	41[b]	10	72	57[a,b,c]	–
Grisby et al., 1987[123]	69	16	–	88	77
Rose et al., 1993[125]	17	–	71	[d]	–
Fishman et al., 1996[126]	39	–	20		80

[a]3-Year survival rate of stage I and II cancer = 78%.
[b]Results by grade: 1, 72%; 2, 59%; 3, 31%.
[c]Significant number (12 of 28) died of unrelated causes
[d]Median disease-free interval = 36 months.
Abbreviation: DFS, disease-free survival.

control than that achieved by radiation alone. Three series indicate 5-year survival rates of approximately 50%.[122,128,129]

Recently, Kucera and colleagues reported their experience with high-dose iridium 192 intracavitary brachytherapy without additional external beam radiation in 228 patients.[130] At 5 years, the overall survival rate was 59.7%. In clinical stage IA disease, the survival rate was 88.6% at 5 years and 82.7% at 10 years—significantly different in comparison with 80.2% and 63.4%, respectively, in stage IB disease. Intrauterine recurrence was 17.5%, but extrauterine pelvic relapse occurred in only 0.4% of patients. Others have also reported high-dose-rate (HDR) brachytherapy with or without external beam radiation,[131,132] and the American Brachytherapy Society published guidelines and recommendations in 2000.[133]

Adjuvant RT for Clinical Stage I Disease ■ The present recommendation to give postoperative RT in surgical stage I is dependent on prognosis as defined by the histologic features of the primary tumor within the endometrium. Extensive staging studies have identified that several of the aforementioned factors predict for the presence of clinically occult extrauterine disease.[54]

Although patients considered to be at high risk of recurrence (eg, those with grade 2 or 3 disease with penetration of the outer 50% of the myometrium) have generally been treated with postoperative adjuvant RT, there is only one randomized trial addressing the benefit of adjuvant RT in surgically staged patients (GOG-99, 147). There are three randomized clinical trials in patients who had incomplete surgical staging (Aalders,[56] Postoperative RT in Endometrial Carcinoma 1 and 2 [PORTEC-1 and -2, respectively]).

Aalders and colleagues reported that 540 patients with clinical stage I endometrial cancer were treated by TAH and BSO (TAH-BSO) and 60 Gy to the vaginal vault postoperatively.[56] Patients were then randomized to either no further therapy or external beam pelvic radiation at a dose of 40 Gy in 20 fractions over 4 weeks. Approximately half of the patients (261) were considered to be in the high-risk category, with greater than 50% myometrial penetration of any grade or grade 3 tumors with any degree of invasion. The authors suggested an improvement in survival achieved only in a defined subset; patients with high risk (poorly differentiation cancers with deep myometrial invasion)

The PORTEC-1 trial reported 741 patients with clinical stage IB, grades 2 to 3 cancer and stage IC, grades 1 to 2 cancer who were randomized to pelvic RT versus no additional treatment (NAT) after TAH-BSO but no lymph node assessment.[134] There was a significant reduction in locoregional recurrence in the RT cohort (4% vs 14%; $p < .001$) but no improvement in overall survival (81% vs 85%; $p = .31$). Treatment-related complications occurred in 25% of RT patients and in 6% of the controls ($p < .0001$).

For intermediate-risk disease (stage IB, grade 3; stage IC, grades 1 and 2), omitting RT would leave the patients with a significant risk of vaginal and pelvic relapse. Because there was a suggestion that vaginal brachytherapy might reduce the risk of vaginal relapse with less morbidity and a better quality of life, the PORTEC-2 trial was conducted randomizing 427 patients between pelvic RT (external beam RT [EBRT]—46 Gy in 23 fractions) and vaginal brachytherapy (VBT) (VBT—21 Gy HDR in 3 fractions, or 30 Gy LDR) after TAH-BSO without full staging. Eligible patients had a high-intermediate risk EC: age > 60 and stage 1C grade 1–2 or stage 1B grade 3; any age and stage 2A grades 1–2 or grade 3 with < 50% invasion. Three-year rates of vaginal, pelvic and distant relapse as first failure were 0%, 1.3%, and 6.4% in the VBT group, and 1.6%, 0.7%, and 6.0% in the EBRT group. There were no significant differences in 3-year overall survival (OS) (90.4% vs 90.8% $p = .55$) and recurrence-free survival (RFS) (89.5% vs 89.1% $p = .38$). The authors suggested that VBT should be the treatment of choice for patients with high-intermediate risk endometrial carcinoma.[135]

The last of the aforementioned trials is the only randomized trial addressing the role of adjuvant RT in surgically staged patients. The GOG reported the results of this phase III randomized trial (GOG 99) of NAT versus 5040 cGy of pelvic RT in patients with intermediate-risk endometrial cancer defined by the GOG 33. A high–intermediate-risk (HIR) subgroup of patients was defined (as an increased recurrent rate of 25% at 5 years based on GOG 33) as those: (1) age under 50 with moderately to poorly differentiated tumor, the presence of lymphovascular invasion, and outer third myometrial invasion; (2) age 50 years or more with any two of the risk factors listed above; or (3) age of at least 70 years with any risk factor listed above. All other eligible participants were considered to be in the low–intermediate-risk (LIR) subgroup. The median follow-up for the study was 69 months. Three hundred ninety-two women were randomized. (202 NAT, 190 RT). The median follow-up was 69 months The estimated 2-year cumulative incidence of recurrence was 12% in the NAT arm and 3% in the RT arm (relative hazard [RH] 0.42; $p = .007$). The treatment difference was particularly evident among the HIR subgroup (2-year cumulative incidence of recurrence in NAT vs RT: 26% vs 6%; RH: 0.42). Overall, radiation had a substantial impact on pelvic and vaginal recurrences (18 in NAT and 3 in RT). The estimated 4-year survival rate was 86% in the NAT arm and 92% for the RT arm, which is not significantly different (RH 0.86; $p = .557$). This HIR subgroup represented about one-third of the patients (132 of 392) and accounted for nearly two-thirds of the recurrences (28) and two-thirds of the cancer-related deaths. The conclusions were that adjunctive RT in early-stage intermediate-risk endometrial carcinoma decreases the risk of recurrence but should be limited to patients whose risk factors fit a HIR definition.[136]

Vault Irradiation ■ The rationale for administering pelvic RT in GOG-99 was to prevent vaginal vault recurrences and to sterilize occult pelvic side wall disease, presumably not excised at surgery. Other occult pelvis side wall disease not found at surgery, such as in the lymphatic channels in the parametrium or in parametrial lymph nodes, occurs infrequently and is an unlikely source of recurrence. Thus, on a theoretic basis, the patient who undergoes thorough staging, ideally with a bilateral pelvic and lower para-aortic lymphadenectomy, might be at low risk of a pelvic side wall recurrence in the absence of lymph node metastasis. This side wall disease, when undetected and untreated, likely would contribute to preventable mortality for this patient population. The major site for possible recurrence within the pelvis for these patients would be the vaginal vault, which is amenable to irradiation with either low-dose-rate (LDR) or HDR applicators with a high probability of local control and, presumably, cure. In addition to the prospective data from PORTEC-2[135] supporting this hypothesis there are several retrospective studies, which have demonstrated rare pelvic recurrences in high-risk patients (stage IB, grade 3 and stage IC) who undergo therapeutic pelvic lymphadenectomy and either no RT[137] or vault brachytherapy[138] alone in the absence of lymph node metastasis.[54,139–141]

Stage III ■ The 1988 FIGO surgical staging for endometrial cancer now includes patients with metastases to pelvic and/or para-aortic lymph nodes as stage IIIC. The current staging classification covers a broad spectrum of prognostic groups that have diverse outcomes after standard surgery with or without adjuvant pelvic irradiation. Unfortunately, many of the published series include patients with microscopic extension to the adnexa (stage IIIA), those with malignant ascites (stage IIIA), and those with gross pelvic side wall disease (stage IIIA or IIIC) without distinction, resulting in widely variable survival data.

Treatment recommendations at this time for patients with stage III disease must be made on an individual basis. Those in whom appropriate surgical staging has been completed without evidence of disease beyond the ovaries should be considered for adjuvant postoperative pelvic irradiation, although the importance of microscopic adnexal invasion in patients without other risk factors is unclear. For those who have had surgical staging and who have pelvic but not para-aortic nodal involvement, it may be appropriate to offer postoperative adjuvant irradiation confined to the pelvis. Disease-free survival rates between 35% and 60% have been reported for patients receiving 45 to 50Gy of external beam irradiation to the para-aortic nodes, usually with pelvic irradiation. Almost in all cases, macroscopic para-aortic nodal disease is not curable with RT without complete cytoreduction first.[54,142–147] Retrospective data from Johns Hopkins Hospital suggest that in patients with stage IIIC endometrial carcinoma, complete resection of macroscopic nodal disease and the administration of adjuvant chemotherapy, in addition to directed RT, are associated with improved survival (Table 99-8).[148]

Some subsets of stage III endometrial cancer patients may be candidates for cytotoxic chemotherapy only. Figure 99-3 presents an algorithm for the postoperative management of endometrial carcinoma.

Table 99-8 ■ **Results of Para-aortic Radiotherapy in Endometrial Cancer**

Study	Complication (%)	*n*	NED (%)	RT Dose (Gy)
Hicks et al., 1993[143]	11[a]	4	36	45
Rose et al., 1992[142]	26	9	35	45
Komaki et al., 1983[144]	–	7	60	50
Feuer and Calanog, 1987[145]	18	8	44	50
Corn et al., 1992[146]		50[b]	46	48
Potish et al., 1985[147]	–	48	52	48
Morrow et al., 1991[54]	–	48	20	40

[a]Three of 17 with macroscopic disease.
[b]Twenty-four of 50 para-aortic nodes diagnosed on radiography.
Abbreviations: NED, no evidence of disease; RT, radiation therapy.

Treatment of Recurrent Disease

Patients who develop locoregional reccurences without previous radiation, can expect a salvage rate of 90% with RT. Those who develop a component of extra pelvic recurrence will require systemic therapy.

In the patient who has had initial adjuvant postoperative pelvic irradiation, there may rarely be a role for interstitial therapy at relapse if there is isolated central pelvic failure. For some systemic therapy may be applicable. For patients with other sites of disease or bony, cerebral, or nodal metastases, short courses of palliative irradiation may be useful in relieving the symptoms of disease. Similarly, palliative irradiation may be used for the uncommon patient (approximately 3% of those at presentation) who has stage IV disease.

Unlike ovarian carcinoma, little is known regarding the role of secondary cytoreduction in recurrent endometrial carcinoma. In a report from an Italian group, 20 women with recurrent endometrial adenocarcinoma were treated with maximal cytoreductive surgery.[149] Sixty-five percent of patients had complete resection of their tumor. Women with no residual tumor had a significantly increased PFS and OS compared with women with residual tumor; however, there was a 10% perioperative death rate in this series. The role of pelvic exenteration was examined in a four-institution retrospective review of 31 patients.[150] Twenty patients underwent exenteration with curative intent, all of whom had previously received pelvic irradiation. The 5-year disease-free survival rate was 45%.

Cytotoxic Chemotherapy

Cytotoxic chemotherapy for patients with endometrial cancer was rarely administered before 1980. In his 1974 literature review, Donovan reported only 126 patients who had been treated with 16 different agents.[151] A combination of complete and partial responses was identified in 34 of 126 patients (27%).

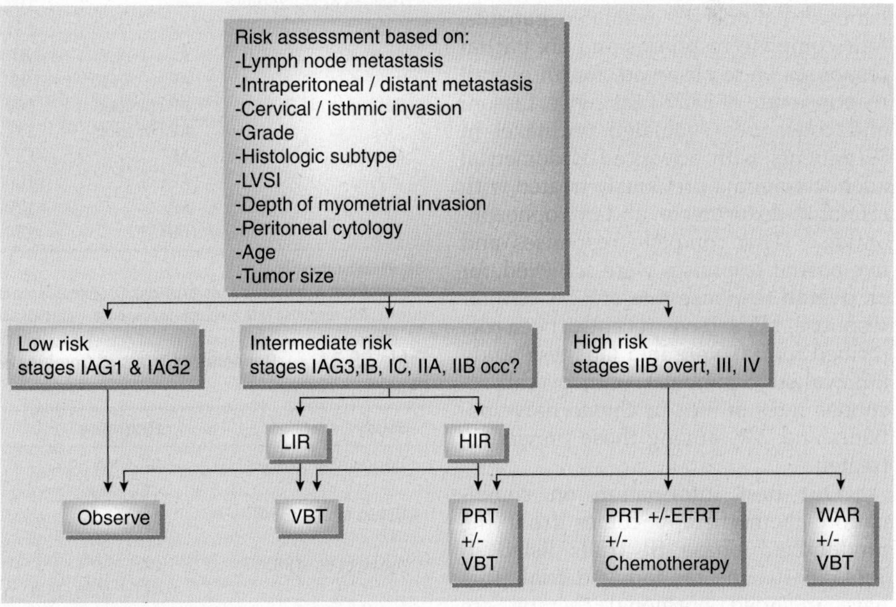

Figure 99-3 ■ Postoperative management of endometrial carcinoma. *Abbreviations*: EFRT, extended field radiation therapy; HIR, high-intermediate risk based on Gynecologic Oncology Group 99: age < 50, 50–70, > 70; LIR, low intermediate risk; LVSI, lymph–vascular space invasion, outer third invasion, grade 2 or 3 (see text); PRT, pelvic radiation therapy; VBT, vaginal brachytherapy; WAR, whole abdominopelvic radiotherapy.

In 1977, Muggia and colleagues reported that doxorubicin (adriamycin, 37.5 mg/m²) in combination with cyclophosphamide (500 mg/m²) intravenously (IV) every 21 days in 11 patients with recurrent endometrial cancer resulted in five objective responses.[152] The GOG studied single-agent doxorubicin at a dose rate of 60 mg/m² IV every 3 weeks and reported a 37% response rate in 43 patients.[153] Although the most frequent adverse effect was on the hematopoietic system, cardiac toxicity occurred in 12%, and there was one cardiotoxic death in a patient who had received more than 500 mg/m² of drug. This study was important because it clearly established the value of doxorubicin as a single agent in the chemotherapy of endometrial cancer. Studies by GOG and The Eastern Cooperative Oncology Group demonstrated no benefit from adding cyclophosphamide.[154,155]

The GOG, in heavily pretreated patients found no efficacy for cisplatin alone,[156] however, Trope in a small series observed four responses (36%) in 11 chemotherapy-naive patients with cisplatin at a dose rate of 50 mg/m².[157]

A combination of cisplatin and doxorubicin in advanced or recurrent endometrial cancer produced response rates of 33% to 80%, depending on the proportion of patients previously treated with either chemotherapy or radiation.[158,159]

If one selects only drugs that have achieved at least a 20% response rate in studies including at least 20 patients, the list is small (Table 99-9). Paclitaxel is an active drug in recurrent endometrial adenocarcinoma. The GOG studied paclitaxel in patients with advanced or recurrent adenocarcinoma of the endometrium.[160] Among 28 evaluable patients, four complete responses and six partial responses were observed, for an overall response rate of 35.7%. Likewise, Lissoni and colleagues evaluated paclitaxel in 19 patients with advanced endometrial adenocarcinoma previously treated with cisplatin, doxorubicin, and cyclophosphamide.[161] Two complete responses and five partial responses were achieved, for an overall response rate of 37%. Similar response rates have recently been described for Taxotere in a Japanese study (32 evaluable patients), with overall response rates of 36% in chemo naïve patients and 23% among those previously treated.[162]

Our best information on combination chemotherapy comes from the randomized phase III trials listed in Table 99-10. The randomized trials that have included hormonal therapy are listed in Table 99-11.

Table 99-10 lists the randomized trials that compared single agents with one or two different combinations. The European Organisation for Research and Treatment of Cancer (EORTC) study reported by Aapro and colleagues, a survival advantage was demonstrated with a response rate of 43% for the doxorubicin and cisplatin combination versus 17% for single-agent doxorubicin ($p < .001$).[163] The GOG found no difference when doxorubicin and cisplatin were administered in a circadian fashion compared with a standard fashion.[164]

The GOG also conducted a phase III study of doxorubicin plus cisplatin versus doxorubicin plus 24-h paclitaxel in primary stage III or IV or recurrent endometrial carcinoma. This study found no difference in response rate, PFS, or OS.[165]

The most recent phase III prospective randomized GOG study (Protocol 177) compared standard doxorubicin (60 mg/m²) and cisplatin (50 mg/m²), that is, AP against TAP with paclitaxel (Taxol 160 mg/m²/3 h), doxorubicin (45 mg/m²), and cisplatin (50 mg/m²).[149] Two hundred sixty-six patients were randomized, and the results indicated that TAP produced a significant improvement in response rate (57% vs 34%; $p < .01$) and PFS (median 8.3 vs 5.3 months; $p < .01$) and overall survival (median 15.3 vs 12.3 months; $p = .037$).[166,167] The GOG is currently randomly assigning patients with advanced (stage IVB) or recurrent disease to either TAP or paclitaxel and carboplatin to determine whether it is possible to drop doxorubicin from the regimen and substitute carboplatin for cisplatin with-

Table 99-9 Single-Agent Cytotoxic Chemotherapy for Endometrial Cancer

Agent	Reference	*n*	Prior Treatment	No CR + PR	%
Paclitaxel	160	28	No	4 + 6	36
Paclitaxel	161	19	Yes	2 + 5	37
Docetaxel	162	19	No	1 + 6	36
Docetaxel	162	13	Yes	0 + 3	23
Cisplatin	194, 198	75	No	3 + 18	28
Carboplatin	199–201	76	No	5 + 18	28
Doxorubicin	153, 163, 168	280	No	31 + 49	29
Epirubicin	202	27	No	2 + 5	26
Fluorouracil	203	34	NS	7	21
HMM	204	30	No	10	33

Reported series with at least 20 patients with a response rate of at least 20%.
Source: Adapted from Muss HB[205] and Thigpen JT.[168]
Abbreviations: CR, complete response; HMM, hexamethylmelamine; NS, not stated; PR, partial response.

Table 99-10 Randomized Trials of Combination Chemotherapy Regimens for Endometrial Cancer

Study	Regimen	Number Evaluable	RR (%)	Median PFS (Mo)	Median Overall Survival (Mo)
Thigpen et al., 1994[155]	A	132	22	3.2	6.7
	AC	144	30	3.9	7.3
Thigpen et al., 2004[168]	A	150	25	3.8	9.2
	AP	131	42[a]	5.7*	9.0
Aapro et al., 2003[163]	A	87	17	7.0	7.0
	AP	90	43[a]	8.0	9.0[a]
Gallion et al., 2003[164]	AP standard	169	46	6.5	11.2
	AP circadian	173	49	5.9	13.2
Fleming et al., 2004[165]	AP	157	40	7.2	12.6
	AT	160	43	6.0	13.6
Fleming et al., 2004[167]	AP	129	34	5.3	12.3
	TAP	134	57[a]	8.3[a]	15.3[a]

[a]Significant difference.
Abbreviations: A, adriamycin (doxorubicin); C, cyclophosphamide; F, 5-fluorouracil; P, platinol (cisplatin); PFS, progression-free survival; RR, response rate = complete response + partial response; T, taxol (paclitaxel).

Table 99-11 Randomized Trials of Combination Chemotherapy + Hormonal Therapy for Endometrial Cancer

Study	Regimen	Number Evaluable	RR (%)
Horton et al., 1982[206]	CA + MA	55	27
	CAF + MA	56	16
Cohen et al., 1984[207]	F-Mel + MA	126	38
	CAF + MA	131	36
Ayoub et al., 1988[187]	CAF	20	15
	CAF + MPA/TAM	23	43[a]
Cornelison et al., 1995[208]	APE + MA	50	54
	F-Mel + MPA	50	48

[a]Significant difference.
Abbreviations: A, adriamycin (doxorubicin); C, cyclophosphamide; F, 5-fluorouracil; MA, megestrol acetate; Mel, melphalan; MPA, medroxypro gesterone acetate; P, platinol (cisplatin); RR, response rate = complete response + partial response; TAM, tamoxifen.

out loss of efficacy and with a marked improvement in toxicity profile (GOG Protocol 209).[168]

In patients with surgical bulk reduction (to residual < 2 cm) for stage III to IVA disease, the GOG in Protocol 122 (a randomized phase III trial) demonstrated that chemotherapy with doxorubicin (60 mg/m^2) and cisplatin (50 mg/m^2) had superior PFS (0.71; 95% confidence interval [CI] = 0.55–0.91; $p < .01$) and overall survival (0.68; 95% CI = 0.52–0.89; $p < .01$) compared with whole-abdomen radiation.[169]

Adjuvant Chemotherapy for High-Risk Early-Stage Disease

Stringer et al. studied 31 patients with high-risk stage I endometrial cancer and 2 patients with occult stage II disease.[170] Postoperatively, the patients were treated with CAP chemotherapy including cisplatin, 50 mg/m^2, doxorubicin, 50 mg/m^2, and cyclophosphamide, 500 mg/m^2, every 4 weeks for six cycles. The 2-year PFI rate was 79%, and the 2-year survival was 83%. The median survival time for patients was not reached at 45 months. These results were considered superior to those of historical controls from the same institution.

The GOG randomized patients with high-risk clinical stage I and stage II disease to postoperative whole-pelvis irradiation with or without doxorubicin and found no difference in PFI and OS.[171]

The Japanese GOG designed a multi-center randomized phase III trial to address the relative efficacy of CAP chemotherapy (cyclophosphamide (333 mg/m^2), doxorubicin (40 mg/m^2) and cisplatin (50 mg/m^2) every 4 weeks for 3 or more courses) versus whole pelvic RT (WPRT) in stage IC to III. Although there was no difference in PFS or OS in the entire cohort—a subgroup analysis of 120 high-intermediate risk patients (defined as (1) stage IC in patients over 70 years old or with G3 endometrioid adenocarcinoma or (2) stage II or IIIA (positive cytology)),found that the CAP group had a significantly higher PFS rate (83.8% vs 66.2%, log-rank test $p = .024$, hazard ratio 0.44) and higher OS rate (89.7% vs 73.6%, log-rank test $p = .006$, hazard ratio 0.24).[172]

In a study of 74 patients with stage I UPSC, Kelly et al. have demonstrated that all patients with residual disease (including disease confined to the endometrium) have improved PRs and OS with adjuvant platinum based chemotherapy. There were no vaginal recurrences in those receiving vaginal brachytherapy. There were no recurrences in the 12 patients with stage IA disease with no residual disease at hysterectomy regardless of treatment and observation in these patients may be considered. Because clear cell carcinoma behaves like UPSC, in spite of the absence of data, they should be treated in a similar fashion.[173]

Hormone Therapy

Progestins Kelly and Baker, in 1961, described six objective responses in 21 patients that lasted from 9 months to 4½ years. This report represents one of the first successes of biologic therapy for cancer patients.[174] Since then, numerous reports described treatment with a variety of progestational drugs: most commonly 17-hydroxyprogesterone caproate, medroxyprogesterone acetate (MPA), and megestrol acetate (MA). Reifenstein analyzed 992 patients treated with hydroxyprogesterone caproate by 113 investigators.[175] He studied the records of 314 patients in detail and found, (1) that there was little response before 7 weeks of treatment, (2) that the longest remissions were achieved with a minimum of 12 weeks of initial therapy, and (3) that there was no relationship between clinical response and patient age when correction was made for tumor differentiation. Kauppila reviewed 1068 patients treated in 17 different trials with either MPA (Provera), MA, or hydroxyprogesterone caproate and found an overall response rate of 34%.[176] The duration of response was approximately 20 months, and the average survival time was approximately 25 months.

The optimum dose for progestational treatment has not been determined and the doses employed in the most recent GOG studies were based on dose seeking studies by Kohorn and Thigpen.[177,178] There is no evidence that lower doses are not equally effective, and therefore selecting lower doses in special circumstances may be permissible in order to avoid complications. Several investigators compared oral and parenteral routes of administration employing a variety of progestational agents and found no advantage for the parenteral route.[175,179] Milligram equivalents of progestational agents frequently do not translate into biologic equivalence, and the dose of a particular progestogen required for tumor control may have to be empirically derived.

Ramirez and colleagues, in reviewing the literature, found that the majority of patients reported with well-differentiated endometrial adenocarcinoma who undergo conservative treatment for primary uterine cancer (in lieu of hysterectomy) with a progestational agent respond to treatment (62 of 81 = 76%).[180] When an initial response is not achieved or when disease recurs after an initial response (15 of 62 = 24%), carcinoma extending beyond the uterus is rare.[180] In addition, Montz and colleagues described the feasibility of using a progesterone-containing intrauterine device to treat presumed FIGO stage IA, grade 1 endometrioid cancer in women at high risk of perioperative complications.[181]

In summary, the following generalizations can be made concerning progestational therapy: (1) the response rate for patients with advanced or recurrent endometrial carcinoma ranges from 10% to 30%, probably relating to the receptor level in the tumor; (2) well-differentiated cancers respond best; (3) the PR level diminishes sharply as the grade of the tumor increases; (4) clinical responses may not occur before 7 weeks to 12 weeks of therapy; (5) two-thirds of patients will not respond; (6) there is no published evidence that progestational agents employed in an adjuvant mode offer any benefit; (7) appropriate oral doses based on GOG studies are 160 mg/day of megestrol or 200 mg/day of MPA, however lower doses can be individualized; and (8) oral progestins and the progesterone-containing intrauterine device are alternatives to consider for primary treatment of selected cases of early-stage, low-grade endometrial cancer.

Tamoxifen ■ Hormonal therapy by agents other than progestogens has been studied by many researchers. Extrapolating from the experience with breast cancer, investigators employed tamoxifen in doses of 20 to 40 mg daily for patients with advanced or recurrent endometrial carcinoma. In a review of eight published studies, Moore and colleagues described an overall response rate of 22%.[182] As one might predict, there is a wide spectrum of reported responses, ranging from 0% to 53%.[183] This variation may be explained by the report of Edmonson and colleagues, who found a 21% response rate in patients naive to hormone therapy and no response in patients who had failed progesterone treatment.[184] Not unlike the progestin experience, it would seem that tamoxifen is more likely to be effective in patients with low-grade tumors, receptor positivity, and either no previous hormone therapy or a previous response to progestin therapy.

Because progestins ultimately downregulate PRs, and because tamoxifen induces these receptors in target tissues, the notion of the combined administration of these hormones has been examined by the GOG with two different strategies. In Whitney and colleagues' report, tamoxifen citrate 40 mg/day combined with alternating weekly cycles of MPA 200 mg/day in 58 patients with recurrent or measurable advanced endometrial carcinoma resulted in a 33% response rate (10.3% complete response and 23.4% partial response), with a median PFI of 3 months and a median overall survival of 13 months.[185] In the Fiorica study, alternating 3-week courses of MA (160 mg/day) and tamoxifen citrate (40 mg/day) in 56 patients with recurrent or measurable advanced endometrial carcinoma produced a 27% response rate (21.4% complete response and 5.4% partial response), with a median PFI of 2.7 months and a median OS of 14.0 months.[186]

The combination of tamoxifen, progestin, and chemotherapy has also been tested. Ayoub and colleagues studied 46 patients with metastatic endometrial cancer, randomly assigning them to receive monthly cycles of cyclophosphamide, adriamycin (doxorubicin), and 5-fluorouracil (CAF) or CAF plus MPA, 200 mg/day for 3 weeks, followed cyclically by tamoxifen, 20 mg/day for 3 weeks.[187] Objective responses of 15 and 43% were seen, respectively, with CAF and CAF plus hormonal therapy ($p = .05$). Because progestational agents have not improved the response to chemotherapy in previously cited studies,[188] it is reasonable to attribute this difference to the addition of tamoxifen. Recently, Pinelli and colleagues evaluated sequential cyclical hormone therapy (MA and tamoxifen citrate) plus the single agent carboplatin.[189] Of 13 evaluable patients, 4 patients had a complete response and 6 had partial responses, for an overall response rate of 77%. The median PFI was 14 months for complete responders. The median survival was 11 months for all patients and 33 months for complete responders.

Other Hormonal and Targeted Therapy

The GOG have conducted several phase II clinical trials to evaluate biologic therapy in endometrial cancer. Gonadotropin-releasing hormone analogues (goserelin and leuprolide) have been tested in small phase II trials of patients with recurrent endometrial carcinoma, with response rates varying from 0% to 35%.[190–192] A GOG-180 trial of danazol showed hepatic toxicity in four patients but no responses among the 25 patients.[193]

Aromatase inhibitors have been tested in a limited fashion. The GOG-168 phase II trial had a 9% response rate (2 partial responses of 23) with anastrozole,[192] whereas the Canadian National Cancer Institute study reported a 9.4% response rate (2 partial responses of 28) with letrozole.[194]

RAD001 a mammalian target of rapamycin (mTOR) inhibitor had no objective responses and a 44% stable disease rate in 25 evaluable patients with recurrent endometrial cancer.[195] Sorafenib (a small molecular inhibitor of Raf kinase, platelet-derived growth factor [PDGF], vascular endothelial growth factor [VEGF] receptor 2 & 3 kinases and c Kit) had a 5% partial response and a 50% stable disease rate in 39 patients with recurrent endometrial cancer.[196] A series of other targeted therapies have recently been tested by the GOG in phase II trials and the results are pending—including iressa (EGFR), trastuzumab (HER-2/NEU), lapatanib (EGFR & HER-2/neu), bevacizumab (VEGF), and VEGF trap.

Increased levels of VEGF and angiogenic markers are associated with poor outcome in endometrioid endometrial cancer patients. Using a novel orthotopic model of endometrioid endometrial cancer, the MD Anderson group showed that combination of antivascular therapy (bevacizumab) with docetaxel is highly efficacious and should be considered for future clinical trials.[197] The notion of combining metronomic chemotherapy and biologic therapy appears quite appealing.

The Future

Efforts must continue to expand information about molecular characteristics to better define patient susceptibilities and therapeutic possibilities.. From a surgical standpoint, laparoscopic staging is offered more frequently but the role of robotic surgery is incompletely defined.[121] For patients with early disease and poor prognostic features, further randomized studies comparing RT with systemic therapy are required.. For patients with advanced or recurrent disease, better systemic therapy including biologic and targeted agents must be identified.. It is obvious that with a cure rate in the United States of approximately 80%, it will be essential that patients with poor prognostic features or recurrent or metastatic disease be entered into collaborative trials to maximize the opportunities for improving survival.

Selected References

The complete reference list can be found at www.CANCERMEDICINE8.com

2. Creasman WT, Odicino F, Maisonneuve P, et al. Carcinoma of the corpus uteri. FIGO 6th Annual Report on the Results of Treatment in Gynecological Cancer. *Int J Gynaecol Obstet.* 2006;95(Suppl 1):S105–S143.
23. Fisher B, Costantino JP, Wickerham DL, et al. Tamoxifen for prevention of breast cancer: report of the National Surgical Adjuvant Breast and Bowel Project P-1 Study. *J Natl Cancer Inst.* 1998;90:1371–1388.
25. Cohen CJ, Rahaman J. Endometrial cancer. Management of high risk and recurrence including the tamoxifen controversy. *Cancer.* 1995;76(10 Suppl):2044–2052.
30. Bokhman JV. Two pathogenetic types of endometrial carcinoma. *Gynecol Oncol.* 1983;15:10–17.
36. Hendrickson M, Ross J, Eifel P, et al. Uterine papillary serous carcinoma: a highly malignant form of endometrial adenocarcinoma. *Am J Surg Pathol.* 1982;6:93–108.
40. Kurman RJ, Scully RE. Clear cell carcinoma of the endometrium: an analysis of 21 cases. *Cancer.* 1976;37:872–882.
42. Cohen CJ, Gusberg SB, Koffler D. Histologic screening for endometrial cancer. *Gynecol Oncol.* 1974;2:279–286.
49. Creasman WT, Morrow CP, Bundy BN, et al. Surgical pathologic spread patterns of endometrial cancer. A Gynecologic Oncology Group study. *Cancer.* 1987;60(8 Suppl):2035–2041.
53. Mariani A, Dowdy SC, Cliby WA, et al., Prospective assessment of lymphatic dissemination in endometrial cancer: a paradigm shift in surgical staging. *Gynecol Oncol.* 2008;109(1)11–18.
54. Morrow CP, Bundy BN, Kurman RJ, et al. Relationship between surgical-pathological risk factors and outcome in clinical stage I and II carcinoma of the endometrium: a Gynecologic Oncology Group study. *Gynecol Oncol.* 1991;40:55–65.
56. Aalders J, Abeler V, Kolstad P, et al. Postoperative external irradiation and prognostic parameters in stage I endometrial carcinoma: clinical and histopathologic study of 540 patients. *Obstet Gynecol.* 1980;56:419–427.
59. DiSaia PJ, Creasman WT, Boronow RC, et al. Risk factors and recurrent patterns in stage I endometrial cancer. *Am J Obstet Gynecol.* 1985;151:1009–1015.
72. Mariani A, Sebo TJ, Webb MJ, et al. Molecular and histopathologic predictors of distant failure in endometrial cancer. *Cancer Detect Prev.* 2003;27:434–441.
89. Caduff RF, Johnston CM, Svoboda-Newman SM, et al. Clinical and pathological significance of microsatellite instability in sporadic endometrial carcinoma. *Am J Pathol.* 1996;148:1671–1678.
90. Tashiro H, Isacson C, Levine R, et al. p53 gene mutations are common in uterine serous carcinoma and occur early in their pathogenesis. *Am J Pathol.* 1997;150:177–185.
94. Ito K, Watanabe K, Nasim S, et al. Prognostic significance of p53 overexpression in endometrial cancer. *Cancer Res.* 1994;54:4667–4670.
99. Enomoto T, Fujita M, Inoue M, et al. Alterations of the p53 tumor suppressor gene and its association with activation of the c-K-ras-2 protooncogene in premalignant and malignant lesions of the human uterine endometrium. *Cancer Res.* 1993;53:1883–1888.
104. Lukes AS, Kohler MF, Pieper CF, et al. Multivariable analysis of DNA ploidy, p53, and HER-2/neu as prognostic factors in endometrial cancer. *Cancer.* 1994;73:2380–2385.
106. Monk BJ, Chapman JA, Johnson GA, et al. Correlation of C-myc and HER-2/neu amplification and expression with histopathologic variables in uterine corpus cancer. *Am J Obstet Gynecol.* 1994;171:1193–1198.
110. Risinger JI, Hayes K, Maxwell GL, et al. PTEN mutation in endometrial cancers is associated with favorable clinical and pathologic characteristics. *Clin Cancer Res.* 1998;4:3005–3010.
114. Prasad M, Wang H, Douglas W, et al. Molecular genetic characterization of tamoxifen-associated endometrial cancer. *Gynecol Oncol.* 2005;96:25–31.
119. Obermair A, Manolitsas TP, Leung Y, et al. Total laparoscopic hysterectomy for endo-

metrial cancer: patterns of recurrence and survival. *Gynecol Oncol.* 2004;92:789–793.

123. Grigsby PW, Kuske RR, Perez CA, et al. Medically inoperable stage I adenocarcinoma of the endometrium treated with radiotherapy alone. *Int J Radiat Oncol Biol Phys.* 1987;13:483–438.
125. Rose PG, Baker S, Kern M, et al. Primary radiation therapy for endometrial carcinoma: a case controlled study. *Int J Radiat Oncol Biol Phys.* 1993;27:585–590.
130. Kucera H, Knocke TH, Kucera E, et al. Treatment of endometrial carcinoma with high-dose-rate brachytherapy alone in medically inoperable stage I patients. *Acta Obstet Gynecol Scand.* 1998;77:1008–1012.
133. Nag S, Erickson B, Parikh S, et al. The American Brachytherapy Society recommendations for high-dose-rate brachytherapy for carcinoma of the endometrium. *Int J Radiat Oncol Biol Phys.* 2000;48:779–790.
134. Creutzberg CL, van Putten WL, Koper PC, et al. Surgery and postoperative radiotherapy versus surgery alone for patients with stage-1 endometrial carcinoma: multicentre randomised trial. PORTEC Study Group. Post Operative Radiation Therapy in Endometrial Carcinoma. *Lancet.* 2000;355:1404–1411.
135. Nout RA, Putter H, Jürgenliemk-Schulz IM, et al. Vaginal brachytherapy versus external beam pelvic radiotherapy for high-intermediate risk endometrial cancer: Results of the randomized PORTEC-2 trial. *J Clin Oncol.* 26: 2008 (May 20 suppl; abstr LBA5503).
136. Keys HM, Roberts JA, Brunetto VL, et al. A phase III trial of surgery with or without adjunctive external pelvic radiation therapy in intermediate risk endometrial adenocarcinoma: a Gynecologic Oncology Group study. *Gynecol Oncol.* 2004;92:744–751.
141. Eltabbakh GH, Piver MS, Hempling RE, et al. Excellent long-term survival and absence of vaginal recurrences in 332 patients with low-risk stage I endometrial adenocarcinoma treated with hysterectomy and vaginal brachytherapy without formal staging lymph node sampling: report of a prospective trial. *Int J Radiat Oncol Biol Phys.* 1997;38:373–380.
148. Bristow RE, Zahurak ML, Alexander CJ, et al. FIGO stage IIIC endometrial carcinoma: resection of macroscopic nodal disease and other determinants of survival. *Int J Gynecol Cancer.* 2003;13:664–672.
158. Seltzer V, Vogl SE, Kaplan BH. Adriamycin and cisdiamminedichloroplatinum in the treatment of metastatic endometrial adenocarcinoma. *Gynecol Oncol.* 1984;19:308–313.
163. Aapro MS, van Wijk FH, Bolis G, et al. Doxorubicin versus doxorubicin and cisplatin in endometrial carcinoma: definitive results of a randomised study (55872) by the EORTC Gynaecological Cancer Group. *Ann Oncol.* 2003;14:441–448.
167. Fleming GF, Brunetto VL, Cella D, et al. Phase III trial of doxorubicin plus cisplatin with or without paclitaxel plus filgrastim in advanced endometrial carcinoma: a Gynecologic Oncology Group study. *J Clin Oncol.* 2004;22:2159–2166.
168. Thigpen JT, Brady MF, Homesley HD, et al. Phase III trial of doxorubicin with or without cisplatin in advanced endometrial carcinoma: a Gynecologic Oncology Group study. *J Clin Oncol.* 2004;22:3902–3908.
169. Randall ME, Filiaci VL, Muss H, et al. Randomized phase III trial of whole-abdominal irradiation versus doxorubicin and cisplatin chemotherapy in advanced endometrial carcinoma: a Gynecologic Oncology Group Study. *J Clin Oncol.* 2006;24(1):36–44.
172. Susumu N, Sagae S, Udagawa Y, et al. Randomized phase III trial of pelvic radiotherapy versus cisplatin-based combined chemotherapy in patients with intermediate- and high-risk endometrial cancer: a Japanese Gynecologic Oncology Group study. *Gynecol Oncol.* 2008;108(1):226–233.
173. Kelly MG, O'Malley M, Hui DP, et al. Improved survival in surgical stage I patients with uterine papillary serous carcinoma (UPSC) treated with adjuvant platinum-based chemotherapy. *Gynecol Oncol.* 2005;98(3)353–359.
180. Ramirez PT, Frumovitz M, Bodurka DC, et al. Hormonal therapy for the management of grade 1 endometrial adenocarcinoma: a literature review. *Gynecol Oncol.* 2004;95:133–138.
185. Whitney CW, Brunetto VL, Zaino RJ, et al. Phase II study of medroxyprogesterone acetate plus tamoxifen in advanced endometrial carcinoma: a Gynecologic Oncology Group study. *Gynecol Oncol.* 2004;92:4–9.
186. Fiorica JV, Brunetto VL, Hanjani P, et al. Phase II trial of alternating courses of megestrol acetate and tamoxifen in advanced endometrial carcinoma: a Gynecologic Oncology Group study. *Gynecol Oncol.* 2004; 92:10–14.
187. Ayoub J, Audet-Lapointe P, Methot Y, et al. Efficacy of sequential cyclical hormonal therapy in endometrial cancer and its correlation with steroid hormone receptor status. *Gynecol Oncol.* 1988;31:327–337.
188. Cohen CJ, Deppe G, Bruckner HW. Treatment of advanced adenocarcinoma of the endometrium with melphalan, 5-fluorouracil, and medroxyprogesterone acetate: a preliminary study. *Obstet Gynecol.* 1977;50:415–417.
189. Pinelli DM, Fiorica JV, Roberts WS, et al. Chemotherapy plus sequential hormonal therapy for advanced and recurrent endometrial carcinoma: a phase II study. *Gynecol Oncol.* 1996;60:462–467.

100 Neoplasms of the Fallopian Tube

Jamal Rahaman, MD ▪ Carmel J. Cohen, MD

Malignant neoplasms of the fallopian tube are the rarest of the gynecologic cancers. Although cancers metastatic to the tube occur frequently from ovarian cancer, endometrial cancer, or other sources, and although there are reports of transitional cell carcinomas, adenosquamous carcinomas, and sarcomas, almost all of the primary cancers of the fallopian tube are papillary adenocarcinomas.

From the first gross description of fallopian tube cancer by Renaud in 1847, fewer than 2500 patients with fallopian tube carcinomas have been reported, and the vast majority of these reports included less than 50 patients analyzed retrospectively over a period of more than 10 years in individual institutions. Recently, collaborative groups and multi-institutional investigators have reported their data.[1] For example, Rosen and colleagues reported 143 women treated from 1980 to 1995 by the Austrian Cooperative Study Group for Fallopian Tube Carcinoma.[2,3] In addition to reports from single institutions with experience in treating 40 or more patients,[4-8] from which conclusions concerning pathophysiology, clinical presentation and course, and treatment patterns can be drawn, several attempts have been made at definitive literature reviews.[9-12]

Epidemiology

Primary fallopian tube carcinoma (PFTC) comprises approximately 0.31-1.11% of cancers of the female genital tract.[9,13,14,15] The most recent epidemiologic study of fallopian tube carcinoma was reported by Stewart and colleagues in 2007. A total of 3051 PFTC cases diagnosed from 1998 to 2003, reported from population-based cancer registries, were analyzed. The incidence rate was 0.41 per 100,000 women from 1998 to 2003. White, non-Hispanic women and women aged 60-79 had the highest incidence rates ($p < 0.0001$). The majorities (88%) of PFTCs were adenocarcinomas; serous adenocarcinomas accounted for 44% and endometrioid adenocarcinomas for 19% of adenocarcinoma diagnoses. Essentially half (49.9%) of PFTCs were poorly differentiated; 89% were unilateral at diagnosis. Stage at diagnosis was fairly evenly distributed among localized (36%), regional (30%), and distant (32%). Overall, rates of PFTC remained stable over time. Among women aged 65-69, incidence rates increased significantly by 3.8% per year from 1998 to 2003 ($p < 0.05$).[16] Etiologic factors for the development of primary fallopian tube carcinoma have not been clearly defined. Chronic tubal inflammation commonly coexists in fallopian tubes that contain carcinoma.[10,17] Whether there is an etiologic relationship or not remains unclear.

The increased risk of fallopian tube carcinoma among breast cancer (*BRCA*)-positive patients was described in recent reports, indicating a need to remove completely the fallopian tube when performing prophylactic surgery in these patients.[18-29] Some cases of occult primary fallopian tube carcinoma have been detected at prophylactic bilateral oophorectomy in *BRCA1* mutation carriers, and this risk should not be ignored.[18,20,21,25,26,28] In addition, cases of fallopian tube carcinoma have been described following prophylactic salpingo-oophorectomy in known *BRCA* carriers 22. As a result, several centers have established surgical-pathologic protocols to increase the ability to detect occult fallopian tube cancers by mandating peritoneal cytologic evaluation and employing serial sectioning of the fallopian tubes.[20,25,26,29]

Clinical Presentation

The most frequently occurring symptoms are vaginal bleeding, unexplained vaginal discharge, and pelvic pain. However, epidemiologic data has suggested that these symptoms are only present in 15% of women with the disease.[30] The discharge may often be serosanguineous, is usually unexplained by microbiologic studies, and is unresponsive to antimicrobial therapy. The uterine bleeding is obviously pathologic because the majority of patients are postmenopausal, and it is almost invariably unexplained by uterine curettage. Thus, primary fallopian tube carcinoma must be considered in the differential diagnosis when postmenopausal bleeding persists after a negative curettage.

The presence of pain is highly significant because cancers of the ovary, endometrium, and cervix do not cause pain until their diagnosis is all too obvious. The syndrome of "hydrops tubae profluens," described by Latzko,[31] in which a patient presents with a pelvic mass, profuse watery or honey-colored vaginal discharge, and pelvic pain that is greatly relieved by the sudden disappearance of the mass, is rarely encountered but is almost pathognomonic. The pain is attributed to distention of the fallopian tube by trapped fluid, and when the fluid is emptied by traversing the tubal-uterine-vaginal channel, the patient is immediately relieved. Pelvic mass is the most common physical finding, occurring in approximately 65% of patients.[12] Ascites accompanies a mass in only 15% of cases, and a variety of less frequent physical findings are attributable to widely metastatic disease at presentation.

Preoperative Diagnosis

Because of the rarity of this disease, with the resultant low level of suspicion by the medical community, a preoperative diagnosis is made in fewer than 3% of the patients described.[8] The presence of a pelvic mass is rarely attributed to tubal carcinoma by the examining physician, and radiography of the urinary and gastrointestinal tracts is useless in making the diagnosis.

The effectiveness of cytologic diagnosis from cervical and/or vaginal pool samples is widely variable and has been reported as positive in 40-60% of women with tubal carcinoma.[10,32] Of greater importance is the presence of adenocarcinoma in cervical or vaginal pool samples in the face of negative fractional dilatation and curettage of the uterus and absent palpable pathology. These patients may have early tubal carcinomas.

During the last decade, there have been increasing numbers of reports of successful diagnosis of fallopian tube carcinoma by ultrasonography.[33,34] The usual ultrasonography findings included a sausage-shaped mass with internal projections into a fluid-filled lumen, giving a characteristic "cogwheel" appearance. The successful preoperative diagnosis of primary fallopian tube carcinoma using transvaginal color and pulsed Doppler ultrasonography was reported by Kurjak and colleagues.[35] Computed tomographic and magnetic resonance imaging features have also been described.[36-38]

In 1984, Niloff and colleagues demonstrated the value of elevated cancer antigen (CA) 125 levels in monitoring four patients with recurrent fallopian tube carcinoma.[39] More recently, Rosen and colleagues determined pre- and postoperative CA 125 values in 13 patients with fallopian tube carcinoma.[40] The median preoperative value was 1220 IU/mL, significantly higher in comparison with postoperative levels (median 194 IU/mL). Correlation analysis with stage and grading failed to achieve statistical significance; however, a trend for a positive correlation with stage and preoperative value could be observed.

Although it is well established that serum levels of CA 125 can be significantly elevated in patients with pelvic inflammatory disease, endometriosis, and early pregnancy, and although neither CA 125 nor CA 19-9 is highly specific, the presence of an adnexal mass in a postmenopausal woman is an indication for serum marker studies preoperatively, at least to establish reference values for measuring therapeutic response.

Clinicopathologic Classification and Staging

Although more than 90% of the fallopian tube cancers are papillary adenocarcinomas, the synchronous presentation of the same histology in multiple pelvic sites recommends the establishment of diagnostic criteria that will identify primary fallopian tube cancer. The criteria established by Hu and colleagues[41] and later modified slightly by Sedlis[42] have been widely accepted (Table 100-1). Hu and colleagues accepted the histologic classification originally proposed by Sanger and Barth in which three grades of tumor were observed (papillary, papillary-alveolar, or alveolar-medullary).[41] This classification is no longer used by many pathologists, and histologic grade is usually simply designated as well, moderately, or poorly differentiated. The degree of differentiation of fallopian tube carcinomas has generally not been related to prognosis.[5,7,43,44]

Table 100-1 Diagnostic Criteria for Carcinoma of the Fallopian Tube

1. Grossly: The main tumor is in the tube and arises from the endosalpinx
2. Histologically: The pattern reproduces the epithelium of tubal mucosa (papillary pattern)
3. Transition from benign to malignant tubal epithelium should be demonstrated
4. The ovaries and endometrium are normal or have a much smaller tumor volume than that of the tube

Source: Adapted from Refs. 41 and 42.

Until 1991, there was no universally accepted staging system for patients with tubal carcinoma. In 1991, International Federation of Gynecologists and Obstetricians (FIGO) officially promulgated a staging system for tubal carcinoma (Table 100-2).[45] The new staging system takes into account the hollow viscus observations, the importance of ascites, and the impact of lymphatic spread. However, recently, Alvarado-Cabrero and colleagues proposed expanding the staging system to permit staging of noninvasive tubal carcinomas and fimbrial carcinomas and that substaging based on depth of invasion merits exploration in future studies.[46] Their recommendations are based on the observation that there was a significant difference in the length of recurrence-free survival of patients with no invasion beyond the epithelium or invasion of the lamina propria versus invasion into the muscularis.

Patterns of Spread

Studies from the literature indicate that the pattern of spread of fallopian tube carcinoma is similar to ovarian carcinoma, with both intraperitoneal and lymphatic spread commonly encountered.[5,42] However, because older staging systems did not mandate lymphadenectomy, there are few data on the incidence of lymph node metastases at the time of presentation.

Tamimi and Figge reviewed 15 patients treated over a 12-year period in their institution.[17] Lymph node sampling was not routine at the time of initial surgery, yet four of their patients had positive paraaortic nodes at the time of presentation and, overall, eight of their patients had lymph node involvement, either at the time of presentation or at the time of recurrence shortly after treatment. Semrad and colleagues, studying patterns of recurrent disease, noted a 71% incidence of extraperitoneal metastases, suggesting a strong probability of unrecognized lymphatic invasion at the time of initial therapy.[47] This observation is strengthened by reports of other investigators.[4,5,43] More recently, di Re and colleagues, studying the lymphatic spread of fallopian tube carcinoma in 17 patients undergoing surgical staging, observed an increase in the rates of nodal metastases with stage of disease and grade.[48] It may be noted that the percentage of patients with positive nodes was 33%, 66%, and 80% for stages I, II, and III-IV disease, respectively. Overall, patients with negative nodes had a median survival of 76 months compared with only 33 months if nodal metastases were found.

Prognostic Factors

In view of the inherent difficulties in studying such a rare disease, the role of prognostic factors assumes a greater importance. Stage is the most consistent prognostic factor associated with survival.[2,3,5,43,49] Although the initial tumor burden does not have predictive significance regarding survival, residual disease after cytoreduction is a strong prognostic factor of survival.[4,5,49,50] Other

Table 100-2 Staging of Carcinoma of Fallopian Tube

Stage 0	Carcinoma in situ (limited to tubal mucosa).
Stage I	Growth limited to the fallopian tubes.
Stage IA	Growth limited to one tube with extension into the submucosa and/or muscularis but not penetrating the serosal surface, no ascites.
Stage IB	Growth limited to both tubes with extension into the submucosa and/or muscularis but not penetrating the serosal surface, no ascites.
Stage IC	Tumor either stage IA or IB with tumor extension through or onto the tubal serosa or with ascites present containing malignant cells or with positive washings.
Stage II	Growth involving one or both fallopian tubes with pelvic extension.
Stage IIA	Extension and/or metastasis to the uterus and/or ovaries.
Stage IIB	Extension to other pelvic tissues.
Stage IIC	Tumor either stage IIA or IIB and with ascites present containing malignant cells or with positive peritoneal washings.
Stage III	Tumor involving one or both fallopian tubes with peritoneal implants outside of the pelvis and/or retroperitoneal or inguinal nodes. Superficial liver metastases equals stage III. Tumor seems limited to the true pelvis with negative nodes but with histologically proven malignant extension to the small bowel or omentum.
Stage IIIA	Tumor grossly limited to the true pelvis with negative nodes but with histologically confirmed microscopic seeding of abdominal peritoneal surfaces.
Stage IIIB	Tumor involving one or both tubes with histologically confirmed implants of abdominal peritoneal surfaces, none exceeding 2 cm in diameter. Lymph nodes negative.
Stage IIIC	Abdominal implants greater than 2 cm in diameter and/or positive retroperitoneal or inguinal nodes.
Stage IV	Growth invading one or both fallopian tubes with distant metastases. If pleural effusion is present, there must be positive cytology to be stage IV. Parenchymal liver metastases equals stage IV.

clinical prognostic factors include the presence of ascites.[5] More recently, Rosen and colleagues reported on prognostic factors in 143 women with primary fallopian tube carcinoma.[2] FIGO stage, histologic grade, and the presence of residual tumor had an independent prognostic impact in multivariate analysis. Several histologic factors are prognostic of survival, most notably the extent of tubal invasion. The observation that the extent of tubal invasion was associated with a poorer prognosis was first reported by Schiller and Silverberg.[10] Peters and colleagues, analyzing stage I disease, observed a statistically significant increase in the risk of death with invasion of more than 50% of the tubal muscularis.[49] No association between grade and survival was observed by several investigators.[5,7,43] *BRCA* status has recently been established as an independent favorable prognostic variable.[25]

Treatment

Initial management of carcinoma of the fallopian tube is surgical. No consensus exists regarding the best adjunctive therapy or whether adjuvant therapy has any value. The absence of surgical staging has probably inflated the number of patients assigned to stage I, thereby obscuring the subset that might not require adjuvant treatment. However, by analogy with ovarian cancer, it is possible that patients with grade 1 and stage I tumors require no further therapy. For the remainder, with 5-year survival rates for patients with stage II disease in the range of 50-60% and for patients with stage III and stage IV disease in the range of 10-20%,[4,5,42,43,51] consideration and investigation of postsurgical therapy are warranted.

The combined analysis of two large international multicenter trials has demonstrated that platinum-based therapy significantly improves the disease-free interval and overall survival of patients with early stage high-risk ovarian cancer, with an 8% survival advantage in the chemotherapy treatment arm.[52] By extrapolation, such adjuvant therapy could also be of benefit to early-stage high-risk fallopian tube carcinoma (Fig. 100-1).[13]

Surgical Therapy

Because fallopian tube cancer is rarely diagnosed preoperatively, the surgeon is usually confronted with the diagnosis intraoperatively. The new FIGO staging system requires a surgical exercise similar to that mandated for ovarian carcinoma. This includes cytologic analysis of either ascitic fluid or pelvic and abdominal washings, abdominal hysterectomy and bilateral salpingo-oophorectomy, omentectomy, and selective (or therapeutic) pelvic and para-aortic lymphadenectomy with selective peritoneal biopsies. In apparent early-stage disease, there may be up to a 33% incidence of nodal metastases,[48] highlighting the importance of performing a selective pelvic and para-aortic lymphadenectomy. For advanced disease, the same principles of cytoreductive surgery for ovarian carcinoma apply to fallopian tube carcinoma as well. The importance of cytoreductive surgery is supported by the observations of Eddy and colleagues, who found that the median survival of patients with no gross residual disease was 30 months, significantly longer than the survival of patients whose largest tumor diameter was greater than 2 cm (17 months).[4]

Several studies examining the role of second-look laparotomy in fallopian tube carcinoma have been performed.[4,7,8,50] Barakat and colleagues reported the largest series of patients undergoing second-look laparotomy.[50] Only 19% of patients whom they observed had a recurrence after negative second-look laparotomy, with a mean follow-up of 50 months. This contrasts with advanced-stage ovarian carcinoma patients who are treated with platinum-based chemotherapy, among whom approximately 50% will experience recurrence following a negative second-look procedure, with a median interval of 14 months to recurrence.[53] However, more recently, Cormio and colleagues observed that 31% of patients with a negative second-look had recurrences, with a mean follow-up of 49 months.[54]

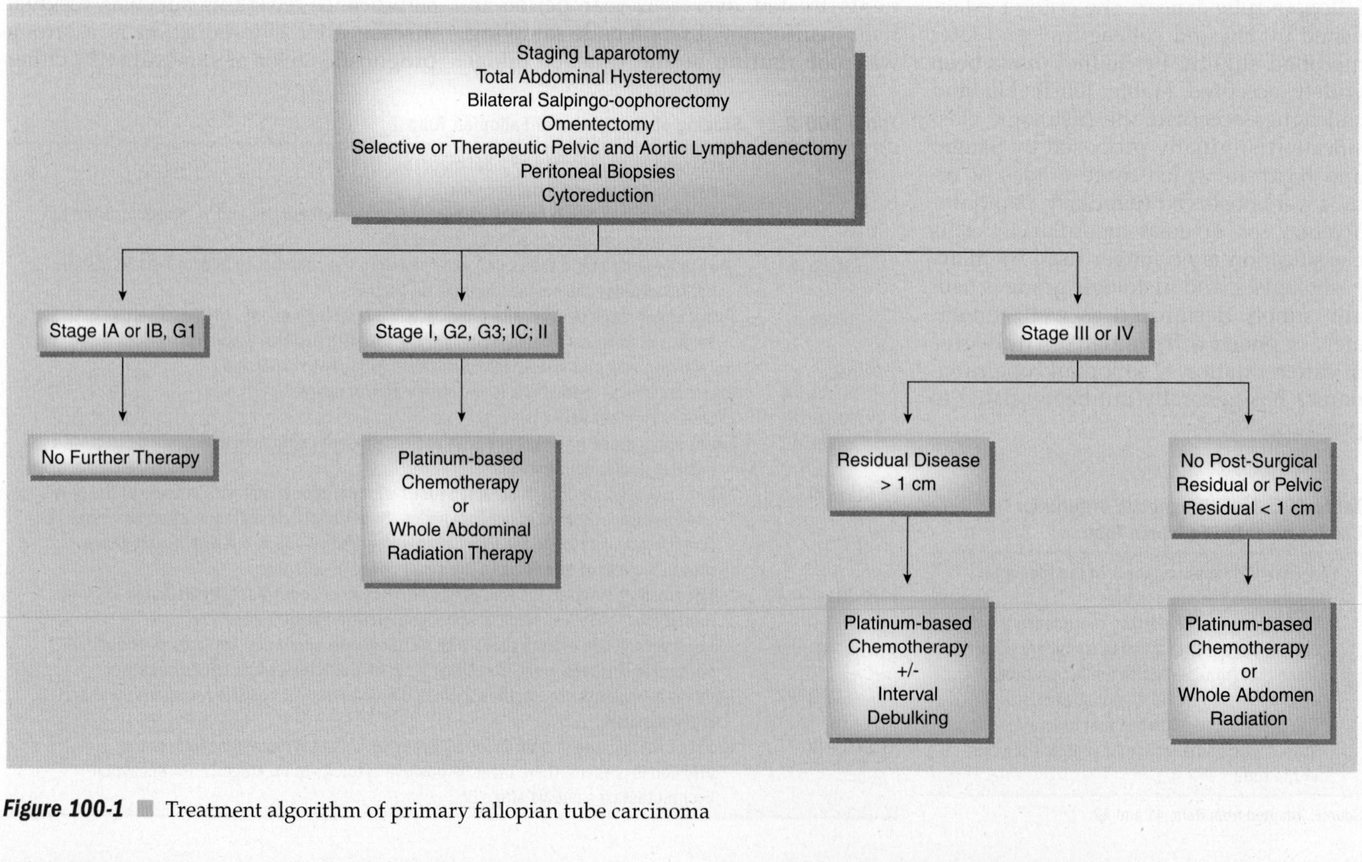

Figure 100-1 Treatment algorithm of primary fallopian tube carcinoma

A randomized trial in Europe demonstrated a survival benefit for interval cytoreductive surgery in ovarian cancer patients initially left with residual disease >1 cm,[55,56] and we would advocate consideration for interval surgery in the same cohort of patients with fallopian tube cancer as illustrated in Figure 100-1. In addition, analogous to the paradigm employed in ovarian cancer, we would consider secondary cytoreductive surgery in highly selected patients who develop recurrences with long disease-free intervals and initial optimal cytoreduction and in whom there is good likelihood of an optimal secondary surgery (residual disease <1 cm).[57,58]

Radiation Therapy

Although abdominal irradiation has been used in treating patients with more advanced disease and varying amounts of postsurgical tumor residuum, it does not appear to be of curative benefit.[5,6,43,59,60] Comparable studies in ovarian cancer suggest that adjuvant whole-abdomen irradiation can cure only when the postoperative residual tumor is less than 1-2 cm in size in the pelvis and there is no macroscopic disease in the upper abdomen. Although fallopian tube cancer is radiosensitive, the dose that may be delivered safely to the upper abdomen will not eradicate macroscopic disease. Thus, postoperative abdominopelvic radiation therapy has been reserved for those with microscopic or no residual disease in the upper abdomen and less than a 1 cm residuum in the pelvis. In 2000 Baekelandt suggested that in view of its low efficacy and high rate of serious complications, the use of postoperative radiotherapy in the treatment of patients with fallopian tube carcinoma should no longer be recommended.[61]

Chemotherapy

Because of similarities in the appearance of papillary carcinomas of the tube and ovary, it was logical to apply to patients with tubal carcinoma the cytotoxic agents known to be active against ovarian carcinoma. Cyclophosphamide, melphalan, doxorubicin, and thiotepa were among the frequently used single agents in the early cytotoxic treatment of tubal carcinoma.[7,8,62,63] Response rates to single alkylating agents were generally less than 20% in small series of patients with disparate stages and prognostic features. With the introduction of cisplatin-containing regimens,[63] complete clinical responses were noted in patients with advanced disease and were confirmed by second-look surgery. Peters and colleagues demonstrated that multiagent chemotherapy with cisplatin achieved an 81% objective response rate, whereas multiagent therapy without cisplatin achieved a 29% response rate and single-agent therapy (other than cisplatin) achieved a 9% response rate.[8] In the cisplatin group, there were 12 complete surgical responses in 20 patients.

Barakat and colleagues reported results of treating 38 patients with cisplatin-based chemotherapy.[64] Although the overall survival rate of the group was 51% at 5 years, patients with bulky disease who had complete cytoreductive surgery had a 5-year survival rate of 83% compared with 28% if there was residual disease postoperatively. Of 21 patients with advanced-stage disease who came to second-look surgery, 11 were found to be without evidence of disease and there was 1 recurrence. Similarly, Cormio and colleagues treated 32 patients with cisplatin, doxorubicin, and cyclophosphamide after primary cytoreductive surgery.[65] The overall clinical response rate was 80%. Ten of 14 patients who underwent second-look laparotomy had a pathologic complete response, but 3 relapsed. The median survival for the entire group was 38 months, and the 5-year survival rate was 35%. Other investigators have reported similar experience with platinum-based regimens in the treatment of fallopian tube carcinoma.[66]

During the past decade, as experience increased, it became obvious from the literature that fallopian tube carcinoma responds well to cytotoxic chemotherapy; multidrug regimens containing cisplatin seem to be more active than nonplatinum single agents or multidrug regimens without cisplatin. The platinum-paclitaxel combination is now employed analogous to its standard application in ovarian cancer, as reflected in a report by Gemignani and colleagues in 23 patients treated from 1993 to 1998.[67] Paclitaxel was administered at 135-175 mg/m^2 in combination with carboplatin in 17 patients and cisplatin in 6 patients.

The European Organisation for Research and Treatment of Cancer (EORTC) reported a phase 2 study of a combination of cyclophosphamide, Adriamycin (doxorubicin), and cisplatin (CAP) in 24 eligible patients with advanced fallopian tube carcinoma (FIGO stages III-IV). The CAP regimen consisted of cyclophosphamide 600 mg/m^2, doxorubicin 45 mg/m^2, and cisplatin 50 mg/m^2 administered intravenously every 28 days. Ten patients had a complete and six patients had a partial response (response rate 67%). The median overall survival was 24 months, and the 1-, 3-, and 5-year survival rates were 73%, 25%, and 19%, respectively.[68]

Second-line and salvage therapy currently uses the same agents employed in ovarian cancer,[13,69] including liposomal doxorubicin,[70] topotecan,[71,72] docetaxel,[73,74] and gemcitabine.[75]

The role of hormonal therapy in the treatment of tubal carcinoma is unclear; however, medroxyprogesterone acetate and megestrol acetate have been employed, usually in combination with cytotoxic agents.[5,7,63] There is no evidence that progestational therapy alone is effective in this disease.

Figure 100-1 proposes an algorithm for the treatment of such patients.

Prognosis

Table 100-3 provides a comparison of studies examining survival for primary fallopian tube carcinoma. Rosen and colleagues, in a retrospective analysis of 143 women in Austria over 15 years, reported a 5-year survival rate of 59% for stages I and II and 19% for stages III and IV.[2] Using the National Cancer Institute's Surveillance, Epidemiology and End Results (SEER) Program, Kosary and Trimble identified 416 women with fallopian tube carcinoma diagnosed between 1990 and 1997.[76] Almost half of those diagnosed with stage I or II disease did not undergo surgical evaluation of lymph nodes. Most women with stage I or II disease were treated with surgery

Table 100-3 Comparison of Studies Reporting Survival for Primary Fallopian Tube Carcinoma

		5-Year Survival Rates				
Series Year (Ref.)	**Patients**	**Stage I**	**Stage II**	**Stage III**	**Stage IV**	**All Patients**
Barakat 1991 (64)	38	-				51%
Rosen 1999 (2)	143	59%		19%		43%
Baekelandt 2000 (61)	151	73%	37%	29%	12%	44%
Gadducci 2001 (85)	88	-				57%
Obermair 2001 (86)	36	63%		53%		-
Kosary 2002 (76)	416	95%	75%	69%	45%	-
Heintz 2006 (15)	175	81%	67%	41%	33%	56%
Singhal 2006 (87)	35	64%	42%	32%	17%	
Moore 2007 (1)	96	95%		-		59%

alone, whereas most women with stage III or IV disease were treated with surgery and chemotherapy. The 5-year relative survival rates by FIGO stage were as follows: stage I (n = 102), 95%; stage II (n = 29), 75%; stage III (n = 52), 69%; stage IV (n = 151), 45%.

In an attempt to identify prognostic features, the Austrian Cooperative Study Group for Fallopian Tube Carcinoma analyzed the 66 patients treated in Austria between 1980 and 1990.[44] The authors found no prognostic impact of degree of differentiation or the presence, absence, or concentration of estrogen and progesterone receptors. Lymphocyte infiltration in the tumor was confirmed as a prognostic factor by multivariate analysis, as was stage of disease. In a separate review of the Austrian experience, 61 specimens of fallopian tube carcinoma were examined by image cytometry for ploidy determination.[3] Forty-eight of the tumors showed an aneuploid pattern. Although patients with a euploid pattern had a median survival of 33.8 months compared with 24.5 months for patients with aneuploid tumors, significance was not reached, nor was there a correlation between ploidy status and the stage or grade of the tumor.

A study was performed of the pathology specimens and clinical case records from 151 patients with fallopian tube carcinoma who were treated consecutively in Norway.[61] In a multivariate analysis, disease stage, the presence of residual tumor, and a hydrosalpinx-like appearance of the fallopian tube were of independent prognostic significance for the whole cohort. For patients with stage I disease, the depth of infiltration in the tubal wall and intraoperative tumor rupture were of independent prognostic significance. Prognostic factors in patients with early-stage (stages 0 and I) fallopian tube carcinoma seem to differ from those in patients with early-stage ovarian carcinoma. For patients with more advanced-stage disease, owing to the striking similarities in prognostic and clinical characteristics between the two diseases, the authors recommended that the treatment and follow-up strategies for patients with ovarian carcinoma be adopted in the management of patients with fallopian tube carcinoma.

Other Malignant Fallopian Tube Neoplasms

Fewer than 150 other fallopian tube cancers have been reported, including less than 55 malignant müllerian mixed tumors of the fallopian tube,[77-82] as well as rare primary leiomyosarcomas,[83] rare examples of immature teratomas, and occurrences of trophoblastic disease, primarily choriocarcinomas.[84] The diagnostic approach for any of these tumors is the same as that for primary adenocarcinoma of the fallopian tube, except that in the case of trophoblastic disease, human chorionic gonadotropin serum levels are useful; and in the case of malignant teratoma, alpha fetoprotein levels are useful. Surgical therapy should be followed by individualized treatment with cytotoxic chemotherapy appropriate to the histology or radiation therapy to postoperative fields according to the primary tumor classification and stage of disease.

Selected References

The complete reference list can be found at www.CANCERMEDICINE8.com

1. Moore KN, Moxley KM, Fader AN, et al. Serous fallopian tube carcinoma: a retrospective, multi-institutional case-control comparison to serous adenocarcinoma of the ovary. *Gynecol Oncol.* 2007;107(3):398–403.
2. Rosen AC, Klein M, Hafner E, et al. Management and prognosis of primary fallopian tube carcinoma. Austrian Cooperative Study Group for Fallopian Tube Carcinoma. *Gynecol Obstet Invest.* 1999;47:45–51.
4. Eddy GL, Copeland LJ, Gershenson DM, et al. Fallopian tube carcinoma. *Obstet Gynecol.* 1984;64:546–552.
5. Podratz KC, Podczaski ES, Gaffey TA, et al. Primary carcinoma of the fallopian tube. *Am J Obstet Gynecol.* 1986;154:1319–1326.
10. Schiller HM, Silverberg SG. Staging and prognosis in primary carcinoma of the fallopian tube. *Cancer.* 1971;28:389–395.
13. Gadducci A. Current management of fallopian tube carcinoma. *Curr Opin Obstet Gynecol.* 2002;14:27–32.
14. Rosenblatt KA, Weiss NS, Schwartz SM. Incidence of malignant fallopian tube tumors. *Gynecol Oncol.* 1989;35:236–239.
16. Stewart SL, Wike JM, Foster SL, et al. The incidence of primary fallopian tube cancer in the United States. *Gynecol Oncol.* 2007;107(3):392–397.
17. Tamimi HK, Figge DC. Adenocarcinoma of the uterine tube: potential for lymph node metastases. *Am J Obstet Gynecol.* 1981;141:132–137.
18. Paley PJ, Swisher EM, Garcia RL, et al. Occult cancer of the fallopian tube in BRCA-1 germline mutation carriers at prophylactic oophorectomy: a case for recommending hysterectomy at surgical prophylaxis. *Gynecol Oncol.* 2001;80:176–180.
19. Aziz S, Kuperstein G, Rosen B, et al. A genetic epidemiological study of carcinoma of the fallopian tube. *Gynecol Oncol.* 2001;80:341–345.
20. Colgan TJ, Murphy J, Cole DE, et al. Occult carcinoma in prophylactic oophorectomy specimens: prevalence and association with BRCA germline mutation status. *Am J Surg Pathol.* 2001;25:1283–1289.
23. Levine DA, Argenta PA, Yee CJ, et al. Fallopian tube and primary peritoneal carcinomas associated with BRCA mutations. *J Clin Oncol.* 2003;21:4222–4227.
24. Dijkhuizen FP, Huisman A, Boonstra H, et al. Carcinoma of the fallopian tube after prophylactic laparoscopic ovariectomy in a patient with a BRCAI mutation. *Ned Tijdschr Geneeskd.* 2003;147:877–879.
25. Cass I, Holschneider C, Datta N, Barbuto D, Walts AE, Karlan BY. BRCA-mutation-associated fallopian tube carcinoma: a distinct clinical phenotype? *Obstet Gynecol.* 2005;106:1327–1334.
26. Carcangiu ML, Peissel B, Pasini B, et al. Incidental carcinomas in prophylactic specimens in BRCA1 and BRCA2 germline mutation carriers, with emphasis on fallopian tube lesions: report of 6 cases and review of the literature. *Am J Surg Pathol.* 2006;30(10):1222–1230.
27. Olivier RI, van Beurden M, Lubsen MA, et al. Clinical outcome of prophylactic oophorectomy in BRCA1/BRCA2 mutation carriers and events during follow-up. *Br J Cancer.* 2004;90(8):1492–1497.
28. Agoff SN, Mendelin JE, Grieco VS, et al. Unexpected gynecologic neoplasms in patients with proven or suspected BRCA-1 or -2 mutations: implications for gross examination, cytology, and clinical follow-up. *Am J Surg Pathol.* 2002;26:171–178.
29. Powell CB, Kenley E, Chen LM, et al. Risk-reducing salpingooophorectomy in BRCA mutation carriers: role of serial sectioning in the detection of occult malignancy. *J Clin Oncol.* 2005;23:127–132.
30. Pectasides D, Pectasides E, Economopoulos T. Fallopian tube carcinoma: a review. *Oncologist*, 2006;11(8):902–912.
35. Kurjak A, Kupesic S, Ilijas M, et al. Preoperative diagnosis of primary fallopian tube carcinoma. *Gynecol Oncol.* 1998;68:29–34.
36. Takagi H, Matsunami K, Noda K, et al. Primary fallopian tube carcinoma: a case of successful preoperative evaluation with magnetic resonance imaging. *J Obstet Gynaecol.* 2003;23:455–456.
37. Mikami M, Tei C, Kurahashi T, et al. Preoperative diagnosis of fallopian tube cancer by imaging. *Abdom Imaging.* 2003;28:743–747.
38. Santana P, Desser TS, Teng N. Preoperative CT diagnosis of primary fallopian tube carcinoma in a patient with a history of total abdominal hysterectomy. *J Comput Assist Tomogr.* 2003;27:361–363.
40. Rosen AC, Klein M, Rosen HR, et al. Preoperative and postoperative CA-125 serum levels in primary fallopian tube carcinoma. *Arch Gynecol Obstet.* 1994;255:65–68.
41. Hu CY, Taylor ML, Hertig AT. Primary carcinoma of the fallopian tube. *Am J Obstet Gynecol.* 1950;59:58–67.
44. Rosen A, Klein M, Lahousen M, et al. Primary carcinoma of the fallopian tube—a retrospective analysis of 115 patients. Austrian Cooperative Study Group for Fallopian Tube Carcinoma. *Br J Cancer.* 1993;68:605–609.
45. Petterson F. Staging rules for gestational trophoblastic tumors and fallopian tube cancer. *Acta Obstet Gynecol Scand.* 1992;71:244–245.
46. Alvarado-Cabrero I, Young RH, Vamvakas EC, et al. Carcinoma of the fallopian tube: a clinicopathological study of 105 cases with observations on staging and prognostic factors. *Gynecol Oncol.* 1999;72:367–379.

48. di Re E, Grosso G, Raspagliesi F, et al. Fallopian tube cancer: incidence and role of lymphatic spread. *Gynecol Oncol.* 1996;62:199–202.
49. Peters WA III, Andersen WA, Hopkins MP, et al. Prognostic features of carcinoma of the fallopian tube. *Obstet Gynecol.* 1988;71:757–762.
50. Barakat RR, Rubin SC, Saigo PE, et al. Second-look laparotomy in carcinoma of the fallopian tube. *Obstet Gynecol.* 1993;82:748–751.
52. Trimbos JB, Parmar M, Vergote I, et al. International collaborative ovarian neoplasm trial 1 and adjuvant chemotherapy in ovarian neoplasm trial: two parallel randomized phase III trials of adjuvant chemotherapy in patients with early-stage ovarian carcinoma. *J Natl Cancer Inst.* 2003;95:105–112.
61. Baekelandt M, Jorunn Nesbakken A, Kristensen GB, et al. Carcinoma of the fallopian tube. *Cancer.* 2000;89:2076–2084.
63. Deppe G, Bruckner HW, Cohen CJ. Combination chemotherapy for advanced carcinoma of the fallopian tube. *Obstet Gynecol.* 1980;56:530–532.
64. Barakat RR, Rubin SC, Saigo PE, et al. Cisplatin-based combination chemotherapy in carcinoma of the fallopian tube. *Gynecol Oncol.* 1991;42:156–160.
65. Cormio G, Maneo A, Gabriele A, et al. Treatment of fallopian tube carcinoma with cyclophosphamide, Adriamycin, and cisplatin. *Am J Clin Oncol.* 1997;20:143–145.
66. Jacobs AJ, McMurray EH, Parham J, et al. Treatment of carcinoma of the fallopian tube using cisplatin, doxorubicin, and cyclophosphamide. *Am J Clin Oncol.* 1986;9:436–439.
67. Gemignani ML, Hensley ML, Cohen R, et al. Paclitaxelbased chemotherapy in carcinoma of the fallopian tube. *Gynecol Oncol.* 2001;80:16–20.
68. Wagenaar HC, Pecorelli S, Vergote I, et al. Phase II study of a combination of cyclophosphamide, Adriamycin and cisplatin in advanced fallopian tube carcinoma. An EORTC gynecological cancer group study. European Organization for Research and Treatment of Cancer. *Eur J Gynaecol Oncol.* 2001;22:187–193.
76. Kosary C, Trimble EL. Treatment and survival for women with fallopian tube carcinoma: a population-based study. *Gynecol Oncol.* 2002;86:190–191.
77. Horn LC, Werschnik C, Bilek K, et al. Diagnosis and clinical management in malignant müllerian tumors of the fallopian tube. A report of four cases and review of recent literature. *Arch Gynecol Obstet.* 1996;258: 47–53.
81. Ebert AD, Perez-Canto A, Schaller G, et al. Stage I primary malignant mixed mullerian tumor of the fallopian tube. Report of a case with five-year survival after minimal surgery without adjuvant treatment. *J Reprod Med.* 1998;43(7):598–600.
83. Jacoby AF, Fuller AF Jr, Thor AD, et al. Primary leiomyosarcoma of the fallopian tube. *Gynecol Oncol.* 1993;51:404–407.
85. Gadducci A, Landoni F, Sartori E, et al. Analysis of treatment failures and survival of patients with fallopian tube carcinoma: a cooperation task force (CTF) study. *Gynecol Oncol.* 2001;81(2):150–159.
86. Obermair A, Taylor KH, Janda M, et al. Primary fallopian tube carcinoma: the Queensland experience. *Int J Gynecol Cancer.* 2001;11(1):69–72.
87. Singhal P, Odunsi K, Rodabaugh K, et al. Primary fallopian tube carcinoma: a retrospective clinicopathologic study. *Eur J Gynaecol Oncol.* 2006;27(1):16–18.
92. Callahan MJ, Crum CP, Medeiros F, et al. Primary fallopian tube malignancies in BRCA-positive women undergoing surgery for ovarian cancer risk reduction. *J Clin Oncol.* 2007;25(25):3985–3990.

101 Ovarian Cancer

Jonathan S. Berek, MD, MMS ■ Michael L. Friedlander, MD, PhD ■ Robert C. Bast, Jr, MD

Epithelial Ovarian Cancer

Ovarian cancer is one of the most treatable solid tumors, as the majority will respond temporarily to surgery and cytotoxic agents. The disease, however, frequently persists and recurs, having the highest fatality-to-case ratio of all the gynecologic cancers. Ovarian cancer represents one-fourth of the malignancies of the female genital tract, but it is the most common cause of death among women who develop cancers of gynecologic origin. Ovarian carcinomas account for 4% of the total cancers in women in the United States, ranked behind malignant neoplasms of the lung, breast, colon and uterus. In 2008, almost 22,000 new cases and more than 15,000 deaths are expected.[1] Despite these discouraging statistics, improvement in 5-year survival has occurred steadily over the past three decades with more aggressive surgical management and the development of more effective chemotherapy. Five-year survival for all stages and histologies combined in the United States has improved significantly ($p < .05$) from 37% in 1974-1976 to 52% in 1992-1998.[1]

Ovarian cancer is predominantly a disease of postmenopausal women, with only 10% to 15% of all cases diagnosed in premenopausal women.[1-3] The median age for diagnosis of women with epithelial ovarian cancer, the most common histologic type, ranges between 60 and 65 years. Less than 1% of epithelial ovarian cancers are found in women younger than 30 years of age, and most ovarian malignancies in these younger patients are germ cell tumors (GCTs).[2-3] Ovarian cancer is neither a common nor a rare disease. The prevalence of ovarian cancer among postmenopausal women in the United States is 40 per 100,000 or 1 in 2500. The lifetime risk for a woman to develop ovarian cancer is approximately 1 in 70 (1.4%), compared to 1 in 8 or 9 for breast cancer.[4] The prevalence of ovarian cancer in the general population impacts substantially on strategies for prevention and early detection. In the absence of better markers for increased risk, strategies for prevention must have few serious side effects and screening strategies must be highly specific. A strong hereditary component contributes to development of the disease in 10% of cases with inherited germline mutations in *BRCA1*, *BRCA2* or mismatch repair genes, but 90% are sporadic.

Etiology and Epidemiology

The cause of ovarian cancer is unknown.[5] Some have speculated that an etiologic agent or a potentiator of oncogenesis could enter the peritoneal cavity through the lower genital canal and spread through the uterus and the fallopian tubes.[3] Possible carcinogens, such as infectious agents and chemical carcinogens have been studied, and although case-control studies have failed to document a specific agent, some studies have linked environmental exposure to asbestos-contaminated talc in douches and contraceptives with the development of epithelial tumors.[3,4] Cigarette smoking has been linked to mucinous ovarian cancers, but not to the more common serous carcinomas.[5] Case-control studies have also pointed to an association of white race, high-fat diet and galactose consumption with a higher incidence of the disease.[4,6]

Among the epidemiologic variables, however, prior reproductive history and the number of ovulatory cycles appear to have the greatest impact on development of the disease, with low parity, infertility, early menarche and late menopause increasing the risk.[6,7] Fertility enhancing drugs, such as clomiphene citrate and gonadotropins used for ovulation induction have been thought to increase the risk of ovarian cancer, but the data have not been consistent and have not adequately distinguished the influence of infertility per se from the use of fertility stimulating agents.[8-12] A pooled analysis of eight case-control studies that included 5207 cases and 7705 controls found an association of fertility stimulating drugs with serous borderline tumors, but not with invasive ovarian cancers.[10-12] The increased incidence of ovarian cancer in single women, nuns, and nulliparous women suggests that continual ovulation, uninterrupted by pregnancy, may predispose women to develop this malignancy.[13] Over many cycles of ovulation, the ovarian surface epithelium undergoes repetitive disruption and repair. Epithelial cells covering the ovarian surface are stimulated to proliferate, increasing the probability of spontaneous mutations in tumor suppressor or proto-oncogenes that might contribute to oncogenesis. Alternatively, trapping of epithelial cells within the stroma following ovulation can lead to the formation of inclusion cysts where epithelial cells are subjected to a unique microenvironment.

Most case-control and cohort studies have failed to link hormone replacement therapy to an increased risk of epithelial ovarian cancer.[14] A large cohort study has recently reopened controversy regarding this issue.[15] Among 44,241 postmenopausal women in the Breast Cancer Detection Demonstration Project, 329 developed ovarian cancer. Women who had received estrogen replacement therapy only for more than 10 years without progestin were at increased risk of developing ovarian cancer. By 20 years the relative risk was 3.2-fold.

The incidence of ovarian cancer varies in different geographic locations throughout the world. Western countries, including the United States and the United Kingdom, have an incidence of ovarian cancer that is 3-7 times greater than in Japan, where epithelial ovarian tumors are considered rare.[2,3] In Asia, the incidence of GCTs of the ovary appears to be somewhat higher than in the West. Japanese immigrants to the United States, however, exhibit a significant increase in the incidence of epithelial ovarian cancer at a rate approaching that of white women from the United States. The incidence of epithelial tumors is about 1.5 times greater in whites than in blacks.

Although it has been widely believed that epithelial ovarian cancers arise from either the surface epithelium of the ovary or from inclusion cysts within the ovary, dysplasia or in situ changes have been very rarely observed in epithelial cells at either location. There is growing evidence to suggest that many high-grade serous carcinomas of the ovary arise from the fimbrial end of the fallopian tube, rather than from the ovary as has previously been thought.[16,17] It has been suggested that epithelial ovarian cancers should be separated into two distinct groups, Type 1 and Type 2 tumors, as they differ considerably in the cells of origin, molecular pathogenesis as well as their biological behavior.[18] Type 1 tumors include low-grade micropapillary serous carcinoma, mucinous, endometrioid, and clear cell carcinomas. They are genetically stable and are characterized by mutations in *K-RAS*, *BRAF*, *PTEN*, and β-catenin. Type 2 tumors are rapidly growing, highly aggressive neoplasms that lack well-defined precursor lesions; most are at advanced-stage, or soon after, their inception and exhibit mutations of *TP53*.[18]

Prevention

As parity is inversely related to the risk of ovarian cancer, having at least one child is protective of the disease with a risk reduction of 0.3 to 0.4. Remarkably, use of oral contraceptives for 5 or more reduces the relative risk to 0.5 (ie, there is a 50% reduction in the likelihood of developing ovarian cancer).[9] Women who have had two children and have used oral contraceptives for 5 or more have a relative risk of ovarian cancer as low as 0.3, or a 70% reduction. Therefore, the oral contraceptive pill is the only documented method of chemoprevention for ovarian cancer, and it should be recommended to women for this purpose. When counseling patients regarding birth control options, this important benefit of oral contraceptive use should be emphasized. This is also important for women with a strong family history of ovarian cancer.[19]

Fenretinide ■ Fenretinide (4-hydroxyphenylall-trans-retinoic acid amide), a vitamin A derivative, has been given to women with unilateral breast cancer in an effort to reduce the risk of contralateral breast cancer. In a prospective, randomized, placebo-controlled trial conducted in Italy, women with unilateral breast cancer were given either oral fenretinide or a placebo for 5 years.[20] In the treatment group, no ovarian cancers developed during the 5 years on study, whereas there were 6 cases of ovarian cancer in the control group ($p < .01$). When participants were followed long-term, however, the protective effect disappeared after discontinuing the drug.[21,22] In cell culture, fenretinide can induce apoptosis in ovarian cancer cells and in normal ovarian surface epithelial cells. Trials are ongoing to determine the effect of fenretinide on the ovaries of women at high-risk for developing ovarian cancer who will receive the drug prior to prophylactic oophorectomy.

Oophorectomy ■ The performance of a prophylactic oophorectomy will reduce, but not eliminate, the excess risk of cancer in women at high-risk for developing ovarian cancer.[22,23] Because the entire peritoneum is at risk, peritoneal carcinomas can occur even after prophylactic oophorectomy in less than 5% of cases. Recent evidence suggests that many so-called "ovarian" cancers actually arise from the fallopian tube and it is essential that women having prophylactic surgery have their fallopian tubes removed as well and that these are carefully assessed by the pathologist as it is easy to miss small cancers, particularly in the fimbrial end of the fallopian tube.[17] Because the ovaries provide protection from cardiovascular disease and osteoporosis, prophylactic bilateral salpingo-oophorectomy (PBSO) should not be routinely performed in premenopausal women at average risk for ovarian cancer.

Genetic Risk for Epithelial Ovarian Cancer

Most epithelial ovarian cancers are sporadic. Familial or hereditary patterns account for 5% to10% of all ovarian malignancies.[24] A recent population-based study from Canada has, however, suggested that *BRCA1* and *BRCA2* mutations may be more common than previously believed. Risch et al.[25] reported BRCA mutations in 13% of ovarian cancers, in 18% of women with high-grade serous cancers, and 21% of women diagnosed were between 40 and 50 years of age. Furthermore, the incidence was much higher in members of specific ethnic groups, such as Ashkenazi Jewish (29%), Indo-Pakistani (29%), and Italian (26%) women. These higher figures need to be confirmed in other large population-based studies. A positive family history is associated with a higher risk of ovarian cancer than that of the general population.[26-36] Most familial ovarian cancer is associated with mutations in *BRCA1*, *BRCA2*, or DNA mismatch repair genes in the human nonpolyposis colorectal cancer (HNPCC, Lynch type II) syndrome.[32-35] A few cases of ovarian cancer have been associated with Li-Fraumeni syndrome that occurs due to *TP53* mutations in the germ line.[35] In the past, it had been thought that there were two distinct syndromes associated with a genetic risk, site-specific hereditary ovarian cancer, and hereditary breast/ovarian cancer syndrome. However, it is now believed that these groups essentially represent a continuum of mutations with different degrees of penetrance within a given family.

BRCA1* and *BRCA2 ■ The majority of ovarian cancer families have mutations in the *BRCA1* gene that is located on chromosome 17.[26-32] A smaller fraction of inherited disease has been traced to another gene, *BRCA2*, located on chromosome 13.[27-32] Discovered through linkage analyses, these two genes are associated with the genetic predisposition to both ovarian and breast cancer.

BRCA1/2 mutations are passed via autosomal dominant inheritance, and a full pedigree analysis (ie, both maternal and paternal sides of the family) must be carefully evaluated. There are numerous distinct mutations that have been identified on each of these genes, and the mutations have different degrees of penetrance which may account for the preponderance of either breast cancer, ovarian cancer, or both, in any given family. Based on analysis of women who have a mutation in the *BRCA1* gene and are from high-risk families, the lifetime risk of ovarian cancer may be as high as 28% to 44% and the risk has been calculated to be as high as 27% for those women with a *BRCA2* mutation.[23-31] The risk of breast cancer in women with a *BRCA1* or *BRCA2* mutation may be as high as 56% to 87%.

Hereditary ovarian cancers generally occur in women about 10 years younger than those with nonhereditary tumors.[25,28] The median age of ovarian cancer in women with *BRCA1* related ovarian cancer is in the mid-40s in contract to the late 50s and early 60s in women with *BRCA2* mutations. As the median age of epithelial ovarian cancer is in the mid-60s to late 60s, a woman with a first-degree or second-degree relative who had premenopausal ovarian cancer may have a higher probability of carrying an affected gene.

Within a given family, a combination of epithelial ovarian and breast cancers can affect a mixture of first-degree and second-degree relatives. Women with this syndrome tend to develop cancers at a young age; breast cancers may be bilateral. If two first-degree relatives are affected, this pedigree is consistent with an autosomal dominant mode of inheritance.[30,31]

Founder Effect ■ More than 100 different mutations of *BRCA1* and *BRCA2* have been cataloged in different families with ovarian and breast cancer. A particularly high carrier rate of *BRCA1* and *BRCA2* mutations has been found in women of Ashkenazi Jewish descent and in Icelandic women.[28,34] Three specific mutations occur repeatedly in the Ashkenazi population and are associated with many of the breast and ovarian cancer families: 185delAG and 5382insC in *BRCA1*, and 6174delT in *BRCA2*. One in 40 or 2.5% of all Ashkenazi Jewish women carry at least one of these three mutations. The prevalence of these specific mutations in the Ashkenazi population is thought to have resulted from a "founder effect," where the mutations can be traced to particular families within a defined geographic area.

Pedigree Analysis ■ The risk of ovarian cancer depends on the number of first-degree and/or second-degree relatives with a history of epithelial ovarian carcinoma and/or breast cancer, and on the number of malignancies that occur at an early age. The degree of risk is difficult to determine precisely unless one performs a full pedigree analysis.

In families with two first-degree relatives (ie, mother, sister, or daughter) with documented premenopausal epithelial ovarian cancer, the risk that a female first-degree relative will have an affected gene could be as high as 35% to 40%.[23] In families with a single first-degree relative and a single second-degree relative (ie, grandmother, aunt, first cousin, or granddaughter) with epithelial ovarian cancer, the risk that a woman will have an affected gene also may be increased. The risk may be 2-fold to 10-fold higher than in those without a familial history of the disease.[27,31,36] In families with a single postmenopausal first-degree relative with epithelial ovarian carcinoma, a woman may not have an increased risk of having an affected gene because the case is most likely to be sporadic. However, if the ovarian cancer occurred in a premenopausal relative, this could be significant, and a full pedigree analysis should be undertaken but even the absence of a family history does not preclude a mutation as demonstrated in the Canadian population study by Risch and colleagues which is discussed above. Women with a primary history of breast cancer have twice the expected incidence of subsequent ovarian cancer.

Lynch Type II Syndrome ■ The HNPCC syndrome includes multiple adenocarcinomas, including familial colon, ovarian, endometrial, and breast cancers, as well as other malignancies of the gastrointestinal (GI) and genitourinary systems.[37] Mutations of DNA mismatch repair genes have been associated with this syndrome including mutations of *MSH2*, *MLH1*, *PMS1*, and *PMS2*. The risk that a woman who is a member of a Lynch type II family will develop epithelial ovarian cancer depends on the frequency of this disease in her first-degree and second-degree relatives, although these women appear to have at least 3 times the relative risk of the general population.

Management of Women at High Risk for Ovarian Cancer

Current recommendations for management of women with high-risk for ovarian cancer have been addressed in many reports and expert guidelines are widely available.[35,36,38-40] Women who appear to be at high-risk for ovarian and or breast cancer should undergo genetic counseling and, if the risk appears to be substantial, may be offered genetic testing for *BRCA1* and *BRCA2*. Women who wish to preserve their reproductive capacity may choose to undergo periodic screening by transvaginal ultrasonography and cancer antigen 125 (CA125) every 6 months, although it should be stressed that there is no evidence to demonstrate that screening is of any value in women at increased genetic risk of ovarian cancer and these women need to be fully informed regarding the lack of evidence for benefit of this approach. The recent data suggesting that the fimbrial end of the fallopian tube is the likely site of origin of many BRCA related "ovarian" cancers make it difficult to believe that screening the ovaries with ultrasound will detect these cancers at an early stage. Prophylactic surgery (BSO with or without a hysterectomy) is the treatment of choice for women who have completed their childbearing. Oral contraceptives should be recommended to young women before undertaking a planned family. Women who do not wish to maintain their fertility, or who have completed their family, may undergo PBSO. The risk should be clearly documented, preferably established by *BRCA1* and *BRCA2* testing, before salpingo-oophorectomy. These women should be counseled that this operation does not offer absolute protection, as peritoneal carcinomas occasionally can occur after BSO. In women who also have a strong family history of breast cancer, annual mammographic screening with MRI and mammograms and possibly also breast ultrasound should be performed commencing at age 30 years. Women with a documented HNPCC syndrome should be treated as above, and in addition, should undergo periodic screening mammography, colonoscopy, and endometrial biopsy.[35]

In a recent study, Markov modeling was performed in a simulated cohort of 30-year old women who tested positive for *BRCA1/2* mutations.[40] Quality adjustment of survival estimates were obtained from a survey of women aged 33 to 50 years. A 30-year old woman could prolong her survival beyond that associated with surveillance alone by 1.8 years with tamoxifen, 2.6 years with prophylactic oophorectomy, 4.6 years with both tamoxifen and prophylactic oophorectomy, 3.5 years with prophylactic mastectomy, and 4.9 years with both surgeries. Quality adjusted survival could be prolonged by 2.8 years with tamoxifen, 4.4 years with prophylactic oophorectomy, 6.3 years with tamoxifen and oophorectomy and 2.6 years with mastectomy or both operations. Benefits would decrease if institution of these preventive measures were delayed beyond age 30.

Biology and Prognosis of Ovarian Neoplasms

The prognosis of ovarian cancer can be correlated with numerous clinical and biologic factors. Tumor stage, grade and size of metastatic disease after resection correlate best with outcome.[41,42] As discussed below, among patients with low-stage disease, tumor grade correlates with prognosis (ie, patients with stage I high-grade lesions have a shorter survival than do those of low-grade).[42] In patients with advanced-stage disease, the size of residual disease after surgery correlates most clearly with survival.[43] The rapidity with which disease regresses during chemotherapy also correlates with survival. A short apparent half life of the serum tumor marker CA125 has correlated with improved survival in more than a dozen studies.[44] Normalization of CA125 by the third course of chemotherapy has been associated with a favorable prognosis.[44]

Several biologic factors have been correlated with prognosis in epithelial ovarian cancer. Using flow cytometry, Friedlander and others have shown that ovarian cancers are commonly aneuploid and that a correlation exists between the International Federation of Gynecology and Obstetrics (FIGO) stage and ploidy, (low-stage cancers tend to be diploid and high-stage tumors tend to be aneuploid).[45,46] Patients with diploid tumors have a significantly longer median survival than those with aneuploid tumors: 5 years versus 1 year, respectively.[46] Multivariate analyses have demonstrated that ploidy is an independent prognostic variable and one of the most significant predictors of survival.[46] Flow cytometric analysis also provides data on the cell cycle, and the proliferation fraction (S-phase) determined by this technique has correlated with prognosis in some studies.[39,45] More recent reports utilizing comparative genomic hybridization suggest that copy number abnormalities for chromosome segments also have prognostic significance.[47]

Most sporadic ovarian carcinomas evolve from a single clone of cells. When primary cancers and metastases have been compared, more than 90% share the same patterns of loss of heterozygosity, inactivation of the same X chromosome and, when present, the same mutations in *TP53*.[48,49] Ovarian cancers can metastasize by multiple routes. Like other epithelial neoplasms, ovarian cancers can spread through lymphatics to the level of the renal hilus and can also spread hematogenously. Most frequently, however, ovarian cancer spreads over the surface of the peritoneum, studding the serosal surface of the bowel and abdominal wall and ultimately producing intestinal obstruction. Ascites formation results from increased leakage of proteinaceous fluid from capillaries under the influence of vascular endothelial growth factor/vascular permeability factor (VEGF/VPF) produced by ovarian cancers and from inhibition of fluid outflow through diaphragmatic lymphatics that have been blocked by metastatic disease.[50] Studies of the immunobiology of the peritoneal cavity suggest that it may function as an immunoprivileged site, with elevated levels of suppressive molecules and growth factors.[51-58]

Epithelial ovarian cancers are thought to arise from a single layer of cells that covers the ovary or that lines cysts immediately beneath the ovarian surface. These cells are generally quiescent, but proliferate following ovulation to repair the defect created by rupture of a follicle. Our understanding of the molecular pathogenesis of ovarian cancer is rapidly increasing. We now recognize that there are at least two different molecular pathways that can lead to the development of ovarian cancers and that these result in tumors which have quite distinct biological behaviors and probably have different cells of origin. There are those tumors (so-called type 1 tumors) that arise from ovarian surface epithelium (OSE)/mullerian inclusions—either from endosalpingiosis/invagination of OSE during repair of ovulation or implantation of cells from endometrium—this typically involves a relatively slow and multistep pathway and accounts for many early-stage cancers such as endometrioid, clear cell, mucinous and low-grade serous cancers. In contrast, the more common high-grade serous cancers have a phenotype that resembles the fallopian tube mucosa and commonly have p53 mutations and these tumors appear to develop rapidly and are almost always at an advanced stage at presentation.

A distinctive profile of genetic and epigenetic alterations has been observed in early and late stage ovarian cancers. A number of oncogenes have been overexpressed and/or activated (Table 101-1) and the function of several tumor suppressor genes has been lost (Table 101-2).[59-78] Among the oncogenes activated, particular attention has been given to the HER family of transmembrane tyrosine kinase growth factor receptors, including the epidermal growth factor receptor (EGFR) and c-erbB-2 (*HER-2*).[59] EGFR is expressed by normal ovarian surface epithelial cells and EGFR expression is lost in approximately 30% of ovarian cancers, associated with an improved prognosis.[73] *HER-2* is overexpressed in approximately 12% to 15% of ovarian cancers and, in some studies, has been associated with a poor prognosis.[59] The *Ras* oncogene is mutated and activated in less than 20% of serous ovarian cancers, but is more frequently mutated in mucinous, borderline and papillary serous low-grade neoplasms.[60,61] In addition, *Ras* may be physiologically activated in a larger fraction of cancers.[63] *Myc* is amplified and overexpressed in approximately 33% of cases.[64] More frequent and consistent abnormalities have been found in the PI3 kinase signaling pathway. The p110 catalytic subunit of the PI3 kinase is amplified, overexpressed, and activated in more than half of ovarian cancers.[65] Downstream within the PI3 kinase signaling pathway, *AKT* is also amplified, overexpressed, and activated in 20% of cases.[66] *PTEN* is mutated in endometrioid ovarian cancers.[67] Overall, abnormalities of the PI3 kinase pathway have been found in more than 70% of ovarian cancers.[65] A majority of tumors contain mutations of *TP53* or loss of *ARHI*. *TP53* is mutated in as much as 70% of ovarian cancers, and although it is not clearly of prognostic value, it is more likely mutated in high-grade, as opposed to low-grade lesions.[62,70,71] When *TP53* is mutated in borderline tumors, their prognosis is worse than the majority of lesions of this histology. Mutation of *TP53* may also be a marker for metastasis, in that mutations are less frequent in stage I. Expression of at least three imprinted genes has been downregulated in ovarian cancers: *LOT1, PEG3* and *ARHI*. Downregulation of ARHI in 60% of ovarian cancers has been associated with decreased disease-free survival.[64,76]

A murine model has been developed that mimics human ovarian cancer and that permits the introduction of multiple genes using an avian retroviral gene delivery technique.[68] When the ovarian target cells were derived from transgenic mice deficient for p53, the addition of any two of the oncogenes *c-Myc, K-Ras* and *AKT* were sufficient to induce ovarian tumor formation when infected cells were injected at intraperitoneal, subcutaneous, or ovarian sites. Another model has been developed from normal human ovarian surface epithelial cells that have also been immortalized with telomerase and with viral T antigen which neutralizes *TP53* and *RB* function. Introduction of activated human *H-ras* or *K-ras* genes transforms these immortalized cells and permits them to grow in immunosuppressed mice with a nodular or papillary histology that resembles human ovarian cancer.[69]

Lysophosphatidic acid (LPA) is a ubiquitous growth factor in ovarian cancer. Normal ovarian cells have very little LPA, but the majority of malignant epithelial ovarian tumors express LPA.[67] IL-8, basic fibroblast growth factor (bFGF), and VEGF are all angiogenic factors, which are frequently found in the ascitic fluid of patients.[79,80] In particular, VEGF, a VPF, is often found in very high levels in ascites.[73]

Upregulation and aberrant glycosylation of extracellular mucins have provided targets for therapy and markers for monitoring disease. MUC-1 is a mucin expressed by more than 80% of ovarian cancers.[81] In transformed cells, aberrant glycosylation exposes peptide determinants recognized by murine monoclonal antibodies that have been used for serotherapy. CA125 is also a mucin (MUC16) associated with cells that line the coelomic cavity during embryonic development. CA125 is shed from 80% of epithelial ovarian cancers[82,83] and can be measured using the murine monoclonal antibody OC125. Regression and progression of disease tend to correlate well with falling or rising CA125 levels. The precise function of the glycoprotein is unknown,[84,85] but knockout of murine MUC16 does not affect the development or fertility of mice.

Table 101-1 Oncogenes in Epithelial Ovarian Cancer

Gene	Chromosome	Amplified (%)	Overexpressed (%)	Mutated (%)	Function
Rab25	1q22	54	80-89	8–12	Cytoplasmic GTPase
Evi -1	3q26	–	–	<1	Transcription factor
elF-5A2	3q26	44	78	2-24	Elongation factor
PKCi	3q26	9-11	32		Cytoplasmic serine-threonine kinase
p110 PI3K	3q26	–	51		Cytoplasmic lipid kinase
FGF-1	5q31	20	41-66		Growth factor for cancer and angiogenesis
Myc	8q24	11-20	9-28		Transcription factor
EGFR	7p12	20-21	62		Tyrosine kinase growth factor receptor
Notch-3	9p13	5	30-52		Cell surface growth factor receptor
K-Ras	12p11-12	6-11	4-12		Cytoplasmic GTPase
HER-2	17q12-21	12-36	42-63		Tyrosine kinase growth factor receptor
p85 PI3K	19q	12-27	12		Cytoplasmic lipid kinase
Cyclin E	19q12	10-15	48		Cyclin
AKT2	19q13.2				Cytoplasmic serine-threonine kinase
BTAK/Aurora A	20q13				Nuclear serine-threonine kinase

Source: From Ref. 72.

Table 101-2 ■ **Putative Tumor Suppressor Genes in Epithelial Ovarian Cancer**

Gene	Chromosome	Downregulated or Inactivated	Mechanisms of Downregulation	Function
ARHI (DIRAS3)	1p31	60%	Imprinting; LOH; promoter methylation; transcription downregulated by E2F1 and E2F4	26 kDa GTPase; inhibits proliferation and motility; induces autophagy and dormancy; upregulates p21; inhibits cyclin D1, PI3K, Ras-MAP, Stat3
RASSF1A	3p21		Hypermethylation	Inhibits proliferation and tumorigenicity in many different cancers. Interacts with *ras* inhibiting downregulating cyclin D and signaling through JNK, stabilizes microtubules, regulates spindle checkpoint and fas- and TNF-induced apoptosis.
DLEC1	3p22.3	73%	Promoter hypermethylation and histone hypoacetylation	166 kDa cytoplasmic protein that inhibits anchorage dependent growth
SPARC	5q31	70-90% decreased expression; 9% lost	Transcription	32 kDa Ca++ binding protein; prevents adhesion
DAB-2 (DOC2)	5q13	58–85% lost	Transcription	105 kDa protein binds GRB2 preventing Ras/MAP activation, prevents c-fos induction and decreases ILK activity, contributing to anoikis and inhibiting proliferation and anchorage independent growth and tumorigenicity
LOT1 (ZAC1)	6q25	39%	Imprinting; LOH; transcription downregulated by EGF, TPA	55 kDa nuclear zinc finger protein inhibits proliferation and tumorigenicity
RPS6KA2	6q27	64%	Monoallelic expression in ovary; LOH	90 k Da ribosomal S6 serine-threonine kinase that inhbits growth, induces apoptosis, decreases pERK and cyclin D1, increases p21 and p27
PTEN (MMAC-1)	10q23	3–8% mutated; expression lost in 27%, particularly in endometrioid and clear cell histotypes	Promoter methylation; LOH; mutation	PI3 Phosphatase; decreases proliferation, migration and survival; decreases cyclin D and increases p27
OPCML	11q25	56–83%	Promoter methylation; LOH; mutation	GPI-anchored IgLON family member; induces aggregation; inhibits proliferation and tumorigenicity
BRCA2	13q12-13	3–6%	Mutation; LOH	Binds RAD51 in repair of DNA double strand breaks (DSBs)
ARLTS1	13q14	62%	Promoter methylation	ADP Ribosylation Factor induces apoptosis
WWOX	16q23	30-49%, particularly in mucinous and clear cell histotypes	LOH; mutation	Decreases anchorage independent growth and tumorigenicity; mouse homolog required for apoptosis
P53	17p13.1	50–70%	Mutation	53 kDa Nuclear Protein induces p21 with cell cycle arrest promoting DNA stability; induces apoptosis
OVCA1	17p13.3	37%	LOH	50 kDa protein; decreases proliferation and clonogenicity; decreased Cyclin D1
BRCA1	17q21	6–8%	Mutation; LOH	E3 ubiquitin ligase that participates directly in repair of DNA DSBs through homologous recombination; regulates c-Abl; induces p53, androgen receptor, estrogen receptor and c-Myc.
PEG3	19q13	75%	Imprinting; LOH; promoter methylation; transcription	Induces p53 dependent apoptosis

Source: From Ref. 72.

Classification and Pathology

Primary ovarian cancers are classified according to the structures of the ovary from which they are derived.[2,86] Most develop from the epithelial cells that cover the ovarian surface or that line inclusion cysts although this concept has recently been challenged and has been discussed above. These cells are ultimately derived from the coelomic epithelium of mesodermal origin and share cytologic markers with mesothelium. Germ cell malignancies constitute the next most common group and the least common tumors are derived from ovarian stromal cells.

Epithelial malignancies account for 85% to 90% of ovarian cancers. The majority of epithelial lesions are seen in patients who are 40 years or older. Under the age of 40 years, epithelial malignancies are uncommon, and most malignancies seen in women under the age of 30 years are of germ cell origin.[2] The histologic types of the epithelial tumors are listed in Table 101-3. The majority of lesions, about 75%, are of the serous type, followed by the mucinous, endometrioid, clear cell, mixed, Brenner, and undifferentiated histologies.[2,86] The cellular patterns of different histotypes resemble different derivatives of the Müllerian duct in different portions of the female reproductive tract. For example, serous epithelial cells resemble cells that line the Fallopian tube, endometrioid epithelial cells resemble the endometrium, and mucinous epithelial cells resemble the uterine endocervix. Expression of *HOXA9*, *HOXA10*, and *HOXA11* drive differentiation of the fallopian tube, uterus, and vagina during normal embryologic development. Re-expression of these genes has been detected in serous, endometrioid and mucinous ovarian cancers and forced expression in transformed ovarian epithelial cells can induce the different histotypes.[87]

Invasive Histologies ■ Serous carcinomas may have a complex admixture of cystic and solid areas with extensive papilla-

Table 101-3 ■ **Epithelial Ovarian Tumors**

Histologic Type	Cellular Type
I. Serous	Endosalpingeal
A. Benign	
B. Borderline	
C. Malignant	
II Mucinous	Endocervical
A. Benign	
B. Borderline	
C. Malignant	
III. Endometrioid	Endometrial
A. Benign	
B. Borderline	
C. Malignant	
IV. Clear cell "mesonephroid"	Müllerian
A. Benign	
B. Borderline	
C. Malignant	
V. Brenner	Transitional
A. Benign	
B. Borderline ("proliferating")	
C. Malignant	
VI. Mixed epithelial	Mixed
A. Benign	
B. Borderline	
C. Malignant	
VII. Undifferentiated	
Anaplastic	
VIII. Unclassified	
Mesothelioma	
Other	

tions, or they may contain a predominantly solid mass with areas of necrosis and hemorrhage (Fig. 101-1) The poorly differentiated tumors may have some areas with a papillary pattern, but other portions may be indistinguishable from the other histologic patterns described below (Fig. 101-2). Stage I or II lesions are most frequently unilateral, with about 10% to 20% involving both ovaries. Conversely, about 50% to 70% of stage III serous carcinomas are bilateral.[2]

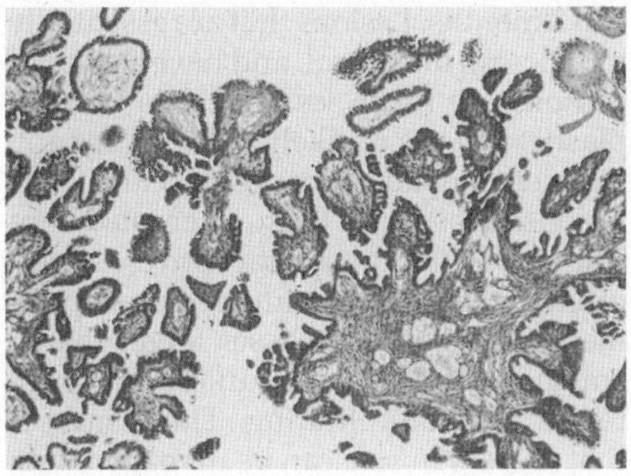

Figure 101-1 ■ Serous cystadenocarcinoma gross with omentum.

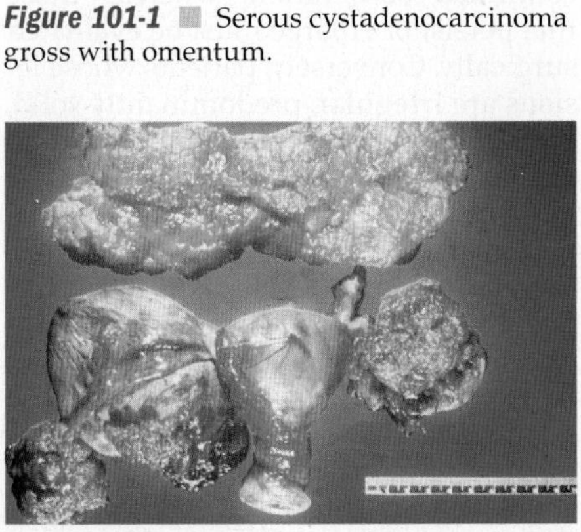

Figure 101-2 ■ Poorly differentiated papillary serous carcinoma of ovary.

Mucinous tumors tend to be large, with many masses over 20 cm in diameter (Fig. 101-3). The histologic pattern resembles uterine endocervical glands. The lesions frequently contain areas of hemorrhage, necrosis, and various quantities of mucin. These tumors are bilateral in 10% to 20% of cases.[2] Occasionally, mucin is secreted into the peritoneal cavity and produces a condition known as pseudomyxoma or myxoma peritonei. A mucocele of the appendix may also be seen in conjunction with this tumor.

Endometrioid carcinomas of the ovary resemble typical carcinomas of the endometrium. These tumors may be seen with synchronous endometrial carcinoma, and when they are, both lesions may be of low-stage. Rarely, endometrioid carcinomas may arise in conjunction with pelvic endometriosis, resulting from malignant transformation of a benign process (Fig. 101-4). Like endometrial cancers, endometrioid ovarian cancers are associated with inactivating mutations of *PTEN* with consequent activation of PI3 kinase signaling. Bilaterality is seen in 10% to 15% of stage I and II disease, and in about 30% of stage III.[2]

Clear cell carcinomas were formerly called mesonephromas, a term that has been abandoned because clear cell tumors are derived from tissues that are embryologically distinct from mesonephrons. About one-fourth of clear cell tumors are associated with endometriosis. Clear cell tumors are only rarely bilateral.[2]

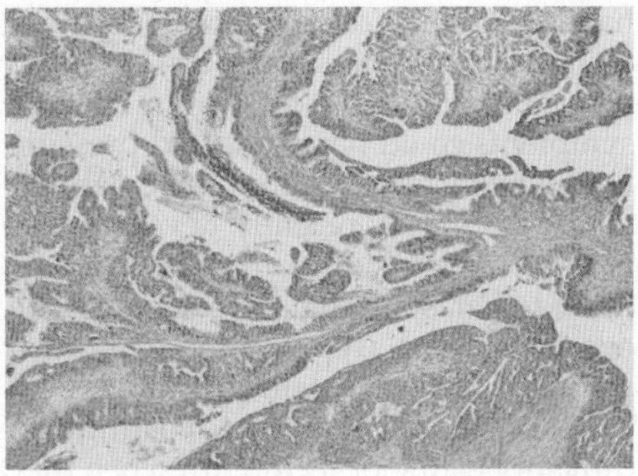

Figure 101-3 ■ Mucinous cystadenocarcinoma.

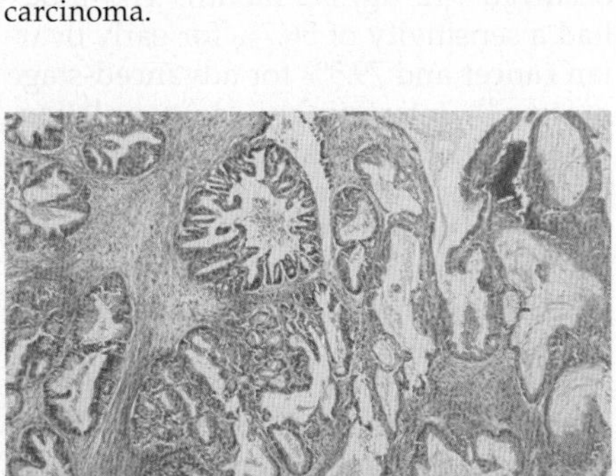

Figure 101-4 ■ Endometrioid carcinoma.

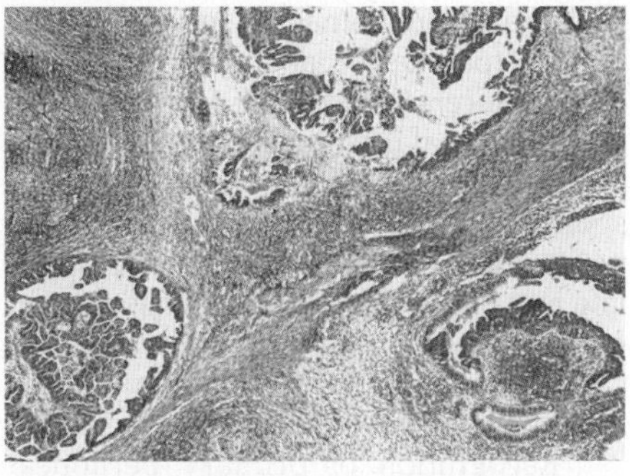

Figure 101-5 ■ Borderline papillary serous tumor.

Brenner tumors are uncommon, representing less than 1% of all epithelial malignancies. Mixed epithelial tumors may contain small areas of Brenner tumor histology, which have a histologic pattern similar to that of transitional cell. Malignant Brenner tumors are unilateral.[2]

Borderline Tumors ■ Borderline tumors, or those of low malignant potential, are important to differentiate from those that are frankly invasive. The treatment and prognosis for borderline lesions are considerably different from those for invasive malignancies. Borderline tumors tend to remain confined to a single ovary at the time of diagnosis, and also tend to occur in younger, premenopausal women (Fig. 101-5). They may be confused with a well differentiated invasive ovarian cancer, and the treatment for the two may be different. Thus, in a young patient who has a lesion confined to the ovary, which is suspected of being an epithelial ovarian cystadenocarcinoma, a borderline tumor must be excluded, because bilateral oophorectomy, hysterectomy, and chemotherapy are unnecessary in these patients. In women under the age of 40 years, about 60% to 70% of non-benign ovarian neoplasms are borderline, whereas in women over 40 years, only 10% are borderline.[2,88] Histologic criteria for borderline tumors include (i) the presence of epithelial cell proliferation with a "piling up" of cells, so-called pseudostratification; (ii) cytologic atypia, but with rare mitoses; and (iii) no evidence of stromal invasion. Borderline tumors tend to remain confined to the ovary, but may be associated with peritoneal disease, which represents either dissemination or the multifocal evolution of the disease. In those rare patients with peritoneal involvement, death can occur by progressive intestinal obstruction.[87,88]

Primary Peritoneal Carcinomas ■ Epithelial malignancies that arise primarily from peritoneal lining cells are referred to as peritoneal carcinomas or primary peritoneal (papillary) adenocarcinomas.[19,89] These cancers are distinct form the very rare peritoneal mesotheliomas that exhibit a different natural history, as well as response to chemotherapy.[90] The cells of the peritoneum have the ability to recapitulate any of the histologic patterns seen in ovarian cancers, although papillary serous carcinomas occur most frequently and the other histologic types are rarely seen.

Recognition of primary peritoneal carcinomas explains the occurrence of ovarian cancer after oophorectomy.[91] Also, primary peritoneal cancers can involve the surface of the ovaries without ovarian enlargement. Thus, ovaries can be innocent bystanders in a process originating in the peritoneal cavity. Therapeutically, primary peritoneal malignancy should be treated as one would manage a primary epithelial ovarian cancer.

Patterns of Spread

Ovarian epithelial tumors spread primarily by direct exfoliation and implantation of cells throughout the peritoneal cavity, but also metastasize via the lymphatic and hematogenous routes. GCTs have a greater predilection for spread via the retroperitoneal lymphatics, which must be evaluated carefully when staging those tumors that appear to be confined to the ovary.[2,92]

Exfoliated ovarian cancer cells spread directly to the pelvic and abdominal peritoneal surfaces, and tend to follow the path of circulation of peritoneal fluid from the right pericolic gutter cephalad to the right hemidiaphragm.[3] At primary surgery, the parietal and visceral peritoneum can be studded with dozens to hundreds of metastatic nodules. The intestinal mesenteries can become involved by peritoneal metastases. Adhesions form between loops of small intestine producing mechanical obstruction, even though involvement of the lumen of the intestine by direct extension is uncommon. The intestinal dysfunction can also result from involvement by tumor of the myenteric plexus, the autonomic innervation of the intestine that is found in the mesentery. This condition has been referred to as "carcinomatous ileus."[3] Large pelvic masses can compress the rectum producing colonic obstruction.

Spread via the lymphatics is common in epithelial ovarian cancer. Apparent stage I and II tumors have retroperitoneal lymphatic dissemination in about 5% to 10% in most series, whereas lymphatic dissemination in stage III has been reported to be as high as 42% to 78% in carefully explored patients.[92,93] Most of these lymph nodes are not enlarged, but are microscopically positive for malignant cells. Spread through the retroperitoneal and diaphragmatic lymphatics can result in metastasis to the supraclavicular lymph nodes on the left and right respectively.

Blood-borne metastasis of ovarian cancer is uncommon at diagnosis and is often a late finding in the disease. Hematogenous dissemination at the time of diagnosis to the parenchyma of the liver or lung is seen in only 2% to 3% of patients. Indeed, most patients who have disease dissemination cephalad to the diaphragm at the time of presentation have a right pleural effusion. Metastasis to the central nervous system is rare and spread to the one is very rare, except for the clear cell histologic type.[2,3] However, in patients who survive many months and years with their disease, involvement of distant sites is more common including parenchymal lung and brain metastases. Distant metastases consistent with stage IV findings were documented in almost two-fifths of patients who died of ovarian cancer originally thought confined to the peritoneal cavity.[3]

Clinical Features

Traditionally, ovarian cancer has been considered a "silent killer" that does not produce symptoms until far advanced. Some patients with ovarian cancers confined to the ovary are asymptomatic, but the majority will have nonspecific symptoms that do not necessarily suggest an origin in the ovary. In one survey of 1725 women with ovarian cancer, 95% recalled symptoms prior to diagnosis, including 89% with stage I/II disease and 97% with stage III/IV disease.[94] Seventy percent had abdominal or GI symptoms, 58% pain, 34% urinary symptoms, and 26% pelvic discomfort. At least some of these symptoms could have reflected pressure on the pelvic viscera from the enlarging ovary. Goff et al. recently developed an ovarian cancer symptom index and reported that symptoms associated with ovarian cancer were pelvic/abdominal pain, urinary frequency/urgency, increased abdominal size or bloating and difficulty eating or feeing full when they were present for less than one year and occurred >12 days a month. The index had a sensitivity of 56.7% for early ovarian cancer and 79.5% for advanced-stage disease.[95] Interestingly, a population-based study from Australia found that there did not appear to be a significant difference in the duration of symptoms or the nature of symptoms in patients with early as opposed to advanced-stage ovarian cancer.[96,97]

Metastatic ovarian cancer is rarely asymptomatic. In addition to the GI and urinary symptoms noted in early-stage disease, formation of ascites can produce an increase in abdominal girth. Pleural effusion may lead to dyspnea as the first complaint. Acute symptoms, such as those of adnexal rupture or torsion, are uncommon. Vaginal bleeding is also an uncommon symptom in postmenopausal women, although premenopausal patients may present with irregular or heavy menses.[3] Detection of an adnexal mass by pelvic examination can permit the early diagnosis of ovarian cancer. Since malignancy is rare and the majority of palpable adnexal masses are benign, an enlarged ovary discovered on pelvic examination is not likely to be an ovarian malignancy. In premenopausal women, ovarian cancer is uncommon and represents less than 7% of all adnexal masses.[2] Even in postmenopausal women, 70% to 80% of adnexal tumors are benign. In some patients who complain primarily of abdominal symptoms, a pelvic examination frequently is omitted and the tumor missed. Signs of advanced disease include abdominal distention and a fluid wave consistent with ascites. These signs are nonspecific and can be associated with many conditions arising in the abdominal cavity, especially malignancies of other primary sites or carcinomatosis from metastatic tumors of the GI tract and breast.

Diagnosis

The diagnosis of ovarian cancer is usually made at laparotomy, but occasionally at laparoscopy. If a pelvic mass is suspicious and the most likely diagnosis is ovarian cancer, surgery should not be unnecessarily delayed. In premenopausal patients, however, simple cystic ovarian lesions can be observed over a period of 1 to 2 months. Lesions that are essentially mobile, are unilateral, and have a smooth contour are much less likely to be neoplastic, and are unlikely to be malignant. In premenopausal patients with cystic lesions of less than 8 cm, attempted suppression with oral contraceptives is indicated. In women who are definitely postmenopausal, cystic masses larger than 5 cm should be removed unless they represent a chronic finding. Those masses that regress in size can be managed with continued observation, whereas those that persist or enlarge must be evaluated surgically. Conversely, patients whose lesions are irregular, predominantly solid, and somewhat immobile should undergo an exploratory laparotomy.[41]

The preoperative evaluation of patients can be aided by the use of CA125. Elevated CA125 levels are most frequently associated with malignant adnexal masses in postmenopausal women. In women over 50 years of age whose serum CA125 level is greater than 35 U/mL the adnexal mass is malignant in about 80% of cases. A CA125 of more than 95 U/mL is associated with a positive predictive value (PPV) of 96% in this setting. Conversely, the majority of premenopausal women with serum CA125 levels greater than 35 U/mL have benign conditions, such as uterine myomata, endometriosis, and benign ovarian tumors.[3,98] Elevation of serum CA125 in a postmenopausal patient with a pelvic mass should prompt exploration by surgeons prepared to undertake complete staging and, if necessary, cytoreductive operations. Greater accuracy has been obtained using a combination of ultrasound, CA125 and menopausal status to create a risk of malignancy index (RMI) that has achieved a sensitivity of 85% with a specificity of 97% for predicting the presence of ovarian cancers in women with pelvic masses.[99] Recently, an algorithm has been derived and validated prospectively in a large trial that utilize CA125, human epididymis protein 4 (HE4) and menopausal status to distinguish malignant from benign pelvic masses with a sensitivity of 94% and specificity of 75% in postmenopausal women and with a sensitivity of 76% and a specificity of 75% in premenopausal women.[100] Overall, 95% of patients with malignant pelvic masses were identified as high-risk.

Ultrasonographic signs of malignancy include an adnexal pelvic mass with areas of complexity, such as irregular borders; multiple echogenic patterns within the mass; and dense, multiple irregular septae. Bilateral tumors are more likely to be malignant, although the individual characteristics of the lesions are of greater significance. Transvaginal ultrasonography may have a somewhat better resolution than transabdominal ultrasonography for adnexal neoplasms. Newer techniques using Doppler colorflow imaging may enhance the specificity of ultrasonography for demonstrating findings consistent with malignancy.[101]

Radiographic techniques, including abdominal radiographs, computed tomography (CT) scans, and nuclear magnetic resonance imaging (MRI), are not useful prior to the surgical diagnosis of ovarian cancer. The preoperative evaluation of patients who have a suspicious pelvic mass can omit these studies when blood chemistries and enzymes suggest normal hepatic and pancreatic function. In patients with ascites and no pelvic mass, however, a CT or MRI may be useful in identifying other potential sites of origin. Paracentesis is not recommended because of the frequency of metastatic implantation and growth in the needle tract. Liver–spleen scans, brain scans, and bone scans are unnecessary unless specific symptoms suggest metastasis to these sites.

In premenopausal women, radiographic studies of the intestines are not required unless there is the finding of occult blood in the rectum or there are symptoms indicating upper or lower intestinal obstruction. A barium enema or endoscopy is appropriate in postmenopausal patients. Mammography should be performed to exclude primary breast cancer, which can coexist with ovarian cancer or spread to the ovaries. Cervical cytology should be performed, although ovarian cancer cells are unlikely to exfoliate through the uterus to the cervix. In patients with irregular or heavy menses, an endometrial biopsy should be performed to exclude primary endometrial pathology.[41]

The differential diagnosis of an adnexal mass includes a variety of functional changes of the ovary, benign neoplasms of the reproductive tract, and inflammatory lesions of these organs. A hydrosalpinx, endometriosis, and pedunculated uterine leiomyomata can simulate an ovarian neoplasm. Non-gynecologic diseases, such as inflammatory processes of the colon and rectum, must be excluded.

Screening ■ There is no well-established strategy for early detection of ovarian cancer.[101] Discovery of a pelvic mass on routine physical examination can lead to surgery prior to the dissemination of a malignancy, but conventional diagnosis detects only 20% of patients in stage I. Given the prevalence of ovarian cancer in the postmenopausal population, any screening strategy must be highly specific (> 99.6%) as well as highly sensitive for early stage disease (> 75%) to achieve a PPV of 10% (ie, 10 laparotomies for each case of ovarian cancer detected). Two approaches have been evaluated for early detection of ovarian cancer: ultrasonography and serum tests such as CA125.

Ultrasonography ■ Transvaginal sonography (TVS) has proven superior to transabdominal sonography (TAU) for the detection of a pelvic mass. In three large studies that screened 66,620 women with TVS, 565 operations were performed to detect 45 ovarian cancers, 34 of which were invasive.[102-104] Overall, the sensitivity for early-stage disease was 78%, but the specificity fell just short of that required for a PPVof 10% with 12 operations per case of ovarian cancer detected. The most promising single study achieved a PPV of 9.9%.[103] Confirmatory tests with Doppler ultrasound have not proven consistent, but additional studies with 3-D power Doppler are underway to improve specificity in distinguishing malignant from benign ovarian abnormalities.

CA125 ■ CA125 is elevated in 50% to 60% of patients with stage I and in 90% with stage II ovarian cancer.[105] CA125 levels can rise 10 to 60 months prior to diagnosis with an average estimated lead time of 1.9 years prior to diagnosis of disease in all stages.[106] In the Prostate, Lung, Colorectal and Ovarian (PLCO) Screening trial, 37,500 postmenopausal women had an annual CA125 and TVS for three years.[107] If either were abnormal, women were referred to a gynecologist. CA125 alone had a PPV of 3.7%, TVS alone had a PPVof 1%. If both were abnormal the PPV rose to 23.5%, but 60% of the invasive ovarian cancers would have been missed. Thus, the specificity for a single determination of CA125 or a single TVS is not adequate to screen a population at average risk, but specificity can be improved with a two-stage strategy that utilizes CA125 followed by ultrasound in a subset of women with elevated CA125. Use of CA125 to trigger ultrasound has been evaluated in trials in Sweden and in the United Kingdom.[108,109] The latter randomized 22,000 women to conventional surveillance or to annual CA125 with TAU if the value were elevated.[109] When TAU was abnormal, surgery was undertaken. Among 10,985 women screened, 29 operations were performed to detect 6 cancers, providing a PPV of 21%. During 7 years of follow-up, 10 more cancers were diagnosed in the screened group. Over the same intervals, 21 ovarian cancers were diagnosed in the control group. Median survival in the screened group (72.9 months) was significantly greater (p = .0112) than that in the control group (41.8 months).

Risk of Ovarian Cancer (ROC) Algorithm ■ A rising CA125 is a more specific indicator of ovarian cancer. Analyzing serum samples stored from screening studies in Stockholm and in the United Kingdom with an improved CA125 II assay, it has been possible to improve the specificity of CA125 as a screening tool by following the values of an individual over time.[110,111] Elevated CA125 levels in women without ovarian cancer remain static or decrease with time, whereas levels associated with ovarian malignancy tend to rise. This finding has been incorporated into an algorithm that uses age, rate of change of CA125 and absolute levels of CA125 to calculate an individual's "risk of ovarian cancer" (ROC). Patients at sufficient risk undergo TVS.[111] In a prospective trial, 6532 women were screened with CA125 and the ROC algorithm.[112] Sixteen patients had abnormal findings prompting operations that detected 4 cases of primary ovarian cancer, yielding a specificity of 99.8% and a PPV of 19%.

Currently, accrual to a trial has been completed in the United Kingdom that includes 200,000 postmenopausal women who were randomized to three groups: a control group (100,000) who have been followed with conventional pelvic examinations; a second group (50,000) who had annual TVS; and a third group

(50,000) who had CA125 determined at least annually. Based on the ROC algorithm, patients in the third group were referred for TVS and/or surgery. Women will be screened for 3 years and followed for 7 years. The anticipated date when the data will mature is 2012. Results from the first year of screening suggest that the ROC algorithm followed by TVS will have substantially higher specificity and no less sensitivity than annual TVS, but data in subsequent years will be required to determine whether screening improves survival.

Complementary Markers ■ Whatever the outcome of the current trial in the United Kingdom, strategies based on CA125 alone are not likely to exceed a sensitivity of 80%, as CA125 is not expressed by 20% of epithelial ovarian cancers. Greater sensitivity might be attained through the use of multiple serum markers in combination, provided that specificity was not compromised.

Altered levels of more than 50 biomarkers have been reported in the serum or urine of ovarian cancer patients. A number of novel markers for ovarian cancer have been identified in recent years including mesothelin, a 110 kD fragment of EGFR (sEGFR), LPA, HE4, prostasin, osteopontin, and human kallikreins 6 and 10.[113-119] Multiplex assays can measure >50 biomarkers with a few hundred microliters of serum.[120] Using the multiplex technology, a combination of CA125, HE4, sEGFR, and soluble vascular cell adhesion molecule-1 (vCAM-1) have distinguished 90% of stage I ovarian cancer patients from 98% of healthy controls. Use of surface laser desorption and ionization (SELDI) with subsequent resolution by mass spectroscopy has demonstrated a pattern of low molecular weight moieties that has been reported to distinguish sera from ovarian cancer patients from those of healthy individuals with 100% sensitivity and 95% specificity.[121] Prospective replication of these results and determination of sensitivity for stage I disease should be available in the near future. Methodological issues have been raised regarding these data.[122] SELDI may also identify a limited number of protein peaks that could be assayed by more conventional techniques.[123] Assay of a combination of apolipoprotein A1, transthyretin, connective tissue activating protein 3 (CTAP3) and CA125 in serum have distinguished 87% of patients with stage I ovarian cancer from healthy individuals with 98% specificity. In a 2-stage strategy, an initial stage with 98% specificity would require ultrasounds to be performed in only 2% of women screened. Mathematical techniques to combine markers, enhancing their sensitivity without sacrificing specificity, have also been developed. Both artificial neural networks and mixtures of multivariate normal distributions have been used to combine values for four serum markers (CA125 II, CA72-4, CA15-3, and macrophage colony-stimulating factor [M-CSF]) from patients with stage I ovarian cancer and from healthy individuals. Using either technique, sensitivity could be increased from 48% using CA125II alone to 72% to 75% using the combination, while maintaining specificity at 98%.

Current Recommendations for Women at Average Risk ■ The application of screening techniques other than pelvic examination for ovarian cancer in the entire female population is unwarranted at this time. The sensitivity and specificity of ultrasound and CA125 are low in premenopausal women, making it unlikely that this approach will be useful in this group. However, with refinements of the transvaginal and flow techniques, as well as the addition of other serum markers, screening could become a reality in the future and this is being addressed in a large randomized trial in the United Kingdom. There is a need for critical studies to define the potential of different screening strategies and to determine whether their application can decrease mortality from the disease.

Current Recommendations for Screening Women at High Risk ■ In screening has been frequently advocated for women at increased genetic risk of ovarian cancer, although the efficacy of such surveillance to reduce risk is unproven. Many of the occult cancers found after PBSO have been in the fimbrial end of the fallopian tube and this consistent finding suggests that ultrasound of the ovaries is unlikely to detect cancers at an early stage in women at high genetic risk. Screening can be problematic because this high-risk population generally includes premenopausal women who have a higher incidence of false-positive CA125 elevations and ultrasound abnormalities. In these high-risk populations, initial screening trials using ultrasound alone or in combination with color-flow Doppler were associated with high false-positive rates (2.5-4.9%). The current trend is to combine ultrasound every 6 to 12 months with CA125 every 3 to 6 months.

There are 5 prospective studies where combined screening has been undertaken in high-risk populations.[124-128] In three, screening programs involving a total of 1228 women with a family history of ovarian cancer, no invasive ovarian cancer was detected and false-positive rates have ranged from 0.4% to 3.9%.[124-136] In one of the remaining two studies, one case of ovarian cancer was detected on screening 137 high-risk women with a false-positive rate of 0.7%; in the other study 9 ovarian cancers were detected in screening 180 women with a false-positive rate of 3.9%.[127,128] The findings of two recent prospective studies of annual transvaginal ultrasound and CA125 screening in 888 *BRCA1* and *BRCA2* mutation carriers in the Netherlands and 279 mutation carriers in the United Kingdom are not encouraging and suggest a very limited benefit of screening in high-risk women.[129,130] Despite annual gynaecological screening, Hermssen et al. reported that a high proportion of ovarian cancers in *BRCA1/2* carriers were interval cancers and the large majority of all cancers are diagnosed were at advanced stage and similar results were reported by Woodward. Therefore, it is unlikely that annual screening will reduce mortality from ovarian cancer in *BRCA1/2* mutation carriers.[97,129]

The model proposed by Kurman and Shih (2008[81]) helps to explain why current screening techniques, aimed at detecting stage I disease, have not been effective. Tumors that remain confined to the ovary for a long period belong to the type 1 group such as clear cell, endometrioid and low-grade serous cancers, but they account for only 25% of the malignant tumors. These tumors generally do not occur in women with *BRCA* mutations. The majority of patients at high genetic risk have high-grade serous cancers with p53 mutations and these are only rarely confined to the ovary at diagnosis. Mutation of p53 has correlated with metastatic potential and can occur at the earliest stage of ovarian oncogenesis in genetically predisposed individuals. In specimens from prophylactic oophorectomies, occult cancers with p53 mutations have been found within small ovarian cysts. Cancers that arise in the fallopian tube or peritoneum are almost always at advanced stage at diagnosis. Kurman has suggested that a more realistic end point for the early detection of ovarian cancer is volume and not stage of disease.

Women in the high-risk population who request screening should be counseled about the current lack of evidence for the efficacy for either CA125 or for sonography as well as the associated false-positive rates. Many will still opt for screening despite the risks and limitations of the available strategies. Screening is best carried out in clinical trials such as those conducted by the Cancer Genetics Network or by several university centers. This important question has been addressed in Gynecologic Oncology Group (GOG)-199, a study of screening with annual transvaginal ultrasound and CA125 ROCA compared to PBSO. Study accrual is complete as of November 2006; with 2605 participants enrolled: 1030 (40%) into the surgical cohort and 1575 (60%) into the screening cohort. Five years of prospective follow-up ends in November 2011.[131] Screening with TVS every 6 to 12 months and with CA125 every 3 to 6 months is currently being evaluated.

Staging of Ovarian Cancer

Ovarian malignancies are staged according to the FIGO system. The FIGO staging system of 1987 (Table 101-4) is based on the findings at surgical exploration. A preoperative evaluation should exclude the presence of extraperitoneal metastases. A thorough surgical exploration is important because subsequent treatment will be determined by the stage of disease. In patients whose exploratory laparotomy does not reveal any macroscopic evidence of disease by inspection and palpation of the entire intra-abdominal space, a careful search for microscopic spread must be undertaken.[41,93] In an earlier series in which patients did not undergo careful surgical staging, the overall 5-year survival for patients with apparent stage I epithelial ovarian cancer was only about 60%.[1,41] Survival rates of 90% to 100% have been reported for properly staged patients found to have stage IA or IB disease.[41,42]

Metastases in apparent stage I or II epithelial ovarian cancer are common. About 30% of patients whose ovarian epithelial cancers appear to be confined to the pelvis have occult metastatic disease in the upper abdomen or in the retroperitoneal lymph nodes.[41] The importance of a comprehensive initial surgical staging is emphasized by the findings of a cooperative national study in which 100 patients with apparent stage I or II disease who were referred for subsequent therapy underwent additional surgical staging.[120] In this series, 28% of patients initially thought to have stage I disease were upstaged, and 43% of patients thought to have stage II disease had more advanced disease. Thus, 31% of patients were upstaged as a result of additional surgery, and 77% were reclassified as stage III. Histologic grade was a significant predictor of occult metastasis, ie, 16% of patients with grade 1 lesions were upstaged, compared to 34% with grade 2 and 46% with grade 3 disease.

Although the literature has emphasized the importance of thorough surgical exploration in patients with disease apparently localized to the ovaries, scant recognition is made of the semantic difficulty presented by the concept of extension to other pelvic (ie, stage II) or abdominal (ie, stage III) organs. No problem exists when the surgeon encounters discrete implants, or seeds, separate from the primary tumor, or when solid tumor is found growing into adjacent structures. A more common situation, however, is the apparently benign adherence of the tumor to adjacent structures in the absence of metastatic implants or obvious direct tumor extension. There is a considerable body of evidence that such benign adherence, when it is dense, is associated with a relapse risk equivalent to stage II, and that these patients should not be included in stage I, but rather in stage II.[133-135] Adherence is considered dense when sharp dissection is required to mobilize the tumor, when a raw area is left at the site of adherence, or when rupture of a cyst results from dissecting free the adhesions. It is the practice at most North American centers to advance the stage of densely adherent tumors to stage II, and this was done in a recent multicenter study of stage I and II disease.[132]

After a comprehensive staging laparotomy, less than half of women are found to have local or regional disease (FIGO stages I and II). Of the 26,600 women diagnosed yearly with epithelial ovarian cancer in the United States, approximately 2000 to 3000 have the disease confined to pelvic structures.[41] The prognosis for these patients depends on clinical-pathologic features, as summarized below.[41,45,132-135]

Although accounting for only 15% to 20% of all cases, approximately one-third to one-half of all cured patients are derived from stage I, highlighting its importance. An in-depth understanding of the management of stage I is hampered by the small fraction of patients with limited disease, as well as by their excellent long-term prognosis (over an 80% 5-year relapse-free rate). Consequently, Phase 3 randomized trials are difficult to conduct with this group due to their small numbers and relatively low rate of recurrence and death. No controlled study to date has been able to establish a curative advantage to postoperative adjuvant therapy.

The most recent FIGO staging classification of stage I, in practice, is descriptive rather than prognostic. The classification recognizes nine subcategories of stage I. Subclasses A (unilateral), B (bilateral), and C (capsular penetration, tumor spillage, or positive peritoneal cytology) are each further subdivided according to differentiation into three grades.[67]

Within each grade, it is incorrect to assume that the factors that assign patients to substages B and C necessarily carry a worse prognosis than substage A, or that rupture, capsular penetration, and positive peritoneal cytology all worsen prognosis to the same degree, or that ascites in the absence of positive cytology is not prognostic. Indeed, several studies have failed to show that bilaterality or iatrogenic intraoperative rupture had any influence on outcome.[132-134] Data on the prognostic significance of positive peritoneal cytology in ovarian cancer are scarce and inadequate.

Treatment of Early-Stage Ovarian Cancer

The treatment of early-stage epithelial ovarian cancer must be individualized. Thorough surgical exploration and stag-

Table 101-4 **FIGO Stages for Primary Carcinoma of the Ovary**

Stage I	Growth limited to the ovaries
Stage IA	Growth limited to the ovary; no ascites. No tumor on the external surface; capsule intact
Stage IB	Growth limited to both ovaries; no ascites. No tumor on the external surfaces; capsule intact
Stage IC	Tumor either stage IA or IB but with tumor on the surface of one or both ovaries; or with capsule ruptured; or with ascites present containing malignant cells or with positive peritoneal washings
Stage II	Growth involving one or both ovaries with pelvic extension
Stage IIA	Extension and/or metastases to the uterus and/or tubes
Stage IIB	Extension to other pelvic tissues
Stage IIC	Tumor either stage IIA or IIB with tumor on the surface of one or both ovaries; or with capsule(s) ruptured; or with ascites present containing malignant cells or with positive peritoneal washings
Stage III	Tumor involving one or both ovaries and/or positive retroperitoneal or inguinal nodes. Superficial liver metastasis equals stage III. Tumor is limited to the true pelvis, but with histologically proven malignant extension to small bowel or omentum
Stage IIIA	Tumor grossly limited to the true pelvis with negative nodes but with histologically confirmed implants of abdominal peritoneal surfaces, none exceeding 2 cm in diameter. Nodes negative
Stage IIIB	Tumor of one or both ovaries with histologically confirmed implants of abdominal peritoneal surfaces, none exceeding 2 cm in diameter. Nodes negative
Stage IIIC	Abdominal implants more than 2 cm in diameter and/or positive retroperitoneal or inguinal nodes
Stage IV	Growth involving one or both ovaries with distant metastasis. If pleural effusion is present, there must be positive cytologic test results to allot a case to stage IV. Parenchymal liver metastasis equals stage IV

These categories are based on findings at clinical examination and/or surgical exploration. The histologic characteristics are to be considered in the staging, as are results of cytologic testing as far as effusions are concerned. It is desirable that a biopsy be performed on suspicious areas outside the pelvis. In order to evaluate the impact on prognosis of the different criteria for allotting cases to stage IC or IIC, it would be of value to know if rupture of the capsule was (1) spontaneous or (2) caused by the surgeon, and if the source of malignant cells detected was (1) peritoneal washings or (2) ascites.

ing are indicated for all patients with early-stage disease. Adjuvant treatment with chemotherapy or radiotherapy is appropriate for those women at highest risk of recurrence.

Surgery ■ Properly staged early disease can be managed conservatively. The primary treatment for invasive stage I epithelial ovarian cancer is surgical, ie, the performance of a total abdominal hysterectomy, BSO, and surgical staging.[66] In certain circumstances, a unilateral oophorectomy may suffice, as discussed below.

Radiotherapy ■ There have been randomized studies of external-beam radiotherapy in stage I epithelial ovarian cancer comparing pelvic radiotherapy with no postoperative treatment. These data suggest that pelvic irradiation reduced the rate of pelvic relapses, but because relapses occurred throughout the peritoneal cavity, there was no therapeutic benefit. Abdominopelvic radiotherapy has not been studied in a randomized phase 3 trial in patients with stage I ovarian cancer. Results of treating a large number of patients at the Princess Margaret Hospital in Toronto over 25 years ago. When abdominopelvic radiotherapy was compared to pelvic radiotherapy or to observation, there was no apparent benefit for grade 1 tumors, where the risk of relapse was under 5%l. With grade 2 and 3 cancers, a nonsignificant reduction in relapse risk was observed. A significant reduction in relapse risk was seen in patients whose tumors were densely adherent to the pelvic wall, but in more recent studies these patients have been classified as stage II.[135]

Chemotherapy ■ *Adjuvant* ■ Based on experience in treating patients with advanced ovarian cancer, cisplatin, carboplatin, cyclophosphamide, and paclitaxel have been administered, individually and in combination, to patients with early-stage disease following surgical resection. Several series reported outcomes when cisplatin and/or cyclophosphamide have been used to treat patients with stage I disease.[136-138] IA GOG trial compared three cycles of cisplatin and cyclophosphamide to intraperitoneal 32P in patients with stage IB and IC disease. Progression-free survival (PFS) of women receiving the platinum-based chemotherapy was 31% higher than that of women who received the radiocolloid.[137] The Gruppo Italiano Collaborativo Oncologica Ginecologica (GICOG) has reported two studies that evaluated treatment with cisplatin for women with early-stage disease.[138] The first study included patients who had stage I cancers of grades 1 and 2, without ascites, positive cytology, rupture, or capsular penetration. When observation was compared to six cycles of cisplatin, the 4-year disease-free rates were 70% and 71% in the bservation group and the group who received to six cycles of cisplatin, respectively. In the second study, patients with all other classes of stage I were randomized to intraperitoneal 32P or six cycles of cisplatin. The 4-year disease-free survival rate with cisplatin was 79% compared to 69% with intraperitonial (IP) radiocolloid, but this difference did not achieve statistical significance.

The GOG reported the results of a randomized study comparing three cycles of carboplatin and paclitaxel with six cycles in 457 patients with early-stage ovarian cancer.[139] An unexpectedly large number of patients (126, 29%) had incomplete or inadequately documented surgical staging in this study. The recurrence rate for six cycles was 24% lower (hazard ratio [HR] 0.76 confidence interval [CI] 0.5-1.13 $p = 0.18$) for six cycles versus three cycles but this was not statistically significant.The estimated probability of recurrence at 5 years was 20.1% for six cycles and 25.4% for three cycles. They concluded that three cycles of adjuvant carboplatin and paclitaxel was a reasonable option for women with high-risk early-stage ovarian cancer, although many oncologists would recommend six cycles, if chemotherapy is given to early-stage patients.

The GOG has subsequently completed an additional trial in which high-risk patients were randomized to three or six cycles of carboplatin and paclitaxel. The results of this trial are currently not available. The current GOG trial provides all patients at high-risk of recurrence with three cycles of carboplatin and paclitaxel and participants are then randomized to observation or 6 months of weekly low-dose (40 mg/m^2) paclitaxel.

Two large parallel randomized phase 3 clinical trials were conducted on women with early-stage disease: the International Collaborative Ovarian Neoplasm Trial 1 (ICON1) and the Adjuvant Chemotherapy Trial in Ovarian Neoplasia (ACTION).[140,141] When the data from the two trials were combined and analyzed,[142] a total of 465 patients were randomized to receive platinum-based adjuvant chemotherapy and 460 to observation until disease progression. After a median follow-up of more than 4 years, the overall survival was 82% in the chemotherapy arm and 74% in the observation arm (HR = 0.67, p = .001). Recurrence-free survival was also better in the chemotherapy arm: 76% vs 65% (HR = 0.64, p = .001). The results of this analysis must be interpreted with caution, because most of the patients did not undergo thorough surgical staging, but the findings suggest that platinum-based chemotherapy should be given to patients who have not been optimally staged.

Management of Invasive Early-Stage Low-Risk Disease (Stages IA and IB, Low-Grade) ■ In patients who have undergone a thorough staging laparotomy where there is no evidence of spread beyond the ovary, the performance of an abdominal hysterectomy and BSO is appropriate therapy. The uterus and contralateral ovary can be preserved in women with stage IA diploid lesions who wish to preserve fertility. These women should be followed carefully with periodic pelvic examinations and CA125 levels. Generally, the other ovary and uterus are removed at the completion of childbearing. In a recent report by Guthrie and colleagues, the outcome of 656 patients with early-stage epithelial ovarian cancer was studied.[143] No patients who had a properly documented stage I, grade 1 cancer died of their disease; ie, there was a 100% survival in this condition when patients were surgically staged, and thus adjuvant chemotherapy is unnecessary in patients with low-risk low-stage ovarian cancer.

Management of Invasive Early-Stage High-Risk Disease (Stage IA and IB, High-Grade, Stage IC and Stage II) ■ High-risk stage I is defined as stages IA or IB, grade 3, stage IC, or clear cell carcinomas. In patients whose disease is more poorly differentiated or in whom there are malignant cells either in ascitic fluid or peritoneal washings, additional therapy is indicated. Patients with grade 2 and grade 3 tumors, with densely adherent tumors, with large-volume ascites, and/or with positive peritoneal cytology, have a relapse risk of 20% to 45%, and postoperative treatment is warranted. Regrettably, it would appear that thorough staging with negative findings, including random peritoneal biopsies and lymph node sampling, does not eliminate the risk of relapse in patients with these characteristics.[143] Chemotherapy for patients with early-stage high-risk epithelial ovarian cancer can be either single-agent carboplatin or a combination of carboplatin and a taxane.. Melphalan is not recommended due to its leukemogenic properties, its long-term compromise of marrow reserve, and its variable oral absorption, despite its ease of administration.[144] We recommend that four to six cycles of chemotherapy with carboplatin (area under the curve [AUC] 5-6) or a combination of carboplatin and paclitaxel be considered in all given to patients with high-risk low-stage ovarian cancer.

Management of Early-Stage Borderline Tumors ■ The principal treatment for borderline ovarian tumors is the surgical resection of the primary tumor. There is no evidence that either subsequent chemotherapy or radiation therapy improves survival. After performing a frozen section and determining that the histology is borderline, premenopausal patients who desire preservation of ovarian function may be managed with a conservative operation, such as a unilateral salpingooophorectomy.[41] Thus, hormonal function and fertility can be maintained. In patients in whom an ovarian cystectomy has been performed and a borderline tumor is documented in the permanent pathology, no additional surgery is warranted.

There has been considerable controversy regarding the optimum treatment of patients with localized borderline ovarian tumors. This has been due, in part, to lack of unanimity regarding the histopathologic criteria for borderline tumors. For all stages of ovarian cancer, borderline tumors have a more favorable natural history than have invasive tumors.[42] There have been conflicting reports regarding the efficacy and necessity of adjuvant chemotherapy for patients with localized stage I or stage II borderline tumors. In the large GOG trial described above, a total of 51 patients were reclassified as having borderline tumors. In these carefully staged patients, there have been no deaths directly attributable to cancer. While a substantial number of patients did receive adjuvant chemotherapy in these trials, there is no evidence that it was necessary or beneficial. If, after careful histologic review of multiple slides sectioned at 1-cm intervals, no evidence of stromal invasion is found, patients with localized borderline tumors should not routinely receive adjuvant therapy.

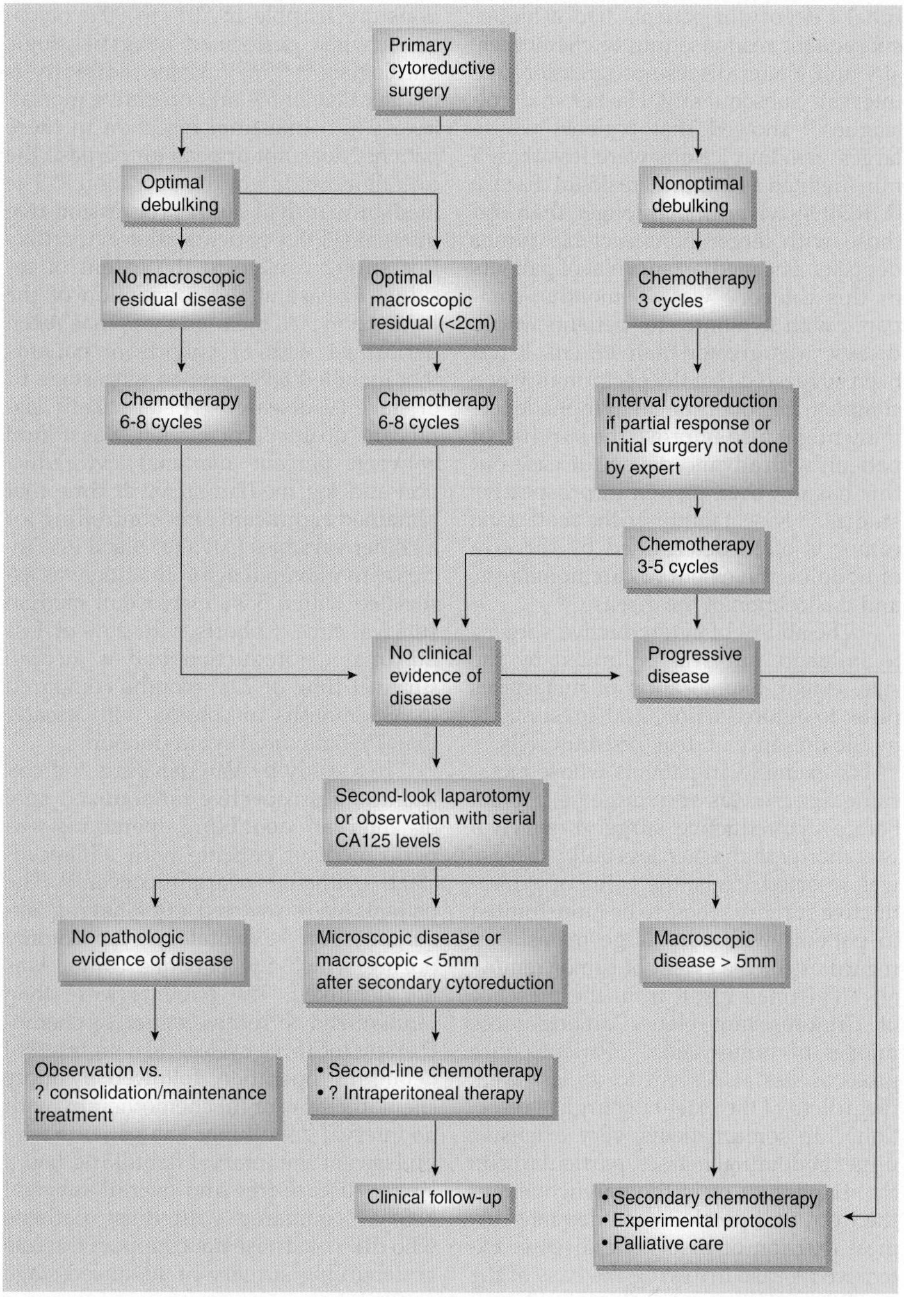

Figure 101-6 Treatment scheme for patients with advanced-stage ovarian cancer. Perform in a research setting where treatment will be based on outcome. *Source*: From Berek JS, Hacker NF. Practical gynecologic oncology, 4th ed. Baltimore, MD: Lippincott Williams & Wilkins; 2005:460.

Treatment of Advanced-Stage Epithelial Ovarian Cancer

A scheme for the management of patients with advanced-stage epithelial ovarian cancer is presented in Figure 101-6. The components of this approach are discussed below.

Cytoreductive Surgery in Ovarian Cancer Patients who have advanced-stage epithelial ovarian cancer documented at initial exploratory laparotomy should undergo cytoreductive surgery to remove as much of the tumor and its metastases as possible in order to facilitate the effectiveness of subsequent therapies.[5-154] The operation usually includes the performance of a total abdominal hysterectomy and BSO, a complete omentectomy, and resection of metastatic lesions on the peritoneal surfaces or from the intestines. In addition, the pelvic tumor may directly involve the rectosigmoid colon, the terminal ileum, and the cecum. In some patients, most or all of their disease is confined to the pelvic viscera and the omentum, so that removal of these organs results in the extirpation of all gross tumor and patients with no macroscopic residual disease, a situation that is associated with a reasonable chance of complete response.

The rationale for cytoreductive surgery relates to the following three general theoretical considerations:

1. potential physiologic benefits from excising the tumor
2. improved tumor perfusion and increased growth fraction, that may increase the likelihood of a response to chemotherapy or radiation therapy
3. enhanced immunologic competence of the patient.[148,151]

The principal goal of cytoreductive surgery is to remove all of the primary cancer and, if possible, its metastases. If resection of all metastases is not feasible, the goal is to reduce the tumor burden by resection of all individual tumors to an optimal status.[68,128,132] The definition of "optimal" was initially proposed by Griffiths, who found that the survival of patients whose metastatic disease was resected to less than 1.5 cm in maximum dimension was significantly longer than the survival of those whose residual lesions were larger than 1.5 cm.[145] The optimal category of patients had a higher subsequent response rate to chemotherapy and longer disease-progression-free interval. Subsequently, Hacker and colleagues[146] showed that patients whose largest residual lesions were less than 5 mm (defined as minimal residual disease [MRD]) survived much longer than did those with larger nonresectable tumor deposits. The median survival of patients in this category was 40 months, compared with 18 months for patients whose disease was greater than 1.5 cm. It has been suggested that the performance of a complete retroperitoneal lymphadenectomy might also improve the survival of patients with advanced-stage disease, but this has not been proven in prospective studies.[149] Resectability of the metastatic tumor is often determined by the size of nodules, the extent of carcinomatosis, and the location of the disease.[155]

The ability of cytoreductive surgery to influence survival is limited by the size, extent, and location of metastases prior to cytoreduction, and presumably by the presence of drug-resistant cells.[152-157] For example, in patients whose metastatic disease was very large (ie, >10 cm before cytoreductive surgery), survival was shorter than when less bulky disease was resected. Thus, the value of cytoreductive surgery seems to be more limited in patients with very large metastases, regardless of the extent of tumor removal.[146] This may result from the presence of drug-resistant clones among large masses of tumor cells.[151] Patients with gross ascites also seem to do less well, regardless of the extent of surgical resection.[154] In some patients, very extensive upper abdominal masses, particularly on the diaphragm or in the parenchyma of the liver, will preclude an adequate surgical excision of metastatic disease. Extensive disease involving the base of the small bowel mesentery, the large bowel mesentery, the lesser omentum, and the porta hepatis, as well as diffuse extraperitoneal metastasis, may prevent the optimal resection of tumor.[153] Thus, the efficacy of cytoreductive surgery is limited. From these and other data, definitions of the patients' status based on the extent of residual disease are presented in Table 101-5.

An analysis of the retrospective data available suggests that these operations are feasible in 70% to 90% of patients when performed by gynecologic oncologists.[146-150,152-157] Major morbidity is in the range of 5% and operative mortality is 1%.[147] Intestinal resection in these patients does not appear to increase the overall morbidity of the operation.[156] The median survival and progression-free interval (PFI)of patients after cytoreductive surgery relate to the extent of residual disease at the completion of the laparotomy. A meta-analysis has been performed with 81 cohorts of patients that included 6885 women with stage III or stage IV disease.[157] A statistically significant positive correlation was found between percent maximal cytoreduction and log median survival time that remained significant after controlling for all other variables ($p < .001$). Each 10% increase in maximal cytoreduction was associated with a 5.5% increase in median survival time. Cohorts with 25% or less maximal cytoreduction had a median survival time of 22.7 months compared to 33.9 months in cohorts with greater than 75% maximal cytoreduction.

In a study by Van der Burg and colleagues, a prospective randomized trial of "interval" debulking operations was performed on patients with advanced-stage epithelial ovarian cancer.[158] The patients were referred after having undergone an exploratory laparotomy during which the patient's tumor was not debulked. The patients were then randomized to receive either (i) chemotherapy for three cycles, then an interval debulking operation, followed by more chemotherapy; or (ii) chemotherapy with no interval debulking. The patients who underwent the interval debulking had a longer disease-free and overall survival (OS) as compared with those patients who did not. These data support the role of debulking surgery in advanced-stage epithelial ovarian cancer and suggest that the sooner the operation can be performed during the course of treatment, the more likely it is that the surgery will improve the survival. In a GOG study of interval cytoreductive surgery, the study design was different because the patients entered on the trial had already undergone a maximal attempt at tumor resection at their initial surgery.[159] The randomized findings showed no difference between the group who had an additional attempt at debulking after three cycles of chemotherapy compared with those who did not (32 months vs 33 months). Therefore, primary cytoreductive should be the standard of care in patients with advanced epithelial ovarian cancer. If the primary operation was not attempted, interval debulking should be performed whenever possible.

Chemotherapy for Advanced-Stage Epithelial Ovarian Cancer ■ Systemic chemotherapy is the standard treatment for metastatic epithelial ovarian cancer.[160-185] Cisplatin was initially used in combination with cyclophosphamide and doxorubicin, but the modest contribution of doxorubicin to the efficacy of the combination prompted simplification of the standard regimen to cyclophosphamide and cisplatin. By the early 1990s a combination of carboplatin and cyclophosphamide was found to be as effective as cisplatin and cyclophosphamide, but substantially less toxic, with less nausea, renal toxicity and neurotoxicity. Paclitaxel was incorporated into combination chemotherapy in the 1990s.[160-164] Over the past decade, a substantial amount of clinical investigation has centered on (i) whether a combination of a platinum compound and a taxane is superior to an optimal dose of a platinum compound alone, (ii) the choice of the optimal platinum compound and taxane, and (iii) the most convenient and effective schedule for taxane administration. Recent studies have focused on the introduction of other compounds into a "triplet" or a "sequential doublet" to eliminate drug-resistant cancer cells.

A variety of regimens containing combinations of cytotoxic drugs have been tested in the treatment of advanced epithelial ovarian cancer. Combination chemotherapy has been shown to be superior to single-agent therapy in most studies in patients with advanced epithelial ovarian cancer.

Platinum Compounds **■** For the past two decades, platinum compounds have been the most active agents against ovarian cancer.[165] In early studies from England, cisplatin was found superior to cyclophosphamide as a single agent. Concurrently, cisplatin was tested in combination with a variety of different drugs. Platinum-containing regimens have proven superior to regimens that lacked platinum compounds.[166] In a meta-analysis performed on 37 randomized studies involving 5667 patients with advanced-stage disease, those patients given cisplatin-containing combination chemotherapy were compared with those treated with regimens that did not include cisplatin.[167,173] Platinum-based chemotherapy was superior to nonplatinum based chemotherapy. A trend favored platinum combinations

Table 101-5 **■ Nomenclature for Patient Status–Residual Ovarian Cancer**

Residual Disease		Status
None	Pathologic	Complete remission
Microscopic disease	Only	Microscopic
Macroscopic disease	<5 mm	Minimal residual
Macroscopic disease	<1-2 cm	Optimal residual
Macroscopic residual disease	>1-2 cm	Suboptimal
Macroscopic disease	>2-3 cm	Bulky residual

Nomenclature for status of patient based on the extent of residual ovarian cancer prior to treatment.

over single-agent platinum. In studies of cisplatin-containing regimens, several trials have compared cyclophosphamide and cisplatin (CP) with cisplatin, doxorubicin, and cyclophosphamide (PAC).[168-172] No study showed a significant difference in survival between treatment arms. The GOG's randomized prospective comparison of equitoxic doses of PAC vs PC showed no benefit to the inclusion of doxorubicin in the combination.[168] While a meta-analysis of the combined data from these four trials showed a 7% survival advantage at 6 years for those patients treated with the doxorubicin-containing regimen, the survival curves converge at 8 years. Consequently, in recent years doxorubicin has not been incorporated in regimens for epithelial ovarian cancer in the United States. It is, however, possible that a small subset of ovarian cancer patients benefit substantially from treatment with anthracyclines. In the future, new technologies may permit the identification of those patients and permit individualization of their treatment.

In the 1980s, the second-generation platinum analogue carboplatin became available, exhibiting greater myelotoxicity, but substantially less nephrotoxicity, ototoxicity, peripheral neurotoxicity, and emetogenic potential than did cisplatin. Initial studies showed that carboplatin and cisplatin had approximately a 4:1 ratio of potency. Thus a standard single-agent dose of about 400 mg/m^2 has been used in most phase 2 trials. The dose is best calculated by using the probable AUC based on the glomerular filtration rate (GFR) according to the Calvert formula.[179] When used as a single agent, a target AUC of 5 to 7 is appropriate for previously untreated patients with ovarian cancer. When used in combination with other myelotoxic drugs, AUCs of 5 to 6 have been used more frequently.

Meta-analyses have suggested that cisplatin and carboplatin are equally effective against epithelial ovarian cancer.[180] Direct comparison of cisplatin and cyclophosphamide to carboplatin and cyclophosphamide demonstrated comparable response rates and survival, but significantly less toxicity for the carboplatin containing regimen.[174,175]

Paclitaxel ■ Paclitaxel was shown to be a very active agent against ovarian cancer.[160-164] The overall response rates for paclitaxel in phase 2 trials was 36% in previously treated patients, which is a higher rate than was seen for cisplatin when it was first tested.[160]

Three large concurrently controlled randomized trials in previously untreated patients with ovarian cancer have compared paclitaxel and a platinum compound to different platinum-containing regimens that did not contain paclitaxel[162,163,176] The GOG randomized 410 women with suboptimally cytoreduced stage III-IV ovarian cancer to six cycles of chemotherapy with a combination of cisplatin (75 mg/m^2) and paclitaxel (135 mg/m^2 over 24 h) or with cisplatin (75 mg/m^2) and cyclophosphamide (750 mg/m^2) (GOG-111).[162] Patients who received the paclitaxel combination had a superior overall response rate (73% vs 60%), clinical complete response rate (51% vs 31%), prolongation of disease-free survival (18 months vs 14 months), and prolongation of overall survival (36 months vs 24 months).

The superiority of paclitaxel-cisplatin was confirmed in a trial (OV-10) conducted jointly by the European Organization for the Research and Treatment of Cancer (EORTC), the Nordic Ovarian Cancer Study Group (NOCOVA), and the National Cancer Institute of Canada (NCIC) in which 680 women with both optimal and suboptimal disease in stages IIB-IV were treated.[163] Patients were randomized to six cycles of cisplatin (75 mg/m^2) and cyclophosphamide (750 mg/m^2) or to six cycles of cisplatin (75 mg/m^2) with a slightly higher dose of paclitaxel (175 mg/m^2) over a shorter interval (3 h) than in GOG-111. In this study, the paclitaxel-containing arm produced a significant improvement in median PFI (15.5 months vs 11.5 months) and overall median overall survival (35.6 months vs 25.8 months) that extended to both optimal and suboptimal groups. Greater neurotoxicity was observed with the combination of paclitaxel and cisplatin when the paclitaxel was infused over 3 h in OV-10 compared to infusion over 24 h in GOG-111.

A third study, the International Collaborative Ovarian Neoplasm-3 (ICON-3), was conducted as 4 parallel trials across 130 centers in eight countries in Europe to compare carboplatin (AUC 5) and paclitaxel (175 mg/m^2 over 3 h) to regimens that did not contain paclitaxel.[176] Prior to randomization, each patient and physician could choose a control arm that included either carboplatin (AUC 5) alone or a combination of cisplatin (50 mg/m^2), doxorubicin (50 mg/m^2) and cyclophosphamide (500 mg/m^2). Of the women on the control arm, 69% received carboplatin. Dose escalation was permitted and occurred in approximately half of patients. Overall, 2074 women participated with ovarian cancer of all stages, including 20% of women with stage I-II disease. A central review of pathology, surgical staging, cytoreduction, or protocol adherence was not performed. No significant difference was found in overall median survival between the paclitaxel-carboplatin group (36.1 months) and the control group (35.4 months). In comparing the three trials, the outcome was no worse in the paclitaxel-carboplatin arm of ICON-3 than in the paclitaxel-cisplatin arms of GOG-111 and OV-10, but the control group in ICON-3 enjoyed a better outcome. The better survival of controls in ICON-3 might relate to the fraction of early-stage patients or possibly to the optimization of carboplatin dosage permitted by dose escalation.[181] A trend ($p = .22$) was noted toward a benefit of paclitaxel-carboplatin in patients who had > 2 cm residual disease, patients comparable to those entered in GOG-111.

The GOG had undertaken a comparison of sequential and simultaneous paclitaxel-cisplatin (GOG-132).[177] A three-arm comparison of equitoxic doses of paclitaxel (200 mg/m^2 over 24 h) vs cisplatin (100 mg/m^2) vs a combination of paclitaxel (135 mg/m^2 over 24 h) and cisplatin (75 mg/m^2) was carried out in 648 suboptimal stage III and IV patients. Crossover was permitted and the three groups exhibited similar median overall survival of 26 to 30 months. The simultaneous regimen was better tolerated than the sequential use of agents at these optimized doses. The overall response rate to cisplatin alone or to the paclitaxel-cisplatin combination was 67%, whereas the response to paclitaxel alone was 42% ($p < .001$). This observation suggests that more than half of patients who are treated arbitrarily with the combination of paclitaxel and a platinum derivative may not benefit from the taxane. To date, laboratory studies do not support any super-additive interaction of platinum compounds and taxanes, arguing against synergy in the clinic. In the future, using molecular markers it may be possible to identify those patients who would respond or not respond to paclitaxel, providing another opportunity to individualize therapy. Some data suggest that *BRCA* related ovarian cancers as well as cancers that have down regulation of *BRCA* function through hypermethylation of the BRCA promoter may be more sensitive to treatment with platinum. In vitro data document that *BRCA* is a DNA damage response gene and appears to play a role in the regulation of mitosis and is involved in modulating response to spindle poisons such as taxanes, but the relevance of BRCA status to choice of chemotherapy is not yet clear.[182,183]

Two randomized, prospective clinical studies have compared the combination of paclitaxel and carboplatin to that of paclitaxel and cisplatin.[161,162,174-175] In both studies, response rates and duration of survival are similar, but the carboplatin containing regimens have more acceptable toxicity. In the first trial conducted by the GOG (GOG-158), patients were randomized to carboplatin (AUC 7.5) and paclitaxel (175 mg/m^2) over 3 h vs the previous standard of cisplatin (75 mg/m^2) and paclitaxel (135 mg/m^2

over 24 h). PFS of the carboplatin containing arm was 22 months vs 21.7 months for the control arm.[161,174] The GI and neurotoxicity of the carboplatin arm were appreciably lower than that of the cisplatin arm. In addition, paclitaxel administration over 3 h is substantially more convenient than administration over 24 h. A similar result was obtained in a large randomized trial in Germany, in which carboplatin (AUC 6) and paclitaxel (185 mg/m^2 over 3 h) were compared to paclitaxel (135 mg/m^2 over 24 h) and cisplatin (75 mg/m^2).[162,175] Thus, the best established regimen in patients with advanced-stage disease is a combination of carboplatin and paclitaxel over 3 h.

Docetaxel ■ Docetaxel is a semisynthetic second-generation taxane with properties that differ from paclitaxel. Docetaxel is a more potent promoter of microtubule assembly and stabilization than paclitaxel.[184] Docetaxel is taken up, bound, and retained more effectively by cancer cells than paclitaxel. Docetaxel has produced a 23% to 28% overall response rate in platinum-resistant ovarian cancer, and a combination of docetaxel and cisplatin or carboplatin has achieved a 66% to 81% overall response rate in phase 2 trials.[184] A combination of docetaxel (75 mg/m^2 over 1 h) and carboplatin (AUC 5) has been compared to paclitaxel (175 mg/m^2) and carboplatin (AUC 5) in the SCOTROC trial.[185] Similar efficacy was observed, but docetaxel/carboplatin was associated with significantly less neurotoxicity. Consequently, a combination of carboplatin and docetaxel should be considered for treatment of ovarian cancer in patients with significant neuropathy.

Other Doublets and Triplets ■ Use of platinum compounds and taxanes has improved median and OS, but the outcome in patients with advanced ovarian cancer is still disappointing. Drug resistance ultimately develops in the majority. A number of drugs have exhibited activity against recurrent disease including liposomal doxorubicin, gemcitabine, topotecan, navelbine, and etoposide. The GOG has conducted a series of phase 1 pilot studies in previously untreated patients to define combinations that are suitable for a group wide phase 3 trial. A five-arm study has now been initiated, administering eight cycles of chemotherapy to women with newly diagnosed stage III/IV ovarian cancer has recently been carried out. GOG-182 compared the standard combination of *carboplatin* and *paclitaxel* with in combination with *gemcitabine, topotecan,* or *liposomal doxorubicin* in sequential doublets or triplets.[186] This was the largest randomized trial ever carried out in women with advanced ovarian cancer and recruited over 4000 patients. The results have been presented and there was no apparent difference between any of the arms in terms of PFS or median survival, but there were differences in the side effects experienced in the different arms. The conclusion was that carboplatin and paclitaxel remain the standard of care.

Dose-Intensification With Intravenous Chemotherapy ■ Higher or more frequent doses of chemotherapy might be more effective than standard dosing, if tolerated. The issue of dose-intensification of cisplatin was examined in a prospective trial conducted by the GOG. In this study, 243 patients with suboptimal ovarian cancer were randomized to receive either 50 mg/m^2 or 100 mg/m^2 cisplatin plus 500 mg/m^2 cyclophosphamide.[177] There was no difference in response rates in those patients with measurable disease and the overall survival was identical. As one might anticipate, there was greater toxicity associated with the high-dose regimen. A group in Scotland performed a similar study and found that patients who received 100 mg/m^2 cisplatin plus 750 mg/m^2 cyclophosphamide had a significantly longer median survival compared with those who received 50 mg/m^2 cisplatin plus the same dose of cyclophosphamide. The overall median survival time was 114 weeks in the high-dose group and 69 weeks in the low-dose group (p = .0008), but this difference disappeared with longer follow-up.[178] Thus, doubling the dose of cisplatin does not improve long-term survival. Dose escalation of paclitaxel and carboplatin require G-CSF because of their combined myelosuppressive effects, but there is no evidence to support more intensive administration of either agent.[174,178]

Intraperitoneal Chemotherapy ■ As ovarian cancer spreads over the surface of the peritoneum and often recurs at this site; investigators have evaluated intraperitoneal (IP) administration of chemotherapy that can achieve high local concentrations of drug. A randomized, prospective trial performed by the Southwest Oncology Group (SWOG) and the GOG compared IP cisplatin (100 mg/m^2) to intravenous (IV) cisplatin (100 mg/m^2), each given with II cyclophosphamide (600 mg/m^2), in patients with disease less than 2 cm in diameter.[187] The IP cisplatin arm had a significantly longer overall median survival than the intravenous arm, 49 months vs 41 months (p = .03). In the patients with the least residual disease (< 0.5 cm maximum residual), however, there was not a statistically significant difference in median survival between the two treatments, 51 months vs 46 months (p = .08).

Results of this randomized trial became available as paclitaxel was being incorporated into clinical practice. In a follow-up trial conducted by the GOG, a standard regimen of IV cisplatin (75 mg/m^2) and IV paclitaxel (135 mg/m^2 over 24 h) was compared to a dose-intense regimen that was initiated by giving moderately high-dose carboplatin (AUC = 9) for two induction cycles followed by IP cisplatin 100 mg/m^2 and IV paclitaxel (135 mg/m^2 over 24 h).[188] The dose-intense arm produced slightly better progression-free median survival (27.6 months vs 22.5 months, p = .02), but there was not a statistically significant difference in overall survival (52.9 months vs 47.6 months, p = .056).

A randomized prospective GOG study[189] compared IP *cisplatin* and *paclitaxel* with IV *cisplatin* and *paclitaxel*[190] and was reported in late 2006. Four hundred and twenty nine patients were randomly assigned and 415 were eligible. The median PFS was 23.8 months in the IP arm vs 18.3 months in the IV arm (p = .05). The median overall survival was 65.6 months in the IP group and 49.7 months in the IV group (p = .03) —90% of patients in the IV arm received the six planned cycles of therapy whereas only 42% of patients received the assigned six cycles of IP therapy with the remainder switching to IV therapy. The reasons for discontinuing were primarily for catheter related problems but there were also significantly more side effects in the IP group with more patients experiencing severe fatigue, abdominal pain, hematological toxicity, nausea and vomiting as well as metabolic and neurotoxicity. It is likely with more training and appropriate dose modifications and better antiemetics that the toxicity can be reduced. The results of this study together with the previous studies led to a NCI Clinical Announcement recommending that women with optimally cytoreduced stage 3 ovarian cancer be considered for IP chemotherapy.

There has been a *Cochrane Review* as well as a separate meta-analysis that concluded that IP chemotherapy was associated with better outcomes than IV chemotherapy.[191,192] The meta-analysis included six randomized trials with a total of 1716 ovarian cancer patients. The pooled HR for PFS of IP cisplatin as compared to IV treatment regimens was 0.792 (95% CI = 0.688-0.912, p= 0.001), and the pooled HR for OS was 0.799 (95% CI: 0.702-0.910, p = 0.0007). The authors conclude that these findings strongly support the incorporation of an IP cisplatin regimen to improve survival in the frontline treatment of stage III, optimally debulked ovarian cancer.[191] Similar conclusions were reached in the *Cochrane Review.* The reviewers concluded that their analysis establishes the benefit of IP chemotherapy and that it is associated with an increased overall survival and PFS in patients with optimally debulked stage III advanced ovarian cancer. However, they also commented on the potential for catheter related complications and increased toxicity with IP therapy and concluded that the optimal dose, timing and mechanism of administration should be addressed in the next phase of clinical trials.[192] The role of IP chemotherapy however is still contentious with some arguing that the trials to date were not pure tests of IP therapy and were flawed and in addition they have raised concerns about the technical difficulties as well as increased toxicity of IP therapy.[193] Although decisions regarding primary therapy must be individualized, IP therapy should be seriously considered for all optimally cytoreduced patients with ovarian cancer, given the difference in overall survival.

Neoadjuvant Chemotherapy ■ Some authors have suggested that, for patients with suboptimal stage III and stage IV disease, chemotherapy may be given in lieu of cytoreductive surgery. A series performed at Yale by Schwartz and colleagues suggested that the survival of patients treated with "neoadjuvant" or cytoreductive chemotherapy was comparable to those patients historically treated with cytoreductive surgery followed by conventional chemotherapy in the same institution.[194] As other authors have shown a benefit to debulking patients prior to chemotherapy, the issue would need to be resolved by a prospective clinical trial. However, two or three cycles of chemotherapy prior to cytoreductive surgery may be helpful in patients with massive ascites or large pleural effusions. Chemotherapy may eliminate the effusions, improve the patient's performance status, and decrease postoperative morbidity, particularly within the chest. Bristow et al. recently reported the results of a systemic overview of neoadjuvant chemotherapy and concluded that neoadjuvant chemotherapy represents a viable alternative management strategy for the limited number of patients felt to be optimally unresectable by an experienced ovarian cancer surgical team; however, currently available data suggest that the survival outcome achievable with initial chemotherapy is inferior to successful up-front cytoreductive surgery. The EORTC have recently completed a large randomized trial of surgery followed by six cycles of carboplatin and paclitaxel vs three cycles of chemotherapy followed by surgical debulking and a further three cycles of chemotherapy and this will help address the value, if any, of neoadjuvant chemotherapy.

Radiotherapy in Advanced Invasive Disease ■ In the past decade, several studies have refined our knowledge of the possible benefits of radiation therapy in ovarian cancer. In particular, subgroups of patients have been identified who are most likely to have a curative benefit when radiation therapy is used as the sole postoperative treatment. In addition, the technical aspects of whole abdominal radiation (WAR) have been worked out, permitting therapy to be delivered with acceptable late toxicity (Table 101-6).[195] Despite this knowledge, WAR is not used widely. The results of these studies are concordant in showing long-term failure-free survivors determined both by the stage at presentation and by the volume of residual disease, as expressed by the largest diameter of the largest remaining lesion. Most of the long-term survivors had stage II disease, in which the postoperative tumor residuum was confined to the pelvis and was encompassed in the boost volume, where radiation doses are significantly higher than can be delivered to the upper abdomen. Although there is evidence that whole abdominal irradiation is therapeutic for patients with small-volume residual ovarian cancer, questions have been raised about the interpretation of these results in the context of more modern surgical techniques and more effective chemotherapy.

Table 101-6 ■ **Whole Abdominal Radiation in Patients With Residual Disease**

Study End Point (Ref. No.)	Volume of Residual Disease Prior to Radiation	
	<2 cm (%)	>2 cm (%)
Percent 10-year RFR[170]	38	6
Percent 15-year FFR[171]	50	14
Percent 10-year RFS[172]	62	0
Percent 10-year survival[173]	42	10
Surviving fraction at 6 years[174]	41	—
Percent 9-yr RFR[175]	62	8

Abbreviations: FFR, failure-free rate; RFR, relapse-free rate; RFS, relapse-free survival.

Chemotherapy and Molecular Targeted Therapies ■ Inhibition of angiogenesis with drugs such as bevacizumab has demonstrated activity and benefit in women with recurrent ovarian cancer and in view of this there are two large randomized trials investigating the impact of the addition of bevacizumab to standard carboplatin and paclitaxel in patients with advanced ovarian cancer. There is evidence in other tumor types such as breast cancer, colon cancer, and lung cancer that the addition of bevacizumab to chemotherapy increases response rates and PFS and also survival in some studies.[196-198] GOG-218 is a phase 3, 3-arm randomized double blind placebo-controlled trial. Patients in arm 1 will receive six cycles of carboplatin and paclitaxel and placebo starting with the second cycle and continuing for 10 additional cycles after the completion of chemotherapy. Patients in arm 2 will receive six cycles of chemotherapy with bevacizumab starting with cycle 2 and administered with chemotherapy followed by 10 cycles of placebo and in arm 3 patients will receive bevacizumab to start with cycle 2 of chemotherapy and will then receive 10 additional cycles after the completion of chemotherapy. This study is designed to investigate the benefit of bevacizumab in combination with chemotherapy as well as a maintenance. The bevacizumab is administered at a does of 15 mg/kg and starts with the second cycle of chemotherapy to decrease the risk of GI perforation which has been a rare complication of this agent in the setting of its use in colorectal cancer. The ICON 7 study is similar but is a 2 arm study of carboplatin and paclitaxel plus or minus bevacizumab 7.5 mg/kg administered every 3 weeks with chemotherapy and then as maintenance therapy. These studies have opened in the last 6 months and it will be a few years before the results are available.

Management of Advanced Invasive Ovarian Cancer

At present, the treatment of choice for patients with advanced invasive epithelial ovarian cancer is cytoreductive surgery followed by six to eight cycles of chemotherapy with a combination of carboplatin (AUC 5-6) and paclitaxel (175 mg/m^2 over 3 h) every 3 weeks (Table 101-7). Paclitaxel is administered before the carboplatin. In patients at risk for severe neuropathy,

Table 101-7 ■ **Combination Chemotherapy for Advanced Epithelial Ovarian Cancer: Recommended Regimens**

Drugs	Dose	Administration (Hours)	Interval	No. of Treatments
Paclitaxel	175 mg/m^2	3	Every 3 weeks	6–8 cycles
Carboplatin	AUC = 5–6			
Docetaxel	75 mg/m^2	1	Every 3 weeks	6–8 cycles
Carboplatin	AUC = 5			

Drugs that can be substituted for Taxol, if hypersensitivity to that drug occurs. Standard regimens are given. *Abbreviation*: AUC, "area under the curve" dose by Calvert formula.

for example, diabetics, a combination of docetaxel (75 mg/m^2) and carboplatin (AUC 5) provides an alternative that is less neurotoxic. As data confirming the SCOTROC trial are obtained, the latter regimen may become a standard option for all patients. In women who cannot tolerate the toxicity of taxanes, carboplatin alone (AUC 6-7) can be given. For the rare patient who cannot tolerate IV chemotherapy, an oral alkylating agent can be used for palliation. For patients who have had complete cytoreduction, IP chemotherapy should be seriously considered.

Management of Advanced Borderline Tumors

The effectiveness of chemotherapy in patients with advanced-stage borderline tumors has not been established. The GOG is evaluating the use of chemotherapy in patients with advanced-stage borderline tumors who have recurrent disease after initial surgery. Until the results of this trial are known, the current approach to treatment is primarily surgical. Patients should undergo cytoreductive surgery and observation. Borderline tumors, even in advanced stage, have a favorable prognosis. The first symptomatic recurrence may be several years after diagnosis. In contrast to the 20% to 25% survival rates for advanced epithelial invasive carcinoma of the ovary, the survival rate for patients with stage III borderline tumors is over 60%.[41,42] Consequently, secondary cytoreductive surgery frequently will lead to another prolonged interval of symptom free survival. Chemotherapy can be administered to the patients in whom cytoreductive surgery is no longer feasible, although its efficacy is uncertain.

Assessment of Response in Patients Who Are Clinically Free of Disease

Many patients who have undergone optimal cytoreductive surgery and subsequent therapy for epithelial ovarian cancer will have no evidence of disease at the completion of treatment. Tumor markers and radiologic assessments have proven to be too insensitive to exclude accurately the presence of subclinical disease.[199-201] A technique used to evaluate residual disease has been the second-look operation.[202,203]

A second-look operation is one performed on a patient who has no clinical evidence of disease after a prescribed course of chemotherapy, in order to determine the response to therapy. Most often, patients have undergone a formal reassessment laparotomy. The laparoscope also has been used in some of these cases but there is a 35% false-negative rate if laparoscopy is used as a second-look procedure.[202]

If a second-look operation is performed, the proper surgery should be carried out to maximize the likelihood of detecting any microscopic residual disease. The technique of the second-look laparotomy is essentially identical to that of the staging laparotomy.[41] The ability to obtain a complete remission with a platinum-based therapy is dependent on the extent of residual disease at the time chemotherapy is initiated. Clinical trials have uniformly demonstrated that patients who have bulky disease (any tumor nodule greater than 2 to 3 cm in diameter) have less than a 10% likelihood of achieving a complete remission with induction chemotherapy with a platinum-based regimen. In contrast, patients who have small-volume disease after the initial laparotomy have a three to four times higher likelihood of achieving a complete remission.[204] There is no evidence that prolonging the number of cycles of induction chemotherapy will increase the complete remission rate.

The levels of CA125 have been correlated with the findings at second-look surgery. Positive levels are useful in predicting the presence of disease, but negative titers are an insensitive marker for the absence of disease. In studies performed to date, the predictive value of a positive test has been 96%, ie, if the level of CA125 is > 35 U/mL, disease is almost always detectable in patients at the second-look.[200] In one such prospective analysis, the predictive value of a negative test was only 56%, ie, if the level was less than 35 U/mL, disease was present in 44% of the patients at the time of the second-look.[200] Therefore, the CA125 is not sensitive enough to exclude subclinical disease in many patients. Serum CA125 levels can be used to follow those patients during chemotherapy whose level was positive at the initiation of therapy.[201] Changes in CA125 level (ie, falling, rising, or plateauing) generally correlates with response. Those patients with persistently elevated levels of CA125 after 3 months of treatment most likely have resistant tumors. Persistently elevated or rising titers on treatment usually indicate treatment failure and suggest that continuation of the current regimen is unlikely to be of value.

Because second-look laparotomies have not been shown to influence patient survival, they should be done only in a research setting, as second-line or salvage therapies in patients with persistent cancer have not yet demonstrated a clear improvement in the overall survival.[41] The findings at a second-look procedure do, however, correlate with subsequent outcome and survival. Patients who have no histologic evidence of disease have a significantly longer survival compared with those who have microscopic or macroscopic disease documented at laparotomy.[180] About 50% to 70% of patients with negative second-look examinations remain free of disease at 5 years, whereas the median survival of patients with any disease (microscopic and macroscopic) is 12 to 18 months. The extent of residual disease documented at the second-look procedure also correlates with patient survival.[41] Patients with microscopic disease only have a 5-year survival of 40% to 50% (median of more than 36 months), compared with 12 months for patients with any evidence of macroscopic disease. Clearly, it is not possible to sample every potential site of disease. In addition, disease can become clinically apparent at sites that are impossible to examine, such as the liver parenchyma. The majority of recurrences after a negative second-look procedure are in patients with poorly differentiated cancers.

Consolidation Chemotherapy and Immunotherapy

The optimal management of patients who do achieve a clinical complete remission after induction chemotherapy remains to be determined. Even patients who achieve a surgically confirmed complete remission have a 30% to 50% recurrence rate.[41,203] Some investigators have suggested that second-look laparotomy should be performed to identify patients who may be candidates for IP therapy.[204] There is, however, currently no evidence that the routine sequential administration of IP chemotherapy after IV induction chemotherapy leads to a prolongation of survival.

Clinical trials are in progress to determine whether consolidation therapies are of benefit in patients who achieve a surgically confirmed clinical complete remission. A study conducted by the GOG and SWOG compared 3 and 12 monthly cycles of "consolidation" chemotherapy with paclitaxel (135-175 mg/m^2 IV over 3 h) for patients who had achieved a clinical remission following primary paclitaxel and carboplatin chemotherapy.[205] PFI was 21 months and 28 months in the 3-cycle and 12-cycle paclitaxel arms (p = .035) respectively. Consequently, 9 months of further chemotherapy provided an additional 7 months of PFS. To date, there is no difference in OS between the two arms. Two placebo-controlled randomized trials have been performed in Europe using consolidation with four cycles topotecan given to patients in clinical remission following chemotherapy with carboplatin and paclitaxel, and in both trials there was no improvement in survival compared with placebo.[206,207]

A number of experimental regimens are being tested including IP chemotherapy, high-dose IV chemotherapy with stem cell support, and immunotherapy with interferon (IFN). A randomized trial of IP administration of 90Y-labeled anti-MUC1 antibody showed no survival advantage.[208] The therapeutic potential of an anti-idiotypic response to an anti-CA125 antibody was discovered in a retrospective analysis of a diagnostic study with MAb-B43.13, where a large group of patients who had been imaged enjoyed unexpectedly long survival. Vaccine trials are ongoing with OvaRex, in an attempt to utilize anti-idiotypic immunity against antibodies reactive with CA125. A randomized placebo-controlled trial of OvaRex was performed in patients who were in clinical remission after platinum and paclitaxel chemotherapy was performed.[209] While there was no difference in survival in the overall group, the subset of optimal chemosensitive patients had a median relapse-free survival of 24 months compared with 10.5 months for those receiving a placebo (p = .06). Based on these results, a large phase 3, placebo-controlled trial was conducted in the optimal patients only, and there was no difference in time to relapse in the group given the OvaRex vss placebo.

Outside of a clinical research setting, a standard approach is to follow patients carefully after the achievement of a clinical complete remission until recurrence.

Consolidation or Salvage Radiotherapy ■ Salvage radiotherapy is inappropriate for most patients with any macroscopic disease after chemotherapy.[210-214] When consolidative radiotherapy has been used, there does not appear to be any curative benefit.

Follow-up Examinations ■ The optimal frequency of follow-up examinations is unknown, but in those patients who have completed chemotherapy and who are in clinical remission it is reasonable to perform a pelvic examination and to obtain a CA125 every 3 months for 1 to 2 years. An elevated CA125 (> 35 U/mL) can provide lead time of approximately 3 to 6 months before there are clinical signs or symptoms of recurrence in detecting recurrent disease. The Gynecologic Cancer Inter Group (GCIG) have developed a standard definition for CA125 progression which is now widely used in clinical trials. Patients with elevated CA125 pretreatment and normalization of CA125 must show evidence of CA125 greater than or equal to 2x the upper normal limit on two occasions at least 1 week apart or patients with elevated CA125 pretreatment, which never normalizes must show evidence of CA125 greater than or equal to 2x the nadir value on two occasions at least 1 week apart.[215]

A rising CA125 may prompt the performance of a CT scan. The role of positron emission tomography (PET) scanning in this setting has not been defined. A recent review conclude that PET has a sensitivity of 90% and a specificity of 85% approximately for the detection of recurrent ovarian cancer, and that it appears to be particularly useful for the diagnosis of recurrence when CA125 levels are rising and conventional imaging is inconclusive or negative although the value of this is debatable. Combined 18fluorodeoxyglucose (FDG)-PET/ CT devices, which perform contemporaneous acquisition of both 18FDG-PET and CT images and may be more valuable to detect recurrent ovarian cancer and this technique may be useful for the selection of patients with late recurrent disease who may benefit from secondary cytoreductive surgery.[216] A rising CA125 level in the absence of changes on physical examination or CT scan in a patient in initial remission poses a dilemma. At present, additional cytotoxic therapy is not recommended based on a rising CA125 alone in the absence of clinical symptoms or radiologic evidence of recurrence. Treatment with tamoxifen has sometimes been given and although stabilization or a fall in CA125 may be observed in approximately 20% of patients, the value of this intervention is uncertain. The GOG has compared tamoxifen to thalidomide in patients with a rising CA125 without other evidence of disease recurrence. Similar efficacy was observed, although tamoxifen was less toxic. There are also trials using a rising CA125 to evaluate a paradigm to evaluate the activity of novel cytostatic targeted drugs. As more effective salvage therapy becomes available, serum markers such as CA125 may have greater utility. In patients whose disease was never found to be metastatic to the chest or who never had a pleural effusion, chest radiograph surveillance is not mandatory. In the absence of a rising CA125, follow-up CT or MRI scans should be used with discretion during the first 3 years after chemotherapy.[41]

Intravenous Second-Line Therapy in Patients With Recurrent or Persistent Advanced Epithelial Ovarian Cancer ■ The majority of women who relapse will be offered further chemotherapy with the likelihood of benefit related in part to the initial response and the duration of response. The goals of treatment include improving control of disease related symptoms, maintaining or improving quality of life, delaying time to progression, and possibly prolonging survival, particularly in women with platinum-sensitive recurrences. Many active chemotherapy agents (platinum, paclitaxel, topotecan, liposomal doxorubicin, docetaxel, gemcitabine, and etoposide) as well as targeted agents(bevacizumab) are available and the choice of treatment is based on many factors including likelihood of benefit, potential toxicity and patient convenience.[217,218] Women who relapse greater than 6 months after primary chemotherapy are classified as "platinum-sensitive" and usually receive further platinum-based chemotherapy with response rates ranging from 27% to 65% and a median survival of 12-24 months.[219,220] Patients who relapse within 6 months of completing first-line chemotherapy are classified as "platinum-resistant" and have a median survival of 6 to 9 months and a 10% to 30% likelihood of responding to chemotherapy. Patients who progress while on treatment are classified as having "platinum-refractory" disease. Objective response rates to chemotherapy in patients with platinum-refractory ovarian cancer are low and are less than 20%.[217]

Platinum-Sensitive Disease ■ Second-line therapies are usually selected according to whether the patients responded to their initial platinum-based chemotherapy and how long the treatment-free interval has been. Although the concept of platinum sensitivity and resistance has been variously defined, platinum sensitivity is generally accepted to be a PFI of > 6 months following primary therapy. In patients who achieve a complete remission on a platinum-based induction regimen and have a disease-free interval of greater than 6 months, second-line treatment with a platinum compound has approximately a 30% response rate.[219-221] The likelihood of response to a platinum-based regimen is greater as the treatment-free interval increases beyond 6 months.[219-221] Patients can be retreated with either cisplatin or carboplatin. Because of its more favorable toxicity profile, carboplatin is the drug of choice for patients who relapse after responding to a platinum-based induction regimen. In contrast, if patients do not achieve a remission on a platinum-based regimen or have a very short response duration, retreatment with a platinum-based regimen is unlikely to be beneficial, and such patients should be encouraged to enter experimental clinical trials.[222]

Platinum plus paclitaxel may be better for second-line therapy than platinum alone. A combination of platinum plus paclitaxel has been compared to single-agent platinum in two multinational randomized phase 3 trials[223] and a randomized phase 2 study.[224] In a report of the ICON4 and the AGO-OVAR-2.2 trials,[223] 802 women with platinum-sensitive ovarian cancer who relapsed after being treatment-free for at least 6 to 12 months were randomized to platinum-based chemotherapy. Two heterogeneous treatment groups were compared: (i) single-agent cisplatin or carboplatin or cisplatin plus cyclophosphamide and/or doxorubicin without paclitaxel; and (ii) a combination of paclitaxel and platinum-based chemotherapy with carboplatin or cisplatin. Combining the trials for analysis, there was a significant survival advantage for the paclitaxel-containing therapy (HR = 0.82) with a median follow up of 42 months. The absolute 2-year survival advantage was 7% (57% vs 50%), and there was a 5-month improvement in median survival (29 months vs 24 months). PFS was better with the paclitaxel regimen (HR = 0.76); there was a 10% difference in 1-year PFS (50% vs 40%) and a 3-month prolongation in median PFS (13 months vs 10 months). The toxicities were comparable, except there was a significantly higher incidence of neurologic toxicity and alopecia in the paclitaxel group, whereas myelosuppression was significantly greater with the non-paclitaxel-containing regimens. In both trials, a significant fraction of the patients had, however, not received paclitaxel as part of their initial chemotherapeutic regimen. Consequently, there is still debate regarding whether retreatment with a combination of paclitaxel plus carboplatin is superior to using these agents sequentially in patients who have had both agents during primary therapy. Many investigators do recommend that combination chemotherapy be used as part of reinduction for patients who have a disease-free interval that extends beyond 12-18 months.[225]

Recently two randomized trials have compared carboplatin alone to carboplatin and gemcitabine or liposomal doxorubicin. There was a higher response rate with the combination therapy and a longer PFS, but the studies were not powered to look at overall survival. In the GCIG study comparing carboplatin and gemcitabine with carboplatin alone, the response rate was 47.2% for the combination and 30.9% for carboplatin with the PFS being 8.6 months and 5.8 months respectively.[224] A SWOG study of carboplatin versus carboplatin and liposomal doxorubicin was closed early with only 61 patients accrued, but the response rate was 67% for the combination and 32% for carboplatin; the PFS was 12 months versus 8 months and intriguingly the OS was 26 months compared to 18 months(p = 0.02).[226] A phase 2 study from France confirmed the high response rate of 67% with carboplatin and liposomal doxorubicin in patients with platinum-sensitive recurrent ovarian cancer and a large GCIG study (CALYPSO) comparing carboplatin and liposomal doxorubicin with carboplatin and paclitaxel has recently completed recruitment and the results are expected in the next 18 months.[227]

Platinum-Resistant and Refractory Disease ■ The management of ovarian cancers that are platinum-resistant ie, progressing within 6 months of completion of chemotherapy or platinum refractory, ie, progress while on treatment is difficult and "non-cross-resistant agents" are usually selected, but there does not appear to be one best treatment. There are a variety of active drugs that are frequently prescribed including paclitaxel, docetaxel, topotecan, liposomal doxorubicin, gemcitabine, oral etoposide, vinorelbine, and bevacizumab.[226-231,235,236-244] All of these second-line agents have a comparable degree of activity with partial response rates of approximately 20%. Older agents such as tamoxifen, ifosfamide and hexamethylmelamine may be somewhat less active. Single-agent therapy is typically used sequentially, because combination regimens are associated with more toxicity without any apparent additional benefit. High response rates of 48% to 64% have, however, been reported with dose-dense combinations of weekly carboplatin (AUC = 4) and paclitaxel (90 mg/m^2).[228,229] Similarly, a combination of cisplatin and gemcitabine produce response rates of 38% and 70% with responses that have been maintained for 3-5 months.[230,235]

Few formal comparisons have been performed among these drugs. Pegylated liposomal doxorubicin has been compared to topotecan in a phase 3 study.[242,243] Similar response rates (19.7% vs 17.0%) and overall survival times (60 weeks vs 57 weeks) were observed for the entire group of patients with recurrent disease. Liposomal doxorubicin was more active than topotecan in the subset of women with platinum-sensitive disease, producing improved PFS (29 weeks vs 23 weeks, $p = .037$) and overall survival (108 weeks vs 71 weeks, $p = .008$).[243]

The modest impact of chemotherapy in patients with platinum-resistant disease is well demonstrated by a trial in 195 patients with platinum-resistant ovarian cancer who were randomized to receive either liposomal doxorubicin or gemcitabine. In the gemcitabine and liposomal doxorubicin groups, median PFS was 3.6 months vs 3.1 months; median OS was 12.7 months vs 13.5 months; overall response rate (ORR) was 6.1% vs 8.3%; and in the subset of patients with measurable disease, ORR was 9.2% versus 11.7%, respectively. None of these differences were statistically significant.[230] Similar results were obtained in the study comparing topotecan with liposomal doxorubicin with low response rates and poor prognosis among women with platinum-resistant ovarian cancer.[242,243] In a subset analysis of platinum-resistant patients, the median time to progression ranged from of 9.1 and 13.6 weeks for topotecan and liposomal doxorubicin respectively. The median survival ($p = .455$) was 35.6 weeks for pegylated liposomal doxorubicin and 41.3 weeks for topotecan. Objective response rates were recorded in 6.5% of patients who received topotecan and in 12.3% of those who received pegylated liposomal doxorubicin ($p = .118$). It is not known whether the treatment improved symptoms control or quality of life as this was not specifically addressed.

The overall prognosis is unfavorable for patients who do not achieve a complete remission with induction chemotherapy or who relapse after an initial response.[218-224,226-231,235] Responses to second-line therapy can, however, be clinically beneficial, but the potential adverse effects associated with chemotherapy, particularly in patient with platinum resistant/refractory ovarian cancer, should not be underestimated and have been well documented.[217,231-234]. The three most commonly used drugs are paclitaxel, topotecan and liposomal doxorubicin. The reported adverse effects associated with paclitaxel included alopecia in 62% to 100%, neurotoxicity (any grade) in 5% to 42% of patients and severe leucopenia in 4% to 24% of patients. Topotecan is associated with significantly greater myelosuppression than liposomal doxorubicin or paclitaxel and is observed in 49% to 76% of patients. Liposomal doxorubicin is associated with palmer-plantar erythrodysesthesia (PPE) of any grade in over 50% of patients and is severe in 23%. In addition; severe stomatitis has been reported in up to 10% of patients.[218] Selection of the appropriate agent for an individual patient is based on prior toxicity, expected toxicities of the second-line agent, patient preference for IV versus oral administration, and quality of life considerations.

High-Dose Chemotherapy and Stem Cell Transplantation ■ The use of high-dose chemotherapy and either autologous bone marrow transplantation (ABMT) or peripheral stem cell support has been evaluated in patients with advanced ovarian cancer.[245-247] In one trial of high-dose mitoxantrone, carboplatin, and cyclophosphamide with stem cell support, 89% of patients responded with clinical complete responses documented in 88% of platinum-sensitive and 47% of platinum-resistant cases.[245] Median PFS was 10.1 months for platinum-sensitive disease and 5.1 months for platinum-resistant disease. In another retrospective analysis of 35 patients treated with high-dose melphalan and stem cell support, 9 of 12 patients with evaluable residual disease had a measurable response. The morbidity of this approach is high, and the survival after this approach in a phase 2 trial has been similar to the survival following second-line paclitaxel. Transplantation earlier in the course of disease may have a greater impact. A study that included 96 patients, many of whom were in clinical response (CR) (43%) or progesterone receptors (PR) (34%), produced 6-year survival of 37%. For patients who received transplantation for remission consolidation, the 6-year survival was 53% and the PFS was 29%.[246]

A European study of high-dose chemotherapy was recently reported.[247] One hundred forty-nine patients with untreated ovarian cancer were randomly assigned after debulking surgery to receive standard combination chemotherapy or sequential high-dose treatment with two cycles of cyclophosphamide and paclitaxel followed by three cycles of high-dose carboplatin and paclitaxel with stem cell support. High-dose melphalan was added to the final cycle. After a median follow-up of 38 months, the PFS was 20.5 months in the standard arm and 29.6 months in the high-dose arm. The median OS was 62.8 months in the standard arm and 54.4 months in the high-dose arm. This is the first randomized trial comparing sequential high-dose versus standard dose chemotherapy in first-line treatment of patients with advanced ovarian cancer and they observed no statistically significant difference in PFS or OS. The investigators concluded that high-dose chemotherapy does not appear to be superior to conventional dose chemotherapy using these particular agents. As non-hematopoietic toxicity of carboplatin and paclitaxel may be dose limiting, other regimens are likely to be more effective.

Immunotherapy ■ The use of IV or subcutaneous immunostimulants in addition to chemotherapy has not improved the response rate or survival of ovarian cancer patients. Based on the response seen with regional nonspecific immunotherapy, several trials of IP cytokines have been performed.[92,248-261] In a phase 2 trial conducted by the GOG, there was a 28% surgically-documented response rate to IFN-α in 25 patients with platinum-sensitive minimal residual tumors.[252] Overall, 53 surgically evaluated patients have been treated in three trials, with 40% responses and 25% complete responses.[248-252] All of the responding patients had microscopic or small macroscopic residual disease. Thus, the use of high-dose IP recombinant IFN-α given frequently can result in the regional control of very small-volume disease confined to the peritoneal cavity. Whether survival is affected is not known. Other cytokines have been evaluated. A phase 1-2 trial of IP IFN-γ also yielded a 30% response rate.[253] Another phase 1 trial with IP IL-2 has been performed, and the optimal dose was defined.[254,260]

Preclinical studies have examined the interaction of cytokines, such as IFN-α, tumor necrosis factor, and IL-2, with various cytotoxic agents, including cisplatin and doxorubicin.[255,256,260] In a phase 2 study of IFN-α alternating with cisplatin in patients with platinum-sensitive minimal residual disease, the surgically-documented response rate was 28%.[257] In a randomized phase 3 trial, Windbichler and colleagues have demonstrated that the use of subcutaneous IFN-γ in women receiving first-line platinum-based chemotherapy in ovarian cancer was well-tolerated.[259] A higher complete clinical response rate (68% vs 56%) and longer disease PFS (48 months vs 17 months, $p = .031$) were observed in women receiving the IFN-γ plus chemotherapy than in women who were treated with chemotherapy alone. Improved PFS was seen in patients with residual disease greater than 2 cm, as well as in those with optimal resection. In a phase 3 study by Alberts and colleagues, the addition of IFN-γ to combination of carboplatin and paclitaxel chemotherapy for primary treatment of advanced-stage ovarian cancer did not result in any difference in survival.[260]

Monoclonal antibodies raised against antigens on the surface of the epithelial ovarian cells have been used in clinical trials. In a phase 2 trial of IP 90Y-labeled anti-human milk fat globulin protein (HMFG) monoclonal antibody reactive with MUC-1 HMFG,[262] the IP administration of radionuclide conjugate significantly prolonged survival relative to historical controls. However, in a multicenter randomized controlled study comparing IP treatment with 90Y-labeled anti-MUC1 antibody to observation in patients without evidence of disease following second-look laparoscopy, no difference in survival was noted.[208]

Trastuzumab (Herceptin) has been studied in a phase 2 trial by the GOG in ovarian cancers that overexpress HER-2. Only 11% of ovarian cancers overexpressed HER-2 and the response rate was only 4%.[263] Thus, trastuzumab alone is not likely to be useful in ovarian cancer patients. As noted above, there is experience with OvaRex, the anti-CA125 monoclonal antibody in the setting of consolidation; however, there are no data regarding its potential usefulness in relapsed patients.[209,264]

Targeted Therapies ■ We are entering a new era of cancer treatment where knowledge of molecular pathways within normal and malignant cells has led to development of agents with specific molecular targets. The greatest success to date in ovarian cancer has been in targeting angiogenesis as VEGF has been found to play a major role in the biology of epithelial ovarian cancer.[265] There have been three main approaches to target angiogenesis—the first has been to target VEGF itself, the second to target the VEGF receptor, and the third is to inhibit tyrosine kinase activation and downstream signaling with small molecules that work at the intracellular level.

Bevacizumab is the first targeted agent to show significant activity in ovarian cancer. It is a humanized monoclonal antibody that targets angiogenesis by binding to VEGF-A, thereby blocking the interaction of VEGF with its receptor. There have been a number of phase 2 studies reported using bevacizumab in patients with platinum-sensitive and resistant ovarian cancer. A response rate as high as 35% was reported by Wright et al.[266] but in most studies response rates have ranged from 16% to 22% in both platinum-sensitive and refractory patients.[267,268] Furthermore, up to 40% of patients have had stabilization of disease for at least 6 months. A recent study of low-dose metronomic chemotherapy with 50 mg of cyclophosphamide daily and bevacizumab 10 mg/kg intravenously every 2 weeks showed significant activity in a study of 70 patients with recurrent ovarian cancer.[269] The primary end point was PFS at 6 months. The probability of being alive and progression free at 6 months was 56%. A partial response was achieved in 17 patients (24%). Median time to progression and survival were 7.2 months and 16.9 months, respectively. The side effects of bevacizumab are now well recognized and include hypertension, fatigue, proteinuria, GI perforation or fistula, and uncommonly vascular thrombosis and central nervous system (CNS) ischemia, pulmonary hypertension, as well as bleeding and wound healing complications. The most common side effects are hypertension which is grade 3 in 7% of patients and is usually readily treatable. The most concerning side effect is bowel perforation[265,267-269] which occurs in approximately 5% of patients overall.[268] Simkins et al.[270] limited bevacizumab treatment to patients without clinical symptoms of bowel obstruction or evidence of rectosigmoid involvement on pelvic exam or bowel involvement on CT scan. Their study included 25 patients with platinum-resistant ovarian cancer who had been heavily pretreated and they observed a response rate of 28% and had no bowel perforations or any other grade 3 or 4 toxicities were reported.

Other forms of anti-angiogenic therapy are being evaluated in clinical trials.[271] VEGF Trap functions as a soluble decoy receptor soaking up ligand before it can interact with its receptor and is also currently being evaluated in phase 2 trials in patients with recurrent ovarian cancer. There are also a number of other oral agents that target angiogenesis through tyrosine kinase inhibition.[271]

Hormonal Therapy ■ Epithelial ovarian tumors frequently contain elevated levels of estrogen and androgen receptors. Some patients with epithelial ovarian tumors have had responses to endocrine therapy, although it appears that the overall response rate is approximately 10% to 20%. Progestational agents and estrogen antagonists, such as tamoxifen, have been used either alone or in combination with cytotoxic chemotherapy in patients with advanced disease, and other studies have used gonadotropin agonists, for example, leuprolide acetate alone or with tamoxifen, or aromatase inhibitors.[272-275] In a study of patients with advanced epithelial ovarian cancer, tamoxifen exhibited only a 13% partial response rate, but disease progression was delayed in 30%.[274] There is a lack of correlative studies comparing the response to endocrine manipulations and the presence of hormone receptors. Hormonal therapy for patients with advanced ovarian cancer should primarily be reserved for those who have failed chemotherapeutic regimens and who are not candidates for aggressive salvage drug regimens or investigative approaches.

Palliative Radiotherapy in Ovarian Cancer ■ Radiotherapy as a palliative modality in ovarian cancer may be very useful if the sole dominant symptomatic problem for the patient is localized to a site and volume that may be safely encompassed in a limited radiation field. For example, a fixed pelvic mass eroding the vaginal mucosa causing bleeding, pain, or bowel or bladder dysfunction may occur without obvious disseminated symptomatic peritoneal disease. Localized masses in the retroperitoneal nodes or in extra abdominal sites such as the supraclavicular or inguinal node regions or bony or brain metastases may benefit from palliative irradiation as would painful hepatomegaly from hepatic capsular distention.

An objective and subjective response rate of patients treated with radiation for recurrent ovarian cancer after resistance to available chemotherapeutic agents has been reported. A study from Memorial Sloan-Kettering Cancer Center documented subjective or objective responses in 70% of patients who had platinum-refractory disease.[276] While the optimal dose for palliation has not been established, it is clear that durable palliation may be achieved with local radiotherapy for ovarian cancer recurring after chemotherapy even in the presence of chemoresistant disease. Palliative whole brain irradiation is indicated for documented cerebral metastases in those whose life expectancy is several weeks to months.

Survival of Patients With Advanced Ovarian Cancer

Cisplatin-based combination chemotherapy regimens have clearly produced higher response rates and, complete remission rates, and an improvement in the median survival of patients with advanced ovarian cancer. The impact on long-term survival has been modest, and the majority of patients with advanced ovarian cancer still die of their disease. Five-year survival rates for patients treated with cisplatin-based regimens for advanced disease are approximately 20% to 25%.[277-281] Although this is a substantial improvement over the 5% to 10% survival rate reported for patients with advanced disease in the preplatinum era, it is obvious that ovarian cancer still remains a formidable challenge and that new treatment approaches are needed.

The prognosis for patients with epithelial ovarian cancer is related to several clinical variables. Survival analyses based on the most commonly used prognostic variables are presented below. Including patients at all stages, patients less than 50 years of age have a 5-year survival rate of about 40%, compared with about 15% for patients older than 50 years.[41,42,281]

The 5-year survival rate for carefully and properly staged patients with stage I disease is 76% to 93%, depending on the tumor grade.[42,137,138] The 5-year survival for stage II is 60% to 74%.36 The 5-year survival rate for stage IIIA is 41%, for stage IIIB about 25%, for stage IIIC 23% and for stage IV disease 11%.[42] An analysis of the National Cancer Institute's Surveillance, Epidemiology and End Results (SEER) database reveals a trend toward improved survival for ovarian cancer in the United States during the last period of analysis (1988-1994). In this cohort, the survival for stage I was 93%, for stage II 70%, for stage III 37% and for stage IV 25%.[281] Compared with the interval 1983 to 1987, there was a statistically significant improvement in survival for stages I, III, and IV disease.

Survival of patients with borderline tumors is excellent, with stage I lesions having a 98% 15-year survival.[42] When all stages of borderline tumors are included, the 5-year survival rate is about 86% to 90%.

For invasive cancers grade affects the prognosis. For invasive stage I disease, the 5-year survival rate for grade 1 epithelial ovarian cancers is about 91%, compared with about 74% for grade 2 and 75% for grade 3.53 For stage II disease, the survivals are 69%, 60% and 51%, respectively, for grades 1, 2, and 3. Examining stage III-IV patients, the 5-year survivals for grade 1, 2, and 3, are 38%, 25%, and 19% respectively. Patients with stage III disease with microscopic residual disease at the start of treatment have a 5-year survival rate of about 40% to 75%, compared with about 30% to 40% for those with optimal disease and only 5% for those with nonoptimal disease. Patients whose Karnofsky index (KI) is low (< 70) have a significantly shorter survival than those with a KI > 70.[281]

Nonepithelial Ovarian Cancer

Nonepithelial cancers of the ovary are uncommon. They include malignancies of germ cell origin, sex cord-stromal cell origin, metastatic carcinomas to the ovary, and a variety of extremely rare ovarian cancers, such as sarcomas and lipoid cell tumors (Fig. 101-7). Nonepithelial malignancies account for about 10% of all ovarian cancers.[2,3,282] Although there are many similarities in the presentation, evaluation, and management of these patients, there are also many unique qualities of these tumors that require a special approach. This is particularly true because many more nonepithelial lesions are germ cell in origin, and they are usually found in young patients.

Germ Cell Malignancies

GCTs are derived from the primordial germ cells of the ovary. Whereas malignant GCTs can arise in extragonadal

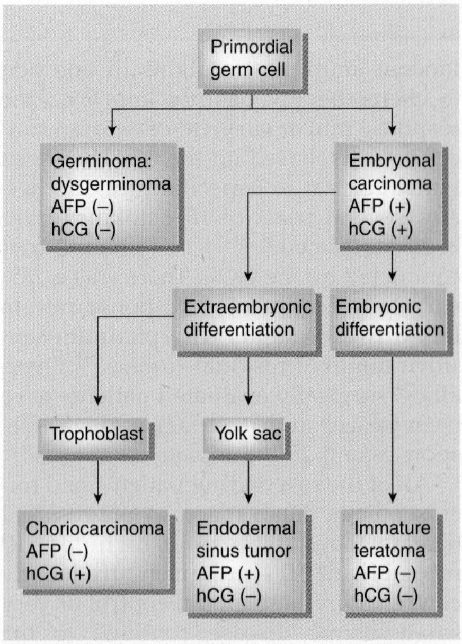

Figure 101-7 ■ Relationship between examples of pure malignant GCTs and their secreted substances. *Abbreviations*: AFP, α-fetoprotein; hCG, human chorionic gonadotropin. *Source*: From Berek JS, Hacker NF. Nonepithelial ovarian cancer. In: Berek JS, Hacker NF, eds. Practical gynecologic oncology. 4th ed. Baltimore, MD: Williams & Wilkins; 2005, p. 513.

sites, such as the mediastinum and the retroperitoneum, the majority of GCTs arise in the gonad from the undifferentiated germ cells. The variation in the sites of these cancers is explained by the embryonic migration of the germ cells from the caudal part of the yolk sac to the dorsal mesentery, prior to their incorporation into the sex cords of the developing gonads.[2,282]

Classification

A histologic classification of ovarian GCTs is presented in Table 101-8.[281-285] Alpha-fetoprotein (AFP) and human chorionic gonadotropin (hCG) are both secreted by some germ cell malignancies and, therefore, the presence of circulating hormones can be clinically useful in the diagnosis of a pelvic mass and in monitoring the course of a patient after surgery. Alpha-1-antitrypsin (AAT) can be detected rarely in association with GCTs. By correlating the histologic and immunohistologic identification of these substances in tumors, a classification of GCTs can be made. In this classification, embryonal carcinoma, which is composed of undifferentiated cells, synthesizes both hCG and AFP, and this tumor is the progenitor of several other germ cell malignancies. More differentiated GCTs, such as the endodermal sinus tumor, which secretes AFP, and the choriocarcinoma, which secretes hCG, are derived from the extraembryonic tissues, whereas the immature teratomas are derived from the embryonic cells that have lost the ability to secrete these substances.[2,282] Pure germinomas do not secrete these markers.

Epidemiology

Although 20% to 25% of all benign and malignant ovarian neoplasms are of germ cell origin, only about 3% of these tumors are malignant. Germ cell malignancies account for less than 5% of all ovarian cancers in Western countries but they represent up to 15% of ovarian cancers in Asian and African societies, where epithelial ovarian cancers are much less common.[5]

In the first two decades of life, almost 70% of ovarian tumors are of germ cell origin, and one-third of these are malignant. GCTs account for two-thirds of the ovarian malignancies in this age group. Germ cell cancers also are seen in the third decade, but thereafter become quite rare.

Table 101-8 Histologic Typing of Ovarian Germ Cell Tumors

I. Dysgerminoma
II. Teratoma
A. Immature
B. Mature
1. Solid
2. Cystic
a. Dermoid cyst (mature cystic teratoma)
b. Dermoid cyst with malignant transformation
C. Monodermal and highly specialized
1. Struma ovarii
2. Carcinoid
3. Struma ovarii and carcinoid
4. Others
III. Endodermal sinus tumor
IV. Embryonal carcinoma
V. Polyembryoma
VI. Choriocarcinoma
VII. Mixed forms

Source: Adapted from Ref. 64.

Clinical Features

The most common symptoms in young patients with a GCT of the ovary are a pelvic fullness, urinary frequency, and dysuria. Rectal pressure, menstrual irregularities in postmenarchal patients, and lower abdominal pain or pressure may be present. Some young patients may misinterpret the early symptoms of a neoplasm as those of pregnancy, and this can lead to a further delay in the diagnosis of the cancer. Acute symptoms associated with the torsion or rupture of the adnexa can develop. These symptoms may be confused with acute appendicitis. In more advanced cases, ascites may develop and the patient can present with extensive abdominal distention.[2,282]

In patients with a palpable adnexal mass, the evaluation should proceed expeditiously. Some patients with GCTs will be premenarchal and may require examination under anesthesia. If the lesions are principally solid or a combination of solid and cystic, as might be noted on an ultrasonographic evaluation, a neoplasm is probable and a malignancy is possible. The rest of the physical examination should search for signs of ascites, pleural effusion, and organomegaly.[285]

Diagnosis

When an adnexal mass is 2 cm or larger in a premenarchal female, or 8 cm or larger in other premenopausal females, surgical exploration is frequently required. In young patients, blood tests should include serum hCG and AFP levels, a complete blood count, and liver function tests. A chest radiograph should be performed because GCTs can metastasize to the lung or mediastinum. A karyotype should be obtained preoperatively on all premenarchal females, because of the propensity for these tumors to arise in dysgenetic gonads.[286] A preoperative CT scan may document the presence and extent of retroperitoneal lymphadenopathy or liver metastases, but because these patients require surgical exploration, a more extensive and time-consuming preoperative evaluation is unnecessary. If postmenarchal patients have predominantly cystic lesions up to 8 cm in diameter, they may undergo a trial of observation.

Dysgerminomas

Dysgerminomas are the most common malignant GCTs, accounting for about 30% to 40% of all ovarian cancers of germ cell origin.[2,282,286,287] The tumor represents only 1% to 3% of all ovarian cancers, but as much as 5% to 10% of ovarian cancer in patients younger than 20 years of age. Seventy-five percent of dysgerminomas occur between the ages of 10 and 30 years, 5% under the age of 10 years, and rarely over the age of 50 years.[2,282] Because these malignancies occur in young women, 20% to 30% of ovarian malignancies associated with pregnancy are dysgerminomas.

Much has been, and continues to be learned about the management of dysgerminoma by analogy with its male counterpart, testicular seminoma (Fig. 101-8).[285] The dominant route of spread in both is lymphatic, via the gonadal lymphatics to the renal hilar and para-aortic nodes. Both are exquisitely radiosensitive and curable with modest doses of radiotherapy, 2500 to 3500 cGy, even when bulk disease up to 5 cm is being treated. For this reason, excellent long-term survival rates were obtained when surgical removal, using oophorectomy or hysterectomy/BSO, is followed by radiotherapy to para-aortic and pelvic nodes although this is not considered standard of care now given the high efficacy of chemotherapy.[285,287]

About 75% of dysgerminomas are stage I at diagnosis ie, confined to one or both ovaries. About 85% to 90% of stage I tumors are confined to one ovary; 10% to 15% are bilateral. In fact, dysgerminoma is the only germ cell malignancy that has this significant rate of bilaterality, other GCTs rarely being bilateral.

Dysgerminomas affect younger women (85% are under 29 years of age) and are present in two-thirds of cases as stage IA. Dysgenetic gonads tend to develop dysgerminoma.[282,287] Therapeutic concepts have changed dramatically

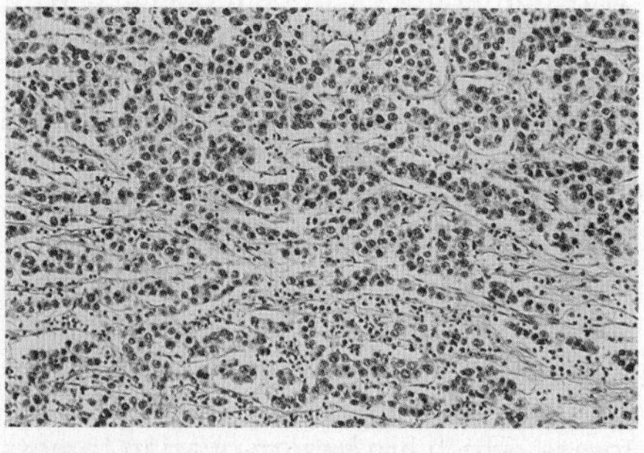

Figure 101-8 Dysgerminoma.

over the past few years, largely because of (i) the recognition of dysgerminomas' chemosensitivity, allowing cure without ovarian ablation by surgery or radiotherapy in many cases; (ii) the advent of improved techniques of imaging the retroperitoneum, with lymphography, and CT and /MRI scanning that allow detection of disease under 3 to 5 cm in diameter when it is eminently curable; (iii) tumor markers, AFP and the β subunit of hCG (β-hCG), which distinguishes pure dysgerminoma from the mixed GCTs; and (iv) the recognition that emerging emphasis in treatment on preservation of childbearing capacity is important and does likely, presumably not compromise the high chance of without compromising cure.

Many aspects of management are controversial: the need for complete surgical staging; the extent of the primary operative procedure in unilateral, bilateral, and metastatic disease; the role of postoperative observation in stage IA; the choice between radiotherapy and chemotherapy; the decision as to which chemotherapy drugs should be used; and the need for second-look procedures and debulking of residual masses. The subject was recently reviewed in greater depth than is possible here.[282]

In the 25% of patients who present with metastatic disease, the tumor most commonly spreads via the lymphatics. It also can spread hematogenously, or by direct extension through the capsule of the ovary, with exfoliation and dissemination of cells over the peritoneal surfaces. Metastases to the contralateral ovary occur and may be present when there is no other evidence of spread. An uncommon site of metastatic disease is bone, and when it does occur here, the lesions are seen principally in the lower vertebrae. Metastases to the lungs, liver, and brain are seen most often in patients whose disease is longstanding or recurrent. Metastatic disease to the mediastinum and supraclavicular lymph nodes is usually a late manifestation of disease.

Dysgenetic Gonads ■ Approximately 5% of dysgerminomas are discovered in phenotypic females with abnormal gonads.[2,282] This malignancy can be associated with patients who have pure gonadal dysgenesis (46XY, bilateral streak gonads), mixed gonadal dysgenesis (45X/46XY, unilateral streak gonad, contralateral testis), or the androgen insensitivity syndrome (46XY, testicular feminization). Therefore, premenarchal patients with a pelvic mass should have their karyotype determined. In most patients with gonadal dysgenesis, dysgerminomas arise in gonadoblastomas, which are benign ovarian tumors that are composed of germ cells and sex cord–stroma. If gonadoblastomas are left in place in patients with gonadal dysgenesis, more than 50% will develop into ovarian malignancies.[286] Also, dysgerminomas that contain significant numbers of syncytiotrophoblastic cells can be hormonally active, producing isosexual precocious pseudopuberty in premenarchal females and menstrual irregularities in older women.[282,284,286]

Surgery ■ The treatment of patients with dysgerminoma is primarily surgical, including the resection of the primary lesion and proper surgical staging. If necessary, radiation or chemotherapy is administered to selected patients. Because the disease principally affects young females, special consideration must be given to the preservation of fertility whenever possible.[2,282]

Ideally, the initial operation should include exploration of the abdominal contents, with careful palpation of the retroperitoneal node-bearing areas, sampling of enlarged nodes, and cytologic examination of peritoneal washings. If these steps were omitted in what was apparently stage I disease, the need for reexploration for restaging purposes is questionable, simply because noninvasive imaging techniques are capable of detecting residual disease or nodal metastases disease of less than 5 cm, and these are highly curable tumors, unlike the cystadenocarcinomas. For the same reason, biopsy of nonpalpable lymph nodes is probably unnecessary. A benefit of cytoreductive surgery has not been shown in this disease.

The minimum operation for ovarian dysgerminoma is a unilateral oophorectomy or salpingo-oophorectomy.[282] If there is a desire to preserve fertility, the contralateral ovary, fallopian tube, and uterus should be conserved to retain childbearing potential. This is probably true even in the presence of metastatic disease, because of the exquisite sensitivity of dysgerminomas to chemotherapy. In patients whose fertility need not be preserved, it is appropriate to perform a total abdominal hysterectomy and BSO. In patients whose karyotype analysis reveals a Y chromosome, both ovaries should be removed, although the uterus might be conserved for possible future embryo transfer.[286] Dysgerminoma is the only GCT that tends to be bilateral, and not all of the bilateral lesions have obvious ovarian enlargement. Therefore, excisional biopsy of any suspicious lesion is desirable.[287]

Postoperative workup should include the serum markers AFP and β-hCG, a chest radiograph, and an abdominopelvic CT or MRI scan. In premenarchal females with an ovarian mass, preoperative karyotyping should be performed, as detection of a Y chromosome is an indication for bilateral oophorectomy, as discussed below. Even with a histologic diagnosis of pure dysgerminoma, the presence of an elevated AFP value or a markedly elevated β-hCG level (over approximately 100 IU/L), indicates the presence of nondysgerminomatous elements, and is reason enough to base treatment on these more aggressive elements. As with seminoma, lower β-hCG levels are sometimes found in the pure form of the disease, produced by syncytial-like giant interstitial cells. Lymphography can be useful, both in detecting nodal involvement and in localizing the nodal chains for radiation treatment.

Management of Stage IA ■ The extent of initial of the initial extirpative surgery can be quite conservative. Long-term survival results in concurrent series reported for a policy of unilateral salpingo-oophorectomy with subsequent treatment withheld until relapse (91% in 145 cases) are not inferior to results of hysterectomy, bilateral adnexectomy, and routine postoperative radiotherapy (85% in 53 cases).[282,287] In these older series, two-thirds of relapses were salvaged by reexcision or radiotherapy. Better results would be expected today: because marker studies would show that some of the patients included did not have pure dysgerminoma from the outset; because relapse would be detected earlier by modern imaging techniques, when tumor bulk was lower; and because chemotherapy and megavoltage radiotherapy would be expected to salvage nearly all first relapses. Radiotherapy is rarely required or used to treat dysgerminomas. However, a conservative approach requires frequent patient monitoring: clinical and tumor marker checks every 2 months, and CT scans every 3 months in the first 2 to 3 years. In patients whose contralateral ovary has been preserved, disease can develop in 5% to 15% of the retained gonads over the next 2 years.[282] This figure includes those not treated with additional therapy, as well as patients with gonadal dysgenesis.

The reasons for a conservative initial approach are (i) to avoid ablative surgery and chemotherapy-radiotherapy in the majority of cases (probably 80% to 85% of properly evaluated stage IA patients are cured by oophorectomy), and (ii) to preserve fertility. Because the morbidity of low-dose radiotherapy is small, and the dollar cost of close surveillance of conservatively managed patients is appreciable, the strongest justification for conservatism is the desire to preserve fertility. This requires a highly compliant patient and a knowledgeable, attentive physician.

Management of Relapsed Stage I The choice of salvage therapy depends on the site and size of the relapse when it is detected, and the desire to maintain fertility. In general, treatment of relapse need not imply loss of fertility if chemotherapy or pelvis-sparing radiotherapy is used.

There is argument as to whether a tumor size over 10 cm at diagnosis is a contraindication to conservative therapy, since a higher relapse rate is associated with larger tumors.[288] The literature does not resolve this issue, but in the opinion of the authors a large tumor size per se does not preclude a conservative approach.

Stages IB, II, III, and IV About 6% of patients present with bilateral ovarian involvement, and a similar number of stage IA patients experience recurrence in the opposite ovary. In general, bilateral oophorectomy is advised for stage IB, possibly with uterus conservation for future embryo transfer, although occasionally some residual normal tissue can be salvaged. The choice of postoperative therapy in stage IB–III is as described above for disease that recurs after primary management of stage IA. In the past when radiation was used, the portals included the pelvic nodes on the affected side(s) and the renal hilar and para-aortic nodes up to the diaphragm, and prophylactic mediastinal/supraclavicular irradiation was not advised, since its value is questionable. Because these tumors are highly chemosensitive, fertility preservation is desirable, and a small fraction (10% to 20%) of abdominal spread is transperitoneal, abdominopelvic, the preferred treatment is chemotherapy as outlined below.[288]

Bleomycin, etoposide, and cisplatin (BEP) is the most frequently used chemotherapeutic regimen for GCTs, although there is some evidence to support carboplatin and etoposide, vinblastine, bleomycin, and cisplatin (VBP), and vincristine, actinomycin, and Cytoxan (VAC) (Table 101-9).[289-302] Encouraging results (long-term disease-free status over 90% in previously untreated patients, and in about 70% of recurrent cases) have been reported in a number of series using cisplatin, vinblastine, bleomycin (PVB), VAC, or variants.

Unlike the nondysgerminomatous ovarian GCTs, whose chemoresponsiveness is not as great as for the nonseminomatous testicular tumors, dysgerminoma may be even more chemosensitive than the testicular tumors. For example, one report cites a sustained complete response in 7 of 10 patients with residual disease treated with a doxorubicin/cyclophosphamide (AC) combination (two of the three relapses were salvaged with PVB).[303] The same report describes an additional eight patients treated with PVB; all eight are alive without disease, although one patient whose disease relapsed in the brain was salvaged by radiotherapy. Of some note is that four patients had residual ovarian or uterine disease; all are disease-free, and one, treated with AC, has subsequently borne a child.

There have been numerous reports of successful control of metastatic dysgerminomas with systemic chemotherapy, and this should now be regarded as the treatment of choice.[288-297] The obvious advantage is the preservation of fertility. The most frequently used chemotherapeutic regimens for GCTs are BEP, VBP, and VAC. The GOG studied three cycles of etoposide (EC) (120 mg/m^2 intravenously on days 1, 2, and 3 every 4 weeks) carboplatin (400 mg/m^2 intravenously on day 1 every 4 weeks) for patients with completely resected ovarian dysgerminoma, stages IB, IC, II, or III.[295] The results showed a sustained disease-free remission rate of 100%.

For patients with advanced, incompletely resected GCTs, the GOG studied cisplatin-based chemotherapy on two consecutive protocols.[294,295] In the first study, patients received four cycles of vinblastine, bleomycin, and cisplatin. Patients with persistent or progressive disease at second-look laparotomy were treated with six cycles of VAC. In the second trial, patients received three cycles of BEP initially, followed by consolidation with VAC, which was later discontinued in patients with dysgerminomas. The VAC consolidation after BEP in patients with tumors other than dysgerminoma is unnecessary still being investigated, and but VAC does not appear to improve the outcome following three cycles of the BEP regimen. A total of 20 evaluable patients with stage III and IV dysgerminoma were treated in these two protocols, and 19 are alive and free of disease after 6 to 68 months (median 26 months). Fourteen of these patients had a second-look laparotomy, and all findings were negative. Another study at MD Anderson Cancer Center used BEP in 14 patients with residual disease, and all patients were free of disease with long-term follow-up.[293] These results suggest that patients with advanced-stage, incompletely resected dysgerminoma have an excellent prognosis when treated with platinum-based combination chemotherapy. The standard regimen is three to four cycles of BEP, based on the data from testicular cancers cancers.[298,299] If bleomycin is contraindicated or omitted because of lung toxicity then consideration should be given to four cycles of cisplatin and etoposide.

Recurrent Disease Recurrences are very uncommon in women with dysgerminomas following platinum-based chemotherapy. About 75% of recurrences occur within the first year after initial treatment, the most common sites being the peritoneal cavity and the retroperitoneal lymph nodes.[2,282,303] These patients should be treated with either radiation or chemotherapy, depending on their primary treatment. Patients with recurrent disease who have had no therapy other than surgery should be treated with platinum-based chemotherapy. If prior chemotherapy with BEP has been given, paclitaxel, ifosfamide and platinum (TIP) is one of the more commonly used salvage regimens. Cisplatin, vincristine, methatrexate, bleomycin, actinomycin D, cyclophosphamide, etoposide (POMB-ACE) may be used in patients with relapsed testicular GCTs. These treatment decisions should be made in a multidisciplinary setting with input of physicians experienced in the treatment of patients with GCTs. Consideration may be given to the use of high-dose chemotherapy with peripheral stem cell support. There are a number of high-dose regimens that have been used in phase 2 studies and the choice depends of prior chemotherapy, the time to recurrence and residual toxicity from prior therapy. Once again these decisions are best made in consultation with an experienced multidisciplinary group (Table 101-10), and consideration should be given to the use of high-dose chemotherapy (eg, with carboplatin and etoposide) and autologous bone marrow transplantation. Alternatively, radiation therapy (RT) is also very effective for this disease, with the major disadvantage being loss of fertility if pelvic and abdominal radiation is required but should be considered if there is a localized nodal recurrence.

Second-Look Laparotomy There appears to be no need to perform a second-look

Table 101-9 **Combination Chemotherapy for GCTs of the Ovary**

Regimens and Drugs	Dosage and Schedule[a]
BEP:	
Bleomycin	30 IU weekly to a maximum of 12 weeks 15 U/m^2/week × 5; then on day 1 of course 4
Etoposide	100 mg/m^2/day × 5 days every 3 weeks
Cisplatin	20 mg/m^2/day × 5 days, or 100 mg/m^2/day × 1 day every 3 weeks

[a]All doses given intravenously.

Table 101-10 **POMB/ACE Chemotherapy for GCTs of the Ovary**

POMB	
Day 1	Vincristine I mg/m^2 IV; methotrexate 300 mg/m^2 as a 12-h infusion
Day 2	Bleomycin 15 mg by 24-h infusion, folinic acid rescue started 24 h after the start of methotrexate in a dose of 15 mg every 12 h for 4 doses
Day 3	Bleomycin 15 mg by 24-h infusion
Day 4	Cisplatin 120 mg/m^2 as a 12-h infusion, given together with hydration and 3 mg magnesium sulfate supplementation
ACE	
Days 1-5	Etoposide (VP16) 100 mg/m^2, days 1 to 5
Days 3-5	Actinomycin D 0.5 mg IV, days 3, 4, and 5
Day 5	Cyclophosphamide 500 mg/m^2 IV, day 5
OMB	
Day 1	Vincristine 1 mg/m^2 IV; methotrexate 300 mg/m^2 as a 12-h infusion
Day 2	Bleomycin 15 mg by 24-h infusion; folinic acid rescue started at 24-h
Day 3	Bleomycin 15 mg by 24-h infusion

The sequence of treatment schedules is two courses of POMB followed by ACE. POMB is then alternated with ACE until patients are in biochemical remission as measured by hCG and AFP, PLAP and LDH. The usual number of courses of POMB is three to five. Following biochemical remission, patients alternate ACE with OMB until remission has been maintained for approximately 12 weeks. The interval between courses of treatment is kept to the minimum (usually 9 to 11 days). If delays are caused by myelosuppression after courses of ACE, the first 2 days of etoposide are omitted from subsequent courses of ACE.

laparotomy in patients with dysgerminoma whose macroscopic disease was all resected at the primary operation.[304] The role of surgery to resect residual masses following chemotherapy for dysgerminomas is not clear and the vast majority of these patients will only have necrotic tissue and nonviable tumor. These patients should in general be closely monitored with scans and tumor markers. PET scan should be considered in patients who have bulky residual masses more than 4 weeks after chemotherapy, as a positive PET scan is a reliable predictor of residual seminoma in males with residual lesions > 3 cm and the same may apply in females with dysgerminomas.[305] If the PET is positive or if there is a suggestion of progressive disease on scans then ideally there should be histological evaluation and confirmation of residual disease before embarking on salvage therapy. In patients with macroscopic residual disease at the start of chemotherapy, we prefer to perform a second-look operation because second-line therapy is available and the earlier persistent disease is identified, the better the prognosis should be.

Coexistent With Pregnancy ■ Because dysgerminomas tend to occur in young patients, they may coexist with pregnancy. When a stage IA cancer is found, the tumor can be removed intact and the pregnancy continued. In patients with more advanced disease, continuation of the pregnancy will depend on gestational age, but chemotherapy can be given in the second and third trimesters of pregnancy if required using the same dosages as given for the nonpregnant patient.[306]

Prognosis ■ In patients whose initial disease is stage IA (ie, a unilateral encapsulated dysgerminoma), the conservative approach outlined above results in 5-year disease-free survivals of greater than 95%. The 5-year survival for patients with all stages of dysgerminoma is in excess of 90-95%.[282,284–306] The features that have been associated with a higher tendency to recur include lesions larger than 10 to 15 cm in diameter, age younger than 20 years, and microscopic characteristics that include numerous mitoses, anaplasia, and a medullary pattern.[303,305]

With current staging methods, the proportion of relapsing patients should be no more than 15% to 20%.[293] The theoretic cure rate of this group is 98%. Although in the past, surgery for advanced disease followed by pelvic and abdominal radiation produced a 5-year survival of 63% to 83%, cure rates approaching 100% of 85% to 90% for this same group of patients are being seen now with combination chemotherapy.[296,304]

Many patients with a dysgerminoma will have a tumor that is apparently confined to one ovary and will be referred after unilateral salpingo-oophorectomy without surgical staging.[301] The options for such patients are repeat laparotomy for surgical staging, regular pelvic and abdominal surveillance with CT scans, or adjuvant chemotherapy. As these are rapidly growing tumors, our preference is to perform regular CT surveillance. Tumor markers (AFP and β-hCG) should also be monitored in case occult mixed germ cell elements are present.

Immature Teratomas

Immature teratomas contain elements resembling tissues derived from the embryo. Immature teratomatous elements may occur in combination with other GCTs as mixed GCTs. The pure immature teratoma accounts for less than 1% of all ovarian cancers, but it is the second most common germ cell malignancy. This lesion represents 10% to 20% of all ovarian malignancies seen in females under 20 years of age and 30% of the deaths from ovarian cancer in this age group [2,282] About 50% of pure immature teratomas of the ovary occur between the ages of 10 years and 20 years, and they rarely are seen in postmenopausal women. Immature teratomas are classified according to a grading system (grades 1 to 3) that is based on the degree of differentiation and the quantity of immature tissue.[282,307-312] Semiquantification of the amount of neuroepithelium correlates with survival in ovarian immature teratoma and is the basis for grading of the these tumors.[309,310,311] Those with less than one lower power field of immature neuroepithelium on the slide with the greatest amount of such tissue (grade 1) have a survival of at least 95%, whereas greater amounts of immature neuroepithelium (grades 2 and 3) appear to have a lower overall survival (approximately 85%).[310,311] This may not apply, however, to immature teratomas of the ovary in children as they appear to have a very good outcome with surgery alone, regardless of the degree of immaturity, in these cases.[312,313] Some authorities have recommended a two tier grading system and have recommended that immature teratomas are categorized as either low-grade or high-grade due to the significant inter and intra-observer difficulty with a 3 grade system[310] and this is what we currently use. Immature ovarian teratomas are associated with gliomatosis peritonei, a favorable prognostic finding if composed of completely mature tissues, with the recent reports, using molecular methods, that these glial "implants" are not tumor derived but represent teratoma-induced metaplasia of pluri-potent mullerian stem cells in the peritoneum.[305,311]

The preoperative evaluation and differential diagnosis are the same as for patients with other GCTs. Some of these lesions will contain calcifications similar to mature teratomas, and these can be detected by a radiograph of the abdomen or by ultrasonography. Rarely, they are associated with the production of steroid hormones and can present with sexual pseudoprecosity.[305] Patients may present with abnormal bleeding, but most frequently the symptoms and signs are nonspecific, usually those of a pelvic mass with or without pelvic pressure or pain. The lesions may be growing rapidly, and thus the symptoms and signs often have a subacute onset. Tumor markers are negative unless a mixed GCT is present.

Surgery ■ As with the dysgerminoma in a young patient whose lesion appears confined to a single ovary, a unilateral oophorectomy or salpingo-oophorectomy and surgical staging should be performed. In older patients who do not desire preservation of fertility, a total abdominal hysterectomy and BSO should be carried out. Contralateral involvement is rare, and in patients whose contralateral ovary reveals no evidence of gross involvement, routine resection or wedge biopsy is unnecessary.[282] Any lesions on the peritoneal surfaces should be sampled carefully and submitted for histologic evaluation. The most frequent site of dissemination is the peritoneum and, much less commonly, the retroperitoneal lymph nodes. Blood-borne metastases to organ parenchyma, such as the lungs, liver, or brain, are uncommon. When present, they are usually seen in patients with late or recurrent disease, and most often in tumors that are poorly differentiated.

Chemotherapy ■ The results of therapy for patients with GCTs other than dysgerminomas (eg, immature teratomas and endodermal sinus tumors of the ovary) have improved with cisplatin-based chemotherapy. The primary prognostic factor in patients with immature teratoma is the tumor grade. There is no evidence that chemotherapy will improve the outcome of patients with stage IA, grade 1 lesions. In patients whose tumors are stage IA, grades 2 and 3, chemotherapy should be used.[306,308,314-316] In patients who have ascites and ruptured tumors, chemotherapy is indicated, regardless of tumor grade. While patients with stage I, grade 1 immature teratoma rarely suffer a relapse, most patients with grade 2 and 3 tumors will not be cured by surgery alone. Similarly, most patients with endodermal sinus tumors will not be cured by surgery alone, as discussed below. Therefore, adjuvant platinum-based chemotherapy is recommended for all patients other than those with stage I, grade 1 immature teratomas. Although nonplatinum-based chemotherapy regimens, such as VAC [308] have been somewhat successful when administered in the adjuvant situation, they have been replaced by platinum-based therapy.[309] The newer approach has been to incorporate cisplatin into the primary treatment of these tumors, and most of the experience has been with the VBP and BEP regimens. Standard therapy in these patients is now the BEP regimen. In a GOG trial, 50 of 52 stage I, stage II, and stage III patients with completely resected tumor remain disease-free after three courses of BEP.[295,307]

No direct comparison of these regimens with VAC has been reported, but the BEP combination can save some patients who have persistent or recurrent disease after VAC. The GOG has evaluated three courses of BEP therapy in patients with completely resected stage I, II, and III ovarian GCTs.[304] Overall, the toxicity has been acceptable, and 91 of 93 patients with nondysgerminomatous tumors treated are clinically free from disease. Thus the BEP regimen, which is used more extensively for testicular cancer, appears to be superior to the VAC regimen in the treatment of completely resected nondysgerminomatous GCTs of the ovary. Because some patients can progress rapidly, treatment should be initiated as soon as possible after surgery, preferably within 7 days to 10 days.

The switch from VBP to BEP has been prompted by the experience in patients with testicular cancer, where the replacement of vinblastine with etoposide has been associated with a better therapeutic index (ie, equivalent efficacy and lower morbidity), especially less neurologic and GI toxicity. Although associated with pulmonary toxicity, use of bleomycin appears to be important in this group of patients. In a randomized study of three cycles of etoposide plus cisplatin without or with bleomycin (EP vs BEP) in 166 patients with GCTs of the testes, the BEP regimen had a relapse-free survival rate of 84% compared with 69% for the EP regimen ($p = .03$).[299] In addition, cisplatin may be slightly better than carboplatin in patients with metastatic GCTs. One hundred ninety-two patients with GCTs of the testes were entered into a study of four cycles of EP vs four cycles of etoposide plus carboplatin (EC). There have been three relapses with the EP regimen and seven with the EC regimen, although the overall survival of the two groups is identical thus far.[298] A German group randomized patients to BEP (three cycles at standard doses (given days 1-5) or the carboplatin, etoposide and bleomycin (CEB) regimen (carboplatin with a target AUC of 5 mg/ml × min on day 1, etoposide 120 mg/m^2 on days 1 to 3 and bleomycin 30 mg on days 1, 8, and 15.[317] Four cycles of CEB were given, with the omission of bleomycin in the fourth cycle the so the cumulative doses of etoposide and bleomycin applied in the two treatment arms were comparable. Fifty-four patients were entered on the trial, 29 were treated with PEB and 25 with CEB chemotherapy. More patients treated with CEB (32% vs 13%) relapsed after therapy, and 4 patients (16%) died of disease progression in contrast to 1 (3%) after BEP therapy. The trial was terminated early after an interim analysis. The inferiority of carboplatin was also confirmed in a larger randomized trial later reported by Horwich et al.[318] These results substantiate that BEP is the preferred treatment regimen for patients with gross residual disease as well as completely resected disease.

Immature teratomas with malignant squamous elements appear to have a poorer prognosis than those tumors without these elements.[311] The treatment in these patients is also the BEP regimen.

Second-Look Procedures ■ A second-look is not necessary in most patients who have received chemotherapy, particularly those who were treated in an adjuvant setting (ie, stage IA, grades 2 and 3 disease) because chemotherapy in these patients is so effective.[304] An enlarged contralateral ovary may contain a benign cyst or a mature cystic teratoma, which may be managed with an ovarian cystectomy.[282] The need for a second-look operation for ovarian GCTs has been questioned [40,41]. It is not justified in patients who have received chemotherapy in an adjuvant setting (ie, stage IA, grades 2 and 3), because these patients have an excellent prognosis. However, we continue to prefer second-look laparotomy in patients with residual disease at the completion of chemotherapy as these patients may have residual mature teratoma and are at risk of "growing teratoma syndrome" a rare complication of immature teratomas.[319,320] Furthermore, cancers can arise at a later date in residual mature teratoma and it is important to resect any residual mass and exclude persistent disease as further chemotherapy may be indicated. The principles of surgery are based on the much larger experience of surgery in males with residual masses following chemotherapy for GCTs with a component of immature teratoma.[321] Matthew et al.[322] reported their experience with laparotomy in assessing the nature of postchemotherapy residue in ovarian GCTs. Sixty-eight patients completed combination chemotherapy with cisplatin regimens, of whom 35 had radiological residual masses. Twenty nine out of these 35 patients underwent laparotomy and three patients had viable tumor, seven immature teratoma, three mature teratoma and 16 only necrosis or fibrosis. None of the patients with dysgerminoma, embryonal carcinoma, absence of teratoma element in the primary tumor and radiological residual mass of < 5 cm had viable tumor whereas all patients with tumors containing teratoma component initially had residual tumor strengthening the case for surgery in patients with immature teratoma and any residual mass.[322]

Prognosis ■ The most important prognostic feature of the immature teratoma is the grade of the lesion.[2,309] Historically the 5-year survivals have been reported to be 82%, 62%, and 30% for patients with grade 1, 2, and 3 lesions respectively prior to the era of CT, tumor markers and optimal chemotherapy.[309] Occasionally, these tumors are associated with mature or low-grade glial elements that have become implanted throughout the peritoneum, and such patients typically have a favorable long-term survival as discussed above. In addition, the stage of disease and the extent of tumor at the initiation of treatment also affect the curability of the lesion. Patients whose tumors have been incompletely resected prior to treatment have a significantly lower 5-year survival than do those patients whose lesions have been completely resected (94% vs 50%).[306] In young women with conserved contralateral ovaries and a uterus, normal reproductive function and pregnancy have been reported in a significant fraction of successfully treated patients.[288] Overall, the 5-year survival of patients with all stages of pure immature teratomas is 70% to 80%, whereas it is 90% to 95% for patients with surgical stage I lesions.[282]

Endodermal Sinus Tumors (ESTs)

ESTs have also been referred to as yolk sac carcinomas, because they are derived from the primitive yolk sac.[2,282,323-332] These lesions are the third most frequent malignant GCT of the ovary. ESTs at a median age of 18 years, and about one-third of the patients are premenarchal at the time of presentation. Like the other nondysgerminomatous ovarian malignancies, abdominal or pelvic pain is the most frequent presenting symptom, occurring in about 75% of patients. An asymptomatic pelvic mass is documented in about 10% of patients.[282]

Most EST lesions secrete AFP. There is a good correlation with the extent of disease and the AFP level, although discordance has been observed. The serum level of AFP is particularly useful in monitoring the patient during and after treatment and the half-life is approximately 5 days.[282]

Surgery ■ The treatment of EST includes a surgical exploration, a unilateral oophorectomy, and a frozen section for diagnosis. Any gross metastases should be removed if possible, but a thorough surgical staging is not necessary because all patients need chemotherapy. The tumors tend to be solid and large, ranging in size from 7 to 28 cm (median is 15 cm).[2,282] The EST is thought never to be bilateral, and the other ovary will have metastasis only when there are other metastases in the peritoneal cavity. Most patients have early-stage disease: 71% have stage I, 6% have stage II, and 23% have stage III. The performance of a hysterectomy and contralateral salpingo-oophorectomy does not alter outcome and is not necessary.[282]

Chemotherapy ■ ESTs are treated in all patients, regardless of stage, with either adjuvant or therapeutic chemotherapy.[315-331] Prior to the routine use of combination chemotherapy for this disease, the 2-year survival was only about 25% but now is over 90%. With conservative surgery and adjuvant chemotherapy, fertility can be preserved as with other GCTs.

As with other nondysgerminomatous GCTs, a cisplatin-containing combination chemotherapy regimen, either BEP or VBP, is most effective in the treatment of EST, particularly in the treatment of measurable or incompletely resected tumors.[330] In the GOG series, only about 20% of patients with residual metastatic disease responded completely to the VAC regimen, whereas about 60% of those treated with VBP had a complete response.[307] However, VBP has salvaged some failures of VAC therapy. BEP is probably the best current primary chemotherapy for this disease. The optimal number of treatment cycles has not been established in ovarian GCTs but it is reasonable to extrapolate from the much larger experience in testicular GCTs where three cycles of BEP is considered optimal for good-prognosis low-risk patients and four cycles for patients with intermediate to high-risk GCTs.[329] In patients, in whom bleomycin is omitted or dropped because of toxicity, four cycles of cisplatin and etoposide are recommended. An alternative approach is to use VIP (etoposide, ifosfamide, and cisplatin) in patients with more advanced disease in whom bleomycin is contraindicated. Four cycles of VIP are equivalent to four cycles of BEP, but it is more myelotoxic and generally requires growth factor support.[330]

The group from the Charing Cross Hospital in London developed the POMB-ACE regimen for high-risk GCTs of any histologic type and their results appeared to be superior to BEP in patients with poor prognostic features (add ref). This protocol introduces seven drugs into the initial management, which is intended to minimize the chances of developing drug resistance. This is particularly relevant in patients with massive metastatic disease, and we have tended to use the POMB-ACE regimen as primary therapy for such cases as well as in patients with liver or brain metastases. The POMB schedule is only moderately myelosuppressive, so the intervals between each course can be kept to a maximum of 14 days (usually 9 to 11 days), thereby minimizing the time for tumor regrowth between courses. When *bleomycin* is given by a 48-hour infusion, pulmonary toxicity is reduced. With a maximum of 9 years of follow-up, the Charing Cross group has seen few long-term side effects in patients treated with POMB-ACE. Children have developed normally, menstruation has been physiologic, and several have completed normal pregnancies. However, it is still not clear if POMB-ACE is superior to BEP but it is unlikely that this will ever be addressed in a randomized trial.

The GOG protocols have used nine treatment cycles of VBP given every 4 weeks, but four to six cycles may be equally effective.[330]

Embryonal Carcinoma

Embryonal carcinoma of the ovary is an extremely rare tumor. It can be distinguished from a choriocarcinoma by the absence of syncytiotrophoblastic and cytotrophoblastic cells. Embryonal carcinomas may be hormonally active, with some patients developing precocious pseudopuberty or irregular bleeding. The presentation is similar to that of the EST. The patient's ages ranged between 4 and 28 years (median 14 years) in one series.[331] The primary lesions tend to be larger than 15 cm in diameter, and about two-thirds are confined to one ovary at the time of presentation. As with the pure EST, these lesions often secrete AFP and hCG, and these markers are useful for following the response to subsequent therapy. The treatment of embryonal carcinomas is the same as for the EST, ie, the performance of a unilateral oophorectomy or salpingo-oophorectomy followed by combination chemotherapy with BEP.[305]

Choriocarcinoma of the Ovary

Pure nongestational choriocarcinoma of the ovary is an extremely rare tumor.[332,333] The majority of patients with this cancer are younger than 20 years. Isosexual precocity has been documented in about 50% of patients whose lesions arise prior to menarche. The presence of hCG can be valuable in monitoring the patient during and after treatment. Because of its rarity, there are only a few series of reports in which chemotherapy was used for these nongestational choriocarcinomas, but there have been complete responses reported to the methotrexate, actinomycin D, and cyclophosphamide (MAC) regimen.[285] However, as BEP or EP is active in gestational choriocarcinoma, these regimens are also a reasonable approach for the nongestational lesions are considered standard of care as for other GCTs The prognosis for ovarian choriocarcinoma has been poor, with the majority of patients having metastatic disease to organ parenchyma at the time of initial diagnosis but this is likely to have improved with more effective platinum-based chemotherapy.[282]

Mixed GCTs

Mixed germ cell malignancies of the ovary contain two or more elements of the lesions described above. In one series, the most common component of a mixed malignancy was dysgerminoma, which occurred in 80%, followed by EST in 70%, immature teratoma in 53%, choriocarcinoma in 20%, and embryonal carcinoma in 16%.[293,328] The most frequent combination was a dysgerminoma and an EST. The mixed lesion may secrete either AFP or hCG, or both or neither, depending on the components.

Because most of these lesions contain poorly differentiated elements, mixed germ cell malignancies should be treated with combination chemotherapy with BEP, probably BEP or VBP. The serum marker, if positive initially, should may become negative during chemotherapy and fall within its half-life, but this may reflect the regression of only a particular component of the mixed lesion. Therefore, in patients with advanced-stage mixed germ cell malignancies that also contain teratomatous elements, consideration should be given to resect any residual masses following the completion of chemotherapy. The rationale for this is discussed in detail above in the section on immature teratomas. A second-look laparotomy may be useful to determine the response to therapy, unless the tumor was confined initially to the ovary.

The most important prognostic features are the size of the primary tumor and the relative amount of its most malignant component.[328] In stage IA lesions smaller than 10 cm, survival is 100%. Tumors composed of less than one-third EST, choriocarcinoma, or grade 3 immature teratoma also have an excellent prognosis, but it is less favorable when these components make up the majority of the mixed lesions.

Surveillance for Stage I Ovarian GCTs ■ Surveillance is a common approach to the management of young men with apparent stage I testicular GCT and there is a large body of evidence to support this approach as well as guidelines on what constitutes appropriate surveillance.[330] Although up to 20-30% of patients will relapse, almost all will be cured with salvage chemotherapy with BEP and the potential adverse effects of chemotherapy can be avoided in most patients. While this is a very common approach to management of young men with stage 1 testicular GCTs has not been widely adopted in females with ovarian GCTs. However, there are now some data available to support surveillance in selected patients who have been surgically staged. Cushing et al.[334] reported a study of 44 pediatric patients with completely resected ovarian immature teratomas who were followed carefully for recurrence of disease with appropriate diagnostic imaging and serum tumor markers. The 4-year disease-free and overall survival for the ovarian immature teratoma group and for the ovarian immature teratoma plus yolk sac tumor group was 97.7% (95% CI, 84.9-99.7%) and 100%, respectively. The only yolk sac tumor relapse occurred in a child with ovarian immature teratoma and yolk sac tumor who was then treated and salvaged with chemotherapy.[334] These findings were supported by another pediatric study which reported a 97% event free survival in young girls with stage I ovarian immature teratomas. Dark et al.[335] reported a study that included 24 patients with malignant stage IA ovarian GCT who were also enrolled onto a surveillance program. The group consisted of nine patients with dysgerminoma, nine with pure immature teratoma, and six with endodermal sinus tumor (with or without immature teratoma). Treatment consisted of surgical resection without adjuvant chemotherapy, followed by a surveillance program of clinical, serologic, and radiologic review, and included a second-look procedure. All but one patient were alive and in remission after a median follow-up of 6.8 years. The 5-year overall survival is 95%, and the 5-year disease-free survival is 68%. Eight patients required chemotherapy for recurrent disease or second primary ovarian GCT. This included three patients with grade 2 immature teratoma and three patients with dysgerminoma, and a further two women with dysgerminoma who developed contralateral (presumed second primary) dysgerminoma 4.5 and 5.2 years after their first tumor. All but one, who died of a pulmonary embolus, have been successfully salvaged with chemotherapy.[335]

More recently Patterson[336] updated the experience of the same group and reported on the safety of their ongoing surveillance program of all stage IA female GCTs. Thirty-seven patients (median age 26, range 14-48 years) with stage I disease underwent surgery and staging followed by intense surveillance, which included regular tumor markers and imaging. The median period of follow-up was 6 years. Relapse rates for stage IA nondysgerminomatous tumors and dysgerminomas were 8 of 22 (36%) and 2 of 9 (22%), respectively, plus one patient with mature teratoma and glial implants also relapsed; 10 of these 11 patients (91%) were successfully cured with platinum-based chemotherapy. Only one patient died from chemoresistant disease. All relapses occurred within 13 months of initial surgery. The overall disease-specific survival of malignant ovarian GCTs was 94%. Over 50% of patients who underwent fertility-sparing surgery went on to have successful pregnancies. They concluded that surveillance of all stage IA ovarian GCTs is safe and that the outcome is comparable with testicular tumors and they questioned the need for potentially toxic adjuvant chemotherapy in nondysgerminoma patients who have greater than 90% chance of being salvaged with chemotherapy if they relapse later. This strategy is appealing and is supported by a larger pediatric literature but there is a much less experience in adults. This is a question that deserves further study but will require international collaboration to answer it. If one is going to embark on a surveillance program it is essential that the protocols used by Dark and Patterson[335,336] are closely adhered to and that the patient understands that the data are limited and that close surveillance is required.

Late Effects of Treatment of Malignant GCTs of the Ovary ■ Although there are substantial data regarding late effects of *cisplatin*-based therapy in men with testicular cancer, much less information is available for women with ovarian GCTs The toxicity of BEP chemotherapy has been well documented and includes significant pulmonary toxicity in 5% of patients with fatal lung toxicity in 1%; acute myeloid leukemia or myelodysplastic syndrome in 0.2% to 1% of patients; neuropathy in 20% to 30%: Raynauds phenomenon in 20%, tinnitus in 24% and high tone hearing loss in up to 70% of patients, as well as late effects on gonadal function as well as an increased risk of hypertension and cardiovascular disease and some degree of renal impairment in 30% of patients.[337,338] These side effects underscore the importance of limiting the number of cycles of chemotherapy and also highlight the need for these patients to be referred to clinicians with experience in managing GCTs.

Sex Cord-Stromal Tumors

Sex cord-stromal tumors of the ovary account for about 5% to 8% of all ovarian malignancies.[2,282] This group of ovarian neoplasms is derived from the sex cords and the ovarian stroma or mesenchyme. The tumors usually are composed of various combinations of elements, including the "female" cells (granulosa and theca cells) and "male" cells (Sertoli and Leydig cells), as well as morphologically indifferent cells. A classification of this group of tumors is presented (Table 101-11).

Granulosa-Stromal Cell Tumors

This group of tumors includes granulosa cell tumors, thecomas, and fibromas. The granulosa cell tumor is a low-grade malignancy, and rarely thecomas and fibromas become malignant and are called fibrosarcomas.[2]

Granulosa cell tumors, which are estrogen secreting, are seen in women of all

Table 101-11 Sex Cord-Stromal Tumors

A. Granulosa-stomal cell tumors
1. Granulosa cell tumor
2. Tumors in the thecoma-fibroma group
a. Thecoma
b. Fibroma
c. Unclassified
B. Androblastomas: Sertoli-Leydig cell tumors
1. Well differentiated
a. Sertoli cell tumor
b. Sertoli-Leydig cell tumor
c. Leydig cell tumor; hilus cell tumor
2. Moderately differentiated
3. Poorly differentiated (sarcomatoid)
4. With heterologous elements
C. Gynandroblastoma
D. Unclassified

Source: Adapted from Ref. 64.

ages (Fig. 101-9). They are found in prepubertal females in 5% of cases, and the rest throughout the reproductive and postmenopausal years.[282] They are bilateral in 2% of patients. In the rare prepubertal lesion, three-fourths are associated with sexual pseudoprecocity because of the estrogen secretion. In the reproductive age group, most patients present with menstrual irregularities or secondary amenorrhea, and cystic hyperplasia of the endometrium may accompany these lesions. In postmenopausal women, abnormal uterine bleeding is frequently the presenting symptom. Indeed, the estrogen secretion in these patients can be sufficient to stimulate the development of endometrial cancer. Endometrial cancer occurs in association with granulosa cell tumors in about 5% of cases; 25% are associated with endometrial hyperplasia.[282] The other symptoms and signs of granulosa cell tumors are nonspecific and are the same as for most ovarian malignancies. Ascites is present in about 10% of cases, and, rarely, a pleural effusion is present. Granulosa tumors tend to be hemorrhagic, and occasionally rupture and produce a hemoperitoneum. Inhibin is secreted by granulosa cell tumors and is a useful marker for the disease.[339-341]

Granulosa cell tumors are usually stage I at diagnosis, but they may recur 5 to 30 years after initial diagnosis.[282]

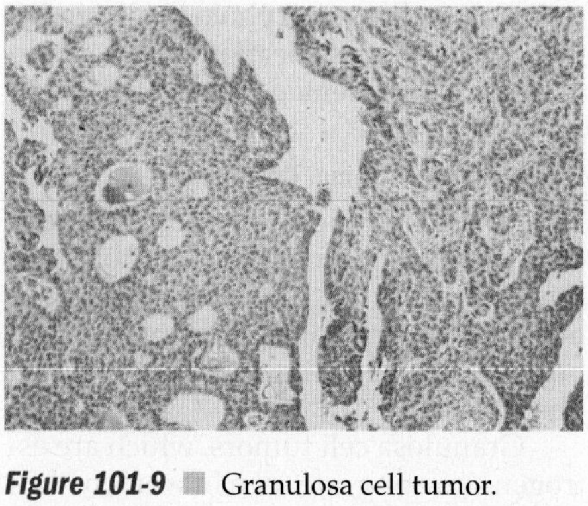

Figure 101-9 Granulosa cell tumor.

The tumors also may spread hematogenously, and patients can develop metastases years after initial diagnosis in the lungs, liver, and brain. When they do recur, they can progress rapidly. Malignant thecomas are extremely rare, and their presentation, management, and outcome are similar to those of the granulosa cell tumors.

Surgery The treatment of a granulosa cell tumor depends on the age of the patient and the extent of disease. For most patients, surgery alone is sufficient primary therapy. The performance of a unilateral oophorectomy or salpingo-oophorectomy is appropriate therapy for stage IA tumors in children or in women of reproductive age.[282] If a granulosa cell tumor is identified by frozen section at laparotomy, a staging operation is performed, including an assessment of the contralateral ovary. If the opposite ovary appears enlarged, it should be biopsied. In perimenopausal and postmenopausal women for whom ovarian preservation is not important, a hysterectomy and BPSO should be performed. In premenopausal patients in whom the uterus is not removed, a dilation and curettage of the uterus should be carried out because of a possible coexistent adenocarcinoma of the endometrium.

Radiotherapy and Chemotherapy There is no evidence to support the use of adjuvant radiation therapy for granulosa cell tumors, although pelvic radiation may help to palliate isolated pelvic recurrences.[342,343] Furthermore, it is unclear that adjuvant chemotherapy will prevent recurrence of disease.[344] However, metastatic lesions and recurrences have been treated with a variety of different chemotherapeutic agents and historically responses have been reported using a number drugs and regimens antineoplastic drugs including VAC and PAC.[345] The actinomycin D, 5-fluorouracil, and cyclophosphamide (AcFuCy) regimen has been used in the past by the GOG and has been associated with approximately a 20% response rate.[342,343] Response rates of about 30% have been reported shown with paclitaxel as a single-agent paclitaxel.[346] The combination of bleomycin, etoposide and platinum is also very active and produced responses in 45%.[343] The use of hormonal agents, such as progestins or anti-estrogens, has been suggested, but there are no data available.[347,348]

The rarity of these tumors has made it impossible to conduct well-designed randomized studies assessing the value of therapy for patients with stage II to IV disease. In retrospective series, postoperative chemotherapy has been associated with a prolonged PFI in women with stage III/IV disease,[343] but a survival benefit has not been shown. Despite the absence of data supporting a survival benefit, some experts recommend postoperative chemotherapy for women with completely resected stage II to IV disease because of the high-risk of disease progression and the potential for long-term survival after platinum-based chemotherapy.[343,344] Among the acceptable options are BEP, EP, PAC, or carboplatin and paclitaxel.

For patients with suboptimally cytoreduced disease, BEP has produced overall response rates of 58% to 83%.[343,344] In one study, 14 of 38 patients (37%) with advanced disease undergoing second-look laparotomy following four courses of BEP had negative findings.[349] With a median follow-up of 3 years, 11 (69%) of 16 patients with primary advanced disease and 21 (51%) of 41 patients with recurrent disease were progression free.[344] There is a need to develop less toxic and equally active regimens for this older group of patients. Paclitaxel is an active agent and the combination of platinum with a taxane has been reported to have a response rate of 60% which makes it a more viable alternative.[346]

Hormonal Therapy About 30% of granulosa cell tumors have estrogen receptors and 100% have PRs.[347] Hormonal agents such as progestins or luteinizing hormone-releasing hormone (LHRH) agonists are therapeutic options, but there are very limited data to suggest effectiveness or who to treat. Small clinical series and case reports indicated that luteinizing hormone-releasing hormone agonists had a 50% response rate in 13 patients [343] while 4 of 5 patients in the literature were reported to respond to a progestational agent.[349] Freeman[348] recently reported two cases of patients with recurrent adult granulosa cell tumors who had received multiple treatment modalities including chemotherapy and had previously progressed on leuprolide. Both patients were started on anastrozole with subsequent normalization of inhibin B levels and clinical exams and have been maintained on treatment for 14 and 18 months, respectively. The numbers are too small to draw any conclusions and it is likely that there has been significant publication bias with more people reporting responses to treatment.

Prognosis Granulosa cell tumors have a prolonged natural history and a tendency for late relapse, reflecting their low-grade. As such, 10-year survivals of about 90% have been reported, with 20-year survivals of 75%.[282,331,350,351] Most histologic types have the same prognosis, but the more poorly differentiated diffuse or sarcomatoid type tends to do worse.[349]

Sertoli-Leydig Cell Tumors

This group of tumors occurs most frequently in the third and fourth decades, with 75% of the lesions seen in women younger than 40 years. They are rare, representing less than 0.2% of ovarian cancers.[282] Sertoli-Leydig cell tumors are usually low-grade malignancies, although a poorly differentiated variety may behave more aggressively.

The tumors typically produce androgens, and clinical virilization is noted in 70% to 85% of patients.[282] Signs of virilization include oligomenorrhea, amenorrhea, breast atrophy, acne, hirsutism, clitoromegaly, a deepening voice, and a receding hairline. Measurement of plasma androgens may reveal an elevated testosterone and androstenedione, with normal or slightly elevated dehydroepiandrosterone sulfate. Rarely, the Sertoli-Leydig tumor can be associated with manifestations of estrogenization, such as, isosexual precocity or irregular or postmenopausal bleeding.

Because these low-grade lesions are only rarely bilateral (under 1%), the usual treatment for patients in their reproductive years is a unilateral oophorectomy or salpingo-oophorectomy and evaluation of the contralateral ovary.[282] In older patients for whom fertility is not an issue, the performance of a hysterectomy and BSO is appropriate. There are insufficient data to document the value of radiation or chemotherapy in patients with persistent disease. The 5-year survival is 70% to 90%, and recurrences thereafter are uncommon.[351] Poorly differentiated lesions account for the majority of fatalities.

Uncommon Ovarian Tumors

There are several types of rare malignant ovarian tumors that together compose about 0.1% of ovarian malignancies. These lesions include small cell carcinomas, lipoid cell tumors, and primary ovarian sarcomas.

Small Cell Carcinomas

This rare tumor occurs at an average of 24 years (range 2-46 years).[352] The tumors are all bilateral. Approximately two-thirds of the tumors are accompanied by paraendocrine hypercalcemia. This tumor accounts for one-half of all of the cases of hypercalcemia associated with ovarian tumors. About 50% of the tumors have spread beyond the ovaries when they are diagnosed.

Management consists of surgery followed by *platinum-based* chemotherapy and or radiation therapy. In addition to the primary treatment of the disease, control of the hypercalcemia may require aggressive hydration, loop diuretics, and the use of bisphosphonates.[352] The prognosis tends to be poor, with most patients dying within 2 years of diagnosis in spite of treatment.

In a collaborative GCIG study of small-cell carcinoma of the ovary, data were collected for 17 patients treated in Australia, Canada and Europe.[353] The median follow-up was13 months for all patients and 35.5 months in surviving patients. Ten patients had FIGO stage I tumors, six stage III tumors and one stage unknown. All underwent surgical resection. Adjuvant platinum-based chemotherapy was given to all patients. Seven received adjuvant radiotherapy with either pelvic and para-aortic radiotherapy, or pelvic and whole abdominal radiotherapy. The median survival for stage I tumors was not reached and was 6 months for stage III tumors. For the ten patients with stage I tumors: six received adjuvant radiotherapy with five alive and disease-free; four received no adjuvant radiotherapy with one alive and disease-free, while three have relapsed with one alive and disease-free after resection. Of the seven patients with stage III or unknown stage tumors, all but one have died. Recurrences were most frequent in the pelvis and the abdomen. Patients receiving salvage treatment with chemotherapy and radiotherapy did poorly. In view of these findings we advocate a multi-modality treatment approach including surgery, chemotherapy with the addition of radiotherapy either sequentially or concurrently.[354] Others have advocated high-dose chemotherapy with stem cell support with a number of long-term survivors reported [353] The optimal approach to management is not known given the rarity of these tumors.

The management of these malignancies consists of surgery followed by platinum-based chemotherapy and/or radiation therapy. In addition to the primary treatment of the disease, control of the hypercalcemia may require aggressive hydration, loop diuretics and the use of phosphates. The prognosis tends to be poor, with most patients dying within 2 years of diagnosis in spite of treatment.

Lipoid Cell Tumor

The lipoid cell tumor is thought to arise in adrenal cortical rests that reside near the ovary. Over 100 cases have been reported, and bilaterality in only a few.[2,282] Most are associated with virilization, and occasionally with obesity, hypertension, and glucose intolerance, reflecting glucocorticoid secretion. Rare cases of hyperestrogenism and isosexual precocity occur.

The majority of lipoid cell tumors have a benign or low-grade behavior, but about 20%, most of which are initially larger than 8 cm in diameter, develop metastatic lesions. Metastases are usually within the peritoneal cavity, and rarely to distant sites.[282] The primary treatment is the surgical extirpation of the primary lesion, and there are no reports of effective radiation or chemotherapy.

Sarcomas

Malignant mixed mesodermal sarcomas of the ovary are rare, and only about 100 cases have been reported.[355-358] Most are heterologous, and 80% occur in postmenopausal women. The presentation is similar to that of most ovarian malignancies, although these tumors are biologically aggressive, and the majority of patients have metastases to organ parenchyma, such as the liver and lung, and to the retroperitoneal lymph nodes.

Such patients should be treated by cytoreductive surgery and postoperative *platinum*-containing combination chemotherapy.[356] Silassi et al.[355] recently reported their experience from Yale in 22 patients all but two of whom presented with advanced-stage disease. The median survival for the entire cohort was 38 months. The median survival was 46 months for 18 optimally debulked (<1 cm) patients and 27 months for 4 patients who were suboptimally debulked (>1 cm). Six patients were treated with optimal cytoreduction and adjuvant cisplatin and ifosfamide and they reported a median PFI of 13 months, and median survival of 51 months.

First-line cisplatin and ifosfamide or carboplatin and paclitaxel can achieve survival rates observed in epithelial ovarian cancer. Leiser et al.[356] reported the Memorial Sloan-Kettering experience with platinum and paclitaxel in 30 patients with carcinosarcomas of the ovary and they also found it was very active. Twelve (40%) had a complete response, 7 (23%) a partial response, 2 (7%) stable disease, and 9 (30%) progression of disease. In the carboplatin and paclitaxel group, the median PFI was 6 months and median survival was 38 months. The difference in survival between the cisplatin and ifosfamide group and the carboplatin and paclitaxel group was not statistically significant (p = 0.48). However, the carboplatin and paclitaxel group had much less toxicity. The median time to progression for responders was 12 months and with a median follow-up of 23 months, the median overall survival was 43 months for survivors. The 3- and 5-year survival rates were 53% and 30%, respectively. The most effective cytotoxic regimen remains to be determined.

Metastatic Tumors

About 5% to 6% of ovarian tumors are metastatic from other organs, most frequently from the female genital tract, the breast, or the GI tract.[359-363] The metastasis may occur from direct extension of another pelvic neoplasm, by hematogenous spread, by lymphatic spread, or by transcoelomic spread, ie, by surface implantation of the peritoneal cavity.

Gynecologic ■ Nonovarian cancers of the genital tract can spread by direct extension or metastasize to the ovaries. Tubal carcinomas involve the ovaries secondarily in 13% of cases usually by direct extension. Under some circumstances, it is difficult to ascertain whether the tumor originates in the tube or in the ovary when both are involved. Cervical cancer spreads to the ovary only in rare cases (<1%), and most of these are of advanced clinical stage or of adenocarcinoma histotype.[282] Although adenocarcinoma of the endometrium can spread and implant directly onto the surface of the ovaries in as many as 5% of cases, two synchronous primaries probably occur with greater frequency. In these cases, there is usually an endometrioid carcinoma of the ovary associated with the adenocarcinoma of the endometrium. Malignant melanoma rarely can metastasize to the ovaries.[361]

Nongynecologic ■ The reported frequency of metastatic breast carcinoma to the ovaries varies, but the phenomenon is common.[360,363] In autopsy data of women who die of metastatic breast cancer, the ovaries are involved in 24% of cases and 80% of the involvement is bilateral.[360] Similarly, when ovaries are removed to palliate advanced breast cancer, about 20% to 30% of cases reveal ovarian involvement, 60% bilaterally. The involvement of ovaries in early-stage breast cancer appears to be considerably lower, but precise figures are not available. In almost all cases, ovarian involvement either is occult or a pelvic mass is discovered after other metastatic disease becomes apparent.

Krukenberg ■ The Krukenberg tumor accounts for 30% to 40% of metastatic cancers to the ovaries and for 1% to 2% of all malignant ovarian tumors reported at some institutions. It involves the ovarian stroma and has characteristic mucin filled, signet ring cells. The primary tumor is most often from the stomach, but less commonly from the colon, breast, or biliary tract, and rarely, from the cervix or bladder. Most are bilateral. The lesions may not be discovered until the primary disease is advanced, and most patients die of their disease within a year. In some cases, a primary tumor is not found.

In other cases of metastasis from the GI tract to the ovary, the tumor does not have the classic histologic appearance of Krukenberg tumor, and most of these are from the colon and, less commonly, the small intestine.[359] As many as 1% to 2% of women with intestinal carcinomas will develop metastases to the ovaries during the course of their disease.[360] Prior to exploration for an adnexal tumor in a woman older than 40 years, a barium enema is indicated to exclude a primary GI carcinoma with metastases to the ovaries. Metastatic colon cancer can mimic a mucinous cystadenocarcinoma of the ovary.[282,360]

Carcinoid ■ Metastatic carcinoid tumors are rare, representing less than 2% of metastatic lesions to the ovaries.[364] Conversely, only about 2% of primary carcinoids have evidence of ovarian metastasis, and only 40% of these patients have the carcinoid syndrome at the time of discovery of the metastatic carcinoid. Therefore, in perimenopausal and postmenopausal women with an intestinal carcinoid, it is reasonable to remove the ovaries to prevent subsequent metastasis. The discovery of an ovarian carcinoid should prompt a careful search for a primary intestinal lesion.

Lymphoma and Leukemia ■ Lymphoma and leukemia can involve the ovary, and when they do, the involvement is usually bilateral.[365] Less than 5% of patients with Hodgkin disease develop lymphomatous involvement of the ovaries, and then typically only with advanced-stage disease. With Burkitt lymphoma, ovarian involvement is very common. Other types of non-Hodgkin lymphoma involve the ovaries more frequently than Hodgkin disease, but leukemic infiltration of the ovaries is uncommon. Sometimes the ovaries can be the only apparent sites of involvement of the abdominal or pelvic viscera with non-Hodgkin lymphoma, and if this circumstance is found, a careful surgical staging is necessary. If a frozen section of a solid ovarian mass reveals a lymphoma, the patient needs a careful operative evaluation, including a palpation of the entire intra-abdominal contents. Treatment for the lymphoma or leukemia involves the use of chemotherapy and/or radiotherapy appropriate for the specific type of primary lesion. Consideration should be given to removal of significantly enlarged ovarian disease to palliate symptoms and possibly to facilitate a response to treatment.

Selected References

The complete reference list can be found at www.CANCERMEDICINE8.com

1. Jemal A, Siegel R, Ward E, et al. Cancer statistics, 2008. *Cancer J Clin.* 2008;58:71–96.
2. Scully RE, Young RH, Clement PB. *Tumors of the ovary, maldeveloped gonads, fallopian tube, and broad ligament.* Third Series, Fascicle 23. Washington, DC: Armed Forces Institute of Pathology; 1998.
8. Franceschi S, La Vecchia C, Booth M, et al. Pooled analysis of three European case-control studies of epithelial ovarian cancer: II. Age at menarche and menopause. *Int J Cancer.* 1991;49:57–60.
9. Negri E, Franceschi S, Tzonou A, et al. Pooled analysis of three European case-control studies of epithelial ovarian cancer: I. Reproductive factors and risk of epithelial ovarian cancer. *Int J Cancer.* 1991;49:50–56.
12. Ness RB, Cramer DW, Goodman MT, et al. Infertility, fertility drugs and ovarian cancer: a pooled analysis of case control studies. *Am J Epidemiol.* 2002;155:217–224.
19. Centers for Disease Control Cancer and Steroid Hormone Study. Oral contraceptives and the risk of ovarian cancer. 1983;249:1596–1607.
23. Kauff ND, Satagopan JM, Robson ME, et al. Risk-reducing salpingo-oophorectomy in women with a BRCA1 or BRCA2 mutation. *New Engl J Med.* 2002;346:1609–1615.
24. Rebbeck TR, Lynch HT, Neuhausen SL, et al. Prophylactic oophorectomy in carriers of BRCA1 or BRCA2 mutations. *New Engl J Med.* 2002;346:1616–1622.
30. Chetrit A, Hirsh-Yechezkel G, Ben-David Y, Lubin F, Friedman E, Sadetzki S Effect of BRCA1/2 mutations on long-term survival of patients with invasive ovarian cancer: the national Israeli study of ovarian cancer. *J Clin Oncol.* 2008 Jan 1;26(1):20–25.
31. Burke W, Daly M, Garber J, et al. Recommendations for follow-up care of individuals with an inherited predisposition to cancer. II. BRCA1 and BRCA2. *Cancer Genetics Studies Consortium.* 1997;277:997–1003.
38. Narod SA, Risch H, Moslehi R, et al. Oral contraceptives and the risk of hereditary ovarian cancer. *N Engl J Med.* 1998;339:424–428.
41. Berek JS. Epithelial ovarian cancer. In: Berek JS, Hacker NF, eds. *Practical Gynecologic Oncology.* 4th ed. Philadelphia: Lippincott Williams & Wilkins; 2005.
42. Heintz APM, Odicino F, Maisonneuve P, et al. Carcinoma of the ovary. 25th Annual report on the results of treatment of gynaecological cancer, International Federation of Gynecology and Obstetrics. Int *J Gynecol Obstet.* 2003;83:135–166.
48. Jacobs IJ, Kohler MF, Wiseman R, et al. Clonal origin of epithelial ovarian cancer: analysis by loss of heterozygosity, p53 mutation and X chromosome inactivation. *J Natl Cancer Inst.* 1992;84:1793.
72. Bast RC Jr, Mills GB. Molecular pathogenesis of epithelial ovarian cancer. In: Mendelsohn J, Howley, Israel M, Gray JW, Thompson CB, eds. *The Molecular Basis of Cancer,* 3rd edition. Philadelphia: Saunders-Elsevier; 2008:441–454.

82. Bast RC Jr, Klug TL, St. John E, et al. A radioimmunoassay using a monoclonal antibody to monitor the course of epithelial ovarian cancer. *N Engl J Med.* 1983; 309:883–887.
84. Yin BW, Lloyd KO. Molecular cloning of the CA125 ovarian cancer antigen: identification as a new mucin, MUC16. *J Biol Chem.* 2001:27371–27375.
87. Cheng W, Liu J, Yoshida H, et al. Lineage infidelity of epithelial ovarian cancers is controlled by *HOX* genes that specify regional identity in the reproductive tract. *Nat Med.* 2005;11:531.
95. Goff BA, Mandel LS, Drescher CW, et al. Development of an ovarian cancer symptom index: possibilities for earlier detection. *Cancer.* 2007 Jan 15;109(2):221–227.
101. Das PM, Bast RC Jr. Early detection of ovarian cancer. *Biomarkers Med.* 2008; In press.
110. Jacobs IJ, Skates SJ, MacDonald N, et al. Screening for ovarian cancer: a pilot randomized controlled trial. *Lancet.* 1999:1207–1210.
124. Burke W, Daly M, Garber J, et al. Recommendations for follow-up care of individuals with an inherited predisposition to cancer. II. BRCA1 and BRCA2. Cancer Genetics Studies Consortium. *JAMA.* 1997;277:997–1003.
129. Hermsen BB, Olivier RI, Verheijen RH, et al. No efficacy of annual gynaecological screening in BRCA1/2 mutation carriers; an observational follow-up study. *Br J Cancer.* 2007 May 7;96(9):1335–1342.
131. Greene MH, Piedmonte M, Alberts D, et al. A prospective study of risk-reducing salpingo-oophorectomy and longitudinal CA-125 screening among women at increased genetic risk of ovarian cancer: design and baseline characteristics: a Gynecologic Oncology Group study. *Cancer Epidemiol Biomarkers Prev.* 2008 Mar;17(3):594–604.
139. Bell J, Brady MF, Young RC, et al. Randomized phase III trial of three versus six cycles of adjuvant carboplatin and paclitaxel in early stage epithelial ovarian carcinoma: a Gynecologic Oncology Group study.
140. Trimbos JB, Vergote I, Bolis G, et al. Impact of adjuvant chemotherapy and surgical staging in early-stage ovarian carcinoma: European Organisation for Research and Treatment of Cancer—Adjuvant Chemotherapy in Ovarian Neoplasm Trial. *J Natl Cancer Inst.* 2003;95:113–125.
141. International Collaborative Ovarian Neoplasm (ICON1) Collaborators. International collaborative ovarian neoplasm trial 1: a randomized trial of adjuvant chemotherapy in women with early-stage ovarian cancer. *J Natl Cancer Inst.* 2003;95:125–132.
142. Trimbos JB, Parmar M, Vergote I, et al. International Collaborative Ovarian Neoplasm Trail 1 and Adjuvant Chemotherapy. In: Ovarian Neoplasm Trial: two parallel randomized phase III trials of adjuvant chemotherapy in patients with early-stage ovarian carcinoma. *J Natl Cancer Inst.* 2003;95:105–112.
157. Bristow RE, Tomacruz RS, Armstrong DK, et al. Survival effect of maximal cytoreductive surgery for advanced ovarian carcinoma during the platinum era: a meta-analysis. *J Clin Oncol.* 2002;20:1248–1259.
158. van der Burg MEL, van Lent M, Buyse M, et al. The effect of debulking surgery after induction chemotherapy on the prognosis in advanced epithelial ovarian cancer. *N Engl J Med.* 1995;332:629–634.
174. Ozols RF, Bundy BN, Greer B, et al. Phase III trial of carboplatin and paclitaxel compared with cisplatin and paclitaxel in patients with optimally resected stage III ovarian cancer. *J Clin Oncol.* 2003;21:3194–3200.
175. Du Bois A, Lueck HJ, Meier W, et al. A randomized clinical trial of cisplatin/paclitaxel versus carboplatin/paclitaxel as first-line treatment of ovarian cancer. *J Natl Cancer Inst.* 2003;95:1320–1330.
176. The International Collaborative Ovarian Neoplasm (ICON) Group. Paclitaxel plus carboplatin versus standard chemotherapy with either single agent carboplatin or cyclophosphamide, doxorubicin and cisplatin: in women with ovarian cancer: the ICON3 randomised trial. *Lancet.* 2002;360:505–515.
180. Aabo K, Adams M, Adnitt P, et al. Chemotherapy in advanced ovarian cancer: four systematic meta—analyses of individual patient data from 37 randomized trials. Advanced Ovarian Cancer Trialists' Group. *Br J Cancer.* 1998;78:1479–1487.
186. Bookman M for the Gynecological Cancer Intergroup. GOG0182-ICON5: 5-arm phase III randomized trial of paclitaxel (P) and carboplatin (C) vs combinations with gemcitabine (G), PEG-liposomal doxorubicin (D), or topotecan (T) in patients (pts) with advanced-stage epithelial ovarian (EOC) or primary peritoneal (PPC) carcinoma *J Clin Oncol.* 2006 ASCO Annual Meeting Proceedings Part I. Vol 24, No. 18S (June 20 Supplement), 2006: 5002.
187. Alberts DS, Liu PY, Hannigan EV, et al. Intraperitoneal cisplatin plus intravenous cyclophosphamide versus intravenous cisplatin plus intravenous cyclophosphamide for stage III ovarian cancer. *N Engl J Med.* 1996;335:1950–1955.
188. Markman M, Bundy B, Benda J, et al. Randomized phase III study of intravenous cisplatin/paclitaxel versus moderately high dose intravenous carboplatin followed by intraperitoneal paclitaxel and intraperitoneal cisplatin in optimal residual ovarian cancer: an Intergroup trial (GOG, SWOG, ECOG). *J Clin Oncol.* 2001;19:921–923.
189. Armstrong D, Bundy B, Wenzel L, et al. Intraperitoneal cisplatin and paclitaxel in ovarian cancer. *New Engl J Med.* 2006; 354:34–53.
191. Hess LM, Benham-Hutchins M, Herzog TJ, et al. A meta-analysis of the efficacy of intraperitoneal cisplatin for the front-line treatment of ovarian cancer. *Int J Gynecol Cancer.* 2007 May-Jun;17(3):561–570.
192. Jaaback K, Johnson N. Intraperitoneal chemotherapy for the initial management of primary epithelial ovarian cancer. *Cochrane Database Syst Rev.* 2006 Jan 25;(1): Intraperitoneal chemotherapy in ovarian cancer remains experimental.
204. Greer BE, Bundy BN, Ozols RF, et al. Implications of second-look laparotomy in the context of optimally resected stage III ovarian cancer: a non-randomized comparison using an explanatory analysis: a Gynecologic Oncology Group study. *Gynecol Oncol.* 2005 Oct;99(1):71–79.
214. Thomas GM. Is there a role for consolidation or salvage radiotherapy after chemotherapy in advanced epithelial ovarian cancer? *Gynecol Oncol.* 1993;51:97–98.
218. Fung-Kee-Fung M, Oliver T, Elit L, Oza A, Hirte HW, Bryson P. Optimal chemotherapy treatment for women with recurrent ovarian cancer. *Curr Oncol.* 2007;14:195–207.
219. Blackledge G, Lawton F, Redman C, Kelly K. Response of patients in phase II studies of chemotherapy in ovarian cancer: implications for patient treatment and the design of phase II trials. *Br J Cancer.* 1989;59:650–653.
220. Gore ME, Fryatt I, Wiltshaw E, Dawson T. Treatment of relapsed carcinoma of the ovary with cisplatin or carboplatin following initial treatment with these compounds. *Gynecol Oncol.* 1990;36:207–210.
221. Markman M, Rothman R, Hakes T, et al. Second-line platinum chemotherapy in patients with ovarian cancer previously treated with cisplatin. *J Clin Oncol.* 1991;9:389–393.
223. Parmar MK, Ledermann JA, Colombo N, et al. Paclitaxel plus platinum-based chemotherapy versus conventional platinum-based chemotherapy in women with relapsed ovarian cancer: the ICON4/AGO-OVAR-2.2 trial. *Lancet.* 2003;361: 2099–2106.
224. Gonzalez-Martin AA, Calvo E, Bover I, et al. Randomised phase II study of carboplatin versus paclitaxel-carboplatin in platinum-sensitive recurrent advanced ovarian carcinoma with assessment of quality of life: a GEICO study (Spanish Group for Investigation on Ovarian Carcinoma) (abst). *Proc Am Soc Clin Oncol.* 2003;22 (abst 1812) (update).
242. Gordon AN, Fleagle JT, Guthrie D, et al. Recurrent epithelial ovarian carcinoma: a randomized phase III study of pegylated liposomal doxorubicin versus topotecan. *J Clin Oncol.* 2001;19:3312–3322.
259. Windbichler GH, Hausmaninger H, Stummvoll W, et al. Interferon-gamma in the first-line therapy of ovarian cancer: a randomized phase III trial. *Br J Cancer.* 2000;82: 1138–1144.
267. Burger RA, Sill MW, Monk BJ, Greer BE, Sorosky JI. Phase II trial of bevacizumab in persistent or recurrent epithelial ovarian cancer or primary peritoneal cancer: a Gynecologic Oncology Group Study. *J Clin Oncol.* 2007 Nov 20;25(33):5165–5171.
294. Williams SD, Blessing JA, Hatch K, Homesley HD. Chemotherapy of advanced ovarian dysgerminoma: trials of the Gynecologic Oncology Group. *J Clin Oncol.* 1991;9:1950–1955.
295. Williams SD, Blessing JA, Liao S, et al. Adjuvant therapy of ovarian germ cell tumors with cisplatin, etoposide, and bleomycin: a trial of the Gynecologic Oncology Group. *J Clin Oncol.* 1994;12:701–706.
305. Ulbright, T, Germ cell tumors of the gonads: a selective review emphasizing problems in differential diagnosis, newly appreciated, and controversial issues. *Mod Pathol.* 2005 Feb;18(Suppl 2):S61–S79. Review. PMID: 15761467 [PubMed - indexed for MEDLINE]
312. Heifetz SA, Cushing B, Giller R, et al. Immature teratomas in children: pathologic considerations: a report from the combined Pediatric Oncology Group/Children's Cancer Group.*Am J Surg Pathol.* 1998 Sep;22(9):1115–1124. PMID: 9737245 [PubMed - indexed for MEDLINE].

102 Molar Pregnancy and Gestational Trophoblastic Neoplasia

Donald P. Goldstein, MD ■ Ross S. Berkowitz, MD

Molar pregnancy and gestational trophoblastic neoplasia (GTN) comprise a group of interrelated diseases that includes complete and partial hydatidiform mole, invasive mole, placental site trophoblastic tumor (PSTT), and choriocarcinoma (CCA). Gestational trophoblastic neoplasms are one of the rare human malignancies that are highly curable, even with widespread metastases.[1,2] Molar pregnancy and GTN produce a distinct tumor marker, the beta subunit of human chorionic gonadotropin (B-hCG). Complete and partial moles are noninvasive, localized tumors that develop as a result of an aberrant fertilization event that leads to a proliferative process. The other trophoblastic tumors represent malignant disease because of their potential for local invasion and metastases. GTN most commonly develops from a molar pregnancy, but can rise *de novo* after any gestation: spontaneous or induced abortion, ectopic, preterm, or term pregnancy.

Most patients with GTN can now anticipate a high cure rate with appropriate therapy and follow-up. Because remission can often be achieved while retaining fertility, many patients have normal subsequent pregnancies. However, patients with protracted delays in diagnosis, particularly after non-molar pregnancies, still present with extensive tumor burdens and are at substantial risk for treatment failure and death. Efforts are, therefore, needed to alert clinicians about the importance of early diagnosis and to develop effective and less toxic chemotherapy regimens.

Epidemiology

The reported incidence of GTN varies substantially in different regions of the world.[3] The incidence of molar pregnancy in Asian countries is 3–10 times greater than the reported incidence in North America or Europe.[4] Variations in the incidence rates of molar pregnancy partly result from differences between reporting hospital-based versus population-based data. The incidence of complete and partial mole has been determined in Ireland by studying all products of conception from spontaneous abortions.[5] Based on a thorough pathologic review, the incidence of complete and partial mole was found to be 1:1,945 and 1:695 pregnancies, respectively.

The high incidence of molar pregnancy in some populations has been attributed to socioeconomic and nutritional factors. Case-control studies have observed that the risk for complete hydatidiform mole (CHM) progressively increased with decreasing levels of consumption of dietary carotene (vitamin A precursor) and animal fat.[6,7] Global regions with a high incidence of vitamin A deficiency correspond to areas with a high frequency of molar pregnancy. Dietary factors such as carotene may therefore partly explain the regional variations in the incidence of molar pregnancy.

Risk Factors

The two main risk factors for molar pregnancy and GTN are extremes of maternal age (especially over 35 and under 16) and a history of previous mole or GTN.[8,9] Parazzini and colleagues noted that the risk for complete mole was increased 2-fold for women older than age 35 years and 7.5-fold for women older than age 40 years.[10] Ova from older women may be more susceptible to abnormal fertilizations. Nevertheless, most cases of molar disease and GTN occur in women under 35 because of the greater number of pregnancies in this age group. The risk for partial mole has not been associated with maternal age.

Studies from the United States and England have found that women with a history of 1 molar pregnancy or GTN have an approximately 1% chance of recurrence in subsequent pregnancies, compared to a 0.1% incidence in the general population. The recurrence rate after 2 molar pregnancies is approximately 25%.[11–15]

Etiology

Complete moles usually have a 46,XX karyotype, and all molar chromosomes are derived from paternal origin (androgenetic).[16] Most complete moles arise from an anuclear ovum that is fertilized by a haploid sperm, which then duplicates its own chromosomes.[17] While most complete moles have a 46,XX karyotype, approximately 10% have a 46,XY chromosomal pattern.[18] The 46,XY complete mole arises from fertilization of an anuclear ovum by 2 spermatozoa. While the chromosomes in the complete mole are entirely of paternal origin, the mitochondrial deoxyribonucleic acid (DNA) is of maternal origin.[19]

Partial hydatidiform moles (PHM) generally have a triploid karyotype resulting from fertilization of an apparently normal ovum by 2 spermatozoa (dispermy).[20] Lage and colleagues and Lawler et al reported that 93% and 90%, respectively, of partial moles were triploid.[21,22] Fetuses with partial moles generally have the stigmata of triploidy, including multiple congenital anomalies and growth retardation. Both complete and partial moles are therefore characterized by an excessive amount of paternal chromosomes, which may induce trophoblastic hyperplasia.

Histopathologic Classification of GTD

Hydatidiform mole may be categorized as either complete or partial based on gross morphology, histopathology, and karyotype.[23] Complete moles have diffuse swelling of the chorionic villi and diffuse trophoblastic hyperplasia. Embryonic or fetal tissues are not identifiable (Figs. 102-1 and 102-2). Partial moles are characterized by the presence of 2 populations of chorionic villi. Some chorionic villi exhibit focal swelling and focal trophoblastic hyperplasia, as well as villous scalloping and stromal trophoblastic inclusions. Fetal and embryonic tissues are commonly present. Locally invasive or metastatic GTN that develops after either a complete or partial mole can have the histologic features of either molar tissue or CCA.

CCA does not contain chorionic villi, but is composed of sheets of both anaplastic cyto- and syncytiotrophoblasts (Fig. 102-3). Although CCA is most commonly preceded by a CHM, it may develop after any gestation. After a non-molar

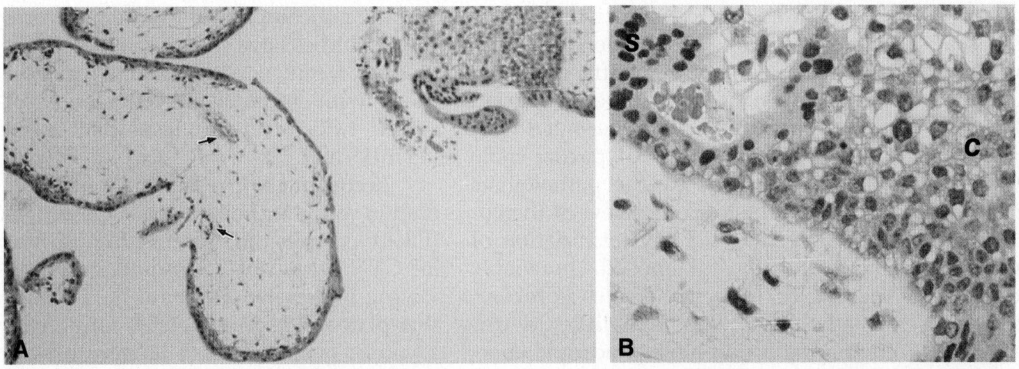

Figure 102-1 First trimester abortion. (**A**) Chorionic villi containing fetal blood vessels *(arrows)* in edematous stroma, lined by 2 layers of trophoblastic cells. Note unipolar trophoblastic proliferation. (H&E; ×100) (**B**) Polar trophoblastic proliferation of cytotrophoblast *(c)* and syncytiotrophoblast *(s)*. (H&E; ×400) *Source:* Courtesy of Liane Deligdisch, MD, Mount Sinai Medical Center, New York.

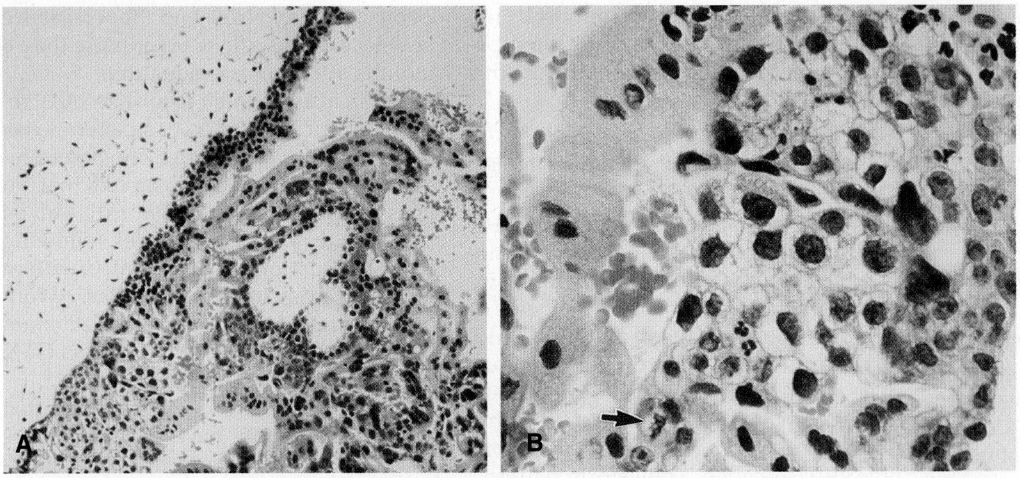

Figure 102-2 Hydatidiform mole. (**A**) Chorionic villi with edema and hydropic degeneration (central cistern; *top left)*. Trophoblastic proliferation is circumferential rather than polar. (H&E; ×100) (**B**) Marked proliferation of cytotrophoblastic and syncytiotrophoblast showing nuclear atypia and mitotic activity *(arrows)*. (H&E; ×400) *Source:* Courtesy of Liane Deligdisch, MD, Mount Sinai Medical Center, New York.

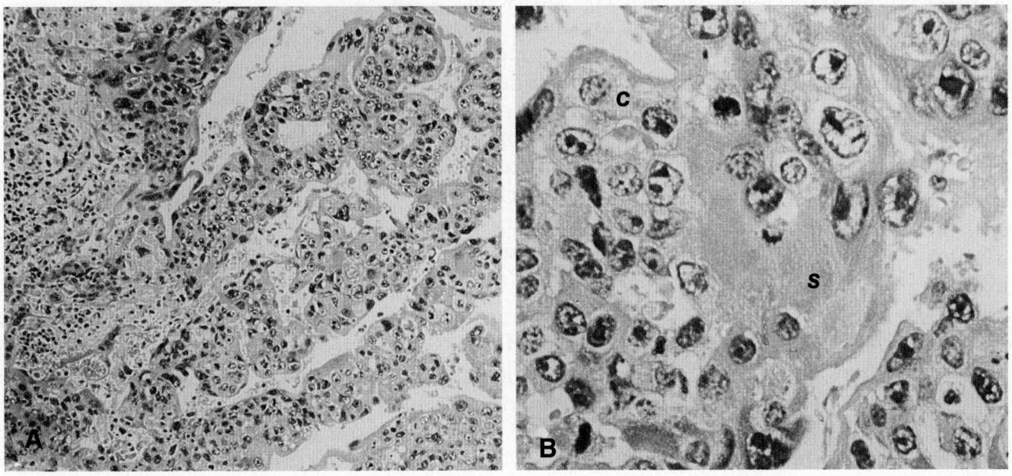

Figure 102-3 Choriocarcinoma. (**A**) No villous structure is present. Tumor shows necrosis and hemorrhage at left. (H&E; ×100) (**B**) Biphasic tumor pattern composed of severely atypical cytotrophoblasts *(c)* and syncytiotrophoblastic *(s)* cells with high mitotic activity. (H&E; ×400) *Source:* Courtesy of Liane Deligdisch, MD, Mount Sinai Medical Center, New York.

pregnancy, persistent GTN usually has the histologic pattern of CCA, but rarely can be present as PSTT. CCA is a highly vascular tumor that disseminates via the blood stream initially to the lungs. Distant sites such as the brain, liver, kidney, gastrointestinal tract, and spleen usually are late manifestations of the disease in patients where there has been a delay in diagnosis.

PSTT is an uncommon variant of CCA, which is composed almost entirely of mononuclear intermediate trophoblast and does not contain chorionic villi.[24] PSTT tends to infiltrate the myometrium, increasing the likelihood of lymphatic spread. In contrast to CCA, metastases are a late manifestation of the disease.

Molecular Pathogenesis

While the precise molecular pathogenesis of molar pregnancy and CCA has not been determined, various growth factors and oncogenes have been studied in these tissues.[25,26] Complete mole and CCA are characterized by overexpression of cmyc, cerbB-2, bcl- 2, TP53, and Rb. These oncoproteins may be important in the pathogenesis of GTN.[27,28] Strong immunostaining of epidermal growth factor receptor and c-erbB-3 in the extravillous trophoblast of complete mole was found to significantly correlate with the development of post-molar tumor.[29]

Familial recurrent molar pregnancy is an infrequent occurrence, but may provide important insights into the molecular biology and genetic pathogenesis of molar pregnancy.[30] 12 families have been reported in which at least 2 close relatives have had molar pregnancies, and consanguinity was observed in about half of the families. Affected women have had 152 pregnancies resulting in 113 (74 %) complete moles, 26 (17 %) spontaneous abortions, 6 (4 %) partial moles, and only 7 (5%) normal pregnancies. Strikingly, the complete moles in these patients were biparental with 1 haploid set of both maternal and paternal chromosomes. In normal gestations, certain genes are parentally imprinted such that they are normally expressed only on the maternal or paternal alleles. Although these moles were biparental, the molar tissue did not express maternally transcribed genes like p57 KIP2 similar to the more usual androgenetic complete moles. Dysregulation of normal parental imprinting of genes with the loss of maternally transcribed genes is likely to be an important event in the pathogenesis of complete mole. Linkage and homozygosity mapping in a large consanguineous family enabled the gene for familial recurrent mole to be mapped to a 1.1 Mb region on chromosome 19 q 13.4.[31] Mutation in this gene or genes likely result in dysregulation of genetic imprinting in the female germ line with abnormal development of extraembryonic and embryonic tissues.

Clinical Presentation and Diagnosis

Clinical Presentation of Complete Mole

Vaginal bleeding is the most common presenting symptom in patients with complete mole, occurring in 97% of the patients.[32] Because the diagnosis of molar pregnancy is being made earlier, patients now less commonly present with signs of marked trophoblastic proliferation, including excessive uterine enlargement, theca lutein ovarian cysts, and toxemia.[33] Theca lutein cysts result from ovarian hyperstimulation due to high serum levels of hCG.

Patients with CHM who present with excessive uterine enlargement and high hCG values are at increased risk for medical complications such as toxemia, hyperthyroidism, and respiratory insufficiency. Patients with "high risk" complete mole also have an increased risk of developing GTN. Because of the homology between the beta-subunits of hCG and TSH, hCG has been shown to have weak thyroid-stimulating activity.[34,35] Although patients who present with markedly elevated levels of hCG may exhibit chemical signs of hyperthyroidism, they do not have severe manifestations of hyperthyroidism such as seen in Graves disease. Nonetheless, patients have been noted to develop thyroid storm because of anesthesia induction. The cause of respiratory insufficiency is usually multifactorial, including trophoblastic embolization, and the cardiopulmonary effects of toxemia, hyperthyroidism, and vigorous transfusion therapy.

Clinical Presentation of Partial Mole

Patients with a PHM usually present with the signs and symptoms of missed or incomplete abortion. Excessive uterine enlargement is noted in only 4–11%.[36,37] We reviewed 81 consecutive patients with partial mole and none of the patients had respiratory insufficiency, hyperthyroidism, or prominent ovarian theca lutein cysts. Only 2 presented with toxemia. The diagnosis of partial mole is frequently made by the pathologists after careful histologic review of the curettage specimens. Early termination of sonographically diagnosed nonviable pregnancies frequently creates a problem for pathologists who have difficulty differentiating a non-molar hydropic abortion from an early PHM or CHM. The use of flow cytometry and immunostaining for maternally expressed, imprinted paternal genes can be very helpful in this differential diagnosis.[38]

Role of Ultrasonography in the Diagnosis of Molar Pregnancy

Complete molar pregnancy is reliably diagnosed by ultrasonography. Sonographic features of complete mole include: (1) the absence of an embryo or fetus; (2) the absence of amniotic fluid; (3) the presence of a central heterogenous mass with numerous discrete anechoic spaces, which correspond to diffuse hydatidiform swelling of the hydropic chorionic villi (so-called "snowstorm pattern"; and (4) theca lutein cysts. The ultrasonic features of a partial mole are much less specific and may be absent. Sonographic features of a partial mole may include: (1) a fetus, which may or may not be viable, but is often growth retarded and abnormal; (2) increased transverse diameter of the gestational sac; and (3) focal anechoic spaces and/or increased echogenicity of chorionic villi; (4) absence of theca lutein cysts.[39]

Clinical Presentation of Post-Molar GTN

After molar evacuation, all patients must be monitored for development of post-molar GTN, defined as those patients who develop persistently elevated hCG levels, require chemotherapy and/or excisional surgery, or have evidence of metastases. In order to rule out the development of post-molar tumor, patients should be monitored with weekly hCG levels until normal for 3 consecutive weeks. Approximately 50% of patients achieve normal hCG levels in 6–14 weeks after molar evacuation.[40] Moreover, patients with complete and partial molar pregnancy were followed with monthly hCG levels for a total of 6 months after achieving 3 consecutive normal weekly values. Many patients find the 6-month period of follow-up difficult to complete. Many women, particularly those over 35, are anxious to begin attempting another pregnancy. Furthermore, gonadotropin follow-up is anxiety-provoking for many women, expensive, and inconvenient, making noncompliance common. Several recent studies have shown that persistent disease rarely occurs (<1/1000) among those with spontaneous regression of serum hCG levels to less than assay (<5 mIU/mL).[41–43]

According to the International Federation of Gynecology and Obstetrics (FIGO) criteria, the presence of post-molar GTN should be diagnosed if the following is present: (1) serum hCG values that plateau (decline of <10% for at least 4 values over 3 weeks); (2) serum hCG levels rise (increase more than 10% over 2 consecutive weeks); and (3) persistence of detectable serum hCG for more than 6 months after molar evacuation.

It is also possible to utilize hCG regression curves to predict a patient's risk of developing GTN after molar evacuation. Growden et al observed that an hCG level greater than 199 mIU/mL in the third through eighth week following PHM evacuation was associated with at least a 35% risk of GTN.[44] Similarly, Wolfberg et al reported that post-evacuation hCG levels could be used to predict GTN within 3 weeks of CHM evacuation.[45]

It is important to emphasize that some patients may have a false positive elevation in their serum hCG concentration due to a number of factors other than GTN. Patients with elevated hCG values should also be considered potentially to have a pregnancy, germ cell tumor of the ovary or other site, a non-trophoblastic gonadotropin-producing tumor (eg, hepatoma), or phantom hCG caused by heterophilic antibody.[46] Post-menopausal women have also been reported with detectable hCG levels of pituitary origin, which can be suppressed by hormone replacement therapy.[47]

Complete moles develop uterine invasion or metastasis in about 15% and 4% of patients, respectively.[48] The risk for post-molar tumor is substantially increased in complete moles with signs of marked trophoblastic proliferation such as excessive uterine size, high serum hCG levels (>100,000 mIU/mL), and theca lutein ovarian cysts. Following evacuation, 31% of these patients developed uterine invasion and 9% developed metastases. The risk of developing post-molar GTN is considerably less for patients without signs of marked trophoblastic growth. After evacuation, only 3.4% of these patients developed invasion and 0.6% developed metastases. Therefore, patients with complete moles, excessive uterine size, and markedly elevated hCG values are categorized as high risk. Older patients with complete moles are also at increased risk of developing a post-molar tumor. Tow and Tsukamoto et al reported that 37% of women older than age 40 years and 56% of women older than age 50 years, respectively, developed persistent tumor after a complete mole.[49,50] Approximately 1–4% of patients with PHM develop persistent tumor, which is generally non-metastatic.[51] Patients who develop GTN following PHM do not have distinguishing clinical or pathologic characteristics.[52]

Clinical Presentation of Non-Metastatic GTN

Locally invasive GTN also occur, albeit infrequently, after non-molar pregnancies.[48] These patients may present with persistently elevated hCG levels, irregular vaginal bleeding, uterine subinvolution, or asymmetric uterine enlargement. Theca lutein ovarian cysts are rare in the absence of high levels of hCG (>100,000 mIU/mL). The trophoblastic tumor may erode into uterine vessels, causing vaginal hemorrhage, or may perforate through the myometrium, producing intra-abdominal bleeding. Bulky necrotic tumors in the endometrial cavity may also serve as a nidus for sepsis, causing pelvic pain and purulent discharge.

Presentation of Metastatic GTN

Metastases develop in approximately 4% of patients after complete mole and infrequently after other gestations.[48] When metastases occur, the pathology is usually CCA because this tumor has a propensity for early vascular invasion and dissemination. The presenting signs and symptoms in these patients depend on the sites of metastasis: hemoptysis from lung lesions, shock from intraperitoneal bleeding from ruptured liver metastases, acute neurologic deficits from intracranial hemorrhage, etc.

The most common site of metastasis is the lungs. 80% patients with metastatic GTN have pulmonary involvement on chest radiographs or computed tomography (CT). Because respiratory symptoms and radiographic findings may be striking, the patient may be thought to have a primary pulmonary process before the diagnosis of GTN is made. Pulmonary hypertension can develop as a result of pulmonary arterial occlusion by trophoblastic emboli. The development of early respiratory failure requiring intubation is associated with a dismal outcome.[53] Gynecologic symptoms may be minimal or absent even when the patient has extensive metastatic disease. *The diagnosis of GTN should be considered in any woman in the reproductive age group with unexplained pulmonary or systemic symptoms.*

Vaginal metastases are present in 30% of patients with metastatic GTN. Because these lesions are highly vascular, they may bleed vigorously if biopsied.

Hepatic and cerebral metastases occur in approximately 10% of patients with metastatic GTN. Hepatic and cerebral lesions invariably have the histologic pattern of CCA, and usually follow a non-molar pregnancy. These patients characteristically have protracted delays in diagnosis and extensive tumor burdens. Virtually all patients with hepatic and cerebral metastases have concurrent pulmonary or vaginal involvement.[54,55]

Staging and Risk Assessment

An anatomic staging system for GTN was adopted by the (FIGO) in 1982:

Stage I: Lesion confined to uterus
Stage II: Lesion outside uterus but confined to vagina and pelvis
Stage III: Lung metastases
Stage IV: Other metastatic sites (brain, liver, kidney, gastrointestinal tract, spleen, etc.)

In addition to anatomic staging, the World Health Organization (WHO) has adopted a prognostic scoring system (Table 102-1) that reliably predicts the risk of drug resistance and assists in selecting the appropriate chemotherapeutic regimen.[56,57] Prognostic scores less than 7 are associated with a low risk of resistance to single agent chemotherapy. When the prognostic score is 7 or greater, the patient is considered to be at high risk of developing drug resistance to single agent therapy, and requires intensive combination chemotherapy to attain remission. Patients with Stage I GTN usually have a low-risk score, and those with Stage IV disease generally have a high-risk score. Therefore, the distinction between low and high risk mainly applies to patients with Stages II and III disease.

Management of Molar Pregnancy

The initial management of both complete and partial mole is evacuation of the uterus by suction curettage. Evacuation is indicated for pathologic confirmation of the diagnosis, relief of symptoms, and to prevent complications related to molar disease. Furthermore, this procedure is definitive therapy for the majority of patients. Suction evacuation is the preferred method because it is less likely to result in uterine perforation or intrauterine adhesions than sharp curettage, and evacuates the uterus more completely than medical methods.[32,58–60] Patients who have completed their childbearing may opt for hysterectomy, which eliminates the risk of local invasion, but does not prevent metastases. The adnexa may be retained; if prominent theca lutein cysts are present, these may be drained at the time of surgery. Theca lutein cysts will slowly resolve as hCG levels fall. Prior to surgery, the patient should be evaluated to identify the presence of medical complications such as anemia, toxemia, electrolyte imbalance, or hyperthyroidism.

Prophylactic Chemotherapy for Complete Moles

Several investigators have reported that prophylactic chemotherapy at the time of evacuation of CHM reduces the frequency of post-molar GTN.[51,61,62] Kim and colleagues and Limpongsanurak reported in prospective randomized trials that prophylactic methotrexate (MTX) or actinomycin D (ACTD), reduced the incidence of post-molar tumor from 47% to 14% and from 50% to 14%, respectively, in patients with high-risk complete mole.[63,64] Chemoprophylaxis may be particularly beneficial in patients with high-risk complete moles when hormonal follow-up is either unavailable or unreliable.

Pretreatment Evaluation and Staging of GTN

Patients who have or who are suspected of having GTN including invasive mole, CCA, or PSTT must undergo a thorough evaluation in order to determine their

Table 102-1 Scoring System for Gestational Trophoblastic Tumors Based on Prognostic Factors

	Score[a]			
	0	1	2	4
Age (years)	<-39	>39		
Antecedent pregnancy	Mole	Abortion	Term	
Interval[b]	<4	4–6	7–12	
hCG (IU/L)	$<10^3$	10^3–10^4	10^4–10^5	
ABO groups (female × male)		O × A A × O	B AB	
Largest tumor, including uterine tumor		3–5 cm	5 cm	
Site of metastases		Spleen, kidney	Gastrointestinal tract, liver	Brain
No. of metastases identified		1–4	4–8	>8
Prior chemotherapy			Single drug	2 or more drug

[a]Interval is the time (months) between end of antecedent pregnancy and start of chemotherapy.
[b]The total score for a patient is obtained by adding the individual scores for each prognostic factor. Total score: <4 = low risk; 5–7 = intermediate risk; >- 8 = high risk.
Source: Data from Ref. 50.

stage and risk status, which will guide the clinician in selecting the appropriate treatment protocol (Fig. 102-4). The physical examination should always include a speculum examination of the vagina to detect vaginal implants, which can hemorrhage. Radiographic evaluation should include a pelvic ultrasound to look for evidence of retained trophoblastic tissue in the uterus, and to evaluate the pelvis for local spread. Chest imaging is also required, as the lungs are the most common site of metastatic disease. Chest CT scans are more sensitive than a chest x-ray; pulmonary metastases can detected by chest CT in up to 40% of patients with a negative chest x-ray.[65] However, chest CT is not mandatory since detection of occult pulmonary metastases does not affect the prognostic score or outcome. In the absence of pulmonary and vaginal metastases, brain and liver involvement are rare. Because of improvements in central nervous system scanning technology, the determination of cerebrospinal fluid hCG levels is no longer indicated. As long as the clinical picture is compatible with a diagnosis of GTN, metastatic lesions need not be biopsied for confirmation because of the vascular nature of these implants and the risk of hemorrhage.

Management of Low-Risk GTN

Primary Therapy of Low-Risk GTN

Low risk GTN includes patients with both non-metastatic (Stage I) and metastatic GTN whose prognostic score is less than 7. In patients with Stage I GTN, the selection of primary therapy is based on the patient's desire to preserve fertility. If the patient has completed her childbearing, hysterectomy may be performed, with one course of adjuvant single-agent chemotherapy for treatment of any occult metastases. Either MTX or ACTD can be used, although MTX is preferred because it is better tolerated. The use of adjuvant chemotherapy in this setting has not been shown to increase the risk of peri-operative complications.[60]

Single-agent chemotherapy with sequential MTX/ACTD is the preferred treatment in patients with Stage I GTN who desire to retain fertility, as well as in patients with low-risk metastatic GTN. MTX with folinic acid (MTX-FA) has been the preferred single-agent regimen at the New England Trophoblastic Disease Center (NETDC).[66] MTX-FA induced complete remission in 147 (90.2%) of 163 patients with Stage I GTN and in 15 (68.2%) of 22 patients with low-risk Stages II and III GTN. One course of MTX-FA induced remission in 132 (81.5%) of these patients. Thrombocytopenia (platelets <100,000/mm³), granulocytopenia (white blood cell count <1,500/mm³), and hepatotoxicity (serum glutamic-oxaloacetic transaminase >50 units) developed in only 3 (1.6%), 11 (5.9%), and 26 (14.1%) patients, respectively. ACTD is used as primary therapy in those patients with pre-existing hepatic dysfunction, who develop hepatic toxicity to MTX, or sequentially in those patients who prove resistant to MTX.[67,68]

In contrast, patients with Stage I PSTT should be treated with hysterectomy because it is relatively chemoresistant.[24] However, patients with metastatic PSTT may still achieve remission with intensive combination chemotherapy and surgical intervention.[24]

Single-agent chemotherapy with either MTX or ACTD has achieved excellent and comparable remission rates in both non-metastatic and low-risk metastatic GTT.[2,48] Several protocols using MTX and ACTD have been used effectively in the treatment of GTN, but no study has compared all of these regimens (Tables 102-2 and 102-3).[69–76] Single-agent chemotherapy is administered either at a fixed time interval, or on the basis of the hCG regression curve. At the NETDC, after the first course of single agent is administered, further chemotherapy is withheld as long as the hCG level is falling progressively. A second course of chemotherapy is administered under the following conditions: (1) the hCG level plateaus for more than 3 consecutive weeks, or re-elevates, or (2) the hCG level does not decline by 1 log within 18 days after completing the first treatment. Subsequent courses are administered based on the hCG regression curve. If a patient's hCG level declines less than 1 log, she is considered to be resistant to that drug and an alternative agent is substituted.

Salvage Therapy of Low-Risk GTN

Patients with low-risk GTN who develop resistance to sequential single-agent chemotherapy can usually achieve remission with combination chemotherapy, either MAC (MTX, ACTD, and cyclophosphamide (Table 102-4), or EMACO (etoposide, MTX, ACTD, cyclophosphamide, and Oncovin (Table 102-5).[77] MAC is preferred as the initial combination

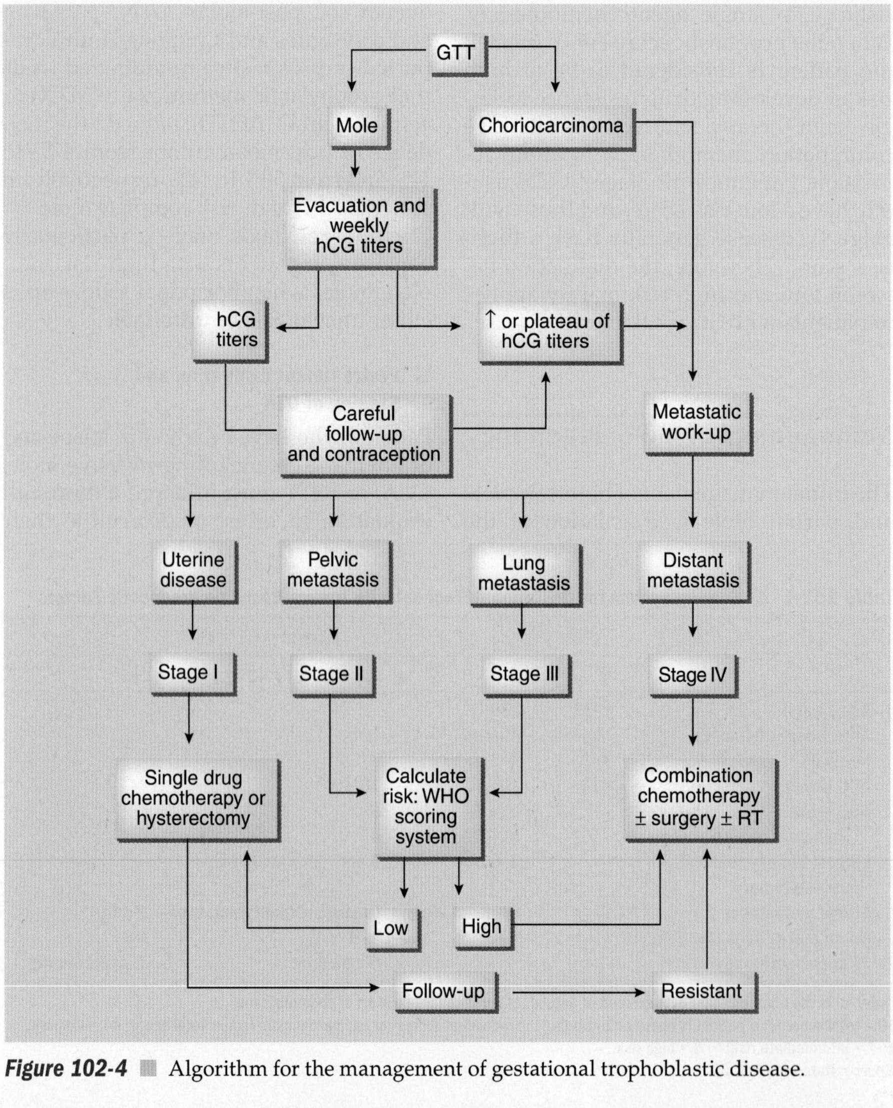

Figure 102-4 Algorithm for the management of gestational trophoblastic disease.

Table 102-2 Single-Agent Regimen

Methotrexate Treatments
MTX-FA
MTX 1.0 mg/kg IM on days 1, 3, 5, and 7
FA 0.1 mg/kg IM or po on days 2, 4, 6, and 8
5-day MTX
MTX 0.4 mg/kg/day IV or IM daily for 5 days
Pulse MTX
MTX 50 mg/m^2 IM weekly
Actinomycin D Treatments
5-day Act-D
Act-D 12 μg/kg/day IV for 5 days
Pulse Act-D
Act-D 1.25 mg/m^2 IV every 2 weeks

Abbreviations: FA, folinic acid; IM, intramuscular; IV, intravenous.

Table 102-3 Results of Single-Agent Regimens in Nonmetastatic GTT

Regimen	No. of Patients	Rate of Remission (%)
MTX–FA[66]	163	90.2
5-Day MTX[67]	58	93.0
Pulse MTX[68]	63	81.0
5-Day Act-D[69]	31	94.0
Pulse Act-D[70]	31	94.0

chemotherapy because etoposide is associated with an increased risk for second tumors.[78] If the disease is resistant to both single-agent and combination chemotherapy, hysterectomy or local resection (if the patient wants to preserve fertility) may be considered. Ultrasonography, MRI scan, pelvic arteriography, and/or PET scan may aid in identifying the site of resistant uterine tumor when local resection is planned.

Management of High-Risk GTN, Stages II and III

Primary Therapy

Women with FIGO Stages II and III and a WHO score of 7 or higher are at high risk for developing chemotherapy resistance and disease recurrence. These patients should be treated with primary combination chemotherapy with EMACO.[79]

Salvage Therapy

Patients with disease resistant to EMACO may be treated by modifying that regimen by substituting cisplatin and etoposide (EMACE) on day 8.[79] Combination MAC is inadequate as primary treatment for patients with high-risk metastatic GTN. MAC induced remission in only half of patients with metastases and a high-risk score.[77] Bower and colleagues and Bolis and colleagues reported that EMACO induced complete remission in 86% and 76%, respectively, of patients with metastases and a high-risk score.[80,81] Combination chemotherapy is administered at 2–3 week intervals, toxicity permitting, until the patient attains 3 consecutive undetectable hCG levels. After undetectable hCG values are achieved, 2–4 additional courses of chemotherapy are administered to reduce the risk of relapse.

Table 102-4 MAC Regimen

Day/Time	Therapy
1	MTX, 1.0 mg/kg, IM Act-D, 12 μg/kg, IV push cyclophosphamide, 3 mg/kg IV bolus
2	FA, 0.1 mg/kg, IM or PO Act-D, 12 μg/kg, IV push cyclophosphamide, 3 mg/kg IV bolus
3	MTX, 1.0 mg/kg, IM Act-D, 12 μg/kg, IV push cyclophosphamide, 3 mg/kg IV bolus
4	FA, 0.1 mg/kg, IM or PO Act-D, 12 μg/kg, IV push cyclophosphamide, 3 mg/kg IV bolus
5	MTX, 1.0 mg/kg, IM Act-D, 12 μg/kg, IV push cyclophosphamide, 3 mg/kg IV bolus
6	FA, 0.1 mg/kg, IM or PO
7	MTX, 1.0 mg/kg, IM
8	FA, 1.0 mg/kg, IM or PO

Abbreviations: Act-D, actinomycin D; FA, folinic acid; IM, intramuscular; IV, intravenous; MTX, methotrexate; PO, per os (by mouth).

Table 102-5 EMACO Regimen

Time	Treatment
Day 1	Etoposide 100 mg/m^2 by IV infusion in 200 mL of saline over 30 min
	Act-D 0.5 mg IV push
	MTX 100 mg/m^2 IV push
	MTX 200 mg/m^2 by IV infusion over 12 h
Day 2	Etoposide 100 mg/m^2 by IV infusion in 200 mL of saline over 30 min
	Act-D 0.5 mg IV push
	FA 15 mg IM or po every 12 h for 4 doses beginning 24 h after starting MTX
Day 8	Cyclophosphamide 600 mg/m^2 IV in saline Oncovin (vincristine) 1.0 mg/m^2 IV push

Abbreviations: Act-D, actinomycin D; FA, folinic acid; IM, intramuscular; IV, intravenous; MTX, methotrexate; po, per os (by mouth).

Management of Stage IV GTN

Patients with Stage IV disease are the highest risk group with a propensity for rapidly progressive disease and chemoresistance. The use of primary combination chemotherapy in conjunction with the selective use of radiation and surgical treatment has resulted in significantly improved survival. At the NETDC, before 1975 only 30% of patients with Stage IV disease survived. After 1975, when the concept of early intensive multi-agent treatment was introduced, a dramatic improvement was observed. At present 80% of patients with Stage IV disease, achieve a complete sustained remission with a relapse rate under 10%. Therefore, these patients should be treated with the intent to cure.

All patients with Stage IV GTN are managed with primary combination chemotherapy with EMACO. When CNS metastases are present, the MTX dosage in the infusion is increased to 1 g/m^2.[82,83] Patients who develop resistance to EMACO should then be treated with EMACE (Table 102-6). A combination of ci-splatin, vinblastine, and bleomycin (BEP) has also been used effectively in patients with drug-resistant tumor.[84–86]

The potential role of autologous bone marrow transplantation or stem cell rescue has yet to be defined. However, individual cases have been reported where high-dose chemotherapy with autologous bone marrow or stem cell support has induced complete remission in patients with otherwise refractory GTN.[87,88]

Despite the efficacy of well-recognized regimens, efforts continue to identify new agents effective in treating resistant disease. Although ifosfamide and paclitaxel have been used successfully, further studies are needed to define their potential role in either primary or second line therapy.[89,90] Osborne and associates have reported that a novel 3-drug doublet regimen consisting of paclitaxel,

Table 102-6 EMACE Regimen

Time	Treatment
Day 1	Etoposide 100 mg/m^2 by IV infusion in 200 mL of saline over 30 min
	Act-D 0.5 mg IV push
	MTX 100 mg/ m^2 IV push
	MTX 1,000 mg/m^2 by IV infusion over 12 h
Day 2	Etoposide 100 mg/m^2 by IV infusion in 200 mL of saline over 30 min
	Act-D 0.5 mg IV push
	FA 30 mg IM or PO every 12 h for 6 doses beginning 32 h after starting MTX
Day 8	Cisplatin 60 mg/m^2 IV with prehydration etoposide 100 mg/m^2 by IV infusion in 200 mL of saline over 30 min

Abbreviations: Act-D, actinomycin D; FA, folinic acid; IM, intramuscular; IV, intravenous; MTX, methotrexate; po, per os (by mouth).
Source: From Ref. 1.

etoposide, and cisplatin (TE/TO) induced complete remission in 2 patients with relapsed high-risk GTN.[91] Wan et al demonstrated the efficacy of floxuridine (FUDR)-containing regimens in drug-resistant patients.[92] Matsui et al found that 5FU in combination with ACTD could also be used effectively as salvage therapy [93]

Role of Surgery

Surgery is performed either to treat complications or excise sites of resistant tumor.[94] Hysterectomy may be necessary to control uterine hemorrhage or sepsis, or to reduce the tumor burden and thereby limit the need for chemotherapy. Bleeding from vaginal metastases may be managed by packing, wide local excision, or arteriographic embolization of the hypogastric arteries.[95] Thoracotomy may be performed to excise persistent viable tumor despite intensive chemotherapy.[96] However, fibrotic nodules may persist indefinitely on chest roentgenograms after complete gonadotropin remission is attained. An extensive metastatic survey should be undertaken to exclude other sites of persistent tumor. A radioisotope-labeled antibody to hCG or a PET scan may be useful to identify occult sites of viable tumor.[97,98] Hepatic resection may be required to manage bleeding metastases although embolization has also been utilized in this setting.[99] Craniotomy may be necessary to provide acute decompression or to control bleeding, in addition to its role in the primary resection of solitary metastatic disease.[100]

Role of Radiation Therapy

When cranial metastases are identified whole-brain irradiation and systemic chemotherapy are promptly instituted at the NETDC to reduce the risk of cerebral hemorrhage. Yordan and colleagues reported that deaths as a result of cerebral involvement occurred in 11 (44%) of 25 patients treated with chemotherapy alone, but in none of 18 patients treated with brain irradiation and chemotherapy.[101]

Results of Therapy

Stage I GTN

Between July 1965 and June 2006, 534 patients with Stage I GTN were treated at the NETDC and all attained remission. 419/460 patients (77%) achieved remission with sequential MTX/ACTD. All 32 patients managed with primary hysterectomy and adjuvant single-agent chemotherapy achieved remission and required no further treatment. The remaining 83 patients resistant to primary treatment were treated successfully with either combination chemotherapy or surgical intervention.

Stages II and III GTN

Complete remission was achieved at the NETDC in all 28 patients with Stage II GTN, and in 160/161 patients with Stage III GTN. Single-agent chemotherapy induced remission in 16 (80%) of 20 patients with low-risk Stage II disease, and in 90 (82%) of 110 patients with low-risk Stage III disease. All patients with disease resistant to single-agent chemotherapy attained remission with combination chemotherapy.

Stage IV GTN

Prior to 1975, only 6/20 patients (30%) with Stage IV GTN achieved remission at the NETDC. However, after 1975, 16 of 20 patients (80%) with Stage IV disease attained remission. This dramatic improvement in survival resulted from the use of intensive multimodal therapy early in the course of treatment. While brain irradiation is commonly employed in the United States for cerebral metastases, excellent remission rates have been reported in patients with cerebral metastases who were treated with chemotherapy alone. 30 of 36 patients (86%) with cerebral lesions attained remission with intensive combination chemotherapy, including high-dose intravenous and intrathecal MTX.[83]

hCG Follow-Up and Relapse

All patients with Stages I, II, and III GTN are followed with weekly hCG values until undetectable for 3 weeks, and then monthly until undetectable for 12 months. Patients with Stage IV GTN are followed monthly for 24 months because they are at greater risk for late relapse. All patients must be encouraged to use effective contraception during the entire interval of monitoring. Relapse rates at the NETDC are as follows: Stage I, 2.9%; Stage II, 8.3%; Stage III, 4.2%; and Stage IV, 9.1%. The mean time to recurrence from the last non-detectable hCG level was 6 months, and this did not differ among the 4 stages.

When relapse occurs, the patient should be restaged, and appropriate therapy begun with a new regimen not previously utilized in this patient. All relapsed patients in the series with Stages I, II, and III achieved remission, whereas both patients with relapsed Stage IV GTN died.

Quiescent GTN

A rare cause of persistent (present for at least 3 months) low-level hCG is quiescent GTN (range 0.5–200 mIU/mL) that most commonly follows a molar pregnancy. Quiescent GTN is thought to be due to the presence of highly differentiated, non-invasive syncytiotrophoblast cells. This condition is characterized by the following: (1) foci of disease are not readily identifiable clinically; and (2) hCG level unresponsive to therapy, presumably because the growth cycle of these cells is long and comparable to normal cells. Patients with quiescent GTN should not be treated with chemotherapy, but close follow-up is indicated because 6–10% will eventually develop active GTN requiring treatment. The presence of low levels of hyperglycosolated hCG indicates the presence of quiescent GTN. Increasing levels of hyperglycosolated hCG indicate the development of active GTN that requires treatment.[46,47]

Subsequent Pregnancies

Patients with complete and partial mole can anticipate normal reproduction in the future.[102] However, these patients are at increased risk of developing molar pregnancy in later conceptions. 35 (1:150) of the patients had at least 2 molar pregnancies. Following 2 episodes of molar pregnancy, the risk of mole in a later gestation is 18–25%. Patients with GTN successfully treated with chemotherapy can also expect normal reproduction in the future.[102] Importantly, the frequency of later major and minor congenital malformations is not increased.

Because the risk of a repeat molar pregnancy is increased 10-fold, an obstetrical ultrasound should be obtained in the late first trimester of subsequent pregnancies to conform normal fetal development. Additionally, an hCG test should be performed 6 weeks after completion of any subsequent pregnancy to rule out occult CCA. Later products of conception should be evaluated by a pathologist following any spontaneous miscarriage or therapeutic abortion.

Second Cancers

The use of etoposide in GTN has been reported to increase the risk of later secondary tumors, including myeloid leukemia, melanoma, colon cancer, and breast cancer. Among all patients treated with etoposide, 1.5% subsequently developed leukemia.[78]

Selected References

The complete reference list can be found at www.CANCERMEDICINE8.com

1. Bagshawe KD. Risks and prognostic factors in trophoblastic neoplasia. *Cancer.* 1976;38:1373–1385.

2. Goldstein DP, Berkowitz RS. *Gestational trophoblastic neoplasms: clinical principles of diagnosis and management.* Philadelphia: WB Saunders; 1982:1–301.
4. Palmer JR. Advances in the epidemiology of gestational trophoblastic disease. *J Reprod Med.* 1994; 39:155–162.
6. Berkowitz RS, Cramer DW, Bernstein MR, et al. Risk factors for complete molar pregnancy from a case-control study. *Am J Obstet Gynecol.* 1985;152:1016–1020.
11. Berkowitz RS, Tuncer ZS, Bernstein MR, Goldsatein DP. Management of gestational trophoblastic disease: subsequent pregnancy experience. *Semin Oncol.* 2000;27:678–682.
15. Sand PK, Lurain JR, Brewer JI. Repeat gestational trophoblastic disease. *Obstet Gynecol.* 1984;63:140–145.
16. Kajii T, Ohama K. Androgenetic origin of hydatidiform mole. *Nature.* 1977;268: 633–634.
17. Yamashita K, Wake N, Araki T, et al. Human lymphocyte antigen expression in hydatidiform mole: androgenesis following fertilization by a haploid sperm. *Am J Obstet Gynecol.* 1979;135:597–600.
20. Szulman AE, Surti U. The syndromes of hydatidiform mole. I. Cytogenetic and morphologic correlations. *Am J Obstet Gynecol.* 1978;131:665–771.
23. Szulman AE, Surti U. The syndromes of hydatidiform mole: II. Morphologic evolution of the complete and partial mole. *Am J Obstet Gynecol.* 1978;132:20–27.
24. Feltmate C, Genest DR, Wise L. et al. Placental site trophoblastic tumor: a 17-year experience at the New England Trophoblastic Disease Center. *Gynecol Oncol.* 2001;82:415–419.
30. Fisher RA, Hodges MD, Newlands ES. Familial recurrent hydatidiform mole—a review. *J Reprod Med.* 2004; 49:595–601
32. Goldstein DP, Berkowitz RS. Current management of complete and partial molar pregnancy. *J Reprod Med.* 1994;39:139–146.
33. Soto-Wright V, Bernstein MR, Goldstein DP, Berkowitz RS. The changing clinical presentation of complete molar pregnancy. *Obstet Gynecol.* 1995;86:775–779.
36. Berkowitz RS, Goldstein DP, Bernstein MR. Natural history of partial molar pregnancy. *Obstet Gynecol.*1986;66:677–681.
37. Szulman AE, Surti U. The clinicopathologic profile of the partial hydatidiform mole. *Obstet Gynecol.* 1982;59:597–602.
38. Kato H, Wake N. Differential diagnosis between complete and partial mole using a T55c3 antibody. *J Reprod Med.* 2006;51:861–867.
39. Fine C, Bundy AL, Berkowitz RS, et al. Sonographic diagnosis of partial hydatidiform mole. *Obstet Gynecol.* 1989;73:414–418.
42. Wolfberg AJ, Feltmate C, Goldstein DP, et al. Low risk of relapse after achieving undetectable HCG levels in women with complete molar pregnancy. *Obstet Gynecol.* 2004;104:551–554.
44. Growdon WB, Wolfberg AJ, Feltmate CM, et al. Postevacuation hCG levels and risk of gestational trophoblastic neoplasia among women with partial molar pregnancies. *J Reprod Med.* 2006;51:871–875.
45. Wolberg AJ, Berkowitz RS, Goldstein DP, et al. Postevacuation hCG levels and risk of gestational trophoblastic neoplasia in women with complete molar pregnancy. *Obstet Gynecol.* 2005;106:548–552.
46. Cole LA, Butler S. Detection of hCG in trophoblastic disease—the USA hCG Reference Service Experience. *J Reprod Med.* 2002;47:433–444.
47. Cole LA, Khanlian SA, Giddings A, et al. Gestational trophoblastic diseases: 4. Presentation with persistent low positive human chorionic gonadotropin test results. *Gynecol Oncol.* 2006;102:165–169.
48. Berkowitz RS, Goldstein DP. Chorionic tumors. *N Engl J Med.* 1996;335:1740–1748.
51. Berkowitz RS, Goldstein DP. Presentation and management of molar pregnancy. In: Hancock BW, Newlands ES, Berkowitz RS, editors. *Gestational trophoblastic disease.* London: Chapman and Hall; 1997:127–142.
52. Feltmate CM, Growdon WB, Wolfberg AJ, et al. Clinical characteristics of persistent gestational trophoblastic neoplasia after partial hydatidiform molar pregnancy. *J Reprod Med.* 2006;51:902–906.
53. Bakri YN, Berkowitz RS, Khan J, et al. Pulmonary metastases of gestational trophoblastic tumor: risk factors for early respiratory failure. *J Reprod Med.* 1994;39:175–178.
54. Newlands ES, Holden L, Seckl MJ, et al. Management of brain metastases in patients with high risk gestational trophoblastic tumours (GTT). *J Reprod Med.* 2002;47:465–471.
56. World Health Organization. *Trophoblastic diseases: technical report series 692.* Geneva: WHO; 1983.
57. Kohorn EI. The new FIGO 2000 staging and risk factor scoring system for gestational trophoblastic disease: description and critical assessment. *Int J Gynaecol Cancer.* 2001;11:73–77.
60. Soper JT. Surgical therapy for gestational trophoblastic disease. *J Reprod Med.* 1994;39:168–174.
63. Kim DS, Moon H, Kim KT, et al. Effects of prophylactic chemotherapy for persistent trophoblastic disease in patients with complete hydatidiform mole. *Obstet Gynecol.* 1986;67:690–694.
64. Limpongsanurak, S. Prophylactic actinomycin D for high risk complete hydatidiform mole. *J Reprod Med.* 2001;46:110–116.
65. Garner EIO, Garrett A, Goldstein DP, Berkowitz RS. Significance of chest computed tomography findings in the evaluation and treatment of persistent gestational trophoblastic neoplasia. *J Reprod Med.* 2004; 49:411–414.
66. Berkowitz RS, Goldstein DP, Bernstein MR. Ten years experience with methotrexate and folinic acid as primary therapy for gestational trophoblastic disease. *Gynecol Oncol.* 1986;23:111–118.
69. Homesley HD, Blessing JA, Rettenmaier M, et al. Weekly intramuscular methotrexate for nonmetastatic gestational trophoblastic tumor. *Obstet Gynecol.* 1998;72:413–418.
70. Osathanondh R, Goldstein DP, Pastorfide GB. Actinomycin D as the primary agent for gestational trophoblastic disease. *Cancer.* 1973;36:863–866.
72. Homesley HD. Single–agent therapy for nonmetastatic and low risk gestational trophoblastic disease. *J Repro Med.* 1998;43:69–72.
73. Garrett AP, Garner EO, Goldstein DP, Berkowitz RS. Methotrexate infusion and folic acid as primary therapy for nonmetatastic and low risk metastatic gestational trophoblastic tumors. 15 years experience. *J Reprod Med.* 2002;47;355–359.
77. DuBeshter B, Berkowitz RS, Goldstein DP, et al. Metastatic gestational trophoblastic disease: experience at the New England Trophoblastic Disease Center, 1965–1985. *Obstet Gynecol.* 1987;69:390–395.
78. Rustin GJS, Newlands ES, Lutz JM, et al. Combination but not single–agent methotrexate chemotherapy for gestational trophoblastic tumors increases the incidence of second tumors. *J Clin Oncol.* 1996;14:2769–2773.
79. Newlands ES, Bower M, Holden L, et al. Management of resistant gestational trophoblastic tumors. *J Reprod Med.* 1998;43:111–118.
82. Newlands ES, Bagshawe KD, Begent RH, et al. Results with the EMA/CO (etoposide, methotrexate, actinomycin D, cyclophosphamide, vincristine) regimen in high risk gestational trophoblastic tumours, 1979 to 1989. *Br J Obstet Gynaecol.* 1991;98:550–556.
91. Osborne R, Covens, Merchandani DE, Gerulath AS. Successful salvage of relapsed high-risk gestational trophoblastic neoplasia patients using a novel paclitaxel-containing doublet. *J Reprod Med.* 2004;49:655–658.
94. Lurain JR, Singh DK, Schink JC. Role of surgery in the management of high-risk gestational trophoblastic neoplasia. *J Reprod Med.* 2006;51:773–777.
96. Jones WB, Romain K, Erlandson RA, et al. Thoracotomy in the management of gestational choriocarcinoma: a clinicopathologic study. *Cancer.* 1993;72:2175–2178.
98. Dhillon T, Palmieri C, Sebire NJ, et al. Value of whole body 18 FDG-PET to identify the active site of gestational trophoblastic neoplasia. *J Reprod Med.* 2006;51: 879–883.
102. Garner EIO, Lipson E, Bernstein MR, et al. Subsequent pregnancy experience in patients with molar pregnancy and gestational trophoblastic tumors. *J Reprod Med.* 2002;47:380–386.

103 Gynecologic Sarcomas

Jamal Rahaman, MD ■ Carmel J. Cohen, MD

Even though the female pelvis is richly endowed with blood vessels, connective tissue, and müllerian elements, sarcomas (including mesenchymal and mixed epithelial–mesenchymal malignancies) of the vulva, vagina, cervix, uterus, and ovaries account for less than 1.5% of the cancers of these organs. The most common site for sarcoma in the female pelvis is the uterus, but uterine sarcomas represent only 4–9% of uterine cancers, with an annual incidence rate of less than 20 per million females.[1,2] The overall incidence for Blacks is twice that of Whites, but there were no differences in survival for women who received similar therapy.[2] The risk of malignant mixed müllerian tumor (MMMT) increases sharply with age.[1] The incidence rate per million women per year was 8.2 for MMMTs, 6.4 for leiomyosarcomas (LMSs), 1.8 for endometrial stromal sarcomas (ESSs), and 0.7 for unclassified sarcomas.[1]

Because of the infrequent occurrence of sarcomas, classification of these cancers was a taxonomic dilemma until Ober, in 1959,[3] proposed a classification that became the basis from which modern modifications have been derived. Table 103-1 presents a detailed classification, adapted from Kempson and Bari[4] and a functional classification developed by the Gynecologic Oncology Group (GOG).

Epidemiologic risk factors for uterine sarcoma have not been clearly defined. An association has been observed between exposure to radiation and development of uterine sarcomas, most of which are MMMTs. Although the relative risk is estimated at 5.4,[5] the percentage of patients with uterine sarcomas who have previously undergone radiation therapy ranges from 12% to 30%.[6] Recent reports have also suggested an increased risk or uterine sarcomas (mostly MMMT) related to previous tamoxifen use.[7,8]

The uterus is the most common site of gynecologic sarcomas. Uterine sarcomas can be assigned to two general categories with an origin from either the endometrial or the myometrial compartment. ESSs are derived only from the endometrial compartment, whereas LMSs arise solely from the myometrial compartment, and the MMMTs have contributions from both derivatives.[4] The homologous tumors include carcinoma plus a sarcoma differentiating toward tissues indigenous to the uterus, and the heterologous tumors include carcinoma plus sarcoma resembling tissue from some extrauterine source (bone, cartilage, striated muscle) with or without homologous elements. Traditionally, authors have reported that MMMT and LMS each account for 35–40% of uterine sarcomas, with ESS accounting for 10–15% and other sarcomas comprising 5%. However, in one of the most detailed clinicopathologic evaluations of clinical stages I and II uterine sarcomas prospectively performed, the GOG, in an analysis of 453 patients, found that 66% had MMMT, 13% had LMS, and the remaining 21% were predominantly adenosarcoma and ESS.[9]

The reason for this apparent change in the ratio of the two most frequently diagnosed uterine sarcomas is unclear; however, several smaller series reported in the past decade have noticed this trend in the histologic analysis performed. The significance of the GOG studies is that a single group of referee pathologists reviewed all of the pathologic material, and surgeons followed common surgical guidelines so that all patients met strict criteria for the acceptability of both the surgical procedure and the adequacy of pathologic specimens submitted.

Table 103-1 ■ **Classification of Uterine Sarcomas**

Classification of Kempson and Bari

- I. Pure sarcomas
  - A. Pure sarcomas
    - 1. Leiomyosarcoma
    - 2. Stromal sarcoma
    - 3. Stromal endometriosis (endometrial stromatosis, endolymphatic stromal myosis)
    - 4. Angiosarcoma
    - 5. Fibrosarcoma
  - B. Pure heterologous
    - 1. Rhabdomyosarcoma (includes sarcoma botryoides)
    - 2. Chondrosarcoma
    - 3. Osteosarcoma
    - 4. Liposarcoma
- II. Mixed sarcomas
  - A. Mixed homologous
  - B. Mixed heterologous with or without homologous elements
- III. Malignant mixed müllerian tumors (mixed meso-dermal tumors)
  - A. Malignant mixed müllerian tumors, homologous type—carcinoma plus one sarcoma or mixture of sarcomas in IA, I through 5, above (carcinosarcoma)
  - B. Malignant mixed müllerian tumors, heterologous type—carcinoma plus heterologous sarcoma with or without homologous sarcoma
- IV. Sarcoma unclassified
- V. Malignant lymphoma

Gynecologic Oncology Group Classification

- I. Leiomyosarcomas
- II. Endometrial stromal sarcomas
- III. Mixed homologous müllerian sarcomas (carcinosarcoma)
- IV. Other uterine sarcomas

Source: Adapted from Ref. 4.

One of the pitfalls in diagnosing sarcomas is the variability in threshold for distinguishing between atypical benign lesions and clearly malignant ones. In general, it is reasonable to conclude that if a mesenchymal tumor of the uterus has 1–4 mitoses per 10 high-power fields, the metastatic potential is virtually nonexistent. If there are 10 or more mitoses per 10 high-power fields, the risk of recurrence is high, irrespective of the presence of atypia. If there are 5–9 mitoses per 10 high-power fields without atypia, the risk of recurrence or metastasis is moderate, but if atypia is also present, the patient should be considered to have a sarcoma.

It is important to realize, however, that there are important exceptions to these generalizations. For example, mitotically active smooth muscle tumors without atypia occurring in young women usually behave in a benign manner. Conversely, myxoid LMSs often have deceptively low mitotic counts.

Clinical Profile

■ Uterine Endometrial Stromal Tumors

Patients with endometrial stromal tumors tend to be perimenopausal and ordinarily present with irregular vaginal bleeding. If the lesion is small, pain may be absent, but on pelvic examination, tumor tissue may be seen protruding through the cervical os because the tumor originates in the endometrium and may grow large without penetrating through the uterine wall. The diagnosis is made by endometrial sampling, which should be done liberally to explain vaginal bleeding. Among the endometrial stromal tumors is the endometrial stromal nodule, usually an expansile, noninfiltrating, unifocal lesion with low mitotic activity and low virulence. Removal of the nodule has resulted in cure, without further therapy. Endolymphatic stromal myosis is a low-grade stromal sarcoma with a worm-like infiltrative pattern that extends beyond the uterus in approximately 40% of patients. It recurs in approximately 50% after surgical removal but is indolent in its course and is often treated by repeated excisions over a long course of months or years. There is evidence of radiosensitivity and hormone sensitivity,[10] with the observation that oophorectomy alone can control the disease in a subset of patients. High-grade ESSs, on the other hand, are more aggressive cancers. Patients survive well when the tumors are small and confined to the uterus at the time of initial treatment; however, poorly differentiated lesions or those with extrauterine extension are usually lethal.

Mixed Tumors

The incidence of MMMT begins to increase at approximately 50 years of age and does not plateau until after age 75 years. The presenting complaints may include vaginal bleeding, heavy discharge, abdominal pain, and sometimes an increase in abdominal girth. The diagnosis is made more frequently by endometrial sampling than in the case of LMS because the latter disease often does not involve the endometrial cavity. Other than previous exposure to ionizing radiation, there is no unusual risk factor for patients with uterine sarcomas.

Uterine Myometrial Tumors

LMS commonly occurs during the fourth and fifth decades of life, with a peak incidence at 45 years of age, after which there is a gradual decline in incidence until the eighth decade. The lesion is frequently associated with benign leiomyomas, although among leiomyomas, sarcoma is found less than 1% of the time.[11] There is considerable debate over whether the lesion "develops" from a benign leiomyoma or occurs independently. Ferenczy and colleagues were unable to demonstrate a developmental relationship,[12] whereas Spiro and Koss found intermediate changes in leiomyomas and indicted[13] these benign lesions in 50% of the cases of LMS they studied. Often LMSs are discovered by chance at the time of myomectomy or hysterectomy. Davids, who removed five sarcomas in a series of 1150 myomectomies, observed that the five patients were well after 5 years and that three of them subsequently became pregnant.[14] No mention was made of virulence indices in the pathologic examination of these tumors.

Diagnosis

Of patients with uterine sarcomas, 75–95% present with abnormal vaginal bleeding.[15,16] Pelvic pain, discharge, and aborting tissue occur frequently. Endometrial biopsy may confirm MMMT in the majority of cases[17]; however, LMS and ESS are missed in at least 40 and 20% of cases, respectively.[10,18,19]

Radiography may be useful in diagnosing uterine sarcomas. Several investigators are currently studying ultrasonography.[20] Kurjak and colleagues evaluated the role of transvaginal color Doppler ultrasonography in differentiating uterine sarcomas from leiomyomas.[20] Computed tomography will identify extrauterine spread, and magnetic resonance imaging can assess the depth of myometrial invasion. The FDG-PET showed a better detection rate than the abdominal CT scan for extrapelvic metastatic lesions.[21]

Sarcoma-Like Variants

Four pathologic entities are abnormal forms of leiomyoma and should be distinguished from uterine sarcomas.

Benign metastasizing leiomyoma is a rare entity in which histologically benign uterine smooth muscle is found in extrauterine deposits, often distant from the uterus, especially in lymph nodes and lungs.[22] Whether the nodules are metastatic or multifocal remains to be resolved. Several observers have noted the hormone dependence of these deposits. After hysterectomy with bilateral salpingo-oophorectomy, the nodules often regress, and if they interfere with performance, they can be individually resected.

Intravenous leiomyomatosis is the growth of histologically benign smooth muscle into venous lumina. Although the pattern is often worm-like, it should not be confused with endolymphatic stromal myosis, which is located primarily extravascularly. Although intravenous leiomyomatosis is histologically benign, deaths have been reported from very long tumor extensions occupying the vena cava and the heart.[23] In this condition, the extension of tumor is contiguous, unlike the widely disparate deposits in benign metastasizing leiomyoma.

Leiomyomatosis peritonealis disseminata is a rare condition in which nodules comprising benign smooth muscle are densely distributed throughout the peritoneal cavity. Much of the peritoneal surface may be occupied by nodules ranging in size from a few millimeters to several centimeters. Treatment requires removal of as much disease as possible and reversal of any estrogenic stimulation, either by removing the ovaries or by treatment with antiestrogen regimens.

Epithelioid leiomyoma or leiomyoblastoma denotes a rare group of benign smooth muscle tumors that are formed by round cells with clear cytoplasm. They are less well circumscribed than a typical leiomyoma and occasionally lack the whorled, cut surface and the discrete borders of a typical leiomyoma. Usually, their mitotic rate is less than three mitoses per 10 high-power fields, and the rate of recurrence or metastasis is low.[24]

Patterns of Spread

Uterine sarcomas can spread by lymphatic and hematogenous routes[25] as well as by local extension and peritoneal spread.[26] Several studies have addressed the metastatic pattern of uterine sarcomas. Chen examined nodal metastases in 20 patients with clinical stage I uterine sarcomas.[27] Fourteen patients had MMMT, four had LMS, and two had ESS. Of nine patients (45%) with lymph node metastases, six had both para-aortic and pelvic node involvement, and three had only pelvic node involvement. Among ESS and MMMT patients, a high frequency of association was observed between nodal spread and deep myometrial invasion. Other sites of extrauterine spread were the ovary (two patients) and the serosa of the uterus (one patient). DiSaia and colleagues reported on 28 patients with clinical stage I and II carcinosarcoma who underwent total abdominal hysterectomy, bilateral salpingo-oophorectomy, and pelvic and para-aortic lymph node sampling.[28] Ten (35%) of the 28 patients had positive pelvic nodes; 4 of these 10 patients also had para-aortic node metastasis (14.5%). In every instance of nodal involvement, the myometrial invasion was to the middle or outer third.

Rose and colleagues studied the autopsy findings of 73 patients with uterine sarcoma, including 43 patients with MMMT, 19 with LMS, 9 with ESS, and 2 with ESM.[25] The peritoneal cavity and omentum were the most frequently involved sites (59%), followed by the lung (52%), pelvic (41%) and para-aortic (38%) lymph nodes, and liver parenchyma (34%). Of note, the presence of lung metastasis was not associated with pelvic or para-aortic nodal metastasis or intraperitoneal disease. In another review of autopsy findings, Fleming and colleagues reviewed the records of 22 patients treated for uterine sarcoma, including 11 MMMTs, 6 ESSs, and 5 LMSs.[26] Fifty-nine percent had lymph node involvement, and 45% died with disease limited to the pelvis and abdomen. The most common site of disease above the diaphragm was the lung. The authors reviewed the autopsy findings of 58 patients from previous reports in the literature and found a similar incidence of nodal involvement (57%) and disease limited to the pelvis and abdomen (31%). In addition, 65.5% of patients had abdominal and distant metastases.

Goff and colleagues examined nodal metastases from uterine LMS and ESS.[18]

Retroperitoneal lymph node sampling revealed lymph node metastases in 4 of 15 women with LMS, and in each instance, there was also disseminated intraperitoneal disease. Seven of 10 women with ESS had lymphadenectomies, and none had positive nodes.

Prognostic Factors and Prognosis

Prognostic factors differ for the three major types of uterine sarcomas. Major and colleagues reported the GOG clinicopathologic study of clinical stage I and II uterine sarcoma, which included 59 patients with LMS and 301 patients with MMMT.[9] Of the 453 patients eligible for analysis, 430 underwent complete surgical staging that included lymphadenectomy. The median survival was 62.6 months for homologous MMMT, 22.7 months for heterologous MMMT, and 20.6 months for LMS. The overall recurrence rate for homologous MMMT was 56%.

In patients with LMS, lymph vascular space involvement and involvement of the cervix and isthmus were common, whereas lymph node metastases, adnexal metastases, and positive peritoneal cytology were infrequent findings. The only surgicopathologic finding that correlated with progression-free interval was the mitotic index. Whereas there were no treatment failures among the three women who had less than 10 mitoses per 10 high-power fields, 61% of women with 10–20 mitoses per 10 high-power fields and 79% of women with greater than 20 mitoses per 10 high-power fields developed recurrences. Fewer mitoses were also associated with longer survival. Other investigators have confirmed these results?[5,29]

In contrast to patients with LMS, surgicopathologic factors of MMMT that related to progression-free interval included adnexal spread, lymph node metastasis, histologic cell type (heterologous versus homologous), and the grade of sarcoma. Of note, patients with MMMT had high rates of nodal and adnexal metastases and positive peritoneal cytology. Pelvic nodes were involved twice as often as aortic nodes (15 vs 7.8%), and both nodal groups were involved in 5% of the patients.

Nonuterine Gynecologic Sarcomas

The Vulva ■ Fewer than 300 patients with vulvar sarcoma have been described in the literature. LMS, rhabdomyosarcoma, and fibrosarcoma are the most frequently diagnosed vulvar tumors. The clinical behavior of these tumors is related to their grade, mitotic count, histology, and stage. For the lowest-grade tumors, wide local excision should suffice. However, for the more aggressive histologic patterns, radical vulvectomy with lymphadenectomy followed by cytotoxic chemotherapy should be considered, although the role of adjuvant chemotherapy has not been studied in these tumors.

The Vagina ■ LMS of the vagina occurs in the same age groups as does LMS of the uterus. Although this tumor is highly virulent, survivors are among those treated by hysterectomy, oophorectomy, and vaginectomy. Embryonal rhabdomyosarcomas, formerly termed sarcoma botryoides, occur most frequently in children and have a typical grape cluster-like appearance. The disease was once uniformly fatal, provoking radical extirpative surgery that resulted in exenteration for young girls. Various multidrug cytotoxic chemotherapy regimens with or without radiation therapy have replaced primary exenteration, and a cure is now expected. Radical surgery is reserved for failures of nonsurgical treatment.

The Ovary ■ Most types of sarcomas described in the vagina, vulva, or uterus have been found in the ovary as well. The diagnosis of ovarian sarcoma is infrequently made prior to laparotomy. The surgical treatment is identical to that for epithelial ovarian cancers. During the past decade, MMMT of the ovary has been described with increasing frequency.[30,31] Survival is better for patients with early-stage disease and those whose tumors have homologous stromal elements.

Fallopian Tube ■ The fallopian tube is the least frequent site of primary sarcomas in the gynecologic tract. From reports in the literature, it would seem that carcinoma of the fallopian tube, itself an unusual entity, is more than 20 times more common than fallopian tube sarcoma. The most common histologic type is MMMT.[32,33] In Imachi and colleagues' 1992 review, there were 39 patients with MMMT of the fallopian tube.[32] Clinical features and difficulty in diagnosis are identical to those for patients with adenocarcinoma of the fallopian tube. Half of the patients had homologous elements and half had heterologous components. The surgical approach is the same as that used for ovarian or fallopian tube epithelial carcinoma, and postoperative treatment has usually included cytotoxic chemotherapy. Combinations of cyclophosphamide, doxorubicin, and cisplatin have been effectively applied, as has the combination of vincristine, doxorubicin, and cyclophosphamide.[33,34] More recently, ifosfamide and cisplatin combination chemotherapy as well as paclitaxel has been employed. Long-term survivors have been reported but are uncommon (Fig. 103-1).[35]

Surgical Treatment

The initial therapy for sarcomas of the gynecologic tract is surgical except for embryonal rhabdomyosarcomas (Fig. 103-2). Patients with uterine sarcoma require total abdominal hysterectomy and careful staging. In patients with MMMT limited to the uterus by pathologic staging, the cytologic presence of malignant cells in the peritoneal washings is a poor prognostic factor.[35]

The ovaries should be retained in premenopausal patients with LMS because this appears to improve their prognosis.[19,36,37] However, a bilateral salpingo-oophorectomy should be performed in all other patients, including those with low-grade ESS, because these tumors may be hormone dependent or responsive and have a propensity for extension into the parametria, broad ligament, and adnexal structures.

For MMMT, a high percentage of patients with clinical stage I or II disease are upstaged at the time of laparotomy;[38,39] thus it appears reasonable to surgically stage these patients. There is a paucity of data regarding the role of lymph node sampling in patients with LMS and ESS, but it appears that almost all patients with these sarcomas who have lymph node metastases also have evidence of intraperitoneal disease spread.[11]

Unlike other gynecologic malignancies, there is a role for thoracotomy or video-assisted thorascopy in patients with uterine sarcoma metastatic to the lung. Levenback and colleagues reviewed 45 patients whose pulmonary metastases from uterine sarcoma were resected at Memorial Sloan-Kettering Cancer Center, the majority of which were LMS (84%).[40] Most lesions were unilateral (71%), 70% were greater than 2 cm, and half were isolated lesions. The mean survival of patients with unilateral disease (39 months) was significantly greater than that of patients with bilateral disease (27 months). No single risk factor was identified that could exclude an individual patient from consideration for pulmonary resection. There is also a role for surgery in the treatment of local and regional recurrences of uterine sarcomas. In The University of Texas M. D. Anderson Cancer Center series of 120 patients with MMMT reported by Spanos and colleagues, 67 patients developed recurrent disease.[41] In the six patients with lesions deemed suitable for resection (one locoregional, two pulmonary, and three abdominal), five complete responses and partial responses

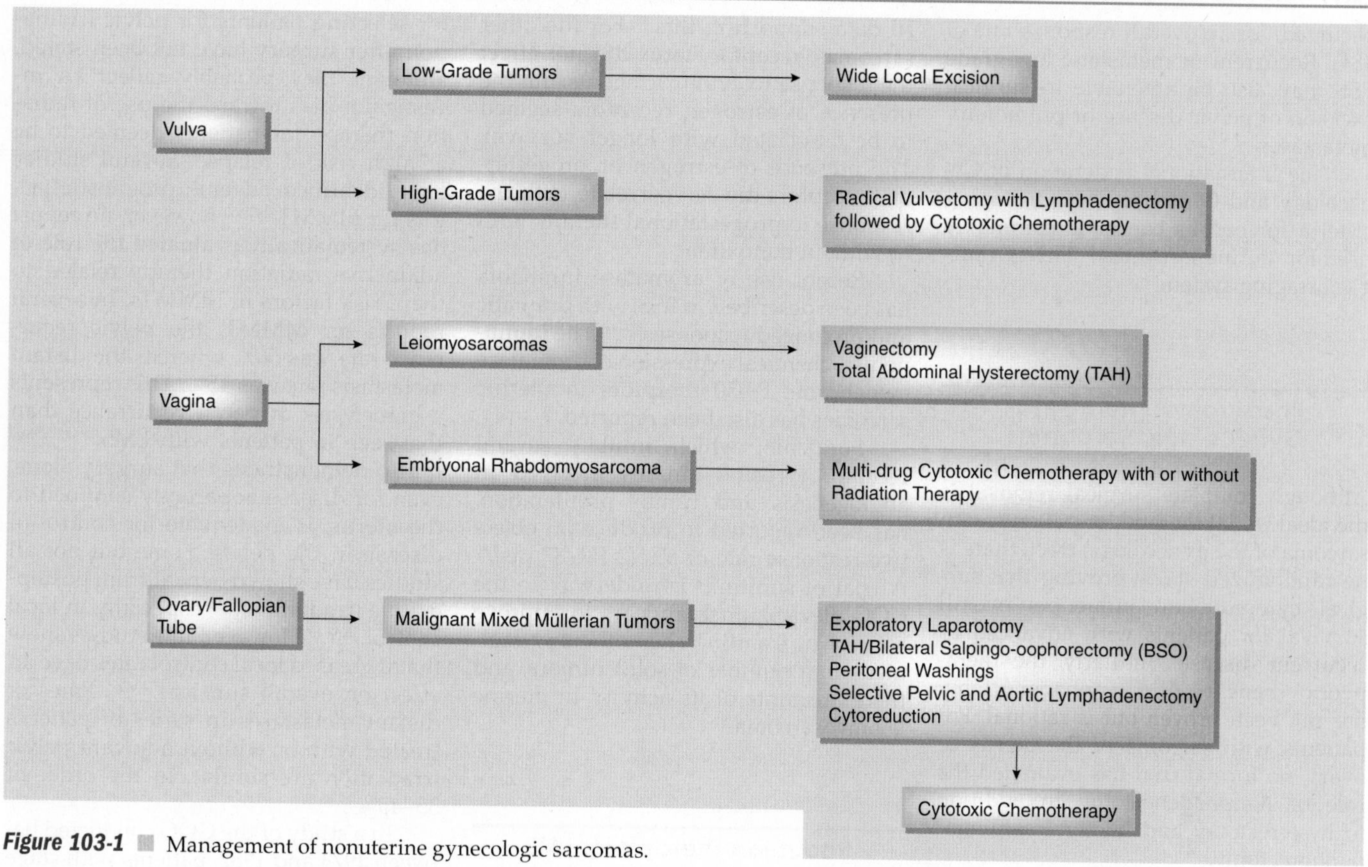

Figure 103-1 ■ Management of nonuterine gynecologic sarcomas.

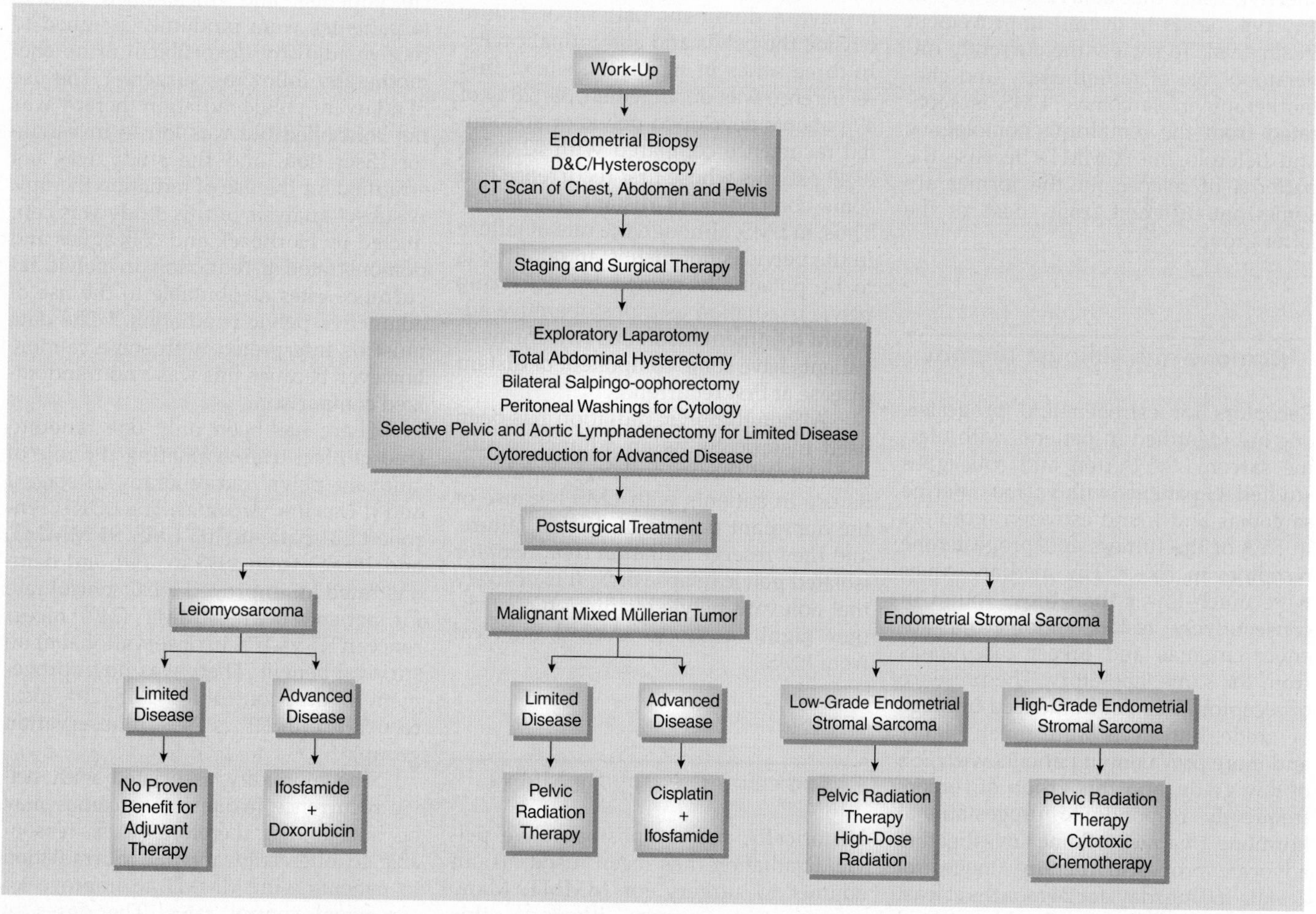

Figure 103-2 ■ Management of uterine sarcomas.

occurred, for an overall response rate of 83%. Recurrent or metastatic low-grade ESS may also be amenable to surgical excision of pelvic disease or pulmonary metastases.

The International Federation of Gynecology and Obstetrics (FIGO) staging criteria for corpus cancer is commonly used for uterine sarcomas.[42] This is a surgical staging system.

Postsurgical Therapy for Gynecologic Sarcomas

Although complete surgical removal is the ideal initial therapy for patients with sarcoma of the gynecologic tract, there is no randomized study proving that surgical cytoreduction influences overall survival for patients with advanced or recurrent disease. Similarly, the therapeutic benefit of lymphadenectomy has not been proven but is rational. For patients with sarcoma of the uterus or ovary, no formal trial has evaluated the role of lymphadenectomy in addition to hysterectomy and bilateral salpingo-oophorectomy.

For patients with uterine sarcoma, there is no definitive evidence from prospective trials that adjuvant therapy of any type leads to overall improvement in survival. To review the currently understood role of radiotherapy and chemotherapy in sarcomas, LMS is separated from the remaining homologous and heterologous MMMTs because the patterns of relapse for the former are somewhat different from those of the latter group.

Hormone and Biologic Therapy

Receptors for estrogen and progesterone are identified in patients with uterine sarcoma.[43,44] Sutton and colleagues studied 43 patients with various uterine sarcomas and found estrogen receptors in 55% of the tumors and progesterone receptors in 55%.[43] The median values were much lower than those found in consecutively tested endometrial adenocarcinomas and breast carcinomas from the same laboratory. The presence of receptors was not influenced by stage or grade, but levels were much higher and more prevalent in patients with ESS of low grade, and this group of tumors frequently responds to progestational hormone treatment. Some investigators advocate progestin therapy (megestrol acetate 160 mg/day) for 24 months at least for patients with completely resected low-grade ESS; however there is no level III data supporting this.[45] For the other sarcomas, receptor status did not affect the response to cytotoxic agents, but the presence of estrogen receptors seemed to be associated with longer survival. The presence of estrogen or progesterone receptors did not correlate with the response to progestational therapy with or without tamoxifen.

Recent use of aromatase inhibitors has been described in ESS, with dramatic and prolonged responses.[46-48] The immunohistochemical expression of aromatase cytochrome P-450 receptors in uterine sarcomas has also been reported.[49]

Sorafenib, which inhibits several receptor tyrosine kinases involved in angiogenesis and tumor proliferation, has been reported to produce an objective response rate of 5% (2 PR/37 pts).[50] A trial of sunitinib is underway in the GOG. Bevacizumab appears to improve activity of frontline chemotherapy regimens in a number of solid tumors, and there are hints of its activity in uterine leiomyosarcoma.[51]

Radiation Therapy for LMS

In contrast to other sarcomas, patients with LMS confined to the uterus appear to have a dominant pattern of failure outside the pelvis and abdominal cavity. In three series in which the site of first recurrence was documented, 14 (28%) of 49 patients developed pelvic or abdominal recurrence compared with 32 (65%) of 49 patients whose first recurrence had some component of distant disease.[52-54] Thus, in LMS, although the rate of failure in the pelvis is not insubstantial, little is to be potentially gained by delivering pelvic irradiation as a postoperative adjuvant treatment insofar as two-thirds of patients have some component of distant disease at first recurrence.

Although pelvic radiation has been used historically as an adjunct to surgery, many therapists have abandoned its use in patients with LMS because of the dominant pattern of distant failure, and they reserve radiation treatment for isolated pelvic relapse only. It is unlikely that adjuvant pelvic irradiation contributes significantly to overall survival from LMS.

Radiation Therapy for MMMT

Historically, pre- or postoperative pelvic irradiation has been used as an adjunct to surgery for MMMT. Many retrospective reviews illustrate this common use.[15,41,55-59] Often the criteria for selecting patients for pelvic irradiation after surgery have not been stated, although they probably reflect an investigator bias toward the use of radiation therapy for patients deemed to be at high risk of relapse. Several studies have identified adverse prognostic factors for MMMT;[15,39,60] however, no report has systematically evaluated the role of adjunctive radiation therapy related to these risk factors in MMMTs. In several reports for MMMT, the pelvic recurrence rate was 56%, whereas the distant metastasis rate was 45%. This represents a higher risk of pelvic recurrence than that seen in patients with LMS.[15,41,55,56,60] It also demonstrates that surgery alone, even for disease apparently confined to the uterus, is inadequate for control of disease in the pelvis. Some but not all studies have shown benefit from postoperative irradiation,[61,62] especially in local control.[58,63-67] However, few studies show that increased local control rates have an effect on overall survival.[15,67,68] Rates of distant metastases in series of patients treated with or without adjuvant pelvic irradiation are similar, in the order of 35–45%.[15,55,58]

In a study of the GOG conducted between 1973 and 1982, patients with stage I or II uterine sarcomas, including LMS (48 patients), MMMT (95 patients), ESS (10 patients), and unclassified tumors (4 patients), were randomly assigned to receive adjuvant doxorubicin or no chemotherapy following surgery.[58] The use of adjuvant pelvic radiation therapy was not controlled but was left to investigator discretion, and the study was not stratified for the use of radiation therapy. A subset analysis of this study was conducted by Hornback and colleagues and demonstrated a reduction in pelvic recurrence rates attributable to the use of adjunctive pelvic irradiation.[58] The data must be interpreted with some caution, however, because this was a nonrandomized comparison.

There has been only one randomized clinical trial evaluating the role of adjuvant pelvic radiotherapy in stage I and II Uterine Sarcomas .The EORTC enrolled 224 patients(103 LMS, 91 MMMT, and 28ESS) from 1998 to 2001 and demonstrated an improved local control rate for patients with MMMT (24% recurrence in RT vs 47% in observation) but no survival benefit. There was no improvement in local control for LMS (20% local recurrence in RT vs 24% in observation group).[69]

The morbidity associated with pelvic recurrence in uterine sarcomas may be substantial; therefore, it is reasonable to offer adjuvant pelvic irradiation to patients with MMMT to improve locoregional control rates. The doses of radiation have not been standardized;

however, it is probable that doses should be at least 50 Gy, fractionated over 5 weeks.

The GOG also conducted a phase III study of whole-abdomen irradiation (WAI) versus three cycles of cisplatin-ifosfamide and mesna (CIM) in 206 eligible patients with optimally debulked stage I–IV MMMT. Although there was no significant advantage the observed difference favored the use of combination chemotherapy. The adjusted recurrence rate was 21% lower for CIM patients (CI 0.53–1.17; p = 0.25) and the adjusted death rate was 29% lower (CI 0.48–1.04; p = 0.085). Moreover there was a significant increase in late adverse events in the WAI patients.[70]

Primary pelvic irradiation has been employed rarely in patients with sarcoma deemed inoperable. The possible additional utility of intracavitary irradiation must be evaluated because radiation dose distribution may be inadequate if the uterus is bulky. Literature reports suggest that in approximately half or two-thirds of patients, pelvic disease could be controlled with standard fractionated irradiation; a small proportion of patients are cured with such treatment.[15,41,55,56]

Finally, radiation may be useful as a palliative measure for recurrent or uncontrolled pelvic tumor causing pain or bleeding.

Chemotherapy

Two characteristics of uterine sarcomas increase the likelihood that systemic therapy will be required: a recurrence rate of at least 50% even in stage I disease and a tendency to recur at distant sites. Nevertheless, the amount of meaningful data on the use of systemic therapy is limited by the low incidence of these lesions. Studies by the GOG first identified the differential sensitivity of MMMT and LMS to drug therapy.[71] Because these two cell types respond differently to chemotherapy, they are discussed separately.

Single-Agent Therapy

Several drugs have been studied in advanced or recurrent MMMT and/or LMS (Table 103-2), including cisplatin,[72-75] ifosfamide,[76-78] doxorubicin,[71,79] liposomal doxorubicin,[80] etoposide,[81-83] mitoxantrone,[84] paclitaxel,[85,86] topotecan,[87] gemcitabine,[88] Trimetrexate,[89] and docetaxel.[90,91]

Malignant Mixed Müllerian Tumor

Ifosfamide is the most active single agent in the treatment of advanced or recurrent MMMT of the uterus. Sutton and colleagues conducted a phase II study of ifosfamide (1.5 g/m^2/day for 5 days every 4 weeks) and mesna in 30 patients with advanced or recurrent MMMT who had no previous chemotherapy.[76] Of 28 evaluable patients, 5 complete responses (17.9%) and 4 partial responses (14.3%) were observed (32.2% overall response rate). However, the response duration ranged from 1.4 to 8.6 months, with a median response duration of only 3.8 months (Table 103-2).

Cisplatin also appears to have significant activity.[72] In patients who had previously received chemotherapy, cisplatin 50 mg/m^2 produced an 18% response rate. Of 28 patients available for evaluation, 2 complete responses and three partial responses were observed. In patients who had not previously received chemotherapy, the same response rate of 19% was observed among a larger group of 63 patients treated with the same dose and schedule.[73] In a separate phase II trial, a higher dose, ranging from 75 to 100 mg/m^2 every 3 weeks, produced one complete response and four partial responses among 12 patients (42%) who had not received chemotherapy.[74] The small number of cases and the lack of a randomized trial permit no conclusions to be drawn about the merits of the higher dose.

The GOG conducted a phase II study of paclitaxel 170 mg/m^2 (135 mg/m^2 in those with prior irradiation) intravenously every 3 weeks in patients with histologic confirmation of MMMT and measurable disease who had failed appropriate local therapy. Among 44 evaluable patients, 8 (18.2%) had a response to paclitaxel: 4 had a complete response and 4 had a partial response.[86]

Leiomyosarcoma

Of the single agents that have been tested in patients with LMS (Table 103-2), doxorubicin is the most active. In the two GOG phase III trials comparing doxorubicin based chemotherapy in combination with dimethyltriazenoimidazole carboxamide (DTIC)[71] or cyclophosphamide[92] in advanced uterine sarcomas, response rates of 25% and 13%, respectively, were observed in patients with LMS treated with doxorubicin alone. Patients with LMS also had a significantly longer survival time than the other histologic cell types studied (12.1 vs 6.0 months). Liposomal doxorubicin at 50 mg/m^2 every 4 weeks had a disappointing respone rate of only 16%.[80] Ifosfamide, 1.5 g/m^2/day for 5 days every 3–4 weeks, exhibited moderate activity (17.2%), with 6 responses among 35 patients.[77] Single agent Gemcitabine had

Table 103-2 Single-Agent Activity in Uterine Sarcomas

Drug	Prior Chemotherapy	Schedule	Response, *n* (%)			Reference
			MMMT	LMS	ESS	
Ifosfamide	No	1.5 g/m^2/d + mesna, 0.3 g/m^2/d, d 1–5 q 4 weeks	9/28 (32)	6/35 (17)	7/21 (33)	68-70
Cisplatin	No	50 mg/m^2 q 3 weeks	12/63 (19)	1/33 (3)		64
	Yes	50 mg/m^2 q 3 weeks	5/28 (18)	1/19 (5)		65, 67
	No	75–100 mg/m^2 q 3 weeks	5/12 (42)			66
Doxorubicin	No	60 mg/m^2 q 3 weeks	4/41 (10)	7/28 (25)		63
	No	50–90 mg/m^2 q 3 weeks	0/9 (0)			71
Liposomal doxorubicin	No	50 mg/m^2 q 4 weeks		5/32 (16)		96
Etoposide	Yes	100 mg/m^2/d, d 1–3 q 4 weeks	2/31 (6)	3/28 (11)		72, 74
	Yes	50 mg/m^2/d, d 1–21 q 4 weeks		2/29 (7)		73
	No	100 mg/m^2/d, d 1–3 q 3 weeks		0/28 (0)		74
Mitoxantrone	Yes	12 mg/m^2 q 3 weeks	0/17 (0)	0/12 (0)		75
Paclitaxel	No	175 mg/m^2 q 3 weeks		3/34 (9)		76
Pacitaxel	Yes	170 mg/m^2 q 3 weeks	8/44 (18.)			95
Topotecan	No	1.5 mg/m^2/d, d 1–5 q 3 weeks		3/36 (8)		77
Gemcitabine	Yes	1,000 mg/m^2 d 1, 8, 15 q 4 weeks		9/44 (20.5)		78
Docetaxel	No	100 mg/m^2 q 3 weeks		0/16 (0)		98

Abbreviations: ESS, endometrial stromal sarcoma; LMS, leiomyosarcoma; MMMT, malignant mixed müllerian tumor.

a 20.5% response rate with 1 complete and 8 partial responses among 44 evaluable patients.[88] There were no responses in 16 LMS patients treated with single agent Docetaxel.[91]

Endometrial Stromal Sarcoma

There are few data in the gynecologic literature regarding the use of chemotherapy for ESS. The GOG conducted a phase II study of ifosfamide as initial chemotherapy in women with metastatic ESS.[78] Of 21 evaluable patients, there were 3 complete responses and 4 partial responses, for an overall response rate of 33.3%. Other agents have also been found to be active in the treatment of ESS, including doxorubicin;[10,18] the combination of vincristine, actinomycin D, and cyclophosphamide[10]; the combination of mitomycin and vinblastine[10]; chlorambucil[93]; and the combination of cyclophosphamide, vincristine, doxorubicin, and dacarbazine.[93]

In summary, the most active single agents against MMMT are ifosfamide, paclitaxil, and cisplatin. In LMS, doxorubicin, gemcitabine, and ifosfamide appear to have significant activity.

Combination Therapy

Randomized Trials

Four randomized trials evaluating combination chemotherapy have been completed to date and form the basis for current conclusions regarding the role of chemotherapy.

Leiomyosarcoma

In the first, patients with advanced (stage III or IV or recurrent) uterine sarcoma received either doxorubicin or doxorubicin plus DTIC (Table 103-3).[71] Although no significant differences between the two regimens were observed, conclusions from the trial were limited by an insufficient number of each histologic type to permit subset analysis.

The second randomized trial studied doxorubicin with or without cyclophosphamide (Table 103-3) and was closed prior to completion of original accrual goals because, based on the early data, the likelihood of identifying a difference in the two treatment regimens was extremely small.[92] The overall response rate was the same for doxorubicin with or without cyclophosphamide (19.2% total response rate). When the data were analyzed by cell type, 3 of the 20 patients with MMMT had complete responses.

Malignant Mixed Müllerian Tumor

With recognition of the difference in response between LMS and MMMT, randomized trials had to consider the two major histologic types as distinct entities requiring separate studies. A third phase III trial (GOG Protocol 108), completed in July 1996, compared ifosfamide with and without cisplatin in patients with advanced or recurrent MMMT.[94] Ifosfamide was given in a dose of 1.5 g/m^2/day for 5 days every 3 weeks for eight courses, with mesna uroprotection. In the combination arm, cisplatin was added at 20 mg/m^2 for 5 days. Early in the study, the dose of the combination regimen was decreased by 20% because of toxicity. Overall, 54% of patients treated with the combination regimen and 36% of patients treated with ifosfamide alone responded to therapy. This combination offered a slight prolongation of progression-free survival (relative risk 0.73; 95% upper confidence limit 0.94; p = .02, one-tailed test) but no significant survival benefit (relative risk 0.80; 95% upper confidence limit 1.03; p = .071, one-tailed test).

The most recent randomized trial by the GOG tested Ifosfamide with or without paclitaxel in advanced , persistent or recurrent MMMT. Random assignment to treatment was between ifosfamide 2.0 g/m^2 intravenously (IV) daily for 3 days (arm 1) or ifosfamide 1.6 g/m^2 IV daily for 3 days plus paclitaxel 135 mg/m^2 by 3-hour infusion day 1 (arm 2). Mesna was administered similarly (both arms); filtrate began on day 4 (arm 2). Of 179 evaluable patients, median PUFFS and OS, respectively, for arm 1 compared with arm 2 were 3.6 vs 5.8 months and 8.4 vs 13.5 months, respectively. There was a 31% decrease in the hazard of death (hazard ratio [HR], 0.69; 95% CI, 0.49–0.97; p = 0.03) and a 29% decrease in the hazard of progression (HR, 0.71; 95% CI, 0.51–0.97; p = 0.03) relative to arm 1 when stratifying by performance status. Toxicities in the combination arm were expected and manageable.[95]

Phase II Trials for LMS

Studies of LMS continue to focus on the identification of active drugs in phase II trials.

As discussed previously, the GOG demonstrated no benefit to the addition of either cyclophosphamide or DTIC to doxorubicin in advanced uterine sarcomas.[71,92] The GOG conducted a phase II study of doxorubicin in combination with ifosfamide-mesna in previously untreated patients with advanced or recurrent uterine LMS.[96] Of 33 patients, there was 1 complete response and 10 partial responses. Although the overall response rate was 33.3%, the toxicity was severe, with 13 patients developing grade 4 neutropenia and 2 patients developing grade 4 cardiotoxicity. Leyvraz and colleagues reported much higher response rates with a higher-dose intensity with the same combination.[97] At the 1998 meeting of the American Society of Clinical Oncology, they presented data on 17 patients with uterine LMS with a 55% response rate using ifosfamide 2–2.4 g/m^2/day on days 1–5, with doxorubicin 20–30 mg/m^2/day on days 1–3. Granulocyte colony-stimulating factor was used for 10 days and toxicity was still significant, with 63% febrile episodes and 40% grade 2–3 mucositis.

The GOG also reported on the results of a phase II trial of hydroxyurea, DTIC, and etoposide in the treatment of advanced or recurrent uterine LMS with an overall response rate of 18.4% in 38 evaluable patients.[94]

Hensley and colleagues reported a phase II trial in patients with unresectable, measurable LMS of the uterus (n = 29) or another (n = 5) primary site who had failed zero to two previous chemotherapy regimens in a single institution study.[98] Patients received gemcitabine 900 mg/m^2 intravenously on days 1 and 8 plus docetaxel 100 mg/m^2 intravenously on day 8, with granulocyte colony-stimulating factor subcutaneously on days 9–15. Cycles were repeated every 21 days. Patients with prior pelvic radiation received 25% lower doses of both agents. Among 34 patients, a complete response was observed in 3 patients and a partial response in 15, for an overall response rate of 53% (95% confidence interval 35–70%). Seven patients had stable disease.

To better define the activity of this combination chemotherapy regimen the GOG conducted two phase II studies with this regimen with gemcitabine at a fixed dose rate of 10 mg/m^2/min as first line and second line therapy for metastatic LMS.[99,100] As first line therapy, objective responses were observed in 15 of 42 patients (35.8% overall; complete response

Table 103-3 Randomized Trials of Chemotherapy in Advanced or Recurrent Uterine LMS

	Regimen, *n* (%)		
Study	**Doxorubicin**	**Doxorubicin + DTIC**	**Doxorubicin + Cytoxan**
GOG Protocol 2161	13/80 (16)	16/66 (24)	
Leiomyosarcoma	7/28 (25)	6/20 (30)	
Mixed mesodermal sarcoma	4/41 (10)	7/31 (23)	
Other sarcomas	2/11 (18)	3/15 (20)	
GOG Protocol 4278	5/26 (19)		5/26 (19)

Abbreviations: DTIC, dimethyltriazenoimidazole carboxamide; GOG, Gynecologic Oncology Group.

Table 103-4 Randomized Trials of Doxorubicin Versus No Further Therapy in Completely Resected Stages I and II Uterine Sarcoma

Cell Type	Recurrences		
	Doxorubicin	No Therapy	Total
Leiomyosarcoma	11/25 (44%)	14/23 (61%)	25/48 (52%)
Mixed mesodermal sarcoma	17/44 (39%)	25/49 (51%)	42/93 (45%)
Other sarcomas	3/6 (50%)	4/9 (44%)	7/15 (47%)
Total	31/75 (41%)	43/81 (53%)	74/156 (47%)

Source: From Ref. 101.

4.8%, partial response 31%, 90% confidence interval 23.5–49.6%), with an additional 11 (26.2%) having stable disease. The median progression-free survival (PFS) was 4.4 months (range 0.4–37.2+ months). Among 15 women with objective response, median response duration was 6 months (range 2.1–33.4+ months). Median overall survival was 16+ months (range: 4–41.3 months). Hensley et al. concluded that fixed dose rate gemcitabine and docetaxel is a reasonable option for first line treatment of uterine LMS.[99] Among 48 evaluable patients in the second line trial, the overall objective response rate is 27%, with complete response in 6.3% (3/48), and partial response in 20.8% (10/48). An additional 50% (24/48) had stable disease (median duration 5.4 months).[100] Of note, the exciting response rates noted in the initial single institution study (53%) was not reproduced in the lager uniform GOG trial.(27%).[100]

Adjuvant Chemotherapy for Limited Disease

The only randomized trial (GOG Protocol 20) of adjuvant chemotherapy in uterine sarcomas to date assigned patients to either doxorubicin 60 mg/m^2 every 3 weeks for eight cycles or no further therapy (Table 103-4).[101] For the overall patient population, there were no significant differences in recurrence rate, progression-free interval, or survival between those who received no further treatment and those who received adjuvant doxorubicin. Although each of the two major histologic subsets contained too few patients for proper analysis, in each subset, a 12% or greater difference in recurrence rate was noted, favoring the group receiving doxorubicin. The overall median survival was 73.7 months for patients given doxorubicin and 55.0 months for those given no further therapy. The major deficiency in this study—its failure to take into account the difference in response of the two major histologic subsets—is the result of a lack of understanding of this distinction when the trial was conducted.

The GOG also reported a study (GOG Protocol 117) of adjuvant ifosfamide, mesna, and cisplatin in patients with completely resected stage I or II MMMT of the uterus in which no postoperative radiotherapy was allowed. Ifosfamide was given in a dose of 1.5 g/m^2 and cisplatin 20 mg/m^2 daily for 5 days every 3 weeks for three cycles, with mesna uroprotection.[102] Early in the study, the regimen was reduced to 4 days because of myelotoxicity. Of the 65 evaluable patients, the median age was 65 years; 50 patients (77%) were stage I and 15 (23%) were stage II. Progression-free survival and overall survival rates, respectively, were 69% and 82% at 24 months and 54% and 52% at 84 months. The overall 5-year survival rate was 62%. Leukopenia was the most commonly reported, but manageable, toxicity.

Seleted References

The complete reference list can be found at www.CANCERMEDICINE8.com

1. Harlow BL, Weiss NS, Lofton S. The epidemiology of sarcomas of the uterus. *J Natl Cancer Inst.* 1986;76:399–402.
2. Brooks SE, Zhan M, Cote T, et al. Surveillance, epidemiology, and end results analysis of 2677 cases of uterine sarcoma 1989–1999. *Gynecol Oncol.* 2004;93(1):204–208.
3. Ober WB. Uterine sarcomas: Histogenesis and taxonomy. *Ann NY Acad Sci.* 1959;75:568
4. Kempson RL, Bari W. Uterine sarcomas. Classification, diagnosis, and prognosis. *Hum Pathol.* 1970;1:331–349.
5. Czesnin K, Wronkowski Z. Second malignancies of the irradiated area in patients treated for uterine cervix cancer. *Gynecol Oncol.* 1978;6:309–315.
6. Norris HJ, Taylor HB. Postirradiation sarcomas of the uterus. *Obstet Gynecol.* 1965;26:689–694.
7. Wickerham DL, Fisher B, Wolmark N, et al. Association of tamoxifen and uterine sarcoma. *J Clin Oncol.* 2002;20(11):2758–2760.
8. Wysowski DK, Honig SF, Beitz J. Uterine sarcoma associated with tamoxifen use. *N Engl J Med.* 2002;346(23):1832–1833.
9. Major FJ, Blessing JA, Silverberg SG, et al. Prognostic factors in early-stage uterine sarcoma. A Gynecologic Oncology Group study. *Cancer.* 1993;71(4 Suppl):1702–1709.
10. Berchuck A, Rubin SC, Hoskins WJ, et al. Treatment of endometrial stromal tumors. *Gynecol Oncol.* 1990;36:60–65.
11. Leibsohn S, d'Ablaing G, Mishell DR Jr, et al. Leiomyosarcoma in a series of hysterectomies performed for presumed uterine leiomyomas. *Am J Obstet Gynecol.* 1990;162:968–974; discussion 974–976.
12. Ferenczy A, Richart RM, Okagaki T. A comparative ultra-structural study of leiomyosarcoma, cellular leiomyoma, and leiomyoma of the uterus. *Cancer.* 1971;28:1004–1018.
13. Spiro RH, Koss LG. Myosarcoma of the uterus. *Cancer.* 1965;18:571–588.
14. Davids AM. Myomectomy surgical technique and results in a series of 1150 cases. *Am J Obstet Gynecol.* 1952;63:592–604.
15. Larson B, Silfversward C, Nilsson B, et al. Mixed müllerian tumours of the uterus—prognostic factors: a clinical and histopathologic study of 147 cases. *Radiother Oncol.* 1990;17:123–132.
16. Wen, BC, Tewfik FA, Tewfick HH, et al. Uterine sarcoma: a retrospective study. *J Surg Oncol.* 1987;34(2):104–108.
17. Ali S, Wells M. Mixed Mullerian tumors of the uterine corpus: a review. *Int J Gynecol Cancer.* 1993;3(1):1–11.
18. Goff BA, Rice LW, Fleischhacker D, et al. Uterine leiomyosarcoma and endometrial stromal sarcoma: lymph node metastases and sites of recurrence. *Gynecol Oncol.* 1993;50:105–109.
19. Berchuck A, Rubin SC, Hoskins WJ, et al. Treatment of uterine leiomyosarcoma. *Obstet Gynecol.* 1988;71(6 Pt 1):845–850.
20. Kurjak A, Kupesic S, Shalan H, et al. Uterine sarcoma: a report of 10 cases studied by transvaginal color and pulsed Doppler sonography. *Gynecol Oncol.* 1995;59:342–346.
21. Sung PL, Chen YJ, Liu RS, et al. Whole-body positron emission tomography with 18F-fluorodeoxyglucose is an effective method to detect extra-pelvic recurrence in uterine sarcomas. *Eur J Gynaecol Oncol.* 2008;29(3):246–251.
22. Cramer SF, Meyer JS, Kraner JF, et al. Metastasizing leiomyoma of the uterus. S-phase fraction, estrogen receptor, and ultrastructure. *Cancer.* 1980;45:932–937.
23. Evans AT III, Symmonds RE, Gaffey TA. Recurrent pelvic intravenous leiomyomatosis. *Obstet Gynecol.* 1981;57:260–264.
24. Kurman RJ, Norris HJ. Mesenchymal tumors of the uterus. VI. Epithelioid smooth muscle tumors including leiomyoblastoma and clear-cell leiomyoma: a clinical and pathologic analysis of 26 cases. *Cancer.* 1976;7:1853–1865.
25. Rose PG, Piver MS, Tsukada Y, et al. Patterns of metastasis in uterine sarcoma. An autopsy study. *Cancer.* 1989;63:935–938.
26. Fleming WP, Peters WA III, Kumar NB, et al. Autopsy findings in patients with uterine sarcoma. *Gynecol Oncol.* 1984;19:168–172.
27. Chen SS. Propensity of retroperitoneal lymph node metastasis in patients with stage I sarcoma of the uterus. *Gynecol Oncol.* 1989;32:215–217.
28. DiSaia PJ, Morrow CP, Boronow R, et al. Endometrial sarcoma: lymphatic spread pattern. *Am J Obstet Gynecol.* 1978;130:104–105.
29. Gadducci A, Fabrini MG, Bonuccelli A, et al. Analysis of treatment failures in patients with early-stage uterine leiomyosarcoma. *Anticancer Res.* 1995;15:485–488.
30. Barakat RR, Rubin SC, Wong G, et al. Mixed mesodermal tumor of the ovary: analysis of prognostic factors in 31 cases. *Obstet Gynecol.* 1992;80:660–664.

31. Plaxe SC, Dottino PR, Goodman HM, et al. Clinical features of advanced ovarian mixed mesodermal tumors and treatment with doxorubicin- and cis-platinum-based chemotherapy. *Gynecol Oncol*. 1990;37:244–249.
32. Imachi M, Tsukamoto N, Shigematsu T, et al. Malignant mixed müllerian tumor of the fallopian tube: report of two cases and review of literature. *Gynecol Oncol*. 1992;47:114–124.
33. Horn LC, Werschnik C, Bilek K, et al. Diagnosis and clinical management in malignant müllerian tumors of the fallopian tube. A report of four cases and review of recent literature. *Arch Gynecol Obstet*. 1996;258:47–53.
34. Jacobs AJ, McMurray EH, Parham J, et al. Treatment of carcinoma of the fallopian tube using cisplatin, doxorubicin, and cyclophosphamide. *Am J Clin Oncol*. 1986;9:436–439.
35. Ebert AD, Perez-Canto A, Schaller G, et al. Stage I primary malignant mixed müllerian tumor of the fallopian tube. Report of a case with five-year survival after minimal surgery without adjuvant treatment. *J Reprod Med*. 1998;43:598–600.
36. Taylor HB, Norris HJ. Mesenchymal tumors of the uterus. IV. Diagnosis and prognosis of leiomyosarcomas. *Arch Pathol*. 1966;82:40–44.
37. Aaro LA, Symmonds RE, Dockerty ME. Sarcoma of the uterus. A clinical and pathologic study of 177 cases. *Am J Obstet Gynecol*. 1966;94:101–109.
38. Peters WA III, Kumar NB, Fleming WP, et al. Prognostic features of sarcomas and mixed tumors of the endometrium. *Obstet Gynecol*. 1984;63:550–556.

104 Neoplasms of the Breast

Gabriel N. Hortobagyi, MD, FACP ■ Laura Esserman, MD ■ Thomas A. Buchholz, MD, FACP

Female breast cancer is a major medical problem with significant public health and societal ramifications. Major advances have been made in the past 40 years in understanding the biologic and clinical nature of the disease, and dramatic changes in treatment have been implemented.[1] Since 1990, there has been a significant reduction in breast cancer mortality in the United States and several Western European countries. Starting in 2001, a significant reduction in incidence was documented in the United States. The National Cancer Institute estimates that there are currently more than 2 million breast cancer survivors in the United States. The lifetime risk for women of being diagnosed with breast cancer is currently between 1 in 7 and 1 in 8 (Table 104-1).[2] The risk is even higher for women with certain risk factors, such as a strong family history or known genetic mutations. As new information accumulates, new paradigms of management compete for acceptance with existing ones. It is axiomatic that good scientific data provides the bedrock for good clinical management. Information obtained from molecular, biologic, and pathologic investigations and from clinical trials provides the major focus of this chapter.

Epidemiology

Breast cancer is the most common malignancy in North American women and for women throughout the industrialized world. In the United States, breast cancer accounts for 26% of all cancers in women.[3] The American Cancer Society estimates that during 2008, 182,460 women will be diagnosed as having breast cancer.[3] In addition, 1990 men will be diagnosed with breast cancer. These figures exclude the 67,770 new cases of in situ breast cancer expected to occur. The incidence rate of breast cancer had increased steadily over 40 years, leveled off in the 1990s to about 110 cases per 100,000, and around 2001 rates started to decrease by 3.5% per year through 2004 (Table 104-2).[2]

Some experts believe that the earlier gradual increase in incidence might have been explained by more frequent and systematic use of screening mammography and the lead-time bias associated with earlier diagnosis. Other significant causes of the increasing incidence of breast cancer include the increasing average age of the population, with more women moving into age ranges where breast cancer is most common, as well as the common use of postmenopausal hormone replacement. The incidence of breast cancer has also increased worldwide. In 1985, it was estimated that more than 500,000 new cases would be diagnosed, with about half of the cases occurring in the Western, industrialized countries and the other half occurring in developing countries. By 1990, it was estimated that close to 900,000 new cases of breast cancer would be diagnosed, and during 2007, more than 1,301,867 women developed breast cancer. Incidence rates vary substantially around the world. The incidence rates reported range 4 and 6 per 100,000 (Mozambique and Gambia, respectively) to 28.61 per 100,000 women (Japan) and contrast with incidence rates higher than 125 new cases per year per 100,000 women from the United States and Northern Europe.[4] Some of these differences have been attributed to diet, whereas others might be related to the changing roles of women in modern industrialized societies (earlier onset of menses, delayed parity, use of oral contraceptives and hormone replacement therapy (HRT), later onset of menopause, longer life-expectancy, and increased consumption of alcohol).[5,6]

The mortality rate of breast cancer in the United States remained essentially stable from the 1950s to 1989. According to the most recent data, however, mortality rates declined significantly since 1990, with the largest decreases in younger women—both white and African American.[2] These decreases are probably the result of earlier detection and improved treatment. The American Cancer Society estimated that in 2008, 40,930 deaths related to breast cancer would be reported, 40,480 of them in women. That figure represents 15% of all cancer-related deaths in American women.[3] National statistics suggest that there has been a decrease in the mortality rate of breast cancer in women of all ages over the past 15 years, being most prominent in white women under the age of 50 years and least notable in African American women older than 50 years. Similar decreases in breast cancer-related mortality obtained from population-based figures have been documented in Canada, Austria, Germany, Sweden, and the United Kingdom. However, these favorable trends are not universal and have not been evident in other countries.[4,7,8] Breast cancer is the second leading cause of cancer-related deaths in women in the United States (after lung cancer), but it is the leading cause of cancer-related deaths in women between the ages of 20 and 59.[3] The relative 5-year survival rates increased from 63% to 90% for white women between 1960 and 2003 and from 46% to 78% for black women during the same period.[3]

Sixty-three percent of new breast cancer cases in the United States are diagnosed while in the localized (node-negative) stage; another 29% are diagnosed in a regional stage, and 6% have metastasized to distant sites at the time of initial diagnosis (stage was unknown

Table 104-1 ■ **Lifetime Probability of Developing Breast Cancer (Females, All Races)**

Age	Cumulative Probability
By age 25	1 in 7692
By age 30	1 in 1639
By age 35	1 in 483
By age 40	1 in 181
By age 45	1 in 80
By age 50	1 in 43
By age 55	1 in 28
By age 60	1 in 19
By age 65	1 in 14
By age 70	1 in 11
By age 75	1 in 9
By age 80	1 in 8
By age 85	1 in 7

Source: Feuer EJ, Wun LM. DEVCAN: Probability of developing or dying of cancer software, Version 6.3.0 National Cancer Institute, April 2008. http://srab.cancer.gov/devcan/canques.html

Table 104-2 ■ **Rates by Race or Ethnicity: United States, 2001-2005**

	All Races	White	African-American	Hispanic-Latino	American Indian/ Alaskan Native	Asian/Pacific Islander
Incidence rates (per 100,000)[2,3]	126.1	130.6	117.5	90.1	75.0	89.6
Mortality rates (per 100,000)[2,3]	25.0	24.4	33.5	15.8	14.3	12.6

for the remaining 2%).[3] The percentage of patients with localized breast cancer is even higher among women who follow a systematic screening strategy; among these patients, between 20% and 30% of breast cancer cases are diagnosed in a noninvasive stage, and of those with invasive breast cancer, up to 79% have negative axillary lymph nodes. In contrast, at least 50% of breast cancer cases in Latin America and other parts of the developing world are reported in stage III or IV at the time of diagnosis.[9] This is a substantial public health challenge for these countries, and, despite lower incidence rates, it results in higher mortality rates than those observed in Western Europe and the United States.[10] The mortality-to-incidence ratios ranged from 0.19 in North America to 0.46 in Southeast Asia to a high of 0.73 in Middle Africa. This could represent late stage diagnosis or a difference in the biology of the tumors that present or a combination of both. In 2000 it was estimated that 471,000 deaths were attributed to breast cancer around the world.[9]

Risk Factors

The incidence of breast cancer varies substantially according to certain well-established risk factors (Table 104-3).[5,11,12] Among these factors, the two most prominent are gender and age.

Gender

The age-adjusted breast cancer incidence rate is approximately 100 times higher in women than in men in the United States, a ratio that is fairly consistent around the world, although some reports suggest that the incidence of male breast cancer might be several fold higher in some African countries.[2,4] A number of risk factors have been identified in women. Because of the small number of male breast cancers, risk factors for male breast cancer are much less well established.

Age

The incidence of breast cancer increases dramatically with age, ranging from fewer than 10 cases per 100,000 women between the ages of 20 and 30 to more than 300 cases per 100,000 women over the age of 60.[2] The probabilities of developing invasive breast cancer are 0.48%, 3.86%, 3.51%, 6.95%, and 12.28% for women aged 39 or younger, 40 to 59, 60 to 69, 70 and older, and lifetime, respectively.[3] However, the correlation of age and increase in incidence is not linear. The slope of the correlation curve is steepest in younger women; it decreases dramatically during and shortly after the menopause, to resume a steeper correlation several years after menopause. The median age at diagnosis of breast cancer in the United States is 64 years. In other parts of the world, where life expectancy is shorter, the median age at which breast cancer develops is 10 to 15 years younger. Age-related mortality rates parallel this pattern.

Table 104-3 Risk Factors Associated With the Development of Breast Cancer

Major increase
Mutations in *BRCA1*, *BRCA2*, Li-Fraumeni syndrome
Increasing age
Western culture
Family history of breast or ovarian cancer in first- degree relatives
Atypical hyperplasia, LCIS before the age of 45
Exposure to ionizing radiation
Moderate increase
Prior diagnosis of breast cancer
Early menarche
Late menopause
Nulliparity or delayed first full-term pregnancy (above age 30)
High socioeconomic status
Alcohol intake
Atypical hyperplasia, LCIS over the age of 45
Obesity (postmenopausal women only)
Unfavorable mammographic parenchymal pattern
Diagnosis of soft-tissue sarcoma in son or daughter
Prior diagnosis of uterine, ovarian, or colon cancer
Modest increase
Benign breast disease with hyperplasia (no atypia)
Oral contraceptives (for longer than 10 years)
Postmenopausal estrogen replacement therapy
Questionable increase (no evidence to support)
Interrupted first pregnancy
Psychosomatic factors
High-fat diet
Complex fibroadenoma
Decrease
Full-term pregnancy before age 20
Multiple pregnancies
Ovariectomy before age 45
Regular exercise, especially during adolescence and early adulthood
Breast feeding
No effect
Breast reduction

Socioeconomic Class

Breast cancer is found more frequently in women of higher economic class and educational status.[11] This finding is probably related to lifestyle factors such as diet, age at first childbirth, exogenous hormonal use, and alcohol consumption. However, mortality is higher in women of underprivileged groups, suggesting that access to care and compliance with treatment remain important obstacles for optimal diagnosis and treatment.

Ethnicity

Multiple reports suggest that there are important differences in breast cancer incidence and mortality rates among various minority groups in the United States (see Table 104-2).[3] The incidence rates of female breast cancer for 1998 to 2002 were 119.4 per 100,000 among African Americans, 89.9 per 100,000 among Hispanic Americans, 54.8 per 100,000 for American Indians/Alaskan Natives, 96.6 per 100,000 for Asians/Pacific Islanders, and 141.1 per 100,000 for white women.[2] These represent increases compared to the previous 5-year period.[2,3] In contrast, the estimated mortality rates for 1995 to 2001 for the same ethnic groups were 34.7, 16.7, 13.8, 12.7, and 25.9, respectively. Although breast cancer was diagnosed in a localized stage in 64% of white women, it was diagnosed in that stage in only 53% of African Americans.[3] Studies of migrant populations have shown that when low-risk groups (eg, Chinese or other Far-Eastern groups) move to high-risk regions (Hawaii or mainland United States), their incidence of breast cancer increases rapidly, approaching the rates of the host population within one or two generations.[13]

Family History/Genetics

Eleven to 30% of women with breast cancer have one or more first-degree relatives with breast cancer, while up to 40% report one relative of any type with breast cancer.[14] About 4% to 9% are considered to have hereditary breast cancer.[15] Individuals with a first-degree relative with a history of breast cancer have a substantially increased risk of developing breast cancer themselves compared to women without such a family history (Table 104-4).[11] The identification and cloning of *BRCA1* and *BRCA2*, two genes associated with familial breast (and other) cancer, have highlighted the importance of taking a careful family history during the initial evaluation of breast cancer risk factors. Linkage analyses localized *BRCA1* to chromosome 17q21, and loss of heterozygosity studies suggested that this gene acts as a tumor suppressor gene. Its physiological function is related to DNA repair. *BRCA2* was localized to chromosome 13q12. *BRCA2* mutations are associated with early-onset breast and ovarian cancer and male breast cancer, as well as prostate and pancreatic cancer.[16-18] The prevalence of *BRCA1* mutations in high-risk families ranges from less than 20% to more than 80% in different countries. The prevalence is higher in families with ovarian cancer or both ovarian and breast cancer. In population-based series of patients who had breast cancer diagnosed before age 35 years, *BRCA1* mutations were detected

Table 104-4 **Risk Model and Associated Relative Risks**[a]

Risk Factor (Code No.)		Associated Relative Risk	No. of Cases (*n* = 2852)	No. of Controls (*n* = 3146)
Age at menarche (yr)				
≥14 (0)		1.000	790	926
12-13 (1)		1.099	1554	1735
<12 (2)		1.207	508	485
No of previous breast biopsies				
Age <50 yr				
0 (0)		1.000	635	794
1 (1)		1.698	113	93
≥2 (2)		2.882	66	24
Age ≥50 yr				
0 (0)		1.000	1551	1817
1 (1)		1.273	312	300
≥2 (2)		1.620	175	118
Age at First Live Birth (Yr)	**No. Relatives With Breast Cancer**			
<20 (0)	0 (0)	1.000	167	285
	1 (1)	2.607	44	40
	≥ 2 (2)	6.798	8	0
20-24 (1)	0 (0)	1.244	708	1042
	1 (1)	2.681	208	123
	≥2 (2)	5.775	25	5
25-29 or nulliparous (2)	0 (0)	1.548	986	1106
	1 (1)	2.756	247	178
	≥2 (2)	4.907	46	20
≥30 (3)	0 (0)	1.927	307	291
	1 (1)	2.834	87	50
	≥ 2 (2)	4.169	19	6

[a]Relative risk compared to an individual of the same age without any risk factors is estimated by locating the person's associated relative risk for AGEMEN, NBIOPS, and the combination AGEFLB and NUMREL and multiplying these three numbers together.

Source: From Ref. 57.

in 6.2%.[19,20] The great majority of *BRCA1* mutations are found in individuals with moderate-risk to high-risk families. For those individuals with *BRCA1* or *BRCA2* mutations, the lifetime risk of developing breast cancer ranges from 40% to 85%. The characteristics of *BRCA1*-related breast cancers include earlier age at onset, lower diploidy rate, higher proliferative rate, higher mitotic counts, higher proportion of estrogen receptor (ER)-negative and progesterone receptor (PR)-negative tumors, and more lymphocytic infiltration than sporadic cancers.[20] BRCA2-associated cancers had lower mitotic counts, higher score for tubule formation, ER positivity and greater proportion of continuous pushing margins than sporadic tumors.[20] Despite the association with adverse prognostic characteristics, *BRCA1*-associated breast cancers have prognoses similar to or better than sporadic tumors of similar stage.[20,21]

Studies have suggested that Jewish women, especially those with a family history of breast cancer in a first-degree relative, have a risk of breast cancer almost four times that of women in other ethnic groups. Characteristic *BRCA1* (185delAG, 5382insC) and *BRCA2* (6174delT) mutations have been identified in Ashkenazi Jews; the combined frequency of these genes in the general population exceeds 2%.[16,22] Similar "founder" mutations have been identified in Belgium, Denmark, Finland, France, Holland, Hungary, Iceland, Norway, Russia and West Africa, among other ethnic communities.[23] Familial breast cancer, however, accounts for less than 10% of all breast cancers, and *BRCA1*-related and *BRCA2*-related familial breast cancers appear to be responsible for only half to two-thirds of these cases. Other genetic abnormalities and less common familial cancer syndromes (Li-Fraumeni and others) are responsible for an additional small number of breast cancers. The cloning of *BRCA1* and *BRCA2* and additional molecular genetic markers of risk brought the issue of genetic screening and counseling to the forefront. Both negative and positive test results are associated with a variety of emotional, economic, and work-related issues. Genetic screening has become an important part of the management of breast cancer patients (see the section on prevention below).

Endocrine and Reproductive Risk Factors

Numerous studies suggest a strong link between the female hormones estrogen and progesterone and the development of breast cancer. In experimental systems, estrogen is required for optimal development of mammary carcinomas. Breast cancer is almost exclusively a disease of women and is rare in males. Ovarian ablation reduces dramatically the risk of mammary cancers in premenopausal women and in experimental animals. Clinical reports suggest that the younger the age when ovarian ablation is performed, the greater the protective effect. This is true even in women who carry a *BRCA1* or *BRCA2* mutation and are genetically predisposed to develop breast cancer. Epidemiologic studies have demonstrated repeatedly that the lack of full-term pregnancies is a risk factor for breast cancer.[12] Early onset of menarche, late onset of menopause, and a greater number of years with ovulatory cycles have all been associated with an increased risk of breast cancer. Thus, women who start menses before the age of 12 have twice the incidence of breast cancer as do those who undergo menarche after age 12.[12] This is probably related to longer exposure of the breast parenchyma to physiologic levels of estrogens. External influences that delay the onset of menses, such as poor nutrition or strenuous physical activity, might, therefore, reduce the incidence of breast cancer.[24] Menopause occurring after age 54 increases risk of breast cancer twofold, compared to the risk of women who have their menopause before age 45. The incidence of breast cancer for women who have their first full-term pregnancy before age 18 is one-third that of women who have their first pregnancy after age 35. This has led to speculation that the initial mutagenic event usually occurs before age 18, probably during the rapid growth of the breast at puberty, and that the hormonal milieu of pregnancy diminishes the oncogenicity of the mutated cells. Women who have their first child after age 30 have a higher risk of breast cancer than nulliparous women. The possible mechanism for this apparent enhancement in risk might be the stimulatory effect of pregnancy (and its altered hormonal environment) on an otherwise involuting epithelium. Most epidemiologic studies have suggested that long periods of lactation reduce breast cancer risk, but that the effect of short periods of lactation that are typical of women in most developed nations is likely to be small. In a recent meta-analysis, each birth decreased the relative risk (RR) of breast cancer by 7%, and each year of breastfeeding decreased the RR by an additional 4.3%.[25] There is now consistent evidence that the addition of progesterone to estrogen is associated with an increased risk of developing breast cancer,[26-28] which will be discussed in greater detail below.

Exogenous Hormones

The relationship of exogenous hormone replacement or oral contraceptives to risk of breast cancer has been under intense scrutiny for the past several decades.[29,30] Until recently, published studies have presented inconsistent and often contradictory conclusions about hormone replacement therapy (HRT). In a large meta-analysis, the Collaborative Group on Hormonal Factors in Breast Cancer found that current or recent use of HRT was associated with a modest increase in risk of breast cancer.[29] The RR was 1.35 (ie, a 35% increase) for women who had used HRT for 5 years or longer. On an annualized basis, this increase is comparable in magnitude with the effect on breast cancer of delaying menopause.

Definitive results were recently provided by the Women's Health Initiative randomized controlled trial. In this study, 16,608 postmenopausal, otherwise healthy women were randomly assigned to conjugated estrogen plus medroxyprogesterone acetate or placebo.[30] The combined estrogen and progesterone arm was stopped in July of 2002 after 5.2 years of followup, because health risks exceeded health benefits. There was a 29% increase in coronary heart disease, a 26% increase in breast cancer, a 41% increase in stroke and a 13% increase in pulmonary embolism associated with HRT. Simultaneously, there was a 47% reduction in colorectal cancer and a 34% reduction in hip fractures among women on hormonal replacement. No protective effects were found for memory loss or other measures of intellectual function. The Million Women Study and the HERS II study reached similar conclusions.[28,31] The increase in the RR of breast cancer was greater for women of lower rather than women of higher weight or body mass index.[29] Combined estrogen-progestin treatments conferred a significantly higher risk than estrogen replacement alone (which was studied in 10,739 women who had undergone hysterectomy). This arm of the trial was not stopped and after 6.8 years, there was no evidence that exposure to estrogen alone increases breast cancer risk.[32] The increase in risk of endometrial cancer associated with estrogen replacement only therapy (the reason why progesterone was added to HRT in the first place) is substantially less than the risk of breast cancer associated with combined HRT. Exposure to combined HRT (in the WHI) led to a 1.26 increase in the incidence of breast cancer.[27] Endometrial cancers that arise after estrogen exposure are almost always low grade and treated with hysterectomy alone. However, the breast cancers that arise after combination HRT were not all low grade, low stage cancers. A substantial fraction was grade 2 and 3 and node-positive. The increased risk associated with HRT appears to be driven by progesterone.

The United States Preventive Services Task Force concluded that the harmful effects of estrogen and progestin exceed the chronic disease prevention effects in most women. Although short-term use of HRT might be beneficial for control of vasomotor symptoms related to menopause, long-term use is not indicated.

The composition of oral contraceptives has changed considerably over the years; the type and dose of estrogens, the presence or absence of a progestin, duration of administration, and age at onset all vary from study to study. Recent, detailed analyses of the many epidemiologic studies correlating oral contraceptive use with risk of breast cancer have reached somewhat similar conclusions.[33] Current or recent users of oral contraceptives have a small increase in the RR of having breast cancer (RR for current users = 1.24), but this excess risk disappears 10 years after stopping use. Women who began using oral contraceptives before age 20 had higher RRs of having breast cancer diagnosed. As was stated in relation to HRT, the cancers diagnosed in association with oral contraceptive use tended to be less advanced clinically than the cancers diagnosed in those who have never used oral contraceptives.[33]

Abortion

There is insufficient evidence to support an association of abortion with breast cancer risk.

Physical Activity

Regular physical activity, especially during adolescence, has been associated with significant reductions in the risk of early onset of breast cancer in some studies.[24] Strenuous exercise has profound effects on menstrual activity during adolescence. Exercise delays menarche and produces amenorrhea in ballet dancers and females participating in college athletic programs. Participation in even moderate levels of physical activity can significantly reduce the frequency of ovulatory cycles.[34] Any factor that reduces the frequency of ovulation, and therefore the cumulative exposure to ovarian hormones, may reduce a woman's lifetime risk of developing breast cancer. On the basis of this information, one might hypothesize that regular physical exercise during adolescence and early adulthood would be beneficial, even if its effect on reducing breast cancer risk remains unproven. Two recent reports suggest that low-fat diet as well as exercise result in reduced risk of recurrence following treatment of primary ER-negative breast cancer.

Insulin-Like Growth Factor

Insulin-like growth factor type 1 (IGF-1) is a mitogenic peptide that enhances the proliferation of breast epithelial cells and is thought to have a role in breast cancer.[35] A recent case-control study within the prospective Nurses' Health Study cohort showed a positive relation between circulating IGF-1 concentration and risk of breast cancer among premenopausal women. This correlation was absent in the postmenopausal group. Additional studies to determine the potential clinical utility of this observation are needed.

Environmental Factors, Obesity, and Diet

There is a six- to ten-fold difference in incidence between the United States and Western Europe (highest incidence) and most middle-African countries (lowest incidence), with Asian, Latin American, and Eastern and Southern European countries reporting an intermediate incidence.[10] The incidence rates in some of the low-risk regions have been increasing over the past several decades. Furthermore, epidemiologic studies have indicated that immigrant groups from low- to high-risk regions evidence increasing incidence rates that approach those of the higher risk host region.[13,34] These observations suggest that environmental factors might influence the risk of developing breast cancer. Variations in weight, height, and reproductive factors represent confounding variables in these studies. In addition, most confounding risk factors point to dietary differences between high- and low-risk regions.[36] Multiple laboratory and epidemiologic studies have provided conflicting data about a correlation between dietary intake of animal proteins, total calories, animal fat, fiber, micronutrients, and risk of breast cancer.[5,36-39] Virtually all these studies were retrospective in nature. More recent and definitive studies have failed to confirm this hypothesis.

On the basis of these conflicting experimental and clinical data, one might conclude that the association between diet and risk of breast cancer is weak, at best, and possibly nonexistent. Dietary interventions have been tested in preclinical animal experiments with mixed results. In some models and animal species used, decreased caloric intake and a low-fat diet have been associated with a decreased risk of breast cancer or no change in the incidence of mammary carcinoma.

Dietary interventions (mostly low-fat diets that limit daily caloric intake from fat to less than 15% to 20%) have proven feasible in clinical studies.[40,41] The Women's Health Initiative is a randomized, placebo-controlled, multicenter trial involving postmenopausal women aged 50 to 79 years. Three different interventions were built into this study, one of which was designed to reduce fat intake to 20% of all caloric intake while increasing the intake of fruits and vegetables. Whether this modest reduction in dietary fat intake can result in a tangible reduction in breast cancer risk or not, the reduction in dietary fat may have salutary effects on the prevention or control of cardiovascular disease, osteoarthritis, endometrial cancer, diabetes, and other chronic illnesses. Because obesity in post-menopausal women is a risk factor that is associated with a greater risk of breast cancer, weight reduction should be encouraged in middle-aged and older adults, even in the absence of demonstrated clear-cut reduction of breast cancer incidence because other health benefits may be associated with this intervention. Additional studies should clarify the role of diet in the etiology of breast cancer. Finally, there is some evidence that women with a high intake of phytoestrogens, particularly the isoflavonic phytoestrogen equol and the lignan enterolactone, have a lower breast cancer risk.

The relation of body weight to breast cancer is complex.[42-44] An inverse association between relative weight and breast cancer risk has been found among premenopausal women in case-control and prospective studies. Obesity may reduce breast cancer risk slightly in premenopausal women through its association with an ovulatory menstrual cycles. In many case-control studies, body mass index has been positively associated with postmenopausal breast cancer.[43] However, prospective studies have generally suggested only a weak, if any, positive association.[42,43] Postmenopausal women who are obese have higher estrogen levels resulting from greater conversion of adrenal androgens to estrogens in adipose tissue, and they have lower levels of sex hormone–binding globulin, resulting in more free estrogen.[44] Dietary fat reduction has been shown to reduce body weight and plasma estradiol concentration in postmenopausal women.[44] This provides additional evidence in support of interventional studies to reduce chances of developing breast cancer. Other studies suggest that total body size, rather than weight-to-height ratio, and increased central-to-peripheral body fat distribution may be more important than degree of adiposity.[42] In summary, the role of specific dietary factors in breast cancer causation is not completely resolved. Results from prospective studies do not support the concept that fat intake in middle life has a major relation to breast cancer risk. However, weight gain in middle life contributes substantially to breast cancer risk. Alcohol is the best-established dietary risk factor, probably by increasing endogenous estrogen levels. Hypotheses relating diet during youth to risk decades later will be difficult to test. Nevertheless, available evidence indicates that breast cancer risk can be reduced by avoiding weight gain during adult years, and by limiting alcohol consumption.

Alcohol Consumption

Epidemiologic studies have consistently found that women who consume alcohol are at increased risk of developing breast cancer.[45,46] In multivariate analyses controlled for age, race, body mass, and smoking, the RR ranged from 1.5, for one to two drinks per day, to 3.3, for six or more drinks per day. There were no significant differences in this association depending on the type of alcoholic beverage. Early exposure to alcohol may be a key risk factor. Alcohol consumption in premenopausal women has been associated with increased total estrogen levels and bioavailable estrogens. The association of alcohol consumption and postmenopausal obesity with subsequent breast cancer risk might be mediated, at least in part, through alteration of plasma estrogen levels. Recent epidemiologic data suggested that the excess risk of breast cancer associated with alcohol consumption may be reduced by adequate folate intake.[47]

Viral Particles

Various investigators have suggested that breast cancer might be associated with oncogenic viruses. Such reports were strengthened by the demonstration that mouse mammary tumor virus (MMTV) caused mammary carcinomas in mice. Recent reports have shown that sequences highly homologous to segments of MMTV are present in human malignant breast tumors.[48] This finding is present in 30% to 40% of breast cancers in Western Europe and the United States, whereas in the Far East it is found in about 10% of breast cancers. Such sequences have not been found in normal breast tissue. Whether these viral particles are causally related to human breast cancer remains to be established.

Radiation Exposure

Exposure to ionizing radiation is a known risk factor for breast cancer. Atomic bomb survivors and patients treated with irradiation for postpartum mastitis, acne, hirsutism, or arthritic conditions all have an increased incidence of breast cancer, even after low or moderate radiation doses. Repeated fluoroscopic chest radiography, as used for monitoring the treatment of tuberculosis in the past, is also associated with increased risk of breast cancer. However, the risk of developing breast cancer as a result of common diagnostic radiologic procedures is minimal, and radiology technologists do not have an increased incidence of breast cancer. The incidence of breast cancer is also increased in patients who received mantle radiotherapy for Hodgkin disease.[49] The adolescent and young adult breast appear most susceptible to the carcinogenic effects of ionizing radiation, but irradiation during infancy and childhood also increases breast cancer risk. The latency period between radiation exposure and the development of breast cancer is long (median, 30 years). Recent evidence suggests that therapeutic radiation administered to treat primary breast cancer increases modestly (about 30%) the risk of developing a contralateral breast cancer more than 5 years after treatment.[50]

Environmental Factors

Cigarette smoking does not appear to increase the overall risk of developing breast cancer, but a recent study showed that there was a significant increase in the risk if young women begin smoking within 5 years of menarche. Although there is substantial interest in evaluating the influence of other occupational and environmental exposures on the risk of breast cancer, no definitive correlation has been found.

Benign Breast Disease

Benign breast disease includes a broad array of different, unrelated pathologic entities. However, a number of studies suggest that the presence (or history) of benign breast disease is associated with an increase in breast cancer risk.[51] Other studies have found that women who have had a previous breast biopsy for benign disease are also at increased risk. This association is limited to a large extent, however, to biopsy-proven lesions with histologic demonstration of atypia or proliferative lesions (atypical ductal or lobular hyperplasia) (Table 104-5).[52] Atypia has emerged as a significant risk factor in almost every study and diagnosed in almost any way, whether by surgical biopsy, random periareolar fine need aspiration, or ductal lavage.[53] Atypia has emerged as a significant risk factor in almost every study and diagnosed in almost any way, whether by surgical biopsy, random periareolar fine need aspiration, or ductal lavage.[53] When compared with women who had never had a breast biopsy, women with benign breast disease without hyperplasia had an odds ratio of breast cancer of 1.5; women with hyperplasia without atypia had an odds ratio of 1.8, and women with hyperplasia and atypia had an odds ratio of 2.6 to 4.3.[52,54] There has been growing consensus among pathologists to adopt the classification of benign breast disease proposed by Page and colleagues.[51] In this system, the joint occurrence of family history of breast cancer and atypical hyperplasia had a strong synergistic

Table 104-5 Relative Risk[a] of Invasive Breast Carcinoma Based on Histologic Examination of Breast Tissue Without Carcinoma

No increased risk (no proliferative disease)
Adenosis
Apocrine change
Duct ectasia
Mild epithelial hyperplasia of usual type
Slightly increased risk (1.5-2 times) (proliferative disease without atypia)
Hyperplasia of usual type, moderate or florid
Papilloma (probably)
Sclerosing adenosis
Moderately increased risk (4-5 times) (atypical hyperplasia or borderline lesion
Atypical ductal hyperplasia
Atypical lobular hyperplasia
High risk (8–10 times) (carcinoma in situ)[b]
Lobular carcinoma in situ–both breasts
Ductal carcinoma in situ (noncomedo)–unilateral, local

[a]Women in each category are compared with women matched for age who have had no breast biopsies for the risk of invasive breast cancer during the ensuing 10 to 20 years. These risks are not lifetime risks.
[b]Only smaller examples of noncomedo ductal carcinoma have consistently been assessed as risk indicators after biopsy only.
Source: From Ref. 51.

effect on breast cancer risk. Importantly, in a recent study from Mayo Clinic on 9087 women with benign breast disease, the combination of young age (under 45) and atypia had hazard ratio of 6.99 for developing breast cancer. [53] The excess risk in the 10 years after biopsy was in the ipsilateral breast, much like with DCIS. This is consistent with observations that women with cancer at a young age have a higher risk of bilateral cancer, and that DCIS at young age is associated with higher risk of progression to invasive disease. What is important is that young women with atypia can be identified as having very high risk, as well as those who may have as much as an 85% risk reduction from chemoprevention with tamoxifen.[55] Most other forms of benign breast disease appear to be unrelated to an increased breast cancer risk. Therefore, the majority of women with lumpy breasts, and most of those with benign breast disease, do not have a significantly increased risk of breast cancer. Cytogenetic and molecular genetic studies have suggested that some alterations found in breast cancer are first detected in the biological continuum between normal breast epithelium and frank carcinoma.[56] Although some abnormalities have been detected more often than others, no characteristic molecular abnormalities for various benign breast syndromes have been determined.

Mammographic Parenchymal Pattern

In 1976, Wolfe proposed that mammographic parenchymal patterns were predictive of breast cancer risk.[57] The P2 pattern, defined as prominent ducts occupying 25% or more of the breast volume, and the DY pattern, characterized by irregular, sheet-like radiographic densities, posed the highest risk. Subsequent studies have been inconsistent in confirming this observation, perhaps because of a lack of standardization and poor reproducibility in accurately classifying mammograms. Much recent research has focused on quantitative measures of breast density. Women with the highest quartile of breast density appear to have significantly elevated risk, 4.5-fold to 5-fold higher than those with the least dense breast tissue. Using the density reported on standard mammography (1, 2, 3, and 4 relating to fatty, scattered fibroglandular densities, heterogeneously dense, and homogeneously dense, respectively), different studies reproducibly show strong correlation with breast cancer risk. In fact, the Gail Risk model for estimating 5-year and lifetime risks for breast cancer has been modified by using a multiplier of breast density and Gail model risk. The density-modified Gail risk is calculated by multiplying the lifetime Gail risk by 0.59, 1.00, 1.41, or 1.94 for a BIRADS of 1, 2, 3, or 4 respectively.[58]

Other Risk Factors

Patients with a previous history of ovarian, uterine, or bowel cancer have a higher breast cancer risk. Mothers of children with soft-tissue sarcoma have been reported to have a two- to threefold increased risk of breast cancer. Caffeine consumption does not increase breast cancer risk, and its ability to exacerbate the symptoms of benign breast disease remains unproven. Recent studies suggesting that various psychosomatic factors increase breast cancer risk lack confirmation, as does the recent report suggesting that exposure to extremely low-frequency electromagnetic fields causes excess mortality from breast cancer.

Breast Cancer Risk Assessment Models Statistical models can be used to estimate a woman's risk of breast cancer. Some models predict the risk of developing breast cancer framing both short-term and lifetime risk. The models are highly dependent on the age of the person; thus, a very low short-term risk for a young woman may be accompanied by a high lifetime risk. The Gail Risk Assessment model[59,60] and the Claus model[61,62] are the most frequently used models to predict a woman's risk of breast cancer.[63] Other models, such as BRCAPRO,[64] Frank,[65] and Couch[66] predict the risk or probability of carrying a genetic mutation. These models should be used to guide decisions to perform genetic testing for the presence of cancer causing mutations in *BRCA1* or *BRCA2*. They do not identify the risk of developing cancer; rather, prediction will depend on the results of the test looking for inherited predisposition for breast cancer. The interpretation of the results of genetic testing results depends on the knowledge of whether the proband (person with a cancer) is the one being tested, and whether or not there is a known cancer causing mutation in the family.

Gail Model The Gail Risk Assessment Model is the most commonly used statistical model for estimating the risk of developing breast cancer in women undergoing annual screening. Gail and colleagues used data from 284,780 predominantly white women in 28 participating centers of the Breast Cancer Detection Demonstration Project to develop the model. This is an unconditional logistic regression model based on the ratio of risk in a woman with specified risk factors compared with the risk in a woman with no risk factors. Risk factors used in this model include age, age at menarche, age at first live birth, number of first-degree relatives with breast cancer (mother, sisters, or daughters only), number of breast biopsies, and breast pathology exhibiting atypical hyperplasia.

The Gail Model is applicable to the largest number of women. A score of 1.67 (which is the average 5-year Gail score for a 60-year-old woman) was used as the minimum risk criterion to join the NSABP P-01 prevention trial in the United States. The Gail Risk model is now widely used for clinical decision making for individual patients, with many forms of access (NCI Web site, handheld and computer applications).[67] It is good at predicting the risk for a population, but a cutoff of 1.67 does not show great discriminatory power.[68] Ozanne and colleagues have developed improved methods for incorporating Gail Risk by comparing a woman's Gail Risk in context with other women. Showing women that they are in the highest quartile or decile of risk is much more discriminatory, and much more helpful in identifying truly high risk women.[69] A limitation of the model is the treatment of family history: neither paternal family history of breast cancer nor age at onset in affected relatives is accounted for in the model. The model is currently being revised to improve the prediction of risk in the African American population. As described above, a multiplier can be used to incorporate breast density with subsequent improvement in predictive performance of the model.[58]

Claus Model The Claus Model estimates the probability that a woman will develop breast cancer based on her family history of cancer. This includes the number of first and second-degree relatives with breast cancer and the age of cancer onset. This model was developed from the Cancer and Steroid Hormone (CASH) population-based, case-control study involving 4730 patients with histologically documented breast cancer and 4688 matched controls.[61]

The statistical calculation of this model is based on the premise that breast cancer risk is transmitted as an autosomal dominant trait, and uses the genetic relationships between the affected relatives and the woman in question to predict risk. Risks can be calculated as lifetime probabilities of developing cancer, or as an estimated risk for a woman to develop cancer over 10-year intervals. A handheld application is also available for clinical use. The main limitation of this model is that it relies only on family history to predict risk and does not include personal risk factors.

Hereditary Models ■ Models such as BRCAPRO,[64] Frank,[65] and Couch,[66] are designed to predict the chance of carrying a BRCA1 or BRCA2 mutation based on an autosomal dominant pattern of inheritance and the incidence of mutations within high-risk populations, but they do not predict the risk of developing a cancer. They are based on both the maternal and paternal cancer history, and include age and number of first-degree relatives with breast cancer. Most women do not fall into this risk category.

The hereditary models are used clinically for women with a positive family history of breast cancer and are discriminatory and well calibrated for predicting the presence of a *BRCA* mutation. It is predicted that at most, 5% to 10% of diagnosed breast cancers are in women with either the *BRCA1* or *BRCA2* mutation. BRCAPRO performs as well in predicting mutations in families of African American descent as it does for Caucasian families. However, it is suspected that approximately 20% of breast cancers are due to unidentified hereditary factors. The remaining 70% are thought to be sporadic or nonhereditary cancers.[70]

Biomarkers ■ The models described above predict risk based on family history and internal hormonal exposure. Mutations in *BRCA1* and *BRCA2* certainly predict lifetime risk, and risk at earlier age, but are not accurate predictors of short-term risk. It is essential to identify biologic markers that can serve as quantifiable markers of risk. The optimal application of biomarkers in the prevention setting is to have markers that both predict an increased short-term risk and benefit from a targeted intervention.[69] The biomarkers that are potentially changeable and that have consistently been shown to be associated with greater risk for breast cancer include atypia,[71] and breast density. As discussed above, atypia has been shown to be associated with a three- to fivefold increase in risk whether detected by histology or cytology. Atypia has also been shown to predict a greater benefit from the use of tamoxifen, with a risk reduction of up to 89% in the NSABP P-1 study.[72] It has been shown that women whose breasts appear mammographically dense in greater than 50% of total breast tissue area have a 3-fold to 5-fold increased risk of breast cancer compared to women who have less than 25% mammographically dense breasts.[73] This relationship has recently been shown to be even stronger in women with a family history of breast cancer. Multiple investigators are conducting biomarker studies to determine if these markers are reliable surrogate markers that change in response to interventions.[75] How would these biomarkers then be used to test prevention interventions? Agents such as selective estrogen modifiers or aromatase inhibitors that are known to target ER positive disease, can be used to treat women with cytologically documented atypia, and the impact of the intervention measured by reduction in atypia. Change in breast density can also be measured over the course of the treatment (6 to 12 months), and used as a surrogate to better define those populations most likely to benefit from preventive interventions.

Regulation of Breast Cancer Growth

Understanding the basis for the development and regulation of breast cancer growth provides us with a foundation for developing strategies for breast cancer prevention and treatment. The adult female breast is composed of epithelial lactiferous ducts terminating in secretory alveoli embedded in a fibrous tissue framework and fat. Normal breast growth and development are regulated by the complex interaction of many hormones and growth factors, some of which are secreted by the mammary cells themselves and may have autocrine functions. Estradiol regulates the expression of several genes corresponding to peptides and proteins involved in mammary cell growth control mechanisms. Binding to specific receptors triggers effects of these growth factors and hormones. Polypeptide hormone receptors are typically located on the cell membrane, whereas receptors of the steroid hormone family are found mostly in the nuclear compartment of the cell.[76] However, steroid hormone receptors can also be found localized to the cell membrane. The interaction of growth factors, cytokines, and hormones with specific membrane receptors triggers a cascade of intracellular biochemical signals, resulting in the activation and repression of various subsets of genes. Several of these hormones have been shown to play an active role in breast epithelial cell growth and development and in lactation. Because these hormones and their receptors regulate normal breast tissue, it is not surprising that malignant cells arising from breast tissue might also express receptors for many of these hormones and might retain some degree of hormonal dependence. Numerous studies using cultured cells, as well as human breast cancer tissue, have demonstrated the presence of receptors for most of these hormones in human breast cancer cells. Genetic aberrations in growth factor signaling pathways, for the most part acquired, are inextricably linked to developmental abnormalities and to a variety of chronic diseases, including cancer. Malignant cells arise as a result of a stepwise progression of genetic events that include the unregulated expression of growth factors or components of their signaling pathways.

Growth regulation of breast cancer cells by hormones and growth factors is shown schematically in Figure 104-1. The biological role of estrogens is mediated through high-affinity binding to ER by molecules belonging to a family of ligand-inducible nuclear receptors that have steroid and thyroid hormones and vitamins as known ligands .[77]

Recent studies suggest that breast cancer cells under estrogen control can synthesize and secrete their own growth factors that could autostimulate breast cancer cells or adjacent stromal tissues through autocrine or paracrine mechanisms. Aromatase is abundantly expressed in many breast cancers, providing the malignant cell with the ability to synthesize its own major growth factor, estrogen. Stromal tissues may also secrete IGF-1 and IGF-2 that can stimulate breast cancer cells. Potential autocrine/paracrine growth factors identified include EGF, TGF-α, IGF-2, platelet-derived growth factor, and fibroblast growth factor. EGF, TGF-α, IGF-1, and IGF-2 have been found to be expressed and secreted by cultured breast cancer cells and by human breast cancer tissue specimens.[76] They are potential mitogens for the epithelial (malignant) component of the tumor. Platelet-derived growth factor and fibroblast growth factor are secreted by breast cancer cells and may be respon sible for the proliferation of the mesenchymal stromal component evident in many breast cancers.

Human breast cancer cells also secrete several peptides that may have autocrine inhibitory activity. TGF-β is a family of growth factors that inhibit the

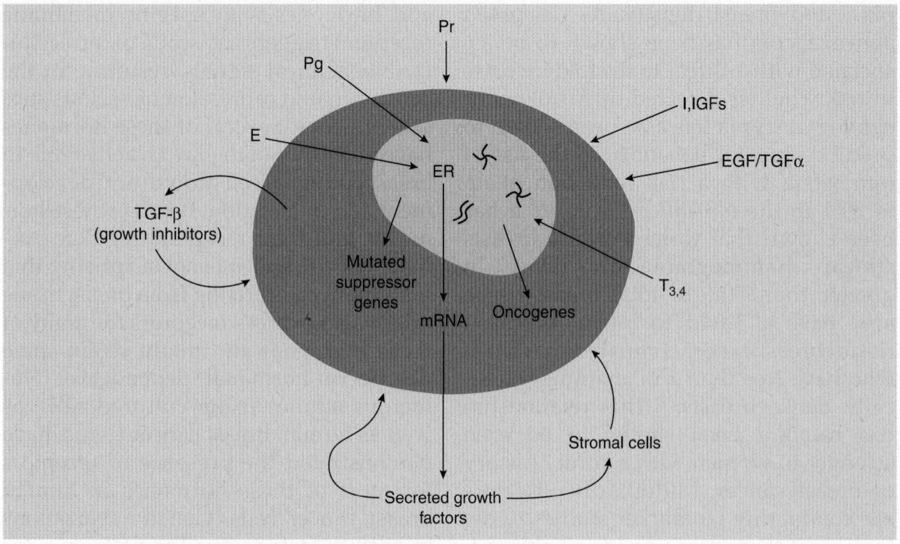

Figure 104-1 Growth regulation of breast cancer by hormones and growth factors. *Abbreviations*: E, Estrogen; EGF, epidermal growth factors; I, insulin; IGFs, insulin-like growth factors; Pg, progesterone; Pr, prolactin; T3,4, thyroid hormones; TGF-α, transforming growth factor alpha; TGF-β, transforming growth factor beta.

proliferation of epithelial tissues and stimulate the proliferation of stromal tissues.[56] Studies suggest that ER-negative breast cancer cells are more sensitive to TGF-β than are cells expressing ER. The malignant potential of breast cancer is likely to depend, in part, on the balance between growth stimulators and growth inhibitors produced by the tumors. The epithelial and/or stromal cells within the tumor also secrete proteases, such as the cathepsins, stromelysins, gelatinases, or urokinase plasminogen activator, which may participate in tumor invasiveness and metastatic potential.

In ER-positive breast cancer cells, expression and secretion of certain autocrine growth factors, such as TGF-α and IGF-2, are stimulated by estrogen and inhibited by antiestrogens. In ER-negative breast cancer cells, secretion of these factors is not estrogen regulated. Investigators have hypothesized that changes in the expression of these secreted factors may mediate to some extent the growth effects of estrogens and antiestrogens. Estrogens and antiestrogens have a variety of other effects on breast cancer cells. Estrogen stimulates RNA, DNA, and protein synthesis and the activity of key regulatory enzymes. Anti-estrogens have the opposite effects in most tissues. Estrogens ultimately regulate movement of the cells through the cell cycle and mitosis.

Disturbance of normal growth control mechanisms within a cell can result in uncontrolled cell division and the development of cancer. Such cellular transformation occurs through the activation of oncogenes, loss or mutation of tumor suppressor genes, or both. The normal counterparts of oncogenes, termed proto-oncogenes, function as growth regulators in normal cells. Alterations of proto-oncogenes are associated with the initiation, promotion, and/or maintenance of tumors in animals and humans. The products of oncogenes are frequently growth factors, growth factor receptors, molecular switching or transcription factors. Oncogenes often found overexpressed in human breast cancer tissue include members of the *myc* and *ras* family (*c-myc, Ha-ras-1*), *int-2*, which is involved in mouse (and, presumably, human) mammary gland carcinogenesis; the members of the EGF receptor (EGFR, *erbB*) family, including *erbB-2* (also known as *HER2* or *neu*), *HER3*, and *HER4*. Overexpression and mutation of growth factor receptors often lead to constitutive activation of these receptors (ie, signaling in the absence of their cognate ligands). Growth-promoting signals may be continuously transmitted into the cells, resulting in activation of multiple intracellular signal transduction pathways and unregulated cell growth. Genes normally involved in cell cycle control, especially members of the cyclin D and E families, may also function as oncogenes. Overexpression of these oncogenes may contribute to the initiation and maintenance of the malignant phenotype. Tissue-specific expression of *myc*, *ras*, and *HER2* in mammary glands of transgenic mice has been shown to result in an increased incidence of both benign and malignant breast pathology. Altered expression of these otherwise normal genes can have profound effects on growth homeostasis of breast epithelium. Recent studies have shown that blockade of these growth factor receptors or pathways has therapeutic implications.[78] These studies have shown that, both in preclinical models and in human breast cancer, monoclonal antibodies to *HER2* have dramatic antitumor effects and downregulate the PI3K signaling pathway. Furthermore, these antibodies have synergistic interactions with cytotoxic agents, such as the anthracyclines, the platinum analogs, vinorelbine and the taxanes. The EGFR, when overexpressed, confers an adverse prognosis to patients with EGFR-overexpressing tumors. However, EGFR does not seem to be a critical driver of malignant behavior in breast cancer, and monoclonal antibodies against this target have had only marginal success in clinical trials. Quantification of the expression of these oncogenes in human breast cancer specimens has been shown to provide valuable information on tumor aggressiveness, prognosis, and sensitivity to therapy.[79] Bcl2 is another gene frequently overexpressed in breast cancer; its overexpression is associated with unfavorable prognosis, resistance to apoptosis and decreased responsiveness to cytotoxic therapy. Signaling molecules downstream from the cell surface receptors are often activated or otherwise altered in malignant cells. Thus, the PI3 kinase pathway, and the MAP kinase pathway are frequently activated in breast cancer, even in the absence of EGFR or HER2 overexpression.

Tumor suppressor genes also play a role in breast carcinogenesis. Loss of the normal "suppressor" function of these genes through mutations or deletion may cause cancer. Alterations in known suppressor genes, such as the retinoblastoma gene (*RB1*) and the human *TP53* gene, have been identified in human breast cancer cells, as well as in other solid tumors. Mutations in the *TP53* gene have been found in families with the Li-Fraumeni syndrome, who have a markedly increased incidence of breast cancer and other neoplasms. In addition, up to 50% of breast cancers have been shown to have mutations in the *TP53* gene. The two mutated genes associated with familial breast cancer, *BRCA1* and *BRCA2*, are also considered tumor suppressor genes. The normal function of the protein products of these genes is to control cell proliferation (*RB1* and *TP53*) or to facilitate/mediate DNA repair (*TP53, BRCA1, BRCA2*). Mutations lead to mutated proteins and thus to dysregulated transit of cells through the cell cycle. Recognition that mutational inactivation of suppressor genes is associated with breast cancer could lead to early recognition of high-risk families, as well as to new treatment strategies to reverse the malignant phenotype by introducing normal gene copies through gene therapy or by treatment with the normal suppressor protein itself. Such strategies are under active investigation, both in the laboratory and in early clinical trials.

Estrogen and Progesterone Receptors

Estrogen receptors are members of the nuclear hormone–receptor superfamily and have several functional domains. There are two subtypes, with each subtype having several isoforms and splice variants. The ERα (alpha) gene has been mapped to the long arm of chromosome 6 (6q24-q27), whereas the ERβ (beta) gene is located on band q22-24 of chromosome 14. `There are at least three PR subtypes and their tissue distribution and function are under active investigation. Other estrogen-induced proteins regulate events leading to cell proliferation. When receptors are bound to antiestrogens, such as tamoxifen, transcription of growth-promoting genes is blocked, although other genes might be activated by tamoxifen.

Assays for ERα and PR α are helpful in selecting the patients most likely to benefit from endocrine therapy, and they provide prognostic information on recurrence and survival, since their expression is related to the degree of tumor differentiation. The role of ERβ and the other subtypes of PR in selecting responders to endocrine therapy is less well understood.

Both ER and PR in their classical form are nuclear proteins that can be measured in intact cells or tumor extracts by several assay techniques. Earlier detection techniques by ligand binding assays have been replaced by immunohistochemical (IHC) or immunocytochemical assays. The availability of monoclonal antibodies that recognize human ER or PR circumvents many of the shortcomings from earlier biochemical assays. In addition, IHC can be performed on small tissue or cytologic specimens; is not affected by endogenous hormone levels, and displays the cellular heterogeneity of receptor expression; most importantly, it can be used on fresh or archival (paraffin-embedded) tissues. The results of IHC assays correlate well with quantitative enzyme-linked immunoassay techniques and those of the older biochemical assays. More important, the results of IHC correlate well with response to hormonal therapy and prognosis. The remaining disadvantage of IHC is that it is only semiquantitative; the scoring of slides is subjective and requires a trained histopathologist. Nevertheless, because of the simplicity and reproducibility of the assay, IHC is considered the assay of choice for ER and PR today. Nuclear localization of ER leads to its genomic effects. Upon binding its ligand, the ER-ligand complex binds to the estrogen responsive element and initiates transcription of estrogen-driven genes. In its cell membrane localization, ER mediates the non-genomic effects of ligand binding, mostly through crosstalk with peptide growth factor receptors (EGFR, HER2). Upon development of antiestrogen resistance, there is marked increase in the non-genomic effects of ER.

ERs are detected (or expressed) in 60% to 80% of breast cancer samples, depending on the assay used and the clinical characteristics of the tumor and patient. The ER concentration varies widely from tumor to tumor (from 0 to more than 1000 fmol/mg protein, or 0 to 100% of cells, depending on the method used). Higher ER levels are seen in postmenopausal patients. ER assays performed on primary tumors are more frequently positive than are assays done on metastatic lesions, especially those obtained from visceral metastases. This probably reflects the greater propensity for ER-negative tumor cells to metastasize to visceral organs. ER positivity also correlates with histologic demonstration of differentiation (ie, low nuclear grade), favorable histologic subtypes (tubular, mucinous, lobular), with diploid DNA content, and with low proliferative indices (low S-phase fraction (SPF) or Ki-67 expression). ER expression is inversely correlated with HER2 and EGFR expression. These associations may explain in part the prognostic significance of ER status.

The most important application of the ER assay is the selection of appropriate patients for endocrine therapy. Approximately 50% to 60% of patients with ER-positive tumors benefit from endocrine therapy. This percentage includes patients with metastatic disease who achieve a major objective remission (partial or complete) and those who derive long-term (>6 months) stability of the disease with endocrine therapy; both groups have equivalent survival expectations. The ER status predicts equally well for all modalities of endocrine therapy. Patients with no detectable ER or PR in their tumors do not benefit from endocrine therapy; however, breast cancers with very low but detectable ER and/or PR respond, albeit infrequently, to endocrine therapy. This may explain why some patients with "ER-negative" tumors have been reported to benefit from adjuvant tamoxifen therapy. Until recently, arbitrary cutoff values were used to differentiate between ER-positive and ER-negative tumors. These values were usually around 10 to 20 fmol/mg protein for ligand-binding assays, or >10% positive cells/hpf in IHC assays. More recently, it has been recognized that virtually any ER expression indicates some probability of benefit from endocrine therapy. For this reason, many laboratories have adopted a semiquantitative method that takes into consideration the percent positive cells as well as the intensity of staining as the basis for determining ER-positivity. Quantitative ER assay and the simultaneous determination of PR expression increase the predictive accuracy of these assays. Tumors with high ER concentration (>100 fmol/mg protein or strong, homogeneous staining) or those positive for both ER and PR have the highest probability of response and clinical benefit from hormonal therapy. PR information is not as widely available as ER information in clinical trials, so the relevance of ER-status on treatment selection is more clearly established than that of PR status. Patients with ER-positive but PR-negative tumors are less likely to benefit from endocrine therapy, although they certainly should be offered a therapeutic trial; the ER--positive, PR-negative phenotype is commonly associated with growth factor receptor (HER1, HER2) activation, and relative resistance to endocrine treatment. Tumor ER and PR status can change over time or with intervening therapy; thus, repeat biopsies of accessible tissue may be helpful in selecting sequential therapies. However, ER status on the primary tumor still predicts reasonably well for endocrine response at the time of relapse. There is a strong trend for higher response rate to chemotherapy in ER-negative tumors, so hormone receptor status might be helpful in predicting response to chemotherapy in a generic way. It is not known why 40% to 50% of ER-positive tumors fail to respond to hormonal therapy despite the presence of receptor. Clearly, an assay that would identify truly hormone-sensitive tumors would be more clinically useful. At least one multigene assay, the Oncotype Dx, is being used increasingly in the United States to characterize the risk of developing distant metastases after 5 years of Tamoxifen for women with ER-positive disease.[80] Ongoing research from neoadjuvant hormonal studies,[81] will lead to the identification of patients less likely to benefit from hormonal intervention and determination of better strategies to treat such women. Variant and/or mutated ERs have been identified in breast cancer tissue. Some of these altered receptors are constitutively active (activate transcription in the absence of estrogen), some are inactive, and some have dominant negative activity. The biologic importance of these variants and their role, if any, in hormone-resistant states remains to be clarified.

Pathology

Recent biologic and clinical advances have made the role of the pathologist in establishing the diagnosis of a breast lesion more, rather than less, important. Today, greater expertise is required of the pathologist to establish the diagnosis of cancer from fine-needle aspiration (FNA) and core biopsy specimens, and to determine the nature of the increasing number of borderline and precancerous lesions. Distinguishing microinvasive from noninvasive lesions, and understanding atypical hyperplasias, all usually diagnosed after discovery by mammography, are new challenges. Pathologic discriminants involving immunohistochemistry are playing a larger role in determining patient prognosis. In increasing number of assays based on gene or protein expression are completing clinical validation and will add to the complexity of diagnosis, prognostication and selection of therapy. Increasingly, novel targeted therapies require the identification and quantitation of the putative target to match patient and treatment, and predict probability of therapeutic benefit. Finally, the pathologist also provides information that can contribute to a better understanding of the biology of the disease.[82]

Histologic Types

Pathologic classifications of mammary carcinoma are frequently confusing to the individual who is not a specialist in breast disease (Table 104-6). If it is appreciated that morphologic studies are based on anatomic or structural units present in an organ, and that in the female breast these units consist of large, medium, and small ducts from which a variety of tumor types arise, a better understanding of breast tumor pathology may ensue. (Only during pregnancy are acinar units present.)

Table 104-6 Incidence of Histologic Types of Invasive Breast Cancers (1000 Cases from NSABP B-04)[82]

Histologic Type	No.	%
Pure tumor groups	526	52.6
Infiltrating duct NOS		
Medullary	62	6.2
Lobular invasive	49	4.9
Mucinous	24	2.4
Tubular	12	1.2
Adenocystic	4	0.4
Papillary	3	0.3
Carcinosarcoma	1	0.1
Paget's disease	23	2.3
With intraductal carcinoma	2	0.2
Infiltrating duct NOS	16	1.6
+ Tubular	4	0.4
+ Mucinous	1	0.1
Combinations with infiltrating duct NOS	280	28.0
Infiltrating duct NOS		
+ Tubular	165	16.5
+ Lobular invasive	33	3.3
+ Mucinous	16	1.6
+ Lobular invasive + tubular	16	1.6
+ Papillary	12	1.2
+ Adenocystic	10	1.0
+ Tubular + adenocystic	8	0.8
+ Tubular + papillary	8	0.8
+ Mucinous + papillary	4	0.4
+ Adenocystic + mucinous	2	0.2
+ Lobular invasive + adenocystic	1	0.1
+ Lobular invasive + mucinous	1	0.1
+ Lobular invasive + papillary	1	0.1
+ Tubular + mucinous	1	0.1
+ Adenocystic + papillary	1	0.1
+ Lobular invasive + tubular	1	0.1
+ Adenocystic + mucinous	16	1.6
Other combinations of tumor types exclusive of NOS		
Tubular + papillary	5	0.5
Lobular invasive + tubular	4	0.4
Tubular + mucinous	2	0.2
Lobular invasive + mucinous	1	0.1
Tubular + adenocystic	1	0.1
Adenocystic + mucinous	1	0.1
Mucinous + papillary	1	0.1
Lobular invasive + tubular + adenocystic + papillary	1	0.1
Total	1000	100.0

Abbreviation: NOS, not otherwise specified.

Tumors arising from ductal epithelium may be found only within the lumen of the ducts of origin; that is, the carcinomas are intraductal and do not penetrate the basement membrane or invade surrounding stroma. Most frequently, such tumors arise from large ducts and may present as several types. If they grow into the ducts with a papillary configuration, they are recognized as papillary carcinomas (Fig. 104-2). Such lesions are rare, accounting for about 1% of breast cancers. Histologically, pleomorphic duct epithelial cells with disturbed polarity can be demonstrated, as can their "heaping up" into papillae. Difficulty may be encountered in differentiating a papillary carcinoma from a benign atypical papilloma.

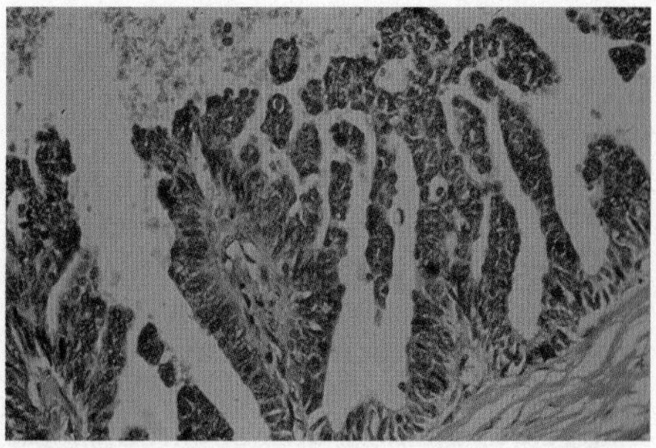

Figure 104-2 Papillary carcinoma of the breast. This uncommon tumor, <1%, rarely infiltrates and has a favorable prognosis.

Papillary carcinomas rarely invade the surrounding stroma. A survival rate approaching 100% may be anticipated upon complete excision of such tumors. When these tumors do invade surrounding tissue, they grow rather slowly and attain considerable bulk. Skin and fascial attachments are unusual, and axillary node involvement is a late feature. Clinically, noninvasive tumors are found to be movable, circumscribed lesions that have a soft consistency not unlike that of fibroadenomas.

The noninvasive variety of ductal carcinoma, referred to as intraductal carcinoma or ductal carcinoma in situ (DCIS), is a proliferation of a subgroup of epithelial cells confined to the mammary ducts without light microscopic evidence of invasion through the basement membrane into the stroma. The histologic diagnosis of DCIS poses certain problems. It is often difficult to distinguish between benign but highly atypical hyperplasia and DCIS, and it is sometimes difficult to identify small foci of stromal invasion. Occasionally, it is difficult to distinguish between DCIS and lobular carcinoma in situ (LCIS), since DCIS may extend into breast lobules and LCIS may involve extralobular ducts. Some lesions may be intermediate between the two. A variety of histologic patterns of DCIS has been recognized. The most frequently encountered are comedo, cribriform, solid, papillary, and micropapillary (Fig. 104-3). The different histologic patterns have been associated with differences in biologic behavior. The proliferative rate has been found to vary according to the histologic characteristics of DCIS. A high proliferative rate has been observed with comedo-DCIS, and a low proliferative rate with cribriform, papillary, and solid DCIS. A type of carcinoma known as comedocarcinoma is characterized by ducts that are dilated and filled with carcinoma cells. These are necrotic and can be expressed as semisolid necrotic plugs. Such cancers are not usually regarded as a separate cell type, but rather represent

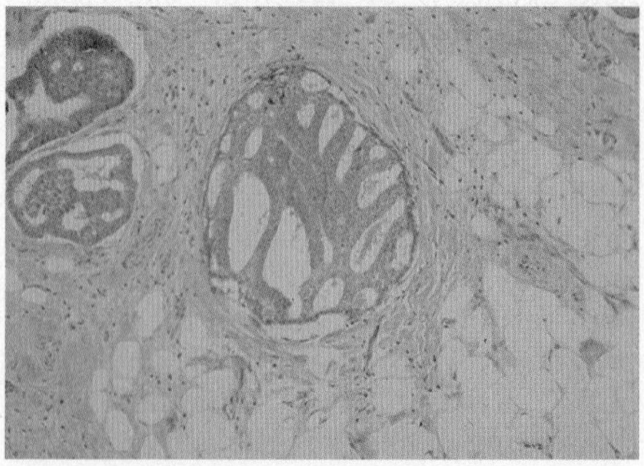

Figure 104-3 Ductal carcinoma in situ (DCIS), cribriform type. Duct spaces are completely involved by a proliferation of ductal cells with relatively uniform nuclei, arranged in back to back (cribriform) glands. The glands are fairly uniform in size and shape and exhibit rigid inner borders (so-called cookie-cutter appearance). *Source*: Courtesy of Dr. Ira Bleiweiss, Mount Sinai School of Medicine.

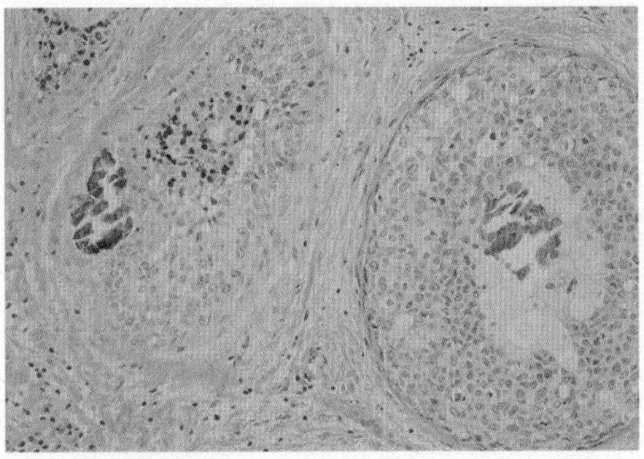

Figure 104-4 Ductal carcinoma in situ (DCIS), comedo type. Two duct spaces contain tumor cells with high nuclear grade, focal necrosis, and calcifications. The combination of high-grade nuclei and central necrosis is diagnostic of comedocarcinoma. *Source*: Courtesy of Dr. Ira Bleiweiss, Mount Sinai School of Medicine.

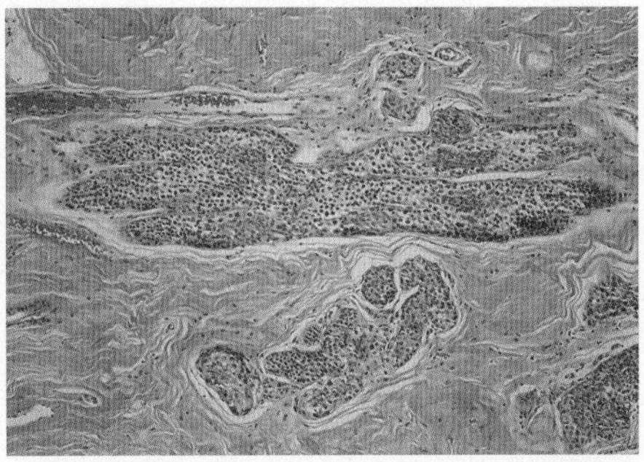

Figure 104-5 Lobular carcinoma in situ (LCIS). Terminal ducts and acini are completely filled and dilated by a uniform small cell proliferation. *Source*: Courtesy of Dr. Ira Bleiweiss, Mount Sinai School of Medicine.

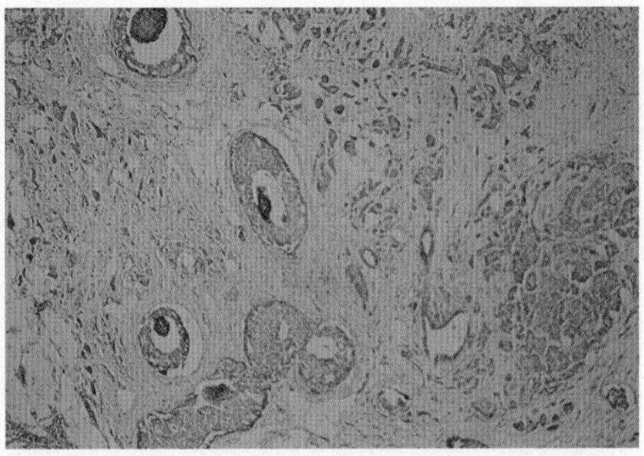

Figure 104-7 Infiltrating ductal carcinoma of the breast, not otherwise specified (NOS). Nearly 80% of breast cancers exhibit this histology, about one-third of the time with additional types of differentiation.

a descriptive variant of intraductal carcinoma. Patients whose DCIS exhibits comedo features have been shown to have increased rates of local recurrence and may progress more rapidly to invasive breast cancer compared to other types (Fig. 104-4). Human EGF-receptor 2 (HER2/neu) protein overexpression has been observed in solid and comedo types of DCIS but not in papillary or cribriform types. Assays for ER are an integral part of assessing DCIS lesions and are necessary to select optimal therapeutic interventions. Attempts to gain consensus on pathological classification for DCIS include the EORTC system, the Van Nuys system, and the Philadelphia consensus conference, and have all produced different systems with some overlapping features.

Lobular carcinoma arises from the small end ducts of the breast. The noninvasive variety—the so-called lobular carcinoma in situ—is characterized by small cells of low nuclear grade that fill and expand lobules without penetration of the basement membrane (Fig. 104-5). When this lesion extends beyond the boundary of the lobule or terminal duct from which it arises, it is known as invasive lobular carcinoma. Often the small cells inter-digitate between collagen bundles in a single line, so-called "Indian file." At other times, lobular car- cinoma may be nearly indistinguishable from the conventional infiltrating ductal carcinoma (Fig. 104-6). Noninvasive mammary carcinomas make up almost 22% of all neoplastic lesions of the female breast and that LCIS accounts for about 60% of these, or 12% of all tumors. Whereas DCIS often accompanies invasive ductal carcinoma, and may well be its usual precursor, LCIS may be followed by invasive ductal or invasive lobular carcinomas in either breast. LCIS thus is more a systemic marker than a local precursor. With the increased use of mammography, a much higher proportion of noninvasive cancers is being detected. though DCIS and LCIS are both called CIS, they are considered and treated somewhat differently.

Infiltrating duct carcinomas in which no special type of histologic structure is recognized are designated "not otherwise specified" (NOS) and are the most common duct tumors, accounting for almost 80% of breast cancers (Fig. 104-7). They are characterized clinically by their stony hardness to palpation. When they are transected, a gritty resistance is encountered, and the tumor retracts below the cut surface. Yellowish, chalky streaks that represent necrotic foci are observed. Histologically, varying degrees of fibrotic response are present. They frequently metastasize to axillary lymph nodes, and their prognosis is the poorest of the various tumor types. More than half (52.6%) of breast cancers are pure infiltrating duct lesions (NOS).

Several other types of invasive carcinomas arise from large ducts, and each has its own distinct histopathologic picture. Medullary carcinoma, composing 3% to 6% of all mammary carcinomas, often attains large dimensions (Fig. 104-8). This tumor is formed by cells of relatively high nuclear grade, and usually exhibits an extensive infiltration of the tumor by small lymphocytes. Medullary carcinomas have a relatively well-circumscribed border, sometimes described as a "pushing" border, in contrast to the NOS tumors in which small nests of cells tend to infiltrate the adjacent stroma more extensively. A study of medullary cancer using 336 typical and 273 atypical medullary breast cancers from 6404 patients enrolled in various stage I and stage II National Surgical Adjuvant Breast Project (NSABP) trials indicated that the survival of patients with typical medullary cancers was better than that for patients with NOS invasive ductal carcinomas. Survival was comparable for those with atypical medullary and NOS types.[83]

Tubular carcinoma is an invasive carcinoma in which tubule formation is highly prominent. This tumor represents 1% to 2% of breast cancers and has a low nuclear grade with some cell polarity (Fig. 104-9). Its prognosis is favorable, and, when combined with small size, it is a curable tumor.

Mucinous or colloid carcinoma, which composes about 1% to 2% of all mammary carcinomas, is characterized on microscopy by its nests and strands of epithelial cells floating in a mucinous matrix. It usually grows slowly and can reach bulky proportions. When the tumor is predominantly mucinous, the prognosis tends to be good (Fig. 104-10).

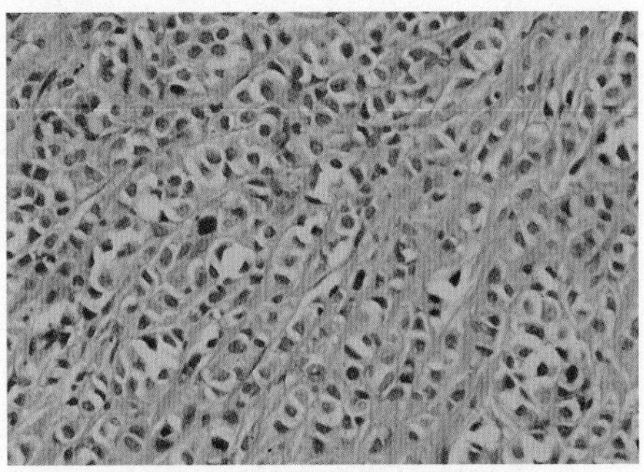

Figure 104-6 Infiltrating lobular carcinoma. Tumor cells with relatively uniform nuclei invade in a single file or linear pattern (so-called Indian file). *Source*: Courtesy of Dr. Ira Bleiweiss, Mount Sinai School of Medicine.

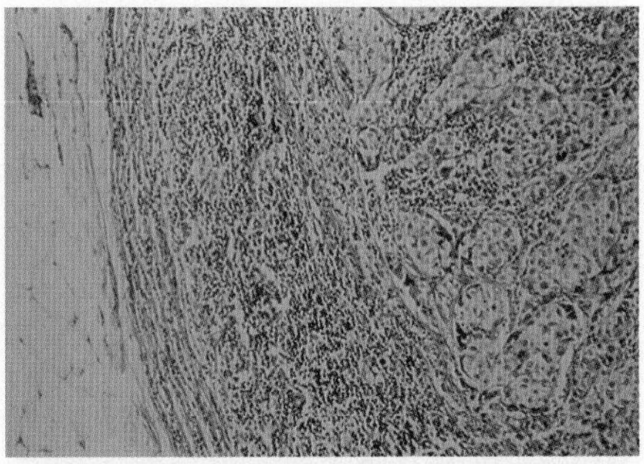

Figure 104-8 Medullary carcinoma of the breast accounts for about 5% to 7% of breast cancers. Despite its relatively poor differentiation, this tumor has a better prognosis than does infiltrating ductal carcinoma.

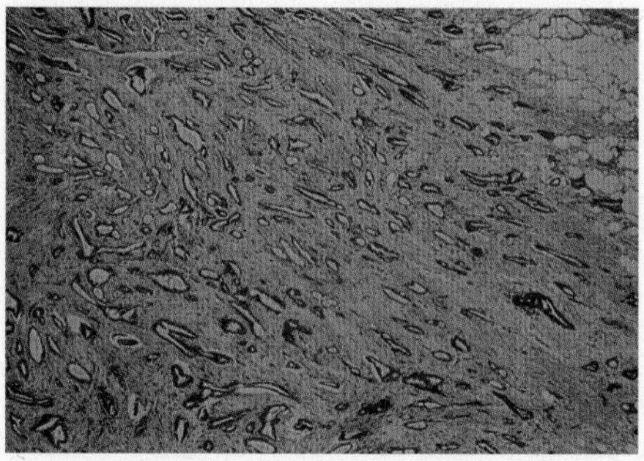

Figure 104-9 Tubular carcinoma of the breast. This tumor is rare in its pure form, less than 1 %, but has a better prognosis than infiltrating duct carcinoma not otherwise specified (NOS). Partial tubular differentiation is seen in 20% of infiltrating duct carcinomas NOS.

Two entities represent special manifestations of mammary carcinoma. Paget disease of the breast occurs in 1% to 4% of all patients with breast cancer. Clinically, the patient presents with a relatively long history of eczematoid changes in the nipple, with itching, burning, oozing, and/or bleeding. The nipple changes are associated with an underlying carcinoma in the breast that can be palpated in about two-thirds of the patients. The subjacent tumor may be either intraductal or of the invasive duct type. Prognosis is related to the invasiveness and histologic type of the associated tumor. Histologically, the nipple epithelium contains nests of carcinoma cells.

Inflammatory breast cancer, or "dermal lymphatic carcinomatosis" of the breast, is characterized clinically by skin redness, warmth, edema (peau d'orange), a visible erysipeloid margin, induration of the underlying breast, and a rapid evolution, usually less than 3 months from first sign to diagnosis. These features must be present at the time of primary diagnosis. Biopsies of the erythematous areas and adjacent normal-appearing skin often but not always reveal poorly differentiated cancer cells filling and obstructing the subdermal lymphatics. Inflammatory cells are rarely present. Patients typically have signs of advanced cancer, including palpable axillary nodes, supraclavicular nodes, and/or distant metastases. Inflammatory breast cancer represents about 1-2 % of breast cancers in the United States and Western Europe, although its incidence is reportedly higher in North Africa and the Middle East.

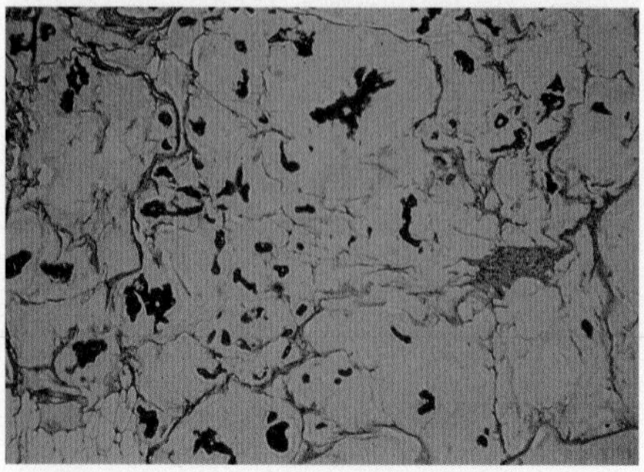

Figure 104-10 Mucinous or colloid carcinoma of the breast. This tumor is uncommon (about 2%) but has a rather favorable prognosis.

Several other histologic types of mammary carcinomas have been described but are rarely (<1%) encountered. Adenocystic carcinoma, carcinosarcomas, pure squamous cell carcinoma, metaplastic carcinomas (carcinoma with osseous or cartilaginous stroma), basal cell carcinomas, and so-called lipid-rich carcinomas have been observed. Because of their rarity, clinical correlates are practically nonexistent.

Nonepithelial Neoplasms of the Breast

A variety of nonepithelial neoplasms of the breast have been described. Fibrosarcomas, leiomyosarcomas, rhabdomyosarcomas, and angiosarcomas are all infrequent.[82] Non-Hodgkin lymphomas can have their initial onset in the breast and can also occur as a focus of generalized disease. These usually have a B-cell phenotype. Some cases resemble carcinoma on routine histology; immunohistochemistry is often helpful in resolving this question. Only a few cases of Hodgkin disease and leukemia have been reported with initial manifestation in the breast.

Phyllodes tumor (cystosarcoma phyllodes) is a biphasic neoplasm that is partially epithelial and partially mesenchymal (Fig.103-11). Phyllodes tumors may achieve a great size and, not infrequently, demonstrate some invasion of adjacent breast tissue. They are best managed by local excision with a rim of normal breast tissue. Phyllodes tumors are classified as benign, borderline or indeterminate, or malignant. Malignant phyllodes tumor has been known to metastasize and to kill. High mitotic rate, cellular atypia, stromal overgrowth, infiltrative margins, hemorrhage, and necrosis are considered features of malignancy. Although it is difficult to determine from clinical or histologic appearance which tumors behave malignantly and will metastasize, malignant histology and stromal overgrowth are predictive of metastasis.[84]

Tumor Characteristics

Tumor Size

In addition to being a determinant for optimal local therapy, tumor size has prognostic significance in the determina-

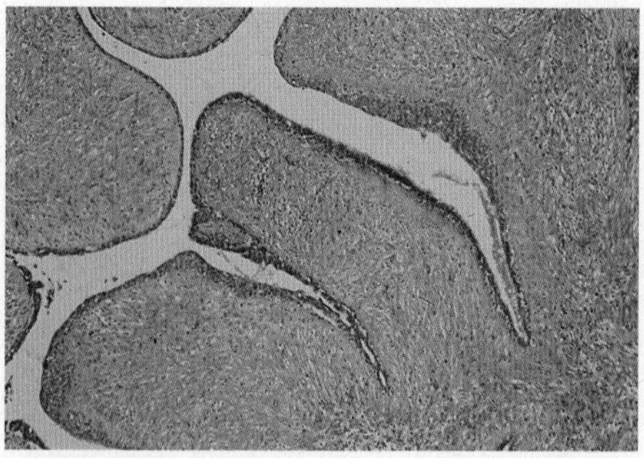

Figure 104-11 Phyllodes tumor (cystosarcoma phyllodes). Leaf-like projections, lined by benign epithelium, contain a hypercellular stroma.

tion of additional therapy (Table 104-7). As the size of the tumor increases, the risk of recurrence or metastasis also increases, for both lymph node-negative and node-positive tumors. Because the risk of treatment failure is already high for patients with node-positive breast cancer, increasing tumor size adds relatively little prognostic value. However, tumor size is often the main prognostic indicator in node-negative breast cancer. This variable is particularly important in the decision to use or not to use adjuvant systemic therapy in patients with node-negative breast cancer. Tumor size refers only to the invasive component and should be determined in all three dimensions by the pathologist. Approximately 25% to 30% of patients with negative lymph nodes and a primary tumor less than 2 cm in diameter will experience a recurrence within 20 years of follow-up.[85] Patients with tumors 1 cm or less in diameter have an excellent prognosis, with fewer than 15% recurring at 10 years in the absence of effective adjuvant therapy. The largest database demonstrating the relationship among tumor size, lymph node status, and breast cancer survival comes from the Surveillance, Epidemiology, and End Results (SEER) program (see Table 104-7).[86] Less than 2% of patients with tumors under 1 cm and negative nodes died of breast cancer within 5 years, and only 4% at 10 years.[87] Considering the excellent prognosis for this group of patients with very small tumors, as well as the expense and toxicity of treatment, routine use of chemotherapy is not indicated. The combination of poor nuclear grade and lymphatic vessel invasion identifies a small subset (approximately 10%) of patients with T1a, b N0 M0 breast cancer with a significant risk of relapse, up to 30%, that warrants systemic adjuvant therapy.[83,88]

Axillary Lymph Node Involvement

Involvement of the ipsilateral axillary lymph nodes is still the most reliable and reproducible prognostic indicator for

Table 104-7 **5-Year Breast Cancer-Specific Mortality Rates According to Tumor Size and Axillary Lymph Node Involvement[a]**

	5-Year Breast Cancer Specific Mortality Rate (%)		
	Positive Nodes		
Tumor Size (cm)	0	1 to 3	More Than 3
<0.5	0.8	4.7	41.0
0.5–0.9	1.7	6.0	45.8
1.0–1.9	4.2	13.4	32.8
2.0–2.9	7.7	16.6	36.6
3.0–3.9	13.8	21.0	43.1
4.0–4.9	15.4	30.2	47.4
>5.0	17.8	27.0	54.5

[a]Information derived from SEER data: Number of positive axillary lymph nodes.

primary breast cancer (see Table 104-7).[89] In general, 50% to 70% of patients with positive lymph nodes have a relapse, whereas only 15% to 45% of patients with all lymph nodes negative for metastatic disease have a relapse after locoregional treatments only. The risk of tumor recurrence in a patient with primary breast cancer is a continuum related to the number of positive axillary lymph nodes.[89] With each additional positive lymph node found, the risk of recurrence and metastasis increases by a few percentage points. Thus, patients with 4 to 10 positive lymph nodes have a greater risk than those with 1 to 3 positive nodes, and those with 10 or more positive nodes have a greater than 80% probability of recurrence and metastasis. Because nodal status cannot be accurately assessed by clinical means, an axillary lymph node dissection, including levels I and II, is considered the standard of care. Clinical studies have demonstrated that lymph node negativity is reliable only if at least 6, but preferably, 10 axillary lymph nodes are removed and examined. Both macro- and micrometastasis within the lymph nodes have similar prognostic significance.[90] In recent years, primary breast cancer has been diagnosed in earlier and mostly localized stages. A classic axillary lymph node dissection has no therapeutic benefit for patients with node-negative axillae and is associated with considerable short- and long-term morbidity. An alternative (diagnostic) staging procedure for these patients is the sentinel lymph node biopsy.[91] This procedure limits considerably the extent of the surgical procedure in the axilla and, for the great majority of patients with negative axillary lymph nodes, precludes the need for formal axillary dissection while providing similar (and in some cases superior) diagnostic and prognostic information. The identification of a single (or just a few) sentinel node also permits the pathologist to perform a more detailed assessment to detect micrometastases by combining light microscopy, IHC, and even more sensitive molecular techniques. The prognostic significance of identifying isolated metastatic cells in histologically negative lymph nodes by more sensitive techniques is still undetermined. Sentinel node biopsy and assessment are under extensive evaluation by large cooperative research groups, including the NSABP and the American College of Surgeons Oncology Group (ACOSOG). Preliminary reports of randomized trials comparing axillary dissection with sentinel lymph node biopsy have demonstrated that the latter is associated with significantly reduced morbidity. Because of these results, sentinel lymph node biopsy has replaced classic axillary dissection for early, localized breast cancer in a substantial percentage of patients with clinically negative axillae.

Although axillary lymph node status is still the most powerful prognostic indicator, 15% to 45% of patients whose lymph nodes do not contain metastases still experience a recurrence and die. Conversely, about 15% of patients with >10 positive lymph nodes treated only with surgery and radiotherapy survive without recurrence or metastases. Because of this limitation, other prognostic markers have been developed to improve prognostic accuracy, particularly in the group of patients with node-negative tumors (Table 104-8). Interestingly, the molecular tests based on gene expression, suggest that biology of the tumor may be more important than stage. Data were recently presented showing that, in women with node-positive breast cancer who were determined to be low risk based on the NKI 70 gene assay, that recurrence-free survival was excellent 95% and 94%, both for those that did not received chemotherapy (39) and those who did (57 women). This contrasted with the recurrence-free survival of those with an NKI 70 gene poor risk determination, which was 69% for the 89 women who did not receive chemotherapy and 77% for the 44 women who did.[92] This will continue to be an important area of research and molecular analysis of tumors is likely to, in the future, become a major tool for determining therapy.

Table 104-8 **Effect of Lymph Node Involvement on Recurrence and Survival**

	Status				
	Relapse Rate %			Survival %	
Axillary Node	18 Months	5 Yr	10 Yr	5 Yr	10 Yr
N−	5	18	24	78	65
N+	33	65	76	47	25
N+ (1-3)	13	50	65	62	38
N+ (≥4)	52	79	86	32	13
All patients	17	40	50	64	46

Source: From Ref. 144.

Histologic Type

Several histologic variables have been reported to have prognostic significance.[82] The prognoses of ductal and lobular carcinomas are similar enough to prompt the same treatment modalities. Several less common cancers, including pure tubular carcinoma, mucinous or colloid carcinoma, papillary carcinoma, and all noninvasive breast cancers, have substantially better prognoses, especially when found in a node-negative stage.[93,94] The more favorable prognosis of these histologic types often justifies omission of adjuvant systemic treatment, especially for small tumors (<3 cm). Because most of these special types have small dimensions when diagnosed and are node-negative, regional treatment is usually all that is required. When stringently defined, medullary carcinoma, when associated with negative axillary lymph nodes, is also considered by some but not all experts to have a better prognosis.[83,94,95] The magnitude of this difference, in terms of 10-year survival, was reported to be 17%. However, the prognoses of atypical medullary carcinomas (those that do not fulfill the necessary histological criteria) or mixed medullary and ductal carcinomas are similar to those of ductal and lobular breast cancers.

Histologic Grade or Differentiation

Tumor grade has been shown to be an important prognostic indicator. In general, tumors expressing features that indicate a high degree of tumor differentiation have the most favorable prognosis. Multiple studies have shown that higher grade is associated with higher rates of recurrence and metastases and poorer survival. These correlations are independent of tumor size and lymph node involvement. High tumor grade is also associated with hormone receptor negativity and increased response to cytotoxic therapy. Conversely, low grade is associated with hormonal sensitivity and lower response to chemotherapy.

The clear definition of various histologic differentiation grades led to the recognition that those grades had reproducible prognostic significance.[96] Trained, experienced breast pathologists can recognize poorly differentiated, moderately well-differentiated, and differentiated tumors without much difficulty; the assessment of the histologic grade for those tumors is quite reproducible. Furthermore, although there is some variation among different pathologists, the concordance rate is quite acceptable. Recent reports based on the SEER tumor registry provided strong evidence supporting the prognostic value of histologic grade determined by "average" pathologists. Something similar can be said for nuclear grade, although some find that histologic grade is a more reliable prognostic indicator because it includes cellular and tissue-related criteria. Nuclear grade can be determined in cytologic specimens. Well-differentiated histologic types, such as tubular, papillary, or colloid (mucinous), have a lower incidence of axillary nodal metastases and a lower risk of distant recurrence than the more common infiltrating ductal carcinomas NOS.[88,94] Less than 20% of patients with negative nodes having well to moderately well-differentiated (grade 1 or 2) tumors experience a recurrence in 5 years, compared to more than 30% for those with poorly differentiated tumors.[97] Smaller tumors are more often well differentiated, whereas larger tumors are predominantly poorly differentiated. Tumor differentiation is also associated with other prognostic indicators such as ER expression, PR expression, ploidy, and SPF.

The grading system most frequently used is the Elston-Ellis modification of the Scarf-Bloom-Richardson system.[98] In this system, invasive ductal breast cancers are categorized into three histologic grades, depending on their degree of tubular and/or gland formation, cellular pleomorphism, and number of mitoses per high-power microscopic field. Within each of these categories, a score of 1 to 3 is assigned, with 1 representing the most favorable findings (for example, prominent gland formation, little cellular pleomorphism, low mitotic rate) and 3 indicating the least favorable. The scores for each of these categories are added together. Grade 1 carcinoma (well differentiated or low grade) is defined as having a total of 3 to 5 points, grade II (moderately differentiated or intermediate grade) is defined as 6 to 7 points, and grade 3 (poorly differentiated or high grade) is defined as 8 to 9 points.

Other Histologic Variables

Tumor Necrosis Tumor necrosis of varying degrees was encountered in 60% of 1539 patients with invasive breast cancer in NSABP protocol B-04. Necrosis, particularly when observed to be of marked degree, was positively correlated with increased rates of treatment failure. Although necrosis was observed to be significantly associated with a number of clinical and histopathologic features purportedly related to an ominous prognosis in this disease, it was not correlated with pathologic nodal status, and multivariate analysis revealed it to influence treatment failure independently of tumor size in lesions less than 5 cm in their greatest diameter.

Circumscription Mammary carcinomas generally assume either a circumscribed structure, or a more infiltrative irregular or stellate configuration. A better prognosis has been ascribed to the former tumor type.

Lymphatic and Blood Vessel Invasion Lymphatic and blood vessel invasion has been associated with poor prognosis in numerous clinical reports. One-third of NSABP patients exhibited extension into lymphatics within the dominant mass, and another 23% were considered questionable (Fig. 104-12). Such a finding was associated with other unfavorable characteristics. Blood vessel invasion was observed in only 5% of patients and was associated with the finding of four or more positive axillary nodes, lymphatic invasion, and certain other unfavorable findings (Fig. 104-13). In other studies, blood vessel invasion has been reported in 5 to 50%. In one report from Memorial Sloan-Kettering Cancer Center 14% of patients with T1 N0 tumors and in 22% of T1 N1 breast cancer evidenced blood vessel invasion.

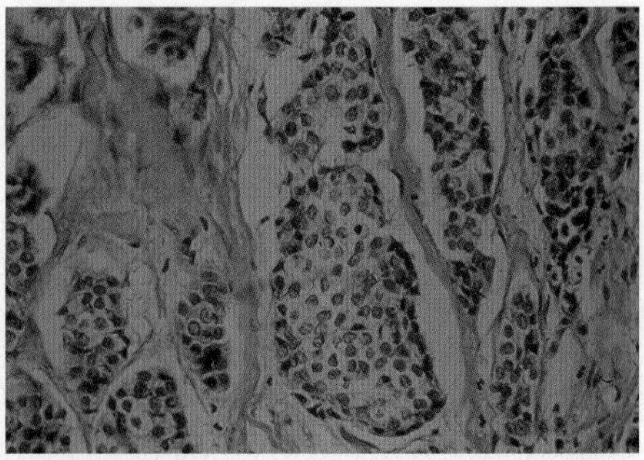

Figure 104-12 Lymphatic invasion by breast cancer. The vessel walls are thin and lined with endothelial cells.

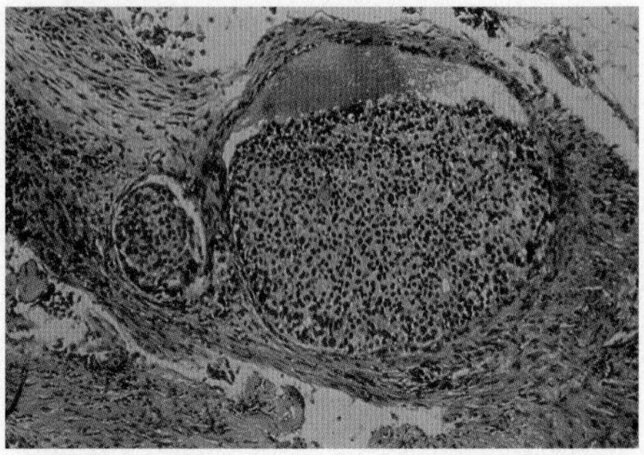

Figure 104-13 Blood vessel invasion by breast cancer. The vessel wall structure is recognizable, together with erythrocytes in the vessel.

Multicentricity Many breast cancers are multicentric in origin. In an examination of 904 NSABP cases, excluding those instances in which the lesion was beneath the nipple or in the tail of the breast, data were collected from only those quadrants in which the primary lesion was not encountered. This method eliminated the difficulty in distinguishing a new focus of carcinoma in the quadrant of the primary from an integral part of the primary lesion. Either invasive or noninvasive cancers regarded as independent were found in 13.4% of the 904 patients. The frequency of invasive and noninvasive multicentric cancers was 4.1% and 9.3%, respectively. The types of noninvasive cancers encountered were intraductal (66.7%), LCIS (22.6%), and a combination of both (10.7%). Increased utilization of magnetic resonance imaging (MRI) of the breast for pre-operative assessment of extent of disease has indicated that multi-centricity is much more common than previously determined by mammography. However, the clinical significance of such an observation remains uncertain because of the finding that lumpectomy with or without breast irradiation is as effective as mastectomy in terms of curability. Results from the randomized trials of breast conservation indicate that tumors that recur in the ipsilateral breast following lumpectomy are, in the vast majority of instances, found at the site of the initial operation rather than elsewhere in the breast.

Despite the significant incidence of multifocal lesions in both breasts in a woman with a primary breast cancer, two or more clinically overt primary cancers in the primary breast are uncommon. Similarly, synchronous bilateral tumors are uncommon, and the incidence of a second asynchronous primary tumor in the uninvolved or opposite breast (about 4% to 6% in 10 years) fails to approach the incidence predicted by the number of occult lesions detected by random biopsy, autopsy or MRI. It has been noted, for example, that the incidence of clinically latent intraductal carcinomas in the breasts of women over the age of 70 who died of causes other than mammary carcinoma is 19 times greater than the reported incidence of clinical breast cancer.[99] Such findings strongly suggest that not all cancers progress to overt clinical lesions and that they may even undergo regression. These conclusions are similar to and gain support from evidence about adrenal neuroblastomas in children, from thyroid carcinomas, and from carcinomas of the prostate, which are found more frequently pathologically in randomly examined material than clinically in comparable populations.

In a report of 950 women with node-negative invasive breast cancer enrolled in NSABP study B-06, 22 pathologic and 4 clinical features were evaluated for their prognostic significance.[100] Their assessment in a Cox regression model demonstrated that only nuclear grade, histologic tumor type, and race were prognostically important. Eighty-six percent of patients having tumors of good nuclear grade treated with loco-regional therapy survived for 8 years as opposed to 64% in whom the nuclear grade was scored as poor. Patients with mucinous, tubular, or papillary cancers fared significantly better than did those with NOS or atypical medullary tumors. Survival for patients with typical medullary, NOS combinations, or lobular invasive cancers was intermediate. African Americans had a worse survival rate than did whites. This experience suggests that as a predictor of survival in node-negative patients, nuclear grade is as good as, if not better than, information derived from other markers, such as HER2 gene expression, cathepsin activity, SPF, ploidy, tumor size, or ERs.

In another report, discriminants for treatment failure by the tenth year in 614 patients treated by radical mastectomy were provided.[101] Nodal metastasis was the most significant prognostic discriminant for disease-free survival in the tenth year. Histologic grade and tumor size were significant discriminants in patients with four or more positive nodes, but no additional factors were found to be significant discriminants in patients with one to three positive nodes.

Natural History and Prognostic Markers

The natural history and prognosis for primary breast cancer vary considerably from patient to patient (Table 104-8). Some patients present with very indolent disease and either are cured by local therapy or survive for many years even after developing metastases. A small percentage of patients survive more than 10 years without any treatment.[102] In other patients, the disease follows an aggressive, rapidly progressive course that is refractory to treatment.

The heterogeneity in the clinical course of breast cancer is mirrored by great variability in measured doubling time and other cell kinetic parameters. In general, human breast cancer has a low growth fraction (proportion of cells in the active cell cycle) compared with many other tumors, with estimated values ranging from 5% to 30%, depending on the method used. The SPF is an indicator of the rate of cell turnover, or growth rate. In rapidly growing tumors, such as testicular cancer or high-grade lymphomas, it may exceed 50%.

Estimated tumor volume doubling times for primary human breast tumors are also prolonged. In one retrospective study, 147 tumors observed to grow on serial mammograms were evaluated.[103] Doubling times ranged from 44 to more than 1800 days, with a mean of 212 days. It is not possible to determine the growth rate of breast cancers in their preclinical (microscopic) stage, but if one assumes that a cancer begins with a single cell and grows with a constant doubling time of 200 days, a tumor would need about 20 years of growth to reach 1 to 2 cm in diameter. A tumor with a faster doubling time of 100 days would still require 10 years to become clinically detectable, and a remarkably fast-growing tumor (doubling time of 20 days) could possibly have originated just 2 years earlier. Similarly, a 2 mm tumor with an average doubling time would require about 4 years of growth to reach a size of 1 cm. These growth calculations assume logarithmic growth, whereas Gompertzian growth models indicate that growth rates are not constant throughout the life history of the tumor and that preclinical latency may not be very long. Metastatic lesions may have a slightly faster average rate of growth than primary tumors. Some tumors, which present as interval cancers, or as a clinical mass, may arise rapidly and the doubling times observed in mammographically detectable tumors would likely not apply.[103 ADD IKEDA REF] Cancers that arise rapidly, which include Her-2 positive tumors, may indeed have a much more rapid doubling time. These observations may explain the relatively poorer prognosis recorded in several studies for very young women (<35 years old) with breast cancer. These women may have a higher proportion of faster growing, more aggressive tumors, since indolent, slowly growing tumors would not have had time to become clinically evident by that age. These data also suggest that for tumors that have had a prolonged preclinical life of at least several years, delays in diagnosis of only a few months from the first symptoms of primary breast cancer are unlikely to have a major impact on the presence or absence of metastases or ultimate patient survival. It has been estimated that only 5% of patients would be adversely affected by delays longer than 3 months. Even if primary tumors were diagnosed and treated a full year earlier, only a 30% reduction in the percentage of patients with metastases would result.[104] These estimates are compatible with the documented benefits of mammography screening programs, which detect microscopic, nonpalpable early breast cancers in many patients.

The heterogeneity of the natural history of breast cancer complicates patient management. Obviously, patients with virulent, fast-growing tumors might be treated aggressively because of their poor prognosis, whereas other patients with indolent tumors might be spared the morbidity and cost of excessive interventions when their disease is unlikely to compromise survival. A major focus of research in recent years has been the identification of tumor or host factors that would accurately predict patient outcome. The ideal prognostic marker would be one that, if expressed by the tumor, signified early metastases and short survival. Tumors not expressing the marker would be associated with an indolent course, the absence of metastases, and prolonged survival in nearly all patients. Although the ideal prognostic factor does not yet exist, a number of new molecular tools have been developed that hold promise to enable us to make better predictions about both prognosis[105-107] and the impact of therapy.[108] These factors attempt to measure and quantify the degree of tumor differentiation, tumor aggressiveness or metastatic potential, rate of growth or sensitivity/resistance to planned treatment.

After surgery has been completed and the surgical specimens have been examined and evaluated by the pathologist, ER, PR, Her-2/neu and grade are the critical prognostic and predictive indicators that are used to determine whether additional therapy is necessary and which treatment(s) will be potentially useful.

Age and Menopausal Status

Both patient characteristics have been extensively evaluated. When other, more important tumor characteristics are considered, age and menopausal status are not important prognostic indicators, although the very young (those under age 35 years) and elderly patients (those over age 75 years) had the worst breast cancer specific survival in several studies.

Angiogenesis Markers

Angiogenesis plays a substantial role in the growth and spread of malignant tumors.[109] Consequently, markers of angiogenic activity have received increasing attention. Counting the number of tumor capillaries immunohistochemically after staining for factor VIII has been shown to have major prognostic value. Tumors with fewer capillaries have a lower metastatic potential and better prognosis.[110] Markers of angiogenesis have also become therapeutic targets.

Markers of Proliferative Capacity

Measurement of the proliferation rates of malignant tissues has strong prognostic value for several types of cancer, including breast cancer. Several techniques are used to evaluate the proliferative capacity of the malignant cell, including mitotic indices, thymidine-labeling indices (TLIs) and SPF. The mitotic index is determined by counting mitotic figures using light microscopy on a tumor specimen stained with hematoxylin and eosin. It has been validated by both univariate and multivariate analyses. Many proteins play a role in the control of the cell cycle or are expressed at higher levels during certain phases of the cell cycle. Ki-67 and proliferating cell nuclear antigen (PCNA) are additional markers for the proliferation rate of malignant tumors.[111,112] Of these, Ki-67 has been more extensively studied, and it correlates strongly with the results of SPF determination and, therefore, long-term prognosis. This technique can be performed on fresh or frozen tissues and on archival paraffin-embedded material. A low value indicates a more slowly proliferating tumor and is associated with a slower rate of recurrence regardless of axillary nodal status. A high Ki-67 fraction is strongly correlated with other adverse prognostic factors, such as high histologic and cytologic grades, aneuploidy, and a negative steroid receptor status. Not surprisingly, the predictive molecular assays that have emerged are driven in part by genes that regulate proliferation.

Steroid Hormone Receptors

Both the ER and the PR have been studied extensively in patients with primary breast cancer.[113] Both clearly have prognostic value, although their ability to discriminate between low- and high-risk patients is quite limited. Patients with ER-positive tumor tend to have a more indolent course and to metastasize preferentially to soft tissue and bone; conversely, those with ER-negative tumors relapse earlier, and metastases to liver, lung, and central nervous system are more likely. ER-positive tumors are more often well differentiated and are associated with other favorable prognostic characteristics. Although patients with ER-positive tumors tend to have better short-term disease-free and overall survival rates than do patients with ER-negative tumors, the differences between the two groups tend to diminish or even disappear with time.[114]

PR appeared in some studies to be a more valuable prognostic indicator than the ER. The best use of steroid hormone receptors is not in the determination of prognosis but in the prediction of response to systemic endocrine therapy and, therefore, the selection of optimal adjuvant systemic treatments. Multiple recent reports have emphasized the strong predictive value of ER negativity for response to chemotherapy, especially in the neoadjuvant setting.

Molecular Genetic Alterations

Malignant tumors develop as a consequence of multiple critical gene abnormalities secondary to oncogene activation, loss of function of tumor suppressor genes, or alterations of other genes critical for cell control mechanisms. Two members of the type 1 growth factor receptor family, the EGFR (or HER1) and *HER2/neu*, are frequently amplified and/or overexpressed in breast cancer.[115,116] Over-expression of the proteins encoded by these genes is associated with a more aggressive clinical course, including a higher risk of developing metastases and more rapid growth and tumor progression. HER2 is overexpressed in 20% to 30% of breast cancers and overexpression is almost always the result of gene amplification. Overexpression is inversely correlated with ER expression and associated with poorly differentiated tumors with high growth rate. Survival is shorter for patients with HER2-overexpressing tumors than for patients with normal HER2 expression. Several recent reports suggest, however, that patients with HER2-overexpressing breast cancer derive greater benefit from anthracycline-containing adjuvant chemotherapy than from other regimens, particularly at higher dose.[117]

Whereas some studies suggest that HER2 overexpression is a marker of tamoxifen resistance, other analyses have provided conflicting results. The most important clinical application of HER2 testing is to identify candidates for HER2-directed therapy with trastuzumab (Herceptin) or lapatinib (Tykerb).[78,118] Reports have suggested that fluorescence in situ hybridization (FISH) is the most definitive testing method to predict response to trastuzumab.[79] The prognostic value of EGFR overexpression is less well established, and there is no FDA-approved diagnostic test for this receptor. It has not been validated as a relevant therapeutic target in breast cancer.

TP53 is frequently mutated in breast cancers.[119] Although some studies have found that *TP53* mutation is associated with poor prognosis and others have found correlations with response or resistance to cytotoxic or endocrine agents, no compelling evidence has emerged yet from large, multivariate analysis to support the routine testing for *TP53* gene mutation or abnormal protein expression as either prognostic or predictive factor. Evidence is even less compelling to support testing for *myc*, *ATM*, *RB*, or others. The prognostic value of gene mutations for *BRCA1* or *BRCA2* remains to be established.

Bone Marrow Involvement

Several investigators have presented data to suggest that the presence of microscopic involvement of the bone marrow, detectable by sensitive IHC analyses or other molecular assays, is a major determinant of prognosis.[120] In fact, some have suggested that this finding is superior to axillary lymph node involvement in its prognostic capability.[121] Although these data are increasingly interesting, this marker of prognosis has not been generally accepted or adopted in clinical practice and one standard test has not emerged as superior. This is an active area of ongoing investigation. There is also ongoing work with detection of circulating cancer cells and its correlation with prognosis or response to systemic therapy. Technological advances allow the reproducible detection and quantification of epithelial cells distinct from other nucleated cells in blood. A recent report of a prospective trial indicated that the presence of 5 or more circulating tumor cells per 7.5 mL blood at baseline was an adverse prognostic indicator in the metastatic setting[122] and that persistence of 5 or more cells after one month of systemic therapy was associated with a very high probability of short-term progressive disease. The clinical utility of quantifying and monitoring circulating tumor cells during treatment of metastatic breast cancer is currently under investigation.

Several other histologic factors, including lymphatic invasion, vascular invasion, tumor necrosis, and mononuclear cell infiltration, have been associated with better or worse prognoses in at least one report. Although extensive clinical experience supports the prognostic value of each of these factors, they have not survived the test of independence in multivariate analysis, nor have they been sufficiently evaluated to date.

Investigational Markers

Many biochemical, molecular, genetic, and immunologic markers have been under investigation for the past several years. All of them were suggested by one or more reports to have prognostic significance. However, evaluation of these markers falls short of determining whether they are independent prognostic factors or valuable additions to other proven, commonly used prognostic indicators. Among the promising investigational markers are heat shock proteins, *nm23*, cathepsin D, urokinase plasminogen activators (Upa), urokinase plasminogen activator receptors (Upar), plasminogen activator inhibitors (PAI-1, PAI-2), *Bcl-2*, *BAX*, laminin receptors, and apoptotic rate. Tumor levels of Upa and PAI-1, or the ratio of these two markers has been shown, in a prospective multicenter trial designed to validate their prognostic value, to be independently associated with prognosis. Furthermore, the European Organization for Research and Treatment of Cancer-Receptor and Biomarker Group also validated these markers in a prospective trial. A standardized ELISA assay exists. However, because of the need for a fresh, larger tumor sample this assay has not gained wide acceptance.

Some markers can be shown to be relevant as predictors of response to chemotherapy or hormone therapy, whereas others may serve to identify tumors using particular targets of biologic intervention (*HER2/neu*, EGFR). Many genes commonly associated with cancer participate in the regulation of cell proliferation and apoptosis. In a recent report, levels of total cyclin E and low molecular-weight cyclin E in tumor tissue, as measured by Western blot assay, correlated strongly with survival in patients with breast cancer.[112] Alterations in these genes may be important in determining the chemosensitivity of cancer cells. For instance, cells that express high levels of cyclin D 1 mRNA and protein have increased resistance to phase-specific agents like methotrexate, but not to doxorubicin or paclitaxel.[111] Mutations or deletions of p53 might be associated with resistance to various DNA-damaging drugs.

Over the years, there have been numerous attempts to reach a consensus on what prognostic factors are of recognized clinical utility. However, with the exception of the basic histopathologic factors, steroid hormone receptors, markers of proliferation, and HER2 expression, the majority of proposed factors fall short of general acceptance as useful clinical tools. The exception to this may be the emerging expression based tools using either array or RT-PCR based techniques.

Prognostic Indices

There have been multiple attempts to integrate prognostic information into standardized prognostic indices. The University of Nottingham index is based on tumor grade, axillary lymph node involvement, and hormone receptor status.[123] It has been validated prospectively and confirmed by an independent center, but it still has limited usefulness in the determination of individual prognosis. The Adjuvantonline program (Fig. 104-14) (https://www.adjuvantonline.com/index.jsp) is the prognostic index in greatest use. This free online software includes patient age, comorbid conditions, tumor size, grade, number of positive axillary nodes, and ER status. With this information, it calculates the 10-year probability of relapse and death for an individual patient.[124] Using this estimated risk level, the program also calculates the absolute benefit the patient would derive from adjuvant tamoxifen, aromatase inhibitors, and various chemotherapy regimens. Investigators from British Columbia recently validated the program, with observed results well within 2% of those predicted. A recent update of the program now includes the possibility to include other, ad hoc prognostic factors.

An emerging area of investigation of prognosis and prediction of sensitivity or resistance to therapy is genomics. cDNA arrays, including 20,000 to 30,000 genes are being used to develop gene expression profiles for improved disease classification and to correlate them with treatment outcome.[106] Although this is an evolving technology, early results suggest great promise in understanding better the biology of cancers, determining prognosis and predicting drug sensitivity.[125] Gene expression profiling using cDNA arrays or oligonucleotide arrays requires at this time the availability of fresh or fresh-frozen tissue. An alternate approach to develop multigene predictors of prognosis or response to therapy was recently presented.[108] This method (Oncotype Dx), based on RT PCR, can be performed on paraffin-embedded archival material. The assay, as presented, consists of 21 genes, including genes related to ER, HER2, proliferation genes and proteases identified from the literature. The results of the assay are expressed as a Recurrence Score, a quantitative estimate of recurrence at 5 years. This test was validated using samples collected prospectively as part of NSABP randomized trials. Updated analyses indicated that the assay had been validated on multiple independent groups of patients, and that the Recurrence Score was also a good predictor of therapeutic benefit from tamoxifen and adjuvant chemotherapy. One study showed that there was minimal or no benefit of tamoxifen in patients with high Recurrence Score, and limited or no benefit for chemotherapy in patients with low or intermediate scores. Conversely, there was a large absolute benefit of chemotherapy if the Recurrence Score was in the high category. The assay was first developed and validated on patient groups with ER-positive, lymph node negative breast cancer. More recently, Oncotype Dx was also validated on ER-positive, lymph node-positive breast cancer.

The new molecular array tests may be able to provide additional discriminatory information over and above what can be gleaned from ADJUVANT. This is true for both Oncotype DX[126] and the NKI 70 gene test (Mammaprint).[107] The NKI 70 gene test uses an index that segregates patients into low risk and high risk based on the expression profile of 70 genes in the tumor, and is FDA approved for the intended use to give prognostic information. The NKI 70 gene test outperforms ADJUVANT! as well as the clinical assessment of low and high risk (by NIH and St. Gallen criteria).[107] The major limitation of applying this assay is that the test requires fresh tissue and must be sent at the time of diagnosis or surgical excision. Both tests are being used in two very large prospective, multicenter randomized trials to test whether the information from the tests should determine whether to give chemotherapy to patients with ER positive breast can-

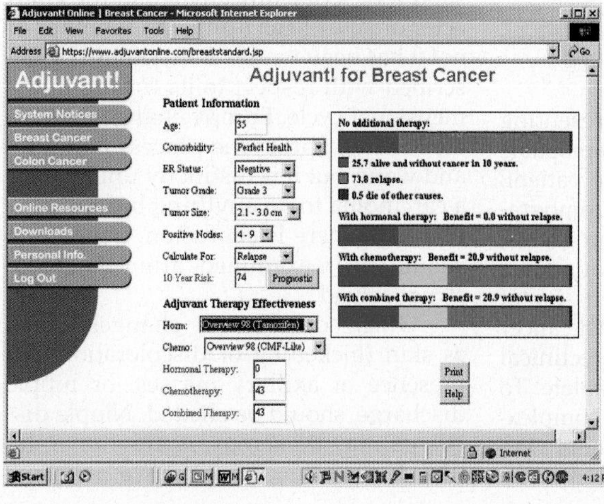

Figure 104-14 On-line prognostic software that predicts 10-year probability of recurrence and mortality, as well as the probability of benefit from various systemic adjuvant treatment options based on individual patient and tumor characteristics.

cer (MINDACT in Europe, Mammaprint, and TailoRX in the US, using Oncotype DX). Both tests also show that the information from the gene arrays may be more important that the involvement in lymph nodes. These tests also show that the measurement of RNA ER expression can differ from, and might be more accurate than the measurement of ER by immunohistochemistry.

Clinical Use of Prognostic Factors

The major objective of prognostic factors is to calculate the individual risk of recurrence and disease-related mortality for patients with primary breast cancer treated with curative intent. It is considered that patients with a risk of relapse lower than 10% would have only marginal benefit from adjuvant chemotherapy. However, calculations of the benefits of tamoxifen or an aromatase inhibitor administered for 5 years to patients with ER-positive breast cancer and the demonstration that the combination of hormonal therapy and chemotherapy has additive effects on reduction of risk of relapse and mortality have prompted a reassessment of these recommendations. Most patients with invasive primary breast cancer larger than 1 cm should be encouraged to receive adjuvant systemic therapy; some with tumors smaller than 1 cm should also be advised to consider adjuvant therapy, because randomized trials have not identified any subgroups that failed to derive benefit from these interventions. The use of prognostic factors, under these circumstances, serves more to place the benefit:risk ratio for individual patients in the context of their own prognosis. The acceptable benefit:risk ratio varies substantially from person to person; therefore, after a best attempt to calculate individual risk of relapse and mortality, treatment options and the probability of benefit from each should be presented in the light of toxicity and cost to facilitate informed treatment decisions.

Diagnosis and Screening

Historically, the primary presenting symptom of breast cancer was a palpable mass, often first detected by the patient. Today, the increasing use of mammography, especially in screening programs, results in many cancers being found at a preclinical stage. A simple discussion of the signs and symptoms of breast cancer without consideration of these preclinical manifestations would be incomplete. To some extent, this means greater complexity in selecting for biopsy patients who are suspected of having carcinoma. The clinical and mammographic signs and symptoms are best understood against the background knowledge of the anatomy and biology of breast cancer—how it grows and extends locally.

Patient History

The patient's history should include standard epidemiologic and reproductive information to assess the RR factors. Information about lumps, pain, or any changes in the breast should be obtained and correlated with physical findings. Although pain is probably the most frequent breast complaint that brings a patient to a physician's office, it is uncommonly the presenting factor in cancer. Breast cancer, especially in its early stages, is usually painless. Most breast pain is related to hormone stimulation and swelling of breast tissue (although these symptoms may draw attention to a mass that proves to be cancer). Careful questioning of the patient usually reveals that the pain is cyclic, beginning any time between ovulation and the onset of menstruation, and that commonly it is most intense a few days before menstruation. Pain usually disappears by the first or second day of the menstrual period, only to return again at the next cycle. Cyclic pain is present at a mild level in more than 50% of women of childbearing age. Less frequently, the pain can reach intense proportions. Some patients report that, during the worst days, it is too painful even to take a shower.

The most effective treatment is explanation and reassurance, although some patients who are extremely symptomatic and incapacitated by the pain may require treatments with hormones or hormone-blocking drugs. There are occasional reports that caffeine limitation or low-fat diets help, but relief seems to be individual, and these reports are not supported by persuasive clinical trials.

A patient who reports a lump or any other physical change in her breast needs careful attention. The history should describe any change in the character or size of the lump and whether or not it has been tender. Pain should be described with respect to its timing in the menstrual cycle. Lumpy changes associated with a fibrocystic process may wax and wane, but it is distinctly unusual for a carcinoma to do anything but increase in size. If there is confusion, the patient should be reexamined after the menstrual period.

Other descriptive changes, such as skin thickening or discoloration, the presence of axillary masses, or nipple discharge, should be elicited. Nipple discharge may be serous, watery, or milk-like. It may be clear or have a yellow or greenish hue, or it may be sero-sanguineous or frankly bloody. Although the latter may indicate a neoplasm, this is most commonly an intraductal papilloma, which is benign. It is possible, but rare, for such a discharge to signal an intraductal papillary carcinoma; all bloody discharges require further investigation.

Clear or serous discharge, especially if it involves more than one major duct opening on a nipple, is likely to be benign. Non-bloody discharge that is not spontaneous but requires manual compression to elicit is also likely to be benign. In an apocrine system such as the breast, there is always some cell desquamation and liquefaction and, therefore, some fluid present in the duct system. If this is not well absorbed, it can make its way through the collecting ducts to the nipple and present as a discharge. Similarly, if the duct is blocked by fibrosis or inspissated material, the pressure of secretion can cause dilation and cyst formation. Cytologic examination of the discharge has poor accuracy and is not very useful.

Physical Examination

The patient should be examined, first in a sitting, then in a supine position. When the patient is sitting erect, more useful information is obtained visually than by palpation. When the arms are raised and stretched upward, the contour of the skin is pulled tight, allowing for easier detection of contour abnormalities in the upper half of the breast. This position also emphasizes dimpling, especially in the lower half of the breast. Because much of the breast tissue coalesces in the sitting position, it is very difficult when palpating to appreciate true masses and often easy to be confused by confluent tissue. The axilla is palpated by relaxing and adducting the patient's arm, but this is best done with the patient in the sitting position.

With the patient supine and the arm raised so that the hand is behind the head and the elbow lies flat on the pillow, the breast tissue can be spread across the chest wall, allowing for proper palpation. The patient should be slightly turned to the contralateral side to aid this process. It is important to proceed in a pattern, but whether it be performed by quadrants or strips is up to the examiner. Skin changes, such as dimpling, peau d'orange (edema), erythema, or areas of fixation and ulceration, suggest advanced cancer that has invaded the skin or the immediate subcutaneous tissue. Skin retraction is often more easily detected when the patient is sitting and the arms are raised or when the patient is leaning forward. Retraction or asymmetry of the nipple is another worrisome sign unless the patient reports that this has been present all her life. A subtle reddish thickening of the nipple and areola or flaking of the superficial epithelium may suggest Paget's disease.

The examination is concluded with a search for axillary, infraclavicular, and supraclavicular nodes and palpation of the liver to detect enlargement. Although palpably enlarged axillary nodes raise the probability of metastases, careful studies have shown that clinical judgment is highly inaccurate. In a study conducted by the NSABP, a group of cancer patients were judged by their clinicians to have normal axillary nodes, but 38% showed histologic evidence of metastatic tumor when the specimens were examined pathologically.[82] Conversely, in 25% of such cases, nodes that appeared enlarged and were judged to contain cancer were found to be normal.

The most difficult clinical decision is differentiating between a pathologic mass and a physiologic density associated with fibroglandular (or fibrocystic) changes. Many women have the latter condition, which is characterized by a rubbery density without clear margins. A true lump has definite margins. Whether these are smooth, as in a gross cyst or fibroadenoma, or somewhat irregular, as in carcinoma, they delineate a discrete mass that requires further investigation. Invasive ductal carcinomas are usually hard, and dominant in the breast, in contrast to multiple firm masses that may exist in benign breast disease. Lobular carcinomas are not usually so hard and thus are more difficult to recognize.

It is important to measure the size of a tumor with a caliper so that subsequent examinations can more accurately establish any change in size. Mobile lesions are usually considered benign, but this is another area of clinical uncertainty. Advanced cancers may be fixed, but early palpable lesions will certainly be mobile with respect to skin or fascia and muscle of the chest wall. There is, however, a subtle difference in mobility (better called "movability") characteristic of cysts or fibroadenomas, which have capsules and move much more easily within the surrounding breast tissue. Carcinoma, on the other hand, which has no capsule and is surrounded by an infiltrating desmoplastic process, tends to move with the neighboring breast tissue rather than within it, because the process "locks" it into the stroma and surrounding glandular tissues, even when it is not fixed to surrounding structures, such as skin or muscle. Even the most experienced examiner can sometimes fail to distinguish correctly between benign and malignant lesions.

Mammography

An ideal screening test should be cheap, easy to administer, and highly sensitive and specific.[127] The current method of screening and diagnosis, mammography, which modestly fits this criteria, is the best tool we currently have and is recommended by most advisory groups including the U.S. Preventive Services Task Force, the American Cancer Society and the National Cancer Institute. Another summit on mammography was conducted and continued to recommend screening on the basis that there is a 20% to 30% reduction in the relative mortality from breast cancer, which translates into a 4% to 6% absolute difference in mortality from screening. Mammography, although the best screening tool we have, is flawed. The prevalence of cancers is 1 to 7 per 1000 women screened, depending on age. Mammographic screening generates many additional procedures (false negatives), identifies many early lesions, some of which might never come to clinical attention, is expensive, and interpretation varies significantly. Part of the problem is that we do not have a way to identify women for whom mammography is most effective. Mammography is more effective when the prevalence of disease is higher in the population (eg, in older women, or women known to be at higher risk), and performs optimally in the setting of relatively fatty breast tissue and less well in the setting of extremely dense tissue.[128] The introduction of digital mammography resulted in some tangible improvements: digital mammography appears more effective in younger women and in those with dense breasts. In addition, the images can be manipulated by the reader, and computerized assist software can identify areas of concern for the reader to focus. Mammography is much more cost effective for women aged 50 to 70 than it is for women aged 40 to 50,[129] and the aggregate cost of mammography is high, in the range of 6 to 10 billion dollars (US) in the United States alone. Mammograms are most accurate when interpreted by experienced, high-volume readers who review their own data and get feedback on their performance[129]; however, there is a shortage of well-trained breast imagers. Another consequence of mammography is that we have dramatically increased our capacity to identify stage 0 or in situ cancers, which has led to an increase in the use of mastectomy. For all of these reasons, the Institute of Medicine recently made recommendations of how to improve the current practice of screening and detection by a number of interventions, and particularly encouraged a change from opportunistic (encounter-based screening) to population-based organized screening such as is found in some European countries.[130]

MRI is increasingly being used in the management of breast cancer. MRI has the advantages of providing a three-dimensional view of the breast, performing with high sensitivity in dense breast tissue and using non-ionizing radiation. MRI has important disadvantages as well, including its high cost, variability in performance, and moderate specificity that in combination with high sensitivity often leads to unnecessary work-up.[131]

MRI is not appropriate as a general screening tool. It is at least 10 times as expensive as mammography, which would drive the cost of screening in the United States into the 100 billion dollar (US) range. MRI should be reserved for those situations where there is a high prior probability of identifying a cancer (high risk) and very high sensitivity is preferred and where other, less expensive, robust screening tools (eg, mammography) are known to be less sensitive,[128,132] such as *BRCA1* or *BRCA2* mutation carriers who have an 85% lifetime risk of developing breast cancer. Although the average 35-year-old would have a 1/10,000 chance of having a cancer, a mutation carrier would have a risk in the range of 1 to 5/100, and MRI would be much more sensitive in this population than mammography. Women with a very high 5-year Gail risk and very dense breast tissue may also fall into this category. Using a density modified Gail Risk score,[58] which combines both risk and breast density as recorded on a mammogram (BIRADS density), enables the identification of women both at high risk and at risk for false negatives with mammography. The density-modified Gail risk is calculated by multiplying the lifetime Gail risk by 0.59, 1.00, 1.41, or 1.94 for a BIRADS of 1, 2, 3, or 4, respectively. Those with a lifetime risk of >50%, as calculated by the density-modified Gail model, are recommended for MRI screening. Consideration can be given to women with a 35-49% lifetime risk using this tool, though there is no current evidence to support the addition of annual MRI screening.

The true measure of a screening test is not whether it finds more cancers, but whether finding the cancers decreases mortality and morbidity from breast cancer. No study has yet shown that cancers found by MRI decrease mortality from breast cancer. However, two large studies have shown that screening using MRI is much more sensitive in high risk women, with remarkably similar results.[133,134] If tumor size and lymph node involvement is used as a surrogate for outcome, MRI does improve the stage at which tumors are identified in women in the highest risk cohort. In the Netherlands study, the cancers found in the 1909 women screened with mammography and MRI were compared to two appropriate control groups of mutation carriers and high-risk patients, none of whom had access to MRI screening. In the highest risk group (50-85% estimated life time risk), 63% of mutation carriers with screened cancers had negative nodes when screened with MRI compared to 47% with negative nodes in the controls. In the moderate risk group (15-30% estimated lifetime risk), only 12% had lymph node involvement and 87% had negative nodes (compared to 52-56% positive nodes and 44-48% negative nodes in the control groups). Therefore, MRI appears to be able to find cancers at an earlier stage. However, the rate of detection of cancer is also important, and MRI should be used where that rate is high, and significantly higher than in the usual screened group. Of note, the cancer detection rate was 26.5, 5.4, and 7.8 per 1000 women years for the mutation carriers, high-risk, and moderate-risk respectively. This should be compared to the detection rate of 5 to 7/1000 women where mammography is most cost-effective, in women aged 50 to 70 years. The only group that had a higher rate of cancer development was the highest risk group, the mutation carriers and we should be careful to restrict the use of MRI for those highest risk women

Screening comes at a price, both financial and psychological. In the Netherlands study of 1909 women screened for 10 years, 1200 extra procedures were performed. In the process of finding the 45 cancers, MRI led to twice as many extra procedures (420) compared to mammography (207), and three times as many unnecessary biopsies, 24 versus 7 for MRI and mammography, respectively.[131] MRI should be applied very judiciously as a screening tool and with rigorous criteria, so that we do not misapply resources and inadvertently cause women anguish over false positives which are both more likely and more difficult to follow and resolve, because MRI-directed biopsy tools are not readily available. It is common to recommend 3-months or 6-months follow-up studies after an abnormal imaging test. However, MR exams cost $1000 to 2000 (US), so it is inappropriate to order these tests unless there truly is a situation where the likelihood of finding an abnormality is much higher than in the general population, and where mammography would be unlikely to be effective. The two key messages are that we need to find ways of stratifying risk to appropriately tailor the use of technology, and MRI screening should be undertaken only in facilities that have the capability of investigating MRI abnormalities, both with ultrasound and MRI-guided biopsy if necessary. The Blue Cross/Blue Shield technology assessment concluded in 2003 that MRI screening was justified in women who carry an inherited predisposition to breast cancer. The Netherlands and Canadian studies[133,135] only strengthened this conclusion. The moderate- and high-risk women probably gain less overall because the risk is not as great, suggesting that MR must become more specific and follow-up of abnormalities easier before we implement widespread screening of intermediate risk women.

Not all MR exams are alike. There is a great deal of variability in technique, sequences, interpretation, and capability for follow-up and biopsy. Although the use of breast MR has proliferated rapidly, standards have not. Clinicians ordering breast MRIs need to know that technique, time of menses (the midcycle is optimal 4-14 days after starting menses), and that the skill in interpretation impact results. Interpreting images performed in different institutions is also a challenge because of the relative inability to transfer and view images electronically. Each of these areas is under active investigation, and further research and technological improvements will substantially improve our ability to appropriately integrate MRI into breast cancer management.

MRI has also been used after a diagnostic test reveals an abnormality. The most definitive study on the performance characteristics of MRI for the evaluation of mammographic abnormalities and palpable masses is the multi-institutional International Breast MRI Consortium (IBMC) study. Eight hundred forty-one patients were evaluated using MRI across 14 institutions. All patients received high resolution scans and 500 women with enhancing lesions were returned for a dynamic scan within 48 hours. High sensitivity and moderate specificity were confirmed in this study. It was also found that the high-resolution technique had the same performance characteristics as dynamic scans. High-resolution scans give greater anatomic detail and do not require specialized computer software to perform kinetic analysis. This is important because high-resolution scans are also easier for clinicians to interpret, and thus high resolution scanning is likely to be included in all MRI exams. Diagnostic characterization of lesions by MRI is improving, but it is not sufficiently specific to substitute a biopsy. MRI after an abnormal diagnostic mammogram significantly increases false positives. Currently, there is no role for MRI in the diagnosis of breast cancer unless suspicious mammographic findings can not be evaluated or localized or unless there is another compelling reason to order MRI (eg, if a patient is a mutation carrier, or has a very high risk of cancer and very dense breast tissue).

Perhaps the most important role for MRI is the staging of known cancer in the breast and monitoring the response to therapy.[131] MRI reveals that tumors form distinct patterns in the breast, and different types of tumors, such as lobular and inflammatory cancers, are more commonly associated with distinct patterns.

Initial imaging characteristics identify women likely to have a particularly poor response, such as diffuse tumors with large volumes.[134] A multicenter trial sponsored by ACRIN, CALGB, and SPORE is underway to validate the role of MRI in predicting and monitoring response to therapy, and to correlate molecular and protein markers to imaging phenotypes.

Biopsy

When a woman presents with a diagnostic abnormality, a decision to intervene should be made in context of the likelihood of the lesion being invasive cancer or in situ cancer, as well as the age, underlying health condition, and life expectancy of the patient. A decision about which type of biopsy to perform is made by thinking about the need for future procedures. The goal should be to minimize the total number of procedures (including definitive cancer surgery), to minimize discomfort and scarring, minimize diagnostic wait time and anxiety, and enable the optimal timing of procedures.

There are a number of options available for the diagnosis of masses and mammographic abnormalities.[132] For palpable lesions, the options include FNA, core biopsy, or excisional biopsy. Minimally invasive techniques, core biopsy and FNA, are quite accurate in experienced hands and when the "triple assessment" is used. Triple assessment is the consideration of the imaging, clinical, and pathologic findings. If there is significant discordance, further evaluation should be pursued. In general, excisional biopsy is not the optimal diagnostic procedure. Minimally invasive biopsy techniques can be performed immediately in the office, and facilitate a rapid diagnosis and discussion of options, and full evaluation of the extent of disease in the breast prior to definitive surgery. FNA or core biopsies can also be used to confirm the suspicion of multi-centric disease and thereby avoid multiple trips to the operating room, and in general, allow the optimal sequencing of interventions.

The type of biopsy performed should depend on the expertise at a given institution. FNA is highly accurate, with sensitivity and specificity of 98% and 99%, respectively, in the hands of experienced operators. FNA both for palpable and mammographic lesions has been used extensively and successfully in Sweden and the UK where it is the standard diagnostic tool. This technique requires practitioners who have training and experience in sampling the lesion (the aspect prone to greatest error), preparing the slides, and interpreting cytology.[136] The advantage is that it can be performed right away and yields results within a day. Both FNA and core biopsy are preferred when there is a high suspicion of invasive cancer and the anticipation that a sentinel lymph node dissection (SLND) will be performed. When an SLND is performed, the type of biopsy performed affects the accuracy of the SLND. Core and FNA have a lower false negative rate than excisional biopsy when a subsequent sentinel node dissection is performed: 8% compared to 14% for incisional biopsy and 15% for excisional biopsy. In the setting of a patient with a large obvious tumor, FNA can facilitate the rapid confirmation of a diagnosis and a discussion of options, including neoadjuvant therapy and clinical trials. For patients who opt for surgical management, no further test is needed. For those who opt for neoadjuvant therapy, a core biopsy should be obtained for histology to confirm invasive disease, to save for future studies in the event of complete pathologic response, and potentially for clinical trials. In the event that cytology expertise does not exist in a given institution, a core biopsy can also be rapidly performed in the office setting.

Recall for mammographic abnormalities is common, and the likelihood of cancer being diagnosed from a mammographic biopsy (cancer to biopsy rate or CBR) is highly variable, anywhere from 10% to 40%. A low CBR is not necessary for high sensitivity, and in fact, the most experienced and highly trained mammographers find more cancers and order fewer biopsies for what turns out to be benign.[137] CBR rates decline over time in settings where quality improvement and feedback on performance is the rule. There are several ways to avoid biopsies of non-cancerous tissue. The first is to take the extra time to get old mammograms for comparison. Circumscribed mass lesions that have been stable for over 2 years will be converted to probably benign and not require a biopsy. If an experienced mammographer has not read the films, a second opinion can always be obtained.

In the event that a biopsy is recommended, it is important to make sure that the lesion is not palpable. If it is, and particularly if the lesion is suspicious for cancer, an FNA not only establishes the diagnosis, but confirms that the palpable mass is indeed the cancer, avoiding the need for wire localization at the time of lumpectomy. An attempt to locate nonpalpable suspicious mammographic masses with ultrasound will enable diagnostic and definitive procedures to be ultrasound guided, which is more comfortable for patients. In the event that a mammographic lesion can only be seen on mammogram, then a stereotactic biopsy can be performed, using digital images to locate the lesion and direct the core biopsy. The sensitivity of this procedure is as high as 98% by experienced practioners.[136] A specimen radiograph is obtained to confirm that the target has been obtained (usually calcifications). If there is a risk that all calcifications will be removed, it is then critical to leave a clip to localize the area later.

It is important to perform procedures in the context of their value to the overall management of the patient. If a cancer is not present, an adequate sampling of the calcifications or lesions should be performed. If cancer is present, the minimal amount to establish the diagnosis is sufficient. At this point, the diagnostic procedure is not definitive and wide excision is needed. Some radiologists take over 30 core biopsy samples. This is not necessary, and can create hematomas, distortion of tissue, and difficulty assessing the true extent of the lesion. It is also unpleasant for the patient.

Some mammographic lesions cannot be biopsied using stereotactic techniques either because the lesion is too close to the chest wall, or the breast compresses to less than 3cm in the direction the biopsy needle would be placed. In this case, an excisional biopsy must be performed. A wire is placed by the radiologists to guide the surgery, with the tip of the wire just under or at the level of the calcifications or mass. The surgeon should use the radiologist's estimate for the likelihood of malignancy to determine the extent of resection. For lesions more likely to be cancer, the lesion and a one-cm rim of tissue should be taken. For low suspicion lesions, a smaller volume of tissue can be taken. To avoid taking unnecessary tissue, an incision should be made near the tip of the wire or the expected location of the abnormality. Starting the excision at the insertion site of the wire only leads to excessive tissue being removed and usually results in a close margin at the end of the wire. Making the incision over the lesion is helpful in locating the biopsy cavity in the event that an additional resection is necessary. All specimens need to be sent to mammography or evaluated using a Faxitron to assure the surgeon that the target lesion has been removed. Mammographers routinely recommend a biopsy of any lesion that is a BIRADS (Breast Imaging Reporting and Data System scale) 4 or greater. However, a BIRADS classification of 4 includes lesions that have a risk of as low as 3% or as high as 75% for being malignant. The lesion may be suspicious for either in situ or invasive cancer—no distinction is implied by the categorization of a BIRADS 4. The surgeon should make sure that they understand both the type of lesion suspected as well as a more specific estimate of risk as it may make a difference in how the patient is evaluated. An older woman with several co-morbidities and a mammogram with a BIRADS 4, if she has a lesion that is approximately 90% likely to be benign and 10% likely to be DCIS, may not need a biopsy. This is the type of lesion that could be followed on mammography. In general, we recommend that a minimally invasive biopsy be used to establish a diagnosis, but excisional biopsy may be the procedure of choice for a woman who has a confined cluster of linear calcifications that are highly suspicious for high grade DCIS. In this situation, a core biopsy would likely reveal DCIS, and a negative biopsy would be discordant and require wire localization and excision. If the likelihood of associated, invasive cancer is low, a sentinel node dissection or axillary sampling will not be necessary, and therefore, there is little value in starting with a stereotactic biopsy.

Role of Breast Self-Examination

In the HIP study, about one-third of breast cancer cases were found using mammography alone; overall, 75% were detectable on clinical examination. Because mammographic techniques have improved since the 1960s, the value of clinical examination and breast self-examination (BSE) seems less clear today. Many studies have shown that women who perform regular BSEs detect breast cancers at an earlier clinical and pathologic stage of the disease.

The Swedish mammography studies did not include either clinical examination or BSE, which raises the question as to whether those results would have been better, had these modalities been included. The Canadian NBSS included instructions in BSE, and the teaching was reinforced at subsequent annual screenings, but it is uncertain whether the practice had any effect since all participants received instruction. Whereas it seems logical to recommend widespread use of BSE as a screening tool that is free and available to everyone, the evidence in support of it is far from solid and remains controversial. Furthermore, BSE can be expected to prompt a significant number of unnecessary biopsies with their attendant anxiety.

On the other hand, most breast masses are still self-discovered, suggesting that women are an important source of detecting their own breast cancers, and self awareness may contribute to diagnosing the disease earlier, or when the lesions are smaller. Perhaps more importantly, women should be given the message that they should be familiar with their breast tissue so that they will be able to recognize a change, and bring it to the attention of a physician. Being aware and doing at least a cursory self exam may be sufficient and a more formal detailed BSE may not be of value.

Prospective randomized studies of BSE from China and Russia have failed to demonstrate a survival benefit.[138] A meta-analysis from Canadian investigators shows no benefit of routinely teaching BSE to women and concludes that the net effect on the population is a harmful one because the potential for unnecessary biopsies and anxiety is not balanced by any gain in mortality reduction.

Differential Diagnosis

In performing breast examinations, the first objective is the detection of potential abnormalities. Discovery of an abnormality is followed by further investigation and evaluation to decide whether intervention is necessary. Mammography and ultrasound can provide additional information, and should be used in most cases. Fibroadenomas cannot be easily distinguished from cysts clinically, but a needle aspiration solves the problem instantaneously. Ultrasonography can also differentiate cysts from solid lesions and is useful when mammography detects small lesions, probably cysts that cannot be palpated.

The most common breast lumps are caused by a process previously called fibrocystic disease, more recently labeled fibrocystic or fibroglandular changes or benign breast disease. The process is usually symmetric, and most often situated in the upper outer quadrants because that is where most of the glandular tissue is found. Microscopically, there is a combination of fibrosis and ductal swelling, which gives the process its classic "fibrocystic" name. Clinically, the tissue feels more dense or rubbery, but focal areas can be quite firm or hard. If a gross cyst is present, it tends to be round, circumscribed, and somewhat movable. The process is usually accompanied by pain or tenderness and tends to be cyclic, with relief as the menstrual period begins. It affects 50% of premenopausal women but usually subsides after menopause (Fig. 104-12). Fibroadenomas are also smooth, round, and mobile and occur from adolescence to menopause.

In older women, the inferior ridge of the breast may be compressed in a crescent-shape pattern due to the weight of the overlying breast. This area represents simple fat compression and is benign. Many poorly defined processes require surgical biopsy to distinguish them from malignancy. Causes of these vague densities include sclerosing adenosis, hyperplasia with or without atypia, and mammary duct ectasia. The last is the end result of the fibrocystic process, with ducts filled with liquid and cellular debris accompanied by fibrous changes and lymphocytic infiltration.

Lesions that are less smooth and less mobile with poorly defined margins, particularly if hard, raise the suspicion of carcinoma. The identification of the nature of a mass requires careful integration of all available information, including imaging. The clinician's responsibility is to establish the diagnosis of cancer when it exists but to minimize the number of unnecessary biopsies. A simplistic approach—biopsy of every clinical abnormality—would certainly identify all of the cancers but would be irresponsible, because of the large numbers of unnecessary operations. Similarly, abstaining from biopsy until the signs are absolutely incontrovertible would be dangerous, even though this approach would minimize unnecessary operations. The proper strategy is to apply all of the available information—history, clinical signs, mammographic and ultrasound information, and needle aspiration cytology—and to biopsy all of those lesions where a reasonable doubt as to their benign nature exists.

Staging and Classification

The purposes of staging are to (1) plan a therapeutic strategy that is most appropriate for the patient, (2) allow for more intelligent projection of outcome based on the disease status of the patient, and (3) permit comparison of therapeutic results obtained from different sources by different means. The common staging methods in use today are clinical and pathologic, but newer methods involving biologic assessments are under development and validation. Regardless of the staging method used, it is important to remember that the stage represents the state of disease or biologic potential of an individual patient's tumor. The usefulness of a particular staging method must be judged against its accuracy in performing this task.

The TNM classification devised by the International Union Against Cancer (UICC) and accepted by the American Joint Commission on Cancer Staging is a world standard.[139] The TNM is based on the clinical features of tumor (T), the regional lymph nodes (N), and the presence or absence of distant metastases (M). The tumor is characterized by its size, so that a T1 is a tumor less than 2 cm, a T2 is 2 to 5 cm, and a T3 is over 5 cm. Similarly, N0 represents negative, or normal, regional lymph nodes, and so on (Table 104-9).

Clinical staging systems generally underestimate the extent of disease. The inclusion of pathologic information improves staging accuracy and is the basis for most modern clinical trials. In all cases, it is wise to remember that the goal is to define the biologic activity of the tumor. Cox regression statistical models demonstrate that the presence of nodal metastases is the most important factor. Furthermore, the number of nodes involved can be used to further subset the prognostic groups (Table 104-7). It is generally acknowledged that nodal metastases that penetrate the capsule and extend into adjacent perinodal tissue carry a worse prognosis.

The complete dissection of levels I and II axillary nodes provides an extremely high degree of confidence in establishing whether axillary metastases exist. A comparison of protocols employing Halsted radical mastectomy, modified mastectomy, and lumpectomy with axillary dissection shows that, essentially, the same number of lymph nodes is retrieved for examination, despite the different procedures. Even with multiple positive nodes, axillary recurrence is not common with today's limited axillary dissection. Identification, mapping and biopsy of the sentinel node is a more limited procedure with a high degree of prognostic accuracy and markedly decreased morbidity when compared to conventional level I and II axillary dissection.

Tumor size was seen in a regression analysis model to be closely related to axillary lymph node involvement.[93,100] Tumor size is not an important discriminant within axillary node groups, except for patients with more than four involved nodes. Thus, size, which can be a function of either time or growth rate, is less useful than axillary node involvement, which is a more specific indicator of biologic aggressiveness. Furthermore, some patients with large masses may have slow-growing tumors, ignored for years, which have not metastasized. A similar problem exists in classifying patients with small but aggressive tumors found by screening mammography in whom distant metastases already exist. These patients may die rapidly despite the initial favorable local clinical features. A biologic classification would identify these women more accurately than does the TNM system.

Biologic Markers

Detection and Staging ■ Modern molecular biologic techniques will probably change

Table 104-9 TNM Stage Definitions

Primary Tumor (T)	
TX	Primary tumor cannot be assessed
T0	No evidence of primary tumor
Tis	Carcinoma in situ
Tis (DCIS)	Ductal carcinoma in situ
Tis (LCIS)	Lobular carcinoma in situ
Tis (Paget's)	Paget's disease of the nipple with no tumor
T1	Tumor 2.0 cm or less in greatest dimension
T1mic	Microinvasion 0.1 cm or less in greatest dimension
T1a	Tumor more than 0.1 but not more than 0.5 cm in greatest dimension
T1b	Tumor more than 0.5 cm but not more than 1.0 cm in greatest dimension
T1c	Tumor more than 1.0 cm but not more than 2.0 cm in greatest dimension
T2	Tumor more than 2.0 cm but not more than 5.0 cm in greatest dimension
T3	Tumor more than 5.0 cm in greatest dimension
T4	Tumor of any size with direct extension to (a) chest wall or (b) skin, only as described below.
T4a	Extension to chest wall, not including pectoralis muscle
T4b	Edema (including peau d'orange) or ulceration of the skin of the breast or satellite skin nodules confined to the same breast
T4c	Both T4a and T4b
T4d	Inflammatory carcinoma
Regional Lymph Nodes (N)	
NX	Regional lymph nodes cannot be assessed (eg, previously removed)
N0	No regional lymph node metastasis
N1	Metastasis to movable ipsilateral axillary lymph node(s)
N2	Metastasis in ipsilateral axillary lymph node(s) fixed or matted, or in clinically apparent ipsilateral internal mammary nodes in the absence of clinically evident axillary lymph node metastasis
N3	Metastasis in ipsilateral infraclavicular lymph node(s) with or without axillary lymph node involvement, or in clinically apparent ipsilateral internal mammary lymph node(s) and in the presence of clinically evident axillary lymph node metastasis; or metastasis in ipsilateral supraclavicular lymph node(s) with or without axillary or internal mammary lymph node involvement
Pathologic Classification (pN)	
pNX	Regional lymph nodes cannot be assessed (previously removed, or not removed for pathologic study)
pN0	No regional lymph node metastasis
pN1	Metastasis in 1 to 3 axillary lymph nodes, and/or in internal mammary nodes with microscopic disease detected by sentinel lymph node dissection but not clinically apparent
pN2	Metastasis in 4 to 9 axillary lymph nodes, or in clinically apparent internal mammary lymph nodes in the absence of axillary lymph node metastasis
pN3	Metastasis in 10 or more axillary lymph nodes, or in infraclavicular lymph nodes, or in clinically apparent ipsilateral internal mammary lymph nodes or in the presence of 1 or more positive axillary lymph nodes with clinically negative microscopic metastasis in internal mammary lymph nodes; or in ipsilateral supraclavicular lymph nodes
Distant Metastasis (M)	
MX	Presence of distant metastasis cannot be assessed
M0:	No distant metastasis
M1	Distant metastasis present
AJCC Stage Groupings	
Stage 0	Tis, N0, M0
Stage I	T1,N1, M0
Stage IIA	T0, N1, M0 T1, N0, M0 T2, N0, M0
Stage IIB	T2, N1, M0 T3, N0, M0
Stage IIIA	T0, N2, M0 T1, N2, M0 T2, N2, M0 T3, N1, M0 T3, N2, M0
Stage IIIB	T4, Any N, M0 Any T, N3, M0
Stage IV	Any T, Any N, M1

Source: From Ref. 139.

the approach to detecting and staging early breast cancer. The advent of mammography resulted in a change in presenting sign from a clinical mass to a subclinical mammographic abnormality. The search is now on for biologic markers that can indicate the presence of early carcinoma or that can be used as prognostic indicators to select patients for adjuvant therapies. These markers are usually substances produced by a cancer cell or by the host.

Nonspecific antigens, such as carcinoembryonic antigen (CEA), and more characteristic antigens, such as MUC1 (measured with monoclonal antibody-based commercial kits CA 15–3 or CA 27–29), were studied. These are more reliably elevated in advanced disease (stage III or stage IV) than in early stages and are more useful in following the course of a patient who has established cancer than in detecting the presence of cancer in a screening program.[140] Levels of these markers do decline with a good response to chemotherapy and are a useful reflection of changing tumor burden; therefore, they help monitor response to therapy.

Ongoing work in this area has concentrated on HER2, receptors for estrogen and progesterone, but EGF, and IGF-1R are among other receptors now being studied. To date, findings are encouraging, but results are not currently applicable to routine clinical practice.

Current practice requires axillary lymph node assessment to determine nodal involvement. This information is used for prognosis and for assignment of patients to adjuvant chemotherapy treatments. Attempts to identify lymph node involvement by radioimmunoscintigraphy or PET scanning have, so far, been of limited usefulness because of the inability to image lesions in the microscopic range. Experience with removing the "sentinel node" and studying serial sections with IHC has shown a high degree of accuracy.[91,141] NSABP protocol B-32, which has completed patient accrual, attempts to answer the question of whether an axillary dissection adds any therapeutic benefit to patients with negative sentinel lymph node. The ACOSOG's protocols Z10 and Z-11 will further determine whether in patients with clinically negative lymph nodes a positive sentinel node is an indication for an axillary dissection or whether no additional axillary surgery is needed.

Such less invasive methodology and, the advent of molecular indicators of tumor aggressiveness have largely supplanted surgical lymph node dissection in patients with clinically negative axillae, but the axillary lymph node dissection remains the most reliable prognostic indicator for patients with positive axillae.

Psychosocial Aspects of Breast Cancer

In recent decades, there has been increasing awareness of the psychosocial needs of cancer patients. These issues arose in breast cancer patients, in particular, because of the many changes that occurred in therapy. Radical breast surgery gave way to breast-conserving surgery at the same time that adjuvant therapies—many of them accompanied by uncomfortable side effects—were introduced. Axillary dissection is being replaced by sentinel lymph node biopsy in clinically node-negative patients. In general, lumpectomy patients report fewer feelings of unattractiveness and loss of femininity and less change in body image. When mastectomy is performed, immediate reconstruction results in a decrease in psychological morbidity.

Multiple surgical interventions and adjuvant chemotherapy are accompanied by an increased fear of recurrence. This fear is probably due to the perception that these additional therapeutic manipulations imply a more worrisome prognosis. Many adjuvant chemotherapy regimens are accompanied by nausea, vomiting, or by hair loss, and it is not surprising that these side effects have an impact on the psychosocial status of patients. Many studies indicate that breast cancer patients suffer from either increased anxiety states or depressive illness, but these analyses suggest that it is the diagnosis rather than the type of treatment that is responsible. Furthermore, the level of psychological distress at the time of initiating adjuvant chemotherapy had no effect on disease-free survival or survival. Lumpectomy patients are not less anxious or depressed but, in general, adapt more favorably to their surgery and exhibit less functional change. There is increasing agreement that counseling services should be provided to help improve the quality of life of breast cancer patients.[142]

Surgery

Over the past three decades, revolutionary changes have occurred in the locoregional management of primary breast cancer. As a result, radical and extended radical mastectomy has been relegated to the archives of surgical history. The publication of a series of randomized controlled clinical trials comparing radical mastectomy to less extensive surgical interventions led an NIH-sponsored consensus development conference (1990) to recommend that breast preservation is the preferable treatment for women with stages I and II breast cancer because it provides survival figures equivalent to those of total mastectomy and axillary dissection while, at the same time, preserving the breast.[143]

Information from various sources indicates that many patients with breast cancer have disseminated disease by the time a clinical diagnosis is established. This is not surprising since a breast tumor of 1 cm has already progressed through 30 of the theoretical 40 doublings that result in a tumor of approximately 1 kg, a size that could be lethal to the patient. However, today we know that breast cancer is a heterogeneous disease, and that some patients have tumors with a low potential for metastatic spread, and that some, even when small and confined to the breast, have a high risk for metastatic spread.[107,108] Molecular profiling is likely to add much to our ability to distinguish these types of tumors and to tailor treatment accordingly.

Three of four patients with positive axillary nodal involvement and almost 9 of 10 patients with four or more involved nodes became treatment failures 10 years after radical mastectomy without adjuvant chemotherapy for what were considered to be clinically "curable" breast cancers. These findings emphasize the systemic nature of some breast cancer[144] and indicate the inadequacy of extensive local and regional surgery when used as sole modalities of treatment in those women at high risk to develop metastases.

Breast Conserving Treatments

The goal of breast conservation is to remove the tumor and a rim of normal tissue while preserving the contour and shape of the breast. Tumor left at a margin will increase the risk of recurrence. Recht and colleagues, in a study of 533 patients, showed that recurrence risk depends on the amount of tumor left at the margin: grossly positive margins, focally positive margins, close margins were associated with a recurrence risk of 27%, 14%, and 7%. Close margins did not materially change the recurrence risk in this study where all women received radiation therapy. The presence of extensive intraductal carcinoma, once thought to be a contraindication to breast conservation, has now been shown not to be associated with higher risk of local recurrence if all of the DCIS has been excised. After breast conservation, 90% of all in-breast recurrences, in the first decade after diagnosis, are in the same quadrant and genetically identical to the primary breast cancer. Long-term follow-up studies of breast conservation surgery versus mastectomy, however, show that there is an ongoing risk for developing new cancers in the breast after 10 years, but these often occur in other quadrants.

Breast Biopsy

Two-Stage Procedure and Fine-Needle Aspiration ■ With the advent of lumpectomy, there was a need to adopt a two-stage approach to biopsy and then to definitive surgery. Preoperative core needle biopsies, either clinically or radiologically directed, should be considered standard, so that the surgeon has a definite diagnosis before any surgery takes place and can better plan the operation. A detailed algorithm describing an optimal surgical strategy for the management of primary breast cancer has been described and is presented in Figure 104-15.

If an open breast biopsy must be carried out, it should be done as if a lumpectomy were being performed. Attention must be given to ensuring that specimen margins are likely to be free of tumor should a malignancy be encountered. In all circumstances where breast conservation is feasible, the operation carried out to establish the definitive diagnosis of a breast lesion becomes the definitive treatment whether axillary surgery is done at that time or later. Most breast cancer operations—biopsy, lumpectomy, axillary dissection, and even mastectomy—can be performed as out-patient procedures with comparable low levels of surgical complications and equal or better personal and social adjustment to the procedure.

Technique and Cosmetic Considerations ■ To achieve the best cosmetic results, the incision should be planned based on the extent of tumor in the breast, the location of the tumor, and the native shape of the breast. Many options now exist for patients who require breast surgery. The extent of tissue that can be resected depends on the breast size. Plastic surgery techniques can be used to improve symmetry, both with and without cosmetic surgery on the contralateral breast. Once breast tissue is removed, undermining the breast tissue at the level of the fascia provides the opportunity to arrange the closure of the breast tissue in a medial to lateral direction, thereby avoiding the displacement of the nipple either superiorly or inferiorly. Mastopexy or reduction can be performed on the contralateral breast to improve symmetry. If there is a significant degree of ptosis in the breast, a partial mastectomy can be accomplished by performing a breast reduction, thereby combining a cosmetic enhancement with the oncologic procedure of removing the breast tissue (Fig. 104-16). In a breast reduction procedure, over half of the breast tissue can be removed, thus this technique can be used for larger tumors, or

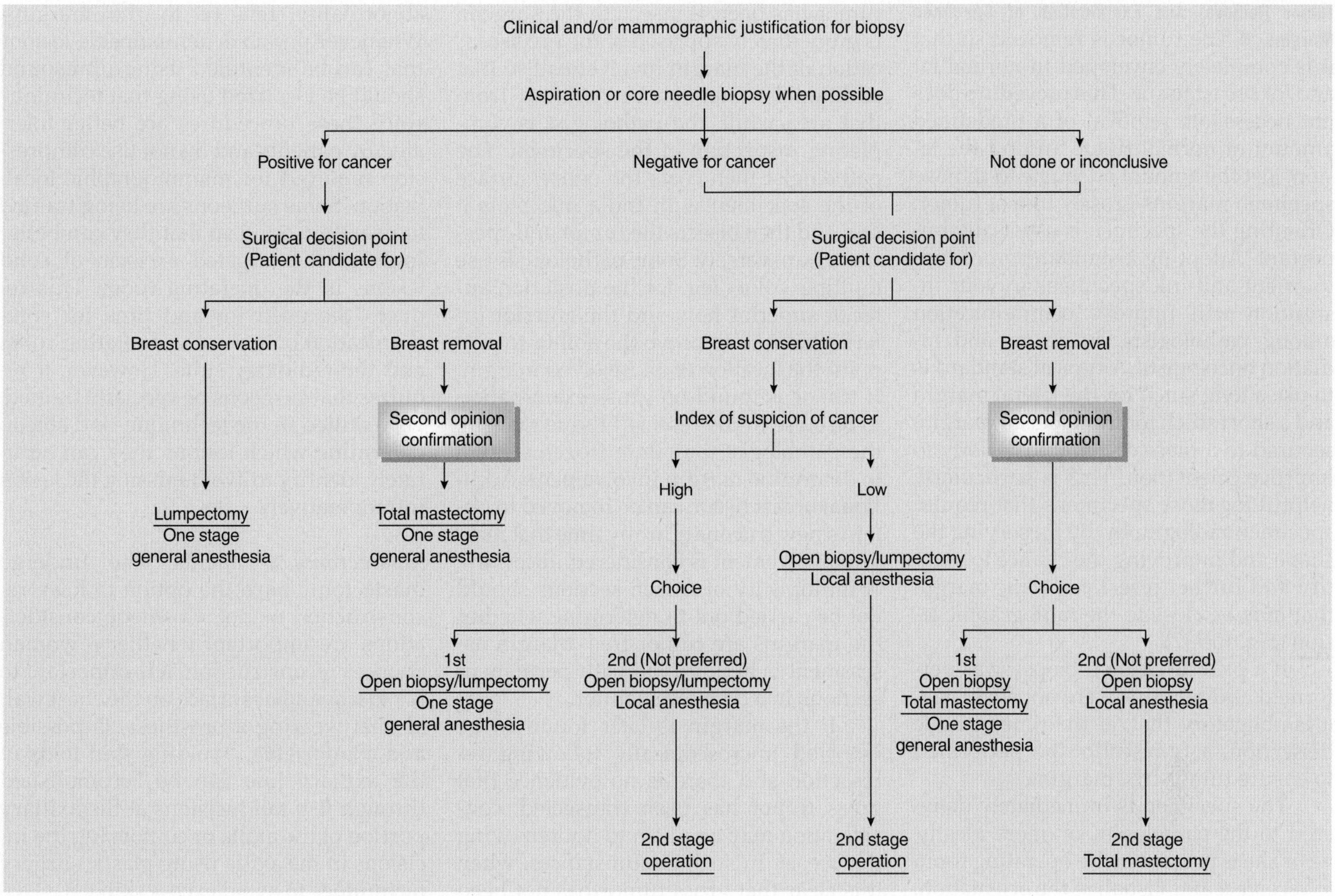

Figure 104-15 ■ Recommended surgical strategy for management of primary breast cancer.

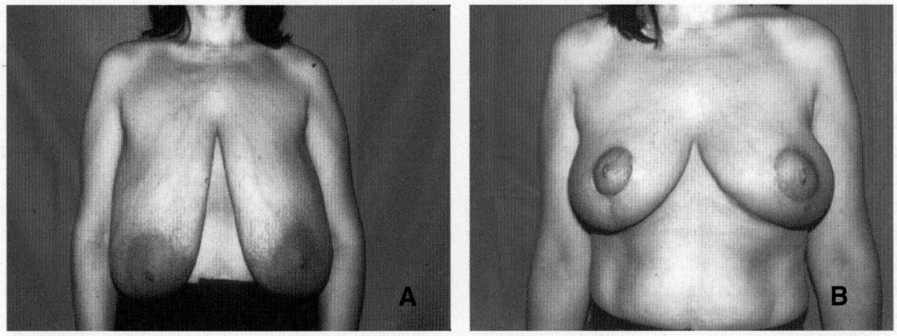

Figure 104-16 ■ Example of a breast reduction technique to accomplish a breast reduction and partial mastectomy in a woman with extremely large, pendulous breasts. (**A**) Preoperative and (**B**) postoperative photographs.

when there is scattered in situ disease in a single quadrant. Figures 104-16A and B show an example of a patient, with significant discomfort from her large breast size, who had always wanted to undergo breast reduction.

Clear margins were easily obtained by removing over a quadrant of the breast tissue, leaving medial and lateral flaps of at least 1 cm, and achieving a very nice cosmetic result. Pre-operative MRI can be very useful for planning the surgical approach. High-resolution scans should be used to maximize the anatomic detail provided by MRI. When breast surgery is required, it provides an opportunity to change the shape and size of the breast, which, if desired by the patient, may make the surgical resection easier and turn an unpleasant procedure to one that is much more tolerable.

To perform a satisfactory lumpectomy, it is essential that the incision be placed directly over the tumor. The use of a circumareolar incision for removal of a lesion that is not in proximity to the areola is not optimal, nor is tunneling through breast tissue to remove a lesion that is not beneath the incision. Tumor-free specimen margins are difficult and often impossible to obtain when such an incision is made. Reexcision of the tumor site to obtain free margins through such an incision is equally difficult. If there is concern that a mastectomy may eventually be necessary, the incision should be made with some thought as to what type of incision would be made if a mastectomy were required. In the instances a lumpectomy cannot be carried out because of the inability to obtain tumor-free margins, the mastectomy incisions can be tailored to accommodate the lumpectomy incision. Preoperative diagnosis with needle biopsy can be of enormous help in planning the incision and should be the standard.

Skin removal is not required for lumpectomy. If a prior biopsy was performed, skin encompassing the biopsy scar can be removed when lumpectomy is done but it is not essential. The quality of cosmesis is inversely related to the amount of skin removed. A special point to be emphasized is that skin edges should not be undermined when the excision is being performed; that is, thin skin flaps are not desirable. Undermining of skin can result in an unfavorable cosmetic result, so removal of skin may be the better cosmetic option in some cases.

Tumor Removal and Examination of Specimen Margins ■ The tumor is removed so that it is completely enveloped in normal fat and/or breast tissue. This procedure does not necessitate removal of a predefined amount of normal tissue around the lesion, just the amount adequate to achieve specimen margins grossly free of tumor. Orienting the specimen is especially important. Adopting a standard procedure to orient and ink specimens in your institution will improve communication among pathologists, surgeons, and radiation oncologists. A typical standard is to use a long stitch for the lateral margin and a short stitch for the superior margin, secured to a piece of Telfa posteriorly to improve orientation. This is particularly helpful for those specimens that require specimen radiography, by preserving the shape and improving the chance to identify and further resect a specific margin that may be close to the radiographic lesion (Fig. 104-17).

If a prior excisional biopsy was performed and margins were not evaluated, it is obligatory that, at the time of node dissection, a re-resection be performed to ensure tumor-free margins.

The specimen is immediately delivered to the pathologist, or, more ideally, he or she is present in the operating room to receive it and visualize the orientation. The pathologist's role is to confirm or establish the diagnosis of cancer (if a needle biopsy was not done), to aid the surgeon in deciding intraoperatively whether the specimen margins are grossly free of tumor, and to take an aliquot of tumor for any special studies.

The pathologist receives the specimen and carefully orients it by means of the suture tags that the surgeon has placed. After measurement, the uncut specimen is inspected for gross margin involvement. If there is evidence that the tumor has been transected, the surgeon is immediately apprised of the precise location of the margin involvement so that additional tissue can be removed from that area while the pathologist is completing inspection of the specimen. The pathologist then coats the entire surface of the specimen with India ink, blots it dry, and then bisects the tumor and specimen transversely. Some pathologists use multiple colors (eg, for the posterior, anterior superior half, and the anterior inferior half), to improve the ability to pinpoint the location of an involved margin. If tumor is found on gross examination to be close to the resected tissue margin, the pathologist may do a frozen section to determine margin involvement. Additional breast tissue can be removed to obtain a new true margin any time that margin involvement is considered uncertain. A multiplicity of frozen sections should not be carried out to determine whether the margins are tumor free. Margin assessment is better done with permanent sections in a detailed manner.

If the margin is later found to be involved microscopically following re-resection and there is no evidence that gross tumor has been transected, consideration may be given to not removing the breast. In such circumstances, when it is clear that gross tumor has not been transected, it is likely that radiation plus systemic therapy will provide adequate locoregional tumor control and that the majority of patients will remain free of local recurrence. An update on their series of reports on margin control from the Joint Center in Boston demonstrates that recurrence rates are the same for focally positive margins as for true negative ones.[145] Similarly, when a breast tumor recurrence occurs following lumpectomy, it is likely that tumor control will be obtained by repeat lumpectomy if such tumors are small and can be removed with tumor-free specimen margins.

Pathologic criteria used for making a decision about whether the tumor involves specimen margins can vary. Many pathologists infer margin involvement by such subjective designations as tumor "very close" to margin. A review of cases showed that there was residual cancer in only 12% of total mastectomy specimens removed because the margin was close. Thus, it is most appropriate to regard lines of resection as involved only when cancer is transected.

For mammographically detected carcinomas that require radiographic guidance, one or more wires are placed in the breast either to bracket calcifications, or pinpoint the center of the lesion or calcifications. Specimen mammography is required once the lesion is removed to confirm the presence of the lesion as well as the location of the mammographic abnormality relative to the margins. Whenever possible, non-palpable lesions that can be identified using ultrasound should be localized using that technique since these procedures are better tolerated by patients and do not use compression required for mammographic localization. Some surgeons are being trained to use ultrasound so that they can better improve the targeted excision of solid lesions in the operating room. This reduces the need for and time for communication between the operating room and the radiology suite. However, it requires that surgeons be specially trained, very skilled in the technique, and able to determine which lesions they can accurately identify to avoid missing the lesion intraoperatively.

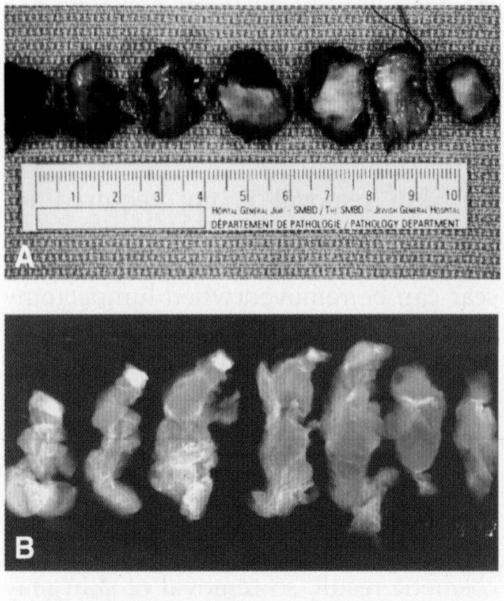

Figure 104-17 ■ (A) Photo of gross specimen. (B) Radiograph of gross specimen showing calcifications.

Mastectomy ■ Patients who undergo mastectomy have the option to have reconstruction or not. Cosmetic considerations are important whether a woman chooses reconstruction. It is important to try to leave a flat surface on the chest wall so that wearing a prosthesis is possible and comfortable. Avoiding skin folds in the axillary line can be accomplished through fish tail incisions at the axillary portion of the axilla or contouring the incisions in the axilla using plastic surgery techniques to avoid excess skin.

Immediate reconstruction has been shown to be safe,[146] even in the setting of locally advanced disease (Fig. 104-18), when appropriate multimodal therapy is used. Therefore, any woman considering mastectomy should also be told about options for reconstruction, both immediate and delayed. Complications after reconstruction are common and should be expected by both the surgeon and the patient. Expectations about outcomes should be appropriately set, and women should be prepared for the possibility of multiple surgical procedures to optimize the reconstructive outcome. If the decision to use chemotherapy does not require additional tissue or definitive resection of the primary tumor, and if chemotherapy if going to be part of multimodal treatment for a given woman, and if a woman is strongly considering mastectomy, based on extent of disease or patient preference, neoadjuvant chemotherapy should be strongly considered. Sequencing the surgery and reconstruction after systemic therapy minimizes the risk that a complication would delay adjuvant therapy, and gives women much more time to consider surgical options and adjust to the diagnosis and consider the surgical options more clearly.

For women who are ambivalent about reconstruction, delayed reconstruction may be optimal. However, cosmetic outcomes are better when reconstruction is performed immediately, and

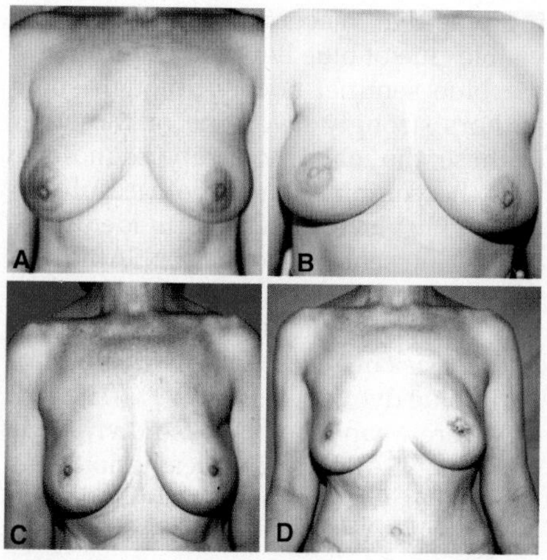

Figure 104-18 ■ Preoperative and postoperative photos of a skin-sparing mastectomy with immediate reconstruction with TRAM flap, delayed nipple reconstruction in a 37-year-old (**A**, **B**) and a 65-year-old. Postoperative photos are 12 weeks (**C**) and 8 weeks (**D**). shows appearance 5 days after nipple reconstruction.

scars can be minimized and tailored to the type of reconstruction that has been chosen. It is difficult to make reconstruction decisions in a matter of days, and women who are deciding should be reassured that an extra week or two to study their options and make good decisions will not affect their survival outcome. They will likely live for decades with the consequence of this decision, so the investment of a few weeks, if necessary, to make sure they are comfortable with their decision is important.

There are two basic types of reconstruction that can be offered. Implant reconstruction or autologous tissue reconstruction. Implants can be placed as expanders or permanent implants. Expanders are the most commonly used form of reconstruction. They are placed under the pectoralis muscle and the pocket is gradually expanded until is it larger than the desired breast size. Then the expander is exchanged for a permanent implant and the breast shape is contoured. The entire process can take 6 to 8 weeks. An alternative technique, used in conjunction with skin sparing mastectomy, is the placement of permanent implants.[146] The majority of implants used for reconstruction are saline. Although silicone implants were pulled off the market because of a concern that they increased the risk for developing autoimmune disease, several large studies have failed to show a definitive connection; as a result, silicone implants are again being used.[147] There are specific instances where silicone products may be preferred (eg, if a permanent implant is placed immediately, but the ability to expand the implant is desired). Autologous tissue flaps include TRAM, or DIEP flaps or, latissimus dorsi flaps (Figs. 104-19 and 104-20).

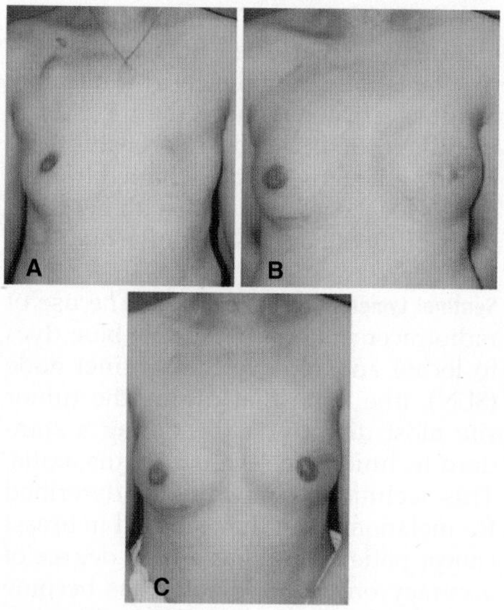

Figure 104-19 ■ Examples of total skin sparing technique combined with various reconstruction techniques. (**A**) Placement of immediate implant, using mastopexy incision, and contralateral mastopexy. Mastectomy is on left, photos are 3 weeks post-operative. (**B**) Bilateral mastectomy with placement of immediate implants in a woman at high risk after recurrence subsequent to lumpectomy for subcentimeter DCIS prior. Pre-operative MRI demonstrated single small focus of lateral recurrence. (**C**) Mastectomy on right followed by immediate reconstruction using TRAM flap.

Decisions about type of reconstruction depend largely on patient preference, although treatment considerations can also play an important role. If radiation is anticipated, complications are less if autologous tissue is used. There is controversy about whether TRAM flaps can tolerate radiation, and several published reports suggest that radiation causes significant deleterious effects on the flap. It may be that free flaps, requiring an anastomosis, tolerate radiation as well as pedicle flaps, or more likely, institutions that use higher doses of radiation (up to 6500 Gy including the boost) may experience more complications. An institution from Dundee, Scotland that limits radiation to the chest wall to 4500-5000 Gy recently reported excellent results in a large series of patients.

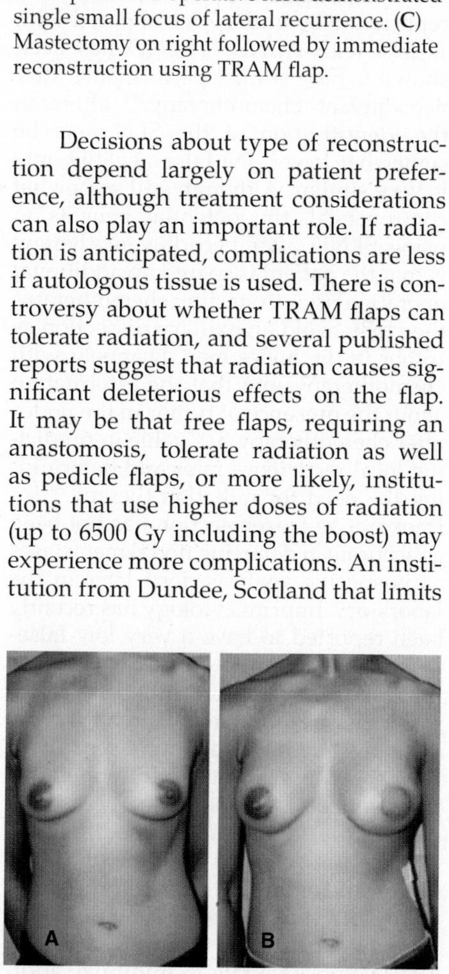

Figure 104-20 ■ Latissimus dorsi reconstruction with bilateral augmentation in a 39-year-old. Pre- (**A**) and (**B**) 12-week postoperative photo.

A new technique for mastectomy is the total skin sparing mastectomy. This technique removes all of the breast tissue, including the tissue of the areola and nipple, but preserves the overlying dermins. A recent report of 171 cases shows that, over time, the technique has become reliable, and that various incisions can be used to achieve excellent results. This technique results in 99% preservation of nipple and areola skin. Although follow-up is limited, early results show that the local recurrence rate is extremely low (<2%), and we anticipate that the total skin sparing technique will not affect recurrence risk. The key is the complete removal of the nipple duct tissue (Figs. 104-19 and 104-20). This technique can be combined with any reconstructive technique except the use of permanent implants. The immediate expansion of the skin significantly increases the risk of skin necrosis. This exciting development in technique, while challenging, offers the safety associated with removal of all of the breast tissue combined with superior cosmetic results. The opportunity to use total skin sparing mastectomy is especially important when considering prophylactic mastectomy for women at highest risk, and may enable women to feel comfortable enough about the cosmetic result to undergo the surgery.

Management of the Axilla

Axillary Dissection

Axillary dissection is not used with the intent of enhancing curability since regional lymph nodes are regarded as indicators of distant metastatic disease rather than as instigators of such tumor.

The incision for axillary dissection should be separate from that used for removal of the tumor in the breast. A longitudinal incision placed along the posterolateral margin of the pectoralis major muscle or a transverse incision just below the axillary hairline may be used. An axillary dissection today includes nodes from axillary levels I and II. The anatomic delineation of this dissection is the latissimus dorsi muscle laterally, the axillary vein superiorly, and the medial border of the pectoralis minor muscle medially. Removal of the pectoralis minor muscle is not required. The nerves to the serratus anterior and latissimus dorsi muscles should be identified and preserved. The axillary vein should be visualized and followed under the pectoralis minor muscle to the medial border. These are the minimal limits for the dissection. The average number of nodes removed is about 15. Although the lumpectomy site in the breast is not drained, a suction drain is present in the axilla for several postoperative days.

The management of the axilla has changed significantly since the introduction of sentinel node dissection. This procedure limits considerably the extent of the surgical procedure in the axilla and, for the great majority of patients with negative axillary lymph nodes, precludes the need for formal axillary dissection while providing similar (and in some cases superior) diagnostic and prognostic information. The identification of a single (or just a few) sentinel node(s) also permits the pathologist to perform a more detailed assessment by assessing multiple level sections of the sentinel node. The detection of micrometastases is significantly increased by combining light microscopy, immunohistochemistry (IHC), and even more sensitive molecular techniques. However, the prognostic significance of identifying isolated metastatic cells in histologically negative lymph nodes by more sensitive techniques is still undetermined; therefore, at this time it is not considered sufficient to constitute stage 2 disease.[139] Sentinel node biopsy and assessment are under extensive evaluation by large cooperative research groups, including the NSABP and the ACOSOG. ACOSOG trial Z-010 required that clinicians not use immunohistochemical analysis in their hospital so that all nodes could be centrally stained and the results blinded in order to assess the prognostic significance of microscopic metastases to the lymph nodes. NSABP B-32 randomized 5611 women with negative SLN to either SLN biopsy alone or SLN biopsy followed by axillary lymph node dissection (ALND). Women found to have positive SLN also proceeded to full ALND. The strength of the study is that it is the largest randomized trial of SLND and that it is representative of a cross section of surgeons across the country with 232 surgeons participating across 80 centers. Although the longer term outcomes, regional control and survival, are not yet known, the technical results are. On average, 3 SLNs were removed per patient; the SLN identification rate was 97.2% and improved with surgeon experience, and 26% of patients had a positive sentinel node. In 61.5% of patients with a positive sentinel node, the additional nodes were negative (38.5% had additional positive nodes). The false negative rate (axillary node involvement when the SLN was negative) was 9.7%, which did not change with experience but was significantly affected by the type of biopsy used for diagnosis; the false negative rate went from 8.0%, to 14.3% and 15.2%, for FNA/core, incisional, and excisional biopsy, respectively. The number of SLNs identified also affected SLN false negative rates. The confidence in a negative result is greater if more than 1 SLN is identified, or if the prior probability of having a negative node is high, but may be less for the woman with a higher prior probability of having a positive node.

Sentinel Lymph Node Dissection ■ The use of radiotracer material or visible blue dyes to locate and remove the sentinel node (SLN), (the node that drains the tumor site most directly), is becoming a standard technique for evaluating the axilla. This technique was initially described for melanoma and then studied in breast cancer patients and has a high degree of accuracy once the operator has become proficient with the technique. The ability to identify a sentinel node ranges in the literature from 85% to 97%. The ACOSOG, in recruiting surgeons to participate in a sentinel node registry trial as well as a trial to determine if full node dissection after SLN removal was of value, required proof that the sentinel node could be identified in 90% of cases and that the false negative rate for SLN was under 5%. Lymphedema rates after SLND are reported to be under 7% compared with 17-25% with ALND.[148] SLND has been shown to have similar performance after neoadjuvant chemotherapy,[149] although the identification of the SLN may be somewhat lower, the false negative rate is very similar. Although still somewhat controversial, the potential benefits to using SLND after neoadjuvant therapy is that the patient is spared an additional operation prior to starting chemotherapy, they may avoid an axillary dissection as tumor in the nodes may disappear with chemotherapy, and that the information about the presence of tumor in the nodes after chemotherapy has value in predicting local recurrence rates and determining the need for radiation therapy.[150] Intraoperative frozen section has not been as accurate in detecting nodal metastases as is specific analysis done later in the laboratory. Imprint cytology has recently been reported to have a very low false-negative rate but the sensitivity is not as high as frozen section. In NSABP B-32, cytology was found to indeed have a low false positive rate, 0.4% but a sensitivity of 61.5%. There is value in intraoperative detection of LN metastases because it enables the surgeon to proceed to a full axillary dissection at the time of SLND, thereby avoiding a second procedure. Clinicians should use the technique in their own institution that yields the lowest false positive rate to minimize additional unnecessary surgery.

Radioisotope injection with a gamma isotope labeled colloid and scanning with a hand-held probe is replacing blue dye injection which provides a visible clue of blue lymphatics leading to the blue sentinel node. Although some authors strongly favor one or the other of these, the majority of reports indicate that the combination of both results in the highest level of successful identification of the sentinel node. In NSABP B32, the radioisotope had a higher SLN identification than blue die. There is a small but real risk of anaphylaxis with lymphosurin blue dye, just less than 1%. The risk of severe anaphylaxis was shown to be 0.2% in NSABP B-32. Anesthesiologists should be aware of this possibility if blue dye is used.

Need for Axillary Dissection ■ It is frequently asked whether all lumpectomy patients require axillary staging. If the need for systemic therapy, as well as the type of systemic therapy, can be determined by patient and tumor characteristics other than the status of the axillary nodes, then the need for axillary staging becomes less clear. Furthermore, if all node-negative and node-positive patients were to be given the same systemic adjuvant therapy, as is the case in trials of preoperative chemotherapy, there would seem to be no reason to know the nodal status, except for predicting patient outcome. The Early Breast Cancer Trialists' Collaborative Group overview suggests that adjuvant chemotherapy benefits women with node-negative and node-positive cancers, and that the proportionate reduction in risk of treatment failure is the same for both groups, and many oncologists offer adjuvant chemotherapy to all women except those that have such a low proportionate reduction as to be of little real gain. However, tailored decision making tools such as Adjuvantonline.com, a well-validated tool for predicting absolute benefit of chemotherapy,[124] or molecular tools which provide a recurrence score, such as the Oncotype DX[108] have increased oncologists' ability to refine recommendations for systemic therapy. The molecular characteristics of the tumor may be more important than stage in determining whether to give adjuvant therapy and which type to use. Two molecular tests in use in the United States and Europe are in clinical trials to better answer these questions (TAILORx trial in the United Sates and MINDACT in Europe). As these data mature, the roles of sentinel node dissection and axillary dissection will need to be clarified. In the molecular age there are situations still where removal of all possible local regional tumor may be very important: for those women where surgical excision is the primary treatment eg, in a setting with a low predicted risk of recurrence; or for women who have undergone neoadjuvant chemotherapy and have residual disease and possibly resistant to best available therapies, In the setting of complete pathologic response after neoadjuvant therapy, less surgery may be necessary, and the increasing use of sentinel node dissection after neoadjuvant chemotherapy in women with clinically N0 disease, regardless of nodal status pre treatment, is an example of tailoring the extent of surgical treatment to response to therapy. The need for axillary dissection may also be questioned specifically in elderly women with ER-positive disease who are planning to take adjuvant hormonal therapy. In this setting, the status of the axillary nodes would not likely alter the decision about administration of adjuvant therapy. In almost all cases with clinically negative axilla, however, sentinel node dissection is a standard part of staging and surgical management, and can be successfully performed in most women with very low morbidity. In the setting of positive sentinel nodes, level I and II axillary dissection is considered to be standard management. Although it is generally accepted that axillary dissection provides optimal local control of the axilla, a randomized trial comparing total mastectomy with and without axillary dissection suggested that not all patients with positive axillary lymph nodes would develop an axillary recurrence in the absence of an axillary dissection: in fact only about half would. We are awaiting the results of the ACOSOG trial Z11, which randomized women with a positive sentinel node to full axillary dissection versus not, to determine if and when some women can be spared full node dissection.

Local-Regional Treatments for Ductal Carcinoma In Situ ■ Ductal carcinoma in situ (DCIS) is defined by cytologically malignant epithelial cells within the ductal system of the breast that have not invaded through the basement membrane into the breast parenchyma. Figure 104-3 shows a histological example of DCIS. Although once a relatively uncommon condition, the incidence of DCIS has dramatically and consistently increased over the past three decades. It is estimated that over 58,000 new cases of DCIS will be diagnosed in 2008, which makes it the fourth most common cancer in females (behind invasive breast cancers, lung cancer, and colon cancer).[3] Furthermore, over the past 30 years, the incidence of DCIS has increased at a rate 5 times that of invasive breast cancer, until the late 1990s, when the number of new cases of has started to stabilize. DCIS was uncommon prior to screening mammography because by the time most malignant breast lesions become palpable they have an invasive component. In contrast, most patients with DCIS diagnosed this year will have asymptomatic, nonpalpable, small lesions detected after a mammogram demonstrates a focal area of pleomorphic calcifications.

DCIS is presumed to be a premalignant condition, which left untreated, has a risk of progressing into an invasive cancer. The genetic and epigenetic events that cause DCIS to develop an invasive phenotype remain unclear and are likely complex. The use of new molecular tools, such as DNA microarray technology, may in the future allow for greater insights into the etiology of disease progression, and help to clarify the risk of subsequent invasive disease in an individual with DCIS. It is clear that DCIS encompasses a spectrum of pathologic disease. High-grade DCIS is defined by frequent cellular mitosis, crowded cellular growth patterns often with comedo necrosis, high rates of genetic mutations, and high proliferative indices. In contrast, well-differentiated DCIS is often very difficult to distinguish from atypical ductal hyperplasia and more frequently grows in a papillary or cribriform pattern. The risk of progressing to an invasive breast cancer and the risk of recurrence after local therapy is in part related to these biological traits.

As DCIS is considered a premalignant condition, the majority of patients currently diagnosed with this disease undergo surgical resection of the disease. Therefore, limited data are available concerning the natural history of untreated DCIS. One of the largest series of untreated DCIS described a group of 28 cases of DCIS followed serially over 30 years.[151] These cases were identified after the initial pathology from an excisional biopsy was subsequently reclassified from a benign condition to low-grade DCIS. All women had small lesions and none had high-grade disease or comedo necrosis. Therefore, it is important to recognize that these patients represent only the most favorable end of the DCIS spectrum. Over the 30-year period 11 patients developed an invasive breast cancer at the site of their DCIS. The risk of developing an invasive breast cancer was about 40%, three to six-fold higher in these patients compared to that of the general population. Interestingly, these risks are very similar for the risks associated with atypia . Furthermore, as many of these patients had an excisional biopsy of their low-grade DCIS, it is possible that some who did not develop invasive ductal carcinoma had been adequately treated by a complete surgical resection. But this is also similar to the situation of a biopsy where atypia is identified. Histologically, the distinction between low grade DCIS and atypia can be difficult to distinguish, and likely represents a spectrum of biologic changes. What is consistent is that the risk for progression appears to be strongly influenced by and is higher in women with young age. This challenging area of diagnosis and management will benefit from further study and by new prevention and treatment approaches.

These data suggest that surgical resection of DCIS is warranted in an effort to reduce the risk of progression to invasive disease. Despite the fact that breast conservation therapy for DCIS has never been formally compared to mastectomy in a randomized trial, breast conservation is currently the standard of care for most patients with DCIS if the region of DCIS can be resected with clear margins. Mastectomy should be considered when the patient prefers this approach, when there is a strong genetic predisposition to the development of subsequent breast primaries, and when the disease is diffusely present throughout the breast. The reason that breast conservation has become the accepted standard is that it allows for organ preservation, excellent long-term local control rates, and survival rates approaching 100%.

The major ongoing therapeutic questions concerning the treatment of DCIS concern the use of radiation and hormonal therapy. Both of these questions have been the focus of a number of completed phase 3 clinical trials. Four trials, conducted by the National Surgical Adjuvant Breast and Bowel Project (NSABP B17 trial), the European Organization for Research and Treatment of Cancer (EORTC), a cooperative effort from the United Kingdom, Australia, and New Zealand (UK/ANZ), and a multi-insitutional trial conducted in Sweden have examined the question of radiation benefit by randomizing patients treated with complete excision of DCIS to either whole breast irradiation or observation.[152-155] A summary of the results of these studies is shown in Table 104-10.

In aggregate, over 4000 patients were enrolled in these studies. Three of the four trials required the achievement of negative margins as an entry criterion and the majority of patients in the trials had mammographically detected, non-palpable disease. In all four studies, the addition of radiation was found to reduce the rate of ipsilateral breast recurrence. The B-17 trial has the longest follow-up, and after 12 years, the overall rates of ipsilateral breast cancer recurrence (DCIS combined with invasive cancer) were 31.7% for patients treated with surgery only versus 15.7% for those treated with surgery and radiation, $p < .000005$.[152] This 58% proportional reduction of recurrence was roughly of the same magnitude as that seen in the other three trials.[153-154] Of note, each trial found that approximately 50% of the recurrences were invasive breast cancer and

Table 104-10 **Phase III Randomized Prospective Clinical Trials Investigating the Use of Radiation After Lumpectomy in Patients With Ductal Carcinoma In Situ**

Study	No. of Patients	Follow-up (Yr)	Treatment	Breast Cancer Recurrences: Noninvasive	Invasive	Overall
NSABP B-17[152]	818	12	Radiation	8%	7.7%	15.7%
			No radiation	14.6%	16.8%	31.7%
			p	.001	.00001	.000005
EORTC 10853[153]	1002	10.5	Radiation	7%	8%	15%
			No radiation	14%	13%	26%
			p	.0011	.0065	<.001
UK/ANZ trial[154]	1701	5	Radiation	2.3%	2.5%	4.8%
			No radiation	8.4%	5.3%	13.7%
			p	.01	.0004	<.0001
SweDCIS[155]	1067	5	Radiation			22%
			No radiation			7%
			p			<.001

Abbreviations: EORTC, European Organization for Research and Treatment of Cancer; NSABP, National Surgical Adjuvant Breast and Bowel Project; UK/ANZ, United Kingdom, Australia, New Zealand.

the risk of developing an invasive breast recurrence within the treated breast was significantly decreased. A recent meta-analysis of these trials concluded that radiation therapy lowers the RR of both invasive and in situ ipsilateral breast recurrence by 60% (95% confidence interval for the meta-effect: 40% to 67% for invasive recurrence, 47% to 69% for in situ recurrence).[156] Radiation use did not impact overall survival or risk of distant metastasis.

Based on the results of these randomized trials, lumpectomy and whole breast radiation should be offered to patients with DCIS. However, in studies that have evaluated the patterns of care in the United States, it is clear that many patients with DCIS are treated with lumpectomy alone. A study using data from the SEER Program found that only 45% of patients treated with lumpectomy for DCIS received radiation in 1992 and this percentage had only increased to 54% by 1999.[157] Furthermore, in a survey of physicians in Australia and New Zealand, only 22% of patients treated with breast conservation surgery for DCIS were referred for radiation oncology consultation.[158]

The lack of radiation use for women with DCIS is in part attributable to the low risk of dying from breast cancer after treatment with surgery alone. In addition, data from single-institution retrospective studies have suggested that highly selected subsets of patients may have low breast recurrence rates after lumpectomy alone. One of the leading proponents of treating favorable DCIS with lumpectomy alone has been Silverstein and colleagues, who in 1995 developed the Van Nuys Prognostic Index (VNPI) to help define selection criteria for cases with low recurrence risk.[159] The original VNPI classes were determined from the retrospective analysis of 333 patients treated at two institutions between 1979 and 1995. Patients received 1 to 3 points for three factors: tumor grade and the presence or absence of necrosis (combined into one category), tumor size, and margin status. Over two-thirds of the patients had an intermediate-risk VNPI (cumulative score of 5–7), and, similar to the randomized data, radiation reduced the probability of breast cancer recurrence in this cohort (32% vs 15%; $p = .0\ 17$).[159] Fewer than one-third of their patients had small, low-grade disease with widely negative surgical margins, and the breast cancer recurrence rate was low after breast conservation surgery alone (3% breast cancer recurrence rate among 76 patients treated without radiation). Subsequently, this group has also incorporated patient age into their prognostic index. Similar data were subsequently reported from a population-based cohort study of 1036 women ≥40 years old in the San Francisco area treated with lumpectomy alone for DCIS. This study found overall a relatively high recurrence rate (20%/10% for all recurrence and invasive recurrence, respectively, at 5 years), but reported that the subset of patients with mammographically detected low-grade disease treated with surgery that achieved widely negative margins had a low risk of recurrence after surgery alone.[160]

Using an expansion of this original cohort, Silverstein and colleagues reanalyzed their data, focusing on the importance of margin status for patients treated with DCIS. In this analysis,[161] they reported that 93 patients with a margin width of 10 mm or more had an 8-year local recurrence rate of only 3%. The 8-year probability of recurrence was much higher after treatment with lumpectomy without radiation when the margin width was 1 to 10 mm (recurrence rate 20%) and when margins were under 1 mm (58%). When this study was updated and expanded to include 212 patients with margin widths of 10mm or more, the breast recurrence rate in this cohort increased to 14%.[162] In addition, the low recurrence rate noted in the setting of 10 mm margins could not be confirmed in a single-arm prospective trial conducted at the Dana-Farber/Harvard Cancer Center. In this study, 157 patients with grade 1 or 2 DCIS, ≤2.5 cm, underwent wide local excision alone with achievement of negative margins of ≥1 cm.[163] The trial was closed early because the recurrence rate met pre-defined stopping rules, with an estimated 5-year local recurrence rate of 12.5% (invasive cancer occurrence of 6%). The authors concluded that even in this highly selected group of patients, there was a substantial local recurrence rate. The Eastern Cooperative Oncology Group (ECOG) has also conducted a prospective study of 711 patients with DCIS treated with surgery plus/minus tamoxifen without radiation. Two different patient strata were enrolled: (1) low- or intermediate-grade DCIS, size <2.5 cm; or (2) high-grade DCIS size less than 1 cm. All patients were required to have a negative post-lumpectomy mammogram and negative margins of 3 mm or more. The five-year risk of IBTR was 7% in the low- or intermediate-grade stratum, and 14% in the high-grade stratum.[164] Given the success of salvage therapies and the low risk of cancer-associated death with surgical only treatment, it is reasonable to inform patients about the available data and have them participate in their local-regional treatment decisions.

The second major area of research and controversy regarding the management of DCIS concerns the use of hormonal therapy. After completion of the B-17 trial, the NSABP conducted the B-24 trial, which randomized 1802 patients treated with lumpectomy and radiation to either receive 5 years of tamoxifen or 5 years of placebo.[165] The eligibility of this trial differed from B-17 in that it included patients with positive surgical margins, which ended up being present in 25% of the study population. In addition, the primary endpoint of the study was not ipsilateral breast recurrence but rather the probability of having an ipsilateral recurrence or developing a contralateral breast cancer. Therefore, this trial was designed to investigate the combined therapeutic benefit of tamoxifen against the index DCIS and the chemopreventive benefit of tamoxifen in reducing subsequent independent breast cancers.

The results of the B-24 trial indicated that patients treated with tamoxifen, surgery and radiation had a 5-year rate of non-invasive or invasive breast cancers of 8.2% compared to a 13.4% rate for the patients treated only with surgery and radiation.[165] Clearly, a component of this benefit was the chemoprevention effects of tamoxifen. In B-24, the use of tamoxifen resulted in a 41% reduction in the 5-year incidence of contralateral breast cancers. These data are consistent with the reduction in second primary breast cancers seen in the adjuvant tamoxifen trials and the NSABP P-1 trial, which found that tamoxifen decreased breast cancer development in women at increased risk for breast cancer by 49%.[72] In a subsequent retrospective analysis of ER expression from stored tumor material from 628 patients (327 placebo, 301 tamoxifen), it was found that the benefit of tamoxifen was limited to 482 patients (77% of those on study) with ER-positive disease.[166] In this cohort, tamoxifen was associated with a significant reduction in both ipsilateral breast recurrence and the development of contralateral breast cancer. There was no apparent benefit of tamoxifen in those with ER-negative tumors, but the sample size precluded detecting a small benefit.

The UK/ANZ trial provides additional information concerning the interaction of radiation and tamoxifen after lumpectomy in patients with DCIS.[154] In this study, tamoxifen use decreased the rate of DCIS recurrence but not invasive recurrence for patients who did not receive radiation. However, in the patients treated with radiation after lumpectomy, tamoxifen provided no benefit in ipsilateral breast events. Unlike the B-24 trial, this study required all patients to have negative surgical margins after lumpectomy and did not include the development of a contralateral breast cancer as an event in their primary outcome measure.

These data suggest that, for patients treated with an adequate lumpectomy that achieves negative surgical margins and subsequently receive radiation, the therapeutic benefits of tamoxifen are likely to be very low in reducing risk of recurrence in the ipsilateral breast but there will be a protective benefit in the contralateral breast. Interestingly, a recent survey found that 56% of United States practitioners routinely recommend tamoxifen for women with DCIS whereas only 22% of European practitioners routinely recommend tamoxifen.[167] Despite the lack of clarity concerning the therapeutic benefits of tamoxifen in DCIS, for patients with ER-positive disease the addition of tamoxifen is likely to have chemopreventive effects and minimize the risks of subsequent new breast cancers. To further evaluate the benefit of hormonal therapy in patients with DCIS, NSABP is currently conducting a phase 3 trial comparing tamoxifen and anastrozole after lumpectomy and radiation in postmenopausal women.

Local-Regional Treatment of Early Stage Invasive Breast Cancer ■ Since the routine use of mammographic screening, the vast majority of patients diagnosed with invasive breast cancer have T1 or T2 primary tumors that are amenable to a breast conserving local-regional treatment. Breast conservation therapy is now firmly established as an appropriate standard of care for women with early stage breast disease.[143] This therapy consists of three important components: removal of the tumor with achievement of negative margins (often called a lumpectomy, tylectomy, or a segmental mastectomy), surgical assessment of axillary lymph nodes with either a sentinel lymph node surgery and/or a level I/II axillary lymph node dissection, and breast irradiation. Most women treated with modern breast conservation approaches achieve excellent outcomes. When combined with systemic therapy, the local recurrence rate after appropriate breast conservation treatments currently is reported to be less than 0.5% per year for women with favorable disease.[168,169] Furthermore, the complication rates of breast conservation therapy are very low and continue to improve with advances in surgical and radiotherapy techniques.

Despite these facts, breast conservation remains underutilized in the United States. In a recent multi-national randomized trial comparing two hormonal therapies for women with early stage disease, the rate of breast conservation in the United States was only 49%.[170] In contrast, the rate of breast conservation in the United Kingdom patients was 58%, and even higher rates were noted in patients from Sweden, Germany or Australia/New Zealand. Previous data had also indicated that the use of breast conservation varies within regions of the United States, with Southern and Midwestern women less likely to be treated with breast conservation compared to women from either the East or West Coast.[171] The reasons for the under-use of breast conservation are likely multifactorial. Unfortunately, some women undergo mastectomy based on a misperception that mastectomy is likely to achieve a superior outcome. Other factors, such as choices celebrity role models make, can influence decisions made by providers and patients. For example, after Nancy Reagan had an early stage breast cancer treated with mastectomy, the rates of breast conservation dropped in the United States. It is critical, therefore, that breast cancer providers understand the data concerning breast conservation so that patients with newly diagnosed disease can be given the option of this treatment if appropriate.

Breast Conservation Therapy Versus Mastectomy ■ Breast conservation has been studied as an alternative local-regional treatment to mastectomy for over 40 years. After initial successful results were obtained in single institutions, a number of phase 3 clinical trials was initiated that directly compared the outcome of patients treated with breast conservation versus those of patients treated with mastectomy.[172-174] One of the more important of these trials was the NSABP B-06 study.[168] This trial began in 1976 and enrolled 1843 women. Patients with T1 or T2, N0, or N1, M0 breast tumors of 4 cm or less were randomly assigned to one of three treatment groups: (1) modified radical mastectomy, (2) lumpectomy and axillary dissection, or (3) lumpectomy, axillary dissection, followed by radiation therapy. With 20 years of follow-up, this trial demonstrated that breast conservation therapy provides survival equivalent to mastectomy.

Contraindications for Breast Conservation Therapy ■ Selected patients with early-stage breast cancer are not suitable for breast conservation therapy because the primary tumor cannot be successfully removed with a lumpectomy. For example, patients presenting with diffuse suspicious calcifications that cannot be resected with a lumpectomy that leaves an acceptable aesthetic result are best treated with a mastectomy. Similarly, patients in whom repeated attempts at breast conservation surgery fail to achieve negative surgical margins are best managed with a mastectomy. Increasingly, however, women who present with stage II and III cancers can be treated with neoadjuvant chemotherapy or hormone therapy, and over 50% have sufficient shrinkage of the primary tumor to enable breast conservation. A second reason why some patients are not candidates for breast conservation is that they are at high risk for radiation complications. Specific examples of such patients include those previously treated with radiation, women who are pregnant, and patients with certain connective tissue diseases. For women early in the course of their pregnancy, internal radiation scatter from irradiation of the intact breast can reach lethal and teratogenic dose levels.[175] Certain collagen vascular diseases, such as systemic scleroderma, polymyositis, dermatomyositis, lupus erythematosus, and mixed-connective tissue disorders have been associated with significant risks, including breast fibrosis and pain, chest wall necrosis, and brachial plexopathy.[176]

The Role of Radiation After Breast Conservation Surgery for Invasive Disease ■ Defining the role of radiation in breast conservation therapy has been the focus of numerous randomized prospective clinical trials conducted over the past 30 years.[173,174] In aggregate, these trials have demonstrated that radiation after breast conserving surgery significantly improves local control, minimizes the risk of subsequent distant metastases, and decreases breast cancer death rates.

The NSABP B-06 trial was one of the first randomized studies to evaluate the benefit of radiation after lumpectomy. This trial showed that for patients treated with breast conserving surgery, radiation offered a significant clinical benefit. After 20 years, the recurrence rates in the breast were 40% for those treated with lumpectomy alone versus 14% for those treated with lumpectomy plus radiation. The almost two-thirds reduction in the risk of recurrence was very similar to reductions observed in other, similarly designed trials.[168]

The data from NSABP B-06 and the other prospective clinical trials assessing the role of radiation for patients with invasive disease treated with breast conservation have been analyzed by the Early Breast Cancer Trialists' Collaborative Group (EBCTCG). In this important meta-analysis, the individual patient data from 7300 women were studied. Breast irradiation after lumpectomy reduced the 10-year rate of in-breast recurrence from 29% to 10% for patients with negative lymph nodes and from 47% to 13% for patients with positive lymph nodes. More importantly, radiation use significantly decreased the 15-year risk of dying from breast cancer. For patients with negative lymph nodes the breast cancer mortality was reduced from 31% to 26% and for patients with positive lymph nodes the breast cancer mortality was reduced from 55% to 48%.[173] Although the meta-analysis and large trials such as the NSABP B-06 provide conclusive data that radiation is beneficial for the majority of patients treated with breast-conserving surgery, there remains an interest as to whether subsets of patients may do well with surgery alone. Therefore, some trials have limited eligibility criteria to patients with more favorable disease characteristics. Investigators from Milan, Italy, conducted a trial to evaluate whether radiation is needed following excision of a small tumor with widely negative margins. In this study, patients with tumors 2.5 cm or less were randomized to undergo quadrantectomy and axillary dissection versus this surgery plus breast radiation. The 10-year results from this trial indicated that radiation reduced the breast recurrence rate from 24% to 6% ($p < .001$).[177]

Patients with stage I disease represent another potentially favorable group. In such patients, data from a Swedish trial indicated that radiation reduced the 5-year breast recurrence rate from 18% to 2% ($p < .0001$).[178] A similar randomized trial from Finland, which was limited to patients with stage I disease who had 1 cm or greater negative margins, also found radiation reduced the breast recurrence rate from 14.1% to 6.2%; $p = .029$.[179]

Data from trials have also indicated that the use of systemic treatment (either chemotherapy or tamoxifen) does not obviate the need for breast radiation. In the NSABP B-06 trial, chemotherapy was used in patients with lymph node–positive disease, and the 20-year breast recurrence rate for these patients was 44% when no radiation was used versus a 9% when radiation was used.[168] A randomized trial from Scotland required systemic treatment for all patients, with approximately 75% of the 589 enrolled patients receiving tamoxifen as the sole systemic treatment.[180] In this trial, the 6-year breast recurrence rates were 6% in the surgery, systemic therapy, and radiation arm versus 25% in the patients randomized to surgery plus systemic therapy without radiation.

Three more recent trials have further refined selection criteria. The results of these three studies are shown in Table 104-14.[168,181,182] In all three of these studies, radiation achieved a statistically significant reduction in breast recurrence rate, although the recurrence rate in some subcategories of patients treated with surgery alone was relatively low. The NSABP B-21 trial enrolled only patients with lymph node–negative breast cancers whose primary tumors measured 1.0 cm or less. All patients underwent lumpectomy and axillary lymph node dissection and were randomized to tamoxifen alone, radiation alone, or tamoxifen and radiation.[183] The Canadian trial had very similar eligibility criteria and very similar results.[182] Finally, the CALGB/Intergroup study focused on patients over the age of 70 with favorable early stage disease.[181] In the latter 2 trials, women with ER-positive tumors on tamoxifen had low recurrence risk. In the CALGB trial, the 5 year recurrence rates were 6% versus 2 % in the tamoxifen only and tamoxifen plus radiation arms, respectively. The distant recurrence risk was 3% in both arms and the mastectomy rate was not altered. In almost all cases of recurrence in the tamoxifen arm, re-excision was achievable. While radiation certainly reduces the chance of recurrence, for many older women planning to take hormonal adjuvant therapy, the risk of recurrence with hormonal therapy alone is low and thus the overall benefit from radiation low.

In conclusion, nearly all of the clinical studies to date have indicated that breast radiation reduces local recurrences following breast conservation surgery and therefore should be considered a standard component of treatment for all women with early stage invasive disease. The most recent trials that have incorporated both the use of systemic therapy and radiation after lumpectomy indicate the probability of having a breast recurrence after such treatment is very low, less that 0.5% per year.[168,181,182] Thus far, most attempts to define favorable subsets of early-stage breast cancer patients who may not require radiation have been unsuccessful with the exception of women over the age of 70 who have disease that is lymph node-negative and ER-positive and who are candidates for tamoxifen. In this cohort, decision as to whether to use radiation or not should be based on the patient's life expectancy and personal preferences.

Factors Affecting Local-Regional Treatment Outcome After Breast Conservation Therapy ■ A number of patient-related, tumor-related, and treatment-related factors have been found to influence local recurrence rates following breast conservation therapy. The most consistent patient factor demonstrated to influence both local and distant recurrence rates is patient age. Young patient age (most commonly defined as ≤40 years old) is associated with an increased risk of distant metastases and lower disease-specific survival[184,185] and an increased risk for ipsilateral breast tumor recurrence following breast conservation therapy.[169,186] Other patient factors, such as African American race/ethnicity have been associated with higher rates of distant metastasis but not clearly been shown to affect ipsilateral breast recurrence rates.[187,188] A number of articles have also indicated that a family history of breast cancer does not predispose to ipsilateral breast recurrence.[189,190] However, breast recurrence rates are likely higher in cases with true familial breast cancer. For example, Haffty and colleagues reported that the breast recurrence rates were 40% or higher for women with *BRCA* mutations treated with breast conservation therapy.[191] A large percentage of these recurrences occurred many years after treatment and may have been second primary tumors that developed independently from the index cancer. Indeed, the rate of ipsilateral breast recurrence was approximately the same as the rate of development of a contralateral breast cancer.[192] A multicenter retrospective study also indicated that the risk of breast recurrence was much less in carriers who had undergone bilateral oopherectomy.

The status of the surgical margins is one of the most important tumor/pathological factors that affect the rates of local control after breast conservation surgery and radiation. In general, the goal of breast conserving surgery should be to achieve complete tumor resection with 2 mm negative margins, although this definition of negative margins is controversial. In a study that evaluated margins according to the density of malignant tissue in addition to distance, margin status highly correlated with breast recurrence risk. This study had the strength of having a central pathology review of 607 cases with mature follow-up and found 12-year recurrence rates of 9% (negative), 6% (near-least), 18% (near-intermediate), 24% (near-greatest), and 30% (positive).[193] Another report suggested that systemic treatment may also influence the prognostic importance of margin status. In this report, the crude local recurrence rate at 8 years was 7% in the 45 patients with focally positive margins treated with systemic therapy versus 18% in the 77 patients with focally positive margins who did not receive systemic therapy.[194] Patients with more extensive margin involvement had unacceptably high local recurrence rates, which were not affected by the use of systemic therapy. A reasonable approach is to recommend re-excision for patients with positive margins and to individualize treatment recommendations for patients with close or focally positive margins, considering breast aesthetics and other factors that also affect recurrence risks.

In addition to complete surgical resection of the primary tumor, there are a number of other treatment-related variables that affect rates of local control. One of these is the use of systemic therapy. In the NSABP B-06 trial, patients with lymph node–positive disease that were treated with radiation and chemotherapy had a 20-year local recurrence rate of 9% compared to a local recurrence rate of 17% in lymph node–negative patients treated with surgery and radiation alone.[168] In NSABP B-21, tamoxifen similarly improved local control rates in patients with lymph node–negative breast cancers measuring less than 1 cm.[183] There was only a 3% crude rate of breast tumor recurrence in women randomized to lumpectomy, radiation, and tamoxifen compared to a 7% rate in women treated with lumpectomy and radiation alone. Data from the University of Texas MD Anderson Cancer Center investigating the impact of systemic therapy on local control following breast conservation therapy in patients with lymph node–negative breast cancer further confirmed these data. In that study, 277 patients treated with systemic therapy had improved 5-year (97.5% vs 89.8%) and 10-year (95.6% vs 85.2%) local control rates compared to the 207 patients who received no systemic treatment (p = .004).[169] Finally, in an analysis of NSABP systemic therapy trials, Fisher and colleagues reported a disease-free survival advantage for the use of systemic therapy in tumors less than 1 cm with negative lymph nodes.[195] Most of this benefit was found to be a reduction in ipsilateral breast tumor recurrences.

Another treatment related factor that has been found to affect local control in breast conservation therapy is the use of a tumor bed boost of radiation following whole breast irradiation. The first randomized trial investigating the impact of a 10 Gy boost following 50 Gy of breast irradiation was performed in Lyons, France. The use of a boost led to a small but statistically significant reduction in the rates of local recurrence at 5 years (3.6% vs 4.5%, p = .04).[196] Subsequently, the EORTC completed a much larger trial that randomized over 5000 patients to 50-Gy delivered to the breast alone or 50 Gy plus a tumor bed boost of 16 Gy. This trial again demonstrated a reduced breast recurrence rate in patients treated with a boost (10.2% vs 6.2% at 10 years; p < .001).[197] In a subset analysis, this benefit was noted across all ages but most pronounced in younger women.

New Radiation Treatment Approaches for Early-Stage Breast Cancer ■ Some patients treated with breast conservation therapy for an early stage breast cancer do not receive radiation as a component of therapy and a number of patients who are excellent candidates for breast conservation therapy elect to be treated with mastectomy in order to avoid radiation. A major factor that contributes to both of these scenarios concerns the inconvenience and expense associated with external beam radiation. Conventional external beam radiation treatments for early-stage breast cancer typically require 1 or 2 days of treatment planning followed by 25 to 33 daily treatment visits. The schedule is particularly burdensome for patients who have to travel many hours for access to the nearest radiation facility. In addition, worldwide, there are too few facilities and equipment to offer this type of treatment schedule to all patients with early-stage breast cancer.

For these reasons and others, a number of strategies are being investigated in order to shorten the radiation treatment schedule. Whelan and colleagues conducted a phase 3 prospective randomized trial comparing a 3-week fractionation schedule to the conventional 5-week course for women ≥ 50 years old with T1 or T2 N0 disease.[198] After a median follow-up of 4.6 years, there was no difference in local recurrences, survival, or breast aesthetics. This trial has affected practice patterns in the United States, predominantly for older women with stage I, ER-positive disease.

A second strategy for shortening the total treatment time is to minimize the volume of breast tissue being irradiated. The rationale for this strategy is that 80% of patients who undergo lumpectomy for small primary tumors have no residual disease after lumpectomy or disease that is within 2 cm of the index cancer.[199] By limiting the volume of breast irradiated, radiation can potentially be delivered at a higher dose rate, allowing for a 1-week course of treatment. Most of the partial breast irradiation outcome data with follow-up of 5 years or greater have been from studies that investigated interstitial brachytherapy alone as a method to deliver the radiation dose. For this procedure, patients typically have catheters surgically placed to create a volume 2 to 2.5 cm around the tumor bed. Subsequently, high–dose-rate radioactive seeds are temporarily placed within the catheters in two sessions a day for 5 days total.

The placement of the catheters geometrically around the tumor bed to assure 2 cm of coverage can be difficult and requires a skill set that may not be available in every radiation facility. Therefore, other attempts at partial breast radiation have been used. In Milan, Veronesi and colleagues are conducting a phase 3 clinical trial comparing a single fraction of intraoperative electron beam radiation to a standard course of whole breast irradiation. From an initial phase 1/2 trial with intraoperative radiation, these authors have reported that there have been minimal complications in the first 100 patients treated.[200] Other commercial vendors have developed intraoperative orthovoltage cones that also can fill the lumpectomy cavity and irradiate the local margin in a single intraoperative fraction.[201] Finally, others have used a similar strategy but deliver therapy through a brachytherapy applicator device, called the Mammosite RTS. The Mammosite utilizes an inflatable balloon within the tumor bed cavity and allows for insertion of a high–dose-rate radioactive source within the center of the balloon.[202]

There are limited data to date concerning the efficacy of partial breast radiation strategies. The most mature data on this subject are single-institution reports of phase 2 brachytherapy trials. To date, the 10-year outcome data for highly selected patients with favorable disease characteristics using this approach have been excellent.[203] However, others have noted higher rates of clinical fat necrosis and poorer efficacy compared to conventional breast external beam radiation.[204,205] The outcome data utilizing the Mammosite is also favorable but the efficacy follow-up to date has been limited to 3 years.[206] These data suggest that this treatment approach warrants additional study in prospective trials with rigid quality assurance to assure proper volumetric coverage. The concept of partial breast radiation has some additional theoretical downsides. Many devices, such as the Mammosite, treat a volume of only 1 to 1.5 cm around the tumor bed.[207] Therefore, these treatments would be expected to have similar efficacy as a surgical procedure that resected an additional 1 to 1.5 cm of tissue circumferentially around the tumor bed. As noted previously, a randomized trial that compared quadrantectomy versus quadrantectomy and radiation for small primary tumors found a significant disadvantage for quadrantectomy alone (failure rates of 23.5% vs 5.8%, respectively).[177] Consequently, the efficacy and toxicity of partial breast radiation needs to be prospectively compared to fully understand the advantages and shortcomings of this approach. To address this, the NSABP and the Radiation Therapy Oncology Group have jointly sponsored a phase 3 trial, which is currently ongoing. The schema of this trial is shown in Figure 104-21. Similar trials are also being conducted in Canada and Europe.

Local-Regional Therapy for Locally Advanced Disease ■ ***Breast-Conservation After Neoadjuvant Chemotherapy*** ■ Modified radical mastectomy followed by adjuvant chemotherapy and postmastectomy radiation has been the historical standard local-regional therapy for patients with locally or regionally advanced primary tumors. However, over the past three decades the use of neoadjuvant chemotherapy (chemotherapy given prior to surgery) has significantly increased in patients with advanced disease. This strategy was first adopted for patients with unresectable or marginally resectable disease and the initial clinical data from such patients indicated that chemotherapy achieved high rates of tumor response. Subsequently, this approach has also been investigated in patients with large, resectable breast cancers at diagnosis. One reason to investigate the sequencing of chemotherapy prior to surgery was to determine whether breast conservation could be offered to selected patients with larger primary tumors whose residual disease after chemotherapy was amenable to a lumpectomy-type resection. To investigate this, the NSABP and EORTC independently conducted clinical trials that compared neoadjuvant chemotherapy with adjuvant chemotherapy for patients with stage II or III breast cancer (Fig. 104-22). Both of these trials found that breast conservation rates were higher in the neoadjuvant chemotherapy arms.[208,209] In the NSABP study, the respective rates of breast conservative surgery were 68% in the neoadjuvant arm and 60% in the adjuvant arm. This increase was directly due to a greater percentage of patients with T3 disease being offered breast conservation after first responding to chemotherapy (22% breast conservation rate vs 8%, respectively).

The goal of breast conservation therapy for patients with advanced disease is to achieve an aesthetically acceptable cosmetic outcome and a low risk of breast recurrence. Accordingly, for patients with large initial primaries, resection must be directed at the post-chemotherapy tumor bed rather than the initial volume of residual disease. However, one concern with resecting only the post-chemotherapy volume of residual disease is that some advanced breast cancers do not shrink concentrically to a solitary nidus in response to neoadjuvant chemotherapy, but rather break up into nests of residual disease over the initially involved volume.[134] In such cases, surgery directed at the primary core may leave a higher burden of microscopic disease around the tumor bed site, which may theoretically be associated with higher rates of breast cancer recurrence.

In the NSABP B-18 trial, the overall rate of breast recurrence did not statistically differ in the patients treated with neoadjuvant chemotherapy compared to those treated with adjuvant chemotherapy (16-year rates of 13% vs 10%, respectively).[210] However, the breast recurrence rate was higher in patients with large primary tumors in whom a response to neoadjuvant chemotherapy permitted a breast conserving surgery. In this subset of patients treated with neoadjuvant chemotherapy, the breast recurrence rate at 8 years was 16%, which was over twice the rate in the patients with smaller tumors who were treated with breast-conserving surgery first.[208] Other multicenter series have also shown relatively high breast cancer recurrence rates in patients who receive neoadjuvant chemotherapy.[211,212] In general, series that include patients with inflammatory carcinoma and those that use radiation therapy alone (without surgery) in patients who achieve a complete clinical response have also noted higher local recurrence rates.

In contrast to these data, single institution studies with careful selection criteria and a high degree of multidisciplinary coordination have reported excellent rates of local control. Investigators at The University of Texas MD Anderson recently published the results of one of the largest studies investigating breast conservation after neoadjuvant chemotherapy.[213] In this study, 340 carefully selected patients who had a favorable response to chemotherapy were treated with breast conserving surgery and radiation. Despite the fact that 72% of patients in the study had clinical stage IIB or III disease, the 5-year and 10-year breast cancer recurrence rates were only 5% and 10%, respectively. Four tumor-related factors were associated with breast cancer recurrence and local-regional recurrence: clinical N2 or N3 disease, lymphovascular space invasion, a multifocal pattern of residual disease, and residual disease greater than 2 cm in diameter.[213] Eighty-four percent of patients had either just one of these factors or none of the factors, and in these patients the 10-year breast recurrence rate was only 4%. In contrast, there was a 45% breast cancer recurrence rate in the 4% of patients with 3 of these factors. Interestingly, having a T3 or T4 tumor did not correlate with breast cancer recurrence overall, but those patients with T3 or T4 disease in which the primary tumor broke up and left a multifocal pattern of residual disease had a 20% breast recurrence risk. These investigators also applied this prognostic index to a cohort of patients treated with neoadjuvant chemotherapy, mastectomy, and postmastectomy radiation. They found that for patients with 0 or 1 of these factors, breast conservation

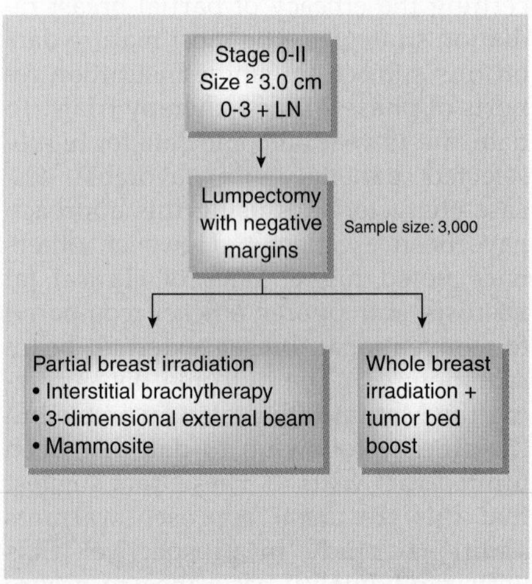

Figure 104-21 ■ Design of the ongoing NSABP/Radiation Therapy Oncology Group phase III trial comparing partial breast irradiation versus whole breast irradiation for patients with stage 0-II breast cancer.

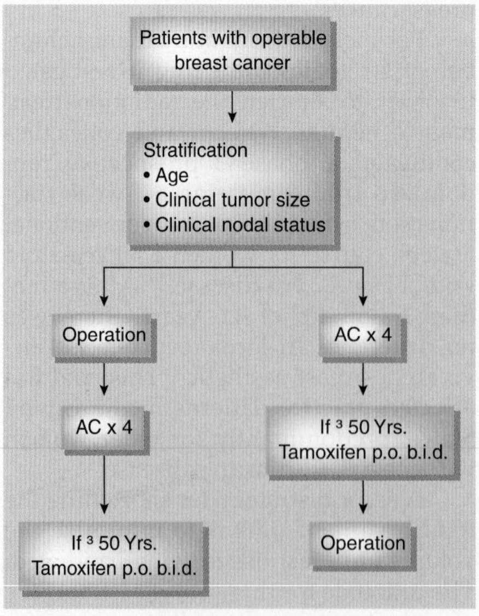

Figure 104-22 ■ NSABP study of B-18 schema.

offer similar excellent outcome as mastectomy and radiation. However, mastectomy and radiation was associated with a lower risk of local-regional recurrence in the patients with at least 3 factors.[214]

In conclusion, the data indicate that breast conservation therapy is an appropriate treatment option for carefully selected patients with advanced primary tumors that have a favorable response to neoadjuvant chemotherapy.

Postmastectomy Radiation ■ There is a strong rationale for combining the beneficial effects of radiation and mastectomy for selected women with breast cancer. For women with locally advanced disease, areas of subclinical disease extending beyond the operative field limit the efficacy of mastectomy. Radiation can often overcome this limitation by treating a larger volume of normal tissue and treating regions such as the supraclavicular fossa, where surgical resections are difficult and can cause significant morbidity. In contrast, the greatest limitation of radiation is its inability to control bulky sites of disease. Fortunately, mastectomy is highly effective in resecting all sites of gross disease for most women with breast cancer.

The initial studies that investigated radiation after mastectomy began in the 1950s and represented some of the first controlled clinical trials in oncology history. It is therefore somewhat surprising that after more than five decades of study there remain significant controversies over the value of post-mastectomy radiation and the proper selection criteria for its use. A number of factors have contributed to the continued uncertainties. First, early radiation techniques were found to be associated with life-threatening toxicities that became apparent 10 to 15 years after treatment.[173] Fortunately, technological improvements have lowered the morbidity of postmastectomy radiation, but decades of follow-up were needed to demonstrate this improvement. A second change that has occurred over time has been the addition of chemotherapy as a routine component of care. This change was important because it decreased the competing risk of distant metastases, thereby allowing improvements in local-regional control to have a positive effect on survival.

There have been several meta-analyses conducted to quantify the value and risk of radiation use after mastectomy. The most comprehensive and important of these has been the work of the EBCTCG. This group was able to obtain the raw data from every randomized prospective trial that has investigated post-mastectomy radiation. The most recently published analysis from this group evaluated 9933 patients treated with mastectomy with axillary clearance and subsequently randomized to postmastectomy radiation therapy versus none. For patients with lymph node-positive disease, radiation reduced the 15-year isolated local-regional recurrence from 29% to 8%. Importantly, this reduction led to a 5% decrease in the 15-year breast cancer mortality rate (60% vs 55%). For patients with lymph node–negative disease, local-regional recurrences were reduced from 8% to 3% and this small improvement in local-regional recurrence was not associated with a difference in overall survival.[173] These data are important in that they clearly indicated that eradication of persistent local-regional microscopic disease that is present after a definitive surgery can be the source of a subsequent distant metastasis, which eventually can lead to death. While the local-regional benefits of radiation were apparent within 5 years, the differences in survival occurred between years 5 and 15. The data from the metaanalysis also suggested that the survival benefit was only manifested in the trials in which there was a 10% or greater improvement in the 5-year local-regional control rate.[173]

Modern Postmastectomy Radiation Trials ■ Three of the more recent randomized trials investigating postmastectomy radiation that contributed to the EBCTCG metaanalysis provided new insights into the potential benefit of radiation but also further fueled the controversy regarding its use. Importantly, all of these studies used more modern radiation techniques and all patients in these studies received systemic therapy.

The Danish Breast Cancer Cooperative Group (DBCCG) 82b trial is perhaps the most important of these three trials. This study randomized 1708 premenopausal women with stage II or III breast cancer to mastectomy followed by 9 cycles of CMF chemotherapy or mastectomy, radiation, and 8 cycles of CMF. Radiation therapy consisted of 50 Gy in 25 fractions delivered to the chest wall and draining lymphatics (including the internal mammary lymph nodes) and used electron beams in the regions over the heart to minimize dose to the cardiovascular structures.[215] The majority of patients entered in this trial had 1 to 3 positive lymph nodes. However, most patients in this trial did not undergo a formal level I/II axillary dissection. The median number of axillary lymph nodes resected was only 7, with only 24% of patients having 10 or more lymph nodes removed and 15% having 3 or fewer lymph nodes removed. The most significant finding of this study was that patients randomized to radiation had an improved overall survival rate (10-year rates: 54% vs 45%, respectively; $p < .001$). This survival advantage was likely a consequence of the reduced rate of local-regional recurrence in the patients receiving radiation (9% vs 32%, $p < .001$).

Simultaneously, investigators in Vancouver, British Columbia conducted a smaller trial of similar design. In this trial, 318 premenopausal women with lymph node–positive disease were randomized to receive mastectomy and CMF, or mastectomy, radiation, and CMF.[216] The results were very similar, with radiation use being associated with an improvement in overall survival (20-year rates: 47% vs 37%, respectively; $p = .03$) and local-regional control (20-year rates: 87% vs 61%, respectively; $p < 0.0001$).

Finally, the DBCCG 82c, randomized 1300 postmenopausal patients to mastectomy and tamoxifen or mastectomy, tamoxifen, and radiation.[217] The stage of disease and extent of axillary surgery were also very similar to the 82b trial. The magnitude of the benefits in overall survival and local control was similar to the two previous studies. The 10-year overall survival rates favored patients randomized to receive radiation (45% vs 36%, respectively; $p = .03$), as did the rates of local-regional control (10-year rates: 92% vs 65%; respectively; $p < .001$).

An 18-year update of the DBCCG 82b&c combined data continued to show that radiation use was associated with continued benefits in local-regional control (86% vs 51%, $p < 0.0001$) and distant metastasis-free survival (47% vs 36%, $p < 0.0001$).[218]

Indications for Postmastectomy Radiation ■ There is a general consensus that a modified radical mastectomy achieves excellent rates of local-regional control for women with stage I breast cancer. In addition, there is consensus that patients with stage III disease, (defined by T3 with involved lymph nodes, T4 primaries, or 4 or more involved lymph nodes) should receive post-mastectomy radiation,[219] because these cohorts of patients have a 20% to 30% risk of local-regional recurrence after mastectomy, standard axillary dissection, and chemotherapy.

For patients with stage II disease with 1 to 3 positive lymph nodes the use of radiation is controversial. Most of the patients in the Danish and British Columbia trials had 1 to 3 positive lymph nodes, and radiation use in this cohort was associated with a reduction in local-regional recurrence and an improvement in overall survival. However, the 18-year local-regional recurrence rate for patients with this stage of disease in the Danish trials who were treated with mastectomy and systemic treatment was 41%.[218] In the British Columbia trial, the 10-year overall rate of local-regional recurrence for patients with 1-3 positive lymph nodes who did not receive radiation was 21.5%, which is much higher than the 12.6% (p = 0.02) rate noted in similarly staged patients treated with mastectomy and chemotherapy at M. D. Anderson Cancer Center.[220] The likely reason for the lower rate of local-regional recurrence in patients with 1-3 positive lymph nodes who are treated in United States centers is that some of the patients in the Danish and Vancouver trials had axillary sampling procedures rather than axillary dissections. This can lead to an underestimation of the true number of positive lymph nodes, such that many of the patients reported to have 1 to 3 positive lymph nodes would likely have had 4 or more lymph nodes if a more extensive surgical procedure had been performed. Second, the more limited dissection led to a high rate of axillary recurrences in the patients randomized to not receive radiation, which likely would have been avoided with a standard axillary dissection.

A number of recent studies has been conducted to assess the risk of local-regional recurrence in patients with 1-3 positive lymph nodes who were treated with a standard modified radical mastectomy and chemotherapy. The data from these studies is shown in Table 104-15 and collectively indicate that the 10-year risk of local-regional recurrence for such patients is approximately 13% to 15%.[215,217,221–223] Within the subgroup of patients with stage II disease with 1-3 positive lymph nodes, selected patients have additional features that increase the risk for local-regional recurrence to over 15%. Table 104-11 highlights these additional factors.[221,223–225]

Table 104-11 ■ **Factors Associated With Higher Local-Regional Recurrence Risk for Patients with 1-3 Positive Lymph Nodes**

Author	Factor
Katz et al.[221]	Extracapsular extension ≥2 mm Tumor size ≥4 cm Fewer than 10 lymph nodes recovered >20% of lymph nodes positive Positive or close margins Pectoralis muscle invasion
Taghian et al.[224]	Age under 50 with tumor size over 2 cm
Wallgren et al.[223]	Premenopausal: lymphovascular space invasion, G2-3 Postmenopausal: tumor over 2 cm, G3
Cheng et al.[225]	Tumor size ≥3 cm

Whether radiation provides a survival benefit for patients with less than a 15% long-term risk of local-regional recurrence is unknown. A randomized trial designed to investigate postmastectomy radiation for patients with stage II breast cancer with 1-3 positive lymph nodes did not successfully accrue in the United States and was closed. It is likely that radiation will decrease local-regional recurrence in such patients, but the absolute magnitude of this benefit will be small. Indeed, a study from M. D. Anderson reported that radiation use decreased the rate of local-regional recurrence in this cohort of patients from 13% to 3%.[226]

Postmastectomy Radiation Therapy After Neoadjuvant Chemotherapy ■ Significantly fewer data are available that address the indications for and efficacy of postmastectomy radiation in patients treated with neoadjuvant chemotherapy. In patients treated with mastectomy first, the decision to administer radiation therapy is predominantly made based on the pathological extent of disease. This is because clinical and radiographic assessment of primary tumor size and number of lymph nodes involved with disease is imprecise. It is clear that neoadjuvant chemotherapy changes the extent of pathological disease in 80 to 90% of cases, and one study found that the correlation between the pathological extent of disease with local-regional recurrence after mastectomy is different for patients treated with neoadjuvant chemotherapy than it is in patients treated with surgery first.[227] These data imply that both the pretreatment clinical stage and the extent of pathologically defined residual disease after chemotherapy need to be considered when assessing the risk of local-regional recurrence in patients treated with neoadjuvant chemotherapy and mastectomy. Indeed, in an analysis of the patients treated with neoadjuvant chemotherapy, mastectomy and no radiation, a multivariate analysis of local-regional recurrence predictors found that both pre- and post-treatment factors were independently associated with local-regional recurrence.[228] The efficacy of radiation in reducing local-regional recurrence in patients treated with neoadjuvant chemotherapy and mastectomy has never been evaluated in a prospective randomized trial. However, one retrospective study compared the outcomes of 579 patients who received neoadjuvant chemotherapy, mastectomy, and radiation therapy with those of 136 patients who were treated with neoadjuvant chemotherapy and mastectomy alone.[229] Radiation therapy was not a randomized variable in this population and there were significant imbalances in the prognostic factors between the two groups. In general, those treated with radiation therapy had more extensive disease and worse disease characteristics than those treated without radiation. Despite this, the local-regional recurrence rate was significantly lower in the patients treated with postmastectomy radiation therapy than in those treated with neoadjuvant chemotherapy and mastectomy alone (10-year local-regional recurrence rates were 8% and 22%, respectively, p = .001). In a multivariate analysis, the hazard ratio for local-regional recurrence associated with not receiving radiation therapy for the endpoint of LRR was 4.7 (95% CI, 2.7– 8.1, p < .0001). In the subgroup of patients with clinical T4 tumors, clinical stage IIIB/C disease, and in those with 4 or more positive lymph nodes after chemotherapy, the absolute improvement in local-regional recurrence risk was approximately 30 to 40%. The use of radiation in these same subgroups was associated with an approximately 15% to 20% improvement in overall and cause-specific survival. In a multivariate analysis of cause-specific survival for the entire cohort, the hazard ratio for no radiation use was 2.03 (95% CI, 1.41–2.92, p < .0001).

In a subsequent analysis from this group that focused just on patients who achieved a pathological complete response, the local-regional recurrence rate for those patients with clinical stage III disease was improved with radiation therapy (33% vs 7%, p = .04). None of the patients with clinical stage II disease who had a pathological complete response had a local-regional recurrence.[230]

Whether to use radiation for patients with clinical stage II disease who have positive lymph nodes after chemotherapy remains less clear. A report of 132 patients with clinical stage II disease who did not receive radiation therapy after neoadjuvant chemotherapy and mastectomy indicated that patients with clinical T3N0 disease or 4 or more positive lymph nodes had high rates of local-regional recurrence.[231] The 5-year local recurrence rates in the remaining patients were less than 10%. In the patients with clinical stage II disease who had 1 to 3 positive lymph nodes after neoadjuvant chemotherapy the 5-year rate of local-regional recurrence was 8%. It is important to recognize that this study had a small sample size and that the studied population was prone to selection biases, in that they represented only those patients for whom the treating physicians elected not to use radiation. Data from patients treated with neoadjuvant chemotherapy, mastectomy, and no radiation on NSABP B-18 and B-27 protocols has been presented but not published. The rate of local-regional recurrences in the cohort of patients who had one or more positive lymphs after neoadjuvant chemotherapy was approximately 15%.[150]

On the basis of the available data, it is reasonable to recommend postmastectomy radiation therapy for all patients with clinical stage III disease at initial presentation. It is also reasonable to assume that patients with clinical stage I or II disease who have 4 or more positive lymph nodes after chemotherapy or who have progressive disease leading to a primary tumor size over 5 cm are at high risk for local-regional recurrence and should receive radiation. It is currently not known whether radiation will benefit patients with clinical stage I or II disease who have 1 to 3 positive lymph nodes after neoadjuvant chemotherapy.[150]

Palliative Radiotherapy ■ There is a well-defined role for palliative radiotherapy in the treatment of metastatic breast cancer. Painful bony metastases and simple pathologic fractures of non–weight-bearing bones respond well to short courses of radiotherapy, such as 3000 to 3500 cGy in 10 to 14 fractions. However, local radiotherapy is no substitute for proper orthopedic fixation in weight-bearing bones. A phase 3 randomized trial from RTOG compared single fraction versus ten fraction treatment and found equivalent results for control of bony metastases. Most still favor multiple fraction therapy for those with a long life expectancy and those treatment in which sensitive normal structure are next to the metastases. However, the single treatment approach minimized time in treatment and is certainly appropriate for palliative treatments in patients who have progressive disease in other sites. Treatment with radiotherapy is the mainstay for multiple intracranial metastases and is preferable to surgical treatment in the presence of widespread, poorly controlled systemic metastases. The generally accepted course of palliative brain irradiation for multiple lesions is 3000 cGy in 10 to 12 fractions administered in conjunction with high-dose corticosteroids with or without phenytoin (Dilantin). The optimal therapy for a solitary intracranial metastasis in the absence of widespread systemic metastases is less clear. A randomized trial comparing surgical removal plus radiotherapy to radiotherapy alone concluded that patients receiving combined therapy lived longer, had fewer recurrences, and enjoyed a better quality of life.[232] In addition, the use stereotactic radiosurgery/gamma knife for patients with 2-3 intracranial metastases with avoidance of whole brain irradiation is becoming an increasing common treatment approach. In such patients, the toxicity associated with whole brain treatment may be reserved for those with multiple brain metastases or for those with recurrent metastases after radiosurgery.

Details of Radiation Treatment ■ The planning and design of the treatment fields and the delivery of radiation treatments for breast cancer are of critical importance and require modern equipment and attention to detail. It is clear that radiation treatments can have serious normal tissue consequences and even cause life-threatening radiation injuries, which can be avoided or minimized with modern treatment techniques.

There have been a number of recent advances in the field of radiation oncology that directly benefit breast cancer patients. One of these major advances has been the use of three-dimensional imaging to assist in field design. Computed tomography (CT)-based simulation allows radiation oncologists to design treatment fields on CT images acquired from patients in their treatment positions, thereby permitting better visualization of the targeted regions and the normal tissues that one wishes to avoid, such as the heart. An example of a field design for a stage I left breast cancer treatment after lumpectomy is shown in Figure 104-23. In this image, the tumor bed has been contoured on individual CT slices and reconstructed for the image. The breast is treated with a medial tangentially oriented beam, with a deep edge that enters near the mid-line and transverses the anterior thorax to exit near the mid axillary line. This field is opposed with a lateral tangent beam to match the fall off of dose as the beam travels through the breast and ultimately provides a homogeneous dose distribution.

Other regions of interest, such as lymph nodes in the axilla, internal mammary chain, or supraclavicular fossa can likewise be contoured in order to visualize their anatomical location with respect to treatment field borders. Figure 104-24 shows a "beam's eye-view" of a medial tangent beam used to treat the breast (including the tumor bed), the upper internal mammary lymph nodes, and level I and a portion of level II of the axilla.

A second major advance has been the development of three-dimensional dose calculation systems, which more accurately calculate and display the dose on the CT images throughout the three-dimensional treatment volume. Finally, modern treatment tools now also allow the dose to be modulated in three-dimensions. The goal of such modulation is to provide a homogeneous dose distribution, which minimizes the risk of normal tissues receiving more than the prescribed dose and the risk of targeted areas receiving less than the prescribed dose.

The treatment planning process is the initial critically important step in radiation treatments of breast cancer. Patients are immobilized in a supine position with the ipsilateral arm abducted and externally rotated. They then undergo a CT scan that acquires the image set used for treatment planning. Reference marks are placed on the patient's skin of the breast. The planning process, in which the fields are designed and the dose distribution optimized typically takes 2 to 3 days and does not require the patient to be present. Following completion of planning, daily treatments begin which typically require 15 minutes each day in the treatment room. The therapy is painless. The most common course of treatment entails 25 to 28 treatments of 180 to 200 cGy per day to the breast or chest wall with or without inclusion of lymphatic regions at risk. This course is typically followed by 5 to 8 supplemental treatments of 180 to 200 cGy per day to the tumor bed

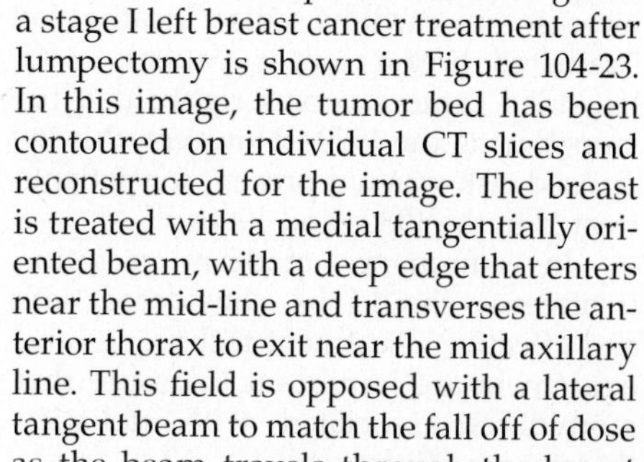

Figure 104-23 ■ Cross-sectional picture of radiation fields used for the treatment of left-sided invasive breast cancer. The red shaded areas represent the volume included within the fields. The solid yellow object represents the tumor bed, which was reconstructed by contouring this region on sequential computed tomography slices. Two opposed treatment fields are used: a medial tangent that obliquely enters the medial breast and exits the lateral breast and an opposed lateral tangent field. The fields are opposed to match the fall-off of radiation dose that occurs as beams travel through tissue.

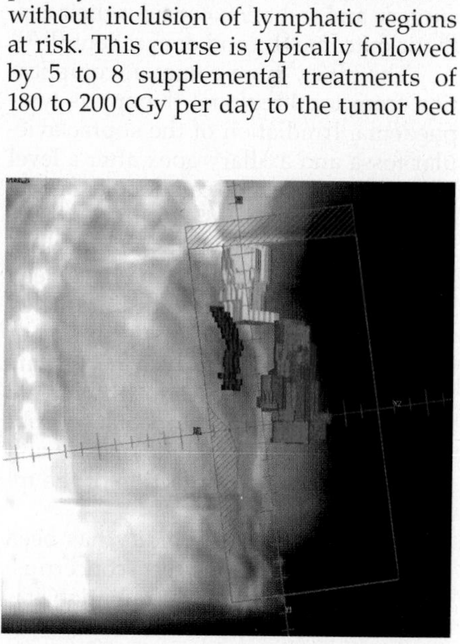

Figure 104-24 ■ A beams' eye-view of a medial tangent radiation treatment field designed to cover the breast, low axilla, and upper internal mammary lymph node chain. The reconstructed contours of a tumor bed (red), upper internal mammary lymph node region (blue) and the low axilla (yellow) are shown.

region (often called a tumor bed or chest wall boost). In total, treatments are given 5 days a week for approximately 6 to 6.5 weeks. However, prospective trials from both Canada and the United Kingdom have suggested that patients with stage I disease with favorable features achieve excellent outcomes with a 16 fraction over 3.5 week approach.

Morbidity of Radiation Treatments for Breast Cancer ■ Modern radiation treatments for breast cancer are relatively well tolerated and have low rates for long-term morbidity. Morbidities from radiation are considered as either acute effects or late effects. Acute effects typically occur during or immediately after treatment and for the most part are self-limited. The usual acute effects associated with breast or postmastectomy radiation include treatment-related fatigue and radiation dermatitis. These effects are usually relatively mild for women with early stage disease and patients typically can continue to work and continue their usual daily routines.

Late effects following treatment are also relatively unusual, particularly for patients treated after breast-conserving surgery for early-stage breast cancer or DCIS. For these patients, the most common late effect is a change in breast aesthetics. The cosmetic results after lumpectomy and breast irradiation are influenced by technique, patient body habitus, use of systemic therapy, and the extent of surgery. Approximately 85% of women treated with breast-conserving surgery and radiation consider their aesthetic outcome as good or excellent.[233,234]

The other, more common complication from local-regional therapy is lymphedema. Irradiation of the supraclavicular fossa and axillary apex after a level I-II axillary dissection can double the rate of lymphedema from 8% to 10% (surgery alone) to 15% to 20%. Rates can increase further if level III dissections have been performed and in cases with unresected involved lymph nodes in the infra- or supraclavicular fossa, which necessitate higher radiation dosages to this region. Other patient-related factors that contribute to lymphedema include obesity and subsequent injury or infection of the ipsilateral arm.

Cardiovascular morbidity has been the most significant long-term concern associated with breast cancer radiation. It is clear that radiation treatments for breast cancer can cause significant cardiovascular-related deaths if high dose is delivered to underlying cardiovascular structures.[173] Modern radiation treatments for breast cancer are associated with less cardiovascular morbidity and mortality than earlier radiation techniques. In the Danish postmastectomy radiation trials an electron beam technique was exclusively used in treating the chest wall to minimize dose to the cardiac structures. After a median follow-up of 117 months, there was no increase in mortality or cardiac-related hospitalizations in the approximately 1500 patients randomized to receive radiation versus the 1500 who were randomized to no radiation.[235] A similar morbidity and mortality analysis was performed in a Canadian study by Vallis and colleagues.[236] The long-term follow-up on 2128 patients treated with radiation as a component of breast conservative therapy, with a median patient follow-up in excess of 10 years, these authors found that cardiovascular morbidity was not increased in women with left-sided breast cancer compared to those with right breast cancer. Most recently, a report analyzing SEER data found an increase in cardiovascular deaths for irradiated breast cancer patients with left-sided tumors versus right-sided tumors during the 1970s. However, this increased risk was not present for patients treated in the 1980s and 1990s.[237]

In summary, modern radiation treatments should be considered safe and effective. Treatment techniques and equipment are important to assure that morbidities associated with radiation therapy are minimized.

Sequencing of Local-Regional Breast Cancer Treatment With Systemic Therapies ■ As the beneficial therapeutic effects of surgery, radiation, chemotherapy, and hormonal therapy have become elucidated, important questions concerning the sequencing of therapies have arisen. Most breast cancer patients benefit from multimodality treatment and decisions concerning the sequencing of these treatments are optimally handled in a multidisciplinary fashion, with input from surgeons, medical oncologists, radiation oncologists, pathologists, and diagnostic radiologists.

Sequencing of Surgery and Chemotherapy ■ Definitive surgical therapy has been the historical initial treatment for most patients with breast cancer. However, an increasing percentage of breast cancer patients is treated with chemotherapy prior to definitive surgery. This approach was initially investigated in patients with advanced or inflammatory breast cancer in an attempt to render the disease operable. Subsequently, neoadjuvant chemotherapy was investigated as a strategy to permit breast conservation therapy for patients with large T2 or T3 disease. Even more recently, neoadjuvant chemotherapy has been explored as a treatment option for any woman who was felt to potentially benefit from chemotherapy. These more recent treatment philosophies have permitted the majority of breast cancer patients to be eligible for neoadjuvant chemotherapy.

There are a number of potential advantages and some possible disadvantages for sequencing chemotherapy prior to surgery. Table 104-12 reviews some of these advantages and disadvantages. Neoadjuvant chemotherapy treatment has high anti-tumor activity: numerous studies have indicated that 80% to 90% of breast cancers respond to neoadjuvant chemotherapy, and in 15% to 30% of the cases there is no evidence of residual disease within the surgical specimen at either the primary site or the lymph nodes (termed a pathological complete response [pCR]).[208,209]

During the 1980s, several randomized and nonrandomized studies were conducted to evaluate the worth of preoperative chemotherapy for primary operable breast cancer.[238] Nonrandomized studies were limited to the evaluation of primary tumor response to preoperative chemotherapy and possibly to the correlation of such response to outcome. All of these studies demonstrated that

Table 104-12 ■ **Potential Benefits and Determinants of Using Neoadjuvant Chemotherapy in Breast Cancer**

Benefits
Facilitates the use of mastectomy for patients presenting with inoperable disease or inflammatory breast cancer
Increases rates of breast conservation surgery for patients presenting with larger primary tumors
Improves the aesthetic result of a breast conservation surgical procedure if less of the breast is resected after the tumor has responded to chemotherapy
Allows for identification of resistance to treatment permitting clinicians to stop ineffective chemotherapy regimens and thereby minimize the continued risk of treatment toxicity
The pathological response of disease to neoadjuvant chemotherapy is prognostic. Therefore, this sequencing strategy has proved to be an invaluable research tool to:
Directly compare the effectiveness of two systemic regimens
Directly study biological factors that influence chemotherapy sensitivity/resistance
Identify patients for clinical studies of new agents because of their high risk for recurrence despite receiving the best available standard regimens
Potential Determinants
Information concerning the pathological extent of disease prior to treatment is unknown. Accordingly, the following are less certain:
Margin status of a breast conservation surgery
Risk of additional lymph node disease when a sentinel lymph node is negative or shows fibrosis and/or treatment-induced changes
Indications for postmastectomy radiation

preoperative chemotherapy results in a high rate of primary tumor response. Some authors indicated that a correlation existed between response of the primary tumor to chemotherapy and outcome. In some of these studies, reduction in tumor size allowed an increased rate of breast-conserving surgery.

The most important assessment of preoperative chemotherapy comes from randomized trials. The NSABP updated protocol B-18, a randomized trial comparing the preoperative and postoperative administration of four cycles of Adriamycin and cyclophosphamide (AC) in patients with operable breast cancer.[210] Patients with palpable operable (T1, T2, T3) breast cancer in whom the diagnosis had been established by FNA cytology were stratified by age, clinical tumor size, and clinical nodal status and randomly assigned to one of two groups. Group I patients underwent a total mastectomy plus axillary dissection, or a lumpectomy plus axillary dissection. They then received four cycles of AC (60 and 600 mg/m^2 every 21 days × 4). Group II patients received four cycles of AC as in group I, followed by a total mastectomy or lumpectomy within 4 weeks of the fourth course of chemotherapy. All patients who were 50 years of age or older received tamoxifen 10 mg twice daily. For patients treated by lumpectomy, breast irradiation was administered after the completion of all chemotherapy.

In the preoperative chemotherapy arm, 36% of patients demonstrated a clinical complete response, and 43% had a clinical partial response, for an overall response rate of 79%. Patients receiving preoperative chemotherapy were more likely to have a lumpectomy than were patients receiving postoperative chemotherapy (68% vs 59%, $p < .01$). Responding patients were significantly more likely to receive a lumpectomy than non-responding patients. Preoperative chemotherapy also resulted in axillary nodal downstaging: 59% versus 42% pathologically negative axillary nodes, for an axillary nodal downstaging of 34%. There was a highly significant correlation between tumor response to preoperative chemotherapy and pathologic nodal status. Eighty-seven percent of patients with a complete clinical response had pathologically negative nodes, versus 57% with partial response, 50% with stable disease, and 38% with progressive disease. Disease-free survival and overall survival were no different in the preoperative chemotherapy group from the postoperative adjuvant therapy group, however, thus failing to confirm the major hypothesis of this study. The EORTC completed a confirmatory trial of very similar design, with results quite similar to those obtained in NSABP B-18.[209] A recently published update of B-18 continued to show no survival advantage for either arm but did report an interaction between age and treatment sequencing, such that younger patients appear to have an improved disease-free survival with neoadjuvant chemotherapy and older patients appeared to have an improved outcome with adjuvant chemotherapy. As the age-treatment sequencing interaction was found in an exploratory analysis, these data need to be confirmed in other studies prior to being considered in patient treatment decisions.[210]

One unanswered question arising from this study concerns the need for further therapy following initial treatment. This question was addressed in the Aberdeen trial,[239] the M. D. Anderson Trial 85-01,[240] and NSABP protocol B27.[210,241] Smith and collaborators reported the results of a multicenter study (the "Aberdeen" trial) in 162 patients with large operable and locally advanced breast cancer. All received four cycles of doxorubicin, cyclophosphamide, vincristine and prednisolone (CVAP); those who responded were randomized to receive four more cycles of CVAP or four cycles of docetaxel (100 mg/m^2). All non-responders received four cycles of docetaxel. The clinical complete remission (CR) and clinical partial remission (PR) rate (94% vs 66%, $p = .001$) and pathologic CR (34% vs 16%, $p = .04$) rates were higher for those who were randomized to receive docetaxel. This improvement in response rates translated into longer relapse-free and overall survival rates. In this small study, treatment was of equal duration in both arms, so the improved outcome could only be attributed to the introduction of docetaxel. The study results confirm that improvements in pathological CR rate are associated with improvement in relapse-free and overall survival.

Thomas and colleagues, from the M. D. Anderson evaluated the use of an alternate, non-cross-resistant adjuvant chemotherapy regimen in women with a poor pathologic response to a preoperative doxorubicin-based regimen.[240] One hundred ninety-three patients with locally advanced breast cancer received three cycles of vincristine, doxorubicin, cyclophosphamide, and prednisone (VACP) every 21 days followed by surgery. Patients with less than 1 cm^3 residual tumor at mastectomy received an additional five cycles of VACP. Those with more than 1 cm^3 residual tumor were randomly assigned to receive an additional five cycles of VACP or five cycles of vinblastine, methotrexate with calcium leucovorin rescue, and fluorouracil (VbMF). Overall clinical response was seen in 83.4% after three cycles of VACP, whereas the pathologic complete response rate was 12.2%. One hundred six patients were randomly assigned to VACP or VbMF. Those receiving VbMF achieved higher relapse-free survival (RFS) and overall survival (OS) than those who received additional VACP, although the differences did not reach statistical significance ($p = .08$). Initial stage of tumor, clinical complete response, and pathologic complete response were all associated with statistically superior survival rates. For patients with a poor response to initial neoadjuvant chemotherapy, treatment with a non-cross-resistant regimen was associated with a trend toward improved RFS and OS compared with those continuing with the doxorubicin regimen.

NSABP B-27 was designed as a three-arm randomized trial where all patients received an initial four courses of preoperative AC therapy. One group received no further adjuvant treatment. A second group received four courses of docetaxel (Taxotere) after surgery, and the third group received four courses of docetaxel before surgery.

Preliminary results indicated that the addition of preoperative docetaxel significantly increased the rate of complete pathological response. In the AC only arms of B-18 and B-27, the clinical complete remission (cCR) rates were 36% and 40%, respectively, in contrast to 65% for the preoperative docetaxel arm in B-27. The pathological CR (pCR) rates were 9% and 9.1% for the two AC arms and 18.9% for the arm with preoperative docetaxel.[241] An update indicated that the administration of preoperative docetaxel following AC was associated with a significant prolongation of relapse-free survival ($p = .03$), although no survival differences had emerged. Since this study confirmed that the rate of pCR predicted relapse-free survival, it also validated the use of pCR as a surrogate marker of long-term benefit from treatment and therefore provided a useful tool for comparing treatment options.

This could provide a useful tool for future chemotherapy regimens. The response to preoperative chemotherapy becomes a prognostic marker for disease-free survival and survival. Thus, response to preoperative chemotherapy can be used as an intermediate end point in testing new regimens or in testing the additional effect of new drugs administered after well-established regimens, without having to wait for several years until disease-free survival and survival end points can be compared. With the demonstration that preoperative chemotherapy is equivalent to postoperative chemotherapy for disease-free survival and survival, new chemotherapeutic regimens can be tested in this setting without fear of putting patients at a disadvantage.

Even if preoperative chemotherapy does not improve disease-free survival and survival, there are several reasons why it may sometimes be preferred over postoperative chemotherapy. The administration of preoperative chemotherapy results in separating patients into five different groups according to their pathologic and clinical response to chemotherapy: (1) pathologic complete responders, (2) clinical complete responders, (3) clinical partial responders, (4) patients with clinically stable disease, and (5) patients with clinically progressive disease.

The observed reduction in the size of the primary tumor following preoperative chemotherapy, resulting in increased rates of breast-conserving surgery, constitutes an additional advantage. There are some advantages for being able to assess disease response to neoadjuvant chemotherapy. For example, studies have indicated the extent of residual disease after neoadjuvant chemotherapy is prognostic, and therefore more clearly stratifies which patients, such as those who achieve a pCR, have an excellent disease-free survival, and which patients remain at high risk of subsequent systemic relapse despite the chemotherapy treatment.[208,209,242] The assessment of disease response is of particular value as a research tool, in that it permits the activity of different chemotherapy regimens to be more easily compared. Response data can also provide insights into the biological determinants of chemotherapy response. For example, a study that used microarray technologies, identified and validated a profile of 70 genes that predicted which patients would achieve a pCR to taxane chemotherapy.[125] These types of studies may improve the understanding of chemotherapy resistance and identify new molecular targets for drug development.

Sequencing of Adjuvant Chemotherapy and Radiation ■ As the majority of breast cancer patients treated in the United States undergo surgery as the initial component of their therapy, the most common treatment-sequencing question concerns the timing of adjuvant chemotherapy and radiation. There has been one relatively small, randomized prospective trial that investigated this question. In this study, patients treated with breast conservation therapy were randomized to radiation followed by 4 cycles of chemotherapy or the same chemotherapy followed by radiation.[243] The final report of this trial noted no differences in local or distant disease control in either arm, or the patterns of first failure. It did appear that patients with close margins did worse with radiation delay, suggesting that such patients may benefit from re-excision. The equivalent first failure pattern noted in this trial was also found in a similar retrospective analysis of patients treated on Southwest Oncology Group trials.[244]

Fewer data are available concerning the sequencing of chemotherapy and radiation for women treated with mastectomy. In the Danish 82b trial, radiation was sequenced very early in the adjuvant course .[215] However, a recent study that examined the timing of radiation delivery in the Cancer and Leukemia Group B 9344 trial, found very low rates of local-regional recurrence after postmastectomy radiation and the rates of local-regional recurrence were lowest in those for whom there was a delay in delivering radiation in order to first treat with taxane chemotherapy.[245]

Until definitive data are obtained in trials, it is reasonable to consider the risks and benefits of any adjuvant sequencing approach according to the particulars of each case. The majority of data suggest that the breast tumor recurrence risk is not increased with radiation delay if negative margins are achieved. Therefore, a reasonable sequencing strategy would be to attempt to achieve negative surgical margins and administer chemotherapy prior to radiation.

Systemic Therapy of Breast Cancer

Endocrine Therapies

Suppression of Steroid Hormone Production ■ This therapeutic objective can be accomplished by the surgical removal of organs that produce and secrete hormones involved in breast cancer growth, radiotherapy-induced ablation, or chemical inhibition of hormone synthesis.

Ovarian Ablation ■ Ovarian ablation is the oldest form of endocrine therapy, first described in 1896. It is ineffective for postmenopausal patients. Ovarian ablation can be performed by surgical removal of the ovaries or by radiotherapy. The latter requires 2 to 3 months for maximal ablation of ovarian function, which is a disadvantage in the treatment of symptomatic patients. Ovarian ablation by radiotherapy is noninvasive, but its effects may not be permanent. Over the short term, ovarian ablation is a safe, well-tolerated procedure. Acute side effects include hot flashes, alterations in mood, and other symptoms of estrogen deprivation. Long-term consequences include accelerated loss of bone mineral density and alterations in the blood lipid profile that indicate an increased risk of coronary artery disease. In the United States, surgical ablation is preferred over radiotherapy-induced ablation. Ovarian ablation has been largely displaced by antiestrogens and LHRH analogs.

Selective Aromatase Inhibitors ■ Aromatase, an enzyme of the cytochrome P-450 superfamily catalyzes the conversion of androgenic precursors to estrogens in peripheral tissues. Aromatase is substantially concentrated in adipose and hepatic tissues and is also found in elevated concentrations in breast cancer.[246] The enzyme has no effect on glucocorticoid, androgen, or mineralocorticoid production. Aromatase inhibitors lower serum and tumor estrogen levels in postmenopausal patients. Therefore, aromatase inhibition is applicable only to postmenopausal (or oophorectomized) women in whom estrogen production is predominantly from peripheral sources. Two types of aromatase inhibitors have been developed: Type 1 aromatase inhibitors (exemestane, formestane) are exclusively steroidal and bind the enzyme covalently and irreversibly; type 2 inhibitors (such as aminoglutethimide, letrozole, anastrozole) reversibly inhibit cytochrome P-450.

Type 1 Aromatase Inhibitors ■ The earliest of the new inhibitors, formestane (or 4-hydroxyandrostenedione), has no estrogenic properties and is rapidly metabolized by the liver. By intramuscular administration, its half-life is 5 to 10 days. It has an excellent therapeutic index and requires no glucocorticoid replacement. It is commercially available in several European countries.

Exemestane (Aromasin) is the most potent and commonly used member of this family.[247] Its potency in inhibiting aromatase is similar to the type 2 inhibitors, and its pharmacokinetic properties make it quite competitive.

Type 2 Aromatase Inhibitors ■ Both anastrozole (Arimidex) and letrozole (Femara) are FDA-approved for treatment of hormone receptor positive breast cancer in postmenopausal women.[247] Both agents inhibit aromatase activity by 96% to 98%, and have excellent antitumor activity and excellent tolerance profile. All three selective AIs are more effective and better tolerated than megestrol acetate and compare favorably with tamoxifen in the metastatic setting. Anastrozole and letrozole are superior to tamoxifen in the adjuvant setting for primary breast cancer. Anastrozole, letrozole, and exemestane have all proven superior to tamoxifen after 2 to 5 years of adjuvant tamoxifen therapy. Fadrozole demonstrated antitumor efficacy similar to that of established AIs or other hormonal agents. It was well tolerated, although nausea, vomiting, anorexia, headache, rash, and other minor adverse effects have been reported. This agent is commercially available in Japan. The major advantage of the selective AIs over their predecessors is a better therapeutic index. Furthermore, anastrozole, exemestane, and letrozole are conveniently administered orally, once daily. There is incomplete cross-resistance between type 1 and type 2 AIs.

Inhibitors of Pituitary Function ■ LHRH analogs (buserelin, goserelin, leuprolide) produce long-lasting inhibition of luteinizing hormone and follicle-stimulating hormone release after a transient initial increase. Their action could also be described as pharmacologic ovarian ablation because they inhibit ovarian estradiol release by about 90%.[248] In addition, some authors have hypothesized that LHRH analogues may have direct effects on breast cancer cells; however, this action remains speculative. LHRH analogs are primarily effective in premenopausal women.

Interference with Hormonal Action

The endocrine therapies described in this section act by interfering with the effects of hormones on the end organ (ie, the breast cancer cell).

Selective Estrogen Receptor Modulators (SERMs or Antiestrogens) ■ Antiestrogens were initially developed in the search for better contraceptives. Although their efficacy as antifertility drugs was limited, they were found to cause regression of breast cancer cells. Tamoxifen is known to bind competitively to the ER, but it also has multiple additional adverse effects on the cancer cell.[249] It can lower the production of IGF-1 and TGF-α; it blocks angiogenesis and induces the production of TGF-β, calmodulin, and protein kinase C. It also has been reported to increase natural killer cell activity. The effects of tamoxifen have been studied mostly in postmenopausal women, although its effects have also been examined in younger patients. The serum estrogen level rises dramatically in some premenopausal patients, but this effect does not mediate tamoxifen resistance. The usual dose of tamoxifen is 20 to 40 mg daily. Higher doses do not appear to be more effective. Tamoxifen and its active metabolites have a prolonged serum half-life (7 days) after reaching steady-state levels. Thus, once-a-day dosing is sufficient, and missing an occasional dose will not alter serum levels dramatically.

Several new SERMs have been extensively tested. Toremifene was approved by the FDA for the management of metastatic, ER-positive breast cancer, based on evidence indicating therapeutic equivalence with tamoxifen.[249] Raloxifene was approved for the prevention of osteoporosis, and more recently for reducing the risk of breast cancer.[250] Limited phase 2 evaluation suggested modest antitumor efficacy in metastatic breast cancer. Both toremifene and raloxifene appear to lack estrogen agonist activity on the uterus. For this reason, raloxifene was compared with tamoxifen in a large, randomized trial of breast cancer prevention (STAR trial).[251] Other SERMs (idoxifene, droloxifene, LY353381, LY357489, EM-652, and GW5638) under development have not shown to be more effective or less toxic, than tamoxifen.[249]

Another important endocrine agent is the selective ER downregulator (SERD), fulvestrant (Faslodex®).[249] This steroidal antiestrogen is a pure estrogen antagonist. Fulvestrant blocks ER transactivation from both the activation function (AF)-1 and AF-2 domains. Fulvestrant also impairs receptor dimerization and induces receptor degradation, resulting in a dramatic reduction of receptor concentration in the cell. Fulvestrant exhibits 100 times greater affinity for the ER than tamoxifen, and it is effective in tamoxifen-resistant cell lines. Furthermore, it is a potent inhibitor of tamoxifen-stimulated breast cancer cells in vivo. Fulvestrant was shown to be equivalent to anastrozole in the treatment of tamoxifen-resistant tumors.

Progestins ■ The synthetic progestational agents megestrol acetate (Megace, 40 mg PO qid), and medroxyprogesterone acetate (Provera, 400 mg/day) were evaluated for the treatment of advanced breast cancer.[252] Although responses to progestin therapy correlated with ER content, there is no evidence that PR content is a better predictor of response for this group of agents than for other hormonal treatments. Toxicity is clearly dose related. At high doses, substantial weight gain, fluid retention, and other toxicities become prominent. At commonly used doses, the efficacy, and tolerance of progestins appear similar to those of tamoxifen. Despite their activity, progestins were rapidly displaced by selective AIs over the past few years. High-dose progestins stimulate appetite and weight gain and have been used with some success for cancer cachexia. For palliative treatment of patients with advanced cancer, progestins can improve a sense of well being. Low doses of progestins were reported to be effective treatment of vasomotor instability-related symptoms in postmenopausal women.

Androgens ■ Androgen therapy also is an effective approach to the endocrine treatment of breast cancer, but the virilizing effects make it intolerable to many women. Semisynthetic testosterone derivatives, such as fluoxymesterone (Halotestin, 10 mg orally bid) and danazol, are better tolerated, with fewer virilizing effects. Nevertheless, with long-term therapy, hirsutism, deepening of the voice, clitoral hypertrophy, male pattern alopecia, and increased libido occur. Like other hormonal agents with intrinsic endocrine effects, androgens also can cause tumor flare. The therapeutic index of the new antiestrogens, AIs, and LHRH analogs is clearly superior to that of androgens. Through their anabolic activity, androgens exhibit an important palliative effect, even in the absence of tumor regression. Increased appetite and weight gain are common. Androgens, like estrogens, can be valuable therapeutic tools when cost is an important consideration, especially when good tolerance can be established in an individual patient.

Estrogens ■ Second to ovarian ablation, estrogens are probably the oldest form of hormonal therapy for breast and other hormone-responsive tumors. It appears paradoxical that both reduction of estrogen levels by ablative therapies and the administration of high doses of estrogen can cause tumor regression. The mechanisms by which high doses of estrogen induce tumor regression are not known, but estrogen therapy is as effective as antiestrogens or progestins for postmenopausal patients. High-dose estrogen therapy was also reported to have therapeutic activity in pre-menopausal women with breast cancer. Diethylstilbestrol 15 mg/day and ethinyl estradiol 1.5 to 3 mg/day are the most common preparations used. The major drawback of estrogen therapy is toxicity. Common side effects include nausea, vomiting, fluid retention, increased risk of thrombotic phenomena, tumor flare, urinary incontinence, and vaginal bleeding. When compared to tamoxifen, estrogens were found to be more toxic and less well tolerated, but also less expensive than tamoxifen or several of the other modern hormonal therapies. Like androgens, estrogens have been largely displaced by SERMs and AIs. For postmenopausal women who have responded to several lines of hormonal therapy (SERMs, SERD, AIs, progestins, and perhaps androgens), estrogen therapy is a viable therapeutic alternative. Starting at a lower dose and escalating to the full therapeutic dose over a 2- to 3-week period lessens gastrointestinal toxicity and improves tolerance.

Corticosteroids ■ The antitumor efficacy of corticosteroids is poorly documented for metastatic breast cancer but is considered to be about 10%. The long-term administration of glucocorticoids is associated with potentially severe and intolerable side effects. Therefore, glucocorticoids are not recommended as antitumor agents for metastatic breast cancer.

Glucocorticoids have a specific role in the management of well-defined complications of breast cancer, however. High-dose glucocorticoid therapy is administered for short periods to patients with central nervous system metastases and those with spinal cord compression, and some experts also use it during the management of acute hypercalcemia of malignancy. This latter indication has been relegated to the management of bisphosphonate-refractory cases in recent years. Its antiemetic effects are also well known.

Antiandrogens (flutamide and cyproterone acetate) and *antiprogestins* (mifepristone, RU 486) have been evaluated in a few clinical trials. Their efficacy against metastatic breast cancer appears limited. At this point, there is no role for these agents in the standard treatment of breast carcinoma.

Side Effects of Hormone Therapy ■ Most types of hormonal therapy can produce hot flashes, mild nausea, fluid retention, and an increase in the incidence of thromboembolic phenomena. Tamoxifen has been associated with an increased risk of endometrial hyperplasia, dysplasia, and carcinoma, as well as the development of ovarian cysts and other benign gynecologic abnormalities. A recent report suggested an increase in the incidence of uterine sarcomas as well. Ocular toxicity has also been attributed to tamoxifen, especially when it is administered at high doses, including cataracts and macular deposits. Progestins are known to cause moderately severe fluid retention, increased appetite, and weight gain, and they can occasionally cause or contribute to glucose intolerance. The newer aromatase inhibitors and LHRH analogs appear to be better tolerated.[247,248] However, since both types of agent produce estrogen deprivation, arthralgias, bone pain, musculoskeletal pain, diarrhea, nausea, headaches, hot flushes, and vaginal dryness and alopecia have been reported in association with these agents. In addition, loss of bone mineral density and increased rate of osteoporotic fractures have been reported with LHRH analogs and aromatase inhibitors.

Cytotoxic Chemotherapy

Breast cancer is moderately sensitive to a number of cytotoxic agents. Several classes of agents with different mechanisms of action and only partially overlapping toxic effects have substantial antitumor activity in patients with metastatic breast cancer. The most active drugs include the anthracyclines (doxorubicin, epirubicin, and liposomal formulations of doxorubicin), alkylating agents (cyclophosphamide, melphalan, thiotepa, and platinum salts), the anthraquinones (mitoxantrone), antimetabolites (methotrexate, 5-fluorouracil, capecitabine and gemcitabine), the vinca alkaloids (vinorelbine, vinblastine, and vincristine), epothilone-derivatives (ixabepilone) and the taxanes (paclitaxel, nab-paclitaxel and docetaxel). Response durations after single-agent therapy are short, in the range of 4 to 6 months and there is no noticeable impact on survival. One of the most important additions in recent years has been capecitabine. This agent is a fluoropyrimidine prodrug, converted to the active compound by thymidine phosphorylase. Many malignant cells produce high concentrations of this enzyme, resulting in preferential activation of the drug at the site of tumor deposits. Some cytotoxic agents, such as the taxanes, induce the production of thymidine phosphorylase, thus further enhancing local drug activation and resulting in a synergistic combination.

Combination Chemotherapy ■ Combination chemotherapy was developed based on the rationale that combining agents with different mechanisms of action and nonoverlapping toxicities would increase treatment benefit, prevent or delay the emergence of drug resistance without significantly worsening morbidity or quality of life. (For details of the strategy and tactics of combination chemotherapy see Chapter 45: Principles of Dose, Schedule, and Combination Chemotherapy.) Combination chemotherapy regimens consisting of cyclophosphamide, methotrexate, 5-fluorouracil (CMF); and 5-fluorouracil, doxorubicin (Adriamycin), cyclophosphamide (FAC) produce higher overall response rates, exceeding 50% in most reports, with remission durations that range from 6 to 12 months and survival that approaches 2 years. Randomized trials demonstrated that these combinations were more effective than single agents such as 5-fluorouracil, cyclophosphamide, and melphalan, resulting in higher response rates and longer times to progression.

Since the introduction of the taxanes into the treatment of advanced breast cancer, two competing hypotheses have directed clinical research in chemotherapy for breast cancer. One, the conventional approach based on the Goldie–Coldman hypothesis, called for concurrent administration of two or more cytotoxic agents to prevent or minimize the development of drug resistance and maximize cytoreduction.[253] The other, based on the Norton–Simon hypothesis, proposed the sequential administration of full-dose, single-agent treatments, to maximize dose-intensity and minimize toxicity.[254] In general, sequential single-agent therapy is better tolerated than simultaneous combinations, provided the same doses of all drugs are used. In the metastatic setting, in the absence of life-threatening or symptomatic disease, the sequential use of single agent therapies is a reasonable alternative to simultaneous combinations. However, there is no obvious benefit for using sequential single agents if the optimal doses of two active drugs can be administered simultaneously. In recent years there has been emphasis on rational combinations. Thus, capecitabine and taxanes represent synergistic combinations, as do taxanes with trastuzumab or bevacizumab (vide infra).

Side Effects of Cytotoxic Chemotherapy ■ Cytotoxic chemotherapy regimens used for breast cancer treatment have produced considerable side effects. Most cytotoxic agents are myelosuppressive. The most serious toxicity is neutropenia, which can lead to severe infection. The correlation of neutropenia with infection appears when the neutrophil counts fall below 500 cells/μL, and the risk of infection rises greatly when neutrophil count drops below 100 cells/μL or severe neutropenia lasts more than 5 days. Sepsis associated with neutropenia is the most common cause of death during chemotherapy. The availability of hematopoietic growth factors allows the administration of myelosuppressive agents with minimal myelosuppressive toxicity and rapid recovery, enhancing on-time administration of chemotherapy. Many drugs produce partial or total alopecia. Most produce some degree of nausea and vomiting, and some can produce oral and gastrointestinal mucositis, diarrhea, constipation, and peripheral neuropathy. Modern antiemetics have dramatically reduced the incidence and severity of nausea and vomiting. Many patients receiving chemotherapy report fatigue. Fatigue is often associated with anemia, which can sometimes be prevented or treated with erythropoietin administration. Recent reports suggested that erythropoiesis-stimulating agents adversely affect the survival of patients with breast cancer: their use in this disease is currently not indicated. Other important side effects of chemotherapy include ovarian ablation in premenopausal women, which brings with it the short- and long-term consequences of premature menopause and the development of infertility. Premature menopause leads to rapid loss of bone density and the development of osteoporosis.

Long-term side effects include a slight increase in the incidence of myelodysplastic syndromes and acute leukemias. Two types of chemotherapy-related myelodysplastic syndromes have been identified. One, which is related to large cumulative doses of alkylating agents, results in the development of acute hematologic malignancies 5 to 15 years after the initiation of therapy. Since long-term alkylating agent therapy is seldom used, this type of acute leukemia has become less common. A second syndrome, which is attributed to topoisomerase II inhibitors, has been reported to include development of myelomonocytic leukemia (M4, M5), mostly within 2 years after the initiation of therapy. This second syndrome has been reported with higher doses of doxorubicin or epirubicin, often in association with an alkylating agent and/or a hematopoietic growth factor. Since anthracycline-containing regimens represent the standard of care for both metastatic and primary breast cancer, this type of leukemia or myelodysplastic syndrome is more commonly seen today.

Targeted Therapies

The rapid expansion of our understanding of the biological changes that lead to malignant transformation and the growth-stimulatory and growth-inhibitory factors that influence this process led to the identification of a number of critical steps that can be targeted for therapeutic intervention.[255] Growth factors and their cognate receptors, intracellular signaling pathways, angiogenesis, the metastatic cascade, have all been recognized as potentially useful targets. A very large number of candidate therapeutics that focus on these putative targets is under preclinical and clinical evaluation. Among these, the type 1 growth factor receptor (human epidermal growth factor receptor or EGFR) family is in a prominent place. There are four members of this family: *EGFR* or *HER1*, *HER2*, *HER3*, and *HER4*. *EGFR* is often overexpressed in colorectal, lung and head and neck carcinomas, and less often (10% to 20%) in breast cancer. HER2 is amplified and/or overexpressed in about 20% to 30% of breast cancers. *HER3* and *HER4* are also found overexpressed, but they have been less extensively studied. *HER2* is a normal gene involved in growth regulation. When overexpressed, the cell surface receptors become constitutively activated, producing uninterrupted signaling that stimulates growth, invasion and metastasis.

The cause of overexpression is gene amplification in the great majority of breast cancers. Patients with *HER2*-overexpressing breast cancers have a higher rate of relapses and relapses tend to occur earlier than in patients with normal *HER2* expression. Mortality is also higher in patients with *HER2*-overexpressing breast cancer. A monoclonal antibody (trastuzumab, Herceptin) that binds to the extracellular domain of the HER2 protein was developed almost 18 years ago. This agent was shown to produce objective regressions in about 11% to 16% of patients with *HER2*-overexpressing breast cancers with extensive previous exposure to chemotherapy.[78] In previously untreated patients, the activity of the antibody was more pronounced, with response rates exceeding 25%. Trastuzumab has increased the response rate to anthracyclines, taxanes, vinorelbine and platinum salts. In combination with paclitaxel, docetaxel or the doxorubicin, AC combination, trastuzumab resulted in significant increases in response rate, time to progression, response duration and survival of patients with metastatic breast cancer in large randomized trials .[256,257] Pertuzumab is a different HER2-directed monoclonal antibody that is also effective against metastatic breast cancer.[258]

Several monoclonal antibodies and small molecules with inhibitory effects on the receptor tyrosine kinase have reached clinical development.[259] Dual inhibitors of HER1 and HER2 (such as lapatinib), inhibitors of protein farnesylation (tipifarnib), ERK-inhibitors, mTOR inhibitors (everolimus, temsirolimus), angiogenesis inhibitors (bevacizumab, sunitinib, sorafenib, and others), protein kinase C-inhibitors, cyclin and cyclin-dependent kinase inhibitors, inhibitors of the proteasome (bortezomib) and modulators of apoptosis are also in clinical development. Lapatinib, a dual inhibitor of EGFR and HER2, has completed phase 3 clinical evaluation in patients with metastatic breast cancer. Used as monotherapy, its activity appears similar to single-agent trastuzumab. In combination with capecitabine, it improves response rate and time to progression over chemotherapy alone.[118] Bevacizumab is a monoclonal antibody that targets the vascular endothelial growth factor (VEGF), and has shown significant clinical activity.[260] In monotherapy, it produces responses in 5% to 10% of heavily pretreated patients with metastatic breast cancer. In combination with paclitaxel, it improves response rate and time to progression (as it does in NSCLC, head and neck and colorectal cancers). Many other signaling inhibitors seem to have modest single-agent activity to date, and their clinical development emphasizes combinations with chemotherapy, radiotherapy or other biological agents. Currently, there is much interest in testing two- and three-drug biological combinations in an attempt to block multiple signaling pathways, or the same pathway in multiple steps. The combination of trastuzumab and bevacizumab produced objective response rates in excess of 50%, and combinations of trastuzumab with lapatinib, lapatinib and pazopanib, trastuzumab and pertuzumab and many others are under careful evaluation. There is also much interest in developing combinations of signaling inhibitors with cytotoxic drugs, hormones or other targeted interventions.

Systemic Adjuvant Therapy

Early Trials

One of the most important advances in oncology came out of the acceptance of evidence that most patients with primary, lymph node-positive breast cancer, and many of those without lymph node involvement, have disseminated tumor at the time of diagnosis and that increased survival results only from effective systemic therapy used in conjunction with surgical therapy and radiation. This concept led to a major conceptual shift of the biology of breast cancer and to the implementation of clinical trials to evaluate the efficacy of systemic treatment regimens as adjuncts to operation.

Ashworth made the earliest observation of tumor cells in the blood in 1869. In 1955, Fisher and Turnbull, and Engell reported the presence of tumor cells in the blood of cancer patients and a surge of interest ensued. Following reports of favorable effects of chemotherapeutic agents on the destruction of disseminated tumor cells in experimental animals, a rationale for embarking on clinical trials of adjuvant therapy was established. As a result of experimental findings, in 1958, under the auspices of the NIH Cancer Chemotherapy National Service Center, the NSABP initiated a trial to determine the efficacy of administering chemotherapy in addition to cancer surgery with curative intent to decrease recurrence and to extend the survival of patients with breast cancer. It was anticipated that such a therapeutic regimen could destroy the tumor cells dislodged into the blood and lymph during surgical manipulation. Participants were treated by either radical mastectomy and triethylene thiophosphoramide (thiotepa) or by radical mastectomy and placebo. Thiotepa was administered at the time of operation and on each of the first 2 postoperative days. The results reported in 1968 indicated a significant increase in the 5-year survival of premenopausal women who received thiotepa. The difference, which was seen only in patients with four or more positive axillary nodes, persisted after 10 years of follow-up. Thus, it was demonstrated for the first time that the natural history of some breast cancer patients could be altered by systemic therapy.

In the 1960s, new concepts were formulated that led to a second generation of chemotherapy trials. The first of this second generation of clinical trials, conducted jointly by the NSABP and the Eastern Cooperative Oncology Group (ECOG) demonstrated that the use of L-phenylalanine mustard (L-Pam) administered orally for 24 months after radical mastectomy to patients with positive nodes could prolong the disease-free interval of patients. Extended follow-up (more than 20 years) has demonstrated not only a significant prolongation of disease-free survival but also a significant benefit in the overall survival of premenopausal patients with the use of this single agent.[261] A similar trend, initially observed in postmenopausal women, was not sustained. Women taking L-Pam reported minimal undesirable side effects; mild nausea and vomiting occurred in about one-third of the patients. In 1973, a second clinical trial begun at the Instituto Nazionale Tumori in Milan demonstrated the effectiveness of a three-drug combination, cyclophosphamide, methotrexate, and 5-fluorouracil (CMF) as an adjuvant to mastectomy: a significant reduction in treatment failure occurred in all subgroups of patients treated with CMF. About two-thirds of patients experienced some toxicity, indicated by nausea, vomiting, anorexia, alopecia, cystitis, or amenorrhea. The 20-year results from the Milan trial continue to indicate a benefit in premenopausal, but not postmenopausal, women.[262]

Over the next 25 years, over 200 controlled clinical trials were initiated to extend the earlier results, define optimal adjuvant systemic therapy, and evaluate a variety of newer treatment regimens. To summarize these results, the NIH organized three consensus development conferences.[143] In addition, the Early Breast Cancer Trialists Collaborative Group (EBCTCG) performed several meta-analyses of all (published and unpublished) prospective randomized trials designed and conducted for operable primary breast cancer.[263] Review of the consensus documents and the reports of the EBCTCG's meta-analyses shows the continuous evolution of this field, based on the maturation of clinical trial results and the availability of new data. The information obtained from the individual clinical trials, the consensus process, and the meta-analyses can be summarized as follows:

1. Adjuvant chemotherapy effectively reduces the risk of recurrence and death from breast cancer.
2. Combination chemotherapy is more effective than single-agent chemotherapy.
3. Adjuvant chemotherapy is more effective for women younger than 50 years of age than for older women, but significant benefit is observed in women in all age groups in which chemotherapy has been adequately evaluated.
4. Adjuvant anthracycline-containing regimens are more effective than other combinations lacking an anthracycline. This is particularly true for regimens that use three or more drugs and are given for longer than four cycles.
5. Adjuvant chemotherapy for longer than 6 months with the same regimen is not more effective than chemotherapy for 6 months.
6. The addition of taxanes to adjuvant chemotherapy regimens significantly improves relapse-free and overall survival rates.
7. The administration of chemotherapy with doxorubicin, cyclophosphamide and paclitaxel with hematopoietic growth factor support at 2-week intervals instead of the conventional 3-week intervals significantly improved relapse-free and overall survival rates.
8. Adjuvant tamoxifen effectively reduces the risk of recurrence and death from breast cancer. This effect is similar for patients in all.
9. Adjuvant tamoxifen is effective only in patients with ER-positive and/or PR-positive breast cancer.
10. The efficacy of adjuvant tamoxifen increases with longer duration of therapy. At this time, data indicate that the optimal duration of adjuvant tamoxifen is 5 years.
11. Adjuvant tamoxifen significantly reduces the incidence of new or contralateral breast cancers.
12. Adjuvant ovarian ablation effectively reduces the risk of recurrence and death from breast cancer.
13. Adjuvant ovarian ablation is effective only for premenopausal women.
14. Adjuvant gonadotrophin (LHRH) analogs produce reversible ovarian function suppression equivalent to surgical ovarian ablation.
15. Adjuvant gonadotrophin (LHRH) analogs produce reductions in odds of recurrence and death similar to six cycles of adjuvant CMF chemotherapy.
16. Adjuvant gonadotrophin (LHRH) analogs combined with tamoxifen for five years produce greater reduction in odds of recurrence and death than six cycles of CMF chemotherapy.
17. Adjuvant anastrozole or letrozole is more effective and better tolerated than adjuvant tamoxifen in postmenopausal women.
18. After receiving 5 years of adjuvant tamoxifen, crossover to letrozole for another 5 years significantly improves relapse-free survival and reduces the risk of second primary breast cancer.
19. After receiving 2 to 3 years of adjuvant tamoxifen, cross-over to anastrozole or exemestane for another 2 to 3 years significantly improves relapse-free survival and reduces the risk of second primary breast cancer compared to continuing tamoxifen until completing 5 years of therapy. For patients with positive lymph nodes crossover to exemestane was associated with a significant improvement in survival.
20. The combination of tamoxifen and adjuvant chemotherapy is more effective than chemotherapy alone or tamoxifen alone for patients with hormone receptor-positive tumors.
21. For optimal results, chemotherapy and tamoxifen should not be administered simultaneously. Rather, chemotherapy followed by tamoxifen appears to be appropriate.
22. Patients with steroid hormone receptor negative tumors benefit from chemotherapy to a greater extent than those with receptor positive tumors.
23. Patients with HER2-positive breast cancer benefit substantially from the concomitant or sequential addition of trastuzumab to adjuvant chemotherapy.

The report of the fourth EBCTCG meta-analysis, conducted in the fall of 2000, included 102 chemotherapy clinical trials (53,353 women), 21 ovarian ablation trials (11,313 women), and 71 tamoxifen trials (80,273 women).[263] The fifth meta-analysis confirmed and extended the conclusions derived from earlier analyses. In addition, it determined that high-dose chemotherapy significantly reduced the odds of recurrence by about 14%, breast cancer mortality by about 8%, but a five-fold increase in non-breast cancer deaths; this resulted in no significant gain in overall mortality. An independent meta-analysis confirmed these findings.[264] The EBCTCG meta-analysis also demonstrated a 23% reduction in the odds of recurrence and a 17% reduction in odds of death from the addition of a taxane to anthracycline-based chemotherapy. Finally, the meta-analysis also demonstrated an 11% reduction in odds of death for aromatase inhibitors compared to tamoxifen. The results of adjuvant chemotherapy trials are summarized on Table 104-13. The summary of adjuvant endocrine therapy trials is found on Table 104-14.

Thirty-five to 85% of patients with lymph node-positive breast cancer will develop metastatic or recurrent breast cancer after optimal loco-regional therapy in the absence of systemic treatments. Tumor recurrence and death due to breast cancer affects a significant percentage of the patients with lymph node-negative breast cancer. In one study, treatment failed in approximately 25%, and 15% died during 5 years of follow-up. Unpublished data from other studies indicate that treatment failed in 43% of the patients; 32% had died by 10 years of follow-up. A review of the literature

Table 104-13 Comparative Efficacy of Adjuvant Chemotherapy Regimens

Therapies	% Reduction in Annual Odds of Recurrence	p	Death	p
CT vs no CT (CMF vs Nil)	23.5	<.00001	17	<.00001
Doxorubicin vs no doxorubicin	12-30	.006	11-35	.02
Taxane vs no taxane	19	<.00001	17	<.00001

Table 104-14 Comparative Efficacy of Adjuvant Hormonal Therapies

Therapies	% Reduction in Annual Odds of Recurrence	p	Death	p
Tamoxifen vs no tamoxifen	50	<.00001	33	<.00001
AI vs tamoxifen	19-22	.007	8	>.1
Tamoxifen × 5 years □ AI	43	.00008	18	.3
Tamoxifen × 2-3 years □ AI	32-64	<.006	21	.004

suggests that with longer follow-up, even patients with small (<1 cm), node-negative tumors have reported recurrence rates ranging up to 20% by 10 years, depending on specific tumor characteristics.[265]

The 1990 NIH consensus conference recommended the routine administration of adjuvant systemic therapy to women with high-risk histologically negative axillary nodes based on newer data.[266-268] High-risk patients include those with tumors larger than 1 cm, high grade, hormone receptor-negativity, high proliferative rates and those with lymphovascular invasion. Subsequent trials have demonstrated that regimens effective for patients with lymph node-positive tumors are also effective for those without lymph node involvement.

Endocrine Therapy

Tamoxifen Starting more than 20 years ago, multiple randomized, controlled trials demonstrated that tamoxifen, 10 to 20 mg twice a day, resulted in about a 50% reduction in odds of recurrence in patients with ER-positive tumors, regardless of age and lymph node status.[263,268] Several individual trials, and the Oxford meta-analysis also reported a significant survival benefit ($p = .0001$). The tamoxifen-treated patients had fewer locoregional and distant metastases. Of particular interest was the reduction by 58% in ipsilateral breast tumor recurrences in patients treated by lumpectomy and breast irradiation and the reduction by 40% in the number of contralateral breast cancers when tamoxifen was administered. Clinical trials testing different durations of tamoxifen concluded that 5 years were superior to shorter durations, while durations exceeding 5 years were not superior to 5 years. There is compelling evidence to limit the use of tamoxifen to patients with ER-positive and/or PR-positive tumors.[268] A number of retrospective analyses have shown that patients with *HER2/neu* overexpression have associated resistance to hormonal therapy. While this observation was initially limited to tamoxifen, it appears to apply to all endocrine agents. Patients with ER-positive and *HER2/neu*-positive tumors, express much lower levels of ER, and ongoing cross-talk between growth factor signaling pathways and the ER-pathway have been amply documented.

Evidence from the EBCTCG meta-analysis and from large randomized trials showed that tamoxifen combined with chemotherapy provides more effective systemic adjuvant treatment to patients with hormone receptor-positive breast cancer than either tamoxifen alone or chemotherapy alone.[268] Recent reports have indicated, however, that the benefit from chemotherapy is greater for patients with ER-negative breast cancer compared to those with ER-positive tumors. Furthermore, there is emerging information to suggest that patients with strongly ER-positive tumors that are well differentiated derive only marginal benefit from chemotherapy, while the effects of chemotherapy are greater for women with ER-negative or weakly positive tumors.[269] SWOG trial S8814 (Intergroup 0100) randomized 1477 patients with hormone receptor–positive breast cancer to receive either tamoxifen alone, concurrent tamoxifen and CAF, or sequential CAF followed by tamoxifen. At a median follow-up of 8.5 years, 8-year disease-free survival (DFS) estimates were 67% for sequential CAF followed by tamoxifen and 62% for concurrent CAF plus tamoxifen ($p = .045$).[270] The 10-year estimated DFS rates were 60%, 53% and 48% for the same three groups ($p = .002$)[271] The 10-year overall survival rates were 68%, 62% and 60% for the sequential, simultaneous and tamoxifen alone arms, respectively ($p = .05$). Both FAC plus tamoxifen arms were superior to tamoxifen alone. There were no differences in toxicity between the two combination arms. These results would indicate that the sequential administration of chemotherapy followed by tamoxifen would be the preferred strategy.

Toxicity Although hot flashes, vaginal discharge, and irregular menses occurred more often in tamoxifen-treated patients than in those given placebo, the differences were not as pronounced as might have been thought if the placebo control had not been present. Thromboembolic events were more frequent in the tamoxifen-treated than in the placebo-treated group (1.3% vs 0.1%, $p < .001$). Pulmonary embolism occurred in 6 of 1422 tamoxifen treated patients versus in 1 of 1439 placebo-treated women ($p = .06$). This excess in thromboembolic complications associated with tamoxifen administration has also been reported in other large controlled trials. Some investigators have reported an increased risk of thromboembolic complications when tamoxifen and chemotherapy are administered simultaneously. Second primary tumors other than endometrial carcinomas occurred equally in the two groups. Liver, gastrointestinal, urinary tract, and non-uterine genital cancers were not increased by tamoxifen treatment.

The relationship of tamoxifen administration to the development of endometrial cancer was investigated retrospectively in several randomized clinical trials. In one of the largest adjuvant tamoxifen trials a 7.5 RR for endometrial cancer was reported in the tamoxifen group, compared to placebo. Subsequent trials indicated a more modest increase in risk. In addition, most cases were of good-to-moderate histologic grade and deaths from endometrial cancer occurred in 4 of 23 women. The cumulative hazard rate for endometrial cancer was 6.3 per 1000 patients. Including all reported endometrial cancers, the annual hazard rate through all follow-up was 0.2 per 1000 in the placebo-treated group and 0.6 per 1000 in the randomized, tamoxifen-treated group. Using population-based rates of endometrial cancer from SEER data, the RRs would be 2.2. The 5-year cumulative hazard rate for relapse from breast or endometrial cancer in the randomized tamoxifen group was 38% lower than that in the placebo group.

Additional information about the risk of developing endometrial cancer for patients receiving tamoxifen can be derived from the results of the BCPT.[72] After a median time on study of 47.7 months, 36 invasive endometrial cancers were reported on the tamoxifen arm, compared to 15 on the placebo arm. The RR was 4 for patients 50 years of age or older, whereas there was no detectable increase in risk for younger women

Although the risk of endometrial cancer increases after tamoxifen therapy, the net benefit vis-à vis breast cancer greatly outweighs the risk. Endometrial cancers occurring after tamoxifen therapy do not appear to be of a different type or of a worse prognosis than such tumors in patients who have not received tamoxifen. The excess risk essentially disappeared after completion of tamoxifen therapy.

Adjuvant Ovarian Ablation

Ovarian ablation lowers the odds of recurrence and death by amounts that are quantitatively similar to those produced by chemotherapy, a benefit that is restricted to premenopausal women.[272] Ovarian ablation is not commonly employed as adjuvant therapy in the United States, however, largely because adjuvant chemotherapy produces a chemical ovarian ablation in the majority of patients anyway and because there is fear of the long-term effects of the premature menopause caused by ovarian ablation. A direct comparison of ovarian ablation and CMF chemotherapy in premenopausal women with primary breast cancer suggested equivalence of the two interventions. Further analysis indicated that for patients with ER-positive tumors, ovarian ablation was significantly more effective than CMF, whereas for patients with ER-negative breast cancer, CMF produced higher disease-free rates. The combination of chemotherapy and tamoxifen appears to provide superior disease control to patients with hormone receptor–positive breast cancer. However, the data in support of the superiority of the combination of chemotherapy and ovarian ablation for women under the age of 50 years are much less compelling.[272] A nonsignificant trend in some studies suggests that the combination of ovarian ablation and chemotherapy might be superior to chemotherapy alone for premenopausal women with ER-positive tumors. Additional studies to clarify the role of combined hormone therapy and chemotherapy are ongoing in this population.

The introduction of luteinizing hormone-releasing hormone (LHRH) analogs has also created new treatment opportunities.[248] In metastatic breast cancer, the efficacy of LHRH analogs has been validated: Their efficacy is similar to surgical or radiotherapy-induced ovarian ablation. An international group of investigators recently reported the results of a prospective randomized trial comparing the efficacy and tolerability of goserelin with IV CMF in premenopausal women with node-positive breast cancer.[273] After a median survival of 6 years, 42% of 1640 women reported an event. In the subgroup with ER-positive tumors, the two treatments were equivalent ($p = .94$). As expected, in the ER-negative group, CMF was therapeutically superior to goserelin ($p = .0006$).

Another randomized trial included 2631 premenopausal patients in a comparison of standard adjuvant therapy, with or without goserelin (ZIPP trial). With follow-up approaching 8 years, a trend favoring the goserelin arm approached statistical significance ($p = .08$). The Cancer Research Campaign conducted a trial comparing tamoxifen to goserelin and to the combination of tamoxifen and goserelin; the International Breast Cancer Study Group (IBCSG VIII) compared goserelin to CMF, and to CMF followed by goserelin; and the North American Intergroup has completed a randomized trial comparing CAF to CAF plus goserelin, and to CAF plus goserelin plus tamoxifen. These studies and others assessing the contribution of LHRH analogs alone or in combination with chemotherapy and/or tamoxifen will provide important guidance for the treatment of premenopausal patients with primary breast cancer. There are three important randomized trials assessing the place of LHRH analogs in the management of ER-positive premenopausal breast cancer. Known by their acronyms, the SOFT, TEXT and PERCHE trials were intended to determine whether the combination of an LHRH analog and tamoxifen or an aromatase inhibitor is superior to tamoxifen alone for chemotherapy treated patients (SOFT), whether an LHRH analog and exemestane is superior to the LHRH analog plus tamoxifen, regardless of prior exposure to chemotherapy (TEXT) and whether chemotherapy adds to optimal combination endocrine therapy (PERCHE). These three studies represent a major international effort conducted in Europe, North America and several other regions of the world. While the SOFT trial has recruited about 50% of the intended population, the TEXT and PERCHE trials closed prematurely due to poor accrual.

Aromatase Inhibitors

Third-generation, selective AIs have potent effects on enzyme activity and reduce estrogen production in postmenopausal women by more than 90%. The updated (100 month) results of the Arimidex, Tamoxifen, Alone or in Combination (ATAC) trial (n = 9366) showed that, after 8 years of follow up, adjuvant anastrozole was significantly superior to tamoxifen in therapeutic efficacy and tolerance in a group of post-menopausal patients with positive or negative nodes.[274,275] Anastrozole was associated with a 15% relative reduction in risk of recurrences, a figure even greater for patients with ER-positive tumors. There was also a significant, 40% reduction in second primary breast cancers compared to the group of patients treated with tamoxifen. No survival differences were reported. Anastrozole was associated with fewer side effects than tamoxifen, although there were more fractures with anastrozole than with tamoxifen. Analysis after a median follow-up of 100 months confirmed the increased separation of the relapse-free survival curves. The absolute difference in recurrences at 9 years was 4.8%, and the carryover effect of anastrozole in years 5 to 9 was about 50%. Similar data were reported from a large clinical trial comparing letrozole to tamoxifen in patients with primary breast cancer (BIG1-98).

The Canadian MA-17 trial randomized postmenopausal patients with ER-positive breast cancer who had completed 5 years of adjuvant tamoxifen to 5 additional years of adjuvant letrozole or placebo.[276] After two and a half years of median follow-up, a 43% reduction in events was observed (HR: 0. 57, 0.43–0.75, $p = .00008$). One year later, a significant survival benefit was reported for patients with positive lymph nodes. Another international group of investigators reported the results of a randomized trial of over 4400 postmenopausal patients with ER-positive breast cancer who had completed 2 to 3 years of adjuvant tamoxifen. At that stage, they were randomly assigned to complete 5 years of tamoxifen or cross over to exemestane for the remainder of the 5 years.[277] After a 42-month median follow-up, there was a 32% reduction in recurrences ($p = .00005$) as well as a significant reduction in contralateral breast cancers, and a trend for a reduction in breast cancer deaths ($p = .08$). A smaller, Italian study of identical design using anastrozole and the combined analysis of an Austrian and a German clinical trial of very similar design provided confirmatory evidence in favor of a crossover to an aromatase inhibitor (anastrozole in these three trials) compared to continued tamoxifen therapy. A recent meta-analysis of all randomized trials comparing adjuvant aromatase inhibitors to no aromatase inhibitors indicated a highly significant disease-free advantage for the aromatase inhibitors and a significant survival improvement. Thus, evidence is overwhelming that a selective aromatase inhibitor must form part of adjuvant endocrine therapy for postmenopausal women with ER and/or PR-positive breast cancer.[278] Whether starting with an aromatase inhibitor is better than crossing over after some time on adjuvant tamoxifen remains to be established. Two large international trials (BIG1-98 and TEAM) will determine whether sequential administration of tamoxifen and AIs is superior to upfront AI administration. Similarly, the role of aromatase inhibitors in the management of premenopausal women with hormone-responsive breast cancer is currently under evaluation in the SOFT trial. An additional trial addressing the role of selective aromatase inhibitors in premenopausal women was reported at the 2008 ASCO meeting by the Austrian

Breast Cancer Trials Group (ABCSG). There were 1801 premenopausal patients with primary breast cancer treated with goserelin for three years in the ABCSG-12 trial. These patients were randomly assigned to receive tamoxifen or anastrozole in this trial. There were no differences in disease-free or overall survival after 60 months of median follow-up. The optimal duration of treatment with aromatase inhibitors is unknown and whether aromatase should be given sequentially or simultaneously with chemotherapy remains to be determined.

Primary Tumors Smaller Than 1 cm

In an ECOG/Intergroup trial, patients with primary tumors <1 cm in largest diameter had a 75% 10-year disease-free survival rate and a 79% overall survival rate. However, other investigators have reported markedly superior survival figures for patients with primary tumors <1 cm and negative nodes, especially patients with tumors < 0.5 cm, negative nodes, and no other unfavorable prognostic indicators.[279] These observations prompted the analysis of data from five NSABP trials that focused on the prognosis of patients with node-negative tumors <1 cm in largest diameter and the therapeutic effect of chemotherapy or hormonal therapy. One thousand, two hundred and fifty-nine patients were identified among the population registered in protocols B-06, B-13, B-14, B-19, and B-20.[280] Relapse-free survival rates were available at 8 years for the 1024 patients with ER-negative tumors. They were 81% for those treated with surgery and 90% for those who received chemotherapy after surgery ($p = .06$). The 8-year relapse-free survival rates for women with ER-positive tumors treated with surgery alone, surgery plus tamoxifen and surgery, tamoxifen and chemotherapy were 86%, 93%, and 95%, respectively ($p = .01$ and .07). The authors concluded that even for this highly selected group of patients with favorable prognosis, the relapse rates were higher than previously reported and no subset could be identified that would not benefit from treatment.

A review of T1a,bN0M0 breast cancer cases registered in the Surveillance, Epidemiology, and End Results (SEER) Program between 1988 and 2001 was recently reported to investigate the impact of prognostic factors on breast cancer-specific (BCSM) and non-breast cancer-related mortality. The investigators identified 57,830 patients with a median follow-up of 56 months (range 0-167 months).[87] Ten-year probabilities of overall mortality and breast cancer specific mortality were 24% and 4%, respectively. High grade, hormone receptor-negative status and age <50 years were associated with increased rates of treatment failure and breast cancer deaths. The reports of the SEER program and several single-institution reports also highlight the excellent prognosis of patients with special, favorable histologic subgroups: those with pure tubular or mucinous carcinomas. Clearly, there are subgroups of patients with excellent prognosis for whom the benefit from adjuvant chemotherapy (and even tamoxifen) might be so minimal as to be matched or exceeded by the risk of serious or life-threatening toxicity of the interventions. The challenge is to develop reproducible methods to identify such patients prospectively. One such approach was recently developed utilizing an RTPCR assay based on 21 genes related to the ER, proliferation, HER2 and several stromal proteases.[80] When this assay was performed on paraffin-embedded tissue blocks from patients who participated in several NSABP clinical trials for node-negative breast cancer, the results identified three prognostic subgroups of patients. About 50% of patients fell in the low-risk category with an estimated 10-year relapse rate of 6.8% when treated with adjuvant tamoxifen. This would suggest that about half of the patients with node-negative breast cancer have a low enough risk of recurrence to spare them the rigors of adjuvant chemotherapy. Subsequent extensions of the evaluation of this assay demonstrated that the benefits of tamoxifen were much greater in the low-risk group and those of chemotherapy in the high-risk group. This assay (Oncotype Dx) was recently applied to paraffin embedded samples of patients with hormone receptor-positive, lymph node-positive breast cancer who participated in a Southwest Oncology Group randomized trail comparing adjuvant tamoxifen to tamoxifen plus chemotherapy with a three-drug regimen (CAF). The Recurrence Score separated three distinct prognostic groups, with a 10-year disease-free survival probabililty of 60%, 49%. and 43% for low, intermediate. and high recurrence score, respectively, after tamoxifen treatment. The benefit from the addition of chemotherapy was clear in the high and intermediate Recurrence Score groups, but not detectable in the low Recurrence Score group. This assay, which is FDA approved and commercially available, is currently being validated in a large, prospective, multicenter, randomized trial led by the Eastern Cooperative Oncology Group to validate its clinical utility (TailoRx trial). Two other assays based on gene expression microarray technology were developed by investigators from Amsterdam and Rotterdam, respectively.[105,107] Based on 76 and 70 genes, respectively, both assays can identify good-prognosis and poor-prognosis groups among patients with lymph node-negative breast cancer. The Amsterdam gene profile (Mammaprint), is also FDA approved and commercially available, and it is under validation in a large, international, multicenter randomized trial (MINDACT Trial) led by the Breast International Group or BIG. The mammaprint assay requires fresh or frozen tissue. These various assays bring us one step closer to personalized medicine, and in addition to identifying patients with such excellent prognosis as to justify foregoing systemic adjuvant therapies, they might help to identify those tumors that do and those that do not benefit with currently used chemotherapy regimens.

Although tamoxifen is successful in reducing local recurrence and distant disease in all categories evaluated, the proportionate reduction remains constant. Therefore, the likelihood of real clinical benefit diminishes as prognosis in general improves. With extremely small and favorable tumors, the use of systemic adjuvant therapies has as much rationale for prevention of new primary cancers as it does for treatment of the index cancer. Until new answers come from ongoing clinical trials, it is probably best in practice to review the available data with each patient concerning whether to use systemic therapy because of their putative "good" prognosis. The Oncotype DX and Mammaprint assays are now available to refine estimates of individual risk and benefit. One reported validation of the Mammaprint assay demonstrated that this gene expression profile based assay was superior to the Adjuvantonline! software available on the Internet for prediction of prognosis.[107]

The use of tamoxifen and other hormonal treatments is not recommended for women with ER-negative tumors.[268]

The routine use of biological markers, such as the estrogen and progesterone receptors and HER2, as well as information derived from gene expression microarrays identifies three distinct types of breast cancer: (1) Hormone-receptor positive, HER2-negative (also referred to as Luminal A subtype), (2) HER2-positive (also referred to as HER2-like), and (3) triple receptor-negative (sometimes referred to as basal-like), These three clinical entities have different clinical courses, risk of recurrence or death after standard treatment and respond differently to available systemic therapies. Therefore, their identification at the time of diagnosis is critical to plan optimal combined modality therapy, especially to select the most effective systemic treatments. Patients with hormone receptor-positive, HER2-negative breast cancer have tumors that are highly sensitive to endocrine treatment: SERMs, AIs, LHRH analogs, etc. The most important systemic treatment for these patients is endocrine therapy, selected on the basis of age and menopausal status. Thus, premenopausal women would benefit the most from tamoxifen (or other SERMs) or ovarian ablation/suppression, or a combination of both. Postmenopausal women with hormone receptor-positive, HER2-negative breast cancer would derive optimal benefit from aromatase inhibitors and SERMs. Large randomized trials and the Oxford meta-analysis have repeatedly shown that patients with hormone receptor-positive tumors derive additional (incremental) benefit from chemotherapy added to tamoxifen or ovarian ablation. More recently, retrospective subset analyses of clinical trials and genomic assays (Oncotype DX and Mammaprint) have suggested that not all patients in this category benefit equally (or perhaps at all) from the addition of chemotherapy to tamoxifen. Ongoing prospective trials will define whether some patients with hormone receptor-positive breast cancer have chemotherapy-unresponsive disease and whether the above mentioned assays (or others being developed) can identify them in a reliable manner. Retrospective review of three cooperative group trials suggested that the benefit from taxane therapy was limited to patients with HER2-positive, ER-negative breast cancers.[281] However, other reports suggest that both ER-positive and ER-negative tumors benefit from taxane treatment.[282,283]

Patients with HER2-positive breast cancer should have a HER2-directed agent (trastuzumab or lapatinib) as the basis of their treatment. These tumors are also substantially chemotherapy sensitive and benefit from treatment with anthracyclines, taxanes, vinca alkaloids and platinum salts. Randomized trials have shown that combined therapy with chemotherapy and HER2-directed therapy produces higher response rates, longer time to progression, and in some trials, superior survival to chemotherapy alone or HER2-directed therapy alone.[256] Whether some combinations are superior to others remains to be established. Suggestive (but not compelling) evidence indicates that continued suppression of HER2 signaling leads to better outcome.

Patients with HER2-positive, hormone receptor-positive tumors have relative resistance to endocrine therapy; this endocrine resistance can be partially overcome with simultaneous blockade of HER2 and the ER (eg, trastuzumab and tamoxifen or an AI). There is also emerging information suggesting that HER2-positive, hormone receptor-positive tumors might be less responsive to lapatinib than HER2-positive, hormone receptor-negative tumors. There is no data about the effect of ER expression on sensitivity to trastuzumab.

Chemotherapy is considered the treatment of choice for patients with triple receptor-negative breast cancer. This is a heterogeneous group of tumors that includes most *BRCA1*-mutated breast cancer, many *p53*-mutated tumors, neoplasms with extensive metaplastic changes and the *claudin*-low subgroup. While all these subgroups share the triple-receptor negative phenotype, they are poorly characterized and much additional investigation is needed to understand the differences and commonalities between the subgroups. Triple receptor-negative breast cancers are by and large highly responsive to standard chemotherapy, although they tend to relapse and die early. *BRCA1* and *p53* mutations are associated with increased sensitivity to platinum salts and somewhat decreased responsiveness to taxanes. *BRCA1*-mutated tumors are also exquisitely sensitive to PARP-inhibitors.

Although the magnitude of the benefit from chemotherapy is greater for younger women, significant reduction in risk of recurrence and death has been documented for women up to age 69 years. Furthermore, a recent retrospective review of four CALGB trials including women up to age 79 indicated that there was no association between age and disease-free survival .[284] The authors concluded that "age alone should not be a contraindication to the use of optimal chemotherapy regimens in older women who are in good general health."

For the first decade of routine use of adjuvant chemotherapy, CMF was broadly employed as the chemotherapeutic regimen of choice. For the past 10-15 years, anthracycline-containing combinations have become more commonly employed and the *de facto* standard of care. Several prospective randomized trials comparing doxorubicin (or epirubicin)–containing regimens versus non–anthracycline-containing regimens in the adjuvant setting for node-positive and also node-negative breast cancer, and the meta-analysis of all randomized trials, have concluded that anthracycline-containing regimens have superior efficacy.[263] Further analysis of existing randomized trials indicated that those anthracycline-containing regimens that included three or more drugs (FAC, CAF, FEC) have demonstrated superiority over CMF, whereas the doxorubicin, AC combination was equivalent to CMF.[285] Whether these differences in the various regimens are related to the additional drugs or the longer duration of therapy common to three-drug regimens are questions currently being investigated in clinical trials.

HER2/neu overexpression has been associated with increased relapse rates after adjuvant therapy, and apparent relative resistance to certain types of cytotoxic treatment—for instance, the CMF regimen. Several retrospective analyses of prospective clinical trials have suggested that patients with HER2/neu overexpressing breast cancer benefit more from treatment with an anthracycline than with the CMF regimen. However, preclinical studies do not show that HER2-amplification or overexpression alters sensitivity to anthracyclines. Rather, it has been hypothesized that, since topoisomerase II is one of the major targets of the anthracyclines, its presence on the short arm of chromosome 17, close to the amplicon that contains *HER2* could explain the association between *HER2*-amplification and increased sensitivity to anthracycline therapy. Some investigators have presented data that supports co-amplification of *HER2* and topoisomerase II. Others, however, have been unable to confirm a correlation between topoisomerase II amplification and sensitivity to anthracyclines.[286]

NSABP protocol B-15 suggested that AC would be preferable to CMF.[287] Although of shorter duration and in general easier to administer than six cycles of CMF, this regimen is not more effective. Bonadonna and colleagues compared, in a randomized trial in high-risk patients, sequential administration of doxorubicin at 75 mg/m^2 for four courses followed by IV CMF for eight courses with alternating chemotherapy (two courses of IV CMF followed by one course of Adriamycin), for a total of 12 courses.[288] Results of this study after a median follow-up of 17 years demonstrated a significant improvement in disease-free survival with the sequential regimen versus the alternating regimen. This difference was translated into a significant difference in survival (Fig. 104-25). Similar results were reported by other groups with sequential, non-cross-resistant chemotherapy. The Milan trial was an important clinical confirmation for the Norton-Simon hypothesis (as distinct from the Goldie-Coldman hypothesis) and stimulated the design of a later cooperative group trial (C9741).

The clinical evaluation of taxanes (paclitaxel [Taxol] and docetaxel [Taxotere]) in patients with metastatic breast cancer indicated that both agents have marked antitumor activity. Both taxanes retain a high degree of activity in anthracycline-resistant tumors. The results of several clinical trials incorporating the taxanes into adjuvant systemic therapy of high-risk primary breast cancer indicated a highly significant improvement in relapse-free survival and overall survival at 7 years. The benefit of adding paclitaxel appeared greater for patients

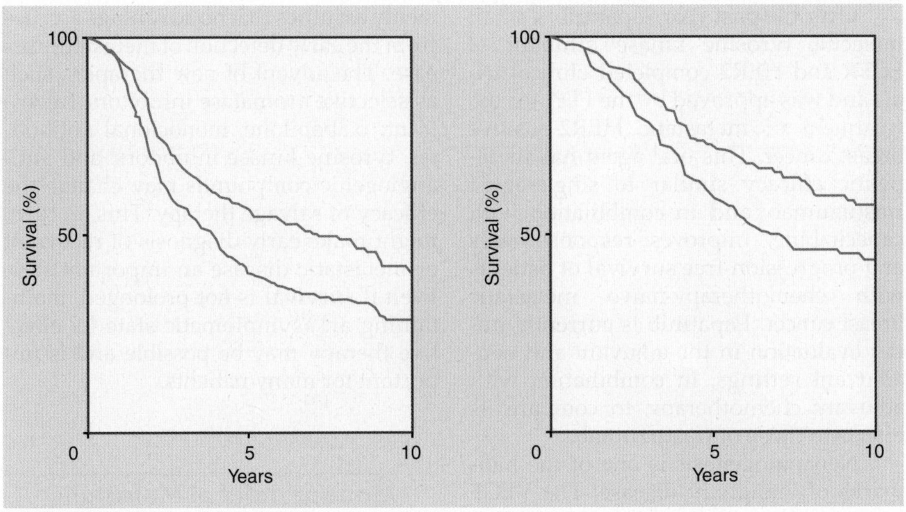

Figure 104-25 Disease-free (left panel) and overall survival (right panel) of patients with more than three metastatic nodes, who were less than 70 years old. They received four courses of moderately high-dose doxorubicin followed by eight cycles of CMF (purple line), or two courses of CMF alternating with a cycle of doxorubicin four times (blue line). This is the best example so far of a comparison of the Norton-Simon hypothesis and the Goldie-Coldman hypothesis. *Source:* From Ref. 288.

with ER-negative breast cancer than for those with ER-positive tumors.[269] However, this was not confirmed in several docetaxel-containing trials.[283] Taxanes improve outcome of adjuvant therapy whether included concomitantly or sequentially with anthracycline-based regimens. A large randomized trial evaluating the contributions of either paclitaxel or docetaxel to the management of primary breast cancer was recently reported. ECOG protocol E1199 randomized patients with operable breast cancer and positive (or high-risk negative) axillary nodes to receive four cycles of AC followed by four cycles of paclitaxel or docetaxel administered at three-week intervals or the same drugs given weekly for 12 weeks.[289] More than 5000 patients were registered. After 5 years of follow-up, a significant difference in relapse-free survival favoring the weekly paclitaxel arm was observed. Docetaxel every 3 weeks was also significantly better than three-weekly paclitaxel. Weekly paclitaxel resulted in a significant prolongation of overall survival.

Taxanes have been included into neoadjuvant chemotherapy in multiple clinical trials. These trials demonstrated that the addition of taxanes significantly increased overall and pathological complete response rates, reducing the extent of residual disease in the breast and regional lymph nodes.

Dose Modulation of Chemotherapy for Patients With Positive Axillary Nodes

Among the hypotheses formulated to design more effective adjuvant treatment strategies, the contention that inadequate drug dose administration is a major factor responsible for the failure to achieve a greater therapeutic effect in responsive tumors led to several important clinical trials.

In 1984, Hryniuk and Bush presented arguments for recognizing the importance of dose intensity in the use of chemotherapy for metastatic breast cancer. They defined dose intensity as the amount of drug administered per unit of time, expressing intensity as milligrams per square meter per week using a single-drug regimen. They concluded that the higher the dose intensity, the higher would be the remission rate of patients with advanced breast cancer. Results from several randomized trials were considered to support the Hryniuk thesis. A prospectively randomized trial conducted by Tannock and colleagues to test the relationship between two dose levels of CMF and the remission rate in patients with advanced breast cancer significantly favored the standard rather than the half-dose regimen.

Using the same approaches that they employed for evaluating dose intensity in advanced disease, Hryniuk and his associates concluded in 1986 that, as in advanced disease, dose intensity of adjuvant chemotherapy correlated with relapse-free survival, and that this correlation was independent of the number of positive nodes or menopausal status.

The CALGB conducted a study comparing three dose-levels of the CAF regimen administered for 4 or 6 months. The results from the study indicated a significant difference in the 3-year disease-free survival between the high or moderate-dose groups and the low-dose group (high-dose group, 75 ± 2%; moderate-dose group, 70 ± 3%; low-dose group, 64 ± 3%; $p < .00001$). A subsequent CALGB study demonstrated no improvement in outcomes when doxorubicin (as part of the AC regimen) was escalated from 60 mg/m^2 to 90 mg/m^2.

When colony-stimulating factors became widely available, even higher intensification of cyclophosphamide could be achieved. NSABP developed two consecutive clinical trials to determine the effects of increasing the dose and dose-intensity of cyclophosphamide in the context of the AC combination. B-22 compared standard-dose AC (60 mg/m^2 and 600 mg/m^2, respectively), with 60 and 1200 for two doses and four doses respectively. B-25 adopted the highest dose level achieved in B-22 as the control arm and further increased the dose of cyclophosphamide to 2400 mg/m^2 for two doses or four doses in the other arms. There were more than 2500 patients randomized in each study, and the average time on study exceeded 4 years; no statistically significant differences were observed for survival or disease-free survival.[290] Toxicity information from B-25 indicated that the maximum acceptable dose of cyclophosphamide given in the outpatient setting had been achieved. Sixteen patients treated on protocol B-25 were diagnosed with myelodysplastic syndrome (MDS) or acute myeloid leukemia (AML). The 4-year cumulative incidence of AML or MDS for patients on protocol B-25 was 0.87%, greater than that observed in previous NSABP studies using standard-dose cyclophosphamide (600 mg/m^2). Thus, the doxorubicin 60 mg/m^2 with cyclophosphamide 600 mg/m^2 regimen proved to be best.

Although dose-intensification has not improved the outcome of adjuvant chemotherapy to date, the application of the Norton-Simon hypothesis provided improved results in CALGB 9741. Patients with lymph node-positive primary breast cancer were randomly assigned adjuvant chemotherapy with doxorubicin, cyclophosphamide and paclitaxel at standard doses given every 3 weeks, or every 2 weeks with filgrastim support.[291] After a median observation period of 2 years significant prolongation of relapse-free survival and overall survival was observed in the groups treated with the dose-dense or accelerated schedule. These improved results persisted after 5 years of follow-up.

The development of autologous hematopoietic stem cell support techniques and of hematopoietic growth factors (G-CSF, GM-CSF, and erythropoietin) made possible testing of the dose-outcome hypothesis along a much broader range of doses. Following the developmental trials of high-dose chemotherapy in metastatic disease and the early and apparently encouraging results in advanced breast cancer, several prospective randomized clinical trials were developed to investigate the contribution of high-dose adjuvant chemotherapy to the management of patients with high-risk primary breast cancer. The results of these trials, and of two meta-analyses of these trials have now been reported. High-dose chemotherapy was associated with a modest decrease in recurrences, but also with higher morbidity and mortality rates, resulting in no improvement in overall survival.[264]

Targeted Therapy

The monoclonal antibody, trastuzumab, represents specific therapy for HER2-positive cancers. After demonstration of its efficacy and safety in the management of HER2-positive metastatic breast cancer (vide infra), prospective trials were initiated to determine its contribution to the management of HER2-positive primary breast cancers. Six randomized trials were initiated: in all four trastuzumab was added, either simultaneously or sequentially, to conventional adjuvant chemotherapy and compared to the same chemotherapy without trastuzumab. After follow-ups ranging from 1 to 2½ years, five trials (NSABP B-31, N9831, BCIRG006, FinHER and HERA) demonstrated such marked benefit that the trials were stopped and the results reported.[292,293] Compared to the arms without trastuzumab, trastuzumab-treated patients had about a 46% to 58% reduction in risk of recurrence in these five trials. These reductions were very highly significant, and translated into a 3-year absolute reduction in recurrences of 8% to 12%. Significant survival benefits have emerged in five of the six trials, with a 33% to 59% reduction in mortality, resulting in absolute differences of 2% to 6% at three years. A sixth trial failed to show a significant benefit from trastuzumab. While one study suggested that simultaneous administration with chemotherapy was more effective than sequential administration after chemotherapy, definitive assessment of this question will require longer follow-up. The recommended duration of adjuvant trastuzumab is one year; shorter and longer durations are under investigation in clinical trials. There was increased cardiac toxicity associated with the administration of trastuzumab, especially in those treatment arms that called for simultaneous administration of chemotherapy and the antibody. Grade III/IV cardiac toxicity (congestive heart failure) was observed in 0.5% to 4.1% of patients in these trials. The reversibility of these cardiac events is uncertain. However, at this time, the therapeutic benefits appear to exceed by far, the adverse events and for high-risk patients with HER2-positive breast cancer, trastuzumab should be incorporated into adjuvant systemic therapy.

Over the past year, lapatinib, a small molecule tyrosine kinase inhibitor of EGFR and HER2 completed clinical trials and was approved by the FDA for the treatment of metastatic HER2-positive breast cancer. This oral agent has therapeutic efficacy similar to single-agent trastuzumab, and in combination with capecitabine, improves response rates and progression-free survival of patients with chemotherapy-naïve metastatic breast cancer. Lapatinib is currently under evaluation in the adjuvant and neoadjuvant settings, in combination with adjuvant chemotherapy, to compare its effects to those of trastuzumab.

Neoangiogenesis is one of the hallmarks of malignant disease. The VEGF is one of the commonly overexpressed pro-angiogenic substances produced by breast cancer. Bevacizumab is a monoclonal antibody with high affinity for VEGF. Clinical trials have shown that, although its therapeutic benefit is modest when used as monotherapy, it improves the outcomes of treatment of advanced colorectal, renal cell, breast and lung cancers. It is commonly administered in combination with taxanes as front-line therapy of metastatic breast cancer.[260] Bevacizumab is currently under evaluation in combination with other targeted agents in advanced breast cancer, and as part of adjuvant and neoadjuvant therapy of primary breast cancer.

In addition to the steroid hormone receptor, HER2 and components of the angiogenic cascade, a number of other molecular targets are under investigation along with multiple new agents that target them. Putative therapeutic targets include the Insulin-like growth factor receptor family, PI3 kinase, AKT, mTOR, SRC, TGF-beta, heat shock proteins, MAP kinase, integrins, cyclins, cycloxygenase-2, PPAR-gamma, PARP, methylation and deacetylation, among others.

Monitoring Disease Status After Adjuvant Therapy

After completion of combined-modality therapy for primary breast cancer, patients are followed at regular intervals to detect recurrent disease, second primary tumors, or complications of therapy. During the first 2 years, patients are seen every 4 months, for the subsequent 3 years every 6 months, and yearly thereafter. A careful history and a complete physical examination are performed at each visit. A yearly mammogram of the remaining breast(s) completes the necessary evaluation for asymptomatic patients. Other tests are performed only if symptoms or physical findings warrant them. No advantage has been demonstrated for performing frequent or extensive imaging studies or tumor markers.[294] Controversy exists on this point, however, because it tacitly assumes that no advantage accrues from the early detection of metastatic disease. The advent of new therapies, such as selective aromatase inhibitors, fulvestrant, ixabepilone, monoclonal antibodies, tyrosine kinase inhibitors, and anti-angiogenic compounds may change the efficacy of salvage therapy. This, in turn, might make early diagnosis of recurrent or metastatic disease an important step. Even if survival is not prolonged, maintaining an asymptomatic state by effective therapy may be possible and is important for many patients.

Management of Metastatic Breast Cancer

General Considerations

Patients with untreated metastatic breast cancer demonstrate considerable heterogeneity in the clinical course of their disease. Some have a rapidly progressing tumor that metastasizes to multiple vital organs and causes death within a few months after detection of the first metastasis. Other patients have an indolent disease course, with slow progression alternating with long periods of stability in metastasis to soft tissues or bone. Some of these patients survive in the absence of active treatment for more than 10 years.[102]

The organ localization of recurrent or metastatic disease and the extent of metastatic breast cancer partially determine the long-term prognosis.[295] The biologic characteristics of the tumor, including its growth rate and relative resistance or sensitivity to available interventions, also contribute to the outcome. Finally, the efficacy of individual treatment modalities determines the success of palliation and the duration of disease control. Most patients with overt distant metastases are presently incurable. However, among those who achieve a complete remission after standard chemotherapy, a few remain progression-free for extended periods of time, occasionally exceeding 20 years.[296] Complete remissions of long duration have also been reported after high-dose chemotherapy programs. The median survival of patients with metastatic breast cancer is 2 to 3 years. It is longer for patients who present with low-volume metastases to skin, lymph nodes, or bone and shorter for patients with multiple organ involvement, especially those with visceral organ (liver, brain, lung) involvement. The survival is longer for patients with ER-positive tumors and for those who achieve a complete remission with chemotherapy (3 to 4 years), compared to patients with hormone receptor-negative tumors or those who fail to respond to systemic treatment.[295]

Diagnostic Evaluation

Patients with a previous diagnosis of primary breast cancer who present with findings suspicious for recurrent metastatic disease should be strongly considered for diagnostic biopsy, especially if there has been a long disease-free interval. A biopsy is helpful in excluding benign processes that frequently masquerade as metastases and in ruling out the development of other cancers. Furthermore, the tissue can be assayed for ER, PR, HER2/neu and other markers, to assist in treatment decisions. These markers may change from the time primary breast cancer was diagnosed and accurate determination will lead to better choice of therapy.

Metastases from breast cancer are usually multiple and frequently involve more than one organ site. Thus, surgical resection of metastatic lesions is not usually indicated for therapeutic purposes in breast cancer patients. However, it is advisable to remove resectable chest wall recurrences, a solitary brain metastasis in the patient with a long disease-free survival, or when histologic confirmation of a recurrence requires an open biopsy. Occasionally, resection of solitary metastasis to lung, liver or other organs can lead to a long recurrence-free period, especially when combined with systemic therapy. Several recent reports have indicated that removing the primary tumor in patients diagnosed with stage IV disease provides a survival advantage. Prospective confirmation of those reports, using randomized simultaneous controls is needed.

Diagnostic tests and staging procedures are directed by the organ sites most frequently involved in metastatic breast cancer and by patient signs and symptoms. Documentation of initial metastatic sites is helpful in treatment planning and in later assessment of response to treatment. History and physical examination should focus on the detection of metastases on the chest wall, skin, remaining breast, regional and distant lymph nodes, axial skeleton, lungs, liver, and central nervous system. Laboratory evaluation should include a complete blood count, a platelet count, serum calcium, and liver and renal function studies. A chest radiograph and bone scan should be obtained in most patients because these sites are commonly involved with metastatic breast cancer. Suspicious lesions on bone scan need confirmation by radiograph or by other diagnostic imaging or biopsy because of the high false-positive rate. CT and MRI are also commonly used for this purpose.[297] In the presence of bone pain unexplained by results of the bone scan, radiographs or MRI of the symptomatic area should be performed. Although bone scans are quite sensitive, they are of limited use in assessing treatment response in the first 2 to 4 months after the start of a new therapy. Increased intensity of uptake in existing lesions or even new lesions can signify either disease progression or disease regression with active bone healing. Bone scan changes must be corroborated by other information. Optimal monitoring of bone lesions during therapy should include symptoms, tumor markers (CA 27–29, CA 15-3, CEA), and radiographs (radiographs, computed tomograms) or MRI of involved areas. Routine brain and liver imaging procedures are expensive and are not indicated in the absence of symptoms, physical findings, or laboratory values suggesting involvement. Patients with ER-positive tumors are especially unlikely to suffer recurrence initially in the brain or liver. Serial blood tumor markers are recommended by some clinicians as an aid for monitoring disease status, especially when no measurable disease exists. The most frequently used markers are CA 15-3, CA 27-29, and carcinoembryonic antigen (CEA). CA 153 and CA 27-29 are more sensitive than CEA and are elevated in more than 70% of metastatic breast cancer patients, compared with 55% for CEA. The extracellular domain (ECD) of the HER2 oncoprotein is often shed into the circulation and can be assayed. In patients with baseline elevated concentrations of HER2 ECD, changes in concentration often reflect the clinical course of metastatic disease. CA 15-3, CA 27-29, and CEA can be moderately increased in certain benign diseases, especially liver disease, and with other neoplasms, including lung, gastrointestinal, and genitourinary cancers. Levels of all three markers do correlate significantly, although not absolutely, with changing disease status. Increasing levels may signal the need to perform more objective diagnostic tests to confirm worsening of the disease. Decreasing levels may provide greater confidence that a treatment is working. Modifying treatment based solely on changing marker levels, however, is often hazardous and in general should be avoided. For optimal utilization of markers, the clinician must be aware of the normal variations in measurements in the laboratory used (ie, the coefficient of variation) and confirm decreasing or increasing values with additional measurements over time. These markers are of limited value in following patients for recurrence after treatment of primary breast cancer and current guidelines do not recommend them. The average lead-time in the diagnosis of a recurrence is only 4 to 6 months, and there are no data to suggest that early institution of presently available systemic therapy at the time the marker rises affects survival. Positron emission tomography (PET) is an additional diagnostic modality with a number of potential advantages. First, it represents functional, as opposed to anatomical, imaging of tumor deposits. Second, PET scanning (like bone scanning) gives a whole body image and might detect previously unsuspected metastatic lesions. PET scanning might serve to differentiate malignant from benign solitary lesions, and might also be useful in monitoring response to therapy. PET scanning might also serve to advance our understanding of biological correlates and behavior of breast cancer. In combination with CT or MRI, PET will lead to more precise anatomical localization and functional imaging of suspected metastatic lesions. PET scanning is usually performed with 18F-fluorodeoxyglucose (FDG), although other radiopharmaceuticals (16-alpha-[^{18}F] fluoroestradiol or ([^{18F}]FES); (18)F-fluorodeoxythymidine) are under active evaluation.[298] FDG PET was recently accepted for reimbursement by the federal health care financing authorities, reflecting its increasing importance in the diagnosis, staging, and monitoring of breast cancer. In this rapidly evolving field combined PET/CT scans are rapidly replacing PET scanning, since they offer more precise anatomical localization combined with functional imaging.

General Therapeutic Guidelines

Over the past four decades, systemic treatment with endocrine or cytotoxic agents became the fundamental treatment approach of the management of metastatic breast cancer.[1] Treatment decisions can be complicated because of the varied clinical courses among different patients and because many different therapies of apparently similar efficacy are available. Improved understanding of the biological heterogeneity of breast cancer and the identification of molecular subsets based on expression of ER, PR and HER2, or microarray-based gene expression profiling has markedly changed our conceptual and therapeutic approach to metastatic breast cancer. Upon diagnosis of metastatic disease, the first task is to assess the location and extent of metastasis and to determine, based on available biological and clinical information, the likely clinical course, potential vital organ failure or other catastrophic complications. In this sense, patients are often classified into low- and high-risk groups on the basis of clinical information and imaging. Those at low risk include patients who have had a long disease-free interval and have limited metastatic disease, often located in soft tissues or osseous sites. Some patients with limited visceral disease may also qualify. Other than bone pain, symptoms attributed to the disease are minimal. The age of the patient, the presence of comorbid conditions, the organ distribution and extent of metastatic disease, and abnormalities in vital organ functional influence the selection of treatments. However, the critical biological information consists of accurate determination of ER, PR and HER2 in high-volume laboratories with stringent quality control.

Whereas some oncologists elect to treat selected patients with solitary metastatic lesions with locoregional therapy, the great majority of patients receive systemic therapy from the onset of overt metastatic disease. Certainly, symptomatic patients with widespread disease or aggressive visceral metastases should receive chemotherapy. In addition to bone pain, common symptoms include anorexia, weight loss, and reduced performance status. The disease-free interval for patients with high-risk or aggressive metastatic disease is typically short (less than 2 years), and the tumor is frequently ER-negative. Carcinomatous meningitis, extensive liver metastases, lymphangitic lung metastases, or brain metastases usually signify aggressive disease that is unresponsive to endocrine therapy. Patients who have been diagnosed with aggressive disease should be treated with combination chemotherapy, even if the tumor contains ER and PR. Endocrine therapy is less likely to induce remission in this setting, and the more rapid response usually seen with chemotherapy is highly desirable. High-risk patients with receptor-positive tumors can be considered for endocrine therapy at a later date or if they fail to respond to chemotherapy. Patients with brain metastases should also receive regional therapy, usually whole brain irradiation or radiosurgery, which are very effective in palliating symptoms of central nervous system involvement.

Symptomatic Management ■ Pain management, appropriate prevention of chemotherapy-related nausea, appropriate dietary intervention, and psychological support complete the multidisciplinary management of metastatic breast cancer. When used judiciously, all of these interventions contribute to the maintenance or improvement of quality of life while delaying the progression of metastatic breast cancer to the utmost.

Management of Endocrine-Sensitive Metastatic Breast Cancer

Patients with ER- and/or PR-positive, HER2-negative tumors and low-risk characteristics are excellent candidates for hormone therapy as the first intervention for metastatic breast cancer.[1] Selection of endocrine therapy should be based on a high quality estrogen and progesterone receptor assay, preferably on tumor tissue obtained at the time the decision needs to be made. In the unusual circumstance an assay is not available or tumor tissue cannot be obtained for the assay, patient and tumor characteristics are helpful in the determination of whether a tumor is likely to respond to hormonal manipulation. Older, postmenopausal patients with disease-free interval that exceeds 3 years, and small volume metastatic disease located predominantly in soft tissue and/or bone are more likely to respond to endocrine therapy than patients with the opposite characteristics. Patients with ER-positive metastatic tumors have a 50% or greater probability of clinical benefit from hormone therapy, whereas those with clearly ER- and PR-negative tumors have marginal or no probability of response. Those with high ER concentrations have higher probabilities of an objective response than those with lower ER concentration, and patients with both ER and PR expression respond better than those with only one receptor expressed. Recently conducted prospective, randomized clinical trials comparing different hormonal agents as first-line therapy for metastatic breast cancer revealed that overall response rates, using strict definitions of complete and partial remission, ranged from 13% to 40%, even in patients with ER- and PR-positive tumors. Prolonged disease stability (including minor responses) was achieved in an additional 20% to 30% of patients during hormonal therapy. Stable disease for longer than 6 months is associated with survival durations similar to those of patients who achieve a partial or complete response with endocrine therapy. In case of an indolent clinical course, a negative ER assay should prompt a repeat assay to make sure a false-negative result does not preclude potentially beneficial endocrine therapy.

Patients who achieve an objective regression or longstanding disease stability after first-line hormone therapy often benefit from second-line and sometimes subsequent hormonal interventions. The hormonal interventions of choice today include selective AIs such as anastrozole, exemestane, formestane, and letrozole, SERMs (tamoxifen, toremifene) and selective ER downregulators (fulvestrant). Selective aromatase inhibitors are at least as effective as (and sometimes more effective than) tamoxifen for postmenopausal women and their safety profile is superior to that of tamoxifen. For premenopausal women, tamoxifen remains the endocrine agent of choice. Although oophorectomy is still practiced, it has largely been replaced by LHRH analogues (goserelin, leuprolide, buserelin, etc.), that provide an effect equivalent to ovarian ablation. Progestins such as megestrol acetate and medroxyprogesterone acetate are also well tolerated when administered at the usual dose and schedule and have displaced estrogens, androgens, and corticosteroids. Since most postmenopausal women with ER-positive metastatic breast cancer will have received a selective aromatase inhibitor in the adjuvant setting, either an aromatase inhibitor of a different class (ie, non-steroidal to steroidal, or vice versa) or fulvestrant would be the first choice for metastatic disease, unless adjuvant endocrine therapy ended more than a year before. Subsequent lines of therapy would include progestins, high-dose estrogens and androgens. For postmenopausal women who received no adjuvant endocrine therapy, an aromatase inhibitor would be the first choice, followed by fulvestrant or an aromatase inhibitor from a different class.

For premenopausal women with hormone receptor-positive metastatic breast cancer, an antiestrogen would be the first choice, unless metastases developed within a year of adjuvant antiestrogen therapy. Ovarian ablation or suppression is also useful for ER-positive tumors in premenopausal women. This effect is permanent, inducing a menopausal state that permits the use of other endocrine therapies, including the selective AIs, for second- and third-line therapy. Although tamoxifen is an effective alternative to surgical ovarian ablation, the two treatments can be used in sequence, since response to one often predicts a high response rate to the other. The LHRH analogs offer another alternative for premenopausal patients by causing a chemical (or medical) castration.[248] Results to date suggest that serum estrogen concentrations are suppressed to postmenopausal levels and that response rates in advanced breast cancer are similar to those obtained after surgical ovarian ablation. Recent randomized trials and a meta-analysis of these trials (including 506 patients) indicated that the endocrine treatment of choice for premenopausal women with hormone-responsive metastatic breast cancer was a combination of tamoxifen with an LHRH analog.[299] The combination resulted in higher response rates and longer time to progression and survival than the LHRH agonist alone. One criticism of these trials is that none of them compared the combination to the sequential use of both components. After ovarian ablation, the same sequence used for postmenopausal women can be followed. However, if an LHRH analogue was used, it should be continued if an aromatase inhibitor is to be used next, since the latter drugs are ineffective in premenopausal women with intact ovarian function.

The time to obtain maximal response with endocrine therapy can be quite prolonged, and treatment should not be abandoned prematurely. Patients should be continued on a therapeutic trial for 6 to 12 weeks in the absence of progressive disease, before other therapies are used. Prolonged stable disease, without objective regression, is one form of clinical benefit associated with endocrine therapy. This effect is particularly acceptable in patients with minimal or no disease-related symptoms. A "tumor flare" with increased bone pain, swelling, or erythema of superficial lesions or hypercalcemia during the first week or two of therapy should not be confused with disease progression. Tumor flare is seen occasionally with endocrine treatments such as high-dose estrogens, tamoxifen, androgens, and progestins, and it frequently reflects hormone-sensitive disease. If tumor flare occurs early, within the first few weeks of starting treatment, endocrine therapy should continue under close observation and appropriate symptomatic support unless life-threatening conditions exist. Management of hypercalcemia with hydration and bisphosphonate therapy and liberal use of analgesics should be applied until the flare resolves.

For patients who initially respond to endocrine therapy, additional responses with second-and third-line endocrine interventions are common. This is especially the case for patients with indolent tumors. These patients should be offered additional endocrine therapies, in the absence of life-threatening disease, before changing to chemotherapy. Some patients derive many months or even years of high-quality life with sequential endocrine therapies. Few patients who fail to benefit from the initial endocrine treatment will respond to second- or third-line hormonal interventions. These patients, those who develop endocrine resistance, and those who manifest life-threatening disease should be offered chemotherapy. Table 104-20 documents the recommended sequence of hormonal treatments. Eventually, most patients with hormone-responsive breast cancer develop resistance to endocrine manipulations and become candidates for cytotoxic chemotherapy.

Management of HER2-Positive Breast Cancer

HER2 is a normal gene involved in cellular proliferation and survival. It codes for a transmembrane growth factor receptor, one of four known members of the family that also includes the EGFR. Amplification (increased number of gene copies) or overexpression (increased cell surface receptor protein) confers on the cell more aggressive characteristics, including increased proliferation, motility, invasion, angiogenesis and metastases. Between 20% and 25% of breast cancers present with HER2 amplification. Inflammatory breast cancer, and cancer in younger women is more frequently HER2-positive than is breast cancer in postmenopausal women. Historically, HER2-positive tumors had a more aggressive course, with increased rate of metastases and death, as well as shortened survival. HER2-positive tumors tend to metastasize early, and spread to visceral organs (liver, lungs and central nervous system) with increased frequency. ER expression is less frequent in HER2-positive tumors, and when present, ER concentration is much lower than in HER2-negative tumors. As a result, HER2-positive, ER-positive breast cancers are less endocrine-responsive, and even responding tumors develop progressive growth early. This relative resistance to endocrine therapy has been documented for tamoxifen and aromatase inhibitors, but probably applies to all endocrine treatments used today. Studies on preclinical models have documented the extensive cross-talk between the hormone receptor signaling pathways and the HER2/EGFR pathways. It is thought that such cross-talk is largely responsible for the relative hormone resistance observed, and that inhibition of signaling in both pathways is necessary to restore therapeutic sensitivity. A recent randomized trial compared anastrozole alone to the combination of anastrozole plus trastuzumab in patients with HER2-positive and ER-positive metastatic breast cancer. Of the 208 patients randomized, response rate was higher with the combination (20% vs 7%, $p = .018$), and the median time to progression was prolonged by the addition of trastuzumab to endocrine therapy (4.8 months vs 2.4 months, $p = .0016$). There was no difference in overall survival. The results of this relatively small trial confirm the relative endocrine resistance of HER2-positive, ER-positive breast cancers and indicate that HER2-inhibition reverses that resistance to some degree. However, the results of the combination are still poor, indicating that chemotherapy and HER2-inhibition might be a better choice for most patients with HER2-positive disease. Trastuzumab, a humanized monoclonal antibody with high binding affinity to the extracellular domain of the HER2 oncoprotein is the first targeted therapy developed against this target.[78] As a single agent, trastuzumab has modest antitumor activity against metastatic, HER2-positive breast cancer: about 25% of patients with untreated metastatic breast cancer will achieve an objective response to trastuzumab, while patients with prior chemotherapy have a 11% to 15% response rate. While the initial studies were based on weekly trastuzumab administration, pharmacokinetic studies have indicated that the long half-life of trastuzumab lends itself to administration at three-weekly intervals. Trastuzumab was also evaluated in prospective, randomized trials of first-line chemotherapy for metastatic breast cancer.[256,257] In these studies, patients were offered treatment with doxorubicin and cyclophosphamide or docetaxel if no prior chemotherapy exposure had occurred, or single-agent paclitaxel, if the patient had received prior anthracycline therapy. In addition, patients were randomly assigned to receive trastuzumab by intravenous administration once a week. Objective response rates were significantly higher with chemotherapy and trastuzumab compared to chemotherapy alone. Time to progression, duration of response, time to treatment failure and overall survival were all significantly improved by the addition of trastuzumab to chemotherapy. On the basis of these data, regulatory agencies in the United States and Europe approved the use of trastuzumab for treatment of patients with HER2-positive metastatic breast cancer. Several other trastuzumab-containing combinations have been reported, with high response rates and prolonged duration of disease control. Trastuzumab also potentiates chemotherapy with platinum derivatives, vinorelbine and gemcitabine. Randomized trials assessing the value of the addition of carboplatin to taxane and trastuzumab have had conflicting results; while the triple drug combination is considered by many the initial treatment of choice for patients with HER2-positive metastatic breast cancer, others are skeptical of its superiority over a taxane plus trastuzumab combination. Combinations of trastuzumab and chemotherapy have been well tolerated, although increased cardiac toxicity has been reported, especially in combination with anthracyclines, or in patients with significant previous anthracycline exposure. Therefore, assessment of cardiac function before initiation of trastuzumab therapy and during treatment with the antibody is customary to prevent cardiac complications. Based on the concept that chronic inhibition of HER2 signaling is necessary for long-term control of active, HER2-positive breast cancer, some oncologists have elected to continue trastuzumab treatment even after the development of progression disease while receiving a trastuzumab-containing treatment regimen. Thus, upon development of progressive disease while receiving a taxane plus trastuzumab combination, trastuzumab would be continued, while chemotherapy would change to vinorelbine or gemcitabine, or another cytotoxic drug. Retrospective analyses to determine the clinical benefit of such an approach have provided conflicting results, and attempts to complete a randomized trial to determine the worth of indefinite trastuzumab administration have failed because of abysmal patient accrual.

A second monoclonal antibody, pertuzumab, targets different epitopes of the receptor, and appears to have complementary antitumor effects to trastuzumab. Pertuzumab is in clinical trials, mostly in combination with trastuzumab, as well as various chemotherapy regimens.

Lapatinib is a small molecule tyrosine kinase inhibitor that targets both HER2 and EGFR. It is active as monotherapy, with antitumor effects similar to those of trastuzumab in HER2-positive breast cancer, but has marginal (<10% response rate) activity in HER2-negative, EGFR-positive metastatic breast cancer. As a result, subsequent clinical development has largely focused on HER2-positive breast cancer. Lapatinib is well tolerated, with dose-dependent diarrhea being its major adverse effect. Cardiac toxicity appears to be rare with this agent. Lapatinib has been combined with various cytotoxic agents, including taxanes, capecitabine, 5-fluorouracil, SN-38 and with other targeted agents, such as LBH589, trastuzumab, bevacizumab, and pazopanib. Lapatinib is also under investigation, in combination with chemotherapy in the adjuvant and neoadjuvant treatment of HER2-positive primary breast cancer.

Management of Triple Receptor-Negative Metastatic Breast Cancer (TNBC)

Fifteen to 20% of breast cancers do not express ER, PR or HER2. These tumors tend to have higher proliferative rates, high grade and a more aggressive course, with higher recurrence rates and shorter survival compared to patients with ER and or PR-positive breast cancer, or HER2-positive breast cancers treated with trastuzumab-containing regimens. Almost half express EGFR, and many carry *p53* mutations. Most *BRCA1*-mutated tumors fall in this group. There are no validated molecular targets in TNBC, so the primary treatment modality for these patients is chemotherapy. TNBC are highly responsive to standard anthracycline- and taxane-containing regimens, and preliminary information suggests that platinum salts are highly effective in this group. Despite high response rates to standard chemotherapy, responses tend to be short, as is median survival.

A recent randomized trial (E2100) compared the combination of bevacizumab (a monoclonal antibody against VEGF and paclitaxel to paclitaxel alone in first-line metastatic breast cancer. Patients treated with the combination fared better: response rate was higher, and time to progression was significantly longer than with paclitaxel alone. There was no difference in overall survival between the two groups. A second randomized trial used docetaxel instead of paclitaxel, and the design was placebo controlled. This trial confirmed the results of the E2100 trial and led to FDA approval of bevacizumab for the treatment of metastatic breast cancer. Interestingly, an earlier trial tested the combination of capecitabine and bevacizumab in patients with metastatic breast cancer previously treated with anthracyclines and taxanes. While response rate was higher with the combination than with capecitabine alone, there was no difference in progression-free survival or overall survival. Bevacizumab seemed to provide the same benefit in all subsets of breast cancer, including TNBC. Although there is no method to select patients who will benefit from bevacizumab therapy, it is reasonable to consider a bevacizumab combination for management of first-line therapy of TNBC.

Cytotoxic Chemotherapy for Metastatic Breast Cancer

Chemotherapy is used in patients with aggressive disease who are not candidates for endocrine therapy and in those with tumors that no longer respond to endocrine therapy. Forty to 50% of previously untreated patients with metastatic breast cancer achieve an objective regression after single-agent anthracycline therapy. Mitoxantrone and the alkylating agents produce partial or complete responses in 30% to 40% of patients, whereas the other drugs are estimated to have a 20% to 30% response rate. Cisplatin was also reported to produce response rates of around 50%, but this information is based on two small studies; the reported response rate with carboplatin was around 30%. Mitomycin is another effective agent, although its use has decreased markedly since the development of the taxanes, vinorelbine, and other new drugs.

Over the past two decades several new, moderately effective cytotoxic agents have completed clinical trials and been approved by the FDA for the treatment of breast cancer. These agents include the taxanes, paclitaxel, nab-paclitaxel and docetaxel, the oral fluoropyrimidine analog, capecitabine, and the epothilone derivative, ixabepilone.[300-302]

The Taxanes ■ Paclitaxel and docetaxel are certainly among the most effective agents for the treatment of breast cancer.[300] Administered as a single agent, paclitaxel has demonstrated activity similar or superior to other first-line chemotherapy regimens. The FDA-approved method to administer paclitaxel is as a 1- to 3-hour infusion every 3 weeks, at the dose of 175 mg/m². However, over the past several years evidence has accumulated to show that the weekly administration of paclitaxel, usually at doses ranging between 80 and 90 mg/m²/week, is more effective and better tolerated than the 3-weekly schedule. The weekly schedule is associated with a different safety profile, with a marked reduction in myelosuppressive and infectious complications, as compared to the 3-weekly schedule of administration. There is no compelling evidence that higher doses or more prolonged durations of administration modify the drug's efficacy in a substantial manner. Paclitaxel and docetaxel are substantially active in previously treated patients with metastatic breast cancer, including a 30% to 50% response rate in patients with anthracycline-resistant breast carcinoma. This degree of activity indicates that these two are the most effective drugs available for anthracycline-refractory breast cancer. Docetaxel and paclitaxel are not completely cross-resistant, and some patients derive clinical benefit from treatment with one taxane after developing resistance to the other. A direct comparison of the two taxanes was recently reported. In a prospective phase 3 trial 372 patients with metastatic breast cancer were randomly assigned to receive docetaxel 100 mg/m² IV every 3 weeks or paclitaxel 175 mg/ m² IV every 3 weeks. Time to progression favored docetaxel (medians, 5.7 and 3.6 months, $p < .0001$), as did overall survival (15.4 vs 12.7, $p = .03$). This study has had minimal impact on practice, since most oncologists use the weekly schedule of paclitaxel, which in the largest comparative study between these two agents performed in the adjuvant setting appeared superior to three-weekly paclitaxel and docetaxel given in two different schedules.

Docetaxel as a single agent produces objective responses in up to 60% of patients with metastatic breast cancer previously unexposed to chemotherapy. The usual method of administering docetaxel is a 1-hour infusion every 3 weeks, at a dose of 75 to 100 mg/m². As for paclitaxel, there is great interest in the weekly administration of docetaxel, since this schedule is associated with less myelosuppressive and musculoskeletal toxicity. However, weekly administration is frequently complicated by asthenia, epiphora, nail changes and fluid retention. Docetaxel as a single agent produced a higher response rate and longer time to progression than full-dose doxorubicin, although survival was equivalent for the two drugs. Docetaxel was superior to the combination of vinblastine and mitomycin for all end points considered and superior to the combination of methotrexate/5-fluorouracil in terms of response rate and time to progression.

Vinorelbine ■ The Vinca alkaloid vinorelbine has undergone extensive clinical evaluation that showed, in addition to excellent tolerability, objective response rates ranging from 40% to 50% in first-line and 20% to 35% in second-line therapy; however, it has not gained FDA approval for treatment of breast cancer, although it is widely used for the treatment of advanced breast cancer. Vinorelbine is effective in patients with anthracycline-refractory tumors, although, based on indirect comparisons it would appear to be less effective in this situation than the taxanes. Vinorelbine is administered intravenously at weekly intervals, and is well tolerated. Myelosuppression and peripheral neuropathy are dose-limiting toxicities.

Capecitabine ■ Capecitabine is a prodrug that is metabolized to 5-fluorouracil upon absorption from the gastrointestinal tract. Its oral bioavailability is excellent and it is a well-tolerated and effective palliative regimen. Capecitabine retains antitumor activity after prior therapy with an anthracycline-containing regimen and a taxane.[301] Capecitabine is under evaluation in comparative trials against other effective single agents (eg, paclitaxel), in combination therapy and in the adjuvant setting. A recent report showed that the addition of capecitabine to single-agent docetaxel resulted in a significant increase in objective response rate, time to progression and overall survival. Other interventions that mimic the continuous intravenous infusion of 5-fluorouracil (S-1) are also under active development.

Gemcitabine ■ Another new drug with considerable antitumor activity in metastatic breast cancer is gemcitabine. This agent was approved by the FDA for the treatment of metastatic breast cancer in combination with paclitaxel. Gemcitabine produces responses in about 40% of patients with untreated metastatic breast cancer and in 20% to 30% of those with previous exposure to chemotherapy, including anthracycline-refractory tumors. The combination of gemcitabine and doxorubicin was recently reported to have substantial antitumor activity and good tolerance. Triple combinations, including gemcitabine, epirubicin and paclitaxel (Taxol) (GET) have also been reported to have very high response rates and overall, excellent antitumor activity.

A new formulation of paclitaxel (nanoparticle albumin-bound paclitaxel, nab-paclitaxel, Abraxane™) does not require solvents, and is largely devoid of allergic reactions.[303] Thus, it requires no premedication. Nab-paclitaxel is administered intravenously, either weekly or every three weeks. Single-agent activity in randomized trials was higher for nab-paclitaxel than for paclitaxel (22% vs 11%, $p = .003$). Weekly nab-paclitaxel was reported to be superior in efficacy to docetaxel in a randomized phase 2 trial. The safety profile of nab-paclitaxel appears better than that of paclitaxel, although at the recommended doses, nab-paclitaxel is associated with higher rates of peripheral neuropathy than paclitaxel.

Ixabepilone (Ixempra™) ■ Ixabepilone is one of several epothilone derivatives, and the first to gain regulatory approval.[302] It is a tubulin-targeting agent, with demonstrate effectiveness in patients with progressive metastatic breast cancer previously treated with anthracyclines, taxanes and capecitabine. Ixabepilone monotherapy produced objective Responses in 12% of such patients. Its efficacy was significantly higher in patients with more limited prior treatment. Peripheral neuropathy, myelosuppression, asthenia, alopecia and stomatitis are common toxicities, although neuropathy appears more rapidly reversible than with taxanes.

Continuous rather than intermittent chemotherapy provided a better quality of life, suggesting that a more substantial antitumor response had a greater influence on quality of life than the negative effects of the regimen-related toxicity. When all published randomized trials addressing the issue of shorter versus longer duration of chemotherapy are pooled in a meta-analysis, there is an important trend for longer duration of survival favoring longer duration of treatment. Over the past few years, retrospective analyses of clinical trials suggested that anthracycline-based regimens were particularly effective in HER2-positive tumors.[304] Since HER2-amplification does not increase sensitivity to anthracyclines, it has been hypothesized that topoisomerase II, a gene in close proximity to HER2 on the short arm of chromosome 17, and one of the targets of anthracycline activity might be co-amplified with HER2 in some tumors, providing the biological basis for increased sensitivity to anthracyclines. Analysis of topoisomerase II amplification/expression in breast cancers, its relationship to HER2 amplification and anthracycline sensitivity has provided conflicting results.[286] At this time there is no convincing evidence that assays for HER2 or topoisomerase II serve to select patients who will (or will not) benefit from anthracycline therapy.

Combination chemotherapy regimens commonly used to treat metastatic breast cancer are shown in Table 104-15. The earliest attempts at combining chemotherapeutic agents were reported by Greenspan in 1958. Subsequently, the five-drug combination consisting of cyclophosphamide, methotrexate, 5-fluorouracil, vincristine, and prednisone (CMFVP, or the "Cooper" regimen) initiated the modern era of combined cytotoxic therapy. Multiple modifications in dose, schedule, and the individual drug components were reported over the next 30 years. The most commonly used modification of the original CMFVP regimen is the three-drug (CMF) combination, without vincristine or prednisone. The intravenous combination previously was shown to be inferior to the "classical" CMF.

Doxorubicin-containing combinations are probably the most commonly used regimens today. The 5-fluorouracil, doxorubicin (Adriamycin), cyclophosphamide (FAC) regimen came into use in 1973; shortly thereafter, other doxorubicin containing combinations were reported. Randomized comparisons between CMF-like and FAC-like regimens have shown a higher response rate and longer time to progression for the anthracycline containing regimens. Some individual studies and a recent meta-analysis of the contribution of doxorubicin to the "Cooper" regimen also showed a significant prolongation of survival.[285] However, anthracycline-containing regimens produce alopecia, nausea, and vomiting with increased frequency and severity, and cardiomyopathy occurs in a dose-dependent manner. Because the added benefits gained with FAC over CMF are modest, the decision about which regimen to choose should be individualized, based on the stated objectives of treatment, understanding and acceptance of a toxicity profile, and the physician's familiarity with a particular regimen.

Paclitaxel has been evaluated in combination with various other cytotoxic agents with demonstrated efficacy against breast cancer. In combination with doxorubicin, it produces a higher response rate and duration of response than either paclitaxel alone, doxorubicin alone, or the combination of doxorubicin/cyclophosphamide. However, schedule-dependent pharmacokinetic interactions and increased myelosuppressive and mucosal toxicity were reported by several investigators. Combinations of bolus doxorubicin and 3-hour paclitaxel were initially reported to have very high response rates, approaching 90%, but a 20% rate of congestive heart failure after six to eight cycles of treatment. Separating the administration of the two drugs by 6 to 18 hours reduces the risk of cardiac toxicity substantially. The initial very high response rates have not been replicated; in most trials with this combination, the overall response rate ranges from 50% to 70%. Other successful two-drug paclitaxel combinations included cisplatin, carboplatin, 5-fluorouracil, or vinorelbine.

Table 104-15 **Commonly Used Combination Chemotherapy Regimens for Metastatic and High-Risk Primary Breast Cancer**

Cytotoxic Agent	Dose (mg/m²)	Route	Schedule and Days	Frequency
>FAC				
5-Fluorouracil	500	IV	Bolus, days 1 + 8	Every 21 days
Adriamycin (doxorubicin)	50	IV	Bolus, day 1, or 72-hr infusion (days 1–3)	
Cyclophosphamide	500	IV	Bolus day 1	
CAF				
Cyclophosphamide	100	PO	Days 1–14	Every 28 days
Adriamycin (doxorubicin)	25	IV	Bolus, days 1 + 8	
5-Fluorouracil	500	IV	Bolus, days 1 + 8	
AC				
Adriamycin (doxorubicin)	60	IV	Bolus, day 1	Every 21 days
Cyclophosphamide	600	IV	Bolus, day 1	
AT				
Adriamycin (doxorubicin)	50	IV	Bolus, day 1	Every 21 days
Taxol (paclitaxel)	220	IV	3-hr infusion, day 2	
AT				
Adriamycin (doxorubicin)	60	IV	Bolus, day 1	Every 21 days
Taxol (paclitaxel)	200	IV	3-hr infusion, day 1	
AT				
Adriamycin (doxorubicin)	60 or 50	IV	Bolus, day 1	
	+ +			
Taxotere (docetaxel)	60 or 75	IV	1-hr infusion, day 1	Every 21 days
CMF				
Cyclophosphamide	100	PO	Days 1–14	Every 28 days
Methotrexate	40	IV	Bolus, days 1 + 8	
5-Fluorouracil	600	IV	Bolus, days 1 + 8	
IV CMF				
Cyclophosphamide	600	IV	Bolus, day 1	Every 21 days
Methotrexate	40	IV	Bolus, day 1	
5-Fluorouracil	600	IV	Bolus, day 1	
CNF				
Cyclophosphamide	600	IV	Bolus, day 1	Every 21 days
Novantrone (mitoxantrone)	12	IV	Bolus, day 1	
5-Fluorouracil	600	IV	Bolus, day 1	
MMM				
Mitomycin	8	IV	Bolus, day 1	Every 42 days
Mitoxantrone	8	IV	Bolus, days 1 + 22	
Methotrexate	35	IV	Bolus, days 1 + 22	
VA				
Vinorelbine	25	IV	30-min IV infusion on days 1 and 8	Every 21 days
Adriamycin (doxorubicin)	50	IV	Bolus, day 1	
TX				
Taxotere (docetaxel)	100	IV	Over 1 hr, day 1	Every 21 days
Xeloda (capecitabine)	2000	PO	Daily for 14 days	
TG				
Taxol (paclitaxel)	175	IV	3 hr, day 1	Every 21 days
Gemcitabine	1250	IV	Bolus, days 1 + 8	
TC				
Taxotere (docetaxel)	75	IV	Over 1 hr, day 1	Every 21 days
Cyclophosphamide	600	IV	Bolus, day 1	

Abbreviations: IV, intravenous; PO, oral.

Docetaxel combinations with doxorubicin or epirubicin have also demonstrated substantial efficacy without an apparent increase in cardiac toxicity. A randomized comparison of docetaxel/doxorubicin with cyclophosphamide/doxorubicin in first-line chemotherapy for metastatic breast cancer showed that the former combination was associated with a higher response rate and longer time to progression than the latter. However, no prolongation in overall survival has been reported. Docetaxel is also under evaluation in combination with cisplatin, carboplatin, cyclophosphamide, vinorelbine, 5-fluorouracil, and other agents.

Nab-paclitaxel has been combined with capecitabine, platinum salts, epirubicin, gemcitabine, and molecularly targeted agents, such as bevacizumab, trastuzumab, and lapatinib.

Vinorelbine has been extensively evaluated in combination with anthracyclines, 5-fluorouracil, cisplatin, and the taxanes. The activity of these combinations appears similar to the activity of CMF or even FAC; however, only the vinorelbine/doxorubicin combination has been directly compared to a standard regimen.

Ixabepilone in combination with capecitabine improved progression-free survival (5.7 months vs 4.1 months, $p < .0001$) compared with capecitabine alone, with increased response rate in patients with metastatic breast cancer previously treated with anthracyclines and taxanes.

Most of these drugs are myelosuppressive, resulting in substantial leucopenia and neutropenia. In addition, they are associated with nausea, vomiting, and, sometimes, mucositis and diarrhea. The anthracyclines produce almost universal (but transient) alopecia, and at high cumulative doses they produce cardiomyopathy. The incidence of cardiomyopathy, nausea, and vomiting decreases markedly when doxorubicin is administered weekly or as a 48- to 96-hour intravenous infusion rather than by bolus. Epirubicin is somewhat less cardiotoxic than doxorubicin; the risk of cardiotoxicity can also be reduced by the co-administration of a cardiac protector, dexrazoxane. Liposome-encapsulated anthracyclines are also considered to have lower cardiac toxicity. The vinca alkaloids and the platinum analogs produce peripheral neuropathy.

Between 50% and 75% of patients with metastatic breast cancer have responses to first-line chemotherapy.[1] In general, patients with a good performance status, normal organ function, and limited extent of disease are more likely to respond than patients with the opposite characteristics. Only 15% to 20% of patients will achieve a complete remission, and most of those patients will develop progressive disease within the subsequent 5 years. Over the past decade, the enthusiasm for using combination chemotherapy to manage metastatic breast cancer has diminished. This change was based on the increased toxicity of combination regimens, and several randomized trials that failed to show a survival benefit of combination chemotherapy over sequential use of the single agent components of the regimens. Thus, many oncologists prefer to use sequential single agents for patients with asymptomatic metastatic breast cancer in the absence of an impending visceral crisis or potential catastrophic complications. This approach reflects the increasing challenge of demonstrating survival benefit in patients with metastatic breast cancer. Since 1970, the median survival of patients with metastatic breast cancer has increased from 12-18 months to 24-36 months, and even longer for patients with endocrine-responsive disease or those with HER2-positive breast cancer treated with HER2-targeting agents. Most patients receive multiple treatment regimens after the first documentation of metastases, and each regimen contributes a relatively short duration of control to the overall survival duration. In that context, a 50% prolongation of progression-free survival by one regimen in a patient who receives five different regimens during the metastatic phase of her illness might effect only a 10% prolongation in survival. None of the randomized trials conducted to date was large enough to have the statistical power to detect such a modest difference in survival. Therefore, and for practical purposes, sequential single-agent therapy is an appropriate approach to manage patients with asymptomatic, low-risk metastatic breast cancer. Patients with higher risk metastatic disease, such as those with visceral crisis, impending serious complications of metastases and those with moderate to severe symptoms would benefit from combination therapy, since it is more likely to produce an objective response. In addition, patients with oligometastases (one or just a few metastatic lesions amenable to surgical resection or radiotherapy) should also be given the benefit of the most effective combination of drugs to maximize their chances of long-term disease control, something akin to adjuvant chemotherapy for high-risk primary breast cancer.

The objections to combination chemotherapy started at a time when there was much emphasis on the importance of dose intensity. In fact, high-dose chemotherapy with hematopoietic stem cell rescue was in vogue at the time. Increasing doses of most cytotoxic drugs are associated with increasingly frequent and severe toxicities. Many commonly used drugs have overlapping toxicities as well. Therefore, it was appropriate in that context to try to increase the dose of each drug to the maximum tolerated, and that often required not administering other drugs at the same time. However, dose-intensive regimens and high-dose chemotherapy were shown to be no more effective than standard doses of the same drugs, and such doses are well tolerated even in two- and three-drug combinations. Increasing understanding of the mechanisms of activity and resistance of commonly used therapeutic agents led to the avoidance of "opportunity-based" combinations, and increasingly toward the development of rational combinations, based on a biological probability of additive or synergistic interaction. Thus, combinations of taxanes and trastuzumab, or platinum salt and trastuzumab, or paclitaxel and capecitabine, or trastuzumab and bevacizumab and currently being explored or have been accepted as "standard". In addition, the improved safety profile of many molecularly targeted agents also led to increased acceptance of combination therapy. Increasingly, whether we select a single agent or a combination, will be based on biological considerations, comorbidity and the major aim of the intervention.

Combined Hormonal Therapy and Chemotherapy

Because hormonal therapy and cytotoxic therapy have different mechanisms of action, and because the two modalities produce different patterns of toxicity, it was hypothesized that their combined use might result in enhanced therapeutic efficacy without increased toxicity. Numerous prospective randomized trials have been conducted using a combination of simultaneous chemotherapy and hormonal therapy. In most cases, the hormonal agent was either ovarian ablation (or LHRH analogues) or tamoxifen, although several trials used progestins or androgens. Some of these trials showed increased response rates, and a few demonstrated a slight prolongation of response duration. However, most individual trials failed to demonstrate an increase in median survival or in long-term survival in patients with metastatic breast cancer. A meta-analysis of randomized clinical trials in the setting of metastatic breast cancer suggested, however, a modest but significant prolongation of survival with simultaneous combination of chemotherapy and endocrine therapy.[285] However, this modest advantage must be considered in the context of increased toxicity with combined therapy. Based on these results, the sequential use of hormonal therapy and chemotherapy is considered the optimal way to provide palliative therapy to patients with metastatic breast cancer.

Targeted Therapies for Metastatic Breast Cancer

One of the hallmarks of malignant disease is neoangiogenesis, or the ability of the tumor to recruit endothelial cells and form a network of blood vessels to provide adequate nutrition and oxygen to the malignant lesion. A number of pro-angiogenic factors are produced and released by malignant cells. The VGEF family and their cognate receptors represent the best studied and understood system. As noted above, a monoclonal antibody with high binding affinity to the VEGF, bevacizumab, was introduced to clinical trials several years ago. As a single agent administered to patients with metastatic breast cancer who had received treatment with conventional therapies, bevacizumab was associated with objective responses in about 10% of patients. Prospective randomized trials to determine its role in the management of metastatic breast cancer were completed. In one phase 3 trial, patients with previously treated metastatic breast cancer were offered capecitabine alone or in combination with the anti-VEGF antibody. While objective responses were almost twice as high in the combination arm compared with capecitabine alone, no differences in time to progression or overall survival were detected. In two additional phase 3 trials, patients with metastatic breast cancer who had received no prior treatment were offered a taxane alone or in combination with bevacizumab. The results showed a highly significant improvement in response rates, as well as significant prolongations in time to progression. No survival differences have been observed. The addition of bevacizumab was associated with hypertension, bleeding, proteinuria, and fatigue in a small number of patients.

Table 104-16 shows a list of molecular targets under active investigation in the area of breast oncology. These represent discrete molecular components of critical signaling pathways often dysregulated in breast cancer, or biological systems (angiogenesis, apoptosis, mitosis, etc) that are critical to the survival and growth of cancer cells. The following paragraphs describe the most prominent molecularly targeted agents that have reached an advanced stage of clinical evaluation.

Angiogenesis Inhibitors ■ A number of small molecule kinase inhibitors target one or several receptors of the VEGFR family. Sunitinib is a potent inhibitor of VEGFR, platelet-derived growth factor receptor (PDGFR), KIT, RET, CSF-1R and flt3. Sunitinib (Sutent™) demonstrated single-agent activity in breast cancer (about 10% response rate) and is in clinical trials for metastatic disease in combination with chemotherapy.

Sorafenib (Nexavar™) inhibits the activity of RAF kinase, VEGFR-2, and PDGFR-beta, among others. It is currently in clinical trials in combination with chemotherapy and aromatase inhibitors.

Pazopanib inhibits multiple kinases, including VEGFR-1, -2 and -3, KIT and PDGFR. It is currently in clinical trials in combination with chemotherapy, lapatinib and various other kinase inhibitors.

Insulin-Like Growth Factor and Receptor ■ This system is frequently dysregulated in breast cancer. Investigations have disclosed extensive cross-talk with endocrine signaling and other growth factor systems. IGFR is believed to be involved in the development of resistance to endocrine therapy as well as HER2-targeted agents. Several monoclonal antibodies targeting IGF1-R and several tyrosine kinase inhibitors are in preclinical or clinical development as monotherapy and in combination with other agents.

PI3 Kinase/AKT/mTOR ■ This signaling network has extensive interaction with

Table 104-16 New Molecular Targets Under Investigation in Breast Cancer

Molecular Targets	Examples of Molecular Therapeutics
Steroid hormone receptor pathway	Tamoxifen (Nolvadex)
	Toremifene
	Raloxifene
	Fulvestrant (Faslodex)
HER-family	Cetuximab (Erbitux)
EGFR (HER1)	Erlotinib (Tarceva)
HER2	Gefitinib (Iressa)
	Trastuzumab (Herceptin)
	Lapatinib (Tykerb)
	XL647
	Neratinib (HKI-272)
IGF/IGFR-family	IMC-A12
	INSM-18
	CP-751871
	NVP-ADW742
	AG1024
	ATL-1101 (antisense)
PI3K, AKT, mTOR	PI3 kinase inhibitors
	XL147
	BEZ235
	GDC-0941
	AKT inhibitors:
	Triciribine
	Perifosine
	INCB-18424
	mTOR inhibitors
	Everolimus
	Temsirolimus
Protein farnesylation	Tipifarnib
	Lonafarnib
Src	Dasatinib
	AP23846
	SKI-606
TGF- β	GC1008
HSP90	17-AAG
	SNX-5422
	IPI-504 (retaspimycin)
	STA 9090
MAPK	VX-702
	SCIO-469
	Pamapimod
	681323
	856553
	KC-706
	Atypical MAP Kinase inhibitors
MEK	PD-325901
	ARRY-142886
Angiogenesis (VEGF, VEGFR)	Axitinib (AG-13736)
	Cediranib (Recentin)
	Pazopanib (GW786034
	Sorafenib (Nexavar)
	Sunitinib (Sutent)
	Vandetanib (Zactima)
	ABT-869
	RTA-402
	SU-14813
	SU-6668
	Bevacizumab (Avastin)
	Aflibercept)VEGF Trap, Regeneron)
Integrins	Integrin inhibitors
	Monoclonal antibodies (Vitaxin)
	Synthetic peptides (cilengitide, EMD 121974, IS20I, ATN-161)
	Peptidomimetics (S247)
PDGF	CP-673,451
	CDP860
	GFB-111
	leflunomide
Proteasome	bortezomib
Apoptosis modulators	rhAPO2L/TRAIL
	ABT-263
	GX 15-070 (Gemin X)
	Mapatumumab (HGS-ETR1)
	AS1A404 (DMXXA)
Cyclins–cdks	Chk 1 inhibitors
	CDK inhibitors
	E7070
	Flavopiridol
	SCH727965
	Seliciclib (Cyclacel)
COX-2	Celecoxib
	Rofecoxib
PPAR-gamma	T0070907
	GW9662
	Badge
RANK, RANK-L	Osteoprotegerin
	Denosumab
Methylation, deacetylation	SAHA
	LBH589
	LAQ824
	Depsipeptide
	CI-994
	MS-275

many transmembrane receptor tyrosine kinases, integrings and mediates energy and nutritional metabolism. Mutations of PI3K and AKT are frequently found in breast cancer. Several inhibitors of PI3K and AKT are in phase 1 and 2 clinical trials in breast cancer. Three mTOR inhibitors have made substantial progress in clinical development: everolimus, temsirolimus and AP23573. While these agents are expected to have modest efficacy against breast cancer in monotherapy, their effects will enhance the efficacy of other signaling inhibitors in combination. Thus, everolimus added to letrozole significantly enhanced the activity of letrozole in the neoadjuvant setting.

Special Issues Regarding Therapy

Management of Isolated Local-Regional Recurrence

If an isolated chest wall or regional lymph node recurrence is detected, biopsy confirmation and surgical resection are recommended. If not irradiated earlier, radiotherapy to the chest wall and involved regional lymph node-bearing area is indicated. Should the tumor be hormone receptor positive, adjuvant endocrine therapy has been shown to reduce the risk of additional recurrences. Although no controlled trial has been conducted to assess its efficacy, some centers advocate the use of "adjuvant chemotherapy" in these situations to reduce the risk of recurrence and death.

Osseous Metastases

Osseous metastases represent the commonest type of metastatic spread in breast cancer: Up to 80% of patients with metastatic breast cancer will develop bone metastases during the clinical course of the illness. Bone metastases are the most frequent source of morbidity and disability related to breast cancer. Orthopedic assessment of metastatic lesions in major weight-bearing sites (hips, femora, humera and shoulders) is recommended to prevent pathological fractures that would lead to disability and frequently death. Radiotherapy to painful sites of bone metastasis or impending fracture sites in weight-bearing bones is commonly used in association with systemic treatments. Bisphosphonates are effective inhibitors of osteoclast activation and, therefore, of bone resorption and the development of osteolytic bone metastases. Treatment with pamidronate, zoledronic acid, or clodronate alone was shown to produce pain relief and radiographic evidence of healing in 20% to 25% of patients with osteolytic bone metastases from breast cancer in several phase 2 clinical trials. Several large randomized clinical trials demonstrated that the administration of pamidronate disodium combined with chemotherapy or hormone therapy delays the appearance and reduces the severity of bone-related complications of breast cancer. Similar data exist for clodronate, another second-generation bisphosphonate, and more recently, for ibandronate and zoledronic acid. Zoledronic acid, 4 mg IV over 15 minutes every 4 weeks is the preferred bisphosphonate regimen for management of patients with bone metastases. Bisphosphonate therapy should start at the first evidence of osteolytic bone metastases and be continued during the clinical course of metastatic breast cancer. Breast cancer and various therapeutic interventions result in rapid decrease of bone mineral density. Bisphosphonates represent the treatment of choice for osteoporosis and osteopenia and have been shown to prevent and reverse iatrogenic osteoporosis. Monitoring bone density during treatment is a necessary component of bone health care and will lead to appropriate preventive or therapeutic interventions with bisphosphonates and other osteoclast inhibitors. Increasing evidence suggests that bisphosphonates reduce the risk of metastases in patients with high-risk primary breast cancer.

Several bone-seeking radionuclides (^{89}Srontium chloride, ^{153}Samarium-EDTMP) were shown to target osseous metastases and provide temporary pain relief for patients with systemic bone metastases. Because of protracted myelosuppression associated with these agents, they are often reserved for third-line therapy and beyond.

Pregnancy and Breast Cancer

Among women with breast cancer, 1% to 2% are pregnant at the time of diagnosis, their average age being around 35 years. There is no evidence that pregnancy is associated with either the development or the progression of breast cancer, since the patient's prognosis is related to the stage of the disease rather than to the pregnancy itself. The generally worse prognosis for women diagnosed with breast cancer during pregnancy can be attributed to the fact that diagnosis in such patients is often delayed so that by the time the disease is detected, it has already progressed to an advanced stage. Changes in the breasts during pregnancy that make cancer difficult to detect, as well as the reluctance of physicians to perform mammography in pregnant patients, may account for the delay in diagnosis. With the use of abdominal shields, however, radiation exposure to the fetus is negligible, and adverse effects to the fetus have not been observed with mammography. Therefore, the diagnostic procedures performed in women who present with suspected breast cancer during pregnancy should be the same as those used for non-pregnant women. Similar results can be obtained with non–radiograph-based imaging techniques, such as sonography. MRI is not recommended during pregnancy as there is no data on the safety of gadolinium, during breast feeding, the diffuse enhancement of the breast tissue makes MR images difficult to interpret. Treatment is generally similar to that prescribed for nonpregnant breast cancer patients. Although modified radical mastectomy might be considered the treatment of choice in order to avoid the need for postoperative radiation, there is a role for lumpectomy followed by breast irradiation after delivery, particularly in late pregnancy. Avoiding chemotherapy during the first trimester of pregnancy, when organogenesis is taking place, is strongly recommended. If chemotherapy is going to be given, it can be given neoadjuvantly and surgery performed after delivery. Doxorubicin based treatments are considered safe and can be started in the second or third trimester, and held after week 35 to enable normal delivery in week 38. In all cases of breast cancer diagnosed during pregnancy, decisions should be based on close interaction between breast surgeon, obstetrician, and medical oncologist, after clear discussions with the patient, to understand and respect her belief and value system, while providing the highest probability of cure (see Chapter 65; Pregnancy and Cancer). Termination of the pregnancy is rarely warranted, since combined modality therapy can usually be delivered with proper care. If the diagnosis occurs during late pregnancy and the tumor is a low-risk malignancy, the patient can be treated after delivery. In a group of women with a similar stage of breast cancer, there is no significant difference in prognosis between those who are pregnant and those who are not. With regard to subsequent pregnancies for patients who have had breast cancer, several authors have suggested a waiting period of 3 to 5 years, depending on the nodal status of the cancer. Findings from recent studies, however, fail to show a worse prognosis in breast cancer patients who subsequently become pregnant; some have even indicated a better prognosis for such patients compared to breast cancer patients who do not have subsequent pregnancy, but this is best explained by self-selection—patients wait to see if they will be well for a time, so early failures are removed from consideration.

Male Breast Cancer

Carcinoma of the breast occurs infrequently in men in the developed countries, the incidence being about 1% of that in women.[2,3] In several African countries, the incidence in hospital registries is 5% to 15% that of female breast cancer. Breast cancer accounts for about 0.1% of all cancers in American men and rarely occurs in males under the age of 40, with the average age at onset about 60 years. Familial associations have been reported. Between 4% and 40% of male breast cancers have recently been reported to have mutations in the BRCA2 gene.[305] Most are frameshift mutations that result in truncated proteins. Several factors have been implicated in the etiology of the disease, including history of prior radiation, hyperestrogenism, and Klinefelter syndrome. The association between gynecomastia and male breast cancer is less clear.

Histologic tumor characteristics in males are similar to those in females, with two-thirds of patients presenting with ductal carcinoma. LCIS, however, is not observed in males. ERs have been found in up to 84% of tumors in males who have the disease. Reports indicate that between 1.7% and 45% of male breast cancers overexpress the HER2 gene. HER2 overexpression adversely affects prognosis. The most common presenting symptoms include breast mass, bloody nipple discharge, nipple retraction, axillary mass, and distant or local pain. Breast cancer usually presents in a more advanced stage in men than in women. However, operability rates of from 74% to 95% have been reported. Surgical treatment with mastectomy is indicated. More extensive surgery may be necessary if there is muscle involvement. However, in the setting of locally advanced breast cancer, chemotherapy can be used to shrink the tumor. Indications for postmastectomy radiation are the same as for women, and combination of tumor size, lymph node and margin involvement, lymphovascular invasion, and skin involvement should dictate the use of radiation. Patterns of metastasis are similar to those in females. The prognosis for breast cancer in men depends on lymph node status, size of the tumor, and ER and HER2 expression.

The treatment for metastatic breast cancer in men has changed during recent years.[305] As noted earlier, breast cancer is more often hormone receptor—positive in men than in women. This also has been confirmed clinically by the more frequent observation of responses to hormonal therapy in men as compared to women. Tamoxifen is the hormonal treatment of choice for male breast cancer today. More than 50% of unselected patients with metastatic breast cancer respond, as do 70% to 80% of patients with ER-positive tumors.

The experience with other SERMs in male breast cancer is quite limited. Other hormonal agents with demonstrated efficacy against metastatic breast cancer in men are progestins, aminoglutethimide, estrogens, and antiandrogens. Selective aromatase inhibitors have not been formally evaluated in male breast cancer. Case reports suggest stability of metastatic disease but no objective responses to date. Anecdotal reports have shown antitumor activity of androgens and corticosteroids in men with breast cancer. However, these reports are based on only a few patients. Combined hormonal therapy has not been extensively evaluated in males.

In cases of progression after an initial remission with tamoxifen, orchiectomy or gonadotropin-releasing hormone agonist treatment is indicated, with other modalities such as chemotherapy being reserved for further failures. Chemotherapy as the initial therapy for metastatic disease has efficacy similar to that observed in women with breast cancer.

Adjuvant therapy decisions are made on the basis of stage, age, ER/PR, HER2 and comorbid conditions. Because no randomized trials have been conducted in male breast cancer, decisions are based largely on extrapolation from female breast cancer.

Inflammatory Breast Cancer

Inflammatory breast cancer (IBC) is a locally advanced and particularly aggressive form of breast cancer.[306] This disease constitutes 1% to 6% of all newly diagnosed breast cancers (probably closer to

2% in the United States). The diagnosis of IBC is based on a clinical triad of erythema, edema of the skin of the breast (peau d'orange), and ridging, a tactile sensation caused by engorged dermal lymphatics. IBC's evolution is usually rapid, usually taking less than 3 months to go from the first detectable abnormality to the establishment of a diagnosis. Because an underlying mass is frequently absent, IBC is often mistakenly treated with antibiotics on the working assumption that the patient has mastitis. The inflammatory process may extend off the breast onto the adjacent chest wall. A core needle biopsy usually provides a definitive diagnosis. Before the advent of systemic adjuvant therapy, the 5-year survival rate for patients with IBC after surgery, radiotherapy, or a combination of the two was reported by multiple investigators to be less than 5%.[238] Median survival seldom reached 1 year, and rapid tumor dissemination to multiple organs was the rule. Since the introduction of primary chemotherapy into the multidisciplinary management for IBC, the prognosis has improved significantly. Most cases of IBC respond dramatically to chemotherapy; in addition, more than 90% of patients with IBC can be rendered free of locoregional disease with a combination of either chemotherapy and surgery or chemotherapy and radiotherapy, and 5-year survival rates now routinely exceed 30% and sometimes 50%. Long-term follow-up of multidisciplinary protocols from several institutions has shown that 25% to 30% of IBC patients survive progression-free for at least 10 and sometimes 15 years. Radiotherapy is a critical component of combined modality therapy for this subset of breast cancer. Although IBC is frequently ER-negative, patients with ER-positive IBC should be offered endocrine therapy after completion of chemotherapy and local-regional treatments. Patients with HER2-positive IBC should receive trastuzumab-containing combination therapy for optimal results. Although no randomized trials have been performed involving patients with IBC, those statistics represent such a dramatic departure from the natural history following locoregional therapy only that they provide reasonably compelling evidence of progress.

Despite improvements in both local and systemic control of locally advanced breast cancer and IBC achieved with modern combined-modality treatments, the majority of patients still die of the disease. Therefore, multiple attempts are under way to improve the odds of eradicating micrometastases. Among them, consolidation therapy with paclitaxel, docetaxel, vinorelbine, and several molecularly targeted agents is being tested.

Treatment of the Elderly

The fastest growing segment of the US population is that aged 65 years or older. Today, this group represents 12% of the population, but 50% of breast cancers occur in this group. As life expectancy of US women approaches 80 years, and as our elders are healthier today, the life expectancy of most breast cancer patients exceeds 10 years. Few studies have been carried out to clearly define the management of elderly women with breast cancer. The definition of "elderly" may be based on chronologic age, physiologic age, or life expectancy. Increasingly, therapeutic decisions in this group are made on the basis of comorbid conditions that usually limit life expectancy to a much greater extent than breast cancer. A healthy 70 year old patient with breast cancer should be treated the same way as someone with the same stage who is twenty years younger. The presence of important comorbid conditions changes life expectancy, and therefore the expected benefits from all our interventions for breast cancer. The standard treatment for "elderly patients with early stage breast cancer should be lumpectomy, sentinel lymph node biopsy and radiotherapy, with adjuvant systemic treatment defined on the basis of prognostic factors, ER, PR, and HER2. Increasingly, molecular profiles that predict tumor behavior will aid us in tailoring treatment. In a recent study of the impact of the NKI 70 gene test on a population where 70% were over the age of 55, the NKI low population experienced no recurrences after 8 years, in spite of no systemic adjuvant treatment. In the future, we will look to the use of molecular tests to define a population of patients where we can test the impact of less intervention.

At present, the use of aromatase inhibitors or tamoxifen has become standard therapy for the management of women with hormone receptor–positive tumors, regardless of age. Endocrine therapy is not indicated for patients with hormone receptor-negative tumors. It should be noted, that in CALGB 9343, women over 70 with ER positive tumors treated with tamoxifen or tamoxifen plus radiation were much more likely to die of other disease. At 8 years, death from breast cancer was 3% and death from other causes was 21%.

Once it is determined that the risk is high enough for chemotherapy to be administered and that the benefit from chemotherapy will exceed its risks, full dose chemotherapy should be given to elderly patients. The use of less than full-dose chemotherapy will usually be ineffective, at the cost of unnecessary toxicity. In a CALGB study, however, women who received doxorubicin in a CAF regimen at a dose of 30 mg/m^2 every 4 weeks × 4, did as well as those who received 60 mg/m^2 × 4 or 40 mg/m^2 × 6 if their HER2/neu assay was negative. Prospective validation of these results is needed. Only recently, has there been interest in devising protocols to evaluate new drugs that may be less toxic in such patients. A recently reported clinical trial compared single-agent oral capecitabine with classical CMF or AC in the adjuvant treatment of patients older than age 65. Capecitabine was clearly inferior to the standard regimens in disease-free survival.

Breast Cancer Prevention Strategies

All women are at risk for developing breast cancer. If a woman lives to the age of 80, she has a 1 in 8 chance of developing breast cancer. This does not tell us what type of breast cancer will develop and whether it will be lethal, only that there is a risk of developing some type of breast cancer. Most women are interested in their risk over the next 5 to 10 years, not just their lifetime risk. The timing of risk is important for thinking about surveillance and treatment of high-risk women. Women have about a 12% lifetime risk of getting cancer, but that risk is distributed differently, depending on age, exposures, and genetic composition. The average 25-year old woman has a 1 in 20,000 chance of developing a cancer. That is in contrast, however, to the extreme of someone who is at very high risk based on an inherited mutation in *BRCA1* or *BRCA2*.

In the setting of a known inherited mutation in *BRCA1* or *BRCA2*, testing a woman family member for the presence of that mutation will update the lifetime probability of developing breast cancer to 40% to 85% if the mutation is found, or to a lifetime risk of 12% if a mutation is not found. More importantly, the risk curve is shifted dramatically to the left, indicating that women with the mutation get cancers at a much earlier age. Therefore, a 30-year-old with a known *BRCA* mutation, who presents with a mass has a much higher likelihood of having a cancer and should be treated accordingly.

Mutations in both *BRCA1* or *BRCA2* result in impaired DNA repair, but the tumors that arise are different. Interestingly, we now know that mutations in the *BRCA1* gene lead frequently to the development of high-grade, circumscribed tumors (medullary carcinomas). We also know something about the pathways that activate the tumors. The tumors in the setting of a *BRCA1* mutation are usually devoid of estrogen and progesterone receptors on the surface and they do not overexpress *HER2/neu*. Expression profiling has confirmed this observation, demonstrating that the gene expression pattern shows that BRCA1 tumors have the basal cell phenotype, also typically ER–/PR–/HER2/neu–, or "triple negative," and are thought to arise from basal cells within the breast ducts.[307] Women who develop BRCA2-mutated tumors are more likely to develop ER-positive tumors that are HER2-negative. The understanding of the biology of the tumors that develop enables us to tailor recommendations for preventive interventions. For example, women with *BRCA2* mutations who are not interested in prophylactic mastectomy can be offered chemoprevention (tamoxifen or raloxifene), known to reduce the risk of ER-positive tumors.

Approximately 15% of breast cancers are considered hereditary, but only 5% to 7% can be explained based on inherited mutations in *BRCA1* or *BRCA 2*. Considerable effort is being devoted to improve our ability to find groups at high risk, especially young women and to develop methods or tools to risk-stratify the population.[308] Genetic testing is an example of a tool that has tremendous risk discrimination. In the setting of a family with a known inherited mutation in *BRCA1* or *BRCA2*, an unaffected family member has a 50% chance of carrying that mutation. Clearly, these results would and often do generate very different choices for breast cancer prevention. Women at highest risk often choose prophylactic mastectomy (17-35%). Women more often choose prophylactic oophorectomy (35-50%) because of the increased lifetime risk for developing ovarian cancer (20-40%, depending on the mutation), the ability to remove the ovaries by laparoscopy, the limited ability to effectively screen for that disease, and because of the significant risk reduction in breast cancer risk (see discussion below). However, it is important to remember that a negative genetic test can only be used to assure women that they have the same risk as the average woman if there is a known mutation in the family. Otherwise, a woman from a family where many members have been affected by cancer must continue to be considered high risk. Genetic testing plays an important role in cancer prevention and identifying women who stand to benefit most from prophylactic surgery (mastectomy and oophorectcomy).[309] Early surgical prophylaxis results in huge improvement in life years gained (over 4 years). In addition, women who present with early onset cancer represent an opportunity to identify mutation carriers, who may carry a significant risk of developing contralateral breast cancers as well as ovarian cancer, and identification of a mutation often will alter surgical treatment.

There are a number of conditions that identify women at "high risk" for developing breast cancer. Table 104-17 shows the risk for progression to invasive cancer for a given diagnosis (CBC, contralateral breast cancer; DCIS, ductal carcinoma in situ; LCIS, lobular carcinoma in situ.[310] The ranges of risk overlap, but the treatment choices are extremely different. As work in the prevention field starts to intersect with the management of cancer, and in particular, in situ cancer, we will begin to merge our ideas of risk and provide a more rational intervention approach for women with a variety of conditions, who now are given very different treatment recommendations. What is the reason for identifying a woman as having high risk? One reason is to tailor screening and surveillance strategies, and the other is to offer chemoprevention, prophylactic surgery, or participation in breast cancer prevention trials. Several risk models have been developed and are being used for counseling in the clinic to help women make decisions about breast cancer. Increasingly, scientists and clinicians are thinking about using biomarkers to identify both an increased risk for breast cancer and increased likelihood that a particular drug/intervention will be successful in lowering risk.[69]

Breast Cancer Screening Options for Women at High Risk ■ The standard recommendations for screening are to begin mammographic screening 10 years prior to the onset of cancer in the youngest first- or second-degree relative with breast cancer. However, another option is emerging that should be considered for very high-risk women, MRI. The appropriate population for MRI screening includes women with known genetic predisposition, or extremely high risk based on family history, dense breast tissue, and deleterious *BRCA1* and mutations. Two large screening studies have now demonstrated that MRI is far more sensitive than mammography in very high risk women.[133,135]

One-third of the mutation carriers with screened cancers had tumors over 2 cm compared to 13% and 19% of the high- and moderate-risk groups, respectively. The mutation carriers have high-grade tumors with an apparently faster potential for metastatic spread and a higher chance of having nodes involved, and perhaps should be screened at different intervals. There did not appear to be a difference in the rate of cancers between the moderate- and high-risk groups, but the biology was not the same. As we go forward, it will be critical to develop tools to improve our ability to predict which cancers women are susceptible to and tailor screening strategies accordingly. For example, *BRCA2* carriers may be able to have annual screening, whereas *BRCA1* carriers might be better served with screening that is more frequent. Interestingly, whereas MRI found many more cancers (20 of 45) that were not seen by mammography, there were eight cancers seen by mammography alone, and one found by clinical exam alone.[311] This suggests that the optimal screening strategy for mutation carriers may be to stagger mammography and MRI at 6-month intervals and a physical exam should be performed at that time as well.

Table 104-17 ■ **Estimated Yearly Rate for Progression to Invasive Breast Cancer Without Treatment**

Predisposing Condition	Annual Rate (%)
DCIS	1-3
Atypical hyperplasia	1-4
LCIS	0.5-2
BRCA1 or *BRCA2* mutation	1-5
5-Year Gail risk of >5	1-2
60-year-old woman with Gail risk ≤2.0	0.3-0.5
CBC invasive cancer	0.5

Abbreviations: CBC, contralateral breast cancer; DCIS, ductal carcinoma in situ; LCIS, lobular carcinoma in situ.[92]

For the purposes of identifying women at sufficiently high risk to justify MRI screening, a reasonable strategy, given the current data, is to evaluate women on the basis of three criteria: age under 50, dense breasts, and at least a threefold higher lifetime risk than the average woman (in the range of 35% or greater). For a mutation carrier, elevated risk and young age (where standard screening has limited value) are sufficient to recommend MRI screening. For women without a known mutation, the modified Gail Risk (described earlier) can be used as a guide. Women with a 50% lifetime risk fall into the recommended guidelines. Those with lifetime risk of 35-50% can be considered for MRI screening, and this approach requires a balanced discussion of the risks (false positives requiring biopsy which may be difficult to perform) and benefits with the patients. The density-modified Gail Risk combines both risk and likelihood of benefit from standard screening, (dense breast tissue decreases the sensitivity of mammography) as women with very dense breast tissue are given a multiplier of 2.5 in this model.[312]

Risk Reduction Options for Breast Cancer ■ The management of high-risk women is challenging. The degree of underlying risk, patient risk tolerance and preference, and the attendant "price to pay" for each intervention is what should drive these decisions. Although many women are concerned about their risk of developing breast cancer, their options for risk reduction are limited.[310] Current preventative or risk-reducing options include prophylactic surgery, ovarian suppression, chemoprevention with tamoxifen, and lifestyle modifications.

Prophylactic Surgery ■ Evidence suggests that prophylactic mastectomy provides the most breast cancer risk reduction, decreasing a woman's breast cancer risk by greater than 90%.[313,314] Although reconstruction options have improved significantly,[315,316] prophylactic mastectomy still comes at high personal cost for most women. Total skin-sparing mastectomy (see section below on mastectomy) provides superior cosmetic results, and is emerging as a safe and reliable technique. Often, the ability to preserve the nipple and areolar skin is very important to young women and is sufficient to enable them to take advantage of the risk reducing benefits of prophylactic mastectomy. Prophylactic oophorectomy for women in their 30s can reduce breast cancer risk by as much as 60%.[315] Early oophorectomy is a particularly good option for women who are at increased risk because of hereditary predisposition (*BRCA1* or *BRCA2* mutation carriers) and who face risk of both breast and ovarian cancer, but the decision is dependent on the timing of childbearing.

Prophylactic mastectomy has been shown, in retrospective cohort studies, to dramatically reduce the risk of developing breast cancer.[313,314] This has now been confirmed in a prospective study. Rebeck and colleagues showed that, in a cohort of 483 mutation carriers, 1.9% of those who had chosen mastectomy developed cancer, vs 98.1% of those who did not, with a 95% reduction in risk.[317] Prophylactic surgery is estimated to extend life expectancy in women with *BRCA1* or *BRCA2* mutations in their 30s and 50s by 1.6 and 0.9-years, respectively.[309] Prophylactic oophorectomy alone will also reduce the risk of developing breast cancer, by 60% if the oophorectomy is performed in the patients' 30s, and 50% if it is performed in their 40s. The risk reduction from prophylactic surgery is shown on Figure 104-26 for a woman with high risk based on an inherited mutation in either *BRCA1* or *BRCA2*. The graphic is taken from a prevention tool used for patient education.

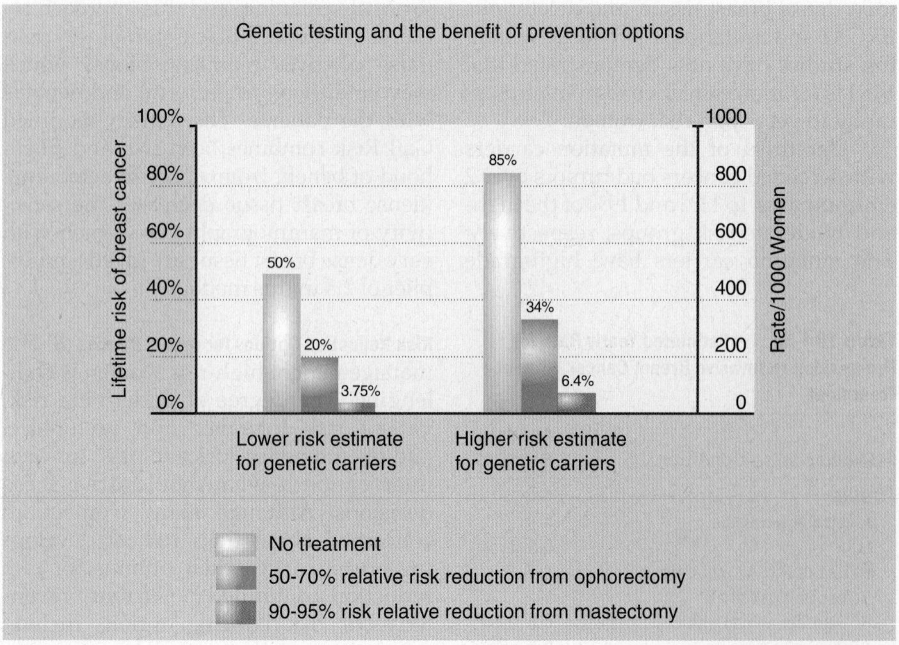

Figure 104-26 ■ Risk reduction from prophylactic surgery for a woman with high risk on the basis of an inherited mutation in either BRCA1 or 2.

Lobular Carcinoma In Situ

The surgical treatment of LCIS has changed in recent years as a result of a better understanding of the biology and natural history of this tumor. Treatment strategies for LCIS evolved from considerations relative to its multi-centricity, its bilaterality, and its tendency to develop into invasive breast cancer. Formerly, the recommended therapy for LCIS included bilateral total mastectomy, total mastectomy with mirror-image biopsy of the opposite breast, or total mastectomy with elective biopsy of the opposite breast. However, better information about the natural history of LCIS indicates that the majority of patients with the disease do not develop invasive cancer. Furthermore, both breasts are at similar risk for the development of invasive cancer. LCIS is a marker for increased risk for the development of invasive breast cancer of any type in either breast and does not represent a marker of risk in a particular region of breast tissue. The likelihood of developing invasive lobular cancer is much higher (40-50%) relative to the frequency of ductal cancers (10%).[318] Because the risk for developing cancer spans a horizon of 5 to 15 years, and because the in situ lesion does not necessarily predict the geographic location for cancer development, further surgery is not considered the appropriate treatment in a patient with a biopsy-proven LCIS, even if the margins of resection are involved. However, since such patients are at higher risk for developing invasive cancer (a risk estimated to be approximately 10 times the normal), close follow-up with mammography and physical examination is recommended. To date, there is no evidence that breast irradiation is effective in preventing the development of invasive cancer in patients with LCIS.

A more rational approach to the management of LCIS would be an attempt to prevent the development of invasive breast cancer in women with this disease. The National Surgical Adjuvant Breast and Bowel Project (NSABP) breast cancer prevention trial[72] demonstrated that tamoxifen reduced the risk of a woman with diagnosed LCIS progressing to invasive cancer reduced by nearly 50%. Because LCIS is the expression of a phenotype carrying a higher than-normal risk of breast cancer, interventions like tamoxifen represent the promise of ultimate biologic control of these conditions.

Chemoprevention ■ ***Tamoxifen*** ■ Anoption for women at increased risk is a 5-year course of tamoxifen therapy. The FDA approved this chemoprevention drug for women with a 5-year breast cancer risk equal to or greater than 1.67% as assessed by the Gail risk assessment model. This relatively arbitrary Gail score was chosen as that of an average 60-year-old woman. Tamoxifen data from the NSABP P-1 Breast Cancer Prevention Trial (BCPT) demonstrated that the use of tamoxifen can decrease a woman's risk of developing breast cancer with an average RR reduction of 49% in a 4 to 5 year period (Table 104-18). Although other tamoxifen prevention studies have not shown as great a reduction in breast cancer, a meta-analysis including the P-1 trial and three other trials utilizing tamoxifen concluded that this agent reduced risk of breast cancer by about 38%, without significantly affecting overall survival yet (Fig. 104-27).[319] Women with a known cancer have an elevated risk of developing a contralateral cancer, and tamoxifen in the adjuvant setting confers approximately a 50% reduction in risk of contralateral cancer.

Decisions about the use of tamoxifen can be very difficult for women who are yet unaffected by breast cancer. The NSABP prevention study demonstrated that of the 13,338 women in the study, only 120 breast cancers were averted. Tamoxifen is associated with both mild and

Table 104-18 **Rates for Invasive Breast Cancer by Age, 5-Year Predicted Breast Cancer Risk, Number of First-Degree Relatives With Breast Cancer, History of Lobular Carcinoma In Situ (LCIS), or History of Atypical Hyperplasia**

Patient Characteristic	Rate per 1000 Women per 5 Years		Risk Ratio	95% Confidence Interval
	Placebo	Tamoxifen		
Age (yr)				
49	33.5	18.9	0.56	0.4-0.9
50–59	31.4	15.5	0.49	0.3-0.8
≥60	36.7	16.6	0.49	0.3-0.7
5-Year predicted risk (%)				
≤2.00	27.7	10.3	0.37	0.2-0.7
≥ 5.01	66.4	22.6	0.34	0.2-0.6
Number of first-degree relatives with breast cancer				
0	32.3	14.9	0.46	0.2-0.8
1	30.0	15.2	0.51	0.4-0.7
2	43.4	23.8	0.55	0.3-1.0
3	68.6	35.1	0.51	0.2-1.6
History of LCIS				
Yes	65.0	28.5	0.44	0.2-1.1
No	32.1	16.5	0.51	0.4-0.7
History of atypical hyperplasia				
Yes	50.6	7.2	0.14	0.0-0.5
No	32.2	18.1	0.56	0.4-0.7

serious side effects. Serious side effects are limited largely to postmenopausal women and include a 1% increase in endometrial cancer (typically low grade) after 5 years and a similar increase in vascular events (in women over 60). The more frequent side effects decrease quality of life but the rare side effects can be life threatening.[72] Current estimates suggest that over 10 million women in the United States are eligible for tamoxifen use by FDA guidelines, but it is rarely prescribed by physicians or accepted by women as a preventive option.[320] Using more rigorous eligibility criteria for tamoxifen use proposed by Gail and colleagues,[321] it is still estimated that over 2 million women in the United States are eligible for tamoxifen treatment.[321] Approximately 200,000 women are expected to develop breast cancer this year, far less than either of the estimated number of women eligible for tamoxifen use.[3] Thus, better ways of identifying women at high

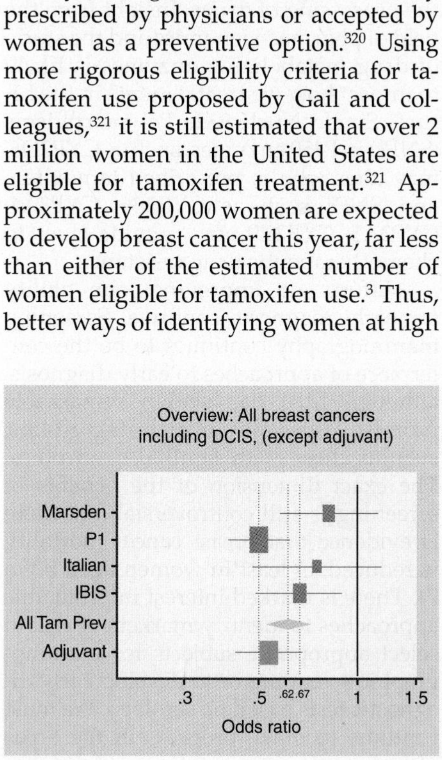

Figure 104-27 Reduction in the incidence of breast cancer by tamoxifen in randomized clinical trials.

risk are needed (see discussion in LCIS section), The presence of atypia found on surgical biopsy is an example of a biomarker that identifies women at higher risk and greater benefit from tamoxifen, and has been shown to motivate women to choose chemoprevention. However, not all women benefit from tamoxifen, and it does not appear to prevent the development of ER-negative disease, so new agents will be necessary. In order to optimize the use of preventive agents and minimize exposure to side effects, stratification by both risk of breast cancer and benefit from available interventions is necessary.

Raloxifene ■ Raloxifene which is a selective ER modifier, similar to tamoxifen, has been shown to significantly reduce the risk of ER-positive breast cancer in women at risk for osteoporosis, yet it does not appear to increase the risk of developing endometrial cancer.[322] It was tested in a large prevention trial by the NSABP (STAR Trial, NSABP P-2) where 19,747 women at high risk (Gail Risk above 1.67) were randomized to tamoxifen versus raloxifene. The numbers of invasive cancers in both groups were statistically equivalent. However, raloxifene seemed less effective in preventing noninvasive breast cancers than tamoxifen. One-third fewer uterine cancers developed in the raloxifene-treated group than the tamoxifen treated arm, and significantly fewer thromboembolic events were reported in the raloxifene arm. Twenty-seven percent of participants took the drug for 5 years. As a result of this and the previous trials indicating the risk-reduction effects of raloxifene, the FDA approved in early 2008 the indication of reduction in risk of invasive breast cancer in postmenopausal women.

Agents Under Investigation ■ Over the past 10 years, selective aromatase inhibitors were shown to be more effective and better tolerated than megestrol acetate and tamoxifen in treating metastatic and primary breast cancer. A significant reduction in second primary breast cancers was observed in randomized adjuvant trials when selective aromatase inhibitors were compared to tamoxifen. It is estimated that, compared to no endocrine treatment, aromatase inhibitors might reduce the risk of second primary breast cancers by up to 75%. Anastrozole is currently under assessment as a chemopreventive agent in three randomized trials: in two, it is being compared to tamoxifen (IBIS II and B-35 DCIS study); in the third, to placebo (IBIS II chemoprevention trial).

Much excitement was generated over the COX-2 inhibitors; however, after several of these agents were pulled from the market because of an associated increased risk in fatal and non-fatal cardiac events, all of the COX-2 inhibitors have come under investigation and most trials have been stopped. This underscores the importance of finding health-promoting or health-neutral interventions for prevention, given the need to expose large populations to the interventions in order to reduce the incidence of cancer. This suggests we should more closely investigate known health promoting drugs such as statins that have been reported to reduce breast cancer risk. It also makes a compelling case for identifying higher risk populations, such as patients with DCIS. We may soon be able to classify pre-malignant and high-risk lesions better by molecular means. Given that high-risk lesions are not an emergency, but rather a marker of predisposition to progress to invasive disease, time can be used to learn more about these lesions. It is possible that the peri-operative period, or a period of neoadjuvant treatment, will help us to learn more about the response characteristics of an individual tumor and lead to better ways of preventing breast cancer.

Lifestyle Changes ■ Lifestyle changes such as increased exercise, decreased consumption of alcohol and animal fat, and refraining from or stopping HRT are thought to have moderate risk reduction potential.[310,323,324] The Nurses' Health Study I and II have demonstrated that lifestyle modifications, especially maintenance of optimal weight after menopause and limiting animal fat intake, can decrease breast cancer risk by 30% to 45%.[325,326] Women thought to be at higher risk for breast cancer should avoid prolonged HRT exposure, and no woman should take it unless there is a specific reason or need. Women who drink excessively should take B vitamins, which have shown to be protective in the setting of alcohol.[47]

Perspectives

With the rapid rate of change in basic and clinical cancer research, it is sometimes difficult to see things in perspective. Some seemingly new ideas have really been around a long time, and some concepts seem to gain acceptance very slowly. For the first half of the twentieth century, breast cancer thinking was stuck in an anatomic mode leading to radical surgical concepts, and clinical research amounted to little more than counting cases and outcomes in tumor registries. With the advent of chemotherapy and modern endocrine therapy and the realization that breast cancer was more likely to be a systemic disease and that it was a disorder of growth regulation, new ideas quickly took hold.

One avenue of research was to determine the optimal amount of surgery necessary, and determine the indications of and the benefits from radiation therapy. A second was to combine surgery with systemic adjuvant systemic treatments to improve cure rates. When attention then focused on metastasis and issues of drug resistance, there began a happy convergence of basic and clinical researchers into what is now called translational research. From today's perspective, it is easy to see that we have made the transition from anatomic to biologic thinking and have many new and exciting avenues for further progress. In this chapter, we reviewed some of the new biologic approaches with adjuvant systemic therapy, including the recent introduction of trastuzumab, lapatinib, and bevacizumab into adjuvant therapy. We also reviewed the potential application of preoperative chemotherapy as a drug sensitivity test, and, perhaps most important for the immediate future, in the use of tamoxifen and raloxifene as a chemopreventative agents. In this sense, the two SERMs are presented not as simple anti-estrogens but as biologic growth factor inhibitors. Another investigative strategy would evaluate other interventions that might interfere with the initiation and/or promotion of breast cancers. Although there are several candidates for evaluation (eg, low-fat diets, other SERMs, COX-2- inhibitors or retinoids), one category that is particularly interesting involves drugs that act as inhibitors of aromatase.

It is clear that systemic therapies have become better tolerated and more effective, and the relative importance of surgery and radiation therapy has shifted. It is easier to obtain local control than it is to control metastases, even the micrometastases at which adjuvant therapies are aimed. Therefore, efforts must be directed at identifying better systemic therapies. New cytotoxic agents, such as capecitabine, gemcitabine, liposomal doxorubicin, vinorelbine and ixabepilone have already been tested and shown to have clear antitumor activity. Other efforts to devise progressively better regimens for systemic treatment, both for adjuvant and advanced disease, should certainly persist. The power of endocrine interventions has become manifest as novel agents are moved into the adjuvant setting. Within the past 5 years, the aromatase inhibitors have changed completely our approach to adjuvant endocrine therapy. As our understanding of the crosstalk between the various growth factor pathways, including the estrogen-driven signaling, HER2, IGF1-R, PI3K/AKT/mTOR and angiogenesis increases, combined therapies will become more effective and better targeted to individual needs.

The emergence of molecular profiling and their evolving role in both prognosis and prediction of response to therapy holds the promise of enabling us to tailor our efforts to improve screening, prevention, and treatment. Clearly, breast cancer is very heterogeneous, and one treatment will not be effective against all tumors. New molecular profiles suggest, as does long term follow-up of patient cohorts, that there is likely to be a population of breast cancers that do not have a significant risk for progression and may be best managed with local regional directed therapy. In contrast, in those cancers with substantial risk for progression, the most critical intervention is identifying the therapy that is most effective against the specific tumor type. As we go forward, we will have the opportunity to apply profiling to better characterize low risk cancers, and to study the impact of eliminating interventions. In women with higher risk tumors, we have the opportunity to study the impact of targeted therapies using the neoadjuvant approach, optimizing interventions based on the biology of the tumors using tumor markers, imaging, and innovative trial design. Using response of the primary tumor has the advantage of dramatically shortening the time to assessing new agents and studies that incorporate biomarkers carry the promise of being able to develop markers that can be used to guide optimal therapy. The neoadjuvant model should be used not only for chemotherapy and cytotoxic therapy, but for endocrine therapy, in women whose cancers appear to respond best to hormonal therapies. Finally, the *in situ* setting can also be used as an opportunity to learn how to tailor prevention interventions, and a neoadjuvant approach to this disease entity, again, incorporating imaging and molecular markers, may also accelerate our ability to learn who is likely to respond to known interventions, test new interventions, and tailor therapy in the future.

In addition to the heterogeneity of tumors, we are starting to understand the heterogeneity of the host, including the microenvironment in which tumors arise. The microenvironment may provide clues to how to develop new treatment approaches. New therapeutic modalities, such as immunomodulators and vaccines, are currently in early clinical trials. Targeted immune cells may be used to introduce cytotoxic agents, such as tumor necrosis factor, directly to tumor cells, or to alter tumor cells genetically in order to suppress their growth. There is emerging interest in targeting the tumor microenvironment and new agents that targeted such cells, such as macrophages, are starting to enter phase 1 trials. Such approaches may be tested alone or in conjunction with chemo- and hormonal therapeutic agents of proven value. Evaluation of methodologies for overcoming drug resistance and for modulating the action of chemotherapeutic agents based on pharmacologic principles should also continue, as should testing of currently available modalities in novel ways.

Other host factors include the consideration of the individual variation in the processing of drugs. Insight from the field of pharmacogenomics and the study of drug metabolizing enzymes is likely to impact how we treat patients in the future. Single Nucleotide Polymorphisms (SNPs) in P450 enzymes, such as CYP2D6, may alter who is prescribed tamoxifen, and SNPs such as CYP2B6, CYP3A4, CYP3A5, CYP2C9 may provide clues to chemotherapeutic drug resistance.

Efforts at improving our ability for early diagnosis continue. Screening mammography continues to be the centerpiece of approaches to early diagnosis, although MRI has shown remarkable promise, especially in high-risk groups, such as those with familial syndromes. The exact dimension of the benefits of screening is still controversial, but there is evidence that breast cancer mortality is reduced, at least in women aged 50 to 74. There is marked interest in proteomic approaches to identify markers of risk to select appropriate subjects for mammographic screening or to develop early diagnostic tests based on serology. We must continue to make progress in the areas of breast cancer prevention and of early treatment of systemic metastases as described above. One happy, but still troubling aspect of successful mammographic screening is the continued increase in the proportion of small tumors at diagnosis. Sorting out how much treatment is appropriate in these cases will continue to occupy our attention.

It is likely that any discussion of breast cancer will have as its major component information regarding the mechanisms and feasibility of chemoprevention. The findings of the tamoxifen and raloxifene prevention trials are arguably some of the most important public health advances in breast cancer, mainly because they demonstrate that it is feasible to intervene and reduce breast cancer incidence with a pharmacologic agent, which opens new avenues for research. Ongoing studies in this area (NSABP B-35 and IBIS II trials) will define the best choice of agents for chemoprevention and identify the role of aromatase inhibitors in primary and secondary prevention. Breast cancer results from DNA damage, and, although it is possible that lifestyle changes can diminish this slightly, it will take intervention with active agents, with their risk of side effects, to control or reverse this fundamental cause.

Last, but probably most important because it brings us to the core of the problem, are all of the new advances in molecular biology and genetics. Better fundamental understanding of the etiology and pathogenesis of breast cancer should provide new approaches that are likely to have a major impact on therapy, diagnosis, and prevention. As it has for decades, the rate of progress continues to increase. New knowledge continues to offer us new possibilities and new challenges.

Selected References

The complete reference list can be found at www.CANCERMEDICINE8.com

1. Hortobagyi GN. Treatment of breast cancer. *N Engl J Med.* 1998;339:974–984.
3. Jemal A, Siegel R, Ward E, et al. Cancer statistics, 2008. *CA Cancer J Clin.* 2008;58:71–96.
4. Garcia M, Jemal A, Ward EM, et al. *Global Cancer Facts & Figures 2007.* Atlanta, GA: American Cancer Society, 2007.
14. Lynch HT, Lynch JF. Breast cancer genetics in an oncology clinic: 328 consecutive patients. *Cancer Genet Cytogenet.* 1986;22:369–371.
18. Blackwood MA, Weber BL. BRCA1 and BRCA2. From molecular genetics to clinical medicine. *J Clin Oncol.* 1998;16:1969–1977.
23. Thompson D, Easton DF. Breast Cancer Linkage Consortium. Cancer Incidence in BRCA1 mutation carriers. *J Nat Cancer Inst.* 2002;94:1358–1365.
27. Chlebowski RT, Hendrix SL, Langer RD, et al. Influence of Estrogen plus Progestin on breast cancer plus mammography in Healthy Postmenopausal women: The Women's Health Initiative Randomized Trial. *JAMA.* 2003;289:3243–3253.
29. Collaborative Group on Hormonal Factors in Breast Cancer. Breast cancer and hormone replacement therapy. Collaborative reanalysis of data from 51 epidemiological studies of 52,705 women with breast cancer and 108,411 women without breast cancer. *Lancet.* 1997;350:1047–1059.
33. Collaborative Group on Hormonal Factors in Breast Cancer. Breast cancer and hormonal contraceptives. Collaborative reanalysis of individual data on 53,297 women with breast cancer and 100,239 women without breast cancer from 54 epidemiological studies. *Lancet.* 1996;347:1713–1727.
45. Schatzkin A, Jones DY, Hoover RN, et al. Alcohol consumption and breast cancer in the epidemiologic follow-up study of the first National Health and Nutrition Examination Survey. *N Engl J Med.* 1987;316:1169–1173.
51. Dupont WD, Page DL. Risk factors for breast cancer in women with proliferative breast disease. *N Engl J Med.* 1985;312:146–151.
53. Hartmann LC, Sellers TA, Frost MH, et al. Benign breast disease and the risk of breast cancer. *N Engl J Med.* 2005;353: 229–237.
59. Gail MH, Brinton LA, Byar DP, et al. Projecting individualized probabilities of developing breast cancer for white females who are being examined annually. *J Nat Cancer Inst.* 1989;81:1879–1886.
67. National Cancer Institute: Breast Cancer Risk Assessment Tool. Available at: http://bcra.nci.nih.gov/brc (last accessed July 30, 2005).
72. Fisher B, Costantino JP, Wickerham DL, et al. Tamoxifen for prevention of breast cancer: report of the National Surgical Adjuvant Breast and Bowel Project P-I Study. *J Natl Cancer Inst.* 1998;90:1371–1388.
73. Wolfe IN, Saftlas AF, Salane M. Mammographic parenchymal patterns and quantitative evaluation of marnmographic densities: a case-control study. *AJR Am J Roentgenol.* 1987; 1148:1087–1092.
78. Baselga J, Tripathy D, Mendelsohn J, et al. Phase II study of weekly intravenous recombinant humanized anti-pl85 HER2 monoclonal antibody in patients with HER2/neu-overexpressing metastatic breast cancer. *J Clin Oncol.* 1996;14:737–744.
80. Paik S, Shak S, Tang G, et al. A multigene assay to predict recurrence of tamoxifen-treated, node-negative breast cancer. *N Engl J Med.* 2004;351:2817–2826.
86. Carter CL, Allen C, Henson DE. Relation of tumor size, lymph node status, and survival in 24,740 breast cancer cases. *Cancer.* 1989;63:181–187.
87. Hanrahan EO, Gonzalez-Angulo AM, Giordano SH, et al. Overall survival and cause-specific mortality of patients with stage T1a,bN0M0 breast carcinoma. *J Clin Oncol.* 2007;25:4952–4960.
91. Mabry H, Giuliano AE. Sentinel node mapping for breast cancer: progress to date and prospects for the future. *Surg Oncol Clin North America.* 2007;16:55–70.
94. Gamel JW, Meyer JS, Feuer E, et al. The impact of stage and histology on the longterm clinical course of 163,808 patients with breast carcinoma. *Cancer.* 1996;77:1459–1464.
95. Pedersen L, Holck S, Schiodt T, et al. Medullary carcinoma of the breast, prognostic importance of characteristic histopathological features evaluated in a multivariate Cox analysis. *Eur J Cancer.* 1994;30:1792–1797.
98. Elston CW, Ellis IO. Pathologic prognostic factors in breast cancer. I. The value of histologic grade in breast cancer: experience from a large study with long-term follow-up. *Histopathol.* 1991;19: 403–410.
105. van't Veer LJ, Dai H, van de Vijver MJ, et al. Gene expression profiling predicts clinical outcome of breast cancer. *Nature.* 2002;415:530–536.
108. Paik S, Tang G, Shak S, et al. Gene expression and benefit of chemotherapy in women with node-negative, estrogen receptor-positive breast cancer. *J Clin Oncol.* 2006;24:3726–3734.
110. Weidner N, Semple JP, Welch WR, et al. Tumor angiogenesis and metastasis—correlation in invasive breast carcinoma. *N Engl J Med.* 1991;324:1–8.
116. Slamon DJ, Clark GM, Wong SG, et al. Human breast cancer. Correlation of relapse and survival with amplification of the HER-2/neu oncogene. *Science.* 1987;235:177–182.
122. Cristofanilli M, Budd GT, Ellis MJ, et al. Circulating tumor cells, disease progression, and survival in metastatic breast cancer. *N Engl J Med.* 2004;351:781–791.
124. Ravdin PM, Siminoff LA, Davis GJ, et al. Computer program to assist in making decisions about adjuvant therapy for women with early breast cancer. *J Clin Oncol.* 2001;19:980–991.
125. Ayers M, Symmans WF, Stec J, et al. Gene expression profiles predict complete pathologic response to neoadjuvant paclitaxel and fluorouracil, doxorubicin, and cyclophosphamide chemotherapy in breast cancer. *J Clin Oncol.* 2004;22:2284–2293.
131. Hylton N. Magnetic resonance imaging of the breast: opportunities to improve breast cancer management. *J Clin Oncol.* 2005;23:1678–1684.
135. Kriege M, Brekelmans CT, Boetes C, et al. Efficacy of MRI and mammography for breast-cancer screening in women with a familial or genetic predisposition. *N Engl J Med.* 2004;351:427–437.
150. Buchholz TA, Lehman CD, Harris JR, et al. Statement of the science concerning locoregional treatments after preoperative chemotherapy for breast cancer: a National Cancer Institute conference. *J Clin Oncol.* 2008;26:791–797.
152. Fisher B, Dignam J, Wolmark N, et al. Lumpectomy and radiation therapy for the treatment of intraductal breast cancer: findings from National Surgical Adjuvant Breast and Bowel Project B-17. *J Clin Oncol.* 1998;16:441–452.
165. Fisher B, Dignam J, Wolmark N, et al. Tamoxifen in treatment of intraductal breast cancer. National Surgical Adjuvant Breast and Bowel Project B-24 randomised controlled trial. *Lancet.* 1999;353:1993–2000.
173. Early Breast Cancer Trialists' Collaborative Group. Favourable and unfavourable effects on long-term survival of radiotherapy for early breast cancer: an overview of the randomised trials. *Lancet.* 2000;355:1757–1770.
192. Pierce LJ, Levin AM, Rebbeck TR, et al. Ten-year multi-institutional results of breast-conserving surgery and radiotherapy in BRCA1/2-associated stage I/II breast cancer. *J Clin Oncol.* 2006;24:2437–2443.

198. Whelan TJ, MacKenzie RG, Levine M, et al. A randomized trial comparing two fractionation schedules for breast irradiation postlumpectomy in node-negative breast cancer. *Proc Am Soc Clin Oncol.* 2000;19:2a (abst 5).
203. Vicini FA, Antonucci JV, Wallace M, et al. Long-term efficacy and patterns of failure after accelerated partial breast irradiation: a molecular assay-based clonality evaluation. *Int J Radiat Oncol Biol Phys.* 2007;68:341–346.
210. Rastogi P, Anderson SJ, Bear HD, et al. Preoperative chemotherapy: updates of National Surgical Adjuvant Breast and Bowel Project Protocols B-18 and B-27. *J Clin Oncol.* 2008;26:778–785.
256. Slamon DJ, Leyland-Jones B, Shak S, et al. Use of chemotherapy plus a monoclonal antibody against HER2 for metastatic breast cancer that overexpresses HER2. *N Engl J Med.* 2001;344:783–792.
263. Early Breast Cancer Trialists' Collaborative Group (EBCTCG). Effects of chemotherapy and hormonal therapy for early breast cancer on recurrence and 15-year survival: an overview of the randomized trials. *Lancet.* 2005;365:1687–1717.
268. Early Breast Cancer Trialists' Collaborative Group. Tamoxifen for early breast cancer: an overview of the randomised trials. *Lancet.* 1998;351:1451–1467.
275. Arimidex, Tamoxifen alone or in Combination ATAC Trialists' Group, et al. Effect of anastrozole and tamoxifen as adjuvant treatment for early-stage breast cancer: 100-month analysis of the ATAC trial. *Lancet Oncology.* 2008;9.1:45–53.
278. Winer EP, Hudis C, Burstein HJ, et al. American Society of Clinical Oncology Technology assessment on the use of aromatase inhibitors as adjuvant therapy for postmenopausal women with hormone receptor-positive breast cancer: status report 2004. *J Clin Oncol.* 2005;23: 619–629.
286. Pritchard KI, Messersmith H, Elavathil L, et al. HER-2 and topoisomerase II as predictors of response to chemotherapy. *J Clin Oncol.* 2008;26:736–744.
307. Sorlie T, Perou C, Tibshirani R, et al. Gene expression patterns of breast carcinomas distinguish tumor subclasses with clinical implications. *Proc Natl Acad Sci U S A.* 2001; 98:10869–10874.
313. Rebbeck TR, Friebel T, Lynch HT, et al. Bilateral prophylactic mastectomy reduces breast cancer risk in BRCAI and BRCA2 mutation carriers: The PROSE Study Group. *J Clin Oncol.* 2004;22(6):1055–1062.

105 Melanoma

Jeffrey E. Gershenwald, MD ■ Patrick Hwu, MD

Epidemiology and Etiology

According to the American Cancer Society, 68,720 new cases of melanoma will have been diagnosed in the United States in 2009, and approximately 8,650 deaths from the disease will have ocurred.[1] Between 1975 and 2005, the annual incidence of invasive cutaneous melanoma in the United States has been rising by an average of 3.1% per year, faster than that of nearly all cancers.[2,3] The lifetime risk for developing cutaneous melanoma is 1 in 50.[2] The age-adjusted annual incidence in the United States is approximately 22.6 per 100,000; some geographic areas have a greater incidence.[2] Trends indicate that the incidence of melanoma continues to increase, particularly in individuals over 65 years. Additionally, recent data demonstrate a real increase for both males and females, including young women.[2,4] Also of concern is the finding that while the incidence of most cancers followed by SEER is decreasing, among those cancers which show increasing incidence between 1995 and 2006, the increase in melanoma incidence rates is the highest.[2] Over the past 30 years, there have been changes in the distribution and stage of melanoma at diagnosis, with an increase in thinner lesions.

Risk Factors

Numerous epidemiologic studies have identified risk factors—including environmental, genetic, and host—that determine melanoma risk. From a clinical standpoint, understanding the nature and complexity of these interacting factors can be useful in determining primary prevention and screening strategies. Patients identified as having a high risk for melanoma can also be recruited to ongoing and future prevention trials.

Environmental Factors

Several observations strongly suggest that ultraviolet (UV) light may be a critical factor leading to the development of cutaneous melanoma.[5,6] The incidence of melanoma increases with increasing distance from the North and South Poles. Adults who migrate to sunny climates are at less risk than similar individuals who were born there, suggesting that duration of exposure to UV radiation may be important in the development of melanoma. Freckles and nevi induced by solar irradiation are risk factors for the development of melanoma. These epidemiologic observations suggest that sunlight, particularly UV light, has an important role in the induction of cutaneous melanoma and that changes in the pattern of sun exposure have substantially contributed to increases in melanoma incidence during the past several decades.

Occasional or recreational exposure to sunlight, especially a history of severe blistering sunburn, has been associated with increased risk of melanoma; these observations are consistent with a hypothesis that the relationship between sun exposure and the risk of developing melanoma is related to acute, intense, and intermittent exposure. However, UV radiation may play different roles for different categories of melanomas. Melanomas on intermittently exposed sites such as the trunk and proximal extremities peak in incidence around 55 years of age, while melanomas on chronically exposed sites such as the face and distal extremities continue to rise with age. The relative incidence drop of melanomas on intermittently exposed skin indicates a period of vulnerability to UV radiation early in life, which is consistent with epidemiologic studies that show migration before puberty into geographic regions with high UV exposure as a major risk factor. Factors other than UV light also contribute to the development of melanoma. Melanoma can occur in relatively or absolutely unexposed areas, such as the palms and soles and even in mucosal sites. These melanoma types account for only a small percentage of melanomas in Caucasian populations, but represent the majority in populations of African or Asian extraction. The effects of sunlight have mainly been attributed to exposure to UV-B radiation. Some evidence also implicates UV-A radiation in the development of melanoma through the production of oxygen radical species capable of inducing DNA mutations.[7] Data also support the fact that the increase in melanoma incidence among young women is observed in the context of overall trends in UV radiation exposure. Trends among adolescents 16-18 years of age demonstrate that both the prevalence of sunburn and average number of days spent at the beach[4] continues to increase, and that tanning bed usage is also increasing among U.S. adults, where it is also most prevalent among young women.[4]

Evolving data support that tanning bed use may increase the risk of melanoma.[8-12] In a systematic review, the International Agency for Research on Cancer Working Group on Artificial Ultraviolet Light and Skin Cancer revealed an association of age at first use of less than 35 years with melanoma risk, with a relative risk of 1.75 (1.35-2.26).[12] The use of a tanning bed more than 10 times per year is associated with a doubling in the risk of melanoma for patients age 30 years or older. Young patients who use tanning booths more than 10 times per year have more than 7 times the melanoma risk of patients who do not use tanning booths. Taken together, these findings also support the concept that childhood exposure to sunlight is associated with melanoma risk in adults.[12]

Host Factors

Although the etiology of melanoma is not entirely understood, case-control studies have shown that it is largely a disease of fair-complected individuals. Individuals with red or blond hair and fair skin, who burn easily or have a history of severe sunburn, or who are unable to tan are at substantially higher risk of developing melanoma than more darkly pigmented, age-matched controls. Individuals with an increased number of nevi or a tendency to develop freckles are also at increased risk for developing melanoma.[13] Several genome-wide association studies have revealed inherited polymorphisms in genes important in constitutive skin pigmentation and the tanning response to be risk factors for melanoma and non-melanoma skin cancers. Recently, the risk of cutaneous melanoma in the presence of increased numbers of nevi, large nevi, and clinically atypical nevi on the body was confirmed in a pooled analysis of melanocytic nevus phenotype, even at different latitudes.[14] Both prior personal history (relative risk 9-10) and family history (relative risk 8) are important risk factors for the development of melanoma.[6] It has been estimated that the cumulative probability of having a second primary diagnosed within 5 years of initial diagnosis is approximately 5%, a 25-fold increase in risk over the general population.[15] Patients who have specific genetic conditions such as xeroderma pigmentosum, retinoblastoma, and Li-Fraumeni syndrome, are also at increased risk.

Genetic Predisposition and Familial Melanoma

Approximately 5-12% of all cases of cutaneous melanoma occur in persons with a familial predisposition to the development of melanoma.[16] Familial human melanoma is characterized by an increased risk of developing a primary tumor, a higher incidence of multiple primary tumors, and typically an earlier age at onset.[6,17] Nonetheless, compared to patients with nonfamilial melanoma, the clinical course and histologic appearance are not appreciably different. Specific genetic alterations have been implicated in the pathogenesis of familial melanoma. Mutations at the CDKN2A locus on chromosome 9p21 which codes for the tumor suppressor p16 and p14/ARF account for about one-third of familial cases. A minority of familial melanomas is caused by inherited mutations in CDK4 at chromosome 12q14.

Nonetheless, since mutations of either of these genes are present in only a subset of familial melanoma kindreds, other melanoma susceptibility genes likely exist. In some families with CDKN2A mutations, an increased risk of developing pancreatic cancer and other cancers is found.[18,19] All patients and their families should undergo surveillance and participate in educational programs as part of their routine medical care.[20] Moreover, due to the low likelihood of identifying mutations even among high-risk individuals, challenges to interpretation of positive test results, and, in particular, the lack of change in medical management, genetic testing other than for research purposes is generally not recommended (see also the section on Molecular Pathology below).

Atypical Mole and Melanoma Syndrome

Previously known as dysplastic nevus syndrome, atypical mole and melanoma syndrome is characterized by the presence of multiple, generally large atypical moles (dysplastic nevi) that represent a distinct clinicopathologic type of melanocytic lesion. They can be precursors of melanoma as well as markers of increased melanoma risk.[6] Although the actual frequency of an atypical mole progressing to melanoma may be low, patients with atypical mole and melanoma syndrome should be observed closely, and family members should be screened. Melanoma may arise from dysplastic nevi or from apparently normal skin remote from nevi in these patients; this latter observation contributes to the argument against resection of all atypical nevi for melanoma prevention. Melanomas associated with dysplastic nevi are generally of the superficial spreading type and are often relatively thin.

Giant Congenital Nevi

A giant congenital nevus has been defined as a nevus that measures at least 15 cm in diameter or at least twice the size of the affected person's palm. Patients with giant congenital nevi have an estimated 4-10% lifetime risk of developing a melanoma.[21-23] For those individuals with a giant congenital nevus greater than 20 cm, the estimated relative risk of developing melanoma is five.[6] It is estimated that approximately half of the melanomas that develop in giant congenital nevi develop within the first 3-5 years of life. However, a considerable proportion of these childhood lesions may represent benign lesions that mimic melanoma histopathologically. Decisions about the management of giant congenital nevi are difficult because such lesions are often so extensive that prophylactic surgical excision may be impossible. When the location and size of a lesion permit prophylactic excision, some experts suggest that excision should be considered before the age of 2 years. Among 170 prospectively followed patients with large congenital melanocytic nevi (LCMN), large LCMN diameter and increasing number of satellite lesions were noted among patients who developed melanoma compared to patients who did not.[24]

Melanocytes and Antecedent Lesions

Melanocytes, pigment-producing cells, arise from the neural crest and migrate to their final destinations in the skin, uveal tract, meninges, and mucosae. Most melanocytes are found at the epidermal-dermal junction of the skin, and the vast majority of melanomas arise from cutaneous sites. However, melanoma has also been reported in the meninges, in the mucosa of the oropharynx, and in the gastrointestinal, respiratory, and urogenital tracts. Clinical and histological observations indicate that a subset of melanomas arise in association with a pre-existing melanocytic lesion.[25] However, the distinction between areas possibly representing a benign nevus and the melanoma portion cannot always be made with certainty on morphological grounds so that the frequency with which a precursor lesion is found varies widely in the literature.

Clinical Presentation

Cutaneous melanoma can occur anywhere on the body; classically, it is most commonly found on the lower extremities in women and on the trunk in men. Clinical features of melanoma include variegated color, irregular raised surface, irregular perimeter, and surface ulceration. A biopsy should be performed on any pigmented lesion that undergoes a change in size, configuration, or color. Pigmented lesions that appear distinctly different from the other moles of a patient also deserve particular scrutiny ("ugly duckling sign"). The so-called ABCDEs of early diagnosis pioneered by Rigel et al.[26] are an easy mnemonic device to help physicians and laypersons remember the classic early signs of melanoma: A denotes lesion asymmetry; B, border irregularity; C, color variegation; D, diameter greater than 6 mm; and E, a lesion that is evolving or enlarging.[26,27] To simplify further, Weinstock succinctly focused the message by emphasizing that the most important warning sign is a new or changing skin lesion.[27] A minority of melanomas lack pigment and are termed amelanotic.

Biopsy

When a patient presents with a lesion suggestive of melanoma, biopsy followed by histologic examination is essential. The choice of biopsy technique varies according to the anatomic site, size, and shape of the lesion. Definitive therapy must be considered in choosing a biopsy technique. Wherever possible, an excisional biopsy of the entire pigmented lesion is preferable to avoid sampling error and allow the histopathological assessment of circumscription, an important diagnostic parameter. If an excisional biopsy is not feasible due to the size or anatomic location of the lesion, one or several incisional biopsies using a scalpel or punch is acceptable. Every pathology requisition sheet should include information on the size of the lesion noted clinically and whether the biopsy is complete or partial. An excisional biopsy allows the pathologist to most accurately determine the maximal thickness of the lesion. Where possible, a narrow margin of normal-appearing skin (1-3 mm) is removed with the specimen. To facilitate closure following subsequent wide local excision (WLE), proper orientation of the biopsy specimen is essential to minimize the subsequent need for complex reconstructive approaches for wound closure. Punch biopsy is generally reserved for lesions that are large, are located on anatomic areas where maximum preservation of surrounding skin is important, or can be completely excised with a 6-mm punch. Punch biopsies should be performed at the most raised or darkest area of the lesion. Full-thickness biopsy into the subcutaneous tissue must be performed to permit proper microstaging of the lesion.

Shave biopsies are discouraged if a diagnosis of melanoma is considered, since failure to obtain a full-thickness specimen may result in inaccurate microstaging if melanoma is diagnosed. If shave biopsy is performed, some expert pathologists recommend that the specimen be placed on a thin piece of cardboard before it is immersed in formalin, to prevent the specimen from rolling, which interferes with processing. Fine-needle aspiration biopsy may be used to document nodal and extranodal melanoma metastases but should not be used to diagnose primary melanomas. In general, all pigmented lesions should be submitted for permanent-section examination and definitive surgery should be performed later. There is no evidence that an interval of 2-3 weeks between excisional biopsy and wide excision adversely affects outcome.

Pathology—"Histogenetic" Subtypes

While the pathologic analysis of a suspected melanoma primarily consists of microscopic examination of hematoxylin-eosin-stained tumor, several melanocytic cell markers may also be useful in confirming the diagnosis of melanoma. Two antibodies widely used in immunohistochemical evaluations are S-100 and HMB-45. S-100 is expressed by more than 90% of melanomas but also by several other tumors and some normal tissues, including dendritic cells. In contrast, the monoclonal antibody HMB-45 is virtually specific (yet not as sensitive) for melanocytic cells. It is therefore an excellent confirmatory stain for neoplastic cells when the diagnosis of melanoma is being considered. Anti-MART-1 (Melan-A) and MITF staining has also been shown to be useful in the diagnosis of melanoma.

The major classical "histogenetic" subtypes of melanoma are based on histopathologic findings, anatomic site, and degree of sun damage.

Superficial Spreading Melanoma

Superficial spreading melanoma (SSM) represents approximately 70% of all melanomas in Caucasians. SSM generally arises in a pre-existing lesion and is the lesion most commonly associated with dysplastic nevi. SSM may have a relatively long natural history. Typically, diagnosis follows an increased rate of change in a precursor lesion. Early in their evolution, SSMs usually appear flat, with irregular borders, and extend radially (radial growth phase). Notching of the border is particularly characteristic. The lesions are multiple shades of tan, brown, black, red, and white (Figure 105-1A). Amelanotic areas may represent areas of regression and typically appear lighter than the surrounding skin. As the lesion evolves, it develops areas with a raised surface that correspond to areas of accelerated growth (vertical growth phase). SSMs tend to occur throughout adulthood, with a peak incidence in the fifth decade of life. Classically, they occur on the trunk in males and on the extremities in females.

Nodular Malignant Melanoma

Nodular malignant melanoma (NM) comprises 10-15% of all cutaneous melanomas. NM may develop on any body surface area but most commonly is diagnosed on the trunk of men. NM is thought to be biologically more aggressive than SSM. Clinically, the lesion can be pigmented or unpigmented. Such amelanotic melanoma can be misdiagnosed as benign lesions resulting in diagnostic delay. Histologically, NM is notable for the absence of a radial growth phase (Fig. 105-1B and C). For this reason, nodular melanomas tend to be thicker, high-risk lesions.

Lentigo Maligna Melanoma

Lentigo maligna melanoma (LMM), which constitutes approximately 4-10% of all melanomas, arises from lentigo maligna (melanotic freckle of Hutchinson or precancerous melanosis of Dubreuilh). LMM is found most commonly on chronic sun-exposed skin in elderly individuals (median age 70 years). The lesions are often large (3-4 cm in diameter at diagnosis) and flat with irregular borders, in variable shades of tan to dark brown (Fig. 105-1C). Hypopigmented areas in the lesion represent areas of regression. The precursor lesion, lentigo maligna, histologically represents in situ melanoma, and it often takes 5-15 years before the development of invasive melanoma. While these lesions have traditionally been believed to be less aggressive, the prognosis of all melanoma types is similar when lesions of similar depth of invasion are compared.

Acral Lentiginous Melanoma

Acral lentiginous melanoma (ALM) occurs on the palms (palmar), soles (plantar), and nail beds; these sites are relatively well protected from UV radiation.[28] It represents approximately 3-5% of all cutaneous melanomas in Caucasian patients, but a substantially higher proportion of melanomas (estimated at 35-60%) occur in darker-skinned patients (Fig. 105-1D). ALM typically occurs in older individuals. ALM is often a tan to dark brown macule with an irregular border, which can reach several

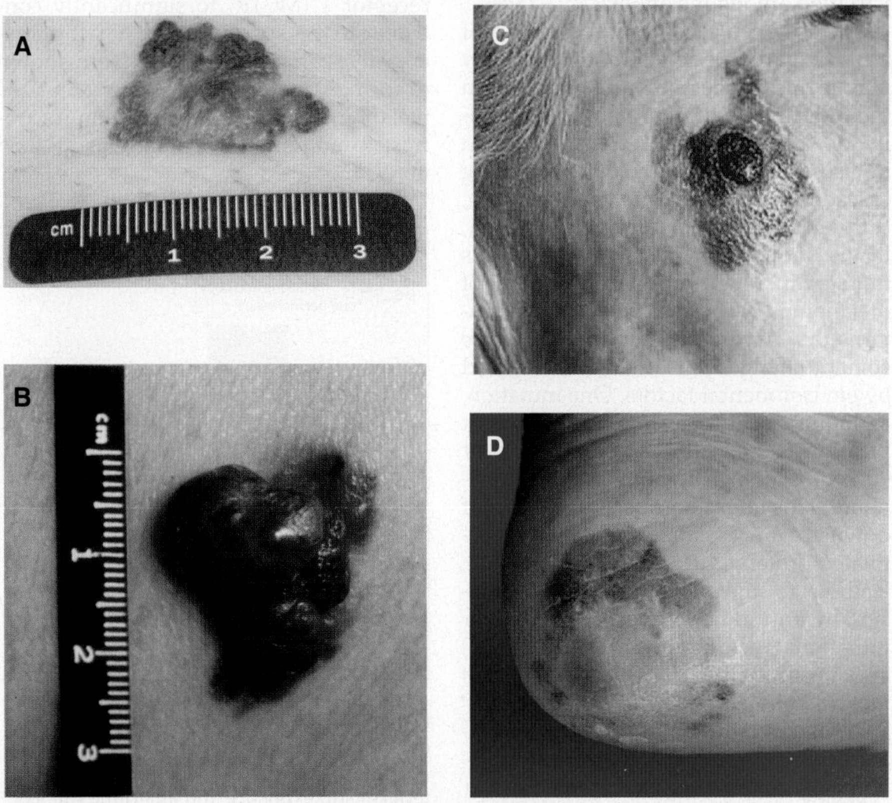

Figure 105-1 (A) Superficial spreading melanoma. Note irregular borders, variegation in color, and size greater than 6 mm. (B) Nodular melanoma. (C) LMM with a nodular area of accelerated growth. (D) Acal lentiginous melanoma of heel. *Source*: Courtesy of Jeffrey E. Gershenwald, MD.

centimeters in diameter. However, lesions can be entirely amelanotic and thus easily misdiagnosed as wart or trophic ulcer. Any non-healing ulcer on acral skin needs, particularly in the elderly, to be evaluated for melanoma. Finally, mucosal lentiginous melanoma (MLM) is similar in appearance to ALM, but is restricted to anatomic sites covered by mucosal membranes. This lesion may develop in a number of mucosal sites, including the oropharynx, paranasal sinuses, esophagus, anorectal areas, urogenital tract, and conjunctiva.

Genetics and Molecular Pathology

Despite the longevity of the "histogenetic" classification system for melanoma described above, significant unresolved complexity exists in the clinical and histopathological presentation, relationship to UV light, and epidemiology of melanoma.[28] Taken together, the myriad associations among features outlined above suggest that melanoma is not a homogeneous disease but instead is composed of biologically distinct subtypes.[28] Intriguingly, evidence is rapidly accumulating that indeed biologically distinct categories of melanoma do exist, and that underlying genetic alterations drive the observed morphologic (phenotypic) variation among melanomas.[28]

It has been recently discovered that a particular genetic alteration that may play a role in melanoma is mutation in the *BRAF* gene. RAF proteins are a family of serine/threonine-specific protein kinases that form part of a signaling cascade that regulates cell proliferation, differentiation, and survival. Recently, it was shown that the *BRAF* isoform is mutated in a high proportion (60-70%) of melanomas.[29] The majority of the mutations that have been found in *BRAF* are somatic changes presumed to be induced by environmental factors. One mutation, a glutamic-acid-for-valine substitution at position 600 (V600E), accounts for over 90% of the BRAF mutations in melanoma. This mutation causes activation of downstream effectors of the mitogen-activated protein kinase-signaling cascade, leading to melanoma tumor progression by an unknown mechanism. Other mutations, including *NRAS*, *c-KIT*, *AKT*, and most recently *GNAQ*, have also been identified in patients with melanoma.[30-33]

Bastian and colleagues differentiated two patterns of UV-induced melanoma by quantifying the degree of solar elastosis in the skin surrounding the melanoma to distinguish melanomas arising on skin with chronic sun-induced damage (CSD) from those melanomas on skin without such damage (non-CSD).[34] *BRAF* muations were shown to be very common in melanomas arising in a background of non-CSD, whereas the frequency of *BRAF* mutations is relatively low in CSD melanomas (approximately 70% vs 15%) (Fig. 105-2). In addition to *BRAF*, other genetic alterations were noted between CSD and non-CSD melanomas—approximately 30% of CSD melanomas had either mutations or increases in DNA copy number of *KIT*,[31] in contrast to the absence of *KIT* mutations in non-CSD melanomas (Fig. 105-2).

Melanomas with *BRAF* mutations have certain morphologic features such as increased pigmentation and upward epidermal scattering of melanocytes in contrast to those with other mutations.[35] The strong association observed between morphology and *BRAF* mutation status suggested that some of the features may be directly caused by *BRAF* mutations. The observation that *BRAF* mutations noted in melanocytic nevi[36] typically arising by early adolescence occurred with the same frequency as in non-CSD melanoma led Bastian and colleagues to propose that patients with acquired nevi and non-CSD melanomas may have a particular susceptibility for developing *BRAF*-mutated melanocytic neoplasms at relatively low doses of UV radiation.[28,31] Remarkably, this concept was supported in subsequent studies that demonstrated a germline variation in the melanocortin receptor 1 (MC1R) to significantly contribute to this susceptibility.[28,37] More specifically, variants of MC1R were shown to strongly increase the risk for non-CSD melanomas with *BRAF* mutation in contrast to non-mutant melanomas also on non-CSD skin.

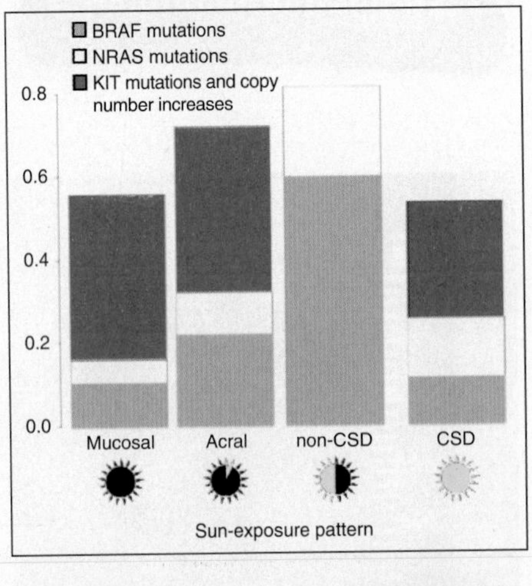

Figure 105-2 Frequency distribution of oncogenic alterations in *BRAF*, *NRAS*, and *KIT* in melanoma stratified based on patterns of sun exposure and anatomic site. For *BRAF* and *NRAS*, point mutations in exon 15 (*BRAF*) and exons 1 and 2 (*NRAS*) are shown. For KIT, mutations and copy number increases are shown. *Source*: From Ref. 3.

These and other data (reviewed in reference 28) clearly demonstrate advances in our understanding of the genetic basis for melanocytic transformation.[28] Overall, these findings may be leveraged to improve the classification of melanoma, possibly leading to an improved ability to predict outcome and, by identification of new targets for antitumor therapy, response to therapy, too.[28]

Melanoma Staging

The AJCC Staging System

The melanoma staging system has been revised numerous times as our understanding of this biologically complex disease has improved.[38-42] The Melanoma Task Force of the American Joint Committee on Cancer (AJCC) published revisions to the melanoma staging system and companion validation prognostic factor analyses in 2001.[38,41] This revised clinical and pathologic staging system was published in 2002 in the sixth edition of the *AJCC Cancer Staging Manual*[40] and was based on an improved understanding of melanoma-associated prognostic factors, including data from the largest multicenter melanoma prognostic factor survival analysis ever conducted at the time.[41] Features of the revised system, introduced in 2002, included new strata for primary tumor thickness, incorporation of primary tumor ulceration as an important staging criterion in both the T and N classifications, revision of the N classification to reflect the importance of regional nodal tumor burden, and new categories for Stage IV disease.

This staging system has been validated over the past several years. Based on a comprehensive 2008 AJCC collaborative melanoma database analysis, minor changes in melanoma staging have been introduced in the seventh edition of the *AJCC Cancer Staging Manual* which was published in October 2009[42] with official implementation set for early 2010. Modifications to the T, N, and M classifications are discussed in detail below.

Highlights of the changes introduced in the seventh edition of the *AJCC Cancer Staging Manual* have recently been summarized and include the following[43]:

1. Mitotic activity (defined as mitoses/mm^2) is an important primary tumor prognostic factor. A mitotic rate at least 1/mm^2 denotes a primary melanoma at higher risk for metastasis.
2. Melanoma thickness and primary tumor ulceration will continue to be used to define strata in the T category, except for T1 melanomas, where mitotic rate is proposed to re-

place level of invasion as a primary criterion for defining T1b lesions (with ulceration).
3. The presence of nodal micrometastases can be defined by either hematoxylin and eosin (H&E) or immunohistochemical staining (previously, only the former was included).
4. There is no lower threshold of tumor burden defining the presence of regional nodal metastasis. Specifically, inclusion of tumor deposits less than 0.2 mm in diameter (an empiric threshold previously used for defining nodal metastasis), reflects the consensus that even small amounts of metastatic tumor are clinically significant. While the concept of isolated tumor cells (especially in subcapsular sinuses) may be valid, no evidence-based lower threshold of "false-positive" or clinically insignificant nodal metastases has yet been defined.
5. Lymphatic mapping and sentinel lymph node (SLN) biopsy are important components of melanoma staging and should be used (and discussed with the patient) in defining occult Stage III disease among patients who present with clinical Stages IB and II melanoma.
6. Survival estimates for patients with intralymphatic regional metastases (satellites and in transit metastasis) are somewhat better than the remaining cohort of Stage IIIB patients; nonetheless, this stage grouping represents the closest statistical fit, so the current stage definition for intralymphatic regional metastasis remains the same.
7. The prognostic significance of microsatellites remains controversial. The AJCC Melanoma Staging Committee recommended that this uncommon feature be retained in the N2c category, although it was noted that previously published studies were insufficient to substantiate revision of the definitions used in the sixth edition staging manual.
8. The site of distant metastases remains the primary component of the M-category (non-visceral [cutaneous, subcutaneous, distant nodal], lung, and visceral metastasis).
9. An elevated serum lactic dehydrogenase (LDH) level remains a powerful predictor of survival and is also to be used in the M category.
10. No subgroups of Stage IV melanoma are recommended.
11. From a staging perspective, the definition of metastatic melanoma from an unknown primary site was clarified; isolated metastases arising in lymph nodes, skin and subcutaneous tissues are to be categorized as Stage III rather than Stage IV.

The melanoma staging system described in the seventh edition of the *AJCC Cancer Staging Manual* is included in this chapter, because the final version of the seventh edition was published in October 2009 just before this chapter went to press. The TNM categories are defined in Table 105-1[40] and the stage groupings in Table 105-2.[40] The melanoma staging recommendations for the seventh edition of the

Table 105-1 Definition of the TNM Staging Categories for Cutaneous Melanoma Based on the *AJCC Cancer Staging Manual*: Seventh Edition

Melanoma TNM Classification		
T Classification	**Thickness**	**Ulceration Status**
Tis	not applicable	not applicable
T1	≤1.0 mm	a: w/o ulceration and mitosis <1/mm^2 b: with ulceration or mitosis ≥1/mm^2
T2	1.01-2.0 mm	a: w/o ulceration b: with ulceration
T3	2.01-4.0 mm	a: w/o ulceration b: with ulceration
T4	>4.0 mm	a: w/o ulceration b: with ulceration
N Classification	**No. of Metastatic Nodes**	**Nodal Metastatic Mass**
N1	1 node	a: micrometastasis[a] b: macrometastasis[b]
N2	2-3 nodes	a: micrometastasis[a] b: macrometastasis[b] c: in transit met(s)/satellite(s) without metastatic nodes
N3	4 or more metastatic nodes, or matted nodes, or in transit met(s)/ satellite(s) *with* metastatic node(s)	
M Classification	**Site**	**Serum LDH**
M1a	Distant skin, SQ or nodal metastases	Normal
M1b	Lung metastases	Normal
M1c	All other visceral metastases	Normal
	Any distant metastasis	Elevated

[a]Micrometastases are diagnosed after sentinel or elective lymphadenectomy.
[b]Macrometastases are defined as clinically detectable nodal metastases confirmed by therapeutic lymphadenectomy or when nodal metastasis exhibits gross extracapsular extension.
Abbreviation: SQ, subcutaneous. *Source*: From Ref. 42.

Table 105-2 Definition of the Stage Groupings for Cutaneous Melanoma Based on the *AJCC Cancer Staging Manual*: Seventh Edition

Stage Groupings for Cutaneous Melanoma							
Clinical Staging[a]				Pathologic Staging[b]			
0	Tis	N0	M0	0	Tis	N0	M0
IA	T1a	N0	M0	IA	T1a	N0	M0
IB	T1b	N0	M0	IB	T1b	N0	M0
	T2a	N0	M0		T2a	N0	M0
IIA	T2b	N0	M0	IIA	T2b	N0	M0
	T3a	N0	M0		T3a	N0	M0
IIB	T3b	N0	M0	IIB	T3b	N0	M0
	T4a	N0	M0		T4a	N0	M0
IIC	T4b	N0	M0	IIC	T4b	N0	M0
III	Any T	N>N0	M0	IIIA	T1-4a	N1a	M0
					T1-4a	N2a	M0
				IIIB	T1-4b	N1a	M0
					T1-4b	N2a	M0
					T1-4a	N1b	M0
					T1-4a	N2b	M0
					T1-4a	N2c	M0
				IIIC	T1-4b	N1b	M0
					T1-4b	N2b	M0
					T1-4b	N2c	M0
					Any T	N3	M0
IV	Any T	Any N	M1	IV	Any T	Any N	M1

[a]Clinical staging includes microstaging of the primary melanoma and clinical/radiologic evaluation for metastases. By convention, it should be used after complete excision of the primary melanoma with clinical assessment for regional and distant metastases.
[b]Pathologic staging includes microstaging of the primary melanoma and pathologic information about the regional lymph nodes after partial or complete lymphadenectomy. Pathologic Stage 0 or Stage IA patients are the exception; they do not require pathologic evaluation of their lymph nodes.
Source: From Ref. 42.

Table 105-3 **5-Year Survival Rates of Pathologically Staged Patients (Based on 2008 AJCC Melanoma Database)[a]**

	IA	IB	IIA	IIB	IIC	IIIA	IIIB	IIIC
Ta:	T1a	T2a	T3a	T4a		N1a,N2a	N1b, N2b	N3
Nonulcerated	97%	91%	79%	71%		78%	48%	47%
Tb:		T1b	T2b	T3b	T4b		N1a, N2a	N1b, N2b
Ulcerated		94%	82%	68%	53%		55%	N3 38%

[a]The presence of tumor ulceration of a primary melanoma (designated Tb) causes upstaging by 1 substage compared with a nonulcerated melanoma (designated Ta).
Source: From Ref. 43.

AJCC Cancer Staging Manual are based on the updated 2008 AJCC collaborative melanoma database that contained prospective data on over 50,000 patients with Stages I, II, and III melanoma, plus almost 10,000 patients with Stage IV melanoma. The 5-year survival rates over the 5-year interval between these analyses demonstrate some improvement in survival rates for melanoma, likely due to the improvements in melanoma staging (ie, more widespread use of lymphatic mapping and sentinel node biopsy for patients with T1b-T2 lesions) and perhaps treatment (Table 105-3).[42] Updated survival rates for patients with Stages I-IV melanoma are shown in Figure 105-3; substages are shown in Figures 105-4-105-6.

Prognostic Factors in Primary Melanoma (Stages I and II)

The overall prognosis for patients with localized melanoma without any nodal or distant sites is generally favorable (Figs. 105-3 and 105-4).[42] In the 2008 AJCC analysis, among 25,734 patients with localized melanoma (documented clinically or pathologically), tumor thickness and ulceration were the two most important independent predictors of survival (Table 105-4).[42] Similar results were obtained in the cohort of 9883 patients without clinical evidence of nodal metastases at initial presentation whose disease was pathologically staged using sentinel or elective lymphadenectomy (Table 105-5).[42] In this latter group, the majority of whom underwent SLN biopsy, nodal status was the most significant independent predictor, and level of invasion was no longer a predictor of outcome.

Tumor Thickness ■ One of the earliest descriptions of the concept of tumor thickness was published by Breslow[44] in 1970, when he theorized that primary melanoma tumor volume correlates with prognosis. Realizing that accurate and reproducible tumor volume measurements are essential yet difficult to perform, he reasoned that the measured maximal thickness of the primary melanoma would be an accurate, reproducible surrogate for tumor volume and a significant predictor of prognosis. This concept was validated in multiple studies, including the AJCC database analysis on which the current version of the staging system is based.[41,44-48] In the seventh edition AJCC staging system, the cutoff points for tumor thickness strata will remain at 1, 2, and 4 mm based on prior statistical best-fit modeling,[49,50] the lack of naturally occurring break points in the analysis,[41] and the fact that they also represent useful thresholds for clinical decision-making (Tables 105-1–105-3) (Fig. 105-4).

Ulceration ■ Primary tumor ulceration is the second most important predictor of survival in clinically node-negative patients.[41] Ulceration is defined as the absence of an intact epidermis overlying the primary tumor on histologic examination of the primary lesion[38,51,52] and is a reproducibly identifiable feature of melanoma.[53,54] Numerous studies have shown that the ulcerated primaries represent a more aggressive subset of melanoma with a higher likelihood of metastases and a worse prognosis.[41,51,52] In the 2008 AJCC prognostic factor analysis, the presence of ulceration at any tumor thickness predicted a significantly worse survival outcome, and patients with ulceration again had outcomes approximately the same as those of patients in the next higher tumor-thickness stratum whose lesions were not ulcerated (Table 105-3).[41] In the T classification, ulceration at each tumor thickness level is categorized as either absent or present. Recently, Spatz et al.[55] developed a clear definition of histologic criteria for traumatic ulceration, an important contribution since this form of ulceration has no prognostic value, but nontraumatic ulceration has important independent prognostic significance.

Mitotic Rate ■ Accumulating data support that primary tumor mitotic rate is an independent prognostic factor in patients with cutaneous melanoma. The value of mitotic rate as a prognostic factor was first identified by Salman and Rogers,[56] who reported that for patients with melanomas less than 0.75 mm thick, those with a mitotic index greater than 5 had a worse prognosis. In the largest single institution study to date, the Sydney Melanoma Unit determined by Cox multivariate analysis that mitotic rate (expressed as the number of mitoses/mm^2) was a highly significant independent prognostic factor,[57] an observation also noted by other investigators.[58-66]

As a result of numerous studies showing an inverse association between primary tumor mitotic rate and survival, this covariate was analyzed for the first time in the 2008 AJCC collaborative melanoma database analysis. The number of mitoses/mm^2 correlated strongly with tumor thickness. Overall,

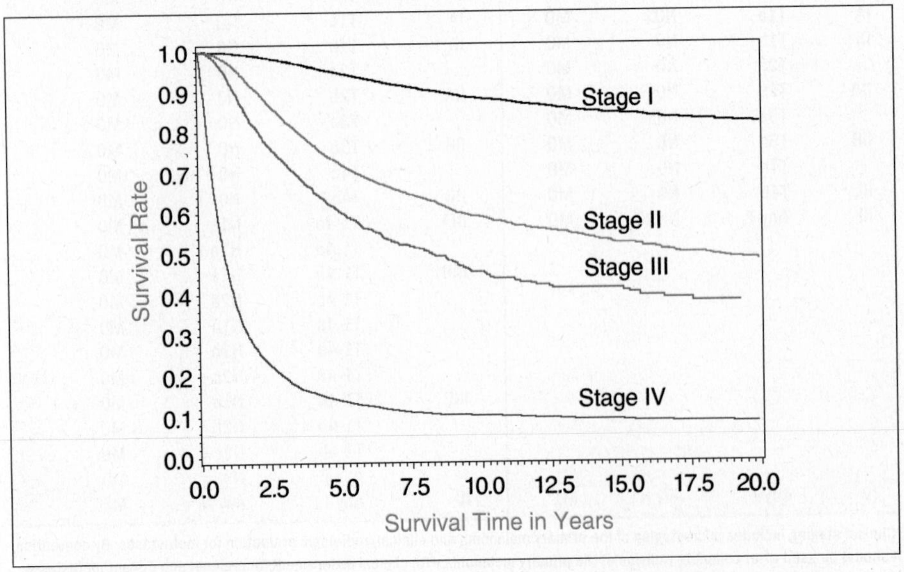

Figure 105-3 Survival curves for patients with localized melanoma (Stages I and II), regional metastases (Stage III), and distant metastases (Stage IV). The differences between the curves are highly significant ($p < 0.0001$). *Source*: From Ref. 42.

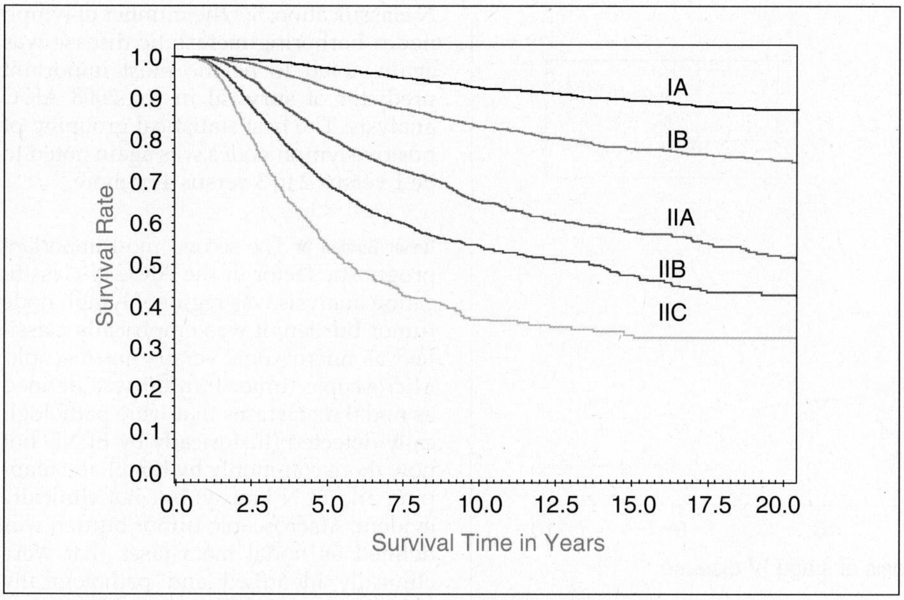

Figure 105-4 AJCC 2008 Melanoma Staging Database: Stage I/II survival curves by substage. Survival rates from the AJCC 2008 Melanoma Staging Database comparing the different stage groupings for Stages I and II melanoma. *Source*: From Ref. 42.

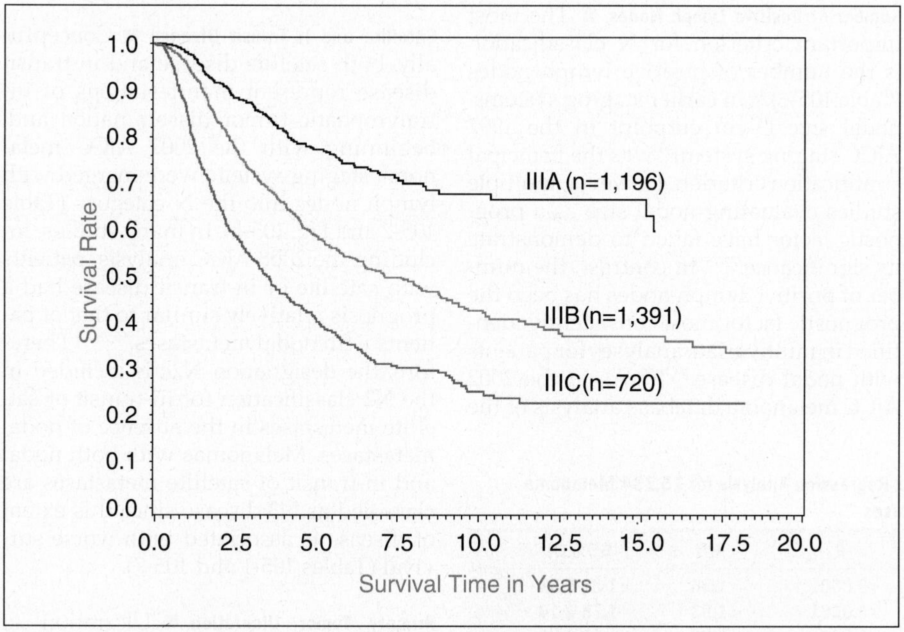

Figure 105-5 Survival rates from the AJCC 2008 Melanoma Staging Database comparing the different stage groupings for Stage III melanoma. *Source*: From Ref. 42.

although only 21.3% of patients whose melanoma tumor thickness was up to 0.5 mm had any mitotic activity (ie, >0 mitosis/mm^2) documented in their primary tumor, the incidence of any mitotic activity increased rapidly up to approximately 2 mm, which corresponds to the approximate primary tumor depth beyond which nearly all patients had at least some mitotic activity.[43]

By univariate analysis, there was a significant, consistent decrement in survival as the number of mitoses/mm^2 increased. Overall, the mitotic rate was a second most powerful independent adverse predictor of survival by multivariate Cox analysis among the 11,664 patients in the 2008 AJCC collaborative melanoma database with Stage I or II melanoma in whom mitotic rate was also known. Tumor ulceration remained highly significant, but level of invasion was only of borderline significance. Recently performed multivariate Cox modeling analyses suggest that among patients with T1 (ie, "thin") melanomas, the presence of at least 1 mitosis/mm^2 is an independent adverse predictor of survival when compared with less than 1 mitosis/mm^2.[42]

Clark Level of Invasion The importance of the Clark level of invasion has been controversial. In 1969, Clark and colleagues[67] described the classification of malignant melanoma by its level of invasion into the dermis as determined by histologic analysis. Five categories of invasion analogous to the current five Clark levels were described. However, the prognostic significance and reproducibility of the Clark level have been debated. In most,[45,68,69] but not all[70] comparative studies, including analyses of large prospective databases,[49,50] tumor thickness was shown to be a more powerful prognostic factor and more reproducible measurement than the Clark level.

More recent analyses confirmed the importance of tumor thickness as a prognostic factor and found that the level of invasion was significant only for melanoma lesions less than or equal to 1 mm thick. Similarly, in the 2002 AJCC database analysis,[41] the level of invasion had greater prognostic significance than ulceration only for tumors less than or equal to 1 mm thick. While Clark level is included in the 2002 staging system for T1 lesions only, it is proposed to be supplanted by mitotic rate as a primary criterion for T1b melanoma (with ulceration) in the seventh edition Melanoma Staging System, except in those rare instances when mitotic rate cannot be determined.[42]

Other Factors Although a detailed discussion is beyond the scope of this chapter, age, sex, primary tumor site, regression, and growth phase have also been associated with prognosis in at least some studies (reviewed in Ref. 71).

Stage I and II Groupings In the current AJCC staging system, primary melanomas without evidence of nodal or distant metastases are grouped into Stage I or II on the basis of the primary tumor characteristics comprising the T classification (Tables 105-1 and 105-2) (Fig. 105-4). A notable finding in the AJCC survival analyses was that the presence of primary tumor ulceration "upstaged" a patient's survival to that of a patient with a nonulcerated melanoma of the next highest tumor-thickness category[40] (Tables 105-2 and 105-3). Stage I includes primary lesions associated with a low melanoma-specific mortality rate (Table 105-3) (Fig. 105-4).[42] Stage II includes lesions associated with an intermediate and somewhat higher risk of metastatic disease and melanoma-specific mortality rate (Fig. 105-4) (Table 105-3).[42] Current stage groupings are summarized in Table 105-2.[40]

N Classification (Stage III)

Regional lymph nodes represent the most common first site of metastasis in melanoma patients. In the 2002 AJCC

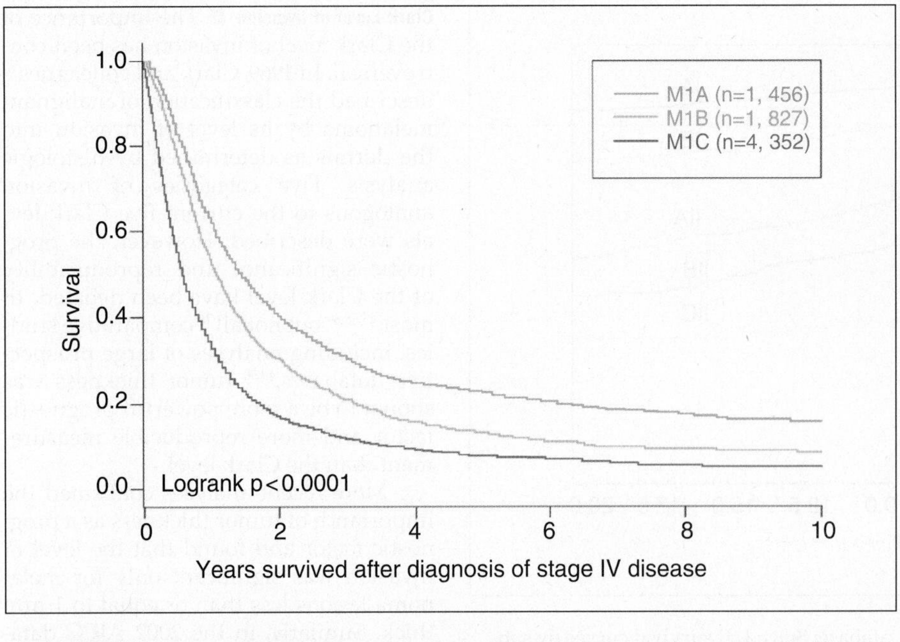

Figure 105-6 ■ AJCC 2008 Melanoma Staging Database Stage IV melanoma survival by site of distant metastases. (Note that the LDH level is NOT included in this graph.) *Source*: From Ref. 42.

melanoma staging system, four criteria were established as significant prognostic factors for survival in patients with regional metastases: (1) the number of lymph nodes harboring metastatic disease, (2) microscopic versus macroscopic tumor burden in the lymph nodes, (3) the presence of satellite or in-transit metastases, and (4) the presence or absence of ulceration in the primary lesion[38] (Table 105-2). Because of the prognostic importance of these criteria, pathologic evaluation of lymph nodes is required to determine a pathologic stage in all patients except those with T0 or T1a disease.[40]

Number of Positive Lymph Nodes ■ The most important criterion for N classification is the number of positive lymph nodes (Table 105-6).[42] In earlier staging systems, nodal size (3-cm cutpoint in the 1997 AJCC staging system)[39] was the principal stratification criterion. However, multiple studies evaluating nodal size as a prognostic factor have failed to demonstrate its significance.[72-75] In contrast, the number of positive lymph nodes has been the prognostic factor most consistently identified in multivariate analyses for patients with nodal disease.[50,76,77] As in the 2002 AJCC melanoma database analysis of the N classification,[38,41] the number of lymph nodes harboring metastatic disease was again noted to be the most important predictor of survival in the 2008 AJCC analysis. The best statistical grouping of positive lymph nodes was again noted to be 1 versus 2 to 3 versus 4 or more.[42]

Tumor Burden ■ The second most important prognostic factor in the AJCC N-classification analysis was regional lymph node tumor burden; it was empirically classified as microscopic versus macroscopic. Microscopic tumor burden was defined as nodal metastases that were pathologically detected (historically by ELND but now more commonly by lymphatic mapping and SLN biopsy) but not clinically evident. Macroscopic tumor burden was defined as nodal metastases that were clinically identified and pathologically confirmed. In the 2008 analysis, survival rates for patients with macroscopic nodal disease were significantly worse than rates for patients with microscopic nodal disease (Tables 105-6 and 105-7).[42]

Satellite and In-Transit Disease ■ Conceptually, both satellite disease and in-transit disease represent manifestations of intralymphatic tumor dissemination and, beginning with the 2002 AJCC melanoma staging system, were merged with lymph nodes into the N category (Table 105-2 and Fig. 105-5). In many studies, including the 2008 AJCC analysis, patients with satellite or in-transit disease had a prognosis relatively similar to that of patients with nodal metastases.[50,78-83] Therefore, the designation N2c is included in the N2 classification for in-transit or satellite metastases in the absence of nodal metastases. Melanomas with both nodal and in-transit or satellite metastases are classified as N3 disease since this extent of disease is associated with worse survival (Tables 105-1 and 105-7).

Primary Tumor Ulceration ■ Ulceration of the primary tumor was included in the Stage III classification because it was the only primary tumor feature that independently predicted survival in patients with nodal metastases (Tables 105-3 and 105-6).[41,42,50,84,85] Similar to the case in patients with Stage I or II disease, the presence of an ulcerated primary melanoma in patients with Stage III disease upstages a patient's survival to that of a patient with a nonulcerated melanoma in a higher nodal-tumor-burden category.

Stage III Groupings ■ Because of the significant heterogeneity of prognoses among patients with Stage III disease, 3 substages were defined: IIIA, IIIB, and IIIC (Tables 105-2 and 105-7).[40,42] The 5-year survival rates for patients with Stages IIIA, IIIB,

Table 105-4 ■ **AJCC 2008 Melanoma Database Cox Regression Analysis for 25,734 Melanoma Patients Without Evidence of Nodal or Distant Metastases**

Variable	Chi-Square Values (1 DF)	*P*	HR	95% CI
Tumor thickness	420.1	<0.0001	1.35	1.31-1.39
Ulceration	257.3	<0.0001	1.93	1.78-2.10
Clark's Level	46.3	<0.0001	1.22	1.16-1.30
Site	75.6	<0.0001	1.41	1.30-1.52
Gender	46.5	<0.0001	0.76	0.71-0.83
Age	90.0	<0.0001	1.16	1.13-1.20

Abbreviations: CI, confidence interval; DF, degree of freedom; HR, hazard ratio, *P*, probability.
Source: From Ref. 71.

Table 105-5 ■ **AJCC 2008 Melanoma Database Cox Regression Analysis for 9,883 Melanoma Patients Without Clinical Evidence of Nodal or Metastases Whose Regional Lymph Nodes Were Pathologically Staged After Sentinel or Elective Lymphadenectomy**

Variable	DF	Chi-Square (Wald)	*P* value	Risk Ratio	95% CI
Nodal status	1	222.5	<.0001	2.52	2.23-2.84
Thickness	1	162.1	<.0001	1.33	1.27-1.38
Ulceration	1	113.4	<.0001	1.93	1.71-2.18
Site	1	36.1	<.0001	1.45	1.28-1.63
Age	1	47.6	<.0001	1.20	1.14-1.26
Gender	1	11.3	0.0008	0.80	0.71-0.91
Clark's level	1	2.1	0.1512	1.11	0.96-1.29

Abbreviations: CI, confidence interval; DF, degree of freedom; *P*, probability.
Source: From Ref. 71.

Table 105-6 AJCC 2008 Melanoma Staging Database Stage III 5-Year Survival According to Number of Involved Lymph Nodes, Nodal Tumor Burden (Macroscopic or Microscopic), and Primary Tumor Ulceration (N = 2,740)[a]

Nodes	Ulceration	5-Year Survival Rate ± SE: Micrometastasis	5-Year Survival Rate ± SE: Macrometastasis
1	No	0.80 ± 0.02 (n = 891)	0.50 ± 0.07 (n = 90)
	Yes	0.56 ± 0.03 (n = 599)	0.44 ± 0.06 (n = 105)
2-3	No	0.71 ± 0.03 (n = 323)	0.47 ± 0.07 (n = 83)
	Yes	0.50 ± 0.04 (n = 269)	0.37 ± 0.06 (n = 107)
≥4	No	0.40 ± 0.07 (n = 74)	0.36 ± 0.08 (n = 58)
	Yes	0.40 ± 0.08 (n = 61)	0.28 ± 0.06 (n = 80)
Total No. of Patients		2,217	523

[a]Includes micrometastasis patients with number of positive nodes, tumor thickness, ulceration, and follow-up information available.
Abbreviation: SE, standard error. *Source*: From Ref. 71.

Table 105-7 AJCC 2008 Melanoma Database: Stage III Substage Survival Rates

Stage	N	Survival Rate ± SE: 5-Year	Survival Rate ± SE: 10-Year
IIIA	1,196	0.78 ± 0.02	0.68 ± 0.02
IIIB[a] (including N2c)	1,391	0.59 ± 0.02	0.43 ± 0.02
IIIB (excluding N2c)	992	0.54 ± 0.02	0.38 ± 0.03
IIIC	720	0.40 ± 0.02	0.24 ± 0.03

[a]399 N2c patients (intralymphatic metastases) had 5- and 10-year survival rates of 69% and 52%.
Abbreviation: SE, standard error. *Source*: From Ref. 42.

and IIIC disease are 78%, 59%, and 40%, respectively (Table 105-7). The distribution of Stage III melanoma patients with regional metastases by stage groupings is shown in Tables 105-3, 105-6, and 105-7.

M Classification (Stage IV)

Patients with Stage IV melanoma generally have a poor prognosis with historical median survival from the time of initial Stage IV diagnosis of 6-7.5 months and an associated 5-year survival of less than 10%.[86-89] Nonetheless, recent multivariate prognostic factor analyses have identified several independent factors that predict survival in the overall poor-prognosis group.[88-90] In an effort to significantly expand previous Stage IV analyses, the AJCC developed a first-in-kind international AJCC Stage IV database in 2008 in which more than 9000 patients with Stage IV melanoma were compiled (Figs. 105-3 and 105-4). In patients with distant metastasis, the site or sites of metastasis and serum levels of LDH are used to delineate the M categories into 3 groups: M1a, M1b, and M1c with 1-year survival rates at 62% for M1a, and 53% for M1b, and 33% for M1c melanoma.[42] Patients with distant metastases in the skin, subcutaneous tissue, or distant lymph nodes are categorized as M1a if their LDH level is normal and have a relatively better prognosis compared to patients with disease located in other anatomic sites. Patients with metastasis to the lung are categorized as M1b and have an "intermediate" Stage IV prognosis when comparing survival rates. Patients with metastases to any other visceral sites, or a combination of any site with an elevated serum LDH are designated as M1c and are associated with the shortest survival estimates.

Building on the initial experience of the 2002 AJCC Melanoma Database analysis, the international AJCC 2008 Stage IV database demonstrated that survival differences among skin, subcutaneous, and distant lymph node metastases (M1a), versus lung metastases (M1b) versus other visceral sites of metastases (M1c) were maintained and were also independently associated with survival by multivariate Cox regression analysis that included elevated LDH level as an important adverse predictor of survival.[91] These data support the current AJCC Stage IV staging system.[42] Other important predictors of survival in patients with Stage IV disease include site of distant metastasis, number of metastatic sites, and number of metastases.[86-89,92-94] The finding by multivariate analysis that both site of metastatic disease and LDH level retained independent prognostic significance strongly supports the current AJCC melanoma M-category criteria. It is anticipated that additional analyses will continue to identify predictors of survival among this highest risk group, not only to facilitate better prognostic assessment, but also to facilitate design and analysis of melanoma clinical trials and potentially to calibrate therapeutic intensity to metastatic risk.

Metastatic Melanoma to Lymph Nodes From an Unknown Primary Site

In 2-9% of patients who present with evidence of melanoma nodal metastasis, no identifiable primary tumor and no history of a primary melanoma is identified. In these cases, the most frequent site of involved nodes when a primary site is not identified is the axilla (47%), followed by the neck and groin.[71] Previous reports have demonstrated that the survival rate appears similar in patients with an unknown primary site and patients matched according to nodal metastasis having a known primary site.[86,95] In a more recent analysis, Cormier et al.[96] conducted a retrospective analysis of consecutive patients with melanoma from an unknown primary (MUP) (N = 71) who underwent surgical resection for metastasis to regional lymph nodes and were classified by N-category after lymph node dissection was performed. With a median follow-up of 7.7 years, the 5- and 10-year overall survival rates were 55% and 44%, respectively, for patients with MUP, compared with 42% and 32%, respectively, for patients with a known primary melanoma (N = 466) (p = 0.04); in multivariate analyses, MUP was identified as a favorable prognostic factor (hazard ratio, 0.61; 95% CI, 0.42-0.86; p = 0.006) for overall survival. More recently, the favorable survival profile in patients with MUP was also noted in a study of 262 patients with MUP by researchers at the John Wayne Cancer Institute,[97] with survival rates remarkably similar to those in the study by Cormier et al.[96] The relatively favorable long-term survival of patients with MUP in this study suggests that patients with MUP have a natural history that is similar to (if not better than) the survival of many patients with Stage III disease.[42] Therefore, the inability to identify the primary tumor in patients with metastatic melanoma to lymph nodes after a thorough search does not appear to be an adverse prognostic factor; these patients should be treated as Stage III with an aggressive surgical approach and considered for Stage III adjuvant therapy protocols.[96]

Treatment of Patients With Primary Melanoma

In planning treatment for patients with early-stage primary cutaneous melanoma, the surgeon must determine: (1) the extent of excision of the primary tumor (ie, WLE) and how the resulting defect will be repaired and (2) whether the patient is a candidate for lymphatic mapping and SLN biopsy, a surgical technique used to assess regional nodal basins at risk for occult Stage III disease (see below).

Treatment of the Primary Lesion—Wide Local Excision

To address the primary tumor, a WLE with radial margins appropriate for tumor thickness is performed (Fig. 105-7). Historically, even thin melanomas were excised with 3-5 cm margins. Guidelines for radial margins for WLE of primary cutaneous melanoma (Table 105-8) are based on primary tumor thickness; overall, these guidelines have been established based on the results of important clinical trials[98-103] (reviewed in reference 104). Failure to perform re-excision after biopsy of a primary melanoma has been associated with a local recurrence rate as high as 40%.

The first randomized study involving surgical margins for melanomas less than 2 mm thick was reported by the WHO Melanoma Group.[103] In an update of the study including 612 evaluable patients randomly assigned to a 1- or 3-cm margin of excision, there were no local recurrences among patients with primary melanomas thinner than 1 mm. There were 4 local recurrences among the 100 patients with melanomas 1-2 mm thick, and all 4 occurred in patients with 1-cm margins.[103] There was no significant difference in survival between the 1- and 3-cm surgical margin groups.[103] These results demonstrate that a narrow excision margin (ie, 1 cm) is safe for thin (<1 mm) melanomas.[102,103]

A randomized, prospective study conducted by the Intergroup Melanoma Committee compared 2- and 4-cm radial margins of excision for intermediate-thickness melanomas (1-4 mm).[98,99] There was no difference in local recurrence rate between the 2 groups. 46% of patients in the 4-cm group required skin grafts, whereas only 11% of patients in the 2-cm group did ($p < 0.001$). Other studies have demonstrated that margins of excision did not influence overall survival.[100,105]

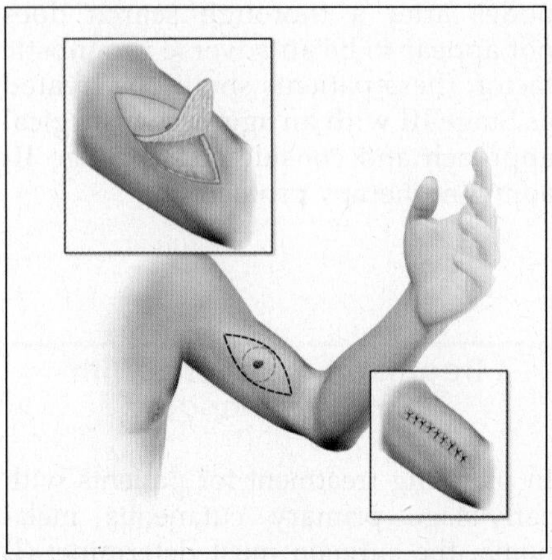

Figure 105-7 Schematic of WLE of primary melanoma. Appropriate radial margin marked schematically (center, purple line) along with proposed axially oriented elliptical incision to facilitate primary closure (inset, bottom right) following wide excision (inset, top left). *Source*: Courtesy of Jeffrey E. Gershenwald, MD.

Table 105-8 Recommendations for Primary Melanoma Excision Margins Based on Tumor Thickness

Tumor Thickness	Margin of Excision
≤1 mm	1 cm
1-2 mm	1-2 cm
2-4 mm	2 cm
>4 mm	2 cm[a]

[a]No randomized prospective trials have specifically addressed this cohort.
Source: From Ref. 104.

These data strongly support the use of a 2-cm margin for intermediate-thickness lesions. Specifically, for patients with tumors 2-4 mm thick, a 2-cm margin is recommended. For patients with an invasive melanoma 1-2 mm thick, development of a simple recommendation is difficult because the data from several trials evaluating excision margins in this patient population are conflicting.[98-103] In general, a 2-cm margin is preferred if anatomically feasible, although in regions of anatomic constraint (eg, the face), a 1-cm margin is sufficient. This recommendation is based on the fact that the overall survival rate was not affected by margin size in the 1-cm vs 3-cm World Health Organization (WHO) trial.[102,103]

In patients with melanoma more than 4 mm thick, only one randomized, prospective trial—the United Kingdom Melanoma Study Group trial—provides relevant data. In the early[101] reports of this trial, excision margins (1 cm vs 3 cm) in patients with melanoma more than 2 mm thick (none of whom underwent SLN biopsy or elective lymph node dissection [ELND]) did not appear to affect the survival rate. However, the lower incidence of local-regional recurrence in patients randomly assigned to the 3-cm excision arm indicates that residual microscopic local disease present after limited margin excision may be the source of at least some regional failures and suggests a potential benefit from wider excision. In a large retrospective trial that included patients with thick melanoma at least 4 mm thick[106] a 2-cm minimum margin was not associated with a decrease in the disease-free survival rate or overall survival rate compared with a larger margin.

Most WLE defects can be closed primarily using routine approximation techniques or mobilization of adjacent tissues (Fig. 105-7). Less commonly, the location of the lesion or the magnitude of the excision creates a defect that requires more complex closure techniques.

Site-Specific Considerations ■ General recommendations regarding the extent of surgical resection are applicable to most areas of the body. However, certain anatomic sites are not amenable to rigid surgical criteria. More than three-fourths of subungual melanomas involve either the great toe or the thumb. A melanoma located on the skin of a digit or beneath the nail (ie, subungual) is usually removed by a partial digital amputation. In general, amputations are performed at the middle interphalangeal joint of the fingers or proximal to the interphalangeal joint of the thumb. More proximal amputations are not associated with improved survival and are rarely indicated. For a melanoma located on a toe, an amputation of the entire digit at the metatarsal-phalangeal joint is indicated; for a melanoma of the great toe, however, amputation can be performed proximal to the interphalangeal joint.

Excision of a melanoma on the plantar surface of the foot often produces a sizable defect in a weight-bearing area. A plantar flap can provide well-vascularized local tissue for weight-bearing areas; more recently, staged closure of some plantar melanomas has been performed with initial use of a wound V.A.C. ® (vacuum-assisted closure device) to stimulate granulation tissue followed by staged skin graft application. Facial lesions usually cannot be excised with more than l-cm margin because of adjacent vital structures; in these cases, the tumor diameter, tumor thickness, and tumor's exact location on the face must all be considered when margin width is planned.

Special Clinical Situations

Mucosal Melanoma ■ Patients with true mucosal primaries—including the head and neck, vagina, and anal canal—represent very uncommon presentations of melanoma; in general, patients have a relatively poor prognosis regardless of surgical therapy, although long-term survival has been observed. An aggressive surgical approach is generally not recommended for patients with clinically localized disease.[107] In particular, local excision of anorectal melanomas is recommended over abdominoperineal resection.[107,108] Abdominoperineal resection is associated with much greater morbidity, leaves the patient with a permanent colostomy, offers no survival advantage, and does not treat at-risk inguinal nodes unless the procedure is combined with groin dissection.[108] Adjuvant radiation therapy following local excision may be administered to patients with mucosal melanoma in an attempt to decrease the risk of locoregional recurrence. While some have historically offered biochemotherapy to many of these patients,[109] based on unique genetic abnormalities observed in a subset of these patients (eg, activating cKIT mutations), new therapeutic approaches are being employed that may successfully target these aberrant pathways. (see targeted therapy section below).[110,111]

Desmoplastic Melanoma

Desmoplastic melanoma is an uncommon histologic variant of melanoma that is characterized by an unusual spindle-cell morphology and the presence of fusiform melanocytes dispersed in a prominent collagenous stroma.[112] Often presenting as a thick primary tumor, desmoplastic melanoma is classically associated with a higher incidence of local recurrence than nondesmoplastic melanoma. Desmoplastic melanoma may display morphologic heterogeneity; specifically, some desmoplastic melanomas are characterized by a uniform desmoplasia that is prominent throughout the entire tumor ("pure" desmoplastic melanoma), whereas other desmoplastic melanomas appear to arise in association with other histologic subtypes ("mixed-type").[113] Distinguishing the phenotypic heterogeneity of desmoplastic melanomas has been reported to be important for stratifying patients with regard to rate of lymph node metastasis and prognosis.[113,114] Recent data indicate that patients with pure desmoplastic melanoma have a lower incidence of positive SLNs than do patients with mixed-type or non-desmoplastic melanoma[115]; studies also suggest that patients with mixed desmoplastic melanoma have a greater risk of death or metastatic disease than patients with the pure form.[114,115]

Pregnancy

The precise influence of pregnancy or hormonal manipulation on the clinical course of melanoma has not been defined. Because historical case reports suggested a poor outcome for pregnant women with melanoma, some investigators suggested that melanoma may be hormonally stimulated and therefore more aggressive in pregnant women. More recently, multiple studies have documented overall good outcomes for women with melanoma during pregnancy. A study from the WHO found that female patients who presented during pregnancy had slightly thicker melanomas (2.38 mm vs 1.49 mm) but, once accounted for, no difference in survival was noted.[116] Other studies found no significant difference in prognostic characteristics or 5-year survival rates between pregnant and nonpregnant females with localized melanoma.[117,118] In a large population-based study of pregnant women conducted over a 9-year period in California, there was no evidence of a more advanced stage, thicker tumors, increased risk of metastasis to lymph nodes, or worse survival in pregnant women. Furthermore, maternal and neonatal outcomes were equivalent to those of pregnant women without melanoma and their newborns.[119] In aggregate, these data support the concept that melanoma is not more common, more aggressive, or more lethal during pregnancy. Surgery is the treatment of choice in pregnant patients with early-stage melanoma. Although opinions differ on planning pregnancy after a diagnosis of melanoma, the weight of evidence does not demonstrate an increased risk of developing metastatic disease with pregnancy. Furthermore, several studies have found no association between oral contraceptive use and survival in melanoma. Recently, Lea et al. did not find any association between melanoma risk and oral contraceptive use and hormone replacement therapy.[120]

Management of Regional Lymph Nodes

Regional lymph nodes are the most common first site of melanoma metastasis. Effective palliation and sometimes cure can be achieved in patients with regional metastases. Fine-needle aspiration or core biopsy can usually yield a diagnosis in patients who develop clinically enlarged regional nodes. Open biopsy is rarely warranted. Surgical excision of the involved lymph nodes is currently the only effective treatment for melanoma metastatic to lymph nodes. Lymphadenectomy for specific regional nodal basins has been described elsewhere in detail.[121]

Although the majority of patients who present with invasive cutaneous melanoma have clinically negative regional lymph node basins, a subset of these patients harbor occult regional lymph node metastases. Surgical treatment of clinically negative regional lymph node basins in patients with melanoma has therefore been controversial. Historically, some surgeons preferred to perform lymphadenectomy only for clinically demonstrable nodal metastases. This type of excision has been termed *delayed* or *therapeutic lymph node dissection* (TLND). Other surgeons choose to excise the nodes even when they appear normal in patients who are at increased risk of developing nodal metastases. This excision has been termed *immediate, prophylactic,* or *elective lymph node dissection.* Advocates of this latter approach argued that "early" identification of histologically positive lymph nodes at ELND was associated with a better chance for long-term survival than if clinically apparent metastases developed in the regional lymph nodes during follow-up.[122-126]

Therapeutic Lymph Node Dissection

With TLND, only patients with known metastases undergo a major lymphadenectomy; this reduces the number of potentially unnecessary lymphadenectomies and may not reduce the chance for cure. The disadvantage of TLND is that delaying treatment until lymph node metastases are clinically evident may result in many patients having distant micrometastases at the time of lymphadenectomy. Chances for cure may therefore be diminished.

Elective Lymph Node Dissection

ELND has the theoretical advantage of treating melanoma nodal metastases at a relatively early stage in the natural history of the disease. The disadvantage of ELND is that many patients undergo surgery when they do not have nodal metastasis. Advocates of ELND argue that patients with clinically negative, histologically positive lymph nodes at ELND have a better chance for survival than do patients in whom the regional lymph nodes are not dissected and who develop clinically apparent metastases in the regional lymph nodes during follow-up.

Although all prospective, randomized clinical trials have failed to show any benefit from routine ELND,[126-129] data from WHO Melanoma Group Trial 14 and the Intergroup Melanoma Surgical Trial suggest that certain subgroups of patients might benefit from this procedure.[130-132] Results from the WHO ELND Trial in patients with truncal melanoma at least 1.5 mm thick indicate that patients with only microscopic regional nodal disease after pathologic analysis of the surgical specimen in the ELND treatment arm had improved overall survival compared with patients in whom lymph node dissection was delayed until palpable adenopathy developed after WLE of the primary melanoma alone[131] (5-year survival 48.2% vs 26.9%, $P = 0.04$) (Fig. 105-8). In the Intergroup Melanoma Surgical Trial, patients who had 1-2-mm-thick primary tumors (vs thicker), nonulcerated primary tumors, or were younger than 60 years also had a survival benefit with ELND.[46] Interestingly, this was the first prospective study to require preoperative lymphoscintigraphy in all patients to identify and surgically address all basins at risk for metastasis. Without such guidance, ELND may be misdirected in many patients.[133] Based on these subset analyses, dissection of clinically undetectable regional node metastases may lead to increased survival compared to nodal observation followed by TLND performed only when nodal metastases become clinically evident.

An argument against a policy advocating ELND in all target populations is

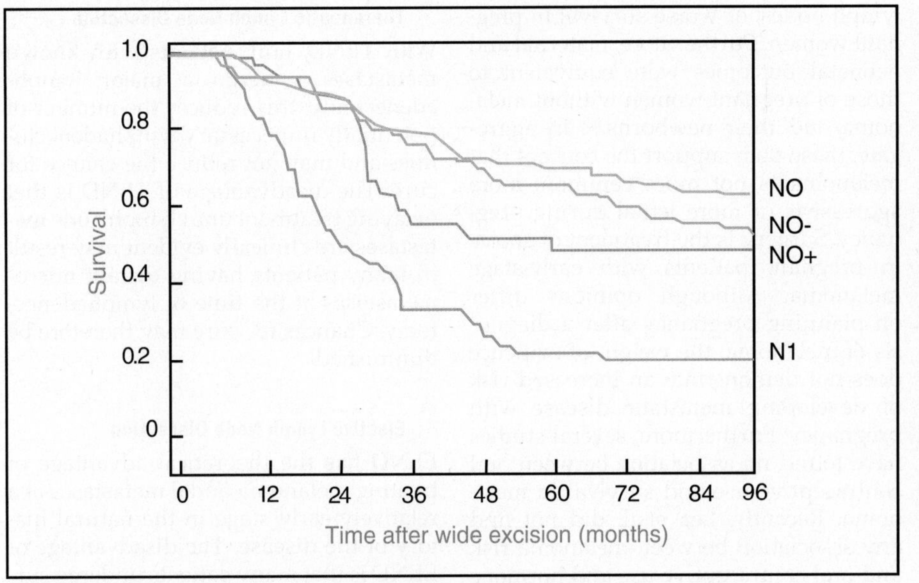

Figure 105-8 WHO Melanoma Programme Trial—Survival according to status of regional nodes. N0, patients who never developed node metastases after wide excision of primary. N0–, patients with clinically and histologically negative nodes at elective node dissection. N0+, patients with clinically negative and histologically positive nodes at elective node dissection. N1, patients who developed node metastases during follow-up and underwent delayed regional node dissection. *Source*: From Ref. 131.

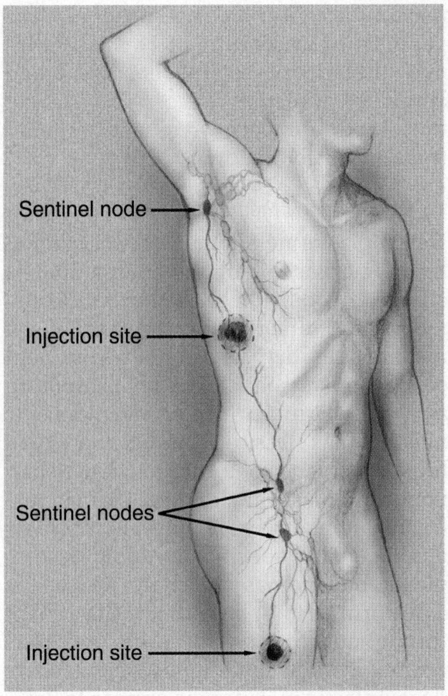

Figure 105-9 Concept of lymphatic mapping and sentinel node biopsy. In this example, "melanoma" of right flank "drains" to both right axilla and right groin, while afferent lymphatics also "drain" to right groin from "melanoma" of right thigh. *Source*: Courtesy of Jeffrey E. Gershenwald, MD.

that the majority of these patients who do not harbor occult metastases would be exposed to a procedure associated with significant morbidity and potential disability. Although the survival advantage of ELND over observation in selected patients is an important finding, it is difficult to recommend a procedure with significant risks of morbid complications to a broad group of melanoma patients when, overall, only 15-20% of patients with clinically negative regional lymph nodes are found to harbor occult metastatic disease. The results of a multicenter retrospective trial from Germany[134] also demonstrated an absolute survival advantage, of at least 13%, for patients with positive nodes detected by SLN biopsy compared to patients with positive nodes detected during observation of the nodal basin.

These data call into question recommendations to delay lymphadenectomy until palpable nodal disease develops; the data also support the use of alternative approaches to permit earlier identification of occult nodal disease. Over the past nearly two decades, many surgeons have adopted a selective approach to regional lymph node dissection—the technique of intraoperative lymphatic mapping and SLN biopsy originally developed by Morton. This technique satisfies many proponents of ELND as well as many proponents of TLND.

Lymphatic Mapping and SLN Biopsy

The technique of lymphatic mapping and SLN biopsy has been proposed as a minimally invasive procedure for identifying patients who harbor occult microscopic disease.[135,136] In a landmark report published in 1992,[135] and based on animal studies in a feline model, Morton and colleagues[137,138] described this technique in melanoma that has subsequently led to a global paradigm shift in the identification of regional nodal metastases in this disease. This technique relies on 2 concepts: (1) different regions of the skin have specific patterns of lymphatic drainage to the regional lymphatic basins; (2) for a given region of the skin there is a specific lymph node(s) (ie, SLN[s]) in the basin to which the cutaneous afferent lymphatic vessels drain first. Subsequent early studies confirmed that the SLN(s) is the most likely first site of metastatic disease and demonstrated that if the SLN(s) is histologically negative, then the remainder of the lymph nodes in the basin are histologically negative as well,[136,139,140] and suggested that patients with melanoma can be accurately staged with procedures that are less extensive than complete dissection.

With lymphatic mapping and SLN biopsy, the specific lymph node or nodes in a regional nodal basin that are the first to receive the afferent lymphatic drainage from a primary cutaneous melanoma—the sentinel nodes—are identified and removed (Figs. 105-9 and 105-10). If the SLN lacks metastasis, the remainder of the regional lymph nodes are unlikely to contain disease, and a completion lymph node dissection need not be performed.[139,141] If, however, the SLN contains metastatic tumor cells, a completion lymph node dissection is recommended to ensure regional basin control. Since this approach limits the number of lymph nodes submitted for pathologic evaluation (ie, fewer nodes compared to complete lymphadenectomy), the SLN(s) can be subjected to a more thorough pathologic analysis—such as use of serial sectioning and immunohistochemical analysis—to assess for the presence of microscopic nodal disease.[76,142-148] Thus, the likelihood of identifying patients who harbor microscopic metastases and thus may benefit from early TLND and adjuvant therapy is improved.

Goals and Benefits of SLN Biopsy The goals of surgical treatment of regional lymph nodes are (1) pathologic regional lymph node staging, (2) regional disease control, and (3) potential cure of Stage III disease.

Role of SLN Biopsy in Pathologic Regional Lymph Node Staging: Prognostic Value of SLN Pathologic Status *Early Results* Over the past 19 years, the SLN biopsy technique has gained increasing acceptance and has been substantially refined and validated.[76,135,139,149-154] In the initial report by Morton et al.,[135,137] SLN biopsy was performed with vital blue dye alone. SLNs were successfully

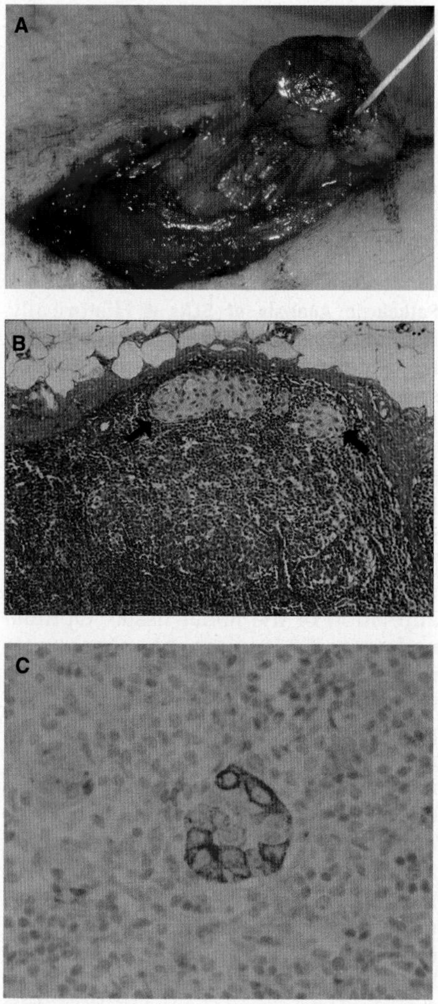

Figure 105-10 ■ (**A**) Intraoperative identification of an SLN. Intradermal injection of a vital blue dye around the intact melanoma or biopsy site leads to uptake of the dye by the lymphatic system and transport of the dye to the draining regional nodal basins, thereby allowing for identification of SLNs. Note isosulfan blue-stained afferent lymphatic vessel leading to blue-stained SLN. *Source*: Courtesy of Jeffrey E. Gershenwald, MD, and M. D. Anderson Cancer Center. (**B**) Example of SLN metastasis. (H&E) *Source*: From Ref. 76. (**C**) Sentinel node stained with HMB-45 (AEC, aminoethylcarbazol, ×40). Light hemotoxylin used as a counterstain. Note that not all melanoma cells are labeled with the antibody. *Source*: Courtesy of Victor G. Prieto, MD, PhD.

identified in 194 (82%) of the 237 lymphatic basins. Of the 40 patients with histologically positive nodes, SLN biopsy successfully identified 38 patients (ie, 5% false-negative rate). SLN metastases were detected either by routine histologic examination with H&E staining (12%) or exclusively by immunohistochemical staining (9%). Remarkably, non-SLNs were the exclusive site of metastasis in only 2 of 3079 nodes from 194 lymph node dissections, for a false-negative rate of 1% (with nodes rather than patients as the unit of analysis). While these early data suggested that this new technique accurately identified patients with occult lymph node metastases,[135,137] significant room for improvement was also evident. Experience at several other institutions[76,85,139,141,149,151,152,155-160] confirmed that nodal metastasis from cutaneous primary sites follows an orderly, nonrandom, progressive pattern and, by performing concomitant lymphadenectomy at the time of SLN biopsy,[139] that SLN status reflects the histology of the nodal basin. Overall, recent studies reflect that the predictive value of a negative SLN approaches 99% and that the SLN procedure has a low false-negative rate (<4%).[159,161]

Prognostic Significance ■ The prognostic significance of SLN pathologic status in patients with cutaneous melanoma has been convincingly demonstrated.[135,136,150,151,159,162-166] In 1999, Gershenwald and colleagues[150] showed that SLN status was the most significant independent clinicopathologic prognostic factor with respect to survival, even when primary tumor thickness and ulceration status were included in the analysis. In an updated analysis of 1,487 patients who underwent SLN biopsy (median tumor thickness, 1.5 mm), the 5-year survival rate for patients with positive SLNs was 73.3%, compared with 96.8% for patients with negative SLNs. Several other multivariate regression analyses have confirmed that regional lymph node status is the most powerful predictor of recurrence and survival,[41,85,150,151,162,163,165,167-177] even among patients with thick melanomas.[167,178-184] According to analyses of the AJCC Melanoma Task Force database, 5-year survival rates for patients with Stage III disease range from 80% for patients with nonulcerated melanomas and only 1 microscopically positive SLN to 28% for patients with ulcerated primary tumors and clinically evident nodal disease with more than 3 pathologically involved nodes (Table 105-6). In an AJCC melanoma database study that compared patients with melanoma greater than or equal to 1 mm who underwent lymphatic mapping and negative sentinel node biopsy to those who had either clinically uninvolved lymph nodes or a negative ELND, survival was better in those patients who underwent SLN biopsy procedures, thus underscoring the improved staging among this latter cohort of patients.[163] Further refinements in AJCC staging criteria will likely occur, potentially providing improved prognostic stratification for patients in the expanding population with microscopic nodal disease.

Tumor burden in the regional nodal basins is an important predictor of survival and, therefore, is an important stage determinant in the current AJCC system (Tables 105-3 and 105-6).[38,41,42] Both the number of positive nodes[41,185] and the burden of disease in the nodes (macroscopic vs microscopic) are significant predictors.[41] Interestingly, recent data indicate that the extent of microscopic disease in SLNs can also be used to stratify disease-specific survival.[165,170-176,181,186-192] Recent data suggest that isolated tumor cells in regional lymph nodes are clinically relevant in patients with melanoma, although others suggest that a lower threshold may exist below which metastatic deposits may not be clinically relevant.[166,170-176,193-196] The concept of microscopic nodal tumor burden will likely be important in the era of SLN biopsy as accurate microscopic staging of SLNs becomes even more widespread and patients are better stratified on the basis of microscopic tumor burden. As our understanding of the significance of microscopic nodal tumor burden is refined, clinical decisions regarding the need for and extent of further surgery or adjuvant therapy may also be based on the extent of microscopic nodal tumor burden.[185,197]

Non-SLN Involvement Following Completion Lymphadenectomy ■ In patients with clinically negative nodal basins, most nodal metastases, when present, are identified by SLN biopsy and are microscopic. Current standard clinical practice for patients with microscopic nodal metastases includes completion lymph node dissection, an approach recommended by an international consensus panel of melanoma experts.[198] However, additional positive non-SLNs are identified in only 8-33% of completion lymph node dissection specimens,[78,140,150,152,164-166,170,172,174,175,181,185,188,191,194,199-210] suggesting that a subset of patients with microscopic nodal disease may not benefit from completion lymph node dissection after a positive SLN biopsy. Understanding which factors predict additional non-SLN disease in patients with positive SLNs may allow better selection of patients who may benefit from completion lymph node dissection and may spare SLN-positive patients at "minimal" risk for additional non-SLN regional metastases from the morbidity of a completion lymph node dissection. In one study, the presence of a thick or ulcerated primary tumor in patients with a positive SLN predicted involvement of non-SLNs at completion lymph node dissection.[199] Other reports have failed to identify clinicopathologic variables that accurately predict the subset with additional disease in the nodal basin.[202,211] In a recent study of 343 patients who had completion lymph node dissection after the discovery of positive SLNs,[185] 14.5% had additional non-SLN disease in the lymphadenectomy specimen. The extent of microscopic tumor burden in the SLN(s) was examined to determine whether tumor burden—defined by several surrogate markers—could be used as a predictor of non-SLN involvement. Interestingly, by multivariable logistic regression analysis, measures of SLN microscopic tumor burden, tumor thickness greater than 2 mm, and number of SLNs harvested also predicted additional disease; a model was also developed that stratified patients according to their risk for non-SLN involvement.[185]

It is important to note that the completion lymph node dissection specimen is not routinely histologically assessed in the same fashion as the SLN; additional disease, if present, may go undetected with standard histologic techniques, and may represent a potential source of subsequent recurrence if it were not removed. Although less than one-fifth of patients with a positive SLN have additional melanoma detected by routine histologic examination of non-SLNs, a completion lymph node dissection remains the standard of care for all patients with a positive SLN. In the future, selection of patients for completion lymph node dissection may be based, at least in part, on the extent of SLN microscopic nodal tumor burden. The MSLT-II trial has been initiated and will explore the role of completion lymphadenectomy in patients with a positive SLN as well as prospective determination of the prognostic significance of micrometastases identified by reverse-transcriptase-polymerase chain reaction (RT-PCR) assessment of SLNs that show no evidence of tumor by conventional histopathologic techniques, including immunohistochemistry.

Predictors of SLN Status ■ Since the histologic status of the SLN is the dominant independent predictor of survival in clinically node-negative patients with melanoma,[150,212] identification of predictors of SLN metastasis has been the subject of intense investigation. In addition to their independent significance in predicting survival, tumor thickness and ulceration are the dominant independent predictors of SLN metastasis in patients with clinically negative regional lymph nodes.[46,151,164,213,214] It is therefore not surprising that the incidence of SLN metastasis increases with AJCC T-category (Table 105-9).[213] In one large series, 4% of patients with tumors less than or equal to 1 mm thick (T1) had positive SLNs, whereas 44% of patients with tumors thicker than 4 mm (T4) had positive SLNs.[213] When patients are stratified solely by the presence of primary tumor ulceration, 35% of patients with ulcerated tumors and 12% of patients with nonulcerated tumors have positive SLNs (Table 105-9).[213] When stratified by both ulceration and tumor thickness, patients with ulcerated primary lesions are more likely to have positive SLNs than are patients without evidence of ulceration within each AJCC T-category.[213] This pattern provides a useful paradigm for preoperative patient counseling. More recently, other factors—including high mitotic rate and younger patient age—have also been shown to increase SLN positivity rates.[215-217] Knowledge of the factors associated with a positive SLN is necessary for appropriate patient counseling regarding treatment options and possible outcomes.

Role of SLN Biopsy in Regional Disease Control ■ The role of SLN biopsy in regional disease control has been the subject of debate. It has been hypothesized that by disrupting lymphatic drainage pathways, the SLN biopsy procedure itself might compromise regional disease control. As such, patients who have a SLN biopsy might have a higher risk of in-transit and regional nodal recurrences. Gershenwald and colleagues[186] showed that SLN biopsy does not compromise regional nodal control in patients with melanoma and a positive SLN. Overall, these low rates of in-basin recurrence after positive SLN biopsy compare favorably with those observed after formal lymphadenectomy in patients with clinically evident nodal disease (9-36%) and are similar to the in-basin failure rates of patients who have undergone ELND and have proven microscopic disease.[186,218-222]

Pathologic Analysis of SLNs ■ Historically, histologic assessment of lymph nodes from formal lymph node dissection specimens has involved conventional H&E examination of 1 section from each lymph node. With the advent of SLN biopsy, however, an average of only 2-3 lymph nodes per nodal basin are submitted for pathologic review. With fewer lymph nodes to analyze, the pathologist can perform a much more intense examination of the nodal tissue. Optimal nodal staging requires not only accurate identification of the SLN but also careful examination of the SLN with special pathologic techniques. It is likely that many false-negative SLN biopsies do not actually reflect true skip metastases but are the result of micrometastases missed on routine pathologic examination. The recurrences could have potentially been prevented if the SLNs had undergone detailed histologic examination initially, the micrometastases had been found, and complete node dissection had been performed.[76,140,143,147,150,159,223-227] Methods to facilitate more intense histologic evaluation of SLNs—serial sectioning and immunohistochemical staining—have therefore been developed and refined to enhance identification of occult nodal disease (Fig. 105-10).[76,223,228-230] In nearly all melanoma centers, SLNs are currently routinely examined using serial sectioning, immunostaining, or both,[142-145,147,148,173,201,223,231,232] although techniques do vary among institutions.[146,147,232-234] Importantly, immunohistochemically detected SLN metastases are considered as evidence of node-positive disease in the seventh edition of the AJCC Melanoma Staging System.

Clinical Relevance of Submicroscopic Disease ■ Molecular techniques such as RT-PCR have also been explored in assessing SLNs to detect submicroscopic disease that might not be detectable by conventional histologic methods.[225,235-242] Early studies with limited follow-up have suggested that the prognosis of patients with an SLN that is positive by RT-PCR but negative by histology or immunohistochemistry is worse than that of patients who have negative results by all techniques. However, when similar questions were addressed after longer follow-up in 2 of these studies, there was

Table 105-9 ■ **Effect of Ulceration on SLN Metastases for a Given Tumor Thickness (n = 1,375)**

		Positive SLN					
			Not Ulcerated		Ulcerated		*P* Value[a]
Tumor Thickness (mm)	Total Patients (%)	All (%)	(%)	AJCC Stage[b]	(%)	AJCC Stage[b]	Ulcerated vs Not
≤1.00	28	4	3	IA	16	IB	0.026
1.01-2.00	38	12	11	IB	22	IIA	0.007
2.01-4.00	23	28	25	IIA	34	IIB	0.115
>4.00	11	44	33	IIB	53	IIC	0.021
All Patients	100	17	12		35		<0.0001

[a]Fisher's exact test for each tumor thickness group.
[b]Stage groupings calculated using tumor thickness and ulceration data only.
Source: From Ref. 213.

no difference in recurrence rates between patients whose SLNs were histologically negative and RT-PCR positive and patients whose SLNs were negative both histologically and by RT-PCR.[243,244] Taken together, these data suggest that the ultimate value of RT-PCR staging of SLNs is not yet clear.[240,245] Despite the absence of survival impact from these long-term follow-up studies, investigators at the JWCI reported intriguing data to support the possibility that these approaches may be used to identify submicroscopic disease[246,247] and are addressing this hypothesis in the MSLT-II. Nonetheless, RT-PCR remains investigational and should not be used to direct adjuvant therapy at this time.[243,244]

Role of SLN Biopsy in Potential Cure ■ With respect to treatment of the primary melanoma, the therapeutic efficacy of sentinel node biopsy is being compared with excision alone as part of a multicenter randomized phase III trial—the Multicenter Selective Lymphadenectomy Trial (MSLT-1).[212] Although interim results of this trial have not thus far demonstrated an overall survival difference after a median follow-up of 5 years (Fig. 105-11B), data indicate that sentinel node biopsy, followed immediately by complete dissection if the sentinel node contains tumor, clearly prolongs disease-free survival (Fig. 105-11A) and spares the patient the psychological trauma of anticipating possible nodal recurrence during the traditional "watch and wait" approach.[212] Interim results also demonstrate improved melanoma-specific survival in patients who underwent early TLND following a positive SLN compared to those who developed clinical recurrence after nodal observation, suggesting that failure to identify and remove occult sentinel node metastases may allow development of more extensive regional node disease (Fig. 105-11D).[212] The prognostic significance of sentinel node biopsy was also validated in this multicenter trial (Fig. 105-11C).[212,248] Additional discussion of this important clinical trial can be found elsewhere.[249,250]

Patient Selection ■ The technique of lymphatic mapping and SLN biopsy has been shown to be highly accurate in representing the status of the regional nodal basin.[135,141,150,159,212] This approach has become a standard of care for melanoma patients,[198] providing an alternative to ELND. In nearly all melanoma centers worldwide, SLN biopsy is routinely offered to patients with primary cutaneous melanoma whose primary tumor thickness is at least 1 mm. However, among the very prevalent group of patients whose primary tumors are less than 1 mm, in many centers, various clinicopathologic factors have been employed in an attempt to identify patients in this overall favorable risk group who may be at increased risk of harboring microscopic Stage III disease and for whom SLN biopsy may be warranted (reviewed

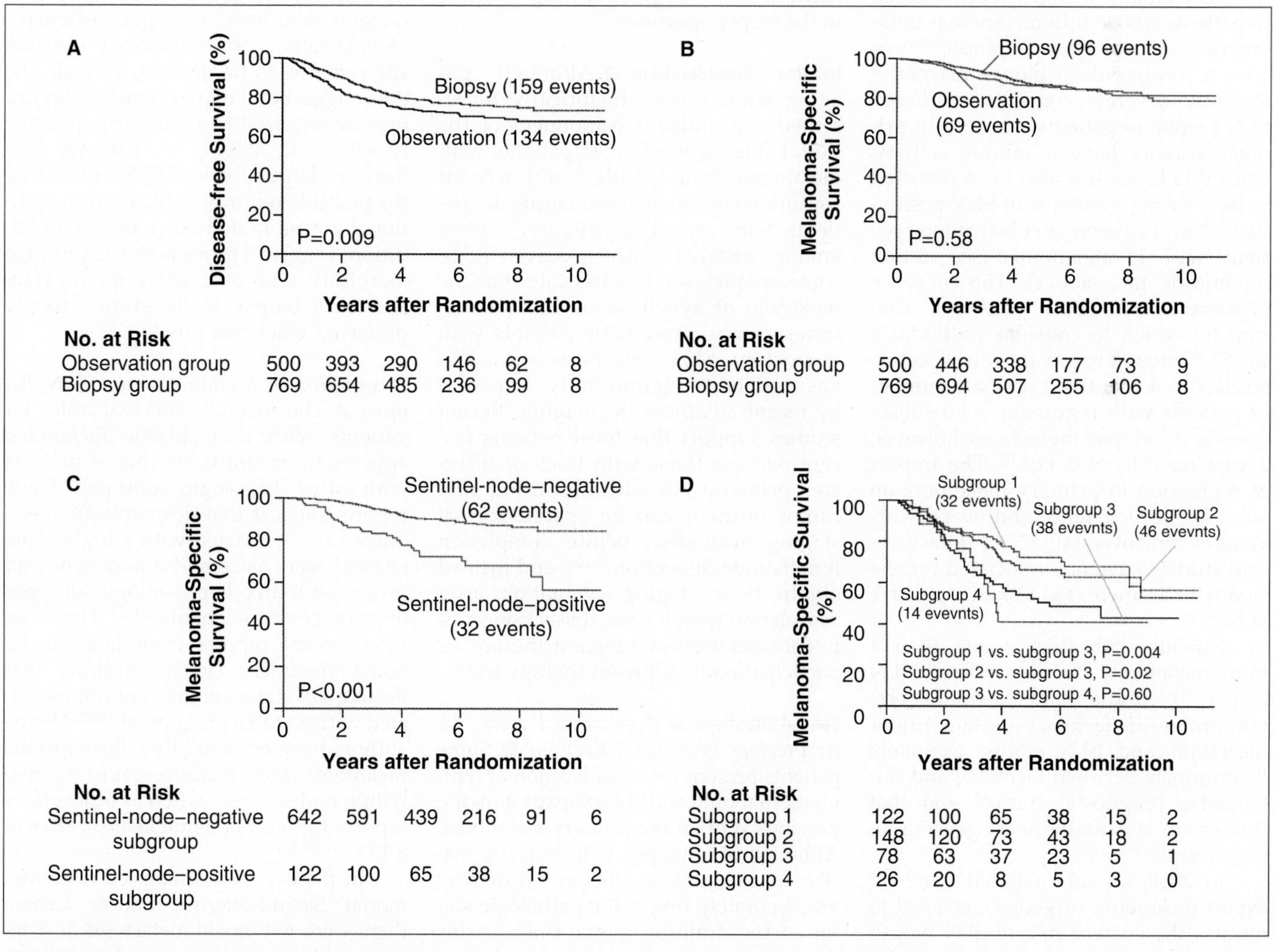

Figure 105-11 Interim results of the Multicenter Selective Lymphadenectomy Trial (MSLT-1). (**A**) Disease-free survival and (**B**) melanoma-specific survival, respectively, according to the type of treatment. (**C**) Melanoma-specific survival according to the tumor status of the sentinel node in patients who underwent sentinel node biopsy. (**D**) Melanoma-specific survival among patients with nodal metastases: subgroup 1 comprised patients with a tumor-positive sentinel node; subgroup 2, the patients in subgroup 1 plus those in subgroup 4 with a nodal recurrence after a negative result on biopsy; subgroup 3, those with nodal recurrence during observation; and subgroup 4, those with nodal recurrence after a negative result on biopsy. *Source:* From Ref. 212.

in reference 251). However, due to the overall low incidence of SLN positivity in this cohort, coupled with the inherent individual institutional bias in the clinicopathologic profile of patients offered SLN biopsy in patients with less than 1 mm melanoma, even large, single-institution analyses have limited potential to unravel this important clinical challenge due to the limitations in the extent to which analyses can be performed. Nonetheless, many centers have also offered SLN biopsy to patients with a melanoma less than 1.0 mm thick, if it is at least Clark level IV or is ulcerated[76,150,198] and if the patient has no evidence of metastatic melanoma in regional lymph nodes and distant sites on physical examination and staging evaluation (chest radiograph and LDH levels).[150] Consistent with the aforementioned inclusion criteria, AJCC melanoma staging system currently recommends lymphatic mapping and SLN biopsy for patients with T1b and greater melanoma (including patients with thick primaries).

SLN biopsy has also been offered to patients whose thin melanomas demonstrate vertical growth phase[252-254] or have a positive deep biopsy margin.[255] Recently, several groups have offered SLN biopsy to patients whose thin primary tumors have a mitotic activity, since this factor has also been reported to be a strong predictor of SLN positivity[215,256] and adverse survival among patients with T1 melanomas (see section on mitotic rate, above). The presence of regression has been used as a criterion by which to consider individuals for SLN biopsy based on retrospective studies that identified a small number of patients with regression who subsequently developed metastases; however, a vast majority did not.[257] The impact of regression in primary melanoma on subsequent recurrence and overall survival is controversial[253,257-261]; in fact, recent studies have not associated regression with an increased risk of a positive SLN.[262,263]

Patients with thick (more than 4 mm) melanoma are also offered SLN biopsy.[178,180] Studies have shown that certain prognostic factors, especially tumor ulceration and SLN status accurately discriminate between favorable and unfavorable prognostic subsets and that this group is actually heterogeneous in prognosis.[178,180,182-184]

In 2008, an international panel of expert melanoma surgeons convened to discuss the current role of SLN biopsy in the management of patients with primary cutaneous melanoma.[198] They further noted that SLN biopsy is valuable because it is a minimally invasive procedure to stage the regional lymph nodes with little morbidity[212,248]; it represents a standard of care, and should be discussed with all appropriate clinically node-negative melanoma patients who will undergo wide excision of a primary melanoma.[198] Most of the panelists also discussed and offered SLN biopsy to patients whose melanomas are not thicker than 1.0 mm but have characteristics that increase the likelihood of regional node micrometastasis. Although unanimous consensus was not reached for all criteria, most panelists would consider recommending the procedure based on primary tumor ulceration, a mitotic rate equal to or greater than 1/mm^2 and/or Clark level IV/V invasion—especially if tumor thickness exceeds 0.75 mm. In fact, some of the panelists would use this tumor thickness as a sole criterion for SLN biopsy. Ulceration, mitotic rate, and Clark level would be especially relevant in patients who have no significant comorbidity, who are younger than 40-45 years, or whose primary tumor depth is uncertain because of tumor-positive deep margins in the biopsy specimen.[198]

Imaging Considerations ■ Although imaging studies have historically represented a prominent component of the initial staging workup of patients with melanoma, there is little, if any, role for routine comprehensive imaging in patients with *early-stage* disease.[264] Even among patients with positive SLNs, contemporary studies indicate that the incidence of synchronous distant metastasis in asymptomatic patients with microscopic SLN metastases is low and has not been siginificantly impacted by recent advances in imaging. Recent studies support that most patients (except perhaps those with thick or ulcerated primaries, or with significant SLN tumor burden) can be spared formal staging evaluation before completion lymph node dissection,[264-266] and instead obtain their staging evaluation after completion lymph node dissection prior to consideration of adjuvant therapy or participation in adjuvant therapy trials.

Special Situations ■ *Approach to Patients After Previous Wide Local Excision* ■ Some patients present for consideration of lymphatic mapping and SLN biopsy following previous WLE of the primary melanoma. Although SLN biopsy is technically feasible in such patients, the procedure may less accurately reflect the pathologic status of the draining lymph node basins due to concern that the patterns of afferent lymphatic flow from a primary tumor site in this setting may be altered because of disruption of the lymphatic vessels from theWLE. Lymphatic mapping may be particularly insensitive when a melanoma was excised with particularly large margins, when a defect was covered with a rotation flap, or when the primary tumor was situated in a region of ambiguous lymphatic drainage. Our experience in 104 patients who had a previous WLE without a significant rotational flap suggests that the approach is technically feasible—the SLN positivity rate was similar to that in 1291 patients mapped during the same time period (with a similar overall pattern of clinicopathologic risk factors) in whom WLE had not previously been performed.[267] At a median follow-up of 51 months, there were no regional lymph node recurrences in any of these 104 patients. Other investigators have also documented the potential utility of SLN biopsy in patients after previous WLE.[268-273] These data support that SLNs can be successfully identified and accurately reflect the status of the regional lymph node basin in carefully selected melanoma patients with a previous WLE; in contrast, the utility of SLN biopsy in patients who have undergone extensive reconstruction of the primary excision site remains to be defined. Overall, the data suggest that more extensive surgery may be required to accomplish accurate lymph node staging in patients who have undergone prior WLE—including the possible removal of SLNs from additional lymph node basins and as an additional surgical procedure; to minimize morbidity and cost, concomitant WLE and SLN biopsy is therefore strongly preferred whenever possible.[267]

Desmoplastic Melanoma and SLN Biopsy ■ The overall survival rate for patients with desmoplastic melanoma appears to be similar to that of patients with other histologic subtypes. Some reports suggest that desmoplastic melanomas are associated with a higher rate of local recurrence and a poorer overall prognosis than other histologic subtypes of cutaneous melanoma.[274-277] However, more recent reports from large melanoma treatment centers indicate that desmoplastic melanomas are not associated with a worse prognosis.[114,277,278] Some authors have reported that desmoplastic melanoma rarely metastasizes to regional lymph nodes,[115,276,279] whereas others have reported lymph node metastasis rates of 8-15%.[274,277,280-286]

In the experience reported from Memorial Sloan-Kettering Cancer Center, there were few nodal metastases at diagnosis or during follow-up, and no patients with desmoplastic melanoma had a positive SLN.[114,115] In contrast, Su and colleagues[286] reported that in a series of 33 patients with desmoplastic neurotropic melanoma undergoing sentinel lymphadenectomy, 4 (12%) were found to harbor micrometastases in the SLN. None of the 4 had any additional non-SLN metastases at completion lymph node dissection. A recent review of the experience at the University of Texas M. D. Anderson Cancer Center, which included 1,850 patients undergoing SLN biopsy, found a low incidence of SLN metastasis (2%) in a group of 47 patients with pure desmoplastic melanoma, despite their having thicker primary tumors at presentation.[115] Interestingly, patients with "mixed" desmoplastic melanoma (*N* = 19) (defined as <90% of the invasive component of the melanoma having desmoplastic features) or non-desmoplastic melanoma (*N* = 1785) had a similar incidence of a positive SLN (15.8% and 17.5%, respectively). Since patients with pure desmoplastic melanoma are unlikely to have metastatic disease in regional lymph nodes, SLN biopsy in patients with pure desmoplastic melanoma may not be warranted[114,115] (see also Radiation Therapy for Locoregional Disease below).

Complications and Morbidity Following Lymphatic Mapping and SLN Biopsy ■ At the same time, SLN biopsy is associated with low morbidity.[212,248,287,288] There are substantially fewer postoperative complications after SLN biopsy than after ELND,[288,289] and the rate of lymphedema, pain, numbness, and loss of active range of motion are lower after SLN biopsy than after full anatomical dissection.[177,212,288,290,291] In addition, recent data have shown that SLN biopsy does not increase the incidence of in-transit recurrence.[248,292-294]

Investigators from the Sunbelt Melanoma Trial reported overall low complication rates following SLN biopsy alone in more than 1,202 trial patients compared to the 277 patients who required a complete lymph node dissection as part of the trial.[288] This observation has been recapitulated by others,[295,296] as well as in the Multicenter Selective Lymphadenectomy Trial, in which an overall complication rate of 10% after lymphatic mapping and SLN biopsy increased to 32.7% after completion lymph node dissection.[212,248] Strategies to reduce the incidence of lymphedema, more common following lymphadenectomy, are also helpful.

Although the SLN biopsy technique has gained widespread acceptance for a number of reasons—accurate nodal staging, enhanced regional control, possible survival benefit, limited surgical morbidity compared to formal lymphadenectomy—some authors have suggested that SLN biopsy may increase the risk of in-transit metastasis (ITM), thereby reducing, eliminating, or reversing any potential survival advantage associated with the SLN biopsy technique.[297] The hypothesis that the SLN biopsy technique and subsequent completion lymph node dissection in SLN-positive patients may disturb lymph flow by mechanical disruption and lead to increased rates of ITM—if accurate—is of particular concern since SLN biopsy has been widely adopted as the standard of care for many patients with clinically localized melanoma. The collective experience at several large academic centers,[292,293,298] including the MSLT-1 trial,[212] provides strong support that the technique of SLN biopsy itself does not increase the risk ofITM.[212,292,293,298] Instead, the risk of in-transit melanoma metastasis depends on tumor biology and not the surgical approach to regional lymph nodes.[294]

Technical Considerations—Lymphatic Mapping and Sentinel Node Biopsy ■ Successful SLN biopsy requires the integration of several disciplines—nuclear medicine, surgery, and pathology. The contemporary approach consists of 3 main components: (1) preoperative cutaneous lymphoscintigraphy to identify the regional nodal basins at risk and the number and location of the SLNs within the basin; (2) excisional biopsy of SLNs in all regional nodal basins at risk as shown by preoperative lymphoscintigraphy and intraoperative localization with vital blue dye and handheld gamma probe detection of ^{99}Tc-labeled sulfur colloid (in the United States); and (3) careful pathologic evaluation of the SLNs. Lymphatic mapping and SLN biopsy is performed at the time of wide excision of the primary tumor or biopsy site. Since the introduction of lymphatic mapping and SLN biopsy, the technique has undergone several refinements that have resulted in improved detection of SLNs.

Use of a vital blue dye (isosulfan blue 1%) to help identify SLNs has been part of the lymphatic mapping and SLN biopsy procedure since its introduction. The blue dye is injected into the patient intradermally around the intact tumor or biopsy site, taken up by the lymphatic system, and carried via afferent lymphatics to the SLN (Figs. 105-9 and 105-10). The draining nodal basin is explored, and the afferent lymphatic channels and first draining lymph nodes (the SLNs) are identified by the uptake of the blue dye. With the use of blue dye alone, an SLN is identified in approximately 85% of cases. Although this initial approach was promising, it left 15% of patients unable to benefit from SLN biopsy because no SLN was identified.

Subsequently, two additional techniques have been incorporated that have significantly improved SLN localization: (1) preoperative lymphoscintigraphy and (2) intraoperative injection of ^{99}Tc-labeled sulfur colloid accompanied by intraoperative use of a handheld gamma probe. Preoperative lymphoscintigraphy using ^{99}Tc-labeled sulfur colloid permits the identification of patients with multiple draining nodal basins and patients with lymphatic drainage to SLNs located outside standard nodal basins, including epitrochlear, popliteal, and ectopic/interval sites.[299-302] For the SLN biopsy technique to be accurate, all true SLNs, regardless of location, must be biopsied.[303,304] Although the number of reported cases is small, SLNs of either the interval or ectopic type can harbor metastatic melanoma. The incidence of ectopic SLN positivity can be as high as 14%.[299,305] In patients with melanomas that drain to multiple regional nodal basins, the histologic status of 1 draining basin does not predict the status of other basins. Therefore, it is particularly important to identify and assess all at-risk regional nodal basins to properly stage the disease.

Perhaps the most important development in the SLN biopsy technique has been the introduction of intraoperative lymphatic mapping using a handheld gamma probe. Preoperative intradermal injection of 0.5-1.0 mCi of ^{99}Tc-labeled sulfur colloid permits intraoperative use of a handheld gamma probe that is used to transcutaneously identify SLNs that will be removed. The use of both blue dye and radiocolloid increases the surgeon's ability to identify the SLN (>96-99% accuracy) compared to the use of blue dye alone (84% accuracy).[151] Overall, radiocolloid and vital blue dye mapping techniques are complementary; to facilitate regional nodal staging, this latter technique represents the preferred approach to SLN biopsy by large academic centers[151,306] and by an international consensus panel.[198] In general, SLNs are subjected to enhanced pathologic analysis that includes both serial sectioning and immunohistochemical analysis (see above). Frozen section analysis of SLNs in patients with cutaneous melanoma is not routinely performed.[307]

When the SLNs are histologically negative, no further surgery is performed, and the remaining regional lymph nodes are left intact. When the SLNs show evidence of metastatic disease, completion lymphadenectomy of the affected nodal basin is the current standard of care. Pathologic evaluation of completion lymphadenectomy specimens often reveals no additional disease. However, it is important to remember that completion lymphadenectomy specimens are routinely assessed with standard histologic techniques rather than the more rigorous examination reserved for SLN biopsy specimens. As a result, there may actually be additional disease in the completion nodal specimen that goes undetected. This disease would represent a potential source of subsequent recurrence if it were not removed. Because such recurrences are difficult to treat surgically and may contribute to significant morbidity, completion lymphadenectomy performed for microscopic disease provides the potential for improved regional control. In addition, identifying patients with minimal disease burden by using the SLN approach may help identify the group of patients who may derive an improved survival benefit from early TLND. Furthermore, knowledge of the pathologic status of the SLNs allows proper staging and facilitates decision-making regarding adjuvant treatment.

Management of Local Recurrence, Satellites, and ITM

Local Recurrence versus Satellites

Classically, local recurrence implies the regrowth of incompletely excised melanoma. However, since most melanoma patients who develop local recurrences have had WLE with relatively extensive negative margins, local recurrence after WLE more accurately represents a form of lymphatic metastasis that is distinct from regrowth of tumor that was incompletely excised from the site of a previous primary melanoma.[50] This is supported by the similar prognosis for patients with "local recurrence"[80,82,308,309] compared with that for patients with satellite, in-transit,[80,83,308,310] and/or regional lymph node metastases,[55,56,64,99-102,132,215,311] in support of these probably being manifestations of the same disease process—that is, lymphatic dissemination.

True local recurrence—defined as recurrence at the primary tumor site of the melanoma, within or contiguous with the scar—is most likely the result of incomplete excision of the primary tumor. It is a relatively rare pattern of recurrence, that in many cases may more appropriately be considered persistence of the primary tumor.[312,313] Since the prognosis after a true local recurrence is significantly better than that associated with in-transit disease (see the next section), correct classification is important in treatment planning. For example, a local recurrence consisting of a single lesion in a patient whose primary melanoma had favorable prognostic features may be appropriately treated with excision alone. Patients with local recurrences consisting of multiple, small and superficial lesions may be treated in a fashion similar to that used to treat patients with in-transit disease (see the next section).

In-Transit and Satellite Metastasis

Traditionally, in-transit and satellite metastases have been described as recurrent locoregional disease found in the dermis or subcutaneous tissue between the primary melanoma and the regional lymph node basin (Fig. 105-12). This pattern of recurrence is unique to melanoma and is reported to occur in 3-12% of melanoma cases.[292] Although the molecular determinants and pathophysiology of in-transit disease are not well-defined, such events most likely represent an intralymphatic manifestation of melanoma metastases. Independent predictors of in-transit recurrence include age greater than 50 years, a lower extremity primary tumor, increasing Breslow depth, ulceration, and positive SLN status.[212,292-294,298] In a study from The University of Texas M. D. Anderson Cancer Center, patients with a positive SLN had a significantly higher rate of in-transit metastases (12%) than patients with a negative SLN (3.5%). Regional nodal metastases occur in about two-thirds of patients with in-transit disease and, if present, are associated with lower survival rates (Table 105-7).[42] Predictors of distant metastasis among patients with in-transit recurrence include positive SLN status, in-transit tumor size of at least 2 cm, and disease-free interval before in-transit recurrence of less than 12 months.[292] Patients who present with synchronous distant and in-transit disease likely have a worse disease-specific survival compared to patients who present with only in-transit or distant disease.[292]

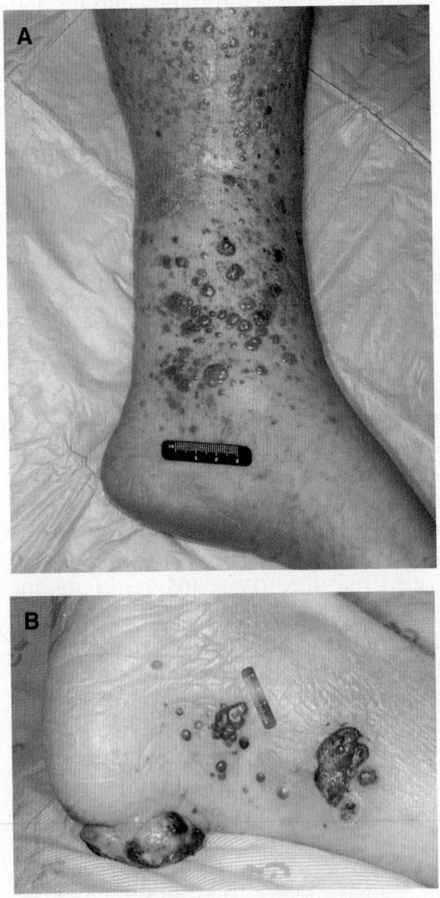

Figure 105-12 **(A)** Example of in-transit metastases. **(B)** Bulky melanoma of posterior heel with synchronous satellite and in-transit metastases. *Source*: Courtesy of Jeffrey E. Gershenwald, MD.

For patients with in-transit metastases confined to a limb that are not amenable to standard surgical measures—eg, patients with recurrent and/or multiple in-transit metastases and patients with large-burden in-transit disease—regional chemotherapy techniques such as isolated limb perfusion or, more recently, isolated limb infusion, may be considered (see below). Amputation is rarely indicated. Intralesional immunotherapy with bacille Calmette-Guérin (BCG) has been reported as an alternate means to control the regional manifestations of recurrent inoperable in-transit melanoma.[314] Systemic therapy with high-dose IL-2 in patients with cutaneous-only disease, including those with inoperable in-transit metastases, has reported response rates of up to 50% (see below).[315] Radiation therapy for locally recurrent and in-transit melanoma has been inadequately investigated, although several reports have suggested encouraging response rates. It may therefore be reasonable to consider palliative radiation in those patients who are not candidates for other approaches noted above. Clinical trial participation is highly encouraged.

Hyperthermic Isolated Limb Perfusion (HILP)

HILP with melphalan has been used to treat in-transit metastases of the extremities since the mid-1950s. Melphalan is currently the most active single agent for use in HILP. Overall response rates of more than 80% have been reported, with a median response duration in patients with a complete response (CR) ranging from 9 to 19 months. Nonrandomized studies of hyperthermic limb perfusion by Leinard et al.[316] reported a high CR rate (over 90%) with a combination of melphalan, tumor necrosis factor-α (TNF-α), and interferon-γ (IFN-γ); Fraker[317] reported a 100% response rate in patients treated with melphalan alone and a 90% response rate in patients treated with melphalan and TNF-α. Based on these and other non-randomized data, a multicenter randomized trial sponsored by the American College of Surgeons Oncology Group comparing melphalan alone to a combination of melphalan and TNF-α for patients with in-transit metastases was conducted; it was ultimately closed to accrual as the interim analysis failed to reveal a benefit for TNF-α.[318] As a result, although TNF-α is available in Europe, TNF-α is not available in the United States for such procedures.

Although HILP may be effective as primary treatment for in-transit metastases, the technique involves a complex and invasive operative procedure entailing expensive equipment, long operating times, and considerable ancillary staff. In an attempt to achieve similar results using less complex techniques, a new regional chemotherapy technique, isolated limb infusion, has been introduced for the management of in-transit metastases.

Isolated Limb Infusion ■ Pioneered by Professor John Thompson at the Sydney Melanoma Unit, isolated limb infusion is essentially a low-flow isolated limb perfusion performed via percutaneously inserted catheters, but without oxygenation of the circuit as employed in HILP.[319] Cytotoxic agents—classically melphalan and actinomycin-D—are infused and circulated in the setting of progressive hypoxia. The hypoxia and acidosis associated with isolated limb infusion are therapeutically attractive because a number of cytotoxic agents, including melphalan, appear to damage tumor cells more effectively under hypoxic conditions.[320]

While at least one study concluded that isolated limb infusion has been shown to yield response rates similar to those observed after conventional HILP (overall response rate of 84%—CR rate, 38%; partial response rate, 46%),[319] others have noted a better response rate by HILP.[321] In ILI, CR rate has been shown to decrease with increasing stage of disease.[319] Nonetheless, because of the simplicity of the isolated infusion technique, ILI may not only be a more attractive option for patients with comorbidities or the elderly, but it may also serve as an excellent platform to investigate new treatments.[322,323]

Toxicity and Morbidity ■ HILP and isolated limb infusion can be associated with potentially significant regional adverse effects, including myonecrosis, nerve injury, compartment syndrome, and arterial thrombosis, sometimes necessitating fasciotomy or even major amputation. Recently, an improved toxicity profile has been reported by adjusting dose to ideal body weight. Systemic toxic effects, including hypotension and adult respiratory distress syndrome, have sometimes been seen with the addition of TNF-α to the perfusion or infusion regimen. Given the high degree of technical expertise required and associated significant risk of complications, the procedure should be performed only in centers that have experience with the technique.

Adjuvant Setting ■ A role for routine use of HILP in the adjuvant setting has not been defined. At present, there is little evidence to justify the use of prophylactic perfusion or infusion, except as part of a clinical trial.

Adjuvant Therapy

For the vast majority of patients presenting with melanoma, complete resection of the primary melanoma lesion along with any locoregional spread will be possible, leaving the patient without evidence of disease. However, the risk of recurrence as discussed above, especially for patients with thick primary lesions or positive lymph nodes, is substantial; so much effort has been spent on adjuvant therapy in this setting in order to decrease recurrence. These studies are challenging to perform, since recurrences, while most common within the first 3 years after diagnosis, can occur at any time following a diagnosis of melanoma. Randomized controlled trials are required to definitively assess adjuvant interventions, requiring large numbers of patients and several years of follow-up. Although challenging, multiple well-designed randomized studies have been performed for the adjuvant therapy of melanoma.

IFN-Alpha in the Adjuvant Setting

Type 1 IFNs, including IFN-alpha, are natural proteins produced by immune cells, including specialized plasmacytoid dendritic cells, in response to pathogens. They are essential to initiate a successful immune response against infectious agents, such as viruses, and lead to the stimulation of a potent T-cell immune response that leads to destruction of the invading organism. In order to harness the immune system against cancer, IFN-alpha has been tested in a number of settings in the clinic against melanoma.

Clinical Trials With IFN-Alpha ■ Multiple randomized studies using recombinant IFN-alpha, a natural cytokine produced by immune cells in response to viral infections, have been performed for the adjuvant therapy of melanoma.

The majority of studies with high-dose IFN have been conducted over the years by the Eastern Cooperative Oncology Group (ECOG). The first randomized study to suggest that high-dose IFN was beneficial to melanoma patients in the adjuvant setting was E1684. In this study, 287 Stage IIB and III melanoma patients were randomized to observation versus high-dose IFN, at a dose of 20 million international units per m^2/day i.v. × 4 weeks followed by 10 million international units per m^2 subcutaneously 3 times per week × 48 weeks. This study revealed a benefit in the IFN arm for recurrence-free survival ($p = 0.0023$) as well as overall survival ($p = 0.0237$). On the basis of results of these Intergroup trials, the U.S FDA approved IFNα-2b as the first postsurgical adjuvant for AJCC Stage IIb and III melanoma. However, the toxicity of high-dose IFN and some inconsistencies in the results of randomized trials have generated controversy regarding its international adoption as the standard of care (see below). Subsequent studies have confirmed the importance of IFN in prolonging recurrence-free survival but have not confirmed unequivocally significant effects on overall survival.[324]

A pooled analysis of studies E1684 and a follow-up study, E1690, of over 900 Stage IIB and III melanoma patients with a median follow-up of 7.2 years revealed that relapse-free survival was significantly prolonged in the group receiving high-dose IFN versus the observation group ($p = 0.006$).[324] A meta-analysis of 12 trials, including E1684 and E1690, found a highly significant improvement in recurrence free survival with IFN therapy ($p = 0.000003$). However, an overall survival benefit was less clear ($p = 0.1$). There appeared to be a dose–response with IFN in relationship to recurrence-free survival.[325]

A large study from the EORTC was recently performed, evaluating pegylated IFN for the adjuvant therapy of melanoma. In this study, 1256 Stage III melanoma patients were randomly assigned to observation or pegylated IFN-alpha-2b at a dose of 6 μg/kg for 8 weeks followed by 3 μg/kg for up to 5 years. Consistent with findings with standard IFN, there was a significant benefit seen in the patients receiving IFN with respect to recurrence-free survival but not overall survival. Interestingly, the patients who most greatly benefited were those with microscopic disease.[326]

IFN-alpha has a number of potential adverse reactions such as fever, fatigue, and hepatotoxicity. Patients receiving high-dose IFN-alpha should have their AST/ALT routinely monitored. Dose modifications or early discontinuation of therapy may be necessary based on toxicity (see Hauschild et al.[327] for a review of potential toxicities and appropriate dose modifications and contraindications to therapy).

While the overall survival benefit of IFN-alpha is debated, it appears to be the only agent thus far that has demonstrated an impact on disease-free survival in the adjuvant setting. Therefore, in the absence of other effective agents, it is currently standard of care for the adjuvant therapy of Stage III melanoma. In addition, IFN has an interesting mechanism of action and may have much potential for enhancing therapeutic results in the setting of both adjuvant and metastatic melanoma as part of combination regimens with other agents.

Mechanism of Action of IFN-Alpha ■ Multiple mechanisms may explain the anti-melanoma effect of type 1 IFNs (Fig. 105-13). IFN can have a direct anti-proliferative effect on tumor cells. In addition, numerous studies have demonstrated that IFNs can have an antiangiogenic effect. However, recent studies suggest that the primary mechanism of action of IFN-alpha in the adjuvant therapy of melanoma may be through activation of the immune system. Gogas et al evaluated 200 patients receiving high-dose IFN-alpha for Stage III melanoma for the development of autoimmunity.[328] Autoimmunity was defined as either development of anti-thyroid, anti-DNA, anti-cardiolipin, or anti-nuclear antibodies, or the development of clinical manifestations of autoimmunity such as vitiligo or hypothyroidism. She found that survival significantly correlated with the development of autoimmunity[329] (Fig. 105-14). Therefore, it appears that an IFN-induced immune response may be primarily responsible for the antitumor effects seen in melanoma patients.

IFN in turn has a number of effects on the immune system (Fig. 105-15), including upregulation of class 1 and class 2 molecules on the surface of melanoma cells, making them better targets for the immune system. In addition, type 1 IFNs can co-stimulate T-cells[330-334] and increase the ability of dendritic cells to process and present antigens to T-cells.[335-337] Further studies to understand the mechanism of the positive effects of IFN-alpha on the immune system in melanoma patients will be helpful in the rational design of combination regimens.

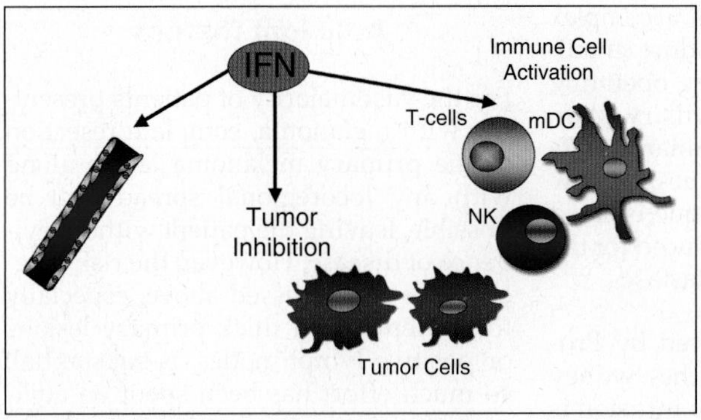

Figure 105-13 IFN-alpha: Mechanisms of action. There are multiple mechanisms by which type 1 IFN, such as IFN-alpha, can exhibit antitumor activity, including (1) inhibition of angiogenesis, (2) direct inhibition of tumor proliferation, and (3) activation of the immune system.

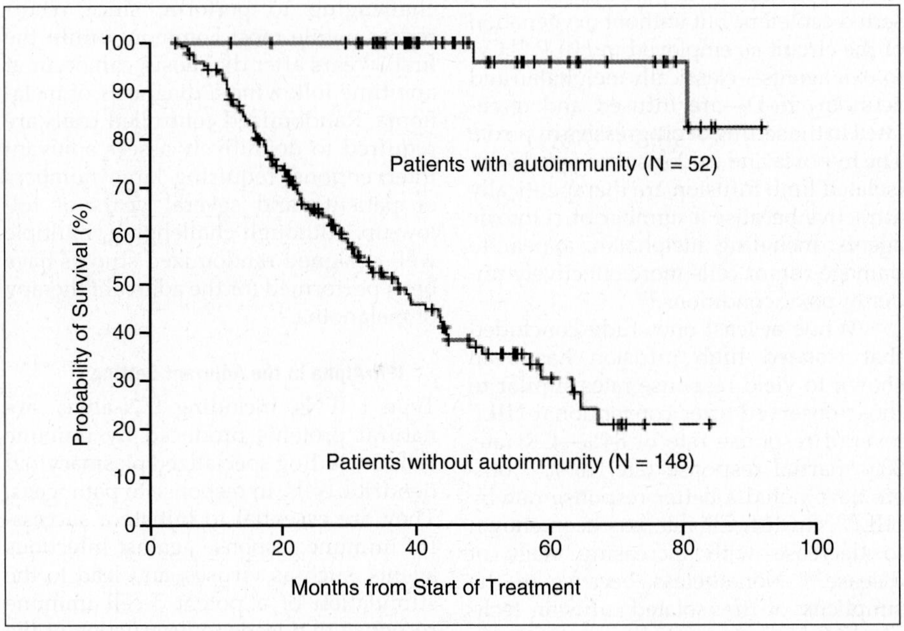

Figure 105-14 Development of autoimmunity correlates with survival in melanoma patients treated with IFN-alpha. Stage III patients receiving IFN-alpha in the adjuvant setting were studied for the development of either clinical or laboratory signs of autoimmunity. Patients who developed autoimmunity while on IFN had longer survival. *Source*: From Ref. 329.

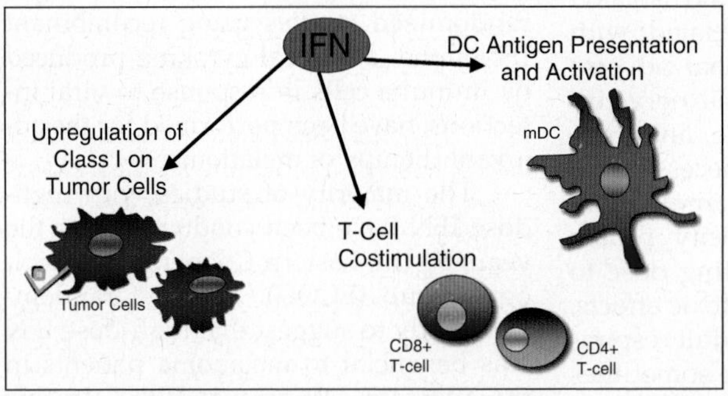

Figure 105-15 How is IFN working to enhance immunity? IFN-alpha may enhance antitumor immune responses by: (1) activating antigen presenting cells, (2) co-stimulating T-cells, and (3) upregulating MHC molecules on tumor cells, thereby making them easier to recognize by T-cells.

Cancer Vaccines in the Adjuvant Setting

Tumor antigens recognized by T-cells were first characterized in melanoma patients. T-cells specific for melanoma were isolated from patients and used to clone the first tumor antigens using a c-DNA library approach.

The antigens uncovered thus far fall into three major categories: (1) tumor differentiation antigens, which are expressed by melanocytes as well as melanoma cells (eg, MART-1, gp100), (2) tumor-testis antigens, which are expressed in some melanomas as well as other tumor types, as well as the testis (eg, MAGE-1), and (3) mutated antigens (eg, beta-catenin).[338]

These antigens have been used in numerous formulations for the study of active vaccination against melanoma, including peptide fragments, recombinant protein, recombinant viral vectors (poxvirus and adenovirus), DNA plasmids, and antigen-pulsed dendritic cells. Despite many patients being treated with these vaccines, the response rate for metastatic melanoma patients remains low.[339] However, using immunomonitoring assays, it is clear that a number of these approaches have demonstrated that it is possible to increase the level of circulating T-cells that recognize the tumor antigens following immunization.[340,341]

As with infectious diseases, it is likely that vaccine therapy will be more useful in preventing recurrences as opposed to treating diffusely metastatic disease. Multiple studies have now shown that the tumor microenvironment can be immunosuppressive. In addition, as with vaccines for infectious diseases, multiple immunizations are required to optimally activate antigen-specific immune cells. Therefore, treating earlier disease with vaccines will likely be more effective than treating metastatic disease, although the randomized studies required to demonstrate benefit will be more challenging to perform.

Another approach to immunizing patients is to take whole tumor cells and modify them or add an immune stimulant to enhance their ability to activate immune cells. For example, one approach has been to gene modify melanoma cells to express GM-CSF in order to attract dendritic cells capable of activating T-cells. Using an alternative whole cell vaccine approach, Morton et al. immunized patients in the adjuvant setting with either BCG, a bacterial extract that stimulates immune cells alone or in combination with allogeneic melanoma cells ("Canvaxin"). Over 1600 patients with completely resected Stage III or Stage IV melanoma were randomized to receive either BCG + allogeneic tumor vaccine or BCG + placebo. No differences were observed between the immunized (BCG + Canvaxin) and control groups (BCG alone).[342] Other vaccine approaches include pulsing tumor antigens onto dendritic cells[343] and the intratumoral administration of immune modulators. In addition, combination with cytokines such as IL-2 or IFN-alpha, or other immune modulators such as anti-CTLA-4 (see below) may enhance vaccine efficacy. Continued research efforts are necessary in order to bring vaccine therapy into common practice.

Radiation Therapy for Locoregional Disease

Although surgery remains the primary treatment modality for patients with localized or regionally metastatic melanoma, available data indicate a need for improved locoregional control in patients with high-risk features or when complete surgical resection may be compromised or impossible.[344,345] Adjuvant radiation therapy has been classically recommended to most patients with desmoplastic melanoma, particularly when neurotrophic. At least two recent studies call into question this previously routine practice.[115,346] Nonetheless, based on available—albeit limited—data, it is reasonable to consider adjuvant radiotherapy to surgery in patients with highest risk for local recurrence—and includes those with primary head and neck melanoma, narrow surgical margins, and neurotropism.[275,328,347] Radiotherapy has also been considered for patients with lentigo maligna melanoma (LMM) when complete excision is not practical,[345] as well as for select patients with mucosal melanoma.[344] Factors associated with a high risk of subsequent regional basin recurrence after lymph node dissection include lymph node size of at least 3 cm, 4 or more positive lymph nodes, the presence of extracapsular extension, and recurrent disease after initial surgical resection. The role of radiation therapy for all patients with nodal disease in the adjuvant setting is somewhat controversial.[344,348] Historically, most reports are small, retrospective comparisons of patients treated at a variety of sites, with varying doses and doses per fraction, usually after surgical resections of varying degrees of completeness.[344,345] Nonetheless, retrospective and phase 2 prospective studies have shown that adjuvant radiation therapy may significantly improve the locoregional control rate in these clinical settings.[344] Although the only randomized, controlled study showed no difference in local control between conventional and hypofractionated schedules, many centers currently employ a hypofractionated regimen that is generally well-tolerated and relatively convenient for patients. The impact of adjuvant radiation therapy on the incidence of distant metastasis and overall survival is less clear. Challenges to accrual in previous randomized trials must also be recognized. While significant improvements in overall patient outcome will require improvements in systemic disease control, the importance of locoregional control in reducing morbidity should not be underestimated. In general, patients with multiple involved or large, matted regional nodes or with extracapsular extension of regional lymphatic metastases should be considered for adjuvant radiation therapy.[344,345,349] Due to increased risk of complications following adjuvant radiation therapy to the groin following lymphadenectomy, some experts recommend radiotherapy in such patients if at least two of these factors are present[350] (see also the section on Radiotherapy).

Management of Distant Metastases

At autopsy, the lung, liver, brain, and lymph nodes are the most common sites of metastasis. However, essentially any visceral site may be involved. Symptoms associated with distant melanoma metastasis vary with the site of involvement. Although some patients have no symptoms, others experience seizures associated with intracranial metastases, gastrointestinal bleeding and/or intusception from small bowel metastases, and/or pain from soft tissue, visceral, and/or bony masses. Because of this variable presentation, the onset of new and persistent symptoms in individuals previously diagnosed with melanoma should be evaluated by standard radiologic studies, including computed tomography (CT) of chest and abdomen/pelvis and magnetic resonance imaging of the brain. Contrast studies of the small bowel in patients with unexplained anemia or with evidence of blood loss from the gastrointestinal tract may reveal evidence of small-bowel metastases. More recently PET/CT has been employed as a complement to conventional imaging.[264] Although evidence-based support is limited,[351] many clinicians routinely screen patients at high risk for melanoma recurrence with imaging studies under the assumption that early detection of recurrence may maximize treatment options and possibly a chance for cure. Further studies are clearly warranted in this regard.

Treatment of Distant Metastatic Melanoma

Although distant metastasis is not yet curable in the majority of patients with melanoma, the clinical course of patients with distant metastatic melanoma may vary widely. Disease progression may be extremely rapid, or existing metastases may remain stable for prolonged periods. For these reasons, careful clinical judgment is required for optimal therapy. Modalities available for the treatment of distant metastasis include surgical resection, systemic chemotherapy, radiation therapy, immunotherapy with vaccines and biologic response modifiers, and other investigational treatment options. The goal of systemic therapy for metastatic melanoma is long-term survival. Unlike many other solid tumors, a subset of patients with advanced melanoma may have dramatic responses to systemic therapy resulting in long-term disease-free remission. Treatments that are associated with these responses include agents that stimulate the immune response, such as IL-2 and anti-CTLA-4. However, because long-term survival is only observed in a minority of patients with metastatic melanoma, treatment of patients on clinical trials is also an important option in order to work towards improving long-term outcome.

Chemotherapy ■ Dacarbazine (DTIC) is the standard, FDA-approved chemotherapy for the treatment of metastatic melanoma. However, response rates are under 10% in most series, and durable responses are not commonly seen.[352] Temozolomide, a derivative of dacarbazine, has also been extensively studied in melanoma patients. Although randomized trials have not identified a difference in survival between dacarbazine and temozolomide,[353] the latter has the advantage of oral administration. Other potential advantages of temozolomide include the fact that it does not require metabolism by the liver to the active form and increased CNS penetration. However, no randomized studies have been performed demonstrating superior efficacy of temozolomide in the treatment of melanoma brain metastases. Combination chemotherapy regimens such as cisplatin, vinblastine, and dacarbazine (CVD) or carboplatin and taxol have demonstrated higher response rates in some series, but no survival advantages have been demonstrated for combination chemotherapy compared to single agent dacarbazine (Table 105-10).[354-356] With the limited success of combination chemotherapy, current efforts are focused on immunotherapy and targeted therapy either alone or in combination with chemotherapy.

High-Dose Interleukin-2 ■ Melanoma is an immunogenic tumor, capable of being recognized and destroyed by immune cells including cytotoxic T-cells. As described above, antigens have been cloned from melanoma cells that are capable of being recognized by T-cells. In addition, dramatic responses can be seen in some patients treated with immune therapies, including cytokines, immunomodulating antibodies, and T-cells. Infusion of interleukin-2 (IL-2), a natural protein produced by T-cells, has a 10-20% response rate in patients with metastatic melanoma. CRs are seen in approximately half of the responding patients and these are highly durable with long-term disease-free intervals in over 50% of patients with CRs (Fig. 105-16).[357] Because of this potential for long-term survival, albeit in a minority of patients, IL-2 is considered a standard frontline therapy for metastatic melanoma. Current studies are aimed at identifying the host and tumor characteristics at the molecular level that will predict responses and in combining IL-2 with other agents to increase the number of long-term survivors.

High-dose IL-2 therapy has a significant number of toxicities, including hypotension, capillary leak syndrome resulting in pulmonary edema, and transient renal toxicity. Therefore, safe administration requires adequate prescreening of patients to insure adequate cardiac and pulmonary function as well as significant training and experience of the health care team. As with IFN, clinical response to IL-2 is associated with autoimmunity. The development of hypothyroidism or vitiligo, an autoimmune destruction of melanocytes following IL-2 therapy, has been correlated with clinical response.[358,359]

In patients with metastatic, nonvisceral disease, response rates from IL-2 are particularly high, and have been reported to be as high as 50% for patients with cutaneous- or subcutaneous-only metastases.[315] Therefore, high-dose IL-2 may be considered as a first-line therapeutic option in some patients with in-transit or cutaneous-only metastases.

Rosenberg et al. reported a 42% response rate in patients treated with a combination of gp100 peptide vaccine and high-dose IL-2.[360] However, phase 2 studies by other groups failed to replicate this response rate.[361] Currently, a randomized multicenter study comparing high-dose IL-2 with vaccine and IL-2 only will help to shed light on whether the combination is beneficial (ASCO 2009).[362]

Table 105-10 ■ **Phase 3 Trials of Chemotherapy**

Author (Year)	Regimens	N	Response (CR + PR)	Median Survival (Months)
Luikart[354] (1984)	DTIC	32	14% (7 + 7)	4.3
	BVP	45	10% (0 + 10)	5.2
Resthoven[355] (1996)	CBD	100	21% (6 + 15)	6.9
	CBDT	104	30% (3 + 27)	7.6
Chapman[356] (1999)	DTIC	118	10% (0 + 10)	6.3
	CBDT	108	17% (0 + 17)	7.7

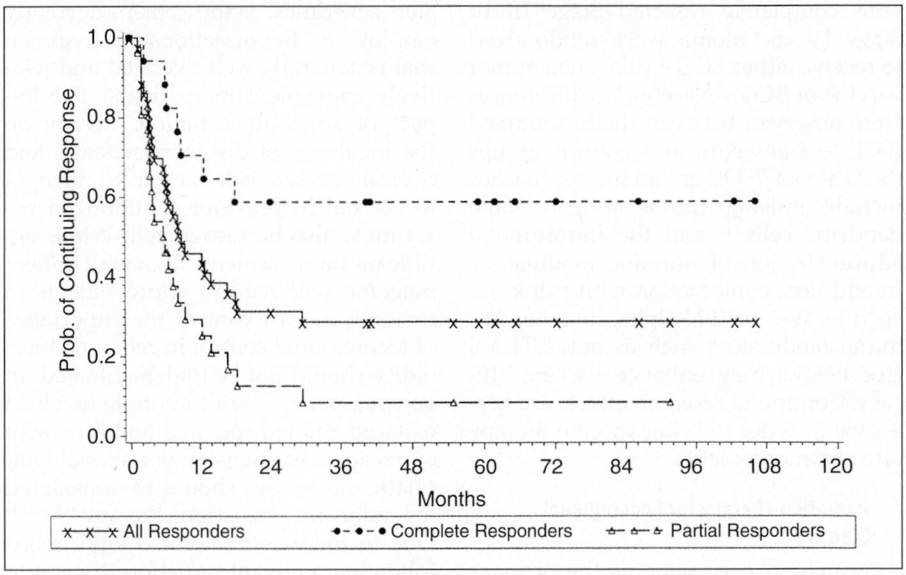

Figure 105-16 ■ Responses are durable following treatment with high-dose IL-2. Complete responses following high-dose IL-2 are most often durable in patients with metastatic melanoma. *Source*: From Ref. 357.

Biochemotherapy ■ Biochemotherapy, the combination of chemotherapy with cytokine therapy, has been extensively studied. Cisplatin, vinblastine, and dacarbazine in combination with interleukin-2 and IFN-alpha has been evaluated with a variety of schedules. Multiple randomized studies have been performed comparing combination chemotherapy with biochemotherapy (Table 105-11).[363-366] While the majority of studies have shown no differences in median survival between patients treated with biochemotherapy versus combination chemotherapy, long-term survival is seen in some patients treated with biochemotherapy. Bedikian et al. recently reported that 10-year survival of patients with metastatic melanoma treated with biochemotherapy was 12.5%.[367,368] For this reason, it is still reasonable to utilize biochemotherapy as a frontline regimen, especially in patients with rapidly progressive disease. In addition, response rates are consistently higher in patients treated with biochemotherapy compared with combination chemotherapy. Therefore, in some patients with aggressive locoregional disease that is borderline resectable, neoadjuvant therapy

Table 105-11 ■ **Phase 3 Trials of Biochemotherapy**

Author (Year)	Regimens	N	Response (CR + PR)	Median Survival (Months)
Rosenberg[363] (1999)	CDT/IL-2, IFN	50	44% (6+38)	10.7
	CDT	52	27% (8+19)	15.8
Eton[364] (2002)	CVD/IL-2, IFN	91	48% (6+42)	11.8
	CVD	92	25% (1+24)	9.5
Ridolfi[365] (2002)	CD/IL-2, IFN	87	25% (3+22)	11
	CD	89	20% (3+17)	9.5
Keilholz[421] (2003)	CD/IL-2, IFN	182	20.8%	9.0
	CD/INF	181	22.8%	9.0
Atkins[366] (2008)	CVD/IL-2, IFN	200	19.5%	9.0
	CVD	195	13.8%	8.7

with biochemotherapy may increase the likelihood that the disease could be rendered surgically resectable.

Although the majority of trials have been performed in patients with metastatic melanoma from a primary cutaneous lesion, response rates are likely similar for patients with mucosal melanoma primaries.[109,369,370]

Anti-CTLA-4 ■ The immune system has evolved a number of regulatory mechanisms to prevent autoimmune tissue damage. One of these is the CTLA-4 molecule, which is expressed on T-cells following activation (Fig. 105-17). CTLA-4 binds strongly to the co-stimulatory molecules CD80 and CD86 (B7-1 and B7-2) on antigen-presenting cells, thereby preventing the binding of these molecules to CD28, which is required for full T-cell activation. Thus, the CTLA-4 molecule acts as a "braking" mechanism to decrease function of activated T-cells. Antibodies blocking CTLA-4 thus release this braking mechanism, allowing increased activation of T-cells. Anti-CTLA-4 therapy has been evaluated in multiple trials in patients with advanced melanoma. Overall response rates are approximately 15% (Table 105-12).[371-373] Importantly, though, some patients receiving this agent have had long-term disease-free survival. Further follow-up will be required to determine how this compares to standard high-dose IL-2 in the ability to induce long-term survival in a subset of patients. In addition, because anti-CTLA-4 has an immune-mediated mechanism of action, delayed, durable clinical responses have been observed in some patients, highlighting a possible need for unique criteria to measure response rates using this class of agents.

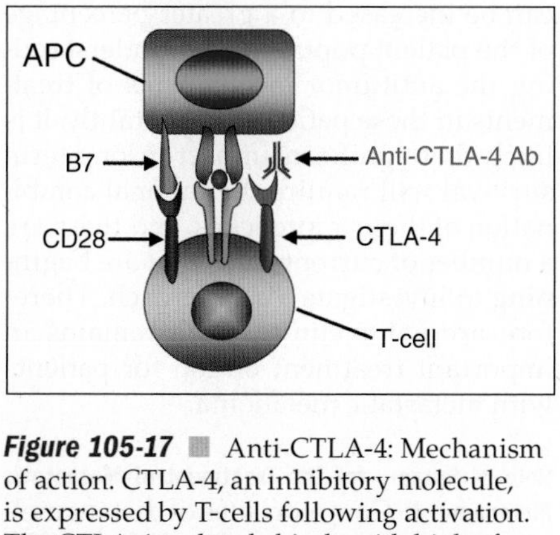

Figure 105-17 ■ Anti-CTLA-4: Mechanism of action. CTLA-4, an inhibitory molecule, is expressed by T-cells following activation. The CTLA-4 molecule binds with high affinity to the co-stimulatory molecules CD80 (B7-1) and CD86 (B7-2) on antigen-presenting cells, thereby preventing their ability to interact with CD28, a receptor on T-cells that requires ligation in order to maintain full T-cell activation. Blocking this CTLA-4 "braking" mechanism using an antibody allows full T-cell activation and the ability to mediate antitumor responses in some patients.

Table 105-12 ■ **Response to Anti-CTLA4**

N	CR	PR	Total Response	Treatment
56	2 (3.5%)	5 (9%)	7 (12.5%)	MDX-010 (3mg/kg, then 3 mg/kg or 1 mg/kg q 3 weeks) + gp100 vaccine; NCI
29	2 (7%)	2 (7%)	4 (14%)	CP-675,206 (0.01 to 15 mg/kg); UCLA, MDACC

Source: From Refs. 372–374.

Because anti-CTLA-4 strongly stimulates activated T-cells throughout the body, autoimmune adverse reactions are frequently seen, including hypophysitis (inflammation of the pituitary gland), rash, diarrhea, and hepatitis. Skin and colonic biopsies demonstrate immune infiltration, thereby suggesting the mechanism of toxicity is release of CTLA-4 regulation on the surface of immune effector cells. As with the general autoimmunity seen with IFN therapy and the vitiligo seen with IL-2 treatment, the development of autoimmunity appears to be linked to clinical response in patients receiving anti-CTLA-4 (Table 105-13).[374] The severity of autoimmune toxicities can range from mild to life-threatening. Severe diarrhea or hepatitis may require treatment with steroids. Diarrhea not responsive to steroids may require administration of anti-TNF agents.

While a small subset of patients benefits from this agent, there is significant potential to improve these results through the rational combination of anti-CTLA-4 with cytokines and vaccines, simulating the complex immune reaction that naturally occurs in the successful resolution of viral infections.[375] Indeed, murine models have demonstrated synergy between vaccines and anti-CTLA-4.[376,377] In addition, the use of anti-CTLA-4 in the adjuvant therapy of melanoma is currently being investigated.

Future work is also focused on the development of antibodies against other positive and negative co-stimulatory molecules of the immune system, such as 4-1BB and PD-1.[378] These approaches are bolstered by significant advances in basic immunology elucidating specific positive and negative receptors in the regulation of the immune response.

Adoptive T-Cell Therapy ■ The infusion of antigen-specific T-cells, often cultured and expanded in the laboratory, termed adoptive T-cell therapy (ACT), has been shown to be successful in treating a number of diseases including CMV infection post-transplant,[379] EBV-induced lymphoproliferative disease post-transplant,[368,380] EBV-induced nasopharyngeal cancer,[381] leukemias treated with donor lymphocyte infusions,[382] and melanoma.[383,384] The most successful T-cell therapies for metastatic melanoma have been reported following treatment with tumor-infiltrating lymphocytes (TIL). In a subset of melanoma metastases, tumor-specific T-cells can be isolated and expanded from the tumor itself, and reinfused into the patient (Fig. 105-18). Response rates have been higher with this approach if the infusion is performed following lymphodepleting chemotherapy, which may enhance the treatment effect by increasing homeostatic proliferation of antigen-specific T-cells (ie, making "space" in the lymphoid compartment prior to infusion) or through the elimination of regulatory T-cells. Response rates for patients receiving lymphodepleting chemotherapy followed by TIL infusion and high-dose IL-2 have been reported to be approximately 50%[383,384] and perhaps even higher if whole body radiation and stem cell transfer is included.[385] With addition of 2 Gy or 12 Gy of total body irradiation, response rates increased to 52% and 72%, respectively.

Table 105-13 ■ **Correlation of Autoimmunity with Response to Anti-CTLA-4**

Grade III/IV Autoimmune Toxicity	*N*	CR + PR
Yes	14	5 (36%)
No	42	2 (5%)

P = 0.008.
Source: From Ref. 374.

Further follow-up is required to determine the impact of adoptive T-cell therapy on long-term survival. Current studies are focused on improving methods to generate tumor-specific T-cells including the use of peripheral blood lymphocytes gene-modified with T-cell receptor genes.[386] In addition, combining alternative cytokines and immune modulating antibodies with T-cell therapy is an important area of study.

Targeted Agents ■ As noted earlier in this chapter, melanomas can now be separated into several distinct molecular subtypes; the signaling pathways that drive proliferation of melanoma cells are becoming more delineated (Fig. 105-19),[387] leading to the opportunities to personalize therapies. 50-70% of metastatic melanomas from cutaneous primaries, particularly those arising from cutaneous sites without chronic sun damage, have a mutated *BRAF* gene at position 600, with a glutamic acid substitution in place of valine.[388] While this mutation is also present in some normal nevi, inhibition of *BRAF* by siRNA in preclini-

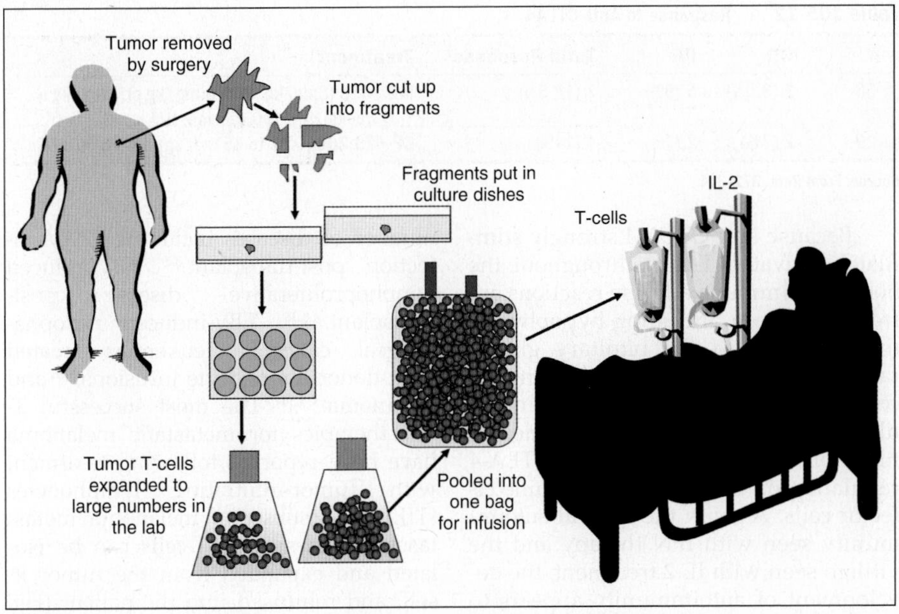

Figure 105-18 ■ Adoptive cell therapy (ACT) with antigen specific T-cells. Tumor-specific T-cells are present in the majority of melanoma deposits. Following tumor resection, these T-cells can be expanded and activated in the laboratory using interleukin-2 (IL-2). The T-cells can then be reinfused into the patient along with systemic IL-2.

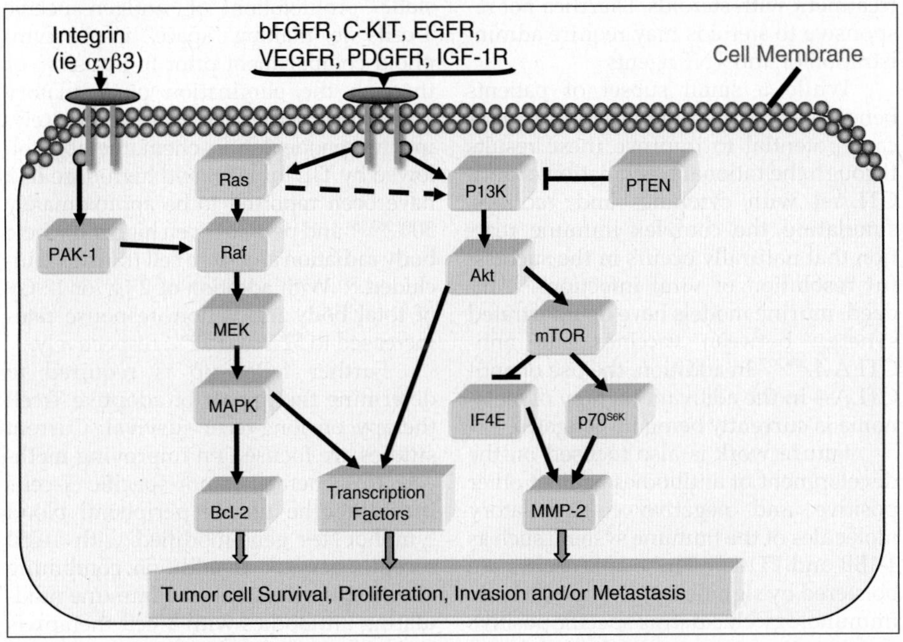

Figure 105-19 ■ Multiple molecular pathways drive melanoma proliferation and survival. A number of pathways, such as the RAF/MEK/MAPK and PI3K/AKT pathways, have been found to support melanoma proliferation and survival. Understanding these pathways will enable the development of targeted therapies for melanoma.

cal studies has resulted in decreased tumorgenicity.[389,390] These and other preclinical studies have led to the use of targeted therapies with specific inhibitors of *BRAF*, as well as other downstream targets in the MAPK and MEK pathways. Initial studies of combination chemotherapy with sorafenib, a weak *BRAF* inhibitor, have not shown any advantage over chemotherapy alone.[391] However, sorafenib is only a weak *BRAF* inhibitor, and newer studies with more specific agents are currently underway. Although *BRAF* mutations are found in over 50% of melanomas arising from cutaneous areas without chronic sun damage, they are rare in melanomas arising from other skin sites, such as acral lentiginous or chronic sun-damaged skin, or from mucosal surfaces.[32]

As noted above, 15-25% of melanomas which derive from acral lentiginous and mucosal primaries, as well as those from chronic sun-damaged skin, have mutations in *c-kit* (Fig. 105-20), mostly point mutations in exons 11 and 13 of the *c-kit* gene, opening the possibility for these tumors to be treated with *c-kit* inhibitors; indeed, case reports have shown that these tumors may be responsive to this approach.[111,392] While still representing a minority of melanomas, this represents one of the clearest examples of personalized targeted therapy for melanoma, and future progress will build on this as other targets and inhibitors are identified and validated.

Other potential important targets based on preclinical studies are in the PI3K/AKT pathway, and studies of mTOR inhibitors, a downstream mediator in this pathway are underway. AKT activation can antagonize the intrinsic apoptotic pathway, leading to increased tumor cell survival.[388] Besides strategies to target the AKT pathway, agents designed to enhance tumor apoptosis and manipulate apoptosis are also currently being studied, such as the use of a *BCL2* antisense oligonucleotide in combination with dacarbazine.[352] Clearly, future progress will rely on adequately inhibiting multiple pathways and personalizing approaches to maximize tumor damage over normal tissue toxicity.

Combination Therapy ■ Multiple approaches have been utilized for the treatment of melanoma metastases. While there are exciting scientific leads for many of these strategies, such as the immunomodulation of positive and negative co-stimulatory molecules with antibodies and targeted therapy of specific pathways using small molecules, there has thus far been limited success with any one approach. The proof of concept that some patients with advanced disease can have long-term survival provides the hope that this can be increased to a greater percentage of the patient population by understanding the antitumor mechanisms of treatments in these patients. Importantly, it is likely that significant impact on long-term survival will require the rational combination of these approaches, and there are a number of current trials that are beginning to investigate this approach. Therefore, accrual to clinical trials remains an important treatment option for patients with metastatic melanoma.

Role of Surgery for the Treatment of Metastatic Melanoma ■ Common sites of distant melanoma metastasis in order of decreasing frequency are skin and subcutaneous tissues, lung, liver, and brain. Patients with systemic metastases have a poor prognosis; no treatment for metastatic melanoma has been proven to unequivocally prolong survival. Morbidity and mortality from melanoma usually results from widespread distant metastases.

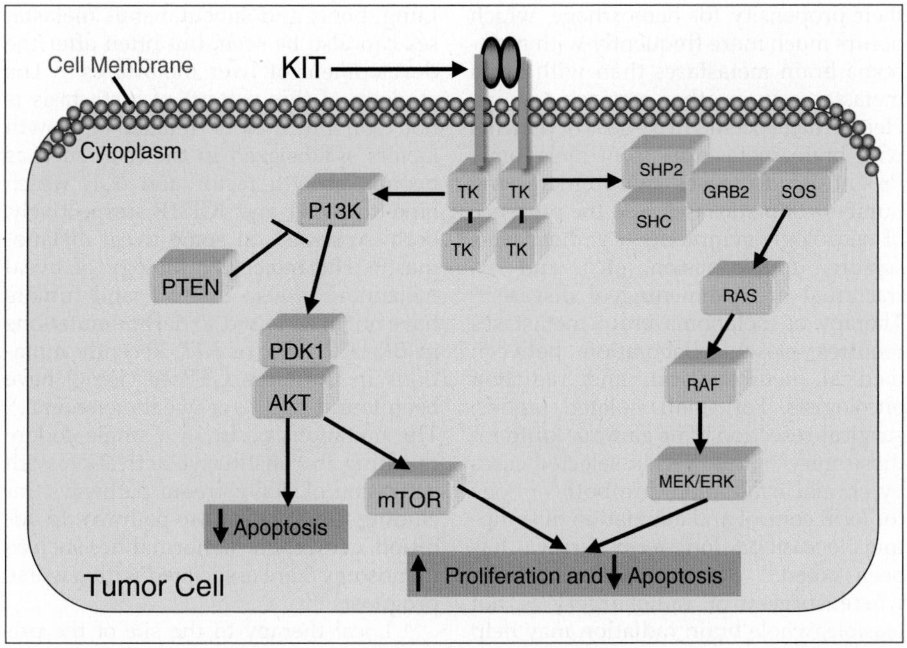

Figure 105-20 ■ The KIT receptor is mutated and activated in some melanomas. In 15-25% of mucosal and acrolentiginous primary lesions as well as melanomas from chronic-sun damaged skin (LMMs), the KIT receptor gene is mutated. This may enable targeted therapies for this population using KIT inhibitors.

In a subset of highly selected patients, resection of metastases can result in long-term disease-free survival[393,394]; if all lesions in the setting of solitary or oligo-distant metastatic disease are resectable with acceptable morbidity, surgery generally represents a reasonable therapeutic option that may even result in long-term survival. Comprehensive imaging studies represent an important component of the overall workup to accurately assess extent of disease, particularly when curative resection is entertained.[264] In this regard, patient selection is clearly of paramount importance, as patients with favorable biology are more likely to benefit from resection. Some hallmarks associated with favorable biology include long disease-free interval, longer tumor-doubling time, site(s) and extent of metastatic disease, stage of initial disease, and ability to achieve complete resection.[395,396] Moreover, some patients with multiple metastases in the same organ, such as the lung, may enjoy long-term survival. A study of 1,574 patients undergoing resection of distant metastases at JWCI revealed a 5-year survival rate of up to 29% for patients with solitary metastases.[397,398] Factors predictive of survival include site and number of metastases, prior stage of disease, and disease-free interval before diagnosis of Stage IV melanoma. In very highly selected individuals, surgical excision of sequentially developing metastases can also be beneficial.[399] Surgery may also offer effective palliative treatment for isolated, accessible, distant metastases. Examples of accessible lesions include isolated visceral metastases, isolated brain metastases, and isolated lung metastases.

Subcutaneous and Lymph Node Metastases ■ Metastatic deposits in subcutaneous sites and lymph nodes are frequent in patients with disseminated melanoma and may represent the only manifestation of disease. Surgical excision of these clinically involved sites can be associated with prolonged disease-free survival.[400]

Pulmonary Metastases ■ The lungs represent one of the most frequent sites of metastatic involvement by melanoma. Occasionally, patients present with a solitary pulmonary nodule as the only manifestation of recurrent melanoma. Thoracotomy in this setting can result in substantial (i.e, up to 35%) 5-year survival. Isolated pulmonary metastases reportedly account for approximately 5% of disseminated melanomas. Some experts consider for pulmonary resection those patients whose tumors have a doubling time greater than 60 days.[396,397,401] Although the best candidates for resection are patients with a solitary pulmonary lesion, no evidence of extrapulmonary intrathoracic metastases, and a tumor doubling time longer than 60 days, patients with multiple metastases and no extrapulmonary intrathoracic disease may still have a 5-year survival rate approaching that for solitary lesions and can therefore be reasonably considered for resection.[397,401]

Gastrointestinal Metastases ■ Gastrointestinal metastases from metastatic melanoma may produce highly symptomatic and immediately life-threatening clinical manifestations. Most commonly, gastrointestinal metastases present as the result of occult blood loss or as obstructing lesions at the lead point of an intussuscepting segment of small bowel. Indications for surgery are most frequently associated with acute bowel obstruction from intussuscepting small bowel or chronic gastrointestinal bleeding. Surgical exploration may reveal multiple sites of involvement. Operative intervention, whether for curative or palliative intent, can often be performed with acceptable morbidity and mortality. Five-year survival rates of 25-41% for patients undergoing curative resection of gastrointestinal tract metastases have been reported.[402,403]

Liver Metastases ■ 15-20% of patients with distant metastatic melanoma develop liver metastases. Historically, the median survival of patients with liver metastases has ranged from 2 to 7 months. Chemotherapy is generally of limited efficacy against hepatic metastases; despite this challenge, many investigators have suggested that resection of hepatic metastasis is not warranted because of the associated dismal prognosis. Other investigators have suggested that resection may be appropriate only in patients with an ocular primary tumor because their clinical course is better than that of patients with liver metastases from cutaneous primary tumors. In a recent series of 40 patients who underwent resection of liver metastases from melanoma, 75% of the patients developed a subsequent recurrence.[404] Patients with cutaneous melanoma were significantly more likely to have a subsequent recurrence outside the liver, suggesting that the disease is systemic at the time of hepatic resection. No patient with cutaneous melanoma metastatic to the liver was alive at 5 years.[404] To further illustrate the limited role of surgical resection on survival in patients with hepatic metastases, only 2% of patients with hepatic metastasis underwent resection among 1,750 patients with hepatic metastasis in the combined JWCI—Sydney Melanoma Unit experience.[405] Taken together, while surgery for GI metastasis has been associated with long-term survival in some patients, long-term survival associated with resection of hepatic or adrenal metastasis is less clear.

Recurrent Distant Metastases ■ Unfortunately, many patients undergoing complete surgical resection of distant metastatic melanoma (Stage IV) develop recurrent disease. A recent study examined whether a second metastasectomy could prolong the survival of patients with recurrent Stage IV melanoma. In this study, the recurrent disease affected soft tissue, pulmonary, gastrointestinal, cerebral, skeletal, and gynecologic sites. Median survival following treatment for recurrent

Stage IV melanoma was 18.2 months after complete metastasectomy, compared to 12.5 months after a palliative surgical procedure and 5.9 months after nonsurgical management. The 5-year survival rate was 20% for patients in the complete metastasectomy group, compared to 7% for those in the palliative surgery group and 2% for those in the nonsurgical group. By multivariate analysis, the two most important prognostic factors for survival following diagnosis of recurrent Stage IV melanoma were a prolonged disease-free interval before recurrence and complete surgical removal of the recurrent disease. These findings indicate that in very *highly selected* patients, repeat metastasectomy can prolong the survival of patients with recurrent Stage IV melanoma and should be considered if all clinically evident tumors can be resected.

Multidisciplinary Approaches involving Surgery Studies are currently evaluating the role that neoadjuvant systemic therapy strategies play in rendering borderline resectable disease amenable to surgery. This approach also facilitates the acquisition of tissue for molecular analysis to determine the effectiveness of targeted therapies on specific pathways. Long-term disease-free intervals have also been seen following surgical resection after partial responses from systemic therapy, such as high-dose IL-2. In these cases, the systemic therapy may have successfully treated distant micrometastases, allowing successful long-term results following resection of remaining disease.[406,407] Surgery also plays an important role in the acquisition of tumor for the expansion of antigen-specific T-cells (TIL) that can be used for systemic therapy.

Radiation Therapy for Metastatic Disease Multiple or recurrent skin or subcutaneous lesions not amenable to surgical resection may be approached with hypofractionated radiation therapy.[344,345] In select patients, radiotherapy can often provide long-term local control and effective palliation. Potential sites include symptomatic bony metastases, bleeding and fungation from cutaneous sites not amenable to other approaches, neurological compromise and spinal cord compression from vertebral metastasis, bleeding from mucosal head and neck sites, and pain and/or bleeding from other soft tissue and visceral sites.[344,345]

Special Considerations

Brain Metastases

Melanoma is one of the most likely solid tumors to metastasize to the brain, and once it does, is one of the most aggressive. An unusual feature of brain metastases is their propensity for hemorrhage, which occurs much more frequently with melanoma brain metastases than with brain metastases from other primary tumors. Hemorrhage occurs in 33-50% of patients with brain metastases from melanoma. Prognosis decreases with increasing numbers of metastases, and the presence of neurologic symptoms (e.g., headache, seizure, double vision, etc.), and extracranial or leptomeningeal disease.[408] Therapy of melanoma brain metastases requires close collaboration between medical, neurosurgical, and radiation oncologists. For small isolated lesions, surgical resection[409] or gamma knife radiosurgery[410] (followed in selected cases by cranial irradiation) are both options for local control and alleviation of symptoms; occasional long-term survival has been noted.[411] For multiple metastases where surgery or radiosurgery is not feasible, whole brain radiation may help to stabilize melanoma progression. The use of whole brain irradiation following resection remains somewhat controversial. While chemotherapeutic agents are often unsuccessful in mediating disease regression of brain metastases, agents such as temozolomide have been used as a radiosensitizer given in combination with radiation therapy. However, a recent study evaluating the combination of temozolomide, thalidomide, and whole brain radiation in 39 chemo-naive patients with brain metastases found a response rate of only 7.6% for the CNS, but with no responses when considering all sites of disease.[412]

Current research is focused on understanding the unique microenvironment in the brain and the interactions between tumor cells and elements of the CNS stroma. This will allow specific therapeutic interventions for melanoma brain metastases. Understanding the specific tumor-stroma interactions present in other sites, as well as bone, liver, and lung, may also provide insights into therapy for melanoma metastases to these sites.[413]

Uveal Melanoma

Melanoma of the uveal tract, which includes the iris, ciliary body, and choroid, represents only 5% of melanoma diagnoses, but is the most common primary intraocular malignancy in adults. Uveal melanoma is quite distinct from melanoma arising from cutaneous or mucosal sites. While cutaneous melanomas commonly metastasize to multiple tissues throughout the body, choroidal melanomas frequently metastasize first to the liver through hematogenous spread. The liver is the exclusive site of systemic metastases in approximately 40% of patients with metastatic uveal melanoma.[414] Lung, bone, and subcutaneous metastases can also be seen, but often after the development of liver metastases.[415] The etiology of this pattern of metastasis is not clear but may be related to growth factors synthesized in the liver such as hepatic growth factor and IGF, which bind to c-met and IGF-1R, respectively, both expressed on some uveal melanomas.[416] The molecular biology of uveal melanoma is also distinct, and tumors have not been found to harbor mutations in *BRAF*, *NRAS*, or *KIT*. Recently mutations in the large GTPase *GNAQ* have been found in 50% of uveal melanoma.[33] The mutations occur in a single codon, resulting in constitutive activation with activation of downstream pathways, including the MAP-kinase pathway. In addition, cytogenetic abnormalities such as monosomy 3 are associated with a worse prognosis.[387]

Local therapy to the site of the primary includes radiation, either by the application of a radioactive plaque or by proton therapy to avoid damage to the optic nerve. Enucleation is also an option for advanced primaries. In a randomized study comparing 125I plaque brachytherapy with enucleation, 85% of patients receiving radiation retained their eye for 5 years or more, and 37% had visual acuity over 20/200 in the irradiated eye 5 years after therapy. No survival differences were seen between the groups.[417,418]

While 99% of cases present localized to the eye, many patients will develop distant metastases, with 30% mortality at 5 years and 45% at 15 years.[414] Currently no adjuvant therapies have been found to be effective and systemic therapeutic options for metastatic disease are limited. Because the majority of patients presenting with metastases have disease isolated to the liver, local treatment approaches to the liver, such as intrahepatic chemoembolization or hepatic perfusion, may be considered. Surgical resection of hepatic metastasis has not, in general, been associated with favorable long-term results.[404] High-dose IL-2 and single agent DTIC or temozolomide have not been found to be effective in patients with metastatic choroidal melanoma. A regimen of bleomycin, Oncovin, lomustine, and DTIC (BOLD) plus IFN has been evaluated in a number of studies with an average response rate of 14%.[414] The discovery of GNAQ mutations may offer new opportunities for targeted therapeutic interventions for this aggressive type of melanoma.

Melanoma Biomarkers

The absence of a dependable biomarker to gauge prognosis and response to therapy has limited the speed with which clinical trials of new agents can be evaluated, especially for adjuvant therapeutic trials. While LDH levels have been associated with poor prognosis in patients with metastatic melanoma and have therefore been incorporated into the staging system as described above, its nonspecific nature does not allow LDH levels to be followed as a biomarker during therapy. A number of studies have evaluated various potential biomarkers including methods to detect tumor DNA released into the serum and PCR of circulating mononuclear cells for the expression of tumor antigens such as MART-1 and gp100. Work has also been performed evaluating serum S100B levels in melanoma patients. In one study evaluating Stage IIB and III melanoma patients, S100B levels were found to correlate with relapse and death, regardless of the cutoff value.[419] Lower S100B values at baseline and over 1 year of follow-up were associated with longer survival, and the worst survival was seen in patients with low levels at baseline that increased to high levels during the follow-up period. Mocellin et al. recently performed a meta-analysis evaluating 22 studies enrolling 3393 Stage I-IV cutaneous melanoma patients to evaluate the relationship between S100B level and survival.[420] Serum S100B levels were associated with poorer survival with a hazard ratio of 2.23 ($p < 0.0001$). While S100B and LDH may add to prognostic information, biomarkers that can be followed to assess response to therapy are still needed. Reliable biomarkers for melanoma may greatly enhance the ability to adequately select patients for specific therapies, manage patients on therapy, and efficiently evaluate new agents.

Summary and Future Directions

As its incidence continues to increase, melanoma represents a growing public health problem. While numerous epidemiologic studies have identified risk factors—including environmental, genetic, and host—that determine melanoma risk, a better understanding of the nature and complexity of these interacting factors will hopefully prove useful in improving primary prevention and screening strategies. Recently, insights into the genetic alterations in melanoma have provided the unique opportunity to refine our approach to classifying melanoma by defining subsets based on biology that has the potential to evolve into better diagnostic, prognostic, and therapeutic approaches to this challenging and devastating disease.

Based on a comprehensive 2008 AJCC collaborative melanoma database analysis, changes in melanoma staging have been recommended for the seventh edition of the *AJCC Cancer Staging Manual* to be published in 2009 and officially implemented in early 2010. While this large analysis largely validated the existing staging system, among the most notable lessons learned include the importance of mitotic rate in primary melanoma and the heterogeneity of Stage III disease, including the significance of tumor burden even at the microscopic level.

Approximately 85% of patients diagnosed with melanoma have clinically localized disease at presentation and in general have a favorable prognosis; nonetheless, it is probable that multiple known and as yet unknown prognostic factors lead to heterogeneity in clinical course and outcome for patients with early stage melanoma. Over the past three decades, the approach to patients with clinically negative regional lymph node basins has undergone considerable evolution. During this time, the technique of lymphatic mapping and SLN biopsy was introduced and subsequently emerged as the standard of care to identify patients with microscopic lymph node involvement using a minimally invasive approach that clearly has obvious advantages over a treatment algorithm that includes routine ELND. Overall, this technique has been shown to reliably identify those patients who are most likely to benefit from completion lymph node dissection while sparing patients with negative nodes the morbidity of an additional surgical procedure; its prognostic power and success is dependent on excellent communication and coordination among the surgeon, nuclear medicine physician, radiologist, and pathologist.

The advent of the SLN biopsy technique has helped to usher in a new era of molecular pathologic analysis of SLNs. Rather than traditional routine histologic examination, SLNs are subjected to more extensive pathologic examination with serial sectioning, immunohistochemical staining, and, in clinical trials, evolving molecular-based strategies. Going forward, developing and maturing technologies may make possible a genomic approach to melanoma classification, potentially allowing the identification of genetic markers or expression profiles that might be important for diagnosis, determination of prognosis, and even therapy. Other frontiers in the treatment of early-stage melanoma include defining the role of SLN biopsy in patients with T1 primary tumors and determining which patients benefit the most and the least from a completion lymph node dissection following identification of a positive SLN. These represent only a few of the many questions that remain unanswered in this complex disease.

For patients with advanced regional and distant metastatic disease, significant challenges exist in effecting a cure in the majority of patients. Insights into the biology of melanoma—from both cancer biology (i.e., signaling pathway) and immunologic standpoints—combined with a rapidly expanding appreciation that melanoma represents not a single, homogeneous entity, but rather multiple distinct subtypes, have together ushered in a new era of potentially promising personalized targeted and immunologic therapies. While significant progress has been made, there is still much to be learned in our quest for effective treatments and ultimately a cure.

Selected References

The complete reference list can be found at www.CANCERMEDICINE8.com

1. Jemal A, Siegel R, Ward E, et al. Cancer statistics, 2009. *CA Cancer J Clin.* 2009;58:225-249.
10. Cokkinides V, Weinstock M, Lazovich D, et al. Indoor tanning use among adolescents in the US, 1998 to 2004. *Cancer.* 2009;115:190–198.
31. Curtin JA, Busam K, Pinkel D, et al. Somatic activation of KIT in distinct subtypes of melanoma. *J Clin Oncol.* 2006;24:4340–4346.
32. Curtin JA, Fridlyand J, Kageshita T, et al. Distinct sets of genetic alterations in melanoma. *N Engl J Med.* 2005;353:2135–2147.
33. Van Raamsdonk CD, Bezrookove V, Green G, et al. Frequent somatic mutations of GNAQ in uveal melanoma and blue naevi. *Nature.* 2009;457:599–602.
38. Balch CM, Buzaid AC, Soong SJ, et al. Final version of the american joint committee on cancer staging system for cutaneous melanoma. *J Clin Oncol.* 2001;19:3635–3648.
41. Balch CM, Soong SJ, Gershenwald JE, et al. Prognostic factors analysis of 17,600 melanoma patients: validation of the American joint committee on cancer melanoma staging system. *J Clin Oncol.* 2001; 19:3622–3634.
42. Balch CM. Melanoma of the skin. In: Edge SB, Byrd DR, Compton CC, et al., eds. *AJCC Cancer Staging Manual*, 7th ed. New York: Springer Verlag; 2009.
57. Azzola MF, Shaw HM, Thompson JF, et al. Tumor mitotic rate is a more powerful prognostic indicator than ulceration in patients with primary cutaneous melanoma: an analysis of 3661 patients from a single center. *Cancer.* 2003;97:1488–1498.
66. Gimotty PA, Elder DE, Fraker DL, et al. Identification of high-risk patients among those diagnosed with thin cutaneous melanomas. *J Clin Oncol.* 2007;25:1129–1134.
76. Gershenwald JE, Colome MI, Lee JE, et al. Patterns of recurrence following a negative sentinel lymph node biopsy in 243 patients with stage I or II melanoma. *J Clin Oncol.* 1998;16:2253–2260.
85. Gershenwald JE, Thompson W, Mansfield PF, et al. Multi-institutional melanoma lymphatic mapping experience: the prognostic value of sentinel lymph node status

in 612 stage I or II melanoma patients. *J Clin Oncol.* 1999;17:976–983.
97. Lee CC, Faries MB, Wanek LA, et al. Improved survival after lymphadenectomy for nodal metastasis from an unknown primary melanoma. *J Clin Oncol.* 2008;26:535–541.
104. Bedrosian I, Gershenwald JE. Surgical clinical trials in melanoma. *Surg Clin North Am.* 2003;83:385–403.
111. Quintas-Cardama A, Lazar AJ, Woodman SE, et al. Complete response of stage IV anal mucosal melanoma expressing KIT Val560Asp to the multikinase inhibitor sorafenib. *Nat Clin Pract Oncol.* 2008;5:737–740.
113. Scolyer RA, Thompson JF. Desmoplastic melanoma: a heterogeneous entity in which subclassification as "pure" or "mixed" may have important prognostic significance. *Ann Surg Oncol.* 2005;12:197–199.
115. Pawlik TM, Ross MI, Prieto VG, et al. Assessment of the role of sentinel lymph node biopsy for primary cutaneous desmoplastic melanoma. *Cancer.* 2006;106:900–906.
131. Cascinelli N, Morabito A, Santinami M, et al. Immediate or delayed dissection of regional nodes in patients. *Lancet.* 1998;351:793–796.
135. Morton DL, Wen DR, Wong JH, et al. Technical details of intraoperative lymphatic mapping for early stage melanoma. *Arch Surg.* 1992;127:392–399.
147. Prieto VG, Clark S. Processing of sentinel lymph nodes for detection of metastatic melanoma. *Ann Diagn Pathol.* 2002;6:257–264.
148. Scolyer RA, Thompson JF, McCarthy SW. Sentinel lymph nodes in malignant melanoma: extended histopathologic evaluation improves diagnostic precision. *Cancer.* 2004;101:2141–2142; author reply 2142–2143.
150. Gershenwald J, Thompson W, Mansfield P, et al. Multi-institutional melanoma lymphatic mapping experience: the prognostic value of sentinel lymph node status in 612 stage I or II melanoma patients. *J Clin Oncol.* 1999;17:976–983.
172. Scolyer RA, Li LX, McCarthy SW, et al. Micromorphometric features of positive sentinel lymph nodes predict involvement of nonsentinel nodes in patients with melanoma. *Am J Clin Pathol.* 2004;122:532–539.
185. Gershenwald JE, Andtbacka RH, Prieto VG, et al. Microscopic tumor burden in sentinel lymph nodes predicts synchronous nonsentinel lymph node involvement in patients with melanoma. *J Clin Oncol.* 2008.
198. Balch CM, Morton DL, Gershenwald JE, et al. Sentinel node biopsy and standard of care for melanoma. *J Am Acad Dermatol.* 2009;60:872–875.
215. Sondak VK, Taylor JM, Sabel MS, et al. Mitotic rate and younger age are predictors of sentinel lymph node positivity: lessons learned forom the generation of a probabalistic model. *Ann Surg Oncol.* 2004;11:247–258.
243. Kammula U, Ghossein R, Bhattacharya S, et al. Serial follow-up and the prognostic significance of reverse transcriptase-polymerase chain reaction-staged sentinel lymph nodes from melanoma patients. *J Clin Oncol.* 2004;22:3989–3996.
244. Scoggins CR, Ross MI, Reintgen DS, et al. Prospective multi-institutional study of reverse transcriptase polymerase chain reaction for molecular staging of melanoma. *J Clin Oncol.* 2006;24:2849–2857.
251. Andtbacka RH, Gershenwald JE. The role of sentinel lymph node biopsy in patients with thin melanoma. *JNCCN.* 2009;7:308–317.
264. Choi EA, Gershenwald JE. Imaging studies in patients with melanoma. *Surg Oncol Clin N Am.* 2007;16:403–430.
265. Aloia TA, Gershenwald JE, Andtbacka RH, et al. Utility of computed tomography and magnetic resonance imaging staging before completion lymphadenectomy in patients with sentinel lymph node-positive melanoma. *J Clin Oncol.* 2006;24:2858–2865.
266. Gold JS, Jaques DP, Busam KJ, et al. Yield and predictors of radiologic studies for identifying distant metastases in melanoma patients with a positive sentinel lymph node biopsy. *Ann Surg Oncol.* 2007;14:2133–2140.
267. Gannon CJ, Rousseau DL Jr, Ross MI, et al. Accuracy of lymphatic mapping and sentinel lymph node biopsy after previous wide local excision in patients with primary melanoma. *Cancer.* 2006;107:2647–2652.
294. Pawlik TM, Ross MI, Thompson JF, et al. The risk of in-transit melanoma metastasis depends on tumor biology and not the surgical approach to regional lymph nodes. *J Clin Oncol.* 2005;23:4588–4590.
303. Uren RF, Howman-Giles R, Thompson JF. Patterns of lymphatic drainage from the skin in patients with melanoma. *J Nucl Med.* 2003;44:570–582.
315. Chang E, Rosenberg SA. Patients with melanoma metastases at cutaneous and subcutaneous sites are highly susceptible to interleukin-2-based therapy. *J Immunother.* 2001;24:88–90.
318. Cornett WR, McCall LM, Petersen RP, et al. Randomized multicenter trial of hyperthermic isolated limb perfusion with melphalan alone compared with melphalan plus tumor necrosis factor: American College of Surgeons Oncology Group Trial Z0020. *J Clin Oncol.* 2006;24:4196–4201.
319. Kroon HM, Moncrieff M, Kam PC, et al. Outcomes following isolated limb infusion for melanoma. A 14-year experience. *Ann Surg Oncol.* 2008;15:3003–3013.
324. Kirkwood JM, Manola J, Ibrahim J, et al. A pooled analysis of eastern cooperative oncology group and intergroup trials of adjuvant high-dose interferon for melanoma. *Clin Cancer Res.* 2004;10:1670–1677.
329. Gogas H, Ioannovich J, Dafni U, et al. Prognostic significance of autoimmunity during treatment of melanoma with interferon. *N Engl J Med.* 2006;354:709–718.
339. Rosenberg SA, Yang JC, Restifo NP. Cancer immunotherapy: moving beyond current vaccines. *Nat Med.* 2004;10:909–915.
352. Bedikian AY, Millward M, Pehamberger H, et al. Bcl-2 antisense (oblimersen sodium) plus dacarbazine in patients with advanced melanoma: the Oblimersen Melanoma Study Group. *J Clin Oncol.* 2006;24:4738–4745.
357. Atkins MB, Lotze MT, Dutcher JP, et al. High-dose recombinant interleukin 2 therapy for patients with metastatic melanoma: analysis of 270 patients treated between 1985 and 1993. *J Clin Oncol.* 1999;17:2105–2116.
367. Bedikian AY, Johnson MM, Warneke CL, et al. Prognostic factors that determine the long-term survival of patients with unresectable metastatic melanoma. *Cancer Invest.* 2008;26:624–633.
371. Weber J. Overcoming immunologic tolerance to melanoma: targeting CTLA-4 with ipilimumab (MDX-010). *Oncologist.* 2008;13(Suppl 4):16–25.
372. Phan GQ, Yang JC, Sherry RM, et al. Cancer regression and autoimmunity induced by cytotoxic T lymphocyte-associated antigen 4 blockade in patients with metastatic melanoma. *Proc Natl Acad Sci USA.* 2003;100:8372–8377.
373. Ribas A, Camacho LH, Lopez-Berestein G, et al. Antitumor activity in melanoma and anti-self responses in a phase I trial with the anti-cytotoxic T lymphocyte-associated antigen 4 monoclonal antibody CP-675,206. *J Clin Oncol.* 2005;23:8968–8977.
383. Dudley ME, Wunderlich JR, Robbins PF, et al. Cancer regression and autoimmunity in patients after clonal repopulation with antitumor lymphocytes. *Science.* 2002;298:850–854.
384. Dudley ME, Wunderlich JR, Yang JC, et al. Adoptive cell transfer therapy following non-myeloablative but lymphodepleting chemotherapy for the treatment of patients with refractory metastatic melanoma. *J Clin Oncol.* 2005;23:2346–2357.
388. Fecher LA, Cummings SD, Keefe MJ, et al. Toward a molecular classification of melanoma. *J Clin Oncol.* 2007;25:1606–1620.
392. Jiang X, Zhou J, Yuen NK, et al. Imatinib targeting of KIT-mutant oncoprotein in melanoma. *Clin Cancer Res.* 2008;14:7726–7732.

106 Other Skin Cancers

Victor A. Neel, MD, PhD ■ Arthur J. Sober, MD

The skin is a heterogeneous organ, consisting of elements of ectodermal, endodermal, and mesodermal origin. Such a diverse group of tissues gives rise to a wide variety of benign and malignant tumors. Many of these tumors are rare and will not be discussed in this chapter. Table 106-1 lists the more common premalignant and malignant tumors, which we discuss in detail. These are tumors relevant to the oncologist because they have the capacity to metastasize and cause serious medical harm. We also touch on several tumor syndromes that may present with unusual benign skin tumors that, if recognized, should prompt the clinician to conduct a detailed search for an internal malignancy. Melanoma, Kaposi sarcoma, the malignant histiocytoses, and the cutaneous lymphomas are discussed elsewhere in this book.

The incidence of nonmelanoma skin cancer (NMSC), which includes squamous cell carcinoma (SCC) and basal cell carcinoma (BCC), is increasing (Table 106-2). In 1983, approximately 480,000 persons were diagnosed with NMSC in the United States.[1] In 2008, over 1 million cases were reported.[2] The ratio of BCC to SCC among whites in the United States, Australia, and the United Kingdom is about 4:1.[1,3,4] Together, these two tumors account for approximately 90% of all skin cancers. In recent years, the role of the sun in the causation of these common skin tumors has received much attention.[5]

Ultraviolet Radiation in the Pathogenesis of Skin Cancers

In the past several decades, research on the relationship between the sun and skin cancer has escalated principally because of fear of the consequences of increased ultraviolet B (UVB) radiation on the earth's surface as a result of ozone depletion in the stratosphere. There is now general consensus over the role of sunlight in the etiology of NMSC.[6,7] Chuang and colleagues[8] reported a 45-fold increase in NMSC skin cancer in the Japanese population in Kauai, Hawaii, as compared with the Japanese population in Japan. Another study showed the incidence of SCC, but not BCC, in Maryland watermen (a group of white men who make a living fishing in the Chesapeake Bay), correlated directly with the amount of sun exposure.[9] A population-based study on nearly 12,000 patients also demonstrated the close correlation between chronic cumulative sun exposure and SCC.[10] Geographically, the incidence of skin cancer in whites increases toward the equator, further supporting the role of sunlight in carcinogenesis.

UVB imprints a unique signature on the DNA it damages. Cellular attempts to repair this damage can lead to CC>TT mutations or C→T transitions. In the precursors of SCC (known as actinic keratoses), Zeigler and colleagues[11] showed that inactivating mutations of the tumor-suppressor p53 harbor these UV-induced errors. Because p53 is involved in the transcriptional regulation of DNA repair genes, cell-cycle control genes, and the induction of cell death, damage to this important regulator by UV irradiation is one mechanism that allows for the overgrowth of damaged cells.

UVB and UVA (320-400 nm) also have direct and indirect effects on the cutaneous immune system, lowering cell-mediated immunity and inducing T-suppressor cell production.[12] Loss of local immunity is thought to be another factor influencing carcinogenesis.

Table 106-1 ■ **Common Premalignant and Malignant Neoplasms of the Skin**

	Premalignant	Malignant
Epidermis	Keratoacanthoma Actinic keratosis Arsenical keratosis HPV-induced premalignant papules (epidermodysplasia verruciformis, bowenoid papulosis) Mucosal leukoplakia	Basal cell carcinoma Merkel cell carcinoma Squamous cell carcinoma
Dermal		Dermatofibrosarcoma protuberans Malignant fibrous histiocytoma Angiosarcoma
Appendageal	Nevus sebaceous	Sebaceous carcinoma Extramammary Paget disease
Benign cutaneous tumors associated with cancer syndromes Trichilemmomas → Cowden disease (breast/visceral tumors) Sebaceous tumors → Muir-Torre syndrome (GI/GU tumors) Mucosal neuromas → MEN type IIB (thyroid carcinoma/pheochromocytoma)		

Abbreviations: GI, gastrointestinal; GU, genitourinary; HPV, human papillomavirus; MEN, multiple endocrine neoplasia.

Table 106-2 ■ **Nonmelanoma Skin Cancer Statistics (U.S. 2008)**

	Basal and SCC	Merkel Cell Carcinoma
Magnitude of the problem (yearly)	>1,000,000 new patients	1000-1500 new patients
Severity of the problem (yearly)	1-2% deaths from SCC Disfigurement Disability	300-500 deaths Incidence increasing

Tumors Arising From the Epidermis

Actinic Keratosis

Definition ■ Actinic keratosis, also known as solar keratosis, is a very common lesion occurring in susceptible persons as a result of prolonged and repeated solar exposures. The action of ultraviolet radiation results in damage to the keratinocytes and produces single or multiple, discrete, dry, rough, adherent scaly lesions. These premalignant lesions may, in time, progress to SCCs.

Epidemiology ■ Actinic keratosis affects predominantly the sun-exposed areas of fair-skinned people. The incidence in elderly whites may approach 100% in some populations.[1] The appearance of actinic keratosis may be at a much younger age (under 30 years) if the susceptible individuals have an outdoor occupation, such as farmers, ranchers, and sailors, or have an outdoor lifestyle in sports or recreation. The lesions are more common in transplant recipients[13] and albinos.[14] It is rare in darker-skinned individuals, and almost never affects blacks, East Indians, or other Asians.

Clinical Features ■ The onset of actinic keratosis is insidious as a rule and therefore often passes unnoticed for some time. The characteristic lesion is rough and gritty to palpation, similar to the feel of coarse sandpaper. On close examination, they appear as round-to-oval lesions, often less than 1.0 cm in diameter. They may be flat to nodular, as in the hypertrophic variety of actinic keratosis (Fig. 106-1). The lesions are usually skin-colored or yellow brown, often with a reddish tinge. There may be single or multiple scattered discrete lesions, typically limited to sun-exposed areas. A pigmented variant of actinic keratosis, named spreading pigmented actinic keratosis, is a brown, slowly growing, slightly scaly lesion that tends to appear on the face and may be larger than 1.5 cm in diameter, making it difficult to distinguish from lentigo maligna.

Diagnosis ■ The diagnosis of flat actinic keratosis is usually based on clinical examination alone. In contrast, the hypertrophic variant may sometimes be confused with an early SCC. Suchniak and colleagues[15] demonstrated histologically the presence of in situ or invasive SCCs in 50% of lesions diagnosed clinically as hypertrophic actinic keratoses.

Treatment ■ The flat actinic keratosis lesions are most easily treated with cryotherapy.[16] Brief applications of liquid nitrogen with either a cotton tipped swab or a spray gun will suffice in the majority of cases. Retreatment may be necessary for the more stubborn lesions. It is not necessary to freeze to the point of blistering. Curettage and electrodesiccation of the lesions are equally effective, but carry a slightly greater risk of scarring and dyspigmentation. The hypertrophic lesions are best evaluated by biopsy to rule out invasive SCC.

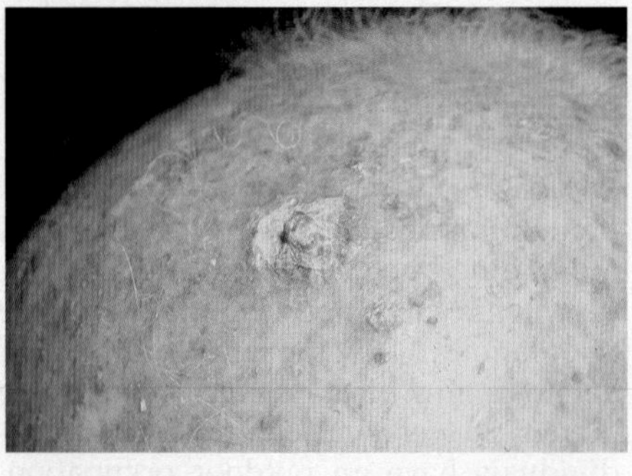

Figure 106-1 ■ Actinic keratosis. Multiple discrete lesions on the scalp. These lesions are "gritty" to palpation. The largest lesion in the center of the picture represents the hypertrophic variant. This must be differentiated from a squamous cell carcinoma in situ.

Where large areas of skin are involved, applications of 5-fluorouracil preparations twice a day to the affected areas may be used for up to 4 weeks. This will result in a brisk reaction in the treated areas, ranging from redness, soreness, and weeping, to shallow ulceration and crusting (Fig. 106-2). The reaction will gradually subside after discontinuation of the cytotoxic cream. Newer formulations containing 0.5% 5-fluorouracil used once daily for 4 weeks may cause less irritation to the skin.[17]

Three additional topical approaches are available. In widest use is 5% imiquimod cream twice weekly for 16 weeks to nonhypertrophic, actinic keratoses of the face/scalp in immunocompetent individuals. Side effects include redness, itch, and/or burning at the local site. Local site hypopigmentation has been observed. Mechanism of action is unknown, but immune modulation likely has a role. Topical 3% diclofenac or sodium gel has been reported to be efficacious for actinic keratoses.[18] The product is used twice daily for 60-90 days. Irritation of the skin can result from treatment. The frequency of complete response seems lower than with the 5-fluorouracil or imiquimod. The third approach, termed photodynamic therapy, employs the use of a topically applied photosensitizer, aminolevulinic acid, which is preferentially absorbed by the premalignant cells. Photoactivation upon exposure to blue light results in clearance of the actinic keratoses. Stinging of the affective skin occurs during light exposure. A sunburn-like reaction follows therapy. Very good results have been observed in patients with extensive actinic keratoses of the face and scalp.

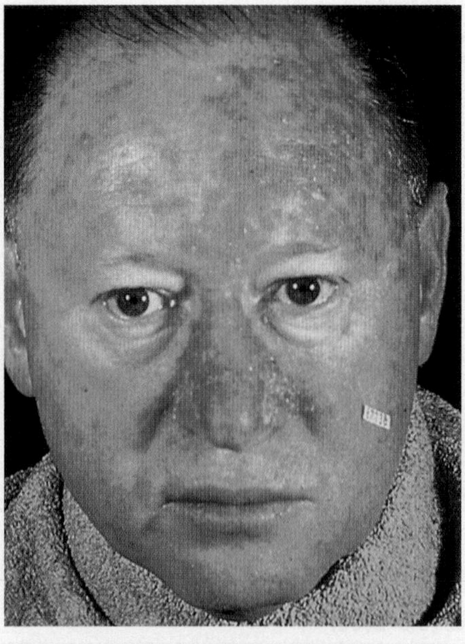

Figure 106-2 ■ Actinic keratosis. Extensive actinic keratosis on the face. Note that the right half has been used as control and the left half of the forehead and the nose were treated with 5% 5-fluorouracil cream for 14 days.

Course and Prognosis ■ The lesions of actinic keratosis may disappear spontaneously, but, in general, they persist if not treated. There is modest lifetime risk (<10%) of an individual actinic keratosis transforming into SCC. Marks and colleagues[19] reported that 60% of SCCs arise from preexisting solar keratoses.

Keratoacanthoma

Definition ■ Keratoacanthoma is a common, rapidly growing but benign tumor that may involute spontaneously, even if untreated. It is believed to originate from the hair follicles.

Epidemiology ■ Few studies have been done on the incidence of keratoacanthoma.[20] Chuang and colleagues[21] reported an incidence rate of 103.6 per 100,000, based on the small population in Kauai, Hawaii. It is most common between the ages of 60 and 65 years and is rare in persons younger than the age of 20 years. In contrast to SCC and BCC, there is no increase in frequency in old age. It is uncommon in blacks or Japanese, and is approximately two to three times more common in males. The majority of patients have a solitary lesion.

Sun exposure and exposure to chemical carcinogens such as tar are thought to be etiologic factors. The possibility of a viral etiology is still being debated. The presence of HPV has been demonstrated by DNA hybridization and polymerase chain reaction (PCR) studies.[22] The possibility of a genetic defect has also been proposed because these tumors are more common in patients with the Muir–Torre syndrome than in the general population.

Clinical Features ■ Keratoacanthomas characteristically arise on hairy skin. The most common areas are the central parts of the face: the cheeks, nose, ears, lips, eyelids, and forehead. The dorsa of the hands, wrists, and forearms are also common sites. The trunk and scalp are uncommon sites. Typically, the lesion presents as a solitary, rapidly growing, firm, dome-shaped, flesh-colored to slightly pink lesion with a plug of keratin in the central crater (Fig. 106-3). The evolving lesion typically grows rapidly for 2-4 weeks to a size of up to 2 cm in diameter. The mature lesion involutes spontaneously after a few months, leaving a scar. The complete cycle of growth to spontaneous resolution takes approximately 4-6 months.[23] Multiple or recurrent lesions may occur, particularly in cases associated with tar exposure. Multiple lesions associated with defects in cell-mediated

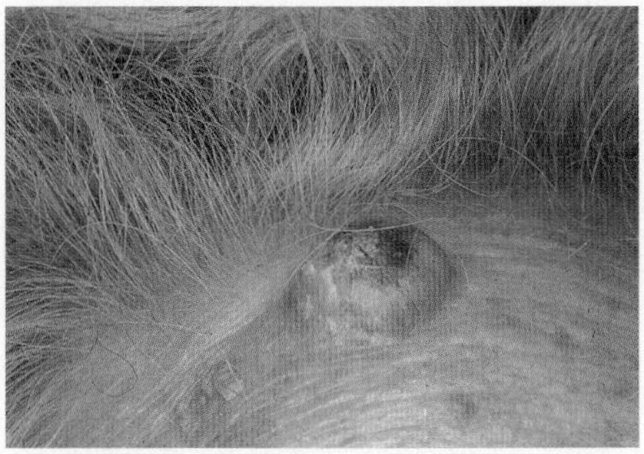

Figure 106-3 ■ Keratoacanthoma. A pink, dome-shaped lesion with a central core of keratin. This rapidly growing lesion is located on the mid-forehead. *Source:* Courtesy of P.L. McCarthy, MD.

immunity and with multiple internal malignant neoplasms and sebaceous adenomas, as part of Muir–Torre syndrome, have been noted. There is no evidence that the solitary type is associated with internal malignancy.

Diagnosis ■ The main differential diagnosis is to distinguish keratoacanthoma from SCC. The rapid evolution and spontaneous involution, the characteristic dome shape with a central plug of keratin, and the relatively young age of the patient are all clues to the diagnosis. In most cases, a wedge biopsy is essential in order to exclude an invasive SCC.

Treatment ■ Keratoacanthomas may resolve spontaneously, leaving behind a scar. Surgical excision of the lesion will produce better cosmetic results as well as provide tissue for histopathologic diagnosis. Radiotherapy[24] has been used successfully in lesions that cannot be distinguished from SCCs, as well as the so-called giant aggressive keratoacanthomas.[25,26] The dosage used, 4000-6000 cGy, is the same as the tumoricidal dosage used for SCCs. A biopsy of the lesion to rule out a squamous cell carcinoma prior to treatment may be prudent.

Course and Prognosis ■ Keratoacanthoma is a benign tumor that carries a very good prognosis. Reports of malignant transformation as well as metastasizing lesions are probably misdiagnosed SCCs.

■ Squamous Cell Carcinoma

Definition ■ SCC is a malignant tumor arising from epidermal or appendageal keratinocytes or from squamous mucosal epithelium. There is often a history of damage by exogenous agents acting as carcinogens, such as sunlight, ionizing radiation, local irritants, or arsenic ingestion. The tumor cells have a tendency toward keratin formation. Bowen disease is an in situ SCC. Verrucous carcinoma is a variant of low grade SCC with a clinicopathologically distinct warty appearance. The Buschke–Loewenstein tumor is the subset of verrucous carcinoma found on the genitals.

Epidemiology ■ The incidence of SCC of the skin varies greatly for different parts of the world and for different races and different people with different life habits and occupations. In 1983, Scotto and colleagues[1] reported an incidence of 41.4 cases per 100,000, and the incidence of cutaneous SCC is increasing.[2]

As previously mentioned, mutations in the p53 tumor-suppressor gene have been found in a number of SCCs.[27] Phototherapy patients who had received UVB or psoralen plus ultraviolet A (PUVA) for the treatment of skin diseases, such as psoriasis or mycosis fungoides, are also at increased risk.[28,29] The incidence of SCC is known to be much higher in immunosuppressed patients, and these patients should be followed very carefully. Many dermatology departments now have dedicated clinics for immunosuppressed and transplant patients.[30] Depending on the dose of immunosuppressive drugs and previous sun exposure, transplant patients have up to a 65-fold increased risk of developing SCC.[31] The SCC to BCC ratio also reverses from 0.25 to 1 in the general population to 1.5-3 to 1 in transplant patients. Tumors in such patients tend to behave more aggressive clinically.[28,32]

Verrucous carcinoma of the skin (epithelioma cuniculatum) is a rare tumor, with more than 100 reported cases.[33] Approximately 80-90% of patients are male, with a mean age of 52-60 years. The Buschke–Loewenstein tumor is considered a verrucous carcinoma of the anogenital mucosa. Penile Buschke–Loewenstein tumor is the most common, with an incidence between 5% and 24% of all penile cancers. Vaginal, cervical, perianal, and perirectal Buschke–Loewenstein tumors are less common than penile ones. The etiology of these tumors is linked to HPV, particularly to HPV 6 and 11.8.[33]

The incidence of Bowen disease has not been extensively investigated. Chute and colleagues[34] reported an incidence of 14 per 100,000 population for Bowen disease in a Rochester, Minnesota, population. In a 5-year prospective study based on the residents of Kauai, Hawaii, Reizner and colleagues[35] reported an incidence of 142 per 100,000 population.

Progress has also been made in the identification of heritable risk factors in NMSC.[36] Polymorphisms of the melanocortin-1 receptor, which are linked to an increased risk of melanoma, segregate with patients at an elevated risk for both SCC and BCC.

Clinical Features ■ SCC often arises in damaged skin or skin that has been subjected to chronic irritation. Thus, the skin adjacent to the carcinoma may show evidence of solar damage, such as actinic keratosis, wrinkling and dryness, telangiectasia, and irregular pigmentation. Alternatively, there may be features of radiodermatitis from previous radiation therapy,[37] a sinus tract associated with an underlying osteomyelitis, or scarring from a burn (Marjolin ulcer).[38] Chronic venous ulcers of the lower extremities are also associated with increased risks of developing squamous cell carcinomas.[39] Chronic ulcer that shows features of proliferation beyond the expected granulation process should raise the suspicion of malignant transformation.

SCC usually evolves faster than BCC, but not as rapidly as keratoacanthoma. The earliest lesion, the so-called intraepidermal SCC or carcinoma in situ, typically appears as a scaly, erythematous plaque on sun-exposed areas. The lesion often has a sharply demarcated but irregular outline (Fig. 106-4). Bowen disease is clinically identical to SCC in situ. Bowen disease on the glans penis is also known as erythroplasia of Queyrat.

Invasive SCC (Fig. 106-5) almost always arises from a preexisting premalignant lesion or from an in situ carcinoma,

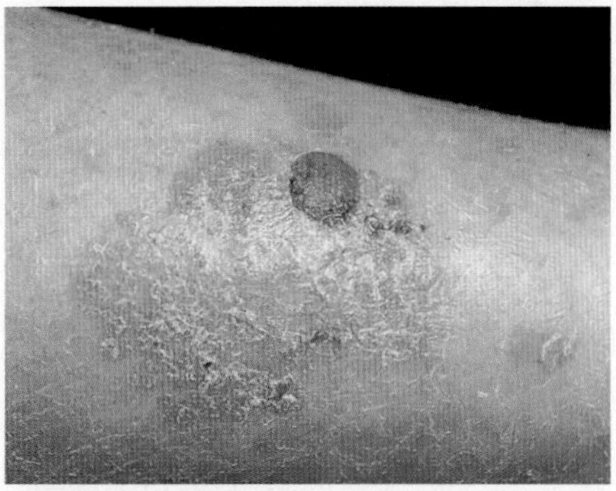

Figure 106-4 ■ Squamous cell carcinoma (SCC) arising in SCC in situ. A nodule of invasive SCC on the lower leg arising within the well-demarcated, erythematous scaly plaque of SCC in situ.

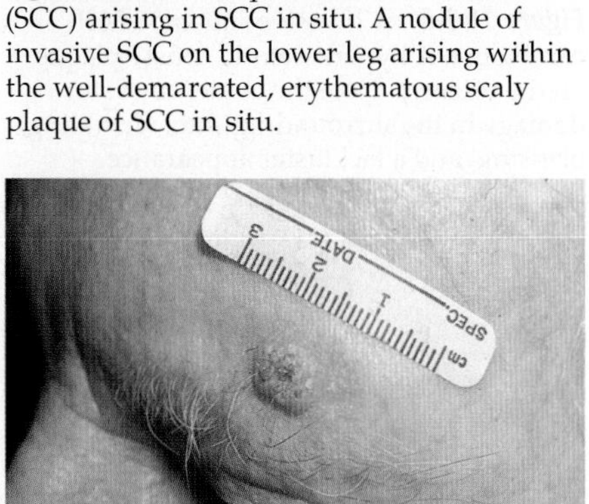

Figure 106-5 ■ Invasive squamous cell carcinoma. Erythematous, hyperkeratotic nodule on the forehead resembling a keratoacanthoma (see Fig. 106-3). An incisional or excisional biopsy is necessary to distinguish the two lesions.

although de novo squamous cell carcinoma has been reported.[40] The lesion is typically an erythematous, indurated papule, plaque, or nodule. The shape of the lesion may be polygonal, oval, round, or verrucous (Figs. 106-6 and 106-7). The tumor tends to increase both in elevation and diameter with time. A hallmark of SCC is its firmness on palpation. The late lesion is often eroded, crusted, and ulcerated with an indurated margin. The ulcer is often covered with a purulent exudate and bleeds easily (Fig. 106-7). Early ulceration is often a marker for anaplastic lesions. Regional lymphadenopathy may be present either as a response to infection of the ulcer or from metastases. In the latter case, they tend to be rubbery and more irregular, and may be fixed to adjacent tissues.

Verrucous carcinoma of the skin is most commonly found on the soles of men.[33] Typically, it presents as a slowly enlarging cauliflower-like mass. It is locally aggressive and may grow to a significant size. The ball of the foot is involved in more than 50% of cases. Other locations include the face, buttocks, oral cavity, trunk, and extremities. The bulk of the tumor is soft and "squashy," and may be foul smelling. If left untreated, the tumor will eventually penetrate the underlying soft tissue and bone. However, metastasis is rare.

The Buschke–Loewenstein tumor most commonly affects the penile glans and prepuce of uncircumcised males, presenting as a cauliflower-like, fungating, foul-smelling tumor on the coronal sulcus. In women, it may present on the vagina, cervix, or vulva. The Buschke–Loewenstein tumor has a tendency to infiltrate deeply, causing destruction of underlying tissues.

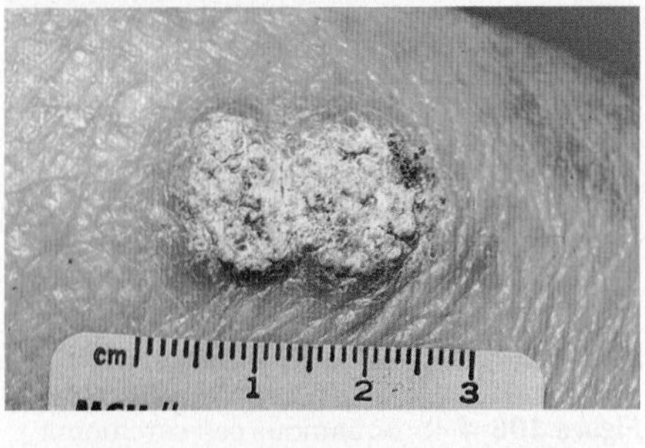

Figure 106-6 ■ Invasive squamous cell carcinoma. A hyperkeratotic, crusty plaque on the forearm. Note the evidence of sun damage in the surrounding skin: wrinkling, bruising, and a lackluster appearance.

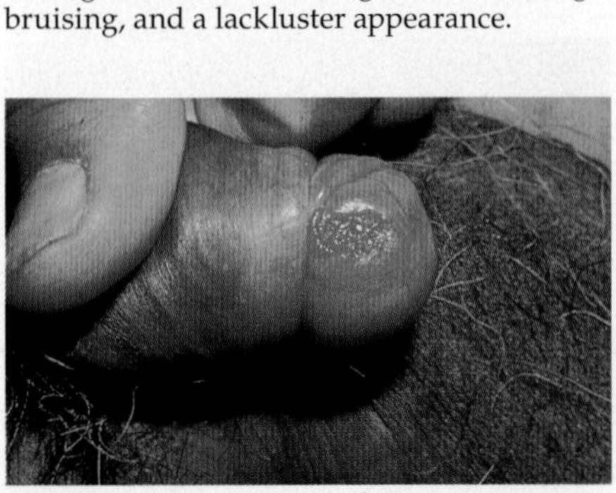

Figure 106-7 ■ Invasive squamous cell carcinoma. An ulcerated lesion on the glans penis with an indurated margin. The ulcer typically bleeds easily.

SCC of the lip may arise from an area of leukoplakia or actinic cheilitis. Approximately 90% of SCCs occur on the lower lip. This tumor is typically much more aggressive than those on glabrous skin and has a high rate of metastasis.

Carcinoma arising in late radiation dermatitis or x-ray keratoses tends to be very anaplastic and extremely aggressive. The rate of metastasis is high in such tumors.[41]

Treatment ■ The choice of treatment modality depends on the degree of differentiation of the tumor and the presence or absence of metastasis. The size, shape, location of the tumor, and the predisposing factors should also be considered. In the case of a localized, well-differentiated tumor with no evidence of metastasis, the goal should be complete eradication of the lesion. In the case of a poorly differentiated, recurrent tumor or the presence of lymph node metastases, palliative treatment may be considered, if complete eradication is deemed impossible. The variety of modalities available for consideration include excisional surgery, Mohs surgery, cryosurgery, electrosurgery, and radiation therapy.[24,42-44] The final result often depends as much on the experience of the surgeon as on the choice of treatment selected. Thus, cooperation among dermatologists, surgeons, and radiotherapists is important.

Excisional Surgery ■ Surgical excision with primary closure or repair with skin graft or flap is the treatment of choice for relatively small lesions with distinct borders. There should be an adequate margin of clearance of 3-5 mm to minimize the risk of recurrence. Brodland and Zitelli[45] reported that margins of 4 mm were required to achieve a 95% tumor clearance rate. For invasive or large tumors (>2 cm), or tumors on high-risk areas such as the scalp, ears, nose, eyelids, or lips, a minimum margin of 6 mm is recommended.

Tumors arising in late radiation dermatitis or x-ray keratosis should also be surgically excised rather than treated with more radiation. Likewise, tumors previously treated with radiation should be excised with the entire radiation scar, if possible, because tumor may exist in multiple foci within the irradiated field.

Large tumors situated near the lip, eyelid, and the anogenital area should be excised in order to preserve the function of the structures and avoid retraction caused by excessive scarring.

Surgery is also preferred for lesions invading bone or cartilage. Treating such lesions with radiation therapy may result in radiation necrosis of the bone or cartilage. Recurrent carcinomas, tumors with indistinct borders, and those arising in scars, ulcers, or sinuses may be treated with surgery to allow histologic examination of the excision margins. Tumors that have metastasized to regional lymph nodes are also best treated with excision surgery and lymph node dissection. Prophylactic lymph node dissection is not recommended because of the relatively low rate of metastasis. The utility of selective lymph node dissection for high-risk tumors is currently being evaluated.

Mohs Surgery ■ Surgery with microscopic control of the excision margins (Mohs micrographic surgery) has become the treatment of choice for extensively invasive and infiltrative tumors or those that are recurrent. This technique allows maximum conservation of "good tissue" while the surgeon can still be reassured of clear margins. This modality of treatment is also associated with a lower local recurrence rate.[45]

Cryosurgery ■ Treatment of SCC by freezing with liquid nitrogen is best restricted to the most superficial tumors and carcinoma in situ. This modality has the advantage of simplicity with an excellent cure rate when employed in the proper situation.[43,46] Because collagen, cartilage, and bone are less sensitive to injury by freezing than the tumor cells, scarring and damage to underlying bony or cartilaginous structures can be minimized.

Radiation Therapy ■ Radiation therapy is often employed for poorly differentiated tumors and for patients who may not be able to tolerate other more invasive treatment modalities. The site of the lesion has to be taken into consideration to minimize the late complications of ionizing radiation. Thus, lesions on the dorsum of the hand and those over bony and cartilaginous structures should not be treated with radiation. Tumors that have a tendency to invade along the planes of embryonic closure, such as those in the nasolabial fold and pre- and postauricular areas, are good candidates for this modality of treatment. Excellent results can also be obtained for small lesions of the nose, lip, eyelid, and canthus. A fractionated dose is usually preferred to a single massive dose for the best cure rate and to minimize the local as well as systemic side effects of radiation.[24] The treatment schedule is determined by the size, depth, and location of the tumor and the particular time-dose-fractionation schedule used. The total dose is typically between 4000 and 6000 cGy.

Chemotherapy ■ The use of oral isotretinoin in patients with large, recurrent or metastatic SCCs resulted in partial to complete regression of the tumors. Isotretinoin also decreased the incidence of a second primary SCC, when given as a chemopreventive agent. However, the benefit from such long-term use has to be weighed against the toxicity. In organ transplant recipients, where the risk of developing skin cancer is increased, the use of retinoids may be justified.[47]

Course and Prognosis ■ The risk factors correlated with local recurrence and metastatic rates include treatment modality, prior treatment, location, size, depth, histologic differentiation, histologic evidence of perineural involvement, precipitating factors other than ultraviolet light, and host immunosuppression. Squamous cell carcinoma in skin carries an overall metastatic rate of 3-6%.[48] Those arising from sun-damaged skin typically have a low risk for metastasis whereas those arising from chronic osteomyelitic sinus tracts, irradiated areas, and burn scars have a much higher metastatic rate (31%, 20%, and 18%, respectively). Carcinoma on the lower lip, although mostly sun induced, has a metastatic incidence of about 15%. Tumor arising in areas such as the glans penis (see Fig. 106-7), the vulva, and the oral mucosa also have a high rate of metastasis.

Histologically, the best prognostic indicators are level of dermal invasion and vertical tumor thickness.[48]

With proper treatment, the overall 5-year remission rate is 90%, including squamous cell carcinoma of the lip. Frankel and colleagues[49] recommended follow-ups at least every 3 months for a year after treatment of SCC, and semiannually thereafter for up to 4 years.

Basal Cell Carcinoma

Definition ■ BCC is a malignant tumor that rarely metastasizes. It is composed of cells that arise from the epidermis and the appendages which resemble the basal layer of the epidermis and is associated with a characteristic stroma. It tends to grow slowly and invade locally over many years, which eventually leads to ulceration, hence the name "rodent ulcer."

Epidemiology ■ BCCs account for more than 75% of nonmelanoma skin cancers diagnosed in the United States each year.[50,51] Incidence of BCC varies from 422 per 100,000 general population in Kauai, Hawaii,[52] to 146 per 100,000 in Rochester, Minnesota.[53] It is the most common form of skin cancer in whites,[1] and is rare in darkly pigmented people. It most frequently occurs in persons older than 40 years of age. The frequency is slightly higher in males. Other risk factors include geographic locations with high solar intensity, exposures to inorganic trivalent arsenic ionizing radiation, and immunosuppression. Photo-therapy patients receiving UVB or PUVA for treatment of certain dermatoses, such as psoriasis or mycosis fungoides, are also at increased risk.[28] Several recent studies suggest a correlation between BCCs and exposures to sunlight in early life and intense intermittent (recreational) sun exposures.[55,56] This is contrary to the previous belief that BCCs result from cumulative lifetime sunlight exposures. Genetic studies show that loss-of-function mutations in the tumor-suppressor gene patched, or gain-of-function mutations in the smoothened gene, lead to the formation of sporadic basal cell tumors.[57,58] Genetically inherited form is described in basal cell nevus syndrome.

Clinical Features ■ The BCC is characteristically slow growing over months to years. It is usually asymptomatic unless ulceration occurs, and then there is bleeding. It most frequently occurs on sun-exposed areas such as the face and upper trunk, and is rare on the palms and soles.

The early lesions are round-to-oval papules or nodules, often with an umbilicated center that may be ulcerated. The color is pink to red and often has a translucent or pearly quality (Fig. 106-8). BCCs are firm to palpation. If left untreated, the lesion enlarges slowly and is destructive to neighboring structures by direct invasion. Longstanding lesions are ulcerated as a rule (Fig. 106-9). There are often telangiectasias in the surrounding skin, which also shows other evidence of solar damage, such as actinic keratosis, atrophy, wrinkling, dryness, and irregular pigmentation. Some BCCs are pigmented and may exhibit a bluish hue.[59] These may be confused with malignant melanoma (Fig. 106-10). The so-called superficial-type BCC usually presents on the trunk as an irregular, atrophic plaque

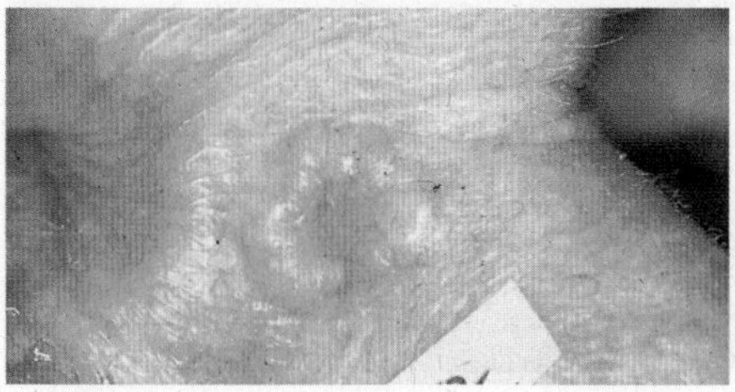

Figure 106-8 ■ Basal cell carcinoma. A pearly nodule with an umbilicated, ulcerated center and telangiectasia.

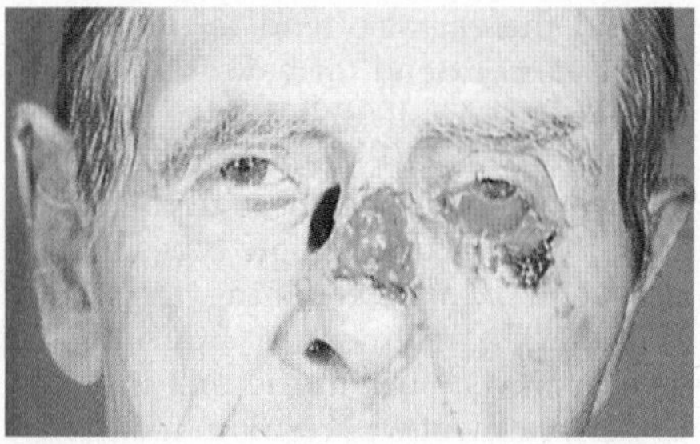

Figure 106-9 ■ Basal cell carcinoma. Note the erosive nature of such a long-standing lesion.

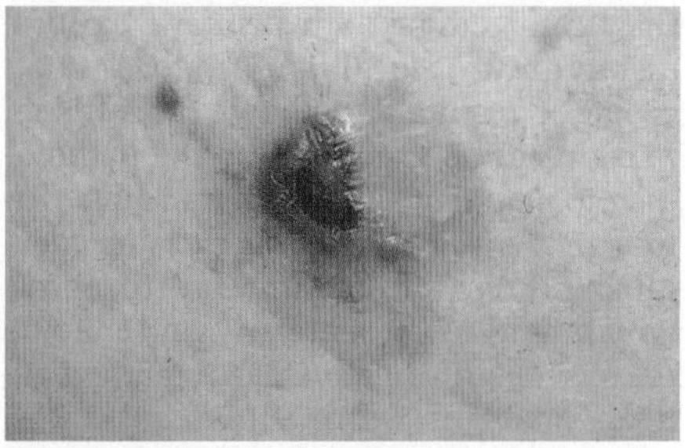

Figure 106-10 ■ Pigmented basal cell carcinoma. A pink, irregular plaque with dark-blue to black pigmentation at the center that mimics a superficial spreading melanoma. The shiny quality is one clue to the diagnosis.

with a slightly raised border (Fig. 106-11). Flat BCCs can be difficult to detect. They are often ivory-white, and may resemble morphea and are therefore called morphea-like BCCs. This type of lesion usually occurs on the face and has a more aggressive behavior.[60]

Treatment ■ The choice of therapy depends on the type and size of the lesion, the location, the general condition of the patient, the cosmetic considerations, and, not least, the experience and skill of the operator.[61] Morphea-like BCCs usually have indistinct borders clinically and may result in underestimation of the extent of the tumor and, consequently, in under-treatment. Lesions situated in the nasolabial crease, around the eye, and

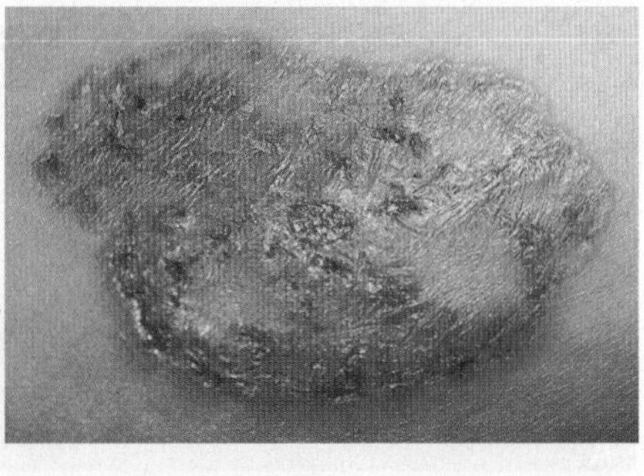

Figure 106-11 ■ Superficial basal cell carcinoma. A large, 5-cm lesion on the abdomen. The pearly, string-like border is the clue to the clinical diagnosis.

behind the ear also tend to undermine deeply and extend far beyond the clinical border (Fig. 106-12). Lesions that ulcerate early tend to be more aggressive. Knowledge of the behavior of the different clinical and pathologic types of BCC is essential in determining the choice of therapy. Treatment of BCCs should be aimed at a cure in the first instance. Undertreatment will result in recurrence and deep invasion, and there is a 50% recurrence rate for the cases that are treated inadequately.

Surgical Excision ■ Surgical excision of the tumor either with primary closure, a skin graft or local flap produces good cosmetic results and allows the surgical margins to be examined by the pathologist to confirm adequate margins. Tumor present at the lateral excision margins will result in marginal recurrences, which tend to present early and may be reexcised with relative ease. Inadequate deep margins result in recurrences, which tend to present late, together with invasion of deep structures. Surgery is the therapy of choice for lesions with indistinct clinical borders and for the morphea-like lesions.

Mohs Surgery ■ Surgery with microscopic control of the excision margins (Mohs micrographic surgery) is the treatment of choice for the morphea-like lesions and for all extensively invasive or recurrent tumors.[62] This technique allows maximum conservation of "good tissue," while the surgeon can still be reassured of clear margins (see Fig. 106-12).

Radiation Therapy ■ Treatment with ionizing radiation may produce excellent therapeutic and cosmetic results, provided care is taken in patient selection. Radiation therapy is preferred for elderly and fragile patients, particularly those with medium-sized lesions between 1 and 5 cm in diameter. Lesions larger than 5 cm have higher recurrence rates as compared with smaller tumors.[63] Atrophy, necrosis, and scarring may be kept to a minimum when the total dose, typically in the range of 4000-6000 cGy, is divided into several smaller fractions over several weeks. The choice of a treatment schedule is chosen according to the type, location, size, and depth of the tumor, the total dose of radiation, and the number of fractions that will be given. The appropriate dose schedule may be determined according to the time-dose-fractionation tables.

Chemotherapy ■ Topical applications of 5% 5-fluorouracil cream to the tumor twice a day for several weeks is best suited only for small, superficial tumors in the elderly patients who will not be able to tolerate other more aggressive forms of treatment. The rate of recurrence, however, is considerably higher. Intralesional 5-fluorouracil has also been tried in nodular lesions.[64,65] Five percent imiquimod cream five times per week for 6 weeks has been shown to be effective therapy for the majority of biopsy proven superficial BCCs in immunocompetent individuals. Lesions greater than 2.0 cm or lesions not located on trunk, neck, or extremities (other than hands and feet) are excluded in the FDA indications.

Course and Prognosis ■ Basal cell carcinomas are slow growing as a rule. However, if left untreated, they may reach a large size, with consequent extensive tissue destruction. In a comprehensive review of recurrence rates for primary BCCs, the results are highly comparable for the various treatment modalities.[62] Most studies reported a 95% or higher cure rate.[66,67] A lower 5-year recurrence rate has been reported with Mohs surgery than with other commonly used modalities. Metastasis, although rare, may occur, particularly in large and late lesions.[68] In such cases, the prognosis is usually poor, with a 1-year survival rate of less than 20%, and a 5-year survival rate of approximately 10%. The 5-year occurrence rate of new BCCs developing in patients with a previous BCC may be as high as 45%.[69] Patients with numerous BCCs, for instance in patients with the inherited syndrome basal cell nevus syndrome, may decrease the onset of tumor formation by taking low-dose isotretinoin.[70]

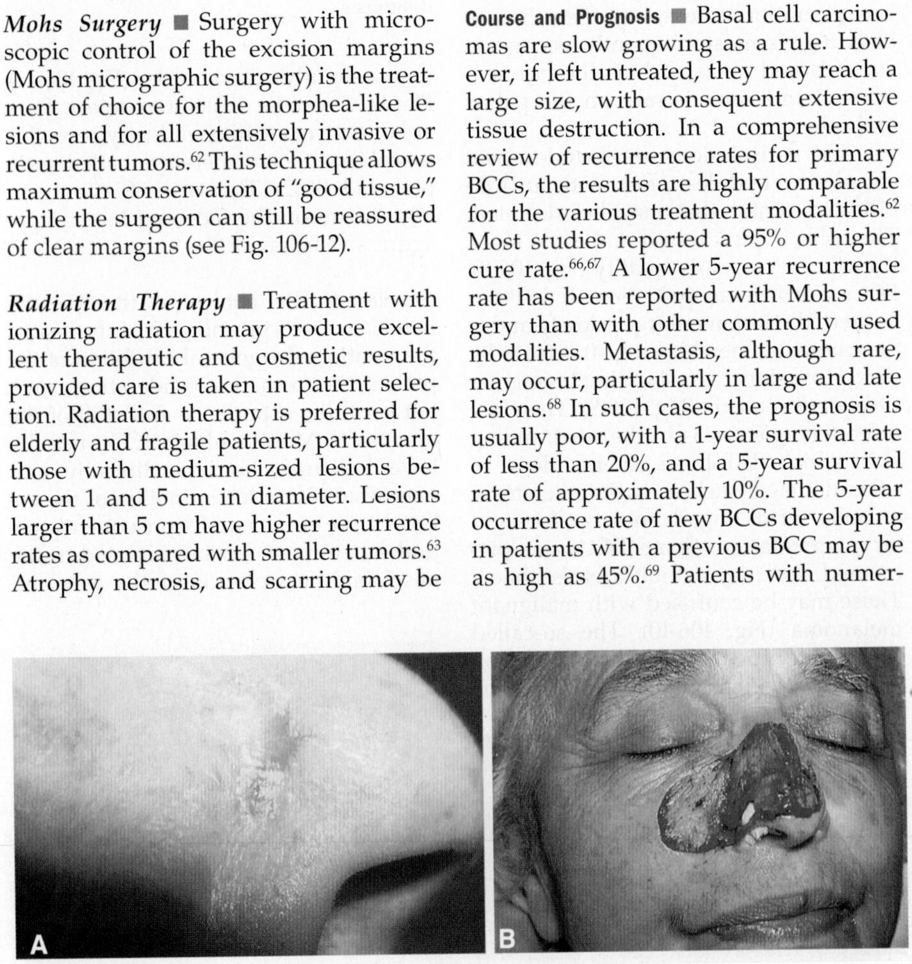

Figure 106-12A-B ■ **(A)** Basal cell carcinoma. The lesion is quite limited clinically. **(B)** Same patient after treatment with Mohs surgery, illustrating the cryptic extension far beyond the clinically evident border.

Merkel Cell Carcinoma

Definition ■ The Merkel cell was first described by Merkel in 1875. It is a nondendritic, nonkeratinocytic epithelial clear cell normally found in the epidermis and dermis of mammals and humans.

The Merkel cell tumor was first described by Toker in 1972. It is thought to arise from the cutaneous Merkel cell. It is a high-grade malignant tumor, with a high rate of local recurrence and metastasis. Mortality of 33% at 3 years exceeds that seen in cutaneous melanoma .

Epidemiology ■ Merkel cell carcinoma is a relatively uncommon neoplasm. Data from SEER show a 3-fold increase in evidence from 1996 to 2001 (0.15-0.44 per 100,000 annually).[71] In the past year it is estimated that 1000-1500 new cases will be diagnosed. The median age at diagnosis is 69 years. Ninety percent of patients with Merkel cell carcinoma are older than 50 years. There is a slight male predominance. Higher rates of Merkel cell carcinoma are seen in patients with HIV, CLL, or solid organ transplantation. A previously unknown polyoma virus was recently identified in 80% of MCC tumors.[72]

Clinical Features ■ The most common sites of involvement are head and neck (49%), extremities (38%), with the lower extremities more frequently involved than the upper extremities, and trunk (13%), mainly lower back and buttocks. The lesions present as papules or nodules, pink to red to violet, often with overlying telangiectasia. Typically, the tumors are less than 2 cm in size. Merkel cell carcinoma can be suspected based on the mnemonic AEIOU (asymptomatic/lack of tenderness, expanding rapidly, immune suppression, older than 50 years, ultraviolet exposed site on a person with fair skin).[71] Cytokeratin 20 immunostaining (perinuclear dot pattern) has greatly assisted the diagnosis of Merkel cell carcinoma.

Treatment ■ Wide local excision is the standard treatment modality.[73] Alternatively, local excision with margin control by frozen-section histology (Mohs surgery) may be of value.[74] Studies have shown that sentinel lymph node biopsy is predictive of nodal involvement.[75] Radiation may be beneficial for either local recurrences or for local control after node dissection.[76] Chemotherapy regimens have not been shown to extend life.

Course and Prognosis ■ Overall mortality by 3 years is approximately 33% for patients with Merkel cell carcinoma. Outcome is based on primary tumor size and stage of disease. Sentinel node biopsy is of value in identifying patients with disease in the nodes (stage III). The AJCC is considering a 4-stage classification for Merkel cell carcinoma (stage I—tumor < 2cm; stage II—Tumor >= 2cm; stage III—nodal involvement; stage IV—distant metastases). Immunosuppression patients have a higher mortality than immunocompetent patients.[77]

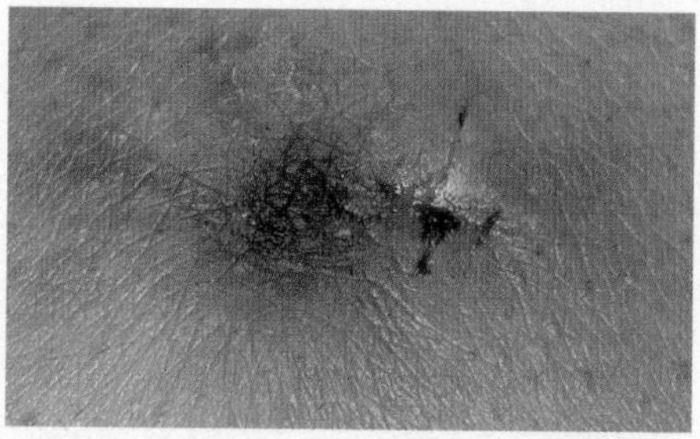

Figure 106-13 ■ Dermatofibrosarcoma protuberans on the back of the neck. Firm papule resembling a dermatofibroma. *Source:* Courtesy of R.A. Johnson, MD.

Tumors Arising From Dermis

Dermatofibrosarcoma Protuberans

Definition ■ Dermatofibrosarcoma protuberans (DFSP) is a locally malignant, slow-growing tumor originating in the dermis. The tumor cells resemble fibroblasts with various degrees of atypia.

Epidemiology ■ This is an uncommon tumor that typically presents during early to mid-adult life. It is reported rarely in children. Males are affected 4 times as often as females. It may be more common in blacks than in whites. Associations with arsenic exposure, burn or surgical scar, acanthosis nigricans, and rapid growth during pregnancy have been reported.

Clinical Features ■ DFSP is most commonly situated on the trunk and proximal extremities. It typically presents as a solitary, slow-growing nodule with multiple palpable surface irregularities.[78] The early lesion may resemble a dermatofibroma, keloid scar, or squamous cell carcinoma (see Fig. 106-13). The lesion is firm to palpation and varies from flesh color to reddish to yellow. The center may be ulcerated. The tumor can achieve an enormous size with multiple satellite nodules, if untreated. The characteristic irregular surface on a firm, plaque-like base may suggest the diagnosis. A biopsy will provide confirmation. The average size at the time of surgery is approximately 5 cm.

Recently, DFSPs were shown to harbor chromosomal translocations that fuse the collagen type I alpha gene with the gene for platelet-derived growth factor B.[79] The presence of this specific t(17;22) translocation permits the diagnosis of DFSP in equivocal cases.

Treatment ■ The treatment of choice is Mohs surgical excision with microscopic evaluation of the excision margins. DFSP has a high recurrence rate after conventional surgical excision, with a range of 30-50%.[80] Lateral surgical margins of at least 3 cm excised through the deep fascia are the current recommendation for conventional excision. In one large series, this yielded a recurrence rate of approximately 10%. Because of the potential for deforming surgical defects, Mohs surgery, which permits microscopic control of the excision margins, has been advocated. This allows the subclinical margins to be mapped at the time of surgery, and, consequently, the surgical margins more precisely determined. Prophylactic lymph node dissection is not recommended because of the low initial risk of metastasis. Recently, the receptor tyrosine kinase inhibitor imatinib has been used with success in treating multiply recurrent and metastatic cases of DFSP.[81]

Course and Prognosis ■ In a review of 136 cases of DFSP treated with Mohs surgery, a local recurrence rate of 6.6% was determined, although smaller studies have shown fewer recurrences.[82] It is clear that the experience of the Mohs surgeon is critical in preventing tumor recurrence. Historically, late recurrences are frequent, thus long-term follow-up is recommended.

Cutaneous Angiosarcoma

Definition ■ Angiosarcoma (AS) is an aggressive malignancy of endothelial cells, arising in the setting of chronic lymphedema, chronic radiation dermatitis or on the face and scalp of the elderly patients.

Epidemiology ■ Cutaneous AS of the face and scalp is a disease in elderly persons, with men affected more often than women. Sun does not appear to be an important factor because the tumor often appears under cover of hair.[83] AS developing in areas of chronic lymphedema (the so-called Stewart–Treves syndrome) is an infrequent complication of mastectomy, axillary node dissection for melanoma, lymphedema secondary to filarial infection and chronic idiopathic lymphedema. Unfortunately, up to 0.5% of women undergoing mastectomy and lymph node dissection develop AS within 1-30 years. Radiation-induced AS is a rare iatrogenic complication of radiation that develops in or near the irradiated site. The incubation period may be up to 40 years in some cases.

Clinical Features ■ In all three presentations, the clinical features can be similar. Bruise-like macules, papules, and nodules develop and tend to enlarge quickly. Ulceration can occur in advanced lesions. On the face, facial edema can be the presenting sign. In all cases, the lesions extend beyond the clinical borders.

Treatment ■ Treatment for AS is not promising. One problem facing clinicians is that by the time a diagnosis is made the tumors have spread several centimeters beyond the clinically appreciated borders. AS of the face and scalp is rarely less than 10 cm in diameter at presentation. Wide surgical resection followed by radiotherapy is the mainstay of treatment. In a study of 24 patients with AS of the face and scalp, local control was obtained in 57%. However, of those patients, 47% developed distant metastases.[84] In surgically unresectable tumors, radiation therapy and adjuvant chemotherapy with intralesional recombinant interleukin-2 and interferon-α-2b[85] or liposomal doxorubicin[86] may extend the life of some patients.

Course and Prognosis ■ Survival at 5 years is approximately 12%.[83]

Tumors Arising From Appendages

Sebaceous Carcinoma

Definition ■ Frequently arising on the eyelid, sebaceous carcinoma is a malignant adnexal neoplasm.

Epidemiology ■ Sebaceous carcinoma is the second most frequent malignancy of the eyelid next to BCC.

Clinical Features ■ Misdiagnosis is frequent with sebaceous carcinoma. The tumor usually appears as a painless, flesh-colored papule, or nodule on the upper or lower eyelid where it is easily dismissed as a chalazion or chronic blepharitis. Ulceration is often the feature that stimulates clinical suspicion and biopsy. Focal loss of eyelashes and a yellowish hue are other diagnostic clues. Sebaceous tumors are frequently associated with the Muir–Torre syndrome, as described later in this chapter.

Treatment ■ In a recent evidence-based review on the management of eyelid malignancies, Mohs micrographic surgery and excision with frozen-section control were shown to be superior to other modalities, including radiation therapy.[87]

Course and Prognosis ■ In a study of 18 patients with sebaceous carcinoma treated with the Mohs technique, Spencer and colleagues found an 11% recurrence rate after an average follow-up of 37 months.[88] One patient had metastatic disease (5.6%). This compared favorably to other published rates of recurrence and metastasis, which had been as high as 30% and 22%, respectively.

Extramammary Paget Disease

Definition ■ Extramammary Paget disease (EPD) is a neoplasm of apocrine glands that clinically resembles Paget disease of the breast, but occurs in areas rich in apocrine glands, including the perineum and axilla.

Epidemiology ■ More frequent in women and whites, EPD usually strikes after the fifth decade.

Clinical Features ■ EPD is a scaly, sharply marginated plaque, most commonly found in the vulva. Because itching and burning are common symptoms, it is often mistaken for intertrigo or flexural eczema, and the diagnosis is delayed. Progressive enlargement of the plaque in the face of topical steroid or antifungal medications is a diagnostic clue.

Treatment ■ Evaluation to identify the presence of underlying malignancy is crucial. Surgical excision is the treatment of choice for primary EPD. Although conventional surgery can yield a recurrence rate of more than 40%, microscopically controlled excision appears to yield at least as good results while sparing tissue loss. High-dose (4000 cGy) radiotherapy produced local regression in one small study. Ablative carbon dioxide laser treatment is palliative, as recurrence rates are very high.

Course and Prognosis ■ When EPD is associated with an adenocarcinoma, the prognosis is poor. However, even primary EPD can eventually ulcerate and become locally invasive and spread to lymph nodes, with depth of invasion > 1 mm being an important prognostic factor . Even after wide excision, local recurrence still approaches 25%.

Benign Cutaneous Tumors Associated with Cancer Syndromes

Trichilemmoma (in Cowden Disease)

Definition ■ Trichilemmoma is a tumor that exhibits features of outer root sheath differentiation of hair. In Cowden disease, multiple trichilemmomas are associated with multiple hamartomatous neoplasms of ectodermal, mesodermal, and endodermal origin.[89]

Epidemiology ■ Cowden disease is a rare autosomal dominant condition with variable expressivity. Less than 100 cases are reported to date. Male patients slightly exceed females among all the cases reported. All reported patients are white, except for one Japanese and two black patients. The age span is between 4 and 75 years, with the median age being 39 years.

Clinical Features ■ In Cowden disease, multiple trichilemmomas are associated with a wide variety of hamartomas and tumors of other organ systems; the most important include fibrocystic disease and carcinoma of the breast, adenoma and follicular adenocarcinoma of the thyroid, gastrointestinal polyps, and lipomas. The trichilemmomas present as small lichenoid, skin-colored to yellow-tan papules with a smooth surface. They are concentrated on the face, especially around the orifices and the ears. Similar papules may appear on the extremities, including palmoplantar surfaces, and the oral cavity, particularly on the gingiva and the tongue (Figs. 106-14 and 106-15). The presentation of these papules usually precedes the appearance of breast cancer and, therefore, can serve as a marker of associated cancer.

Genetics ■ Germ line mutations in the protein tyrosine phosphatase PTEN have been linked to multiple families with Cowden disease.[90]

Treatment ■ Therapies are directed toward achieving good cosmetic appearance and treatment of the various associated benign and malignant tumors, as indicated. In view of the high incidence of breast cancer in female patients, which may be as high as 50%, frequent breast examination and mammography are indicated.

Sebaceous Adenoma (in Muir–Torre Syndrome)

Definition ■ Sebaceous adenoma is a rare, benign tumor consisting of incompletely differentiated sebaceous lobules within the dermis. In Muir–Torre syndrome, multiple sebaceous adenomas and carcinomas are associated with multiple visceral malignant neoplasms. These sebaceous tumors are rare enough that the presence of a single lesion in an otherwise healthy patient warrants an investigation for internal neoplasms.

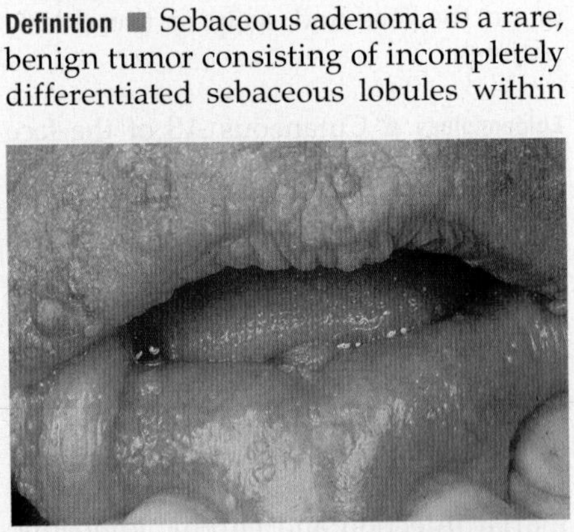

Figure 106-14 ■ Cowden disease. Multiple trichilemmomas on the upper lip. Similar papules are present on the mucosal surface of the lower lip.

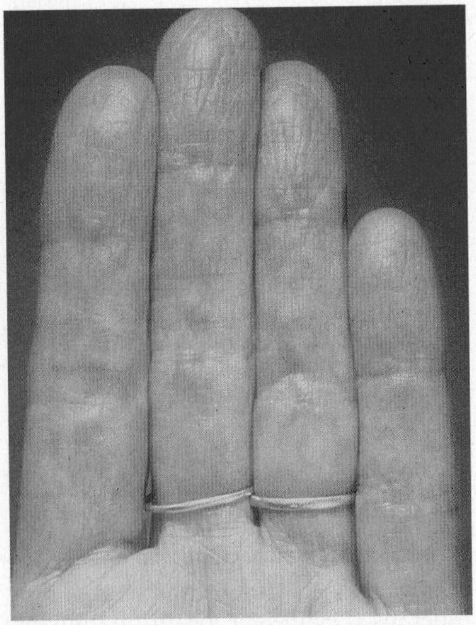

Figure 106-15 ■ Cowden disease. Translucent keratotic papules on the palmar surface. *Source:* Courtesy of R.A. Johnson, MD.

Epidemiology ■ Solitary sebaceous adenoma is a rare tumor that occurs in elderly patients of both sexes. The multiple type, associated with Muir–Torre syndrome, is familial, with more than 50% of reported patients having an immediate family member with a history of internal cancer, most frequently of the colon.[91]

Clinical Features ■ Sebaceous adenoma typically appears as a firm, flesh-colored to waxy-yellow papule or pedunculated lesion, usually less than 1 cm in size. The surface may be smooth or verrucous. Older lesions may be plaque-like or ulcerated. It is usually located on the face or scalp and is usually slow growing.

In Muir–Torre syndrome, multiple sebaceous tumors, including adenomas and carcinomas, and keratoacanthomas are associated with multiple visceral carcinomas, most commonly carcinoma of the colon and carcinoma of the ampulla of Vater.

Genetics ■ Overlap between Muir–Torre syndrome and kindreds with hereditary nonpolyposis colon cancer allowed the identification of the DNA mismatch repair gene hMSH2 as one of the genes disturbed in Muir–Torre syndrome.[92]

Treatment ■ The treatment of choice is surgical excision. The tumor is also radiosensitive.

Multiple Mucosal Neuromas (Multiple Endocrine Neoplasia 2B, MEN2B)

Definition ■ Mucosal neuromas present as small, discrete and coalescing, painless nodules, usually involving the lips, and sometimes studding the margins of the tongue. The association of multiple mucosal neuromas, medullary thyroid carcinoma and pheochromocytoma has been established as a familial syndrome.

Epidemiology ■ Discrete mucosal neuromas are common and often result from direct trauma, as in the typical bite neuroma. More than 150 cases of multiple neuromas associated with endocrine tumors have been described in the literature.[93]

Clinical Features ■ In MEN2B, diffusely enlarged lips are an early feature. Diffuse and symmetric fleshy papules and nodules occur on the tongue by the end of first decade. Any mucosal surface may be involved. Patients often develop a Marfanoid habitus. Most importantly, medullary thyroid carcinoma may develop in early adulthood. These tumors produce calcitonin and can stimulate parathyroid hyperplasia. Pheochromocytomas are frequently present as well.

Genetics ■ In all cases studied to date, mutation in the protooncogene RET, a receptor tyrosine kinase, has been uncovered.[94]

Course and Prognosis ■ Medullary thyroid carcinoma is often the cause of death. Routine screening for this tumor with ultrasonography and by measuring serum calcitonin levels is useful, but current recommendations suggest prophylactic thyroidectomy in cases where a RET mutation is documented.[95]

Metastatic Tumors to the Skin

Cutaneous metastases of internal cancers are uncommon. In a report of 7316 nonmelanoma cancer patients by Lookingbill and colleagues,[96] only 1% of patients had cutaneous metastases at the time of diagnosis. In Gates' study of 2298 patients reported as having died of visceral carcinoma, only 2.7% had evidence of cutaneous metastases. In a more recent retrospective study by Lookingbill and colleagues of 4020 patients with metastatic carcinomas and melanoma, 10% had cutaneous metastases. In general, the incidence of the various cancers metastatic to the skin correlates well with the incidence of the particular primary tumor.

Hence, the spectrum of metastatic tumors differs slightly between the 2 sexes.[97]

In Lookingbill and colleagues' study, the most common primary sources of metastatic carcinoma to the skin in males were malignant melanoma (32%), lung (12%), large intestine (11%), carcinoma of the oral cavity (9%) and larynx (5.5%), and kidney (5%). In females, breast is by far the most common source (70%), followed by melanoma (12%), and ovary (3%), and large intestine, lung, and oral cavity, each accounting for 1.3-2.3% of the cases. In recent years, the incidence of carcinoma of the lung has increased dramatically in females, resulting in a corresponding rise in the incidence of cutaneous metastatic lung carcinoma deposits in females . Other carcinomas that metastasize to the skin include thyroid, pancreas, liver, gallbladder, urinary bladder, endometrium, prostate, and testis. However, these are quite rare.

Typically, metastatic cancer presents as multiple, firm, nonulcerated nodules. When solitary, they may be misdiagnosed as primary skin tumors. Inflammatory skin metastases mimicking cellulitis may occur in 10% of metastases from breast cancer. The most common sites for skin metastases are chest and abdomen, followed by head and neck; metastasis to the extremities is rare. Those metastases situated in the scalp can be associated with alopecia ("alopecia neoplastica"). Dissemination may be via the bloodstream or via the lymphatics. Carcinomas of the breast and of the oral cavity tend to spread through the lymphatics, whereas other carcinomas tend to be hematogenous in their spread. Lymphatic dissemination may explain the observation that skin metastases tend to be close to the site of the primary tumor: chest in lung carcinoma, abdominal wall in gastrointestinal tumors, and lower back in renal cell carcinoma.

The prognosis for patients with cutaneous metastases is generally poor. In Lookingbill and colleagues[97], the average time from diagnosis of skin metastases to death for the various primary tumors varies from 1 to 34 months. The variability in prognosis may be the result of advances in cancer therapy during the past decades. Some patients with metastatic melanoma to skin as the sole site of metastasis may have prolonged disease-free survival.

Selected References

The complete reference list can be found at www.CANCERMEDICINE8.com

2. American Cancer Society. *Cancer Facts & Figures 2008*. Atlanta: American Cancer Society; 2008.
7. Weinstock MA. Death from skin cancer among the elderly: epidemiological patterns. *Arch Dermatol*. 1997;133:1207.
8. Chuang T-Y, Reizner GT, Elpern DJ, et al. Non-melanoma skin cancer in Japanese ethnic Hawaiians in Kauai, Hawaii: an incidence report. *J Am Acad Dermatol*. 1995;33:422.
10. Franceschi S, Levi F, Randimbison L, La Vecchia C. Site distribution of different types of skin cancers: new aetiological clues. *Int J Cancer*. 1996;67:24.
12. Clydesdale GJ, Dandie GW, Muller HK. Ultraviolet light induced injury: immunological and inflammatory effects. *Immunol Cell Biol*. 2001;79:547-568.
13. Ramsay HM, Fryer AA, Hawley CM, et al. Non-melanoma skin cancer risk in the renal transplant population. *Br J Dermatol*. 2002;147:950.
14. Lookingbill DP, Lookingbill GL, Leppard B. Actinic damage and skin cancer in albinos in northern Tanzania: findings in 164 patients enrolled in an outreach skin care program. *J Am Acad Dermatol*. 1995;32:653.
15. Suchniak JM, Baer S, Goldberg LH. High rate of malignant transformation in hypertrophic actinic keratoses. *J Am Acad Dermatol*. 1997;37:392.
16. Clark DP, Feinstein RJ, Graham G. Guidelines of care for actinic keratoses. *J Am Acad Dermatol*. 1995;32:95.
17. Gupta AK, Weiss JS, Jorizzo JL. 5-Fluorouracil 0.5% cream for multiple actinic or solar keratoses of the face and anterior scalp. *Skin Therapy Lett*. 2001;6:1-4.
18. Jarvis B, Figgitt DP. Topical 3% diclofenac in 2.5% hyaluronic acid gel: a review of its use in patients with actinic keratoses. *Am J Clin Dermatol*. 2003;4:203-213.
22. Hsi ED, Svoboda-Newman SM, Stern RA, et al. Detection of human papilloma virus DNA in keratoacanthomas by polymerase chain reaction. *Am J Dermatopathol*. 1997;19:10.
28. Katz, KA, Marcil I, Stern RS. Incidence and risk factors associated with a second squamous cell carcinoma or basal cell carcinoma in PUVA-treated psoriasis patients. *J Invest Dermatol*. 2002.118:1038.
29. Nijsten TE, Stern RS. The increased risk of skin cancer is persistent after discontinuation of PUVA: a cohort study. *J Invest Dermatol*. 2003;121:252.
30. Christenson LJ, Geusau, A, Ferrandiz F, et al. Specialty clinics for the dermatologic care of solid-organ transplant recipients. *Dermatol Surg*. 2004;30:598-603.
31. Jensen P, Hansen S, Moller B, et al. Skin cancer in kidney and heart transplant recipients and different long-term immunosuppressive therapy regimens. *J Am Acad Dermatol*. 1999;40:177-186.
32. Martinez JC, Otley CC, Stasko T, et al. Defining the clinical course of metastatic skin cancer in organ transplant recipients: a multicenter collaborative study. *Arch Dermatol*. 2003;139:301.
33. Schwartz RA. Verrucous carcinoma of the skin and mucosa. *J Am Acad Dermatol*. 1995;32:1.
35. Reizner GT, Chuang T-Y, Elpern DJ, et al. Bowen's disease (squamous cell carcinoma in situ) in Kauai, Hawaii: a population-based incidence report. *J Am Acad Dermatol*. 1994;31:596.
40. Lebwohl M. Actinic keratosis: epidemiology and progression to squamous cell carcinoma. *Br J Dermatol*. 2003;149 (Suppl 66):31.

41. Maalej M, Frikha H, Kochbati L, et al. Radio-induced malignancies of the scalp, 98 patients and 150 lesions, and literature review. *Cancer Radiother.* 2004;8:81.
47. De Graaf YG, Euvrard S, Bouwes Bavinck JN. Systemic and topical retinoids in the management of skin cancer in organ transplant recipients. *Dermatol Surg.* 2004;30:656.
48. Cherpelis BS, Marcusen C, Lang PG. Prognostic factors for metastasis in squamous cell carcinoma of the skin. *Dermatol Surg.* 2002;28:268.
51. Hoy WE. Nonmelanoma skin carcinoma in Albuquerque, New Mexico: experience of a major health care provider. *Cancer.* 1996;77:2489.
56. Kricker A, Armstrong BK, English DR, Heenan PJ. Does intermittent sun exposure cause basal cell carcinoma? A case-control study in Western Australia. *Int J Cancer.* 1995;60:489.
57. Johnson RL, Rothman AL, Xie J, et al. Human homolog of patched, a candidate gene for the basal cell carcinoma syndrome. *Science.* 1996;272:1668-1671.
58. Lam CW, Xie J, To KF, et al. A frequent activated smoothened mutation in sporadic basal cell carcinomas. *Oncogene.* 1999;18:833-836.
64. Newman MD, Weinberg JM. Topical therapy in the treatment of actinic keratosis and basal cell carcinoma. *Cutis.* 2007;79 (Suppl 4):18.
71. Heath M, Jamies N, Lemos B, et al. Clinical characteristics of Merkel cell carcinoma at diagnosis in 195 patients: the AEIOU features. *J Am Acad Dermatol.* 2008; 58:375.
72. Feng H, Shuda M, Chang Y, et al. Clonal integration of polyomavirus in human Merkel cell carcinoma. *Science.* 2008;319:1096.
73. Allen PJ, Zhang ZF, Colt DG. Surgical management of Merkel cell carcinoma. *Ann Surg.* 1999;229:97-105.
74. O'Connor WJ, Roenigk RK, Brodland DG. Merkel cell carcinoma: comparison of Mohs micrographic surgery and wide excision in eighty-six patients. *Dermatol Surg.* 1997;23:929.
75. Messina JL, Reintgen DS, Cruse CW, et al. Selective lymphadenectomy in patients with Merkel cell (cutaneous neuroendocrine) carcinoma. *Ann Surg Oncol.* 1997;4:389-395.
77. Skelton HG, Smith KJ, Hitchcock CL, et al. Merkel cell carcinoma: analysis of clinical, histologic, and immunohistologic features of 132 cases with relation to survival. *J Am Acad Dermatol.* 1997;37:734.
79. Wang J, Hisaoka M, Shimajiri S, et al. Detection of COL1A1-PDGFB fusion transcripts in dermatofibrosarcoma protuberans by reverse transcription polymerase chain reaction using archival formalin-fixed, paraffin-embedded tissues. *Diagn Mol Pathol.* 1999;8:113-119.
80. Parker TL, Zitelli JA. Surgical margins for excision of dermatofibrosarcoma protuberans. *J Am Acad Dermatol.* 1995;32:233.
81. Maki, RG, Awan RA, Dixon, RH, et al. Differential sensitivity to imatinib of 2 patients with metastatic sarcoma arising from dermatofibrosarcoma protuberans. *Int J Cancer.* 2002;100:623-626.
82. Snow SN, Gordon EM, Larson PO, et al. Dermatofibrosarcoma protuberans: a report on 29 patients treated by Mohs micrographic surgery with long-term follow-up and review of the literature. *Cancer.* 2004;101:28-38.
84. Sasaki R, Soejima T, Kishi K, et al. Angiosarcoma treated with radiotherapy: impact of tumor type and size on outcome. *Int J Radiat Oncol Biol Phys.* 2002;52:1032-1040.
85. Ulrich L, Krause M, Brachmann A, et al. Successful treatment of angiosarcoma of the scalp by intralesional cytokine therapy and surface irradiation. *J Eur Acad Dermatol Venereol.* 2000;14:412-415.
86. Wollina U, Fuller J, Graefe T, et al. Angiosarcoma of the scalp: treatment with liposomal doxorubicin and radiotherapy. *J Cancer Res Clin Oncol.* 2001;127:396-399.
88. Spencer JM, Nossa R, Tse DT, Sequeira M. Sebaceous carcinoma of the eyelid treated with Mohs micrographic surgery. *J Am Acad Dermatol.* 2001;44:1004-1009.
89. Gustafson S, Zbuk KM, Scacheri C. Cowden syndrome. *Semin Oncol.* 2007;34:428.
90. Liaw D, Marsh DJ, Li J, et al. Germline mutations of the PTEN gene in Cowden disease, an inherited breast and thyroid cancer syndrome. *Nat Genet.* 1997;16:64-67.
91. Pettey AA, Walsh JS. Muir-Torre syndrome: a case report and review of the literature. *Cutis.* 2005;75:149.
94. Santoro M, Carlomagno F, Romano A, et al. Activation of RET as a dominant transforming gene by germline mutations of MEN2A and MEN2B. *Science.* 1995;267:381-383.
95. Sanso GE, Domene HM, Garcia R, et al. Very early detection of RET proto-oncogene mutation is crucial for preventive thyroidectomy in multiple endocrine neoplasia type 2 children: presence of C-cell malignant disease in asymptomatic carriers. *Cancer.* 2002;94:323-330.

107 Bone Tumors

Timothy A. Damron, MD, FACS ■ David G. Murray, MD

Introduction

As a group, bone tumors are uncommon lesions arising from a wide array of cells, affecting all ages of patients, and involving any bone in the body. They include benign lesions, primary bone sarcomas, metastatic carcinomas to bone, myeloma, and lymphoma. The benign bone lesions may behave in an inactive, active, or aggressive fashion. Despite the broad spectrum of bone tumors, each individual entity has a distinct clinical and radiographic presentation, with a predilection for specific locations, which lends itself to narrowing the differential diagnosis and selecting appropriate management.

Bone sarcomas account for less than 0.2% of all cancers.[1] During 2008, approximately 2380 new cases of primary bone sarcomas were diagnosed and approximately 1470 deaths occurred. The three most common bone sarcomas are osteosarcoma (45%), chondrosarcoma (36%), and Ewing sarcoma (18%).[2] However, the most common primary malignancy of bone is myeloma, and the most common cancer that involves bone is metastatic carcinoma. Malignancies of bone as a group are only the tip of the iceberg, as the vast majority of bone lesions are benign.

The pathologic classification of bone tumors continues to evolve. To a large extent, classification continues to be according to the cell of origin or tissue type. Primary bone tumors may derive from cartilage cells—chondrocytes (enchondromas, periosteal chondromas, chondroblastomas, chondromyxoid fibromas, chondrosarcomas), bone cells—osteoblasts and osteocytes (osteoma, osteoid osteoma, osteoblastoma, osteosarcoma), and vascular cells (hemangioma and angiosarcoma), among others, but for some tumors, the cell of origin is unknown. The most widely accepted pathologic classification system to date is that of the WHO, and their terminology is used to a large degree in this chapter, although some tumors, such as benign fibrous tumors, are grouped differently.[3]

The introductory sections of this chapter deal with the pretreatment phase (evaluation, staging, and biopsy), the middle sections with surgical treatment (surgical margins through reconstructive options), radiation therapy and medical management, and the final sections with the specific benign and malignant bone tumors as well as congenital syndromes related to bone tumors.

Evaluation

Crucial information about bone lesions is derived from the history, physical examination, and radiographic features. The goal of evaluation of any bone lesion is to arrive at a narrow differential diagnosis which will guide subsequent action. In some cases, a specific diagnosis may be determined, and, depending upon the diagnosis, the action may include observation (eg, non-ossifying fibroma, enchondroma), biopsy confirmation (eg, aneurysmal bone cyst, chondroblastoma, giant cell tumor, osteosarcoma), irrigation/debridement (eg, osteomyelitis), aspiration/injection (eg, unicameral bone cyst), radiofrequency ablation (eg, osteoid osteoma), excision (eg, osteochondroma), or prophylactic stabilization (eg, established metastatic carcinoma, myeloma). In other cases, the lesion may only be categorized according to a general category of biologic behavior: latent, active, or aggressive. Latent bone tumors may be observed. Active lesions often require biopsy and curettage with or without grafting. Aggressive bone tumors almost always require biopsy confirmation prior to treatment and include both benign aggressive lesions (eg, aneurysmal bone cyst, chondroblastoma, and giant cell tumor of bone) and malignancies (eg, primary bone sarcomas, metastatic carcinoma, myeloma, lymphoma).

Important historical features are the patient's age and the means by which the lesion was discovered. Age divisions are particularly helpful when the patient is less than 5 years old, where metastatic neuroblastoma occurs almost exclusively, and when the patient is older than 40, where the differential diagnosis, in order of decreasing frequency, includes metastatic carcinoma, myeloma, lymphoma, and primary bone sarcomas such as chondrosarcoma, secondary osteosarcoma, malignant fibrous histiocytoma of bone, and fibrosarcoma.

The means of discovery of a bone lesion are variable. Bone lesions discovered incidentally during evaluation for other reasons are usually latent lesions that require nothing further than observation. In adult patients, the most common lesion discovered incidentally is an enchondroma; in pediatric patients, it is a non-ossifying fibroma. Painless bony masses are usually osteochondromas, but other surface bone lesions may present in this fashion. The broadest category is the painful bone lesion, and this includes a wide variety of active and aggressive bone lesions. Pathologic fractures may be divided into those preceded by pain, which are usually associated with active or aggressive bone tumors, and those not preceded by pain, which are more commonly latent lesions.

Plain radiographs are standard for the radiologic evaluation of any bone tumor. These should be evaluated for location (epiphyseal, metaphyseal, diaphyseal, surface, or intracortical), lesional border characteristics (geographic, moth-eaten, or permeative), bone response to the lesion (periosteal reaction), and matrix mineralization pattern (cartilaginous, osseous, ground glass) when present (Table 107-1). Putting these radiographic features together with the clinical features will often yield a narrow differential diagnosis.

Bone scans help to determine whether the lesion shows uptake of the Tc^{99} radionuclide, indicating an active or aggressive lesion, and whether the lesion is solitary or only one of numerous lesions. Myeloma deposits in bone serve as an exception to the rule, often being cold on bone scan. Some aggressive lesions, such as renal carcinoma metastases, may not be hot on bone scan if tumor destruction outpaces the bone's ability to form bone in response.

Magnetic resonance imaging (MRI) of bone tumors is indicated when the diagnosis is not evident from the plain radiographs and for determining the local extent of bone sarcomas. Specific bone tumors that may be confirmed with MRI include simple bone cysts (rim enhancement of a fluid-filled lesion) and aneurysmal bone cysts (septations separating multiple loculated areas filled with blood, as indicated by fluid-fluid levels). Perilesional edema is common surrounding bone sarcomas, but may also be seen in certain benign conditions, including osteomyelitis, osteoid osteoma, chondroblastoma, Langerhans cell histiocytosis, and chondromyxoid fibroma. Computed tomography (CT) is indicated to find the

Table 107-1 **Classic Examples of Bone Tumors Fitting Specific Patterns of Lesional Borders, Bone Response, and Lesional Matrix on Plain Radiographs**

Radiographic Category	Type	Classic Examples[a]
Lesional border	Geographic (well-defined)	Nonossifying fibroma Unicameral bone cyst
	Moth-eaten (blurred)	Aneurysmal bone cyst Chondroblastoma Giant cell tumor
	Permeative (poorly defined)	Osteosarcoma Ewing sarcoma Metastatic carcinoma Lymphoma
Bone response	Marginal sclerosis	Nonossifying fibroma Fibrous dysplasia
	Cortical thickening	Osteoid osteoma Osteomyelitis
	Laminar periosteal response	Stress fracture
	Endosteal expansion and scalloping	Low-grade to intermediate grade chondrosarcoma
	Periosteal rimming	Aneurysmal bone cyst Giant cell tumor of bone
	Codman's triangle Cumulus cloud reaction	Osteosarcoma
	Onion-skinning periosteal response	Ewing sarcoma
Lesional matrix	Punctate rings and arcs	Hyaline cartilage tumors (enchondromas/chondrosarcomas)
	Ground glass appearance	Fibrous dysplasia
	Osteoblastic	Osteoid osteoma Osteoblastoma Osteosarcoma Metastatic carcinoma (prostate, breast) Lymphoma

[a]None of the radiographic findings here are specific, and there is considerable overlap; hence, those lesions listed may be considered classic but by no means the only ones that may present with such findings.

Source: Adapted from Damron TA, editor. *Orthopaedic Surgery Essentials: Oncology and Basic Science*. Lippincott: Williams and Wilkins; 2008.

radiolucent nidus of an osteoid osteoma within the surrounding reactive bone, to assess for endosteal scalloping in a cartilage tumor to distinguish enchondroma from chondrosarcoma, to find the pattern of lesional mineralization when it is unclear, and to supplement MRI in difficult anatomic locations such as the sacrum, pelvis, and scapula.

Staging

Staging of bone sarcomas requires assessment of both the primary site and distant disease. For assessment of the primary site, radiographs and MRI of the entire involved bone should be obtained in order to check for other "skip" lesions. The two most common sites of metastases from bone sarcomas are lung followed by bone. Hence, the most crucial staging studies to obtain are chest radiograph and CT to evaluate the lungs as well as a total body bone scan to evaluate the rest of the skeleton. The role of positron emission tomography (PET) scans continues to evolve, but current indications in the setting of musculoskeletal tumors are limited.

Traditionally, the staging system most commonly used for musculoskeletal sarcomas was that originally described by William Enneking and adopted by the Musculoskeletal Tumor Society (MSTS) (Table 107-2). Variables incorporated into the MSTS staging system include the presence or absence of metastases, grade (high or low), and local extent of the tumor (intraosseous or with extension into the soft-tissues). The typical chondrosarcoma is low-grade and intra-compartmental (confined to the bone), so it is usually stage IA. The conventional high-grade osteosarcoma usually extends into the soft-tissue, and since 80% present without evidence of distant metastases, the typical stage is IIB. Evidence of metastases equates to a stage III in this system.

The current most widely accepted staging system for bone sarcomas is that of the American Joint Commission on Cancer (AJCC)[5] (Table 107-3). This system has more well-documented prognostic significance (Fig. 107-1). Variables incorporated into the AJCC system include presence or absence of metastases (with multiple/discontinous bone tumors separated from distant metastases), grade (grade 1 or 2 vs grade 3 or 4), and size (8 cm or smaller versus larger than 8 cm). This system is similar to the MSTS system in separating Stage I from II based on grade, but the A-B designation is based upon size here. For osteosarcoma and Ewing sarcoma, Stage IIB patients have higher rates of metastases than Stage IIA patients. Patients with "skip lesions" (discontinuous lesions in the same bone) are designated as Stage III. Distant metastases in this system are Stage IV, but since metastases to sites other than the lung (such as bone) may carry a worse prognosis than lung metastases alone, a separate designation is reserved for those two groups (IVA and IVB). Hence, for a less than 8 cm low-grade chondrosarcoma, the typical staging would be Stage IA. For a larger than 8 cm high-grade osteosarcoma without skip lesions or metastases, the typical staging is Stage IIB.

Table 107-2 **Musculoskeletal Tumor Society Staging System**

Stage	Grade	Local Extent	Metastases
I	Low	A-Intracompartmental B-Extracompartmental	None
II	High	A-Intracompartmental B-Extracompartmental	
III	Any	Any	Present

Source: Adapted from Enneking WF, Spanier SS, Goodman MA. A system for the surgical staging of musculoskeletal sarcoma. *Clin Orthop Relat Res*. 1980;153:106–120.

Biopsy

Biopsy of bone tumors is indicated when a specific benign diagnosis cannot be determined based by radiographic evaluation alone. When the clinico-radiographic diagnosis of a latent lesion such as nonossifying fibroma, unicameral bone cyst, or enchondroma can be made, biopsy is generally unnecessary. Some active lesions, such as fibrous dysplasia, intraosseous lipoma, and osteochondroma do not always require biopsy if the diagnosis can be established radiographically. For most other active and all aggressive lesions, biopsy should be done to determine or confirm the diagnosis. Suspected high-grade sarcomas should be biopsied prior to initiating treatment neoadjuvant.

Careful consideration must be given when metastases are suspected, because the treatment of metastatic carcinoma to bone differs dramatically from that of a primary bone tumor. Hence, even for patients with a history of a known carcinoma with predilection to bone (breast, prostate, lung, renal, thyroid), the first bone metastases should generally be established by biopsy. When dealing with

Table 107-3 **American Joint Commission on Cancer Staging System for Bone Sarcomas**

Primary tumor [T]	
TX	Primary tumor cannot be assessed
T0	No evidence of primary tumor
T1	Tumor 8 cm or less in greatest dimension
T2	Tumor more than 8 cm in greatest dimension
T3	Discontinuous tumors in the primary bone site
Regional lymph nodes [N]	
NX*	Regional lymph nodes cannot be assessed
N0	No regional lymph node metastasis
N1	Regional lymph node metastasis
Distant metastasis [M]	
MX	Distant metastasis cannot be assessed
M0	No distant metastasis
M1	Distant metastasis
M1a	Lung
M1b	Other distant sites
Histologic grade [G]	
GX	Grade cannot be assessed
G1	Well differentiated—low-grade
G2	Moderately differentiated—low-grade
G3	Poorly differentiated—high-grade
G4	Undifferentiated—high-grade

Stage	Tumor [T]	Node [N]	Metastasis [M]	Grade [G]
Stage IA	T1	N0	M0	G1, 2 low grade
Stage IB	T2	N0	M0	G1, 2 low grade
Stage IIA	T1	N0	M0	G3, 4 high grade
Stage IIB	T2	N0	M0	G3, 4 high grade
Stage III	T3	N0	M0	Any G
Stage IVA	Any T	N0	M1a	Any G
Stage IVB	Any T	N1	Any M	Any G
	Any T	Any N	M1b	Any G

*Because of the rarity of lymph node involvement in sarcomas, the designation NX may not be appropriate and could be considered N0 if no clinical involvement is evident. Ewing's sarcoma is classified as G4.
Source: Adapted from Ref. 3.

suspected metastatic disease requiring a biopsy, reamings are not the best way to submit a biopsy specimen, because once the intramedullary canal to and through the lesion has been breached, all associated bone and soft-tissue has been potentially contaminated with tumor. If the pathology shows sarcoma, rather than metastatic disease, unnecessary contamination of previously uninvolved tissue will have already occurred.

There are four general biopsy techniques applicable to bone tumors: (1) Fine needle biopsy, (2) core needle biopsy, (3) incisional open biopsy, and (4) excisional biopsy. Fine needle aspiration (FNA) biopsy provides only cells for cytology and it is usually done by interventional radiologists. An FNA is useful in two general clinical situations where bone tumors are involved: (a) when the diagnosis of a bone lesion is strongly suspected (metastatic carcinoma, recurrent sarcoma) and (b) for difficult to access lesions (spine, pelvis, scapula). Core needle biopsies allow for interpretation of the tissue architecture in addition to the cytological detail. For bone lesions, core biopsies may be done in the same situations as FNA and for bone lesions with soft-tissue extension. Incisional open biopsy is the workhorse biopsy tool for bone lesions, as it provides adequate tissue for histological interpretation. However, there are numerous pitfalls to open biopsy which must be considered, and for most incisional biopsies, the surgeon who will be doing the definitive surgery, no matter what the final diagnosis, is the person who should do the biopsy.[6,7] Excisional biopsy is usually only used for bone tumors such as osteochondromas, where the radiographic features establish the diagnosis, the morbidity of excision is small, and the surface location of the lesion lends itself to excision.

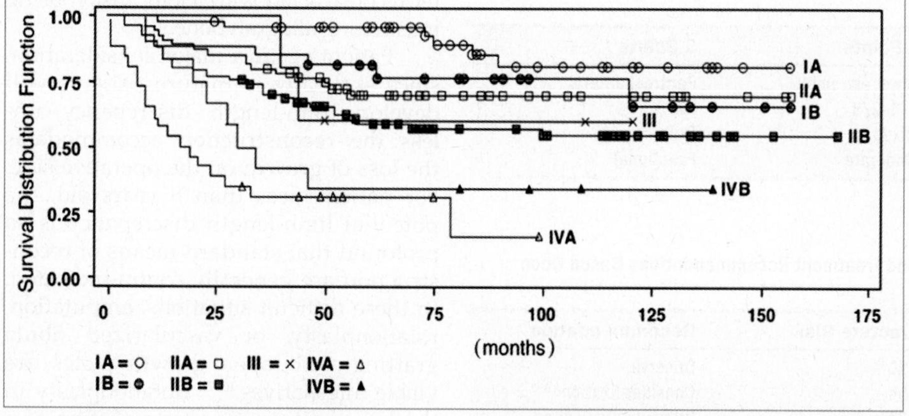

Figure 107-1 Survival according to staging by the new American Joint Commission on Cancer staging system for bone sarcomas. *Source:* From Ref. 1.

Surgical Margins

Surgical margins depend upon the type of excision done, and the appropriate type of excision varies according to bone tumor type. There are four types of excisions: (1) intralesional, (2) marginal, (3) wide, and (4) radical.[8] For most benign bone lesions, an intralesional excision by way of a curettage is appropriate. When necessary, metastatic bone lesions undergoing surgery for stabilization may be treated by curettage. For aggressive benign lesions (aneurysmal bone cyst, chondroblastoma, and giant cell tumor), an extended intralesional curettage is indicated. This differs from a simple curettage in that it utilizes mechanical (high-speed burr, pulsatile lavage) and adjunctive (phenol, laser, liquid nitrogen) techniques to extend the margin into normal bone. Recent trends suggest that most extremity low-grade chondrosarcomas may also be treated in this way. Marginal en bloc excision (through the pseudocapsule surrounding the tumor, is appropriate for osteochondromas, but wide resection (excision with a cuff of normal tissue) is indicated for most bone sarcomas.

Limb Salvage Versus Amputation

Two issues must be considered in making the decision regarding limb salvage versus amputation: oncologic safety and function. First, in order for a patient to be a candidate for limb salvage, the oncologic procedure should not lower the expected survival beyond that which could be achieved with an amputation. This question has been addressed prospectively, and—in properly selected patients—survival is no less with limb-sparing surgery when compared to amputation.[9,10] However, this decision still needs to be made carefully for each patient. Oncologic safety considers two variables: response to chemotherapy (when applicable) and surgical margin. The poorer the response to chemotherapy, the greater the likelihood of local recurrence for any given margin achieved intra-operatively. Hence, for a poor response to chemotherapy (tumor progression), limb salvage surgery is a relatively strong contraindication. A wide surgical margin is the goal of bone sarcoma surgery, and it can usually be achieved with the appropriately planned level of amputation but not always with limb-sparing surgery. If vital structures (major vessels and nerves) are encased by the soft-tissue extent of the sarcoma, necessitating their resection along with the tumor, limb salvage is contraindicated and amputation is preferable.

As with oncologic safety, if limb salvage is to be done, the expected function of the planned reconstruction should be at least equivalent to that of a comparable level amputation. In the lower extremity, function with a below-knee amputation is generally thought to be better than a distal tibia reconstruction, so a distal tibial location is a relative indication for amputation. In the upper extremity, it is preferable to be able to preserve two of the three major nerves (radial, ulnar, median) for limb salvage. Tumor encasement of more than one major upper extremity nerve and/or the axillary or brachial vessels is an indication for amputation.

Operative Management of Metastatic Carcinoma, Myeloma, Lymphoma

There are four settings that potentially require operative management for patients with bone lesions from metastatic carcinoma, myeloma, and lymphoma: (1) biopsy to establish diagnosis, (2) prophylactic stabilization of impending pathologic fracture, (3) operative fixation of pathologic fracture, and (4) en bloc resection of isolated lesions. Biopsy issues have been previously discussed but cannot be emphasized enough: the diagnosis should be established before embarking upon an operative treatment plan. Prediction of impending fracture risk is evolving. Currently, fractures are predicted based upon clinical and radiographic criteria. A rating system devised by Mirels has been devised based upon four variables[11] (Tables 107-4 and 107-5). The Mirels system is valid across experience levels, but it still has a low specificity of approximately 33%.[12] Evaluation of CT-based biomechanical analyses for this purpose is under study.[13]

When pathologic fractures occur in the setting of disseminated malignancies, they usually warrant operative fixation in order to improve function since these patients have limited life expectancy. Exceptions include moribund immediately preterminal patients, those who cannot tolerate operative intervention, and fractures that are usually managed by nonoperative means. In order for the patient to benefit from the procedure, life expectancy should be longer than the expected time required to recover from any proposed procedure.

The principles of operative fixation for fractures in this clinical situation differ from those of standard fracture fixation. Since later lesions may develop elsewhere in the bone, intramedullary nail fixation, as opposed to plate/screw fixation, is preferred in the long bones in order to protect the remainder of the bone. Immediate stability is the goal in order to avoid prolonged recovery that diminishes patient function, so bone cement is much more commonly used to supplement fixation in this situation. Fracture healing in the setting of metastatic carcinoma and myeloma is notoriously slow, so the fixation should be planned assuming there will be no fracture healing. Postoperative radiotherapy has been shown to improve function and reduce reoperation rates.[14]

Table 107-4 ■ Mirels' Scoring System for Predicting Risk of Pathologic Fracture in Metastatic Disease

	1 Point	2 Points	3 Points
Site	Upper extremity	Lower extremity	Peritrochanteric
Size	<1/3	1/3-2/3	>2/3
Nature	Blastic	Mixed	Lytic
Pain	Mild	Moderate	Functional

Source: Mirels H, CORR 1982;166:193–198.

Table 107-5 ■ Mirels' Definitions, Fracture Risk, and Treatment Recommendations Based Upon Point Totals

Definition	Points	Fracture Risk	Recommendation
Non-impending	<7	<10%	Observe
Borderline	8	15%	Consider fixation
Impending fracture	9	33%	Prophylactic fixation
	>10	>50%	Prophylactic fixation

Source: Mirels H, CORR 1982;166:193–198.

Reconstructive Alternatives

Benign Bone Tumors

The defects created after curettage of benign bone tumors can be filled with autologous bone graft, allograft bone, synthetic filler material, or bone cement.[15] Bone cement is usually reserved for defects created after extended intralesional curettage of giant cell tumors of bone. Bone cement provides immediate stability that allows full weight bearing, solidifies with an exothermic reaction that extends the margin, and provides a clear radiographic border to facilitate diagnosis of local recurrence. In cases where large lesions have been curetted, prophylactic stabilization with pins or plates/screws may be used to minimize the chance of fracture.

Primary Bone Sarcomas

Following resection of bone sarcomas, numerous alternatives are available to reconstruct the large bone and associated soft-tissue deficits that result. Selection of the appropriate reconstruction in each instance requires consideration of the patient age and expectations, prognosis, adjuvant treatments, type of resection, and anatomic site. In general, reconstructive techniques include endoprostheses, structural allografts, allograft-prosthetic composites, and vascularized bone grafts. Over time, the use of endoprosthetic and allograft-prosthetic composite reconstructions following resections that include a joint has increased, while the indications for structural allografts have continued to decline. Apart from allograft-prosthetic composite reconstructions, the main role for structural allografts has been for intercalary reconstructions (when the joints above and below the diaphyseal segment can be preserved). The most frequent type of resection for sarcomas is intra-articular (removal of the bone up to and including the joint surface), requiring reconstruction of the joint surface, usually with a joint replacement. When the tumor invades the joint, an extra-articular resection (removal of both sides of the joint) is indicated, and this is often better reconstructed with a joint fusion using intervening allograft bone.

Patient age is a major consideration, since skeletally immature patients will develop limb-length discrepancy unless the reconstruction accommodates the loss of growth on the operative side. For patients less than 8 years old, the potential limb-length discrepancy is so profound that standard means of reconstruction are generally contra-indicated. In these difficult situations, amputation, rotationplasty, or vascularized fibula grafting with open growth plates are viable alternatives.[16–22] Rotationplasty in the lower extremity after resection of a tumor around the knee involves fixing the foot and ankle in a position rotated

180 degrees from normal so that the heel points forward and the ankle is situated at the level of and functions as the patient's knee. In this situation, the patient is able to function as a below-knee amputee rather than having to settle for a higher above knee amputation. In patients older than 8 years old, expandable endoprosthetic reconstructions are available.[23–27] In recent years, the availability of such growing prostheses with a noninvasive mechanism has increased their attraction.[26] However, the complication rate may be high, and their durability once the patient reaches skeletal maturity has been questioned.

Upper Extremity ■ For reconstructions following bone sarcoma resection about the shoulder, function is most dependent on whether the deltoid muscle may be preserved during resection of the tumor.[28,29] If a tumor of the proximal humerus extends into the deltoid, and the deltoid has to be removed to achieve a wide margin, function of the shoulder will be poor regardless of the reconstruction. When the deltoid can be preserved, consideration is often given to using an allograft-prosthetic composite reconstruction.[30] In this way, the patient's remaining rotator cuff tendons can be repaired to the allograft tendons, and there is potential for improved function. If an osteoarticular allograft reconstruction is chosen, there is an increased risk of nonunion of the allograft-host junction, fracture, and subchondral collapse. The scapula and all portions of the humerus may be reconstructed with an endoprosthesis. The distal upper extremity is an unusual site for bone sarcomas.

Lower Extremity ■ Following limb-preserving bone sarcoma resection of the pelvis (internal hemipelvectomy), no reconstruction is needed when the hip joint can be preserved (eg, anterior pubic/ischial rami and supra-acetabular iliac resections), and some surgeons do not reconstruct even following resection of the acetabular portion of the pelvis. The numerous reconstructive alternatives for the acetabulum and hip joint following internal hemipelvectomy are fraught with complications.[31,32] For the proximal femur, reconstruction is often done with either an endoprosthetic hemi-arthroplasty (replacing the femoral head side but without a cup in the pelvis) or an allograft-prosthetic composite.[33–35] The latter reconstruction allows attachment of the patient's hip abductors to the allograft tendon, which may improve stability and gait.

Most reconstructions of the distal femur utilize a distal femoral replacement endoprosthetic total knee reconstruction. Because of the attachment of the extensor mechanism through the patellar tendon to the tibial tuberosity, resection of the proximal tibia necessitates consideration of extensor mechanism reconstruction. Here, the primary alternatives are endoprosthetic proximal tibial total knee reconstruction or allograft-prosthetic composite reconstruction. For both reconstructions, the medial head of the gastrocnemius muscle is often used both to cover the allograft and/or prosthesis and to reconstruct the extensor mechanism. With an allograft-prosthetic composite reconstruction of the proximal tibia, the patient's remaining patellar tendon may be sutured to the allograft tendon, further augmenting the extensor mechanism reconstruction.

Complications ■ Complications after resections and reconstructions for bone sarcomas are numerous and frequent. Infection is a concern with all reconstructions, particularly considering the large dead space created following these procedures, the prolonged wound healing while receiving adjuvant treatments, and the prevalence of chemotherapy-induced neutropenia. However, certain complications are associated with specific anatomic sites and types of reconstructions. The proximal tibia is an anatomic site particularly prone to infection given the paucity of soft-tissue coverage. For endoprosthetic reconstructions of the shoulder and hip, joint instability and frank dislocation are relatively common complications. All endoprosthetic reconstructions are prone to loosening, but prosthetic survival is acceptable (proximal femur-90%, distal femur-60%, proximal tibia-50%).[36] Exciting new developments in alternative means of fixation other than those commonly used with joint arthroplasties have been reported and warrant close follow-up.[37] Allografts, particularly when used alone, are prone to nonunion at the allograft-host junction and to fracture.

Radiotherapy for Bone Tumors

Radiotherapy plays a limited role in the treatment of primary tumors of bone, but it is a mainstay of local treatment for bone lesions resulting from metastatic carcinoma, myeloma, and lymphoma. Radiotherapy should generally be avoided in the treatment of benign bone tumors, but low-dose radiotherapy has been advocated in recalcitrant symptomatic spine cases of Langerhans cell histiocytosis.[38] For bone sarcomas, radiotherapy may be considered for the treatment of Ewing sarcoma, but it is not part of standard treatment for osteosarcoma or chondrosarcoma.

Potential complications of bone irradiation include post-radiation sarcoma, spontaneous and fragility fracture, osteonecrosis, and—in pediatric patients—growth arrest or angular deformities. Post-radiation sarcomas typically occur at a minimum of 3 years following the radiation exposure and after mean doses of 50 Gy.[39] Risk factors for post-radiation fracture include periosteal stripping, neoadjuvant chemotherapy, femoral location, higher dose irradiation, and circumferential irradiation.[40] Post-radiation fractures are gaining increasing attention because of their difficulty in management, prolonged healing times and high nonunion rates (45–67%), and the frequent need for surgical treatment, multiple operations, radical bone resection/reconstruction, and/or amputation.[40]

Medical Management of Bone Tumors

The roles for medical management of bone tumors continue to expand. As a rule, high-grade bone sarcomas warrant chemotherapy to address systemic microscopic disease. Chemotherapy for bone sarcomas is usually initiated prior to (neoadjuvant chemotherapy) and completed after local surgical or radiation treatment. Hence, the treatment of both conventional high-grade osteosarcoma and Ewing sarcoma begins with neoadjuvant chemotherapy. There is no established role for chemotherapy in the treatment of low-grade chondrosarcoma.

Use of bisphosphonates to inhibit osteoclast-mediated bone destruction has become standard of care for myeloma and many metastatic carcinomas, including breast, prostate, and lung.[41] Recently, bisphosphonates drugs have also been used off-label for specific benign bone lesions, including fibrous dysplasia and giant cell tumor, but their efficacy has not been established. Of concern, however, is the risk of bisphosphonates related osteonecrosis of the jaw.[41]

Specific Benign Bone Tumors

■ Cartilage Tumors

Cartilage tumors can be divided into those that derive from mature hyaline cartilage (chondromas and osteochondromas) versus those that derive from immature cartilage (chondroblastoma and chondromyxoid fibroma).

Chondromas ■ The WHO classification lists enchondromas, periosteal chondromas, and enchondromatosis under the general heading of "chondromas".[42] Enchondromas are the intramedullary variety of these benign hyaline cartilage tumors, and periosteal chondromas are the variety that resides on the bone surface. Enchondromatosis (multiple enchondromas/Ollier's disease and Maffucci's syndrome) is discussed under the congenital syndromes section.

Enchondromas are relatively common among primary bone tumors, representing up to 17% overall. They likely represent residual rests of hyaline growth plate cartilage left behind during skeletal immaturity. Most of these lesions are asymptomatic and incidentally noted on imaging studies done for other causes of pain.[43] Enchondromas represent the most common bone lesion seen in the small bones of the hand. In the long bones, they are most commonly located in the femur (where they are frequently picked up on x-rays of patients with hip or knee pain) and the humerus (where they are picked up during radiologic evaluation of patients with common causes of shoulder pain). Solitary enchondromas of the flat bones are rare, and the possibility of chondrosarcoma needs to be considered when a cartilage lesion occurs there. Because the radiographic characteristics of hyaline cartilage are typical, the primary challenge is distinguishing enchondromas from chondrosarcomas.

The natural history of enchondromas is that they become more calcified over time. Hence, mature lesions in adults almost always display a characteristic punctate pattern of calcified arcs and rings which is so distinctive as to often allow the diagnosis to be confirmed radiographically without biopsy (Fig. 107-2). They can be associated with some endosteal scalloping. However, when they have periosteal reaction, expansion of the surrounding bone, more extensive cortical destruction, or soft-tissue extension, they have to be considered chondrosarcomas. MRI characteristics of enchondromas are a lobular pattern of organization, which is dark on T1-weighted (T1W) images and bright on T2-weighted (T2W) images. Increased uptake on bone scan is typical of enchondromas and it should not be considered a sign of malignancy; it is likely due to ongoing remodeling of the surrounding bone.

Under the microscope, enchondromas are comprised of benign, sparsely cellular hyaline cartilage, but the degree of cellularity and atypia is variable. In certain locations, such as the fingers and other small bones, the histologic features often appear more aggressive despite their benign behavior.

The vast majority of enchondromas, especially when they present as asymptomatic lesions with typical radiological findings, can simply be observed to ensure that they do not progress. However, when either the radiographic features or associated pain cast doubt on the diagnosis, the lesion may require a complete curettage and complete histological review to differentiate from chondrosarcoma. Cartilage lesions rarely recur after curettage.

Periosteal chondromas, by contrast, are distinctly unusual benign hyaline cartilage lesions. They more commonly present as a bump on a digit or as a low-grade painful lesion elsewhere. Radiographically, the usually show a typical "saucerization" of the underlying cortex of this surface lesion. They need to be distinguished from periosteal chondrosarcoma. Smaller lesions (less than 7 cm) are usually chondromas. Depending upon the location, periosteal chondromas may be removed by curettage or en bloc excision.

Chondroblastoma ■ This immature cartilage derived tumor is an uncommon benign process that typically presents with joint pain, is difficult to diagnosis, and occurs in the epiphysis of the long bones.[44] The vast majority of cases occur in skeletally immature patients, and their presentation with joint pain (due to their location at the end of long bones), mimicking symptoms of far more common processes, and their initially subtle radiographic findings may lead to a prolonged course prior to diagnosis. Although they may occur in numerous bones, their most common locations are the proximal humerus, distal femur, and proximal tibia.

Radiograph appearance can be subtle, since its immature cartilage usually does not cause the calcification seen so characteristically with hyaline cartilage lesions. Furthermore, the subtle epiphyseal round radiolucency of chondroblastoma is not usually surrounded by an obvious sclerotic rim. Easier to recognize on MRI, chondroblastoma is dark on T1W and bright on T2W images and shows extensive perilesional edema. Bone scans are hot at the site of the lesion.

Chondroblastoma histology shows a preponderance of rounded cells with distinct folded "coffee-bean" nuclei arranged in a pseudolobulated "cobblestone" pattern of organization. Giant cells and chondroid matrix may also be seen.

Treatment of chondroblastoma must take into account the fact that while it usually behaves only as an active lesion, it may also behave in an aggressive fashion. An extended intralesional curettage is indicated. Chondroblastoma is also one of two benign bone lesions (along with giant cell tumor) that carry the potential to develop pulmonary metastases, so initial screening and subsequent surveillance of the lungs should be considered.

Chondromyxoid Fibroma ■ Like chondroblastoma, chondromyxoid fibroma is a benign tumor of immature cartilage.[45] Unique from chondroblastoma, however, is the metaphyseal eccentric location in long bones, often immediately adjacent to

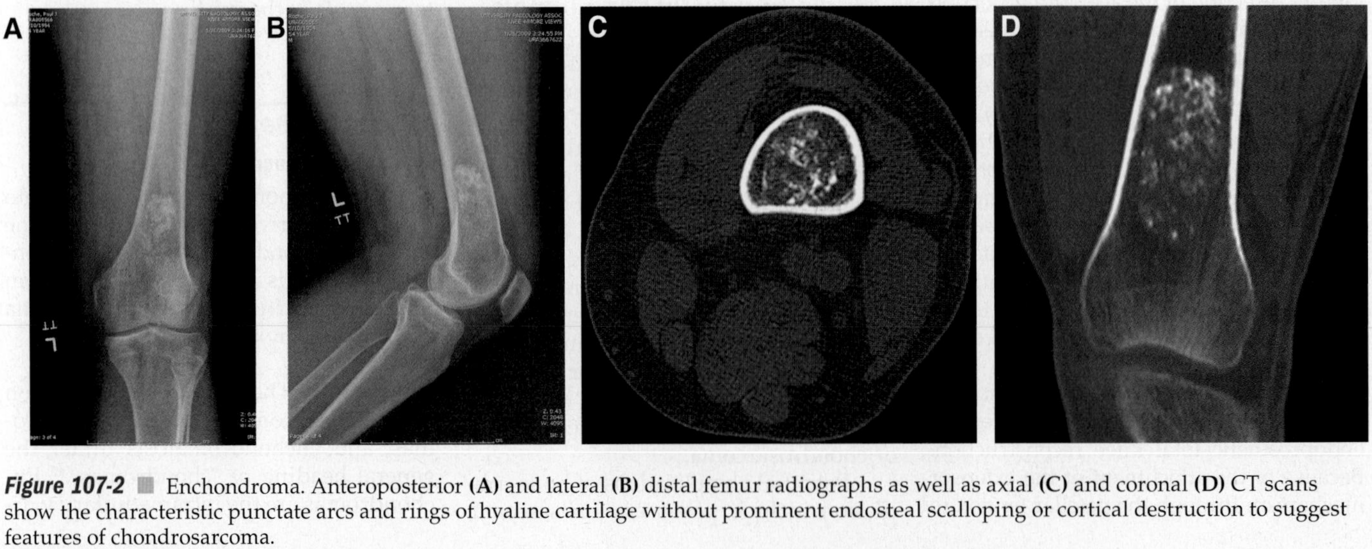

Figure 107-2 ■ Enchondroma. Anteroposterior **(A)** and lateral **(B)** distal femur radiographs as well as axial **(C)** and coronal **(D)** CT scans show the characteristic punctate arcs and rings of hyaline cartilage without prominent endosteal scalloping or cortical destruction to suggest features of chondrosarcoma.

the growth plate. It is a rare tumor, representing less than 1% of bone tumors. The most common long bone involved is the tibia. One-third of these tumors occur in flat bones. Chondromyxoid fibromas usually present with pain.

Radiographic features of chondromyxoid fibroma include its eccentric metaphyseal location, lytic lobulated, soap-bubble appearance usually without matrix mineralization, and associated cortical thinning. In some cases, the appearance may be of an aggressive tumor, with cortical breakthrough and even soft-tissue extension (Fig. 107-3). Under the microscope, the tumor is arranged in lobules, which are more cellular around the periphery than the sparsely cellular myxoid center. The characteristic cells are "stellate" in shape.

Treatment is typically by curettage and grafting. Local recurrence rates range from 15% to 25%. Chondromyxoid fibromas do not metastasize.

Osteochondroma ■ The most common tumor of bone, osteochondroma, is an exophytic growth of physeal cartilage away from the growth plate and joint but paralleling the temporal course of long bone growth.[46] As the cartilage grows, it leaves behind either a sessile or pedunculated bony prominence. These tumors form and grow during the period of skeletal immaturity, cease growing at or around the time of skeletal maturity, and remain throughout a patient's life unless excised. They may present as a painless mass or with pain. Pain is usually from irritation of the overlying soft-tissues or bursitis, but may also result from fracture of the stalk or malignant degeneration. Malignant degeneration is rare in solitary osteochondromas, but it occurs somewhat more commonly in patients with the hereditary form (see Congenital Syndrome section).

Osteochondromas may be diagnosed radiographically with confidence. They are an exophytic metaphyseal projection characterized by continuity of the cortical and underlying medullary bone. When they have a stalk, the cap of the osteochondroma is directed away from the nearest joint. MRI is sometimes used to assess the thickness of the cartilage cap, which may be up to 3 cm in children. In adults, however, the cap should be less than 1.5 cm; thicker caps should cause suspicion for chondrosarcoma arising from the underlying osteochondroma. Under the microscope, osteochondromas have a benign hyaline cartilage cap overlying normal trabecular bone.

Treatment of osteochondromas is based on symptoms and clinical presentation. When they are asymptomatic, they may be observed. When they are painful in children, they may be excised, but the older the child and the farther away from the growth plate, the lower the risk of recurrence. In adults, any symptomatic or enlarging osteochondroma should be investigated further with an MRI to make sure that it has not developed into a chondrosarcoma.[46]

■ Fibrous Tumors

These three lesions are grouped together based on their histologic similarity in being comprised of fibrous tissue. In the latest WHO classification system for bone lesions, fibrous dysplasia and osteofibrous dysplasia are listed together under "miscellaneous lesions." Non-ossifying fibroma and fibrous cortical defect, being non-neoplastic lesions, are not included in the current WHO outline of bone tumors.[42]

Fibrous Dysplasia ■ The etiology of fibrous dysplasia has been identified to be a mutation of the GNAS gene, creating a developmental anomaly of bone formation. It is a relatively common bone process, which has its onset in children but may also be diagnosed in adults. The spectrum of clinical presentation is broad and depends upon age, number of lesions, and site(s) of involvement. Patients may present with incidental lesions, painful lesions, or pathologic fracture. Monostotic (solitary) fibrous dysplasia is most commonly located in the skull, followed by the femur, tibia, and ribs. Polyostotic lesions (less common than the monostotic form) most often involve the femur, pelvis, and tibia. The polyostotic form may also present as McCune-Albright syndrome (see Congenital Syndrome section) or Mazabraud's syndrome (associated intramuscular myxomas).

Radiographically, lesions of fibrous dysplasia usually present as geographic lytic lesions. In long bones, they are frequently described as "long lesions in long bones." They affect any portion of the bone (epiphysis, metaphysis, or diaphysis) and have a characteristic "ground glass" appearance of the matrix. In the proximal femur, extensive involvement may lead to a "shepherd's crook" deformity. Uptake on Tc99 bone scan is usually intense. Under the microscope, immature woven bone classically described as taking the form of "Chinese characters" lacks the osteoblastic rimming seen with osteofibrous dysplasia and is surrounded by bland appearing fibroblasts.

Treatment is based upon age, location, and symptoms. When the radiographic appearance is classic, asymptomatic lesions may be observed. For some symptomatic lesions, curettage and grafting may be done, but structural bone graft is usually preferred, as particulate graft materials are usually resorbed. Prophylactic stabilization is often considered in the proximal femur, where the disorganized trabecular bone of fibrous dysplasia predisposes to stress fracture and remodeling. For symptomatic patients with polyostotic fibrous dysplasia, bisphosphonates have been used with some success.[47]

Non-Ossifying Fibroma and Fibrous Cortical Defect ■ Non-ossifying fibromas and fibrous cortical defects are variants of a spectrum of developmental abnormalities of skeletally immature bone.[48] Fibrous cortical defects are smaller and generally confined to the cortex while non-ossifying fibromas are larger, extending into the medullary canal. They are so common as to almost be considered variants of normal. Fully 1/3

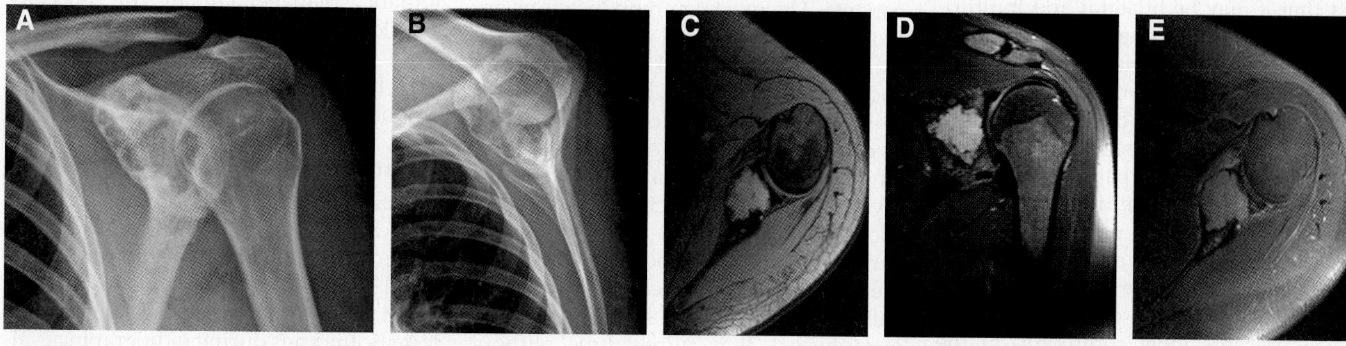

Figure 107-3 ■ Chondromyxoid fibroma. Anteroposterior shoulder **(A)** and scapular-Y **(B)** radiographs and T2-weighted axial **(C)**, coronal **(D)**, and proton-density axial **(E)** MRI images show the features of a chondromyxoid fibroma, in this case involving a flat bone, the scapula. Note the cortical thinning and focal cortical destruction that characterizes aggressive behavior and may lead to confusion with chondrosarcoma.

of children seen in the emergency room for knee injuries will show evidence of one or more of these lesions. They are almost always an incidental, asymptomatic finding. In the rare instance where they are discovered after a fracture has occurred through one, the characteristic history is the absence of pain leading to the time of fracture. This absence of pain underscores their latent nature without active features. The metaphyses of long bones are affected most frequently, particularly around the knee.

These lesions may be diagnosed with confidence on plain x-rays in nearly all cases. Their characteristic features are an at least partially intracortical, eccentric metaphyseal position, a soap-bubble lytic geographic appearance, and a thin rim of sclerotic bone around the periphery of the lesion. Magnetic resonance imaging, when necessary, shows a low signal center on both T1W and T2W sequences that is also characteristic. Perilesional edema is absent in the absence of fracture. Rarely, biopsy is needed to establish the diagnosis, and in those instances, the histopathology features a storiform, whirling background of fibroblasts with scattered giant cells.

Treatment of the vast majority of fibrous cortical defects and non-ossifying fibromas should be observation alone. The unusual associated pathologic fracture should be treated according to the location and type of fracture, combining curettage and grafting of the lesion when operative management is indicated.

Osteofibrous dysplasia ■ In the past, osteofibrous dysplasia has been referred to as ossifying fibroma and Campanacci's disease.[48] It is unique among fibrous tumors in its location (anterior tibial shaft almost exclusively) and histology (bone islands surrounded by osteoblastic rimming and separated by a bland fibrous background). It is almost exclusively a tumor of children, and most cases occur in patients less than 8 years old. It's restricted sites of occurrence within bones that have a relatively superficial location (tibia, fibula, ulna, radius) is distinctive, as is the fact that it may be bilateral and multifocal within a single bone. It should be distinguished from adamantinoma, a bone sarcoma that also occurs most frequently in the anterior aspect of the tibia. Clinical presentation of osteofibrous dysplasia is variable, with some patients noticing a painless lump over the tibia, others presenting with episodic pain from associated stress fractures, and rare patients developing progressive tibial bowing.

Radiographically, osteofibrous dysplasia presents most commonly in the tibia within the middle or proximal third in an eccentric anterior position with a lytic, soap-bubble or saw-toothed appearance. In older patients, there is radiographic overlap with adamantinoma, from which it must be distinguished. Unlike in adamantinoma, soft-tissue extension is not seen on MRI in osteofibrous dysplasia. As an active lesion, osteofibrous dysplasia shows increased uptake on bone scan. Under the microscope, osteofibrous dysplasia must be distinguished from both fibrous dysplasia and adamantinoma. While both osteofibrous dysplasia and fibrous dysplasia have woven bone islands within a sea of benign fibrous tissue, only osteofibrous dysplasia has osteoblastic rimming around those islands. The distinction from adamantinoma is that osteofibrous dysplasia does not show islands of epithelioid cells seen in the more aggressive condition.

Treatment of osteofibrous dysplasia varies according to age, symptoms, and radiographic appearance. Prior to closure of the growth plate, an asymptomatic and radiographically classic lesion may be observed. If stress fractures occur, bracing should be considered. When the radiographic features are atypical, biopsy should be undertaken to establish the diagnosis. Surgical excision with or without grafting is only indicated for progressive deformity or in symptomatic patients after skeletal maturity.

Giant Cell Tumors

Giant cell tumor of bone is a relatively common (5–10% of all bone tumors) benign tumor of bone characterized by its distinct histology and behavior.[49] It is one of four benign bone tumors (along with aneurysmal bone cyst, chondroblastoma and osteoblastoma) that have the potential to behave in an aggressive fashion. In addition, along with chondroblastoma, it is unique in its potential to create pulmonary metastases despite its benign designation. Because giant cell tumor typically behaves in an active or aggressive fashion, it presents clinically with pain, swelling, limited range of motion at the associated joint, and sometimes with pathologic fracture. It is a tumor of adulthood, peaking in young adults aged 20–40, and it is very unusual in skeletally immature patients. The most common locations are around the knee (distal femur and proximal tibia), wrist (distal radius), sacrum, and shoulder (proximal humerus).

Radiologically, giant cell tumor has its epicenter within the metaphysis of the long bones but almost always extends to involve the epiphysis, creating an eccentric radiolucency with moth-eaten borders that abuts the subchondral bone of the adjacent joint. In skeletally immature patients, however, the lesion is usually metaphyseal. It is purely lytic without matrix mineralization, and it may show radiographic signs of aggressive behavior complete with cortical destruction and an associated soft-tissue extension.

Local treatment of giant cell tumor depends upon location. In expendable locations, such as the proximal fibula or distal ulna, en bloc excision is appropriate. For most sites, however, the recommended treatment is extended intralesional curettage and either grafting or cementing of the defect. Extended curettage involves mechanical removal (curettes) combined with a high-speed burr and additional means of extending the margin (eg, phenol, liquid nitrogen, or laser). The local recurrence rate for intralesional curettage of giant cell tumor varies from 30% to 47% after simple curettage but is less than 25% with extended curettage. An integral part of the care of patients with giant cell tumor is assessment for potential pulmonary metastases and extended follow-up for early diagnosis of local recurrence. Recurrences have been described up to 20 years later.[49]

Hemangioma of Bone ■ The most common benign bone tumor of the spine, hemangioma of bone is a proliferation of blood vessels that may rarely be seen in other locations. The vast majority of hemangiomas of bone, particularly in the spine, are asymptomatic incidental findings, and the true source of any presenting symptoms should be sought apart from this tumor. Rarely, they may cause expansion of the bone or pathologic fracture. In the spine, these problems may cause neurologic compromise.

In the spine, the radiographic characteristics of hemangioma of bone are so typical that in the majority of cases, no biopsy is needed for confirmation. Radiographs show "jailbar" vertical striations. Axial CT and MRI scans show a "polkadot" pattern. On T2-weighted MRI images, hemangiomas show high signal; after contrast administration, these lesions enhance markedly. When radiographic features are atypical, biopsy will usually show variably sized benign blood vessels, but numerous histologic subtypes have been described. In non-spinal sites, appearances are variable, and biopsy is often needed.

Since most hemangiomas are asymptomatic, management in the majority should simply be observation. For the rare truly symptomatic lesion, consideration may be given to excision, radiotherapy, embolization, and sclerosing therapy.

Osteogenic Tumors

Enostosis ■ Enostosis, or bone island, is a localized region of dense lamellar bone within cancellous bone of the medullary canal.[50] Enostoses are uniformly benign latent lesions that are incidental asymptomatic findings during radiographic evaluation of other problems. They are most concerning when they occur in adults as part of the autosomal dominant condition osteopoikilosis, where they present as multiple lesions and must be distinguished from osteoblastic metastatic disease.

On plain radiographs and CT scans, enostoses are densely sclerotic areas within medullary bone that are distinguished by the lack of a central nidus (as seen in osteoid osteoma), radiating spicules emanating from the periphery of the lesion, and absence of uptake on bone scan (except in giant enostoses) (Fig. 107-4). They usually do not require biopsy, but under the microscope, the histology is that of mature lamellar bone.

No treatment is necessary. Once the diagnosis is established, nothing more than observation is warranted.

Osteoid Osteoma ■ A benign bone-forming condition that typically presents with a unique and distinctive pain pattern, osteoid osteoma is most common in adolescents and young adults.[51] The pain pattern is that of pain that is worse at night and relieved (in 70% of patients) dramatically and completely over a very short time course (20–30 min) with nonsteroidal anti-inflammatory drugs (NSAID's). Relief with NSAID's is theorized to be due to the beneficial effect these agents have on lowering the elevated prostaglandin levels known to be present within the nidus of osteoid osteoma. Osteoid osteomas occur with greatest frequency in the femur and tibia, but they are also one of the three most common tumors of the posterior elements of the spine (along with osteoblastoma and aneurysmal bone cyst). In the spine, they may cause painful scoliosis, where they are located in the concavity of the curve. In juxta-articular locations, they may cause an arthropathy, with associated effusion and synovitis.

The characteristic radiographic finding in an osteoid osteoma is the radiolucent nidus, which is less than 2 cm in diameter and usually surrounded by dense sclerotic reactive bone. The lesion is usually intracortical; appearing eccentrically in the bone, so the reactive bone may extend both into the medullary canal and also cause expansion of the bone externally. The reactive bone may be so dense that the nidus is only evident on CT or MRI evaluation. On MRI, the extensive perilesional edema associated with osteoid osteoma is characteristic. Osteoid osteomas are always intensely hot on bone scan. Histologically, the nidus of an osteoid osteoma is characterized by irregularly arranged seams of variably mineralized osteoid surrounded by both osteoblasts and osteoclasts within a vascular fibrous stroma.

Treatment of osteoid osteoma has evolved considerably over time. The mainstay of operative treatment currently is radiofrequency ablation (RFA).[52] Success of first-time RFA in eliminating symptoms is approximately 90%. When RFA is not feasible (spinal lesions close to nerve roots, juxta-articular or difficult to access sites), surgical excision of the nidus will eliminate the symptoms. However, the nidus is sometimes difficult to localize intraoperatively, and numerous techniques have been described. The third option is medical management with NSAID's, but the mean duration of treatment needed before the lesion ceases to cause symptoms is 2.5 years.

Osteoblastoma ■ Osteoblastoma shares a great deal of similarity with osteoid osteoma, and to a large degree, the primary distinguishing feature of osteoblastoma is the larger size of its nidus.[51] Similarities include their peak occurrence in adolescent and young adult patients, predilection for the posterior elements of the spine and their underlying histology. Differences include the absence of the typical pain pattern of osteoid osteoma, the potential for aggressive behavior, and a nidus of larger than 2 cm in osteoblastoma. In addition, a much higher proportion of osteoblastomas (up to 70%) are located in the spine, making the long bones an unusual site.

Radiological features are similar to osteoid osteoma but with a larger nidus that typically shows some faint calcifications. The microscopic appearance overlaps considerably with that of osteoid osteoma, showing irregularly arranged seams of variably mineralized osteoid surrounded by both osteoblasts and osteoclasts within a highly vascular fibrous stroma.

Because of its larger size and potential for more aggressive behavior than osteoid osteoma, treatment of osteoblastoma involves excision, usually by extended intralesional curettage. Recurrence rates range from 10% to 30%. Radiation should be reserved for recurrent lesions in difficult locations such as the spine.

Cysts and Other Tumors

Aneurysmal Bone Cyst ■ Aneurysmal bone cyst may occur as a primary or a secondary lesion.[53] Primary aneurysmal bone cysts are neoplastic proliferations characterized by gene rearrangements involving the oncogene USP6 and the promoter CDH11.[54,55] Secondary aneurysmal bone cysts occur in association with other primary bone lesions and do not carry the same chromosomal abnormalities.[55] Along with chondroblastoma, giant cell tumor, and osteoblastoma, aneurysmal bone cyst is one of the four benign bone tumors that have the potential to behave in an aggressive manner. Peak age range is from 1 to 20 years. They typically present with pain and sometimes with swelling and/or pathologic fracture. Anatomic distribution is predominately within the long bones, with the femur and tibia being the most common, but aneurysmal bone cyst is also one of the three most common tumors of the posterior elements of the spine (along with osteoid osteoma and osteoblastoma).

Radiographically, the classic appearance of an aneurysmal bone cyst is that of an eccentric, osteolytic, aneurysmal-like "blown-out cortex" surrounded only by

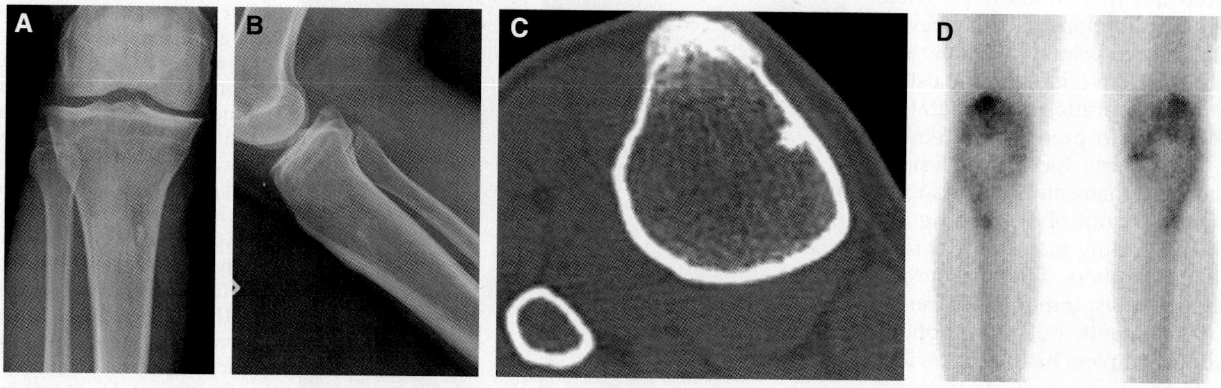

Figure 107-4 ■ Enostosis (bone island). Anteroposterior **(A)** and lateral **(B)** radiographs of the knee show an incidental small radiodense bone lesion. Axial CT **(C)** shows the characteristic radiating spicules that extend from the periphery of the sclerotic bone island and interdigitate with the surrounding bone trabeculae. As in this case **(D)**, there is usually absence of uptake on bone scan.

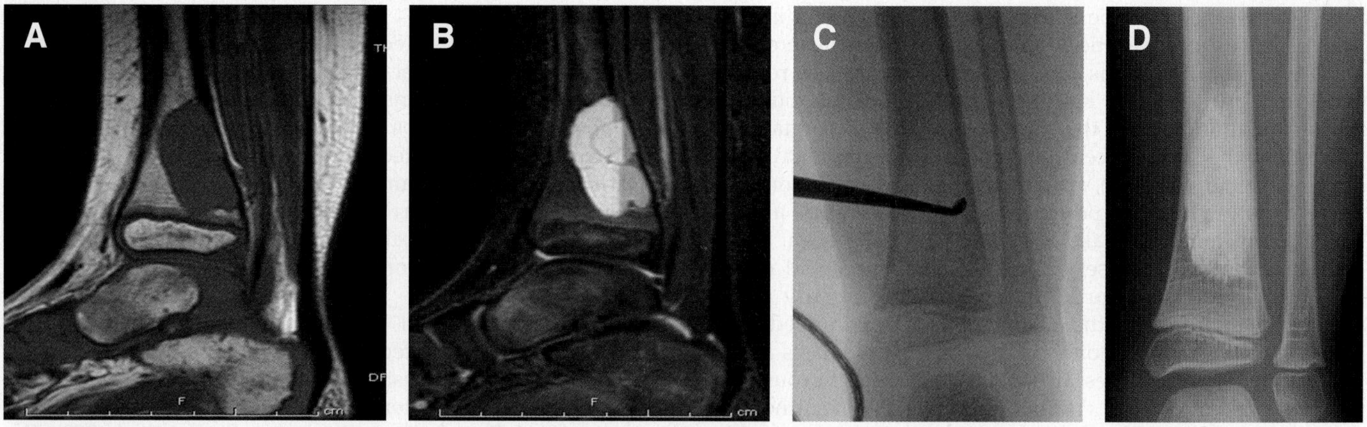

Figure 107-5 ■ Aneurysmal bone cyst. Magnetic resonance images of this radiolucent bone lesion that presented with pain in a 4 year old show fluid signal characteristics on T1-weighted sagittal images **(A)**, but the septations and fluid-fluid levels characteristic of aneurysmal bone cyst are best seen in this case on the T2-weighted sagittal images **(B)**. Intraoperative fluoroscopic images **(C)** show that this lesion does not show aggressive features seen with many aneurysmal bone cysts (ballooned out cortex). This lesion was curetted completely and filled with synthetic graft material **(D)**.

an "eggshell thin rim" of reactive bone. However, these features are not present in all cases, and the plain films may show an appearance that overlaps with other benign conditions such as simple bone cyst, non-ossifying fibroma, and fibrous dysplasia (Fig. 107-5). In those cases, MRI of aneurysmal bone cyst will show septations separating loculated regions filled with blood, manifest as fluid-fluid levels. The radiographic presence of these characteristic findings, however, does not clinch the diagnosis, and underlying primary lesions should be sought. Biopsy is indicated to establish the diagnosis and to distinguish from telangiectatic osteosarcoma, which has an overlapping radiographic appearance. The microscopic appearance of aneurysmal bone cyst is that of blood-filled lakes separated by bland fibroblastic septa with evidence of hemosiderin deposition and scattered giant cells.

Because of its potential for aggressive behavior and its highly vascular tissue, treatment of aneurysmal bone cyst is challenging, and the natural history is sometimes difficult to predict.[56] In most cases, an initial thorough curettage is preferred in order to allow complete histologic examination that may reveal other underlying primary lesions and to distinguish from telangiectatic osteosarcoma. Before curettage, consideration should be given to preoperative embolization, particularly for central lesions that do not lend themselves to intraoperative tourniquet control of bleeding. Intraoperative bleeding may be life threatening. Some authors have suggested embolization or aspiration/injection as definitive treatments, but these options do not allow complete histologic review. Local recurrences do not always progress in an aggressive fashion, so these may sometimes be observed closely. Low-dose irradiation should be reserved for incompletely excised, aggressive, recurrent lesions in difficult to access locations such as the spine.

Simple Bone Cyst ■ In contrast to aneurysmal bone cyst, simple (or unicameral) bone cyst is usually an inactive lesion and at worst an active lesion. Without a prior fracture, it is a single cavity within bone filled with serous or serosanguinous fluid. Most simple bone cysts are diagnosed during childhood and are located in the proximal humerus, proximal femur, or calcaneus. In young adults, they are more common in the calcaneus and ilium. Simple bone cysts are usually asymptomatic until fracture, and many present with pathologic fracture following minimal trauma.

Radiographically, simple bone cysts are usually centrally located within the metaphysis or metadiaphysis of a long bone, are purely radiolucent in the absence of prior fracture, lack prominent marginal sclerosis, thin and sometimes slightly expand the surrounding cortex, and may rarely demonstrate the pathognomonic "fallen fragment sign" after fracture. The fallen fragment (or leaf) sign is a thin wafer of cortical bone that is situated at the caudad aspect of the bone cyst because it passed through the fluid in the cyst to reach that position. MRI of simple bone cyst shows homogenous fluid signal within the lesion, dark on T1W and bright on T2W sequences. Peripheral rim enhancement without any central enhancement is the norm. In some cases after fracture, blood products mixed with the serous fluid may produce a single low fluid-fluid level, but the lack of septations and numerous fluid levels should distinguish a simple bone cyst. When aspirated, clear serous fluid is obtained unless there has been a fracture, in which case, the fluid can be bloody. After curettage, histologic findings reveal only a bland fibrous membrane with scattered histiocytes.

Treatment of simple bone cysts depends upon location, age, and presentation. In the proximal humerus, pathologic fractures should be allowed to heal first. Approximately one of seven simple bone cysts will heal after fracture (Fig. 107-6). If

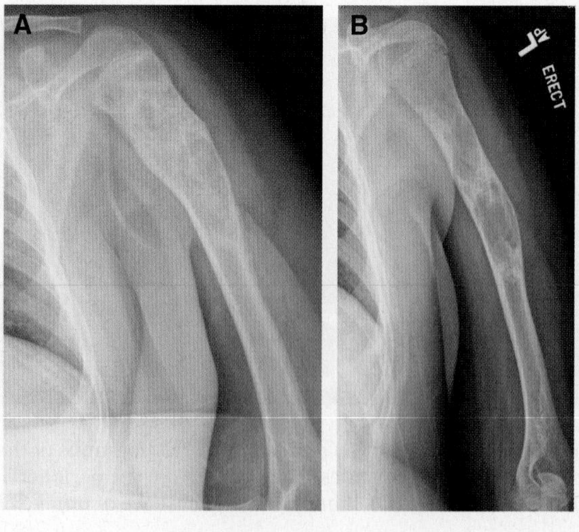

Figure 107-6 ■ Unicameral bone cyst (simple bone cyst). Plain radiographs of the left humerus of a 9 year old **(A)** who has incurred two prior fractures with minimal trauma through this lytic geographic proximal humeral bone lesion abutting the proximal humeral growth plate. At this point, there is evidence of healing within the cyst, which occurs in approximately 1/7th of simple bone cysts after fracture. However, 2 years later **(B)**, the cyst shows signs of recurrence, with increased radiolucency in the mid-diaphysis. Note that the proximal humeral growth plate has grown away from the bone cyst. These lesions are only active during skeletal immaturity.

the cyst does not heal with fracture healing, then definitive treatment options usually employ some form of aspiration and injection. Various agents have been used in the injection, including methylprednisolone, demineralized bone matrix, bone marrow, and combinations of agents, but none has been proven superior.[57] In the proximal femur, the risk of fracture through unicameral bone cysts is higher and the consequences potentially more devastating, so consideration should be given to open curettage and grafting here in order to prevent fracture. When a proximal femoral simple bone cyst has caused a pathologic fracture, open reduction and internal fixation of the fracture should be accompanied by curettage and grafting. In some locations, such as the calcaneus and ilium, observation may be elected if the cyst is asymptomatic, since pathologic fractures in these sites are very unusual. Regardless of the means of treatment, approximately 60% respond with progressive healing of the lesion. Partial healing may occur in another 30%, but 10% persist or recur. The natural history of simple bone cyst must always be borne in mind, as those in the typical locations resolve after skeletal maturity. Hence, the closer the patient is to skeletal maturity, the less aggressive the approach should be.

Langerhans Cell Histiocytosis ■ Langerhans cell histiocytes, the cells of origin of this disease entity, are a component of the reticuloendothelial system involved in phagocytizing foreign debris and originating in the bone marrow.[38] The group of disease entities encompassed by Langerhans cell histiocytosis includes solitary eosinophilic granuloma, Hand-Christian-Schuller disease (may include classic triad of multifocal bone lesions, exophthalmos and diabetes insipidus), and Litterer-Siwe disease (disseminated, often fatal form). The younger the patients at clinical presentation, the more likely they are to have disseminated disease, with most disseminated disease patients being less than 2 years, and most patients with eosinophilic granuloma being between 5 and 20 years of age. Solitary eosinophilic granuloma is more common in flat bones such as the skull, pelvis, ribs, and vertebral bodies; in the long bones, it occurs as a diaphyseal or metaphyseal lesion. In multifocal disease, the skull and jawbones as well as bones of the hands and feet are more commonly involved.

Clinical presentation varies depending upon the stage of the disease. Patients with solitary or isolated multifocal bone disease often present with pain localized to the site of involvement or a limp with involvement in the lower extremity, but the bone lesions may also be asymptomatic and discovered as incidental findings. Systemic manifestations of this disease spectrum may include diabetes insipidus, exophthalmos, fevers, infections, hepatosplenomegaly, lymphadenopathy, and papular rash, among others.

Radiological presentation is variable, and hence bone lesions in Langerhans cell histiocytosis are "great mimickers" (along with osteomyelitis), often simulating more aggressive processes including sarcomas (Fig. 107-7). They typically show a lytic appearance with permeative margination and soft-tissue extension, and they are often mistaken for Ewing sarcoma. In the spine, they create a "vertebra plana" appearance, with profound flattening of the vertebral body. On MRI, these lesions will also show considerable perilesional edema. Bone scan has a 30% false negative rate, so a skeletal survey should always be performed in patients with any form of Langerhans cell histiocytosis. Because of the overlap in clinical presentation with other entities, including Ewing sarcoma and lymphoma, biopsy is indicated in order to establish the diagnosis. Under the microscope, the characteristic Langerhans histiocyte (large, basophilic, coffee-bean shaped nucleus) predominates, often accompanied by numerous eosinophils.

Treatment of biopsy-proven Langerhans cell histiocytosis depends upon the stage and the symptoms, location, size, and number of bone lesions. Systemic involvement warrants consideration of chemotherapy. Low-dose radiotherapy is sometimes employed for vertebral lesions at risk for collapse. Surgical treatment may involve curettage alone, curettage and grafting, prophylactic stabilization, and aspiration/injection. Patients with solitary eosinophilic granuloma generally do well with little treatment, and in some cases, the bone lesions resolve after biopsy alone. Patients with systemic disease have prognosis inversely proportional to age at presentation and extent of involvement.

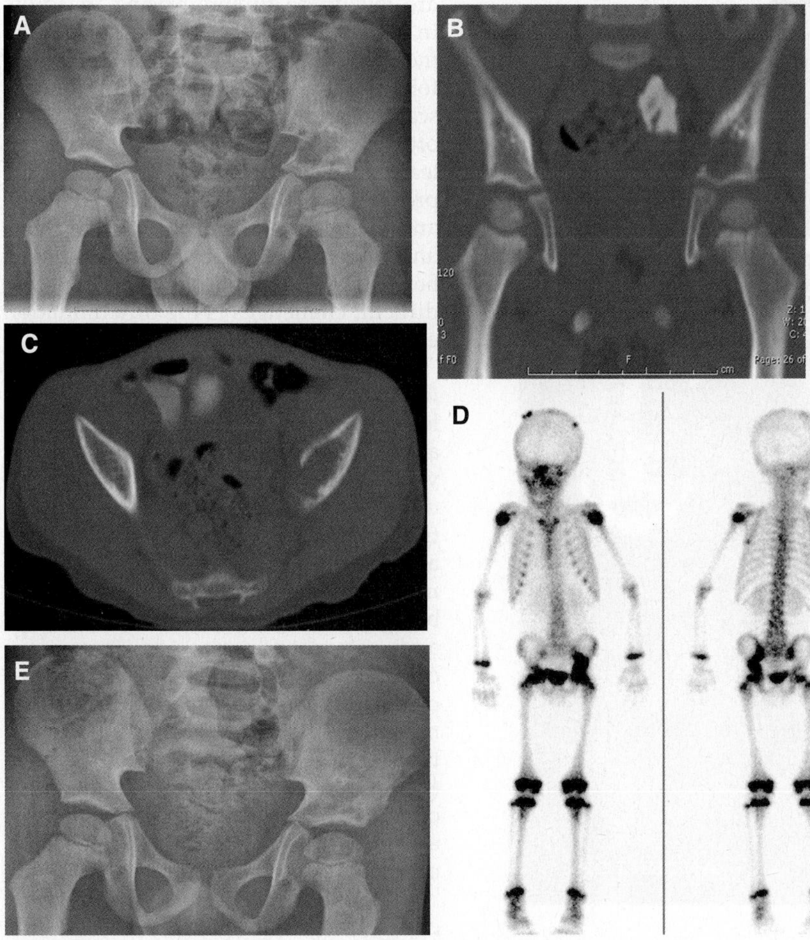

Figure 107-7 ■ Langerhans cell histiocytosis (eosinophilic granuloma). This anteroposterior pelvis radiograph **(A)** of a 4 year old boy shows a left supra-acetabular lytic bone lesion with moth-eaten borders. Cortical destruction seen on coronal **(B)** and axial **(C)** CT scans cause concern for metastatic neuroblastoma or Ewing's sarcoma, but biopsy showed sheets of Langerhans cells interspersed with eosinophils. Bone scan **(D)** showed increased uptake in this lesion, and a skeletal survey was done to exclude other lesions that might not show up on bone scan. In this case, there was only a solitary lesion and no visceral involvement. One year after biopsy and curettage, the lesion is less apparent on radiograph **(E)**, and the patient remains asymptomatic.

Primary Bone Sarcomas

Adamantinoma

An epithelial neoplasm, adamantinoma is a rare primary bone sarcoma of low-grade that is thought to be derived from ectopic rests of epithelial cells.[58] It represents approximately 0.4% of all bone tumors. Older children and young adults are most commonly affected, and 95% affect the tibia, particularly the anterior aspect, or both the tibia and fibula. The most common presentation is of progressive pain and swelling localized to the middle third of the lower leg.

Radiographically, adamantinoma is an eccentric destructive lytic process that usually destroys the anterior cortex of the mid-tibia and leads to an associated soft-tissue mass. The medullary border usually has a rim of sclerotic reactive bone surrounding the radiolucenct areas. On MRI, the lesion is dark on T1W and bright on T2W sequences with soft-tissue extension commonly and sometimes multifocal disease. Under the microscope, it shows a biphasic arrangement with epithelial groups of cells often forming glandular structures and surrounded by a background of fibrous tissue.

Treatment of adamantinoma is surgical and involves achieving a wide surgical resection of all involved bone and soft-tissue with a margin of uninvolved tissue. Although cure is achieved in 85% of cases, long-term follow-up is necessary, as these tumors may recur or metastasize years later.

Chondrosarcoma ■ Chondrosarcomas derive from chondrocytes, the cartilage cells that are crucial to bone growth and development.[59–62] Among bone tumors, they are relatively common, representing the second most common bone sarcoma. The vast majority of chondrosarcomas are low-grade tumors arising in adults in a wide variety of anatomic sites. The most common locations are the pelvis, followed by the femur, ribs, humerus, scapula, and tibia. Chondrosarcomas are often painful, and this symptom often leads to their discovery. Because of the prevalence of cartilage neoplasms of bone and the overlap in clinical, radiographic, and even histologic appearance between benign and malignant, one of the most difficult challenges is the differentiation enchondromas from chondrosarcomas.

Chondrosarcomas may be classified in other ways than grade. Specific histologic subtypes (clear cell, dedifferentiated, and mesenchymal) other than conventional low-grade chondrosarcoma are discussed individually below. Conventional low-grade chondrosarcomas may arise de novo as "primary chondrosarcomas" or in association with preexisting benign cartilage lesions (enchondromas and osteochondromas) as "secondary chondrosarcomas" (Fig. 107-8). Further, chondrosarcomas that arise within the medullary bone are "central" whereas those arising on the surface of the bone (periosteal/juxtacortical chondrosarcoma or secondary chondrosarcoma arising within a preexisting osteochondroma) are "peripheral."

On plain radiographs, conventional chondrosarcomas usually show the same sort of hyaline cartilage mineralization in the forms of arcs and rings that typify enchondromas. However, a number of features that accompany this mineralization pattern point towards a malignant diagnosis. These include cortical destruction with soft-tissue extension, progressive enlargement over time,

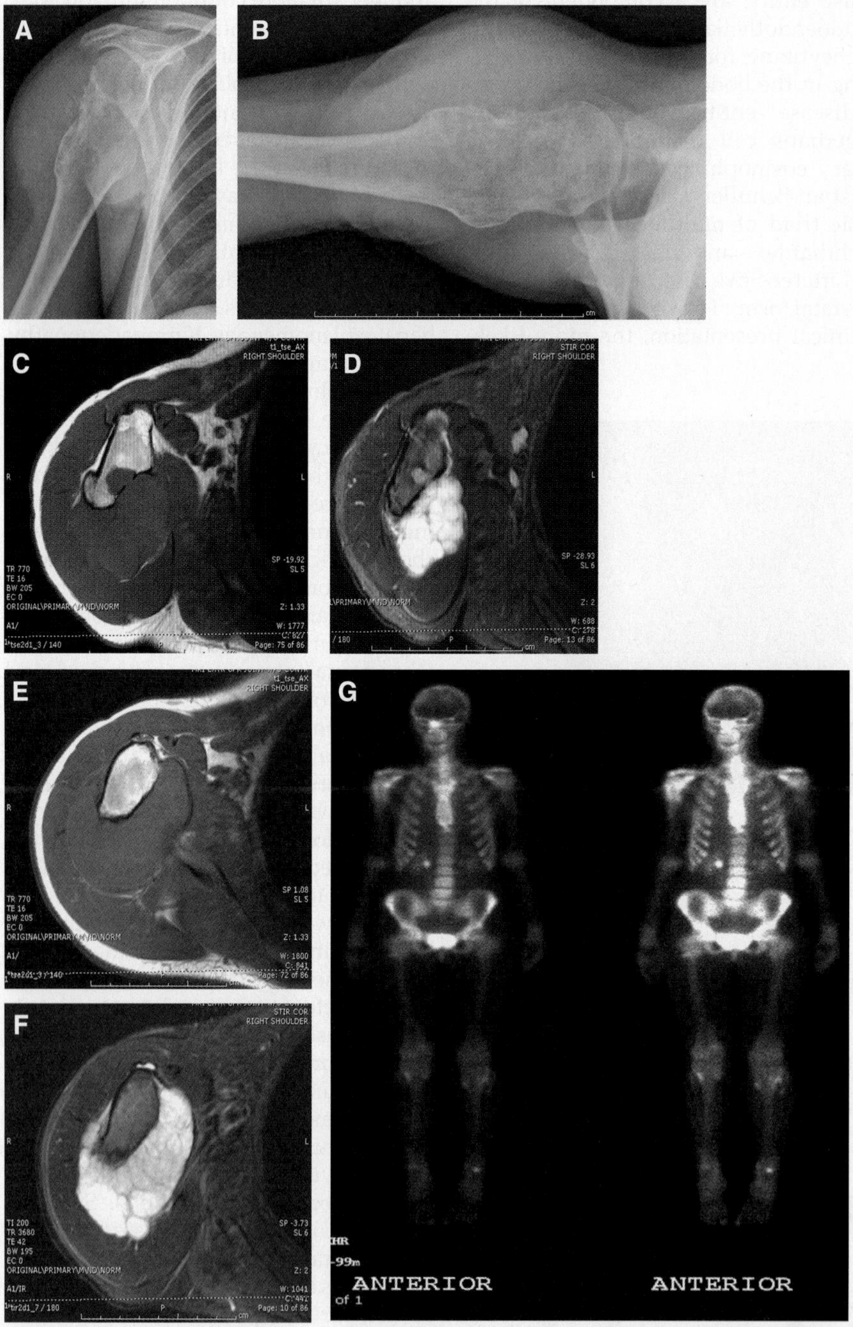

Figure 107-8 ■ Secondary peripheral chondrosarcoma. This 26 year old woman with underlying multiple osteochondromatosis developed pain and swelling in her right shoulder. Anteroposterior **(A)** and axillary lateral **(B)** right shoulder radiographs show numerous osteochondromas arising from the proximal humeral metaphysis but also a large soft-tissue shadow associated with the bone. In addition, particularly on the lateral view, there is cortical irregularity. Magnetic resonance axial T1-weighted **(C,E)** and T2-weighted **(D,F)** images show that there is a cartilage cap measuring more than 2 cm thick, indicative of a chondrosarcoma arising from the underlying osteochondroma and extending into the underlying bone as well. Uptake is noted in the right proximal humerus on bone scan. This patient underwent proximal humeral resection and prosthetic reconstruction.

cortical expansion and >50% endosteal scalloping, enlarging regions of radiolucency, and periosteal reaction. MRI may be more sensitive at showing soft-tissue extension and perilesional edema, but the pattern of being dark on T1W images and bright on T2W images holds true for both benign and malignant cartilage tumors. CT scan is often best at delineating the degree of scalloping and cortical destruction. Bone scans usually show increased uptake in any hyaline cartilage tumor, so they do not play a major role in distinguishing benign from malignant cartilage tumors. The classic histologic distinction between enchondromas and chondrosarcomas is the presence of "encasement" (hyaline cartilage lobules isolated and surrounded by rimming reactive bone) in enchondromas compared to "permeation" (cartilage tumor permeating around preexisting bone trabecular) in chondrosarcomas. In addition, increased cellularity, cytologic atypia, and binucleation favor chondrosarcoma. The anatomic site has to be considered as well. The histologic appearance of enchondromas arising in the hand or in the setting of Ollier's disease may have a malignant histologic appearance but nonetheless have a benign course. Overall, the histologic distinction between benign and low-grade malignant cartilage tumors is fraught with difficulty, and this process should always take into account the clinical presentation and radiographic features. In many hyaline cartilage tumors, a firm diagnosis may be established based largely on clinical and radiographic grounds.

Because of the large amount of matrix and relatively low cellularity, current treatment is usually restricted to surgical means. There is no standard role for either radiotherapy or chemotherapy in most low-grade chondrosarcomas. In recent years, there has been a shift to performing extended intralesional curettage with local adjuvants (phenol, liquid nitrogen, or laser) for grade I intramedullary chondrosarcomas rather than the classic treatment recommendation, which was to perform a wide resection of the tumor. However, this less aggressive approach has been limited to chondrosarcomas without soft-tissue extension and generally does not apply to grade II or grade III chondrosarcomas. Prognosis for chondrosarcoma is closely related to grade (Table 107-6). As with other predominately low-grade tumors, long-term follow-up is recommended.

Clear Cell Chondrosarcoma ■ Similar to conventional chondrosarcoma in being a low-grade sarcoma, clear cell chondrosarcoma has a distinctive location (the epiphysis of long bones) and histology (large cells with abundant clear cytoplasm in a cartilage matrix). The most common locations of this rare tumor are the proximal epiphysis of the femur, tibia, or humerus. Peak ages are 20–40 years. Pain is the usual presenting symptom.

Given its epiphyseal location, clear cell chondrosarcoma should be considered in the differential diagnosis of chondroblastoma but in older patients (since most chondroblastomas are in skeletally immature patients). On plain radiographs, clear cell chondrosarcoma is seen as a radiolucent lesion that extends to subchondral bone and can have an appearance very similar to that of giant cell tumor of bone. The large clear cells are distinctive under the microscope and the permeative pattern belies its malignant behavior.

Wide en bloc resection is the standard of care for clear cell chondrosarcoma. Prognosis is very good with appropriate treatment. Overall recurrence rate is approximately 15%.

Dedifferentiated Chondrosarcoma ■ Among chondrosarcomas, dedifferentiated chondrosarcoma is the most aggressive and carries the worst prognosis. By definition, it consists of a conventional low-grade chondrosarcoma adjacent to a region of high-grade sarcoma, often osteosarcoma. The most common locations are the femur, pelvis, humerus, ribs, and scapula. Radiographically, a lytic region developing within an otherwise typical chondrosarcoma may signify a dedifferentiated chondrosarcoma. Treatment for chondrosarcoma should be directed at the high-grade component, but the role for chemotherapy remains to be established, and prognosis is uniformly poor, with less than a 10% 5-year survival rate.[59]

Mesenchymal Chondrosarcoma ■ The rarest of all chondrosarcomas of bone, mesenchymal chondrosarcoma is a highly aggressive chondrosarcoma, which predominately affects teenagers and young adults. The most common locations are in the axial skeleton, and the tumor is usually eccentric. Under the microscope, mesenchymal chondrosarcomas show nodules of cellular chondroid tissue surrounding vascular spaces. As with most chondrosarcomas, surgery is the mainstay of treatment, although recent reports continue to explore the potential benefits of chemotherapy.[60] Prognosis has been reported as ranging from <30% to 52% 5-year survival.[63]

Chordoma ■ Chordoma is a low-grade malignancy arising from vestigial notochord remnants that exist in the midline of the spine. Following the distribution of those remnants, chordoma is a midline tumor involving the sacrococcygeal, spheno-occipital, and other mobile spine regions. Chordoma predominately involves adults, and in adults, the sacrum is the most common location. It is very rare in African-Americans. In younger patients, the skull is the most common location. It accounts for only 3–4% of all primary bone tumors. Clinical presentation is dependent upon location, although pain is usually a presenting symptom. In the sacrum, bowel, bladder, or sexual symptoms may be present. In the skull, cranial nerve deficits may be present. In the mobile spine, back or leg pain predominates.

Radiographs of chordoma may be difficult to interpret, as the findings of lytic destruction are often subtle in these anatomically complex sites. Only CT or MRI will show the extensive anterior soft-tissue mass that usually accompanies the bone destruction in chordoma. Under the microscope, chordoma is composed of nests or cords of physaliferous cells, distinctive large cells with bubbly vacuolated cytoplasm.

Treatment of chordoma involves wide surgical resection when possible, but irradiation improves the disease-free interval in patients with marginal or contaminated margins.[64] Chemotherapy does not play a role in this low-grade malignancy. Local recurrence is common (up to 70%), and overall survival drops from 75–85% at 5 years to 40–50% at 10 years.

Ewing Sarcoma ■ Overall, Ewing sarcoma is the third most common bone sarcoma after osteosarcoma and chondrosarcoma.[63] In patients 5–30 years old (the peak ages for Ewings), Ewings is second only to osteosarcoma. Thought to be derived from primitive mesenchymal cells, Ewing sarcoma is a poorly differentiated malignant small round blue cell tumor closely related to other tumors within the Ewings family of tumors.[65] The Ewings family of tumors includes Ewing sarcoma, PNET/primitive neuroecto-

Table 107-6 ■ **Chondrosarcoma Survival, Metastatic Potential, and Local Recurrence Rates According to Grade**

Type	5-Year Survival	Metastatic Potential	Recurrence Rate
Grade I	90%	0%	Low
Grade II	81%	10–15%	Intermediate
Grade III	29%	>50%	High

Source: Modified from Randall RL, Hunt KJ. 6.3 Chondrosarcoma. In: Damron TA, editor. *Orthopaedic Surgery Essentials: Oncology and Basic Science*. Lippincott Williams, and Wilkins, Philadelphia, PA (Table 6.3–4, p. 201).

dermal tumor, and Askin's tumor, all of which have translocations involving the EWS gene on chromosome 22. The most common locations are the femur and pelvis, but vertebral body and rib involvement is relatively common. Presenting symptoms usually include both pain and swelling, but in approximately 20%, the symptoms may be accompanied by fever and malaise. In 10%, pathologic fractures are present at diagnosis. Increased ESR is common, and some patients may also have anemia and leukocytosis.

Radiographically, Ewing sarcoma has a varied presentation depending upon the location. Within the long bones, it has a predilection of diaphyseal involvement, and onion-skinning periosteal reaction (numerous layers of reactive new bone a few millimeters apart formed as the periosteum is lifted off by the expanding tumor and repetitively forms reactive bone) is frequent, accompanied by permeative poorly defined borders, cortical destruction, and usually an associated soft-tissue mass. The radiographic pattern is almost always lytic. Under the microscope, Ewing sarcoma is a prototypical small round blue cell tumor and is difficult to distinguish from other such entities (such as lymphoma and metastatic neuroblastoma) without special studies. Immunohistochemistry is positive for CD-99 (the MIC2 protein) in 95% of cases. The most definitive test is demonstration of the t(11;22)(q24;q12) or similar translocation (t(21;22)) by fluorescent in-situ hybridization (FISH). Resulting fusion proteins that result from these translocations are EWS-FLI1 and EWS-ERG.

Treatment of Ewing sarcoma involves neoadjuvant multiagent chemotherapy for systemic disease and either wide surgical resection or irradiation for local disease.[65] Active chemotherapeutic agents in Ewing sarcoma include adriamycin, vincristine, cytoxan (cyclophosphamide), and actinomycin D. It has been chemotherapy that has led to the greatest improvement in survival. The latest trend is for increased surgical resection, but historically Ewing sarcoma has been considered a radiosensitive tumor. Radiotherapy is still utilized for unresectable central locations (some pelvic tumors, sacrum, spine, cranium), for metastatic disease, and as a surgical adjuvant if margins of resection are close or microscopically positive. Surgical resection has evolved from being used initially only for expendable bones (iliac wing, rib, fibula, proximal radius, distal ulna) to now being used more frequently for reconstructable anatomic sites (femur, tibia, humerus). There have been no randomized studies comparing radiotherapy to surgical resection in Ewings patients, and retrospective studies suffer from selection bias, as radiotherapy has traditionally been used for the worst centrally located tumors. Currently, some trials have suggested that the prognosis is as good as 65–70% 5-year survival, but based on minimum 5-year follow-up for 3225 Ewing's sarcomas collected in the National Cancer Database, 5-year survival was only 50.6% for Ewing sarcoma.[63]

Table 107-7 ■ **Osteosarcoma Variants According to Grade**

Low Grade	Intermediate Grade	High Grade

Low-grade intramedullary
Parosteal
	Periosteal	Conventional
		High-grade surface
		Secondary
		  Pagetoid
		  Post-radiation
		Small cell

Osteosarcoma ■ The most common bone sarcoma, osteosarcoma comprises a somewhat heterogeneous group of sarcomas that are predominately high-grade but with three low-grade to intermediate grade variants (Table 107-7). The common thread is that they are felt to be derived from the osteoblast cell line and are bone-forming sarcomas.[66,67] Ninety percent of osteosarcomas are conventional high-grade. Classically, the age distribution has been described as bimodal, but the peak age is during the second and third decades of life; cases in older adults usually occur in the setting of Paget's disease (Pagetoid osteosarcoma) or following irradiation (post-radiation osteosarcoma). Clinical presentation almost always involves progressively worsening pain and sometimes associated swelling. The most common locations reflect the most active areas of growth in skeletally immature patients … the distal femur followed by the proximal tibia and proximal humerus. Overall, there is a 1.5:1 male to female ratio.

Radiographically, osteosarcomas in general are bone-forming, relatively poorly defined metaphyseal tumors that frequently have associated soft-tissue extension accompanied by cumulus cloud type bone formation (Fig. 107-9). Some histologic subtypes, especially the fibroblastic and telangiectatic osteosarcomas, form radiolucent tumors without the classic bone formation. Telangiectatic osteosarcoma, due to its blood-filled lakes, can closely resemble a benign aneurysmal bone cyst (ABC) on imaging studies, so this tumor should always be considered in the differential diagnosis of an apparent ABC. On MRI, the tumor is dark on T1W and bright but heterogeneous on T2W sequences, usually shows soft-tissue extension, and may show skip lesions within the medullary canal. They show increased uptake on bone scan. Under the microscope, there is some variation, particularly between the low and high-grade variants, but the key element is malignant osteoid production. The most common histologic subtype is osteoblastic, followed by chondroblastic, fibroblastic, and—rarely—telangiectatic.

Treatment depends upon grade and extent of the tumor. For all high-grade variants, neoadjuvant multidrug chemotherapy is the key, and this involves adriamycin, ifosfamide, cisplatin, and methotrexate.[68] The advantage of neoadjuvant chemotherapy is that it allows determination of percent tumor necrosis after resection and often reduces the size of the soft-tissue extension of the tumor, facilitating surgical resection. Tumor necrosis >95% is strongly predictive of disease-free and overall survival. Drug resistance is sometimes seen due to the p-glycoprotein membrane bound pump (coded for by the MDR-1 gene), which pumps the chemotherapeutic agents out of the cell. Local disease is addressed by wide surgical resection. There is no role for radiotherapy in standard treatment of osteosarcoma. For low-grade central and parosteal osteosarcoma (the low-grade variants), treatment only involves wide surgical resection; neither chemotherapy nor radiotherapy play a role.

Features unique to the various clinicopathologic subtypes will be presented below.

Conventional Osteosarcoma ■ As the classic osteosarcoma, conventional high-grade osteosarcoma has the typical radiographic appearance of a metaphyseal tumor most common in the distal femur, proximal tibia, and proximal humerus. It usually demonstrates a cloud-like bone formation with permeative borders on plain radiographs and often has cortical breakthrough with an associated soft-tissue extension bordered by Codman's triangles (reactive bone formed by the bordering periosteum as it is lifted away from the bone surface by the expanding tumor) (Fig. 107-9).

Histologically, osteosarcoma is comprised of pleomorphic cells with frequent mitoses forming lace-like pink osteoid. Conventional osteosarcoma may show a predominance of bone formation (osteoblastic), chondroid matrix (chondroblastic), fibrous background (fibroblastic), or

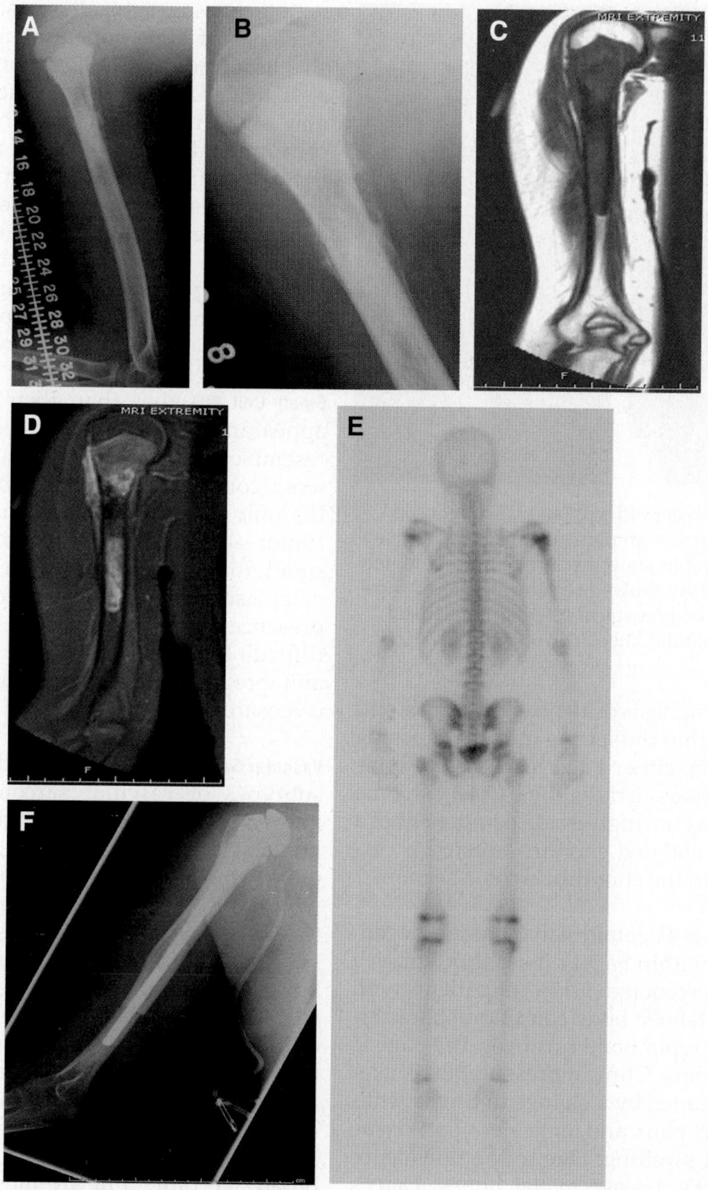

Figure 107-9 ■ Conventional osteosarcoma. A 13 year old girl with right shoulder pain and swelling has shoulder radiographs **(A-B)** showing a radiodense proximal humeral metaphyseal lesion with permeative borders and Codman triangle periosteal reaction and soft-tissue extension. Coronal T1-weighted **(C)** and T2-weighted **(D)** MRI images show the soft-tissue extension and extent of the tumor within the medullary canal. Bone scan **(E)** shows increased uptake in the proximal humerus. In a young patient, these features are nearly diagnostic of osteosarcoma, and a biopsy confirmed the diagnosis of high-grade osteosarcoma. After neoadjuvant chemotherapy, the patient underwent wide resection and proximal humeral allograft-prosthetic reconstruction **(F)**.

blood-filled pools (telangiectatic). Differentiation of chondroblastic osteosarcoma from chondrosarcoma and fibroblastic osteosarcoma from fibrosarcoma is based upon the presence of malignant osteoid.

Prognosis for osteosarcoma has improved considerably over the years due primarily to the use of multiagent chemotherapy. Clinical trials involving patients with non-metastatic disease report actuarial 5-year survival rates of 75–80%. For all comers, including all ages and those with metastatic disease, data from the National Cancer Database of the American College of Surgeons suggests a less optimistic outlook.[2] Based upon 8104 osteosarcomas cases with a minimum 5-year follow-up from 1985 to 1998, the relative 5-year survival rate for high-grade was 52.6%. For osteosarcoma patients younger than 30 years, the relative 5-year survival rate was 60%; for those aged 30–49 years, it was 50% and for those aged 50 years or older it was 30%. For the approximately 20% of patients with osteosarcoma that present with metastases, aggressive treatment leads to 5-year survival in 30–40%, but for patients who develop metastases after treatment, 5-year survival is only 15–20%.

High-Grade Surface ■ Although the other two surface osteosarcomas (parosteal and periosteal) are low or intermediate grade, this surface variant is defined by its more aggressive radiographic and histologic appearance and clinical behavior. Otherwise, the clinical presentation, demographic features, pathology, and treatment are identical to those of conventional high-grade osteosarcoma.

Low-Grade Intramedullary ■ Along with parosteal osteosarcoma, low-grade central intramedullary osteosarcoma is the only other low-grade osteosarcoma. In contrast to the two other low to intermediate grade osteosarcomas (parosteal and periosteal, respectively), this one is not a surface tumor; conversely, this is the only intramedullary low-grade osteosarcoma. A rare tumor, it represents only 1–2% of all osteosarcomas. Clinical presentation usually involves pain. The typical patient is slightly older than classic osteosarcoma, often being in the third decade of life.

Radiographically, the well-demarcated radio density that characterizes low-grade intramedullary osteosarcoma is often confused with fibrous dysplasia (Fig. 107-10). Under the microscope, the appearance is distinctly different from high-grade conventional osteosarcoma. Like parosteal osteosarcoma, low-grade central osteosarcoma is comprised of bands of osteoid trabecular separated by a hypocellular fibroblastic stroma with minimal atypia and rare mitoses.

As for both of the low-grade osteosarcomas, low-grade intramedullary osteosarcoma is treated by wide surgical resection alone without chemotherapy or radiotherapy. Overall prognosis is quite good, with local recurrences in only approximately 5% following appropriate surgery and a 90% 5-year survival rate, which drops, slightly, to 85% at 10 years. In rare cases, dedifferentiation may occur by way of an adjacent high-grade sarcomatous component.

Parosteal ■ The low-grade surface osteosarcoma, parosteal osteosarcoma is a distinct clinical, radiographic, and pathologic entity that accounts for 5% of osteosarcomas. Similar to its intramedullary counterpart, the peak age is in the third decade of life. Females are affected more commonly than males (M:F 1:2). Parosteal osteosarcoma has a strong predilection for the posterior aspect of the distal femur (80% of cases); the proximal tibia and proximal humerus are other relatively common locations. It usually presents as a painless posterior distal thigh mass that may decrease knee range of motion.

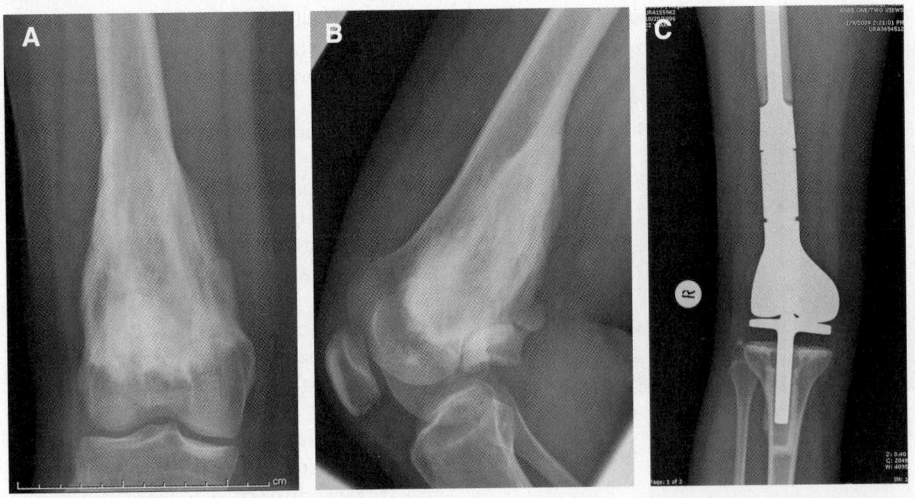

Figure 107-10 ■ Low-grade central osteosarcoma. This 26 year old woman was diagnosed with low-grade central osteosarcoma after a prolonged course with pain and swelling over several years. Plain anteroposterior **(A)** and lateral **(B)** radiographs show a sclerotic predominately intramedullary lesion of the distal femoral metaphysis. Biopsy showed streaming osteoid separated by a relatively bland fibrous background. Following wide surgical resection, the distal femur was reconstructed with a distal femoral replacement total knee arthroplasty **(C)**.

Radiographically, parosteal osteosarcoma usually shows a lobulated, fairly densely ossified mass that has the appearance of being "stuck-on" the underlying bony cortex. In unusual cases, the tumor may encircle the bone, and the underlying cortex may show reactive changes. Under the microscope, parosteal osteosarcoma looks like low-grade central osteosarcoma, with a sparsely cellular fibroblastic stroma between bands of osteoid trabeculae.

Treatment for parosteal osteosarcoma involves wide surgical resection alone; there is no established role for chemotherapy or radiotherapy. In rare instances, dedifferentiated areas may arise. Overall prognosis is 86% 5-year survival.[2]

Periosteal ■ Another surface tumor, periosteal osteosarcoma accounts for only 1–2% of osteosarcomas. Clinical presentation and peak age are the same as for conventional osteosarcoma, but it has a predilection for the tibial diaphysis and the femoral diaphysis. Radiographically, in addition to its diaphyseal surface predilection, periosteal osteosarcoma is characterized by mineralization, which may present as a sunburst periosteal reaction or patchy calcification reflecting it's often chondroblastic histology. Under the microscope, periosteal osteosarcoma is similar to conventional osteosarcoma except for being intermediate grade and usually having a chondroblastic pattern. Treatment usually employs conventional neoadjuvant chemotherapy followed by wide surgical resection. Prognosis is intermediate between parosteal and conventional osteosarcoma.

Secondary ■ Secondary osteosarcomas have a peak age in older patients, have the worst prognosis of all osteosarcomas, and arise within the setting of a predisposing condition, either Paget's disease of bone or previous irradiation. Osteosarcoma arising as the high-grade component of a dedifferentiated chondrosarcoma is discussed in the chondrosarcoma section.

Pagetoid ■ Pagetoid sarcomatous degeneration within Paget's disease occurs in a small percentage (1–15%) of patients with this metabolic bone condition characterized by rapid bone turnover. Peak age is 55–85 years. Clinical presentation is usually heralded by a change in the patient's baseline pain and/or a new soft-tissue mass or swelling. Due to the prevalence of Paget's disease in flat bones, Paget's osteosarcoma has a predilection for the scapula, pelvis, and ribs. Radiographic presentation is usually of an aggressive osteoblastic or osteolytic area arising within Pagetoid bone. Treatment involves chemotherapy—if the patient can tolerate it—and wide surgical resection. The benefits of chemotherapy in this group remain unproven. Prognosis is poor, with 5 year survival 5–18%.[2]

Post-Radiation ■ The criteria for defining post-radiation sarcoma is that the sarcoma arises within a previously irradiated area without a preexisting sarcoma of the same histologic type and that a latent period of at least 3–4 years has elapsed since the initial radiotherapy and the development of the sarcoma. Post-radiation osteosarcoma arises within previously irradiated bone and represents 70% of post-radiation bone sarcomas. Other pathologies include malignant fibrous histiocytoma and fibrosarcoma. Clinical presentation is that of swelling and pain arising within the previously irradiated region. Radiographically, post-radiation sarcomas of bone appear as an aggressive lesion within the previously irradiated field. Under the microscope, they may show the histology of high-grade conventional osteosarcoma, malignant fibrous histiocytoma, or fibrosarcoma. Treatment is by surgical resection and adjuvant chemotherapy when the patient can tolerate it, although the benefits of chemotherapy in this group are unproven.[69] Prognosis is extremely poor, ranging from 5% to 30% 5-year survival.

Small Cell ■ Other than their histologic appearance, small cell osteosarcomas resemble high-grade conventional osteosarcomas. Under the microscope, the only feature that distinguishes this tumor—comprised predominately of small round blue cells with indistinct cytoplasm—from Ewing sarcoma is the presence of osteoid, which is sometimes difficult to identify on biopsy. Treatment and prognosis are as for conventional osteosarcoma.

Vascular Sarcomas ■ There are three major subtypes of vascular sarcomas which may involve bone: hemangioendothelioma, hemangiopericytoma, and angiosarcoma.[70] Hemangiopericytoma, which has classically been included in this category, has been reclassified as a solid fibrous tumor in the latest WHO scheme.[42] These tumors represent a spectrum of disease, with hemangioendothelioma at the less aggressive end of the spectrum and angiosarcoma at the aggressive end. These are rare tumors, as a group representing less than 1% of bone sarcomas. Clinically, they have a broad age range but are most common in middle aged and older adults. As with most bone sarcomas, presenting symptoms include pain and swelling. Rarely, pathologic fracture may occur, more commonly with angiosarcoma. One-third of patients with vascular sarcomas will have multifocal disease, either "skipping joints" in a single limb or involving disseminated sites throughout the body. Any bone may be affected, but long bones predominate.

Radiographically, these tumors are typically lytic and destructive, but a combination of osteolysis and sclerosis may be seen. Soft-tissue extension is not usually seen in these tumors. Under the microscope, each tumor has a characteristic appearance with some evidence of rudimentary vascular channels. In hemangiopericytoma, the channels form "staghorn spaces."

Treatment of vascular sarcomas may involve wide surgical resection or radiotherapy. Hemangioendothelioma is a particularly radiosensitive tumor and may be treated primarily with radiotherapy. The role of chemotherapy for this group of tumors is not well established. For extensive or multifocal disease, radiotherapy has efficacy.

Metastatic Disease to Bone

The most common malignancy to affect bone is metastatic carcinoma. It is far more common than bone sarcoma or myeloma. The most common "osteophilic" primary tumors to affect bone arise from primaries of the breast, prostate, lung, kidney, and thyroid. Patients with breast and prostate cancer have usually had their primary cancer treated and then develop delayed metastatic disease to bone. Patients with metastatic lung carcinoma more commonly present with metastatic bone disease as the presenting symptom of their lung cancer. Patients with kidney and thyroid cancer may present with either concurrent or delayed metastatic disease. For a primary carcinoma metastatic to bone in a patient with no history of cancer, the most common sources are lung and kidney primaries. Metastatic carcinoma to bone most commonly involves patients older than 40 years. In patients less than 5, metastatic neuroblastoma predominates, and in older pediatric patients, rhabdomyosarcoma is the most common primary source. Presenting symptoms may involve pain, swelling, or pathologic fracture, but in some cases, the bone lesions are asymptomatic and are discovered on routine staging studies. In the spine, neurologic symptoms and even paraplegia may be seen. The most common sites are the spine, proximal femur, pelvis, ribs, sternum, proximal humerus, and skull. Metastases distal to the elbow and knee are unusual, and when they are present, the most common source is lung carcinoma.

Evaluation of bone lesions suspected of being due to metastatic disease involves a comprehensive physical examination, laboratory parameters, and a radiographic evaluation of common sites of primary disease. Since myeloma is often in the differential diagnosis of metastatic carcinoma in adults, serum and urine protein electrophoresis is often requested. Lactate dehydrogenase may be elevated in lymphoma, although it is nonspecific. Prostate specific antigen is usually elevated in prostate cancer. Renal cell carcinoma may cause hematuria. Standard radiographs of any involved bone, a total skeleton bone scan, and CTs of the chest, abdomen, and pelvis comprise the radiographic evaluation.

Radiographically, metastatic carcinoma may have a myriad of appearances. Some tumors, such as prostate metastases, are typically osteoblastic. Breast cancer metastases usually show a combination of osteolysis and sclerosis. Metastases from lung, kidney, and thyroid cancer are usually purely osteolytic. Bone scans usually show increased uptake at multiple sites, but solitary metastatic lesions are quite common, and certain very aggressive bone metastases, such as those from renal or thyroid carcinoma, may not show increased uptake. Pathology often falls into a general descriptive category, such as adenocarcinoma, squamous cell carcinoma, or poorly differentiated carcinoma. In these cases, immunohistochemistry markers are of greater importance in identifying the source (Table 107-8). Some tumors have specific histopathology patterns, such as clear cell carcinoma of the kidney, well-differentiated follicular carcinoma of the thyroid, and metastatic pigmented malignant melanoma of the skin.

Treatment of metastases can be viewed as systemic and local. Systemic treatment is directed both at the primary tumor (discussed in other chapters throughout the text) and at the mediator of bone destruction, the osteoclast. Bisphosphonates have become widely accepted in the setting of metastatic bone disease to inhibit the osteoclastic bone destruction. Operative management of metastatic carcinoma, myeloma, and lymphoma has been discussed in a previous section. Once bone metastases are diagnosed, prognosis is poor, but survival varies according to the underlying primary tumor (Table 107-9).

Table 107-8 **Examples of Immunohistochemistry Markers for Evaluation of Metastatic Disease to Bone**

Immunohistochemistry Marker	Primary tumor Source
Prostate specific antigen (PSA)	Prostate carcinoma
Thyroid transcription factor (TTF-1)	Lung carcinoma
Leukocyte common antigen (LCA)	Lymphoma

Table 107-9 **Common Primary Tumors Metastatic to Bone: Frequency of Bone Involvement and Survival After Metastases**

Primary Tumor	(%) of Patients That Develop Metastatic Disease	Patients (%) with Metastatic Who Have Bone Involvement Clinically	Median Survival After Diagnosis of Metastatic (Months)	Mean 5-Year Survival (%)
Breast carcinoma	65–75%		24	20
Prostate carcinoma	65–75%	30–40%	40	25
Lung carcinoma	30–40%	20–40%	<6	<5
Renal carcinoma	20–25%	15–25%	6	10
Thyroid carcinoma	60%	20–40%	48	40

Source: Data from Coleman RE. *Cancer.* 1997;80(suppl 8):1588–1594. Table from Damron TA. Metastatic disease (Chapter 8). *Orthopaedic Essentials: Tumor and Basic Science.* 2008, Table 8–2, p. 231.

Myeloma

Myeloma represents the most common primary bone malignancy. As it is covered elsewhere in this text, only the details related to bone will be presented here. Myeloma predominately affects adults aged 50–80 and has a propensity to affect blacks greater than Caucasians by a ratio of 2:1. Clinical presentation may involve pain, pathologic bone fracture, bone marrow failure (manifesting as fatigue and weakness from anemia, bruising and bleeding from thrombocytopenia, recurrent infections from neutropenia), renal failure, or hypercalcemia. A solitary plasmacytoma in the bone does not clinch the diagnosis of myeloma. Diagnostic criteria for myeloma include at least 10% plasma cells in the bone marrow, monoclonal protein in the serum (monoclonal gammopathy on serum protein electrophoresis) or urine (Bence-Jones proteins on urine protein electrophoresis), and end-organ failure (hypercalcemia, renal insufficiency, anemia, or bone lesions).

Radiographic manifestations of myeloma include single or multiple "punched-out" small lytic lesions sometimes coalescing into much larger lesions. Since 80% of myeloma bone lesions do not show increased uptake on bone scan, a skeletal survey should be considered to search for other lesions during the initial evaluation. Under the microscope, myeloma is comprised of sheets of plasma cells with large round, clock face, eccentric nuclei, and perinuclear clearing.

Bone lesions from myeloma are very sensitive to radiotherapy but for large lesions or those with pathologic fracture, surgical fixation is warranted. For surgical management of myeloma bone manifestations please refer to the earlier section.

Bone Lymphoma

Primary lymphoma of bone was first described as "reticulum cell sarcoma" and it is comprised of malignant lymphoid infiltrate within bone in the absence of concurrent lymph node or visceral involvement. Just about any age may be affected, and the most common locations are the femur, ilium, and ribs. Clinical presentation may include pain, an associated soft-tissue mass or pathologic fracture. Unlike diffuse lymphoma, these patients rarely have systemic symptoms.

Radiographically, lymphoma may be diaphyseal or metaphyseal and typically has a permeative, poorly defined border on plain films. Many cases are osteolytic, but in some cases, a sclerotic appearance may simulate osteosarcoma. Under the microscope, primary lymphoma of bone is a small round blue cell tumor, which requires immunhistochemistry in order to distinguish it from Ewing sarcoma. Ninety percent of primary bone lymphomas are large B-cell type. Immunohistochemical markers for B-cells include CD19 and CD20.

Treatment of primary bone lymphoma requires a multidisciplinary approach. Chemotherapy and radiotherapy play the primary role, with surgery reserved for biopsy, fracture fixation, and prophylactic fixation of impending fractures. Chemotherapy often involves cyclophosphamide, doxorubicin, vincristine, and prednisone (CHOP) and rituximab (monoclonal antibody against CD20).

Congenital Syndromes

A number of congenital syndromes either involve bone lesions, predispose to development of bone malignancies, or both. Some of these syndromes are covered in this section.

Enchondromatosis

Enchondromatosis may involve simply multiple enchondromas (Ollier disease) or the combination of multiple enchondromas with multiple soft-tissue hemangiomas (Maffucci syndrome). Both syndromes occur sporadically. Neither has a known cause. They are uncommon and are typically diagnosed in childhood. Radiographically, the enchondromas individually are not different from those of solitary disease. The most important distinguishing feature of these two syndromes is the risk of developing malignancy.

Ollier Disease

Multiple enchondromatosis carries up to a 20–30% risk of developing one or more chondrosarcomas. Hence, these patients should be followed on an annual basis for surveillance. The most common locations for chondrosarcomas in Ollier disease are the pelvis, proximal femur, and proximal humerus.

Maffucci Syndrome

Patients with Maffuci syndrome are also at risk of developing chondrosarcomas, but they are at increased risk of developing numerous other types of malignancies as well. In fact, the risk of malignancy in Maffuci patients approaches 100%. Common primaries include acute lymphocytic leukemia, astrocytoma, and gastrointestinal malignancies. Vigilant surveillance is essential for early diagnosis of these tumors.

Familial Adenomatous Polyposis

The early onset of multiple colorectal polyps characterizes this autosomal dominant condition caused by a mutation in the adenomatous polyposis coli (APC) gene. The only bone lesion associated with familial adenomatous polyposis (and the related Gardner syndrome) is osteoma. These lesions do not require specific treatment nor do they predispose to bone malignancy. The only malignancy associated with this familial adenomatous polyposis is colon cancer.

Polyostotic Fibrous Dysplasia, McCune-Albright's Syndrome, and Mazabraud's Syndrome

While most fibrous dysplasia lesions occur in a single location (monostotic), some involve multiple bones (polyostotic fibrous dysplasia). In addition, polyostotic fibrous dysplasia may be accompanied in 30–50% of cases by distinctive pigmented cutaneous markings with a "coast-of-Maine" irregular border, precocious puberty, or endocrinopathies, a syndrome named McCune-Albright (or Albright's syndrome). Rarely, fibrous dysplasia may occur in the setting of soft-tissue myxomas (Mazabraud's syndrome). The common etiologic thread for these conditions is the presence of activating mutations of the GNAS1 gene. Usually these patients are diagnosed in childhood or adolescence either with manifestations of their underlying bone disease (pain, limp, swelling, angular deformity, limb-length discrepancy, or craniofacial abnormalites), the characteristic skin lesions, precocious puberty, or one of numerous endocrinopathies (hyperparathyroidism, hyperthyroidism, Cushing's syndrome, acromegaly, diabetes, rickets, osteomalacia, hyperprolactinemia).

Radiographically and histologically, the individual fibrous dysplasia lesions are the same as those described previously for solitary fibrous dysplasia. Treatment should address any associated condition (particularly the endocrinopathy) as well as the bone manifestations. Since polyostotic fibrous dysplasia is more often associated with progressive deformity, particularly in the proximal femur, more aggressive prophylactic treatment—

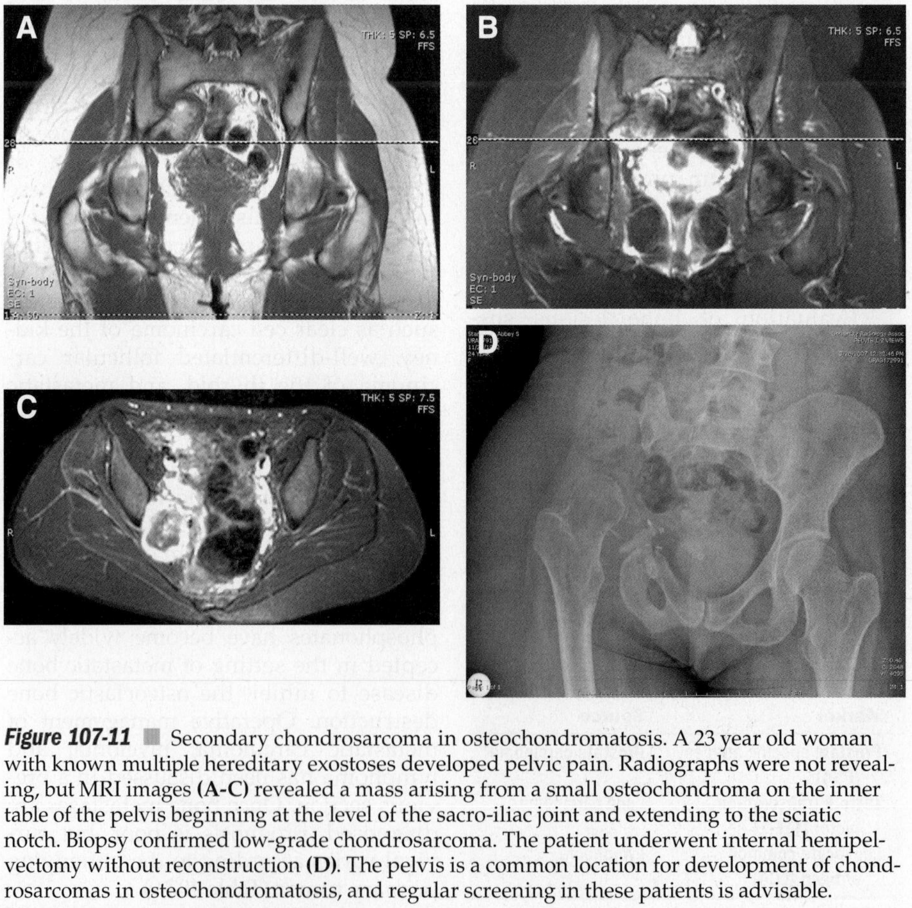

Figure 107-11 ■ Secondary chondrosarcoma in osteochondromatosis. A 23 year old woman with known multiple hereditary exostoses developed pelvic pain. Radiographs were not revealing, but MRI images **(A-C)** revealed a mass arising from a small osteochondroma on the inner table of the pelvis beginning at the level of the sacro-iliac joint and extending to the sciatic notch. Biopsy confirmed low-grade chondrosarcoma. The patient underwent internal hemipelvectomy without reconstruction **(D)**. The pelvis is a common location for development of chondrosarcomas in osteochondromatosis, and regular screening in these patients is advisable.

including surgical intervention and bisphosphonate therapy—should be considered. Malignancy in these conditions is rare and usually preceded by radiotherapy.

Multiple Osteochondromatosis

An autosomal dominant condition attributable to mutation of either the EXT1 or EXT2 gene, multiple osteochondromatosis (multiple hereditary exostoses) is rare compared to the solitary occurrence of osteochondromas, the most common benign bone tumors. The condition is usually diagnosed in early childhood between ages 2 and 10. Typical manifestations include "knobby" protuberances near joints, short stature, shortened limbs, coxa valga, genu valgum, radial head dislocation, and pain. Radiologic features consist of multiple osteochondromas, each of which has the characteristic features of a solitary osteochondroma. As for solitary osteochondromas, excision is recommended only for symptomatic tumors. Risk of malignant degeneration has been estimated at between 3% and 10% and typically involves a low-grade chondrosarcoma (Fig. 107-11).

Retinoblastoma Syndrome

Patients with a germline mutation of the RB1 gene are predisposed to develop not only retinoblastoma but also—via a "second hit" somatic mutation—other malignancies, the most common of which is osteosarcoma. Hence, this syndrome has also been referred to as "retinoblastoma/osteogenic sarcoma syndrome." Patients with retinoblastoma are usually diagnosed before age 3, and the potential for osteosarcoma peaks in the adolescent age range. Radiographic presentation, histology, and treatment of the osteosarcoma are the same as for conventional high-grade osteosarcoma, discussed previously.

Rothmund-Thomson Syndrome

This rare syndrome is important in the context of bone tumors because of its predisposition for development of osteosarcoma. An autosomal recessive genetically transmitted syndrome attributable to mutation in the RECQL4 helicase gene on chromosome 8, Rothmund-Thomson syndrome is usually diagnosed within the first 6 months of life based on a characteristic sun-sensitive erythematous rash that eventually leaves a hyper-pigmented and hypo-pigmented poikiloderma. Genetic testing confirms the disorder in a substantial number of cases, but related conditions such as Werner syndrome and Bloom syndrome should be excluded. Other orthopedic associated manifestations include osteoporosis, clavicular hypoplasia, syndactyly, patellar aplasia, genu valgum, and benign osseous lesions. There is no specific treatment for Rothmund-Thomson syndrome. High vigilance should be maintained to diagnosis musculoskeletal malignancies such as osteosarcoma.

Werner Syndrome

A syndrome related to Rothmund-Thomson syndrome by gene homology and clinical overlap, Werner syndrome (adult progeria) is another autosomal recessive disorder and is caused by mutation in the WRN gene on chromosome 8. The resultant RECQ helicase deficiency predisposes to development of a wide variety of malignancies, including osteosarcoma, although soft-tissue sarcomas, thyroid cancer, and melanomas are much more common. Diagnosis is not usually made until adulthood due to manifestations of premature aging (scleroderma, premature graying and alopecia, nonsenile cataracts, calcific valvular deposits, atherosclerosis, diabetes, and hypogonadism) confirmed by genetic testing and elevation of urinary hyaluronic acid level. Orthopedic associated conditions include osteoporosis, muscle wasting, calcific deposits, and pes planus. For patients with an established diagnosis of Werner syndrome, vigilance should be maintained for the early diagnosis of malignancy.

Selected References

The complete reference list can be found at www.CANCERMEDICINE8.com

1. Detailed Guide: Bone Cancer. What Are the Key Statistics About Bone Cancer? http://www.cancer.org/docroot/CRI/content/CRI_2_4_1X_What_are_the_key_statistics_for_bone_cancer_2.asp
2. Damron TA, Ward WG, Stewart A. Osteosarcoma, chondrosarcoma, and Ewing's sarcoma: National Cancer Data Base Report. *Clin Orthop Relat Res.* June 2007;459:40–47.
4. Enneking WF, Spanier SS, Goodman MA. A system for the surgical staging of musculoskeletal sarcoma. *Clin Orthop Relat Res.* 1980;153:106–120.
5. Heck, RK, Jr., Peabody, TD, Simon, MA. Staging of primary malignancies of bone. *CA Cancer J Clin.* 2006;56:366–375.
6. Mankin HJ, Lange TA, Spanier SS. The hazards of biopsy in patients with malignant primary bone and soft tissue tumors. *J Bone Joint Surg Am.* 1982;64:1121–1127.
8. Wolf RE, Enneking WF. The staging and surgery of musculoskeletal neoplasms. *Orthop Clin North Am.* 1996;27(3):473–481.
9. Lindner NJ, Ramm O, Hillmann A, et al. Limb salvage and outcome of osteosarcoma. The University of Muenster experience. *Clin Orthop.* 1999;358:83–89.
10. Gherlinzoni F, Picci P, Bacci G, Campanacci D. Limb sparing versus amputation in osteosarcoma. Correlation between local control, surgical margins and tumor necrosis: Istituto Rizzoli experience. *Ann Oncol.* 1992;3:S23–S27.
12. Damron TA, Morgan H, Prakash D, Grant W, Aronowitz J, Heiner J. Critical evaluation of Mirel's rating system for impending pathologic fractures. *Clin Orthop Relat Res.* 2003;415S:S201–S207.
13. Snyder BD, Hauser-Kara DA, Hipp JA, Zurakowski D, Hecht AC, Gebhardt MC. Predicting fracture through benign skeletal lesions with quantitative computed tomography. *J Bone Joint Surg Am.* 2006;88:55–70.
14. Townsend PW, Smalley SR, Cozad SC, Rosenthal HG, Hassanein RE. Role of postoperative radiation therapy after stabilization of fractures caused by metastatic disease. *Int J Radiat Oncol Biol Phys.* January 1, 1995;31(1):43–49.
15. Kelly C. Benign tumors of bone. In: Damron TA, editor. *Orthopaedic Essentials: Oncology and Basic Science.* Lippincott: Williams and Wilkins; 2008:54–60, Chapter 4.2.
16. Cammisa FP, Jr, Glasser DB, et al. The Van Nes tibial rotationplasty. A functionally viable reconstructive procedure in children who have a tumor of the distal end of the femur. *J Bone Joint Surg Am.* 1990;72(10):1541–1547.
17. Hanlon M, Krajbich JI. Rotationplasty in skeletally immature patients. Long-term followup results. *Clin Orthop.* 1999;1(358):75–82.
18. Hillmann A, Rosenbaum D, et al. Rotationplasty type B IIIa according to Winkelmann: electromyography and gait analysis. *Clin Orthop.* 2001;384:224–231.
20. Innocenti M, Delcroix L, et al. Vascularized proximal fibular epiphyseal transfer for distal radial reconstruction. *J Bone Joint Surg Am.* 2004;86-A(7):1504–1511.
22. Van Nes CP. Rotation-plasty for congenital defects of the femur. Making use of the ankle of the shortened limb to control the knee joint of a prosthesis. *J Bone Joint Surg Am.* 1950;32-B(1):12–16.
23. Ward WG, Sr, Yang RS, et al. Endoprosthetic bone reconstruction following malignant tumor resection in skeletally immature patients. *Orthop Clin North Am.* 1996;27:493–502.
24. Eckardt JJ, Kabo JM, et al. Expandable endoprosthesis reconstruction in skeletally immature patients with tumors. *Clin Orthop.* 2000;1(373):51–61.
25. Eckardt JJ, Safran MR, et al. Expandable endoprosthetic reconstruction of the skeletally immature after malignant bone tumor resection. *Clin Orthop.* 1993;297:188–202.
27. Hoffman C, Hillmann A, et al. Functional results and quality of life measurements in patients with multimodal treatment of a primary bone tumor located in the distal femur. Rotationplasty versus endoprosthetic replacement. *Med Pediatr Oncol.* 1998;31:202–203.
28. Damron TA, Rock MG, O'Connor MI, et al. Distal upper extremity function following proximal humeral resection and reconstruction for tumors: contralateral comparison. *Ann Surg Oncol.* April–May 1997;4(3):237–246.
29. Damron TA, Rock MG, O'Connor MI, et al. Functional laboratory assessment after oncologic shoulder joint resections. *Clin Orthop.* March 1998;(348):124–134.

30. O'Connor MI, Sim FH, Chao EY. Limb salvage for neoplasms of the shoulder girdle. Intermediate reconstructive and functional results. *J Bone Joint Surg Am*. December 1996;78(12):1872–1888.
32. Abudu, A, Grimer RJ, Cannon SR, Carter SR. Surgical complications and functional results of prosthetic reconstruction of the pelvis. In: *Proceedings of the 8th International Symposium on Limb Salvage*, Florence 1995:66.
33. Chao EYS, Sim FH. Composite fixation of salvage prostheses for the hip and knee. *Clin Orthop*. 1992;276:91–101.
34. Malkani AL, Sim FH, Chao EYS. Custom-made segmental femoral replacement prosthesis in revision total hip arthroplasty. *Orthop Clin North Am*. 1993;24:727–733.
36. Malawer MM, Chou LB. Prosthetic survival and clinical results with use of large-segment replacements in the treatment of high-grade bone sarcomas. *J Bone Joint Surg Am*. 1995;77:1154–1165.
37. Bini SA, Johnston JO, Martin DL. Compliant prestress fixation in tumor prostheses: interface retrieval data. *Orthopedics*. July 2000;23(7):707–711; discussion 711–712.
38. Azouz EM, Saigal G, Rodriguez MM, et al. Langerhans' cell histiocytosis: pathology, imaging and treatment of skeletal involvement. *Pediatr Radiol*. 2005;35:103–115.
39. Sheppard DG, Libshitz HI. Post-radiation sarcomas: a review of the clinical and imaging features in 63 cases. *Clin Radiol*. January 2001;56(1):22–29.
40. Cannon CP, Lin PP, Lewis VO, Yasko AW. Management of radiation-associated fractures. *J Am Acad Orthop Surg*. September 2008;16(9):541–549.
41. Body JJ. Bisphosphonates for malignancy-related bone disease: current status, future developments. *Support Care Cancer*. May 2006;14(5):408–418.
42. Fletcher CDM, Unni KK, Mertens F. *World Health Organization Classification of Tumours. Pathology and Genetics. Tumours of Soft Tissue and Bone*. Lyon, France: IARC Press; 2002.
43. Levy JC, Temple HT, Mollabashy A, et al. The causes of pain in benign solitary enchondromas of the proximal humerus. *Clin Orthop Relat Res*. 2005:181–186.
44. Springfield DS, Capanna R, Gherlinzoni F, et al. Chondroblastoma: a review of seventy cases. *J Bone Joint Surg [Am]*. 1985;67:748–755.
45. Wu CT, Inwards CY, O'Laughlin S, et al. Chondromyxoid fibroma of bone: a clinicopathologic review of 278 cases. *Hum Pathol*. 1998;29:438–446.
47. Lane JM, Khan SN, O'Connor WJ, et al. Bisphosphonate therapy in fibrous dysplasia. *Clin Orthop Relat Res*. 2001;382:6–12.
48. Marks KE, Bauer TW. Fibrous tumors of bone. *Orthop Clin North Am*. 1989;20(3):377–393.
49. O'Donnell RJ, Springfield DS, Morwani HK, et al. Recurrence of giant cell tumors of the long bones after curettage and packing with cement. *J Bone Joint Surg [Am]*. 1994;76(12):1827–1833.
51. Greenspan A. Benign bone-forming lesions: osteoma, osteoid osteoma, and osteoblastoma. Clinical, imaging, pathologic, and differential considerations. *Skel Radiol*. 1993;22:485–500.
52. Rimondi E, Bianchi G, Malaguti MC, et al. Radiofrequency thermoablation of primary non-spinal osteoid osteoma: optimization of the procedure. *Eur Radiol*. 2005;15:1393–1399.
53. Ramirez AR, Stanton RP. Aneurysmal bone cyst in 29 children. *J Pediatr Orthop*. 2002;22(4):533–539.
54. Oliveira AM, Perez-Atayde AR, Dal Cin P, et al. Aneurysmal bone cyst variant translocations upregulate USP6 transcription by promoter swapping with the ZNF9, COL1A1, TRAP150, and OMD genes. *Oncogene*. May 12, 2005;24(21):3419–3426.
55. Oliveira AM, Perez-Atayde AR, Inwards CY, et al. USP6 and CDH11 oncogenes identify the neoplastic cell in primary aneurysmal bone cyst and are absent in so-called secondary aneurysmal bone cysts. *Am J Pathol*. November 2004;165(5):1773–1780.
56. Papagelopoulos PJ, Choudhury SN, Frassica FJ, et al. Treatment of aneurysmal bone cysts of the pelvis and sacrum. *J Bone Joint Surg [Am]*. 2001;83(11):1674–1681.
57. Wright JG, Yandow S, Donaldson S, Marley L, Simple Bone Cyst Trial Group. A randomized clinical trial comparing intralesional bone marrow and steroid injections for simple bone cysts. *J Bone Joint Surg Am*. April 2008;90(4):722–730.
58. Keeney GL, Unni KK, Beabout JW, Pritchard DJ. Adamantinoma of long bones: a clinicopathologic study of 85 cases. *Cancer*. 1989;64:730–737.
59. Chow WA. Update on chondrosarcomas. *Curr Opin Oncol*. July 2007;19(4):371–376.
60. Gelderblom H, Hogendoorn PC, Dijkstra SD, et al. The clinical approach towards chondrosarcoma. *Oncologist*. March 2008;13(3):320–329.
61. Seo SW, Remotti F, Lee FY. Chondrosarcoma of bone. In: Schwartz HS, editor. *Orthopaedic Knowledge Update: Musculoskeletal Tumors 2*. Chicago, IL: AAOS; 2007:185–195.
63. Damron TA, Ward WG, Stewart A. Osteosarcoma, chondrosarcoma, and Ewing's sarcoma: National Cancer Data Base Report. *Clin Orthop Relat Res*. June 2007;459:40–47.
64. Fuchs B, Dickey ID, Yaszemski MJ, Inwards CY, Sim FH. Operative management of sacral chordoma. *J Bone Joint Surg*. 2005;87: 2211–2216.
66. Klein MJ, Kenan S, et al. Osteosarcoma. Clinical and pathological considerations. *Orthop Clin North Am*. 1989;20(3):327–345.
67. Gibbs CP, Weber KL, Scarborough MT. Malignant bone tumors. *JBJS*. 83-A, 2001;Num 11:1728–1745.
68. Benjamin R, Chawla S, et al. Preoperative chemotherapy for osteosarcoma: a treatment approach facilitating limb salvage with major prognostic indications. In: Jones S, Salmon S, editors. *Adjuvant Therapy of Cancer IV*. Philadelphia: Grune and Stratton; 1984:601–610.
69. Lewis VO, Raymond K, Mirza AN, Lin P, Yasko AW. Outcome of postradiation osteosarcoma does not correlate with chemotherapy response. *Clin Orthop Relat Res*. 2006;450:60–66.

108 Soft Tissue Sarcomas

Peter W.T. Pisters, MD, FACS ▪ Brian O'Sullivan, MD, FRCPI ▪ Robert G. Maki, MD, PhD

Sarcomas of nonosseous tissues, known traditionally as soft tissue sarcomas (STS), comprise a group of relatively rare malignancies that exhibit tremendous diversity of anatomic site and histopathologic characteristics. These tumors share a common embryologic origin, arising primarily from mesodermal tissues. The notable exceptions are sarcomas of the neural tissues and possibly the Ewing sarcoma/primitive neuroectodermal tumor (PNET) family of tumors, which are believed to arise from ectodermal tissues. Despite the fact that the somatic nonosseous tissues account for as much as 75% of total body weight, primary neoplasms of these connective tissues are comparatively rare, accounting for 1% of adult malignancies and 15% of pediatric malignancies. About 10,700 new cases of STS are diagnosed in the United States each year, with 3,800 deaths annually.[1] Despite their rarity, a thorough understanding of these tumors is important because patients' outcomes might be compromised if initial management is anything less than ideal. Furthermore, biologic insights about sarcomas are providing new strategies for the detection, treatment, and prevention of other, more common malignancies.

This chapter reviews current concepts in the diagnosis, staging, and multidisciplinary management of patients with sarcomas of nonosseous tissues. The evolving contributions of molecular biology and basic scientific principles underlying the varied differentiation and clinical behavior of these tumors will also be reviewed. Although histopathologic aspects of sarcomas are increasingly important in categorizing these tumors, the anatomic site of primary disease remains an important variable on which treatment and outcome may depend. Extremity sarcomas account for approximately 50% of all sarcomas and are the focus of the therapy sections of the chapter. Retroperitoneal sarcomas (RPS), gastrointestinal stromal tumors (GIST), and dermatofibrosarcoma protuberans (DFSP) are addressed separately later in the chapter. Sarcomas at other anatomic sites are not discussed because of their rarity. Throughout the chapter, the emphasis is on identifying what is known from definitive data and what requires additional research.

Etiology

The causes of sarcoma remain obscure in the vast majority of cases. The conceptual frameworks that address the neoplastic transformation of mesenchymal stem cells are in rapid evolution owing to new insights from the molecular analysis of sarcomatous and normal tissues from STS patients and family members. Genetics and environmental factors each appear to play a role in the neoplastic transformation of soft tissues into sarcomas.

It has been recognized for more than 30 years that sarcomas can arise in persons with certain genetic predispositions to cancer development. One of the earliest observations of familial cancer development (ie, genetically transmitted predisposition to malignancy) was the development of sarcoma and other tumor types (such as breast cancer) in certain families.[2,3] This autosomal dominant genetic predisposition has now become known as the Li-Fraumeni syndrome, and it has been characterized at the molecular level as a germline mutation of the *TP53* gene, which presumably acts in this context as a faulty tumor suppressor.[4,5]

Other genetic disorders are also associated with an increased risk of developing certain types of sarcoma. The best studied example of this is the predilection of patients with neurofibromatoses to develop malignant peripheral nerve sheath tumors (MPNSTs, also referred to as neurofibrosarcomas or malignant schwannomas).[6] Type 1 neurofibromatosis (von Recklinghausen disease) is an autosomal dominant disease that can disrupt the function of the *NF1* gene, located on chromosome 17q11.2. The endogenous function of the *NF1* gene product, neurofibromin, is incompletely understood, but it appears to act as a tumor suppressor via stimulation of guanosine triphosphatase activity. This, in turn, may control *ras* oncogene signaling pathways. Common mutations in *NF1* include truncations, with loss of function leading to uncontrolled signaling through *ras* pathways.[7-9] This may be a fundamental process that facilitates the development of MPNSTs over time in patients with neurofibromatosis. Patients with type 1 neurofibromatosis have up to a 10% cumulative lifetime risk of developing sarcoma (usually MPNST).[10]

Survivors of childhood retinoblastoma have also been noted to have an increased risk of sarcoma development later in life. This provides yet another molecular model of a dysfunctional or deleted tumor suppressor genetic element (in this case, the product of the *Rb* gene on chromosome 13q14).[11-16] The risk of STS in retinoblastoma patients and their families is accompanied by the risk of developing several other types of neoplasms, including osteosarcomas, breast cancer, and lung cancer. No reasons have been convincingly posited for the development of one type of malignancy over another in patients with *Rb* mutations, and this remains an important question to be addressed by future research on mechanisms of neoplastic transformation.

Gardner syndrome represents an important genetic connection between dysfunctional regulation of epithelial and of mesenchymal cells. Gardner's syndrome represents a subset of familial adenomatous polyposis disorders of the bowel (usually the colon); patients with the syndrome also have extracolonic abnormalities such as epidermoid cysts and osteomas. The molecular lesion has been identified as a defect within the *APC* (adenomatous polyposis coli) gene on chromosome 5q21. Patients with Gardner syndrome are at much increased risk of developing mesenteric and intraperitoneal desmoid tumors. Desmoid tumors are mesenchymal cells proliferating in a pattern of aggressive fibromatosis, characterized by bland cells that—although histologically benign—act in a malignant fashion with uncontrolled proliferation and infiltration of vital structures. It remains poorly understood why some patients with Gardner syndrome develop desmoid tumors whereas others do not, and the lifetime risk of developing desmoid tumors has been estimated at approximately 10-20%, representing a nearly 1000 times greater risk than that of the general population.

Certain environmental exposures have also been associated with the development of sarcomas. One of the most important is ionizing radiation. Radiation-associated sarcoma is most often a late effect of radiotherapy (RT) given to treat another condition (often a prior malignancy). Sarcomas have been noted as a late effect of RT for breast cancer,

Hodgkin disease, non-Hodgkin lymphomas, and other tumor types.[12] The radiation dose appears to be correlated with the later development of sarcoma, with a very low risk in patients who received less than 10 Gy.[12] However, the molecular mechanisms may be complex, since it has been noted clinically that sarcomas appear at the margins of prior RT fields. This suggests that the mutagenic effect may be maximal at the edges of prior RT where scatter radiation leads to a dose sufficient to induce mutations but insufficient to kill the mutated cells. Traditionally, radiation-associated sarcomas were thought to arise several years following RT, although newer data indicate that a shorter latency period of 2-4 years may also be possible.[17-20] MPNSTs, angiosarcomas, and other high-grade unclassifiable histopathologic subtypes comprise the majority of radiation-associated sarcomas. Although they are aggressive, radiation-associated sarcomas may not behave truly differently from other high-grade sarcomas. Clinical outcomes have been reported to be poor in patients with radiation-associated sarcomas, perhaps because of their typically high-grade and because of the inability to use full multimodality treatment (eg, because the patient has already received the maximum tolerable radiation dose or has had extensive prior doxorubicin exposure). Radiation-associated sarcomas should be approached as new primary disease and treated appropriately to optimize the patient's outcomes.

Certain chemical exposures have also been documented to induce sarcomas, and chemical-induced development of sarcomas in animal models has been one of the more widely employed models of studying neoplastic transformation in the laboratory. Hepatic angiosarcomas have been associated with exposure to several classes of chemicals, including polyvinyl chloride, arsenic compounds, and the thorium dioxide colloid Thorotrast (an antiquated contrast agent).[21-29] The possible relationship between exposure and development of sarcoma is less clear for other compounds, including dioxins (such as Agent Orange and other phenoxyacetic acid-based herbicides) and chlorophenols used in wood preservatives.[30]

Chronic irritation of tissues is a controversial potential cause of sarcomas. Certainly, there is an increased sarcoma risk in the lymphedematous arms of women who have undergone radical mastectomy, often with the additional complicating variable of prior RT (the Stewart-Treves syndrome).[31,32] Limited data also suggest that other sources of chronic tissue irritation and inflammation might be associated with the development of sarcoma.[33] Although a history of trauma is not infrequently elicited from patients with STSs, the impact of such trauma on sarcoma development is in doubt.

Severe and chronic immunosuppression following solid organ transplantation represents yet another risk factor for the development of sarcomas. Sarcomas represent a disproportionate percentage of tumors (10%) in patients following solid organ transplantation, with Kaposi sarcoma comprising the majority of these.[34]

Screening

Given the rarity of sarcomas in the general population, no general screening is indicated beyond routine health care surveillance. However, it is important for physicians to be aware of the predisposing genetic tendencies and environmental exposures that might increase patients' risk of sarcoma development. A complete family history should reveal clues about genetic predispositions, including a family history of polyposis, neurofibromatosis, retinoblastoma, any cancer at a young age in first-degree relatives, or sarcomas. Genetic counseling would be appropriate to discuss issues relating to these predispositions. In patients at increased risk of sarcoma, a more detailed clinical evaluation might be required at a lower threshold of intervention than one might use in general practice. Rapidly growing masses, especially symptomatic ones, in patients with neurofibromatosis should be considered for surgical removal to rule out the potential of sarcomatous transformation of a neurofibroma. Similarly, any superficial or deep abnormalities of skin or soft tissues in patients with a history of prior RT should be evaluated very thoroughly.

Clinical Presentation, Classification, and Diagnosis

Sites of Origin

Sarcomas of nonosseous tissues have been noted to arise at virtually all anatomic sites. The anatomic sites and site-specific histologic subtypes of more than 5113 sarcomas treated at a single referral institution are outlined in Figure 108-1. Approximately one-third to one-half of all sarcomas of nonosseous tissues occur in the lower extremities, where the most common histopathologic subtypes have traditionally been noted to include liposarcomas as well as the vaguely defined entity "malignant fibrous histiocytoma." With improved pathologic tools to categorize sarcomas (eg, immunohistochemistry and molecular analyses), it is increasingly recognized that sarcomas previously referred to as malignant fibrous histiocytoma (MFH) are often more accurately categorized as poorly differentiated liposarcomas or leiomyosarcomas, as well as other histologic subtypes.[35] RPSs comprise 15-20% of all STSs, with liposarcoma and leiomyosarcoma being the predominant histologic subtypes. The visceral sarcomas make up an additional 24%, and the head and neck sarcomas approximately 4% of sarcomas.

Clinical Presentation

The majority of patients with nonosseous sarcomas present with a painless mass,

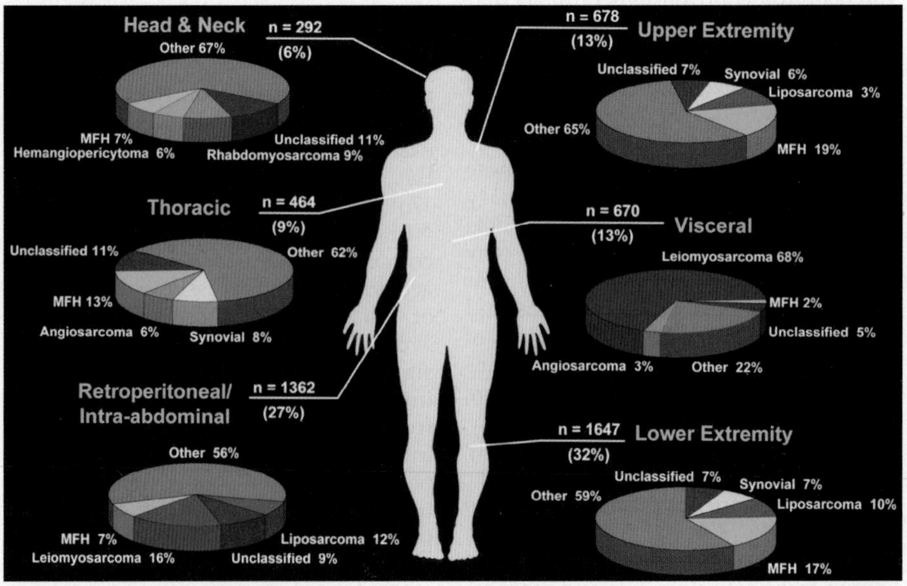

Figure 108-1 Anatomic distribution and site-specific histologic subtypes of 5113 consecutive STSs seen at the University of Texas MD Anderson Cancer Center Sarcoma Center (MDACC Sarcoma Database, June 1996 to June 2005).

although pain is noted at presentation in up to one-third of cases.[36] Delay in diagnosis of sarcomas is common, with the most common incorrect diagnosis for extremity and trunk lesions being hematoma or "lipoma." Late diagnosis of RPS is extremely common, since tumors in this area can grow to massive size before causing any symptoms (such as abdominal distention or psoas irritation with back or groin discomfort).

Physical examination should include an assessment of the size and mobility of the mass. Its relationship to the fascia (superficial vs deep) and nearby neurovascular and bony structures should be noted. A site-specific neurovascular examination and assessment of regional lymph nodes should also be performed.

Histopathologic Classification

Methods of Classification In broad terms, sarcomas can be classified as neoplasms arising in bone versus those arising from the nonosseous or periosseous soft tissues. Sarcomas of nonosseous tissues can be further grouped into those that arise from the viscera (eg, gastrointestinal or gynecologic organs) and those that originate in nonvisceral soft tissues such as muscle, tendon, adipose tissue, pleura, synovium, and other connective tissues.

The most universally applied classification scheme for STS is based on histogenesis, as outlined in the recent WHO classification system for sarcomas.[37,38] This classification system is reproducible between pathologists for the better differentiated tumors. However, as the degree of histologic differentiation declines, the determination of cellular origin becomes increasingly difficult. In particular, despite advanced immunohistochemical techniques[39] and electron microscopy, determining the cellular origin for some spindle cell and round cell soft tissue tumors is difficult to impossible.[39] A discrepancy between the original histologic assessment and that of a subsequent expert review has been noted in as many as 25% of cases of some subgroups of STS.[40,41]

Difficulties in establishing the specific cellular origin of STS have occasionally been viewed as having limited clinical importance because clinical investigators have not had sufficient data to tie the histologic subtype directly to biologic behavior or to specific therapeutic interventions. Important exceptions to this generalization include epithelioid sarcoma, clear cell sarcoma, angiosarcoma, and embryonal rhabdomyosarcoma, all of which have a greater risk of regional lymph node metastasis.[42,43] In 1 single-institution study, the overall rate of nodal metastasis at the time of presentation was only 2.7%; however, the rate was much higher for the histologic subtypes: angiosarcoma (13.5%), embryonal rhabdomyosarcoma (13.6%), and epithelioid sarcoma (16.7%).[42] Thus, treatment strategies may differ for these histologic subtypes. For the remaining histologic subtypes, biologic behavior appears to be determined more by histologic grade than by histologic subtype.[44] However, as the fundamental biologic and molecular understanding of the mechanisms of malignant transformation in sarcomas increases, in-depth categorization may well prove to have important clinical ramifications. The tools required to categorize or identify sarcomas at the molecular level are now present for certain types, including synovial sarcomas, liposarcomas, GIST/myofibroblastic sarcomas, Ewing sarcoma/PNET, and rhabdomyosarcomas (Table 108-1). Future studies will need to take histologic subtype into account in a more sophisticated manner than in the past three decades of research when molecular markers were not available. Recently, there has also been a tendency to significant redefinition within the pathological classification of STS. Thus, MFH has traditionally been regarded as the most common STS in adults, but the true nature and validity of this entity have increasingly been questioned. Available data suggest that most patients with MFH can be subclassified into specific STS types. Specifically, pleomorphic STS showing myogenic differentiation are significantly more aggressive than other subtypes.[28,35] Recent evaluations have shown very profound changes to the classification of previously diagnosed cases with more than 50% of cases undergoing significant modification.[29,45] Of note, Daugaard recently studied a series of cases where the number of MFHs was reduced from 72 to 2, with 22 renamed myxofibrosarcomas and 20 cases (7%) were found not to be sarcomas.[29,45] Contributing reasons are recent advances in immunohistochemistry in addition to changes in nomenclature. The findings are important for several reasons, including the implications they have for retrospective research and potentially also on treatment approaches for some patients.

Histologic Grade Biologic aggressiveness can often be predicted based on histologic grade.[44,46] The spectrum of grades varies among specific histologic subtypes (Fig. 108-2). In careful comparative multivariate analyses, histologic grade has been the most important prognostic factor in assessing the risk of distant metastasis and tumor-related death.[44,46] Several grading systems have been proposed, but there is no consensus regarding the specific morphologic criteria that should be employed in the grading of STS.

Two of the most commonly employed grading systems are the US National Cancer Institute (NCI) system developed by Costa and colleagues and the system developed by the Federation Nationale des Centres de Lutte Contre le Cancer (FNCLCC) Sarcoma Group.[47,48] The NCI system is based on the tumor's histologic subtype, location, and amount of tumor necrosis, but cellularity, nuclear pleomorphism, and mitosis count are also to be considered in certain situations. The FNCLCC system employs a score generated by the evaluation of 3 parameters: tumor differentiation, mitotic rate, and amount of tumor necrosis. In a retrospective comparison of these 2 grading systems, in a population of 410 adult patients with nonmetastatic STS, univariate and multi-

Table 108-1 Cytogenetic Aberrations in Nonosseous Sarcomas

Histologic Subtype	Cytogenetic Finding	Genes
Myxoid liposarcoma	t(12;16)	TLS/CHOP
Well-differentiated liposarcoma	Rings and giant markers	Amplified 12q13-15
		HMG1-C
		CDK4
		MDM2
Lipoma (minimal atypia)	12q abnormalities	Amplified 12q13-15
Lipoma	12q14-15 abnormalities	
	6p abnormalities	
Synovial sarcoma	t(X;18)	SYT/SSX1 or SSX2
Ewing's family/PNET	t(11;22) and others	EWS/FLI1 (and others)
Rhabdomyosarcoma	t(2;13) or t(1;13)	PAX3 (or 7)/FKHR (alveolar)
Clear cell sarcoma	t(12;22)	EWS/ATF1
Extraskeletal myxoid chondrosarcomas	t(9;22)	EWS/CHN
	t(9;17)	RPB56/CHN
Dermatofibrosarcoma protuberans	t(17;22)	
Collagen type I alpha1 ring(17;22)	PDGF-B	
Endometrial stromal sarcoma	t(7;17)	
Uterine leiomyosarcoma	t(12;14)	
	7q-	
Desmoplastic small round-cell tumor	t(11;22)	EWS/WT1
Alveolar sarcoma of soft parts	t(X;17)	

Abbreviation: PNET, primitive neuroectodermal tumors.

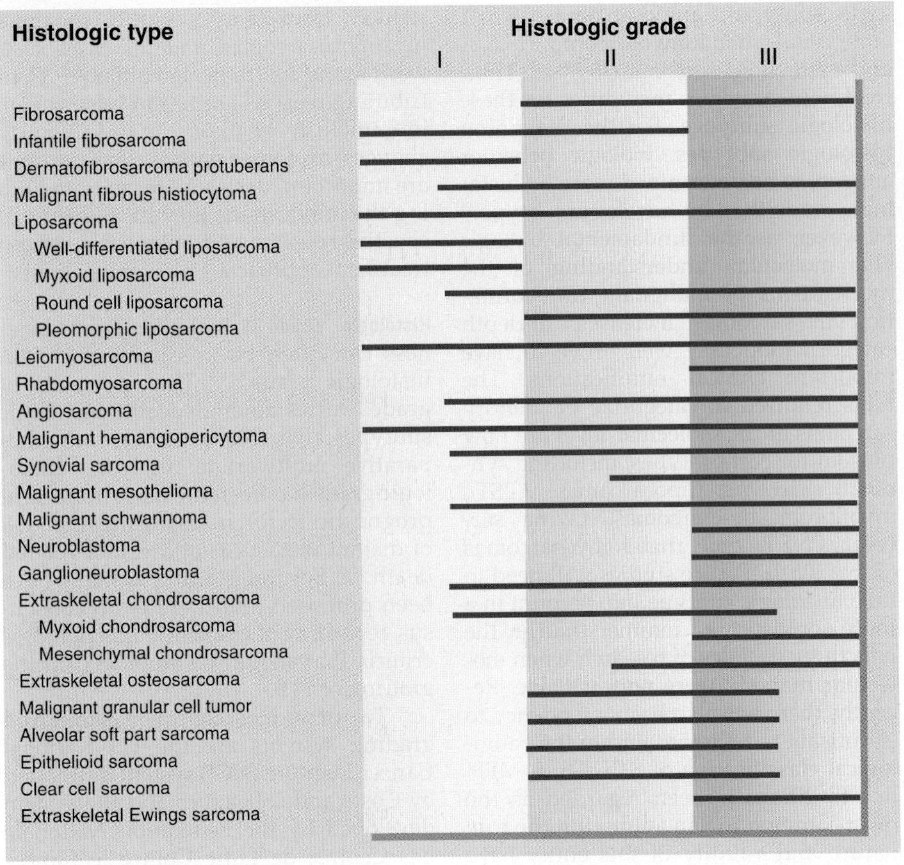

Figure 108-2 ■ Spectrum of grades observed among histologic subtypes of STS. *Source*: From Enzinger FN and Weiss SW, editors. Soft tissue tumors. 3rd ed. Mosby-Year Book Inc; 1995.

variate analyses suggested that the FNCLCC system has a slightly better ability to predict distant metastasis and tumor-related death.[49] Significant discrepancies in assigned grade were observed in one-third of cases. An increased number of grade 3 tumors, reduced number of grade 2 tumors, and better correlation with overall and metastasis-free survival were observed in favor of the FNCLCC system.[49] Thus, in the absence of other comparative data, the FNCLCC system may be the best presently available grading system.

In discussing grade, it is important to note 2 well-described characteristics of sarcomas. First, there is often tremendous intratumoral heterogeneity within individual sarcomas. Therefore, diagnoses based on very limited amounts of tumor may be inaccurate (eg, diagnoses based only on fine-needle aspiration biopsy specimens). This is particularly true for such histopathologic subtypes as de-differentiated liposarcomas, where one area of the tumor might have a relatively low-to-intermediate grade appearance and another area within the same tumor might have more evident high-grade components. Any discussion of the clinical relevance of grading must take into account this variability inherent in the diagnostic process, which will add to the clinical variability in outcomes among patients with any given grade of sarcomas.

Second, the grade of tumors may change over time. This process is best described in the evolution of de-differentiated liposarcoma arising in conjunction with well-differentiated liposarcoma in the same patient. Additional examples include the fibrosarcomatous degeneration that can accompany multiple recurrent DFSPs.

Imaging

Optimal imaging of the primary tumor is dependent on the anatomic site. For soft tissue masses of the extremities, magnetic resonance imaging (MRI) has been regarded as the imaging modality of choice (Figs. 108-3 and 108-4) because MRI enhances the contrast between tumor and muscle and between tumor and adjacent blood vessels and provides multiplanar definition of the lesion.[50,51] However, a study by the Radiation Diagnostic Oncology Group that compared MRI and computed tomography (CT) in patients with malignant bone (n = 183) and soft tissue (n = 133) tumors demonstrated no specific advantage of MRI over CT.[52] On the other hand, although it may be true that the diagnostic evaluation is equally served by both modalities, surgery and RT planning may require additional information provided by the multiplanar capability of MRI and the ability to perform MRI/CT image fusion.[53,54] For pelvic lesions, the multiplanar capability of MRI may provide superior single-modality imaging (Fig. 108-4), whereas in the retroperitoneum and abdomen, CT usually provides satisfactory anatomic definition of the lesion. Occasionally, MRI with gradient sequence imaging can better delin-

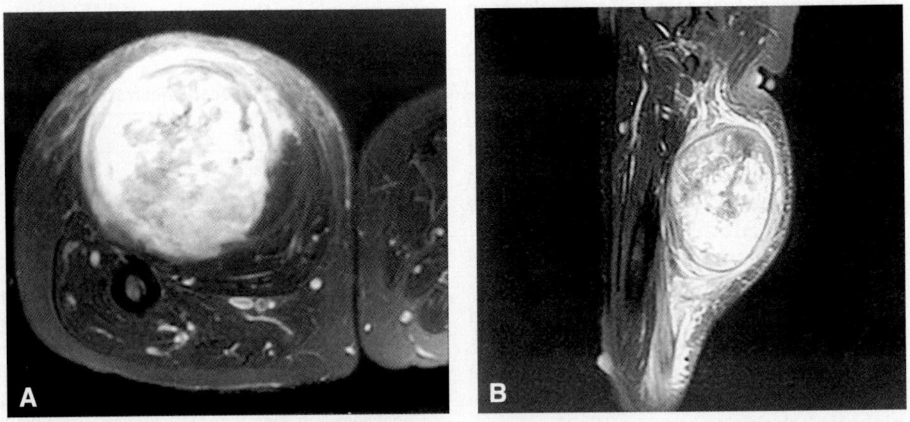

Figure 108-3 ■ (A) Weighted T2-fat-saturated magnetic resonance image of a TNM T2b high-grade sarcoma in the posterior thigh compartment of a 55-year-old woman. Note the containment by the superficial fascia overlying the posterior thigh muscles, where there is a "strip" of peritumoral edema. Anteriorly, the lesion can be seen to be separate from the femur, but the edge of the tumor is less clearly defined than its superficial component, presumably because of muscle infiltration. (B) Sagittal MRI of the same patient. The main lesion manifests a well-defined border. However, a clear zone of peritumoral edema is evident tracking proximally toward the head of the femur, seen at the top of the figure. Inferiorly, the edema seems to be even more pronounced as evidenced by the triangular signal enhancement pointing inferiorly. Whether the zone of edema harbors microscopic disease is uncertain, and this uncertainty can complicate accurate treatment planning (see text).

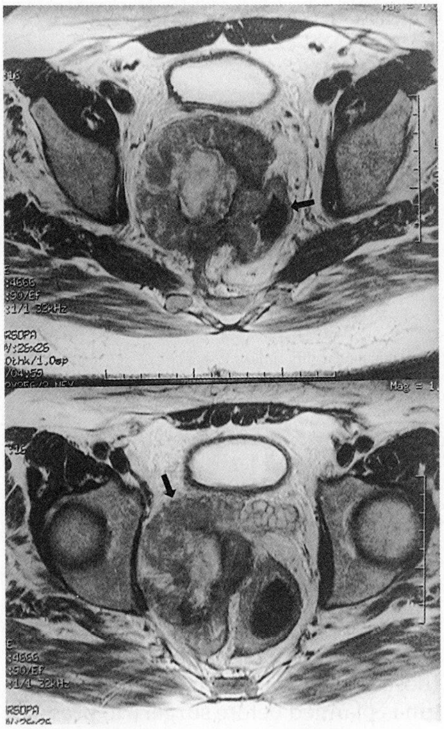

Figure 108-4 A 57-year-old man with T2 pelvic leiomyosarcoma. **(A)** Axial T2-weighted fast-spin echo MRI reveals a heterogeneous mass involving the rectum (*arrow,* air in rectal lumen). **(B)** Note abutment of mass to right seminal vesicle (*arrow*).

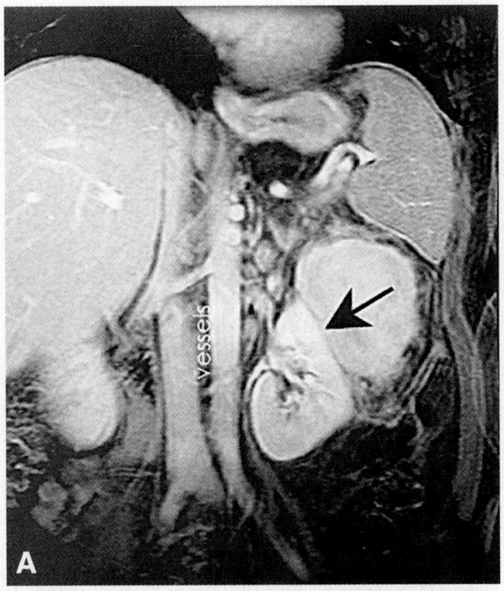

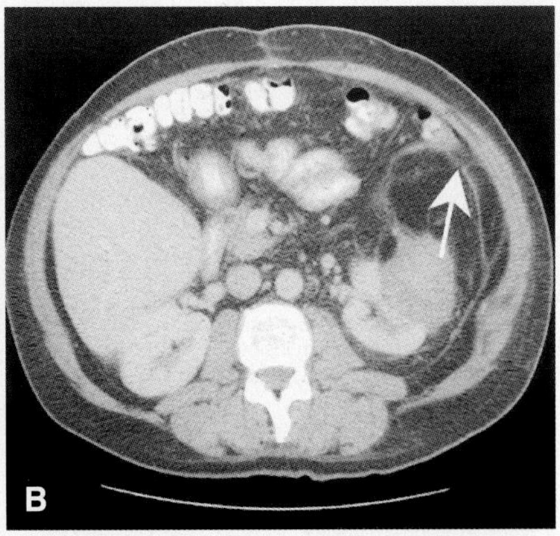

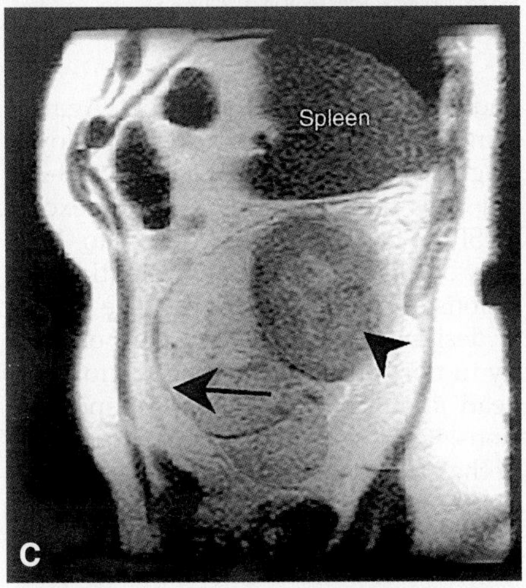

Figure 108-5 (**A**) Coronal fat-saturated gadolinium-enhanced MRI showing a solid liposarcoma, 8.3 cm × 6.6 cm, adjacent to and compressing the upper pole of the left kidney. The mass lies below the spleen and is separate from the kidney (line of demarcation, *arrow*), but is part of a larger fatty tumor. The midline vessels are well visualized. (**B**) CT image of the same lesion. The mass can be seen adjacent to the kidney, as before. An additional mass of fatty attenuation with gray areas of edema, inflammation, or increased cellularity can be seen bounded by a rim anteriorly (*arrow*). This mass has the appearance of abnormal fat, which must be considered in treatment planning. Note the displacement of bowel containing contrast. (**C**) Sagittal MR image of the same case but without gadolinium. The potential advantage of MR imaging in separating the anterior edge of the retroperitoneal sarcoma (*long arrow*) from the normal fat anteriorly is seen. The more solid component can also be seen (*arrowhead*) inferior to the spleen. In addition, these images can be exported digitally to a three-dimensional RT treatment planning workstation or CT simulator workstation where the MR images can be fused to the CT planning slices. This can provide more accurate demonstration of tumor in selected cases for contouring the gross tumor volume and clinical target volume than may be possible with CT images alone. This is particularly helpful in situations where CT does not show tumor as well as MRI.

eate the relationship of a tumor to midline vascular structures, particularly the inferior vena cava and aorta (Fig. 108-5). More invasive studies such as angiography or cavography are almost never required for the evaluation of STS.

Cost-effective imaging to exclude the possibility of distant metastatic disease is dependent on the size, grade, and anatomic location of the primary tumor. In general, patients with low- and intermediate-grade tumors or high-grade tumors 5 cm or less in diameter require only a chest radiograph for satisfactory staging of the chest. This directly reflects the comparatively low risk of presentation with pulmonary metastases in these patients.[55] However, patients with high-grade tumors larger than 5 cm (T2) should undergo more thorough staging of the chest by CT owing to the increased risk of presentation with established metastatic disease in this group.[56,57] Patients with RPS and intra-abdominal visceral sarcomas should undergo imaging of the liver to exclude the possibility of synchronous hepatic metastases; the liver is a more common site of first metastasis from these lesions. CT is usually adequate in these patients to assess the liver, although the increased sensitivity of MRI of the liver may be valuable if any questionable findings are noted on initial CT.

Biopsy

Biopsy of the primary tumor is essential for most patients presenting with soft tissue masses. In general, any soft tissue mass in an adult that is enlarging (even if asymptomatic), is larger than 5 cm, or persists beyond 4-6 weeks should be biopsied. The preferred biopsy approach is generally the least invasive technique required to allow a definitive histologic diagnosis and assessment of grade. In most centers, core-needle biopsy provides satisfactory tissue for diagnosis and results in substantial cost savings compared with open surgical biopsy.[58-60] However, incisional biopsy may still be required to yield optimal amounts of tissue to assess histopathology over a larger area of tumor volume, given the known heterogeneity of sarcomas, as well as to provide sufficient material for detailed molecular and cytogenetic assays. Direct palpation can be used to guide needle biopsy of most superficial lesions, but less accessible sarcomas often require imaging-guided biopsy for safe percutaneous sampling of the most radiographically suspicious area(s) of the mass. Tumor recurrences within the needle track after percutaneous biopsy are rare but have been reported, leading some physicians to advocate tattooing the biopsy site for subsequent excision.[61] In some centers, fine-needle aspiration may be an acceptable biopsy technique for primary soft tissue masses provided that an experienced sarcoma cytopathologist is available.[62-65] However, because of the frequent difficulty in accurately diagnosing these lesions, even when adequate tissue is available, the major utility of fine-needle aspiration in most centers is in the diagnosis of suspected recurrences of sarcoma.

A practical approach for biopsy and staging of the patient who pres-

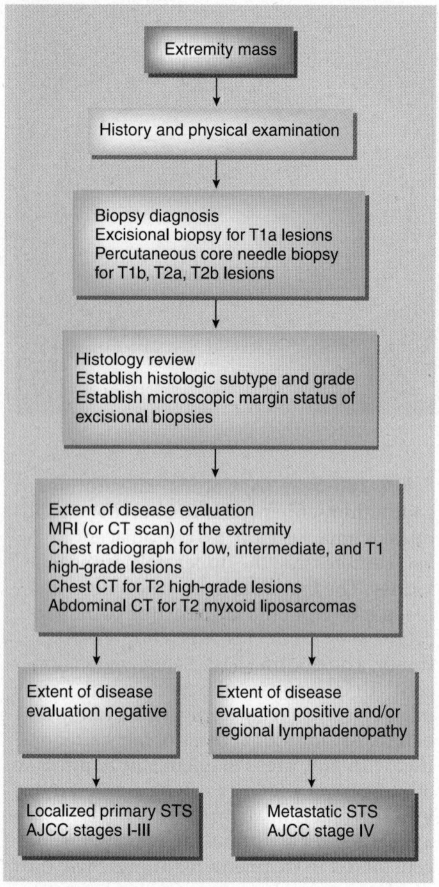

Figure 108-6 Approach for pretreatment evaluation and staging of the patient presenting with a primary extremity soft tissue mass. AJCC, American Joint Committee on Cancer. *Source*: From Pisters PWT, Ann Surg Oncol 1998;5:464–72.

Table 108-2 **American Joint Committee on Cancer Staging System for STSs**

TX	Primary tumor cannot be assessed					
T0	No evidence of primary tumor					
T1	Tumor 5 cm or less in greatest dimension					
T1a	Superficial tumor					
T1b	Deep tumor					
T2	Tumor more than 5 cm in greatest dimension					
T2a	Superficial tumor					
T2b	Deep tumor					
N1	Regional lymph node metastasis					
G1	Well differentiated					
G2	Moderately differentiated					
G3	Poorly differentiated					
G4	Poorly differentiated or undifferentiated (four-tiered systems only)					
Stage I	T1a, 1b, 2a, 2b	N0	M0	G1-2	G1	Low
Stage II	T1a, 1b, 2a	N0	M0	G3-4	G2-3	High
Stage III	T2b	N0	M0	G3-4	G2-3	High
Stage IV	Any T	N1	M0	Any G	Any G	High or Low
	Any T	N0	M1	Any G	Any G	High or Low

Source: From Freene FL, Page DL, Fleming ID, et al, editors. American Joint Committee on Cancer AJCC cancer staging manual. 6th ed. New York: Springer-Verlag; 2002.

ents with a primary extremity soft tissue mass is outlined in Figure 108-6. Small superficial lesions on an extremity where the morbidity of excisional biopsy is minimal (ie, remote from joints, tendons, and neurovascular structures that would compromise the surgical margin) are easily biopsied by excisional biopsy with microscopic assessment of surgical margins. T2 lesions, T1 lesions located beneath the investing fascia of the extremity, or superficial T1 lesions situated in proximity to joints, tendons, or neurovascular structures are best biopsied by percutaneous core-needle biopsy.

Staging and Prognostic Factors

Staging

The relative rarity of STS, the anatomic heterogeneity of these lesions, and the presence of more than 50 recognized histologic subtypes of variable grades have made it difficult to establish a functional system that can accurately stage all forms of this disease. The staging system (6th edition) of the American Joint Committee on Cancer (AJCC) and the International Union Against Cancer is the most widely employed staging system for STS (Table 108-2).[66] All STS subtypes are included except DFSP, a condition considered to have only borderline malignant potential, and lesions of the hollow viscera. The system is designed to optimally stage extremity tumors but is also applicable to torso, head and neck, and retroperitoneal lesions; it should not be used for sarcomas of the gastrointestinal tract.

A major limitation of the present staging system is that it does not take into account the anatomic site of STS. Anatomic site, however, has been recognized as an important determinant of outcome.[67,68] Therefore, although site is not a specific component of any present staging system, outcome data should be reported on a site-specific basis.

Conventional Prognostic Factors

A thorough understanding of the clinicopathologic factors known to impact outcome is essential in formulating a treatment plan for the patient withSTS. Several multivariate analyses of prognostic factors for patients with localized sarcoma have been reported.[48,69-83] However, with few exceptions, most studies have analyzed fewer than 300 patients (range, 82-297 patients).[44,46,69,75]

The more recent, larger reports have established the clinical profile of what is now accepted as the high-risk patient with extremitySTS: the patient with a large (≥5 cm), high-grade, deep lesion.[44,46,69] In addition, the previously unappreciated prognostic significance of certain histologic subtypes and the increased risk of adverse outcome associated with a microscopically positive surgical margin or presentation with locally recurrent disease were noted. The type of microscopically positive surgical margins also appears important. Patients with low-grade liposarcomas have a relatively low risk of local recurrence as do those patients in whom the positive margin is planned before surgery to preserve critical structures and RT can sterilize the small amount of residual disease. However, patients with 2 categories of positive margin are at relatively higher risk of local recurrence. These include patients who underwent "unplanned" excision and still have positive margins on re-excision and those with unanticipated positive margins after primary resection.[84] An "unplanned excision" is defined as an excisional biopsy or resection carried out without adequate preoperative staging or consideration of the need to remove normal tissue around the tumor.

Unlike for other solid tumors, the adverse prognostic factors for local recurrence of a STS are different from those that predict distant metastasis and tumor-related death (Table 108-3).[44] In other words, patients with a constellation of adverse prognostic factors for local recurrence are not necessarily at increased risk of distant metastasis or tumor-related death. Therefore, staging systems that are designed to stratify patients for risk of distant metastasis and tumor-related death will not necessarily stratify patients for risk of local recurrence.

Kattan and colleagues from the Memorial Sloan-Kettering Cancer Center (MSKCC) have utilized a database of over 2,000 prospectively followed adult patients with STS to predict the probability of sarcoma-specific death by 12 years.[67] The results have been used to construct and internally validate a nomogram to predict sarcoma-specific death (Fig. 108-7) This tool is available at www.nomograms.org and may be used for patient counseling, follow-up scheduling, and clinical trial eligibility determination.

Table 108-3 Multivariate Analysis of Prognostic Factors in Patients With Extremity STS

Endpoint	Adverse Prognostic Factor	Relative Risk
Local recurrence	Fibrosarcoma	2.5
	Local recurrence at presentation	2.0
	Microscopically positive margin	1.8
	Malignant peripheral nerve sheath tumor	1.8
	Age > 50 years	1.6
Distant recurrence	High grade	4.3
	Deep location	2.5
	Size 5.0-9.9 cm	1.9
	Leiomyosarcoma	1.7
	Nonliposarcoma histology	1.6
	Local recurrence at presentation	1.5
	Size ≥ 10.0 cm	1.5
Disease-specific survival	High grade	4.0
	Deep location	2.8
	Size ≥ 10.0 cm	2.1
	Malignant peripheral nerve sheath tumor	1.9
	Leiomyosarcoma	1.9
	Microscopically positive margin	1.7
	Lower extremity site	1.6
	Local recurrence at presentation	1.5

Adverse prognostic factors identified are independent by Cox regression analysis.
Source: From Ref. 44.

Potential Molecular Prognostic Factors

Specific molecular parameters evaluated for prognostic significance in STS have included *TP53, mdm2* mutations, *Ki-67* status, altered expression of the RB gene product in high-grade sarcomas, and the presence of specific molecular subtypes of *SYT-SSX* fusion transcripts in synovial sarcoma or *EWS-FL11* fusion transcripts in Ewing's sarcoma.[16,85-89] Recently, however, conflicting evidence for a relationship to the presence of *SYT-SSX* fusion transcripts in synovial sarcoma has emerged.[90] Histologic grade, but not *SYT-SSX* fusion type, is an important prognostic factor in patients with synovial sarcoma.[90] Complete discussion of the extensive literature on molecular prognostic factors in sarcoma is beyond the scope of this chapter. Readers are referred to recent detailed reviews.[91,92] Data evaluating the prognostic significance of the most widely studied molecular factor, Ki-67, are summarized below.

Ki-67, an antigen expressed throughout the majority of the cell cycle, is used as a measure of the fraction of cells undergoing division.[93] Preliminary reports of series of heterogeneous sarcomas in adults suggested that the proliferation index as measured by Ki-67 nuclear staining correlated with histologic grade but was not of independent prognostic significance when histologic grade was taken into account.[94,95] However, additional studies in larger numbers of patients have demonstrated that Ki-67 status is an independent prognostic factor.[85,96,97] An initial immunohistochemical analysis of a cohort of 65 STSs and a subsequent analysis of 132 STSs by the FNCLCC Sarcoma Group demonstrated the adverse prognostic significance of increased Ki-67 activity.[96,97] More recently, Heslin and colleagues evaluated the potential prognostic significance of Rb, *TP53, mdm2*, and *Ki-67* by immunohistochemical techniques in a population of 121 patients with primary, high-grade extremity sarcomas and compared these factors with conventional clinicopathologic prognostic factors (median follow-up, 64 months).[85] Clinicopathologic and molecular factors found to be statistically significant adverse prognostic factors in both univariate and multivariate analyses for the separate end points of distant metastasis and tumor-related death included T2 tumor size, microscopically positive surgical margin, and a Ki-67 score greater than 20 (>20% nuclear staining). Overexpression of *TP53* or *mdm2* or absence of the Rb gene product did not correlate with an increased risk of distant metastasis or tumor-related death.

Although specific cellular and molecular parameters have been identified as having independent prognostic significance, there is presently no consensus on how these prognostic factors should be used in clinical practice. Until more data are available, molecular prognostic factors proven to be of prognostic significance (eg, *Ki-67*) should be considered for inclusion as stratification criteria in clinical trials.

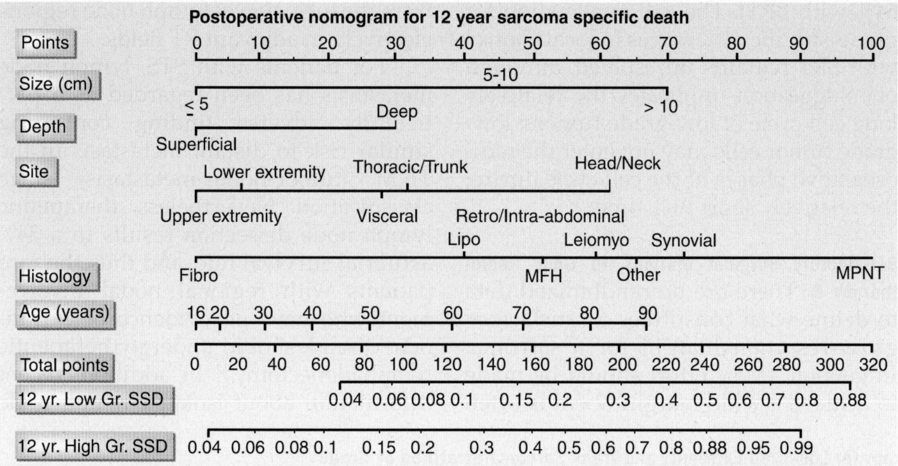

Instructions for physicians: Locate the patient's tumor size on the size axis. Draw a line straight upwards to the points axis to determine how many points towards sarcoma-specific death the patient receives for his tumor size. Repeat this process for the other axes, each time drawing straight upward to the points axis. Sum the points achieved for each predictor and locate this sum on the total points axis. Draw a line straight down to either the low grade or high grade axis to find the patient's probability of dying from sarcoma within 12 years assuming he or she does not die of another cause first.

Instructions for patients: If we had 100 patients exactly like you, we would expect between (predicted percentage from nomogram - 8%) and (predicted percentage + 8%) to die of sarcoma within 12 years if they did not die of another cause first, and death from sarcoma after 12 years is still possible.

Figure 108-7 Postoperative nomogram for 12-year sarcoma-specific deaths in 2163 patients treated at Memorial Sloan-Kettering Cancer Center. *Abbreviations*: Fibro, fibrosarcoma; Lipo, liposarcoma; Leiomyo, leiomyosarcoma; MFH, malignant fibrous histiocytoma; MPNT, malignant peripheral-nerve sheath tumor; GR, grade; SSD, sarcoma-specific death. *Source*: From Kattan MW et al. *J Clin Oncol*. 2002;20:791–796.

Treatment of Localized Primary Disease of the Extremities

Surgery

General Issues ■ Surgical resection remains the cornerstone of therapy for localized primary STS. The discussion that follows focuses on STSs in the limbs, the most common site of origin, but the principles are equally applicable to sarcomas at other anatomic sites.

Over the past 20 years, there has been a marked decline in the rate of amputation as the primary therapy for extremity STS. With the widespread application of multimodality treatment strategies, the vast majority of patients with localized STS of the extremities undergo limb-sparing treatment; less than 10% of patients presently undergo amputation.[98,99] In selected patients, limb sparing can be approached with surgery alone.

Amputation Most surgeons consider definite major vascular, bony, or nerve involvement by STS as relative indications for amputation. Complex en bloc bone, vascular, and nerve resections with interposition grafting can be undertaken, but the associated morbidity is high. Therefore, for a few patients with critical involvement of major bony or neurovascular structures, amputation remains the only surgical option, but offers the prospect of prompt rehabilitation with excellent local control and survival rates.[100]

Combined-Modality Limb-Sparing Treatment Currently, at least 90% of patients with localized extremity sarcomas can undergo limb-sparing procedures.[98,101] The use of limb-sparing multimodality treatment approaches for extremity sarcoma is based largely on a phase 3 trial from the NCI, in which patients with extremity sarcomas amenable to limb-sparing surgery were randomly assigned to receive amputation or limb-sparing surgery with postoperative RT.[100,102] Both arms of this trial included postoperative chemotherapy with doxorubicin, cyclophosphamide, and methotrexate. With greater than 9 years of follow-up evaluation, this study established that for patients for whom limb-sparing surgery is an option, limb-sparing surgery combined with postoperative RT and chemotherapy yields disease-related survival rates comparable to those for amputation while simultaneously preserving a functional extremity.[100,102]

Satisfactory local resection involves resection of the primary tumor with a margin of normal tissue around the lesion. Dissection along the tumor pseudocapsule (enucleation) is associated with local recurrence rates ranging between 33% and 63%.[103-105] In contrast, wide local excision with a margin of normal tissue around the lesion is associated with local recurrence rates in the range of 10-31%, as noted in the control arms (surgery alone) of randomized trials evaluating postoperative RT and in single-institution reports.[106-108]

In the modern era, a discussion of limb-preserving approaches must be linked to a discussion of the role of adjuvant therapies, most commonly RT. Several randomized controlled trials have addressed issues surrounding the use of adjuvant therapy and collectively have established important milestones in the evolution of the local management of STS. With 1 exception, these trials have focused on extremity lesions and the themes of surgery and adjuvant RT.

Yang and colleagues randomized 91 patients with high-grade extremity lesions following limb-sparing surgery to receive adjuvant chemotherapy alone or concurrent chemotherapy and RT.[107] An additional 50 patients with low-grade tumors were to receive adjuvant RT or no further treatment following limb-sparing surgery. The local control rate for those who received RT was 99% compared with 70% in the no-RT group (p = .0001).[107] The results were similar for high- and low-grade tumors (Table 108-4).

Adjuvant RT was also evaluated at MSKCC in a randomized trial of 126 cases treated between 1982 and 1987 (Table 108-4).[106] Brachytherapy (BRT) was administered postoperatively, via an iridium-192 implant that delivered 42-45 Gy over 4-6 days. At 5 years, the local control rate for high-grade tumors was 91% with BRT compared with 70% in surgery-alone controls (p = .04). Of note, no improvement in local control with BRT was evident for the low-grade tumors (the local control rate was 74% with surgery alone and 64% with BRT). The full explanation for grade-specific differences in local control with BRT remains unresolved, although one suggestion implicates the relatively long cell cycle of low-grade tumors: low-grade tumor cells may not enter the radiosensitive phases of the cell cycle during the relatively short BRT time.[106]

Satisfactory Surgical Margins to Omit Radiotherapy There are no randomized data to define what constitutes a satisfactory gross resection margin for a sarcoma. In general, every effort should be made to achieve a wide margin (2 cm is often an arbitrary choice) around the tumor mass, except in the immediate vicinity of functionally important neurovascular structures, where, in the absence of frank neoplastic involvement, dissection is performed in the immediate perineural or perivascular tissue planes. Technical details of the surgical approach to extremity sarcomas are beyond the scope of this chapter, but are reviewed in Bland and colleagues' *Atlas of Surgical Oncology*.[109] However, the principle remains that adequate clearance of potential tumor-bearing tissues can be achieved if there is sufficient distance between the surgical margin and the edge of any grossly evident tumor (eg, at least 2 cm for the closest margin), or where an intact barrier to tumor spread is excised en bloc with the tumor. In such cases, there is little evidence that RT is required even when potential adverse prognostic factors, such as large high-grade tumors are present. The exception in cases of "unplanned" excision where significant contamination of surrounding tissues may have taken place and the precise extent of the tumor is essentially unknown.

Management of Regional Lymph Nodes Given the low (2-3%) prevalence of lymph node metastasis in adults with sarcomas, there is no role for routine regional lymph node dissection in most patients.[42,43] However, patients with angiosarcoma, embryonal/alveolar rhabdomyosarcoma, and epithelioid sarcoma have an increased incidence of lymph node metastasis and should be carefully examined for lymphadenopathy. These patients may benefit from the inclusion of lymph node regions electively in adjuvant RT fields.

For patients with STS, lymph node metastasis has been regarded as a particularly adverse finding conferring similar risk to distant metastasis in the TNM (tumor-nodes-metastasis) stage classification. Nevertheless, therapeutic lymph node dissection results in a 34% actuarial survival rate, and thus the rare patients with regional nodal involvement who have no evidence of extranodal disease should undergo therapeutic lymphadenectomy.[42] In addition, recent information about isolated lymph node

Table 108-4 **Phase 3 Trials of Adjuvant Radiotherapy for Localized Extremity and Trunk Sarcoma Stratified by Grade**

Histologic Grade	First Author/Institution	Treatment Group	Radiation Dose, Gy	No of Patients	No. Local Failure (%)	LRFS (%)	OS (%)
High grade	Pisters/MSKCC(104)	Surgery + BRT	42-45	56	5 (9)	89	27
		Surgery	–	63	19 (30)	66	67
	Yang(105)/NCI	Surgery + XRT	45 + 18 (boost)	47	0 (0)	100	75
		Surgery	–	44	9 (20)	78	74
Low grade	Pisters(104)/MSKCC	Surgery + BRT	42-45	22	8 (36)	73	96
		Surgery	–	23	6 (26)	73	95
	Yang(105)/NCI	Surgery + XRT	45 + 18 (boost)	26	1 (4)	96	NR
		Surgery	–	24	8 (33)	63	NR

Abbreviations: BRT, brachytherapy; LRFS, local recurrence-free survival; MSKCC, Memorial Sloan-Kettering Cancer Center; NCI, National Cancer Institute; NR, not reported; OS, overall survival; XRT, external-beam radiotherapy.

metastasis (as opposed to synchronous distant metastasis) indicates that isolated lymph node metastasis, if treated intensively, appear to have a prognosis similar to patients with Stage III tumors (ie, those with high-grade, deep lesions and lesions larger than 5 cm). This questions whether the impact of nodal disease should be reconsidered in the future editions of the staging system.[110,111]

Radiotherapy

Rationale for Combining Radiotherapy With Surgery ■ The use of RT in combination with surgery for STS is supported by 2 phase 3 clinical trials (Table 108-4) and is based on 2 premises: microscopic nests of tumor cells can be destroyed by RT, and less radical surgery can be performed when surgery and RT are combined.[106,107] Although the traditional belief was that STSs were resistant to RT, radiosensitivity assays performed on sarcoma cell lines grown in vitro have confirmed that the radiosensitivity of sarcomas is similar to that of other malignancies; this confirmation supports the first premise.[112,113] The second premise stresses the philosophy of preservation of form (including cosmesis where possible) and function as a goal for many patients with extremity, truncal, breast, and head and neck sarcomas.[114-116] Similar principles govern the frequent use of RT for sarcomas at problematic sites, for example, RPS, high-risk sarcomas of the head and neck with skull base invasion, or spinal canal invasion by paravertebral lesions.

Visceral sarcomas are not ordinarily managed with RT, in part because of the mobile nature of these structures within the pelvic, abdominal, or thoracic compartments. After resection of visceral sarcomas, accurate identification of the field at risk of residual disease is particularly problematic. Contaminated loops of bowel or mesentery may relocate remotely within the abdominal cavity after surgery, and pleural contamination and mediastinal shift may occur following intrathoracic resections. Fixed tumors in the pelvis or tumors attached to internal truncal walls may occasionally be suited to preoperative or postoperative RT. Typically, however, the vast size of the radiation fields needed to cover entire body cavities, coupled with the limited RT doses that can be safely administered to the organs within the cavities, and the overwhelming risk of distant rather than local recurrence, confines adjuvant RT for the investigational setting.

Essential Elements in Treatment Planning of External Beam Radiotherapy ■ Accurate tumor localization is the first essential for RT planning. It primarily uses CT for dosimetric reasons, but MRI can provide complementary information about the tumor extent and can be assimilated in the computer planning workstation through image fusion technology.[53,54] Further essential information is obtained from the pathology and operative reports, and metallic clips placed at the time of surgery may also help define the tumor bed.

It is often helpful to secure the targeted area to minimize set-up variations and eliminate movement during treatment. Simple maneuvers such as comfortable limb positioning or fashioning of customized thermoplastic molds for immobilization will facilitate reliable and consistent treatment setups. RT of superficial tissues, including the scar following definitive resection, with appropriate application of tissue-like bolus material should be considered, but with the recognition that fibrosis, atrophy, and telangiectasis may result. Dose uniformity within irregular volumes can be optimized using beam segmentation, compensators, or wedge filters. Whenever possible, the entire limb circumference, whole joints, or pressure areas (eg, elbow or heel) should not be treated with the full RT dose as this may adversely affect limb function and cause distal edema.

It is also prudent to assess baseline function before initiating RT. This is especially important with paired organs, such as eyes or kidneys, if the functional ablation of one organ by RT is expected.

Three-Dimensional Treatment Planning ■ Very complex modulation of the beam is becoming available in many centers with the introduction of intensity-modulated RT (IMRT), but until recently such intensity modulation is reserved for situations in which the target volume is adjacent to critical normal tissues as found at the skull base or within the abdomen.[117-119] This is discussed briefly in the RT sections below. Although there is potential advantage in approaching sarcoma with more precise targeting, clinical trials are only just commencing to assess the validity and efficacy of these approaches.

Dose-Volume Histograms ■ The treatment of sarcoma often requires large volumes of normal tissue to be irradiated, frequently to high doses. Fortunately, because most sarcomas arise in the limbs, the likelihood of life-threatening sequelae from RT damage to critical organs is low. However, the potential for serious damage to neurologic tissues in the head and neck or intra-abdominal organs including liver and small bowel remains for tumors adjacent to these structures. Because the tolerance of many normal tissues to radiation depends on the irradiated volume, the development of three-dimensional treatment planning has provided tools to quantify the relationships between dose, volume, and normal-tissue complications. Models permit normal-tissue complication probability to be determined for different irradiated volumes of organs or tissues and varying dose levels.[120,121]

These concepts are helpful when treating certain tumors in the retroperitoneum. If right-sided or of great size, an RPS may infiltrate the liver capsule or be "hooded" by the liver, making RT access to an appropriate tissue volume surrounding the tumor extremely difficult. This area may be particularly appropriate for IMRT approaches because of the exquisite conformality that is possible with this approach and permits liver and other normal tissue to be excluded from the irradiated volume.[122,123] Fortunately, although the tolerance of the entire liver to radiation is low, the normal-tissue complication probability model has shown that part of the liver may be safely treated to much higher doses.[124] The "volume effect" can be exploited and cases may be planned more readily and safely using dose-volume histograms.[114] In these instances, if a subsequent liver resection is needed because of tumor infiltration or adherence to the capsule, detailed consultation between the surgical and radiation oncology teams is needed to ensure that an adequate volume of nonirradiated liver is left in situ.

Dose Fractionation Issues ■ Total radiation doses administered postoperatively for sarcoma depend on the tumor grade and involvement of the surgical margin.[107,125,126] Typical total doses are 60 Gy for low-grade and 66 Gy for high-grade tumors, respectively. When RT is given preoperatively, the total dose used in most institutions is approximately 50 Gy in daily fractions administered over 5 weeks.[126,127] However, data regarding radiation dose response are very limited and based on underpowered retrospective studies. Based on current data, higher doses of RT are probably indicated in the postoperative setting (compared with preoperative RT), but the search for an alternative lower dose postoperative schedule seems desirable.

The fraction size used in conventional fractionation schemes varies (usually 1.8 or 2.1 Gy).[126,128] Absence of late effects can be expected with smaller fraction size; this tissue is particularly important when critical structures are irradiated. Several altered fractionation schemes have been described including hyperfractionated, hypofractionated, and accelerated schedules.[129-132] As yet, no apparent benefit from these various strategies is evident compared with conventional RT.

Radiation Target Volume ■ STS generally respect barriers to tumor spread in the axial plane of the extremity, such as bones,

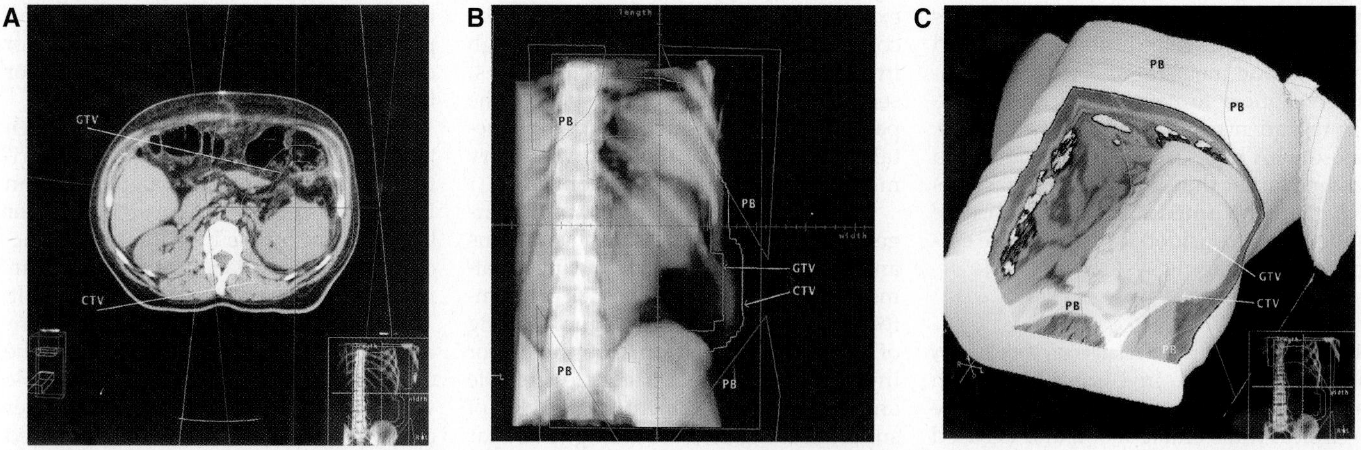

Figure 108-8 (**A**) The GTV has been contoured on a CT simulator workstation (red outline). This includes the anterior abnormal fat shown earlier (Fig. 108-5 B and C). This process is performed with many thin CT slices to permit reconstruction of the image later for three-dimensional treatment planning. The CTV is outlined in yellow to account for potential microscopic spread beyond the GTV. An additional margin will also be added to account for set-up variation and organ motion. Note the displacement of bowel loops by the tumor mass. The straight lines show the path of the beam for a conventional setup with opposed anterior and posterior fields. (**B**) The contoured GTV and CTV information displayed in a beam's eye view (BEV) using a digitally reconstructed radiograph created by the CT simulator. Shielding (Pb) can be placed once the path of the beam within the target areas defined is seen on the BEV. One can also discern the opaque tumor partially displacing bowel from target area. (**C**) A three-dimensional reconstruction with the GTV, CTV, and areas to be shielded (Pb) shown and abdominal wall and anterior structures cut away. Generally, these "cut-away" images are most useful for visualizing the edge of the target volume adjacent to critical anatomy that must be protected and when the spatial relationship cannot be verified precisely with conventional imaging.

interosseous membranes, or major fascial planes. Consequently, extremity STS tend to spread longitudinally within the specific muscle groups of the extremity. Therefore, the margins of the RT volume must be wide in the cephalocaudal direction. In the cross-section, there may be much greater security in defining nontarget structures, especially those delimited by an intact barrier to tumor spread. For nonextremity lesions, the preferred direction of spread is also along the direction of the involved musculature, but care must be taken to ensure that the fascial planes are appropriately recognized and encompassed in the radiation target volume.

Earlier, this chapter summarized principles concerning anatomic planes and the preferential pathways for sarcomas to spread within tissues. This information facilitates the design of target areas for RT. The basic elements in RT planning are to first define a gross tumor volume (GTV) and then place a margin around it to encompass tissues at risk of harboring microscopic residual disease (clinical target volume [CTV]) (Figs. 108-8 A-C and 108-9).[133] Generally, RT is phased so that an initial volume (phase 1) around the risk zone is treated to doses that are capable of sterilizing microscopic amounts of tumor cells (eg, 50 Gy in 1.8 or 2.0 Gy fractions). It is then customary to have at least one field reduction to permit an augmented dose to a smaller volume surrounding the highest risk zone (phase 2). This dose is usually 15-16 Gy but can be higher if there is gross residual disease. This postoperative "boost" is generally restricted to patients who received preoperative RT and have margin-positive disease at surgery. This is because the local control rate for margin-negative cases is in excess of 90% even when a boost is not provided.[126,134,135] A positive margin is declared when the tumor reaches the inked surface of the specimen, and clear margins can be declared if the tumor does not reach the ink irrespective of how close it is.[126] In the preoperative RT setting, the GTV typically represents the radiologically defined tumor. Some sarcomas have extensive peritumoral edema that extends along fascial planes for some distance beyond the main tumor mass.[136] It is uncertain whether the edema contains viable tumor cells.[137] The inclusion of edema within the GTV can influence the magnitude of the RT field, especially its length. There is no uniform policy or guideline as to whether this area should be considered part of the GTV. Studies to correlate the radiologic imaging appearances of sarcomas with the pathologic findings are needed and would be very relevant in the contemporary era of conformal treatment planning.

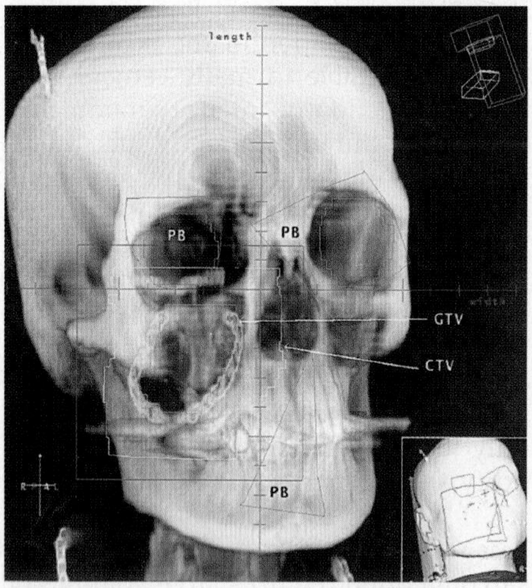

Figure 108-9 A digitally reconstructed radiograph of the head and neck of a young woman with a STS of the right cheek. Because of the proximity to the right eye, preoperative radiotherapy has been chosen because of its ability to permit maximal restriction of the CTV to the local environment of the tumor. The same process was followed using a CT simulator as described in Figure 108-7. The GTV on the cheek can be seen with the surrounding CTV. Shielding (Pb) is also evident. A hair clip, which the patient was wearing during the CT slice acquisition, is evident in the right parietal area; one can also see her necklace. The smaller insert shows a three-dimensional image of the patient with potential beams applied.

When postoperative RT is administered, there is no GTV if one strictly follows the conventions of the International Commission on Radiation Units and Measurements.[133] However, for RT planning, it is still helpful to represent a theoretic GTV as the surgical field comprising all of the tissues handled during the surgical procedure, including undermined skin flaps, drain sites, and scars. A putative zone of potential microscopic residual disease beyond this represents the CTV.

Bone, interosseous membranes, and fascial planes are considered barriers to tumor spread in the axial direction, and, therefore, descriptions of radiation margins employed are principally in the cephalocaudal direction. The RT protocol in the NCI of Canada Clinical Trial performed by the Canadian Sarcoma Group (SR2), which compared preoperative and postoperative RT (see below), required a field margin of 5 cm around the GTV for the initial phase of treatment (50 Gy in 25 fractions).[138] Generally, the GTV included any peritumoral edema seen on MRI, irrespective of tumor grade or size. Subsequently, a reduced volume field was treated to a total combined dose of 66 Gy in all patients who had postoperative RT and in preoperative RT patients with positive resection margins. However, there is variability among centers about what constitutes optimal coverage of tissues at risk of harboring microscopic disease.[128] BRT protocols use margins of only 2 cm around the surgical bed.[106] Despite these differences, the local control rates reported are approximately 90% if low-grade lesions are excluded from the BRT data. This suggests that the zone of microscopic involvement may be less than was previously realized. Recent improvements in surgical technique may lessen the degree of intraoperative tumor dissemination, and irradiation of all surgically handled tissues, scars, and drain sites may be unnecessary. This seems particularly relevant for major centers where surgery is performed by teams with extensive experience in sarcoma management. One must also consider the possibility that case selection factors may explain apparent variations in practice between BRT and external beam RT approaches.

Sequencing of Radiotherapy and Surgery ■ Preoperative RT is delivered to an undisturbed and potentially better oxygenated tumor site, which may be one reason why lower preoperative radiation doses do not appear to compromise local control.[139,140] Nielsen and colleagues repeated RT planning in patients who had undergone preoperative RT and surgery and observed that the field size and number of joints irradiated in preoperative RT were significantly less than if the treatment had been administered postoperatively.[141] This observation was recently validated in a prospective randomized trial and there is evidence that smaller treatment volumes may result in improved limb function.[130,138,142]

Another advantage of preoperative RT is that it promotes collaboration between the surgical and radiation oncologists and facilitates the formulation of a coordinated management plan prior to any treatment. In some circumstances, preoperative RT may provide better tumor control compared to postoperative RT, although this has not yet been substantiated by prospective randomized trial data. A retrospective series from Massachusetts General Hospital suggested that preoperative RT may be more efficacious for larger lesions (>5 cm).[143] More recently, Pollack and colleagues suggested that preoperative RT is preferable in patients presenting with locally advanced primary disease.[127] Finally, although much of the discussion about preoperative RT is focused on extremity lesions, patients with RPS tolerate preoperative RT substantially better than postoperative RT. This is because the tumor acts as a tissue expander to exclude the bowel from the RT volume (Figs. 108-8A-C). This is discussed in detail later in the section "Retroperitoneal Sarcomas."

Preoperative RT also has certain disadvantages. Definition of the target volume relies almost completely on the imaging characteristics of the tumor, and this may underestimate the true extent of the tumor. In addition, preoperative RT is delivered based on the results of only partially representative biopsy specimens and may interfere with future histopathologic analysis. However, these 2 concerns are more academic and theoretical than practical. One clinical concern with the preoperative delivery of RT remains the increased risk of serious wound complications following definitive resection (discussed below).

Which approach—preoperative or postoperative RT—is more "correct" is thus controversial.[144] Many competing issues are involved, and the treatment decision algorithm is complex. It is also important to appreciate that conclusions from much of the available data are liable to bias because of the nonrandomized fashion in which treatment was allocated. Often preoperative RT is chosen for patients with more adverse presentations of disease who are therefore in need of more extensive surgery.[140]

The NCI of Canada/Canadian Sarcoma Group SR2 clinical trial represents the only prospective randomized comparison of preoperative versus postoperative RT.[138] The RT parameters for this protocol were briefly addressed earlier. The trial found that wound complications are twice as common with preoperative RT as with postoperative RT (35% vs 17%), although the increased risk is almost exclusively confined to patients with sarcomas of the upper extremity. Of interest, a recent report from the University of Texas M.D. Anderson Cancer Center, using the same criteria for classifying wound complications as were used in the Canadian NCI trial, found almost identical results.[145]

The SR2 trial also found, as anticipated, that larger field sizes are also needed with postoperative RT. In addition, preliminary data concerning RT toxicity rates in the Canadian trial after 2 years differed between the 2 arms of the study with a tendency to manifest greater fibrosis in the postoperative arm of the study compared to those treated with preoperativeRT.[146] This observation is potentially important because patients with significant fibrosis, joint stiffness, or limb edema, all late treatment responses, had significantly lower limb-function scores at these later time points.[146] Moreover this subsequent analysis also suggested strongly that field size was predictive of greater degrees of fibrosis and joint stiffness and also may be related to edema.[147]

In the initial report of the SR2 trial with 3.3 years median follow-up, an improvement in overall survival (p = .0481) in the preoperative RT arm was noted and partially explained by increased deaths in the postoperative RT unrelated to sarcoma.[138] The local failure rate was identical in the 2 arms (7%) (Fig. 108-10). However, updated results were recently presented and the preliminary survival difference has disappeared.[148] The 5-year results for preoperative versus postoperative, respectively, were, local control: 93% versus 92%; metastatic relapse-free: 67% versus 69%; recurrence-free survival: 58% versus 59%; overall survival: 73% versus 67% (p = .48); cause-specific survival: 78% versus 73% (p = .64). Cox modeling showed only resection margins as significant for local control. Tumor size and grade were the only significant factors for metastatic-relapse, overall survival, and cause-specific survival. Grade was the only consistent predictor of recurrence-free survival.[148]

For the present, decisions about preoperative versus postoperative RT should be individualized, taking into account tumor location, tumor size, RT field size, comorbidities, and risks. In general, preoperative RT provides some advantages over postoperative RT, but exposes the patient to significantly increased risks of serious postoperative wound complications. A summary of the relative indications that can be used to select patients for preoperative RT is provided in Table 108-5.

Methods of Radiotherapy Delivery ■ No randomized trials directly comparing external beam RT and BRT have been undertaken, but both forms of RT have been compared with surgery alone. BRT has several advantages over external beam, including a shorter overall treatment time (4-6 days vs 5-6.5 weeks) and quicker initiation of RT after surgery while clonogen numbers are at a minimum. Because of its brevity, BRT is also more easily integrated into protocols that include systemic chemotherapy than is external beam RT, with its protracted courses. The irradiated volume is also smaller with BRT, which may confer functional advantages.

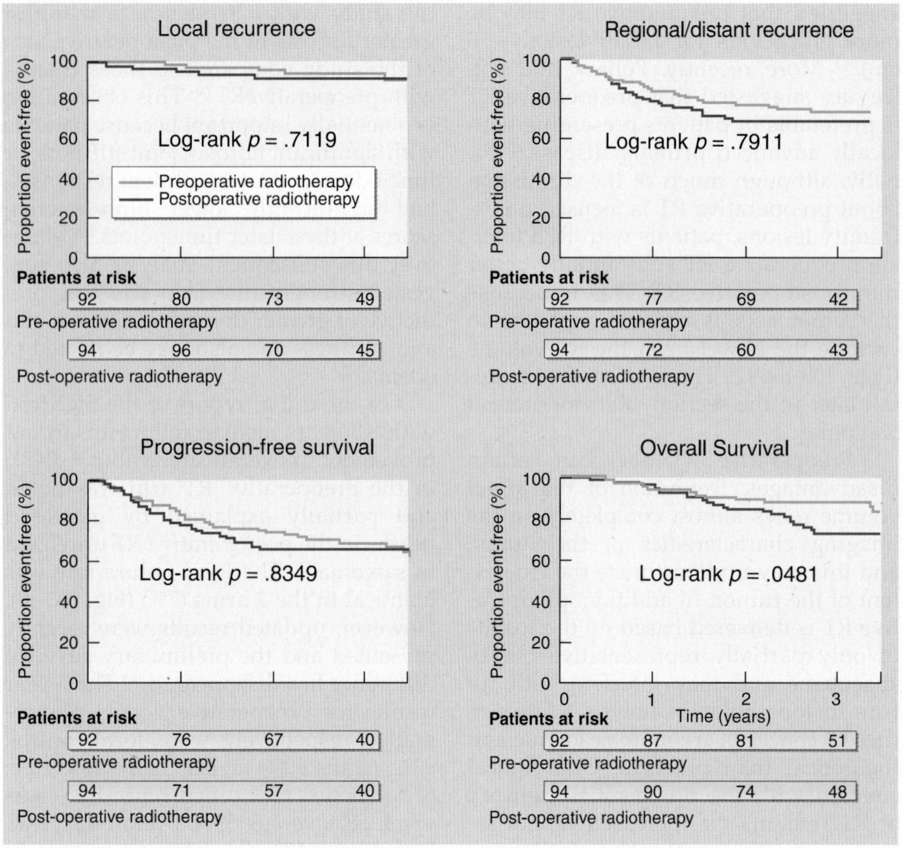

Figure 108-10 Kaplan-Meier plots for probability of local recurrence, metastasis (local and regional recurrence), progression-free survival, and overall survival in the Canadian Sarcoma Group randomized trial of the NCI of Canada Clinical Trials Group comparing preoperative and postoperative radiotherapy. *Source*: From Ref. 138.

Furthermore, BRT costs $1,000 US per patient less than external beam.[149] BRT may also have an advantage in situations in which normal-tissue tolerance to RT is compromised. One such scenario would be when a postoperative RT boost to the operative bed is desired in patients who received preoperative RT. The use of BRT with surgery in previously irradiated tissues is another situation to achieve limb salvage.[150-153] As noted earlier, no apparent benefit for BRT over surgical excision alone is evident with low-grade lesions, and external beam appears more effective for these tumors (Table 108-4).[107,143,154]

As noted earlier, an alternative method of delivering RT to a complex shaped target is by means of external beams designed with variable intensity across their profiles, in contrast to the uniform flat profile used in traditional RT. Such variable intensity beams, when shaped according to the needs of the target and in combination with numerous other uniquely characterized beams, all taking account of the dose provided by each other, comprise IMRT. IMRT is capable of exquisite dose conformation around targets and permits conformal avoidance of structures that would otherwise be damaged by conventional beams, even if delivered by conformal techniques. It may be particularly valuable for tumors of complex shape, such as sarcomas, and has recently been used to treat large intra-abdominal targets such as RPS.[119] Clinical results are awaited from studies of these exciting improvements in RT planning and delivery.

In addition to external beam RT, BRT, and IMRT, several other approaches for RT delivery exist. These include particle beam RT (electrons, protons, pions, or neutrons), intraoperative RT (IORT) using external beam or BRT approaches, and combinations of other techniques (eg, hyperthermia) with RT. IORT has been used most often in the management of RPSs and will be discussed later. Some

Table 108-5 **Relative Indications for Preoperative RT, Despite Concerns Related to Wound Complications**

Treatment Context/Sarcoma Site	Issues of Concern	Comments
Head and neck		
Paranasal sinus	Proximity to optic apparatus (eye, orbit, chiasma)	Major visual functional deficit can be minimized
Skull base	Proximity to spinal cord, brain stem	Other "lesser" morbidities (dental, xerostomia) may also be less due to reduced doses and volumes
Cheek and face	To TS: check earlier edition.	To TS: check earlier edition.
Split thickness skin graft reconstruction (especially lower limb)	Skin graft breakdown and consequent infection	Many months to years of recreational and/or vocational disability may occur during healing (rare)
Large volume GTV or CTV occupying coelomic cavities	To TS: check earlier edition.	To TS: check earlier edition.
Retroperitoneum	Proximity to bowel, liver, kidney	Critical organs may be displaced by tumor or not fixed or adherent as is likely in postoperative setting Entire tumor treated prior to possible contamination of cavity
Some small bowel lesions	Proximity to critical anatomy, especially intestine with side wall adherence	Contamination of abdominal cavity renders postoperative RT unsuitable
Thoracic wall/pleura	Proximity to lung or cardiac structures	Lung may be displaced by chest wall or pleural tumor and can be avoided with preoperative RT, or permits GTV to be treated prior to operative contamination
Abdominal trunk walls, pelvic side wall	Proximity to kidney, bowel, liver, ovaries	Avoid CTV encroachment on vulnerable anatomy GTV adjacent to dose limiting critical anatomy
Thoracic inlet/upper chest	Proximity to brachial plexus	Dose limitation of critical anatomy lends itself to preoperative wall low neck RT. Additional volume considerations
Medial thigh (young male)	Proximity to testes	Permanent infertility may be avoided
Central limb tumor	Proximity to other compartments	Permits partial circumferential sparing, which would not be feasible in postoperative setting

Abbreviations: CTV, clinical target volume; GTV, gross tumor volume; RT, radiotherapy.
Source: Reproduced with permission from *Semin Radiat Oncol*. 1999;9:335.

reports also describe IORT for extremity sarcomas.[155,156] Formal clinical trials have not compared the relative merits of these approaches, and their use may be governed as much by the availability of an approach at a given center as by any special advantage that it may confer. In the case of proton beam RT, its ability to achieve accurate targeting provides an advantage when tumors lie in proximity to critical structures.[157,158] In general, however, although reports on the use of many of these approaches exist, the problems of selection bias need to be considered in interpreting these small series in which treatments were not randomly assigned.[159-163]

Chemotherapy

Chemotherapy is used widely in the metastatic setting for patients with STSs. The use of chemotherapy in the adjuvant setting remains controversial. However, if chemotherapy is going to have the same impact as radiation and surgery in the management of sarcomas, effective drugs will have to be identified that help improve the cure rate for patients with primary tumors and unseen microscopic metastatic disease. This section will review the use of chemotherapy in the adjuvant and metastatic settings. A brief discussion of chemotherapy combined with radiation therapy is also included in this section.

Chemotherapy Following Primary Surgical Resection Although local or locoregional recurrence is a problem for a small subset of patients following primary therapy, the major risk to life in sarcoma patients is uncontrolled systemic disease. The availability of systemic therapy with proven, albeit often limited, ability to induce shrinkage of advanced sarcomas has raised the question of whether the early use of systemic treatment might affect microscopic metastatic disease and yield improvements in overall survival and disease-free survival (DFS).

Certainly for Ewing sarcoma/PNET, rhabdomyosarcoma, and osteogenic sarcoma, adjuvant or neoadjuvant chemotherapy are an appropriate standard of care.[164-166] However, for more common STSs such as leiomyosarcoma, liposarcoma, and high-grade undifferentiated pleomorphic sarcoma (formerly known as MFH), the benefit of chemotherapy, if there is one, is small.[167] Since adjuvant therapy is utilized by many practitioners for more common diseases where the benefit is a relatively small one, such as Stage I breast cancer and Stage II colon cancer, this small potential benefit is an issue that needs to be discussed on an individualized basis. Certainly the lack of available effective agents for metastatic sarcoma have impeded progress in this area, but the utility of imatinib in GIST gives hope that new agents will contribute to the ultimate goal of any type of systemic therapy specifically increasing the cure rate for people with new diagnoses.

There have been over a dozen studies of anthracycline-based adjuvant chemotherapy for STSs that date back nearly as long as the initial development of doxorubicin.[168,169] These will not be reviewed here, since anthracycline/ifosfamide-based therapy constitute a better standard of care in patients offered adjuvant chemotherapy, and only one of the studies completed by 1992 had used ifosfamide. The best summary of anthracycline-containing adjuvant-based chemotherapy for extremity sarcomas to date was the 1997 meta-analysis of 14 studies encompassing sarcomas of all anatomic sites.[170] In this study, 23 potential studies were considered, and 14 ultimately selected, constituting 1,568 patients with STSs of extremity and nonextremity sites with a median follow-up of 9.4 years. Pathology review was not centralized. The results of the meta-analysis, including the actuarial outcome probabilities and the hazard ratios, are summarized in Figure 108-11 and Table 108-6.

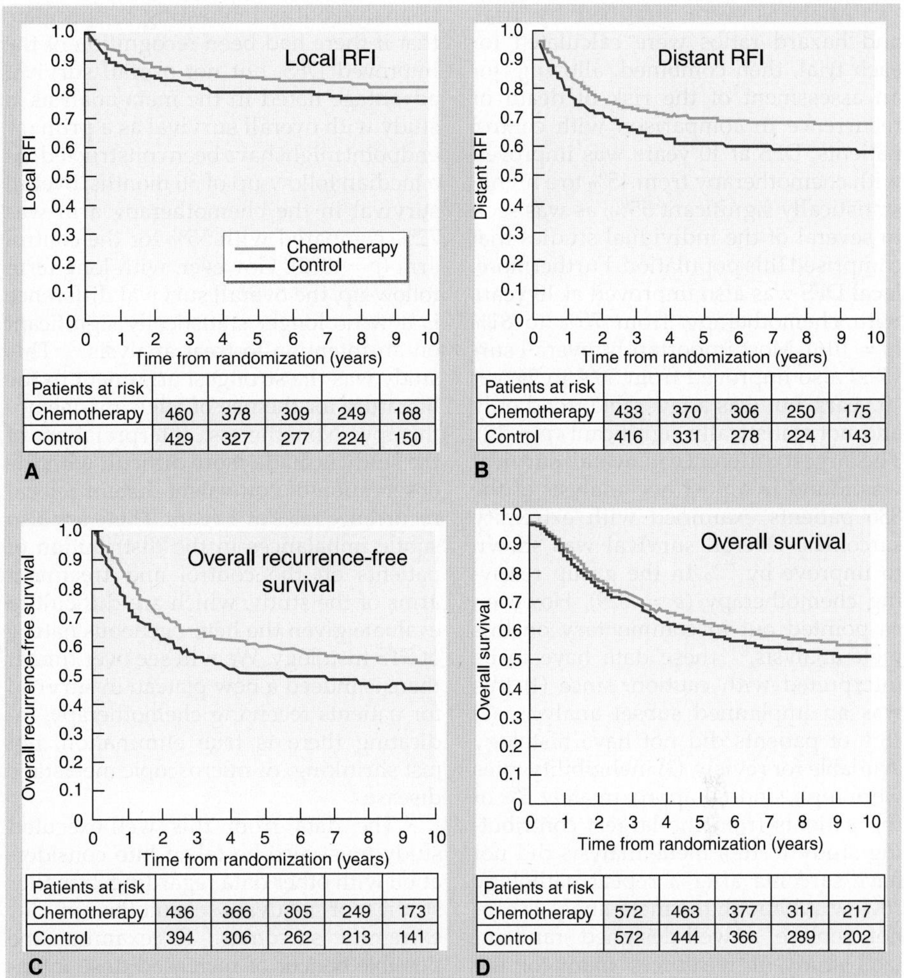

Patients at risk (A)					
Chemotherapy	460	378	309	249	168
Control	429	327	277	224	150

Patients at risk (B)					
Chemotherapy	433	370	306	250	175
Control	416	331	278	224	143

Patients at risk (C)					
Chemotherapy	436	366	305	249	173
Control	394	306	262	213	141

Patients at risk (D)					
Chemotherapy	572	463	377	311	217
Control	572	444	366	289	202

Figure 108-11 Actuarial curves from individual patient data meta-analysis: (**A**) local recurrence-free interval (RFI), (**B**) Distant recurrence-free interval, (**C**) overall recurrence-free survival, and (**D**) overall survival.[178] *Source*: From Ref. 178.

Table 108-6 **Hazard Ratios for Individual Patient Data Meta-Analysis in 1568 Adults from 14 Trials of Doxorubicin-Based Chemotherapy for STS**

Hazard Ratio	Outcome	95% Confidence Intervals	*p* Value
Local RFI	0.73	0.56-0.94	.016
Distant RFI	0.70	0.57-0.85	.0003
Overall recurrence-free survival	0.75	0.64-0.87	.0001
Overall survival	0.89	0.76-1.03	.12

Abbreviation: RFI, recurrence-free interval.
Source: Data from the Sarcoma Data Base Meta-Analysis Collaboration and *Semin Radiat Oncol.* 1999;9:352-359.

Analyses were stratified by trial, and hazard ratios were calculated for each trial, then combined, allowing for an assessment of the risk of death or recurrence in comparison with control patients. DFS at 10 years was improved with chemotherapy from 45% to a highly statistically significant 55%, as was seen in several of the individual studies that comprised this population. Furthermore, local DFS was also improved at 10 years with chemotherapy, from 75% to 81% (p = .016). Most importantly, overall survival also improved from 50% to 54% at 10 years, but was a favorable trend only and not statistically significant (p = .12). The largest difference in overall survival was found in a post hoc analysis of the 886 patients examined with extremity sarcomas. Overall survival was shown to improve by 7% in the group receiving chemotherapy (p = .029). However, as pointed out in commentary on this meta-analysis,[171] these data have to be interpreted with caution, since (1) this was an unplanned subset analysis, (2) 18% of patients did not have histology available for review, (3) ineligibility rates were high, and (4) approximately 6% of the patients from the largest contributing study to this meta-analysis did not have sarcoma after a repeat pathology review. Although the meta-analysis cannot replace a well-designed randomized study, it reinforces many of the findings from smaller studies that local and distant recurrence-free survival is definitely improved, but not necessarily overall survival.

Adjuvant and Neoadjuvant Studies Since the 1997 Meta-Analysis ■ Given that the relevance of these older data to more modern practice may be limited, owing to improved imaging, widespread acceptance of limb-sparing surgery, better pathological classification of sarcomas, and the introduction of ifosfamide and supportive care such as offered by hematopoietic growth factors, other groups have re-examined the question of the utility of adjuvant chemotherapy in randomized studies.

In the largest of such studies, the Italian Sarcoma Study Group (ISSG) examined patients with primary or recurrent resected STS of the extremity or limb girdle treated or not treated with radiation.[172] 104 patients were randomized to receive no chemotherapy or to receive ifosfamide (1,800 mg/m^2/day for 5 consecutive days with mesna) and epirubicin (60 mg/m^2 on 2 consecutive days), with filgrastim support. Interim analysis in 1996 led to early conclusion of the trial because the study had reached its primary endpoint, that of improved DFS. This study was started before the publication of the above-described meta-analysis. It is interesting to speculate that if there had been recognition of the improved DFS, but not overall survival advantage noted in the meta-analysis, a study with overall survival as a primary endpoint might have been constructed. At a median follow-up of 36 months, overall survival in the chemotherapy arm was 72%, compared with 55% for the control arm (p = .002). However, with long-term follow-up, the overall survival difference is now no longer statistically significant on an intention-to-treat analysis.[173] This study was the strongest argument in the literature for the use of adjuvant chemotherapy. Nonetheless, interpretation of the study is made more difficult with the observation of equivalent distant ± local recurrence rates at 4 years. There are also subtle imbalances in the distribution of patients on the control and treatment arms of the study, which are difficult to evaluate given the heterogeneous nature of STS histology. We will see over time if there is indeed a new plateau in survival for patients receiving chemotherapy, indicating there is true elimination, not just shrinking, of microscopic metastatic disease.

The data from this well-executed study must also be taken into consideration with other data regarding 2 smaller studies of adjuvant chemotherapy for extremity sarcomas. To examine the possible benefit of increased dose intensity in an adjuvant setting, an Austrian group studied 59 patients receiving no chemotherapy or doxorubicin 50 mg/m^2/cycle, dacarbazine 800 mg/m^2/cycle, and ifosfamide 6 g/m^2/cycle every 2 weeks with mesna and filgrastim support following surgical resection of the primary sarcoma. Overall survival and relapse-free survival did not differ significantly between the treatment arms at a mean follow-up of 41 months.[174] There were trends to improved recurrence-free survival, but the study was underpowered to detect a small difference in overall survival or DFS. A randomized phase 2 neoadjuvant study of doxorubicin 50 mg/m^2 and ifosfamide 5 g/m^2 by the EORTC and NCI-Canada also failed to show a survival advantage for the use of chemotherapy (estimated 5-year overall survival 64% for the control arm, 65% for the treatment arm).[175] Neoadjuvant chemotherapy is discussed in greater detail below. Finally, the EORTC have completed accrual in December 2003 to an adjuvant trial (Study 62931) of high-grade STSs for all sites, utilizing doxorubicin 75 mg/m^2 and ifosfamide 5,000 mg/m^2 with filgrastim. Analysis will not be feasible until there has been sufficient follow-up.

Preoperative (Neoadjuvant) Chemotherapy ■ Preoperative chemotherapy has theoretical advantages over postoperative treatment. First, preoperative chemotherapy provides an in vivo test of chemotherapy sensitivity. Patients whose tumors show objective evidence of response are presumed to be the subset that will benefit most from further postoperative systemic treatment. In contrast, it is assumed that the population of nonresponding patients will derive minimal or no benefit from further chemotherapy and can therefore be spared its toxicity. On the other hand, it is conceivable that the patients whose tumors respond to chemotherapy may not be those who would derive the most from chemotherapy, because these lesions with favorable biology might be those destined to do well irrespective of any systemic treatment. In contrast, those who do not respond may be those with unfavorable disease who could derive the greatest benefit from the discovery of highly effective systemic treatments.

A second potential advantage of preoperative chemotherapy is that it treats occult microscopic metastatic disease as soon as possible after the cancer diagnosis. This may theoretically prevent the development of chemotherapy resistance by isolated clones of metastatic cells or prevent the postoperative growth of microscopic metastases, but given the nature of growth of sarcomas, at most one or two doublings of the tumor would be affected, far fewer than the greater than 35 typically required in the development of a greater than 1-cm tumor. Chemotherapy-induced cytoreduction may permit a less radical and consequently less morbid surgical resection than would have been required initially. In patients with large STS of the extremities, cytoreduction may reduce the morbidity of limb-sparing surgical procedures and possibly even allow patients who might otherwise have required an amputation to undergo limb-sparing surgery.

Investigators from the MD Anderson Cancer Center reported long-term results with doxorubicin-based preoperative chemotherapy for AJCC Stages IIC and III (formerly AJCC Stage IIIB) extremity STS.[176] In a series of 76 patients treated with doxorubicin-based preoperative chemotherapy, radiologic response rates were as follows: complete response, 9%; partial response, 19%; minor response, 13%; stable disease, 30%; and disease progression, 30%. The overall objective major response rate (complete plus partial responses) was 27%. At a median follow-up of 85 months, 5-year actuarial rates of local recurrence-free survival, distant metastasis-free survival, DFS, and overall survival were 83%, 52%, 46%, and 59%, respectively. The event-free outcomes reported from MD Anderson are similar to those observed with chemotherapy in the phase 3 postoperative chemotherapy trials. Furthermore, comparison of responding patients (complete and partial responses) and non-responding patients did not reveal any significant differences in event-free outcome.

In a prospective study from MSKCC, 29 patients with AJCC (4th edition) Stage IIIB STSs larger than 10 cm were treated with 2 cycles of a doxorubicin-based regimen prior to local therapy.[177] Subjective changes in the degree of primary tumor firmness and in imaging characteristics of the tumor (intratumoral necrosis and hemorrhage) were observed in many patients but were not quantifiable. Only one patient met the standard criteria for a partial response. Survival results in this population of high-risk patients were similar to those in historic controls treated with postoperative doxorubicin or patients treated with local therapy alone. The reasons for the apparent discrepancy in response rates between the reports from M.D. Anderson and MSKCC remain unclear. Possible explanations include the fact that the population treated at MSKCC appears to be a higher risk population, with all patients having high-grade lesions larger than 10 cm, as is discussed below in studies examining retrospective data from both institutions. Moreover, the patients treated at MSKCC received a lower doxorubicin dose (60 mg/m^2) for fewer cycles (2). This may be important given the known dose-response relationship with doxorubicin.[178]

Recently, ifosfamide-containing combinations have been used in the preoperative setting. Selected patients treated with aggressive ifosfamide-based regimens have had major responses, and preliminary results suggest that response rates may be higher than in historic controls treated with nonifosfamide-containing regimens.[179] However, as noted above, the randomized phase 2 neoadjuvant study of doxorubicin and ifosfamide chemotherapy showed no benefit for the treatment arm, although the study was not specifically designed to determine a survival advantage.[175]

Modifying Chemotherapy ■ It has been theorized that the antisarcoma action of adjuvant chemotherapy might be improved by modifying factors related to drug delivery. One such modification is administering chemotherapy regionally rather than systemically. To a great extent, the rationale is based on work in other malignancies that spread predominantly within one segment of the body, such as ovarian cancer, which tends to remain within the peritoneal cavity. Certain sarcomas, such as GIST and some gastrointestinal leiomyosarcomas, have the tendency to recur repeatedly within the peritoneum, without development of widespread hepatic or lung metastases. For such patients, several investigators have examined intraperitoneal chemotherapy. Limited single-institution data have shown it to be feasible, although the efficacy cannot be rigorously assessed because comparisons have been only with historic controls.[180] Decreases in locoregional recurrence rates have been suggested, but the impact of such treatment on overall survival, if any, may be quite limited since it will not effect the development of hepatic metastases. Accordingly, intraperitoneal chemotherapy remains an investigational modality.

Some investigators have promulgated the use of heated chemotherapy instilled into the peritoneal cavity following resection, based on studies of hyperthermic perfusion for extremity lesions.[181,182] However, no clinical data have been generated to assess objectively the potential contribution of heat in this setting. Others have evaluated whole-body hyperthermia to enhance the efficacy of combination chemotherapy, using methods to increase the temperature of the entire body or a specific region alone to 41°C.[183-185] Despite some limited data regarding clinical responses, this technique remains highly investigational. Given the observed toxicities of hypotension and nephrotoxicity, the clinical outcomes associated with this approach would have to represent significant improvements over conventional treatments in order to be widely accepted.[186] Hyperthermia is not routinely employed in the adjuvant therapy of sarcomas.

Combined Preoperative Chemotherapy and RT

With the advances made with combined-modality treatment of other solid tumors, there has been interest in combined-modality preoperative treatment (concurrent or sequential chemotherapy and RT) for patients with localized STSs. One putative advantage of preoperative chemo-radiation is the potential to shrink selected lesions resectable only by amputation sufficiently that they become amenable to a limb-sparing approach.

Concurrent chemotherapy and radiation has been employed extensively by Eilber and colleagues at UCLA and has been modified and examined by other groups.[187-189] The initial chemo-radiation treatment protocol typically involved intra-arterial doxorubicin with unusually high dose per fraction RT (35 Gy of external beam radiation delivered in 10 daily fractions, which was reduced to 17.5 Gy in 5 daily fractions to minimize local toxicity). Although the intra-arterial route delivers chemotherapy more directly to the tumor, it is more complex, expensive, and prone to complications than intravenous chemotherapy.[190] Indeed, a prospective randomized trial comparing preoperative intra-arterial doxorubicin with intravenous doxorubicin, both followed by 28 Gy of radiation delivered over 8 days and then surgical resection, showed no differences in local recurrence or survival.[191]

The largest study to date directly studying systemic chemotherapy combined with RT examined razoxane as the radiation-sensitizing agent in a randomized study of drug versus no drug in combination with radiation therapy for resectable or unresectable STSs. Acute skin reactions were enhanced in the razoxane arm, but late toxicity was not greater than in the control arm. Although there are imbalances in the arms of the study, for the 82 of 130 evaluable cases examined with gross disease RT (median dose 56-58 Gy) with razoxane (daily oral doses of 150 mg/m^2 throughout RT) showed an increased response rate (74% vs 49%), and improved local control rate (64% vs 30%; $p < .05$) compared with external beam radiation alone.[192]

Ifosfamide and cyclophosphamide have been routinely combined with radiation therapy as part of the definitive therapy for Ewing sarcoma and rhabdomyosarcoma in an attempt to continue systemic therapy at the same time as maximizing local control.[165,166] In general, toxicity does not appear to be greater than that seen for radiation alone. However, skin toxicity from the combination was greater in one study than that seen with radiation alone.[193]

An alternative sequential chemotherapy and radiation strategy in patients with localized, high-grade, large (>8 cm) extremity STSs has been examined.[165,166] This treatment protocol involved 3 courses of doxorubicin, ifosfamide, mesna, and dacarbazine with two 22-Gy courses of radiation (11 fractions each) for a total preoperative radiation dose of 44 Gy. This was followed by surgical resection with careful microscopic assessment of surgical margins. An additional 16-Gy (8 fractions) boost dose was delivered for microscopically positive surgical margins. The outcomes of 48 patients treated with this regimen have been compared with those of matched historic controls and was superior to that of the historical control patients. The 5-year actuarial local control, freedom from distant metastasis, DFS, and overall survival rate were 92% vs 86% ($p = .1155$), 75% vs 44% ($p = .0016$), 70% vs 42% ($p = .0002$), and 87% vs 58% ($p = .0003$) for the MAID and control patient groups, respectively. Febrile neutropenia was a complication in 25% of patients. Wound healing complications were substantial and occurred in 14 (29%) patients receiving the chemotherapy/radiation sequential therapy. One patient who received chemotherapy developed late fatal myelodysplasia. Given the favorable results of this study in comparison to historical controls, the Radiation

Therapy Oncology Group is conducting a multi-institutional trial, modifying the chemotherapy in an attempt to address the local toxicity issue.

Although significant toxicity was observed, local control was improved in the prior study, raising the possibility that combined chemotherapy and radiation could be combined safely to decrease local control risk. Pisters and colleagues examined concurrent doxorubicin and irradiation in the neoadjuvant setting in 27 patients with extremity STS.[194] Preoperative external beam radiation was administered in 25 fractions of 2 Gy each. Doxorubicin was administered in escalating doses with a bolus followed by 4-day continuous infusion weekly. Radiographic restaging was performed 4-7 weeks after chemoradiation. Patients with localized disease underwent surgical resection. The maximum tolerated dose of continuous infusion doxorubicin combined with standard preoperative radiation was 17.5 mg/m^2/week; 7 of 23 (30%) patients had grade 3 dermatologic toxicity at this dose level. Macroscopically complete resection (R0 or R1) was performed in all 26 patients who underwent surgery. For 22 patients who were treated with doxorubicin at the maximum tolerated dose and subsequent surgery, an encouraging 11 patients (50%) had 90% or greater tumor necrosis, including 2 patients who had complete pathologic responses. This approach is being further studied with other radiation-sensitizing agents, such as gemcitabine.[195] Further studies of combination therapy are also discussed later in the section "Retroperitoneal Sarcomas."

Recent Analyses of Multicenter Data Regarding Adjuvant Therapy for STS

It is well recognized that different sarcoma subtypes have different chemotherapy sensitivity patterns. For example, MPNSTs are typically resistant to doxorubicin, and leiomyosarcomas are typically less sensitive to ifosfamide than other forms of sarcoma. Synovial sarcoma and myxoid/round-cell liposarcoma appear to be more sensitive to chemotherapy in the metastatic setting than other subtypes of sarcoma, and may well be 2 subtypes that respond to both anthracyclines and ifosfamide.[196] This argues that adjuvant chemotherapy should be examined on a subtype-specific basis. Combined nonrandomized data from UCLA and MSKCC showed that adjuvant chemotherapy may indeed be useful in the setting of synovial sarcomas and myxoid/round-cell liposarcoma, and argued for the use of chemotherapy in the neoadjuvant setting for all types of STS, based on MSKCC and Dana-Farber institutional databases.[197-199] Interestingly, data of all patients treated or not treated with chemotherapy from MD Anderson and MSKCC indicated in the adjuvant or neoadjuvant setting that there was no statistical difference in overall survival in the group of patients who received chemotherapy versus those who did not.[200] However, these data are inherently biased in that it is likely that younger, healthier patients with larger high-grade tumors were those selected to receive chemotherapy. Even though there was no statistically significant difference between the group of patients who received chemotherapy and those who did not, there were still shifts in the frequency of patients with larger sarcomas with a predominance of liposarcoma toward receiving chemotherapy, perhaps representing the selection bias that allowed a group of patients with an inherently poorer outcome to do as well as those with a better outcome.

In summary, for AJCC Stage III STS, if there is a benefit to chemotherapy in the adjuvant setting, it appears to be a small one. In such a situation, it is the authors' practice to attempt to compare benefits and risks of systemic therapy and individualize the plan of treatment for a given clinical setting. Younger patients with relatively chemotherapy-sensitive subtypes such as myxoid/round-cell liposarcoma and synovial sarcoma may be those who benefit most among this very heterogeneous patient population. Certainly, the finding of 20% or more of STS with specific genetic translocations or mutations brings hope that the benefit seen with imatinib and GIST will carry over to the adjuvant setting for a subset of patients with STS of the extremities and trunk when adjuvant chemotherapy is combined with one of the new protein kinase-targeted inhibitors.

"Pediatric" Sarcomas and Adjuvant Therapy

The standard of care for nearly all sarcomas specific to the pediatric population involves chemotherapy. It is of proven benefit in patients with osteogenic sarcoma, Ewing sarcoma, and rhabdomyosarcoma. A few brief comments on these chemotherapy-sensitive tumors follow.

Neoadjuvant chemotherapy, established by Rosen and colleagues, is the standard of care for the initial treatment of osteogenic sarcoma.[201] In the era before chemotherapy, cure rates, even in the setting of amputation for primary disease, was only on the order of 15%. With chemotherapy, the survival rate is on the order of 70%. Yet the 30% of patients who relapse remain a frustrating problem because the addition of new agents has changed the chance for cure comparatively modestly. The outcome of adjuvant chemotherapy (degree of tumor necrosis after chemotherapy) is directly associated with improved clinical outcome, and provides the opportunity for changing chemotherapy for a poor initial response. The standard of care for adjuvant chemotherapy is a backbone of cisplatin and doxorubicin, with more centers adding ifosfamide in newer regimens. High-dose methotrexate is used in most pediatric patients and is an active drug in metastatic disease. The benefit for multiagent adjuvant therapy was called into question in a 1997 paper in which the combination of doxorubicin and cisplatin alone was shown equivalent to a more complicated and toxic regimen (Rosen T10-like) containing high-dose methotrexate as well.[164] However, the methotrexate component of neoadjuvant therapy has been observed to be an important component of the chemotherapy used for osteosarcoma in some studies.[202]

Through a careful series of international clinical studies, the adjuvant program for rhabdomyosarcoma typically involves an induction course of chemotherapy, followed by combination chemotherapy and radiation, followed by the completion of chemotherapy, which will last approximately 48 weeks in pediatric population. The standard of care is the combination of vincristine, dactinomycin, and cyclophosphamide, since this combination was shown as effective as VAI and VIE and less toxic.[166] The addition of doxorubicin to the vincristine, dactinomycin, and cyclophosphamide regimen did not appear to improve overall survival and is usually omitted in the treatment of rhabdomyosarcoma.[203] The frequent dosing of vincristine is extremely difficult to complete for adults and requires dose adjustment or shorter courses of therapy for adults than for children with this diagnosis. Children with this diagnosis appear to fare better than adults with the same diagnosis stage for stage in most studies.[204]

For patients with Ewing sarcoma, in distinction from rhabdomyosarcoma, the addition of additional agents (ifosfamide and etoposide) to an existing backbone of vincristine, doxorubicin, and cyclophosphamide chemotherapy improved outcome for localized disease,[165] while data regarding metastatic disease remain unpublished as of January 2005. This 5-drug regimen is a good standard of care for patients with a new diagnosis of Ewing sarcoma. It is often difficult to administer the entire 48 weeks of chemotherapy to adults, and abbreviation to the adjuvant therapy program is often necessary. As with rhabdomyosarcoma, children with this diagnosis appear to fare better than adults with the same diagnosis, stage for stage.[205]

Treatment of Locally Advanced Disease

Hyperthermic Isolated Limb Perfusion

Hyperthermic isolated limb perfusion (HILP), an investigational technique in the United States (although recently approved by regulatory agencies in other parts of the world), has received considerable attention in the treatment of locally advanced, unresectable sarcomas of nonosseous tissues. HILP has been evaluated in 2 settings: (1) attempted limb preservation in cases of locally advanced extremity lesions surgically amenable only to amputation and (2) function extremity preservation for the short survival duration anticipated in cases of locally advanced extremity lesions with synchronous pulmonary metastases (Stage IV disease).

A multicenter phase 2 trial has evaluated a series of 55 patients with radiologically unresectable extremity STSs using HILP with high-dose tumor necrosis factor-α, interferon-α, and melphalan.[206] A major tumor response was seen in 87% of patients: complete responses in 20 (36%) and partial responses in 28 (51%). Limb salvage was achieved in 84% of patients. Regional toxicity was limited, and systemic toxicity was minimal to moderate. There were no treatment-related deaths. This approach is being further evaluated in ongoing trials in Europe.

Radiation Alone

Apart from patients with some very radiosensitive subtypes of sarcomas, most patients who undergo RT as the sole treatment modality for sarcoma have been deemed to have locally advanced unresectable disease. RT alone is a rare treatment choice that should be done only at centers skilled in the management of sarcomas; medically fit patients with grossly "unresectable" but nonmetastatic disease should always be referred to a specialty center for multidisciplinary management, which may combine surgery, RT, and possibly chemotherapy. For example, proximal inguinal or axillary tumors that encircle major vascular structures in the proximal leg or arm may be resected along with the involved vasculature and the vessels reconstructed. Adjuvant RT is also generally used. Rarely, a patient with truly inoperable locally advanced disease may require RT alone, with either photon or particle (proton, neutron, or pion) beams.[157,161,207-209] No formal clinical trials have been performed to compare these strategies with each other, and they are generally administered in an adverse clinical setting. Local control has been reported in 40-70% of such cases treated with neutrons; treatment with photons is reported to produce local control in approximately 30% of cases.[161,207]

Treatment of Metastatic Disease

Clinical Problem of Metastases

The diagnosis of recurrent or metastatic disease in patients with STSs is devastating. Patients and physicians are aware that, in general, such a diagnosis significantly worsens the expected outcomes. The role of the multidisciplinary sarcoma team in the management of patients with metastatic sarcoma is to recognize opportunities in which multimodality care might still improve important outcomes such as survival or quality of life. Both surgery and systemic chemotherapy can play an important role in improving these outcomes in selected patients. Overall, it is important to recognize that unresectable metastatic sarcomas of soft tissues are—with rare exceptions—eventually fatal, and that chemotherapy is given with the palliative aim of prolonging life and improving quality of life.

The most common site of metastasis from STS of the extremities is the lungs. Indeed, the lungs are the only site of metastasis in approximately 80% of patients with metastases from primary extremity and trunk STS.[210,211] Primary visceral and gastrointestinal sarcomas commonly metastasize to the liver as well as the lungs. Extrapulmonary metastases are uncommon forms of first metastasis from extremity sarcomas and usually occur as a late manifestation of widely disseminated disease.[211] The median survival after development of distant metastases is 11.6 months (Fig. 108-12).[212] The optimal treatment of patients with metastatic STS requires an understanding of the natural history of the disease and individualized selection of treatment options based on patient factors, disease factors, and limitations imposed by prior treatment.

The approach to patients with advanced or metastatic sarcomas is changing over time. We are recognizing that clinical trials must be stratified rationally for data of value to be derived. Studies of "sarcomas" without stratification will soon seem as naïve as studies of "cancer" without further qualification: These mesenchymally derived diseases lumped under the heading of "sarcomas" can be quite different, and studies need to take that into account. To do that and to generate studies of sufficient size and power, large-scale collaborations on a national and international level will be required. Such collaborations are already in place among the nations of Europe (the Soft Tissue and Bone Sarcoma Group of the EORTC), Scandinavian centers, Italian centers, and Canadian centers, and new collaborations are beginning in the United States under the auspices of the American College of Surgeons Oncology Group (ACOSOG). With these collaborations, it is hoped that further research will rapidly translate research findings into the novel therapeutics that are so desperately required by patients with sarcomas.

Resection of Metastatic Disease

Multiple investigators have reported their experience with pulmonary metastasectomy for metastatic STS in adults.[213-222] 3-year survival rates following thoracotomy for pulmonary metastasectomy range

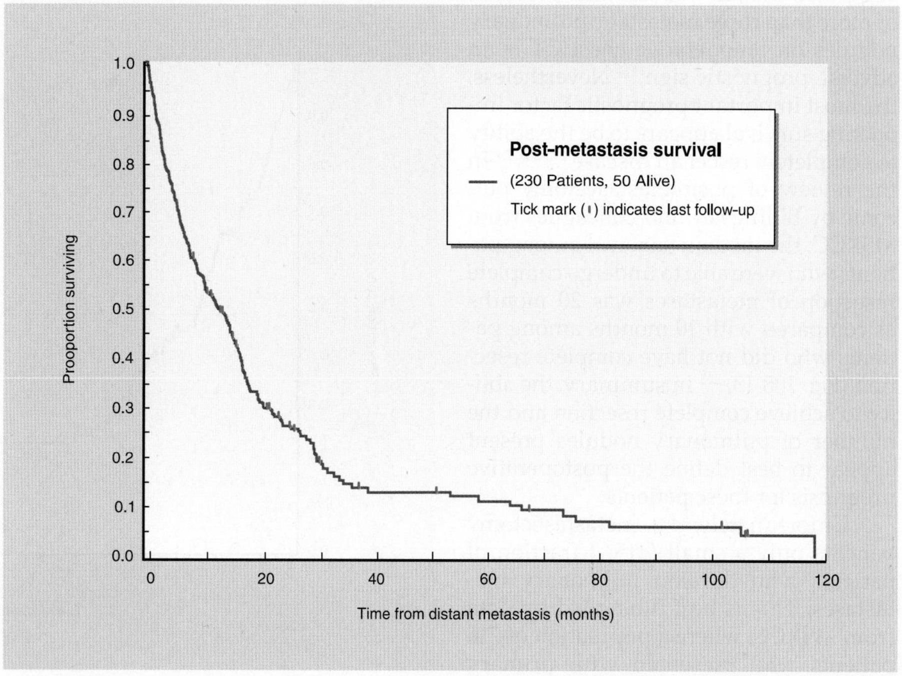

Figure 108-12 Postmetastasis survival (from time of diagnosis of M1 disease) in a cohort of 230 patients with primary STS of the extremities. The median postmetastasis survival was 11.6 months. *Source*: From Ref. 208.

Table 108-7 **Survival Following Complete Resection of Pulmonary Metastases from STS in Adults**

	No. of Patients					
First Author/Institution	Pulmonary Metastases	Total Metastases	Surgical Treatment	Complete Resection (%)	Median Survival, (mo)	3-Year Survival (%)
Creagan[213]/Mayo	112	112	112	64 (57)	18	29
Putnam[223]/NCI	487	93	68	51 (75)	23	32
Jablons[224]/NCI	74	57	57	49 (86)	27	35
Casson[214]/MDACC	68	68	68	58 (85)	25	42
Verazin[231]/Roswell	78	78	78	61 (78)	21	21.5 (5 yr)
Gadd[215]/MSKCC	716	135	78	65 (83)	19	23
van Geel[222]/EORTC	255	255	255	255 (100)	NR	54

Abbreviations: Mayo, Mayo Clinic; Roswell, Roswell Park Cancer Institute; NCI, U.S. National Cancer Institute; MDACC, M. D. Anderson Cancer Center; MSKCC, Memorial Sloan-Kettering Cancer Center; EORTC, European Organization Table for Research and Treatment of Cancer.

from 23% to 54% (Table 108-7).[213-215,222-225] Since the ability to completely resect all metastatic disease is an important determinant of outcome, the reported interinstitution variability in postmetastasectomy survival rates is partially a function of whether survival was reported for all patients who underwent thoracotomy or only for the subset who underwent complete resection.[212,215,224]

It remains difficult to predict which patients with pulmonary metastases will benefit from pulmonary resection. A number of clinical criteria have been evaluated by univariate analysis in this regard, including the disease-free interval, number of metastatic nodules, and tumor doubling time.[213,223,225-230] Multivariate analyses from both the NCI and Roswell Park Cancer Institute confirm that a short disease-free interval and incomplete pulmonary resection are adverse prognostic factors for survival for patients with pulmonary metastases.[224,231] A multivariate analysis from MD Anderson suggested that, in addition, the presence of more than three metastatic pulmonary nodules on preoperative chest CT is an adverse prognostic sign.[214] Nevertheless, the most important prognostic factor impacting survival appears to be the ability to completely resect all disease.[212,215,224] In the review of postmetastasectomy outcome by Billingsley and colleagues from MSKCC, the median survival among patients who were able to undergo complete resection of metastases was 20 months as compared with 10 months among patients who did not have complete resection (Fig. 108-13).[212] In summary, the ability to achieve complete resection and the number of pulmonary nodules present appear to best define the postoperative prognosis for these patients.

Unfortunately, metastasectomy benefits only a small (<15%) fraction of patients who develop pulmonary metastases. This is best illustrated by data from MSKCC, where a population of 716 patients who presented with primary extremity sarcoma were followed for the subsequent development and treatment of pulmonary metastases (Fig. 108-14).[210] Of the initial cohort of 716 patients, 148 patients (21%) developed pulmonary metastases. Isolated pulmonary metastases occurred in 135 (91%) of these 148 patients. Of the 135 patients with pulmonary-only metastases, 78 (58%) were considered to have operable disease, and 65 (83%) of those taken to thoracotomy were able to undergo complete resection of all of their pulmonary metastatic disease. Thus, 44% of all patients with pulmonary metastases were able to undergo complete metastasectomy. The median survival from the time of complete resection was 19 months, and the 3-year survival rate was 23%. All patients who did not undergo thoracotomy died within 3 years. For the entire cohort of 135 patients developing pulmonary-only metastases, the 3-year survival rate was only 11% (Fig. 108-14).

Many investigators believe that repeat thoracotomy to render patients free of disease from pulmonary STS metastases is justified in the absence of effective systemic therapy. Several series of repeat pulmonary metastasectomy have been published.[232,233] In a series of 43 patients thus treated at the NCI, 72% of patients could be rendered free of disease at the second thoracotomy, with a median survival duration from the time of second thoracotomy of 25 months.[232] In a report from MD Anderson of a series of 39 patients undergoing reoperation for a second pulmonary metastasis after successful initial metastasectomy, factors predicting long-term survival included the presence of a solitary metastasis and the ability to perform a complete resection.[233] The MD Anderson study also illustrates the significant survival duration many of these patients enjoy: The median survival in the 19 patients who had complete resection of unifocal recurrent metastatic disease was 65 months as compared with 14 months in the 15 patients who had complete resec-

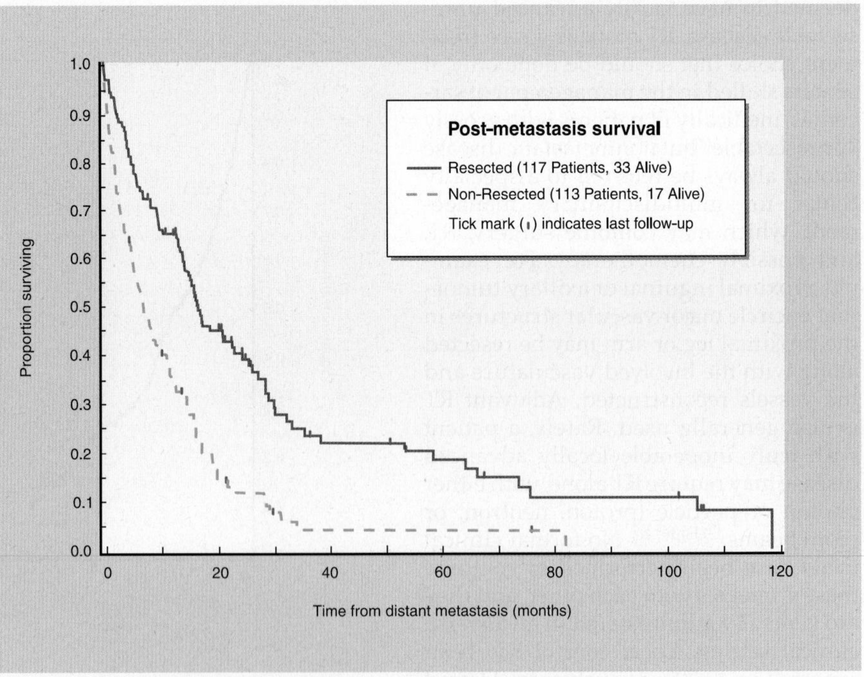

Figure 108-13 Postmetastasis survival stratified by resection of pulmonary metastatic disease. The median survival among patients undergoing complete resection of pulmonary metastatic disease was 20 months. *Source*: From Ref. 212.

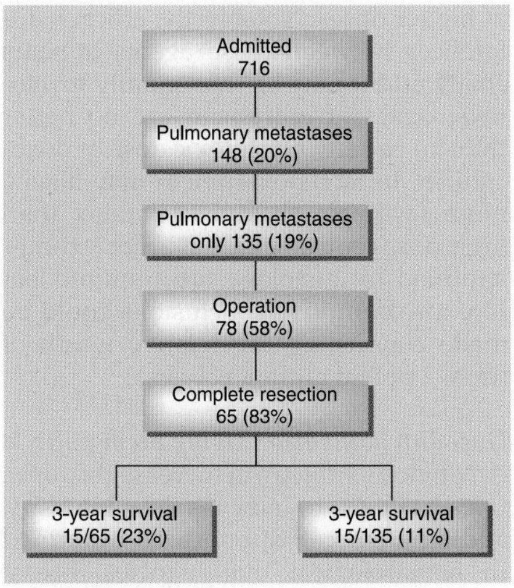

Figure 108-14 Risk and subsequent management of pulmonary metastases in 716 patients with primary or locally recurrent extremity STS. *Source:* From Ref. 210.

tion of two or more sites of recurrent disease.

The rather disappointing overall results of treatment of metastatic disease underscore the importance of careful patient selection for resection of pulmonary metastases. The following criteria are generally agreed upon: (1) the primary tumor is controlled or is controllable, (2) there is no extrathoracic disease, (3) the patient is a medical candidate for thoracotomy and pulmonary resection, and (4) complete resection of all disease appears possible.[234] With careful patient selection, the morbidity of thoracotomy (or repeated thoracotomies) can be limited to the subset of patients who are most likely to benefit from this aggressive treatment approach. The potential role of systemic adjuvant chemotherapy following complete metastasectomy is discussed below in the section "Individualized Therapy" on individualizing chemotherapy for metastases.

Chemotherapy for Metastatic Disease

Natural History of Metastases A good place to begin a discussion of chemotherapy for unresectable metastatic sarcoma is the expected course of the disease. The EORTC has made a major contribution in defining the expected course of unresectable metastatic sarcoma by publishing its large series of more than 2,000 patients with advanced sarcomas of soft tissues to describe prognostic features and the response to anthracycline-based chemotherapy.[235] In this study reviewing more than 20 years of experience, the median overall survival was approximately 1 year for the group as a whole. However, a subset of patients had longer median survival. Such patients were typically those who were younger, had a better performance status, had low-grade sarcoma, had no liver metastases, and had developed metastatic disease following a longer interval from initial diagnosis. Importantly, this study concluded that the variables predicting improved survival were actually different from variables predicting objective response to chemotherapy (the latter variables including such items as high-grade tumor and liposarcoma subtype). Thus, one interpretation that is reasonable is that the most important predictors of survival with metastatic sarcoma are variables dependent on the tumor biology itself, as well as certain patient factors such as age and comorbid disease. These data are critical to understand so that information regarding the impact of new drugs and treatments can be interpreted appropriately, based on a comparison with the correct expectations for the natural or treated history of the disease in past clinical trials.

Individualized Therapy The approach to patients with advanced or metastatic sarcomas is evolving. We increasingly recognize that clinical trials must be stratified rationally for data of value to be derived. Studies of "sarcomas" without stratification will soon seem as naïve as studies of "cancer" without further qualification; each of the greater than 50 mesenchymal cancers lumped under the heading "STSs" has a distinct biological behavior, and studies need to take that into account. To generate studies of sufficient size and power, large-scale collaborations on a national and international level will be required. Such collaborations are already well established among the nations of Europe (the Soft Tissue and Bone Sarcoma Group of the EORTC), Scandinavian centers, Italian centers, and Canadian centers, and new collaborations are forming in the United States under the auspices of the ACOSOG, Intergroup Committee Against Sarcomas (ICAS), and Sarcoma Alliance for Research through Collaboration (SARC). With these collaborations, it is hoped that further research will rapidly translate research findings into the novel therapeutics that are so desperately required by patients with sarcomas.

Tremendous effort has gone into testing multiple, commercially available and experimental agents in STS. Nonetheless, with the exception of imatinib in GIST, no new medication has been accepted widely for use in sarcomas since the introduction of ifosfamide. Nonetheless, new data regarding a gemcitabine/docetaxel combination provides a new option for certain subtypes of sarcoma. The data discussed below are a synopsis of many studies, most of which cannot be referenced owing to constraints of space. Special attention to specific subtypes that are sensitive or resistant to particular chemotherapy drugs is noted.

Anthracyclines and Ifosfamide With the caveat that specific sarcomas demonstrate differential sensitivity to different chemotherapy agents, doxorubicin and ifosfamide remain the 2 most active agents for metastatic sarcoma, with RECIST-defined response rates in the 10-20% range for each drug.[236] Depending on the ratio of sensitive versus less sensitive subtypes of STSs in past studies, the response rate can be significantly higher. For example, synovial sarcoma and myxoid/round-cell liposarcomas are relatively sensitive to ifosfamide (as well as doxorubicin), while GIST, alveolar soft parts sarcoma, and hemangiopericytoma/solitary fibrous tumor are notoriously resistant to both agents. Certain studies have recognized that conventional doxorubicin plus ifosfamide-based chemotherapy is suboptimal for gastrointestinal leiomyosarcomas, and patients with these tumors are excluded from studies of such treatments. However, when this iscompleted, it is impossible to tell whether high rates of response are due to the treatment under study or due to the exclusion of groups of patients who have had lower response rates in other trials.[179]

It is also important to recognize that response rates per se are increasingly being criticized as possibly poor surrogates of clinical benefit. Many sarcomas have densely hyalinized desmoplastic stromal tissues associated with them. Even when chemotherapy successfully induces massive tumor cell kill in vivo, this hyalinized tissue remains unchanged, leading to falsely negative imaging findings of tumor response to chemotherapy. Thus, objective response rates based on imaging may actually underestimate the antitumor efficacy of chemotherapy. Conversely, simply shrinking a tumor and achieving a nondurable response may not be worth the toxicities of aggressive multiagent chemotherapy. Thus, from both standpoints, RECIST-defined responses may not be an ideal indicator of antitumor efficacy in sarcoma management in general, with GIST an excellent case in point.[237] Increasing attention in the field of sarcoma drug development is thus being paid to other important indicators of clinical outcomes, such as progression-free survival duration, percentage survival at a given time point, and overall survival rate.

Some drugs may slow disease progression and prolong survival even if objective response rates are low, although the clinical data to support those claims must be generated with rigor and careful attention to consistency of follow-up. Nonetheless, despite observations that clinical benefit might be underestimated by RECIST, it remains the yardstick by which clinical responses are measured. The measurement of clinical benefit will be an increasingly important question as molecular protein kinase inhibitors such as antiangiogenic agents become more widely used. It may well be that tumor stasis or "euangiogenesis" is the best possible outcome achieved by some of these newer agents, although it is hoped in and of itself normalization of blood vessels within tumors may allow for reactivation of apoptotic mechanisms within the cell that are suppressed by hypoxia through the action of HIF-alpha.[238] It will be difficult to prove the activity of such agents in comparison with historical control groups because of selection bias issues, and careful statistical designs will be necessary to help identify which newer agents are useful or not.

Notably, taxanes or gemcitabine alone (in the typical 30-minute bolus infusion) were largely inactive.[239,240] However, with gemcitabine given as a controlled rate infusion of 10 mg/m^2/min in combination with docetaxel, activity increased to 40-50% in a group of patients with leiomyosarcoma as a dominant histology.[241,242] These data both point out the importance of examining different schedules of drugs as well as the differential sensitivity of different subtypes of sarcomas to different chemotherapy agents.

Dose-Response Relationships ■ The sensitivity of sarcomas to chemotherapy was first convincingly demonstrated with doxorubicin in the early 1970s.[178] Subsequent studies of doxorubicin in sarcomas have widely been viewed as supporting a dose-response relationship, with doses of 50 mg/m^2/cycle or less producing far less antitumor activity than doses of 60 mg/m^2/cycle or higher. Although a dose-response relationship may exist, it is important to recognize that other variables may affect antitumor efficacy, such as histopathologic subtype of sarcoma, as noted above. Nonetheless, since a dose threshold for optimal activity has been documented with doxorubicin in another chemotherapy-sensitive solid tumor, specifically breast cancer, it seems reasonable to conclude that doxorubicin is best used at doses above 60 mg/m^2/cycle. Also analogous to breast cancer, improved response rates above the conventional 60-75 mg/m^2/cycle dose range are difficult to demonstrate.

A wide variety of dose- and schedule-ranging studies have been performed with ifosfamide. It is clear that antitumor response is improved by higher doses of ifosfamide.[179] This point has been made most convincingly by the responses to high-dose ifosfamide (>10,000 mg/m^2/cycle) in patients who had previously failed to respond to the same drug at lower doses (ie, <6,000 mg/m^2/cycle). However, given the potential toxicities of this drug at high doses, high-dose ifosfamide is best reserved for a small subset of patients with disease that is expected to be highly chemotherapy sensitive to achieve meaningful responses (eg, prior to planned surgical extirpation of metastases).

Single-Agent vs. Combination Chemotherapy ■ A continuing controversy is whether the optimal approach to patients with advanced sarcomas is combination chemotherapy regimens or sequential single agents. One of the best prospective randomized trials of combination chemotherapy for advanced disease came from a U.S. intergroup study in which ifosfamide was or was not given to previously untreated patients with metastatic or advanced STS receiving doxorubicin plus dacarbazine. This study demonstrated no survival advantage for the group receiving ifosfamide in combination with doxorubicin plus dacarbazine, although this group had a statistically significant increase in objective response rate.[243] The role of combination chemotherapy is further called into question for broad use given the statistically significant increase in toxicities when ifosfamide was added. Thus, despite the increased anticancer activity as evidenced by the small but significant improvement in response rates, no survival benefit was obtained by adding a third drug. These data are widely interpreted as supporting aggressive combination chemotherapy for patients with bulky locally advanced disease who may be candidates for limb-sparing surgery after preoperative chemotherapy. However, for patients with widespread advanced disease, such combination chemotherapy may be appropriate only if a rapid induction of response is required to control acute symptoms such as tumor-related pain or obstruction. It is hoped that the advent of less toxic kinase-directed therapy will decrease the overall toxicity burden for many patients receiving palliative treatment.

Strategies to Improve the Therapeutic Index of Chemotherapy ■ ***Epirubicin vs. Doxorubicin*** ■ Advances in pharmacology and other supportive care have yielded significant changes in the delivery of active chemotherapy for sarcoma patients. The impact of these advances may not yet have been recognized in widespread practice. One of the first such strategies was modifying the chemical structure of the most potent agent, doxorubicin, into another anthracycline, epirubicin. Epirubicin has diminished cardiac toxicity on a milligram-for-milligram basis compared with doxorubicin, allowing the delivery of higher doses. Notably, the efficacy differences between these agents appears small, and it may be that equally myelotoxic doses of epirubicin are no better than an equally myelotoxic dose of doxorubicin. In fact, doxorubicin may have a more favorable therapeutic index than high-dose epirubicin.[244] Larger studies stratified by histology are required before any definitive conclusions could be made concerning the relative worth of these 2 potent anthracyclines.

Dose Intensification Using Stem Cells ■ An obvious strategy to increase response rates has been to increase dose intensity, adding stem cell support, as examined in hematological malignancies, breast adenocarcinoma, and other malignancies. This was initially attempted solely with provision of autologous bone marrow support and in the past decade has been significantly facilitated by the availability of hematopoietic cytokines to improve hematologic tolerance to myelosuppressive chemotherapy. It is clear that peripheral blood progenitor cells can be mobilized and harvested following standard chemotherapy for sarcoma supported by granulocyte colony-stimulating factor.[245] However, even in chemotherapy-sensitive diseases such as Ewing sarcoma, dose intensification with autologous stem cell support does not appear to be beneficial for improving survival, although contamination of stem cells with tumor cells may be a contributing factor to its lack of efficacy. The use of high-dose chemotherapy with stem cell and cytokine support remains investigational for sarcomas.

Encapsulated Anthracyclines ■ Another strategy to increase the therapeutic index of anthracyclines is to encapsulate the drug within a liposomal vehicle. At least three liposomal preparations of anthracyclines have been tested, and all have shown some efficacy against sarcomas. Notably, the most widely used agent has decreased cardiac risk in comparison to older preparations of larger liposomes containing doxorubicin. Pegylated liposomal doxorubicin (Doxil/Caelyx) is a small liposome with polyethylene glycol anchored within the lipid bilayer, acting as a hydrophilic coating to preserve the circulating half-life of the liposome and prevent degradation within the reticuloendothelial system. This preparation, given at a dose rate less than that of unencapsulated doxorubicin, is better tolerated than doxorubicin, with substantially less myelotoxicity, cardiac toxicity, and alopecia at the cost of hand-foot syndrome and idiosyncratic reactions to the first dose of therapy. In 1 randomized phase 2 study, pegylated liposomal doxorubicin was as effective as doxorubicin.[246]

A less toxic anthracycline preparation has yielded a way to extend systemic therapy to patients with poorer performance status and in principle is a novel way of treating very slowly growing connective tissue lesions such as myxoid liposarcomas or desmoid tumors.

New Agents ■ Sarcomas represent a fertile ground for the field of drug development. Doxorubicin was first recognized as an effective agent against sarcomas and subsequently was developed into one of the most widely used anticancer agents ever discovered. A few of the new agents and their utility in sarcoma are noted below, in particular trabectedin (ET-743), which shows specific activity against liposarcomas and leiomyosarcomas. The next edition of this chapter will no doubt contain much more information on small molecule kinase inhibitors and other small molecule inhibitors, many of which are just beginning to be tested now.

Trabectidin (ET-743, Ecteinascidin) ■ Trabectedin (Yondelis) is a marine-derived drug from the marine tunicate *Ecteinascidia turbinata*. It covalently binds to the minor groove of the DNA and blocks the cell cycle in late S and G2, and affects the transcription in part by prevention of binding of transcription factor NF-Y, thus decreasing expression of a variety of genes, including multidrug resistance genes.[247] After initial promising results in phase 1 studies, multiple phase 2 trials were performed examining GIST (in which it was inactive), osteogenic sarcoma, and untreated and previously treated metastatic STS patients.[248-252]

In the first study of previously treated sarcoma patients, ET-743 was administered at a dose of 1.5 mg/m^2 over 24 hours by ambulatory infusion pump every 3 weeks.[252] 52 patients were assessable for response. Tumor histology included leiomyosarcoma (26 nonuterine, 15 uterine), liposarcoma (n = 11), GIST (n = 7), synovial sarcoma (n = 6), MFH (n = 6), fibrosarcoma (n = 7), and other sarcomas (n = 22). Patients received a median of three cycles of ET-743. 2 partial responses and 4 minor responses were observed, as well as 9 patients with stable disease as best response. Median progression-free survival was 1.9 months. 24% of patients were progression-free at 6 months. 30% of patients were alive at 2 years, with an overall median survival of 12.8 months. 2 patients died of treatment-related causes, but both were attributed to protocol eligibility violations. Toxicity included reversible grade 3-4 elevations in AST or ALT in half of patients, and 61% of patients had grade 3-4 neutropenia, with 6 episodes of febrile neutropenia.

A confirmatory phase 2 study of ET-743 was performed in pretreated patients, excluding GIST patients.[251] Patients again received ET-743 as a 24-hour IV continuous intravenous at 1.5 mg/m^2 every 3 weeks. Tumor histology included leiomyosarcoma (n = 13), liposarcoma (n = 10), synovial sarcoma (n = 6), malignant schwannoma (n = 2), and other (n = 5). Overall response rate was 8% (95% confidence interval, 2-23%), with 1 complete response and 2 partial responses. The most significant finding was that responses lasted up to 20 months. Including two patients with minor responses, the "clinical benefit rate" was 14%. The most common significant toxicities were again grade 3-4 neutropenia and grade 3-4 transaminitis. 1-year estimates for time to progression and overall survival rates were 9% and 53%, respectively. Similar response rates are seen in previously untreated patients. A phase 2/3 study of ET-743 in patients with metastatic leiomyosarcoma and liposarcoma comparing a weekly schedule of ET-473 with the 24-hour infusion schedule noted above is open and should complete accrual in 2005.

9-Nitrocamptothecin ■ A phase 2 study of topoisomerase I inhibitor 9-nitrocamptothecin (9NC) was recently completed, examining patients with gastrointestinal (GI) leiomyosarcomas and other STSs.[253] 9-NC was given by mouth at 1.5 mg/m^2 daily, 5 days every week. A total of 56 patients were enrolled on this study. Only 1 of 17 patients with GI leiomyosarcoma responded, so that arm of the study was closed; of 39 patients with other sarcomas 3 partial responses were observed, lasting 4, 6, and 13 months. 4 patients required hospitalization for nausea, vomiting, and dehydration; other toxicities included anorexia, diarrhea, fatigue, and neutropenia. Its relative lack of activity was consistent with a phase 2 study of irinotecan in sarcomas (several of which were GIST and therefore resistant to chemotherapy). It should be noted that topoisomerase I agents are active in rhabdomyosarcoma and Ewing's sarcoma/PNET.

Bortezomib ■ Bortezomib (PS-341, Velcade), a therapy targeting the proteasome of the cell, is active against myeloma as well as previously difficult to treat malignancies such as mantle-cell lymphoma. It is believed that disruption of the many physiological processes dependent on protea-some function is the reason for activity of bortezomib in these malignancies, such as regulation of cell-cycle proteins, TP53, and NF kappa B signaling pathways. A two-arm phase 2 study was performed examining sarcomas with histologies more commonly seen in adults or in children. Bortezomib was given as a 1.5 mg/m^2 intravenous push twice weekly, 2 weeks on, 1 week off. Only 1 response (leiomyosarcoma) was seen in 21 evaluable patients and the study was closed.[254] Side effects were significant, and included myalgias, persistent neuropathy, abdominal pain, and fatigue. The authors concluded if bortezomib were to be studied further, it should be in combination with other chemotherapy agents.

Management of Local Recurrence

If an isolated local recurrence is identified, the treatment goals are the same as for patients with primary tumors, namely, optimal local control while maintaining as much function and cosmesis as possible.[152] Early identification of local relapse may improve the chance of successful salvage therapy, and, like newly diagnosed patients, these patients are probably best managed in specialized multidisciplinary sarcoma centers. An approach to the evaluation and management of locally recurrent STS is summarized in Figure 108-15. The initial evaluation must include a full review of previous therapy because this will have a bearing on the therapeutic options available. Therefore, all prior surgery and pathology reports should be examined, as should reports on previous chemotherapy and previous RT, especially volume treated, dose, and energy of radiation.

Staging should be performed in the same way as for new cases. The areas adjacent to the original lesion and potentially contaminated by previous surgical interventions should be scrutinized carefully. Both these areas and tissues adjacent to the recurrent tumor, containing potential tumor extensions, should be considered at risk and candidates for resection and/or inclusion in radiation fields.

Several distinct groupings are evident under the rubric of "locally recurrent" disease: (1) cases in which prior treatment did not include RT, (2) cases treated with RT in the past, (3) cases in which distant metastases are also present, and (4) cases in which it is difficult to distinguish between recurrence and secondary tumors induced by RT. Although the therapeutic options available are more limited in recurrent disease and the challenge posed by these cases are much more formidable, a proportion of these patients can be cured. Clinical experience is needed to determine which therapeutic options are appropriate in a given case of recurrent disease.

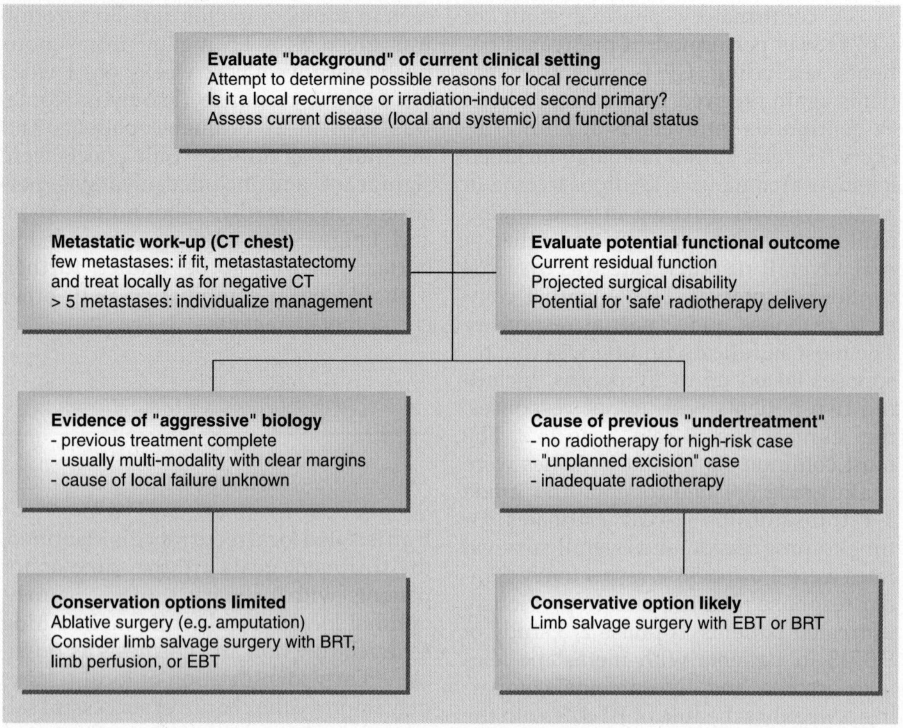

Evaluate "background" of current clinical setting
Attempt to determine possible reasons for local recurrence
Is it a local recurrence or irradiation-induced second primary?
Assess current disease (local and systemic) and functional status
Metastatic work-up (CT chest)
few metastases: if fit, metastastatectomy
and treat locally as for negative CT
> 5 metastases: individualize management
Evaluate potential functional outcome
Current residual function
Projected surgical disability
Potential for 'safe' radiotherapy delivery
Evidence of "aggressive" biology
- previous treatment complete
- usually multi-modality with clear margins
- cause of local failure unknown
Cause of previous "undertreatment"
- no radiotherapy for high-risk case
- "unplanned excision" case
- inadequate radiotherapy
Conservation options limited
Ablative surgery (e.g. amputation)
Consider limb salvage surgery with BRT,
limb perfusion, or EBT
Conservative option likely
Limb salvage surgery with EBT or BRT

Figure 108-15 Schema for approaching the patient with local recurrence of STS. The schema is oriented toward extremity lesions but is equally applicable to other anatomic sites (eg, head and neck and retroperitoneum). *Abbreviations*: BRT, brachytherapy; EBT, external beam radiotherapy. *Source*: From Catton CN et al. *Semin Radiat Oncol*. 1999;9:378–388.

Gastrointestinal Stromal Tumors

No discussion of sarcomas would be complete without noting the remarkable advances made with one particular sarcoma subtype, GIST, which has changed the way people think about sarcomas. With the recognition of c-*kit* as a good marker for GIST to distinguish it from other sarcomas and the recognition of c-*kit* or PDGFR activating mutations that are likely responsible for the constitutive activation of c-*kit*,[255] clinical studies followed rapidly, and have been done in parallel to studies investigating the biology of GIST. Of note, Ewing sarcomas can mark positive for c-*kit* but kit is not mutated in these tumors and Ewing sarcomas do not respond to imatinib.

After the recognition of in vivo efficacy of imatinib against a GIST cell line, treatment of metastatic disease has rapidly advanced from treating a single patient (Fig. 108-16) to phase 1, 2, and 3 studies for patients with metastatic disease.[256-260] The results have been remarkably consistent. Imatinib is at least 10-fold more active than any agent ever examined for treatment of GIST (formerly called GI leiomyosarcoma). The response rate to imatinib is approximately 60%, 20% with stable disease, and 20% with overt progression on therapy. U.S. phase 3 data indicate that 400 mg and 800 mg yield equivalent time-to-progression curves, but the European/Australian phase 3 study indicates that time to progression is improved with the higher dose (800 mg daily) arm.[259] Remarkably, patients' c-*kit* genotype determined their response rate (Fig. 108-17).[261] Patients with exon-11 mutation (just inside the cell membrane) had an 80-90% response rate, while patients with exon-9 mutation had a high response rate only one-third to one-half. Patients with no mutation in c-*kit* had a much lower response rate, but still higher than that observed for other chemotherapy drugs. For the time being, regardless of mutation status, imatinib is the standard of care for metastatic GIST. A dosage of 400 mg daily is a reasonable starting point for most patients, with increase toward 800 mg if there is evidence of progression of disease or the presence of exon 9 mutation.[262] Therapy should not be interrupted if apparent new hypodense lesions appear in the liver; these likely represent occult metastatic disease.[263]

The median time to progression for patients with metastatic GIST on imatinib is approximately 18-22 months. Patients with progression on a lower dose of imatinib can respond again with dose increases. The phase 1 study of imatinib indicated that the maximum tolerated dosage is 800 mg daily (400 mg by mouth bid). Patients with progression of disease have had unusual patterns of progression.[263] In some cases, tumor regrowth in an apparently necrotic tumor is observed, and in others only one metastatic deposit is seen to progress instead of the multiplicity of lesions seen in many patients with advanced GIST. As a result some patients have been treated with carefully planned operations to remove problematic single sites of metastatic disease.

The rationale for consideration of metastasectomy for patients with respoidning or stable metstatic disease on Imatinib is based on the observations that: (1) pathologic complete response to imatinib is very rare (<5%) and many (perhaps most) patients will eventually develop secondary resistance to imatinib owing chiefly to development of secondary resistance mutations. Reports from high volume centers demonstrate that carefully selected patients treated by imatinib and subsequent metastasectomy appear to have very favorable progression-free survival rates. Whether this is due to case selection or bona fide clinical benefit related to surgery is unclear.[264,265] A randomized controlled trial evaluation of the impact of metasectomy in patients with stable or responding disease is planned in Europe. Results of this trial or similar design studies will help to better define what role surgery should play in the management of patients with metastatid GIST.

In the era of imatinib resistance, new agents are coming to the fore. The addition of mTOR inhibitor RAD001 was examined in imatinib-resistant patients, since RAD001, like rapamycin, blocks a step downstream from the c-kit molecule and could again inhibit an important pathway keeping the GIST cell alive. Early data are not particularly encouraging, but the study was in its early stages.[266] Better results to date have been observed with c-kit (and flt3 and VEGF receptor) inhibitor SU11248. SU11248 can only be taken intermittently owing to cumulative toxicity, typically mucositis, toxic epidermal necrolysis (deep-seated blister-like rash of the palms and soles), inanition, and thus presently is being investigated in a 4-week-on, 2-week-off daily schedule starting at 50 mg daily. Although the RECIST response rate is only approximately 10% in the imatinib refractory setting from early phase 1/2 data, a significant proportion of patients (~50%) are able to remain without progression of disease for more than 6 months, and often have some decrease in size of tumor lesions.[267] PET scan will often indicate inactivation of the tumor, but CT scan responses have been slow to develop in comparison to those seen with imatinib. A similar compound, AMG706, is under investigation in the imatinib refractory setting, as are other newer "targeted therapies."

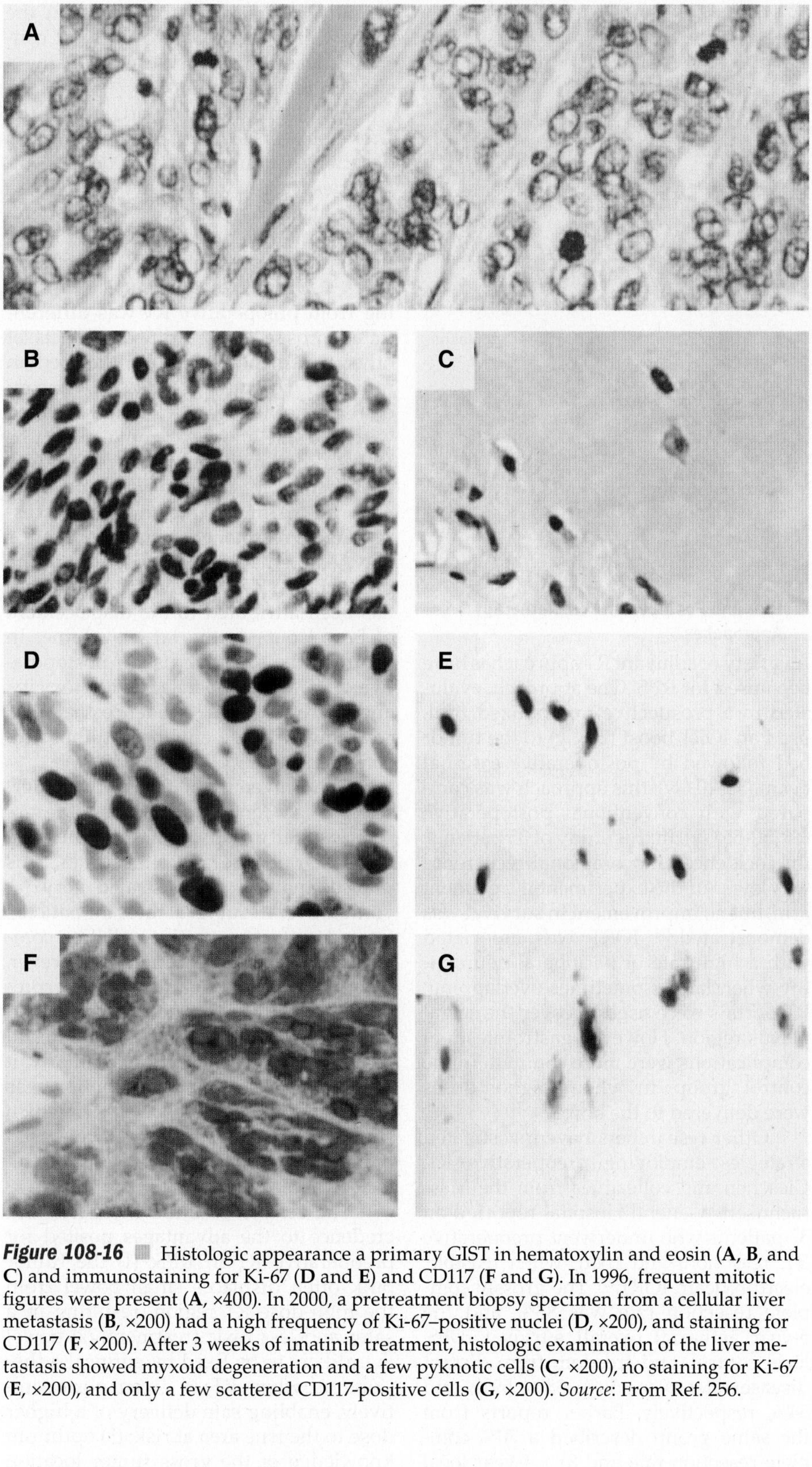

Figure 108-16 ■ Histologic appearance a primary GIST in hematoxylin and eosin (**A**, **B**, and **C**) and immunostaining for Ki-67 (**D** and **E**) and CD117 (**F** and **G**). In 1996, frequent mitotic figures were present (**A**, ×400). In 2000, a pretreatment biopsy specimen from a cellular liver metastasis (**B**, ×200) had a high frequency of Ki-67–positive nuclei (**D**, ×200), and staining for CD117 (**F**, ×200). After 3 weeks of imatinib treatment, histologic examination of the liver metastasis showed myxoid degeneration and a few pyknotic cells (**C**, ×200), no staining for Ki-67 (**E**, ×200), and only a few scattered CD117-positive cells (**G**, ×200). *Source*: From Ref. 256.

Given the remarkable activity of imatinib in the metastatic setting, there has been considerable interest in its possible role as adjuvant treatment after primary tumor resection. The ACOSOG has recently reported results of a phase 3 trial that compared adjuvant imatinib (400 mg/daily) to placebo following complete resection of GISTs greater than 3 cm in size. This study was halted to further accrual after accruing 762 patients when a planned interim analysis for the primary endpoint demonstrated superior progression-free survival in the imatinib arm (97% vs 83% in the placebo arm).[268] 2 additional randomized trials have completed accrual in Europe. These studies compare 1 versus 3 years of adjuvant imatinib and observation versus 2 years of imatinib. These studies will shed more light on the optimal duration of adjuvanttherapy. At this juncture, the only recommendation that can be made is that 1 year of adjuvant treatment be considered for patients with intermediate- and high-risk resected primary GISTs.

Dermatofibrosarcoma Protuberans

DFSP is a nodular "protruberant" lesion arising from the dermis with characteristically slow but persistent growth over many years. Although histologically of low grade or borderline malignant potential, DFSP has a propensity for local recurrence after simple excision. Typical manifestations of DFSP are a red to purple lesion on the upper trunk, especially the shoulder and supraclavicular regions of the head and neck. Not infrequently, small satellite lesions are evident at the site of a prior excision or bordering a skin graft following an unsuccessful previous excision. Surgical resection with wide surgical margins or more conservative surgery (facilitating cosmesis) with adjuvant external beam RT results in extremely low recurrence rates. Adjuvant RT should be considered in cases of recurrence. Recurrent DFSP can be associated with secondary fibrosarcomatous histologic changes, thereby reinforcing the need to achieve primary tumor control as well as to optimize cosmesis. In rare instances, metastasis may result in association with fibrosarcomatous transformation.

Imunohistochemical staining for the CD34 antigen is a hallmark of DFSP. In addition, chromosomal translocation and gene fusion products (Table 108-1) result in the expression of a COL1A1-PDGF-B fusion protein that is processed to mature PDGF-B, resulting in autocrine or paracrine interaction with the PDGF-B receptor on the cell surface of DFSP. Of importance, imatinib inhibits the PDGF tyrosine kinase receptor in the same way that it inhibits the BCR-ABL tyrosine kinase receptor of chronic myeloid leukemia and the *c-Kit* tyrosine kinase receptor of GISTs. Recent clinical data have shown substantial responses to imatinib in patients with metastatic DFSP.[269,270] This suggests the opportunity for targeted molecular therapies, particularly for metastatic or locally advanced DFSP.

Retroperitoneal Sarcomas

RPSs comprise about 15% of STS. They present late and are located in regions where the administration of both surgery and RT is often compromised

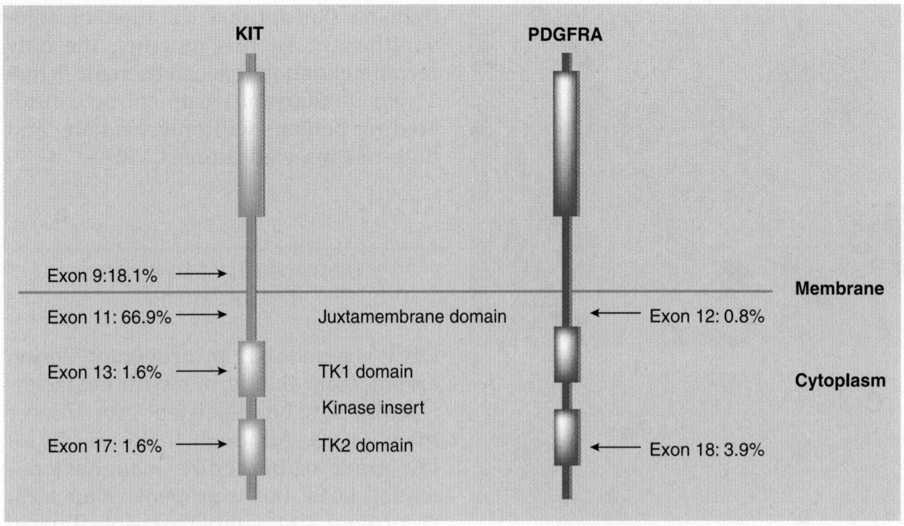

Figure 108-17 Mutation status of gastrointestinal stromal tumors and location on the c-kit or PDGFRA protein. *Source*: From Ref. 26.

(eg, adjacent to the small bowel and liver). Consequently, the local control rates achieved with combined-modality treatment of extremity STSs are not seen in RPS. In a series of 102 RPS patients treated at Princess Margaret Hospital, complete excision was achieved in only 45, gross disease remained in 29, and only a biopsy was possible in 28.[271] The overall locoregional relapse-free rates were 28% and 9% at 5 and 10 years, respectively. RT did not improve survival but appeared to significantly lengthen the time to locoregional relapse, especially with higher doses. Complete tumor resection was the only significant prognostic variable for survival and locoregional and distant failure. These results are similar to those reported from MSKCC.[272] Patients with RPS should be evaluated in a multidisciplinary clinic prior to treatment so that patients can benefit from the expertise and investigational approaches available in such centers.

Recently, 2 reports from Europe have explored extended surgery termed compartmental resection as a strategy to improve local control for patients with RPS.[273,274] These retrospective reports from France and Italy have suggested that local control may be enhanced by resecting adjacent involved viscera—primarily the kidney and colon. Interpretation of these reports is complicated by significant selection bias and, as outlined in an editorial that accompanied these papers,[275] no specific therapeutic recommendation can be made based on these data. At this time, there are no clinical trials demonstrating improved local control with more radical surgery that involves resection of adjacent uninvolved viscera.

Pre- and Postoperative Radiotherapy Approaches

A variety of adjuvant RT approaches have been used for RPS. One approach, evaluated in a prospective randomized trial, used an IORT boost (20 Gy) to the tumor bed followed by postoperative external beam (35-40 Gy); this approach was compared with conventional postoperative RT (50-55 Gy). In this study of 35 patients, the incidence of locoregional recurrence was lower in the experimental treatment arm, but no improvement in survival was demonstrated.[276] IORT was associated with a high rate of peripheral neuropathy when large, sometimes overlapping, RT portals were used to cover the sacral plexus region. However, gastrointestinal complications were more common in the control group, in whom higher doses were delivered to the bowel.

Other researchers have investigated strategies employing preoperative RT. Gieschen and colleagues from the Massachusetts General Hospital reported on 37 patients who underwent preoperative RT, resection, and then, when feasible, electron beam IORT.[277] The grossly complete resection rate was 83%, and the 5-year actuarial overall survival, DFS, local control, and freedom from distant disease rates were 50%, 38%, 59%, and 54%, respectively. Earlier reports from the same group described a 70% complete resection rate and 81% 4-year local control rate.[278] The more recent report also indicates that complete resection and IORT improved overall survival and local control rates (74% and 83%, respectively) compared with no IORT (30% and 61%, respectively). However, the study was not randomized, and potentially more favorable and accessible lesions may have been chosen for IORT. More recently, Petersen and colleagues at the Mayo Clinic found improved local control, at least of primary tumors, using a similar treatment approach.[279]

Another recent report (from the University of Toronto Sarcoma Group) described an unusually favorable outcome, especially for primary lesions, in a single-arm prospective trial of preoperative RT (median dose of 45 Gy in 25 fractions) plus postoperative BRT in selected cases.[280] Of interest, acute toxicity resulting from preoperative RT was differentiated prospectively from the effects of other treatments. Although the median radiation volume exceeded 7L, preoperative external beam RT was associated with extremely low gastrointestinal toxicity scores. Furthermore, no patient was hospitalized for acute toxicity, and there were no treatment interruptions or cessations of treatment because of acute toxicity. The remarkably low toxicity of the preoperative RT with enormous volumes has been attributed to the displacement of bowel outside the target volume. In contrast, the selective use of postoperative BRT was associated with toxicity, and there was little evidence that BRT contributed to the enhanced tumor outcome reported.[280]

The University of Texas MD Anderson Cancer Center and Princess Margaret Hospital groups combined the data from their phase 2 and pilot studes. This pooled analysis demonstrated very favorable overall survival rates for patients treated with preoperative radiation combine with surgical resection.[281] However, we again caution against overinterpretation of results that could be explained by surgical technique at major referral centers or by case selection. Similarly, it remains unclear what contribution was provided by the BRT or IORT, which should probably remain protocol-based or be reserved for nonstandard use in selected cases.

The results of these 3 reports add credence to the advantages posited for preoperative RT in RPS: (1) the tumor bulk often displaces small bowel from the high-dose RT region, resulting in a safer and less toxic treatment; (2) bowel is unlikely to be fixed by surgical adhesions as when RT is given postoperatively, enabling safe delivery of a higher dose to the true area at risk; (3) optimum knowledge of the gross tumor location is possible, permitting better radiation targeting; (4) the tumor is contained by an intact peritoneal covering, providing a physical barrier to immediate tumor dissemination; (5) the risk of intraperitoneal tumor dissemination at the time of surgery may be reduced by the biologic impact of preoperative RT; and (6) using traditional principles of sarcoma RT, the radiation dose believed to be biologically effective is lower in the preoperative setting. Although RT planning for RPS can be complex, the use of conformal techniques or intensity modulation usually permits the RT dosage to be administered safely to the critical organ preoperatively. It is imperative that members of both the surgical and radiation oncology teams be present in the operating room when a significant amount of liver has been irradiated preoperatively to evaluate the planned residual liver volume. We cannot overemphasize the detailed evaluation of dosimetry and treatment planning films are needed to be certain that a sufficient volume of unirradiated liver is left unresected at the time of surgery.[114]

The only standard that exists at present for RPS treatment is that complete surgery should be performed wherever possible. The adjuvant RT approaches described above should be considered experimental and be the subject of further assessment. Recently, it was also suggested that a more scientifically sound approach to study design should be undertaken in RPS, particularly exploring the role of external beam RT through a randomized controlled trial.[282] An intergroup phase 3 trial of preoperative radiation plus surgery versus surgery alone is currently in the planning stages.

Chemoradiation Approaches

Although chemotherapy alone has not been associated with obvious improvements in outcome of RPS, chemoradiation, as in other solid tumors, is a subject of interest as a treatment strategy for RPS. This is especially relevant in high-grade RPS, which have a more adverse prognosis than the more common low-grade lesions.

Pilot studies using preoperative idoxuridine and doxorubicin plus external beam radiation have been reported, often in patients with extremely large tumors, with acceptable toxicity and with achievement of local control in patients in whom a negative-margin resection was possible.[190,283,284] These reports demonstrate that chemoradiation approaches are feasible. Additional phase 2 studies will be necessary to clarify response rates and toxicity profiles and determine whether chemoradiation should be tested in phase 3 trials. The Radiation Therapy Oncology Group has completed phase 2 study of preoperative doxorubicin and ifosfamide followed by preoperative RT and then by surgical resection with an intra- or postoperative radiation boost in patients with intermediate- and high-grade RPS. This study demonstrated significant toxicities and event-free outcomes that were considered modest.[285,286]

Additional Issues in STS Management

Functional Outcome and Morbidity of Treatment

The functional result of extremity sarcoma management has become an important component of outcome assessment. Assessing the functional result is difficult, as it requires methods that are valid and reproducible. Many centers have yet to become experienced in the development and use of these methods, and much of the literature contains significant heterogeneity in patient samples.

Thus far, the variables associated with poorer functional outcome include large tumor size, higher doses and larger volumes of radiation, nerve sacrifice, postoperative fracture, and wound-healing complications.[142,289-289] To evaluate and compare functional outcome, it is imperative that functional data be reported consistently. Three disease-specific scoring scales have been reported as useful in assessing functional outcome.[290] This area has been discussed in detail by Davis, who observed that "function" has many meanings in the literature.[290] The concepts of impairment, disability, and handicap following extremity STS are likely misunderstood and certainly not used consistently. Davis noted that impairment is a disorder of structure or function whereas disability is a restriction or lack of ability to perform an activity. Handicap results from impairment and disability and prevents or restricts an individual from performing in a role that is normal for the individual. For sarcoma patients, impairments can be manifested as soft tissue fibrosis, loss of motion at a joint, and decreased muscle strength; disability can be manifested as limited mobility and difficulty performing routine self-care and activities of daily living; and handicap can be evident in limitation in family roles, social functioning, and the capacity for employment.

Impairments are the most frequently reported deficits following limb-preserving therapy for extremity STS, and up to 50% of patients appear to experience significant impairments.[290] Disability occurs less frequently, although reports are contradictory. It seems likely that many sarcoma patients learn to accommodate their impairments. Handicap has received little attention in the literature. However, the limited data suggest that up to 50% of patients may experience changes in their employment and vocation status after treatment of extremity STS.[290]

The future challenge in treating sarcomas is to define the therapeutic ratio for the patient with sarcoma of the extremity. Specifically, the aim of the multidisciplinary team will be to minimize the amount of treatment while maintaining or improving current standards of disease control to reduce treatment morbidity and enhance patient outcome.[290]

Wound Complications ■ Considerable variability in reporting wound-healing complications exists in the literature. Wound complications have been reported in up to 40% of patients undergoing extremity sarcoma surgery.[129,291-293] Differences in the definition of wound complications probably account for some of the variability in reporting. The retrospective data suggest that factors associated with compromised wound healing include advanced patient age, poor nutritional status, lower extremity tumor location, large tumor size, and preoperative adjuvant treatment, especially RT.[294-297] Particularly high complication rates were noted recently with a protocol using preoperative RT and hyperthermia.[163] Although many authors have reported an association of wound complications with preoperative RT, reports of high rates of surgical complications without RT or chemotherapy also exist.[298] Most likely, these relate to the risk of major wound complications associated with extensive tumor resection, particularly in the lower extremities. The use of vascularized tissue transfers to replace resected tissues and optimize wound closure may decrease the risks of major wound complications and allow for more extensive limb-sparing surgical approaches.[294,299,300] As noted earlier, the SR2 trial results have confirmed the adverse effect of preoperative RT on wound healing in a prospective manner, but did not resolve the contribution of tissue transfer for wound reconstruction as its use was determined on an individual basis at the surgeon's discretion.[138]

Molecularly and Pathobiologically Based Sarcoma Management

Management of sarcomas is increasingly being driven by the specific nature of the disease entity, most importantly the pathophysiologic subtype. The work of Pasteur and Koch was fundamental for the recognition and definition of pathogenic microbes; similarly, many laboratories today are identifying molecular and cellular lesions that will redefine the field of sarcoma research. An example of this work is in the recognition of the Ewing's sarcoma/PNET family of tumors as extraosseous STSs rather than sarcomas of bone. These tumors should be treated with curative intent using an aggressive multimodality approach that begins with multi-agent chemotherapy. If primary surgery has removed measurable disease, adjuvant chemotherapy is definitely indicated, with consideration of adjuvant RT if surgical margins were suboptimal. By adopting similar strategies for PNETs and Askin tumors as for conventional Ewing sarcomas, outcomes have improved.[205,301] The molecular similarities between tumors of this family have led to the current convention of considering them morphologic and clinicopathologic variants of the same underlying molecular disease process.[89,302]

Molecular diagnostics are also becoming very relevant in synovial sarcomas. Synovial sarcomas have been identified in most series as a very chemotherapy responsive subset of sarcomas.[179,196] Of note is the fact that clinically relevant histologic differences appear to exist even within this subclass of sarcomas, with poorly differentiated synovial sarcomas typically having a far worse prognosis than do synovial sarcomas that exhibit a more well-differentiated histologic profile. Most important, the specific chromosomal breakpoint and rearrangement appear to be important in predicting the clinical behavior of synovial sarcomas, with a rearrangement in the *SSX1* gene conveying a worse prognosis.[87,303] The mechanisms by which translocations transform cells via the chimeric fusion proteins are an area of important scientific inquiry with therapeutic potential.

Finally, the multiple histopathologic subtypes of liposarcomas are becoming increasingly well researched and well understood.[304] Myxoid and round-cell liposarcomas exhibit a characteristic chromosomal rearrangement T(12;16)(q13;p11). These liposarcomas tend to be quite sensitive to doxorubicin-based chemotherapy. Well-differentiated liposarcomas exhibit ring and giant marker chromosomes on cytogenetic analysis and these karyotypic abnormalities carry through even in de-differentiated liposarcomas, which arise from well-differentiated liposarcomas. Targeting the PPAR-γ nuclear receptor is a particularly promising therapeutic strategy to force the differentiation of sarcoma cells and to decrease the proliferative thrust.[305] Initial proof-of-concept data have been published in a clinical trial using this strategy, and larger randomized trials are planned to assess the clinical worth of this approach.[306]

Summary

It is clear that STS management has come a long way in a short time. In less than three decades, the standard of care has shifted toward coordinated multimodality care in specialty centers, with increased rates of function-sparing surgery and better outcomes for patients. Judicious use of aggressive multimodality approaches shows promise to decrease relapse rates and improve survival rates. New scientific approaches are furthering the fundamental understanding of these unusual diseases and providing novel approaches for diagnostic techniques, which will banish the vagaries and lack of consistency that have plagued this field of clinical investigation. Already new therapeutic initiatives are attacking the basic mechanisms of sarcomatous transformation of cells in some subtypes of STS, and it is hoped that these initiatives will improve outcomes for patients with less morbidity than current treatments entail. Large collaborative studies will further this work tremendously.

Selected References

The complete reference list can be found at www.CANCERMEDICINE8.com

1. Jemal A, Siegel R, Ward E, Hao Y, Xu J, Thun MJ. Cancer statistics, 2009. *CA Cancer J Clin.* 2009;49:8–31.
2. Li FP, Fraumeni JF Jr. Soft-tissue sarcomas, breast cancer, and other neoplasms. A familial syndrome? *Ann Intern Med.* 1969;71:747–752.
10. Pollack IF, Mulvihill JJ. Neurofibromatosis 1 and 2. *Brain Pathol.* 1997;7:823–836.
11. Cavenee WK, Hansen MF, Nordenskjold M, et al. Genetic origin of mutations predisposing to retinoblastoma. *Science.* 1985;228:501–503.
12. Tucker MA, DAngio GJ, Boice JD Jr, et al. Bone sarcomas linked to radiotherapy and chemotherapy in children. *N Engl J Med.* 1987;317:588–593.
13. Hansen MF, Koufos A, Gallie BL, et al. Osteosarcoma and retinoblastoma: a shared chromosomal mechanism revealing recessive predisposition. *Proc Natl Acad Sci USA.* 1985;82:6216–6220.
14. Draper GJ, Sanders BM, Kingston JE. Second primary neoplasms in patients with retinoblastoma. *Br J Cancer.* 1986;53:661–671.
27. MacMahon HE, Murphy AS, Bates MI. Endothelial cell sarcoma of liver following Thorotrast injections. *Am J Pathol.* 1947;23:585–587.
36. Lawrence WJ, Donegan WL, Natarajan N, et al. Adult STSs. A pattern of care survey of the American College of Surgeons. *Ann Surg.* 1987;205:349–359.
42. Fong Y, Coit DG, Woodruff JM, Brennan MF. Lymph node metastasis from STS in adults. Analysis of data from a prospective database of 1772 sarcoma patients. *Ann Surg.* 1993;217:72–77.
43. Weingrad DN, Rosenberg SA. Early lymphatic spread of osteogenic and soft-tissue sarcomas. *Surgery.* 1978;84:231–240.
46. Coindre JM, Terrier P, Bui NB, et al. Prognostic factors in adult patients with locally controlled STS. A study of 546 patients from the French Federation of Cancer Centers Sarcoma Group. *J Clin Oncol.* 1996;14:869–877.
59. Ball AB, Fisher C, Pittam M, et al. Diagnosis of soft tissue tumours by Tru-Cut biopsy. *Br J Surg.* 1990;77:756–758.
60. Skrzynski MC, Biermann JS, Montag AG, Simon MA. Diagnostic accuracy and charge-savings of outpatient core needle biopsy compared with open biopsy of musculoskeletal tumors. *J Bone Joint Surg Am.* 1996;78:644–649.
61. Schwartz HS, Spengler DM. Needle tract recurrences after closed biopsy for sarcoma: three cases and review of the literature. *Ann Surg Oncol.* 1997;4:228–236.
89. de Alava E, Kawai A, Healey JH, et al. EWS-FLII fusion transcript structure is an independent determinant of prognosis in Ewing's sarcoma. *J Clin Oncol.* 1998;16:1248–1255.
90. Guillou L, Benhattar J, Bonichon F, et al. Histologic grade, but not SYT-SSX fusion type, is an important prognostic factor in patients with synovial sarcoma: a multicenter, retrospective analysis. *J Clin Oncol.* 2004;22:4040–4050.
98. Williard WC, Collin CF, Casper ES, et al. The changing role of amputation for STS of the extremity in adults. *Surg Gynecol Obstet.* 1992;175:389–396.
99. Williard WC, Hajdu SI, Casper ES, Brennan MF. Comparison of amputation with limb-sparing operations for adult STS of the extremity. *Ann Surg.* 1992;215:269–275.
100. Yang JC, Rosenberg SA. Surgery for adult patients with STSs. *Semin Oncol.* 1989;16:289–296.
101. Brennan MF, Casper ES, Harrison LB, et al. The role of multimodality therapy in soft-tissue sarcoma. *Ann Surg.* 1991;214:328–337.
102. Rosenberg SA, Tepper JE, Glatstein EJ, et al. The treatment of soft-tissue sarcomas of the extremities: prospective randomized evaluations of (1) limb-sparing surgery plus radiation therapy compared with amputation and (2) the role of adjuvant chemotherapy. *Ann Surg.* 1982;196:305–315.
103. Bowden L, Booher RJ. The principles and techniques of resection of soft parts for sarcomas. *Surgery.* 1958;44:963–977.
104. Cantin J, McNeer GP, Chu FC, Booher RJ. The problem of local recurrence after treatment of STS. *Ann Surg.* 1968;168:47–53.
105. Gerner RE, Moore GE, Pickren JW. STSs. *Ann Surg.* 1975;181:803–808.
135. Tanabe KK, Pollock RE, Ellis LM, et al. Influence of surgical margins on outcome in patients with preoperatively irradiated extremity STSs. *Cancer.* 1994;73:1652–1659.
136. Panicek DM, Schwartz LH. Soft tissue edema around musculoskeletal sarcomas at magnetic resonance imaging. *Sarcoma.* 1997;1:189–191.
190. Eilber FR, Eckardt J, Rosen G, et al. Preoperative therapy for STS. *Hematol Oncol Clin North Am.* 1995;9:817–823.
191. Eilber FR, Giuliano AE, Huth JF, et al. Intravenous (IV) vs. intraarterial (IA) Adriamycin, 2800 Gy radiation and surgical excision for extremity STSs: a randomized prospective trial. *Proc Am Soc Clin Oncol.* 1990;9:309.
192. Rhomberg W, Hassenstein EO, Gefeller D. Radiotherapy vs. radiotherapy and razoxane in the treatment of STSs: final results of a randomized study. *Int J Radiat Oncol Biol Phys.* 1996;36:1077–1084.

193. Cormier JN, Patel SR, Herzog CE, et al. Concurrent ifosfamide-based chemotherapy and irradiation. *Cancer.* 2001;92:1550–1555.
194. Pisters PW, Ballo MT, Fenstermacher MJ, et al. Phase I trial of preoperative concurrent doxorubicin and radiation therapy, surgical resection, and intraoperative electron-beam radiation therapy for patients with localized retroperitoneal sarcoma. *J Clin Oncol.* 2003;21:3092–3097.
195. Pisters PW, Ballo MT, Bekele N, et al. Phase I trial using toxicity severity weights for dose finding of gemcitabine combined with radiation therapy and subsequent surgery for patients with extremity and trunk STSs [abstract 9008]. ASCO Meeting 2004.
196. Rosen G, Forscher C, Lowenbraun S, et al. Synovial Sarcoma. Uniform response of metastases to high dose ifosfamide. *Cancer.* 1994;73:2506–2511.
197. Eilber FC, Eilber FR, Eckardt JJ, et al. Impact of ifosfamidebased chemotherapy on survival in patients with primary extremity synovial sarcoma [abstract 9017]. ASCO Meeting 2004.
198. Eilber FC, Eilber FR, Eckardt J, et al. The impact of chemotherapy on the survival of patients with high-grade primary extremity liposarcoma. *Ann Surg.* 2004;240:686–695.
199. Grobmyer SR, Maki RG, Demetri GD, et al. Neo-adjuvant chemotherapy for primary high-grade extremity STS. *Ann Oncol.* 2004;15:1667–1672.
200. Cormier JN, Huang X, Xing Y, et al. Cohort analysis of patients with localized, high-risk, extremity STS treated at two cancer centers: chemotherapy-associated outcomes. *J Clin Oncol.* 2004;22:4567–4574.
232. Pogrebniak HW, Roth JA, Steinberg SM, et al. Reoperative pulmonary resection in patients with metastatic STS. *Ann Thorac Surg.* 1991;52:197–203.
233. Casson AG, Putnam JB Jr, Natarajan G, et al. Efficacy of pulmonary metastasectomy for recurrent STS. *J Surg Oncol.* 1991;47:1–4.
239. Okuno S, Ryan LM, Edmonson JH, et al. Phase II trial of gemcitabine in patients with advanced sarcomas (E1797): a trial of the Eastern Cooperative Oncology Group. *Cancer.* 2003;97:1969–1973.
240. Patel SR, Jenkins J, Papadopoulos N, et al. Preliminary results of a two-arm phase 2 trial of gemcitabine in patients with gastrointestinal leiomyosarcomas and other soft-tissue sarcomas (STS). *Proc Am Soc Clin Oncol.* 1999;18:2091a.
261. Heinrich MC, Corless CL, Demetri GD, et al. Kinase mutations and imatinib response in patients with metastatic gastrointestinal stromal tumor. *J Clin Oncol.* 2003;21:4342–4349.
262. 262. Chacon et al. Meta GIST abstract from ASCO 2008.
275. Pisters PWT, et al. editorial *JCO.* 2009 in press.
276. Sindelar WF, Kinsella TJ, Chen PW, et al. Intraoperative radiotherapy in retroperitoneal sarcomas. Final results of a prospective, randomized, clinical trial. *Arch Surg.* 1993;128:402–410.
292. Ormsby MV, Hilaris BS, Nori D, Brennan MF. Wound complications of adjuvant radiation therapy in patients with STSs. *Ann Surg.* 1989;210:93–99.
293. Arbeit JM, Hilaris BS, Brennan MF. Wound complications in the multimodality treatment of extremity and superficial truncal sarcomas. *J Clin Oncol.* 1987;5:480–488.

109 The Myelodysplastic Syndrome

Lewis R. Silverman, MD

The existence of a hematopoietic disorder characterized by anemia and dyspoiesis preceding the onset of acute myelocytic leukemia (AML) has been recognized since the early part of the twentieth century. Initially designated as preleukemia, the syndrome was ill defined and could only be established with certainty retrospectively. Moreover, the terminology itself conveyed an unwarranted confidence in predicting the outcome that often belied the facts. The more accurately descriptive and appropriate designation as a myelodysplastic syndrome (MDS) was adopted in 1976 by the French-American-British[1] (FAB) Study Group.[2] The FAB classification permitted the prospective identification of patients within this heterogeneous clonal disorder.

MDS, derived from a multipotent hematopoietic stem cell, is characterized clinically by a hyperproliferative bone marrow, reflective of ineffective hematopoiesis, and is accompanied by one or more peripheral blood cytopenias. Bone marrow failure results, leading to death from bleeding and infection in the majority, while transformation to acute leukemia occurs in up to 40% of patients. The evolution of the disease proceeds in accordance with the multistep pathogenesis theory of carcinogenesis and can thus serve as an important model in furthering our understanding of the processes involved in neoplastic transformation.

This constellation of findings raises the question of whether MDS represents a frank neoplastic state or is merely a preneoplastic condition in transition. The syndrome appears to represent a spectrum, where the initial lesion in the genome, though clinically undetectable, subsequently evolves, with the acquisition of additional lesions, to a state of frank neoplasia.

The designation of this disorder as the MDS, rather than preleukemia, permits its distinction from other abnormalities that are known to be associated with the development of acute leukemia. These latter include the classic myeloproliferative syndromes (polycythemia vera, chronic myelocytic leukemia, agnogenic myeloid metaplasia, essential thrombocythemia), aplastic anemia, paroxysmal nocturnal hemoglobinuria (PNH), as well as Fanconi, Bloom, and Down syndromes. These particular "preleukemic states," which can lead to leukemia, are beyond the scope of this chapter.

MDS can be further divided into primary and secondary syndromes. The former arise de novo and are of indeterminate etiology, while the latter are induced by identifiable environmental, occupational, or iatrogenic causes.

Estimates of the incidence of MDS range from 1 case per 100,000 per year to a frequency equal to that of AML, or approximately 14,000 new cases per year in the United States. One recent population-based study demonstrated an incidence almost twice that of AML.[3,4] The SEER database now tracks the disease, thus more accurate data will be available in the future. The consensus is that the incidence is increasing owing to a number of factors, including greater awareness, greater diagnostic precision, and the aging of the population.

History

Luzzatto first described a case of chronic anemia associated with bone marrow erythroid hyperplasia, which he designated as "pseudo-aplastic anemia."[5] It was not until Rhoads' and Bomford's description of this entity, however, that the designation of the disease as refractory anemia became generally accepted.[6,7]

In the early 1950s, it became apparent that some patients with refractory anemia could develop leukemia, which led to the term preleukemia, coined by Hamilton-Peterson and Block and colleagues.[8,9] In 1956, a special subclass of patients with refractory anemia and ringed sideroblasts, a proportion of whom developed leukemia, was described.[10] Subsequent reports led Dameshek to speculate that sideroblastic anemia might represent an early form of erythroleukemia.[11,12] In patients with sideroblastic anemia, Dacie described one population of hypochromic normocytic cells and another of normochromic macrocytic cells in the blood, suggesting the possibility of a clonal origin for this disorder. Although the clinical features of preleukemia lacked specificity, certain identifiable features could make the diagnosis easier.[13,14] These included frequent cytopenias in the peripheral blood, with morphologic evidence of dyshematopoiesis, associated with a hyperproliferative bone marrow, without clear findings of acute leukemia.

The plethora of terminology applied to the disorder, however, made it difficult to determine whether investigators were describing patients with the same disease. The designation as "preleukemia" often seemed erroneous, since many patients succumbed as a result of bone marrow failure without developing leukemia. In 1976, the FAB established diagnostic criteria for MDS that would permit prospective diagnosis.[2,15]

Classification

Based on bone marrow cellularity, the syndrome was divided into three groups: acquired sideroblastic anemia, refractory anemia with excess blasts, and chronic myelomonocytic leukemia. In 1982, the FAB group updated and expanded their classification to include five categories of MDS based on morphologic characteristics and the percentage of blasts in the bone marrow and peripheral blood.[16] These included (1) refractory anemia (RA), (2) refractory anemia with ringed sideroblasts (RARS), (3) refractory anemia with excess blasts (>5% to <20% blasts) (RAEB), (4) chronic myelomonocytic leukemia (CMML), and (5) refractory anemia with excess blasts "in transformation" (20% to <30% blasts) (RAEBT). Concerns that the classification might result in an underdiagnosis of M6 myeloid leukemia (erythroleukemia) led to further revision and refinement in 1985.[17]

Some debate focuses on the category of chronic myelomonocytic leukemia and whether this truly represents a subgroup of MDS or should more appropriately be considered a subgroup of the myeloproliferative disorders (MPD). Some patients with CMML have features of both MDS and MPD, and thus an overlap syndrome with characteristics of both.[18,19] The biologic behavior appears related most closely to the percentage of blasts in the bone marrow.[20-26]

The International Prognostic Scoring System (IPSS) has been advanced based on the percentage of bone marrow blasts, cytogenetics, and degree of cytopenias.[27] The IPSS has predictive value for both survival and risk of transformation to acute leukemia and classifies patients into four subgroups according to risk: low, intermediate-1, intermediate-2,

Table 109-1 **International Prognostic Scoring System (IPSS) Classification of MDS According to Prognostic Risk Subgroups**

International Prognostic Scoring System (IPSS)	Risk of Transformation to Acute Myelod Leukemia (in 25% of Patients) (Years)	Median Survival (Years)
Low	9.4	5.71
Intermediate-1	3.3	3.5
Intermediate-2	2.1	1.2
High	0.2	0.4

Source: Modified after Ref. 27.

Table 109-2 **IPSS Score**

	Score Value				
Prognostic Variable	**0**	**0.5**	**1.0**	**1.5**	**2.0**
Bone marrow blasts (%)	< 5	5–10	–	11–20	21–29
Karyotype	Good	Interm	Poor		
Cytopenias	0/1	2/3			

Scores	Cytogenetics
Low: 0	Good: Normal
Intermediate-1: 0.5–1.0	-y
Intermediate-2: 1.5–2.0	del (5q)
High: > 2.5	del (20q)
	Poor: Chromosome 7 abnormalities
	Complex ≥ 3 abnormalities
	Intermediate: Other

Source: Modified after Ref. 27.

and high risk (Table 109-1). This system has been validated and has become, along with the World Health Organization (WHO) classification (see below; REF – 2008), the standard classification (Table 109-2). If cytogenetic data are not available, however, the predictive power of the model diminishes significantly.

In 1999, another classification system was published by a working group of the WHO, relying more closely on the FAB system's conventional morphologic criteria, but also considering cytogenetic markers[28] (Table 109-3). Data from 1,600 patients with primary MDS were evaluated, expanding the FAB system by two categories for a total of seven, all having a high degree of correlation with prognosis. CMML with WBC > 13 × 10^9/L was eliminated from the WHO categories and included with MPDs, while those with WBC < 13 × 10^9/L are still classified as MDS/MPD. RA was split into pure refractory anemia (PRA) and refractory cytopenia with multilineage dysplasia (RCMD). Some conditions previously classified as RARS were placed in the pure sideroblastic anemia[29] group, while those with additional dysplastic features were put into the RCMD category, along with refractory anemias without ringed sideroblasts. RAEB was divided into RAEB I and RAEB II, based on medullary and peripheral blast counts. RAEB in transformation (RAEB-T) was included under AML.

Additionally, MDS associated with karyotypic abnormality 5q- was separated as a distinct entity, although its relatively benign nature prevails only if the proportion of medullary blasts is less than 5%. The WHO classification has been updated with some modification as noted in Table 109-3.

Etiology

Although the etiologic agent cannot be identified in the majority of patients with MDS, in some, exposure to ionizing radiation, chemicals, drugs, or other environmental agents can be implicated.

Radiation exposure has been clearly linked to the development of stem cell abnormalities.[30] Dogs that survive the transient hematopoietic failure following exposure to continuous total-body gamma irradiation often develop a preleukemic syndrome.[31] In addition, the leukemias that developed in survivors of atomic bomb explosions were often preceded by a preleukemic state.[32] Atomic bomb survivors continue to exhibit an increased incidence of genetic instability seen as structural and numerical chromosomal abnormalities long after the initial exposure, which may contribute to the development of MDS and AML.[33] Furthermore, long-term population studies demonstrate an increased incidence of MDS and AML among patients exposed to thorium dioxide.[34]

Table 109-3 **World Health Organization (WHO) Classification**

Refractory anemia (RA)
with ringed sideroblasts
without ringed sideroblasts
Refractory cytopenia with multilineage dysplasia (RCMD)
with ringed sideroblasts
without ringed sideroblasts
Refractory anemia with excess blasts
RAEB - I (6–10% blasts)
RAEB - II (11–19% blasts)
5q-syndrome
CMML (MDS/MPD)
Myelodysplastic syndrome, unclassifiable

Source: Modified after Ref. 28.

Chemical injury to the marrow is a well-established phenomenon, and an increased risk of leukemogenesis has been noted among workers exposed to petrochemicals, benzene, and the rubber industry.[35,36] The link between leukemia and exposure to benzene is the most strongly established.[37] Many of the initial cases of benzene-induced leukemia were associated with a preleukemic syndrome.[38] Exposure of human cell lines to hydroquinone, a benzene metabolite, is associated with the development of abnormalities of chromosomes 5, 7, and 8 and may be responsible, in part, for the DNA damage associated with the chemical exposure.[39] Farrow and colleagues have demonstrated, in an age and sex matched case-control study of occupational and environmental factors in patients with or without ringed sideroblasts that exposure to diesel oil fumes ($p < .01$), diesel oil liquids ($p < .01$), or ammonia ($p < .05$) was associated with the development of MDS.[40] A careful history of exposure to environmental and occupational hazards should be an integral part of the work-up of all patients with MDSs. Additional environmental factors may include use of hair dye and cigarette smoking.[41] Further studies will be required to better define the risk.

Enzymatic pathways such as glutathione S-transferase (GST) play an important metabolic role in the detoxification of certain mutagens and carcinogens. Genetic differences among individuals in the effects of environmental toxins may contribute to the development of MDS. In one study, patients with MDS had a higher incidence of the GST theta 1 null genotype compared with a population-based control group.[42] This translated to a 4.3-fold higher risk of developing MDS, thus raising the possibility that inability to detoxify certain environmental or endogenous toxins may contribute to the development of MDS. Additional studies have found conflicting results, which may reflect different study populations.[43–45] Larger population-based prospective studies will be required.

Therapy-related myelodysplasia and leukemia following treatment with radiation and/or chemotherapy has been recognized, since this was initially observed in patients treated for Hodgkin's disease.[46] A hematologic disorder characterized by trilineage dysplasia, cytopenias, and panmyelosis following chemotherapy constitutes the least ambiguous cause of MDS.[47–49] Since the initial reports following treatment of Hodgkin's disease, therapy-induced MDS has been reported following treatment of cancers of the breast, lung, ovary, gastrointestinal tract, non-Hodgkin's lymphomas, seminoma, multiple myeloma, polycythemia vera, chronic lymphocytic leukemia (CLL), as well as nonmalignant conditions. The leukemogenic potential is greatest for alkylating agents, nitrosoureas, and procarbazine.[49] The risk associated with exposure to these particular agents is further substantiated by the increased frequency of abnormalities involving chromosomes 5 and 7 in comparison with the much lower frequency of abnormalities involving these chromosomes in patients treated with anthracyclines which nonetheless carry risk, or antimetabolites.[49] Leukemogenicity appears to be a function of both dose and time of exposure, as observed in patients with ovarian cancer treated with melphalan or chlorambucil.[49] The use of etoposide in combination with cisplatin or other alkylating agents in patients treated for germ cell tumors is associated with an increased risk of MDS or AML.[50] The relationship of the cumulative dose of etoposide or teniposide to development of MDS or therapy-related AML remains to be determined.[51,52] Abnormalities involving deletions of a portion of the short arm of chromosome 17 (17p) associated with either mutations or overexpression of the TP53 oncogene have also been described related to prior chemotherapy.[53] This has been identified in both patients with lymphoid neoplasms treated with alkylating agents as well as in those with MPDs treated with either hydroxyurea or p.32. Recently, treatment-related MDS has been reported in association with both fludarabine and cladribine.[54]

It has long been debated whether the increase in leukemogenic potential derives as a direct result of exposure to radiation and/or chemotherapy, or more simply reflects a natural predisposition related to the underlying disease. The risk of developing MDS and/or metachronous leukemia has been reported to be increased in association with certain cancers, such as multiple myeloma, lymphoma, carcinoma of the lung, and CLL.[55,56] However, the difference in the rates of developing leukemia after various treatments for polycythemia vera or Hodgkin's disease point to treatment as the most critical etiologic factor. In patients with polycythemia vera, the risk of developing leukemia is significantly elevated in those treated with chlorambucil, compared with those treated with phlebotomy alone.[57] Similarly, patients with Hodgkin's disease treated with ABVD (doxorubicin, bleomycin, vinblastine, and dacarbazine) have a much lower incidence of therapy-related leukemia than those treated with the MOPP (nitrogen mustard, vincristine, procarbazine, and prednisone) regimen.[58] The recognition of this potential risk has led to efforts to develop equally potent, but less leukemogenic therapies, particularly in diseases with the potential for long-term survival. In a registry review of patients with chronic neutropenia treated with filgrastim, 9% of patients with congenital neutropenia developed MDS and/or leukemia compared with none of the patients with cyclical or idiopathic neutropenia.[59] The relationship of the use of filgrastim and the development of MDS in these patients is uncertain.

High-dose chemotherapy with stem cell support is being applied as a curative approach in a number of malignancies, non-Hodgkin's lymphoma among them. As noted above, an increased risk of developing MDS or metachronous leukemia in association with lymphoma has been suggested.[55,56] Although therapy-induced MDS in patients with non-Hodgkin's lymphoma treated with standard doses of chemotherapy has been identified, MDS has now been recognized as a late complication of treatment with high-dose chemotherapy regimens.[51,60,61] The reported actuarial risk ranges from 6.4% up to 18% at 6 years.[62–64] The role that the pretransplant chemotherapy and the high-dose regimen (which often includes total body irradiation or high-dose alkylating agents) contribute to the emergence of the MDS clone are the subject of prospective studies.[65] Strategies currently under study that use high-dose myeloablative treatments earlier in the course of this disease in patients with poor prognosis make the identification of the magnitude of this problem an increasingly important issue.[51,66,67] Studies that track the emergence of abnormal hematopoietic clones poststem cell infusion may provide further insight into the pathogenesis of MDS following high-dose treatments.

Pathobiology

Clonal Origin

Since originally suggested by Dacie, a substantial body of evidence has accumulated that points to a clonal origin for MDSs. The identification of nonrandom chromosomal abnormalities detectable in 30–70% of patients with MDS confirmed the likelihood that these were clonal disorders.[68–73] Evidence that these disorders originate from pluripotent stem cells was suggested by reports of patients developing biphenotypic and lymphoid leukemias following MDS.[74–77]

Analysis of the patterns of inactivation of an X-linked polymorphic enzyme such as glucose-6- phosphate dehydrogenase (G6PD) has proven to be a useful tool in the analysis of the clonal origin of tumors.[78] Raskind and colleagues have demonstrated that 21 of 24 B lymphoblastoid lines transformed by Epstein-Barr virus expressed a single light chain immunoglobulin and contained only one of the G6PD isoenzymes. In contrast, the T cells expressed both the A and B G6PD isoenzymes.[79] The frequency with which the lymphoid lineage is involved as part of the abnormal clone in MDS is quite variable, as demonstrated in a number of studies.[80–84]

Subsequent studies using more refined and sensitive molecular techniques have also suggested that cells of lymphocytic origin belong to the abnormal clone, with B lymphocytes being involved more regularly than T cells.[80,81,83] Other studies have found evidence that only cells committed to the myeloid lineage are involved in the clone, but that lymphocytes are of polyclonal origin.[80–84] Fluorescent in situ hybridization (FISH) or polymerase chain reaction analysis of loss of heterozygosity has confirmed the involvement of an early stem cell that can give rise to CD34+ cells as well as those of erythroid, megakaryocytic, and myelomonocytic lineage, but not lymphocytes.[85] Subsequently, in a study using combined techniques of immunophenotyping and FISH, B-lymphocytes were found to be involved in patients with the 5q- syndrome.[86] Molecular and flow cytometric analysis of T-cell clonality has also suggested involvement of T cells in the MDS clone of some patients.[87] The reason for the discrepant findings is unclear, but may reflect the heterogeneity of the disease and interpatient variability. This is further suggested in one study where the bone marrow from 2 of 5 patients with MDS manifests evidence of residual polyclonal hematopoiesis.[88] Thus, the diverse heterogeneity of disease biology at the clinical level may simply reflect the degree of heterogeneity of the disease at the cellular level. Stromal cells do not share in the clonal abnormalities, and where studied have a normal karyotype.

In Vitro Progenitor Growth Characteristics

A variety of abnormalities in the growth of hematopoietic progenitors has been detected in colony assays in vitro of both bone marrow and peripheral blood from patients with all categories of MDS.[89–93] In a series of studies, 74% of 170 patients had abnormal bone marrow myeloid progenitor growth colony forming units—granulocyte macrophage (CFU-GM). The pattern of colony growth can be classified as either a leukemic or nonleukemic pattern.[90–92] The former are characterized by increased formation of micro- and macroclusters, defective maturation of the colonies formed with the persistence of blasts, or decreased or absent colony formation (<2 colonies/10^5 bone marrow cells plated). A leukemic type growth pattern is more commonly associated with shortened survival and an increased risk of transformation to acute leukemia than a nonleukemic pattern.[91,92] Reports have also indicated decreased to absent colony or burst growth of progenitors, including those of erythroid (CFU-E, BFU-E),[80,94,95] mixed lineage (CFU-GEMM),[96–98] and megakaryocytic(CFU-Mk)[99,100]precursors. Chronic myelomonocytic leukemia is often distinguished by increased CFU-GM growth, even in the absence of exogenous growth factor supplementation.[97]

Production of endogenous regulatory factors influencing the growth of myeloid, erythroid, and megakaryocytic precursors is diminished.[98,99,101] Bone marrow conditioned medium from patients with MDS had both decreased CFU-GEMM colony stimulating activity and burst promoting activity (BPA) compared with conditioned medium from normal marrow. Both of these activities were completely neutralized by anti–IL-3 antibodies, suggesting that MDS conditioning did not produce IL-3.[98] In addition, accessory cells, including macrophages and NK cells, appear to be capable of directly or indirectly inhibiting bone marrow CFU-GM through the production of soluble factors.[94,102] T cells, although abnormal in number and in their response to mitogens, appear to produce normal levels of growth factors.[103] Partial restoration of colony growth can be accomplished through the addition of exogenous growth factors or other agents to the culture.[95] The addition of rhGM-CSF can result in an increase in CFU-GM, but has little effect on the growth of CFU-GEMM, BFU-E, or CFU-Mk.[93,96] Colony growth of CFU-E and BFU-E in some subgroups of MDS improved with the addition of a recombinant human erythropoietin (rhEpo) or *kit* ligand.[104] Addition of rhG-CSF in vitro partially restored the abnormal function of neutrophils derived from patients with MDS.[105]

Studies of cytokine production by the bone marrow stroma have produced variable results. Stromal cell production of a variety of cytokines, including GM-CSF, IL-3 IL-6, IL-1 β, TNF-α, and IL-8, has been reported to be impaired in some patients with MDS and can be restored, at least in part, by in vitro or in vivo administration of hematopoietic growth factors.[106,107] However, the level of G-CSF, IL-1β, IL-6, IL-8, or stem cell factor messenger ribonucleic acid (mRNA) in a small series has been reported to be normal or increased.[108] Serum cytokine levels have for the most part been found to be normal or increased except for stem cell factor, which in one series was decreased.[109–112]

Bone Marrow Microenvironment

Histologic examination of bone marrow trephine biopsies by Tricot and colleagues have pointed to abnormalities of the microenvironment.[113] They noted the presence of clusters of immature precursor cells in the central intertrabecular region of the marrow, rather than along the endosteal surfaces. They cited this as evidence of abnormal localization of immature precursors (ALIP).[113] In a series of 40 patients, the presence of ALIP correlated significantly with shortened survival and was associated with an increased risk of transformation to AML. These findings were independent of the FAB subtype and were detected even in patients with refractory anemia. However, care must be applied to differentiate true ALIP from pseudo-ALIP. In the latter case, the clusters of cells are either of erythroid or megakaryocytic origin and do not convey the same prognostic information compared with the former, where the immature cells are of myeloid origin. The determination of the immature precursor phenotype by immunohistochemical methods may be helpful in distinguishing pseudo- and true ALIP, and thus permit identification of specific subgroups with a poor prognosis.[114] ALIP is not, however, specific to patients with MDS and, therefore, not helpful as a diagnostic tool.[114]

Investigations to define the potential role of the bone marrow stroma in MDS have been limited and have yielded conflicting data to date. Some studies, however, have suggested that abnormalities of the stroma contribute to the pathophysiology of MDS. In vitro stromal cells either fail to reach confluent growth or their growth is absent in the majority of patients. Furthermore, stromal cell support of normal hematopoiesis in long-term bone marrow cultures can be impaired.[115–118] Cytokine production of leukemia inhibitory factor (LIF) and TNF-α by MDS stroma is also impaired. In vivo labeling techniques have demonstrated that the ineffective hematopoiesis in MDS is accompanied by a high cell turnover with an increase in apoptosis of both hematopoietic progenitors and stromal cells. In vitro analyses indicate that the areas of apoptosis are associated with high levels of TNFα and low levels of GM-CSF.[118–120] Characterization of cellular subsets of bone marrow stroma indicates that fibroblasts and macrophages from some patients with MDS are functionally abnormal, with increased production of TNF-α and IL-6 and an increased apoptotic index.[121]

Signal Transduction

Whether the primary pathophysiologic defect(s) resulting in disordered maturation and function are intrinsic to hematopoietic progenitor cells or derive from their interaction with accessory cells and other microenvironmental factors or a combination thereof is uncertain. Hematopoietic cell defects may relate not only to quantitative abnormalities of progenitors, but also reflect abnormalities in signal transduction in response to cytokines or other regulatory molecules that trigger proliferation and differentiation pathways.

Hematopoietic cells from MDS patients display impaired responses to a number of cytokines and are unable to respond to external signals owing either to abnormalities in number or function of cytokine receptors or to dysfunctional postbinding signal transduction.[101]

Hematopoietic progenitors have impaired responses to cytokine stimulation with decreased CFU-GM, CFU-GEMM, and BFU-E colony number.[95,103,122,123] Purified blast cells from MDS patients proliferate but do not mature in response to G-CSF and GM-CSF. Purified populations of CD 34+ cells from MDS patients also demonstrate impaired responses to G-CSF.[124] Receptor abnormalities in MDS are not commonly observed,[125–128] although in some patients their number is either diminished or their structure aberrant.[129] In a small series of patients with congenital neutropenia, analysis of the G-CSF receptor demonstrated a common deletion in 3 nucleotides in the juxtamembrane domain of the G-CSFR. This was associated with an increase in proliferative response to G-CSF but not GM-CSF or IL-3 in cells expressing the mutated G-CSFR. Treatment of these cells with G-CSF was associated with increased and prolonged expression of STAT3.[130] Further studies will be necessary to determine the role of this mutation in the pathogenesis of the transformation to AML.

In patients with a truncated erythropoietin receptor progenitor differentiation to erythropoietin is blocked and cells undergo apoptosis.[129] On the other hand, defects in signal transduction appear to play a larger role in the aberrant response of hematopoietic progenitors to regulatory molecules.[131,132] This pertains both to the cytokine signal transduction pathways and factors which regulate apoptosis.[131,133] Patients with MDS have defective activation of STAT5 in response to erythropoietin but not IL-3 suggesting a defect in the erythropoietin signaling pathway. Despite the relative impairment, increasing concentrations of cytokines can partially correct the defects.[134,135] Epigenetic changes resulting in transcriptional silencing is another potential mechanism affecting cytokine signaling. Recent evidence demonstrates aberrant hypermethylation of the SOCS-1 gene in 31% of MDS patients associated with increased activity of the JAK/STAT pathway.[136] Hypermethylation which occurs in other genes such as p15 may be explained in part by the over-expression of DNA methyltransferase 1 and 3A that has been identified in bone marrow of MDS patients.[137]

The majority of patients with MDS have hypercellular bone marrows with evident proliferation of various cellular lineage components. One interpretation of this finding is a compensatory response in the marrow to feedback signals secondary to the peripheral blood cytopenias. Yet, the response does not translate into effective hematopoiesis; a role for increased apoptosis has been suggested.[133,138–140] A deficiency in cytokines or relative resistance to their effects could explain this phenomenon of ineffective hematopoiesis. In several recent studies, bone marrow cells from MDS patients have demonstrated increased expression of Fas and Fas-ligand. In marrow cultures, strategies that block TNF-mediated signals, such as the use of anti–TNF-α antibody, significantly increased the numbers of hematopoietic colonies compared with untreated cells.[139] Additional studies have implicated a dysregulated Fas pathway and TNF-α as contributing to ineffective hematopoiesis.[138,140,141] Inhibition of the TGF-B signaling pathway, which is overexpressed in some patients, can restore hematopoiesis suggesting a negative regulatory role for TGF-B.[142] Increased apoptosis may be related to mitochondrial encoded cytochrome c-oxidase I gene mutations.[143] Spontaneous release of mitochondrial cytochrome c results in activation of caspase -9 with activation of the apoptotic pathway in patients with low-risk MDS. G-CSF can suppress the spontaneous cytochrome c release and reduce apoptosis, particularly in patients with RARS.[144] Iron accumulation in mitochondria in patients with RARS may be secondary to reduced gene expression of ABCB7 where the reduction in the levels of gene expression is proportionately related to iron accumulation.[145]

Increased apoptosis was identified in both mature cells and immature CD34+ cells by assays for annexin V, measurements of mitochondrial membrane potential, and caspase 3 activity from cell lysates in patients with MDS compared with patients with de novo AML. These results demonstrated that the patients with MDS had increased apoptosis in all FAB subcategories, which was distinctive compared with patients with AML and was equally applicable to the RAEB-T alone group.[146]

The role of cytokine signaling with apoptosis is not well delineated, but may contribute.[131,147] Progenitors with impaired signal transduction, thus constituting a refractory target cell, could undergo accelerated apoptosis analogous to withdrawal of obligate survival factors. Alternatively, the apoptotic pathway itself may be dysregulated with direct activation of the fas pathway.[147] As MDS evolves to AML, the acceleration of apoptosis declines and AML is characterized by increasing progenitor survival.[148]

Patients may also have myelofibrosis as a component of MDS and another manifestation of the MDS-MPD overlap syndrome. Recent reports suggest that in these patients the increased fibrosis may be secondary to increased production of TGF-β by bone marrow blasts, resulting in fibroblast proliferation.[149]

Cytogenetics

Chromosomal abnormalities, found in 30–70% of MDS patients, are similar to those seen in patients with AML and involve complete or partial deletions, most frequently involving chromosomes 5(-5,5q-), 7(-7,7q-), and 8(8+) (Table 109-4).[22,27,72,73,150–152] Certain karyotypic abnormalities that are associated with core binding factor rearrangements, such as t(15;17) in acute promyelocytic leukemia (M3), t(8;21) in AML (M2), and inv 16 in AML (M4), have only rarely been identified in MDS.[80,153–155] Moreover, patients with these AML subtypes have good prognoses with potential for cure. Thus, they should be viewed as having AML and should be managed accordingly. Furthermore, abnormalities involving partial deletions of the long arm of chromosome 20 (20q-), seen frequently in MDS, particularly RARS, polycythemia vera, and myeloproliferative syndromes, are usually not seen in patients with de novo AML.[22] Abnormalities are identified most frequently in patients with RAEB and RAEB-T compared to those with RA and RARS.[152,156] Although specific chromosomal abnormalities have been identified, unlike AML, no specific abnormality has been associated with any specific FAB category.[22,73,152] Newer techniques using FISH have identified additional chromosomal abnormalities in patients beyond those with banding alone and are complementary to standard techniques.[157]

Many studies have demonstrated that the presence of karyotypic abnormalities is an independent prognostic variable.[22,27,73,152] Several studies have demonstrated that patients with abnormalities present in 100% of the mitoses(AA) examined, or a mix of normal and abnormal mitoses (AN) have poorer survival than patients with normal karyotypes (NN).[22,72,73,156,158] Furthermore, more complex abnormalities are associated with shortened survival compared with either single clonal abnormality or a normal karyotype.[27,73,151,152,156] Certain specific clonal subtypes have varying prognostic significance for both survival and the risk of leukemic transformation. Monosomy 7 or 5 and 7q- are associated with shortened survival, while deletions of the long arms of chromosome 20 (20q-) and 5(5q-syndrome) and deletion of y[159] as the sole abnormality are associated with longer survival.[27,73,151,156,158] In the IPSS, cytogenetic findings are an independent prognostic variable classifying patients according to 3 subgroups: good, intermediate, and poor risk.[27]

Genetic instability as demonstrated by clonal evolution occurs in a substantial percentage of patients. Around 20–35% have been found to undergo clonal evo-

Table 109-4 Cytogenetics in MDS

	No. With Abnormal Karyotype (%)[a]						Frequency (%)						
No. of Patients	No. of Abnormal (%)	RA	RARS	RAEB	RAEB-T	CMML	5q-	-5	7q-	-7	20q-	8+	Ref.
167	64(38)	13(29)	8(21)	30(43)	6(50)	5(45)	17	7	0	4	8	20	132
244	125(51)	NR	NR	NR	NR	NR	17	9	2	22	8	21	66
77	55(71)	26(63)	4(57)	17(89)	8(73)	2(29)	27	8	0	9	0	13	133
120	50(42)	10(36)	2(14)	25(56)	9(19)	4(29)	11	0	3	3	1	9	134
31	17(55)	NR	NR	12(55)	NR	5(50)	0	5	0	6	0	1	137
49	19(39)	4(29)	1(13)	8(89)	4(80)	2(20)	4	1	2	2	4	5	21
56	44(79)	11(86)	4(31)	21(95)	4(100)	3(100)	5	1	9	9	6	6	67
744	374(50.2)	64(11)	19(3)	113(19)	31(5)	21(4)	81(22)	31(8)	16(4)	55(15)	27(7)	75(20)	

[a]Percent of all patients with FAB subtype specified. *Abbreviation*: NR, not reported.

lution during the course of the disease, independent of karyotypic status at the outset.[72] The significance of clonal evolution with respect to leukemic transformation and survival is contradictory at the outset.[72,152,158,160] In some studies, clonal evolution was associated with a poor prognosis without an increased risk of leukemic transformation.[158] In contrast, Glenn and colleagues have demonstrated karyotypic changes in clinically stable patients.[160] One study of 31 patients evolving to AML from MDS suggests that additional abnormalities involving chromosomes 1, 7, 8, 11, and 17 may contribute to the transformation process.[161] Subclonal evolution suggests genomic instability. Microsatellite instability involving defects in the DNA mismatch repair system has been identified in some MDS patients, particularly those with therapy-related disease.[162] After autologous transplantation for lymphoma, patients who develop secondary MDS/AML are found to have reduced regenerative capacity in marrow progenitors and accelerated telomere shortening just preceding the transformation.[163]

One particular abnormality involving a deletion of part of the long arm of chromosome 5 (5q-) deserves special note. As originally described, the del 5q- syndrome is associated with a refractory macrocytic anemia, a normal or increased platelet count, giant thrombocytes, dyserythropoiesis, hypolobulated megakaryocytes, female predominance, prolonged survival, and a low rate of leukemic transformation.[73,156,164,165] It is important to differentiate the del 5q- syndrome from instances where this deletion is found in combination with other chromosomal abnormalities or in association with FAB subtypes other than refractory anemia. It is clear that those patients with the del 5q-abnormality, without the characteristic clinical and morphologic features, have a more aggressive clinical course associated with shorter survival.

Patients with MDS secondary to exposure to mutagenic or carcinogenic agents have similar findings in terms of the types and significance of the chromosomal abnormalities.[68,166,167] Patients treated with epidophyllotoxins (etoposide and teniposide) can develop specific translocations involving the breakpoint at 11q23.[50,168] This leads to transcription of a fusion protein involving the mixed lineage leukemia (MLL) gene.[169,170]

Newer techniques are being explored that can detect abnormalities in the genome not identifiable by normal metaphase cytogenetics (MC) (Gondek, Dunbar et al. 2007). Single nucleotide polymorphism arrays (SNP-A) reveal a higher percentage of genetic abnormalities than indicated by MC. Moreover, in 20% of patients in one series, uniparental disomy was detected with copy-neutral loss of heterozygosity suggesting that loss of gene function could be playing an important role in MDS pathophysiology (Mohamedali, Gaken et al. 2007; Tiu, Gondek et al. 2007; Gondek, Tiu et al. 2008).

Gene Mutations and Dysregulation ■ Alterations in the control and expression of proto-oncogenes in the cellular genome, leading to abnormalities of cellular proliferation and differentiation, are thought to contribute to the molecular basis of neoplastic transformation.[171] Point mutations of the ras family of oncogenes have been identified in association with a number of human tumors, including lung, pancreatic, colorectal, and hematopoietic neoplasms.[153–155,172] Activated ras genes with specific point mutations involving codons 12, 13, and 61 have been identified in 20–30% of patients with AML and 9–48% of patients with MDSs (Table 109-5). These findings have suggested that activation of ras genes either may contribute to the development of MDS or, once established, to the process of transformation of the commonly affected stem cell. Ki-ras, with H-ras are involved in only a few cases. CMML was the FAB subtype most frequently associated with a ras mutation. The abnormality was found in 40% of cases.[173] However, the association may be a function of the monocytosis, since other FAB subcategories with ras mutations were often associated with increased monocyte counts.[174]

In the initial reports, the presence of a mutant ras gene was associated with transformation of MDS to AML.[175,178] Overall, 47% (65 of 137) of patients with a ras mutation transformed to AML, compared with only 14% (89 of 628) of those without a mutation.[155,161,175–185] A significantly shortened survival of patients with MDS who transformed to AML has been associated with the presence of a ras mutation in most but not all patients.[73,178,186] It is unclear whether the presence of a ras mutation is an independent prognostic variable.

The ras mutation may confer a selective growth advantage to cells and appears to occur after initiation of leukemogenesis.[180,182,184] These mutations can appear in either the early or late stages of MDS (Figure 109-1). In the early stages, the mutation is present in all bone marrow and peripheral blood cells and involves a totipotent stem cell.[174,182] In other cases, it appears later in the disease and tends to be associated with an evolving and expanding clone of cells.[158,177,180] Its appearance in association with evolving karyotypic changes indicates an underlying genetic instability and suggests that ras mutations are neither the first nor the last step in the transformation pathophysiology.[179] It is also unclear whether ras mutations contribute to the transformation from MDS to AML, or merely represent a genetic epiphenomenon in the emergence of a new clone.

CD34+ progenitors modified to express a mutated N-ras were found to have defective differentiation in response to erythropoietin. This was manifest as reduced proliferation, increased doubling time, and decreased number of cells in S/G2M, leading to a failure to express the differentiation program in the late erythroblast stage. These cells also tended to undergo accelerated apoptosis, suggesting that expression of a mutated N-ras could be partially responsible for the pathophysiology underlying MDS.[187] A recent report suggests that activating mutations of FLT3 with internal tandem duplication of fms-like tyrosine kinase 3 at the tyrosine kinase domain may interact with ras mutations and contribute to the transforming events of MDS to AML.

Deletion of all or part of chromosome 5 in a substantial number of patients with either de novo or secondary MDS has led to the hypothesis of a tumor suppressor

Table 109-5 ■ ***ras* Oncogene Activation and Mutation in Relation to Leukemic Transformation in Myelodysplastic Syndromes**

Oncogene	No. with Activated or Mutated Gene/Tot. No. Pts. Studied	Pts. Transformed to AML (*ras* (+)/*ras* (-)	Ref.
N-*ras*	1/15	-	147
N-*ras*	3/8	3/0	149, 154
Ki-*ras*	2/4	2/0	153
N-*ras*	5/61	2/3	159
ras	0/4	0/4	157
Ki-*ras* or N-*ras*	3/34	0/4	155
N-*ras* or Kiras or Ha-*ras*	20/50	8/4	156
N-*ras*	5/21	1/-	160
N-*ras* or Ki-*ras*	11/27	8/3	158
N-*ras*	6/35	4/8	150
N-*ras*	19/193	13/38	151
N-*ras*	21/50	6/2	161
ras	36/75	14/6	152
ras	5/51	4/17	162
Total	137/628	65/89	

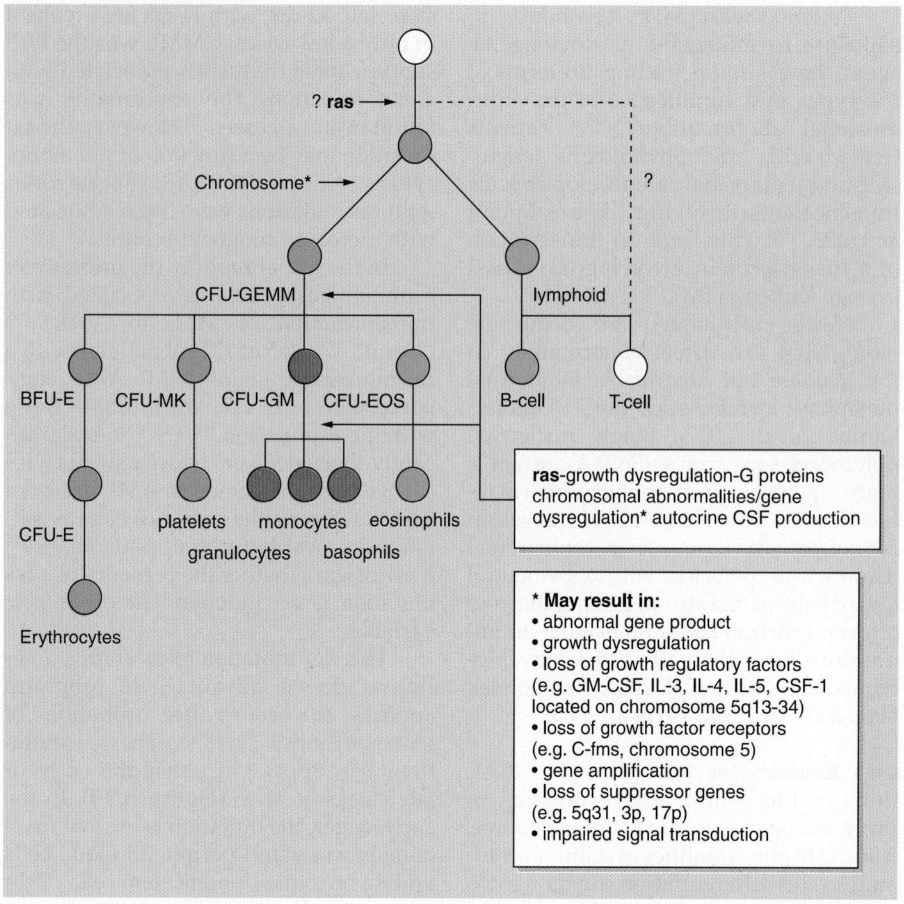

Figure 109-1 Multiple steps involved in the pathogenesis of MDS affecting a pluripotent hematopoietic stem cell (white circle). Chromosomal abnormalities and ras mutations may occur as early or late events in the pathogenesis of the disease. In younger patients, disease appears to originate in a stem cell committed along a more restricted lineage pathway (●) and is similar to the stem cell origin in some patients with de novo AML. In most patients with MDS the disease originates from a multi-potent stem cell affecting progeny involving multiple hematopoietic lineages (● ●). *May result in abnormal gene product; growth dysregulation; loss of growth regulatory factors (eg, GM-CSF, IL-3, IL-4, IL-5, CSF-1 located on chromosome 5q13–34); loss of growth factor receptors (eg, cfms, chromosome 5); gene amplification; loss of suppressor genes (eg, 5q31, 3p, 17p); impaired signal transduction. *Abbreviations*: IL, interleukin; CSF, colony-stimulating factor.

gene located within a short segment of the long arm in the so-called critical region at 5q21-5q34.[188] This region has been the focus of intensive study, and candidate genes either deleted or dysregulated have been identified, narrowing the region of interest.[189] The interferon regulatory factor-1 (IRF-1) is a DNA binding regulatory factor that regulates, in part, expression of interferon and interferon-inducible genes by binding to promoter regions. It functions as an activator, has antiproliferative and antioncogene activity, and can reverse a transformed phenotype.[190] The *IRF-1* gene has been mapped to the 5q31 region.[191] A loss of one or both IRF-lalleles in patients with MDS[192] or AML with a del 5q has been described.[191,193,194] In vitro studies have suggested that loss of the *IRF-1* gene is associated either with a transformed phenotype and/or with chemo- and radiation-induced apoptosis. Although these data suggest a potential role for the *IRF-1* gene, studies have not confirmed these observations. A recent study suggests a role for over-expression of IRF-1 leading to upregulation of Toll-like receptors resulting in an activated apoptotic pathway (Maratheftis, Giannouli et al. 2007). The lack of identification of a definitive tumor suppressor gene responsible for the disease has led to other approaches investigating the underlying mechanism. Ebert and colleagues used RNA-mediated interference (RNAi) to identify genes that might be involved. They identified a partial loss of function of the ribosomal subunit protein, *RSP14* gene, that was associated with a block in erythroid differentiation in progenitor cells from patients with the del 5q-. Using the RNAi in vitro, they were able to recapitulate the phenotype of cells from patients with del 5q-. Over-expression of the *RSP14* gene in cells from patients with del 5q- was able to rescue the phenotype and restore normal erythropoiesis, suggesting that this gene is causal for the del 5q- hematopoietic picture. The loss of function of the RSP14 results in reduction in processing of the 18s pre-rRNA levels. This is similar to the mechanism involved in the Diamond-Blackfan anemia, the congenital bone marrow failure state (Ebert, Pretz et al. 2008).

Point mutations in the TP53 tumor suppressor gene have been reported in 8% of MDS cases.[195,196] In one series, patients with secondary MDS (sMDS) or therapy-related AML (tAML) were found to have a higher than expected prevalence of TP53 mutations in leukemic, but not germline tissues. Accumulation of TP53 abnormalities with sequential follow-up was identified in patients as they transform to AML.[197] Microsatellite instability was identified and was consistent with a mutator phenotype, suggesting that these patients were at higher risk of developing therapy-related MDS/AML.[159] Recently, patients have been described with a 17p- syndrome characterized by dysgranulopoiesis with pseudo–Pelger-Huet hypolobulation and small vacuoles in neutrophils. In one series, 15 of 16 patients with this deletion had an associated deletion of TP53, suggesting a potential role for loss of a tumor suppressor gene as a contributing factor to the morphologic, cytogenetic, and molecular phenotype of this syndrome.[198] The expression of several other genes, including EVI-1, c-mpl, PDGF, MLL, and the CSF-1 receptor have recently been described to be dysregulated in some patients with MDS.[170,193,199,200] The EVI-1 gene, located on chromosome 3, has been shown to play a role in both myeloid and erythroid differentiation. Dysregulation of gene expression is associated with blocks in myeloid and erythroid maturation.[201,202]

The V617F JAK 2 mutation has been described in patients with the MPDs, polycythemia vera, myelofibrosis, and essential thrombocythemia. There is also a small subset of patients with MDS with the mutation. These patients usually have high platelet counts and may have sideroblastic anemia. Some have designated this small subset RARS-T (T= thrombocytosis) (Wardrop and Steensma 2009).

Clinical and Laboratory Features

The clinical and laboratory picture in patients with MDS is dominated by and derives from the defect involving a multipotent hematopoietic stem cell. Although the disease has occasionally been described in children and adolescents, it is primarily encountered in adults in their sixth decade or older.[203] In most reports, the median age is over 65, and there appears to be a male predominance. The clinical presentation is nonspecific. The symptoms relate primarily to the cytopenias, with those attributable to anemia being most common. These include fatigue, weakness, pallor, dyspnea, angina pectoris, and cardiac failure. Other signs and symptoms encountered less frequently include easy bruising, ecchymosis, epistaxis, gingival bleeding, petechiae, and bacterial infections, particularly respiratory and dermal. Physical findings are nonspecific. Hepatic and/or splenic enlargement is reported in 10–40% of patients and is most commonly found in CMML. Lymphadenopathy and skin infiltration are uncommon,[21,23,24,26,204,205] although the appearance of leukemia cutis in patients with MDS may herald a transformation to leukemia by weeks or months. Its identification may suggest the development of a more aggressive clinical course and in one study appeared to be associated with a poor prognosis.[206] Non-therapy-related MDS has been reported in association with other neoplasms, including lymphoproliferative and plasma cell disorders as well as carcinomas.[23]

The characteristic hematologic findings include peripheral blood cytopenias associated with dysmyelopoietic morphology and functional abnormalities involving one or more of the cell lines and are detailed in Table 109-6. The bone marrow is hypercellular in the majority and features the dysmyelopoietic morphology of part of all of the progenitors. Abnormalities involving erythrocyte enzymes, surface antigens, hemoglobin production, and iron metabolism have been described. Some of the changes in enzyme activity, such as pyruvate kinase, may affect red cell survival.[207,208] Impaired activity of A and H transferase and galactosyltransferase has resulted in changes in blood types.[209,210] Hemoglobin production is affected with increased fetal hemoglobin, aberrant globin chain synthesis, and disordered ferrokinetics.[211,212]

The myeloid series often reveals leukopenia with immature forms and increased numbers of large unstained cells (LUC). Neutropenia is more commonly found in patients with RAEB and RAEB-T than RA and RARS.[23] Leukocytosis most often accompanies CMML, and by definition, requires an absolute monocytosis (>1 × 10^9/L) for diagnosis. Monocytosis may, however, also be present in the other MDS subtypes.[23] Cytoplasmic abnormalities result in cells with hypo- or defective granule formation, Auer rods, or abnormal azurophilic granules. Histocytochemical studies reveal cells with increased or decreased levels of leukocyte alkaline phosphatase,[213] decreased myeloperoxidase staining, and loss of granule membrane glycoproteins.[208,214] Surface antigen analysis has shown loss of lineage-specific antigens, with persistent or increased expression of inappropriate antigens and lineage infidelity.[212–215] In some instances, the abnormal persistence of antigens or an increased proportion of cells expressing those antigens was associated with an increased risk of leukemic transformation and shortened survival. Abnormal expression of an activated surface phenotype on monocytes has been demonstrated in patients within all FAB subtypes, while expression of activated surface antigens on granulocytes was almost exclusively seen in patients with excess blasts.[219] Impaired granulocyte function includes impaired respiratory burst, deficit in chemotaxis and superoxide release, as well as a defect in neutrophil stimulation signaling.[219,220] Nuclear and functional abnormalities are outlined in Table 109-6.[102,221]

Table 109-6 Morphologic and Functional Cellular Abnormalities in Myelodysplastic Syndromes

Erythrocytes
Morphology
anisocytosis
poikilocytosis
oval macrocytes
microcytes
basophilic stippling
Howell-Jolly bodies
circulating nucleated red cells
megaloblastoid maturation
multinucleated precursors
nuclear budding
karryohexis
defective hemoglobinization
ringed sideroblasts
increased stainable iron
Enzymes
increased hexokinase
decreased pyruvate kinase
decreased 2,3 diphosphoglycerate mutase
decreased phosphofructokinase
increased adenosine deaminase
increased pyruvate kinase
Decreases or loss of blood group antigens
Increased fetal hemoglobin
Aberrant globin chain synthesis
Disordered ferrokinetics
Leukocytes
Morphology
pseudo–Pelger-Huet cells
abnormal chromatin clumping
abnormal nuclear bridging
monocytosis
defective granule formation (hypogranulation)
megaloblastoid maturation
Auer rods
Increased LAP
Decreased myeloperoxidase
Increased muramidase (CMML)
Loss of granule membrane glycoproteins
Inappropriate surface antigens
Lineage infidelity
Decreased adhesion
Defective chemotaxis
Deficient phagocytosis
Impaired bacteriocidal activity
Megakaryocytes
Morphology
micromegakaryocytes
hypolobulated nuclei
large mononuclear forms
circulating megakaryocyte fragments
giant thrombocytes
Defective platelet aggregation
Deficiency in thromboxane A2
Bernard-Soulier-like defect
Immune Deficiencies
Decreased T-cell IL-2 receptors
Decreased IL-2 production
Decreased NK activity
Decreased NK response to gamma interferon
Decreased response to mitogens
Decreased T4 cells
Immunoglobulin abnormalities
Autoantibodies
Autoimmune phenomenon
Impaired self-recognition

Megakaryocytes can be decreased and their morphology is often bizarre (see Table 109-6). Patients with RAEB and RAEB-T more commonly have thrombocytopenia, decreased megakaryocytes, and greater degrees of dysmegakaryopoiesis.[23] Megakaryocyte fragments and giant thrombocytes may circulate in the peripheral blood. Hemorrhagic symptoms in these patients may be due not only to thrombocytopenia, but to functionally defective platelets as well. Dysfunction can result from defective platelet aggregation, deficiencies in thromboxane A2 activity, or the development of a Bernard–Soulier-type platelet defect. This latter defect has developed from a deficiency in the membrane glycoprotein GP lb-IX complex.[222,223]

A small percentage of patients present with hypoplastic bone marrows and cytopenias that morphologically may be difficult to distinguish from aplastic anemia.[224] Cytogenetic analysis with or without interphase FISH may be helpful in establishing a diagnosis.

The relationship of MDS to abnormalities of the immune system is of particular interest given the broad range of abnormalities described. There is a decrease in the number of T-cell interleukin-2 (IL-2) receptors, as well as IL-2 production. The latter is due, in part, to a failure of immunoregulatory B cells.[225] NK cell activity and responsiveness to α-interferon is decreased, as is α-interferon production, while total numbers of NK cells are variable.[94,225] There are decreases in the number of T cells, responsiveness to mitogenic stimulation, the total number of cells, and the T4/T8 ratio.[212,226,227] The latter is due predominantly to a decrease in T4 cells.

Immunoglobulin abnormalities manifest as autoantibodies or a positive direct Coombs' test is often present.[226,228] The relationship of the disease to the immune abnormalities is poorly understood. A general dysregulation of the immune system appears prevalent in many patients. Consistent with this is the finding of altered antibody repertoires of self-reactive IgM and IgG in MDS patients, indicating a disturbance in self-recognition mechanisms.[229] Whether some abnormalities relate, in part, to the number of red cell transfusions, or whether they are reversible with effective treatment is unknown. Given the nature of the defect in a multipotent stem cell with potential to differentiate along multiple pathways,[230] the dysregulation of T and B cells should not be surprising. A report of 20 patients with nontherapy-related MDS and concurrent lymphoid or plasmacytic malignant neoplasms contributes further evidence to the multi-potency of the stem cell affected and to the derivative generalized immune dysregulation.[226]

Establishing a Diagnosis

The diagnosis in most patients is readily established with standardized testing, which should include history and physical examination, complete blood count, and review of the peripheral blood smear. The findings of cytopenias in the absence of explanation from biochemical, vitamin deficiency, hemorrhage, toxin/drug, or infectious etiology should lead to a bone marrow aspirate and biopsy. Routine cytogenetic evaluation should be included as well. The diagnosis of MDS is based primarily on morphologic criteria demonstrating dysmorphic features in the peripheral blood and bone marrow precursors (see Table 109-6). Although some of the classification systems include cytogenetic information (IPSS and WHO), they are based primarily on bone marrow and peripheral blood morphology. Analysis of the marrow population using flow cytometric analysis has become standard for the diagnosis and subtyping in patients with acute leukemia. It is more routinely being applied to establish a diagnosis of MDS as well. Abnormal populations and skewed antigen expression can be identified.[231–237] However, comparative studies of bone marrow morphology and flow cytometry results have not been conducted, and thus one cannot be certain if used alone whether flow cytometry results can reliably establish a diagnosis and classification of MDS. Accurate classification according to FAB, IPSS, or WHO criteria must be based, at least in part, on bone marrow morphology. Thus, flow cytometry should be viewed as a complementary examination but not sufficient to establish the diagnosis and classification.

Diagnostic Dilemmas

Some patients with MDS present with features also suggestive of a MPD, representing an "overlap syndrome."[238,239] In these patients, cytopenias may present simultaneously with elevated white or platelet counts. In some patients, an increased leucocyte count may be accompanied by monocytosis. Under current classification systems, some of these patients will be clearly defined as MPD, while others are still categorized as MDS, depending on the upper limit of WBC permitted in the classification system. Others may have myelofibrosis with or without marked splenomegaly and peripheral blood cytopenias,[239–242] yet also have dysplastic features suggesting MDS. These patients are more difficult to classify. Those with myelofibrosis with markedly enlarged spleens and a leucoerythroblastic peripheral smear are more likely classic myelofibrosis with myeloid metaplasia, while patients without significant splenomegaly and/or the peripheral leucoerythroblastic picture may be considered to have primary MDS with fibrosis. The presence of V617F Jak2 mutation would favor a diagnosis of a MPD over MDS except in patients with RARS-T (Wardrop and Steensma 2009).

The hypoplastic MDS variant is often indistinguishable from aplastic anemia and may have many features in common.[235,243–246] Those patients with increased expression of HLA-DR 15 and the PNH phenotype (decreased expression of CD59), whether MDS or aplastic anemia, may respond to immunomodulatory treatments. Cytogenetic abnormalities, if present, involving chromosomes frequently abnormal in MDS, may suggest the diagnosis of MDS, but do not completely exclude aplastic anemia.[245] In these patients, therapeutic options may be the determinants in the orientation of the diagnosis in the absence of other criteria.

Finally, there are patients who present with severe pancytopenia and bone marrow findings that are nondiagnostic (ie, minimal, if any, dysmorphic changes; no increase in myeloblasts) and without any cytogenetic abnormalities. Some of these patients may have MDS, and only with continued observation and testing will a diagnosis be unequivocally established. Others may have been exposed to a bone marrow insult (toxin, infectious agent, etc.), which may never be identified, but which may permit eventual complete or partial marrow recovery, which takes months or years. In these latter individuals, in the absence of clear diagnostic evidence, patience, continued observation, and supportive care (SC) maybe the best approach pending a declarative diagnosis. One other consideration for these patients would be an immune-mediated injury to hematopoietic stem cells. The differential in these patients would include large granular lymphocytic leukemia (LGL), where T-cell receptor and immunoglobulin gene rearrangement studies may be informative.[247]

Pathogenesis and Relation to Leukemic Transformation

Initiation and promotion of an abnormality affecting a multipotent stem cell may be related to a variety of factors, including chemical insult, radiation, or infection, leading to modification of gene expression. Since most patients with MDS are in the sixth, seventh, or eighth decades, cell senescence may also play a role. Once established, the clonal lesion follows the multistep process of oncogenesis and results in the transformation to acute leukemia in up to 40% of patients. It is likely that multiple events occur and lead to evolution of the disease and ultimate emergence of a dominant clone of cells.[230] Based on the knowledge of a number of abnormalities that do occur, one may speculate on the possible interrelationship of these events that contribute to the pathogenesis. Mutations of the ras oncogene, either as an early or late event in the development of the disease, may be one of the steps in this process.[174,180,182] One model of ras mutation results in impaired growth and differentiation along with impaired response to erythropoietin and increased apoptosis, similar to the response of the in vivo phenotype.[187] Such mutations may serve to confer a growth advantage to the mutated cells, resulting in their progressive expansion.[175] As a late event, the selective growth advantage may be sufficient to trigger a leukemic transformation. However, when alteration of the *ras* gene occurs as an early event, it may be insufficient to trigger further progression and may require the concerted action of other factors such as those accompanying chromosomal abnormalities and the attendant gene dysregulation that occurs.

The impaired response of hematopoietic progenitors suggests an underlying abnormality of signal transduction. Mutations of cytokine receptors can result in a signal that is muted or overexpressed. Mutations have been identified of the FLT3 and G-CSF receptor in association with transformation to AML in patients with MDS.[248] Most studies, however, have not identified abnormalities of cytokine receptors, suggesting a defect further downstream from the ligand-receptor interaction. The increase in apoptosis in the bone marrow with apparent dysregulation of TNF-α and TGF-β further suggest cytokine dysregulation. Hematopoietic progenitors with impaired cellular response to cytokine signals could behave as though deprived of obligate survival factors, and thus undergo accelerated apoptosis. This would be the predominant phenotype until further genetic or growth regulatory changes occurred that would trigger a proliferative advantage and transformation to AML. In patients with severe congenital neutropenia, evolution to a MDS or acute leukemia is usually accompanied by acquired mutations in the G-CSF receptor.[249] Point mutations of the G-CSF receptor gene cause truncation of the C-terminal cytoplasmic region of the receptor. Cells with this defect fail to undergo terminal maturation to granulocytes in response to the G-CSF.[250] In a mouse model, the equivalent G-CSF receptor mutation leads to expansion of the G-CSF receptor responsive progenitor population.[251] Treatment with G-CSF leads to neutrophilia, accompanied by increased activation of transcription factors and prolonged external cell surface expression owing to defective internalizaiton. Further genetic mutations in the face of clonal expansion can contribute to leukemogenesis.

Karyotypic abnormalities have been described in up to 79% of patients with MDS[73] and appear to be a later phenomenon. This is suggested by the identification of karyotypic abnormalities in cells belonging to already established clones derived from a multipotent stem cell[81,223] and by their greater frequency in patients with increased bone marrow blasts.[152,156] The association in some studies of complex karyotypic abnormalities with an increased risk of leukemic transformation[22,27,152] further suggests that these anomalies confer a growth advantage to a clone, as well as reflecting underlying genetic instability. This instability, manifest by clonal evolution with the subsequent acquisition of additional chromosomal abnormalities, has also been associated with disease progression, either to a more malignant subtype or frank AML.[25,27] Finally, most of the karyotypic abnormalities involve complete or partial deletions of chromosomes and suggest that gene loss may play a role in the pathogenesis.[167,188,252,253] The critical region on the long arm of chromosome 5, in the interstitial region q13-q34, contains genes encoding a number of important proteins, including GMCSF, IL-3, IL-4, IL-5, CSF-1, and the oncogene *cfms*, which codes for the CSF-1 receptor.[252–254] Changes in this critical region may result in the production of an abnormal gene product or a point mutation. Deletion or loss of chromosomal material may result in a cell hemizygous for a mutant allele, which can be expressed, or loss of a tumor suppressor gene. Several chromosomal regions that are commonly deleted in patients with MDS have been identified, including del 1q, del 5q, del 17p, and del 3p, and may contain tumor suppressor genes whose loss may contribute to the transformation process.[255,256]

Dysregulation of the cell cycle may occur and contribute to the leukemic transformation. The cyclin-dependent kinase inhibitor (CDKI) gene p1 5INK4B undergoes aberrant methylation of the CpG islands in up to 50% of patients with MDS studied in one series. Patients with high-risk MDS had the highest frequency of hypermethylation, compared to those with low-risk MDS. In addition, hypermethylation became more prominent as disease progressed.[257] The EVI-1 gene, with a role in the regulation of erythroid and myeloid maturation, is another involved gene. In patients with translocation t(3;21), a novel chimeric transcription factor, AML1/EVI-1 is formed that appears to block granulocytic differentiation, and thus may play a role in the transformation process.[258] Additionally, unknown factors, including the influence of growth factors on cells, probably participate in leukemogenesis. Additional mutations involving other genes such as the *EVI-1* gene, resulting in impaired cell maturation, or of the *MLL* gene, leading to altered fusion proteins, may be part of the pathogenic process.[170,202] Other candidate tumor suppressor genes may be harbored on chromosomes lq, 3p, or 17p.

Treatment

For many years, the management of patients with MDS was a frustrating and daunting task, compounded by the age of the patients, their debility secondary to bone marrow failure, comorbidities, and a lack of effective treatments. The mainstay of therapy was primarily SC, consisting of transfusions and antibiotics in an effort to alleviate symptoms, but without impact on the disease outcome. Therapeutic efforts are complicated by the heterogeneity of the disease, which determines individual prognosis. Additional complicating features, including the general lack of randomized trials and the lack of uniform response criteria, made the interpretation of therapeutic results more difficult. The last decade has witnessed an expanded interest in the treatment of MDS, with the identification of new potentially useful therapeutic strategies.

Differentiation-Inducing and Novel-Acting Agents

There has been great interest in the potential of differentiation therapy as an antitumor modality since Charlotte Friend and her colleagues first demonstrated that dimethylsulfoxide (DMSO) could induce differentiation of murine erythroleukemic cells in vitro, thus altering their malignant phenotype.[259] The phenomenon although readily achieved in vitro, is more difficult to demonstrate in the clinical setting. A number of agents that have effectively induced differentiation in vitro were tested in MDS without significant success (eg, cis- and trans-retinoic acid, vitamin D3, butyrate, and hexamethylene bisacetamide [HMBA]).

The hypomethylating agent azacitidine (AzaC) has produced significant benefit (Table 109-7).[260,261] The promoter region of genes that are not expressed are often associated with hyper-methylated CpG islands. Aberrant acquired changes in methylation, or epigenetic events, resulting in gene silencing can have important effects on genes regulating the cell cycle and differentiation programs. A series of experiments by Christman, Acs, and colleagues led to the development of a biochemical model that provided an explanation for the action of AzaC as an inducer of differentiation through its effects on DNA methylation.[262,263] AzaC, once incorporated into DNA, covalently binds to DNA methyltransferase, the enzyme in mammalian cells responsible for methylation of newly synthesized DNA. This binding results in hypomethylated DNA distal to the binding point and leads to transcription of previously quiescent methylated genes. In patients with β-thalassemia,[264] treatment with AzaC resulted in an increase in fetal hemoglobin production, which was associated

Table 109-7 Randomized Controlled Trials in Patients with MDS Drug vs Supportive Care +/– Placebo

Agent	Response to Treatment	Quality of Life	Frequency of Transformation to AML	Time to Progression	Time to AML or Death	Survival at 24 Months	Ref.
Cis-retinoic acid	NSSD	–	–	–	–	NSSD	217, 273, 275
Low-Dose Cytarabine	Cytarabine	–	NSSD	NSSD	NSSD	NSSD	270, 271
G-CSF	G-CSF	–	NSSD	NSSD	SC[a]	SC[a]	311
GM-CSF	GM-CSF	–	NSSD	–	–	NSSD	308
Azacitidine	Azacitidine[b]	Azacitidine[c]	Azacitidine[b]	Azacitidine[d]	Azacitidine[e]	Azacitidine[f]	260, 261
Decitabine	Decitabine	Decitabine	NSSD	NSSD	NSSD	NR	SABA

[a]Differences are for patients with RAEB. For those with RAEB-T, there was NSSD between G-CSF and SC. [b]$p < .001$ [c]fatigue ($p = .001$); physical functioning ($p = .002$); dyspnea ($p = .0014$); mental health index ($p = .0077$). [d]$p < .0001$. [e]$p = .004$. [f]$p = .03$

Abbreviations: NSSD, no statistically significant difference between agent tested and placebo or supportive care (SC); —, endpoint not assessed in trial; NR, not reported.

with hypomethylation in the region of the gamma globin chain gene. Based on this model, a trial testing the efficacy of AzaC in MDS was undertaken by the Cancer and Leukemia Group B (CALGB).[265] AzaC was administered at 75 mg/m2/d continuous IV infusion for 7 days repeated in 28- day cycles. Of 43 evaluable patients, 21(49%) achieved a response. In a second study in the CALGB, AzaC was administered subcutaneously at the same dose and schedule in an ambulatory regimen with comparable efficacy and toxicity profiles.[266] This led to the conduct of a phase III trial of AzaC compared with SC in the CALGB. In a crossover design, patients with progression could crossover to treatment after a minimum of 4 months in the SC group. Responses occurred in 60% on the AzaC arm (7% CR, 16% PR, 37% improved) compared with 5% (improved) for SC ($p <$ .0001). The median time to leukemic transformation or death was significantly delayed for those on AzaC (21 mos vs 13 mos for SC [p = .007]) (Figure 109-2). Probability of transformation to AML as the first event was lower on AzaC (15%) than SC[192] (p = .001). The quality of life (QOL) of patients on the AzaC arm was significantly superior to that experienced by individuals in the control group as measured by several test methods. On crossover to AzaC treatment, the same individuals were evaluated according to the same serial interviews, and striking improvement in their QOL ensued. Patients on the AzaC arm experienced significantly greater improvement over time than patients in the SC group in fatigue, physical functioning, dyspnea, psychosocial distress, and positive affect. Significant differences persisted after controlling for RBC transfusions. Prior to crossover, the QOL of patients on SC was stable or worsening. After crossover to AzaC, significant improvements occurred in fatigue, physical functioning, dyspnea, and general well-being.[45,46] Detailed analyses make placebo or Hawthorne effects an unlikely explanation for improvements in QOL by AzaC. Median survival for AzaC and SC (analyzed by intent to treat regardless of crossover) was 20 and 14 months, respectively (p = .1). The probability of survival at 24 months was 41% for AzaC compared with 25% for SC (p = .03), In order to eliminate the confounding effect caused by including the 49 crossover patients in the survival analysis, a landmark analysis was done in which the survival of three subgroups of patients were compared from a 6-month landmark date. These subgroups were 189 SC patients who never crossed over or who crossed over only after 6 months,[260] SC patients who crossed over before 6 months, and[192] patients who were initially randomized to AzaC. The 36 patients who died before the landmark date were excluded. The additional median survival (after the 6-month landmark date) for these three groups was 11, 14, and 18 months, respectively. The AzaC group was significantly different from the SC subgroup who crossed over late or never (p = .03). SC patients who crossed over early (subgroup 2) had a longer median survival than the patients who crossed over late or never (subgroup 1), though this did not reach statistical significance (p = .11). Results demonstrate that patients treated with AzaC had significantly higher response rates, improved QOL, delayed time to progression, improved survival at 24 months, delayed time to leukemic transformation or death, and significantly reduced risk of transformation to AML compared with SC.[260,261] as the first event was lower on AzaC (15%) than SC 189 (p = .001). The quality of life (QOL) of patients on the AzaC arm was significantly superior, according to several test methods, to that experienced by individuals in the control group. On crossover to AzaC treatment, the same individuals were evaluated for quality of life according to the same serial interviews. Striking improvement in their QOL ensued. Patients on the AzaC arm experienced significantly greater improvement over time in fatigue (EORTC, p = .001), physical functioning (EORTC, p = .002), dyspnea (EORTC, p = .0014), psychosocial distress (MHI, p = .0 15), and positive affect (MHI, p = .0077) than patients in the SC group. Significant differences persisted after controlling for RBC transfusions. Prior to crossover, the QOL of patients on SC was stable or worsening. After crossover to AzaC, significant improvements occurred in fatigue (EORTC, p = .0001), physical functioning (EORTC, p = .004), dyspnea (EORTC, p = .0002), and general well being (MHI, p = .016).[260] Detailed analyses make unlikely placebo or hawthorne effects as explanations for improvements in QOL by AzaC. Median survival for AzaC and SC (analyzed by intent to treat regardless of crossover) was 20 and 14 months, respectively (p = .1). The probability of survival at 24 months was 41% for AzaC compared with 25% for SC (p = .03), respectively. In order to eliminate the confounding effect caused by including the 49 crossover patients in the survival analysis, a landmark analysis was done in which the survival of three subgroups of patients were compared from a 6-month landmark date. These subgroups were SC patients who never crossed over or who crossed over only after 6 months,[260] SC patients who crossed over before 6 months, and patients who were initially randomized to AzaC. The 36 patients who died before the landmark date were excluded. The additional median survival (after the 6-month landmark date) for these three groups was 11, 14, and 18 months, respectively. The AzaC group was significantly different from the SC subgroup who crossed over late or never (p = .03). SC patients who crossed over early (subgroup 2) had a longer median survival than the patients who crossed over late or never (subgroup 1), though this did not reach statistical significance

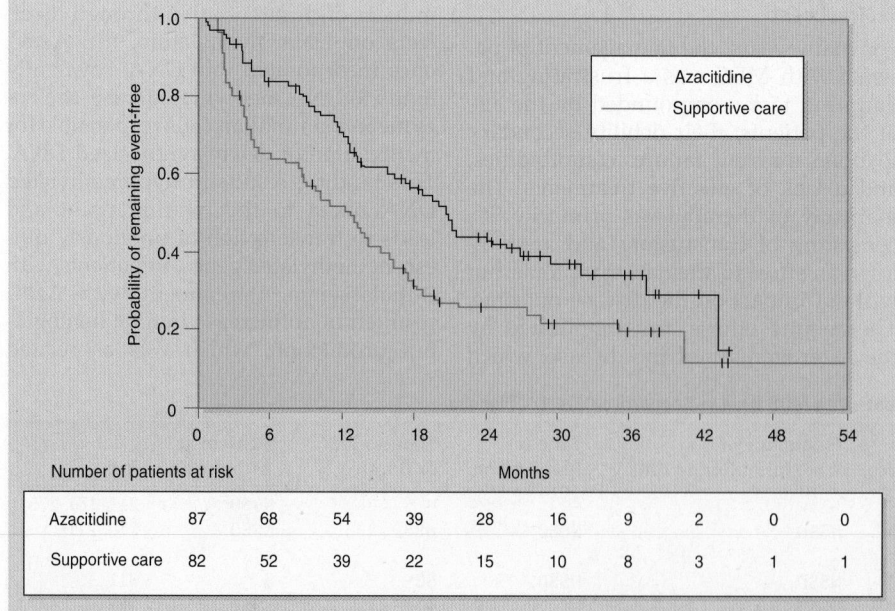

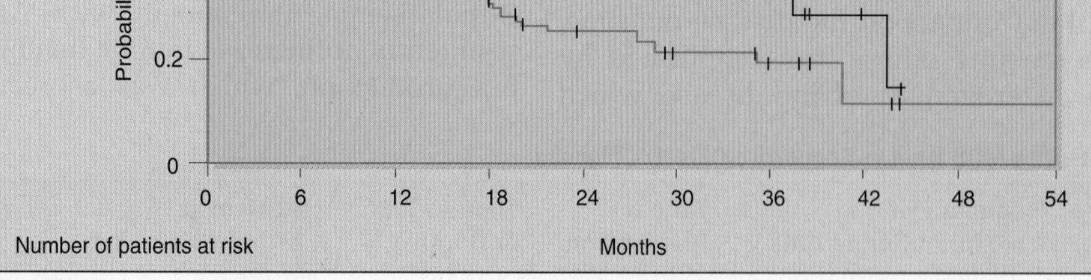

Azacitidine	87	68	54	39	28	16	9	2	0	0
Supportive care	82	52	39	22	15	10	8	3	1	1

Figure 109-2 Time to transformation or death in patients treated with azacitidine compared to supportive care. Measured from time of study entry to first event, either transformation to AML or death, and estimated according to the method of Kaplan–Meier. Median time 21 vs 13 months, respectively (p = .007). *Source*: From Ref. 261.

(p = .11). Results demonstrate that patients treated with AzaC had significantly higher response rates, improved QOL, delayed time to progression, improved survival at 24 months, delayed time to leukemic transformation or death, and significantly reduced risk of transformation to AML compared with SC.[260,261] Additional analyses demonstrated that AzaC results in transfusion independence in 45% of patients and is effective in producing responses in patients according to the WHO AML classification (blasts > 20%) with a median survival of 19.3 months suggesting a potential benefit in this patient population (Silverman, McKenzie et al. 2006). Thus, AzaC is the only agent other than allogeneic bone marrow transplantation to alter the natural history of MDS. Furthermore, AzaC is not age restricted, as is marrow transplantation. A second randomized controlled trial has confirmed and extended these observations demonstrating a significant survival advantage for patients treated with AzaC compared to a conventional care regimen (a physician directed choice of either best SC, low dose evtarabine or induction chemotherapy with an anthraeycline and eytarabine) with median OS for AzaC of 24.4 months compared to 15 months for the conventional care regimen (Fenaux, Mufti et al. 2009). Time to AML or death, and time to AML, were significantly delayed for patients in the AzaC treated group. Transfusion independence occurred in 45% of patients and there was a reduction by 33% in the infections requiring intravenous antibiotics in the AzaC treated patients. Additional analyses suggest that maintenance therapy with AzaC is beneficial (Silverman ASII 08) (Silverman McKenzie et al. 2006).

AzaC acts via a number of mechanisms. It can be a cytotoxic agent, but in vitro data indicate that it also functions as a biologic response modifier, affecting cytokine signal transduction pathways.[265,267] Another hypomethylating agent, decitabine, (2-deoxy-5-AzaC) has also been evaluated.[268,269] Although response criteria are different, decitabine, like AzaC, produces responses. In a randomized North American randomized trial of decitabine compared to SC, decitabine was superior with a response rate of 17% CR+PR compared to 0% for SC. However, there was no difference in the second co-primary endpoint of time to AML or death between the 2 groups (Kantarjian. Issa et al. 2006). In a second randomized trial conducted in Europe by the EORTC of decitabine compared to SC in patients with intermediate-2 or high-risk disease, there was no difference in time to AMI or death or survival between the 2 groups. An alternative dosing regimen of 20 mg/m2/d × 5 days every 4 weeks has yielded response rates that are comparable but maybe less myelosuppressive (Kantarjian. Oki et al. 2007). However, this was not a controlled trial and the effects on modifying disease outcome are uncertain.

Cytosine arabinoside has been extensively tested. In a review of the literature, low-dose cytosine arabinoside was reported to produce 16% CR in 170 patients.[270] Median duration of CR was 10.5 months, but achievement of a response appeared to have little effect on overall survival. In a randomized trial conducted by Eastern Cooperative Oncology Group (ECOG) and Southwest Oncology Group (SWOG), patients with MDS were treated with either low-dose cytarabine or SC. Patients in SC who progressed could cross over and receive treatment with cytarabine. There was no significant difference between the cytarabine and SC groups with respect to overall survival, time to progression, or frequency of transformation to AML (see Table 109-7).[271] In a subset analysis in the most recent randomized trial of AzaC compared to a conventional care regimen was superior to low-dose eytarabine improving survival significantly in patients with intermediate-2 and high-risk MDS (Fenaux, Mufri et al. 2009).

Retinoic acid and related compounds, highly effective inducers of differentiation in vitro,[272] have been disappointing in their lack of efficacy in several clinical trials.[217,273–276]

The observations regarding the potential role of TNF in the pathophysiology of MDS (described above in the section "Signal Transduction") have led to therapeutic strategies targeting TNF in small pilot studies. Etanercept, an anti-TNF fusion protein, caused erythroid response of 30% in one trial and a lower response in the other.[277,278] Thalidomide has been tested based on potential anti-TNF activity, but also because of effects on vascular endothelial growth factor (VEGF). Responses, predominantly in the erythroid lineage ranged from 10% to 19%.[279,280] Somnolence and neuropathy forced withdrawal of patients from treatment. Lenalidomide, an analog without sedative or neuropathic side effects and with more potent in vitro anti-TNF and anti-VEGF effects was tested in a phase II trial. Of the 148 patients with low and intermediate-1 disease with del 5q either isolated or combined with other cytogenetic abnormalities, 67% patients became red cell transfusion independent (List. Dewald et al. 2006). The median duration of transfusion independence was 115 weeks (List 2008). In a second study of low and intermediate-1 disease in patients without a deletion 5q, 26% patients achieved transfusion independence for a median of 41 weeks.[281]

Hormones ■ Although used as a nonspecific stimulant of erythropoiesis in aplastic anemia with some benefit, androgens have not proven to be useful in MDS. Initial observations suggesting that treatment with androgens accelerated the disease and were associated with an increased rate of leukemic transformation were not confirmed in subsequent studies, nor was any efficacy identified.[285,286]

Glucocorticoid therapy yielded an overall response rate of only 9% and 24% of nonresponding patients experienced significant deleterious side effects.[287]

Danazol has been reported to produce improvements in the thrombocytopenia and anemia in patients with MDS. The effects appear to be mediated, in part, through inhibition of Fc receptor expression on monocytes, which alter the clearance of immunoglobulin-coated platelets and red cells from circulation, rather than a direct stimulatory effect on hematopoiesis. Danazol may be helpful in those patients where immune-mediated cell destruction contributes to the deficit.[288]

Chemotherapy ■ Chemotherapeutic agents, alone and in combination, have been used to treat patients with MDS. These agents have been employed in a variety of regimens ranging from attenuated low-dose schedules[92] to the more conventional antileukemic myelotoxic-type strategies. These have been employed to treat patients at all stages of disease. Antileukemic-type treatments have not substantially altered the outcome of the disease for most patients and have been associated with significant toxicity in many.

The pharmacologic interaction between fludarabine and cytosine arabinoside increases intracellular ara-CTP and has been exploited in a regimen with activity in patients with relapsed AML. Subsequently, the combination with (FLAG) or without (FA) G-CSF has been tested in patients with MDS and de novo AML.[289] The two regimens yielded comparable complete response rates of 60% and 55%, respectively, with the response rate generally higher in the subgroups of MDS with excess blasts. Overall, 27% of patients (MDS and AML) died during induction. The median projected survival was 29 weeks for FAand 39 weeks for FLAG. These differences were not statistically significant. In patients with deletion of chromosome 5 or 7, FLAG produced a response rate of 64% versus 36% for FA. However, the differences were attributed by the authors to factors other than an effect of treatment. Use of G-CSF was associated with a more rapid recovery of neutrophil count, but this did not translate into decreased rates of infection or infection-related mortality.[289] Overall, there were no differences in treatment outcome for patients with MDS compared with AML.

In a successor study, 215 patients (153 AML and 62 RAEB/RAEB-T) were treated with fludarabine (F), cytarabine (A), and idarubicin (I) with or without either G-CSF or all-trans-retinoic acid (ATRA) (FAI; FAI + G-CSF; FAI + ATRA; FAI + G-CSF +ATRA).[290] The response was 51%, and the median survival was 28 weeks. Addition of G-CSF ± ATRA to FAI did not affect overall outcome.

In general, results from earlier studies indicated that responses to treatment of patients with either MDS or AML following MDS are less favorable than treatment of de novo AML.[291–293] Age appears to influence the rate and duration of response, with younger patients achieving CR more frequently[294] and remaining in remission longer compared with older patients. Achievement of a CR in MDS is associated with improved survival in comparison to nonresponding patients,[288,290] but the duration of the response is substantially shorter in comparison with patients with de novo AML who achieve response. Treatment prior to the transformation to AML,[292] and patients with shorter intervals between the diagnosis of MDS and leukemic transformation,[290] are associated with higher response rates. However, aggressive antileukemic-type treatment is associated with high rates of morbidity and mortality, with up to 30% of the patients dying from drug-related complications. Addition of topotecan to chemotherapy regimens does not appear to modify these results.[295,296]

Bone Marrow Transplantation ■ Results of allogeneic and syngeneic bone marrow transplantation from a series of reports containing small numbers of MDS patients have suggested that 35–40% can achieve durable long-term disease-free remissions when treated with this modality.[297,298] This has been substantiated with the results from two larger single-institution series.[299,300] In one large series, 251 patients treated between 1981 and 1996 were evaluated.[297] Appelbaum and colleagues reported an estimated (Kaplan-Meier) 5-year disease-free survival (DFS) of 40%. Younger age, shorter duration of disease, female gender, and de novo MDS were predictors of better DFS. Patients under the age of 20 years had a 60% DFS rate, compared with 40% and 20% for those 20–50 years old or over the age of 50, respectively. Patients with low-risk MDS had a 55% DFS at 6 years compared with only 30% for those with high-risk MDS. This difference correlated with a higher rate of relapse among those with more advanced disease. Among patients with low and intermediate-1 risk according to the IPSS score, there were almost no relapses. The 5-year DFS for those in the low and intermediate-1 groups was 60%, 36% for those in intermediate-2, and 28% for those in the high-risk group. Patients undergoing matched unrelated donor (MUD) marrow transplants fare less well. In an analysis of results from the National Marrow Donor Program, patients receiving MUD transplants during the first 4 years of registry data (1986–1990) had a disappointing DFS of only 18% at 2 years and 24% an overall survival at 2 years[301] In one study, patients with primary MDS demonstrated a survival advantage over those with secondary MDS (56% vs 27%).[302]

The exact role and timing of bone marrow transplantation remains to be determined, as does the optimal conditioning regimen. A recent analysis of patients with low-risk disease, suggests that watchful waiting until evidence of disease progression increases life expectancy compared with immediate transplantation. For patients with high-risk disease, transplantation shortly after diagnosis was associated with better life expectancy.[303] For patients 40 years or younger with a compatible related donor, however, transplantation should be favored, since no other therapy thus far is curative. However, selection of transplant candidates for patients under the age of 50 remains problematic. There are some younger patients with low-risk MDS with a median survival greater than 15 years treated with SC alone (Kuengdeng). Fewer patients over the age of 40 have been transplanted, but limited data for those with related donors suggest that up to 30% may survive disease free.[302] Transplantation for those without a related donor is a more difficult choice in view of the data noted above. Given the age of most patients with MDS and the availability of donors, transplantation in the foreseeable future is likely to be of limited value, benefiting only about 5–10% of all patients with MDS (Oliansky, Antin et al. 2009).

Because of the age of most MDS patients and the potential toxicity of fully ablative transplantation regimens, interest has developed in reduced-intensity conditioning hematopoietic stem cell transplantation as an alternative. These treatment strategies use conditioning regimens, often fludarabine-based, which are better tolerated and not intended to be fully ablative. They permit chimerism to be established with either sibling or volunteer unrelated matched donors. Recent reports demonstrate that this strategy can be used in patients over the age of 60 years with mortality rates ranging from 0% to 21%. Chimerism was established in 83% of patients. Duration of remission and relapse are dependant on the IPSS classification, similar to fully ablative transplantation.[304] Thus, this is a feasible approach that can be extended to older patients, but further studies will be necessary to determine its potential role in therapy (Oliansky. Antin et al. 2009).

The use of high-dose chemotherapy with either autologous bone marrow or peripheral blood stem cell (PBSC) infusion has been used in a limited fashion. The European Group reported on 79 patients treated with intensive chemotherapy and autologous bone marrow transplantation in first CR. Fifty-five of the 79 in whom the duration of first CR was known were matched with 110 patients with de novo AML. The 2-year survival for all 79 patients was 39%, and the DFS at 2 years was 28% for the 55 patients with MDS/sAML versus 51% for patients with de novo AML. Relapse rates were 69% for MDS/sAML and 40% for de novo AML (p = .007).[213] Use of PBSC infusion is more problematic given that adequate collection from patients with MDS is obtained in only half the patients.[305]

Growth Factors The hematopoietic growth factors are regulatory glycoproteins that control the proliferation and differentiation of bone marrow stem cells.[306] Several studies have defined the effects of GM-CSF in MDS. In a controlled study, patients were randomized to observation or treatment with rhGM-CSF.[307,308] Those treated had significant increases in neutrophils, eosinophils, monocytes, and lymphocytes, while the frequency of infections was decreased in comparison with those observed in the absence of this cytokine. There were no differences in platelet count, hemoglobin, or transfusion requirements between the two groups. The risk of leukemic transformation appeared greatest for those patients with greater than 15% blasts in the bone marrow and may be a critical level with respect to leukemic transformation.[309]

Maintenance therapy, administering GM-CSF on a chronic basis, has met with mixed results, with some reports of benefit or even continued improvement in the granulocyte count, while other reports have shown a progressive deterioration in counts despite continued treatment.[310,311]

Filgrastim (G-CSF) has also been evaluated. In a randomized controlled trial, 102 patients with RAEB or RAEB-T were treated with either G-CSF or SC.[312] No differences in frequency or time to progression to AML were seen between the two groups. There was no difference in survival for those with RAEB-T. However, among patients with RAEB, those in the treatment group had a significantly shortened survival compared with patients in the control group, resulting in early termination of the study.

Human recombinant erythropoietin has also been studied in patients with MDS, with red cell responses being demonstrated in 20–25% of the patients tested.[312-316] Responses were confined to the erythroid lineage. A meta-analysis suggests that efficacy declines as bone marrow failure progresses.[317] Those who have lower serum erythropoietin levels and less transfusion need are more likely to respond. The observation that in vitro erythropoiesis improved in patients treated in vivo with G-CSF led to two clinical trials of erythropoietin and G-CSF in combination. The response rate ranged from 35% to 40% and appeared to enhance the activity of erythropoietin. Serum erythropoietin levels in these trials, as in others, are of predictive value with few responses in patients with levels above 500 U/L. In another report, the response-enhancing effect of G-CSF was not substantiated.[318] In a series of 191 patients treated with the combination, the overall response was 39%. Low-risk disease was associated with a higher response, and patients achieving a CR had a longer duration of response.[319] An algorithm based on transfusion need and serum erythropoietin levels maybe a useful guide for patient selection.[320] Effects of erythropoietin therapy on survival suggests that elimination of a transfusion requirement may be beneficial (Jadersten, Malcovati et al. 2008).

For patients with a variant of MDS characterized by severe hypoplasia and pancytopenia, which may resemble severe aplastic anemia (hypoplastic MDS), administration of antithymocyte globulin produced responses in 11 of 25 patients treated (9 of 14 RA; 2 of 6 RAEB).[321] Responses were characterized predominantly by loss of transfusion requirement and 3 of 25 had normalization of their counts. There were no changes in the dysplastic features or in bone marrow cellularity. In the completed study, 61 patients were treated, with 21(34%) responding. Transfusion requirement was eliminated in 76% of responding patients or 25% overall.[332] The effect may be mediated, in part, through an immunosuppressive effect alleviating a T-cell suppression of hematopoietic progenitors.[323] Patients who are younger, have more cytopenias, shorter duration of red cell transfusion dependence, and the presence of HLA-DRB1–15, appear more likely to respond.

Clinical Management

The management of patients with MDS presents a series of difficult choices (Figure 109-3). For patients with RA or RARS, low- or intermediate-1–risk groups, who have better prognoses and in whom the disease is manifest predominantly as asymptomatic anemia, observation and SC should be the mainstay. For those who require red cell transfusions, a trial of erythropoietin with or without GCSF appears reasonable. Those patients with a karyotypic abnormality (other than the 5q- syndrome, del 20q, or del y) have a less favorable prognosis. Such patients warrant closer follow-up and are candidates for investigational studies, particularly if they manifest an increasing number of blasts in the bone marrow or develop significant neutropenia or thrombocytopenia. Patients with low-risk disease who fail therapy with erythropoietin with or without G-CSF for anemia or who have severe cytopenias in other lineages can be considered for treatment with AzaC, which has demonstrated efficacy in low-risk disease with amelioration of symptoms. Lenalidomide will likely be of benefit in the future for patients with -5q abnormalities. For patients 40 years or younger who have a compatible donor, allogeneic bone marrow transplantation should be considered, since it is the only therapy that has so far achieved cures. For patients between 41 and 60 years old, the risks associated with bone marrow transplantation appear to be increased, though fewer MDS patients have been treated in this age category. Patients over 60 years may still be considered for bone marrow transplantation, although data are limited, efficacy is low, and complication rates high.

Patients with RAEB or RAEB-T or intermediate-2–or high-risk disease have a poorer prognosis and are candidates for treatment. Those with RAEB 1 (5–10% blasts) without other poor prognostic features (ie, abnormal karyotype, severe thrombocytopenia) could be closely observed to determine the relative stability of the disease. Those with evidence of progression are candidates for immediate intervention.

Patients with RAEB and RAEB-T can benefit from treatment with AzaC. It has demonstrated significant benefit compared with SC, induces remission, decreases transfusion requirements, extends survival, and improves the quality of life.[260,261] This therapy may now represent the standard of care.[324] Alternatively, they can be treated as part of an investigational program. Stem cell transplantation is a consideration for those patients as a potential curative strategy and should be considered early in the evaluation process after the diagnosis is established, if a donor is available, and dependent on the patient's age. However, the rate of relapse is high, and many centers will not consider these patients as candidates. Strategies aimed at inducing a remission prior to transplantation may be useful.

For patients who have transformed to leukemia, aggressive antileukemic chemotherapy can be undertaken. The CR rate ranges between 30% and 60%, but is associated with a high rate of treatment-related morbidity and mortality. Most patients relapse. Patients with hypoplastic MDS, particularly if younger, may benefit from antithymocyte globulin with or without cyclosporin.

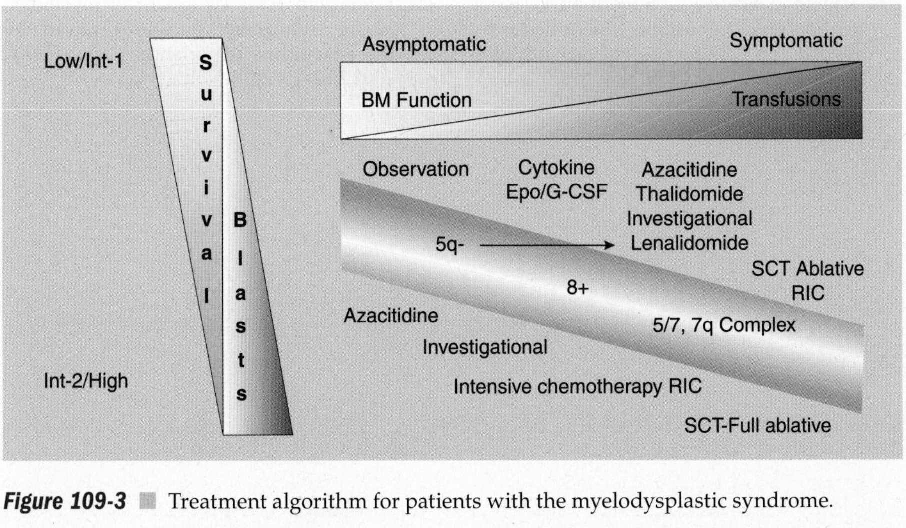

Figure 109-3 Treatment algorithm for patients with the myelodysplastic syndrome.

Future Directions

Progress in the prevention and therapy of MDS depends on a better understanding of the basic biochemical and molecular defects that contribute to the development of this syndrome. Well-designed clinical trials using clearly defined biologic end points are critical. Survival is the ultimate goal, but too global a composite to serve as the sole working criterion. Quality of life assessments have gained favor as useful tools in the measure of the effects of treatment. These assessments should be included routinely in phase II and III studies and help as a critical measure of a palliative treatment. Finally, cost analysis is another useful gauge of treatment efficacy. Pharmacoeconomic studies should also be included in future phase III studies.

In a disease characterized by the development of a progressive uncoupling of cellular maturation and proliferation, induction differentiation is an attractive approach. This has proven to be a highly provocative strategy in the treatment of acute promyelocytic leukemia with trans-retinoic acid. AzaC, which may act in part as a biologic response modifier with effects on signal transduction, may be advantageously combined with other agents. Drugs that interfere with or block abnormal signal transduction (eg, farnesyl transferase inhibitors) may prove beneficial. Tumor vaccines and the use of allogeneic T cells will be explored in the coming years.

Selected References

The complete reference list can be found at www.CANCERMEDICINE8.com

2. Bennett JM, Catovsky D, Daniel MT, et al. Proposals for the classification of the acute leukaemias. French-AmericanBritish (FAB) Co-operative Group. *Br J Haematol*. 1976;33: 451–458.
3. Aul C, Gattermann N, Heyll A, et al. Primary myelodysplastic syndromes: analysis of prognostic factors in 235 patients and proposals for an improved scoring system. *Leukemia*. 1992;6:52–59.
7. Bomford PR, Rhoads CP. Refractory anaemia. I. Clinical and pathological aspects. *Q J Med*. 1941;10:175.
9. Block M, Jacobson LO, Bethard WF. Preleukemic acute human leukemia. *JAMA*. 1953;152:1018–1028.
16. Bennett JM, Catovsky D, Daniel MT, et al. The FrenchAmerican-British Cooperative Group. Proposals for the classification of the myelodysplastic syndromes. *Br J Haematol*. 1982;51:189–199.
27. Greenberg P, Cox C, LeBeau MM, et al. International scoring system for evaluating prognosis in myelodysplastic syndromes [comments] [published erratum appears in Blood 1998;91:1100]. *Blood*. 1997;89:2079–2088.
28. Harris N, Jaffe E, Diehold J, et al. World Health Organization classification of neoplastic diseases of the hematopoietic and lymphoid tissues: report of the Clinical Advisory Committee Meeting—Airlie House, Virginia, November 1997. *J Clin Oncol*. 1999;17:3835–3849.
32. Kamada N, Uchins H. Preleukemic states in atomic bomb survivors. *Blood Cells*. 1976;2:57–65.
40. Farrow A, Jacobs A, West RR. Myelodysplasia, chemical exposure, and other environmental factors. *Leukemia*. 1989;3:33–35.
49. Kantarjian HM, Keating MJ. Therapy-related leukemia and myelodysplastic syndrome. *Semin Oncol*. 1987;14:435–443.
57. Berk PD, Goldberg JD, Silverstein MN, et al. Increased incidence of acute leukemia in polycythemia vera associated with chlorambucil therapy. *N Engl J Med*. 1981;304:441–447.
60. Fisher RI, Gaynor ER, Dahlberg S, et al. Comparison of a standard regimen (CHOP) with three intensive chemotherapy regimens for advanced Non-Hodgkin's lymphoma. *N Engl J Med*. 1993;328:1002–1006.
72. Second International Workshop on Chromosomes in Leukemia. Chromosomes in preleukemia. *Cancer Genet Cytogenet*. 1980;2:108.
116. Coutinho L, Will A, Radford J, et al. Effects of recombinant human granulocyte colony-stimulating factor (CSF), human granulocyte macrophage-CSF, and gibbon interleukin-3 on hematopoiesis in human long-term bone marrow culture. *Blood*. 1990;75:2118–2129.
118. Zinzar S, Silverman LR, Holland JF. Stromal defects in the myelodysplastic syndrome (MDS) contribute to the hematopoietic abnormalities. *Proc Am Assoc Cancer Res*. 1997;38:146.
179. Padua RA, Guinn BA, Al-Sabah Al, et al. RAS, FMS and p53 mutations and poor clinical outcome in myelodysplasias: a 10-year follow-up. *Leukemia*. 1998;12:887–892.
181. Lyons J, Janssen JWG, Bartram C, et al. Mutation of Ki-ras and N-ras oncogenes in myelodysplastic syndromes. *Blood*. 1988;71:1707–1712.
216. Baumann MA, Keller RH, McFadden PW, et al. Myeloid cell surface phenotype in myelodysplasia: evidence for abnormal persistence of an early myeloid differentiation antigen. *Am J Hematol*. 1986;22:251–257.
225. Sorskaar D, Forre O, Albrechtsen D, Stavem P. Decreased natural killer cell activity versus normal natural killer cell markers in mononuclear cells from patients with smouldering leukemia. *Scand J Haematol*. 1986;37:154–161.
255. Sankar M, Tanaka K, Kumaravel TS, et al. Identification of a commonly deleted region at 17pl3.3 in leukemia and lymphoma associated with 17p abnormality. *Leukemia*. 1998;12:510–516.
256. Najfeld V, Scalise A, Silverman L. Three regions on chromosome 1 identified to be involved in pathogenesis of myelodysplasia. *Leuk Res*. 1999;23:S9.
258. Tanaka T, Mitani K, Kurokawa M, et al. Dual functions of the AML1/Evi-1 chimeric protein in the mechanism of leukemogenesis in t(3;21) leukemias. *Mol Cell Biol*. 1995;15:2383–2392.
265. Silverman LR, Holland JF, Weinberg RS, et al. Effects of treatment with 5-azacytidine on the in vivo and in vitro hematopoiesis in patients with myelodysplastic syndromes. *Leukemia*. 1993;7(Suppl):21–29.
269. Wijermans P, Lubbert M, Verhoef G, et al. Low-dose 5-aza-2'-deoxycytidine, a DNA hypomethylating agent, for the treatment of high-risk myelodysplastic syndrome: a multicenter phase II study in elderly patients. *J Clin Oncol*. 2000;18:956–962.
297. Appelbaum FR, Anderson J. Allogeneic bone marrow transplantation for myelodysplastic syndrome: outcomes analysis according to IPSS score. *Leukemia*. 1998;12(Suppl 1):S25–S29.
298. Bunin NJ, Casper JT, Chitambar C, et al. Partially matched bone marrow transplantation in patients with myelodysplastic syndromes. *J Clin Oncol*. 1988;6:1851–1855.
300. O'Donnell MR, Nademanee AP, Snyder DS, et al. Bone marrow transplantation for myelodysplastic and myeloproliferative syndromes. *J Clin Oncol*. 1987;5:1822–1826.
301. Kernan NA, Bartsch G, Ash RC, et al. Analysis of 462 transplantations from unrelated donors facilitated by the National Marrow Donor Program. *N Engl J Med*. 1993;328:593–602.
303. Cutler CS, Lee SJ, Greenberg P, et al. A decision analysis of allogeneic bone marrow transplantation for the myelodysplastic syndromes: delayed transplantation for low-risk myelodysplasia is associated with improved outcome. *Blood*. 2004;104:579–585.
308. Vadhan-Raj S, Keating M, LeMaistre A, et al. Effects of recombinant human granulocyte-macrophage colony-stimulating factor in patients with myelodysplastic syndromes. *N Engl J Med*. 1987;317:1545–1552.
310. Rose C, Wattel E, Bastion Y, et al. Treatment with very low-dose GM-CSF in myelodysplastic syndromes with neutropenia. A report on 28 cases. *Leukemia*. 1994;8:1458–1462.
323. Molldrem JJ, Jiang YZ, Stetler-Stevenson M, et al. Haematological response of patients with myelodysplastic syndrome to antithymocyte globulin is associated with a loss of lymphocyte-mediated inhibition of CFU-GM and alterations in T-cell receptor Vbeta profiles. *Br J Haematol*. 1998;102:1314–1322.
324. Kantarjian HM. Treatment of myelodysplastic syndrome: questions raised by the azacitidine experience. *J Clin Oncol*. 2002;20:2415–2416.

110 Acute Myeloid Leukemia in Adults: Mast Cell Leukemia and Other Mast Cell Neoplasms

Charles A. Schiffer, MD ■ Richard M. Stone, MD

Acute myeloid leukemia (AML) is the most common variant of acute leukemia occurring in adults, comprising approximately 80% of acute leukemia cases diagnosed in individuals greater than 20 years of age. Striking advances in transfusion medicine and the treatment of infections, the development of potent antiemetics, as well as improved chemotherapeutic approaches, have eradicated the therapeutic nihilism that characterized many editorials and reports as late as the 1970s and early 1980s. Currently, more than 80% of young adults and 60% of all patients can achieve complete remission (CR) defined as a morphologically normal bone marrow with normal neutrophil and platelet counts.[1] Varying with patient age and other biologic factors, from 10% to 70% of these complete responders can be expected to achieve long-term survival with the likelihood that most of these individuals are cured of their disease (Fig. 110-1). However, the chemotherapeutic approach to this disease has remained largely static for two decades and it is hoped that more targeted therapies based on molecular pathophysiology will improve upon these results in the future.

AML affects adults of all ages but is especially common in older adults. The median age of patients with de novo AML entered on recent cooperative group studies is approximately 55 years, and the median age at diagnosis is probably 65-70 years. AML can present either as a de novo leukemia without an apparent antecedent illness or as an evolution from marrow disorders such as myelodysplasia, aplastic anemia, and Fanconi anemia, or after the administration of therapy for other types of cancers or nonmalignant disorders. An acute leukemic phase morphologically indistinguishable from AML uniformly terminates chronic myelogenous leukemia (CML) and, less often, other myeloproliferative disorders. De novo AML in young adults is believed usually to derive from stem cells that are more committed to myeloid lineage than the more primitive stem cells that give rise to secondary AML or AML in older patients.[2]

The proper care of patients with AML is a multidisciplinary effort, benefiting from a team approach. Expertise in transfusion medicine, infectious disease, placement and care of indwelling catheters, nutrition, and antineoplastic drug pharmacology are required as well as the availability of sophisticated diagnostic laboratory facilities and psychosocial counseling for both patients and their families. These disciplines are described elsewhere in this text, but their critical

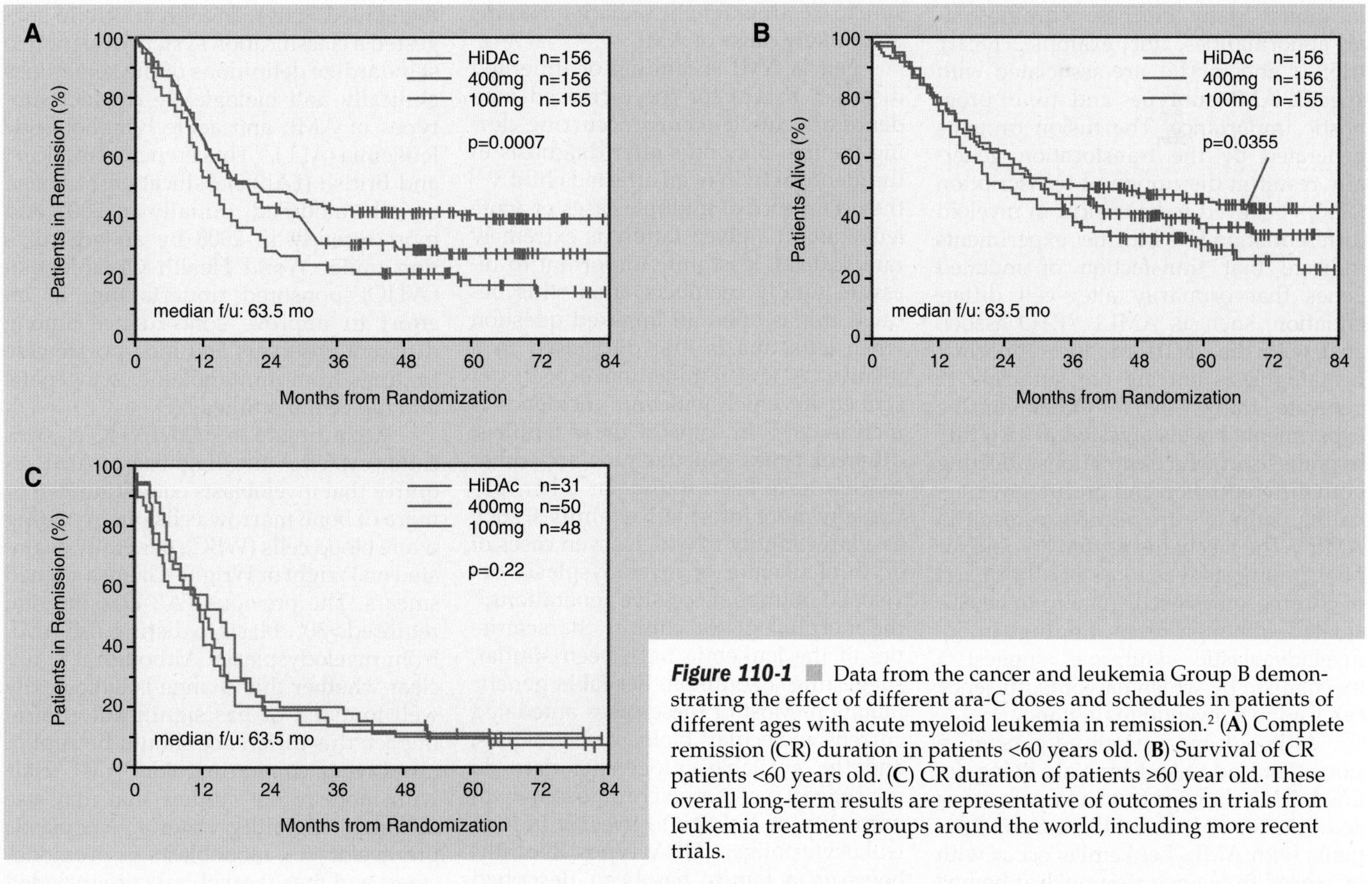

Figure 110-1 ■ Data from the cancer and leukemia Group B demonstrating the effect of different ara-C doses and schedules in patients of different ages with acute myeloid leukemia in remission.[2] (**A**) Complete remission (CR) duration in patients <60 years old. (**B**) Survival of CR patients <60 years old. (**C**) CR duration of patients ≥60 year old. These overall long-term results are representative of outcomes in trials from leukemia treatment groups around the world, including more recent trials.

importance in the care of the leukemia patient cannot be overestimated.

Pathogenesis and Etiology

The pathophysiology of AML can be explained by the acquisition of genetic changes in bone marrow stem cells that both promote self-renewal and impair normal hematopoietic differentiation, resulting in an accumulation of immature cells. The genetic changes may involve mutations that lead to activation of growth-promoting proto-oncogenes, inactivation of tumor suppressor genes, or alterations in transcription factors.[3,4] For example, mutations in codons 12, 13, or 61 of the *N-ras* gene that encodes a 21 kDa guanosine nucleotide binding protein involved in signal transduction have been noted in up to 30% of those with AML.[5] Mutations of the FLT3 growth-factor receptor are also common, occurring in as many as 30% of patients with normal karyotypes,[6-8] resulting in a constitutive proliferation signal. A number of other discrete mutations described later have been identified in subsets of AML patients, some of which may be involved in leukemia pathogenesis while others influence outcome after treatment.

Initial insights regarding AML pathogenesis were provided by the identification of genes at cytogenetic breakpoints involved in balanced translocations. Many of these chromosomal abnormalities, for example, t(8;21), t(15;17), and inv(16), are associated with specific AML subtypes and are of prognostic importance. The fusion proteins generated by the translocation generally result in disruption of transcription factors believed to be critical in myeloid differentiation.[4,9,10] Murine experiments indicate that transfection of mutated genes that primarily alter cell differentiation, such as AML1 /ETO associated with the t(8;21), produce abnormal hematopoiesis but are not sufficient to generate frank AML.[11] Other murine experiments have suggested a "two hit" hypothesis in which mutations affecting both differentiation and proliferative signaling pathways are needed to result in AML.[12] The mechanisms that account for poor prognosis when loss of all or parts of chromosomes occur remain to be elucidated, although recent findings in 5q- myelodysplastic syndrome, suggest a mechanism by which haploinsufficiency can lead to a myeoild malignancy.[13]

Although more acquired genetic lesions that lead to leukemia are being defined, DNA damage from a known cause accounts for only a small fraction of patients with AML. Leukemias occur with increased frequency after nuclear bomb[14] or therapeutic radiation exposure,[15] after certain types of chemotherapy, and with heavy and continuous occupational exposures to benzene or petrochemicals.[16,17] It is now recognized that there are two types of chemotherapy-related leukemias: (1) the classic alkylating agent-induced type[18] in which the leukemia is usually preceded by a myelodysplastic prodrome and is characterized by clonal abnormalities, often with loss of chromosome 5 and/or 7 and (2) an epipodophyllotoxin/topoisomerase II inhibitor associated type with a shorter (median 2- vs 5-year) incubation period, which is usually associated with myelomonocytic or monocytic differentiation and abnormalities at the 11q23 region.[19]

There have been a number of epidemiologic studies that have attempted to link a variety of environmental exposures to leukemia incidence. Many of these studies contain relatively small sample sizes and identify modest, if any, increases in risk ratio. Older and retrospective studies may be suspect in that the pathologic diagnoses were not usually reviewed and classified using contemporary criteria, and, therefore, the distinctions between myeloid, lymphoid, and perhaps even acute vs chronic leukemia may not be accurate. Furthermore, as in many epidemiologic studies, it is difficult to quantify the degree of exposure to various environmental insults. There may be a small increased risk associated with cigarette smoking,[20] whereas exposure to electromagnetic radiation[21] seems an unlikely cause of AML.

Nor is AML a familial or inherited disorder. Except for the increased incidence of acute leukemia occurring during the first 6 months after diagnosis in the identical twin of an affected child,[22,23] the occurrence of multiple cases of acute leukemia in a given family is extremely rare. Indeed, it is quite important to reassure family members about this because this is often an unasked question when leukemia is first diagnosed in a relative. A few families have been described in which leukemia incidence is increased.[24-27] In some of these families, different types of leukemias and other cancers have been found. In other, potentially more informative families, such as a large family in which seven cases of erythroleukemia or myelodysplasia developed in three successive generations;[26] the morphologic or clinical characteristics of the leukemia have been similar, suggesting a common, heritable genetic mutation. Most of these cases antedated current molecular biologic techniques, and the available cytogenetic data do not suggest a common chromosomal abnormality or linkage to specific human leukocyte antigen (HLA) types. Recently, however, a family has been described in which three patients with AML had identical inherited mutations in *CEBPA*,[27] a gene involved in granulocytic differentiation, while another large kindred with a familial platelet disorder with a predisposition toward AML had been shown to be associated with mutations in the gene encoding *CBF-α*(formerly *AML1*).[28] Lastly, there seems to be a predisposition toward evolution to AML in individuals with inherited polymorphisms in the receptor for granulocyte colony stimulating factor.[29] It is likely that other such associations will be identified as gene array technology is applied to other familial aggregates and that some of these mutations will be detected in "sporadic" cases as well.

Morphologic Classification and Clinical and Laboratory Correlates

The diagnosis of AML depends on the examination of well-prepared specimens of peripheral blood and bone marrow. Both bone marrow aspirates and biopsies should be evaluated. Although the biopsy is usually not helpful in identifying individual cells, it provides the best assessment of cellularity, can occasionally identify aggregates of leukemic cells not seen on aspirate, and is necessary to evaluate marrow fibrosis. In 1976, a group of morphologists from France, the United States, and Great Britain suggested a classification system designed to standardize definitions of the sometimes clinically and biologically distinct subtypes of AML and acute lymphoblastic leukemia (ALL).[30] This French, American, and British (FAB) classification has been serially modified, initially in 2002 and most recently in 2008 by an organization under World Health Organization (WHO)-sponsored undertaking, in an effort to improve concordance among different observers and incorporate new findings from immunologic, cytogenetic and molecular studies.[31,32]

According to the 2002 WHO classification system,[32] the diagnosis of AML requires that myeloblasts constitute 20% or more of bone marrow cells or circulating white blood cells (WBC), generally evaluated on Wright or Wright–Giemsa stained smears. The previous FAB classification required >30% blasts to distinguish AML from myelodysplasia. Although it is unclear whether this change is biologically well founded or has significant clinical impact, this difference should be kept in mind when comparing older AML trials with more recent studies that may use different eligibility criteria. Neoplastic promyelocytes, monoblasts or promonocytes, and megakaryoblasts are included in this percentage, and their presence defines the various morphologic subtypes described later. An assortment of histochemical stains is used to aid in subclassification and to distinguish AML from ALL. Monoclonal antibodies directed against antigen groups (termed cluster designations [CD]) considered to be restricted to cells committed to myeloid differentiation are also helpful in making this diagnostic distinction. Antibodies against CD11b, CD13, CD14, CD33, and C117 are used most commonly. These antigens are found on normal hematopoietic elements, are not leukemia-specific or unique to different AML FAB subtypes. They, generally, do not correlate with prognosis,[33] with the possible exception of CD34. The antigen CD34 is detected on undifferentiated hematopoietic progenitors and can be found on the blasts of patients with either AML or ALL. There is a suggestion that patients with AML whose blasts strongly express CD34 have an inferior outcome because of chemotherapy-resistant leukemia,[34,35] particularly in patients with less morphologically differentiated leukemias in which other myeloid-associated antigens are less strongly expressed.

The FAB and WHO nomenclature classify the subtypes of AML according to the normal marrow elements that the blasts most closely resemble. This does not mean, however, that the leukemic event exclusively involves the cell lineage that is most prominently represented morphologically. Until recently, the involvement of other hematopoietic lineages could be inferred only by the presence of prominent morphologic abnormalities in these other cell lines. Thus, in patients with myelodysplasia or erythroleukemia, there is usually morphologic evidence of trilineage dysplasia with the inference that the initial cell that was malignantly transformed was a hematopoietic precursor with capability of multilineage maturation. The ability to pinpoint the lineages involved in an individual patient's leukemia has been enhanced by cytogenetic and in situ hybridization techniques using specific molecular probes capable of detecting abnormalities in morphologically identifiable cells, as well as in vitro studies of colonies of different lineages. For example, Fialkow and colleagues,[36] studying female patients with X chromosome-linked polymorphisms of glucose-6-phosphate dehydrogenase, were able to demonstrate involvement of myeloid but not erythroid or megakaryocytic progenitors in some patients with AML. In contrast, using specific chromosomal probes, others demonstrated multilineage involvement in patients with erythroleukemia and myelodysplasia.[37,38] There are relatively few studies of this type, and it is unknown how many lineages are affected in most patients with AML. In particular, patients with more differentiated types of AML such as acute promyelocytic leukemia (APL) or monocytic leukemia have not been systematically evaluated, although in a few patients with APL there is a suggestion that the mutation is restricted to the myeloid series.

Representative examples of different subtypes of AML are shown in Figures 110-2 to 110-11. The immunologic, cytogenetic, and (where they exist) clinical correlates of these morphologic subtypes are reviewed in Table 110-1.

Peripheral Blood

Most patients with AML present with anemia (median hemoglobin 8 gm%), thrombocytopenia (median platelet count 40,000-50,000/μL), and leukocytosis (median WBC count 10,000-20,000/μL). The red blood cell morphology is usually relatively normal. Large, sometimes hypogranular, platelets can be seen and functional defects can contribute to hemorrhagic manifestations. Most patients are neutropenic, and morphologic abnormalities (nuclear hyperlobulation, hypogranulation, Pelger–Huet anomaly) are often noted in the remaining neutrophils. Careful examination will detect blasts in most patients, although it can be difficult to distinguish among leukemia subtypes (or occasionally even to be confident of the diagnosis of acute leukemia) in patients with a low number of circulating blasts. In occasional patients, marked leukopenia at presentation (so-called aleukemic leukemia) may obscure the diagnosis until a marrow examination is performed.

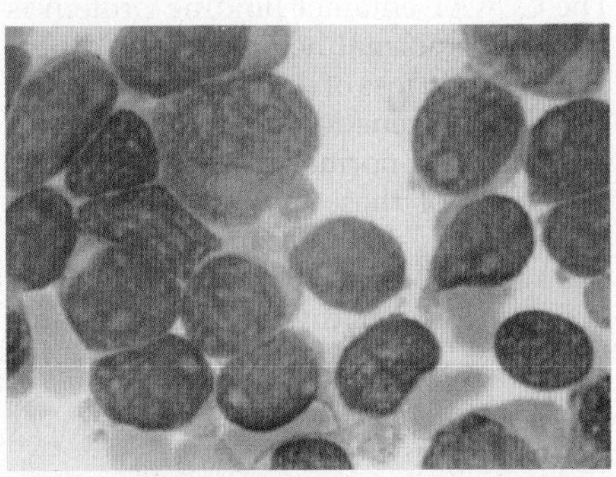

Figure 110-2 M0. Marrow blasts from patients with this undifferentiated type of acute myelogenous leukemia can have variable amounts of agranular cytoplasm. Cells are peroxidase- and Sudan black-negative and can be confused with FAB M7 or FAB L2. Myeloid commitment of these blasts can be confirmed by immunophenotyping with antibodies against myeloid antigens and/or demonstration of ultrastructural peroxidase-positive granules using transmission electron microscopy.

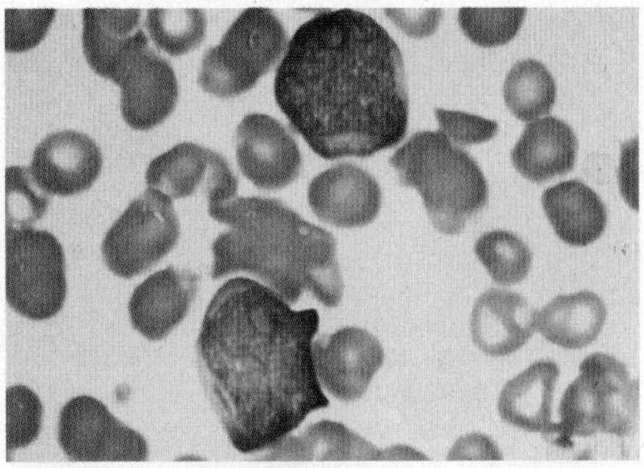

Figure 110-3 One of the blasts from a patient with M1 acute myeloid leukemia contains a prominent Auer rod.

2008 WHO Classification

The most recent WHO classification incorporates features of the older FAB morphologic categories with the recognition of distinct entities associated with certain cytogenetic and molecularly detected mutations.[39] Some biologic and clinical implications of these categories are summarized herewith.

AML with Recurrent Genetic Abnormalities

Cytogenetic

The clinical findings associated with t(8;21), inv(16), and t(15;17) have been appreciated for decades and are described in the sections on M2, M4 with eosinophilia, and M3 (APL) later. AML with t(8;21) and inv(16) are referred to as "core binding factor" (CBF) leukemias because of the molecular abnormalities in transcription produced by these translocations. Mutations of the C-KIT tyrosine-kinase receptor, which result in a constitutive proliferative signal, have recently been described in a subset of patients with CBF AML with data suggesting a poorer outcome in patients with this additional mutation.[40] These *C-KIT* mutations are generally insensitive to treatment with imatinib mesylate[41] and

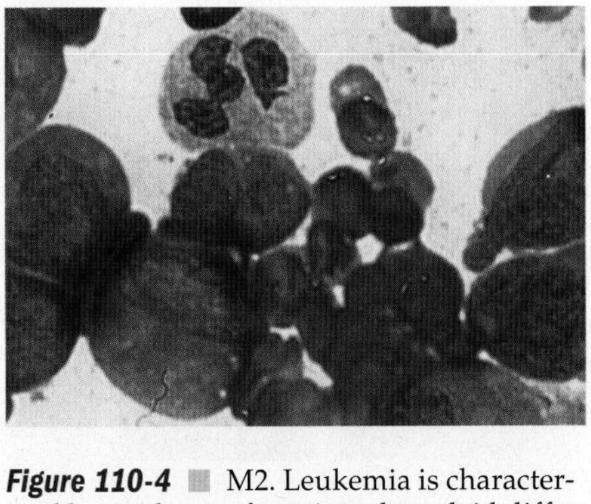

Figure 110-4 M2. Leukemia is characterized by evidence of continued myeloid differentiation with myelocytes and more mature myeloid elements present.

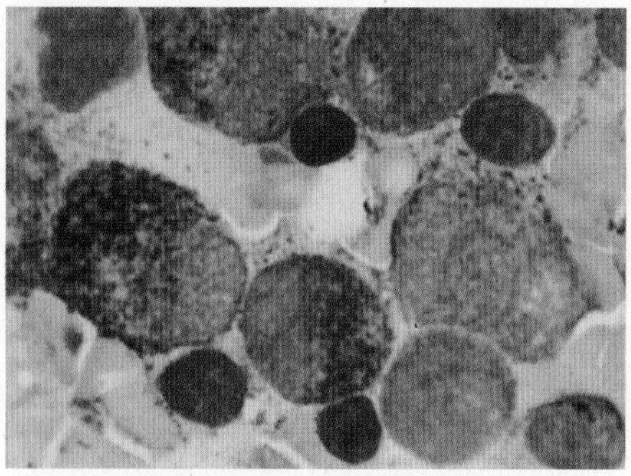

Figure 110-5 ■ M3—Promyelocytic leukemic cells usually have round nuclei with heavily granulated cytoplasm. Extracellular granules are often noted, and blasts with multiple Auer rods (not shown) are common. This leukemia has typical 15;17 translocation and a characteristic clinical picture of disseminated intravascular coagulation.

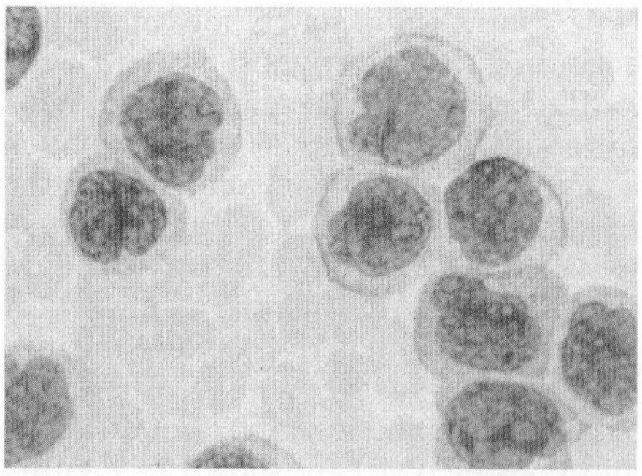

Figure 110-7 ■ M5. Monocytic leukemia. Prominent nuclei filled with nucleoli in some cells, light granulation, and large amounts of lightly basophilic cytoplasm give these cells the appearance of promonocytes.

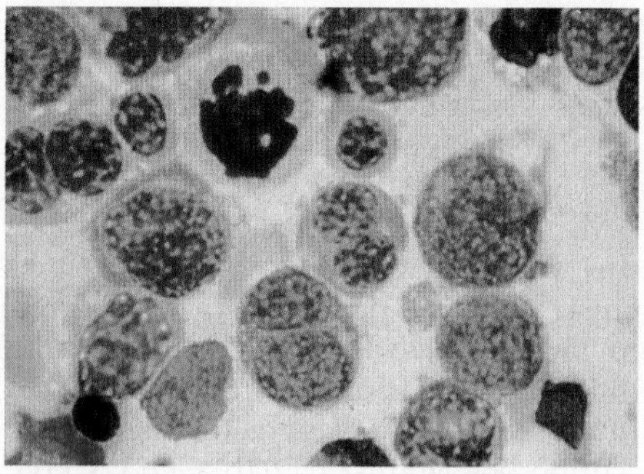

Figure 110-9 ■ M6. Erythroleukemia is characterized by the presence of bizarre megaloblastic and often multinucleated erythroid precursors. Karyorrhexis is seen in some cells. The somewhat arbitrary distinction between FAB M6 and myelodysplastic syndrome with excess blasts in transformation is made by quantification of the fraction of myeloid blasts.

trials with "second generation" tyrosine kinase inhibitors are in progress.

The new classification has added inv3(q21;q26.2), t(3;3)(q21;26.2), and t(1;22)(p13;q13) [RBM15-MLK1] usually found in infants (see M7 later) as well as t(6;9)(p23;q23)[DEK-NUP214] to this group. The t(6;9) is very uncommon, may occur more frequently in younger patients and can be found in association with a variety of AML morphologies, often with prominent basophilia. *ITD* mutations are found in approximately two-thirds of patients with t(6;9). The outcome with chemotherapy alone is poor and allogeneic transplantation should be considered in appropriate patients.[42]

Molecularly Detected Abnormalities

Molecular analyses have identified a large number of recurrent abnormalities in patients with AML, with a recent focus on patients with normal karyotypes.[10,43,44] As noted earlier, FLT3 is a transmembrane–tyrosine kinase receptor, which when activated initiates a signal pathway stimulating cell proliferation. Approximately 30% of patients with "normal" karyotypes have a repeat of between 3 and greater than 33 amino acids in the juxtamembrane region (internal tandem duplication [ITD] or length mutation) and 10% have a point mutation in the tyrosine kinase domain. Mutations of the *FLT3* gene are detected by PCR and seem to confer an inferior outcome.[6,7] *FLT3* mutations can also be detected in other types of AML including those with t(6;9) and APL. Activating mutations may manifest as an in-frame base pair repeat in the region encoding the juxtamembrane part of the molecule (internal tandem duplication), or as a point mutation in the C-terminal activation loop. Small molecule inhibitors of *FLT3* are available[45,46] and randomized studies comparing standard chemotherapy with and without these inhibitors are in progress.

Mutations in the nucleophosmin gene, which codes for a nuclear/cytoplasmic shuttling protein (NPM1)[47] and in the transcription factor CCAAT entamer binding protein encoded by the *CEBPα* gene at 19q13[48] have been added as "provisional" entities in the WHO classification with further correlative studies needed. The CCAAT entamer binding protein is critical for normal hematopoietic differentiation and loss of activity either by mutation or epigenetic silencing can result in a block in normal differentiation.[49,50] Mutations of these genes are found in 50-60% and 7-10% of patients with normal karyotypes, respectively. Both mutations are associated with more favorable outcomes with chemotherapy treatment but can occur in combination with other mutations, including those that may reduce the positive impact of an NPM1 mutation.[51] The diagnostic evaluation of newly diagnosed patients is likely to include molecular analyses to detect these mutations in the future.

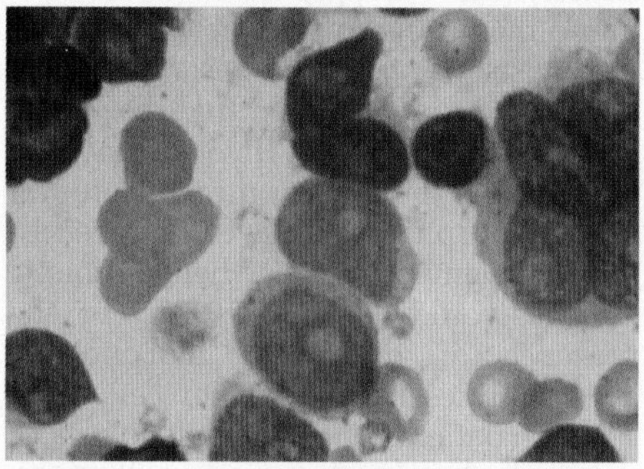

Figure 110-10 ■ M7. Megakaryocytic leukemia. Blasts in this category are often morphologically undifferentiated. The presence of multinucleated cells, dysplastic micromegakaryocytes, and cytoplasmic budding can be helpful diagnostic clues. The diagnosis is confirmed by immunophenotyping or ultrastructural studies.

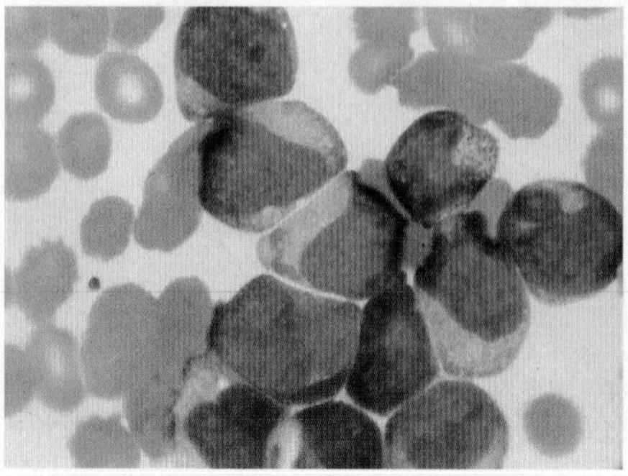

Figure 110-6 ■ M4. Myelomonocytic leukemia has blasts with both myeloid and monocytoid appearance.

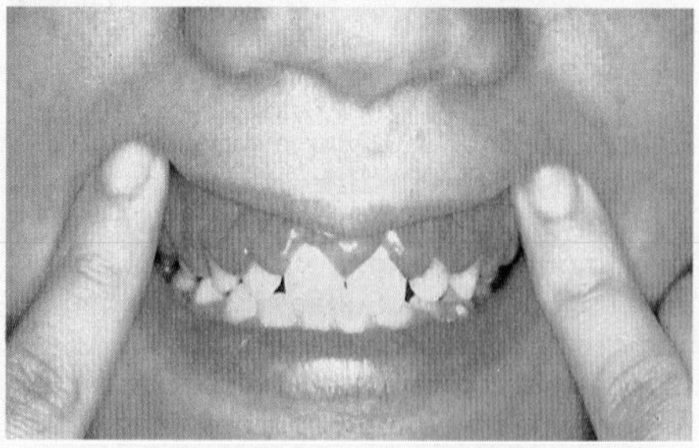

Figure 110-8 ■ M5. Gingival hypertrophy due to infiltration by leukemic cells in acute monocytic leukemia.

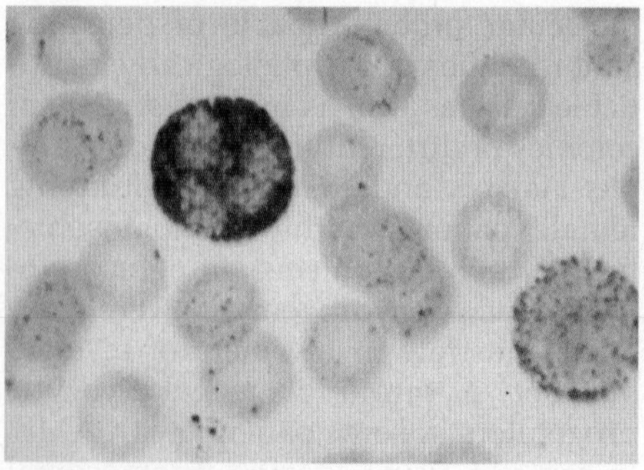

Figure 110-11 ■ Typical granular staining with Sudan black B of a blast and a neutrophil from a patient with FAB M1 acute myeloid leukemia.

Table 110-1 Recurring Karyotypic and Molecular Abnormalities in AML

Cytogenetic Abnormality	FAB Morphology	Affected Genes	Median Age	Approximate Incidence in De Novo AML	Prognostic Effects	Comments
t (8;21)	M2	*AML1/ETO*	30 yrs	5-7%	Favorable	Auer rods usually present
t (15;17)	M3	*PML-RARa*	40	5-8%	Favorable-high cure rate with ATRA-based therapy	DIC
t(11;17)	Similar to M3	*PLZF/ RARa*	?	<1%	Poor response to ATRA-based therapy	
abn 16q22	M4 with eosinophilia	*CBFA/MYH11*	35-40	5%	Favorable	High reinduction rate post relapse
abn11q23	M5	*MLL* + many partners	>50	3%	Poor except t(9;11)	Hyperleukocytosis, extra medullary disease
+8	Varied		>60	5-10%	Poor	
del 5, del 7, 5q-, 7q-, or combinations	Varied; common in FAB M6		>60	15-20%	Poor	Common in patients with secondary AML, prior MDS
Inv 3	Abnormal megakaryocytes	Ribophorin/*EVI1*	?	<1%	Poor	Increased platelet count; other abnormalities common(del 5, del 7)
+13	Varied; sometimes undifferentiated		Probably > 60	~1-2%	Poor	Higher frequency of hybrid features
t(6;9) (p2;q34)	M2/M4 with basophilia	*DEK/CAN*	?	<1%	Poor	Prominent basophilia
t(9;22)	Usually M1	*BCR/ABL*	Probably > 50	~1%	Poor	Splenomegaly
t(1;22)	Often M7	*MOZ/CBP*	Infants	<1%	Poor	Organomegaly
t(8;16)	M4,5		?	<1%	Poor	Erythrophagocytosis
Molecular Abnormality						
Fms-related tyrosine kinase gene mutations[8]	Varied—most common in CN-AML; can be found with (6;9); t(15;17)	Internal tandem repeat or point mutation of	?	~30% in CN-AML	Adverse	
Nucleophosmin (*NPM1*)—(5q35) mutation[47]	Varied	Nucleophosmin (NPM1); often found with other mutations	?	~35% of AML, ~50% of CN-AML	Favorable DFS except when associated with mutation	
CEBPα gene[48]	Varied	Mutation results in decreasing levels of CEBPα (CCAAT entamer binding protein)	?	~15% of CN-AML	Favorable except when associated with mutation	
Overexpression of BAALC (Brain and Acute Leukemia Cytoplasmic) protein[375]	Varied	Overexpression of BAALC	?	Studied most extensively in CN-AML	Adverse—further studies needed	
Partial tandem duplication of MLL (mixed lineage leukemia) gene[57]	Varied	Affects *HOX* gene function	?	~8% of CN-AML	Unclear—further studies needed	

Abbreviations: AML, acute myelogenous leukemia; ATRA, all *trans* retinoic acid; DIC, disseminated intravascular coagulation; FAB, French, American, and British; MDS, myelodysplastic syndrome.

Although data are not yet sufficient to include in diagnostic classifications, overexpression of BAALC (Brain and Acute Leukemia Cytoplasmic) protein,[52,53] the ETS-related gene (*ERG*)[54,55] and meningioma-1 proteins may be negative prognostic factors.[56] Mutations involving the *MLL* gene at 11q23 present a more complicated scenario in that most translocations affecting this locus confer a poor outcome while partial tandem duplications (*MLL-PTD*) in this gene in patients with normal karyotypes may be associated with prolonged disease free survival, if this is the sole molecular abnormality.[57,58]

Gene expression array studies[59] will undoubtedly identify other prognostically important mutations or gene expression patterns, presenting the opportunity to develop appropriately selected therapies and new agents aimed at these specific changes. Recently, the expression of certain microRNA species, especially those that downregulate the immune response, has been shown to be associated with an adverse prognosis in the normal chromosome subset.[60] An additional formidable challenge will be to elucidate how combinations of these mutations and molecular changes interact both biologically and clinically, since it is common to detect more than a single mutation in an individual patient.[43,44]

AML With MDS-Related Changes

The addition of this category reflects the recognition that a substantial fraction of AML, particularly in older patients, evolves from a prior myelodysplastic disorder. This group includes patients with a prior history of MDS, those with >50% dysplasia in at least two cell lines and patients with so-called "MDS cytogenetics" including, -5, -7, i(17)/t(17p), -13, del 11q, del (12p), del 9q and complex karyotypes, which may include these changes as well as the presence of marker chromosomes. These leukemias seem to arise in a very early hematopoietic stem cell and tend to have low response rates with short durations of response. It is important to recognize that some of these patients can have a smoldering clinical course and do not require immediate treatment.

Therapy-Related AML

This category includes patients whose AML followed treatment with chemotherapy and/or radiation therapy for other disorders. Morphology and karyotypes are similar to those seen in MDS with the addition of a group of patients with abnormalities of 11q23 associated with prior treatment with topoisomerase II inhibitors and often with a short interval until the development of AML. Therapy-related AML tends to be more resistant to chemotherapy, and allogeneic transplant should be considered in suitable patients who achieve remission. Of note is that occasional patients with therapy-related AML can have inv(16), t(8;21), and t(15;17) (APL) and can respond well to standard approaches for these subtypes.[61]

Myeloid Sarcoma

Occasionally patients will present for medical attention because of lesions identified to be AML by histochemical staining but without apparent bone marrow involvement. Masses can involve the skin, gastrointestinal tract, ovaries, central nervous system, and virtually every body organ. There is little systematic literature about the management of such patients although there is a high rate of eventual systemic relapse without treatment and most clinicians consider induction and consolidation treatment in medically fit patients after the diagnosis is established. Despite such "early" treatment, the recurrence rate is high; the role of stem cell transplant is unclear.

AML Not Otherwise Specified

This category includes the large group of patients whose AML does not fall into the previously listed groups and in general, bears similarities to the older FAB classification.

M0—Minimally Differentiated AML

In most patients, it is relatively simple to distinguish between AML and ALL on morphologic grounds. In general, the blasts from patients with AML are larger, with more abundant cytoplasm and more prominent, often multiple, nucleoli. The definitive diagnosis depends, however, on the presence of Auer rods, which are linear bundles of myeloid-containing granules, or demonstration of at least 3% granulated precursors in AML,[30] usually visible on Wright stain and confirmed by staining with either myeloperoxidase or Sudan black B. It can occasionally be difficult to distinguish between positivity in blasts vs staining in residual maturing myeloid elements in patients with ALL; careful correlation with the Wright stain is mandatory.

As shown in Figure 110-2, some patients have blasts that resemble myeloid blasts but are negative at the light microscopic level when examined with myeloperoxidase, Sudan black B or other histochemical stains. The myeloid nature of these leukemias can be detected, however, by immunologic means or by election microscopy of peroxidase stained preparations. Electron micrographs reveal ultrastructural peroxidase-positive granules, whereas immunologic phenotyping demonstrates reactivity with antibodies directed against myeloid antigens and nonreactivity with antibodies that characterize lymphoid differentiation.[62,63] The cells are often reactive with antibodies directed against CD34. Terminal deoxynucleotidyl transferase (TdT) is generally absent but can sometimes be detected in a minority of blasts.

Approximately 7% of patients with untreated AML have minimally differentiated AML (so-called M0 AML), which is relatively treatment resistant.[63-65] This undifferentiated leukemia can easily be confused with ALL and it is therefore critically important to obtain immunophenotyping of blasts from patients with morphologically undifferentiated leukemias. Other than resistance to chemotherapy, this M0 variant does not appear to be associated with specific clinical findings. Many M0 patients have complex karyotypic abnormalities.[63,64] No distinctive cytogenetic pattern has been noted, with the possible exception of trisomy 13, which has been reported to occur in some patients with morphologically less differentiated leukemias.[66]

M1—Myeloid Leukemia Without Maturation

The blasts from patients with M1 morphology have round nuclei with moderate amounts of sometimes lightly granulated cytoplasm, which can contain Auer rods (Fig. 110-3). In contrast to M2, there is little evidence of myeloid maturation, with <10% of cells beyond the level of the promyelocyte. There is no particular age, gender, clinical feature, or characteristic cytogenetic abnormality associated with this morphologic variant.

M2—Myeloid Leukemia With Maturation

In contrast to M1, there is obvious continued maturation in the myeloid series with the presence of promyelocytes, myelocytes, and often more mature myeloid elements. Granulation is generally more obvious, Auer rods are often prominent, and there is virtually never any difficulty in distinguishing this variant from ALL (Fig. 110-4). Approximately 20-25% of patients with M2 AML have a characteristic translocation between chromosomes 8 and 21 [t(8;21)(q22;22)]; this translocation is seen almost exclusively in patients with M2 and Auer rods. Such patients have a lower median age (approximately 30 years), a very high initial complete response rate (>85% in most series), a lower relapse rate, and improved long-term disease-free survival, particularly when treated with high-dose cytarabine-based consolidation therapy,[67,68] except for a subset with an activating mutation of *c-kit* or an adverse gene signature.[40] The incidence of extramedullary granulocytic sarcomas, often in unusual sites, may be increased in patients with t(8;21) M2 AML whose blasts express the adhesion molecule CD56 on their surface.[69] These can present as discrete tumor masses, sometimes in paraspinous locations, confer a poor prognosis, and are distinct from the gingival and cutaneous involvement found in monocytic leukemia.

The t(8;21) involves what has been termed the *AML1* gene on chromosome 21 and the *ETO* gene on chromosome 8. The *AML1* gene has homology to the *Drosophila runt* gene and encodes the alpha chain of the heterodimeric transcriptional apparatus, core binding factor (CBF).[70] Normal CBF function is critical for mammalian hematopoietic development. The AML1-ETO protein recruits nuclear corepressor molecules including histone deacetylase, which prevents transcription of genes required for myeloid differentiation.[71,72] The AML1-ETO fusion product can be detected by reverse transcriptase polymerase chain reaction (RT-PCR), which is used for both diagnostic testing and monitoring for minimal residual disease. Of note is that the AML1-ETO has been detectable in the peripheral blood cells of some patients in long-term complete remission (CR) after treatment, suggesting that molecular detection by highly sensitive RT-PCR may not necessarily presage relapse.[73]

M3—Acute Promyelocytic Leukemia

APL is one of the most distinctive subtypes of AML with regard to morphologic, clinical, cytogenetic features, and response to differentiating agent therapies, such as all-trans-retinoic acid (ATRA).[74,75] In most patients, the morphologic diagnosis is straightforward, with the marrow being replaced by blasts that resemble unusually heavily granulated progranulocytes. The nuclei are round, with obvious nucleoli, and the cytoplasm is filled with multiple, large, and often coalesced azurophilic granules (Fig. 110-5). Auer rods are usually seen, and multiple Auer rods (so-called faggot cells) are frequently noted. In a minority of patients, the blasts are hypogranular and granules sometimes can only be seen with electron microscopy.[76] This hypogranular variant often has cells with bilobed or lobulated nuclei, which can sometimes be confused with monocytic variants of AML. In contrast to the typical leukopenic presentation of APL, patients with the hypogranular variant tend to have higher white cell counts. In both types of APL, staining with either Sudan black B or myeloperoxidase is strongly positive. Class II HLA antigens (HLA DR), which are found on all hematopoietic precursors, are usually not detected on the surface of the malignant progranulocytes. The explanation for and biologic implications of this finding are not known. In contrast, CD33 is consistently strongly expressed.

Patients with APL tend to be somewhat younger, with a median age of 30-40 years, although APL is seen in patients of all ages. APL accounts for approximately 10% of AML and may be more prevalent in Latinos[77] and obese people.[78] APL is almost uniformly characterized by hypofibrinogenemia, variable depletion of other coagulation factors, elevated levels of fibrin degradation products, and accelerated consumption of endogenous and transfused platelets. The granules contain potent procoagulants, and disseminated intravascular coagulation (DIC) is generally accelerated following lysis of blasts by chemotherapy, often with increased bleeding. In some patients, there is evidence that accelerated fibrinolysis may be the primary event triggering the coagulopathy. APL is associated with the highest frequency of hemorrhagic morbidity and mortality, the latter usually related to intracranial hemorrhage. During chemotherapeutic treatment with accelerated cell lysis, these patients need aggressive platelet transfusion support and can require platelet transfusions 2-3 times per day during the first few days of treatment. Except for patients with very severe hypofibrinogenemia who may require supplementation with cryoprecipitate, most patients do not require infusion of clotting factors other than the plasma accompanying the platelet transfusion. Aggressive blood product support is probably as effective as heparin, once frequently used to interrupt the clotting cascade during drug therapy.[79] Indeed, the heparin- vs transfusion- vs antifibrinolytic-[80,81] therapy debate has been largely silenced in recent years, because treatment with ATRA ameliorates DIC within hours of its administration.[82]

Almost all patients with APL have a characteristic translocation involving chromosomes 15 and 17 [t(15;17)(q22;q12)],[83] which may be associated with additional cytogenetic abnormalities, such as trisomy 8.[84] RT-PCR can be used to detect the fusion transcript, is useful for assessing for minimal residual disease[85] and permits the proper classification of the occasional patient with clinically and morphologically typical APL but with an apparently normal karyotype. The breakpoint on chromosome 17 is in an intron of the retinoic acid receptor alpha gene. A gene that has been termed *PML*, also with DNA-binding capability, is translocated from chromosome 15, resulting in the formation of a fusion protein that functions in a dominant fashion to block transcription of genes controlled by *RAR*-α, probably by recruiting nuclear corepressor activity. Retinoic acid treatment relieves the corepression activity, allowing transcription of genes involved in differentiation.[86-88] There is also interest in the use of histone deacetylase inhibitors in patients with APL as another means of enhancing gene expression.[89] *ITD* mutations can be detected in approximately a third of patients with APL. Although further analyses are needed, these mutations seem to be associated with higher WBC counts and M3 variant morphology. The initial response rate is similar in patients with ITD mutations, although there may be a poorer long term outcome.[90]

A group of patients with a leukemia similar in morphology to APL but with a t(11;17)(q23;q21) have been described. Although *RAR*-α is rearranged, these patients fail to respond to ATRA. A novel zinc finger gene termed PZLF from chromosome 11 is translocated to the *RAR*-α, rather than the *PML* gene from chromosome 15, creating a fusion protein that does not allow the ATRA-mediated release of transcriptional corepression activity.[91]

Historically, the remission rate in patients with APL treated with chemotherapy was quite high. Initial drug resistance was very unusual, and most failures of therapy were related to hemorrhagic or infectious deaths. APL is uniquely sensitive to anthracycline therapy, and CR rates in excess of 80% can be seen with anthracycline therapy alone.[74,75] In contrast to other types of AML, remission can be attained with chemotherapy in APL without producing bone marrow aplasia.[92,93] Post-treatment bone marrows frequently remain cellular with abnormal progranulocytes, with follow-up marrows demonstrating disappearance of these cells and return of normal hematopoiesis without additional chemotherapy. DIC does not reappear despite the persistence of morphologically abnormal cells. Undoubtedly, this unique feature of APL is related to the equally unique sensitivity of APL to agents that have a differentiating and noncytotoxic mechanism of action (see the section "Therapy of Acute Promyelocytic Leukemia" later in this chapter).

M4—Myelomonocytic Leukemia

Myelomonocytic leukemia is characterized morphologically by a mixture of myeloid and monocytic elements and represents about 15-20% of newly diagnosed patients with AML. According to the FAB criteria, greater than 20% of the leukemic cells must be monocytic in morphology to distinguish this variant from FAB M1 and particularly from FAB M2. The monocytic elements often resemble partially differentiated monocytes with lightly granulated, grayish cytoplasm and folded nuclei, which are frequently seen in the peripheral blood (Fig. 110-6). Monocytic derivation can be confirmed by staining with nonspecific esterases such as α-naphthyl acetate or α-naphthyl butyrate.

There is no distinct clinical picture associated with this variant, perhaps because this classification encompasses a wide spectrum of patients owing to the generous morphologic criteria for inclusion. The median age tends to be somewhat higher, and there may be an increased incidence of hyperleukocytosis and extramedullary leukemic involvement, as can be seen with monocytic leukemia (see later). There is no particular cytogenetic clustering, and it is impossible to reliably predict short- or long-term outcome in patients with M4.

M4EO—Myelomonocytic Leukemia With Eosinophilia

Approximately 5% of patients with de novo AML have typical morphologic features of myelomonocytic leukemia with the presence of variable numbers of dysplastic eosinophils at various stages of maturation. The distinctive eosinophils usually represent only 5-10% of the cells of the marrow.[94,95] These cells generally contain large basophilic granules in addition to typical eosinophilic granules. Occasional patients with M2 morphology with eosinophilia have also been described.

M4Eo tends to occur in patients of younger age (median age 35-40 years) and is associated with an excellent prognosis.[96] CR rates are high (generally >85%) and failure due to initial drug resistance is unusual. In some series, this variant represents the subtype with the most favorable long-term prognosis. Mutations of the *C-KIT* tyrosine-kinase receptor have recently been described in some patients with CBF AML with data suggesting a poorer outcome in this subset.[40] In addition to long initial CRs, second remissions, which are often quite sustained, are generally easier to accomplish in patients with FAB M4Eo.[97,98] Older series suggested that there may be a high rate of central nervous system (CNS) relapse in patients with bone marrow eosinophilia. With more intensive regimens using higher doses of cytosine arabinoside (ara-C), CNS relapse in AML is now an unusual occurrence and patients with FAB M4Eo do not require prophylactic CNS therapy.

Essentially all patients with FAB M4Eo have a cytogenetic abnormality involving chromosome 16 at band q22. In most patients, the cytogenetic changes involve a pericentric inversion (inv16), although translocations between the two chromosomes 16 with homologous deletions at 16q22 have also been noted.[94,95] This breakpoint involves a fusion between the CBF-β chain and the gene encoding the smooth muscle myosin heavy chain. The fusion protein thus generated may recruit nuclear corepressor activity (in the form of histone deacetylase), which prevents transcription of genes required for myeloid differentiation in a fashion analogous to the CBF-α ETO fusion in t(8;21) M2 AML.[99] Although it is clear that patients with inv(16) leukemia respond very well to intensive chemotherapy (>60-70% 3 year DFS rate in those receiving high-dose ara-C),[68,96] the reason for this is uncertain. One group has suggested that the gene coding for the multidrug-resistance protein (MRP) is mutated as a consequence of this translocation, hypothesizing that the enhanced chemosensitivity may be related to a decrease in the normal amounts of this resistance factor.[100]

M5—Monocytic Leukemia

Two variants of monocytic leukemia have been described; in both, >80% of the blasts are of monocytic derivation. Less common is so-called M5a, in which the monocytic blasts have round nuclei and small amounts of sometimes deeply basophilic cytoplasm without evidence of morphologic differentiation. In monocytic leukemia with differentiation (M5b), at least 20% of the blasts resemble promonocytes with folded nuclei and abundant, lightly granulated cytoplasm, generally without Auer rods. The nuclear folding can often be quite marked with rarification of the nuclear chromatin (Fig. 110-7). Phagocytosis of other hematopoietic elements by these cells is frequently noted in bone marrow preparations. These monocytic elements stain prominently with nonspecific esterase that is inhibited by fluoride.

Although seen in patients of all ages, monocytic leukemias are somewhat more common in older adults. Patients with FAB M5 have higher blast counts at diagnosis, and problems with hyperleukocytosis are most common in this morphologic variant (see the section "Complications" later in this chapter).[101] In addition, the incidence of extramedullary leukemia is highest in M5, particularly in those with evidence of morphologic differentiation.[102] For example, it is common for patients to present to the dentist with gingival hypertrophy, an example of which is seen in Figure 110-8. Skin infiltration is common both at diagnosis and relapse and frequently represents the initial site of recurrence, sometimes while the bone marrow is still morphologically normal. Other less common areas of extramedullary involvement include the gastrointestinal tract, conjunctivae and the CNS. It is likely that extramedullary infiltration is related to active migration of the leukemic promonocytes to these sites. These partially differentiated cells are capable of migration to skin windows in vivo as well as phagocytosis of microorganisms and adherence to nylon fibers in vitro.[103]

Serum levels of lysozyme are elevated in most patients with AML, but are generally much higher in patients with monocytic leukemia.[104] Lysozyme can affect renal tubular function, and severe, symptomatic hypokalemia can occur in patients with FAB M4 and M5 leukemia. This problem generally resolves with cytoreduction, but can also be additive to the hypokalemic side effects of antibiotics and amphotericin B, vomiting, and diarrhea.

In addition to the initial problems presented by complications of hyperleukocytosis, patients with monocytic leukemia tend to have lower complete response rates related to drug-resistant disease. Although older studies indicated that CR durations tended to be shorter with consequent very low rates of long-term disease-free survival, a recent analysis of a large number of patients treated by the Eastern Cooperative Oncology Groups (ECOG) suggested similar outcomes to other morphologic subtypes of AML when other risk factors are accounted for.[105] A variety of cytogenetic abnormalities can be detected, although the most common findings involve abnormalities of chromosome 11 at band q23. This break point, at what has been termed the mixed lineage leukemia (*MLL*) gene, can be involved in leukemias of myeloid or lymphoid origin as well as in leukemias associated with therapy with epipodophyllotoxins and other drugs directed at topoisomerase II.[19,106] The *MLL* gene, also called *All-1* or *HRX*, may partner with at least 16 different genes in balanced translocation.[4] *MLL* is homologous to a gene important in Drosophila development and includes DNA binding elements.[107,108] The t(9;11) is a relatively common translocation involving the MLL gene, which may actually confer a better prognosis than formerly thought, with higher initial CR rates.[109-111] There is an association between M5b with extensive erythrophagocytosis and the t(8;16)(p11;p13), a translocation involving the CBP class of translocation factors that are positive regulators of myeloid differentiation.[112,113]

M6—Erythroleukemia

Erythroleukemia, often termed de Guglielmo syndrome in earlier literature, is the variant of AML in which morphologic abnormalities of erythropoiesis are most prominent. Cases of pure erythroleukemia, in which the predominant malignant cell is clearly identified as a pronormoblast, are rare. Rather, this is a disease of the myeloid stem cell with marked dysplastic changes in all three hematopoietic lines. Along with the increase in myeloid-appearing blasts, there is persistence of morphologic abnormalities in the erythroid series with profound megablastosis, multinuclearity, karyorrhexis, increased numbers of mitoses, and staining with periodic acid-Schiff (PAS), often in a block pattern (Fig. 110-9). Increased iron stores are usually seen, often with ringed sideroblasts. These changes are morphologically identical to those seen in patients with myelodysplasia, and many observers feel that most cases of erythroleukemia are biologically similar, if not identical, to patients with refractory anemia with excess blasts. This contention is supported by the very poor response to therapy in both groups, the tendency for the disease to occur in patients of older age, and the presence of similar cytogenetic abnormalities (complex karyotypic abnormalities, loss of part, or all of chromosomes 5, and/or 7, and marker chromosomes).[114] Nonetheless, in order to provide some consistency in terms of protocol entry and reports of clinical trials, the FAB and WHO groups, somewhat arbitrarily distinguished among M6, myelodysplasia (RAEB), and other FAB subtypes with significant numbers of erythroblasts by quantification of the number of erythroblasts and myeloblasts. Most of these patients will now be placed in the "AML with MDS-related Changes" in the most recent WHO iteration. M6 is defined by the presence of >30% blasts among non-erythroid cells when >50% of the marrow nucleated elements are erythroid. Antibodies against glycophorin A are lineage-specific for erythroblasts, but immunologic phenotyping is rarely needed to identify these morphologic subtypes. In occasional patients, transfusion of red blood cells can result in a marked decrease, if not elimination, of the marrow erythroid elements, suggesting the continued response to normal feedback mechanisms.

M7—Megakaryocytic Leukemia

Morphologic abnormalities of megakaryocytopoiesis, usually characterized by the presence of mono- or binucleated micromegakaryocytes, are common in many variants of AML and can be particularly prominent in patients with M6 or myelodysplasia. A minority of these patients have thrombocytosis and abnormalities of chromosome 3 [inv(3)(q21;q26)]. This cytogenetic abnormality is often found in association with other chromosomal deletions, with a variety of primary morphologies (M1, M2, M4),and in patients with a prior background of MDS.[115] These patients have a poor response to initial treatment and low overall survival. Thrombocytosis is not unique to patients with the inv(3) karyotype but can also be present in other patients with AML at the time of diagnosis.[116] The gene at the chromosome 3q21 break point is associated with the activation of EVI1 transcription factor.[117,118]

The diagnosis of FAB M7 is reserved for those patients in whom the predominant leukemic cell is of megakaryocytic lineage.[119] In some patients, there is obvious evidence of megakaryocytic dysplasia or multinucleated cells that strongly points toward principal involvement of the megakaryocyte (Fig. 110-10). In others, however, the leukemia is undifferentiated morphologically, with variable amounts of generally agranular cytoplasm and can sometimes be confused with M1 or even ALL. Sudan black B (Fig. 110-11), myeloperoxidase, and α-naphthyl butyrate stains are negative, whereas PAS and acid phosphatase may be positive, usually in a diffuse, speckled pattern. Histochemical staining is nondiagnostic, however, and the definitive diagnosis depends on either the detection of platelet-specific peroxidase by ultrastructural techniques or, more commonly, by the demonstration of a variety of platelet antigens (usually glycoprotein IIb/IIIa [CD41] or von Willebrand's factor) on the surface of the blasts.[120] At times, the diagnosis can be quite difficult to confirm, particularly because there is increased marrow reticulin in most patients, rendering the marrow fibrotic and inaspirable. Careful evaluation of peripheral blood blasts is necessary in such patients. It is likely that most patients with what has been termed acute myelosclerosis actually have acute megakaryocytic leukemia. Acute megakaryocytic leukemia should not be confused with the late stages of agnogenic myeloid metaplasia, and, indeed, prominent splenomegaly is not a clinical feature of M7. Although an uncommon variant of AML, most series suggest that this subtype is associated with a very poor prognosis. Prolonged aplasia is common following induction chemotherapy, and, because of the marrow fibrosis, it is often difficult to follow the results of therapy with repeated marrow aspirations. There have been relatively few cytogenetic evaluations of this variant, and except for the inv(3) and cases of t(1;22) (p13;q13) [RBM15/MKL1 gene fusion] found in infants,[121] no consistent abnormality has been identified.

Acute Panmyelosis With Myelofibrosis (APMF)

This is a very rare variant of AML felt to derive from the hematopoietic stem cell, in which the marrow demonstrates a marked increase in reticulin fibers with evidence of morphologically abnormal trilineage hematopoiesis and a variable number of blasts with an immature myeloid immunophenotype.[122,123] Patients usually present with pancytopenia and constitutional symptoms. It can sometimes be difficult to distinguish APMF from acute megakarypcytic leukemia or myelodysplastic syndromes with myelofibrosis. APMF responds poorly to standard chemotherapy.

Hybrid Leukemias

Morphologists have long been perplexed by cases that defy easy categorization or seem to have features of both lymphoid and myeloid histology. A variety of terms have been used to describe such cases including hybrid leukemia, mixed lineage leukemia, biclonal leukemia, lineage infidelity or promiscuity, and biphenotypic leukemia. The serial application of biochemical, immunologic, and molecular biologic techniques has demonstrated that sharing of myeloid and lymphoid characteristics may be a relatively common feature of both myeloid and lymphoid leukemia. In most such patients, individual cells coexpress myeloid and lymphoid features rather than the simultaneous occurrence of two apparently separate leukemias.

The mechanism of expression of TdT or other lymphoid markers in those with typical myeloperoxidase-positive AML is unclear. Although up to 25% of AML patients may express TdT, there are conflicting data about whether such a feature confers an adverse prognosis.[124,125] In adults with AML treated on Cancer and Leukemia Group B (CALGB) clinical trials, lymphoid antigen expression had no effect on outcome.[126] T-cell antigen expression or T-cell gene rearrangement in children with AML may or may not correlate with a higher level of resistance to regimens designed for AML patients.[127] The significance of a T-cell receptor rearrangement, a finding not uncommon in the AML patient, is even less clear. In fact, CD7 expression is not uncommon in t(8;21) AML, which responds well to chemotherapy.[128,129] Although the phenotypic features of the leukemic blasts are generally constant throughout the patient's course (eg, at diagnosis and relapse), examples of lineage switch, usually AML followed by ALL, have been noted.[130,131]

For patients whose blasts are myeloperoxidase and/or nonspecific esterase positive and express mainly myeloid antigens, but who also display TdT positivity or express one lymphoid antigen, an AML regimen is appropriate. For those ALL patients whose blasts express one or two myeloid antigens, treatment with an ALL protocol is indicated. For the very occasional patient who truly has equal myeloid and lymphoid features or even less commonly, seems to have two distinct populations of cells, one approach would be to combine AML and ALL regimens, although there are few data concerning the outcome of this strategy.

Presenting Signs and Symptoms

Patients with AML generally present with symptoms related to complications of pancytopenia including combinations of weakness, easy fatigability, infections of variable severity or hemorrhagic findings such as gingival bleeding, ecchymoses, epistaxis, or menorrhagia (Table 110-2). Occasional patients present because of prominent extramedullary sites of leukemia usually related to either cutaneous or gingival infiltration by leukemia cells. Bone pain is infrequent in adults with AML, although some individuals describe sternal discomfort or tenderness, occasionally with aching in the long bones, particularly of the lower extremities. It is generally difficult to date the onset of AML precisely, at least in part because individuals have different symptomatic thresholds for choosing to seek medical attention. It is likely

Table 110-2 Initial Diagnostic Evaluation

History and physical examination—In addition to an overall comprehensive evaluation, emphasis should be placed on the following:
• Duration of symptoms
• Menstrual history
• Prior pregnancies, transfusions, history of transfusion reactions
• Drug allergies (antibiotics)
• Sites of infection: rectum, vagina, oropharynx, gingiva, skin
• Signs of hemorrhage
• Signs of extramedullary leukemia—skin, gingiva
• Dentition status
Bone marrow aspirate and biopsy
• Morphologic classification
• Cytochemistry
• Immunophenotyping
• Cytogenetics
• Terminal deoxynucleotidyl transferase
Blood chemistries
• Blood urea nitrogen, creatinine, electrolytes, uric acid
• Transaminases, alkaline phosphatase, bilirubin, lactate dehydrogenase, calcium, phosphorus
Coagulation studies
• Prothrombin time, activated partial thromboplastin time, fibrinogen, fibrin split products
Chest radiograph, electrocardiogram, left ventricular ejection fraction if clinically indicated
HLA typing (patient and family); lymphocytotoxic (anti-HLA) antibody screen
Herpes simplex and cytomegalovirus serology
Lumbar puncture (only if symptomatic)

Abbreviation: HLA, human leukocyte antigen.

that most patients have had more subtle evidence of leukemia for weeks, to perhaps months, before diagnosis. This can sometimes make the distinction between de novo leukemia and leukemia associated with prior hematologic disorders arbitrary.

The findings on physical examination are variable and generally nonspecific. If fever is present, it is almost always related to infection, and an infectious site must be vigorously sought and treated empirically with broad-spectrum antibiotics. A small minority of patients have fever related solely to the underlying leukemia, which abates with appropriate chemotherapy; there is a suggestion that this may be more common in patients with promyelocytic leukemia.[92] Examination of the skin can reveal pallor, infiltrative lesions suggestive of leukemic involvement, cutaneous sites of infection, which may be either primary or embolic, or, most commonly, petechiae or ecchymoses related to thrombocytopenia and/or coagulopathy. Examination of the fundus reveals hemorrhages and/or exudates in the majority of patients (see the section "Ophthalmic Complications" later in this chapter). The conjunctivae may be pale, according to the magnitude of the anemia. Careful examination of the oropharynx and teeth is important because of the occasional occurrence of leukemic involvement and the value of applying effective dental prophylaxis with antibiotic coverage, if time permits, prior to chemotherapy. Palpable adenopathy is uncommon in patients with AML, and significant lymph node enlargement is rare. Similarly, hepatomegaly and splenomegaly are uncommon and, if found, may suggest the possibility of ALL or chronic myeloid leukemia in blast crisis. None of these findings is diagnostic of acute leukemia, and the final diagnosis and categorization depends on appropriate evaluation of peripheral blood and bone marrow.

Because of the rigorous nature of the chemotherapy required for the successful treatment of AML, particular attention should be paid to other medical problems that could complicate the patient's management. A history of congestive heart failure or other heart disease may preclude therapy with anthracyclines and mandates careful monitoring of the large amounts of intravenous fluids, including antibiotics, blood and platelet transfusions, hydration for nephrotoxic antimicrobial agents and sometimes parenteral nutrition, given during the 3-4 weeks of chemotherapy-induced pancytopenia. Prior transfusion for other disorders or multiple previous pregnancies may presage difficulties with platelet transfusions or herald the occurrence of transfusion reactions after red blood cell or platelet administration. Careful appraisal for possible drug allergies is critical, since virtually every patient will require antibiotic therapy. A history of prior herpes simplex infections (or the presence of an elevated antibody titer) provides justification for prophylactic administration of acyclovir.[132] In premenopausal women, menses should be suppressed with a GNRH agonist or estrogens and/or progestational compounds until thrombocytopenia is resolved.

After the diagnosis is established, the physician and staff must present the goals of therapy and the side effects of treatment to the patient and family. For almost all patients, this discussion can rightfully emphasize the potential benefits of treatment with regard to both the short- and long-term outcome. It is frequently appropriate and necessary to repeat this discussion and counsel later during the patient's course. Sometimes, intensive treatment with the intent to achieve CR may be less advisable because of advanced patient age, debility, or prior myelodysplasia. Particularly with de novo leukemia, this represents the exception, and the administration of chemotherapy with the intent to achieve CR affords the greatest potential for both short and longer term benefit for most patients.

Therapy

The therapy of AML has traditionally been divided into stages: induction, postremission therapy of varying intensity and duration, and postrelapse therapy. In newly diagnosed patients with AML, the goal of induction therapy is to achieve CR, which then permits the administration of subsequent therapy that for most patients is designed to maximize the probability of disease-free survival and cure. Currently, CR is defined primarily on morphologic grounds and includes the development of a morphologically normal bone marrow containing less than 5% blast elements, absence of any signs of extramedullary leukemia, and return of normal neutrophil (>1500/μL) and platelet (>150,000/μL) counts.[1] Even if the bone marrow contains <5% blasts, patients are not considered to be in remission if distinctive morphologic signs of leukemia, such as Auer rods, are noted. Low hemoglobin levels and the presence of symptoms unrelated to leukemia no longer exclude CR since they are often treatment-related and slow to normalize.

It has been assumed that CR is accomplished because the cytotoxic chemotherapy markedly decreases the number of cells in the leukemic clone, thereby allowing repopulation of the bone marrow by residual normal progenitors whose proliferation had been suppressed. This explanation is supported by observations that cytogenetic abnormalities present in the original leukemia cells are not detectable in patients in remission. However, in some patients, intensive chemotherapy appears to eliminate the block in differentiation such that the apparently normal cells seen in the bone marrow and peripheral blood during a CR are actually progeny of the leukemic clone.[133-135] Studies of female patients in CR using X chromosome-linked polymorphisms (glucose-6-phosphate dehydrogenase isoenzymes or restriction fragment-length polymorphisms) have suggested that as many as 20% of adult patients in CR have monoclonally derived hematopoiesis with the same genotype as the leukemic clone. The frequency of this "clonal CR," its possible association with particular subtypes of AML or remission duration, the mechanism by which this important biologic phenomenon occurs, and a number of important technical issues need to be defined further.[136]

Prognostic Factors

A number of clinical and laboratory factors have been described that help predict the likelihood of attaining CR and disease-free survival. In general, prognostic factors provide only relative guidelines to be used when discussing the probabilities of treatment outcome with individual patients. Conversely, they are of critical importance in focusing clinical and laboratory research efforts directed toward improving outcome. Most clinical factors are associated with decreased response to initial chemotherapy because they result in poor tolerance of the complications of prolonged pancytopenia. Advanced age (and particularly age > 70 years), renal insufficiency, congestive heart failure, concurrent infection, decreased serum albumin, and history of alloimmunization to blood products are examples.[137] Many can be summed in the assessment of the patient's performance status at the time of presentation.

As supportive care improves and in younger patients in whom some of these issues are less critical, the intrinsic biologic characteristics of the patient's leukemia become the dominant factors. Because the major cause of treatment failure is associated with drug resistance, these biologic predictive factors usually are associated with both decreased complete response rates as well as shorter durations of remission. A number of large multivariable analyses have consistently demonstrated that patients with age > 60 years, hyperleukocytosis, increases in serum lactate dehydrogenase, prior history of myelodysplasia or other hematologic disorder, and M6 or M7 and probably M0 morphology are associated with poor initial response rates and shorter durations of response. In contrast to patients with ALL, immunologic phenotyping using currently available reagents does not appear to identify distinct biologic or prognostic groups.

Major attention has focused on the prognostic impact of the nonrandom cytogenetic abnormalities and more recently molecular abnormalities detectable in AML blasts. Clonal abnormalities can be identified in 60-75% of patients.[68,111,138-141] As described earlier, certain recurring abnormalities have a very tight relationship with both morphology and treatment outcome (Table 110-1). These findings have produced considerable interest in the possibility of specific therapy directed according to different risk groups, and some such approaches were described previously. Although it is tempting to apply the knowledge of karyotypes and molecular changes to therapeutic decisions, a number of important and unanswered questions remain. In order for cytogenetic or molecular findings to represent more than a simple addition to the descriptive list of clinical factors, dissection of the mechanisms by which these changes are associated with leukemia cell resistance are required. Interestingly, there is little understanding of the factors resulting in *sensitivity* to chemotherapy and virtually no insight as to why certain patients are cured. With the extraordinary pace of development of molecular, proteomic, and immunologic techniques in the past few years, it is this aspect of the impact of leukemia biology that is most exciting.

Induction Therapy: General Principles

Induction therapy is designed to produce rapid clearing of leukemic cells from the peripheral blood with subsequent marrow aplasia. Perhaps the only exception to this principle occurs in patients with acute promyelocytic leukemia (FAB M3), in whom remission can be achieved despite the persistence 2-3 weeks later of what appear morphologically to be viable leukemia cells.[92,93] Approximately 1 week after standard induction therapy is completed (generally 2 weeks after the initiation of treatment), bone marrow aspirates and biopsies are done to evaluate the magnitude of cytoreduction. If the marrow is profoundly hypoplastic, the marrow is repeated at approximately weekly intervals to assess whether there is return of normal hematopoiesis, leukemia cells, or a mixture of both. If the marrow is not hypoplastic and only leukemia cells are noted on the day 14 marrow, then a second course of therapy is generally administered, although if high-dose cytarabine was used as induction chemotherapy, it is not repeated if leukemia is persistent.

At times, particularly if the marrow is hypocellular, it can be difficult to distinguish between residual leukemia cells and normal undifferentiated hematopoietic progenitors. In this instance, it is advisable to delay retreatment and perform another marrow aspirate in a few days. If there is no evidence of further maturation, then a second course of treatment is indicated. The presence of erythroid precursors, juvenile megakaryocytes, or increases in the peripheral blood platelet or neutrophil counts, serve as clues that normal regeneration is occurring and that a second course of treatment should be delayed. With standard regimens, approximately 30% of patients with AML require two courses of treatment to enter remission. Despite these guidelines, there remains considerable variability and imprecision as to when a second course of therapy is indicated. Some clinicians have advocated performing bone marrow aspirates and biopsies on the day after chemotherapy is completed because of a suggestion that evidence of residual leukemia at this time may be a signal of inadequate cytoreduction and a decreased probability of CR.[142,143] Although it has been suggested that further therapy be administered immediately to such patients, there is no evidence that this approach increases the rate of CR or improves survival; bone marrows that have been so recently exposed to intensive chemotherapy are also often difficult to interpret.

Most papers report results as complete response or no response. It is helpful, however, in investigations of prognostic factors or assessment of the cytotoxic activity of different regimens, to more rigorously classify the causes of failure to achieve remission. One such classification divides nonresponders into those with apparent chemotherapy-resistant leukemia, those who die with aplastic bone marrows in whom the response to chemotherapy cannot be determined, and those in whom either early death or failure to obtain adequate bone marrow studies prior to death preclude determination of whether persistent leukemia was present. Patients with drug-resistant leukemia include those patients who survive treatment and those who die but have morphologic evidence of leukemia in the bone marrow or blood antemortem or at autopsy. This categorization is relatively simple to perform in most patients and can be helpful in distinguishing between failure due to drug resistance and failure related to inadequacies of supportive care.[144]

The overall rate of CR in large cooperative group studies is approximately 65%. Patient age and cytogenetics are the most critical clinical variables, with CR rates of 75-80% in younger patients and ~50% in patients >60 years of age. The reasons for treatment failure vary according to patient age. With improved supportive care, it is uncommon for patients less than 50 years of age to die from complications of treatment and most of the approximately 25% induction failure rate is a consequence of drug-resistant leukemia. In contrast, in patients >60 years of age, failures are divided equally between drug-resistant leukemia and deaths occurring during marrow aplasia as a consequence of reduced end organ tolerance.

Comparisons among studies can be difficult because of imbalances in age and other prognostic factors. In addition, many reports do not stipulate whether patients with secondary leukemias or prior myelodysplasia were included in the trial. Exclusion of such patients, who represent approximately 5-10% of adult AML patients overall, and a higher fraction of older patients, can produce apparently improved results. It is preferable to present results in these patients and in patients with de novo leukemia separately. The criteria for CR are generally reached a median of 30-35 days after treatment has begun, although patients achieve adequate levels of circulating neutrophils (>500/μL) and no longer require platelet transfusion (at counts of approximately 10-20,000/μL), at least 7-10 days earlier.

Although there have been gradual improvements in the CR rates worldwide during the past 10-15 years, much of this can be attributed to better supportive care and not to changes in therapy. With the exception of the use of ATRA for patients with APL (see below), relatively few changes in therapy have been made since the introduction of combined therapy with daunorubicin and ara-C, the so-called "7 and 3" regimen.[145] This two-drug combination was derived from observations of single agent activity with either compound. Daunorubicin is generally administered by intravenous push at dosages of 45-60 mg/m^2/day for 3 days; ara-C is administered at dosages of 100-200 mg/m^2/day by continuous infusion for 7 days (Table 110-3). A series of randomized studies[145-151] by the Cancer and Leukemia Group B (CALGB) demonstrated that:

1. Results were superior using the 7 and 3 regimen compared with 5 days of ara-C and two doses of daunorubicin.
2. The addition of oral 6-thioguanine (DAT regimen) to the 7 and 3 program did not increase the CR rate.
3. Continuous infusions of ara-C produced slightly better outcome than twice-daily short intravenous infusions when combined with daunorubicin.
4. Results were not improved when 10 days of ara-C by continuous infusion were administered compared with 7 days.
5. Substitution of doxorubicin for daunorubicin produced almost identical CR rates, although mucosal toxicity was greater with doxorubicin.
6. There was no overall benefit from doubling the dosage of ara-C from 100 mg/m^2 to 200 mg/m^2/day.

Other Modifications of the 7 and 3 Regimen

Other attempts to improve the 7 and 3 induction regimen have also been relatively disappointing. Alternative anthracyclines or other agents such as mitoxantrone, rubidazone, aclacinomycin, amsacrine, mitoxantrone, and idarubicin have been used in several trials.[152-156] None of these studies demonstrated a survival or disease-free survival advantage with these different agents, perhaps because most are relatively similar in structure and mechanism of action and hence, become susceptible to the same mechanisms of resistance. The largest reported experience has been with idarubicin, where three initial trials demonstrated that induction results are at least equivalent to results achieved with daunorubicin and ara-C.[153,155,156] More recent randomized trials have not shown an advantage for idarubicin compared with daunorubicin, particularly in older patients.[157] In addition, the duration of myelosuppression was greater in the idarubicin cohorts, calling into question the equitoxicity of the arms. Therefore, the substitution of these compounds has not had a major impact on the long-term disease-free survival rate of patients with AML.

Another trial from Australia added etoposide to the 7 and 3 regimen.[158] The CR rate was similar in older patients when compared with daunorubicin and ara-C alone and possibly slightly increased with a modest prolongation of CR duration in younger patients receiving the etoposide. This was a relatively small study and requires confirmation, since the overall disease-free survival in the group receiving the etoposide during both remission induction and postremission therapy was similar to other larger studies using daunorubicin and ara-C alone. Large phase I studies from the CALGB in which etoposide was added to 7 and 3 had outcomes similar to the past experience with the two drugs alone.[159]

Because high-dose ara-C (HIDAC) is a beneficial postremission therapy (see below), several groups have tested the concept of using this approach during induction in younger patients. Studies have compared standard 7 and 3 to daunorubicin plus intermediate- or high-dose ara-C (2-3 g/m^2 for 8-12 doses).[160-162] These studies failed to show an improved CR rate for the recipients of HIDAC, although one study documented a more prolonged duration of CR (but no change in overall survival) in the patients randomized to HIDAC.[161] The addition of HIDAC to standard daunorubicin/ara-C during induction has also been studied. Although a small trial demonstrated an 87% remission rate in patients under 60 years old,[163] a cooperative group trial failed to confirm those positive results.[164] In addition, a recent randomized trial demonstrated similar results if HIDAC was used either as part of induction or only as postremission therapy.[165]

So-called "double –induction" strategies in which a second high dose ara-C based regimen is given on day 21, regardless of whether marrow recovery has occurred, have also failed to have an impact on CR rates or long term outcome.[166] Although the addition of other agents, such as topotecan have been evaluated,[167] unfortunately, there are few convincing data to suggest that alternative induction regimens have made a significant difference in either the CR or cure rates. A possible exception is the addition of gemtuzumab ozogamicin, an anti-CD33 monoclonal antibody that serves as a delivery agent for calicheamicin, a toxin linked to the antibody, to the standard 7 and 3 regimen. In a recent randomized study, there was no improvement in the CR rates but a suggestion of improved disease free survival with the three drug combination.[168] Updates of this trial and others which are in progress are awaited with interest.

Induction Therapy of Secondary AML

CR can be achieved in approximately 20-30% of patients whose leukemia followed treatment of another cancer. Responses may be better in patients who do not have an extended pancytopenic or myelodysplastic period prior to developing frank leukemia. Although responses tend to be short in such patients, intensive induction should be offered, particularly to younger patients in whom subsequent stem cell transplantation may be an option.[169,170] Some younger patients with apparent secondary leukemia have been found to have cytogenetic findings associated with good prognosis de novo AML, such as t(8;21) or t(15;17), and may have a more favorable clinical course than expected.[61,171] These patients

Table 110-3 Representative Chemotherapy Regimens for Acute Myeloid Leukemia

	Dose	Route	Days
Induction			
Cytarabine	100-200 mg/m^2	Continuous IV infusion	1-7
+			
Daunorubicin	45-60 mg/m^2	IV	1-3
or			
Idarubicin	12 mg/m^2	IV	1-3
or			
Mitoxantrone	12 mg/m^2	IV	1-3
Postremission			
Cytarabine	3 g/m^2 q12h (over 3 h)	IV (6 doses)	1, 3, 5
or			
Cytarabine	1.5-2 g/m^2 q12h (over 1 h)	IV (8 doses)	1-4 (12 doses)
or			
Cytarabine	100 mg/m^2	Continuous IV infusion	1-5

See text for details about number of courses and patient selection for different regimens.

should be treated in the same fashion as those with de novo disease.

Whether and how to treat patients with well-documented prior myelodysplastic syndrome (MDS) and leukemia evolving from RAEB can be problematic. CR rates are lower, sustained responses are unusual, prolonged periods of aplasia are common, and such patients are usually older and less able to tolerate pancytopenic complications. Although data from the University of Texas M. D. Anderson Cancer Center suggest that the absolute number of marrow blasts (eg, whether a patient has RAEB, RAEB-T [now categorized as AML] or frank AML) is not of itself of prognostic significance,[172] the presence of major cytogenetic abnormalities and a truly prolonged history of MDS have a profoundly negative prognostic impact. If a histocompatible donor is readily available, initial therapy with allogeneic stem cell transplantation should be considered for selected younger patients with prior MDS,[173,174] although there is concern that the relapse rate is increased in patients with circulating blasts and/or a higher percentage of bone marrow blasts and some patients may benefit from induction chemotherapy prior to transplantation.[175] There has been some interest in using very low-dose ara-C (10-20 mg/m^2/day) in older patients to decrease acute side effects. Although responses can be seen with low-dose ara-C, many weeks of therapy can be required with consequent pancytopenic complications equivalent to those seen with higher-dose treatment. In addition, the CR rate is low, and although median survivals may be similar using the two different dosage approaches, the prospect for longer-term survival is greater when the intent of treatment is to achieve CR.[176,177] Clinical trials in which such patients receive novel agents such as the alkylating agent, cloretazine, the nucleoside analog, clofarabine, or the DNA hypomethylating agent, decitabine, have shown CR rates similar to those obtained with standard chemotherapy, possibly with lower levels of treatment-related mortality.[178-180] Whether these initial results will be confirmed and/or lead to significantly longer leukemia-free surivival await the performance of larger, comparative studies.

Postremission Therapy

Morphologic assessments of CR are subjective and relatively insensitive. It is estimated that as many as 10^9 leukemia cells may still be present in patients in apparent CR. Rare patients can remain in CR for 1-2 years without further treatment, but it is generally accepted that some form of therapy after CR is required to achieve long-term disease-free survival. In a trial conducted by the German Cooperative Leukemia Group, a subset of 37 patients did not receive postremission therapy for a variety of protocol and medical reasons; all of these individuals relapsed.[181] The Eastern Cooperative Oncology Groups (ECOG) reported a randomized study in which patients achieving CR were randomized to either no therapy, lower-dose maintenance therapy, or an intensive postremission program.[182] All of the patients in the no-treatment arm relapsed rapidly, with a median CR duration of 4 months, resulting in early termination of this arm of the trial. Similar results were noted in a smaller randomized study reported by Embury and colleagues.[183] Although timed sequential therapy, in which patients receive additional chemotherapy during the early postinduction recovery phase, has been associated with prolonged remissions in the absence of postremission chemotherapy,[184,185] this treatment regimen is more analogous to consolidation therapy. It therefore remains standard practice to administer chemotherapy with or without subsequent stem cell transplantation after remission is achieved with conventional regimens.

Chemotherapeutic Approaches ■ Considerable uncertainty and controversy remain about which chemotherapy-based postremission approach is preferable. These different approaches can be generally categorized according to the intensity of the therapy administered. The terms "consolidation" and "intensification" have been used to describe therapies that are of equal and greater intensity than the regimens used in initial induction therapy. These phrases are used rather loosely, however, and readers are advised to assess carefully the stipulated doses as well as the doses actually delivered, and the periods of aplasia experienced by the recipients. The term "maintenance" has generally referred to lower-dose outpatient therapy administered on an intermittent basis for months to years, patterned on the model successfully used in childhood ALL. Again, however, the ability to deliver such regimens as scheduled varies considerably.

A variety of agents have been used for postremission therapy, including the agents successfully administered in initial induction, with a particular focus on high-dose ara-C (HIDAC) as consolidation, as well as different classes of compounds, some of which have proven activity in AML, and others of which may have had only limited activity. Since a variety of prognostic factors significantly affect ultimate outcome, independent of the type of therapy administered, good results in small nonrandomized studies may reflect inadvertent patient selection and must ultimately be confirmed by multi-institutional applicability.

Overall, in adults, it can be expected that the administration of some sort of postremission therapy will result in a median CR duration of 12-18 months with approximately 20-25% of complete responders remaining as long-term disease-free survivors (Fig. 110-12). A large review of CALGB patients who achieved CR demonstrated a relatively constant relapse rate of 4.7% per month during the first 6 months following CR. The failure rate decreased in subsequent 6-month intervals (3.5% per month in months 7-12 and 2.4% per month in months 13-18), with a flattening of the curves after 3+ years of CR.[186] In general, patients relapsing earlier have leukemia that is more drug-resistant than those who relapse late. Older randomized trials of postremission therapy conducted by the CALGB failed to demonstrate long-term benefits from: (1) an alternate month compared with a monthly schedule of maintenance therapy; (2) 3 years of relatively low-dose maintenance therapy compared with 8 months of a similar program (indeed, there was a modest survival advantage for patients randomized to stop therapy

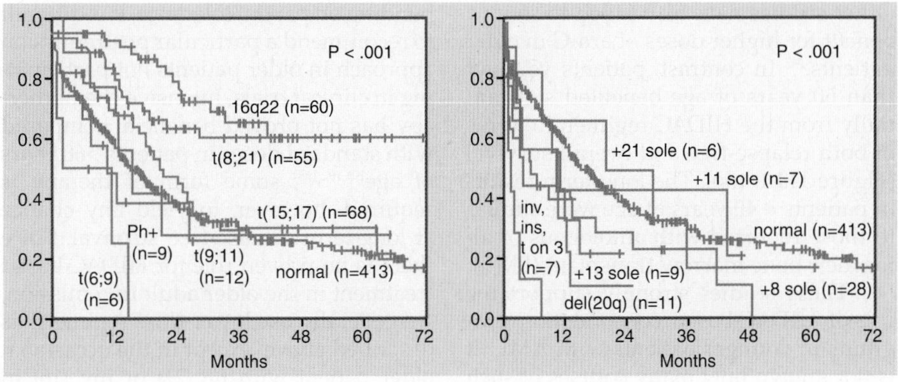

Figure 110-12 ■ Overall survival according to cytogenetic findings in patients with de novo acute myeloid leukemia treated with intensive induction and postremission chemotherapy on CALGB studies.

after 8 months); (3) doubling of the dose of ara-C from 100 to 200 mg/m² during maintenance therapy; and (4) addition of nonspecific immunotherapy in the form of methanol-extractable residue of Bacille Calinette Grain (MER) to maintenance therapy.[146-149]

With regard to the role of maintenance chemotherapy, an older ECOG study demonstrated no benefit from the addition of 2 years of maintenance therapy following two courses of postremission treatment with DAT (daunorubicin, ara-C, thioguanine).[187] Earlier studies from Germany reported by Buchner and colleagues[181] suggested a modest prolongation of CR duration when long-term maintenance therapy was administered after a single course of postremission DAT, although with a questionable effect on long-term survival. There was less effect of maintenance in later studies when more intensive postremission consolidation was used before the maintenance.[188,189]

Two important randomized trials have shown that HIDAC in the postremission setting is better than lower doses of the drug in younger patients. In an ECOG study, patients randomized to receive one course of very intensive postremission consolidation with a HIDAC-type regimen had a longer median duration of remission than patients receiving 2 years of lower-dose maintenance therapy.[190] The CALGB randomized 596 AML patients in CR to receive four courses of ara-C administered at three different dose levels (100 mg/m² by continuous IV infusion [CIV] for 5 days, 400 mg/m² CIV for 5 days, 3 g/m² IV for 3 hours q12h on days 1, 3, and 5 [total 6 doses/course]). There was no benefit from the higher-dose arms in patients > 60 years of age (Fig. 110-1, bottom) with a median duration of CR of approximately 13 months and with only 10-12% long-term disease-free survival.[191] In addition, there was a substantial incidence of CNS neurotoxicity in the older patients, manifested primarily as cerebellar dysfunction. Other studies have also failed to show a benefit for higher doses of ara-C in older patients.[192] In contrast, patients younger than 60 years of age benefited substantially from the HIDAC regimen in terms of both relapse-free and overall survival (Figure 110-1, top). The long-term results in patients < 40 years of age were similar to those reported with autologous or allogeneic bone marrow transplant (BMT).

These studies strongly support the use of HIDAC-based consolidation programs in younger patients with AML. It is not known how many courses of such therapy are needed, the optimal dose and schedule of HIDAC and whether the addition of other active agents will improve on these results. In a recent randomized study, the use of other potentially non-cross-resistant regimens substituted for HIDAC was not superior to 3 cycles of HIDAC[193] and studies from the Medical Research Council in Britain which used multiple post remission courses using a variety of different drugs produced similar overall outcomes.[194,195] The CALGB data suggest that the benefit from HIDAC was most pronounced in patients with favorable cytogenetic findings [t(8;21); and inv (16)] with much less effect in patients with unfavorable karyotypes typically associated with drug resistance.[68,111] When medically feasible, most clinicians attempt to administer at least three courses of reasonably intensive HIDAC-based therapy postremission regimens. Programs that use HIDAC in the range of 2-3 g/m² for 8-12 doses are often only able to administer one to two courses of such treatment (Table 110-3).

The decision about the type of postremission therapy must take into consideration the patient's medical condition and the possible persistence of infection (particularly with fungal organisms) acquired during induction, as well as the ability to provide adequate platelet transfusion therapy, in an attempt to balance the risk of intensive postremission approaches with the potential benefit. Depending on the intensity of the consolidation program, a 5% mortality rate in CR is to be expected and must be carefully explained to the patient, although the use of myeloid growth factors after consolidation can appreciably shorten the duration of severe neutropenia and therefore make the administration of this therapy safer.[196,197]

Between 5% and 15% of patients achieving CR do not receive intensive postremission programs because of concerns about the patient's ability to tolerate and survive this therapy. Such patients should receive some sort of lower-dose treatment if possible, and we frequently use ara-C (100-200 mg/m²/day by CIV for 5 days or sometimes on a bid, subcutaneous schedule), with or without 1-2 doses of an anthracycline for 2-4 courses, depending on patient tolerance. It is difficult to recommend a particular postremission approach in older patients not participating in clinical trials. Intensive chemotherapy has not proved beneficial compared with standard doses in patients >60 years of age[191,192,198]; some form of therapy is required, however, to yield any chance at long-term disease-free survival. Since there is no proven role for HIDAC-based treatment in the older adult in remission, we generally use lower-dose regimens as described above, except in the occasional older patient with t(8; 21) or inv (16) in whom HIDAC is preferred, if medically feasible. In view of the lack of proven benefit and the expense and morbidity associated with long-term maintenance therapy, prolonged treatment cannot be recommended for patients of any age.

Stem Cell Transplantation ■ Stem cell transplantation (SCT) represents the other major therapeutic option for postremission therapy for younger patients, although increasingly, nonmyeloablative transplant is being considered in selected older patients. Syngeneic SCT, using identical twins as donors,[199] and allogeneic SCT, using HLA-identical siblings,[200] were first evaluated in patients with advanced, refractory AML. After demonstrating an approximately 10% rate of long-term disease-free survival in this refractory group of patients and a 40-50% disease-free survival in patients in first remission receiving syngeneic transplants, studies of allogeneic transplantation in first remission AML were begun.[201] Early small series were promising, demonstrating a low rate of relapse with most of the mortality related to complications of acute and chronic graft-vs-host disease (GVHD).

At least in part because of difficulties in identifying suitable donors for many patients, as well as the complications of GVHD, considerable attention has also been focused on the use of autologous SCT. Cryopreserved autologous bone marrow can rapidly reconstitute recipients of ablative regimens, although marrow recovery may be delayed compared with allogeneic BMT.[202] More recent experience using cytokine mobilized peripheral blood stem cells (PBSC) indicates that the durations of neutropenia and particularly thrombocytopenia are shortened compared with the use of bone marrow.[203] Because of the absence of GVHD, the autologous procedure is much better tolerated and can be readily applied to patients up to 65 years of age and perhaps older. The major disadvantages include the absence of a graft-versus-leukemia effect, as well as concern that viable leukemic progenitors will be administered with the autologous stem cells. A number of purging techniques have been used including monoclonal antibodies directed against myeloid blasts, as well as incubation with high concentrations of cytotoxic agents[202] that rather remarkably spare hematopoietic progenitors, although delayed marrow reconstitution is not uncommon.[204] It is unknown whether these in vitro manipulations are necessary and randomized trials have not been reported. More recently, when unpurged autologous BMT was harvested after high-dose consolidation therapy, retrospective comparisons did not suggest an increased rate of relapse. A number of centers and groups have reported relapse-free survival rates in excess of 40% following autologous SCT in first CR.[205-207] Historically, syngeneic transplant experience in this situation demonstrated relapse rates of approximately 50%, which is probably the best that can be expected with the autologous approach. Other evidence of the potential of this approach derive from reports of apparent cure rates of 20% in patients transplanted in second and third remissions of AML.[202]

Following these initial results, the suggestion was made that all suitable patients with AML in first CR with available donors should be considered for transplant. Contentious debate ensued, eventually resulting in several large prospective trials which "genetically" assigned patients with histocompatible siblings to allogeneic BMT (usually only in those 45 years old or less) while randomizing the others to either autologous BMT or chemotherapy.[194,195,208-210] In the first of these trials which included 422 patients < 45 years of age (median 33 years), disease-free survival was similar in patients undergoing allogeneic BMT (55% projected at 4 years) and autologous BMT (48%) and superior to the chemotherapy group (30%), which received a second course of consolidation chemotherapy with intermediate-dose ara-C and m-amsacrine.[208] Overall survival was similar, however, because many patients relapsing after chemotherapy could be successfully re-induced and then undergo SCT in second CR. Many patients did not undergo treatment as randomized, and no information was provided about responses to the three treatments in different cytogenetic risk groups.

Another similarly designed trial performed in France failed to show a benefit for either type of BMT compared with patients receiving intensive postremission chemotherapy.[209] More recently, a large study from Germany failed to demonstrate a benefit from autologous transplantation given as a component of consolidation therapy.[166] The Medical Research Council (MRC) 10 trial conducted in Great Britain[194] appeared to show that autologous BMT was beneficial. All patients not assigned to allogeneic BMT received three cycles of post-CR chemotherapy and were then randomized to nonpurged autologous BMT or observation. The *addition* of the autologous transplant prolonged CR duration but there was no significant difference in overall survival between the two groups. Allogeneic BMT was not significantly better than autologous BMT; no modality was clearly better than another in different cytogenetic risk groups. The MRC trials were recently updated with intent to treat analysis of results in patients with and without matched sibling donors.[195] Again, there was no apparent survival benefit compared with chemotherapy for patients who had available donors in whom a transplant could have been performed, and no advantage when patients with donors who were and were not transplanted were compared.

The trial conducted by the North American Intergroup[210] found that chemotherapy was at least as good as autologous or allogeneic BMT in leading to cure, based on the intent to treat analysis. As in all the other studies, many patients assigned to autologous BMT did not receive this therapy for a variety of reasons. Randomized trials evaluating allogeneic or autologous PBSC have not been reported.

Some general points can be made concerning the role of allogeneic BMT in the management of patients with AML in first CR:

1. The applicability of the technique is limited by patient age. Mortality from GVHD increases from decade to decade, and many centers do not perform myeloablative allogeneic transplantation in patients older than 60 years, thereby excluding most patients with AML. Improvements in supportive care and the increased use of reduced intensity transplants using nonmyeloablative conditioning regimens and peripheral blood stem cells may allow increased use of transplantation to older individuals. Early side effects are markedly decreased by the nonablative approach, although it appears that the severity and duration of chronic GVHD is increased and further follow-up is needed to assess the ultimate rate of overall survival. The nonmyeloablative approach is medically feasible in selected older patients,[211] although a recent, more systematic prospective study from the same group demonstrated that because of clinical, administrative and donor availability issues, only a small fraction of older patients in first CR can actually proceed to transplantation.[212] Nonetheless, several US cooperative groups are assessing the feasibility and outcome of this approach in older adults because of the predicted poor outcome using chemotherapy alone.
2. Less than one-third of potential recipients have suitable HLA-matched family donors. Although alternatives include the use of matched unrelated donors or partially mismatched family donors, GVHD is increased with both approaches, and administrative delays in identifying suitable donors remain problematic despite the availability of millions of HLA-typed donors throughout the world.[213,214] This is particularly true for patients from ethnic minority groups with less common HLA types and also indicates that there is considerable selection bias in reports of unrelated donor transplants, since some higher risk patients relapse while awaiting for a donor to be identified. Nonetheless, with the use of molecular histocompatibility typing, the results following unrelated allogeneic transplant is equivalent to those with matching sibling transplant potentially extending the use of allogeneic transplant for a much larger group of patients with AML in first remission.[215] Umbilical cord blood may offer an alternative source of stem cells for those without matched siblings or unrelated donors. The incidence of graft- versus-host disease is much lower following cord blood transplants with better tolerance of mismatched transplants. Engraftment can be delayed, however, and dosage considerations represent an issue for many adult recipients.[216,217]
3. Although allogeneic SCT can cure some patients with chemotherapy-resistant disease, there remains an appreciable relapse rate and at least some of the factors predictive of drug resistance and relapse after chemotherapy also apply to SCT recipients.[218,219]
4. The antileukemic effect following BMT correlates with the occurrence and severity of GVHD, presumably as a result of a graft-versus-leukemia effect. Attempts to attenuate GVHD with a variety of immunosuppressive approaches are associated with a decrease in GVHD, but also an increase in the relapse rate.[220] Selective T-cell depletion approaches and other immunologic manipulations of the graft are being evaluated in an attempt to make allogeneic SCT safer without an increased relapse risk.[221,222]
5. Although important advances in supportive care directed against cytomegalovirus have been made, the consequences of the immunosuppression and direct organ sequelae of GVHD still represent formidable barriers.
6. As many as 10-20% of surviving patients may have significant symptoms and impairment of performance status because of chronic GVHD. There is also a small increase in the frequency of secondary tumors in long-term survivors.[223]

It is hoped that additional ongoing studies, perhaps requiring meta-analysis of results, will clarify many of these issues, particularly with regard to optimal treatments for different risk subgroups of patients. Contradictory results in different cytogenetic subgroups were noted in the randomized trials.[209,224] It would appear, however, that all approaches are in need of considerable improvement. Although the causes of failure are different (high rate of relapse with chemotherapy, lower rate of relapse but high mortality owing to GVHD for allogeneic SCT), historic results suggest that the overall outcomes may be similar with the inevitable conclusion that improved cytoreductive approaches are needed in both arenas.

This assessment begs the question about what to recommend to individual patients. Because of the low but real potential for cure following allogeneic transplant for some highly resistant diseases such as MDS and blast crisis CML, most clinicians consider allogeneic transplantation in first CR for suitable patients with AML and high risk features, while reserving transplant for second CR in those with more favorable molecular or cytogenetic subtypes.[51] The best approach for the large group with "intermediate" risk and the molecular subgroups of patients within the normal cytogenetics group remains unclear. For example, there are conflicting data from retrospective analyses about whether allogeneic transplantation is of benefit for patients with ITD mutations.[44,225] It should be kept in mind that overall the long term outcome of allogeneic transplantation was never worse than chemotherapy in the randomized trials although an unsuccessful allogeneic transplant could result in an inferior short-term survival.

Therapy of Relapsed and Refractory AML

There are a number of agents available that have clear-cut activity when used alone or in combination in patients with relapsed or refractory AML, including amsacrine, mitoxantrone, diaziquone, idarubicin, fludarabine, 2-chlorodeoxyadenosine, etoposide, homoharringtonine, topotecan, carboplatin, and most recently, clofarabine, cloretazine and troxacitabine.[226-235] There is considerable heterogeneity among relapsed patients, and a number of factors in addition to the specific drugs used influence the outcome of treatment.[97,236-238] Some consistent trends are evident: (1) Response rates are uniformly low in patients with primarily refractory leukemia, in those with short initial CR durations, or in those who relapsed while receiving postremission chemotherapy; (2) secondary leukemias, leukemias that evolved from a prior hematologic disorder, and patients with poor-risk cytogenetics are particularly resistant to further therapy; (3) patients in second and subsequent relapse have a poorer prognosis than patients in first relapse, and the durations of subsequent remissions tend to decrease progressively.

Results from the MRC in Britain, which prospectively followed all patients entered on an induction AML trial, are supportive of these conclusions[238] (Table 110-4). In another study, patients whose initial remission was greater than 18 months had a re-induction rate of 64% (37 of 58) compared with a 29% CR rate in 278 patients with shorter initial remissions. Furthermore, the duration of second CR was longer in the former group (8 months vs 3 months). Patient age and cytogenetic findings are also important prognostic factors, emphasizing the enormous influence of patient selection on the results of reported phase II trials. In the absence of comparative trials, differing results may very well be the consequence of patient selection rather than the superiority of a particular regimen.[237,239]

Table 110-4 ■ Treatment of AML in Relapse

Duration of First CR	Frequency of Second CR (%)
>2 years	61
1.5-2 years	53
1-1.5 years	30
7-12 months	19
1-6 months	10
Total	29 (155 of 531 patients)

Patients received a variety of different reinduction regimens.
Abbreviations: AML, acute myeloid leukemia; CR, complete response.
Source: Adapted from Ref. 191.

The type and timing of therapy for relapsed patients should be individualized. Patients with other medical problems who have had poor responses to initial therapy have a small likelihood of sustained benefit from re-induction therapy and, indeed, may have life shortened by intensive therapy. Some such patients can be supported for many months, with maintenance of a reasonable quality of life, with a more conservative approach using red blood cell and platelet transfusions and oral hydroxyurea to control elevated WBC counts or symptoms such as bone pain. However, there is no potential for long-term benefit. Conversely, younger patients with longer initial responses may derive prolonged benefit from intensive re-induction therapy.

Recurrence of leukemia is often detected when the patient is asymptomatic, blood counts are normal, and there is modest marrow infiltration by blasts. Although it is logical to begin re-induction therapy at the earliest sign of relapse, when tumor burden is presumably the lowest, there are no data to demonstrate the validity of this approach except possibly as preparation for subsequent SCT.[240] The drawback to early treatment is that re-induction therapy is often unsuccessful and may result in excessive early morbidity and premature patient death. Our general policy is to observe such patients until there has been a pattern of deterioration in blood counts, but to initiate therapy while adequate numbers of circulating granulocytes and platelets are still present, prior to the development of symptoms or infection. An important exception is patients who are candidates for allogeneic transplantation (see below). Other patients have relapse diagnosed when bone marrows are done because of falls in blood counts. Such patients usually require re-induction therapy more immediately. In occasional patients, relapse develops in an explosive fashion with high circulating blast counts, fever, and infection. It is likely that the outcome in this group of patients is poorer.

There are essentially no comparative trials providing guidance about the choice of agents to be used. The initial decision is generally between reuse of drugs that have previously been effective in a given patient, compared with the use of new drugs, some of which may be investigational. If a patient has relapsed while receiving chemotherapy, it makes little sense to use these same agents for re-induction. The oft-quoted exception to this guideline is the use of HIDAC (2-3 g/m^2 q12h for 8-12 doses), even in patients who had recently received more conventional doses of this agent. Although CR can be achieved in this setting, the duration of CR appears to be short, and it is not clear that the HIDAC approach is of long-term value in such patients.

In contrast, in patients who have longer first remissions, there is logic to reusing initial treatment. Many centers have arbitrarily felt that patients relapsing more than a year after completion of therapy should again receive the standard treatment. Although the CR rate in such patients is probably in excess of 50% when the original drugs are reused, it is not clear whether the same results could have been achieved in this favorable group using other tactics, including new investigational agents.

Gemtuzumab ozogamicin was recently approved for use in older patients with AML in first relapse whose first CR was greater than 3 months in duration.[241] Although it is clearly an active agent with few acute side effects, it produces prolonged myelosuppression and may be associated with an increased incidence of hepatic veno-occlusive disease, particularly in patients who go on to receive allogeneic transplantation.[242,243] CR rates have also been lower than initially reported when its use was expanded to other patient populations; further studies are required to assess its long-term role in AML therapeutics.[168,244,245]

There is no proven benefit of postremission chemotherapy in patients achieving second or third remissions. The obvious downside is that one is potentially depriving patients of time when they would be asymptomatic and out of hospital by the administration of therapy of variable toxicity but no proven long-term efficacy. At the moment, most re-induction studies do not specify that patients in second or later remission receive either maintenance or consolidation therapy.

It is unclear whether SCT should be offered at the time of initial relapse or whether patients should be re-induced and transplanted when a second remission is achieved. Unfortunately, most patients do not achieve second remission, and some develop medical problems during re-induction therapy that preclude subsequent transplantation. Enthusiasm for transplantation in relapse derives from reports from Seattle indicating that the results of allogeneic transplantation in early relapse were equivalent to or better than those achieved in patients transplanted in second or subsequent remission.[240] It is often a practical problem to identify patients during early relapse and to be able to refer such patients for transplantation rapidly. Nonetheless, it would probably be best to consider allogeneic transplantation for patients in early relapse if a suitable donor is available and the patient is under the age of 55-60 years. Similarly, allogeneic BMT can produce long-term survival in some patients with primary refractory leukemia, and it is advisable to HLA-type patients and their families at diagnosis to allow for this possibility. It is more difficult to use nonrelated donors for these purposes because of delays caused by tissue typing, identification of donors, and stem cell procurement. Currently, most transplant centers recommend that patients in more florid relapse receive induction chemotherapy first because of poor results with SCT as primary therapy in such patients.

Patients who achieve second remission probably have a greater chance of long-term survival if transplanted in second remission. Hence, relapsed patients who are candidates for allogeneic transplantation should have donor searches done while they are undergoing reindcution treatment. Data using both allogeneic and autologous approaches are promising in this regard, although it should be kept in mind that all such reports include highly selected patient populations, most of whom have had second remissions lasting a few months prior to transplantation. These patients have thereby identified themselves as having more chemotherapy-sensitive disease. A few centers cryopreserve bone marrow from patients in first CR for use in either early relapse or as consolidation in second CR. This is an expensive, administratively cumbersome approach, although it merits study in investigational settings, particularly in high-risk patients, prior to its more widespread application. Lastly, selected patients who relapse following BMT can derive benefit from lymphocyte infusions from their donor or a second BMT and, in general, can receive and tolerate further chemotherapy.[246]

Therapy of Acute Promyelocytic Leukemia (APL)

The treatment of APL differs substantially from that for other subtypes of AML and will be considered separately. In theory, if leukemic progenitors could be forced to undergo terminal differentiation in vivo, then the leukemic clone could lose the capacity for self-renewal and be eliminated, with fewer side effects than occur with intensive cytotoxic chemotherapy. With the exception of the HL-60 cell line and blasts obtained from patients with APL, it has been difficult to reproducibly induce fresh leukemia cells to differentiate in vitro.

Limited clinical trials evaluating "differentiating" therapies, including vitamin D and low-dose ara-C, have produced disappointing results except for occasional patients with APL who derived transient benefit from treatment with *cis*-retinoic acid.[247] The differentiation paradigm was verified, however, by dramatic responses in patients with APL reported from China with all-trans-retinoic acid (ATRA) administered orally for 30-90 days.[248] CRs were seen in >80% of both relapsed and previously untreated individuals. Marrow aplasia did not occur and serial bone marrows demonstrated what appeared to be maturation of the abnormal, hypergranulated promyelocytes.[249,250] Disseminated intravascular coagulation resolved promptly, with a profound reduction in the requirement for platelet transfusions following ATRA treatment. Although the hemorrhagic complications are decreased, approximately 20-30% of patients treated with ATRA alone develop significant side effects that can include fever, rapidly evolving pulmonary insufficiency, pericarditis, and pleurisy. This syndrome can occur independently of the leukocytosis frequently observed with ATRA therapy and can be fatal. Optimal management includes the prompt administration of corticosteroids at the first signs of the "ATRA" syndrome.[251,252] Resistance to ATRA eventually develops in patients treated in relapse, and virtually all patients treated with ATRA alone relapse. Possible pharmacokinetic mechanisms include induction of more rapid metabolism of the ATRA and induction of cytoplasmic retinoic acid binding protein in normal tissues that bind the ATRA, thereby decreasing the exposure of residual APL cells to the drug.[253]

A randomized study conducted in Europe first demonstrated the superiority of ATRA (with the addition of chemotherapy as needed) to chemotherapy alone in newly diagnosed patients with APL, both in terms of response to induction therapy and disease-free survival.[254] A large North American trial compared initial ATRA therapy versus chemotherapy as well as ATRA versus observation in the late postremission period.[255] Patients who never received ATRA did very poorly compared with patients receiving ATRA during induction or maintenance. Subsequent studies have demonstrated that optimal results are achieved when ATRA and anthracycline-based chemotherapy are administered concurrently during induction.[256-259] The frequency of the "ATRA syndrome" is also substantially lower when concurrent chemotherapy is added.

Approximately 70% of patients are cured with ATRA and anthracycline induction followed by anthracycline-based consolidation therapy. Results are less satisfying in older patients and in those presenting with WBC count > 10,000/μL.[260] There is some controversy as to whether the addition of ara-C in induction and consolidation improves upon these results with a suggestion that ara-C may add benefit only in the patients in higher risk groups.[261,262] There appears to be a role for intermittent administration of ATRA as maintenance therapy and possibly further benefit from oral maintenance treatment given for 1-2 years with methotrexate and 6-mercaptopurine, although one study suggests that maintenance may not be needed in patients in whom RT-PCR for PML/RAR-α is negative.[263] Although large numbers of multi-national randomized trials have been completed, there are subtle and often major differences in the post remission and maintenance programs as well as differences in the sensitivities of the PCR assays for minimal residual disease, and it hoped that ongoing trials will finally settle some of these issues. A representative approach is summarized in Table 110-5.

An exciting new development in APL has been the demonstration, again in China, that arsenic trioxide administered intravenously, produces a high rate of CR and major tumor burden reduction (four to five orders of magnitude based on PCR testing) even in patients with advanced, multiply relapsed disease.[264,265] Although the precise mechanism of action and the explanation for its relative specificity for APL remain to be elucidated, arsenic trioxide serves to accelerate apoptotic cell death in APL. Recently, tetra-arsenic tetra-sulfide has been shown to be very active in both newly diagnosed and relapsed APL patients with the great advantage of oral administration.[266] While arsenic trioxide is now the standard therapy for relapsed APL, there is considerable interest in using arsenic as part of the induction and postremission treatment of APL. Investigators from China demonstrated high response

Table 110-5 **Representative Regimen for Acute Promyelocytic Leukemia**

	Dose mg/m^2	Route	Days
Induction			
ATRA	45	PO	1-until CR is achieved
Daunorubicin[a]	50	IV	1-4
Cytarabine[b]	200	CIV	1-7
Consolidation (2 courses)[c]			
ATRA	45	PO	7 days
Daunorubicin	50	IV	1-3
Maintenance			
ATRA	45	PO	1-7, alternate wks for 1-2 yrs
6-mercaptopurine	60	PO	Daily for 1-2 yrs
Methotrexate	20	PO	Weekly for 1-2 yrs

Note: The therapy of APL is in evolution but this represents a treatment program in common use in North America. See section on "Treatment of APL" for additional comments.
[a]Other regimens use idarubicin 12 mg/m^2 days 2, 4, 6, 8 for induction and idarubicin and mitoxantrone during consolidation.[259,260]
[b]The need for cytarabine for lower risk patients has been questioned by some studies.[376]
[c]One study suggests a benefit from adding two courses of arsenic trioxide (0.15 mg/kg/day for 5 days/week × 5 weeks) before this consolidation (see text).[270]
Source: From Ref. 255.

rates using ATRA and arsenic as initial treatment,[267] while other studies from India and Iran reported high molecular CR rates which were durable using arsenic alone. Using only ATRA and arsenic in patients not deemed to be candidates for anthracycline-based therapy, with gemtuzumab ozogamicin added for patients with high WBC or insufficient response, the MD Anderson group has demonstrated a leukemia-free survival rate, albeit with short follow-up, as high as that seen in cooperative trials employing more standard therapy.[268,269] Finally, the North American Intergroup evaluated the addition of two courses of arsenic as consolidation therapy post remission and showed a survival benefit compared to the standard treatment without arsenic. This study has been criticized however, because the control group fared more poorly than expected.[270]

It is thus clear that arsenic and ATRA based regimens are likely to become the backbone of future treatment approaches with the hope of eliminating the need for chemotherapy and particularly high dose anthracyclines because of the concerns about late cardiotoxicity. The combination is now used frequently in older patients with cardiac disease who cannot receive anthracyclines and additional trials are in progress in both standard and higher risk patients.[81]

Treatment of Relapsed APL ■ Although sustained second remissions can be seen following multiple courses of arsenic,[265] most clinicians recommend the addition of stem cell transplantation in suitable patients. There are studies demonstrating long term disease free survival with autologous transplantation in patients in second remission who become PCR negative for the PML/RAR-α, although allogeneic transplant should be considered in PCR + patients because of the high rate of relapse following autologous transplant in these patients.[271] Relapse in the CNS is unusual during the initial course of APL, but is more common and can be very difficult to treat in relapsed patients. Therefore, prophlaxis with intrathecal chemotherapy is recommended when patients achieve second CR.[81]

Other Supportive Care and Therapeutic Approaches

Hematopoietic Growth Factors

Because myelosuppression-associated mortality is so high, particularly in older adults with AML, the development of hematopoietic growth factors (HGFs) held promise to ameliorate such side effects. Granulocyte-macrophage colony-stimulating factor (GM-CSF), granulocyte colony-stimulating factor (G-CSF), and interleukin (IL)-3 have been evaluated as well as the thrombopoietic factors, megakaryocyte growth and development factor (MGDF) and IL-11. The use of these agents in AML lagged behind that in solid tumors because of the concern that pharmacologic doses would lead to blast proliferation and a poor clinical outcome. Although fears regarding this clinical problem have proven unfounded, the HGFs have not lived up to their promise for other reasons.

Multiple randomized studies have been completed in which older patients received an HGF or placebo following the completion of initial induction therapy with the goal of improving CR rate by reducing infectious complications as a consequence of shortened durations of severe myelosuppression.[196,272-279] All trials noted a decrease on the order of 2-5 days in the number of days of neutropenia < 500/μL, sometimes in association with a smaller 1- to 2-day reduction in the duration of hospitalization, but with the exception of a smaller trial reported by the ECOG, there was no significant difference in the incidence of severe infection, deaths from infections, CR rate, or survival.[272] One randomized trial using G-CSF after induction therapy for older patients with AML showed an improved CR rate for the G-CSF recipients.[277] Somewhat unexpectedly, the infectious mortality was similar in the two groups of patients, and the reason for the increased CR rate is unclear. There was no difference in overall survival.

In aggregate, it would appear that the benefits of growth factors administered after the completion of induction therapy are modest at best.[280] In contrast, G-CSF following intensive consolidation therapy has appreciably shortened the duration of neutropenia, albeit without improvement in CR duration or survival.[196,197] Because of the potential for eliminating the need for hospitalization, the use of HGF can be recommended following consolidation therapy. Smaller studies with pegylated thrombopoietin failed to demonstrate reduced needs for platelet transfusions during the induction or consolidation treatment of AML.[281,282]

Although in vitro evidence suggests that HGFs can increase the cytotoxic effects of ara-C, at least in part by increasing the fraction of cells in S-phase,[283,284] clinical results with the priming strategy have been disappointing. An early study from the M. D. Anderson group suggested that GM-CSF administered before and during chemotherapy produced lower response rates and survival than seen in a historical control group treated with chemotherapy alone.[285] Most subsequent studies that randomized patients to receive GMCSF/G-CSF or no marrow stimulants, before, during, and/or after induction chemotherapy[286-288] also failed to show an advantage for patients primed with growth factor. Some of these studies used HIDAC, whereas others evaluated more conventional continuous-infusion schedules.

Immune Modulation ■ A critical component of the therapeutic benefit associated with allogeneic SCT is related to the graft-versus-leukemia effect. Although this is a complex, multifactorial set of events, further studies may enable the rational application of lymphokines to stimulate the appropriate cells in patients treated with chemotherapy alone. Circulating natural killer (NK) cells that can be cytotoxic to leukemia cell lines, and autologous leukemia cells in vitro, can be detected after both autologous and allogeneic transplantation, but not after chemotherapy.[289] The numbers of NK cells can be expanded by the post-transplant administration of IL-2.[290] IL-2 itself has some antileukemic effect in patients with AML in relapse.[291,292] Pilot trials have documented the feasibility of administering IL-2 in the postchemotherapy setting but unfortunately, a large randomized trial failed to demonstrate any benefit from the use of IL-2 given after completion of consolidation chemotherapy in older patients with AML.[293] A similar trial in younger adults documented a trend toward improved LFS and OS in patients randomized to IL-2, but many patients refused randomization or refused IL-2 if they randomized to receive it.[282] Another randomized trial showed that a combination of histamine plus IL-2 was beneficial in the late post-remission setting,[294] but has been criticized because of the heterogeneity of the pre-randomization chemotherapy. Vaccine-based approaches using dendritic cell fusions to present leukemia-associated antigens such as WT1 and PR1, or transducing AML cells to express proteins capable of stimulation of immune response, are under development.[295,296]

Circumvention of Drug Resistance ■ The sum of complex and interacting mechanisms determine whether sufficient cytoreduction occurs in a given patient. The pharmacokinetics of antineoplastic agents vary widely among patients receiving the same calculated dose of drug, resulting in marked differences in drug exposure. Cell-cycle kinetics also differ widely, potentially modulating the effectiveness of agents such as ara-C that are largely S-phase–specific.[297] Similarly, there are potential differences in drug transport across leukemia cell membranes and variations among patients, and among individual leukemia cells within a given patient, in the cellular pharmacology of different antineoplastic agents. The ability of individual leukemia cells to repair sublethal damage is a critical variable as well. It is also likely that ultimately drug resistance is conferred by properties of a small fraction of leukemia cells, presumably that fraction capable of efficient self-renewal.[298,299] Investigations of these leukemia "stem cells" have been hampered by difficulties in reliably and repeatedly cloning leukemic cells from individual patients to allow serial studies to be performed. In addition, a potential sampling bias exists in that the in vitro results are a reflection only of the characteristics of cells obtained at a single point in time that can grow in an artificial environment. Nonetheless, there is considerable interest in the development of drugs which may preferentially target these cells.[300]

Despite these problems, there have been many important studies done in the area of leukemia drug resistance. Changes in ara-C dose and schedule as well as modifiers of nucleotide metabolism or the cell cycle such as thymidine, l-asparaginase, and fludarabine[301-303] have been evaluated as a means of increasing the amount and rate of incorporation of ara-C into DNA, which appears to be the ultimate lethal event. Except for the apparent beneficial effects of very high-dose ara-C, these maneuvers have not resulted in unequivocal improvement in the therapeutic index.

The multidrug resistance (MDR) phenotype is associated in most cases with increased amounts of a membrane glycoprotein (p-170), which serves as a pump accelerating the efflux of a wide variety of agents, including the anthracycline antibiotics, vincristine, taxanes, and mitoxantrone.[304] Levels of p-170 can be assessed by immunoperoxidase studies of individual AML cells, Western blots of cell preparations, and indirectly by mRNA levels and gene expression and are increased in patients refractory to chemotherapy.[305,306] The MDR phenotype is most common in patients with relapsed or refractory disease, older patients, and those with other adverse prognostic factors.[307-309]

Incubation with a variety of compounds in vitro, including calcium channel blockers verapamil, quinine, and cyclosporine A, can reverse the effect of the p-170.[309] Cardiotoxicity occurs at the doses of verapamil required to produce this effect. Cyclosporine can reverse the MDR phenotype in vitro at drug levels that are likely to be clinically acceptable in terms of toxicity. A randomized trial of the addition of cyclosporin A to an ara-C plus continuous-infusion daunorubicin regimen for patients with relapsed AML suggested an overall survival benefit for adults in the experimental arm.[310] PSC–833 is a more potent nonimmunosuppressive cyclosporine analogue, which has been evaluated in randomized trials as an adjunct to standard therapy. Unfortunately, no improvement in CR rates was seen, with some trials demonstrating increased toxicity in the PSC833 recipients.[311-314] Because of their effects on normal tissues such as the liver and kidney, these modulators also affect the pharmacokinetics of antineoplastic agents, such that the dosage of anthracyclines or etoposide usually have to be attenuated if given with an MDR modulator.[315]

P-glycoprotein is unlikely to represent the only mechanism of drug resistance in patients with AML. Preliminary evidence suggests over-expression of the multidrug-resistance protein (MRP) and breast cancer resistance protein (BCRP) in cells from some patients with AML, particularly in samples from patients in relapse.[316,317] Thus, intervention to circumvent resistance might best be applied during initial treatment prior to the enrichment of subpopulations resistant by other mechanisms. Additional trials with these and other MDR modulators, some of which have less effect on chemotherapy drug metabolism,[318,319] are in progress but overall, attempts to modify drug efflux mechanisms of resistance have been disappointing.

Minimal-Residual Disease (MRD)

A number of techniques can detect residual leukemia cells in patients in morphologic CR, including (in approximate descending order of sensitivity) conventional cytogenetics,[320] Southern blotting for known gene rearrangements, fluorescent in situ hybridization (FISH), multiparameter flow cytometry, and RT-PCR.[321,322] Serial measurement of MRD is an important component of the management of APL[86] and chronic myelogeneous leukemia, is being used more frequently in childhood ALL, but is not sufficiently standardized to be used in other patients with AML.[323] Technical problems abound, including the requirement for a known and already cloned abnormality when applying molecular techniques and the potential for changes in antigen expression over time when using immunologic monitoring. There are few large prospective studies available. Although preliminary data tend to be compatible with the logical premise that persistence of detectable disease presages eventual relapse, false-positive (see comments on t(8;21) above)[73] and false-negative rates may be appreciable and could result in incorrect decisions about further treatment. Serial monitoring is cumbersome, and it is hoped that future studies will determine specific time points after completion of therapy when detection of MRD is prognostically significant. It is also likely that different sampling strategies will be needed for different AML subtypes. The key clinical question is whether intervention with further therapy or allogeneic SCT will be of value if applied earlier, prior to gross relapse. There are no data addressing this issue. Because of the presence of residual disease, autologous collection and high-dose therapy may be predicted to be of less value in this circumstance. Indeed, patients with APL who are in morphologic and cytogenetic CR but are positive for PML/ RAR-α by RT-PCR have a high rate of relapse after autologous transplantation.[271]

Complications

Hyperleukocytosis

Leukemic blasts are considerably less deformable than mature myeloid cells[324] and are "stickier" than lymphoblasts because of the expression of cell surface adhesion molecules. With increasing blast counts, usually at levels greater than 100,000/μL in the myeloid leukemias, blood flow in the microcirculation can be impeded by plugs of these more rigid cells. Local hypoxemia may be exacerbated by the high metabolic activity of the dividing blasts, with endothelial damage and hemorrhage. The situation can be worsened by red blood cell transfusions that rapidly increase whole-blood viscosity in the presence of hyperleukocytosis, thereby further compromising local blood flow. Red blood cell transfusions should, therefore, be administered very slowly or, if possible, withheld until the blast count is reduced. Coagulation abnormalities, including disseminated intravascular coagulation, further increase the risk of local hemorrhage. Liberal use of platelet transfusions is recommended, particularly since the platelet count is frequently overestimated because of the presence of fragments of blasts on blood smears, which can be mistakenly counted as platelets by automated blood cell counters.[325]

Although pathologic evidence of leukostasis can be found in most organs in patients with extremely high blast cell counts, clinical symptomatology is usually related to CNS and pulmonary involvement.[101,326,327] Occasionally, dyspnea with worsening hypoxemia can occur following therapy and lysis of trapped leukemic cells. Spurious elevation of serum potassium can occur because of the release from WBCs during clotting, and it is sometimes necessary to measure potassium levels on heparinized plasma. Similarly, pO2 can appear falsely decreased because of the enhanced metabolic activity of the WBCs, even when the specimen is appropriately placed on ice during transport to the laboratory. Pulse oximetry provides an accurate assessment of O2 saturation in such circumstances. Hyperleukocytosis is more common in patients with myelomonocytic or monocytic leukemia, and it is possible that the clinical manifestations are exacerbated by the migration of leukemic promonocytes into tissue where further proliferation occurs.[103]

The initial mortality rate for patients with AML and symptomatic hyperleukocytosis is high.[101,327] If patients survive the initial period, they tend to have somewhat lower remission rates and shorter CR durations. Symptomatic hyperleukocytosis in AML (and rarely in ALL) constitutes a medical emergency, and efforts should be made to lower the WBC count rapidly. In most patients, rapid cytoreduction can be achieved by chemotherapy, with either standard induction agents or with high doses of hydroxyurea (3 g/m^2/day). Some centers also advocate low-dose cranial irradiation, including the retina, in order to prevent further proliferation of leukemic cells in CNS sites where drug delivery may theoretically be compromised. This treatment is well tolerated, although there are no comparative studies to determine whether the results are superior to chemotherapy alone.

In some patients, it is impossible to initiate chemotherapy immediately because of renal insufficiency, metabolic problems, delays in initiating allopurinol therapy so as to prevent hyperuricemia, or similar considerations. In such patients, emergency leukapheresis has been used to lower or stabilize the white count.[328,329] Although intensive leukapheresis, with procedure times often lasting many hours, can produce improvement of pulmonary and CNS symptomatology, there are theoretic and practical limitations to its benefits. It is difficult, for example, for leukapheresis to affect already established vascular plugs, particularly if vascular invasion has taken place. In such cases, chemotherapy is the primary modality, although theoretically, leukapheresis could decrease further accumulation of leukocytes at these sites. Furthermore, it is precisely the patient in whom leukostasis is most likely to occur, that is, the patient with high and rapidly rising blasts counts, in whom the technical limitations of leukapheresis are apparent, in that it is often difficult, even with highly efficient cell separators, to reduce the rising count. In such patients with a high proliferative thrust, cycle-specific chemotherapeutic agents are more likely to be most immediately effective. Leukapheresis is also of modest benefit to patients who develop pulmonary problems during cytotoxic treatment, since in some such patients the symptoms are related at least in part to a local inflammatory response following leukocyte lysis.

Central Nervous System Leukemia

Involvement of the CNS is considerably less common in patients with AML than in both adults and children with ALL. Most clinicians have the impression that the incidence has decreased even further in recent years, perhaps related to the use of higher doses of ara-C, which can penetrate into the CNS. The incidence of CNS leukemia has been less than 5% in large AML clinical trials in recent years. Therefore, diagnostic lumbar punctures are not routinely indicated in the absence of CNS symptoms, and chemotherapy regimens do not include CNS prophylaxis. The most common symptoms are consequences of increased intracranial pressure and usually consist of a constant headache, sometimes associated with lethargy or other mental changes. Cranial nerve signs (most commonly cranial nerves III or VI) and, occasionally, peripheral nerve manifestations are secondary to nerve root involvement and can be accompanied by headaches or occur alone.[330]

The diagnosis is usually easily confirmed by examination of cytocentrifuge preparations of cerebrospinal fluid (CSF) after lumbar puncture. Cell counts can vary from as few as 5/μL to >1000. Most patients have moderate elevations in CSF protein with a moderate decrease in glucose. After the administration of intrathecal therapy, cytocentrifuge preparations can demonstrate reactive ependymal cells that can be difficult to distinguish from leukemia cells, particularly if the leukocyte count is low. Treatment consists of the administration of intrathecal chemotherapy, with the addition of cranial radiation (usually 2400 cGy), to patients who do not respond fully to chemotherapy or in whom cranial nerve involvement is present.[330] Either methotrexate (15 mg/dose when administered by lumbar puncture) or ara-C (50 mg/dose) can be used as initial therapy, with a crossover to the other agents in the event of refractoriness or relapse. A typical schedule includes treatment 2-3 times a week until the CSF has cleared, generally occurring after a few injections. Treatment is then given at weekly intervals for two more doses to be followed by monthly administration for a total of a year. An Ommaya reservoir to permit intraventricular drug administration is frequently needed either because of difficulties in performing repeated lumbar punctures or because of concern that in some individuals, the CSF flow does not deliver sufficient amounts of the drug from the lumbar space to the entire CNS. Successful therapy with systemically administered agents that penetrate the CNS, such as diaziquone (AZQ), high-dose methotrexate, or high-dose ara-C, have also been reported.[331] Slow-release ("depo") preparations of ara-C may be an alternative.[332] Unfortunately, the relapse rate is high, either in association with bone marrow relapse or independently, even after initial successful therapy.

It has been suggested that the incidence of CNS leukemia is higher in patients with FAB M4 E0 morphology and possibly in patients with monocytic leukemia and high circulating blast counts.[333] This may no longer be the case using more contemporary treatment regimens, and prophylactic therapy is not indicated in such individuals. Recent studies have suggested that CNS involvement occurs frequently in patients with APL in relapse and some clinicians administer CNS prophylaxis when second CR is achieved.

Ophthalmic Complications

Essentially every ocular structure can be involved in the leukemias, sometimes dominating the clinical picture in the prechemotherapy era.[334] Leukemia cells can infiltrate the conjunctiva and lacrimal glands, producing obvious masses that may require treatment with radiation therapy. Involvement of the choroid and retina is most common, however. A prospective study of 53 newly diagnosed adults with AML documented retinal or optic nerve abnormalities in 64% of patients.[335] Hemorrhage and cotton-wool spots (a consequence of nerve fiber ischemia) were most frequent, and the occurrence of these findings was unrelated to patient age, FAB type, WBC count or hematocrit. Initial platelet counts were lower in patients with retinopathy. Ten patients had decreased visual acuity, including five with macular hemorrhages. It was felt that many of the cotton-wool spots were either a consequence of or exacerbated by ischemia due to anemia. Definite leukemic infiltrate of the retina could not be confirmed. All patients received aggressive chemotherapy and platelet transfusion support; no patient received cranial or ocular irradiation. All ocular findings resolved in patients achieving CR and there was no residual visual deficit in any patient. Infectious ocular problems were not noted and seem to be uncommon, perhaps because the prompt empiric use of antibacterial and antifungal antibiotics has decreased the possibility of hematogenous spread of infections to the eye.

Pregnancy

AML is occasionally diagnosed during pregnancy, either because of clinical manifestations or as an incidental finding during blood count checks. If detected during the first trimester, termination of pregnancy followed by treatment of the leukemia is advisable. The management of patients diagnosed later in pregnancy, such as late in the second trimester or during the third trimester, is more problematic. If the leukemia is relatively indolent, it is sometimes possible to manage patients conservatively with leukapheresis and/or transfusion with induction of labor and delivery of the fetus as soon as possible.[336] There have also been many reports of patients treated with chemotherapy later in their pregnancy.[337,338] The majority of these women have not aborted, and there have been no reports of leukemia occurring in the children or an increased incidence of abnormalities in the infants.

Metabolic Abnormalities

Patients receiving therapy for AML can experience a wide range of metabolic problems as a consequence like vomiting, diarrhea, impaired nutrition, or renal dysfunction, usually because of side effects from antibiotics, particularly amphotericin B. Some metabolic disorders are related to the leukemic process itself. Hyperuricemia, occasionally accompanied by urate nephropathy with renal insufficiency, is the most frequent metabolic accompaniment of AML. All patients should receive allopurinol, 300 mg/day or more, as soon as the diagnosis of acute leukemia is established, so that chemotherapy can be administered as soon as is medically appropriate. In most patients, urate nephropathy can be avoided or ameliorated with vigorous hydration and urinary alkalization with systemic or oral administration of sodium bicarbonate. Allopurinol can usually be discontinued within a day or two after chemotherapy is completed. In occasional patients with markedly elevated levels of uric acid, the use of recombinant urate oxidase, which can rapidly lower levels within a few hours, may be advisable.[339] A single dose is almost always sufficient with the decision about subsequent doses dependent on serial monitoring of uric acid.[340]

Tumor lysis syndrome occurs more frequently in patients with ALL, although some AML patients experience hyperphosphatemia, hypocalcemia, hyperkalemia, and renal insufficiency as a consequence of massive leukemic cell death. The inciting cause seems to be release of large amounts of phosphate from lyzed blasts, which coprecipitates with calcium in the kidneys, leading to hypocalcemia and sometimes to oliguric renal failure. Hyperuricemia further contributes to this problem, which is usually self-limited and responds to judicious hydration.

Despite markedly hypercellular marrows, hypercalcemia is extremely unusual in patients with AML. Severe, occasionally symptomatic, hypokalemia is not infrequent, particularly in patients with monocytic leukemias. The mechanism appears to be renal potassium loss because of tubular damage induced by the high levels of lysozyme often noted in these patients.[104] Aggressive replacement with parenteral potassium is required; the syndrome usually abates after cytoreduction by chemotherapy. Lastly, rare patients have been described in whom lactic acidosis has been a constant metabolic accompaniment of the leukemia both at the time of presentation and relapse.[341] The mechanism is unclear, although anaerobic metabolism by the leukemia cells at sites of leukostasis has been postulated.

Summary

Largely because of improvements in supportive care and the anticipatory management of complications of the treatment and underlying disease, the overall outlook for adults with AML has improved throughout the world. It is equally clear, however, that results have leveled off and that new approaches are needed to increase the fraction of patients cured. Dramatic advances in molecular genetics offer promise both because of increased understanding of leukemia biology and the production of small molecules, monoclonal antibodies, cytokines and HGF with potential clinical utility. Further clarification of mechanisms of drug resistance with the possibility of enhancement of the effectiveness of currently available drugs is also an exciting and achievable prospect. These strategies, as well as clinical trials designed to assess the appropriate use of SCT and newer chemotherapeutic drugs, provide the hope that therapy for AML will be both more successful and less empiric in the future.

Mast Cell Leukemia and Other Mast Cell Neoplasms

Mast cell disorders are classified amongst the myeloproliferative diseases and produce a wide spectrum of clinical findings, ranging from reactive benign syndromes with cutaneous involvement to malignant variants with mast cell infiltration of multiple organs, including the bone marrow.[342,343]

Reactive Mast Cell Hyperplasia

Mast cell hyperplasia frequently occurs in tissues involved in immediate or delayed-type hypersensitivity reactions, such as in the nasal mucosa during allergic rhinitis. Increased numbers of mast cells in the bone marrow have been noted in association with a wide range of malignant disorders, including lymphoproliferative disorders,[344] hairy cell leukemia,[345] and myeloid neoplasms.[346,347] The mast cells in such patients appear to be reactive rather than derived from the malignant clone.

Neoplastic Mast Cell Disease

Urticaria pigmentosa is by far the most common manifestation of neoplastic mast cell proliferation.[348] The typical eruption of urticaria pigmentosa consists of multiple discrete hyperpigmented nodulopapular lesions and portends a benign clinical course, especially in children. Cutaneous symptoms may include the classic urticarial wheals that result from mast cell degranulation in response to mechanical insult (Darier's sign), pruritus or episodic flushing. A blurred distinction exists between cutaneous mastocytosis (CM)[349] and systemic mast cell disease (SMCD), an indolent disorder in which mast cells may also be found in extracutaneous sites. The serum tryptase level is higher in SMCD than in CM.[350] Systemic mastocytosis may present with a variety of constitutional and/or gastrointestinal symptoms, each of which can be attributed to excessive elaboration of mast cell mediators. Such symptoms, which may also present to a lesser degree in patients with urticaria pigmentosa, include rhinitis, asthma, nausea, vomiting, diarrhea, syncope, chest pain, bone pain, and rectal discomfort.[351] The bony skeleton, the gastrointestinal tract and the spleen can also be sites of mast cell infiltration.

Malignant mastocytosis is more aggressive subset of SCMD characterized by a much less favorable clinical course.[351] Unlike indolent systemic mastocytosis, in which an affected patient has a normal life expectancy, survival beyond 1-2 years after diagnosis of malignant mastocytosis is uncommon. The bone marrow is always involved, eosinophilia and cytopenias are common, and adenopathy and/or organomegaly are frequently noted.[352] In the early 1990s, it was recognized that mast cells from patients with systemic mastocytosis are capable of growing independent of stimulation with C-KIT ligand, the critical mast cell growth factor.[353] Cell lines and patient samples demonstrated that the basis for this growth independence was constitutive activation of C-KIT,[354,355] most often associated with a mutation at codon 816 in the kinase domain, although juxtamembrane region mutations have also been described.[356] The ASP-816 VAL mutation has been detected in both B cells and monocytes from patients, suggesting that systemic mastocytosis is a clonal disorder evolving from an early hematopoietic stem cell.[356,357] In contrast, blasts from patients with mast cell leukemia do not have this mutation, suggesting an alternative derivation of the leukemia.[358]

Mast cell leukemia represents a rare and aggressive subtype of malignant mastocytosis characterized by the presence of large numbers of atypical mast cells in the peripheral blood.[359-361] Patients with mast cell leukemia have a median survival of less than 6 months, in contrast to those with the nonleukemic type of malignant mastocytosis, who tend to survive for a longer time. The majority of reported cases of mast cell leukemia arise in patients with preexisting malignant mast cell disease. Criteria required for the diagnosis of mast cell leukemia are: (1) the percentage of mast cells in the peripheral WBC differential must be 10% or greater; (2) the leukemic mast cells should display features of morphologic atypia; and (3) cytochemical properties of the leukemic cells must be typical of mast cell derivation (presence of metachromatic granules staining with chloroacetate esterase, but not with peroxidase).[360]

Although bone marrow infiltration with atypical mast cells is always present in mast cell leukemia, hematologic findings at the time of diagnosis can vary widely. A mild to moderate degree of anemia is always present; initial leukocyte counts can range from normal to >50,000/µL.[360] The percentage of atypical mast cells (hypogranulated metachromatically staining cells with fragmentation, cytoplasmic tails, and multiple nuclei) may be relatively low (but greater than 10%), but almost always increases substantially with time. Karyotypic studies in several patients with mast cell leukemia have been normal, although the lack of dividing cells for metaphase analysis frequently precludes cytogenetic evaluation. Bone marrow cells from patients with systemic mastocytosis often display cytogenetic abnormalities, such as trisomy 8, monosomy 7/7q-, 20q-, typical of those with myeloproliferative disorders.[359,361] Particularly in patients with concomitant eosinophilia, it is important to exclude cytogenetic abnormalities affecting PDGFR (involving chromosome 5q31-32), since such patients can benefit from treatment with imatinib.

Treatment

Treatment of mast cell neoplasms is based on the disease subtype and clinical manifestations. Patients with cutaneous mastocytosis usually require no treatment. Systemic mast cell disease, however, has protean clinical manifestations. For example, those with hematological abnormalities may require supportive care, which could include transfusions or the empiric use of hematopoietic growth factors. Avoidance of mast cell stimulants such as anesthesia, alcohol, aspirin and morphine may diminish flushing, pruritus and diarrhea, symptoms that may be histamine related.[362-364] H1 and H2 antihistamines or disodium chromoglycolate may offer palliative benefit. Radiation therapy may control localized disease without causing histamine release.[365]

Unfortunately, the typical ASP-816 VAL mutation is insensitive to the C-KIT inhibitors imatinib mesylate[355,366,367]and nilotinib,[368] although in vitro studies suggest that there this mutated C-KIT may be sensitive to dasatinib[369] and clinical trials with dasatinib and other tyrosine kinase inhibitors are in progress.[370,371] Preclinical data suggest that the multitargeted-kinase inhibitor, PKC412, may also inhibit the product of this activating mutation and early reports suggest potential clinical activity.[372,373]

Cladribine and alpha interferon have cytoreductive activity in systemic mastocytosis and should be considered in patients with active systemic symptoms.[371,374] Responses are usually transient however, and subsequent therapy for those with malignant mastocytosis or frank mast cell leukemia (activating mutations of c-kit are not believed to occur in this entity) is not at all standardized, although induction therapy with an anthracycline in combination with cytarabine for patients with leukemia could be followed by consolidation with high-dose ara-C. Allogeneic hematopoietic stem cell transplantation could be considered in the appropriate patient, although there is limited experience with this approach.

Selected References

The complete reference list can be found at www.CANCERMEDICINE8.com

1. Cheson BD, Bennett JM, Kopecky KJ, et al. Revised recommendations of the International Working Group for Diagnosis, Standardization of Response Criteria, Treatment Outcomes, and Reporting Standards for Therapeutic Trials in Acute Myeloid Leukemia. *J Clin Oncol*. 2003;21:4642–4649.

8. Bacher U, Haferlach C, Kern W, Haferlach T, Schnittger S. Prognostic relevance of FLT3-TKD mutations in AML: the combination matters—an analysis of 3082 patients. *Blood*. 2008;111:2527–2537.

17. Austin H, Delzell E, Cole P. Benzene and leukemia. A review of the literature and a risk assessment. *Am J Epidemiol*. 1988;127:419–439.

27. Smith ML, Cavenagh JD, Lister TA, Fitzgibbon J. Mutation of CEBPA in familial acute myeloid leukemia. *N Engl J Med*. 2004;351:2403–2407.

32. Vardiman JW, Thiele J, Arber DA, Brunning RD, Borowitz MJ, Porwit A, Harris NL, Le Beau MM, Hellström-Lindberg E, Tefferi A, Bloomfield CD. *Blood. 2009 Jul 30;114:937-51.*

36. Fialkow PJ, Singer JW, Adamson JW, et al. Acute nonlymphocytic leukemia: heterogeneity of stem cell origin. *Blood*. 1981;57:1068–1073.

44. Schlenk RF, Dohner K, Krauter J, et al. Mutations and treatment outcome in cytogenetically normal acute myeloid leukemia. *N Engl J Med*. 2008;358:1909–1918.

53. Langer C, Radmacher MD, Ruppert AS, et al. High BAALC expression associates with other molecular prognostic markers, poor outcome and a distinct gene-expression signature in cytogenetically normal acute myeloid leukemia: a Cancer and Leukemia Group B (CALGB) study. *Blood*. 2008.

59. Valk PJ, Verhaak RG, Beijen MA, et al. Prognostically useful gene-expression profiles in acute myeloid leukemia. *N Engl J Med*. 2004;350:1617–1628.

60. Marcucci G, Radmacher MD, Maharry K, et al. MicroRNA expression in cytogeneti-

cally normal acute myeloid leukemia. *N Engl J Med*. 2008;358:1919–1928.
68. Bloomfield CD, Lawrence D, Byrd JC, et al. Frequency of prolonged remission duration after high-dose cytarabine intensification in acute myeloid leukemia varies by cytogenetic subtype. *Cancer Res*. 1998;58:4173–4179.
70. Downing JR, Head DR, Curcio-Brint AM, et al. An AML1/ETO fusion transcript is consistently detected by RNA-based polymerase chain reaction in acute myelogenous leukemia containing the (8;21)(q22;q22) translocation. *Blood*. 1993;81:2860–2865.
81. Sanz MA, Tallman MS, Lo-Coco F. Tricks of the trade for the appropriate management of newly diagnosed acute promyelocytic leukemia. *Blood*. 2005;105:3019–3025.
83. Larson RA, Kondo K, Vardiman JW, Butler AE, Golomb HM, Rowley JD. Evidence for a 15;17 translocation in every patient with acute promyelocytic leukemia. *Am J Med*. 1984;76:827–841.
95. Hogge DE, Misawa S, Parsa NZ, Pollak A, Testa JR. Abnormalities of chromosome 16 in association with acute myelomonocytic leukemia and dysplastic bone marrow eosinophils. *J Clin Oncol*. 1984;2:550–557.
96. Byrd JC, Ruppert AS, Mrozek K, et al. Repetitive cycles of high-dose cytarabine benefit patients with acute myeloid leukemia and inv(16)(p13q22) or t(16;16)(p13;q22): results from CALGB 8461. *J Clin Oncol*. 2004;22:1087–1094.
98. Schlenk RF, Benner A, Krauter J, et al. Individual patient data-based meta-analysis of patients aged 16 to 60 years with core binding factor acute myeloid leukemia: a survey of the German Acute Myeloid Leukemia Intergroup. *J Clin Oncol*. 2004;22:3741–3750.
111. Byrd JC, Mrozek K, Dodge RK, et al. Pretreatment cytogenetic abnormalities are predictive of induction success, cumulative incidence of relapse, and overall survival in adult patients with de novo acute myeloid leukemia: results from Cancer and Leukemia Group B (CALGB 8461). *Blood*. 2002;100:4325–4336.
115. Bitter MA, Neilly ME, Le Beau MM, Pearson MG, Rowley JD. Rearrangements of chromosome 3 involving bands 3q21 and 3q26 are associated with normal or elevated platelet counts in acute nonlymphocytic leukemia. *Blood*. 1985;66:1362–1370.
118. Suzukawa K, Parganas E, Gajjar A, et al. Identification of a breakpoint cluster region 3′ of the ribophorin I gene at 3q21 associated with the transcriptional activation of the EVI1 gene in acute myelogenous leukemias with inv(3)(q21q26). *Blood*. 1994;84:2681–2688.
137. Estey E, Smith TL, Keating MJ, McCredie KB, Gehan EA, Freireich EJ. Prediction of survival during induction therapy in patients with newly diagnosed acute myeloblastic leukemia. *Leukemia*. 1989;3:257–263.
141. Grimwade D, Walker H, Harrison G, et al. The predictive value of hierarchical cytogenetic classification in older adults with acute myeloid leukemia (AML): analysis of 1065 patients entered into the United Kingdom Medical Research Council AML11 trial. *Blood*. 2001;98:1312–1220.
145. Yates JW, Wallace HJ, Jr., Ellison RR, Holland JF. Cytosine arabinoside (NSC-63878) and daunorubicin (NSC-83142) therapy in acute nonlymphocytic leukemia. *Cancer Chemother Rep*. 1973;57:485–488.
150. Preisler HD, Anderson K, Rai K, et al. The frequency of long-term remission in patients with acute myelogenous leukaemia treated with conventional maintenance chemotherapy: a study of 760 patients with a minimal follow-up time of 6 years. *Br J Haematol*. 1989;71:189–194.
152. Arlin Z, Case DC, Jr., Moore J, et al. Randomized multicenter trial of cytosine arabinoside with mitoxantrone or daunorubicin in previously untreated adult patients with acute nonlymphocytic leukemia (ANLL). Lederle Cooperative Group. *Leukemia*. 1990;4:177–183.
156. Wiernik PH, Banks PL, Case DC, Jr., et al. Cytarabine plus idarubicin or daunorubicin as induction and consolidation therapy for previously untreated adult patients with acute myeloid leukemia. *Blood*. 1992;79:313–319.
160. Weick JK, Kopecky KJ, Appelbaum FR, et al. A randomized investigation of high-dose versus standard-dose cytosine arabinoside with daunorubicin in patients with previously untreated acute myeloid leukemia: a Southwest Oncology Group study. *Blood*. 1996;88:2841–2851.
176. Burnett AK, Milligan D, Prentice AG, et al. A comparison of low-dose cytarabine and hydroxyurea with or without all-trans retinoic acid for acute myeloid leukemia and high-risk myelodysplastic syndrome in patients not considered fit for intensive treatment. *Cancer*. 2007;109:1114–1124.
191. Mayer RJ, Davis RB, Schiffer CA, et al. Intensive postremission chemotherapy in adults with acute myeloid leukemia. Cancer and Leukemia Group B. *N Engl J Med*. 1994;331:896–903.
197. Moore JO, Dodge RK, Amrein PC, et al. Granulocyte-colony stimulating factor (filgrastim) accelerates granulocyte recovery after intensive postremission chemotherapy for acute myeloid leukemia with aziridinyl benzoquinone and mitoxantrone: Cancer and Leukemia Group B study 9022. *Blood*. 1997;89:780–788.
201. Thomas ED, Buckner CD, Clift RA, et al. Marrow transplantation for acute nonlymphoblastic leukemia in first remission. *N Engl J Med*. 1979;301:597–599.
202. Yeager AM, Kaizer H, Santos GW, et al. Autologous bone marrow transplantation in patients with acute nonlymphocytic leukemia, using ex vivo marrow treatment with 4-hydroperoxycyclophosphamide. *N Engl J Med*. 1986;315:141–147.
210. Cassileth PA, Harrington DP, Appelbaum FR, et al. Chemotherapy compared with autologous or allogeneic bone marrow transplantation in the management of acute myeloid leukemia in first remission. *N Engl J Med*. 1998;339:1649–1656.
219. Tallman MS, Kopecky KJ, Amos D, et al. Analysis of prognostic factors for the outcome of marrow transplantation or further chemotherapy for patients with acute nonlymphocytic leukemia in first remission. *J Clin Oncol*. 1989;7:326–337.
224. Slovak ML, Kopecky KJ, Cassileth PA, et al. Karyotypic analysis predicts outcome of preremission and postremission therapy in adult acute myeloid leukemia: a Southwest Oncology Group/Eastern Cooperative Oncology Group Study. *Blood*. 2000;96:4075–4083.
237. Schiffer CA, Lee EJ. Approaches to the therapy of relapsed acute myeloid leukemia. *Oncology (Williston Park)*. 1989;3:23–27; discussion 8.
245. Larson RA, Sievers EL, Stadtmauer EA, et al. Final report of the efficacy and safety of gemtuzumab ozogamicin (Mylotarg) in patients with CD33-positive acute myeloid leukemia in first recurrence. *Cancer*. 2005;104:1442–1452.
248. Huang ME, Ye YC, Chen SR, et al. Use of all-trans retinoic acid in the treatment of acute promyelocytic leukemia. *Blood*. 1988;72:567–572.
255. Tallman MS, Andersen JW, Schiffer CA, et al. All-trans-retinoic acid in acute promyelocytic leukemia. *N Engl J Med*. 1997;337:1021–1028.
257. Fenaux P, Chevret S, Guerci A, et al. Long-term follow-up confirms the benefit of all-trans retinoic acid in acute promyelocytic leukemia. European APL group. *Leukemia*. 2000;14:1371–1377.
265. Soignet SL, Frankel SR, Douer D, et al. United States multicenter study of arsenic trioxide in relapsed acute promyelocytic leukemia. *J Clin Oncol*. 2001;19:3852–3860.
269. Estey E, Garcia-Manero G, Ferrajoli A, et al. Use of all-trans retinoic acid plus arsenic trioxide as an alternative to chemotherapy in untreated acute promyelocytic leukemia. *Blood*. 2006;107:3469–3473.
273. Stone RM, Berg DT, George SL, et al. Granulocyte-macrophage colony-stimulating factor after initial chemotherapy for elderly patients with primary acute myelogenous leukemia. Cancer and Leukemia Group B. *N Engl J Med*. 1995;332:1671–1677.
280. Schiffer CA. Hematopoietic growth factors as adjuncts to the treatment of acute myeloid leukemia. *Blood*. 1996;88:3675–3685.
312. Baer MR, George SL, Dodge RK, et al. Phase 3 study of the multidrug resistance modulator PSC-833 in previously untreated patients 60 years of age and older with acute myeloid leukemia: Cancer and Leukemia Group B Study 9720. *Blood*. 2002;100:1224–1232.
335. Karesh JW, Goldman EJ, Reck K, Kelman SE, Lee EJ, Schiffer CA. A prospective ophthalmic evaluation of patients with acute myeloid leukemia: correlation of ocular and hematologic findings. *J Clin Oncol*. 1989;7:1528–1532.
339. Pui CH, Jeha S, Irwin D, Camitta B. Recombinant urate oxidase (rasburicase) in the prevention and treatment of malignancy-associated hyperuricemia in pediatric and adult patients: results of a compassionate-use trial. *Leukemia*. 2001;15:1505–1509.
343. Valent P, Akin C, Escribano L, et al. Standards and standardization in mastocytosis: consensus statements on diagnostics, treatment recommendations and response criteria. *Eur J Clin Invest*. 2007;37:435–453.
356. Garcia-Montero AC, Jara-Acevedo M, Teodosio C, et al. KIT mutation in mast cells and other bone marrow hematopoietic cell lineages in systemic mast cell disorders: a prospective study of the Spanish Network on Mastocytosis (REMA) in a series of 113 patients. *Blood*. 2006;108:2366–2372.
371. Tefferi A, Verstovsek S, Pardanani A. How we diagnose and treat WHO-defined systemic mastocytosis in adults. *Haematologica*. 2008;93:6–9.

111 Chronic Myeloid Leukemia

Jorge Cortes, MD ■ Richard T. Silver, MD ■ Hagop M. Kantarjian, MD

Chronic myeloid leukemia (CML) is a clonal proliferative disorder of a pluripotent stem cell involving myeloid, erythroid, megakaryocytic, B, and sometimes T, lymphoid cells, but not marrow fibroblasts. Like polycythemia vera, agnogenic myeloid metaplasia, and essential thrombocythemia, CML is classified as a myeloproliferative disorder, but is distinguished from these diseases by specific cytogenetic and molecular abnormalities. CML is associated with the Philadelphia chromosome (Ph) involving a balanced translocation t(9;22) (q34, q11.2), and the related BCR-ABL chimeric gene.

Advances in understanding the disease pathophysiology and molecular genetics have yielded a wealth of information regarding CML. The efficacy of imatinib mesylate therapy has radically changed the prognosis of CML. With imatinib, the survival in CML has improved from a median of 3-6 years with hydroxyurea and interferon-alpha to an estimated 8-year survival rate of 80-90% (Fig. 111-1). In this chapter we review the hematologic and clinical aspects of CML, its biology, standard therapy including the roles imatinib and allogeneic stem cell transplant (SCT), and new generation tyrosine kinase inhibitors (TKIs; dasatinib, nilotinib, bosutinib) in patients with CML post-failure of imatinib therapy.

Incidence and Epidemiology

The annual incidence of CML is about 10 cases per million. It accounts for 15% of all leukemias.[1,2] It is estimated that 4830 new cases of CML were diagnosed in the United States in 2008 for an incidence of 1.1-1.9:100,000. The prevalence, with older therapies, based on a median survival of 3-6 years was 15,000-30,000 cases. With imatinib, the annual mortality has decreased from 15-20% to 2%, and the estimated median survival may exceed 20 years. Thus, the prevalence of CML in the United States in the next three decades may exceed 200,000 cases. CML will then change from a rare cancer to a relatively common one.

Etiology

In most patients with CML, a causative factor cannot be identified. Ionizing radiation is leukemogenic. The most common type of leukemia following radiation is acute myeloid leukemia, but CML has also been observed in studies following the atomic bomb explosions in Japan in 1945, and in earlier studies in radiologists and in patients with ankylosing spondylitis treated with radiation therapy.[3,4]

Clinical and Hematologic Characteristics

The median age of onset of CML is 55-65 years, and the incidence increases with age. There is slight male preponderance (ratio 1.3:1). CML typically follows a bi- or triphasic course with a chronic phase, followed by an intermediate or accelerated phase, and finally a blastic phase. Approximately 90% of patients are diagnosed in the chronic phase, which is frequently asymptomatic.[5] Symptoms usually develop insidiously and may be due to splenomegaly (pain, abdominal fullness, early satiety) or anemia (fatigue). Less commonly, patients may present with symptoms of gout, anorexia, weight loss, unexplained fever, or signs of platelet dysfunction (eg, petechiae, ecchymoses, or hemorrhage). Leukocytosis is common, with white cell counts frequently higher than 100×10^9/L and occasionally leading to retinal hemorrhage and signs of hyperviscosity (priapism, cerebrovascular accidents, tinnitus, confusion, stupor). Historically, the median survival for patients in chronic phase has been 3-6 years, with an estimated annual risk of transformation to the blastic phase of 5-10% in the first 2 years, and 15-20% subsequently. Accelerated-phase CML is characterized by increasing maturation arrest heralding transformation to the blastic phase. Different criteria have been used to define the accelerated phase. One common classification defines accelerated phase as the presence of any of the following features: 15% or more blasts, 30% or more blasts plus promyelocytes, 20% or more basophils, platelets lower than 100×10^9/L unrelated to therapy, or cytogenetic clonal evolution.[6] Other criteria have been proposed but some of these classifications, such as the World Health Organization (WHO) proposal,[7] have not been clinically validated. The median survival for patients in accelerated phase is 1-2 years,[8] but the criteria used and the therapy implemented (eg, imatinib) may affect the expected survival. Symptoms associated with the accelerated phase may include fever, night sweats, or weight loss, or bleeding associated with thrombocytopenia. Occasionally, blood and bone marrow changes that herald transformation to the accelerated phase occur even in patients who are asymptomatic and identified only during routine follow-up. The blastic phase is defined by the presence of at least 30% of blasts in the peripheral blood or the bone marrow, or the presence of extramedullary disease.[9] The WHO classification has proposed this to be changed to 20% blasts or more, but this may not be justified based on clinical data.[10] The blastic phase of CML is associated with constitutional symptoms (night sweats, weight loss, fever, bone pain), anemia, an increased risk of infections, and/or bleeding. The blastic phase

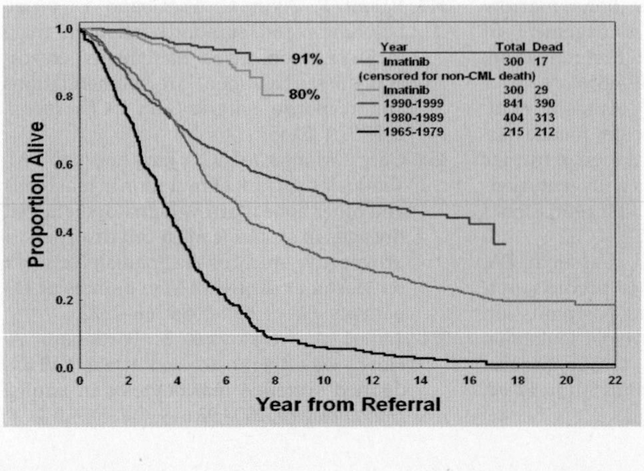

Figure 111-1 ■ Survival of patients with newly diagnosed CML in chronic phase referred to MD Anderson Cancer Center (*N* = 1760; 1965 to present). Censoring from non-CML death (*n* = 12): second cancers—3; old age, Alzheimer—2; cardiac—3; car accident—2; pneumonia, surgical complications—2.

can be classified according to the immunophenotype as myeloid or lymphoid, but biphenotypic or mixed lineage (lymphoblastic-myeloblastic) blastic phase can be observed. Lymphoid blastic phase occurs in 20-30% of patients, myeloid in 50%, and undifferentiated in 25%.[11] The median survival in blastic phase CML is 3-6 months. Patients with lymphoid blastic phase have a better prognosis, with a response rate of 60% to acute lymphoblastic leukemia (ALL)-like therapy, and a median survival of 9-12 months. With imatinib therapy, the median survival in blastic phase has improved to a range of 6-24 months.

Laboratory features in the chronic phase include leukocytosis and a left maturation shift (Fig. 111-2). Basophilia and eosinophilia may be prominent. Thrombocytosis is common but thrombotic phenomena are unusual. A slight degree of anemia is common. There is a reduction in leukocyte alkaline phosphatase (LAP) activity, and a marked elevation of serum B12 levels. An increase in circulating basophils may occur, and it is asociated with poor-prognosis CML or with transformation. Occasionally, with severe basophilia, high histamine levels may be associated with skin rashes, diarrhea, and other histamine-related problems.

The bone marrow is hypercellular. In chronic phase, all stages of differentiation are present, but the myelocytes predominate, whereas myeloblasts and promyelocytes account for <10% of marrow cells (Figs. 111-3 and 111-4). Megakaryocytes may be increased. Cells morphologically indistinguishable from Gaucher cells can be seen in 10% of cases. There is increased reticulin fibrosis, which may worsen with disease progression, and is reversed with imatinib therapy.[12] Marrow fibrosis may be a secondary phenomenon resulting from an abnormal interaction between the proliferative clone of megakaryocytes and elements regulating marrow fibrosis and collagen, including platelet-derived growth factor, transforming growth factor-β, basic fibroblastic growth factor, and other cytokines.[13] End-stage marrow fibrosis is very uncommon in the era of imatinib therapy.

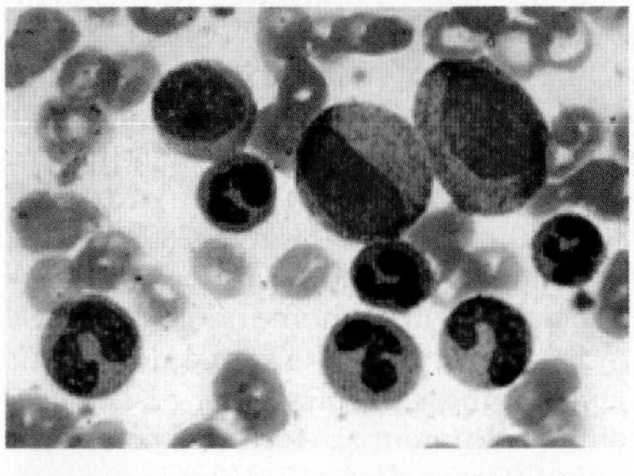

Figure 111-2 Chronic myeloid leukemia. Leukocytosis with myelocytes, metamyelocytes, band cells, and polymorphonuclear leukocytes are characteristics of the peripheral blood in the chronic phase of this disease.

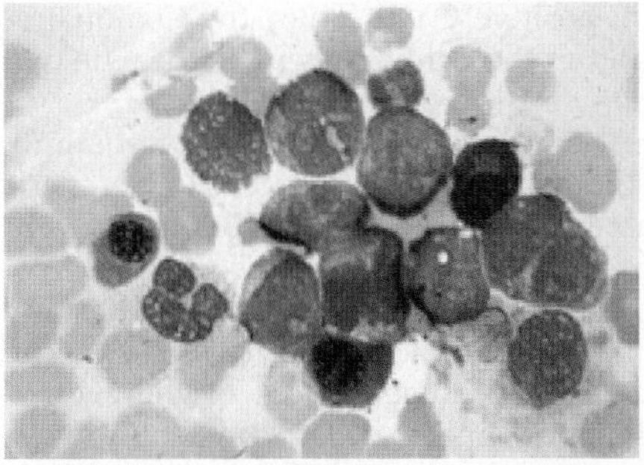

Figure 111-3 Chronic myeloid leukemia, myeloid blast crisis. The marrow aspiration shows predominance of blast forms, which have a myeloid appearance.

In the blastic phase, blasts are increased to 30% or more. Lymphoid blastic cells contain terminal deoxynucleotidyl transferase (TdT), an enzyme that catalyzes the polymerization of deoxynucleoside triphosphates. Lymphoblasts express CD10, CD19, and CD22 or other B-cell markers.[11] T-cell blastic phase occurs in a small proportion of patients. The myeloid blastic phase may mimic acute myeloid leukemia. The myeloblasts stain with myeloperoxidase and express myeloid markers, including CD13, CD33, and CD117.

Rarely, patients may present in lymphoid or myeloid blastic phase without a recognized antecedent chronic phase. The differentiation between this presentation and Ph-positive acute lymphoblastic or myeloid leukemias may be impossible, but the distinction has no clinical value as the treatment and prognosis would be the same. Megakaryoblastic and erythroblastic transformations and blastic phases marked by basophilia and high blood histamine levels are uncommon.

The mechanisms of CML transformation are not understood. Cytogenetic abnormalities, in addition to the Ph chromosome, often develop prior to, or at the time of, transformation, but they may not necessarily be causally related to blastic transformation. Other molecular events, such as alterations of the *TP53* and *p16* genes, may be associated with disease transformation.[14] It has been suggested that granulocyte-macrophage progenitors may be the candidate stem cells in blastic phase CML; activation of β-catenin may enhance the self-renewal activity and leukemic potential of these cells.[15]

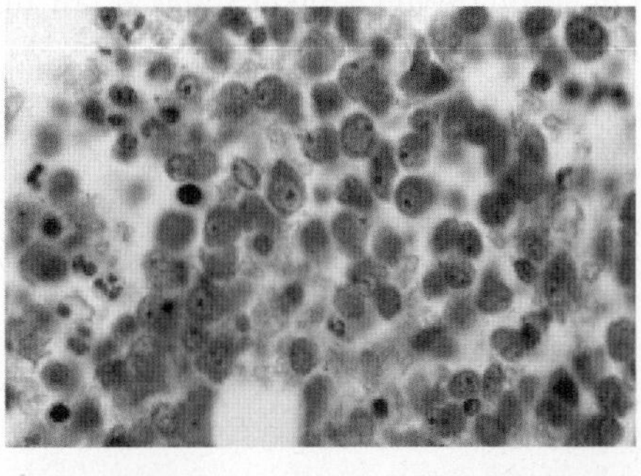

Figure 111-4 Chronic myeloid leukemia, blast phase. This bone marrow biopsy shows "blasts" with prominent nucleoli comprising about 75% of the marrow cells.

In approximately 5-10% of morphologically typical cases of CML the Ph chromosome cannot be identified. A third of these has the associated BCR-ABL molecular abnormality and has similar characteristics, response to imatinib, and prognosis as Ph-positive CML.[16] The other two-thirds lack the BCR-ABL rearrangement and have less characteristic clinical and hematologic features, including lower initial white cell and platelet counts These Ph-negative BCR-ABL negative cases (called "atypical CML" in the WHO classification) have a median survival of 18-24 months.[17] This type of leukemia is not further discussed in this chapter.

Prognostic Classification

Prognosis in CML is variable. Risk classifications have been proposed to stratify patients and assist in treatment decisions. The Sokal model is most frequently used[18] and defines three risk groups, low risk (about 40-50% of all patients), intermediate risk (about 30%), and high risk (10-20%), with median survivals of 4.5, 3.5, and 2.5 years, respectively, with busulfan or hydroxyurea. The model still predicts response to therapy and progression-free survival with imatinib therapy, although outcomes for all risk groups are significantly better than in the past. Other classifications have been proposed that are more applicable to patients treated with interferon-alpha (the Harford score),[19] or specific for transplant (the Gratwohl score).[20] Common poor prognostic factors in CML include older age, splenomegaly, increased blasts or basophils, thrombocytosis, clonal evolution, and fibrosis. With imatinib therapy, the significance of several of these factors (older age, fibrosis, and deletion of derivative 9q) has been reduced or eliminated.[21-23]

Pathophysiology

The characteristic abnormality in CML is an increase in the myeloid component, with a total granulocyte pool 10-150 times normal. This appears to be related to a shift in the number of self-renewal cells toward differentiating cells. The primary biologic defect in CML may be unregulated proliferation of leukemic stem cells, discordant maturation wherein a slight delay in cell maturation within the myeloid compartment results in increased myeloid mass, and a decreased in apoptosis of myeloid cells. Defective adherence of immature CML cells to marrow stromal cells in vitro, increased levels of or sensitivity to granulocyte-macrophage colony-stimulating factor (GMCSF), or decreased levels of sensitivity to inhibitors of myelopoiesis, (acid lactoferrin or prostaglandin E) may also be contributory events.[24-26]

Cytogenetics

The cytogenetic hallmark of CML is the Ph chromosome.[27] This results from a reciprocal translocation following a break on chromosome 9 at band q34.1 that transposes the 3′ segment of the *ABL* gene to the 5′ segment of the *BCR* gene on chromosome 22 at band q11.21, t(9;22)(q34.1;q11.21).[28] This chromosomal abnormality creates the chimeric BCR-ABL oncogene (Fig. 111-5).

The Ph chromosome is found in ~95% of patients with CML. It is also observed in 5% of children and 15-30% of adults with acute lymphoid leukemia and in 2% of patients with newly diagnosed acute myeloid leukemia.[29] In addition, some patients have variant translocations, which may occur in a simple form (involving 22q11 and one additional breakpoint) or a complex form (involving 22q11, 9q34, and at least one additional breakpoint).[30] These patients historically were reported to have an inferior outcome, but with imatinib therapy they have a similar prognosis to patients with the classic Ph chromosome.[31] Approximately 5% of patients with typical morphologic CML lack the Ph chromosome but demonstrate the BCR-ABL rearrangement.[32] The clinical and hematologic characteristics as well as the response to treatment and the course with Ph-negative, BCR-ABL-rearranged CML are the same as that of Ph-positive CML. Thus, the demonstration of the chimeric gene is the sine qua non for the diagnosis of CML.

Progression of CML is frequently accompanied by additional cytogenetic abnormalities. The most common abnormalities include a second Ph chromosome, isochromosome 17, trisomy 8, trisomy 19, and deletion 20q.[33] The molecular consequences of these cytogenetic abnormalities are not always known. Mutations or deletions of tumor-suppressor genes such as p16 and TP53, and hypermethylation or promoter genes such as ABL, BCR, p15, and cadherin-13 are associated with and may contribute to transformation.[34-37]

After successful treatment with imatinib, chromosomal abnormalities may be found in the Ph-negative cells. The most frequently observed abnormalities are trisomy 8, monosomy 7 or 5, and deletion 20q.[38,39] These occur in 5-10% of patients treated with imatinib, and may regress spontaneously (70% of cases). The clinical significance of this finding is unclear. Rare instances of "secondary" acute leukemia or myelodysplastic syndrome have been reported in <1% of all patients treated with imatinib.[40-42] This phenomenon (ie, chromosomal abnormalities in Ph-negative cells) differs from clonal evolution where the same cell expresses both the Ph chromosome and additional chromosomal abnormalities. It may represent a form of karyotypic instability of the primitive marrow stem cell that predisposed to the initial development of CML.

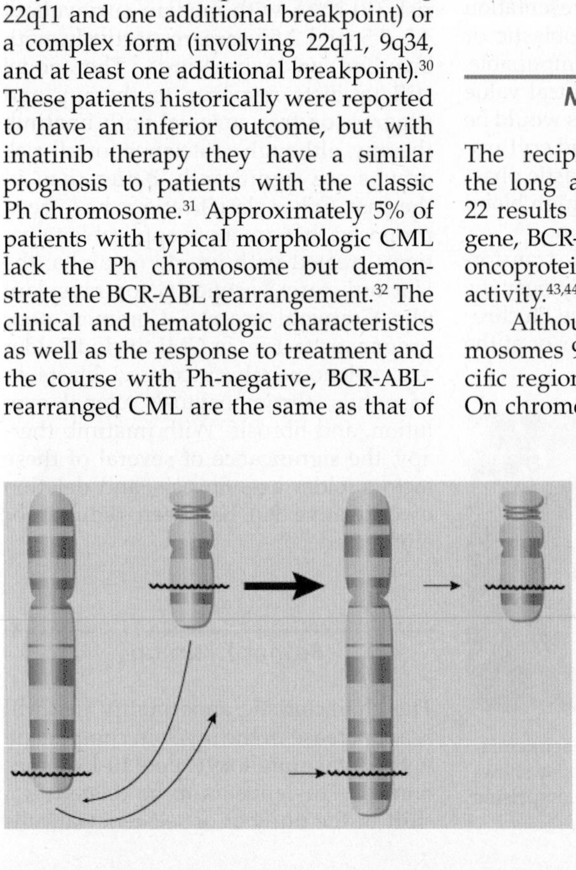

Figure 111-5 ■ Schematic of 9.22 chromosome translocation.

Molecular Biology

The reciprocal translocation between the long arms of chromosomes 9 and 22 results in a fusion or chimeric oncogene, BCR-ABL, that codes for a Bcr-Abl oncoprotein with altered tyrosine kinase activity.[43,44]

Although the breakpoints on chromosomes 9 and 22 are restricted to specific regions, some heterogeneity exists. On chromosome 9, breaks may occur in a region 200 kb or more in length, resulting in most of the c-*abl* gene being translocated.[43] The breakpoints within the *ABL* gene occurs either upstream of exon Ib, downstream of exon Ia, or more frequently, between exons Ib and Ia. Breakpoints occur in most instances in what is known as the major breakpoint cluster region that includes exons e12-e16 (formerly called b1-b5), giving rise to fusion transcripts with either b2a2 or b3a2 junctions both of them generating a 210-kDa protein (p210*BCR-ABL1*). In few patients with CML (but more frequently in Ph-positive ALL) the breakpoint may occur in the minor breakpoint cluster region, resulting in an e1a2 fusion. Less frequently, the breakpoint may occur in a different, more distal breakpoint region, μ-bcr. Variability in the chromosome 9 breakpoints, at least within the major breakpoint cluster region, has no clinical or prognostic consequences.

Depending on the breakpoint in the *BCR* gene, the fusion protein can vary in size from 185 (190) kDa to 230 kDa. Each fusion gene encodes the same portion of the *ABL* gene but differs in the length of *bcr* sequence. Transcription of the fusion BCR-ABL oncogene results in a chimeric BCR-ABL mRNA that is translated into three fusion proteins of varying sizes $p190^{Bcr\text{-}Abl}$, $p210^{Bcr\text{-}Abl}$, and $p230^{Bcr\text{-}Abl}$, according to the breakpoint of the *BCR* gene (Fig. 111-6). These cytoplasmic proteins have unregulated constitutive tyrosine kinase activity and activate a number of intracellular signaling pathways that affect cell proliferation, differentiation, and apoptosis rendering the cell independent of cytokine regulation.[44,45] Among the recognized target proteins are STAT, RAS, RAF, JUN kinase, MYC, AKT, and other signal transducers.

Most patients with typical chronic phase CML express the 210-kDa Bcr-Abl oncoprotein. Two types of BCR-ABL mRNAs occur as a result of bcr breakpoint heterogeneity: b2a2 or b3a2. The clinical features, response to treatment, and prognosis are similar in both groups. Patients with Ph-positive acute lymphocytic leukemia may express either $p210^{Bcr\text{-}Abl}$ (30-50%) or $p190^{Bcr\text{-}Abl}$ (50-70%). Rare patients with CML in chronic phase may express $p190^{Bcr\text{-}Abl}$ and may have a worse prognosis than those with typical $p210^{Bcr\text{-}Abl}$.[46] The larger $p230^{Bcr\text{-}Abl}$ has been rarely reported in CML and may be associated with a more indolent disease and a phenotype more similar to chronic neutrophilic leukemia. That fusion proteins of different sizes can be correlated with different clinical outcomes suggests that $p190^{Bcr\text{-}Abl}$ has more tyrosine kinase activity than $p230^{Bcr\text{-}Abl}$, thus affecting the clinical manifestations of the illness.[47]

Reverse transcriptase-polymerase chain reaction (RT-PCR) can detect the

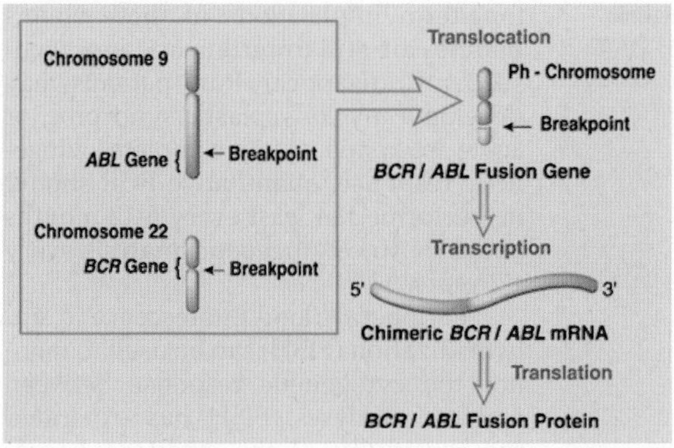

Figure 111-6 Summary of the cytogenetic and molecular effects of the Ph chromosome.

BCR-ABL transcript with a sensitivity of 10^{-5}.[48] Interestingly, using a more sensitive RT-PCR (sensitivity ~10^{-8}) the BCR-ABL chimerism has been identified in as many as 25-30% of normal adults.[49] This suggests the presence of BCR-ABL-positive cells in a sizable number of individuals who never develop CML, indicating that clonal disease requires a critical number of cells and/or a second oncogenic event. Abundant experimental evidence suggests that BCR-ABL is causally related to the clinical development of CML. When murine hemopoietic stem cells are transfected with a retrovirus encoding $p210^{Bcr-Abl}$ and transplanted into irradiated syngeneic mice, they develop several hematologic malignancies including a syndrome resembling human chronic myeloid leukemia.[50] A causal relationship between the BCR-ABL chimeric gene and human leukemia supported the concept that elimination of the Ph chromosome may improve prognosis in CML, and the need to develop BCR-ABL-targeted therapies for CML.

Treatment

Imatinib mesylate, a selective Bcr-Abl tyrosine kinase inhibitor introduced in the 1990s, has revolutionized the treatment and prognosis of CML.[51-56] With long-term follow-up, the solid benefits of imatinib therapy are sustained: the 7-year estimated incidence of durable complete cytogenetic response (Ph-positive metaphases 0%) is ~70%; the estimated 7-year survival is close to 90%, and 94% if only CML-related deaths are counted.[57] These results have established imatinib as optimal frontline therapy in newly diagnosed chronic phase CML. Among patients who present with accelerated or blastic phase CML, or who develop imatinib resistance, allogenic stem cell transplant (SCT), second-generation tyrosine kinase inhibitors, and imatinib combinations are treatment options and will be discussed later. Hydroxyurea, busulfan, interferon-alpha, cytarabine, and other agents (homoharringtone, decitabine) are still relevant in CML therapy and will be reviewed briefly.

Imatinib Mesylate

The deregulated or constitutively active tyrosine kinase of the Bcr-Abl chimeric fusion oncoprotein is the causative molecular abnormality in CML. Thus, the Bcr-Abl tyrosine kinase is an ideal molecular target. Imatinib mesylate is a potent selective Bcr-Abl tyrosine kinase inhibitor.[51,52] By preventing tyrosine phosphorylation, downstream effectors that influence cell death, cell signaling, adhesion, and other vital cellular functions cannot be activated, thus disrupting the pathway to CML cell survival.

Today, imatinib is the standard therapy for CML.[58] It was first used in CML after failure or intolerance to interferon-alpha.[59,60] Imatinib 400 mg orally daily, given to 454 patients, resulted in a complete cytogenetic response of 57%. The estimated 5-year survival rate was 76%.[59]

The efficacy of imatinib in previously untreated patients was demonstrated in a multicenter randomized trial comparing imatinib to the combination of interferon-alpha plus low-dose cytarabine (IRIS trial).[58,61] This study showed significantly higher rates of hematologic and cytogenetic response, improved tolerance, and prolonged progression-free survival with imatinib compared with the combination of interferon-alpha and cytarabine. After 60 months of follow-up, among 553 patients treated with imatinib 400 mg daily, the projected rate of complete cytogenetic response was 87%.[55] The estimated 5-year overall survival was 89%. Survival was significantly improved with imatinib compared with past experiences[62,63] (Fig. 111-1).

The standard starting dose of imatinib in chronic phase is 400 mg daily. Higher doses of imatinib (600-800 mg daily) may result in improved response rates that may be achieved sooner. Among patients in chronic phase who progress on imatinib 400 mg daily therapy, imatinib 800 mg daily recaptured some complete cytogenetic responses and complete molecular response.[64] Whether using high-dose imatinib in newly diagnosed CML will translate into long-term benefit remains to be determined in ongoing randomized studies.[65]

The response to imatinib at early time points is indicative of the longer-term outcome and should be used for treatment decisions. Among patients receiving imatinib as first-line therapy, patients who are not in CHR after 3 months, who are still 100% Ph-positive after 6 months of therapy, who have less than a major cytogenetic response (Ph-positive ≥ 35%) at 12 months, or who are not in complete cytogenetic response after ≥18 months should be considered to have imatinib failure and undergo treatment modifications.[58,66]

Management of Adverse Events In general, imatinib is well tolerated. The most common adverse event is myelosuppression. In early chronic phase, grade 3 or higher neutropenia (ie, neutrophils $<1 \times 10^9$/L) occurs in up to 20% of patients, thrombocytopenia (ie, platelets $<50 \times 10^9$/L) in 10%, and anemia in 5%. The current recommendation is to interrupt therapy in patients who develop grade 3 or higher neutropenia or thrombocytopenia and not to immediately lower the dose. Upon recovery, treatment is restarted with the same dose if recovery takes <2 weeks or with a reduced dose if it takes longer than this time. The use of hematopoietic growth factors (G-CSF for neutropenia, erythropoietin for anemia) has been reported to be effective in patients with recurrent or persistent cytopenias.[67,68] Myelosuppression is most frequently seen during the first 2-3 months of therapy as leukemic hematopoiesis is replaced by normal hematopoiesis. A brief treatment interruption is frequently sufficient to allow recovery, and most patients will not require dose reductions or growth factor support.

Nonhematologic adverse events are relatively common but usually mild and dose-related. Grade 3 or higher adverse events are rare; only 2-3% of patients require permanent discontinuation of therapy because of toxicity. These include skin rash, muscle cramps, gastrointestinal toxicity (nausea, diarrhea), bone aches, liver dysfunction, weight gain, fluid retention, and rare cardiotoxicity. Suggestions for the management of the most common adverse events are presented in Table 111-1.[68,69]

Monitoring Effect of Therapy; Role of Molecular and Mutational Studies Experience with interferon therapy showed that achievement of complete cytogenetic response was associated with a significant survival benefit, a 10-year survival rate of 70-80%.[70] This then became the new goal of therapy and cytogenetic

Table 111-1 **Suggested Management of Most Common Adverse Events Associated With Imatinib**

Adverse Events	Management
Nausea/vomiting	Take with food, fluids
	Antiemetics
Diarrhea	Loperamide
	Diphenoxylate atropine
Peripheral edema	Diuretics
Periorbital edema	Steroid-containing cream
Skin rash	Avoid sun exposure
	Topical steroids
	Systemic steroids (early intervention important)
Muscle cramps	Tonic water or quinine
	Electrolyte replacement as needed
	Calcium gluconate
Arthralgia, bone pain	Nonsteroidal anti-inflammatory agents
Elevated transaminases (uncommon)	Hold therapy and monitor closely
	Dose reduction upon resolution
Myelosuppression	
Anemia	Treatment interruption/dose reduction usually not indicated
	Consider erythropoietin or darbepoietin[a]
Neutropenia	Hold therapy if grade ≥ 3 (ie, ANC < 1 × 10^9/L)
	Consider filgrastima if recurrent/persistent, or sepsis
Thrombocytopenia	Hold therapy if grade ≥ 3 (ie, platelets <50 × 10^9/L)
	Consider IL 11[a] 10 mcg/kg 3-7 days/week

[a]The use of erythropoietin, darbepoietin, filgrastim, and interleukin-11 (IL-11) in this setting is not standard and should be considered investigational.

monitoring became mandatory. With imatinib, most patients achieve complete cytogenetic response.[58] The goal of therapy is now shifting toward achieving a major or complete molecular response that hopefully would translate into further improvement in survival.

The significance of molecular monitoring in CML was first documented with SCT. Patients who had BCR-ABL detectable by polymerase chain reaction (PCR) 6 months after transplant have a significantly higher probability of relapse; those with the highest level of transcripts had the highest risk.[71] Molecular monitoring with quantitative PCR (QPCR) is now routine after SCT, and early intervention (eg, imatinib, donor lymphocyte infusion) is indicated based on increasing levels of BCR-ABL transcripts. It should also be considered a routine test for all patients treated with imatinib or second-generation tyrosine kinase inhibitor.

Real-time PCR has become a routine test to evaluate the effect of imatinib therapy. The IRIS trial demonstrated a significantly improved molecular response with imatinib compared with interferon at each time point from the achievement of complete cytogenetic response.[72] After 18 months of therapy, 35-40% of patients treated with imatinib had a 3-log reduction of BCR-ABL transcripts, and 4-10% had undetectable BCR-ABL. This depth of response had been rare with interferon-alpha. Among patients who achieved a complete cytogenetic response with imatinib, those with ≥3-log reduction in BCR-ABL transcripts at 18 months from the start of therapy had a significantly better probability of transformation-free survival at 6 years compared with those who had <3-log reduction (100% vs 96%, $p < .001$).[73] In other studies, increases of molecular disease by twofold up to 1-log and/or loss of a major molecular response have been correlated with a higher probability of detection of imatinib-resistant mutations and with a high probability of loss of cytogenetic response and CML progression.[74-77]

Thus, the objective of therapy in the imatinib era is to achieve a major molecular response that increases the probability of long-term durable responses.

A recommended algorithm for monitoring patients includes a cytogenetic analysis and quantitative PCR (real-time PCR) for all patients at diagnosis.[78] During the first 12 months of therapy, it is appropriate to monitor the patients every 3 months with marrow studies for cytogenetic analysis or peripheral blood FISH (see below) until complete cytogenetic response, then with quantitative PCR every 3 months in the first 2 years and every 6 months once in stable cytogenetic CR, with cytogenetic analysis every 1-2 years. This last test, although inconvenient, is the only one that gives reliable information regarding the presence of other chromosomal abnormalities. The presence of additional chromosomal abnormalities may reduce the probability of response to imatinib and overall survival.[79] Also, 10% of patients who respond to imatinib may develop chromosomal abnormalities in the Ph-negative metaphases.[38,39,42] The long-term implications of these abnormalities are still uncertain and most subsequently disappear. Rare patients may develop a myelodysplastic syndrome, or acute leukemia. After complete cytogenetic response, quantitative PCR should be performed at least every 6-12 months and a routine cytogenetic analysis every 1-2 years.[66,78]

Peripheral blood fluorescence in situ hybridization (FISH) can be used to monitor the cytogenetic response between marrow analyses. FISH has expanded the sensitivity of the standard karyotype because it can survey many more cells. This technique uses peripheral blood (avoiding painful marrow aspirations), and is useful if cytogenetic studies are unsuccessful because of insufficient metaphases (10-20% of cases) as it can be done in interphase.

FISH has some disadvantages[80,81]: (1) even with the newest probes there is a small percentage of false positivity with FISH; (2) routine FISH does not provide information on every chromosome; and (3) although it surveys more cells for the Ph chromosome than a cytogenetic analysis, it is not as sensitive as PCR. A 100% negative FISH test corresponds to only approximately a 2-log reduction in transcript levels, whereas with PCR the limit of detection extends to approximately 4.5-5 logs. A 3-log reduction of QPCR is equivalent to an absolute QPCR value of 0.1% on the international scale.

A subset of patients treated with imatinib will develop resistance. Among those treated in chronic phase, the rate of resistance is <4% per year; for those who achieve a complete cytogenetic response, the rate of resistance beyond year 3 of imatinib therapy is 1% or less, suggesting the durable stability of a complete cytogenetic response on imatinib and the predictability of the CML course once such a response is obtained. Several mechanisms of resistance have been identified; the most common are mutations in the BCR-ABL kinase domain (KD). More than 50 different mutations have been reported, and involve any of the important domains in the BCR-ABL structure, including the P-loop (the area where ATP binds), the activation loop, and the catalytic domain, as well as the amino acids where imatinib makes contact with BCR-ABL. In one study, an increase in BCR-ABL of more than twofold was found in 34 of 35 patients with a mutation.[75] Different mutations have considerable variability with respect to resistance to imatinib. Some mutations are inhibited by slightly higher concentrations of imatinib than required to inhibit the wild-type form; others are completely insensitive to imatinib. Mutational analysis is useful in patients with imatinib resistance for several reasons[78,82-84]: (1) to identify patients with the T315I mutant that do not respond to imatinib or the second-generation TKIs (dasatinib, nilotinib, bosutinib) and who should consider immediate allogeneic SCT or therapy with T315I-selective inhibitors; (2) knowledge of the sensitivity of the different mutant, as determined by the IC_{50} for particular agents, can help select the TKI: an $IC_{50} > 3$ nM to dasatinib suggests a poor-response and short-response durations to dasatinib, and a similar correlation is found with an $IC_{50} > 150$ nM to nilotinib. Mutational studies may be helpful in patients who develop cytogenetic or hematologic resistance or relapse on imatinib therapy and those with significant increasing of BCR-ABL transcript levels on imatinib therapy. Recent trends are to consider the significance of mutations by their IC_{50} values to different agents rather than their geographic locations. A list of such mutations is shown in Table 111-2.

Treatment Options After Imatinib Failure

Allogeneic SCT is considered a standard treatment option in post-imatinib failure, and is discussed in detail later. Several new agents are being developed to treat patients with CML and imatinib resistance or intolerance.[85-89] Two of them, dasatinib and nilotinib have received regulatory approval and are now commercially available.

Dasatinib is a dual Src-Abl inhibitor that is 300 times more potent than imatinib in vitro. Following encouraging phase I studies,[90] pivotal trials post-imatinib failure established its efficacy in all CML phases. In chronic phase CML, dasatinib induced complete cytogenetic response in 50-60% of patients; the estimated 2-year survival post-imatinib failure was 90%. Dasatinib is approved for the treatment of CML in all phases post-imatinib failure and for the treatment of Ph-positive ALL.[91-94] Results of dasatinib are summarized in Table 111-3. Dasatinib was initially approved at an oral dose of 70 mg twice daily. Common side effects of dasatinib at this dose include myelosuppression in 50-60% and pleural effusions in 20-30% (severe in 5-10%). Subsequent randomized trials showed that a single dose of dasatinib 100 mg daily has equivalent efficacy and less toxicity than 70 mg twice daily. Dasatinib 100 mg single daily dose is now the standard drug dose schedule post-imatinib failure.[94]

Nilotinib is a selective BCR-ABL inhibitor that is 30 times more potent than nilotinib. Following encouraging phase I trials,[95] pivotal studies showed its activity post-imatinib failure.[96,97] In chronic phase, nilotinib 400 mg orally twice daily was associated with a complete cytogenetic response rate of 40-50%; the estimated 18-month survival post-imatinib failure was 91%.[96] Nilotinib is approved for the treatment of CML in chronic and accelerated phases post-imatinib failure (Table 111-3). Nilotinib side effects include myelosuppression in 20-30%, liver function abnormalities in 10-15%, and elevated (usually asymptomatic) lipase and amylase levels in 10-15%. Rare cases (<1%) of pancreatitis have been reported. Patients with QTc prolongation >450 msec or with serious cardiac problems should not be treated with nilotinib. Drugs that prolong QTc should be avoided during nilotinib therapy.

Bosutinib, another dual Src-Abl inhibitor 30-50 times more potent than nilotinib, is under investigation with favorable efficacy and toxicity profiles.[98]

None of these agents is active in patients with CML and T315I mutations. Other investigational agents of interest include tyrosine kinase inhibitors with activity against T315I, homoharrintonine, decitabine, and different vaccines (for minimal residual disease). There is interest in reintroduction of pegylated forms of interferon, in combination with TKIs in higher risk CML, or at the time of minimal residual disease.

Table 111-2 In Vitro Sensitivity of Different BCR-ABL Mutants to Tyrosine Kinase Inhibitors

	IC_{50}-Fold Increase (WT = 1)			
	Imatinib	Bosutinib	Dasatinib	Nilotinib
WT	1	1	1	1
L248V	3.54	2.97	5.11	2.80
G250E	6.86	4.31	4.45	4.56
Q252H	1.39	0.31	3.05	2.64
Y253F	3.58	0.96	1.58	3.23
E255K	6.02	9.47	5.61	6.69
E255V	16.99	5.53	3.44	10.31
D276G	2.18	0.60	1.44	2.00
E279K	3.55	0.95	1.64	2.05
V299L	1.54	26.10	8.65	1.34
T315I	17.50	45.42	75.03	39.41
F317L	2.60	2.42	4.46	2.22
M351T	1.76	0.70	0.88	0.44
F359V	2.86	0.93	1.49	5.16
L384M	1.28	0.47	2.21	2.33
H396P	2.43	0.43	1.07	2.41
H396R	3.91	0.81	1.63	3.10
G398R	0.35	1.16	0.69	0.49
F486S	8.10	2.31	3.04	1.85

Abbreviations: Mutations can be classified as sensitive (IC50-fold increase ≤ 2), resistant (between 2.01 and 10), or highly resistant (>10). T315I mutation

Source: From Ref. 82.

Stem Cell Transplantation

From 1980 until 2000, allogeneic SCT was the centerpiece of the management of CML.

Allogeneic SCT may be curative in 40-80% of patients who receive a transplant from an HLA-identical sibling or an unrelated donor.[99] Because of the requirements for age, adequate organ function and performance status, availability of donor, and other factors, only a fraction of patients (10-30%) are eligible, particularly because the median age of patients with CML is 55-65 years, and because only one-third of patients have an HLA-matched sibling. The number of potential donors may be increased by using matched unrelated donors, but the cure rate and graft-versus-host disease (GVHD) rate are worse. These may be improved by careful molecular typing, especially HLA-A, -B, and -DRB1.[100]

The expected results with modern SCT techniques are illustrated by a recent series from Seattle,[99] which used a conditioning regimen with cyclophosphamide plus targeted oral busulfan for 131 patients in early chronic phase (median age of 43 years; range 14-66 years). At 3 years, the projected non-relapse mortality rate was 14%; 78% of patients were projected to be alive and free of disease. However, 60% had extensive chronic graft-versus-host disease (GVHD).

Cure with allogeneic SCT usually refers to the 5- to 6-year EFS rate. Few series have analyzed the very long-term results of SCT and the magnitude of complications, relapse, or death beyond this period. The availability of imatinib therapy has now accentuated the need for a more critical evaluation of risk versus benefit of allogeneic SCT. In the long-term International Bone Marrow Treatment Registry (IBMTR) studies, the 5-year EFS was 60% for sibling SCT in

Table 111-3 Response to Dasatinib, Nilotinib, and Bosutinib After Imatinib Resistance

	Percent Response										
	Dasatinib				Nilotinib				Bosutinib		
	CP[93]	AP[92]	MyBP[91]	LyBP[91]	CP[119]	AP[120]	MyBP[121]	LyBP[121]	CP[98]	AP[122]	BP[122]
Response	*n* = 387	*n* = 174	*n* = 109	*n* = 48	*n* = 321	*n* = 137	*n* = 105	*n* = 31	*n* = 146	*n* = 51	*n* = 38
Median follow-up (mo)	15	14	12[b]	12[b]	19	9	3	3	7	6	3
% Resistant	74	93	91	88	70	80	82	82	69	NR[a]	NR[a]
Hematologic		79	50	40	94	56	22	19	85	54	36
CHR	91	45	27	29	76	31	11	13	81	54	36
NEL	-	19	7	6	-	12	1	0	-	0	0
Cytogenetic	NR	44	36	52	NR	NR	NR	NR		NR	NR
Complete	49	32	26	46	44	20	29	32	34	27	35
Partial	11	7	7	6	15	12	10	16	13	20	18
% Survival (at *x* months)	96 (15)	82 (12)	50 (12)	50 (5)	88 (24)	67 (24)	42 (12)	42 (12)	98 (12)	60 (12)	50 (10)

[a]48% had previously received dasatinib and/or nilotinib in addition to imatinib.
[b]Minimum follow-up.
Abbreviations: NR, not reported; CP, chronic phase; AP, accelerated phase; MyBP, myeloid blastic phase; LyBP, lymphoid blastic phase; BP, blastic phase; CHR, complete hematologic response; NEL, no evidence of leukemia.

chronic phase, but the 20-year EFS was 40-45%, only partly due to relapse.[101] Thus, the expected annual mortality (beyond year 5) may not be the same as for normal individuals, perhaps because of subtle but serious effects of SCT or GVHD on organ funtions. Allogeneic SCT affects quality of life because of the development of infertility, cataracts, hip necrosis, chronic lung disease, immune disorders, GVHD complications, second cancers, and others.[102] Thus, the role of allogeneic SCT as therapy of CML, even in younger patients, must be evaluated critically.

Patients transplanted in more advanced stages of CML (accelerated or blastic phase) have significantly worse outcomes, with 5-year survival probabilities of 40% accelerated phase and 10-15% blastic phase. Patients in blastic phase transplanted after induction of a second chronic phase may have long-term outcomes similar to accelerated phase.[103,104]

Patients who do not have a sibling donor may undergo a matched unrelated donor transplantation. This procedure is associated with higher rates of early mortality and GVHD. The long-term disease-free survival rate after such transplants for patients younger than 30 years of age transplanted within 1 year from diagnosis is 61% compared with 68% for matched siblings.[105] Patients age 30-40 years have long-term disease-free survival rates of 57% and 67%, respectively.[105] The results with unrelated transplants are improving with the use of molecularly matched donors.

Nonmyeloablative transplants have been used for older patients or those with health considerations that prevent them from receiving a SCT. Early results (frequently including mostly young patients with short follow-up) report disease-free survival rates as high as 85% at 70 months.[106] There is, however, a higher rate of residual CML after nonablative SCT. The use of alternative donors such as cord blood or haplo-identical donors remains investigational.

Another important consideration is the possible effect that prior therapy may have on SCT. Recent studies suggest that prior imatinib therapy has no adverse impact on SCT outcome.[107]

Patients who relapse after transplant can frequently be reinduced into remission with imatinib, other TKIs, or donor lymphocyte infusion (DLI).[108,109] In patients who relapse in the chronic phase, a complete remission is achievable in 70%, and may be higher if treated at the time of molecular relapse (compared with cytogenetic or hematologic relapse). The response rate is 20% for those who relapse in accelerated phase and <10% for patients in blastic phase. Toxicity includes myelosuppression in 20-30%, GVHD in 40%, and a mortality of 10-20%. The risks of myelosuppression and GVHD are lower with imatinib than with DLIs.

Hydroxyurea and Busulfan

Hydroxyurea and busulfan were historically the main drugs used to treat CML. In randomized trials, hydroxyurea yielded better results than busulfan: the median survival was 59 months with hydroxyurea and 45 months with busulfan.[110] Presently, the main use of hydroxyurea is as an initial CML debulking agent in newly diagnosed CML, as an interim measure in-between established therapies, or in combination with TKIs. The usual dose is 0.5-5 g orally daily, to keep a WBC count between 2 and 10 × 10^9/L. The main use of busulfan in modern times is as part of preparative regimens for allogeneic SCT. Neither agent produces significant durable cytogenetic remissions. Hydroxyurea side effects include stomatitis, nausea and vomiting, rashes, and skin ulcers. Side effects of busulfan include marrow hypoplasia or aplasia amenorrhea, increased skin pigmentation, a wasting syndrome with features of Addison disease, cataracts, "busulfan lung," and endocardial fibrosis.

Interferon

Recombinant interferon alpha-2a and alpha-2b, alone or combined with cytarabine, can induce durable complete cytogenetic responses in 5-30% of patients and prolong survival in CML.[111-114]

The achievement of a cytogenetic remission is good surrogate endpoint for survival.[70] Patients who achieve a complete cytogenetic remission but have high levels of minimal residual disease by quantitative PCR have a high probability of relapse, whereas 80% of those with low transcript levels (ie, BCR-ABL/ABL <0.045%) have remained in remission after 3 years.[115] Approximately 30% of patients who achieve a complete cytogenetic remission have undetectable disease by PCR (ie, complete molecular remission); none of these patients has relapsed after a median follow-up of 10 years and may be cured.[70,115] However, even among those with residual disease by PCR, 40-60% have remained in cytogenetic remission after 10 years. This has been called an "operational" or "biological" cure. These data emphasize the importance of achieving a complete cytogenetic response with CML therapy.

In a study comparing interferon-alpha to hydroxyurea, the time to progression from chronic phase to accelerated blastic phase was 72 months with interferon compared with 45 months with hydroxyurea ($p < .001$). Overall, median survival was 72 months with interferon and 52 months with hydroxyurea. Major cytogenetic responses correlated with improved survival.[114] Other randomized trials have confirmed the superiority of interferon over hydroxyurea in low-risk patients.[112]

The side effects of interferon include fever, chills, malaise, fatigue, headache, anorexia, joint pain, vomiting, low backache, myalgia, neuropathy, changes in mood and concentration, abnormalities of liver enzymes, retinal vein thrombosis, leukopenia, thrombocytopenia, and autoimmune effects, including immune-mediated thrombocytopenia, hypothyroidism, and hemolytic anemia.

Treatment Recommendations in CML in 2009

A new treatment algorithm in CML has been established in the past decade. The results with imatinib to date have been excellent and durable. With complete cytogenetic responses of 82%, major molecular responses of 40-70%, and annual mortality of 1-2%, the estimated median survival may become 20-30 years,[116,117] and a significant proportion of patients may have long-term EFS. While allogeneic SCT is curative in a significant proportion of eligible patients, limiting factors include availability of a donor and age of the patient, the risk of early mortality, and considerable morbidities affecting the quality of life of patients. Most studies with allogeneic SCT emphasize the results of the first 5 years, but late relapses, higher than average mortality, and complications should also be taken into consideration. With current knowledge, it is reasonable to offer all patients with newly diagnosed chronic phase CML initial therapy with imatinib, and consider allogeneic SCT only after imatinib failure (eg, no CHR after 3 months, 100% Ph-positive after 6 months, or ≥35% Ph-positive after 12 months, or no complete cytogenetic response after ≥18 months imatinib therapy) or resistance to imatinib.

Changing therapy should be considered for patients who have CML post-imatinib failure as defined earlier. Several treatment alternatives are now available. Increasing the dosage of imatinib to 800 mg daily and new tyrosine kinase inhibitors should be considered. An important recent question arising from the success of new generation TKIs is whether allogeneic SCT should be always considered as the optimal second-line therapy post-imatinib failure or whether one can resort to new generation TKI as a definitive second-line therapy before considering allogeneic SCT. The decision should rely on several factors: (1) the CML phase at the time of imatinib failure; (2) the patient age and source of SCT (matched related, unrelated, mismatched); (3) the presence of particular mutations; and (4) the initial response to the new generation TKIs. In general, patients who progress on imatinib with accelerated or blastic phase should consider allogeneic SCT immediately, regardless of the risk, and use new generation TKIs as a temporary approach to debulk CML disease hoping to improve outcome post-allogeneic SCT; these patients should be considered for TKI maintenance post-allogeneic SCT. Patients with imatinib failure who remain in chronic phase may consider allogeneic SCT as second-line therapy if its risks are acceptable (younger age, fully matched sibling donor). Otherwise, they may consider new generation TKIs as a more definitive therapy and evaluate this choice based on the particular identified mutations, early response to the new TKIs, and the general condition and age of the patients. Older patients (age ≥ 65-70 years) and those with significant comorbiditis may elect to continue on the new generation TKIs and forgo the potential of a cure with allogeneic SCT, in favor of a durable control of the disease (functional cure) and a better quality of life. Failure to achieve a cytogenetic response and particular mutations with high IC_{50} are associated with shorter durations of disease control.

Finally, patients with T315I mutations (10% to 20% of patients post-imatinib failure; 1-3% of all patients) should consider immediate allogeneic SCT.[118]

Selected References

The complete reference list can be found at www.CANCERMEDICINE8.com

6. Kantarjian HM, Dixon D, Keating MJ, et al. Characteristics of accelerated disease in chronic myelogenous leukemia. *Cancer*. 1988;61:1441–1446.
7. Vardiman JW, Harris NL, Brunning RD. The World Health Organization (WHO) classification of the myeloid neoplasms. *Blood*. 2002;100:2292–2302.
9. Kantarjian HM, Keating MJ, Talpaz M, et al. Chronic myelogenous leukemia in blast crisis. Analysis of 242 patients. *Am J Med*. 1987;83:445–454.
14. Ahuja H, Bar-Eli M, Arlin Z, et al. The spectrum of molecular alterations in the evolution of chronic myelocytic leukemia. *J Clin Invest*. 1991;87:2042–2047.
17. Onida F, Ball G, Kantarjian HM, et al. Characteristics and outcome of patients with Philadelphia chromosome negative, bcr/abl negative chronic myelogenous leukemia. *Cancer*. 2002;95:1673–1684.
18. Sokal JE, Cox EB, Baccarani M, et al. Prognostic discrimination in "good-risk" chronic granulocytic leukemia. *Blood*. 1984;63:789–799.
19. Hasford J, Pfirrmann M, Hehlmann R, et al. A new prognostic score for survival of patients with chronic myeloid leukemia treated with interferon alfa. Writing Committee for the Collaborative CML Prognostic Factors Project Group. *J Natl Cancer Inst*. 1998;90: 850–858.
20. Gratwohl A, Hermans J, Goldman JM, et al. Risk assessment for patients with chronic myeloid leukaemia before allogeneic blood or marrow transplantation. Chronic Leukemia Working Party of the European Group for Blood and Marrow Transplantation. *Lancet*. 1998;352:1087–1092.
27. Nowell PC, Hungerford DA. A minute chromosome in human chronic granulocytic leukemia. *Science*. 1960;132:1497–1501.
38. Deininger MW, Cortes J, Paquette R, et al. The prognosis for patients with chronic myeloid leukemia who have clonal cytogenetic abnormalities in philadelphia chromosome-negative cells. *Cancer*. 2007;110:1509–1519.
45. Sawyers CL. Chronic myeloid leukemia. *N Engl J Med*. 1999;340:1330–1340.
50. Daley GQ, Van Etten RA, Baltimore D. Induction of chronic myelogenous leukemia in mice by the P210bcr/abl gene of the Philadelphia chromosome. *Science*. 1990;247:824–830.
51. Druker BJ, Tamura S, Buchdunger E, et al. Effects of a selective inhibitor of the Abl tyrosine kinase on the growth of Bcr-Abl positive cells. *Nat Med*. 1996;2:561–566.
52. Beran M, Cao X, Estrov Z, et al. Selective inhibition of cell proliferation and BCR-ABL phosphorylation in acute lymphoblastic leukemia cells expressing Mr 190,000 BCR-ABL protein by a tyrosine kinase inhibitor (CGP-57148). *Clin Cancer Res*. 1998;4:1661–1672.
53. Druker BJ, Sawyers CL, Kantarjian H, et al. Activity of a specific inhibitor of the BCR-ABL tyrosine kinase in the blast crisis of chronic myeloid leukemia and acute lymphoblastic leukemia with the Philadelphia chromosome. *N Engl J Med*. 2001;344:1038–1042.
54. Druker BJ, Talpaz M, Resta DJ, et al. Efficacy and safety of a specific inhibitor of the BCR-ABL tyrosine kinase in chronic myeloid leukemia. *N Engl J Med*. 2001;344:1031–1037.
58. Druker BJ, Guilhot F, O'Brien SG, et al. Five-year follow-up of patients receiving imatinib for chronic myeloid leukemia. *N Engl J Med*. 2006;355:2408–2417.
60. Kantarjian H, Sawyers C, Hochhaus A, et al. Hematologic and cytogenetic responses to imatinib mesylate in chronic myelogenous leukemia. *N Engl J Med*. 2002;346:645–652.
61. O'Brien SG, Guilhot F, Larson RA, et al. Imatinib compared with interferon and low-dose cytarabine for newly diagnosed chronic-phase chronic myeloid leukemia. *N Engl J Med*. 2003;348:994–1004.
62. Kantarjian HM, Talpaz M, O'Brien S, et al. Survival benefit with imatinib mesylate versus interferon-alpha-based regimens in newly diagnosed chronic-phase chronic myelogenous leukemia. *Blood*. 2006;108:1835–1840.
63. Roy L, Guilhot J, Krahnke T, et al. Survival advantage from imatinib compared with the combination interferon-alpha plus cytarabine in chronic-phase chronic myelogenous leukemia: historical comparison between two phase 3 trials. *Blood*. 2006;108: 1478–1484.
70. Kantarjian HM, O'Brien S, Cortes JE, et al. Complete cytogenetic and molecular responses to interferon-alpha-based therapy for chronic myelogenous leukemia are associated with excellent long-term prognosis. *Cancer*. 2003;97:1033–1041.
72. Hughes TP, Kaeda J, Branford S, et al. Frequency of major molecular responses to imatinib or interferon alfa plus cytarabine in newly diagnosed chronic myeloid leukemia. *N Engl J Med*. 2003;349:1423–1432.

75. Branford S, Rudzki Z, Parkinson I, et al. Real-time quantitative PCR analysis can be used as a primary screen to identify patients with CML treated with imatinib who have BCR-ABL kinase domain mutations. *Blood.* 2004;104:2926–2932.
77. Press RD, Galderisi C, Yang R, et al. A half-log increase in BCR-ABL RNA predicts a higher risk of relapse in patients with chronic myeloid leukemia with an imatinib-induced complete cytogenetic response. *Clin Cancer Res.* 2007;13:6136–6143.
78. Kantarjian H, Schiffer C, Jones D, Cortes J. Monitoring the response and course of chronic myeloid leukemia in the modern era of BCR-ABL tyrosine kinase inhibitors: practical advice on the use and interpretation of monitoring methods. *Blood.* 2008;111:1774–1780.
81. Lesser ML, Dewald GW, Sison CP, Silver RT. Correlation of three methods of measuring cytogenetic response in chronic myelocytic leukemia. *Cancer Genet Cytogenet.* 2002;137:79–84.
82. Redaelli S, Piazza R, Rostagno R, et al. Determination of the activity profile of bosutinib, dasatinib and nilotinib against 18 imatinib resistant Bcr/Abl mutants. *Blood.* 2008;112:Abst# 3220.
83. O'Hare T, Eide CA, Deininger MW. Bcr-Abl kinase domain mutations, drug resistance and the road to a cure of chronic myeloid leukemia 10.1182/blood-2007-03-066936. *Blood.* 2007:blood-2007-2003-066936.
85. Weisberg E, Manley PW, Breitenstein W, et al. Characterization of AMN107, a selective inhibitor of native and mutant Bcr-Abl. *Cancer Cell.* 2005;7:129–141.
87. Weisberg E, Manley PW, Cowan-Jacob SW, Hochhaus A, Griffin JD. Second generation inhibitors of BCR-ABL for the treatment of imatinib-resistant chronic myeloid leukaemia. *Nat Rev Cancer.* 2007;7:345–356.
88. O'Hare T, Walters DK, Stoffregen EP, et al. In vitro activity of Bcr-Abl inhibitors AMN107 and BMS-354825 against clinically relevant imatinib-resistant Abl kinase domain mutants. *Cancer Res.* 2005;65:4500–4505.
89. Shah NP, Tran C, Lee FY, Chen P, Norris D, Sawyers CL. Overriding imatinib resistance with a novel ABL kinase inhibitor. *Science.* 2004;305:399–401.
90. Talpaz M, Shah NP, Kantarjian H, et al. Dasatinib in imatinib-resistant Philadelphia chromosome-positive leukemias. *N Engl J Med.* 2006;354:2531–2541.
91. Cortes J, Kim DW, Raffoux E, et al. Efficacy and safety of dasatinib in imatinib-resistant or -intolerant patients with chronic myeloid leukemia in blast phase. *Leukemia.* 2008;22:2176–2183.
92. Guilhot F, Apperley J, Kim DW, et al. Dasatinib induces significant hematologic and cytogenetic responses in patients with imatinib-resistant or -intolerant chronic myeloid leukemia in accelerated phase. *Blood.* 2007;109:4143–4150.
93. Hochhaus A, Baccarani M, Deininger M, et al. Dasatinib induces durable cytogenetic responses in patients with chronic myelogenous leukemia in chronic phase with resistance or intolerance to imatinib. *Leukemia.* 2008;22:1200–1206.
94. Shah NP, Kantarjian HM, Kim DW, et al. Intermittent target inhibition with dasatinib 100 mg once daily preserves efficacy and improves tolerability in imatinib-resistant and -intolerant chronic-phase chronic myeloid leukemia. *J Clin Oncol.* 2008;26:3204–3212.
95. Kantarjian H, Giles F, Wunderle L, et al. Nilotinib in imatinib-resistant CML and Philadelphia chromosome-positive ALL. *N Engl J Med.* 2006;354:2542–2551.
96. Kantarjian HM, Giles F, Gattermann N, et al. Nilotinib (formerly AMN107), a highly selective BCR-ABL tyrosine kinase inhibitor, is effective in patients with Philadelphia chromosome-positive chronic myelogenous leukemia in chronic phase following imatinib resistance and intolerance. *Blood.* 2007;110:3540–3546.
97. le Coutre P, Ottmann OG, Giles F, et al. Nilotinib (formerly AMN107), a highly selective BCR-ABL tyrosine kinase inhibitor, is active in patients with imatinib-resistant or -intolerant accelerated-phase chronic myelogenous leukemia. *Blood.* 2008;111:1834–1839.
98. Cortes J, Kantarjian H, Kim D-W, et al. Efficacy and safety of bosutinib (SKI-606) in patients with chronic phase (CP) Ph+ chronic myelogenous leukemia (CML) with resistance or intolerance to imatinib. *Blood.* 2008;112:Abst# 1098.
99. Radich JP, Gooley T, Bensinger W, et al. HLA-matched related hematopoietic cell transplantation for chronic-phase CML using a targeted busulfan and cyclophosphamide preparative regimen. *Blood.* 2003;102:31–35.
106. Or R, Shapira MY, Resnick I, et al. Nonmyeloablative allogeneic stem cell transplantation for the treatment of chronic myeloid leukemia in first chronic phase. *Blood.* 2003; 101:441–445.
107. Lee SJ, Kukreja M, Wang T, et al. Impact of prior imatinib mesylate on the outcome of hematopoietic cell transplantation for chronic myeloid leukemia. *Blood.* 2008;112: 3500–3507.

112 Acute Lymphoblastic Leukemia

Stefan Faderl, MD ■ Ching-Hon Pui, MD ■ Susan O'Brien, MD ■ Hagop M. Kantarjian, MD

Introduction

Acute lymphoblastic leukemia (ALL) is a heterogeneous disease. Identification of cytogenetic-molecular features in ALL has translated into more accurate classifications of disease subtypes, institution of risk-adapted therapies, and emergence of new drugs. Most impressively, advances in ALL therapy over only a few decades have led to cures for most children with ALL. Adaptation of successful pediatric ALL treatment strategies into therapeutic algorithms of adult ALL have also resulted in significant improvement, although long-term disease-free survival (DFS) rates of around 40% are still inferior. Nonetheless, ongoing molecular dissection of ALL subtypes, refinements of mulitagent chemotherapy in combination with the development of new and targeted drugs, comprehension of the kinetics of residual disease, and an increasing grasp of the impact of pharmacogenomic features and drug resistance is expected to contribute to further improvement of the prognosis of adult patients with ALL in due time as well.

Epidemiology and Etiology

ALL is predominantly a disease of children where it constitutes about 80% of all childhood leukemias and 25% of all childhood cancers, peaks between ages 2–5, and is diagnosed at an incidence of 3.5–4/100,000. In contrast, it makes up less than 3% of malignancies in adult patients. The age-adjusted overall incidence of ALL in the United States is about 1.5/100,000 and it is diagnosed annually in nearly 4,000 patients in the United States.[1] Although the average age of patients with ALL who enter clinical trials is between 30 and 35 years, older patients are likely underrepresented, which is also underlined by a second peak beyond age 50 where the incidence may exceed 2/100,000.

ALL is more frequent among Caucasians. Geographic variations in its frequency have been described with higher rates among Hispanic populations in Spain and Latin America.[2,3] While there is a slightly higher incidence rate in males than in females among childhood ALL, the rate is much more predominant in males among patients older than 20 years (1.3:1). A higher incidence of ALL has also been observed in industrialized and urban areas giving rise to speculation about socioeconomic factors in the etiology of ALL.[2–5]

In most cases no etiology can be established. Among children, only a few cases (<5%) are associated with inherited, predisposing genetic disorders (eg, Down syndrome, Klinefelter syndrome, Fanconi anemia, Bloom syndrome, ataxia-telangiectasia, Nijmegen breakage syndrome).[6–9] There are an extensive list of conflicting or isolated reports purported to confer an increased risk of childhood ALL, including parental occupation, maternal reproductive history, parental tobacco or alcohol use, maternal diet, prenatal vitamin use, exposure to pesticide or solvents, and exposure to the highest levels (>0.3 or 0.4 μT) of residential, power-frequency magnetic fields.[10,11] Investigations have also focused on genetic variability in drug metabolism, DNA repair, cell-cycle checkpoints that might interact with environmental, dietary, maternal, and other external factors to affect leukemogenesis. Preliminary data suggested a possible role for polymorphisms of genes encoding cytochrome P450, NAD(P)H quinone oxidoreductase, glutathione S-transferase, methylenetetrahydrofolate reductase (MTHFR), thymidylate synthase, and cell-cycle inhibitors.[12–15] To date, however, no direct gene-environment interactions have been established convincingly.

Observations of a peak age of development of childhood cases of 2–5 years, an association of industrialization and modern or affluent societies with increased risk, and the occasional clustering of childhood ALL (especially in new towns) have fueled two parallel-based hypotheses: population-mixing hypothesis and delayed infection hypothesis.[16,17] The first theory suggests that clusters of childhood cases result from exposure of susceptible (nonimmune) individuals to common, fairly nonpathological infections after population-mixing with carriers.[16] The second theory is based on a minimal two-hits model and suggests that some susceptible individuals with a prenatally acquired preleukemic clone had low or no exposure to common infections early in life because of their affluent hygienic environment.[17] Such infectious insulation predisposes the immune system of these individuals to aberrant or pathological responses to common infections at an age commensurate with increased lymphoid proliferation. Indeed, retrospective studies of archived neonatal blood spots and monozygotic twin pairs have identified preleukemic clones, and support the notion that additional postnatal transforming events are needed for full leukemic transformation.[18–20]

Clinical Presentation and Laboratory Abnormalities

The clinical signs and symptoms of ALL are quite variable. While the initial signs and symptoms appear insidiously and persist for months in some cases, they occur suddenly in most cases and derive from expansion of the leukemic cells in the marrow, involvement of the peripheral blood and extramedullary sites such as lymph nodes, liver, spleen, and the central nervous system (CNS). Common symptoms include fatigue, lack of energy, constitutional symptoms (fevers, night sweats, weight loss), easy bruising or bleeding, dyspnea, dizziness, and infections. Extremity and joint pain may be the only presenting symptoms in children, especially the very young. Diffuse osteopenia or lytic bone lesions are rare. Less than 10% of patients have overt CNS involvement at diagnosis, although CNS disease occurs more often in patients with mature B-cell ALL (Burkitt leukemia/lymphoma). Cranial nerve palsy (especially cranial nerves VI, III, IV, and VII) can lead to double vision, abnormal ocular movements, facial dysesthesias and facial droop. Nausea and vomiting, headaches, or papilledema may point towards meningeal infiltration and raised intracranial pressure. Chin numbness due to mental nerve involvement may be subtle and can be easily missed unless solicited.[21] Diagnosis of CNS involvement is made from cytospin slides from the cerebrospinal fluid (CSF). Whereas previous guidelines required the presence of >5 WBC/μL of CSF plus identifiable blasts, controversy arose around cases with <5 WBC/μL, but presence of blasts.[22] A more recent approach has been to define four diagnostic scenarios with no detectable blast cells in CSF (CNS 1), <5 WBC/μL and blasts (CNS 2), >5 WBC/μL and blasts or cranial nerve symptoms, and traumatic lumbar puncture with blasts.[23] T-lineage ALL presenting with a mediastinal mass can result in stridor and wheezing, pericardial effusions, and superior vena cava syndrome. Testicular involvement occurs with a low frequency predominantly in infant and adolescent boys. It typically presents as an indolent unilateral mass although bilateral involvement is commonly found on biopsies. It should be distinguished from hydrocele (resulting from lymphatic obstruction) by ultrasonography. Except for mature B-cell ALL where it may cause bleeding or rupture, involvement of the gastrointestinal tract is infrequent.

The physical examination is notable for pallor, ecchymoses or petechiae, generalized lymphadenopathy and hepatosplenomegaly. Physical examination findings are rarely specific for ALL and can be elicited in other forms of leukemia as well.

Tumor lysis syndrome is common in patients with mature B-cell ALL, but can also occur in any other subtype with hyperleukocytosis.[24] It is characterized by hyperuricemia, hyperphosphatemia, hypocalcemia, and hypo- or hyperkalemia. Disseminated intravascular coagulation (DIC) is a frequent laboratory finding, but rarely manifests as clinical DIC. Table 112-1 summarizes the clinical and laboratory characteristics of patients with adult ALL presenting to a tertiary referral center.[25]

Table 112-1 **Features of Adult Acute Lymphocytic Leukemia at Presentation (*N* = 204)**

Characteristic	Variable
Median age (yr)	39.5
Range	16–79
≥60 yr (%)	22
ECOG performance status >2 (%)	7
Organ involvement (%)	1
Lymphadenopathy	32
Splenomegaly	25
Hepatomegaly	16
Median WBC (x 10^9/L)	7.7
WBC >30 x 10^9/L (%)	26
Chemistry abnormalities (%)	
↑ Lactic dehydrogenase	59
Creatinine ≥1.3 mg/dL	16
Bilirubin ≥1.3 mg/dL	13
Immunophenotype (%)	
Precursor B	67
Mature B	9
T cell	12
Other (null, biphenotypic)	12
Myeloid marker positive (%)	54
Karyotype (%)	
Diploid	22
Ph-positive	16
t(8;14); t(8;2); t(8;22)	4
Hyperdiploid	4
Hypodiploid	5
Risk assignment (%)	
Standard	22
High	78

Abbreviations: BCM, below costal margin; CNS, central nervous system; ECOG, Eastern Cooperative Oncology Group; LDH, lactate dehydrogenase; ULN, upper limit of normal; WBC, white blood cells.
Source: From Ref. 25.

Diagnosis of ALL

The diagnosis of ALL requires identification of blast cells either in the blood, marrow, or both. Use of biopsy sections becomes important in cases with few circulating blasts or where the marrow is inaspirable. A thorough morphologic, cytochemical and immunologic assessment of ALL blasts remains essential in the work up. Identification of distinct cytogenetic-molecular abnormalities has contributed to a more complex view of the leukemic blasts and thus has enabled a more accurate assessment of the prognosis. Ongoing efforts are focused on genomic profiling leading to a new definition of ALL subtypes and, through it, to the identification of subgroups of patients with different treatment outcomes and prognoses that are only partially discriminated by currently available diagnostic tools.[26,27]

Morphology and Cytochemistry

ALL blasts are heterogeneous in size and shape and one of the first attempts to classify ALL was based on this observation. The French American British (FAB) Cooperative Group thus distinguished three subgroups of lymphoblasts: L1 blasts are smaller, have a high nuclear-to-cytoplasmic ratio and inconspicuous nucleoli. The cytoplasm is sparse and variably basophilic. L2 blasts are larger and more pleomorphic, have moderately abundant cytoplasm, a lower nuclear-to-cytoplasmic ratio, and more prominent nucleoli. L1 morphology is more common in children than in adults, whereas L2 morphology is more common in adults. L3 blasts are more homogenous, medium in size, with dispersed chromatin, prominent nucleoli, typically deep blue cytoplasmic basophilia, and sharply demarcated vacuoles.[28] L3 morphology is mostly associated with mature B-cell ALL or Burkitt lymphoma. Mature B-cell ALL is characterized by a high rate of cell turnover, which is reflected morphologically by the so-called starry sky appearance in marrow biopsy specimens.

The distinction into L1, L2, and L3 morphologies has been largely abandoned as with the exception of L3 and its association with mature B-cell ALL, it is no longer prognostically or therapeutically relevant.

Although no cytochemical stain is diagnostic for ALL, the key diagnostic cytochemical feature of ALL is lack of myeloperoxidase (MPO) and nonspecific esterase (NSE) activity. Low-level MPO positivity (3–5%) can occur in patients with lymphoid blast phase of chronic myeloid leukemia and other rare cases.[29,30] Sudan black B staining closely resembles those of myeloperoxidase itself, but lack of specificity and the ease with which myeloperoxidase stains can be applied has limited its use. Terminal deoxynucleotidyl transferase (TdT) is a useful marker to distinguish between reactive versus malignant lymphocytosis and is usually positive in ≥40% of ALL blasts. L3 ALL is characteristically TdT-negative.[31] About 10% of ALL blasts are positive for periodic acid-Schiff (PAS) showing a large, globular pattern. It is not specific as it may also be positive in cases of AML such as erythroblastic leukemia.

The WHO Classification of Neoplastic Diseases of Hematopoietic and Lymphoid Tissues emphasizes the importance of both immunologic and cytogenetic-molecular features over morphologic characteristics.[32,33]

Immunophenotyping

Immunophenotyping by flow cytometry is the essential next step to accurately diagnose ALL, resolve difficult differential diagnoses, and to define subtypes further.[34] Although there is no uniformly accepted panel, commonly used markers as listed in Figure 112-1 are usually sufficient to establish the diagnosis and confirm lineage affiliation in >95% of the cases.[35]

The majority of cases of ALL (70–85%) are of B-lineage. Based on their stage of maturation, they can be divided into: (i) pre-pre-B ALL (pro-B-ALL); (ii) early pre-B (common ALL); (iii) pre-B ALL; and (iv) mature B-ALL. In their earliest identifiable stage, pre-pre-B-ALL blasts are positive for CD19, CD79a, or CD22, but no other B-cell differentiation antigens. CD19-positive, CD10-negative, cytoplasmic immunoglobulin-negative B-lineage ALL with myeloid marker coexpression is common among infants with ALL, is typically associated with translocation t(4;11) and *MLL* gene rearrangements, and has a poor prognosis. Common ALL (cALL, early pre-B-ALL) represents an intermediate stage in blast development, and is the most common immunophenotype in adults and children. It is characterized by expression of CD10 (common ALL antigen, CALLA) and is a frequent immunophenotype with Philadelphia chromosome (Ph)-positive ALL. In their more mature stages, pre-B-ALL blasts express TdT, HLA-DR, CD19, CD79a, and cytoplasmic immunoglobulins. A high proportion of pre-B-ALL cases have the translocation t(1;19) which is more common in black than in white patients.[36,37] Mature B-cell ALL (Burkitt leukemia) blasts express surface immunoglobulins (sIg, usually IgM), are clonal for κ or λ light chains, and lack expression of TdT. About 50% are CD10 positive, which may

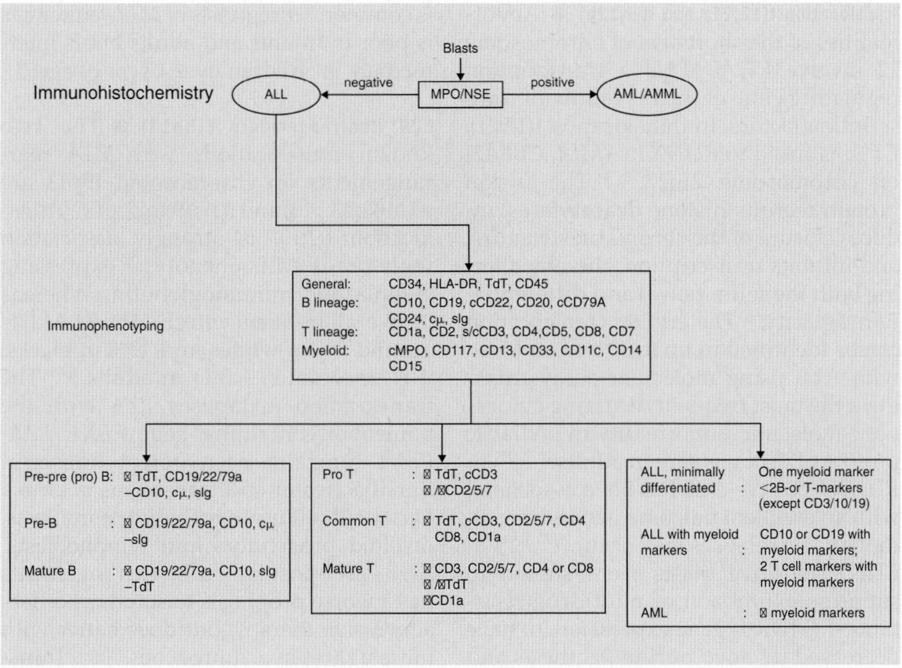

Figure 112-1 Diagnostic approach to ALL. *Abbreviations*: MPO, myeloperoxidase; NSE, nonspecific esterase; c, cytoplasmic; s, surface.

be associated with a better prognosis. Expression of CD20 is almost ubiquitous in mature B-cell ALL, where as it occurs in only about 40–50% of other ALL subtypes.

T-cell ALL accounts for only 15–20% of cases, is more common in black than in white patients,[37] and similar to B-lineage ALL can be further stratified into subtypes based on different stages of intrathymic differentiation.[38,39] T-cell ALL expresses various levels of CD1a, CD2, CD3, CD4, CD5, CD7, and CD8. CD4 and CD8 are either double-positive or double-negative. CD7 is the most sensitive T-cell marker but lacks specificity because cases of AML-cell or NK-cell leukemia are sometimes CD7-positive as well. Expression of cytoplasmic CD3 (cCD3) is the most lineage-specific marker for T-cell differentiation. Mature T-ALL expresses both surface CD3 (sCD3) and cCD3, CD2, and either CD4 or CD8 but not both. T-cell ALL of the earlier stages of differentiation (precursor T-ALL corresponding to a "prothymocyte" or "immature thymocyte" type) expresses cCD3 but not sCD3. sCD3- and CD7-postive T-ALL may suggest poor prognosis. T-cell ALL with the lack of CD1a and CD8 expression (in association with low expression of CD5 and frequent coexpression of myeloid-associated markers-CD13 and CD33) appear to be especially aggressive.[40]

Coexpression of myeloid-associated markers is common (15–50% in adult ALL; 5–35% in children), but does not automatically indicate bilineage potential. Frequently found myeloid-associated markers include CD13 and CD33, CD14, CD15, and CDw65.[41,42] Myeloid-associated marker expression is more frequent in ALL with translocation t(9;22), t(4;11), and t(12;21) with *TEL-AML1* fusion, and is generally absent in mature B-cell ALL.[42,43] Myeloid-associated marker expression has no prognostic significance,[41,43–47] but is useful to distinguish leukemic cells from normal progenitor cells, thereby enabling detection of minimal residual leukemia.[43] To identify the rare cases of bilineage ALL several scoring systems have been developed in which lineage-specific markers are weighed according to their discriminatory value of myeloid versus lymphoid.[36,48,49] Their practical clinical value is however limited.[50]

Cytogenetic and Molecular Abnormalities

Cytogenetic-molecular abnormalities are common in ALL (Table 112-2).[51–55] Their identification are important as they provide pathobiological insights, serve as targets for drug development, and furnish prognostic information, which has been translated into risk-adapted therapies.[55,56] Conventional karyotype analysis remains a cornerstone for the detection of chromosome abnormalities. In addition, fluorescence insitu hybridization (FISH), Southern blotting of genomic DNA, and real-time reverse transcriptase polymerase chain reaction (RT-PCR) assays of mRNA are applied to detect minimal residual disease and to monitor patients after therapy.[43] Oligonucelotide or cDNA microarray technology is currently being tested to identify previously unrecognized molecular ALL subtypes and as a complement to the other methods.[27,57–59]

Numerical Abnormalities Numerical abnormalities have an important prognostic impact in ALL, in children even more so than in adult patients. Hypodiploidy defines a karyotype with less than 46 chromosomes. The incidence of hypodiploidy is <10% without significant differences by age.[60] Among hypodiploid cases, only those with <44 chromosomes have inferior treatment outcome, especially cases with near-haploidy or its multiplication.

Table 112-2 **Cytogenetic and Molecular Abnormalities in ALL**

Cytogenetics	Gene Involved	Frequency (%) Adult	Frequency (%) Child
t(1;14)(p32;q11)	*TAL-1*	10-15	5-10
del(5)(q35)	*HOX11L2*	<2	<2
t(5;14)(q35;q32)	*HOX11L2*	1	2-3
del(6q), t(6;12)	?	5	<5
del(7p)	?	5-10	<5
+ 8	–	10-12	2
t(8;14), t(8;22), t(2;8)	*c-MYC*	5	2-5
t(9;22)(q34;q11)	*BCR-ABL*	15-25	2-6
del(9)(p21-22)	*CDKN2A and CDKN2B*	6-30	20
del(9)(q32)	*TAL-2*	<1	<1
Extrachromosome 9q	*NUP214/ABL*	<5	?
t(10;14)(q24;q11)	*HOX11*	5-10	<5
del(11)(q22)	*ATM*	25-30[a]	15[a]
del(11)(q23)	*MLL/AF4*	5-10	<5
del(12p) or t(12p)	*ETV6-AML1*	<1[b]	20-25[b]
del(13)(q14)	*miR15/miR16*	<5	<5
t(14q11-q13)	*TCR* α *and* δ	20-25[c]	20-25[c]
t(14q32)	*IGH, BCL11B*	5	?
t(1;19), t(17;19)	*E2A-PBX1, E2A-HLF*	<5	4-5
Hyperdiploidy	–	2-15	10-26
Hypodiploidy	–	5-10	5-10

[a] As determined by LOH (loss of heterozygosity).
[b] As determined by PCR (polymerase chain reaction).
[c] In T-ALL, overall incidence < 10%.
Abbreviations: IgM, immunoglobulin M; Igκ, immunoglobulin kappa; Igλ, immunoglobulin lambda; TdT, terminal deoxynucleotidyl transferase.

A range of structural abnormalities have been associated with hypodiploidy, but the prognostic impact of these remains unclear.[61–63]

Hyperdiploidy is defined by chromosome numbers of more than 46. It is detected more commonly in children than in adults (~25% vs 5%).[64,65] The range of added chromosomes is not random. Most commonly increased chromosomes are 4, 8, 10, and 21 followed by chromosomes 5, 6, 14, and 17. Gene expression profiles in pediatric patients demonstrated that 70% of the genes that defined this group belonged to either chromosomes X or 21 irrespective of whether or not these chromosomes were increased in the leukemic blasts.[27] Hyperdiploid blasts from patients with ALL have been shown to accumulate more methotrexate and methotrexate polygluatamate, and to be more sensitive to other drugs such as mercaptopurine, thioguanine, cytarabine, and L-asparaginase.[66–68] Response duration and survival is more favorable for patients with hyperdiploid chromosomes. Discrepancies between some studies may be based on inclusion of patients with additional structural abnormalities.

Structural Abnormalities ■ Translocation t(9;22). The translocation between the long arms of chromosome 9 and 22, t(9;22)(q34;q11) Ph is the most common abnormality in adult ALL (15–30%), but is rare in children (<5%).[65,69] On a molecular level, the *BCR* gene on chromosome 22q11 is fused to the *ABL* gene on 9q34. The chimeric *BCR-ABL* gene is translated into hybrid BCR-ABL oncoproteins of different sizes and molecular weights depending on the exact location of the breakpoint location within *BCR*.[70] Whereas $p210^{BCR\text{-}ABL}$ is the most frequent oncoprotein in CML, $p190^{BCR\text{-}ABL}$ occurs in 60–80% of patients with Ph-positive ALL. *BCR-ABL* proteins are distinguished by constitutively active tyrosine kinase activity leading to activation of downstream signaling pathways such as Ras/Raf, Jak-Stat, PI3-kinase, Crkl and AKT, adhesion kinases, and others. Secondary chromosomal abnormalities may accompany t(9;22) in up to more than 80% of the patients and are contributing to worse outcome. ALL with t(9;22) typically affects older patients, presents with higher white blood cell and blast counts at diagnosis, is of a pre-B-cell immunophenotype, and often demonstrates coexpression of myeloid markers.[71] Whereas Ph-positive ALL used to be one of the subtypes with the worst long-term DFS, use of inhibitors of BCR-ABL kinase activity (tyrosine kinase inhibitors, reviewed below) in combination with multiagent chemotherapy appear to be achieving better outcomes nowadays.

Translocation t(12;21) and del(12p) ■ Abnormalities of the short arm of chromosome 12 involve *ETV6* (*TEL*) a transcription regulating gene of the Ets family of transcription factors. In translocation t(12;21), *ETV6* is fused to *RUNX1* (*AML1, CBFA2*) on chromosome 21q22.[72,73] The fusion protein recruits histone deacetylases, induces closure of the chromatin structure, and inhibits transcription, thereby altering both the self-renewal and differentiation capacity.[65] The cryptic translocation can be identified in up to 30% of children with ALL using molecular assays making it the most frequent recurring cytogenetic-molecular abnormality in pediatric pre-B ALL; but it is rare in adults.[74] *ETV6-RUNX1*-positve ALL has been associated with an excellent outcome in children, although late relapses may occur.[75,76] *ETV6-RUNX1*-positive blasts were shown to suppress expression of multidrug resistance-1 (MDR-1) gene expression, to have decreased de novo purine synthesis and to suppress genes involved in purine metabolism.[77]

del(9p21) ■ Abnormalities of 9p21 occur in up to 15% of patients with ALL.[78] The ALL blasts are predominantly of T-cell lineage. Prognosis in these patients is generally unfavorable, and characterized by higher rates of relapse and shorter survival. The prognostic associations are stronger in children and are less well defined in adult ALL.[79–82] Commonly involved genes with del(9p21) include the cyclin-dependent kinase inhibitor genes *CDKN2A* (*MTS1, p16*INK4a) and *CDKN2B* (*MTS2, p15*INK4b). Using FISH or PCR, heterozygous and/or homozygous deletions of *CDKN2A* have been described in up to 80% of children with T-ALL and 20% of pre-B ALL. Hypermethylation of promoter regions of these genes has been described.[83]

***MLL* Rearrangements (11q23)** ■ The common denominator of 11q23 abnormalities is involvement of the mixed lineage leukemia gene *MLL* (*ALL-1, HRX, HTRX1*). It encodes a nuclear protein that maintains the expression of particular members of the *HOX* family and is frequently involved in reciprocal rearrangements with other genes located on chromosomes 4q21, 9p22, 19p13, 1p32, and many others.[65,84] The fusion of *MLL* with *AF4* on chromosome 4q21 is a frequent abnormality in infant ALL, accounting for up to 85% of the cases, but is detected in only 3–8% of adults.[85–87] Adults with this translocation tend to be older, have higher white blood cell counts and organomegaly; sanctuary sites such as the CNS are involved more frequently. CD10-negative, cytoplasmic immunoglobulin-positive pre-B ALL was described to have a high *MLL* rearrangement rate.[88] Myeloid antigen coexpression is common.[52] Prognosis of *MLL* leukemias is poor in infants and adults but is intermediate in children over 1 year of age.[89]

***E2A* Rearrangements (19p13)** ■ The two known translocations with *E2A* rearrangements on chromosome 19p13 are t(1;19)(q23;p13) and t(17;19)(q21;p13). Translocation t(1;19) is strongly association with pre-B ALL phenotype expressing cytoplasmic immunoglobulin. Whereas its overall frequency in childhood ALL is around 3% in whites and 12% in blacks, it is uncommon (<3%) in adults.[37,65] The translocation juxtaposes *E2A* with the homeobox-containing gene *PBX1*. *E2A-PBX1* functions as a potent transcriptional activator and transforms *in vitro* a variety of cell types including fibroblasts, myeloid progenitors and lymphoblasts. *E2A-PBX1*-positive ALL rearrangements has a worse prognosis to standard or less aggressive therapy, but does better with more aggressive approaches.[15,90,91] Translocation t(17;19) is a rarer variant in association with hypercalcemia and DIC at diagnosis and generally poor outcome.[92]

8q24 Rearrangements ■ The *c-MYC* gene, located on 8q24, is involved in one of the three translocations with kappa or lambda immunoglobulin (Ig) light chain locus in mature B-ALL: (i) The t(8;14)(q24;q32), with a frequency of 80%, is the most common translocation. In this translocation, *c-MYC* is juxtaposed to the immunoglobulin heavy chain (IgH) gene locus on 14q32; (ii) The t(8;22)(q24;q11),occurs in about 15% of B-ALL patients and involves the Ig lambda gene locus on 22q11; and (iii) the t(2;8)(p12;q24)] is the least frequent of translocation and involves the Ig kappa gene locus on 2p12. Translocations of *c-MYC* into the T-cell receptor alpha/delta gene on 14q11 have been described and lead to the same effect of increasing transcription of *c-MYC*.[93]

***T-Cell Receptor (TCR)* ■ *Gene Rearrangements*.** TCR gene rearrangements define the majority of cytogenetic abnormalities in T-lineage ALL. Genes for T-cell receptors are located on chromosomes 14q11 (TCR α/δ), 7q15 (TCR γ), and 7q35 (TCR δ). Although no specific cytogenetic abnormality can be linked to a specific clinical subtype of T-lineage ALL, a number of distinct chromosomal translocations have been identified. The clinical relevance of the translocations depends on the partner genes involved. In most cases, partner genes are deregulated and come under the influence of promoter/enhancer regions of TCRs.[65]

Other Molecular Abnormalities

More than 50% of cases of T-cell ALL have activating mutations that involve *NOTCH1*, a gene encoding a transmembrane receptor that regulates normal T-cell development.[15] In fact, activating mutations of *NOTCH1* could be the instigating event in most T-cell leukemias. In childhood T-cell ALL, this genetic abnormality was associated with a favorable prognosis in one study.[94] Smad3 is an intermediate in the chain of transforming growth factor (TGF)-β dependent signaling pathways from cell surface to nucleus. Loss of Smad3 protein was recently identified in samples of children with T-linage ALL and together with loss of p27Kip1 was found to act synergistically in T-cell leukemogenesis in mice.[95] Activating mutations of *fms-like tyrosine kinase 3* (*FLT3*) are rare in ALL, but have been detected with higher frequency in some subtypes (eg, ALL with rearrangements of *MLL*, hyperdiploid ALL, some T-cell subsets). In contrast to AML, internal tandem duplications of *FLT3* have not been identified. Use of FLT3 inhibitors may have therapeutic activity in some of these cases.[96] About 2% of childhood ALL cases have intrachromosomal amplification of chromosome 21, which is associated with a B-cell precursor immunophenotype, older age, low leukocyte count and more importantly, an increased risk of relapse.[97]

Gene Expression Microarrays

Microarray technology is used to establish gene expression profiles that further distinguish subtypes of ALL, stratify patients according to risk and response, identify genetic markers associated with drug sensitivity and resistance pathways, and yield useful insights into pathogenesis and biology of ALL.[27,57,65,98–100] Gene expression profiling has also a significant potential to facilitate the identification of new diagnostic markers, therapeutic targets and to propel novel drug development.[65,101]

In a study of 360 children with ALL, 6 subtypes of ALL could be identified that corresponded to known genetic subtypes (t(12;21) [*TEL-AML1*], t(1;19) [*E2A-PBX1*], t(9;22) [*BCR-ABL*], 11q23 rearrangements [*MLL*], hypderdiploidy, and T-cell ALL).[27] An additional subtype was identified that did not fit any of the described cytogenetic categories and whose clinical relevance needs to be determined. Gene expression profiling has demonstrated different signature patterns in T-lineage ALL.[102,103] In a study using high-resolution single nucleotide polymorphism arrays, deletions, amplifications, point mutations, and other structural rearrangements were identified in genes encoding regulators of B-lymphocyte development in 40% of cases of B-cell precursor ALL.[98] The *PAX5* gene was the most frequent target, involving in a third of the cases. Some of the pathways seemed to have prognostic relevance; however these findings require confirmation.

The possibilities of gene expression profiling are inriguing; however, numerous issues related to reproducibility, statistical significance, and practical application of such an approach still need to be resolved before gene expression profiling is ready for clinical use. In addition, proteomics has been an evolving field generating questions about the significance of gene expression versus protein expression profiles.

Epigenetic Alterations in ALL

Aberrant methylation of promoter-associated CpG islands and silencing of genes related to the tumor phenotype is an important step in the process of malignant transformation of cells.[104] Epigenetic silencing of cancer-related genes is common in ALL at diagnosis and relapse where abnormal methylation patterns are found in up to 80% of patients.[105] Genes frequently involved include p73, the cyclin-dependent kinase inhibitors p15, and p57^{KIP2}, which play a crucial role in cell cyle regulatory pathways. It seems that methylation of at least 2 genes is required to be associated with an unfavorable prognosis.[106–108] In recent years, the interplay between methylation changes and organization of histone complexes has become a focus of attention, not least because many drugs (eg, DNA methyltransferase inhibitors, histone deacetylase inhibitors) are now available targeting these various aspects of epigenetic alterations.

The Therapy of ALL

Starting in the 1960s, physicians and researchers at St. Jude Children's Research Hospital were the first to design a series of Total Therapy treatment for pediatric ALL, that would make ALL to become the first disseminated cancer to be cured, and later on also lead to substantial improvements in the prognosis of adults with ALL.[109] The design was based on a combination of all available antileukemia drugs that were delivered in a sequence of extended courses of therapy. The goal was to prevent emergence of resistant subclones and to rapidly restore normal hematopoiesis. Therapeutic strategies in adult ALL have been patterned after the pediatric regimens and although various combinations with differences in treatment sequence and choice of agents are being used, the same basic principles apply: induction therapy followed by early intensification and consolidation, specific CNS treatment, and a prolonged maintenance phase.[25,45] Given the high remission rates with these regimens, the focus of current ALL programs is concentrated on improvement of remission duration and survival of adult patients and to improve quality of life of pediatric patients. With this goal in mind, validation of subtype-specific prognostic models and development of risk-adapted and targeted therapy designs have become the major objectives of clinical trials.[110–112]

Treatment of Newly Diagnosed Patients

As complex as ALL treatment programs are and as much variations are found in many of its details, an easily recognizable framework is common to all of them and is presented in Figure 112-2. Because therapy is becoming increasingly subset-specific and depends on proper risk-stratification, the section on prognostic factors is discussed first prior to proceeding to therapy programs in more detail.

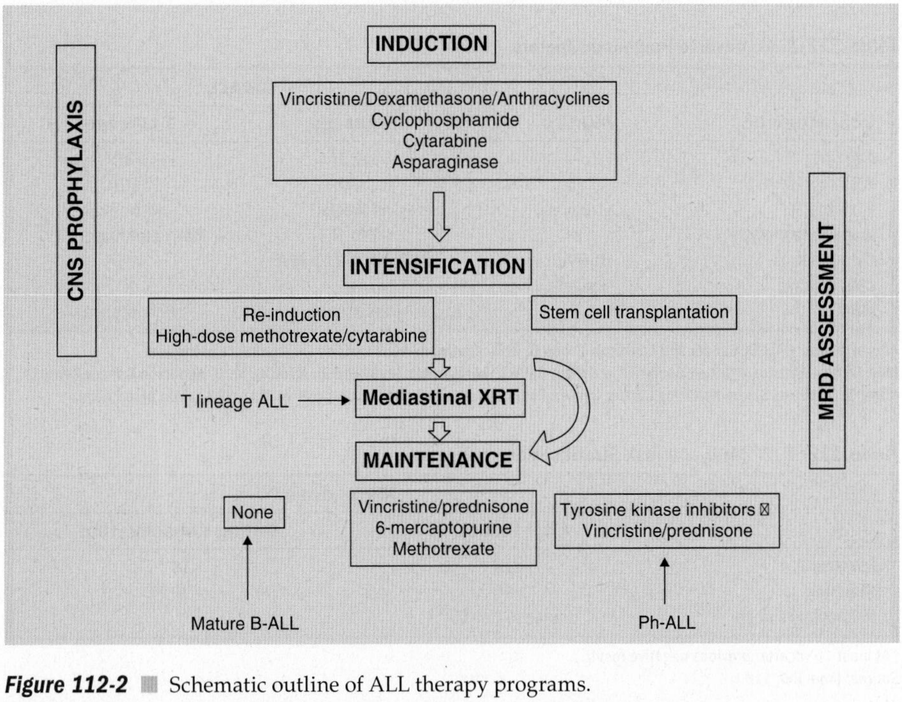

Figure 112-2 Schematic outline of ALL therapy programs.

Prognostic Factors

Efforts to describe risk models for ALL date back to the 1980s and have since experienced continued improvements as a result of the accumulating experience from a sequence of clinical trials.[44,55,113,114] Although remission rates are high with current induction regimens and can hardly be increased, prognostic models are still useful for risk-directed postremission therapy to improve the DFS rates in adults and children with high-risk leukemia, and to avoid overtreatment of those with favorable disease. It should be noted that improved treatment has abolished the prognostic impact of many clinical, laboratory, or biological variables. For example, once associated with poor prognosis, T-cell ALL has long-term DFS of over 50% in adults and 80% in children with current therapies including cyclophosphamide and cytarabine, and mature B-cell ALL have complete response (CR) rates of 90% and DFS rates >50% in adults and >80% in children with short-term dose-intense treatment regimens.[55] Information from morphological assessment, immunophenotyping, karyotype analysis, molecular genetics, and, increasingly, measurements of minimal residual disease (MRD), has contributed to a more comprehensive risk-stratification of patients (Table 112-3).[25,44,,52,55,115,116] Gene expression analysis in T-lineage ALL has demonstrated high expression of *ERG* and *HOX11L2* as unfavorable features and associations with other molecular markers have been established.[117–119]

Monitoring of MRD after induction and during consolidation has emerged as one of the most powerful predictors of relapse and has been most helpful to further stratify standard-risk patients.[44,55,120,121] The German Multicenter Study Group for Adult ALL (GMALL) prospectively monitored 196 standard-risk ALL patients at up to 9 time points in the first year of therapy with quantitative polymerase chain reaction.[120] MRD was predictive for relapse and according to the rapidity of eradication of MRD or persistence of MRD over time, three risk groups could be defined with the 3-year relapse risk varying between 0% (low-risk group) to 94% (high-risk group) (Table 112-4).

Other factors with impact on prognosis have been identified (eg, time to platelet recovery during induction, expression of drug resistance markers, pharmacogenetics). Their validation in the context of prognostic models is lacking and they are not generally accepted in the assignment of risk-adapted therapies.[122–124]

Induction Therapy

Vincristine, corticosteroids, and a third agent (anthracyclines in adults and asparaginase in children) have long been the backbone of ALL induction therapy.[55,125] No difference in outcome has been established based on the use of different anthracyclines. Whether higher doses of anthracyclines during induction improve outcome remains disputed.[126–129] Todeschini et al[128] used daunorubicin at total doses of 270 mg/m^2 during induction and high-dose cytarabine during consolidation. The CR rate was 93%, the induction mortality 8%, and the 6-year event-free survival 55% in 60 patients with adult ALL. On the other hand, the CALGB could not demonstrate an improvement of DFS with intensified daunorubicin.[129] CALGB study 19802 included 163 adults with untreated ALL. For patients <60 years, the daunorubicin dose of the induction module was increased from 45 to 60 mg/m^2 and then 80 mg/m^2 daily for 3 days. Outcome was determined primarily by age, with patients over 60 years doing significantly worse, but not by the dose of daunorubicin.

Additional drugs have become part of ALL induction and intensification cycles. These include cytarabine, methotrexate, cyclophosphamide, L-asparaginase, and less frequently etoposide, tenposide, m-amsacrine or other agents. With CR rates at around 90%, it will be difficult to demonstrate further improvement. Yet, intensification of induction and intensification has shown a positive impact on remission duration and survival, and this effect has been most obvious for specific subtypes. Cytarabine and cyclophosphamide have increased response rates and DFS in T-cell ALL.[111,130] Another important drug has been L-asparaginase. Large randomized pediatric ALL trials have demonstrated improved survival rates where L-asparaginase was given throughout the remission and/or postremission phase.[131,132] L-asparaginase is a bacterial enzyme, which efficiently depletes serum asparagine. ALL cells require asparagine for protein production, but, in contrast to normal cells, are unable to produce it themselves so that they depend on sufficiently high serum levels for their survival. The most commonly used form of asparaginase is derived from *E.coli*, whose major limitation is development of hypersensitivity and worse tolerability in adults than in children. Pegasparaginase is a modified form of *E.coli* asparaginase with longer serum half-life and reduced risk of hypersensitivity reactions and several studies have been reported in adults.[133–135] CALGB study 9511 investigated pegasparaginase as a replacement for *E.coli* asparaginase in previously untreated adult patients with ALL.[134] Pegasparaginase was given at 2000 units/m^2 subcutaneously or intramuscularly during each of the first three courses. Asparagine depletion occurred in up to 80% of patients, antibodies to pegasparaginase developed in only three patients, and the risk of hypersensitivity reactions or pancreatitis was low.

Fractionation of cyclophosphamide and high doses of methotrexate have improved the outcome in mature B-cell ALL.[111,136–138]

Monoclonal antibodies have been included in adult ALL induction programs. Most experience exists with the anti-CD20 chimeric antibody rituximab. Expression of CD20 has been associated with a higher relapse rate in adult patients with pre-B ALL,[139] although the association of outcome with CD20 expression remains more disputed in children.[140] Several studies have shown improvement in prognosis with chemotherapy plus rituximab combina-

Table 112-3 Adverse Prognostic Factors

		GMALL	
Characteristic	**MDACC**	**B-lineage**	**T-Lineage**
Age (yr)	–	>35	>35
WBC (× 10^9/L	>5	>30	>100
Time to CR	>1 course	>4 weeks	>4 weeks
Immunophenotype	B	Pro-B	Early and mature T
Cytogenetics	*BCR-ABL*	BCR-ABL; ALL1-AFA	–
CNS disease	Present	–	–
MRD	–	Persistence	Persistence

Abbreviations: CALGB, Cancer and Leukemia Group B; CNS, central nervous system; CR, complete remission; FAB, French-American-British Cooperative Group; GMALL, German ALL Study Group; MDACC, M. D. Anderson Cancer Center; MSKCC, Memorial Sloan-Kettering Cancer Center; Ph, Philadelphia chromosome-positive ALL; WBC, white blood cells.

Table 112-4 MRD and Risk Stratification

	MRD Levels	
	After Induction	**During Consolidation**
Low risk	$<10^{-4}$	$<10^{-4}$
High risk	$>10^{-4}$	$>10^{-4}$
Molecular relapse	Increase to $>10^{-4}$ [a]	

[a] At least 16 wk after previous negative result.
Source: From Ref. 110.

tions especially in mature B-cell ALL where CD20 expression is virtually ubiquitous.[141–143] The picture in pre-B ALL is more complicated. A recent update of the modified hyper-cyclophosphamide, vincristine, adriamycin, dexamethasone (-CVAD) regimen from the group at MD Anderson Cancer Center showed improved DFS in favor of rituximab in patients younger than 30 years, but not older ALL patients. Overall survival (OS) was not affected.[143]

Steroids are a standard part of ALL induction and prednisone or prednisolone is the most commonly used steroid, particularly during the maintenance phase. Compared to prednisone and prednisolone, dexamethasone has shown better in vitro antileukemic activity and achievement of higher drug levels in the CSF. Using a dose of 6 mg/m^2 or 6.5 mg/m^2 throughout therapy, the Children Oncology Group and UK Medical Research Council randomized trials demonstrated a significant reduction in isolated CNS relapse and a significant improvement of event-free survival.[144,145] On the other hand, a smaller study from the Tokyo Children's Cancer Study Group including 231 children with standard- and intermediate-risk ALL showed no difference between dexamethasone (8 mg/m^2 during induction and 6 mg/m^2 during intensifications) and prednisolone (60 and 40 mg/m^2, respectively).[146]

Given the intensity of induction combinations, supportive care has become an important part of ALL therapy. The rationale for hematopoietic growth factors includes shortening of the duration of myelosuppression and therefore associated infectious complications. In addition, a rapid recovery of the marrow function following chemotherapy allows timely administration of dose-intense treatment regimens.[147] Three randomized adult trials have demonstrated advantages of using hematopoietic growth factors such as granulocyte-colony stimulating factor (G-CSF).[148–150] In the double-blinded, randomized Cancer and Leukemia Group B (CALBG) trial 9111, as compared to the 102 patients receiving supportive care alone, the G-CSF treated group (n = 96) had faster neutrophil recovery to >1 × 10^9/L (16 vs 22 days, p < .001), platelet recovery (16 vs 19 days, p = .003), shorter duration of hospital stays (p =.02), higher CR rates (87% vs 71%, p = .01), and less mortality (5% vs 11%, p = .04).[150] G-CSF therapy reduced induction mortatlity from 25% to 10% (p = .24) in patients older than 60 years. G-CSF was not associated, however, with longer remission duration or OS. In a pediatric randomized trial, G-CSF treatment has limited clinical utility.[151] A possible role of erythropoietic growth factors in the decrease of transfusion requirements is being studied.

Prophylactic antibiotics including antibacterials (eg, levofloxacin, ciprofloxacin, trimethoprim-sulfamethoxazole), antifungals (eg, fluconazole, itraconazole, voriconazole), and antivirals (eg, acyclovir) should accompany induction therapy until recovery of the neutrophil count to at least 1000/μL in adults.[152] Tumor lysis and in some cases DIC should be anticipated in patients wih significant leukocytosis and be treated appropriately. Organ involvement and dysfunction may respond to high-dose steroids (eg, hyperbilirubinemia related to ALL).

Post-Remission Therapy

Postremission therapy consists of an intensified consolidation followed by maintenance therapy, and stem cell transplantation for some patients. Following the experience from children with ALL, an intensification of post-remission therapy has improved outcome, particularly in patients with high-risk disease. There is no consensus, however, on the optimal type or duration of consolidation. Consolidation programs typically consist of a repetition of the induction sequence or rotational programs including additional agents, which may benefit particular ALL subtypes. As dose, schedule, and combinations of cytostatic drugs vary considerably between studies, it remains difficult to assess the value of the individual components of various programs.

Table 112-5 details the hyper-CVAD program as one example. During hyper-CVAD, hyperfractionated cyclophosphamide alternates with high doses of cytarabine and methotrexate for 8 courses, which equals about 6 months of intensified post-remission therapy.[25] Compared with the earlier and less intense VAD program, there has been a significantly better CR rate (91% vs 75%) and survival. In CALGB study 8811, patients underwent early and late intensification courses with eight drugs following a five-drug induction regimen.[45] Maintenance therapy was given until 2 years after diagnosis. The median remission duration was 29 months and the median survival 36 months, considerably better than the outcome observed with earlier less intense trials. In a UK study (MRC UKALL XA), patients were randomized to either early intensification at 5 weeks, late intensification at 20 weeks, both, or neither.[153] Early intensification prevented relapses although DFS at 5 years was increased only slightly. In the GIMEMA ALL 0288 trial, patients were randomized to early post-CR intensification versus maintenance therapy.[154] Of 388 patients, 201 had maintenance alone and 187 received consolidation followed by maintenance. Intensification of post-CR treatment did not influence the continuous CR rate. At 8 years, 36% of patients on consolidation-maintenance and 37% of patients on maintenance alone remained in CR. Furthermore only 35% of the patient who were randomized to the intensified consolidation completed their treatment in the expected time frame, raising doubts as to the feasibility of prolonged intensified consolidation in adults because of toxicities and compliance problems.

Most adults with ALL are considered to be at high risk of disease recurrence and hence one trend of current treatment programs is a further intensification as adapted from pediatric protocols.[155,156] On the other hand, since a few patients do well with less intense therapies, many contemporary studies use sophisticated prognostic models to optimize therapy as discussed before. The GRAALL-03 trial included intensive steroid pretreatment, high-dose and earlier use of L-asparaginase, and delayed intensifications.[157] The CR rate in 144 patients was 91% with an estimated 18-month event-free survival and OS of 65% and 74%, respectively. Evaluation of morphological early response correlated closely with postinduction MRD measurement. In GMALL study 06/99 a shortened and intensified induction regimen was developed and included dexamethasone, a cyclophosphamide prephase, intensive daunorubicin, and pegaspargase. Two induction cycles were then followed by consolidation and then maintenance, which was adapted according ot the course of MRD levels.[110,158] A total of 843 patients with a median age of 36 years participated. The CR rate was 83%. After modifications of the dexamethasone doses for early toxicities, an optimized induction regimen achieved 89% CR with an early mortality of 4%. Shortened, intensified induction, intensified consolidation, risk-adapted and extended stem cell transplant indications and MRD based treatment stratification are now the basis of the GMALL 07/03 trial.[159] A preliminary analysis of 713 patientes confirmed the high CR rate of 89% and demonstrated an improved survival of 54% (above 70% for standard-risk patients). Implications of this study for stem cell transplantation are discussed below.

Most maintenance schedules include 6-mercaptopurine, methotrexate, and monthly pulses of vincristine and prednisone, and extend over 2–3 years. Further intensifications during maintenance are being studied, but remain investigational. Maintenance therapy has become subset-specific: it is of little value in mature B-cell ALL as these patients relapse within the first year of remission and rarely later;[136] tyrosine kinase inhibitors have become an integral component in Ph-positive ALL (where treatment with kinase inhibitors may even be

Table 112-5 ■ **The Hyper-CVAD Program in ALL**

Component	Drug	Subtype: Unspecified	CD20-Positive	Mature B Cell	T-Lineage	Ph-Positive
		INDUCTION and INTENSIFIED CONSOLIDATION				
Hyper-CVAD (cycles 1, 3, 5, 7)	Cyclophosphamide, Doxorubicin, Vincristine, Dexamethasone	✓	✓	✓	✓	✓
	Rituximab	–	✓[a]	✓	–	✓[a, b]
	Dasatinib	–	–	–	–	✓[c]
Methotrexate + HD cytarabine (cycles 2, 4, 6, 8)	Methotrexate, Cytarabine	✓	✓	✓	✓	✓
	Rituximab	–	✓[a]	✓	–	✓[a, b]
	Dasatinib	–	–	–	–	✓[c]
		CNS PROPHYLAXIS				
Intrathecal therapy[d]	IT, methotrexate[e]; IT cytarabine	✓	✓	✓	✓	✓
		PRE-MAINTENANCE				
Mediastinal XRT	–	–	–	–	✓[f]	–
Nelarabine	Nelarabine	–	–	–	✓[g]	–
		MAINTENANCE				
POMP	6-mercaptopurine, Oral methotrexate, Prednisone, Vincristine	✓[h]	✓[h]	–	✓[h]	✓[i]
Intensification	Oral methotrexate/L-asparaginase (months 6 and 18)	✓	✓	–	✓	✓
	Hyper-CVAD (months 7 and 19)	✓	✓	–	✓	✓
Dasatinib	Dasatinib	–	–	–	–	✓[j]

[a] During cycles 1 to 4.
[b] If CD20-positive.
[c] On days 1 to 14 of each of the first 8 courses (dose 50 mg orally twice daily). Chest x-ray prior to each course to evaluate for pleural effusions.
[d] Number of intrathecal therapies depending on risk for CNS disease (4 for lowrisk, 8 for intermediate risk, 16 for highrisk including mature B cell). Two intrathecals are given with each induction/intensified consolidation course).
[e] Dose of intrathecal methotrexate should be reduced by 50% if administered via Omaya reservoir.
[f] If bulky mediastinal adenopathy (≥7 cm).
[g] Two cycles of 28 to 35 days each.
[h] Total duration 30 months.
[i] Total duration 24 months.
[j] Continuous administration beyond maintenance.

considered life long); and other more T-cell specific drugs such as nelarabine are studied in T-lineage ALL.

Stem cell transplantation (SCT) has improved outcome for patients with high-risk ALL in first CR (Table 112-6).[160–167] Although there has been resistance to apply SCT for standard-risk patients in CR1, recent reports suggest that the benefit of SCT extends also to some standard-risk patients, in some cases possibly based on MRD levels or other features not captured by traditional prognostic markers.[159,168] Studies have also compared the results of allogeneic versus autologous SCT or chemotherapy in patients with ALL in first CR. Unbiased comparisons between treatments remain difficult for several reasons. Most patients lack a matched related sibling and cannot be allocated to allogeneic SCT in the first place. Furthermore, significant heterogeneity exists with regard to transplant preparative regimens, source of stem cells (peripheral blood, marrow), the role of T-cell depletion, and uniform application of prognostic markers.[169]

In a French multicenter trial (LALA 87) patients with a matched sibling donor were allocated to receive allogeneic SCT if they were in CR and younger than 40 years (n = 116), or were randomized to chemotherapy (n = 96) or autologous SCT (n = 95) if they were older or had no sibling donor.[166] The 5-year survival rates were not significantly different (48% vs 35%, p = .08), except for patients with high-risk ALL (Ph-positive ALL, undifferentiated ALL, age > 35 years, leukocyte count > 30 × 10^9/L, time to CR > 4 weeks), where allogeneic SCT achieved better 5-year survival (44% vs 20%, p = .03) and DFS (39% vs 14%, p =.01). In an update of the LALA 87 study, OS rates at 10 years were 44% in the allogeneic SCT arm versus 11% with chemotherapy (p =.009) in the high-risk group, and 49% and 39%, respectively (p = .6), for standard-risk patients.[170]

The LALA-94 study focused on a more risk-adapted postremission strategy and the role of allogeneic SCT in ALL.[171] A total of 922 patients were divided into standard-risk, high-risk, Ph-positive, and CNS-positive. All patients received a standard 4-week induction and then divided

Table 112-6 ■ **Outcome of Allogeneic SCT in First Remission**

N	Median Age (Yr) (Range)	DFS in % (Yr)	Ref.
18	24 (5-36)	42 (3)	160
25	22 (4-36)	71 (3)	161
151	31 (15-52)	60.3 (5)	162
41	22 (18-50)	61 (5)	163
184	25 (15-44)	49.5 (6)	164
29	24 (16-41)	62 (8)	167
22	15-51	58 (3)	165

either postremission chemotherapy (standard-risk group) or allogeneic SCT (all other risk groups) if an HLA-identical sibling was identified. Autologous SCT was offered to patients without donor, or they were randomized between autologous SCT and chemotherapy in the absence of Ph or CNS disease. The study confirmed better DFS for high-risk ALL patients in first CR. On the other hand, autologous transplant did not confer a significant benefit over chemotherapy.

The Groupe Ouest-Est des Leucémies Agiuës et Maladies du Sang (GOELAMS) has evaluated the impact of allogeneic SCT for high-risk patients in first CR versus delayed autologous SCT for patients without matched donors and those older than 50 years.[172] On an intent-to-treat analysis for patients younger than 50 years, 6-year OS was significantly improved with allogeneic SCT compared with autologous stem cell transplant (75% vs 40%, $p = .0027$).

The MRC UKALL XII/ECOG E2993 trial was a collaborative effort to address if allogeneic SCT could be beneficial for all suitable adult patients; and if a single autologous SCT could be as effective as postremission chemotherapy.[168] The study enrolled 1929 patients between 15 and 59 years of age. All patients who had an HLA-matched sibling donor were assigned to receive an allogeneic SCT, whereas those who did not or were over age 55, were randomized to receive an autologous SCT versus chemotherapy. Any randomization was preceded by induction chemotherapy and intensification with high-dose methotrexate. High-risk was defined as age > 35 years, leukocytosis (≥30 × 10^9/L for B-lineage and 100 × 10^9/L for T-lineage) and Ph-ALL. CR rate was 90% and 5-year survival 43% for all patients. The following results emerged: (1) survival at 5 years was 53% for Ph-negative patients with a donor, versus 45% for those without a donor ($p = .02$); (2) 5-year survival for Ph-negative standard-risk patients was superior for patients with a donor compared to those without (62% vs 52%, $p = .02$); (3) 5-year survival for high-risk patients was not significantly different whether patients had a donor or not (41% vs 35%, $p = .2$). In this group, transplant-related toxicity prevented a better outcome and abrogated the effect of a reduction in relapse rate; (4) postremission chemotherapy resulted in superior event-free and OS when compared to autologous SCT ($p = .02$ and .03, respectively).

The the GMALL 07/2003 trial applied a more refined risk assignment including assessment of MRD levels during various stages of therapy, and resulted in a referral of a proportion of standard-risk patients to transplant, although the intention was not to allocate every standard-risk patients to receive an allogenetic SCT.[159] Further updates are needed to draw conclusions.

Although a broader role of allogeneic SCT for patients with ALL in first CR is now emerging, optimal timing remains challenging. Novel therapies (eg, tyrosine kinase inhibitors for Ph-ALL) may affect outcome requiring a redefinition of SCT in some of the risk groups. Nonmyeloablative SCT has been successfully used in older or debilitated patients.[173] The major impediment for SCT remains the fact that less then 30% of patients have a matched sibling donor. Much work is therefore invested in improving transplants from partially matched related donors, matched unrelated donors (MUD), and umbilical cord blood (UCB). Bishop et al[174] determined outcomes between autologous SCT and MUD SCT in 260 adult patients in CR1 or CR2. Although treatment-related mortality was higher with MUD SCT, relapse risk was lower and 5-year leukemia-free and OS rates were similar (37% vs 39%, 38% vs 39%, respectively). Similar results were reported by other groups.[175]

Allogeneic SCT clearly benefits several pediatric subgroups such as Ph+ ALL and T-cell ALL with poor early response[176,177] but its benefits in infants with the t(4;11) remains controversial.[15]

CNS Prophylaxis

CNS involvement is rare at diagnosis (<5% in children and <10% in adults). Nonetheless, in the absence of CNS prophylaxis, CNS disease occurs in 40–50% of the patients and has been a major obstacle to cure.[178] CNS relapse can occur as isolated CNS disease, follow marrow recurrence, or occur concomitantly with a marrow or testicular relapse or both. As CNS relapse confers a poor prognosis irrespective of the intensity of retreatment, with the possible exception of late CNS relapses, effective CNS prophylaxis is the more important.[23,179,180] CNS prophylaxis should start early and extend through the induction and intensified consolidation phase as delayed CNS prophylaxis has been associated with an increased incidence of CNS disease.

Risk factors for CNS involvement include younger age, T-lineage and mature B-cell ALL immunophenotype, a high white blood cell count and the presence of blasts in cerebrospinal fluid at diagnosis.[23] Expression of CD7, CD56 and interleukin-15 was found to have prognostic implications with regard to extramedullary manifesfions of ALL.[181–183] Elevated serum LDH levels and a high proliferative index (S + G2M >14%) proved to be sensitive predictors of the risk of CNS disease.[184] In a multivariate analysis the risk of CNS involvement was 4% with normal LDH levels and low proliferative index, 13% with a high proliferative index only, 29% with an elevated LDH only, and 56% if both LDH and proliferative index were high.[184]

Therapeutic modalities for CNS prophylaxis include intrathecal (IT) chemotherapy (methotrexate, cytarabine, steroids), high-dose systemic chemotherapy (methotrexate, cytarabine, L-asparaginase, dexamethasone, 6-thioguanine), and craniospinal irradiation (XRT).[21,23,179] Combined triple modality IT therapy is more effective for CNS control than IT methotrexate alone, but carries a higher risk of treatment-related CNS morbidity and unexpectedly was associated with an increased risk of bone marrow and testicular relapse in one randomized trial.[185] One explanation for this paradoxical finding is that an "isolated" CNS relapse may in fact be an early manifestation of system relapse, and that better CNS control favors leukemic relapse in other sites at a later time. Several studies in children in adults have demonstrated that IT therapy is equivalent to craniospinal XRT, so that the role of cranial XRT has become controversial.[23,25,154,186] Adverse effects of XRT can be severe and disabling leading to seizures, dementia, and intellectual dysfunction, as well as other complications such as multiple endocrinopathies and growth retardation in children. CNS prophylaxis based on high-dose systemic therapy alone is not sufficient. During the hyper-CVAD regimen, CNS prophylaxis (in addition to systemic high-dose chemotherapy) consisted of 4 intrathecal treatments in the low-risk category (based on a normal LDH and low proliferative index), 8 intrathecal treatments with high-risk disease, and 16 intrathecal treatments for mature B-cell ALL or Burkitt disease.[25] Patients with cranial nerve root involvement may benefit from selective irradiation to the base of the skull.

Pharmacogenetics and Mechanisms of Drug Resistance

By affecting pharmacodynamics, the cytogenetic-molecular characteristics of leukemic cells can influence treatment outcome.[65,187] For example, hyperdiploidy cases accumulate higher intracellular methotrexate polyglutamates because they have extra copies of the gene encoding reduced folate carrier, an active transporter of methotrexate.[188] Blasts with a t(12;21) and *ETV6-RUNX1* fusion are more sensitive to asparaginase.[189] Cells harboring *MLL* rearrangements have increased sensitivity to cytarabine possibly by overexpression of cellular cytarabine receptors.[190]

In addition to acquired genetic abnormalities, an association between germ line genetic characteristics (involving genes encoding drug-metabolizing enzymes, transporters, and drug targets) and drug metabolism and sensitivity to chemotherapy is being recognized as well.[191] Rocha et al[192] determined whether ALL outcome was related to 16 genetic polymorphisms affecting the pharmacodynamics of antileukemic agents. They found that among 130 children with high-risk disease, the glutathione *S*-transferase (*GSTM1*) nonnull genotype had a higher risk of relapse, which was further increased by the thymidylate synthetase (*TYMS*) 3/3 genotype.[192] Homozygosity for the triple-tandem repeat polymorphism of the thymidylate synthase gene has been associated with increased levels of the enzyme, and with inferior outcome in children with ALL in another study as well.[193] Other polymorphisms of relevance in response to ALL therapy involve *MTHFR* and thiopurine methyltransferase (*TPMT*) gene.[194–196] It is noteworthy that in some cases, polymorphisms cause increased sensitivity to therapy agents and may thus predict for a higher probability of side effects (including second cancers) as much as higher sensitivity and improved outcome.[55] Interestingly, pharmacogenetics of bone marrow mesenchymal cells can also affect treatment outcome, such that high levels of asparagine synthetase can protect ALL cells from asparaginase treatment.[197]

Most of these studies have been conducted in children with ALL and knowledge about pharmacokinetic variables and how they contribute to outcome in adult ALL remains sparse. There is however growing interest in designing programs, which monitor pharmacogenetic properties and individualize dose and schedule of therapy accordingly.

Minimal Residual Disease (MRD)

In children and adults relapse is thought to result from residual leukemia cells, which persist following achievement of a morphologic and cytogenetic remission, but remain undetectable by conventional methods such as microscopy and cytochemical stains. A number of sensitive techniques have been developed including multicolor flow cytometry and and PCR assays. Whatever the assay, detection of residual leukemia cells depends on identification of unique leukemia cell markers. For flow cytometry, aberrant expression of surface marker combinations can be followed, whereas for PCR, leukemia-specific fusions genes (eg, *BCR-ABL, MLL-AF4, ETV6-RUNX1*) or patient-specific junctional regions of rearranged immunoglobulin and T-cell receptor genes constitute appropriate markers.[44,198–201]

A plethora of studies in both children and adults has provided convincing evidence for the usefulness of MRD monitoring to assess relapse risk.[202–207] There is general consensus from pediatric studies that high levels of MRD at the end of induction therapy, persistently high levels during consolidation and maintentance, and continuous increases of MRD levels at any point, are associated with a high risk of relapse.[44] Whereas more adults have higher levels of MRD at the completion of induction, and the relapse risk is higher even with low levels of MRD compared to children, continuous MRD assessment along several time points has proved predictive for relapse in adult patients as well.[202,203]

Assessment of MRD status has been included in a number of current studies to decide about intensification of postremission therapy. Several questions, however, still remain: (1) what is a clinically relevant threshold of residual disease upon which clinical decisions should be based?; (2) which are the most appropriate time points to measure MRD following induction, and how do they change in the context of the specific treatment administered?; (3) does intervention based on a molecular relapse improve outcome, and if so, do response criteria upfront need to be modifed to include molecular responses? (4) how reproducible are MRD assays across a multitude of laboratories and how reliably can MRD data from different institutions be compared? In this respect some progress of standardiziation has been accomplished trhough initiatives such as Europe Against Cancer (EAC) and BIOMED.[208] Finally, the conundrum remains that many patients with residual disease will never relapse, whereas vice versa molecular responders are not safe from disease recurrence. Beyond being a helpful tool for risk-adapted treatment stratifications, the study of residual disease will hopefully also reveal more about the biology of ALL itself.

Salvage Therapy

Prognosis of adult patients with relapsed ALL remains poor. In the MRC UKALL12/ECOG 2993 study, OS at 5 years after relapse was only 7%.[209] Factors predicting for better outcome (indicating 5-year survival rates of 11–12%) included age younger than 20 years and remission durations of more than 2 years. Treatment received during first CR had no impact on outcome. Although there is no standard approach to salvage therapy, there is general consensus, that allogeneic SCT should be first choice in this situation. For patients who have achieved a second remission, long-term leukemia-free survival rates of 14–43% have been reported with subsequent SCT.[169,210,211] Allogeneic SCT has also proved successful in some patients with primary refractory ALL even without undergoing a second attempt of induction therapy. In a study of the outcome of 314 patients with adult ALL, 29 patients underwent allogeneic SCT with durable remission rates of 38% and 31% in patients with primary refractory leukemia and second CR, respectively.[212]

For most patients, SCT is not an option for lack of a suitable donor, other ongoing comorbid conditions (eg, infections, poor performance status), or simply uncontrollable disease. Most nontransplant salvage attempts are modeled after patterns familiar from frontline therapy and include: (1) combinations of vincristine, steroids, and anthracyclines; (2) asparaginase and methotrexate combinations; or (3) high-dose cytarabine.[213] Direct comparisons of various regimens are difficult because of differences in patient characteristics, prior drug exposure and sensitivity, number of salvage attempts, variations in dose and schedule of agents, the use of SCT as consolidation in some patients, and not least because of the overall poor outcome.

Exploration of new agents for ALL therapy remains important (Table 112-7).[214] Rituximab, a chimeric monoclonal antibody against the cell surface protein CD20, has been combined with chemotherapy and improved outcome in nonHodgkin's lymphoma and subsets of patients with ALL.[143] The role of alemtuzumab, a humanized CD52-directed monoclonal antibody, in CD52-positive ALL and in combination with chemotherapy in aggressive T-lymphocytic malignancies is being explored.[215,216] Other monoclonal antibodies are in earlier stages of their clinical assessment and are summarized in Table 112-7. A continuous source of active drugs in leukemias is the vast group of nucleoside analogs. Clofarabine is a new generation purine nucleoside modeled after fludarabine and cladribine, but with different mechanisms of action and spectrum of activity.[217] In a phase 2 trial of clofarabine in 61 pediatric patients with relapsed or refractory ALL, 30% responded including seven patients with complete remissions, five with marrow remissions but lack of platelet recovery (CRp), and six children with partial remissions.[218] Median remission durations for children who did not proceed to SCT was 6 weeks, but sustained remissions for up to 64 weeks have been reported in some patients.[219] Clofarabine has been approved by the FDA for children with ALL relapse in December of 2004. Nelarabine is a soluble prodrug of 9-β-D-arabinofuranosylguanine (ara-G) with activity predominantly in relapsed T-lineage lymphoid malignancies and approval by the FDA for this indication in October of 2005. Response

Table 112-7 New Agents in ALL

Class	Examples
Nucleoside analogs	Clofarabine Nelarabine
Liposomal and pegylated compounds	Liposomal vincristine (Marqibo) Liposomal doxorubicin Liposomal annamycin Pegasparaginase
Monoclonal antibodies	Rituximab Alemtuzumab CAT-3888 (BL22) - anti-CD22 immunotoxin mAb216 - human IgM monoclonal antibody
Antifolates	Pemetrexed
Histone deacetylase inhibitors and DNA methyltransferase inhibitors	LBH589 PDX101 (Belinostas) Decitabine Azacitidine
Tyrosine kinase inhibitors	Imatinib Dasatinib Nilotinib
mTOR inhibitors	RAD001 (Everolimus)
Microtubule destabilizing agents	ENMD-1198

rates of 33% and up to 41% have been achieved in a group of 121 children and 39 adults with relapsed T-lineage leukemia/lymphoma, respectively.[220,221] Median OS in the adult group was 20 weeks.[221] Neurotoxicity is the major adverse event of nelarabine, which is both dose and schedule dependent and can be limited with every other day administration rather than daily. Of interest are other established compounds which have been modified to achieve more advantageous pharmacokinetic properties such as pegylated asparaginase, liposomal doxorubicin, or liposomal vincristine. Experience of 52 patients who have been treated with liposomal vincristine on two different studies demonstrated an overall response rate 21% with another 23% of the patients achieving hematologic improvement.[222,223] A larger multicenter study of liposomal vincristine in ALL relapse is currently ongoing.

Among what is considered small molecular targeted therapies, tyrosine kinase inhibitors have had the biggest impact and are discussed below.

Disease Subtypes

Ph-Positive ALL

Historically, Ph-positive ALL has had the worst survival rates with standard chemotherapy and, being much more frequent in adults than children, was attributed to some degree with the overall worse prognosis of adult patients.[224] It has therefore long been concluded that in almost all cases of Ph-positive ALL chemotherapy alone is insufficient to cure and SCT required.[225] In one of the largest prospective studies to date by the International ALL trial group, 167 patients with Ph-positive ALL received either a matched related SCT (n = 49), a matched unrelated donor transplant (n = 23), or an autologous SCT (n = 7), or continued with chemotherapy alone (n = 77).[226] Although the treatment-related mortality was higher with SCT (37% for matched sibling transplants, 43% for matched unrelated donor transplants, 14% with autologous SCT, 8% with chemotherapy), the risk of relapse at 5 years was lower with allogeneic SCT (29%) compared with autologous SCT/chemotherapy (81%). Likewise, the 5-year survival probability was 43% with allogeneic SCT, and 19% with autologous SCT or chemotherapy. Experience with alternative stem cell sources (unrelated, haploidentical, umbilical cord) is more limited. Nonetheless, transplant outcome with fully matched unrelated donors with respect to toxicity and transplant-related mortality appears similar to matched sibling SCT. Comparisons of antileukemic activity remain difficult due to the retrospective nature and small and heterogeneous patient populations in most studies.

Since the discovery of imatinib and several newer generation tyrosine kinase inhibitors in its wake, an array of new treatment possibilities in Ph-positive ALL have become available. Imatinib competitively binds to the ATP binding site of BCR-ABL and inhibits autoactivation of the oncoprotein as well as phosphorylation of downstream intracellular proteins. Imatinib has single-agent activity in Ph-positive ALL with hematologic response rates in the range of 20–30%, but response durations are not maintained and short so that many investigators have combined imatinib with multiagent chemotherapy.[227,228] Single-agent kinase inhibitor therapy possibly combined with low-intensity therapy (vincristine, steroids) is of particular benefit in elderly and frail patients not considered candidates for more aggressive therapy.[229]

Several studies have successfully combined imatinib with intensive chemotherapy programs.[230–232] The group at MDACC combined imatinib with hyper-CVAD.[230] Imatinib 600 mg was given daily for 14 days with the induction cycle and then continuously thereafter until the dose was again increased to 800 mg for indefinite maintenance therapy. Of the 54 patients with a median age of 51 years (range 17–84 years) treated, 93% achieved a complete remission with a median time to response of 21 days. The molecular response rate based on nested PCR was 52%. Sixteen patients proceeded to allogeneic SCT within a median of 5 months from start of therapy, though survival at 3 years did not seem improved whether or not patients received a SCT (63% vs 56%). Outcome is superior to hyper-CVAD alone: 3-year OS rates were 55% versus 15% ($p < .001$).There is a general consensus that imatinib is more effective when started early during induction and when given concurrently with and subsequent to induction and consolidation rather than alternating with chemotherapy.[233]

Dasatinib and nilotinib are two second generation tyrosine kinase inhibitors, which are many times more potent than imatinib in in vitro models, which includes activity against most imatinib-resistant kinase domain mutations. Both have shown activity in imatinib-resistant Ph-positive ALL.[234,235] Experience in frontline Ph-positive ALL remains limited to early studies with dasatinib where rapid hematologic clearance of marrow blasts and residual disease was observed in all patients, and in combination with hyper-CVAD, high early remission rates were associated with a manageable toxicity profile.[236,237]

Mature B-ALL (Burkitt Leukemia)

Mature B-cell ALL is a rare entity of ALL and predominates in children. The difference between the ALL variety and its lymphoma counterpart appears mostly semantic. A diagnosis of ALL is considered when the marrow blasts exceed 25% in the absence of significant extramedullary disease. Conventional ALL therapy was not successful. Only adaptation of intensive pediatric protocols for adults has substantially improved prognosis of these patients. Complete remission rates now exceed 80%, with 2-year DFS rates of 60–80%. Relapses are rare after the first year in remission. Intensive early prophylactic intrathecal therapy (with or without cranial irradiation), in addition to intensive systemic administration of methotrexate and ara-C, significantly reduced the systemic and CNS relapse rates.[238,239]

Thomas et al[239] combined hyper-CVAD with rituximab to treat 31 newly diagnosed patients with mature B-ALL or lymphoma and a.median age of 46 years (29% older than 60 years). The overall CR rate was 86%. The 3-year OS and DFS rates were 89% and 88%, respectively, which was similar in the elderly patients. Younger age and treatment with rituximab were identified as independent favorable factors.

Treatment of HIV-related mature B-cell ALL/lymphoma remains challenging.[240,241] Short and intensive ALL protocols have proved more effective for these patients than conventional lymphoma therapies such as CHOP.[241] Using the same combination of hyper-CVAD with rituximab in combination with highly active antiretroviral treatment (HAART), a complete remission rate of 92% has been reported with nearly 50% of the patients living longer than 2 years from diagnosis.[240]

Summary

Progress in the understanding of the biology of ALL and refinements of prognostic systems have led to increasing sophistication of therapy. Patients with mature B-cell ALL do best with short-term dose-intensive therapies, whereas outcome in T-cell ALL has improved with the addition of cyclophosphamide and cytarabine. It is now widely accepted that treatment for Ph-positive ALL should include tyrosine kinase inhibitors, ideally from the start and probably best maintained for many years thereafter. The role of transplantation is modified according to better and more predictable risk-stratification. Transplantation should be considered in first remission in any high-risk patients without prohibitively serious comorbidities, or any patients beyond a first remission. Its expansion into standard-risk groups is being discussed, but not a standard approach.

As for any other malignancy, the key to improving prognosis of ALL, especially for adult patients, lies in continuously better definitions of the many subtypes of ALL. Elaboration of the biologic characteristics will lead to more accurate risk-stratification. Treatment programs in ALL are complex and will continue to be. Although development of new drugs and agents is vital, to understand modes of action and pharmacokinetic properties of existing drugs and to know how to include new agents remains an ongoing challenge.

Selected References

The complete reference list can be found at www.CANCERMEDICINE8.com

1. Jemal A, Siegel R, Ward E, et al. Cancer statistics. *CA Cancer J Clin*. 2006;56:106–130.
3. Wartenberg D, Groves FD, Adelman AS: Acute lymphoblastic leukemia: epidemiology and etiology. In: Estey EH, Faderl S, Kantarjian H, editors. *Acute Leukemias*, 1st ed. Berlin: Springer; 2008:77–93.
15. Pui CH, Robinson LL, Look AT: Acute lymphoblastic leukaemia. Lancet 2008 Mar 22; 372(9617):1030–43.
21. Alvarez RH, Cortes JE. Central nervous system involvement in adult acute lymphocytic leukemia. In: Estey EH, Faderl S, Kantarjian H, editors. *Acute Leukemias*, 1st ed. Berlin: Springer; 2008:263–274.
22. Mahmoud HH, Rivera GK, Hancock ML, et al. Low leukocyte counts with blast cells in cerebrospinal fluid of children with newly diagnosed acute lymphoblastic leukemia. *N Engl J Med*. 1993;329: 314–319.
23. Pui C-H, Howard SC. Current management and challenges of central-nervous-system disease in paediatric leukaemia. *Lancet Oncol*. (in press).
25. Kantarjian HM, Thomas D, O'Brien S, et al. Long-term follow-up results of hyperfractionated cyclophosphamide, vincristine, doxorubicin, and dexamethasone (Hyper-CVAD), a dose-intensive regimen, in adult acute lymphocytic leukemia. *Cancer*. 2004;101:2788–2801.
26. Albitar M, Giles FJ, Kantarjian H. Diagnosis of acute lymphoblastic leukemia. In: Estey EH, Faderl S, Kantarjian H, editors. *Acute Leukemias*, 1st ed. Berlin: Springer; 2008:119–130.
33. WHO. In:Jaffe ES, Harris NL, Stein H, Vardiman JW, editors. *World Health Organization Classification of Tumours. Pathology and Genetics of Tumours of Haematopoietic and Lymphoid Tissues*. Lyon: IARC Press; 2000:111–187.
37. Pui C-H, Sandlund JT, Pei D, et al. Results of therapy for acute lymphoblastic leukemia. *JAMA*. 2003;290:2001–2007.
44. Pui C-H, Campana D, Evans WE. Childhood acute lymphoblastic leukemia: current status and future perspectives. *Lancet Oncol*. 2001;2:597–607.
45. Larson RA, Dodge RK, Burns CP, et al. A five-drug remission induction regimen with intensive consolidation for adults with acute lymphoblastic leukemia: Cancer and Leukemia Group B Study 8811. *Blood*. 1995;85:2025–2037.
47. Pui CH, Rubnitz JE, Hancock ML, et al. Reappraisal of the clinical and biologic significance of myeloid-associated antigen expression in childhood acute lymphoblastic leukemia. *J Clin Oncol*. 1998; 16:3768.
51. Armstrong SA, Look AT. Molecular genetics of acute lymphoblastic leukemia. *J Clin Oncol*. 2005;23:6306–6315.
52. Faderl S, Kantarjian HM, Talpaz M, Estrov Z. Clinical significance of cytogenetic abnormalities in adult acute lymphoblastic leukemia. *Blood*. 1998;91:3995–4019.
53. Wetzler M, Dodge RK, Mrozek K, et al. Prospective karyotype analysis in adult acute lymphoblastic leukemia: The Cancer and Leukemia Group B experience. *Blood*. 1999;93:383.
54. Mancini M, Scappaticci D, Cimino G, et al. A comprehensive genetic classification of adult acute lymphoblastic leukemia (ALL): analysis of the GIMEMA 0496 protocol. *Blood*. 2005;105:3434–3441.
55. Pui CH, Williams WE. Treatment of acute lymphoblastic leukemia. *N Engl J Med*. 2006;354:166–178.
56. Moorman AV, Harrison CJ, Buck GA, et al. Karyotype is an independent prognostic factor in adult acute lymphoblastic leukemia (ALL): analysis of cytogenetic data from patients treated on the Medical Research Council (MRC) UKALLXII/Eastern Cooperative Oncology Group (ECOG) 2993 trial. *Blood*. 2007;109:3189–3197.
57. Ebert BL, Golub TR. Genomic approaches to hematologic malignancies. *Blood*. 2004;104:923–932.
63. The Groupe Français de Cytogenetique Hematologique: Cytogenetic abnormalities in adult acute lymphoblastic leukemia: Correlations with the hematologic findings and outcome. A collaborative study of the Groupe Français de Cytogenetique Hematologique. *Blood*. 1996; 88:3135–3142.
104. Issa JP. DNA methylation as a therapeutic target in cancer. *Clin Cancer Res*. 2007;13:1634–1637.
105. Garcia-Manero G, Daniel J, Smith TL, et al. DNA methylation of multiple promoter-associated CpG islands in adult acute lymphoblastic leukemia. *Clin Cancer Res*. 2002;8:2217–2224.
106. Shen L, Toyota M, Kondo Y, et al. Aberrant DNA methylation of p57KIP2 identifies a cell-cycle regulatory pathway with prognostic impact in adult acute lymphoblastic leukemia. *Blood*. 2003;103:4131–4136.
107. Roman-Gomez J, Jimenez-Velasco A, Castijello JA, et al. Promoter hypermethylation of cancer-related genes: a strong independent prognostic factor in acute lymphoblastic leukemia. *Blood*. 2004;104:2492–2498.
108. Roman-Gomez J, Jimenez-Velasco A, Barrios M, et al. Poor prognosis in acute lymphocytic leukemia may relate to promoter hypermethylation of cancer-related genes. *Leuk Lymphoma*. 2007;48: 1269–1282.
110. Gökbuget N, Arnold R, Böhme A, et al. Treatment of adult ALL according to protocols of the German Multicenter Study Group for adult ALL (GMALL). In Estey EH, Faderl S, Kantarjian H, editors. *Acute Leukemias*, 1st ed. Berlin: Springer; 2008:166–176.
111. Larson RA, Yu D, Sanford BL, Stock W. Recent clinical trials in acute lymphoblastic leukemia by the Cancer and Leukemia Group B. In Estey EH, Faderl S, Kantarjian H, editors. *Acute Leukemias*, 1st ed. Berlin: Springer; 2008:137–144.
112. Thomas X, Fiere D. Conventional therapy in adult acute lymphoblastic leukemia: review of the LALA program. In Estey EH, Faderl S, Kantarjian H, editors. *Acute Leukemias*, 1st ed. Berlin: Springer; 2008:144–159.
114. Hoelzer D, Thiel H, Löffler H, et al. Prognostic factors in a multicenter study for treatment of acute lymphoblastic leukemia in adults. *Blood*. 1988;71:123–131.

120. Brüggemann M, Raff T, Flohr T, et al. Clinical significance of minimal residual disease quantification in adult patients with standard-risk acute lymphoblastic leukemia. *Blood*. 2006;107:1116–1123.
121. Holowiecki H, Krawczyk-Kulis M, Giebel S, et al. Minimal residual disease status is the most important predictive factor in adults with acute lymphoblastic leukemia. Prospective, multicenter PALG 4–2002 MRD Study. *Blood*. 2007;110:830a.
133. Graham ML. Pegaspargase: a review of clinical studies. *Adv Drug Deliv Rev*. 2003;55:1293–1302.
135. Douer D, Yampolsky H, Cohen LJ, et al. Pharmacodynamics and safety of intravenous pegaspargase during remission induction in adults aged 55 years or younger with newly diagnosed acute lymphoblastic leukemia. *Blood*. 2007;109:2744–2750.
136. Hoelzer D, Ludwig W-D, Eckhard E, et al. Improved outcome in adult B-cell acute lymphoblastic leukemia. *Blood*. 1996;87:495–508.
139. Maury S, Huguet F, Pigneux A, et al. Prognostic significance of CD20 expression in adult B-cell precursor acute lymphoblastic leukemia. *Blood*. 2007;110:832a.
140. Jeha S, Behm F, Pei D, et al. Prognostic significance of CD20 expression in childhood B-cell precursor acute lymphoblastic leukemia. *Blood*. 2006;108:3302–3304.
142. Thomas DA, Faderl S, O'Brien S, et al. Chemoimmunotherapy with hyper-CVAD plus rituximab for the treatment of adult Burkitt and Burkitt-type lymphoma or acute lymphoblastic leukemia. *Cancer*. 2006;106:1569–1580.
143. Thomas DA, Kantarjian H, Faderl S, et al. Update of the modified Hyper-CVAD regimen with or without rituximab as frontline therapy of adults with acute lymphocytic leukemia (ALL) or lymphoblastic lymphoma (LL). *Blood*. 2007;110:831a.
150. Larson RA, Dodge RK, Linker CA, et al. A randomized controlled trial of filgrastim during remission induction and consolidation chemotherapy for adults with acute lymphoblastic leukemia: CALGB study 9111. *Blood*. 1998;92:1556–1564.
168. Goldstone AH, Richards SM, Lazarus HM, et al. In adults with standard-risk acute lymphoblastic leukemia, the greatest benefit is achieved from matched sibling allogenic transplantation in first complete remissions, and an autologous transplantation is less effective than conventional consolidation/maintenance chemotherapy in all patients: final results of the International ALL Trial (MRC UKALL XII/ECOG E2993). Blood 2008 Feb 15:111(4):1827–33.
179. Pui CH. Central nervous system disease in acute lymphoblastic leukemia: prophylaxis and treatment. *Hematology Am Soc Hematol Educ Program*. 2006; 142–146.
187. Pui CH, Relling MV, Evans WE. Role of pharmacogenomics and pharmacodynamics in the treatment of acute lymphoblastic leukemia. *Best Pract Res Clin Haematol*. 2003;15:741–756.
209. Fielding AK, Richards SM, Chopra R, et al. Outcome of 609 adults after relapse of acute lymphoblastic leukemia (ALL); an MRC UKALL12/ECOG 2993 study. *Blood*. 2007;109:944–950.
213. Lamanna N,von Hassel M, Weiss M. Relapsed acute lymphoblastic leukemia. In: Estey EH, Faderl S, Kantarjian H, editors. *Acute Leukemias*, 1st ed. Berlin: Springer; 2008:275–279.
214. Pui C-H, Jeha S. New therapeutic strategies for the treatment of acute lymphoblastic leukaemia. *Nat Rev Drug Discov*. 2007;6:149–165.
217. Jeha S, Kantarjian H. Clofarabine for the treatment of acute lymphoblastic leukemia. *Expert Rev Anticancer Ther*. 2007;7:113–118.
221. DeAngelo DJ, Yu D, Johnson JL, et al. Nelarabine induces complete remissions in adults with relapsed or refractory T-lineage acute lymphoblastic leukemia or lymphoblastic lymphoma: Cancer and Leukemia Group B study 19801. *Blood*. 2007;109:5136–5142.
222. Thomas DA, Sarris AH, Cortes J, et al. Phase II study of sphingosomal vincristine in patients with recurrent or refractory adult acute lymphocytic leukemia. *Cancer*. 2006;106:120–127.
223. Thomas DA, Kantarjian HM, Stock W, et al. Safety and efficacy of Marqibo (vincristine sulfate liposomes injection, OPTISOME™) for the treatment of adults with relapsed or refractory acute lymphocytic leukemia (ALL). *Blood*. 2007;110:263a.
236. Foa R, Vignetti M, Vitale A, et al. Dasatinib as front-line monotherapy for the induction treatment of adult and elderly Ph+ acute lymphoblastic leukemia (ALL) patients: interim analysis of the GIMEMA prospective study LAL1205. *Blood*. 2007;110:10a.
237. Ravandi F, Thomas D, Kantarjian H, et al. Phase II study of combination of the HyperCVAD regimen with dasatinib in patients with Philadelphia chromosome (Ph) or BCR-ABL positive acute lymphoblastic leukemia (ALL) and lymphoid blast phase chronic myeloid leukemia (CML-LB). *Blood*. 2007;110:828a.

113 Chronic Lymphocytic Leukemia

Kanti R. Rai, MD ■ Matthew Kaufman, MD

Chronic lymphocytic leukemia (CLL) is a monoclonal B-cell lymphoproliferative disease. It is a clinically heterogeneous disorder derived from antigen-experienced B lymphocytes that differ in their level of immunoglobulin (Ig) V gene mutations.[1] It is characterized by a progressively increasing accumulation of leukemic B lymphocytes; however, there is also evidence that there is a higher rate of leukemic cell proliferation than was previously recognized. Table 113-1 summarizes some of the important differences between the way CLL is defined now and in the past.[1]

Brief History of Identification of CLL as Distinct Entity

The history of CLL is linked with case reports of chronic leukemias of any nature first recorded in 1845—independently and virtually simultaneously—by Virchow[2] and Bennett.[3,4] Within a decade thereafter, several other observers also reported similar cases with excessively "white" blood containing colorless corpuscles. Bennett called this condition "leukocythemia" in 1852; Virchow coined the term "leukemia" in 1847, and published a classic paper on the subject in 1856.[5] Gowers,[6] in 1879, identified the differences in the roles of spleen and lymph nodes in what he termed "splenic leukocythemia" and "lymphadenosis." In 1893, Kundrat[7] provided a detailed description of lymphosarcoma and distinguished it from leukemia based on the major evidence of disease in the lymphoid organs in the former and in the bloodstream in the latter. In 1903, Turk[8] was able to describe the interrelationships of various acute and chronic malignant disorders of the lymphatic system under the umbrella term "lymphomatoses."

The pace of research in leukemia received a major boost at the beginning of the 20th century, following the introduction in 1891 of staining methods for blood cells by Ehrlich.[9] In 1924, Minot and Isaacs[10] provided the first comprehensive description of the clinical features and natural history of CLL; it remained a standard reference for more than four decades. Clinical reviews that help to illuminate the variable nature of CLL have also been provided by Boggs and colleagues[11] and by Hansen.[12] An understanding of the pathophysiology of CLL in relation to the function of lymphocytes was heralded independently and simultaneously by Galton[13] and Dameshek.[14] Methods of clinical staging of CLL introduced by Rai and colleagues[15] in 1975 and by Binet and colleagues[16] in 1981 enabled many others to examine numerous additional prognostic factors and to initiate controlled clinical trials to deal with this disease.

The "modern" era in CLL research dawned near the end of the 20th century when the heterogeneity of CLL was discovered to be associated with the mutation status of IgV genes.[1,17-19] Those investigations have generated renewed interest in learning more about the molecular biology of CLL and new attempts to further refine prognostic characteristics and therapeutic approaches to the disease.

Table 113-1 ■ B-Cell Chronic Lymphocytic Leukemia as Viewed Then and Now

Previously	Currently
• A clinically heterogeneous disease with a homogeneous cellular origin • A disease derived from naïve B lymphocytes • Leukemic cell accumulation occurs because of an inherent apoptotic defect involving the entire mass of leukemic cells • A disease of accumulation • Prognostic markers identify patients at low/intermediate/high (Rai) or A/B/C (Binet) risk with an acknowledged heterogeneity (vis-à-vis clinical outcomes) among patients in the low/A and intermediate/B risk categories • Therapy based largely on clinical observations and trial-and-error methods	• A clinically heterogeneous disease originating from B lymphocytes that may differ in activation and maturation state or cellular subset • A disease derived from antigen-experienced B lymphocytes that differ in the level of immunoglobulin V gene mutations • An inherent apoptotic defect involving the entire mass of leukemic cells is unlikely to exist initially. Cell accumulation occurs because of survival signals delivered to a subset of leukemic cells from the external environment through a variety of receptors (eg, *BCR*, chemokine and cytokine receptors, etc.) and their cell-bound and soluble ligands • A disease of accumulation with an associated level of proliferation that exceeds that previously appreciated • Newer molecular and protein markers separate patients within the low/A and intermediate/B risk categories that follow different clinical courses • Above-noted newer findings provide clues to discover discrete targets for developing hypothesis-driven and effective therapeutic agents

Evolution over the past 10 years of our understanding of the biology and derivation of chronic lymphocytic leukemia cells and the effects of this knowledge on predicting and hopefully altering the natural history of this currently incurable leukemia.

Incidence and Epidemiology

Among the adult populations of the Western world, CLL is the most common form of leukemia and—because of its relatively longer survival—the one with the highest prevalence rate among all leukemias. The cancer incidence statistics prepared by the American Cancer Society indicate that, in 2008, an estimated 15,110 new CLL cases were diagnosed and 4390 deaths occurred among patients suffering from CLL.[20] CLL accounted for >33% of all leukemias diagnosed that year.

The male:female incidence ratio of CLL is approximately 1.5:1. The disease usually affects adults over the age of 60 years; the median age at diagnosis is 70 years. In recent years, however, an increasing number of younger people, even some between 30 and 39 years of age, have been diagnosed with CLL. The incidence increases rapidly with age after 55 years. Based on data from the Surveillance, Epidemiology and End Results (SEER) Program for the period 1983-1991,[21,22] Figure 113-1 depicts the incidence of CLL according to age at diagnosis. Age-specific SEER data from 1987 to 1991 show 12.8 and 22.0 cases per year per 100,000 population in the age groups 65-69 years and 75-79 years, respectively.[21] A study in Olmsted County, Minnesota during the period from 1975 to 1989 demonstrated a trend of more patients being diagnosed while asymptomatic because of routine examinations or routine testing for other illnesses.[23] Many of these patients remain stable for years without evidence of developing clinical features of disease progression. These "smoldering" CLL[24] patients have

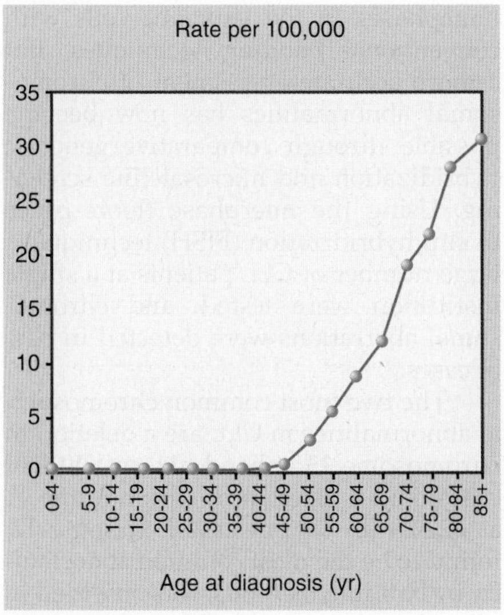

Figure 113-1 Incidence of chronic lymphocytic leukemia per 100,000 population according to age at diagnosis. From Surveillance, Epidemiology and End Results (SEER) Program data, 1983-1987. *Source:* Adapted from Ref. 21.

minimal organomegaly, a normal hemoglobin and platelet count, and a survival rate that is the same as an age- and sex-matched population. Many could indeed be considered to have monoclonal B lymphocytosis[25] (see below).

The incidence of CLL in the African population is nearly the same as in the white population.[26] For reasons still unknown, the incidence of CLL is extremely low in Asian countries such as China and Japan, where the disease is estimated to occur at a frequency that is only 10% of that in countries of the Western world.[27,28] Genetic rather than environmental factors are the most likely explanation for these geographic and ethnic differences in incidence: it has been observed that Japanese emigrants who settled in Hawaii do not have a higher incidence of CLL than that seen in native Japanese.[29]

Population studies of farm workers and industrial workers exposed to benzene and other solvents reveal no clearly discernible occupational or environmental risk factors (including chronic antigenic stimulation) that predispose to CLL.[30,31] The role of exposure to herbicides, especially Agent Orange, in increasing the risk of developing CLL has been under review for several years. In a report released in 2003, a committee of the Institute of Medicine of the National Academy of Science stated that there is evidence of an association between exposure to herbicides such as Agent Orange and CLL.[32] In addition, the Tecumseh Community Health Study,[33] initiated in 1959 to study the cancer incidence in a Midwestern rural farming community (which has a higher than-average exposure to agricultural chemicals, insecticides, and herbicides), showed a high standardized incidence ratio of lymphopoietic neoplasms (including CLL) among both males and females. The combined standardized incidence ratio[33] was 1.40. The lifespan cohort of atomic bomb survivors studied during the period 1950-1987 showed no increase in incidence of CLL, although increases in all other types of leukemia were seen.[34] These results suggest that the reported cancer pattern is an expression of risk from sustained environmental exposure to agricultural chemicals, perhaps in conjunction with familial or genetic factors.

Pathogenesis and Causation

Familial CLL and Monoclonal B-Cell Lymphocytosis

The Tecumseh study[33] also showed that the relative risk of a family history of lymphoma, leukemia, or myeloma was significantly increased among patients with lymphoproliferative neoplasms (odds ratio 3.81). Other observers have confirmed the somewhat increased incidence of CLL or related disorders among the family members of people known to have CLL.[35,36]

In this context, it is noteworthy that Rawstron and colleagues[37] found monoclonal B-cell lymphocytosis (MBL) of CLL phenotypes but not meeting the criteria for diagnosis of CLL among 13.5% of normal first-degree relatives of people known to have CLL. That incidence is much higher than 3.5% that Rawstron and colleagues discovered among adults with normal blood counts and who did not have first-degree relatives with CLL.[25] Whether the presence of MBL in family members of CLL patients is indicative of an inherited predisposition for the disease is also not clear, but these observations are likely to stimulate research to discover a putative CLL predisposition gene and a possible CLL carrier state.

Exploring the concept of MBL further, Rawstron's group compared the incidence of MBL in patients with normal blood counts with those with a history of a lymphocytosis. They found an incidence of 5.1% of MBL in the former group, compared to 13.9% in the latter.[38] Similar to Kyle's MGUS data in multiple myeloma,[39] the rate of progressing to CLL requiring treatment in these MBL patients was 1.1% per year.[38] A prospective cohort study found that 44 of 45 CLL patients had a circulating monoclonal B-cell population up to 77 months prior to developing CLL, suggesting that MBL precedes virtually all CLL cases.[40] This finding has led some investigators to call for the codification of MBL in the International Classification of Diseases, similar to MGUS.[41]

CLL in Monozygotic Twins

In 1987, deoxyribonucleic acid (DNA) analysis of a set of monozygotic twins with CLL revealed that the malignant cells were genetically distinct between the two individuals.[42] However, we studied another set of monozygotic twins with CLL and found that the two were concordant for CLL, but that the disease course is indolent in one twin and progressive in the other.[43] Blood lymphocytes from the twin with a progressive clinical course expressed ZAP-70 (the gene for zeta-associated protein 70), but lymphocytes from the twin with indolent disease did not.[43] These observations suggest that the differences in leukemia-cell characteristics between monozygotic twins with CLL cannot be explained by genetic polymorphism.

Immunobiology and Immunophenotype of CLL Cells

CLL lymphocytes are clonal B cells arrested in the B-cell differentiation pathway at some intermediate stage between pre-B cell and mature B cell. Morphologically, B-cell chronic lymphocytic leukemia (B-CLL) cells resemble mature lymphocytes in the normal peripheral blood.

Perhaps as a result of the functional incompetence of the accumulated monoclonal B lymphocytes, CLL patients become immunocompromised and, with advancing disease, profoundly hypogammaglobulinemic. CLL patients tend to develop autoimmune hemolytic anemia (AIHA), characterized by the presence of polyclonal autoantibodies to self-antigens expressed only by blood cells.[36,44]

Several other malignancies of mature-appearing lymphocytes (Table 113-2) sometimes present with clinical features overlapping those of CLL. Immunophenotyping of lymphocytes, usually by flow cytometry,[45-47] is extremely helpful in distinguishing CLL from other diseases (Table 113-3).

Table 113-2 **Malignancies of Morphologically Mature-Appearing B Lymphocytes**

Chronic lymphocytic leukemia/small lymphocytic lymphoma (CLL/SLL)
B-prolymphocytic leukemia (PLL)
Hairy cell leukemia (HCL)
Follicular lymphoma in leukemic phase (FL-L)
Mantle cell lymphoma in leukemic phase (MCL-L)
Splenic lymphoma with villous lymphocytes (SLVL)
Lymphoplasmacytoid lymphoma

Table 113-3 ■ CD19+/CD20+ Lymphoid Malignancies

	sIg	CD19	CD20	CD5	CD23	Others
B-CLL	Dim	+	+	+	+	CD79b, CD38
PLL	Bright	+	+	–	–	CD79b
HCL	Bright	+	+	FMC7+; CD103+, CD25+		
MCL-L	Bright	+	+	+	–	t(11;14), cyclin D1
SLVL	Bright	+	+	±	–	

Abbreviations: B-CLL, B-cell chronic lymphocytic leukemia; HCL, hairy cell leukemia; MCL-L, mantle cell lymphoma in leukemic phase; PLL, B-prolymphocytic leukemia; sIg, surface immunoglobulin; SLVL, splenic lymphoma with villous lymphocytes.

As stated earlier, the malignant lymphocytes in CLL bear scanty quantities of sIgs, usually IgM or IgM and IgD, and express either kappa or lambda light chain. In some cases, the quantity of sIg or light chain may be so small that it is undetectable by flow cytometry. CLL cells always express pan-B immunophenotypic markers, such as CD19 and CD20, along with a T-cell marker CD5.1 The activation antigen CD23, a low-affinity receptor for IgE, is characteristically overexpressed on CLL lymphocytes. On the other hand, mantle cell lymphoma (MCL), the other CD5+ B-cell malignancy, is known to be CD23-negative.[45-47]

CLL-B cells express low levels of B-cell receptor and of CD79b, both known to be critical for signaling, proliferation, and differentiation of B cells.[1,18,19,48,49] Defective B-cell receptor signaling is also associated with low levels of CD38 on subsets of B-CLL cells.[50,51]

Whether CLL-B cells coexpress CD38 has become a topic of considerable interest in recent years, because this finding has independent prognostic value for CLL patients. CD38 is a modulator of intracellular signaling. Cross-linking of CD38 up-regulates BCL-2 and inhibits apoptosis in normal mature B cells.[48,51] Damle and colleagues provided evidence that CLL leukemic cells coexpressed CD38 in approximately half of the CLL patients they studied, and also showed that those patients had a significantly worse prognosis, independent of other prognostic factors, than did patients whose leukemic cells did not express CD38.[51] Several subsequent investigators confirmed both observations: that CD38 is coexpressed on leukemic cells in a number of B-CLL patients, and that this finding is an independent indicator of a worse prognosis.[52-55]

Some reports[55,56] have suggested that CD38 expression may vary during the course of the disease. But for 29 patients who were repeatedly studied, D'Arena and colleagues reported that some patients showed progression of their clinical disease without change in CD38 expression.[57] We conclude that whether CD38 expression does or does not change with disease progression, it should be included in the flow cytometric analysis of leukemic cells in CLL patients because of its prognostic value.

Clinical Consequences of Defective B- and T-Cell Functions

Although the mechanisms underlying the various clinical manifestations of disordered immunity associated with CLL are not yet clearly defined, defects in the functions of B and T lymphocytes and natural killer cells are considered to be the key elements. Hypogammaglobulinemia, autoimmune complications, and monoclonal gammopathy are the most frequently observed immune complications of CLL.[45,58-60]

The incidence of hypogammaglobulinemia is ~8% at the time of initial diagnosis, but may increase significantly—reaching up to 65% with disease progression.[45] Infection is the most frequent cause of death in CLL patients, and profound hypogammaglobulinemia undoubtedly plays a major role in development of infections.

AIHA in CLL is most often associated with warm antibodies. Although cold AIHA, autoimmune pure red-cell aplasia, and immune thrombocytopenia also occur, they are seen less frequently than is AIHA.[61-63] By positive direct antibody test, the antibodies in AIHA patients are almost always polyclonal and not directly the products of the malignant CLL cells. These antibodies are of the IgG subclass. In cold AIHA, the antibody is of the IgM class and fixes complement more readily than does IgG.[64] The incidence of positive direct antibody test and AIHA increases with disease progression, and there is some evidence that the introduction of purine analogs, such as fludarabine, into CLL treatment is associated with an increased incidence of AIHA.[65,66] Italian investigators reported that the incidence of AIHA in a large number of CLL patients seen at a single institution was only ~4%.[66] The incidence of other nonhematologic autoimmune diseases, such as rheumatoid arthritis, systemic lupus erythematosus, and Sjögren's syndrome, is believed to be somewhat higher in CLL, but available corroborative data are scant.

Cytogenetics

Cytogenetic analysis of CLL used to be limited because of an inability to induce metaphases in the leukemic cells with conventional banding techniques. But a more accurate assessment of chromosomal abnormalities has now become possible through comparative genomic hybridization and microsatellite screening. Using the interphase fluorescence in situ hybridization (FISH) technique, a large number of CLL patients at a single institution were tested, and chromosomal aberrations were detected in 82% of cases.[67]

The two most common chromosomal abnormalities in CLL are a deletion in chromosome 13 at band q14 (in >50% of cases) and a deletion in chromosome 11 at q22-23 (in 18% of cases). Trisomy 12, found to be the most common abnormality by banding methods, was observed in 16% of cases by FISH. Other abnormalities noted less frequently are deletions in chromosome arms 17p (7%) and 6q (6%).[67] By FISH techniques, the investigators observed normal karyotype in 18% of cases.[68]

Deletions in chromosome 11 at q22-23 are thought to result in inactivation of a tumor suppressor gene. The ataxia telangiectasia mutation (ATM) gene is located at 11q22-23 within the minimal region of loss described in CLL. There is some evidence that 11q deletions in CLL may result in ATM gene inactivation.[69] The 11q22-23 abnormality is associated with a clinical subgroup of CLL patients characterized by extensive lymph node enlargement and poor survival.[69]

Trisomy 12 seems to be associated with advanced or atypical cases of CLL, and its functional effects remain undefined.[69]

A systematic study of a large number of CLL patients has revealed that del 13q, when observed as the only chromosomal abnormality (noted in 36% of cases), is associated with good prognosis, while patients with del 6q and 12+; del 17p and del 11q are known to have worse prognosis.[68]

Molecular Genetics

Although chromosomal translocations involving the *BCL-2* gene are rare in CLL, high levels of *Bcl-2* protein have been noted in about 85% of cases. Hypomethylation of the promoter region of the *BCL-2* gene was found in almost all of these cases.[70] *BCL-2* is a known suppressor of apoptosis, and high amount of *Bcl-2* protein contributes to the longevity of CLL lymphocytes, resulting in the hallmark of this disease (ie, progressive accumulation of the cells).

Tumor Protein p53 ■ The tumor protein p53 (*TP53*) gene resides on chromosome 17p. Mutations that inactivate *TP53* occur in a small percentage of CLL patients.[67] The loss of *TP53* activity can promote both prolonged cell survival and accelerated cell proliferation, which are noted in the advanced stage and in the transformation of CLL to the aggressive disease phase.[67]

IgV Gene Mutation ■ It was previously believed that, in all cases of CLL, the leukemic CD5+ B lymphocytes did not generate immunologic memory, did not carry mutations in their Ig genes, and did not pass through a follicle center. Investigations in the past decade suggest, however, that there are at least two subsets of CLL patients: in about half of the patient population, leukemia cells express Ig molecules that closely resemble the germ-line sequence without mutation; in the other half, tumor cells express Ig proteins with somatic mutations, which they likely accrued in the germinal center. Cases with and without mutations were similar in all other respects. Patients with a mutated Ig gene had a better prognosis and more benign disease course than did patients without mutations.[51,71] Several subsequently published studies have confirmed the validity of these observations.[55,72,73]

CLL Lymphocytes May Not Be "Resting" Cells ■ Although the notion that leukemic lymphocytes in CLL were "resting" cells, not in active proliferation, was accepted for decades, recent observations using in vivo labeling with deuterium (2H), a nonradioactive isotope of hydrogen, have clearly demonstrated that these cells have a rather high rate of proliferation.[74] CLL patients participating in that study drank heavy water (^2H_2O). Using mass spectrometry to measure the emergence of B lymphocytes carrying the deuterium label, the researchers observed surprisingly brisk rates of birth, accounting for a renewal rate ranging from 0.1% to 1.0% of the CLL clone per day.[74] If these findings are confirmed by a currently ongoing larger trial, the high lymphocyte counts in CLL patients will be understood to reflect the net result of inhibited apoptosis (and resultant longevity of leukemic cells), together with a concurrent proliferation process of leukemic cells. That understanding might also lead to renewed attempts to use antimetabolite agents-based chemotherapy in CLL. The "higher" than previously considered proliferative rate of leukemic lymphocytes would also explain why telomeres, which cap the ends of chromosomes, but which shorten with each cell division, are smaller in leukemic lymphocytes of CLL than in normal lymphocytes.[75,76]

Clinical Aspects

Diagnosis

Absolute Lymphocytosis in Blood ■ CLL is suspected whenever absolute lymphocytosis occurs in the peripheral blood of an adult. Blood lymphocytosis may also occur with viral or other infections (eg, infectious mononucleosis, pertussis, toxoplasmosis) and with neoplastic conditions other than CLL (eg, leukemic phase of lymphomas, hairy cell leukemia, prolymphocytic leukemia [PLL], and large granular cell leukemia).

The International Workshop on CLL (IWCLL), in 2008, updating the National Cancer Institute Working Group's 1996 Guidelines for CLL, requires the presence of at least 5 × 10^9 B lymphocytes per liter (5000/µL) in the peripheral blood for diagnosing CLL.[77] By flow cytometry these lymphocytes must have the phenotype CD19+, CD20+, CD23+, and CD5+.

Lymphocyte Morphology ■ Lymphocytes must have the morphologic appearance of normal, mature cells. These are typically uniform populations of small lymphocytes (median volume: 211.5 fL).[78] The nucleus virtually fills the cell, leaving only a thin rim of visible cytoplasm. The nuclear chromatin is clumped, and a nucleolus is usually not discernible (Figs. 113-2 and 113-3). A small proportion of cells may be larger lymphocytes with a large, somewhat notched nucleus, lacy-appearing nuclear chromatin, and a clearly visible nucleolus. These prolymphocytes may account for a minority of the overall population of lymphocytes in B-CLL. Most of the other conditions associated with blood lymphocytosis such as hairy cell leukemia, PLL (Fig. 113-4), and large granular lymphocytic leukemia have their own characteristic morphologic features, which are distinct from those seen in CLL.

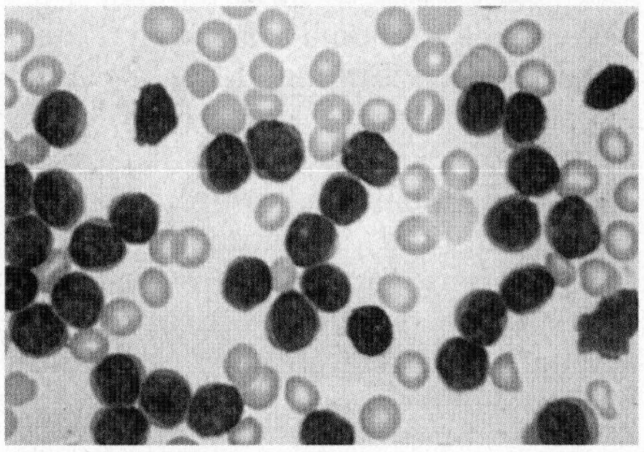

Figure 113-2 ■ Chronic lymphocytic leukemia morphology in peripheral blood smear. Leukocyte count: 100 × 10^9/L. Most of the lymphocytes are mature-appearing. One smudge cell is present. Platelets are absent in this thrombocytopenic patient (Wright-Giemsa stain; ×100 original magnification).

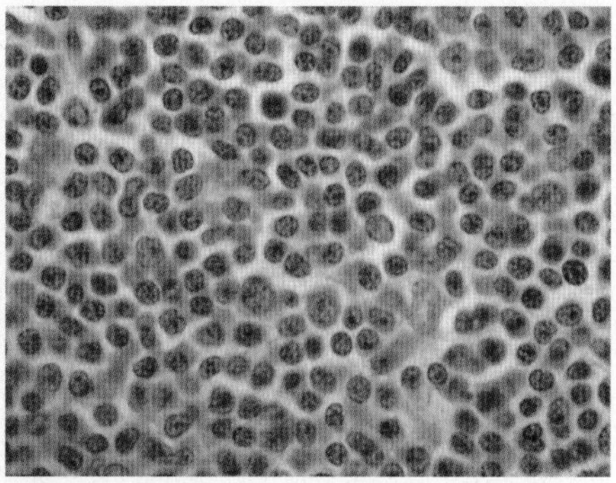

Figure 113-3 ■ Chronic lymphocytic leukemia (CLL). Marrow biopsy with diffuse infiltration by CLL cells (hematoxylin and eosin stain; ×600 original magnification).

Blood Lymphocytosis Sustained Over Time

The requirement that the blood lymphocytosis must be sustained to diagnose CLL was introduced to exclude conditions in which blood lymphocyte counts return to normal after a few weeks (eg, infectious mononucleosis, pertussis, and toxoplasmosis). However, it has not been possible to reach consensus on how often or over how long a period of time blood counts should be repeated to document "sustained" lymphocytosis. Some physicians recommend monthly blood counts for 3-6 months; others perform counts weekly for 4-6 weeks. This imprecise diagnostic criterion for CLL has now been eliminated altogether because of the recently developed requirement of at least 5000/µL B lymphocytes whereas previous definition included all (B and T) lymphocytes.

Only in CLL and similar lymphoid malignancies is lymphocytosis in the blood accompanied by bone marrow lymphocytosis. In small lymphocytic lymphoma (SLL), a disease virtually identical to CLL, but diagnosed by lymph node biopsy, increased lymphocytes may or may not be found in the bone marrow. As opposed to CLL and most cases of SLL, in infectious mononucleosis and pertussis, bone marrow lymphocytosis does not occur. Thus, even though

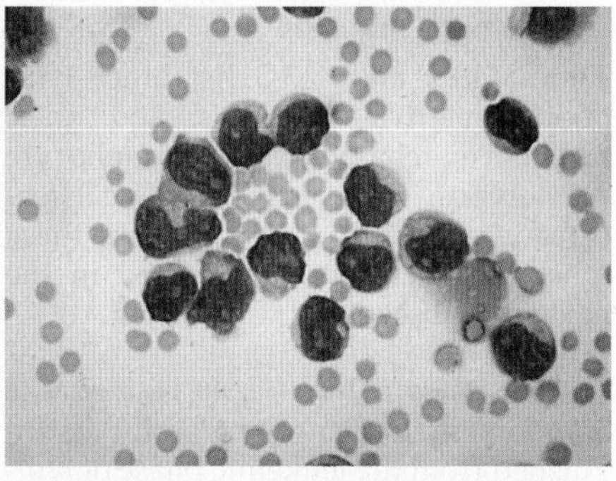

Figure 113-4 ■ Prolymphocytic leukemia. Peripheral blood smear shows cells with prominent nucleoli and abundant cytoplasm (Wright-Giemsa stain; ×1000 original magnification).

blood lymphocytosis is recognized to be persistent and not transient in CLL, empiric and arguable recommendations for requiring sustained lymphocytosis for a certain period of time can be obviated by requiring that a bone marrow examination be performed to document lymphocytosis in cases where any doubts persist concerning the cause.

The characteristic findings of a bone marrow aspirate smear at the time of initial diagnosis of CLL include either hypercellularity or normocellularity (ie, not hypocellularity), with lymphocytes accounting for >30% of all nucleated cells (Fig. 113-3). A bone marrow biopsy examination is not required for establishing the diagnosis of CLL, but as discussed in "Criteria Predictive of Course of Disease in the Low- and Intermediate-Risk Groups" later in this chapter,[77,79] it has considerable prognostic value.

Minimum Diagnostic Requirements

Minimum requirements for the diagnosis of CLL include an absolute count in the peripheral blood of at least 5 × 109/L (5000/μL) B lymphocytes, with the majority appearing morphologically mature (Fig. 113-2).

These lymphocytes must demonstrate the following phenotype characteristics by flow cytometry:

- Extremely low levels of surface membrane immunoglobulin (SmIg) and either kappa or lambda light chains (but not both)
- CD19, CD20, CD23, and CD5 positivity.

The presence of the T-cell antigen CD5 is a distinguishing property of B cells in B-CLL; CD23 positivity distinguishes CLL from another CD5+ lymphoid malignancy, mantle cell lymphoma.

In addition, although not required for the diagnosis, a bone marrow examination, if performed, should show hypercellular or normocellular bone marrow with lymphocytes accounting for >30% of all nucleated cells.

Differential Diagnosis

Tables 113-2 and 113-3 list other lymphoproliferative disorders and their respective characteristic lymphocyte phenotypes. The pertinent clinical features distinguishing CLL from these other disorders are highlighted in the next few subsections.

Leukemic Phase of Non-Hodgkin Lymphomas ■ Sometimes CLL cannot be easily distinguished from the leukemic phase of lymphomas because of overlapping clinical features. In contrast to the phenotypic features of CLL, however, the amount of SmIg is abundant in lymphoma, and the lymphocytes are usually CD5−.

Hairy Cell Leukemia ■ When hairy cell leukemia[80] is associated with an elevated lymphocyte count in the peripheral blood, the distinction from CLL is possible because of the typical morphologic features of hairy cells with cytoplasmic projections. A bone marrow biopsy will show diffuse infiltration by hairy cells in a characteristic loose fashion, with a well-defined rim of cytoplasm, leaving a clear zone around the cells (Fig. 113-2). Cytochemically, a moderately strong acid phosphatase reaction, not inhibited by tartaric acid, will be seen. Characteristically, the hairy cell phenotype consists of CD11c+, CD25+, and CD103+.

Prolymphocytic Leukemia ■ The main feature distinguishing PLL[80,81] from CLL is the morphology of blood lymphocytes: large cells with somewhat immature-appearing nuclear chromatin, a prominent vesicular nucleolus, and abundant cytoplasm (Fig. 113-4). Other characteristics include a very large spleen and hyperlymphocytosis (usually more than 100 × 109/L). Phenotypically, prolymphocytes are B cells that are CD19+, CD20+, CD22+, and CD79b+, and yet are distinct from CLL lymphocytes, having normal amounts of SmIg, and most often being CD5−.

T-Cell Chronic Lymphocytic Leukemia ■ Lymphocytes in T-cell chronic lymphocytic leukemia (T-CLL)[80,82] are large cells with slightly eccentrically placed nuclei and moderately abundant cytoplasm with fine azurophilic granules. These cells are also described as large granular lymphocytes. They express a mature postthymic phenotype: CD31+, CD42+, CD81+, and CD21+.

Sézary Cells ■ In the leukemic manifestation of cutaneous T-cell lymphoma, the lymphocytes have a cerebriform nucleus (Sézary cells), which are usually CD41+ and CD82+.

Adult T-Cell Leukemia/Lymphoma ■ Adult T-cell leukemia/lymphoma[80] is a viral neoplasm totally different from all other lymphoproliferative disorders. It has a unique incidence in certain parts of the world (Japan and countries of the Caribbean) and in immigrants from those regions. In this disease, the cells have a characteristic cloverleaf nucleus, and patients are rarely asymptomatic at presentation.

Clinical Presentation

Like other human neoplasms, CLL can produce a wide range of symptoms and physical and laboratory abnormalities at the time of its initial discovery in an individual patient.

Symptoms

It is not unusual for a patient to feel entirely healthy, with no symptoms whatsoever, when a routine blood count reveals an absolute lymphocytosis requiring additional follow-up investigations that establish a diagnosis of CLL. At the other end of the spectrum is the patient who presents with many or all of the typical "B" symptoms of lymphoma (ie, marked weakness, profuse night sweats, unintended weight loss, and fever without infection). Each of these extremes accounts for ~20% of cases at presentation. The remaining 60% have varying symptomatology, with milder constitutional symptoms. Most patients consult a physician because they have noted painless swelling of lymph nodes, often in the cervical area (but also at times in other lymph node–bearing sites), that spontaneously wax and wane but do not altogether disappear. Occasionally, the presenting features relate to CLL as an acquired immunodeficiency disorder manifested by infection from opportunistic organisms or herpes zoster virus, or by exaggerated reactions to bee stings or insect bites, or by autoimmune complications such as hemolytic anemia or thrombocytopenia.

Physical Findings at Initial Diagnosis

Lymph Nodes

The most consistent abnormal finding on physical examination is lymphadenopathy. Lymph node enlargement may be generalized or localized, and the size of the enlarged nodes may be as small as a few millimeters in diameter or as large as an orange. When cervical nodes are extremely enlarged, they may be easily discernible by simple inspection and may give the patient a "jowly" appearance.

Characteristically, enlarged nodes in CLL are firm, rounded, discrete, nontender, and freely mobile upon palpation. Exceptions to these generalizations are encountered, particularly when the nodes have grown rapidly. Occasionally, several enlarged nodes in the same anatomic site (cervical triangle, axilla, or femoral-inguinal areas) may become confluent with each other, forming large spherical lymphoid masses. New lymph nodes may appear, sometimes in places other than the usual lymph node–bearing sites, such as over the sacrum or the thorax.

Spleen

Next to lymph nodes, the spleen is the lymphoid organ most frequently enlarged. It may be palpably enlarged in

30-40% of cases. The extent of enlargement varies from an organ barely palpable upon deep inspiration to one so large as to occupy the entire left side of the abdomen and pelvis, to cross the midline, and to encroach upon the right side of the abdomen. As is the case with enlarged lymph nodes, an enlarged spleen in CLL is usually painless. Upon palpation it is nontender, with a sharp edge and a smooth, firm surface. Painful or infarcted splenic enlargement is an unusual presenting feature for CLL.

Liver

Enlargement of the liver may be noted at the time of initial diagnosis of CLL in ~20% of cases. The liver in CLL generally is not greatly enlarged, ranging from 2 to 6 cm below the right costal margin, with a span of dullness on percussion of 10-16 cm. Upon palpation, the liver is usually nontender and firm, with a smooth surface.

Other Tissues

In addition to palpably enlarged peripheral lymph nodes, liver, and spleen, virtually any other lymphoid tissue in the body—for example, Waldeyer's ring or the tonsils—may be enlarged at diagnosis. In addition, infiltration with CLL cells may occur in any organ. At the time of diagnosis, skin lesions are the most obvious, but are seen in fewer than 5% of cases. In contrast to lymphoma, gastrointestinal mucosal involvement is rarely seen in CLL. Similarly, meningeal leukemia is unusual in CLL at the time of initial presentation.

Radiologic Findings

Radiologic examinations are not required, nor should they be utilized, as part of evaluation at the time of initial diagnosis or follow-up. CT scans or chest films will often reveal adenopathy not detected on examination, but these findings do not change the clinical Rai or Binet stage. A recent study showed that abdominal lymphadenopathy revealed on CT scan in Rai stage 0 patients may indicate a more aggressive disease course[83] while another study demonstrated no added benefit.[84] In the setting of a therapeutic research protocol, computed tomography imaging is recommended, but in clinical practice it has no role unless there is a specific clinical question that requires imaging for the answer.

Laboratory Abnormalities

Lymphocytosis

The most noteworthy abnormalities among laboratory findings in CLL are lymphocytosis in the blood and bone marrow. A few additional features related to lymphocytosis are considered here.

Although the absolute blood lymphocyte threshold for diagnosing CLL was placed at 5×10^9/L, most patients present with considerably higher counts, usually in excess of 15×10^9/L, and occasionally as high as 200×10^9/L. Upon examination of a peripheral blood smear, mature-appearing small lymphocytes may be preponderant in the population of leukocytes, ranging from 50% to as much as 99% or 100%. Lymphocytes that appear flattened or smudged in the process of being spread on the glass slide may also be seen. Such "smudge" cells, perhaps reflecting some fragility or vulnerability to distortion upon mechanical manipulation, are considered characteristic of CLL (Fig. 113-2). When blood leukocyte counts are in excess of 200×10^9/L, the increased number of cellular elements may result in abnormally high whole-blood viscosity.

In addition to an increased ratio of mature-appearing lymphocytes in the smears of aspirated morrows, three patterns of infiltration by lymphocytes are recognized in trephine biopsy specimens of the bone marrow (Fig. 113-3): nodular, interstitial, and diffuse. Sometimes a given biopsy sample may show a mixture of nodular and interstitial or of nodular and diffuse patterns. It has been observed that patients with diffuse infiltration tend to have advanced disease and relatively worse outlook. For prognostic purposes, nodular and interstitial patterns, which are associated with less-advanced disease and better prognosis, may be grouped together and termed "nondiffuse."[85-87]

Other abnormalities, anemia and thrombocytopenia may be observed at the time of initial diagnosis, but usually they are of relatively mild degree. Low hemoglobin and platelet levels (below 110 g/L and 100×10^9/L respectively) are observed at diagnosis in ~20% of CLL patients and herald an overall poor prognosis. A direct antiglobulin (Coombs) test may be positive in ~25% of cases, but overt autoimmune hemolytic anemia occurs less frequently. In the absence of a reliable test to demonstrate antiplatelet antibodies, autoimmune thrombocytopenia is most often diagnosed on the basis of the presence of adequate numbers of megakaryocytes in the bone marrow with an abnormally low platelet count in the blood. Agranulocytosis or neutropenia may be encountered. Hypogammaglobulinemia may be present at the time of initial diagnosis, but in most cases it is observed only later in the course of the disease. All three immunoglobulin classes (IgG, IgA, and IgM) are usually decreased, but in some patients, only one or two classes may be low. Significant hypogammaglobulinemia and neutropenia result in increased vulnerability of CLL patients to major bacterial infections.

Blood lymphocyte phenotype characteristic of CLL were detailed earlier in this chapter. It should be noted, however, that the normal T:B ratio (2:1) is altered. Instead, a large proportion of cells are B lymphocytes.

No abnormalities in blood chemistry are characteristic of CLL, but elevated levels of serum lactate dehydrogenase, uric acid, hepatic enzymes (alanine aminotransferase [ALT] or aspartate aminotransferase [AST]), and (rarely) calcium may be observed.

Natural History and Terminal Events

It is a generally held belief that CLL is an indolent disease with a prolonged chronic course and that the eventual cause of death may be co-morbidities unrelated to CLL; however, this observation is true for fewer than 30% of all CLL cases. The natural history is heterogeneous in most patients. Many patients live for 5-10 years with an initial course that is relatively benign, but that is almost always followed by a terminal phase lasting 1-2 years, during which considerable morbidity ensues both from the disease itself and from complications of therapy. During the initial asymptomatic phase, the patients are able to maintain their usual lifestyle, but during the terminal phase, performance status is poor, with recurring need for hospitalization. Other patients die rapidly, within 2-3 years of diagnosis, from complications or causes directly related to CLL. In patients with progressive disease, the cause(s) of death are directly related to CLL. These are most frequently severe systemic infection (especially pneumonia and septicemia), bleeding, and inanition with cachexia.

In ~3% of CLL patients, a diffuse large-cell immunoblastic lymphoma supervenes terminally[88] (Richter transformation; Fig. 113-5). Richter syndrome is associated with a rapidly progressive

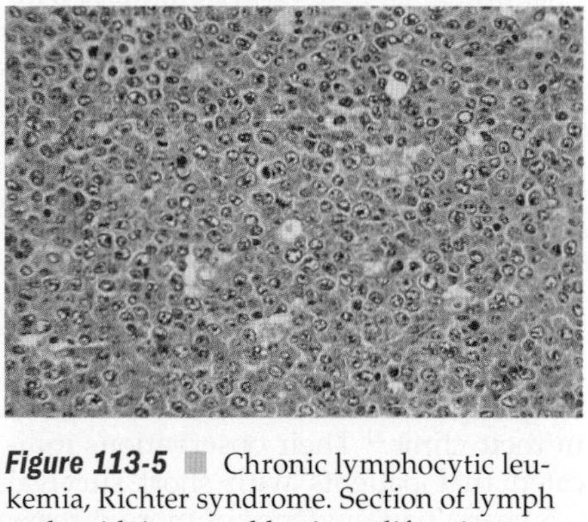

Figure 113-5 Chronic lymphocytic leukemia, Richter syndrome. Section of lymph node with immunoblastic proliferation consisting of large cells with prominent nucleoli (hematoxylin and eosin stain; ×600 original magnification).

course, refractoriness to all currently known chemotherapy, and death within 6 months.[89] The diagnosis of Richter's syndrome requires histopathologic examination of a lymph node.

In an equally small minority of patients, the terminal event is a morphologic transformation of blood lymphocytes from the typical small, mature-appearing cell to somewhat larger cells with distinct nucleoli and a somewhat less-dense chromatin in the nucleus. This event is called "prolymphocytoid transformation," and it is associated with refractoriness to the usual chemotherapeutic agents.[80]

Acute leukemia is observed only extremely rarely as a terminal event in CLL. When it does occur, it is myeloid in origin (myelocytic, myelomonocytic, or acute erythroleukemia). Prior therapy with alkylating agents has not been clearly implicated in the causation of terminal acute leukemia because a few cases have been observed in patients who did not previously receive such therapy for CLL. Acute leukemia developing in patients with CLL is treated with any of the acute leukemia therapy regimens, but almost invariably with poor outcome.

Patients with CLL have been found to have over twice the risk of developing another cancer than is the general population.[89] Skin cancers occur with considerably greater frequency among CLL patients than among the general population, as do other hematologic malignancies, prostate and breast cancers. Those cancers do not result in higher mortality.

Clinical Staging and Other Prognostic Features

The natural history of CLL can be extremely variable, with survival times from initial diagnosis that range from 2 to 20 years. Until the mid-1970s, no reliable clinically applicable criteria were available to physicians to enable them to prospectively separate patients with a poor outlook for survival from those with an excellent prognosis. Understandably, this difficulty forced physicians to make decisions almost exclusively on an empiric basis about the need for (and timing of) therapeutic interventions in their CLL patients.

With the objective of finding prognostic criteria, Boggs and colleagues published an analysis of the clinical features of a large series of patients with CLL who were continuously followed in their clinic.[11] Their observations indicated that patients with short survival (<5 years) had evidence of more disease (eg, larger lymphoid masses, more abnormalities in blood counts) at the time of initial diagnosis of CLL than did the patients whose survival time was longer than 5 years. Soon thereafter, Galton[13] and Dameshek[14] almost simultaneously presented their respective ideas, which are remarkably similar and which have since become the classic tenets for understanding the pathophysiology of CLL. These investigators observed that, in CLL, functionally inert lymphocytes progressively accumulate and that the rate and extent of increase of these nonfunctional lymphocytes influence the overall activity of the disease and the outlook for survival of patients. These observations were subsequently confirmed in a study performed by Hansen,[12] in which case histories of a large series of CLL patients followed and treated at a single institution were reported with meticulous precision.

Those reports, published between 1966 and 1973, constituted the basis on which Rai and colleagues[15] developed a system for staging CLL that could prospectively distinguish patients according to their overall outlook for survival. This method of staging was recognized as a simple yet accurate predictor of survival; consequently, it rapidly gained wide acceptance by clinicians. With the advent of reliable criteria for stratification according to survival outlook, the Cancer and Leukemia Group B (CALGB) was able to initiate clinical trials in patients at various stages of CLL to test various therapeutic strategies.[90-93] During the ensuing years, several additional systems of clinical staging were proposed by investigators around the world, each having certain merits. A few of these staging systems are summarized below, but only two—the Rai system[15] and the Binet system[16]—are in wide use in both clinical practice and research.

Staging System of Rai and Colleagues

The Rai system is based on the concept that in CLL a gradual and progressive increase in the body burden of leukemic lymphocytes occurs, resulting in sequential clinical manifestations of the disease. Those manifestations start in the blood and bone marrow; then affect the lymph nodes, spleen, and liver; and eventually compromise bone marrow function to a significant degree. The earliest stage is the one in which no stigmata of disease are seen other than the minimum diagnostic requirements for CLL (ie, lymphocytosis in blood and marrow [stage 0]), as detailed in Table 113-4. It is important to note that anemia and thrombocytopenia in the context of staging refer to those caused by bone marrow infiltration by CLL, and exclude AIHA and ITP.

At the time of initial diagnosis of CLL, approximately 20-25% of patients are in the earliest clinical stage (stage 0), ~25% are in the advanced stages (stages III and IV), and the remaining 50% are in stage I or II. Table 113-4 shows the exact stage distributions from various series, revealing a consistent pattern.

The median survival times from the time of diagnosis in the series of patients studied by Rai and coworkers were 150 months for stage 0, 101 months for stage I, 71 months for stage II, 19 months for stage III, and 19 months for stage IV.[15] Although Rai and colleagues noted in their 1975 paper that only three (and not five) distinct actuarial survival patterns emerged from the data (stage 0, stages I and II combined, and stages III and IV combined), they recommended that the five-stage system be maintained to investigate prospectively whether biologic and clinical differences would emerge between stages I and II and between stages III and IV. However, in the 1980s, it became apparent that it was impractical to stratify patients in five categories for prospective randomized trials of CLL therapy. In 1987, therefore, the staging system was modified to consist of three groups: low (Rai stage 0), intermediate (Rai stages I and II combined), and high (Rai stages III and IV combined) risk categories.[94] Figure 113-6 depicts the actuarial survival curves according to clinical stage at the time of diagnosis.

The modified Rai staging system was used for stratification of patients according to their risk category in a large Intergroup comparative study in the front-line therapy of CLL conducted in the 1990s.[92,93]

Table 113-4 Distribution of Cases in Various Series According to Rai Staging

References	Cases (*n*)	Series (Years)	Stage (% of Cases) 0	I	II	III	IV
Rai et al. (1975)	125	18	23	31	17	11	14
Geisler and Hansen (1981)	102	20	36	19	17	8	31
Baccarini et al. (1982)	188	26.5	26.5	21	9	17	9
Skinnider (1982)	745	19	21	31	16	13	31
MRC CLL-1[a] (1989)	660	28	18	29	10	15	31

[a]The hemoglobin level for stage III in Medical Research Council of Great Britain Chronic Lymphocytic Leukemia Trial I was <110 g/L. *Source:* From Ref. 80.

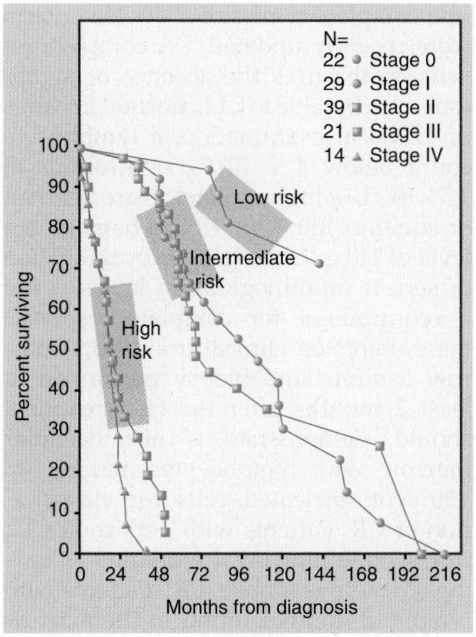

Figure 113-6 Five stages of chronic lymphocytic leukemia modified into a three-stage system: low risk, intermediate risk, and high risk. *Source:* Adapted from Refs. 15, 94.

Method of Binet and Colleagues

Binet's method classifies all patients with anemia (defined as hemoglobin below 100 g/L) and/or thrombocytopenia (platelets less than 100 × 10^9/L), or both, as stage C.[16] All of the remaining (non-C) patients are divided into two groups, depending on the presence of fewer than three (stage A) or three or more (stage B) sites of palpable enlargement of lymphoid organs. This staging takes into consideration five sites: cervical, axillary, and inguinal lymph nodes (whether unilateral or bilateral, each area is counted as one), and the spleen and liver. This system has been found to be of great value in dividing patients into three types of survival curves, with A, B, and C corresponding, respectively, to the Rai low-, intermediate-, and high-risk groups.

Criteria Predictive of Course of Disease in the Low- and Intermediate-Risk Groups

Virtually all patients in the high-risk group (stages III and IV) have a relatively rapid clinical course and have a short survival; however, in the other risk groups, the course of disease is not uniform. Patients in the low- and intermediate-risk groups (stage 0 and stages I and II, respectively) may have a benign clinical course in which the disease remains indolent and is associated with a long overall survival measurable in years or even decades. On the other hand, the course of disease in patients in the low- and intermediate-risk groups may also progress rapidly and have a relatively short overall survival time. The need to prospectively predict the clinical course of CLL in these risk groups is therefore obvious, and even crucial; however, neither Rai nor Binet, nor any other currently available method of staging, is of value for this purpose.

Several prognostic factors have been tested and found to be of limited usefulness in predicting the course of disease in non-advanced stages of CLL.[95] These prognostic factors include extent of blood lymphocytosis; morphologic features of blood lymphocytes (ie, the relative proportion of prolymphocytes); presence of normal or abnormal chromosomal karyotype; phenotypic profile of B lymphocytes; age, gender, and levels of serum immunoglobulins; molecular genetics markers; and β-2-microglobulin.[96]

Smoldering CLL

In the low-risk group, several investigators have discovered certain clinical criteria that may identify patients whose disease will remain indolent or smoldering, as distinct from those whose disease will progress to higher-risk groups. Spanish workers observed that a relatively low absolute lymphocyte count in blood (below 30 × 10^9/L), a long projected or actual time of doubling of blood lymphocyte count in low-risk group patients not receiving cytotoxic therapy, a hemoglobin level above 12 g/dL, and a bone marrow biopsy showing a non-diffuse (interstitial or nodular) pattern of lymphoid infiltration are associated with smoldering CLL and survival statistics similar to those of an age- and sex-matched Spanish population.[95,97] French workers found that stage A patients with hemoglobin in excess of 12 g/dL and blood lymphocytosis below 30 × 10^9/L had a survival time equal to that of the age- and sex-matched French population.[98] This concept is related to but distinct from monoclonal B lymphocytosis (MBL) (see above).

Cytogenetics

Cytogenetic abnormalities discovered by applying FISH (and not the conventional banding) techniques can be of immense clinical value in the management of an individual CLL case. The observations of Dohner and colleagues[68] revealed that patients with 13q deletion as the sole abnormality had a median survival duration of 133 months, patients with normal karyotype had 111 months, those with trisomy 12 had 114 months, those with 11q deletion had 79 months, and those with 17p deletion had 32 months. Their relative frequencies in CLL patients are the following: 7% have 17p deletion, 18% have 11q deletion, 16% have trisomy 12, 55% have 13q14 deletion, and 18% have no detectable cytogenetic abnormality. These abnormalities often correlate with particular clinical profiles. Patients with 17p deletion are often refractory to fludarabine-based therapy. Deletion of 11q is associated with massive lymphadenopathy and is typically associated with males and a relatively young age. Importantly, patients can acquire new cytogenetic abnormalities over time, and they often correlate with increasing clinical aggressiveness of the disease. The incidence of 17p deletion has been found to be significantly higher in patients who have undergone treatment than in patients who are treatment-naïve.[99] The prognostic significance of these cytogenetic findings is independent of the markers discussed below.

IgVH Mutation ■ More recent discoveries of promising new prognostic markers have been the subject of current investigations in predicting the clinical course of CLL in all non-advanced stages of the disease (ie, stages 0, I, and II). The mutational status of Ig genes on CLL lymphocytes is one such marker. Multiple studies have confirmed that the presence of somatic mutations in the IgVH gene (mutated) correlates with significantly longer survival and a relatively more benign disease course than are seen when such mutations are lacking (unmutated).[51,71,100] Testing for mutation status is rapidly becoming more widely available in clinical laboratories. Additional markers have been examined as possible surrogates for the mutation status.

CD38 ■ Investigators showed that increased CD38 expression had a high correlation with the lack of somatic mutation and could potentially be used as a more readily obtainable surrogate marker.[49,52,53,55,72,73] However, additional data showed that CD38 may change over the course of disease,[55] and its predictive value of disease course may be inconsistent.[101]

Zap-70 Expression ■ Zap-70 is an intracellular protein involved in activation signaling. It is normally present in T lymphocytes and natural killer cells and is rarely present in normal B cells.[102] In spite of the fact that ZAP-70 testing can be performed by flow cytometry, the methodology and reproducibility of these tests have yet to be standardized, so like mutation status its testing remains reliable only in very specialized centers. Studies demonstrated its aberrant expression in leukemic B lymphocytes correlates with unmutated IgVH genes.[43,103] Subsequent investigations demonstrated Zap-70 positivity in CLL as an independent predictor of disease progression and inferior clinical outcome.[102-106] A recent study suggested that ZAP-70 was actually superior to mutation status in predicting time to treatment, and that CD38 was only useful if the other two factors were unknown.[100] Taken together, these studies demonstrate that the data of mutation status, CD38, and Zap-70 are convincing but the issue continues to evolve; their respective powers to predict disease course remains unclear, particularly when the markers have conflicting results. These issues are further confounded by the continued lack of standardized testing methods. For the above reasons, in addition to the lack of proof that earlier treatment of high-risk patients will be beneficial, the utility of these markers in clinical practice remains undefined. Current clinical trials will help to answer these questions, evaluating the benefit of treating patients with high-risk markers earlier in their disease course. In current practice, however, the clinical picture must still ultimately dictate the treatment plan. Table 113-5 summarizes these newly identified prognostic markers.

Newer Prognostic Tools

More recently, investigators have identified a microRNA signature that differentiates Zap-70 expression, mutation status, and disease progression that may add yet another useful prognostic tool in the future.[107] High expressions of beta-2 microglobulin is yet another potentially useful markers, with data showing its correlation with poor prognosis.[108] In addition, increased expression of activation-induced cytidine deaminase (AID) mRNA has been shown to be associated with unmutated disease and high-risk cytogenetic aberrations.[109]

Treatment

Initiation of early treatment is considered crucial in most malignant diseases. In CLL, treatment is rarely started immediately at the time of diagnosis. The lack of evidence that CLL can be cured with currently available modalities[97] has resulted in a "watch and wait" in the initial approach to most patients. However, the development of new regimens with significant activity in CLL—namely, purine analogs, monoclonal antibodies, and application of autologous and allogeneic hematopoietic stem cells transplantation—has led to consideration of curative attempts in younger patients. Moreover, the recognition of new prognostic markers (CD38, ZAP-70, IgVH mutation status, FISH genetic abnormalities, p53 mutations, and thymidine kinase) has led to consideration of earlier intervention in early-stage, low tumor burden, asymptomatic patients. Currently this approach is not recommended outside of a clinical trial.[110] Well-designed clinical trials are underway, however, to examine the effect of early intervention on high-risk patients.

Indications for Treatment

The International Workshop on CLL, updating the NCI-Working Group 1996 guidelines, recommends treatment to be initiated for the following[77]:

1. Rai stage I or II (Binet stage B) in patients with disease-related symptoms
2. Rai stage III or IV (Binet Stage C)
3. Massive or rapidly enlarging, symptomatic lymphadenopathy, or splenomegaly
4. Lymphocyte doubling time of <6 months
5. AIHA or thrombocytopenia (or both) that is poorly responsive to corticosteroid therapy.

A short period of time with enlarging lymph nodes and/or rapid lymphocyte doubling should be assessed cautiously; such events can be transient. Only when a true trend is established should a decision to treat be made based on these criteria.

No data exist determining a particular threshold of lymphocyte count that warrants treatment. However, theory and anecdotal evidence suggests that an extremely high counts can cause complications secondary to hyperviscosity. An acceptable value is ~250,000 lymphocytes, beyond which treatment may be recommended.

Goals of Therapy

Traditionally, treatment of CLL continued until symptoms resolved or clinically troubling lymphadenopathy and splenomegaly were controlled. Complete remission was not an objective of treatment.

In recent years, the availability of regimens with higher complete remission rates in CLL has led both the NCIWG and the IWCLL to develop criteria to define complete remission.[111] These criteria were recently updated.[77] A complete remission requires the absence of symptoms attributable to CLL, normal findings on physical examination, a lymphocyte count below 4×10^9/L, neutrophils at 1.5×10^9/L or higher, platelets greater than or equal to 100×10^9/L, and hemoglobin level of 110 g/L or higher. Normalization of serum immunoglobulin levels is not a requirement for complete response. For patients on clinical trials, bone marrow aspirate and biopsy performed at least 2 months after the last treatment should demonstrate a normocellular marrow with lymphocytes making up <30% of nucleated cells for classification of CR. Patients with persistent CLL in the bone marrow are defined as having a partial response (PR). Patients with lymphoid nodules found in the marrow following treatment are categorized as nodular PR. New guidelines recommend that these nodules be further characterized by immunohistochemistry staining to determine if these are CLL cells or T-lymphocyte clusters. Those patients without evidence of CLL but persistent cytopenias after treatment should be considered to be in a CR with incomplete bone marrow recovery (CRi).

Other criteria for PR were defined as a reduction in previously elevated lymphocyte counts, enlarged nodes, spleen, or liver by 50% or more. Peripheral blood should also show one of the following: a neutrophil count of 1.5×10^9/or higher, a platelet count of 100×10^9/L or higher, or a hemoglobin level of 110 g/L or higher (or a 50% or better improvement over pre-therapy deficits in these counts). These responses must persist for a minimum period of 2 months.

Another concept relevant to clinical trials is that of minimal residual disease (MRD). Eradication of (MRD) refers to the complete eradication of leukemic cells by either four-color flow cytometry or by allele-specific oligonucleotide PCR. This determination must be made at least 3 months after the completion of therapy. Whereas absence of MRD may indicate a more favorable prognosis, its value as a therapeutic goal remains unclear. This issue is discussed further below. The efforts of the NCIWG and IWCLL in standardizing criteria for clinical research protocols and for evaluating response have allowed results of different trials to be compared and have greatly enhanced the quality of clinical research in CLL.

Chemotherapy

For 50 years, the backbone of chemotherapy in CLL was the use of alkylating agents such as chlorambucil or cyclophosphamide, with or without the addition of corticosteroids. Despite evidence that chlorambucil is associated with a

Table 113-5 Recently Identified Molecular and Cytogenetic Markers of Prognosis in Chronic Lymphocytic Leukemia (CLL)

	Markers of		
	Good Prognosis	Worse Prognosis	References
IgVH mutation status	Mutated	Unmutated	51,71
ZAP-70 on CLL-B Lymphocytes	Negative	Positive	103–106
CD38 on CLL-B lymphocytes	Negative	Positive	51,72,73
FISH cytogenetics	Sole abnormality is 13q del	11q del, 17p del	68

lower response rate and shorter response duration than that achieved with purine analogs, chlorambucil is still widely used in older patients because it is a convenient and easy to administer oral drug, well-tolerated, and inexpensive.

Great variability in the dose and schedule of chlorambucil has been observed. Two commonly used schedules are a daily dose of 0.08 mg/kg (4-8 mg total dose per day) and a pulsed intermittent dose of 0.8 mg/kg (40-80 mg in a single day) given every 3-4 weeks.[111,112] The intermittent schedule was an attempt to prevent myelosuppression, which is the main toxicity. A CALGB study revealed that chlorambucil is equally effective when given daily or on an intermittent basis.[90]

Chlorambucil is usually administered for a period of several weeks until maximum clinical response is reached. Maintenance therapy is uncommon, and recurrence of disease is followed by resumption of therapy. A substantial fraction of patients achieve second and third responses. Chlorambucil is more likely than cyclophosphamide to cause thrombocytopenia. Oral cyclophosphamide can be given, but it is more frequently administered intravenously, at a dose of 750 mg/m^2 in intervals of 3-4 weeks, and often in combination with another agent (see below). These two alkylating agents generally get similar results.

Corticosteroids

Prednisone has been administered to CLL patients as a single agent, usually in an initial dose of 20-60 mg, with dose reductions occurring in a graduated fashion.[112,113] One-third of patients so treated had shrinkage of lymph nodes or spleen. Often, in the first 1-2 months, an increase in the lymphocyte count was followed by a subsequent decline, caused by a shift of lymphocytes from lymph nodes and bone marrow into the blood. Anemia and thrombocytopenia improved in approximately two-thirds of patients. Usually, 3-6 months of treatment were required. The major side effects were those of chronic corticosteroid therapy and infections.

At the present time, the major indication for prednisone appears to be management of antibody-mediated (autoimmune) anemia and thrombocytopenia. In addition, high-dose methylprednisolone has been shown to be effective in shrinking large lymph node masses.[114]

Combinations Using Alkylating Agents

A study of daily high-dose chlorambucil (15 mg/day) until complete remission or toxicity was compared to 6 doses of chlorambucil 75 mg once weekly, combined with prednisone.[114] A significantly higher response rate was noted for the chlorambucil arm versus the combination regimen. The cumulative dose in the chlorambucil-alone arm was five to six times that in the combination arm, with substantial marrow toxicity. A survival advantage was noted for the chlorambucil-alone arm. The COP (cyclophosphamide, vincristine (Oncovin), and prednisone) and CHOP regimens have not shown superiority over chlorambucil.[115-117]

Past Trials for Early-Stage CLL

In two clinical trials by the French Cooperative Group on CLL (FCGCLL) involving patients with Binet stage A CLL, immediate treatment with chlorambucil (first trial) or with chlorambucil plus prednisone (second trial) was compared with delay of treatment until progression was noted.[98] The delayed treatment groups each had a slightly superior survival with fewer second malignancies. In Binet stage B patients, the FCGCLL compared chlorambucil with cyclophosphamide, vincristine (Oncovin), and prednisone (COP); similar survival and rate of disease progression were observed between the two groups.[117]

Purine Analogs

Purine analogs have become the major treatment class for CLL. Fludarabine monophosphate (Fludara), 2-chlorodeoxyadenosine (2-CdA), and pentostatin (2′-deoxycoformycin, DCF) are highly active in CLL and have changed the standard of care.

Early Studies Using Purine Analogs

In phase 2 trials of fludarabine, response rates of 40-60% were noted in previously treated patients, with 15% achieving complete remission. Higher response rates were seen in earlier-stage disease.[118,119] The addition of prednisone did not improve the response rate and was associated with an increased incidence of substitute and *Listeria* infections.[120] The major side effects associated with purine analogues were myelosuppression and episodes of fever and infection. Subsequent studies have evaluated fludarabine with and without prednisone in previously untreated patients, with complete remission rates of 25-30% and an overall response rate of 80% being achieved.[120]

The drug cladribine (2-CdA), which is potent in hairy cell leukemia, has been studied in CLL with an overall response rate of 30-70% in advanced-stage disease.[121-123] Studies in previously untreated patients demonstrated response rates of 56-85%, with complete response rates varying between 10% and 47%.[124] Both fludarabine and 2-CdA are 50-60% bioavailable by mouth and are effective clinically when administered by the oral route. Although historical comparisons show lower response rates for single-agent pentostatin than those of fludarabine and cladribine, pentostatin-based combination therapy has a substantial role in current treatment (see below).[125,126]

As found in the above studies, the major causes for concern in using purine analogs are infections and myelosuppression.[124,127] With fludarabine therapy, CD4 and CD8 T-cell counts in CLL patients fall to ~200/µL for prolonged periods. Nevertheless, patients in remission of therapy have a very low incidence of infections: approximately one febrile episode or infection for every 2.5 patient-years at risk. Serious infections such as pneumonia occurred at a frequency of one for every 16 patient-years at risk. Herpes zoster appears to occur more frequently in patients treated with purine analogs: approximately 15-20% of patients experienced an outbreak at some time during their course.

Comparative Studies Using Purine Analogs

In an Intergroup study, a prospective, randomized trial in previously untreated CLL patients in North America showed significantly higher rates of overall response and complete response, as well as longer durations of response and progression-free survival in patients randomized to fludarabine than in patients who received chlorambucil. However, there was no significant difference in overall survival between the two arms, though this may have been due to the crossover design of the study.[92] A third arm of the study, combining fludarabine and chlorambucil, was discontinued because of excessive infections. Major infections as well as herpes virus infections occurred more often on the fludarabine arm than on CLB arm. Advanced stage and low serum levels of immunoglobulin were associated with an increased incidence of infections. More therapy-related myeloid leukemias were noted in the fludarabine arm than in the chlorambucil arm.[127]

These results were confirmed in a comparative German CLL Study Group (GCLLSG) study of intravenous fludarabine versus oral chlorambucil in patients older than 65 years. They demonstrated significantly higher rates of complete response and overall response, and improved quality of life measurements for the purine analog.[128] Finally, a randomized comparative trial of 2-CdA or chlorambucil plus prednisone demonstrated a significantly higher complete response rate for the 2-CdA arm (47% vs 12%), and significantly longer remission duration, but no difference in survival.[123]

Several Europeans studies found purine analogs superior to combination therapies containing anthracyclines as well. Fludarabine was compared with cyclophosphamide, doxorubicin (adriamycin), and prednisone (CAP) in a randomized fashion.[129] In untreated patients, the response rate was 70% for fludarabine versus 58% for CAP; in previously treated patients, it was 45% versus 26%, respectively. No survival difference was observed, although time to progression was significantly longer for the fludarabine-treated patients. French investigators evaluated fludarabine versus CAP versus French CHOP.[130] A higher response rate was found with fludarabine (71%) and with CHOP (72%) than with CAP (58%). Complete responses were more frequent with fludarabine. No difference in survival was noted. The incidences of infections and autoimmune hemolytic anemia were similar in the three groups.

Bendamustine

Bendamustine has been used in eastern Europe since the 1970s in various hematologic malignancies. It is an alkylating agent with potential antimetabolite properties associated with its benzimidazole ring. The FDA recently approved this agent in CLL based on a randomized trial comparing it to chlorambucil in previously untreated patients.[131] Bendamustine, given at a dose of 100 mg/m^2 IV for 2 days every 4 weeks, was found to be superior to chlorambucil in overall response rate (67% vs 30%), and progression-free survival (21 months vs 8 months). The bendamustine arm had more myelosuppression, but not more infections. Its role in CLL treatment is still evolving.

Monoclonal Antibodies

Monoclonal antibodies have been evaluated in CLL because of potential target antigens on the surface of CLL cells. Monoclonal antibodies, rituximab against CD20 and alemtuzumab (Campath-1H) against CD52, have become important components in CLL treatment.

Rituximab is more active in follicular than in diffuse SLL or CLL; in the latter relapsed or refractory diseases, the response rate is only 12-15%.[132,133] Dose-intensive regimens demonstrated a dose-response relationship; high doses of rituximab in CLL gave higher response rates than did conventional doses.[134,135] Even in the higher dose, though, single-agent rituximab does not typically provide durable responses. This agent, however, has been of great utility when used in combination with other drugs (see below). Its activity in CLL is poorly understood and its efficacy in this disease is somewhat puzzling. CD20 is typically expressed in low levels on CLL cells. Moreover, CLL patients have been shown to have soluble CD20 in their plasma that may bind rituximab and hasten its clearance.[136]

Alemtuzumab has been shown to be effective in a number of settings. It has impressive activity in clearing disease in blood, bone marrow, and spleen but is relatively ineffective in treating bulky lymph nodes.[137] In fact, there is an inverse relationship between the size of lymph nodes and probability of response. Its efficacy at clearing the bone marrow has led to its investigation as a potential consolidation agent (discussed below under chemoimmunotherapy). Another important characteristic of alemtuzumab in CLL therapy is its effectiveness in treating high-risk populations. A German study demonstrated a response rate of 54% in fludarabine-refractory patients with 17p deletions or p53 abnormalities.[137] This benefit was confirmed in subsequent trials and additional data showed its benefit in 11q-deleted patients as well (see below).[138,139]

The initial FDA approval of alemtuzumab was based on a pivotal trial in 93 fludarabine-refractory patients in which alemtuzumab demonstrated a response rate of 33%.[140] In early studies alemtuzumab was administered intravenously but subcutaneous administration is now widely accepted and effectively avoids infusion-related complications. Local reactions can be dose-limiting in some patients, but are usually manageable after the first 1-2 weeks. This shift to subcutaneous injection was supported by a GCLLSG study that demonstrated equal response rates for subcutaneous and intravenous administration of alemtuzumab in fludarabine-refractory patients.[141]

Recently published results of the CAM307 trial led to alemtuzumab's approval in the front-line setting.[138] The CAM307 trial was an international, prospective, randomized trial comparing alemtuzumab to chlorambucil. The alemtuzumab arm was superior in response rate (83% vs 55%), complete responses (24% vs 2%), and time to alternative treatment (23 months vs 15 months). Perhaps most interesting was the further evidence of alemtuzumab's activity in high-risk groups such as 17p-deleted patients and 11q-deleted patients.[138]

Alemtuzumab has well-known infectious complications and in early trials ~50% of patients had major infections.[142] These complications were more often found in non-responders. All patients should receive prophylaxis against *P. carinii* pneumonia, jeroveci DNA viruses, and undergo close monitoring for CMV antigenemia by PCR testing for 6 to 8 months (at least until T-cell recovery) following treatment with alemtuzumab. Cytomegalovirus (CMV) reactivation is the most common infection associated with alemtuzumab and occurs in 15-25% of patients. This typically responds quickly to gancyclovir or foscarnet. With these aggressive measures, the infectious complications are generally manageable and this agent can be extremely valuable tool for CLL therapy.

The complementary effects of these two monoclonal antibodies, with rituximab's efficacy on treating bulky lymph nodes, and alemtuzumab's activity on the bone marrow and spleen, provided the rationale for recent studies of alemtuzumab plus rituximab, which have response rates of 50% or more in patients with relapsed and refractory CLL.[143]

Combinations

Purine Analog-Alkylating Agent Combinations

Based on the ability of fludarabine to inhibit repair of alkylator-induced DNA cross-linking,[144] these two drug groups were combined to theoretically potentiate their respective activities. This combination has been reported to have high response rates and acceptable tolerance in both previously treated and untreated patients.[145,146] In the initial phase 2 study, patients with fludarabine-refractory disease had a response rate of 41% to the fludarabine/cyclophosphamide combination.[145] Three major phase 3 trials demonstrated that the combination therapy with fludarabine and cyclophosphamide was superior to fludarabine alone. The US Intergroup E2997 phase 3 Trial compared fludarabine to fludarabine combined with cyclophosphamide in previously untreated patients. The combination group had a superior complete response (23.4% vs 4.6%) and overall response rates (74.3% vs 59.5%) than single-agent fludarabine. Progression-free survival was also higher in the combination arm (31.6 months vs 19.2 months).[147]

The LRF CLL4 Trial from the United Kingdom confirmed these results.[148] Patients received either a combination of fludarabine and cyclophosphamide, single-agent fludarabine, or single-agent chlorambucil. The combination was superior in complete response, overall response, and progression-free survival. These advantages were found in all ages and prognostic groups as determined by mutation status. Interestingly, the combination arm had significantly less hemolytic anemia than either the fludarabine or chlorambucil arms.[148] The German CLL4 trial provided yet additional supporting evidence for combination therapy.[149] This trial compared fludarabine + cyclophosphamide to fludarabine single agent as front-line therapy in patients younger than 66 years. Again, combination therapy showed higher complete responses, overall responses, and progression-free survival.[149] All three trials demonstrated that the combination arm had more hematologic toxicities, including neutropenia. In two of the three trials there was no increase in infections.[147-149] Combinations of 2-CdA and cyclophosphamide (Cytoxan) and pentostatin and cyclophosphamide are also effective.[150,151]

Fludarabine and cyclophosphamide combined with mitoxantrone has been developed as a salvage and front-line regimen in CLL.[152-154] High rates of complete response and overall response were demonstrated in previously treated patients, with many responders showing no minimal residual disease (MRD) by flow cytometry and polymerase chain reaction (PCR). Despite these results, this combination is rarely used in current clinical practice.

Chemoimmunotherapy Combinations

Multiple trials have proven a potentiating effect of adding immunotherapy to chemotherapy. This phenomenon is incompletely understood though several known characteristics of these agents may explain this effect. Rituximab may sensitize lymphoid cell lines to a variety of chemotherapeutic agents, including fludarabine and cyclophosphamide by down-regulating antiapoptotic proteins, Bcl-2 and Bcl-x_L.[155] Fludarabine, on the other hand, down-regulates complement-resistant proteins, CD55 and CD59 on CLL cells.[156] This may thereby enhance cytotoxicity mediated by complement lysis with rituximab or alemtuzumab therapy.

Fludarabine-Rituximab (FR)

Three chemoimmunotherapy programs using rituximab have been developed (Table 113-6).[93,157,158] In the CALGB 9712 study, fludarabine was combined with either simultaneous or sequential rituximab, followed by consolidation rituximab in both arms.[93] The complete remission rate was higher with the simultaneous protocol (47% vs 33%), with no additional toxicity apart from neutropenia. No increase in infections was noted. These results were retrospectively compared with patients, from a prior CALGB study (9011) with similar clinical characteristics, who received single-agent fludarabine.[159] The group that received fludarabine plus rituximab had significantly better progression-free survival and overall survival than those who received fludarabine alone. Though this retrospective comparison does not provide definitive evidence, it does suggest that the addition of rituximab to fludarabine yields a significant benefit. A head-to-head trial from Germany, described below, showed a definitive benefit of adding rituximab to a combination of fludarabine and cyclophosphamide.[160]

Table 113-6 Front-Line Therapy (Chemoimmunotherapy) for Chronic Lymphocytic Leukemia

References	Regimen	Pts.	%CR	%OR	Resp. Duration Med. (Months)
Rai et al.[92]	FLU	170	20	63	251
	CLB	181	4	37	14
FCSG[129]	FLU	52	23	71	NR
	CAP	48	17	60	7
Leporrier et al.[130]	FLU	336	40	71	32
	CHOP	351	30	71	30
	CAP	237	15	58	27
Robak[200]	CDA+PRED	126	47	87	21
	CLB+PRED	103	12	45	18
Robak et al.[150]	CDA+C	62	30	88	NR
Flynn et al.[147]	FLU + CYT	141	23	74	32
	FLU	137	5	60	19
Kay et al.[158]	PCR	65	41	91	NR
Byrd et al.[159]	FLU	53	47	90	NR
	FLU+RIT	51	28	72	
Hallek et al.[160]	FCR	408	52	95	NR
	FLU + CYT	409	27	88	NR
Keating et al.[154]	FCR Q 4 weeks (FLU 25 mg/m² d1-3 CYT 600 mg/m² d1-3 RIT 375 mg/m² d1, cycle 1 then 500 mg/m² d1 subsequent cycles)	224	70	95	NR
Reynolds et al.[161a]	PCR	92	7	45	NR
	FCR	92	17	58	NR
Hillmen et al.[138]	ALEM	149	24	83	15
	CLB	148	2	55	12
Knauf et al.[131]	BEN	162		67	21
	CLB	157		30	8
O'Brien et al.[218]	FLU+ ALEM	36	42	92	NR
Bosch et al.[152]	FLU + CYT + MIT	69	64	90	37

[a]Trial included some relapsed patients.

Abbreviations: Alem, alemtuzumab; CAP, cyclophosphamide, doxorubicin, prednisone; CDA, chlorodeoxyadenosine; CHOP, cyclophosphamide, hydroxydaunomycin (doxorubicin), Oncovin (vincristine), prednisone; CLB, chlorambucil; CR, complete response; CYT, cyclophosphamide; F, fludarabine; FC, fludarabine, cyclophosphamide; FLU, fludarabine; NR, not reported; OR, overall response; PCR, pentostatin, cyclophosphamide, rituximab; PRED, prednisone; Pts. = patients; RIT, rituximab; FCR= fludarabine + cyclophosphamide + rituximab; BEN, bendamustine; MIT, mitoxantrone.

Fludarabine-Cyclophosphamide-Rituximab (FCR)

Several single-arm studies have combined purine analogs with an cyclosphosphamide and rituximab in both the up-front and refractory settings. In a single institution, single-arm study, one group successfully treated 224 previously untreated patients with fludarabine, cyclophosphamide, and rituximab (FCR).[157] Seventy-two percent of these patients achieved a CR and the overall response rate was 95%. Moreover, many of the patients with complete responses had no detectable disease in the bone marrow as measured by flow cytometry. Grade 3-4 neutropenia occurred in over 50%. These results, while encouraging, provide no head-to-head data in evaluating the benefit of adding cyclophosphamide. A multi-institution, prospective trial directly comparing FCR to FR is currently under way and will provide more definitive evidence as to which regimen is superior.

In a well-designed, phase 3 trial of 817 previously untreated patients, the German CLL Study Group evaluated the benefit of adding rituximab to FC. Preliminary results of 761 evaluable patients demonstrated that FCR was superior to FC in OR rate (95% vs 88%; p = 0.001), CR rate (52% vs 27%; $p < 0.0001$), and PFS (76.6% vs 62.3% at 2 years; $p < 0.0001$).[160] Interestingly, these benefits were more pronounced in the earlier-stage patients. The FCR arm had a greater incidence of neutropenia, but not of grade 3 or 4 infections. We currently recommend FCR in the front-line for the majority of patients, though FR is also acceptable. FCR as well as other purine analog-alkylator-rituximab (see below) regimens should all be given with antibiotic prophylaxis against *Pneumocystis*, varicella, and *Candida*.

Pentostatin-Cyclophosphamide-Rituximab (PCR)

Pentostatin, cyclophosphamide, and rituximab (PCR) is yet another front-line treatment in CLL. A smaller single-arm study demonstrated an overall response rate of over 90%[158] in previously untreated patients. The CR rate was 41%, with many achieving MRD negativity as well. The US Oncology group recently presented early results from a phase 3 study comparing PCR to FCR.[161] The FCR had a superior CR rate, and there was no statistical difference in terms of infectious toxicities. Importantly, this trial used 4 mg/m^2 of pentostatin, as opposed to the 2 mg/m^2 dose in the aforementioned study, and patients included both treated and untreated. Taken together, these results demonstrate that PCR is a reasonable alternative to FCR in the up-front setting, though no solid conclusions about comparative safety and efficacy can be drawn. Both FCR and PCR regimens have been shown to be effective in the relapsed setting as well.[162,163]

Bendamustine-Rituximab (BR)

The combination of bendamustine + rituximab (BR) is already being used in clinical practice. Early results presented at the 2008 Annual meeting of the American Society of Hematology demonstrated a 77% overall RR and 14.5% CR rate in relapsed patients.[164] This promising combination will likely become more widely accepted as data from this and other clinical trials mature.

Alemtuzumab Consolidation and Eradication of Minimal Residual Disease (MRD)

Following successful treatment with fludarabine-based regimens, the bone marrow is typically the site of residual disease. Due to its potency in treating marrow-based CLL, alemtuzumab has been examined as a consolidation therapy to eradicate persistent disease in the bone marrow in this setting. A CALGB study demonstrated that patients treated with alemtuzumab following fludarabine improved the quality of responses significantly, with many patients upgrading from a partial response to a complete response.[165,166] An Italian group showed a similar upgrade in responses, improving from 35% CRs after fludarabine to 79% following alemtuzumab consolidation.[167] A German trial randomized patients to receive alemtuzumab consolidation versus observation following fludarabine-based therapy. Although the trial was stopped early due to infectious complications, preliminary results showed an improvement in PFS in the consolidation arm.[168]

The effectiveness of alemtuzumab at achieving a greater degree of disease eradication has led to the concept of eliminating minimal residual disease (MRD). MRD elimination, or negativity, refers to the complete eradication of leukemic cells either by four-color flow cytometry or by allele-specific oligonucleotide PCR. Recent consolidation studies using alemtuzumab were designed to evaluate the ability to achieve, and the benefits of attaining MRD negativity. In a single-arm trial from the United Kingdom, alemtuzumab was given in 91 previously treated patients.[169] It was observed that those patients who achieved MRD negativity (20%) had significantly improved PFS and overall survival when compared to those who achieved CRs but still had evidence of disease in their bone marrow. These results initiated a discussion as to whether or not achievement of MRD negativity should be the new goal of treatment.[170] To date, it is unclear if the attainment of MRD negativity itself results in improved outcomes, or if the successful clearing of the bone marrow simply represents a group of patients with more treatment-sensitive disease. Whereas intuitively MRD negativity is expected to correlate to improved PFS and OS, giving additional therapy in its pursuit may result in unnecessary toxicity without true benefit. In current clinical practice MRD negativity should not be used as a therapeutic end point until clinical trials resolve this debate.

Salvage Therapy and New Agents

Treatment options available for salvage therapy in CLL are shown in Table 113-7. Single-agent purine analogs have overall response rates of ~50% in relapsed and refractory CLL (10-15% complete response). In one comparative study, fludarabine had a higher response rate than did CAP.[171] Increasingly, combinations of purine analogs with DNA-active agents such as cyclophosphamide, doxorubicin, or mitoxantrone are being explored, with the achievement of high overall response rates.[151,153,154,162-166,171] Comparison of such studies is difficult because of the diversity of patients entered in the protocols, but several combinations have shown promise in single-arm studies.

The addition of rituximab or alemtuzumab (or both) appears to increase response rates in salvage regimens.[165-169] A combination of oxaliplatin, fludarabine, cytarabine, and rituximab (OFAR) showed significant activity in the settings of fludarabine-refractory disease and Richters transformation, with response rates of 33% and 50%, respectively, in each patient-group.[172]

Lenalidomide, an immunomodulatory agent approved for multiple myeloma and 5q del-myelodysplastic

Table 113-7 **Salvage Therapy for Relapsed Chronic Lymphocytic Leukemia**

Regimen	References	Patients	%CR	%OR
FLU	Keating et al.[119]	68	13	57
ALEM	Keating et al.[140]	93		33
FLU+CYT	O'Brien et al.[145]	94	10	70
2-CdA	Robak et al.[219]	184	13	48
FLU+ ALEM	Elter et al.[220]	36	30	83
CFAR	Wierda et al.[221]	44	27	65
FCR	Wierda et al.[162]	177	25	73
PCR	Lamanna et al.[163]	32	25	75
OFAR	Tsimberidou et al.[172]	30 (CLL) 20 (Richter)		33 50
FLU + CYT + Oblimersen	O'Brien et al.[222]	120	17 (CR + nodular PR)[a]	
Bendamustine + RIT	Fischer et al.[164]	81	15	77
Ofatumumab	Osterborg[180]	59 (DR)[b] 79 (BR)[c]		58 47
Lenalidomide (25 mg/day)	Chanan-Khan et al.[174]	45	18	57
Lenalidomide (10-25 mg/day)	Ferrajoli et al.[175]	44	7	32
Flavopiridol	Byrd et al.[183]	117		48

[a]Two-arm study: FLU + CYT arm had 7% CR.
[b]DR, double refractory(FLU and ALEM).
[c]BR, bulky nodes + FLU refractory.
Abbreviations: CR, complete response ; OR, overall response; 2-CdA, 2-chlorodeoxyadenosine; Alem, alemtuzumab; CAP, cyclophosphamide, doxorubicin, prednisone; CYT, cyclophosphamide; DCF, 2′-deoxycoformycin; Doxo, doxorubicin; FLU, fludarabine; Mitox, mitroxitrone; RIT, rituximab: FCR= fludarabine + cyclophosphamide + rituximab; OFAR, oxaliplatin, fludarabine + cytarabine + rituximab; CFAR, fludarabine + cyclophosphamide + rituximab + alemtuzumab.

syndrome, has shown promise in CLL. In CLL its activity may be due to the upregulation of costimulatory molecules (CD40, CD80, CD86), inhibition of prosurvival cytokines (vascular endothelial growth factor, TNF alpha, IL-6), as well as activation of T and NK cells.[173] Two single-arm studies showed impressive response rates (57% and 32%) and complete responses (18% and 7%) in relapsed or refractory patients.[174,175] Another trial demonstrated activity of lenalidomide in the front-line setting as well.[176] However, significant tumor lysis and tumor flare were seen with this agent, particularly in previously untreated patients, and even at relatively small doses. Larger trials are underway to further refine the dosing schedule and explore lenalidomide's potential role in CLL as a single agent, and in combination with other drugs.

New monoclonal antibodies, lumiliximab and ofatumumab, also show promise in CLL. Lumiliximab, a macaque-human primatized monoclonal antibody targeting CD23, showed impressive CR rates in a phase 2 trial in combination with FCR.[177] A larger trial evaluating this combination is underway. Ofatumumab, a fully humanized anti-CD20 monoclonal antibody, targets a distinct epitope on CD20[178] from that of rituximab. A phase 1/2 trial demonstrated safety and clinical activity of ofatumumab.[179] A large trial evaluating its activity in CLL patients who were either fludarabine-refractory with bulky lymph nodes or refractory to both alemtuzumab and fludarabine-based therapies had 51% overall response rate.[180]

Among many other new agents being investigated in CLL are cyclin-dependent kinase (CDK) inhibitors, BCL-2 inhibitors, and Hsp90 inhibitors.[181] Studies with flavopiridol, a CDK inhibitor, have been encouraging. After various dosing schedules, a recent trial employed a 30 min IV bolus followed by a 4-h continuous IV infusion.[182] One hundred seventeen with relapsed CLL/SLL had a 48% RR, many of whom had high-risk genetic abnormalities, such as 17p and 11q deletions.[183] The hyperacute tumor lysis syndrome remains a concern with this agent and has been a dose-limiting toxicity in trials. Preclinical studies have also suggested that telomeres would be a viable target in CLL.[184] GRN163L, a telomerase inhibitor, is currently in clinical trials in CLL.

Immunotherapy

The success of cellular therapy in nonablative (minimal) stem cell transplantation (see below) encouraged exploration of other approaches to immunotherapy. The administration of expanded autologous T cells resulted in a reduction in nodes and spleen in one-third of patients.[185] Autologous CLL cells have been transfused to induce expression of CD154 (CD40 ligand). Such infusions can induce CLL-specific T-cell responses and have been associated with clinical improvement.[186] Likewise, cells expressing both CD40L (or CD154) and interleukin 2 have been studied.[175] Use of agents such as interferon-β, tumor necrosis factor receptor–binding agents, interleukin 2, and interleukin 4 has been disappointing.[187-189] A recent trial involving a vaccine against the idiotype (anti-Id, or antigen recognition site) on CLL cells had disappointing results. Nevertheless, researchers continue to explore these concepts.

Stem Cell Transplantation

Autologous stem cell transplantation (SCT) has been conducted in several series.[179,180] The technique is safe and shows a lower relapse rate in patients transplanted at first response as an intensification procedure, as compared with patients transplanted in the presence of active disease as a salvage regimen.[190] In either case, these patients typically relapse and autologous transplant has proven no clear benefit in CLL.

In the past, allogeneic SCT had not been widely performed in CLL because of the relatively advanced age of most patients. Recently, allogeneic SCT is being more seriously considered as an option for an increasing number of younger age CLL patients. Allogeneic transplantation patients have a significantly longer survival if the transplantation procedure occurs while their disease is chemosensitive rather than after their CLL becomes refractory.[191,192] Nevertheless, results of myeloablative allogeneic stem cell transplants have shown high treatment-related mortality and should be reserved for very specific cases.

Reduced-intensity transplantation has shown promise in CLL. This procedure is based on nonmyeloablative conditioning, and relies on the graft-versus-leukemia effect for efficacy. PCR negativity can, in fact, be achieved with nonablative transplantation—and this result is attributed to the graft-versus-leukemia effect. Importantly, these transplantations can be performed in patients older than 70 years of age.[193-195] Early results show significantly reduced treatment-related mortality,[196] moderate evidence of long-term disease control,[197] and effectiveness in high-risk groups such as those patients with unmutated IgVH, or 11q or 17p cytogenetic abnormalities.[198,199] Patients with sensitive disease[183] and less bulky lymph nodes (smaller than 5 cm) tend to have superior outcomes.[199] Though these initial results are encouraging, this method is still investigational and future studies will establish the place of this transplantation modality in the context of CLL.

Radiation Therapy

The major indication for radiation therapy in CLL is large, bulky lymphoid masses causing compression symptomatology, especially if the bulky masses are unresponsive to chemotherapy. CLL lymphocytes are sensitive to radiation, and shrinkage of lymphoid masses is usually possible to achieve symptomatic relief.[200] Splenic irradiation has been performed in patients with painful splenic enlargement or cytopenias related to hypersplenism as well. This does not typically provide long-term control; if the patient is in a satisfactory clinical state, splenectomy is the preferred option.

Leukapheresis

Apheresis is seldom necessary for leukocytosis per se, because leukostasis rarely causes symptoms such as shortness of breath associated with pulmonary infiltrates or neurologic symptoms unless the white cell count is extremely high (>400 × 10^9/L). In such cases, chemotherapy is typically effective at reducing lymphocyte counts to a safe level. Nevertheless, leukapheresis can provide relief, albeit transiently, in the setting of active symptomatology.

Splenectomy

A number of patients with advanced CLL develop splenomegaly and pancytopenia. This syndrome often responds to effective chemotherapy. A number of studies have suggested hematologic and survival benefits from splenectomy in patients with CLL. Suggested benefits include removal of the major site of disease, control of hypersplenism, and improvement in immune-mediated cytopenias.

In a series of 55 patients, perioperative mortality (9%) was more common in patients with poor performance status. Improvements in platelet count, neutrophil count, and hemoglobin occurred in 81%, 59%, and 33% of patients, respectively. The mortality of splenectomy (formerly 20%) has decreased in modern times, especially with laparoscopic procedures.[201] Among Rai stage IV patients, a trend toward improved survival was noted using a case-control method of analysis. Despite the benefits suggested in this study, the evidence does not support splenectomy as a routine treatment modality, particularly with the introduction of modern therapies such as purine analogs and immunotherapy. As such, splenectomy should be reserved for those patients with massive splenomegaly and cytopenias not responsive to other treatments.

Clinical Management of Patients

Psychosocial Aspects of CLL

A diagnosis of leukemia is a major emotional challenge to patients. Many doctors tell patients that they have CLL but need not be concerned, and that the recommended approach is no treatment. Careful explanation of this approach should be based on the natural history of the disorder, emphasizing that some patients never need treatment and that early treatment has not been shown to be beneficial. Patients need to be reassured that effective treatments are available when treatment becomes necessary because of progressive disease or symptoms. Knowledge that survival in many early-stage (smoldering) CLL patients is the same as in the age- and sex-matched general population is comforting to patients. Explanation of newer prognostic factors must also be made with care. Favorable markers can reassure that observation is appropriate but many patients have difficulty accepting this initial approach when the markers indicate high risk. Development of a close relationship with patients, particularly those in the early phases of disease, and careful responses to questions raised are important in providing psychological and emotional support to the patient and family. The rapidly increasing range of options for therapy, particularly for younger patients, provides a basis for optimism when treatment becomes necessary.

Infections

Progressive tumor burden can lead to bone marrow and immune system failure resulting in major episodes of infection. Immune defects can be both inherent and treatment-related. The inherent immune deficiencies of CLL—hypogammaglobulinemia, impaired T-cell function, and impaired opsonization—have led to the fallacious concept that patients with CLL are immunologic cripples.[202,203] Patients who receive intravenous gamma globulin experience a reduction in the frequency of infections, mainly moderate ones, and the infections that do occur can then be easily controlled with outpatient antibiotics.[204] Nevertheless, a low IgG laboratory value should not result in an automatic implementation of this therapy. Rather, a reasonable clinical recommendation is to treat with prophylactic gamma globulin only those patients with a history of repeated infections, particularly major ones such as pneumonia or septicemia. The usual dose is 200-400 mg/kg by intravenous infusion given at 4-week intervals. If no change is noted in the frequency of infections, the treatment should be discontinued. If a substantial decrease in the incidence of infections is seen, treatment at gradually extended intervals might be considered.

The approach to management of the most common sinobronchial infections is to use broad-spectrum conventional antibiotics such as penicillins, cephalosporins, quinolones, or sulfamethoxazole-trimethoprim. Most patients respond to such treatment, but some develop chronic sinusitis, which may require referral to an ear, nose, and throat specialist. CLL infiltrates of the sinonasal mucosa are common. Despite the immunosuppression that occurs in CLL, mycobacterial infections are uncommon. They should be considered, however, in any patient who develops persistent fever or unexplained pulmonary infiltrates. In patients receiving prophylaxis, early investigation by bronchoalveolar lavage of unexplained or unresponsive pulmonary infiltrates is recommended to identify opportunistic pathogens such as CMV, herpes simplex virus, *P. carinii*, or mycobacteria. The use of growth factors such as granulocyte colony–stimulating factor (G-CSF) or granulocyte macrophage colony–stimulating factor (GM-CSF) in patients with CLL who have neutropenia should follow established guidelines for management of infections in such patients.

Some clinicians routinely give sulfamethoxazole-trimethoprim or aerosolized pentamidine prophylaxis when patients are off-treatment. No clinical trial has substantiated the efficacy of this approach. While the incidence of opportunistic infections is low, vigilant observation and early initiation of treatment appears reasonable. Routine prophylaxis may be more cost-effective than expensive diagnostic testing, however. Structured clinical trials to address the efficacy of prophylaxis against bacterial and viral infections should be encouraged.

Most infections occur late in the disease, after therapy has been initiated, when progressive CLL with neutropenia and possible worsening of immune function occur. During this phase, herpes zoster and herpes simplex infections in particular may occur, and early institution of treatment with antivirals is effective in dealing with these problems. Herpes zoster is usually dermatomal and rarely becomes disseminated.

The spectrum of treatment-related infections has increased with the introduction of purine analogs to include many opportunistic infections such as *Nocardia*, *Pneumocystis*, aspergillosis, and CMV. Purine analogs' profound impact on T cells likely accounts for this. Immunotherapy with alemtuzumab results in yet a greater degree of immunosuppression. The addition of steroids to these agents increases risks of infections and is not recommended. As described earlier, certain treatment combinations such as FCR and single agents such as alemtuzumab warrant antimicrobial prophylaxis both during and after treatment. G-CSF has a role in CLL treatment as well. Adding G-CSF to fludarabine in advanced stage, previously treated patients reduced the incidence of neutropenia and pneumonia as compared with the incidence in a historical population.[205]

Anemia

Anemia in CLL can be caused by a number of different mechanisms. In some cases, extensive marrow infiltration is likely to be a cause. A number of patients develop anemia without proportional decrease of other counts that would typically be seen in progressive infiltration of the bone marrow. Autoimmune hemolytic anemia (AIHA) must always be considered in such cases. This often manifests as a rapid decline in hemoglobin and is usually associated with a positive Coombs test, hyperbilirubinemia, low haptoglobin, and elevation of serum lactic dehydrogenase. In other cases, there may be an inhibitory effect of the leukemia on red-cell production such as the one occurs in other malignant diseases. Shortened red-cell survival (as is common in other cancers) may also be a factor and may be accentuated in patients with major splenomegaly. Other patients (usually Coombs-negative) develop pure red-cell aplasia with disappearance of red-cell precursors from the bone marrow.

Management of anemia depends on the cause. Anemia secondary to progressive bone marrow infiltration should be treated with an established CLL chemo- or chemoimmunotherapy regimen. Treatment of AIHA should follow established patterns, with the initial use of corticosteroids to try to achieve disease remission. Historically, splenectomy was typically used as a second-line option. Though splenectomy remains an important option, a trial, first, with rituximab-based treatment is reasonable. Rituximab has demonstrated effectiveness in this setting as a single agent,[206] combined with steroids, and combined with cyclophosphamide and dexamethasone (RCD).[207] High-dose intravenous gamma globulin can also be useful in treating refractory AIHA. CLL-associated red-cell aplasia can be effectively treated with cyclosporine, though results can take up to several weeks.[208] Recombinant human erythropoietin may have a role in CLL patients with Coombs-negative anemia. A randomized comparative trial demonstrated that recombinant human erythropoietin therapy in this setting resulted in an increase in hemoglobin level in some patients.[209] As compared with only one in six patients in the placebo group, half of the erythropoietin-treated group experienced a hematocrit increase of 6%. Treatment was well-tolerated and was associated with significant improvement in energy level. The dose administered was 150 U/kg subcutaneously three times per week. Response was usually seen within the first 6-8 weeks of therapy. Single weekly doses of erythropoietin were demonstrated to be as effective as three times-per-week dosing. Darbepoetin (Aranesp) has been demonstrated to be effective in anemia of CLL.[210] However, changing guidelines for use of erythropoietin often dictate its use in clinical practice.

Transfusion of packed red cells is indicated when patients are clinically symptomatic from anemia. No particular level of hemoglobin requires transfusion, but many clinicians use a cutoff of 9 g/dL. This number is somewhat arbitrary and the decision should be made on clinical grounds. The risks of transfusion in patients with CLL are similar to the risks seen in other patients. Leukocyte-trapping filters are useful for patients who have repeated episodes of fever.

Thrombocytopenia

Patients can develop thrombocytopenia by mechanisms similar to those for anemia, with suppression of production in the presence of modest or extensive tumor burden or antibody-mediated mechanisms. In addition, dilutional effects associated with splenomegaly are not uncommon. The thrombocytopenia that occurs initially is usually modest. Severe thrombocytopenia (<50,000/μL) usually occurs only late in the disease process and signals poor prognosis.

Response to treatment of CLL is usually associated with improvement in thrombocytopenia. However, if patients fail to respond to alkylating agent or purine analog treatment with a reduction in tumor burden, thrombocytopenia is often aggravated. When the thrombocytopenia is immune-mediated, approach is similar to that of AIHA. Treatment with corticosteroids, danazol, high-dose intravenous gamma globulin, and rituximab all have been used judiciously, with variable results. Cyclosporine is often useful in cases with megakaryocytic hypoplasia.[208] Finally, splenectomy may be useful in refractory-thrombocytopenic patients with or without clinical splenic enlargement.[201] Improvement in platelet count occurs in most patients, and for patients with severe thrombocytopenia, platelet transfusion frequency is usually reduced. It has been suggested that splenectomy improves prognosis in Rai stages III and IV disease, but significant evidence for this is lacking.[201]

CLL Variants

The major variants of CLL seen in practice are PLL, which may be of the B- or T-cell type, and splenic lymphoma with circulating villous lymphocytes (SLVL) or marginal zone leukemia (MZL). In addition, patients with mantle cell lymphoma (MCL) can present in a leukemic phase; the differential diagnosis from CLL is sometimes difficult. MCL patients usually have a chromosomal translocation, t(11;14), and an increase in cyclin D1 levels, MCL patients can also present with massive splenomegaly.[211]

The response to treatment and the prognosis in PLL and MCL are much less satisfactory than in CLL, with only transient responses to alkylating agent regimens, CHOP, or purine analogs. Intensive regimens such as hyper-CVAD (fractionated cyclophosphamide, vincristine, Adriamycin, dexamethasone) followed by transplant are useful in MCL.[211] Bortezomib, a proteasome inhibitor, is a promising new agent in MCL.[212] Complete and partial responses have been noted.

The management of SLVL often involves splenectomy, with most patients responding satisfactorily.[213] Purine analogs and rituximab are both active in SLVL and MZL. Rituximab appears to have resulted in a major improvement in prognosis.

Occasionally, patients with follicular lymphoma in a leukemic phase are misdiagnosed as CLL. However, when the correct diagnosis is subsequently made, this disease should be treated as any low-grade lymphoma.

Large granular lymphocytosis characterized by monoclonal proliferation of a T-suppressor cell subset, immunophenotypically characterized as CD3+, CD8+, CD56+, and CD57+, often does not need treatment for substantial periods of time.[214] Antitumor treatment is usually not indicated; the use of G-CSF or GM-CSF for neutropenia is usually satisfactory. Alkylating agents, purine analogs, and cyclosporine all show some activity.

The management of true T-cell CLL (T-CLL) is less satisfactory than that of B-cell CLL.[215] Although purine analogs are highly effective in reducing the number of normal T cells, they are less effective in the management of T-CLL. The drug 2-CdA appears to be more effective than fludarabine.[215] Campath-1H is associated with a high response rate in T-CLL/PLL. Two separate studies have demonstrated that alemtuzumab achieves the highest complete remission rates in patients with T-cell CLL/PLL.[216,217] A number of patients have had remissions even if extensively previously treated with other regimens, including pentostatin.

Recommended Approach to Therapy

It was noted earlier in this chapter that immediate treatment is recommended for patients with advanced-stage disease or large tumor burden, and for patients with symptoms related to their disease or to repeated infections.[77] Otherwise, a period of observation is recommended. During observation, it can be determined whether the patient is developing progressive disease or a rapid doubling time. If the doubling time for the patient's lymphocyte count is <12 months, survival is significantly shorter than if the patient shows a longer doubling time. Treatment in such cases will likely be required in the near future. The exact time of initiating treatment is dependent on several factors. First, as mentioned earlier, if the patient has symptoms attributable to CLL treatment is warranted. Second, if the disease burden begins to compromise normal systemic functions, treatment should be initiated. Typically this refers to bone marrow, but it is true of other sites as well (lung, kidney, or CNS infiltration can occur in CLL). A third scenario is when there is evidence of accelerating disease with a rapid doubling time and lymph node enlargement. Often a gray area exists when no clear symptomatology is present and cytopenias are only beginning to manifest. If the patient prefers, it is reasonable to continue observation at this point, monitoring counts and revisiting the issue prior to when cytopenias drop to levels of concern. Finally, as earlier noted, leukocytosis to the level of 250,000 raises concern for the theoretical possibility of hyperviscosity. Although no evidence exists to treat at any particular leukocyte count, therapy should be considered around this level.

The choice of regimen depends on the patient and clinical presentation. Typically, a purine analog-based regimen should be considered in front-line. Fludarabine has the most data supporting its use in CLL, though pentostatin and cladribine are effective as well. Mature data show that purine analogs have a higher response rate than do alkylating agent regimens. Combining a purine analog with rituximab has been shown to optimize response without significant increase in toxicity, making this combination a good choice for first-line treatment.

The addition of cyclophosphamide to a purine analog + rituximab (FCR or PCR) has shown impressive response and CR rates in single-arm studies. In many scenarios, such as the presence of extensive bulky disease, these triple combinations may be a reasonable initial choice. However, no evidence exists showing superiority of triple combinations over double in head-to-head studies. Moreover, if the desired response is not seen in the initial cycles of FR or PR, cyclophosphamide is easily added. Before solidly proven recommendations can be made for one approach over another, additional studies must be completed.

In patients with Coombs positivity or a history of AIHA, avoiding a purine analog may be preferable. However, this issue is controversial and many report their safe use in these settings. There also exists a theoretical lack of efficacy of purine analogs in patients with p53 deletions. Though a trial with a purine analog is reasonable in these cases, other options also exist. Early but growing data of the efficacy of alemtuzumab in high-risk cytogenetic groups make a regimen containing this agent a consideration. Recent results from CAM307 trial showed its utility as a first-line alternative.[138]

Relapsed disease is typically more difficult to treat. Patients may respond again to previously used agents and combinations, but responses are usually shorter in duration. If a patient has not been exposed to an alkylating agent, its addition to a purine analog and rituximab is often effective. Alemtuzumab has an important role in refractory disease, particularly when the disease is marrow- or spleen-based.

The goals and duration of therapy for CLL are poorly defined. There is no clear evidence that maintenance therapy in CLL is of benefit, and the optimal duration of treatment with purine analogs has not yet been established. However, if patients are responding to and tolerating therapy, it appears reasonable to continue until the maximum clinical benefit is achieved, or toxicity supervenes. No predetermined number of cycles can be set. Continued treatment after complete remission is of no proven clinical benefit.

High complete remission rates with chemoimmunotherapy regimens, as well as the attainability of MRD negativity, have been promising advancements. But long-term benefit of these successes remains unproven and MRD negativity should be considered a treatment goal only in the setting of a clinical trial. Nonmyeloablative stem cell transplants have introduced the possibility of cures with less (though still significant) toxicity, and this option should be considered in younger patients who are in otherwise good health.

Selected References

The complete reference list can be found at www.CANCERMEDICINE8.com

1. Chioriazzi N, Rai KR, Ferrarini M. Mechanism of disease: chronic lymphocytic leukemia. *N Engl J Med.* 2005;352:804–815.
11. Boggs DR, Sofferman SA, Wintrobe MM, Cartwright GE. Factors influencing the duration of survival of patients with chronic lymphocytic leukemia. *Am J Med.* 1966;40:243–254.
12. Hansen MM. Chronic lymphocytic leukaemia clinical studies based on 189 cases followed for a long time. *Scand J Haematol Suppl.* 1973;18:3–286.
13. Galton DAG. The pathogenesis of chronic lymphocytic leukemia. *Can Med Assoc J.* 1966;94:1005–1010.
14. Dameshek W. Chronic lymphocytic leukemia: an accumulative disease of immunologically incompetent lymphocytes. *Blood.* 1967;29:566–584.
15. Rai KR, Sawitsky A, Cronkite EP, et al. Clinical staging of chronic lymphocytic leukemia. *Blood.* 1975;46:219–234.
16. Binet JL, Auquier A, Dighiero G, et al. A new prognostic classification of chronic lymphocytic leukemia derived from a multivariate survival analysis. *Cancer.* 1981;48:198–206.
17. Schroeder HW Jr, Dighiero G. The pathogenesis of CLL: analysis of the antibody repertoire. *Immunol Today.* 1994;15:288–294.
18. Chiorazzi N, Ferrarini M. B-cell chronic lymphocytic leukemia: lessons learned from studies of the B-cell antigen receptor. *Annu Rev Immunol.* 2003;21:841–894.
25. Rawstron AC, Green MJ, Kuzmick A, et al. Monoclonal B-lymphocytes with characteristics of "indolent" chronic lymphocytic leukemias are present in 3.5% of adults with normal blood counts. *Blood.* 2002;100:635–639.
38. Rawstron AC, Bennett FL, O'Connor SJ, et al. Monoclonal B-cell lymphocytosis and chronic lymphocytic leukemia. *N Engl J Med.* 2008;359:575–583.
40. Landgren O, Albitar M, Ma W, et al. B-cell clones as early markers for chronic lymphocytic leukemia. *N Engl J Med.* 2009;360:659–667.
51. Damle RN, Wasil T, Fais F, et al. Immunoglobulin V gene mutation status and CD38 expression as novel prognostic indicators in chronic lymphocytic leukemia. *Blood.* 1999;94:1840–1847.
61. Fais F, Ghiotto F, Hashimoto S, et al. Chronic lymphocytic leukemia B cells express restricted sets of mutated and unmutated antigen receptors. *J Clin Invest.* 1998;102:1515–1525.
68. Dohner H, Stilgenbauer S, Benner A, et al. Genomic aberrations and survival in chronic lymphocytic leukemia. *N Engl J Med.* 2000;343:1910–1916.
71. Hamblin TJ, Davis Z, Gardiner A, et al. Unmutated IgVH genes are associated with a more aggressive form of chronic lymphocytic leukemia. *Blood.* 1999;94:1848–1854.
74. Messmer B, Messmer D, Allen SI, et al. In vivo measurements document the dynamic cellular kinetics of chronic lymphocytic leukemia B cells. *J Clin Invest.* 2005;115:755–764.
75. Damle RN, Batliwalla FM, Ghiotto F, et al. Telomere length and telomerase activity delineate distinctive replicative features of the B-CLL subgroups defined by immunoglobulin V gene mutations. *Blood.* 2004;103:375–382.
77. Hallek M, Cheson BD, Catovsky D, et al. Guidelines for the diagnosis and treatment of chronic lymphocytic leukemia: a report from the International Workshop on Chronic Lymphocytic Leukemia updating the National Cancer Institute–Working Group 1996 guidelines. *Blood.* 2008;111:5446–5456.
91. Shustik C, Mick R, Silver R, et al. Treatment of early chronic lymphocytic leukemia: intermittent chlorambucil versus observation. *Hematol Oncol.* 1988;6:7–12.
92. Rai KR, Peterson BL, Appelbaum FR, et al. Fludarabine compared with chlorambucil as primary therapy for chronic lymphocytic leukemia. *N Engl J Med.* 2000;343:1750–1757.
99. Lozanski G, Heerema NA, Flinn IW, et al. Alemtuzumab is an effective therapy for chronic lymphocytic leukemia with p53 mutations and deletions. *Blood.* 2004;103:3278–3281.
102. Chan AC, Iwashima M, Turck CW, Weiss A. Zap-70 a 70 kD protein–tyrosine kinase that associates with the TCR zeta chain. *Cell.* 1992;71:649–662.
104. Rassenti LZ, Huynh L, Toy TZ, et al. ZAP-70 compared with immunoglobulin heavy-chain gene mutation status as a predictor of disease progression in CLL. *N Engl J Med.* 2004;351:893–901.
107. Calin GA, Ferracin M, Cimmino A, et al. A MicroRNA signature associated with prognosis and progression in chronic lymphocytic leukemia. *N Engl J Med.* 2005;353:1793–1801.
108. Tam CS, O'Brien S, Wierda W, et al. Long-term results of the fludarabine, cyclophosphamide, and rituximab regimen as initial therapy of chronic lymphocytic leukemia. *Blood.* 2008;112:975–980.
131. Knauf, Wolfgang Ulrich, Lissitchkov, Toshko, Aldaoud, et al. Bendamustine versus chlorambucil as first-line treatment in B cell chronic lymphocytic leukemia: an updated analysis from an international phase III study. *ASH Annual Meeting Abstracts.* 2008;112:2091.
137. Stilgenbauer, S; Cohner, H. Campath-1H induced complete remission of chronic lymphocytic leukemia despite p53 gene mutation and resistance to chemotherapy. *N Engl J Med.* 2002;347:452–453.
138. Hillmen P, Skotnicki AB, Robak T, et al: Alemtuzumab compared with chlorambucil as first-line therapy for chronic lymphocytic leukemia. *J Clin Oncol.* 2007;25:5616–5623.
140. Keating MJ, Flinn I, Jain V, et al. Therapeutic role of alemtuzumab (Campath-1H) in patients who have failed fludarabine: results of a large international study. *Blood.* 2002;99:3554–3561.
141. Lundin J, Kimby E, Bjorkholm M, et al. Phase II trial of subcutaneous anti-CD52 monoclonal antibody alemtuzumab (Campath-1H) as first-line treatment for patients with B-cell chronic lymphocytic leukemia (BCLL). *Blood.* 2002;100:768–773.

147. Flinn IW, Neuberg DS, Grever MR, et al. Phase III trial of fludarabine plus cyclophosphamide compared with fludarabine for patients with previously untreated chronic lymphocytic leukemia: US Intergroup Trial E2997. *J Clin Oncol*. 2007;25:793–798.
148. Catovsky D, Richards S, Matutes E, et al. Assessment of fludarabine plus cyclophosphamide for patients with chronic lymphocytic leukemia (the LRF CLL4 Trial): a randomized controlled trial. *Lancet*. 2007;370:230–239.
149. Eichhorst BF, Busch R, Hopfinger G, et al. Fludarabine plus cyclophosphamide versus fludarabine alone in first-line therapy of younger patients with chronic lympho-cytic leukemia. *Blood*. 2006;107:885–891.
158. Kay NE, Geyer SM, Call TG, et al. Combination chemoimmunotherapy with pentostatin, cyclophosphamide, and rituximab shows significant clinical activity with low accompanying toxicity in previously untreated B chronic lymphocytic leukemia. *Blood*. 2007;109:405–411.
159. Byrd JC, Rai K, Peterson BL, et al: The addition of rituximab to fludarabine may prolong progression-free survival and overall survival in patients with previously untreated chronic lymphocyticleukemia: an updated retrospective comparative analysis of CALGB 9712 and CALGB 9011. *Blood*. 2005;105:49–53.
173. Chanan-Khan AA, Cheson BD. Lenalidomidefor the treatment of B-cell malignancies. *J Clin Oncol*. 2008;**26**:1544–1552. doi: 10.1200/JCO.2007.14.5367.
175. Ferrajoli A, O'Brien S, Faderl SH, et al. Lenalidomide induces complete and partial remissions in patients with relapsed and refractory chronic lymphocytic leukemia. *Blood*. 2008;111:5291–5297.
176. Chen, Christine, Paul, Harminder, Xu, Wei, et al. A Phase II Study of Lenalidomide in Previously Untreated, Symptomatic Chronic Lymphocytic Leukemia (CLL). *ASH Annual Meeting Abstracts*. 2008;112:44.
177. Byrd JC, Castro JE, Flinn IW, et al. Lumiliximab in combination with FCR for the treatment of relapsed chronic lymphocytic leukemia (CLL): results from a phase I/II multicenter study. *J Clin Oncol*. 2008;26:372s.
179. Coiffier B, Lepretre S, Pedersen LM, et al. Safety and efficacy of ofatumumab, a fully human monoclonal anti-CD20 antibody, in patients with relapsed or refractory B-cell chronic lymphocytic leukemia: a phase 1-2 study. *Blood*. February 1, 2008;111(3):1094–1100.
180. Osterborg, Anders, Kipps, Thomas J., Mayer, Jiri, et al. Ofatumumab (HuMax-CD20), a Novel CD20 Monoclonal Antibody, Is An Active Treatment for Patients with CLL Refractory to Both Fludarabine and Alemtuzumab or Bulky Fludarabine-Refractory Disease: Results from the Planned Interim Analysis of An International Pivotal Trial. *ASH Annual Meeting Abstracts*. 2008;112:328.
182. Byrd JC, Lin TS, Dalton JT, et al. Flavopiridol administered using a pharmacologically derived schedule is associated with marked clinical efficacy in refractory, genetically high-risk chronic lymphocytic leukemia. *Blood*. 2007;109:399–404.
196. Dreger P, Brand R, Milligan D, et al. Reduced-intensity conditioning lowers treatment-related mortality of allogeneic stem cell transplantation for chronic lymphocytic leukemia: a population-matched analysis. *Leukemia*. 2005;19:1029–1033.
207. Gupta N, et al. Rituximab-based chemotherapy for steroid-refractory autoimmune hemolytic anemia of chronic lymphocytic leukemia. *Leukemia*. 2002;16(10):2092–2095.
222. O'Brien S, Moore JO, Boyd TE, et al. Randomized phase III trial of fludarabine plus cyclophosphamide with or without oblimersen sodium (Bcl-2 antisense) in patients with relapsed or refractory chronic lymphocytic leukemia. *J Clin Oncol*. March 20, 2007;25(9):1114–1120.

114 Hodgkin Lymphoma

Peter M. Mauch, MD ▪ Lawrence Weiss, MD ▪ James O. Armitage, MD

History

The life and accomplishments of Thomas Hodgkin have been detailed in an excellent biography of this distinguished physician and scientist.[1] Briefly, in his historic paper entitled "On Some Morbid Appearances of the Exorbant Glands and Spleen," presented to the Medical Chirurgical Society in London on January 10, 1832, Thomas Hodgkin described the clinical history and postmortem findings of the massive enlargement of lymph nodes and spleens of patients studied at Guy's Hospital in London.[2] Hodgkin recognized that these patients had suffered from a disease that started in the lymph nodes located along the major vessels in the neck, chest, or abdomen.

Hodgkin began his work at Guy's Hospital in London, in 1825, after graduating from Edinburgh Medical School in Scotland. At Guy's, he assembled and cataloged anatomic specimens relevant to specific diseases that led to his discovery in 1832. Although Hodgkin is best known for his study of malignancy and the abnormalities of the spleen and lymph nodes, he also contributed to the study of heart disease, promoted the use of the microscope, and advocated reforms in medical education and public health. Despite these achievements, Hodgkin was passed over for a teaching position and left Guy's Hospital in 1837, ending his academic career.[1] For the remainder of his life, he devoted himself to the plight of the native populations of colonial countries and their treatment by Western civilization.

It was not until 1865, a year before his death, that Hodgkin was credited with his discovery. This occurred as a result of the work of two physicians at Guy's Hospital. Dr. Richard Bright, an expert on kidney disease, had written a paper on abdominal tumors in 1838.[3] This included the history and postmortem findings of Hodgkin's cases 1 and 2, specifically citing his original discovery. Independently, in 1856, Sir Samuel Wilks, a Guy's Hospital pathologist, described 10 postmortem cases that had "a peculiar enlargement of the lymphatic glands frequently associated with disease of the spleen." Unknown to him, his report included Hodgkin's original cases 1, 2, 3, and 4, which had been preserved in the Gordon Museum at Guy's Hospital. Before completing his work, Wilks came across Bright's reference to Hodgkin's original cases, and he credited Hodgkin with the initial discovery. By 1865, Dr. Wilks had collected 15 cases that were published in a second paper entitled "Cases of the Enlargement of the Lymphatic Glands and Spleen (or Hodgkin disease) with Remarks."[4]

Wilks was one of the first physicians to use the microscope to study Hodgkin lymphoma. Although he and other physicians noted the characteristic giant cells present in the lymph nodes and spleens of patients with Hodgkin lymphoma, Dr. W.S. Greenfield, in 1878, was the first to contribute drawings of them from a low microscopic magnification of a lymph node specimen.[5] (Providing more detailed descriptions of these cells, Dr. Carl Sternberg, in 1898, and Dr. Dorothy Reed, in 1902, are credited with the first definitive microscopic descriptions of Hodgkin lymphoma.[6,7])

Both Sternberg and Reed, along with many other physicians, believed that Hodgkin lymphoma was caused by an associated infection rather than by a separate malignant process of the lymph nodes. Eight of Sternberg's 13 cases of Hodgkin lymphoma had coexistent tuberculosis, and he believed Hodgkin lymphoma to be a variant of tuberculosis. In contrast, Reed believed that Hodgkin lymphoma was an independent illness with which tuberculosis might sometimes be associated. Still, Reed considered Hodgkin lymphoma to be an inflammatory illness rather than a malignancy. Other physicians believed that Hodgkin lymphoma was a cancer of the lymph nodes. Clinical and pathologic studies, available in the early twentieth century, helped to confirm the view that Hodgkin lymphoma was a malignant neoplasm.[8]

Radiation Therapy

The early treatment of Hodgkin lymphoma with crude x-rays in 1901 soon followed the discovery of radiographs by Roentgen, radioactivity by Becquerel, and radium by the Curies at the end of the nineteenth century. Prior to this time, serum and other biologic preparations, arsenic, iodine, and surgery, were ineffective in the treatment of Hodgkin lymphoma. Thus, the first reports of x-ray radiograph treatments that would dramatically shrink enlarged lymph nodes produced great excitement and premature predictions for the curability of Hodgkin lymphoma.[9,10]

The development of modern radiation therapy techniques for the treatment of Hodgkin lymphoma began in the 1920s with the work of Gilbert, a Swiss radiotherapist. Being one of the first physicians to point out certain clinical patterns in the behavior of Hodgkin lymphoma, Gilbert attempted to adapt his radiation therapy techniques to these patterns. He began to advocate treatment of apparently uninvolved adjacent lymph node chains that might contain suspected microscopic disease, as well as of the evident sites of lymph node involvement.[11]

Peters used a similar technique to treat patients at the Ontario Institute of Radiotherapy in the late 1930s and early 1940s. In her historic paper, published in the *American Journal of Roentgenology* in 1950, Peters provided evidence that patients with limited Hodgkin lymphoma could be cured with high-dose radiation therapy that treated involved nodal disease and adjacent nodal sites.[12] She reported 5- and 10-year survival rates of 88% and 79%, respectively, for patients with stage I Hodgkin lymphoma, rates that were notably high for a disease in which virtually no one survived 10 years. Despite these results, the concept that early stage Hodgkin lymphoma might be curable with radiation therapy was slow to be accepted. Prior to the 1960s, most patients with limited Hodgkin lymphoma were not treated at all, or only with small doses of radiation.

No one deserves greater credit than Henry Kaplan for the development of successful modern treatment for Hodgkin lymphoma. His accomplishments are many. He pioneered work on the development of the linear accelerator, defined radiation field sizes and doses for a curative approach for early Hodgkin lymphoma, refined and improved diagnostic staging techniques, developed models for translating laboratory findings into clinical practice, and promoted early randomized clinical trials in the United States.[13,14]

The development of the linear accelerator that allowed for the use of higher doses and larger radiation fields, the proposal of new classification systems for histologic subtyping[15] and staging, the pioneering of methods for more precise radiographic and surgical staging (bipedal lymphangiography and staging laparotomy), and the development of an effective multiagent chemotherapy regimen,[16] all contributed to the development of curative treatment for early stage Hodgkin lymphoma. From these advances, the philosophy and practice of managing early stage Hodgkin lymphoma changed dramatically by the late 1960s. Early stage patients who 10 years earlier would not have been treated now received extensive staging and radiation therapy with wide fields and high doses, resulting in the cure of a high proportion of patients.

Chemotherapy

The management of Hodgkin lymphoma using chemotherapy represents one of the first major accomplishments in medical oncology. Although patients with localized Hodgkin lymphoma could occasionally be cured with radiotherapeutic techniques available in the mid-twentieth century, advanced Hodgkin lymphoma was uniformly fatal. Even though mechlorethamine was shown to be an active drug in the 1940s, and numerous other active agents were discovered over the next 20 years,[17] it was not until the 1960s that combination chemotherapy was used for patients with Hodgkin lymphoma.[18] By using single agents, fewer than 5% of patients survived for 5 years.[19] In the mid-1960s, investigators at the National Cancer Institute of the United States first treated patients with a four drug combination chemotherapy regimen using mechlorethamine, vincristine, methotrexate, and prednisone (MOMP).[18] When procarbazine became available, this drug was substituted for methotrexate (MOPP).[16] The initial results with this regimen demonstrated an improved complete remission rate and prolonged survival, overcoming the concerns that "using up" all active drugs at one time would shorten survival.[20] Since the curability of advanced Hodgkin lymphoma with MOPP became accepted, numerous other chemotherapy regimens have been developed. These have been aimed at improving the effectiveness of therapy and at reducing toxicity. In recent years, combination of increasing numbers of drugs, combined modality therapy, and high-dose therapy with autologous hematopoietic stem cell transplantation have all been studied in an attempt to improve cure rates.

Early in the use of chemotherapy, the model of leukemia in which maintenance therapy was used was often applied. However, randomized trials documented the lack of benefit of maintenance chemotherapy in Hodgkin lymphoma.[21] It also became clear that comparatively brief courses of chemotherapy could effect cure in Hodgkin lymphoma. Between 6 and 12 cycles of treatment have frequently been used. One randomized trial demonstrated that eight cycles of ABVD was comparable to 12 cycles of alternating ABVD and MOPP.[22] Reduced toxicity and increased efficacy have made ABVD the favored chemotherapy regimen.[23] At present, the most frequently used duration of therapy is six to eight cycles of biweekly ABVD with the goal of treating two cycles after achieving remission.

Epidemiology and Etiology

There are approximately 7600 new cases of Hodgkin lymphoma diagnosed each year in the United States. The incidence has been stable over the last two decades. Slightly more men than women develop this malignancy. In economically developed countries, there is an age-related bimodal incidence for Hodgkin lymphoma. The first peak occurs in the third decade of life, with a second rise in incidence occurring after the age of 50 years.[24]

The incidence of Hodgkin lymphoma by age differs by histologic subtype. Mixed cellularity disease is more common in patients 40-45 years of age or older; the nodular sclerosis subtype occurs more frequently in patients between 15 and 45 years of age.[25] Lymphocyte predominant histology is more frequently seen in persons younger than age 16 years and in persons 40-45 years of age or older, and has a high male to female predominance (4:1), as compared to the other subtypes. The epidemiologic significance of the age- and gender-related differences remains unknown.

Several different theories have been proposed for the epidemiology and etiology of Hodgkin lymphoma. Historically, *Mycobacterium tuberculosis* was first suspected to be the etiologic organism for Hodgkin lymphoma because of the high coexistence of tuberculosis. Later, it was appreciated that Hodgkin lymphoma was associated with deficits in the immune system, making the presence of associated infections more likely.[26] Several reports in the 1970s suggested that Hodgkin lymphoma might be contagious because of reports of clustering of the disease. The studies, by Vianna and Poln, noted clustering among high-school students exposed to Hodgkin lymphoma.[27] However, population-based studies, using cancer registries in Connecticut and California, convincingly made the argument that the reported clusters occurred by chance alone. A study that repeated the methodology of Vianna and Poln in a different location failed to confirm their findings.[28]

A number of studies have suggested that, under certain circumstances, there is a genetic predisposition for Hodgkin lymphoma. There is an increased incidence in Jews and among first-degree relatives. Siblings appear to have a two- to fivefold increased risk; in siblings of the same sex, there is as much as a ninefold increased risk.[29,30] An even higher risk has been reported in monozygotic twins of Hodgkin lymphoma cases.[29] There is an increased risk among parent-child pairs but not among spouses, again suggesting a genetic rather than an infectious etiology. In addition, Hodgkin lymphoma has been linked with certain human leukocyte antigens (HLAs).[30]

There is increasing evidence to suggest a viral etiology for Hodgkin lymphoma. In economically developed countries, there is an association between Hodgkin lymphoma in younger patients and increased maternal education, decreased numbers of siblings and playmates, early birth order, and single-family dwellings in childhood.[31,32] This association between Hodgkin lymphoma and childhood factors that decrease exposure to infectious agents at an early age has led to the proposal that Hodgkin lymphoma appears to mimic a viral illness that has an age-related host response to infection (such as seen with polio and infectious mononucleosis). Under this circumstance, a viral infection that would be mild in young children but more persistent and severe in young adults, perhaps with prolonged immunogenic stimulation, would trigger development of Hodgkin lymphoma.[31,32] Supporting this theory is the infrequent occurrence of Hodgkin lymphoma in children younger than 10 years old in economically developed countries.

Epstein-Barr virus (EBV) is a leading candidate as the causative agent for Hodgkin lymphoma.[33,34] EBV is the causative agent in African Burkitt lymphoma, and EBV-associated lymphomas are documented in patients with immunodeficiency disorders and following organ transplantation. There is a two- to threefold excess in the incidence of Hodgkin lymphoma among patients with a prior history of mononucleosis, a disease caused by EBV. In addition, there appears to be an altered antibody pattern to EBV in patients prior to clinically presenting with Hodgkin lymphoma with elevated titers against the viral capsid antigen and against the EBV nuclear antigen (EBNA).[34] This suggests that these patients may have had more severe initial EBV infections or more frequent viral replication associated with the development of Hodgkin lymphoma.

Recent cellular and molecular biology data have provided additional support for the association of EBV and classic forms of Hodgkin lymphoma. Through the use of sensitive molecular probes, 30-50% of Hodgkin lymphoma specimens have been found to contain EBV genome fragments in the diagnostic Reed-Sternberg cells.[35] EBV genome status appears to be stable over time when studied in initial biopsies and at relapse. EBV genome-positive Reed-Sternberg cells express the so-called type II latency profile, with expression of latent membrane protein (LMP)-1, LMP-2a, EBNA-1, and Epstein-Barr encoded ribonucleic acid (EBER). LMP-1 is critical in transformation and acts as an oncogene in transfection studies, whereas EBNA-1 is essential for the replication of the episomal viral genome.

Despite these compelling data, direct evidence for EBV as a causative agent for development of Hodgkin lymphoma remains to be obtained. The lack of an animal model and the difficulties in studying the malignant cells in Hodgkin lymphoma continue to frustrate investigators. Additional epidemiologic, serologic, and molecular data are needed to determine the precise role of EBV in Hodgkin lymphoma.

There is less support for other proposed causes of Hodgkin lymphoma. Although there are scattered reports of the association of Hodgkin lymphoma with environmental exposure to toxic agents, the data have not been confirmed in case-control studies. It has been suggested that Hodgkin lymphoma might be caused by an altered immune response. Although there are theories that this might occur based on biologic data, there is no clinical evidence that Hodgkin lymphoma is an illness of chronic immune suppression. In contrast to other malignancies, Hodgkin lymphoma is rarely seen as a second malignancy and does not appear to be increased in patients with illness- or treatment-related chronic immunosuppression.

Pathology

Histopathology

Hodgkin lymphoma is unique among lymphomas for its histologic diversity. Involved lymph nodes contain varying degrees of normal reactive and inflammatory cells, fibrosis, and a scattering of the characteristic malignant cells of Hodgkin lymphoma, the Reed-Sternberg cells, and their mononuclear variants. The typical Reed-Sternberg cell has abundant cytoplasm and two or three nuclei, each with a single prominent nucleolus. The large size and unusual appearance of the Reed-Sternberg cell sets it apart from the adjacent smaller background cells. The mononuclear variants have nuclear and cytoplasmic features of Reed-Sternberg cells, but have only a single nucleus. Although the diagnosis of Hodgkin lymphoma should rarely be made in the absence of Reed-Sternberg cells, the presence of these cells alone is not sufficient to make the diagnosis. Reed-Sternberg-like cells have been found in infectious mononucleosis, non-Hodgkin lymphomas, and in nonlymphoid malignancies, including carcinomas and sarcomas. Thus, criteria for the diagnosis of Hodgkin lymphoma include both the presence of the Reed-Sternberg cell and the characteristic background of normal lymphocytes, plasma cells, and eosinophils.

In the early twentieth century, physicians began to describe different cellular patterns of Hodgkin lymphoma and to suggest microscopic classifications. But it was not until 1944 that the division of Hodgkin lymphoma, as proposed by Jackson and Parker, into the three subcategories of paragranuloma, granuloma, and sarcoma gained wide acceptance.[36] This classification was not challenged for 20 years, despite its limited clinical utility, perhaps because of the lack of effective treatment. The Jackson-Parker classification identified 10% of patients with the most favorable and 10% with the least favorable prognoses as paragranuloma and sarcoma, respectively; the remaining 80% of patients had the granuloma subtype. An alternative classification, devised by Lukes and Butler, was proposed for international adoption at a conference entitled "Obstacles to the Control of Hodgkin's Disease" held in Rye, New York, in September 1965. Their proposal contained six histologic subtypes. Later, this was simplified to four subtypes. The classification appeared to correlate well with clinical stage and aggressiveness of disease[15] and, as a result, rapidly replaced the Jackson and Parker classification. Most of the Rye classification has been included as part of the newer Revised European-American Lymphoma (REAL) and World Health Organization (WHO) classifications. The REAL classification proposed modest changes in the histopathologic classification of Hodgkin lymphoma.[37,38] These changes mainly reflect the distinct entity of nodular lymphocyte predominant Hodgkin lymphoma (NLPHD) and the new classification of lymphocyte-rich classical Hodgkin lymphoma. The new system includes (1) classical Hodgkin lymphoma: nodular sclerosis, mixed cellularity, lymphocyte depletion, and lymphocyte-rich classical Hodgkin lymphoma (predominance of lymphocytes but Reed-Sternberg cell morphology and immunophenotype of classic Hodgkin lymphoma); (2) NLPHD; and (3) Hodgkin lymphoma unclassifiable.

Although the subtypes proposed in the Rye classification initially correlated with aggressiveness of disease, with modern treatment, subtyping of Hodgkin lymphoma has become less important in guiding clinical management, prognosis, and therapy. Nevertheless, the histologic subtypes of Hodgkin lymphoma are associated with different sites of presentation, distinct natural histories, and variable prognoses. These differences are most evident in the nodular lymphocyte predominance subtype.

Classical Hodgkin Lymphoma ■ Mixed cellularity Hodgkin lymphoma (MCHD) has an inflammatory background abundant in normal cells as well as frequent in malignant Reed-Sternberg cells and their mononuclear variants with 5 to 15 malignant cells per high-power field (Figs. 114-1 and 114-2). Lymphocytes, plasma cells, eosinophils, and histiocytes are frequent. Patients with mixed cellularity histology are older, are more likely to have symptoms of fever, sweats, or weight loss, and often have abdominal involvement or advanced disease. Approximately 25% of patients with Hodgkin lymphoma in the United States present with MCHD. The subtype is more commonly seen in underdeveloped countries. Because of the background cellular pattern, mixed

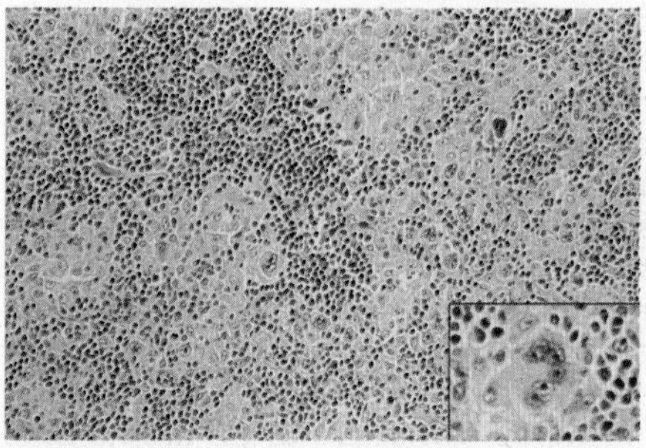

Figure 114-1 ■ Hodgkin disease, mixed cellularity type. Reed-Sternberg cells in histiocyte-rich cellular background. Inset: Multinucleated Reed-Sternberg cell at higher magnification.

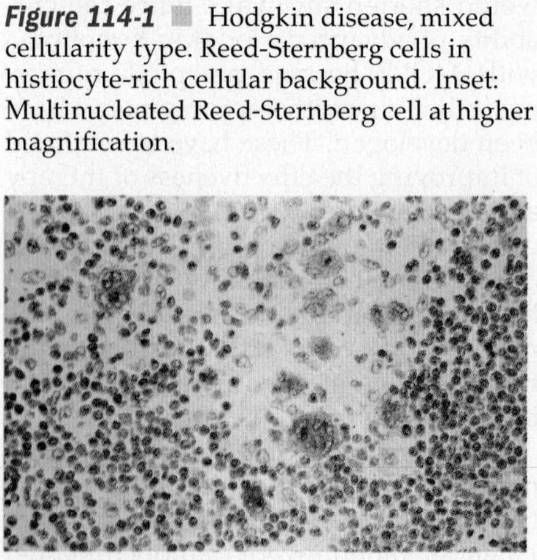

Figure 114-2 ■ Immunostain for Epstein-Barr virus-latent membrane protein in Hodgkin disease, mixed cellularity type (same biopsy as Fig. 114-1).

cellularity Hodgkin lymphoma can be confused with peripheral T-cell lymphoma. Immune markers may help to distinguish the two entities.

The diagnosis of lymphocyte-depleted Hodgkin lymphoma is rarely made today and accounts for less than 1% of Hodgkin lymphoma in economically advanced countries. Generally, patients with lymphocyte-depleted Hodgkin lymphoma present with advanced disease. With advances in immunohistochemistry, some patients with a prior diagnosis of lymphocyte-depleted Hodgkin lymphoma would now be classified as having non-Hodgkin lymphoma. In lymphocyte-depleted Hodgkin lymphoma, Reed-Sternberg cells and "pleomorphic" variant cells are more frequently seen in comparison to normal lymphocytes. Most cases have only sparse numbers of normal lymphocytes.

Nodular sclerosis Hodgkin lymphoma is morphologically and clinically distinct from the other subtypes. Two histologic features differentiate this form of Hodgkin lymphoma from all others: (1) a proliferation of collagenous bands divide the lymph node into circumscribed nodules and (2) these nodules contain a variant of the Reed-Sternberg cell called the lacunar cell. In formalin-fixed tissue, this cell's abundant pale cytoplasm often retracts and gives the appearance of a cell in space (Figs. 114-3, 114-4, and 114-5).

Nodular sclerosis is the only subtype of Hodgkin lymphoma as common in women as in men. It occurs in adolescents and young adults and is unusual in patients older than age 50 years. It has a striking propensity to involve lower cervical, supraclavicular, and mediastinal lymph nodes and has an orderly pattern of spread.[25] It makes up 60-70% of Hodgkin lymphoma in economically developed countries, but is less commonly seen in underdeveloped countries. Patients with this histology, particularly those with localized disease, have a good prognosis.

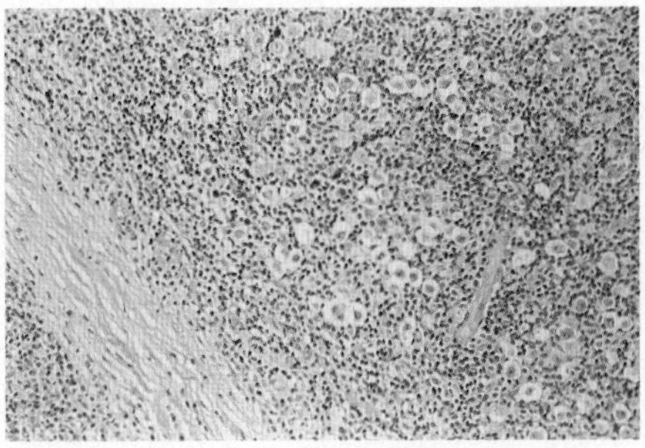

Figure 114-4 Hodgkin disease, nodular sclerosis. A fibrous band is present in the left lower part of the field. Neoplastic lacunar cells having abundant, clear cytoplasm stand out against the lymphocytic background.

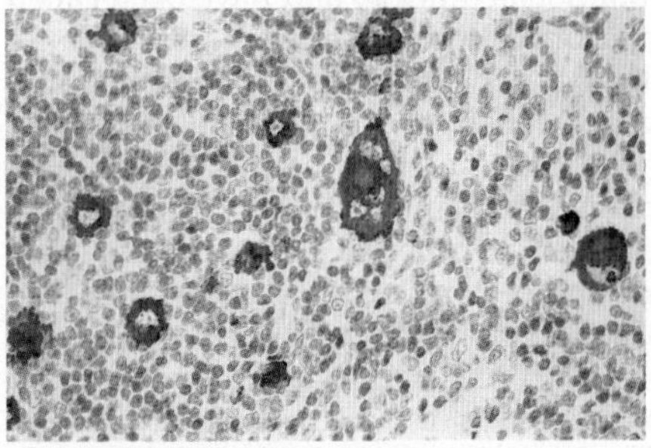

Figure 114-5 Immunostain for CD15 in Hodgkin disease, nodular sclerosis type. Neoplastic Reed-Sternberg cells and mononuclear Hodgkin cells show positive immunoreactivity.

The British National Lymphoma Investigation subclassified nodular sclerosis (NS) Hodgkin lymphoma into two subtypes—NS I and NS II—based on the number of Reed-Sternberg cells and variants, the degree of atypia, and the quality and quantity of fibrosis (Figs. 114-6 and 114-7).[39] In the British National Lymphoma Investigation study, patients with NS I histology had a better prognosis than patients with NS II histology. The adverse prognosis of NS II histology has been supported by some studies, but not by others, and rarely plays a part in current patient management.

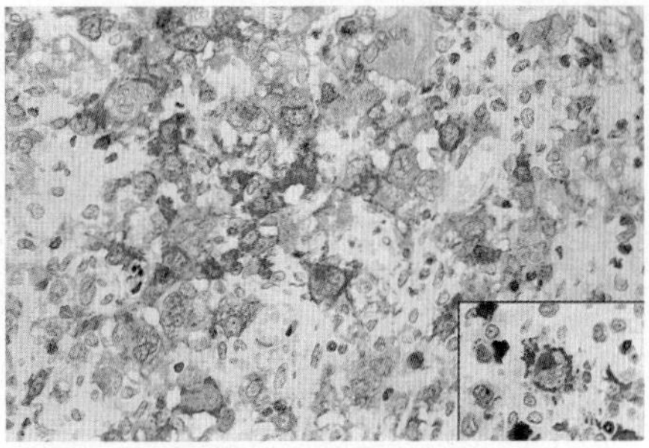

Figure 114-7 Hodgkin disease, nodular sclerosis, British National Lymphoma Investigation grade 2 (same biopsy as Fig. 114-7). Neoplastic large cells show diffusely positive immunoreactivity for CD30, positive immunoreactivity for CD15 (inset), and variable immunoreactivity for CD20 (not shown).

Lymphocyte-rich classical Hodgkin lymphoma, nodular or diffuse, was newly proposed by the REAL classification in 1994. Several recent reports have described the histopathologic and clinical characteristics of nodular lymphocyte predominant Hodgkin lymphoma and lymphocyte-rich classical Hodgkin lymphoma.[40,41] Lymphocyte-rich classic Hodgkin lymphoma may resemble either mixed cellularity, nodular sclerosis, or nodular lymphocyte predominant Hodgkin lymphoma and may be nodular or diffuse. Many cases have a vaguely nodular appearance on low magnification. Reed-Sternberg cells are relatively rare and the background is dominated by small mature lymphocytes (Figs. 114-8 and 114-9). Eosinophils and neutrophils are usually restricted to blood vessels. Some cases of lymphocyte-rich classical Hodgkin lymphoma may show a distinctly nodular appearance that may closely mimic nodular lymphocyte predominant Hodgkin lymphoma. The nodules of lymphocyte-rich classic Hodgkin lymphoma often contain small reactive germinal centers, with Hodgkin and Reed-Sternberg cells present in and near the mantle zones, a pattern that has been called follicular Hodgkin lymphoma.

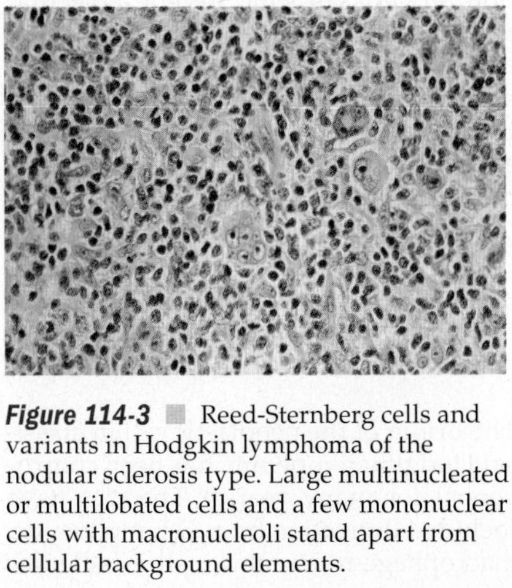

Figure 114-3 Reed-Sternberg cells and variants in Hodgkin lymphoma of the nodular sclerosis type. Large multinucleated or multilobated cells and a few mononuclear cells with macronucleoli stand apart from cellular background elements.

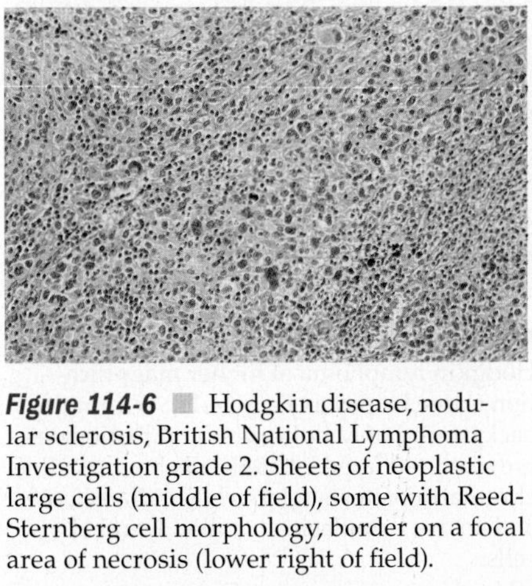

Figure 114-6 Hodgkin disease, nodular sclerosis, British National Lymphoma Investigation grade 2. Sheets of neoplastic large cells (middle of field), some with Reed-Sternberg cell morphology, border on a focal area of necrosis (lower right of field).

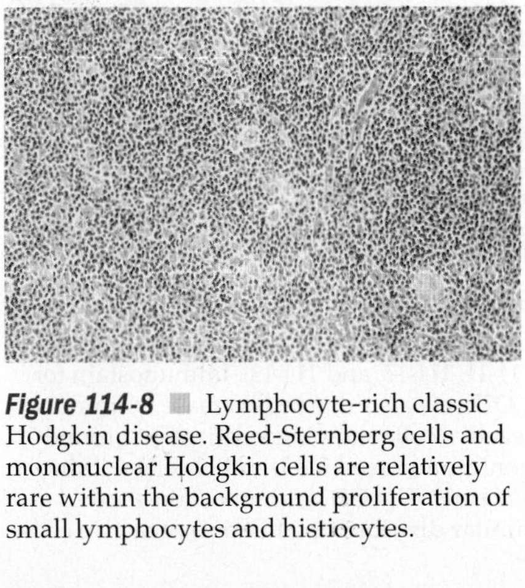

Figure 114-8 Lymphocyte-rich classic Hodgkin disease. Reed-Sternberg cells and mononuclear Hodgkin cells are relatively rare within the background proliferation of small lymphocytes and histiocytes.

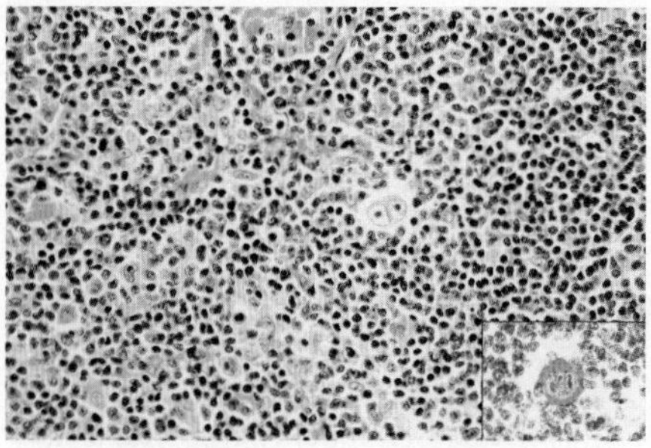

Figure 114-9 ■ Lymphocyte-rich classic Hodgkin disease. Binucleated Reed-Sternberg cell in center of field. In same biopsy, Reed-Sternberg cells immunostained positively for CD15 (inset).

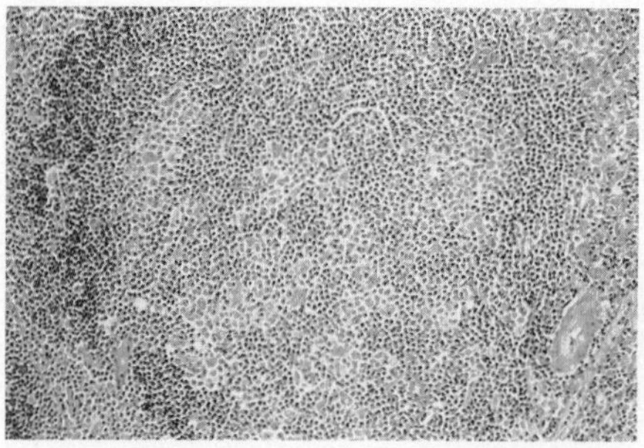

Figure 114-11 ■ Lymphocyte predominant Hodgkin disease. The vaguely nodular histologic pattern is apparent.

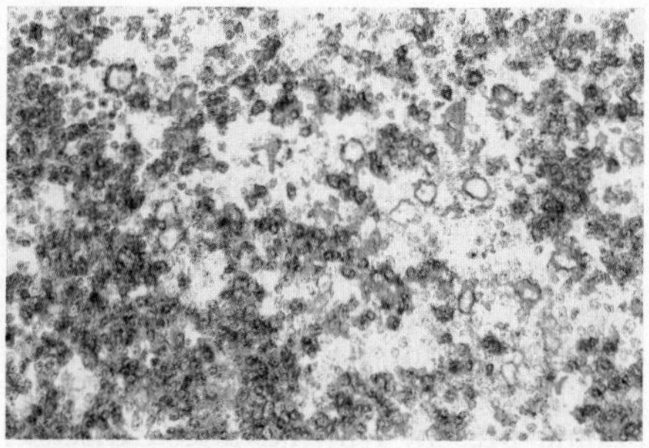

Figure 114-13 ■ Lymphocyte predominant Hodgkin lymphoma (same biopsy as Figs. 114-11 and 114-12). Immunostain for CD20 demonstrates positive staining of L and H cells as well as a high percentage of lymphocytes within a nodule.

The immunophenotype of the neoplastic cells in lymphocyte-rich classical Hodgkin lymphoma is identical to that of classic Hodgkin lymphoma, that is, CD15+ and CD30+, whereas that of nodular lymphocyte predominant Hodgkin lymphoma are CD20+ and lack CD15 and CD30. There are, however, differences in the background cells, as many cases of lymphocyte-rich classical Hodgkin lymphoma present with a B-cell-rich infiltrate, in contrast to the marked T-cell predominance usually found in other types of classic Hodgkin lymphoma. This immunohistochemical staining pattern of lymphocytes and follicular dendritic cells of lymphocyte-rich classic Hodgkin lymphoma is similar to that of nodular lymphocyte predominant Hodgkin lymphoma: the nodules are composed predominantly of B cells with nodular meshworks of follicular dendritic cells.

In nodular lymphocyte predominant Hodgkin lymphoma, the lymph node architecture is usually effaced, although a remnant of normal nodal architecture may remain. Nodular lymphocyte predominant Hodgkin lymphoma contains an abundance of benign-appearing cells. True diagnostic Reed-Sternberg cells are not seen, but variant lymphocytic and histiocytic (L and H) cells are typical (Figs. 114-10 and 114-11). These cells often have multilobated nuclei and have been called popcorn cells because of their resemblance to a popped kernel of corn. Fibrosis is not usually seen. In the nodular subtype of lymphocyte predominant Hodgkin lymphoma, the L and H or "popcorn" variants of Reed-Sternberg cells occur in background of polyclonal B lymphocytes (Fig. 114-11).[42,43] L and H cells are usually positive for B-cell CD20, but negative for CD15 and negative or weakly positive for CD30 (Figs. 114-12 and 114-13).[43,44] EBV is rarely detected in the nodular LP subtype.[45]

Progressive transformation of germinal centers is often associated with lymphocyte predominant Hodgkin lymphoma. The architecture of nodes undergoing progressive transformation of germinal centers is altered by large nodules that contain dispersed follicular center cells in clusters.

Reed-Sternberg cells and L and H variants are absent. Progressive transformation of germinal centers can also be seen in association with nodular lymphocyte predominant Hodgkin lymphoma in the same lymph node specimen or follows it in other sites.[44] It is important to distinguish nodular lymphocyte predominant Hodgkin lymphoma from progressive transformation of germinal centers, which is a benign disorder.[44]

Nodular lymphocyte predominant Hodgkin lymphoma makes up 5-10% of Hodgkin lymphoma in the United States. It often presents with a long natural history and has the longest time to recurrence of any of the subtypes of Hodgkin disease. Death from this subtype of Hodgkin lymphoma is rare. Nodular lymphocyte predominant Hodgkin lymphoma has distinct patterns of presentation when compared to the other subtypes.

It is often localized to a single peripheral nodal region (high cervical, submandibular, epitrochlear, or inguinal or femoral nodes) and infrequently involves (8%) mediastinal or abdominal nodes. Nodular lymphocyte predominant Hodgkin lymphoma is distinctive, clinically and histologically, from other subtypes of Hodgkin lymphoma; it should be reported separately in clinical studies.

Sometimes Hodgkin lymphoma morphologically resembles certain large-cell non-Hodgkin lymphomas, including anaplastic large-cell lymphoma, T-cell lymphoma, and T-cell/histiocyte rich large B-cell lymphoma. Immunohistochemical markers can aid in distinguishing between these entities; however, in some cases, such differentiation remains difficult. Recent molecular profiling studies have shown a close relationship between primary mediastinal large B-cell lymphoma and classical Hodgkin lymphoma, and there may be a true "gray-zone" neoplasm that combines features of both neoplasms.[46]

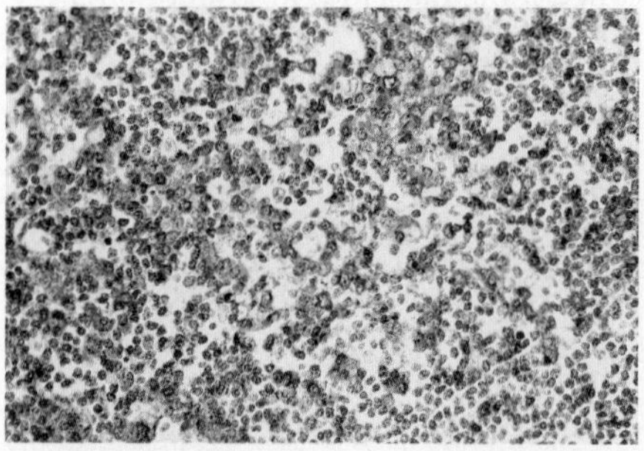

Figure 114-10 ■ Lymphocyte predominant Hodgkin lymphoma (same biopsy as Figs. 114-11, 114-12, and 114-13). Immunostain for CD57 reveals a marked increase in immunoreactive cells showing localization around nonimmunoreactive L and H cells within a nodule. The CD3 immunostain showed a similar distribution of immunoreactive cells.

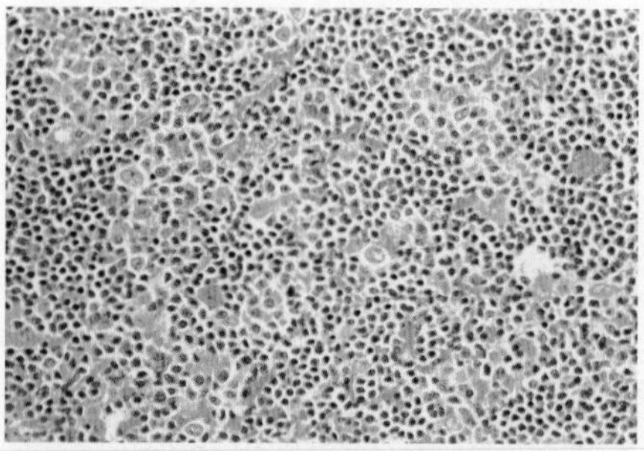

Figure 114-12 ■ Lymphocyte predominant Hodgkin lymphoma at higher magnification (same biopsy as Fig. 114-11). Within the background of lymphocytes and histiocytes are scattered large lobated cells having a fine chromatin pattern, relatively small nucleoli, and sparse cytoplasm so-called L and H cells.

Nature of the Reed-Sternberg Cell Surface Antigens

The origin of the neoplastic cell in classical Hodgkin lymphoma has been controversial for many years.[47] Theories have included derivation from B-lymphocytic, macrophage-reticulum cell, follicular center dendritic cell, or histiocytic lineages. However, more recent evidence indicates a lymphocyte origin for the Reed-Sternberg cells. Reed-Sternberg cells of classical Hodgkin lymphoma may express antigens found on resting or activated lymphocytes, most often B-cell (CD20, PAX5, CD79a) or, more rarely, T-cell surface (CD3, CD4, CD8, T-cell receptor 0 chain) antigens, although Reed-Sternberg cells express neither phenotype in many cases. The L and H cells of nodular lymphocyte predominant Hodgkin lymphoma consistently express B-cell antigens, indicating derivation from B cells. Both CD30 and CD15 antigens are on the surface of most Reed-Sternberg cells and can be detected in paraffin-embedded sections. Nearly all cases of classical Hodgkin lymphoma are CD30+ and approximately 80% of cases are CD15+, whereas CD45 (leukocyte common antigen) is usually negative. In contrast, the Reed-Sternberg cells in nodular lymphocyte predominant Hodgkin lymphoma are CD15–, CD30– or only weakly positive, and CD45+ (leukocyte common antigen).[45]

Molecular Biology

Microdissection studies performed on single Hodgkin cells obtained from cases of classical Hodgkin lymphoma have clearly demonstrated clonal immunoglobulin gene rearrangements in the vast majority of cases, confirming the clonality of the cells and moreover definitely establishing a B-cell lineage, despite the aberrant absence of immunoglobulin gene expression.[48,49] In addition, these studies have shown that the Hodgkin cells possess somatically mutated V genes, implying a germinal center or post-germinal center origin. However, the pattern of mutations suggests that many of them are nonfunctional. Normal germinal center B cells that develop such "crippling" mutations are usually eliminated within the germinal center through apoptosis; thus, there is some mechanism in Hodgkin cells that renders them resistant to the usual apoptotic mechanism. Unsuccessful germinal center cells usually undergo apoptosis via the FAS/CD95 pathway, a process that is inhibited by c-FLIP, a gene that is constitutively expressed by Hodgkin cells.[50] Several hypotheses have been generated to explain this phenomenon, including activation of the NF-κB pathway, general lineage promiscuity, and Epstein-Barr infection. Evidence favoring the NF-κB pathway includes the observation of constitutive expression of NF-κB in Hodgkin lymphoma-derived cell lines, the finding that suppression of NF-κB impairs tumor growth in severe combined immunodeficient mice and growth of cell lines,[51] and an epidemiology study showing that regular aspirin use is associated with a reduced risk of developing Hodgkin lymphoma, presumably through inhibition of NF-κB transcription.[52] LMP-2a expression may substitute for a functional B-cell receptor in EBV-associated cases (see above). Rare cases of classical Hodgkin lymphoma studied by singecell techniques show clonal rearrangements of the T-cell receptor genes.

Microdissection studies have shown that L and H cells of lymphocyte predominant Hodgkin lymphoma also undergo clonal immunoglobulin gene rearrangements, again definitively establishing clonality of the process and providing confirmation of a B-cell lineage.[48] In addition to demonstrating somatically mutated V genes, intraclonal sequence diversity can also be detected, providing strong evidence that lymphocyte predominant Hodgkin lymphoma is a germinal center lymphoma. In contrast to classical Hodgkin lymphoma, the mutations are compatible with functional antigen receptors.

Cytogenetics ■ Cytogenetic abnormalities are common in Reed-Sternberg cells; however, no consistent pattern has been described. The t(14:18) translocation, common in follicular, small cleaved cell B-cell lymphomas, is unusual in Hodgkin lymphoma (less than 2% of cases studied). Comparative genomic hybridization studies demonstrate recurrent gains on chromosomal arms 2p (the site of NF-κBREL and BCL1 1a), 9p (the site of JAK2), and 12q (the site of MDM2), and amplifications on chromosomal bands 4p16, 4q23-q24, and 9p23-p24. Recently, recurrent imbalances have been demonstrated in a majority of cases of classical Hodgkin lymphoma using genome-wide GeneScan technology.[53]

Cytokine Secretion ■ It has been hypothesized that cytokines are responsible for the marked inflammatory component, fibrosis, and the diverse histologic patterns of Hodgkin lymphoma, as well as clinical symptoms such as fever, weight loss, and night sweats.[54-56] Many cases of Hodgkin lymphoma are associated with up-regulation of tumor necrosis factor receptor (TNFR) and ligand family members, Th2 and to a lesser extent Th1 cytokines, and a variety of chemokines. Necrosis factor receptor (NFR) members may lead to constitutive activation of nuclear factor kappaB (NF-κB), an important factor in proliferation and survival of B lymphocytes. Preferential expression of Th2 cytokines and chemokines may explain the frequent presence of eosinophils and fibroblasts, as well as local suppression of the cellular immune response. EBV may contribute to the production of cytokines, for example, via LMP-1-induced activation of NF-κB and stimulation of interleukin (IL)-10, a potent inhibitor of cellular immunity. In some cases, specific cytokines may be associated with specific histologic features. For example, transforming growth factor (TGF), a known stimulus for fibroblast proliferation and collagen formation, is associated with the formation of nodular sclerosis Hodgkin lymphoma,[57] and TARC (CCL27), a lymphocyte-directed CC chemokine secreted by Hodgkin cells, may be responsible for the infiltration by CD4+ T cells.[58] Tissue eosinophilia may be due to expression of IL-5, IL-9, CCL11, and CCL28. Other cytokines, such as IL-13, may play a role in autocrine stimulation of Hodgkin cells.[59]

Immunologic Abnormalities in Patients

Hodgkin lymphoma is characterized by functional deficits in cellular immunity and in T-cell-mediated immune responses that exist prior to treatment. These deficits persist in cured patients and include impairment of delayed cutaneous hypersensitivity, depressed proliferative responses to T-cell mitogen stimulation, enhanced immunoglobulin production, and decreased natural killer cell cytotoxicity.[58-60] These abnormalities suggest an immunosuppression secondary to chronic overstimulation by cytokines. In patients with active Hodgkin lymphoma, these findings are consistent with increased cytokine secretion by Reed-Sternberg cells. However, it has been difficult to explain the persistence of these abnormalities in patients after successful treatment.

Hodgkin lymphoma is characterized by the presence of Hodgkin and Reed-Sternberg cells surrounded predominantly by CD4+ T lymphocytes. These cells express a variety of activation markers but are incapable of mounting an effective immune response against tumor cells.[60] There appear to be three potential causes of immune suppression after treatment for Hodgkin lymphoma: residual effects from radiation therapy and chemotherapy, immunocompromise from splenectomy after staging laparotomy, and persistence of abnormalities present at diagnosis biologically related to Hodgkin lymphoma.

Treatment-induced immunosuppression returns to normal at varying times after Hodgkin lymphoma but appears to have its greatest effect over the first few years after treatment.[61] One of the clinical consequences of this immunosuppression is the development of herpes zoster. There is an excess of herpes zoster infections during the first year after initiation of treatment for Hodgkin lymphoma. More than 75% of Hodgkin lymphoma-associated herpes zoster cases occur within the first year. Few cases occur after the third year (only 6% of all cases).[62] In addition, the risk of zoster appears highest in patients receiving intensive radiation therapy and alkylating agent chemotherapy (50-57%).[62] In contrast, the risk of zoster is only 14-23% for patients receiving radiation therapy or chemotherapy alone. The incidence of zoster appears less with the ABVD regimen than with the more immunosuppressive MOPP chemotherapy.

Unlike the deficits in delayed hypersensitivity, most patients with Hodgkin lymphoma at diagnosis appear to have relatively normal B-cell numbers and function.[61] However, B-cell function is adversely affected by treatment with chemotherapy or combined chemotherapy and radiation therapy, and the ensuing consequences may be greater after prior splenectomy.

To counteract the risks of bacterial sepsis, patients in the past were vaccinated prior to staging laparotomy and splenectomy. Antibody response to the 14-valent (and 23-valent) pneumococcal vaccine, combined with *Haemophilus influenzae* type B and meningococcus type C, is normal in patients with untreated Hodgkin lymphoma and similar to that of healthy controls, asplenic controls, and patients treated with radiation therapy alone.

Rarely do patients with Hodgkin lymphoma undergo splenectomy as part of treatment in current practice. However, patients who have had a splenectomy or splenic irradiation in the past as part of management for Hodgkin lymphoma should be revaccinated every 6 years.[63] Even with improvements in vaccines, neither immunization nor antibiotic prophylaxis can be guaranteed to prevent the development of sepsis from encapsulated microorganisms in patients with Hodgkin lymphoma whose staging included splenectomy or who have been heavily treated with combined modality therapy (CMT). Both physicians and patients should remain alert to this risk.

Staging

Natural History and Patterns of Spread ■ The Swiss radiotherapist Gilbert is credited with first reporting that Hodgkin lymphoma spread by contiguity from one lymph node chain to adjacent regions.[11] Peters, and later Kaplan and others, extended Gilbert's work by employing the use of prophylactic radiation therapy to lymph nodes adjacent to those involved with disease.[64,65] The development of new radiographic studies and the routine use of staging laparotomy improved understanding of the presentation, distribution, and evolution of Hodgkin lymphoma.[66,67] Although there is strong evidence that Hodgkin lymphoma begins in a single group of lymph nodes and then spreads to contiguous lymph nodes, eventually the malignant cells become more aggressive, may invade blood vessels, and spread to organs by hematogenous dissemination.

One study of more than 700 patients evaluated continuous nodal involvement from a combination of clinical and laparotomy staging.[25] Evidence for contiguous spread was most convincing for patients with classic Hodgkin lymphoma. The mediastinum, left side of the neck, and right side of the neck were each involved in more than 60% of patients. These sites were four or more times as common as other nodal sites above or below the diaphragm, suggesting that most cases of classical Hodgkin lymphoma begin in the chest or neck. Significant associations were found between the mediastinum and the right or left neck, the neck and the ipsilateral axilla, the mediastinum and the hilum, and the spleen and abdominal nodal involvement. There was a negative association between the right and left neck if the mediastinum was not involved, suggesting that spread from one neck to the other occurred through the mediastinum.

Most patients with classical Hodgkin lymphoma have a central pattern of lymph node involvement (cervical, mediastinal, paraaortic). In contrast, certain nodal chains (mesenteric, hypogastric, presacral, epitrochlear, popliteal) are seldom involved. The spleen is involved more frequently with adenopathy below the diaphragm, systemic symptoms, and in patients with mixed cellularity histology variants. Involvement of the liver in an untreated patient is rare and almost always occurs with splenic involvement. Infiltration of the bone marrow is usually focal and almost invariably associated with extensive disease and systemic symptoms. The same observation applies to bony involvement, which is a rare event early in the course of the disease. In the great majority of patients, the initial pattern of spread occurs nonrandomly and predictably via lymphatic channels to contiguous lymph node chains. This important observation, first made more than 50 years ago, formed the basis for prophylactic irradiation of adjacent lymph node-bearing regions in patients with apparently localized Hodgkin lymphoma treated with radiation therapy alone in the 1970s, 1980s, and early 1990s.

Patterns of Relapse ■ A relapse is a new manifestation of disease documented after complete tumor remission. In more than 80% of patients, initial relapses occur within the first 5 years of treatment for Hodgkin disease. The median time to relapse is stage- and treatment-dependent; recurrences occur earlier in patients with large mediastinal adenopathy than in patients without bulky disease.[68] Late relapses, for example, those occurring beyond the first 5 years, are uncommon and range from 5% to 15% of all recurrences.[69] Relapses among patients treated with radiation therapy generally occur outside the radiation field, whereas relapses among patients treated with chemotherapy occur at previous sites of involvement. True recurrence, that is, relapse within a treated field, is a rare finding when a tumoricidal dose of radiation therapy of greater than 30 Gy or greater is applied. Clinical trials are now testing whether 20 Gy is a sufficient dose to control Hodgkin lymphoma in favorable prognosis patients when administered after ABVD.

Marginal recurrence or relapse appearing at or immediately adjacent to the margin of the irradiated field is more frequent and related to treatment and extent of disease. The risk of a marginal recurrence is partially related to the radiation technique used and to the response to chemotherapy and number of cycles of chemotherapy delivered. Trials are being developed in Europe to test the concept of treating the initially involved nodes as opposed to the initially involved nodal regions.

The sites of initial recurrence after chemotherapy alone correlate with the sites of largest disease prior to therapy;[70] however, recurrences occur even with chemotherapy alone in patients with less-bulky disease. To date, there are no reliable estimates for the risk of nodal recurrence after chemotherapy alone by number of sites or size of disease in patients with less-bulky disease. As standard practice, adjuvant radiation therapy is usually recommended in patients with localized disease after treatment with chemotherapy to reduce the risk of recurrence. In patients who have a favorable prognosis, this has allowed a reduction of the number of cycles of chemotherapy needed.

Staging Classification ■ The advent of new imaging modalities and the frequent use of combined modality treatment have made staging procedures simpler and less invasive in recent years. The latest international staging classification was proposed in 1989, during a meeting held in Cotswolds, England.[71] The Cotswolds classification (Table 114-1) is a modification of the Ann Arbor classification using information from staging and treatment obtained in the 1970s and 1980s.

Some of the recommended modifications include adding criteria for clini-

Table 114-1 The Cotswolds Staging Classification for Hodgkin Disease

Stage I	Involvement of a single lymph node region or lymphoid structure (eg, spleen, thymus, Waldeyer ring) or involvement of a single extralymphatic site (IE)
Stage II	Involvement of two or more lymph node regions on the same side of the diaphragm (hilar nodes, when involved on both sides constitute stage II disease); localized contiguous involvement of only one extranodal organ or site and lymph node region(s) on the same side of the diaphragm (IIE). The number of anatomic regions involved should be indicated by a subscript (eg, II3)
Stage III	Involvement of lymph node regions on both sides of the diaphragm (III), which may also be accompanied by involvement of the spleen (IIIS) or by localized contiguous involvement of only one extranodal organ site (IIIE) or both (III SE)
III1	With or without involvement of splenic, hilar, celiac, or portal nodes
III2	With involvement of paraaortic, iliac, and mesenteric nodes
Stage IV	Diffuse or disseminated involvement of one or more extranodal organs or tissues, with or without associated lymph node involvement
Designations applicable to any disease stage	
A:	No symptoms
B:	Fever (temperature, >38°C [100.4°F]), drenching night sweats, unexplained loss of >10% of body weight within the preceding 6 months
X:	Bulky disease (a widening of the mediastinum by more than one-third of the presence of a nodal mass with a maximal dimension greater than 10 cm)
E:	Involvement of a single extranodal site that is contiguous or proximal to the known nodal site
CS:	Clinical stage
PS:	Pathologic stage (as determined by laparotomy)

Source: Adapted from Ref. 71.

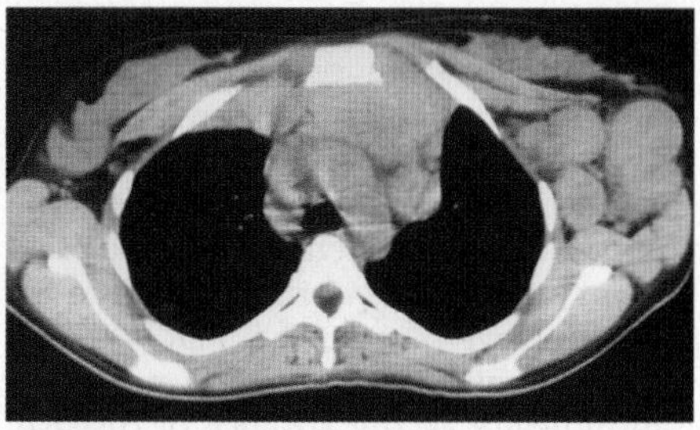

Figure 114-14 Thoracic computed tomography image from a patient with nodular sclerosis Hodgkin disease. Note the very large involvement of the left axillary nodes, involvement of the right pleura, and the anterior mediastinal disease.

cal involvement of the spleen and liver to include evidence of focal defects with two separate imaging techniques and eliminating the findings of abnormal liver function as evidence of liver involvement. The suffix "X" was added to designate bulky disease (greater than 10 cm maximum dimension). A new category of response to therapy, that is, unconfirmed/uncertain complete remission, was introduced to accommodate the difficulty evaluating persistent radiologic abnormalities of uncertain significance following primary therapy. A category of localized extranodal disease (eg, lung, pleura, chest wall, bone) contiguous to involved nodes was added and classified in the appropriate lymph node system stage followed by the subscript E. Patients with localized extranodal disease have a more favorable prognosis than patients with disseminated involvement (stage IV).

Table 114-2 lists recommended staging procedures. An adequate surgical biopsy is required for histopathologic examination. When the diagnosis of Hodgkin lymphoma is made from biopsy of an extranodal site, a concomitant node biopsy confirmation of diagnosis is desirable unless the diagnosis is considered unequivocal.

Radiographic Staging Above the Diaphragm The radiologic assessment of patients with newly diagnosed Hodgkin lymphoma is summarized below. More than 60% of patients have radiographic evidence of intrathoracic involvement. Although frontal and lateral chest radiographs represent an easy means for subsequent surveillance, computed (axial) tomography (CT) scanning should be performed on all patients as it provides a much more accurate assessment of the extent and distribution of thoracic disease. CT scanning is especially apt in detecting pulmonary disease, pleural or pericardial involvement, apical cardiac nodal enlargement, and extension into the chest wall, and in defining the extent of involved axillary lymph nodes (Fig. 114-14). Such information has considerable potential to influence clinical management. Identification of the extent of thoracic disease will help to define the extent of combination chemotherapy and the dose, extent, and need for radiation therapy.

Massive mediastinal adenopathy (large mediastinal adenopathy) has been variously defined as the ratio greater than one-third between the largest transverse diameter of the mediastinal mass and the transverse diameter of the thorax at the diaphragm on a standing posterior-anterior chest radiograph (Fig. 114-15),[72] as greater than 35% of the thoracic diameter at T5-T6, or as measuring greater than 5 or 10 cm in width. Patients with large mediastinal adenopathy have an increased risk of relapsing in nodal and extranodal sites above the diaphragm following radiation therapy alone; this risk is reduced with the use of combined radiation therapy and chemotherapy.[68] These patients make up 20-25% of clinical stage I-II patients, generally present with involvement of multiple supradiaphragmatic nodal chains, and may have extension of tumor into the lung, pericardium, or chest wall. Systemic symptoms are frequently present.

Baseline nuclear medicine imaging studies are also routinely recommended both in the initial staging and response assessment of Hodgkin lymphoma patients. Most centers currently

Table 114-2 Recommended Staging

Adequate surgical biopsy reviewed by an experienced hemopathologist
Detailed history with attention to the presence or absence of systemic symptoms
Careful physical examination, emphasizing node chains, size of liver and spleen, and Waldeyer ring inspection
Routine laboratory tests: complete blood count, erythrocyte sedimentation rate, and liver function tests
Chest radiograph (posteroanterior and lateral) with measurement of mass/thoracic ratio
Chest, abdominal, and pelvic computed tomography scans
Radioisotopic evaluation with positron emission tomography
Core-needle biopsy of bone marrow from the posterior iliac crest in patients with stages IIB to IV disease
Needle or surgical biopsy of any suspicious extranodal (eg, hepatic, osseous, pulmonary, cutaneous) lesion(s)
Cytologic examination of any effusion

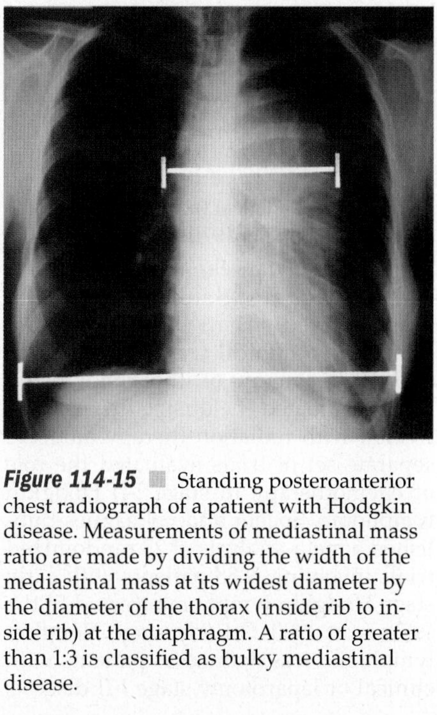

Figure 114-15 Standing posteroanterior chest radiograph of a patient with Hodgkin disease. Measurements of mediastinal mass ratio are made by dividing the width of the mediastinal mass at its widest diameter by the diameter of the thorax (inside rib to inside rib) at the diaphragm. A ratio of greater than 1:3 is classified as bulky mediastinal disease.

use fluorine-18-fluorodeoxyglucose positron emission tomographic (FDG-PET) scanning.[73,74] Negative follow-up FDG-PET scanning supports the supposition that there is no active disease after the completion of treatment even in the presence of a residual abnormality on the CT scan. However, a negative FDG-PET after treatment is a relative and not absolute indicator of the absence of disease. In the absence of adjuvant involved field radiation therapy, recurrences may occur in the initially involved site after chemotherapy alone despite negative gallium or FDG-PET scanning post-chemotherapy. At present there is no information supporting the use of FDG-PET scanning to guide whether to use adjuvant involved field radiation in patients with early stage disease.

Radiographic Staging Below the Diaphragm CT scanning and FDG-PET have limitations in the radiologic evaluation of the abdominal nodes. No single study is reliable for detecting Hodgkin lymphoma in normal-size nodes, and there is a 20-35% false-negative rate primarily as a consequence of the inability to detect occult Hodgkin lymphoma in the spleen.[71,72] Most centers currently use a combination of FDG-PET and frequent uptake of FDG-PET in sites of inflammation, both the CT scan and the FDG-PET should be clearly positive to consider that there is evidence of Hodgkin lymphoma in the abdomen.

In contrast to the value of the CT/PET scan in the initial diagnosis of Hodgkin lymphoma, there is less certainty about the value in the routine follow-up of patients because of the false-positive rates seen. An alternative is to follow patients with contrast CT scans once treatment has been completed.

Treatment of Stage I-II Hodgkin Lymphoma

Randomized Clinical Trials: Meta-analysis of Trials From the 1970s

Significant advances in the treatment of early stage Hodgkin lymphoma have been derived from information obtained from clinical trials. In the 1970s and 1980s, many of the randomized trials evaluated field size in patients treated with radiation therapy alone. A separate set of trials evaluated the role of chemotherapy in stage I-II Hodgkin lymphoma. Specht and colleagues published a meta-analysis of 23 randomized trials involving 3888 patients with early stage Hodgkin lymphoma treated in the 1970s and 1980s.[75] Early stage Hodgkin lymphoma was defined as patients with clinical or laparotomy stage I-II disease; in some cases, patients with stage III disease were included. Patients with B symptoms and patients with extensive thoracic Hodgkin lymphoma were also included. Specht and colleagues divided the randomized trials into two groups: eight trials compared more extensive radiation therapy to less extensive radiation therapy and 13 trials compared multiagent chemotherapy and radiation therapy to radiation therapy alone. Individual patient data including age, stage, date of entry, treatment allocation, date of recurrence, and date and cause of death or date last seen were collected for each patient randomized.

In the radiation alone trials evaluating field size, a significant advantage in disease-free survival was seen with larger field compared to smaller field irradiation. The combined risk of failure by treatment, in the eight trials at 10 years, was 43.4% for patients treated with less extensive radiation therapy alone, as compared to 31.3% for those treated with more extensive radiation therapy alone ($p < .00001$). No difference was seen in the 10-year actuarial survival rates suggesting that salvage chemotherapy for relapse after initial radiation therapy alone may be effective enough to minimize the impact of the increase in relapse. In addition, the small increased mortality from recurrent Hodgkin lymphoma in patients receiving smaller field irradiation appeared to be balanced by an increased mortality from treatment-related causes in patients receiving more extensive radiation therapy.

In the trials evaluating treatment with multiagent chemotherapy (usually MOPP or an equivalent regimen) and radiation therapy compared to radiation therapy alone, there was a significant advantage in disease-free survival with combined chemotherapy and radiation therapy.

Long-Term Outcome After Treatment for Early Stage Hodgkin Lymphoma

Much of the long-term follow-up data for early stage Hodgkin lymphoma are derived from laparotomy staged patients treated with radiation therapy alone in the 1970s and 1980s. Large, single institutional studies demonstrate approximately an 80% actuarial 10- to 20-year freedom from relapse and less than a 10% mortality from Hodgkin lymphoma following mantle and paraaortic irradiation for PS IA-IIA patients. This approach was used in part to avoid the use of MOPP chemotherapy whenever possible, a regimen that was associated with loss of fertility, significant marrow toxicity and immunosuppression, and a risk of treatment-related leukemia.

The treatment of early stage Hodgkin lymphoma in these studies was so successful that at 15-20 years posttreatment, the overall mortality rate from treatment-related causes exceeded than that seen from Hodgkin lymphoma.[76-78] Thus, it is in the second and third decades after Hodgkin lymphoma that improved survival of early stage patients might be seen with modern era reduced treatment regimens.

There are a number of published reports that detail causes of mortality after Hodgkin lymphoma.[76,78-80] Deaths from Hodgkin lymphoma occur most frequently in the first 5-10 years; causes of death other than Hodgkin lymphoma are most common after 5-10 years. In one recent study, the absolute excess risk of mortality by 5-year interval ranged from 87 to 158 per 10,000 person-years.[76] Thus, on average, these patients had approximately a 1% excess risk of mortality per year over the first 25-30 years after Hodgkin lymphoma (Table 114-3).[76] Much of this data is from laparotomy staged patients treated with wide field radiation therapy with or without MOPP or MOPP-like regimens. Current clinical trials are based on the data that suggest that reduction of field size and dose of radiation and the use of modified nonalkylating agent regimens results in a reduction of this late mortality incidence.

The three most common causes of death after treatment for Hodgkin lymphoma (Hodgkin lymphoma, secondary malignancy, cardiac disease) are discussed below. Patients who develop recurrent Hodgkin lymphoma after radiation therapy alone are as likely to be cured with combination chemotherapy as if the chemotherapy were used as part of initial treatment. The 10-year actuarial survival rate of patients initially treated with radiation therapy alone after relapse and treatment with multiagent chemotherapy is 57-89%.[81-82]

Survival rates are significantly worse for patients who relapse after chemotherapy alone or combined radiation therapy and chemotherapy; most of the data are from patients who initially had advanced Hodgkin lymphoma. Treatment with similar or alternative chemotherapy regimens after relapse from chemotherapy alone yields 5- to 10-year survival rates of only 20-32%,[83-84] suggesting cross-

Table 114-3 **Excess Mortality After Hodgkin Disease**

Time after Hodgkin Lymphoma (Years)	Absolute Excess Risk per 10,000 Person-Years
0-5	117
5-10	89
10-15	87
15-20	100
≥20	158

Source: Adapted from Ref. 76.

resistance among different chemotherapy regimens. Because of the poor overall prognosis of patients who relapse after standard chemotherapy, many centers recommend high-dose chemotherapy and autologous bone marrow rescue at first relapse for patients initially treated with chemotherapy or combined chemotherapy and radiation therapy. Although the results of high-dose therapy are promising, many patients with recurrent disease are not eligible for this approach because of poor tumor response, or occasionally co-morbid disease, or advanced age. Patients who undergo transplant, and who are subsequently cured of Hodgkin lymphoma, face significant long-term treatment-related morbidity and mortality risks. Current information suggests that when chemotherapy is used as definitive treatment for early stage Hodgkin lymphoma, treatment should be designed to minimize relapse. This is probably best achieved with the combined use of both chemotherapy and radiation therapy.

Many years after chemotherapy and/or radiation therapy, patients with Hodgkin lymphoma have an increased risk of developing acute nonlymphoblastic leukemia, non-Hodgkin lymphoma, and second solid tumors.[85-88] This increased risk may be multifactorial, resulting both from the immune dysregulation associated with Hodgkin lymphoma and from its treatment and the carcinogenic effects of radiation therapy and chemotherapy. Certain cytotoxic agents, especially those contained in the MOPP and ChlVPP (chlorambucil, vinblastine, procarbazine, and prednisone) regimens, are associated with a marked increase in acute nonlymphoblastic leukemia after Hodgkin lymphoma.[89-90] The total incidence of acute leukemia, usually occurring within 10 years of treatment, ranges from 2% to 6%.[89,91] The routine use of ABVD has dramatically reduced the risk of leukemogenesis, but there remains concern for secondary leukemia with alternating or hybrid regimens. Regimens that contain significant amounts of alkylating agents known to cause leukemia should not be used in treating favorable prognosis CS I-II patients.

Nearly all cases of non-Hodgkin lymphoma occurring after Hodgkin lymphoma are of intermediate or high-grade histology. The histologies represented are similar to lymphomas seen in patients with immunodeficiency diseases or under chronic immunosuppression for organ transplantation or autoimmune disorders. These lymphomas have a cumulative risk of 1.2-2.1% at 15 years.[91-92] The risk is probably not treatment-related.

The absolute excess risk of developing a solid tumor is greater than that of developing leukemia or non-Hodgkin lymphoma after Hodgkin lymphoma. Solid tumors constitute 55-75% of the second malignancies in long-term studies.[85-87,90,92] The relative risk of solid tumors continues to be elevated more than 20-30 years after Hodgkin lymphoma.[85] Risk factors for developing a solid tumor after treatment for Hodgkin lymphoma include initial treatment with radiation therapy (solid tumors), treatment with chemotherapy (lung cancer), age at treatment (female patients younger than 35 years of age at treatment and increased breast cancer risk), and environmental factors (ie, smoking and lung cancer).[93] Volume and dose of radiation therapy and type of chemotherapy may all be independent risk factors for the development of second tumors. Additional data are needed to determine the extent to which current treatment reduction strategies will result in a lower second tumor mortality. However, reduction in the radiation field size will almost certainly result in a lower second tumor risk, as many of the radiation-induced tumors occur within or on the edge of the treatment field. Techniques to combine chemotherapy and radiation limited to involved fields should reduce this risk. In addition, prevention and surveillance strategies are becoming increasingly important in the routine follow-up of long-term survivors of Hodgkin lymphoma and a number of efforts are ongoing to help define these strategies.[94]

Complications related to cardiac irradiation (arrhythmias, myocardial infarction and coronary artery disease, pericarditis, myocarditis, pericardial effusion, and tamponade) have been carefully documented after radiation therapy to the mediastinum. In many of the earlier studies, these complications are related to treatment techniques that resulted in a high radiation doses to the anterior mediastinum and heart. Current practice that permits lower radiation dose and volume by the use of preradiation chemotherapy has yielded fewer late cardiac complications. However, even with advances in treatment, patients will continue to be at some increased risk for cardiac disease years after Hodgkin lymphoma. Four recent studies detail cardiac risks in long-term survivors of Hodgkin lymphoma and provide recommendations for surveillance.[95-98] Data are now emerging that indicate that patients who received mediastinal irradiation, and have other classic cardiac risk factors, are at significantly increased risk for cardiac disease compared to patients without risk factors.[99] This may allow development of surveillance and prevention strategies for these patients.

Other complications that have factored into the development of clinical trials include pulmonary toxicity and loss of fertility. Radiation pneumonitis typically occurs 1-6 months after completion of thoracic irradiation. Symptomatic radiation pneumonitis is characterized by a mild, nonproductive cough, low-grade fever, and dyspnea on exertion and occurs in less than 5% of patients. Infection and recurrent Hodgkin lymphoma must also be considered in the diagnosis. Radiographically, pneumonitis is characterized by the formation of infiltrates confined to the original radiation fields. Infection, rather than pneumonitis, is more likely if the infiltrates extend into areas of the lung initially protected from radiation by lung shielding. Severe pneumonitis may require treatment with steroids. If the symptoms do not respond to steroid treatment, the presence of a superimposed infection, such as *Pneumocystis carinii*, should be considered. Patients who develop pneumonitis usually do not have long-term pulmonary dysfunction after the acute effects subside.

After bleomycin-containing regimens, a reticulomicronodular pattern located generally at the lower lung zones occurs in 10-15% of patients when the cumulative dose of bleomycin exceeds 200 mg/m^2. For lower cumulative doses, such as those used in the delivery of four to six cycles of ABVD, early pulmonary toxicity occurs 5% or less of the time, and radiologic findings are reversible with the help of corticosteroids. If left undetected, particularly when bleomycin-containing chemotherapy is administered after prior pulmonary irradiation, the initial findings often evolve into a coarse striking reticulation. In turn, this can evolve into restrictive lung fibrosis.

Gonadal dysfunction is an important iatrogenic toxicity that considerably affects the quality of life in patients after Hodgkin lymphoma. MOPP or MOPP-like combinations induce azoospermia in 90-100% of men. Only 10-20% of patients eventually show recovery of spermatogenesis, even after long periods. Following MOPP alternated with ABVD, where the cumulative doses of MOPP are 50% of those in full-course MOPP, the incidence of permanent azoospermia is still nearly 50%. Approximately 50% of women become amenorrheic after six courses of MOPP, and premature ovarian failure appears to depend on age (older than age 30 years, 75-85%; younger than age 30 years, approximately 20%). In contrast, it has been reported that the administration of ABVD chemotherapy produces only transient germ cell toxicity in men and no drug-induced amenorrhea.[100] Thus, to circumvent chemotherapy-induced sterility, the use of non-alkylating agent regimens is recommended. An alternative for men undergoing MOPP or MOPP-ABVD involves sperm storage prior to chemotherapy. However, approximately one-third of male patients with Hodgkin lymphoma have low sperm count or sperm motility before starting cytotoxic treatment; this may affect the success of the procedure.

Prognostic Factors for Stage I-II Hodgkin Lymphoma

Prognostic factors such as age, size of nodal involvement, and presence of systemic symptoms help to determine initial treatment strategies. Patients with stage I-II Hodgkin lymphoma with favorable prognostic factors are candidates for modified chemotherapy and involved field irradiation, or in some cases for chemotherapy alone or radiation therapy alone. Patients with unfavorable prognostic factors should receive chemotherapy and radiation therapy as initial treatment. Although many of the adverse prognostic factors have lost significance as more intensive combined radiation therapy and chemotherapy regimens have been used, these factors continue to be very important in the design of clinical trials that evaluate reduction of radiation therapy and chemotherapy for early stage Hodgkin lymphoma.

Prognostic Factors for Freedom From Treatment Failure and Survival in Stage I-II Patients

Prognostic factors have been identified for stage I-II Hodgkin lymphoma that predict for a higher risk of relapse or a lower rate of survival. Many factors predict for recurrence after treatment with radiation therapy alone; fewer predict for relapse after chemotherapy and radiation therapy. Only older age at diagnosis has been consistently reported as a significant adverse factor for survival, both after radiation therapy alone and after combined radiation therapy and chemotherapy.[101-103]

All studies report large mediastinal adenopathy or large tumor burden as a major factor predicting an increased risk of relapse. Most reports also have identified B symptoms as an important factor for recurrence and survival. A large retrospective study combining data from PS IB-IIB patients treated at Stanford University Medical School and Harvard Medical School suggested that patients with night sweats without other B symptoms treated with radiation therapy alone had a prognosis similar to that of patients with PS IA-IIA disease. However, the presence of fevers, weight loss, large mediastinal adenopathy, and age 40 years or older all independently predicted for an increased risk of relapse, and survival was impaired in patients who had both fevers and weight loss.[104]

Two other factors, large number of regions involved and elevated erythrocyte sedimentation rate (ESR), have been identified as adverse factors for freedom from treatment failure in clinically staged patients.[102,103] In current clinical trials, B symptoms are often combined with an elevated ESR in defining an unfavorable prognosis.

Older patients appear to have a lower survival rate, but if treated as younger patients, do not have a higher recurrence rate. Older patients appear to be less successfully treated at relapse[81,105] and they have a greater absolute excess risk of mortality from causes other than Hodgkin lymphoma, such as second tumors and cardiac disease. Thus, their reduced survival is both disease- and treatment-related. Age older than 50 years is used as the criterion for unfavorable prognosis in current EORTC trials.

Prognostic Factors Determine Treatment in Clinical Trials

Cooperative groups identify favorable and unfavorable prognostic groups for different clinical trials in stage I-II patients. Prognostic factors for the current European Organization for the Research and Treatment of Cancer (EORTC) and the German Hodgkin Study Group (GHSG) are listed below. Favorable prognostic factors are listed in Table 114-4 and unfavorable prognostic factors are listed in Table 114-5. For the EORTC and GHSG, favorable prognosis means the absence of each of the factors listed in Table 114-4.

Approximately 55% of patients with CS I-II Hodgkin lymphoma will fall into the favorable prognosis group. For the EORTC and GHSG, unfavorable prognosis means the presence of any of the factors listed in Table 114-5. Approximately 35% of patients with CS I-II Hodgkin lymphoma will have either B symptoms or large mediastinal adenopathy, and approximately 10% will have four or more sites involved without B symptoms or large mediastinal disease. The International Prognostic Factor Project analyzed additional prognostic factors in patients with advanced stage Hodgkin lymphoma to determine poor prognostic groups of patients who might need more aggressive initial treatment (Table 114-6).[106] This international prognostic index is especially valuable for patients with advanced Hodgkin lymphoma.

Reduction of Staging or Treatment: Ongoing and Recently Completed Trials for Favorable Prognosis CS I-II Hodgkin Lymphoma

Increasing concern for the long-term consequences of treatment has prompted many investigators to reexamine the aggressive approaches developed for the staging and treatment of early stage Hodgkin lymphoma in the 1970s and 1980s. Many of the ongoing and recently completed studies were developed in an attempt to reduce the long-term complications of treatment without increasing mortality from Hodgkin lymphoma. These include studies that (1) evaluate

Table 114-4 **Favorable Prognosis Stage I-II Hodgkin Disease**[a]

EORTC	GHSG
No large mediastinal adenopathy, ESR <50 without B symptoms, ESR <30 with B symptoms, age ≤50, 1–3 lymph node sites involved	No large mediastinal adenopathy, ESR <50 without B symptoms, ESR <30 with B symptoms, no E disease, and 1–2 lymph node sites involved

[a]See Ref. 107

Abbreviations: EORTC, European Organization for the Research and Treatment of Cancer; GHSG, German Hodgkin's Study Group.

Table 114-5 **Unfavorable Prognosis Stage I-II Hodgkin Disease**

EORTC	GHSG
Any one of the following:	
Large mediastinal adenopathy, ESR ≥50 without B symptoms, ESR ≥30 with B symptoms, age >50, or ≥4 lymph node sites involved	Large mediastinal adenopathy, ESR ≥50 without B symptoms, ESR ≥30 with B symptoms, E disease, or ≥3 lymph node sites involved

Abbreviations: EORTC, European Organization for the Research and Treatment of Cancer; GHSG, German Hodgkin's Study Group.

Table 114-6 **Final Cox Regression Model, International Prognostic Factor Project**

Factor	Log Hazard Ratio	Relative Risk
Serum albumin <4 g/dL	0.40 ± 0.10	1.49
Hemoglobin <10.5 g/dL	0.30 ± 0.11	1.35
Male sex	0.30 ± 0.09	1.35
Stage IV disease	0.23 ± 0.09	1.26
Age ≥45 years	0.33 ± 0.10	1.39
White cell count (WCC) ≥15,000/mm^3	0.34 ± 0.11	1.41
Lymphocyte count <600/mm^3 or <8% of WCC	0.31 ± 0.10	1.38

combined radiation therapy and chemotherapy and attempt to identify the optimal chemotherapy regimen, identify the optimum number of cycles of chemotherapy, or determine the optimal radiation volume and dose when combined with chemotherapy; (2) evaluate combination chemotherapy alone; and (3) define circumstances for radiation therapy alone and define radiation dose and field size in this setting. Most of the studies discussed in the following sections have relatively short follow-up or are ongoing and would not be expected to demonstrate survival differences. High relapse rates and significant acute toxicity are the main criteria for adverse outcome.

Combination Radiation Therapy and Chemotherapy: Randomized Clinical Trials Using Modified Chemotherapy and Radiation Therapy

Randomized trials of combined modality therapy are based on the premise that this approach results in a very high freedom from recurrence in early stage Hodgkin lymphoma, and that the efficacy of combined chemotherapy and radiation can be maintained even when using modified and less toxic regimens. Listed in Tables 114-7 and 114-8 are selected trials using modified chemotherapy regimens and radiation therapy. In the Southwest Oncology Cancer Group (SWOG)/Cancer and Leukemia Group B (CALGB) trial and the German Hodgkin Study Group (GHSG) HD7 trial, subtotal nodal and splenic irradiation was used in the combined chemotherapy and radiation therapy arm because extended field irradiation was standard at the time the trials were developed. More recent trials have restricted the radiation fields to the involved regions. Analysis of patterns and frequency of failure will eventually provide better guidelines for such modified regimens to control occult Hodgkin lymphoma not appreciated on physical examination or radiographic evaluation either in adjacent nodes or below the diaphragm.

SWOG/CALGB Study of Three Cycles of Adjuvant Doxorubicin and Vinblastine Plus Subtotal Nodal and Splenic Irradiation Versus Subtotal Nodal and Splenic Irradiation Alone in CS IA-IA Hodgkin Lymphoma Patients ■ The trial met stopping rules at the second interim analysis after 348 of the initially planned 420 patients had been enrolled, with the radiation alone group having significantly more recurrences than the combined chemotherapy and radiation group (Table 114-7). No overall survival differences were seen. There was significantly higher-grade 3-4 hematologic toxicity in the patients receiving both radiation therapy and chemotherapy.[107] Subsequent trials have been designed to use more limited involved field irradiation when combined with chemotherapy.

The German Hodgkin Study Group HD7 Trial (1994-1998) ■ The GHSG HD7 study randomized patients to subtotal nodal and splenic irradiation alone or to two courses of ABVD and the radiation therapy regimen. In the 627 patients, there is a significantly improved 7-year freedom from treatment failure in the radiation therapy and chemotherapy arm (88%) versus radiation therapy alone (67%, $p < .0001$). No survival differences are seen.[108]

European Organization for the Research and Treatment of Cancer (EORTC) H7F Trial (1988-1993) ■ This trial compared EBVP (epirubicin, bleomycin, vinblastine, and prednisone) and involved field irradiation (n = 168) to mantle and paraaortic-splenic irradiation (n = 165) for favorable prognosis CS IA-IIA patients. The EORTC-EBVP regimen (one dose per cycle) was proposed as a potentially less toxic but similarly effective regimen when compared to ABVD. In the H7F trial with 333 patients enrolled, six cycles of EBVP were combined with involved field radiation and randomly compared with subtotal nodal and splenic irradiation. The 10-year event-free survival rate was significantly higher for patients on the combined chemotherapy and radiation therapy arm than for those on the radiation therapy alone arm (88% vs 78%, respectively, p = .0113). The 10-year survival rate was excellent in both treatment arms (92% vs 92%, respectively, p = .156).[109] In contrast, in the H7U trial for the 389 patients with unfavorable disease, EBVP and involved field radiation therapy was inferior to MOPP/ABV (Adriamycin [doxorubicin], bleomycin, and vinblastine) and involved field radiation therapy both in 10-year event-free survival (68% vs 88%, $p < .001$) and in overall survival (79% vs 87%, p = .0175) demonstrating that defining prognostic factors is crucial in selecting patients for modified chemotherapy and radiation therapy regimens.

BNLI Trial (1996-2001) ■ This trial compared VAPEC-B chemotherapy (vincristine, doxorubicin [Adriamycin], prednisolone, etoposide [VP-16], cyclophosphamide, and bleomycin) for 4 weeks and involved field irradiation to mantle irradiation alone. With a median follow-up time of 51 months, the 5-year relapse-free survival was 87% for the chemotherapy and involved field irradiation versus 70% for mantle irradiation alone (p = .002). The 5-year survival rates were 98% and 92%, respectively (p = .036).[110]

Modified Stanford V for Early Stage Favorable Prognosis Hodgkin Lymphoma

The relatively short but intensive Stanford V chemotherapy regimen, given for 12 weeks to patients with poor prognosis stage I-II disease,[111] was modified for favorable prognosis CS IA-IIA patients to 8 weeks of the Stanford V regimen and modified involved field irradiation. The

Table 114-7 ■ Randomized Clinical Trials in Favorable Prognosis Stage I-II Hodgkin Disease: Trials to Identify the Optimum Chemotherapy Combination

Trial	Eligibility	Treatment Regimens	No. of Patients	Outcome
EORTC H7F[109]	CS IA-IIB without: age >50, ESR ≥50 mm/h in A; ≥30 mm/h in B, 4 or more sites of disease, large mediastinal disease (? 0.35 m/t ratio), CS IA, NS/LP, <40, ESR <50 mm/h	A. EBVP X 6 + IFRT (36 Gy) B. STLI (S)	168 165	Relapse-free survival (10 years): A = 88%; B = 78%; p = .014 Survival (10 years): A = 92%; B = 92%; p = .156
SWOG 9133/ CALGB 9391[107]	CS IA-IIA without: age <16, large mediastinal disease	A. Doxorubicin and vinblastine for three cycles and STLI (S) (36-40 Gy) B. STLI (S) (36-40 Gy)	348	Failure-free survival (3 years) A = 94%; B = 81%, $p < .001$ Overall survival (3 years) No difference
Stanford V for favorable prognosis[111]	CS I-II without B symptoms for favorable age <16 and >60, large mediastinal disease, two extranodal sites initial involvement	Stanford V for 8 weeks and modified FRT	86 (open)	Freedom from progression (5.7 years) 96% Overall survival (5.7 years) 98%

Abbreviations: CS, clinical stage; EBVP, epirubicin, bleomycin, vinblastine, and prednisone; EORTC, European Organization for the Research and Treatment of Cancer; ESR, erythrocyte sedimentation rate; IF, involved field; LP, lymphocyte predominance histology; NS, nodular sclerosis histology; RT, radiation therapy; Stanford V regimen, echlorethamine, doxorubicin, vinblastine, prednisone, vincristine, bleomycin, VP- 16; STLI (S), subtotal nodal irradiation (splenic irradiation).

Table 114-8 **Randomized Clinical Trials in Favorable Prognosis Stage I-II Hodgkin Disease: Trials to Identify the Optimal Number of Chemotherapy Cycles**

Trial	Eligibility	Treatment Regimens	No. of Patients	Outcome
GHSG HD7[108]	CS IA-IIB without large mediastinal mass, massive splenic disease, localized extra-nodal disease, ESR ≥50 mm/h in A, ≥30 mm/h in B, ≥3 involved areas	A. RT alone (STLI-spleen) (30 GY) + IFRT (40 Gy) B. ABVD × 2 + RT (RT regimen as in A)	571	FFTF (7 years) A = 67%; B = 88%; $p < .001$ Survival (7 years) A = 92%; B = 94%; p = NS
GHSG HD10[112]	CS IA-IIB without large mediastinal mass, massive splenic disease, localized extra-nodal disease, ESR ≥50 mm/h in A, ≥30 mm/h in B, ≥3 involved areas	A. ABVD × 2 + IFRT (30 Gy) B. ABVD × 2 + IFRT (20 Gy) C. ABVD × 4 + IFRT (30 Gy) D. ABVD × 4 + IFRT (20 Gy)	1131	FFTF (28 mo) = 97% OS (28 mo) = 99%
EORTC/GELA[113] H8F	CS IA-IIB without age: 50, ESR 50 mm/h in A, 30 mm/h in B, four or more sites of disease large mediastinal disease	A. MOPP/ABV × 3 + IFRT (36 Gy) B. STLI (S)	543	FFS (8 years) A = 98%; B = 74%; $p < .001$ Survival (8 years) A = 97%; B = 92%; $p < .001$

Abbreviations: ABVD, Adriamycin (doxorubicin), bleomycin, vinblastine, and dacarbazine; CS, clinical stage; EORTC, European Organization for the Research and Treatment of Cancer; ESR, erythrocyte sedimentation rate; FFS, failure-free survival; FFTF, freedom from treatment failure; GELA, French Adult Lymphoma Group; GHSG, German Hodgkin Study Group; IF, involved field; MOPP, mechlorethamine, vincristine, procarbazine, prednisone; NS, no significant difference; RT, radiation therapy; STLI (S), subtotal nodal irradiation (splenic irradiation).

chemotherapy regimen includes mechlorethamine (6 mg/m^2 on weeks 1 and 5), doxorubicin (25 mg/m^2 on weeks 1, 3, 5, and 7), vinblastine (6 mg/m^2 on weeks 1, 3, 5, and 7), prednisone (40 mg/m^2 on days 1-36, then taper off), vincristine (1.4 mg/m^2 on weeks 2, 4, 6, and 8), bleomycin (5 U/m^2 on weeks 2, 4, 6, and 8), and VP-16 (60 mg/m^2 on days 15 and 16 and days 43 and 44). With a median follow-up of 5.7 years, the freedom from progression (FFP) is 96% and overall survival (OS) is 98%.

The German Hodgkin Study Group HD10 Trial (1998-2002) ■ This study randomized 1370 patients to four treatment arms: two cycles of ABVD followed by 30 Gy involved field radiation therapy; two cycles of ABVD followed by 20 Gy involved field radiation therapy; four cycles of ABVD followed by 30 Gy involved field radiation therapy; and four cycles of ABVD followed by 20 Gy involved field radiation therapy. At a median follow-up of 28 months, the 2-year freedom from treatment failure was 96.6% and the 2-year overall survival was 98.5%, with no significant differences between the number of cycles of chemotherapy or in the involved field radiation dose.[112] However in a third interim analysis with 41-month median follow-up, although there were no differences in the FFTF curves at 4 years, there appears to be a near significant increase in the recurrence rates in the 20 Gy arms (versus the 30 Gy arms) with separation of the curves after 4 years (p = .076) (data presented in the plenary session of the American Society of Therapeutic Radiation Oncology meeting held in Denver, Colorado, October 2005). Comparison data between the four individual arms are not available and we are awaiting published peer-reviewed data from the trial to see if these differences persist.

EORTC/Groupe d'Etude des Lymphomes de l'Adulte (GELA) H8F Trial (1993-1998) ■ This trial compared three cycles of MOPP/ABV hybrid and involved field irradiation to mantle and paraaortic-splenic irradiation for favorable prognosis CS IA-IIA patients. With a medium follow-up of 92 months, this trial shows a significant advantage in 5-year event-free survival with three cycles of MOPP/ABV and involved field radiation as compared to subtotal nodal and splenic irradiation alone (98% vs 74% $p < .001$).[113] The 10-year overall survival estimates were 97% and 92%, respectively (p = .001). In both the H7UF and H8F trials, significant differences in event-free survival did not appear to confer a survival difference at 4 to 5-year follow-up, but did translate into a significant survival advantage in both studies with 10-year follow-up for the patients who were in the arms that had fewer recurrences. These trials thus demonstrate the importance of disease-free or event-free survival differences in trials even when the early follow-up data do not show survival differences. This suggests that when large enough EFS differences are seen, eventually significant overall survival differences will also be noted.

The GHSG 13 trial is an ongoing four-arm study comparing two cycles of ABVD, AVD, ABV, and AV, all followed by 30 Gy of involved field irradiation in CS I-II patients without risk factors. This trial is designed to determine the most important drugs in the ABVD regimen, with special focus on the dacarbazine and the bleomycin.

Randomized Clinical Trials Identifying the Appropriate Radiation Volume and Dose When Combined With Chemotherapy

Two trials in favorable prognosis early stage Hodgkin lymphoma evaluate radiation dose to involved sites after chemotherapy. The GHSG HD10 trial (Table 114-8) evaluates the number of cycles of chemotherapy and radiation dose. Patients are randomized to two or four cycles of ABVD. Patients in complete remission will be randomized to either 20 Gy or 30 Gy involved field radiation. Four groups of patients were randomized: ABVD × 2 and 20 Gy, ABVD × 2 and 30 Gy, ABVD × 4 and 20 Gy, and ABVD × 4 and 30 Gy (see above). The EORTC H9F trial is evaluating 36 Gy, 20 Gy, or no radiation to involved sites in patients who have achieved a complete remission after six cycles of EBVP (see below).

Summary of Combined Chemotherapy and Radiation Therapy Alone Trials ■ Combined radiation therapy and chemotherapy trials have focused on maintaining a low risk of relapse while minimizing late complications of treatment through systematic reduction of both modalities in clinical trials. The success of these trials depends in part on the careful selection of patients with favorable prognostic features. Quality control in the details of delivery of radiation therapy are increasingly important with the reduction in the amount of chemotherapy and both the EORTC and the GHSG have built quality controls into their early stage trials. Most trials use relapse-free or event-free survival as endpoints. With longer follow-up available in some trials overall survival differences are sometimes seen when initially only event-free survival differences were seen.

Chemotherapy Alone

Randomized Clinical Trials of Chemotherapy Alone Versus Radiation Therapy Alone ■ Two randomized trials in PS I-II patients evaluating MOPP chemotherapy alone versus subtotal lymph node irradiation alone have been published. The National Cancer Institute (NCI) study was initially designed to include patients with both favorable and unfavorable prognosis early stage Hodgkin lymphoma. However, the most favorable patients with PS IA Hodgkin lymphoma in peripheral sites were not included in the trial and were treated with radiation therapy alone, and patients with an unfavorable prognosis (B symptoms, large mediastinal adenopathy, and limited stage III disease) were included in the trial so that many of the patients did not have favorable prognosis early stage disease.[114] Patients were randomized to 6 months of MOPP chemotherapy alone or subtotal nodal irradiation alone. After researchers recognized that patients with massive mediastinal involvement and PS IIIA disease were not optimal candidates for the radiation therapy alone arm, the eligibility criteria were changed while the study was ongoing. Table 114-9 shows the data for the IA (central sites), IB, IIA, and IIB patients without large mediastinal involvement. No difference in disease-free or overall survival is seen at 10 years.

The Italian prospective randomized study randomized patients with PS IA-IIA Hodgkin lymphoma to receive either 6 months of MOPP alone or subtotal nodal irradiation alone.[115] There were no differences in freedom from progression (Table 114-9). However, the survival rate was significantly higher in patients treated with radiation therapy alone (93%) than in those treated with chemotherapy alone (56%). The difference in survival was attributed to the inability to salvage patients relapsing after MOPP chemotherapy.

Both the NCI and the Italian studies demonstrated greater acute toxicities in patients who received MOPP chemotherapy. Both trials demonstrate freedom from treatment failure rates of only 64-82% with MOPP alone. More modern trials are being conducted in clinically staged patients using ABVD or similar regimens without alkylating agent chemotherapy.

The National Cancer Institute of Canada (NCIC) and Eastern Cooperative Oncology Group CTG HD6 Study is a modification of the NCI and Italian studies with the randomization of clinically staged patients and the use of ABVD as the chemotherapy regimen. Patients with nonbulky CS I-II disease were stratified into low-risk (LP/NS, age <40, ESR <50, and <3 sites of disease) and high-risk groups.[116] Low-risk patients were randomized to extended field irradiation versus four to six cycles of ABVD, and high-risk patients were randomized to two cycles of ABVD followed by radiation therapy versus four to six cycles of ABVD. At a median follow-up of 4.2 years, patients treated with chemotherapy alone had a significantly inferior 5-year progression-free survival of 87% versus 93% in patients treated with either extended field irradiation or combined modality therapy (p = .006). There were no significant differences in overall survival. The trial has not reported separately the results among favorable prognosis versus unfavorable prognosis patients. A problem with this trial is the long time to completion of the patient accrual so that the "standard arm" of extended field irradiation, which has been shown to be inferior to combined modality therapy in several randomized trials even among favorable patients, is currently no longer viewed as standard treatment.

Randomized Clinical Trials of Chemotherapy Alone Versus Combined Modality Therapy ■ The EORTC three-armed trial (H9F) for favorable prognosis CS I-II patients compares six cycles of the EBVP II regimen alone to the same regimen with different doses of involved field irradiation. Patients who achieve a complete remission after the chemotherapy are randomized to 36 Gy involved field irradiation versus 20 Gy involved field irradiation versus no radiation therapy (4-year event-free survival rates were 87%, 84%, and 70%, respectively) (Table 114-10). This trial is designed to evaluate the role of involved field irradiation in favorable prognosis early stage Hodgkin lymphoma and to evaluate potential differences in the dose of radiation delivered. At the most recent interim analysis, the chemotherapy alone arm was closed due to a higher than expected number of relapses that met stop-

Table 114-9 ■ **Randomized Clinical Trials in Favorable Prognosis Stage I-II Hodgkin Disease: Trials of Chemotherapy Alone Versus Radiation Therapy Alone**

Trial	Eligibility	Treatment Regimens	No. of Patients	Outcome
Italian Prospective	PS IA-IIA	A. STLI	45	FFP (8 years): A = 76%; B = 64%; p > .05
Randomized Trial[91]		B. MOPP × 6	44	Survival (8 years): A = 93%; B = 56%; p < .001
NCI242122	PS IA-IIB without large mediastinal disease	PS IA peripheral nodes STLI	30	30/30 FFFR; 28/30 alive
		PS IA (central), IB, IIA, IIB		
		A. STLI	41	FFP (10 years) A = 67%; B = 82%; p = .27
		B. MOPP × 6	41	Survival (10 years) A = 85%; B = 90%; p = .68
NCIC	CS IA-IIA without MC or LD histology, age	A. STLI (S) or inverted Y RT		PFS (5 years) RT ± CT = 93%
CTG	≥40, ESR ≥50 mm/h, four or more sites	B. ABVD × 4-6		CT alone = 87%
	of involvement			
HD6[116]				(p = .006)

Abbreviations: ABVD, Adriamycin (doxorubicin), bleomycin, vinblastine, and dacarbazine; CS, clinical stage; ESR, erythrocyte sedimentation rate; FFFR, freedom from first relapse; FFP, freedom from progression; LD, lymphocyte depletion; MC, mixed cellularity; MOPP, mechlorethamine, vincristine, procarbazine, prednisone; NCI, National Cancer Institute; NCIC, National Cancer Institute of Canada; PS, laparotomy staged; RT, radiation therapy; STLI (S), subtotal nodal irradiation (splenic irradiation).

Table 114-10 ■ **Randomized Clinical Trials in Favorable Prognosis Stage I-II Hodgkin Disease: Trials of Chemotherapy Alone Versus Combined Modality Therapy**

Trial	Eligibility	Treatment Regimens	No. of Patients	Outcome
EORTC[117]	CS IA-IIB without age ≥50, ESR 50 mm/h	A. EBVP II × 6 + IFRT (36 Gy)	783	EFS; A. 87%, B. 84%, C 70%.
H9F	in A, ≥30 mm/h in B, four or more sites	B. EBVP II × 6 + IFRT (20 Gy)		
	of disease, large mediastinal disease	C. EBVP II × 6 alone (closed because of		
	(? 0.35 m/t ratio)	stopping rules)		
CCG 5942[118]	All stages	Patients stratified by stage into one of three	501	EFS
		treatment regimens. Patients in complete		A = 93%; B = 85%; p = .024
		remission randomized to A. IFRT or B.		
		no rx		
MSKCC[119]	CS/PS IA-IIB, IIIA without large mediasti-	A. ABVD ×6		FFS A. 81% B. 86%, p = NS
	nal disease, peripheral or retroperito-	B. ABVD × 6 + Mantle or inverted Y RT		OS A. 90% B. 97% p = NS
	neal nodes >10 cm	(36 Gy); STLI/TLI for stage IIIA		

Abbreviations: ABVD, Adriamycin (doxorubicin), bleomycin, vinblastine, and dacarbazine; CS, clinical stage; EBVP, epirubicin, bleomycin, vinblastine, prednisone; ESR, erythrocyte sedimentation rate; EORTC, European Organization for the Research and Treatment of Cancer; IFRT, involved field radiation therapy; MSKCC, Memorial Sloan-Kettering Cancer Center; PS, laparotomy staged; RT, radiation therapy; STLI/TLI, subtotal nodal/total nodal irradiation.

ping rules.[117] A potential criticism of this study is whether inadequate chemotherapy was employed. However, this study was restricted to selected patients with favorable features, and the EBVP II regimen was chosen since its efficacy in combination with involved field radiation therapy had been proven in the earlier EORTC H7F trial.

The Children's Cancer Group (CCG) randomized 501 patients who received a complete response to chemotherapy to involved field radiation or no further treatment. All stages were included. The chemotherapy alone arm in this trial has been stopped. The interim analysis showed increased recurrences in the no radiation arm that met the stopping rules.[118] At 3 years, based on treatment received, the event-free survival was 93% with involved field radiation and 85% without radiation ($p = .024$).

The Memorial Sloan-Kettering Cancer Center trial randomized CS I-IIIA patients who achieved a complete remission after six cycles of ABVD to either mantle irradiation (35 Gy) or no further treatment. Patients with large mediastinal adenopathy and nodes greater than 10 cm were not eligible; however, CS IIB and all other CS IIA patients were included; thus, this trial was not restricted to early stage favorable prognosis Hodgkin lymphoma. After 152 patients were accrued at 10 years, the trial was closed due to slow accrual. No significant differences in freedom from progression, for radiation therapy versus on radiation therapy (86% vs 81%, respectively), and overall survival (97% vs 90%, respectively) were found at a median follow-up of 60 months. The trial, however, was underpowered to determine if the two treatment approaches are truly equivalent, but preliminary analysis predicts no greater than an 18% point difference in recurrence-free survival favoring the radiation arm.[119]

Pavlovsky and colleagues from the Grupo Argentino de Tratamiento de la Leucemia Aguda (GATLA) randomized 277 patients with CS I-II Hodgkin lymphoma to receive six monthly cycles of cyclophosphamide, vinblastine, procarbazine, and prednisone (CVPP) followed by involved field radiation therapy to 30 Gy, versus six cycles of CVPP alone.[120] At 84 months, the disease-free survival (DFS) of the combined modality therapy arm was significantly higher than that of the chemotherapy alone arm (71% vs 62%, $p = .01$). On subgroup analysis, the difference between the two arms was highly significant among patients with unfavorable features (age >45, >2 sites or bulky disease), with DFS of 75% in the combined modality therapy arm versus 34% in the chemotherapy alone arm ($p = .001$). Among favorable patients, the difference in DFS was not significant (77% vs 70%).

Laskar and colleagues reported results of a randomized trial from Tata Memorial Hospital with six cycles of ABVD. Complete responders were randomized to involved field radiation therapy or no further treatment.[121] Patients of all stages were included; 55% had CS I-II disease. Significant differences in 6-year event-free survival (88% vs 76%, $p = .01$) and overall survival (100% vs 89%, $p = .002$) were observed, favoring the combined modality therapy arm. The trial contained a high proportion of pediatric patients. Seventy-one percent of cases were of mixed cellularity histology, reflecting the high proportion of Epstein-Barr virus-related cases in developing countries.

Summary of Chemotherapy Alone Trials ■ Nearly all of the chemotherapy alone trials are in favorable prognosis patients. These trials have had a number of problems in design, in patient accrural, and in variations in the type of chemotherapy and field size of radiation therapy utilized. None-the-less, most of the trials have demonstrated significantly higher recurrence rates in the chemotherapy alone arms versus the chemotherapy and radiation therapy arms. Low-dose involved field radiation therapy is considerably safer than the higher-dose larger field treatments used in the past and that on balance the use of the adjuvant radiation may reduce toxicity by limiting the risk of relapse and allowing the use of shorter course chemotherapy.

Radiation Therapy Alone Trials

Risk of Occult Abdominal Involvement in Patients With Clinical Stage I or II Hodgkin Lymphoma

Combination chemotherapy and limited field irradiation or in some cases chemotherapy alone have largely replaced radiation therapy for early stage Hodgkin lymphoma. This has occurred due to the availability of effective and relatively safe chemotherapy (such as ABVD), and because of the concerns for the increased risk of late second malignancies and cardiac disease after high-dose wide field irradiation. The routine use of chemotherapy has allowed a reduction of both the dose and field size of radiation therapy. The additional benefits of the approach have been the replacement of surgical staging with radiographic staging, and the improved freedom from treatment failure with the use of both chemotherapy and radiation therapy. Included below is a discussion of the use of radiation therapy alone in the modern era, especially as it pertains to very early stage disease and to nodular lymphocyte predominant Hodgkin lymphoma.

Dose-Response Data

Only one prospective randomized study has been completed.[122] The multicenter trial by the GHSG evaluated the tumoricidal doses for subclinical involvement by Hodgkin lymphoma. A total of 376 laparotomy staged favorable prognosis IA-IIB Hodgkin lymphoma patients were enrolled. Only patients without adverse risk factors were included in the trial. Patients were randomized to receive either 40 Gy extended field radiation therapy or 30 Gy extended field radiation therapy followed by an additional 10 Gy to involve lymph node regions. The 5-year freedom from treatment failure results favored the 30 Gy extended field plus 10 Gy arm over the 40 Gy extended field arm (81% vs 70%, respectively, $p = .026$). The 5-year survival results also favored the 30 Gy extended field arm (98% vs 93%, respectively, $p = .067$), suggesting that 30 Gy is sufficient for treating subclinical involvement of Hodgkin lymphoma with radiation therapy alone.

Field Size: Mantle Irradiation Alone in PS IA-IIA Patients ■ To determine the role of prophylactic abdominal irradiation in early stage Hodgkin lymphoma, the EORTC H-5 trial (1977-1982) compared the use of mantle and paraaortic-splenic pedicle irradiation to mantle irradiation alone in laparotomy-negative patients with favorable early stage Hodgkin lymphoma.[123,124] This study included only patients with nodular sclerosis or lymphocyte predominant histology, age 40 years or younger, PS I or PS II with mediastinal adenopathy, and an ESR less than 70 mm/h. With 15-year follow-up, no differences were seen between the two treatment arms, either for cumulative treatment failure probability or overall survival. These excellent results with mantle irradiation alone in laparotomy staged patients have been corroborated in another retrospective study.[125] In the single-arm Harvard University Medical School trial for laparotomy staged IA-IIA Hodgkin lymphoma patients, the freedom from treatment failure at 5 years was 89% for stage IA and 80% for stage IIA disease (Figure 114-4).[126] The 10-year survival was 98%.

Mantle Irradiation Alone in CS IA-IIA Patients ■ Results from prospective and retrospective studies of mantle irradiation alone for unselected CS I-II patients have been disappointing. The EORTC H-1 trial, one of the first studies to evaluate the role of chemotherapy in early stage Hodgkin disease, randomized clinically staged I-II patients to receive mantle irradiation alone or combined with vinblastine chemotherapy. All CS I-II patients were enrolled. Fewer recurrences were seen in patients who received both mantle irradiation and vinblastine chemotherapy. However, relapse rates were high in both groups (freedom from recurrence was only 38% in the mantle alone group; the 15-year survival rate was only 58%), suggesting that mantle irradiation alone was not adequate treatment for unselected patients with CS I-II Hodgkin disease. These high recurrence rates in unselected patients are not surprising, as more than 20% of CS I-II patients have occult abdominal involvement, and absence of treatment (with radiation therapy or chemotherapy) to cover potential abdominal disease therefore results in higher recurrence rates than achieved with more extensive treatment. When mantle irradiation was restricted to clinically staged, asymptomatic patients with a single lymph node region involved (CS IA), better results have been seen with 10- to 15-year freedom from recurrence rates of 58-81%.[125,127]

Mantle Irradiation Alone in Patients With a Low Risk of Abdominal Involvement ■ The EORTC defined a subgroup of CS I-II patients (women younger than 40 years of age with CS IA nodular sclerosis Hodgkin disease or nodular lymphocyte predominant Hodgkin disease and an ESR <50 mm/h) who were treated with mantle irradiation alone without staging laparotomy in the EORTC H7VF (VF, very favorable) and H8VF trials. This was a group of patients who would have been expected to have a low risk of abdominal involvement by prognostic factors. In the H7VF trial, 40 patients were treated according to this concept and complete remission was reached in 95%. However, 23% of patients relapsed, yielding a 6-year event-free survival rate of 66%, a relapse-free survival rate of 73%, and overall and cause-specific survival rates of 96%.[108] The relapse rates were thought to be unacceptably high in this selected subgroup of stage IA patients. Most patients relapsed primarily in the abdomen.

In summary, in most trials the freedom from treatment failure with mantle irradiation alone in clinically staged patients is inferior to results with more extensive radiation therapy or combined radiation therapy and chemotherapy. In contrast, following a negative laparotomy, early stage patients have a very good outcome after mantle irradiation alone. In an era when staging laparotomy is rarely performed, most patients should be treated with combined radiation therapy and chemotherapy.

Regional Radiation Alone for Nodular Lymphocyte Predominant Hodgkin Lymphoma (NLPHL) ■ The preferred treatment for NLPHL is regional radiation alone. This subtype of Hodgkin disease has the lowest disease-related mortality of all the subtypes, and studies suggest that ABVD may not be as effective for NLPHL as for classic Hodgkin lymphoma.[41,128] In an attempt to reduce the risk of treatment-related second cancers, we and others have suggested treatment with radiation therapy alone with limited fields, usually defined as the involved nodal and adjacent prophylactic nodal regions. For patients with disease above the diaphragm, it may be feasible to avoid treating the mediastinal nodes as the mediastinum is rarely involved.

Recommendations and Future Directions

Standard care currently provides a number of treatment options for patients with early stage favorable prognosis Hodgkin lymphoma (see the NCCN guidelines on Hodgkin disease), although the most commonly used approach uses combination chemotherapy and radiation therapy, often with a modified number of cycles of chemotherapy and some modification of radiation field sizes and doses. Reasonable modification of chemotherapy off-study includes giving ABVD for 3-4 cycles. Reasonable modifications of radiation therapy off-study include involved fields to 30 Gy after a complete remission or an uncertain complete remission. Alternatively, patients can be treated to an involved field to 30 Gy in the involved region (involved field by definition) followed by a cone down to the residual disease to 36 Gy.

Current clinical trials are evaluating the use of alternative chemotherapy combinations, shortened courses of chemotherapy, chemotherapy with smaller radiation fields or lower radiation doses, and chemotherapy without radiation therapy. Fortunately, death from Hodgkin lymphoma in favorable prognosis early stage patients is unusual and mortality from causes other than Hodgkin lymphoma occurs many years later; however, this means that survival is not always the most useful parameter to evaluate results in early stage Hodgkin lymphoma. Current trials must be judged also by freedom from first recurrence rates, acute morbidity, and by quality of life and cost-effectiveness. Long-term data allows assessment of mortality risk both from Hodgkin lymphoma and from the treatment and thus every effort must be taken to reanalyze trials as data become more mature. New methods in decision analysis should also help in the design of trials and in the analysis of retrospective data.

Despite the increasing availability of guidelines for the treatment of Hodgkin lymphoma, there must remain room for individualization of treatment. With different treatment options, some of which may result in a higher recurrence risk at the gain of less toxic initial treatment (without any difference in long-term survival), patient preferences must be assessed. In addition, treatment should be individualized when a particular treatment approach might result in a higher risk of serious late complications (ie, treatment of young female patients with large radiation fields and the risk of late breast cancer; heavy smoking history and risk of lung cancer).

Unfavorable Prognosis CS I-II Hodgkin Lymphoma

A number of clinical trials comparing radiation therapy alone to combined modality therapy for unfavorable prognosis stage I-II Hodgkin lymphoma were conducted in the 1970s and 1980s. The high recurrence rates with radiation therapy alone led to the development of strategies in current trials that use various combinations of both combination chemotherapy and radiation therapy. To illustrate, the large EORTC (H5U) trial randomized patients with unfavorable prognostic factors to total nodal irradiation versus MOPP chemotherapy (six cycles) and mantle irradiation. There were differences in treatment failure (35% vs 16%, $p < .001$) favoring the combined chemotherapy and radiation therapy arm, but no overall survival differences (69% in both groups at 15 years).[124]

Trials to Identify the Best Combination of Chemotherapy and Radiation Therapy ■ The evolution of studies to identify the best chemotherapy combination for unfavorable early stage Hodgkin lymphoma paralleled trials to identify the optimal chemotherapy for advanced Hodgkin lymphoma. Early trials evaluated MOPP versus MOPP-like combinations; later trials compared these combinations with ABVD, and, finally, the most recent trials compare new intense chemotherapy combinations with ABVD. Table 114-11 shows representative trials.

The first combined modality trial to test MOPP versus ABVD in unfavorable prognosis patients was the Milan study conducted between 1974 and 1982. Split-course treatment was employed, with three cycles of chemotherapy preceding and following subtotal nodal irradiation. There was no significant difference in 5-year freedom from progression; however, the number of patients enrolled was too small to definitively rule out a difference in outcome.[129] The EORTC H6U trial (1982-1988) also used split-course chemotherapy and radiation therapy and compared MOPP and ABVD.[130] Three hundred sixteen patients were randomized. The 10-year survival was equivalent in both arms, but the freedom from treatment failure rate was significantly higher with ABVD than with MOPP.

Table 114-11 Randomized Clinical Trials in Unfavorable Prognosis Stage I-II Hodgkin Disease: Trials to Identify the Optimal Chemotherapy Combination

Trial	Eligibility	Treatment Regimens	No. of Patients	Outcome
EORTC H6U 1982–1988[130]	CS I-II with large mediastinal mass or ESR ≥50 mm/h in A; ≥30 mm/h in B or ≥3 involved areas	CT ×3 + Mantle + CT ×3 A. MOPP B: ABVD	165 151	FFTF (10 years) A = 68%; B = 90%; $p < .0001$ Survival (10 years) A = 87%; B = 87%; $p = .52$
GATLA 1986–1992[131]	Score of age, B symptoms, stage, number of sites, and bulky disease	A: CVPP × 3 + IFRT (30 Gy) + CVPP × 3 B: AOPE × 3 + IFRT (30 Gy) + AOPE × 3	92 84	EFS (5 years) A = 85%; B = 66%; $p = .009$ Survival (5 years) A = 95%; B = 87%; $p = .16$
EORTC H7U[108] 1988–1992	CS IA-IIA with age >50 years or ESR ≥50 mm/h in A; ≥30 mm/h in B or large mediastinal mass (≥0.33 m/t)	A: EBVP II × 6 + IFRT (36 Gy) B: MOPP/ABV × 6 + IFRT	160 156	EFS (6 years) A = 68%; B = 88%; $p < .001$ Survival (6 years) A = 769%; B = 87%; $p = .017$
EORTC H9U[117]	Same as H7U	A: ABVD × 6 + IFRT (30 Gy) B: ABVD × 4 + IFRT C: BEACOPP × 4 + IFRT		EFS A. 96% B. 95%. C. 93%
GHSG HD11[132] 1998–	CS IA-IB, IIA with ESR 50 mm/h or CS IIB and ESR >30 mm/h or large mediastinal disease	A: ABVD × 4 + IFRT (30 Gy) B: ABVD × 4 + IFRT (20 Gy) C: BEACOPP × 4 + IFRT (30 Gy) D: BEACOPP × 4 + IFRT (20 Gy)	1363	Completed
ECOG 2496 1998–	Large mediastinal disease	A: ABVD × 6 + IFRT (36 Gy) to bulky sites (>5 cm) B: 12 weeks Stanford V + IFRT to bulky sites		

Abbreviations: ABVD, Adriamycin (doxorubicin), bleomycin, vinblastine, and dacarbazine; BEACOPP, bleomycin, etoposide, doxorubicin, cyclophosphamide, vincristine, procarbazine, and prednisone; CS, clinical stage; CVPP, cyclophosphamide, etoposide, procarbazine, and prednisone; ECOG, Eastern Cooperative Oncology Group; EFS, event-free survival; EORTC, European Organization for the Research and Treatment of Cancer; ESR, erythrocyte sedimentation rate; FFTF, freedom from treatment failure; GATLA, Grupo Argentina de Tratamiento de Leucemia Aguda; GHSG, German Hodgkin Study Group; IFRT, involved field radiation therapy; MOPP, Mustargen (mechlorethamine), Oncovin (vincristine), procarbazine, and prednisone; Stanford V, mechlorethamine, doxorubicin, vinblastine, prednisone, vincristine, bleomycin, and etoposide.

A large randomized trial was designed to test whether four cycles of combination chemotherapy and radiation therapy is sufficient treatment compared to six cycles of chemotherapy and radiation therapy. The EORTC H8U study randomized patients to combined modality therapy with four or six cycles of MOPP/ABV, and between involved field and extended field irradiation (Table 114-12). At 10 years there are no differences in failure-free survival or overall survival between the three arms of the trial with four cycles of ABVD and involved field irradiation having the same outcome as the two arms with more extensive treatment.[113]

The Grupo Argentino de Tratamiento de la Leucemia Aguda (GATLA) trial and the EORTC H7U trial (Table 114-11) studied modified nonalkylating agent regimens versus standard alkylating agent regimens in unfavorable prognosis early stage patients. All patients received combined radiation therapy and chemotherapy. In both trials, the arms using modified chemotherapy were associated with significantly higher recurrence rates. In the GATLA trial, the event-free survival was 66% for doxorubicin, vincristine, prednisone, and etoposide and involved field radiation therapy versus 85% ($p = .009$) for CVPP (cyclophosphamide, etoposide, procarbazine, and prednisone) and involved field radiation therapy.[131] In the H7U trial for the 389 patients with unfavorable disease, EBVP and involved field radiation therapy was inferior to MOPP/ABV (Adriamycin [doxorubicin], bleomycin, and vinblastine) and involved field radiation therapy both in 10-year event-free survival (88% vs 68%, $p < .001$) and in overall survival (87% vs 79%, $p = .0175$).[109] The recurrence rate in this trial was high enough to result in early closure of the trial. These trials illustrate the importance of careful assessment of prognostic factors prior to treatment for early stage Hodgkin lymphoma. Minimal combined chemotherapy and radiation therapy approaches

Table 114-12 Randomized Clinical Trials in Unfavorable Prognosis Stage I-II Hodgkin Disease: Trials to Identify the Appropriate Radiation Volume

Trial	Eligibility	Treatment Regimens	No. of Patients	Outcome
French Cooperative Trial 1976–1981[134]	CS I- II without age >45 years, three or more regions of disease, bulky disease	A. MOPP × 3 + IFRT (40 Gy) + MOPP × 3 B. MOPP × 3 + EFRT (40 Gy) + MOPP × 3	82 91	DFS (6 years) A = 87%; B = 93%; p = NS Survival (7 years) A = 92%; B = 91%; p = NS
Milan[133]	All CS I-II	A. ABVD × 4 + STLI B. ABVD × 4 + IFRT	65 68	FFP (5 years) 1990-1997 A = 96%; B = 93%; p = NS
EORTC/GELA H8U 1993–1998[113]	CS IA-IIB with age >50 years, ESR ≥50 mm/h in A; >30 mm/h in B, four or more sites of disease, large mediastinal disease	A. MOPP/ABV × 6 + IFRT (36 Gy) B. MOPP/ABV × 4 + IFRT (36 Gy) C. MOPP/ABV × 4 + STLI	995	FFS (5 years); p = NS A = 84%; B = 88%; C = 87% Survival (5 years); p = NS A = 90%; B = 94%; C = 93%
GHSG HD8 1993–1998	CS IA-IIB with ESR >50 mm/h in A; ≥30 mm/h in B, three or more sites of disease, large mediastinal disease	COPP/ABVD × 4 months + IFRT COPP/ABVD × 4 months + EFRT	Not reported	Not reported

Abbreviations: ABV, Adriamycin (doxorubicin), bleomycin, and vinblastine; ABVD, Adriamycin (doxorubicin), bleomycin, vinblastine, and dacarbazine; CS, clinical stage; DFS, disease-free survival; EFRT, extended field radiation therapy; EORTC, European Organization for the Research and Treatment of Cancer; ESR, erythrocyte sedimentation rate; FFP, freedom from progression; FFS, failure-free survival; GELA, Groupe d'Etude des Lymphomes de l'Adulte; GHSG, German Hodgkin Study Group; IFRT, involved field radiation therapy; MOPP, Mustargen (mechlorethamine), Oncovin (vincristine), procarbazine, and prednisone; STLI, subtotal nodal irradiation.

may not be ideal for patients with unfavorable prognosis CS I-II disease.

Based mainly on trials in advanced Hodgkin lymphoma, ABVD has become the standard regimen used in patients with CS I-II disease. A number of current trials compare combined modality therapy using ABVD with more intense, novel regimens. Both the EORTC H9U and GHSG HD11 studies of combined modality therapy are comparing four cycles of ABVD with four cycles of BEACOPP-baseline (bleomycin, etoposide, Adriamycin [doxorubicin], cyclophosphamide, vincristine, procarbazine, and prednisone).

The EORTC H9U trial randomizes patients between six and four cycles of ABVD or four cycles of the BEACOPP regimen, all followed by involved field irradiation.[117] The most recent interim analysis showed 4-year event-free survivals of 94%, 89%, and 91%, respectively, and an overall 4-year survivals of 96%, 95%,and 93%, respectively. None of the differences were statistically significant.

The GHSG HD 11 trial randomized patients into four arms comparing two doses of involved field radiation therapy (20 vs 30 Gy) and four cycles of ABVD versus four cycles of BEACOPP.[132] A total of 1363 patients have been entered on to the trial. At 2 years, there are no differences in treatment outcome between chemotherapy regimens and between doses of radiation therapy. The 2-year freedom from treatment failure rate is 90%. In the ECOG 2496 trial of combined modality therapy, six cycles of ABVD are being compared to 3 months of Stanford V. In the recently opened GHSG HD 15 trial, patients with CS I-II disease with risk factors are randomized to four cycles of ABVD versus two cycles of dose-escalated BEACOPP and two cycles of ABVD, followed by involved field irradiation to 30 Gy.

Trials to Identify the Appropriate Radiation Therapy Volume ■ Several randomized trials have studied radiation field size when combined with chemotherapy for unfavorable prognosis early stage Hodgkin lymphoma. The French Cooperative Trial reported by Zittoun and colleagues randomized 218 stage I-II unfavorable prognosis patients to six cycles of MOPP sandwiched around involved field (40 Gy) or extended field (40 Gy) irradiation.[133] The 6-year disease-free survival rates were 87% and 93%, respectively (p = .15), for the involved field and extended field arms. The Milan study reported by Santoro incorporated only 4 months of chemotherapy (ABVD), followed by involved field (36 Gy) or subtotal nodal irradiation (30-36 Gy). One hundred thirty-three patients were treated; 20% had bulky disease.[134] The 5-year freedom from progression rates were 96% and 93%, respectively (Table 114-12). The EORTC/GELA H8U trial, reported above, randomized patients to four cycles of MOPP/ABV plus involved field versus subtotal nodal irradiation. The GHSG HD8 trial, conducted between 1993 and 1998, used two cycles (4 months) of cyclophosphamide, Oncovin (vincristine), procarbazine, and prednisone (COPP)/ABVD followed by either involved field or extended field irradiation to 30 Gy (Table 114-12). Evidence from these randomized trials suggests that radiation fields may be safely limited to involved regions in most combined chemotherapy and radiation therapy programs.

Trials of Chemotherapy Alone Versus Combined Modality Therapy ■ Only one prospective trial of chemotherapy alone versus combined modality therapy in unfavorable prognosis stage I-II has been reported. The GATLA randomized 104 patients with unfavorable disease characteristics to six cycles of CVPP alone or six cycles of CVPP sandwiched around involved field irradiation (30 Gy). The 7-year survival rates were 66% and 84%; the freedom from relapse rates were 34% and 75% ($p < .001$), both favoring combined modality treatment.[120]

The ongoing NCIC HD6 trial evaluates patients with unfavorable disease characteristics but excludes patients with large mediastinal adenopathy or nodes greater than 10 cm. Patients are randomized to receive combined modality therapy with two cycles of ABVD followed by irradiation (an extended mantle plus splenic irradiation or mantle plus paraaortic and splenic irradiation) or four to six cycles of ABVD alone (depending on the rapidity of response). Data have not been separately reported for these two groups of patients.[116]

Recommendations and Future Directions ■ The outcome of treatment for patients with unfavorable prognosis stage I-II Hodgkin lymphoma has improved dramatically in the past three decades. Mainly, this is a result of the use of combined modality therapy, because historically fewer than 50% of patients in some subgroups remain free in first remission when radiation therapy alone is used as initial treatment. Combined radiation therapy and chemotherapy not only enhances the likelihood of local tumor control, but also it should control occult nodal and extranodal disease in the majority of patients. Current clinical trials are exploring new combinations of radiation therapy and chemotherapy to try to reduce late morbidity and mortality while maintaining a high probability of freedom from first recurrence.

Treatment of Advanced Hodgkin Lymphoma

For many years, the most popular chemotherapy regimen used in the treatment of advanced Hodgkin lymphoma was MOPP (Table 114-13). DeVita and colleagues reported 198 patients treated with this regimen.[16] The complete remission rate was 81%. Eventually, 36% of the complete responders relapsed, giving a 52% 10-year disease-free survival rate. The overall survival at 10 years was 50%, reflecting some deaths from treatment-related toxicity. Several subsequent trials using MOPP[23,135,136] have shown disease-free survivals of 36-47%.

A number of variations on the MOPP regimen have been reported. The most popular have been MVPP (mechlorethamine, vinblastine, procarbazine, and prednisone)[137,138] ChlVPP,[139,140] and BCVPP (carmustine, cyclophosphamide, vinblastine, procarbazine, and prednisone).[136] These regimens have led to disease-free survival rates approximately comparable to MOPP. The ChlVPP regimen has been reported to have less immediate toxicity and frequently has been used for the treatment of older patients.

The first major alternative to the MOPP regimen was reported by Bonadonna and colleagues in 1975.[141] This regimen used ABVD. Whereas MOPP was administered for 14 days and then no treatment for 14 days, ABVD was administered every other week with all of the drugs given intravenously. Several randomized trials have compared MOPP and ABVD.[23,129] In no case has MOPP been found to be superior; it was generally found to have an inferior outcome. In addition, ABVD appeared to have less toxicity.[129,142] A study by Cancer and Leukemia Group B showed a failure-free survival of 61% for ABVD and 50% for MOPP.[22] The results of this study have caused ABVD to be, by far, the most frequently used regimen for treating advanced Hodgkin lymphoma in the United States. Bonadonna and colleagues first reported using a combination of MOPP and ABVD to treat patients with Hodgkin lymphoma.[135] The two regimens have been combined in a variety of ways in subsequent trials. Some patients receive alternating cycles of MOPP and ABVD.[136] Other studies combined MOPP and ABVD in a single cycle with the first 7 days of the cycle using the drugs from MOPP, with the drugs in ABVD being given on day 8. In these studies, the dacarbazine was frequently deleted.[143] Some studies found no difference between the two approaches, whereas others identified superiority to using MOPP/ABV in a "hybrid" regi-

Table 114-13 **Chemotherapy Regimen Used for Hodgkin Disease**

Drug	Dose (mg/m²)	Route	Schedule (Days)	Cycle Length (Days)
MOPP				
Mechlorethamine	6	IV	1.8	21
Vincristine	1.4	IV	1.8	
Procarbazine	100	PO	1-14	
Prednisone	40	PO	1-14	
BCVPP				
Carmustine	100	IV	1	28
Cyclophosphamide	600	IV	1	
Vinblastine	5	IV	1	
Procarbazine	50	PO	1	
	100	PO	2-10	
Prednisone	60	PO	1-10	
ChlVPP				
Chlorambucil	6	PO	1-14	28
Vinblastine	6	IV	1.8	
Procarbazine	100	PO	1-14	
Prednisone	40 total	PO	1-14	
COPP				
Cyclophosphamide	650	IV	1.8	28
Vincristine	1.4	IV	1.8	
Procarbazine	100	PO	1-14	
Prednisone	40	PO	1-14	
MVPP				
Nitrogen mustard	6	IV	1.8	42
Vinblastine	6	IV	1.8	
Procarbazine	100	PO	1-14	
Prednisone	40 total	PO	1-14	
LOPP				
Chlorambucil	10 total	PO	1-10	28
Vincristine	1.4	IV	1.8	
Procarbazine	100	PO	1-10	
Prednisone	25	PO	1-14	
CVPP				
Lomustine	75	PO	1	28
Vinblastine	4	IV	1.8	
Procarbazine	100	PO	1-14	
Prednisone	40	PO	1-14	
ABVD				
Adriamycin (doxorubicin)	25	IV	1.15	28
Bleomycin	10	IV	1.15	
Vinblastine	6	IV	1.15	
Dacarbazine	375	IV	1.15	
MOPP/ABVD hybrid				
Mechlorethamine	6	IV	1	28
Oncovin (vincristine)	1.4[a]	IV	1	
Procarbazine	100	PO	1-7	
Prednisone	40	PO	1-7	
Adriamycin (doxorubicin)	25	IV	15	
Bleomycin	10	IV	15	
Vinblastine	6	IV	15	
Dacarbazine	35	IV	15	
MMOPP/ABV hybrid				
Mechlorethamine	6	IV	1	28
Oncovin (vincristine)	1.4[a]	IV	1	
Procarbazine	100	PO	1-7	
Prednisone	40	PO	1-14	
Adriamycin (doxorubicin)	35	IV	8	
Bleomycin	10	IV	8	
Vinblastine	6	IV	8	

[a]No more than 2.0 mg Oncovin total dose to be delivered.

men. A randomized trial comparing the alternating or hybrid regimens to ABVD alone did not show an advantage to the more complex regimen.[143] This has further solidified the place of ABVD as the "standard" regimen for the treatment of advanced Hodgkin lymphoma.

Unfortunately, 30-40% of patients with advanced Hodgkin lymphoma treated with ABVD fail to achieve an initial remission or relapse from remission. The proportion of patients with a large number of adverse risk factors that fail ABVD is even higher. These results have led to attempts at identifying improved treatment regimens. The most popular of these have been Stanford V and BEACOPP (Table 114-14).[144,145] The Stanford V regimen uses doxorubicin, vinblastine, mechlorethamine, bleomycin, vincristine, etoposide, and prednisone. The drugs are administered weekly for 12 weeks.[111] The regimen is followed by adjuvant radiation therapy to sites of initial bulky disease of 5 cm or greater. One hundred forty-two patients with stage III or IV or locally extensive mediastinal stage I or II disease who received Stanford V were reported with a median follow-up of 5.4 years. The overall failure-free survival was 89% and the overall survival was 96%.[146] There were no treatment-related deaths. Patients with 0 to 2 adverse risk factors in the International Prognostic System for Hodgkin lymphoma had a failure-free survival of 94% versus 75% for patients with a score of 3 or higher. No secondary leukemias were observed. In a recent update for these data[147] 86% of patients treated with stage III or IV Hodgkin lymphoma were free from progression at 8 years follow-up and 83% of the patients were free from progression at 12 years follow-up. The 12-year overall survival was 95%. Fertility seems to be preserved with 72 posttreatment conceptions. A study from the United Kingdom compared the Stanford V regimen to ABVD and found similar anti-Hodgkin lymphoma efficacy with less toxicity using the Stanford V regimen.[149]

Investigators in Germany have developed a dose-intense regimen named BEACOPP (Table 114-14).[145] BEACOPP has been given at two dose levels, with the higher-dose level requiring hematopoietic growth factors and more intensive supportive care. When compared to COPP/ABVD in a randomized trial, the BEACOPP regimen (ie, both the standard dose BEACOPP and the escalated dose BEACOPP) had a superior freedom from treatment failure at 5 years (69% COPP-ABVD, 76% standard dose BEACOPP, and 87% escalated dose BEACOPP). The overall survival rates at 5 years were 83%, 88%, and 91%, respectively, favoring the BEACOPP regimens but not significantly so. However, when the two BEACOPP regimens were combined, there was a significant difference in overall survival. A recent update of these data confirmed the superiority of escalated dose BEACOPP in eradicating Hodgkin lymphoma with an 85% 82-month freedom from treatment failure, which was significantly better than COPP-ABVD, or standard dose BEACOPP.[149] However, secondary acute myeloid leukemia/myelodysplasia was more frequent with the escalated

Table 114-14 New Chemotherapy Regimen for Hodgkin Disease

Drug	Dose (mg/m²)	Route	Schedule (Days)	RT	Cycle Length
BEACOPP (Escalated BEACOPP)				Bulky, residual	21 days
Bleomycin	10	IV	8		
Etoposide	100 (200)	IV	1-3		
Adriamycin (doxorubicin)	25 (35)	IV	1		
Cyclophosphamide	650 (1250)	IV	1		
Oncovin (vincristine)	1.4[a]	IV	8		
Procarbazine	100	PO	1-7		
Prednisone	40	PO	1-14		
G-CSF	– (+)	SQ	8+		
Stanford V					
Mechlorethamine	6	IV	Weeks 1, 5, 9	Bulky	12 weeks
Adriamycin (doxorubicin)	25	IV	Weeks 1, 3, 5, 9, 11		
Vinblastine	6	IV	Weeks 1, 3, 5, 9, 11		
Vincristine	1.4[a]	IV	Weeks 2, 4, 6, 8, 10, 12		
Bleomycin	5	IV	Weeks 2, 4, 6, 8, 10, 12		
Etoposide	60 × 2	IV	Weeks, 3, 7, 11		
Prednisone	40	PO	Weeks 1-10 q.o.d.		
G-CSF			Dose reduction or delay		

[a]No more than 2.0 mg Oncovin total dose to be delivered.

dose BEACOPP arm occurring in 11 of 466 patients versus 5 of 469 patients with standard dose BEACOPP and one of 260 patients with COPP-ABVD.

The place of combined modality therapy in advanced Hodgkin lymphoma is clear in only few instances. Patients with bulky mediastinal masses certainly benefit from adjuvant radiation therapy. The Stanford V regimen is a combined modality regimen and has initially been shown to have excellent results. The BEACOPP regimen also uses radiation therapy for bulky sites of disease at the completion of chemotherapy. In patients without bulky disease most clinicians would avoid radiation therapy in an attempt to minimize long-term toxicity.

However, the role of radiation therapy in advanced Hodgkin lymphoma remains somewhat controversial. In part, this is because of the potential morbidity from the large fields of radiation that often are required, the increased risk of extranodal recurrences outside of the radiation fields as the stage of disease increases, and the lack of survival differences in randomized studies. Some randomized trials suggest an improvement in freedom from treatment failure with the use of adjuvant (often low-dose) radiation therapy. In the SWOG trial, when the analysis was restricted to patients of all histologic subtypes who received their randomly assigned therapy, the remission duration of those who received consolidation radiation therapy was significantly better than that of the patients who were treated with chemotherapy alone (85% vs 67%; $p < .002$).[150] In addition, significant improvements in freedom from recurrence were seen in patients with nodular sclerosis histology and in patients with bulky disease. Similar results were reported in a meta-analysis of randomized trials where adjuvant radiation therapy resulted in an 11% advantage in freedom from recurrence, but no overall survival differences when compared to the same chemotherapy regimen alone.[151] In contrast, a recently reported EORTC trial showed no significant difference in event-free survival with adjuvant involved field irradiation in patients who were in complete remission prior to the randomization to radiation or no further treatment. However, the trial suggested a benefit to radiation therapy in patients who did not achieve a complete remission.[152]

Given the above data and guidelines from standard practice, the following are circumstances in which adjuvant radiation therapy should be considered for use in the management of advanced or recurrent Hodgkin lymphoma: in patients with stage III-IV disease who have not achieved a complete remission with chemotherapy; to sites of large bulky disease such as the mediastinum following a complete response to chemotherapy in other sites;[153] when using chemotherapy regimens that have published data with radiation therapy as part of the up-front management such as Stanford V,[192] and as part of systemic treatment (standard dose or high-dose chemotherapy) for localized recurrent disease.

The use of PET scans might modify the use of radiation therapy in advanced Hodgkin lymphoma. Patients who achieve a PET negative status are much more likely to be cured than those whose PET scans remain abnormal, a finding that seems to apply for both patients studied at the end of treatment and those studied earlier after several cycles of treatment.[154-156] It is possible that becoming PET negative will make the use of adjuvant radiation therapy unnecessary, even with residual masses. At present this is a topic for clinical trials.

The optimal chemotherapy regimen for the treatment of patients with advanced Hodgkin lymphoma remains unknown. All regimens fail to cure some patients and long-term toxicity is a significant concern. The risk of secondary leukemia seems to be a reflection of the dose of alkylating agents in the treatment regimen. Secondary acute leukemia or myelodysplasia is an unusual complication of treatment with ABVD, but occurs more frequently in patients treated with MOPP-like regimens.[157] The risk of secondary solid tumors seems to be primarily related to the use of radiation therapy in the treatment regimen, although alkylating agents are associated with an increased risk of lung cancer, especially in patients who smoke.[93,158] Other toxicities, including heart disease, lung disease, endocrine dysfunction, and infertility, are seen in a subset of patients. However, in patients with poor-risk Hodgkin lymphoma, the cure rate does not seem to be high enough with available treatments to reduce dose intensity, although in good-risk patients with advanced disease this might be a reasonable consideration.

Very-high-dose therapy and autologous bone marrow transplantation have also been tested as part of the primary therapy in patients with very poor-risk Hodgkin disease. One problem in applying this treatment approach has been the difficulty in identifying patients with Hodgkin lymphoma who have a very poor survival with modern therapies. Italian[159] and Spanish[160] investigators have reported encouraging results in pilot studies. The European Group for Bone and Marrow Transplantation compared 56 patients transplanted in complete remission with 168 patients who were matched by risk factors from the GHSG. Freedom from relapse was superior in patients undergoing transplantation, but overall survival did not differ. An international study of 163 patients with poor-risk Hodgkin lymphoma who achieved a complete or partial remission with four courses of a doxorubicin containing chemotherapy regimen were randomly assigned to four more courses of standard chemotherapy or autotransplant. At a median follow-up of 48 months, the freedom from failure and overall survival rates were not different. At present, the value of bone marrow transplantation in the primary therapy of patients with Hodgkin lymphoma remains unproven.

Elderly Patients With Hodgkin Lymphoma

Elderly patients with Hodgkin lymphoma have not benefited from chemotherapy to the same degree as younger patients. Patients older than 60 years of age with Hodgkin lymphoma had a very poor outlook, with 5-year failure-free survival rates less than 50%, and even poorer results in those patients with high stage, symptomatic disease. A recent study retrospectively comparing patients older than 60 years of age who were treated with ChlVPP with those receiving the hybrid regimen ChlVPP/ABV showed an advantage in 5-year overall survival (87% vs 39%) and 5-year event-free survival (75% vs 31%) for ChlVPP/ABV.[161] It may be that the addition of doxorubicin to the treatment regimen is even more important in elderly patients. A similar regimen (ChlVPP/EVA) in the study of patients of all ages was found to be superior to a weekly chemotherapy regimen in high-risk patients.[162]

Hodgkin Lymphoma in Patients With HIV Infection ■ The association of Hodgkin lymphoma and infection by the human immunodeficiency virus (HIV) was first noted in 1984.[163] Subsequent studies have shown that Hodgkin lymphoma is 5 to 20 times more frequent in patients with HIV infection. Patients with HIV infection who develop Hodgkin lymphoma are more likely to have the mixed cellularity as opposed to the nodular sclerosis subtype when compared to patients without HIV infection. Patients with HIV infection are more likely to present with advanced stage, extranodal involvement, and B symptoms. Before the development of highly active antiretroviral therapy (HAART), the treatment outcome was poorer than in patients without HIV infection. However, paradoxically, the incidence of Hodgkin lymphoma in patients with HIV infection appears to have increased since the development of HAART.[164]

The development of HAART and its use in HIV-infected patients being treated for Hodgkin lymphoma has improved the treatment outcome. In a report of 59 patients treated with the Stanford V regimen while simultaneously receiving HAART and hematopoietic growth factor support, 69 patients were able to complete treatment with no dose reduction or treatment delays.[165] The 3-year overall survival was 51%, 3-year disease-free survival 68%, and 3-year freedom from progression 60%. Patients with a higher International Prognostic Score (IPS) had a poorer outcome (ie, 83% freedom from progression with an IPS score of 2 or lower versus 41% with an IPS score of 3 or higher).

Investigators from Germany treated 12 patients with Hodgkin lymphoma and HIV infection utilizing the standard dose BEACOP regimen.[166] Eight of the 12 patients completed the planned six courses of BEACOPP. Two patients died of opportunistic infections and one relapsed. The remaining nine patients were in complete remission at a median of 49 months at the time of the report. Most but not all the patients in this series were receiving antiretroviral therapy. Another series from Germany comparing patients who did or did not receive HAART with chemotherapy regimens for Hodgkin lymphoma showed an improved 2-year overall survival (ie, 88% vs 19%) in patients who received HAART.[167]

A combination of HAART and chemotherapy for Hodgkin lymphoma is practical and achieves treatment outcomes almost as good as seen in HIV negative patients. Except for patients who are seriously ill with opportunistic infections, patients with Hodgkin lymphoma who are HIV-positive should be treated with standard regimens and most of these patients can be cured of Hodgkin lymphoma.

Salvage Therapy

For the purposes of this section, salvage therapy refers to treatment administered to patients with Hodgkin lymphoma who fail to achieve an initial complete remission or relapse after achieving an initial complete remission. Although seemingly straightforward, the diagnosis of treatment failure is not always easy. Patients with bulky mediastinal or retroperitoneal masses regularly have residual, albeit smaller, masses on imaging studies at the completion of successful therapy. In these patients, previously abnormal PET scans and elevated ESR usually revert to normal, but this may take some time. In many cases, a biopsy will be required to prove persistent lymphoma. Biopsy should always be done in the patient who achieves a complete remission and then develops new adenopathy or imaging abnormalities. A patient with Hodgkin lymphoma can develop non-Hodgkin lymphoma, other malignancy, and tuberculosis or other infections. Failure to establish a firm diagnosis of relapse can be tragic.

Patients, who are treated initially with radiation therapy alone and who progress, have an excellent outcome with salvage chemotherapy.[81-82] When compared to patients who are treated with chemotherapy from the outset, those receiving similar chemotherapy regimens for relapse after radiation therapy have an equivalent or superior outlook.[81] The use of radiation therapy to rescue patients who fail chemotherapy is occasionally an effective treatment maneuver.[168] In patients with localized relapse, extended field radiation therapy can achieve durable remissions in 25-50% of cases. It must be emphasized that only occasional patients with nonbulky disease confined to a few node-bearing areas and who do not have systemic systems are candidates for this treatment approach.

Unfortunately, 30-40% of patients with advanced Hodgkin lymphoma will either fail to achieve a remission with chemotherapy or relapse after complete remission. Those patients, who are primarily refractory and never achieve an initial remission to an effective chemotherapy regimen, have a particularly poor outlook. Early experience with ABVD showed that some patients who failed MOPP could be successfully treated, whereas the converse was less often true.[88] Even so, the durable remission rate in this setting is less than 20%.[169]

New treatment regimens such as Stanford V and BEACOPP seem to cure a high proportion of patients with advanced Hodgkin lymphoma but expose patients to more drugs and/or higher doses than seen with ABVD. It is possible that salvage therapies after these regimens will not be as effective as have been described for patients treated with ABVD or other earlier treatment regimens.

Early autologous bone marrow transplantation in patients who are primarily refractory to an excellent chemotherapy regimen for Hodgkin lymphoma can produce durable remissions in a significant proportion of patients. The North American Autologous Blood and Marrow Transplant Registry reported 103 such patients. The overall in progression-free survival at 5 years was 40%.[170] The European Group for Blood and Marrow Transplantation described 290 patients with primary refractory Hodgkin lymphoma and reported a 5-year failure-free survival of 30%.[171] Investigators from GELA found that patients with at least a partial response to induction chemotherapy had a better 5-year survival (72%) than did patients with no response or progressive disease (30%).[172] Investigators at Stanford University performed a case-control study for primary chemotherapy failures. They found an event-free survival at 4 years of 52% for transplantation, in contrast to 10% for alternate standard chemotherapy regimens.[173] Patients who fail to achieve remission with primary chemotherapy are best treated with autologous bone marrow transplantation, and this probably represents the clearest indication for autologous transplantation in patients with Hodgkin lymphoma.

Patients who achieve an initial complete remission and relapse represent a heterogeneous group of patients. In general, the longer the initial complete remission, the better the outlook with any form of salvage therapy.[84,174] A follow-up analysis of the original MOPP-treated patients from the NCI found that those patients who had an initial remission longer than 12 months achieved second complete remissions 74% of the time, in contrast to only 28% of the time in patients with initial remissions lasting less than 12 months.[89] However, even in patients with long initial remissions, the eventual survival after first relapse was only 24%. Similar results have been reported from Milan,[174] Vancouver,[175] and Paris.[176] In addition to a brief initial remission, other adverse prognostic factors include advanced age, more extensive initial disease, systemic symptoms, and elevated serum lactate acid dehydrogenase level.[176]

A variety of treatment regimens have been used for patients with relapsed Hodgkin lymphoma. In addition to MOPP or ABVD in patients who received the opposite regimen initially, a number of other treatments have been used. Unfortunately, the number of patients achieving extended survival free of Hodgkin lymphoma is quite poor, although patients with no adverse risk characteristics (see above) have been reported to have 5-year failure-free survival as high as 50%.[90,174]

An encouraging new drug in the treatment of Hodgkin lymphoma is gemcitabine.[177-179] Gemcitabine has a significant response rate as a single agent in patients with refractory Hodgkin lymphoma and is now being tested in combinations. It is possible that gemcitabine will some day be used earlier in the treatment of patients with Hodgkin lymphoma. Treatment with the monoclonal antibody rituximab produced objective responses in five of 22 patients with nodular sclerosing classical Hodgkin lymphoma and alleviated system symptoms in a larger number of patients.[180,181] The studies suggested that the responses might be related to the depletion of normal B cells rather than a direct anticancer effect. Biologic therapies using monoclonal antibodies directed against CD30 have shown early activity in relapse patients and are undergoing clinical trials.[182]

In patients with multiple treatment failures, long remissions are rare. In these patients, there is often a point where further intensive chemotherapy regimens are more likely to do harm than good, and a palliative treatment approach should be adopted. Treatment approaches such as low to moderate doses of vinblastine administered weekly[183] and the judicious use of involved field radiotherapy can alleviate symptoms and produce a reasonable quality of life. Asymptomatic patients might be best followed without therapy. Patients with fevers refractory to other treatment approaches can sometimes be effectively palliated with nonsteroidal anti-inflammatory drugs such as naproxen or indomethacin.

Autologous bone marrow transplantation can rescue occasional patients with multiply relapsed Hodgkin lymphoma. Unfortunately, the results in this setting are usually disappointing. Because of the superior results in patients treated early in the course of the disease, most advocates of bone marrow transplantation would prefer to use it as part of the treatment of the initial relapse after an effective initial chemotherapy regimen. Patients who receive an alternate standard chemotherapy regimen and achieve at least a partial remission then undergo autologous transplantation. The results in this setting have yielded durable remissions in 47-85% of patients.[184-186] In a randomized trial conducted in Europe, patients with relapsed, chemosensitive Hodgkin lymphoma had a significantly better failure-free survival with transplantation rather than continuing standard dose chemotherapy.[187] Patients with long initial remissions had a better failure-free survival, but both early and late relapsers had significant improvement in failure-free survival with the transplant. However, there was not a significant improvement in overall survival. It appears that the International Prognostic Score predicts outcome for patients undergoing autologous transplantation, and that patients with four or more adverse risk factors are probably poor candidates.[188]

Allogeneic bone marrow transplantation has been performed in patients with relapsed Hodgkin lymphoma, but the results have been disappointing. Treatment-related mortality rates have varied from 31% to 61%, but there does seem to be a lower relapse rate in patients surviving allogeneic transplantation in comparison to those surviving autologous transplantation.[189] The explanation for the high treatment-related mortality with allogeneic transplantation might relate to patient selection or other, as yet unidentified, factors making these patients more susceptible to treatment toxicity. At the present time, allogeneic bone marrow transplantation should rarely be selected as the primary salvage treatment for patients with Hodgkin lymphoma. However, one report of patients who had failed an autotransplant for relapsed Hodgkin lymphoma and then underwent a full intensity allotransplant using the BEAM regimen followed by early withdrawal of immunosuppression had a surprisingly good outcome.[190] Ten patients, four of whom received unrelated donor hematopoietic stem cells, were treated with no early deaths. Seven of the ten patients remained in continuous complete remission at 12 months follow-up although the majority had chronic graft versus host disease. The lower mortality associated with nonmyeloablative allogeneic transplantation seen in some early trials might lead this form of allotransplant to be more widely used.[191]

Summary

Tremendous progress has been made in the last three decades toward the cure of Hodgkin lymphoma. Additional work, however, is needed to further minimize the morbidity and mortality associated with the disease and its treatment. This includes the need to better understand the etiology and pathology of Hodgkin lymphoma, to optimize control rates, especially in patients with unfavorable prognosis or advanced stage disease, to modify therapeutic approaches to reduce the long-term complications, and to increase the awareness of physicians and patients to the potential late effects of treatment so that patients will receive appropriate follow-up care.

Selected References

The complete reference list can be found at www.CANCERMEDICINE8.com

1. Kass A, Kass E. *Perfecting the World: The Life and Times of Thomas Hodgkin (1798–1866).* New York: Harcourt Brace Jovanovich; 1988.
2. Hodgkin's T. On some morbid appearances of the absorbent glands and spleen. *Medico-Chirugical Trans.* 1832;17:68–97.
12. Peters M. A study of survivals in Hodgkin's disease treated radiologically. *Am J Roentgenol.* 1950;63:299–311.
20. DeVita VJ, Simon R, Habbard S, et al. Curability of advanced Hodgkin's disease with chemotherapy: longterm follow up of MOPP-treated patients at the National Cancer Institute. *Ann Intern Med.* 1980;92:587–95.
22. Canellos GP, Anderson JR, Propert KJ, et al. Chemotherapy of advanced Hodgkin's disease with MOPP, ABVD, or MOPP alternating with ABVD [see comments]. *N Engl J Med.* 1992;327:1478–1484.
23. Bonadonna G, Zucali R, Monfardini S, et al. Combination chemotherapy of Hodgkin's disease with Adriamycin, bleomycin, vinblastine, and imidazole carboxamide versus MOPP. *Cancer.* 1975;36:252–259.
24. MacMahon B. Epidemiological evidence of the nature of Hodgkin's disease. *Cancer.* 1957;10:1045–1054.

34. Mueller N, Evans A, Harris N, et al. Hodgkin's disease and Epstein-Barr virus, altered antibody pattern before diagnosis. *N Engl J Med.* 1989;320:689.
35. Weiss L, Movahed L, Warnke R, et al. Detection of Epstein-Barr viral genomes in Reed-Sternberg cells of Hodgkin's disease. *N Engl J Med.* 1989;320:502–506.
41. Diehl V, Sextro M, Franklin J, et al. Clinical presentation, course, and prognostic factors in lymphocyte predominant Hodgkin's Disease and lymphocyte rich classical Hodgkin's disease: report form the European Task Force in Lymphoma on lymphocyte predominant Hodgkin's Disease. *J Clin Oncol.* 1999;17:776.
76. Ng A, Bernardo M, Weller E, et al. Long-term survival and competing causes of death in patients with early stage Hodgkin's disease treated at age 50 or younger. *J Clin Oncol.* 2002;20:2101.
90. van Leeuwen FE, Swerdlow AJ, Travis LB. Second cancers after treatment of Hodgkin lymphoma. In: Hoppe RT, Mauch PM, Armitage JO, et al, eds. *Hodgkin Lymphoma.* Philadelphia: Lippincott Williams & Wilkins; 2007:347–370.
94. Mauch P, Ng A, Aleman B, et al. Report from the Rockefeller Foundation Sponsored International Workshop on reducing mortality and improving quality of life in long-term survivors of Hodgkin's disease: July 9-16, 2003, Bellagio, Italy. *Eur J Haematol.* 2005(suppl 66):68–76.
106. Hasenclever D, Diehl V. A prognostic score for advanced Hodgkin's disease. International Prognostic Factors Project on Advanced Hodgkin's Disease. *N Engl J Med.* 1998;339:1506–1514.
108. Engert A, Franklin J, Eich HT, et al. Two cycles of ABVD plus extended field radiotherapy is superior to radiotherapy alone in early-favorable Hodgkin lymphoma: final results of the GHSG HD7 trial. *J Clin Oncol.* 2007;25:3495–3502.
109. Noordijk EM, Carde P, Dupouy N, et al. Combined-modality therapy for clinical stage I or II Hodgkin's lymphoma: long-term results of the European Organization for Research and Treatment of Cancer H7 Randomized Controlled Trials. *J Clin Oncol.* 2006;24:3128–3135.
113. Ferme C, Eghbali H, Meerwaldt JH et al. Chemotherapy plus involved-field radiation therapy in early-stage Hodgkin's disease. *New England J Med.* 2007;357:1916–1927.
130. Carde, P. Hagenbeek, A. Hayat, M et al. Clinicalstagingversuslaparotomyandcombined modality with MOPP versus ABVD in early-stage Hodgkin's disease: the H6 twin randomized trials from the European Organization for Research and Treatment of Cancer Lymphoma Cooperative Group. *J Clin Oncol.* 1993;11:2258–2272.
146. Horning SJ, Hoppe RT, Breslin S, et al. Stanford V and radiotherapy for locally extensive and advanced Hodgkinís disease: mature results of a prospective clinical trial. *J Clin Oncol.* 2002;20:630–637.
149. Eiehl V, Franklin J, Pfreundschuh M, et al. Standard and increased-dose BEACOPP chemotherapy compared with COPP-ABVD for advanced Hodgkinís disease. *N Engl J Med.* 2003;348:2386–2395.
161. Weekes C, Vose J, Hynch J, et al. Hodgkin's disease in the elderly: improved treatment outcome with a doxorubicin containing regimen. *J Clin Oncol.* 2002;20:1087–1093.
186. Poen JC, Hoppe RT, Horning SJ. High-dose therapy and autologous bone marrow transplantation for relapsed/refractory Hodgkin's disease: the impact of involved field radiotherapy on patterns of failure and survival [see comments]. *Int J Radiat Oncol Biol Phys.* 1996;36:3–12.
187. Schmitz N, Pfistner B, Sextro M, et al. Aggressive conventional chemotherapy compared with high-dose chemotherapy with autologous haemopoietic stem-cell transplantation for relapsed chemosensitive Hodgkin's disease: a randomised trial. *Lancet.* 2002;359:2065–2071.

115 Non-Hodgkin Lymphoma

Arnold S. Freedman, M.D.

The malignant lymphomas are neoplastic transformations of cells that reside predominantly within lymphoid tissues. Although Hodgkin and non-Hodgkin lymphomas (NHLs) both infiltrate lymphohematopoietic tissues, their biologic and clinical behaviors are distinct. They differ with regard to the neoplastic cells of origin, sites of disease, presence of specific symptoms, and response to treatment. Although both are among the most sensitive malignancies to radiation and cytotoxic therapy, their cure rates markedly differ. Hodgkin lymphomas are cured in nearly 75% of all patients employing both conventional and salvage treatment strategies whereas NHLs are cured in less than 50% of patients.

Epidemiology and Etiology

Incidence and Mortality

In 2007 there were 63,190 new cases of NHL in the United States, 4% of all new cancers in males, 4% in females.[1] This is more than seven times the incidence of Hodgkin lymphoma. There is a slight male-to-female predominance and a higher incidence for Caucasians than for African Americans. The incidence rises steadily with age, especially after age 40 years. The malignant lymphomas are among the most common neoplasms in patients between the ages of 20 and 40 years. Moreover, the incidence of NHL nearly doubled between 1970 and 1995, but the rate of increase has slowed since the mid-1990s.

There are striking differences in the age-dependent incidence of NHL by histologic subtype. In children, Burkitt, lymphoblastic, and diffuse large B-cell lymphoma (DLBCL) are the most common. Histologic subtypes commonly diagnosed in adults, specifically the indolent lymphomas (small lymphocytic and follicular lymphomas [FL]) are extremely rare in children. With increasing age, the incidence of FLs and other aggressive lymphomas continues to rise. Small lymphocytic and FLs are most commonly diagnosed in patients over age 60.

NHL ranks as the seventh most common cause of cancer-related death in the United States. In 2007, 18,660 deaths from NHL were predicted.[1] In the decades between 20 and 39 years, it ranks fourth for males, and for females 80 or greater, it ranks fifth. The 5-year survival rates for NHL is 64% for Caucasians and 56% for African Americans.

Exposures and Diseases Associated With Increased Risk of Developing NHL

Infectious agents are involved in the pathogenesis of some NHLs (Table 115-1). Epstein-Barr virus (EBV) has a strong association with development of Burkitt lymphoma and human immunodeficiency virus-1-related lymphoma.[2] Between 45% and 70% of human immunodeficiency virus-1-related NHLs are EBV-related. Essentially, 100% of the primary central nervous system (CNS) lymphomas are EBV-related in human immunodeficiency virus-1-infected individuals. The natural killer cell and natural killer-like T-cell lymphomas that involve the upper aerodigestive tract as well as other extranodal sites also are EBV-associated.[3] Human T-cell leukemia virus (HTLV)-1 is responsible for adult T-cell leukemia/lymphoma that is endemic to the Caribbean and southern Japan.[4] The gastric marginal zone lymphomas (MZLs) are associated with *Helicobacter pylori* infection.[5] Splenic MZL has been associated with hepatitis C infection.[6] Chronic hepatitis B infection has also been associated with an increased risk of NHL.[7] The ocular adnexal MZL are linked with *Chlamydia psittaci* infection although this remains controversial[8] and immunoproliferative small intestinal disease (Mediterranean lymphoma, alpha heavy chain disease) has been associated with *Campylobacter jejuni*.[9] *Borrelia burgdorferi* infection has been associated with extranodal MZLs of the skin in cases from Europe.[10] The Kaposi sarcoma-associated herpes virus, also known as HHV-8, has been isolated from the neoplastic cells in patients with primary effusion lymphomas in primarily human immunodeficiency virus (HIV)-1-infected individuals, but also HIV-negative patients and rarely cardiac transplant patients.[11,12]

Table 115-1 ■ **Exposures and Diseases Associated With Increased Risk of Developing Non-Hodgkin Lymphoma**

Infectious agent association (other than human immunodeficiency virus [HIV])
Epstein-Barr virus
Human T-cell leukemia/lymphoma virus
Helicobacter pylori
HHV-8
Hepatitis C
Chlamydia psittaci
Campylobacter jejuni
Borrelia burgdorferi
Drug or chemical exposures
Diphenylhydantoin
Dioxin, phenoxyherbicides
Radiation
Prior chemotherapy
Prior radiation therapy
Inherited immunodeficiency diseases
Klinefelter syndrome
Chédiak-Higashi syndrome
Ataxia telangiectasia syndrome
Wiskott-Aldrich syndrome
Common variable immunodeficiency syndrome
Acquired immunodeficiency disease
Iatrogenic immunosuppression
Acquired immunodeficiency virus (HIV-1)
Acquired hypogammaglobulinemia
Autoimmune diseases
Sjögren syndrome
Celiac sprue
Rheumatoid arthritis and systemic lupus erythematosus

An increased risk of NHL has been associated with a number of exposures and/or disease states (Table 115-1). There is controversial evidence that certain chemical exposures, specifically the herbicide phenoxyacetic acid, increase the risk of NHL.[13] Other potential environmental associations include exposure to arsenic, pesticides, fungicides, chlorophenols, or organic solvents, halomethane, lead, vinyl chloride, or asbestos.[14,15] Occupational exposures associated with an increased risk include agricultural work, welding, and work in the lumber industry.[16] NHL has been observed as a late complication of prior chemotherapy and/or radiation therapy. Specifically, patients with Hodgkin lymphoma treated with radiation therapy and chemotherapy exhibit an increased risk of developing secondary DLBCL.[17]

Diseases of inherited and acquired immunodeficiency as well as autoimmune diseases are associated with an increased incidence of lymphoma. The association between immunosuppression and induction of NHLs is compelling because if the immunosuppression can be reversed, a percentage of these lymphomas regress spontaneously.[18] The incidence of NHL is increased nearly 100-fold for patients undergoing organ transplantation necessitating chronic immunosuppression, and is greatest in the first-year post-transplant. About 30% of these arise as a polyclonal B-cell proliferation that evolves into a clonal B-cell malignancy. The NHLs that occur in the context of immunosuppression or immunodeficiency, including human immunodeficiency virus-1 infection, are frequently associated with EBV.[19] Histologically, DLBCLs are most frequently associated with immunosuppression and autoimmune diseases. The rare inherited immunodeficiency diseases like X-linked lymphoproliferative syndrome, Wiskott-Aldrich syndrome, Chédiak-Higashi syndrome, ataxia telangiectasia, and common variable immunodeficiency syndrome are complicated by highly aggressive lymphomas. The incidence of lymphoma in iatrogenic immunosuppression, AIDS, and autoimmune disease (Felty syndrome, Sjögren syndrome, celiac disease, Crohn disease, rheumatoid arthritis and systemic lupus, non-hepatitis C-related mixed cryoglobulinemia) argues strongly for immune dysregulation contributing in the pathogenesis of some lymphomas.[20,21] The outcome of treatment of NHL in patients with rheumatoid arthritis is associated with a decreased risk of death due to lymphoma and relapse as compared to unaffected patients with NHL.[22] An increased risk of NHL has been observed in first-degree relatives with NHL, Hodgkin lymphoma, or leukemia.[23]

Pathology, Immunobiology, and Natural History of NHL

In 1995, the Society for Hematopathology and the European Association of Hematopathologists jointly developed a classification of hematologic neoplasms for the WHO. The goals of the WHO project, in part, were to update and revise the WHO classification of the lymphoid neoplasms, using a combination of morphology, immunotyping, genetic features, and clinical syndromes.[24] To provide a context for this classification, the large numbers of entities will be grouped in "indolent," "aggressive," and "highly aggressive" categories (Table 115-2).

Table 115-2 ■ **Classification of Non-Hodgkin Lymphoma**

Indolent lymphomas
Follicular lymphoma
B-chronic lymphocytic leukemia/small lymphocytic lymphoma
Lymphoplasmacytic lymphoma
Marginal zone lymphoma (nodal, extranodal, splenic)
T/natural killer large cell granular lymphocyte leukemia
T-chronic lymphocytic leukemia/prolymphocytic leukemia
Aggressive lymphomas
Mantle cell lymphoma
Diffuse large B-cell lymphoma
Peripheral T-cell lymphoma (unspecified)
Peripheral T-cell lymphoma (angioimmunoblastic, angiocentric)
T/natural killer cell, hepatosplenic γ/δ, intestinal T-cell lymphoma
Anaplastic large-cell lymphomas
Highly aggressive lymphomas
Precursor T- or B-lymphoblastic leukemia/lymphoma
Burkitt and Burkitt-like lymphoma
Adult T-cell leukemia/lymphoma (HTLV-1+)

■ Indolent Lymphomas

The indolent NHLs are generally associated with reasonably long survival, measured in years, even if left untreated, but they are usually not curable with conventional treatment. Indolent lymphomas represent 35-40% of the NHLs diagnosed in Western countries. The most common subtypes are FL, small lymphocytic lymphoma, and MZL, comprising 22%, 6%, and 5% of all NHLs, respectively. In comparison, lymphoplasmacytic lymphoma, mycosis fungoides/Sézary syndrome, and splenic MZLs are rare diseases, comprising 1% or less of all NHLs.

Follicular lymphomas (FLs) are the most common type of indolent NHL, and morphologically recapitulate normal germinal centers of secondary lymphoid follicles[25] (Fig. 115-1). The WHO classification includes three grades; grade I (0–5 large cells/high power field) (Fig. 115-2); grade II (6–15 large cells/high power field); and grade III (>15 large cells/high power field).[24] Although the grading system remains in place, clinically, grade I and II FLs are approached similarly. Similar to normal germinal centers, small numbers of T cells and follicular dendritic cells are present in the malignant follicles; however, tingible body macrophages, which are macrophages that have ingested apoptotic cells, are not observed. Involvement of the peripheral blood with malignant cells is commonly seen, and morphologically these cells have notches and have been referred to as "buttock cells."

Early studies suggested that FL and normal follicular center B cells were regulated by their expression of cell surface antigens. Virtually all FLs express monoclonal surface immunoglobulin. Virtually all cases express the B-cell antigens CD19, CD20, CD10, CD79a, but lack CD5. Cytoplasmic bcl-2 protein is overexpressed in essentially all cases of grade I and II, whereas nuclear bcl-6 is expressed by at least some of the neoplastic cells. The most common cytogenetic abnormality in FL is t(14;18) that leads to overexpression of the antiapoptotic protein bcl-2 in over 85% of cases (see Chapter 8: Genomic Alterations and Chromosome Aberrations in Human Cancer). Additional chromosomal abnormalities are present in FL, most frequently involving 1p and 6p.[26] A small number of cases are CD10-negative, and often MUM1- or IRF4-positive. These cases lack bcl-2/IgH, occur in older patients, and have grade III (a and b) histology.[27]

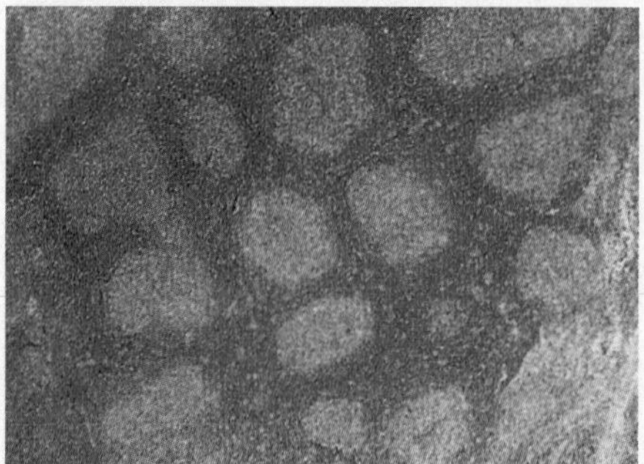

Figure 115-1 ■ Follicular lymphoma grade I (low power).

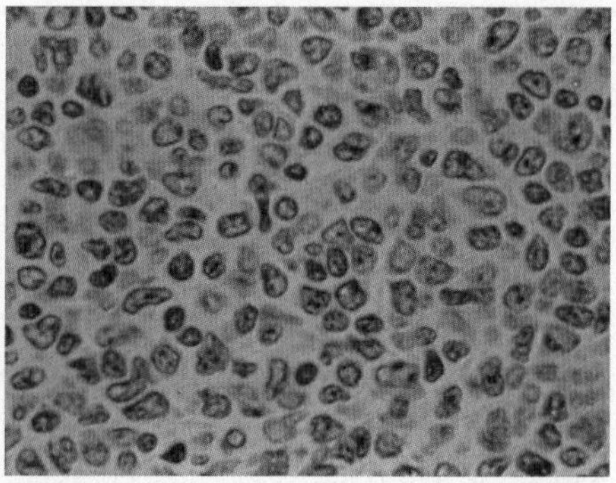

Figure 115-2 ■ Follicular lymphoma grade I (high power).

FLs account for about 22% of NHLs, with the grade I subtype being most common.[28] Although uncommon until the third and fourth decades, the median age at diagnosis is 60 years. This histologic subtype is less common in Asians and blacks. Patients usually present with painless peripheral adenopathy in cervical, axillary, inguinal, and femoral regions. Often lymph node enlargement has been present for long periods, and the nodes have waxed and waned. Hilar and mediastinal nodes are often involved, but large mediastinal masses are rare. Some patients present with asymptomatic large abdominal masses with or without evidence of gastrointestinal and/or renal obstruction. Staging studies usually demonstrates widely disseminated disease with involvement of spleen (40%), liver (50%), and bone marrow (70%). Bone marrow involvement in FL reveals a unique pattern of paratrabecular infiltration. Very few patients present with extranodal extramedullary disease, and only about 20% present with B symptoms or lactate dehydrogenase (LDH) elevation. Central nervous system involvement is uncommon although peripheral nerve compression and epidural tumor masses causing cord compression may develop.

Many cases of primary cutaneous B-cell lymphomas have features of FL.[29] These tumors are bcl-2-positive in only 30-40% of cases. They occur on the head and trunk, and tend to remain localized to the skin, where they are amenable to local therapy.

The course of FL is quite variable. Some patients can be observed with waxing and waning disease for 5 years or more without the need for therapy.[30] Others present with more disseminated disease and rapid growth, and require treatment because massive nodal or organ enlargement leads to pain, lymphatic obstruction, or organ obstruction. A recent analysis using SEER data suggests that overall survival for these patients has improved when comparing outcome for patients treated from 1983 to 1989 to those treated from 1990 to 1999.[31] The median survival for patients with stages III and IV disease is between 7 and 10 years. Regardless of the long natural history, it should be stressed that except for a subset of patients with stage I disease, virtually all patients eventually die of this disease.

Histologic transformation to aggressive lymphoma, usually DLBCL, occurs in up to 60% of patients with FL and is characterized by rapid progression of lymphadenopathy, infiltration of extranodal sites, development of B symptoms, elevated LDH, and often a poor prognosis.[32-35] The progression from follicular to DLBCL occurs regardless of whether the FL is treated aggressively or conservatively, and occurs at a rate of 3% per year. Specific genes have been identified as being altered in transformation, including deletions of the cyclin-dependent kinase inhibitors p15 and p16, mutations of p53 and bcl-2, as well as the noncoding regulatory region of the *BCL-6* gene.

FL grade III has been subdivided into grade IIIa, in which centrocytes are present, and grade IIIb in which there are predominantly centroblasts.[36] Although controversial, grade IIIa can behave as a more indolent disease, whereas grade IIIb behaves very similar to DLBCL.[37,38] In contrast to DLBCL, the relapse rate of FL grade III is higher following combination chemotherapy, but the survival is longer.

Small Lymphocytic Lymphoma ■ Small lymphocytic lymphoma and B-cell chronic lymphocytic leukemia are viewed as the same entity by the WHO classification. Although the major population of cells resembles small normal lymphocytes, larger cells resembling those seen in prolymphocytic leukemia are seen in the nodal tissue in areas known as proliferation centers (Fig. 115-3, and Figs. 147-2, 147-3). The small lymphocytic lymphomas are phenotypically nearly identical to B-cell chronic lymphocytic leukemias, by the expression of HLA-DR, B-cell antigens CD19, CD20, CD23, weak surface immunoglobulin, and CD5. Cytogenetic abnormalities include trisomy 12 present in about 40% of cases, and 13q in 45-55%, 11q abnormalities in 17-20%, and 17p abnormalities in 7-10% of cases. Cases with 13q deletions have the most favorable prognosis, whereas those with 11q or 17p abnormalities have an unfavorable prognosis.[39]

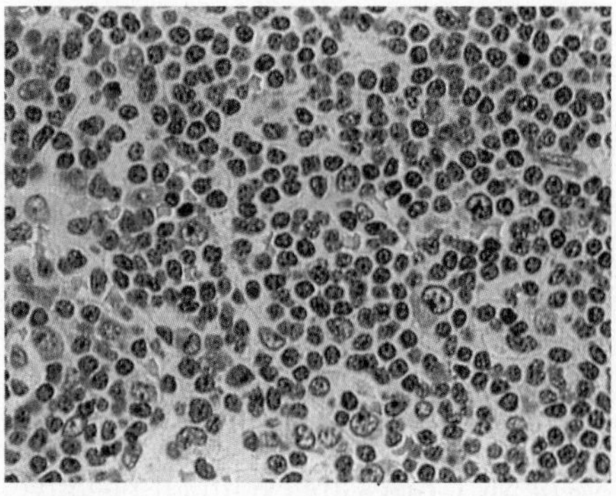

Figure 115-3 ■ Small lymphocytic lymphoma.

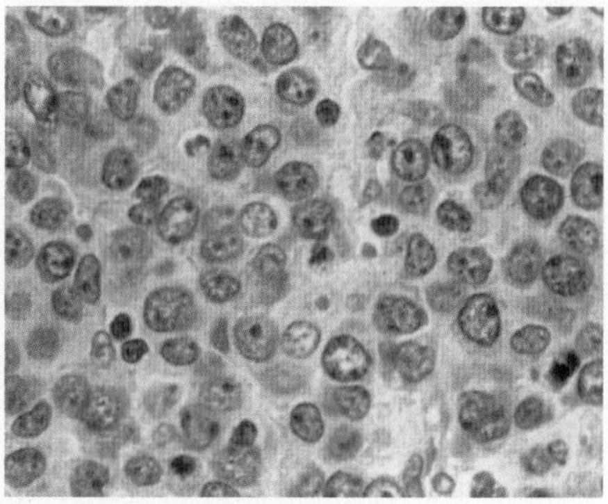

Figure 115-4 ■ Diffuse large B-cell lymphoma.

Recent studies suggest that 30-50% of these diseases have non-mutated immunoglobulin variable region genes and correspond to naïve B cells. These cases often express CD38 and the tyrosine kinase ZAP-70, and have a worse prognosis.[40] The remaining 50-70% of cases have mutated immunoglobulin variable region genes and are derived from germinal center or post-germinal center B cells. These mutated immunoglobulin variable region gene cases are more likely to lack CD38 and ZAP-70, and have a favorable prognosis.

Small lymphocytic lymphomas makes up about 6% of all NHLs.[28] The clinical presentation is similar to FL. Unlike B-cell chronic lymphocytic leukemia, the peripheral blood may be normal or reveal only a mild lymphocytosis (60% have absolute lymphocytosis of <4000 per microliter at diagnosis). In contrast, the bone marrow is positive in 70-90% of cases. A serum paraprotein is found in about 20% of cases and hypogammaglobulinemia is present in about 40%. Small lymphocytic lymphomas and B-cell chronic lymphocytic leukemia can convert to DLBCL (Richter syndrome, Fig. 115-4).[41]

Lymphoplasmacytic Lymphoma ■ Lymphoplasmacytic lymphoma is an indolent lymphoma composed of diffuse proliferation of small lymphocytes with evidence of maturation to plasma cells.[42] Evidence of immunoglobulin is seen in these cells by special stains or inclusions. These tumors express B-cell antigens CD19, CD20, and surface immunoglobulin M isotype, and in general do not express CD5, CD10, or CD23. Up to 50% of the lymphoplasmacytic lymphomas have t(9;14)(p13;q32).

Lymphoplasmacytic lymphoma represents about 1% of all NHLs. Clinically this disease is similar to small lymphocytic lymphomas. The median age is early 60s, and virtually all patients have stage IV disease by virtue of bone marrow involvement. B symptoms and elevated serum LDH are uncommon. Lymph node and splenic involvement are common. A serum M component is commonly seen. As with B-CLL, the paraprotein may have autoantibody or cryoglobulin activity. However, most cases with mixed cryoglobulinemia have been shown to be related to concurrent hepatitis C virus infection.[43,44] In these cases, treatment with interferon to reduce viral load is associated with regression of the lymphoma. In the WHO clinical study, 5-year overall survival (58%) and failure-free survival (25%) were identical to that of small lymphocytic lymphomas.

Marginal Zone Lymphomas

MZLs are a group of distinct entities including nodal MZL; extranodal MZL also known as the lymphomas of mucosal-associated lymphoid tissues; and the splenic MZL.[45-47] In the nodal MZL, the tumor cells cytologically resemble "normal" monocytoid B cells and often involve lymph node sinuses. Phenotypically these tumors express surface immunoglobulin M and B-cell antigens (CD19, CD20). Similar to other indolent lymphomas, MZL can transform into a higher-grade lymphoma. The nodal MZLs constitute 1% of all NHLs. Over 70% of patients present with stage III/IV disease and the majority are asymptomatic. Bone marrow involvement is less common than in most indolent lymphomas, and gastrointestinal involvement unusual. The median survival of these patients is in excess of 10 years.

The extranodal MZL tumor cells express B-cell antigens (CD19, CD20) and surface immunoglobulin M. It is hypothesized that these are malignancies of memory B cells. Cytologically, these tumor cells resemble monocytoid B cells. A feature of extranodal MZL is a lymphoepithelial lesion associated with centrocytes. These tumors do not form follicles but the malignant cells surround reactive follicles. When the extranodal MZL spread to lymph nodes, the neoplastic cells involve the marginal zones. The most common cytogenetic abnormality is trisomy 3, occurring in up to 60% of cases (particularly the gastric extranodal MZL) and t(11;18), with t(11;18) occurring in 25-40% of cases.[48]

Extranodal MZLs constitute about 5% of all NHLs, and almost 50% of all gastric lymphomas. B symptoms are uncommon[19] and most patients present with stage I or II disease. There is no age predilection for these tumors that most commonly involve the gastrointestinal tract (stomach most commonly), lung, dura, lacrimal and salivary glands, skin, thyroid, and breast. Less than 25% of cases have lymph node or bone marrow involvement. Patients can present with peptic ulcer disease, abdominal pain, and sicca syndrome, or a mass at the site of involvement. These lymphomas can disseminate to other mucosal-associated lymphoid tissue sites or bone marrow in about 30% of cases, typically later in the course of the disease. This is more commonly seen in non-gastric MZLs.[49] These diseases have high complete remission rates and potentially long survival, as high as 80% at 10 or more years.[50]

The splenic MZLs constitute less than 2% of all NHLs, with a median age of 65, uncommon before age 50.[28] In splenic MZL there is expansion of marginal zones in the spleen. Bone marrow and peripheral blood involvement (referred to as splenic lymphoma with villous or non-villous lymphocytes) can also be present. In splenic MZL trisomy 3 is present in 39% of cases. The survival of patients is in excess of 70% at 10 years. A prognostic model based on three risk factors: hemoglobin less than 12 g/dL, LDH level greater than normal, and albumin level less than 3.5 g/dL could identify patients with 5-year cause-specific survival of 88% for patients with 0 risk factors, 73% for patients with 1 factor, and 50% for patients with 2 or 3 factors.[51]

Aggressive Lymphomas

Mantle Cell Lymphoma ■ Mantle cell lymphoma (MCL) is generally an aggressive disease.[52-54] These tumors are neoplastic counterparts of naive "mantle zone" B cells. Morphologically, MCL can have either diffuse architecture, or a vaguely nodular appearance, occasionally with expansion of the mantle zone of secondary lymphoid follicles. Cytologically, the neoplastic cells are medium-sized, with irregular nuclei. Some cases of MCL have a predominance of "blastic" cells with a high mitotic rate. The cells express B-cell antigens, surface immunoglobulin M with or without immunoglobulin D, CD5, and CD43, but lack CD10 and CD23, respectively. Overexpression of cyclin D1 protein further distinguishes these tumors from other entities. Approximately 70% of MCLs have t(11;14)(q13;q32) that is rearrangements of *bcl-1* (cyclin D1) gene. About 8% of MCL cases are cyclin D1-negative. These cases overexpress cyclin D2 and 4 or cyclin D3, without chromosomal rearrangements. They are clinically similar to cyclin D1-positive cases.[55] MCL constitutes about 7% of all NHLs. About 75% of patients are males, with median age of 63. Approximately 70% of patients have stage IV disease and B symptoms are observed in approximately one-third of patients. Typical sites of involvement are lymph nodes, spleen,liver, Waldeyer ring, and bone marrow. Peripheral blood involvement is present in 25-50% of patients at presentation. MCL can involve any region of the gastrointestinal tract, occasionally presenting as multiple intestinal polyposis. The median survival of patients with MCL is 3-4 years and patients with the blastic variant at diagnosis have a median survival of 18 months. Blastic transformation occurs in 35% of patients, with a risk of 42% at 4 years, and once occurring the median survival is 3.8 months.[56]

Diffuse Large B-Cell Lymphoma ■ The DLBCLs consist of a diffuse proliferation of large cells that have a high mitotic rate. The cells have a moderate amount of cytoplasm with either cleaved or non-cleaved nuclei often with multiple nucleoli, although there can be great variability in the morphology (Fig. 115-4). Rare cases contain only scattered large cells in a background of small T cells and epithelioid histiocytes, called T-cell/histiocyte-rich large B-cell lymphoma.[57] Gene expression profiling has been applied to DLBCL.[58-61] These studies have subdivided DLBCL into distinct genetic entities. There is evidence that DLBCLs correspond to germinal center B cells or activated B cells.[58,59] The tumor cells generally express B-cell antigens (CD 19, CD20), monoclonal surface immunoglobulin M, but occasionally other heavy chain isotypes CD5-positive cases are uncommon and may have a worse prognosis.[62] CD10 and bcl-6 support a GC origin, whereas expression of MUM1 a non-GC origin. Twenty-five to 80% of DLBCLs are reported to express bcl-2 protein, but impact on prognosis is controversial.[45] Approximately 70% express bcl-6 protein, consistent with a germinal center origin.[63]

Several chromosomal abnormalities have been observed in DLBCL. Bcl-6 is associated with chromosomal rearrangements involving 3q27.[64] Rearrangements of the *gene* are found in a small proportion of FLs (6–13%) but occurs in 20-40% of diffuse aggressive lymphomas.[48] t(14;18) is not specific for FLs and has been observed in approximately 30% of patients with DLBCL. Some of these cases may represent histologic transformations of prior FL.

DLBCL constitutes 31% of all NHLs, and is the most common histologic subtype. Patients who are generally middle-aged or older (median age 64 years) present with either nodal enlargement or extranodal disease. DLBCL presents in a localized (stage I or IE) manner approximately 20% of the time. The disease is confined to one side of the diaphragm (stage I or II) in approximately 30-40% of patients. Stage IV disease is seen in approximately 40% of patients. B symptoms are occurring in 30% of patients, and unlike most NHLs, LDH is elevated in over half the patients. During the course of the disease, the liver, kidneys, and lung may be involved. DLBCL is highly invasive, with local compression of vessels or airways, involvement of peripheral nerves, and destruction of bone. Bone marrow involvement is initially found in only 10-20% of patients, and has strong correlation with risk of spread to the central nervous system.[65] Extranodal disease, specifically testicular and paranasal sinus, multiple extranodal sites, and elevated LDH are other risks for central nervous system dissemination.

Within the DLBCL is a distinct clinical entity known as primary mediastinal large B-cell lymphoma (7% of all cases of DLBCL).[66] Histologically the cellular infiltrate is heterogeneous, and sclerosis is frequently present. The immunophenotype of these lymphomas includes B-cell antigens (CD19, CD20), but they are often negative for surface and cytoplasmic immunoglobulin. Gene expression profile studies suggest that this is a distinct entity from germinal center or activated B-cell types of DLBCL. Recent studies suggest that the gene expression profile pattern of primary mediastinal large B-cell lymphoma closely resembles Hodgkin lymphoma Reed-Sternberg cell lines.[67,68]

Primary mediastinal large B-cell lymphomas have a female predominance, with median age of 40. Over 70% of these patients present with stage I/II bulky disease involving the mediastinum, pleural, and pericardial effusions in about one-third of the patients. Superior vena cava syndrome is common in these patients. Similar to DLBCL, an elevated LDH is present in the majority, whereas bone marrow involvement is infrequent.

The prognosis of patients with primary mediastinal large B-cell lymphoma is similar to patients with DLBCL.

Rare cases of DLBCL present with a disseminated intravascular proliferation of large lymphoid cells, involving small blood vessels, without an obvious tumor mass. The organs most commonly involved are the central nervous system, kidneys, lungs, and skin, but virtually any site may be involved. Patients present with a variety of symptoms related to organ dysfunction secondary to vascular occlusion. Onset with fever, skin rash, or prominent and rapidly progressive neurologic signs is common. The prognosis for intravascular large B-cell lymphoma is poor, with 10% of patients surviving at 3 years.[69,70]

Peripheral T-Cell Lymphomas ■ The category of peripheral T-cell lymphomas (PTCLs) includes a number of entities, which constitute 15% of all NHLs in adults.[71] Among these, in decreasing frequency, are the PTCL, not otherwise unspecified (NOS); anaplastic large-cell lymphoma (ALCL); angioimmunoblastic T-cell lymphoma; the extranodal NK/T-cell lymphoma, nasal type; and the much rarer entities, panniculitis-like T-cell lymphoma; enteropathy type T-cell lymphoma; and hepatosplenic γ/δ T-cell lymphoma.

PTCLs can be nodal or extranodal-based diseases. The diffuse cellular infiltrates range from a mixture of small and large cells; infiltrates of pleomorphic cells, often with a background of epithelioid histiocytes, plasma cells, eosinophils, and Reed-Sternberg-like cells; or predominantly large cells. In contrast to B-cell lymphomas, the pattern of expression of T-cell surface antigens is highly variable. The majority of them will express CD2, CD3, and CD4, with a subset of tumors expressing CD8.[72] In most cases, one or more "mature" T-cell antigens, such as CD5 or CD7, is lost. Many cases of PTCL express are EBV-positive, especially the extranodal NK/T-cell lymphomas, nasal type.[73] EBV positivity is associated with a poor prognosis.

Abnormal metaphases are seen in 90% of T-cell lymphomas. The most commonly seen translocations in peripheral T-cell lymphomas are t(7;14), t(11;14), inv(14), and t(14;14). These translocations involve genes for the T-cell receptor (TCR) at 14q11, 7q34-35, and 7p15. Young patients with ALCL have t(2;5) and less commonly t(1;2).[74] ALCL in adults generally lack t(2;5) in the tumor cells but cases with the t(2;5) have a significantly better prognosis than cases lacking the t(2;5). Hepatosplenic γ/δ T-cell lymphomas are associated with isochromosome 7q and trisomy 8.[75]

Histologically, there are uncommon subtypes of PTCL that have unique histologic features. The angioimmunoblastic T-cell lymphoma in addition to a pleomorphic heterogeneous cellular infiltrate, has increased amounts of high endothelial venules present, giving a hypervascular appearance. In this subtype, Ig heavy chains may be rearranged in 10% cases, and EBV genomes are detected in most cases and may be in either T or B cells.[76] The subcutaneous panniculitis-like T-cell lymphoma is characterized by subcutaneous nodules with cellular infiltrates in the subcutaneous fat, with generally sparing of the overlying skin. Intestinal T-cell lymphoma, often associated with gluten enteropathy, is characterized by mucosal ulceration or masses in the small bowel. The neoplastic infiltrate consists of anaplastic large cells. Often the adjacent mucosa shows changes seen in celiac disease, with villous atrophy and a lymphocytic infiltrate. These tumor cells are generally CD4–, and express CD103, which is an adhesion receptor on intestinal lymphocytes. Hepatosplenic γ/δ T-cell lymphoma is an extremely rare disease presenting with hepatosplenomegaly, often with marrow involvement and occasionally with peripheral blood involvement.[75] The tumor cells infiltrate the red pulp of the spleen and liver sinusoids. The tumor cells are CD2+, CD3+, variably CD8+, but also CD7+ and CD56+. In contrast to most PTCL, which express the α/β T-cell receptor, a unique feature of these tumors is expression of the γ/δ T-cell receptor.

Patients with PTCL have a similar median age as patients with DLBCL. However, 80% of patients with PTCL have stage III/IV disease, and more frequently have B symptoms, hepatosplenomegaly, and extranodal disease, such as the skin. PTCL generally have a worse prognosis than DLBCL.[77,78] Angioimmunoblastic T-cell lymphoma usually affects older adults who present with the acute onset of generalized lymphadenopathy, hepatosplenomegaly, skin rash, and B symptoms.[76] Immunologic abnormalities are common and include plasmacytosis polyclonal hypergammaglobulinemia, and a positive Coombs test. The median survival is 30 months. Infection is the most common cause of death, followed by the aggressive T-cell lymphoma or development of EBV-positive DLBCL.

Subcutaneous panniculitis-like T-cell lymphoma is also a rare disease that presents with subcutaneous nodules, developing into progressive disseminated disease. Many of these patients have hemophagocytic syndrome either at diagnosis or later on. Hepatosplenic γ/δ T-cell lymphoma is a highly aggressive lymphoma. It typically presents in younger males with hepatosplenomegaly, bone marrow, and peripheral blood involvement. These patients are pancytopenic and have a median survival of 1-2 years. The enteropathy type T-cell lymphomas are rare aggressive diseases that are generally associated with a history of gluten enteropathy.[79,80] These patients present with intestinal obstruction, perforation, and bleeding. In some patients, there is a brief history of gluten sensitivity or worsening gluten enteropathy. Uncommonly, there is extraintestinal disease with dissemination to the lungs or skin. These patients have a very poor prognosis, with only occasional patients cured with surgical resection.

The extranodal NK/T-cell lymphomas, nasal type are characterized by vascular invasion and extensive tissue destruction.[3,81] EBV is present in the tumor cells in virtually all cases. The tumor cells express the phenotype of natural killer cells CD2, CD56, CD45RO, CD43, but lack surface CD3 and TCR. Occasional cases are reported, which express CD4 or CD8. The extranodal NK/T-cell lymphomas, nasal type are rare, typically present in males with average age of 60. The vast majority of patients have localized disease with nasal obstruction and a destructive mass. Occasionally, the aerodigestive and gastrointestinal tracts and testis are involved. B symptoms are uncommon. Over 60% of patients with stage I disease remain in long-term remission with treatment, whereas patients with stage II to IV disease have a poor prognosis, with extranodal relapses.[82,83]

ALCL is a T-cell NHL that can have nodal, soft tissue or cutaneous involvement. When involving nodes, ALCL characteristically involves the sinusoids of lymph nodes with bizarre large cells. Neoplastic cells derived from patients with ALCL also generally express the phenotype of mature activated T cells (HLA-DR, CD30, CD25). The ALK protein (anaplastic lymphoma kinase) is detected in 40-60% of cases using the ALK1 monoclonal antibody, showing both nuclear and cytoplasmic staining in cases with the t(2; 5). ALK-positive cases are more common in children and younger adults and have a better prognosis than ALK-negative cases.[84]

ALCL constitutes 2% of all NHLs in adults, but is the second most common T-cell lymphoma. The median age of patients with ALCL is 34 with a male predominance. There is a bimodal distribution of this disease, with peaks in childhood, young adults, and late adulthood. In adults, B symptoms, peripheral and retroperitoneal adenopathies are common. Skin is a common site of extranodal disease (about 25% of patients), whereas bone marrow involvement is infrequent. The prognosis of these adult patients with systemic ALCL is similar to patients with DLBCL.[85] When ALCL, PTCL NOS, and angioimmunoblastic T-cell NHL are compared, ALCL had the highest OS, whereas angioimmunoblastic cells had the lowest, largely due to the IPI score.[86]

Highly Aggressive Lymphomas

Precursor T- or B-Lymphoblastic Leukemia/Lymphoma ■ There is a significant overlap between lymphoblastic lymphoma and acute lymphoblastic leukemia (see Chapter 112). Cytologically, lymphoblastic lymphoma cells are identical to acute lymphoblastic leukemia cells, the majority L1 morphology in the FAB classification. These cells have a high nuclear to cytoplasmic ratio, scant cytoplasm, and nuclei with fine chromatin with multiple small nucleoli, and have a high mitotic rate. The nuclei can have folds or convolutions. Typically, nodes involved with lymphoblastic lymphoma are effaced by malignant cells (Fig. 115-5).

The vast majority of lymphoblastic lymphomas are of T-cell lineage. Several investigators have noted that most T-cell lymphoblastic lymphomas correspond to stages of thymocyte differentiation. From a clinical point of view, as well as by cell surface markers, T-cell ALL and T-cell lymphoblastic lymphomas have considerable overlap. Approximately 10-15% of lymphoblastic lymphomas have a precursor B-cell phenotype.

Although lymphoblastic lymphomas represent a major subgroup of childhood NHLs, they are unusual in adults (2% of adult NHLs). Patients are usually males in their 20s or 30s who present with lymphadenopathy in cervical, supraclavicular, and axillary regions (50%) or with a mediastinal mass (50-75%). These masses can be associated with superior vena cava syndrome, tracheal obstruction, and pericardial effusions. Less commonly, patients present with extranodal disease (eg, skin, testicular, or bony involvement). More than 80% of patients present with stage III or stage IV disease, almost 50% have B symptoms, and the majority have elevated LDH. Although the bone marrow is frequently normal at presentation, virtually all patients develop bone marrow infiltration and a subsequent leukemic phase indistinguishable from T-cell acute lymphoblastic leukemia. Patients with bone marrow involvement have a very high incidence of central nervous system infiltration. B-cell lymphoblastic lymphoma is a very rare variant, affecting patients with a median age of 39.[87] B-cell lymphoblastic lymphomas present without a mediastinal mass but instead involve lymph nodes and extranodal sites.

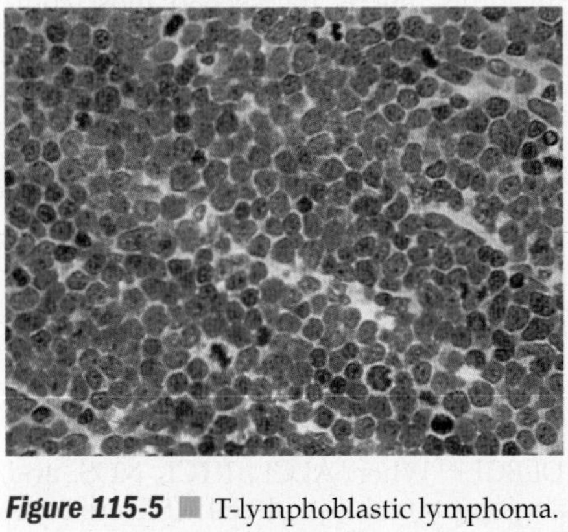

Figure 115-5 ■ T-lymphoblastic lymphoma.

Burkitt and Burkitt-Like Lymphoma ■ Burkitt lymphoma cells resemble the small noncleaved cells within normal germinal centers of secondary lymphoid follicles. Because of the high mitotic rate, frequent mitotic figures are seen and, analogous to normal germinal centers, tingible body macrophages are seen, giving the classical "starry sky" appearance. Burkitt-like lymphoma cells are more pleomorphic with fewer nucleoli. The pathologic distinction between many cases of Burkitt-like lymphoma and DLBCL remains a challenge. It is generally agreed that the fraction of Ki-67 (proliferating cells) in Burkitt-like lymphoma should be 99% or greater.[24]

Burkitt lymphoma is a tumor of B-lineage derivation identified by the expression of a variety of B-cell-restricted antigens including CD19, CD20, surface immunoglobulin M, CD10, and nuclear bcl-6 protein.[88] The endemic Burkitt lymphoma is EBV-positive, whereas the vast majority of non-endemic Burkitt lymphoma is EBV-negative. The immunophenotype of Burkitt-like lymphomas is similar to Burkitt lymphomas, although expression of CD10 and CD21 is more variable. Burkitt lymphoma cells lack bcl-2 protein, whereas Burkitt-like lymphomas are bcl-2-positive.

Burkitt lymphoma involves a translocation of chromosome 8q24 in 90% of the cases studied with either chromosome 14, 2, or 22. In contrast, the Burkitt-like lymphomas have c-myc translocations in approximately one-third of cases; dual translocations of bcl-2 and c-myc rearrangements are reported in one-third of cases, and no other abnormality is noted in the remaining one-third of cases. Pathologically identified Burkitt or atypical Burkitt had gene expression profile associated with overexpression of *myc* target genes, differential expression of normal germinal center genes, and decreased expression of MHC class I and NF-kB target genes. These studies will help refine the histologic diagnosis of difficult to classify cases.[89-91] Burkitt lymphoma is in general a pediatric tumor that has three major clinical presentations. The endemic (African) form presents as a jaw or facial bone tumor that spreads to extranodal sites including ovary, testis, kidney, breast, and especially to the bone marrow and meninges. The non-endemic form has an abdominal presentation with massive disease, ascites, renal, testis, ovarian involvement, and, like the endemic form, also spreads to the bone marrow and CNS. Immunodeficiency-related cases more often involve lymph nodes and may present as acute leukemia. Burkitt lymphoma has a male predominance and is typically seen in patients less than 35 years of age. Burkitt-like lymphoma, a rare disease, occurs in patients with a median age of 55, with a male predominance. This is an aggressive disease involving lymph nodes, the nasopharynx and gastrointestinal tract are involved as well. Occasionally Burkitt-like lymphomas presents as a solitary bone tumor. These tumors have a high propensity to invade the bone marrow and central nervous system.

Adult T-Cell Leukemia/Lymphoma ■ Adult T-cell leukemia/lymphoma (ATLL) is a highly aggressive disease that is associated with infection by the human T-cell lymphotropic virus, type 1.[92,93] ATLL is endemic in southern Japan, Caribbean basin, Africa, and the southeastern United States. These cells are neoplastic counterparts of normal activated CD4+ T cells, expressing CD2, CD3, CD5, and CD25. The median age of patients is 55. The disease can present as four variants: acute (most common), lymphomatous, chronic, and smouldering. The median survival of these variants is 6 months, 10 months, 24 months, and not reached, respectively. Patients present with BM and peripheral blood involvement, high white blood cell count, hypercalcemia (due to PTH-related protein, TGF-β, RANK ligand), lytic bone lesions, lymphadenopathy, hepatosplenomegaly, skin lesions, and interstitial pulmonary infiltrates.

Differential Diagnosis and Sites of Disease at Presentation

More than two-thirds of patients with NHL present with persistent painless peripheral lymphadenopathy. At the time of presentation, differential diagnosis of generalized lymphadenopathy necessitates the exclusion of infectious etiologies including bacteria, viruses (eg, infectious mononucleosis, cytomegalovirus, hepatitis B, and human immunodeficiency virus), and parasites (toxoplasmosis) (Table 115-3). It is generally agreed that a firm lymph node larger than 1.5 × 1.5 cm that is not associated with a documented infection and that persists longer than 4-6 weeks and that is progressing should be considered for biopsy. However, lymph nodes in several histopathologic subtypes of NHLs frequently wax and wane.

Table 115-3 ■ **Generalized Lymphadenopathy Potentially Confused With Non-Hodgkin Lymphoma**

Infectious
Bacterial (syphilis, brucellosis)
Viral (infectious mononucleosis, cytomegalovirus, human immunodeficiency virus, cat scratch fever)
Mycobacterial (tuberculosis)
Parasitic (toxoplasmosis)
Autoimmune
Systemic lupus erythematosus
Sjögren syndrome
Hydantoin derivatives
Granulomatosis
Sarcoidosis
Neoplasms
Hodgkin disease
Small cell carcinoma of the lung
Malignant histiocytosis
Melanoma
Germ cell neoplasms
Other conditions
Reactive lymphoid hyperplasia
Lymphomatoid granulomatosis
Dermatopathic lymphadenopathy
Angioimmunoblastic lymphadenopathy
Castleman disease

Table 115-4 ■ **Sites of Disease at Presentation Correlated With Working Formulation**

Disease Site	Low Grade	Intermediate Grade	High Grade
Peripheral nodes	Common	Common	Common
Abdominal nodes	Common	Less frequent	Less frequent
Mediastinal nodes	Common	Less frequent	Less frequent
Bone marrow	Common	Less frequent	Common
Liver	Common	Less frequent	Common
Spleen	Common	Less frequent	Less frequent
Extranodal	Uncommon	Common	Common

In teenagers and young adults, infectious mononucleosis and Hodgkin lymphoma should be placed high in the differential diagnosis. Involvement of Waldeyer ring, epitrochlear, and mesenteric nodes are more frequently observed in patients with NHL than Hodgkin disease. Unlike patients with Hodgkin lymphoma who frequently present with weight loss, fever, or night sweats, about 40% of all patients with NHL present with systemic complaints. B symptoms are more common in patients with aggressive histologies approaching 50%. Less frequent presenting symptoms, occurring in less than 20% of patients, include complaints such as fatigue, malaise, and pruritus.

NHLs also present with thoracic, abdominal, and/or extranodal symptoms (Table 115-4). Although much less common than with Hodgkin lymphoma, approximately 20% of patients with NHL present with mediastinal adenopathy. These patients most frequently present with persistent cough, chest discomfort, or without clinical symptoms but have an abnormal chest radiograph. Occasionally, a superior vena cava syndrome accompanies presentation. Differential diagnosis of mediastinal presentation includes infections (eg, histoplasmosis, tuberculosis, infectious mononucleosis), sarcoidosis, Hodgkin lymphoma, as well as other neoplasms. Involvement of retroperitoneal, mesenteric, and pelvic nodes is common in most histologic subtypes of NHL. Unless massive or leading to obstruction, nodal enlargement in these sites usually does not produce symptoms. In contrast, patients with an abdominal mass, massive splenomegaly, or primary gastrointestinal lymphoma present with complaints similar to those caused by other space occupying lesions. These complaints include chronic pain, abdominal fullness, and early satiety—symptoms associated with visceral obstruction, or even acute perforation and gastrointestinal hemorrhage. Rarely, patients present with symptoms of unexplained anemia. Those with aggressive NHLs can present with primary cutaneous lesions, testicular masses, acute spinal cord compression, solitary bone lesions, and rarely lymphomatous meningitis. Symptoms of primary NHL of the central nervous system include headache, lethargy, focal neurologic symptoms, seizures, and paralysis.

When NHL presents in an extranodal site, the differential diagnosis is more difficult. NHL uncommonly presents in the lung as bronchovascular, lymphangitic, nodular, or alveolar patterns of involvement.[94] Between 25% and 50% of patients with NHLs present with hepatic infiltration although relatively few present with large hepatic masses. Of the advanced stage indolent lymphomas, nearly 75% of patients have microscopic hepatic infiltration at presentation. In contrast, primary hepatic lymphoma is rare and is nearly always an aggressive histology. Primary lymphoma of bone is another extranodal site of presentation occurring in less than 5% of patients, presenting as a painful bony site. Most frequently, lytic lesions are observed on standard radiographs. The most common sites of primary lymphoma of bone include femur, pelvis, and vertebrae. Approximately 5% of NHLs present as primary gastrointestinal lymphoma. These patients present with hemorrhage, pain, or obstruction since the stomach is most frequently infiltrated followed by small intestine and colon, respectively. Most gastrointestinal lymphomas are of the diffuse aggressive histologies, specifically DLBCL, MCL, and the intestinal T-cell lymphoma. The most common site for extranodal MZLs to involve is the stomach. A subset of MCLs presents as multiple intestinal polyposis involving any sites in the gastrointestinal tract. An uncommon presentation (2-14%) of NHL is in renal infiltration, and even less common is localized presentation in the prostate, testis, or ovary. The typical histologic subtypes of these sites are DLBCL, Burkitt or Burkitt-like lymphomas. Rare sites of primary lymphoma include the orbit, heart, breast, salivary glands, thyroid, and adrenal gland.

Staging and Disease Detection

The Ann Arbor staging system developed in 1971 for Hodgkin lymphoma was adapted for staging NHLs.[95] This staging system focuses on the number of tumor sites (nodal and extranodal), location, and the presence or absence of systemic symptoms. Table 115-5 summarizes the essential features of the Ann Arbor system. Because NHLs most frequently disseminate hematogenously, this staging system has proven to be much less useful than for Hodgkin lymphoma.

The concept of staging has less impact in NHL than in Hodgkin lymphoma. Only 10% of patients with FL have localized disease at diagnosis and the majority of patients with aggressive lymphomas have advanced stage disease. There is little therapeutic benefit to distinguishing between stage III and stage IV disease,

Table 115-5 ■ **Ann Arbor Staging System for Non-Hodgkin Lymphoma**

Stage I	Involvement of a single lymph node region or of a single extranodal organ or site (IE)
Stage II	Involvement of two or more lymph node regions on the same side of the diaphragm, or localized involvement of an extranodal site or organ (IIE) and one or more lymph node regions on the same side of the diaphragm
Stage III	Involvement of lymph node regions on both sides of the diaphragm, which may also be accompanied by localized involvement of an extranodal organ or site (IIIE) of spleen (IIIS) or both (IIISE)
Stage IV	Diffuse or disseminated involvement of one or more distant extranodal sites. Fever >38°C, night sweats, weight loss >10% of body weight in 6 months preceding admission are defined as systemic symptoms and denoted by the suffix B. Other patients are denoted by the suffix A

since the treatment options are identical. Multiple studies have demonstrated that prognosis is more dependent on histology and clinical parameters than stage at presentation. Staging is undertaken in NHLs to identify the small number of patients who can be treated with local therapy or combined modality treatment and to stratify within histologic subtypes to determine prognosis and assess the impact of treatment.

Diagnosis and Initial Evaluation

Staging must be undertaken in the context of the histology. After the initial biopsy, blood tests should be obtained, including complete blood count, routine chemistries, liver function tests, and serum protein electrophoresis to document the presence of circulating monoclonal paraproteins. The serum beta-2 microglobulin level is useful in patients with indolent lymphomas, for prognostic purposes, as a surrogate measure of disease volume, and for monitoring response to therapy. Serum concentrations of LDH are an important independent predictor of survival in NHL. Isolated Waldeyer ring involvement is associated with intestinal involvement in 20% of cases and endoscopy should be considered. Chest, abdominal, pelvic computed tomography scan is essential for accurate staging to assess lymphadenopathy. Unilateral bone marrow biopsies should be performed, since the likelihood of lymphomatous involvement of the marrow is relatively high, especially in most indolent lymphomas where marrow involvement occurs in most cases. In patients with aggressive lymphomas with marrow involvement, paranasal sinus involvement, paraspinal masses, testicular or if clinically indicated, examination of the cerebral spinal fluid (CSF) by lumbar puncture should be performed. Radionuclide scans have clinical utility as diagnostic and monitoring studies. Gallium scans are positive in virtually all of the aggressive lymphomas and in about 50% of indolent lymphomas, but gallium scanning has been largely superceded by positron emission tomography (PET) using 18F-fluorodeoxyglucose. FDG PET scanning is a highly sensitive and specific scanning modality for detecting NHL in both nodal and extranodal sites. PET scanning is very useful for DLBCL, mantle cell lymphoma, and follicular lymphoma, not as sensitive for PTCL and MZL.[96] The intensity of 18F-FDG uptake or SUV correlates with histologic aggressiveness.[97,98] PET scanning detects actively metabolizing tumor in residual masses following or during chemotherapy, and that persistent abnormal uptake predicts for early relapse and/or reduced survival.[99]

Recently an International Harmonization Project has provided consensus recommendations for PET scanning. Among the recommendations are: PET can only be used for DLBCL and HL; scanning during therapy can be only part of clinical trials; and the scan after all therapy is completed can be done at least three but preferably 6–8 weeks after chemotherapy and 8–12 weeks after radiation or chemoradiotherapy. There is no evidence that long-term follow-up should include PET scanning.[100] Magnetic resonance imaging is most valuable for evaluation of the brain and spinal cord.

Immunologic and Molecular Studies

Biologic studies including cell surface markers, cytogenetics, and molecular techniques are used in diagnosis, staging, and minimal disease detection. Monoclonal antibodies directed against cell surface antigens expressed on lymphoid cells, and molecular techniques to define immunoglobulin and T-cell receptor gene rearrangements are sensitive tools with which to assess tumor cell infiltration. Immunophenotypic and cytogenetic studies can help to determine histologic subtypes of lymphomas. For those NHLs with known chromosomal translocations, it is possible to identify unique chromosomal breakpoints that can be studied with fluorescent in situ hybridization (FISH), cytogenetics, and polymerase chain reaction (PCR). For example, PCR can be used to detect the t(14;18) of FLs.[101] With this approach, one tumor cell in 10^5-10^6 cells can be detected. Studies of minimal disease are providing important insights into whether patients are in molecular remission and whether further therapy is required.

Disease Parameters That Influence Prognosis and Assessment of Disease Response

Clinical Prognostic Factors in Aggressive NHL

The analysis of a large group (2031 patients) with diffuse aggressive NHLs treated with an anthracycline containing regimen led to the establishment of a prognostic model of predicting outcome known as the International Prognostic Index (IPI) (Table 115-6).[102] Of a large number of factors examined for all patients, age (≤60 vs >60); serum LDH (≤normal vs >normal); performance status (0 or 1 vs 2–4); stage (I or II vs III or IV); and extranodal involvement (≤site vs

Table 115-6 The International Index and Age-Adjusted Index

Risk Group	Risk Factors	Distribution of Cases (%)	CR Rate	RFS of CRs (%) 2-Year Rate	RFS of CRs (%) 5-Year Rate	Survival (%) 2-Year Rate	Survival (%) 5-Year Rate
International index (patients of all ages)							
Low (L)	0.1	35	87	79	70	84	73
Low-intermediate (LI)	2	27	67	66	50	66	51
High-intermediate (HI)	3	22	55	59	49	54	43
High (H)	4.5	16	44	58	40	34	26
Age-adjusted index applied to patients <60 years of age							
Low (L)	0	22	92	88	86	90	83
Low-intermediate (LI)	1	32	78	74	66	79	69
High-intermediate (HI)	2	32	57	62	53	59	46
High (H)	3	14	46	61	58	37	32
Age-adjusted index applied to patients >60 years of age							
Low (L)	0	18	91	75	46	80	56
Low-intermediate (LI)	1	31	71	64	45	68	44
High-intermediate (HI)	2	35	56	60	41	48	37
High (H)	3	16	36	47	37	31	21

Abbreviation: RFS of tcf, relapse-free survival of patients who sustained complete remission.

>1 site) were independently prognostic for overall survival. These data permitted the identification of four risk groups based on the number of risk factors: low-risk with 0 or 1 factor; low-intermediate with two factors; high-intermediate with three factors; and high with four or five factors. The 5-year overall survival rates for patients with scores of 0 to 1, 2, 3, and 4 to 5 were 73%, 51%, 43%, and 26%, respectively. For the patients aged 60 or less, only stage, LDH, and performance status were of prognostic significance. Patients ≤60 with 0, 1, 2, or 3 risk factors had 5-year survival rates of 83, 69, 46, and 32%, respectively. Survival rates for those >60 with the same scores were 56, 44, 37, and 21%, respectively.

The IPI has been adapted following treatment with rituximab plus CHOP therapy for DLBCL. Within that model, the 4-year progression-free survival is 94%, 80%, and 53% for 0 and 1, 2, or 3 or more risk factors, respectively.[103]

The IPI has been modified for patients with stage I or II aggressive NHLs[77] with age >60, LDH, stage II and performance status ≥2 being significant factors. When this was applied to patients treated with three courses of cyclophosphamide, adriamycin, vincristine, and prednisone (CHOP), plus involved region radiation therapy, the 10-year overall survival rates for patients with 0, 1 or 2, and 3 or 4 factors were 90%, 56%, and 40% respectively.[104]

Clinical Prognostic Factors in Indolent NHL

A predictive model based on over 4000 patients with follicular NHL has been developed, known as the follicular lymphoma IPI or FLIPI. This study identified the following prognostic factors: age >60; stage III/IV, more than four nodal sites; elevated serum LDH concentration; and hemoglobin less than 12. The 10-year survival rates for patients with zero to one (low-risk), two (intermediate-risk), or three or more (high-risk) of these adverse factors averaged 71%, 51%, and 36%, respectively (Table 115-7).[105] Analogous to DLBCL, rituximab therapy has improved outcome for patients with follicular NHL. The FLIPI remains clinically relevant with this improvement in therapy.[106]

Gene Expression Profiling

Gene expression profiling using DNA microarrays has been used to examine DLBCL with one goal of identifying patients with different prognoses.[58-60,107] Based on gene expression, DLBCLs have been subclassified into "germinal center" or "activated" B-cell types. Patients with germinal center B-like DLBCL had significantly better overall survival than those with the activated B-like variant. There is a suggestion that with rituximab added to chemotherapy, that the significance of cell of origin on prognosis in DLBCL may be less important than the IPI.[108]

Based on finding from gene expression profiling, immunohistochemistry using tissue microarrays has been used for a limited number of gene products as prognostic markers.[107] Germinal center and non-germinal center B-cell derivation can be determined by expression of CD10 and bcl-6, and MUM1. Using tissue microarrays, 42% of DLBCLs are considered germinal center B-cell derivation and 58% are non-germinal center B-cell derivation.

In FL, gene expression profiling has been examined in pretreatment tissue and correlated with survival. This study has shown that genes associated with the nonmalignant cell infiltrate segregate patients into subgroups with favorable and unfavorable prognoses. Immune response 1 signature (gene associated with certain T-cell and macrophage markers) was favorable, whereas immune response 2 signature (genes highly expressed in macrophages) was unfavorable.[109]

Table 115-7 ■ **Follicular Lymphoma International Prognostic Index**

Risk Group	No. Risk Factors	5-Year Survival%	10-Year Survival
Low	0 or 1	97	71
Intermediate	2	78	51
High	3, 4, 5	52	36

Cell Surface Phenotype

With IPI stratification, PTCL patients generally have worse prognoses than DLBCL. More recently, a modification of the IPI was reported for patients with PTCL (not otherwise specified).[110] In this model, four prognostic factors were identified: age >60; PS >1; LDH greater than normal; and bone marrow involvement. The 10-year overall survivals for patients with 0, 1, 2, and 3 or 4 risk factors were 50%, 32%, 30%, and 9%, respectively. Patients with DLBCL whose tumors do not express HLA-DR had a significantly shorter survival duration compared to HLA-DR-positive patients. The HLA-DR-negative cases had fewer CD8+ T cells infiltrating the tumor tissue. A multivariate analysis, adjusting for prognostic factors of known clinical significance, confirmed the importance of the expression of HLA-DR as a prognostic factor.[111]

Therapeutic Approaches According to WHO Classification

Indolent Lymphomas

Therapy of Early Stage Indolent Lymphoma ■ Patients having localized indolent lymphoma should be treated with local radiotherapy with curative intent. However, the majority of patients with indolent NHL present with advanced disease. Only 10-20% of patients have clinical stage I/II disease and less than 10% have pathologic stage I/II. In a study of 177 patients from Stanford, 44% of patients had stage I and 56% had stage II disease.[112] Patients were treated with either involved field, extended field, with a limited number receiving total lymphoid irradiation. Survival rates at 10, 15, and 20 years were 64%, 44%, and 35%, respectively. The relapse-free survival rates at 10, 15, and 20 years were 44%, 40%, and 37%, respectively. The freedom from recurrence was significantly better for patients under age 60, and for patients who received radiation to both sides of the diaphragm (although there was no difference in overall survival). This analysis has been extended to outcome after relapse.[113] Most patients (76%) had stage I/II disease at relapse. Actuarial survival rates 5, 10, 15, and 20 years after relapse were 56%, 35%, 17%, and 17%, respectively. The progression-free survival rate for the entire group at 5 years was 44%, and remained at 22% 10, 15, and 20 years following relapse. The development of second solid tumors had been noted in 17% of the patients treated with extensive radiotherapy, whereas the incidence of second solid tumors was 6.8% in patients who received involved- or extended-field radiation. Several studies have employed local radiotherapy with adjuvant chemotherapy, and there appears to be no significant advantage of combined modality over local radiotherapy.

The extranodal MZLs often present with localized disease involving the gastrointestinal tract, salivary glands, thyroid, orbit, conjunctiva, breast, and lung. Since many cases of gastric MZL appear to be a B-cell clonal expansion in response to *H. pylori*, treatment has been directed at the chronic gastritis. Therapy with antibiotics (metronidazole, amoxicillin, clarithromycin) and a proton pump inhibitor induce regression of superficial low-grade MZL of the stomach in over 80% of patients. The long-term remission status of these patients remains uncertain. The presence of bcl-10 nuclear expression and/or t(11;18) may be useful to prospectively identify those patients with gastric MZL lymphomas who do not benefit from anti-*H. pylori* treatment.[114] Non-gastric MZLs have been also associated with *H. pylori*; however in contrast to gastric MZL, therapy directed at *H. pylori* is generally ineffective.[115] Antibiotic therapy (doxycycline) against *Chlamydophila* has been reported with variable results in ocular MZLs.[8] For patients with localized disease who progress after antibiotic therapy or are *H. pylori*-negative, involved-field radiotherapy with or without surgical resection has a 10-year disease-free survival of over 90%.[116,117] For other sites of extranodal MZL, since these diseases tend to remain localized for long periods of time prior to systemic spread, surgery remains a highly effective approach, often with adjuvant involved-field radiotherapy. In a retrospective study of patients with stage IE or IIE MZL, most were treated with involved-field radiation therapy alone.[118] The 5-year disease-free and overall survival for the entire group was 76% and 96%, respectively. Patients with gastric and thyroid disease had 5-year disease-free survival of 93%, whereas disease-free survival for other sites of involvement was 69% ($p = .006$). The response rate for chemotherapy with alkylating agents, fludarabine or rituximab alone, for MZL is high.[119,120]

Treatment of Advanced Stage Indolent NHL ■ Asymptomatic patients with low-volume disease can be monitored closely without active therapy. The long natural history of indolent NHLs and the lack of symptoms in some patients at diagnosis have fostered close observation as the initial approach to many of these patients. Moreover, spontaneous remissions of longer than 1 year have been reported in 23% of patients, making treatment unnecessary in this subgroup of patients.[30] In studies from Stanford and the British National Lymphoma Investigation[121] where asymptomatic patients were randomized either to initial therapy or to deferred treatment until the time of symptoms (usually progressive bulky disease), there was no difference in the actuarial survival between the two groups. In the Stanford study, the median time until therapy was needed was 3 years.[122]

The initial treatment of choice for patients with indolent NHL who are not eligible for clinical trials has historically included either alkylating-based regimens (single agent or combinations such as cyclophosphamide, vincristine, and prednisone) or purine analogs such as fludarabine. Although more aggressive regimens such as CHOP have been used in the initial treatment of FL, there is no evidence that a superior response rate or duration of remission is seen as compared to CVP.[123] Other randomized trials have looked at the impact of combination chemotherapy in patients with advanced FL. CHOP with bleomycin was compared to cyclophosphamide alone in patients with FL. There was no difference in disease-free survival or overall survival for the entire population or the grade I FL patients, but there was a survival advantage for the patients with FL grade II.[124] Fludarabine-based regimens are highly effective, but not superior to CVP in terms of remission duration or overall survival.[125]

The treatment paradigm for treating advanced stage FL has changed with the use of the anti-CD20 monoclonal antibody, rituximab. Phase III randomized trials have demonstrated a significant improvement in outcome by combining chemotherapy regimens with the anti-CD20 monoclonal antibody rituximab. This has been the major innovation in treating these diseases in the past three decades. In an international study of 321 patients randomized to CVP or rituximab plus CVP, the overall (81% vs 57%) and complete (41% vs 10%) response rates were higher in the CVP-R treatment arm.[126] At a median follow-up of 30 months, the median times to progression (32 vs 15 months) and treatment failure (27 vs 7 months) were significantly longer in the CVP-R arm. A nonstatistically significant increase in overall survival was seen. Similar findings were observed by the German Low Grade Lymphoma Group where rituximab was combined with CHOP and compared to CHOP alone with improvement in both remission duration and overall survival.[127] Another study using mitoxantrone, chlorambucil, and prednisolone with or without rituximab, saw similar improvement in RR, PFS, and a statistically significant improvement in overall survival.[128] The efficacy of rituximab maintenance in patients with advanced stage FL following initial induction with chemotherapy plus rituximab is uncertain at present.

Phase II trials have employed rituximab alone as initial therapy in patients with indolent lymphoma with overall response rates of 54–73%.[129-132] At a median follow-up of 30 months, median progression-free survival was 34 months in one of the trials. Moreover extended treatment with rituximab increased PFS compared to observation.[132] Longer-term follow-up of these studies is necessary before rituximab alone can be recommended as initial therapy. Radioimmunotherapy has been studied in a limited fashion in previously untreated patients with FL. The overall response rate and CR rate of 131-I tositumomab were 95% and 75%, respectively and a 5-year progression-free survival of 59% in treatment naïve patients.[133]

Following relapse, these indolent lymphomas continue to be sensitive to single agents and combination chemotherapy; but the median relapse-free survival progressively decreases with each subsequent relapse. A randomized trial compared fludarabine to CVP in previously treated patients with FL. Although the response rates (62% vs 52%) and 2-year overall survival (70% vs 75%) were similar, 2-year progression-free survival was significantly improved with fludarabine (32% vs 14%).[134] Single agent rituximab has a 50-60% response rate, with 6% CR, in patients with previously treated FL.[135] In small lymphocytic lymphoma the response rate is only about 10%. The median duration of responses is about 11 months. A phase II trial studied the safety and efficacy of retreatment with rituximab in patients with relapsed indolent NHL all of whom had previously responded to rituximab.[136] The overall response rate was 40%, with 11% complete remissions and the estimated median time to progression after treatment was 18 months. Rituximab has been combined with other agents (eg, fludarabine, CVP, CHOP), with encouraging results in patients with relapsed/resistant disease. An international randomized phase III study evaluated the role of rituximab in induction as well as maintenance therapy in relapsed FL patients who had not previously received an anthracycline or rituximab.[137] Patients received six cycles of CHOP or CHOP-R. Those pateints who achieved complete or partial remission underwent a second randomization to maintenance rituximab (375 mg/m^2 IV once every 3 months) for a maximum of 2 years or observation. The overall (85% vs 72%) and complete (30% vs 16%) remission rates were significantly higher for CHOP-R than for CHOP. The median progression-free survival from first randomization was significantly longer after CHOP-R than after CHOP (33 vs 20 months). The median progression-free survival from the time of second randomization was longer for those receiving rituximab maintenance (52 vs 15 months), both after induction with CHOP or CHOP-R. Moreover, maintenance rituximab, as compared with observation, also significantly improved 3-year overall survival (85% vs 77%). Since patients with relapsed FL who have not had prior treatment with rituximab are becoming uncommon, it is unclear whether data from this study can be extrapolated to relapsed patients with FL receiving CHOP-R as their initial induction therapy.

Radioimmunoconjugates are FDA-approved therapies for patients with relapsed follicular NHL. 131-I tositumomab is a murine anti-CD20 mAb conjugated to 131-I. The overall response rate in previously treated patients was 65% with 20% CRs.[138] The median duration of remission had not been reached by 47 months. A murine anti-CD20 antibody conjugated to 90-yttrium, ibritumomab, has an 82% response rate with 26% CR, and median duration of response of greater than 12 months in patients with relapsed disease.[139] In a phase III study of 143 patients with relapsed or refractory low-grade, follicular, or transformed CD20+ NHL, patients were randomized to receive either rituximab or rituximab plus 90-yttrium ibritumomab tiuxetan.[140]

The overall response rates to rituximab or the rituximab 90-yttrium ibritumomab tiuxetan combination were 56% and 80%, respectively. Radioimmunotherapy following chemotherapy has been investigated in previously untreated patients with FL. Patients with advanced stage FL were treated with six cycles of CHOP followed 4–8 weeks later with 131-I tositumomab. At a median follow-up of 5.1 years, estimated PFS and OS were 67% and 87%, respectively.[141] The precise role for radioimmunotherapy in the treatment paradigm of indolent lymphoma continues to be evaluated in randomized trials.

Allogeneic stem cell transplantation in relapsed FL. In 176 patients with FL, 67% of whom had chemosensitive disease at the time of transplantation, estimates of treatment-related mortality, recurrence rates, and overall survival at 5 years following allogeneic bone marrow transplantation were 30%, 21%, and 51%, respectively. During this same period, 597 patients with FL received unpurged autologous transplantation; 82% were chemosensitive at the time of transplant. The estimates of treatment-related mortality, recurrence rates, and overall survival at 5 years following unpurged autologous bone marrow transplantation were 8%, 58%, and 55%, respectively.[142] In an effort to have lower treatment-related mortality and to exploit the graft versus lymphoma effect of allogeneic transplantation, non-myeloablative allogeneic transplants are being actively studied in indolent NHLs, with encouraging results to date. Non-relapse mortality is about 15-25%, with progression-free survival approximately 60-70%.[143]

Autologous Stem Cell Transplantation for Relapsed Indolent NHL ■ Long-term follow-up of phase II studies suggest that a subset of patients with relapsed FL, with chemosensitive disease, who undergo high-dose therapy and ASCT are long-term survivors with disease-free survival of 48% at 12 years.[144] A randomized trial compared conventional chemotherapy to autologous stem cell transplantation with purged or unpurged bone marrow, referred to as the European CUP trial.[145] In this study, 89 patients with relapsed or progressive FL received three cycles of CHOP. Those patients who achieved a CR or PR, and had less than 20% bone marrow involvement with FL, were randomized to three further cycles of CHOP chemotherapy or to high-dose therapy and autologous stem cell support with anti-B cell antibody purging or high-dose therapy and autologous stem cell support without purging. At a median follow-up of 69 months, the overall 5-year survival for all registered patients was 50%, but the median survival had not yet been reached for the subset of patients treated with high-dose therapy and autologous stem cell transplantation (either purged or unpurged). Both progression-free and overall survival favored the transplantation arms, but there was no difference between those patients receiving a purged autograft and those receiving an unmanipulated graft.

Histologic Transformation ■ The prognosis for patients following histologic transformation of indolent NHL is generally poor.[32] The median survival of a large series of patients with follicular NHL undergoing histologic conversion was 11 months.[34] In a report from Stanford, the median survival for the entire group of patients was only 22 months, except for patients who achieved a CR with treatment who had an actuarial survival of 75% at 5 years.[35] There have been several reports of ASCT in patients with chemosensitive disease and a good performance status after histologic transformation for FL. In the series from Dana-Farber Cancer Institute, where 21 patients have undergone anti-B-cell purged autologous bone marrow transplantation for transformed FL, the estimate of the percentage of patients alive and disease-free at 5 years is 46%, with follow-up from 12 to 120+ months.[146] When pathology at relapse was available, all patients recurred with DLBCL. Similar results were reported from St. Bartholomew's Hospital, Stanford University, and the European Bone Marrow Transplant Registry.[147-150] Aggressive therapy with ASCT is a reasonable treatment option for selected patients who have chemosensitive disease.

Aggressive Lymphomas

The aggressive lymphomas within the WHO classification include diffuse large B cell; MCL; the peripheral T-cell lymphomas (nonspecified and the specific subtypes); anaplastic large-cell lymphoma; MCL; and FL grade III (follicular large cell) (Table 115-2).

Therapy of Early Stage Aggressive Lymphoma ■ Less than 20% of patients with diffuse large-cell lymphoma have truly localized disease. The recommended treatment for localized disease outside of clinical trials is abbreviated, combination chemotherapy plus involved-field radiotherapy, or combination chemotherapy alone. The benefit of adding radiotherapy to six to eight cycles of chemotherapy is of unclear survival benefit. The SWOG randomized trial of patients with localized diffuse aggressive lymphoma compared eight cycles of CHOP to three cycles of CHOP plus involved-field radiotherapy.[104] Patients treated with three cycles of CHOP plus radiotherapy had a significantly better 5-year progression-free survival and overall survival than patients treated with eight cycles of CHOP (77% vs 64% for progression-free survival, 82% vs 72% for overall survival). Overall, life-threatening toxicity and cardiac toxicity were significantly higher in the patients receiving CHOP alone. The benefit of attenuated chemotherapy was largely found in patients over the age of 60. Another randomized trial compared eight courses of CHOP with or without involved-field radiotherapy in patients with previously untreated bulky or extranodal stage I or stage II diffuse aggressive NHL. The disease-free survival was greater for CR patients who received radiotherapy (73% vs 56%) although 10-year overall survival was similar in the two treatment arms (68% vs 65%).[151] The role of radiation therapy remains uncertain in some patients with stage I or II disease. In patients aged 60 or less with low-risk disease, an aggressive regimen (ACVBP) was superior to CHOP plus radiation.[152] Similarly, in patients over age 60, the addition of radiation therapy did not improve disease-free or overall survival for patients who received four cycles of CHOP alone.[153] These studies raise the question of the necessity of radiotherapy for patients with early stage disease. The role of rituximab in early stage disease has not been studied in phase III trials.

Therapy of Advanced Stage Aggressive Lymphoma ■ The current recommendation for treatment of advanced stage DLBLC or PTCL if a clinical trial is not available is combination chemotherapy with CHOP plus rituximab or CHOP, respectively for both patients under age 60 as well as over age 60. A major question in recent clinical trials has been the number of cycles and the interval for those cycles. In patients with DLBCL ages 60-80, the GELA group reported that eight cycles of CHOP plus rituximab was superior to CHOP alone in terms of PFS, DFS, and overall survival with no added toxicity.[154,155] A United States Intergroup study compared in a similar population, administering CHOP or CHOP plus rituximab given on a different schedule.[156] Responding patients were randomly assigned to receive either rituximab maintenance therapy or no maintenance. A beneficial impact of rituximab added to CHOP chemotherapy on event-free and overall survival was observed; however, no benefit was seen for maintenance rituximab following CHOP plus rituximab induction. Similarly, in patients less than 60, CHOP-R with IPI of 0 and 1, the addition of rituximab to CHOP improved time to treatment failure and overall survival. This benefit was greater in the patients with an IPI of 1.[157]

The number of cycles of therapy has been examined in the RICOVER trial, in patients over age 60. This study compared six to eight cycles of CHOP or CHOP plus rituximab administered every 14 days. R-CHOP was superior to CHOP given for six or eight cycles (70% vs 57%) and there was no benefit of eight cycles of CHOP-R over six cycles.[158] It remains undetermined whether CHOP plus rituximab administered every 3 weeks for six or eight cycles compared to CHOP-R[14] given for six cycles.

For PTCL, similar treatment approaches to DLBCL have been taken for patients with localized and advanced stage disease. When patients are stratified by the IPI, the disease-free survival and overall survival is generally inferior for patients with PTCL than for patients with DLBCL. There is presently no evidence to support superiority of different treatment regimens for PTCL.[159] ALCL has the most favorable prognosis of the T-cell lymphomas.[86] The prognosis for patients who express the ALK protein is particularly favorable with 5-year overall survival of 79%.[84] For patients with NK/T nasal type T-cell lymphoma with stage IE/IIE disease, radiotherapy is central to optimal treatment, and the role of combined modality therapy is controversial.[160]

Autologous Stem Cell Transplantation for NHL in First Remission ■ Several studies have examined the role of high-dose therapy and autologous stem cell transplantation (ASCT) in first CR/PR for patients with aggressive NHL, and to date no definitive recommendation can be made. ASCT following abbreviated induction therapy generally does not improve outcome when compared to standard induction. The LNH93-3 study included patients younger than 60 years with high-intermediate/high-risk IPI scores who were then randomized to ACVBP plus consolidation or three cycles of dose-escalated cyclophosphamide, epirubicin, vindesine, bleomycin, and prednisone followed by BCNU, etoposide, cytarabine, cyclophosphamide, and ASCT. CR rates were not different between the two treatment arms. The 5-year overall survival and event-free survival rates for ACVBP and ASCT were 60% and 46% ($p = .007$) and 52% and 39% ($p = .01$), respectively.[161] In contrast, ASCT after full or very intensive induction may improve outcome for selected patients. Patients with aggressive NHL who obtained a CR with standard therapy were randomly assigned to receive either consolidative sequential therapy (ifosfamide, etoposide, asparaginase, and cytarabine) or high-dose chemotherapy with ASCT. A superior, durable, DFS was observed only in the subgroup of higher-risk patients who underwent ASCT.[162] A GOELAMS study of CHOP for eight cycles versus intensive combination chemotherapy induction followed by consolidation then high-dose BCNU, etoposide, cytarabine, melphalan, and ASCT, found event-free survival at 5 years, was 46% vs 63% ($p = .037$), respectively, but no difference in OS (56% vs 71%). Only patients with high-intermediate IPI, but not low or low-intermediate, had significantly higher event-free and overall survival with high-dose therapy.[163] The overall benefit of autologous stem cell transplant in first remission for patients with diffuse aggressive lymphomas remains uncertain despite many randomized trials. Given the generally inferior prognosis of patients with PTCL, autologous SCT has been investigated in first remission. There are reports of patients with enteropathic T-cell lymphoma and angioimmunoblastic T-cell lymphoma undergoing autologous stem cell transplantation in first remission with encouraging results.[164,165]

FL Grade III (Follicular Large Cell) ■ A subset of patients with follicular large-cell lymphoma have disease that behaves clinically similar to diffuse large-cell lymphoma.[37,38] It is generally agreed that these patients should be treated with aggressive combination chemotherapy, with complete remission rates of about 80% and 50%, and overall survival of approximately 70% and 60% for stage I/II and III/IV patients, respectively.[37] A study of 100 patients with follicular large-cell lymphoma from a single institution supported this strategy, suggesting prolonged disease-free survival, and an overall favorable prognosis.[38]

Mantle Cell Lymphomas (MCL) ■ The median survival of patients with MCL is 3-4 years. The treatment of MCL generally involves alkylating agents to which 30-50% of patients will have a CR, with median duration of 1-3 years.[52] Generally, single alkylating agents offer similar results as combination chemotherapy.[166] In the randomized German Low Grade Lymphoma Group trial, CHOP plus rituximab had an overall response rate of 94% with CR rate of 34%. In contrast, CHOP alone had overall response rates of 75% and CR rates of 7%.[167] A recent meta-analysis of three studies of chemotherapy versus rituximab with chemotherapy, there was improved disease control, and nonsignificant improvement in OS.[168] Autologous transplant for patients less than 65, in first CR or PR, has shown improvement in PFS as compared to interferon-α maintenance, but a nonstatistically significant improvement in overall survival.[169]

The HyperCVAD regimen, with escalated doses of cyclophosphamide, high-dose methotrexate and cytarabine has a very high response rate (38% CR).[170] In this report, all patients went on to either autologous or allogeneic stem cell transplantation. The results for previously untreated patients was encouraging with 5-year disease-free survival of 43%, with overall survival of 73%.

High-Grade Lymphomas

Lymphoblastic, Burkitt, and Burkitt-Like Lymphomas ■ The treatment of lymphoblastic lymphoma is detailed in Chapter 112: Acute Lymphoblastic Leukemia.

The Burkitt and Burkitt-like lymphomas in human immunodeficiency virus-1-negative adults have been similarly treated with regimens designed for the pediatric populations with 2-year EFS and OS of 65% and 70%, respectively.[171] Using the Magrath regimen (CODoxM for low-risk patients, or CODoxM/IVAC for high-risk patients), the event-free survival was 92% at 2 years in 39 adults.[172] A study of 14 patients with median age of 47 reported 64% of patients disease-free at 29 months with a similar intensive regimen.[173] There is presently no evidence that first remission autologous transplant is indicated for adult Burkitt lymphoma.[174]

Adult T-cell leukemia/lymphoma are approached with intensive multiagent chemotherapy regimens.[175] Overall response rate was reported to be 81%, but the median survival was 13 months, with estimated 2- and 4-year survivals of 31% and 21%, respectively. Although the results of treatment have been poor, recently a very aggressive multiagent regimen has been shown to have an improved outcome when compared to CHOP.[176] Antiretroviral therapy has been reported but follow-up has been lacking.[177] Similarly, conventional and nonmyeloablative allogeneic stem cell transplants have shown limited success in this disease.[178]

Treatment of Recurrent Aggressive NHL

Following relapse, at least 50% of patients' disease remain sensitive to conventional treatment, but less than 10% of patients with aggressive NHL experience prolonged disease-free survival with second-line treatment regimens, and essentially all patients with indolent disease relapse. Following relapse, the current curative approach for patients with relapsed NHL involves high-dose therapy and stem cell transplantation.

Conventional Salvage Therapy ■ The vast majority of patients with relapsed or refractory NHL have limited benefit from conventional salvage regimens. A number of regimens have been developed for patients with relapsed, aggressive NHL.[179-181] The response rates for these salvage regimens have ranged from 20%

to 77% with 20-30% CRs reported. The duration of these responses and overall survival of these patients is about 6 months. Although a higher response is seen in indolent NHLs, the response rate of patients with relapsed aggressive NHL to single agent rituximab is 37% (9% CR) and the median duration is 8 months.[182] In relapsed mantle cell lymphoma, fludarabine-based regimens have response rates of about 60%, improved by combining rituximab, and further improved for selected patients with maintenance rituximab.[183] Bortezomib is active single agent in relapsed MCL, with a 33% response rate.[184]

Allogeneic Bone Marrow Transplantation in NHL ■ Allogeneic stem cell transplantation has been applied to patients with relapsed and refractory NHL. Nearly all patients had relapsed disease, many of whom were resistant to conventional dose therapy. In the European Bone Marrow Transplant registry, the recurrence rate after allogeneic transplantation for aggressive NHL was lower than autologous transplantation but there was no difference in OS, due to higher transplant-related mortality with allogeneic transplantation.[185] The EFS and OS at 5 years was 43%, with treatment-related mortality 25% at 1 year. Patients who underwent allogeneic transplant following lymphoma relapse less than 12 m after initial chemo had a significantly higher risk of relapse following transplant.[186] Non-myeloablative transplants have been performed in patients with aggressive NHL; most patients had a prior autologous transplant, with the 2-year event-free survival only 17%.[187]

Autologous Stem Cell Transplantation for Relapsed Aggressive NHL ■ The disease sensitivity at the time of ASCT has remained the most significant prognostic variable for predicting treatment outcome.[188] Several large series have shown that patients who undergo ASCT when the disease is resistant to the initial induction therapy have less than 10% probability of disease-free survival. Those relapsed patients whose disease remains sensitive to chemotherapy have a 30-60% probability of long-term disease-free survival. In contrast, only 10-15% of patients with resistant disease are long-term survivors.

ASCT has been compared to conventional salvage therapy for relapsed aggressive NHL in a multicenter trial known as the PARMA trial.[189] Patients with relapsed aggressive NHL (largely DLBCL) received two cycles of cisplatin, cytarabine, solumedrol, and if responsive, were randomized to continued chemotherapy for four additional cycles or high-dose chemotherapy and autologous bone marrow transplantation. With median follow-up in excess of 5 years, patients randomized to the high-dose arm had superior event-free survival (46% vs 12%) and overall survival (53% vs 32%).

New Therapeutic Approaches for NHL

Significant improvements have been made in the treatment of NHL, with the major impact in B-cell malignancies, largely due to monoclonal antibody therapy. However the majority of patients are not cured, and less progress has occurred in therapy of many disease entities, such as peripheral T-cell lymphoma and mantle cell lymphoma. There are a vast number of new agents that are undergoing evaluation many of which go under the auspices of rational targets. These include new monoclonal antibodies focused on antigens besides CD20, improved antibodies with enhanced cytotoxicity. Several small molecules developed to antagonize bcl-2, kinases, or pathways involved in cell survival are also in clinical trials. Further ways to enhance host immunity against the patient's own tumor cells have involved vaccination studies with the immunoglobulin idiotype to induce specific immunotherapy against residual tumor cells. Several randomized trials will provide important insights as to whether this will be a useful adjunct to treatment. The most significant advance is our understanding of the genetic events and pathways that are aberrant in lymphoma cells as compared to normal cells, and the differences that have been recognized within histologic subtypes of lymphomas. Novel targets may potentially be identified which are more specific to the neoplastic event and less toxic to normal cells.

Selected References

The complete reference list can be found at www.CANCERMEDICINE8.com

10. Goodlad JR, Davidson MM, Hollowood K, et al. *Borrelia burgdorferi*-associated cutaneous marginal zone lymphoma: a clinicopathological study of two cases illustrating the temporal progression of B. burgdorferi-associated B-cell proliferation in the skin. *Histopathology.* 2000;37:501–508.
24. Harris NL, Jaffe ES, Diebold J, et al. World Health Organization classification of neoplastic diseases of the hematopoietic and lymphoid tissues: report of the Clinical Advisory Committee meeting-Airlie House, Virginia, November 1997. *J Clin Oncol.* 1999;17:3835–3849.
25. Staudt LM. A closer look at follicular lymphoma. *N Engl J Med.* 2007;356:741–742.
28. Armitage JO, Weisenburger DD. New approach to classifying non-Hodgkin's lymphomas: clinical features of the major histologic subtypes. Non-Hodgkin's Lymphoma Classification Project. *J Clin Oncol.* 1998;16:2780–2795.
29. Willemze R, Jaffe ES, Burg G, et al. WHO-EORTC classification for cutaneous lymphomas. *Blood.* 2005;105:3768–3785.
30. Horning SJ, Rosenberg SA. The natural history of initially untreated low-grade non-Hodgkin's lymphomas. *N Engl J Med.* 1984;311:1471–1475.
31. Swenson WT, Wooldridge JE, Lynch CF, et al. Improved survival of follicular lymphoma patients in the United States. *J Clin Oncol.* 2005;23:5019–5026.
32. Freedman AS. Biology and management of histologic transformation of indolent lymphoma. *Hematology Am Soc Hematol Educ Program.* 2005:314–320.
39. Grever MR, Lucas DM, Dewald GW, et al. Comprehensive assessment of genetic and molecular features predicting outcome in patients with chronic lymphocytic leukemia: results from the US Intergroup Phase III Trial E2997. *J Clin Oncol.* 2007;25:799–804.
40. Rassenti LZ, Huynh L, Toy TL, et al. ZAP-70 compared with immunoglobulin heavy-chain gene mutation status as a predictor of disease progression in chronic lymphocytic leukemia. *N Engl J Med.* 2004;351:893–901.
53. Rosenwald A, Wright G, Wiestner A, et al. The proliferation gene expression signature is a quantitative integrator of oncogenic events that predicts survival in mantle cell lymphoma. *Cancer Cell.* 2003;3:185–197.
60. Monti S, Savage KJ, Kutok JL, et al. Molecular profiling of diffuse large B-cell lymphoma identifies robust subtypes including one characterized by host inflammatory response. *Blood.* 2005;105:1851–1861.
66. van Besien K, Kelta M, Bahaguna P. Primary mediastinal B-cell lymphoma: a review of pathology and management. *J Clin Oncol.* 2001;19:1855–1864.
69. Ponzoni M, Ferreri AJ, Campo E, et al. Definition, diagnosis, and management of intravascular large B-cell lymphoma: proposals and perspectives from an international consensus meeting. *J Clin Oncol.* 2007;25:3168–3173.
71. Rizvi MA, Evens AM, Tallman MS, et al. T-cell non-Hodgkin lymphoma. *Blood.* 2006;107:1255–1264.
86. Sonnen R, Schmidt WP, Muller-Hermelink HK, et al. The International Prognostic Index determines the outcome of patients with nodal mature T-cell lymphomas. *Br J Haematol.* 2005;129:366–372.
88. Blum KA, Lozanski G, Byrd JC. Adult Burkitt leukemia and lymphoma. *Blood.* 2004;104:3009–3020.
89. Dave SS, Fu K, Wright GW, et al. Molecular diagnosis of Burkitt's lymphoma. *N Engl J Med.* 2006;354:2431–2442.
100. Juweid ME, Stroobants S, Hoekstra OS, et al. Use of positron emission tomography for response assessment of lymphoma: consensus of the Imaging Subcommittee of International Harmonization Project in Lymphoma. *J Clin Oncol.* 2007;25:571–578.
102. A predictive model for aggressive non-Hodgkin's lymphoma. The Inter-

national Non-Hodgkin's Lymphoma Prognostic Factors Project. *N Engl J Med.* 1993;329:987–194.

103. Sehn LH, Berry B, Chhanabhai M, et al. The revised International Prognostic Index (R-IPI) is a better predictor of outcome than the standard IPI for patients with diffuse large B-cell lymphoma treated with R-CHOP. *Blood.* 2007;109:1857–1861.
104. Miller TP, Dahlberg S, Cassady JR, et al. Chemotherapy alone compared with chemotherapy plus radiotherapy for localized intermediate- and high-grade non-Hodgkin's lymphoma. *N Engl J Med.* 1998;339:21–26.
105. Solal-Celigny P, Roy P, Colombat P, et al. Follicular lymphoma international prognostic index. *Blood.* 2004;104:1258–1265.
109. Dave SS, Wright G, Tan B, et al. Prediction of survival in follicular lymphoma based on molecular features of tumor-infiltrating immune cells. *N Engl J Med.* 2004;351: 2159–2169.
110. Gallamini A, Stelitano C, Calvi R, et al. Peripheral T-cell lymphoma unspecified (PTCL-U): a new prognostic model from a retrospective multicentric clinical study. *Blood.* 2004;103:2474–2479.
117. Tsai HK, Li S, Ng AK, et al. Role of radiation therapy in the treatment of stage I/II mucosa-associated lymphoid tissue lymphoma. *Ann Oncol.* 2007;18:672–678.
119. Thieblemont C, Berger F, Dumontet C, et al. Mucosa-associated lymphoid tissue lymphoma is a disseminated disease in one third of 158 patients analyzed. *Blood.* 2000;95:802–806.
126. Marcus R, Imrie K, Belch A, et al. CVP chemotherapy plus rituximab compared with CVP as first-line treatment for advanced follicular lymphoma. *Blood.* 2005;105:1417–1423.
127. Hiddemann W, Kneba M, Dreyling M, et al. Frontline therapy with rituximab added to the combination of cyclophosphamide, doxorubicin, vincristine, and prednisone (CHOP) significantly improves the outcome for patients with advanced-stage follicular lymphoma compared with therapy with CHOP alone: results of a prospective randomized study of the German Low-Grade Lymphoma Study Group. *Blood.* 2005;106:3725–3732.
130. Colombat P, Salles G, Brousse N, et al. Rituximab (anti-CD20 monoclonal antibody) as single first-line therapy for patients with follicular lymphoma with a low tumor burden: clinical and molecular evaluation. *Blood.* 2001;97:101–106.
132. Ghielmini M, Schmitz SF, Cogliatti SB, et al. Prolonged treatment with rituximab in patients with follicular lymphoma significantly increases event-free survival and response duration compared with the standard weekly × 4 schedule. *Blood.* 2004;103:4416–4423.
133. Kaminski MS, Tuck M, Estes J, et al. 131I-tositumomab therapy as initial treatment for follicular lymphoma. *N Engl J Med.* 2005;352:441–449.
135. McLaughlin P, Grillo-Lopez AJ, Link BK, et al. Rituximab chimeric anti-CD20 monoclonal antibody therapy for relapsed indolent lymphoma: half of patients respond to a four-dose treatment program. *J Clin Oncol.* 1998;16:2825–2833.
137. van Oers MH, Klasa R, Marcus RE, et al. Rituximab maintenance improves clinical outcome of relapsed/resistant follicular non-Hodgkin lymphoma in patients both with and without rituximab during induction: results of a prospective randomized phase 3 intergroup trial. *Blood.* 2006;108:3 295–3301.
138. Kaminski MS, Estes J, Zasadny KR, et al. Radioimmunotherapy with iodine (131) I tositumomab for relapsed or refractory B-cell non-Hodgkin lymphoma: updated results and long-term follow-up of the University of Michigan experience. *Blood.* 2000;96:1259–1266.
144. Rohatiner AZ, Nadler L, Davies AJ, et al. Myeloablative therapy with autologous bone marrow transplantation for follicular lymphoma at the time of second or subsequent remission: long-term follow-up. *J Clin Oncol.* 2007;25:2554–2559.
145. Schouten HC, Qian W, Kvaloy S, et al. High-dose therapy improves progression-free survival and survival in relapsed follicular non-Hodgkin's lymphoma: results from the randomized European CUP trial. *J Clin Oncol.* 2003;21:3918–3927.
151. Horning SJ, Weller E, Kim K, et al. Chemotherapy with or without radiotherapy in limited-stage diffuse aggressive non-Hodgkin's lymphoma: Eastern Cooperative Oncology Group study 1484. *J Clin Oncol.* 2004;22:3032–3038.
152. Reyes F, Lepage E, Ganem G, et al. ACVBP versus CHOP plus radiotherapy for localized aggressive lymphoma. *N Engl J Med.* 2005;352:1197–1205.
153. Bonnet C, Fillet G, Mounier N, et al. CHOP alone compared with CHOP plus radiotherapy for localized aggressive lymphoma in elderly patients: a study by the Groupe d'Etude des Lymphomes de l'Adulte. *J Clin Oncol.* 2007;25:787–792.
155. Feugier P, Van Hoof A, Sebban C, et al. Long-term results of the R-CHOP study in the treatment of elderly patients with diffuse large B-cell lymphoma: a study by the Groupe d'Etude des Lymphomes de l'Adulte. *J Clin Oncol.* 2005;23:4117–4126.
156. Habermann TM, Weller EA, Morrison VA, et al. Rituximab-CHOP versus CHOP alone or with maintenance rituximab in older patients with diffuse large B-cell lymphoma. *J Clin Oncol.* 2006;24: 3121–3127.
157. Pfreundschuh M, Trumper L, Osterborg A, et al. CHOP-like chemotherapy plus rituximab versus CHOP-like chemotherapy alone in young patients with good-prognosis diffuse large-B-cell lymphoma: a randomised controlled trial by the MabThera International Trial (MInT) Group. *Lancet Oncol.* 2006;7:379–391.
158. Pfreundschuh M, Schubert J, Ziepert M, et al. Six versus eight cycles of bi-weekly CHOP-14 with or without rituximab in elderly patients with aggressive CD20+ B-cell lymphomas: a randomised controlled trial (RICOVER-60). *Lancet Oncol.* 2008;9:105–116.
163. Milpied N, Deconinck E, Gaillard F, et al. Initial treatment of aggressive lymphoma with high-dose chemotherapy and autologous stem-cell support. *N Engl J Med.* 2004;350:1287–1295.
167. Lenz G, Dreyling M, Hoster E, et al. Immunochemotherapy with rituximab and cyclophosphamide, doxorubicin, vincristine, and prednisone significantly improves response and time to treatment failure, but not long-term outcome in patients with previously untreated mantle cell lymphoma: results of a prospective randomized trial of the German Low Grade Lymphoma Study Group (GLSG). *J Clin Oncol.* 2005;23:1984–1992.
169. Dreyling M, Lenz G, Hoster E, et al. Early consolidation by myeloablative radiochemotherapy followed by autologous stem cell transplantation in first remission significantly prolongs progression-free survival in mantle-cell lymphoma: results of a prospective randomized trial of the European MCL Network. *Blood.* 2005;105:2677–2684.
172. Magrath I, Adde M, Shad A, et al. Adults and children with small non-cleaved-cell lymphoma have a similar excellent outcome when treated with the same chemotherapy regimen. *J Clin Oncol.* 1996;14:925–934.
188. Philip T, Armitage JO, Spitzer G, et al. High-dose therapy and autologous bone marrow transplantation after failure of conventional chemotherapy in adults with intermediate-grade or high-grade non-Hodgkin's lymphoma. *N Engl J Med.* 1987;316:1493–1498.
189. Philip T, Guglielmi C, Hagenbeek A, et al. Autologous bone marrow transplantation as compared with salvage chemotherapy in relapses of chemotherapy-sensitive non-Hodgkin's lymphoma. *N Engl J Med.* 1995;333:1540–1545.

116 Mycosis Fungoides and Sézary Syndrome

Richard T. Hoppe, MD ■ Youn H. Kim, MD ■ Ranjana Advani, MD

Mycosis fungoides (MF) is a cutaneous lymphoma first described by the French dermatologist Alibert in 1806. The mushroom-like appearance of the cutaneous tumor nodules of MF gives the disease its name. MF is included in the spectrum of diseases referred to as cutaneous T-cell lymphomas (CTCL). This group of diseases also includes Sézary syndrome (SS), which is an erythrodermic, leukemic variant of MF.[1]

Epidemiology and Etiology

MF is a rare lymphoma. The estimated annual incidence rate in the United States is 0.64 per 100,000, or less than 1,000 new cases annually.[2] It accounts for only 2% of new cases of NonHodgkin's lymphoma (NHL). It commonly affects older adults (median age 55-60 years); however, it does not spare younger patients.[3] There is a 2:1 male predominance, without racial predilection.

The etiology of MF is unknown. Some retrospective studies have suggested an etiologic role for environmental chemical exposure. However, a large case-controlled study refutes the hypothesis.[4] A viral etiology was once proposed, based on the isolation of human T-cell leukemia/lymphoma virus 1 (HTLV-1) from the peripheral blood lymphocytes of a patient with a cutaneous lymphoma resembling MF. The clinical characteristics of this entity, HTLV-1–associated T-cell lymphoma, have now been described more precisely[5] and are quite different from those of typical MF. Despite many years of probing patient blood and tissues for HTLV-1, there has not been any conclusive evidence to support an association between the virus and MF.[6]

Pathology/Pathogenesis

The classical histopathology of MF includes abnormal cells infiltrating the epidermis (epidermotropism) as single cells or in clusters (Pautrier microabscesses) (Fig. 116-1). Typically, there is also an upper dermal infiltrate of similar cells, as well as variable proportions of histiocytes, eosinophils, and plasma cells. The neoplastic cells of MF are mononuclear cells. Under oil immersion, the nuclei of these cells have a hyper-convoluted surface. Electron microscopic studies demonstrate marked infolding of the nuclear membrane, which on three-dimensional reconstruction simulates a cerebriform appearance.

Functional studies and monoclonal antibody staining indicate that the majority of cases of MF are associated with the helper T-cell phenotype (CD4+).[7] Immunophenotyping studies demonstrate that the neoplastic cells of MF usually retain the CD4 antigen but lose other mature T-cell antigens, such as Leu-8 or Leu-9 (CD7). This loss of mature T-cell antigens may help in the differential diagnosis of MF from benign dermatoses. Occasional cases of MF have been demonstrated to be CD8+ (cytotoxic/suppressor T-cell phenotype).

Analysis of the abnormal cells in MF using the Southern blot and polymerase chain reaction (PCR) methods to assess rearrangements of the T-cell receptor (TCR) have been reported. These studies indicate monoclonal rearrangements of the TCRs in the skin, lymph nodes, and peripheral blood of patients with MF.[8] In general, biopsies performed on multiple lesions in a patient at the same time, or different biopsies sequentially performed on lesions in the same patient, demonstrate consistent rearrangements.

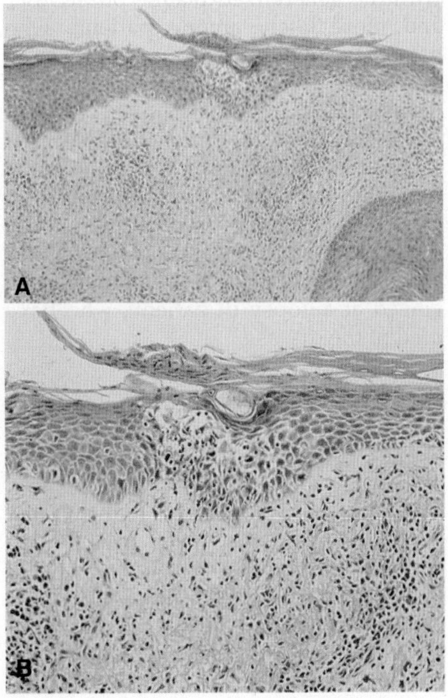

Figure 116-1 ■ **(A)** Histopathology of MF showing upper dermal infiltrate and characteristic epidermotropism of atypical lymphocytes (H&E; × 80). **(B)** Higher magnification of the same field demonstrating cluster of epidermotropic, pleomorphic cells, and Pautrier microabscess, diagnostic of MF (H&E; × 120).

The pathology of extracutaneous disease poses special problems. Most commonly, enlarged lymph nodes demonstrate changes of dermatopathic lymphadenitis, including the presence of sinus histiocytosis and an abundance of pigment-laden macrophages. There may also be a variable number of atypical lymphocytes with cerebriform nuclei. The prognostic relevance of the degree of infiltration by these abnormal cells led to the development of a lymph node classification system. In this system, lymph nodes are classified as LN-0 to LN-4. These lymph node designations may be combined into 3 groups, category 1 (LN-0-2), which includes dermatopathic nodes and nodes with clusters of as many as 6 atypical cells, category 2 (LN-3), with clusters of 10 or more atypical cells, and category 3 (LN-4) with partial or complete effacement of the node by atypical cells.[9] Detection of abnormal cells in the lymph node is facilitated by the use of Southern blot or PCR analysis. Potential neoplastic involvement with clonal TCR rearrangement may be demonstrated even in lymph nodes that show only dermatopathic changes on routine evaluation.[10]

Natural History

MF often has a long natural history. The disease may present in a premycotic phase with nonspecific, slightly scaling skin lesions that wax and wane for years. Biopsies are generally nondiagnostic during this phase, and patients may respond to topical corticosteroids. Some of these patients will experience an evolution of their disease and develop more typical patches or infiltrated plaques, from which a definitive biopsy may be obtained. The median duration from the onset of skin symptoms to a diagnosis of MF may be 5 years or longer.

The initial presentation of MF may be as patches, plaques, tumors, or generalized erythroderma. A patient may present with more than one morphologic type of skin disease or change from one type to another during the course of disease. The typical patches of MF are slightly scaling and mildly erythematous. Many patients present with involvement in a "bathing trunk" distribution, although lesions may be present on any part of the body. Pruritus is the most common symptom, even in the early phases of the disease and is often the problem that prompts a visit to the dermatologist.

More infiltrated lesions become palpable plaques. These are erythematous, slightly scaling, with well-defined borders. The shape is variable, and the distribution may vary. Infiltrated plaques may eventually develop into ulcerating or fungating tumors (Fig. 116-2). Tumors may become infected, and sepsis secondary to infection is often the cause of death in individuals affected. Generalized dermal thickening from infiltrative disease may cause the classic but rare leonine facies of MF.

Another cutaneous manifestation is generalized erythroderma (Fig. 116-3). Plaques or tumors may be superimposed over the erythroderma. These patients suffer from intense pruritus. Patients with erythroderma may also have lymphadenopathy and circulating abnormal cells in the peripheral blood. These cells may have the same microscopic appearance, immunophenotypic, and genotypic characteristics as the cells that infiltrate the epidermis. Patients with this complex of findings have SS.[11]

Other clinical presentations of MF include the follicular-tropic variant,[12] pagetoid reticulosis,[13] granulomatous MF,[14] and hypopigmented MF.[15]

Although MF is usually an indolent disease, and many patients demonstrate only the patch or plaque phase of skin involvement throughout the duration of their disease,[16,17] some will progress to develop cutaneous tumors. The rapidity of this progression is unpredictable. Most patients with MF demonstrate only cutaneous disease throughout the course of their illness. Only 15-20% develop clinical problems related to extracutaneous disease. This likelihood is related to the extent of skin involvement. It is exceedingly rare among patients who have only the limited plaque phase of skin involvement, relatively uncommon among those with the generalized plaque phase (8%), and more likely among patients who have developed tumorous involvement of the skin (30%) or generalized erythroderma (25%).[18]

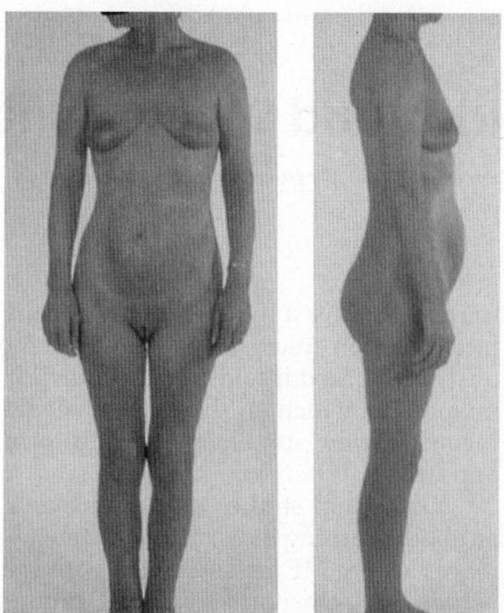

Figure 116-3 ■ Generalized erythroderma (or "l'homme rouge"), often with very atrophic skin, is typical of patients with SS.

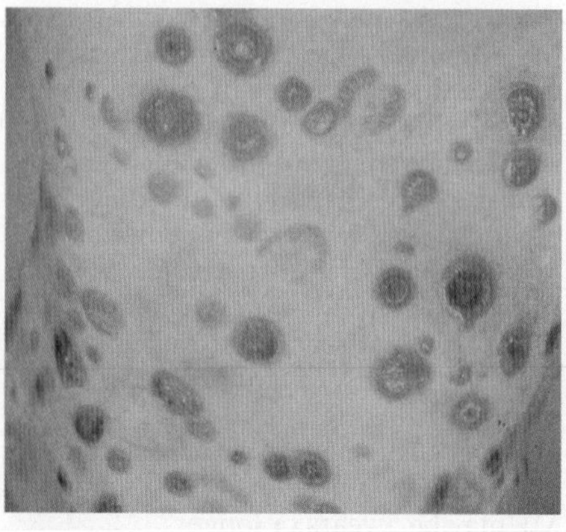

Figure 116-2 ■ The flank of a patient with typical plaques of MF, many of which have evolved into tumors with central ulceration.

The most commonly identified route of extracutaneous spread is to the regional lymphatics and secondarily to viscera. The organs most commonly involved include the spleen, liver, and lungs, but virtually any organ may be involved at autopsy in patients who have died of the disease.[19]

Diagnosis

A diagnosis of MF or SS may be suspected in patients who present with chronic nonspecific dermatitis or generalized erythroderma. Similar skin lesions can be seen in benign skin conditions, such as psoriasis, parapsoriasis, eczematous dermatitis, photodermatitis, or drug reactions. For patients with tumorous lesions, the differential includes non-MF CTCL or primary cutaneous B-cell lymphoma.

Skin biopsy with routine histology is the most important laboratory tool to assist in establishing the diagnosis. Neoplastic cells must be present in the epidermis (epidermotropism or Pautrier's microabscesses) in order to make a definitive diagnosis of MF (Fig. 116-1). Although such collections are characteristic of the disease, they may not be present in early patch-stage lesions. As lesions evolve from patches to plaques, the density of neoplastic cells within the dermis increases, and the degree of epidermotropism becomes more notable. In tumorous lesions, the dermal infiltrate is very dense, involving the full breadth of the dermis, often extending into the subcutaneous fat, and epidermotropism tends to be less marked.

Immunophenotyping is used to support the routine histology. Occasionally, when the routine histology is equivocal, the immunophenotyping results may help to confirm or refute the diagnosis. However, results of immunohistochemical studies must be interpreted with caution. There may be discordant expression of antigens between intraepidermal and intradermal T cells in MF and SS.[20] In addition, significant differences of antigen expression in biopsies obtained from different sites from the same patient have been observed.

Evaluation of skin biopsies to detect TCR gene rearrangements, or genotyping, may also be helpful. TCR gene rearrangements can be detected by Southern blot analysis[21] or by methods utilizing PCR amplification.[8] PCR amplification methods for frozen or paraffin tissue analysis are widely available and affordable.[22] Genotyping is becoming an integral diagnostic procedure for patients in whom the routine histology or immunophenotyping is equivocal but whose clinical presentation is strongly suggestive of MF.

Blood and lymph nodes may also be probed for malignant cells. Flow cytometry studies of the peripheral blood may show expansion of the CD4+CD7– population reflective of circulating atypical lymphocytes of Sézary type.[23] PCR methods can be helpful in determination of blood[24] or lymph node involvement.[10]

Staging and Prognosis

The intensity of the staging studies performed is dictated by the extent of skin involvement and the results of screening staging procedures. Patients with the limited plaque phase of skin involvement typically will require only a good physical examination, careful mapping of the skin lesions, a complete blood count, Sézary cell detection, screening chemistries, and a chest radiograph. If these are all within normal limits, additional studies need not be performed. Routine imaging studies in patients who have limited disease

Table 116-1 Tumor-Node-Metastasis-Blood Classification for MF

T (Skin)	
T1	Limited patch, papules, or plaques covering <10% of the skin surface
T2	Patches, papules, and/or plaques covering ≥10% of the skin surface
T3	1or more tumors (>1 cm in diameter)
T4	Confluence of erythema >80% of body surface area
N (Nodes)	
N0	No clinically abnormal peripheral lymph nodes; biopsy not required
N1	Clinically abnormal peripheral lymph nodes; histopathology Dutch Gr 1 or NCI LN0-2
N2	Clinically abnormal peripheral lymph nodes; histopathology Dutch Gr 2 or NCI LN3
N3	Clinically abnormal peripheral lymph nodes; histopathology Dutch Gr 3-4 or NCI LN4
NX	Clinically abnormal peripheral lymph nodes; no histologic confirmation
M (Viscera)	
M0	No visceral organ involvement
M1	Visceral involvement (must have pathology confirmation and organ involved should be specified
B (Blood)	
B0	Absence of significant blood involvement: <5% of peripheral blood lymphocytes (PBL) are atypical (Sézary) cells
B1	Low blood tumor burden: >5% of PBLs are atypical (Sézary), but does not meet criteria for B2
B2	High blood tumor burden: >1,000/mcL Sézary cells with positive clone

Source: From Ref. 26.

without peripheral lymphadenopathy is unproductive, however, patients with cutaneous tumors, erythroderma, or palpable adenopathy should undergo CT or PET/CT imaging.[25] Any blood or radiographic abnormalities should be evaluated further. Patients who have palpable lymphadenopathy should have a biopsy of the enlarged nodes. Significant bone marrow disease is usually reflected by the presence of readily detectable Sézary cells in the peripheral blood. Therefore, bone marrow biopsy is not routinely used as part of the initial staging.

A tumor-node-metastasis-blood (TNMB) staging system has proved useful for MF and was introduced at the Workshop on Mycosis Fungoides held at the National Cancer Institute (NCI) in 1978. This staging system has been revised to reflect the updated prognostic information and is more consistent with current practice and management.[26] Tables 116-1 and 116-2 summarize the staging classification and TNMB categories for the revised classification. The T-classification reflects the extent of skin involvement. The N-classification indicates the presence of lymph node involvement. Enlarged lymph nodes should be biopsied, since palpable enlargement is often associated only with changes of dermatopathic lymphadenitis; however, recent studies suggest that patients with lymph nodes exhibiting rearranged TCR genes by molecular methods have a worse prognosis, regardless of the histologic grade.[26] In the M-classification, suspected disease should also be documented and treatment programs for visceral disease should be considered only if definite proof of disease exists. In the B- (blood) classification, the presence of a significant proportion of abnormal, cerebriform (Sézary) cells should be noted; however, low levels of Sézary-like cells can be detected in the peripheral blood of patients with benign skin conditions. The current practice is to use the criterion of an expanded peripheral blood CD4+ population with increased ratio of CD4 to CD8 T lymphocytes (greater than 10:1), expanded populations of abnormal T-cells with CD4+/CD7– or CD4+/CD26– phenotype, and molecular evidence of a relevant TCR gene rearrangement in the peripheral blood.[26]

The T-classification and presence of extracutaneous disease are the most important indicators predictive of survival (Fig. 116-4).[18] Patients with limited patch/plaque (T1, overall Stage IA) disease have an excellent prognosis with a long-term life expectancy that is similar to an age-, sex-, and race-matched control population.[16] According to a retrospective study of 122 Stage IA patients at Stanford, the median survival had not yet been reached at 33 years. Nearly all patients with Stage IA disease die from causes other than MF. Furthermore, only 9% of treated patients at this stage will ever progress to a more advanced stage of disease.

Patients with generalized patch/plaque disease without evidence of extracutaneous involvement (T2, Stage IB or Stage IIA) have a median survival greater than 11 years.[17] Patients with T2 disease have a greater likelihood of disease progression (24%), and nearly 20% die of causes related to MF.

Patients with cutaneous tumors (T3, Stage IIB) or generalized erythroderma (T4, Stage III) without extracutaneous disease have median survivals of 3.2 and 4.6 years, respectively. The majority of these patients will die of MF. The long-term outcome in patients with erythroderma (T4) is quite variable and is dependent on patient age at presentation (<65 years vs >65 years), overall Stage (III vs IV), and peripheral blood involvement (B0 vs B1).[27] The median survival can vary widely depending on the combinations of these independent prognostic factors: distinct prognostic subgroups have been identified, based on the number of adverse fac-

Table 116-2 Clinical Staging System for MF/SS

	T	N	M	B
IA	1	0	0	0,1
IB	2	0	0	0,1
II	1-2	1,2	0	0,1
IIB	3	0-2	0	0,1
III	4	0-2	0	0,1
IIIA	4	0-2	0	0
IIIB	4	0-2	0	1
IVA1	1-4	0-2	0	2
IVA2	1-4	3	0	0-2
IVB	1-4	0-3	1	0-2

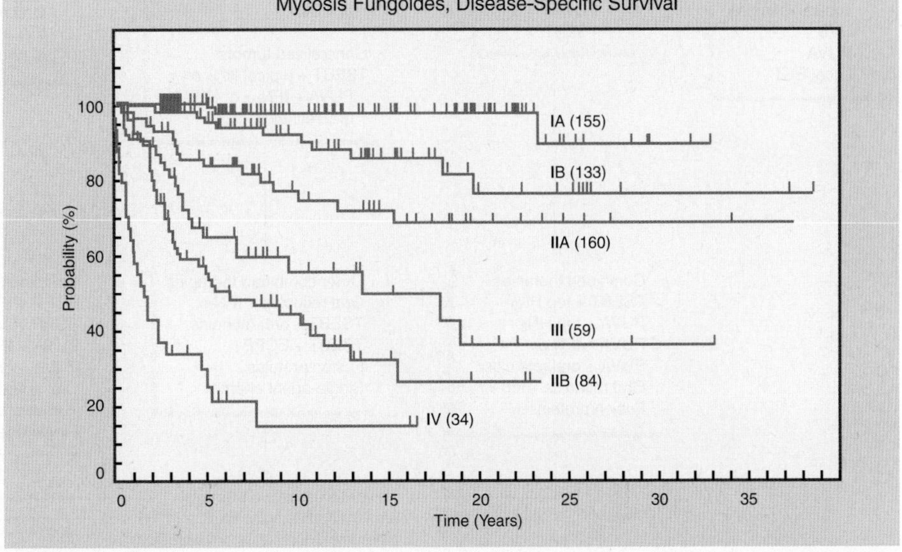

Figure 116-4 Disease-specific survival by initial disease stage for 525 patients with MF treated at Stanford University.

tors present, with median survivals of 10.2, 3.7, and 1.5 years.

Patients with extracutaneous disease at presentation involving either lymph nodes (Stage IVA) or viscera (Stage IVB) have a median survival of less than 1.5 years.[28] The presence of significant Sézary cells in the peripheral blood usually correlates with more advanced T-classification (usually T4) and the presence of extracutaneous disease.[29]

In a study of patients at the NCI, patients with lymph node biopsies showing dermatopathic changes or just a small number of atypical cells (category 1) had a 5-year survival of 80%. Those patients with large clusters of paracortical atypical cells (category 2) had a 5-year survival of 30%, and those with effaced nodes (category 3) had a 5-year survival of only 15%.

Patients with plaque-type or erythrodermic MF may develop cutaneous tumors with large cell histology. Large cell transformation is defined on the basis of either an infiltrate of large atypical lymphocytes that comprise greater than 25% of the dermal infiltrate, or nodular expansile aggregates of atypical large lymphocytes.[30,31] These large cells may often express CD30 (Ki-1), but shares a common clonal origin with the pre-existing MF, and this evolution does not represent a new lymphoma.[32] An increased mitotic activity is readily observed, and the Ki-67 proliferation rate by immunohistochemistry is greater than 25%.[30] Immunophenotypically, the transformed large lymphocytes can exhibit variable loss of one or more T-cell–associated antigens such as CD3, CD5, CD4, CD8, CD45RO, or CD43.[30,31] These patients may have more rapid disease progression and require more intensive local or systemic therapy.[33]

Therapy

The National Comprehensive Cancer Network (NCCN) has established consensus guidelines for the therapy of MF and the SS.[34] Nearly all patients with MF will require treatment directed at their skin. Common therapies include topical corticosteroids, psoralen plus ultraviolet A (PUVA), topical chemotherapy, topical retinoids, and irradiation. A minority of patients (10-20%) will also require treatment for systemic disease. There are multiple therapeutic options for MF and SS. Selection of a specific treatment plan is based primarily on the clinical stage of disease (Fig. 116-5).

Topical Chemotherapy

Topical nitrogen mustard (mechlorethamine, HN2) is a very effective form of management for patients with MF.[35] The mechanism of action has not been defined and may not be related simply to its alkylating agent properties. The activity of HN2 may be mediated by immune mechanisms or by interaction with the epidermal cell–Langerhans cell–T-cell axis. HN2 may be applied locally, regionally, or to the entire skin. It may be mixed in water or in an ointment base. Nitrogen mustard ointment is prepared by the pharmacist at an initial concentration of 10-20 mg of HN2 per 100 g of Aquaphor (10-20 mg%). For the aqueous preparation, which is not commonly used, patients prepare the solution themselves at a concentration of 10-20 mg/100 mL of water and apply it to their skin with a cloth or brush. The aqueous and ointment preparations appear to have similar clinical efficacy, although a prospective comparison has not been performed. Topical HN2 is applied at least once daily during the clearing phase. The concentration and frequency of application may be altered, depending on tolerance and response. Skin clearance may require 6 months or longer, and is followed by maintenance therapy (≥2 months). There is no evidence that more prolonged maintenance is beneficial.

If response is particularly slow, the concentration of the HN2 may be increased to 30-40 mg/100 mL, especially to small areas, or the frequency of application may be increased to twice a day. The complete response (CR) rate for topical HN2 for limited patch/plaque (T1) disease is 70-80%. The median time to skin clearance is 6-8 months. When treatment is discontinued, more than half of patients will relapse in the skin, but most will respond to a resumption of therapy. The proportion of patients treated with topical HN2 who have a durable complete response (>10 years) is 20-25%.

The primary acute complication of HN2 is a cutaneous hypersensitivity reaction. This may occur in as many as

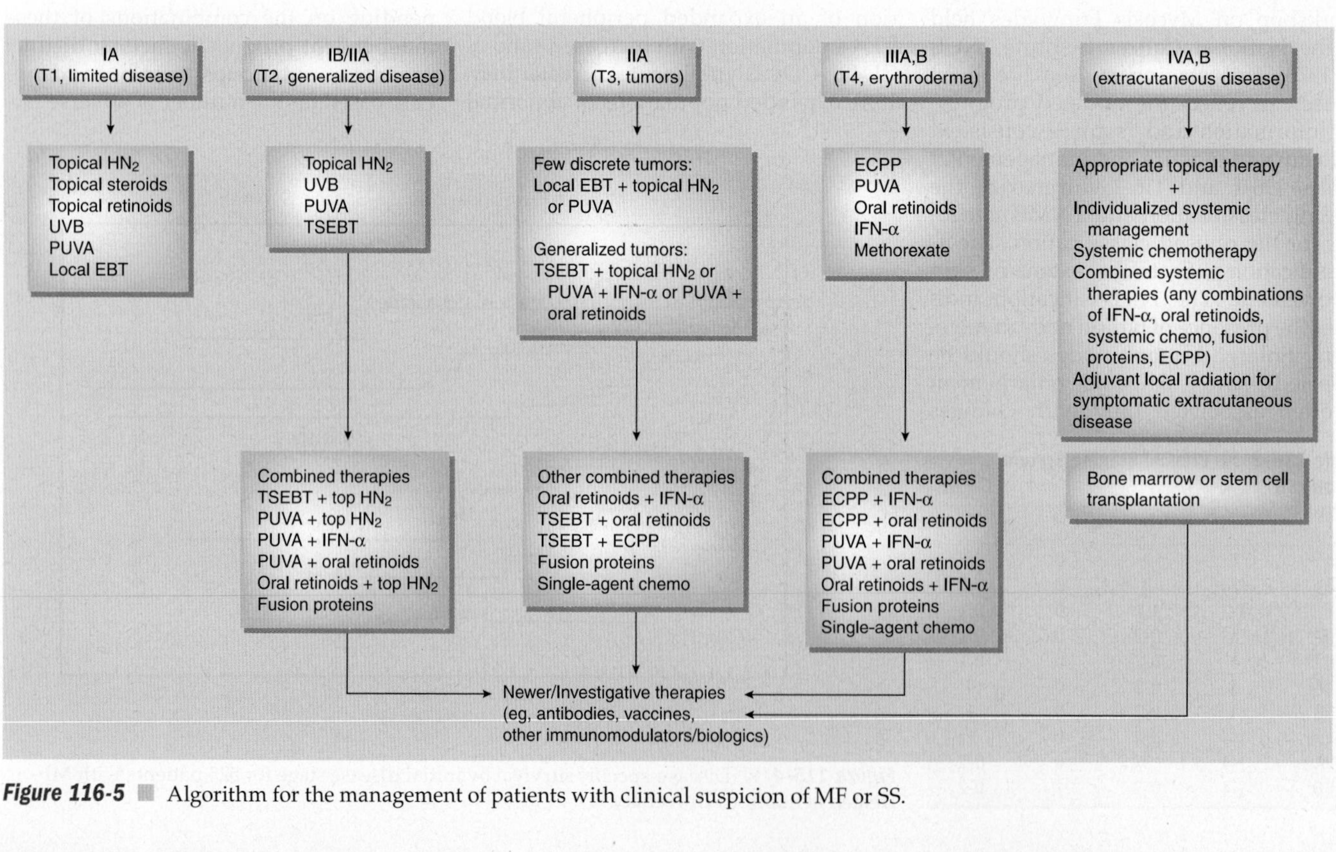

Figure 116-5 Algorithm for the management of patients with clinical suspicion of MF or SS.

60% of patients treated with the aqueous preparation but in only about 5% of those treated with the ointment-based preparation. Desensitization may be achieved by a variety of topical or systemic desensitization programs. There is no systemic absorption of topical HN2, so hematologic monitoring is not necessary, there are no effects on fertility, and it is safe to use even in children.[35] Occasionally, patients treated with topical HN2 develop secondary squamoproliferative lesions. This risk is the greatest among patients who have had long-term sequential therapy with multiple topical modalities. There is no increased risk for developing secondary skin cancers among patients who have used topical HN2 as monotherapy.

Because of its efficacy and ease of application, topical HN2 is employed commonly, especially among patients who have T1 or T2 disease (Fig. 116-5). For patients with a discrete number of tumors or refractory lesions, treatment may be supplemented with local irradiation.

Topical Retinoids

Bexarotene (Targretin) 1% gel, an RXR-selective synthetic retinoid, is the most commonly used topical retinoid for treating MF. Bexarotene gel is applied with a thin application to the patches or plaques and is most effective and best-tolerated when used twice daily. Due to the irritant effect of the retinoids, it is only feasible to use this agent when there are a discrete number of patches or plaques. It is not intended for generalized application. A phase 3 trial of Bexarotene included 50 patients with refractory or persistent early stage disease (Stages IA-IIA).[36] Responses were seen in 62% of patients with Stage IA and 50% of patients with Stage IB disease. 3 patients with Stage IIA or IIB disease did not respond. The most common toxicity of bexarotene gel is irritation at the sites of application, which occurs in the majority of patients. Because of the erythema from the irritant reaction, it may be necessary to withhold therapy for a few weeks to assess disease activity. Bexarotene gel is approved by the FDA for patients with Stages IA and IB disease who have refractory or persistent disease after other therapies or who have not tolerated other therapies.

Phototherapy

Phototherapy includes ultraviolet (UV) radiation in the UVA or UVB wavelengths. The long-wave UVA has the advantage over UVB in its greater depth of penetration into the dermal infiltrates of MF. For early limited diseases, UVB alone[37] or home UV phototherapy (UVA + UVB)[38] may be effective. UVB therapy is initiated as a daily or three times per week regimen with gradual incremental dose delivery. After complete clearance is achieved, the frequency of therapy is gradually reduced during the maintenance period and then discontinued. A CR rate of 83% has been reported using UVB phototherapy in patients with patch-type Stage IA disease.[38] More recently narrow-band UVB (nb-UVB) phototherapy has been shown to be more effective than the traditional broadband UVB. Nb-UVB is associated with less toxicity than broadband UVB or PUVA. The clinical efficacy of nb-UVB may also be superior to broadband UVB.[39]

UVA may be used with psoralen, a photosensitizing agent, as PUVA, referred to as photochemotherapy. In the presence of UVA, psoralen intercalates with DNA, forming monofunctional and bifunctional adducts, which inhibit DNA synthesis. This results in cytotoxic and antiproliferative effects. There may also be immunomodulatory effects, either through a direct effect on T-cells or indirectly by modulating cytokine production. The technique of treatment is for the patient to ingest the psoralen drug (usually 8-methoxypsoralen) followed by controlled exposure to UVA in a specially designed light box, usually commencing 1-2 hours later. Only the eyes are shielded routinely. All other body surfaces may be treated; however, selected areas can be shielded to minimize undesired photo damage. Certain "shadowed" areas such as the scalp, perineum, axillae, and other skin fold areas will not receive adequate exposure.

PUVA treatment is initiated thrice weekly until skin clearance is achieved, after which the frequency of treatment is gradually decreased to as infrequently as once every 2 weeks. Maintenance therapy should be discontinued within 1 year in order to minimize the risks of cutaneous carcinogenesis. The usual time to skin clearance is 2-6 months and the likelihood of clearance is related to the extent of skin involvement. The complete clearance rate is 50- 90% in patients with patch or plaque disease.[40] Indications for PUVA treatment include its use as the primary therapy for patients with limited or generalized patch or plaque disease or as a secondary therapy following the failure of other topical modalities (Fig. 116-5). PUVA may also be effective for patients with erythroderma, provided that very low daily exposures are utilized to avoid photo-toxicity reactions. In patients with SS, PUVA may be supplemented by systemic therapies; such as interferon alpha[41] or systemic retinoids.[42] The treatment of patients with more advanced cutaneous disease may be facilitated by the addition of localized irradiation to particularly refractory plaques or tumors.

The primary acute complication of PUVA therapy is a phototoxic reaction, with erythroderma and blistering. Patients should shield their skin and eyes for at least 24 hours following psoralen ingestion. The potential long-term complications of PUVA therapy include cataract formation and secondary cutaneous malignancies.[40] .

Radiation Therapy

MF is an extremely radiosensitive neoplasm. Individual plaques or tumors of MF may be treated with electron beam radiation therapy (EBT) to total doses of 15-25 Gy in 1-3 weeks, with a high likelihood of achieving long-term local control.

Techniques have been developed to treat the entire cutaneous surface with electrons (total skin EBT, or TSEBT).[43] Conventional linear accelerators may be modified to treat patients in the standing position at an extended distance. By having the patient stand in multiple positions, the entire skin surface may be irradiated. The treatment technique employed at Stanford (and adopted at many other centers) uses a six-field technique (anterior, posterior, and 4 opposed oblique fields). Treatment is administered 4 times a week, to a total dose of 30-36 Gy. Supplementary treatment is required for the soles of the feet, the perineum, and under the breasts. Only the eyes are shielded routinely, but other areas may be shielded during part of the treatment to help control localized cutaneous reactions.

Several centers have developed expertise in the use of TSEBT.[44,45] Overall response rates (ORR) are nearly 100%, with CR rates ranging from 40% to 98%, depending on the extent of skin involvement. As many as 50% of patients with limited plaque disease and 25% of patients with generalized plaque disease may remain free of disease for more than 5 years after completion of a single course of EBT. Although the curative potential of this treatment remains disputed, there is no doubt that it provides an important palliative benefit, especially for patients with extensive disease. Often, when disease recurs, it is in a more limited distribution and may be controlled more readily with localized topical therapies. The use of EBT is often indicated in the primary or secondary management of patients with generalized plaque or tumorous involvement of the skin. After complete skin clearance, adjuvant therapy with topical HN2 may be utilized. Repeat courses of TSEBT may be administered in selected situations.[46]

The complications of TSEBT include acute erythema, desquamation, and temporary epilation. Patients also experience temporary loss of their fingernails and toenails, as well as an impaired ability to sweat for up to 12 months. There is an increased risk of secondary squamous and basal cell cancers of the skin, but this is most noticeable in patients who have received protracted therapy with a variety of topical agents, including PUVA and topical HN2.[47]

In patients who have lymph node involvement, traditional megavoltage (4-15 MeV) photon irradiation may be helpful in providing important additional palliation. Doses of 30-36 Gy in 3-4 weeks are often sufficient to achieve local control of lymph node or other extracutaneous disease.[44]

Systemic Chemotherapy

Systemic chemotherapy is appropriate for patients with extracutaneous, advanced, or refractory disease or when biological therapies have failed. Virtually all drugs that are effective as single agents or in combination therapy in the treatment of patients with NHL have been tested in MF/SS. Unfortunately, most of these regimens result in only temporary palliative responses. Recently, the NCCN published guidelines which recommend stage-based therapy and using this algorithm, only a minority of patients with MF (10-20%) require systemic management.[48]

For single agent chemotherapy, no particular drug is clearly superior and no large, randomized studies comparing agents have been reported. In 526 patients reported in single agent chemotherapy trials, the response rates were 20-80% and the median duration of responses ranged from 3 to 22 months.[49] The largest study is with methotrexate, which has activity in many doses and schedules.[50-52] It is not clear that high-dose methotrexate is superior to low-dose methotrexate therapy. With low-dose methotrexate, the ORR ranges from 33% to 58 %, and the time to treatment failure is 15-32 months, depending on the extent of prior therapy.[53] Another commonly used single agent is chlorambucil, administered daily or intermittently with corticosteroids, titrating the dose according to hematologic toxicity.[54,55] Some newer drugs have shown encouraging single activity in early clinical trials and are summarized in Table 116-3.

The purine analogs are a class of drugs that have demonstrated activity in MF. T-cells have a high level of adenosine deaminase (ADA), a key enzyme in the purine degradation pathway. The purine analogs pentostatin (deoxycoformycin), fludarabine, and cladribine (2-CDA) are a group of structurally similar agents that were developed to target ADA. They have different interactions with ADA but all result in DNA damage. The largest overall experience has been with pentostatin, although each individual study is small. The response rates vary from 14% to 70%.[56,57] 2- CDA,[58,59] and fludarabine[60,61] have reported response rates of 20-40%. Hematologic toxicity and opportunistic infections are the most common complications associated with this class of drugs. Prophylactic antibiotics against *Pneumocystis carinii* and antivirals to prevent *herpes* virus infection are indicated routinely. Combinations of purine analogs with interferon have also been used in small studies and show increased response durations compared with series using these agents alone.[62] The combination of fludarabine and cyclophosphamide is associated with a longer response duration of 10 months but with a significant increase in hematologic toxicity.[63] A higher response rate of 63% has been suggested when fludarabine is combined with extracorporeal photopheresis.[60]

Gemcitabine (2′2′-difluorodeoxycytidine, Gemzar) is a deoxycytidine analog with excellent antitumor activity against a number of solid tumors and lymphoproliferative disorders.[64] It must be activated by deoxycytidine kinase and other kinases to its triphosphate form, gemcitabine triphosphate, that can then be incorporated into RNA and DNA. The latter action causes masked chain termination and inhibition of DNA repair and is considered responsible for its antitumor effect. Response rates as high as 70%[65,66] have been reported, but the complete remission rate is low. This agent has also been used in the front line setting with a median duration of complete remission of 10 months (range 4-22 months).[67]

Pegylated liposomes are stable, long-circulating carriers useful for delivering doxorubicin to tumor sites with a lower toxicity than the free drug. In a study of patients who had refractory or relapsed CTCL, pegylated doxorubicin (Doxil) was given at a dose of 20 mg/m^2 every month until a CR was achieved or a total dose of 400 mg was achieved.[68] An ORR of 80% and response duration of 15 months were reported. The most frequent side effects were mild anemia, lymphopenia, and palmoplantar erythrodysaesthesia. These results were subsequently confirmed in a larger retrospective multi-center study of 34 patients.[69] An ORR of 33% has also been reported in refractory patients with Stage IVB disease.[70] Recently, another pegylated agent (Caelyx) has been evaluated prospectively in patients with refractory or relapsed MF or SS at doses of 40 mg/m^2 administered IV once every 4 weeks with a ORR of 56% and PFS of 5 months.[71] In this prospective study the ORR was lower than those reported by prior retrospective reports. This may be due to the inclusion of a larger number of patients with transformed disease or prior chemotherapy exposure.

Another new cytotoxic agent is temozolomide. Temozolomide has shown encouraging activity in MF and needs further prospective testing. Its mechanism of action is similar to other alkylating agents. It induces DNA damage by cross-linking and resistance has been associated with high levels of the scavenger protein O 6-alkylguanine DNA alkyltransferase in tumor cells. Response rates from 26% to 33 % have been reported in patients with relapsed Stage IB-IVA disease.[72,73]

Proteosome inhibition with bortezomib is a novel effective strategy in NHL and multiple myeloma. Recently it has been suggested that NF-κB may play a key role in CTCL resistance to apoptosis.[74] This observation supports a potential therapeutic role for bortezomib

Table 116-3 ■ Results of Chemotherapy Treatment in MF

Study	Therapy	Patients (N)	ORR (%)	CR (%)	Response Duration (Months)
Single agent chemotherapy					
Bunn et al.[49]	Single agent chemotherapy	528	329 (62)	91 (33)	3-32
Zackheim et al.[53]	Low dose methotrexate	69	20 (33)	13 (22)	15
Holmes et al.[54]	Chlorambucil + prednisone	21	11 (57)	3 (14)	Not reported
Coors et al.[55]	Chlorambucil + fluocortone	13	13 (100)	7 (54)	16.5
Tsimberidon et al.[57]	Pentostatin	32	13 (54.8)	6 (14)	4.3
Von Hoff et al.[61]	Fludarabine	33	6 (19)	1 (5)	Not reported
Saven et al.[58]	2 CDA	15	7 (47)	3 (20)	5
Kuzel et al.[59]	2 CDA	21	6 (28)	3 (14)	2-16
Zinzani et al.[65]	Gemcitabine	30	21 (70)	5 (11)	6-22
Duvic et al.[66]	Gemcitabine	32	22 (68)	3 (9)	Not reported
Marchi et al.[67]	Gemcitabine	32	24 (78)	7 (22)	10
Wollina et al.[69]	Liposomal doxorubicin (Doxil)	34	30 (88)	15 (44)	10-13
Quereux et al.[71]	Liposomal doxorubicin (Caleyx))	25	14 (56)	5 (20)	5
Rosen et al.[72]	Temozolomide	22	6(26)	–	Not reported
Tani et al.[73]	Temozolomide	9	3 (33)	1 (11)	Not reported
Zinzani et al.[75]	Bortezomib	12	8 (67)	2 (17)	7-14
Combination chemotherapy					
Bunn et al.[49]	Combination	331	(81)	(38)	5-41
Greim et al.[80]	CAVE	52	47 (90)	20 (38)	Not reported
Fierro et al.[78]	VICOB-P	25	20 (80)	9 (36)	8-7

in the treatment of patients with CTCL. This agent has shown encouraging activity with a ORR of 67% and was well tolerated.[75]

There are no randomized trials comparing combination chemotherapy with single agent regimens. It is also difficult to compare results across studies, since inclusion criteria and response assessment have varied considerably. The largest experience is with combinations that include cyclophosphamide, vincristine, and prednisone with or without doxorubicin.[76,77] CR rates are generally about 25% (range 11-57%) and response duration 3 to 20 months. Most of the patients treated with combination chemotherapy have advanced disease (IIB-IV), although a few patients with early stage disease (IA-IIA) who had a CR were disease free (with short follow-up) at the time of the reports.[49]

An intensive regimen as front line therapy has been reported using VICOB-P (etoposide, idarubicin, cyclophosphamide, vincristine, prednisone, and bleomycin).[78] This intensive regimen was administered weekly for 12 weeks with a response rate of 80% (CR 36%). The median duration of response was 6-7 months, similar to that reported for CHOP chemotherapy. No response was seen in patients with SS. Other intensive salvage regimens active in relapsed aggressive NHL such as ESHAP (etoposide, high dose cytarabine and methylprednisone) has also been used without significant durable remissions and poor tolerance due to prolonged myelosuppression and infectious complications.[79]

At one time, based on uncontrolled studies, combined modality therapy with combination chemotherapy and total skin irradiation was proposed as a preferred treatment.[80-82] This concept was then tested in a prospective randomized trial at the NCI, which compared an aggressive program of combination chemotherapy (cyclophosphamide, doxorubicin, vincristine, and etoposide) and total skin electron beam irradiation with sequential conservative therapies.[83] The objective response rates (90 vs 65%) and CR rates (38 vs 18%) were higher with the combined therapy. However, there was no difference in overall survival and considerably greater toxicity in the combination therapy group. There are several reports of combining chemotherapy with biological agents such as targeted toxins and immunomodulating agents that appear encouraging and need to be confirmed in large prospective studies.[84]

High-Dose Chemotherapy With Hematopoietic Stem Cell Transplant (HSCT)

Recent interest has been shown in using high-dose chemotherapy followed by peripheral stem cell support (autologous or allogeneic) in MF. Despite the broad experience with HSCT in other forms of refractory lymphoma, the experience in CTCL is limited. The number of patients is small and there are no well-defined prognostic factors to identify patients suitable for this therapy. Recent studies are summarized in Table 116-4.

The overall experience with autologous HSCT is limited, only about 20 cases have been reported.[85] Bigler and associates[86] reported that 5 of 6 patients achieved a CR with an autologous transplant. 3 of the responses lasted less than 100 days and 2 patients were disease-free at 1 year. In another study,[87] 8 of 9 patients achieved a CR of brief duration, 2 months in 4 of the patients, but 3 others were disease-free at 11 months. Eventually all patients in those 2 studies relapsed, suggesting that autologous transplant is not a curative approach. Overall the experience with autologous transplant suggests that there an anti-MF effect, however responses are short lived with a median estimated time to progression of only 2.3 months.[85]

One of the limitations of an autologous approach, which might account for the short-lived responses, is the potential reinfusion of contaminating malignant T-cells. In an attempt to overcome this problem, auto-transplantation with T-cell depletion has been evaluated. In a pilot study, 9 patients had their apheresis products treated with immunomagnetic methods for T-cell depletion.[88] 8 of 9 patients engrafted and 7 achieved a CR. Although all patients relapsed, at a median of 7 months, it appears that they may have relapsed with less advanced disease that responded to conventional therapy.

The concept of allogeneic hematopoietic cell transplantation is provocative, since even in the absence of a CR an allogeneic graft versus tumor effect may provide an immune mechanism to control the malignant T-cell process. Eligibility and preparatory regimens have varied across studies. In a report by Guitart and associates,[89] 3 patients received an allograft from HLA-matched siblings. Complete and sustained clinical and histologic remissions were achieved in 2 patients that continued for 4.5+ years, and 15+ months. The third patient was in CR for 9 months followed by a limited cutaneous recurrence. Molina and associates[90] reported a CR in all 6 patients transplanted for refractory disease. 5 patients remained in CR at a median follow-up of 17 months (range 3-65 months). Mild acute and chronic graft versus host disease (GVHD) developed in all patients and chronic GVHD was ongoing in patients with sustained remissions, suggesting a possible graft versus lymphoma (GVL) effect. Thus, it appears that in contrast to autologous HSCT, allogeneic HSCT may result in durable long-term remissions.

Although the results of allogeneic transplant are encouraging and appear durable, it has limited applicability due to toxicity related issues in older patients. Emerging data using non-myeloablative approach with reduced intensity conditioning regimens have been reported.[85] The first published report from Italy suggested that all 3 patients achieved a durable CR although with a high incidence of infection and chronic skin GVHD.[91] Other reports also suggest a role of GVL with relapses post transplant responding to reducing the immunosuppression and donor lymphocyte infusion.[92] Another large series from Italy treated 15 patients with refractory MF who had failed three prior regimens. With a median follow-up of 41 months, 9 were still in CR with a 5-year PFS of 60%.[93]

Thus, it appears that compared to autologous HSCT, allogeneic HSCT (myeloablative or with reduced intensity conditioning regimes) and resultant GVL may result in durable long-term remissions. Larger prospective studies will be required to identify the optimal timing of transplant, the best conditioning regimen, and resultant efficacy and safety of the therapy. With numerous biological agents showing promising activity with tolerability there may also be a role for post maintenance therapies with the ultimate goal of influencing the quality of life. With better understanding of the disease biology and with newer molecular characteristics it may be possible to identify patients and develop prognostic factors so that these aggressive approaches can be offered to suitable patients most likely to benefit.

Table 116-4 Results of High-Dose Therapy and HSCT in MF

Study	Stage	N	No. CR	Response Duration
Autologous hematopoietic cell transplantation				
Bigler et al.[86]	IIB-IV B	5	4	4 pts < 1 y, 1 pt >1 y
Russel-Jones et al.[87]	IIB-IV B	9	8	4 pts <3 mo, 3 pts 11 mo
Olavarria et al.[88]	IIB-IV B	9	7	All in 1 y
Allogeneic hematopoietic cell transplantation				
Soligo et al.[91]	IV	3	3	16 mo, 12 mo
Guitart et al.[89]	IIB-IV A	3	3	10 m, 26 mo +, 67 mo +
Molina et al.[90]	IIB-IV	8	8	6 pts NED at median of 56 mo
Onida et al.[93]	IIB-IV	15	9	9 pts NED at median of 41 mo

Extracorporeal Photopheresis

Photopheresis (extracorporeal photopheresis [ECP] or systemic photochemotherapy) is a method of delivering PUVA systemically by using an extracorporeal technique.[94] The patient's white blood cells are collected via leukapheresis, exposed to a photoactivating drug (8-methoxypsoralen, Uvadex), and then irradiated with UVA. The irradiated cells are then returned to the patient intravenously. The mechanism of action of photopheresis remains unclear. The treatment is believed to induce apoptosis of circulating tumor cells (Sézary cells). The released tumor antigen is then processed by the peripheral dendritic cells leading to the augmentation of systemic antitumor responses.[95] Photopheresis is usually given every 4 weeks, but in patients with severe disease, it can be given as often as every 2 weeks. Once complete clearance is achieved, the frequency can be gradually reduced and then discontinued. The most important application of this procedure is for patients with erythroderma (T4 classification). The majority experience some level of response to ECP, with an ORR of 83%. The CR rate is only 21%, but 41% of patients showed at least a 50% improvement in their disease.[96] The efficacy of ECP in T1, T2, and T3 disease remains unclear.

When using ECP in some situations, such as in SS with high-peripheral blood Sézary burden, it can be combined with other systemic biologic agents such as interferons or retinoids (eg, bexarotene).[97] In addition, skin-directed therapies such as topical steroid, topical nitrogen mustard, phototherapy, or total skin electron beam therapy can be combined with ECP if additional skin-directed treatment is needed.[48,98]

ECP has minimal adverse effects. Some patients may experience nausea, mostly due to the ingested psoralen, and some have a transient low-grade fever or slight malaise after treatment. There are no reports of significant organ damage or bone marrow or immune suppression.[99]

IFN-alpha is indicated for the palliative management of refractory or advanced disease. It may be used alone, but more often with other topical or systemic therapies. Administration is usually initiated at a low dose of 3-5 million units subcutaneously 3 times a week. This dose is gradually increased, depending on the clinical response and the severity of adverse effects. Reported ORR when used as monotherapy are 53-74%, with CR rates of 21-35%.[100,101] The clinical response and response duration appear to be better with the combined regimen of PUVA and IFN, as compared with either treatment alone, but randomized prospective clinical trials are needed to confirm this impression.[41]

Systemic Retinoids

Systemic retinoid therapy, most commonly bexarotene, has been shown to be beneficial in the management of MF and SS.[102] The initial dose of bexarotene is 100-300 mg/m^2/day, which can be adjusted according to the severity of the disease, clinical response, and the degree of adverse effects, especially hyperlipidemia. Systemic retinoids are indicated for palliative therapy for refractory or advanced disease, often in combination with other topical or systemic therapies, including PUVA (RePUVA), IFN-α, or total skin electron beam therapy. The reported response rate is approximately 45-55%, with a 10-20% CR rate.[103] Retinoids may be used in combination with other skin-directed or systemic therapies, including PUVA, IFN-α, or total skin electron beam therapy.[104-106]

Combinations of systemic biologic therapies have been used successfully and with potential synergistic effects when individual therapies fail to attain adequate responses.[97,107] For example, when retinoids are used in combination with PUVA, the response rate is similar to that of PUVA alone; however, the responses may be achieved with fewer PUVA treatments and with a lower cumulative UVA dose.[42] The duration of remission tended to be prolonged if retinoids were given as maintenance therapy.

The most common complications of systemic bexarotene therapy include photosensitivity, xerosis, myalgia, arthralgia, headaches, and impaired night vision. The well-known teratogenic effects of retinoids must be considered in women of childbearing age. Because of its potential hepatotoxic and hyperlipidemic effects, liver function and serum lipid levels should be monitored in each patient during treatment. In addition, central hypothyroidism is often induced, so patients are routinely started on levothyroxin immediately before bexarotene and lipid-lowering agents are administered. Most toxicities due to systemic retinoids are reversible after cessation of therapy.

Recombinant Fusion Proteins

Recombinant fusion protein therapy, such as the IL-2–diphtheria toxin fusion protein (Ontak, denileukin diftitox), involves the use of growth factor–diphtheria toxin fusion proteins designed specifically to kill defined neoplastic cell populations. Ontak has undergone a multicenter phase 3 trial in patients with IL-2 receptor (CD25+)-expressing MF.[108] Patients with Stage IB-III MF who failed to respond to multiple prior therapies, or Stage IVA MF who failed to respond to at least 1 prior therapy, were included in the phase 3 trial. The ORR was 30%, with CR and PR rates of 10% and 20%, respectively. The main complication related to a "capillary leak" syndrome, which may be ameliorated by pretreatment with corticosteroids. Ontak was approved by the FDA for patients with CTCL who have persistent or recurrent disease and whose malignant cells express CD25.

Histone Deacetylase Inhibitors

Histone deacetylase (HDAC) inhibitors are a novel class of agents that can induce growth arrest, differentiation, or apoptosis by affecting gene expression and protein function. Vorinostat (suberoylanilide hydroxamic acid) is an orally available pan-HDAC inhibitor that has activity in patients with MF and SS. This agent has been approved by the FDA for the treatment of cutaneous manifestations of MF in patients with refractory disease.[26] The ORR was 30% ($n = 74$); however, only one patient achieved complete response. Vorinostat is available as 100 mg capsules and the recommended starting dose is 400 mg daily.

The most common side effects of vorinostat included fatigue, diarrhea, nausea, anorexia, and dysgeusia, and thrombocytopenia. Other hematologic abnormalities were less common and mild. QTc interval prolongation has been observed but none were considered clinically significant or associated with new cardiac symptoms.

Novel Therapies

Knowledge of the immunology of MF and its incurability, especially in the advanced stages, has led to the development of a variety of newer therapies. The efficacy of anti–T-cell antibodies has been studied in MF. Early trials using murine monoclonal antibodies were unsuccessful due to the development of human anti–mouse antibodies (HAMA). A chimeric anti–helper-T-cell (anti-CD4) antibody was been used in order to provide more specific treatment against the MF subset of T-cells, and to avoid the development of HAMA.[109] (In addition, humanized anti-CD3 and anti-CD4 antibodies have been developed.[110]

The safety and efficacy of alemtuzumab (Campath-1H), a humanized monoclonal antibody directed against CD52, was tested in 22 previously treated patients, most of whom had Stage III or IV disease, reduced performance status, and severe pruritus.[108] Complete and partial responses were noted in 32% and 23%, respectively, with a median time to treatment failure of 12 months. Serious infections (CMV, generalized herpes simplex, fatal aspergillosis, and mycobacterium pneumonia) were noted, especially in patients who had received more than 3 prior treatment regimens. These patients require antibiotic and antiviral prophylaxis and close observation for the development of infection and cardiac toxicity.

Photodynamic therapy, using nonionizing laser light after topical or systemic application of a photosensitizing agent, such as 5-aminolevulinic acid, has been used for the local treatment of cutaneous lesions in a small number of patients with MF.[111,112] Most of these reports have involved successful treatment of single lesions resistant to treatment with other agents. Toxicity is minimal, and has been limited to local pain, erythema, or blistering.

Selected References

The complete reference list can be found at www.CANCERMEDICINE8.com

1. Kim YH, Hoppe RT. Mycosis fungoides and the Sézary syndrome. *Semin Oncol.* 1999; 26:276–289.
3. Crowley JJ, Nikko A, Varghese A, et al. Mycosis fungoides in young patients: clinical characteristics and outcome. *J Am Acad Dermatol.* 1998;38:696–701.
4. Whittemore A, Holly E, Lee I, et al. Mycosis fungoides in relation to environmental exposures and immune response: a case-control study. *J Natl Cancer Inst.* 1989;81:1560–1567.
7. Wood GS, Weiss L, Warnke R, et al. The immunopathology of cutaneous lymphomas: Immunophenotypic and immunogenotypic characteristics. *Semin Dermatol.* 1986;5:334–345.
9. Ralfkiaer E. Mycosis fungoides and Sézary syndrome. In: Jaffe ES, Harris NL, Stein H, et al., eds. *Pathology and genetics of tumours of haematopoietic and lymphoid tissues.* IARC Press: Lyon; 2001:216–220.
11. Willemze R, Jaffe ES, Burg G, et al. WHO-EORTC classification for cutaneous lymphomas. *Blood.* 2005;105:3768–3785.
16. Kim YH, Jensen RA, Watanabe GL, et al. Clinical stage IA (limited patch and plaque) mycosis fungoides. A long-term outcome analysis. *Arch Dermatol.* 1996;132:1309–1313.
17. Kim YH, Chow S, Varghese A, et al. Clinical characteristics and long-term outcome of patients with generalized patch and/or plaque (T2) mycosis fungoides. *Arch Dermatol.* 1999;135:26–32.
18. Kim YH, Liu HL, Mraz-Gernhard S, et al. Longterm outcome of 525 patients with mycosis fungoides and Sézary syndrome at Stanford: clinical prognostic factors and risks of disease progression and second cancer *Arch Dermatol.* 2003;139:857–866.
19. Epstein EH Jr, Levin DL, Croft JD Jr, et al. Mycosis fungoides. Survival, prognostic features, response to therapy, and autopsy findings. *Medicine (Baltimore).* 1972;51:61–72.
21. Weiss L, Hu E, Wood GS, et al. Clonal rearrangements of T-cell receptor genes in mycosis fungoides and dermatopathic lymphadenopathy. *J Invest Dermatol.* 1985;85:199–202.
22. Kohler S, Zehnder JL. Use of the polymerase chain reaction in the evaluation of cutaneous T-cell infiltrates. *Dermatol Clin.* 1999;17:657–666.
25. Tsai E. Staging accuracy in mycosis fungoides/Sézary syndrome using integrated positron emission tomography and computed tomography. *Arch Dermatol.* 2006;142:577–584.
27. Kim YH, Bishop K, Varghese A, et al. Prognostic factors in erythrodermic mycosis fungoides and the Sézary syndrome [see comments]. *Arch Dermatol.* 1995;131:1003–1008.
28. de Coninck EC, Kim YH, Varghese A, et al. Clinical characteristics and outcome of patients with extracutaneous mycosis fungoides. *J Clinical Oncol.* 2001;19:779–784.
29. Sausville EA, Eddy JL, Makuch RW, et al. Histopathologic staging at initial diagnosis of mycosis fungoides and the Sézary syndrome. Definition of three distinctive prognostic groups. *Ann Intern Med.* 1988;109:372–382.
32. Wood GS, Bahler DW, Hoppe RT, et al. Transformation of mycosis fungoides: T-cell receptor beta gene analysis demonstrates a common clonal origin for plaque-type mycosis fungoides and CD30+ large-cell lymphoma. *J Invest Dermatol.* 1993;101:296–300.
34. www.nccn.org Non-Hodgkin Lymphoma MF/SS practice guidelines.
35. Kim YH, Martinez G, Varghese A, et al. Management with topical nitrogen mustard in mycosis fungoides: update of the Stanford experience. *Arch Dermatol.* 2003;139:165–173.
36. Heald P, Mehlmauer M, Martin AG, et al. Topical bexarotene therapy for patients with refractory or persistent early-stage cutaneous T-cell lymphoma: results of the phase III clinical trial. *J Am Acad Dermatol.* 2003;49:801.
38. Resnik KS, Vonderheid EC. Home UV phototherapy of early mycosis fungoides: long-term follow-up observations in thirty-one patients. *J Am Acad Dermatol.* 1993;29:73–77.
41. Kuzel TM, Roenigk HH Jr, Samuelson E, et al. Effectiveness of interferon alfa-2a combined with phototherapy for mycosis fungoides and the Sézary syndrome. *J Clin Oncol.* 1995;13:257–263.
43. Jones GW, Hoppe RT, Glatstein E. Electron beam treatment for cutaneous T-cell lymphoma. Hematol/Oncol Clin North Amer 1995;9:1057–1076.
44. Hoppe R. Mycosis fungoides: radiation therapy. *Dermatologic Therapy.* 2003;16:347–354.
46. Becker M, Hoppe RT, Knox SJ. Multiple courses of high-dose total skin electron beam therapy in the management of mycosis fungoides. *Int J Radiat Oncol Biol Phys.* 1995;32:1445–1449.
48. Horwitz SM, Olsen EA, Duvic M, Porcu P, Kim YH. Review of the treatment of mycosis fungoides and Sezary syndrome: a stage-based approach, *J Natl Compr Canc Netw.* 2008;6:436–442.
53. Zackheim HS, Kashani-Sabet M, McMillan AK. Low dose methotrexate to treat mycosis fungoides: a retrospective study in 69 patients. *J Am Acad Dermatol.* 2003;49:873–878.
57. Tsimberidon AM, Giles F, Duvic M, et al. Phase II study of pentostatin in advanced T-cell lymphoid malignancies: update of an M.D. Anderson Cancer Center series. *Cancer.* 2004;100:342–349.
59. Kuzel T, Hurria A, Samuelson E, et al. Rose Phase II trial of 2-chlorodeoxyadenosine for the treatment of cutaneous T-cell lymphoma. *Blood.* 1996;87:906–911.
61. Von Hoff D, Dahlberg S, Hartsock R, et al. Activity of fludarabine monophosphate in patients with advanced mycosis fungoides: Southwest Oncology Group study. *J Natl Cancer Inst.* 1990;82:1353–1355.
65. Zinzani PL, Baliva G, Magagnoli M, et al. Gemcitabine treatment in pretreated cutaneous T-cell lymphoma: experience in 44 patients. *J Clin Oncol.* 2000;18: 2603–2606
71. Quereux G, Marques S, Nguyen JM, et al. Prospective multicenter study of pegylated liposomal doxorubicin treatment in patients with advanced or refractory mycosis fungoides or Sézary syndrome *Arch Dermatol.* 2008;144:727–733.
73. Tani M, Fina M, Alinari L, Stefoni V, Baccarani M, Zinzani PL. Phase II trial of temozolomide in patients with pretreated cutaneous T-cell lymphoma. *Haematologica.* 2005;90:1283–1284.
75. Zinzani PL, Musuraca G, Tani M, et al. Phase II trial of proteasome inhibitor bortezomib in patients with relapsed or refractory cutaneous T-cell lymphoma. , 2007;25:4293–4297.
81. Winkler CF, Sausville EA, Ihde DC. Combined modality treatment of cutaneous T cell lymphoma: Results of a 6- year follow up. *J Clin Oncol.* 1986;4:1094–1100.
83. Kaye FJ, Bunn PA Jr, Steinberg SM, et al. A randomized trial comparing combination electron-beam radiation and chemotherapy with topical therapy in the initial treatment of mycosis fungoides. *N Engl J Med.* 1989;321:1784–1790.
84. Duvic M, Apisarnthanarax M, Cohen DS, et al. Analysis of long-term outcomes of combined modality therapy for cutaneous T-cell lymphoma. *J Am Acad Dermatol.* 2003;49:35–49.
85. (Duarte RF, Schmitz N, Servitje O, Sureda A. Haematopoietic stem cell transplantation for patients with primary cutaneous T-cell lymphoma. *Bone Marrow Transplant.* 2008;4:597–604.
91. Soligo D, Ibatici A, Berti E, et al. Treatment of advanced mycosis fungoides by allogeneic stem-cell transplantation with a nonmyeloablative regimen. *Bone Marrow Transplant.* 2003;31:663–666.
92. Herbert KE, Spencer A, Grigg A, Ryan G, McCormack C, Prince HM. Graft-versus-lymphoma effect in refractory cutaneous T-cell lymphoma after reduced-intensity HLA-matched sibling allogeneic stem cell transplantation. *Bone Marrow Transplant.* 2004;34:521–525.
96. Heald P, Rook AH, Perez M, et al. Treatment of erythrodermic cutaneous T-cell lymphoma with extracorporeal photochemotherapy. *J Am Acta Dermatol.* 1992;27:427–433.
100. Chiarion-Sileni V, Bononi A, Fornasa CV, et al. Phase II trial of interferon-alpha-2a plus psoralen with ultraviolet light A in patients with cutaneous T-cell lymphoma. *Cancer.* 2002;95:569.
103. Duvic M, Martin AG, Kim Y, et al. Phase 2 and 3 clinical trial of oral bexarotene (Targretin capsules) for the treatment of refractory or persistent early-stage cutaneous T-cell lymphoma. *Arch Dermatol.* 2001;137:581–593.
108. Olsen E, Duvic M, Frankel A, et al. Pivotal phase II trial of two dose levels of denileukin diftitox for the treatment of cutaneous T-cell lymphoma. *J Clin Oncol.* 2001;19:376–88.
109. Knox S, Levy R, Hodgkinson S, et al. Observations on the effect of chimeric-anti-CD4 monoclonal antibody in patients with mycosis fungoides. *Blood.* 1991;77:20–30.
110. Kim Y et al., *Blood.* 2007;109:4655–4662.

117 Plasma Cell Tumors

Noopur Raje, MD ■ Teru Hideshima, MD, PhD ■ Kenneth C. Anderson, MD

Multiple Myeloma

Multiple myeloma (MM) is a malignant proliferation of plasma cells and plasmacytoid cells in the bone marrow (BM) characterized nearly always by the presence, in the serum and/or urine, of a monoclonal immunoglobulin (Ig) or Ig fragment.[1-4] This disease has probably been recognized since 1845, when the first patient was noted with bone pain and heat soluble "animal matter" in urine.[5,6] The term MM was coined in 1873, reflecting distinct sites of BM involvement. The plasma cell was discovered in 1890 and MM associated with plasmacytosis shortly thereafter, in 1900. The application of electrophoresis in 1939 and immunoelectrophoresis in 1953 allowed for the identification of monotypic Ig characteristic of MM.[7,8]

Diagnostic Criteria

Both major and minor criteria for the diagnosis of MM have been defined (Table 117-1).[9] These include the presence of excess monotypic marrow plasma cells, monoclonal Ig in serum and/or urine, decreased normal serum Ig levels, and lytic bone disease. Active MM must be distinguished from other disorders characterized by monoclonal gammopathies, both malignant and otherwise, in particular monoclonal gammopathy of undetermined significance (MGUS) and smoldering MM.[10,11] Other conditions include macroglobulinemia, non-Hodgkin lymphoma, primary amyloidosis, idiopathic cold agglutinin disease, essential cryoglobulinemia, and heavy chain disease. Active MM is defined by the presence of a monoclonal spike in the serum and/or urine, with ≥10% plasma cells in the BM with associated hypercalcemia, renal dysfunction, anemia, and/or bone disease related to the MM.

Table 117-1 ■ **Durie and Salmon Criteria**

Major criteria
1. Plasmacytomas on tissue biopsy
2. Bone marrow plasmacytosis (>30% plasma cells)
3. Monoclonal immunoglobulin spike on serum electrophoresis immunoglobulin G (IgG) >3.5 g/dL or immunoglobulin A (IgA) >2.0 g/dL; kappa or lambda light chain excretion >1 g/day on 24 hour urine protein electrophoresis
Minor criteria
1. Bone marrow plasmacytosis (10 to 30% plasma cells
2. Monoclonal immunoglobulin present but of lesser magnitude than given under major criteria
3. Lytic bone lesions
4. Normal IgM < 50 mg/dL, IgA < 100 mg/dL or IgG < 600 mg/dL
Any of the following sets of criteria will confirm the diagnosis of multiple myeloma:
Any two of the major criteria
Major criterion 1 plus minor criterion 2, 3, or 4
Major criterion 3 plus minor criterion 1 or 3
Minor criterion 1, 2, and 3 or 1, 2, and 4

Monoclonal Gammopathy of Unclear Significance ■ MGUS is present in 3.2% of persons 50 years of age or older and 5.3% of persons 70 years of age or older.[11] Patients have <3.5 g/L monoclonal Ig, little or no proteinuria, fewer than 5% monoclonal marrow plasma cells, and no bone lesions, anemia, hypercalcemia, or renal dysfunction. In a large experience of 1384 patients diagnosed at the Mayo Clinic, 115 patients progressed to MM, *IgM* lymphoma, primary amyloidosis, macroglobulinemia, chronic lymphocytic leukemia, or plasmacytoma with relative risk of progression of 25.0, 2.4, 8.4, 46.0, 0.9, and 8.5, respectively.[12] The risk of progression of MGUS to MM or related disorders is about 1% per year, and the initial concentration of serum monoclonal protein was a significant predictor of progression at 20 years. Similar results have been published by Cesana and colleagues.[13] Independent prognostic factors associated with MGUS transformation to MM include: (1) >5% BM plasmacytosis, (2) Bence Jones proteinuria, (3) decrease in polyclonal serum immunoglobulin, and (4) an elevated erythrocyte sedimentation rate.[13] More recently, risk factors for progression include an abnormal serum kappa–lambda free light chain ratio, a high serum monoclonal protein level, and non-IgG.[14] The risk of progression from smoldering MM to symptomatic disease is related to the proportion of BM plasma cells and serum monoclonal protein level at diagnosis.[15] In some cases, MGUS can be associated with symptomatology requiring therapy. For example, plasma exchange appears to be efficacious in neuropathy associated with IgG or IgA MGUS.[16]

Epidemiology

In addition to MGUS, a potential risk factor for the development of MM includes exposure to irradiation or petroleum products. Unlike leukemia, there is no increased risk of MM with benzene exposure.[17] Families with two or more affected individuals have been reported, suggesting a possible genetic predisposition.[18] MM has also been found to occur with somewhat greater frequency (but less than twofold) in farmers, paper producers, furniture manufacturers, and wood workers.

There are two major misconceptions regarding MM. The first is that MM is a rare disease. MM is the second most common hematologic malignancy, accounting for 19,920 new cancer cases in the United States in the year 2008 and approximately 2% of cancer-related deaths.[19] The highest incidence rates have been reported for African Americans and Pacific Islanders; Europeans and North American white people have intermediate rates, while generally low rates have been reported for Asians living in Asia and the United States.[20] Although it has been suggested that the incidence of MM is increasing, data from Olmstead County, Minnesota, demonstrate that the incidence of MM has not changed significantly during the past 46 years.[21] A second misunderstanding is that MM is solely a disease of the old. In a large Mayo Clinic series, the mean age was 62 years for men and 61 years for women.[4] Although 98% of MM patients were 40 years of age or older, 35% of men and 41% of women were less than 60 years old. Importantly, 75% of men and 79% of women were younger than age 70. The fact that a significant population of affected individuals is younger than age 70 and therefore can tolerate more aggressive therapeutic approaches influences potential treatment strategies.

Clinical Features

The presenting features in 869 cases of MM evaluated from 1960 to 1971 are summarized in Tables 117-2A and B.[4] Although there was a slight predominance of men (61%) in this series, other studies suggest that incidence in men and women may be equivalent. Symptoms of bone pain and anemia remain the most common presenting features.

Laboratory Features

Laboratory evaluation identifies roentgenographic abnormalities in bone and monoclonal Ig in serum and/or urine in the majority of cases. In most series,

Table 117-2A **Presenting Features of Multiple Myeloma**

Percentage of Patients	Presenting Feature
98	More than 40 years old
88	Proteinuria
79	Skeletal roentgenographic abnormalities
68	Bone pain
62	Anemia
61	Male
55	Renal insufficiency
49	Bence Jones proteinuria
30	Hypercalcemia
21	Hepatomegaly
5	Splenomegaly

Source: From Ref. 4.

Table 117-2B **Presenting Features of Multiple Myeloma**

Percentage of Patients	Presenting Feature
83	Monoclonal heavy chain on serum immunoelectrophoresis (IEP)
76	Spike on serum protein electrophoresis (SPEP)
75	Spike on urinary electrophoresis
15	Minor or no abnormalities
9	Hypogammaglobulinemia (SPEP)
8	Monoclonal light chain (IEP)
7	Amyloidosis
0.3	Nonsecretory

Source: From Ref. 4.

50-60% of patients with MM have both serum and urinary monoclonal protein; 20-30% of patients have serum without urinary protein; 15-20% of patients have monoclonal protein in urine only; and only 1-2% of patients do not secrete monoclonal protein in blood and/or urine.[22] IgG or IgA monoclonal proteins are most common, and IgD or IgE are rare. A biclonal process is much more common than previously appreciated, often only documented by immunofixation techniques. Thirty-three percent are IgG and IgA; 24% are IgM and IgG. It appears that patients with biclonal and IgD disease have prognoses similar to those patients with monoclonal disease.[23] Laboratory evaluation of quantitative immunoglobulins can distinguish MGUS from smoldering, indolent, and overt MM (Table 117-3). It provides the basis for staging systems to predict both response and survival. No therapy is an appropriate choice for patients with MGUS, or smoldering and indolent MM, whereas multiple regimens have been employed for therapy of individuals with overt MM.[24] The natural history of MM is a progressive increase in tumor growth. The M protein doubling time, a measure of the MM growth rate, shortens with each relapse. Eventually, marrow failure develops, with sideroblastic anemia, leukopenia, and thrombocytopenia. The median interval from marrow failure to death is 3 (range 1–9) months.[25] Infection and renal failure account for 52% and 21% of deaths, respectively, in patients with MM.[26] Acute myeloid leukemia develops in a small fraction of patients, but far in excess of the anticipated baseline incidence.[25]

Table 117-3 **Classification of Monoclonal Gammopathies**

A. Monoclonal gammopathy of unclear significance:
M-component level
IgG < 3.5 g/dL
IgA < 2.0 g/dL
Bence Jones protein < 1.0 g/24 h
Bone marrow plasma cells < 10%
No bone lesions
No symptoms
B. Indolent myeloma as in a except:
No bone lesions or only limited bone lesions (<3lytic lesions); no compression fractures
M-component levels
(a) IgG <7 g/dL
(b) IgA <5 g/dL
No symptoms or associated disease features; ie:
Performance status >70%
Hemoglobin >10 g/dL
Serum calcium normal
Serum creatinine <2.0 mg/dL
No infections
C. Smoldering myeloma as in B except:
No bone lesions
Bone marrow plasma cells <30%

Abbreviation: Ig, immunoglobulin.

Biology

Cell Surface Phenotype B-cell–restricted and associated antigens (Ags) have been used to delineate stages of normal and malignant B-cell differentiation.[27]Moreover, antigenic profiles are useful not only to identify stages of malignant B-cell differentiation, but also to categorize B-cell tumors. MM cells share cell surface expression of some Ags, for example, CD38 and PCA-1, which are also present on normal plasma cells, suggesting that the normal cellular counterpart of MM is the normal plasma cell. However, a number of other Ags to date have been described on the surface of MM cells, which in some cases react with B cells at stages of differentiation earlier than the plasma cell, but also react with non-B cells.[28-33] Harada and colleagues have shown that normal plasma cells are CD19+CD56–, whereas no MM cells have this phenotype.[34] The core protein of MUC- 1 antigen is expressed on MM cells.[35] The expression and function of adhesion molecules on MM cells is described below. This observed heterogeneity in cell surface phenotype has led to controversy as to the cellular origin of MM.

Cellular Origin of MM

As is well known, the cells that accumulate in the BM of patients with MM have plasma cell or plasmablast morphology. However, it has been known since the 1970s, based on studies using anti-idiotypic antibodies, that unique idiotypic determinants can identify clones of peripheral blood lymphocytes in patients with macroglobulinemia, MM, MGUS, and chronic lymphocytic leukemia.[36] The presence of idiotypic determinants on cytoplasmic μ-containing pre-B cells in MM BM provided further evidence that the oncogenic event may occur at the pre–B-cell stage. Studies identified B and T cells bearing identical idiotypic determinants, suggesting that target cells for oncogenic transformation could be precursor cells for both B and T-cell clones.[37] Aneuploid marrow MM cells can express mRNA for cell surface proteins characteristic of myeloid, erythroid, and platelet lineages, also supporting the view that the malignant clone can extend from an early stage of differentiation.[38] Moreover, monoclonal B-lineage cells in peripheral blood of MM patients, which are late-stage B cells (low CD19 and CD20, moderate CALLA and PCA-1, with strong CD45RO antigen expression) are continuously progressing toward the plasma cell stage.[31] However, it remains unclear as to which cell within the malignant clone is "clonogenic" and capable of self-renewal. Some evidence suggests that pre-B and naive B cells migrate from the BM to the lymph node (LN) where antigen recognition, selection, and somatic hypermutation occur. The memory–B-cell compartment is thought to contain the cytoplasmic μ-positive precursor cell of MM, which then undergoes Ig class switching in the LN.[39] *Ig*-variable (*VH*) gene sequence analysis has shown MM tumor cells to be postfollicular, with the mutated homogeneous clonal sequences indicating no continuing exposure to somatic hypermutation mechanism.[40] *VH* gene analysis of IgM MM indicates an origin from a memory cell undergoing isotype switch events.[41] Mutated heterogeneous sequences in MGUS suggest that tumor cells remain under the influence of the mutator.[42] Abnormalities of 14q (the location of IgH) are most common in MM. Since proto-oncogenes are translocated to this region and overexpressed in B-cell malignancies including follicular lymphoma, Burkitt lymphoma, and chronic lymphocytic leukemia, they may also play a role in the oncogenesis of MM. In addition, translocations involving switch regions indicate that the final oncogenic molecular event in MM occurs late in B-cell ontogeny.[42] More recently, CD138-cells with a memory B-cell phenotype are thought to be the clonogenic MM 'stem' cells, although this concept needs further validation.[43]

Role of Adhesion Molecules, Cytokines, and BM Stromal Cells in MM

Adhesion molecules mediate both homotypic and heterotypic adhesion of tumor cells to either extracellular matrix (ECM) proteins or BM stromal cells (BMSCs) (Fig. 117-1).[44] Moreover, they play a critical role in pathogenesis of disease progression. After class switching in the LN, adhesion molecules (eg, CD44, VLA-4, VLA-5, LFA-1, CD56, syndecan-1, and MPC-1) mediate homing of MM cells to the BM.[44-47] Subsequently, binding of MM cells occurs to BMSCs, for example, via VLA-4 to VCAM-1, and to ECM, for example, via syndecan to type I collagen and VLA-4 to fibronectin. Such binding not only localizes tumor cells in the BM microenvironment, but also stimulates interleukin-6 (IL-6) transcription and secretion from BMSCs with related paracrine growth of MM cells.[48-50] Moreover, triggering via CD40 found on tumor cells induces IL-6 transcription and secretion, with related autocrine MM cell growth (Fig. 117-2).[51] Tumor necrosis factor-α (TNF-α) up-regulates adhesion molecules on MM cells and BMSCs, thereby increasing binding and cell adhesion-mediated (CAM) drug resistance.[52] Syndecan-1 is a multifunctional regulator of tumor cell growth and survival as well as of bone cell differentiation, and elevated serum syndecan1 correlates with increased tumor cell mass, decreased metalloproteinase-9 activity, and poor prognosis.[53-55] Adhesion also induces matrix metalloproteinase-1, which favors bone resorption and tumor invasion.[56] Syndecan-1 is shed from the surface of most MM cells, induces apoptosis, and can inhibit the growth of MM cells; it also mediates decreased osteoclast and increased osteoblast differentition.[53] As the disease progresses, the development of plasma cell leukemia (PCL) is characterized by decreased expression of certain adhesion molecules (eg, CD56, VLA-5, MPC-1, and syndecan-1), which in turn facilitates tumor cell mobilization. Furthermore, the acquisition of other adhesion molecules on PCL cells, such as CD11b, CD44, and RHAMM, assists transit through endothelium during egress from the BM. Extramedullary spread of MM cells is facilitated by the reappearance of CD56, VLA-5, MPC-1, and syndecan-1. Since adhesion molecules play a central role in the pathogenesis of MM, therapeutic strategies targeting these molecules have been developed and tested in animal models; for example, anti-ICAM-1 antibodies have been shown to inhibit tumor development in severe combined immunodeficient (SCID) mice.[57] Moreover, a model of MM in SCID mice bearing fetal bone grafts (SCID-hu mice) provides for the first time an in vivo model for the evaluation of homing of human MM cells to human BM ECM proteins and BMSCs, the biologic sequelae of binding, as well as testing of novel treatments based on interruption of this process.[58,59] MM cells resistant to melphalan and doxorubicin typically overexpress VLA-4, and adherence to ECM proteins like fibronectin induces CAM drug resistance, with upregulation of p27 in tumor cells.[55] As we will discuss below, novel agents, including thalidomide (Thal) and its immunomodulatory derivatives (IMiDs) such as lenalidomide, as well as the proteasome inhibitor bortezomib can target both the tumor cell and its BM microenvironment and thereby overcome CAM drug resistance.[60-64]

We have characterized the mechanisms whereby MM cells home to the host BM and adhere to BMSCs and ECM proteins, as well as the functional sequelae of this binding, in order to identify targets for novel therapies. Importantly, our past studies have identified those adhesion molecules mediating MM cell binding to fibronectin and BMSCs, as well as the MM cell growth and survival advantage conferred by this binding.[44,50,65-67]

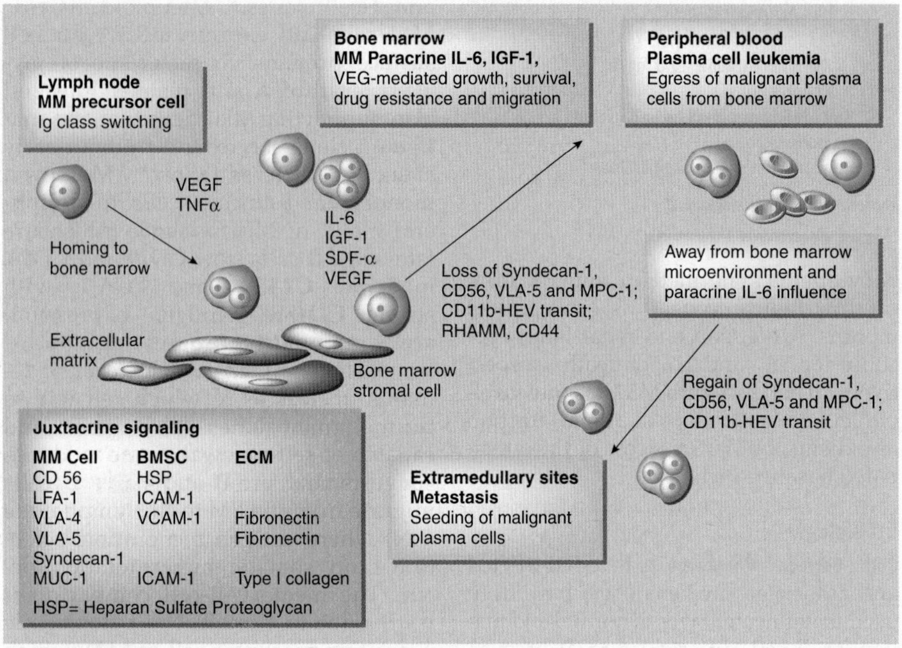

Figure 117-1 ■ Role of adhesion molecules in myeloma pathogenesis.

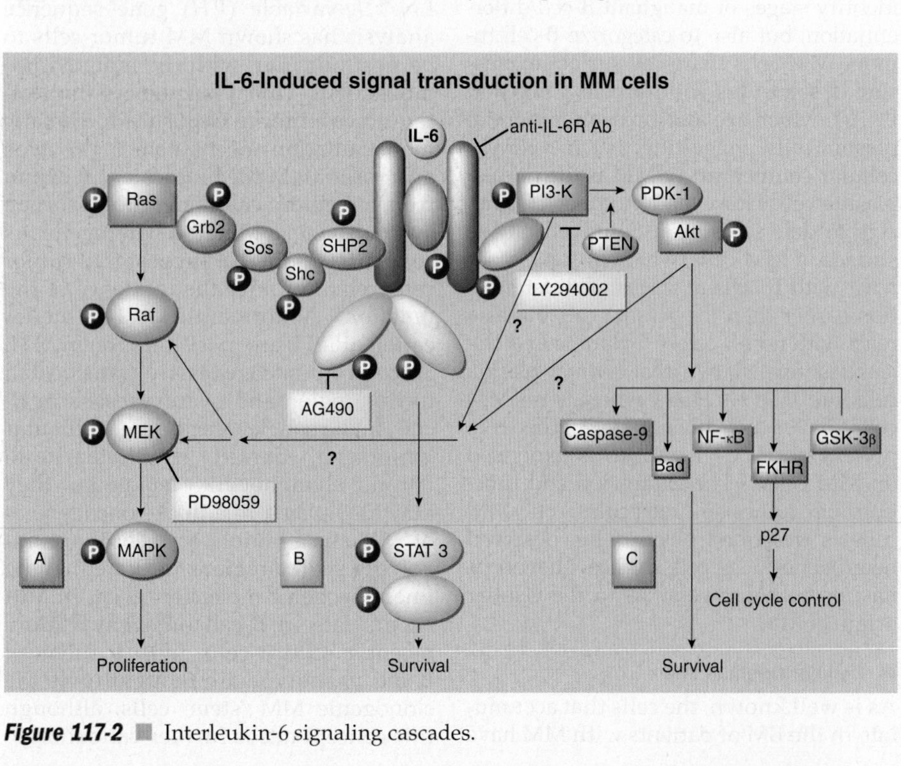

Figure 117-2 ■ Interleukin-6 signaling cascades.

Our studies show that BMSCs secrete cytokines, such as IL-6,[3] insulin-like growth factor-1 (IGF-1),[68] vascular endothelial growth factor (VEGF),[69,70] stromal cell derived growth factor (SDF-1)α,[71] and B-cell activating factor (BAFF),[72,73] which augment MM cell growth, survival, drug resistance, and migration in the BM milieu (Fig. 117-3). Besides localizing tumor cells in the BM microenvironment, our studies demonstrate that adhesion of MM cells to BMSCs also triggers the paracrine NF-κB-dependent transcription and secretion in BMSCs of IL-6, the major cytokine mediating MM cell growth, survival, and resistance to dexamethasone (Dex)-induced apoptosis via MAPK and PI3-K/Akt, Jak/STAT, and PI3-K/Akt signaling cascades, respectively.[48,50,67,68,74-85] VEGF is secreted by both MM cells and BMSCs, and its secretion is similarly upregulated by binding of MM cells to BMSCs; it augments MM cell growth angiogenesis, although the pathophysiologic significance of angiogenesis in MM BM is undefined.[86,87] It induces migration via PKC signaling.[70] Although TNF-α does not directly alter MM cell growth and survival, our studies show that it induces NF-κB-dependent upregulation in cell surface expression of adhesion molecules (ICAM-1, VCAM-1) on both MM cells and BMSCs, resulting in increased binding and related induction of IL-6 transcription and secretion in BMSCs.[52] Recombinant IL-1β stimulates MM cells to produce IL-6, which consequently augments proliferation of MM cells.[88] Transforming growth factor-β (TGF-β) is secreted by MM cells and triggers IL-6 secretion in BMSCs,[89] thereby augmenting paracine IL-6 mediated tumor cell growth. TGF-β secreted by MM cells likely also contributes to the immunodeficiency characteristic of MM by downregulating B cells, T cells, and natural killer cells, without similarly inhibiting the growth of MM cells. IL-10 is a proliferation factor, but not a differentiation factor, for human MM cells.[90] IGF-1 has been shown to augment MM cell growth, survival, and drug resistance.[68] Macrophage inflammatory protein-1α (MIP-1α) is an osteoclast stimulating factor in MM.[91,92] BAFF is produced by the BMSCs, and specifically by osteoclasts. It signals through several receptors including BAFF-R, transmembrane activator, calcium modulator and cyclophilin ligand interactor (TACI), B-cell maturation Ag (BCMA).[72,73] The level of TACI gene expression in MM cells is associated with microenvironment dependence.[93] This signaling cascade has a prosurvival effect on MM cells. Autocrine growth mediated by IL-15,[94] and most recently IL-21,[95] has been demonstrated in both MM cell lines and patient cells.

Wnt signaling regulates various developmental processes and can lead to malignant formation and has been recently studied in the context of MM. Wnts are a family of secreted glycoproteins that bind to frizzled seven-transmembrane span receptors. Intracellularly, the Wnt signaling cascade blocks degradation of β-catenin in proteasomes, thereby leading to accumulation of β-catenin in the cytoplasm. In MM, a canonical Wnt signaling pathway is activated following treatment with Wnt-3a, associated with accumulation of β-catenin. Wnt-3a treatment further led to significant morphological changes in MM cells, accompanied by rearrangement of the actin cytoskeleton.[96] Derksen and colleagues[97] demonstrated that MM cells overexpress β-catenin, including its N-terminally unphosphorylated form, consistent with active β-catenin/T-cell factor-mediated transcription. Further accumulation and nuclear localization of β-catenin, and/or increased cell proliferation, was achieved by stimulation of Wnt signaling with either Wnt-3a, LiCl, or the constitutively active mutant of βcatenin. Interestingly, MM cells in BM-biopsy specimens contained detectable dickkopf 1 (DKK1), a negative regulator of Wnt signaling cascade and a target of the β-catenin/TCF pathway.[98] Moreover, elevated DKK1 levels in BM plasma and peripheral blood from patients with MM correlated with the DKK1 gene-expression patterns and was associated with the presence of focal bone lesions.[99]

Most importantly, adhesion of MM cells to the BM induces changes in gene profile: ie, upregulation of growth, survival, and drug resistance genes in tumor cells; upregulation of adhesions molecules on MM cells and BMSCs; and changes in cytokines in BMSCS both in vitro and in our in vivo models of human MM in mice.[100-102] Interaction of MM cells with BMSCs activates Notch signaling, which induces melphalan resistance.[103] Others have shown that MM cell adhesion to fibronectin confers conventional cell adhesion mediated (CAM) drug resistance with induction of p27 and G1 growth arrest.[60] Excitingly, novel agents including thalidomide (Thal) and derivatives (IMiDs) including lenalidomide,[61,62] as well as proteasome inhibitor Bortezomib (velcade, PS-341),[52,63] can target both the tumor cell and its BM microenvironment, thereby overcoming CAM) conventional drug resistance. Induction of proteasome activity when MM cells bind to BMSCs may sensitize them to therapy.

We have shown that IMiDs (lenalidomide) inhibit VEGF and IL-6, which are known to downregulate antigen presenting function of dendritic cells (DCs) in MM.[104] Moreover, lenalidomide directly activates CD28 on T cells, thereby stimulating transcription and secretion of IL-2, with resultant upregulation of T and NK cell anti-MM activity.[104,105] Lenalidomide can upregulate antibody dependent cellular mediated cytotoxicity.[106]

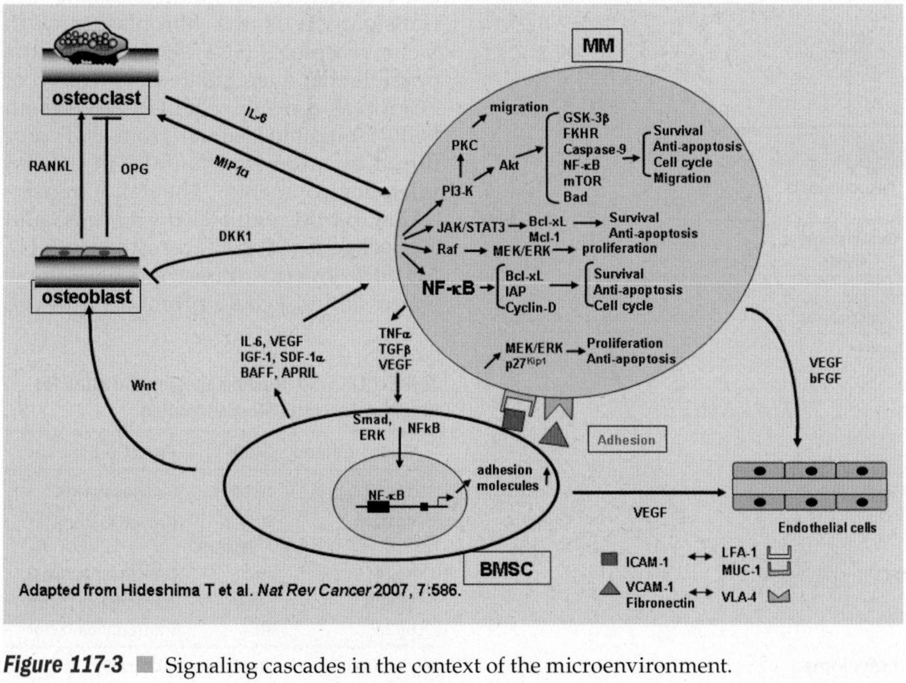

Figure 117-3 Signaling cascades in the context of the microenvironment.

Molecular Pathogenesis of MM

The malignant plasma cells in MM are localized to the BM in close association with BMSCs. They are long-lived cells with a very low labeling index (LI = 1–2%). The rearranged *Ig* genes are extensively somatically hypermutated in a manner compatible with antigen selection, with no evidence that the process of hypermutation is continuing (Fig. 117-4).[40] However, MM cells have a significantly lower rate of Ig secretion than normal plasma cells. Thus it appears that the critical oncogenic events in MM cells either occur after or do not interfere with most of the normal differentiation process involved in generating a long-lived plasma cell.

Gene microarray profiling has recently been used to characterize changes associated with the progression from normal plasma cells to MGUS toMM.[107-109] The mRNA profile of MGUS and MM is similar yet distinct from that of normal plasma cells.[109] These studies may not only enhance understanding of basic pathophysiology, but also identify novel therapeutic targets.

By conventional analyses, karyotypic abnormalities are detected in MM at a frequency of 30 to 50% in large studies of MM tumors (Table 117-4).[110-112] The frequency and extent of karyotypic abnormalities correlates with the stage, prognosis, and response to therapy. For example, approximately 20% are abnormal in stage I disease, 60% in stage III patients, and >80% for extramedullary tumor. This analysis is dependent on obtaining reliable metaphase preparations and greatly underrepresents the extent of DNA alterations in these infrequently dividing cell populations. By interphase FISH analysis, two studies report that at least one chromosome is trisomic in 96% or 89% of MM tumor samples, respectively.[113,114] Although conventional karyotypes are not routinely reported for MGUS, it appears that a substantial fraction of MGUS plasma cells are aneuploid as well. By FISH analysis, the incidence of trisomy for at least one chromosome was 43% and 53% in two studies of MGUS cells; in the former, 61% of the cells had an aneuploid DNA content by image analysis.[113,115] The characteristic numerical abnormalities are monosomy 13 and trisomies of chromosomes 3, 5, 7, 9, 11, 15, and 19. Nonrandom structural abnormalities most frequently involve chromosome 1 with no apparent locus specificity; 14q32(IgH) locus occurs in 20-40%; 11q13(bcl-1 locus) in about 20%, but mostly translocated to 14q32; 13q14 interstitial deletion in 15%; and 8q24 in about 10%, with about half of these involved in a translocation. Importantly, a recent report documents similar translocations in MGUS and MM, including t(4;14)(p16.3;q32) and t(14;16)(q32;q23), without any obvious clinical or biologic correlation.[116]

Table 117-4 ■ **Myeloma Chromosomal Alterations**

Chromosome anomaly: Incidence
Conventional banding: 30–50% of patients
Interphase FISH: > 90% of cases
SKY: ? ~100%
Specific chromosome changes
14q32: majority of cases
11q13: most common (Bcl-1 locus, 30%)
4p16 (FGFR3, MMSET, 25%)
8q24 (c-myc, 5%)
16q23 (c-maf, 1%)
6p25 (IRF4, rare)
13 deletion (Rb)

Abbreviations: FISH, fluorescence in situ hybridization; SKY, spectral karyotyping.

The hallmark genetic lesion in many B-lymphocyte tumors involves dysregulation of an oncogene as a consequence of a translocation involving the IgH locus (14q32.3); less frequently, variant translocations involve one of the IgL loci (2p12, kappa or 22q11, lambda) (see Tables 117-4 and 117-5). From conventional karyotypic analyses, translocations involving 14q32 appear to occur in about 20 to 40% of MM with an abnormal karyotype.[3] The incidence of these translocations is significantly higher in the extramedullary phase of the disease and in cell lines, perhaps because of a higher number of metaphase spreads that are examined. In about 30% of these translocations, the partner chromosomal locus is 11q13 (bcl-1, cyclin D1), but in most cases the partner is not identified (14q32+). Transcriptional activation of cyclin D1 has recently been confirmed in some primary tumors, as has cyclin D3 activation associated with t(6;14)(p21;q32) translocation.[116-118] Other recurrent partner loci have been identified infrequently, including 8q24(c-myc) in less than 5%, 18q21(bcl-2), 11q23(MLL-1), and 6p21.1. By combining conventional karyotypic analysis with a comprehensive Southern blot assay, which detects translocations involving IgH switch regions, it has become apparent that most MM cell lines and one primary tumor fully examined have IgH translocations that mainly involve IgH switch regions.[42,119] Recent FISH studies have also shown that IGH gene rearrangements are present in 73% of MM patients.[120] The apparent oncogene dysregulated by the 4;14 translocation is the fibroblast growth factor receptor 3 (*FGFR3*) gene, and it is possible that dysregulated expression of *FGFR3*, as a result of t(4;14), receives an FGFR3-mediated signal from FGF produced by stromal cells (SCs) in the BM microenvironment.[121] The t(4;14) translocation in MM regulates both *FGFR3* and a novel gene, MMSET, resulting in IgH/MMSET hybrid transcripts.[122] Ectopic expression of *FGFR3* promotes MM cell

Table 117-5 ■ **Nonimmunoglobulin Sites for Illegitimate Switch Recombination**

Chromosome	Gene	Function
11q13	cyclin D1	Induces growth
4p16	FGFR3, MMSET	Growth factor R
8q24	myc	Growth/apoptosis
16q23	c-maf	Transcription factor
6p25	IRF4	Transcription factor

Source: Kuehl WM. Natl Rev Cancer 2002;3:175.

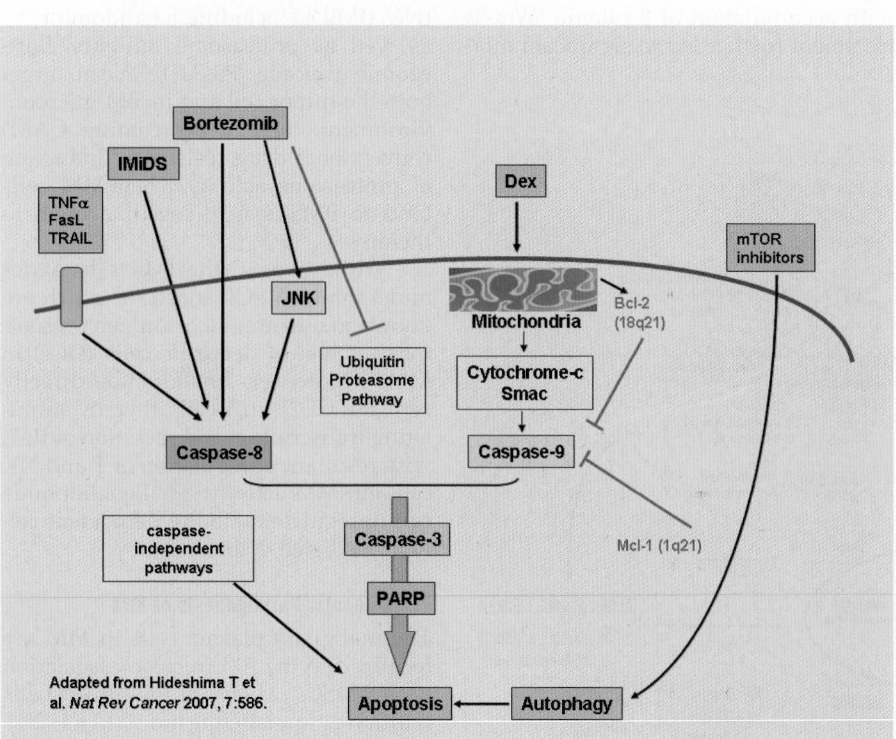

Figure 117-4 ■ Identification of the tumor cell in myeloma.

proliferation and prevents apoptosis, and its oncogenic potential has been tested in a murine model, confirming its capacity to transform hemopoietic cells.[123,124] Finally, there is evidence that elevated expression of c-myc and selective expression of one c-myc allele may occur frequently in MM, although structural genetic changes near c-myc have been identified in only 10-20% of tumors.

Ras mutations occur in about 39% of newly diagnosed MM patients, and the frequency of ras mutations increases with disease progression. Mutations of *N*- and *K-ras* are rarely detected in solitary plasmacytoma and MGUS, but occur more frequently in MM (9-30%) and in the majority of terminal disease or PCL patients (63-70%).[125,126]Activating mutations of the *ras* oncogenes may also result in growth-factor independence and suppression of apoptosis in MM.

Although translocation (14;18) occurs at a low frequency (0–15%) in MM, an overexpression of *Bcl-2* is seen in the majority of MM patients and in MM cell lines.[127,128] High levels of Bcl-2 protein are likely to mediate the resistance of MM cells to apoptosis induced by IL-6 deprivation, staurosporine, or other drugs.[129] In a murine MM cell line, Bcl-XL showed a predominant role in preventing apoptosis in response to cycloheximide treatment or IL-6 withdrawal.[130] Similarly, overexpression of *Bcl-2* or *Bcl-XL* could prevent apoptosis induced by IL-6 withdrawal in the B-9 IL-6–dependent cell line.[131] *Mcl-1* is overexpressed in MM cells, up-regulated by IL-6, and mediates potent resistance to apoptosis, whereas antisense oligonucleotide to Mcl-1 triggers apoptosis (Fig. 117-5).[132]

Chromosome 13 deletions are present in over 50% of MM and are associated with poor prognosis.[116,133-135] However, these deletions are also associated with MGUS, and their role in transformation to MM is therefore at present undefined.[116,136,137]

Recent understanding of the molecular pathogenesis of MM has resulted in a new proposed classification of MM.[138,139] Majority of MM tumors have chromosomal abnormalities and are broadly classified into hyperdiploid (HRD) or nonhyperdiploid (NHRD) tumors. Nearly half of MM tumors are HRD, the remaining being categorized as NHRD, which includes tumors which are hypodiploid, pseudodiploid, or subtetraploid. These NHRD tumors have been associated with a poorer prognosis. Five recurrent IgH translocations have been seen in MM including MMSET and FGFR3 (15%), cyclin D3 (3%), cyclin D1 (15%), c-maf (5%), and MAFB (2%) accounting for a prevalence of 40%. Recent evidence suggests that three of these five translocations are predominant in NHRD tumors.

With the advent of cDNA microarrays, an expeditious and comprehensive gene expression profiling is possible to better define disease biology, highlight prognostic factors, and identify potential targets for novel therapies.[117,136,137,140] These studies will also identify mechanisms of sensitivity vs resistance to conventional and novel MM therapies.[141,142] Known target antigens likely represent only the tip of the iceberg. Most recently, aCGH has been correlated with gene profiling to identify chromosomal amplifications and transcript overexpresssion, respectively. Then classical overexpression and knock down experiments are done, first in cancer models and then in MM models, to identify potential novel targets for monoclonal antibody (cell surface) or small molecule inhibitor (intracellular) therapies.[143]

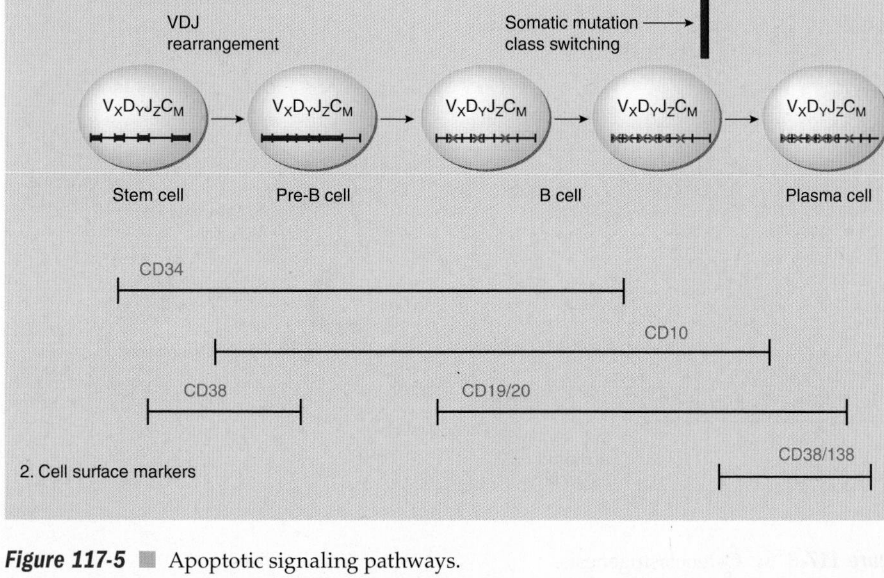

Figure 117-5 ■ Apoptotic signaling pathways.

Prognostic Factors

Staging Systems ■ Multiple attempts have been made to define clinical and laboratory parameters that have prognostic significance.[9,144-146] Of the many staging systems, the Durie–Salmon system was most commonly used (Table 117-6).[9] Tumor cell mass for patients in stage I is low at <0.6 × 10^{12} cells/m^2, intermediate for patients with stage II disease at 0.6 to 1.2 × 10^{12} cells/m^2, and high for patients with stage III disease with > 1.2 × 10^{12} cells/m^2. In this system, survival duration is 61.2, 54.5, 30.1, and 14.7 months for patients with stage IA, stage IB + IIA + IIB, stage IIIA, and stage IIIB disease, respectively.

Single Risk Factors ■ Many additional single parameters have been examined for their value as prognostic features. Higher labeling indices, serum IL-6 receptor levels, more ras mutations, more aggressive disease, and shortened survival has been reported in patients with plasmablast morphology.[147] Serum β2M represents the light chain of the major histocompatibility complex of the cell membrane, and increased serum β2M results from release by tumors with high growth fraction and cell turnover rates. In patients with MM and normal renal

Table 117-6 ■ **Durie-Salmon Myeloma Staging System Criteria**

Stage I
All of the following:
Hemoglobin value > 10 g/L
Serum calcium value normal (< 12 mg/dL)
On roentgenogram, normal bone structure (scale) or solitary bone plasmacytoma only
Low M-component production rates
IgG value < 5 g/dL, IgA value < 3 g/dL
Urine light chain M-component on electrophoresis < 4 g/24 hours
Stage II
Overall data as minimally abnormal as shown for stage I and no single value as abnormal as defined for stage III
Stage III
One or more of the following:
Hemoglobin value < 8.5 g/dL
Serum calcium value > 12 g/dL
Advanced lytic bone lesions (scale 3)
High M-component production rates
IgG value > 7 g/dL, IgA value >> 5 g/dL
Urine light chain M-component on electrophoresis 12 g/24 hours
Subclassification
A = Relatively normal renal function (serum creatinine value < 2.0 mg/dL
B = Abnormal renal function (serum creatinine > 2.0 mg/dL)

Abbreviation: Ig, immunoglobulin.
Source: From Ref. 203.

function, rising serum β2M predicts for progression.[148] The labeling index (LI), a measure of DNA synthesis by MM cells, predicts for survival. It is usually low (<1%) at diagnosis, higher at relapse, and lower in MGUS and indolent MM.[149] Chromosome 13 deletions are present in over 50% of MM and are associated with poor prognosis;[133-135,150] however, these deletions are also associated with MGUS,[116,136,137] and their role in transformation to MM is therefore at present undefined. Hyperdiploid MM has improved outcome and distinct clinical features, and chromosome 13 deletion does not have adverse impact.[151] Moreover, it is not prognostic for response to Bortezomib, highlighting the importance of prognostic factors for particular therapies.[152] Gene expression profiling will not only define disease pathogenesis, but also identify both novel prognostic factors and potential therapeutic targets.[117,123] These studies will also identify mechanisms of sensitivity vs resistance to conventional and novel MM therapies.[141,142] Serum IL-6 levels in some studies appear to correlate both with stage of disease and survival.[153,154] IL-6 stimulates hepatocytes to produce acute phase proteins, such as CRP. This therefore may reflect the IL-6 level and proliferative status of BM plasma cells. Indeed, CRP levels are significantly lower in patients with MGUS than in those with MM, and survival can be correlated with serum CRP level.[155] High serum soluble IL-6 receptor (sIL-6R),[156] hepatocyte growth factor,[157] and syndecan-1[158] levels, as well as low serum hyaluronate levels,[159] are independent prognostic factors predicting poor outcome. The percentage of circulating plasma cells in peripheral blood and their labeling indices are independent prognostic factors for survival in MM after both conventional and high-dose therapy.[160,161] Circulating endothelial cells also correlate with disease course and response to thalidomide.[162] Finally circulating proteasome levels are an independent prognostic factor for survival.[163]

Combinations of Factors ■ Many of these factors are interrelated and, therefore, of limited independent value. Using multivariate analysis, several groups have found that the best combination of variables to predict outcome was serum β2M, reflecting both the tumor burden and the renal function; and the proliferative activity of plasma cells, evaluated by the LI or number of tumor cells in S-phase. Age and performance status also improves the prognostic assessment.[164,165] Three recent prognostic staging systems have been proposed to better predict patient outcome. First, an international staging system based upon serum β2m and albumin has provided a new three stage International Staging System (ISS).[146] Second, cyclin D dysregulation has been identified as an early and unifying event in MM. Using gene expression profiling to identify five recurrent translocations, specific trisomies, and expression of cyclin *D2* genes, MM can prognostically be divided into eight TC (translocation/cyclin D) groups.[166] Additional molecular classifications have been proposed,[167] with high-risk myeloma defined by deregulated expression of genes mapping to chromosome 1.[168] Most recently, the first DNA-based classification scheme has been proposed to predict outcome to high-dose therapy.[143]

Complications

Complications of MM include bone disease and hypercalcemia, hyperviscosity, recurrent infections, renal failure, and cardiac dysfunction.

Bone Disease and Hypercalcemia ■ As noted earlier, 80% of patients with MM present with bone pain. Bone lesions can be isolated, discrete lytic abnormalities, or diffuse osteopenia. Bone scans and serum alkaline phosphatase are usually not abnormal. Evaluation with roentgenographs is standard; magnetic resonance imaging (MRI) is more sensitive and demonstrates bone healing with bisphosphonate therapy. Active osteoclastic bone resorption is usually evident when >20% MM cells are present, and lytic bone lesions occur when $>10^{12}$ cells are present. Bone resorption leads to increased calcium in extracellular fluid. Although patients with normal renal function can increase urine calcium excretion, those with renal failure develop hypercalcemia. Therefore, hypercalcemia is more likely to occur in the setting of Bence Jones proteinuria, MM kidney, chronic infection, or uric acid nephropathy. Overall, hypercalcemia occurs in 20-40% of patients with MM.[169] Osteosclerosis occurs in <1% of patients, who may have POEMS syndrome.[170] The differentiation of the POEMS syndrome from so-called osteosclerotic MM with peripheral neuropathy appears to have no clinical value.

Pathogenesis ■ MM cell lines, MM cells, and explants of bone containing MM cells, produce osteoclast-activating factors that are similar biologically and chemically to bone-resorbing activity in normal activated leukocyte culture supernatants (Fig. 117-6).[169] These include lymphotoxin (LT), TNF-α, hepatocyte growth factor (HGF), IL-6, IL-1, metalloproteinases (MMP1, MMP2, MMP9), RANKL, and insulin-like growth factor binding protein 4 (IGF-IV).[171-175] IL-6 can induce TNF-α and IL-1 production in marrow cells and cause bone resorption and hypercalcemia in vivo. MIP-Iα has been shown to increase osteoclast stimulatory activity in patients with MM.[91,92,176] MIP-Iα mRNA is present in freshly isolated BM from MM patients. More importantly, recombinant hMIP1α induces OCL formation in human BM cultures.[177] Conversely, blocking MIP-1α in the ARH-77 cell line inhibits tumor growth in an in vivo model of bone disease.[91,92,176] The levels of RANKL/osteoprotegerin ligand (OPGL), an OCL

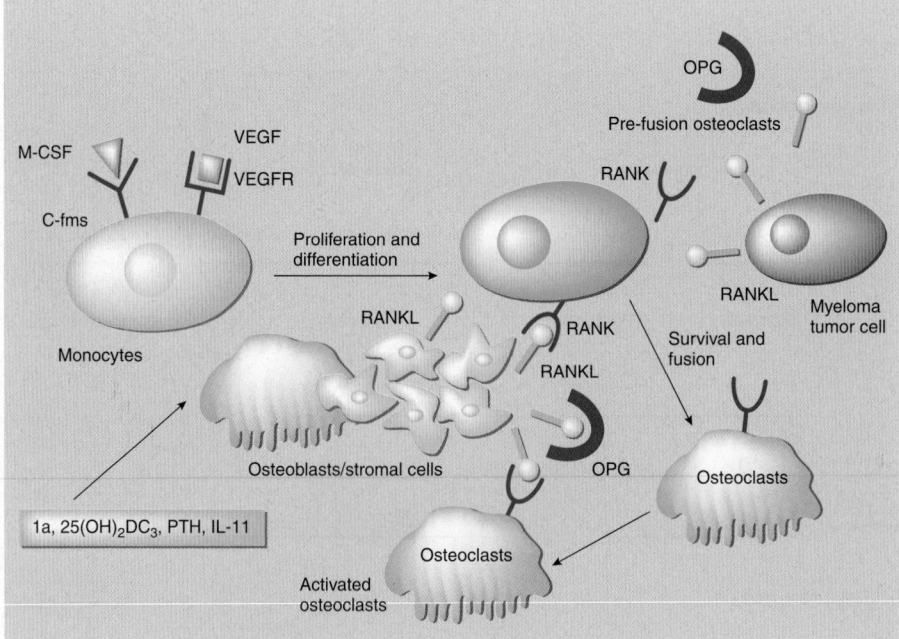

Figure 117-6 ■ Osteoclastogenesis.

activation and differentiation factor, and of osteoprotegerin (OPG), which is a decoy receptor for OPGL, modulate osteoclast formation; furthermore, an imbalance favoring osteoclast activation has been seen in MM patients.[178-180]Although OPG levels are decreased in MM patients with osteolytic lesions, the levels do not correlate with clinical stage or survival. OPG, which neutralizes OPGL, may have therapeutic application in MM bone disease.[175]

An in vivo model of MM bone disease has been developed in which SCID mice injected with ARH-77 tumor cells develop radiologically detectable lytic bone lesions, and their marrow plasma contains a bone-resorbing activity that stimulates osteoclastic bone resorption in bone organ cultures and in human and murine marrow cultures.[181] It appears that a novel cytokine mediates osteoclast activation in this model. Hjorth-Hansen and colleagues have used a different human MM cell line in this model and found similar results.[182] The use of OPG to inhibit osteolytic bone disease has been demonstrated in an in vivo model by Croucher and colleagues.[183] Another antagonist of OPGL is RANK-Fc molecule, a fusion of the Fc portion of immunoglobulin to a soluble form of the RANK receptor. RANK-Fc alone or in combination with bisphosphonates has been evaluated using in vivo models and also blocks bone destruction.[60,184]

Treatment ■ Prior to the advent of effective bisphosphonate therapy, bone healing in MM occurred uncommonly and was delayed in treated patients despite responses to chemotherapy. In this context, a major effort over the last 30 years has been made to either prevent or inhibit further bone resorption in patients with MM. A double-blind randomized trial of clodronate vs placebo in 350 patients revealed that the proportion of patients with progression of osteolytic lesions was twice as high in the placebo group as in the clodronate-treated group.[185] Another randomized trial demonstrated that oral clodronate slowed progressive skeletal disease and associated morbidity but achieved no benefit in survival. Pamidronate has been shown in a prospective randomized trial to reduce skeletal-related events, including pathologic fractures, radiation therapy to bone, and spinal cord compression in patients with Durie–Salmon stage III MM and ≥1 lytic bone lesion.[186] This benefit was maintained until 21 months, and formed the basis of previous ASCO recommendations suggesting that MM patients remain on intravenous bisphosphonates indefinitely to reduce skeletal events and pain, regardless of their response to chemotherapy.[187,188] Interestingly, patients in this study who had failed first-line chemotherapy also had improved survival, suggesting that bisphosphonates may have anti-MM activity.[189] Recent evidence supports the view that bisphosphonates may down-regulate IL-6 production from BMSCs as well as induce apoptosis of both osteoclasts and tumor cells. Pamidronate has been studied in patients with indolent MM. Bone turnover was reduced in treated patients,[190,191] but no significant antitumor activity was noted.[192] More potent bisphosphonates, such as zoledronate, have undergone clinical evaluation and offer the benefit of shorter infusion times than pamidronate.[193-195] On the other hand, ibandronate, a third-generation bisphosphonate, failed to enhance survival or reduce morbidity from bone disease in patients with stage II and III MM.[196] A word of caution should however be exercised with the use bisphosphonate therapy because of reported cases of osteonecrosis of the jaw.[197-199] This newly recognized complication in a small percentage of patients, led ASCO to update their guidelines and now recommend discontinuing bisphosphonates in patients with responsive or stable disease at two years, with further use at the discretion of the physician.[200] Other supportive care measures such as vertebroplasty or kyphoplasty can restore supine stability and relieve pain for patients with localized disease.[201,202]

The treatment of hypercalcemia consists of treatment of the underlying MM, as well as inhibition of osteoclastic bone resorption with corticosteroids, calcitonin, mithramycin, and/or bisphosphonates. Corticosteroids may impair formation of new osteoclasts; mithramycin is toxic to osteoclasts, but it is also nephrotoxic. Calcitonin and corticosteroids are almost always effective for the short term and useful even in the setting of renal failure. Bisphosphonates bind to the bone surface and inhibit osteoclast activity, and they constitute a mainstay of treatment. Therapeutic recommendations at present, therefore, include initial cytotoxic therapy for MM and cautious forced saline diuresis and bisphosphonate therapy, with the use of calcitonin, prednisone, or mithramycin only for nonresponders to these first-line treatments. In a randomized trial of 287 patients with hypercalcemia of malignancy, zoledronate was found to be superior to pamidronate.[203] A prominent problem exacerbating hypercalcemia relates to patients' becoming immobile because of bone pain or other reasons. Therefore, an important approach is to keep the patient, whenever possible, physically active.

Hyperviscosity ■ Hyperviscosity is characterized clinically by spontaneous bleeding with neurologic and ocular disorders. Hyperviscosity occurred in 4.2% of 238 patients with IgG MM and in 22% of 46 patients with serum IgG M components >5.0 g/dL.[204] The IgG3 subclass produces hyperviscosity at lower levels than other IgG paraproteins.[205] The severity of the syndrome is not directly related to the serum viscosity. Clinical findings improve with vigorous plasmapheresis, which reduces both MM protein concentration and serum viscosity.

Recurrent Infections ■ Patients with MM had 15 times more infections than a control group of patients with arteriosclerotic heart disease.[206] *Streptococcus pneumoniae* and *Haemophilus* infections usually occur early and typically during response to chemotherapy. Gram-negative infections occur in refractory, advancing disease; in the setting of previous antibiotic therapy; instrumentation; immobilization; colonization with hospital flora; and azotemia. Fatal infections may be hospital-acquired, emphasizing the need to minimize indwelling foreign bodies such as catheters in patients with MM. There is lack of correlation between bacteremia (either gram-negative or positive) and chemotherapy-induced febrile neutropenia. Fungal, herpes, mycobacterial, and Pneumocystis infections are only rarely described in MM patients. Infection is the most common cause of death (20–50% of cases).[26]

The evidence of increased clinical infections in MM has led to attempts at prophylaxis. Although MM patients have normal-fold rises in antibody titers after pneumococcal vaccination, preimmunization titers are markedly diminished.[207] Post-immunization titers are therefore low and considered nonprotective. Nonetheless, because of its low cost and possible benefit to some patients, the use of pneumococcal vaccination has been recommended. In a double-blind randomized trial of gammaglobulin prophylaxis in patients with MM, no benefit of gammaglobulin prophylaxis at reducing infection was noted.[208] At present, gammaglobulin is reserved for those patients with recurrent or life-threatening infections.

Renal Failure ■ Renal failure in MM can predict for adverse outcome. One series found that 22% of patients had a serum creatinine >2 mg/dL at diagnosis; renal function normalized with treatment in 50% of those with creatinine >2 but <3.9 mg/dL. The causes of renal failure in MM are often multifactorial and include hypercalcemia; MM kidney, with distal and proximal tubules obstructed by large, laminated casts containing albumin, IgG, and κ and λ light chains surrounded by giant cells; hyperuricemia; toxicity from intravenous urography;

dehydration; plasma cell infiltration; pyelonephritis; and amyloidosis. The most important predisposing factor is dehydration; aggressive hydration is therefore crucial to avoid irreversible renal dysfunction. Otherwise, treatment is for the underlying disease, along with avoidance of intravenous urography. Combination chemotherapy should be used because of the more rapid response that is observed with melphalan and prednisone. The type and quantity of proteinuria can distinguish MM kidney, with larger amounts of light chains and less albuminuria; light chain deposition disease, characterized by low levels of both light chains and albumin in urine; and amyloidosis, in which large amounts of albuminuria and less light-chain proteinuria occur.[209]

The renal manifestations associated with the production of monoclonal light chains in MM, light-chain deposition disease, and amyloidosis result from the deposition of certain Bence Jones proteins (BJP) as tubular casts, basement-membrane precipitates, or fibrils, respectively.[210-212] For unknown reasons, the severity of the renal manifestations varies greatly from patient to patient. BJP from 40 patients were injected into mice, and 26 (65%) were deposited in mouse kidneys as tubular casts, basement-membrane precipitates, or crystals in a pattern similar to those noted in patients.[212] This experimental model has potential value for the identification and differentiation of nephrotoxic or amyloidogenic light chains. The development of progressive kidney damage and MM kidney has been demonstrated in IL-6 transgenic mice, shedding additional insight into the role of IL-6 in the pathogenesis of MM.[213]

Cardiac Failure ■ The mean and median age of patients with MM is approximately 60 years, and affected patients are also frequently at risk of cardiovascular disease. However, patients can be uniquely susceptible to cardiac ischemia and/or congestive heart failure (CHF) because of myocardial infiltration with amyloid, causing dilated or restricted cardiomyopathy, hyperviscosity syndrome, and/or anemia. MM patients are also susceptible to high output CHF of unclear etiology.[214]

Anemia ■ Anemia in MM can be due to a number of factors, including tumor infiltration of the BM, renal impairment, the myelosuppressive effects of chemotherapy, and a deficient production of erythropoietin (EPO) relative to the degree of anemia. Pilot studies demonstrated efficacy of exogenous EPO administration in MM.[215-217] Osterborg and colleagues have carried out a randomized study of EPO therapy at 10,000 U/day, a titrated dose of EPO starting with 2000 U/ day and escalating stepwise until response, or no EPO for 24 weeks; response was defined as an increase in Hb > 2 g/dL and elimination of transfusion need.[218] Sixty percent of EPO-treated groups responded, 72% of those with low EPO levels, and only 20% of those with normal EPO levels. 10,000 units SC three times weekly was the optimal starting dosage, although more recently 40,000 units SC once weekly is a commonly used approach.

Neuropathies ■ A variety of malignant and paraproteinemic disorders can be associated with neuropathies.[219] In MM, a symmetric, distal sensory or sensorimotor neuropathy is most common and is associated with axonal degeneration, with or without amyloid deposition; there is no specific therapy. In some cases, this is associated with monoclonal antibodies directed against peripheral nerve myelin.[220]

Associated Diseases ■ MM has been described in association with both hematologic disorders and solid tumors. Acute leukemia either is induced by leukemogens, such as radiation and alkylating agents, or is part of the natural history of MM. The mean interval from diagnosis of MM to occurrence of acute leukemia is 60 (17–147) months, consistent with either possibility. The occurrence of acute leukemia in untreated MM patients suggests that it may be part of the natural history of the disease.[221] Furthermore, acute leukemia has been reported in 6 of 125 (4.8%) MM patients treated with alkylating agents, which is significantly higher than the incidence of acute leukemia in ovarian cancer patients treated with irradiation and alkylators.[25] Actuarial risk of leukemia in MM patients treated with melphalan and prednisone or with melphalan, cyclophosphamide, carmustine, and prednisone has been reported to be as high as 17.4% at 50 months from initiation of therapy.[222] Gonzalez and colleagues described 11 of 476 patients with MM who developed myeloid leukemia or sideroblastic anemia.[221] All had received melphalan-prednisone for a median of 3 years and had major cytogenetic abnormalities. This study suggests that leukemia is predominantly treatment related. Finally, in 628 patients with MM, the incidence and diversity of solid tumors were similar to those observed in otherwise healthy persons of the same age.[223]

Treatment

Patients undergoing therapy for MM should have clinical and laboratory assessment to assure both safety and efficacy of treatment. Before each course of treatment, a complete blood count, including differential and platelets, should be done. Serum chemistries should be measured at least every 3 months or more often if clinically indicated. Concomitantly, monoclonal protein in the serum and/or urine should be measured by immunoelectrophoresis or, preferably, using more sensitive immunofixation techniques. A skeletal survey should be done annually, with BM examination reserved for diagnosis and time of subsequent change in clinical status, in monoclonal Ig, or in hemogram. It is important to remember that reduction of serum or urine M component as objective evidence of tumor response could reflect increased protein catabolism, decreased protein production, or both. Moreover, non-M protein-secreting MM clones may emerge during treatment, so that even a marked reduction in monoclonal Ig may not correlate with decrease in tumor burden.

Two major definitions of response in MM have been widely used, that of the Chronic Leukemia–MM Task Force and that of the Southwest Oncology Group (SWOG).[224,225] The former requires ≥50% decrease in monoclonal serum or urine protein, ≥50% decrease in cross-sectional areas of plasmacytoma, and some recalcification of bone lesions (without new lesions); whereas the latter requires a 75% or greater reduction in production of MM protein. However, the frequencies of response by either definition are similar in previously untreated patients receiving melphalan and prednisone. Response rates of 32-53% were noted by SWOG criteria, and 33-56% responses were recorded by Task Force criteria. Need for, and response to, treatment may be a more important determinant of survival than initial tumor stage. For example, a low IL may define patients who may not need therapy irrespective of stage; such patients may have a long course prior to need for therapy, a gradual response to treatment, and prolonged survival. The Blade criteria to assess response post-transplant were developed for the European Group for Blood and Marrow Transplant (EBMT), the International BM Transplant Registry (IBMTR), and the Autologous Blood and Marrow Transplant Registry (ABMTR).[226] These criteria include a more sensitive and rigorous definition of complete response, including absence of paraprotein assayed by immunofixation, and excludes transient responses (Table 117-7). Most recently, serum free light chain assays have been incorporated into response criteria[227-229] and the International myeloma working group response criteria are being universally used.

Conventional Therapy Initial Treatment ■ Oral administration of melphalan and prednisone (MP) is a standard form of ther-

Table 117-7 **Response Comparison of Southwest Oncology Group (SWOG) and Blade Criteria**

Response Criteria	SPEP Reduction (%)	IF (Serum and Urine)	UPEP Reduction (%)	Bone Marrow	Bone Disease	Calcium	Confirmation
CR							
SWOG	75	Not required	90	Not required	Not required	Not required	Yes (3 weeks)
Blade	100	Negative	100	<5% PC	Stable	Normal	Yes (6 weeks)
PR							
SWOG	50	Not required	Not required	Not required	Not required	Not required	Yes (3 weeks)
Blade	50	Not required	90% or <200 mg	Not required	Normal	Normal	Yes (6 weeks)

Abbreviations: CR, complete response; IF, immunofixation; PC, plasma cells; PR, partial response; SPEP, serum protein electrophoresis; UPEP, urine protein electrophoresis.
Source: Alexanian R. Cancer 1972;30:382; Blade J, Samson D, Reece D, et al.

apy that produces objective response in up to 50-60% of patients.[1,230] The dosage of melphalan, due to the variability of absorption, should be modified if necessary so that some reduction in leukocytes and platelets occurs 3 to 4 weeks after the beginning of each cycle. Unless there is disease progression, MP should be given for at least 1 year until the monoclonal Ig levels in the serum and/or urine have been stable for at least 6 months (plateau state), and then discontinued if the patient has no other evidence of active disease. Typical doses are melphalan daily in a dosage of a 0.15 mg/kg daily for 7 days (8-10 mg/day) and 20 mg of prednisone 3 times daily for the same period. Melphalan must be given before meals because food reduces absorption. It is important to remember that the natural course of MM is one of progression, so that alleviation of pain and lack of progressive disease may be beneficial even in the absence of an objective response.

Multiple studies have examined whether MP is as effective as combination chemotherapy (CCT). In an attempt to determine which patients, if any, do better with more aggressive therapy, Gregory and colleagues examined published reports of 18 randomized controlled trials comparing MP with CCT in the primary treatment of 3814 patients.[231] The overall results suggested that there was no difference in efficacy between these treatment modalities. Those studies with a high MP 2-year survival rate showed a survival difference in favor of MP, whereas those with a low rate suggested a difference in favor of CCT. These results imply that, rather than there being no difference between MP and CCT, MP is superior for patients with an intrinsically good prognosis and inferior for those patients with a poor prognosis. A second overview of 6633 patients from 27 randomized trials of CCT vs MP confirmed higher response rates to CCT, but equivalent mortality and survival (Table 117-8).[232]

There has been a shift in treatment paradigm in MM moving away from conventional chemotherapy and incorporating the use of novel agents. Two studies combined thalidomide

Table 117-8 **Myeloma Therapies vs. Combination Chemotherapy (CCT)**

3814 patients in 18 trials of CCT vs MP[a]
No difference overall: MP superior for good prognosis, inferior for poor prognosis patients
6333 patients in 27 trials of CCT vs MP[b]
Higher response rates to CCT but equivalent mortality and survival

[a]Gregory WJ. Clin Oncol 1992;10:334.
[b]Myeloma Trialists' Collaborative Group. J Clin Oncol 1998;16:3832.

with dexamethasone as initial therapy for MM and achieved rapid responses in two-thirds of patients, allowing for successful harvesting of PBSCs for transplantation.[233,234] Recently Thal/Dex has been compared with VAD and Dex, as initial therapy for patients prior to collection of autologous stem cells and transplantation. In a case control analysis, Cavo et al showed that Thal/Dex achieved higher overall response rates[235] whereas a randomized phase 3 (EGOG) trial showed statistically significantly higher response rates for Thal/Dex than Dex treated patient cohorts.[236] This study provided the rationale for FDA approval of this regimen for initial treatment of MM. Moreover, early studies show 91% responses, including 6% complete and 32% near complete/very good partial responses to lenalinamide combined with Dex.[237] Based on these promising results, a phase 3 trial in the United States headed by ECOG investigated the role of Len/Dex in newly diagnosed MM. The study design allowed all patients to stay on-study for the first 4 cycles only for response assessment, after which patients could go off-study to proceed with stem cell transplant. Provisional safety data from this trial found that combining Len with the low-dose dexamethasone regimen was preferable to the combination with high-dose dexamethasone, with a reduction in grade 3 or higher nonhematologic adverse events (32% vs 49%), including thromboembolism (9% vs 25%), and infections (6% vs 16%) in the two treatment arms of the trial. 238The low-dose dexamethasone-containing regimen did lead to an increased occurrence of grade ≥3 neutropenia (19% vs 10%). Importantly, the combination with low-dose dexamethasone had a survival benefit over combination with high-dose dexamethasone, with a 1-year OS of 96% and 87%, respectively.[238] Prophylaxis against clotting with aspirin, coumadin, or subcutaneous heparin, is needed when patients are treated with lenalidomide therapy.[239,240]

Richardson and colleagues examined single agent Bortezomib,[241] Jagganath et al[242] tested Bortezomib combined with Dex as initial therapy, in both cases, high frequency and extent of response, were noted. A recent observation however highlights the concerns surrounding ability to collect adequate stem cells following lenalidomide based treatments.

Although multiple prior studies of combination chemotherapy regimens have not significantly improved over melphalan and prednisone, including a recent French study showing its superiority over dexamethasone alone in older patients.[243] Palumbo et al recently compared oral daily Thal plus melphalan and prednisone to melphalan and prednisone alone. Both the frequency (>90%) and extent (28% CR) of response were remarkably increased and both progression free and overall survival (OS) improved.[244,245] Importantly, Facon and colleagues in IFM compared melphalan and prednisone; melphalan, prednisone and thalidomide; and melphalan 100 mg/m^2 × 2 followed by autologous stem cell transplant, a regimen which they previously showed to be superior to melphalan and prednisone.[244] Overall and extent of response, as well as progression-free and OS, were superior with melphalan prednisone, and thalidomide.[246] Melphalan, prednisone, and lenalidomide,[247] as well as melphalan prednisone and Bortezomib,[248] are similarly showing very high overall and extent of response when used as initial therapy for older patients who are not transplant candidates.

Radiation Therapy Radiation therapy for MM is used for treatment of localized disease, including plasmacytoma or spinal cord compression syndrome, and is frequently used for palliation. Hemibody radiation therapy has been utilized, either as a consolidation following induction combination chemotherapy or as salvage therapy for chemotherapy resistant MM.[249,250] Total body irradiation (TBI) has been used as a component of ablative therapy prior to hematopoietic stem cell grafting, but is rarely used since high-dose melphalan has equivalent efficacy and less toxicity.[251]

High-Dose Therapies ■ The rationale for the administration of alkylating agents (melphalan, cyclophosphamide, busulfan) in a higher-than-conventional dose with or without TBI, followed by transplantation of syngeneic, allogeneic, and autologous BM or peripheral blood progenitor cells (PBPCs) is as follows: plasma cell dyscrasias remain uniformly fatal; multiple studies document sensitivity of MM cells to chemotherapy and radiotherapy; and CRs can be obtained with high-dose therapy.

Autologous Stem Cell Transplantation ■ High-dose chemoradiotherapy followed by transplantation of either autologous BM or PBPCs has also achieved high (40%) CR rates, but the median duration of these responses has unfortunately only been 24-36 months.[252,253] Patients with sensitive disease and who are less heavily pretreated have the most favorable outcomes. Most importantly, a national French trial of 200 patients with MM who received two courses of VMCP alternating with VBAP and were then randomized to receive either conventional chemotherapy (8 additional courses of VMCP/VBAP) or high-dose therapy (melphalan and TBI) followed by autologous BMT has demonstrated significantly higher response rates, event free survival (EFS) and OS for those patients treated with high dose compared to those receiving conventional therapy.[254] A second randomized trial in MM examined the relative merits of high-dose therapy either early vs late as salvage therapy for relapse after conventional therapy.[255] The OS was 64 months in both groups, but the Quality Adjusted Time without Symptoms and Toxicity (Q-TWIST) strongly favored the early transplant cohort. The United States Intergroup Trial supports this view.[256] The IFM has conducted a randomized trial comparing high-dose melphalan at 200 mg/m^2 vs melphalan at 140 mg/m^2 plus TBI as ablative therapies.[251] Although response rates and EFS were comparable, toxicity and OS was superior in the high-dose melphalan alone arm, suggesting that TBI should not be considered part of the ablation regimen. A Scandinavian population-based study demonstrated prolonged survival for patients with MM < 60 years of age treated with intensive therapy compared with historical controls who received conventional therapy.[257] An additional randomized MRC trial confirmed a 12 month survival benefit in patients receiving high dose compared to conventional therapies.[258] Although these studies are encouraging, it is unlikely that patients are cured after a single high dose and stem cell autografting regimen. In all studies the median event free survival was prolonged; in 4 of 5 studies, transplant led to higher CR rate; and in 3 of 5 trials OS was improved (Table 117-9).

Improving Outcome of Autografting ■ Attempts to improve the outcome of high-dose therapy followed by autografting include the use of autologous BM or PBPCs either depleted of tumor cells,[259-261] or processed to select normal hematopoietic progenitor cells by virtue of CD34 expression.[262,263] These have not translated to improved outcome. Barlogie and colleagues are performing multiple high-dose therapies and stem cell transplantation.[264-266] Response rates are higher relative to historically matched controls, but the impact on long term disease free survival requires further follow-up. A recent comparison of tandem transplant with or without thalidomide has not prolonged OS.[139] In a French randomized trial comparing a single vs double high-dose therapy and stem cell transplantation, there was no significant difference in the CR rate between single and double transplantation arms, and EFS and OS curves separated only after 3 years.[267] This suggests that only a subset of patients may benefit, and indeed only those patients who did not achieve a CR to the first transplant appeared to benefit from the second. A second French trial found no difference in EFS or OS in patients receiving single vs double autotransplants,[268] whereas Dutch HOVON, Bologna-96, and GMMG trials all show prolonged event free survival in favor of double autografting. However, HOVON trial suggests benefit only in those not responding to first transplant with CR or nCR. Further follow-up and additional studies are therefore required to identify those patients who benefit before double autografting is adopted as standard therapy in MM. The addition of anti-IL-6 antibody to ablative regimen of the second transplant did not improve the outcome (Table 117-10).[269]

Champlin and colleagues have reported on the use of cyclosporine to induce GVHD post-autografting in an attempt to generate associated autologous graft vs MM effect.[270] It may be possible to stimulate autologous immunity to MM to treat MRD post autografting and thereby improve outcome. We are also attempting to generate and expand anti-MM–specific autologous T-cells ex vivo for adoptive immunotherapy of MRD in the patient postautotransplant. It is now possible to clone the gene for the patient's specific id-

Table 117-9 ■ **Autologous Transplantation vs Conventional Chemotherapy for Newly Diagnosed Myeloma**

Author	Therapy	Patients (*n*)	CR (%)	EFS (Median, Months)	OS (Median, Months)
Barlogie et al[387]	Conventional[a]	116	–	22	48
	HDT	123	40	49	62
Lenhoff et al[386]	Conventional[a]	274	–		46% at 48
	HDT	274	34	27	61% at 48
Attal et al[377]	Conventional	100	5	18	37
	HDT	100	22	27	52% at 60
Fermand et al[383]	Conventional	96	–	18.7	50.4
	HDT	94	–	24.3	55.3
Blade et al[388]	Conventional	83	11	34.3	66.9
	HDT	81	30	42.5	67.4
Child et al[385]	Conventional	200	8.5	19.6	42.3
	HDT	201	44	31.6	54.8

[a]Historical controls.
Abbreviations: CR, complete response; EFS, event free survival; HDT, hgih dose therapy; OS, overall survival.

Table 117-10 ■ **Single vs Double Autologous Transplantation for Newly Diagnosed Myeloma**

Author	Therapy	Patients (*n*)	CR (%)	EFS (Median, Months)	OS (Median, Months)
Attal et al	Single	88	42	10% at 84	21% at 84
	Double	92	50	20% at 84	42% at 84
Fermand et al	Single	94	37	No difference	No difference
	Double	99	42		
Cavo et al	Single	81	34	21.5	71% at 48
	Double	97	41	29.5	74% at 48

Abbreviations: CR, complete response; EFS, event free survival; OS, overall survival.
Sources: Attal et al. Single vs double autologous stem-cell transplantation for multiple myeloma. N Engl J Med. 2004 Jun 17;350(25):2628. Fermand et al. High-dose therapy and autologous peripheral blood stem cell transplantation in multiple myeloma: up-front or rescue treatment? Results of a multicenter sequential randomized clinical trial. Blood. 1998 Nov 1;92(9):3131-6. Cavo et al. Proc VIII Intl Myeloma Wkshp 2001:516:29.

iotypic protein, use computer programs to identify gene sequences encoding for peptides predicted to be presented within the groove of Class I HLA of a given patient's HLA type, and expand peptide-specific T-cells ex vivo.[271] A similar strategy can be used to expand T cells against peptides within shared antigens that are overexpressed on MM cells, such as the telomerase catalytic subunit (hTERT), MUC-1, or the cytochrome cyp 1B 1.[272-274] Immunologic responses are also being tested to enhance the immunogenicity of the whole tumor cell. For example, our laboratory studies have shown that autologous T cells do not proliferate in response to the patients' own tumor cells as targets. However, CD40 activation of MM cells up-regulates class I and II HLA, costimulatory, GRP94, and other molecules; and CD40-activated MM cells also trigger a brisk autologous T-cell response.[275] Although T cells can be harvested from MM patients before autografting, expanded ex vivo using CD40-activated autologous MM cells as a stimulus, and given as adoptive immunotherapy to treat MRD post-transplant, this is logistically complex. Therefore, we and others are developing and examining the clinical use of a variety of MM vaccines. First, based upon our observation that CD40-activated MM cells trigger a brisk autologous T-cell response, we are examining the use of vaccinations of patients with autologous CD40-activated tumor cells. Second, based on our demonstration of the expression of MUC-1 core protein on freshly isolated MM cells, we are evaluating two vaccines: recombinant vaccinia virus containing the *MUC-1* gene and autologous DCs transduced using adenoviral vectors with MUC-1.[272] Of interest, we have recently shown that MM cells can be fused to DCs and that the use of the MM DC fusion as an antigen-presenting cell presents the entire MM cell as foreign. In a syngeneic murine MM model, vaccinations with MM cell–DC fusions, but not with either MM cells or DCs alone, demonstrate both protective and therapeutic efficacy.[276] Most important, we have shown that patient MM cells can be fused to autologous DCs, which are readily isolated from either patient BM or peripheral blood, and that autologous MM cell–DC fusions can trigger specific cytolytic autologous T-cell responses in vitro.[277,278] We are translating these findings into clinical trials of MM-DC fusion vaccines to assess in vivo MM-specific T-and B-cell responses, as well as clinical efficacy.

Immunization protocols at other centers have already demonstrated a transient anti-Id T-cell response in 3 of 5 patients by injection of autologous Id. Moreover, 5 of 5 patients injected with autologous Id and GM-CSF had long-lasting MHC class I-restricted Id-specific T-cell responses.[279,280] Massaia and colleagues have also shown generation of T-cell proliferative responses and delayed type hypersensitivity to Id after immunization with Id conjugated to KLH with GM-CSF or IL-2 as immunoadjuvants.[281] Vaccination after autologous peripheral blood stem cell transplantation for MM using idiotypepulsed DCs can achieve idiotype-specific T-cell responses in a minority of patients.[282] Other strategies currently under evaluation are immunization with idiotypic DNA vaccines as well as DCs pulsed with idiotype.[283,284] MAGE antigens and the catalytic subunit of telomerase are expressed by MM and contain peptides that can be effectively presented by HLA class I molecules to generate autologous-specific cytolytic T-cell responses.[273,285] Finally, MM cells can be efficiently transduced with adenoviral vectors, and accessory molecules, for example, CD80 or GM-CSF, are currently being transfected into tumor cells prior to vaccination.[286,287]

Multiple reports suggest that patients may mount an anti-MM immune response.[279,283,288] Further studies are needed to optimize the immunization schedule to achieve long-lasting T-cell immunity against idiotypic and other determinants on the MM cell and determine its effect on clinical outcome. Finally, as discussed subsequently, trials are now ongoing evaluating thalidomide and lenalidomide to prolong time to progression post transplant. Thalidomide post tandem transplant did prolong EFS and OS in patients who had not received prior thalidomide;[289] in the total therapy program, it increased CR and EFS, but not OS.[139]

Allogeneic Stem Cell Transplantation ■ Syngeneic transplantation has been done infrequently in MM, but some patients reported from Seattle[290] and in European Bone Marrow Transplant Group (EBMT)[291] remain progression-free at long intervals post BMT. The EBMT has reported on allografting in MM.[292-294] Actuarial OS was 32% at 4 years, and 28% at 7 years for the 72 (44%) patients who achieved CR after BMT. However, overall progression free survival (PFS) was 34% at 6 years, and few patients remain in continuing CR at >4 years post allograft. Favorable pre-BMT prognostic factors for both response to and survival after BMT were female sex, IgA MM, low serum β2M, stage I disease at diagnosis, one line of previous treatment, and being in CR prior to BMT. Of major concern is the early 40% transplant-related mortality (50% in males) in the EBMT report,[295] which has subsequently been reduced to 20-30% due to better patient selection, early transplantation, and less pretransplant treatment.[294] In the allografting experience in Seattle, actuarial probabilities of OS and EFS for the 36% patients achieving CR were 0.50, 0.21, and 43, 0.17, respectively, at 4.5 years. Adverse prognostic factors included: transplantation >1 year from diagnosis; serum β2M > 2.5 mg/dL at transplant; female patients transplanted from male donors; having received >8 cycles of chemotherapy, and Durie Salmon Stage III disease at presentation. Again toxicity was common, with 35 (44%) patients dying of transplant-related causes within 100 days of BMT.[296,297] In an attempt to improve the outcome of allografting in MM by avoiding TRM, we carried out T (CD6) depleted allografting using histocompatible sibling donors in 61 patients with MM whose disease remained sensitive to conventional chemotherapy.[261,298-301] There were 17 (28%) CR and 34 (57%) PR, 2 (3%) NR and only 3 (5%) transplant-related deaths. However, disease free survival (DFS) after allo BMT was 1 year, with only 20% patients disease free at >4 years post-transplant (Table 117-11).

Molecular remissions are more common after allografting than after autografting,[302-305] and donor lymphocyte infusions (DLI) can treat relapsed MM post allografting,[306-308] indicating a clinically significant graft-vs MM (GVM) effect. At our center, relapses post autografting vs the higher toxicity and lower relapse rates in allograft recipients result in equivalent long-term outcomes.[309] In an effort to reduce toxicity and exploit GVM, we have used CD4+ DLI at 6 months post CD6 depleted BM allografting in order to enhance GVM and thereby improve outcome.[301] Although prophylactic DLI induces significant GVM responses after allogeneic BMT, only 58% of patients were able to receive DLI despite T-cell depleted BMT.

Table 117-11 ■ **Representative Studies of Allogeneic Transplantation for Newly Diagnosed Myeloma**

	No. of Patients	TRM (%)	CR (%)	OS (Actuarial, Months)	EFS (Actuarial, Months)
Gahrton et al	162	41	44	28% at 84	45% at 60
Bensinger et al	80	44	36	20% at 54	24% at 54
Alyea et al	61[a]	5	28	40% at 36	20% at 38

[a]T-cell depleted.
Abbreviations: CR, complete response; EFS, event-free survival; OS, overall survival; TRM, transplant-related mortality.
Sources: Gahrton G. Br J Haematol 2001;98:934; Bensinger W. Semin Hematol 2001;38:934; Alyea E, Weller E, Schlossman R, et al.

The use of non ablative transplantation is an alternative strategy to preserve GVM while avoiding the toxicity of allografting.[310] Melphalan at a dose of 100 mg/m^2 has been used in combination with DLI in high-risk MM patients.[311] Although disease control was achieved in some patients, significant GVHD was noted in this group of patients. Autografting has been performed prior to non myeloablative transplant by several investigators, demonstrating the feasibility of this approach to cytoreduce tumor and then enhance anti-MM immunity.[312,313] For example, Maloney et al[314] report an overall response rate of 83% with 57% CRs. Chronic GVHD, transplant-related toxicity, and relapse of disease remain a problem (Table 117-12). One randomized trial in high-risk MM showed that the combination of autologous stem cell transplant followed by dose reduced allogeneic transplant (IFM 99-03) was not superior to tandem autotransplant (IFM 99-04),[315] but a second randomized trial showed superior survival in those patients receiving autologous followed by allogeneic grafts.[316]

Maintenance Therapy ■ The potential mechanisms of action of alpha-2b interferon (IFN-α) include direct cytotoxicity on MM cells; synergism with chemotherapy; a change in the pharmacokinetics of melphalan; inhibition of IL-6; downregulation of IL-6 receptor on MM cells, downregulation of activated oncogenes; an increase in natural killer cells; an increase in tumor cell surface antigens, and/or expansion of specific cytotoxic T-cells.[317] A meta-analysis of 16 randomized trials involving 2286 patients receiving combined IFN-α–chemotherapy for induction treatment yielded higher response rates in the IFN-α arms, but the average gain was only approximately 10%.[318] Similarly, significant but only marginal gains were detected in the IFN-α arms in remission duration (median 7 months) and survival (median 5 months). Moreover, a survey of U.S. patients found a 6-month risk/benefit trade off preferred by the majority of interviewed MM patients with regard to IFNα treatment.[319] Q-TWIST analysis showed that patients treated with maintenance IFN-α gained an average of 9.8 months without disease relapse and 5.8 months of OS vs the control groups; however, the IFN-α group suffered an average of 4.1 months of moderate or worse toxicity.[320] IFN-α maintenance treatment therefore appears to benefit a subset patients who have achieved low tumor burden, and its marginal benefit needs to be balanced against side effects even in this patient group. In a recent SWOG study alternate day prednisone at a dose of 50mg was noted to improve OS and EFS after induction treatment with a VAD like induction regimen.[321]

Although there is no standard maintenance regimen, novel therapies are now being evaluated to prolong PFS. For example, 3 year median PFS and overall PFS were prolonged by the use of thalidomide posttransplant.[289] Thalidomide with or without prednisone have been evaluated as maintenance. Although promising,[322] dose reductions were required with chronic use.[323] Since it is oral and has few side effects, making it an ideal candidate for a maintenance medication, lenalinamide/Revlimid is now under evaluation to prolong PFS post high-dose therapy.

■ Relapsed Disease

Almost all patients with MM who initially respond to chemotherapy eventually relapse. Patients who progress with initial therapy have a 40% response to high-dose or pulsed corticosteroid therapy.324 Thalidomide and dexamethasone achieves high-response rates.233,234 Patients who relapse during therapy or within 6 months of stopping initial treatment have a 75% response rate to VAD chemotherapy.324-326 Patients who relapse >6 months after stopping therapy have a 60-70% response rate when initial therapy is reinstituted;230 if no response is achieved, then VAD or alternate regimens can be used. Unfortunately, even in those patients who respond to salvage therapy, the duration of response is limited. A major advance in the treatment of resistant MM has been the emergence of Thal as an effective therapy,86,327 which achieves an overall 32% response rate in patients with advanced and refractory MM. The 2 year event free survival (EFS) and OS were 20% and 48%, respectively; low PCLI, normal cytogenetics, and a β2microglobulin of <3 mg/L were good prognostic factors for survival. Based on the impressive results of single agent Thal in refractory relapsed MM and in vitro data suggesting its synergy with Dex, Thal has been coupled with Dex to treat patients with disease refractory to either agent alone; even in this setting, half of patients treated respond.328 Thal has also been combined with chemotherapy and bisphosphonates in the treatment of refractory MM.329,330

In order to overcome resistance to current therapies and improve patient outcome, novel biologically-based treatment approaches are needed that target mechanisms whereby MM cells grow and survive in BM.[331] To achieve this goal, we have developed systems for studying growth, survival, and drug resistance mechanisms intrinsic to MM cells. Importantly, we have also developed both in vitro systems and in vivo animal models to characterize mechanisms of MM cell homing to BM, as well as factors (MM cell-BMSC interactions, cytokines, angiogenesis) promoting MM cell growth, survival, drug resistance, and migration in the BM microenvironment.[69,76,81-83,332-334] These model systems have allowed for the development of several promising biologically-based therapies which can target the MM cell and its BM microenvironment, those which target the MM cell only, and those which target only the BM microenvironment.

Drugs that target the MM cell and its BM milieu and thereby can overcome classical drug resistance in vitro include: Thal/IMiDs;[61] proteasome inhibitors Bortezomib[63] and NPI-0052;[335] As2O3;[336] 2 methoxyestradiol;[337,338] VEGF receptor tyrosine kinase inhibitors PTK 787[339] and GW654652;[340] and histone deacetylase inhibitors SAHA;[341] LAQ824[342] and LBH,[343] and mitogen-activated protein kinase kinase (MEK) inhibitor AZD6244.[344] Novel agents that target the MM cell directly and trigger cytotoxicity in the BM milieu include IGF inhibitors;[345] CD40 monoclonal antibody;[346] CS1 monoclonal antibody HuLuc63;[347] Hsp90 inhibitor;[348] Smac mimetics; and telomerase targeting therapies.[349] Drugs acting on the BM milieu and indirectly impacting the MM cell include p38MAPK inhibitors[350,351] and IKK inhibitors (Fig. 117-7).[352 353]

The bench to bedside translation of the immunomodulatory drug lenalinamide (Revlimid) has been very rapid. It was shown to target both the MM cell and BM microenvironment in vitro and in vivo in 2000;[61,354] completed phase I testing that identified an MTD, lack of

Table 117-12 ■ **Representative Studies of Miniallogeneic Transplantation in Myeloma**

Source	Conditioning	Sample Size (*n*)	TRM (%)	Response Rate (%)	Acute GVHD (%)	Chronic GVHD (%)	PFS (%)	OS (%)
Badros et al[313]	Mel or Mel/TBI/Flu	31	10% early, 20% late	CR 6l, PR 10	58	32	86 (1 year)	86 (1 year)
Kroger et al[312]	PBSCT + Mel/Flu/ATG	17	18	CR 73, PR 20	63	40	56 (2 year)	74 (2 year)
Maloney et al[311]	PBSCT + TBI/MMF/cyc	31	16	CR 43, PR 31	45	55	–	81 (1 year)

Abbreviations: CR, complete response; GVHD, graft-vs-host disease; OS, overall survival; PFS, progression free survival; PR, partial response; TRM, transplant-related mortality.

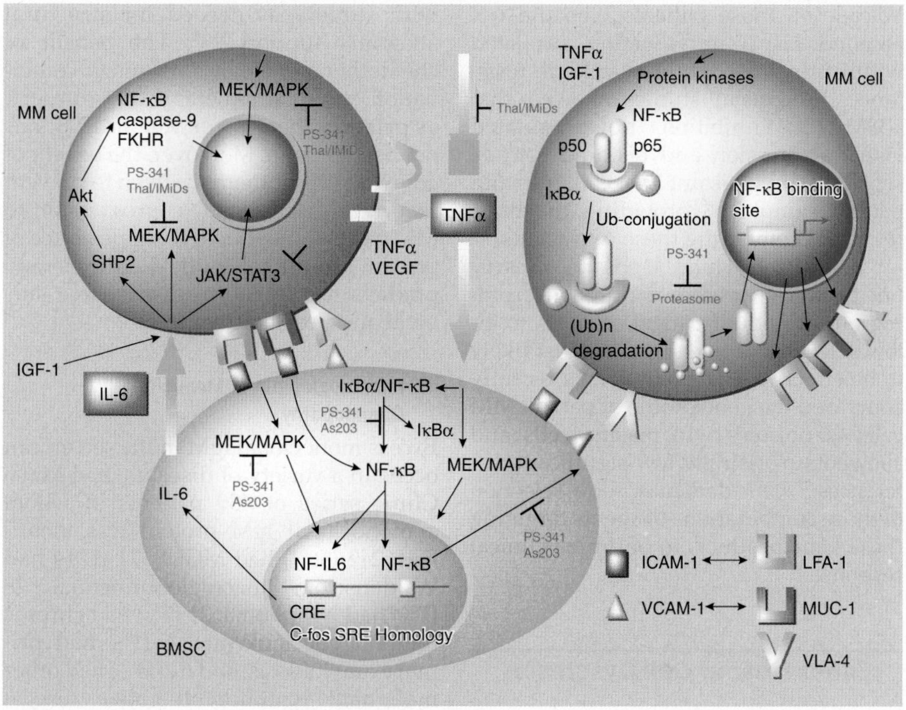

Figure 117-7 ■ Inhibition of signaling pathways by novel therapeutic agents in multiple myeloma.

toxicity, and remarkable anti-MM activity in 2001;[355] and completed phase II testing in 2002.[356] Two large phase III trials comparing Revlimid/Dex with Dex/placebo were unblinded because of statistically significantly higher response rates, as well as increase in time to progression and OS in the lenalidomide/Dex treated cohort, providing the basis for its FDA approval to treat relapsed MM after one prior therapy.[357,358]

The bench to bedside translation of Bortezomib and FDA approval was also very rapid. NF-κB was identified as a target in MM since it conferred drug resistance, modulated adhesion molecule expression on MM cells and BMSCs, and modulated constitutive and MM binding-induced transcription and secretion of cytokines.[48] Phase I trials showed tolerability and early evidence of anti-MM activity.[359] The phase II SUMMIT trial demonstrated responses, including CRs; prolongation of time to progression and survival; and associated clinical benefit, forming the basis for accelerated FDA approval for treatment of relapsed refractory MM.[360] The APEX trial compared Dex vs Bortezomib therapy of relapsed MM was unblinded due to a statistically significant prolongation in time to progression in the Bortezomib treated cohort, forming the basis for its FDA approval extending to relapsed MM.[241] With follow-up, time to progression and OS is significantly improved with Bortezomib, and neurological complications manageable.[361] Which of its many activities account for its MM cytotoxicity is unclear. As noted above, Thal, lenalidomide, and Bortezomib all were initially used to treat relapsed MM, but now are combined with high-dose Dex or with melphalan and prednisone to treat newly diagnosed transplant or nontransplant candidates, respectively, and improving OR, CR, EFS and OS.[242,245,362-364]

■ Future Directions

Evolution of a New Treatment Paradigm for MM ■ Our in vitro and animal model studies have demonstrated the importance of the BM in promoting MM cell growth, survival, drug resistance, and migration in the BM microenvironment and have already derived very promising therapies based on targeting the MM cell in its BM milieu. These studies provide the framework for development of a new treatment paradigm in MM, targeting both the tumor cell and its microenvironment, which is urgently needed since MM remains incurable despite all available therapies.

Identification and Validation of Novel-Targeted MM ■ Therapies Importantly, in our in vitro gene array studies with conventional Dex[141] and novel (Bortezomib)[142] therapies, samples obtained from patients treated on these protocols help to identify *in vivo* targets and mechanisms of novel drug action on the one hand, vs mechanisms of drug resistance on the other, and also aid in determining whether in vivo targets of these novel therapies correlate with their in vitro anti-MM activities. Excitingly, preclinical studies suggest enhanced activity when these novel agents are combined with conventional agents or with each other. These studies have established a new treatment paradigm targeting the MM cell in its BM microenvironment to further elucidate MM pathogenesis as well as overcome drug resistance and improve patient outcome.

Novel single agents of great promise include new proteasome inhibitor NPI-0052 and PR-171, FGFR3 inhibitors,[365,366] humanized anti-CD40 antibodies,[106,346] anti-CS1 antibody,[347] MEK inhibitor AZD6244,[344] and Hsp90 inhibitors.[348] NPI0052[335] and PR-171[367] are next generation proteasome inhibitors and active against Bortezomib resistant MM and nontoxic in preclinical models, and are already in clinical trials in relapsed MM. FGFR3 inhibitors is specifically targeting those 15-20% patients with t(4:14) translocation. CD40 humanized antibodies have demonstrated early activity against MM, and Hsp90 inhibitors as single agents can achieve responses in relapsed refractory MM.

Profiling of gene and protein expression can also provide the preclinical rationale for clinical protocols combining novel targeted therapies. For example, our studies demonstrate that Bortezomib treatment of MM cells in vitro induces death signaling, downregulates survival signaling, and upregulates both ubiquitin/proteasome and stress response gene transcripts.[142] Specifically, Bortezomib induces Hsp90, which not only is a stress response protein but also plays a major role in protein unfolding required before proteins can be degraded by the proteasome. Our in vitro studies show that Hsp90 inhibitor 17AAG can block the Hsp90 stress response induced by Bortezomib and thereby increase MM cell apoptosis. These gene microarray studies therefore provided the framework for a clinical trial coupling these agents in MM which shows that Hsp90 inhibitor KOS953 can sensitize to and even overcome resistance to Bortezomib,[368] and a phase III clinical trial of bortezomib vs bortezomib with KOS953 in relapsed MM is ongoing.

Proteomic studies can also provide the preclinical basis for clinical application of novel targeted therapies. For example, our in vitro studies demonstrate that exposure of MM cells to Bortezomib induces cleavage of DNA repair kinases such as DNA PKcs in a dose and time dependent manner.[369] This observation for the first time suggested that Bortezomib inhibited DNA repair. Subsequent in vitro studies demonstrated that coupling Bortezomib with DNA damaging agents (alkylating agents and anthracyclines) can enhance sensitivity or even restore sensitivity to these agents in resistant MM cells.[370] Already clinical protocols coupling Velcade with Doxil[371] and with melphalan[370] have demonstrated promising clinical results. Specifically, a large randomized trial of Doxil and Bortezomib vs Bortezomib in relapsed MM showed significantly increase OR, EFS and OS in the patients receiving combined therapy, setting the stage for its FDA approval in June 2007.

In order to provide the framework for coupling these novel agents in rational clinical trials, we have also characterized the apoptotic signaling cascades triggered in MM cells by both conventional and these novel agents.[67] For example, use of IMiDs with TRAIL provides dual triggering of caspase 8 death signaling, whereas treatment with IMiDs (lenalidomide/Revlimid) and Bortezomib triggers both caspase 8 and caspase 9-mediated MM cell death. An ongoing clinical trial has demonstrated remarkable activity in patients treated with Revlimid/Velcade, even in patients resistant to either agent alone.[372]

mTOR inhibitor rapamycin sensitizes MM cells to both conventional (dexamethasone) and novel therapies;[373,374] CC-779 has anti-MM activity in xenograft models.[375] Bortezomib inhibits growth (MEK/ERK) and survival (Jak/STAT) signaling, but activates Akt, providing the preclinical rationale for combining Bortezomib with the Akt inhibitor perifosine.[376]

Our recent signaling studies have defined the role of the aggresome in degrading ubiquitinated protein in MM, and specifically used the HDAC6 inhibitor tubacin to inhibit its transport to the aggresome for degradation. Blocking the aggresome with tubacin induces a compensatory upregulation of the proteasome; conversely, blocking the proteasome with Bortezomib triggers a compensatory upregulation of the aggresome. Importantly, blocking both the proteasome and aggresome with Bortezomib and tubacin, respectively, induces synergistic toxicity.[377] This strategy may also have activity against pancreatic cancer.[378]

It is also possible to combine monoclonal antibodies with novel drugs. Lenalidomide, for example, can markedly augment antibody-dependent cellular cytotoxicity (ADCC) induced by anti-CD40 in MM.[106] Finally, gene expression profiling in correlative science studies of patients on clinical protocols will both identify targets of drug sensitivity vs resistance, and allow for predicting those patients most likely to respond to conventional and novel targeted therapies. For example, gene expression profiling of patient tumor samples showed genes upregulated in patients responding to Velcade vs those patients who did not respond. Hsp27 upregulation correlated with intrinsic or acquired velcade resistance. Preclinical studies showed that p38MAPK inhibition downregulated Hsp27 expression and restored velcade sensitivity in resistant MM cell lines and patient samples,[351] providing the basis for a trial combining these two agents.

Ultimately it may be possible to carry out gene and protein expression profiling on individual patient samples to allow selection of those agents most likely to be effective. For example, we recently compared the gene profile of patient MM cells to normal twin plasma cells and showed surprisingly few significant differences.[379] This data may allow selection of those combinations of agents targeting these gene products to optimize clinical response.

Other Plasma Cell Dyscrasias

Plasmacytomas

Clinical Characteristics ■ Plasmacytomas are collections of monoclonal plasma cells originating either in bone (solitary osseous plasmacytoma, SOP) or in soft tissue (extramedullary plasmacytoma, EMP). They comprise <10% of plasma cell dyscrasias. MM must be excluded before the diagnosis of either SOP or EMP can be made. Magnetic resonance imaging can be useful to show additional marrow abnormalities consistent with MM.[380] The median age of diagnosis of either SOP or EMP is approximately 50 years, nearly 10 years younger than that for MM.[381-383] Although patients with SOP and EMP can both progress to MM, persons with SOP progress in the majority of cases, in contrast to EMP, where only up to 50% eventually develop MM. The median survival of 86.4 months and 100.8 months for patients with SOP and EMP, respectively, is similar; however, PFS is markedly different, 16% for SOP patients vs 71% for EMP patients. The persistence of stable monoclonal Ig in serum and/or urine after primary treatment of plasmacytoma does not necessitate additional therapy, since it does not influence survival or disease-free survival.[381] In contrast, rising monoclonal Ig levels in a patient with a history of either SOP or EMP should trigger a work-up for either recurrent plasmacytoma or MM. It has been suggested, as is true for MM, that serum β2M has prognostic value in patients with SOP. Specifically, 17 of 19 patients with elevated serum β2M had transformation to MM and shorter survival (31 months) than those with normal serum β2M levels.[384]

Treatment ■ Treatment of SOP and EMP is local therapy, primarily radiotherapy with surgery as needed for structural anatomic support.[381-383] The benefit of chemotherapy, either alone or in combination with radiotherapy and surgery, as primary therapy for SOP or EMP has not been proven. Moreover, the benefit of adjuvant chemotherapy, given to prevent recurrent disease and/or progression to MM, is also undefined. Disappearance of protein after involved-field radiotherapy predicts for long-term disease-free survival and possible cure.[385]

Immunoglobulin M Monoclonal Gammopathy

Excess monoclonal IgM in the serum can occur in a variety of diseases. In a Mayo Clinic series of 430 patients in whom a monoclonal IgM protein was identified, 242 (56%) had MGUS, 71 (17%) had Waldenström macroglobulinemia, 28 (7%) had lymphoma, 21 (5%) had chronic lymphocytic leukemia, 6 (1%) had primary amyloidosis, and 62 (14%) had other malignant lymphoproliferative diseases.[386] The duration of time from the recognition of the M protein to the development of a malignant lymphoid disease ranged from 4 to 9 years, suggesting that long-term follow-up of such patients is necessary.

Waldenström Macroblobulinemia

The diagnosis of Waldenström macroglobulinemia (WM) requires an IgM serum level of at least 3.0 gm/dL in association with an increase in lymphocytes or plasmacytoid lymphocytes in the marrow.[386-388] WM corresponds most closely to the lymphoplasmacytic lymphoma (LPA) under the World Health Organization (WHO) classification of lymphoid tumors (LPL/immunocytoma of the Revised European–American [REAL] classification of lymphoma). WM accounts for approximately 2% of all hematologic malignancies and is more common in men than in women. Its incidence increases with age, and it is more common among whites than among African Americans.[389,390] Although the etiology of WM is unclear, genetic factors may contribute to the pathogenesis of this disease, since there are reports of families with WM in association with other lymphoproliferative and immunologic disorders.[391] Cytogenetic abnormalities occur in 15-90% of cases, but none are specific for WM.[392,393]The WM B-cell clone demonstrates interclonal differentiation from small lymphocytes with large focal deposits of surface immunoglobulins, to lymphoplasmacytic cells and mature plasma cells that contain intracytoplasmic immunoglobulin. This morphologic heterogeneity is reflected by variable expression of phenotypic markers. All WM cells express monoclonal IgM and most cells are CD19, CD20, CD22, and FMC7 positive. High density of CD38 is also detected with variable intensity of the PCA-1 antigen. Predictably, CD45 isoform expression is heterogenous, probably reflecting ongoing monoclonal B-cell differentiation. In approximately 20% of cases, CD5 and CD23 expression are seen, but their coexpression is uncommon.[394] Circulating clonal B cells in WM increase in patients who fail to respond to therapy or who progress.[395] Recent studies suggest that WM originates from a postgerminal center B cell that has undergone somatic mutations and antigenic selection in the lymphoid follicle and has the characteristics of an IgM-bearing memory B cell.[396-398]

The median age of onset of WM is 61 years. Symptoms are characteristically vague and nonspecific, with the most common being weakness, anorexia, and weight loss. Symptoms due to peripheral neuropathy and Raynaud's phenomenon can precede more serious manifestations. Lymphadenopathy, splenomegaly, and/or hepatomegaly are present in 30-40% of cases, and at least 20-25% lymphoplasmacytoid cells are usually present in the marrow. Visceral involvement of small bowel and peripheral nerves can cause the clinical sequelae of malabsorption and neuropathy, respectively. Hemorrhagic complications are common, attributable to abnormal bleeding times, decreased platelet adhesiveness, or direct interference by the IgM protein with the release of platelet factor 3 and with coagulation factors. An important part of the differential diagnosis is to exclude the less common entity of IgM MM, which is characterized by lytic bone disease and an absence of organomegaly and/or lymphocytic involvement; rarely, WM can itself progress to IgM MM.[399] Amyloidosis occurs rarely in Waldenström macroglobulinemia.[400] Hyperviscosity syndrome, described earlier as a rare complication in MM, occurs more commonly in the setting of excess IgM and is characterized by mucosal bleeding and neurologic, ocular, and cardiovascular abnormalities.[204] Therapy with plasmapheresis is more useful to remove excess IgM than it is in the setting of excess IgG monoclonal proteins and related hyperviscosity in MM.

Plasmapheresis can be considered as only an adjunctive therapy. Treatment regimens used are similar to those used to treat low-grade lymphomas and MM, including chlorambucil, cyclophosphamide, melphalan, and corticosteroids, either as single agents or in combinations.[401] Just as for MM, there is no evidence that combined drug regimens are superior to single therapies. The median survival is approximately 50 months, not that dissimilar from the best reported series of patients with MM. In contrast to persons with MM, however, many individuals with WM have indolent disease requiring no therapy for long periods of time, with survivals in excess of 20 years. Pretreatment parameters, including older age, male gender, general symptoms, and cytopenias, define a high-risk population that could perhaps benefit from newer therapeutic approaches.[402,403] Acute leukemia has developed in patients with WM, emphasizing a potential complication of premature and prolonged low-dose therapy with alkylating agents.[404] Nucleoside analogs, including fludarabine and 2-chlorodeoxyadenosine, have been shown to be effective in newly diagnosed as well as in refractory patients with WM and may achieve more rapid cytoreduction than oral chlorambucil.[401,405-407] Prospective randomized trials are needed to assess the effect of nucleoside analogs on survival.[408] In a recent multicenter trial, 92 patients with WM resistant to first-line treatment were treated with fludarabine or combination chemotherapy, including cyclophosphamide, doxorubicin, and prednisone.[409] Although response rates and EFS were significantly higher in patients treated with fludarabine, no survival difference was noted.

Several reports describe responses in patients with WM using recombinant IFN-α or -γ.[410,411] Interestingly, patients who had been treated with prior chemotherapy had an equivalent response rate to those who had not. Future studies are needed to assess its effect as a remission therapy or as part of other strategies.[412] Although high-dose therapy with autologous stem cell support has been shown to be effective in many patients with MM or with low-grade lymphoma, relatively few patients with WM have undergone transplant. Nonetheless, preliminary data suggest that high-dose therapy is associated with a high complete response rate and acceptable toxicity, and this approach therefore warrants further investigation, particularly in younger patients with poor prognostic features.[413] Splenectomy has been reported to be effective in chemotherapy-resistant patients with WM and results in a major decrease in monoclonal protein concentration and durable remission.[414,415] Monoclonal antibody therapy with rituximab, a chimeric anti-CD20 monoclonal antibody, produces responses in both treated and untreated patients with low-grade lymphoma. Given that the CD20 antigen is typically present in WM, rituximab has been given to patients and a clinical response was seen in about one-third of previously treated patients in early studies.[416,417] Ongoing studies are looking at combining rituximab with fludarabine in the treatment of WM. Salvage strategies for WM include re-use of first line agents, combination chemotherapy (eg, CHOP, CVP, CAP), thalidimide and bortezomib based therapies.

Heavy-Chain Diseases

Since the original description by Franklin and colleagues of a patient with malignant lymphoma whose serum and urine contained large amounts of the Fc fragment of IgG, the clinical and immunochemical scope of gamma heavy–chain disease (γHCD) has broadened.[418] These diseases are characterized by the presence of a portion of the Ig heavy chain in the serum or urine or both. The median age at diagnosis is similar to that for MM, approximately 60 years[419] The clinical and laboratory features can be heterogeneous. Most common presenting symptoms are weakness, fatigue, and fever, associated with lymphadenopathy and hepatosplenomegaly. In addition to Ig heavy chain in serum or urine, a lymphoplasmacytic marrow infiltrate is noted in most cases. The clinical course can be fulminant and rapidly progressive; alternatively, the monoclonal heavy chain can persist for years in otherwise asymptomatic patients. Thus, survival is variable, but the median is only 12 months. Treatment options for patients with active disease are similar to those used for lymphoma or MM, whereas patients with indolent disease should be followed expectantly without therapy. Cases of αHCD, μHCD, and δHCD have also been described. HCD is typically associated with non-Hodgkin lymphoma in the gastrointestinal tract, beginning with plasma cells that produce a heavy chain and aggregate in the intestinal tract and subsequent transformation into a malignant non-Hodgkin lymphoma of the immunoblastic type, probably arising from the more mature plasma cells.[420] The ideal therapy for heavy-chain disease is not known because of its rarity, but intensive chemotherapy including intravenous cyclophosphamide, doxorubicin, vincristine, and oral prednisone appears to offer some patients long-term remissions.

Amyloidosis

Amyloidosis is relatively rare as a clinically significant disease. It has been classified into five categories. These include (1) primary, with or without plasma cell and lymphoid neoplasms; (2) secondary, associated with chronic infections or autoimmune disease; (3) hereditary, associated with familial Mediterranean fever, Portuguese lower limb neuropathy, and others; (4) amyloidosis associated with aging; and (5) amyloidosis of endocrine glands, with medullary thyroid carcinoma and multiple endocrine neoplasia type 2.[400,421] The amyloid found in most cases of amyloidosis can be assigned to one of two types, according to whether the fibrils consist mainly of the variable region of Ig light chains (AL, or primary amyloidosis) or protein A (AA, or secondary amyloidosis). Protein A has a molecular weight of 8500 daltons and consists of 76 amino acids; it is not related to any known immunoglobulin. In AL, amyloid primarily involves the heart, tongue, gastrointestinal tract, and skin, whereas AA primarily results in fibril deposition in liver, kidney, and spleen. A review of 229 patients with AL documented MM in 47 (21%) patients.[421] Initial presenting symptoms were fatigue and weight loss, with pain more common in those who also had MM. Hepatomegaly and macroglossia were present in up to one-third of patients with AL; renal insufficiency was present in one-half of patients, and proteinuria (defined as albuminuria with immune globulin seen, only in MM) was documented in 82% of patients. Nephrotic syndrome, congestive heart failure, orthostatic hypotension, carpal tunnel syndrome, and peripheral neuropathy were all more common in those without MM (30-70% of patients studied) than in persons with MM (<20%). Overall median survival was 12 months, 5 months for those with MM in contrast to 13 months for individuals without MM. Although it has been difficult to monitor the distribution and progression of disease, it has been shown that radiolabeled serum amyloid P component, which has specific binding affinity for amyloid fibrils, can be given intravenously and localizes rapidly and specifically in amyloid deposits.[422] This technique may therefore facilitate diagnosis and monitoring of the extent of systemic amyloidosis, including the effects of therapeutic interventions.

Treatment of AL is unsatisfactory. Only 27 of 153 (18%) patients responded to MP, although median survival for responders was prolonged at 89.4 months; only 5% of patients with primary AL survive ≥ 10 years.[421,423] A prospective randomized trial has concluded that MP was superior to colchicine when analyzed from time of entry into the study to time of death or progression of disease.[424] Other retrospective studies suggest that colchicine is superior to placebo for patients with AL.[425] Alkylating agent-based chemotherapy may therefore be beneficial for a subset of patients and result in prolonged survival. One randomized trial of colchicine, MP, or a combination of the three drugs in patients with primary amyloidosis found that therapy with MP results in objective responses and prolonged survival as compared with colchicine.[426] However, therapy with multiple alkylating agents did not achieve either higher response rate or longer survival time than MP.[427] Early reports suggest that dose-intensive melphalan with blood stem cell support can achieve CRs, with improvement in performance status and clinical remission of organ-specific disease.[428] Guidelines have been developed for patient selection to maximize benefit and minimize treatment-related mortality.[429,430] As in MM, a randomized trial is required to assess the true efficacy of high-dose therapy, since those patients eligible for high-dose treatments may also do well with chemotherapy.[431] Attempts to improve outcomes for patients with symptomatic and advanced multisystem disease may require both solid and stem cell transplantation, as well as the use of less intensive conditioning regimens. [432] Novel drugs with promise in the treatment of MM, including Thal, IMiDs, and PS-341, are also being tested in patients with amyloidosis.

Selected References

The complete reference list can be found at www.CANCERMEDICINE8.com

3. Hallek M, Bergsagel PL, Anderson KC. Multiple myeloma: Increasing evidence for a multistep transformation process. *Blood.* 1998;91:3–21.
9. Durie BGM, Salmon SE. A clinical staging system for multiple myeloma. Correlation of measured cell mass with presenting clinical features, response to treatment and survival. *Cancer.* 1975;36:842–854.
11. Kyle RA, Therneau TM, Rajkumar SV, Larson DR, Plevak MF, Offord JR, Dispenzieri A, Katzmann JA, Melton LJ, 3rd. Prevalence of monoclonal gammopathy of undetermined significance. *N Engl J Med.* 2006;354:1362–1369.
22. Pruzanski W, Ogryzlo MA. Abnormal proteinuria in malignant diseases. *Adv Clin Chem.* 1970;13:335–382.
44. Teoh G, Anderson KC. Interaction of tumor and host cells with adhesion and extracellular matrix molecules in the development of multiple myeloma. *Hematol Oncol Clin North Am.* 1997;11:27–42.
61. Hideshima T, Chauhan D, Shima Y, et al. Thalidomide and its analogues overcome drug resistance of human multiple myeloma cells to conventional therapy. *Blood.* 2000;96:2943–2950.
63. Hideshima T, Richardson P, Chauhan D, et al. The proteasome inhibitor PS-341 inhibits growth, induces apoptosis, and overcomes drug resistance in human multiple myeloma cells. *Cancer Res.* 2001;61:3071–3076.
67. Hideshima T, Anderson KC. Molecular mechanisms of novel therapeutic approaches for multiple myeloma. *Nat Rev Cancer.* 2002;2:927–937.
86. Singhal S, Mehta J, Desikan R, et al. Antitumor activity of thalidomide in refractory multiple myeloma. *N Engl J Med.* 1999;341:1565–1571.
96. Qiang YW, Endo Y, Rubin JS, Rudikoff S. Wnt signaling in B-cell neoplasia. *Oncogene.* 2003;22:1536–1545.
99. Tian E, Zhan F, Walker R, et al. The role of the Wnt-signaling antagonist DKK1 in the development of osteolytic lesions in multiple myeloma. *N Engl J Med.* 2003;349:2483–2494.
138. Bergsagel PL, Kuehl WM. Molecular pathogenesis and a consequent classification of multiple myeloma. *J Clin Oncol.* 2005;23:6333–6338.
139. Barlogie B, Tricot G, Anaissie E, et al. Thalidomide and hematopoietic-cell transplantation for multiple myeloma. *N Engl J Med.* 2006;354:1021–1030.
146. Greipp PR, San Miguel J, Durie BG, et al. International staging system for multiple myeloma. *J Clin Oncol.* 2005;23:3412–3420.
168. Shaughnessy JD, Jr., Zhan F, Burington BE, et al. A validated gene expression model of high-risk multiple myeloma is defined by deregulated expression of genes mapping to chromosome 1. *Blood.* 2007;109:2276–2284.
169. Mundy GR, Bertolini DR. Bone destruction and hypercalcemia in plasma cell myeloma. *Semin Oncol.* 1986;13:291–299.
186. Berenson J, Lichtenstein A, Porter L, et al. Pamidronate disodium reduces the occurrence of skeletal events in patients with advanced multiple myeloma. *N Engl J Med.* 1996;334:488–493.
198. Raje N, Woo SB, Hande K, Yap JT, et al. Clinical, radiographic, and biochemical characterization of multiple myeloma patients with osteonecrosis of the jaw. *Clin Cancer Res.* 2008;14:2387–2395.
226. Blade J, Samson D, Reece D, et al. Criteria for evaluating disease response and progression in patients with multiple myeloma treated by high-dose therapy and haemopoietic stem cell transplantation. Myeloma Subcommittee of the EBMT. European Group for Blood and Marrow Transplant. *Br J Haematol.* 1998;102:1115–1123.
229. Durie BG, Harousseau JL, Miguel JS, et al. International uniform response criteria for multiple myeloma. *Leukemia.* 2006;in press
231. Gregory WM, Richards MA, Malpas JS. Combination chemotherapy versus melphalan and prednisolone in the treatment of multiple myeloma: an overview of published trials. *J Clin Oncol.* 1992;10:334–342.
232. Group MTsC. Combination chemotherapy versus melphalan plus prednisone as treatment for multiple myeloma: an overview of 6,633 patients from 27 randomized trials. *J Clin Oncol.* 1998;16:3832–3842.
241. Richardson PG, Sonneveld P, Schuster MW, et al. Bortezomib or high-dose dexamethasone for relapsed multiple myeloma. *N Engl J Med.* 2005;352:2487–2498.
245. Palumbo A, Bringhen S, Caravita T, et al. Oral melphalan and prednisone chemotherapy plus thalidomide compared with melphalan and prednisone alone in elderly patients with multiple myeloma: randomised controlled trial. *Lancet.* 2006;367:825–831.
246. Facon T, Mary J, Harousseau, H, et al. Superiority of melphalan-prednisone (MP) + thalidomide (THAL) over MP and autologous stem cell transplantation in the treatment of newly diagnosed elderly patients with multiple myeloma. *J Clin Oncol.* 2006;24:1.
254. Attal M, Harousseau JL, Stoppa AM, et al. Autologous bone marrow transplantation versus conventional chemotherapy in

multiple myeloma: a prospective, randomized trial. *New Eng J Med*. 1996;335:91–97.
255. Fermand J-P, Ravaud P, Chevret S, et al. High-dose therapy and autologous peripheral blood stem cell transplantation in multiple myeloma: Up-front or rescue treatment? Results of a multicenter sequential randomized clinical trial. *Blood*. 1998;92:3131–3136.
256. Barlogie B, Kyle RA, Anderson KC, et al. Standard chemotherapy compared with high-dose chemoradiotherapy for multiple myeloma: final results of phase III US Intergroup Trial S9321. *J Clin Oncol*. 2006;24:929–936.
258. Child JA, Morgan GJ, Davies FE, et al. High-dose chemotherapy with hematopoietic stem-cell rescue for multiple myeloma. *N Engl J Med*. 2003;348:1875–1883.
267. Attal M, Harousseau JL, Facon T, et al. Single versus double autologous stem-cell transplantation for multiple myeloma. *N Engl J Med*. 2003;349:2495–2502.
290. Bensinger WI, Demirer T, Buckner CD, et al. Syngeneic marrow transplantation in patients with multiple myeloma. *Bone Marrow Transplant*. 1996;18:527–531.
291. Gahrton G, Svensson H, Bjorkstrand B, et al. Syngeneic transplantation in multiple myeloma—a case-matched comparison with autologous and allogeneic transplantation. *Bone Marrow Transplant*. 1999;7:741–745.
292. Gahrton G, Tura S, Ljungman P, et al. Allogeneic bone marrow transplantation in multiple myeloma. *New Eng J Med*. 1991;325:1267–1273.
297. Bensinger WI, Maloney D, Storb R. Allogeneic hematopoietic cell transplantation for multiple myeloma. *Semin Hematol*. 2001;38:243–249.
331. Anderson KC. Targeted therapy for multiple myeloma. *Semin Hematol*. 2001;38:286–294.
332. Chauhan D, Anderson KC. Apoptosis in multiple myeloma: therapeutic implications. *Apoptosis*. 2001;6:47–55.
335. Chauhan D, Catley L, Li G, et al. A novel orally active proteasome inhibitor induces apoptosis in multiple myeloma cells with mechanisms distinct from Bortezomib. *Cancer Cell*. 2005;8:407–419.
341. Mitsiades N, Mitsiades CS, Richardson PG, et al. Molecular sequelae of histone deacetylase inhibition in human malignant B cells. *Blood*. 2003;101:4055–4062.
348. Mitsiades CS, Mitsiades NS, McMullan CJ, et al. Antimyeloma activity of heat shock protein-90 inhibition. *Blood*. 2006;107:1092–1100.
357. Weber DM, Chen C, Niesvizky R, et al. Lenalidomide plus dexamethasone for relapsed multiple myeloma in North America. *N Engl J Med*. 2007;357:2133–2142.
358. Dimopoulos M, Spencer A, Attal M, et al. Lenalidomide plus dexamethasone for relapsed or refractory multiple myeloma. *N Engl J Med*. 2007;357:2123–2132.
360. Richardson PG, Barlogie B, Berenson J, et al. A phase 2 study of bortezomib in relapsed, refractory myeloma. *N Engl J Med*. 2003;348:2609–2617.
361. Richardson PG, Briemberg H, Jagannath S, et al. Frequency, characteristics, and reversibility of peripheral neuropathy during treatment of advanced multiple myeloma with bortezomib. *J Clin Oncol*. 2006;24:3113–3120.
362. Rajkumar SV, Hayman SR, Lacy MQ, et al. Combination therapy with lenalidomide plus dexamethasone (Rev/Dex) for newly diagnosed myeloma. *Blood*. 2005;106:4050–4053.
369. Hideshima T, Mitsiades C, Akiyama M, et al. Molecular mechanisms mediating antimyeloma activity of proteasome inhibitor PS-341. *Blood*. 2003;101:1530–1534.
387. Dimopoulos MA, Alexanian R. Waldenstrom's macroglobulinemia. *Blood*. 1994;83: 1452–1159.
408. Dimopoulos MA, Panayiotidis P, Moulopoulos LA, Sfikakis P, Dalakas M. Waldenstrom's macroglobulinemia: Clinical features, complications, and management. *J Clin Oncol*. 2000;18:214–226.
419. Kyle RA. The heavy chain diseases. In: Wiernick PH, Canellos GP, Kyle RA, Schiffer CA, eds. *Neoplastic Diseases of the Blood*. New York: Churchill Livingston; 1985:593.
421. Kyle RA, Greipp PR. Amyloidosis (AL)—clinical and laboratory features in 229 cases. *Mayo Clin* Proc. 1983;58:665–683.
428. Comenzo RL, Vosburgh E, Simms RW, et al. Dose-intensive melphalan with blood stem cell support for the treatment of AL amyloidosis: one-year follow-up in five patients. *Blood*. 1996;88:2801–2806.
432. Comenzo RL, Vosburgh E, Falk RH, et al. Dose-intensive melphalan with blood stem-cell support for the treatment of AL (amyloid light-chain) amyloidosis: survival and responses in 25 patients. *Blood*. 1998;91:3662–3670.

118 Myeloproliferative Neoplasms: Essential Thrombocythemia, Primary Myelofibrosis, and Polycythemia Vera

Ayalew Tefferi, MD

The chronic myeloid neoplasms are a diverse group of malignant bone marrow conditions that originate in a transformed multipotential hematopoietic progenitor cell.[1] This heterogeneous group of diseases shares an initially indolent clinical course with a variable degree of risk to evolve into overt acute leukemia. Even in the absence of leukemic transformation, the consequences of the cellular excesses or deficiencies characteristic of these disorders are troublesome for patients and all too frequently fatal; some of these disease complications include thrombosis, bleeding, marked hepatosplenomegaly, profound constitutional symptoms, and cachexia.

Under the revised 2008 World Health Organization (WHO) classification system the broad category of chronic myeloid neoplasms includes the myelodysplastic syndromes (MDS, discussed in Chapter 109), myeloproliferative neoplasms (MPN; formerly referred to as chronic myeloproliferative diseases), "MDS/MPN overlap," and a new subcategory that is characterized by both prominent blood eosinophilia and a mutation involving either platelet-derived growth factor receptor (PDGFRA or PDGFRB) or fibroblast growth factor receptor (FGFR).[2] The 2008 WHO MPN category includes the four classic "myeloproliferative disorders," which includes chronic myelogenous leukemia (CML), polycythemia vera (PV), essential thrombocythemia (ET) and primary myelofibrosis (PMF) as well as chronic neutrophilic leukemia (CNL), chronic eosinophilic leukemia not otherwise specified (CEL-NOS), and mastocytosis. The "MDS/MPN" category displays features that are characteristic of both MDS (dyserythropoiesis or dysgranulopoiesis) and MPN (peripheral blood granulocytosis, monocytosis, eosinophilia, or thrombocytosis).[3] Included in this category are chronic myelomonocytic leukemia (CMML), juvenile myelomonocytic leukemia (JMML), "atypical chronic myeloid leukemia, *BCR-ABL1*-negative" (aCML) and "MDS/MPN, unclassifiable" (Table 118-1).[2] "MDS/MPN, unclassifiable" includes the WHO provisional entity of "refractory anemia with ring sideroblasts associated with marked thrombocytosis (RARS-T)."[3]

The first clear descriptions of ET, PV, and PMF were relatively recent; credit for priority is customarily given to Epstein and Goedel (Vienna, 1934) for ET, Vaquez (Paris, 1892) for PV, and Heuck (Heidelberg, 1879) for PMF.[4] Since 1960, CML has been defined by the presence of the Philadelphia chromosome, t(9;22)(q34q11).[5] In the 1980s, the aberrant *BCR-ABL* translocation—the molecular equivalent of the Philadelphia chromosome—was found to be diagnostic of CML and sufficient to cause the disease in a mouse model. Today, CML is the most well-defined and molecularly characterized of Dameshek's original MPD group.[6] The current chapter considers the three *BCR-ABL*-negative classic MPNs (ie, ET, PV, and PMF).

Essential Thrombocythemia

Epidemiology

ET is an uncommon disorder; estimates of its age- and gender-adjusted incidence range widely, from 0.2 to 2.5 cases per 100,000 persons per year.[7-9] Among

Table 118-1 ■ Clinical Properties of Platelet-Lowering Agents Used in Chronic Myeloproliferative Disorders

	Drug (Class)				
	Hydroxyurea (Myelosuppressive)	Anagrelide (Platelet Specific)	Interferon-α2a (Myelosuppressive)	Phosphorus 32 (Myelosuppressive)	Pipobroman (Myelosuppressive)
Mechanism of action	Antimetabolite	Unknown	Biologic agent with immunomodulatory actions	Radionucleide	Alkylating agent
Pharmacology	Half-life 5 h, renal excretion	Half-life ≈ 1.5 h, renal excretion	Kidney is main site of metabolism	Half life ≈ 14 d	Insufficient information
Suggested starting dose	500 mg PO bid	0.5 mg PO tid	3 million units SC 3 times per week (peginterferon can be given weekly)	2.3 mCi/m^2 IV	1 mg/kg/d PO (comes in 25 mg tablets) ≈ 16 d
Onset of action	≈3-5 d	≈6-10 d	1-3 week	4-8 weeks	
Frequent side effects	Leukopenia, oral ulcers, anemia, hyperpigmentation, nail discoloration, xerodermia	Headache, palpitations, diarrhea, fluid retention, anemia	Flu-like syndrome, fatigue, malaise, anorexia, weight loss, alopecia	Transient mild cytopenia	Nausea, abdominal pain, diarrhea
Infrequent side effects	Leg ulcers, nausea, diarrhea, alopecia, skin atrophy	Arrhythmias, lightheadedness, nausea	Confusion, depression, autoimmune thyroiditis, myalgia, arthritis	Prolonged pancytopenia in elderly patients	Leukopenia, thrombocytopenia, hemolysis
Rare side effects	Fever, cystitis platelet oscillations	Cardiomyopathy	Pruritus, hyperlipidemia, transaminasemia	Leukemogenic	
Absolute contraindications	Pregnancy	Pregnancy		Pregnancy	Pregnancy
Relative contraindications		Cardiomyopathy		Young age	
Cost[a]	Annual ≈ $1,752 for 500 mg tid dose	Annual ≈ $10,512 for 0.5 mg qid dose	Annual ≈ $7,488 for 3 million units 3 day/week	Approximately $1025 for 4 mCi	Not available in USA

Abbreviations: bid, twice daily; IV, intravenously; PO, orally; qid, 4 times daily; SC, subcutaneously; tid, 3 times daily.

[a]Approximate cost to patient for brand name drug purchased from a typical hospital pharmacy (except for phosphorus 32).

younger people (ages 30-50), the disease appears to be more common in women, but this gender imbalance is not as clearly found in other age groups. No clear environmental risk factor has been identified. The incidence of ET (and also of PV and PMF) appears to be increased among Ashkenazi Jews.[10] The median age at diagnosis for all three MPN is approximately 60 years. Familial clustering of ET has been described but is exquisitely rare; some familial cases are associated with mutations in the thrombopoietin (*TPO*) gene that result in increased Tpo production (a megakaryocyte growth factor) with consequent megakaryocyte hyperstimulation.[11,12]

Diagnosis

The chief clinical challenge with respect to ET diagnosis is differentiating genuine autonomous thrombocytosis from the myriad causes of "secondary" or "reactive" thrombocytosis (RT). In more than 80% of routine cases of thrombocytosis, the elevated platelet count is polyclonal and represents a reaction to the presence of a nonmyeloid disorder.[13,14] The thrombocytosis associated with inflammatory, infectious, and malignant conditions is thought to be due to the action of megakaryocyte stimulatory cytokines such as interleukin-6 (IL-6), whereas the peculiar thrombocytosis seen occasionally in iron-deficient states remains poorly understood and may be mediated by erythropoietin (Epo) cross-stimulation of precursor cells committed to platelet production.[15]

The distinction between ET and RT is clinically important because there is an increased risk of thrombosis and bleeding associated with ET, but the risk with RT appears to be much lower.[13] If the presence of RT is not obvious, serum ferritin and C-reactive protein (CRP—a surrogate marker for IL-6 levels) may be diagnostically useful in excluding iron deficiency and inflammation, respectively.[15] Elevated CRP levels suggest RT and should prompt a more thorough search for an obscure source of reactive cytokines. Of course, an elevated CRP does not strictly rule out ET, for a patient may potentially have ET and a co-morbid inflammatory condition, but this is uncommon.[15] Ferritin levels must also be interpreted with caution: although a low value is consistent with iron deficiency, and a high value suggests RT, neither definitively excludes ET.

Surgical hyposplenism is usually obvious from a patient's history, but functional hyposplenism due to amyloidosis, celiac sprue, or another cause may not be so blatant.[16] Therefore, examination of a blood smear, searching specifically for Howell–Jolly bodies, should be made during the initial evaluation of each patient with chronic thrombocytosis.

Once these steps have been taken and there is no evidence for RT or hyposplenism, ET increases in likelihood. However, another diagnostic hurdle remains: it is important to distinguish ET from other myeloid disorders that may have a very different prognosis and require different therapy. Clonal ET look-alike disorders include some cases of MDS, CML, and the other two non-ET classic MPN (ie, PV and PMF, including the potentially confusing "cellular phase" of PMF). If conventional cytogenetic analysis in a suspected ET patient does not reveal a Philadelphia chromosome, it is prudent to obtain peripheral blood or bone marrow fluorescent in situ hybridization (FISH) studies at least once to exclude the possibility of karyotypically occult CML.

Distinguishing ET from PMF is usually not difficult, but there can be exceptions. Mild (grade 1 or 2) reticulin fibrosis can be found in approximately 15% of ET cases.[17] However, the cellular phase of PMF, characterized by marrow hypercellularity with florid atypical megakaryocytic hyperplasia but not heavy fibrosis, can mimic ET in presentation.[18] Abnormal megakaryocyte clusters on the bone marrow biopsy are characteristic of all three *BCR-ABL*-negative PMF (Fig. 118-1). Cytogenetic abnormalities are present in fewer than 10% of patients at diagnosis.[19]

Pathogenesis

As mentioned above, clonal myeloproliferation involving the megakaryocytic lineage and sometimes other myeloid lineages (even in cases where the white count and hematocrit are normal) is demonstrable in the majority of female patients with ET via X chromosome–linked DNA or gene product analysis.[20,21]

In 2005, a *JAK2* gain-of-function mutation (*JAK2*V617F) has been described in the majority of patients with ET as well as those in PMF and PV.[23-26] A much smaller proportion of patients with ET (approximately 5%) carry a *MPL* mutation.[27-30] However, the precise pathogenetic contribution of these mutations is not clear.

In ET, megakaryocyte proliferation and platelet production are apparently autonomous, and normal regulatory pathways are apparently defective. The mechanism remains obscure in most cases. Megakaryocytes from ET patients are not inhibited by antibodies against key growth and differentiation cytokines, including IL-3, IL-6, granulocyte-monocyte colony-stimulating factor (GM-CSF), and Tpo.[31,32] Tpo and its receptor, c-Mpl, comprise the major feedback loop controlling megakaryocyte growth and development, but Tpo and c-Mpl dynamics in ET and related disorders appear to be complex. Tpo levels are often normal or elevated in ET despite the increased megakaryocyte mass, but are not reproducibly different among normal marrow and ET or RT cases, while c-Mpl expression is often (but not always) markedly downregulated in ET (Fig. 118-2). However,

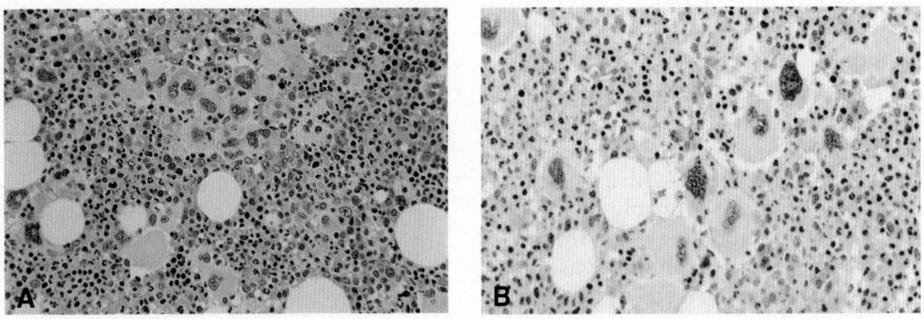

Figure 118-1 (**A, B**) Bone marrow megakaryocytic clusters in essential thrombocythemia. *Source*: From Ref. 22.

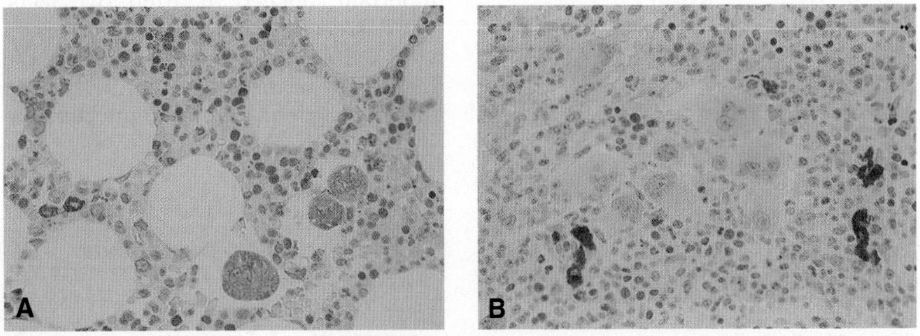

Figure 118-2 (**A**) Normal megakaryocyte c-Mpl immunohistochemical staining and (**B**) decreased megakaryocyte c-Mpl staining in a myeloproliferative disorder. *Source*: From Ref. 37.

c-Mpl expression is also down-regulated in other MPNs, so its diagnostic utility for ET is limited.[33,34] The specific cytokines driving megakaryocyte proliferation in ET have not been worked out in detail, but megakaryocyte progenitors from ET patients may display unexplained hypersensitivity to both IL-3 and Tpo.[35,36]

Clinical Manifestations

At least half of the patients with ET are asymptomatic at presentation; with appropriate therapy many can remain asymptomatic throughout the course of their illness and enjoy a normal life expectancy.[37,38] At presentation, microvascular and vasomotor symptoms are found in 25-50% of ET patients. Major thrombosis is seen in 11-25% of patients at diagnosis and 10-22% during follow-up, while major hemorrhage is observed in 2-5% at diagnosis and 1-7% during follow-up.[9,38-40] Bleeding complications can be exacerbated by the use of aspirin (ASA) and nonsteroidal anti-inflammatory drugs (NSAIDs), which have platelet inhibitory effects. In contrast to other MPN, where splenomegaly is very common, less than 25% of ET patients have palpable splenomegaly at the time of initial presentation.[37]

Vasomotor disturbances (eg, headaches, lightheadedness, visual symptoms such as blurring and scotomata, palpitations, chest pain, erythromelalgia, and distal paresthesias) are troublesome but not generally life threatening. The proximate cause of such symptoms remains poorly defined; speculation has focused on abnormal platelet-endothelium interactions in the microvasculature, which can be associated with inflammation and transient thrombotic occlusion.[41] Various platelet products such as thromboxane A2 are vasoactive, and some of these probably also play a role in the pathobiology. Erythromelalgia is the most dramatic vasomotor symptom, characterized by erythema, warmth, and pain in distal extremities; this symptom is rare but not entirely specific for ET (Fig. 118-3).[42] The presence of vasomotor microvessel disturbances does not clearly predict hemorrhage or thrombosis in large vessels.

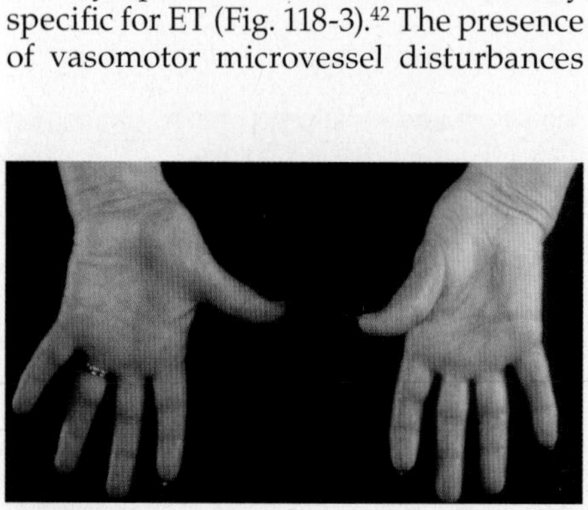

Figure 118-3 Erythromelalgia. Dramatic acral erythema associated with pain and warmth and easily relieved by aspirin. *Source*: From Ref. 22.

There are several potentially life-threatening complications of ET: large-vessel thrombosis (both arterial and venous), hemorrhage, and transformation of the disease into either a fibrotic phase resembling PMF or acute myeloid leukemia (AML). Arterial thrombosis can lead to cerebrovascular events, cardiovascular ischemia, organ infarction, and digital gangrene. Venous thrombosis in ET occurs not only in sites common to other thrombotic diatheses (eg, pulmonary embolism and lower extremity deep venous thrombosis) but also in more unusual sites (eg, cerebral sinus thrombosis, retinal vein thrombosis, and hepatic and portal vein thrombosis).[38]

Mucocutaneous bleeding (epistaxis, gingival bleeding, ecchymoses, and petechiae) can be a major nuisance. This is the most common hemorrhagic problem in ET.[43] Because epistaxis and easy bruising are very common in the general public, it can be difficult to assess the contribution of ET to these symptoms in afflicted patients. If careful control of the platelet count controls the mucocutaneous symptoms, it is reasonable to assume that thrombocytosis was contributory. Serious hemorrhage in ET is most common in the gastrointestinal tract and may be precipitated by ASA or NSAID use.[44] Hemorrhage also occurs in the central nervous system (CNS) and the retina, but such events are fortunately uncommon. Paradoxically, patients with extreme thrombocytosis may be at special risk for bleeding, in part related to the development of an acquired von Willebrand factor (vWF) deficiency that is thought to be related to platelet adsorption of large multimers of vWF. This phenomenon can be seen with extreme thrombocytosis of any cause.[45]

Fibrotic and leukemic evolution of ET are rare events (<5% of patients) during the first 10 years after diagnosis.[37,38]

Prognosis and Therapy

When considering therapy for ET, it is important to keep in mind two facts: (1) ET is generally an indolent disorder, with a life expectancy (at least in the first decade of the disease) quite close to that of an age- and gender-matched control population, and (2) no treatment to date has been shown to influence overall survival.[37,46] Therefore, the maxim primum non nocere should not be forgotten. Therapy for ET is usually initiated to palliate microvascular symptoms or to prevent thrombotic or hemorrhagic complications. Vasomotor disturbances in ET can often be relieved with low dose ASA; 81 mg per day is usually enough. When ASA does not alleviate these symptoms, it is reasonable to add a platelet-lowering agent (Table 118-1) and this is often successful.

Table 118-2 Risk Stratification in Polycythemia Vera and Essential Thrombocythemia

Low risk	Age below 60 years *and* No history of thrombosis *and* Platelet count below 1 million/μL
Indeterminate risk	Age below 60 years *and* No history of thrombosis *and* Platelet count above 1 million/μL
High risk	Age 60 years or older *or* A positive history of thrombosis

There are only a few randomized trials assessing the most appropriate therapy for diminishing the thrombotic risk in patients with ET, so clinical decisions must usually be based on prospective cohort studies and large retrospective analyses. Therapy should be guided by an individualized assessment of thrombotic risk. Two clinical parameters appear to be quite important in making this judgment: a history of thrombosis and age above 60 years.[40,47] Based on the presence or absence of these two risk factors, patients with ET have been grouped into low-risk, high-risk, and indeterminate-risk groups and therapeutic decisions are made accordingly (Tables 118-2 and 118-3).[48] This classification will need to be refined as more data on thrombotic risk become available, but it is useful to guide management at present. The presence or allele burden of *JAK2V617F* has limited relevance in ET prognosis.

The use of ASA (81-325 mg/day) to decrease thrombotic risk in all classes of patients with ET seems reasonable in view of the recently demonstrated antithrombotic benefit in PV,[49] especially if there are other compelling indications for its use (eg, coexisting cardiovascular disease).[50] The more common approach for high-risk ET patients is to try to lower

Table 118-3 Proposed Risk-Adjusted Therapy in Essential Thrombocythemia

Risk Category[a]	Cytoreductive Therapy	Aspirin Therapy	Childbearing Potential[b]
Low	No	Yes	ASA
High	Yes	Yes	Interferon-α + ASA
Indeterminate	Sometimes	Yes (unless aVWD)	ASA (unless acquired VWD)

[a]See Table 118-2 for algorithm regarding risk category assignment.
[b]Suggestions for drug therapy in women of childbearing potential are based on anecdotal evidence of safety.
Abbreviations: ASA, acetylsalicylic acid (low-dose aspirin); aVWD, acquired von Willebrand's disease.

the platelet count into the normal range. One important randomized trial demonstrated a 20% absolute risk reduction (24-3.6%) in thrombotic events with the use of hydroxyurea (HU) in ET patients in a high-risk group.[51] Other cytoreductive agents have not yet been shown in a randomized fashion to reduce thrombotic events. It is not clear precisely how low the goal platelet count should be in the high-risk group—thrombotic events can happen even with a platelet count in the normal range—but <400,000/μL seems to be a reasonable target and is supported by retrospective data.[52,53] For low-risk and indeterminate-risk patients, it is not clear that platelet-lowering agents are of any benefit, as thrombotic events are much less common in this group.

Table 118-1 summarizes information regarding currently used platelet-lowering agents in CMPD. HU should be the first choice in ET because of the high-quality evidence supporting its use. There has been concern about the leukemogenicity of HU, but in two recent studies of HU-treated patients with ET, no cases of leukemia were reported after 5-14 and 2-12 years of therapy.[54,55] It is reasonable to substitute anagrelide or pipobroman (where available) for patients intolerant to HU.[56,57] Interferon-α2A (IFNα) and, more recently, longer-acting pegylated forms of interferon provide therapeutic alternatives, but interferon's well-known toxicity limits use, especially since many high-risk ET patients are elderly and have a difficult time tolerating the necessary doses.[58-60] IFNα is the drug of choice for ET patients requiring cytoreduction during pregnancy (see below).

Major bleeding (ie, enough blood loss to drop hemoglobin level or cause bleeding in a critical organ, like the CNS) occurs in less than 10% of ET patients.[37,38] Extreme thrombocytosis (eg, platelet count >1 million/μL) appears to be a risk factor for bleeding, in part because of the acquired von Willebrand factor deficiency described above. Therapy designed to lower the platelet count and indirectly raise vWF levels may be indicated in the presence of a substantial reduction in large vWF multimers. In an emergency situation, platelet apheresis is the fastest way to lower the platelet count, but its utility has not been proven conclusively.

Special Considerations

Pregnancy in ET is associated with increased risk (approximately 35%) of first trimester spontaneous abortions.[61] There does not appear to be a postpartum thrombosis risk.[62] There is no clear association between the increased risk of spontaneous abortion and the degree of thrombocytosis, nor is there any clear benefit from prophylactic platelet apheresis.[61] High-risk pregnant women with ET (ie, women with previous thrombosis) require cytoreductive therapy just like other high-risk patients. There is anecdotal evidence of the safety of IFNα in pregnancy, but no controlled data. HU and pipobroman are considered teratogenic (FDA pregnancy class D) and anagrelide also crosses the placenta and has unknown effects on the developing fetus (FDA pregnancy class C). The teratogenicity of HU, however, does not appear to be severe enough to justify elective abortion in cases of inadvertent early fetal exposure.[63]

Primary Myelofibrosis

Epidemiology

Among the three classic MPN, PMF is the most aggressive. Fortunately, PMF is a rare scourge; the incidence is only 0.4-1.5 cases per 100,000 persons per year, with a median age at diagnosis above 60 years and a slight male predominance.[7,8] PMF has been associated with exposure to ionizing radiation (eg, in Hiroshima survivors), heavy exposure to petroleum derivatives, and thorium dioxide (Thorotrast) contrast medium, but in the vast majority of cases there is no such exposure history.[64,65]

Pathogenesis

As with other MPN, myeloid-derived cells in PMF have been shown to be monoclonal by analysis of X-linked genes and gene products.[66] In contrast, the marrow fibroblasts in PMF are polyclonal.[66,67] The florid bone marrow stromal reaction that is so characteristic of PMF includes fibroblast hyperproliferation, a dramatic increase in extracellular matrix proteins such as collagen (mostly type I and type III), increased blood vessel formation (angiogenesis), and increased bone synthesis and osteoblast activity (osteosclerosis).[68,69] Such marrow microenvironmental changes are mediated by a cytokine storm elaborated by the clonal myeloid cells. Indeed, increased cellular and extracellular levels of multiple cytokines with fibrogenic, angiogenic, and/or osteogenic potential have been detected in PMF, lending support to this hypothesis.[70]

There are several murine models in which marrow fibrosis and/or extramedullary hematopoiesis have been observed. Mice forced to overexpress TPO develop marrow fibrosis and osteosclerosis, which may be due to hypersecretion of osteoprotegerin, an osteoclast inhibiting factor.[71,72] Mice that underexpress the transcription factor *GATA-1*, which is important in the development and differentiation of hematopoietic cells, suffer impaired megakaryocyte differentiation and diminished platelet production and eventually develop extramedullary hematopoiesis and marrow fibrosis.[73] However, it is not clear to what extent these germline mouse mutants are faithful models of the neoplastic disorder in humans, where any mutations would be expected to be restricted to hematopoietic cells. Mutations or expression changes in TPO or its receptor (c-Mpl) or *GATA-1* have not been found in human PMF, and mutations in FOG-1, the major GATA-1 co-factor, are also generally absent.[74]

The molecular lesions underlying PMF are beginning to become apparent. Most notable is the 2005 report of a *JAK2* gain-of-function mutation (*JAK2*V617F) that was discovered in the majority of patients with PMF, ET, and PV.[23-26] In 2006 and 2007, other *JAK2* (in PV) and *MPL* (in ET and PMF) mutations were described in *JAK2*V617F-negative cases.[27-30] However, the precise pathogenetic contribution of these mutations is not clear. Recurrent karyotypic abnormalities seen in PMF include del(13q), del(20q), trisomy 8, trisomy 9, del(12p), and abnormalities of chromosomes 1 and 7; all of which are found in other chronic myeloid disorders and have no specificity for PMF.[75] About half of the patients with PMF have a cytogenetic abnormality at diagnosis, but there is no predominant lesion and no individual cytogenetic abnormality that affect more than 15-20% of patients.

Diagnosis

Characteristic features of PMF include a hypercellular marrow with fibrosis; extramedullary hematopoiesis (EMH), which is most often manifest as splenomegaly; anemia; and a so-called myelophthisic peripheral blood picture.[70] Marrow fibrosis and a myelophthisic blood picture alone are not diagnostic of PMF, as myelofibrosis is associated with a diverse litany of conditions, including metastatic cancer, other hematologic disorders, and rheumatologic and granulomatous diseases (Table 118-4). Myelophthisic peripheral blood findings include marked anisocytosis, poikilocytosis, teardrop-shaped red cells (dacryocytes), and left-shifted granulocytopoiesis (Fig. 118-4). The mechanism is unclear. Even EMH is not completely specific for PMF, as it can be observed in other conditions where the bone marrow is replaced (eg, metastatic cancer) or marrow hematopoiesis is inadequate (eg, β-thalassemia).[76,77]

Table 118-4 ■ **Causes of Bone Marrow Fibrosis**

Myeloid Disorders	Nonhematologic Disorders	Other Hematologic Disorders
Myelofibrosis with myeloid metaplasia	Metastatic cancer	Hairy cell leukemia
Chronic myeloid leukemia	Connective tissue disorders (eg, lupus and systemic sclerosis)	Multiple myeloma
Essential thrombocythemia	Infections (eg, granulomatous disease, tuberculosis, kala-azar)	Lymphoproliferative disorders
Atypical chronic myeloid disorders	Vitamin D deficiency (rickets)	Gray platelet syndrome
Hypereosinophilic syndromes	Renal osteodystrophy	
Polycythemia vera	Paget's disease	
Myelodysplastic syndrome with fibrosis	Hyperparathyroidism	
Malignant histiocytosis		
Systemic mastocytosis		
Acute myelofibrosis		
Acute megakaryoblastic leukemia (AML-M7)		
Other acute myeloid leukemias		

Because of hypercellularity and fibrosis, the bone marrow in PMF is often difficult to aspirate, resulting in a dry tap. Core marrow biopsy usually shows heavy collagen fibrosis, osteosclerosis, intra-sinusoidal hematopoiesis, and atypical megakaryocyte hyperplasia (Fig. 118-5). Marrow fibrosis can be difficult to assess on standard hematoxylin and eosin stains, and may be better estimated by the use of special stains, such as that for reticulin (a silver impregnation technique that stains a glycoprotein elaborated by stromal cells) or the trichrome stain for collagen. In some cases of PMF, the degree of bone marrow fibrosis may initially be minimal. This finding is often called the "cellular phase" of PMF and can be diagnostically challenging. Fibrosis grading schemes have been developed but are of relatively limited clinical utility.[78]

The bone marrow morphologic features of PMF may sometimes be difficult to distinguish from those of MDS with fibrosis (MDS-*f*) and so-called "acute myelofibrosis." The latter entity has substantial overlap with megakaryocytic acute leukemia (AML-M7).[78] Megakaryocytes alone often appear dysplastic in routine cases of PMF, but significant dysplasia in other cell lines favors a diagnosis of MDS-*f*.[78] Acute myelofibrosis (also known as malignant myelosclerosis or acute myelosclerosis) is suggested when constitutional symptoms are prominent, development of the illness is rapid (ie, over the course of a few weeks), and the spleen is not palpable. Special stains for megakaryoblasts (eg, CD61 or von Willebrand Factor) may reveal the presence of an otherwise unrecognized cell population. Sometimes, despite the best efforts of clinicians and pathologists, the diagnosis is simply not clear and patients must be treated expectantly.

■ Clinical Manifestations

About 25% of patients with PMF are asymptomatic at diagnosis. Most patients have anemia and at least some degree of splenomegaly at presentation. The anemia of PMF is multifactorial. Contributing problems include replacement of normal hematopoietic tissue with fibrosis, ineffective hematopoiesis in the remaining myeloid tissue, and hypersplenism. Splenomegaly in PMF may be massive, and the spleen is usually very firm (Fig. 118-6). Spleen and liver enlargement in PMF is secondary to EMH and may be associated with hypercatabolic symptoms (profound fatigue, weight loss, night sweats, low-grade fever), peripheral edema (from venous compression), diarrhea, early satiety (from gastric compression), and, occasionally, portal hypertension.

Splenomegaly in PMF may be complicated by infarction, an event heralded by moderate to severe pain that may be referred to the left shoulder and often requires opiate analgesics to control.[79] CT imaging in such cases can be unremarkable, or may show wedge-shaped or rounded low-attenuation lesions in the spleen. EMH occurs in a great diversity of sites throughout the body. Common sites besides spleen and liver include lymph nodes, skin, pleura, peritoneum, lung, and the paraspinal and epidural spaces. The latter may result in spinal cord and/or nerve root compression, which is a medical emergency requiring corticosteroids to reduce edema and immediate radiotherapy.[80] It is fortunate that localized EMH responds promptly to low doses of gamma irradiation (100-150 cGy).

Red cell transfusion dependence in PMF is widespread. Serum levels of LDH are often elevated, reflecting both ineffective hematopoiesis and injury to the liver by EMH. Hyperuricemia and consequent episodes of gout are not uncommon and reflect ineffective hematopoiesis with high cell turnover. Bone pain is seen and is multifactorial, related to mar-

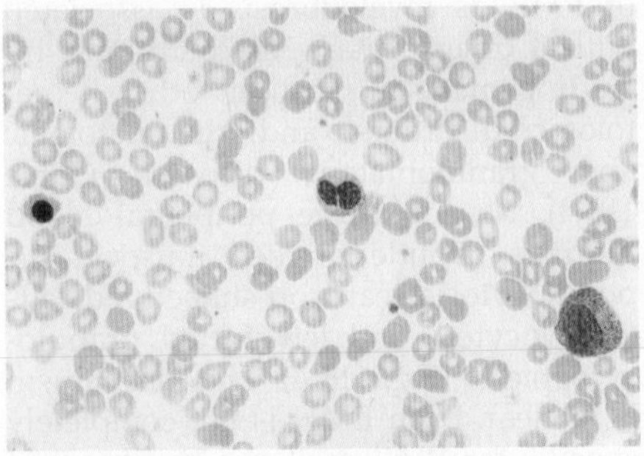

Figure 118-4 ■ Typical peripheral blood findings in myelofibrosis with myeloid metaplasia: erythrocyte poikilocytosis, dacryocytes, a nucleated red blood cell, and an immature myeloid precursor cell (myelocyte).

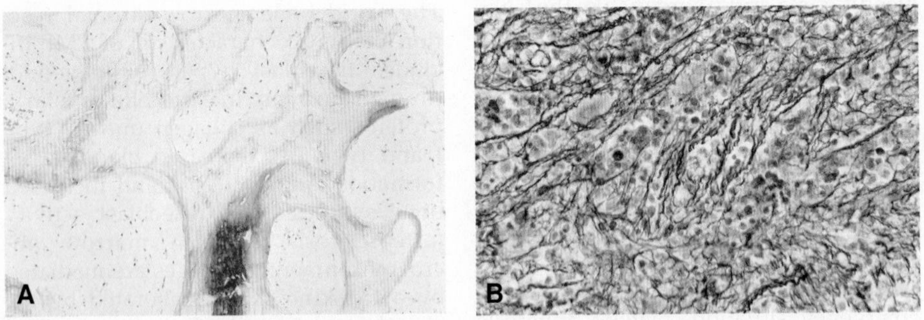

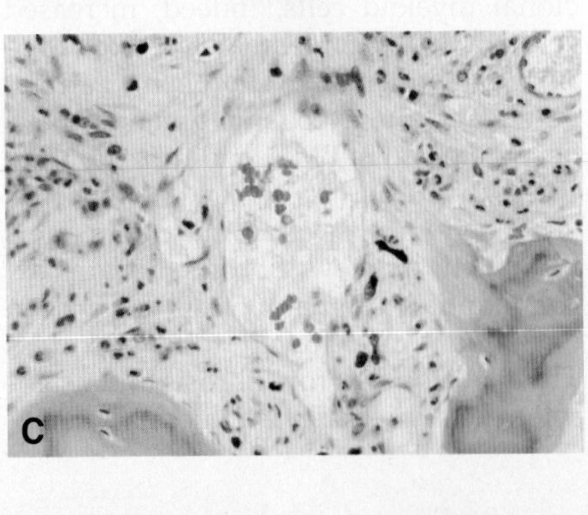

Figure 118-5 ■ Bone marrow biopsy findings in myelofibrosis with myeloid metaplasia, demonstrating osteosclerosis and reduced hematopoietic progenitors (**A**) reticulin fibrosis (**B**) and intrasinusoidal hematopoiesis (**C**). *Source:* From Ref. 70.

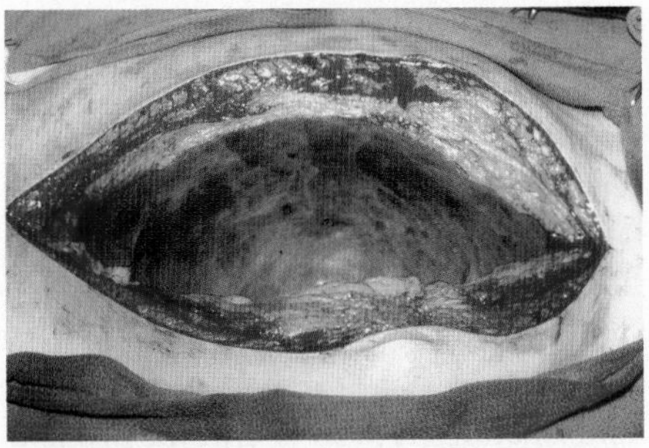

Figure 118-6 Splenomegaly in myelofibrosis with myeloid metaplasia is a result of extramedullary hematopoiesis and can be massive. *Source*: From Ref. 70.

row replacement and periostitis. Sweet syndrome (neutrophilic dermatosis) is sometimes associated with PMF, and this lesion must be distinguished from cutaneous extramedullary hematopoiesis since treatment differs.[81]

Death in PMF can come from many directions. Fatal infection and transformation to a resistant myeloid leukemia are common. Overt leukemia occurs in approximately 20% of patients over the first 10 years.[82] Less frequent causes of death include thrombohemorrhagic events and heart failure, often secondary to pulmonary hypertension.

Prognosis

Survival in PMF is substantially affected by the presence or absence of risk factors that have been used to construct several prognostic scoring systems (PSS).[83-86] The most recent PSS was developed at the Mayo Clinic and four adverse prognostic features were considered: a platelet count of $<100 \times 10^9$/L, hemoglobin level of <10 g/dL, leukocyte count of <4 or $>30 \times 10^9$/L, and an absolute monocyte count of $>1 \times 10^9$/L. In the absence of any of these four poor prognostic indicators (low-risk category), median survival in patients younger than 60 years of age was 14.4 years as opposed to 5 years in the intermediate-risk category (presence of one adverse feature) and 2.2 years in the high-risk category (presence of two or more adverse features). In addition to the aforementioned, circulating immature granulocytes of ≥10%,[87] circulating blast count of ≥3%,[85] advanced age,[85,88,89] male sex,[85] and cytogenetic abnormalities either in the bone marrow[90-92] or splenic tissue[93] have also been identified as adverse prognostic features in some studies. In terms of cytogenetics, the presence of solitary abnormalities involving either 13q- or 20q- were associated with significantly better prognosis compared to all other abnormalities.[92] Of note, the degree of either splenomegaly or bone marrow fibrosis did not appear to affect the overall survival.[83,84,87,90]

Therapy

Conventional therapy for PMF is largely palliative and has not been shown to improve survival. Patients should be considered for clinical trials of new treatments whenever feasible. Older treatments for anemia include androgen preparations (eg, oral fluoxymesterone 10 mg 2 times a day or danazol 400-600 mg per day), which, given the older age of the typical male PMF patient, should be initiated only after ruling out occult prostate cancer.[94] Corticosteroids may also give transient benefit in this setting (eg, oral prednisone at a starting dose of 30-40 mg/day for one month, and then taper off over the second month). Unfortunately, responses to androgens and steroids are uncommon; they occur in less than one-third of PMF patients and are usually of brief duration. In the case of an endogenous Epo level that is less than 100 mIU/mL, it is tempting to consider a brief trial of treatment with erythropoiesis stimulating agents (ESAs).[95] However, such therapy exacerbates PMF-associated splenomegaly, does not work for transfusion-dependent patients, and may be associated with increased risk of leukemic transformation.[96] For symptomatic splenomegaly in PMF, HU is the first choice.[97] An initial dose of 500 mg of HU 3 times per day typically brings salutary results within 1-2 weeks, and the dose can then be adjusted to optimal effect.

Thalidomide can improve cytopenias and reduce spleen size in PMF.[98] Reported response rates range between 20-62% for anemia, 25-80% for thrombocytopenia, and 7-30% for splenomegaly.[98,99] In conventional doses similar to those used for multiple myeloma (eg, 200 mg/day and above), thalidomide has been associated with severe myeloproliferative reactions, including accelerated extramedullary hematopoiesis.[100] Lower doses of thalidomide (eg, 50 mg/day) appear to be better tolerated and responses are often durable.[99,101] The addition of prednisone to the lower dose schedule improves tolerance and may enhance the erythropoietic activity of the drug.[99,101]

Splenectomy can be considered for patients with refractory splenic pain, disabling constitutional symptoms, symptomatic portal hypertension, and/or a need for frequent red cell transfusions. In one series of 223 PMF patients who underwent splenectomy, durable remissions in constitutional symptoms, transfusion-dependent anemia, portal hypertension, and severe thrombocytopenia were achieved in 67%, 23%, 50%, and 0% of patients, respectively.[102] However, even in experienced centers the perioperative mortality rate of splenectomy in PMF may be as high as 9%, and overall survival may not be affected; the median post-splenectomy survival is about 2 years.[102] An elevated D-dimer, even in the absence of overt disseminated intravascular coagulopathy, may predict a higher surgical risk. Up to 25% of surgical survivors will develop marked hepatomegaly or extreme thrombocytosis.[102] Pre-splenectomy thrombocytopenia correlates with the risk of post-splenectomy leukemic transformation, for unclear reasons. Extreme post-splenectomy thrombocytosis is significantly associated with perioperative thrombosis. HU can be used perioperatively to prevent a post-splenectomy rise in platelet count. In poor surgical candidates with symptomatic splenomegaly, the palliative use of splenic irradiation is reasonable, but success is irregular and of brief duration.[103]

The use of allogeneic hematopoietic stem cell transplantation (allo-SCT) in PMF was initially limited because of concerns regarding potential failure of stem cells to engraft in the fibrotic marrow. This concern has not been substantiated. Marrow fibrosis delays post-transplantation platelet recovery by about 3 days and increases platelet transfusion needs slightly, but is not clearly associated with graft failure or other unique transplant-related problems.[104] Interest in allo-SCT in patients with PMF is now growing, but appropriate patient selection and timing remain challenging. While engraftment has not been especially problematic, toxicity continues to be a major issue, even with the newer reduced-intensity "nonmyeloablative" conditioning regimens.[105] In one study of allo-SCT in myelofibrosis, the 5-year survival was only 14% for patients older than 44 years, and in another study the 2-year survival was just 41%.[106,107] Rates of chronic graft vs host disease of up to 59% have been reported.[108] Younger patients do somewhat better, with post-transplant survival rates of up to 60%, but the decision to proceed to transplant must only be made after careful deliberation, and patients chosen should be those with particularly limited life expectancy.[106,108]

Polycythemia Vera

Epidemiology

The incidence of PV is 0.8-2.6 cases per 100,000 persons per year, with most studies giving figures at the upper end of that range, and this incidence appears to be relatively stable over time.[109,110] As is the case with the other MPN, the incidence of PV increases with age. The median age at diagnosis is approximately 60 years; the disease can also be seen in young people, and 7% of cases are diagnosed before the age of 40.[111,112] There may be a slight male preponderance (on the order of a 1.2:1 male-to-female case ratio) and the disease is more common in Jews, especially Ashkenazi Jews.[10,113] In a few cases, true PV may be familial, but apparently familial erythrocytosis is often proven to be a result of a shared high–oxygen-affinity hemoglobin or a common exposure (eg, a residence at high altitude or cobalt intoxication).[114,115]

Pathogenesis

X-linked (G6PD) enzyme analysis first demonstrated the clonal nature of hematopoietic cells in PV in 1976.[116] In 2005, a *JAK2* gain-of-function mutation (*JAK2*V617F) that was discovered in the majority of patients with PV.[23-26] In 2007, other *JAK2* mutations were described in *JAK2*V617F-negative cases.[29] *JAK2*V617F is an exon 14 G to T somatic mutation. The nucleotide change at position 1849 results in the substitution of valine to phenylalanine at codon 617. *JAK2*V617F is also present in patients with PV, ET, and PMF.[23-26] The mutation has also been described in other myeloid neoplasms.[117,118] As of the time of this writing, JAK2V617F has not been reported in lymphoid disorders,[119-122] solid tumor,[123-125] or secondary myeloproliferation.[126,127] In general, mutational frequency is estimated at over 95% in PV, 50% in ET or PMF, 20% in certain other MPNs including refractory anemia with ringed sideroblasts and thrombocytosis (RARS-T), and less than 5% in AML or MDS.[128-131]

*JAK2*V617F induces a PV-like phenotype in murine transplant models.[25,132,133] Mutant allele burden in patients with ET is significantly lower than that seen in patients with either PV or PMF.[134-138] At least in PV, a higher allele burden is the result of *JAK2*V617F homozygosity, which is accomplished by mitotic recombination.[23,26,139] In humans, *JAK2*V617F occurs at a primitive stem cell level and is chronologically an early event.[140-142] Some, but not all,[143] studies have suggested *JAK2*V617F clonal involvement of NK,[144] T,[145] and B[145] lymphocytes. Regardless, there is evidence to suggest that *JAK2*V617F may not be the initial clonogenic event in either PV or other MPNs and that its presence might not be mandatory for endogenous colony formation.[146-148] The recent demonstration of *JAK2*V617F-negative leukemia clones arising in *JAK2*V617F-positive MPN patients lends further support in this regard.[149,150]

In 2007, a set of *JAK2* exon 12 mutations were described in *JAK2*V617F-negative patients with PV in whom erythrocytosis was the predominant feature.[151] Because of the latter feature, some of the cases were assigned the diagnosis of "idiopathic" erythrocytosis, although their serum Epo level was almost always below the reference range and EECs were demonstrated in every instance when tested. The majority of the cases (10 of 11) in the original report[151] were found to harbor one of four exon 12 *JAK2* mutant alleles: N542-E543del (4 cases), F537-K539delinsL (3 cases), K539L (2 cases), H538QK539L (1 case). All four exon 12 mutant alleles induced cytokine-independent/hypersensitive proliferation in erythropoietin receptor-expressing cell lines and constitutive activation of JAK-STAT signaling.[151] In addition, *JAK2*K539L induced a PV phenotype in a mouse transplant model. Many other studies have now confirmed the observations from the above-mentioned study[29,152-156] and in the process, most[29,152,153] but not all[154,156] of the studies suggested that exon 12 mutations occurred in virtually all *JAK2*V617F-negative PV cases (ie, approximately 3% of all PV cases). Furthermore, several other exon 12 mutation variants were added to the list including R541–E543delinsK, I540–E543delinsMK, V536-I546dup11, F537-I546dup10+547L, and E543-D544del.[153-155]

The erythroid colony-forming progenitor cells (BFU-E and CFU-E) in PV are very sensitive to or independent of normal growth and differentiation signals, including Epo, GM-CSF, stem cell factor, and IL-3.[157,158] Although this finding is characteristic of PV, it is not specific and is also observed in ET and PMF. Serum Epo levels in PV patients are generally very low or inappropriately normal in the setting of erythrocytosis, and excessive Epo-independent BFU-E and CFU-E proliferation leads to an increased red cell mass (RCM).[159,160] As is the case with the Tpo receptor in ET, some families with recurrent PV have been found to harbor Epo receptor mutations, but structural changes in the Epo receptor have been diligently sought in nonfamilial PV but not found.[161,162] Epo receptor expression patterns may be abnormal in PV (eg, loss of the normal high-affinity Epo receptor) but this finding is not consistent.[163] Cells from patient with PV are consistently observed for hypersensitive to insulin-like growth factor-1 (IGF-1), which appears to be due to alterations in IGF-1 binding proteins, including increased baseline phosphorylation of the IGF-1 receptor.[164] Decreased activity of the SHP-1 phosphatase (which associates with the receptors for Epo, stem cell factor, and IL-3, and is a negative regulator of signals generated during ligand binding), constitutive activation of STAT-3, increased levels of antiapoptotic proteins such as Bcl-XL, and several other biochemical abnormalities have been reported in subsets of patients; their general pathobiologic relevance is yet unclear.[165-167]

Karyotypic abnormalities are found in about 10-20% of untreated patients.[168,169] The lesions seen are those nonspecific abnormalities typical of chronic myeloid disorders, such as trisomy 8, trisomy 9, del(20q), del(13q), loss of the Y chromosome in men, and abnormalities of chromosomes 5 and 7.[169]

Clinical Features

Signs and symptoms frequently associated with PV are listed in Table 118-5. Many of the clinical features of PV are a direct consequence of the increased RCM and are common to all causes of erythrocytosis, but pruritus and splenomegaly strongly suggest PV. Increased RCM can lead to blood hyperviscosity, which leads to a plethora of symptoms and signs. Headaches are frequent, but blurry vision, altered hearing, mucous membrane bleeding, shortness of breath, and malaise are also observed. Hypertension may be a consequence of increased RCM. At least two-thirds of PV patients have splenomegaly, so the combination of splenomegaly and erythrocytosis should strongly suggest PV.[170] Thrombosis occurs in about 40% of patients, most commonly arterial thrombosis.[111] Clots occur at a rate of about 3.9% of patients per year.[113] Arterial thromboses are more likely to be fatal than venous thromboses. As in ET, venous thrombosis can occur in unusual sites, such as mesenteric or hepatic vessels. Bleeding, especially gastrointestinal, is seen in PV but less often than thrombosis.[111] Pruritus is a common and

Table 118-5 Polycythemia Vera–Related Clinical and Laboratory Features

Symptoms and Physical Findings	Frequency, %
Systolic hypertension	72
Splenomegaly	70
Skin plethora ("ruddy cyanosis")	67
Conjunctival plethora	59
Headache	48
Weakness	47
Engorged retinal veins	46
Pruritus	43
Dizziness	43
Palpable liver	40
Sweating	33
Diastolic hypertension	32
Visual disturbances	31
Weight loss	29
Paresthesias	29
Dyspnea	26
Joint symptoms	26
Epigastric distress	24

Source: Adapted from Ref. 170.

classic PV-associated complaint, may be provoked by warm water ("aquagenic"); its pathogenesis is unclear.[171,172] Erythromelalgia (described above under ET) might also trouble patients with PV, as do other vasomotor symptoms; paresthesias and headaches. Leukocytosis and thrombocytosis are present in less than half of PV patients.

Diagnosis

The major diagnostic difficulty with respect to PV is distinguishing PV from the many other causes of erythrocytosis (Table 118-6).

The 1975 Polycythemia Vera Study Group diagnostic criteria[170] were an advancement in their time, but are now chiefly of historical interest.[173,174] These criteria included the direct measurement of the RCM, which is a cumbersome procedure that is no longer strictly necessary in most cases. The availability of new diagnostic tools, as well as better appreciation of the tight relationship between hematocrit and RCM, have undermined the use of RCM measurement in the diagnosis of PV.

Because more than 95% of patients with PV carry the *JAK2*V617F mutation, one could initiate the workup of a patient with suspected PV with peripheral blood mutation screening for *JAK2*V617F. In order to minimize the consequences of false positive or false negative test results, as well as capture the few cases that are *JAK2*V617F-negative PV, I recommend concomitant measurement of serum Epo level, which is abnormally low in more than 90% of patients with PV.[175] If the results of both tests are suggestive of PV (ie, mutation-positive and low serum Epo), then the diagnosis is likely and bone marrow examination is encouraged but not essential for making the diagnosis. If the *JAK2*V617F and serum Epo test results are both not consistent with the diagnosis of PV (ie, mutation-negative and either normal or increased Epo), then further investigation is not advised unless dictated otherwise by the clinical scenario. If there is discrepancy between the molecular test and serum Epo level, one should first repeat both tests and then proceed with bone marrow examination, provided the results are unchanged. In this regard, the possibility of exon 12 *JAK2* mutations should be entertained in *JAK2*V617F-negative cases with low serum Epo level.

When congenital polycythemia is suspected, initial laboratory testing should include measurement of the oxygen tension at which hemoglobin is 50% saturated (p50). Left-shifted oxygen dissociation curve, suggested by decreased p50, suggests the presence of either high oxygen-affinity hemoglobinopathy (autosomal dominant)[176] or 2,3-bisphosphoglycerate (2,3-BPG) deficiency, usually a consequence of BPG mutase mutation (autosomal recessive).[177] If the p50 is normal, then the possibility of *VHL* mutations should be considered first because they constitute the most frequent mutations in congenital polycythemia. In this regard, Russian ethnic origin would suggest Chuvash polycythemia, which is characterized by increased serum Epo.[178] However, Chuvash-type or other *VHL* mutations have also been described in other ethnic groups and therefore worth considering in the presence of any congenital polycythemia associated with increased serum Epo. There is currently limited information on *HIF-1α* prolyl hydroxylase gene mutation,[179] which incidentally is associated with normal serum Epo level. On the other hand, *EPOR* mutations are well described and should be considered in congenital polycythemia associated with either low or normal serum Epo level.[180]

Table 118-6 Classification of Erythrocytosis

Apparent Polycythemia
Relative polycythemia due to major fluid shifts
Extreme "high normal" values
True Polycythemia
Polycythemia vera
Secondary polycythemia
Erythropoietin (EPO)-mediated
Hypoxia-driven
Central hypoxic process
Chronic lung disease
Right-to-left cardiopulmonary vascular shunts
High-altitude habitat
Carbon monoxide poisoning and smoker's polycythemia
Hypoventilation syndromes including sleep apnea
Peripheral hypoxic process
Localized
Renal artery stenosis
Diffuse
High-oxygen-affinity hemoglobinopathy (congenital; autosomal-dominant)
2,3-Diphosphoglycerate mutase deficiency (congenital; autosomal-recessive)
Hypoxia-independent (pathologic EPO production)
Malignant tumors
Hepatocellular carcinoma
Renal cell cancer
Cerebellar hemangioblastoma
Parathyroid carcinoma
Nonmalignant conditions
Uterine leiomyomas
Renal cysts (polycystic kidney disease)
Pheochromocytoma
Meningioma
Abnormally elevated set point for EPO production (congenital)
Chuvash polycythemia (congenital; abnormal oxygen homeostasis?)
Intentional EPO doping
EPO receptor-mediated
Activating mutation of the erythropoietin receptor
Some cases of autosomal-dominant congenital polycythemia
Drug-associated
Treatment with androgen preparations
Treatment with novel erythropoietic agents such as CERA
Unknown mechanisms
Most cases of autosomal-dominant congenital polycythemia
Some forms of autosomal-recessive congenital polycythemia
Post-renal transplant erythrocytosis

Abbreviation: CERA, continuous erythropoiesis receptor activator.

Prognosis

The median life expectancy for patients diagnosed with PV exceeds 10 years but is worse than a gender- and age-matched control population.[46] Thrombohemorrhagic complications and transformation into AML account for much of the inferior survival.[181] As with ET, older age (>60 years) appears to be a risk factor for thrombosis.[182] Other clearly prognostic factors in PV beyond old age and a history of thrombosis have not been determined. In about 15% to 20% of cases, PV terminates in a "spent phase," a PMF-like state. This transition is usually characterized by worsening anemia and increasing white count and spleen size.

Treatment

As is the case with ET, PV-associated vasomotor symptoms are usually alleviated by low doses of ASA. PV-associated pruritus can be treated with selective serotonin reuptake inhibitors, such as paroxetine.[171] Antihistamines such as hydroxyzine and diphenhydramine are less effective.

The primary goal of treatment in PV is to prevent disastrous thrombotic events without increasing the risk of other life-threatening problems, such as bleeding, or altering the potential for transformation to a fibrotic marrow or acute leukemia. The main tool used to accomplish this goal is therapeutic phlebotomy. The importance of regular phlebotomy as part of a successful treatment program for PV cannot be overemphasized; marrow-suppressing drugs play only a supplementary role. In the first few decades after the disease's description, before aggressive phlebotomy became de rigueur, the median survival for patients with PV was on the order of 2 years, and most deaths were due to thrombotic events.[183,184] Today, most PV-related deaths are still due to thrombosis, but patients treated initially with phlebotomy alone have a median survival of more than 15 years.[111]

Based on studies that have shown an improved cerebral blood flow and normalization of blood viscosity with a hematocrit below 45%, as well as less thrombosis in patients with hematocrits in this range, dropping the hematocrit to below this level and keeping it there should be the goal of phlebotomy-based treatment in PV.[185,186] It has also been widely recommended that females be reduced to a hematocrit of less than 42% because their normal hemoglobin range is lower, but this has not been rigorously tested and whole blood viscosity should not depend significantly on gender.

There has been a long-standing interest in the addition of other therapies to try to further decrease thrombotic risk. When these other agents should be added to phlebotomy is controversial. An elevated platelet count does not appear to be a major thrombotic risk factor in PV, and a very elevated platelet count (eg, >1 million/μL), as in ET, is a risk factor for bleeding in PV.[187] Therefore, young PV patients without a history of thrombosis and with a near-normal platelet count are probably quite safe with phlebotomy alone.

In view of a recent large randomized placebo-controlled study that showed a large reduction in thrombotic events (but not an overall survival improvement) with low-dose aspirin (100 mg/day—a dose not available in the United States) aspirin, all patients with PV who do not have a contraindication should receive aspirin.[49] In this trial the combined endpoint of nonfatal myocardial infarction, nonfatal stroke, or death from cardiovascular causes and the risk of the combined end point of nonfatal myocardial infarction, nonfatal stroke, pulmonary embolism, major venous thrombosis, or death from cardiovascular causes were both reduced (relative risk 0.41 and 0.40 compared with placebo, respectively). The risk of bleeding at this dose was elevated slightly above those treated with placebo (relative risk 1.6).[49]

There has been interest in myelosuppressive agents in PV for several decades, and opinion about the optimal regimen continues to evolve. In a landmark three-arm randomized study that originated in the 1960s, two specific agents, oral chlorambucil and intravenous radioactive phosphorus (^{32}P) were each found to decrease the risk of thrombosis when added to phlebotomy.[181] However, overall survival was inferior with either of the additional treatments because of an increased incidence of acute leukemia compared with phlebotomy alone. The incidence of acute leukemia over 13-19 years was 1.5%, 9.6%, and 13.2% for phlebotomy, ^{32}P, and chlorambucil, respectively, and the corresponding median survivals were 12.6, 9.1, and 10.9 years.[181] Several cases of lymphoma were seen in patients treated with chlorambucil, and the incidence of gastrointestinal and skin cancer was also increased.

Other agents have the potential to decrease thrombosis without the same degree of leukemia risk as ^{32}P or alkylators. One of these agents is HU, which decreases thrombotic risk when used as a supplement to phlebotomy, but which appears less leukemogenic than chlorambucil and ^{32}P. In one PVSG study, HU was associated with lower risk of thrombosis in the first 2 years after diagnosis (6.6% vs 14%) when compared to a historical cohort of patients treated with phlebotomy alone, and only 5.9% of patients had transformed to acute leukemia after a median follow-up of 8.6 years.[188] Because the true leukemogenic risk of HU is unknown, it is used most often as a supplement to phlebotomy for groups at especially high risk for thrombosis, such as the elderly and those with prior thrombosis (Table 118-7). Alternatives to HU include pipobroman, which is not available in the US, and busulfan.

IFNα2A has salutary effects in PV and is the drug of choice for PV patients who wish to become pregnant, because of anecdotal reports of successful maternal and fetal outcomes. This drug controls erythrocytosis in approximately 80% of the patients who can tolerate the necessary dose, which ranges from 4.5 to 27 mil-lion units per week (the usual starting dose is 3 million units subcutaneously 3 times per week), and IFNα2A has a beneficial effect on thrombocytosis.[58,189,190] IFN can also reduce spleen size and frequently gives relief from intractable pruritus. However, at least 20% of patients discontinue therapy because of drug side effects, including fatigue, malaise, fevers, psychological effects, myalgias, and arthralgias.[190] IFNα2A is also more expensive than HU. In addition to women of childbearing potential, it is reasonable to choose IFNα2A for high-risk patients who need a supplement to phlebotomy where the potential benefit of relief from refractory pruritus is desired, or for patients who are particularly concerned about the potential leukemogenicity of HU.

Table 118-7 **Suggested Treatment Algorithm for Patients With Polycythemia Vera**

Risk Category[a]	Age <60 Years	Age ≥60 Years	Women of Childbearing Age
Low	Phlebotomy + ASA	Not applicable	Phlebotomy + ASA
Indeterminate	Phlebotomy + ASA if no aVWD	Not applicable	Phlebotomy + ASA if no aVWD
High	Phlebotomy + ASA + HU or IFNα	Phlebotomy + HU + ASA	Phlebotomy + ASA + IFNα

[a]See Table 118-2 for risk stratification algorithm.
Abbreviations: ASA, acetylsalicylic acid (low-dose aspirin; if no contraindications); HU, hydroxyurea; IFNα, Interferonα2A; aVWD, acquired von Willebrand disease

Selected References

The complete reference list can be found at www.CANCERMEDICINE8.com

2. Tefferi A, Vardiman JW. Classification and diagnosis of myeloproliferative neoplasms: the 2008 World Health Organization criteria and point-of-care diagnostic algorithms. *Leukemia*. 2008;22:14–22.
7. Mesa RA, Silverstein MN, Jacobsen SJ, Wollan PC, Tefferi A. Population-based incidence and survival figures in essential thrombocythemia and agnogenic myeloid metaplasia: An Olmsted County study, 1976–1995. *Am J Hematol*. 1999;61:10–15.
8. Kutti J, Ridell B. Epidemiology of the myeloproliferative disorders: essential thrombocythaemia, polycythaemia vera and idiopathic myelofibrosis. *Pathol Biol (Paris)*. 2001;49:164–166.
9. Jensen MK, de Nully Brown P, Nielsen OJ, Hasselbalch HC. Incidence, clinical features and outcome of essential thrombocythaemia in a well defined geographical area. *Eur J Haematol*. 2000;65:132–139.
10. Chaiter Y, Brenner B, Aghai E, Tatarsky I. High incidence of myeloproliferative disorders in Ashkenazi Jews in northern Israel. *Leuk Lymphoma*. 1992;7:251–255.
11. Kondo T, Okabe M, Sanada M, et al. Familial essential thrombocythemia associated with one-base deletion in the 5′-untranslated region of the thrombopoietin gene. *Blood*. 1998;92:1091–1096.
18. Dickstein JI, Vardiman JW. Hematopathologic findings in the myeloproliferative disorders. *Semin Oncol*. 1995;22:355–373.
19. Steensma DP, Tefferi A. Cytogenetic and molecular genetic aspects of essential thrombocythemia. *Acta Haematol*. 2002;108:55–65.
20. Elkassar N, Hetet G, Briere J, Grandchamp B. Clonality analysis of hematopoiesis in essential thrombocythemia—advantages of studying T lymphocytes and platelets. *Blood*. 1997;89:128–134.
21. Fialkow PJ, Faguet GB, Jacobson RJ, Vaidya K, Murphy S. Evidence that essential thrombocythemia is a clonal disorder with origin in a multipotent stem cell. *Blood*. 1981;58:916–919.
22. Tefferi A. Thrombocytosis. In: Michelson A, ed. *Platelets*. London: Academic Press; 2003.
23. Baxter EJ, Scott LM, Campbell PJ, et al. Acquired mutation of the tyrosine kinase JAK2 in human myeloproliferative disorders. *Lancet*. 2005;365:1054–1061.
24. Kralovics R, Passamonti F, Buser AS, et al. A gain-of-function mutation of JAK2 in myeloproliferative disorders. *N Engl J Med*. 2005;352:1779–1790.
30. Scott LM, Tong W, Levine RL, et al. JAK2 exon 12 mutations in polycythemia vera and idiopathic erythrocytosis. *N Engl J Med*. 2007;356:459–468.

31. Li Y, Hetet G, Maurer AM, Chait Y, Dhermy D, Briere J. Spontaneous megakaryocyte colony formation in myeloproliferative disorders is not neutralizable by antibodies against IL3, IL6 and GM-CSF. *Br J Haematol.* 1994;87:471–476.
32. Taksin AL, Couedic JPL, Dusanter-Fourt I, et al. Autonomous megakaryocyte growth in essential thrombocythemia and idiopathic myelofibrosis is not related to a c-mpl mutation or to an autocrine stimulation by Mpl-L. *Blood.* 1999;93:125–139.
39. Besses C, Cervantes F, Pereira A, et al. Major vascular complications in essential thrombocythemia: a study of the predictive factors in a series of 148 patients. *Leukemia.* 1999;13:150–154.
40. Cortelazzo S, Viero P, Finazzi G, A DE, Rodeghiero F, Barbui T. Incidence and risk factors for thrombotic complications in a historical cohort of 100 patients with essential thrombocythemia. *J Clin Oncol.* 1990;8:556–562.
41. Michiels JJ, Abels J, Steketee J, van Vliet HH, Vuzevski VD. Erythromelalgia caused by platelet-mediated arteriolar inflammation and thrombosis in thrombocythemia. *Ann Intern Med.* 1985;102:466–471.
42. van Genderen PJ, Michiels JJ. Erythromelalgia: a pathognomonic microvascular thrombotic complication in essential thrombocythemia and polycythemia vera. [Review] [23 refs]. *Semin Thromb Hemost.* 1997;23:357–363.
43. Randi ML, Stocco F, Rossi C, Tison T, Girolami A. Thrombosis and hemorrhage in thrombocytosis: evaluation of a large cohort of patients (357 cases). *J Med.* 1991;22:213–223.
49. Landolfi R, Marchioli R, Kutti J, et al. Efficacy and safety of low-dose aspirin in polycythemia vera. *N Engl J Med.* 2004;350:114–124.
50. van Genderen PJ, Mulder PG, Waleboer M, van de Moesdijk D, Michiels JJ. Prevention and treatment of thrombotic complications in essential thrombocythaemia: efficacy and safety of aspirin. *Br J Haematol.* 1997;97:179–184.
57. Mazzucconi MG, Francesconi M, Chistolini A, et al. Pipobroman therapy of essential thrombocythemia. *Scand J Haematol.* 1986;37:306–309.
58. Elliott MA, Tefferi A. Interferon-alpha therapy in polycythemia vera and essential thrombocythemia. *Semin Thromb Hemost.* 1997;23:463.
88. Strasser-Weippl K, Steurer M, Kees M, et al. Age and hemoglobin level emerge as most important clinical prognostic parameters in patients with osteomyelofibrosis: introduction of a simplified prognostic score. *Leuk Lymphoma.* 2006;47:441–450.
89. Kvasnicka HM, Thiele J, Werden C, Zankovich R, Diehl V, Fischer R. Prognostic factors in idiopathic (primary) osteomyelofibrosis. *Cancer.* 1997;80:708–719.
90. Reilly JT, Snowden JA, Spearing RL, et al. Cytogenetic abnormalities and their prognostic significance in idiopathic myelofibrosis: a study of 106 cases. *Br J Haematol.* 1997;98:96–102.
91. Tefferi A, Mesa RA, Schroeder G, Hanson CA, Li CY, Dewald GW. Cytogenetic findings and their clinical relevance in myelofibrosis with myeloid metaplasia. *Br J Haematol.* 2001;113:763–771.
92. Tefferi A, Dingli D, Li CY, Dewald GW. Prognostic diversity among cytogenetic abnormalities in myelofibrosis with myeloid metaplasia. *Cancer.* 2005;104:1656–1660.
93. Mesa RA, Li CY, Schroeder G, Tefferi A. Clinical correlates of splenic histopathology and splenic karyotype in myelofibrosis with myeloid metaplasia. *Blood.* 2001;97:3665–3667.
94. Levy V, Bourgarit A, Delmer A, et al. Treatment of agnogenic myeloid metaplasia with danazol: a report of four cases. *Am J Hematol.* 1996;53:239–241.
95. Rodriguez JN, Martino ML, Dieguez JC, Prados D. rHuEpo for the treatment of anemia in myelofibrosis with myeloid metaplasia. Experience in 6 patients and meta-analytical approach. *Haematologica.* 1998;83:616–621.
109. Ania BJ, Suman VJ, Sobell JL, Codd MB, Silverstein MN, Melton LJ, 3rd. Trends in the incidence of polycythemia vera among Olmsted County, Minnesota residents, 1935-1989. *Am J Hematol.* 1994;47:89–93.
110. Najean Y, Rain JD, Billotey C. Epidemiological data in polycythaemia vera: a study of 842 cases. *Hematol Cell Ther.* 1998;40:159–165.
111. Anonymous. Polycythemia vera: the natural history of 1213 patients followed for 20 years. Gruppo Italiano Studio Policitemia. *Annals of Internal Medicine.* 1995;123:656–664.
119. Melzner I, Weniger MA, Menz CK, Moller P. Absence of the JAK2 V617F activating mutation in classical Hodgkin lymphoma and primary mediastinal B-cell lymphoma. *Leukemia.* 2006;20:157–158.
120. Lee JW, Soung YH, Kim SY, et al. JAK2 V617F mutation is uncommon in non-Hodgkin lymphomas. *Leuk Lymphoma.* 2006;47:313–314.
121. Sulong S, Case M, Minto L, Wilkins B, Hall A, Irving J. The V617F mutation in Jak2 is not found in childhood acute lymphoblastic leukaemia. *Br J Haematol.* 2005;130:964–965.
122. Levine RL, Loriaux M, Huntly BJ, et al. The JAK2V617F activating mutation occurs in chronic myelomonocytic leukemia and acute myeloid leukemia, but not in acute lymphoblastic leukemia or chronic lymphocytic leukemia. *Blood.* 2005;106:3377–3379.
128. Steensma DP, McClure RF, Karp JE, et al. JAK2 V617F is a rare finding in de novo acute myeloid leukemia, but STAT3 activation is common and remains unexplained. *Leukemia.* 2006;20:971–978.
129. Renneville A, Quesnel B, Charpentier A, et al. High occurrence of JAK2 V617 mutation in refractory anemia with ringed sideroblasts associated with marked thrombocytosis. *Leukemia.* 2006;20:2067–2070.
130. Verstovsek S, Silver RT, Cross NC, Tefferi A. JAK2V617F mutational frequency in polycythemia vera: 100%, >90%, less? *Leukemia.* 2006;20:2067.
142. Delhommeau F, Dupont S, Tonetti C, et al. Evidence that the JAK2 G1849T (V617F) mutation occurs in a lymphomyeloid progenitor in polycythemia vera and idiopathic myelofibrosis. *Blood.* 2007;109:71–77.
143. Lasho TL, Mesa R, Gilliland DG, Tefferi A. Mutation studies in CD3+, CD19+ and CD34+ cell fractions in myeloproliferative disorders with homozygous JAK2(V617F) in granulocytes. *Br J Haematol.* 2005;130:797–799.
150. Campbell PJ, Baxter EJ, Beer PA, et al. Mutation of JAK2 in the myeloproliferative disorders: timing, clonality studies, cytogenetic associations, and role in leukemic transformation. *Blood.* 2006;108:3548–3555.
151. Scott LM, Tong W, Levine R, et al. Somatic mutations of JAK2 exon 12 in polycythemia vera and idiopathic erythrocytosis. *NEJM.* 2007;in press.
157. Casadevall N, Vainchenker W, Lacombe C, et al. Erythroid progenitors in polycythemia vera: demonstration of their hypersensitivity to erythropoietin using serum free cultures. *Blood.* 1982;59:447–451.
158. Dai CH, Krantz SB, Dessypris EN, Means RT, Jr., Horn ST, Gilbert HS. Polycythemia vera. II. Hypersensitivity of bone marrow erythroid, granulocyte-macrophage, and megakaryocyte progenitor cells to interleukin-3 and granulocyte-macrophage colony-stimulating factor. *Blood.* 1992;80:891–899.

119 Neoplasms in Acquired Immunodeficiency Syndrome

Jeremy S. Abramson, MD ■ David T. Scadden, MD

Immunodeficiency of multiple etiologies is associated with an increased risk of malignancy, particularly lymphoma. The risk is variable, dependent on the severity and extent of the immunologic abnormality. In the setting of the acquired immunodeficiency syndrome (AIDS) secondary to human immunodeficiency virus type 1 (HIV-1) infection, the range of tumor types is more extensive. Yet, the tumors are generally associated with oncogenic viruses and may be considered secondary, opportunistic neoplasms. Etiologic factors contributing to them include poor control of oncogenic viruses, altered cytokine regulation owing to HIV effects on immune cells and tissue stimulation from other AIDS-associated events. The interplay of immunity, infection and oncogenesis is central to AIDS-related malignancies.[1]

The spectrum of the tumor types seen in the context of immunodeficiency extends beyond that of lymphoma, but is quite limited. There appears to be little interaction between the conditions that predispose to the emergence of epithelial malignancies seen in the general population and immunodeficiency. Rather, immunodeficiency tumors represent a narrow subset of neoplasms, some of which are seen with only very low incidence in the general population. For example, primary central nervous system (PCNS) lymphoma and Kaposi sarcomas (KS) are extremely rare entities in all but the immunodeficient population, where they compose a large proportion of tumors. In addition, the incidence of specific tumor types varies according to the immunodeficient state. Non-Hodgkin lymphoma (NHL) is a common theme among all of the immunodeficiencies, yet in AIDS there is a broader spectrum of histologic subtypes than are seen in other immunodeficient states. KS is increased in subgroups of patients with HIV-related and pharmacologically induced immunodeficiency. Cutaneous tumors are common in many immunodeficient states, but the increase in squamous cell tumors of the skin is higher in the post solid-organ-transplantation population than in those with HIV-related immunodeficiency. In the latter, papillomavirus-related squamous cell neoplasia of the anogenital region predominates (Table 119-1).

Shared among the tumors related to immunodeficient states is the frequent association with an infectious pathogen. The presence of Epstein–Barr virus (EBV) in immunodeficiency-related lymphomas is well known and likely a result of the direct stimulation that virus provides to B-cell proliferation. In the absence of effective immunologic targeting of cells expressing EBV latency gene products, the overgrowth of cells may proceed unchecked, with the subsequent emergence of a transformed cell. This model for the direct ability of viruses to induce cell proliferation is a paradigm that may be applied to human papilloma virus (HPV)-related tumors as well. However, the model is less easily applied to the Kaposi sarcoma-associated herpesvirus/human herpes virus-8 (KSHV/HHV8)-related tumors. The tumors associated with KSHV/HHV8 are more varied and are of less clear pathophysiologic relationship to viral gene products-issues that are discussed in greater depth in sections that follow. In general, the tumors that do emerge in immunodeficiency are those in which a secondary pathogen can be implicated (Table 119-2). Immunodeficiency further leads to a failure of innate host tumor surveillance. In essence, the concept of inadequate immunologic control provides a unifying mechanism, and these tumors may be considered opportunistic malignancies, much the way in which specific infections are considered opportunistic infections. Indeed, the opportunistic malignancies of the immunocompromised patient represent the overlap between infectious diseases and oncology and provide unique insight into the intersection of immune function and tumor development.

Table 119-1 ■ Tumor Types With Increased Incidence in HIV Disease

Definite	
	Kaposi sarcoma
	Non-Hodgkin lymphoma
	Squamous cell neoplasia
	Hodgkin lymphoma
	Leiomyosarcoma (in children)
	Plasmacytoma
Possible	
	Seminoma
	Skin cancers
	Lung cancer
	Osopharyngeal cancer
	Prostate cancer

Table 119-2 ■ Secondary Virus Infections Associated With AIDS-Related Malignancies

Virus	Tumor
EBV	NHL (PCNS; most systemic DLBCL; PBL; oropharyngeal T cell);
	HL
	Leiomyosarcoma (children)
KSHV/HHV8	KS
	NHL (PEL)
HPV	Squamous cell neoplasia

Abbreviations: ARL, AIDS-related lymphoma; EBV, Epstein-Barr virus HL, Hodgkin lymphoma; HPV, human papillomavirus; KS, Kaposi sarcoma; KSHV, Kaposi sarcoma herpesvirus; NHL, non-Hodgkin lymphoma; PCNS, primary central nervous system; PBL, plasmablastic lymphoma; PEL, primary effusion lymphoma; DLBCL, diffuse large B-cell lymphoma.

Epidemiology

The spectrum of tumors in the context of HIV-1 infection varies on the basis of risk group and is substantially affected by the use of potent or highly active antiretroviral therapy (HAART).

Pre-HAART

The use of HAART is largely restricted to the developed world and did not become available until 1996, with the introduction of the protease-inhibitor class of anti-HIV medications. Widespread use of protease inhibitors occurred rapidly in the United States, Western Europe, and Australia, altering the death rate and complication rate of HIV disease. The spectrum of opportunistic diseases also changed,[2] with an impact on malignant disease, discussed below in the section "Post-HAART." Given the lack of access to HAART in much of the developing world, the unclear durability of HAART efficacy, and the number of patients unable to take or having failed HAART, the profile of AIDS-related malignancies in the pre-HAART era is still of considerable importance.

One of the first manifestations of the AIDS epidemic was the cluster of cases of a rare malignancy among men who have sex with men in the coastal cities of United States. That tumor, KS, was identified as an AIDS-defining illness with the first attempt at classifying the immunodeficiency syndrome by the Centers for Disease Control and Prevention (CDC).[3] The prevalence of KS among HIV infected patients was approximately 20% early in the AIDS epidemic, but clearly was noted to be highest among patients whose risk factor for HIV transmission was men having sex with men.[4] KS prevalence was substantially lower in the groups infected by blood products or through parenteral drug use.[5] Subsequent behavioral studies indicated that specific types of sexual practice, including promiscuity and oral–fecal contact,[6] had the highest risk and substantiated the impression that KS might be a manifestation of a secondary, transmissible pathogen. Indeed, it was strong epidemiologic data that galvanized efforts to identify a pathogen and that led to the molecular cloning of the KSHV, also known as HHV8.[7]

The second most common malignancy, which was recognized in 1984 to be increased among young men who have sex with men, was NHL. This disease was added to the list of AIDS-defining complications in the first revision of the CDC criteria for AIDS. It was noted that the lymphomas that occurred in this population were generally of high-grade histology and followed extremely aggressive clinical courses. Unlike KS, this complication was much more broadly based in the risk groups for HIV infection. All groups had a high relative risk, estimated to be approximately 60-fold above that of the general population.[6,8-10] Subsets of infected individuals have been noted to have somewhat greater or lesser risk, such as the hemophiliac population, in which at least one study has noted an increased risk.[6,10] Similarly, it has been noted that risk among intravenous drug users or those from the Caribbean basin may be lower, but concern about confounding issues of care and surveillance complicate that analysis. However, the potential for important cofactors of lymphomagenesis within these subsets remains, and attention to this possibility may yield important information about the process of lymphocyte transformation.

The third most common oncologic complication of HIV disease is anogenital squamous cell neoplasms. These are invariably associated with HPV infection of oncogenic serotypes.[11,12] The impact of antiretroviral therapy on these neoplasms is at present unclear, but with the improved survival of patients with HIV disease, it is considered likely that HPV-related neoplasms will become increasingly problematic.

Post-HAART

The introduction of HAART has resulted in profound and dramatic changes in the nature of HIV disease. The inexorable decline in immune function and its attendant ravaging secondary infections and tumors in many cases is stopped and indeed reversed when combination therapy with protease inhibitors is introduced. The improvement in those patients with advanced disease has led to widespread use of the agents, including among those individuals who have recently acquired HIV-1 infection. The result has been a precipitous decline in the rate of death from AIDS in populations with access to the medications. Although death and debility from AIDS has decreased dramatically, there has not been a similar decline in new cases of HIV infection. Therefore, the total population with HIV infection in the West is rising, and those infected are living longer; globally, the epidemic goes unabated. Some changes in the epidemiology of malignancies in HIV infection have been immediately evident since HAART was introduced, but the impact of longer periods of more modest immune dysfunction or even of the antiretroviral drugs themselves remains to be fully defined.

An observation immediately evident in the clinical care of patients with advanced HIV disease was the regression of KS following successful HIV suppression on HAART. The impact on new cases of KS was also rapidly noticeable, and epidemiologic data have substantiated the magnitude of those clinically apparent effects. Multiple studies from sites in the United States, Europe, and Australia indicate the widespread decline in KS, with estimates of decline in incidence as high as 80-fold.[13-15] The risk for development of KS, both pre-and post-HAART, correlates directly with the depth of CD4 count suppression,[16] though cases of KS in patients with increased CD4 counts are being increasingly reported in the post-HAART era.[17,18]

As with KS, changes in the incidence of primary CNS lymphoma are dramatic. Although this complication of advanced HIV disease was much less common than KS, and its decline was therefore less well documented, the impact in clinical terms has been comparable in magnitude. Cases are rarely seen except among those who have failed or have not been receiving antiretroviral therapy. This is a complication of severe immune suppression that, like the post-transplantation setting, is virtually uniformly associated with EBV detectable in tumor tissue. In general, the EBV latency genes expressed in these tumors are type III or those of lymphoproliferative disease (EBNA1-6, LMP1, and LMP2).[19,20] These and other features distinguish PCNS lymphoma from other AIDS-related lymphomas and may be the basis for clear differences in the impact of HAART.

The incidence of systemic AIDS-related NHL appears to be more modestly affected by the introduction of HAART and is approximately two- to threefold reduced.[21] One large study involved a cohort of 8500 HIV-positive individuals across much of Europe.[22] The incidence of all subtypes of lymphoma in this observational study was significantly reduced after the use of combination antiretroviral therapy was commonplace (March 1999), as compared with those followed prior to the introduction of potent antiretroviral therapy (September 1995). Similarly, additional international cohort studies found a reduction of approximately threefold following the introduction of HAART.[23,24] Of note, there is significant variability among lymphoma subtypes, with the greatest difference seen in immunoblastic diffuse large B-cell lymphoma and PCNS lymphoma; Burkitt lymphoma (BL) and Hodgkin lymphoma (HL) appear to be largely unaffected.[23,25] The risk for most HIV-related systemic NHL and PCNS lymphomas likewise correlates directly with decline in CD4 count, while risk for BL shows no such correlation.[16] The changes evident within only some lymphoma subsets highlights biologic differences between these tumor types and suggests differential immune participation in tumor development.

Kaposi Sarcoma (KS)

It was the announcement of clustered cases of KS in Los Angeles and New York that made headlines and first brought the AIDS epidemic to public awareness in 1981.[26] Having originally been described by the Hungarian dermatologist Moritz Kaposi in 1872,[27] KS was regarded as a tumor that generally had an indolent course in elderly men of Mediterranean extraction, but which could be problematic in the context of immunosuppressive medication for organ transplantation. It was this latter association that helped focus attention on an immune alteration spreading among sub communities in urban centers. Recognized as a common entity among HIV-positive men who have sex with men, but not among groups with other risk factors for HIV infection (such as blood product exposure),[5,25] it was long suspected as being related to a second cofactor.[28] A number of potential culprits were examined; none proved tenable until the identification of KSHV/HHV8. This virus was first recognized through the use of a genetic comparison of tissues from individuals with and without KS. A deoxyribonucleic acid (DNA) fragment was consistently noted that had partial homology with other members of the gamma-herpesvirus family.[7] This subset of the herpesviruses includes several viruses with oncogenic potential, such as EBV, associated with a number of tumors and *herpesvirus saimiri*, associated with the ability to transform T cells. Because of the company KSHV/HHV8 kept and the high frequency of detectable signature DNA sequences in KS lesions, this virus rapidly and justifiably became the focus of investigation for a pathophysiologic basis of KS.

Viral Epidemiology

KSHV/HHV8 is a 165-kilobase (kb) double-stranded DNA virus with features strongly supporting its causative role in clinical KS. There are data indicating that KSHV/HHV8 infection precedes tumor formation,[28,29] that populations with high seroprevalence for KSHV/HHV8 are also those with a high incidence of KS,[25] and that the virus infects cell types within tumors.[28]

The definition of prior exposure to KSHV/HHV8 depends on documentation of antibodies specifically reactive against the virus. There have been a number of assays that have been tested with variable results. Current data indicate seropositivity estimated at 3.5% in North America, up to 25% in the peoples of the Mediterranean basin, and up to 89% in sub-Saharan African populations.[30-32]

The much-suspected role of sexual transmission has been convincingly demonstrated in a longitudinal study of men in San Francisco over a 10-year period. Among exclusively heterosexual men, no KSHV/HHV8 seropositivity was detected; however, among men who have sex with men, the incidence of seroconversion was linearly related to the number of male sexual-intercourse contacts.[33] Men who had more than 250 sexual partners in the preceding 2 years had a seropositivity rate of 65%. Yet, sexual transmission is not the exclusive basis of virus spread. KSHV/HHV8 can be identified in saliva, and it is thought that oral transmission can rarely occur.[34] The higher incidence of KSHV/HHV8 seropositivity among family members in areas of endemic KS, and given that children are often infected in sub-Saharan Africa indicate that nonsexual means of transmission do occur, but the specific basis is still to be fully defined.

Clinical Manifestations

KS characteristically appears as pigmented macular-papular lesions on mucocutaneous surfaces (Figs. 119-1 and 119-2). It is typically violaceous or erythematous in hue and may be associated with an ecchymotic halo. Typically, the lesions are multifocal and do not have a predictable order or pace of progression. Lesions may present as solitary nodules or plaques, but may also occur in clusters or simultaneously in multiple well-segregated sites. Although classic or endemic KS often favors the lower extremities, the pattern of involvement is much less predictable in the setting of HIV infection. Virtually any mucocutaneous site may be involved. On the face, the ears and nose are often affected, resulting in profound disfigurement. In addition to the disabling cosmetic effects of KS, lesions do occasionally become thick, uncomfortable plaques and can ulcerate with possible super-infection. Lesions are not generally destructive, however. The integument or mucous membrane overlying a lesion is most often intact, and deep invasion into muscle or bone generally does not occur.

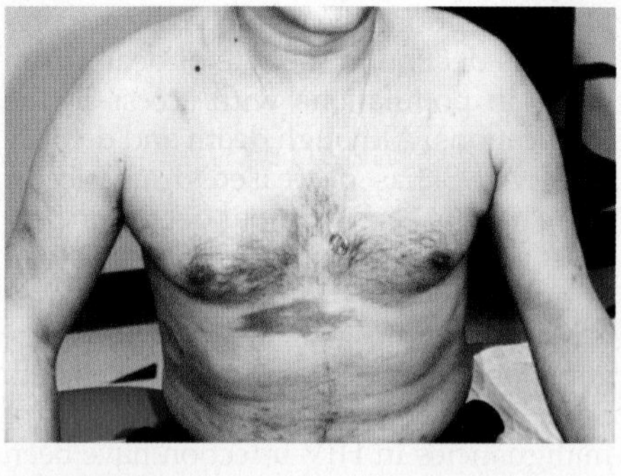

Figure 119-1 Cutaneous Kaposi sarcoma in a white patient with advanced HIV disease. The violaceous plaques on the chest are of characteristic appearance. These lesions entirely resolved on paclitaxel chemotherapy and antiretroviral medication.

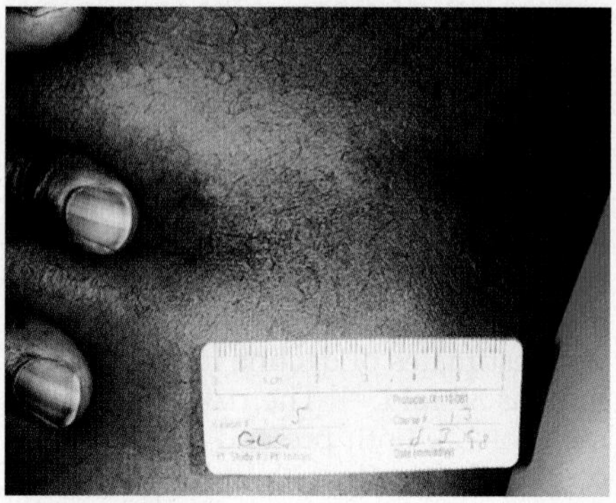

Figure 119-2 Kaposi sarcoma in an African American male with HIV-1 infection. Skin tone can make the lesions less readily distinguishable from other cutaneous processes and quite distinct from the appearance in lighter-skinned individuals.

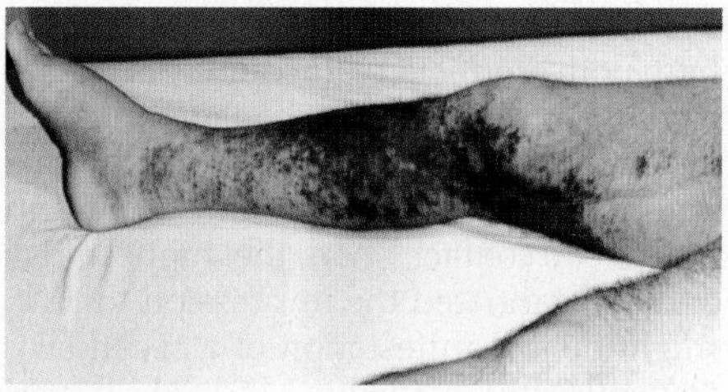

Figure 119-3 Lower extremity involvement by Kaposi sarcoma can result in marked edema and limited mobility. This patient had pedal edema that had limited response to chemotherapy despite marked improvement in the circumferential Kaposi sarcoma.

Edema often accompanies KS either locally or at a dependent site distal to KS lesions (Fig. 119-3). The edema can be marked, with profound compromise of extremity mobility or occasionally with periorbital, peripubic, or genital edema. Two mechanisms are thought to contribute to the development of edema. One is the involvement of lymphatic vessels or lymph nodes with KS, thereby causing a mechanical obstruction to lymphatic flow. The other is the elaboration of permeability factors by KS lesions. The vessels that compose a KS lesion are themselves leaky with extravasation of plasma proteins and cells into surrounding soft tissue. In addition, the vascular endothelial growth factor (VEGF) produced by KS lesions can alter the integrity of surrounding otherwise-normal vessels, increasing their permeability, and thus, their contribution of fluid to interstitial fluid. The increased demand on lymphatic drainage and the compromised egress of lymph results in thickened skin locally and frank edema distally.

Involvement of organs other than lymph nodes and skin occurs frequently. The most common site is the gastrointestinal (GI) tract, where mucosal-based lesions are commonly observed in the course of endoscopic examination. The physiologic significance of these lesions is often minimal, however. Most patients will be unaware of GI involvement, and serendipitous observation of a mucosal KS lesion should not trigger a reflex to undertake aggressive therapy. However, there are some individuals for whom GI KS can be a symptomatic and even life-threatening complication. Massive bleeding has been observed, as has intussusception.

Pulmonary involvement may take several forms. Pleural-surface studding with KS lesions can result in pleural effusions, which are often bloody, but which do not have a characteristic set of diagnostic findings or cytologic abnormalities. Bronchial mucosa may be involved and, like GI mucosal surfaces, may be incidentally noted during bronchoscopic examination. The lesions are generally not destructive, but depending on location, they may be responsible for bronchial irritation, coughing, and hemoptysis. Involvement of the parenchyma of the lung occurs and is arguably the most serious complication of KS, because it is associated with life-threatening respiratory compromise and a high mortality rate if unsatisfactorily treated.[35] Radiographically, involvement often takes the appearance of peribronchiolar cuffing on computed tomography (CT). Pathologically, this infiltration may extend into fine interstitial tissue and affect airspace function. This results in either a patchy or diffuse reticulonodular appearance on x-rays. The diagnosis of KS involvement of the lung is often difficult to firmly establish short of parenchymal thoracoscopic or open biopsy. Bronchoscopy is useful in assessing alternative infectious explanations for clinical findings and may identify mucosal lesions. However, mucosal lesions do not necessarily coincide with parenchymal infiltration, and transbronchial biopsy is often unrevealing. Nuclear medicine scans have some usefulness, with a negative gallium scan and a positive thallium scan reportedly having a high specificity for pulmonary KS.[36,37] In some circumstances, the use of a therapeutic trial may also be helpful in establishing a presumptive diagnosis. If thorough microbiologic evaluation has been unrevealing, the chemotherapeutic agents discussed below have been well tolerated and associated with high rates of response, such that their use in select patients may be justified as a test for chemotherapy responsiveness of a parehhnchymal infiltrate. Such a strategy is generally reserved for those patients in whom (1) there is a diagnosis of KS already established from involvement of other sites, (2) there are no symptoms suggesting infection, or (3) aggressive assessment for infection is negative and there are no other contraindications to cytotoxic chemotherapy.

In addition to lung, GI tract, and lymph nodes, special sites of concern are areas of the upper airway. Involvement of the mucosa of the mouth, sinuses, pharynx, and larynx can result in distortion of soft tissues such that airway compromise or alteration of food ingestion can occur. These are lesions that generally respond rapidly to therapy and do not invade deeper structures. Therapeutic approaches are discussed below in the section "Treatment."

Given the common occurrence of involvement beyond the readily apparent skin or oral mucous membranes, extensive staging evaluations are often considered. Although the bulk of tumor does influence prognosis, other characteristics of the patientís immune and general health were incorporated into a KS staging system by the AIDS Clinical Trials Group (ACTG), based on pre-HAART data on KS patients[38] (Table 119-3). In the HAART era, tumor extent and concomitant systemic illness appear to the most powerful predictors of prognosis in this model, with limited tumor involvement and lack of opportunistic infections predicting a 3-year overall survival of approximately 90%, compared to only 50% with extensive or visceral disease and presence of other HIV-related complications.[39] An alternative prognostic model has been proposed in the HAART era based on multivariate analysis in 326 AIDS-associated KS patients which identified four favorable prognostic variables by multivariate analysis: (1) having KS as the AIDS-defining illness, (2) increasing CD4 count, (3) age less than 50 years, and (4) absence of another AIDS-associated illness.[40] These variables generated risk scores predicting for 5-year overall survival ranging from 98% in the most favorable cohort, to only 8% in the least.

The staging performed at diagnosis is often based on clinical presentation, with radiographic studies limited to a chest x-ray unless symptoms dictate otherwise. Testing of stool for fecal occult blood is a reasonable screening test for gastrointestinal involvement, though specificity is poor. If localizing symptoms do suggest organ involvement, then more extensive radiographic and procedural interventions are appropriate, but they cannot be recommended routinely. Criteria for staging do include assessment of the underlying HIV infection, and all patients should have a careful history regarding medications, other complications of HIV infections, and documentation of the CD4 count in the blood.

Table 119-3 **Staging Classification for AIDS-Related Kaposi Sarcoma**

	Good Risk[a]	Poor Risk (1)[b]
Tumor (T)	Small tumor burden with limited involvement of one or more Lymph nodes Skin Other[c]	Large tumor burden Oral Gastrointestinal Pulmonary Other visceral with involvement of tumor associated edema or ulceration
Immune system (I)	CD^{4+} cells >200 mm^3	CD^{4+} cells <200 mm^3
Systematic illness (S)	No opportunistic infection (including thrush), or B symptoms[d]	History of opportunistic infection or thrush B symptoms[d] Other HIV-related illness (eg, NHL or other malig-nancy, neurologic disease, wasting syndrome)

[a] All the parameters listed.
[b] Any of the parameters listed.
[c] Limited oral disease is confined to the palate and is not nodular.
[d] B symptoms are unexplained fever, night sweats, weight loss of more than 10% of body weight, or diarrhea persisting for more than 2 weeks.

Abbreviations: HIV, human immunodeficiency virus; NHL, non-Hodgkin lymphoma.

Source: Modified from Krown SE, Metroka C, Wernz JC. Kaposi's sarcoma in the acquired immunodeficiency syndrome; a proposal for uniform evaluation, response, and staging criteria. *J Clin Oncol*. 1989;7:1201–1207.

Establishing the diagnosis of KS generally depends on simple punch biopsy of the skin or a snip biopsy of mucosal surfaces. The CDC criteria for an AIDS-defining diagnosis of KS do not require histologic confirmation if assessment is by an experienced clinician. However, biopsy is strongly recommended, given the broad differential diagnosis for nonblanching lesions resembling KS,[38] including bacillary angiomatosis (usually caused by *Bartonella* infection, with increased frequency in advanced HIV-infection patients); hematoma; purpura; sarcoid plaques; lichen planus; pyogenic granuloma[41]; mycosis fungoides; secondary syphilis; pityriasis rosea; drug-related erythema multiforme; prurigo nodularis; nevi; vascular lesions of the phakomatoses; epithelioid hemangioendothelioma; angiosarcoma; melanoma; and basal cell carcinoma.

Pathology and Pathogenesis

The histologic appearance of KS belies its unclear association with the term "sarcoma." No monomorphic array of mesenchymally derived cells is seen. Rather, the lesions are composed of endothelial cells lining ectatic vascular spaces surrounded by spindle cells of variable extent admixed with mononuclear immune cells and extravasated red blood cells. It is the red blood cells that provide the pigment to KS lesions and their breakdown that leads to the ecchymotic halo seen in actively growing lesions. The hemosiderin deposited locally yields a pigmented lesion that may remain even after effective therapy reverses the proliferative spindle and endothelial cell components. Cutaneous lesions are generally within the dermis and deep invasion to muscle is generally not seen.

The origins of the endothelial and spindle cell components remain controversial. The endothelial cells of KS lesions express the VEGF-C receptor characteristic of lymphatic endothelium[42] and do not have detectable nitric oxide synthase, generally present in vascular endothelium.[43] The finding that the spindle cell expresses the mannose-binding receptor and CD68 suggests that the origin may be a macrophage-like cell type, perhaps emanating from the sinuses of secondary lymphoid organs and circulating in the blood before ultimately assuming its role in a KS lesion.[44]

The difficulty in defining the cell of origin emanates from its complex histology and the limitations of the available in vitro or in vivo models. In vitro culture has been established for some cell types, and outgrowth of cell lines has been documented, although the relationship to the primary disease process is unclear. In vivo transplantation of KS tissue into immunodeficient mice has resulted in tumors, but these are of murine origin. The potential for cytokine elaboration driving lesion development was hypothesized, and studies have extensively characterized cytokine production by KS lesions.[45-48] The cytokines, particularly VEGF and basic fibroblast growth factor (bFGF), may play a role in the paracrine or autocrine sustenance of KS. Antibodies to bFGF block the proliferation of KS cells and prevent them from entering the S-phase of the cell cycle, even in the presence of exogenous growth factors like the interleukin (IL)-6–IL-6R complex, IL-10, tumor necrosis factor (TNF)-α, and oncostatin M.[49] But exogenous growth factors do not completely explain the phenotype and growth potential of KS cells, which overexpress the antiapoptotic *bcl-2* gene independently of any factors contained in conditioned medium from these cells.[50]

KSHV/HHV8 appears necessary for the induction of KS and is found in KS lesions regardless of whether the underlying context is HIV disease, organ transplantation, or endemic KS. However, the specific mechanism by which the virus participates in the oncogenic process is unclear and does not readily fit into paradigms established by other virus-related neoplastic disease. The latent genes implicated in EBV-induced transformation do not have homologs in KSHV/HHV8. The genes of *herpesvirus saimiri* (HVS), which are known to transform cells, have homology only in the genome of a KSHV/HHV8 gene, *K1*, that is capable of transforming an immortalized cell line.[51] However, this gene is not expressed in the latent phase of the KSHV/HHV8 life cycle. Similarly, a chemokine receptor-like KSHV/HHV8 gene product, open reading frame (ORF 74), is constitutively activated and is capable of transforming cells when transduced as a single gene; but it is also a lytic-phase gene.[52] The encoded viral G protein-coupled receptor activates multiple signaling pathways including the phosphatidylinositol-3 kinase (PI3K)/AKT, mitogen-activated protein kinase (MAPK), and Janus kinase/signal transducer and activator of transcription (JAK/STAT) pathways.[53-55] These pathways exert protean antiapoptotic and proliferative effects that promote tumorigenesis. Two other gene products, K9 (a homolog of the interferon regulatory factor family) and K12 (with no clear gene family homology), are capable of transforming cell lines when transduced but are not expressed in latent phase.[56-59] The lack of clear association with the latent phase would suggest that these gene products are not transforming in *cis*, but whether they may transform in *trans* cannot be excluded. A number of other mechanisms, including those that may be capable of acting at a distance, have been raised as possibilities for KSHV/HHV8. These include the chemokine-related gene products, vMIP-I (K6) and vMIP-II (K4), or the IL-6 homolog, K2. Each is capable of interacting with cognate receptors on target cells, either acting as agonists (K2 and K6) or antagonists (K4).[60,61] Finally, there are KSHV/HHV8 gene products that have antiapoptotic effects and that may enhance tumorigenicity. ORF 16 encodes a bcl-2–related gene product,[62] and ORF 71 (K131) encodes a functional member of the Fas-associated death domain-like IL-10–converting enzyme-inhibitory protein (FLIP) family of antiapoptotic genes.[63] The vFLIP of KSHV/HHV8 protects cells from Fas-mediated cell death and can enhance tumor progression of cell lines transplanted in vivo. KSHV/HHV8 further induces transcription of hypoxia-induced factor 1 alpha (HIF1alpha) and HIF2alpha resulting in upregulation of the proangiogenic factor, VEGF, as well as other proangiogenic and antiapoptotic factors.[64,65] VEGF and VEGF receptors are richly expressed within KS lesions and appear to play a critical role in pathogenesis.[66,67] KSHV/HHV8 has further been shown to encode a microRNA that down-regulates thrombospondin 1, a negative regulator of angiogenesis and tumor suppressor.[68] Thus, KSHV/HHV8 encodes a range of gene products with potential for altering the growth, death, and immunologic characteristics of infected cells. It is not clear which of these mechanisms will be seen to play a dominant role in oncogenesis; further investigations into the process will certainly lead to new insights into viral-induced tumors and open new avenues for therapeutic attack.

The prevalence of KS in populations, (1) that are HIV-infected, (2) that have undergone solid organ transplantation, (3) that are aged, and (4) that are of Mediterranean extraction, or live in economically disadvantaged parts of tropical Africa, suggests that expression of a KS disease phenotype requires a degree of immunosuppression. The advent of HAART for HIV infection treatment offers dramatic support to a central role for immune suppression: Complete remissions of cutaneous[69] and pulmonary KS are well recognized in the context of increases in CD4 count and declines in HIV load induced by HAART.[70] Although HIV-induced immunodeficiency is only one type of immune abnormality that may predispose to KS, the relative risk among the population co-infected with HIV and KSHV/HHV8 is strikingly high, suggesting the potential for interaction between the two viruses in the pathogenesis of tumor. The HIV gene product, *tat*, affects KSHV/HHV8 replication itself,[71] alters cytokine and cytokine receptor expression in target cells, and leads to proangiogenic effects.[72,73] Expression of *tat* may induce the lytic phase of KSHV/HHV8, resulting in increased viral transcripts, IL6 production, and stimulation of the JAK/STAT proliferation pathway, which offers a pathophysiologic rationale for the preferential occurrence of KS in HIV-infected patients vs solid-organ transplant recipients and other immunosuppressed populations.[53] Retrospective analysis of the incidence of KS among HIV-infected patients receiving antiherpesvirus medications has suggested a direct role of replicating KSHV/HHV8 in the pathologic process. In several studies, there was a decreased incidence of KS in patients treated with ganciclovir[74-76] or foscarnet.[77] In one such treatment program, it was shown that those patients who received systemic ganciclovir had a lower incidence of KS compared with those in whom the drug was delivered by intraocular implant.[74] Therefore, suppression of replicating virus appears to lower the risk of KS. Although transformation is generally associated with the latent phase of herpesvirus infection, control of the lytic phase (the only time at which the anti-herpesvirus medications have known activity) may limit the potential for transformation.

Control of virus by immunologic means also appears to be highly relevant to the risk of developing KS. It has long been known that there is an increased risk of KS in the context of multiple types of immunologic deficiency. The recent definition of epitopes of the virus that are recognized by cytotoxic T lymphocytes will allow for further definition of this important point and potentially lead to vaccine strategies.

Treatment

Treatment of KS should be guided by the impact of the tumor on the patient. The goals of treating this disease are to palliate symptoms, alleviate organ compromise, reduce edema, and improve quality of life in affected patients. The variability in the course of HIV-infected patients with KS and the lack of clear association of tumor control with mortality suggests that aggressive therapy may not always be an appropriate response to the diagnosis of KS. This is particularly true among patients with advanced HIV disease or untreated HIV disease. In that setting, the toxicity of cytotoxic therapy may be daunting, and the potential therapeutic effect of anti-HIV medications is considerable. Suppressing HIV replication is associated with a rise in CD4 count, with attendant improvement in immunologic function, and also reduction in whatever the direct contribution of HIV to the pathophysiology of KS might be. The net result is a high frequency of clinical improvement among patients with established KS and, occasionally, complete eradication, simply by the introduction of antiretroviral therapy. Therefore, for patients in whom the impact of KS is not organ threatening or profoundly symptomatic, a therapeutic trial of antiretroviral therapy alone is appropriate first-line therapy (Fig. 119-4). In patients with highly symptomatic or organ-threatening disease, a more aggressive approach is warranted, concurrent with antiretroviral therapy. Though anti-HIV therapy is an important component in the treatment of HIV-related KS, it should be recognized that not all patients will experience an improvement in their KS with antiretroviral therapy, and that improvement, when it occurs, may only be noted only after 4-8 weeks of therapy. If the patients do not show an improvement in KS by 12 weeks after initiation of anti-HIV therapy, it is unlikely that their disease will be controlled by that intervention alone; additional treatment options must then be considered.

In contrast to antiretroviral drugs, anti-herpesvirus medications have a less-clear role in the management of KS. Although the studies mentioned above do indicate an impact of certain antiviral drugs on KS, the overall impact is modest and does not offset the considerable toxicity and cost of these therapies. Antiherpesvirus agents currently available, therefore, cannot be recommended as anti-KS therapy at this time.

Local Antitumor Chemotherapy ■ Therapies directed at KS tumors can be divided into either local or systemic therapies. Local therapies offer the benefit of deferring systemic chemotherapies and their attendant risks of increased immunosuppression in an already vulnerable patient population. The selection of a local therapy may be influenced by certain factors, such as the extent and location of the lesions (eg, small, singular lesions on the trunk or on an extremity) and the rapidity of clinical change (eg, indolent development of new lesions over months rather than weeks). Options for local therapy include intralesional injection of vinblastine, topical retinoid, radiotherapy and cryotherapy, among others.

For patients who have a small number of lesions that are unresponsive to anti-HIV medications, or who require more rapid improvement than the anti-HIV medications may offer, intralesional injection of vinblastine is a reasonable first-line approach. In particular, palatal or buccal mucosa lesions respond promptly to intralesional vinblastine.[78] Practitioners most commonly use vinblastine at 0.1-0.4 mg/mL, injecting approximately 0.1-0.2 mL into a 1 cm^2 lesion. Local discomfort may be considerable, and so the vinblastine may be admixed 1:1 with lidocaine to improve tolerability. Local reaction is generally modest, but skin breakdown can occur. Unfortunately, responses are usually short lived with most lesions progressing after a few months.

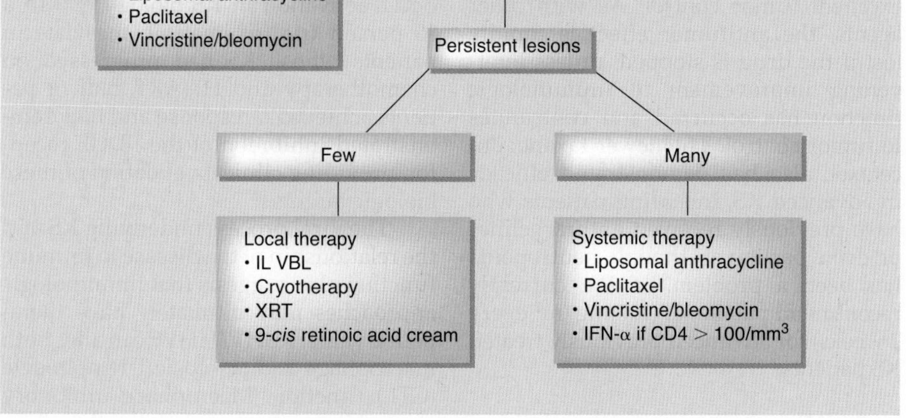

Figure 119-4 ■ Treatment schema for patients with Kaposi sarcoma. *Abbreviations*: HAART, highly active antiretroviral therapy; IFN-α, interferon-α; IL, interleukin; VBL, vinblastine; XRT, radiation therapy.

Topical 9-cis-retinoic acid (alitretinoin) gel has also been approved for treatment of cutaneous KS based on a randomized placebo-controlled trial in 139 patients which demonstrated a sixfold higher response rate in the retinoic acid-treated group, as compared with the placebo-treated group.[79] The difficulty with this medication is its potential for inducing an irritating local reaction when applied to normal skin. Consequently, patients must be counseled to be fastidious in their application of the compound exclusively to affected skin. Even with such care, some patients develop local reactions that may be troubling. Responses are not immediate, and may not be observed for 1-2 months after initiation of treatment, so patience is required. Of note, the same compound appears to have activity when given systemically. In two open-label multicenter trials, the tumor response rate was nearly 40%.[80] Headache, dry skin, hyperlipidemia, and pancreatitis were notable toxicities.

Radiation Therapy ■ Radiation therapy using either orthovoltage or electron beam may provide highly effective locoregional control of KS, even at relatively low doses. The great majority of treated patients will experience an objective response, many of which will be complete. A French study of 643 patients with AIDS-associated KS found a complete response rate of 92% when 20 Gy was delivered over 2 weeks, followed 2 weeks later with 10 Gy over 1 week.[81] Modifications in dose schedule may reduce the complexity for patients. A 36 person study administered a total of 21 Gy in thrice weekly fractions for 2 weeks, achieving an overall response rate of 91% with complete response rate of 80%.[82] Treatment with as little as one 8 Gy fraction has been reported to achieve a response in approximately three quarters of patients.[83,84] Tolerance of therapy is generally good, though acute and late toxicities may occur including increased edema, ulceration, and chronic skin injury. Caution must be used when targeting mucous membranes, as the sensitivity of patients with AIDS to mucositis from radiation therapy appears to be heightened, and debilitating complications can occur.

Photodynamic therapy is an experimental modality employing light activation photosensitizing drugs to result in local tumor necrosis. A study of the photosensitizer photophrin in nearly 350 KS lesions yielded a 96% response rate, one third of which were complete.[85]

Systemic Antitumor Chemotherapy ■ Systemic therapy for KS is appropriate for advanced symptomatic disease, particularly for those patients with edema, extensive mucocutaneous disease, and pulmonary or symptomatic GI involvement. Type 1 interferons have demonstrated efficacy owing to their antiviral, antiproliferative, antiangiogenic, and pro-immunologic activities, though this treatment is rarely employed due to the slow onset of action and poor tolerability.[86] Single agent and combination cytotoxic chemotherapies are most commonly employed for those patients with symptomatic or organ threatening disease who are not candidates for local therapy or HAART alone. Effective agents in this disease include doxorubicin, bleomycin, etoposide, taxanes, and the vinca alkaloids. Combination strategies with either bleomycin and vincristine,[87] or doxorubicin, bleomycin, and vincristine[88] initially demonstrated tumor response rates of 57% to 88%.[89] The definition of response to chemotherapy in KS has historically been more ambiguous than with most other tumors because of the limitations of the bidimensional measurement in cutaneous, mucosal and visceral lesions. KS can undergo complete regression of identifiable tumor on histology, yet the region of hyperpigmentation may not change in size. What does change is the nodularity of the lesion, the color characteristics (from a violaceous or salmon color to a gray-brown hemosiderin stain), and when present initially, associated edema. Responses in the early literature are difficult to assess due to lack of uniform response criteria, while more recent studies have benefited by the introduction of standard response criteria initially defined within the AIDS Clinical Trials Group (ACTG) and refined by a joint effort of the AIDS Malignancy Consortium, the National Cancer Institute, and the US Food and Drug Administration (FDA).

Combination cytotoxic therapy with doxorubicin, bleomycin, and vincristine has served as a standard for comparison with newer treatment regimens. Although combined doxorubicin-bleomycin-vincristine has a substantial response rate, side effects are common, most prominently nausea, alopecia, fatigue, peripheral neuropathy, acral cyanosis, Raynaud phenomenon, cytopenias and infection.[90] These toxicities can be quite debilitating in a patient population on numerous other medications and often dealing with numerous other medical problems. The impetus for an active but more easily tolerated treatment program has therefore been particularly acute in KS. The liposomal encapsulated anthracyclines have provided that option and have emerged as a highly effective and tolerable treatment option. The leaky vasculature composing KS lesions predisposes to deposition of the drug, and lesion concentrations of drug have been shown to be almost an order of magnitude higher than in noninvolved tissue.[91] Furthermore, the side-effect profiles of these agents are more favorable. Two phase III studies with roughly 250 HIV-related KS patients in each found liposomal doxorubicin monotherapy superior to traditional cytotoxic combinations of either doxorubicin-bleomycin-vincristine or vincristine-bleomycin. Liposomal doxorubicin achieved responses in 46% to 58% of patients, compared to 25% with the traditional 2- and 3-drug combinations.[92,93] Time to response and tolerability were both improved in the liposomal doxorubicin treated patients, as was health-related quality of life.[94] No survival differences were observed. A large randomized study comparing the traditional doxorubicin-bleomycin-vincristine combination with liposomal daunorubicin found that liposomal drug to have less toxicity, but the tumor response rate was equivalent and not as high as that found for liposomal doxorubicin.[95] A small trial has compared the liposomal formulations of doxorubicin and daunorubicin, with the liposomal doxorubicin appearing superior, but the trial is too small to draw definitive conclusions.[96] The overall body of evidence supports the use of liposomal doxorubicin as the initial chemotherapy of choice in advanced symptomatic KS; standard dosing is 20 mg/m^2 every 2-3 weeks for a total of 6 cycles.

Taxanes act upon neoplastic cells by stabilizing microtubules, and have emerged as highly active, well-tolerated agents for KS. After showing encouraging activity and safety in a phase I trial,[97] two phase II studies in previously treated patients with KS showed response rates of 56-71% with median durations of response of 9-10 months, longer than has been seen with any other therapy.[98] Responses are seen in anthracycline-treated patients, and patients can tolerate low-dose paclitaxel (100 mg/m^2 every 2 weeks) extremely well. Some patients have received this therapy for over 2 years at our center and have maintained excellent tumor control. As with other agents, the antitumor effect is rapidly lost if the drug is stopped, unless intervening improvement in immunologic function has occurred and contributes to tumor control. The newer taxane, docetaxel, also has demonstrated efficacy in advanced KS, including patients who have previously received anthracyclines or even paclitaxel, though neutropenia has been a problem.[99,100] We currently recommend paclitaxel (100 mg/m^2 every 2 weeks) for advanced previously treated KS patients.

Novel Therapies

The highly vascular nature of KS lesions and their ready accessibility to study have made KS a candidate disease for assessment of antiangiogenesis agents. A number of clinical trials involving a range of different agents have occurred or are under way. The agent thalidomide has a number of properties, including inhibiting angiogenesis, and has been assessed in early phase studies in patients with KS. A phase II study with 20 patients demonstrated partial responses in 8 patients and a median time to progression of 7 months.[101] Neutropenia, depression, somnolence and neuropathy were notable toxicities. Given the role of VEGF and VEGF-receptor signaling in this disease, the anti-VEGF monoclonal antibody bevacizumab is an appealing prospect for therapy that is currently in clinical trials.

Membrane metalloproteinases (MMP) are overexpressed in KS cells and may facilitate tumor invasion and metastasis.[102] The MMP inhibitor COL-3 demons trated efficacy and safety in a 75 patient randomized phase II trial of low dose and high dose oral COL-3.[103] The overall response rate was 41% in the low dose and 29% in the high dose group with responses correlating with decline in plasma MMP levels. Rash and photosensitivity were the most frequent adverse events.

KSHV/HHV8 induces the PI3K/AKT/mTOR pathway resulting in proproliferative and anti-apoptotic effects which contribute to KS pathogenesis.[55] Targeting of the mTOR pathway has therefore garnered attention as a rational therapeutic target in this disease. Enthusiasm for this strategy was generated by a report of 15 patients with KS post renal transplantation who had a striking 100% complete response rate when immunosuppression was changed from cyclosporine to sirolimus.[104] Investigation of sirolimus in HIV-related KS is currently underway.

Tyrosine kinase inhibitors have attracted attention as a possible treatment strategy in KS due to the role of platelet derived growth factor (PDGF) and c-KIT activation in KS biology.[105,106] In a 10 person trial of imatinib mesylate in patients whose KS had progressed on chemotherapy and HAART, half of patients achieved a response and had demonstrated inhibition of the PDGF receptor, providing clinical validation of these biologic targets.[107]

The viral process underlying KS and the relationship of the disease to immune function also suggests that immunologic approaches may ultimately have therapeutic value. KSHV/HHV8 can alter both macrophage and cytotoxic T lymphocyte (CTL) function. Macrophage inhibitory chemokines are encoded by the virus and produced in KSHV/HHV8-infected cells. The cells also produce an OX-2 homologue termed K-14. OX-2 receptors are present on monocyte/macrophages and stimulation dampens the ability of macrophages to be activated by other stimuli. K14 is capable of reducing activated macrophage production of inflammatory cytokines, possibly restricting host response to KSHV/HHV8.[108] In addition, KSHV/HHV8 encodes genes that alter the ability of infected cells to be targeted by CTLs. The K3 and K5 viral gene products limit CTL engagement of MHC class I molecules, and K5 also inhibits interaction with the coreceptor (B7) complex necessary for CTL activation.[109] However, a number of reports have defined epitopes within KSHV/HHV8 gene products that are recognized by CTLs.[110,111] Definition of whether reactivity to certain epitopes associates with protection from disease and whether immune inhibitory pathways can be altered will pave the way for the development of vaccine or adoptive cell therapies of the future.

Non-Hodgkin Lymphoma (NHL)

Lymphoproliferation occurs in the context of immunodeficiency of many different types. It is a common complication of individuals born with congenital abnormalities of T-cell function, of individuals receiving immunosuppressive medications for organ transplantation, and of individuals with HIV infection. The common theme among these is the role of EBV going unchecked in its ability to induce B-cell proliferation. However, only a minority of AIDS-related lymphomas (ARL) resembles the lymphoproliferative disease of the congenital or post-transplantation setting. ARL comprises a complex set of tumors with challenging clinical scenarios. It has been and remains the most lethal complication of HIV infection, demanding new approaches and new understanding of the pathophysiology underlying it. The most common ARL is diffuse large B-cell lymphoma, particularly the immunoblastic variant, followed by Burkitt lymphoma (BL), primary CNS (PCNS) lymphoma, primary effusion lymphoma (PEL) and plasmablastic lymphoma (PBL). These entities show significant variation in incidence based on the depth of HIV-related immunosuppression.

Epidemiology

The association of NHL with HIV infection was evident within the first half-decade of the AIDS epidemic, when an unusual number of lymphomas among young men became evident in cancer registries in California. The first revision of the definition of AIDS by the Centers for Disease Control and Prevention, in 1987, included NHL, and it has remained an important and devastating manifestation of HIV infection. Unlike KS, in which select subsets of HIV-infected individuals have a unique risk, NHL is more uniformly distributed among risk groups for HIV, with little variation. What variation is present may be attributable partly to issues of care.

The risk of NHL among HIV-infected individuals is in part determined by the level of immunosuppression, with higher risk noted among those with low CD4 cell counts; however, specific subsets of lymphoma have a stronger association with severe immunosuppression than others. The occurrence of PCNS lymphoma is restricted to those with very advanced immunodeficiency, as are the PEL and PBL subsets of systemic ARLs. These manifestations of profound immune dysfunction appear to have decreased in incidence since the advent of HAART. Among the other ARLs, diffuse large B-cell lymphoma (DLBCL) appears to occur more commonly in those with more profound immunosuppression, whereas BL is often seen in a group with more preserved immune function.[112] The median CD4 counts in most treatment reports of ARLs are in the range of 50-100 cells/mm^3, with the BL group often having a CD4 count greater than 200 cells/mm^3. In contrast, reports of patients with PCNS lymphomas demonstrate a profound CD4 count depression (30 cells/mm^3 in one study).[113] Thus, NHL may occur across a broad range of contexts in HIV disease, including those with virtually no other manifestations of immunosuppression, and may be the presenting illness of HIV infection. Possible unrecognized HIV infection should therefore be considered in any person presenting with a highly aggressive B-cell lymphoma. The duration and severity of persistent immunosuppression is important in determining risk for developing an ARL, with a relative hazard of approximately 1.4 for each 50% decline in CD4 count. Reassuringly, as the CD4 count responds to HAART, the risk of lymphoma reduces, but there is a lag time of approximately 1 year, somewhat longer than for other opportunistic diseases.[22] Interestingly, the reduction in risk appears to proceed with longer time on HAART in parallel and likely reflects the gradual repair in immune function seen over long periods of time on HAART. Immune function is accompanied by HIV RNA level as a predictor of ARL risk. In the EuroSIDA study, each log of HIV ribonucleic acid (RNA) was associated with a relative hazard of 1.51.[22] Therefore, controlling HIV is a critical determinant of ARL, presumably because of the immunologic alterations it engenders, though other pathophysiologic mechanisms may also participate.

Pathology and Pathogenesis

The development of lymphoma among HIV-infected patients is virtually always associated with transformation of a B cell, a cell type that HIV itself is unable to infect. Thus, HIV does not play a direct role in the development of most ARL; rather, it provides the background immunosuppression either for transforming viruses or for proliferative triggers for B cells to go unabated. The rare exception to this is a small subset of tumors of T-cell origin.

T-cell malignancies in HIV infection are uncommon, but include a spectrum of clinicopathologic entities.[114-123] In one subset, the HIV genome has been identified either in the T cells or in tumor-associated macrophages. Definition of the HIV chromosomal integration site revealed a preferential localization to a region upstream of the c-*fes* proto-oncogene, a finding that suggests a direct role for HIV in tumor pathogenesis.[124]

Although HIV may not be present in any but the rare T-cell malignancy, other viruses often are present. Most notably, EBV is common in certain systemic ARLs and virtually all PCNS lymphomas. The biology by which this gamma-herpesvirus exerts its effects is being unraveled through molecular analyses and perhaps is most clearly defined for the PCNS lymphomas and post-transplantation lymphoproliferative diseases (PTLDs). In that context, specific expression of latent virus genes is characteristic of a so-called type III pattern. These genes include the *LMP1*, *LMP2*, and *EBNA1* through *EBNA6*. The *LMP1* gene has been extensively studied as a potentially direct mediator of B-cell proliferation and has been shown to interact with the tumor necrosis factor receptor (TNFR)-signaling pathway.[125,126] LMP1 is expressed in primary tumor tissue from patients with PTLD and ARL and is associated with activation of NFκB, a critical regulator of survival in normal and malignant B-cells.[127] LMP1 is a six-transmembrane-spanning molecule with a cytoplasmic carboxy terminus capable of interacting with the TNFR II-associated factors (TRAFs) that mediate downstream transcription factor activation.[126,128-131] Aggregation of the cytoplasmic domains of *LMP1* mimic activated TNFR II, thereby providing a stimulus resembling constitutively activated receptor.[132] The activated pathways are similar to those of the TNFR family member CD30, involving the transcriptional regulators NFκB and cjun.[132,133] Potential downstream targets of these regulators are the proproliferative cytokines, IL-6 and IL-10.

A number of mutations within the carboxy terminus of LMP1 have been noted, and there are some data to support the possibility that these are associated with ARL- or HIV-related Hodgkin lymphoma (HL).[131-136] However, other studies have indicated that the frequency of such mutations is no greater among those with lymphoproliferative disease than it is among patients in an unaffected control group.[134] The concept that molecular evolution of persistent EBV infection may lead to alteration in the malignant potential of select latently infected B cells is an appealing hypothesis that remains speculative at this time.

The proportion of tumors associated with EBV varies by histologic subtype. EBV is present in virtually all cases of PCNS lymphoma and plasmablastic lymphoma, and in approximately 80% and 30% of HIV-related DLBCL and BL, respectively.[137-142] This finding leaves a large fraction of systemic ARLs without a clear association with an oncogenic virus; among these, a small proportion is linked to KSHV/HHV8. The clinicopathologic entity, PEL, is typically seen in those patients with profound immunosuppression and presents as fluid without tumor mass in the involved body cavity, which may be the pleural space, peritoneum, or pericardium.[143,144] The tumor cells generally do not express B-, T-, or even hematopoietic-cell surface markers (they are CD45, CD3, and CD19 negative). Molecular analysis of the cells demonstrates that they have undergone immunoglobulin gene rearrangement consistent with an origin in the B-cell lineage. All such tumors identified to date include the KSHV/HHV8 genome, and most have evidence of EBV co-infection.[145,146]

The ability of KSHV/HHV8 to infect B cells in vitro has been shown, whereas the impact of that infection has been difficult to discern in vitro. No clear association of virus infection with altered B-cell growth kinetics, as with EBV, has been noted with KSHV/HHV8. However, the close clinical and pathologic relationship of KSHV/HHV8 to PEL is compelling evidence for a direct relationship between KSHV/HHV8 and B-cell oncogenesis. PEL cells are latently infected with KSHV/HHV8, and so latent gene products likely play a dominant role in disease pathogenesis. Specifically, LANA-1, LANA-2, v-cyclin, v-FLIP, and viral IL6 are all transcribed from a common promoter and are constitutively expressed in PEL cells, where they promote cellular proliferation and survival through various mechanisms.[147]

Among the possible contributions of viruses to malignant transformation is alteration in the immunologic reactivity to neoplastic cells. Mechanisms include the ability of EBV EBNA1 to alter antigen-processing pathways and thereby potentially mask EBV-infected cells from CTL reactivity.[148-150] Although the specific details of the mechanism remain to be elucidated, it appears that KSHV/HHV8 exerts a similar effect on infected transformed cells. In addition, viral gene products may be elaborated by infected cells and may impact immune effector cells. For example, EBV encodes a viral IL-10 homolog (BRCF-1) with biologic activity mimicking that of endogenous IL-10.[151-153] Cell lines and tumors from AIDS patients and animal models of ARL indicate that IL-10 is produced,[151,153-156] and that it potentially exerts an inhibitory influence on the T-helper cell (TH1) response. IL-10 potently suppresses interferon-α and IL-2 production by effector cells of the TH1 response and is a B-cell mitogen.[152]

Other cytokines potentially participating in altered reactivity to malignant cells include IL-6, which in addition to serving as a proliferative stimulus to B cells, may act to alter cell sensitivity to immune killing. Specifically, IL-6 has been shown to reduce the ability of EBV-positive cells to be lysed by antigen-specific CTL from HIV-1–positive individuals.[157] IL-6 levels have been noted to be elevated in the serum of patients with AIDS and may be associated with the development of NHL.[158] The CD40 and CD40 ligand (CD40L) interaction has also been hypothesized to participate in the development of HIV-related lymphomas. Activation of this TNFR family pathway alters the proliferation, differentiation, and survival of B cells that serve as a key mechanism of interaction of the B- and T-cell–mediated immune mechanisms. The infection of microvascular endothelial cells from the bone marrow and CNS has been shown to result in altered CD40 signaling that up-regulates adhesive interactions with B cells and possibly explains the potential for extranodal lymphoma in HIV-infected individuals.[159]

Chemokine pathways may also contribute to the unique susceptibility of HIV-infected patients for lymphomagenesis. Patients with a genetic variant in the CXC chemokine, stroma-derived growth factor-1 (SDF-1), have an excess risk of developing the BL subtype of ARL.[160] This chemokine is a known B-cell mitogen and by exerting chemokinetic effects, may contribute to a proliferative stimulus for patients with the genetic variant. The presence of this variant has been suggested to possibly provide a method of identifying those patients with increased risk of lymphoma, although the potential for this risk factor remains speculative at this time.

Genetic mutations in the tumor cells have been well characterized and are related to the specific histologic subtype. Diffuse large B-cell lymphomas exhibit a Bcl-6 rearrangement in approximately 33% of cases, a c-*myc* rearrangement in 40%, and a TP53 mutation in 25%.[161-163] In contrast, BL seen in AIDS have c-*myc* rearrangements but not *Bcl-6*, and rarely have TP53 mutations.[161,163-166] The presence of EBV is variably associated with either the c-*myc* or *Bcl-6* rearrangements in BL and DLBCL respectively.[163-166] The finding that rearranged c-*myc* gene juxtaposes with the immunoglobulin gene heavy chain switch region suggests that the malignant event is occurring proximate to the time of immunoglobulin class switching.[165,167-170] This relatively late event in B-cell ontogeny is indicative of transformation in a relatively mature germinal center B cell.

Clinical Manifestations

AIDS-related lymphomas are generally extremely aggressive, high-grade lymphomas, most commonly of B-cell origin. The presenting clinical features of systemic ARLs are similar to those of aggressive lymphomas in the immunocompetent host, though HIV-infected patients are likelier to present with advanced-stage disease with most patients' disease involving extranodal sites. Extranodal involvement occurs in up to 95% of patients,[164,171-187] and lymphoma restricted to extranodal sites may be seen in up to 56% of patients.[187] Particular sites of involvement are favored by specific histologic types. Among those patients with Burkitt histology, bone marrow and meningeal disease occurs in approximately one-quarter, while large-cell tumors favor the GI tract and liver as well as brain parenchyma and leptomeninges, though no extranodal site is immune from lymphoma involvement. A summary of the sites of involvement reported in three series is presented in Table 119-4, and indicates the frequency of involvement of the

Table 119-4 Sites of Extranodal Involvement for AIDS High-Grade B-Cell Lymphomas

Author	No. of Patients	% Extranodal	% CNS	% GI	% Marrow	% Liver
Ziegler et al.	90	98	42[a]	17	33	9
Kaplan et al.	84	76	17	4	31	26
Knowles et al.	89	74	21	28	21	16

[a]Meningeal and primary CNS involvement.

Abbrevations: CNS, central nervous system; GI, gastrointestinal.

most common sites: bone marrow, CNS, GI tract, and liver.

Systemic "B" symptoms of significant weight loss, fevers and drenching night sweats are common. Given the immunosuppressed nature of these patients, a thorough microbiologic evaluation is required to exclude concomitant bacterial, mycobacterial, viral, fungal or parasitic disease. KSHV/HHV8-associated multicentric Castleman disease (MCD) should also be considered in the differential diagnosis, as discussed below.

PEL is an end-stage complication of HIV-induced immunosuppression and has been observed in other types of immunosuppression, including that associated with organ transplantation, and rarely occurs at a CD4 count above 50 cells/mm^3.[188] The common sites of involvement with this tumor are the peritoneum, the pleural space, and the pericardium.[189] Involvement of the bone marrow has been observed with progressive disease, and rare cases of solid extracavitary PELs have been reported.[190,191] The approach to this patient population is similar to any other systemic ARL, including evaluation of the CNS.

Plasma cell disorders are increased in the setting of HIV infection and are also fairly heterogeneous. Rare cases of highly aggressive PBL of the jaw and oral cavity may occur in profoundly immunosuppressed patients with CD4 counts below 50 cells/mm^3.[192] Histopathology has indicated that these tumors mark as plasma cells with MUM1, CD138, and CD38 and are often negative for typical lymphoid markers, such as CD45 (leukocyte common antigen) and CD20. EBV is uniformly present with a lower frequency of KSHV/HHV8.[140,193,194] Extramedullary plasmacytomas and overt multiple myeloma with paraprotein specific for HIV antigens have been reported.[195,196] The clinical course of these disorders is highly variable, and the clinical approach should be based on standard guidelines for these diseases outside the context of HIV infection. Rare cases of PBL have responded to antiretroviral therapy alone; however, such a treatment approach is discouraged given the highly aggressive nature of these neoplasms.

PCNS lymphoma represents 15-20% of all HIV-related lymphomas, and is generally a manifestation of severe immunosuppression. Mean CD4 counts are < 30 cells/mm^3, there is commonly a previous history of an AIDS-defining complication, and the EBV genome is invariably present in the tumor.[113] Histologically, these tumors have an immunoblastic diffuse large B-cell appearance and express a type III pattern of EBV latent gene products.[197] The clinical approach to these patients is detailed in a later section.

MCD, or angiofollicular lymph node hyperplasia, may occur in patients with advanced HIV disease and mimic the presentation of an ARL or infectious disease.[198] MCD is a polyclonal disease that is uniformly associated with KSHV/HHV8 in the HIV-infected patient and may exhibit a rapidly progressive, lethal course. Both the hyaline-vascular and plasma cell subtypes of MCD have been reported in AIDS, but the multicentric plasma cell histology type is far more common. KSHV/HHV8 is found in the involved nodes, and there is a high prevalence of co-incident or subsequent KS.[143,198-200] The findings show that fever, hepatosplenomegaly, and anemia are present in virtually all patients. Lymphadenopathy occurs in ~90% and marked weight loss in 70%; pancytopenia is seen in 35%.[198] Some have hypothesized that this syndrome represents an acute or subacute KSHV/HHV8 infection.[201] Acute KSHV/HHV8 infection can also be accompanied by bone marrow failure resembling aplastic anemia.[202] IL-6 is abundantly produced in MCD and plays a critical role in the pathophysiology via activation of the JAK/STAT pathway, and promotion of angiogenesis and proliferation.[203-206] A monoclonal antibody against IL-6 has shown clinical efficacy in treatment of MCD.[207] Patients with MCD may present with a synchronous ARL, and an ARL may occur subsequent to the diagnosis of MCD, so diagnostic vigilance is required with a low threshold for repeat biopsy in the setting of progression or relapse, or based on a change in clinical behavior.

Clinical Approach

Evaluation of patients with ARL follows staging procedures for other types of NHL, with several caveats specific to the HIV-infected population. First, the frequent involvement of the CNS mandates a more thorough assessment of the CNS than in HIV-negative counterparts, including sampling of the cerebrospinal fluid (CSF) in all patients at diagnosis, and consideration of neuroimaging, particularly in the presence of neurologic signs or symptoms. Second, the potential for co-incident opportunistic infection must be kept in mind when evaluating a patient with "B" symptoms. Microbiologic evaluation is particularly important for that population with CD4 counts < 200 cells/mm^3 in whom the risk of opportunistic disease is increased, and is a necessity for those with < 50 cells/mm^3. Depending on the clinical scenario, particular concern should be paid to the possible presence of active Pneumocystis jiroveci (formerly *Pneumocystis carinii*), Cytomegalovirus, *Toxoplasma gondii*, *Mycobacterium avium complex*, *Mycobacterium tuberculosis*, and *Cryptococcus*. Hepatitis B and C serologies should be evaluated in all patients since co-infection may occur. Third, assessment of the status of the HIV disease is critical in defining the therapeutic approach. CD4 cells should be measured as well as plasma HIV RNA, and a detailed history of previous antiretroviral therapy and opportunistic disease should be obtained. Those patients for whom NHL represents a manifestation of end-stage, treatment-refractory HIV disease should be considered for palliative intent. For the majority of patients, however, viral suppression on HAART offers an open-ended prognosis from HIV-1 infection, and the emphasis should be on curing the lymphoma—a concept not realistically considered in the pre-HAART era, but of substantial importance since the availability of HAART in 1996. Experience with long-term ARL survivors now free of any clinical evidence of HIV disease emphasizes the importance of that perspective. Selecting a regimen appropriate for the patient involves weighing where the patient may lie in the continuum of HIV disease.

Prognostic Factors

Prognosis in patients with ARL has generally been poor, but with the advent of HAART, the improved prognosis from HIV-1 itself, as well as the improved tolerance of chemotherapy, long-term outcome in patients with ARL has substantially improved. Prior to the advent of HAART, the median survival for patients with HIV-associated DLBCL was 8 months compared to 43 months in the setting of HAART.[208] Poor prognostic factors in ARL prior to the introduction of HAART included age > 35 years, intravenous drug use, and stages III/IV disease, which predicted overall survival ranging from 46 weeks in the most favorable subgroup to 18 weeks in the least.[209] The International Prognostic Index (IPI) is the most commonly used risk stratification tool in the setting of non-HIV related aggressive lymphoma,[210] and has been evaluated in ARL. In the pre-HAART era, outcome was poor in all IPI subgroups[211,212] though since the advent of HAART, the IPI separates three risk groups with risk scores of 0-2, 3, and 4-5 predicting a 3 year overall survivals of 64%, 50%, and 13%, respectively.[212] Additional studies have also identified failure to achieve a complete response, increase in lactate acid dehydrogenase (LDH),[213] age > 40 years, prior AIDS-defining illness, poor performance status, presence of extranodal disease, and plasmablastic or primary effusion histology to be predictive of risk. Postgerminal center marker expression (BCL-6 and CD10 negative, MUM1/IRF4, or CD138 positive) have been associated with a shorter disease-free survival, analogous to HIV-negative DLBCL.[214]

Remarkably, only a single study has shown the BL histology to be of prognostic importance, and histologically guided therapies have historically not been applied to this population. Recent data suggests that HIV-related BL patients fare just as well as their HIV-negative counterparts when treated with intensive combination therapy.[215] In considering prognosis of ARL patients, the status of HIV disease itself must always be carefully considered given that tolerance of therapy is significantly poorer in patients with advanced AIDS failing antiretroviral therapy.

Treatment

Low-Dose Therapy ■ Early in the AIDS epidemic, the aggressive nature of the lymphomas observed was met with an aggressive clinical approach to therapy. The result was severe toxicity and frequent treatment-related death. Prophylactic therapy for opportunistic infections has improved, and with the advent of growth factors, the tolerability of chemotherapy has also improved. However, given the overall poor prognosis of patients with HIV-1 infection and the frequent necessity of concurrent treatment of other opportunistic illnesses, there was an effort to identify a low-intensity antitumor regimen. This effort resulted in the modified methotrexate, bleomycin, Adriamycin (doxorubicin)cyclophosphamide, Oncovin (vincristine), dexamethasone (mBACOD) regimen,[176] which was tested in a randomized phase III trial comparing it directly with the full-dose regimen.[216] The modified m-BACOD was essentially half dose (Table 119-5), and the full-dose regimen was given with concurrent granulocyte-macrophage colony-stimulating factor (GM-CSF). Surprisingly, the results revealed no statistically meaningful differences in the incidence of complete remission (50% vs 46%), relapse after complete remission (19% vs 23%), time to progression (22 weeks vs 28 weeks), overall median survival (31 weeks vs 34 weeks), death from AIDS (20 patients vs 12 patients), and death from lymphoma (24 patients vs 36 patients). The major difference between the two arms of the trial was that grade 4 neutropenia occurred with greater frequency in patients receiving the standard-dose regimen, notwithstanding the fact that all such patients received GM-CSF as a part of their treatment program. The utility of this regimen has been called into question, however, with the better tolerability of full-dose regimens in the era of HAART and the demonstration in the non-HIV–infected population that a regimen of cyclophosphamide, hydroxydaunomycin (doxorubicin), Oncovin (vincristine), and prednisone (CHOP) to be at minimum as effective as m-BACOD, but with less side effects in a randomized phase III trial.[217] For those patients in whom advanced HIV disease precludes use of full-dose chemotherapy, a low-dose regimen may still be appropriate, but the majority of patients in the HAART era should now be treated with standard-dose regimens.

Standard-Dose Therapies ■ For patients with control of HIV-1, the options are those of standard chemotherapy regimens such as CHOP (Table 119-5), in which response rates slightly lower than that of the uninfected population have been observed.

European investigators have evaluated more chemotherapy-intensive regimens for patients with ARL. The French-Italian Cooperative Group tested the ACVB regemen (adreamycin [doxorubicin], cyclo-phosphamide, Nindesine, biomycin, and prednitsolore) regimen in 140 patients and observed a complete remission rate of 65%, with a relapse rate of 24%.[218] A follow-up study of patients with CD4 count > 100 cells/mm^3, no prior AIDS-defining illnesses, and good performance status has been conducted comparing standard dose CHOP chemo-

Table 119-5 ■ **Commonly Used Therapy Regimens for AIDS-Related Lymphoma**

Therapy Regimen	Standard-Dose Therapy	Low-Dose Therapy
m-BACOD		
Methotrexate (IV)	200 mg/m^2, day 15	200 mg/m^2, day 15
Bleomycin (IV)	4 U/m^2, day 1	4 U/m^2, day 1
Doxorubicin (IV)	45 mg/m^2, day 1	25 mg/m^2, day 1
Cyclophosphamide (IV)	600 mg/m^2, day 1	300 mg/m^2, day 1
Vincristine (IV)	1.4 mg/m^2, day 1	1.4 mg/m^2, day 1
Dexamethasone (po)	6 mg/m^2, days 1-5	3 mg/m^2, days 1-5
GM-CSF (SC)	5 mcg/kg, days 4-13	5 µg/kg, days 4-13, prn
Pneumocystic prophylaxis	Trimethoprim-sulfamethoxazole, dapsone, atovaquone or inhaled pentamidine	
	Standard	**Modified**
CHOP (+/− Rituximab)		
Cyclophosphamide	750 mg/m^2, IVPB, day 1	375 mg/m^2, day 1
Doxorubicin	50 mg/m^2, IVPB day 1	25 mg/m^2, day 1
Vincristine	1.4 mg/m^2 (not to exceed 2 mg), IVPB, day 1	1.4 mg/m^2 (max 2 mg), day 1
Prednisone (each cycle q 21-28 d)	100 mg, po, days 1-5	50-100 mg po, days 1-5
Rituximab (if included)	375 mg/m^2, day 1	
CDE		
Cyclophosphamide	187.5 mg/m^2, CI, days 1-4	
Doxorubicin	12.5 mg/m^2, CI, days 1-4	
Etoposide	60 mg/m2, CI, days 1-4	
ACVBP dose-intensive chemotherapy		
Induction		
Adriamycin	75 mg/m^2, day 1	
Cyclophosphamide	1200 mg/m^2, day 1	
Vindesine	2 mg/m^2, days 1, 5	
Bleomycin	10 mg, days 1, 5	
Prednisolone	60 mg/m^2, days 1-5	
Consolidation		
Methotrexate (IV)	3 g/m^2, days 1,5	
Folinic acid rescue (po)	25 mg × 4, days 1-3, 15-17	
Ifosfamide (IV)	1.5 g/m^2, days 29,33	
VP-16 (IV)	300 mg/m^2, days 29,33	
L-Asparaginase (IM)	50,000 U/m^2, days 57, 64	
Ara-C (SC)	50 mg/m^2 q12 h × 8, days 78, 92	
CNS prophylaxis		
Methotrexate (IT)	12 mg, days 1, 15, 29	
CNS treatment		
Methotrexate (IT)	12 mg 2 × week, for 5 weeks	
RT	24,000 cGy	
EPOCH regimen (+/− Rituximab)		
Etoposide	50/m2, CI, days 1-4	50/m^2, CI, days 1-4
Vincristine	0.4 mg/m^2, CI, days 1-4	0.4 mg/m^2, CI, days 1-4
Doxorubicin	10 mg/m^2, CI, days 1-4	10 mg/m^2, CI, days 1-4
Prednisone	60 mg/m^2, po, days 1-5	60 mg/m^2, po, days 1-5
Cyclophosphamide	375 mg/m^2, IV, day 5	187 mg/m^2, IV, days
Rituximab (if included)	375 mg/m^2, day 1	

Abbreviations: ACVBP, Adriamycin (doxorubicin), cyclophosphamide, vindesine, bleomycin, prednisolone; CDE, cyclophosphamide, doxorubicin, eto-poside; CHOP, cyclophosphamide, hydroxydaunomycin, Oncovin, prednisone; CNS, central nervous system; GM-CSF, granulocyte macrophage colony-stimulating factor; IM, intramuscularly; IV, intravenously; po, per os (orally); prn, pro re nata (according as circumstances may require); RT, radiation therapy; SC, subcutaneously.

therapy with the more intensive ACVBP regimen with granulocyte colony-stimulating factor (G-CSF) support and CNS prophylaxis with intrathecal methotrexate. Toxicity was significantly greater in the ACVBP arm without any difference in outcome, arguing against the use of a dose-intensive regimen, even in favorable risk ARL patients.[219] The 6-year overall survival was only 30%, though less than 40% of enrolled patients received HAART, with those patients receiving antiretrovirals experiencing an improved outcome regardless of treatment group.

Standard Cytotoxic Chemotherapy Plus Antiretroviral Therapy ■ The idea of combining antiretroviral and antitumor therapy has advocates who suggest that the ability of the immune system to participate in combating the malignancy will be maximized by suppressing HIV-1 replication. This view is balanced by the opinion of those who regard the viral infection as a secondary priority in the setting of life-threatening tumor growth and believe that adding the potential risks of drug-related toxicity and drug–drug interactions do not justify combining these two groups of agents. This dichotomous opinion is reflected in two clinical trials; one study employed a three drug, protease inhibitor-containing antiretroviral regimen in combination with CHOP chemotherapy and the other administered continuous-infusion chemotherapy (dose adjusted etoposide, prednisone, Oncovin [vincristine], cyclophosphamide, and hydroxydaunomycin [doxorubicin] [EPOCH]), and held antiretroviral therapy until the completion of chemotherapy.

The trial of CHOP plus indinavir, d4T, and 3TC was conducted by the United States National Cancer Institute-supported AIDS Malignancy Consortium and involved a cohort of patients receiving low-dose CHOP and a subsequent cohort receiving full-dose CHOP plus the same antiretroviral regimen. This study indicated that the combination did not result in unexpected severe or more-frequent toxicities. Pharmacologic analysis tested the possibility both of antineoplastic drugs affecting protease inhibitor levels and of antiviral therapies altering cytotoxic drug metabolism. No alterations in levels of indinavir or doxorubicin were noted, although a reduction in cyclophosphamide clearance of approximately 50% was observed.[220]

The United States National Cancer Institute tested infusional dose adjusted EPOCH without concomitant HAART.[221] The etoposide, vincristine and doxorubicin were given as a 96 h continuous infusion, followed by bolus cyclophosphamide on day 5; the cyclophosphamide dose was modified based on baseline CD4 count and neutropenia during the prior cycle. Intrathecal methotrexate was administered with each cycle for CNS prophylaxis. Holding antiviral therapy resulted in a rise in HIV RNA during cancer chemotherapy that reverted to entry levels when antivirals were resumed following completion of chemotherapy. Clinical outcome was the best reported to date in ARL patients with 74% of patients achieving a complete response and 5-year disease-free and overall survivals of 92% and 60%, respectively. Continuous-infusion regimens have also been combined with antiviral therapy as initial treatment of ARL. The CDE regimen (cyclophosphamide 800 mg/m^2, doxorubicin 50 mg/m^2, etoposide 240 mg/m^2, by continuous 96 h infusion) was tested in 98 patients with concomitant HAART (dideoxy inosine [ddi] monotherapy was used in the first 43 patients) resulted in a complete response rate of 45%, with 43% of patients alive after 2 years.[222] Patients treated with concomitant HAART vs ddi had an improved overall survival owing to decreased hematologic toxicity and treatment-associated death. These trials suggest that combining antivirals and antitumor therapy appears safe and effective. The short-term consequences of holding antiretroviral therapy appear to be acceptable in selected patients with reasonable immune function; but this should be done cautiously.

BL patients have traditionally been included in trials with other ARLs and have not clearly had a worse outcome from HIV-related DLBCL, though the majority of these trials were conducted prior to HAART when outcomes were uniformly poor. Modern evidence suggests that patients with HIV-related BL experience similarly encouraging outcomes to non-HIV infected patients when treated with intensive multi-agent chemotherapy.[215]

Monoclonal Antibody Therapy ■ Efforts to improve the outcome for patients with ARL have included the addition of the humanized anti-CD20 antibody rituximab, which has shown a survival benefit when combined with CHOP chemotherapy in HIV-negative aggressive B-cell lymphomas.[223] A multicenter randomized phase III trial testing CHOP vs CHOP plus rituximab (R-CHOP), however, demonstrated that in the setting of AIDS, patients did not have an improvement in overall outcome with the addition of rituximab.[224] There was a trend toward improved response (58% vs 47%) with rituximab that did not reach statistical significance, however this was outweighed by an increased rate of infectious-related death (14% vs. 2%). Most deaths in the rituximab arm were in patients with CD4 counts less than 100 cells/mm^3, with 60% of deaths occurring at a CD4 count less than 50 cells/mm^3. Further complicating analysis of this trial is a 3 month maintenance rituximab period following initial R-CHOP, during which time 40% of infectious related deaths occurred. In light of these data, the use of rituximab with CHOP must be carefully considered, especially in patients with significantly decreased CD4 counts. When rituximab is included, white cell growth factor support should be provided along with consideration of prophylactic antibiotics in highly immunocompromised individuals. An ongoing randomized trial is studying the question of whether rituximab administered following completion of CHOP therapy will offer benefit while minimizing infectious-related toxicity.

CNS Prophylaxis ■ The role of CNS prophylaxis has been much debated. Although early studies indicated a very high incidence of CNS involvement or relapse (8 of 12 patients in one study[178]), the usefulness of routine CNS prophylaxis has never been rigorously studied in this patient population. Approach to this issue is very center-dependent, and some centers treat all patients with 4 weekly doses of intrathecal ara-C or methotrexate, or include an intrathecal injection with every cycle of systemic chemotherapy. The practice at other centers has been to reserve this treatment for patients with Burkitt histology or bone marrow, testicular, or Waldeyer ring involvement. However, data from Cingolani and colleagues suggest that other features may be associated with risk of CNS relapse. In particular, the presence of EBV in the primary tumor and extra-nodal involvement were highly associated with eventual CNS involvement ($p = .003$ and $p = .006$, respectively).[225] Whether CNS prophylaxis can be restricted to such patients is not clear and it would be prudent to add these features to those that raise particular concern and should prompt serious consideration of prophylactic therapy. It is our practice to include intrathecal methotrexate as CNS prophylaxis in the treatment program for all patients with ARL.

Treatment of Relapsed or Refractory Disease ■ Treatment of relapsed aggressive lymphoma in non-HIV infected individuals incorporates the use of high dose chemotherapy with autologous stem cell rescue (ASCT), an approach which has been proven to cure more patients than standard dose chemotherapy alone.[226] Myeloablative chemotherapy in the setting of HIV infection carries substantially increased risks of morbidity and mortality, though evidence suggests it can be performed effectively in the post-HAART era. In one study including 16 patients with relapsed ARL, a remarkable 81% of patients were alive and free from progression at 3 years.[227] Independent studies from other sites have reported less impressive disease-free survival statistics (65%, 50%, and 28%, respectively), but all studies noted excellent engraftment and safety outcomes.[227-230] ASCT should therefore be considered the treatment of choice for relapsed ARL patients considered fit enough to undergo high dose therapy. Such transplants should only be performed at centers experienced in stem cell transplantation for this uniquely high-risk population of patients.

Allogeneic stem cell transplantation in HIV-infected patients using fully myeloablative conditioning has been reported and carries marked infectious-related toxicity in addition to graft versus host disease and progressive lymphoma.[231-238] Non-myeloablative allogeneic stem cell transplantation using a reduced intensity conditioning regimen has been reported to be feasible in a small series of patients with HIV and relapsed hematologic malignancy.[230] With these adoptive stem cell transplant approaches, genetic modification of the transferred cells to render the cell insensitive to HIV infection is now being explored. Trials performed to date have been disappointing,[239,240] but methods of stem cell gene transfer are still in evolution and it is too early to determine the real potential of this approach. At present, allogeneic stem cell transplantation in HIV-infected patients can only be recommended in the context of a clinical trial.

Supportive Care ■ All patients should be considered for prophylaxis for opportunistic infections. Reduction in CD4 count by approximately half can be expected during chemotherapy, and *Pneumocystis jiroveci* prophylaxis is recommended even if entry CD4 counts exceed 200 cells/mm^3. The other prophylactic therapies standardly used in advanced HIV disease are also applied to this population.

Growth factor use is often required, given the noted increased sensitivity to myelotoxic injury in patients with HIV disease. A single randomized trial of CHOP versus CHOP plus GM-CSF found a significant decrease in the incidence of fever and neutropenia and days of hospitalization in the cohort receiving prophylactic growth factor,[241] though this trial antedated the use of protease inhibitors, which has generally improved patients' tolerance of chemotherapy. Therefore, many practitioners use guidelines similar to those for other patients receiving chemotherapy when deciding about growth factor use.[242] The use of growth factors in the HIV-1–infected population has been of some concern, however, because of the potential for growth factor stimulation of HIV-1 replication.[243,244] This issue has been raised particularly for GM-CSF, in which direct activation of the HIV-1 transcriptional control regions has been documented in vitro. Data regarding the increase in viral load in vivo, however, have been conflicting. Some studies have demonstrated a rise in markers of viral load (HIV p24 at the time of these studies),[241,245] and others show either no increase or a transient increase.[246-248] The trial involving GMCSF and CHOP observed an increase in HIV-1 p24 that was noted in the early cycles but that by the end of the trial was not different compared with controls. The data with G-CSF use are similarly conflicting. G-CSF does not have effects on inflammatory cytokine release or notable induction of HIV-1 in vitro seen with GM-CSF, but has been shown to induce increases in HIV RNA in half the patients receiving it at doses sufficient for stem cell mobilization.[249] These increases were transient and returned to baseline following cessation of the growth factor. The long-term consequences of growth factor use and its relationship to control of virus replication by antiretroviral drugs are not known at present. In general, concerns regarding long-term consequences do not discourage use of growth factors in the context of patients with otherwise strong indications for their benefit.[242]

PCNS Lymphoma

A brain mass in the context of HIV infection can be caused by a number of infectious and neoplastic processes, and thereby poses a substantial diagnostic challenge. Most commonly seen in AIDS patients are *Toxoplasma gondii* abscess, PCNS lymphoma, mycobacterial or bacterial abscess, and progressive multifocal leukoencephalopathy (PML). Criteria for distinguishing among these entities remain imperfect without tissue sampling, but for those patients in whom biopsy is not possible or is refused, certain parameters can raise or lower the likelihood of a lymphoma diagnosis, and the use of PCR analysis for EBV DNA in the cerebrospinal fluid has greatly improved the reliability of a diagnosis without histologic confirmation.

In general, PCNS lymphoma, PML, and toxoplasmosis are complications of far advanced immunosuppression with CD4 counts of <50 cells/mm^3. This patient population is often on trimethoprim-sulfamethoxazole prophylaxis for *Pneumocystis*, which provides excellent protection against *Toxoplasma*. For those patients in whom a *Toxoplasma* antibody titer is negative and who have been on such prophylaxis, the likelihood of a lymphoma diagnosis in the setting of a CNS mass lesion has been documented to be 74%.[250] Additional information can be gained from PCR analysis for the EBV genome in CSF samples. Detection of EBV in the CSF has been reported to have specificity for lymphoma approximating 100%.[250,251] Sensitivity may be only 80% and there are rare cases of EBV+ CSF where no lymphoma is diagnosed, but this test has become extremely useful in assessing the patient who is unable or unwilling to undergo a definitive histologically defining procedure.

Radiographic features more suggestive of lymphoma include central location, lack of multifocality, and size > 2 cm.[177,252] In addition, a lesion that crosses the midline is highly likely to be a neoplastic process. Single-photon emission computed tomography (SPECT) or positron emission tomography (PET) can also help distinguish lymphoma from abscess. The combination of one of these imaging techniques with a positive DNA PCR for EBV is now often considered sufficient evidence for initiation of therapy. If these tests do not clearly delineate the process and a biopsy is not feasible, empiric anti-Toxoplasma therapy may be used as a diagnostic as well as therapeutic tool. Initiation of sulfadiazine or clindamycin with pyrimethamine generally halts the progression by 5 days and results in clinical or radiographic improvement by 14 days.[253,254] For those in whom these milestones are not met, the likelihood of toxoplasmosis is low.

Therapy for PCNS lymphoma remains very limited, and with poor outcome. Radiation therapy, usually with concomitant glucocorticoids, has been the mainstay of care, with response rates ranging from 60% to 79%, but durable remissions are uncommon.[177,255-257] There are some encouraging reports, however, that the control of HIV replication with antiretroviral therapy associated with a subsequent increase in CD4+ cells may provide therapeutic benefit above that of radiation therapy alone and prolong survival.[257]

Alternative antitumor approaches such as high-dose methotrexate have limited experience in this population, but reports of small trials have been encouraging.[258] Combination of cytotoxic chemotherapy and radiation therapy has been tested, with disappointing effect on the tumors and unacceptable toxicity. In spite of the fact that EBV genome is associated with PCNS lymphoma it is generally noted to be in latent phase, and therefore unlikely to be sensitive to lytic-phase-specific antiviral agents. Nonetheless, limited experience with the use of ganciclovir in combination with zidovudine and IL-2 has suggested antitumor activity.[259] The ultimate use of these agents or other EBV-directed genetic[260] or chemical[261] manipulations awaits careful assessment in clinical trial. The relationship of the disease to poor immunologic function does provide rationale, however, for emphasizing optimization of anti-HIV therapy as a component of antitumor therapy. The overall poor outcome for these patients also strongly advocates the encouragement of patients to participate in clinical protocols testing novel approaches.

The use of steroids in this patient population has engendered concern because of the potential worsening of immunosuppression. There is an absence of data regarding this point, but the opportunity to reduce edema and mass effect should not be avoided out of concern for immunosuppression. Rather, the tapering of steroids should be as rapid as is tolerated, and vigilance regarding the development of concurrent infection should be maintained. In the era preceding HAART, death was as commonly caused by secondary events as by tumor.[262] For those patients who present with PCNS lymphoma who have not been receiving HAART, initiating antiretroviral therapy should be considered a priority, as anecdotal reports have emerged of long-term survivors among the group gaining control of HIV-1.[263]

Multicentric Castleman Disease (MCD)

Unlike unicentric Castleman disease where surgical excision is the treatment of choice, there is no accepted standard for treating AIDS-related MCD. Small series have reported efficacy with single agent alkylators, vinblastine, oral etoposide, thalidomide, or liposomal doxorubicin.[264-268] The majority of patients respond to treatment, but relapses are common. Sustained remissions have been observed after anthracycline-containing combination chemotherapy regimens like CHOP, but only in a minority of patients.[269,270] A monoclonal antibody against IL-6 has demonstrated encouraging clinical efficacy in non-HIV patients with MCD, and warrants investigation in the setting of HIV infection.[207,271] Rituximab monotherapy has become increasingly used in MCD for several reasons. First, the B cell is clearly a target of KSHV/HHV8 and is involved in the pathologic process of MCD. Second, early reports of this rare tumor type indicate antitumor activity of rituximab even among patients who have failed more aggressive cytotoxic chemotherapies, and have been associated with an early decrease in viral DNA in peripheral blood and a decline in C-reactive protein and IL-6.[272-277] A prospective trial of rituximab monotherapy in 24 patients with chemotherapy-dependent MCD reported sustained remissions in 71% of patients after 1 year; responses to rituximab in patients previously treated with rituximab have been reported as well.[278,279] Given the efficacy and tolerability, rituximab have emerged as the preferred initial treatment of choice for MCD. There are, however, some reports of KS worsening with rituximab therapy of MCD, so caution must be used.[276]

The association of MCD with KSHV/HHV8 infection has led some to use antiviral medications with varying success. These agents are generally active only in the lytic phase of the viral life cycle, as opposed to the latent phase that characterizes KSHV/HHV8 infection in MCD, therefore, anti-herpesvirus medication can be endorsed only as an experimental approach at this time. There are reports of MCD responses after initiation of HAART, so this should be considered in all patients with HIV-associated MCD. In caring for patients with MCD, attention must also be paid to the high incidence of these patients ultimately developing full blown lymphoma. Either PBL or PEL may occur in these patients and are extremely difficult to treat.[280,281]

Hodgkin Lymphoma (HL)

Although not officially an AIDS-defining tumor, HL is increased in frequency in HIV-infected patients and has a number of unique characteristics distinguishing it from HL outside the context of AIDS.

Epidemiology

The risk of HL in patients infected with HIV-1 is estimated to be 2.5- to 8.5-fold above that of the uninfected population.[282,283] Several analyses of cancer registries have confirmed this increase, including a linkage analysis of cancers and AIDS surveillance data collected by registries in several regions of the United States.[284] A 7.6-fold increased risk of HL was observed in patients with AIDS. In Australia and Italy, similar types of analyses have indicated up to an 18.3-fold increase in the risk of HL. The risk of HL appears to be uniformly increased across the risk groups for HIV infection, independent of age or gender.[285] Notwithstanding the increase in relative risk in the HIV-infected population, the overall magnitude of the problem is still relatively small compared with that of NHL. Unlike most AIDS-associated NHL, the incidence of HL in HIV infection has actually increased since the introduction of HAART.[286] The cause of this surprising increase is speculative, but it may be due to the critical role host CD4 positive T-cell signaling plays in the microenvironment of HL. Indeed, HL is more likely to occur at moderately decreased CD4 counts than in the setting of severe immunodeficiency.

Pathology and Pathogenesis

HL in the context of HIV infection has pathologic features that distinguish it from the seronegative population. In particular, there is a much higher frequency of the mixed-cellularity subtype, with a corresponding reduction in the relative proportion of patients with nodular sclerosis histology.[224] The overall frequency of mixed-cellularity or lymphocyte-depleted histology was found to be two-thirds of the cases in the HIV-1–positive context compared with only 29% in uninfected patients.[287]

In addition, the presence of EBV in HL tissue is markedly increased in HIV-infected individuals. Estimates ranged from 80% to 100% in contrast to the HIV-negative population.[288-290] Of note, expression of the EBV LMP1, but not EBNA2, latency genes is in a type 2 pattern.[290] Thus, the EBV genome is identified with high frequency in HIV-infected HL and is considered likely to play an etiologic role.

In addition to the presence of EBV, there are other molecular characteristics of HL unique to the HIV-infected population. The transcription factor Bcl-6 expressed in germinal-center B cells, is present on Reed–Sternberg cells from both HIV-1-infected and uninfected individuals whereas, syndecan-1 (a proteoglycan associated with the post-terminal center) is restricted to the HIV-1–positive population.[291,292] Therefore, the postgerminal-center B cell may be the cell of origin in HIV-1–related HL, as opposed to the germinal-center cell of origin presumed to be the source of Reed–Sternberg cells in the uninfected population.

Clinical Features

HL in patients with HIV is typically of advanced stage and associated with B symptoms.[293] Stage III or IV disease has been documented in 91% of patients with HIV-associated HL at the time of diagnosis, as compared with 46% in HL patients without HIV.[132] Like ARL, the location of HL in the setting of HIV-1 infection is often extranodal, involving the bone marrow in up to 50% of patients.[294,295] Other sites include the tongue, rectum, skin, and lung,[293] and extra-nodal disease may be the site of presentation. Staging strategies should be the same as those in HL patients outside the context of HIV-1, with particular attention to possible microbiologic explanations for B symptoms.

Treatment

The clinical treatment approach to patients with HL in the setting of HIV infection is similar to that in other contexts, and radiation therapy, chemotherapy, or combined radiation and chemotherapy should be applied as appropriate for stage, similar to guidelines for treatment outside the setting of HIV infection.

Though pre-HAART outcomes of AIDS-associated HL were quite poor, with a median survival of less than 2 years,[296] modern treatment in the setting of antiretroviral therapy has shown encouraging rates of cure. Patients with advanced stage disease treated with standard Adriamycin (doxorubicin), bleomycin, vinblastine and dacarbazine (ABVD), and concomitant HAART were reported to achieve complete responses in 87% of cases with 5 year event-free and overall survivals of 71% and 76%, respectively.[297] Favorable outcomes have also been observed with the bleomycin, etoposide, Adriamycin (doxorubicin), cyclophosphamide, Oncovin (vincristine), procarbazine and prednisone (BEACOPP), and Stanford V (doxorubicin, vinblastine, mechlorethamine, etoposide, vincristine, bleomycin, prednisone, and radiotherapy) regimens, when given with concomitant HAART.[298,299]

The underlying level of immunosuppression and overall performance status of the patient must be considered before embarking on these therapies, and in general, prophylaxis for *Pneumocystis jiroveci* is recommended for all patients regardless of CD4 count. Treatment complications, including myelosuppression and opportunistic infections, may be expected to be more severe among patients with advanced AIDS; however, cure of HL is a realistic aim in the setting of HIV infection, and antitumor therapy dose reduction should be contemplated only in patients with advanced AIDS who have demonstrated intolerance to the standard-dose regimens.

Squamous Cell Neoplasia

The issue of human papillomavirus-related disease is an increasing concern in the HIV epidemic for several reasons, including (1) the increasing frequency of women infected by HIV, (2) the rampant progression of HIV disease in parts of the world where there is already a high incidence of cervical cancer and limited screening for cervical disease, and (3) the extension in overall survival of HIV-infected individuals. The nature of the abnormalities is fairly broad in scope and includes anogenital, conjunctival, oropharyngeal, and cutaneous neoplasia.

Epidemiology

The increased frequency of squamous cell neoplasia in HIV-infected individuals has been well documented, and has not decreased since the introduction of HAART.[300,301] The single AIDS-defining disease among the HPV-related tumors is that of invasive cervical carcinoma, though there is controversy as to whether this malignancy is increased in frequency in the setting of HIV infection. However, it is very clear that intraepithelial neoplasia of both the uterine cervix and the anus is increased. HIV-infected men who have sex with men have a particularly high incidence of squamous cell abnormalities and a markedly increased risk of anal cancer. Whether the incidence of invasive cancer is greater in the HIV-infected as compared with the HIV-seronegative cohort of men who have sex with men also remains controversial. Indirect evidence that immune suppression augments this cancer risk comes from an analysis of AIDS and cancer registries. In a retrospective study of more than 300,000 HIV patients, the incidence of in situ and invasive cancers was significantly higher in the 5 years following an AIDS-defining illness than in the 5 years preceding it.[300] Among women, cervical, vulvar/vaginal, and anal cancers were increased, while among men, anal, penile, tonsillar, and conjunctival cancers were increased.

Pathology and Pathogenesis

The association of specific subtypes of HPV with a potential for epidermal cell transformation has been long established, and the frequency of HPV-16, -18, and -19, is reported to be increased in HIV-infected individuals.[302] The frequency of multiple subtypes of HPV has also been assessed and found to be markedly increased in the HIV-infected population (73% of HIV-1–infected men who have sex with men, as compared with 23% of uninfected men).[302,303] The incidence of high-grade intraepithelial neoplasia of the anus has been estimated to be as high as 48% among HIV-1–positive men who have sex with men over a 4-year interval and was associated with the presence of multiple HPV subtypes, persistent anal infection, and high-level infection with oncogenic HPV subtypes.[304] Screening for intraepithelial neoplasia among HIV-1–infected men who have sex with men has demonstrated a prevalence of high-grade anal intraepithelial neoplasia (or carcinoma in situ [CIS]) of 36% compared with 7% of HIV-1–negative men who have sex with men.[305] Most often, these lesions on the anus and uterine cervix are not solitary sites but rather represent one of multiple areas of dysplasia and are therefore difficult to satisfactorily treat,[306] particularly on the anus. Patients with a history of high-grade intraepithelial neoplasia may often have recurrence following attempts at excision, cryotherapy, or topical treatment because of the ubiquitous nature of the HPV infection locally and the tendency of that virus to continue to have effects on local tissue.

A critical issue in evaluating the magnitude of this problem is the risk of progression of intraepithelial neoplasia to frank invasive cancer. This issue remains ill defined and highly controversial. If the risk is estimated at 1% or above, cost-benefit analyses have indicated that ongoing screening is justified.[307] The lack of large increases in the frequency of invasive anogenital cancer among HIV risk groups suggests that the risk is relatively small. However, the potential for frank invasion is not zero, and therefore, vigilance among patients with HIV disease is warranted.

The risk of some opportunistic neoplasms is clearly diminished in the context of aggressive therapy for HIV and suppression of HIV replication. There have been conflicting reports of whether HPV-related tumors are among those responsive to improved anti-HIV therapy. Some reports have indicated that some individuals may experience improvement in HPV-related neoplasia[308]; however, the bulk of data suggests that antiretroviral therapy has little impact on the incidence of dysplasia or invasive anal cancer.[309,310] At present, the complete suppression of HIV should not be regarded as fail-safe defense against the development of HPV-related tumors.

Clinical Presentation

HPV disease may present anywhere along the continuum of condyloma acuminatum to invasive anal cancer. Patients who have anal dysplasia may or may not have symptoms associated with it. Common practice with patients with a history of high-grade anal dysplasia is to perform an anoscopic examination and possible biopsy, even if the diagnostic lesion is on the anal verge, to assess for possible invasive disease out of the external examination field. Some centers are initiating anal Papanicolaou (Pap) evaluation for HIV-infected individuals, but this approach remains controversial. One study in 245 men found that 96% of anal Pap smears were interpretable with two-thirds of men screened having an abnormal cytology.[311] High-resolution anoscopy and biopsy demonstrated a positive predictive value of 96% for detection of anal dysplasia by cytologic screening. The clinical relevance of early cytologic detection is unclear, though early lesions may benefit from local therapy.

For women with HIV infection, the standard practices and recommendations for cervical screening are to be followed, with increased vigilance for those with severe immunosuppression. For HIV-infected women with CD4 counts of <200 cells/mm^3, the recommendation is for Pap smears to be performed semiannually.

Treatment

Treatment guidelines for dysplasia and carcinoma of the uterine cervix are well defined and should be followed in the setting of HIV infection. Management of anal disease is less clear.

High-grade intraepithelial neoplasia or CIS at the anal verge may be treated with topical imiquimod or 5-fluorouracil, while lesions in the anal canal may be treated with surgical excision, cryotherapy, or laser ablation. Given the ambiguity of risk for progression to frank invasive cancer, these lesions may be followed with vigilant monitoring alone. For patients with invasive carcinoma of the anus, treatment guidelines recommending a combination of chemotherapy and radiation therapy should be followed as in non-HIV infected individuals; this treatment has been reasonably well tolerated in the HIV-infected population.[312,313] There is a distinct increased sensitivity to mucosal injury with radiation in HIV disease, and, therefore, close interaction of the medical and radiation oncologist is essential. If patients have very advanced HIV disease failing antiretrovirals, a conservative approach to management of the malignancy may be warranted, but this requires case-by-case assessment.

Other Non-AIDS Defining Cancers

A number of other non-AIDS defining malignancies occur at a relatively increased risk in HIV-infected individuals; these include cancers of the lung, oropharynx, prostate, testes, and skin.[314-318] Among skin cancers, melanoma, basal cell, and squamous cell cancers all occur at increased rates. Merkel cell carcinoma (MCC) is a very rare neural-crest derived skin cancer that has also been shown to be increased in the setting of AIDS, as well as in solid organ transplant recipients.[319,320] Though generally a disease of the aged, MCC in immunosuppressed patients tends to occur at a significantly younger age and carries an aggressive natural history. The association of this rare skin cancer with immunosuppressed patients prompted a search for an underlying infectious pathogen, which recently resulted in the identification of a previously unknown polyomavirus, now called Merkel cell polyomavirus (MCV).[321] MCV DNA was found to be integrated into the tumor cell genome in the majority of MCCs but not in control tissues, and the pattern of integration suggested that infection preceded clonal expansion of the tumor cells. These data suggest a pivotal role for this novel polyomavirus in the pathogenesis of MCC, though the exact nature of this role has yet to be determined. Identification of the MCV highlights the potential role of other undiscovered viruses in immunosuppression-related malignancies where a pathogen has not yet been identified, and remains an area of ongoing investigation.

Selected References

The complete reference list can be found at www.CANCERMEDICINE8.com

7. Chang Y, Cesarman E, Pessin MS, et al. Identification of herpesvirus-like DNA sequences in AIDS-associated Kaposi's sarcoma. *Science*. 1994;266:1865–1869.
16. Biggar RJ, Chaturvedi AK, Goedert JJ, Engels EA. AIDS-related cancer and severity of immunosuppression in persons with AIDS. *J Natl Cancer Inst*. 2007;99:962–972.
22. Kirk O, Pedersen C, Cozzi-Lepri A, et al. Non-Hodgkin lymphoma in HIV-infected patients in the era of highly active antiretroviral therapy. *Blood*. 2001;98:3406–3412.
24. Besson C, Goubar A, Gabarre J, et al. Changes in AIDS-related lymphoma since the era of highly active antiretroviral therapy. *Blood*. 2001;98:2339–2344.
25. Kedes DH, Operskalski E, Busch M, Kohn R, Flood J, Ganem D. The seroepidemiology of human herpesvirus 8 (Kaposi's sarcoma- associated herpesvirus): distribution of infection in KS risk groups and evidence for sexual transmission [published erratum appears in *Nat Med* 1996 Sep;2(9):1041]. *Nat Med*. 1996;2:918–924.
38. Krown SE, Testa MA, Huang J. AIDS-related Kaposi's sarcoma: prospective validation of the AIDS Clinical Trials Group staging classification. AIDS Clinical Trials Group Oncology Committee. *J Clin Oncol*. 1997;15:3085–3092.
39. Nasti G, Talamini R, Antinori A, et al. AIDS-related Kaposi's Sarcoma: evaluation of potential new prognostic factors and assessment of the AIDS Clinical Trial Group Staging System in the Haart Era J Virol the Italian Cooperative Group on AIDS and Tumors and the Italian Cohort of Patients Naive From Antiretrovirals. *J Clin Oncol*. 2003;21:2876–2882.
40. Stebbing J, Sanitt A, Nelson M, Powles T, Gazzard B, Bower M. A prognostic index for AIDS-associated Kaposi's sarcoma in the era of highly active antiretroviral therapy. *Lancet*. 2006;367:1495–1502.
78. Ramirez-Amador V, Esquivel-Pedraza L, Lozada-Nur F, et al. Intralesional vinblastine vs. 3% sodium tetradecyl sulfate for the treatment of oral Kaposi's sarcoma. A double blind, randomized clinical trial. *Oral Oncol*. 2002;38:460–467.
79. Bodsworth NJ, Bloch M, Bower M, Donnell D, Yocum R. Phase III vehicle-controlled, multi-centered study of topical alitretinoin gel 0.1% in cutaneous AIDS-related Kaposi's sarcoma. *Am J Clin Dermatol*. 2001;2:77–87.
83. Kigula-Mugambe JB, Kavuma A. Epidemic and endemic Kaposi's sarcoma: a comparison of outcomes and survival after radiotherapy. *Radiother Oncol*. 2005;76:59–62.
84. Harrison M, Harrington KJ, Tomlinson DR, Stewart JS. Response and cosmetic outcome of two fractionation regimens for AIDS- related Kaposi's sarcoma. *Radiother Oncol*. 1998;46:23–28.
92. Northfelt DW, Dezube BJ, Thommes JA, et al. Pegylated-liposomal doxorubicin versus doxorubicin, bleomycin, and vincristine in the treatment of AIDS-related Kaposi's sarcoma: results of a randomized phase III clinical trial. *J Clin Oncol*. 1998;16:2445–2451.
93. Stewart S, Jablonowski H, Goebel FD, et al. Randomized comparative trial of pegylated liposomal doxorubicin versus bleomycin and vincristine in the treatment of AIDS-related Kaposi's sarcoma. International Pegylated Liposomal Doxorubicin Study Group. *J Clin Oncol*. 1998;16:683–691.
97. Gill P, Tulpule A, Espina B, et al. Paclitaxel is safe and effective in the treatment of advanced AIDS-related Kaposi's sarcoma. *J Clin Oncol*. 1999;17:1876–1883.
101. Little RF, Wyvill KM, Pluda JM, et al. Activity of thalidomide in AIDS-related Kaposi's sarcoma. *J Clin Oncol*. 2000;18:2593–2602.
104. Stallone G, Schena A, Infante B, et al. Sirolimus for Kaposi's sarcoma in renal-transplant recipients. *N Engl J Med*. 2005;352:1317–1323.
123. Arzoo KK, Bu X, Espina BM, Seneviratne L, Nathwani B, Levine AM. T-cell lymphoma in HIV-infected patients. *J Acquir Immune Defic Syndr*. 2004;36:1020–1027.
142. Carbone A, Gloghini A. AIDS-related lymphomas: from pathogenesis to pathology. *Br J Haematol*. 2005;130:662–670.
189. Nador RG, Cesarman E, Chadburn A, et al. Primary effusion lymphoma: a distinct clinicopathologic entity associated with the Kaposi's sarcoma-associated herpes virus. *Blood*. 1996;88:645–656.
192. Delecluse HJ, Anagnostopoulos I, Dallenbach F, et al. Plasmablastic lymphomas of the oral cavity: a new entity associated with the human immunodeficiency virus infection. *Blood*. 1997;89:1413–1420.
198. Oksenhendler E, Duarte M, Soulier J, et al. Multicentric Castleman's disease in HIV infection: a clinical and pathological study of 20 patients. *AIDS*. 1996;10:61–67.
207. Nishimoto N, Kanakura Y, Aozasa K, et al. Humanized anti-interleukin-6 receptor antibody treatment of multicentric Castleman disease. *Blood*. 2005;106:2627–2632.
208. Lim ST, Karim R, Tulpule A, Nathwani BN, Levine AM. Prognostic factors in HIV-related diffuse large-cell lymphoma: before versus after highly active antiretroviral therapy. *J Clin Oncol*. 2005;23:8477–8482.
209. Straus DJ, Huang J, Testa MA, Levine AM, Kaplan LD. Prognostic factors in the treatment of human immunodeficiency virus-associated non-Hodgkin's lymphoma: analysis of AIDS Clinical Trials Group protocol 142-low-dose versus standard-dose m-BACOD plus granulocyte-macrophage colony-stimulating factor. National Institute of Allergy and Infectious Diseases. *J Clin Oncol*. 1998;16:3601–3606.
212. Lim ST, Karim R, Nathwani BN, Tulpule A, Espina B, Levine AM. AIDS-related Burkitt's lymphoma versus diffuse large-cell lymphoma in the pre-highly active antiretroviral therapy (HAART) and HAART eras: significant differences in survival with standard chemotherapy. *J Clin Oncol*. 2005;23:4430–4438.
214. Hoffmann C, Tiemann M. Schrader C, et al. Blood. 2005;106:1762–1769.
219. Mounier N, Spina M, Gabarre J, et al. AIDS-related non-Hodgkin lymphoma: final analysis of 485 patients treated with risk-adapted intensive chemotherapy. *Blood*. 2006;107:3832–3840.
220. Ratner L, Lee J, Tang S, et al. Chemotherapy for human immunodeficiency virus-associated non-Hodgkin's lymphoma

in combination with highly active antiretroviral therapy. *J Clin Oncol.* 2001;19: 2171–2178.

221. Little RF, Pittaluga S, Grant N, et al. Highly effective treatment of acquired immunodeficiency syndrome-related lymphoma with dose-adjusted EPOCH: impact of antiretroviral therapy suspension and tumor biology. *Blood.* 2003;101:4653–4659.
224. Kaplan LD, Lee JY, Ambinder RF, et al. Rituximab does not improve clinical outcome in a randomized phase 3 trial of CHOP with or without rituximab in patients with HIV-associated non-Hodgkin lymphoma: AIDS-Malignancies Consortium Trial 010. *Blood.* 2005;106:1538–1543.
229. Re A, Cattaneo C, Michieli M, et al. High-dose therapy and autologous peripheral-blood stem-cell transplantation as salvage treatment for HIV-associated lymphoma in patients receiving highly active antiretroviral therapy. *J Clin Oncol.* 2003;21:4423–4427.
251. Cingolani A, De Luca A, Larocca LM, et al. Minimally invasive diagnosis of acquired immunodeficiency syndrome-related primary central nervous system lymphoma. *J Natl Cancer Inst.* 1998;90:364–369.
255. Baumgartner JE, Rachlin JR, Beckstead JH, et al. Primary central nervous system lymphomas: natural history and response to radiation therapy in 55 patients with acquired immunodeficiency syndrome. *J Neurosurg.* 1990;73:206–211.
257. Hoffmann C, Tabrizian S, Wolf E, et al. Survival of AIDS patients with primary central nervous system lymphoma is dramatically improved by HAART-induced immune recovery. *AIDS.* 2001;15:2119–2127.
258. Jacomet C, Girard PM, Lebrette MG, Farese VL, Monfort L, Rozenbaum W. Intravenous methotrexate for primary central nervous system non-Hodgkin's lymphoma in AIDS. *AIDS.* 1997;11:1725–1730.
269. Chronowski GM, Ha CS, Wilder RB, Cabanillas F, Manning J, Cox JD. Treatment of unicentric and multicentric Castleman disease and the role of radiotherapy. *Cancer.* 2001;92:670–676.
278. Gerard L, Berezne A, Galicier L, et al. Prospective study of rituximab in chemotherapy-dependent human immunodeficiency virus associated multicentric Castleman's disease: ANRS 117 CastlemaB Trial. *J Clin Oncol.* 2007;25:3350–3356.
285. Franceschi S, Dal Maso L, Arniani S, et al. Risk of cancer other than Kaposi's sarcoma and non-Hodgkin's lymphoma in persons with AIDS in Italy. Cancer and AIDS Registry Linkage Study. *Br J Cancer.* 1998;78:966–970.
286. Biggar RJ, Jaffe ES, Goedert JJ, Chaturvedi A, Pfeiffer R, Engels EA. Hodgkin lymphoma and immunodeficiency in persons with HIV/AIDS. *Blood.* 2006;108: 3786–3791.
297. Xicoy B, Ribera JM, Miralles P, et al. Results of treatment with doxorubicin, bleomycin, vinblastine and dacarbazine and highly active antiretroviral therapy in advanced stage, human immunodeficiency virus-related Hodgkin's lymphoma. *Haematologica.* 2007;92:191–198.
300. Frisch M, Biggar R, Goedert J. Human papillomavirus-associated cancers in patient with human immunodeficiency virus infection and acquired immunodeficiency syndrome. *J Nat Can Inst.* 2000;92:1500–1510.
301. Palefsky JM, Holly EA, Efirdc JT, et al. Anal intraepithelial neoplasia in the highly active antiretroviral therapy era among HIV-positive men who have sex with men. *AIDS.* 2005;19:1407–1414.
308. Heard I, Schmitz V, Costagliola D, Orth G, Kazatchkine MD. Early regression of cervical lesions in HIV-seropositive women receiving highly active antiretroviral therapy. *AIDS.* 1998;12:1459–1464.
311. Cranston RD, Hart SD, Gornbein JA, Hirschowitz SL, Cortina G, Moe AA. The prevalence, and predictive value, of abnormal anal cytology to diagnose anal dysplasia in a population of HIV-positive men who have sex with men. *Int J STD AIDS.* 2007;18:77–80.
313. Peddada AV, Smith DE, Rao AR, Frost DB, Kagan AR. Chemotherapy and low-dose radiotherapy in the treatment of HIV-infected patients with carcinoma of the anal canal. *Int J Radiat Oncol Biol Phys.* 1997;37:1101–1105.
314. Burgi A, Brodine S, Wegner S, et al. Incidence and risk factors for the occurrence of non-AIDS-defining cancers among human immunodeficiency virus-infected individuals. *Cancer.* 2005;104: 1505–1511.
315. Clifford GM, Polesel J, Rickenbach M, et al. Cancer risk in the Swiss HIV Cohort Study: associations with immunodeficiency, smoking, and highly active antiretroviral therapy. *J Natl Cancer Inst.* 2005;97:425–432.
316. Engels EA, Brock MV, Chen J, Hooker CM, Gillison M, Moore RD. Elevated incidence of lung cancer among HIV-infected individuals. *J Clin Oncol.* 2006;24: 1383–1388.
317. Engels EA, Pfeiffer RM, Goedert JJ, et al. Trends in cancer risk among people with AIDS in the United States 1980–2002. *AIDS.* 2006;20:1645–1654.

120 Neoplasms of Unknown Primary Site

John D. Hainsworth, MD ■ F. Anthony Greco, MD

Cancer of unknown primary site is a common clinical entity, accounting for 2% of all cancer diagnoses in the Surveillance, Epidemiology, and End Results (SEER) registries.[1] In spite of the frequency of this syndrome, relatively little attention has been given to this group of patients, and systematic study of the entity has lagged behind that of other areas in oncology. Widespread pessimism concerning the therapy and prognosis of these patients has been the major reason for the lack of effort in this area. The patient with carcinoma of unknown primary site is commonly stereotyped as an aged, debilitated individual with metastases at multiple visceral sites. Early attempts at systemic therapy yielded low response rates and had a negligible effect on survival, thereby strengthening arguments for a nihilistic approach to these patients. The heterogeneity of this group has also made the design of therapeutic studies difficult; it is well recognized that cancers with different biologies from many primary sites are represented.

Several treatable subgroups of patients within this heterogeneous group have been characterized, and initial identification of these patients is imperative for optimal management. Treatable subsets of patients are recognized either on the basis of specific clinical presentations, or by the use of specialized pathologic techniques that aid in tumor characterization. Empiric chemotherapy for patients who do not fit into any of the specific subsets has also improved, and a trial of therapy should be considered for all patients with good performance status.

The typical patient with cancer of unknown primary site develops symptoms at a metastatic site, but routine history, physical examination, chest radiography, and laboratory studies fail to identify the primary site. The initial light microscopic diagnosis usually identifies one of four histologies and should be used as the initial guideline for further evaluation of these patients. These four light microscopic diagnoses include poorly differentiated neoplasm, adenocarcinoma, squamous cell carcinoma, and poorly differentiated carcinoma. These four groups are discussed separately, because they vary with respect to clinical characteristics, recommended diagnostic evaluation, treatment, and prognosis.

Poorly Differentiated Neoplasms

The diagnosis of poorly differentiated neoplasm implies the inability of the pathologist to distinguish between carcinoma and other cancers, such as lymphoma, melanoma, and sarcoma. Establishing a more precise diagnosis is essential in this group of patients, because highly treatable cancers are common. The most frequent tumor for which specific, highly effective therapy is available is non-Hodgkin lymphoma (NHL); in reported series, 34-66% of poorly differentiated neoplasms were found to be lymphomas after further pathologic evaluation.[2-4] A second important and potentially treatable group comprises of patients with poorly differentiated neuroendocrine carcinoma, accounting for another 10-15% of this group. Most of the remaining patients have poorly differentiated carcinoma; other tumors, including melanoma and sarcoma, and collectively account for less than 15% of all cases.

The evaluation of the poorly differentiated neoplasm requires specialized pathologic studies. Immunoperoxidase staining, electron microscopy, and chromosomal analysis are techniques of proved value in the differential diagnosis of these tumors. However, it is important to remember that an inadequate biopsy specimen is a common cause of a nonspecific light microscopic diagnosis. Fine-needle aspiration (FNA) biopsy provides adequate amounts of tissue for definitive diagnosis of differentiated tumors (eg, squamous carcinoma, adenocarcinoma), but is frequently inadequate for definitive characterization of poorly differentiated cancers.[5] When recognition of a tumor's pattern of growth or the ability to perform special studies is limited by a FNA specimen's small size, a specific diagnosis can often be made simply by obtaining a larger biopsy. Close communication with the surgeon and the pathologist is important if repeat biopsy is performed, because some pathologic studies require special tissue processing. Some neoplasms remain unclassifiable by light microscopy, however, even with an adequate biopsy specimen; in these cases, additional evaluation is essential.

Immunoperoxidase Staining

Immunoperoxidase staining is the most widely available adjunctive tool for the classification of neoplasms. In contrast to most other pathologic techniques, immunoperoxidase staining can be performed on formalin-fixed, paraffinized tissue, which broadens its applicability. Immunoperoxidase methods use monoclonal or polyclonal antibodies directed at specific cell components or products, which can include enzymes (eg, prostatic acid phosphatase, neuron-specific enolase), intermediate filaments and other normal tissue components (eg, keratin, desmin, vimentin, neurofilaments, common leucocyte antigen), hormones (eg, chorionic gonadotropin), oncofetal antigens (eg, alpha-fetoprotein, carcinoembryonic antigen), and other tumor markers (eg, S-100 protein). Specific diagnoses cannot be made on the basis of immunoperoxidase staining alone, because none of these reagents are directed at tumor-specific antigens. Therefore, results must be interpreted in conjunction with the light microscopic appearance. At times, clinical features can also be used to support a diagnosis. Clinical information (eg, gender, age, location of metastases and symptoms) may help the pathologist narrow the differential diagnosis, thereby reducing the number of special stains required to reach a diagnosis.

Specific staining patterns associated with several types of neoplasms are summarized in Table 120-1. In the evaluation of poorly differentiated neoplasms, several important questions can usually be answered by immunoperoxidase staining. First, and most important, these stains can be used to make the distinction between lymphoma and carcinoma.[6-8] Second, staining for chromogranin or synaptophysin can suggest a neuroendocrine carcinoma (eg, small cell lung cancer, carcinoid, islet cell tumor).[9] Third, staining for prostate-specific antigen (PSA) strongly suggests prostate carcinoma in a male patient with metastatic adenocarcinoma.[10] Fourth, certain staining characteristics can suggest amelanotic melanoma (positive staining for S-100 protein, Hmb-45 antigen, and vimentin) or sarcoma (positive staining for desmin, vimentin, or factor VIII antigen).[11,12]

Several potential problems must be recognized when interpreting immunoperoxidase stains. Considerable technical expertise is required to perform these tests accurately and reproducibly, and proper interpretation requires an experienced pathologist. In addition, care

Table 120-1 **Examples of Immunoperoxidase Staining Patterns Useful in the Differential Diagnosis of Poorly Differentiated Neoplasms**

Tumor Type	Cyto-keratin	Epithelial Membrane Antigen	Leukocyte Common Antigen	S-100 Protein	Vimentin	Human Chorionic Gonado-trophin	α-Feto-protein	Prostate-Specific Antigen	Estrogen/Proges-terone Receptor	Desmin	Factor VIII Antigen	Chromo-granin/Synapto-physin
Carcinoma	+	+[a]	–	–	–	±	±	±	±	–	–	±
Lymphoma	–	±[b]	+	–	–	–	–	–	–	–	–	–
Melanoma	–	–	–	+	+	–	–	–	–	–	–	–
Sarcoma	–	±[c]	–	–	+	–	–	–	–	+[d]	+[e]	–
Neuroendo-crine tumor	+	+	–	–	–	–	–	–	–	–	–	+
Germ cell tumor	+	+	–	–	–	+	±	–	–	–	–	–
Prostate cancer	+	+	–	–	–	–	–	+	–	–	–	–
Breast cancer	+	+	–	–	–	–	–	–	+	–	–	–

[a]Adenocarcinoma; [b]anaplastic large cell lymphoma (Ki-1 or CD30-positive lymphoma); [c]epithelioid sarcoma, synovial sarcoma; [d]leiomyosarcoma, rhabdomyosarcoma; [e]angiosarcoma.

must be taken to avoid overinterpretation, because no staining pattern is entirely specific. Certain stains, particularly leukocyte common antigen and PSA, are quite specific; however, false-positive or false-negative staining is more frequent with most of the other stains.

Some data now exist to verify that diagnoses based on immunoperoxidase staining in patients with poorly differentiated neoplasms can be used to plan therapy and predict outcome. Undifferentiated neoplasms that are identified as lymphoma on the basis of positive leukocyte common antigen staining respond well to the combination chemotherapy treatments used for aggressive NHL.[4] In a group of 35 such patients, treatment with a variety of standard lymphoma regimens resulted in an actuarial disease-free survival of 45% at 30 months. This treatment outcome was similar to that for a group of concurrently treated patients who had aggressive lymphomas with typical histology (ie, diagnosed by light microscopy). On the basis of this evidence, aggressive NHLs can be reliably identified using immunoperoxidase staining, and specific treatment can be administered with confidence to these patients. In addition to lymphoma, immunoperoxidase staining can identify patients with poorly differentiated neuroendocrine carcinoma. This group of patients has a high response rate to first-line chemotherapy, similar to patients with other high-grade neuroendocrine tumors (eg, small-cell lung cancer).[13] Limited data exist concerning the treatment of poorly differentiated neoplasms given other diagnoses on the basis of immunoperoxidase staining (see "Poorly Differentiated Carcinoma of Unknown Primary Site").

Electron Microscopy

The identification of specific ultrastructural features by electron microscopy enables a definitive diagnosis in some poorly differentiated neoplasms. Because it is less widely available, requires special tissue fixation at the time of biopsy or rebiopsy, and is relatively expensive, electron microscopy should be reserved for the study of neoplasms whose lineage is unclear after routine light microscopy and immunoperoxidase staining. Like immunoperoxidase staining, electron microscopy is extremely reliable in distinguishing lymphoma from carcinoma and is probably superior in the identification of poorly differentiated sarcoma. Other specific structures, such as neurosecretory granules (neuroendocrine tumors) or premelanosomes (melanoma), are also seen in some poorly differentiated neoplasms and allow specific diagnoses to be made. However, undifferentiated tumors often lose specific ultrastructural features in addition to typical histology; therefore, the absence of a particular ultrastructural finding cannot be used to rule out a specific diagnosis.

In some cases, electron microscopy provides evidence for adenocarcinoma or squamous cell carcinoma. Features of adenocarcinoma include intercellular and intracellular lumina and surface microvilli. Squamous cell carcinomas are characterized by frequent and prominent desmosomes and prominent bundles of prekeratin filaments in the adjacent cytoplasm. It is impossible, however, to pinpoint the origin of poorly differentiated adenocarcinoma or squamous carcinoma by electron microscopic features. Treatment implications for adenocarcinoma and squamous cell carcinoma diagnosed only by ultrastructural features are currently unclear (see "Adenocarcinoma of Unknown Primary Site").

Molecular Genetic Analysis

Tumor-Specific Chromosomal Abnormalities

The analysis of chromosomal abnormalities associated with neoplasms is increasingly important in diagnosis, prognosis, and treatment. Several tumor-specific chromosal abnormalities are occasionally important in the diagnosis of unknown primary cancer. Most B-cell and T-cell NHLs are associated with detectable tumor-specific rearrangements of immunoglobulin genes or T-cell antigen-receptor genes.[14] In the unusual case when the diagnosis of lymphoma cannot be definitively established with either immunoperoxidase staining or flow cytometric immunophenotyping, the detection of these specific gene rearrangements provides definitive diagnostic information. Specific abnormalities associated with solid tumors include a chromosomal translocation (rcp [11:22] [q 24; q 12]) found in all peripheral neuroepitheliomas and most Ewing tumors,[15,16] and an isochromosome of the short arm of chromosome 12 (i12p) found in a large percentage of testicular and extragonadal germ cell tumors in men.[17]

The clinical relevance of molecular and cytogenetic studies in identifying treatable neoplasms has been studied in young patients with poorly differentiated carcinoma or adenocarcinoma involving primarily midline structures or having elevated serum levels of human chorionic gonadotropin (hCG) or alpha-fetoprotein.[18] Specific diagnoses were suggested by genetic studies in 17 of 40 patients (42%): germ cell tumor (12); melanoma (2); lymphoma (1); peripheral neuroepithelioma (1); and desmoplastic small-cell tumor (1). Patients with the diagnosis of germ cell tumor had 75% overall and 45% complete response rates to cisplatin-based therapy, as compared with 17% and 0% overall and complete response rates in the remaining patients.[18] The diagnosis of germ cell tumor based on typical cytogenetic abnormalities, therefore, accurately identifies patients with highly responsive neoplasms. The recent development of a comparative genomic hybridization technique that can detect extra 12p material using paraffin-embedded tissue specimens may make this procedure more clinically applicable, by avoiding the need to obtain fresh tissue by repeat biopsy.[19] Likewise, fluorescence in situ hybridization (FISH) can be applied to fresh or paraffin-embedded tissue for detecting translations and gain or loss of specific chromosomes.

Molecular Profiling

Gene expression profiles specific to the tissue of origin have been identified for many tumor types. Identification of key tissue type-specific gene markers has allowed development of several multigene assays for the purpose of identifying the tissue of origin in patients with tumors of unknown primary site.[20-23] When applied in metastatic tumor tissue from patients with advanced cancers of known primary, these molecular assays correctly identified the tissue of origin in 78-85%.[21-23]

At present, there is limited validation of these molecular assays in patients with cancer of unknown primary site. In a retrospective study of 104 patients with carcinoma of unknown primary site, a 10-gene RT-PCR assay assigned a positive tissue of origin in 61%.[24] In general, the clinical features and response to treatment were consistent with the molecular assay diagnosis. However, the use of the molecular assay diagnosis to guide therapeutic decisions has not been evaluated. Although molecular profiling appears to offer great promise in diagnosis, prospective studies are necessary before this procedure can be recommended as part of routine patient management.

Adenocarcinoma of Unknown Primary Site

Clinical Characteristics

Adenocarcinoma is the most frequent light microscopic diagnosis in patients with neoplasms of unknown primary site and accounts for approximately 70% of cases. The incidence of this diagnosis increases with age; most patients have metastatic tumor at more than one site. The clinical presentation is determined by the sites of tumor involvement, which frequently include the liver, lungs, nodes, and bones.

The clinical course is usually dominated by symptoms related to the sites of metastases. During the clinical course, the primary site becomes obvious in only 15-20% of patients.[25] Even at autopsy, 20-30% of patients have no primary site detected. Unfortunately, large autopsy series in patients evaluated with modern radiologic techniques (eg, CT) are not available; therefore, the primary sites detected may not accurately represent the current patient population. The most common primary sites identified in historical autopsy series included the pancreas, hepatobiliary tree, and lung, accounting for approximately 40-50% of all cases.[26,27] Other gastrointestinal sites were also frequent, and adenocarcinomas from a wide variety of other primary sites were occasionally encountered. Adenocarcinomas of the breast and prostate were identified infrequently in this group of patients, in spite of being common cancer types.[27]

Many patients with adenocarcinoma of unknown primary site have widespread metastases and poor performance status at the time of diagnosis. The outlook for most of these patients is poor, with median survival of 4 months to 6 months. However, subsets of patients with a much more favorable outlook are contained within this large group, and optimal initial evaluation enables the identification of these treatable subsets. In addition, empiric chemotherapy incorporating newer agents has produced higher response rates and probably improves the survival of patients with good performance status.

Pathology

The light microscopic diagnosis of adenocarcinoma is usually made without difficulty based on the formation of glandular structures by neoplastic cells. Because this histologic feature is shared by most adenocarcinomas, the site of the primary adenocarcinoma cannot usually be ascertained by routine histologic examination. Certain histologic features are typically associated with a particular tumor type ("papillary features" with ovarian and thyroid cancer, "signet ring cells" with gastric cancer); however, even these are not specific enough to be used as definitive evidence of the primary site. Immunoperoxidase stains are also of limited utility in identifying the site of origin of most adenocarcinomas. One exception is the stain for PSA, which is quite specific for prostate cancer and should be included in the evaluation of men with adenocarcinoma of unknown primary site. Positive immunoperoxidase staining for estrogen receptor suggests metastatic breast cancer in women with metastatic adenocarcinoma. Other "tumor-specific" immunoperoxidase stains (eg, CK20+/CK7- or CDX2 for colon cancer; TTF-1 for lung cancer) can be used to direct diagnostic evaluation, but are not specific enough to guide therapy.[28-30]

The diagnosis of poorly differentiated adenocarcinoma should be interpreted with caution, since criteria for this diagnosis may vary among pathologists. Additional pathologic evaluation with immunoperoxidase staining should be performed. Evaluation and treatment of patients with poorly differentiated adenocarcinoma should follow the guidelines outlined for poorly differentiated carcinoma (see "Poorly Differential Carcinoma of Unknown Primary Site").

The identification of increasing numbers of oncoproteins that define the malignant phenotype and are prognostically important marks an emerging focus in the characterization of tumors. Some of these substances (eg, epidermal growth factor receptor [EGFR], HER-2 receptor) are now targets for novel therapeutic agents. Although information is currently limited in unknown primary cancer, a substantial percentage of these tumors overexpress p53, Bcl-2, Cmyc, Ras, and EGFR.[31,32] Overexpression of HER-2 is less common: in a group of 94 patients with poorly differentiated carcinoma or poorly differentiated adenocarcinoma, only 10 patients (11%) had 27 or 37 HER-2 staining by using communopreoxidase methods.[33] The value of these markers in predicting prognosis or determining therapy is currently undefined.

Diagnostic Evaluation

The detection of a primary site is unusual in a patient presenting with adenocarcinoma of unknown primary site; initial staging evaluation, therefore, should be performed to evaluate any clinical signs or symptoms and to determine the extent of metastatic disease. Routine initial evaluation should include a thorough history and physical examination (including pelvic examination in women), standard laboratory screening tests (complete blood count, channel biochemistry profile, urinalysis, stool examination for occult blood), and chest radiography. All men should have a serum PSA determination, and women with a clinical presentation compatible with metastatic breast cancer should undergo mammography, because palliative therapy is available for patients with advanced prostate or breast cancer. CT of the abdomen can identify a primary site in 10-35% of patients; in addition, it is frequently useful in identifying additional sites of metastatic disease.[34,35] Positron emission tomography (PET) identifies a primary site in approximately 30% of patients, and is therefore a useful diagnostic procedure.[36] Additional signs or symptoms should be evaluated with appropriate radiologic studies. Extensive radiologic evaluation of asymptomatic areas is rarely useful in identifying a primary site and often results in confusing or false-positive information. Colonoscopy should be considered in patients with intra-abdominal metastases and suggestive pathologic findings (eg, CK20+/CK7- or CDX2+ staining). Otherwise, endoscopy of the stomach and colon is of low yield in asymptomatic patients, although small, occult primary sites are occasionally identified. Commonly used tumor markers (carcinoembryonic antigen [CEA], cancer antigen [CA] 19-9, CA 15- 3, CA 125, hCG, α-fetoprotein) are not useful as diagnostic or prognostic tests; however, they are commonly elevated and may be useful in monitoring response to therapy.[37,38]

Treatment

The group of patients with adenocarcinoma of unknown primary site contains several clinically defined subgroups for which specific therapy is available. Patients who do not fit into one of these subgroups should be considered for a trial of empiric chemotherapy.

Women With Peritoneal Carcinomatosis ■ In women, adenocarcinoma causing diffuse peritoneal involvement usually originates in the ovary, although carcinomas arising in the gastrointestinal tract or breast can occasionally produce this syndrome. However, peritoneal carcinomatosis also occurs in women with normal ovaries and no other evident intra-abdominal primary site. This syndrome has occasionally developed in women from families at high risk for ovarian cancer despite prophylactic oophorectomy,[39] and is increased in incidence in women with BRCA1 mutations.[40] Many of these patients have histologic features typical of ovarian carcinoma, such as papillary configuration or psammoma bodies. Clinical features are typical of advanced ovarian cancer, with tumor involvement limited to the peritoneal surfaces and elevated serum levels of CA 125 antigen. When histologic features suggest ovarian carcinoma, this syndrome has been termed "multifocal extraovarian serous carcinoma" or "peritoneal papillary serous carcinoma." Occasionally, men with peritoneal carcinomatosis, papillary adenocarcinoma, and elevated serum CA 125 levels have also been reported.[41]

Patients with this syndrome often respond well to the chemotherapy regimens effective in the treatment of advanced ovarian carcinoma. Several investigators documented initial response rates of 39-66%, with long-term remissions in 15-20% of patients.[42-47] In the early series, most patients received cisplatin and cyclophosphamide; however, subsequent reports documented the activity of platinum/paclitaxel regimens.[47] As in ovarian cancer, most long-term remissions have been observed in patients who had successful surgical cytoreduction prior to receiving chemotherapy.

The peritoneal epithelium is now accepted as a site of origin for some of these carcinomas. The contiguity of the peritoneal and ovarian epithelial surfaces may explain the similar biology and response to treatment observed in these two tumor types. In fact, these tumors are now thought to be similar enough that women with peritoneal papillary serous carcinoma are routinely included in clinical trials for stage III ovarian carcinoma. Optimal management of women with peritoneal carcinomatosis should therefore include initial maximal surgical cytoreduction followed by taxane/platinum chemotherapy.[48,49] Some patients in this group can be expected to have a complete response to therapy, and a minority will have a prolonged disease-free survival.

Women With Axillary Lymph Node Metastases ■ Metastatic breast cancer should be suspected in women who have axillary lymph node involvement with adenocarcinoma.[50] Breast MRI scanning can identify a primary site even when mammography is normal, and should be performed.[51,52] PET scanning may also be a useful procedure, but further evaluation is required.[53] Initial lymph node biopsy should include measurement of estrogen and progesterone receptors and HER-2; elevated levels provide strong evidence for the diagnosis of breast cancer.[47]

Women who have metastases isolated to axillary lymph nodes after completion of routine staging evaluation are potentially curable and should be managed according to standard guidelines for stage II breast cancer. Primary therapy should include either modified radical mastectomy or axillary lymph node dissection followed by radiation therapy to the breast.[54-56] When mastectomy is performed, an occult breast cancer is identified in 44-82% of patients, even when physical examination and mammograms are normal.[55] Primary tumors are usually less than 2 cm in diameter; in occasional patients, only carcinoma in situ is identified in the breast.[57] Axillary dissection alone is not recommended, because primary breast tumors will subsequently become manifest in approximately 50% of patients.[54-56] Selection of adjuvant therapy should also follow standard guidelines for patients with node-positive breast cancer.

Women with metastatic sites in addition to axillary lymph nodes may also have metastatic breast cancer. These women should receive a trial of systemic therapy using the guidelines for the treatment of metastatic breast cancer. Determination of estrogen receptor status is of particular importance in these patients, because those with positive estrogen receptors may derive major palliative benefit from hormonal therapy. Testing for overexpression of the HER-2 gene using FISH techniques defines a group who are likely to benefit from treatment with trastuzumab.[58]

Men With Skeletal Metastases ■ Metastatic prostate carcinoma should be suspected in men with adenocarcinoma predominantly involving bone, particularly if the metastases are blastic. Elevated serum levels of PSA or tumor staining with PSA provides confirmatory evidence of prostate cancer in this clinical setting, and treatment should follow guidelines for advanced prostate cancer.

Occasionally, patients have been reported with clinical presentations atypical for prostate cancer, in whom the diagnosis was suggested either by elevated serum PSA levels or by tumor staining for PSA.[59,60] These patients usually presented with metastases to the lung, mediastinal lymph nodes, or upper abdominal lymph nodes, with no concomitant involvement of bone or pelvic lymph nodes. Even in the absence of a demonstrable primary tumor in the prostate, initial treatment should include androgen deprivation therapy, according to treatment guidelines for advanced prostate cancer.

Most men with adenocarcinoma of unknown primary site and bone involvement have lytic lesions and normal serum PSA levels. Such patients are unlikely to respond to androgen deprivation therapy; potential occult primary sites include lung, kidney, colon, and thyroid. A trial of empiric chemotherapy should be considered (see "Empiric Chemotherapy for Adenocarcinoma of Unknown Primary Site").

Adenocarcinoma Presenting as a Single Metastatic Lesion ■ Occasionally, only a single metastatic lesion can be identified after a complete staging evaluation. Such single lesions have been described in a variety of sites, including lymph nodes, brain, lung, adrenal gland, liver, bone, and skin. The possibility of an unusual primary site (eg, primary cutaneous apocrine, eccrine, or sebaceous carcinoma) mimicking a metastatic lesion should be considered, but this possibility can usually be excluded on the basis of clinical or pathologic features.

In most of these patients, other metastatic sites become evident within a relatively short time. However, local treatment sometimes results in long disease-free intervals, and occasional patients have prolonged survival. Prior to initiating local treatment, a PET scan is useful to rule out the presence of other metastatic sites.[61] If no other metastases are detectable, resection of the solitary lesion should be undertaken, if technically feasible. In some instances (eg, after resection of a solitary brain metastasis), local radiation therapy may also be appropriate to maximize the chance of local control.[62] The role of systemic chemotherapy in addition to definitive local therapy is undefined; however, patients with poorly differentiated adenocarcinoma may benefit from platinum-based therapy (see "Poorly Differentiated Carcinoma of Unknown Primary Site").

Empiric Chemotherapy for Adenocarcinoma of Unknown Primary Site ■ Most patients with adenocarcinoma of unknown primary site do not fit into any of the specific clinical subgroups outlined above. Empiric chemotherapy with 5-fluorouracil (5-FU) or doxorubicin-based regimens developed for the treatment of gastrointestinal primary tumors produced relatively low response rates and few complete responses. Various cisplatin-based regimens have also been evaluated, but were more toxic and showed no greater efficacy than other non-cisplatin-containing treatments. Table 120-2 summarizes results with various empiric chemotherapy regimens.[63-88] Results of small phase II studies using similar or identical regimens have been pooled in this summary.

The recent introduction of several novel antineoplastic agents with broad-spectrum clinical activity has changed the standard treatment of several common epithelial cancers. These drugs include the taxanes, the topoisomerase I inhibitors irinotecan and topotecan, gemcitabine, and vinorelbine. Although none of these agents has been thoroughly evaluated, experience with various taxane-platinum regimens suggests improved response rates and survival when compared retrospectively to earlier regimens. Our initial experience with the combination of paclitaxel, carboplatin, and oral etoposide gave a 47% response rate and 13-month median survival in a group of 53 patients.[89] Table 120-3 summarizes and updates results with this regimen and other combinations containing newer chemotherapeutic agents. Although response rates vary, median survival in most reports is between 9 and 11 months, with 2-year survivals ranging from 14% to 24%.[89-100] The addition of a third drug to a taxane/platinum-based combination does not appear to improve efficacy. Unfortunately, the lack of comparative trials and the marked heterogeneity of this patient population prevents confident determination of the most efficacious regimen.

Experience with second-line empiric chemotherapy is limited. Single-agent gemcitabine (1000 mg/m² weekly 3 of 4 weeks) has modest activity in this setting.[101] The combination of gemcitabine (1000 mg/m² days 1 and 8) and irinotecan (100 mg/m² days 1 and 8, repeated every 21 days) also has modest activity. In a group of 31 patients, most of whom had previously received a taxane/platinum combination, a response rate of 15% was observed.[102]

The role of various targeted agents in the treatment of patients with carcinoma of unknown primary site has received little attention. The combination of bevacizumab and erlotinib was tested in a group of 51 patients, most of whom had received previous chemotherapy.[103] Although the objective response rate was low (10%), a total of 71% of patients had disease control at 2 months, and the median survival of 7.4 months was better than reported with other second-line therapy. Further evaluation of targeted agents, both alone and in combination with chemotherapy, is indicated.

Retrospective analyses by several investigators have identified clinical and pathologic features associated with a favorable response to treatment with empiric chemotherapy. These features include tumor location in lymph nodes or soft tissue, fewer sites of metastatic disease, female sex, and poorly differentiated carcinoma histology.[104-106] Patients with involvement of the liver or bones have relatively poor prognosis.[104]

At present, all patients with good performance status should be considered for a trial of empiric chemotherapy. Although the most effective combination regimen has not been defined by means of randomized trials, the taxane/platinum combinations recently evaluated have produced higher response rates and have probably prolonged median survival. With these regimens, a substantial minority (approximately 20%) of patients is alive at 2 years, and a small fraction has prolonged disease-free survival. Patients with poor performance status are much less likely to benefit from chemotherapy, and optimal management may include supportive measures only.

Table 120-2 ■ **Empiric Chemotherapy for Patients With Adenocarcinoma of Unknown Primary Site: Pooled Results of Phase II Trials Using Traditional Regimens**

Regimens	No. of Patients	Median Response Rate, % (Range)	Median Survival Months (Range)	Refs.
Single agents				
5-FU ± leucovorin	190	9 (0-16)	4 (3-5)	25, 63-65
Cisplatin	21	19	5	66
Etoposide (oral)	24	8	5	67
Mitomycin C	40	17	5	68
5-FU or anthracycline-based combinations				
AM	159	28 (7-39)	5 (4-8)	68-71
FAM	99	25 (13-37)	9 (5-11)	72-76
CAV	54	33 (24, 50)	6 (5,8)	77,78
CAF/CmeF	51	4 (0-8)	4 (3-7)	25, 72, 79
Platinum-based combinations				
CAP + F	70	24 (17, 28)	7 (6, 7)	80, 81
PveB	50	39	5	71
PE	52	21 (19-25)	5 (4-6)	82, 83
PEF	36	22	5	84
PFL	31	32	18	85
PF Epi	36	28	9	86
CaE	33	23	6	87
CaE Epi	62	43	10	88

Abbreviations: A, doxorubicin; B, bleomycin; C, cyclophosphamide; Ca, carboplatin; Epi, epirubicin; F, fluorouracil; M, mitomycin C; L, leu-covorin; Me, methotrexate; NA, not available; P, cisplatin; V, vincristine; Ve, vinblastine.

Table 120-3 ■ **Summary of Treatment Results Using Newer Chemotherapeutic Agents**

Regimen (Ref.)	No. of Patients	Response Rate	Median Survival (Mo)	2-Year Survival
PC(90)	77	39%	13	20%
DC(91,92)	92	43%	10	24%
PCE(89,93)	71	48%	11	20%
PCG(94,95)	146	30%	9	23%
GC(96)	40	55%	8	NA
IC(96)	40	38%	6	NA
DG(97)	35	40%	10	7%
PCE/GI(98)	132	30%	9	16%
GCCape(99)	33	39%	8	14%
GCV(95)	33	42%	13	NA

Abbreviations: C, cisplatin or carboplatin; D, docetaxel; E, etoposide; G, gemcitabine; I, irinotecan; P, paclitaxel; Cape, capecitabine; V, vinorelbine.

Squamous Carcinoma of Unknown Primary Site

Squamous cell carcinoma at a metastatic site is unusual in the absence of an obvious primary site. Effective treatment is available for patients who fit certain clinical syndromes, and, therefore, appropriate evaluation of these patients is essential.

Squamous Cell Carcinoma Involving Cervical Lymph Nodes

The cervical lymph nodes are the most common metastatic site for squamous cell carcinoma of unknown primary origin. Patients are usually middle-aged or elderly, and many have a history of substantial tobacco and alcohol use. Diagnostic evaluation results in identification of the primary site in the large majority of these patients.[107] When the upper or midcervical lymph nodes are involved, a primary tumor in the head and neck region should be suspected. Optimal evaluation includes a thorough examination of the oropharynx, hypopharynx, nasopharynx, larynx, and upper esophagus by direct vision and fibroscopy, with biopsy of any suspicious areas. Computed tomography of the neck is useful in defining the extent of disease and occasionally in identifying a primary site. PET scanning identifies a primary site in 25% of patients even after other procedures are unrevealing, and should be included as a standard diagnostic procedure.[108] When the lower cervical or supraclavicular lymph nodes are involved, a primary lung cancer should be suspected. Fiber-optic bronchoscopy is indicated if chest radiography and head and neck examination are unrevealing.

Several molecular diagnostic assays have been described that may assist in identifying a head and neck primary site. First, detection of the Epstein-Barr viral genome in tumor tissue is specific for a nasopharyngeal primary site.[109] This assay is of particular importance in young patients with poorly differentiated squamous carcinoma in cervical lymph nodes. Second, presence of human papillomavirus-16 in the lymph node biopsy specimen is specific for a primary site in the oropharynx.[110] Both of these assays can be performed on tissue obtained by fine-needle aspiration biopsy. Finally, chromosomal abnormalities may be detected in histologically benign tissue taken from normal areas during endoscopy.[111] These abnormalities are predictive of subsequent tumor development at that site.

When no primary site is identified, patients should be treated according to guidelines for locally advanced squamous carcinoma of the head and neck. Treatment with definitive local radiation therapy to the pharyngeal axis and bilateral neck, radical neck dissection, or a combination of these local modalities has resulted in long-term disease-free survival for 30-60% of these patients.[112-116] Combined modality therapy with concurrent chemotherapy and radiation therapy is now the treatment of choice for patients with locally advanced head and neck cancer.[117] Although there is limited experience using combined modality therapy in patients with cervical adenopathy and an occult primary site,[118-120] this approach seems reasonable in these patients. As in patients with known primary sites in the head and neck, extensive involvement in neck nodes and poorly differentiated tumor histology are poor prognostic features.[116,121]

Patients with low cervical or supraclavicular lymph nodes are more likely to have a primary lung cancer, and treatment results are inferior in this group of patients. Nevertheless, patients with no detectable disease below the clavicle should be treated with the same approach as are patients with higher cervical nodes, since occasional patients will have long-term disease-free survival.

Squamous Cell Carcinoma Involving Inguinal Lymph Nodes

Most patients with squamous cell carcinoma involving inguinal lymph nodes have a detectable primary site in the genital or anorectal area. In women, careful examination of the vulva, vagina, and cervix is important, with biopsy of any suspicious areas. Men should undergo a careful inspection of the penis. Digital examination and anoscopy should be performed in both sexes to exclude lesions in the anorectal area. Identification of a primary site in these patients is important, since potentially curative therapy is available for carcinomas of the vulva, vagina, cervix, and anus even after they spread to regional lymph nodes. For the occasional patient in whom no primary site is identified, definitive local therapy with inguinal lymph node dissection or radiation therapy sometimes results in long-term survival.[122] Because platinum-based chemotherapy administered concurrently with radiation therapy has improved survival of patients with squamous cancer arising in this region (eg, cervix, anus, bladder), the addition of similar chemotherapy should be considered in patients with an unknown primary site.

Squamous Cell Carcinoma Metastatic to Other Sites

Metastatic squamous cell carcinoma in areas other than the cervical or inguinal lymph nodes usually represents metastasis from a primary lung cancer. Computed tomography of the chest and fiber-optic bronchoscopy should be undertaken if other clinical features suggest the possibility of lung cancer. Chemotherapy with regimens employed in the treatment of non-small-cell lung cancer may be considered in patients with good performance status.

Patients with the diagnosis of "poorly differentiated squamous cell carcinoma" should be evaluated carefully, particularly if other clinical features are unusual for lung cancer (ie, young patient, nonsmoker, unusual metastatic sites). Additional pathologic evaluation with immunoperoxidase stains or electron microscopy should be considered. When the diagnosis remains unclear, such patients should be considered for a trial of therapy for poorly differentiated carcinoma (see below).

Poorly Differentiated Carcinoma of Unknown Primary Site

Patients with poorly differentiated carcinoma account for approximately 20% of patients with carcinoma of unknown primary site; an additional 10% of patients have poorly differentiated adenocarcinoma. Most early empiric chemotherapy trials included these patients along with the more common patients with adenocarcinoma of unknown primary origin, since no clinical differences between these two groups were recognized. It is now clear that some patients with poorly differentiated carcinoma of unknown primary site have extremely responsive neoplasms, and some are curable with combination chemotherapy. Appropriate clinical and pathologic evaluations, therefore, are critical in patients with poorly differentiated carcinoma, so that optimal therapy can be administered.

Pathologic Evaluation

Examination of poorly differentiated carcinoma using routine light microscopy alone is inadequate to assess these tumors optimally. No histologic features have been identified that can distinguish chemotherapy-responsive from nonresponsive tumors.[123] Moreover, it is clear that even with careful retrospective reviews of these cases, some responsive tumors of well-defined types (eg, germ cell tumor, lymphoma) cannot be identified.[123]

Patients with the light microscopic diagnosis of poorly differentiated carcinoma should therefore undergo additional pathologic studies, as described in the section on poorly differentiated neoplasms. Because the initial diagnosis of poorly differentiated carcinoma is more specific than "poorly differentiated neoplasm," the frequency of identifying unsuspected tumors of other types (particularly lymphoma) is much lower in this group. However, unsuspected diagnoses may still be suggested; in a series of 87 patients with poorly differentiated carcinoma in whom a large battery of immunoperoxidase stains was performed, other diagnoses were suggested in 16 patients (18%).[124]

Diagnostic Evaluation

The initial diagnostic evaluation of these patients is similar to that described for patients with adenocarcinoma of unknown primary site. A thorough history, physical examination, routine laboratory testing, and chest radiograph should be obtained in all patients. Computed tomography of the chest and abdomen should be performed in all patients in this group, because of the frequency of mediastinal and retroperitoneal involvement. Serum levels of hCG and α-fetoprotein should be obtained in all patients, because significant elevations of these markers suggest the diagnosis of germ cell tumor. Other serum tumor markers, such as carcinoembryonic antigen, CA 125, CA 19-9, and CA 15-3, are often elevated but are not helpful in predicting response to therapy.

Treatment

When specialized pathologic studies identify a treatable neoplasm, therapy should be administered following guidelines established for the specific tumor identified. Examples of treatable tumor types occasionally identified in this group of patients include lymphoma, Ewing tumor, neuroendocrine carcinoma, and a variety of primitive sarcomas.

It is now well recognized that a few patients in this heterogeneous group have extragonadal germ cell tumors that are unrecognizable by standard pathologic criteria. These patients are usually young males with predominant tumor location in the mediastinum or retroperitoneum. Some also have marked elevations of the serum tumor markers hCG or α-fetoprotein. In some of these patients, molecular genetic analysis enables definitive diagnosis by detecting the i(12p) chromosomal abnormality specific for germ cell tumors.[18] Most young males with poorly differentiated carcinoma and clinical features of extragonadal germ cell tumor have excellent responses to chemotherapy, and some are cured with treatment following guidelines for extragonadal germ cell tumors.[105,125,126] Therefore, all patients with poorly differentiated carcinoma or poorly differentiated adenocarcinoma of unknown primary site who also have clinical characteristics suggestive of an extragonadal germ cell tumor should be treated according to the guidelines established for poor-prognosis germ cell tumors.

Treatment of patients with poorly differentiated carcinoma of unknown primary site who do not have characteristics of extragonadal germ cell tumor remains a subject of controversy. In a group of 220 patients prospectively identified and treated between 1978 and 1989, we reported a 62% overall response rate with 26% complete responses.[105] These patients were treated with intensive cisplatin-based combination regimens used in the treatment of advanced testicular cancer (ie, cisplatin, vinblastine, and bleomycin [PVB] or cisplatin, etoposide, and bleomycin [PEB]). A minority of patients (14%) remained tumor free after a minimum follow-up of 8 years.[127] Most of the patients in this group did not have clinical characteristics strongly suggestive of extragonadal germ cell tumor. However, many patients were young (median age, 39 years), and approximately 40% had predominant tumor location in the mediastinum or retroperitoneum. In a multivariate analysis, clinical features predictive of a favorable treatment outcome included tumor location in the retroperitoneum or peripheral lymph nodes, fewer sites of metastases, younger age, and no history of cigarette smoking.

In a retrospective analysis of a large series of patients with unknown primary cancer, Lenzi and colleagues could not identify a subset of patients with poorly differentiated carcinoma and long-term survival following chemotherapy.[128] In this group, patients with clinical features of extragonadal germ cell tumor were excluded. Patients received a wide variety of treatments, and only a minority of patients with poorly differentiated carcinoma received cisplatin-based therapy used in the treatment of germ cell tumors. Although no long-term survivors were identified, several of the same favorable prognostic factors were detected and included tumor location in lymph nodes, fewer metastatic sites, younger age, female sex, and poorly differentiated carcinoma histology (vs poorly differentiated adenocarcinoma). Other investigators have also documented higher response rates in patients with poorly differentiated carcinoma (vs adenocarcinoma) when treated with cisplatin-based chemotherapy.[106,129]

At present, a trial of combination chemotherapy should be considered for patients with poorly differentiated carcinoma or poorly differentiated adenocarcinoma of unknown primary site. Patients with clinical features of extragonadal germ cell tumor should receive intensive cisplatin-based chemotherapy with a regimen used for the treatment of poor-prognosis germ cell tumors. For the remaining patients in this group, cisplatin-based regimens have also yielded relatively high response rates. Substitution of carboplatin for cisplatin decreases toxicity while producing similar treatment results.[89-91,93,94,97-99] Taxane-based combination regimens have also yielded high response rates with moderate toxicity and are also a good choice for this group of patients.[89-95]

Neuroendocrine Carcinoma of Unknown Primary Site

A broad spectrum of neuroendocrine neoplasia is now recognized, in part due to improved pathologic methods for making the diagnosis. Most well-described adult neuroendocrine tumors have indolent biologies and typical histologic features (eg, carcinoid tumors, islet cell tumors, paragangliomas, pheochromocytomas). A second group of neuroendocrine tumors, typified by small-cell lung cancer, has high-grade tumor biology and a typical "small-cell" anaplastic appearance by light microscopy. A third group of neuroendocrine tumors has high-grade biology and no distinctive neuroendocrine features by light microscopy. In this group, the initial diagnosis is usually "poorly differentiated carcinoma" or "poorly differentiated adenocarcinoma"; neuroendocrine features are only recognized when immunoperoxidase staining or electron microscopy is performed. Neuroendocrine tumors of unknown primary site occur in each of these three categories and are considered separately.

Low-Grade Neuroendocrine Carcinoma

Metastatic carcinoid or islet cell tumors are occasionally found at metastatic site without an obvious primary site. In this situation, the metastatic tumor almost always involves the liver. Some patients have clinical syndromes produced by tumor secretion of bioactive substances. Primary sites in the intestine or pancreas are occasionally identified during the clinical course.

Carcinoid or islet cell tumors of unknown primary site usually exhibit an indolent biology, and management should follow guidelines established for metastatic tumors of these types with known primary sites. Depending on the clinical situation, appropriate management may include local therapy (resection of isolated metastasis, radiofrequency ablation, hepatic artery chemoembolization), treatment of associated syndromes with somatostatin analogues, 5-FU-based systemic therapy, or symptomatic management. Platinum-based chemotherapy has not been useful in these patients.

Small Cell Carcinoma

Patients with small-cell anaplastic carcinoma at a metastatic site usually have a bronchogenic primary. Computed tomography of the chest and fiber-optic bronchoscopy should be performed, as they often identify the primary site. A large number of extrapulmonary primary sites have also been described (eg, salivary gland, esophagus, bladder, prostate, ovary, cervix), and patients with localizing symptoms should have appropriate diagnostic studies performed.

Most patients in this group have tumors with a high mitotic rate and aggressive biology. Many patients have disseminated cancer at the time of diagnosis. Unlike carcinoid-type neuroendocrine tumors, these tumors are responsive to chemotherapy, and all patients should be considered for a trial of treatment at the time of diagnosis. Although the "optimum" chemotherapy regimen is not defined, combination regimens effective in the treatment of small cell lung cancer are recommended.

Poorly Differentiated Neuroendocrine Carcinoma

In 10-15% of poorly differentiated carcinomas, immunoperoxidase staining or electron microscopy identifies neuroendocrine features; these tumors are called "poorly differentiated neuroendocrine tumors" or "primitive neuroectodermal tumors" on this basis. Neuroendocrine features are observed by light microscopic examination in some of these tumors, whereas in others, the light microscopic diagnosis is "poorly differentiated carcinoma." In the original description of this syndrome, 51 patients were retrospectively identified, most of whom had received combination chemotherapy effective in the treatment of small-cell lung cancer.[130] Most patients had clinical evidence of a high-grade tumor, and most had metastases in multiple sites. The retroperitoneum, lymph nodes, and mediastinum were frequently involved. None of these patients had carcinoid syndrome or other syndromes associated with low-grade neuroendocrine carcinoma. Thirty-three of 43 evaluable patients responded to chemotherapy; 13 patients had complete responses and eight remained continuously disease-free more than 2 years after completion of therapy. Five patients with involvement at only one site received local modalities only (three received surgical excision; two received radiation therapy), and four have had long-term disease-free survival. A few similar patients, some with long-term survival following chemotherapy, have been reported by other investigators and have been classified as "extrapulmonary small-cell carcinoma of unknown primary site."[131,132]

In a recent prospective phase II trial, 48 patients with poorly differentiated or small-cell neuroendocrine carcinoma of unknown primary site were treated with paclitaxel/carboplatin/etoposide.[13] The chemosensitivity of these tumors was confirmed: the overall response rate was 55%, with median survival of 14 months and 3-year survival of 20%.

The origin of these poorly differentiated neuroendocrine tumors remains unclear, but it is likely that the group is heterogeneous. Some patients may have small-cell lung cancer with an "occult" primary site. However, many of these patients have no smoking history, and the absence of pulmonary involvement makes this diagnosis unlikely in most patients. As previously discussed, the clinical behavior and histologic appearance of these poorly differentiated tumors are also atypical of most of the other recognized adult neuroendocrine tumors, which are well-defined clinical entities with indolent biologies. However, some of these tumors probably are undifferentiated variants of well recognized neuroendocrine tumors (eg, carcinoid tumor), albeit without a recognizable primary site. In the undifferentiated form, the clinical as well as the pathologic characteristics no longer resemble the characteristics of the more differentiated counterpart. Metastatic anaplastic neuroendocrine carcinomas of gastrointestinal origin have also demonstrated sensitivity to cisplatin-based chemotherapy.[133,134] It is also possible that some of these neoplasms may represent a previously unrecognized type of neuroendocrine tumor.

Although the nature of these tumors remains undefined, the diagnosis of poorly differentiated neuroendocrine carcinoma identifies a highly treatable subgroup. All of these patients should be considered for a trial of therapy with a platinum/etoposide-based regimen. Some patients with a single tumor site may be curable with local treatment modalities alone; however, a course of adjuvant chemotherapy should be considered in these patients, if clinically feasible.

Summary and Future Directions

The recognition of treatable subsets within the large heterogeneous population of patients with carcinoma of unknown primary site represents a definite advance in the management and

Table 120-4 **Carcinoma of Unknown Primary Site: Recommended Evaluation and Treatment of Subsets**

Histopathology	Clinical Evaluation (in Addition to History, Physical Exam, Routine Laboratory, Chest Radiography)	Special Pathologic Studies	Specific Subsets for Therapy	Therapy
Adenocarcinoma (well-differentiated or moderately differentiated)	CT scan of abdomen, chest PET scan Men: Serum PSA Women: Mammograms Additional studies to evaluate signs, symptoms	Men: PSA stain Women: ER, PR stain	1) Women, axillary node involvement	Treat as primary breast cancer
			2) Women, peritoneal carcinomatosis	Treat as stage III ovarian cancer
			3) Men, blastic bone metastases, or high serum PSA or tumor PSA staining	Treat as stage IV prostate cancer
			4) Solitary metastatic lesion	Definitive local therapy
Squamous carcinoma	Cervical presentation: Direct laryngoscopy, nasopharyngoscopy, bronchoscopy, PET scan	–	Cervical adenopathy	Treat as locally advanced head/neck cancer
			Inguinal adenopathy	Inguinal LND + radiation therapy
Poorly differentiated carcinoma	CT abdomen, chest PET scan Serum HCG, AFP Additional studies to evaluate signs, symptoms	Immunoperoxidase staining, electron microscopy, cytogenetic studies	1) Features of EGCT	Treat as nonseminomatous EGCT
			2) Other patients	Empiric platinum or paclitaxel/platinum regimen
Neuroendocrine carcinoma	CT scan of abdomen, chest Additional studies to evaluate signs, symptoms	Immunoperoxidase staining	1) Low-grade	Treat as advanced carcinoid tumor
			2) Small-cell carcinoma or poorly differentiated	Empiric platinum/etoposide regimen

Abbreviations: AFP, α-fetoprotein; CT, computed tomography; EGCT, extragonadal germ cell tumor; ER, estrogen receptor; HCG, human chorionic gonadotropin; LND, lymph node dissection; PR, progesterone receptor; PSA, prostate-specific antigen.

treatment of these patients. Treatable subsets can be defined with appropriate clinical and pathologic evaluation; Table 120-4 provides a summary of the subsets and outlines the recommended evaluation and treatment.

Empiric chemotherapy for patients who do not fit into any defined subset has improved. Treatment with taxane/platinum-based chemotherapy has produced median survival of 9-11 months and 2-year survival of approximately 20%, and should be considered in all patients with adequate performance status. Several other combinations containing newer agents have also shown activity and require further evaluation. Randomized trials to better define a treatment standard are indicated.

During the next few years, further improvements are likely in the diagnosis and treatment of patients with carcinoma of unknown primary site. Molecular profiling of tumors will almost certainly aid in the diagnosis of unknown primary tumors. Several prospective studies are currently evaluating the utility of molecular profiling assays in guiding treatment. In addition, the continued development of effective targeted agents will improve treatment in various cancer types. Many of these targeted agents are likely to have a role in the treatment of unknown primary cancer, but their evaluation is only just beginning. Continued improvement in the treatment of patients with carcinoma of unknown primary site will almost certainly parallel improvements in treatment of other relatively resistant epithelial tumors.

Selected References

The complete reference list can be found at www.CANCERMEDICINE8.com

4. Horning SJ, Carrier EK, Rouse RV, et al. Lymphomas presenting as histologically unclassified neoplasms: characteristics and response to treatment. *J Clin Oncol.* 1989;7:1281–1287.
13. Hainsworth JD, Spigel DR, Litchy S, Greco FA: Phase II trial of paclitaxel, carboplatin, and etoposide in advanced poorly differentiated neuroendocrine carcinoma: a Minnie pearl Cancer Research Network study. *J Clin Oncol.* 2006;24:3548–3554.
15 Turc-Carel C, Philip I, Berger MP, et al. Chromosomal translocation in Ewing's sarcoma. *N Engl J Med.* 1983;309:497–498.
16. Whang-Peng J, Triche TJ, Knutsen T, et al. Chromosome translocation in peripheral neuroepithelioma. *N Engl J Med.* 1984;311:584–585.
17. Bosl GJ, Ilson DH, Rodriguez E, et al. Clinical relevance of the i(12p) marker chromosome in germ cell tumors. *J Natl Cancer Inst.* 1994;86:349–355.
18. Motzer RJ, Rodriguez E, Reuter VE, et al. Molecular and cytogenetic studies in the diagnosis of patients with mid-line carcinomas of unknown primary site. *J Clin Oncol.* 1995;13:274–82.
21. Talantov D, Baden J, Jatkoe T, et al. A quantitative reverse transcriptase-polymerase chain reaction to identify metastatic carcinoma tissue of origin. *J Mol Diagn.* 2006;8:320–329.
22. Ma XJ, Patel R, Wang X, et al. Molecular classification of human cancers using a 92-gene real-time quantitative polymerase chain reaction assay. *Arch Pathol Lab Med.* 2006;130:465–473.
23. Tothill RW, Kowalczyk A, Rischin D, et al. An expression-based site of origin diagnostic method designed for clinical application to cancer of unknown origin. *Cancer Res.* 2005;65:4031–4040.
24. Varadhachary GR, Talantov D, Raber MN, et al. Molecular profiling of carcinoma of unknown primary and correlation with clinical evaluation. *J Clin Oncol.*, 2008;26:4442–4448.
26. Mayordomo JI, Guerra JM, Guijarro C, et al. Neoplasms of unknown primary site. A clinicopathological study of autopsied patients. *Tumori.* 1993;79:321–324.
27. Nystrom JS, Weiner JM, Heffelfinger-Juttner J, et al. Metastatic and histologic presentations in unknown primary cancer. *Semin Oncol.* 1977;4:53–58.
40. Schorge JO, Muto MG, Welch WR, et al. Molecular evidence for multifocal papillary serous carcinoma of the peritoneum in patients with germ-line BRCA1 mutations. *J Natl Cancer Inst.* 1998;90:841–845.
42. Strnad CM, Grosh WW, Baxter J, et al. Peritoneal carcinomatosis of unknown primary site in women. *Ann Intern Med.* 1989;111:213–217.
44. Ransom DT, Patel SR, Kenney GL, et al. Papillary serous carcinoma of the peritoneum: a review of 33 cases treated with cisplatin-based chemotherapy. *Cancer.* 1990;66:1091–1094.
47. Piver MS, Eltabbakh GH, Hempling RE, et al. Two sequential studies for primary peritoneal carcinoma: induction with weekly cisplatin followed by either cisplatin/doxorubicin/cyclophosphamide or paclitaxel/cisplatin. *Gynecol Oncol.* 1997;67:141–146.
52. Schorn C, Fischer U, Luftner-Nagel S, et al. MRI of the breast in patients with metastatic disease of unknown primary. *Eur Radiol.* 1999;9:470–473.
53. Block EF, Meyer MA. Positron emission tomography in diagnosis of occult adenocarcinoma of the breast. *Am Surg.* 1998; 64:906–908.
54. Ellerbroek N, Holmes F, Singletary E, et al. Treatment of patients with isolated axillary nodal metastases from an occult primary carcinoma consistent with breast origin. *Cancer.* 1990;66:1461–1467.
61. Rades D, Kuhnel G, Wildfang I, et al. Localised disease in cancer of unknown primary (CUP): The value of positron emission tomography (PET) for individual therapeutic management. *Ann Oncol.* 2001;12:1605–1609.
62. Nguyen LN, Maor MH, Oswald MJ. Brain metastases as the only manifestation of an undetected primary tumor. *Cancer.* 1998;83:2181–2184.
73. Goldberg RM, Smith FP, Ueno W, et al. Fluorouracil, Adriamycin, mitomycin in the treatment of adenocarcinoma of unknown primary. *J Clin Oncol.* 1986;4:395–399.
89. Hainsworth JD, Erland JB, Kalman LA, et al. Carcinoma of unknown primary site: treatment with one-hour paclitaxel, carboplatin, and extended-schedule etoposide. *J Clin Oncol.* 1997;15:2385–2393.
90. Briasoulis E, Kalofonos H, Bafaloukos D, et al. Carboplatin plus paclitaxel in unknown primary carcinoma: a Phase II Hellenic Cooperative Oncology Group study. *J Clin Oncol.* 2000;18:3101–3107.
93. Greco FA, Burris HA, Erland JB, et al. Carcinoma of unknown primary site: long-term follow-up after treatment with paclitaxel, carboplatin, and etoposide. *Cancer.* 2000;89:2655–2660.
94. Greco FA, Burris HA, Litchy S, et al. Gemcitabine, carboplatin and paclitaxel for patients with carcinoma of unknown primary site: a Minnie Pearl Cancer Research Network study. *J Clin Oncol.* 2002;20:1651–1656.
95. Palmeri S, Lorusso V, Palmeri L, et al. Cisplatin and gemcitabine with either vinorelbine or paclitaxel in the treatment of carcinomas of unknown primary site. *Cancer.* 2006;107:2898–2905.
96. Culine S, Lortholary A, Voigt JJ, et al. Cisplatin in combination with either gemcitabine or irinotecan in carcinomas of unknown primary site: Results of a randomized phase II study—trial for the French Study Group in Carcinomas of Unknown Primary (GEFCAPI 01). *J Clin Oncol.* 2003;21:3479–3482.
97. Pouessel D, Culine S, Becht C, et al. Gemcitabine and docetaxel as front-line chemotherapy in patients with carcinoma of an unknown primary site. *Cancer.* 2004; 100:1257–1261.
98. Greco FA, Rodriguez GI, Shaffer DW, et al. Carcinoma of unknown primary site: sequential treatment with paclitaxel/carboplatin/etoposide and gemcitabine/irinotecan: a Minnie Pearl Cancer Research Network phase II trial. *Oncologist.* 2004;9:644–652.
99. Schneider BJ, El-Reyes B, Muler JH, et al. Phase II trial of carboplatin, gemcitabine, and capecitabine in patients with carcinoma of unknown primary site. *Cancer.* 2007;110:770–775.
100. Greco FA, Gray J, Burris HA, et al. Taxane-based chemotherapy for patients with carcinoma of unknown primary site. *Cancer J.* 2001;7:203–212.
101. Hainsworth JD, Burris HA, Calvert SW, et al. Gemcitabine in the second-line therapy of patients with carcinoma of unknown primary site: a Phase II trial of the Minnie Pearl Cancer Research Network. *Cancer Invest.* 2001;19:335–339.
102. Hainsworth JD, Spigel DR, Raefsky EL, et al. Combination chemotherapy with gemcitabine and irinotecan in patients with previously treated carcinoma of unknown primary site: a Minnie Pearl Cancer Research Network phase II trial. *Cancer.* 2005;104:1992–1997.
103. Hainsworth JD, Spigel DR, Farley C, et al. Phase II trial of bevacizumab and erlotinib in carcinomas of unknown primary site: the Minnie Pearl Cancer Research network. *J Clin Oncol.* 2007;25:1747–1752.
104. Abbruzzese JL, Abbruzzese MC, Hess KR, et al. Unknown primary carcinoma: natural history and prognostic factors in 657 consecutive patients. *J Clin Oncol.* 1994;12:1272–1281.

105. Hainsworth JD, Johnson DH, Greco FA. Cisplatin-based combination chemotherapy in the treatment of poorly differentiated carcinoma and poorly differentiated adenocarcinoma of unknown primary site: results of a 12- year experience. *J Clin Oncol.* 1992;10:912–922.
108. Rusthoven KE, Koshy M, Paulino AC. The role of fluorodeoxyglucose positron emission tomography in cervical lymph node metastases from an unknown primary tumor. *Cancer.* 2004;101:2641–2649.
110. Begum S, Gillison ML, Nicol TL, Westra WH. Detection of human papillomavirus-16 in fine-needle aspirates to determine tumor origin in patients with metastatic squamous cell carcinoma of the head and neck. *Clin Cancer Res.* 2007;13: 1186–1191.
116. Grau C, Johansen LV, Jakobsen J, et al. Results from a national survey by the Danish Society for Head and Neck Oncology. *Radiother Oncol.* 2000;55:121–129.
117. Salama JK, Seiwert TY, Vokes EE. Chemoradiotherapy for locally advanced head and neck cancer. *J Clin Oncol.* 2007;25: 4118–4126.
118. de Braud F, Heilbrun LK, Ahmed K, et al. Metastatic squamous cell carcinoma of an unknown primary localized to the neck. Advantages of an aggressive treatment. *Cancer.* 1989;64:510–515.
122. Guarischi A, Keane TJ, Elhakim T. Metastatic inguinal nodes from an unknown primary neoplasm. A review of 56 cases. *Cancer.* 1987;59:572–577.
124. Hainsworth JD, Wright EP, Johnson DH, et al. Poorly differentiated carcinoma of unknown primary site: clinical usefulness of immunoperoxidase staining. *J Clin Oncol.* 1991;9:1931–1938.
126. Greco FA, Vaughn WK, Hainsworth JD. Advanced poorly differentiated carcinoma of unknown primary site: recognition of a treatable syndrome. *Ann Intern Med.* 1986;104:547–553.
128. Lenzi R, Hess KR, Abbruzzese MC, et al. Poorly differentiated carcinoma and poorly differentiated adenocarcinoma of unknown origin: favorable subsets of patients with unknown primary carcinoma? *J Clin Oncol.* 1997;15:2056–2062.
130. Hainsworth JD, Johnson DH, Greco FA. Poorly differentiated neuroendocrine carcinoma of unknown primary site: a newly recognized clinicopathologic entity. *Ann Intern Med.* 1988;109:364–372.

121 Principles of Pediatric Oncology

Maura O'Leary, MD ■ Gregory H. Reaman, MD

Introduction

In children, in the age group of 0–15 years, cancer differs considerably from cancer in adults. This chapter seeks to provide a broad overview of pediatric oncology. The differences in pediatric oncology extend from the diagnostic type (which ultimately influences etiology, biology, and natural history), relative incidence and distribution frequency, clinical presentation and manifestations and response to therapy and outcome.[1] The overwhelming majority of children less than 15 years of age are treated in a comprehensive pediatric cancer center as outlined by the American Society of Pediatric Hematology Oncology and the American Academy of Pediatrics.[2,3] These centers are also members of the Children's Oncology Group (COG) which is a National Cancer Institute (NCI) sponsored cooperative group primarily to cure and prevent childhood and adolescent cancer through scientific discovery and compassionate care. The emergence of the COG has resulted in a consolidated, unified North American-based clinical trials consortium, providing an extraordinary opportunity for a focused, coordinated, international agenda to maintain, and hopefully exceed, past progress toward increased survival and cure with increased attention to quality of life and survivorship alike. In addition, there is an unprecedented opportunity for population-based clinical trials and research in pediatric cancer; the success of the pediatric cancer cooperative groups has resulted in protocol-directed therapy as standard of care.

In adults, epithelial malignancies are frequently observed but they rarely develop in children. In pediatric malignancies there is an age-dependent variation in frequency.[4,5] The relative incidence in children of cancers arising from the embryonic mesenchyme appropriately suggest the extremely close connection between oncogenesis and developmental biology in childhood malignancies. In general, childhood malignancies tend to be associated with shorter latency periods, grow rapidly and are often disseminated at the time of presentation. They are generally not amenable to surgical removal as a primary treatment modality.[6]

Acute leukemia—more specifically, acute lymphoblastic leukemia—is the most common form of malignancy seen in the pediatric age group. With respect to solid tumors, primary neoplasms of the central nervous system outnumber all other solid tumors in this age group and usually arise in the posterior fossa. Their origin is primarily primitive neuroectodermal rather than glial as in adults. Figure 121-1 shows the distribution frequency of pediatric cancer types as well as their relationship to age, separating the adolescent and young-adult population from the rest of the pediatric age group.[7]

The last several decades of the twentieth century have been a period of enormous accomplishment in pediatric clinical cancer research. Since the 1950s, cancer has moved from being a nearly uniformly fatal disease to being one in which more than 78% of children can be expected to achieve disease-free survival (DFS) in excess of 5 years and, presumably, will be cured of their disease. Data from the Surveillance Epidemiology and End Results (SEER) publications of the NCI demonstrate a consistent reduction in the rate of childhood cancer mortality through the year ending 2003.[8] As shown in Figure 121-2; the past 28 years have seen an improvement of 22% in survival rates. A 24% decrease in childhood cancer mortality has been observed since the mid 1990s alone.[9] Despite the dramatic improvements in outcome, cancer remains the leading cause of death from disease in children and adolescents.

The high-risk childhood cancers in which current 5-year survival rates are near or less than 50% include acute myelogenous leukemia[10]; relapsed acute lymphoblastic leukemia[11,12]; acute lymphoblastic leukemia with specific structural chromosomal abnormalities [t(9;22), t(4,11), and other MLL gene rearrangements][13-15]; biologically unfavorable subgroups of neuroblastoma (age >18 months)[16]; chromosome 1p deletions, *mycN* amplified, *TrkC* expression increased)[17-19]; supratentorial high-grade and brainstem gliomas[20,21]; and metastatic sarcomas of bone and soft tissue.[22-24] These diseases represent an area for focused, coordinated, basic, translational, and clinical research to elucidate mechanisms of resistance and to explore the potential of novel therapeutic approaches, especially those directed at unique molecular targets. An exploitable consequence of targeted molecular therapy in pediatric cancer is the equally important diminution of nonspecific collateral acute and long-term toxicity associated with conventional, cytotoxic anticancer therapy.

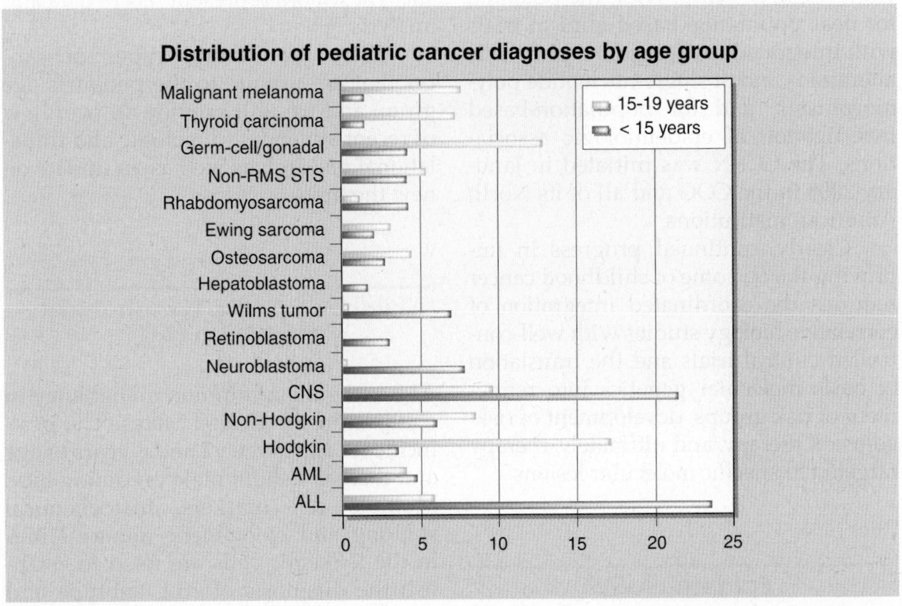

Figure 121-1 ■ Distribution of pediatric cancer diagnoses by age group. *Abbreviations*: ALL, acute lymphoblastic leukemia; AML, acute myelogenous leukemia; CNS, central nervous system; RMS, rhabdomyosarcoma; STS, soft-tissue sarcoma.

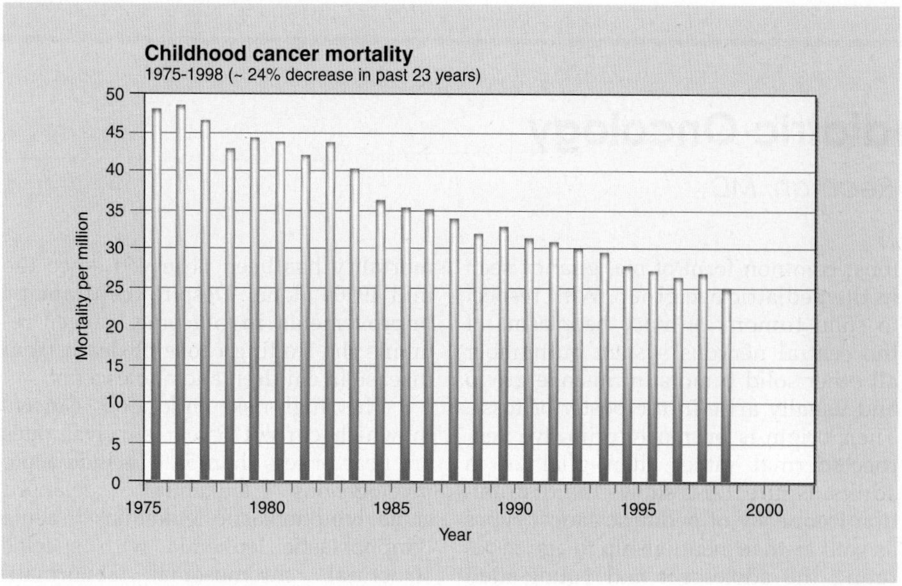

Figure 121-2 Childhood cancer mortality. *Source*: Data from the Surveillance Epidemiology and End Results Program of the National Cancer Institute.

Exploiting specific genetic alterations to design novel treatments for pediatric cancer is critical to the success for achieving improved childhood cancer survival rates in the next decade.[25] Continued progress is much more likely to come from such exploitation than from further intensification of currently available chemotherapy agents, because the chemotherapy approach has nearly reached its maximum potential as a result of limitations imposed by short-term and long-term cumulative toxicities.

Given that most children with cancer will be treated at institutions that are members of the COG, its North American Childhood Cancer Research Network (CCRN) will provide the potential for near population-based clinical trials with integrated investigations of genetic alterations and of single-nucleotide polymorphisms, and for population-based investigation of epidemiologic associations. The CCRN was initiated in January 2008 in the COG and all of its North American institutions.

Clearly, continued progress in improving the outcome of childhood cancer requires the coordinated integration of correlative biology studies with well-controlled clinical trials and the translation of basic molecular genetics into refinement of risk groups, development of risk-adjusted therapy, and ultimately, therapy targeted to specific molecular lesions.

Epidemiology

In 2004, according to United States Cancer Statistics (USCS), 13,421 children and adolescents (0-19) were of diagnosed with cancer, 9165 were under 15 years of age.[26] Pediatric cancers; represent approximately 2% of all cancers diagnosed in the United States each year, they remain the leading cause of death in children as a result of disease.[27] While in the United States and Canada, leukemia and central nervous system (CNS) cancers are the most common in other areas of the world such as South America and India other cancers predominate.[28,29] Incidence data for pediatric cancers have been summarized in a monograph by the NCI's SEER: The SEER pediatric monograph (http://www.seer.nci.nih.gov). There is a follow-up monograph for adolescents and young adults available through the same website. These both represent recent data and analysis.[30,31]

There are several types of cancer that are unique to the pediatric age group and we will provide an overview of recent advances in biologic and translational research as well as an update on new therapies.

Childhood Acute Lymphoblastic Leukemia (ALL)

ALL is the most common malignancy in children in the United States. The peak incidence is between 2 and 6 years of age and there is a slight male predominance. Multiple cell markers, histochemical staining and cytogenetic abnormalities in the leukemic cells are used to establish the diagnosis of ALL subtype and result in specific therapeutic decisions.[32] About 85% of cases of childhood ALL express membrane markers consistent with B-precursor lineage, and about 15% express T-lineage markers. Contemporary therapies include several components, namely, induction, presymptomatic central nervous system therapy, post induction intensification, and maintenance therapy. This design of current treatments will cure more than 80% of patients overall.[33] Gains in outcome in childhood ALL equal or surpass gains in other areas of childhood cancer. Very high-risk disease patients defined as failure to achieve initial remission, Ph+ ALL, hypodiploidy, 11q23 rearrangement, infants less than 12 months and early relapse patients, however, require more innovative strategies. The recent report of the COG on PH+ pediatric ALL which was treated with aggressive chemotherapy and concomitant targeted therapy (imatinib) demonstrated an improvement in event-free survival (EFS).[34]

Additional recent advances in therapy include:

- The substitution of dexamethasone for prednisone, which has improved the survival for SR patients, is currently under investigation in patients with HR disease. Morbidity from dexamethasone, however, has been a factor in the treatment of the HR patient.[35]
- Initial response to therapy determined by day 8 blood and/or bone marrow flow cytometry assessment of minimal residual disease (MRD) is an important predictor of outcome[36] and is now utilized by the COG in risk-adjusted treatment approaches.
- Postinduction intensification (or delayed intensification) improves outcome for both high and standard risk, B-precursor and T-lineage patients particularly when augmented regimens were utilized.[37,38]
- Improved outcome associated with specific cytogenetic aberrations including hyperdiploidy, trisomy 4, 10, and t(12;21)(TEL/AML1).[39]
- Current systemic therapy particularly with dexamethasone in standard risk patients allows elimination of cranial irradiation for most patients.[40]
- Current frontline therapy regimens are tailored to risk category as assessed by clinical features and biologic profile.[41]

The heterogeneity of childhood ALL is reflected in emerging gene-expression microarray data. Such data are currently under evaluation to determine if they will help further profile the newly diagnosed patient for more effective therapy.[42]

Review of comparative outcome results of adolescents and young adults treated with pediatric or adult protocol-based therapy has shown improved outcomes for those treated utilizing the pediatric approach. Stock and colleagues compared the outcome of adolescents, age 16-21 years, with ALL treated on either Cancer and Leukemia Group B (CALGB) or the Children's Cancer Group (CCG) protocols. One hundred three patients treated on adult protocols achieved a 6-year EFS of 38%, similar to that obtained for young adults aged 21–29 years on CALGB protocols; however, 196 patients treated on pediatric protocols achieved a 6-year EFS of 64%.[43] Findings from the French and Dutch groups are similar.[44,45] Adolescents and young adults achieve better outcomes when treated on pediatric protocols at pediatric centers. However, treatment mortality comprises a larger percentage of adverse events than in younger children.[46]

Treatment outcome depends on disease, host, and treatment factors. Treatment factors are paramount and may alter the clinical significance of disease and host factors. Disease factors include features apparent at diagnosis, features that may appear in response to therapy, and factors that become apparent only at relapse. Host factors refer to differences among patients with regard to drug absorption, metabolism, and sensitivity. Considerable heterogeneity has been described with respect to host pharmacology of thiopurines[47] and vincristine.[48,49] Population variability has been described with respect to sensitivity to glucocorticoids.[50,51] Better understanding of the biology of ALL and it relation to early and late marrow and extramedullary relapses will lead to new insights and new treatment strategies. Lessons that are learned in the treatment of childhood ALL might have value in the treatment of other cancers in other populations.

Acute Myeloid Leukemia (AML) in Children

AML comprises about 20% of pediatric leukemia and subacute or chronic myeloid leukemia about 1-2%. Compared with ALL, pediatric AML is less responsive to available chemotherapy.[52] AML survival has recently with marked intensification of both therapy and supportive care attained cure rates of 50% in the pediatric population.[53-55] This disease is covered elsewhere in this text.

AML protocols are becoming increasingly intensive. Since the more intensive induction regimens may have been maximally intensified, new active agents and strategies are needed. These agents and strategies may include histone deacetylase inhibitors, translocation break-point targeted therapy, monoclonal antibody therapy targeted to membrane antigens, and differentiation therapy. Use of differentiation therapyhas worked well with acute promyelocytic leukemia (APL).[56] Finally, development of predictive models of relapse risk may allow for individualization of therapy.[57]

Non-Hodgkin Lymphoma in Children (NHL)

Approximately 15% of all childhood cancers diagnosed in the United States are lymphomas. Sixty percent of all childhood lymphomas have been classified as NHLs, representing 3% of all childhood malignancies for children younger than 5 years, and 8–9% for children and adolescents 5-19 years of age. There are four major subtypes of childhood NHL: (1) Burkitt lymphoma (classic and atypical), (2) lymphoblastic lymphoma, (3) diffuse large B-cell lymphoma (DLBCL), and (4) anaplastic large-cell lymphoma (ALCL). The distribution of these four main histologic subtypes includes approximately 40% Burkitt lymphoma, 30% lymphoblastic lymphoma, 20% diffuse large B-cell, and 10% anaplastic large-cell lymphoma.[58-60]

The primary modality of treatment of all histologic types and stages of childhood NHL is multiagent chemotherapy. The exact regimen of chemotherapy with or without intrathecal therapy and the intensity and length of treatment are usually dictated by the extent of disease and the histologic subtype. The role of surgery is critically important in the diagnosis and staging process, but has a limited role in the overall treatment of childhood NHL.[58,61]

The prognosis for children and adolescents with NHL, both with limited-stage and advanced-stage disease, has improved significantly over the past two decades. Except for rare subtypes, the chance of being alive and disease free at 5 years for limited-stage and advanced-stage disease B-NHL is 95% and 80%, respectively.[62] The prognosis for advanced lymphoblastic NHL in children and adolescents has now increased to over 85% survival.[63] The prognosis, however, for the most advanced childhood and adolescent ALCL is still less than 70% at 7-year follow-up.[64]

Future therapeutic strategies for childhood NHL will likely incorporate immunophenotyping, cytogenetics, and molecular genetic features. Surface, intracellular, and molecular targets will likely be identified that will alter our treatment approach over the next decade. Furthermore, prevention of the development of childhood NHL and the reduction of acute and long-term complications resulting from the treatment of childhood and adolescent NHL will be two major strategies to pursue in years to come.

Hodgkin Disease (HD)

HD accounts for approximately 5% of pediatric malignancies in developed countries. The cure rate for pediatric patients with HD is greater than 90%. Standard therapy for pediatric patients with HD includes combination chemotherapy and low-dose involved-field radiotherapy (RT). Clinical research in pediatric HD aims to delineate minimal treatment necessary for cure[65] and eliminate or minimize late sequelae of treatment.[66] Study of the biology of the RS cell in an effort to identify new therapeutic targets is also receiving significant attention.

In the ongoing CO GHD trial, patients who show a rapid response to 2 cycles of ABVE-PC and a complete response after 4 cycles will be randomized to receive or not receive low-dose involved-field RT. PET scans have been demonstrated to be useful biomarkers of early response and useful in response-based therapy approaches at the end of systemic therapy to determine which patients would be eligible for treatment with chemotherapy alone. In the new German HD study, stage I and II patients with a negative PET scan at the end of chemotherapy will receive no radiation.

Neuroblastoma

Neuroblastoma is a common solid malignancy of childhood and is an embryonal malignancy of the postganglionic sympathetic nervous system. Some tumors undergo spontaneous regression or differentiation to a benign neoplasm, whereas others exhibit a malignant phenotype that is resistant to intensive therapy. There has been substantial improvement in the overall outcome of children with neuroblastoma in the last 30 years but mostly in the treatment and management of low and intermediate stage disease. While there has been some improvement in the treatment of higher stage disease with stem cell transplant and retinoids, the overall survival (OS) remains below 50% with OS for all stages of neuroblastoma at 68.5% (SEER).

Neuroblastoma accounts for 7.2% of all cancers diagnosed between the ages of 0-14 years (http://seer.cancer.gov). The prevalence is approximately 1 case per 7000 live births, and there are about 600–650 new cases of neuroblastoma per year in the United States corresponding to an incidence of 10.4 per million per year.[67]

Neuroblastoma is almost exclusively a pediatric neoplasm. Considerable progress has been made in the past decade toward understanding human neuroblastoma at a cellular and molecular level. The factors responsible for regulating normal differentiation in the sympathetic nervous system are not completely understood, but they at least in part involve the neurotrophin receptor pathways. The expression pattern of the *Trk* neurotrophin receptors is correlated with biological and clinical features of neuroblastoma. High *TrkA* expression has been shown to be associated with younger age (<1 year), lower stage (stage I, II, and IVS), and a favorable outcome.[68-71] There is an inverse correlation between *TrkA* expression and *MYCN*-amplification and that the combined assessment of *MYCN* copy number and *TrkA* expression provides additional prognostic information over either variable alone.[68,72] Flow cytometric analysis of DNA content is a method of measuring total cell DNA content, which correlates well with modal chromosome number. Tumors that have a hyperdiploid DNA content are more likely to have lower stages of disease and to respond to initial therapy, whereas those with a diploid DNA content are more likely to have advanced stages of disease and not to respond to therapy.[73,74] Cytogenetic analyses of neuroblastoma frequently show extra chromosomal double minutes or chromosomally integrated homogeneously staining regions, both of which are manifestations of gene amplification. The region amplified is virtually always derived from the distal short arm of chromosome 2 and contains the protooncogene *MYCN*.[75] Brodeur, Seeger, and colleagues originally demonstrated that *MYCN*-amplification occurs in about 20–25% of primary neuroblastoma from untreated patients; and amplification is associated with advanced stages of disease, rapid tumor progression and a poor prognosis.[76]

Unbalanced gain of distal 17q material is perhaps the most common genetic abnormality detected in primary neuroblastoma tissue specimens and is associated with adverse prognostic features and is present in the vast majority of neuroblastomas with *MYCN* amplification.[77-80]

Deletions of the short arm of chromosome 1 (1p) are found in approximately 25–35% of primary tumors and are highly correlated with the presence of *MYCN* amplification.[81-83] It appears likely that a neuroblastoma suppressor gene is located on the short arm of chromosome 1, and that this gene is inactivated in at least one-third of primary neuroblastomas. The majority of 1p deletions are large and the proximal breakpoints heterogeneous, however, suggesting that distal 1p may contain more than one suppressor gene critical for malignant transformation or progression.[84-87]

Hemizygous deletions of the long arm of chromosome 11 occur in about 40% of human neuroblastomas.[88-91] In addition, constitutional rearrangements of chromosome 11q, including interstitial deletions, have been observed in neuroblastoma patients.[88,89] Thus, 11q also likely harbors a neuroblastoma suppressor gene, but in contrast to 1p deletions, there is a striking inverse relationship of 11q LOH with *MYCN*-amplification, despite the fact that this abnormality is correlated with advanced stage disease.[91] In a recent study of almost 1000 patients registered on COG studies, unbalanced deletions of 11q (11q loss with either retention or gain of 11p material) was independently prognostic for outcome in a multivariate analysis that included all other currently used prognostic markers.[94]

Recent evidence suggests that 3p deletions often occur coincident with 11q deletions and help define the subset of patients with aggressive disease without the oncogenic influence of deregulated *MycN*.[95,96] Array-based genomic studies have recently revealed the true complexity of chromosomal alterations in neuroblastoma, with multiple other areas of recurrent deletions (and gains) scattered throughout the genome.[97-99] However, homozygous deletions are only very rarely identified in this disease,[100,101] thus complicating traditional approaches for identifying the tumor-suppressor genes postulated to be targeted by the hemizygous deletions noted above. An International Neuroblastoma Pathology Classification (INPC) is based primarily on the Shimada system but incorporates other features that should permit improved concordance among pathologists around the world. A standard set of recommended tests to define the clinical stage and extent of disease has been established that includes urinary catecholamines, bone scans, CT scanning and magnetic resonance imaging (MRI). MIBG is an adrenergic neuron blocking agent that is selectively concentrated in more than 90% of neuroblastomas making radiolabeled MIBG scintigraphy a highly specific method for assessment of the primary tumor and metastatic disease.[102,103] MIBG scintigraphy may be performed with either ^{131}I or ^{123}I isotopes, with the latter giving enhanced sensitivity. Immunocytochemical analysis of bone marrow aspirates with monoclonal antibodies directed against neural-specific antigens (eg, GD2, NCAM) increases the sensitivity of detecting marrow involvement to at least 1:100,000 nucleated cells.

An International Neuroblastoma Staging System (INSS) has been established based on clinical, radiographic, and surgical evaluation of children with neuroblastoma.[104,105] The INSS has gained acceptance worldwide and will be used by all major cooperative groups prospectively.

It is important to note that determination of overall response requires assessment of both primary and metastatic sites.

The most important clinical variables predictive of disease outcome are the age of the patient and stage of disease at diagnosis.[106-109] Traditionally, age has been analyzed as a binary function, with a cut point at the first birthday being used by most groups, and this has proven clinical utility. Nonetheless because age is continuous variable, alternative ages have recently been explored as surrogates for tumor behavior. A recent review of 3666 patients by London and colleagues reached the conclusion that 18 months of age more clearly discriminated outcome in patients with INSS stage IV disease and no MYCN amplification.[110] It is important to recognize that the children aged 12-18 months in the studies cited here were all treated with significant chemotherapeutic dose intensity and many received myeloablative chemotherapy. The COG will continue to treat most stage III patients with adjuvant chemotherapy, and will likely develop a response-based algorithm to determine the duration of therapy. These systems are being replaced by a new INSS system that should provide worldwide uniformity in the application of these many variables[111,112] which include homovanillic/vanillylmandelic acid ratios, serum marks such as serum ferritin, neuron-specific enolase (NSE), the cell membrane ganglioside GD2, and lactate dehydrogenase (LDH),[113-117] genetic prognostic markers include tumor cell DNA index, *MYCN* gene copy number, deletion of 1p, 3p, 11q or 14q, unbalanced gain of 17q, and relative expression of the neurotrophin receptor *TrkA*.[118]

The treatment modalities traditionally employed in the management of neuroblastoma are surgery, chemotherapy, and radiotherapy. The role of each is determined by the anticipated clinical behavior of the tumor in individual cases considering age, stage, and biological features. A large body of data supports the hypothesis that the clinical behavior of human neuroblastoma may be reliably predicted based upon the analysis of a panel of prognostic variables.[118,119] Thus, most pediatric oncology clinical trials groups currently stratify patients into "risk groups" based upon analysis of well-defined prognostic factors. The COG Risk Stratification System is based on the experience of both the Pediatric Oncology Group (POG) and CCG uses the INSS system to risk stratify patients along with clinical factors of patient age at diagnosis,[118] the biological factors of tumor histopathology, DNA index and *MYCN*-amplification status, to assign patients to one of three distinct risk groups (low, intermediate, and high), with dramatically different OS probabilities. A major goal of ongoing clinical trials is to prospectively validate the existing risk stratification schema as well as integrate newly discovered prognostic markers with independent prognostic impact into future risk assignment algorithms. There is also movement toward creating an international risk-group system, similar to the INSS, based on the combined worldwide experience.

Treatment of patients with low-risk localized neuroblastoma (INSS 1 and 2) consists of surgical removal of the primary tumor. Unlike other cancers, a complete resection is not necessary in the setting of neuroblastoma that is localized and shows favorable biological features. Patients with INSS 1 tumors (gross total resection) can be expected to have an outstanding probability of RFS and OS.[120-122] A prospective CCG study reported a 93% EFS rate and a 99% OS rate for 141 Evans stage I patients.[123] Surgery alone followed by close observation is also the initial treatment for patients with INSS 2 neuroblastoma with greater than 50% initial tumor resection. The recent prospective CCG study included 233 Evans stage II patients (56% INSS 2) with single-copy *MYCN* and showed a 4-year EFS of 81% with surgery alone and a 4-year OS of 98%.[124] INSS 2 patients with <50% surgical resection at diagnosis are currently treated with 4 cycles of intermediate-risk style chemotherapy, although upcoming cooperative group studies will examine a further reduction in therapy in these patients who have biologically favorable features. Local recurrences in low-risk patients can be managed with second surgeries, and metastatic recurrences are rare but often salvageable with chemotherapy.

The majority of patients with INSS 4S disease fall into the low-risk category (hyperdiploid, favorable Shimada, and single-copy *MYCN*). Retrospective analyses have shown OS rates ranging from 57% to 97% for stage 4S patients taken as a whole.[125-132] Recent prospective analyses have confirmed these observations and show OS probabilities of 85% (n = 110) to 92% (n = 80).[133]

Retrospective comparison of intermediate-risk treatment strategies is difficult because the group of patients currently defined as INSS 3 were treated in a heterogeneous fashion in the past, mainly owing to differences in the staging systems used by the various cooperative groups. Implementation of a standardized staging and risk stratification system should allow a more-uniform approach to treatment planning for this subset of patients.

Matthay and colleagues reported the CCG experience with Evans stage III disease (92% INSS 3). One hundred fifty-one of 228 Evans stage III patients prospectively evaluated for risk status by analysis of age, stage, *MYCN*-amplification status, Shimada pathology, and serum ferritin[143] met the current criteria for intermediate-risk disease. These patients were treated with moderately dose-intensive chemotherapy including cyclophosphamide, doxorubicin, cisplatin, and etoposide, as well as local radiation for any gross residual disease following delayed surgery. Patients with Evans stage III disease and normal *MYCN*, favorable Shimada and low serum ferritin had a 4-year EFS of 100%. Infants with Evans stage III disease and at least one unfavorable biological feature had 4-year EFS and OS rates of 90% and 93%, respectively. In summary, the current approach to intermediate-risk neuroblastoma centers on moderately intensive chemotherapy—and avoids radical surgery and external beam radiotherapy in the majority of patients with the goal of a greater than 90% EFS rate and minimal treatment-related morbidity.[125]

Treatment of High-Risk Disease

Children with metastatic neuroblastoma diagnosed after 18 months remain one of the greatest challenges to pediatric oncologists. Before the mid-1980s, this group of patients had a dismal prognosis with little hope for cure.[135-140] With the advent of comprehensive treatment approaches that include (1) intensive induction chemotherapy; (2) myeloablative consolidation therapy with stem cell rescue; and (3) targeted therapy for minimal residual disease, OS rates have improved. Nonetheless, the current survival rates remain poor and have come at the expense of significant immediate and long-term morbidity.[141]

The vast majority of neuroblastoma patients classified as high-risk are over 1.5 year of age with stage IV disease. The COG also includes any INSS stage III patients with amplified MYCN, INSS stage III patients over 1 year at diagnosis with unfavorable Shimada pathology, INSS stage II patients with amplified MYCN and unfavorable Shimada pathology, and INSS stage IVS patients with amplified MYCN. These latter categories are relatively rare, and the approach to some (INSS stage 3 disease with unfavorable Shimada histology) remains controversial. Most induction-chemotherapy regimens prescribed 5-7 dose-intensive cycles of therapy using alternating combinations of agents including cisplatin, etoposide, vincristine, doxorubicin, cyclophosphamide, and perhaps ifosfamide, carboplatin or more recently topotecan. The efficacy of induction-chemotherapy regimens is assessed by the response rate, typically determined after a second surgical procedure. Initial limited success with chemotherapy in the 1980s led investigators to hypothesize that myeloablative chemotherapy could consolidate a remission and eradicate chemotherapy resistant minimal residual disease. Since the first published trial of myeloablative consolidation therapy using high-dose melphalan alone,[142] multiple single arm trials and registry reviews have been reported in the literature.[143-159] These studies are difficult to compare due to the heterogeneity of induction and consolidation regimens as well as varying strategies for stem cell harvesting and reinfusion. On the other hand, the majority of studies reported at least a trend towards improved survival probabilities compared with nonrandomized control groups and historical controls.[160]

Matthay and colleagues completed the first randomized trial of myeloablative consolidation with immunomagnetically purged bone marrow support compared to intensive consolidation chemotherapy.[160] An intent-to-treat analysis showed a significant improvement in 3-year EFS probability for the patients assigned to myeloablative therapy (34 ± 4% vs 22 ± 4%; p = .03; Fig. 121-3). The follow-up study that compared purged peripheral blood stem cells to unpurged PB stem cells has been completed and no benefit to date has been shown for the purged cells.[161]

It has recently become clear that using peripheral blood stem cells provides superior engraftment kinetics compared to conventional bone marrow grafts, and this technique likely abrogates some transplant-related morbidity.[158,162] All current clinical trials for high-risk neuroblastoma patients use autologous peripheral blood stem cells for postmyeloablative rescue. The current COG clinical trial is a randomization testing the hypothesis that tandem stem cell procedures are superior to a single transplant. The main theoretical advantage of a tandem transplant approach is providing multiple noncross resistant agents at maximal doses in a relatively rapid sequence. Grupp and colleagues showed that a tandem myeloablative consolidation with peripheral blood stem cell support was feasible with rapid myeloid engraftment in a limited institution pilot study of 39 patients.[158] Transplant-related mortality was 8% (3/39) and the 3-year EFS was estimated at 58%.

Minimal Residual Disease Therapy

Relapse occurs all too frequently after autologous transplantation, suggesting that chemotherapy resistant malignant stem cells can survive dose-intensive therapy. Because the original observations that retinoids and other agents can induce differentiation of neuroblastoma

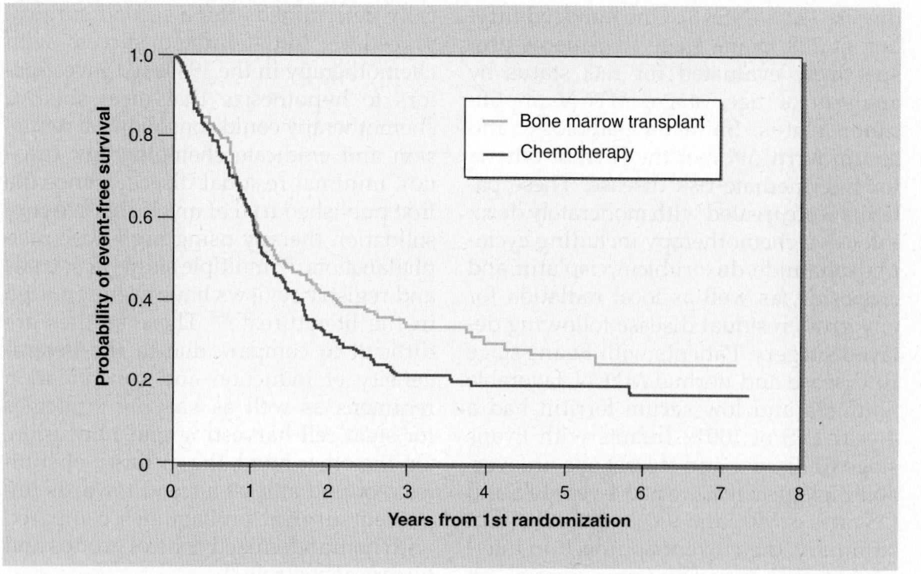

Figure 121-3 Comparison of overall survival of 2196 patients treated at Children's Oncology Group (COG) institutions stratified by risk group. Low-risk, $n = 916$; intermediate-risk, $n = 431$; high risk, $n = 849$. *Source*: Courtesy of W.B. London, Children's Oncology Group Statistical Office, Gainesville.

cells in vitro, a biological-based therapy against minimal residual disease has been sought.

The retinoids are a class of compounds that have been known for two decades to induce cellular differentiation with a concomitant decrease in proliferation of neuroblastoma cells in vitro.[262] The efficacy of 13-*cis*-retinoic acid (CRA) was recently tested. The cohort of patients assigned to receive post transplant therapy with 13-*cis*-retinoic acid had a significantly improved EFS probability (46 ± 6% vs 29 ≤6%) from second randomization; $p = .03$.[160]

An alternative or complementary strategy that appears promising for application during the minimal residual disease phase of therapy is targeted molecules directed against neuroblastoma-specific cellular antigens. Murine, chimeric, and humanized antibodies specific to the cell surface ganglioside GD2, either alone or with cytokines, have shown activity in preclinical models[163-166] as well as phases 1[167-172] and 2[173,174] clinical trials. The murine monoclonal antibodies 3F8276 and GD2a272 and the human-mouse chimeric monoclonal antibody ch14.18 have received the most clinical attention. Measurable responses have been observed in refractory neuroblastoma patients[175-177] justifying further examination in phase 3 clinical trials.[175-177] The COG has recently reported the results of the clinical trial of CRA versus CRA plus ch14.18, IL-2 and GM-CSF. The multi-agent combination with ch 14.18 antibody showed a 20% improvement in EFS (p=0.0115) over CRA alone.(personal communication A. Yu and W. London).

Considerable progress has been made in understanding the genetic basis of clinical heterogeneity observed in neuroblastoma. Patients can now be more reliably categorized as being low-, intermediate-, or high-risk for disease relapse, and this has resulted in more rational treatment choices. High-risk disease remains a significant pediatric problem. It is apparent that although short-term improvements in outcome are likely to come from more effective use of existing treatment modalities, including newer cytotoxic agents and stem cell support, further dose intensification of conventional chemoradiotherapeutics is unlikely to be tolerated in young children. Thus, the challenge for the future is to translate new insights concerning the biology of neuroblastoma into novel treatment approaches that target critical signaling pathways involved in tumor cell survival or maintenance of the malignant state.

Renal Tumors of Childhood

Wilms Tumor is the most common primary malignant renal tumor of childhood and a paradigm for multimodal treatment of a pediatric malignant solid tumor. Developments in surgical techniques and postoperative care, recognition of the sensitivity of Wilms tumor to irradiation, the availability of several active chemotherapeutic agents, and a multidisciplinary approach to clinical research have led to excellent outcomes with progressively less therapy for most children. The annual incidence of Wilms tumor is approximately 7.6 cases per million children under 15 years of age.[178] Wilms tumor represents 6% of childhood cancers in the United States with approximately 500 new cases per year.

Children with Wilms tumor may have associated genitourinary tract abnormalities, aniridia, hemihypertrophy, cryptorchidism, and hypospadias.[179] The first evidence that a specific chromosomal locus was associated with Wilms tumor was the demonstration that patients with WAGR (Wilms, aniridia, ambiguous genitalia and mental retardation) syndrome had a constitutional interstitial deletion encompassing the short arm of chromosome 11, region 1, band 13.5. The underlying tumor-suppressor gene, WT1, appears to be a transcription factor, although its in vivo targets have still not been conclusively identified.[180] The normal function of WT1 is required for normal genitourinary development[181,182]; it is important for differentiation of the renal blastema.[183] Constitutional mutations of single base pairs within the WT1 gene result in the rare Denys–Drash syndrome.[184] However, mutations of WT1 have been found in only about 10% or fewer of sporadic Wilms tumors.[185]

Involvement of the Wnt signaling pathway is suggested by the discovery of activating β-catenin mutations in some Wilms tumors.[186] Intriguingly, these mutations are restricted to tumors with inactivation of the WT1 gene.[187]

In association with Beckwith–Wiedemann syndrome, a second Wilms tumor locus (WT2) maps to an imprinted region of chromosome 11 (11p15.5).[188] It now seems apparent that inactivation of the maternally imprinted, expressed untranslated mRNA gene (H19), whether by genetic or epigenetic mechanisms, is the critical tumorigenic event.[189,190] In summary, Wilms tumor, like many other cancers, is characterized by alterations in multiple genes, some that regulate cell growth, others differentiation, and yet others the cell's proliferative potential, although it is not clear how many genes are involved in each tumor. Although most Wilms tumors are single lesions, 7% are bilateral, and 12% are multifocal within a single kidney.

Microscopically, the classic nephroblastoma consists of varying proportions of three cell types: blastemal, stromal, and epithelial. The absence of anaplastic nuclear changes allows Wilms tumor to be classified as "favorable-histology." Anaplasia, which may be focal or diffuse, is characterized by the presence in cells of markedly enlarged nuclei (diameter more than three times that of nuclei in neighboring cells), and the presence of multipolar or obviously polyploid mitotic figures.[191] Resected tumors with circumscribed, small areas of anaplasia confined to the kidney and surrounded by nonaplastic tissue are defined as focal anaplasia; otherwise, the anaplasia is defined as diffuse. Because anaplasia adversely affects prognosis, meticulous documentation and photographs should be part of the pathology examination.[192] Clear cell sarcoma of the kidney (CCSK) must enter the differential diagnosis.[193] Rhabdoid tumor of the kidney (RTK) is a highly malignant tumor previously not distinguished from Wilms tumor. RCCs may present in childhood and in fact constitute approximately 6% of pediatric renal tumors.[194] They often show histologic and genetic features that are different from carcinomas of the same kind found in adults.

Stage is determined by the results of the imaging studies and both the surgical and pathology findings at nephrectomy. The staging system developed by the former National Wilms Tumor Study (NWTS) Group and now used by the COG is outlined below.[195]

1. In stage I disease, the tumor is limited to the kidney and has been completely resected.
2. In stage II disease, the tumor extends beyond the capsule of the kidney; but it has been completely resected with no evidence of tumor at or beyond the margins of resection.
3. In stage III disease, residual tumor (gross or microscopic) is present but confined to the abdomen. "Residual tumor" includes unresectable primary tumor, lymph node metastases, positive surgical margins, biopsy of the tumor or tumor spillage before or during surgery, or transected tumor thrombus.
4. In stage IV disease, hematogenous metastases (lung, liver, bone, or brain) or lymph node metastases outside the abdominopelvic region are present.
5. In stage V disease, bilateral renal involvement is present at diagnosis. Each side is then staged according to the preceding criteria (I-III) at the time of nephrectomy.

The treatment of children with renal tumors begins with removal of the kidney and the tumor and is determined by the stage and histology of the tumor.

Approximately 7% of children with Wilms tumor present with bilateral tumors. The treatment of such children must be individualized. The two goals of therapy are to eradicate all tumors and to preserve as much normal renal tissue as possible, with the hope of reducing the risk of chronic renal failure among these children.[196,197]

Category of Rhabdoid Tumor of the Kidney

Wilms tumor is a very radiosensitive tumor. The NWTS trials 1-3 demonstrated that use of irradiation could be eliminated in children with stage I or II favorable-histology tumors and that, in children with stage III tumors, only 10.8 cGy was required when combined with three-drug chemotherapy.[198-200] Abdominal radiation is also used for all stages of anaplastic Wilms tumor, CCSK, and RTK.

Unilateral Favorable-Histology Tumors NWTS-4 demonstrated that pulse-intensive regimens using single-dose dactinomycin and doxorubicin produce less hematologic toxicity than the previous standard regimens[201] can be administered at less cost[202] and result in equivalent outcomes.[203] NWTS-4 also demonstrated that approximately 6 months of chemotherapy resulted in outcomes equivalent to the previously standard 15 months of treatment.[204] NWTS-3 and -4 demonstrated that the addition of cyclophosphamide to the DD-4A regimen resulted in significantly better RFS and OS for stages II-IV diffuse, but not focal, anaplastic tumors.[205] Thus, tumors with focal anaplasia may be treated with regimen DD-4A. NWTS-5 sought to build on these results by alternating vincristine/doxorubicin/cyclophosphamide with cyclophosphamide/etoposide (regimen I) for patients with stages II-IV diffuse anaplastic Wilms tumor. Although the analysis of regimen I is ongoing, preliminary results suggest that the regimen is well tolerated and that, in the absence of a clinical trial, it provides a reasonable guideline for the treatment of patients with stages II-IV anaplastic Wilms tumor.

Clear Cell Sarcoma of the Kidney (CCSK)

The use of doxorubicin has appeared to be particularly effective for CCSK.[206,207] But because the ifosfamide/etoposide combination has demonstrated activity against other sarcomas,[208,209] CCSK patients in NWTS-5 were treated with an experimental regimen (I) identical to that for tumors with diffuse anaplastic histology. Although the follow-up duration is currently too short to draw firm conclusions regarding the efficacy of this regimen, regimen I appears to compare favorably to the prolonged vincristine/dactinomycin/doxorubicin regimen used in NWTS-4, and, in the absence of a clinical trial, it is recommended as an appropriate treatment regimen for patients with CCSK.

Rhabdoid Tumor of the Kidney (RTK)

The outcomes for children with RTK treated on NWTS trials with regimens used for the treatment of Wilms tumor have been very poor; no standard treatment regimen has been defined.

Renal Cell Carcinoma (RCC) ■ Historically, patients with RCC were not included in cooperative group trials for pediatric renal tumors, and so knowledge of treatment regimens is based on retrospective case series and literature reviews. Like adult RCC, pediatric RCC is not very chemosensitive; complete surgical resection remains the mainstay of therapy. The distinction between favorable and anaplastic histology Wilms tumor has been identified as the most important determinant of prognosis.[210] Recent analyses have also confirmed the importance of lymph node involvement. The prognostic significance of previously identified factors, such as age and tumor size, has lessened as treatment efficacy has improved.[211]

The results of NWTS-4 predicted that the 4-year RFS and OS percentages that can be expected with use of the its therapy regimens are: (1) 92% and 98% for stage I favorable-histology Wilms tumor, (2) 85% and 96% for stage II favorable-histology Wilms tumor, (3) 90% and 95% for stage III favorable-histology Wilms tumor, and (4) 80% and 90% for stage IV favorable-histology Wilms tumor.[212,213] Current research is focused on identifying additional prognostic factors that could be used to further stratify therapy according to risk of recurrence. NWTS-5 demonstrated that tumor-specific LOH for chromosome arms 1p and 16q, present in 5% of Wilms tumors, is associated with a significantly increased risk of relapse and death. In the current COG study, this criterion is used for treatment stratification to attempt to improve the outcome for this subset of patients.

Soft Tissue Sarcomas of Childhood

The soft tissue sarcomas are a heterogeneous group of connective tissue neoplasms that arise in soft tissues throughout the body. These tumors represent 7.4% of cancer cases in children and adolescents ages 0-20 years.[214] SEER data estimate that 850-900 new cases of soft tissue sarcomas are diagnosed in children each year in the United States. Rhabdomyosarcoma is the most common soft tissue sarcoma in children ages 0-14 years, with an annual incidence of 4.6 cases per million children, representing nearly 50% of soft tissue sarcomas in this age range The nonrhabdomyosarcoma soft tissue sarcomas include fibrosarcoma, synovial sarcoma, leiomyosarcoma, liposarcoma, and others; each histology is rare in children and adolescents.

Since the inception of the pediatric cooperative group process, over 4000 patients with rhabdomyosarcoma have been enrolled in therapeutic trials in North America. Rhabdomyosarcoma can occur in almost any soft tissue site in the body. Rhabdomyosarcoma has been reported in association with neurofibromatosis type 1, 8 and 9 Beckwith–Wiedemann syndrome,[215,216] Li–Fraumeni syndrome,[217,218] cardio-facio-cutaneous syndrome,[219] Costello syndrome,[220] Noonan syndrome,[221,222] a variety of congenital anomalies,[223] and parental use of cocaine and marijuana.[224] The vast majority of cases appear to be sporadic.

Accurate and specific diagnosis of rhabdomyosarcoma is critical for appropriate treatment assignment and analysis of outcome data. The hallmark for diagnosis of RMS is the demonstration of malignant skeletal muscle differentiation. Embryonal RMS (ERMS) is most common, comprising over half of all RMS cases. Alveolar histology tumors comprise about 25% of RMS. This histology is more common in tumors arising in adolescents and in extremity primary tumors. Numerous studies have demonstrated that fusions of PAX3 or PAX7 and the FKHR (FOXO1 a) gene that are generated by t(2;13) and t(1;13) chromosomal translocations are specific and consistent features of the alveolar subtype of RMS.[225,226] Only about 15-20% of patients will have clinically detectable metastatic disease at diagnosis; however, all patients are considered to have micrometastatic disease, providing the rationale for universal chemotherapy. The most common sites for metastatic disease are lungs, bone marrow, and bones.

Extent of disease is among the strongest predictors for long-term outcome. Complete surgical excision of tumor is correlated with better outcome and, for embryonal tumors, obviates the need for local irradiation. However, rhabdomyosarcoma arises in many sites that do not permit primary surgical excision without significant morbidity or loss of function. Fewer than 20% of patients have tumors that are completely excised with negative tumor margins (Clinical Group I). Multiagent chemotherapy is indicated for all patients with rhabdomyosarcoma. Combination therapy including vincristine, dactinomycin, and cyclophosphamide (VAC) continues to be the mainstay of effective, curative therapy. Several other antineoplastic agents are active against RMS, but to date have not improved outcome. The overall 5-year survival for the most favorable subset of patients with low-risk RMS is 95% when treated with vincristine and dactinomycin chemotherapy administered for 48 weeks. The combination of ifosfamide and etoposide is active in patients with recurrent RMS.[227] The highest-risk population comprises patients who have metastatic disease at diagnosis. Fewer than one-third of these children will survive,[228] although some lower-risk subsets have been identified.[229] For patients with embryonal RMS and microscopic or gross residual disease after surgical excision (Clinical Groups II-IV) and for all patients with alveolar RMS, radiation therapy plays a critical role for successful local tumor control. Most children and adolescents with favorable and intermediate-risk rhabdomyosarcoma can be cured with presently available multidisciplinary therapeutic approaches.

Further refinements of risk-group assignment are needed to better identify patient subsets at lower-risk of disease recurrence and potentially to identify new targets for therapeutic intervention for patients with higher-risk soft tissue sarcomas. This may be accomplished by analyzing clinical, pathologic, and new gene-expression profile features that will better characterize these tumors. For patients with rhabdomyosarcoma identified to be at the lowest risk of treatment failure, the goal is to maintain excellent cure rates while decreasing treatment intensity. For patients at highest risk of tumor recurrence and ultimate treatment failure, new therapeutic interventions that ultimately will improve cure rates need to be identified. The NRSTS are much more heterogeneous, and appropriate therapeutic interventions are more controversial. Research efforts should be directed at enabling risk-directed therapeutic interventions for children and adolescents with soft tissue sarcomas that are based on leads from preclinical models adult sarcoma results and on the identification of potential molecular targets for therapeutic intervention.

Pediatric Bone Tumors

Malignant primary bone tumors that occur in both younger and older patients have important differences in pathophysiology, presentation, and treatment, and these differences will be highlighted. Although primary bone tumors are rare, they are the sixth most common malignant neoplasm in children and the third most frequent neoplasm in adolescents and young adults.[230] Malignant bone tumors occur in the United States at an annual rate of approximately 8.7 cases per million children and adolescents younger than 20 years. Only half the bone tumors in childhood are malignant, and of these, osteosarcoma is the most frequent, accounting for approximately 35% of all primary sarcomas of bone. Ewing sarcoma (ES), the second most frequent primary bone cancer, is more common than osteosarcoma in children younger than 10 years.

Osteosarcoma

Osteosarcoma, the most common primary malignant bone tumor, is composed of spindle cells producing osteoid. It is a highly aggressive neoplasm for which dramatic progress has been made in treatment and outcome during the past several decades. Osteosarcoma is primarily a disease of adolescents and young adults; although it can also occur in older patients.[231] The most common clinical presentation is pain with or without an associated soft tissue mass in the involved region of bone. Among young patients, the most common location is the metaphysis of a long bone. Approximately half of all osteosarcomas originate around the knee joint.

Similar to other sarcomas in young patients (typically high-grade), osteosarcoma metastasizes very early in its evolution. Approximately 20% of patients present with radiographically detectable metastases, most frequently to the lung. Death from osteosarcoma is almost always the result of progressive pulmonary metastasis with respiratory failure, pulmonary hemorrhage, pneumothorax, or superior vena cava obstruction. The diagnosis of osteosarcoma is typically suspected by the radiographic appearance of the affected lesion. Osteosarcoma can present as a lytic, sclerotic, or a mixed lytic-sclerotic lesion. The diagnosis of osteosarcoma is dependent on a biopsy for histologic examination providing a pathological diagnosis. Osteosarcoma is a pleomorphic, spindle cell tumor that forms an extracellular matrix consisting mostly of osteoid. Patients with osteosarcoma should undergo a staging work-up to determine the extent of disease at presentation (local and distant).

Osteosarcoma has a bimodal age distribution, with the first peak in the second decade of life during the adolescent growth spurt, and the second among older adults.[232] It is estimated that approximately 400 children and adolescents less than 20 years of age are diagnosed each year in the United States. It is extremely rare before the age of 5 years.

The peak age coincides with a period of rapid bone growth in young people, suggesting a correlation between rapid bone growth and the evolution of osteosarcoma. Radiation exposure is another well-documented etiologic factor. The incidence of osteosarcoma is dramatically increased among survivors of retinoblastoma. In the hereditary form of this disorder, germ-line mutations of the retinoblastoma gene are common. This is the likely basis for the increased frequency of secondary cancers in this population, since the rate in survivors of unilateral sporadic retinoblastoma is much less.[233] Germ-line mutations in the P53 gene can

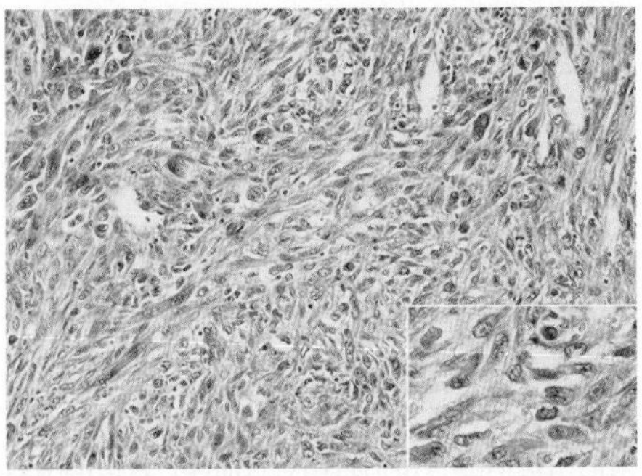

Figure 121-4 Chondroblastic osteosarcoma.

lead to a high risk of developing malignancies, including osteosarcoma, which has been described as the Li–Fraumeni syndrome. Most osteosarcomas, including those in children and adolescents, are of the osteoblastic subtype. The current WHO classification recognizes two additional subtypes of conventional osteosarcoma: chondroblastic (Fig. 121-4) and fibroblastic based on the predominant pattern of differentiation. Telangiectatic osteosarcoma is a rare subtype, which appears as a purely lytic lesion on plain radiographs and thus, may be confused with aneurysmal bone cyst or giant cell tumor.[234] Almost all newly diagnosed patients with osteosarcoma have at least micrometastatic disease as evidenced by the fact that if treated by surgical resection alone, 80% will relapse in the lung within 2 years.[235] These findings suggested the need for systemic chemotherapy, which has now become the standard of care.[236] Osteosarcoma is resistant to radiation therapy; therefore, local control usually consists of surgical resection. Advances made in surgical techniques have significantly improved the clinical practice and functional limb salvage options available for patients.

Rosen introduced the concept of chemotherapy prior to surgical resection.[237] A strong correlation between the degree of necrosis and the probability of subsequent DFS was observed,[238] which has subsequently been confirmed in multiple clinical trials. Soon after the identification of the prognostic value of the degree of necrosis following induction chemotherapy, it was suggested that chemotherapy be modified for the patients with less necrosis. Despite an early report of benefit, changed and intensified regimens have not improved outcome for poor responders.[239,240] The standard treatment of patients with nonmetastatic osteosarcoma, although variable, includes the use of cisplatin and doxorubicin with the addition of high-dose methotrexate in North American countries, and the addition of ifosfamide in Cooperative Osteosarcoma Studies (COSS). The survival of patients with osteosarcoma appears to have reached a plateau.

The standard management for patients with metastatic disease at the time of initial diagnosis follows the same general principles as those who present with localized disease.[240] The outcome of osteosarcoma patients depends on several factors. The most consistent prognostic factor at diagnosis is the presence of clinically detectable metastases, which confers an unfavorable prognosis. In patients with metastatic disease at diagnosis, the number of pulmonary nodules, as well as, whether they are unilateral or bilateral is also of prognostic significance. With currently available regimens, approximately 60-70% of patients with nonmetastatic osteosarcoma of the extremity will survive without evidence of recurrence. In most large reported studies, only 10–20% of patients who present with clinically detectable metastatic disease survive.[241]

Ewing Sarcoma

In the early 1980s, ES and peripheral primitive neuroectodermal tumor (PPNET) were both found to contain the same reciprocal translocation between chromosomes 11 and 22, t(11;22)(q24;q12).[242,243] Later that decade, similar patterns of oncogene expression (c-myc, N-myc, c-myb, and c-mil/raf-1) were seen among these tumors.[244] The combination of the shared translocation, cellular physiology, and clinical response has led to categorizing these tumors into the Ewing sarcoma family of tumors (ESFT). The ESFT includes ES, peripheral primitive neuroectodermal tumor, neuroepithelioma, atypical ES, and Askin tumor (an ESFT of the chest wall).

Based on the SEER data, the incidence of ESFT in persons less than 20 years of age is 2.9 per million per year.[245] The incidence of ESFT peaks in the latter half of the second decade of life. An enigma in ESFT is its racial distribution. The incidence in whites is at least 9-fold higher than in blacks. Frequent primary sites include the pelvis (25%), femur (16%), ribs (12%), and spine (8%).

Approximately 25% of patients present with metastatic disease. Of these, 37% (or 9% of all patients) have metastases confined to the lung or pleura. The remaining patients have bone and/or bone marrow metastases, either alone or in addition to pulmonary/pleural disease. Rarely, patients with bone marrow metastases have extensive infiltration and present with petechiae or purpura from thrombocytopenia. The presence of a pelvic tumor, a high LDH, fever, an interval between onset of symptoms and diagnosis >3 months, and age older than 12 years are risk factors for clinically evident metastatic disease.

The cause of ESFT is unknown. Cases are thought to be sporadic, but family members of ESFT patients have an increased incidence of neuroectodermal and stomach malignancies.[246,247] ESFT are thought to derive from cells of neuroectodermal origin, possibly postganglionic cholinergic neurons, although the exact cell of origin has yet to be identified. The translocation t(11;22)(q24;q12), or another related translocation, occurs in greater than 95% of ESFT. Some argue that such a translocation is pathognomonic and is both necessary and sufficient for a diagnosis of ESFT. The classic t(11;22)(q24;q12) translocation joins the Ewing sarcoma (EWS) gene located on chromosome 22 to an ets-family gene, FLI1 (Friend Leukemia Insertion), located on chromosome 11.[248]

The EWS/FLI1 fusion transcript encodes a 68-kDa protein with two primary domains. The EWS domain is a potent transcriptional activator, while the FLI1 domain contains a highly conserved ets DNA-binding domain. The EWS/FLI1 fusion protein thus acts as an aberrant transcription factor and transforms mouse fibroblasts. To effect this transformation, both the EWS and FLI1 functional domains must be intact.[249] In addition, the IGF-I receptor (IGF-IR) is required for EWS/FLI1 to transform fibroblasts.[250] Thus, the EWS/FLI1 fusion protein is implicated in the pathogenesis of ESFT. Effective strategies for reducing the activity of EWS/FLI1 in ESFT patients through novel delivery systems of small interfering (si) RNA are in development.[251,252] ESFT is one of the small round blue cell tumors and spans a spectrum from undifferentiated (ES) to differentiated (peripheral primitive neuroectodermal tumor). Pseudorosette formation is seen with increasing differentiation. The immunohistochemical hallmark of ESFT is diffuse membranous staining for CD99 (MIC2),[253] which is present in greater than 90% of ESFT. Undifferentiated tumors are negative for other markers except vimentin and FLI-1, whereas more differentiated tumors variably express additional markers, including neuron-specific enolase, S-100, neurofilaments, CD57, and synaptophysin. Muscle and lymphoid markers are negative. A Kiel modified classification proceeds from the least to the most differentiated: ES (0-2 markers), atypical ES (3-5 markers), and PPNET (requires rosettes or 4-5 markers).[256] The current WHO classification does not distinguish between these entities[257] because many statistically mature patient cohorts do not identify a prognostic advantage to classification based on differentiation or diagnosis of ES versus PPNET.[254,256,257]

Identifying an ESFT specific translocation is pathognomonic for the diagnosis. This includes chromosomal break points t(11;22), t(21;22), and t(7;22). Standard cytogenetics and fluorescence in situ hybridization (FISH) can reveal this anomaly and additional karyotypic abnormalities, including trisomies 8 and 12, and chromosomes 1 and 16 abnormalities.[258] Some of the t(21;22) translocations remain cryptic by standard cytogenetic techniques and require reverse transcription polymerase chain reaction (RT-PCR) or FISH.

The most consistent prognostic factor is the presence of metastatic disease at diagnosis. Alkylating agents (cyclophosphamide, ifosfamide, melphalan, and busulfan) and doxorubicin are the most active single agents in ESFT, while the combination of ifosfamide plus etoposide showed significant activity in a classic phase II setting.[259] Platinum derivatives have not shown significant efficacy in ESFT.[260]

The successful management of patients with ESFT requires the use of both local and systemic therapy. In 1973, the first Intergroup Ewing's Sarcoma Study (IESS-1) evaluated the efficacy of VAC compared with VAC plus lung radiation or VAC plus doxorubicin (D). This study showed that for patients with localized disease, VAC alone provided 24%, VAC and lung RT 44%, and VAC plus D 60% 5-year DFS.[261] Besides the dramatic improvement in OS, IESS-1 identified patients with large primary tumors, particularly pelvic, as having a shorter survival. The addition of ifosfamide and etoposide to the three-drug VDC regimen produced further improvement in outcome.[262] The COG study which examined the role of dose-intensive therapy administered every 2 weeks with filgrastin support compared with the conventional every-3-week therapy for patients with initially localized disease has been completed and the intensive timing arm was superior to the standard arm.[263] The current European study, Euro-EWING 99, randomly assigns patients with initially localized, small (<200 mL) primary tumors to ifosfamide or cyclophosphamide in combination with vincristine and actinomycin following standard induction therapy with vincristine-ifosfamide-doxorubicin-etoposide.

ESFT patients with disease metastatic at initial diagnosis have been identified as having a poor outcome since early multiagent trials.[264] Patients with multiple sites of metastases have the lowest survival rates. Patients with metastases confined to the lungs may represent a group of patients with better prognosis than patients with bone or bone marrow metastases. More recently, poor-prognosis patients were treated with melphalan, busulfan, and thiotepa with or without total-marrow irradiation in a pilot study using a tandem autologous stem cell rescue. This study, which included patients with recurrent disease (who historically have had dismal survival chances), showed encouraging results, with a 36% 2-year DFS.[265]

As suggested in earlier studies, the role of mega therapy with stem cell support for ESFT is best evaluated in the context of controlled clinical trials. Toxicity is an important consideration in the therapy of ESFT and late effects including second malignancy will be discussed later in the chapter. ESFT, unlike osteosarcoma, is quite radioresponsive, and radiotherapy is considered a standard option for definitive local control. Radiotherapy can be used as an alternative to disfiguring surgery such as amputation. In large prospective studies, patients who receive radiotherapy for local control have a similar DFS and OS to those patients treated with surgery. If surgery is performed and adequate (≥10 mm of bone or 5 mm of soft tissue) surgical margins are obtained, postoperative radiotherapy is not indicated.[266] Postoperative radiotherapy should be administered when surgical margins are close or positive. ESFT survival is highly dependent on the initial presentation and, therefore, potentially the biologic properties of the disease. OS in patients with ESFT is 60%. For patients with localized disease, it approaches 70%, while patients with metastatic disease have less than a 25% likelihood of long-term survival. The presence of metastatic disease at initial presentation is the most significant adverse prognostic factor despite aggressive chemotherapy.[267] Molecular markers as prognostic indicators in patients with ESFT are under study. Several of these include translocation breakpoint regions, other chromosomal abnormalities, cell-cycle/checkpoint genes and p-glycoprotein expression. The t(11;22) in any individual patient fuses one of many observed combinations of exons together form EWS and FLI1 to form the fusion message. The most common combination is the EWS exon 7 fused to FLI1 exon 6 (type 1 translocation), which occurs in approximately 50-64% of ESFT. Retrospective analyses have shown that patients with localized tumors and the 7/6 fusion have a 70% 4-year survival, while patients with the other variants had a 20% 4-year survival.[268]

Loss of chromosome segment 1p36 has been associated with poor prognosis in patients with localized disease. Additional abnormalities including +8 and +12 may portend a better prognosis.[269] Cell-cycle and checkpoint genes have been evaluated as prognostic markers in ESFT. Although particular checkpoint genes have been found mutated or deleted in small numbers of tumors, as a group, these abnormalities are found in over 50% of ESFT. In patients with ESFT, 80% of p16INK4a mutations or deletions were found in patients with metastatic disease. Other studies confirmed that patients with p16INK4a abnormalities had a poor prognosis. P53 mutations are often identified by over expression (or delayed catabolism) of TP53 measured by increased immunoreactivity in tissues. Increased TP53 occurs in approximately 10% of ESFT samples.[270] In retrospective studies the presence of TP53 has been shown to identify patients with a poor prognosis. In order to improve survival and reduce morbidity, novel combinations of established chemotherapeutic agents and molecular targeted therapies are being tested in ESFT.

The tumor necrosis factor-related apoptosis inducing ligand (TRAIL) can activate tumor necrosis factor-modulated apoptotic pathways in ESFT. TRAIL-activated apoptosis occurs through caspase-8 in ESFT, and most ESFT cell lines express caspase-8. TRAIL may represent a biologic approach to inducing apoptotic cell death in ESFT.[271-273]

The insulin-like growth factor type I receptor is critical for transformation and growth of ESFT.[274,275] New small molecule inhibitors of IGF-IR, either alone or in combination with established chemotherapeutic agents deserve study.

Central Nervous System (CNS) Tumors

Significant differences in epidemiology, molecular genetics, and biology distinguish CNS tumors of the infant and child from those arising in adulthood. Because of these differences, important aspects of clinical presentation, treatment and outcome are uniquely related to childhood CNS tumors.

Malignant CNS tumors are the most common solid tumor of childhood, with 2200 new cases per year in the United States. Pediatric brain tumors vary considerably in their histological, topographical, and gender distribution throughout childhood and adolescence. Boys are 24% more commonly affected than girls in all age groups, but this increase is accounted for mostly by medulloblastoma, PNET, and ependymoma. Over 90% of CNS tumors in children are primary brain tumors. Survival has improved from 60% in 1975 to 1984 to 65% in 1985-1994, and survival is noted to improve with increasing age: 45% in those aged less than 1 year, 59% in those aged 1-4 years, 64% in 5- to 9-year-olds, 70% in 10- to 14-year-olds, and 77% in 15- to 19-year-olds.[276] The main histological entities are pilocytic astrocytomas (23.5%), followed by medulloblastomas (16.3%), ependymomas (10.1%), anaplastic astrocytomas and glioblastomas (7.2% each), and craniopharyngiomas (5.6%).[277]

In the United States, CNS tumors are the most common cause of death due to cancer in childhood, accounting for 24% of cancer related deaths.[276] Morbidity as a result of increasingly successful treatment approaches remains high and includes cognitive, memory and learning impairment, neuroendocrine deficiencies, hearing deficits, sterility, and secondary cancers.

The etiology of CNS tumors remains mostly unknown. The known risk factors include (1) gender (male), (2) therapeutic doses of ionizing radiation to the head (ie, leukemia or prior brain tumor), and (3) genetic syndromes such as neurofibromatosis, tuberous sclerosis, nevoid basal cell carcinoma syndrome (Gorlin syndrome), Turcot's syndrome, and Li–Fraumeni syndrome.

Approximately 10% of medulloblastomas harbor amplification of the *MYCN* oncogene and/or the expression of the tyrosine kinase receptor ERBB2 both of which have been associated with the LCA phenotype and are poor prognostic indicators.[278] Small molecule inhibitors of ERBB2 are currently under clinical investigation.

The most common chromosomal event in medulloblastoma, 17p deletion, occurs in 35-50% of tumors.[279,280] The minimal area of deletion at 17p13.3 encompasses regulatory elements of HIC1, a tumor-suppressor gene that is epigenetically inactivated in the majority of medulloblastoma tumors.[279-281] Atypical teratoid/rhabdoid tumor (AT/RT) has been misdiagnosed as medulloblastoma or PNET; however, mutation of the hSNF5/INI1 gene is observed in most AT/RT and can now be used as a molecular diagnostic tool for this tumor.[282]

The incidence of cortical astrocytomas increases with age, having a first peak at age 5 and again at age 13.[276] In children, brain stem and cerebellar astrocytomas are as common as cortical tumors.

Cerebellar astrocytoma is found almost exclusively in children, occurring most frequently between ages 4 and 9. Juvenile pilocytic astrocytoma (JPA) is the most common subtype, accounting for 85% of cerebellar astrocytomas.[277] Diffuse astrocytoma is the next most common, whereas malignant astrocytoma is rare in this location. Total surgical resection is curative in 95-100%.[283,284] JPAs may stabilize for long periods of time or even spontaneously regress; however, the behavior of cerebellar astrocytomas in children with neurofibromatosis type I (NF-1) may be more aggressive. Gliomas of the visual pathway, hypothalamus, and thalamus comprise a relatively common form of childhood astrocytoma. Tumors of the optic chiasm and hypothalamus are usually low-grade, whereas thalamic tumors tend to be more variable. Twenty percent of children with NF-1 will develop visual pathway tumors, predominantly JPA, during childhood.[285] These tumors present most frequently between 5 and 10 years of age.[286,287]

Brain stem gliomas (BSG) comprise 10–15% of all pediatric CNS tumors and are generally uncommon in the adult population. Peak incidence is between the ages of 5–9 years of age, but may occur anytime during childhood.[276]

BSGs most commonly arise in the pons (diffuse intrinsic), in which location they typically resemble adult glioblastomas multiforme (GBM) and have an almost uniformly dismal prognosis. In contrast, those arising from midbrain or medulla are likely to be low-grade lesions that have a more indolent course and better outcome.[288,289]

Embryonal tumors of the central nervous system comprise a group of tumors that share a histologically similar, undifferentiated morphology, and represent the most common malignant brain tumor group in children (21%). The incidence is constant from infancy to 3 years of age (11.6–10.2 per million) and then a steady decline is observed thereafter.[276] This group includes the PNETs, ependymoblastoma, and AT/RT. PNETs are further subdivided by anatomic location into medulloblastoma (posterior fossa) and supratentorial PNET. Controversy has existed regarding the class division between supratentorial PNET and medulloblastoma but the preponderance of molecular genetic, biologic and clinical evidence validates this division.[290]

AT/RT is an aggressively malignant, primitive tumor most often arising in children younger than 2 years of age.[291,292] These tumors have only recently been recognized as an entity distinct from PNET due to their histological similarity with two-thirds containing foci morphologically indistinct from PNET. Approximately half of AT/RTs arise in the infratentorial compartment with a propensity to invade the cerebello-pontine angle.[293] Because of its association with chromosome 22 deletion and INI1-mutation, analysis of these markers in infants with presumed MB/PNET should be considered for all children with brain tumors who are less than 1 year of age. No effective treatment for AT/RT has yet been found.

Although surgery (preferred gross total resection) and cranio-spinal irradiation have been essential elements of successful therapy for medulloblastoma to reduce late effects, especially in very young children, incorporating chemotherapy permit reduction in radiation dose. Investigational approaches with repeated high-dose chemotherapy and stem cell resue demonstrate even further benefit.

As the third most common CNS tumor of childhood, ependymoma makes up 9% of childhood CNS tumors with approximately two-thirds occurring infratentorially. Greater than half of these tumors occur in children less than 5 years of age with a peak during the second year of life (8.6 per million).[276] The addition of chemotherapy to surgery and radiotherapy for childhood ependymoma has not been proven effective.

Intracranial germ-cell tumors (IGCTs) account for less than 5% of pediatric CNS tumors but are primarily seen in children and adolescents, with 90% occurring in those less than 20 years.[294] Incidence peaks at age 10–12 years. They account for nearly 50% of all pineal region tumors of childhood.

Rare Tumors: Less-Frequently Encountered Tumors of Childhood

Individually, retinoblastoma, GCTs, liver tumors and carcinomas are relatively rare in pediatric patients.[295,296] Collectively, however, these neoplasms account for up to 18% of all cancers seen in young people (ie, those younger than 20 years old). Furthermore, the incidence of some of these tumors, such as germ-cell (GCT) malignancies and certain carcinomas, is significantly higher in older patients, those aged between 15 and 19 years, a population that has been under-represented in prospective cooperative national trials.[297]

Retinoblastoma

Retinoblastoma is the most frequent neoplasm of the eye in childhood and represents 3% of all pediatric cancers. The average incidence of retinoblastoma in the United States is 1 in 14,000-18,000 live births. Thus, an estimated 200-300 children develop retinoblastoma each year.[296] Retinoblastoma presents in two distinct clinical forms: (1) bilateral or multifocal, hereditary (40% of cases), characterized by the presence of germ-line mutations of the RB1 gene [multifocal retinoblastoma may be inherited from an affected survivor (25%) or be the result of a new germ-line mutation (75%)], and (2) unilateral or unifocal, usually nonhereditary (60% of cases).

The human retina is far from having completed its maturation at the completion of gestation, and it is not considered to be terminally differentiated until 3 years of age. It is during this period of time, in which primitive photoreceptor cells are stimulated to differentiate into the mature retina, that cells are at high risk of sustaining oncogenic events that result in the development of a neoplasm.

Retinoblastoma is among the best understood of human neoplasms and has served as an important model for understanding tumorigenesis.[298] The RB1 gene, located in chromosome 13q14, was identified and cloned in 1986.[299,300] Its product (pRb) is a 110 kd nuclear phosphoprotein that acts by binding and inhibiting several proteins with growth-stimulatory activity, and it appears to function as a tumor suppressor by inhibiting cell-cycle progression past the G1-S restriction point. Thus, pRb stands as the major gatekeeper to control this critical point in growth regulation. The lack of pRb or its inactivation removes the pRb constraint on cell-cycle control, with the consequence of deregulated cell proliferation. The RB1 gene is a large gene, containing 27 exons over about 200 kb of DNA, and mutations ("first hit") have been described in almost every exon. Nonsense and frameshift are the most common germ-line and somatic mutations, although deletions and duplications are also frequently encountered.[301] There are no mutational hotspots, although new germ-line mutations have an overwhelming preference for the paternal allele, suggesting that deamination of methylated CpG pairs has an important role in mutagenesis.[302] In both hereditary and nonhereditary retinoblastoma, the second tumorigenic event ("second hit") is chromosomal in nature, often as a result of mitotic recombination errors.[303] This second hit occurs at a much higher frequency than the first hit, and it is more sensitive to environmental factors such as ionizing radiation, thus the increased risk of radiation-induced malignancies in survivors of retinoblastoma. After the "second hit" has taken place, retinoblastoma cells rapidly accumulate additional genetic damage.[304] In fact, it is possible that an additional mutation ("third hit"), probably involving a gene of the apoptotic pathway, is necessary for final retinal tumor formation.[301]

Retinoblastoma is a unique neoplasm, in which the hereditary type shows an autosomal dominant inheritance, with almost complete penetration (85-95%).[305] Although most patients with bilateral retinoblastoma carry a germ-line mutation of the RB1 gene, a small proportion (5-6%) carry a deletion involving the 13q14 locus.

Germ Cell Tumors

GCTs are rare in children, with an incidence of 2.4 cases per million children per year, accounting for less than 3% of all pediatric malignancies.[296] This incidence, however, underestimated, since most tumor registries are biased in favor of malignant types, excluding most mature teratomas. The age distribution follows a bimodal pattern, with a peak during the first 3 years of life and a second peak in late adolescence. In general, females have a higher overall incidence of GCT, although males are more at risk of malignant GCT.[306] The only two well-established predisposing factors are males with cryptorchidism and patients with gonadal dysgenesias. In children, GCT comprises a variety of distinct entities that differ in their histology, molecular biology, and clinical behavior.

GCTs arise from primitive pluripotential germ cells, and thus represent a very heterogeneous group of tumors that range from benign teratomas to very aggressive neoplasms.[307] Close to half of the tumors present at extragonadal sites.[306] A GCT may have many different types of tissue, both benign and malignant, and the most malignant component always dictates the behavior. Therefore, the tumor must be sampled very extensively before the final diagnosis and the treatment plan are made.

Benign GCTs

- Mature teratomas are usually composed of mature representatives of all three embryogenic-germ cell layers. They most commonly occur in ovaries, sacrococcygeal area, and mediastinum, in this order. Sacrococcygeal teratomas occur almost exclusively in neonates, whereas ovarian and mediastinal teratomas occur during the second decade.
- Gonadoblastomas represent a mixture of immature germ cells and gonadal sex cord cells. They are always located in a dysgenetic gonad in patients with aberrant sexual differentiation. They may be associated with germinomas.

GCTs of Indeterminate Behavior

- Immature teratomas, in which immature components are identified. The immature component is almost always of neuroepithelial origin, but can also be immature mesenchyma or renal blastema. Immature teratomas usually occur in the ovaries, and rarely in extraovarian sites. They are graded into four different grades according to the degree of maturation. Grades 0–2 usually have a benign behavior.[308]

Malignant GCTs

- Malignant childhood GCTs differ significantly from their adult counterparts in composition, distribution, and site. For example, more than 40% of malignant GCTs in children occur in extragonadal sites.
- Germinomas are the least aggressive tumors of this group, and they are very chemosensitive and radiosensitive. They can occur in the ovaries (dysgerminomas), central nervous system (pineal region), or very rarely in the testes (seminomas). They are composed of large cells with clear cytoplasm, arranged in nests separated by bands of fibrous tissue.
- Yolk sac tumor (YST) or endodermal sinus tumor is the most common malignant GCT in prepubertal children, and it is usually the only malignant germ-cell component in sacrococcygeal and infantile testicular malignancies.[309] An elevation of alpha-fetoprotein (AFP) is diagnostic of this malignancy.
- Embryonal carcinoma seldom occurs in children. It is often a major component of a mixed GCT of the testes or the mediastinum in adolescents and much less likely a part of an ovarian tumor. Microscopically, embryonal carcinomas are very similar to YST, but cells are larger, with a major epithelial pattern.
- Choriocarcinomas are very rare, may be pure in infants, but in older children usually occurs as a component of a mixed GCT. In infants choriocarcinoma usually represents a maternal or placental metastasis, and thus is actually a gestational trophoblastic tumor rather than a GCT.[32] Both cytotrophoblast and syncytiotrophoblast cells must be present for diagnosis. Elevated serum levels of beta-HCG (B-HCG) are usually diagnostic of this malignancy.

Mixed Malignant GCTs

- In younger children, teratomas usually have YST or germinoma components. In older, usually postpubertal children, more malignant components are seen, usually embryonal carcinoma, YST, germinoma, and choriocarcinoma.

Cytogenetic and molecular studies have confirmed that childhood GCTs constitute a group of distinct entities. A distinct chromosomal aberration, i(12p), is often seen in adult GCT.[310] In children, however, the i(12p) is found almost exclusively in gonadal and extragonadal (usually mediastinal) tumors of adolescent males.[311] As in adults, the i(12p) has also been found in hematopoietic malignancies in adolescents with extragonadal GCT.[312] Contrary to their adult counterparts, in children there is a wide array of cytogenetic abnormalities that appear to define biologically distinct subgroups that cluster based on age and sex and site of origin.[313] Gains in chromosomes 1q, 2, 3, 7, 8, 12, and 14 have been described in tumors originating in prepubertal females, whereas tumors in prepubertal males have been found to have gains in chromosomes 1q, 7, and 21, and losses in chromosome 1p.[311] Central nervous system germinomas have a high frequency of sex chromosome abnormalities, usually increased number of copies of chromosome X. Finally, del 1p36 is a common finding in extragonadal and testicular tumors in young children withYST.[314]

The successful treatment of GCT must include a multimodal strategy, where surgery, chemotherapy, and radiotherapy play a role. The histological subentities differ in their response to chemotherapy and radiotherapy:

- *Low risk:* Patients with stage I immature teratomas (with or without malignant elements) and gonadal malignant GCTs, which can be cured with surgery alone. However, a close follow-up observation to document a normalization of the tumor markers after surgery is mandatory.
- *Intermediate risk:* Patients with stages II-IV gonadal, and stages I-II extragonadal tumors have an excellent outcome (survival > 90%) with the standard PEB44 or JEB46 regimens.
- *High risk:* Patients with stage III/IV extragonadal tumors. For these patients, survival with the standard PEB or JEB regimens is not better than 80%.

Tumors of the Liver

Approximately 60% of all liver tumors are malignant[315] accounting for 1.1% of all childhood cancers. Of the estimated 150 new cases of liver cancer seen in children under the age of 20 years each year in the United States, hepatoblastoma accounts for two-thirds of these.[295,296]

Hepatoblastoma preferentially affects boys and occurs in infants or very young children with a median age of presentation of 16 months.[295,315] The incidence of this disease has steadily increased over the past 30 years, but has been most marked over the past 10 years, and more rapidly among those aged 1-4 years of age.[316] Most cases of hepatoblastoma are sporadic. Hepatoblastoma is strongly associated with premature birth, particularly among neonates that weigh <1000 g, where an excess risk of up to 21-fold has been described.[316-318] Hepatoblastoma occurs in children from families affected by familial adenomatous polyposis, which is associated with an inherited germ-line mutation of the adenomatous polyposis coli (APC) gene.[319,320] Hepatoblastoma is also seen in association with Beckwith–Wiedemann syndrome (BWS), where the relative risk of developing this disease is 2280 times higher than that for other embryonal tumors.[321] Finally, hepatoblastoma has also been observed in patients with Li–Fraumeni syndrome and trisomy.[322-324]

Hepatocellular carcinoma is rare during the first 20 years of life, but its incidence is substantially higher among those aged 15-19 years and is the most common malignant hepatic tumor in adolescents.[295] Patients with hepatocellular carcinoma commonly have a preexisting parenchymal liver disorder or a history of hepatitis B. Other diseases associated with hepatocellular carcinoma include hereditary tyrosinemia type 1, glycogen storage disease type 1, a1-antitrypsin deficiency, ataxia-telangiectasia, neurofibromatosis type 1, Alagille syndrome, and Fanconi anemia.[325-329]

Hepatoblastomas are embryonal neoplasms akin to Wilms' tumors, embryonal rhabdomyosarcomas, and pancreatoblastomas that recapitulate embryonic and fetal hepatocyte development. They are most often unifocal and nonencapsulated, and they can contain epithelial and mesenchymal elements and undifferentiated small cells. The epithelial element can include fetal or embryonal cells; most hepatoblastomas contain both types of cell. Patients with tumors containing only fetal cells, as shown by histology of resected material, appear to have a better prognosis than do those whose tumors contain small undifferentiated cells, the presence of which has been associated with an increased risk of recurrence of the tumor.[330]

Cytogenetic abnormalities of hepatoblastoma cells are seen in half of the cases. Seventy-three percent of cases with an abnormal karyotype have numerical anomalies, most commonly trisomies of chromosomes 2, 8, and 20. A chromosomal translocation, t(1;4)(q12;q34), unique to hepatoblastoma cells has also been reported. The genetic locus for BWS is at chromosome 11p15.5, a region of the genome containing several key genes known to undergo genomic imprinting (ie, silencing of gene-expression from one specific parental chromosome).[321] Loss of heterozygosity at chromosome 11p15.5, with a consistent loss of alleles derived from maternal DNA, has been described in hepatoblastoma. In tumor cells that do not demonstrate loss of heterozygosity at chromosome 11p15.5, loss of imprinting with subsequent gene-expression from both parental alleles may occur.[331,332]

A specific TP53 mutation has been reported in association with aflatoxin B exposure in hepatocellular carcinoma, and the presence of TP53 mutations or serum antibodies against TP53 has been reported to be associated with a reduced survival probability in these patients.[333,334]

Carcinomas and Melanoma

Carcinomas and melanoma account for approximately 9% of all cases of cancer in children.[295] In the SEER database, the distribution of these malignancies is as follows: thyroid carcinoma, 35%; common melanomas, 31%; adrenocortical carcinomas, 1.3%; nasopharyngeal carcinoma, 4.5%; and other skin carcinomas, 0.5%. Most carcinomas (75%) occur in the 15- to 19-year-old age group. In patients aged 15-19 years, thyroid cancer and melanoma account for more than 14% of the malignancies seen in this age group. Melanoma accounts for approximately 1.3% of all cases of cancer among persons younger than 20 years in the United States, and more girls or young women are affected by melanoma than boys or young men (ratio of female to male patients 1:6). At initial examination, most patients (89%) have localized disease, the most common site being the trunk, although patients younger than 20 years are more likely than adults to have disease primarily in the head and neck. Survival rates are similar for patients younger than 20 and older than 20 years of age, and the prognosis appears to be stage dependent.[335] There is a higher incidence of melanoma among those aged between 10 and 19 years in the southern registries, but the incidence of melanoma among patients younger than 10 years does not vary geographically. In the 15- to 19-year-old age group, the incidence of cutaneous melanoma increased at a rate of 2.6% per year between 1975 and 1995 (SEER).

Conclusion and Quality of Survivorship

This brief review cannot provide a full comparison of tumors that arise in adults and those presenting during childhood. Nonetheless, pediatric neoplasms differ in a number of fundamental ways that separate them as a class from adult cancers. These features include their histologic and biologic characteristics, frequent resemblance to embryonal tissues and composition of undifferentiated cells, consistent molecular aberrations, association with congenital malformation, and relative paucity of morphologically recognizable precursor lesions. Proper diagnosis and management of childhood cancers require recognition of these unique features and are thus best accomplished by pathologists and clinicians familiar with them. Thankfully, survival rates for childhood cancer have markedly improved during the past several decades, and proper clinical management esulting from controlled clinical trials has been key to this success. Liberal involvement of pediatric specialists is therefore advisable when generalists are confronted with the many pathologic and clinical issues that arise when dealing with this group of diseases.

Table 121-1 **Age-Adjusted and Age-Specific Annual Incidence Rates per Million Population for Childhood Cancer**

	Age at Diagnosis						
Cancer Type (ICCC Group)	**0–14**	**0–19**	**<1**	**1–4**	**5–9**	**10–14**	**15–19**
All groups combined	139.5	154.3	223.9	188.3	107.9	118.0	198.4
All leukemia	42.2	37.5	35.7	77.2	35.0	24.2	23.5
Acute lymphoblastic leukemia (ALL)	32.9	27.6	18.1	65.2	28.3	15.8	11.9
Acute nonlymphocytic leukemia	6.3	6.8	11.2	8.0	4.4	6.1	8.1
All other leukemias	2.9	3.1	6.4	4.0	2.3	2.3	3.6
All CNS	29.7	27.0	29.4	35.4	30.4	24.6	19.2
Ependymoma	2.7	2.3	4.4	5.3	1.6	1.5	0.9
Astrocytoma	14.6	13.9	11.3	15.1	15.2	14.4	11.9
PNET	6.6	5.5	8.5	9.1	7.1	3.8	2.2
All other CNS	6.8	5.3	5.2	5.9	6.5	4.8	4.3
Hodgkin lymphoma	5.9	13.4	0.3	0.5	4.0	12.9	35.8
NHL	5.6	7.2	1.3	4.1	5.6	7.5	12.1
Burkitt lymphoma	2.3	2.1	0.0	1.9	2.7	2.5	1.6
Neuroblastoma and ganglioneuro blastoma	10.3	7.9	61.9	19.7	3.0	0.8	0.6
Retinoblastoma	4.0	3.0	26.8	8.2	0.5	0.1	0.1
Wilms' tumor	8.3	6.3	20.2	18.8	5.6	0.9	0.3
Hepatoblastoma	1.5	1.2	8.7	3.3	0.3	0.1	0.1
Osteosarcoma	3.5	4.7	0.0	0.5	2.4	7.4	8.3
Ewing sarcoma	2.4	3.0	0.2	0.7	2.3	4.3	4.8
Soft tissue sarcomas	10.1	11.5	14.6	9.7	8.7	10.9	15.6
Rhabdomyosarcoma and embryonal sarcoma	4.8	4.5	5.7	6.7	4.9	3.0	3.6
All other soft tissue sarcomas	5.3	7.0	8.9	3.0	3.8	8.0	12.1
Germ-cell	4.5	9.4	14.8	3.8	1.8	6.0	25.9
Carcinomas	5.4	14.8	3.3	1.1	3.1	11.3	42.7
Adrenocortical carcinoma	0.2	0.2	0.8	0.3	0.2	0.1	0.3
Thyroid carcinoma	1.8	5.3	0.0	0.1	0.9	4.3	15.7
Nasopharyngeal carcinoma	0.3	0.5	0.2	0.1	0.0	0.7	1.4
Malignant melanoma	1.6	4.8	1.3	0.5	1.1	2.9	14.4

Source: From Ref. 8.

Table 121-2 **5-Year Relative Survival Rates (Percent)**

Site (Ages 0-14)	**1975-77**	**1978-80**	**1981-83**	**1984-86**	**1987-89**	**1990-92**	**1993-95**	**1996-02**
All sites	58	62.6	66.7	68.2	71.4	75.4	77.0	79.4
Bone and joint	51.3	48.7	56.8	59.4	66.8	66.8	73.9	71.6
Brain and CNS	56.9	57.7	56.0	61.8	63.8	64.0	70.1	74.1
Hodgkin lymphoma	80.3	87.7	87.7	90.8	87.1	96.7	94.6	95.3
ALL	57.6	66.4	71.3	72.5	77.7	83.0	83.8	87.0
AML	18.8	25.8	26.7	30.0	36.2	41.0	41.0	53.1
Neuroblastoma	52.4	56.9	54.5	52.0	61.9	76.6	67.2	68.7
NHL	42.6	52.7	66.9	70.3	70.7	75.9	80.6	86.0
Soft tissue	61.0	74.3	69.2	73.4	65.4	79.2	76.4	71.7
Wilms tumor	73.1	78.6	86.4	90.7	92.2	91.9	91.4	92.1
Site (Ages 0–19)	**1975-77**	**1978-80**	**1981-83**	**1984-86**	**1987-89**	**1990-92**	**1993-95**	**1996-02**
All sites	61.5	65.2	68.0	70.6	73.3	76.0	77.4	79.5
Bone and joint	51.1	48.4	51.2	57.2	63.5	68.2	68.6	68.0
Brain and CNS	58.7	58.1	57.6	64.0	65.9	66.1	71.0	75.1
Hodgkin lymphoma	86.0	88.7	85.4	90.8	88.9	94.2	93.9	95.1
ALL	54.1	62.4	67.1	70.1	75.0	79.7	81.3	83.5
AML	18.7	26.2	26.4	31.7	36.9	41.0	39.4	48.4
Neuroblastoma	52.7	57.0	53.4	52.0	60.5	76.3	67.0	69.0
NHL	43.4	53.9	63.5	68.1	70.3	72.1	77.8	81.9
Soft tissue	65.2	68.8	68.2	72.4	67.2	68.9	73.8	70.9
Wilms tumor	72.6	78.0	86.5	91.0	92.2	91.3	91.5	92.1

Source: From Ref. 8.

With the use of multimodal and risk-based treatment, the overall 5-year survival rate of the more than 12,500 children and adolescents (age 0-19) diagnosed with cancer each year in the United States is approaching 80%.[336] The improvement in survival has resulted in about 1 in 810 individuals under the age of 20 and 1 in 640 individuals between the ages 20 and 39 years representing childhood cancer survivors.

The late sequelae of cancer treatment or late effects can cause chronic medical problems and involve all organ systems. Overall mortality among childhood cancer survivors has been described to be 10-fold that of the general population.[337,338] The Childhood Cancer Survivor Study (CCSS) assessed overall and cause-specific mortality in a retrospective cohort of 20,227 5-year survivors and demonstrated a 10.8-fold excess in overall mortality.[337] Risk of death was statistically significantly higher in females, individuals diagnosed with cancer before the age of 5 years, and those with an initial diagnosis of leukemia or brain tumor. The excess mortality was due to death from primary cancer, second cancer, cardiotoxicity and noncancer death, and existing up to 25 years after the initial cancer diagnosis.

The more commonly reported second primary cancers are breast, bone, and thyroid cancers, therapy-related myelodysplasia, and acute myeloid leukemia. Female survivors who were treated with chest or mantle radiation for a pediatric malignancy face a significantly increased risk of breast cancer.

Genetic predisposition was first noted to have a substantial impact on the risk of secondary sarcomas among patients with the genetic form of retinoblastoma. This risk is further increased by radiation treatment and increases with the total dose of radiation delivered. Patients with a family history of early-onset cancers have also been shown to be at an increased risk of developing a second cancer. Members of families with Li–Fraumeni syndrome have been reported to be at increased risk of multiple subsequent cancers, with the highest risk observed among survivors of childhood cancer.[339] The subsequent cancers reported in this population were characteristic of Li–Fraumeni syndrome. It therefore appears that germ-line mutations in tumor-suppressor genes, as occurring in Li–Fraumeni syndrome, might interact with therapeutic exposures to result in an increased risk of second cancers.

Several genetic polymorphisms of enzymes capable of metabolic activation or detoxification of anticancer drugs, such as NAD(P)H:quinone oxidoreductase (NQO1), glutathione S-transferase (GST)-M1 and -T1, and CYP3A4, have been examined for their role in the development of therapy-related leukemia or myelodysplasia. These studies indicate that NQO1 polymorphism is significantly associated with the genetic risk of therapy-related acute leukemia and myelodysplasia. In addition, individuals with CYP3A4-W genotype may be at increased risk of treatment-related leukemia, presumably by increasing the production of reactive intermediates that damage DNA.[340-346]

Because subsequent malignancies remain a significant threat to the health of survivors treated for cancer during childhood, vigilant screening is important for those at risk. Risk of secondary acute myeloid leukemia is associated with exposure to topoisomerase II inhibitors (ie, epipodophyllotoxins and anthracyclines) for up to 10 years and with alkylating agents for up to 15 years.

Neurocognitive sequelae of treatment of childhood cancer occur because of radiation to the whole brain, systemic therapy with high-dose methotrexate or cytarabine, or with intrathecal methotrexate and other agents. Children with a history of brain tumors, ALL, or NHL are most likely to be affected. Risk factors include increasing radiation dose, young age at the time of treatment, treatment with both cranial radiation and systemic or intrathecal chemotherapy, and female gender.[347] Severe deficits are most frequently noted in children with brain tumors treated with radiation therapy, and in children who were less than 5 years of age at the time of treatment.

Chronic cardiotoxicity usually manifests itself as cardiomyopathy, pericarditis, and congestive heart failure. Childhood cancer survivors in the CCSS who were treated with chest or spinal radiation had a more than 2-fold increased risk of death related to cardiac disease in comparison with the standard US population.[348] The anthracyclines doxorubicin and daunomycin are well-known causes of cardiomyopathy.[349-351] The incidence of cardiomyopathy is dose-dependent and may exceed 30% among patients who received cumulative doses of anthracyclines in excess of 600 mg/m^2. A cumulative dose of anthracyclines greater than 300 mg/m^2 was associated with an increased risk of clinical heart failure (relative risk 11.8) compared with a cumulative dose lower than 300 mg/m^2. The estimated risk of clinical heart failure increased with time, and approached 5% after 15 years. These studies and others emphasize that cardiomyopathy can occur many years after completion of therapy (15-20 years) and that the onset may be spontaneous or coincide with exertion or pregnancy.

Pulmonary fibrosis and pneumonitis can result from pulmonary radiation. Thus, these problems are seen most often in patients with thoracic malignancies, notably Hodgkin disease. Following hematopoietic cell transplantation (HCT), both restrictive and obstructive lung disease, including bronchiolitis obliterans are well described.[352] In addition to radiation therapy, a growing list of chemotherapeutic agents appears to be responsible for pulmonary disease in long-term survivors. Bleomycin toxicity is the prototype for chemotherapy-related lung injury. Although interstitial pneumonitis and pulmonary fibrosis have been reported in children,[353] clinically apparent bleomycin pneumonopathy is most frequent in older adults.[354] The chronic lung toxicity usually follows persistence or progression of abnormalities developing within 3 months of therapy. Alkylating agents also are believed to cause chronic lung injury.

Chronic fibrosis of the liver is associated with radiation. Chemotherapy, even in the absence of radiation therapy, may be a cause of chronic hepatopathy. Viral hepatitis, most often related to transfusion of blood products prior to 1992, is another cause of chronic liver disease in long-term survivors.[355-357]

Damage to the proximal renal tubule from chemotherapy can cause Fanconi renal syndrome (hypokalemia, hypophosphatemia, glucosuria, proteinuria, renal tubular acidosis, and rickets).[358] Children at particular risk include those who received treatment with more than one nephrotoxic agent and those with concomitant renal damage related to surgery or radiation. Electrolyte wasting associated with ifosfamide therapy and hypomagnesaemia associated with cisplatin therapy appear to persist in some children.[359,360] Cyclophosphamide and ifosfamide are both capable of inducing hemorrhagic cystitis as a result of accumulation of acrolein in the bladder.[361] Radiation to the pelvis or bladder can result in fibrosis and scarring, with resultant decreased bladder capacity and predisposition to urinary tract infections.[362] Bladder cancer has developed in some patients who received bladder-toxic agents during treatment of childhood cancer.[361] Yearly urinalysis should be done in these patients to evaluate for the presence of microscopic hematuria.

Decreased linear growth is a common problem during therapy in children with cancer. Although catch-up growth may occur, such that the premorbid growth status is regained, in some instances short stature is permanent or even progressive. Severe growth retardation, defined as a standing height below the fifth percentile, has been observed in as many as 30-35% of survivors of childhood brain tumors[363-365] and in 10-15% of patients treated with some antileukemia regimens.[366-368] Whole-brain irradiation is a major risk factor for short stature,[367,369] especially in doses exceeding 18 Gy.[370]

Observational studies indicate that obesity as measured by weight or body mass index (BMI) has been reported in small groups of children with ALL and brain tumors treated with conventional therapy or BMT.[371-373] This problem has its onset either during therapy or within the first year after discontinuation of therapy and may either progress or stabilize.

Hypothyroidism is a common late effect and usually is due to radiation to the neck for a nonthyroid malignancy. All therapeutic modalities (radiation, surgery, or chemotherapy) cause both germ-cell depletion and abnormalities of gonadal endocrine function among male cancer survivors. Radiation to the testes is known to result in germinal loss with decreases in testicular volume and sperm production, and increases in follicle-stimulating hormone (FSH). Effects are dose-dependent, following fractionated exposures of 0.1-6 Gy.[374] All males treated with inverted-Y radiation for HD at a cumulative testicular dose of 1.4-3.0 Gy become azoospermic without recovery after 2-40 months of follow-up, despite lead shielding of the scrotum.[375] At doses of 4-6 Gy, azoospermia may persist for at least 3-5 years, and at doses above 6 Gy, usually appears to be irreversible.[376,377] In Seattle, the Bone Marrow Transplantation Team has monitored gonadal function in a large group of male patients who were past puberty at the time of total-body irradiation at a dose of 10 Gy delivered in a single fraction. Azoospermia was universal, although 2 of 41 patients had recovery of sperm production 6 years after HCT.[378]

Alkylating agents decrease spermatogenesis in long-term survivors of cancer, and the effects are dose-dependent. Gonadal damage following cumulative doses lower than 7.5 mg/m^2 of mechlorethamine or 200 mg/kg of cyclophosphamide as used in HCT has been shown to be reversible in up to 70% of patients after therapy-free intervals of several years.[379,380]

The gonadal toxicities are of serious concern to patients and their families. This concern has popularized pretreatment sperm banking. Unlike the males, germ-cell failure and loss of ovarian endocrine function usually occur concomitantly in females. Following radiation therapy, manifestations are both age-dependent and dose-dependent.[381] Prepubertal ovaries are relatively radioresistant, and despite higher doses (12–50 Gy), primary amenorrhea and delayed puberty eventually occurred in 68% of patients treated at a mean age of 6.9 years .[382] Premature menopause also has been reported in the setting of HCT. Ovarian failure has also been associated with chemotherapy, such as single alkylating agents (cyclophosphamide, busulfan, nitrogen mustard) or as combination therapy (MOPP).[383-385] and case reports have suggested that intensive chemotherapy completed before pregnancy, including myeloablative chemotherapy prior to HCT,[386] is compatible with normal offspring.[387] A recent report from the CCSS of 4029 pregnancies in 1915 female 5-year survivors of childhood cancer did not identify excess adverse outcomes for chemotherapeutic agents.[388] A companion study of 2323 pregnancies in partners of 1427 male survivors reported 69% live births, 1% stillbirths, 13% miscarriages, and 13% abortions (5% of outcomes were not accounted for).[389] The probability of a pregnancy ending in a live birth was significantly less than that for partners of male sibling controls (RR 0.8, $p = .007$).

Patients who desire to have children after completion of therapy may require care in high-risk obstetrical clinics, especially those who have a discussion of sperm banking storage received abdominal or pelvic irradiation.[390] Because much remains unknown about the problems of children born to survivors of childhood cancer, long-term general follow-up should be emphasized.

Several potentially ototoxic agents are commonly used in the treatment of children with malignancies, including platinum-based chemotherapy, aminoglycoside antibiotics, loop diuretics, and radiotherapy. These agents are all capable of causing sensorineural hearing loss. Very young children who received ototoxic agents during their cancer treatment and whose speech has not yet developed should undergo audiologic evaluations to determine whether they require intervention.

Interventions to assist children experiencing hearing loss because of cancer treatment include the use of hearing aids and other assistive devices, along with preferential seating in the front of the classroom. Musculoskeletal problems after childhood cancer involve bony abnormalities, such as scoliosis, atrophy, or hypoplasia; avascular necrosis (AVN); and osteoporosis (bone density ≥2.5 SD below mean)/ osteopenia (bone density 1-2.5 SD below mean).

Providing appropriate health care for survivors of cancer is emerging as one of the major challenges in medicine. Childhood cancer survivors, an especially high-risk population, seek and receive care from a wide variety of health care professionals, including oncologists, medical and pediatric specialists, surgeons, primary care physicians, gynecologists, nurses, psychologists, and social workers. The challenge arises from the heterogeneity of this patient population treated with numerous therapeutic modalities in an era of rapidly advancing understanding of late effects. The Institute of Medicine has recognized the need for a systematic plan for lifelong surveillance that incorporates risks based on therapeutic exposures, genetic predisposition, lifestyle behaviors, and comorbid health conditions.[391] The COG has recently updated our risk-based, exposure-related guidelines (Long-Term Follow-Up Guidelines for Survivors of Childhood, Adolescent, and Young-adult Cancers, [Landier, 2004 #741]) specifically designed to direct follow-up care for patients who were diagnosed and treated for pediatric malignancies. These guidelines represent a set of comprehensive screening recommendations that are clinically relevant and can be used to standardize and direct the follow-up care for this group of cancer survivors with specialized health care needs. <www.survivorshipguidelines.org>.

Acknowledgments

The authors acknowledge the previous contributors to this chapter since their work enabled the summary present here and the bibliography. They are Les Robison, PhD; Smita Bhatia, MD, MPH; Paul Gaynon, MD; Anne Angiolillo, MD; Janet Franklin, MD; Richard Aplenc, MD, MSCE; Beverly Lange, MD; Tobey McDonald, MD; Brian Rood, MD; James Nachman, MD; Mitchell Cairo, MD; Elizabeth Raetz, MD; Sherrie Perkins, MD; Carlos Rodriguez-Galindo, MD; Alberto Pappo, MD; Paul Grundy, MD; Jeffrey Dome, MD; John Kalapurakal, MD ; Elizabeth Perlman, MD;Michael Ritchey, MD; John Maris, MD Suzanne Shustermann, MD ; William Meyer,; MD; Kadria Sayed, MD; David Parham, MD; Richard Gorlick, MD, FAAP; Mark Bernstein, MD, FRCP(C); Jeffrey Toretsky, MD; R. Lor Randall, MD,FACS; Mark Gebhardt, MD; Lisa Teot, MD; Suzzane Wolden, MD; Neyssa Marina, MD.

Selected References

The complete reference list can be found at www.CANCERMEDICINE8.com

4. Gurney JG, Davis S, Severson RK, et al. Trends in cancer incidence among children in the US. *Cancer.* 1996;78:532–541.
5. Adamson P, Law G, Roman E. Assessment of trends in childhood cancer. Lancet 2005;365:753.
10. Woods WG, Neudorf S, Gold S, et al. A comparison of allogeneic bone marrow transplantation, autologous bone marrow transplantation, and aggressive chemotherapy for children with acute myeloid leukemia in remission. *Blood.* 2001;97:56–62.
11. Gaynon PS, Qu RP, Chappell RJ, et al. Survival after relapse in childhood acute lymphoblastic leukemia: impact of site and time of first relapse—the Children's Cancer Group experience. *Cancer.* 1998;82:1387–1395.
16. London WB, Castleberry RP, Matthay KK, et al. Evidence for an age cut-off greater than 365 days for neuroblastoma risk group stratification in the Children's Oncology Group (COG). *J Clin Oncol.* September 20, 2005;23(27):6459–6465.
17. Brodeur GM, Ambros PF. Genetic and biological markers of prognosis in neuroblastoma. In: Brodeur GM, Sawada T, Tsuchida Y, Voute PA, editors. *Neuroblastoma.* Amsterdam: Elsevier Science; 2000:355–369.
31. Bleyer A, O'Leary M, Barr R, Ries LAG, editors. *Cancer Epidemiology in Older Adolescents and Young Adults 15 to 29 Years of Age, Including SEER Incidence and Survival: 1975-2000.* National Cancer Institute, NIH Pub. No. 06-5767. Bethesda, MD 2006.
53. Creutzig U, Ritter J, Zimmerman M, et al. Improved treatment results in high-risk pediatric acute myeloid leukemia patients after intensification with high-dose cytarabine and mitoxantrone: results of Study Acute Myeloid Leukemia—Berlin-Frankfurt-Munster 93. *J Clin Oncol.* 2001;19:2705–2713.
54. Stevens RF, Hann IM, Wheatley K, Gray RG. Marked improvements in outcome with chemotherapy alone in pediatric acute myeloid leukemia: results of the United Kingdom Medical Research Council's 10th AML trial. MRC Childhood

Leukaemia Working Party. Br *J Haematol.* 1998;101:130–140.

57. Wheatley K, Burnett AK, Goldstone AH, et al. A simple, robust, validated and highly predictive index for the determination of risk-directed therapy in acute myeloid leukaemia derived from the MRC AML 10 trial [In Process Citation]. *Br J Haematol.* 1999;107:69–79.
64. Rosolen A, Pillon M, Garaventa A, et al. Anaplastic large cell lymphoma treated with a leukemia-like therapy: report of the Italian Association of Pediatric Hematology and Oncology (AIEOP) LNH-92 protocol. *Cancer.* November 15, 2005;104(10):2133–2140.
65. Mason D, Banks P, Chan J, et al. Nodular lymphocyte predominance Hodgkin's disease: a distinct clinico-pathological entity. *Am J Surg Pathol.* 1994;18:526–530.
66. Harris N, Jaffe E, Stein, et al. A revised European-American classification of lymphoid neoplasms: a proposal from the International Lymphoma Study Group. *Blood.* 1994;84:1361–1392.
81. Fong CT, Dracopoli NC, White PS, et al. Loss of heterozygosity for the short arm of chromosome 1 in human neuroblastomas: correlation with N-myc amplification. *Proc Natl Acad Sci USA.* 1989;86:3753–3757.
82. White PS, Maris JM, Beltinger C, et al. A region of consistent deletion in neuroblastoma maps within 1p36.2-.3. *Proc Natl Acad Sci USA.* 1995;92:5520–5524.
83. Maris JM, Weiss MJ, Guo C, et al. Loss of heterozygosity at 1p36 independently predicts for disease progression, but not decreased OS probability, in neuroblastoma patients: a Children's Cancer Group Study. *J Clin Oncol.* 2000;18:1888–1899.
95. Breen CJ, O'Meara A, McDermott M, et al. Coordinate deletion of chromosome 3p and 1 1q in neuroblastoma detected by comparative genomic hybridization. *Cancer Genet Cytogenet.* 2000;120:44–49.
96. Beheshti B, Braude I, Marrano P, et al. Chromosomal localization of DNA amplifications in neuroblastoma tumors using cDNA microarray comparative genomic hybridization. *Neoplasia.* 2003;5:53–62.
107. Cheung NK, Heller G, Kushner BH, et al. Stage IV neuroblastoma more than 1 year of age at diagnosis: Major response to chemotherapy and survival durations correlated strongly with dose intensity. *Prog Clin Biol Res.* 1991;366:567–573.
123. Matthay KK, Sather HN, Seeger RC, et al. Excellent outcome of stage II neuroblastoma is independent of residual disease and radiation therapy. *J Clin Oncol.* 1989;7:236–244.
132. Hsu LL, Evans AE, D'Angio GJ. Hepatomegaly in neuroblastoma stage 4s: criteria for treatment of the vulnerable neonate. *Med Pediatr Oncol.* 1996;27:521–528.
142. Pritchard J, McElwain TJ, Graham-Pole J. High dose melphalan with autologous marrow for treatment of advanced neuroblastoma. *Br J Cancer.* 1982;45:86–94.
143. Philip T, Zucker JM, Bernard JL, et al. Improved survival at 2 and 5 years in the LMCE 1 unselected group of 72 children with stage IV neuroblastoma older than 1 year of age at diagnosis: is cure possible in a small subgroup? *J Clin Oncol.* 1991;9:1037–1044.
150. Matthay KK, Seeger RC, Reynolds CP, et al. Allogeneic versus autologous purged bone marrow transplantation for neuroblastoma: a report from the Children's Cancer Group. *J Clin Oncol.* 1994;12:2382–2389.
170. Frost JD, Hank JA, Reaman GH, et al. A phase I/IB trial of murine monoclonal anti-GD2 antibody 14.G2a plus interleukin-2 in children with refractory neuroblastoma: a report of the Children's Cancer Group. *Cancer.* 1997;80:317–333.
185. Varanasi R, Bardeesy N, Ghahremani M, et al. Fine structure analysis of the WT1 gene in sporadic Wilms tumor. *Proc Natl Acad Sci USA.* 1994;91:3554–3558.
189. DeBaun MR, Niemitz EL, McNeil E, et al. Epigenetic alterations of H19 and LIT1 distinguish patients with Beckwith–Wiedemann syndrome with cancer and birth defects. *Am J Hum Genet.* 2002;70: 604–611.
190. Bliek J, Maas SM, Ruijter JM, et al. Increased tumour risk for BWS patients correlates with aberrant H19 and not KCNQ1OT1 methylation: occurrence of KCNQ1OT1 hypomethylation in familial cases of BWS. *Hum Mol Genet.* 2001;10:467–476.
191. Bonadio JF, Storer B, Norkool P, et al. Anaplastic Wilms tumor: clinical and pathologic studies. *J Clin Oncol.* 1985;3:513–520.
192. Faria P, Beckwith JB, Mishra K, et al. Focal versus diffuse anaplasia in Wilms tumor—new definitions with prognostic significance. *Am J Surg Pathol.* 1996;20:909–920.
193. Argani P, Perlman EJ, Breslow N, et al. Clear cell sarcoma of the kidney (CCSK): a review of 351 cases from the National Wilms Tumor Study Group Pathology Center. *Am J Surg Pathol.* 2000;24:4–18.
200. Thomas PR, Tefft M, Compaan PJ, et al. Results of two radiotherapy randomizations in the third National Wilms' Tumor Study (NWTS-3). *Cancer.* 1991;68:1703–1707.
206. Argani P, Perlman EJ, Breslow N, et al. Clear cell sarcoma of the kidney (CCSK): a review of 351 cases from the National Wilms Tumor Study Group Pathology Center. *Am J Surg Pathol.* 2000;24:4–18.
218. Heyn R, Haeberlen V, Newton WA, et al. Second malignant neoplasms in children treated for rhabdomyosarcoma. Intergroup Rhabdomyosarcoma Study Committee. *J Clin Oncol.* 1993;11:262–270.
220. Gripp KW, Scott CIJ, Nicholson L, et al. Five additional Costello syndrome patients with rhabdomyosarcoma: proposal for a tumor screening protocol. *Am J Med Genet.* 2002;108:80–87.
229. Carli M, Colombatti R, Oberlin O, et al. European intergroup studies (MMT4-89 and MMT4-91) on childhood metastatic rhabdomyosarcoma: final results and analysis of prognostic factors. *J Clin Oncol.* 2004;22:4735–4742.
241. Meyers PA, Heller G, Healey JH, et al. Osteogenic sarcoma with clinically detectable metastasis at initial presentation. *J Clin Oncol.* 1993;11:449–453.
247. Buckley JD, Pendergrass TW, Buckley CM, et al. Epidemiology of osteosarcoma and Ewing's sarcoma in childhood: a study of 305 cases by the Children's Cancer Group. *Cancer.* 1998;83:1440–1448.
257. Terrier P, Henry-Amar M, Triche TJ, et al. Is neuro-ectodermal differentiation of Ewing's sarcoma of bone associated with an unfavourable prognosis? *Eur J Cancer.* 1995;31A:307–314.
263. Womer RR, West DC, Krailo MD et al Randomized comparison of every-two-week vs every-three-week chemotherapy in Ewing sarcoma family tumors(EFST). *J Clin Oncol.* 2008;26(15S Part I of II) #10504.
267. Cotterill SJ, Ahrens S, Paulussen M, et al. Prognostic factors in Ewing's tumor of bone: analysis of 975 patients from the European Intergroup Cooperative Ewing's Sarcoma Study Group. *J Clin Oncol.* 2000;18:3108–3114.
278. Gajjar A, Hernan R, Kocak M, et al. Clinical, histopathologic, and molecular markers of prognosis: toward a new disease risk stratification system for medulloblastoma. *J Clin Oncol.* 2004; 22:984–993.
288. Farmer JP, Montes JL, Freeman CR, et al. Brainstem Gliomas. A 10-year institutional review. *Pediatr Neurosurg.* 2001;34: 206–214.
301. Brantley MA Jr, Harbour JW. The molecular biology of retinoblastoma. *Ocul Immunol Inflamm.* 2001;9:1–8.
314. Perlman EJ, Hu J, Ho D, et al. Genetic analysis of childhood endodermal sinus tumors by comparative genomic hybridization. *J Pediatr Hematol Oncol.* 2000;22:100–105.
330. Haas JE, Feusner JH, Finegold MJ. Small cell undifferentiated histology in hepatoblastoma may be unfavorable. *Cancer.* 2001;92:3130–3134.
343. Smith G, Stanley LA, Sim E, et al. Metabolic polymorphisms and cancer susceptibility. *Cancer Surv.* 1995;25:27–65.
359. Neglia JP, Nesbit ME. Care and treatment of long-term survivors of childhood cancer. *Cancer.* 1993;71:3386–3391.
374. Rowley MM, Leach DR, Warner GA, Heller CG. Effect of graded doses of ionizing radiation on the human testes. *Radiat Res.* 1974;59:665–678.
382. Stillman RJ, Schinfeld JS, Schiff I, et al. Ovarian failure in long-term survivors of childhood malignancy. *Am J Obstet Gynecol.* 1981;139:62–66.
390. Chapman RM, Sutcliffe SB, Malpas JS. Male gonadal dysfunction in Hodgkin's disease: a prospective study. *JAMA.* 1981;245:1323–1328.
391. Hewitt M, Weiner SL, Simone JV, editors. *Childhood Cancer Survivorship: Improving Care and Quality of Life.* Washington, DC: National Academies Press; 2003.

122 Anorexia and Cachexia

Takao Ohnuma, MD, PhD

Introduction

Cachexia and anorexia are commonly associated with a number of acute and chronic diseases, including cancer, acquired immunodeficiency syndrome, sepsis, chronic heart failure, kidney failure, burn injury, severe trauma, and chronic arthritis.[1]

Cachexia is a complex syndrome presenting as wasting of muscle and adipose tissues, weight loss, anorexia, early satiety, fatigue, anemia, hyperlipidemia, systemic inflammatory responses including elevated proinflammatory cytokines and often a hypercatabolic state.

In a study to establish factors influencing survival of cancer patients after diagnosis of terminal cancer of the lung, breast, or gastrointestinal (GI) tract, shorter survival was independently associated with a weight loss of greater than 8.1 kg in the previous 6 months.[2] In addition to a reduction in survival time, patients had a reduced quality of life. Chronic pain and fatigue were common, and there was a poor tolerance to surgery, chemotherapy and radiotherapy.[3]

Extensive loss of skeletal muscle mass and adipose tissue in cachexia may be contrasted with simple starvation in which fat replaces glucose as the preferred fuel to spare lean body mass.[4-6] Cancer cachexia results from altered metabolism rather than just an energy deficit, and it cannot be reversed by forced feeding.*[7-9]

Etiology and Mechanisms

The causes of cancer-related cachexia are multifold and can be grouped into three interrelated categories: anorexia and early satiety, mechanical obstruction of the alimentary tract, and metabolic derangement.

Anorexia and Early Satiety

Anorexia in cancer patients can be divided into disease related, treatment related and emotional distress related. Anorexia may result from early satiety, nausea or dysgeusia, a change in taste.

Abnormalities of taste sensation and olfaction for food aromas have been demonstrated in cancer patients.[10,11] Patients displayed distaste for sweet compared to healthy subjects, which correlated with a loss of taste sensation. Patients experiencing food aversion found the odors of chocolate, pork, roast beef, and chicken significantly less pleasant than controls.[11]

Etiologic Factors of Anorexia and Early Satiety ■ Animal studies and clinical trials have identified many factors as causes of cancer anorexia. Examples are listed in Table 122-1, which illustrates that cancer anorexia is likely multifactorial. Among these factors, serotonin, cytokines as well as neuropeptidergic circuit dysfunction are worthy of additional comments.

Serotonin ■ Abnormal tumor cell utilization of tryptophan, the precursor of serotonin, with resultant excess free tryptophan levels in plasma has been reported in cancer patients.[12] Increase in blood tryptophan results in elevated tryptophan levels in the cerebrospinal fluid, which appears to induce increased serotonin synthesis/secretion in the ventromedial hypothalamic (VMH) serotonergic system. A close relationship between elevated plasma-free tryptophan and anorexia was observed in patients with cancer.[13] Increases in urinary excretion of 5-hydroxyindoleacetic acid, the main metabolite of serotonin, have been identified after cisplatin treatment in cancer patients.[14] As described below, studies of cytokines and neuropeptide circuits have led to identification of central nervous system (CNS) serotonin as a major mediator of cancer anorexia.[15]

Table 122-1 ■ **Possible Causes of Cancer Anorexia**

- Bombesin, a neuropeptide produced by small-cell lung cancer[339]
- Certain cytokines, eg, TNF-α and IL-1[13]
- Emetogenic anticancer agents, eg, cisplatin, nitrogen mustard, doxorubicin[14]
- Glucagon or glucagon-like peptides[340]
- Hypercalcemia, a common paraneoplastic syndrome[341]
- Increases in serum lactate, known to be produced abundantly by tumor[342]
- Dysfunction of neuropeptidergic circuits in the brain[28]
- Satietins, proteins isolated from human plasma[343,344]
- Increases in serotonin levels in serum and CNS in cancer patients.[12-15]
- Toxohormone-L, a lipolytic factor purified from ascitic fluid of patients with hepatoma[95]

Cytokines ■ Certain cytokines, such as tumor necrosis factor-α (TNF-α) and interleukin-1 (IL-1) are shown to be mediators of anorexia. While TNF-α induces IL-1, both cytokines appear to be operative in mediating their anorectic effect through the brain as well as directly on the GI tract, eg, decrease in gastric emptying time.[16,17] Peripherally infused IL-1 increased brain tryptophan and serotonin concentrations, whereas intracerebrally infused IL-1 increased neural firing rate and serotonin release in the VMH, suggesting that IL-1 production during tumor growth facilitated tryptophan conversion in the brain.

Using methylcholanthrene-induced tumors in rats, various specific components of the cytokine-induced anorectic reactions were examined in the tumor tissue, the liver and the brain including: IL-1β system components (ligand, signaling receptor, receptor accessory proteins, and receptor antagonist), TNF-α, TGF-β1, and IFN-γ. IL-1β, TNF-α, and interferon-γ (IFN-γ) mRNA were detected in the tumor tissue of anorectic tumor-bearing rats, whereas in brain regions, anorexia was associated with the upregulation of only IL-1β and its receptor mRNA. All other mRNA's remained unchanged in the brain regions examined. This observation suggests that IL-1β and its receptor played a major role in this model of cancer-associated anorexia.[18]

While IFN-γ infusion produced anorexia in patients with renal cell cancer, the appearance of anorexia in mice associated with tumor growth was similar whether mice were IFN-γ knockout or intact, suggesting that endogenous IFN-γ plays little role in producing anorexia in the tumor-bearing host.[19,20] IL-6 appears to have no direct anorectic effect.[21,22]

Immunohistochemical image analyses of the time course of various proinflammatory cytokines in the CNS of tumor-bearing mice did not find that upregulation of brain cytokines could explain cancer anorexia.[23]

Animal studies showed development of tolerance to injections of TNF-α and IL-1.[24] IL-1 infusion was not anorexigenic in food-deprived rats.[25]

---

*A portion of this review appeared in *Supportive Care in Cancer Therapy* Ettinger, D. (ed.), Cancer Drug Discovery and Development Series, Humana Press, 2009.[9]

Serum levels of circulating TNF-α, IL-1, IL-6, and IFN-γ did not correlate with the anorexia/weight loss syndrome in cancer patients.[26,27] These studies imply that anorexigenic actions of these cytokines are processed by intermediate mediator molecules, such as melanocortins.[28] Cytokines not only produce anorectic effects but also exert direct catabolic activity on muscle and adipose tissues. The direct catabolic effects and cytokine-mediated signaling pathways are discussed in separate sections on "Cytokines" and "Signaling Pathways Involved in Cancer Cachexia and Identification of Muscle Atrophy Genes."

Dysregulation of Neuropeptidergic Circuits ■ Both insulin, secreted from the exocrine pancreas, and leptin, produced primarily by adipocytes, circulate at levels proportional to body fat content and enter the CNS in proportion to their plasma levels. As weight increases insulin secretion is increased both at the basal state and in response to meals to compensate for insulin resistance. As obesity progresses increased insulin secretion promotes insulin delivery to the brain, where it helps to limit further weight gain. Insulin also promotes both fat storage and leptin synthesis by fat cells. Leptin has a more important role than insulin in the CNS control of energy homeostasis. Thus, leptin deficiency causes severe obesity with hyperphagia that persists, despite high insulin levels. In contrast, obesity is not induced by insulin deficiency.[29,30] Several studies have dealt with the role of leptin in cancer-induced anorexia. In cachectic tumor-bearing animals, lower circulating levels of leptin together with decreased adipose tissue leptin mRNA content have been described.[31] Similarly, serum leptin levels were reduced in patients with both advanced lung cancer and colon cancer, suggesting that cancer anorexia and cachexia are not solely due to the dysregulation of leptin production.[32,33] Plasma leptin levels showed gender-dependent associations, and significantly lower levels were found among cachectic women but not among cachectic men.[34]

Ghrelin, a 28-amino acid peptide produced by the oxyntic cells of the stomach, is the natural ligand for the growth hormone secretagogue receptor (GHS-R) in the pituitary gland. It exists in two major molecular forms, ghrelin and des-n-octanoyl ghrelin (des-acyl ghrelin). In vitro, both exhibit similar GHS-R-independent biological activities. It has profound orexigenic, adipogenic, and somatotrophic properties, thereby increasing food intake and body weight.[35] The brain–gut axis is the effector of anabolism, regulating feeding, metabolism, and growth via vagal efferents mediating ghrelin signaling. Animal studies suggested that ghrelin's prime metabolic function is to modulate glucose sensing and insulin sensitivity, rather than directly regulating energy homeostasis.

Studies of ghrelin and of IL-6 levels in cancer patients provided conflicting data. Ghrelin and IL-6 levels were either increased, equal, or lower in cachectic cancer patients than those in noncachectic groups.[36–39]

Both insulin and leptin interact with several distinct hypothalamic neuropeptide-containing pathways.[29,40,41]

Neuropeptides implicated in the control of energy homeostasis are divided into orexigenic (anabolic) and anorexigenic (catabolic) signaling molecules (Table 122-2). Peripheral leptin enters into the CNS where leptin receptors exist in the hypothalamus. Leptin interacts with numerous hypothalamic neuropeptidergic–effector molecules, which are downstream of the leptin signal. Leptin suppresses hypothalamic orexigenic neuropeptides, which include neuropeptide Y (NPY), agouti-related protein (AgRP), melanin-concentrating hormone (MCH), and orexin. Leptin also stimulates anorexigenic neuropeptides including α-melanocytes-stimulating hormone (α-MSH), corticotropin-releasing hormone (CRH), cocaine, and amphetamine-related transcript (CART). The arcuate nucleus transduces leptin signals from the periphery. The leptin receptor is coexpressed with NPY and AgRP in the arcuate nucleus neurons, and is also expressed in pro-opiomelanocortin/CART neurons. NPY/AgRP neurons are inhibited by leptin and activated by a decrease in leptin levels. NPY stimulates food intake and decreases energy expenditure, primarily from a reduction in thermogenesis in brown adipose tissue (BAT) and by facilitating fat deposition in white adipose tissue, partly through increased insulin activity. Both insulin and leptin have been shown to activate the hypothalamic phosphoinositol-3-kinase pathway.[42] From this apparently contradictory observation, possible mechanisms of insulin- and leptin-resistance were inferred.[43] While synthesis and secretion of leptin appear to be stimulated by cytokines such as IL-1, circulating leptin levels are not elevated in cachectic cancer patients.[44,45]

Table 121-2 ■ **Orexigenic (Anabolic) and Anorexigenic (Catabolic) Neuropeptides**

Orexigenic molecules
Neuropeptide Y (NPY)
Agouti-related protein (AGRP)
Melanin-concentrating hormone (MCH)
Hypocretin 1 and 2 (Orexin A and B)
Galanin
Norepinephrine
Opioids
Anorexigenic molecules
Melanoxyte-stimulating hormone (MSH)
Coricotropin-releasing hormone (CRH)
Thyrotropin-releasing hormone (TRH)
Cocaine- and amphetamnine-regulated transcript (CART)
Urocortin
Glucagon-like peptide 1 (GLP-1)
Oxytocin
Neurotensin
Serotonin

Source: Adapted from Ref. 29.

Dysregulation of the neuropeptidergic circuit controlling food intake, energy expenditure, and thus energy homeostasis may play a role in the development of the cancer anorexia–cachexia syndrome.[46] Thus, rats bearing methylcholanthrene-induced sarcomas were refractory to intrahypothalamic injection of NPY as an orexigen compared to controls.[47] NPY mRNA levels are not always increased in anorectic tumor-bearing rats when compared with pair-fed or control animals.[48] Reduced affinity of hypothalamic NPY receptors as well as refractory adenylate cyclase in response to NPY suggested that the postsynaptic NPY-signaling systems were altered in the hypothalamus of tumor-bearing rats.[49,50]

Cytokines produce a more potent effect on feeding and metabolism when injected directly into the CNS rather than peripherally. A central mechanism of action in the production of cachexia has been postulated for many cytokines, including IL-1, IL-6, IL-8, TNF-α, IFN-α, and other chemokines.[40,51]

TNF-α acts peripherally to increase leptin mRNA and centrally upon neural activity of glucose-sensitive neurons within the ventromedial nucleus and the lateral hypothalamic area. Episodic TNF administration has been reported to induce anorexia but does not appear to be able to induce cachexia. Tolerance to the cytokine eventually develops and food intake and body weight returns to normal.[52]

IL-1β blocked hypothalamic NPY mRNA levels and decreased NPY-induced feeding, whereas it stimulated CRH in parallel with suppression of food intake.[52,53] Conversely, at different doses NPY blocked and reversed IL-1β-induced anorexia.[54] IL-1 induced anorexia is mainly due to development of early satiety, and such early satiety has long been linked to enhanced serotonergic activity.[55] In addition, TNF-α and IFN-γ were also shown to stimulate CRH expression and/or release.[56] Cytokines may play an important role in long-term inhibition of feeding by mimicking the hypothalamic effect of excessive negative feedback signaling from leptin by persistent stimulation of anorexigenic neuropeptides such as CRH or by inhibition of the NPY orexigenic network.[46]

In summary, a number of factors have been proposed as putative mediators of cancer anorexia, including hormones (eg, leptin), neuropeptides (eg, NPY), cytokines (eg, IL-1, TNF), and neurotransmitters (eg, serotonin and dopamine). Rather than representing separate and distinct pathogenic entities, it appears that close inter-relationships exist among these factors. Indeed, many studies suggest that different anorexia-related factors converge on a common final pathway as a major target, ie, hypothalamic monoaminergic neurotransmission and serotonergic activity.[57–59]

Alimentary Tract Dysfunction

Abnormalities in perception of taste and smell have been described in cancer patients. Tumors of the mouth, oropharynx, esophagus, stomach, pancreas, liver, and peritoneum may compromise oral intake from mechanical interference with anatomical structures. Intestinal obstruction is a common complication of cancer. Malabsorption secondary to pancreatic insufficiency due to pancreas carcinoma or secondary to the infiltration of the intestine or mesentery by lymphoma has been described.[60,61]

Direct encroachment of a tumor on the GI tract, atrophic changes in the mucosa, and muscles of the stomach, a reduction in the duration or activity of digestive enzymes that may lead to delayed gastric emptying, and slowing of peristalsis are all pathogenic mechanisms that may contribute to early satiety.[62,63] Early satiety is common in patients with decreased upper GI motility.[64]

Major surgery for cancer, particularly on the GI tract, may produce abnormalities in taste, and difficulties in swallowing, digestion, or absorption that may contribute indirectly to anorexia. Chemotherapy commonly induces abnormal perception of taste, mucositis, and nausea and vomiting. Radiotherapy to the head and neck can induce stomatitis, xerostomia, and alterations in taste and smell. Radiotherapy to the abdomen can induce anorexia, nausea, vomiting, diarrhea, and malabsorption.

Biochemical and Metabolic Derangement

Increased Glucose Utilization and Futile Substrate Cycles ■ High rates of glucose utilization with production of lactic acid are characteristic features of the neoplastic cell. In mice bearing transplantable colon tumors, glucose utilization by the tumors was second only to that by the brain.[65] Hexokinase, which catalyzes the first step of the glycolytic pathway and which is often highly overexpressed in tumor cells, is a major player in this process. Binding of tumor hexokinase to the outer mitochondrial membrane provides the enzyme with preferential access to ATP generated in the mitochondrion and increases the activity and stability of the enzyme.[66] The end product of the hexokinase reaction, glucose-6-phosphate, serves not only as a source of ATP via glycolysis but is also a key intermediate in the metabolic processes essential for cell growth and proliferation. Alteration of an isozyme appears closely linked to this process. Thus, the promoter activity of the type II isoform of hexokinase, the dominant form expressed in AS-30 hepatoma cells, was found to be resistant to normal hormonal control.[67] The distal region of the promoter was found to display consensus motifs for hypoxia-inducible factor (HIF-1). Subjecting transfected hepatoma cells to hypoxic conditions activated the type II hexokinase promoter almost 7- fold in the presence of glucose.[68] The tumor cell was able to maintain glycolysis regardless of the metabolic state of surrounding normal cells.

Lactic acid produced via glucose metabolism may be used by other tissues for energy purposes or may be transported to the liver for resynthesis to glucose. The cyclic metabolic pathway, in which glucose is converted to lactic acid by glycolysis in tumor tissue and then reconverted to glucose in the liver, is referred to as the Cori cycle. Conversion of glucose to lactate in cancer cells yields two ATPs, whereas lactate to glucose conversion in the liver requires six ATPs. Thus a systemic energy-losing or futile substrate cycle, involving this interplay of tumor glycolysis and host gluconeogenesis may be an important cause of cancer cachexia.[69] Assuming that all lactate produced is recycled to glucose, the cancer cell acts as an energy parasite. It may be calculated, however, that if 85% of lactate passes through the gluconeogenic pathway and 15% is oxidized, the host's handling of tumor-produced lactate would be energetically neutral. It has been suggested that the increase in the Cori cycle is insignificant in terms of energy expenditure and that increased glucose catabolism itself is responsible for weight loss and development of cachexia.[70]

Cytokines ■ TNF-α, IL-1, IL-6 (and its subfamily members such as ciliary neurotrophic factor (CNTF) and leukemia inhibitory factor (LIF)), and IFN-γ produced by host immune cells and/or tumor cells have all been implicated as mediators of cancer cachexia.[71-73] These cytokines are characterized by the induction of anorexia, weight loss, an acute-phase protein response, protein and fat breakdown, rises in levels of cortisol and glucagon and falls in insulin level, insulin resistance, anemia, fever, and elevated energy expenditure in animals. Direct interaction with leptin, neuropeptides, or serotonin as mechanisms of induction of cancer anorexia has been described earlier.

TNF-α ■ TNF-α was independently and simultaneously discovered as cachectin because it caused systemic suppression of lipoprotein lipase and development of hypertriglyceridemia, a state frequently seen in cachectic animals.[74] One mechanism by which TNF-α induces a net catabolic state in the host is by mediating increased catabolism at the level of specific tissues such as muscle and fat.[75] TNF-α increases activities of both phosphofructokinase and fructose bisphosphate phosphatase in myocytes in culture, producing an increased substrate cycling between fructose-6-phosphate and fructose-1,6-bisphosphate. Each of the fructose-6-phosphate/fructose-1,6-bisphosphate cycles loses one ATP. TNF also increased ubiquitin gene expression in isolated rat muscle.

Elevation of serum TNF-α and/or TNF-α-receptor levels has been associated with the clinical status of patients with B-cell chronic lymphocytic leukemia and with endometrial carcinoma and other solid tumors.[76,77] Administration of TNF-α in humans induced anorexia, negative nitrogen balance, and increases in serum triglycerides and in very low-density lipoprotein.[78,79] In contrast, TNF-α was rarely detected in patients with clinical cancer cachexia, and administration of recombinant TNF-α did not produce demonstrable cachexia.[26,27,80] Patients with type I hyperlipidemia caused by an inherited deficiency in lipoprotein-lipase have normal fat stores and are not cachectic. These observations suggest neither TNF-α nor suppression of lipoprotein-lipase alone can explain loss of adipose tissue and cachexia in cancer patients.

IL-1 ■ The genotype for a diallelic polymorphism of the *IL-1β* gene was examined in patients with pancreatic cancer.[81] The possession of a genotype resulting in increased *IL-1β* production was associated with shortened survival and increased serum C-reactive protein (CRP) level. This may reflect the role of *IL-1β* in inducing an acute phase protein response and cachexia in cancer.

IL-6 ■ A significant role of IL-6β in cancer anorexia is detailed in the earlier section. Involvement of IL-6 in the development of cancer cachexia has been suggested from a number of animal models. Prevention of muscle atrophy in tumor-bearing mice by anti-IL-6 receptor antibody appears to be mediated by modulation of lysosomal and ATP-ubiquitin-dependent proteolytic pathways.[82] The influence of IL-1 on cachexia appears to be mediated through IL-6, and IL-6 seems to act in concert with other cytokines in a final common pathway of cachexia.[83,84]

In patients with lung cancer, increased IL-6 levels were correlated with extensive disease, impaired performance status, enhanced acute phase response, weight loss, and malnutrition.[85,86]

Serum IL-6 concentrations were significantly elevated in tumor bearing animals but only minimally in patients with cancer.[87] IL-1 and IL-6 serum levels were not always measurable.[88] IL-6 administration produced no changes in ubiquitin gene expression, and no effect on body weight or food intake, despite being associated with increased acute-phase protein production.[22] Likewise, transgenic mice constitutively expressing IL-6 did not develop cachexia.[89,90] It has been suggested that IL-6 is necessary but not sufficient for the induction of cachexia, and that additional factor(s) besides IL-1β control production of IL-6 and other cachexigenic factors.[18]

The superfamily of IL-6 includes LIF and CNTF. LIF will be discussed in the section on "Tumor Byproducts." The role of CNTF in cancer anorexia/cachexia in humans has not been established.

IFN-γ ■ IFN-γ may have a bearing on the development of cancer cachexia. IFN and TNF were shown to have similar catabolic effects on NIH 3T3 cells in vitro.[91] Monoclonal antibody against IFN-γ given prior to injection of Lewis lung tumor cells prevented cachexia from developing.[92] IFN-γ was found to be increased in 51% of patients with multiple myeloma.[93] The levels of IFN-γ had no correlation with clinical parameters, however.

As to the link between inflammatory cytokines and energy expenditure, involvement of the transcriptional coactivator, peroxisome proliferator-activated receptor (PPAR) gamma coactivator-1 (PGC-1) has been suggested. Thus, many cytokines activate PGC-1 through phosphorylation by p38 kinase, resulting in stabilization and activation of PGC-1 protein. Cytokine-induced activation of PGC-1 in cultured muscle cells or muscle tissue in vivo caused increased respiration and expression of genes linked to mitochondrial uncoupling and energy expenditure. These data illustrated a direct thermogenic action of cytokines through PGC-1.[94] The role of various cytokines as the initiating signals in the development of cancer cachexia is discussed in the section on "Signaling Pathways Involved in Cancer Cachexia and Identification of Muscle Atrophy Genes."

Tumor Byproducts ■ Various pharmacologically active tumor byproducts have been reported as causal factors of cachexia.

Lipolytic Factors ■ Three different lipolytic factors have been characterized or purified. First, a lipolytic factor termed Toxohormone-L was found in pleural effusions of patients with malignant lymphoma as well as in ascites from patients with ovarian carcinoma and hepatoma.[95] It is an acidic protein with a molecular weight of 65-75 kDa. Toxohormone-L elicited fatty acid release in rat adipose tissue in vitro and injections into rat resulted in suppression of food and water intake. Toxohormone-L and related substances were considered responsible for the cancer cachexia syndrome in nude mice bearing human cancer cell lines.[96]

Second, LIF (leukemia inhibitory factor) was originally isolated from conditioned medium of Krebs II ascites tumor cells. This factor has a differentiation-inducing activity on myeloid leukemia cell lines. In an independent work the identical material was purified from conditioned medium of human melanoma cell line SEKI. The substance was found to be an effective lipoprotein-lipase inhibitor.[97] Comparisons among nude mice bearing various human melanoma cell lines revealed that the degree of LIF mRNA expression correlated with the development of cachexia.[98] LIF caused smaller increases in lipolysis and catabolic effects than those of TNF.[98,99]

Third, British workers purified and characterized what they termed lipid-mobilizing factor (LMF), which was derived from MAC16 murine adenocarcinoma and from urine of cancer patients with cachexia.[100,101] LMF, an acidic peptide, lacked triglyceride lipase activity and was different from natural lipolytic hormones, which were all basic. LMF isolated from either the murine tumor or from patients' urine had an apparent MW of 43 kDa and was homologous to the plasma protein Zn-α2-glycoprotein (ZAG).[100] Both caused direct lipolysis in isolated murine adepocytes and caused selective loss of adipose tissue in male mice.[101] Both caused stimulation of adenylate cyclase in murine adipocyte plasma membranes in a GTP-dependent process, and release of glycerol from isolated adipocytes. Adenylate cyclase stimulation and thus oxygen consumption in BAT by LMF is mediated by a β3-adrenergic receptor.[102,103] Brown adipocytes express abundant amounts of β3-adrenergic receptors. An increase in oxygen uptake by interscapular BAT suggested that LMF exerted its effect by increases in energy expenditure.[102] This increase may be related to changes in expression of uncoupling proteins (UCP) because mice bearing MAC16 tumor showed higher UCP-1 mRNA levels in BAT than did controls.[104] Three types of UCPs are known. UCP1 is present only in BAT, UCP2 is expressed ubiquitously and UCP3 is expressed abundantly and specifically in skeletal muscle in humans and also in BAT of rodents. LMF increased expression of UCP1, 2, and 3 in BAT and UCP-2 in liver and skeletal muscle.[105] UCPs function as mitochondrial protein carriers that stimulate heat production by dissipating the proton gradient generated during respiration across the inner mitochondrial membrane, thereby uncoupling respiration from ATP synthesis. In rodents UCP2 and UCP3 mRNAs were elevated in skeletal muscle during tumor growth; TNF was able to mimic this increase in gene expression.[106]

Recent studies showed that ZAG is produced not only by certain tumors, but also by BAT and white adipose tissue.[107] Glucocorticoids stimulate lipolysis through an increase in ZAG expression, and they are responsible for the increase in ZAG expression seen in adipose tissue of cachectic mice.[108] These findings suggest that increased cortisol levels seen in cachectic cancer patients may lead to an increased lipolysis through ZAG overexpression.

In cancer patients with weight loss, LMF/ZAG levels found in serum and urine were much higher than those in noncancer control patients with comparable weight loss and were proportional to the degree of weight loss.[109] Patients who responded to therapy showed a decrease in the plasma levels of LMF/ZAG, which correlated, with the levels of response.[110]

Proteolysis-Inducing Factor (PIF) ■ Serum from cachectic mice bearing MAC16 adenocarcinoma as well as urine and plasma from cancer patients with weight loss contained factors that induced proteolysis in skeletal muscles.[6,111,112] These factors are termed PIF. The PIFs derived from murine and human sources are identical: both are characterized as a sulfated glycoprotein with a molecular weight of 24 kDa, with a unique amino acid sequence. A murine monoclonal antibody can attenuate weight loss induced by human PIF in mice. PIF was readily detected in the urine of cachectic cancer patients, whereas it was absent in the urine of normal subjects and of patients with weight loss due to trauma or sepsis. Weight loss was associated with loss of skeletal muscles, but there was no effect on the heart and increase in liver weight.[112] Protein degradation induced by PIF appears to be mediated through the ubiquitin-proteasome pathway specifically in skeletal muscles.[113] Increased muscle proteasome activity was correlated with disease severity in gastric cancer patients.[114] Effects of PIF on increased expression of proteasome subunits and the ubiquitin-conjugating enzyme (E214k) were also demonstrated in vitro. The action of PIF on the protein degradation was mediated by the phospholipase A2 catalyzed release of arachidonic acid from membrane phospholipid and its conversion to the lipoxygenase product 15-hydroxyeicosatetraenoic acid.[113]

Production of PIF appears to be associated specifically with cancer cachexia and it was not found in the urine of patients undergoing major surgery or in those with burns, multiple injuries, sepsis, or sleeping sickness, even though the rate of weight loss exceeded that found in cancer patients.[115] Patients with cancer of the pancreas, lung, colon, breast, rectum, liver, and ovary in whom the rate of weight loss was greater than or equal to one kg/month showed evidence of PIF excretion in the urine.[116] Eighty percent of patients with pancreas cancer excreted PIF in the urine.[115]

Signaling Pathways Involved in Cancer Cachexia and Identification of Muscle Atrophy Genes (Table 122-3) ■ ***Nuclear Factor Kappa B-Dependent Pathway*** ■ Research in recent years has elucidated essential functions of the nuclear factor kappa B (NF-κB) family of transcription factors in skeletal myogenesis and muscle disease. The first hint that NF-κB was relevant in cancer cachexia came from studies showing that NF-κB by cachectic factors TNF plus IFN-γ caused a block in muscle differentiation by targeting the myogenic transcription factor MyoD in mouse myocytes. Both TNF and IFN-γ signaling were required for NF-κB-dependent downregulation of MyoD and dysfunction of skeletal myofibers. MyoD mRNA was also downregulated by TNF and IFN-γ expression in mouse muscle in vivo.[117]

In myogenic cell cultures, treatment with a combination of TNF-α and IFN-γ resulted in selective and progressive depletion of myosin heavy chain, whereas, none of other core myofibrillar proteins, troponin T, tropomyosin a and b, actin or actinin were affected.[118] Again treatment with TNF-α alone or IFN-γ alone had negligible effect on the myosin heavy chain depletion. Depletion of myosin heavy chain of cultured myotubes with TNF-α and IFN-γ was associated with a decrease in MyoD. These results imply that TNF-α and IFN-γ selectively trigger a reduction in the expression of the myosin heavy chain through a MyoD-mediated block in gene transcription. The implantation of cells expressing both TNF-α and IFN-γ into muscles of mice led to a similar, specific reduction in the synthesis of the myosin heavy chain relative to that of other myofibrillar proteins such as actin and tropomyosin.

Interestingly, transplantation of C-26 adenocarcinoma, which is known to produce IL-6 rather than TNF-α and IFN-γ resulted in downregulation of myosin heavy chain, but through a different mechanism, via ubiquitin-dependent proteasome mediated protein degradation.[22,82] These observations highlight the importance of myosin heavy chain as a target of cachexia, which occurs through different pathways.

In resting conditions, NF-κB is sequestered in the cytoplasm bound to its inhibitor, I-κB. TNF-α, IL-β, and PIF induce degradation of the wild type (but not the mutant) I-κBα. This degradation leads to nuclear accumulation of NF-κB, which mediates proteolytic loss of the myofibrillar protein myosin in myotubes.[119] PIF also induces expression of the ubiquitin-proteasome pathway. PIF is able to activate the transcription factor NF-κB and NF-κB inducible genes in isolated human Kupffer cells and in monocytes, resulting in production of proinflammatory cytokines, TNF-α, IL-8, and IL-6. PIF also activates the transcription factor STAT3 in Kupffer cells. The proinflammatory effect of PIF, mediated via NF-κB and STAT3 may contribute to the inflammatory procachectic process in the liver.[120]

NF-κB is a dynamic transcription factor family involved in the regulation of innate immune response, cellular proliferation, differentiation, and cell survival. It exists as a homodimer and heterodimer made up of five family members: RelA/p65, c-Rel, RelB, p50/p105 (NF-κB1), and p52/p100 (NF-κB2). The prototypic form of NF-κB consists of the p50/p65 heterodimer. In most cells, the majority of NF-κB resides in the cytoplasm, bound to the IκB, inhibitory protein family. These proteins function as inhibitors through ankyrin repeats, which bind to the REL domain of NF-κB and mask the nuclear localization signal (NLS) site thus preventing NF-κB's nuclear translocation.[121,122]

To gain greater insight on the role of NF-κB in cytokine-induced muscle wasting, regulation of NF-κB in response to TNF and IFN signaling in differentiated skeletal muscle was studied using differentiated C2C12 muscle cultures. Since IFN has not been demonstrated on its own to activate NF-κB, a question was raised whether IFN signaling could synergize with TNF to activate NF-κB to a threshold level required for muscle decay. IFN did not potentiate TNF-induced activation of NF-κB, suggesting that the synergistic interaction of TNF and IFN to induce muscle loss occurs downstream from the initial point of NF-κB activation. It was observed that treatment of C2C12 myotubes with TNF alone caused a clear and pronounced biphasic activity of NF-κB. In contrast to the first phase, which was potent but transient, the activity of the second phase was equally potent but persisted, lasting an additional 24-36 hours following TNF treatment. This type of NF-κB activity profile was unlike the classical scheme represented by a single transient phase. It also differed from the more commonly described chronic or persistent activity of NF-κB.[123]

Ubiquitin-Proteasome Pathway and Muscle Specific Ubiquitin Ligases ■ The ubiquitin–proteasome pathway is one of the three known proteolytic systems involved in muscle protein breakdown, it has been shown to mediate a large part of the degradation of either short-lived proteins or long-lived myofibrillar proteins in skeletal muscle. The addition of ubiquitin to a protein substrate is believed to be an exquisitely modulated process. This process requires three distinct components: an El ubiquitin-activating enzyme, an E2 ubiquitin-conjugating enzyme, and an E3 ubiquitin ligating enzyme.[124] Ubiquitin is first activated by ubiquitin activating enzyme (El). This activated ubiquitin is then transferred to E2. E3 transfers an activated form of ubiquitin from E2 to a lysine residue on

Table 122-3 ■ **Signals Involved in Cancer Cachexia**

Signals	Expression	Function	References
NF-κB dependent pathway p50, c-Rel, Bcl-3	↑	Promotes protein degradation	119-120, 123
Ubiquitin-proteasome pathway and muscle-specific ubiquitin ligases MAFbx/atrogin-1, MuRF1	↑	Promotes protein degradation	118, 125-126
IGF-1/PI3K/AKT pathway eIF3-f	↓	Promotes protein degradation Inhibits protein synthesis	127-130, 132
FOXO-1, FOXO-3	↑	"Disinhibition" of protein degradation	130, 133, 134
MAPKs, PGC-1, p38, ERK ½, JNK, caspase 8	↑	Promotes protein degradation	94, 135
Cathepsin	↑	Promotes protein degradation	136
ROS, oxidative stress, nitric oxide		NF-κB activation, upregulation of ubiquitin-poteasome pathway, and increased apoptosis	137-141
Myostatin, ActIIB	↑	Promotes protein degradation	142-152
Dystrophin-glycoprotein complex (DGC)	↑	Muscle membrane damage and muscle wasting	153-162

the substrate. Individual E3s ubiquitinate specific classes of proteins; hence the E3s play an important role in determining which proteins are targeted for degradation by the proteasome.

There are significant increases in the expression of various components of the ubiquitin pathway during muscle atrophy. Two groups of investigators simultaneously identified muscle atrophy F-box (MAFbx)/atrogin-1 gene.[125,126] MAFbx contained a functional F-box domain that binds to Skpl and thereby to Rocl and Cull, the other components of SCF-type Ubiquitin-protein ligases (E3s), as well as a nuclear localization sequence and PDZ-binding domain. On fasting, MAFbx/atrogin-1 mRNA levels increased specifically in skeletal muscle and before atrophy occurred. MAFbx/atrogin-1 was one of the few examples of an F-box protein or Ub-protein ligase (E3) expressed in a tissue-specific manner and appeared to be a critical component in the enhanced proteolysis leading to muscle atrophy in diverse diseases.

Another novel muscle-specific ubiquitin ligase, muscle ring finger 1 (MuRF1), was also upregulated in several models of muscle atrophy including cancer, diabetes, inflammatory cytokins, unloading, denervation, and disuse.[126] MuRF1 encodes a protein, that contains three domains: a RING-finger domain required for ubiquitin-ligase activity; a "B-box", and a coiled-coil domain required for the formation of heterodimers between MuRF1 and a related protein, MuRF2. Although the triggers that cause atrophy are different the loss of muscle mass in each case involves a common program that stimulates muscle proteolysis.

In the following sections involvements of other upstream signals leading to MuRF1 and MAFbx activation and additional signals leading to muscle atropy will be discussed.

Insulin-Like Growth Factor/Phosphatidyl-Inositol-3-OH Kinase/Akt/Mammalian Target of Rapamycin Pathway ■ The IGF-1/PI3K/Akt/mTOR/P70S6K pathway is a crucial intracellular regulator of muscle hypertrophy.[127] Activation of phosphatidylinositol 3 kinase (PI3K) by upstream ligands such as IGF-1 phosphorylates the membrane phospholipids phosphatidylinositol-4,5-bisphosphate to phosphatidylinositol-3,4,5-trisphosphate, creating a lipid binding site on the cell membrane for a serine/threonine kinase called Akt (or PKB—protein kinase B). Activation of Akt phosphorylates and activates the mammalian target of rapamycin (mTOR) kinase, which in turn increases protein synthesis by phosphorylation and activation of p70S6 kinase, and phosphorylation of eukaryotic translation initiation factor 4E binding protein 1 (4E-BP-1), key regulatory proteins involved in translation and protein synthesis.[128,129]

Although skeletal muscle atrophy is not simply the converse of hypertrophy, recent studies have shown there are important connections between the deactivation of the IGF-1/PI3K/Akt pathway and proteolytic activity/expression of proteolytic genes. Thus, in addition to stimulate muscle protein synthesis through activation of PI3K and Akt, IGF-1 and insulin also reduced the expression of MuRF1 and MAFbx/atrogin-1.[130] Myotubes atrophy induced by dexamethasone was accompanied by the specific increased expression of MAFbx and MuRF1, and this upregulation of MAFbx and MuRF1 was antagonized by simultaneous treatment with IGF-1, acting through the PI3K/Akt pathway. Moreover, in cultured myotubes undergoing atrophy, the activity of the PI3K/AKT pathway decreased, while inhibition of PI3K and expression of a dominant-negative Akt reduced the mean size of myotubes in culture. Therefore, in controlling muscle mass, the IGF-1/PI3K/Akt pathway not only increases overall synthesis but also suppresses proteolysis and the expression of atrophy-related ubiquitin ligases.[131] It appears that Akt lies at the cross-point of multiple cellular signaling pathways and acts as a critical downstream mediator of the growth factor receptors and other receptors that activate PI3K.

Recently, eIF3-f, a regulatory subunit of the eukaryotic translation factor eIF3, a mTOR/S6Kl scaffolding protein in the IGF-1/Akt/mTOR dependent control of protein translation was found to be a key target that accounts for MAFbx/Atrogin-1 function in muscle atrophy. eIF3-f appeared to act as a "translational enhancer" that increases the efficiency of the structural muscle proteins synthesis leading to both in vitro and in vivo muscle hypertrophy.[132]

FOXO-1, FOXO-3 ■ The forkhead box O (FOXO) transcription factor FOXO-1, a member of the forkhead box-containing transcription factors are involved in various cellular processes including cell cycle regulation, differentiation, stress responses, and apoptosis.[133] FOXO-1 is markedly upregulated in skeletal muscle in energy-deprived states such as fasting, cancer, and severe diabetes.

A hierarchy between the signals, which mediate hypertrophy and those which mediate atrophy has now been elucidated.[134] The IGF-1/PI3K/Akt pathway, which has been shown to induce hypertrophy, prevents induction of requisite atrophy mediators, namely MAFbx and MuRF1. Moreover, the mechanism for this inhibition involves Akt-mediated inhibition of the FOXO family of transcription factors; a mutant form of FOXO-1, which prevents Akt phosphorylation, thereby prevents Akt-mediated inhibition of MuRF1 and MAFbx upregulation. In cultured myotubes undergoing atrophy, the activity of the PI3K/ATK pathway decreases, leading to activation of FOXO transcription factors and MAFbx/atrogin-1 induction indicating requirement of FOXO for PI3K/Akt in muscle atrophy. IGF-1 treatment or Akt overexpression inhibits FOXO and MAFbx/atrogin-1 expression. Moreover, constitutively active FOXO-3 acts on the MAFbx/atogin-1 promoter to cause MAFbx/arogin-1 transcription and dramatic atrophy of myotubes and muscle fibers.[133]

The activity of proteins in this pathway in muscle and liver biopsies was assessed from 16 patients undergoing pancreatectomy for possible carcinoma. Patients were divided into a noncachectic or cachectic group according to their weight loss before operation. Extracts of skeletal muscle and liver tissue from eight cachectic patients with pancreas carcinoma and eight noncachectic patients were analyzed by western blotting using pan- and phospho-specific antibodies directed against eight important signal transduction proteins of the PI-K/Akt pathway. Muscle samples from cachectic patients revealed significantly decreased levels of myosin heavy chain and actin in comparison to noncachectic samples. Akt protein level was decreased. The abundance and/or phosphorylation of the transcription factors FOXO-1 and FOXO-3a were reduced by up to fourfold in muscle biopsies from cachectic patients. Various decreases of the phosphorylated forms of the protein kinases mTOR and p70S6K were found. In contrast to skeletal muscle, cachexia is associated with a significant increase in phosphorylated Akt level in the liver samples with a general activation of the PI3-K/Akt cascade. This study demonstrated a cachexia-associated loss of Akt-dependent signaling in human skeletal muscle with decreased activity of regulators of protein synthesis and a disinhibition of protein degradation.[134]

Mitogen-Activated Protein Kinase (MAPK), PPAR Gamma Coactivator-1 (PGC-1), and Caspase Activation ■ In order to elucidate how inflammatory cytokines mediate cachectic states, studies were undertaken to evaluate whether the target of cytokine activation could be PGC-1, the transcriptional PPAR gamma coactivator-1. Many cytokines were found to stimulate phosphorylation and activation of PGC-1 through p38 MAP kinase. Cytokine or lipopolysaccharide (LPS)-induced activation of PGC-1 in cultured muscle cells or muscle in vivo caused increased respiration and expression of genes linked to mitochondrial uncoupling and energy expenditure. These data illustrated a direct thermogenic action of cytokines and p38 MAP kinase through PGC-1.[94]

Using an in vitro model to mimic muscle wasting, the multifaceted roles that one such cytokine, TNF-α, invokes in the degeneration process was elucidated. Treatment of C2 skeletal myoblasts with TNF-α not only suppressed morphological and biochemical differentiation, but following an initial wave of proliferation, and of survival (24 h), induced apoptosis. Investigating the mechanisms underlying these diverse actions of TNF-α, it was demonstrated that cell replication was dependent on rapid and sustained activation of MAP kinases: p38, ERK1/2, and Jun kinase (JNK). MAP kinase was not, however, central to the death process, which was associated with a progressive rise in caspase-8 activity, and was accompanied by sustained activation of JNK1 and transient activation of JNK2. Caspase inhibition caused a dose-dependent reduction in cell death, while inhibition of the JNKs caused a significant increase in apoptosis. PI3 kinase was not involved in conferring early protection against TNF-α-induced death. By contrast, inhibition of NF-κB in the presence of TNF-α culminated in increased cell cycle progression, decreased *gadd45b* expression, and significant and precociously increased cell death, when compared with TNF-α alone. These results begin to characterize the mechanisms underlying the acute mitogenic and antiapoptotic roles of TNF-α, which appeared to be defined by a balance between MAP kinase, JNK, NF-κB, and gadd45b. They established that inhibition of any one of these molecules, as may occur following caspase activation, could eliminate vital stem cells required for skeletal muscle regeneration during chronic catabolic conditions.[135]

Cathepsin B ■ Muscle protein degradation in humans may not always be mediated though the ubiquitin-proteasome pathway. Thus, mRNA levels of the lysosomal protease cathepsin B were shown to be much higher in patients with early stages of lung cancer who had weight loss and muscle wasting.[136]

Reactive Oxygen Species (ROS), Oxidative Stress, and Nitric Oxide (NO) ■ In search of direct effects of cytokines against muscles, the effects of TNF-α on the mouse-derived C2C12 muscle cell line and on primary cultures from rat skeletal muscle were evaluated. TNF-α treatment of differentiated myotubes stimulated time- and concentration-dependent reductions in total protein content and loss of adult myosin heavy chain (MHCf) content; these changes were evident at low TNF-α concentrations (1-3 ng/mL) that did not alter muscle DNA content and were not associated with a decrease in MHCf synthesis. TNF-α activated binding of NF-κB to its targeted DNA sequence and stimulated degradation of I-κBα, an NF-κB inhibitory protein. TNF-α stimulated total ubiquitin conjugation whereas a 26S proteasome inhibitor (MG132) blocked TNF-α activation of NF-κB. Catalase inhibited NF-κB activation by TNF-α; exogenous hydrogen peroxide activated NF-κB and stimulated I-κBa degradation. Thus, TNF-α can directly induce skeletal muscle protein loss; NF-κB is rapidly activated by TNF-α in differentiated skeletal muscle cells; and TNF-α/NF-B signaling in skeletal muscle is regulated by endogenous ROS.[137]

ROS are indicated as crucial players in the onset of muscle protein hypercatabolism by upregulating elements of the ubiquitin–proteasome pathway. Involvement of oxidative stress in the pathogenesis of skeletal muscle wasting was evaluated in two different experimental models: rats rendered hyperglycemic by treatment with streptozotocin and rats bearing the Yoshida AH-130 ascites hepatoma. For this purpose, both tumor bearers and diabetic animals have been treated with dehydroepiandrosterone (DHEA), a multifunctional steroid endowed with multitargeted antioxidant properties. Diabetic rats and AH-130 rats shared several features, hypoinsulinemia, occurrence of oxidative stress, and positive response to DHEA administration, although the extent of the effects of DHEA largely differed between diabetic animals and tumor-bearing rats. The hypercatabolism, evaluated in terms of proteasome activity and expression of atrogin-1 and MuRF1, was activated in AH-130 rats, whereas it was lacking in streptozotocin-treated rats. Moreover, the role of oxidative stress could interfere with muscle wasting through different mechanisms, not necessarily involving NF-κB activation. Although skeletal muscle wasting occurred in both diabetic rats and tumor-host rats, the underlying mechanisms were different. Moreover, despite oxidative stress being detectable in both experimental models, its contribution to muscle wasting was not comparable.[138]

The role of oxidative stress in cancer cachexia may be extended in humans. Thus, neopterin is produced by monocytes/macrophages upon stimulation with IFN-γ. Increased neopterin concentrations in human serum and urine indicate activation of cell-mediated (Thl-type) immune response, eg, during virus infections, autoimmune diseases, allograft rejection, and in certain types of malignancy. In various groups of patients with malignant diseases neopterin concentrations correlate to the stage of disease, and higher neopterin concentrations in serum, urine, or ascitic fluid were shown to significantly predict worse prognosis regarding relapse and survival. The amounts of neopterin produced by activated monocytes/macrophages correlate with their capacity to release ROS. Neopterin concentrations in body fluids can be regarded as an indirect estimate of the degree of oxidative stress emerging during cell-mediated immune response. Moreover, neopterin was found itself to be capable of enhancing toxic effects induced by ROS. In vitro, neopterin derivatives were able to interfere with intracellular signal transduction pathways involved in, eg, programmed cell death and the induction of protooncogene c-fos or nuclear factor-chi B. The data support the view that increased production of ROS indicated by increased neopterin concentrations could modulate the development, the proliferation and the survival of malignant cells.[139]

Various biological parameters relevant to cancer cachexia, such as serum levels of proinflammatory cytokines (IL-1β, IL-6, TNFα), IL-2, acute-phase proteins (C-reactive protein and fibrinogen), leptin, and relevant to oxidative stress, such as ROS, body antioxidant enzymes glutathione peroxidase (GPx) and superoxide dismutase (SOD) were evaluated in a wide population of advanced cancer patients. ROS levels were significantly higher and GPx and SOD activities significantly lower in cancer patients than controls. Serum levels of IL-1β, IL-6, and TNF-α were significantly higher and serum levels of IL-2 and leptin significantly lower in cancer patients than controls. Serum levels of C-reactive protein and fibrinogen were significantly higher in cancer patients than controls. A significant correlation was found in laboratory parameters only between serum levels of leptin and body mass index. Patients with advanced cancer thus exhibited both a high grade of oxidative stress and a chronic inflammatory condition. Antioxidant agents α-lipoic acid, *N*-acetyl cysteine, and amifostine enhanced PBMCs progression through the cell cycle, thus providing evidence of their potential role in the functional restoration of the immune system in advanced cancer patients. These data appears to warrant further investigation with adequate clinical trials.[140]

In using cDNA microarrays of mouse myoblasts, the NO synthase gene was demonstrated to be an important downstream target of NF-κB, suggesting that NO production might be a direct cause of MyoD mRNA degeneration.[141]

Myostatin ■ Myostatin belongs to the transforming growth factor-β superfamily and negatively regulates skeletal muscle mass. Its deletion induces muscle overgrowth, while, its overexpression or systemic administration cause muscle atrophy. Myostatin has been proposed to negatively regulate the skeletal muscle mass.[142,143] Active myostatin circulates in the blood complexed with and inhibited by the propeptide itself or other binding-proteins such as follistatin,[144–146] suggesting that myostatin bioactivity is regulated by the balance with the physiological inhibitors. Binding of free myostatin to the Activin type IIB receptor (ActRIIB), and, to a lesser extent, to the related ActRIIA, results in recruitment and phosphorylation of the low affinity type I receptors ALK (activin receptor like-kinase)-4, or ALK-5.[144,146] This is followed by activation of transcription factors belonging to the SMAD family [mammalian homologue of *Drosophila* MAD (mothers-against-decapentaplegic gene)],[147–150] although myostatin also signals through different pathways, such as the extracellular signal-regulated kinase (ERK)/mitogen activated protein kinase (MAPK) cascade.[151] Mature myostatin induces FOXO-1 and E3 ubiquitin ligase gene, and MAFBx/atrogen-1 independent of NF-κB.

In order to test whether cancer-induced muscle wasting is associated with modulation of myostatin signaling and whether the TNF-α is relevant, protein levels of myostatin, follistatin, and ActRIIB, the major players in myostatin signaling, and the DNA-binding activity of SMAD proteins, their target transcription factors, were measured with western blotting in the gastrocnemius of rats bearing the Yoshida AH-130 hepatoma, a well known cachexia-inducing tumor model. Circulating myostatin and follistatin in tumor hosts were measured by immunoprecipitation, while the DNA-binding activity of the SMAD transcription factors was determined by electrophoretic-mobility shift assay. Muscle myostatin expression and bioactivity were upregulated in experimental cancer cachexia.[152]

Dystrophin Glycoprotein Complex (DGC) ■ Another group of muscle disorders also characterized by severe muscle wasting is the muscular dystrophy. Duchenne/Becker and several forms of limb-girdle muscular dystrophy are linked to mutations in genes that encode components of the DGC, a multiprotein structure associated with myofiber membranes.[153-155] At the core of the DGC is dystrophin, a large 427 kDa protein associating with the cytoskeleton through interaction with F-actin at its amino terminus and connection to the sarcolemma by binding to β-dystroglycan (β-DG) at its carboxyl end.[156,157] β-DG is bound to -dystroglycan (-DG), which itself is linked to the extracellular matrix by its interactions with laminin-2. The DGC therefore forms a strong mechanical link between the cytoskeleton and the extracellular matrix, protecting cells from contraction-induced injuries.[158] In addition, the DGC maintains an active signal transduction pathway by interacting with Grb2 and nNOS.[159] Mutations in dystrophin or other members of the DGC disrupt the mechanical linkage and/or signaling pathway(s), resulting in membrane damage, necrosis, and eventual muscle wasting.[160] Although the underlying mechanisms of muscle cachexia appear nonoverlapping to those in muscular dystrophy, a dysfunctional DGC appeared to be a common link between these two disease states.[142,161]

Tumor-induced alterations in DGC represent a key early event in cachexia.[146] Muscles from tumor-bearing mice exhibited membrane abnormalities accompanied by reduced levels of dystrophin and increased glycosylation on DGC proteins. Wasting was accentuated in tumor *mdx* mice lacking a DGC but spared in dystrophin transgenic mice that blocked induction of muscle E3 ubiquitin ligases. In patients with GI cancers, DGC was examined in muscle biopsies. Compared to healthy controls, cancer patients with marked weight loss had dramatic reduction in dystrophin. Dysrophin reduction in patients was linked with hyperglycosylation of DGC proteins. Further analysis revealed tat DGC deregulation was completely absent in controls but present in 60% ACC samples in cancer patients, thus, the deregulation correlating positively with cachexia. Based on these results, the authors proposed that, similar to muscular dystrophy, DGC dysfunction played a critical role in cancer-induced wasting.[161]

Complexity of Cancer-Related Signaling Molecules Leading to Muscle Wasting ■ It seems that the more we learn about the cancer cahexia the more we become aware of its complexity and highly regulated nature. It is clear that several signaling pathways involved in muscle atrophy interact or are interdependent. Activation or inhibition of a single pathway may have cascade effects on muscle protein balance. In addition, there is no evidence to prove that a pathway is the sole regulator of the process. For instance, activation of NF-κB could lead to increased expression of the muscle-specific ubiquitin ligase MuRF1 and a consequent increase in ubiquitin-dependent proteolysis. Akt has been shown to activate NF-κB in various cell types. It has been reported that activation of the Akt kinase not only enhances protein synthesis pathways, but also suppresses the upregulation of both MuRF1 and MAFbx. Thus, a potential linkage between Akt and NF-κB signaling in muscle can be drawn from the literature. Similarly, in muscle cells, ROS (via H202 treatment) induced activation of both the NF-κB and the FOXO signaling pathway, the latter promoted the expression of another ubiquitin ligase MAFbx/atrogin-1. It appears possible that the increased ROS in cancer cachexia may trigger either the NF-κB, or the FOXO signaling pathway, or both, leading to increased proteolysis through the ubiquitin–proteasome pathway. Expression of a constitutively active form of FOXO-1 increased myostatin mRNA and increased activity of a myostatin promoter reporter construct in differentiated C2C12 myotubes. Examination of the communications among scaffolding two or more signaling pathways may help us to obtain a comprehensive understanding of the complexity of muscle atrophy. Nevertheless, attempts to block the signaling remain a daunting task.[162]

Hormonal Aberration ■ Hormonal aberration may be a contributory factor to cancer cachexia. In a unique endocrine animal tumor model, estrogen was incriminated as the cause of cancer cachexia.[163] Abnormally low levels of testosterone or hypogonadism have been described in male patients with advanced cancer; these findings correlated with weight loss and adverse outcome.[164,165] Plasma cortisol values and arterial glucagon levels in patients with malignant tumors were significantly increased, however, compared with patients with benign surgical disorders.[166,167] This finding is in accord with the hypothesis that glucocorticoids are involved in the increased protein catabolism of skeletal muscles and other organs in cachectic cancer patients.

Prostaglandin Elevation ■ Marked weight loss and wasting of muscle and adipose tissue after tumor transplantation to rats were associated with the presence of circulating TNF-α and high levels of prostaglandin E2.[168] Indomethacin reduced weight loss and increased survival of mice with transplantable tumors receiving chemotherapy, and ibuprofen, a cyclooxygenase inhibitor, abrogated IL-1 induced anorexia in rats.[169,170] Close interaction of host- and tumor-derived cytokines and prostaglandins in the CNS were suggested by these animal models.[170] Recent work showed that prostaglandin E and prostaglandin I receptor levels in the CNS seemed to have little role in cancer anorexia/cachexia, however. Rather, expression of overall prostaglandin E receptors in the liver, fat and skeletal muscles appeared to be directly contributory to metabolic alterations in cancer cachexia.[171]

Tumor Parasitism ■ Selective parasitism of the host by the tumor in the form of a successful competition for substrates with limited availability may be a cause of cachexia. Some animal studies suggest that translocation of nitrogen from host to tumor constitutes nearly the total nitrogen depletion of the host.[172] Tumors are effective nitrogen traps independent of protein intake, despite the wasting of normal host tissue.[173] Since cachexia can appear in patients with very small tumors, however, and the total tumor mass in the majority of cancer patients at death rarely exceeds 0.5 kg, it is unlikely that a simple competition of available nitrogen between tumor and host is responsible for the development of cachexia, especially in early stage cancer.

Dysfunction of Neuropeptidergic Circuit ■ Dysfunction of neuropeptidergic circuits as the mechanism of the cancer anorexia–cachexia syndrome has been discussed in the section on "Anorexia."

Metabolic Derangement Produced by Treatment ■ Postoperative weight loss is a result of increase in energy expenditure due to the stress response and decreased dietary intake.[174] Pancreatic resection can result in pancreatic exocrine and endocrine insufficiency creating major nutritional problems such as steatorrhea and hyperglycemia. Major hepatic resections can cause metabolic abnormalities in the immediate postoperative period. Extensive resection of the small bowel can lead to malabsorption of many nutrients.

A majority of chemotherapeutic agents are toxic, producing a variety of metabolic effects. L-asparaginase and IL-12 exemplify this: profound weight loss and/or hypoalbuminemia are among the common manifestations in patients treated with these compounds.[175-177]

Treatment of Cancer Anorexia/Cachexia

The definitive treatment of cancer cachexia is removal of the causative tumor. Short of achieving this goal various measures have been undertaken with limited success.

Supportive Care

Patients with anorexia from decreased physical activity, concomitant infection and toxicities to the alimentary tract from chemotherapy and radiotherapy are managed symptomatically for maintenance of nutritional status and quality of life. Such management includes the use of mouthwash for stomatitis, frequent small volume feedings, antiemetics, antibiotics, transfusions of blood components, and/or oral and parenteral nutritional supplement. Consideration of the patient's food preferences and service of food in a dining room atmosphere may also be important to stimulate appetite. When a patient is unable to consume a regular diet to obtain adequate nutrition, food supplements, both home-made and commercially available, are an effective means of providing additional calories, protein, fat, vitamins, and minerals, although overall consumption may not increase much. In specific instances such as the malabsorption syndrome secondary to pancreas carcinoma, exogenous pancreas extract improves fat and protein absorption.

Frequent nutritional counseling may increase daily energy and protein intake as well as triceps skinfold measurements. However, response rates and overall survival can not be improved by counseling alone.

Pharmacologic Management

Corticosteroids ■ A number of uncontrolled studies have suggested that corticosteroids can diminish such symptoms as anorexia, asthenia, and pain in patients with cancer. The mechanism of action may include an euphoriant activity, anti-inflammatory action through the inhibition of TNF release and suppression of IL-1β activity, as well as inhibition of prostaglandin metabolism. Significant improvements in appetite and a sense of well-being have been reported in randomized trials with prednisolone, methylprednisolone, or dexamethasone.[178-181] Unfortunately, the improvements were not long lasting and upon completion of the studies all nutritional parameters returned to their baseline. There were no differences in mortality rate or in survival.

In a randomized comparison of dexamethasone and megestrol acetate, both drugs caused a similar degree of appetite enhancement and similar changes in nonfluid weight status, but dexamethasone was found to be less favorable.[182] Dexamethasone had more corticosteroid-type toxicity and a higher rate of drug discontinuation because of toxicity and/or patient refusal than megestrol acetate.

Although corticosteroids have been postulated to be responsible for muscle wasting and cancer cachexia, studies involving treatment with RU38486, a glucocorticoid receptor antagonist, of experimental animals bearing cachexia-producing tumors suggested that glucocoricoids are not involved in skeletal muscle wasting associated with cancer cachexia. Receptor blockade did not abrogate tumor-induced cachexia.[183,184]

Megestrol Acetate and Medroxyprogesterone Acetate ■ Megestrol acetate, a progestational agent, is frequently used in the treatment of patients with metastatic breast cancer. It is generally well tolerated, except that it may cause undesirable weight gain. Subsequently, it was shown that megestrol acetate produced weight gain in a variety of cachectic cancer patients. Significant reduction in serum levels of IL-la and b, IL-2, IL-6, and TNF-α were observed in cancer patients treated with megestrol acetate, which may bear on the mechanism of improved appetite and body weight gain.[185] It has also been postulated that the effect is, at least in part, mediated by NPY, a potent central appetite stimulant.[186]

In a review of 15 randomized clinical trials including more than 2,000 patients, there was a statistically significant advantage for high-dose progestins in regards to improved appetite and gain of body weight.[187] Treatment morbidity was low, due to the brief period of the treatment in most of the studies. A meta-analysis of 26 studies confirmed the usefulness of megestrol acetate in gaining appetite and body weight of cancer patients with anorexia–cachexia syndrome.[188]

Weight gain produced by megestrol acetate was found to be mainly from increased body fat stores rather than accretion of lean tissue.[189,190] It has been argued that the gain of adipose tissue as opposed to lean tissue during treatment with megestrol acetate, although suboptimal, should not be disparaged because depletion of body fat is generally an undesirable outcome of cancer.

The addition of megestrol acetate to chemotherapy for patients with melanoma resulted in higher objective responses and prolonged median survival compared to historical controls with chemotherapy alone.[191] Megestrol acetate is contraindicated in pediatric cachectic patients, since a significant proportion of such patients developed adrenal insufficiency.[192] Megestrol acetate should also be used with caution in geriatric cancer patients because they are prone to develop deep vein thrombosis because of immobility and increases in serum fibrinogen levels.

Medroxyprogesterone acetate is a more widely used synthetic progestagen. Medroxyprogesterone reduced production of cytokines and serotonin.[193] Two placebo-controlled randomized studies have been reported in which increased appetite was described.[194,195] In one study significant increases in rapid turnover proteins such as serum thyroid binding prealbumin and retinol binding protein were reported.[195] In spite of increased appetite, no weight gain was produced in either study.

Anabolic Steroids ■ Anabolic androgenic steroids have been used by athletes to promote muscle growth and strength. In MCG sarcoma-bearing mice with progressive cachexia, administration of nandrolone propionate resulted in significant weight gain.[196] The weight gain was, however, mainly attributed to water retention, and food intake and survival were not affected. Randomized clinical trials were carried out to test whether supplements of nandrolone decanoate influenced the outcome of chemotherapy in patients with nonsmall-cell lung cancer.[197,198] Although the treated group experienced less weight loss, response to chemotherapy and survival were comparable. In a three-arm phase III randomized clinical trial for the treatment of cancer anorexia/cachexia, fluoxymesterone, an anabolic steroid, showed significantly less appetite enhancement and did not have as favorable a toxicity profile as megestrol acetate, a progestational agent, or dexamethasone, a corticosteroid.[182]

Cannabinoids (Dronabinol) ■ While using dronabinol (Delta 9-tetrahydocannabinol, THC) as an antiemetic, it was found that the agent enhanced appetite in healthy individuals and in cancer patients. To study this phenomenon further, an open dose-ranging study was carried out in patients with cancer.[199,200] All patients reported improvement in appetite. Higher doses, 5.0 mg or 7.5 mg/day, were more effective than the low dose of 2.5 mg/day. Patients in all groups nonetheless continued to lose weight although the rate of weight loss decreased with therapy. It is of note that these effects were observed at doses lower than those producing antiemetic effects and without overt psychotropic symptoms.

Recently, a randomized study was carried out to compare dronabinol, megestrol acetate and the combination for palliating cancer-associated anorexia.[201] Megestrol acetate provided superior anorexia palliation among advanced cancer patients compared with dronabinol alone. The combination of megestrol and dronabinol did not appear to confer additional benefit.

Growth Hormone (GH), Somatostatin, and GHRH (GHRP-2) ■ Anabolic properties of GH have been examined in animals. Administration of GH to tumor-bearing rats resulted in increased muscle weight, muscle protein content and preserved host-body composition.[202] GH did not stimulate tumor growth.[203] The effect of a combination of insulin, GH, and somatostatin on tumor growth, metastasis, and host metabolism was evaluated in rats bearing MAC-33 mammary tumor.[204] The triple therapy supported host anabolism, increased hamstring muscle weight and protein content, and inhibited tumor growth kinetics. The rationale for including somatostatin in the treatment was based on the fact that insulin treatment alone led to limited success in treating cancer cachexia due to insulin-induced hypoglycemia and subsequent glucagon secretion. Somatostatin alone is known to have antitumor activity, however, and the contribution of each component to the observed changes was not clear.

The effect of recombinant-human GH and insulin administration on protein kinetics was examined in 28 cancer patients.[205] Whole-body protein net balance was higher in patients treated with both GH and insulin than in insulin only or GH only controls. Skeletal muscle protein net balance in GH/insulin group was higher than in no-treatment controls. Recombinant-human GH and insulin reduced whole-body and skeletal muscle protein loss in cancer patients. Simultaneous use of these agents during nutritional therapy may benefit cancer patients.[205]

In another study, 30 patients undergoing surgery for upper GI tract malignancies were prospectively randomized into one of the three nutritional support groups after surgery: standard TPN, TPN plus GH, and TPN, GH, and systemic insulin. Patients who received standard TPN only were in a state of negative skeletal muscle protein net balance. Those who received GH and insulin had improved skeletal muscle protein net balance. Whole-body protein net balance was improved in the GH and the GH and insulin groups compared with the TPN only group. GH and insulin combined did not improve whole body net balance more than GH alone. GH administration significantly increased serum IGF-1 and GH levels. Insulin infusion significantly increased serum insulin levels and the insulin/glucagon ratio. Thus, GH and GH plus insulin regimens improved protein kinetic parameters in patients with upper GI tract cancer who were receiving TPN after undergoing surgery. The study was carried out for only 5 days. It is unknown whether the TPN plus GH improved wound healing and shortened hospital stay.[206] Whether prolonged use of TPN plus GH would play any role in reversal of cancer cachexia in humans has not been tested.

Daily subcutaneous injections of a more stable synthetic ghrelin receptor agonist GHRP-2 (growth hormone releasing peptide-2) in mice produced dose-dependent increases in food intake and body weight.[207] Pre- and post-treatment analysis of body composition indicated increased fat and bone masses but not lean mass. GHRP-2-induced positive energy balance leading to fat gain occurred in the absence of involvement of hypothalamic NPY neurons. Indeed, GHRP-2 administration to healthy volunteers resulted in increased food intake.[208] Further studies are needed to ascertain whether ghrelin receptor agonists offer a treatment option for syndromes like anorexia nervosa, cancer cachexia, or AIDS wasting.

As a more recent approach, a myogenic plasmid that expresses GH releasing hormone ($GHRH^{1-40}$) was tested in dogs for prevention and/or treatment of cancer anorexia and cachexia. Seventeen geriatric and five cancer-afflicted companion dogs were enrolled. Effects of the treatment were documented for at least 180 days posttreatment, with 10 animals followed for more than 1 year posttreatment. Treated dogs showed increased IGF-1 levels, and increases in scores for weight, activity level, exercise tolerance, and appetite. No adverse effects associated with the GHRH plasmid treatment were found. Most importantly, the overall assessment of the quality of life of the treated animals improved. Hematological parameters such as red blood cell count, hematocrit, and hemoglobin concentrations were increased and maintained within their normal ranges. It was concluded that intramuscular injection of a GHRH-expressing plasmid was both safe and capable of improving the quality of life in animals for an extended period of time in the context of aging and disease.[209]

Insulin-Like Growth Factor-1 (IGF-1) ■ IGF-1, also known as somatomedin-C, mediates many of the anabolic properties of GH including stimulation of amino acid uptake and protein synthesis. In experimental animal cancer cachexia model IGF-1 administration resulted in either host preservation of lean tissue and attenuation of host muscle–protein depletion[210] or was unable to prevent cachexia.[211]

Ten subjects with AIDS-associated cachexia received either low- or high-dose iv recombinant IGF-1 daily for 10 days.[212] Cumulative nitrogen retention was positive for both dosage groups, but a significant increase in daily nitrogen retention occurred only in the low-dose group. The anabolic response was transient, however. Repeated administration of IGF-1 decreased IGF-binding protein-3 levels, producing lower intrainfusion levels of IGF-1 and limiting its therapeutic efficacy. The basal metabolic rate increased with high-dose IGF-1 and may have contributed to the lack of anabolic effect. The authors concluded that partial growth hormone resistance occurred in AIDS-associated cachexia.

A randomized placebo-controlled 12-week trial of combination of recombinant human GH (rhGH, Nutropin) and rhIGF-1 was carried out in 142 subjects with HIV wasting.[213] At 3 weeks, the treatment group had a significantly larger weight increase, but this difference was not observed at any later time point. Similarly, fat-free mass, calculated from skinfold measurements, increased transiently in the treatment group at 6 weeks. No significant differences in isokinetic muscle strength, or endurance testing, or in quality of life were observed between the groups. Authors concluded that the combination of rhIGF-I and low-dose rhGH had no significant anabolic effect in HIV wasting. IGF-I has not been tested in patients with cancer cachexia.

Metoclopramide and Cisapride ■ In advanced cancer patients with delayed gastric emptying or gastroparesis, oral administration of a prokinetic agent, metoclopramide, 10 mg orally 4 times daily before meals and at bedtime, was shown to be effective in stimulating appetite and relieving other dyspeptic symptoms associated with anorexia.[214,215] A controlled release preparation appears to be more effective than immediate release drug due to its control of nausea associated with advanced cancer even without demonstrated abnormalities of the GI tract.[216] Patients with head and neck cancer undergoing radiotherapy were randomized to three groups: megestrol acetate, cisapride, and placebo. Megestrol significantly prevented body weight loss and deterioration of appetite, whereas cisapride lacked these clinical benefits.[217]

Hydrazine Sulfate ■ Hydrazine sulfate, an inhibitor of the enzyme phosphoenolpyruvate carboxykinase, has been shown to interrupt gluconeogenesis in animals.[218] Based on a theory that increased gluconeogenesis and enhanced Cori-cycle activity were the central mechanism of tumor-induced cachexia, clinical studies of hydrazine sulfate were carried out in attempts to prevent or reverse cancer-related cachexia and weight loss. Three multicenter group studies were reported in patients with nonsmall-cell lung cancer or colorectal cancer.[219-221] All three studies failed to show beneficial results in appetite, body weight, quality of life, or survival from hydrazine sulfate.

Indomethacin, Ibuprofen, and Celecoxib ■ It has been proposed that cell growth may be controlled by the interconversion of different types of prostagladins.[222-224] In animal studies, ability of prostagladin biosynthesis inhibitors to reverse cancer cachexia is not universally positive. In one study, indomethacin, ibuprofen, or aspirin inhibited growth of Walker 256 carcinoma in rats.[225] All drug-treated rats partially recovered body weight and food intake compared to a saline-treated group. In another study using the same tumor system, indomethacin and ibuprofen retarded tumor growth and lowered body temperature compared with controls, but these agents had no effect on food intake or body weight of tumor-bearing animals.[226] Celecoxib, a COX-2 inhibitor, was reported to rapidly reverse weight loss in two murine models, colon 26, which induced high levels of circulating IL-6, and a human head and neck tumor 1483 HNSCC xenograft.[227]

In clinical trials indomethacin reduced fever and granulocytosis and was claimed to have improved the well being of cancer patients.[228,229] In cachectic cancer patients indomethacin or ibuprofen was reported to decrease resting energy expenditure and C-reactive protein values, to produce body weight gain and to improve survival.[230-232] In a randomized study in patients with advanced GI cancer with more than 5% weight loss, megestrol acetate alone resulted in weight loss and deterioration of quality of life, whereas the combination of megestrol/ibuprofen appeared to reverse weight loss and appeared to improve quality of life.[233] Impact of erythropoietin was studied in a randomized fashion in unselected weight-losing cancer patients who were treated with indomethacin. The combination resulted in an improvement of hematocrit together with increased serum albumin levels, decreases in C-reactive protein, improved body weight and greater exercise capacity compared to indomethacin alone controls.[234,235] Study and control patients did not differ in survival, however. Well-designed randomized clinical studies are needed to assess therapeutic values of prostaglandin inhibitors alone and in combination with other anticachectic agents.

Pentoxifylline and Lisofylline ■ These agents are methylxanthine analogues with anti-inflammatory properties. They were shown to have profound stimulatory effects on vascular endothelial production of the noninflammatory prostaglandins I2 and E2, while inhibiting TNF-α synthesis by blocking gene transcription.[236] Pentoxifylline, originally used for the treatment of vascular insufficiency because of its hemorheological properties, prevented muscle atrophy and suppressed increased protein breakdown in tumor-bearing rats. Pentoxifylline suppressed the enhanced expression of ubiquitin, the 14-kDa ubiquitin conjugating enzyme E2, and the C2 20S proteasome subunit in muscle from cancer-bearing rats and inhibited the activation of a nonlysosomal, Ca(2+)-independent ubiquitin-proteasome proteolytic pathway.[237]

Prophylactic oral administration of pentoxifylline in allograft recipients together with chemotherapy and radiotherapy resulted in significant reduction in the incidence and severity of treatment-related complications: mucositis, hepatic veno-occlusive disease, renal insufficiency, and the incidence of graft versus host disease.[238]

In an initial study in cancer patients, pentoxifylline suppressed TNF-α mRNA levels, increased the sense of well-being, improved appetite, and improved the ability to perform activities of daily living. Patients who normalized their TNF levels had a weight gain. In a randomized controlled trial in patients with solid tumors, however, pentoxifylline failed to provide improvements in appetite or body weight compared to a placebo group.[239] Likewise, for patients with acute myelocytic leukemia or myelodysplastic syndrome once in complete remission with idarubicin/ara–C chemotherapy, lisofylline provided no favorable effects in terms of rates of infection, overall mortality rates, or outcome.[240] Lisofylline did not alter the toxicities of high-dose IL-2 and thus did not impact the overall dose intensity in the treatment of advanced renal cancer and malignant melanoma.[241]

Proteasome Inhibitors and NF-kB Inhibitors ■ As detailed earlier the ubiquitin-proteasome pathway plays an important role in muscle protein catabolism during cancer cachexia and may be a potential therapeutic target for muscle wasting. Arginine methylester and alanine methylester, selective inhibitors of ubiquitin ligase E3a have not been evaluated clinically.[242] Bortezomib, a direct inhibitor of the protease complex is reportedly under examination in cachectic cancer patients in phase I studies.[243]

Activation of NF-κB leads to the induction of proteasome expression and protein degradation by PIF.

SN50, a synthetic cell permeable peptide NF-κB inhibitor, attenuated the expression of 20S proteasome a-subunits, two subunits of the 19S regulator MSS1 and p42, and the ubiquitin-conjugating enzyme, E2(14k).[244] SN50 also decreased myosin expression in murine myotubes.

The potential for curcumin, a natural product from turmeric, and resveratrol, a natural phytoalexin found in red wine, to act as inhibitors of muscle protein degradation in cancer cachexia, because they are inhibitors of NF-κB activation, has been evaluated in vitro and in vivo.[244,245] Both agents completely attenuated total protein degradation in murine myotubes at all concentrations of PIF, and attenuated the PIF-induced increase in expression of the ubiquitin-proteasome proteolytic pathway. Curcumin was ineffective in preventing weight loss and muscle protein degradation in the animal tumor model, however; whereas resveratrol significantly attenuated weight loss and protein degradation in skeletal muscle, and produced a significant reduction in NF-κB DNA-binding activity.[244,245] The inactivity of curcumin was probably due to low bioavailability. Incubations of isolated extensor digitorum longus muscles in the presence of resveratrol caused a significant decrease in the rate of protein degradation. However, administration of resveratrol in vivo to both rats bearing the Yoshida AH-130 ascites hepatoma and mice bearing the Lewis lung carcinoma had no effect on skeletal muscle mass or body weight in tumor-bearing rodents. In addition, a combination of resveratrol and fish oil was also unable to induce any changes in skeletal muscle weights. This study concluded that resveratrol was unable to influence muscle mass in vivo and had no potential role as anticachectic agent for the treatment of muscle wasting associated with tumor growth.[246]

Administration of dehydroxymethyl-epoxyquinomicin, another NF-κB inhibitor, was reported to have ameliorated cachexia in tumor bearing mice.[247] It was also shown to inhibit IL-6 production in patients with prostate cancer. In follow-up studies, dehydroxymethylepoxyquinomicin was found to reduce atherosclerosis in ApoE-deficient mice and suppressed anti-Thyl.1-induced glomerulonephritis in rats. No confirmatory reports as to its benefit in cancer cachexia have appeared, however.

Pyrrolidine dithiocarbamate (PDTC), is another inhibitor of NF-κB, IL-6 synthesis, and cachexia that was tested in colon 26 tumor-bearing mice. Administration of PDTC dose dependently inhibited the NF-κB activation in tumor tissues, inhibited IL-6 synthesis of the tumor cells, and attenuated the wasting of carcass weight, gastrocnemius muscle, and epididymal fat. Tumor growth was also inhibited by PDTC. These results suggested that PDTC, an inhibitor of NF-κB, can attenuate the development of cachexia in colon 26 tumor-bearing mice through inhibition of IL-6 synthesis regulated by NF-κB.[248] Confirmatory studies showing reversal of cancer cachexia is eagerly awaited.

Antioxidants and Antioxidant Combinations ■ Several mechanisms may lead to oxidative stress in cancer patients: one might hypothesize that the body redox systems, which include antioxidant enzymes and low molecular weight antioxidants, may be unregulated in cancer patients, and that this imbalance might enhance disease progression and induce cancer cachexia.[249]

To test the efficacy and safety of an integrated treatment based on a pharmaconutritional support, antioxidants and drugs, all given orally, were administered in a population of advanced cancer patients with cancer-related anorexia/cachexia and oxidative stress. An open early phase II study was designed according to the Simon two-stage design. The integrated 4-month treatment consisted of diet with high polyphenol content, antioxidant treatment (alpha-lipoic acid + carbocysteine lysine salt + vitamin E + vitamin A + vitamin C), and pharmaconutritional support enriched with (n-3)-PUFA (eicosapentaenoic acid and docosahexaenoic acid), medroxyprogesterone acetate, and selective cyclooxygenase-2 inhibitor celecoxib. Of 44 patients enrolled, 39 completed the treatment and were assessable. Body weight increased significantly from baseline as did LBM and appetite. There was an important decrease of proinflammatory cytokines (IL-6) and TNF-α, and a negative relationship worthy of note was only found between LBM and IL-6 changes. As for quality of life evaluation, there was a marked improvement in the European Organization for Research and Treatment of Cancer QLQ-C30, Euro QL-5D(VAS), and multidimensional fatigue symptom inventory-short form scores. At the end of the study, 22 of the 39 patients were "responders" or "high responders." The minimum required was 21; therefore, the treatment was effective and more importantly was shown to be safe. The efficacy and safety of the treatment have been shown by the study. A randomized phase III study appears warranted.[250]

Myostatin Inhibitors ■ The association between muscle depletion and increased myostatin has led to considering this factor as a potential therapeutic target. Indeed, myostatin blockade by means of specific antibodies, myostatin propeptide administration, or transgenic expression of a myostatin inhibitor improved muscle mass and function in *mdx* mice. These observations suggested that myostatin pathway should be regarded as a potential therapeutic target in cancer cachexia.[251-253]

Clenbuterol ■ Clenbuterol is a β2-adrenoceptor agonist. It prevented muscle protein wasting in tumor-bearing animals and increased muscle mass and function in healthy animals.[254-256] There was no change in food intake or tumor growth. A combinations of naproxen, clenbuterol, insulin, and eicosapentaenoic acid ameliorated cancer cachexia and reduced tumor growth in Walker 256 tumor-bearing rats.[257,258] In a randomized trial clenbuterol was able to improve muscle strength of patients after knee surgery.[259] Its effects on muscle preservation appeared to occur without the need for exercise. Clenbuterol has not yet been studied in patients with cancer cachexia. There are also pitfalls associated with beta-agonist administration and clinical applications have so far been limited, largely because of cardiovascular side effects.

Thalidomide ■ Thalidomide, a drug associated with over 10,000 cases of severe malformation in newborn children, has been revived because of its ability to suppress TNF production in monocytes in vitro and to normalize elevated TNF levels in animals. The drug also possesses antiangiogenic properties. Thalidomide inhibited TNF-α production in patients with leprosy, tuberculosis, AIDS and cancer.[260-264]

In a randomized placebo controlled trial, 50 patients with advanced pancreatic cancer who had lost at least 10% of their body weight received thalidomide 200 mg daily or placebo for 24 weeks.[264] At 4 weeks, patients who received thalidomide had gained on average 0.37 kg in weight and 1.0 cm^3 in arm-muscle mass compared with a loss of 2.21 kg and 4.46 cm^3, respectively, in the placebo group. At eight weeks, patients in the thalidomide group had lost 0.06 kg in weight and 0.5 cm^3 in arm-muscle mass compared with a loss of 3.62 kg and 8.4 cm^3, respectively, in the placebo group. Improvements in physical function correlated positively with weight gain. Thalidomide was well tolerated and appeared effective at attenuating loss of weight and lean body mass in patients with cachexia due to advanced pancreatic cancer. Beneficial effects of thalidomide have not been compared with other anticachexia agents such as megestrol acetate. Lenalidomide, a newer analogue of thalidomide, has not been tested in patients with cancer cachexia.

Adenosine Triphosphate (ATP) ■ Extracellular ATP is involved in the regulation of a variety of biologic processes, including neurotransmission, muscle contraction, and hepatic metabolism of glucose, via purinergic receptors. In nonrandomized studies involving patients with different tumor types ATP infusion appeared to inhibit loss of weight and deterioration of quality of life and performance status.

Patients with nonsmall-cell lung cancer, stage IIIB or IV, were randomized to receive either 10 intravenous, 30-hour ATP infusions every 2-4 weeks, or no ATP.[265,266] In the ATP group no change in body composition occurred over the 28-week follow-up period, whereas, the control group lost 0.6 kg of fat mass, 0.5 kg of fat-free mass, 1.8% of arm muscle area, and 0.6% of body cell mass/kg body weight per 4 weeks. Appetite remained stable in the ATP group but decreased significantly in the control group, by 568 KJ/day in energy intake. These effects were ascribed to maintenance of energy intake by exogenous ATP.

These reports contrast with a strategy of ATP suppression as a means of cancer therapy. ATP suppression in tumor tissue by means of direct intra-arterial delivery of 3-bromopyruvate, a potent inhibitor of ATP production, to the site of the primary tumor, or by a combination of 6-methylmercaptopurine riboside, a purine de novo synthesis inhibitor, and 6-aminonicotinamide, an inhibitor of glycolysis, which were given concomitantly with *N*-(phosphonacetyl)-L-aspartic acid (PALA), a pyrimidine synthesis inhibitor was reported to show marked therapeutic enhancement.[267,268]

5'-Deoxy-5-Fluorouridine (5-dFUrd) ■ The fluorinated pyrimidine nucleoside, 5-dFUrd was shown to effectively attenuate the progress of cachexia in mice bearing the murine adenocarcinomas MAC16 or colon 26, as well as in the human uterine cervical carcinoma xenograft, Yumoto. The anticachexia effect of 5-dFUrd was shown to be independent of its antitumor activity and appears to be at least in part related its inhibition of proteolysis-inducing factor (PIF), thought to be responsible for the development of cachexia in the murine MAC16 model.[269,270] 5-dFUrd has not yet been evaluated as an anticahectic agent in humans.

Proinflammatory-Cytokine Inhibitors, Proinflammatory-Cytokine Antibodies, and Anti-inflammatory-Cytokines ■ In addition to pentoxifylline and thalidomide, a number of cytokine inhibitors and antibodies have been developed.

Anti-TNF-α antibody, anti-IL-1 antibody, and anti-IL-1 receptor antibody were reported to have attenuated the cachexia produced by either chronic TNF-α administration or implantation of a tumor in experimental animals.271,272 Administration of TNF-α antibody to tumor-bearing rats decreased protein degradation rates in skeletal muscle, heart, and liver as compared to controls; the antibody was unable to prevent a reduction in body weight, however.273 Decreases in protein degradation in skeletal muscle by TNF-α antibody appear to be due to inhibition of tumor-induced increases in muscle ubiquitin gene expression.[273]

Randomized clinical trials using anti-TNF antibody failed to increase survival or reverse the protein catabolism associated with severe sepsis or septic shock compared to those who received standard supportive care and antimicrobial therapy.[274] Similarly, clinical trials involving anti-TNF strategies such as etanercept (a dimeric fusion protein consisting of the extracellular ligand-binding portion of the human tumor necrosis factor receptor [TNFR] linked to the Fc portion of human IgG1) or infliximab (monoclonal antibody against TNF-α) in patients with chronic heart failure showed no improvements in clinical outcome as compared to placebo controls.[275]

Suramin, an antitrypanosomal polyanion, prevented the binding of IL-6 to its cell surface receptor subunits in vitro and inhibited colon-26 mediated cancer cachexia in mice.[276] Treatment of mice bearing AB 22 mesothelioma with anti-IL-6 antibody curtailed the clinical symptoms, as did treatment with recombinant human (rhu) IFN-α.[277] Neither anti-IL-6 antibody nor rhuIFN-α had a direct growth-inhibitory effect on the tumor cell line in vitro; however, in vivo rhuIFN-α attenuated both IL-6 mRNA expression in the tumors and serum IL-6 levels, ameliorated the depression of lymphocyte activities, and enhanced the number of tumor-infiltrating lymphocytes and macrophages. A combination therapy of rhuIFN-α and anti-IL-6 antibody may be beneficial in the palliative treatment for patients with malignant mesothelioma.[277]

Administration of an anti-IL-6 antibody in patients seropositive for human immunodeficiency virus-1 and suffering from an immunoblastic or a polymorphic large-cell lymphoma resulted in partial remission or stabilization of the disease.[278] The neutralizing effect of the anti-IL-6 antibody as measured by C-reactive protein levels in the serum was accompanied by abrogation of B clinical symptoms including fever and cachexia.

Production of anti-inflammatory cytokine IL-12 and type 2 immune responses is markedly decreased in cachectic patients with colorectal and gastric cancer.[279] Administration of IL-12 was reported to reduce serum levels of IL-6 in mice bearing colon 26 carcinoma and prevented development of cachexia.[280] The IL-12 activity was T-cell-dependent and the anticachexia effect resulted from at least two mechanisms; the downregulation of IL-6 and the upregulation of IFN-α. Similarly, a gene transfer of IL-10, another IL-6 inhibitor, prevented cachexia in an animal model.[281] IL-15 treatment partly inhibited skeletal muscle wasting in AH-130-bearing rats by decreasing protein degradation rates to values even lower than those observed in non-tumor-bearing animals.[282] These alterations in protein breakdown rates were associated with an inhibition of the ATP-ubiquitin-dependent proteolytic pathway. Administration of IL-15 to rats bearing ascites hepatoma resulted in a significant reduction of muscle wasting and reversal of the increased DNA fragmentation observed in skeletal muscle.[283] IL-15 decreased apoptosis apparently by affecting TNF-α signaling. Administration of IL-15 decreased the inducible NO synthase protein levels by 73%, suggesting that NO formation and muscle apoptosis during tumor growth could be related. IL-12, IL-10, and IL-15 have not been evaluated as anticachectic agents in humans.

Eicosapentaenoic Acid (EPA) ■ ω-3 polyunsaturated fatty acids are an essential component of the diet and are involved in the synthesis of eicosanoids (prostaglandins, leukotriens, and thromboxanes) and in membrane, receptors, and enzyme functions. EPA, an ω-3 polyunsaturated fatty acid found in oily fish such as sardines, salmon, and mackerel, has been shown to possess antitumor as well as anticachexia activities in animal cachexia models.[284,285] EPA-induced inhibition of weight loss was accompanied by increases in total body fat and muscle mass. EPA administration resulted in downregulation of ZAG (see section on "Tumor Byproducts") expression in both white and BAT and suppression of well-characterized mediators of cancer-associated wasting, including IL-6, as well as an attenuation of protein degradation by the ubiquitin-proteasome proleolytic pathway mediated by PIF (see section on "Tumor Byproducts") in cachectic mice.[286-288] PIF in skeletal muscle releases arachidonic acid, which is rapidly metabolized to prostaglandins E2 and F2a as well as 5-, 12-, and 15-hydroxyeicosatetraenoic acids (HETEs). Of all the metabolites, only 15-HETE produces a significant increase in protein degradation. EPA induced inhibition of arachidonic acid release and subsequent decreases in 15-HETE, which serves as a second messenger, abrogate the enhancer effect on the promoter region of the proteasome C3 subunit gene.[289] EPA also decreased glucose utilization of skeletal muscle, inhibited lipolysis in adipocytes by preventing prostaglandin synthesis, and by a rising cyclic AMP in response to the LMF (see section on "Tumor Byproducts"). EPA also inhibited translocation of the nuclear transcription factor NF-κB, by preventing degradation of the inhibitor protein I-κB in the cytosol.[290-292]

Early clinical trials of fish oils were encouraging. Patients with pancreas cancer treated with supplements of fish oil capsules (EPA and docosahexaenoic acid) showed body weight gain accompanied by significant reduction in acute phase protein production and by stabilization of resting energy expenditure.[293] While nutritional supplements alone did not attenuate the development of weight loss in cachectic cancer patients, nutritional supplements enriched with EPA produced significant weight gain along with an improvement in appetite and performance status.[294] Significant increases of lean body mass were noteworthy among various therapeutic interventions reported. A randomized controlled study was carried out to investigate the effects of dietary EPA plus vitamin E on the immune system and survival of well nourished and of malnourished cancer patients.[295] EPA had a considerable immunomodulating effect by increasing the ratio of T-helper cells to T-suppressor cells in the subgroup of malnourished patients. EPA doubled the survival of patients compared with the placebo arm.

More recent randomized clinical studies, however, cast a serious doubt on any unique benefit of EPA. No significant differences in symptomatic or nutritional parameters were found in 60 patients with advanced cancer and loss of both weight and appetite who were randomized to fish oil capsules or placebo.[296] The majority of the patients were not able to swallow more than 10 fish oil capsules per day. After 2 weeks of treatment fish oil did not significantly improve appetite, tiredness, nausea, well-being, caloric intake, nutritional status or function. In an international multicenter randomized double blind trial, 200 patients with weight-losing inoperable pancreas cancer were randomized to receive EPA (2.2 g/day) plus nutritional supplement or the nutritional supplement alone for 8 weeks.[297] Enrichment with EPA did not provide advantage over nutritional supplement alone. Both treatment groups equally benefited in arresting weight loss, but no differences were seen in body mass index, lean body mass, quality of life or survival. In a third trial, 221 patients with cancer associated wasting were randomized to either EPA supplement alone, megestrol acetate alone, or EPA plus megestrol acetate for a median of 3 months.[298] Weight gain of ≥10% was seen in a higher percentage of patients with megestrol acetate than EPA. Overall weight gain, functional assessment of anorexia/cachexia therapy (FAACT), and QOL were essentially identical among the three groups. To meet the criticisms of too short a treatment period in some studies, and of compliance issues of taking large amounts of EPA in randomized trials, a new randomized study comparing placebo versus two doses of EPA, 2 g or 4 g per day for 8 weeks, were undertaken in 518 patients with weight-losing advanced GI or lung cancer. There were no statistically significant improvements in survival, weight, or other nutritional variables.[299]

Recently, clinical use of anti-inflammatory polyunsaturated fatty acids (PUFAs), eicosapentaenoic acid (EPA), and docosahexaenoic acid (DHA), in cancer-associated anorexia–cachexia syndrome (ACS) was reviewed.[300] Seven randomized controlled trials (RCTs) were identified in literature. Except for one trial showing a positive effect on weight, none of the trials found a clinically or statistically significant difference in outcome measures reviewed. EPA and DHA alone have not shown significant clinical effect in altering weight, lean muscle mass, survival, or QOL in patients with ACS associated with cancer.

Thus, available data do not support a value of EPA/DHA in the treatment of cancer cachexia in humans.

β-Hydroxy-β-Methylbutyrate (HMB)/L-arginine/L-glutamine ■ HMB, a metabolite of the amino acid leucine, interferes with the activation of NF-κB. HMB inhibited PIF-induced protein degradation and attenuated the increased protein degradation during cachexia in tumor-bearing mice. In a randomized study the effects of HMB were examined during exercise training. Regardless of gender or training status, HMB increased upper body strength and minimized muscle damage when combined with an exercise program.[301] In a randomized study of patients with AIDS, supplements containing HMB, arginine and glutamine were shown to produce weight gain mainly as a lean body mass.[302] Immune status was also improved as evidenced by an increase in CD3 and CD8 cells and a decrease in the HIV viral load.

A total of 32 patients with solid tumors who had demonstrated a weight loss of at least 5% were randomly assigned in a double-blind fashion to either an isonitrogenous control mixture of nonessential amino acids or an experimental treatment containing HMB (3 g/day), L-arginine (14 g/day), and L-glutamine (14 g/day) (HMB/Arg/Gln).[303] The primary outcomes measured were the change in body mass and fat-free mass (FFM), which were assessed at up to 6 months. The patients supplemented with HMB/Arg/Gln gained 0.95 ± 0.66 kg of body mass in 4 weeks, whereas control subjects lost 0.26 ± 0.78 kg during the same time period. This gain was the result of a significant increase in fat-free mass (FFM) in the HMB/Arg/Gln-supplemented group (1.12 ± 0.68 kg), whereas the control subjects lost 1.34 ±0.78 kg of FFM ($P = 0.02$). The effect of HMB/Arg/Gln on FFM increase was maintained over 24 weeks. The exact reason for this improvement was unclear. The increases of FFM were attributed to the observed effects of HMB on slowing the rate of protein breakdown, with improvements in protein synthesis observed with arginine and glutamine. For the last 6 years no follow-up or confirmatory studies have been published. Whether this combination improved survival or improved tolerance to chemotherapy is unclear. Additional randomized studies are needed to fully assess the benefit of the combination.

Enteral and Parenteral Nutrition ■ Cancer cachexia is different from simple starvation, in that nutritional support, either enteral or parenteral, has only limited value. For the correction of cancer-related malnutrition, therefore, enteral and parenteral administration of nutrient solutions must be used discreetly. In patients with oropharyngeal dysfunction from head and neck neoplasm or esophageal obstruction, blenderized food and liquid supplement can often achieve an adequate level of nutritional repletion. When necessary, percutaneous gastrostomy or jejunostomy offer bypass feeding. For patients who cannot tolerate the use of the GI tract because of nausea, vomiting, obstruction, malabsorption, or absence, it may be necessary to begin total parenteral nutrition (TPN, "hyperalimentation").

The needs of nutritional support in cancer patients during tumor progression and the role of TPN in cancer surgery, chemotherapy, and radiotherapy should be considered at several different levels. Benefits of TPN in patients who underwent cancer surgery have been reported to include improved wound healing, a decreased rate of infection, fewer major complications, and a decrease in postoperative mortality. In other studies, however, no advantage of TPN was found; one report described an increase in the rate of major postoperative complications.[304] TPN in cancer patients with obstructions of the GI tract, GI fistulae, evisceration, and intra-abdominal infection appears justified during and after surgery, however, since it constitutes a treatment for starvation, not cancer cachexia.[305]

No significant benefit of TPN has been demonstrated in patients undergoing chemotherapy and/or radiotherapy in terms of treatment tolerance, response to chemotherapy or radiotherapy, or in survival.[306,307] Furthermore, other authors have reported that TPN is detrimental. Controversies related to TPN in the treatment of cancer cachexia have been reviewed.[308-310]

Recently, in a randomized trial of more than 300 patients with malignant neoplasms who experienced progressive cachexia, indomethacin, and epogen, or these drugs plus oral or parenteral nutritional support were compared.[311] Patients in the latter group had significant improvements in food intake, energy balance, and overall survival. It is unclear, however, whether improved survival was due to combined effects of two drugs plus nutritional intervention or nutritional intervention alone. This question is relevant because a large percentage (92.1%) of patients had GI cancer, suggesting that many patients might have had nausea and vomiting, GI obstruction, ascites, diarrhea, or other GI-specific causes of weight loss rather than simply cancer cachexia. Confirmatory studies are needed, specifically accruing patients with non-GI malignancies.

Branched-Chain Amino Acids ■ Branched–chain amino acids (leucine, isoleucine, and valine) are used by skeletal muscle but not by the liver. They have been shown to be uniquely effective in regulating nitrogen balance in muscle by reducing protein catabolism and increasing protein synthesis in both injured and tumor-bearing animals. Randomized studies have shown improved nitrogen retention, improved protein utilization, and increased protein and albumin synthesis in patients who received parenteral nutritional support with a high content of branched–chain amino acids.[312,313] In contrast, in another randomized study the effects of a balanced amino acid solution with or without supplementation of α-ketoisocaproate or a branched–chain amino acid solution were compared in patients with GI cancer who underwent surgery.[314] The balanced amino acid solution itself with an adequate energy supply had an optimal nitrogen-sparing effect. Branched–chain amino acids or α-ketoisocaproate did not improve nitrogen balance or reduce protein degradation.

Interestingly, the tryptophan (precursor of serotonin) uptake into the brain is competitive with that of branched–chain amino acids.[315] A trial to reduce tryptophan uptake by increasing plasma levels of branched–chain amino acids resulted in a decrease in the severity of anorexia in cancer patients.[316]

Glutamine ■ Tumor cells are major glutamine consumers both for protein synthesis and for oxidation.[317] A glutamine-enriched solution has been used to compensate for the uptake of the amino acid by the tumor to enhance host immune response against tumor growth.[318] In patients undergoing bone marrow transplantation for hematological malignancies, glutamine supplementation was found to be beneficial, improving nitrogen balance and diminishing the incidence of clinical infection.[319] Role of glutamine supplement on cancer cachexia has not been reported.

Orexigenic and Anorexigenic Mediators Insulin ■ Some of the metabolic alterations associated with cancer cachexia include glucose intolerance, increased gluconeogenesis, and Cori-cycle activation. These metabolic changes are accompanied by insulin resistance. These observations led to the study of exogenous insulin administration. Animal studies show that insulin administration has improved the food intake, the host preservation of nitrogen, fat, and potassium and decreased muscle wasting.[320,321] Indeed, daily subcutaneous insulin administration resulted in a marked weight gain in AIDS patients.[322] Insulin administration alone has not been evaluated in the treatment of cancer cachexia (see "Growth Hormone [GH], Somatostatin, and GHRH [GHRP-2]" and "Clenbuterol").

Ghrelin, an orexigenic mediator has recently been reported to have a key role in increasing appetite and food intake. The circulating levels of ghrelin have been reported to be increased in patients with chronic heart failure and muscle wasting, and in patients with cancer cachexia.

In studies examining whether ghrelin counteracted tumor-induced anorexia in animal system, ghrelin treatment increased food intake and body weight gain.[323-326]

Seven cancer patients who reported loss of appetite were subjected to a short-term randomized crossover clinical trial examining whether ghrelin stimulated appetite in cancer patients with anorexia.[327] A marked increase in energy intake was observed with ghrelin infusion compared with saline control, and every patient ate more. The meal appreciation score was greater with ghrelin treatment. No side effects were observed.

In an another study, 21 adult patients were randomized to receive ghrelin on days 1 and 8 and placebo on days 4 and 11 or vice versa, given intravenously over a 60-minute period before lunch: 10 received 2 μg/kg (either lower-dose) ghrelin; 11 received 8 μg/kg (or upper-dose) ghrelin. Active and total ghrelin, growth hormone (GH), and IGF-1 levels were monitored at baseline, during treatment and at end of study. No grade 3/4 toxicity or stimulation of tumour growth was observed. The peak increase of GH was dose-dependent. At day 8, 81% of patients preferred ghrelin to placebo as against 63% at the end of study. Nutritional intake and eating-related symptoms did not differ between ghrelin and placebo. Ghrelin is well tolerated and safe in patients with advanced cancer.[328]

An oral ghrelin mimetic and GH secretagogue, RC-1291, a novel, ghrelin mimetic, and GH secretagogue was administered in a randomized, placebo-controlled, multiple-dose, dose-escalation phase I study in healthy volunteers. Results indicate that RC-1291 produces dose-related increases in body weight with no dose-limiting adverse effects.[329] Studies of long-term effects are needed to examine whether ghrelin improved performance status, maintained lean body mass or overall survival.

Melatonin ■ Melatonin is an indole amine primarily secreted from the pineal gland during the hours of darkness. The functions of melatonin are obscure but it has been claimed to modulate sleep, cardiac rhythms, sexual behavior, the reproductive system, immunologic functions, as well as antioxidative and anti-inflammatory activities. Melatonin has been reported to decrease the level of circulating TNF in patients with advanced cancer, prevent weight loss and reduce chemotherapy-induced malaise and asthenia as well as thrombocytopenia.[330-333]

Based on observations that melatonin amplified IL-2 induced antitumor effects in animals, a randomized study was carried out in patients with metastatic solid tumors comparing a combination of low dose IL-2 plus melatonin with best supportive care.[334] In the treated group the percentage of patients with improved performance status as well as overall survival were significantly higher than the controls. Another randomized study of chemotherapy with cisplatin and etoposide plus/minus melatonin was carried out in poor risk patients with advanced nonsmall-cell lung cancer.[335] There was no significant difference in survival between the two groups, but the melatonin group had less frequent myelosuppression, neuropathy, and cachexia. In a recent Swedish trial, the effect of fish oil, melatonin, or the combination of the two were investigated in 24 patients with advanced GI cancer. None induced major biochemical changes indicative of a strong anticachectic effect. Nonetheless, the interventions may have produced a weight-stabilizing effect.[336] Additional clinical studies appear indicated to define the role of melatonin in the treatment of cancer cachexia.

Cyproheptadine ■ As has been discussed above, anorexia may be mediated by an increased serotonergic activity in the brain. Cyproheptadine is a serotonin antagonist with antihistaminic properties, usually prescribed for allergies. In several clinical situations the agent produced appetite stimulation and weight gain. A randomized trial in patients with advanced malignant neoplasms showed that cyproheptadine produced a decrease in nausea and mild enhancement in appetite. The agent did not abate progressive weight loss in these patients, however.[337] Additional studies are needed with use of other antiserotogenic drugs.

Combination of Anticachexia Agents ■ In 2005, Italian investigators started a phase III randomized study to establish which was the most effective and safest treatment of cancer-related anorexia/cachexia syndrome and oxidative stress in improving identified primary endpoints: increase of lean body mass, decrease of resting energy expenditure (REE), increase of total daily physical activity, decrease of IL-6 and TNF-α, and improvement of fatigue assessed by the Multidimensional Fatigue Symptom Inventory-Short Form (MFSI-SF). All patients were given as basic treatment polyphenols plus antioxidant agents alpha-lipoic acid, carbocysteine, and vitamins A, C, and E, all orally. Patients were then randomized to one of the following five arms: (1) medroxyprogesterone acetate/megestrol acetate; (2) pharmacologic nutritional support containing eicosapentaenoic acid; (3) l-carnitine; (4) thalidomide; or (5) medroxyprogesterone acetate/megestrol acetate plus pharmacologic nutritional support plus l-carnitine plus thalidomide. Treatment duration was 4 months. The sample comprised 475 patients. By January 2007, 125 patients, well balanced for all clinical characteristics, were included. An interim analysis on 125 patients showed an improvement of at least one primary endpoint in arms 3, 4, and 5, whereas arm 2 showed a significant worsening of lean body mass, REE, and MFSI-SF. Analysis of variance comparing the change of primary endpoints between arms showed a significant improvement of REE in favor of arm 5 versus arm 2 and a significant improvement of MFSI-SF in favor of arms 1, 3, and 5 versus arm 2. A significant inferiority of arm 2 versus arms 3, 4, and 5 for the primary endpoints lean body mass, REE, and MFSI-SF was observed on the basis of t test for changes. The interim results obtained thus far seemed to suggest that the most effective treatment for cancer-related anorexia/cachexia syndrome and oxidative stress should be a combination regimen. The study is still in progress and the final results should confirm these data.[338]

Future Directions

Patients with cancer cachexia are characterized by the presence of anorexia, early satiety, anemia, weakness, and weight loss accompanied by muscle and adipose tissue loss. Patients with gastric cancer may present weight-loss as an initial and only sign of the disease; whereas, in patients with lymphoma weight loss and cachexia may be simply a terminal event. Cachexia occurs to a variable extent in different types of cancer at different stages, likely from different mechanisms. The multifactorial nature of cachexia precludes a uniform pathophysiological definition. Inability to translate animal studies to human may lie in this context. These factors have hindered clinical studies not only at a biochemical and molecular levels, but also in terms of the introduction of effective therapy. The advent of novel therapeutic targets (eg, neuropeptidergic circuit, ubiquitin-proteasome pathway and NF-κB) and biological response modifiers (eg, thalidomide) has opened possibilities for new clinical research in cachexia. Regulatory authorities feel it is important not only to demonstrate efficacy in terms of patients' nutritional status (eg, lean body mass) but also functional status (eg, performance status, tolerance to treatment, and survival).

In spite of extensive research on the mechanisms of cachexia, there has been little success in developing effective agents. Differences in therapeutic targets among cachectic cancer patients suggest no single agent will be able to treat all kinds of cachexia. There will likely be no all-in-one panacea for cancer cachexia. Combined anticachectic treatments and individualized approaches based on targets in individual patients are today's standard.

Several potentially promising leads beg for well designed clinical trials. The following agents, with suggestive activity in animal experiments or preliminary clinical explorations deserve critical clinical investigation: TPN plus GH or TPN/GH plus insulin, GHRP-2, megestrol plus ibuprofen, resveratrol, dehydroxymethyl-epoxyquinomicin, pyrrolidine dithioocarbamate, myostatine propeptide, clenbuterol, thalidomide/lenalidomide, 5'-deoxy-5-fluorouridine, IL-12, IL-10, IL-15, HMB/Arg/Gln, ghrelin (and Ghrelin-mimic RC-1291), antioxidant combinations, and antiserotogenic agents.

Effective prevention or control of cachexia would significantly improve cancer therapy.

Summary

Cachexia is a complex syndrome presenting wasting of muscle and adipose tissues, weight loss, anorexia, early satiety, fatigue, anemia, hyperlipidemia, systemic inflammatory responses, and often a hypercatabolic state. Cachexia differs from starvation, where visceral proteins are also depleted. Profound anorexia and early satiety are partly responsible, but metabolic abnormalities are the major cause of cachexia. Mechanisms of cachexia include production of inflammatory cytokines including TNF-α, Interleuken-1 (IL-1), IL-6, and IFN-γ; secretion of tumor byproducts which include lipolytic factors and PIF; hormonal aberration; prostaglandin elevation; possible dysfunction of neuropeptidergic circuits, and metabolic derangement produced by treatment. Recently, examinations of signaling pathway involved in cancer induced muscle atrophy has have identified several cachexia genes. A variety of agents have been used in attempts to reverse cachexia, including corticosteroids, megestrol acetate and medroxyprogesterone acetate, anabolic steroids, cannabinoids, growth hormones, somatostatin and GHRP-2, insulin-like growth factor 1, metoclopramide and cisapride, hydrazine sulfate, anti-inflammatory agents such as indomethacin and ibuprofen, pentoxifylline and lisofylline, proteasome inhibitors and NF-KB inhibitors, clenbuterol, thalidomide, adenosine triphosphate, 5(-deoxy-5-fluorouridine, proinflammatory-cytokine inhibitors including proinflammatory-cytokine antibodies and anti-inflammatory cytokines, eicosapentaenoic acid, enteral and parenteral nutrition, branched–chain amino acids, orexigenic mediators, melatonin, and cyproheptadine. Currently, the most commonly used agent is megestrol acetate. In early studies, ghrelin, thalidomide, NF-κB inhibitors, and combinations of anticancer agents appear effective at attenuating loss of weight and lean body mass in patient with cancer cachexia. Development of agents, which prevent or reverse lean body weight mass are eagerly awaited.

Selected References

The complete reference list can be found at www.CANCERMEDICINE8.com

2. Vigano A, Bruera E, Jhangri GS, et al. Clinical survival predictors in patients with advanced cancer. Arch Intern Med. 2000;160:861–868.
12. Krause R, Humphrey C, von Meyenfeldt M, et al. A central mechanism for anorexia in cancer: a hypothesis. *Cancer Treat Res.* 1981;65(Suppl 5):15–21.
20. Cahlin C, Korner A, Axelsson H, et al. Experimental cancer cachexia: the role of host-derived cytokines interleukin (IL)-6, IL-12, interferon-gamma, and tumor necrosis factor alpha evaluated in gene knockout, tumor-bearing mice on C57 Bl background and eicosanoid-dependent cachexia. *Cancer Res.* 2000;60:5488–5493.
28. Wisse BE, Schwartz MW, Cummings DE. Melanocortin signaling and anorexia in chronic disease states. *Ann NY Acad Sci.* 2003;994:275–281.
29. Schwartz MW, Woods SC, Porte D Jr, et al. Central nervous system control of food intake. *Nature.* 2000;404:661–671.
35. Wu JT, Kral JG. Ghrelin: integrative neuroendocrine peptide in health and disease. *Ann Surg.* 2004;239:464–474.
40. Ramos EJ, Suzuki S, Marks D, et al. Cancer anorexia-cachexia syndrome: cytokines and neuropeptides. *Curr Opin Clin Nutr Metab Care.* 2004;7:427–434.
46. Inui A. Cancer anorexia-cachexia syndrome: are neuropeptides the key? *Cancer Res.* 1999;59:4495–4501.

59. Laviano A, Russo M, Freda F, Rossi-Fanelli F. Neurochemical mechanisms for cancer anorexia. *Nutrition.* 2002;18:100–105.
66. Pedersen PL, Mathupala S, Rempel A, et al. Mitochondrial bound type II hexokinase: a key player in the growth and survival of many cancers and an ideal prospect for therapeutic intervention. *Biochim Biophys Acta.*. 2002;1555:14–20.
67. Mathupala SP, Rempel A, Pedersen PL. Glucose metabolism in cancer cells: Isolation, sequence, and activity of the promotor for type II hexokinase. *J Biol Chem.* 1995;270:16918–16925.
71. Ramos EJ, Suzuki S, Marks D, et al. Cancer anorexia-cachexia syndrome: cytokines and neuropeptides. *Curr Opin Clin Nutr Metab Care.* 2004;7:427–434.
74. Beutler B, Greenwald D, Hulmes JD, et al. Identity of tumour necrosis factor and the macrophage-secreted factor cachectin. *Nature (London).* 1985; 316:552–554.
82. Fujita J, Tsujinaka T, Yano M, et al. Anti-interkeukin-6 receptor antibody prevents muscle atrophy in colon-25 adenocarcinoma-bearing mice with modulation of lysosomal and ATP-ubiquitin-dependent proteolytic pathways. *Int J Cancer.* 1996;68:637–643.
94. Puigserver P, Rhee J, Lin J, et al. Cytokine stimulation of energy expenditure through p38 MAP kinase activation of PPARgamma coactivator-1. *Mol Cell.* 2001;8:971–982.
101. Hirai K, Hussey HJ, Barber MD, et al. Biological evaluation of a lipid-mobilizing factor isolated from the urine of cancer patients. *Cancer Res.* 1998;58:2359–2365.
116. Todorov PT, McDevitt TM, Cariuk P, et al. Induction of muscle protein degradation and weight loss by a tumor product. *Cancer Res.* 1996; 56:1256–1261.
117. Guttridge DC, Mayo MW, Madrid LV, et al. NF-kappaB-induced loss of MyoD messenger RNA: possible role in muscle decay and cachexia. *Science.* 2000;289:2363–2366.
118. Acharyya S, Ladner KJ, Nelsen LL, et al. Cancer cachexia is regulated by selective targeting of skeletal muscle gene products. *J Clin Invest.* 2004;114:370–378.
120. Watchorn TM, Dowidar N, Dejong CH, Waddell ID, Garden OJ, Ross JA. The cachectic mediator proteolysis inducing factor activates NF-kappaB and STAT3 in human Kupffer cells and monocytes. *Int J Oncol.* 2005;27:1105–1111.
123. Ladner KJ, Caligiuri MA, Guttridge DC Tumor necrosis factor-regulated biphasic activation of NF-kappa B is required for cytokine-induced loss of skeletal muscle gene products. *J Biol Chem.* 2003 Jan 24;278:2294–2303.
124. Hershko A, Ciechanover A. The ubiquitin system. *Annu Rev Biochem.* 1998;67:425–479.
125. Gomes MD, Lecker SH, Jagoe RT, Navon A, Goldberg AL. Atrogin-1, a muscle-specific F-box protein highly expressed during muscle atrophy. *Proc Natl Acad Sci USA.* 2001;98:14440–14445.
126. Bodine SC, Latres E, Baumhueter S, et al. Identification of ubiquitin ligases required for skeletal muscle atrophy. *Science.* 2001;294:1704–1708.
127. Glass DJ. Signalling pathways that mediate skeletal muscle hypertrophy and atrophy. *Nat Cell Biol.* 2003;5(2):87–90.
128. Sartorelli V, Fulco M Molecular and cellular determinants of skeletal muscle atrophy and hypertrophy. *Sci STKE.* 2004 27;2004(244):rell.
129. Sacheck JM, Ohtsuka A, McLary SC, Goldberg AL. IGF-I stimulates muscle growth by suppressing protein breakdown and expression of atrophy-related ubiquitin ligases, atrogin-1 and MuRF1. *Am J Physiol Endocrinol Metab.* 2004 Oct;287:E591–E601.
130. Sandri M, Sandri C, Gilbert A, et al. Foxo transcription factors induce the atrophy-related ubiquitin ligase atrogin-1 and cause skeletal muscle atrophy. *Cell.* 2004 Apr 30;117(3):399–412.
132. Frescas D, Pagano M. Deregulated proteolysis by the F-box proteins SKP2 and -TrCP: tipping the scales of cancer. *Nat Rev Cancer.* 2008;8:438–449.
133. Stitt TN, Drujan D, Clarke BA, et al. The IGF-1/PI3K/Akt pathway prevents expression of muscle atrophy-induced ubiquitin ligases by inhibiting FOXO transcription factors. *Mol Cell.* 2004 May 7;14(3):395–403.
134. Schmitt TL, Martignoni ME, Bachmann J, et al. Activity of the Akt- dependent anabolic and catabolic pathways in muscle and liver samples in cancer-related cachexia. *J Mol Med.* 2007;85:647–654.
135. Stewart CEH, Newcomb PV, Holly JMP. Multifaceted roles of TNF-α in myoblast destruction: a multitude of signal transduction pathways. *J Cell Physiol.* 2004;198:237–247.
138. Mastrocola R, Reffo P, Penna F, et al. Muscle wasting in diabetic and in tumor-bearing rats: role of oxidative stress. *Free Radic Biol Med.* 2008 Feb 15;44(4):584–593.
140. Mantovani G, Macciò A, Madeddu C, et al. Antioxidant agents are effective in inducing lymphocyte progression through cell cycle in advanced cancer patients: assessment of the most important laboratory indexes of cachexia and oxidative stress. *J Mol Med.* 2003 Oct;81(10):664–673).
141. Di Marco S, Mazroui R, Dallaire P, et al. NF-kappa B-mediated MyoD decay during muscle wasting requires nitric oxide synthase mRNA stabilization, HuR protein, and nitric oxide release. *Mol Cell Biol.* 2005;25:6533–6545.
142. Lee SJ. Regulation of muscle mass by myostatin. *Annu Rev Cell Dev Biol.* 2004;20:61–86.
152. Costelli P, Muscaritoli M, Bonetto A, et al. Muscle myostatin signalling is enhanced in experimental cancer cachexia. *Eur J Clin Invest.* 2008 Jul;38(7):531–538.
161. Acharyya S, Butchbach ME, Sahenk Z, et al. Dystrophin glycoprotein complex dysfunction: a regulatory link between muscular dystrophy and cancer cachexia. *Cancer Cell.* 2005 Nov;8(5):421–432.
182. Loprinzi CL, Kugler JW, Sloan JA, et al. Randomized comparison of megestrol acetate versus dexamethasone versus fluoxymesterone for the treatment of cancer anorexia/cachexia. *J Clin Oncol.* 1999;17:3299–3306.
187. Pascual Lopez A, Roque i Figuls M, Urrutia Cuchi G, et al. Systematic review of megestrol acetate in the treatment of anorexia-cachexia syndrome. *J Pain Symptom Manag.* 2004;27:360–369.
207. Tschop M, Statnick MA, Suter TM, Heiman ML. GH-releasing peptide-2 increases fat mass in mice lacking NPY: indication for a crucial mediating role of hypothalamic agouti-related protein. *Endocrinology.* 2002;143:558–568.
250. Mantovani G, Madeddu C, Macciò A, et al. Cancer-related anorexia/cachexia syndrome and oxidative stress: an innovative approach beyond current treatment. *Cancer Epidemiol Biomarkers Prev.* 2004 Oct;13:1651–1659.
252. Bogdanovich S, Perkins KJ, Krag TO, Whittemore L-A, Khurana TS. Myostatin propeptide-mediated amelioration of dystrophic pathophysiology. *FASEB J.* 2005;19:543–549.
264. Gordon JN, Trebble TM, Ellis RD, et al. Thalidomide in the treatment of cancer cachexia: a randomised placebo controlled trial. *Gut.* 2005;54:540–545.
300. Mazzotta P, Jeney CM. Anorexia-cachexia syndrome: a systematic review of the role of dietary polyunsaturated fatty acids in the management of symptoms, survival, and quality of life. *J Pain Symptom Manage.* 2008 Dec 1 [Epub ahead of print].
311. Lundholm K, Daneryd P, Bosaeus I, et al. Palliative nutritional intervention in addition to cyclooxygenase and erythropoietin treatment for patients with malignant disease: Effects on survival, metabolism, and function. *Cancer.* 2004;100:1967–77.
327. Neary NM, Small CJ, Wren AM, et al. Ghrelin increases energy intake in cancer patients with impaired appetite: acute, randomized, placebo-controlled trial. *J Clin Endocrinol Metab.* 2004;89:2832–2836.
328. Strasser F, Lutz TA, Maeder MT, et al. Safety, tolerability and pharmacokinetics of intravenous ghrelin for cancer-related anorexia/cachexia: a randomised, placebo-controlled, double-blind, double-crossover study. *Br J Cancer.* 2008 Jan 29;98(2):300–308.
329. Garcia JM, Polvino WJ. Effect on body weight and safety of RC-1291, a novel, orally available ghrelin mimetic and growth hormone secretagogue: results of a phase I, randomized, placebo-controlled, multiple-dose study in healthy volunteers. *Oncologist.* 2007 May;12(5):594–600.
338. Mantovani G, Macciò A, Madeddu C, et al. Randomized phase III clinical trial of five different arms of treatment for patients with cancer cachexia: interim results. *Nutrition.* 2008 Apr;24(4):305–313.

123 Antiemetic Therapy

Aditya Bardia, MBBS, MPH ▪ David S. Ettinger, MD

Overview

Chemotherapy-induced nausea and vomiting (CINV) remains a significant problem for many cancer patients despite recent advances in pharmacologic therapy.[1] It may have a dramatic impact on a patient's quality of life, in addition to physical consequences, including dehydration, nutritional compromise, and metabolic disturbances.[2] Despite the publication of guidelines for preventive antiemetic therapy, some patients continue to receive suboptimal prophylaxis against CINV. Nausea and vomiting occurring after chemotherapy may be more difficult to manage than if the symptoms had been prevented with appropriate pharmacologic intervention. In addition, patients may develop a psychological component to their nausea and vomiting as a result of inadequate management in the past. Thus, optimal control of CINV is a crucial aspect of symptom management among cancer patients.

Historically, approximately 70-80% of all cancer patients receiving chemotherapy experienced emesis,[3] and, fortunately, there have been dramatic improvements since the introduction of effective antiemetic therapy.[1] Studies over the last 20 years have attempted to quantify the impact of chemotherapy side effects on cancer patients. Repeatedly, nausea and vomiting are mentioned as "major physical,"[4] "most troublesome and unpleasant" side effects associated with chemotherapy.[5] Although there have been recent advances in pharmacologic prevention of CINV, a 1997 study by de Boer-Dennert and colleagues revealed that nausea and vomiting ranked as the first and third most distressing side effects of chemotherapy, despite a decrease in the overall incidence and severity with the introduction of 5-hydroxytryptamine 3 (5-HT3) antagonists.[6] Grunberg and colleagues surveyed patients, medical oncologists, and oncology nurses in 2001-2002 to assess the frequency and provider perception of CINV.[1] Although improvements in the prevention of acute nausea and vomiting were seen (acute nausea in approximately 35% and acute emesis in 13%), delayed symptoms were seen more frequently (50-60% with nausea and 30-50% with emesis, depending on the chemotherapy used). Strikingly, more than 75% of physicians and nurses underestimated the occurrence of delayed nausea and vomiting. Progress in relieving the symptoms of CINV will only come with greater awareness of the problem and more aggressive use of current medications.

This chapter highlights the pathophysiology of CINV, the emetogenic potential of common chemotherapeutics, classes of antiemetic therapy including complementary therapies, and guidelines for prevention and acute management of CINV.

Pathophysiology of Nausea and Vomiting

Vomiting is controlled by the central nervous system via a complex pathway of varied afferent inputs and neurotransmitters (Fig. 123-1). In the 1950s, studies by Borison and Wang identified two areas of the brainstem involved in nausea and vomiting: the chemoreceptor trigger zone (CTZ) and the emetic center.[7] The CTZ is located in the area postrema in the floor of the fourth ventricle. Because it lies outside the blood-brain barrier, the CTZ is susceptible to emetogenic stimuli from the bloodstream, such as chemotherapeutic drugs or, more likely, their metabolites.[8] Muscarinic, dopamine D2, serotonin (5-HT3), neurokinin 1 (NK-1) and histamine H1 receptors have been identified in the CTZ. Impulses from the CTZ are then transmitted to the emetic center. In addition to those from the CTZ to the emetic center, afferent pathways from the gastrointestinal tract and pharynx via the vagus and splanchnic nerves are coordinated in the emetic center.[9] Inputs from the cerebral cortex may also be involved, especially in anticipatory emesis. The emetic center receives afferent impulses and coordinates the efferent activities of the salivation center, abdominal muscles, respiratory center, and autonomic nerves that result in vomiting. The emetic center, composed of these indistinct receptor and effector nuclei, is located in the nucleus tractus solitarius of the brainstem.[8]

The most critical neurotransmitters involved in these afferent and efferent pathways are serotonin (5-HT3), dopamine, and substance P. Others include acetylcholine, corticosteroid, histamine, cannabinoid, opiate, and gamma-aminobutyric acid (GABA).[10] Blockade of these neurotransmitters and their receptors form the basis of action of various antiemetic drugs. The most significant advance in antiemetic therapy came in the early 1990s when the 5-HT3 receptor antagonists became available.[6] Substance P, which binds to the NK-1 receptor, is an emerging target in antiemetic therapy,[11] and one Food and Drug Administration (FDA)-approved NK-1 receptor antagonist, aprepitant, has shown clinical utility.[12-14] Drugs such as prochlorperazine, haloperidol and metoclopramide exert their antiemetic effects by inhibiting dopamine. However, it is not fully known how and where along these pathways chemotherapy and its metabolites have their emetic effects. Metabolites may stimulate the CTZ directly. Serotonin and other neurotransmitters may be released from intestinal cells damaged by chemotherapy. Sensory neurons release substance P, and numerous NK-1 receptors have been identified in both the CTZ and the nucleus tractus solitarius. Despite increasing knowledge of the central nervous system and pathways involved in control of vomiting, no single common pathway has been discovered, and it is unlikely that any single agent will be able to provide complete antiemetic protection from chemotherapy.

Types of Emesis

Three distinct types of chemotherapy-induced emesis have been identified: acute, delayed, and anticipatory.

Acute emesis is defined as nausea and vomiting within 24 h of chemotherapy. It has its onset within 1-2 h of chemotherapy and peaks in the first 4-6 h without adequate prophylaxis.

Delayed emesis refers to symptoms that start more than 24 h after chemotherapy. It typically peaks at 48-72 h and may last for 6-7 days. Although delayed emesis may be less frequent and severe than acute emesis, it is less well controlled than acute emesis. Cisplatin is most frequently associated with delayed emesis, and it is also seen with carboplatin, cyclophosphamide, and anthracyclines.

Anticipatory emesis is seen in patients who have previously experienced significant nausea and vomiting following chemotherapy. In these patients, symptoms develop as a conditioned response before

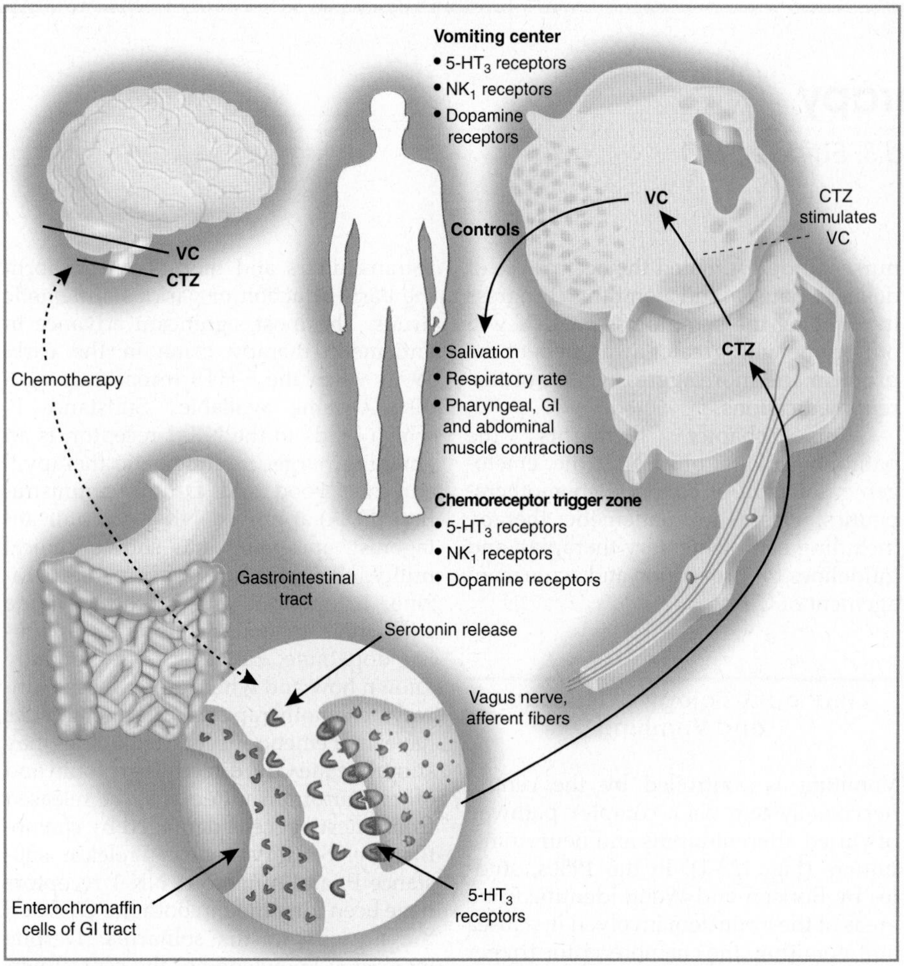

Figure 123-1 Two sites in the brainstem—the vomiting center and the chemoreceptor trigger zone—are important to emesis control. The vomiting center consists of an intertwined neural network in the nucleus tractus solitarius that controls patterns of motor activity. The chemoreceptor trigger zone, located in the area postrema, is the entry point for emetogenic stimuli. Enterochromaffin cells in the gastrointestinal tract respond to chemotherapy by releasing serotonin. Serotonin binds to 5-HT3 receptors, which are located not only in the gastrointestinal tract but also on vagal afferent neurons and in the nucleus tractus solitarius and area postrema. The activated 5-HT3 receptors signal the chemoreceptor trigger zone via pathways that may include the afferent fibers of the vagus nerve. Serotonin may also bind with 5-HT3 receptors in the brainstem. Other neurotransmitters, including dopamine and substance P, also influence the chemoreceptor trigger zone. Afferent impulses from the chemoreceptor trigger zone stimulate the vomiting center, which initiates emesis. *Source*: Grunberg SM, Hesketh PJ. Control of chemotherapy-induced emesis. *N Engl J Med*. 1993;329:1790–1796. Reproduced with permission of MGI Pharma.

the chemotherapy is administered. It may be triggered by sights and activities associated with the chemotherapy (eg, driving to the treatment center). As anticipatory emesis is a conditioned reflex, it is predominantly mediated by the cerebral cortex. As control of CINV has improved, the incidence of anticipatory emesis has declined.[15]

In addition to chemotherapy-induced emesis, other potential causes of nausea and vomiting in cancer patients include partial or complete bowel obstruction, brain metastases, uremia, electrolyte disturbances (ie, hyperglycemia, hypercalcemia, hyponatremia), and gastroparesis. Other medications commonly prescribed in cancer patients, such as opiates, may cause emesis as well.

Emetogenic Chemotherapy

The severity and frequency of CINV are affected by variables of both the patient and the chemotherapy. Patient-related factors predicting a higher incidence of CINV include a history of chemotherapy, a history of CINV, female sex, younger age, a history of motion sickness, and no history of alcohol use. Chemotherapy-related factors include the route and rate of administration and drug dosage. The most predictive factor is the specific chemotherapy agent used.[16]

There is no universally accepted classification system of chemotherapy agents by emetogenic potential (Table 123-1). The most widely accepted, devised by Hesketh and colleagues, divides chemotherapy into five levels of emetogenicity based on the percentage of patients who experience nausea and vomiting following each without any antiemetic prophylaxis. Level 1 drugs result in emesis in less than 10% without antiemetic therapy; level 2, 10-30%; level 3, 30-60%; level 4, 60-90%; and level 5, more than 90% of patients experiencing emesis without prophylaxis.[17] A recently proposed modification would classify chemotherapy into four risk categories[18]:

High risk (level 5): more than 90%
Moderate risk (levels 3 and 4): 30-90%
Low risk (level 2): 10-30%
Minimal risk (level 1): less than 10%

It should be noted that these classification systems were developed with a focus on acute emesis. It is clear from recent data that the frequency and severity of delayed emesis are often underestimated and remain a significant problem for many patients.[1] Adequate antiemetic prophylaxis is required for the duration of days that symptoms are anticipated.

Classes of Antiemetics

Our knowledge of the known neurotransmitters involved in the central nervous system pathways that regulate the vomiting response has provided targets for antiemetic therapy (Table 123-2). In return, successful clinical application of these agents has confirmed the importance of these neurotransmitters and receptors in the vomiting pathway. Neuroreceptors involved in the control of emesis include muscarinic (M1, receptor site for acetylcholine), dopamine (D2, receptor site for dopamine), histamine (H1, receptor site for histamine), 5-HT3 (receptor site for serotonin), NK-1 (receptor site for substance P), and GABA (receptor site for benzodiazepines).[19,20] The most effective and most commonly used antiemetics are the 5-HT3 receptor antagonists, the dopamine antagonists, and corticosteroids. An emerging class of agents, the NK-1 receptor antagonists, further expands the repertoire of antiemetic agents.

Serotonin/5-HT3 Receptor Antagonists

Since the early 1990s, four 5-HT3 receptor antagonists have been approved in the United States: ondansetron, granisetron, dolasetron, and, most recently, palonosetron. These agents revolutionized the antiemetic prophylaxis of highly and moderately emetogenic chemotherapy. Studies of 5-HT3 receptor antagonists used alone demonstrated superior efficacy compared with high-dose metoclopramide alone[21] and equivalence to the combination of

Table 123-1 **Emetogenic Potential of Single Antineoplastic Agents**

Level	Agent
High risk, level 5 (>90% predicted frequency of emesis without prophylaxis)	Carmustine >250 mg/m² Cisplatin ≥50 mg/m² Cyclophosphamide >1500 mg/m² Dacarbazine Mechlorethamine Streptozocin
Moderate risk, level 4 (60-90% predicted frequency of emesis without prophylaxis)	Amifostine >500 mg/m² Busulfan >4 mg/d Carboplatin Cisplatin <50 mg/m² Cyclophosphamide >750 mg/m² and ≤1500 mg/m² Cytarabine >1 g/m² Dactinomycin Doxorubicin >60 mg/m² Epirubicin >90 mg/m² Melphalan >50 mg/m² Methotrexate >1000 mg/m² Procarbazine (oral dosing)
Moderate risk, level 3 (30-60% predicted frequency of emesis without prophylaxis)	Amifostine >300 mg/m²and ≤500 mg/m² Arsenic trioxide Bendamustine Cyclophosphamide ≤750 mg/m² Cyclophosphamide (oral dosing) Doxorubicin 20 and <60 mg/m² Epirubicin ≤90 mg/m² Ifosfamide Interleukin-2 >12-15 million units/m² Irinotecan Lomustine Methotrexate 250-1000 mg/m² Mitoxantrone <15 mg/m² Oxaliplatin >75 mg/m²
Low risk, level 2 (10-30% predicted frequency of emesis without prophylaxis)	Amifostine ≤300 mg/m² Bexarotene Cytarabine 100-200 mg/m² Capecitabine Docetaxel Doxorubicin (liposomal formulation) Etoposide 5-Fluorouracil <1000 mg/m² Gemcitabine Methotrexate >50 and <250 mg/m² Mitomycin Mitoxantrone Paclitaxel Pemetrexed Temozolomide Topotecan
Minimal risk, level 1 (<10% predicted frequency of emesis without prophylaxis)	Alemtuzumab Asparaginase Bevacizumab Alpha Interferon Bleomycin Bortezomib Cetuximab Chlorambucil (oral dosing) Cladribine Dasatinib Dexrazoxane Denileukin diftitox Erlotinib Fludarabine Gefitinib Gemtuzumab ozogamicin Hydroxyurea Imatinib mesylate Melphalan (low dose, oral dosing) Methotrexate ≤50 mg/m² Pentostatin Rituximab Sorafinib Sunitinib Thioguanine (oral dosing) Trastuzumab Valrubicin Vinblastine Vincristine Vinorelbine

high-dose metoclopramide and dexamethasone, the previous standard of care for these patients.[22] However, the combination of 5-HT3 receptor antagonist and dexamethasone was the most effective combination tested.[23] The 5-HT3 antagonists remain the cornerstone of prophylaxis for both highly and moderately emetogenic chemotherapy.

Before 2003, there were three 5-HT3 receptor antagonists approved by the FDA: ondansetron, granisetron, and dolasetron. Numerous subsequent clinical trials demonstrated the clinical equivalence of these three agents, despite differences seen in preclinical models.[24-29] A single-dose prechemotherapy was shown to be as effective as repeat dosing.[30-32] In addition, there was no significant difference whether the agent was given orally or intravenously.[33,34]

In July 2003, a new 5-HT3 receptor antagonist, palonosetron, was approved by the FDA for antiemetic prophylaxis. Palonosetron may have advantages over the other serotonin antagonists because of its higher binding affinity to the 5-HT3 receptor and its longer half-life. Two phase 3 randomized clinical trials demonstrated the superiority of palonosetron compared with ondansetron and dolasetron, particularly in preventing delayed nausea and vomiting.[35,36] In the first, 592 patients were randomized to receive palonosetron at either 0.25 or 0.75 mg or dolasetron at 100 mg 30 min prior to moderately emetogenic chemotherapy. Less than 5% of patients received concomitant corticosteroids. A statistically significant difference was observed between the palonosetron 0.25 mg and dolasetron arms in complete response (CR), defined as absence of emesis and no rescue medication in the first 24 h). CR rates were 63% in the palonosetron 0.25 mg arm vs 52.9% in the dolasetron arm (p = .049) and 57% for the palonosetron 0.75 mg arm (p = .412). For complete control (defined as no emesis, no need for rescue medication, and no symptoms other than mild nausea) of delayed nausea and vomiting (24-120 h), palonosetron 0.25 and 0.75 mg demonstrated statistically significant improvements compared with dolasetron 100 mg (48.1% for palonosetron 0.25 mg compared with 36.1% for dolasetron, p = .027; 51.9% for palonosetron 0.75 mg, p = .016). There was no difference among the groups in observed adverse effects, including headache, constipation, and fatigue.[35] In the second study, palonosetron was compared with ondansetron 32 mg. Five hundred seventy patients receiving moderately emetogenic chemotherapy were randomized to one of two doses of palonosetron (0.25 or 0.75 mg) or ondansetron 32 mg on day 1 of chemotherapy. No patients received corticosteroids. CR rates were superior

Table 123-2 Classes and Recommended Doses of Selected Antiemetics

Agent	Class	Route	Dose
Ondansetron	5-HT3 receptor antagonist	IV	8-12 mg
		PO	12-24 mg
Granisetron	5-HT3 receptor antagonist	IV	1 mg or 0.01 mg/kg
		PO	2 mg
Dolasetron	5-HT3 receptor antagonist	IV	100 mg or 1.8 mg/kg
		PO	100 mg
Palonosetron	5-HT3 receptor antagonist	IV	0.25 mg
Aprepitant	NK-1 receptor antagonist	PO	125 mg day 1
			80 mg day 2, 3
Dexamethasone	Steroid	IV	8-20 mg
		PO	8-20 mg
Prochlorperazine	Dopamine receptor antagonist	IV	10 mg
		PO	10 mg
		Rectal suppository	25 mg
Metoclopramide	Dopamine receptor antagonist	IV	1-2 mg/kg
		PO	20-40 mg
Haloperidol	Dopamine receptor antagonist	IV	1-3 mg
		PO	1-2 mg
Dronabinol	Cannabinoid	PO	5-10 mg

Abbreviations: IV, intravenous; 5-HT3, 5-hydroxytryptamine 3; NK, neurokinin; PO, orally.

for the palonosetron 0.25 mg arm compared with the ondansetron group in prevention of both acute (81% vs 68.6%, $p = .009$) and delayed (74.1% vs 55.1%, $p < .001$) symptoms. Although palonosetron 0.75 mg demonstrated numeric improvement over ondansetron, the results were not statistically significant. Side effects were similar in all groups and included headache, diarrhea, constipation, and fatigue.[36] While palonosetron might be superior to other 5-HT3 agents, particularly in the prevention of delayed symptoms, further studies are needed to evaluate this further. All of the 5-HT3 antagonists are well tolerated; the most common adverse effect is headache, occurring in 15-20% of patients. Less common side effects include constipation and dizziness.

More recently, granisetron has been incorporated in a transdermal system (*Sancuso*) for the prevention of CINV. In a phase 3 study, the transdermal granisetron patch was compared to oral granisetron in the management of CINV. The patch formulation contained 34.3 mg of granisetron with the active ingredient being released slowly over 7 days. In a multicenter study involving 641 patients receiving highly or moderately emetogenic chemotherapy, the granisetron patch was not inferior to repeat doses of oral granisetron.[37]

Dopamine Receptor Antagonists

Three classes of dopamine receptor antagonists are effective in the prevention and treatment of nausea and vomiting: phenothiazines, butyrophenones, and benzamides. In the 1960s, the phenothiazines were the first drugs proven to have efficacy in the prevention of CINV. *Prochlorperazine* is the most commonly used in this class and has efficacy in all classes except the most highly emetogenic chemotherapy.[38] Extrapyramidal effects, including dystonia, may be seen. These are treated with diphenhydramine and cessation of the drug. The butyrophenones, including *haloperidol*, are less frequently used for CINV and have adverse effects similar to those of the phenothiazines. They may be effective in the treatment of breakthrough nausea and vomiting.

Of the benzamides, *metoclopramide* is the best studied and most widely used in CINV. It blocks central and peripheral dopamine (D2) receptors at low doses and exhibits weak 5-HT3 inhibition at high doses. In addition, it speeds gastric emptying and increases sphincter tone at the gastroesophageal junction. Prior to the introduction of the 5-HT3 antagonists, a combination of high-dose intravenous metoclopramide and dexamethasone was the most effective antiemetic prophylaxis for highly emetogenic chemotherapy.[39] Because metoclopramide crosses the blood-brain barrier, side effects, including dystonia and tardive dyskinesia, may be seen, particularly at high doses and in aged patients. Diphenhydramine was commonly given as part of the combination regimen to prevent these adverse effects. This regimen has generally been replaced by a combination containing a 5-HT3 receptor antagonist because of its improved efficacy and safety profile.[21-23] The regimen of metoclopramide, dexamethasone, and diphenhydramine may be useful in patients intolerant of 5-HT3 receptor antagonists or those who have failed first-line treatment.

Corticosteroids

Corticosteroids, most commonly *dexamethasone*, are effective in preventing nausea and vomiting when used alone or in combination for all emetogenic classes of chemotherapy. For moderately to highly emetogenic chemotherapy, dexamethasone plus a 5-HT3 receptor antagonist is used. A meta-analysis of 32 randomized clinical trials including 5613 patients from 1984 to 1998 demonstrated the efficacy of dexamethasone in both moderately and highly emetogenic chemotherapy either alone or in combination with other agents.[40] Later studies revealed the superiority of a combination of 5-HT3 receptor antagonist and dexamethasone compared with either agent alone in highly emetogenic chemotherapy.[41] The site of action of corticosteroids along the vomiting reflex pathway is unknown. Side effects include insomnia, increased energy, and mood disturbances.

NK-1 Receptor Antagonists

NK-1 receptors are found in the nucleus tractus solitarius and the area postrema and are activated by substance P.[11] Inhibitors of the NK-1 receptor have demonstrated antiemetic effects and represent a new target for antiemetic therapy. The first approved medication in this class, *aprepitant*, has been shown to prevent both acute and delayed emesis resulting from highly emetogenic chemotherapy.[13,14]

Following promising preliminary data, two randomized phase 3 multicenter trials demonstrated the efficacy of aprepitant for the prevention of both acute and delayed nausea and vomiting. Five hundred twenty-three patients receiving highly emetogenic chemotherapy (cisplatin >70 mg/m^2) received as emetic prophylaxis either aprepitant in combination with 5-HT3 receptor antagonists and dexamethasone (aprepitant 125 mg PO, ondansetron 32 mg IV, and dexamethasone 12 mg PO on day 1, followed by aprepitant 80 mg PO and dexamethasone 8 mg PO on days 2-3 and dexamethasone 8 mg PO on day 4) or a regimen of a 5-HT3 receptor antagonist and dexamethasone alone (ondansetron 32 mg IV plus dexamethasone 20 mg PO on day 1, followed by dexamethasone 8 mg PO twice daily on days 2-4). In the first study, the overall CR (absence of emesis and no need for rescue medication in the first 24 h) was 62.7% in the aprepitant arm versus 43.3% in the standard therapy arm ($p < .001$). CR rates for the aprepitant arm and the standard therapy arm, respectively, for acute (82.8% vs 68.4%, $p < .001$) and delayed (67.7% compared with 46.8%, $p < .001$) symptoms demonstrated the superiority of the aprepitant arm.[13] The second study, which evaluated the same regimens in 521 patients receiving high-dose cisplatin chemotherapy, confirmed these results. Overall CR rates were 72.7% in the aprepitant group versus 52.3% in the standard arm ($p < .001$). CR rates in both acute and delayed emesis were also superior in the aprepitant arm (89.2% vs 78.1%, respectively, $p < .001$, and 75.4% vs 55.8%, respectively, $p < .001$).[14] These data led to the FDA approval of aprepitant in 2003.

Fosaprepitant is a water soluble phosphoryl prodrug for aprepitant. Fosaprepitant at a dose of 115 mg has been approved by the FDA as a parenteral alternative on day 1 of a 3-drug oral aprepitant regimen.[42]

Aprepitant is a substrate for and moderate inducer and moderate inhibitor of the cytochrome P-450 enzyme 3A4 (CYP3A4).[43] Chemotherapy and other drugs are metabolized by this enzyme, and caution must be used when adding aprepitant in these patients. Docetaxel, paclitaxel, etoposide, irinotecan, ifosfamide, imatinib, vinorelbine, vinblastine, and vincristine are metabolized by CYP3A4. Although, in clinical trials, aprepitant was given to patients receiving these agents without any alteration in dose and no observed adverse effect or decreased efficacy, caution is urged. In addition, aprepitant may interact with other, nonchemotherapy agents. It may induce metabolism of warfarin, leading to reduced levels. Aprepitant appears to increase the active levels of oral dexamethasone and methylprednisolone, and reduced dosing of prophylactic dexamethasone is recommended when used in combination with aprepitant. Other drugs with interactions include oral contraceptives, midazolam, ketoconazole, erythromycin, carbamazepine, rifampin, and phenytoin.

Casopitant is a new orally available potent NK-1 receptor antagonist. Two phase 3 studies have demonstrated complete response rates of 86% for those patients receiving a single dose of casoprepitant together with ondasetron and dexamethasone in a highly emetogenic chemotherapy trial, and 73% of the patients given either a single oral or 3-day oral doses of casoprepitant together with ondasetron and dexamethasone in the moderately emetogenic chemotherapy study compared to ondasteron and dexamethasone respectively.[44,45] The agent is currently under FDA review for potential approval in the United States.

Other Classes of Antiemetics

Additional classes of antiemetic agents that may be useful in patients include the benzodiazepines, anticholinergics, and cannabinoids. The most commonly used benzodiazepines, lorazepam and alprazolam, block GABA receptors, particularly in the cerebral cortex, and have their greatest utility in the treatment of anticipatory nausea and reduction in the anxiety associated with chemotherapy.[46]

Anticholinergics such as promethazine or diphenylhydramine and, less frequently, transdermal scopolamine may be used for treatment of breakthrough CINV. There are fewer randomized clinical trial data to recommend the use of cannabinoids such as marijuana or its synthetic versions, nabilone and dronabinol,[47] although there is anecdotal evidence to support their use in patients who do not respond to conventional antiemetics.

Complementary and Alternative Medicine (CAM) Therapies

The past decade has witnessed a great interest in CAM therapies, particularly among cancer patients. Various CAM therapies such as acupuncture, hypnosis, massage, music and herbal supplements such as ginger have been tried to control nausea. Of these, acupuncture and certain mind-body therapies appear promising,[48] but further research is needed before they can be recommended in routine clinical practice.

Acupuncture has been traditionally used in China for symptom management of various conditions, including nausea. A recent meta-analysis involving 11 randomized trials ($N = 1247$), evaluated the effect of acupuncture in controlling CINV among patients received moderate to high emetogenic chemotherapy.[49] The study found that patients receiving acupuncture had lower acute vomiting than control group (22% vs 31%, $p = 0.04$). Nonetheless, there was no benefit for delayed CINV. It should be noted that all these studies were done before aprepitant was approved, and thus utility of acupuncture in the current era is not well established.

Mind-body therapies such as *hypnosis*, *guided imagery*, and *progressive muscle relaxation therapy* (PMRT) have been reported to significantly reduce CINV.[50-53] In a randomized clinical trial in Hong Kong 71 breast cancer patients receiving antiemetic therapy with metoclopramide and dexamethasone were randomized to progressive muscle relaxation training and imagery (1 h before chemotherapy and then daily for 5 days), versus no intervention. Patients in the intervention arm had decreased duration of CINV ($p = 0.05$) and lower frequency of CINV ($p = 0.07$) as compared to controls. However, the study participants did not receive standard prophylaxis with either 5-HT3 inhibitors or NK-1 inhibitors limiting the clinical applicability of the study.

Other relaxation therapies such as *music* and *massage* have also been reported to be successful as adjunct antiemetic therapies, in small clinical trials involving about 30 patients.[54,55] These relaxation therapies affect the cerebral cortex, and thus are particularly helpful for decreasing the perception of nausea and in anticipatory nausea.

On the other hand, two trials evaluating efficacy of *ginger* for treatment of CINV were negative.[56,57] A number of clinical trials assessing various CAM therapies are currently underway and would provide further useful information regarding efficacy of these therapies (or lack thereof), facilitating optimal inclusion of these therapies in traditional clinical oncology practice (integrative oncology).[48]

Recommendations for Prevention and Treatment of Chemotherapy-Induced Emesis

The goal of antiemetic therapy is complete prevention of CINV (Table 123-3). In patients receiving highly and moderately emetogenic chemotherapy, the period of risk for nausea and vomiting lasts at least 4 days following chemotherapy, and protection with antiemetics is needed throughout this period. The choice of antiemetic prophylaxis is driven by the emetogenic potential of the specific chemotherapy agents as outlined below.[18]

Highly Emetogenic Chemotherapy

Cisplatin and cyclophosphamide are the most frequently used highly emetogenic chemotherapy agents. Nausea and vomiting are virtually ensured without adequate prophylaxis. Prior to the approval of the NK-1 receptor antagonist aprepitant, the previous recommendation was a combination of a 5-HT3 antagonist and dexamethasone. A regimen of a 5-HT3 receptor antagonist, aprepitant (125 mg PO) or fasaprepitant 115 mg IV, and dexamethasone (12 mg PO or IV) on day 1 followed by aprepitant (80 mg PO) and dexamethasone (8 mg PO or IV) on days 2-4 is recommended in all patients receiving highly emetogenic chemotherapy. All prophylaxis should begin prior to the administration of chemotherapy.

Moderately Emetogenic Chemotherapy

A combination of a 5-HT3 receptor antagonist and dexamethasone is rec-

Table 123-3 Guidelines for Prevention of Acute and Delayed Nausea and Vomiting in Patients Depending on Emetic Risk

Emetic Risk	Acute	Delayed
High (>90%)	Aprepitant + 5-HT3 antagonist + dexamethasone	Aprepitant + dexamethasone
Moderate (30-90%)	5-HT3 antagonist + dexamethasone	Dexamethasone
Low (10-30%)	Dexamethasone or phenothiazine or metoclopramide	None
Minimal (<10%)	None	None

Abbreviations: 5-HT3, 5-hydroxytryptamine 3.

ommended in all patients receiving moderately-emetogenic chemotherapy. Given recent data and its superior efficacy in preventing delayed symptoms, palonosetron (0.25 mg on day 1 only) is the preferred 5-HT3 receptor antagonist. If others are used, they should be given on day 1 prior to chemotherapy and then repeated daily on days 2-4. Dexamethasone is given as 12 mg IV or PO on day 1 and then at a daily dose of 8 mg on days 2-4 (either 8 mg daily or 4 mg in divided doses twice daily). In selected patients (those with breakthrough nausea and vomiting despite adequate prophylaxis or those with other patient variables that suggest a higher risk of symptoms), aprepitant (125 mg PO or fasaprepitant 115 mg IV on day 1 followed by 80 mg PO on days 2-3) should be considered.

Low-Risk Chemotherapy

Options for antiemetic prophylaxis in patients receiving chemotherapy of low emetogenic potential include dexamethasone (12 mg PO or IV) or prochlorperazine (10 mg PO or IV every 4-6 h) or metoclopramide (20-40 mg PO every 4-6 h or 1-2 mg/kg IV every 3-4 h with diphenhydramine to prevent extrapyramidal symptoms). All prophylaxis should be given prior to the administration of chemotherapy.

Minimally Emetogenic Chemotherapy

No routine prophylaxis is recommended. If nausea and vomiting do occur, the use of dexamethasone, prochlorperazine, or metoclopramide is recommended. Prophylactic use of these medications should be considered prior to the next cycle of therapy.

Special Situations

Breakthrough Nausea and Vomiting

Ideally, the best treatment for breakthrough nausea and vomiting is to prevent it from occurring at all. At times, despite aggressive prophylaxis, symptoms still occur. The best therapy for breakthrough symptoms is the addition of agents from another class of antiemetics. In addition, an alternative route other than oral, such as intravenous or rectal, may need to be used. These medications work best if taken on a schedule rather than on an as-needed basis. When breakthrough nausea and vomiting occur, the prophylactic regimen should be reevaluated and enhanced prior to the next cycle of therapy.

Anticipatory Nausea and Vomiting

The key to preventing anticipatory nausea and vomiting is preventing symptoms from occurring with each cycle of chemotherapy. Once the symptoms have developed, agents such as the benzodiazepines may be added to the prophylactic regimen.[46] As outlined above, mind-body therapies such as behavioral therapy, systemic desensitization, and hypnosis have also been proven useful.[50-54]

Radiation-Induced Nausea and Vomiting

Radiation-induced nausea and vomiting (RINV) is seen in nearly all patients receiving total body irradiation prior to bone marrow transplantation and in more than 80% of those receiving radiation to the upper abdomen.[58] Studies have demonstrated the efficacy of prophylactic 5-HT3 receptor antagonists compared with placebo[59] and the superiority of prophylaxis with 5-HT3 receptor antagonists compared with combinations with metoclopramide and prochlorperazine.[60,61] The recommendation is for all patients undergoing either upper abdominal radiation therapy or total body irradiation to receive prophylaxis with an oral 5-HT3 receptor antagonist dosed either 2 or 3 times daily with or without oral dexamethasone.[62]

Conclusions

Dramatic progress has been made in the prevention and treatment of chemotherapy-induced emesis, especially since the introduction of the 5-HT3 receptor antagonists in the early 1990s and the 2003 introduction of the NK-1 receptor antagonist, aprepitant. Recent surveys indicate the need for heightened awareness of the frequency and severity of acute and, especially, delayed nausea and vomiting from chemotherapy. Fortunately, new agents have been added to the antiemetic arsenal to further enhance the efficacy of antiemetic prophylaxis. Complementary therapies such as acupuncture, and mind-body interventions appear promising in controlling nausea, and are being explored further. Appropriate implementation of guidelines for prophylaxis based on the specific chemotherapy agents used will ensure that fewer patients experience these most distressing of side effects.[63]

Selected References

The complete reference list can be found at www.CANCERMEDICINE8.com

1. Grunberg SM, Deuson RR, Mavros P, et al. Incidence of chemotherapy-induced nausea and emesis after modern antiemetics. *Cancer.* 2004;100:2261–2268.
2. Mitchell EP. Gastrointestinal toxicity of chemotherapeutic agents. *Semin Oncol.* 1992;19:566–579.
6. de Boer-Dennert M, de Wit R, Schmitz PI, et al. Patient perceptions of the side-effects of chemotherapy: the influence of 5HT3 antagonists. *Br J Cancer.* 1997;76:1055–1061.
9. Carpenter DO. Neural mechanisms of emesis. *Can J Physiol Pharmacol.* 1990;68:230–236.
14. Hesketh PJ, Grunberg SM, Gralla RJ, et al. The oral neurokinin-1 antagonist aprepitant for the prevention of chemotherapy-induced nausea and vomiting: a multinational, randomized, double-blind, placebo-controlled trial in patients receiving high-dose cisplatin—the Aprepitant Protocol 052 Study Group. *J Clin Oncol.* 2003;21:4112–4119.
15. Moher D, Arthur AZ, Pater JL. Anticipatory nausea and/or vomiting. *Cancer Treat Rev.* 1984;11:257–264.
17. Hesketh PJ, Kris MG, Grunberg SM, et al. Proposal for classifying the acute emetogenicity of cancer chemotherapy. *J Clin Oncol.* 1997;15:103–109.
18. Koeller JM, Aapro MS, Gralla RJ, et al. A. Antiemetic guidelines: creating a more practical treatment approach. *Support Care Cancer.* 2002;10:519–522.
19. Mitchelson F. Pharmacological agents affecting emesis. A review (part I). *Drugs.* 1992;43:295–315.
20. Bountra C, Gale JD, Gardner CJ, et al. Towards understanding the aetiology and pathophysiology of the emetic reflex: novel approaches to antiemetic drugs. *Oncology.* 1996;53(Suppl 1):102–109.
21. Chevallier B, Cappelaere P, Splinter T, et al. A double-blind, multicentre comparison of intravenous dolasetron mesilate and metoclopramide in the prevention of nausea and vomiting in cancer patients receiving high-dose cisplatin chemotherapy. *Support Care Cancer.* 1997;5:22–30.
22. Warr D, Wilan A, Venner P, et al. A randomised, doubleblind comparison of granisetron with high-dose metoclopramide, dexamethasone and diphenhydramine for cisplatin-induced emesis. An NCI Canada Clinical Trials Group phase III trial. *Eur J Cancer.* 1992;29A:33–36.
23. Heron JF, Goedhals L, Jordaan JP, et al. Oral granisetron alone and in combination with dexamethasone: a doubleblind randomized comparison against high-dose metoclopramide plus dexamethasone in prevention of cisplatin-induced emesis. The Granisetron Study Group. *Ann Oncol.* 1994;5:579–584.
26. Martoni A, Angelelli B, Guaraldi M, et al. An open randomised cross-over study on granisetron versus ondansetron in the prevention of acute emesis induced by moderate dose cisplatin-containing regimens. *Eur J Cancer.* 1996;32A:82–85.
27. Hesketh P, Navari R, Grote T, et al. Double-blind, randomized comparison of the antiemetic efficacy of intravenous dolasetron mesylate and intravenous ondansetron in the prevention of acute cisplatin-induced emesis in patients with cancer. Dolasetron Comparative Chemotherapy Induced Emesis Prevention Group. *J Clin Oncol.* 1996;14:2242–2249.
28. Audhuy B, Cappelaere P, Martin M, et al. A double-blind, randomised comparison of the antiemeticefficacy of two intravenous doses of dolasetron mesilate and granisetron in patients receiving high dose cisplatin chemotherapy. *Eur J Cancer.* 1996;32A:807–813.

124 Neurologic Complications

Lisa M. DeAngelis, MD

Disorders of the central or peripheral nervous system affect approximately 15% of patients with cancer.[1] The disorders usually appear in patients with advanced metastatic disease, often as only one of several organ systems involved by the cancer. However, sometimes the neurologic disorder is the first symptom of cancer; eg, approximately 10% of patients with lung cancer present with symptoms of brain metastasis. Regardless of whether neurologic complications occur early or late in the course of the patient's cancer, they uniquely threaten the patient's quality of life by causing such distressing symptoms as dementia, paralysis, incontinence, and pain; in addition, neurologic dysfunction itself often shortens survival.

Neurologic complications of cancer are increasing in frequency. In part, this represents increased opportunity for metastases to the nervous system to develop because systemic tumors are better controlled for longer periods.[2,3] Part of the increase also results from more vigorous treatment of the primary tumor with modalities that cause toxicity to the nervous system. Because these toxic effects are often delayed (eg, radiation-induced dementia), the longer the patient lives, the more likely the toxicity is to appear.

Early diagnosis and appropriate treatment of the neurologic symptoms significantly lessen the impact of neurologic complications on many patients. Thus, it is important for the physician to recognize these complications early. This requires knowledge of those disorders associated with cancer that are likely to affect the nervous system, and also the symptoms and signs that distinguish one neurologic disorder from another. This chapter systematically approaches the diagnosis and treatment of nervous system complications of systemic cancer.

Neurologic complications of cancer can be either metastatic or nonmetastatic (Table 124-1). Metastatic lesions affect the nervous system by direct invasion (eg, brachial plexus metastasis), by compression (eg, epidural spinal cord compression), or by compromise of vascular supply (eg, sagittal sinus occlusion from skull metastases). Brain metastases are discussed in Chapter 71. Although any tumor can metastasize to the nervous system, certain tumors have a predilection for causing particular central or peripheral nervous system disorders, (eg, leukemias and lymphomas frequently metastasize to the leptomeninges, but rarely to the brain). Tumors arising in the pelvis are less likely to metastasize to the brain than lung cancer, but when they do, they have a predilection for involving the cerebellum rather than the cerebral hemispheres.[4] Prostate cancer commonly causes epidural spinal cord and cauda equina compression because of its tendency to metastasize to the vertebral bodies, but leptomeningeal or brain involvement is much less common.[5,6]

Table 124-1 ■ Neurologic Complications of Cancer

Metastatic
Intracranial (usually to brain)
Spinal (usually epidural)
Leptomeningeal (usually base of brain and cauda equina)
Cranial nerves (usually from base of skull lesions)
Peripheral nerves (usually brachial or lumbosacral plexus)
Muscle (rare)
Nonmetastatic
Complications of treatment (radiation, chemotherapy)
Vascular disorders (hemorrhage, infarcts)
Metabolic, nutritional disorders
Paraneoplastic syndromes
Infections

Nonmetastatic neurologic complications are often tumor specific. Metabolic derangements are more likely to occur with tumors that metastasize widely to vital organs, such as liver (colon cancer), or that cause changes in fluid and electrolyte balance, such as hypercalcemia (breast cancer) or inappropriate antidiuretic hormone secretion (small-cell lung cancer). Central nervous system (CNS) infections are more common in patients whose cancer is associated with immune suppression, as in Hodgkin disease. Vascular complications are more common in hematologic malignancies than in solid tumors.[7] Paraneoplastic syndromes affecting the nervous system are much more frequent with certain tumors, such as small-cell lung cancer and ovarian cancer, than with the more common adenocarcinomas of lung, colon, and breast.[8]

The physician encountering a cancer patient with neurologic symptoms may begin by considering the disorders listed in Table 124-1. From a more practical point of view, it is often easier to identify the site of neurologic dysfunction by its signs and symptoms and to consider first only those neurologic complications likely to affect that particular site. This approach to diagnosis is listed in Table 124-2.

Metastases

Spinal Metastases

Metastatic lesions compressing the spinal cord or cauda equina are, after brain metastases, the most common symptomatic neurologic complication of metastatic cancer.[1,9,10]

The spinal cord ends at the L-1 or L-2 vertebral body but compression of the cauda equina below that level is usually also considered spinal cord compression (SCC) because the diagnosis and treatment are identical.[1] SCC causes pain and, if untreated, paralysis and incontinence. Patients who become paraplegic as a result of cancer usually die within a matter of months. On the other hand, clinical studies indicate that early diagnosis (while the patient is still ambulatory) and prompt treatment maintain a patient's independent ambulation, and usually result in longer survival.[1,11,12]

Approximately 5% of patients dying of cancer have evidence of SCC at autopsy, suggesting 18,000-20,000 new cases of SCC annually in the United States.[1,13] Approximately 10% of new patients referred to a large cancer center have metastases to the spinal column. Breast, lung, prostate, and lymphoma are the most common primary cancers causing SCC (Table 124-3). SCC usually occurs in the late stages of metastatic cancer, but in up to 20% of patients being treated for neoplastic SCC, cancer was unsuspected prior to the neurologic symptoms.

Vertebral metastases are common in patients with metastatic cancer, but skeletal complications, including SCC, have been reduced by the use of bisphosphonates.[14] The cancer usually spreads hematogenously to the vertebral column, via either the arterial system or Batson venous plexus.[15] SCC then results when the vertebral body metastasis extends into the spinal canal or paraspinal tumor invades the epidural space through a neural foramen (Fig. 124-1). Lymphomas and neuroblastomas often invade the spinal canal through neural foramina without destruction of bone. Epidural lesions may also result when tumors in the

Table 124-2 Neurologic Complications in Cancer Patients by Site

Site	Usual Causes	Typical Symptoms and Signs
Brain	Metastasis Leptomeningeal metastasis Metabolic/toxic encephalopathy Infection (meningitis, brain abscess) Radiation encephalopathy Cerebral hemorrhage or infarction Paraneoplastic (limbic encephalopathy)	Headache Confusion Hemiparesis Seizures Ataxia
Spinal cord and cauda equina	Epidural metastasis Leptomeningeal metastasis Intramedullary metastasis Epidural abscess or hematoma Radiation myelopathy Myelopathy following intrathecal chemotherapy Paraneoplastic myelopathy	Back pain Paraparesis Sensory level Incontinence
Cranial and peripheral nerves	Extrinsic compression by tumor or other mass (eg, hematoma) Direct infiltration by tumor Drug toxicity Varicella-zoster infection Radiation plexopathy Paraneoplastic neuropathy	Focal pain Sensory loss Motor weakness Decreased reflexes in nerve distribution (focal lesion) or distally in hands and feet (polyneuropathy)
Neuromuscular junction	Drugs (aminoglycoside antibiotics) Paraneoplastic disorders (Lambert-Eaton myasthenic syndrome, myasthenia gravis)	Diffuse weakness without sensory loss Respiratory insufficiency
Muscle	Metastasis Steroid myopathy Cachectic myopathy Paraneoplastic polymyositis or dermatomyositis	Proximal weakness Weakness without sensory loss

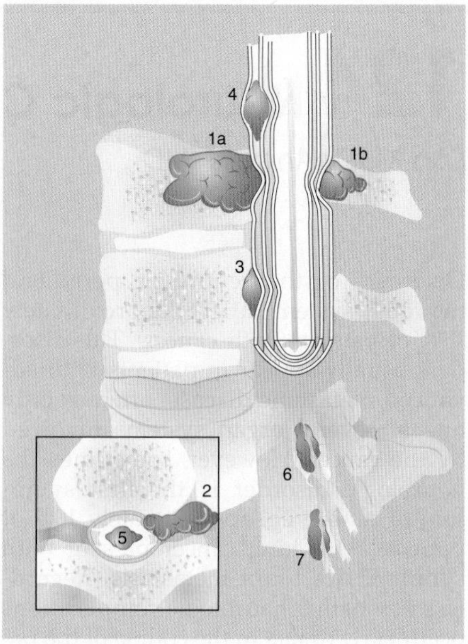

Figure 124-1 Neoplastic epidural spinal cord compression results from direct extension of a bony metastasis to the vertebral body (1a) or posterior elements (1b), by paraspinal neoplasm infiltrating through neural foramina (2), or a direct metastasis to the epidural space (3). Unusual causes of spinal metastases include subdural metastasis (4), intramedullary metastasis (5), and paraspinal metastasis to the radicular vessels (6) or root (7).

Table 124-3 **Primary Cancer Causing Symptomatic Spinal Cord Compression in 583 Patients at Memorial Sloan-Kettering Cancer Center (MSKCC)**

Primary Tumor	No. of Patients
Breast	127
Lung	90
Prostate	58
Lymphoreticular	56
Sarcoma	52
Kidney	39
Gastrointestinal	29
Melanoma	23
Unknown primary	21
Head and neck	19
Miscellaneous	69
Total	583

colon, kidney, prostate, or head and neck area grow directly into vertebral structures. Less-common causes of spinal cord dysfunction result from metastases to a vertebral pedicle, lamina, or arch, or hematogenous metastasis to the epidural space, or to the spinal cord itself. When a metastasis causes the vertebral body to collapse, bone, tumor, and ligament may extend into the spinal canal to compress the spinal cord.

The thoracic spine is the most common location of SCC, followed by the lumbosacral and cervical spine in a ratio of about 4:2:1. Colon cancer preferentially involves the lumbosacral spine. Two or more contiguous vertebral bodies are involved by metastatic disease in approximately 25% of patients with SCC, but, unlike infection, the intervertebral disc space is preserved. As many as 32% of patients have other sites of SCC in addition to the clinically suspected location,[16] emphasizing the importance of imaging the entire length of the spinal canal when evaluating a patient for suspected epidural disease. Multiple sites of vertebral metastases predict a poor prognosis.

Pathophysiology of Spinal Cord Compression The mechanism(s) by which neurologic symptoms and signs are caused by SCC are not fully understood. The symptoms and signs depend on the level of compression (eg, cervical vs thoracic), but not on the site of compression in the transverse plane (eg, anterior, posterior or lateral).[1] In almost one-half of patients, epidural tumor is found both anterior and posterior to the spinal cord; in approximately one-fifth of patients, the tumor is circumferential.[17] Histologic studies show changes limited mainly to the lateral and posterior columns, while the central gray matter shows few abnormalities. The common abnormality is demyelination with infiltration by lipid-laden macrophages, interstitial edema, and focal axonal swelling, but infarction is rare, even in patients who develop the sudden onset of paraplegia. Compression of the epidural venous plexus (possibly contributing to spinal cord edema) occurs early in SCC, whereas obliteration of cord parenchymal vessels with decreased spinal cord blood flow takes place much later. These data suggest that cord ischemia is not a critical factor, at least in the early phases of SCC. Animal models of SCC demonstrate a disrupted blood–spinal cord barrier with vasogenic cord edema that decreases after corticosteroid administration. It is likely that mechanical pressure on the cord and its venous drainage in some manner produces a conduction block, with demyelination and spinal cord edema, resulting in symptomatic spinal cord dysfunction. Increasing evidence also suggests that release of potentially neurotoxic substances, including prostaglandins and serotonin, by compressed neural tissue may play a role in the development of neurologic disability.

Clinical Findings and Diagnosis Back pain is the first symptom of SCC in virtually all patients (Table 124-4).[1,13] The pain may be local (at the involved area of the spine), radicular (radiating into arm, trunk, or leg), or both. The local pain is dull and aching; it is progressive and usually localizes within one or two segments of the involved area of the spine. Local pain caused by movement implies spinal instability. Radicular pain may be constant or brought on by movement. In the

Table 124-4 Symptoms and Signs of Spinal Cord Compression in 213 Patients at Memorial Sloan-Kettering Cancer Center (MSKCC)

	First Symptom		Present at Diagnosis	
	No.	%	No.	%
Pain	201	94	207	97
Weakness	7	3	157	74
Autonomic dysfunction	0	0	111	52
Sensory loss	1	0.5	112	53
Ataxia	2	0.9	8	4

cervical and lumbosacral regions, radicular pain is often unilateral, but in the trunk, it is bilateral (band-like), a finding that is highly suggestive of epidural disease. Pain from SCC is typically worse when the patient is supine, so the patient may sleep sitting up. This feature may help to distinguish epidural tumor from a herniated disc where the pain improves when the patient is supine. The pain of SCC is exacerbated by coughing, straining, or flexion of the neck. During the examination, an attempt should be made to reproduce the patient's pain by spine percussion, gentle neck flexion, and straight leg raising. Pain may be absent in those patients whose SCC is identified incidentally on chest or abdominal computed tomography (CT) or magnetic resonance imaging (MRI) scans done to evaluate the patient's primary cancer.

Weakness is the second most common initial feature of epidural SCC; it usually follows the onset of pain by weeks to months. The weakness is most obvious in proximal muscles of the legs so that the patient may complain of difficulty when arising from a low chair or the toilet seat or when climbing stairs. By the time weakness occurs, tone in the lower extremities is usually increased, deep tendon reflexes are hyperactive, and the plantar responses are extensor. If the SCC occurs below the cord involving the cauda equina, hyporeflexia or areflexia is found. Proximal weakness might at first suggest a myopathy, but in that disorder, the proximal upper extremities are usually also weak, the tendon reflexes and muscle tone are normal, and sensory changes are absent. If the patient can easily walk on their heels, toes, and do a deep knee bend, it is unlikely the patient has significant weakness. If pain limits strength testing, analgesics should be administered to permit adequate evaluation.

Bowel and bladder dysfunction usually occur late in SCC. However, when the conus medullaris is the site of compression (vertebral lesions from T-10 to L-1), bladder dysfunction may be the first and only sign. Both the patient and the physician may fail to recognize that frequent small voidings may be a sign of urinary retention. The patient may be unaware of urinary retention because bladder sensation is lost. Palpation of the abdomen often reveals a distended bladder, and a postvoid ultrasound reveals urinary retention. The anal sphincter is usually flaccid, with loss of both voluntary and reflex constriction (anal wink).

Sensory symptoms include numbness and paresthesias that usually begin in the toes and spread proximally. Except in conus compression, the sacral segments may be spared, even when a sensory level to pinprick is found on the trunk. In a few patients, gait or truncal ataxia mimicking cerebellar disease may be the only neurologic finding although back pain usually precedes the ataxia. Varicella-zoster eruption may occur at the dermatomal level of epidural metastasis. If it precedes the diagnosis of the spinal metastasis, it can delay recognition of SCC.

None of the clinical signs or symptoms of epidural SCC are specific. Table 124-5 lists some of the disorders that can mimic SCC in patients with cancer. Some, such as lumbar strain, herniated disc, or spinal stenosis, are common in patients without cancer and may confuse the initial evaluation of an individual cancer patient. Others, such as epidural hematomas and abscesses, may be directly related to the cancer or its treatment. Metastases generally do not involve the intervertebral disc, and abnormalities at the disc space should raise the question of vertebral osteomyelitis or herniated disc. In most instances, evaluation with magnetic resonance imaging MRI is necessary and sufficient to establish the diagnosis.

Patients with cancer who develop back pain have SCC until proved otherwise. Evaluation should proceed urgently because patients with high-grade compression may develop abrupt compromise of the spinal cord and severe neurologic dysfunction. Risk factors for high-grade compression include: (1) myelopathy on examination, or (2) the presence of local and radicular pain (one-half of these patients have epidural disease).

The most sensitive and specific and usually the only necessary diagnostic test for spinal lesions caused by cancer is an MRI (Fig. 124-2).[18-20] The entire spine should be imaged, but contrast is not necessary to detect spine metastasis or epidural tumor. However, contrast is essential to identify intramedullary spinal metastasis or leptomeningeal tumor. Patients unable to have an MRI (eg, pacemaker) should be imaged by CT-myelography where full reconstructed images can provide excellent views of the spine in all dimensions. MR scans also distinguish malignant lesions from benign ones, such as disc herniation.

Treatment ■ Spinal epidural disease requires urgent therapy directed at reduction of tumor mass and prevention of regrowth.[1,21] Radiation therapy (RT) is the primary treatment for most patients, but surgery and chemotherapy are important modalities in individual patients

Table 124-5 Differential Diagnosis of Epidural Spinal Cord Compression

Diagnosis	Example(s)	Diagnostic Test
Intramedullary tumor	Glioma Metastasis	MRI with gadolinium
Extramedullary-intradural tumor	Meningioma Neurofibroma Drop metastasis from primary brain tumor Metastasis from systemic primary	MRI with gadolinium
Leptomeningeal tumor	Primary lymphoma Metastasis	MRI with gadolinium, CSF cytology
Radiation myelopathy	Previous RT to spine	MRI with gadolinium
Arteriovenous malformation		MRI with gadolinium, myelogram, arteriogram
Transverse myelopathy	Postinfectious myelopathy, multiple sclerosis	MRI with gadolinium
Epidural hematoma	Thrombocytopenia (history of lumbar puncture)	MRI or CT
Epidural abscess	Sepsis, epidural catheter (for pain control)	MRI with gadolinium/culture
Degenerative spinal disorder	Herniated disc, spinal stenosis	MRI
Osteoporosis	Vertebral collapse	MRI/biopsy

Abbreviations: CSF, cerebrospinal fluid; CT, computed tomography; MRI, magnetic resonance imaging; RT, radiation therapy.
Source: Adapted from Ref. 1.

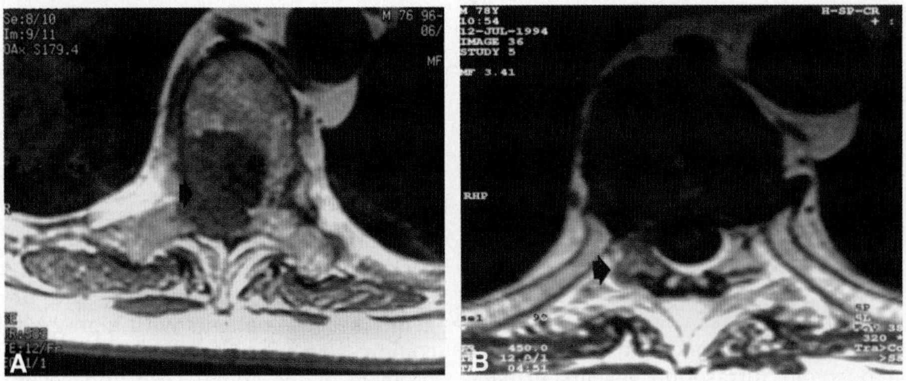

Figure 124-2 ■ MRI demonstrating spinal cord compression from metastatic breast cancer. (**A**) Tumor in the vertebral body compressing the spinal cord arteriorly. (**B**) Axial image at the same level demonstrating anterior and lateral compression and distortion of the cord.

(see below). Re-evaluation during and following treatment is essential. Delay in diagnosis compromises therapy. Many patients present on Fridays suggesting that referral is often delayed.[22]

The initial treatment for all patients is corticosteroids. Corticosteroids have two effects: their oncolytic effect may relieve cord compression by shrinking tumors, especially lymphoma, but in most instances, their salutary effects probably result from their reduction of spinal cord edema. In experimental models, corticosteroids decreased cord edema and improved neurologic function, and higher doses have been found to be more effective than lower doses,[23,24] although not all clinicians agree.[25] In humans, because other treatment is usually started concurrently, the effect of corticosteroids is difficult to evaluate. In one study, 40 mg of dexamethasone per day, followed by RT, resulted in "improvement" in neurologic function within 24 hours in 18 of 29 patients; 5 of the responders had lymphoma. Such improvement occurring within the first 24 hours is unlikely to represent an effect of RT, except possibly in patients with lymphoma.

For patients without neurologic symptoms except pain, one can begin with the standard dose of dexamethasone (16 mg every 24 h), increasing the dose if pain persists or new symptoms develop. For patients with severe pain, or evidence of myelopathy, an intravenous bolus of 100 mg of dexamethasone should be administered, followed by 100 mg every 24 hours in divided doses. The drug should be tapered as the patient is treated with more definitive modalities (see below). Intravenous dexamethasone is infused slowly over a period of 5-10 min; some patients complain of severe genital burning as the drug is infused, but this lasts only a few minutes and is easily tolerated, particularly if the patient is forewarned.

Corticosteroids cause side effects, and some may be more prominent in patients with epidural SCC. Perforation of the gastrointestinal (GI) tract may occur in as many as 1% of patients; constipation, a frequent complication of SCC, appears to increase the risk of GI rupture. Postoperative infections may be more frequent in patients treated with corticosteroids.

RT is the most common treatment for patients with SCC, many of whom are poor surgical candidates because of advanced cancer or multiple vertebral body metastases.[1,10,13] RT is administered to a port that includes the site of compression and one or two vertebral bodies above and below that level. The width of the port depends on the amount of paraspinal disease. Variations in fractionation schedule do not influence outcome, and the standard schedule is 300 cGy for 10 fractions to a total of 3000 cGy. A second course of RT for patients who respond initially but then relapse may be helpful and carries only modest risk.[26] Recent experience suggests that intensity-modulated stereotactic radiotherapy (IMRT) is effective and safe and can be administered with good results to a previously irradiated site or in place of standard external beam RT.[27]

Traditionally, surgery[28] was restricted to; (1) patients who develop SCC at sites already irradiated, (2) patients with SCC in whom a diagnosis of cancer has not been established, (3) when epidural defects result from displaced bone or disc fragments, (4) when spinal instability results from vertebral destruction, and (5) patients with radio-resistant tumors (eg, renal cancer). However, results from a prospective phase III trial have demonstrated the superiority of surgery for SCC.[29] Patients with SCC were randomized to receive focal RT alone or surgery followed by RT. The surgical procedure was left to the discretion of the surgeon, but the goal was to do a complete resection of the local disease; this usually required an anterior approach with resection of the vertebral body. The patients who had surgery had a superior outcome with significantly better neurologic function for longer, including a greater proportion of patients who regained ambulation and continence. Length of survival was not significantly different between the two groups, but there was a trend towards longer survival with surgery (129 days vs 100 days, $p = .08$). These data suggest that surgery should be a consideration in all patients with SCC. However, the patients enrolled in the study were highly selected and it is not clear that the excellent outcome reported here can be expected for all patients with SCC.

The surgical approach depends in part on the location of the tumor, type of reconstruction necessary and general condition of the patient. In addition, vertebroplasty and kyphoplasty may be effective for treating pain, and are emerging options in the treatment of selected patients with SCC.[30,31]

Regardless of treatment type, the majority of patients who are ambulatory at the beginning of therapy remain ambulatory. Some paraparetic patients will recover sufficient function to walk again, but only a few patients who are paraplegic recover useful function.

Chemotherapy, with or without radiation therapy, is useful in some patients with tumors that are sensitive, especially lymphoma and occasionally other solid tumors.[32-34] Excellent responses of SCC from chemosensitive tumors to appropriate chemotherapy are seen, but this approach is limited to those patients who have pain as the only symptom. If myelopathy is present, corticosteroids and RT or surgery must be the primary therapy.

Leptomeningeal Metastasis

Leptomeningeal metastasis (LM), also called carcinomatous or neoplastic meningitis, is less frequent than brain metastasis or SCC, but is becoming increasingly common, particularly in patients with small-cell lung, breast, and ovarian cancers.[35] Quality of life and duration of survival are both severely compromised by LM, and fewer than one-half of those treated by currently available therapy receive benefit.

Reliable estimates of the incidence of LM are difficult to obtain. Few studies of LM give incidence figures and the diagnosis is heavily dependent on the diligence with which it is pursued. Autopsies may double the number of clinically diagnosed cases of LM, but a routine autopsy may miss focal LM. Recognizing these limitations, Table 124-6 lists the reported frequency of LM in patients with various cancers. Overall, LM is probably found in approximately 5% of patients with metastatic cancer.

Pathophysiology ■ Malignant cells may enter the subarachnoid space by several routes (Fig. 124-3). Direct infiltration of the subarachnoid space from dural and bone-based lesions has been well documented. In an autopsy study of children with acute lymphocytic leukemia (ALL), early findings of subarachnoid invasion included infiltration of the wall of veins and of the marrow trabeculae[1]; infiltration via the bridging veins from the marrow of the skull also occurs. Studies with B16 melanoma clones that metastasize to the meninges of mice show that malignant cells attach to the walls of leptomeningeal capillaries and then move directly into the subarachnoid space. Brain parenchymal lesions can erode into the ventricle or into the subarachnoid space or be spilled at surgery, causing LM.[36] LM develops in 40% of patients following resection of a cerebellar metastasis, but in only 2-3% of those who had resection of a supratentorial lesion presumably due to the large cerebrospinal fluid (CSF)-containing spaces in the posterior fossa. The choroid plexus is a route of entry in a few cases. Malignant cells may invade the subarachnoid space by direct infiltration along nerve roots, and possibly via epineural lymphatics.

Leptomeningeal metastasis is probably not a random metastatic event. Infiltrating lobular breast cancer often causes LM, whereas infiltrating ductal carcinoma metastasizes to the brain more commonly. Specific chromosomal abnormalities and eosinophilia in acute myelogenous leukemia (AML) appear to correlate with meningeal chloromas. Experimental B16 melanoma clones derived by serial re-inoculation of meningeal deposits eventually produce predominantly LM.

At autopsy, the leptomeninges may be opacified by tumor, and the sulci may be obliterated. The inferior surface of the brain and the dorsal surface of the spinal cord and the cauda equina are commonly involved areas. Nodular deposits may be visible on nerve roots, especially in the cauda equina. Frequently, however, there is no grossly visible evidence of LM. Communicating hydrocephalus is present in some patients. Microscopically, tumor growth may be focal in any location of the subarachnoid space, or may infiltrate the leptomeninges diffusely. Blood vessels are often ensheathed by tumor, and superficial nodular deposits often form in the parenchyma of the brain and spinal cord via perivascular (Virchow–Robin) spaces. Ischemic changes may be seen superficially in the brain and cerebral infarction has been reported. Nerve roots may be either encased in tumor or directly infiltrated. Fibrosis of the arachnoid membranes is common. Inflammation may be florid but is often sparse or absent.

Leptomeningeal metastasis causes nervous system dysfunction by several

Table 124-6 **Frequency of Leptomeningeal Metastases (LM) in Various Cancers**

Cancer	Percent Developing LM	Features
Carcinoma		
Breast	5	Incidence may be increasing, more common with infiltrating lobular carcinoma
SCLC	9–25	Incidence is increasing, risk increases with duration of survival
NSCLC	?	Less common than breast, probably more common overall than SCLC LM
Melanoma	23	50% at autopsy
Leukemia		
AML	<5	10% without prophylaxis, associated with high white blood count, elevated LDH, extramedullary disease at diagnosis, and with monocytic morphology
ALL	11	30% without prophylaxis, associated with T-cell phenotype, Burkitt's morphology and high white blood cell count at diagnosis
CLL	Rare	May occur during blast crisis
Lymphoma		
NHL	4–10	Associated with diffuse large B-cell and lymphocytic histology, bone marrow involvement
HD	Rare	
Overall	8.6	LM present at autopsy in 56 of 649 brains examined at Memorial Sloan-Kettering Cancer Center

Abbreviations: ALL, acute lymphocytic leukemia; AML, acute myelogenous leukemia; CLL, chronic lymphocytic leukemia; HD, Hodgkin disease; LDH, lactic acid dehydrogenase; NHL, non-Hodgkin lymphoma; NSCLC, non-small-cell lung cancer; SCLC, small-cell lung cancer.

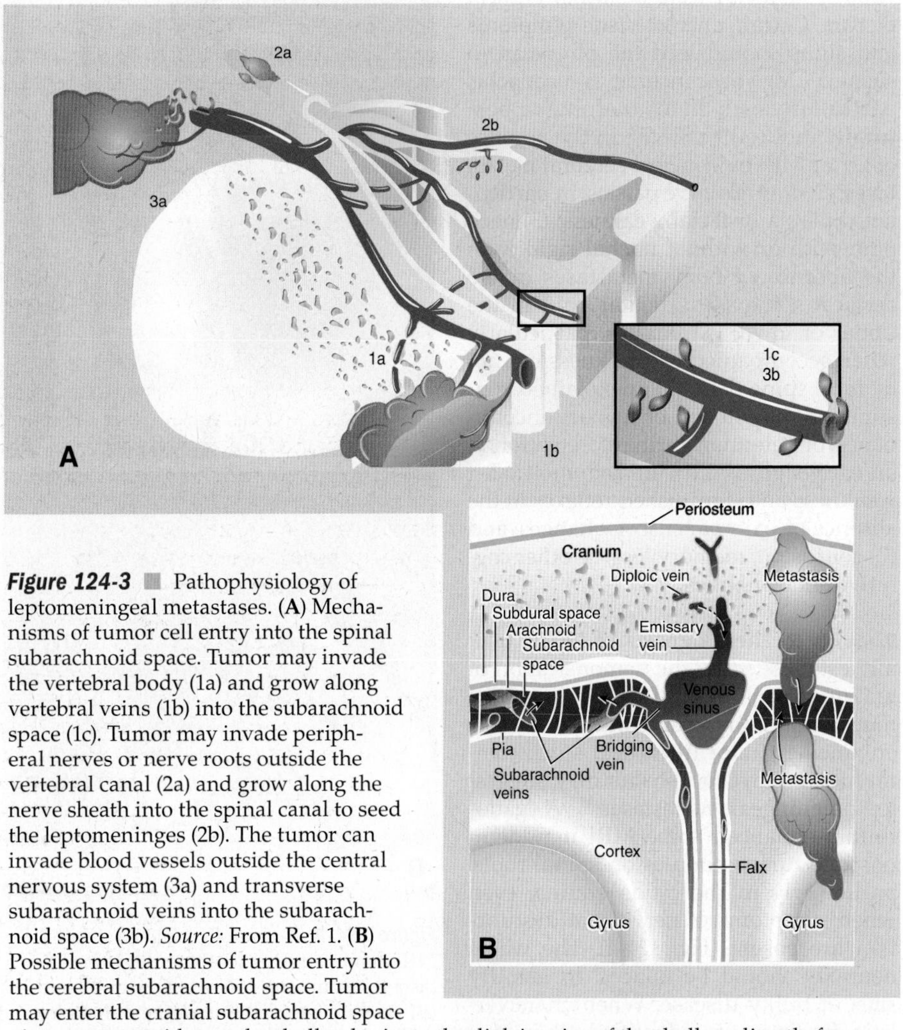

Figure 124-3 Pathophysiology of leptomeningeal metastases. (**A**) Mechanisms of tumor cell entry into the spinal subarachnoid space. Tumor may invade the vertebral body (1a) and grow along vertebral veins (1b) into the subarachnoid space (1c). Tumor may invade peripheral nerves or nerve roots outside the vertebral canal (2a) and grow along the nerve sheath into the spinal canal to seed the leptomeninges (2b). The tumor can invade blood vessels outside the central nervous system (3a) and transverse subarachnoid veins into the subarachnoid space (3b). *Source:* From Ref. 1. (**B**) Possible mechanisms of tumor entry into the cerebral subarachnoid space. Tumor may enter the cranial subarachnoid space via metastases either to the skull or brain, to the diploic veins of the skull, or directly from subarachnoid veins. The choroid plexus (not shown) is also an occasional site for the formation of leptomeningeal tumor.

mechanisms.[1] (1) There is often direct infiltration of malignant cells into the brain, spinal cord, or cranial nerves and spinal roots as they traverse the subarachnoid space. Such infiltration interferes with neural function. (2) Infiltration of the subarachnoid space by tumor interrupts CSF absorption and leads to hydrocephalus with its attendant symptoms of cognitive dysfunction, gait abnormalities, and incontinence. (3) Infiltration of tumor along the Virchow–Robin spaces may reduce blood supply to the brain, and cerebral infarction has been reported.[37]

Symptoms and Signs ■ Two clinical findings suggest LM. The first is synchronous symptoms or signs at multiple sites of the neuraxis.[1,35] This clinical pattern is a result of the multifocal or disseminated nature of the disease. The second is the presence of findings on neurologic examination without symptoms. An example is finding leg weakness or an absent ankle reflex in a patient complaining of diplopia or headache. Multifocal findings are not pathognomonic of LM, however, because multiple parenchymal metastases involving the central or peripheral nervous system can yield a similar clinical picture. Certain characteristic symptoms and signs should lead the physician to suspect LM. These include: (1) headache, particularly early in the morning or posturally induced headache in the absence of CT or MRI evidence of cerebral metastases; (2) cranial nerve palsies, in particular, diplopia or facial weakness; (3) neck pain with or without nuchal rigidity in the absence of bony metastases of the cervical spine; (4) radicular pain in the upper or lower extremities, particularly when accompanied by weakness but not by local spine pain; (5) unexplained constipation, impotence, or urinary incontinence or retention (urinary retention is an early sign of LM); (6) asymmetric leg weakness and diminished reflexes in the absence of pain or sensory changes; and (7) confusion, memory loss, or other cognitive abnormalities.

Diagnosis ■ The diagnosis of LM is usually established by the demonstration of malignant cells in the CSF. A cranial MRI may reveal enhancing cranial nerves or enhancing tumor in cortical sulci; communicating hydrocephalus may suggest leptomeningeal metastases.[38] A gadolinium-enhanced spine MRI may demonstrate tumor nodules on spinal roots, particularly in the cauda equina, even when symptoms of nerve root dysfunction are absent (Fig. 124-4). The whole neuraxis should be imaged to identify sites of bulky disease. When characteristic findings are identified, this may suffice to establish the diagnosis.[1,38] MRI is 76% sensitive and 77% specific. Occasionally, FDG-PET imaging may identify leptomeningeal metastases.[39] When a lumbar puncture is performed, opening pressure measurement, cell count, protein, glucose, and bacterial and fungal studies should be obtained. The cytology specimen should contain at least 10 mL of CSF optimally, and should be processed quickly according to the laboratory's protocol.

Malignant cells are found in the initial CSF sample in 50-60% of patients with LM.[1] False-positives are rare, except in patients with lymphoma or leukemia, where the distinction between reactive and malignant cells may be difficult. Cytologic examination is 75% sensitive, but almost 100% specific. In patients with subsequently documented LM and a negative first cytology, one or two additional samples increase the yield. In a few patients, cisternal CSF may be positive when lumbar CSF is negative. Likewise, cytology may be positive in ventricular fluid but negative in lumbar fluid or vice versa.[40] In the remaining patients, the diagnosis must be supported by other tests. It is rare for a patient with LM to have an entirely normal initial lumbar puncture. Increased opening pressure, pleocytosis, increased CSF protein, and decreased CSF glucose are almost always present in some combination.

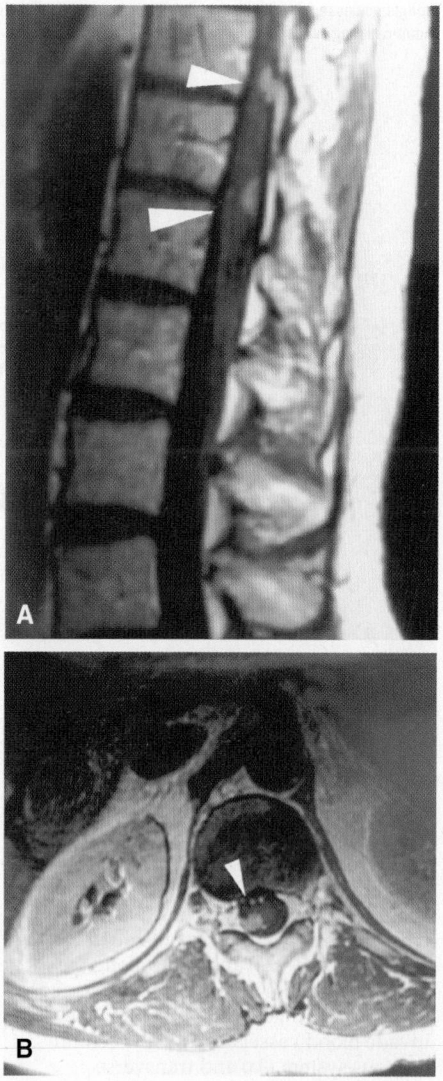

Figure 124-4 ■ Gadolinium enhanced MRI demonstrating leptomeningeal metastases from lung cancer. (**A**) Sagittal and (**B**) axial images demonstrating enhancing nodules within the thecal sac. This patient had a positive cerebrospinal fluid cytology for malignant cells.

Tumor markers, deoxyribonucleic acid (DNA) studies, and immunocytochemistry may help confirm LM when cytologic studies are negative.[35,41] A tumor-associated antigen in the spinal fluid is virtually pathognomonic of LM. In the presence of a normal blood–brain barrier (suggested by a normal CSF protein concentration), the level of tumor antigens, such as carcinoembryonic antigen (CEA), beta human chorionic gonadotropin (βHCG), cancer antigen (CA) 125, CA 19-9, and prostate-specific antigen (PSA), should be no greater than 1% of the serum level. When that amount is exceeded, and particularly if the CSF level is higher than the serum level, the diagnosis is established, even in the absence of a positive cytology. Other markers, such as β-glucuronidase and β2-microglobulin, are less specific because inflammatory conditions frequently elevate these markers as well. If tumor markers are elevated in a patient with documented LM, they can also be used to follow disease status, provided the samples are always taken from the same site (ie, values from ventricular CSF cannot be compared with those from lumbar CSF). Table 124-7 lists tumor markers commonly employed in CSF studies.

An abnormal DNA content of cells in the CSF measured by flow cytometry or in situ hybridization[41] supports the diagnosis of LM. Fewer than 500 cells are necessary for analysis, so data can be obtained on almost all CSF samples (4-5 mL). When LM is suspected in patients with lymphoma or leukemia and the CSF contains cytologically nondiagnostic lymphocytes, immunohistochemistry, flow cytometry, or molecular markers[42] may demonstrate a clonal excess of cells similar to the phenotype of the systemic neoplasm, suggesting LM.

Treatment ■ If untreated, LM usually causes relentless progression of neurologic dysfunction and death within weeks. Treatment is not very effective, and some believe that it does not reverse fixed neurologic deficits. Nevertheless, therapy alters the clinical course in about one-half of patients and often improves symptoms.[1] Occasionally, the course may be indolent especially in patients with LM from lymphoma or breast cancer.

Table 124-7 ■ **CSF Tumor Markers**

CSF Tumor Marker	Comments
CEA	Above 1% of serum CEA[a] in colon, lung and breast carcinoma
β-HCG	Choriocarcinoma, embryonal carcinoma, germ cell tumor
α-FP	Teratocarcinoma, yolk sac tumor, endodermal sinus tumor, embryonal carcinoma
CA 125	Ovarian carcinoma
CA 15-3	Breast cancer
β2-microglobulin	Above 2.0 mg/L[a] lymphoma (not specific), elevated by infection
β-glucuronidase	Above 80 mU/L[a] (not specific)
LDH	Isoenzyme 5 above 10% of total LDH[a] (not specific)
PSA	Prostate cancer

[a]Values suggestive of leptomeningeal metastasis.
Abbreviations: α-FP, α-fetoprotein; CEA, carcinoembryonic antigen; CSF, cerebrospinal fluid; HCG, human chorionic gonadotropin; LDH, lactic dehydrogenase; PSA, prostate specific antigen.

The type of primary cancer is the best predictor of response to treatment; the majority of lymphoma and breast cancer patients respond because these tumors are relatively sensitive to RT and the few chemotherapeutic agents that can be safely instilled into the CSF (see below). Patients with lung cancer or melanoma respond in about one-third and one-fifth of cases, respectively. Patients with severe neurologic disability from LM are less likely to derive benefit because neural damage is often irreversible. Correlations between CSF findings at diagnosis and subsequent response to therapy have been contradictory. Chemotherapy administered intraventricularly has better distribution and greater ease and reliability of delivery than drug administered by lumbar puncture. Because LM disrupts the blood–brain barrier, systemic chemotherapy, particularly when administered in high doses, may also be effective.[43] If symptomatic elevation of intracranial pressure occurs, with or without hydrocephalus, a ventriculoperitoneal shunt should be placed.

Among patients receiving therapy for LM, survival is prolonged only in those whose disease responds to treatment.[1] Although this is not surprising, the inability to predict which patients will respond to treatment makes prognostication difficult. In addition to surviving longer (4-6 months median vs 1-2 months median in nonresponders), patients who respond to therapy are less likely to die as a result of their LM than are patients whose disease progresses despite therapy.

Radiation Therapy ■ RT should be administered to symptomatic or radiologically involved areas of LM.[35] Symptomatic sites should be treated even if subarachnoid tumor is not evident radiographically at the symptomatic location. Entire neuraxis RT is rarely used because of its acute morbidity and myelosuppression that interferes with subsequent chemotherapy. Neuraxis RT is not used even when bulky LM is seen on MRI along the entire spinal axis; RT is still restricted to symptomatic areas. The brain is the most common site to which RT is administered, usually in a dose of 3000 cGy, but the cauda equina is also a common location that produces symptoms requiring RT. Treatment ports should be generous, and for brain, RT should include the cribriform plate and the skull base. During cranial RT, patients often benefit symptomatically from dexamethasone, but corticosteroids do not relieve spinal symptoms. In a study of response of cranial nerve deficits from lymphoma and leukemia LM, early RT (3 days or less after onset of symptoms) resulted in more rapid improvement than treatment later in the course (more than 3 days), but the ultimate response rate was equal between the two treatment groups.[44]

Chemotherapy ■ Intrathecal chemotherapy is used in conjunction with RT in the treatment of LM.[1,45] The most commonly used agent is methotrexate (MTX), which is active against breast cancer, lymphoma, and leukemia, but has poor activity against some of the other common cancers that cause LM, such as lung cancer.

MTX is administered intrathecally to adults in doses of 12-15 mg, diluted in preservative-free saline. With this dose, MTX levels in the CSF exceed the therapeutic concentration of 10^{-6} M and remain above this level for about 36-48 hours.[46] Normal flow patterns of CSF may be altered by intradural deposits of tumor. Studies of CSF flow dynamics using indium[111]-DPTA (diethylenetriamine penta-acetic acid) cisternography have found some obstruction to CSF flow in a high percentage of patients with LM, raising the question of whether flow studies are required before starting treatment. Indium[111] studies predict CSF MTX distribution and indicate that drug reaches all areas of the subarachnoid space unless a complete block is present.[36,47] Patients with impaired CSF flow have a worse prognosis, likely reflecting the extent of subarachnoid tumor, and increased incidence of leukoencephalopathy due to impaired egress of drug out of the ventricular system. Obstruction of CSF flow should be suspected in patients with LM who develop focal leukoencephalopathy around the ventricular catheter track (see Methotrexate).

MTX appears in the serum for prolonged periods following intrathecal administration, and myelosuppression and stomatitis may result. Oral leucovorin can be administered to avert these complications starting 12 hours after MTX injection. Leucovorin does not appear in the CSF in appreciable amounts, but the active conversion product, 5-methyltetrahydrofolate (5-methylTHFA), does; however, the CSF levels of 5-methylTHFA are very low after oral leucovorin administration and are incapable of rescuing tumor cells in the CSF. High-dose intravenous MTX (eg, 3-8 g/m^2) may result in CSF MTX levels that exceed 10^{-6} M, and may represent an alternative to intrathecal delivery, particularly in patients with impaired CSF flow. Systemic drugs may also treat bulky LM, whereas intrathecal chemotherapy has insufficient penetration into tumor nodules. Other agents that can reach the CSF or have been reported effective for LM include high-dose cytarabine for hematologic malignancies and capecitabine for breast cancer.[48] Agents, including the new small molecules, should be chosen on the basis of the likely sensitivity of the primary to a given drug.[49]

Two studies have found that intrathecal MTX as a single agent is equal in efficacy to multiagent intrathecal chemotherapy and has significantly less systemic toxicity. Patients treated with MTX plus RT respond more often than those treated with either alone. Cytarabine (cytosine arabinoside [ara-C]) and thiotepa may also be useful, particularly in LM from lymphoma, leukemia, or breast cancer. Liposomal cytarabine has a long CSF half-life and can be given every 14 days; it has been reported effective against LM from solid tumors not usually considered sensitive to cytarabine.[50] However, it can cause a severe chemical meningitis and patients must receive prophylactic steroids beginning one day before a dose is administered and continued for at least 2 days following the dose. Other agents have been used experimentally.[51-53]

Our approach is to irradiate symptomatic or radiologically involved areas, usually to 3000 cGy over 2 weeks. An Ommaya reservoir is placed in the right lateral ventricle, either before or after RT.[54] After completion of RT, MTX (12 mg) is administered twice per week for six treatments, then once weekly for several weeks, depending on the clinical and CSF response. The treatments are then stretched out to once per month until relapse occurs or for a total treatment time of 6 months. At relapse, cytarabine (50 mg) or thiotepa (10 mg) can be considered for the appropriate primaries. There are few data to guide decisions regarding the duration of therapy in patients who are clinically stable and whose CSF remains free of malignant cells after 6 months of therapy. Neurotoxicity from intrathecal drug can occur and is discussed later in this chapter.

Cranial and Peripheral Nerve Metastases

Lesions of cranial or peripheral nerves often cause severe pain and, depending on the nerve involved, substantial neurologic disability.[55] The frequency of metastatic disease causing cranial and peripheral nerve dysfunction is unknown because only a few studies address this issue in particular tumors. For example, facial nerve paralysis occurs in 5-25% of malignant parotid neoplasms, the lower figure associated with acinous cell carcinomas and the higher with undifferentiated neoplasms. Primary lung cancer arises in the superior sulcus in approximately 3% of patients, the vast majority presenting with pain caused by infiltration of the brachial plexus (Pancoast syndrome). Abdominal and pelvic tumors may involve the lumbar or sacral plexus during the course of disease, but the precise incidence is unknown. Individual nerves either alone or in combination (mononeuritis multiplex) may be compressed or invaded by tumor.

Pathogenesis ■ Tumors affect cranial and peripheral nerves either by compression without directly breaching the epineurium or by invasion along perineurial and endoneurial planes. Pancoast tumors and breast carcinoma metastatic to supraclavicular lymph nodes compress the brachial plexus but usually do not invade it, whereas squamous cell carcinoma of the face, certain melanomas, and prostate cancer can be neurotropic, tracking microscopically along the course of a nerve, often reaching the spinal canal or even the brainstem.[55] The biologic factors that make these tumors neurotropic have not been established. A blood–nerve barrier similar to the blood–brain barrier may exclude water-soluble chemotherapeutic agents from nerve and provide a "sanctuary" for tumor cells.

Symptoms ■ The specific symptoms and signs of cranial and peripheral nerve dysfunction depend on the nerves involved and the mechanism of involvement. With compressive lesions of nerves or plexuses, pain is usually the first symptom. The pain may be felt locally at the site of compression or more distantly in the sensory distribution of the nerve involved. Pain usually precedes other neurologic dysfunction by weeks to months. In invasive lesions of nerves, pain and neurologic dysfunction often occur simultaneously. In general, when mixed nerves are involved, motor function is affected out of proportion to sensory loss, no matter what the mechanism of nerve involvement. Examination of both motor and sensory functions will usually identify the nerves involved and pinpoint the location of the offending lesion. Compressive lesions of nerves can generally be identified by MR imaging studies directed at the area of dysfunction (Fig. 124-5).[1,55] When the lesion is infiltrative instead of compressive, all imaging studies may be normal and the diagnosis must be established clinically or by biopsy. Occasionally infiltration of large nerves such as a plexus or root can be imaged by an enhanced MRI.

Cranial and peripheral neuropathies also occur as side effects of radiation or chemotherapy or as paraneoplastic syndromes (see section on nonmetastatic complications). It is frequently difficult to distinguish these nonmetastatic peripheral nerve lesions from those caused by metastases, but, in general, the latter tend to be painful whereas the former are usually painless. Furthermore, most paraneoplastic and drug-induced neuropathies are bilateral and symmetric, whereas metastatic neuropathies are unilateral or at least asymmetric. Recognizing that any nerve in the body can be affected by metastatic cancer, the following describes some of the more commonly encountered cranial and peripheral neuropathies associated with cancer, and the approach to diagnosis and treatment.

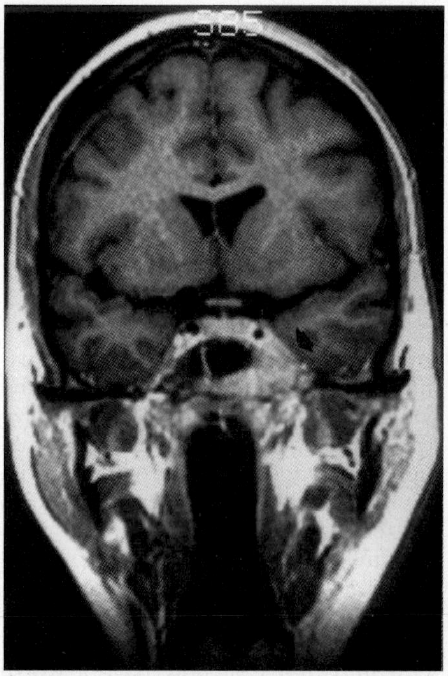

Figure 124-5 ■ Coronal-enhanced MRI demonstrating a metastasis to the left cavernous sinus (*arrowhead*) from breast carcinoma. Patient presented with retro-orbital pain and had evidence of a partial third, sixth, and V1 palsy.

Cranial Neuropathies ■ Cranial nerves may be affected by metastases at any point, from within the brainstem to their end organ (Table 124-8). Brainstem metastases occasionally cause isolated cranial nerve dysfunction, especially of the sixth cranial nerve, but usually other brainstem signs reveal the central location of the lesion. Leptomeningeal metastasis is a common cause of cranial neuropathies that are often multiple. Base of skull metastases often cause recognizable patterns of cranial nerve dysfunction that localize the lesion.[1] Finally, the cranial nerves may be damaged after exiting their foramina.

New-onset cranial neuropathy in a cancer patient should not be ascribed to toxic or idiopathic causes without thorough evaluation (Table 124-9). Evaluation should include an enhanced MRI to visualize the involved cranial nerve along its entire course.[56,57] Lumbar puncture should be performed in the evaluation of cranial neuropathies, and should be considered even when an appropriately placed skull metastasis is discovered, because LM may occur by local invasion from the skull metastasis or by extension along the nerve. If no diagnosis is apparent, empiric radiation therapy to the site of disease (eg, cavernous sinus syndrome) may be advisable in patients with rapidly advancing metastatic disease or with a primary that frequently metastasizes to bone or leptomeninges (eg, lymphoma, breast cancer).

Radiation therapy is usually employed for skull base and orbital metastases. Radiosurgery or charged particle irradiation is used in selected instances.[58,59] Benefit can occasionally be obtained from surgical resection of a calvarial metastasis, but is almost never performed for a skull base metastasis. Chemotherapy can be used in appropriate circumstances.

Brachial Plexopathy ■ Brachial plexopathy in cancer patients usually results from metastatic cancer in axillary or cervical lymph nodes or local bony structures (eg, clavicle), or from superior sulcus lung tumors.[1,60] Because most metastatic tumors compress the plexus from below, the initial symptom is usually pain in the posterior shoulder or pain radiating down the medial aspect of the arm, elbow, and forearm to the fourth and fifth fingers (C-8 or T-1 distribution). Weakness usually begins in the hand and sensory loss begins in the fourth and fifth fingers; both may progress to affect the entire arm. This initial presentation is helpful in distinguishing tumor from the more common

Table 124-8 Metastatic Lesions Causing Cranial Neuropathies

Lesion Site	Findings	Comments
Eye	Decreased visual acuity; retinal detachment	Choroidal lesions are more common than retinal: pain, proptosis and diplopia are rare; breast and lung cancer are common causes
Orbit	Pain, proptosis, diplopia; sensory loss V1; decreased visual acuity in one-third of cases, usually late	Equally as common as choroidal metastases; breast and prostate cancer and lymphoma and neuroblastoma are common causes
Parasellar	Unilateral frontal headache, oculomotor palsies (III, IV, VI), sensory loss V1	Vision rarely affected, no proptosis; lymphoma common
Sella	Diabetes insipidus	Anterior pituitary insufficiency and visual loss are rare; when present, they suggest a primary pituitary tumor. Breast cancer is a common cause
Middle cranial fossa	Facial numbness (V2, 3), abducens palsy in some (VI)	Lightning-like facial pains (trigeminal neuralgia) rare in patients with neoplastic compression
Jugular foramen	Hoarseness, dysphagia, pain in pharynx (IX, X), sternocleidomastoid weakness (XI), occasionally tongue weakness (XII)	Papilledema may occur if a dominant jugular vein is compressed. Glossopharyngeal neuralgia is uncommon
Occipital condyle	Unilateral occipital pain and neck stiffness, unilateral tongue weakness (XII)	Pain may radiate to forehead
Mandible	Unilateral numb chin and gum ("mental neuropathy")	Also results from meningeal or skull base metastases; breast cancer and lymphoma are common causes
Carotid sinus or glosso-pharyngeal nerve	Syncope, pharynx or neck pain on swallowing	Cardioinhibitory, vasodepressor syncope, or both; head and neck cancer, indicates recurrent tumor; may be life-threatening

Table 124-9 Nonmetastatic Causes of Cranial Neuropathy in Cancer Patients

Cranial Nerve (Symptom)	Causes
II (unilateral vision loss)	Gallium, intra-arterial cisplatin, interferon alpha, RT, temporal arteritis, retinal diseases including hemorrhage
III (diplopia, ptosis)	Diabetes (usually spares pupil), aneurysm, increased intracranial pressure (uncal herniation); myasthenia gravis + Grave's disease[a]
IV (jaw pain; facial pain)	Vincristine, trigeminal neuralgia (sudden, lancinating pains without sensory loss)
VI (diplopia)	Vincristine, increased intracranial pressure, head trauma, diabetes, drug toxicity (eg, narcotics, anticonvulsants), strabismus
VII (facial weakness)	Bell's palsy (idiopathic), varicella-zoster infection (Ramsay Hunt syndrome), diabetes
VIII (hearing loss, dysequilibrium)	Cisplatin, aminoglycosides, degenerative disease, acoustic neuroma, RT-induced serous otitis
X (weak phonation, laryngeal paralysis)	Vincristine

[a]Common causes of diplopia, but are not cranial nerve diseases.
Abbreviation: RT, radiation therapy.

cervical disc herniation where pain commonly affects the outer arm and dorsal surface of the forearm, with weakness in the triceps and wrist extensors (C-7 radiculopathy). Tumor masses are occasionally palpable in the axilla or supraclavicular area. When present, an ipsilateral Horner syndrome (ptosis, miosis, and anhydrosis) indicates the tumor has involved the stellate ganglion in the paraspinal region and, therefore, epidural extension must be sought on cervical MRI.

The differential diagnosis includes radiation-induced plexopathy,[61] trauma (eg, intraoperative positioning, or following central line placement), idiopathic plexopathy, and radiation-induced malignant peripheral nerve sheath tumor.[62] A common diagnostic dilemma is the differentiation of metastatic from radiation-induced plexopathy.[1,60] Clinical features that are helpful in distinguishing these two conditions include: (1) initial symptom of pain in metastatic plexopathy, and paresthesias in RT-induced plexopathy; the pain of metastatic disease may be accompanied by vasomotor and trophic changes in the arm[63]; (2) Horner syndrome, which is more consistent with metastatic plexopathy; (3) more rapid progression of symptoms and signs in metastatic plexopathy; (4) supraclavicular fullness in metastatic plexopathy; and (5) lymphedema, which suggests RT-induced plexopathy. Either CT or MRI may demonstrate a mass in the plexus (metastatic plexopathy) or loss of soft-tissue planes from fibrosis (RT-induced plexopathy). When findings are equivocal, a PET scan may help.[64]

Surgical exploration of the brachial plexus, once an important diagnostic procedure, is rarely necessary now that CT and MRI are available. Biopsy of the brachial plexus is still indicated when radiation-induced malignant peripheral nerve sheath tumors are suspected. Diagnostic imaging has also lessened the usefulness of electromyogram (EMG) studies, although the discovery of repetitive spontaneous motor unit discharges (myokymia) is pathognomonic of radiation-induced plexopathy and distinguishes it from metastatic plexopathy.[65] When metastases are paraspinal in location, epidural extension is common and should be excluded by MRI. The design of radiation treatment ports will also depend in part on this information.

RT is the best available treatment for metastatic plexopathy; chemotherapy may be useful for some previously irradiated patients (eg, those with breast cancer or lymphoma). Some superior sulcus lung tumors that invade the brachial plexus can be resected with a combined thoracic and neurosurgical approach. There is no satisfactory treatment for radiation-induced plexopathy. Surgical lysis of fibrotic tissue surrounding the nerves has not been helpful, nor has systemic corticosteroid or local steroid injection. Treatments for pain include carbamazepine, opioids, gabapentin, and neurosurgical ablative procedures. Amputation of the limb does not relieve pain.

Lumbosacral Plexopathy The lumbosacral plexus is formed from spinal nerve roots L-2 to S-5. The upper lumbar portion (L-2 to L-4) exits the pelvis mainly as the obturator (adductor muscles) and femoral (quadriceps muscles) nerves, whereas the remainder of the leg is innervated by the sciatic nerve (L-5 to S-1). The bladder, rectum, and anus are innervated by roots S-3, S-4, and S-5. The lumbosacral plexus may be involved at any point along its course.[1] The femoral nerve may be compressed at the femoral canal by lymph node metastasis, the sciatic nerve may be affected by tumor extending from the pelvis into the sciatic notch, and the obturator nerve compressed in the pelvis or obturator foramen. The sacral plexus is often affected by a sacral bone metastasis or by a soft-tissue mass directly anterior to the sacrum. A difficult but critical problem with localization is differentiating between lesions of the lumbosacral plexus and the cauda equina resulting from epidural or meningeal metastases. Cauda equina involvement is more likely than plexopathy to cause bilateral symptoms and signs, although 25% of metastatic plexopathies were bilateral in one study.[66] Incontinence requires bilateral loss of innervation and, therefore, its presence suggests central (ie, cauda equina) or sacral involvement. Clear differentiation requires enhanced spinal MRI and CSF analysis. Local extension of pelvic and abdominal tumors is the predominant cause of metastatic lumbosacral plexopathy. The differential includes herniated lumbar disc, epidural and meningeal metastases to the cauda equina, radiation-induced plexopathy (usually from brachytherapy for pelvic neoplasms), plexus injury from intra-arterial chemotherapy, intraoperative trauma, hematoma, abscess, and diabetic or idiopathic lumbosacral plexopathy. The differential features of metastatic and radiation-induced plexopathy are similar to those for brachial plexopathy. CT or MRI often demonstrates a mass in the region of the lumbosacral plexus, and may also demonstrate hydronephrosis from ureteral obstruction. Biopsy is indicated if an abscess or a secondary tumor is suspected. RT is the most commonly employed treatment for metastatic lumbosacral plexopathy. If metastatic disease approaches the spine, epidural disease may be present and should be included in the RT port.

Peripheral Neuropathy ■ Single peripheral nerves are sometimes damaged by metastatic cancer, and more widespread invasion of peripheral nerves, causing either a mononeuritis multiplex or diffuse polyneuropathy, may complicate the course of leukemia or lymphoma. However, when polyneuropathy occurs in cancer patients, it usually results from toxin exposure or paraneoplastic disorders, both of which are discussed below.

Table 124-10 ■ **Neurotoxicity of Agents Commonly Used in Cancer Patients**

Acute encephalopathy (delirium)	Headache without meningitis
Corticosteroids	Retinoic acid
Methotrexate (high-dose IV, IT)	Trimethoprim-sulfamethoxazole
Cisplatin	Cimetidine
Vincristine	Corticosteroids
Asparaginase	Tamoxifen
Procarbazine	Ondansetron
5-Fluorouracil (± levamisole)	Seizures
Cytarabine (high-dose IV, IT)	Methotrexate
Nitrosoureas (high-dose of arterial)	Etoposide (high-dose)
Ifosfamide/mesna	Cisplatin
Interferons	Vincristine
Chronic encephalopathy (dementia)	Asparaginase
Methotrexate	Nitrogen mustard
Carmustine	Carmustine
Cytarabine	Dacarbazine (intra-arterial or high-dose)
Fludarabine	Busulfan (high-dose)
Visual loss	Beta-lactam antibiotics
Tamoxifen	Iodinated contrast material (IV or IT)
Gallium nitrate	Myelopathy (intrathecal drugs)
Cisplatin	Methotrexate
Interferon alpha	Cytarabine
Cerebellar dysfunction/ataxia	Thiotepa
5-Fluorouracil (± levamisole)	Peripheral neuropathy
Cytarabine	Vinca alkaloids
Phenytoin	Cisplatin
Procarbazine	Etoposide
Aseptic meningitis	Teniposide
Trimethoprim-sulfamethoxazole (Cotrimoxazole)	Misonidazole
IVIg	Paclitaxel
NSAIDs	Suramin
Monoclonal antibodies	Docetaxel
Bortezomib	Bortezomib
Metrizamide	
Carbamazepine	
Cytarabine (IT)	
Methotrexate (IT)	
Corticosteroids (IT)	

Abbreviations: IV, intravenous; IVIg, intravenous gammaglobulin; IT, intrathecal; NSAID, nonsteroidal anti-inflammatory drugs.
Source: Modified from Ref. 1.

Nonmetastatic Complications of Cancer Therapy

Many cancer treatments are neurotoxic (Table 124-10). Some drugs (eg, vincristine) cause neurotoxicity even at low doses, whereas others (eg, cytarabine) cause neurotoxicity only during intensive therapy. Neurologic toxicity is a dose-limiting factor in several cancer treatments, such as RT, and patients may suffer more from these toxicities than from the cancer itself.[1,67,68] The more commonly encountered neurologic toxicities from cancer treatment are discussed below.

Chemotherapy

Vinca Alkaloids ■ Vinca alkaloids cause nerve damage by binding tubulin in peripheral nerves and disrupting the formation of microtubules that mediate fast axonal transport. Neurotoxicity is a dose-limiting side effect of all the vinca alkaloids, but especially of vincristine; vinorelbine can also cause peripheral neuropathy particularly when combined with or following other neurotoxic agents. Central neurotoxicity is rare because vincristine does not penetrate the normal blood–brain barrier[69]; however, accidental instillation directly into the CSF causes rapid axonal damage that is usually fatal.[70]

Vinca alkaloid neurotoxicity is age (more severe in adults) and dose dependent, and appears to be more prominent in patients with hepatic dysfunction, and in those who have received other potentially neurotoxic therapies.[71] Tingling paresthesias develop in the fingertips, and usually in the toes, of virtually all patients treated with vincristine, although clinically detectable sensory loss is often absent. Loss of ankle stretch reflexes is an early and almost universal sign, and with continued therapy, all reflexes may diminish or disappear. Weakness may occur as therapy continues. Weakness is of two types: (1) A generalized distal axonal neuropathy is the more common. When that weakness is mild, patients lose the ability to walk on their heels and lose strength in wrist extensors. More severely affected patients develop foot drop and slap their feet when they walk. Weakness can become severe enough to render the patient immobile or bed-bound, but the drug should be discontinued prior to the development of such marked weakness. Pre-existing peripheral nerve diseases, especially Charcot–Marie–Tooth neuropathy and probably other neuropathies (eg, diabetic polyneuropathy), increase the severity of vincristine neuropathy.[72] (2) Some patients develop focal weakness, (eg, unilateral foot drop or cranial nerve palsies, such as ptosis or extraocular muscle, facial, or laryngeal paralysis.)[73] Although symptomatic toxicity is usually reversible after discontinuation of the drug, significant weakness may persist in severely affected patients. Autonomic dysfunction, particularly abdominal cramping and constipation, often occurs within hours to days of each dose. Adynamic ileus may result and can be life-threatening. A prophylactic bowel regimen or metoclopramide may reduce the severity of this complication. Impotence has been reported.

Less common complications of vincristine administration include aching bone pain, sharp stabbing pain in the jaw or throat, or an increase in any pre-existing pain. These symptoms typically occur within hours of injection and subside over several days. The symptoms appear with the first or second dose, and rarely recur with subsequent doses. Hyponatremia from inappropriate secretion of antidiuretic hormone occurs within days of drug administration and may recur with subsequent doses. Encephalopathy and seizures not related to hyponatremia have been reported to occur after vincristine administration, but are very rare. There is no effective treatment.

Methotrexate ■ There are several clinically distinct forms of MTX toxicity.[1,67] An acute reaction with meningismus, confusion, fever, and CSF pleocytosis occurs 4-6 hours after intrathecal injection and resolves over several days. This syndrome is often confused with infectious meningitis, but the onset is too rapid after the injection for bacterial contamination; antibiotics are unnecessary unless Gram stain or cultures demonstrate organisms. Dexamethasone may relieve or prevent some of these symptoms. Mild acute toxicity occurs in as many as 10% of patients, but further doses of intrathecal MTX are usually uneventful. The cause of this syndrome is unknown, although high CSF MTX levels may accompany the reaction.

An early delayed reaction follows high-dose intravenous infusion of MTX in about 4% of patients so treated.[74,75] The disorder usually occurs 7-10 days after the third or fourth treatment and is characterized by stupor or coma, often associated with lateralizing neurologic signs that change from hour to hour. Most patients recover completely and the disorder usually does not recur even if MTX is reinstituted. The pathogenesis of this syndrome is unknown.

Paraplegia may follow instillation of MTX or cytarabine by lumbar puncture.[76] The disorder is characterized by weakness and sensory loss in the legs, which evolves over several days to complete transverse myelopathy. Some patients recover, but most remain paraplegic. Extensive necrosis of the spinal cord is found at autopsy. The pathogenesis of the disorder is unknown, but it appears to be idiosyncratic rather than dose related.

MTX leukoencephalopathy occurs in patients who have received a high cumulative dose of intrathecal or systemic MTX or MTX in combination with cranial RT.[35,77] Symptoms begin weeks or months after treatment and appear as focal neurologic deficits that sometimes progress to seizures, coma, and death. Such a severe outcome is uncommon and tends to occur in the pediatric population. More commonly in adults, progressive cognitive impairment in the absence of lateralizing signs may be seen in patients who survive >6 months following treatment with systemic or intrathecal MTX ± RT. Leukoencephalopathy is always found on neuroimaging of these patients, but occasionally it may be found on MRI or at autopsy in asymptomatic patients. The neuropathologic findings consist of multifocal areas of coagulative necrosis in the white matter, often with extensive calcification. Unlike cerebral radionecrosis, fibrinoid necrosis of blood vessels is absent. The areas of necrosis may be distributed randomly in the white matter or be predominantly periventricular. The latter pattern may occur when MTX is injected into the ventricles of patients with abnormal outflow of ventricular CSF.

Alternatively, focal leukoencephalopathy may develop around the catheter track.[78] When MTX is injected into ventricles with elevated pressure, the drug tracks along the outside of the catheter, producing focal leukoencephalopathy that mimics a mass lesion; MRI may show a hypointense enhancing mass (Fig. 124-6). This may resolve on its own or require removal of the catheter.

Platins ■ Peripheral neuropathy is a dose-limiting toxicity of some platins, particularly cisplatin and oxaliplatin.[67,79] Neuropathic symptoms begin as tingling paresthesias in the toes and fingers; loss of stretch reflexes and reduced vibratory and position sensation are found. Pain and temperature sensation and strength are unaffected. These findings and loss of sural (sensory) nerve conduction with preservation of motor nerve conduction indicate a large, myelinated sensory fiber neuropathy that impairs position sense and vibration. Severe, disabling sensory ataxia may result. Symptoms often begin after treatment has been completed, and can progress for months before stabilizing. Gradual resolution follows, although some patients are permanently disabled. Neurotrophic agents and amifostine have both been reported to decrease cisplatin neurotoxicity, but the data are inconclusive.[80,81] Lhermitte sign, an electric sensation in the arms, back, or legs upon neck flexion, is an occasional manifestation of platin neurotoxicity. Oxaliplatin may cause cold-induced paresthesias either during or shortly after an infusion.[79,82]

Ototoxicity caused by cisplatin is a result of damage to the organ of Corti. Toxicity severe enough to interfere with speech perception is uncommon, but hearing loss may or may not resolve. Cisplatin has been associated with optic neuropathy, especially after intracarotid infusion. Seizures and encephalopathy have been reported in patients receiving cisplatin. Cisplatin induces renal magnesium and calcium wasting, and although these disorders must be excluded when seizures or encephalopathy occur, they rarely contribute to platinum neurotoxicity.

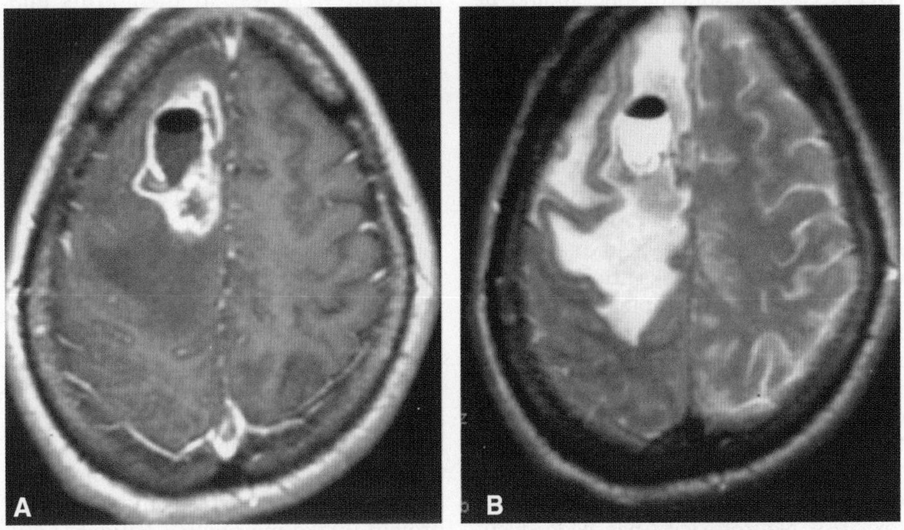

Figure 124-6 ■ Gadolinium enhanced T1-weighted (**A**) and T2-weighted (**B**) MRIs of focal leukoencephalopathy in a patient with a malfunctioning Ommaya reservoir. This reservoir was obstructed but unrecognized. Multiple courses of methotrexate were instilled into the catheter. The drug dissected around the catheter and into the frontal lobe, causing a region of necrosis with prominent surrounding edema. Air can be seen in the central cavity of the lesion after a recent instillation. The patient presented with seizures and a left hemiparesis, both of which resolved with corticosteroids.

Vascular disease producing neurologic symptoms has been reported as a late delayed effect of cisplatin-based chemotherapy. Many such patients develop Raynaud phenomenon, and a few have developed transient ischemic attacks or cerebral infarctions. Other platinum drugs are less neurotoxic.[83]

Taxanes ■ Paclitaxel and docetaxel both bind tubulin where they stabilize and promote microtubular assembly. Both cause a predominantly sensory peripheral neuropathy, beginning with paresthesias of the toes and then fingers.[1,84] More severe sensory impairment and loss of reflexes develop with increasing duration of drug administration. Symptoms usually recover with drug discontinuation. Weakness is seen occasionally, but can be predominantly proximal, mimicking a myopathy, but this is likely secondary to neuropathy.[85] Because taxanes are often used concurrently with or following other neurotoxic agents such as cisplatin, patients may develop significant symptoms with the first few doses because of additive neurotoxic effects.

5-Fluorouracil ■ Generalized encephalopathy has been seen in association with severe systemic toxicity during therapy, and may indicate an inherited deficiency of dihydropyrimidine dehydrogenase, the enzyme responsible for pyrimidine catabolism.[86]

Cytosine Arabinoside ■ Intrathecal cytarabine can cause an acute chemical meningitis with confusion, fever and CSF pleocytosis. This occurs in almost all patients who receive the liposomal preparation (DepoCyt).[50] Dexamethasone should be administered prior to and after every DepoCyt injection.

Intravenous high-dose cytarabine (eg, 3 g/m^2 every 12 hours for six doses) causes neurotoxicity in 10-25% of patients. The common form is pancerebellar dysfunction starting several days after the initiation of therapy and worsening for several more days.[87] Gradual recovery begins about 2 weeks after onset, but recovery may be incomplete in approximately 20% of patients, especially those in whom the neurologic disorder was severe. Pathologic changes include loss of cerebellar Purkinje cells and neurons in the deep cerebellar nuclei.

Encephalopathy and seizures also occur, usually in the setting of cerebellar toxicity.[88] Neurotoxicity has been documented with minimum cumulative doses of 18 g/m^2, but higher doses (eg, 30-40 g/m^2) are associated with increasingly severe toxicity. Age older than 50 years and renal insufficiency predispose patients to more severe toxicity. A recrudescence of neurologic symptoms may occur with retreatment. Peripheral neuropathy is also a rare complication of high-dose cytarabine; in most patients, high-dose cytarabine was given with other potentially neurotoxic agents, such as fludarabine.[1]

Other Drugs ■ Other commonly used drugs that cause neurotoxicity include bortezomib,[89] suramin, and procarbazine, all of which can cause peripheral neuropathy, although procarbazine does so rarely. High-dose busulfan therapy, used to prepare patients for bone marrow transplantation, can cause seizures. At standard doses the drug is not neurotoxic. Gemcitabine, in combination with abdominal radiation, has been reported to cause myositis with acute muscle pain and tenderness.[1,90] It is responsive to steroids. The drug has also been reported to cause a reversible posterior encephalopathy, but this syndrome, characterized by headache, somnolence, seizures, and posterior hemisphere hyperintensities on MRI scans, is associated with a number of anticancer agents, including vincristine and cyclosporin.[1,91] The clinical symptoms, which are usually reversible, are often associated with the development of severe hypertension that is likely critical to the pathophysiology of this disorder which is similar to hypertensive encephalopathy.

Corticosteroids ■ Corticosteroids cause neurotoxicity in the form of myopathy and alterations of mental status.[1]

Myopathy affects most patients taking steroids for brain or spinal cord metastases. Patients develop symmetric, proximal weakness in their arms and legs within weeks after the institution of steroids. The weakness may progress, but very rarely renders the patient nonambulatory. Early symptoms include difficulty arising from chairs or toilet seats and climbing stairs. Muscle stretch reflexes are normal and sensation and bowel and bladder function are not affected. Respiratory function may be compromised, resulting in exercise intolerance and dyspnea. The serum creatine phosphokinase (CPK) is not elevated. The differential diagnosis includes hypokalemia, thyroid dysfunction, polymyositis, Lambert–Eaton myasthenic syndrome (LEMS), and spinal cord compression. The only treatment is reduction or discontinuation of the steroids. Exercise and adequate protein intake may help.[92] Patients with hypoalbuminemia may be at higher risk for steroid myopathy.

Psychosis, delirium, euphoria, or dysphoria may complicate steroid therapy. Dose reduction or discontinuation is usually necessary, although neuroleptics or sedatives can be used in patients for whom continued therapy is critical.

Radiation Therapy

Despite the fact that cells in the CNS turn over slowly or not at all, the brain, spinal cord, and, to a lesser degree, peripheral nerves are susceptible to damage by ionizing radiation that usually causes symptoms months or years after the radiation has been completed (Table 124-11).[1,67,93-95] With patients living longer after initial treatment, the problem of delayed radiation damage to the CNS is increasingly important.

Brain Toxicity ■ Acute reactions, occurring within hours of a dose of RT, are rare with current fractionation schedules when patients are pretreated with dexamethasone.[1] Patients with large or multifocal tumors and cerebral edema, especially those with symptoms of increased intracranial pressure, are more likely to experience this side effect. Symptoms and signs of acute RT toxicity include worsening of existing deficits, headache, nausea and vomiting, lethargy, and somnolence. These are usually transient and respond to increased doses of corticosteroids. The etiology has been ascribed to radiation-induced disruption of the blood–brain barrier with resulting cerebral edema. Occasionally, worsening perilesional edema may be seen on MRI scan.

Early delayed encephalopathy occurs a few weeks to a few months after RT. Patients may develop worsening of lateralizing signs or somnolence in the absence of focal deficits; the former predominates in adults treated for brain tumors and the latter in children treated prophylactically. Symptoms may persist for days to weeks, and are often relieved by corticosteroids; complete resolution is usual. Early delayed encephalopathy is often confused with progression of the primary brain tumor or metastasis being irradiated, and is sometimes called pseudo-progression. An MRI scan reveals an enhancing lesion indistinguishable from progressive tumor. Clinical suspicion and resolution of symptoms over time may be the only real clue to the cause of the deterioration. The pathogenesis of early delayed encephalopathy is probably demyelination resulting from radiation injury to oligodendroglia.[1]

Delayed radiation toxicity is the most serious complication of brain RT,[1,9] and radionecrosis is its most common manifestation, arising months to years after treatment.[1,96-98] In one study, cerebral radionecrosis occurred in 6% of patients treated with 4500 cGy or more.[98] The total dose is the most important factor in the development of cerebral radionecrosis; there is a threshold near 6000

Table 124-11 **Neurologic Complications of CNS Irradiation**

Complication	Latency	Symptoms and Signs	Comments
Brain			
Acute	Hours	Increase in existing deficits, headache, nausea, vomiting, confusion, somnolence	Transient, corticosteroids help
Early	Weeks to months	Malaise, increase in existing signs, increased seizures, somnolence	Resolves over days to weeks, steroids help
Delayed			
a. Radionecrosis	6 months to years	Focal mass lesion	Treatment includes steroids and surgery, tumor often coexists
b. Dementia	1 year	Loss of cognitive function	May be subtle
c. Endocrine	Years	Hypothyroidism, amenorrhea/galactorrhea, changes in libido, growth failure	Hypothalamic or pituitary in origin
d. Secondary tumors	10–40 years, earlier if radiated as a child	Symptoms of brain tumor	Meningioma, sarcoma, malignant glioma
e. Stroke	Years	Abrupt onset of neurologic dysfunction	Large or branch vessels
Spinal cord			
Early	Weeks to months	Electric shocks with neck movement (Lhermitte sign)	Usually transient
Delayed			
a. Myelopathy	Weeks to years	Progressive cord dysfunction, starts with sensory symptoms	Often fatal
b. Lower motor neuron syndrome	Months to years	Focal weakness and atrophy	May improve spontaneously

cGy above which radionecrosis becomes common. However, high daily fraction schedules also carry increased risk for radionecrosis. Headache, focal deficits, and seizures are the usual symptoms. CT/MRI reveals a contrast-enhancing lesion with surrounding edema producing mass effect; this radiographic appearance is indistinguishable from CNS tumor. PET or single-photon emission computed tomography (SPECT) scans may differentiate tumor that is hypermetabolic from necrosis that is hypometabolic. However, the differentiation between radionecrosis and tumor is often difficult, and biopsy may be required. Marked symptomatic improvement follows treatment with dexamethasone, and some patients remain well after steroids are discontinued. Surgical resection of the necrotic material is often necessary. Reports that anticoagulation or hyperbaric oxygen relieve symptoms require confirmation.[99,100] Radiation may also cause dementia unassociated with evidence of necrosis.[101,102] The MRI may show only ventricular dilatation, sulcal atrophy, and white matter hyperintensity. Some of these patients respond to ventriculoperitoneal shunting albeit incompletely and temporarily.[103] This disorder is most common in patients who have received both RT and intensive systemic chemotherapy, and is likely a variant of delayed leukoencephalopathy.

Cerebral infarction may result from occlusion of cervical or intracranial arteries that have received large doses of RT.[104] Vascular malformations may appear and bleed many years after brain radiation therapy.[105] Complicated migraine-like episodes may occur in children after cranial irradiation.[106] Endocrinologic dysfunction may arise years after RT, resulting from either hypothalamic or pituitary failure.[107] Brain tumors may occur decades after cranial RT or radiosurgery administered in adulthood, but latency is often much shorter (median 6 years) in those irradiated in childhood.[108] Radiation-induced brain tumors include meningioma, sarcoma, and malignant glioma.[1]

Spinal Cord Toxicity ■ Spinal cord damage caused by RT is uncommon. Transient, electric shock-like sensations following neck flexion (Lhermitte sign) may occur weeks to months after RT to the cervical cord, including mantle RT for Hodgkin disease.[1] Spontaneous resolution is the rule. Progressive radiation myelopathy, on the other hand, is a devastating complication with onset months to years (median 20 months) following RT.[109] The incidence of radiation myelopathy is affected by the total RT dose and dose per fraction; an estimate of the ED5 (5% incidence of complication) is between 5700 and 6100 cGy for RT delivered in 200 cGy fractions. Symptoms of radiation myelopathy usually begin with sensory changes in the legs and gradually progress to sensory loss, weakness, and sphincter dysfunction. Pain may be present at the level of the cord damage. Dysesthetic pain below the level of cord injury may be prominent. Unlike epidural spinal cord compression, sensory and motor findings are often asymmetric at onset and a Brown-Séquard syndrome is often present. The MRI scan reveals either a normal, enlarged, or atrophic cord that may contrast enhance, but extrinsic compression is absent (Fig. 124-7). Steroids do not reverse the neurotoxic deficits. Anticoagulants and hyperbaric oxygen have been reported to be effective, but this has not been verified.[1] Spontaneous improvement sometimes occurs.[109]

A lower motor neuron syndrome with weakness and muscle atrophy can occur after irradiation of the spinal cord.

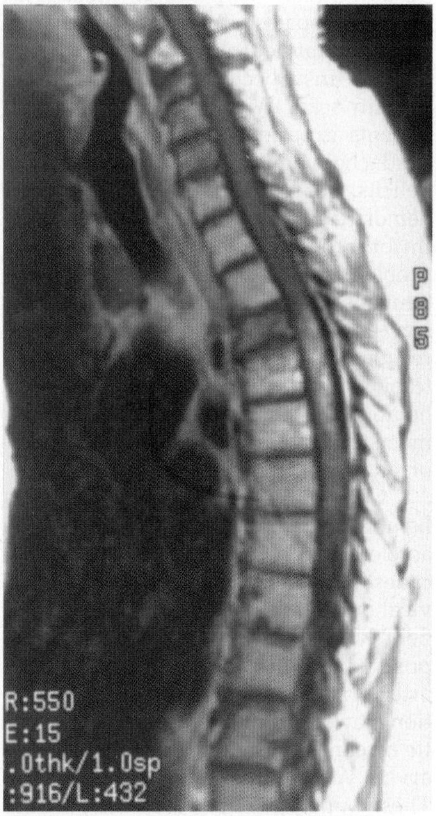

Figure 124-7 ■ MRI demonstrating radiation myelopathy. The hypodense thoracic vertebral body is the site of a bone metastasis from breast cancer for which the patient was radiated. Some months later, the patient developed a myelopathy, and the contrast-enhancing lesion seen in the spinal cord represents radiation damage.

Although weakness is prominent, patients usually remain ambulatory; spontaneous improvement is occasionally seen.[110] Radiation-induced plexopathies were discussed in a previous section (see brachial plexopathy).

Cerebrovascular Complications of Cancer

Cerebrovascular lesions are the second most common neuropathologic finding, after metastases, in postmortem studies of cancer patients. Of 3426 brains studied at autopsy, 15% contained vascular lesions.[1]

Cerebral hemorrhage can develop in any metastasis.[111] It is most commonly seen in lung cancer, but occurs proportionately more frequently in melanoma, thyroid, renal, and germ cell metastases. Intracerebral hemorrhages that are not associated with metastases are seen in patients with leukemia, thrombocytopenia, or coagulopathy. Intravascular leukostasis is not required for hemorrhage in leukemic patients.

Subdural hemorrhage may occur in association with dural metastases or coagulopathy. A hemorrhage may cause abrupt neurologic deterioration or may be unsuspected prior to obtaining a brain scan. With large hemorrhages, patients experience an abrupt onset of headache, vomiting, lethargy, and focal deficits. For patients with intracerebral hemorrhage resulting from coagulopathy or thrombocytopenia, the underlying problem should be treated and the patient observed. Subdural hematomas and some hemorrhages into metastases may respond to surgical evacuation. Corticosteroids are useful in those patients who hemorrhage into an underlying brain metastasis but probably do not help hemorrhage into an otherwise normal brain.

Cerebral infarction is as common as hemorrhage.[1] Infarctions secondary to accelerated atherosclerosis take place decades following RT that has included cervical or cerebral vessels in the irradiated field. RT for head and neck cancer predisposes to carotid stenosis, and intracranial arterial stenosis with subsequent infarction may occur following cranial RT. Septic cerebral infarction is usually secondary to Aspergillus, Candida, or Mucor. These opportunistic organisms produce a vasculitis, and the infarctions are often multiple and hemorrhagic. Aspergillus is the most common causative agent and is always associated with pulmonary infection; discovery of the latter may be a clue to the correct diagnosis. Antifungal therapy is usually unsuccessful, and the outcome is often fatal.

Cerebral venous thrombosis (eg, superior sagittal sinus thrombosis) may result from compression or invasion of vascular structures by a metastasis, or from a coagulopathy.[112] Clinical features include worsening headache, focal deficits, and seizures. The diagnosis can be made by MRI combined with magnetic resonance venography. Lumbar puncture reveals an elevated opening pressure, and frequently red cells in the CSF. Spontaneous resolution usually occurs unless dural metastasis is the cause, in which case RT is required. Anticoagulation is safe and should be considered for progressive neurologic symptoms, even when due to hemorrhage from venous infarction; however, most patients recover fully without treatment.

Cerebral embolism accounts for more than half of strokes in patients with cancer.[113] It may be cardioembolic or result from nonbacterial thrombotic endocarditis (NBTE, marantic endocarditis).[114] Lung and GI carcinomas are the primary cancers most commonly associated with NBTE. Infarctions in patients with NBTE are often multiple and hemorrhagic. Diffuse encephalopathy and focal deficits usually coexist. Approximately one-third of patients with NBTE also have laboratory evidence of disseminated intravascular coagulation (DIC). Two-dimensional echocardiography is rarely helpful, but transesophageal echocardiography can demonstrate the valvular vegetations. Cerebral angiography demonstrates multiple arterial branch occlusions. Anticoagulation with heparin should be considered. Anecdotal evidence suggests that warfarin is not helpful. Tumor emboli originate from pulmonary metastases in most circumstances.[115] The patient develops a neurologic deficit, followed weeks to months later by progressive deficits referable to the same area of brain due to growth of the embolized tumor.

DIC may result in cerebrovascular thrombosis.[7] Neurologic symptoms, which usually begin abruptly with diffuse encephalopathy and fluctuating multifocal deficits, often precede laboratory evidence of DIC. Enhanced MRI is usually negative, although small foci of ischemia are occasionally seen and may be evident on diffusion-weighted sequences. Anticoagulation with heparin, but not warfarin, may prevent progressive neurologic dysfunction.[116]

Metabolic Encephalopathy

Diffuse encephalopathy with or without focal signs is a common and prominent sign of many of the neurologic complications of cancer, including brain (usually multiple) or leptomeningeal metastases; neurotoxicity of many chemotherapeutic agents; vascular complications, particularly DIC; intracranial infections, and some paraneoplastic syndromes. However, most patients with encephalopathy do not suffer from one of these causes; instead, the disorder results from metabolic or nutritional abnormalities related to the underlying cancer or its treatment.[117-119] Table 124-12 lists some of the causes of diffuse encephalopathy in cancer patients, but in most instances the disorder is either multifactorial or the underlying cause is never identified. Opioids or sedative drug overdose, hypoxia, or vital organ failure are the most frequently identified causes. In patients with multiple contributory causes, effective treatment of one factor may reverse the encephalopathy even though others cannot be treated. In patients in whom the cause is not identified, the symptoms often resolve spontaneously; however, the presence of delirium is associated with an overall poor prognosis.[120]

Metabolic encephalopathy usually causes global impairment of attention, alertness, and cognition in the absence of lateralizing signs.[121,122] Focal neurologic findings may occur in metabolic encephalopathy, but their presence should prompt a search for structural lesions. The possibility of structural disease even in nonfocal, encephalopathic cancer patients should always be kept in mind; (eg, multiple brain metastases may present only as a recent change in mental status.) Nonconvulsive status epilepticus may cause encephalopathy without focal signs, although careful observation will

Table 124-12 **Causes of Encephalopathy in Cancer Patients**

Metabolic
Hypoxemia
Fever
Severe anemia
Uremia
Electrolyte imbalance—hypoglycemia
Metabolic acidosis
Hyperammonemia, hepatic failure
Hypercarbia (CO_2 narcosis)
Postanoxic encephalopathy
Thiamine deficiency (Wernicke's encephalopathy)
Thyroid disorders
Toxic
Sedative or opioid intoxication or withdrawal
Sepsis
Corticosteroids
Alcohol withdrawal
Anticholinergics
Chemotherapy agents (high-dose MTX, ifosfamide)
Anticonvulsants

usually detect repetitive movements of eyes or extremities.[123]

Investigation and treatment should proceed simultaneously. When the history does not immediately suggest the etiology (eg, opioid toxicity, sepsis), a stepwise investigation should be carried out to identify the cause. If the examination reveals focal neurologic findings, or if the patient is stuporous, an MRI with and without contrast should be obtained. The tests should cover each of the areas listed in Table 124-12. If no cause is apparent from these tests, a lumbar puncture should be considered.

Simultaneously with evaluation, treatment should be undertaken. General medical measures of oxygenation, blood pressure, temperature control, and hydration often improve mental function. In diabetic patients, dextrose should be administered while awaiting the results of laboratory tests. Medications that are not critical should be stopped. During the initial evaluation, symptomatic treatment with sedatives or neuroleptics should be avoided when possible, because these agents cloud the clinical picture and may hamper diagnosis. Haloperidol or risperidone may help to control symptoms of agitation and hallucinations, if present, but should not be used in alcohol or sedative withdrawal (risk of seizures) or in anticholinergic intoxication; benzodiazepines can be used in the former conditions and physostigmine in the latter. If opioid intoxication is suspected, and the patient's respiratory status is not compromised, it is best to let the intoxication resolve without specific treatment because naloxone administration may precipitate severe, abrupt withdrawal and its effect is short-lived. If naloxone is administered, the initial dose should be 0.2 mg (one-half vial) diluted in saline and administered slowly. Thiamine should be given intravenously to patients with severe malnutrition. Once identified, the underlying cause of the encephalopathy should be treated promptly. However, improvement of the encephalopathy may lag behind improvement in laboratory values, especially if the abnormality was gradual in development.

Paraneoplastic Neurologic Syndromes

Paraneoplastic syndromes refer to disorders of unknown etiology that occur with increased frequency in patients with cancer.[1,8] Compared with known complications of cancer, paraneoplastic syndromes are rare, seen in less than 1% of patients with cancer. As paraneoplastic syndromes precede the diagnosis of cancer in about two-thirds of cases, prompt recognition may lead to early diagnosis and cure of the underlying neoplasm. These disorders often debilitate the patient to a greater degree than does the malignancy, but some of the syndromes improve with successful treatment of the cancer. Table 124-13 lists some paraneoplastic syndromes. The primary cancers most commonly associated with each syndrome are also listed, but these associations are not absolute, because each syndrome has been observed with a variety of cancer types.

The etiologies of these syndromes are not well understood, but most are suspected to have an autoimmune basis. The strongest evidence for an autoimmune disorder is for the Lambert–Eaton myasthenic syndrome in which autoantibodies inhibit the function of presynaptic calcium channels at the neuromuscular junction, resulting in weakness. Examination demonstrates an increase in muscle power after repetitive muscle contraction (the opposite of myasthenia gravis), and absent deep tendon reflexes. These findings, along with autonomic and sensory complaints of dry mouth, impotence, and thigh paresthesias, point to a nerve disorder. Electrodiagnostic tests of repetitive nerve stimulation reveal an increasing amplitude of the muscle action potential that is pathognomonic. Several other paraneoplastic syndromes are associated with the presence of specific antibodies, including subacute sensory neuronopathy, limbic encephalitis, subacute cerebellar degeneration, and gammopathy associated neuropathies. These specific antibodies serve as markers that not only identify the syndrome as paraneoplastic, but suggest the site of the underlying tumor.[8] The antibodies have not been proved to have an etiologic role in the pathogenesis of such syndromes.

A variety of therapies directed at immunomodulation, including plasmapheresis, corticosteroids and intravenous immunoglobin, have failed to reverse the neurologic impairment associated with paraneoplastic disorders. The exception is the LEMs, which responds well to immunosuppressive treatments. Some patients with paraneoplastic neurologic disorders have reversal or stabilization of their neurologic dysfunction when the underlying malignancy is treated effectively and this should be a therapeutic priority for all of these patients.

Table 124-13 **Paraneoplastic Neurologic Syndromes**

Syndrome	Associated Cancer[a]	Clinical Features
Brain		
Limbic encephalopathy[b]	SCLC	Depression, memory loss, confusion, abnormal CSF
Brainstem encephalopathy[b]	SCLC	Ataxia, cranial nerve dysfunction, corticospinal dysfunction, abnormal CSF
Subacute cerebellar degeneration	Breast, ovary, SCLC, Hodgkin	Ataxia, dysarthria, nystagmus, normal CSF
Opsoclonus, myoclonus	Lung	Jerky, irregular movements of eyes and skeletal muscles
Optic neuritis, retinal degeneration	SCLC	Painless loss of vision, transient visual obscuration
Spinal cord		
Necrotizing myelopathy	SCLC, lymphoma, leukemia	Ascending myelopathy
Subacute motor neuronopathy	Hodgkin and NHL	Patchy weakness, atrophy, and fasciculations
Dorsal root ganglia		
Subacute sensory neuronopathy[b]	SCLC	Dysesthesias, sensory ataxia, areflexia
Peripheral nerve		
Gammopathy associated neuropathy	Myeloma	Sensory loss, weakness, reflex loss
Acute polyradiculitis (Guillain–Barré)	Lymphoma	No cells in CSF; high CSF protein
Neuromuscular junction		
Lambert-Eaton myasthenic syndrome	SCLC	Proximal weakness, decreased reflexes, ocular muscles spared
Myasthenia gravis	Thymoma	Weakness, ocular muscles often involved
Muscle		
Dermatomyositis, polymyositis	Lung, breast, ovary, GI	Weakness, elevated CPK

[a]The most commonly associated tumors are listed.
[b]Often occur in association with each other.
Abbreviations: CPK, creatine phosphokinase; CSF, cerebrospinal fluid; GI, gastrointestinal; NHL, non-Hodgkin lymphoma; SCLC, small-cell lung cancer.

Selected References

The complete reference list can be found at www.CANCERMEDICINE8.com

1. DeAngelis LM, Posner JB. *Neurologic Complications of Cancer*, 2nd ed. New York: Oxford Press; 2008.
2. Lin NU, Winer EP. Brain metastases: the HER2 paradigm. *Clin Cancer Res.* 2007;13:1648–1655.
3. Schiff D, Kesari S, Wen PY, eds. *Cancer Neurology in Clinical Practice. Neurologic Complications of Cancer and Its Treatment*, 2nd ed. Totowa, New Jersey: Humana Press; 2007.
5. Osborn JL, Getzenberg RH, Trump DL. Spinal cord compression in prostate cancer. *J Neurooncol.* 1995;23:135–147.
7. Levi M, ten Cate H. Review articles: disseminated intravascular coagulation. *N Engl J Med.* 1999;341:586–592.
8. Darnell RB, Posner JB. Paraneoplastic syndromes affecting the nervous system. *Semin Oncol.* 2006;33:270–298.
9. Abrahm JL, ACP ASIM End Life Care Consensus Panel. Management of pain and spinal cord compression in patients with advanced cancer. *Ann Intern Med.* 1999;131:37–46.
10. Solberg A, Bremnes RM. Metastatic spinal cord compression: diagnostic delay, treatment, and outcome. *Anticancer Res.* 1999;19:677–684.
11. Helweg-Larsen S, Sorensen PS, Kreiner S. Prognostic factors in metastatic spinal cord compression: a prospective study using multivariate analysis of variables influencing survival and gait function in 153 patients. *Int J Radiat Oncol Biol Phys.* 2000;46:1163–1169.
12. Kovner F, Spigel S, Rider I, et al. Radiation therapy of metastatic spinal cord compression—multidisciplinary team diagnosis and treatment. *J Neurooncol.* 1999;42:85–92.
13. Cole JS, Patchell RA. Metastatic epidural spinal cord compression. *Lancet Neurol.* 2008;7:459–466.
17. Wang JC, Boland P, Mitra N, et al. Single-stage posterolateral transpedicular approach for resection of epidural metastatic spine tumors involving the vertebral body with circumferential reconstruction: results in 140 patients. Invited submission from the Joint Section Meeting on Disorders of the Spine and Peripheral Nerves, March 2004. *J Neurosurg Spine.* 2004;1:287–298.
19. Johnson AJ, Ying J, El Gammal T, Timmerman RD, Kim RY, Littenberg B. Which MR imaging sequences are necessary in determining the need for radiation therapy for cord compression? A prospective study. *AJNR Am J Neuroadiol.* 2007;28:32–37.
20. Venkitaraman R, Sohaib SA, Barbachano Y, et al. Detection of occult spinal cord compression with magnetic resonance imaging of the spine. *Clin Oncol.* 2007;19:528–531.
21. Loblaw DA, Laperriere NJ. Emergency treatment of malignant extradural spinal cord compression: an evidence-based guideline. *J Clin Oncol.* 1998;16:1613–1624.
24. Sorensen PS, Helweg-Larsen S, Mouridsen H, Hansen HH. Effect of high-dose dexamethasone in carcinomatous metastatic spinal cord compression treated with radiotherapy: a randomized trial. *Eur J Cancer.* 1994;30A:22–27.
27. Yamada Y, Bilsky MH, Lovelock DM, et al. High-dose, single fraction image-guided intensity-modulated radiotherapy for metastatic spinal lesions. *Int J Radiat Oncol Biol Phys.* 2008;71:484–490.
28. Bilsky M, Smith M. Surgical approach to epidural spinal cord compression. *Hematol Oncol Clin North Am.* 2006;20:307–317.
29. Patchell R, Tibbs PA, Regine WF, et al. Direct decompressive surgical resection in the treatment of spinal cord compression caused by metastatic cancer: a randomised trial. *Lancet.* 2005;366:643–648.
33. Trinh QD, Cardinal E, Gallina A, Perrotte P, Saad F, Karakiewicz PI. Sunitinib relieves renal cell carcinoma spinal cord compression. *Eur Urol.* 2007;51:1741–1743.
34. Wong ET, Portlock CS, O'Brien JP, DeAngelis LM. Chemosensitive epidural spinal cord disease in nonHodgkin's lymphoma. *Neurology.* 1996;46:1543–1547.
36. Van der Ree TC, Dippel DWJ, Avezaat CJJ, et al. Leptomeningeal metastasis after surgical resection of brain metastases. *J Neurol Neurosurg Psychiatr.* 1999;66:225–227.
40. Chamberlain MC, Kormanik PA, Glantz MJ. A comparison between ventricular and lumbar cerebrospinal fluid cytology in adult patients with leptomeningeal metastases. *J Neurooncol.* 2001;3:42–45.
44. Gray JR, Wallner KE. Reversal of cranial nerve dysfunction with radiation therapy in adults with lymphoma and leukemia. *Int J Radiat Oncol Biol Phys.* 1990;19:439–444.
47. Mason WP, Yeh SD, DeAngelis LM. 1 1 1Indium-diethylenetriamine pentaacetic acid cerebrospinal fluid flow studies predict distribution of intrathecally administered chemotherapy and outcome in patients with leptomeningeal metastases. *Neurology.* 1998;50:438–444.
48. Ekenel M, Hormigo AM, Peak S, DeAngelis LM, Abrey LE. Capecitabine therapy of central nervous system metastases from breast cancer. *J Neurooncol.* 2007;85:223–227.
49. Ranze O, Hofmann E, Distelrath A, Hoeffkes HG. Renal cell cancer presented with leptomeningeal carcinomatosis effectively treated with sorafenib. *Onkologie.* 2007;30:450–451.
51. Groves MD, Glantz MJ, Chamberlain MC, et al. A multicenter phase II trial of intrathecal topotecan in patients with meningeal malignancies. *Neurooncol.* 2008;10:208–215.
52. Bernardi RJ, Bomgaars L, Fox E, et al. Phase I clinical trial of intrathecal gemcitabine in patients with neoplastic meningitis. *Cancer Chemother Pharmacol.* 2007 [Epub ahead of print].
54. Sandberg DI, Bilsky MH, Souweidane MM, et al. Ommaya reservoirs for the treatment of leptomeningeal metastases. *Neurosurgery.* 2000;47:49–54.
60. Jaeckle KA. Neurological manifestations of neoplastic and radiation-induced plexopathies. *Semin Neurol.* 2004;24:385–393.
61. Johansson S, Svensson H, Denekamp J. Dose response and latency for radiation-induced fibrosis, edema, and neuropathy in breast cancer patients. *Int J Radiat Oncol Biol Phys.* 2002;52:1207–1219.
66. Jaeckle KA, Young DF, Foley KM. The natural history of lumbosacral plexopathy in cancer. *Neurology.* 1985;35:8–15.
70. Dettmeyer R, Driever F, Becker A, et al. Fatal myeloencephalopathy due to accidental intrathecal vincristine administration: a report of two cases. *Forensic Sci Int.* 2001;122:60–64.
71. Gillies J, Hung KA, Fitzsimons E, Soutar R. Severe vincristine toxicity in combination with itraconazole. *Clin Lab Haematol.* 1998;20:123–124.
72. Hildebrandt G, Holler E, Woenkhaus M, et al. Acute deterioration of Charcot–Marie–Tooth disease IA (CMT IA) following 2 mg of vincristine chemotherapy. *Ann Oncol.* 2000;11:743–747.
73. Rezvani K, Bain BJ, Coulter CA. Loss of singing ability caused by vincristine. *Clin Lab Haematol.* 1998;20:47–48.
78. Stone JA, Castillo M, Mukherji SK. Leukoencephalopathy complicating an Ommaya reservoir and chemotherapy. *Neuroradiology.* 1999;41:134–136.
82. Wilson RH, Lehky T, Thomas RR, et al. Acute oxaliplatin induced peripheral nerve hyperexcitability. *J Clin Oncol.* 2002;20:1767–1774.
84. Argyriou AA, Koltzenburg M, Polychronopoulos P, Papapetropoulos S, Kalofonos HP. Peripheral nerve damage associated with administration of taxanes in patients with cancer. *Crit Rev Oncol Hematol.* 2008;66:218–228.
87. Smith GA, Damon LE, Rugo HS, et al. High-dose cytarabine dose modification reduces the incidence of neurotoxicity in patients with renal insufficiency. *J Clin Oncol.* 1997;15:833–839.
89. O'Connor OA, Wright J, Moskowitz C, et al. Phase II clinical experience with the novel proteasome inhibitor bortezomib in patients with indolent non-Hodgkin's lymphoma and mantle cell lymphoma. *J Clin Oncol.* 2005;23:676–684.
91. Russell MT, Nassif AS, Cacayorin ED, et al. Gemcitabine associated posterior reversible encephalopathy syndrome: MR imaging and MR spectroscopy findings. *Magn Reson Imaging* 2001;19;129–132.
93. Belka C, Budach W, Kortmann R, Bamberg M. Radiation induced CNS toxicity—molecular and cellular mechanisms. *Br J Cancer.* 2001;85(9):1233–1239.
95. Steen RG, Spence D, Wu SJ, Xiong XP, et al. Effect of therapeutic ionizing radiation on the human brain. *Ann Neurol.* 2001;50:787–795.
96. Regine WF, Scott C, Murray K, Curran W. Neurocognitive outcome in brain metastases patients treated with accelerated-fractionation vs accelerated-hyperfractionated radiotherapy: an analysis from Radiation Therapy Oncology Group study 91-04. *Int J Radiat Oncol Biol Phys.* 2001;51:711–717.
97. Duffey P, Chari G, Cartlidge NEF, Shaw PJ. Progressive deterioration of intellect and motor function occurring several decades after cranial irradiation—a new facet in the clinical spectrum of radiation encephalopathy. *Arch Neurol.* 1996;53:814–818.
98. Ruben JD, Daily M, Bailey M, Smith, McLean A, Fedele P. Cerebral radiation necrosis: incidence, outcomes, and risk factors with emphasis on radiation parameters and chemotherapy. *Int J Radiat Oncol Biol Phys.* 2006;65:499–508.
112. Raizer JJ, DeAngelis LM. Cerebral sinus thrombosis in cancer patients. *Neurology.* 2000;54:1222–1226.
113. Cestari DM, Weine DM, Panageas KS, Segal AZ, DeAngelis LM. Stroke in patients with cancer. Incidence and etiology. *Neurology.* 2004;62:2025–2030.
117. Tuma R, DeAngelis LM. Altered mental status in patients with cancer. *Arch Neurol.* 2000;57:1727–1731.

125 Dermatologic Complications of Cancer Chemotherapy

Cindy Berthelot, MD ■ Joy H. Kunishige, MD ■ Narin Apisarnthanarax, MD ■ Madeleine M. Duvic, MD

Dermatologic complications of cancer chemotherapy have become increasingly significant, especially with the continued development of new antineoplastic agents. The frequency of mucocutaneous complications in cancer chemotherapy is a reflection of the increased proliferative nature of affected tissues, such as the mucous membranes, skin, hair, and nails, which renders them particularly susceptible to the actions of chemotherapeutic drugs. Diagnosis of cutaneous reactions in the cancer patient is complicated by the degree of their malignancy, concomitant diseases, polypharmacy, and immunosuppression. With the advances in bone marrow transplantation, graft vs host disease (GVHD) is also being seen more frequently and may mimic and complicate the diagnosis of chemotherapy-induced reactions. Thirteen major cutaneous reactions and a variety of miscellaneous reactions are discussed in this chapter and are listed in Table 125-1. As seen in Table 125-2, these reactions occur in varying degrees of frequency and severity among the classes of chemotherapeutic drugs. Although dermatologic complications are rarely fatal, it is important to recognize potential reactions as they may result in significant morbidity, cosmetic disfigurement, and psychological distress. Proper treatment of potentially dose limiting cutaneous toxicity may also allow ideal schedules of chemotherapy administration, and optimization of response.

Table 125-1 ■ Major Cutaneous Reactions Associated With Chemotherapy

1. Alopecia
2. Stomatitis
3. Nail reactions
4. Extravasation reactions
5. Hyperpigmentation
6. Radiation-associated reactions
7. Photosensitivity
8. Inflammation of keratoses
9. Hypersensitivity
10. Acral erythema
11. Neutrophilic eccrine hidradenitis
12. Eccrine squamous syringometaplasia
13. Cutaneous eruption of lymphocyte recovery
14. Miscellaneous reactions

Alopecia

Alopecia is the most common dermatologic complication associated with chemotherapy. Whereas most drug-induced alopecias involve a telogen effluvium pattern by inducing normal hairs into a premature resting phase, the anagen effluvium pattern of hair loss is the most common type of alopecia produced by chemotherapeutic agents, with the exception of interleukin-2 (IL-2) and interferon-α (IFN-α) therapy. In chemotherapy, anagen effluvium is caused by the abrupt cessation of the high mitotic activity of hair matrix cells in the anagen phase of hair follicles.[1] This type of alopecia can be seen to some degree in most antineoplastic therapies, depending on dosage and route of administration.[2,3] However, there are certain agents, such as doxorubicin, which induce alopecia more frequently and severely (Table 125-3).[2-6] These agents display a synergistic effect when used in combination and may cause severe and complete alopecia.[6] Anagen effluvium manifests within 1-2 weeks after the beginning of chemotherapy but is most noticeable 1-2 months later.[3] Initially, there may not be total hair loss, since approximately 10% of follicles will not be in anagen phase at the start of chemotherapy. However, total hair loss eventually occurs with prolonged therapy, which can also induce hair loss in other areas of the body. Hair regrowth can usually be expected 5 months after the end of chemotherapy, although hair color and texture may change.[7] Permanent alopecia has been reported with busulfan/cyclophosphamide therapy.[8]

Hair loss often has emotional impact on patients receiving chemotherapy. Unfortunately, there are currently no widely accepted methods of prevention and treatment for alopecia. To prevent alope-

Table 125-2 ■ Most Common Mucocutaneous Reactions of the Major Classes of Chemotherapeutic Drugs

Alkylating Agents	Antibiotics
Hyperpigmentation Hypersensitivity	Alopecia Stomatitis Chemical cellulitis Hyperpigmentation Radiation-associated reactions
Vinca Alkaloids	**Antimetabolites**
Alopecia Chemical cellulitis Inflammation of keratoses Neutrophilic eccrine hidradenitis	Acral erythema Alopecia Hyperpigmentation Radiation-associated reactions

Table 125-3 ■ Chemotherapeutic Agents Associated With Alopecia

Most Common or Severe		Least Common or Severe	
Bleomycin	Ifosfamide	Amsacrine	Melphalan
Cisplatin	Interferon-a	Busulfan	Mercaptopurine
Cyclophosphamide	Irinotecan	Carboplatin	Methotrexate
Cytarabine	Mechlorethamine	Carmustine	Mitomycin
Dacarbazine	Nitrosoureas	Chlorambucil epirubicin	Procarbazine
Dactinomycin	Paclitaxel	Gemcitabine	Teniposide
Daunorubicin	Thiotepa	Hydroxyurea	Vinorelbine
Docetaxel	Topotecan		
Doxorubicin	Vinblastine		
Etoposide	Vincristine		
Fluorouracil	Vindesine		
Idarubicin			

Source: Adapted from Ref. 5.

cia, scalp hypothermia and tourniquets have been used with some demonstrated success. Drugs such as doxorubicin, vincristine, vinblastine, dactinomycin, and mechlorethamine, which have short administration periods and half-lives, are particularly well suited for scalp hypothermia.[2] Despite a reported 47% rate of success in preservation of hair, scalp cooling has been controversial. Widespread use of hypothermia has been limited by the possibility that the decreased scalp perfusion and thereby decreased drug exposure could increase the risk of scalp metastasis in certain patients with solid tumors.[7,9] However, confirmatory reports of this risk are lacking.[9] In patients with hematologic malignancies, scalp hypothermia is contraindicated. A small group of women with breast cancer applied topical 2% minoxidil and reported hastened regrowth (duration of alopecia decreased by an average of 50 days); unfortunately, the drug has no preventative effect.[10] Other therapies under investigation include cyclosporine A, FK506, 1,25-dihydroxyvitamin D3 and parathyroid hormone antagonists.

Stomatitis

Stomatitis and other oral complications of cancer chemotherapy are discussed in Chapters 132: Gastrointestinal Complications and Chapter 133: Oral Complications.

Nail Reactions

Hyperpigmentation is the most common nail abnormality encountered in patients receiving chemotherapy, particularly in dark-skinned patients.[2] Vertical bands, horizontal bands, or diffuse hyperpigmentation of nails has been associated with the following medications: bleomycin, cyclophosphamide, daunorubicin, doxorubicin, fluorouracil, hydroxyurea, aminoglutethimide, busulfan, cisplatin, dacarbazine, docetaxel, idarubicin, ifosfamide, melphalan, methotrexate, mitomycin, and mitoxantrone (Fig. 125-1).[5] Hyperpigmentation due to chemotherapy-induced melanocyte stimulation should be distinguished from yellow nail syndrome (YNS). YNS nails have increased transverse curvature, absent lunulae, and no cuticle. Suggested etiologies include paraneoplastic process, AIDS-association, and drug-induction.[12]

Other common nail manifestations include horizontal depressions of the nail plate scalled Beauís lines (Fig. 125-2), horizontal white discoloration of the entire width of the nail plate called Mees lines,

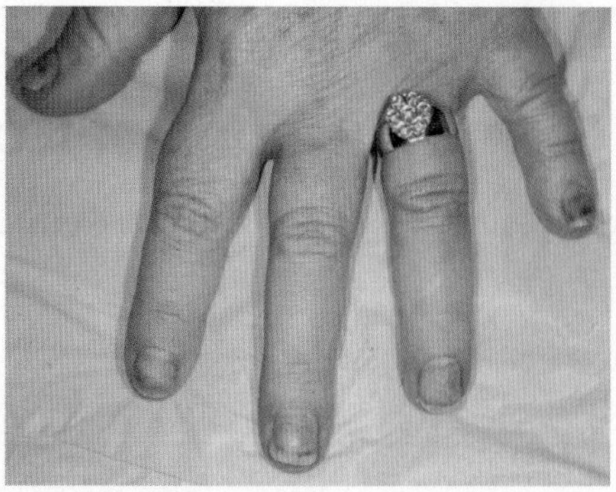

Figure 125-1 Docetaxel-induced nail hyperpigmentation and onychodystrophy.

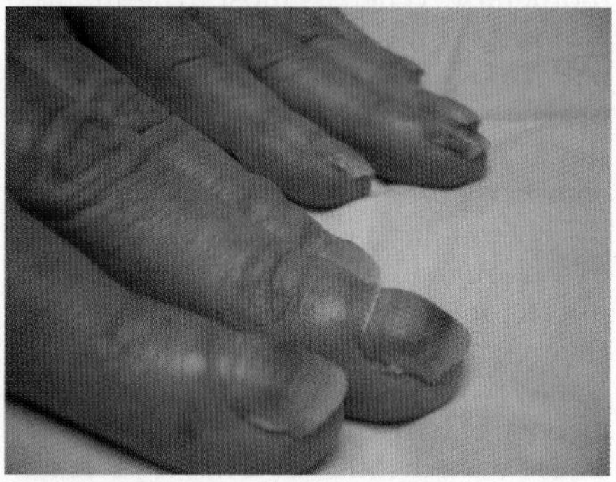

Figure 125-2 Hyperpigmentation and Beauís lines.

horizontal white discoloration involving partial nail width called leukonychia, onycholysis, and onychodystrophy. Associations between bleomycin and nail loss; hydroxyurea and brittle nails; etoposide and nail bed pigmentation have also been reported in the literature.[2,5] Other onychopathies and their associated chemoagents are summarized in Table 125-4. Patients can be reassured that these nail changes are generally benign and resolve after discontinuation of the causative agent and the affected nails grow out. However, nails damaged by chemotherapy are more susceptible to infection by yeast, dermatophytes, and pseudomonas. Infections may cause lasting damage to the matrix that will not resolve.

Extravasation Reactions

Extravasation injury is a well-known adverse event that occurs when offending drugs escape from the veins or intravenous catheters into subcutaneous tissues. Accidental extravasation occurs in approximately 0.1-6% of patients receiving intravenous chemotherapy.[13] Cancer patients are inherently at high risk of extravasation for three reasons. First, these patients often require multiple venipuncture sites and have thin and fragile veins. Second, they may have concomitant peripheral vascular disease and be malnourished. Third, the number of optimal intravenous sites may be reduced due to previous chemotherapy, radiation therapy, or surgery-related lymphedema.[2,14] The cutaneous manifestations of extravasation may range from discomfort and mild erythema to severely painful skin necrosis, ulcerations, and damage to deep tissue structures.

Nerve and tendon damage leads to neurologic deficits, contractures, and joint stiffness. The extent of tissue damage in extravasation largely depends on the concentration, volume, and vesicant nature of the extravasated agent.[13,14]

Extravasated cytotoxic agents generally cause two types of local cutaneous reactions: irritant and vesicant reactions. Irritants cause a shortlived and self-limited phlebitis and tender, warm, erythematous reaction along the vein or at the site of intravenous administration. A variant of this local irritation is an erythematous and urticarial hypersensitivity flare reaction that has been associated with the anthracyclines. Vesicants initially cause a similar reaction; however the irritation may worsen, depending on the amount of drug that has extravasated.

Whereas small-volume extravasations cause limited erythema that resolves over a few weeks, large-volume extravasations may induce necrosis within a matter of days. Eschars are fol-

Table 125-4 Summary of Nail Abnormalities and Associated Chemoagents

Onychopathy	Associated Chemoagents
Beau's lines	Taxanes, bleomycin, cisplatin, doxorubicin, melphalan, vincristine
Transverse leukonychia	Adriamycin
Muehrcke lines	Doxorubicin, cyclophosphamide, vincristine, leucovorin, levamisole, methotrexate
Onycholysis	Taxanes, doxorubicin, fluorouracil, mitoxantrone, bleomycin,
Onychomadesis, defluvium unguium	Taxanes, bleomycin, fluorouracil, mercaptopurine, mitoxantrone
Ischemic changes	Bleomycin, taxanes doxorubicin methotrexate nitrogen mustard etoposide cyclophosphamide busulfan melphalan
Melanonychia	
Non-melanotic pigmentation	5-FU
Acute paronychia	Methotrexate taxanes
Pyogenic granuloma	Cetuximab (C225), gefitinib (Iressa)

Table 125-5 Chemotherapeutic Agents Associated With Chemical Cellulitis

Most Common	Least Common		
Dactinomycin	Amsacrine	Esorubicin	Plicamycin
Daunorubicin	Bisantrene	Etoposide	Pyrazofurin
Doxorubicin	Bleomycin	Fluorouracil	Streptozocin
Mitomycin	Carmustine	Idarubicin	Vinblastine
	Chlorozotocin	Melphalan	Vincristine
	Cisplatin	Mechlorethamine	Vindesine
	Dacarbazine	Mitoxantrone	Vinorelbine
	Epirubicin	Paclitaxel	

lowed by painful ulcerations with red, raised edges. Antibiotics, such as doxorubicin, dactinomycin, daunorubicin, and mitomycin, are the most common, potent, and well documented vesicants (Table 125-5). Though almost all vesicants cause some degree of irritation on a spectrum of injury, carboplatin, cyclophosphamide, docetaxel, ifosfamide, menogaril, and thiotepa are known to produce irritation.[5] Paclitaxel can induce an extravasation recall reaction, in which extravasation of the agent at one site has induced a cutaneous reaction, ranging from erythema to ulcerations, at a previous extravasation site.[15] Drug administration through central venous catheters (CVCs) is less prone to extravasation; however, central lines may dislodge, or venous vessels may be perforated with potentially disastrous consequences, including mediastinitis.[16] Thus, CVC extravasation should be considered in the setting of fever, severe pleuritic pain, upper extremity and neck swelling, and a widened mediastinum.

Vesicant injury is sometimes referred to as chemical cellulitis. It displays poor healing and often continues to worsen, necessitating surgical intervention.[14] Vesicants delay fibroblastic wound contraction and have the ability to bind to DNA, possibly allowing them to be recycled and retained in the tissue to induce damage for a longer duration.[14]

As it has been estimated that about one-third of all vesicant extravasations will develop into ulcerations, vigilant recognition and management of extravasation plays a major role in limiting tissue injury.[17] When extravasation is suspected, prompt discontinuation of the infusion is recommended, followed by aspiration of residual drug and removal of the catheter. Local cold application and elevation of the affected extremity are commonly used and helpful.[14] Intermittent local cooling alone has an 89.1% success rate in preventing ulceration.[18] For the vinca alkaloids, heat application is recommended instead, as cold application may actually induce ulceration.[17]

The use of antidotes is controversial, and some antidotes such as sodium bicarbonate may be harmful or ulcerative. Sodium thiosulfate and hyaluronidase have been recommended for mechlorethamine and vinca alkaloids, respectively. The success of locally injected corticosteroids has also been variable. As few inflammatory cells are involved in extravasation reactions, these reactions may not be inflammatory and would not, hypothetically, benefit from locally injected corticosteroids.[19]

Locally injected granulocyte macrophage colony-stimulating factor, which has been used to promote healing of doxorubicin ulcerations, and pyridoxine, used to treat mitomycin extravasation, are both worthy of further study.[20,21] Whether a local antidote has a specific effect or acts as a diluent is hard to determine. Locally injected saline alone has proven successful in resolving extravasation reactions and preventing ulceration.[22] Although conservative treatment is preferable for most vesicant extravasations, early excision is sometimes favored, especially when the most potent vesicants are involved.[22,23] Surgical consultation for wide local excision and flap reconstruction is invariably necessary when ulcerations become evident, or if extravasation lesions prove unresponsive to therapy. For topical therapy, the free-radical scavenger dimethyl sulfoxide (DMSO) has shown consistent therapeutic success. In 1995, an analysis of 96 cumulative patients from multiple studies showed that DMSO protected 98.3% of extravasation cases from ulceration.[24]

Hyperpigmentation

Hyperpigmentation is a common cutaneous manifestation that may be of cosmetic concern to patients. The skin, mucous membranes, hair, teeth, and nails may be affected, and the reaction may be diffuse or localized. Hyperpigmentation most commonly accompanies use of alkylating agents, antitumor antibiotics, and gemcitabine (Table 125-6).[5] Agents commonly associated with oral mucosal hyperpigmentation include busulfan, fluorouracil, tegafur, doxorubicin, hydroxyurea, cisplatin, and cyclophosphamide.[5] Among the antimetabolites, methotrexate may produce a characteristic hair "flag sign" with horizontal hyperpigmented bands alternating with normal hair color in light-haired individuals.[5] Tegafur can induce hyperpigmentation of the palms, soles, nails, and glans penis in a third of patients receiving the drug. A flagellate, bandlike hyperpigmentation in areas of trauma also occurs with high incidence in 8-20% of patients receiving bleomycin (Fig. 125-3). Busulfanís hyperpigmentation can mimic Addison disease, with symptoms of weakness, weight loss, and diarrhea, but with normal melanocyte-stimulating hormone and adrenocorticotropic hormone serum levels.[7] Hyperpigmentation in areas of occlusion, such as cutaneous areas under electrocardiograph pads, tape, or dressings, with or without preceding erythema, has been reported with ifosfamide, topical carmustine, thiotepa, docetaxel, and combinations of etoposide and carboplatin with either cyclophosphamide or ifosfamide.[5] Finally, localized, serpentine, supravenous hyperpigmentation is often seen at the intravenous administration

Table 125-6 Chemotherapeutic Agents Associated With Hyperpigmentation

Alkylating Agents	Antibiotics	Nucleoside Analogues Antimetabolites	Miscellaneous Combined Regimens
Busulfan	Bleomycin	Fluorouracil	Bleomycin/doxorubicin/vincristine
Cisplatin	Dactinomycin	Methotrexate	Busulfan/cyclophosphamide
Cyclophosphamide	Daunorubicin	Tegafur	Cyclophosphamide/doxorubicin/vincris-tine/prednisone
Fotemustine	Doxorubicin	Brequinar sodium	Cyclophosphamide/etoposide/carboplatin
Ifosfamide	Mitoxantrone	Docetaxel	Doxorubicin/bleomycin/vinblastine/ dacarbazine
Thiotepa	Plicamycin	Hydroxyurea	Ifosfamide/carboplatin/etoposide
Topical carmustine	Gemcitabine	Procarbazine	Methotrexate/cytarabine/ lasparaginase/daunorubicin/ mercaptopurine/cyclophosphamide
Topical mechlor-ethamine	Troxacitabine	Vinorelbine	

Source: Adapted from Ref. 5.

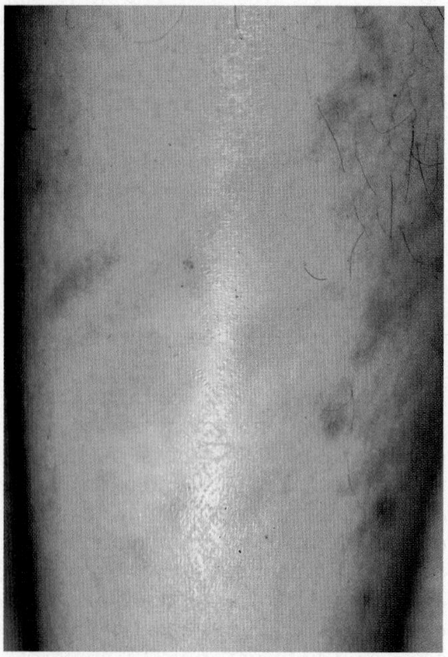

Figure 125-3 ■ Cutaneous flagellate hyperpigmentation of bleomycin.

sites of fotemustine, fluorouracil, vinorelbine, and various combined chemotherapy regimens. The mechanism of chemotherapy-induced hyperpigmentation reactions is currently unknown but may involve direct toxicity, melanocyte stimulation, and postinflammatory changes. Although these reactions may occasionally be permanent, in most cases, discoloration will gradually resolve after the discontinuation of the chemotherapy.

Radiation-Associated Reactions

With the widespread use of regimens combining chemotherapy and radiotherapy, two types of radiation-associated cutaneous reactions have been well described: radiation enhancement and radiation recall (Table 125-7). Radiation enhancement refers to the augmentation of radiation therapy effects, which may occur when both chemotherapy and radiation therapy are given within 1 week of each other. The agents most commonly involved include bleomycin, dactinomycin, doxorubicin, fluorouracil, hydroxyurea, and methotrexate. Although other organs are also affected in this potentiation, the skin is the most common site of this toxicity. The reaction may appear as dry or moist desquamation, or as erythema and edema. When bullae, erosions, and ulcerations accompany erythema, *Staphylococcus* is usually the causative factor.[25] The degree of enhancement of radiation damage depends on, and is inversely related to, the time interval between administration of the drug and radiation. The less time there is between chemotherapy and irradiation, the greater the enhancement effect.[26] Enhancement is also dependent on drug dosage and the pharmacologic mechanism of the drug.[2]

Radiation recall is an erythematous inflammatory reaction in areas of previously irradiated skin. Severe radiation dermatitis can even spread to areas outside the portal as an id reaction. Radiation recall occurs from 8 days up to 15 years after radiation therapy and may also occur in other organs.[5] The most commonly associated agents are the antitumor antibiotics dactinomycin and doxorubicin.[27] Other agents are less frequently the culprit of radiation recall, including the new nucleoside analogue gemcitabine.[28,29] The radiation dosage and the time interval between radiation and chemotherapy determine the occurrence and severity of recall, respectively.[27]

The mechanism of the recall reaction is currently unknown, although it has been theorized that impaired tissue repair may be a result of inadequate stem cell reserve or mutations in cells that survived radiation.[30] Generally, the treatment for radiation-associated reactions is symptomatic with an effort to avoid or treat secondary infections with appropriate antibiotics. Severe ulcerative and necrotic reactions may necessitate debridement. Topical mupirocin and systemic corticosteroids are mainstays in the treatment of radiation recall, and may even allow continuation of the offending drug without further recall effects.[30]

Table 125-7 ■ **Chemotherapeutic Agents Implicated in Radiation-Associated Reactions**

Radiation Enhancement	Radiation Recall	
Bleomycin	Bleomycin	Hydroxyurea
Camptothecins	Cyclophosphamide	Idarubicin
Chlorambucil	Cytarabine	Lomustine
Cisplatin[a]	Dactinomycin	Melphalan
Cyclophosphamide[a]	Daunorubicin	Methotrexate
Dactinomycin	Doxorubicin	Oxaliplatin
Doxorubicin	Docetaxel	Paclitaxel
Fluorouracil	Edatrexate	Tamoxifen
Hydroxyurea	Etoposide	Triazinate
Interferons	Fluorouracil	Trimetrexate
Mercaptopurine	Gemcitabine	Vinblastine
Methotrexate		
Triazinate		
Vincristine[a]		

[a]Reported only in combination drug regimens.
Source: Adapted from Ref. 5.

Photosensitivity Reactions

Cutaneous reactions related to chemotherapy and ultraviolet (UV) light exposure have been well documented, though they are relatively infrequent. Generally, most of these reactions involve exogenous phototoxicity with the agents acting as chromophores. Dacarbazine, fluorouracil, methotrexate, and vinblastine are the most common phototoxic antineoplastic agents (Table 125-8).[31] Both clinically and histologically, these phototoxic reactions appear as exaggerated sunburns. Phototoxicity has also been reported to affect the nails in the form of mercaptopurine-induced photo-onycholysis, which is tender and usually involves the distal third of the nail. Hussain and colleagues reported onycholysis in five patients receiving paclitaxel that resolved when nails were shielded from the sun.[32]

Another form of photosensitivity is the photoallergy that has been described with flutamide and tegafur, in which the cutaneous reaction recurs with readministration of the implicated agent.

A third type of photosensitivity, the UV recall reaction, is observed with suramin (35% incidence), methotrexate, and etoposide/cyclophosphamide therapy, which causes a sunburn reactivation if the drugs are administered within 1 week of obtaining a sunburn.[33] Photosensitivity is suspected when an eruption involves sun-exposed areas. Susceptibility to phototoxic reactions depends on both host and environmental factors and is hard to predict, with the exception of porphyrin drugs, such as hematoporphyrin derivative (74% incidence) and photofrin polypophyrin (20-40% incidence).[31,34,35] Therapy for photosensitivity reactions is symptomatic with topical corticosteroids and antipruritics. Severe cases may require systemic steroids. Chloroquine and beta carotene

Table 125-8 ■ **Chemotherapeutic Agents Associated With Phototoxicity**

Brequinar sodium	Methotrexate
Dacarbazine	Mitomycin C
Dactinomycin	Porphyrins
Doxorubicin	Procarbazine
Fluorouracil	Tegafur
Flutamide	Thioguanine
Hydroxyurea	Vinblastine

have been used for prophylaxis but were not effective in controlled studies.[36] Besides, as the agent may remain in the patientís skin for several weeks, patients should be advised to take sun-avoidance measures.

Inflammation of Keratoses

Several chemotherapeutic agents (Table 125-9) have been known to induce inflammation of preexisting skin disease. Inflammation of actinic keratoses (AKs) is known as an AK recall reaction and is common in elderly patients with fair complexion and history of sun damage. Suramin and cytarabine-induced inflammation of seborrheic keratosis and fludarabine-induced squamous cell carcinoma have also been reported. The association between systemic fluorouracil and the irritation of clinical and subclinical AKs is well- known and resembles the effect produced by topical application of 5-fluorouracil (5-FU). AK recall reactions usually appear 1 week following the initiation of drug administration; reactions usually resolve 1-4 weeks following the end of therapy, although they may regress during therapy as well.[37] This recall reaction may be due to a process similar to radiation recall or increased DNA synthesis in AK lesions and consequently higher chemoagent uptake.[37,38] Although these lesions are self-limiting, superficial ulceration and staphylococcal colonization can occur and necessitate antibiotics or corticosteroids. The reaction may or may not recur with drug readministration. Similar to the effect of topical 5-FU on AKs, systemic fluorouracil often clears the affected AKs after the inflammatory reaction resolves.[39]

Hypersensitivity Reactions

Hypersensitivity reactions, mediated by types I, II, III, and IV immune-mediated allergy, can become dose limiting and are reported with most chemotherapeutic drugs. Although they are generally infrequent, these reactions occur more commonly with L-asparaginase, paclitaxel, docetaxel, teniposide, cisplatin (intravesical), procarbazine, and cytarabine.[40]

The only cytotoxic drugs without reported hypersensitivity when used as single agents are the nitrosoureas, vinca alkaloids, altretamine, and dactinomycin.[40]

Most reactions involve type I hypersensitivity with associated urticaria, angioedema, flushing, and pruritus. Severe anaphylactic reactions also occur, frequently causing shock, hypotension, and, occasionally, death.

L-asparaginase is most commonly associated with hypersensitivity, occurring in 10-25% of patients receiving the drug.[40] Hypersensitivity occurs less frequently when the drug is given in combination drug regimens, especially with vincristine and prednisone.[41] In up to 40% of patients, paclitaxel and docetaxel induce mild rashes and flushing, although premedication with antihistamines and corticosteroids reduces this frequency. Intravesically administered cisplatin in patients with bladder cancer seems to be more allergenic than when the drug is given intravenously and occurs with a 20% incidence.[42]

Maculopapular rashes are the most common manifestation of procarbazine hypersensitivity, although urticaria and angioedema, and type III hypersensitivity with immune complex deposition, manifesting as toxic epidermal necrolysis, may also occur. Maculopapular rash is also the most common manifestation of cytarabine type I hypersensitivity (5-30% incidence). The cytarabine syndrome presents with high fever, rigors, myalgia, arthralgias, and a diffuse erythematous maculopapular rash, and is postulated to be a type III hypersensitivity reaction.[43,44] Hypersensitivity reactions are generally responsive to corticosteroid therapy.

Acral Erythema

Acral erythema (AE) was first reported in association with chemotherapy by Zuehlke in 1974.[45] Other names include palmoplantar erythrodysesthesia, palmoplantar erythema, hand-foot syndrome, peculiar AE, and Burgdorf reaction. It commonly occurs with fluorouracil, capecitabine, cytarabine, clofarabine,[46] and doxorubicin and doxil (Table 125-10). There is a prodrome of dysesthesia of the palms and soles, evolving into painful, tingling, symmetric, well-demarcated swelling and erythema (Fig. 125-4), followed by a desquamative phase on resolution. Erythema and swelling usually appear on the thenar and hypothenar eminences, lateral aspect of the fingers, and the pads of the distal phalanges. The hands are more often affected than the feet. In its various manifestations, AE may appear as alternating bands of erythema and sparing and may also be accompanied by a mild erythema or a morbilliform eruption on the trunk, neck, chest, scalp, and extremities.[47] Methotrexate and cytarabine can reportedly induce a bullous variant of AE, which may progress to full-thickness epidermal necrosis before resolving.[48]

AE occurs with an incidence of 6-42% in different series, and occurs mostly in adults.[46] AE appears to be dose-dependent on peak levels and total cumulative dose, as it occurs earlier and more severely after bolus infusions (24 h to 3 weeks), as compared with continuous low-dose administration (2-10 months).[47,49] AE tends to persist and worsen with further continuation of chemotherapy and may be dose limiting, as the associated pain may progress to become physically and functionally limiting. Cyclosporine infusions have been shown to worsen the pain, possibly due to the therapyís high alcohol content.[50] With long-term chemotherapy, reversible palmoplantar keratoderma can also develop.[51] Cessation of the causative agent will allow resolution of AE in 1-2 weeks, with desquamation and re-epithelialization (Fig. 125-5). AE may or may not recur with readministration. The treatment of AE is symptomatic, aimed at increasing tolerability to allow continued chemotherapy. Corticosteroids have shown variable success. Supportive treatment includes topical wound care, elevation, and pain medication. Similar to the concept of scalp hypothermia for alopecia, the cooling of hands and feet may help prevent AE.[49] Celecoxib, a cy-

Table 125-9 **Chemotherapeutic Agents Associated With Inflammation of Actinic Keratoses**

Dactinomycin/vincristine/dacarbazine
Docetaxel
Doxorubicin
Doxorubicin/cytarabine/thioguanine
Doxorubicin/vincristine
Fluorouracil
Fluorouracil/cisplatin
Pentostatin

Table 125-10 **Chemotherapeutic Agents Associated With Inflammation of Acral Erythema**

Most Common	Least Common		
Capecitabine	Cisplatin	Idarubicin	Paclitaxel
Cytarabine	Cyclophosphamide	Lomustine	Pegylated liposomal doxorubicin
Doxorubicin	Daunorubicin	Melphalan	Floxuridine
Fluorouracil	Docetaxel	Mercaptopurine	Suramin
	Doxifluridine	Methotrexate	Troxacitabine
	Etoposide	Mitomycin	Tegafur
	Hydroxyurea	Mitotane	Vincristine

Source: Adapted from Ref. 5.

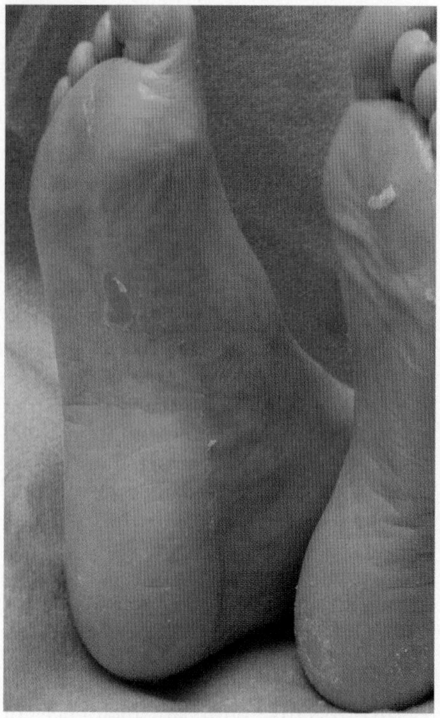

Figure 125-4 Chemo-induced acral erythema of the palms.

clooxygenase 2 (COX-2) inhibitor, was shown to decrease the incidence of AE in a retrospective study of 67 patients with metastatic colorectal cancer who took capecitabine.[52] Celecoxib also attenuated capecitabine-induced diarrhea, increased tumor response, and increased median time to tumor progression compared with capecitabine alone. Pyridoxine may also reduce dysesthesia and pain to allow continuation of therapy.[53]

The pathogenesis of AE is currently unknown, but it is likely multifactorial. Theories are based on the fact that the reaction is usually limited to the palms and soles. Temperature gradients, vascular anatomy, the existence of rapidly dividing epidermal cells, and high concentration of eccrine glands are characteristics of these regions of the body and may play a role in pathogenesis. It is conceivable that AE may be related to a direct toxic effect. Biopsies of AE appear histologically nonspecific but are consistent with a toxic reaction.[49] In the setting of chemotherapy, diagnosis of AE is a relatively simple matter. However in bone marrow transplant (BMT) patients, it may be difficult to differentiate from acute GVHD. There is a 35% incidence of AE in BMT patients, which may be due to the use of higher doses of chemotherapy and total body irradiation.[54] There is a 10-80% incidence of acute GVHD in BMT patients, depending on degree of histoincompatibility between donor and recipient, the number of T cells in the graft, the patient's age, and the GVHD prophylactic regimen.[55] Histologically and clinically, AE may resemble acute GVHD in the first 3 weeks: As in AE, the palms are commonly affected in acute GVHD although it usually progresses with involvement of other areas of the body. Since early biopsies of acute GVHD mimic AE, serial biopsies at 3 to 5-day intervals are helpful in establishing patterns of progression supportive of acute GVHD.[54] Distinguishing AE from acute GVHD is important because the latter requires greater intervention with further immunosuppression; without treatment it usually progresses and may be fatal.

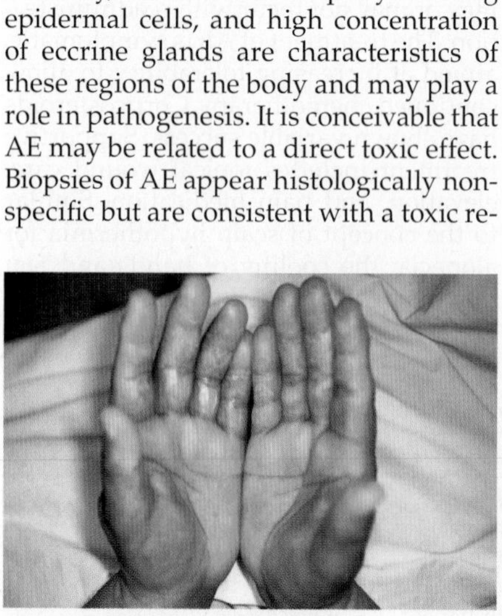

Figure 125-5 Desquamation phase of hand-and-foot syndrome, secondary to capectabine.

Neutrophilic Eccrine Hidradenitis

Neutrophilic eccrine hidradenitis (NEH) has been associated with a variety of drugs and conditions including zidovudine, acetaminophen, granulocyte colony-stimulating factor, infections, and acute myelogenous leukemia.[5,56,57] NEH is most often observed with chemotherapy, and cytarabine is most frequently cited along with bleomycin, chlorambucil, cyclophosphamide, doxorubicin, lomustine, and mitoxantrone.[5]

NEH manifests as erythematous to violaceous macules, papules, plaques, nodules, and pustules, which may be multiple or solitary, and painful or asymptomatic. Unusual presentations occur with involvement of the ears or periorbital inflammation.[57,58] NEH usually begins 2 days to 3 weeks following the initiation of chemotherapy, although it may occur as long as 2 years following therapy.[5] Fever may also accompany the reaction. Given the clinical variability of NEH, a skin biopsy is required for diagnosis. The histopathology shows necrosis of eccrine epithelial cells, and neutrophilic infiltrates centered on eccrine sweat glands and ducts, and possibly apocrine glands.[54] In neutropenic patients, these neutrophilic infiltrates may be sparse. Electron microscopic studies by Brehler and colleagues plus evidence of chemotherapeutic drug levels in sweat in a study by Madsen support the theory that chemotherapy-induced NEH is caused by direct toxicity of the sweat glands.[59,60] NEH is self-limited and resolves spontaneously without scarring within 1-4 weeks after the cessation of therapy. However, there is a 60% recurrence rate with the readministration of the same drug or regimen.[5] Although therapy is rarely needed for NEH, treatment with ibuprofen and corticosteroids may alleviate the discomfort of fever and painful lesions. Dapsone, which has effects on neutrophil migration, has successfully prevented the recurrence of NEH in a case report.[58]

Eccrine Squamous Syringometaplasia

Eccrine squamous syringometaplasia (ESS) is a relatively uncommon and benign cutaneous reaction, which is defined by pathognomonic noninflammatory metaplasia of the cuboidal epithelial cells of the eccrine sweat ducts. It differs from NEH by the absence of neutrophils on skin biopsy. Like NEH, the cutaneous manifestation of ESS is thought to result from a direct toxic effect. Clinically, ESS may give a presentation that is similar to NEH with erythematous macules, papules, plaques, or vesicles, which may be generalized or localized to the intertriginous areas or the palms and soles. Given these similarities to NEH, ESS is thought to represent the noninflammatory end of the spectrum of chemotherapeutic eccrine gland reactions.[61]

ESS reportedly appears 2-39 days after the initiation of chemotherapy and resolves spontaneously in 7-10 days.[62] It is not associated with any one particular cytotoxic agent. A histologic confirmation of ESS changes on biopsy can be a diagnostic aid in differentiating a chemotherapy-induced reaction from acute GVHD or other drug reactions. ESS deserves consideration in any erythematous eruption during chemotherapy.

Cutaneous Eruption of Lymphocyte Recovery

The cutaneous eruption of lymphocyte recovery (ELR) may be seen in patients receiving intensive marrow aplasia–inducing chemotherapy.[63] As with ESS, the ELR phenomenon has been observed with various cytotoxic agents but is not associated with a particular agent. Clinically, ELR has the appearance of variably distributed erythematous and pruritic macules, papules, and plaques, which may become confluent and erythrodermic, and is often associated with a couple days of fever. In the setting of chemotherapy, this reaction has been found to occur

6-21 days after the chemotherapy-induced nadir of the leukocyte count, which correlates with the time of the initial recovery of peripheral lymphocytes. ELR may reflect the return of highly alloreactive immunocompetent lymphocytes to the peripheral circulation and skin.[63] ELR is self-limited and resolves over several days with desquamation and mild residual hyperpigmentation. Given the nonspecific clinical manifestation of ELR, other causes of an erythematous exanthem must be considered in the differential diagnosis, particularly acute GVHD, sepsis, viral exanthem, leukemia or lymphoma cutis, ESS, and drug hypersensitivity. Of these types of eruptions, acute GVHD is similar in time of onset to ELR in the setting of bone marrow transplantation. The similarity with ELR is especially true in the case of autologous GVHD, as both involve a lymphocytic recovery in which histocompatibility is present. However, acute autologous GVHD cannot be reliably distinguished from ELR by skin biopsy.[64] As theorized by Horn, GVHD may represent a form of ELR.[65]

Miscellaneous Reactions

A large number of miscellaneous cutaneous reactions have been reported in the literature as case reports. The reactions are uncommon or their incidence rates are mostly unknown. Table 125-11 lists and updates many of these reactions, including reactions to cytokines, novel pegylated and liposomal drugs, nucleoside analogues, and tyrosine kinase inhibitors.[5,66] This list continues to grow as new and investigational drugs continue to be developed.

Cytokines

With recent advances in biotechnology, there has been increased development of cytokines and immunotherapeutic agents, which target cancer at the cellular level. Roles have already been established for IL-2 as alternative treatment for advanced metastatic melanoma and renal cell cancer and for IFN-α as standard treatment for chronic myelogenous leukemia, hairy-cell leukemia, cutaneous T-cell lymphoma, melanoma and Kaposi sarcoma (KS). In addition to significant toxicities such as capillary leak syndrome, there is a 72% incidence of cutaneous reactions reported with IL-2.[67] Commonly, a pruritic diffuse erythroderma occurs 1-3 days after administration and resolves with desquamation 2 days after cessation of therapy (Fig. 125-6).[67] This reaction is clinically similar to toxic shock syndrome and has been associated with staphylococcal sepsis in some patients. Intra-arterial IL-2 also causes hypersensitivity to iodine-containing contrast dyes in up to 30% of patients.[66] Of potential importance, one study of IL-2 for metastatic melanoma has reported a possible correlation between the development of vitiligo and good prognosis.[68] Although IFN-α is relatively less toxic than IL-2, several cutaneous reactions have been reported in the literature. Perhaps one-third of patients will develop a local injection-site reaction. In a study

Table 125-11 Miscellaneous Reactions and Reactions Associated With Cytokine Therapy

Acneiform eruptions	Raynaud Phenomenon	Sclerodermoid Reaction	Exfoliative Dermatitis
Flushing	Dermatitis herpetiformis	Telangiectasia	Other IL-2 reactions
L-Asparaginase	Flare	Carmustine (BCNU)	Erosions in surgical scars
Bleomycin	Cyclophosphamide/doxorubicin/vincristine	Fluorouracil (topical)	Hypersensitivity to iodine contrast dye
Carboplatin	Bleomycin	Hydroxyurea	Linear IgA bullous dermatosis
Carmustine (BCNU)	Cisplatin	IFN-α	Pemphigus vulgaris (de novo, recurrent)
Cisplatin	Vincristine	Erythema nodosum	Poly/dermatomyositis exacerbation
Cyclophosphamide	Drug-induced SLE	Busulfan	Psoriasis exacerbation
Dacarbazine	Aminoglutethimide	Diethylstilbestrol	Staphylococcal infections
Didemnin B	Diethylstilbestrol	IL-2	TEN-like bullous desquamation
Diethylstilbestrol	Hydroxyurea	Exacerbation of seborrheic dermatitis	Vitiligo
Docetaxel	Leuprolide	Fluorouracil	Fludarabine reactions
Doxorubicin	Tegafur	IL-2	Paraneoplastic pemphigus68
Etoposide	IFN-α	INF-α	Erythema multiforme66
Fluorouracil	Dermatomyositis-like reaction	Increased nonmelanoma skin cancer	Grover disease
Flutamide	Hydroxyurea (long term)	Nitrogen mustard (topical)	Pustular psoriasis
IL-2	Tamoxifen	Acquired cutaneous adherence	Aminoglutethimide
Leuprolide	Tegafur	Doxorubicin/ketoconazole	Pegylated liposomal doxorubicin65
Lomustine	Bleomycin	Porphyria	Cutaneous ulcers
Paclitaxel	Docetaxel	Cisplatin	Hydroxyurea
Plicamycin	Bullous pemphigoid	Porphyria cutanea tarda	IFN-α, pegylated IFN-α
Procarbazine	Dactinomycin/MTX	Busulfan	IL-2
Suramin	Keratotic papules	Cyclophosphamide	Methotrexate
Tamoxifen	Suramin	Diethylstilbestrol	Hirsutism
Teniposide	Chlorambucil/busulfan	Methotrexate	Diethylstilbestrol
Trimetrexate	Cisplatin	Acute intermittent porphyria	Fluoxymesterone
Folliculitis	Methotrexate	Chlorambucil	Tamoxifen
Dactinomycin	Mitomycin-C (intravesical)	Cyclophosphamide	Hair color change
Daunorubicin	Lichenoid eruptions	Other INF-α reactions	Bleomycin
Fluorouracil	Hydroxyurea	Eosinophilic fasciitis	Cisplatin
Methotrexate	Tegafur	Exacerbation of herpes labialis	Cyclophosphamide
Furunculosis	Capillaritis	Increased growth of eyelashes	Methotrexate
Fluoxymesterone	Aminoglutethimide	Necrotizing vasculitis	Tamoxifen
Methotrexate		Paraneoplastic pemphigus	Fixed-drug eruption
Dactinomycin		Psoriasis exacerbation and de novo	Dacarbazine
Medroxyprogesterone		Thyroiditis	Hydroxyurea
Procarbazine			Paclitaxel (bullous)
Vinblastine			Procarbazine
Cetuximab71			
Erlotinib70			

Abbreviations: EGFR, epidermal growth factor receptor; IFN-α, interferon-α; IgA, immunoglobulin A; IL-2, interleukin-2; MTX, methotrexate; SLE, systemic lupus erythematosus.

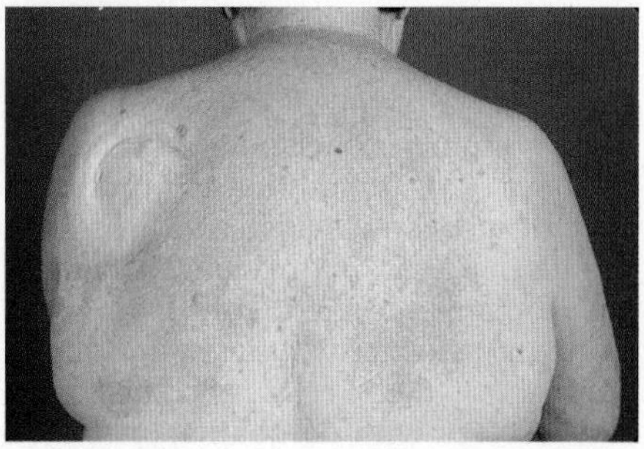

Figure 125-6 Erythematous rash associated with IL-2 therapy in a melanoma patient.

of 1000 patients receiving IFN-α, alopecia and herpes labialis exacerbation were common with 10% and 5% incidence, respectively.[66,69] Both IFN-α and IL-2 also induce and/or exacerbate seborrheic dermatitis and psoriasis.[66]

Pegylated and Liposomal Modified Drugs

Pegylation (polyethylene glycol) and liposomal modification of drugs are relatively recent innovations that are thought to increase the half-life of drugs and offer improved side-effect profiles. Pegylated IFN-α and pegylated liposomal doxorubicin are among the most well studied. Similar to non-modified recombinant IFN-α, pegylated IFN-α has been shown to cause local cutaneous ulcerations at sites of subcutaneous injection.[70] Cutaneous reactions have also been frequent with pegylated liposomal doxorubicin therapy, which has been shown to cause AE in 40%, diffuse follicular rash in 10%, intertrigo-like eruption in 8%, and melanotic macule development in 5% of cases.[71] There has also been a report of the drug causing psoriasiform pustular eruptions.[72]

Nucleoside Analogues

Some of the more recently developed nucleoside analogues have also been shown to produce reactions, particularly with 2-chlorodeoxyadenosine (2-CDA) or fludarabine, which may be associated with Grover disease and severe adverse cutaneous reactions such as erythema multiforme, and paraneoplastic pemphigus.[73-75] In phase I trials, the new nucleoside analogue troxacitabine has been associated with drug eruptions, hyperpigmentation, and acral erythema.[76] At MD Anderson Cancer Center, there have been a number of cases of gemcitabine-induced hyperpigmentation, radiation recall, and cutaneous ulcerations in cutaneous T-cell lymphoma patients.[28,29]

Epidermal Growth Factor Receptor Inhibitors (EFGR)

In recent years, EGFR has been recognized as a significant regulator of cancer cell proliferation, apoptosis, angiogenesis, and metastasis. Ligand binding to the receptor causes receptor dimerization, which activates the intracellular tyrosine kinase domain.[77] EGFR also plays a significant role in normal skin homeostasis.[78] Activation of EGFR in epidermal keratinocytes promotes cell cycle progression, differentiation, migration, which are all critical for normal skin function and wound healing.[79] The tolerability of profile for EGFR inhibitors is characterized by unique cutaneous reactions, including acneiform eruption, hypersensitivity drug reaction, xerosis, eczema, and changes in the hair and nails. Acne folliculitis was frequently observed during clinical trials of erlotinib (OSI774), an EGFR tyrosine kinase inhibitor, and cetuximab (C225), a monoclonal EGFR antibody. It generally appears on the face and upper trunk 8-10 days after treatment initiation. In phase I trials, erlotinib at the maximally tolerated dose induced a pustular acneiform eruption in 50% of cases during the second week of therapy.[80] While the reaction usually resolves by the fourth week of therapy, the eruption is occasionally dose limiting. It may occur most severely in patients who have previously experienced cystic acne vulgaris. The presence and severity of acne folliculitis has been correlated with tumor response and survival, suggesting that it may be a good pharmacodynamic marker of tumor inhibition. Standard acne treatments, including benzoyl peroxide, topical or oral antibiotics, and retinoic acid, may provide some benefit. Superinfection with *Staphylococcus aureus* may require treatment with topical or oral antibiotics.

Likewise, cetuximab commonly produces an acneiform follicular eruption of the face, chest, and upper back, and is thought to be due to a direct follicular toxic effect (Fig. 125-7).[81,82] Other cetuximab cutaneous reactions include paronychial inflammation of the toes and fingers and small oral aphthous ulcers.

Another tyrosine kinase inhibitor, imatinib mesylate (STI571, Gleevec), targets the *BCR-ABL* gene and has been used in the treatment of chronic myeloid leukemia and acute lymphoblastic leukemia. Gleevec has been shown to frequently cause dose-dependent cutaneous reactions, including urticaria, dermatitis, and acute generalized exanthematous pustulosis (AGEP).[83,84] One patient developed an eczematous rash with histologic features of mycosis fungoides.[85]

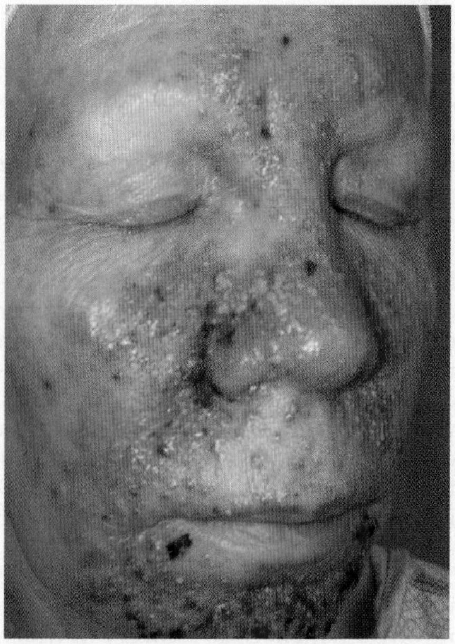

Figure 125-7 Severe acneiform eruption of the face associated with cituximab therapy.

In 18 patients with metastatic breast cancer treated with daily oral erlotinib, phosphorylated mitogen-activated protein kinase (pMAPK) was significantly associated with not developing a rash and may have a predictive utility for skin toxicity in patients treated with erlotinib and possibly with other anti-EGFR agents.[86]

Acute Generalized Exanthematous Pustulosis

Acute generalized exanthematous pustulosis (AGEP) is a cutaneous drug reaction characterized by acute development of dozens or hundreds of nonfollicular sterile pustules on an erythematous background. It usually begins on the face or intertriginous areas, perhaps with burning and itching. It can be accompanied by fever, neutrophilia, and eosinophilia.[87] Ninety percent of cases are drug-induced, mostly with antibiotics such as betalactams, cephalosporins, fluconazole, nystatin, and terbinafine. Other reported triggers include imatinib, the histone deacetylase inhibitor bryostatin (personal observations by Duvic), mercury, thallium, iohexol, patch testing, pseudoephedrine, diltiazem, furosemide, and viral infections. Because of its severe appearance, it can be alarming. Confluence of pustules may mimic the positive Nikolskyís sign seen in toxic epidermal necrolysis (TEN). Rarely, AGEP can manifest as vesicles or targetoid lesions raising suspicion for Stevens-Johnson syndrome (SJS). However unlike

SJS, AGEP affects the mucous membranes less often (only 20% of cases); involvement is usually mild and confined to the oral mucosa. Treatment of AGEP is to simply discontinue the offending agent and monitor for superinfection of the pustules. The macrophage migration inhibition factor (MIF) test, mast cell degranulation (MDC) test, and patch testing can help determine the causative agent. Lesions will spontaneously resolve in 4-14 days.[86]

Selected References

The complete reference list can be found at www.CANCERMEDICINE8.com

1. Crounse RG, Van Scott EJ. Changes in scalp hair roots as a measure of toxicity from cancer chemotherapeutic drugs. *J Invest Dermatol.* 1960;35:83–90.
2. Fischer D, Knobf M, Durivage H. *The Cancer Chemotherapy Handbook.* St. Louis: Mosby; 1997.
3. Hood AF. Dermatologic toxicity. In: Perry MC, ed. *The Chemotherapy Source Book*, 2nd ed. Baltimore: Williams & Wilkins; 1996:595–606.
4. Fitzpatrick JE, Yokel BE, Hood AF. Mucocutaneous complications of antineoplastic therapy. In: Freedberg IM, Eisen AZ, Wolff K, et al., eds. *Fitzpatrickís Dermatology in General Medicine*, 5th ed. New York: McGraw-Hill; 1999:1642–1653.
5. Susser WS, Whitaker-Worth DL, Grant-Kels JM. Mucocutaneous reactions to chemotherapy. *J Am Acad Dermatol.* 1999;40:367–398.
6. Pillans P, Woods D. Drug-associated alopecia. *Int J Dermatol.* 1995;34:149–158.
7. DeSpain JD. Dermatologic toxicity of chemotherapy. *Semin Oncol.* 1992;19:501–507.
8. Baker B, Wilson C, Davis A, et al. Busulfan/cyclophosphamide conditioning for bone marrow transplantation may lead to failure of hair regrowth. *Bone Marrow Transplant.* 1991;7:43–47.
9. Ron IG, Kalmus Y, Kalmus Z, et al. Scalp cooling in the prevention of alopecia in patients receiving depilating chemotherapy. *Support Care Cancer.* 1997;5:136–138.
10. Duvic M, Lemak N, Valero V, et al. A randomized trial of minoxidil in chemotherapy-induced alopecia. *J Am Acad Dermatol.* 1996;35:74–78.
11. Hesketh PJ, Batchelor D, Golant M, et al. Chemotherapy induced alopecia: psychosocial impact and therapeutic approaches. *Support Care Center.* 2004; 12:543–549.
12. Skarin A. Diagnosis in oncology: skin lesions in malignancy. *J Clin Oncol.* 2001; 19:2098–2102.
13. Clamon GH. Extravasation. In: Perry MC, ed. *The Chemotherapy Source Book*, 2nd ed. Baltimore: Williams & Wilkins; 1996:607–611.
14. Rudolph R, Larson DL. Etiology and treatment of chemotherapeutic agent extravasation injuries: a review. *J Clin Oncol.* 1987;5:1116–1126.
15. duBois A, Kommoss FG, Pfisterer J, et al. Paclitaxel induced "recall" soft tissue ulcerations occurring at the site of previous subcutaneous administration of paclitaxel in low doses. *Gynecol Oncol.* 1996;60:94–96.
16. Anderson CM, Walters RS, Hortobagyi GN. Mediastinitis related to probable central vinblastine extravasation in a woman undergoing adjuvant chemotherapy for early breast cancer. *Am J Clin Oncol.* 1996;19:566–568.
17. Dorr RT. Antidotes to vesicant chemotherapy extravasations. *Blood Rev.* 1990;4: 41–60.
18. Larson DL. Treatment of tissue extravasation by antitumor agents. *Cancer.* 1982;49:1796–1799.
19. Luedke DW, Kennedy PS, Rietschel RL. Histopathogenesis of skin and subcutaneous injury induced by Adriamycin. *Plast Reconstr Surg.* 1979;63:463–465.
20. Shamseddine AI, Khalil AM, Kibbi AG, et al. Granulocyte macrophage-colony stimulating factor for treatment of chemotherapy extravasation. *Eur J Gynaecol Oncol.* 1998;19:479–481.
21. Rentschler R, Wilbur D. Pyridoxine: a potential local antidote for mitomycin-C extravasation. *J Surg Oncol.* 1988; 37:269–271.
22. Scuderi N, Onesti MG. Antitumor agents: extravasation, management, and surgical treatment. *Ann Plast Surg.* 1994;32:39–43.
23. Heitmann C, Durmus C, Ingianni G. Surgical management after doxorubicin and epirubicin extravasation. *J Hand Surg [Am].* 1998;23:666–668.
24. Bertelli G, Gozza A, Forno GB, et al. Topical dimethylsulfoxide for the prevention of soft tissue injury after extravasation of vesicant cytotoxic drugs: a prospective clinical study. *J Clin Oncol.* 1995;13:2851–2855.
25. Hill A, Hanson M, Bogle MA, Duvic M. Severe radiation dermatitis is related to *Staphylococcus aureus. Am J Clin Oncol.* 2004;27:362–363.
26. Houtee PV, Danhier S, Mornex F. Toxicity of combined radiation and chemotherapy in non-small cell lung cancer. *Lung Cancer.* 1994;10:S271–S280.
27. Yeo W, Leung S, Johnson P. Radiation-recall dermatitis with docetaxel: establishment of a requisite radiation threshold. *Eur J Cancer.* 1997;33:698–699.
28. Fogarty G, Ball D, Rischin D. Radiation recall reaction following gemcitabine. *Lung Cancer.* 2001;33:299–302.
29. Talpur R, Apisarnthanarax N, Ward S, et al. Phase II evaluation of Gemcitabine as a single agent for cutaneous T-cell lymphoma. Poster presented to the American Society of Hematology, 2003.
30. Schweitzer VG, Juillard GJF, Bajada CL, Parker RG. Radiation recall dermatitis and pneumonitis in a patient treated with paclitaxel.
31. Gould JW, Mercurio MG, Elmets CA. Cutaneous photosensitivity diseases induced by exogenous agents. *J Am Acad Dermatol.* 1995;33:551–573.
32. Hussain S, Anderson DN, et al. Onycholysis as a complication of systemic chemotherapy: report of five cases associated with prolonged weekly paclitaxel therapy and review of the literature. *Cancer.* 2000; 88:2367–2371.
33. Lowitt M, Eisenberger M, Sina B, Kao G. Cutaneous eruptions from suramin: a clinical and histopathologic study of 60 patients. *Arch Dermatol.* 1995;131:1128–1153.
34. Wooten RS, Smith KC, Ahlquist DA, et al. Prospective study of cutaneous phototoxicity after systemic hematoporphyrin derivative. *Lasers Surg Med.* 1988;8:294–300.
35. Dougherty TJ, Cooper MT, Mang TS. Cutaneous phototoxic occurrences in patients receiving Photofrin. *Lasers Surg Med.* 1990;10:485–488.
36. Corbett MF, Hawk JLM, Herxheimer A, Magnus IA. Controlled therapeutic trials in polymorphic light eruption. *Br J Dermatol.* 1982;107:571–581.
37. Johnson T, Rapini R, Duvic M. Inflammation of actinic keratoses from systemic chemotherapy. *J Am Acad Dermatol.* 1987;17:192–197.
38. Hardwick N, Murray A. Inflammation of actinic keratoses induced by cytotoxic drugs. *Br J Dermatol.* 1986;114:639–640.
39. Bataille V, Cunningham D, Mansi J, Mortimer P. Inflammation of solar keratoses following systemic 5-fluorouracil. *Br J Dermatol.* 1996;135:478–480.
40. Weiss RB. Hypersensitivity reactions. In: Perry MC, ed. *The Chemotherapy Source Book*, 2nd ed. Baltimore: Williams & Wilkins; 1996:595–606.
41. Harris RE, McCallister JA, Provisor DS, et al. Methotrexate/L-asparaginase combination chemotherapy for patients with acute leukemia in relapse: a study of 36 children. *Cancer.* 1980;46:2004–2008.
42. Blumenreich MS, Needles B, Yagoda A, et al. Intravesical cisplatin for superficial bladder tumors. *Cancer.* 1982;50:863–865.
43. Castleberry RP, Crist WM, Holbrook T, et al. The cytosine arabinoside (Ara-C) syndrome. *Med Pediatr Oncol.* 1989;9:257–264.
44. Williams SF, Larson RA. Hypersensitivity reaction to highdose cytarabine. *Br J Haematol.* 1989;73:274–275.
45. Zuehlke RL. Erythematous eruption of the palms and soles associated with mitotane therapy. *Dermatologica.* 1974;148:90–92.
46. Chiao N, Bumgardner A, Duvic M. Clofarabine-induced acral erythema during the treatment of patients with myelodysplasia and acute leukemia: a report of two cases. *Leuk Lymphoma.* 2003;44:1405–1407.
47. Demircay Z, Gurbuz O, Alpdogan T, et al. Chemotherapy induced acral erythema in leukemic patients: a report of 15 cases. *Int J Dermatol.* 1997;36:593–598.
48. Hellier I, Bessis D, Sotto A, et al. High-dose methotrexateinduced bullous variant of acral erythema. *Arch Dermatol.* 1996;132:590–591.
49. Baack BR, Burgdorf WHC. Chemotherapy-induced acral erythema. *J Am Acad Dermatol.* 1991;24:457–461.
50. Kampmann KK, Graves T, Rogers SD. Acral erythema secondary to high-dose cytosine arabinoside with pain worsened by cyclosporin infusions. *Cancer.* 1989;63:2482–2485.
51. Jucgla A, Sais G, Navarro M, Peyri J. Palmoplantar keratoderma secondary to chronic acral erythema due to tegafur. *Arch Dermatol.* 1995;131:364–365.
52. Lin E, Morris JS, Ayers GD. Effect of celecoxib on capecitabine-induced hand-foot syndrome and antitumor activity. *Oncology (Williston Park).* December 2002;16 (12 Suppl No 14):31–37.

126 Skeletal Complications

Samuel Kenan, MD ■ Jeffrey I. Mechanick, MD ■ Michael A. Via, MD

Cancer-associated morbidity remains a major public health problem. The development of bone metastases indicates that cure is unlikely, and management of symptoms becomes the focus of treatment. Following metastases to nodes, lung, and liver, the skeleton is the fourth most common site for metastases. A number of orthopedic complications may arise as a direct result of metastatic disease or as a result of the treatment itself, but skeletal metastases are by far the most common type of complication. Over the past several decades, an increase in the survival of patients with bone metastases has been achieved through earlier detection using improved diagnostic modalities and radiographic imaging techniques and through treatment advances in chemotherapy regimens and radiation therapy combined with better surgical approaches. In this chapter, the early and late skeletal complications of cancer are considered, as well as skeletal metastases and hypercalcemia of malignancy (HCM).

Skeletal Metastases

Skeletal metastases represent the major orthopedic complication of failed cancer treatment and are commonly associated with disabling pain and pathologic fracture. Treatment of all patients with metastatic disease involves a multidisciplinary team approach including a medical oncologist, radiation oncologist, and orthopedic surgeon. Advances in surgical techniques and internal fixation modalities have resulted in great improvement in pain control and management of patients with skeletal metastases. The main goals of treatment are to relieve pain, improve function, and return patients, as soon as possible, to their previous environment.

The vast majority of skeletal cancers are of metastatic origin rather than primary bone tumors. In the United States, it is estimated that there will be 1.5 million new cancer cases in 2009. It is estimated that one-third of these new cases eventually will develop metastatic bone disease. In contrast there will be only above 5,000 primary soft tissue sarcomas and 2,000 cases of primary malignant bone tumors. In most cases, metastatic lesions are multifocal and show variable radiographic features, while primary bone tumors demonstrate a typical presentation by their anatomic site and radiographic features. The surgical approach for primary bone tumor is curative by wide surgical resection, while for metastatic disease, the surgical approach is palliative to restore function and relieve pain. In most instances of skeletal metastatic disease, the best treatment may not appreciably extend the life span of the patient.

Within the skeleton, the site of a metastatic lesion can be correlated with the activity of the bone marrow. The axial skeleton contains active hematopoietic (red) marrow, while the peripheral skeleton contains relatively avascular fatty (yellow) marrow.[1] The axial skeleton, especially the thoracolumbar spine, represents the most common site for metastases.[2] This is in part related to the paravertebral venous plexus system described by Batson.[3] Because of the relatively avascular marrow, metastases below the elbow and knee are relatively rare. At autopsy, 70% of patients who die of cancer have been shown to have skeletal metastases.[4] Many of these lesions are asymptomatic and are too small to be recognized radiographically. The proximal femur was found to be the site of metastatic lesions in 11% of all patients: however, when involved, they are often likely to fracture. Approximately 40% of all pathologic fractures occur in the proximal femur. The risk of pathologic fracture is correlated to the extent of the lesion, the type of destruction, and the anatomic location. Lesions in high-stress areas such as the lesser trochanter are very often associated with subsequent pathologic fracture. A high risk of fracture is particularly associated with highly anaplastic and rapidly growing vascular lesions, which are usually osteolytic.

Metastatic lesions that result in a net loss of bone are described as osteolytic, as can be seen in myeloma, metastatic renal cell carcinoma, and metastatic thyroid carcinoma (Fig. 126-1). The mechanism of bone resorption is primarily osteoclast-mediated.[5] Several known osteoclastic stimulating factors associated with cancer play a significant role in the process of bone resorption.[6] Parathyroid hormone-related protein (PTHrP) is the most important molecule leading to bone resorption by transforming osteoblasts to osteoclasts. When the process involves bone formation as observed in metastatic prostate carcinoma, the net increase in bone results in blastic, selerotic lesions (Fig. 126-2). Transforming growth factor-β (TGF-β), expressed in abundant amount in prostate cancer cells has the ability to stimulate osteoblastic proliferation and increase bone formation. In cases in which there are lytic and blastic areas, as can be seen in some metastatic breast carcinomas, lesions are described radiographically as of mixed osteolytic-osteoblastic type.

Pathogenesis of Metastases

Numerous pathologic events are required for a tumor cell to metastasize to bone and develop either osteolytic or osteoblastic lesions. The metastatic process depends on a successful interaction between tumor cells and bone marrow cells. 3 events must occur to establish skeletal metastases:

1. A tumor cell must leave the primary site, travel to the skeleton, and occupy the osseous bone cavity.

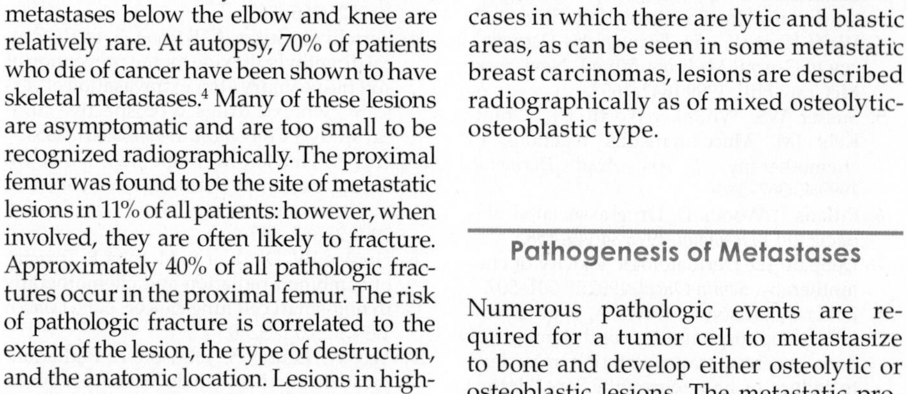

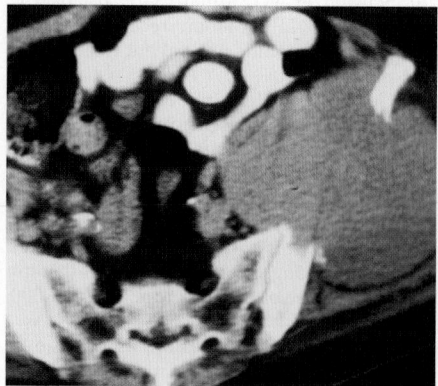

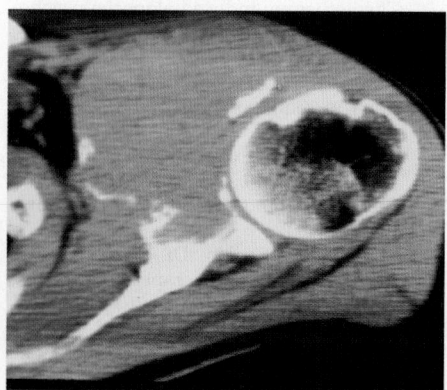

Figure 126-1 ■ Metastatic thyroid carcinoma. Lytic lesions.

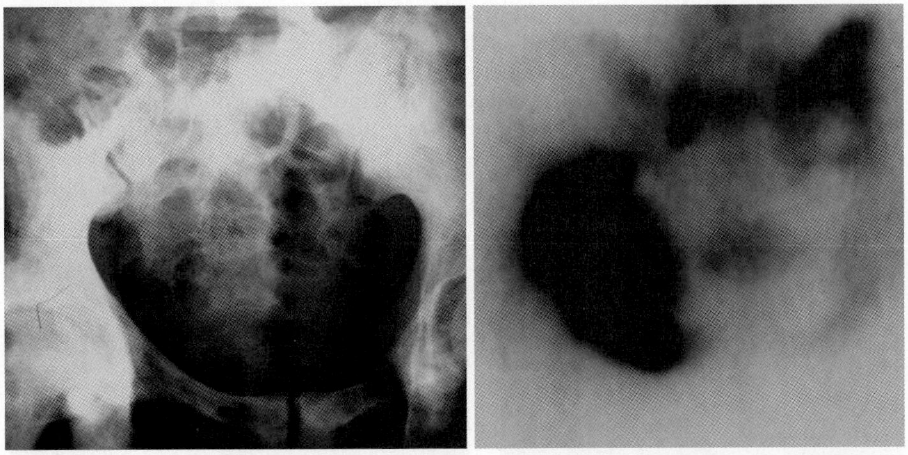

Figure 126-2 Metastatic prostate carcinoma. Sclerotic osteoblastic lesion of the acetabulum and corresponding bone scan.

2. The tumor cell within the osseous cavity must adhere to extracellular matrix and cause bone destruction within the bone marrow compartment.
3. Tumor cells must interact with host cells to enhance tumor cell growth.

Several gene products have been identified in different tumors that have unique expression profiles that predict aggressiveness. Overexpression of gene products that facilitate cell cycling, angiogenesis, and invasion imply a more aggressive tumor. Bone marrow stromal cells and osteoblasts are important targets of tumor-derived factors. Osteoclasts are derived from hematopoietic monocytic macrophage precursors that are stimulated by macrophage colony-stimulating factors. Tumor cells interact with osteoblasts, which in turn stimulate osteoclasts to differentiate from hematopoietic precursors, resulting in increased osteoclastic bone resorption. Osteoclasts are the principal bone resorbing cell. Bone metastases involve a vicious cycle between tumor cells and bone. The main participants in this process are tumor cells, bone forming osteoblasts, bone destroying osteoclasts, and organic mineralized bone matrix.

Despite the fact that tumors originate from a single cell that lacks normal control mechanisms, tumors consist of vast numbers of cells that are not homogeneous. Only a limited number of cells may have the genetic potential to metastasize. Although numerous tumor cells gain access to the systemic circulation, only a small number of cells, probably less than 0.1%, survive the transport.[7] Although random sites of metastasis can occur, selectivity of the metastatic site depends on adhesion of molecules specific to the endothelium within the arterioles, capillaries, and postcapillary venules of particular organs.[8,9]

Complementary molecules characteristic of individual tumor types are permissive for attachment to the specific endothelium, initiating the metastatic cascade. Organ selectivity has been demonstrated in mice by the propensity of harvested metastatic tumor to return, after sequential transplantation, to the organ from which it had been harvested. The differential frequency with which human cancers metastasize to how presumably hypresants the interaction between adhesiem molecules on vascular endothelium of the skeleton and tumor cells of particular types.

Surgical Management

Treatment of patients with metastatic bone disease requires a multidisciplinary team approach, including the medical oncologist, radiation oncologist, and orthopedic oncologist. Patients should be analyzed based on the type of the tumor, anatomic location, and neurologic status. Surgical treatment should be individualized to each patient's medical circumstance and with consideration given to the anticipated impact on longevity. Good judgment and considerable experience are necessary in the selection of patients for surgery.

The patient's general condition must allow the surgical procedure to be performed with reasonable expectation that the patient will survive long enough to benefit from the surgery. Patients should be informed and prepared prior to surgery concerning realistic expectations regarding relevant issues such as functional recovery, longevity, and cure. Preoperatively, patients should be evaluated and treated for dehydration, coagulopathies, anemia, and HCM.

The primary goals of treatment of patients with painful skeletal metastatic lesions are to relieve pain, restore function, allow early mobilization, and ease nursing care. In general, before any surgical intervention, the underlying process must be confirmed as metastatic disease and not a primary malignant bone tumor. The diagnosis cannot be assumed and must be confirmed by biopsy before any irreversible procedure. The surgical modality should take into consideration the natural progress and biologic behavior of the underlying process. A reliable and reproducible fixation modality

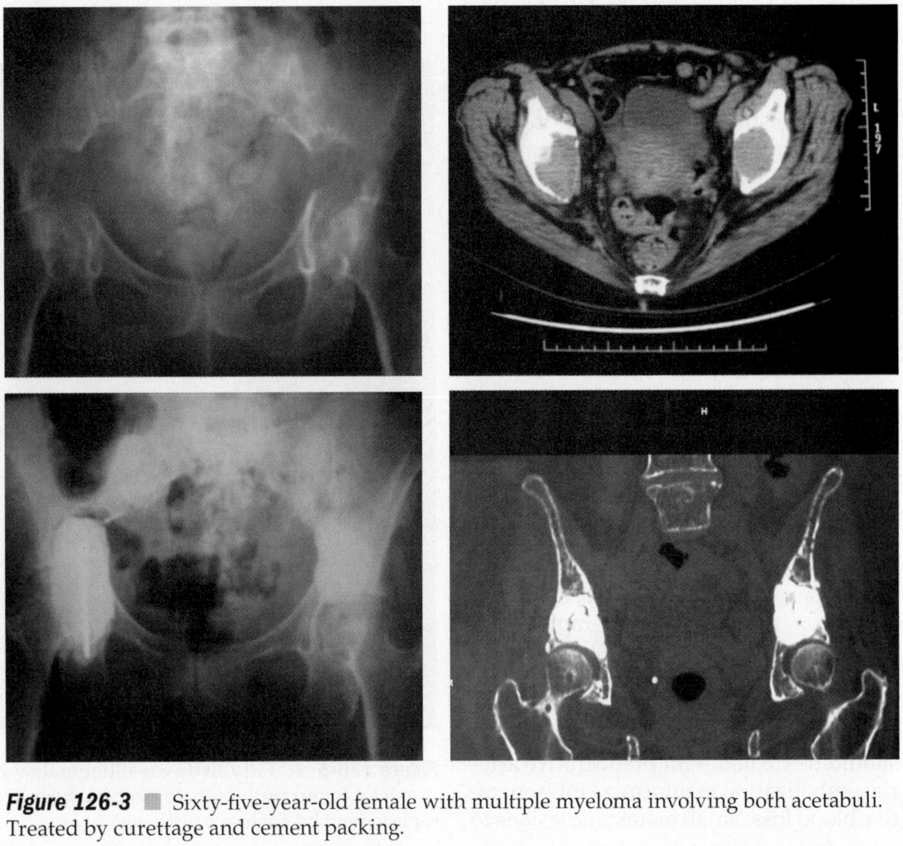

Figure 126-3 Sixty-five-year-old female with multiple myeloma involving both acetabuli. Treated by curettage and cement packing.

should be selected to allow immediate full weight bearing. It is prudent to intervene electively for impending fracture. Patients whose limbs were stabilized preventively had shorter hospitalizations and longer survival than patients with pathologic fractures. Pathologic fracture seems to be associated with an increased incidence of subsequent pulmonary metastases. Prophylactic fixation may reduce the incidence of lung metastases.[10]

Small lesions that do not present with an impending fracture, and which are radiosensitive, can be treated by radiotherapy alone to relieve pain[11] and to diminish progression of the radiated lesion.

Radiation may cause hyperemia at the periphery of treated bone with short-lived softening. which may temporarily increase the risk of fracture.[11] In lesions that may progress to impending fracture, blind intramedullary nailing with local irradiation may give good local control with pain relief. Irradiated pathologic fractures that lack rigid fixation show a higher rate of nonunion. In a larger osteolytic lesion, blind intramedullary nailing may not be sufficient because of mechanical failure and telescoping migration of the bone fragments.[12,13] In a significant number of patients with extensive destruction affecting the joint, particularly the hip or knee, segmental resection and prosthetic replacement may be indicated to allow immediate full weight hearing. The nature of metastatic cancer and the often relatively short survival generally make long-term durability of the prosthesis unimportant.

The most common metastatic tumors arise from carcinoma of the breast, a tumor that accounts for more than 50% of the cases requiring orthopedic intervention, followed by cancers of the lung, kidney, prostate, gastrointestinal tract, thyroid, and other miscellaneous sites. In patients who present with metastatic cancer of unknown primary site, the presence of bone metastases represents a sign of advanced disease with poor life expectancy.[14-16]

Metastatic Tumors to the Acetabulum

The pelvis and acetabulum are common sites for skeletal metastasis. Periacetabular tumors may cause severe debilitating pain with hip dysfunction. Pathologic fractures often lead to protrusio acetabuli. Metastatic lesions to the acetabulum require a computed tomography (CT) scan for better evaluation of the extent of the lesion and to provide a guideline for the surgical approach. Highly vascular tumors such as renal cell carcinoma should be treated with preoperative arterial embolization to minimize intraoperative blood loss. Small metastatic lesions to the acetabulum may be managed by radiation alone. Larger lesions can be treated by intralesional curettage and cement packing (Fig. 126-3). Joint instability with significant acetabular defect may require total hip replacement augmented by cement and screw fixation (Fig. 126-4).

Metastatic Lesions to the Femur

The femur is a common place for metastatic lesions and pathologic fractures. The proximal femur is subjected to axial bending and shearing forces applied

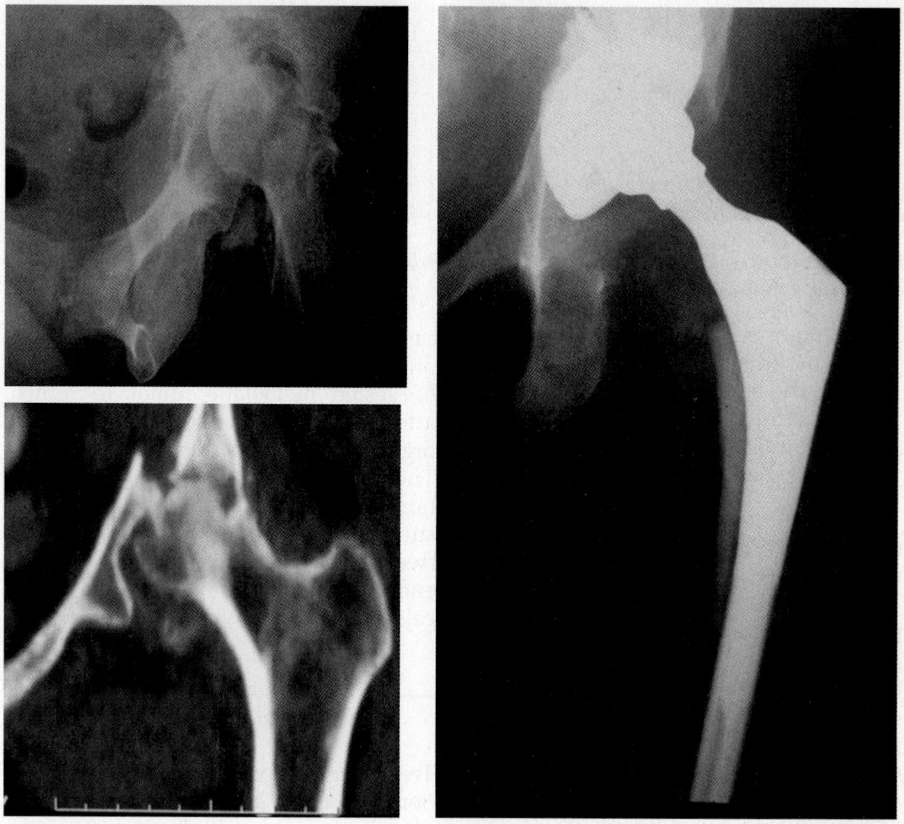

Figure 126-4 Fifty-eight-year-old female with a metastatic lesion of the left acetabulum. Treated by total hip replacement.

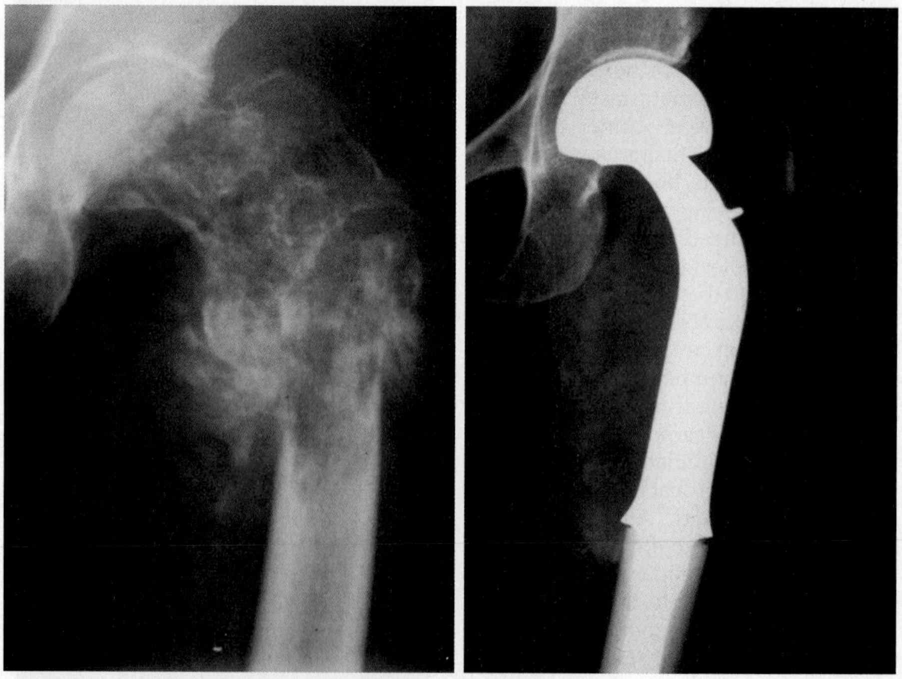

Figure 126-5 Fifty-five-year-old female with metastatic breast carcinoma to the left proximal femur with pathological fracture. Treated by wide proximal femur resection and replacement by custom prosthesis.

directly to any fixation device. Conventional fixation devices ultimately may fail. Surgical management should provide pain relief and immediate restoration of ambulation with unrestricted full weight bearing. A fracture is considered to be impending whenever there is a lesion greater than 50% of the bone diameter, or bigger than 2.5 cm, or whenever there is pathologic avulsion of the lesser trochanter or persistent pain. Methylmethacrylate is very resistant to compressive loading and provides an ideal substitute for deficient bone. Internal fixation of femoral neck fractures is often successful. Metastatic lesions to the femoral neck are best treated by resection and a bipolar prosthesis. Intralesional curettage and cement packing, supplemented by pin and plate fixation can treat metastatic disease to the trochanteric region. Larger lesions of the proximal femur with pathologic fracture are best treated by wide resection and proximal femur replacement (Fig. 126-5).

Impending fractures of the femoral shaft are best treated by closed intramedullary locking nail, which provides rotational stability (Fig. 126-6). Metastatic disease to the femoral condyle may be treated by intralesional curettage and cement packing (Fig. 126-7). In those cases in which there is pathologic fracture, distal femur replacement may be indicated (Fig. 126-8).[17]

The same could be applied to the tibia, where metastatic lesions could be treated by wide segmental resection, internal fixation, and cement spacer (Fig. 126-9).

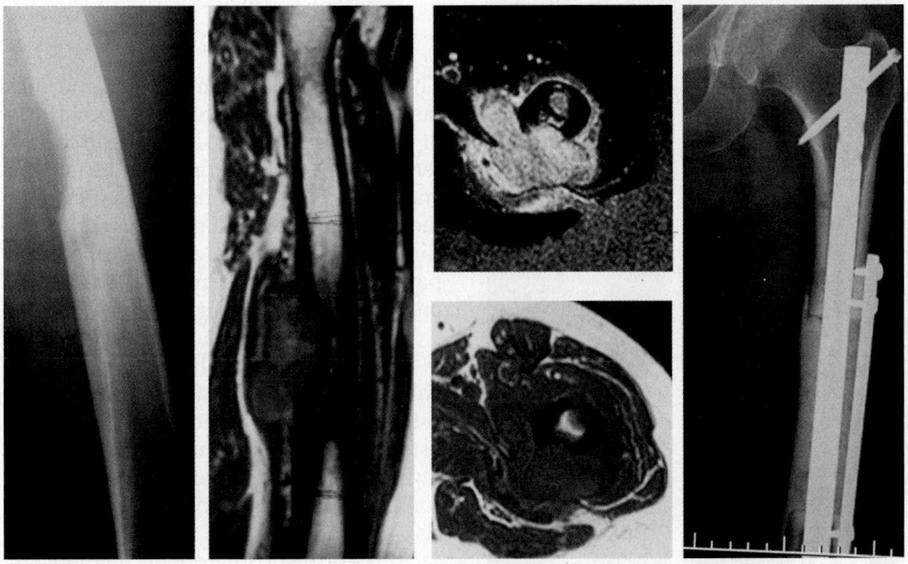

Figure 126-6 Sixty-year-old female with metastatic lung carcinoma to the midshaft of the femur with associated soft tissue mass. Treated by wide segmental resection and intramedullary rod augmented by cement spacer.

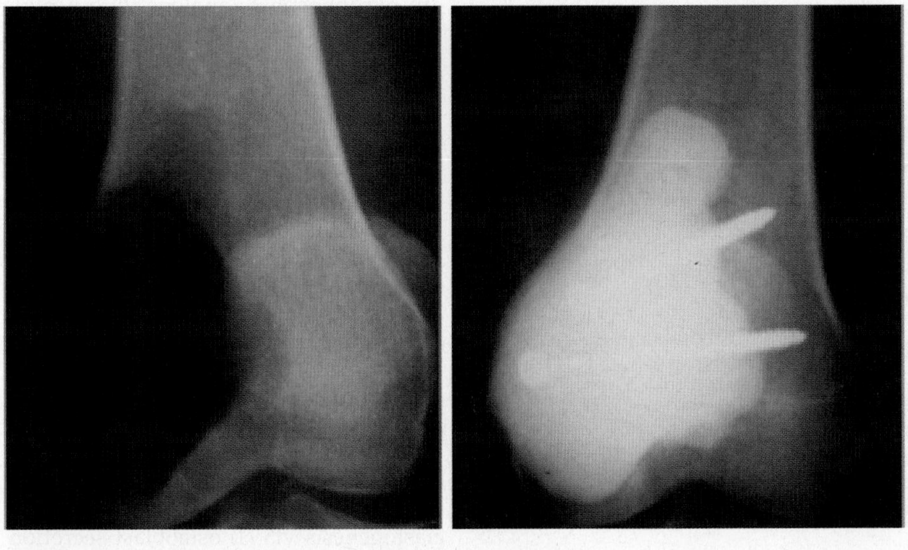

Figure 126-7 Sixty-seven-year-old female with metastatic renal cell carcinoma to the femoral condyle. Treated by intralesional curettage and cement augmentation.

Metastatic Lesions to the Scapula and Upper Extremity

Conservative treatment of pathologic fracture of the humerus is often associated with persistent pain and shoulder stiffness. To provide immediate pain relief and restore shoulder mobility, internal fixation is recommended. Metastatic lesions to the scapula can be treated by partial or total scapulectomy (Fig. 126-10). Pathologic fracture of the humeral head is best managed by endoprosthesis (Fig. 126-11). Large lesions of the proximal humerus with or without pathological fracture are best treated by wide resection and replacement using a custom prosthesis (Fig. 126-12). Cases with large segmental defects are best treated with wide resection and internal fixation using an intramedullary rod augmented by cement spacer (Figs. 126-13 and 126-14). For better local control, radiation can be given 2 weeks postsurgery.[18] Metastatic tumors of the proximal ulna are best treated by wide segmental resection and internal fixation and cement augmentation (Fig. 126-15). For metastatic tumors of the radius or ulna shaft, an intramedullary rod is recommended (Fig. 126-16).

Metastatic Lesions to the Spine

The vertebral bodies are the most common site for metastatic lesions. Most vertebral metastases initially are occult and painless. The majority can be detected on routine bone scan. Metastatic lesions that do not compromise stability may remain asymptomatic. Pain typically occurs when a significant amount of bone destruction has occurred, leading to microfractures. Pathologic fractures of the vertebral bodies are of a compressive type and are usually stable. Patients with metastatic disease to the spine commonly develop back pain before any neurologic sequelae. MRI scan has replaced myelography as the method of choice to demonstrate local extension and extradural compression. In the absence of impingement on spinal cord or cauda equina, back pain may be alleviated by radiotherapy or by percutaneous vertebroplasty with polymethyl-methacrylate. Spinal cord compression at the level of the cervical or thoracic spine can cause hyperreflexia and spasticity with complete paraplegia. Corticosteroids are indicated to reduce edema until emergency treatment is initiated for neurologic salvage. A radiosensitive metastatic

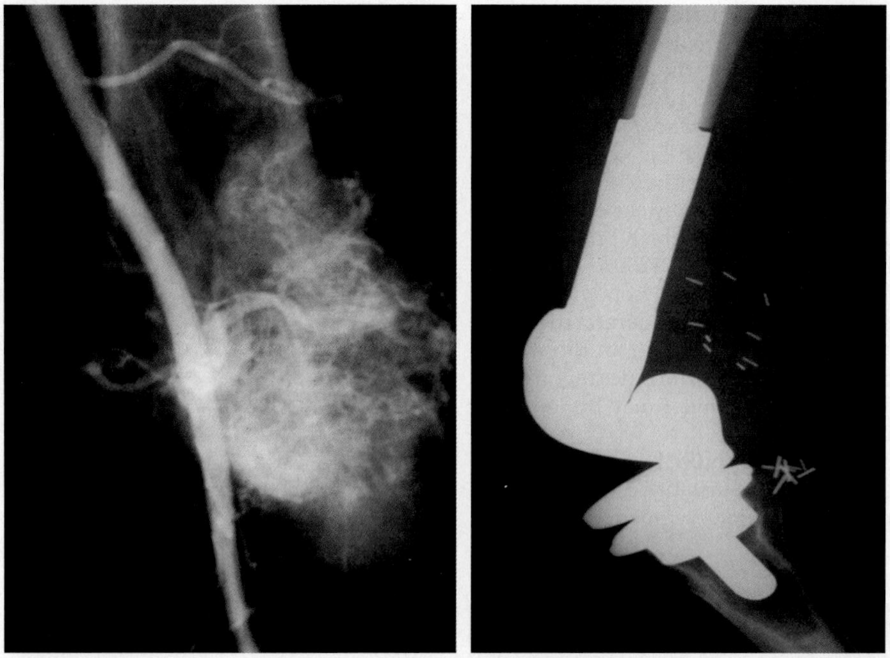

Figure 126-8 Seventy-year-old female with metastatic renal cell carcinoma of the distal femur. Treated by wide resection and prosthesis replacement.

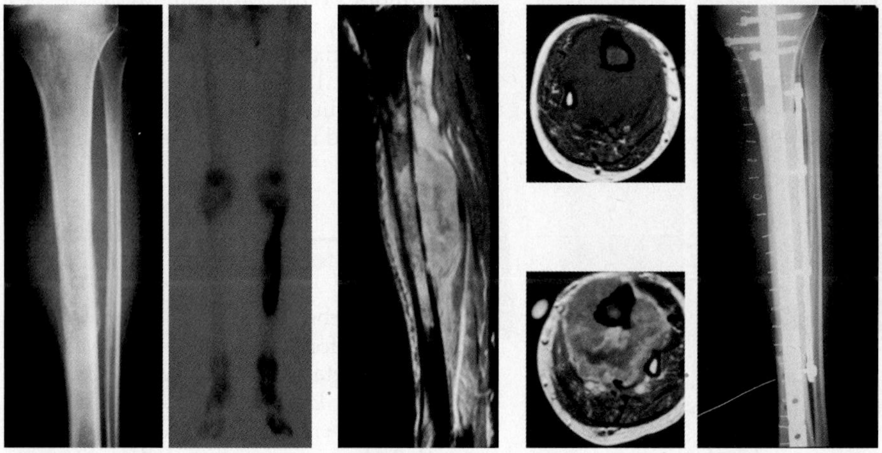

Figure 126-9 Fifty-year-old male with metastatic lung carcinoma of the midshaft tibia. Treated by wide segmental resection, internal fixation, and cement spacer augmentation.

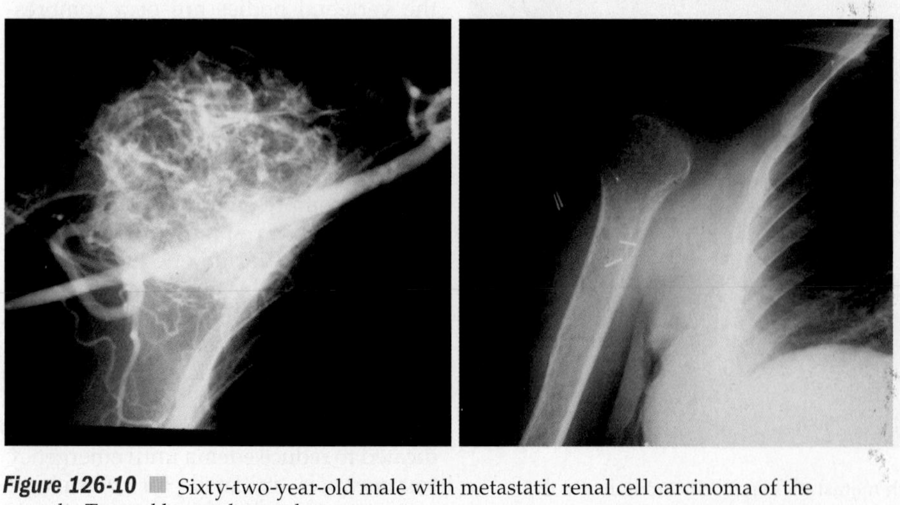

Figure 126-10 Sixty-two-year-old male with metastatic renal cell carcinoma of the scapula. Treated by total scapulectomy.

condition, such as lymphoma, may be treated effectively by radiation therapy or chemotherapy. Surgical decompression may be indicated in those patients who do not respond to radiation therapy and who subsequently develop neurologic deterioration or where cord compression is already critical. Surgical treatment of metastatic conditions to the spine has improved significantly with the introduction of new surgical techniques and instrumentation. The result of anterior spinal decompression with vertebral body resection, replacement by a cement spacer, and bracing has proved to be very effective in stabilizing the spine and preventing further neurologic deterioration[19,20] (Fig. 126-17).

Medical Management of Bone Metastases

The optimal management of bone metastases requires the coordinated efforts of various disciplines. In addition to systemic chemotherapy for bone metastases, endocrine interventions directed at bone metabolism have demonstrated effectiveness in controlling oncogenic bone pain, fracture risk, metastatic growth, and even in prolonging survival.

Bone metabolism is governed by a delicate, though highly regulated, balance between bone formation (by osteoblasts) and bone resorption (by osteoclasts). This results in an ongoing process of bone remodeling, which confers strength and decreased fracture risk. Bisphosphonates are the most efficacious antiresorptive agents available in the management of metabolic bone disease and bone metastases. These agents inhibit osteoclast function and interfere with recruitment and differentiation of osteoclast precursors. Bisphosphonates are pyrophosphate analogs with a high affinity for bone.[21] The non-nitrogen–containing bisphosphonates (etidronate and clodronate are metabolized into cytotoxic analogs of ATP and are not considered to have antitumoral activity.[22] A growing body of experimental animal data demonstrates, however, antitumoral activity of the nitrogen-containing bisphosphonates (n-BP; pamidronate, ibandronate, zoledronate, risedronate, and alendronate). Their effect results in inhibition of tumor cell adhesion, inhibition of tumor cell invasion through the extracellular matrix, antiangiogenic effects (via vascular endothelial growth factor [VEGF]), and induction of tumor cell apoptosis[21,23,24] n-BPs induce apoptosis of osteoclasts and antagonize osteoclastogenesis via (1) osteoblast secretion of an inhibitor of osteoclast recruitment; (2) altering osteoblast secretion of TGF-β,

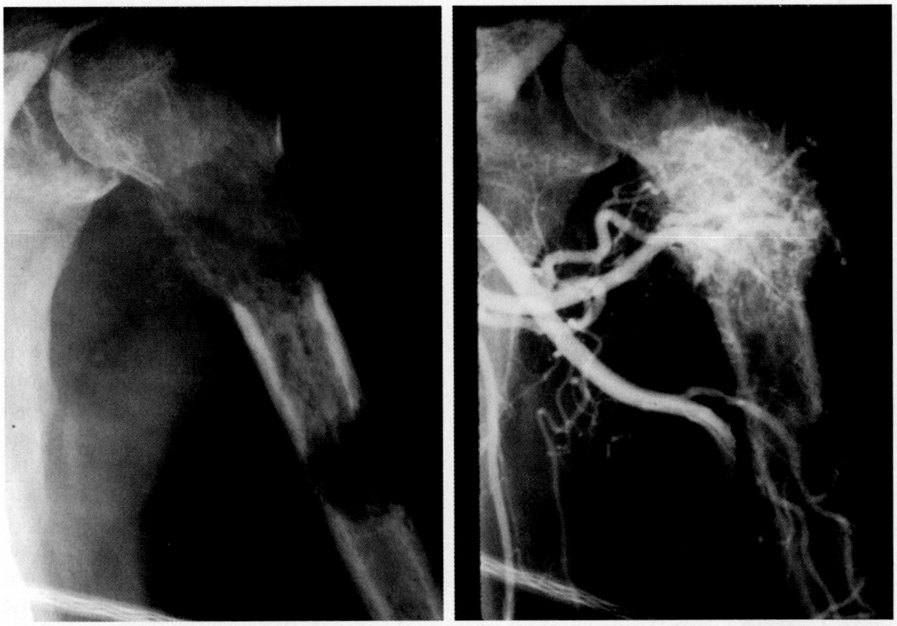

Figure 126-11 Metastatic renal cell carcinoma. Arteriogram demonstrates a highly vascular tumor, for which arterial embolization before surgery is recommended.

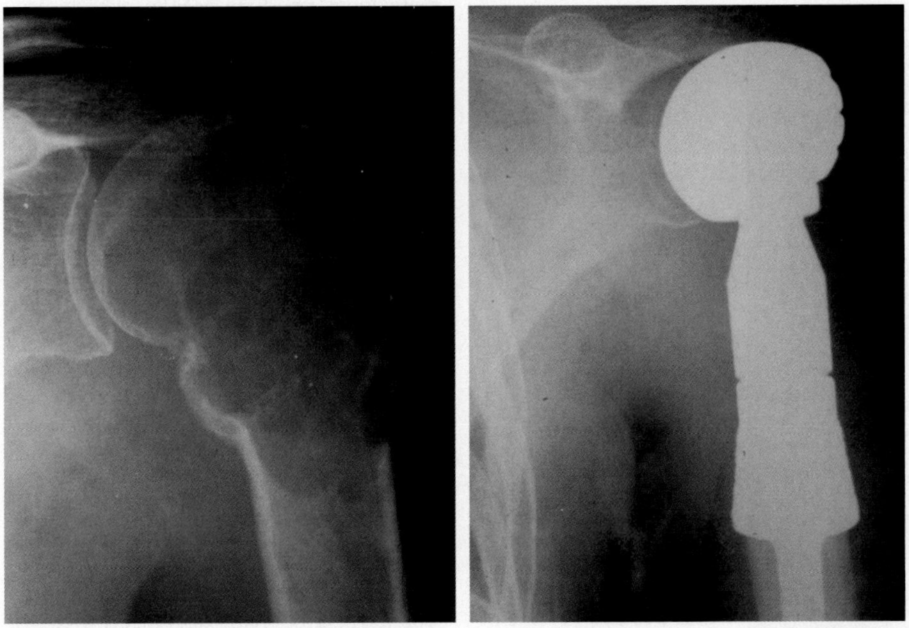

Figure 126-12 Metastatic breast carcinoma proximal humerus. Treated by wide resection and prosthesis replacement.

an osteoclast apoptosis signal; (3) inhibition of farnesyl diphosphate synthase, a key enzyme in the mevalonate pathway; (4) impaired prenylation (farnesylation) causing interference with small GTPases and intracellular signals such as Ras, Rho, and Rac (important for cancer cell migration and invasion); and (5) released mitochondrial cytochrome C and caspase activation.[25,26] Of interest, statins may potentiate n-BP inhibition of the mevalonate pathway.[27] n-BPs also affect expression of the antiapoptotic protein bcl-2, activate the p38 mitogen-activated protein kinase (MAPK) pathway, down-regulate integrins, and increase expression of osteoprotegerin.[23,28] Furthermore, n-BPs are broad-spectrum matrix metalloproteinase (MMP) inhibitors, which may prevent metastases into soft and hard tissue.[29]

In clinical studies, bisphosphonates are well tolerated with minimal acute side effects.[30] Patients may develop nausea, vomiting, and, with pamidronate, a posterior uveitis. Fever may occur after owing to tumor necrosis factor (TNF)-α and IL-6 elaboration by γ/δ T cells, which may also be associated with antitumor activity.[31,32] Nephrotoxicity may be observed but is uncommon. Hypocalcemia and hypophosphatemia may also occur, particularly in patients with a vitamin D deficiency. The safety of long-term bisphosphonate administration (over 2 years) has been well documented.[23,33,34] ONJ was also more common in those receiving intravenous bisphosphonates compared to those on oral bisphosphonates.

Majority of the intravenously administered dose is deposited in the bone where it remains for extended periods of time. Bisphosphonates are not metabolized and are eliminated by renal excretion. In patients with renal failure, pamidronate may be dosed during, or within 24 hours before, hemodialysis. The antiresorptive response to bisphosphonates is best assessed with urine N-telopeptide (NTx) levels.[35] NTx is a bone-specific collagen that is also highly predictive of skeletal complications from metastatic bone disease, as well as of mortality.[36]

In malignant osteolytic bone disease, bisphosphonate administration has been associated with reduced skeletal-related events (SREs), including pain. Treatment protocols include (1) etidronate. 400 mg/day PO × 2 weeks; (2) alendronate, 70 mg PO weekly; (3) pamidronate 60-90 mg IV every 3-4 weeks; (4) zolendronate 4 mg IV every 3-4 weeks.[37-41] The shorter and more convenient infusion protocols, with comparable safety and potential advantages favor zolendronate as the agent of choice. In a large meta-review of 30 randomized controlled trials involving 3,682 patients, bisphosphonate use was significantly more effective than placebo in providing pain relief from bone metastases.[37] Since pain relief might be delayed, bisphosphonate use should be combined with analgesics and/or radiotherapy when appropriate.[42] Moreover, various radiopharmaceuticals, such as rhenium-188, samarium-153, strontium-89, phosphorus-32, and tin-117m, show promise for palliation of bone pain from osseous metastases, albeit with varying levels of hematopoietic toxicity.[43]

The standard of care for the management of osteolytic lesions from breast cancer includes the use of intravenous pamidronate or zoledronate. Pamidronate 45 mg IV every 3 weeks increased the median time to bone progression, improved pain control, reduced the need for radiotherapy, and increased the median time to radiotherapy with no serious adverse effects or worsening of chemotherapy-related toxicities.[44] These results were confirmed in a larger study of Stage IV breast cancer patients with at least one lytic bone lesion given pamidronate, 90 mg IV over 2 hours every month for 12 cycles.[45] Furthermore, the effects of IV pamidronate in decreas-

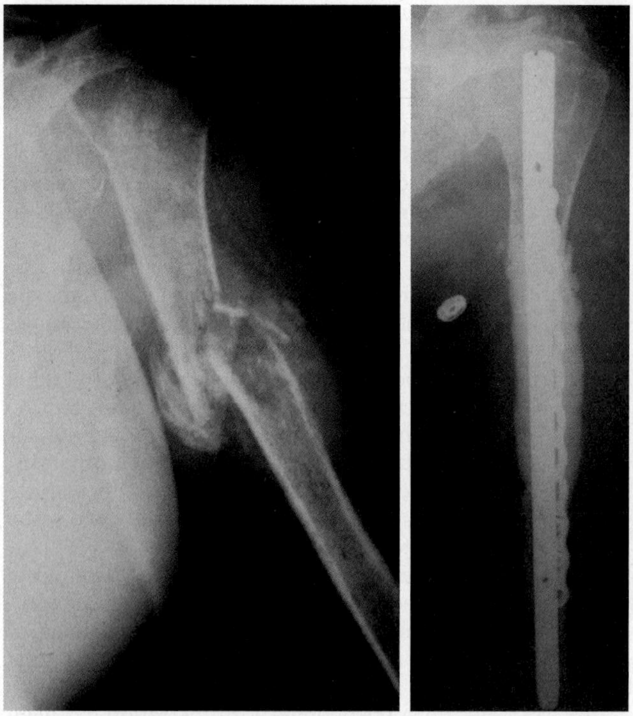

Figure 126-13 ■ Seventy-year-old female with metastatic breast carcinoma midshaft humerus, associated with pathological fracture. Treated by wide segmental resection, intramedullary rod, and cement augmentation.

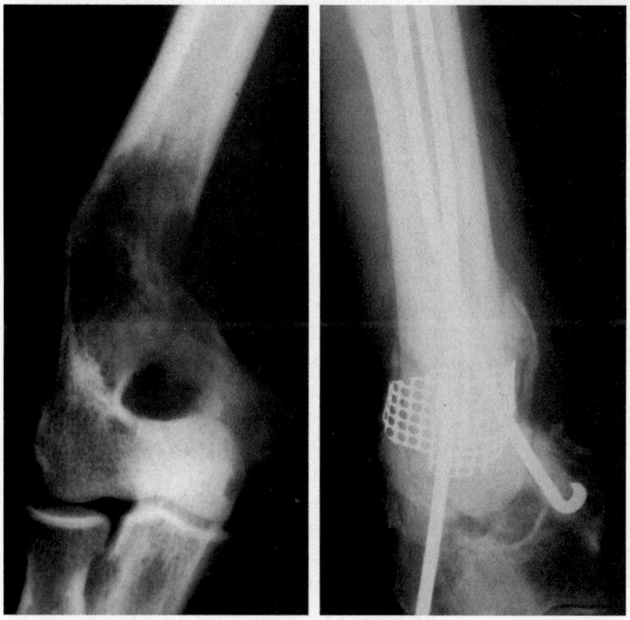

Figure 126-14 ■ Seventy-year-old male with multiple myeloma. Pathological fracture of distal humerus. Treated by curettage, intramedullary rods, and cement augmentation.

ing the risk of osteolytic bone lesion complications in women with breast cancer persists for at least 2 years.[46] On the other hand, in a study of 1,648 patients with either Stage III multiple myeloma or advanced breast cancer, zoledronate, 4 mg IV over 15 minutes, was associated with more sustained beneficial effects on osteolytic bone lesions than 90 mg of IV pamidronate.[47] In a subsequent prospective randomized controlled study of 1,130 patients with breast cancer with at least one osteolytic lesion, 4 mg IV zoledronate was more effective than 90 mg IV pamidronate in reducing skeletal complications.[48] Overall, based on phase 3 studies involving over 3,000 patients with breast cancer, prostate cancer, lung cancer, multiple myeloma, and other cancers, 4 mg IV zoledronate dosing was safe and effective[49] and in women with breast cancer, associated with increased health-related quality of life.[50]

Bisphosphonates are also used to manage cancer-treatment induced bone loss (CTIBL). This has particular application to patients undergoing hormonal therapies for breast and prostate cancers. Average rates of CTIBL owing to ovarian ablation are 1.4-5.9% (lumbar spine [LS]) and 0.34-2.7% (femoral neck [FN]); owing to LHRH agonist therapy, 5.3% (LS) and 3.2% (FN): owing to aromatase inhibitors, 2.6% (LS) and 1.7% (FN): and owing to androgen deprivation therapy for prostate cancer, 0.98-8% (LS) and 0.92-9.6% (FN).[51,52] Oral risedronate, 30 mg/day × 2 weeks followed by 10 weeks of no drug, repeated for 8-12-week cycles, has been associated with prevention of trabecular and cortical bone loss.[53] Standard protocols for the use of bisphosphonates in the treatment of postmenopausal osteoporosis include alendronate. 70 mg/week PO or risedronate, 35 mg/week PO, with calcium, 1,200-1,500 mg/day and vitamin D, to units/day.[54] Clinical trials have also demonstrated efficacy of pamidronate, 60-90 mg IV every 1-3 months[55,56] or zoledronate, 4 mg IV every 3-6 months[57-59] to manage CTIBL.[60]

In prostate cancer, metabolic bone disease can result from direct effects of bone metastases, which have osteoblastic and osteoclastic components, or CTIBL. Fractures are an independent and adverse predictor of survival in prostate cancer patients.[55] Prostate cancer bone metastases produce MMPs, which promote osteolysis, and also the protein receptor activator of nuclear factor-κB ligand (RANKL), PTHrp, and interleukin (IL)-6, all of which induce osteoclastogenesis.[61] Of interest, osteoprotegerin is a soluble decoy receptor for RANKL that inhibits tumor-induced osteolysis.[61] The process of tumor-mediated local bone resorption can facilitate micrometastasis, tumor cell hiding, and eventual macrometastases.[62] Bisphosphonates can target this osteoclastic component of prostate cancer bone metastases as well as promote caspase dependent apoptosis via G-protein geranylgeranylation.[63] However, pamidronate, 90 mg IV q 3 weeks × 27 weeks, was found to lack significant effects on skeletal-related events in men with metastatic prostate cancer.[64] On the other hand, zoledronate, 4 mg over 15 minutes every 3 weeks for 15 months was associated with decreased SREs in a prospective randomized controlled trial of 122 patients with metastatic hormone-refractory prostate cancer.[65] Nevertheless, in patients with progressive prostate cancer receiving zoledronate, 4 mg IV q month, the use of adjuvant calcitriol, with or without dexamethasone, was shown to have no antitumor effect.[66] Calcitriol has been shown to have differentiating and antiproliferating effects, as well as inducing apoptosts in experimental models of prostate cancer.[67,68] In small clinical trials, calcitriol slows the rate of prostatic-specific antigen rise.[69] This topic has led to an unresolved controversy: Is the antitumor effect of bisphosphonates mitigated by the antiresorptive (via RANKL stimulation) and tumor growth-promoting effects of

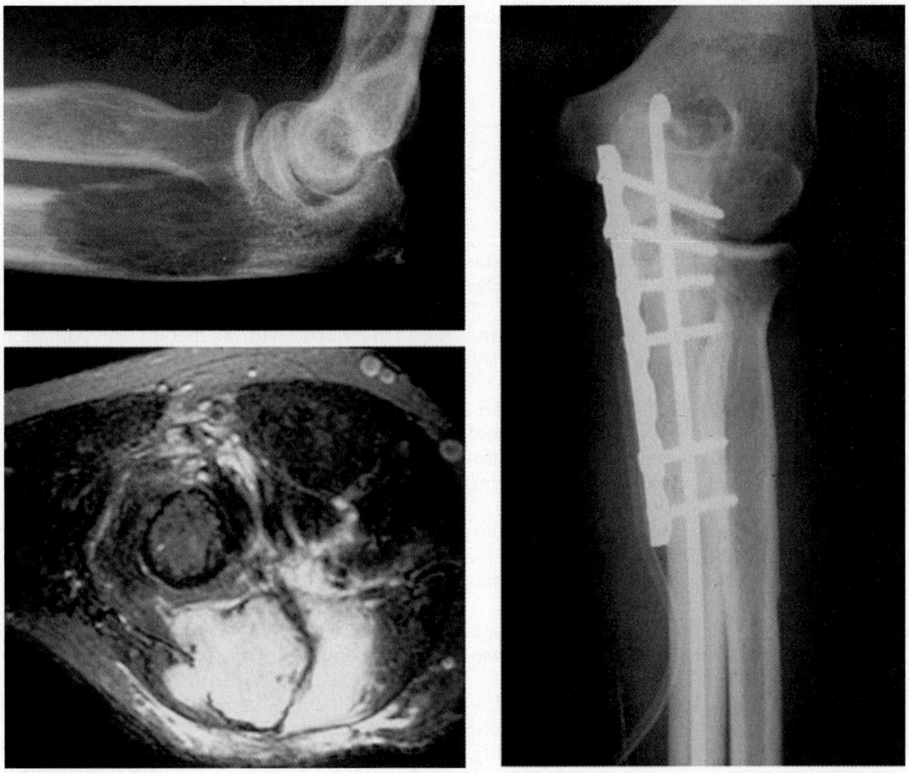

Figure 126-15 ■ Fifty-five-year-old female with metastatic thyroid carcinoma of the proximal ulna with pathological fracture. Treated by wide resection, intramedullary nailing, and cement augmentation.

calcitriol, or do bisphosphonates simply lack significant antitumor effects in prostate cancer?

Intravenous pamidronate or zoledronate has been used to reduce SREs in patients with multiple myeloma, as well as other malignancies.[70] Bisphosphonates may induce apoptosis in plasma cells; this antitumor effect is enhanced by dexamethasone and thalidomide,[71] but may diminish over time because of increased farnesyl pyrophosphate synthase activity.[72,73] Pamidronate, 90 mg over 4 hours IV every 4 weeks for 9 cycles, was associated with decreased bone pain without deterioration in performance status or quality of life in patients with multiple myeloma.[74] However, pamidronate therapy had no effect on progression-free survival in multiple myeloma.[75] Zoledronate, 2-4 mg over 5 minutes, demonstrated comparable efficacy in the management of multiple myeloma bone lesions.[76] Zoledronate has also been found to augment the antileukemic activity in vitro of several chemotherapeutic agents.[77–81]

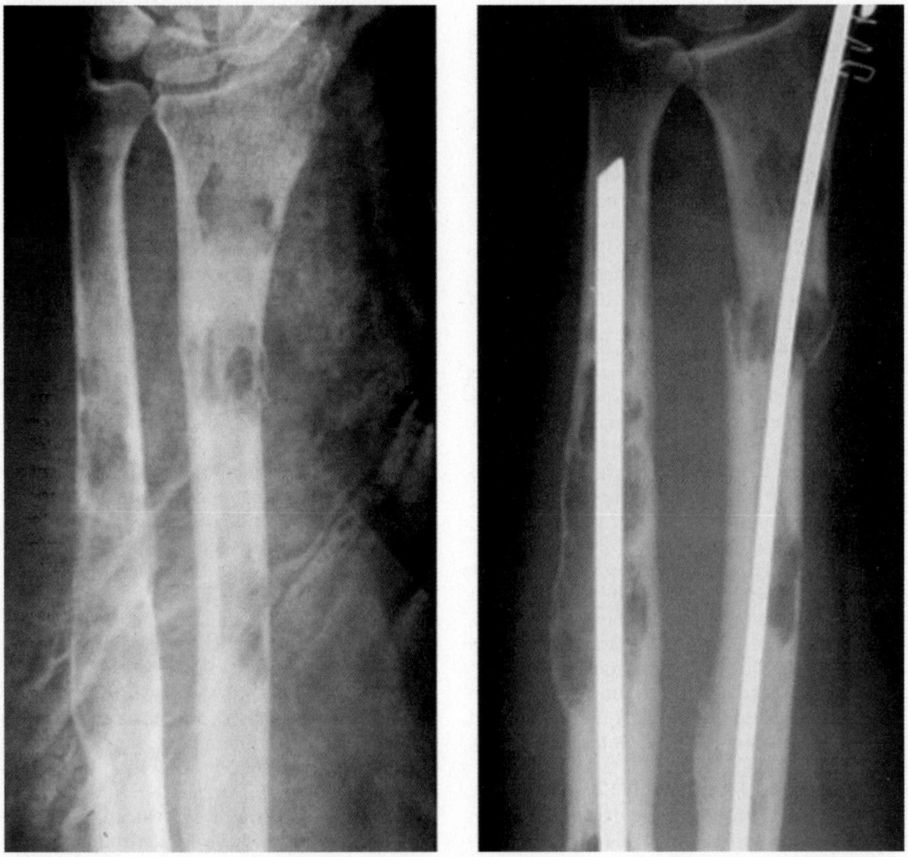

Figure 126-16 ■ Multiple myeloma of radius and ulna with pathological fractures. Treated by intramedullary nailing.

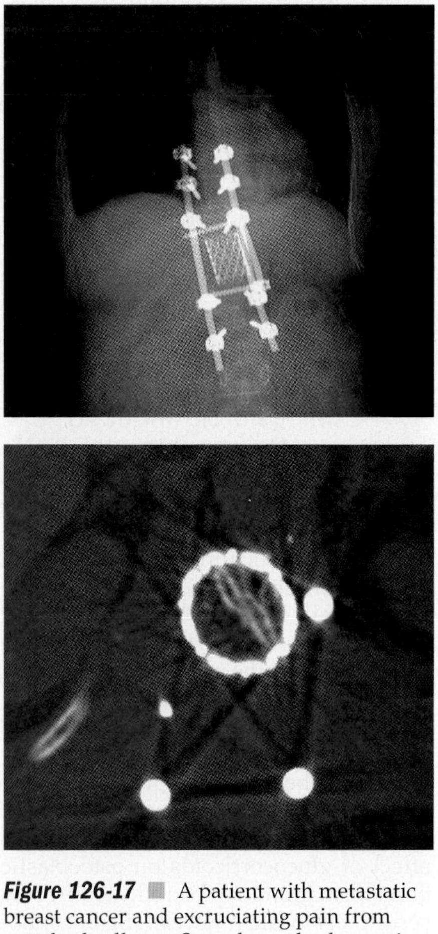

Figure 126-17 ■ A patient with metastatic breast cancer and excruciating pain from vertebral collapse. Staged vertebral resection, posterior support first, with reconstruction of vertebral height with cage, cement, and external rods. The patient lived 4 more years.

Hypercalcemia of Malignancy

Hypercalcemia associated with skeletal metastases is a common metabolic complication and a life-threatening disorder. Symptoms include weakness, nausea, vomiting, anorexia, polyuria, dehydration, lethargy, confusion, stupor, and coma. HCM is due to direct effects of local osteolytic factors derived from skeletal metastases (IL-1, TNF, TGF, and prostaglandins) or is due to production of systemic factors (PTHrp) secreted by the tumor that influence bone physiology. HCM is most common with multiple myeloma or breast cancer, but it can also occur with renal, ovarian, lung, and other cancers. The hypercalcemia associated with lymphomas is generally due to cytokines that stimulate osteoclastic bone resorption or is due to activation of ectopic lα-hydroxylase activity, which converts 25-hydroxyvitamin D into the activated 1,25-dihydroxyvitamin D. The resultant hypervitaminosis D state causes increased gastrointestinal absorption of calcium. Medical management of HCM consists of the following strategies: (1) promoting calciuresis with IV saline and using loop diuretics only if excessive fluid retention occurs; (2) using bisphosphonate (pamidronate. 90 mg over 4-24 hours IV) to inhibit bone resorption,[82] (3) discontinuing calcium and vitamin D supplementation (if any); and (4) consideration of glucocorticoids, which increase the effective circulatory volume, glomerular filtration rate, and calciuresis and suppress ectopic vitamin D activation. Calcitonin may also be used and can inhibit bone resorption to a lesser degree.

Corticosteroid-Induced Osteopenia

When glucocorticoids decrease the intestinal absorption of calcium, the 24-hour urinary calcium excretion rate will be low and calcium (1,200-1,500 mg/day) and vitamin D (400-800 units/day) may be provided orally. If glucocorticoids are increasing the urinary excretion of calcium, hydrochlorothiazide, 25-50 mg once or twice daily, may be used to reduce calciuresis. Negative calcium balance may be reflected by an elevated parathyroid hormone level (secondary hyperparathyroidism). The suppressive effect of glucocorticoids on osteoblastic bone formation may be reflected by low serum osteocalcin levels. Bisphosphonates can also prevent osteocyte and osteoblast apoptosis induced by glucocorticoids in experimental models.[83] Oral alendronate, 70 mg/week, or risedronate 35 mg/week, retards glucocorticoid-induced bone loss.[84,85]

Selected References

The complete reference list can be found at www.CANCERMEDICINE8.com

1. Boland PJ, Lane JM, Sundaresan N. Metastatic disease of the spine. *Clin Orthop.* 1982;169:95–102.
3. Batson OV. The role of the vertebral veins in metastatic processes. *Ann Intern Med.* 1992;16:38–45.
5. Nakchbandi IA, Weir EE, Insogna KL, Philbrick WM, Broadus A. Parathyroid hormone-releted protein induces spontaneous osteoclast formation via a paracrine cascade. *PNAS.* 2000;97:7291–7300.
7. Folkman J. Tumor angiogenesis. *Adv Cancer Res.* 1985;43:175–203.
9. Springfield DS. Mechanisms of metastases. *Clin Orthop.* 1982;169:15–19.
11. Schocker JD, Brady LW. Radiation therapy for bone metastases. *Clin Orthop.* 1982;169:38–43.
13. Ryan JR, Rowe DE, Salciccioli GG. Prophylactic internal fixation of the femur for neoplastic lesions. *J Bone Joint Surg.* 1976;58A:1071.
15. Moertel CG, Reitemeir RJ, Schutt AJ, Hahn RG. Treatment of patients with adenocarcinoma of unknown origin. *Cancer.* 1972;30:1469–1472.
17. Harrington KD, Sim FH, Ennis JE, et al. Methy lmethacrylate as an adjunct in internal fixation of pathological fractures. *J Bone Joint Surg.* 1976;58A:1047.
19. Leving SA, Perin LA, Hayes D, Hayes WS. An evidence-based evaluation of percotaneors vertehroplasty. *Maney Care.* 2000;7:56–60.
21. Sebbah-Louriki M, Colombo BM, et al. A new phenylacetate-bisphosphonate inhibits breast cancer cell growth by proapoptotic and antiangiogenic effects. *Anticancer Res.* 2002;22:3925–3931.
23. Weinstein RS, Roberson FK, Manolaggs SC. Grant osteoclast formation and long-term oral bisphasphenate therapy. *N Engl J Med.* 2009;360:53–62.
25. Senaratne SG, Mansi JL, Colston KW. The bisphosphonate zoledronic acid impairs Ras membrane localization and induces cytochrome c release in breast cancer cells. *Br J Cancer.* 2002;86:1479–1486.
27. Vincenzi B, Santini D, Avvisati G, et al. Statins may potentiate bisphosphonates anticancer properties: a new pharmacological approach? *Med Hypoth.* 2003;61:98–101.
29. Heikkila P, Teronen O, Moilanen M, et al. Bisphosphonates inhibit stomelysin-1 (MMP-3), matrix metalloelastase MMP-12), collagenase-3 (MMP-13), and enamelysin (MMP-20), but not urokinase-type plasminogen activator, and diminish invasion and migration of human malignant and endothelial cell lines. *Anticancer Drugs.* 2002;13:245–254.
31. DiCuonzo G, Vincenzi B, Santini D, et al. Fever after zoledronic acid administration is due to increase in TNFα and IL-6. *J Interferon Cytokine Res.* 2003;23:649–654.
33. Mundy GR. Martin TJ. The hypercalcemia of malignancy: pathogenesis and management. *Metabolism.* 1982;31:1247–1277.
36. Brown JE, Thomson CS, Ellis SP, et al. Bone resorption predicts for skeletal complications in metastatic bone disease. *Br J Cancer.* 2003;89:2031–2037.
39. Iwamoto J, Takedo T, Ichimura S. Treatment relief of metastatic cancer bone pain by oral administration of etidronate. *J Bone Miner Metab.* 2002;20:228–234.
41. Groff L, Zecca E, De Conno F, et al. The role of disodium pamidronate in the management of bone pain due to malignancy. *Palliat Med.* 2001;15:297–307.
43. Pandit-Taskar N, Batraki M, Divgi CR. Radiopharmaceutical therapy for palliation of bone pain from osseous metastases. *J Nucl Med.* 2004;45:1358–1365.
45. Hortobagy GN, Theriault RL. Porter L, et al. Efficacy of pamidronate in reducing skeletal complications in patients with breast cancer and lytic bone metastases. Protocol 19 Aredia Breast Cancer Study Group. *N Engl J Med.* 1996;335:1785–1791.
47. Rosen LS, Gordon D, Kaminski M, et al. Zoledronic acid versus pamidronate in the treatment of skeletal metastases in patients with breast cancer or osteolytic lesions of multiple myeloma: a phase III, double-blind, comparative trial. *Cancer J.* 2001;7:377–387.
49. Cameron D. Proven efficacy of zoledronic acid in the treatment of bone metastases in patients with breast cancer and other malignancies. *Breast.* 2003;12(suppl 2):S22–S29.
51. Lipton A. Toward new horizons: the future of bisphosphonate therapy. *Oncologist.* 2004;9(suppl 4):38–47.
53. Delmas PD, Balena R, Confravreux E, et al. Bisphosphonate risedronate prevents bone loss in women with artificial menopause due to chemotherapy of breast cancer: a double-blind, placebo-controlled study. *J Clin Oncol.* 1997;15:955–962.
55. Smith MR, McGovern FJ, Zietman AL, et al. Pamidronate to prevent bone loss during androgen-deprivation therapy for prostate cancer. *N Engl J Med.* 2001;345:948–955.
57. Smith MR, Eastharn J, Gleason DM, et al. Randomized controlled trial of zoledronic acid to prevent bone loss in men receiving androgen deprivation therapy for nonmetastatic prostate cancer. *J Urol.* 2003;169:2008–2012.
59. Gnant M, Hausmaninger H, Samonigg H, et al. Changes in bone mineral density caused by anastrozole or tamoxifen in combination with goserelin (± zoledronate) as adjuvant treatment for hormone receptor-positive premenopausal breast cancer: results of a randomized multicenter trial. Presented at the *25th Annual San Antonio Breast Cancer Symposium*. December 11–14, 2002, San Antonio, TX.
61. Keller ET. The role of osteoclastic activity in prostate cancer skeletal metastases. *Drugs Today (Barc).* 2002;38:91–102.
63. Coxon JP, Oades GM, Kirby RS, et al. Zoledronic acid induces apoptosis and inhibits adhesion to mineralized matrix in prostate cancer cells via inhibition of protein prenylation. *Br J Urol.* 2004;94:164–170.
65. Saad F, Gleason DM, Murray R, et al. Long-term efficacy of zoledronic acid for the prevention of skeletal complications in patients with metastatic hormone-refractory prostate cancer. *J Natl Cancer Inst.* 2004;96:879–882.

127 Hematologic Complications and Blood Bank Support

Richard M. Kaufman, MD ▪ Kenneth C. Anderson, MD

Hematologic complications occur commonly in patients with cancer, related either to the underlying disease or to its treatment.[1,2] Abnormalities in the red blood cell (RBC), leukocyte (WBC), and platelet number and function require transfusion medicine expertise for the provision of appropriate blood component support.[3,4] Indeed, the therapeutic advances made using high-dose combination chemotherapeutic approaches to date would not have been possible without the parallel development of technology to support patients through the hematologic complications of therapy. In addition, the blood component laboratory plays an increasingly central role in the cellular therapy of cancer, including the collection, processing, cryopreservation, infusion, and quality control of hematopoietic stem cells, donor lymphocytes, and dendritic cells for treatment protocols.[5]

Normal Hematopoiesis

When considering the optimal strategy for supporting cellular blood component needs, a basic understanding of normal hematopoiesis, as well as the impact of cancer and its treatment on this process, is essential.[6] In human marrow, the most primitive clonogenic cell forms a colony of undifferentiated blasts in methylcellulose culture and is referred to as the *CFU-Blast*, the majority of which are noncyclic under normal circumstances.[7] The individual cells of a blast cell colony can form a colony of granulocytes, erythroid cells, monocytes, and megakaryocytes (CFU-GEMM), which can give rise to secondary colonies of granulocytes and macrocytes (CFU-GM), of erythroid cells arranged in clusters known as burst-forming units (BFU-E), of megakaryocytes (CFU-Meg), of eosinophils (CFU-Eo), or of basophils (CFUBas) (Fig. 127-1).

Hematopoiesis

Although the CFU-GEMM is a cell that is multi-potent by virtue of its ability to give rise to multiple cell lineages, it has very limited capacity for self-renewal and does not represent a true stem cell. This is further supported by the observation that CFU-GEMM may be almost eradicated from human bone marrow by in vitro purging with the active metabolite cyclophosphamide, 4-hydroperoxy-cyclophosphamide, yet the ability of that marrow to reconstitute a lethally irradiated recipient is unimpaired.[8] Colony-forming cells with a more restricted commitment status than the CFU-GEMM, such as the BFU-E or CFU-GM, lack self-renewal potential and are normally in an active cell cycle. Based on these observations, it has been proposed that normal hematopoiesis is characterized by the proliferation and commitment of small numbers of self-renewing, pluripotent, relatively quiescent progenitor cells that give rise to a succession of highly proliferative cells with more restrictive capacity for self-

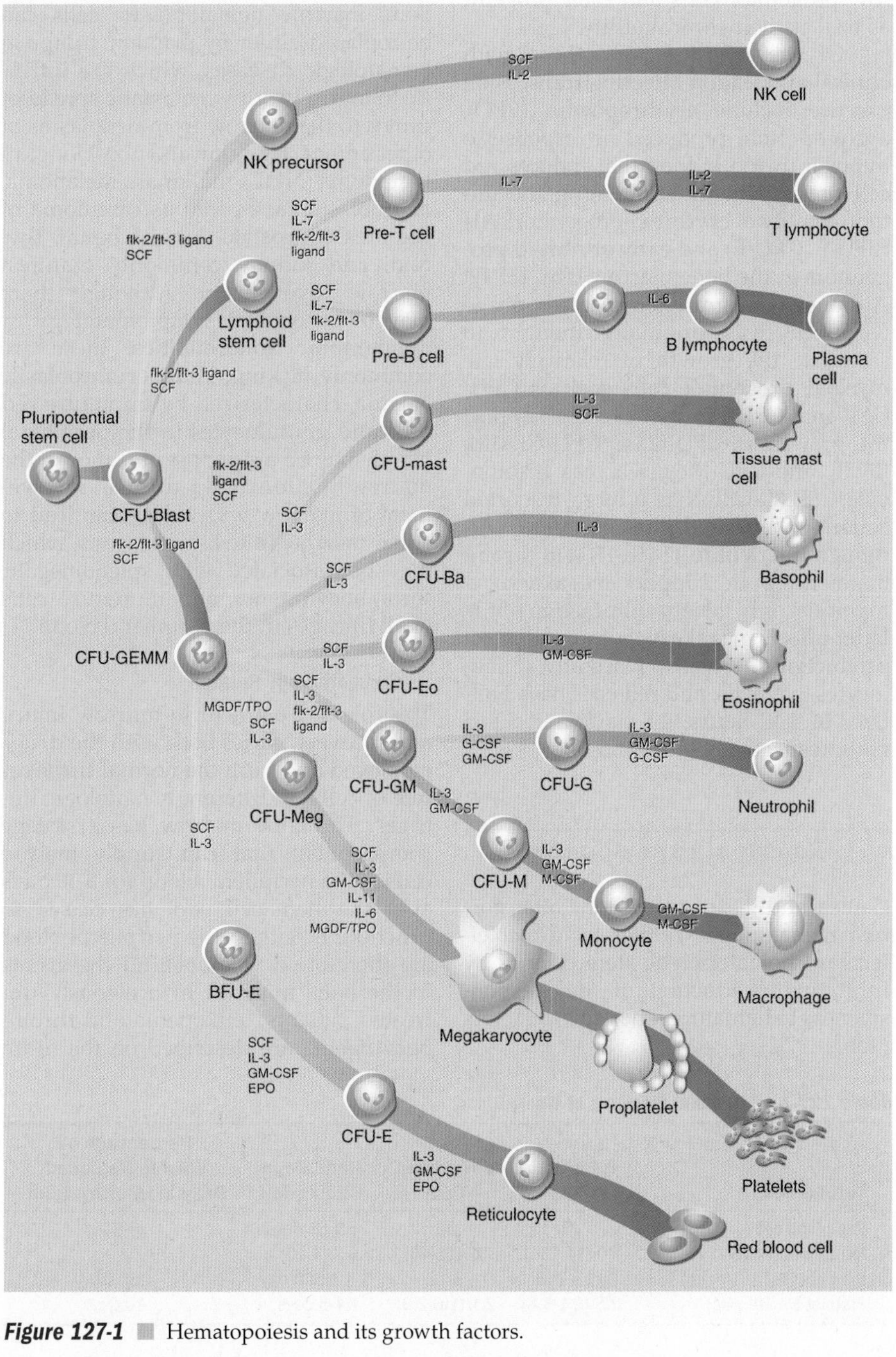

Figure 127-1 ▪ Hematopoiesis and its growth factors.

renewal (CFU-GEMM) and/or commitment (BFU-E, CFU-GM).

Hematopoietic progenitor cells proliferate and become committed to differentiate within a specialized environment that provides a supporting stroma on which the stem cells bind and receive regulatory signals required for stem cell growth. The viability and proliferation of bone marrow progenitor cells to form colonies of mature cells in semisolid medium requires the presence of one or more structurally heterogeneous glycoproteins termed *colony stimulatory factors* (CSFs). The cDNA for many of these factors have been cloned, their genes localized, and large amounts of purified factor have been produced through recombinant technology, thereby permitting delineation of their effects on marrow progenitor cells and their progeny, as well as their clinical utility.[6]

Of the many factors, those with clinical application affecting transfusion practice include erythropoietin (EPO), a glycoprotein produced in response to hypoxia in the kidney that induces red cell production by stimulating the mitotic activity of erythroid progenitor cells (BFU-E, CFU-E) and early erythroid progenitors in the bone marrow (Fig. 127-1).[9] Although granulocyte/macrophage (GM)-CSF was originally thought to stimulate the growth of relatively late myeloid progenitor cells such as CFU-GM and CFU-Eo, it may also support the growth of CFU-Blast, CFU-GEMM, BFUE, and CFU-Meg, whereas granulocyte-CSF (G-CSF) has a more restricted action on myeloid lineage cells.[10] Although interleukin-11 (IL-11) and thrombopoietin both support megakaryocytopoiesis, only genetic elimination of the latter affects megakaryocyte and platelet production in vivo.[11-13] Normally, granulocytes, platelets, and red cells have half-lives of 4-10 hours, 4-5 days, and 50-65 days, respectively (Table 127-1).

Causes of Pancytopenia

Cancer and its treatment may alter normal hematopoiesis either by direct effects on hematopoietic stem cells or by inhibiting production of and responsiveness to hematopoietic growth factors (Table 127-2).

Table 127-1 ■ Cellular Elements of Whole Blood

Total Blood	Total Body Pool	Circulating Pool	Half-Life in Circulation	Percentage of Volume Replaced Daily in Healthy Adult
Red blood cell (× 10^{10}/kg)	33	33	50-65 days	0.8
Neutrophil (× 10^7/kg)	70 (14-160)	31 (11-46)	6.7 (4-10) h	
Lymphocyte (× 10^7/kg)	133-266	8-12	1 h-1,500 days	230.0
Platelet (× 10^{10}/kg)	2.8 (2.1-3.8)	2.1 (1.6-2.9)	4-5 days	10.0

Table 127-2 ■ Causes of Anemia, Thrombocytopenia, and Leukopenia in Cancer

- Bone marrow replacement by primary tumor (eg, leukemia)
- Bone marrow involvement by metastatic tumor (eg, breast, prostate)
- Derangement of normal physiology
  - Nutritional (eg, folate, iron, negative nitrogen balance)
  - Abnormal feedback (eg, stimulation/inhibition of hematopoiesis)
  - Bone marrow reaction (eg, fibrosis)
  - Peripheral destruction (eg, immune hemolysis, diffuse intravascular coagulation, splenomegaly)
  - Blood loss
- Myelosuppression by chemotherapy or radiotherapy

Disease Related

Bone marrow hematopoietic cells can be replaced either by primary tumor in hematologic diseases, which are intrinsic to marrow, or by metastatic spread of tumor to the marrow from neoplasms of other organs. Hodgkin and non-Hodgkin lymphoma (NHL), malignant melanoma, neuroblastoma, as well as carcinoma of the breast, prostate, lung, adrenal, thyroid, and kidney commonly manifest marrow involvement. Although there may be associated symptomatology or radiographic abnormalities, these are commonly lacking. Leukoerythroblastic anemia, characterized by immature red cells and granulocytes in the peripheral blood, may be a signpost of tumor in the marrow.[14] Ultimately, diffuse involvement of marrow with tumor can lead to either marrow fibrosis or necrosis, which may be associated with splenomegaly, thrombocytopenia, and immature cells of all lineages in the peripheral blood.[15]

Chemotherapy Related

The role of treatment in marrow injury and recovery varies both with the drugs employed and with the normal turnover rate of cells of different hematologic lineages. The bone marrow has a storage compartment that can supply mature cells to the peripheral blood for 8-10 days after the stem cell pool has ceased to function. Events in the peripheral blood are therefore a week behind the events in the bone marrow. In previously untreated patients, leukopenia and thrombocytopenia are described on the ninth or tenth day after treatment, with the nadir of counts on days 14-18. Recovery of counts is evident by day 21 and complete by day 28. The cytotoxic dose–response effect is usually related to the nadir WBC and platelet count, not the duration of cytopenia. This is due to the resting state of the stem cells of normal bone marrow, which protects them from damage.

Route and schedule of drug administration, drug metabolism, and pattern of cell sensitivity may influence the pattern of marrow damage. Drugs act at specific points in the cell cycle and are classified on that basis; thus, hematopoietic stem cells may rebound after short-term exposure to a cell cycle–specific agent, but prolonged administration results in permanent bone marrow suppression. For cell cycle–specific agents, such as ara-C or methotrexate, recovery occurs rapidly (7-14 days), whereas stem cell or G0 active agents, such as carmustine (BCNU) and busulfan, cause a much more delayed nadir (4-5 weeks) and recovery (6 weeks). Moreover, a chronic deficit in marrow reserve occurs quickly with sequential BCNU therapy but rarely, if ever, occurs after cell cycle–specific agents such as ara-C. Bone marrow involvement with tumor may compromise bone marrow reserves, thereby shortening the time to leukopenia and thrombocytopenia and prolonging the recovery time. The characteristic effects of several drugs on marrow are shown in Table 127-3.

Gamma Radiation Related

Cells damaged by irradiation may divide one time or more before all progeny are rendered reproductively sterile; thus, an irradiated cell will not appear damaged until it divides.[16] At the time of the first postirradiation subdivision, the cell may die, divide aberrantly and produce unusual forms, be unable to divide and remain physiologically functional, or give rise to one or more generation of progeny until cells become sterile. Since bone marrow stem cells have a very low capacity for repair of sublethal irradiation damage, multiple smaller radiation fractions may preserve other normal tissues (eg, lung, intestine) but will not spare bone marrow. During a course of fractionated irradiation, the ultimate effect on normal bone marrow will depend on whether there has been proliferation in the irradiated field between the fractions or migration of cells from unirradiated adjacent sites. Localized irradiation can cause a chronic lymphopenia (Table 127-3). Finally, the effects of whole body irradiation are qualitatively and quantitatively different from localized therapy. In particular, total body irradiation causes profound suppression of humoral and cellular immune function.

Table 127-3 **Characteristic Effects of Drugs and Treatments on Bone Marrow**

Treatment	Hematologic Complication
Most chemotherapeutic agents	Leukopenia and thrombocytopenia at 9-10 days; nadir counts at 14-18 days; recovery of counts at 21-28 days
Nitrosourea	Myelosuppression at 4-6 weeks
Vincristine, l-asparaginase, bleomycin, myelo-suppression methotrexate with leucovorin	No myelosuppression
Gamma irradiation	Chronic lymphopenia
Whole-body irradiation	Profound suppression of humoral and cellular immune response

Associated Processes

It is essential to remain cognizant of derangements in normal physiology that may be occurring in the setting of cancer and/or treatment and that contribute to pancytopenia. These include nutritional factors, such as folate, iron, or vitamin deficiencies. There may be abnormal feedback loops in hematopoiesis, such as cell-mediated suppression of hematopoiesis in aplastic anemia or stimulation of thrombopoiesis in the setting of antibody-mediated platelet destruction.[17] Fibrosis can occur either as part of a disease process or as a reaction to therapy, thereby compromising bone marrow reserve. Immunologically mediated destruction of cells and other factors, such as splenomegaly, can result in cytopenias. Moreover, occult bleeding must always be considered as a cause of persistent anemia and refractory thrombocytopenia. These clinical examples emphasize the importance of carefully assessing patients with cancer for treatable medical etiologies of their hematologic complications prior to attributing these effects to their underlying neoplasms.

Abnormalities of Red Cells and Red Cell Support

Anemia

Anemia in patients with cancer can be mild to severe and may be attributable to many causes. Hematopoiesis in patients with early stages of cancer may be normal. On the other hand, replacement of marrow cells by tumor is not essential for the development of anemia, even in patients with metastatic cancer. Most commonly, the incidence and magnitude of anemia in patients with cancer increase as the disease progresses. This anemia is designated as anemia of chronic disease only if the cellular pattern in the marrow is nearly normal, the serum iron and iron-binding capacity are low, the iron content of the marrow is normal or increased, and the serum ferritin is elevated.[18] The coexistence of low plasma iron levels with adequate amounts of storage iron helps distinguish anemia of chronic disease from iron-deficiency anemia. Moreover, other causes of anemia, for example, overt hemolysis, bleeding, nutritional deficiency, or marrow replacement, must be ruled out. Finally, ^{51}chromium-labeled RBC studies suggest that RBC survival in patients with advanced cancer can be significantly shortened without classic clinical or laboratory evidence of hemolysis. In some patients, such as those with histiocytic medullary reticulosis or Hodgkin disease (HD), erythrophagocytosis, or hypersplenism may account for this decrease in red cell survival, but in others its etiology is unclear.

Red Cell Growth Factors

Serum EPO levels may be low for a given level of anemia in patients with cancer compared to a control population with anemias of other etiologies.[19] Moreover, increases in EPO serum levels expected for a given degree of anemia can be further blunted by chemotherapy regimens, with or without cisplatin. The inability to produce EPO in cancer patients is not absolute, however, since hypoxemia can restore EPO response. The exact nature of the EPO-producing cells in the kidney and liver is unclear, but it is possible that the EPO-producing cells are damaged by the chemotherapy and radiation therapy. This has been suggested as the etiology of the anemia associated with cisplatin chemotherapy, although direct erythroid marrow toxicity may play a role.[20] Since the endogenous EPO response is inappropriate in patients with cancer, treatment of the anemia of cancer with recombinant human (rH) EPO may be of value.[21,22] Randomized trials demonstrated that rHEPO corrected anemia and reduced homologous red cell transfusion requirements in patients receiving chemotherapy with and without cisplatin.[23-25] In addition to reducing transfusion requirements, a study of 2370 outpatients with a variety of cancers who were also treated with rHEPO demonstrated a beneficial impact on patient-reported functional capacity and quality of life in patients who received chemotherapy independent of tumor response.[26] Endogenous EPO levels may also be low after autologous and allogeneic marrow transplantation and treatment with EPO in this setting is also useful to accelerate erythropoiesis and reduce homologous red cell requirements.[27-30] One study suggests that patients with cancer who do not increase serum EPO levels to more than 100 mU/mL and hemoglobin (Hb) by at least 0.5 g/dL after 2 weeks of rHEPO therapy are likely to be unresponsive to treatment.[31]

Immune hemolytic anemias are associated with neoplasms of the lymphocytic and reticuloendothelial systems. Anemia is usually moderate to severe and is associated with jaundice, splenomegaly, and increased urine and fecal urobilinogen excretion. Red cell survival is decreased and the reticulocyte count increased unless erythropoiesis is profoundly impaired. Hemolytic anemia may be due to a warm-reacting immunoglobulin (Ig)G with a positive direct antiglobulin (Coombs) test and positive reaction to antisera specific for IgG on the red cell. This occurs most commonly in chronic lymphocytic leukemia (CLL) but has also been reported in patients with lymphomas, acute leukemias, myeloproliferative disorders, or carcinoma. Alternatively, IgM antibody can bind and cause agglutination in the cold. In either case, anemia occurs because of reticuloendothelial sequestration of red cells that are coated with antibody or complement components (extravascular hemolysis). Hemoglobinemia and hemoglobulinuria (intravascular hemolysis) occurs very rarely and has been attributed to cold-reacting antibody. The production of inflammatory cytokines by phagocytes may mediate the symptomatology of IgG-mediated hemolytic transfusion reactions.[32]

Microangiopathic anemia, characterized by red cell distortion and fragmentation on smear (schistocytes) and intravascular hemolysis with associated thrombocytopenia, is uncommon, but when observed in oncology, it is usually evident in patients with metastatic adenocarcinomas of the stomach, breast, prostate, lung, pancreas, gall-bladder, and colon and in those with angiosarcomas.[33] Intravascular coagulation with low clotting factor levels, fibrinolysis, increased fibrin degradation products, and increased fibrin catabolism may be present. Red cell fragmentation may be due to deposition of fibrin within vessels, and/or intravascular coagulation may be initiated by the release of thromboplastins by the tumor cells. Finally, anemia may be related to pure red cell aplasia without associated leukocyte or platelet marrow abnormalities commonly associated with thymoma and rarely present in the setting of lymphoma or CLL.[34]

Red Cell Transfusion

Red cell transfusions are indicated to increase oxygen carrying capacity in patients with anemia that is not adequately compensated by normal physiologic mechanisms. Sufficient oxygen-carrying capacity to maintain cardiopulmonary function can be met by a hemoglobin of 7 g/dL (a hematocrit of approximately 21%) when the intravascular volume is adequate for perfusion.[35] In a randomized multicenter study of critical care patients, a restrictive transfusion strategy (maintaining hemoglobin levels between 7 and 9 g/dL) was demonstrated to be at least as safe as a more liberal transfusion strategy, with the possible exception of patients with acute myocardial infarction or unstable angina.[36] However, there is no single hemoglobin level that can be universally applied as a "transfusion trigger." In deciding whether to transfuse a specific patient, the physician should consider the patient's age, degree of anemia, the intravascular volume, and the presence of coexisting cardiac, pulmonary, or vascular conditions.[37] To meet oxygen needs, some patients may require RBC transfusions at higher hemoglobin levels. In particular, hemoglobin levels are commonly maintained at levels of 8 g/dL in the setting of cancer and its therapy. Transfusing one unit of RBC will usually increase the hemoglobin by 1 g/dL and the hematocrit by 2-3% in the average adult weighing 70 kg.

Packed red blood cells (PRBC) are prepared either from whole blood (WB) by the removal of plasma or by erythrocytapheresis. Whole blood is rarely transfused, except to restore both volume and oxygen carrying capacity in the setting of massive hemorrhage. Red cells can be depleted of leukocytes by filtration to produce leukoreduced red cells (LRBC). Leukoreduction can prevent a significant percentage of febrile nonhemolytic transfusion reactions, alloimmunization, and cytomegalovirus (CMV) infection in transfusion recipients.[38] Leukocyte reduction prior to storage can abrogate cytokine release and decrease transfusion reactions.[39] In the United States and around the world, there is a trend to universally transfuse leukoreduced cellular components to avoid the multiple adverse sequelae of leukocytes. Washed red blood cells (WRBC) are prepared by further removal of plasma from PRBCs. These products are sometimes indicated to prevent allergic reactions to plasma proteins.[40] WRBC may be useful in rare patients who are IgA deficient and have circulating anti-IgA antibodies, since these patients may have anaphylactic reactions if transfused with blood components containing IgA. PRBCs are currently stored for up to 42 days at 4°C. Retrospective studies have suggested that transfusing older stored PRBC units may be associated with adverse consequences for the recipient.[41] However, this is a highly controversial notion. Prospective randomized studies are currently being planned to investigate this issue.

Abnormalities of White Cells and White Cell Support

Leukocytosis

Peripheral blood leukocyte counts are usually normal in patients with cancer but may be slightly elevated in patients with lung cancer. Elevated circulating leukocyte counts greater than 50,000/mm^3 may occur in patients with cancer, are termed *leukemoid reactions*, and can consist either of mature leukocytes or of early forms, such as myeloblasts and promyelocytes, in the peripheral blood.[42] Such reactions have been described most commonly in patients with metastatic tumors of the breast, lung, and stomach. They are distinguished from leukoerythroblastic reactions by the absence of nucleated red cells and the immature white cells. Lymphocytic leukemoid reactions occur most often in children and young adults with viral infections but rarely have been reported in association with cancer. Basophilia, frequently present in patients with myeloproliferative syndromes, is also uncommonly evident in patients with leukemoid reactions. Finally, eosinophilia has been reported in association with HD and mycosis fungoides, carcinomatosis, epithelial tumors, brain tumors, melanoma, lymphoma, acute lymphocytic leukemia, eosinophilic granuloma, and myeloproliferative disorders.

Leukopenia

Leukopenia may occur related to cancer and its treatment. In 1965, Hersh and colleagues summarized the causes of death in patients with acute leukemia treated at the National Cancer Institute and noted a marked decline in fatal hemorrhage, due to the availability of platelet transfusions, with a concomitant increase in the occurrence of infection alone as a cause of death.[43]

A quantitative relationship between circulating leukocytes and infection was established in patients with leukemia; in particular, the probability of being infected is proportional to both the severity and duration of leukopenia.[44]

Associated Processes

After profound marrow injury, monocytosis usually precedes neutrophilic recovery. Overshoot in the leukocyte count to 20,000-30,000/mm^3 can occur before leveling out and return to normal leukocyte counts. The overshoot of leukocytes and platelets occurs much more frequently and is of greater magnitude in pediatric patients and young adults than in elderly patients, presumably reflecting marrow reserve capacity, differentiation rapidity, and hematopoietic homeostasis. Otherwise, elevated leukocyte counts in a cancer patient under observation should trigger an evaluation for an infectious cause. Defects in leukocyte function may be present with or without abnormalities in cell numbers. Patients with acute myelogenous leukemia (AML), for example, have defects in phagocytosis or microbial killing that is not present in patients with acute lymphoblastic leukemia (ALL).[45]

Leukocyte Transfusion

Therapeutic granulocytes were first utilized nearly 30 years ago in leukemic patients with leukopenia and serious infection. The earliest trials, which demonstrated the potential value of granulocyte transfusions, utilized granulocytes harvested from patients with chronic granulocytic leukemia and achieved cell dosages never approached when normal donors were utilized.[46] The importance of dose was defined: less than 10^{10} granulocytes were ineffective whereas greater than 10^{11} cells were effective. Indeed, in an afebrile, uninfected man, the half-life of granulocytes in the circulation is 6.7 (4-10) hours and the daily turnover rate is 230%; in the setting of fever and/or infection, this turnover rate can be several-fold higher.[47] Parallel work in canine models had also demonstrated that dogs deliberately made leukopenic by irradiation and given gram-negative bacteremia and pneumonia could be successfully treated with granulocyte transfusions.[48]

Clinical Studies

The randomized prospective clinical trials of therapeutic leukocyte trans-fusions for leukopenic patients with established infections have been reviewed.[49] Early studies demonstrated benefit from leukocyte transfusions and defined several factors to be predictors of outcome: type of infecting organisms, the interval to bone marrow recovery; and the dose of granulocytes transfused. Granulocyte transfusion was not beneficial in the most controlled study, in which recipients were not tested for antileukocyte antibodies, lower numbers of leukocytes were transfused, and a much better survival was noted in the group treated with antibiotics alone.[50] Because of improved efficacy of antibiotics, therapeutic granulocytes are presently utilized only rarely, to treat refractory bacterial or invasive fungal infection in a leukopenic patient who has reasonable expectation of marrow recovery. Five studies indicated a protective effect for leukocyte transfusions, although differences observed were significant in only two trials. Even this finite clinical need may be decreased with the use of recombinant growth factors, for example, GMCSF or G-CSF, to stimulate normal myeloid recovery. Indeed, a recent retrospective analysis did not show a benefit for granulocyte transfusions for treatment of fungal infections in neutropenic patients following bone marrow transplantation (BMT).[51]

There have been six randomized prospective trials of prophylactic leukocyte transfusions, given to prevent infections in leukopenic recipients.[47,49] However, none of the studies demonstrated improved survival because alloimmunization, transfusion reactions, CMV infection, and pulmonary infiltrates occurred more frequently in the transfused group. These studies have been criticized methodologically due to inadequate donor-recipient matching and inadequate doses of granulocytes transfused. A large randomized trial of high-dose granulocytes collected from G-CSF mobilized donors is currently in progress.[49]

Leukocyte Collection and Administration

Granulocytes are harvested in a leukopheresis procedure utilizing hydroxyethyl starch and sodium citrate, which usually takes 90 minutes to remove adequate granulocytes (>10^{10}) while returning RBCs to the donor. The recent use of myeloid growth factors can facilitate the collection of large numbers of granulocytes from normal donors and warrant further study of the utility of granulocyte transfusions.[47,52-54] These leukocytes are obtained from ABO-compatible donors. A test for leukoagglutination using freshly obtained patient serum and donor white cells can be done prior to transfusion to assure compatibility and avoid leukoagglutinin-mediated pulmonary reactions in the recipient. Post-transfusion CMV interstitial pneumonitis is avoided by using only CMV-seronegative donors. Leukocytes are irradiated to prevent proliferation of T cells within the transfused product, which could potentially either engraft or induce graft-versus-host disease (GVHD) when transfused to an immunocompromised host.[55] It is important to note that despite earlier allegations, patients receiving amphotericin therapy are not at increased risk for transfusion-related pulmonary reactions.

Myeloid Growth Factors

The development of recombinant myeloid growth factors, GM-CSF and G-CSF, has significantly shortened the period of leukopenia after high-dose therapies.[10] In particular, GM-CSF was first shown to accelerate myeloid recovery in patients with NHL, ALL, and HD undergoing autologous BMT.[56] G-CSF was shown to decrease the incidence of infection, as manifested by febrile neutropenia, in patients with nonmyeloid malignancies receiving myelosuppressive anticancer drugs associated with a significant incidence of severe neutropenia with fever.[57] Both have also been used, either alone or at the time of recovery from chemotherapy, to enhance collection of both autologous and allogeneic peripheral blood stem cells (PBSC) for transplantation, and ongoing studies are evaluating their cost efficacy to enhance reconstitution posttransplantation.[10,58-61] As noted above, their availability has further decreased the need for therapeutic granulocyte transfusions, but they may facilitate collection of granulocytes from normal donors.[47,52,53] They should not be used in otherwise uncomplicated neutropenia and fever but reserved for appropriate, approved clinical settings.[59-62] Novel applications of these factors are emerging, that is, GM-CSF in vaccine and dendritic cell cancer therapies.[10]

Abnormalities of Platelets and Platelet Support

Thrombocytosis

Primary thrombocytosis is noted not only in essential thrombocythemia but also in polycythemia rubra vera, agnogenic myeloid metaplasia, and chronic myelogenous leukemia (CML).[63] Related hemorrhage is usually from the skin or mucous membranes, and thrombosis involving the arterial and/or venous systems can also occur. Although an elevated whole-blood viscosity, intrinsic defects in platelets, and elevated platelet counts may all predispose to bleeding, it is difficult to assess risks in an asymptomatic patient. Therapy should be utilized for the symptomatic patient (eg, phlebotomy to correct polycythemia), which primarily consists of cytoreductive therapy of the underlying disorder.

Secondary or reactive thrombocytosis can also occur in other cancers but is characterized by only mild elevations of platelet counts without associated changes in platelet morphology and function.[64] This can sometimes serve as a diagnostic clue and is not associated with Trousseau syndrome of migratory thrombophlebitis. Indeed, persons with thrombocytosis over 400,000/mm^3 should be evaluated for chronic or acute inflammatory disorders, acute hemorrhage, anemia, iron deficiency, or neoplasm. After splenectomy, the platelet count rises in the first week to levels of 1×10^6/mm^3 or more and then falls slowly to normal over 3 months.

Thrombocytopenia

Thrombocytopenia in cancer patients is usually attributable to treatment with chemotherapy and radiotherapy. Impaired production of platelets due to a decrease or absence of megakaryocytes is therefore the most common cause of thrombocytopenia in patients with cancer (Table 127-4). However, thrombocytopenia may also be due to splenic sequestration in patients who have splenomegaly as part of their primary neoplastic process. In this setting, increased numbers of megakaryocytes are evident unless extensive marrow infiltration is present. Immune-mediated thrombocytopenia may also occur related to anti–human leukocyte antigen (anti-HLA) or antiplatelet-specific alloantibodies. Interestingly, combination chemotherapy and pulsed high-dose dexamethasone therapy have been shown to be beneficial in some patients in whom immune thrombocytopenia is refractory to corticosteroids and splenectomy.[65,66] Finally, thrombocytopenia may be related to diffuse intravascular coagulation (DIC), especially in patients with acute myelocytic leukemias, lymphomas, and carcinoma of lung, breast, gastrointestinal, or urologic origin. DIC most commonly complicates acute promyelocytic leukemia due to the presence of both thromboplastic material and fibrinolytic proteases in the promyelocytic subcellular components.[67]

Abnormalities in Platelet Function

Platelet function can be abnormal in several chronic myeloproliferative disorders. Although most bleeding in patients

Table 127-4 Causes of Thrombocytopenia

Acute thrombocytopenia due to increased platelet depletion (utilization, sequestration, or destruction)
Massive blood replacement
Cardiac surgery
Splenomegaly
Immune destruction of platelets
Self-limited acute idiopathic thrombocytopenia purpura (ITP)
Posttransfusion purpura
Drug purpura
Chronic idiopathic thrombocytopenia purpura
Consumptive thrombocytopenia
Hereditary defects
Thrombocytopenia with decreased platelet production
Aplastic anemia
Acute leukemia
Idiopathic megakaryocytic aplasia
Marrow infiltration
Malignant
Nonmalignant—Gaucher disease, granulomatous diseases
Following radiation or myelosuppressive drugs
Drugs producing specific suppression of platelet production (eg, thiazides, ethanol, estrogens)
Nutritional deficiency—megaloblastic anemia, severe iron deficiency (rare)
Viral infections
Paroxysmal nocturnal hemoglobinuria

with AML is related to thrombocytopenia, intrinsic abnormalities in platelet function have been described including decreased platelet pro-coagulant activity and decreased aggregation and serotonin release responses to ADP, epinephrine, or collagen.[68] These defects may reflect the fact that megakaryocytes have originated from a leukemic stem cell. Platelet transfusions, coupled with treatment of the underlying disease, remain the mainstay of therapy.

Platelet dysfunction is evident in a fraction of patients with IgA myeloma or Waldenstrom macroglobulinemia, multiple myeloma, and monoclonal gammopathy of undetermined significance.[69] In addition to thrombocytopenia, the following factors may also predispose to bleeding: hyperviscosity, acquired factor X deficiency in the setting of amyloidosis, a circulating heparin-like anticoagulant, fibrinolysis, and interference by myeloma protein with fibrin polymerization and with the function of other coagulation proteins. Cytoreductive therapy is primary, with plasmapheresis reserved for acute bleeding.

Platelet Transfusion Support

In 1910, fresh whole blood was first transfused to thrombocytopenic patients, resulting in a significant rise in the platelet count, hemostasis, and improvement of the bleeding time.[70] In the 1950s, platelets were first used for the treatment of thrombocytopenia related to combination chemotherapeutic treatments of leukemias.[71] Data from the National Cancer Institute in the early 1960s clearly demonstrated that leukemia patients died of hemorrhage during induction of remission with chemotherapy and established the quantitative relationship between platelet count and hemorrhage.[43,72] It was shown that platelet therapy could modify the course of hemorrhage in both pediatric and adult settings, the only difference being the doses required. In the 1970s, studies in children and adults confirmed the efficacy of platelet transfusion to prevent rather than control hemorrhage.[73,74]

Single- and Multiple-Donor Platelets

One unit of platelet concentrate is obtained from one unit of whole blood by centrifugation, and contains approximately 5.5 × 10^{10} platelets/unit. Concentrates from multiple (6-8) donors are pooled to produce a single component for transfusion. Currently, individual platelet concentrates can be stored for up to 5 days prior to pooling and transfusion. Apheresis technology has permitted harvesting the equivalent of several platelet concentrates from a single donor during a single donation.[75,76] A single-donor platelet unit typically contains at least 3 × 10^{11} platelets/unit. The major advantage of multiple-donor platelet concentrates is their availability, since they are derived from conventional whole blood donations. However, some studies suggest that alloimmunization can occur early in patients receiving multiple-donor platelets and that limiting the number of donors per transfusion may postpone the development of refractoriness to platelet transfusions in thrombocytopenic patients.[77] A second potential advantage of single-donor platelets stems from the decreased risk of infection when exposed to fewer donors. Indeed, the Retrovirus Epidemiology Donor Study demonstrated that the prevalence of any viral infection was 50% higher in whole blood donors as compared to apheresis donors.[78] The use of single-donor platelets is increasing; they are generally are considered to be the platelet product of choice for patients being treated for malignancy.[79] Single-donor platelet collections are utilized to provide HLA-matched donors for alloimmunized recipients who have not responded to platelets from random donors.

Indications for Therapeutic and Prophylactic Platelet Transfusion

A minority of patients with cancer require platelet transfusions; however, platelets are more commonly transfused to patients with cancer than to patients with any other category of disease. The majority of platelet transfusions are given prophylactically to prevent bleeding, as opposed to therapeutically, to treat active bleeding.[80] The appropriate indications for transfusion of platelets have been the subject of a National Institutes of Health Consensus Development Conference as well as a more recent American Society of Clinical Oncology clinical practice guideline.[81,82] At present, 6-8 units of random-donor platelet concentrates, or the equivalent platelet dose in the form of a single-donor apheresis platelet product, are often routinely transfused to cancer patients with platelet counts less than 10,000-20,000/mm^3 to prevent hemorrhage. Gmur and colleagues demonstrated that the threshold for prophylactic platelet transfusion can safely be set at 5 × 10^9/L in patients with acute leukemia without fever or bleeding manifestations and at 10 × 10^9/L in patients with such signs.[83] More recently, they have shown this policy to be safe in the outpatient management of patients with aplastic anemia. Prospective clinical trials have shown that the risk of major bleeding was similar whether 10 × 10^9/L or 20 × 10^9/L was used as the platelet-transfusion threshold in patients with acute leukemia, and that the lower threshold reduced platelet use.[84-86] The implications of thrombocytopenia as a risk factor for hemorrhage and therefore the timing and dose of prophylactic platelets may vary in different clinical settings. Moreover, the use of higher doses of platelets per transfusion may extend the interval until additional transfusions are needed.[87]

The risk of bleeding at a given platelet count may vary in distinct clinical settings. For example, patients with thrombocytopenia due to acute myelocytic leukemia were reported to have increased bleeding at less than 10,000/mm^3 platelets, in contrast to patients with ALL, who had similar risk of hemorrhage at less than 20,000/mm^3 platelets.[88] Young platelets are more efficient at controlling hemorrhage, so the need for platelet transfusion will be greater if the count is falling after chemotherapy compared to a similar level during a rise from a nadir.[89] Patients with chronic thrombocytopenia due to decreased platelet production (ie, myelodysplastic disorders) may require transfusions, in contrast to patients with accelerated destruction but active production of platelets (ie, idiopathic thrombocytopenic purpura), who may notrequire routine platelet transfusions. Moreover, patients with chronic thrombocytopenia may tolerate lower absolute platelet counts without transfusion. In patients with abnormalities of platelet function, it is not the absolute platelet count but rather the number of functional platelets that is important for the prevention of bleeding. Thus, it is difficult to define an absolute platelet threshold for transfusion for all patients, and both the timing and the dose of prophylactic platelet transfusion must therefore be determined on a clinical basis.[87,90-93] The multicenter randomized PLADO (PLAtelet DOsing) study demonstrated that prophylactic transfusion with low-dose platelets does not increase the risk of Grade 2 or higher bleeding as compared with standard-dose prophylaxis. Patients receiving low-dose prophylaxis do require more frequent platelet transfusions, although fewer total platelets are required overall.[92]

Clinical and Laboratory Assessment of the Effectiveness of Platelet Transfusion

The effectiveness of platelet transfusion can be assessed by laboratory parameters, the corrected count increment (CCI) in platelet count 1 hour or 10 count to 15 minutes after transfusion and the bleeding time, as well as by the observed clinical outcome after transfusion.[94-97] The corrected platelet increment is defined as the increment in platelet counts from pre- to posttransfusion corrected for the number of units transfused and for the body surface area of the recipient. When low numbers of platelets are transfused, regression analysis of posttransfusion increments may provide a more accurate assessment than CCI.[98] Measurement of the bleeding time after transfusion serves as a measure of the number of functional platelets, particularly in patients known to have dysfunctional platelets. Techniques such as radiolabeling platelets can be utilized to diagnose and identify the site of accelerated platelet destruction, but the most important monitor of the effectiveness of platelet transfusion is critical clinical assessment for the presence and extent of hemorrhage.

Factors Adversely Affecting Platelet Recovery

If an inappropriately low corrected platelet increment is noted at 1 hour after transfusion, the status of both the platelet product transfused and of the recipient must be examined for potential explanations. A CCI of 15,000-20,000/mm^3 is usual at 18-24 hours, provided fresh, properly stored platelets have been transfused.[94] This translates into an absolute increment at 1 hour of approximately 7,000-11,000/mm^3 for each unit of platelet concentrate administered to an average-sized person with body surface area of 1.0 m^2.

Laboratory Factors

Several factors involved in the harvesting and storage of platelets prior to transfusion might result in poor posttransfusion platelet survival: pH, number of contaminating leukocytes, concentration of platelets, plasma volume, temperature, time, and agitation during storage. With the quality control measures currently in practice in most blood banks, it is uncommon to identify a problem either in the harvesting or donation to account for a poor posttransfusion increment.

Clinical Factors

If the survival of transfused platelets is compromised, several conditions in the transfusion recipients may be responsible.[99-103] First, patients with fevers and/or infections have increased consumption of platelets, even when there is no evidence of consumptive coagulopathy. Second, posttransfusion increments in platelet count may also be less than expected due to splenic sequestration, especially in the setting of splenomegaly.[104] Third, drug-induced platelet antibodies, which mediate immune destruction of platelets, have been demonstrated. Antibodies responsible for drug-induced thrombocytopenia may bind to platelets by their fragment-antigen binding (Fab) regions rather than by attaching nonspecifically as immune complexes.[105] Platelet membrane glycoproteins gpIb and gpIIb/IIIa appear to be the preferred targets, although gpV has also been implicated.[106-108] Drugs apparently bind to the platelet membrane, inducing a reversible structural change that provokes an antibody response. Drugs may also induce antibodies that mediate thrombocytopenia without direct drug–platelet interaction, for example, methyldopa.[109] Alter-natively, drugs such as penicillin may bind covalently to the platelet membrane and induce hapten-dependent antibodies.[110] The survival of transfused platelets can be compromised if the recipient possesses antibodies against donor antigens (Ags) of HLA-A and HLA-B loci, the AB-H system, or platelet alloantigens. Response to platelet transfusion in recipients of hematopoietic stem cell transplantation has been specifically studied. One report identified high total bilirubin, total body irradiation, and high serum cyclosporin A levels to be predictive of low CCI, whereas another found irradiation, posttransplant fever, and hepatic venoocclusive disease to be associated with delayed platelet recovery.[101,102] A third study in patients who had undergone hematopoietic stem cell transplantation associated presence of lymphocytotoxic antibodies, male gender, large body surface area, concomitant red cell transfusion, concurrent steroids, major ABO incompatibility, and history of multiple recipient pregnancies with poor CCI post–platelet transfusion.[103]

Alloimmunization

Platelets bear HLA-A and -B but lack HLA-C and -DR Ags, and there is a high correlation between the development of lymphocytotoxic anti-HLA antibodies in the recipient and refractoriness to random-donor platelets.[111] Anti-HLA antibodies are most easily detectable using the patient's serum and a panel of lymphocytes representing known HLA specificities. The incidence and the timing of production of anti-HLA antibodies after platelet transfusion remain controversial and may vary with the recipient population. Most studies document alloimmunization in 50-90% of multitransfused patients.[112] Some studies demonstrate that the rate of alloimmunization increases with the number of transfusions, whereas other reports find no relationship between the number of platelet transfusions given and the rate of alloimmunization.[113,114] Moreover, a fraction of patients with cancer never become sensitized.[115,116] Nonetheless, it is crucial to test for anti-HLA antibodies whenever recipients become refractory to random-donor platelet transfusion, since response to random-donor platelet transfusion is poor in the sensitized host, and HLA-matched or family-member platelets may be useful in this setting.[117] The panel reactive antibody (PRA) screen is usually performed in this context.

Yankee and colleagues first demonstrated that platelets obtained from HLA-identical siblings or from unrelated donors matched at the HLA-A and -B loci (grade A or B matches) could result in satisfactory posttransfusion increments in alloimmunized recipients who were refractory to random-donor platelet transfusions.[117,118] Subsequently, Duquesnoy and colleagues found that donors whose HLA antigens were the same (B match) or crossreactive with the patient's Ags (BX match) were equivalent.[119]

The evaluation of donors for the same or crossreactive Ags became even more complex. For example, platelets from donors lacking HLA-A2 who bear one of two (grade C match) or three of four (grade D match) Ags not present in the recipient may have favorable posttransfusion outcomes in alloimmunized recipients; in contrast, platelets from HLA-A2+ donors who were HLA-A and -B matches were unsuccessful.[119] Weak anti-HLA antibodies, which can cause platelet destruction in vivo, may not be detected by standard assays, and, alternatively, excellent platelet transfusion recoveries have been observed despite a positive lymphocytotoxicity crossmatch.[111,119] Additional cross-matching techniques may be required in those 20% of sensitized patients who remain refractory even to HLA-matched platelets.

The recognition of the refractoriness associated with the development of anti-HLA antibodies led to attempts to either avoid or delay alloimmunization by modifying the platelets to be transfused. Since HLA antigens are expressed on leukocytes, and platelets themselves are poor immunogens, investigators have attempted to (1) remove WBC from platelets or treat platelets with ultraviolet irradiation (UV) to abrogate the leukocyte antigen–presenting function; (2) use single rather than multiple donor platelets to minimize exposure to HLA; and (3) transfuse only HLA-matched or leukocyte-depleted HLA-matched platelets. Leukocyte-reduced platelets are prepared by filtration, which deplete white cells by 3 logs, with varying associated losses of platelets. Filtered platelets with no more than 10^6 contaminating leukocytes were found to reduce the likelihood of formation of anti-HLA antibodies; in contrast, transfusions of similar numbers of non–leukocyte-reduced platelets did sensitize recipients.[38,120] The multicenter prospective Trial to Reduce Alloimmunization to Platelets (TRAP) study confirmed that the incidence of anti-HLA and platelet-specific antibodies alone, as well as the incidence of antibodies associated with platelet refractoriness, were reduced in leukemic recipients who received either filtered or UV-treated pooled random-donor concentrates or filtered single-donor platelets compared to similar patients who received nonfiltered pooled random-donor concentrates (Table 127-5).[121] Only 13% of patients developed platelet refractoriness associated with lymphocytotoxic antibodies, suggesting that the majority of unresponsiveness to transfusion is related to other factors. A meta-analysis of seven randomized controlled trials published between 1983 and 1995 supports the TRAP findings and suggests that these findings can be extended to other than leukemic patients and applied to the prevention of platelet transfusion refractoriness.[120,122]

When sensitized recipients remain refractory to HLA-matched platelets, attempts have been made to carry out additional cross-matching to identify more compatible platelet donors.[108,123-125] These include leukoagglutination,[52] chromium lysis, immunofluorescence, enzyme-linked immunosorbent assay (ELISA), assays of iodine-labeled platelet-associated IgG, and platelet aggregometry. They have enjoyed variable success determining which platelets will be effective in refractory patients, and no one assay or combination of methods has been universally accepted to predict response to transfusion.

Potential mechanisms to explain unexpectedly suboptimal posttransfusion recoveries in patients receiving HLA-matched ABO-compatible platelet transfusions include unrecognized HLA specificities, circulating immune complexes, and antibodies to platelet-specific Ags. Plasma exchange or intravenous immunoglobulin therapy has been used prior to platelet transfusion in those patients who remain refractory to ABO compatible HLA-matched platelets, with mixed benefit.[126,127]

ABO blood group determinants are intrinsic to platelet membranes.[128] Major Ags of the Rh, Duffy, Kidd, Kell, and Lutheran systems, in contrast, are not expressed on the surface of human platelets.[129] Unlike the case with RBC transfusion, ABO mismatch between donor and recipient is not an absolute contraindication to platelet transfusion.[130] That said, ABO-identical platelet transfusions are preferred. Transfused ABO major-incompatible platelets (eg, A donor, O recipient) demonstrate recoveries that are about 1/3rd lower than those seen with ABO-identical transfusions.[131]

Additionally, hemolytic reactions caused by very high titers of isohemagglutinins present within the plasma in the transfused platelet concentrates (eg, donor O, recipient A) have occasionally caused severe hemolysis. The U.K., notably, has instituted routine screening of platelet units for anti-A/B to prevent this problem. Other countries, including the United States., have not adopted a uniform strategy of prevention.[131]

Platelet Alloantigens

There is now a variety of alloantigens implicated in alloimmune thrombocytopenia that have important biologic functions: platelet activation–dependent fibrinogen binding (gpIIb:IIIa complex), platelet–von Willebrand factor interactions (gpIb:IX complex), and platelet/collagen interactions (gpIa:IIa complex).[132,133] Antibodies directed at these Ags can cause immune-mediated destruction of platelets in the presence or absence of anti-HLA antibodies. Sensitization to these Ags is rarely the cause of refractory thrombocytopenia in patients with cancer.[108,121]

One clinical sequela of antibodies to platelet alloantigens is posttransfusion purpura, resulting from antibody directed at the PL^{A1} Ag. In posttransfusion purpura, profound thrombocytopenia develops approximately 1 week after transfusion, primarily in women who have been immunized either by earlier pregnancies or, less frequently, by a previous transfusion.[134,135] Almost all patients have been PL^{A1} negative with anti-PL^{A1} antibody in their plasma at the time of thrombocytopenia. Partial exchange transfusion, plasmapheresis, and high-dose IV immunoglobulin have all been used to accelerate recovery from posttransfusion purpura.[135] The abrupt onset of thrombocytopenia after transfusion can be related to passive alloimmune thrombocytopenia to HPA-1a and HPA-5b, and transplantation-associated alloimmune thrombocytopenia can result from residual host cells producing antibodies against donor platelet Ags (HPA-1).[133]

Alternatives to Platelet Transfusion

Studies to date have not shown reproducible effects of G-CSF or GM-CSF on recovery of platelets. However, numerous molecules have shown thrombopoietic effects in vitro and in vivo.[6,11,13] Examples of these include IL-1, IL-3, IL-6, IL-11, leukemia inhibitory factor (LIF), and *c-kit* ligand (KL). Additionally, with the tools of recombinant DNA, there is the ability to "cut and splice" novel recombinant hybrid molecules that may possess thrombopoietic activity, such as the PIXY 321 molecule, which is a recombinant hybrid of the coding regions from the human GM-CSF and IL-3 genes. Although these growth factors do elevate platelet counts in patients, studies in humans to date suggest that fever and constitutional symptoms may be dose limiting for IL-1, IL-3, and IL-6. Interleukin-11 is now approved by the U.S. FDA as a platelet growth factor.[12] A most exciting development is the recent isolation of thrombopoietin, the *c-mpl* ligand.[11,13] This promotes both megakaryocyte progenitor expansion and megakaryocyte differentiation, and its injection in nanogram quantities raises platelet levels of mice to three or four times the normal. Moreover, mice that are deficient in the *c-mpl* receptor have few megakaryocytes and are profoundly thrombocytopenic but have normal numbers of other hematopoietic cell types.[136] Thrombopoietin may be useful to enhance collection of PBSCs and for ex vivo expansion of stem cells, but its future development to enhance platelet recovery is unclear, since its use in normal donors induced antibodies and related thrombocytopenia.

Attempts have also been made to develop alternatives to platelet transfusion.[137] Klein and colleagues have administered lyophilized whole platelets to treat thrombocytopenic bleeding in

Table 127-5 Trial to Reduce Alloimmunization to Platelets in Patients Undergoing Myeloablative Therapy for Acute Myelocytic Leukemia

	Pooled Random Donor Concentrates (%)	Pooled Random Donor Concentrates Treated with UVB Irradiation (%)	Pooled Random Donor Platelets, White Cell Reduced by Filtration (%)	Single-Donor Platelets[a] (%)
Lymphocytotoxic antibodies and refractoriness to transfusion	13	5	3	4
Lymphocytotoxic antibodies only	45	21	18	17
Alloantibodies and refractoriness to transfusion	13	5	3	4
Alloantibodies only	11	7	6	7

[a]Prepared by apheresis in a white cell reduction protocol and further filtered to reduce white cell contamination to the lowest possible amount.

pediatric patients and observed clinical improvement in 50% of patients, suggesting that morphologic integrity of platelets might not be essential for their in vivo function.[138] Platelets preserved in gelatin also retain hemostatic efficacy.[139] New technologies for cryopreservation of platelets that achieve satisfactory platelet recovery after transfusion are being described.[140] Aldehyde-fixed, dried, and rehydrated platelets adhere to exposed subendothelium and may therefore remain hemostatically active.[141] By crosslinking arginineglycine-aspartic acid (RGD) tripeptides to erythrocytes, Coller and colleagues have produced "thromboerythrocytes" that interact with gpIIb:IIIa receptors on activated platelets.[142] Synthetic liposomes, composed of phospholipids and platelet glycoprotein complexes, can shorten prolonged bleeding times in thrombocytopenic animals.[140] Platelet membrane particles can normalize prolonged bleeding times in animal models and will soon undergo clinical testing.[143,144] Finally, synthetic phospholipids promote procoagulant activity on damaged vessels, suggesting their potential utility as platelet substitutes.[141,145] It is likely that cytokines and/or new products will be developed in the future to substitute for platelet transfusion therapy. The availability of new technology will then allow more effective strategies to both prevent thrombocytopenic hemorrhage and avoid the potential immunohematologic complications of platelet transfusion.

Other Therapeutic Modalities

Transfusion of Fresh Frozen Plasma

Fresh frozen plasma is the fluid portion of 1 unit (450 mL) of whole blood that is centrifuged, separated, and frozen at −18°C or lower. It contains physiologic levels of coagulation factors. Fresh frozen plasma is utilized to correct coagulation factor deficiencies; to reverse warfarin effect; to correct coagulopathy of passive transfusion; for antithrombin III replacement; and to treat thrombotic thrombocytopenic purpura, disseminated intravascular coagulation, coagulopathy of liver disease, thrombolytic agent overdose, protein C or S deficiency, and hemolytic uremic syndrome.[142,146] In addition to the plasma obtained from donated whole blood, it can be collected using plasmapheresis procedures for the production of derivatives: coagulation factors (factors VIII and IX), immunoglobulin, and albumin preparations.

Therapeutic Pheresis

Therapeutic cytapheresis is used in the setting of hyperleukocytic leukemias and lymphomas and in thrombocythemia to remove excess cells. In addition, therapeutic plasmapheresis or plasma exchange is useful in disorders associated with excess abnormal proteins in plasma. Therapeutic pheresis in a cancer patient does not alter the underlying condition; rather, it is utilized as an adjunct to conventional therapy.

Therapeutic leukopheresis can be done when hyperleukocytosis is present when first encountering a patient with leukemia who has clinical evidence of leukostasis or is threatened by a catastrophe from the hyperleukocytosis. Pulmonary sludging with related tachypnea and dyspnea, often with hypoxia and radiographic diffuse infiltration, is one indication. Torpor, headache, or confusion, suggesting the possibility of vascular invasion and related intracerebral hemorrhage, is another. Leukopheresis is also used to reduce tumor mass prior to chemotherapy and thereby to avoid treatment-related hyperuricemia and renal failure. It is indicated for patients with AML or ALL and white cell counts greater than 100×10^9/L and for patients with CML and counts greater than 300 × 109/L.[147] Leukopheresis has also been used to treat patients with CLL, hairy cell leukemia, and Sezary syndrome.[148-150] However, leukopheresis remains expensive and time consuming and therefore is rarely utilized in place of cytotoxic therapy.

Plateletpheresis is commonly used to provide single-donor platelets for patients undergoing therapy for leukemia or cancer. Plateletpheresis can also be utilized to reduce the elevated platelet counts present in the setting of thrombocythemia.[151] In these cases, there can be rapid relief of clinical sequelae, including cerebral and myocardial ischemia, gastrointestinal bleeding, and pulmonary embolism, before the effects of cytotoxic therapy become apparent.

Plasma exchange has been utilized in several oncologic settings. In patients receiving ABO-incompatible allogeneic marrow transplants, plasmapheresis has been utilized to remove high-titer isohemagglutinins.[148] Plasmapheresis has also been utilized to remove leukocyte antibodies from patients receiving granulocyte transfusions.[149] In patients refractory to platelet transfusion by virtue of sensitization to HLA, plasmapheresis has had variable success.[148] Finally, plasmapheresis has been used to deplete paraproteins and relieve hyperviscosity-related sludging and/or hemorrhage.[150] It is more commonly used to deplete IgM in Waldenstrom macroglobulinemia than to remove paraprotein in myeloma, which is almost always non-IgM. Since the paraprotein reaccumulates, plasmapheresis is considered only an adjunct to cytotoxic therapy of the underlying disease.

Effects of Transfusion on the Immune System

It is essential to emphasize that patients with cancer may be immunocompromised due to the neoplastic disease and/or its treatment. This may make any effects of transfusion on recipient immunity of particular importance in this patient population.

Alloimmunization

The most firmly established effect of transfusion is the stimulation of antibodies in the recipient against Ags in the transfused products. Both cellular and plasma Ags in transfused blood expose the recipients to hundreds of known alloantigens.

Over 400 RBC Ags have been identified, yet we routinely ensure compatibility for only three of them: A, B, and D. More than 100 HLA Ags, as well as granulocyte- and platelet-specific Ags, have also been identified. Genetic alleles can result in structural and therefore antigenic differences among all plasma proteins, leading to recipient alloantibodies to the donated immunoglobulins. Most alloantigens are ignored in transfusion therapy, since they are poor immunogens. However, studies clearly demonstrate that the development of recipient antibodies to Ags in transfused products relates not only to the number of transfusions but also to their timing. Specifically, individuals who receive equal numbers of transfusions are more likely to develop antibodies if the transfusions are given repeatedly over a longer period than if given within a shorter interval. Some cancer patients, by virtue of receiving repeated transfusions over a longer period, may therefore be more likely to become alloimmunized. Alloantibodies to RBCs can lead to recipient morbidity and shortened RBC survival; antibodies to leukocytes are associated with febrile transfusion reactions and can impair effectiveness and survival of transfused granulocytes.[152] Anti–HLA-A and -B antibodies as well as platelet-specific alloantibodies impair survival of transfused and autologous platelets.[120,122] Finally, anti-IgA sometimes causes anaphylactic reactions in IgA deficient recipients, but anti-IgG or -IgM or antilipoproteins are not clinically significant.[153]

Immunosuppression

Transfusions may also have immunosuppressive effects on recipients. Animal models have demonstrated immune suppression and accelerated tumor growth in rats that received allogeneic transfusion.[154] In humans, patients who received multiple transfusions have decreased numbers of natural killer (NK) cells and increased circulating Ia+ T cells. T4:T8 ratios may also be decreased.[155,156] The decrease in NK cells is directly related to the number of RBC units received and is seen only in patients transfused within the past year. It has been reported that soluble HLA class I and II and well as Fas ligand accumulate in blood components, in relation to both the number of leukocytes and length of storage.[157] They may be immunoregulatory, evidenced by inhibition of in vitro allogeneic mixed lymphocyte responses and antigen-specific cytotoxic T-cell activity, as well as induction of apoptosis in Fas+ cells.

Research has demonstrated increased renal graft survival in patients who had been previously transfused with blood from donors who share at least one HLA-DR antigen.[158] More recently, both increased cancer recurrence rates and an increased incidence of postoperative infection have been noted following transfusion.[159] Specifically, nontransfused patients with a variety of stages and sites of large bowel cancer fared better in 11 of 14 retrospective studies; when multivariate analysis was done, transfusion was an independent unfavorable predictor of earlier recurrence or cancer-related deaths in 7 of 12 studies. Some studies suggest that recipients of homologous transfusions have higher recurrence rates than have recipients of autologous transfusion.[160]

Transfused patients undergoing surgery for colorectal cancer have also been reported to have higher rates of postoperative infection than those who are not transfused, although this remains an area of investigation.[161,162] Overviews and meta-analyses confirm a lack of significant effect of perioperative transfusion on colorectal cancer recurrence or on postoperative septic complications.[163,164] However, given that patients are often immunosuppressed due to their disease and/or its therapy, any immunosuppressive effect of transfusion further highlights the importance of justifying the medical and surgical indication for all transfusions.

Although the mechanisms of any transfusion-associated immunosuppressive effect in humans is unknown, cancer patients receiving only a small number of RBCs had fewer recurrences and improved survival compared to those receiving only whole blood or larger numbers of RBCs, suggesting that a factor present in whole blood, for example, plasma, is implicated.[159,165] However, in an animal model, transfused allogeneic lymphocytes appear to mediate an immunosuppressive effect, and prestorage, but not poststorage. Leukodepletion abrogates this immunosuppressive effect, suggesting that a cytokine is the mediator of this effect.[166] Future studies are needed to define the precise relationship between transfusion, immunosuppression of the recipient, and cancer recurrence.

Transfusion-Associated GVHD

Historic Perspective

GVHD is commonly observed after allogeneic BMT but is rarely recognized after transfusion or transplantation of other organs. Transfusion associated (TA)-GVHD usually occurs in the immunosuppressed recipient (eg, BMT recipients), but recent reports also involve more nearly immunocompetent recipients.[55,167] The clinical manifestations include fever and skin rash, anorexia, nausea, vomiting, and watery or bloody diarrhea with or without elevated liver enzymes and hyperbilirubinemia. Since there are no pathognomonic features of GVHD, this syndrome is sometimes difficult to distinguish from viral infections or drug eruptions. TA-GVHD is usually severe, and, unlike the situation after allogeneic BMT, it frequently results in pancytopenia secondary to marrow aplasia. The majority of reported cases of TA-GVHD have not responded to immunosuppressive therapies and have been fatal.

TA-GVHD has been reported after transfusion of unirradiated blood components to patients with severe combined immunodeficiency, thymic hypoplasia, and Wiskott-Aldrich syndrome; premature newborns and those with erythroblastosis fetalis; patients with hematologic neoplasms, including Hodgkin and non-Hodgkin lymphomas, acute myelocytic and lymphoblastic leukemias, CLL, and aplastic anemias; patients with carcinomas and sarcomas, including neuroblastomas, glioblastoma, rhabdomyosarcoma, cervical carcinoma, small-cell lung cancer, and germ cell tumor; patients after cardiac surgery and cholecystectomy; and pregnant women.[55,167] This syndrome has developed following exchange and intrauterine transfusions, and after transfusion of whole blood, plasma, RBCs, and platelets. Leukocytes harvested from normal donors and from donors with chronic myelocytic leukemia have also been transfused to patients with hematologic neoplasms and been implicated in TA-GVHD.

Definition of Those at Risk

In 1986, the National Institutes of Health Consensus Development Conference defined patients who have undergone BMT or those with other forms of immunodeficiency as candidates for irradiated platelet concentrates to avoid GVHD.[80] Patients with leukemias and other cancers who may be immunosuppressed secondary to chemotherapy and/or radiation therapy or due to intrinsic immune dysfunction (eg, HD), may be at risk for TA-GVHD.[168] Among patients with HD, it had previously been assumed that combined radiation and chemotherapy were necessary as predisposing factors for the development of TA-GVHD, but several cases of TA-GVHD have recently been documented in patients with HD who were treated with chemotherapy alone.[169] Patients receiving high-dose chemotherapy followed by autologous bone marrow support are also at risk for TA-GVHD.[170] Finally, immunocompetent patients who share an HLA haplotype with HLA-homozygous blood donors also appear to be at risk for TA-GVHD.[171,172] Homozygosity for HLA types is more likely to occur among first-degree family members (eg, parents, children, and siblings). It has, therefore, recently been recommended that cellular blood components from such donors be irradiated with at least 2500 cGy prior to transfusion. Indeed, products from all family member–directed donors should be irradiated, given that TA-GVHD has now been reported after transfusion of blood from a second-degree relative.[173] Reports of TA-GVHD after transfusion of cellular blood components from homozygous blood donors to heterozygous non–blood relatives suggest that indications for gamma irradiation may need to be broadened.[172,174] The risk of transfusion of blood from HLA homozygous donors to unrelated HLA heterozygous patients is 1 in 874 in Japan and may be as high as 1 in 7174 in the United States.[175] Finally, reports confirm that all HLA-matched cellular components should be irradiated.[55,171,172,176]

Strategies for Prevention

The only currently effective method to prevent TA-GVHD is gamma irradiation of blood products prior to transfusion. Studies suggest that irradiation at 1500-2000 cGy can reduce mitogen-responsive lymphocytes by 5-6 logs compared to unirradiated controls.[177] However, the observation that a small percentage of lymphocytes survive irradiation at these doses, coupled with a single reported case of apparent TA-GVHD in a bone marrow transplant recipient who received only blood components irradiated at 2000 cGy, suggest that existing blood product irradiation guidelines require reassessment.[178] Indeed, the standards of the American Association of Blood Banks (AABB), as well as those of the FDA, now require that blood and cellular components be irradiated with a midplane dose of a minimum of 2500 cGy.[179] Studies to date suggest no adverse effects of irradiation on storage of platelets, but the clinical significance of potassium release on storage of irradiated red cells is not yet defined, and posttransfusion red cell recovery of irradiated units may be decreased.[180,181]

A potential alternative method to prevent TA-GVHD would be to deplete lymphocytes from blood products prior to transfusion; however, the number and precise T cells required to mediate TA-GVHD remain undefined, and it is unknown whether depletion of leukocytes using these currently available techniques would decrease the risk of TA-GVHD. Moreover, cases of TA-GVHD in recipients of filtered components have been reported.[175] Using a well-characterized parent-F1 hybrid murine transfusion model, it was shown that the depletion of recipient CD4+ cells increased the number of donor cells needed to induce GVHD, whereas depletion of recipient CD8+ cells decreased the number of donor cells need to induce GVHD, suggesting the importance of CD8+ cells for their protective effect.[182] In this model, photochemical treatment with psoralen followed by long-wavelength UV treatment or cellular components before transfusion has been shown to prevent TA-GVHD, suggesting its potential clinical utility.[183]

Conclusions and Recommendations

Patients who have congenital immunodeficiencies or those who undergo BMT should routinely receive only irradiated (2500 cGy) blood components. Patients with cancer may be immunocompromised secondary to their underlying disease and/or chemoradiotherapy, but the frequency of occurrence and degree of immunosuppression predisposing to TA-GVHD in this population is not precisely defined. Within this group, however, patients receiving high-dose chemoradiotherapy (eg, in preparation for autologous BMT), those with HD, and patients receiving donations of cellular blood components from first-degree blood relatives should receive only irradiated blood components. Whole blood, packed red cells, granulocytes, platelets, and fresh plasma have all caused TA-GVHD, but fresh frozen plasma and frozen deglycerolized red cells have not yet been implicated. Platelets can be irradiated at the time of collection without adverse consequences, but the effects of irradiation and prolonged storage of red cells is not yet defined.

Transfusion-Related Infectious Diseases (Table 127-6)

Hepatitis B

Although hepatitis B (HB) was formerly a common transfusion-related infection, the use of several generations of HB surface antigen assays to screen potential donors and the use of volunteer versus commercial donors has markedly reduced the incidence of HB transmitted by transfusion.[184,185] It is of note that since the use of antibody to HB core (anti-HBc) as a surrogate test to screen potential donors for their ability to transmit non-A non-B hepatitis, the incidence of transfusion-related hepatitis B has fallen even further.[186,187] The current estimated per-unit risk of hepatitis B is approximately 1 in 200,000.[188]

Non-A Non-B Hepatitis

Following the identification of hepatitis A virus and hepatitis B virus, it was quickly appreciated that neither agent was responsible for most cases of post-transfusion hepatitis. Thus, the term non-A non-B Hepatitis (NANBH) was introduced. In the mid-1980s, donors were screened for alanine aminotransferase (ALT) as well as anti-HBc; these served as "surrogate" markers for individuals having a 20% chance of transmitting NANBH.[189] The advantage of surrogate marker testing was the potential reduction of transfusion-related NANBH cases by one-third; the disadvantage was that 70-80% donors with anti-HBc or elevated ALT do not transmit NANBH; moreover, 1-3% and 4-8% of donors are deferred due to elevated ALT and anti-HBc, respectively.[190]

Table 127-6 **Risks of Transfusion**

Complication	Frequency (Episodes:Unit)
Reactions	
Febrile nonhemolytic	1-4:100
Allergic	1-4:100
Transfusion-related acute lung injury	1:5,000
Acute hemolytic	1:250,000
Delayed hemolytic	1:1,000
Anaphylactic	1:150,000
Infections	
Hepatitis C	1:2,000,000
Hepatitis B	1:200,000
HIV-1	1:2,000,000
HIV-2	None reported
HTLV-I and II	1:250,000 to 1:2,000,000
Malaria	1:4,000,000
Bacteria red cells	1:500,000
Bacteria platelets	1:75,000
Other complications	
RBC allosensitization	1:100
HLA sensitization	1:10
Graft-versus-host disease	Rare

Abbreviations: HIV, human immunodeficiency virus; HLA, human leukocyte antigen; HTLV, human T-cell leukemia/lymphoma virus; RBC, red blood cell.

The causative agent of NANBH was finally discovered by cloning a fragment of viral cDNA from a chimpanzee infected with NANBH.[191] Subsequently, the entire genome of what is now called hepatitis C virus (HCV) was cloned. A specific assay was developed for blood-borne NANBH, in which a recombinant HCV polypeptide is used to capture viral antibodies.[192] Subsequent testing using multiple-antigen HCV enzyme assays confirmed that nearly all cases of post-transfusion NANBH are caused by HCV. Uniform screening of blood donors for anti-HCV antibodies was implemented in 1990. Given that 90% of blood donors with anti-HCV have infective virus in their blood and that new generation assays for anti-HCV with enhanced sensitivity are available, look back studies are currently under way to test patients who were transfused prior to the availability of current screening tests.[186,192,193] Nucleic acid amplification technology (NAT) is also being employed to enhance sensitivity in detecting infection.[194] Along with HIV (discussed below) all blood donations in the United States are now screened for HCV.[195] By narrowing the preseronconversion window period from about 75 days to less than 30, the use of NAT has reduced the per-unit risk of HCV to approximately 1 in 2,000,000.[188]

Hepatitis C can have important adverse sequelae in patients with cancer. Long-term leukemia survivors with chronic HCV infection may have more rapidly progressive liver disease.[196] As with blood transfusion, studies now document high rates of transmission of HCV from allogeneic marrow donors at the time of transplantation.[197] A retrospective review noted that patients with liver disease caused by HCV infection are at high risk of developing lethal venoocclusive disease after BMT, demonstrating the importance of this pathogen in patients undergoing high-dose therapy.[198] Guidelines for the management of patient and donor in the setting of hepatitis infection have been reviewed.[199]

Hepatitis GB Virus

Hepatitis GB virus (GBV) and GBV-C are ribonucleic acid (RNA) viruses of the Flaviviridae family, which are also transfusion transmitted.[197,200] However, studies suggest that this infection does not have significant clinical sequelae.[201]

Cytomegalovirus

Cellular blood components transfused from CMV-seropositive donors to CMV-seronegative transplant recipients and neonates can cause CMV seroconversion and infection. In allogeneic BMT, transfusion with seronegative blood products (frozen deglycerolized RBCs and platelets drawn from CMV-seronegative donors) or treatment with immunoglobulin both appear to lessen CMV infection after allogeneic BMT when both donor and patient are seronegative but not when either is seropositive[202]; utilizing both immunoglobulin and CMV-seronegative blood products appears to confer no additional benefit. CMV infection is strongly associated with acute GVHD and may become less frequent due to the development of effective prophylaxis for GVHD.[199,203] In seropositive allogeneic BMT recipients, acyclovir therapy can lessen the incidence of CMV infection and related morbidity.[204] Although equivalent numbers of autologous and allogeneic BMT recipients either seroconvert to or excrete CMV, recipients of autologous BMT rarely develop clinical sequelae.[199]

Methods of CMV prophylaxis have therefore been reserved for allogeneic BMT when both donor and recipient are seronegative; they have not been used in autologous BMT. It should be noted, however, that CMV pneumonia developed in 11 of 159 autologous BMT recipients and was fatal in 9 cases, suggesting that these patients are also at risk for CMV visceral infection.[200]

The traditional CMV-seronegative blood products are red cells and platelets harvested from CMV-seronegative donors. Leukoreduced red cells and platelets have been shown to decrease transfusion-acquired CMV infection in infants, in patients undergoing treatment for acute leukemia, and in autologous and allogeneic BMT recipients.[202,205-207] The ability to utilize filtered blood products as if they were CMV seronegative would markedly expand the donor pool and thereby the supply of noninfectious components.[208] A multicenter randomized trial compared seronegative with filtered cellular blood components in CMV-seronegative patients undergoing autologous BMT and seronegative patients receiving allografts from CMV seronegative donors (Table 127-7).[202] Rates of CMV seroconversion and infection were equivalent in recipients of seronegative and filtered components, but significant clinical sequelae were noted only in those patients receiving filtered, unscreened components. These results suggest that filtering can markedly reduce CMV transmission, and filtered components are now considered "CMV safe"; however, it may be premature to conclude that filtered and seronegative components are equivalent. Transfer of CMV-specific clones of CD8+ T cells from the marrow donor has been shown to be a safe and effective way to reconstitute cellularimmunity against CMV after allogeneic BMT.[209]

West Nile Virus

West Nile virus (WNV) is a mosquito-borne flavivirus that can be transfusion-transmitted. The vast majority of WNV infections result from mosquito bites. About 80% of individuals infected with WNV are asymptomatic. Of the 20% who manifest symptoms, the vast majority will have a mild illness (WNV fever). Less than 1% of infected individuals develop a severe meningo-encephalitis, with advanced age being the strongest risk factor.[210] WNV first appeared in the United States in 1999. In 2002, over 4,000 clinically significant cases of WNV were reported, including 23 cases determined to have been transfusion-associated. In 2003, nucleic acid testing of blood products was begun nationwide under an FDA investigational new drug (IND) protocol. This testing has eliminated most, although not all[210] of the risk of transfusion-transmitted WNV.

Bacterial Sepsis

Bacteria very rarely survive in whole blood stored at 4°C. In contrast, platelets are stored at room temperature on an agitator and are a potential source of bacterial contamination, which can result in transfusion-related sepsis.[211] It is essential to systematically evaluate for transfusion-transmitted bacterial infections, whenever a febrile transfusion reaction occurs. In vitro studies demonstrate that deliberate contamination of platelets with as few as 1/mL on day 0 (either gram negative or positive) can result in 10^8/mL or plateau phase growth after 48-72 hours of incubation. Storage of platelets for 5 days between harvest and transfusion is permitted; however, platelets should be utilized as soon after harvest as possible because of considerations related to in vitro function and recovery, as well as concern for bacterial contamination. Prestorage leukodepletion of platelet concentrates does not appear to increase the likelihood of transfusion-induced septicemia.[212] Screening platelets before transfusion using Gram staining has been shown to reduce transfusion-related infection in some, but not all, centers.[213,214] Blood collection facilities in the United States are now required by AABB to both detect and limit bacterial contamination of platelets.[179] A variety of techniques to address bacterial contamination within platelets, such as automated culture systems, are in use or are under development.[211,215-223]

Bacterial sepsis is a recognized but quite rare complication of red cell transfusion, owing to the fact that red cells, unlike platelets, are stored under refrigerated conditions. Pathogens such as *Yersinia enterocolitica* have been implicated in causing toxemia following transfusion of red cells.[219] Minimizing the storage time of red cells prior to transfusion or extending the screening process to exclude all potential donors with gastrointestinal symptoms or illness in the 4-week period before donation have been suggested as possible methods to minimize this problem, but it is felt to be a rare event.

Table 127-7 Incidence and Actuarial Probability of CMV Infection and Disease by Study Arm

CMV Event	Seronegative Blood (*n* = 252)	Filtered Blood (*n* = 250)	Value
Primary analysis (day 21-100)			
All CMV infections and disease	2 (1.3%)	3 (2.4%)	1.00
CMV disease only	0 (0%)	3 (1.2%)	0.25
Secondary analysis (day 0-100)			
All CMV infections and disease	4 (1.4%)	6 (2.4%)	0.5
CMV disease	0 (0%)	6 (2.4%)	0.03
Survival	79%	82%	0.56

Abbreviation: CMV, cytomegalovirus.

Acquired Immune Deficiency Syndrome (AIDS)

With the recognition in 1983 that AIDS may be transmitted via transfusion, several measures were implemented: (1) physicians were educated about the risk/benefits of transfusion, (2) autologous transfusion was recommended for elective surgery, and (3) questionnaires were used for anonymous self-deferral of high-risk donors. By mid-1983, pressures for "directed" donations from friends or family increased; however, directed donations are not safer than other donations. The use of autologous blood, especially in elective surgeries, is an effective way to avoid infections and other risks of transfusions; however, autologous blood in patients with cancer is not widely utilized due to fear of contaminating tumor cells.

Since 1985, all American blood donors have been screened for anti-HIV antibody using ELISA. Transfusion-transmitted HIV is now exceedingly rare; the few cases that do occur result almost exclusively from seronegative window period donations. Following the initial implementation of HIV antibody screening, improvements in the sensitivity of the HIV-1 and HIV-2 ELISA limited the seronegative window period to approximately 22 days.[221] HIV p24 antigen screening was begun in 1996, shortening the window period to approximately 16 days.[221] The yield of HIV p24 antigen testing has been lower than predicted, perhaps because seroconverting donors may delay repeat donation because of symptoms of acute infection or concern over high-risk behavior.[222] All units donated in the United States are now tested by minipool nucleic acid testing (NAT). NAT testing is performed on pools of 16-24 samples; this technology shortens the window period to approximately 10 or 11 days from the time of exposure. In just over 1 year of testing, only 4 NAT-reactive, p24 antigen-negative/ELISA-negative units were identified out of 12.6 million donations screened (1/3,150,000).[195] It is estimated that the current residual per-unit risk of HIV transmission is less than 1 in 2,000,000.[188]

Human T-Cell Lymphotrophic Virus Type 1

Human T-cell lymphotrophic virus type 1 (HTLV-1) is associated with adult T-cell leukemia/lymphoma (ATL) and tropical spastic paresis (TSP)/HTLV-1–associated myelopathy (HAM), and clusters geographically in endemic areas such as parts of Japan and the Caribbean.[220,223] In the United States, ATL incidence is similar to that in the Caribbean, since the cases in the United States are all among African Americans or in patients born outside the United States.[224,225] Most important, recent studies have found antibodies to HTLV-1 in intravenous drug users in New York and have shown that anti-HIV antibodies do not identify all individuals infected with HTLV-1.[226] Moreover, Minamoto and colleagues documented anti-HTLV-1 antibodies in 6 of 211 multitransfused patients with cancer: None of the HTLV-1–seropositive patients were HIV-1 seropositive; conversely, 18 patients were HIV-1 seropositive and HTLV-1 seronegative.[227]

In Japan, deferral of blood donors with antibodies to HTLV-1 has resulted in a lowering of the HTLV-1 seroconversion rate in transfusion recipients from 53.6% to 0.9%.[228] In the United States, screening of sera from 39,898 blood donors at eight blood centers in geographically distinct areas of the United States defined 10 donors (.025%) to have anti–HTLV-1 antibodies by ELISA, immunoblot, and radioimmunoprecipitation.[229] In accordance with FDA guidelines, blood collection agencies, in November 1988, initiated testing of all blood donors for anti–HTLV-1 antibodies at the time of all donations, with permanent deferral of individuals with confirmed seropositivity. In addition, high-risk individuals who should not donate blood include patients with ATL or TSP; persons from HTLV-1–endemic areas; female sexual partners of infected men; IV drug abusers; recipients of seropositive cellular blood products; and homosexual men. Studies in the United States do, in fact, document that HTLV-1 has been transmitted via transfusion and demonstrate the efficacy of screening.[218,220,230] The risk per unit transfused is between 1 in 250,000 and 1 in 2,000,000.[231-233]

Other Viruses

HTLV-2 is a retrovirus that was discovered in 1982 in a patient with hairy cell leukemia of T cells.[232] No disease association (except for occasional cases of diverse malignant lymphoproliferative disease) or natural reservoir of infection (except drug abusers) has been found. Although there is serologic crossreactivity between HTLV-1 and HTLV-2, type-specific identification of HTLVs can be achieved using the polymerase chain reaction.[234] HIV-2 screening of blood and plasma donated is routinely done in the United States, and no cases of transfusion-transmitted HIV-2 have occurred. It is now known that other herpes viruses, including human herpesviruses types 6, 7, and 8, are present in normal blood donors, and future studies will determine their pathogenic potential in immunocompromised recipients.[235]

Parasitic Diseases

Since there is no practical laboratory screening test for malaria, exclusion of donors who have either traveled to or emigrated from endemic areas is the only effective measure to prevent transfusion-related infection. Other parasitic diseases, such as babesiosis or Lyme disease, can be transmitted by an asymptomatic donor who has been bitten by a tick and may be of particular importance in immunocompromised or asplenic patients. Although transmission of syphilis by transfusion is possible, it requires that blood be drawn during the rather short period of spirochetemia and that the organ-isms remain viable at the time of transfusion. Although performing a serologic test for syphilis does not prevent transmission of syphilis because this test does not become positive until well after the brief period of infectivity, US federal regulations do require its use as a screening test of potential donors.

Another recognized transfusion-related infection is Chagas disease.[236] In Latin America, the risk of transmission is 13-23% for each unit of contaminated blood transfused, and most cases of illness associated with transfusion are mild. In the majority of cases, spontaneous resolution occurs, and patients enter the indeterminate phase with lifelong, low-grade parasitemia, antibodies to parasite antigens, and absence of symptoms. Between 10% and 30% of persons in the indeterminate phase eventually develop symptoms. However, in immunocompromised patients, this illness may take a more fulminant course. The diagnosis of acute infection is made by detection of parasites on blood smear and the diagnosis of chronic infection by the detection of serum antibodies. Neither test has the sensitivity or specificity necessary to be useful for screening blood donors at present. Potential blood donors immigrating from areas endemic for Chagas disease are currently deferred.

Creutzfeldt–Jakob Disease

Although there have been no cases of Creutzfeldt–Jakob disease (CJD) related to blood transfusion, prospective donors of blood products who have a familial history of dementia and have undergone corneal or brain surgery are deferred.[236-238] Due to the identification in 1996 of a variant CJD (vCJD), which may be associated with bovine spongiform encephalopathy (BSE), or "mad cow disease," potential donors who resided in the United Kingdom for 3 months from 1980 to 1996 are deferred from donating. Donors residing in Europe for 5 years cumulatively from 1980 onward are also deferred. These travel restrictions are expected to eliminate 90% of person-days of exposure to the causative agent of vCJD at a cost of eliminating 5% of U.S.1 blood donors.[239] BSE has been transmitted from an infected sheep to a single other sheep by whole blood transfusion.[240] In the United Kingdom, a small number of human cases of transfusion-transmitted vCJD have been reported. Universal use of leukoreduced components for transfusion is being recommended in many countries, based on the fact that the vector for transmission of vCJD appears to be the B lymphocyte.

Future Directions in Blood Component Therapy

Increased Role in Primary Treatment of Cancer (Table 127-8)

The blood component laboratory plays a role in the collection, cryopreservation, thawing, re-infusion, and quality control of PBSCs.[5] A variety of strategies have been evaluated in the blood component laboratory evaluating the use of growth factors and standard versus large volume apheresis to collect autologous and, more recently, allogeneic PBSC.[6,58,241-243] Once collected, cryopreservation and thawing should be done so as to maintain both viability and sterility of PBSCs.[243-247] The blood component laboratory is also central to novel immune therapies based on adoptive immunotherapy and/or vaccines.[248,249] It is also the center for recruitment of donors for the National Marrow Donor Program to provide unrelated donor bone marrow and, more recently, PBSCs for transplantation. The blood component laboratory has also assumed an integral role in the management of programs for unrelated cord blood transplantation, which may permit partially matched unrelated donor transplantation, with less GVHD than has been noted after unrelated BMT.[249-253]

Hematopoietic Stem Cell Transplantation

Blood Component Support Before Transplantation Since many patients undergoing allogeneic BMT have received previous transfusions, sensitization to HLA may have occurred. The effect of HLA sensitization on marrow engraftment is most evident in the setting of aplastic anemia: reported graft rejection rates range from 25% to 60% in multitransfused patients with aplastic anemia given HLA identical sibling marrow grafts.[254] The likelihood of sensitization to HLA after transfusion varies in different patient populations and, in some studies, appears to correlate with the number of donor exposures.[255] When HLA-matched allogeneic BMT is to be done, prior transfusions from family members and especially from the potential marrow donor should be avoided because of the risk of sensitization of the patient to both HLA and non-HLA antigens. Most studies also suggest that a patient's pretransplantation CMV status predicts for the likelihood of infection following transplantation, and efforts should be made not to infect the patient via transfusion, especially if both patient and donor are seronegative.

Blood Component Support Posttransplantation After BMT, there is a period of pancytopenia, when patients require multiple RBC and platelet transfusions.

Table 127-8 **Role of the Blood Bank in Cellular Cancer Therapies**

Allogeneic stem cell transplantation
HLA-matched sibling donors
Donor lymphocyte infusions
HLA-matched unrelated donors
Cord blood transplantation
Autologous stem cell transplantation
Optimal selection
Quality control
Positive selection
Negative selection
Posttransplantation immune therapies

Abbreviation: HLA, human leukocyte antigen.

For example, patients with aplastic anemia undergoing allogeneic BMT received a median of 9 (1-82) and 44 (6-468) units of RBCs and platelets, respectively, primarily during the first 4 weeks after grafting.[256] Several donor and/or patient factors may influence hematologic engraftment and required blood product support after BMT.[5] In all recipients, engraftment may be compromised by disease- and/or treatment-related effects on the marrow microenvironment. Reconstitution after allogeneic BMT may be relatively enhanced since the donor marrow is healthy; however, the graft may be adversely affected by prophylaxis and treatment of GVHD. Moreover, in vitro T-cell depletion of donor marrow has in some patients resulted in failure to engraft and graft rejection. Autologous marrow may be intrinsically compromised by the patient's underlying disease and cytotoxic therapy received prior to marrow harvesting, in vitro techniques utilized for removal of tumor cells, or cryopreservation. In syngeneic BMT, donor marrow is histocompatible and healthy and is neither manipulated nor cryopreserved. However, the underlying disease and prior treatment of the recipient may, as is true in other types of BMT, compromise the marrow microenvironment and thereby adversely affect engraftment.

Testing for HLA compatibility between donor and recipient, combined with treatments to minimize and treat GVHD, has resulted in widespread utilization of allogeneic BMT. Although only 40% of patients have histocompatible related donors, the National Marrow Donor Program has recruited and collected unrelated histocompatible marrow for transplantation and shown very promising preliminary results.[257] Allogeneic PBSCs collected from normal donors are now in widespread use, suggesting an even more primary role of the blood bank in allograft stem cell transplantation.[58,235,258]

ABO incompatibility between marrow donor and recipient may be either major, with isohemagglutinin in the recipient directed against donor RBC antigens, or minor, with isohemagglutinin in the donor directed against recipient RBC antigens. Major ABO incompatibility has the potential risk of severe hemolytic reactions, graft rejection, or delayed engraftment.[259,260] Attempts to overcome major ABO incompatibility have included depletion of RBCs from the bone marrow graft prior to BMT and/or removal of isohemagglutinin from the recipient by large-volume plasma exchanges or immunoadsorption. In addition, some investigators have supplemented these techniques with pre-BMT transfusions of donor type blood or purified A or B substance to completely adsorb recipient isohemagglutinins. Although studies suggest that major ABO incompatible HLA-matched transplants have resulted in no increase in patient mortality, incidence of rejection, delayed reconstitution, or GVHD compared to ABO compatible controls, some reports suggest that RBC reconstitution can be delayed in this setting.[259,261-263] Red cell engraftment may be especially delayed in the setting of major ABO-incompatible nonmyeloablative stem cell transplantation, where host anti-donor isohemagglutinin levels tend to decrease more slowly than in myeloablative BMT.[264] The current standard practice in major ABO-incompatible HLA-matched BMT is to deplete RBCs from marrow before BMT, to anticipate possible delayed erythropoiesis and hemolysis after BMT, and to utilize methods to deplete recipient isohemagglutinins when present in high (> 1:128) titer.

Potential adverse outcomes of minor ABO incompatibility between marrow donor and recipient include rapid immune hemolysis at the time of infusion of donor marrow resulting from passive transfer of isohemagglutinin in the marrow plasma, or delayed immune hemolysis caused by anti-RBC antibodies produced by donor lymphocytes.[5] There is no effect of minor ABO incompatibility on graft rejection, the incidence and severity of GVHD, or patient survival. Although exchange transfusion of the recipient before BMT using red cells of the donor's blood group has been utilized to prevent hemolysis caused by passive transfer of isohemagglutinin in the marrow product, this is rarely a clinically significant problem and can more easily be avoided by removing plasma from the marrow prior to infusion. Minor ABO incompatibility can result in adverse reactions due to the production of anti-A and/or anti-B antibodies by donor marrow lymphocytes early (1-3 weeks) following transplantation, particularly in patients on cyclosporine therapy or those receiving T cell–depleted allografts.[265,266] In this setting, transfusions of either group O or donor group RBCs are utilized to dilute the recipient red cells; in some cases, exchange transfusion has been required due to very rapid engraftment of donor lymphocytes and production of anti-RBC antibodies.

PBSC Autotransplantation

The blood component laboratory plays a role in the collection, cryopreservation, thawing, re-infusion, and quality control of autologous hematopoietic stem cells for transplantation.[5] A variety of strategies have been analyzed in the blood component laboratory, evaluating the use of growth factors and standard versus large-volume apheresis to collect autologous PBSCs.[6,241,242] PBSCs must be collected, processed, cryopreserved, and thawed so as to maintain both their viability and their sterility.[243-247,267] Hematopoietic cell processing may consist of several steps: concentration and washing; sedimentation with hydroxyethyl starch, Ficoll-Hypaque, or Percoll; purging and washing; cryopreservation and storage; and thawing and re-infusion. The goal of hematopoietic cell processing is depletion of RBC, plasma, and fat (from marrow), with minimal loss of progenitor cells. Although originally done manually by simple centrifugation, cell separators are now utilized for preferential concentration of progenitor cells with increased elimination of other hematopoietic cells. In addition, much work has been done to utilize large-volume leukapheresis and fewer procedures, or to compare various PBSC collection and processing technologies.[268-270] Processing may either purge tumor cells or enrich for normal hematopoietic progenitor cells within autografts, or deplete T lymphocytes from allografts. Techniques have been developed to enrich and/or deplete cellular subsets via either positive or negative selection, increasing both the duration and complexity of the procedures performed in the cell processing laboratory, as well as the requirements for quality control. Moreover, specific cell populations are isolated for immune and gene-mediated therapies.[271]

Principles of current good manufacturing practice (cGMP) and total quality management (TQM) can be applied to HPC component processing. In 1991, the 14th edition of the AABB *Standards for Blood Banks and Transfusion Services* was extended to include hematopoietic stem cells. In 1996, the AABB published a separate *Standards for Hematopoietic Progenitor Cells* to expand and replace Section Q of the *Standards for Blood Banks and Transfusion Services*.[272] These standards include sections concerning donor selection, component collection, processing, testing, labeling, storage, transportation, issue, infusion, and record keeping for hematopoietic progenitor cells, including autologous as well as allogeneic bone marrow, peripheral blood progenitor cells, and cord blood. Furthermore, the Foundation for the Accreditation of Cellular Therapy (FACT), formed in 1993, has programs for inspection and accreditation of HPC collection and processing facilities as well as transplantation programs. The FACT Standards represent a consensus document of several organizations working together in the field of clinical conduct of hematopoietic progenitor cell transplantation, including the International Society for Hematotherapy and Graft Engineering (ISHAGE) and the American Society for Blood and Marrow Transplantation (ASBMT).[273] The FDA is currently reviewing the regulation of hematopoietic progenitor cell components and issued in February 1997 a comprehensive draft document concerning its approach to regulation.[274] The FDA has not yet finalized its approach to the regulation of this rapidly developing field but, as a first step, has proposed that all cell and tissue processing facilities register and report their activities.[275]

Leukopoor/Single-Donor Blood Components

As noted above, potential adverse effects in recipients of transfused cellular blood components that have been attributed to WBCs include FNHTRs, alloimmunization, transmission of infectious diseases (eg, CMV), GVHD, transfusion-related acute lung injury, and immunomodulation.[79] Exclusive use of leukoreduced (leukopoor) components can decrease alloimmunization, CMV transmission, and FNHTRs.[120,202,276,277] Recent advances in filtration as well as apheresis techniques have allowed improvement in the extent of WBC reduction achievable in RBCs and platelets so that components with less than 10^6 contaminating WBC can be readily available. In addition, studies have examined the importance of the timing of WBC reduction. For example, in an animal model, prestorage WBC reduction of donor blood was associated with a significantly higher platelet survival and lower rate of refractoriness to allogeneic platelet transfusions than was poststorage WBC reduction. It has been reported that storage of platelet concentrates for 5 days results in highly increased levels of tumor necrosis factor-a (TFN-a) and IL-6, whereas prestorage WBC reduction by filtration, current apheresis technology, or buffy coat preparation of platelet concentrates resulted in leukoreduction and no increase in either TNF-a or IL-6.[278-283] Moreover, Stack and Snyder detected IL-8 in 59% of platelet concentrates sampled, at levels ranging from 30% of 2-day-old units to 83% of 5-day-old units.[284] Cytokines released from WBCs during component storage may, either directly or indirectly, mediate FNHTRs in transfusion recipients by acting on recipient cells and releasing pyrogens. Heddle and colleagues have shown first that IL-6 and IL-1B accumulate within the plasma of stored platelets, that FNHTRs are more common to plasma than to cellular fractions of stored products, and, more recently, that plasma depletion is more effective than poststorage leukoreduction in avoiding FNHTR, confirming the in vivo relevance of transfused cytokines in mediating adverse consequences in transfusion recipients.[277] Poststorage leukoreduction is not quality controlled and is ineffective, further supporting the use of prestorage leukodepleted components. In addition, severe hypotension and respiratory distress have been observed after transfusion of components leukoreduced using negatively charged filters at the bedside (ie, poststorage), further limiting their utility. Interestingly, this reaction may be related to bradykinin release, which is of particular concern in patients on ACE inhibitors.[285,286] Another advantage of prestorage leukoreduction may be in the avoidance of transfusion-related infections. Since the concentration of bacteria in asymptomatic blood donors is thought to be very low, prestorage filtration of blood shortly after collection may represent a method by which the subsequent proliferation of organisms may be reduced or prevented.[287] Finally, B lymphocytes appear to be a vector of CJD infection in animal models, and therefore leukoreduction may decrease the risk of any theoretical transfusion-related infection.[231,237] On the basis of these multiple advantages, the United States and many countries around the world will likely utilize universally and exclusively prestorage leukoreduced components for transfusion.

Conclusion

The development and implementation of new and aggressive therapies for patients with cancer to date would not have been possible without parallel developments for the provision of blood component support. In the future, the blood component laboratory will provide specialized components, such as bone marrow and PBSC, to facilitate the use of new and promising transplantation and cellular therapies for patients with hitherto incurable diseases. Moreover, the advent of growth factor technology holds even greater potential for future treatment strategies, allowing more aggressive and specific therapies while minimizing the need for homologous donor exposures.

Selected References

The complete reference list can be found at www.CANCERMEDICINE8.com

2. *Scientific Basis of Transfusion Medicine. Implications for Clinical Practice*, 2nd ed. Philadelphia: WB Saunders; 1999.
9. Cazzola M, Mercuriali F, Brugnara C. Use of recombinant human erythropoietin outside the setting of uremia. *Blood.* 1997;89:4248–4267.
10. Armitage JO. Emerging applications of recombinant human granulocyte-macrophage colony-stimulating factor. *Blood.* 1998;92:4491–4508.
12. Du XX, Williams DA. Interleukin-11. A multifunctional growth factor derived

from the hematopoietic microenvironment. *Blood*. 1994;83:2023–2030.

15. Kiraly JF III, Wheby MS. Bone marrow necrosis. *Am J Med*. 1976;60:361–368.
16. Mauch PM, Loeffler JS. *Radiation Oncology. Technology and Biology*. Philadelphia: WB Saunders; 1994:594.
20. Rothmann SA, Paul P, Weick JK, et al. Effect of cisdiaminodichloro-platinum on erythropoietin production and hematopoietic progenitor cells. *Int J Cell Cloning*. 1985;3:415–423.
28. Beguin Y, Clemons GK, Oris R, Fillet G. Circulating erythropoietin levels after bone marrow transplantation. Inappropriate response to anemia in allogeneic transplants. *Blood*. 1991;77:868–873.
29. Ayash L, Elias A, Hunt M, et al. Recombinant human erythropoietin for the treatment of the anemia associated with autologous bone marrow transplantation. *Br J Hematol*. 1994;87:153–161.
35. Audet AM, Goodnough LT. Practice strategies for elective red blood cell transfusion. *Ann Intern Med*. 1992;116:403–406.
40. Goldfinger D, Lowe C. Prevention of adverse reactions to blood transfusion by the administration of saline washed red cells. *Transfusion*. 1981;21:277–280.
46. Freireich EJ, Leven RH, Whang J, Carbone PP, Bronson W, Morse EE. The function and fate of transfused leukocytes from donors with chronic myelocytic leukemia in leukopenic recipients. *Ann N Y Acad Sci*. 1964;113:1081.
59. Antman KS, Griffin JD, Elias A, et al. Effect of recombinant human granulocyte-macrophage colony-stimulating factor on chemotherapy-induced myelosuppression. *N Engl J Med*. 1988;319:593–598.
66. Levin J, Conley CL. Thrombocytosis associated with malignant disease. *Arch Intern Med*. 1964;114:497.
67. Figueroa M, Gehlsen J, Hammond D, et al. Combination chemotherapy in refractory immune thrombocytopenic purpura. *N Engl J Med*. 1993;328:1226–1229.
71. Lackner H. Hemostatic abnormalities associated with dysproteinemias. *Semin Hematol*. 1973;10:125–133.
74. Gaydos LA, Freireich EJ, Mantel N, et al. The quantitative relation between platelet count and hemorrhage in patients with acute leukemia. *N Engl J Med*. 1962;266:905–909.
82. Schiffer CA, Anderson KC, Bennett CL, et al. Platelet trans-fusion for patients with cancer: clinical practice guidelines of the American Society of Clincal Oncology. *J Clin Oncol*. 2001;19:1519–1538.
94. Daly PA, Schiffer CA, Aisner J, Wiernik PH. Platelet trans-fusion therapy. One-hour post-transfusion increments are valuable in predicting the need for HLA-matched preparations. *JAMA*. 1980;243: 435–438.
101. Ishida A, Handa M, Wakui M, et al. Clinical factors influencing posttransfusion platelet increment in patients undergoing hematopoietic cell transplantation—a prospective analysis. *Transfusion*. 1998;38:839–847.
116. Holohan TV, Terasaki PI, Deisseroth AB. Suppression of transfusion-related alloimmunization in intensively treated cancer patients. *Blood*. 1981;58:122–128.
117. Lohrmann HP, Bull MI, Decter JA, et al. Platelet transfusions from HLA-compatible unrelated donors to alloimmunized patients. *Ann Intern Med*. 1974;80:9–14.
118. Yankee RA, Graff KS, Dowling R, Henderson ES. Selection of unrelated compatible platelet donors by lymphocyte HLA matching. *N Engl J Med*. 1973;288:760–764.
120. Vamvakas EC. Meta-analysis of randomized controlled trials of the efficacy of white cell reduction in preventing HLA-alloimmunization and refractoriness to random-donor platelet transfusions. *Transfus Med Rev*. 1998;12:258–270.
123. Moroff G, Garratty G, Heal JM, et al. Selection of platelets for refractory patients by HLA matching and prospective cross-matching. *Transfusion*. 1992;32:633–640.
124. Friedberg RC, Donnelly SF, Boyd JC, et al. Clinical and blood bank factors in the management of platelet refractoriness and alloimmunization. *Blood*. 1993;81:3428–3434.
125. Friedberg RC, Donnelly SF, Mintz PD. Independent roles for platelet crossmatching and HLA in the selection of platelets for alloimmunized patients. *Transfusion*. 1994;34:215–220.
126. Bensinger WI, Buckner CD, Clift RA, et al. Plasma exchange for platelet alloimmunization. *Transplantation*. 1986;41:602–605.
127. Lee EJ, Norris D, Schiffer CA. Intravenous immune globulin for patients alloimmunized to random donor platelet transfusion. *Transfusion*. 1987;27:245–247.
128.Cooling LL, Kelly K, Barton J, et al. Determinants of ABH expression on human blood platelets. *Blood*. 2005;105:3356–3364.
129. Dunstan RA, Simpson MB, Rosse WF. Erythrocyte antigens on human platelets. Absence of Rh, Duffy, Kell, Kidd and Lutheran antigens. *Transfusion*. 1984;24:243–246.
130. Julmy F, Ammann RA, Mansouri T, et al. Transfusion efficacy of ABO major-mismatched platelets (PLTs) in children is inferior to that of ABO-identical PLTs. *Transfusion*. 2009;49:21–33.
132. Thompson CB, Jakubowski JA. The pathophysiology and clinical relevance of platelet heterogeneity. *Blood*. 1988;72:1–8.
133. Warkentin TE, Smith JW. The alloimmune thrombocy-topenic syndromes. *Transfus Med Rev*. 1997;11:296–307.
134. Shulman NR, et al. A new syndrome of posttransfusion purpura. *J Clin Invest*. 1960;39:1928.
135. Cimo PL, Aster RH. Post-transfusion purpura. Successful treatment by exchange transfusion. *N Engl J Med*. 1972;289:290–292.
138. Klein E, Farber S, Djerassi I, et al. The preparation and clinical administration of lyophilized platelet material to children with acute leukemia and aplastic anemia. *J Pediatr*. 1956;49:517.
140. Angelini A, Dragani A, Berardi A, et al. Evaluation of four different methods of platelet freezing. *Vox Sang*. 1992;62:146–151.
141. Alving B. Potential for synthetic phospholipids as partialplatelet substitutes. *Transfusion*. 1998;38:997–998.
142. Braunstein AH, Oberman HA. Transfusion of plasma components. *Transfusion*. 1984;24:281–286.
152. McCullough J, Weiblin BJ, Clay ME, Forstrom L. Effect of leukocyte antibodies on the fate in vivo of indium-111-labeled granulocytes. *Blood*. 1981;58:164–170.
161. Tartter PI, Quintero S, Barron DM, et al. Perioperative blood transfusion associated with infectious complications after colorectal cancer operations. *Am J Surg*. 1986;152:479–482.
182. Fast LD, Valeri CR, Crowley JP. Immune responses to major histocompatibility complex homozygous lymphoid cells in murine F1 hybrid recipients. Implications for transfusion-associated graft-versus-host disease. *Blood*. 1995;86:3090–3096.
187. Stevens CE, Aach RD, Hollinger FB, et al. Hepatitis B virus antibody in blood donors and the occurrence of non-A, non-B hepatitis in transfusion recipients. An analysis of the transfusion-transmitted viruses study. *Ann Intern Med*. 1984;101:733–738.
207. Sayers MH, Anderson KC, Goodnough LT, et al. Reducing the risk for transfusion-transmitted cytomegalovirus infection. *Ann Intern Med*. 1992;116:55–62.
250. Gluckman E, Rocha V, Boyer-Chammard A, et al. Outcome of cord-blood transplantation from related and unrelated donors. *N Engl J Med*. 1997;337:373–381.
252. Kurtzberg J, Laughlin M, Graham ML, et al. Placental blood as a source of hematopoietic stem cells for trans-plantation into unrelated recipients. *N Engl J Med*. 1996;335:157–166.
264. Bolan CD, Leitman SF, Griffith LM. Delayed donor red cell chimerism and pure red cell aplasia following major ABO-incompatible nonmyeloablative hematopoietic stem cell transplantation. *Blood*. 2001;98:1687–1694.
300. Read MS, Bode AP, Reddick RL. Studies with dried and rehydrated platelets for transfusion products. *FASEB J*. 1991;1:903a.
311. Macedo de Oliveira A, Beecham BD, Montgomery SP, et al. West Nile virus blood transfusion-related infection despite nucleic acid testing. *Transfusion*. 2004;44:1695–1699.

128 Coagulopathic Complications of Cancer Patients

Maria T. DeSancho, MD ■ Jacob H. Rand, MD

Bleeding and thrombotic complications remain important causes of morbidity and mortality in cancer patients. As a result of advances in cancer treatment, the prevalence of these complications has been progressively rising in recent years. Bleeding is common in patients with leukemias, particularly those with acute promyelocytic leukemia (APL), where up to 90% of patients develop hemorrhage.[1] In general, bleeding complications occur relatively infrequently in patients with solid tumors, except those with melanoma, germ cell tumors, carcinoma of the cecum, and prostate cancer.[2] Similarly, thrombotic complications are common and may be a result of prothrombotic hemostatic changes that occur in more than 90% of cancer patients.[3]

This chapter reviews the physiology of normal hemostasis, and then discusses the relationship of the coagulation system and cancer, and the pathophysiology of bleeding and thrombosis in the cancer patient. Next, the diagnostic and treatment approaches to the disorders most frequently encountered in cancer patients are described. Finally, potential novel anticoagulants such as anti-Factor Xa inhibitors and the oral direct thrombin inhibitors are reviewed.

Physiology of Normal Hemostasis

Hemostasis is the physiologic mechanism that halts bleeding after injury to the vasculature. Normal hemostasis depends on both cellular components and soluble plasma proteins. Circulating platelets adhere and aggregate at sites of blood vessel injury. The adhesion is dependent on the presence of the von Willebrand factor (vWF) and is followed by an aggregation response. Activation of platelets results in exposure of anionic phospholipids that serve as platforms for the assembly of blood coagulation enzyme complexes. The extrinsic pathway of blood coagulation is initiated when blood is exposed to tissue factor (TF), a transmembrane protein expressed in the deeper portions of the blood vessel wall that may also be present in stimulated endothelial cells. Thrombus propagation occurs via incorporation of active, blood-borne TF into the growing clot.[4] TF binds activated factor VII (factor VIIa) and the resulting complex activates factors X and IX. Activated factor IX (factor IXa) combines with factor VIIIa to provide a second pathway to activate factor X. Factor Xa complexes with factor Va and prothrombin to form prothrombinase, which cleaves prothrombin to generate thrombin, the key enzyme in hemostasis. In the final step of the coagulation cascade, thrombin cleaves fibrinogen to generate fibrin monomers, which then polymerize (Fig. 128-1). This polymer is covalently cross-linked by factor XIIIa (itself generated from factor XIII by thrombin) to form a chemically stable clot. Thrombin also feeds back to activate cofactors V, VIII, and XI further amplifying the coagulation system (Fig. 128-2).

Fibrin deposition is limited by an endogenous anticoagulant system. Antithrombin (AT) is a plasma protein member of the serpin (serine protease inhibitor) family that inhibits the activities of all the activated coagulation enzymes. Protein C is a vitamin K-dependent protein that proteolyses factor Va and factor VIIIa to inactive fragments. Protein C binds to an endothelial cell protein C receptor (EPCR)[5] and is activated by thrombin bound to thrombomodulin, another endothelial cell membrane-based protein, in a reaction that is modulated by a cofactor, protein S. TF pathway inhibitor is a plasma protein that forms a quaternary complex withTFs, factor VIIa, and factor Xa, thereby inhibiting the extrinsic coagulation pathway.[6]

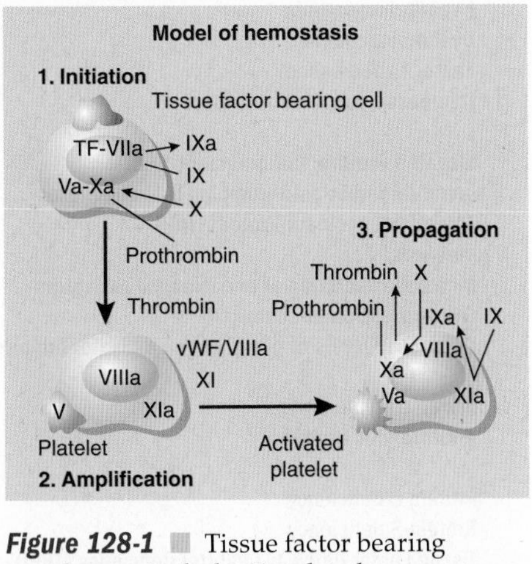

Figure 128-1 ■ Tissue factor bearing membranes include stimulated monocytes, endothelial cells, circulating microparticles, vascular smooth muscle cells, brain cells, lung cells, placental mesenchymal cells and keratinocytes at the level of stratum granulosum.

Finally, fibrin is digested by the fibrinolytic system, the major components of which are plasminogen and tissue-type plasminogen activator (tPA). Both of these proteins are incorporated into polymerizing fibrin, where they interact to generate plasmin, which, in turn, acts on fibrin to dissolve the preformed clot.[6,7] The fibrinolytic system is regulated by three serine proteinase inhibitors, namely, antiplasmin, plasminogen activator inhibitor-1 (PAI-1), and plasminogen activator inhibitor-2 (PAI-2).[7]

Relationship of Coagulation System and Cancer

The relationship between blood coagulation and cancer was first described in the medical literature during the latter half of the nineteenth century when Trousseau reported the association of migratory thrombophlebitis and gastric carcinoma.[8] In 1878, Billroth demonstrated cancer cells within a thrombus and theorized that tumor cells were spread by thromboembolism.[9] The interaction between blood coagulation, tumor angiogenesis and growth is supported by the involvement of several coagulation factors, specifically TF and thrombin in cancer neoangiogenesis, growth, and dissemination. Cancer cells or host cells in response to the neoplastic process cause local and systemic inflammatory stimuli that can switch the endothelium to a prothrombotic surface.[10] Endothelial damage leads to exposure of subendothelial vWF and TF. VWF in turn, induces platelet and tumor cell adhesion, with subsequent platelet activation and aggregation. Tissue factor plays a key role in the initiation of the coagulation cascade. TF is aberrantly expressed on the surface of activated endothelial cells, monocytes, and on tumor cells.[11] TF is up regulated in endothelium in pathologic states such as cancer as evidenced by the expression of TF and cross-linked fibrin on the endothelium of newly formed blood vessels within human tumors.[12] It appears that TF can enhance tumor growth and metastases by both coagulation-dependent mechanisms mediated by its binding to factor VIIa and by coagulation-independent mechanisms via the protease-activated receptor 2 (PAR2), a G protein-coupled receptor that is important in angiogenesis and inflammation. Following TF-mediated clotting activation, fibrin and platelets provide a transient matrix for tumor cell migration and new vessel formation (neoangiogenesis).[12] Additionally, local platelets and fibrin deposits surrounding a new micrometastasis protect tumor cells from immune surveillance mediated by natural killer cells.[13] PAR2 stimulates angiogenesis and enhances cancer cell migration via interleukin-8 and cofilin as well as tumor cell adhesion, thus stabilizing metastatic tumor foci. Tissue factor also has anti-apoptotic effects and upregulates the expression of vascular endothelial growth factor (VEGF), a major regulatory molecule involved in neoangiogenesis. Activated platelets also release VEGF and thus play a role in neoangiogenesis and tumor spread.[12]

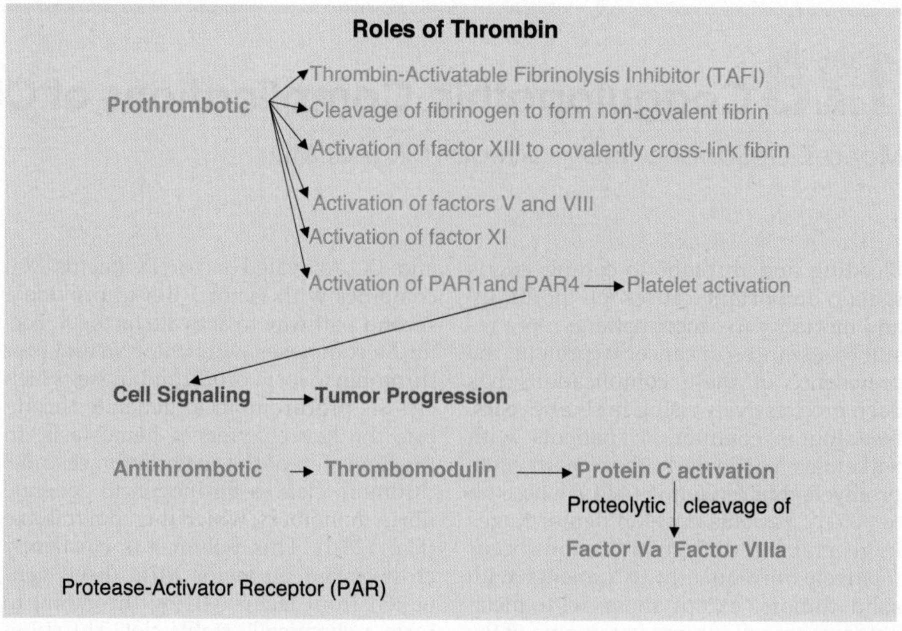

Figure 128-2 Central prothrombotic roles of thrombin.

Bleeding Disorders

Cancer can cause both quantitative and qualitative changes in platelets.[13] Reactive thrombocytosis occurs in approximately 60% of cancer patients, while thrombocytopenia occurs in up to 11% of patients with untreated malignancy (Table 128-1).

The major bleeding problems are commonly caused by tumor invasion of blood vessels and adjacent organs, complications of treatment, and vitamin K deficiency. Bleeding in the cancer patient may present as either localized bleeding usually as a result of tumor invasion or as generalized bleeding diathesis caused by thrombocytopenia, thrombocytopathies, specific coagulation factor deficiencies, disseminated intravascular coagulation (DIC), or hyperfibrinolysis.[14] Appropriate treatment of bleeding in cancer patients depends on the underlying disorder responsible for the bleeding.

Thrombocytopenia

Thrombocytopenia is the most frequent hemostatic disorder in cancer patients, occurring in approximately 10% of cases, even prior to starting chemotherapy.[14] In the acute setting, thrombocytopenia is usually caused by decreased production either secondary to chemotherapy and/or radiation therapy, or bone marrow infiltration, platelet sequestration in the spleen, or increased peripheral destruction, such as in sepsis, DIC, and thrombotic thrombocytopenic purpura (TTP)/hemolytic uremic syndrome (HUS)[15] (Table 128-2). Bortezomimib a proteasome inhibitor used in newly diagnosed and relapsed multiple myeloma causes a transient, cyclical, and reversible thrombocytopenia.[16] Thrombocytopenia as a result of bone marrow infiltration commonly occurs in patients with small-cell

Table 128-1 **Hemostatic Abnormalities in Cancer Patients**

Abnormality	Mechanism
Platelets	
Thrombocytopenia	Marrow infiltration by tumor
	Chemotherapy effects
	Biological response modifiers
	Monoclonal antibodies and immunotoxins
	Proteasome inhibitor (bortezomib)
	Disseminated Intravascular Coagulation
	Hypersplenism
	Immune mediated (autoimmune, alloimmune)
	Microangiopathic hemolytic anemia (TTP and HUS)
Thrombocytosis	Increased production: reactive primary
	Myeloproliferative disorders
Platelet function abnormalities	Uremia
	Acquired von Willebrand syndrome
	Myeloproliferative disorders
Abnormalities in coagulation factors and coagulation activation markers	
Hypofibrinogenemia	Asparaginase, DIC
Dysfibrinogenemia	Hepatocellular carcinoma
Factor X (decreased)	Amyloidosis
Decreased coagulation factors	Impairment in hepatic synthesis, DIC, vitamin K deficiency
Elevated Prothrombin fragment 1+2	Disseminated malignancies, DIC
Elevated thrombin-antithrombin (TAT) complexes	Disseminated malignancies, DIC
Thrombus precursor Protein (TpP)	Measures fibrin soluble polymers
Fibrinolysis	
Increased secretion of plasminogen activators	Acute promyelocytic leukemia (APL)
Overexpression of annexin II	APL
Decreased levels of plasminogen activator inhibitors	Increased fibrin(ogen)degradation products and D-dimer
Acquired thrombophilias	
Antithrombin deficiency	Impaired hepatic synthesis of anticoagulant proteins, DIC, L-asparaginase
Protein C deficiency	Impaired hepatic synthesis, DIC
Protein S deficiency	Impaired hepatic synthesis, DIC
Tissue Factor Pathway Inhibitor deficiency (TFPI)	Impaired hepatic synthesis, DIC
Cytokines and Hemostasis	
Proinflammatory cytokines (IL-1, IL-6, TNF)	Key role in tissue factor expression in monocytes and endothelial cells

Abbreviations: DIC, disseminated intravascular coagulation; HUS, hemolytic uremic syndrome; IL, interleukin; TNF, tumor necrosis factor; TTP, thrombotic thrombocytopenic purpura.

Table 128-2 **Differential Diagnosis of Thrombocytopenia in Cancer Patients**

Decreased platelet production
Metastases to bone marrow
Acute and chronic leukemias
Lymphomas
Plasma cell dyscrasias
Cytotoxic chemotherapy
Radiation therapy
Platelet destruction
Medications
Immune mediated
Bacterial sepsis
Viral, fungal, and protozoal infections
DIC
TTP/HUS
Splenic sequestration
Myeloproliferative disorders
Lymphomas
Chronic lymphocytic leukemias
Combination of the above mechanisms

Abbreviations: DIC, disseminated intravascular coagulation; HUS, hemolytic uremic syndrome; TTP, thrombotic thrombocytopenic purpura.

Table 128-3 **Critical Platelet Counts and Recommendations for Transfusion in Cancer Patients**[a]

Mucocutaneous or gastrointestinal bleeding	>50,000
Leukemias	
Pre-induction chemotherapy	>20,000
Acute promyelocytic leukemia	>5,000-10,000
Prophylaxis	
Asymptomatic	>5,000
Major surgery	>50,000
Invasive procedures	
Major	>50,000
Minor	>20,000

[a]These are intended to serve as general guidelines. Actual treatment will vary depending on specific circumstances.

lung cancer, breast cancer, and prostate cancer, as well as in patients with acute leukemia. On the other hand, thrombocytopenia secondary to splenic sequestration is usually observed with myeloproliferative disorders and less commonly with lymphomas and chronic lymphocytic leukemia. Clinically evident bleeding episodes are more likely to occur when thrombocytopenia is caused by diminished production of megakaryocytes rather than by immune destruction.

The most common clinical manifestation of thrombocytopenia is mucocutaneous bleeding. This can occur in the form of petechiae, ecchymoses, epistaxis, oral, gastrointestinal, or genitourinary bleeding. Spontaneous bleeding usually does not occur unless the platelet count is less than 10,000/mm^3. However, in the presence of sepsis, uremia, trauma, or surgery, bleeding complications may occur with a higher platelet count.

The clinical history, physical examination, review of medications, and timing of prior chemotherapy, immunotherapy, or radiation therapy must be reviewed. In addition, examination of the peripheral blood smear is vital in the diagnostic work-up of thrombocytopenia. Spurious thrombocytopenia manifested by platelet clumping on the peripheral smear or platelet satellitism (platelets surrounding the polymorphonuclear leukocytes) must be excluded.

The treatment of bleeding associated with thrombocytopenia in the cancer patient is often managed empirically even when a specifically defined cause cannot be identified. Table 128-3 lists the critical platelet counts in various situations and general guidelines for platelet transfusion.[17] Prophylactic transfusion of platelets is not indicated in patients who are asymptomatic for bleeding unless the platelet count is below 5,000/mm^3. However, in cancer patients undergoing chemotherapy and those with leukemia, prophylactic platelet transfusions are generally beneficial in decreasing the risk of bleeding when the platelet count is below 10,000/mm^3.[18] For cancer patients undergoing major surgery or invasive procedures such as central venous catheterization, bronchial or endoscopic biopsy, lumbar puncture, thoracentesis, thoracostomy tube placement, and abdominal paracentesis, it is generally recommended that platelet transfusions should be administered in thrombocytopenic patients to a target level greater than 50,000.[18] For minor invasive procedures such as arterial puncture or cannulation, prophylactic transfusion is not necessary if the platelet count is at least 20,000/mm^3 and local pressure is applied at the puncture site until hemostasis is achieved.[15] Platelet transfusions are usually indicated in thrombocytopenic patients to keep the platelet count above 50,000/mm^3 when evidence of microscopic or gross bleeding is detected, as manifested by either occult blood on stool guaiac tests and mucocutaneous bleeding. The risk of central nervous system bleeding is generally low and bleeding depends on several factors such as etiology of thrombocytopenia, coagulation abnormalities, impaired renal or hepatic function, severe sepsis, trauma, and the use of mechanical ventilation. Subdural and intracerebral hematomas occur in approximately 2.5-5%[19] and 2%, respectively of leukemic patients following hematopoeitic stem cell, transplantation.[20,21] Comparative studies show that platelets derived from single or random donors produce similar post-transfusion increments, hemostatic benefits, and side effects.[18]

Thrombocytopathies

In addition to quantitative platelet changes, cancer can also cause qualitative platelet abnormalities. The main disorders are described below.

Acquired von Willebrand Syndrome Several types of cancer have been reported in association with acquired von Willebrand syndrome (aVWS). Among the lymphoproliferative disorders, monoclonal gammopathy of undetermined significance (MGUS) is the condition most frequently associated with aVWS, It can also be associated with multiple myeloma, Waldenstrom macroglobulinaemia, chronic lymphocytic leukemia, hairy cell leukemia and non-Hodgkin lymphoma. Among the myeloproliferative disorders, essential thrombocythemia (ET) is the most common while polycythemia vera (PV) and chronic myeloid leukemia are less frequent. Solid tumors including Wilms tumors and carcinomas have also been associated with aVWS.[22]

The clinical manifestations of aVWS are similar to those seen in patients with the hereditary form of the disease except for the notable absence of a family history or lifelong personal history for bleeding. Spontaneous mucocutaneous and gastrointestinal bleeding may be present. Postsurgical bleeding may also occur. Laboratory screening tests generally reveal a prolonged activated partial thromboplastin time (aPTT) and a normal , borderline prolonged bleeding time, or by prolonged closure times of in vitro testing with the PFA-100. Plasma vWF antigen, vWF ristocetin cofactor activity, ristocetin-induced platelet aggregation, and vWF collagen binding activity are generally decreased. Laboratory tests usually fail to demonstrate inhibitory activity against vWF or factor VIII. Treatment is directed to the underlying malignancy and supportive measures such as corticosteroids, deamino-8-D-arginine vasopressin (desmopressin acetate or DDAVP), factor VIII/vWF concentrate, and intravenous immunoglobulin and intravenous immunoglobulin.[22,23]

Acquired Hemophilia (Factor VIII Autoantibodies) Patients with solid tumors, plasma cell dyscrasias, and lymphoproliferative disorders may develop an acquired hemophilia because of inhibitors against factor VIII, also referred to as acquired inhibitors. The inhibitors are autoantibodies and almost always are immunoglobulin G (IgG) molecules. The most common presenting complaint is bleeding into the skin or muscles in patients with no previous history of bleeding diathesis. Most patients present with severe bleeding; life-threatening hemorrhage is more commonly seen in the first several weeks of presentation but can occur at any time if treatment is not initiated.[24] The hallmark finding is a prolongation of the aPTT in the presence of a normal prothrombin time (PT) along with plasma mixing studies that demonstrate an aPTT that remains prolonged after incubation at 37°C for 1-2 h. In contrast, in patients with coagulation factor deficiencies, plasma mixing studies normalize the aPTT. Contamination of the blood sample with heparin, which frequently is the inadvertent result of instillation for maintaining vascular access line patency, may artifactually prolong the aPTT and affect the mixing tests. Heparin that has entered the sample may be removed with the enzyme reptilase or resin absorption, after which the plasma may be retested. A prolonged thrombin time (TT) in the presence of a normal reptilase time (RT) confirms the suspicion of heparin contamination. After a mixing study confirms the presence of an inhibitor and other nonspecific inhibitors have been ruled out, the factor VIII activity should be measured. If the factor VIII activity is low, the titer of the factor VIII antibody should be ascertained. The strength of an inhibitor can quantified by using the Bethesda assay, which measures residual factor VIII activity after incubation of normal plasma with serial dilutions of patient plasma for 2 h at 37°C. The inhibitor titer in Bethesda units represents the reciprocal of the dilution of the patient's plasma that leads to 50% inhibition in the assay described. The titers can be followed during treatment as a measure of efficacy. The objectives in the treatment of acquired factor VIII inhibitors in patients with cancer are twofold: (1) management of the acute bleeding and (2) elimination of the autoantibody against factor VIII. The acute bleeding can be managed with desmopressin acetate if there is a low inhibitor titer (<5 Bethesda units [BU]) or with human or porcine factor VIII. Factor VIII bypassing agents such as recombinant human factor VIIa, or activated prothrombin complex concentrate are used in case of moderate- to high-titer inhibitor (>5 BU). Immunosuppressive therapy such as corticosteroids, cyclophosphamide, vincristine, cyclosporine, and intravenous immunoglobulin (IVIg) may be used in addition to the treatment of the underlying neoplasm. Rituximab should be considered in patients who are resistant to first-line therapy or cannot tolerate standard immunosuppressive therapy. It has been proposed that rituximab should be included as first-line therapy in combination with prednisone for patients with an inhibitor titer greater than 5 but less than 30 and in addition to prednisone and cyclophosphamide for those patients with a titer greater than 30.[25]

Uremia ■ Platelet dysfunction is common in cancer patients with chronic renal failure and causes significant bleeding. The pathophysiology of uremic bleeding is multifactorial and includes dysfunctional vWF, increased levels of cyclic adenosine monophosphate and nitric oxide generated by platelets, uremic toxins, and anemia. This causes the platelets to be displaced from the vascular endothelium thereby decreasing their ability to adhere and aggregate in response to endothelial damage.[26] Treatment is recommended for patients with active bleeding or for those undergoing an invasive procedure, such as placement of hemodialysis catheters. Patients usually respond to hemodialysis and administration of DDAVP at a dose of 0.3 micrograms/kg intravenously; cryoprecipitate (10 bags given intravenously over 30 min) and conjugated estrogens (0.6 mg/kg over 30-40 min once daily for 5 consecutive days) may occasionally be required. Erythropoietin stimulating agents such as recombinant human erythropoietin and darbepoietin have been shown to reduce and prevent bleeding in uremic patients and has a more sustained effect than either DDAVP or conjugated estrogens.[26]

Myeloproliferative Disorders ■ Among the myeloproliferative conditions, PV and ET are the most likely to be associated with hemorrhagic and thrombotic complications. In a series of 74 young women with ET, the incidence of hemorrhage was 26%. Most of these episodes were minor; however, major hemorrhagic events occurred in 4%.[27] Some patients with ET may have reduced levels of high molecular weight von Willebrand protein in the plasma during extreme thrombocytosis (>1,500 $\times 10^9$/L) and this may play a role in their bleeding diathesis.[28] These patients can have an acquired form of von Willebrand disease. In these cases, prolonged bleeding time and abnormal multimeric pattern of vWF on electrophoresis are useful for diagnosing and monitoring this acquired hemorrhagic disease.[29]

Thrombosis represents the initial manifestation for 12-39% of patients with ET and PV.[28] Increasing age (>65), and a previous history of thrombosis were identified as major risk factors for thrombosis.[28] An acquired point mutation in the pseudokinase domain of Janus kinase 2 (JAK2 (V617F)) is found in approximately 97% and 50% of patients with PV and ET respectively. Retrospective data have identified JAK2(V617F) as a risk factor for thrombosis in ET, and have shown a close association with abdominal vein thrombosis. JAK2 (V617F) is variably associated with thrombosis and, more consistently, with elevations in blood cell counts. A clear link appears to exist between leukocytosis, JAK2(V617F), and the hemostatic system activation in patients with Bcl-negative myeloproliferative disorders.[30,31]

Other potential determinants of thrombotic risk include cardiovascular risk factors. Leukocytosis was found to be an independent risk factor for thrombosis and survival both in PV and ET. Patients participating in the ECLAP study with a leukocyte count greater than 15 $\times 10^9$ per liter had a significant increase in the risk of thrombosis mainly due to a higher rate of myocardial infarction.[32] Patients with either PV or ET can be stratified in "high-risk" or "low-risk" categories according to their age and previous history of thrombosis. All patients with PV are managed with phlebotomy and low-dose aspirin. The recommended HCT target is below 45%, however a randomized clinical study (CYTO-PV) is addressing the issue of the optimal target of cytoreduction in PV. ET patients at low risk for major vascular complications are left untreated. Low-dose aspirin is given in the presence of microvascular symptoms. A careful correction of concomitant cardiovascular risk factors should be pursued. In high-risk patients, HU remains the first choice drug for most PV and ET patients requiring a cytoreductive therapy because it is the only treatment proven effective in reducing life-threatening thrombotic complications.[33] Cautious use of HU should be taken in young patients and in those previously treated with other myelosuppressive agents or carrying cytogenetic abnormalities. IFN-α and anagrelide are considered in younger patients, pregnancy (for IFN-α), and in cases resistant or intolerant to HU. JAK2(V617F) inhibitors have been recently developed; some of these small molecules suppress growth of progenitors carrying JAK-activating mutations and show significant clinical activity. Indications for the use of these drugs are dependent on their expected side effects. JAK2 inhibitors with limited side effects can be considered for patients with PV and/or ET if therapy is required.[34]

Coagulation Factor Deficiencies

Cancer patients may develop various coagulation factor abnormalities resulting from vitamin K deficiency as a consequence of malnutrition, diarrhea, liver disease, biliary obstruction, use of oral anticoagulants, and antibiotic therapy. Patients with primary or metastatic hepatocellular carcinoma have deficiency of vitamin K-dependent factors (factors II, VII, IX, X, protein C, and S), similar to that seen with liver cirrhosis. These patients usually have increased levels of fibrinogen, unlike patients with cirrhosis or acute liver failure who have decreased fibrinogen levels. Acquired inhibitors of coagulation factors are frequently seen in multiple myeloma and other plasma cell dyscrasias.

The treatment of cancer patients with coagulation factor deficiencies, aside from the treatment of the underlying neoplasm, is generally supportive, and consists of vitamin K, fresh-frozen plasma (FFP), and cryoprecipitate. Oral vitamin K is the treatment of choice, and its administration is predictably effective and has the advantages of safety and convenience over parenteral routes. Occasionally, a rapid response may be achieved by administering 1-2 mg of vitamin K by slow IV infusion (over at least 30 min) to minimize the risk of anaphylactic reactions and fatty emboli resulting from the lipid emulsion.[35] FFP (10-15 mL/kg by IV infusion) should be transfused when immediate correction of coagulation factor deficiencies is required either because of bleeding or in patients undergoing an invasive procedure, but dose may be higher in patients with massive bleeding. Cryoprecipitate is the cryoglobulin fraction of plasma obtained by thawing a single donation of FFP. Cryoprecipitate is rich in factor VIII, vWF, fibrinogen, fibronectin, and factor XIII. It is indicated for dysfibrinogenemia and hypofibrinogenemic states and for some patients with renal failure. Cryoprecipitate is administered IV, generally at a dose of 1 unit of cryoprecipitate for every 5 kg of body weight.[36]

Amyloidosis

Haemostatic disorders are common in amyloidosis. Clinical history of bleeding is found in about 28% of patients and bleeding is the presenting complaint in 3%. Cutaneous ecchymoses and purpura are the most common manifestations, although clinically significant bleeding from the gastrointestinal and renal tracts is common. Bleeding at sites other than the skin is significantly associated with prolongation of the PT.[37] Acquired factor X deficiency has been particularly described in patients with primary amyloidosis although acquired deficiencies of factors II, V, IX, and X have all been reported. In addition small vessel fragility due to amyloid deposits and paraprotein interference with fibrin polymerization may contribute to bleeding in amyloidosis. Factor X deficiency is believed to be caused by adsorption of factor X on amyloid fibrils in the liver and the spleen.[38] Functional impairment of plasma factor X may arise in AL-amyloidosis from a defect in post-translational modification, especially glycosylation,[39] or from inactivation of the factor X active site in the circulation by a soluble ligand such as a monoclonal antibody or antibody fragment. Laboratory abnormalities include a prolongation of the PT and the aPTT. Moreover, prolongations of the TT, which have been associated with hepatic amyloid infiltration and RT have also been found. The PT, but not the TT, appears to be a clinically useful predictor of bleeding tendency.[37]

Drug Effects (L-Asparaginase)

L-Asparaginase is used in combination with other agents, for induction of remissions in acute lymphocytic leukemia. L-asparaginase can cause depletion of many of the coagulation factors with an associated risk for thrombosis and hemorrhage. Vitamin K-dependent proteins are significantly decreased during L-asparaginase therapy. The timing and severity of decrease vary among the proteins. The decrease in protein C, and factors IX and X occur earlier than the decrease in protein S and factor II. This transient imbalance in the levels of plasma vitamin K-dependent proteins may contribute to the risk of thrombosis associated with L-asparaginase therapy.[40] Treatment with L-asparaginase also induces a marked decrease in fibrinogen, plasminogen and α2-antiplasmin levels.[41] Moreover, L-asparaginase causes an acquired and transient type 1 deficiency of AT increasing the risk of thrombosis. Replacement therapy with AT concentrates appears to have a beneficial effect by decreasing the rate of thrombosis in adult patients with acute lymphoblastic leukemia (ALL) treated with L-asparaginase.[42] Levels of tissue-type plasminogen activator and plasminogen activator inhibitor were increased during treatment while cross-linked fibrin degradation products remained within normal limits, excluding the presence ofDIC.[43]

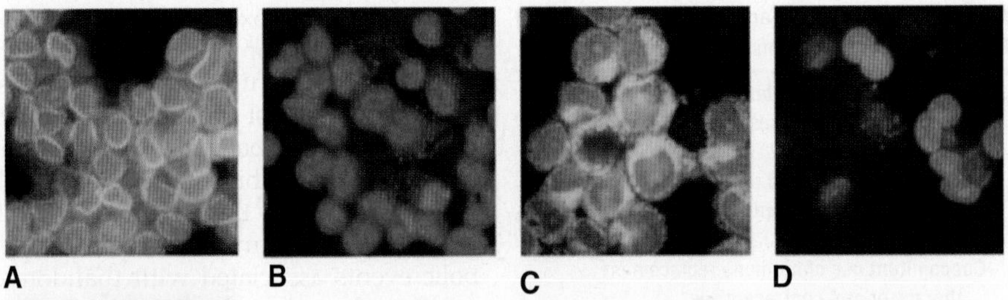

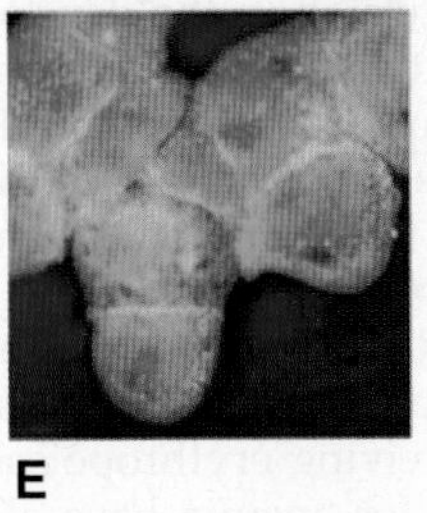

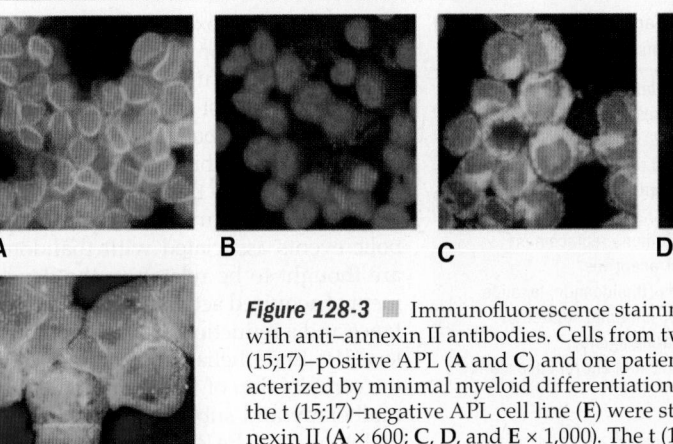

Figure 128-3 Immunofluorescence staining of APL cells with anti–annexin II antibodies. Cells from two patients with t (15;17)–positive APL (**A** and **C**) and one patient with AML characterized by minimal myeloid differentiation (**D**) and cells from the t (15;17)–negative APL cell line (**E**) were stained with anti–annexin II (**A** × 600; **C**, **D**, and **E** × 1,000). The t (15;17)–positive APL cells shown in **A** were also stained with preimmune IgG (**B** × 600). Cells were counterstained with propidium iodide (**A**, **B**, **D**, and **E**) or Evans blue (**C**).

Acute Promyelocytic Leukemia

APL-associated hemostasis disorders result from at least two distinct mechanisms, the release of procoagulant activities and of plasminogen activators from the leukemic cells. The T15-17 translocation induces hyperexpression of TF and renders the patient hypercoagulable. Elevated levels of markers of hypercoagulability such as prothrombin fragment 1þ2, thrombin-antithrombin complexes, fibrinopeptide A and B, and fibrin D-dimer demonstrate that thrombin and fibrin generation occur constantly in this condition.[44] It appears that plasmin-dependent primary fibrinogenolysis is the major etiologic factor for low fibrinogen levels in APL patients. In vivo differentiation therapy with all-transretinoic acid induces a rapid decrease in plasmin activation and a normalization of fibrinogen level, and was associated with a significant decrease in TF gene expression in bone marrow cells.[45] Annexin A2 is a calcium-dependent, phospholipid-binding profibrinolytic protein found on the surface of APL cells and other leukemic cell lines (Fig. 128-3). Overexpression of annexin A2, with the resultant increased production of plasmin, appears to be a mechanism for the excessive fibrinolysis and hemorrhagic complications in APL.[46]

Thrombotic Complications

The pathogenesis of thrombotic complications in cancer patients is multifactorial. In addition to the common predisposing factors for thrombosis such as immobility, advanced age, history of previous thrombosis, venous stasis, sepsis and the use of central venous access devices, tumor cells have unique prothrombotic characteristics. Transformed malignant cells can induce platelet abnormalities, abnormal activation of the coagulation cascade, decreased hepatic synthesis of anticoagulant and coagulant proteins, fibrinolytic abnormalities, acquired thrombophilias, and expression of inflammatory and angiogenic cytokines (Table 128-1). Each of these factors enable tumor cells to become thrombogenic, and increase by coagulation dependent and coagulation-independent mechanisms, the ability of tumor cells to proliferate, migrate, and metastasize.[47]

Several factors´ contribute to the increased risk for bleeding and thrombotic complications in the cancer patient (Table 128-4). Thrombotic manifestations in cancer patients may present as one of the following: migratory thrombophlebitis or Trousseau syndrome, venous thromboembolism (VTE), thrombotic microangiopathy (TTP/HUS), arterial thrombosis, and DIC.

Table 128-4 Risk Factors for Bleeding and Thrombotic Complications in Cancer Patients

Use of indwelling catheters
Systemic inflammatory response syndrome (SIRS)
Sepsis
Prior chemotherapy and radiation treatment
Selective estrogen receptor modulators (SERMs): tamoxifen, raloxifene
Concomitant use of hormone replacement therapy or oral contraceptives
Anti-angiogenic agents (thalidomide, lenalidomide, bevacizumab, sunitinib, sorafenib)
Erythropoiesis-stimulating agents
Metastatic disease to the liver and/or bone marrow
Vitamin K Deficiency
Acute peptic ulcer
Slipped ligatures from recent surgery

Migratory Thrombophlebitis (Trousseau Syndrome)

Trousseau syndrome is a classically described variant form of venous thrombosis characterized by a recurrent and migratory pattern preferentially involving superficial veins of the arms and chest.[8] This syndrome should precipitate the search for an occult malignancy, especially in patients with recurrent and migratory venous thrombosis affecting unusual sites such as subclavian veins, or veins of upper extremities, axilla, or neck. Trousseau syndrome is highly associated with mucin-producing adenocarcinomas.[48] Its clinical manifestations also include chronic disseminated intravascular coagulopathy associated with microangiopathy verrucous endocarditis, and arterial emboli in patients with cancer. Migratory thrombophlebitis has also been associated with the use of somatostatin or octreotide therapy for malignant carcinoid syndrome.

Venous Thromboembolism

VTE, as manifested by deep vein thrombosis (DVT) and pulmonary embolism (PE), may occur in 4-20% of cancer patients and is one of the leading causes of death.[49] The overall incidence of cancer-related VTE in postmortem studies however, has been reported as high as 50%.[50] In patients presenting with de novo idiopathic VTE there is a high risk for a concurrent cancer, especially within the first year after the diagnosis for the thromboembolism.[50] Cancer patients at greatest risk for VTE include those with mucin-secreting tumors (eg, pancreatic and gastrointestinal cancer), cancers of the lung, brain, prostate, breast, and ovary, and patients with APL and myeloproliferative disorders, specifically PV and ET.[50] VTE often complicates the care of cancer patients undergoing major surgery and of patients receiving chemotherapy and/or hormonal therapy.[51]

The risk of developing thrombosis in cancer patients is influenced by the age and hormonal status of the patient. Postmenopausal women with advanced breast cancer receiving tamoxifen in addition to adjuvant chemotherapy have a higher risk for thrombotic events than do premenopausal women with breast cancer.[52] Thromboembolic events have been also reported with angiogenesis inhibitors (thalidomide, lenalidomide, and bevacizumab).[12,53] The pathogenic mechanisms of thromboembolic events associated with thalidomide are thought to be related to the development of acquired activated protein C resistance and a reduction in thrombomodulin level.[12,54] Endothelial injury produced by the combination of thalidomide with chemotherapy and subsequent restoration of endothelial cell PAR-1 expression are probably factors that promote thrombosis.[55] Cancer patients receiving erythropoiesis-stimulating agents for anemia have also been reported to have increased risks of thrombotic complications.[56]

Recent major advances in the diagnosis of VTE include the development and validation of a standardized clinical model (Wells criteria) to determine the pretest probability of VTE and the measurement of plasma D-dimer. The integration of these two advances has resulted in the formulation of safe, diagnostic algorithms that decrease the need for serial and/or invasive testing.[57] In a clinical trial where the Wells clinical model was combined with compression ultrasonography, the need for venography and serial compression ultrasonography testing was decreased[58]; D-dimer levels can be measured by enzyme-linked immunosorbent assay, latex agglutination assay, or by a rapid bedside whole-blood assay. Of the three assays, the whole-blood assay reportedly has the best predictive value with sensitivity rates in symptomatic general medical patients ranging from 85% to 95% and specificity rates of 65-68%.[59] A recent study has shown that d-dimer results have high negative predictive value (NPV) and sensitivity for PE in oncologic patients and, if negative, can be used to exclude PE in this population.[60]

As with other patients, the majority of DVT in cancer patients originate in the ileofemoral venous system. Diagnostic imaging modalities for DVT include ascending contrast venography, compression ultrasonography, and magnetic resonance venography. Ascending contrast venography remains the gold standard for diagnosing DVT, but this procedure is invasive and requires contrast material, which is frequently irritating and may result in complications. The finding of an intraluminal filling defect caused by thrombus surrounded by contrast is diagnostic for DVT. Noncompressibility of a proximal lower limb vein on compression ultrasonography has a diagnostic sensitivity rate of 97% and a specificity rate of 94%.[61] Although compression ultrasonography is highly sensitive for detecting proximal DVT, it is not as accurate for diagnosing isolated calf DVT. Magnetic resonance venography, a relatively new imaging modality that does not use contrast, has sensitivity and specificity rates greater than 95% for proximal DVT. It is potentially useful in diagnosing pelvic vein DVT, especially isolated iliac vein thrombosis, which is difficult to diagnose with compression ultrasonography.

Several studies conducted in cancer patients with suspected DVT have demonstrated that the combination of the following studies can reliably exclude DVT and decrease the need for invasive testing: a normal D-dimer level and a normal compression ultrasonogram, a low pretest probability and normal compression ultrasonogram,[58] and a low pretest probability and a normal D-dimer level.

The standard treatment of VTE outside the setting of malignancy is to initiate anticoagulation with either intravenous or subcutaneous unfractionated heparin (UFH) or subcutaneous low-molecular-weight heparin (LMWH) or fondaparinux (an indirect Xa inhibitor) at therapeutic doses followed by oral warfarin therapy for a minimum of 3 months to achieve an international normalized ratio (INR) between 2.0 and 3.0.[62] However, in patients with active cancer, continued anticoagulation is recommended following the first episode of VTE.[62] Intravenous UFH is usually started with an initial bolus of 80 U/kg followed by a continuous IV infusion of 18 U/kg/h, adjusted to maintain the aPTT at 1.5-2.5 times the control value.[62] Alternatively, LMWH can be administered in weight-adjusted, once or twice-daily subcutaneous doses without the need for laboratory monitoring. Warfarin therapy is commenced within 24 h after heparin treatment is started. Heparin therapy is continued for at least 5 days until the INR is within the therapeutic range for 2 consecutive days. However, in patients with large ileofemoral vein thrombosis or major PE, some investigators have recommended extending heparin treatment to 7-10 days.

Retrospective and prospective clinical trials have demonstrated a survival advantage in cancer patients treated with LMWH for established thrombosis.[63,64] LMWHs have several advantages when compared to UFH: laboratory monitoring is not required, only subcutaneous injection is necessary, and there are lower incidences of bleeding, heparin-induced thrombocytopenia (HIT),[65] and osteoporosis.[66] The use of long-term LMWH as an alternative to warfarin therapy in cancer patients with acute VTE has been analyzed in 2 clinical trials. The CANTHANOX trial compared 3 months of warfarin versus enoxaparin anticoagulation in cancer patients with DVT and/or PE. Although the risk of recurrent VTE was lower in the enoxaparin group, the difference was not statistically significant. Warfarin was associated with a high bleeding rate.[67] In the CLOT trial, the cumulative risk of recurrent VTE at 6 months was reduced from 17% in the oral anticoagulant group to 9% in the LMWH group resulting in a statistically significant risk reduction for VTE.[68] Overall, there were no differences in bleeding between the groups. Current guidelines recommend the use of LMWH for the first 3-6 months as long-term treatment of VTE in cancer patients.[62] Cancer patients with recurrent VTE have a short median survival. Escalating the dose of LMWH can be effective for treating cases that are resistant to standard, weight-adjusted doses of LMWH or a vitamin K antagonist warfarin.[69]

The use of thrombolytic agents such as streptokinase and tPA should be restricted to patients with massive ileofemoral DVT or massive PE and hemodynamic instability because of the significant risks of bleeding associated with thrombolysis.[62] Furthermore, despite the proven efficacy of thrombolytic agents in achieving more rapid resolution of radiologic and hemodynamic abnormalities in patients with PE, studies to date have not shown any survival benefit with thrombolysis. Catheter-directed thrombolysis for initial treatment of VTE should be confined to selected patients requiring limb salvage. In general, thrombolytic therapy is contraindicated in cancer patients with brain metastases who develop VTE because of their significant risk for intracranial bleeding.[70] However, risk stratification may help to identify subgroups of patients at high risk of death that might benefit from systemic thrombolysis.[71] Surgical thromboembolectomy is restricted to patients with massive PE who have contraindications to or who do not respond to thrombolysis, in centers that have the available resources.[62] For cancer patients with VTE who have contraindications to anticoagulant therapy or those with recurrent VTE despite anticoagulation, placement of a (retrievable or permanent) inferior vena cava (IVC) filter is generally recommended. However, IVC filters are associated with undesirable side effects, such as debilitating leg symptoms caused by filter-related thrombosis.[72] A recent study reported that IVC filters were safe and highly effective in preventing PE-related deaths in cancer patients with VTE disease.[73] Additionally, patients with a history of DVT and bleeding or metastatic/disseminated stage of disease had the lowest survival after IVC filter placement.

The major concern about treatment of VTE in cancer patients is the higher risk of bleeding and VTE recurrence compared to non-cancer patients. A prospective cohort study demonstrated that the 12-month cumulative incidence of recurrent VTE in cancer patients was 20.7% versus 6.8% in patients without cancer, and the parallel estimate for major bleeding was 12.4% versus 4.9%, respectively.[74] Recurrence and bleeding were both related to cancer severity and occurred predominantly during the first month of anticoagulant therapy but could not be explained by sub- or over-anticoagulation. The risk of recurrent VTE has been reported to be 2-3 fold higher and the risk of major bleeding is 3-6 fold higher in cancer patients than in patients without cancer.[68]

Previous studies reported that prophylaxis with low-dose warfarin (1 mg daily) or LMWH (dalteparin 2,500 anti-Xa U daily) was efficacious in cancer patients with indwelling central venous catheters.[75,76] It appears however, that the incidence of catheter-related thrombosis (CRT) in cancer patients is much lower than previously reported.[77] Thus, routine prophylaxis with either warfarin 1 mg daily or LMWH (dalteparin 2,500IU SC once a day) is not recommended.[78] Alteplase, a recombinant tPA, is effective in restoring flow to indwelling catheters occluded by thrombus; 1-2 mg per lumen of tPA is a suitable dose for catheter instillation.[79] Perioperative cancer patients, particularly those with breast cancer undergoing chemotherapy or on selective estrogen receptor modulators and patients with advanced cancers that are associated with high risk of VTE such as brain tumors, and colorectal, pancreatic, lung, renal cell, and ovarian adenocarcinomas, should receive antithrombotic prophylaxis with intermittent pneumatic compression devices or compression elastic stockings and either subcutaneous unfractionated heparin or LMWH. The recommended doses are low-dose unfractionated heparin 5,000 U SC every 8 h or LMWH, either dalteparin 5,000 U SC daily, or enoxaparin 40 mg SC daily, or fondaparinux 2.5 mg SC starting 8-12 h postoperatively.[78] 2 trials in cancer patients undergoing surgery reported that continuation of LMWH prophylaxis for 3 weeks after hospital discharge reduced the risk of late venographic DVT by 60%.[80-82] Finally, cancer patients who are immobile or bedridden with an acute medical illness also should receive antithrombotic prophylaxis with low-dose UFH or LMWH. However, ambulatory cancer patients require no VTE prophylaxis. However, in cancer patients receiving chemotherapy or hormonal therapy, routine primary thromboprophylaxis is not indicated.[78] Moreover, thromboprophylaxis with aspirin, warfarin, or LMWH is widely used by clinicians for patients with multiple myeloma receiving thalidomide or lenalidomide in combination with chemotherapy or high-dose steroids.[83,84]

Anticancer Effects of Anticoagulation Treatment

Experimental and indirect clinical evidence suggests that anticoagulants, particularly LMWH may have antineoplastic effects. It has been suggested that anticoagulants can interfere with tumor angiogenesis, proliferation potential of cancer cells and with the immune system by augmenting the anti-tumor activity of tumor necrosis factor and of interferon mediated by NK cells.[85] Anticoagulants may also interfere with the various stages of the metastatic cascade. Recent clinical trials have shown a trend toward improved survival in a subgroup of cancer patients with early disease who received dalteparin.[86,87] Further research is needed to investigate the effects of heparin (UFH and LMWH) and other anticoagulants in patients with different types and stages of cancers.[88]

Heparin-Induced Thrombocytopenia (HIT)

HIT is an immune-mediated thrombocytopenia that occurs in approximately 1-5% of patients receiving heparin.[89] The decrease in platelet count typically occurs 5-10 days after starting heparin but may develop within 24 hours if there has been exposure to heparin during the preceding 3 months. Occasionally, the platelet count starts to fall only after heparin has been stopped (delayed-onset HIT). The frequency of HIT varies according to the type of heparin preparation (bovine UFH > porcine UFH > LMWH) and the exposed patient population (postoperative > medical > pregnancy).[89] HIT is caused by heparin-dependent, platelet-activating antibodies that recognize platelet factor 4 (PF4) bound to heparin. The resulting platelet activation is associated with increased thrombin generation. Venous or arterial thromboses includingDVT, PE, limb artery thrombosis, thrombotic stroke, and myocardial infarction can occur. A clinical pretest probability score known as the 4Ts (degree of thrombocytopenia, timing of thrombocytopenia, other etiologies of thrombocytopenia, and thrombosis) is useful in clinical practice. HIT should be suspected and treatment rapidly instituted in a patient with an intermediate or high test probability.[90] The "gold standard" test for laboratory diagnosis is the platelet serotonin release assay; however, this test is cumbersome and is performed only in a few specialized coagulation laboratories. In clinical practice, the laboratory diagnosis of HIT is made with a positive platelet factor 4-dependent immunoassay. Management consists of discontinuing all forms of heparin and using direct thrombin inhibitors such as lepirudin or argatroban, which do not have any cross-reactivity to HIT antibodies. Lepirudin is excreted by the kidney and should not be used in patients with severe renal failure (creatinine clearance < 20 mL/min). The approved dose is 0.4 mg/kg (IV bolus) followed by an initial infusion rate at 0.15 mg/kg/h targeting the aPTT to 1.5 to 2.5× baseline. Argatroban is metabolized by the liver and the dose should be reduced in patients with hepatic impairment. The usual dose is 2 μg/kg per minute targeting the aPTT to 1.5 to 3× baseline. The starting dose should be reduced by 75% in a patient with significant liver dysfunction. In countries where danaparoid, a heparanoid, is available, this agent may also be used for the prevention and treatment of HIT complicated by thrombosis.[89] Warfarin should be avoided during the acute HIT episode because it decreases the level of protein C and predisposes to microvascular thrombosis including warfarin-induced venous limb gangrene and skin necrosis syndromes. For patients receiving warfarin at the time of diagnosis of HIT, reversal of warfarin anticoagulation with vitamin K is recommended.

Thrombotic Thrombocytopenic Purpura and Hemolytic Uremic Syndrome (TTP/HUS)

TTP/HUS is characterized by a microangiopathic hemolytic anemia (Fig. 128-4), thrombocytopenia, neurologic symptoms, renal dysfunction, and fever. The majority of TTP/HUS cases are reported in patients with adenocarcinoma, particularly gastric cancer; however, TTP/HUS also occurs in patients with breast cancer and lung cancer, and in Hodgkin and non-Hodgkin lymphomas.[91] TTP/HUS also occurs in association with cancer chemotherapy, especially with mitomycin C, bleomycin, cisplatin, and tamoxifen,[92] use of cyclosporine,[93] and interferon,[94] as well as after hematopoeitic stem cell transplantation.[95]

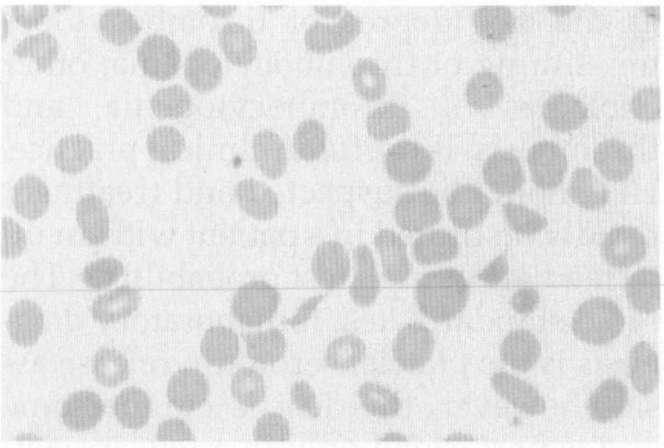

Figure 128-4 Peripheral blood smear in TTP/HUS showing microangiopathic changes. Numerous schistocytes are present along with significantly reduced platelets.

The pathophysiology of cancer-associated TTP/HUS is postulated to be similar to that of usual primary TTP/HUS. It involves injury to vascular endothelium with release of ultralarge vWF multimers due to a deficiency of a vWF–cleaving protease (ADAMTS-13) causing platelet aggregation.[96,97]

The Clinical manifestations of TTP/HUS in cancer patients are Clinical manifestations of TTP/HUS in cancer patients are occur in patients who also have other reasons for thrombocytopenia such as chemotherapy and/or radiation therapy, along with other comorbidities that may obsc the diagnosis. Typically, the microangiopathic hemolytic anemia and thrombocytopenia are severe and reticulocytosis is usually present, with increased levels of lactic acid dehydrogenase, reflecting intravascular hemolysis. The peripheral blood smear demonstrates numerous schistocytes. Renal failure and neurologic and pulmonary dysfunction are common. Neurologic signs and symptoms include headache, confusion, hemiplegia or hemiparesis, and coma. Rarely, severe acute respiratory distress syndrome may occur late in the disease process and is usually fatal. Standard treatment of TTP is plasmapheresis. Other treatment modalities that may be used in refractory cases include vincristine, intravenous gamma globulin, rituximab, and splenectomy.[98,99] Platelet transfusions are usually contraindicated because infused platelets may amplify the extent and severity of the formation of microvascular thrombi. Regardless of treatment, the prognosis of cancer patients with TTP/HUS is generally poor.

Arterial Thrombosis and Nonbacterial Thrombotic Endocarditis (NBTE)

The association between cancer and arterial thrombosis is less well described. Isolated cases have been reported and chemotherapy has been implicated as a cause.[100] Arterial thrombosis in cancer patients is less frequent than venous thrombosis. It usually occurs as a complication of nonbacterial endocarditis and rarely, in patients receiving chemotherapeutic agents such as cisplatin. Arterial thromboses including peripheral arterial thrombosis and cerebrovascular accidents have been reported in breast cancer patients receiving adjuvant chemotherapy and in patients with metastatic colorectal, breast, or non-small-cell lung carcinoma receiving combination treatment with bevacizumab and chemotherapy.[101] The selective estrogen receptor modulators tamoxifen and raloxifen increases the risk of stroke[102] especially in postmenopausal women at increased risk for coronary events and in current smokers.[103]

Nonbacterial thrombotic endocarditis (NBTE) represents a form of consumptive coagulopathy most commonly seen with adenocarcinomas of the lung and pancreas. The diagnosis should be suspected in any cancer patient who presents with ischemic embolic events. Echocardiography is diagnostic with the finding of sterile thrombotic vegetations on cardiac valves. In addition to valvular vegetations, ventricular segmental wall motion abnormalities resulting from silent embolization to the coronary arteries has been reported in 18% of cancer patients with NBTE. Management is essentially supportive and consists of treatment of the underlying cancer and anticoagulant therapy with unfractionated or low-molecular weight heparin.

Disseminated Intravascular Coagulation (DIC)

DIC is a clinicopathological syndrome that complicates patients with malignancy. Patients with solid tumors (prostate, pancreas, lung, stomach, colon, and breast) and those with leukemia, especially APL, may be complicated by DIC that is manifested primarily by bleeding. Patients with hematologic malignancies often present with a state of chronic DIC in the absence of active thrombosis and/or bleeding. The bleeding disorder in APL is thought to be due to the abnormally high levels of expression of annexin A2 on APL cells, which leads to increased production of plasmin and ensuing bleeding from unopposed fibrinolysis (140). Annexin A2 is a phospholipid-binding protein on the surface of endothelial cells that serves to bind plasminogen and its activator, tPA. In APL cells the *t*15–17 translocation, induces hyperexpression of TF in the leukemic cell, linking the primary oncogenic event with induction of hypercoagulability.[104]

Plasma microparticles associated TF procoagulant activity may play an important pathogenic role in the evolution of overt DIC in various types of malignancy.[105]

The thrombotic disorders associated with DIC include recurrent venous thrombosis, peripheral arterial thrombosis, cerebrovascular thrombosis, disseminated arterial disease with organ failure, peripheral limb ischemia, and gangrene. Chronic forms of DIC are characterized by less florid clinical findings and more subtle, but persistent, laboratory abnormalities. Metastatic cancer is a common cause of chronic DIC. Over time, approximately 25% of patients with metastatic cancer develop a thrombotic event. In cancer patients, the diagnosis of DIC is made clinically and corroborated by a constellation of laboratory abnormalities (Table 128-5).[106] There is no single laboratory test that can establish or exclude the diagnosis of DIC. In most cases, a combination of tests in a patient with a clinical condition that is associated with DIC can be used to diagnose the disorder with reasonable certainty. In the presence of an underlying disease associated with DIC, an initial platelet count of less than 100,000/mm^3 or a rapid decline in the platelet count; prolongation of the PT and aPTT is seen in about 50-60% of cases of DIC; and the presence of fibrin(ogen) degradation products in plasma, and D-dimers. Fibrinogen levels may remain in the normal range in the face of its consumption because of increased synthesis of this acute-phase reactant. A finding of hypofibrinogenemia is only useful diagnostically in very severe cases of DIC. The peripheral blood smear may also demonstrate the presence of red cell fragmentation or schistocytes, but rarely >10% of the red cells. Soluble fibrin monomer (SF), which is only generated intravascularly is a sensitive but not specific test for the diagnosis of DIC.[107] There appears to be no added value measuring the natural anticoagulants protein C and/orAT.[108] The International Society of Thrombosis and Hemostasis (ISTH), subcommittee of the Scientific and Standarization Committee (SCC) on DIC has recommended the use of scoring system for overt DIC.[108] The sensitivity and specificity of the ISTH overt DIC score is 91% and 97% respectively.[109] It is important to repeat the tests to monitor the dynamically changing scenario based on the laboratory results and clinical manifestations.

Table 128-5 **Abnormalities in Cancer Patients with DIC**

Thrombocytopenia
Prolongation of PT and aPTT
Hypofibrinogenemia[a]
Decreased levels of factor V and factor VIII[b]
Presence of fibrin(ogen) degradation products and D-dimer[c]
Presence of schistocytes or fragmented red blood cells in the peripheral blood smear indicating microangiopathic hemolysis

[a]Fibrinogen levels may remain in the normal range: a finding of hypofibrinogenemia is only useful diagnostically in very severe cases of DIC.

[b]Factor VIII levels may be increased in some patients with early DIC because of thrombin activation of factor VIII.

[c]Plasma D-dimers are specific cross-linked fibrin derivatives generated when the endogenous fibrinolytic system degrades fibrin.

In general, the treatment of DIC is directed against the underlying cancer but supportive management to the bleeding or thrombotic manifestations is required. Cancer patients with DIC who are bleeding or at high risk for bleeding (patients undergoing surgery or invasive procedures) should receive platelet transfusions to maintain the platelet count greater than 50,000/µL and FFP (initial doses of 15 mL/kg, although a dose of 30 mL/kg produces a more complete correction of coagulation factor levels) if the PT or aPTT are prolonged. The administration of purified coagulation factor concentrates in DIC is not generally recommended unless patients are fluid overloaded and cannot receive FFP. Coagulation factor concentrates contain only specific factors whereas in DIC there is a global deficiency in coagulation factors. Severe hypofibrinogenemia (<1 g/L) needs to be treated with cryoprecipitate or fibrinogen concentrates if available. A dose of 3 g would raise plasma fibrinogen by 1 g/L, this can be given as two cryoprecipitate pools (10 donor units) or as a 3 g of a fibrinogen concentrate. The response to the supportive transfusion therapy should be monitored clinically and with laboratory tests.[106] The bleeding associated with DIC in APL often responds dramatically to treatment with all-trans-retinoic acid.[110]

Although there are no clinical randomized controlled trials demonstrating that the use of heparin in patients with DIC results in improved clinical outcome, intravenous heparin may be used in cancer patients with DIC-associated thrombosis for stabilization while the cancer is being treated unless moderate to severe thrombocytopenia or bleeding is present. The recommended dose of heparin is 10 U/kg/h by continuous IV infusion without a loading dose, monitoring aPTT may be complicated, but monitoring for signs of bleeding is important. In critically ill, non-bleeding patients with DIC pharmacological thromboprophylaxis with either unfractionated or low molecular weight heparin is recommended.[106] In general, patients with DIC should not be treated with antifibrinolytic agents. However in patients with DIC and bleeding secondary to primary fibrinolysis (eg, prostate cancer), the fibrinolytic inhibitor, epsilon aminocaproic acid can be administered with an initial IV loading dose of 4-6 g over 1 h followed by an IV infusion of 1 g/h while monitoring the clinical response. The recommended oral dose of aminocaproic acid is 50-60 mg/kg every 4-6 h.[111] However, in those patients with a primary thrombotic presentation and secondary fibrinolysis, fibrinolytic inhibitors should be avoided until the thrombotic process is controlled.[106]

Novel Drugs for Treatment of Bleeding and Thrombotic Disorders

Recombinant Factor VIIa

Recombinant Factor VIIa (rFVIIa) is FDA approved for patients with bleeding secondary to hemophilia A or B who have inhibitors against factors VIII and IX.[112] It has also been shown to be effective in controlling bleeding due to thrombocytopenia, thrombocytopathies, hereditary factor VII deficiency, acquired coagulation factor deficiencies and in patients undergoing cancer surgery. There is increasing evidence on the use of rFVIIa in patients with hematological malignancies and in patients who develop critical bleeding associated with hematopoietic stem cell transplantation.[113,114] By enhancing thrombin generation on activated platelets, rFVIIa promotes the formation of a stable fibrin clot that is resistant to premature lysis. rFVIIa has a short half-life and is administered at doses of 90-120 micrograms/kg every 2 h and repeated as clinically warranted.[115] Caution should be undertaken in administering rFVIIa to patients with DIC, coronary artery disease, and severe sepsis because of their higher risk for vascular thrombosis.

Thrombopoietic Agonists

Thrombopoietic stimulating agents: romiplostim and eltrombopag are promising agents that have recently demonstrated the ability to increase platelet counts in patients with chronic immune thrombocytopenic purpura (ITP). They have shown benefit in splenectomized and nonsplenectomized patients. There is insufficient data on the long-term risk associated with continued use of thrombopoietic agents beyond 6 months. The risk of thrombosis, myelofibrosis, and development of hematologic malignancies with continued use of thrombopoietic stimulating agents is unknown.[116]

Novel Anticoagulants

Clinical trials of orally administered direct Factor X a inhibitors such as rivaroxaban and apixaban and oral direct thrombin inhibitors like dabigatran for the prevention and treatment ofVTE are being completed. These oral agents can be given in fixed doses without routine monitoring.[117] Rivaroxaban has a half-life of 9 hours and is eliminated by the renal and intestinal routes. Apixaban has a half-life of 12 hours and is cleared by the fecal and renal routes. Phase 2 trials of apixaban in cancer patients are ongoing. Dabigatran etexilate is a prodrug that once absorbed is converted to its active metabolite dabigatran. Peak plasma level occurs at 2 hours and its half-life is 8 hours after a single dose administration and 17 hours after multiple doses. As 80% of dabigatran is excreted by the kidney, this drug is contraindicated in patients with renal failure.[118] Idraparinux is an indirect Factor Xa inhibitor, which binds with high affinity to AT and has a plasma half-life of 80 hours, allowing for subcutaneous administration once a week. Idraparinux can cause excessive bleeding therefore a biotynilated form of idraparinux has been developed that has the same pharmacokinetics and pharmacodynamic properties as idraparinux but can be neutralized by avidin. Avidin binds biotin with high affinity and the complex is cleared renally.[113]

Summary

Bleeding and thrombotic complications are common in cancer patients. Significant advances in the understanding of the interrelationship between cancer, blood coagulation, and tumor angiogenesis have occurred in recent years. Bleeding complications usually result from abnormalities in platelets or deficiency of coagulation factors and require specific blood or coagulation factor replacement. Thromboembolic events including DVT and PE are not only common but also serious complications seen in cancer patients. Advances in diagnostic imaging and availability of newer and more potent anticoagulant agents have greatly facilitated the care of these patients. Ongoing research in the understanding of the various disturbances in hemostasis, application of innovative treatment modalities, and use of appropriate thromboprophylaxis in cancer patients should ultimately lead to decreased morbidity and improved survival.

Selected References

The complete reference list can be found at www.CANCERMEDICINE8.com

1. Tallman MS, Brenner B, Serna Jde L, et al. Meeting report. acute promyelocytic leukemia-associated coagulopathy, 21 January 2004, London, United Kingdom. *Leuk Res.* March 2005;29(3):347–351.
5. Esmon CT. The endothelial protein C receptor. *Curr Opin Hematol.* September 2006;13(5):382–385.
8. Trousseau A. Phlegmasia alba dolens. Lectures on clinical medicine, delivered at the Hotel-Dieu, Paris, New Sydenham Society. 1877.
10. Falanga A. Mechanisms of thrombosis in cancer. *Thromb Res.* February 2005;115 (Suppl 1):21–24.
13. Palumbo JS, Talmage KE, Massari JV, et al. Platelets and fibrin(ogen) increase metastatic potential by impeding natural killer cell-mediated elimination of tumor cells. *Blood.* January 1, 2005;105(1):178–185.
15. DeSancho MT, Rand JH. Bleeding and thrombotic complications in critically ill patients with cancer. *Crit Care Clin.* July 2001;17(3):599–622.
17. Stanworth SJ, Hyde C, Heddle N, Rebulla P, Brunskill S, Murphy MF. Prophylactic platelet transfusion for haemorrhage after chemotherapy and stem cell transplantation. *Cochrane Database Syst Rev.* October 18, 2004;4(4):CD004269.
18. Slichter SJ. Evidence-based platelet transfusion guidelines. *Hematology Am Soc Hematol Educ Program.* 2007;2007:172–178.
22. Franchini M, Lippi G. Acquired von willebrand syndrome: an update. *Am J Hematol.* May 2007;82(5):368–375.
23. Federici AB, Budde U, Rand JH. Acquired von willebrand syndrome 2004: international registry—diagnosis and management from online to bedside. *Hamostaseologie.* February 2004;24(1):50–55.
24. Ma AD, Carrizosa D. Acquired factor VIII inhibitors: pathophysiology and treatment. *Hematology Am Soc Hematol Educ Program.* 2006:432-7.
26. Hedges SJ, Dehoney SB, Hooper JS, Amanzadeh J, Busti AJ. Evidence-based treatment recommendations for uremic bleeding. *Nat Clin Pract Nephrol.* March 2007;3(3):138–153.
33. Harrison CN, Campbell PJ, Buck G, et al. Hydroxyurea compared with anagrelide in high-risk essential thrombocythemia. *N Engl J Med.* July 7, 2005;353(1):33–45.
35. Ansell J, Hirsh J, Hylek E, et al. Pharmacology and management of the vitamin K antagonists: American college of chest physicians evidence-based clinical practice guidelines (8th edition). *Chest.* June 2008;133(6 Suppl):160S–198S.
37. Mumford AD, O'Donnell J, Gillmore JD, Manning RA, Hawkins PN, Laffan M. Bleeding symptoms and coagulation abnormalities in 337 patients with AL-amyloidosis. *Br J Haematol.* August 2000;110(2):454–460.
41. Legnani C, Palareti G, Pession A, et al. Intravascular coagulation phenomena associated with prevalent fall in fibrinogen and plasminogen during L-asparaginase treatment in leukemic children. *Haemostasis.* 1988;18(3):179–186.
46. Menell JS, Cesarman GM, Jacovina AT, McLaughlin MA, Lev EA, Hajjar KA. Annexin II and bleeding in acute promyelocytic leukemia [see comments]. *N Engl J Med.* 1999 04/01/;340(13):994–1004.
47. Falanga A, Barbui T, Rickles FR. Hypercoagulability and tissue factor gene upregulation in hematologic malignancies. *Semin Thromb Hemost.* March 2008;34(2):204–210.
48. Varki A. Trousseau's syndrome: multiple definitions and multiple mechanisms. *Blood.* September 15, 2007;110(6):1723–1729.
49. Lyman GH, Khorana AA, Falanga A, et al. American society of clinical oncology guideline: Recommendations for venous thromboembolism prophylaxis and treatment in patients with cancer. *J Clin Oncol.* December 1, 2007;25(34):5490–5505.
52. Levine MN, Gent M, Hirsh J, et al. The thrombogenic effect of anticancer drug therapy in women with stage II breast cancer. *N Engl J Med.* February 18, 1988;318(7):404–407.
53. Zangari M, Anaissie E, Barlogie B, et al. Increased risk of deep-vein thrombosis in patients with multiple myeloma receiving thalidomide and chemotherapy. *Blood.* 2001 09/01/;98(5):1614–1615.
55. Kaushal V, Kaushal GP, Melkaveri SN, Mehta P. Thalidomide protects endothelial cells from doxorubicin-induced apoptosis but alters cell morphology. *J Thromb Haemost.* February 2004;2(2):327–334.
56. Bennett CL, Silver SM, Djulbegovic B, et al. Venous thromboembolism and mortality associated with recombinant erythropoietin and darbepoetin administration for the treatment of cancer-associated anemia. *JAMA.* February 27, 2008;299(8):914–924.
60. King V, Vaze AA, Moskowitz CS, Smith LJ, Ginsberg MS. D-dimer assay to exclude pulmonary embolism in high-risk oncologic population: correlation with CT pulmonary angiography in an urgent care setting. *Radiology.* June 2008;247(3):854–861.
64. Lee AY. Cancer and venous thromboembolism: prevention, treatment and survival. *J Thromb Thrombolysis.* February 2008;25(1):33–36.
67. Meyer G, Marjanovic Z, Valcke J, et al. Comparison of low-molecular-weight heparin and warfarin for the secondary prevention of venous thromboembolism in patients with cancer: a randomized controlled study. *Arch Intern Med.* August 12–26, 2002;162(15):1729–1735.
68. Lee AY, Levine MN, Baker RI, et al. Low-molecular-weight heparin versus a coumarin for the prevention of recurrent venous thromboembolism in patients with cancer. *N Engl J Med.* July 10, 2003;349(2):146–153.
74. Prandoni P, Lensing AW, Piccioli A, et al. Recurrent venous thromboembolism and bleeding complications during anticoagulant treatment in patients with cancer and venous thrombosis. *Blood.* November 15, 2002;100(10):3484–3488.
78. Geerts WH, Bergqvist D, Pineo GF, et al. Prevention of venous thromboembolism: American college of chest physicians evidence-based clinical practice guidelines (8th edition). *Chest.* June 2008;133(6 Suppl):381S–453S.
82. Agnelli G, Bergqvist D, Cohen AT, Gallus AS, Gent M, PEGASUS investigators. Randomized clinical trial of postoperative fondaparinux versus perioperative dalteparin for prevention of venous thromboembolism in high-risk abdominal surgery. *Br J Surg.* October 2005;92(10):1212–1220.
83. Niesvizky R, Martinez-Banos D, Jalbrzikowski J, et al. Prophylactic low-dose aspirin is effective antithrombotic therapy for combination treatments of thalidomide or lenalidomide in myeloma. *Leuk Lymphoma.* December 2007;48(12):2330–2337.
84. Palumbo A, Rajkumar SV, Dimopoulos MA, et al. Prevention of thalidomide- and lenalidomide-associated thrombosis in myeloma. *Leukemia.* February 2008;22(2):414–423.
86. Lee AY, Rickles FR, Julian JA, et al. Randomized comparison of low molecular weight heparin and coumarin derivatives on the survival of patients with cancer and venous thromboembolism. *J Clin Oncol.* February 7, 2005;23(10):2123-9.
87. Kakkar AK, Levine MN, Kadziola Z, et al. Low molecular weight heparin, therapy with dalteparin, and survival in advanced cancer: the fragmin advanced malignancy outcome study (FAMOUS). *J Clin Oncol.* May 15, 2004;22(10):1944–1948.

129 Urologic Complications

Christopher J. Logothetis, MD ■ Diana M. Hey Cauley, PharmD

The appropriate anticipation and management of urologic complications of cancer and its therapy may significantly improve the opportunity for the treatment of patients with metastatic disease. The management of obstructive uropathy, the criteria for detection of drug-induced renal toxicity, and the management of such toxicity without excessive dose reduction are important ingredients that contribute to the successful treatment of cancer patients. Adjustment of the dose of different chemotherapeutic agents on the basis of renal function and interaction with other agents that may be delivered concomitantly is an essential component of oncologic practice. Furthermore, it is increasingly recognized that successful strategies require optimum control of the site of origin. Thus, for urologic malignancy, control of the primary site does not only avoid local complication of cancer progression but may also be an essential component of a successful treatment strategy. This chapter reviews the most frequent urologic complications of cancers and therapy.

Complications Resulting From Primary Cancer Progression

Urinary Tract Obstruction

Obstruction of the urinary tract may occur at multiple levels (ureter, bladder, and urethra). Large retroperitoneal tumors can produce ureteral obstruction, whereas urethral and outlet obstruction results from cancers involving the bladder, distal urethra, or prostate. Such involvement can be by direct extension, encasement, or invasion of these structures. Obstruction can also occur from metastatic deposits involving these same sites. The course and management of obstructive uropathy are determined by the primary tumor causing the obstruction. Factors that influence the treatment of obstructive uropathy include the anticipated benefit from therapy and the curability of the patient, sensitivity of the neoplasm to cytotoxic therapy, rapidity of response to therapy, and anatomic access to the obstruction. The development of newer imaging techniques and less invasive surgical approaches has increased the accuracy of our assessment and expanded the opportunities for intervention. These advances allow early discovery and intervention and have reduced the need for extensive surgery to palliate distal ureteral obstruction.

Ureteral Obstruction

Ureteral obstruction most commonly occurs due to progressive growth of large periaortic nodal metastases in the retroperitoneal space adjacent to the ureters. Such obstructive uropathy is most frequently the result of either primary nodal diseases (lymphomas) or urologic neoplasms metastasizing to the periaortic nodes, particularly prostate cancer and germ cell tumors. Advanced retroperitoneal germ cell tumors and lymphomas are a unique subset of chemotherapy-sensitive tumors that frequently result in obstructive uropathy. These cancers best illustrate the different approaches that can be used to treat a particular urologic complication produced by different tumors. When the cancer has the typical pathologic and serologic markers of a seminoma, obstructive uropathy is frequently observed with regionally advanced disease, in the absence of distant metastases. Application of effective therapy targeting the cancer (radiation therapy or chemotherapy) can relieve obstruction rapidly without requiring surgical intervention to relieve obstruction. Another curable germ cell tumor, teratoma, is less likely to exhibit a rapid, gratifying reduction in size. Percutaneous nephrostomy is needed to ensure adequate renal function during cisplatin-based chemotherapy. Surgical resection of the teratoma can then follow. In both instances, high cure rates can be achieved.[1,2] The rapidity of the anticipated response and the degree of compromise in renal function often govern whether percutaneous nephrostomy is necessary or whether a reasonable expectation exists that relief of obstruction can be achieved with cytotoxic chemotherapy. Similar approaches can be used for the treatment of lymphomas in which one can anticipate a rapid response to therapy. For curable cancers that require therapies with essential components that are nephrotoxic, such as cisplatin, ifosfamide, and methotrexate (MTX). Attention to the prompt reversal of obstructive uropathy is important to permit renal excretion of the drug. Although a unilateral percutaneous nephrostomy may preserve adequate renal function, patients whose long-term disease-free survival is dependent on nephrotoxic therapy require maximal preservation of renal function. Bilateral percutaneous nephrostomy is often required in these settings. It should, however, be recognized that percutaneous nephrostomies are a source of infection that may complicate, delay, and, ultimately, force modification of treatment plans. To avoid this undesired effect on therapy, attention to detail in the placement and care of nephrostomies is required. This includes the optimal placement of catheters to reduce pain, frequent changes of the catheter (approximately at 3-month intervals), and care of the insertion site to reduce the impact on treatment.

In most patients with acute urinary tract obstruction treated with urinary diversion, retrograde stent placement is attempted initially. Large prostate or bladder tumors, multiple sites of ureteric obstruction, long occlusions, or a tortuous ureter may be indications to proceed directly with percutaneous nephrostomy.[3] During nephrostomy tube placement, the intrarenal collecting system must be properly imaged to select a site of renal entry. Unless the patient is azotemic or allergic to contrast material, the site of entry can be best determined fluoroscopically after intravenous urographic contrast. In experienced hands, an appropriate nephrostomy tract can be established in 98% of cases, with major complications occurring in approximately 4%.[4] Major complications include renal hemorrhage requiring transfusion (1-3%), vascular injury (0.5-1.0%), sepsis (1-2.5%), bowel injury (0.1%), lung injury (0.5-1.0%), and mortality (0.046-0.3%).[3] After the intrarenal collecting system and dilated ureter are allowed to decompress, an internal double-J stent is placed if cystoscopic management of the stent is anticipated. This is performed in an antegrade fashion using the nephrostomy. When cystoscopic management of the stent is inadequate or the stent fails rapidly after placement, permanent percutaneous nephrostomy with external drainage or an internal-external stent is preferred. Complications from such procedures may include infections, tube obstruction, and dislodgment.

Ureteral obstruction caused by retroperitoneal metastases from cervical or breast cancer or from retroperitoneal radiation fibrosis is often treated by stenting. The decision to stent the ureters is influenced by other considerations, including the potential response of the disease to available treatment and the presence of pain. The neoplasm causing the retroperitoneal ureteral obstruction often invades the lumbar or sacral nerve roots, leading to excruciating pain. The wisdom of substituting a prolonged painful death in a setting in which limited therapy options exist should be considered. It is clear that optimum use of this intervention will improve survival and avoid permanent renal compromise in patients with curative prospects. In settings in which limited therapy options exist, it is very clear that the optimum use of this intervention will improve survival and avoid permanent renal compromise in patients with curative prospects. Fortunately, with improved surgical technology and early detection of localized cancer, this challenge is becoming less frequent.

Bladder Outlet Obstruction

Bladder outlet obstruction as a result of a large prostate carcinoma can be rapidly palliated by hormonal therapy or radiation therapy. In a patient with prostate cancer who exhibits androgen-independent growth or progression after radiation therapy or in patients with primary urethral cancer, effective palliation is a much greater challenge. The symptoms resulting from small bladder capacity, bladder irritability, or outlet obstruction can substantially reduce the quality of life for such patients. If a decision has been made to attempt palliation with cytotoxic therapy, the judicious use of a percutaneous nephrostomy can be considered. If the cytotoxic agents used are not nephrotoxic or primarily dependent on renal metabolism for excretion, a unilateral nephrostomy is usually required to preserve sufficient renal function. If agents considered for use are either nephrotoxic or metabolized in the kidney, bilateral nephrostomy may be considered.

The decision to place percutaneous nephrostomies is simple for patients who have reversible and highly curable lesions obstructing the kidneys (lymphomas, seminomas, embryonal carcinomas, and other germ cell tumors). In addition, nephrostomies are a logical choice for patients in whom excellent and sustained palliation can be achieved (breast carcinoma and urothelial malignancies).[5,6] In patients with refractory tumors with limited therapeutic options, the implication of percutaneous nephrostomy placement without control of the primary tumor should be discussed before placement. Although obstructive uropathy can be relieved, control of symptoms related to the continued growth of the cancer within the pelvis is more challenging.

Pathologically, acute urinary tract obstruction results in increased central renal pressure and dilation of the ureter. This is reflected in the increased size and weight of the kidney. With persistent and progressive obstructive uropathy, irreversible injury finally manifests itself with renal cortical atrophy. The selection of a patient for percutaneous nephrostomy should be based, in part, on the cortical thickness. In the absence of significant atrophy, the obstructed kidney most likely will regain significant function, and percutaneous nephrostomy should be considered. Small atrophic kidneys caused by long-standing obstructive uropathy frequently do not benefit from percutaneous drainage. Placement of a percutaneous nephrostomy in a markedly atrophic kidney results in significant morbidity without benefit.

Following relief of obstructive uropathy, metabolic problems may occur. Difficulties in maximum concentration of urine and other tubular defects can result in a brisk postobstructive diuresis. This occurs most often after high-grade acute obstruction. Replacement of fluid and electrolytes is important until normal renal function returns.

Metastatic cancers that invade the urethra or primary urethral, prostatic, or bladder tumors are frequently drained unsatisfactorily by placement of Foley catheters or suprapubic tubes. In general, a suprapubic tube is contraindicated in patients with urothelial malignancies when there is curative intent, because it violates the normal anatomic barriers and increases the probability of regional spread of the disease. Urothelial malignancies that diffusely involve the bladder have a propensity to recur in surgical wounds. The inability to place a Foley catheter is sometimes a complication of primary urethral or prostatic tumors. In such instances, suprapubic catheter drainage can be used to relieve symptoms of acute obstruction. In patients with urinary frequency caused by bladder invasion or with bladder irritability as a consequence of treatment, Foley catheter placement to relieve symptoms can be attempted, but this has limited success.

Poorly controlled primary cancers of the bladder, prostate, or urethra frequently result in a debilitating dysuria, frequency, and nocturia that compromise the quality of life. The palliation of severe urinary tract symptoms infrequently requires permanent urinary diversion. Urethral and suprapubic catheters are sometimes associated with urethral discomfort, however. Under such circumstances, urinary diversion to reduce these symptoms is helpful. Because of the limited overall benefit patients can expect to achieve when they require diversion for advanced cancer, the method of diversion with the least morbidity is chosen. Thus, percutaneous nephrostomies are used more frequently than surgically constructed urinary diversion.

We attribute the apparent reduction in the frequency with which we encounter these events to earlier detection, improved anticipation of local progression, and more effective surgical techniques. The problem of locally advanced cancer limiting bladder outlet and resulting in symptoms has few effective palliative measures and is best avoided; this justifies early intervention in properly selected patients. Locally advanced cancer is a major source of morbidity, the best solution being early effective intervention.

Diagnostic studies for the radiologic and urologic assessment of the lower urinary tract have changed little and provide detailed assessment of anatomic determinants of obstruction. The first indication of obstructive uropathy is frequently a rising serum creatinine level. Urinalysis may reveal isosthenuria, and the blood urea nitrogen (BUN) level may rise. Proteinuria is not uncommon in obstructive uropathy.[7] Difficulties sometimes exist in detecting small degrees of low-grade obstructive uropathy with equivocal radiographic abnormalities. In such rare circumstances, radionuclide scans with the use of diuretics may help distinguish between a vascular and an obstructive lesion. The mainstays for the study of obstructive uropathy are ultrasonography and computed tomography (CT). When ultrasonography cannot be effectively performed because of gaseous distension, CT scans can be helpful. The superiority of ultrasonography in such patients lies in its value for marking the area for percutaneous drainage of the kidney and in the absence of contrast material, which could be injurious to renal function. More recently, endoureteral ultrasonography has been used to define the anatomy of the obstruction.

Algorithm for the Management of Urinary Obstruction

Pelvic tumors can produce urinary symptoms, obstruction, and renal failure. Urinary obstruction often requires palliation or urinary diversion before systemic therapy can be delivered. An algorithm for management of these complications based on factors such as sensitivity to chemotherapy and expected survival can be used to develop a reasoned approach to the management of pelvic disease. Before intervening in urinary obstruction, the first question that should always be asked is "To what end?" Relief of urinary obstruction does not relieve pelvic symptoms attributed to infiltration of tumor. Thus, the relief of urinary obstruction should principally be used in those subsets of patients in whom cancer control can be expected, or, at a minimum, the origin of the symptoms is judged to arise from the obstruction itself as opposed to pelvic or retroperitoneal infiltration of the cancer.

Methods for relief of urethral obstruction are principally retrograde or antegrade. In the era of interventional radiology, open surgical diversion is rarely considered a treatment option. Retrograde placement of urethral stents by cystoscopy is frequently used. The advantage of this approach is the avoidance of external catheters and urinary diversion. The success of such an approach is, however, often difficult to assess. In some subsets of patients, ureteral stents cannot be placed because of acute angulation and lack of control of the primary tumor. The approach that is frequently used by many physicians is a percutaneous nephrostomy. Percutaneous nephrostomies are safe and reliable procedures when performed by experienced radiologists in properly selected patients. Bilateral percutaneous nephrostomies are best placed in renal failure when a delay in response to therapy is expected or nephrotoxic cytotoxic agents are used. Coagulopathy and patient preference are the two major contraindications to percutaneous nephrostomies. The risk of such procedures is exceedingly low, and complications as a consequence of malplacement occasionally occur, such as bleeding into the pelvicaliceal system producing an obstructive uropathy. Both the percutaneous nephrostomy and retrograde ureteral stents often result in urinary tract infection.

On some occasions, even with obstructive uropathy from urethral obstruction, expectant management could be considered, as in situations in which highly responsive tumors are expected to respond quickly and result in relief of urinary obstruction. Examples include lymphomas and germ cell tumors for which the placement of nephrostomy can be delayed in the hope of an excellent response of the tumor. Patients with tumors of an intermediate response rate can be initially relieved of their obstruction; therapy then follows.

Lower Urinary Tract Obstruction

Distal outlet obstructions by locally advancing tumors produce obstructive uropathy and in which a nephrostomy is often considered are ovarian tumors, urothelial tumors, and, rarely, breast cancers. If bilateral obstructive uropathy is present, relief with percutaneous nephrostomy is generally recommended.

For patients with urethral obstruction, the symptoms are often more difficult to relieve. Although percutaneous nephrostomies can divert urinary drainage, they do not result in relief of the pelvic symptoms related to urgency, hematuria, dysuria, and frequency. In such instances, transurethral resection of the prostate can be considered, as can a simple placement of a percutaneous nephrostomy or suprapubic tube. Although relieving the urinary obstruction, such management often fails to relieve the severe pelvic symptoms related to progressive disease at this site. The management of these severe symptoms is a therapeutic challenge for clinicians.

Hemorrhagic Cystitis

Hematuria is frequently a striking and frightening event in the course of cancer and its treatment. Hematuria can be a result of bleeding anywhere along the entire urinary tract. Gross hematuria frequently requires palliation. The characteristics of the hematuria often permit physicians to suspect the origin of the bleeding. Long, vermiform clots typically indicate upper tract bleeding and are a result of a ureteral cast (broader clots are occasionally difficult to evacuate and cause ureteral colic or are indicative of lower tract bleeding). Bright red blood without a clot that clears partially during urination usually indicates a lower tract bleed. Hemorrhage can be a result of drug-induced or radiation-induced effects or of progressive cancer.

Drug-Induced Hematuria ■ Cyclophosphamide and ifosfamide are the most commonly used oxazaphosphorines. Both agents are metabolized to acrolein, the main urothelial toxic metabolite.[8,9] In addition to acrolein, thrombocytopenia tends to exacerbate the bleeding. Sterile hemorrhagic cystitis has been reported in up to 20% of patients receiving high doses of cyclophosphamide and in approximately 8% of patients receiving ifosfamide.[10] With conventional doses of cyclophosphamide, cystitis can be prevented by encouraging aggressive oral hydration at the time of chemotherapy. In the case of ifosfamide, this complication can be reduced with intravenous hyperhydration and the use of uroprotective mesna. Mesna is given as an intravenous bolus equal to 20% of the ifosfamide dose 15 min before ifosfamide administration, as well as 4 and 8 h later (the total dose of mesna should be equivalent to 60% of the ifosfamide dose).[11] Mesna can also be given as a continuous infusion at a dose equal to the ifosfamide dose. Continuous infusion of mesna should be maintained for 4-8 h after completion of the ifosfamide infusion. In the case of cyclophosphamide, mesna is given mainly with high-dose chemotherapy in bone marrow transplantation. The dose of mesna used is approximately 60-160% of the cyclophosphamide dose and is given intravenously in 3 to 5 divided doses or by continuous infusion.[10] Other agents that can produce gross hematuria include intravesical treatment with doxorubicin, mitomycin, and bacillus Calmette-Guérin.[11]

With the use of high-dose chemotherapy, hemorrhagic cystitis occurs in approximately 2% of conditioning regimens without cyclophosphamide. This bleeding is most commonly associated with thrombocytopenia.[12] When cyclophosphamide is used, up to 20% of patients may develop macrohematuria.[13] Moreover, the use of busulfan in addition to cyclophosphamide in high-dose chemotherapy tends to increase the risk of bleeding.[14] Hemorrhagic cystitis in bone marrow transplantation can also be associated with infection from adenovirus[15] or BK human polyomavirus.[16]

Care must be taken to ensure optimal delivery of the potentially offending agents and to avoid these feared complications.

Radiation-Induced Hematuria ■ Approximately 5.7-11.5% of patients treated with pelvic irradiation (median toxic dose 80 Gy) can develop bladder complications.[17] Although less common, hemorrhagic cystitis can be seen in the treatment of pelvic neoplasms with both external beam radiation and brachytherapy. Up to 9% of these patients can develop hematuria,[18] and approximately 10% will have bleeding more than 6 months after treatment.[19] Total-body irradiation for bone marrow transplantation is associated with hemorrhagic cystitis in 10-17% of patients.[14,20] Symptoms include recurrent hemorrhage, urinary urgency, and pain. The patients at highest risk are those with previous operations and those receiving cyclophosphamide. It is important to note that approximately 85% of the patients who develop macrohematuria after radiation actually have a recurrence of their tumor.[19] The pathophysiology of radiation-induced cystitis involves damage to the vascular endothelium and endarteritis, causing progressive ischemia, inflammation, and fibrosis, with the end result being tissue necrosis. This is also complicated by infections that prevent proper healing.

Recurrence of Tumor

Another important cause of gross hematuria is related to recurrence of bladder tumors or invasion by other pelvic neoplasms. Most of these patients have advanced disease. In many, the treatments are palliative and directed to the underlying malignancy and symptoms.

Treatment

Clot retention is a painful complication of lower urinary tract bleeding. Intermittent bladder injections or constant 2-channel bladder irrigation with antibiotic-containing saline or water usually can dissolve or dissociate clots. Cystoscopic evacuation of clots is sometimes required for palliation. In patients who have not been treated with radiation therapy for their bleeding tumors, radiation is a useful approach. Cyclophosphamide-, ifosfamide-, or radiation-induced cystitis and bleeding are far more challenging problems. Embolization of bladder vessels or instillation of steroids has occasionally palliated such patients, but treatment is frequently unsatisfactory. Diluted formaldehyde may denature and fix superficial tissue layers. Emergency cystectomy has been undertaken to avoid exsanguination. Other treatments include hyperhydration, bladder irrigation, intravesical alum,[20] and intravesical prostaglandins.[21] Experimental approaches include amifostine,[22] hyperbaric oxygenation,[23] conjugated estrogens,[24] and glucose mannose–binding plant lectins.[25]

Radiation Nephritis

Radiation is frequently delivered to control nodal metastasis from radiation-sensitive tumors (eg, lymphomas and seminomas). The dose of radiation delivered to the kidneys can sometimes result in significant renal compromise from radiation-induced nephritis. The kidney is an important dose-limiting organ in radiation therapy. When both kidneys are radiated, the dose tolerance (TD5/5) is 20 Gy in adults, and approximately 17% of patients will develop symptomatic renal disease. When only one kidney is irradiated, the tolerance increases. Glomerular function starts to decrease at 15 Gy, and function is completely lost at 25-30 Gy. Radiosensitizers such as cisplatin, carmustine (BCNU), and actinomycin D tend to lower normal tissue radiation tolerance. Symptoms are rarely seen acutely within 6 months of treatment. Subacute symptoms, such as anemia, hypertension, edema, albuminuria, active urinary sediment, and an increase in BUN and creatinine, are seen 6-12 months after radiation. In the chronic phase (>12 months), benign or malignant hypertension is the most common finding. Eventually, the patient may develop hyperreninemic hypertension related to renal scarring, atrophy of cortical tubules, and glomerulosclerosis. Management involves decreasing the renal workload with salt and fluid restriction and a low-protein diet. Some patients may develop progressive deterioration of renal function requiring hemodialysis or renal transplantation.[26] Avoiding the debilitating complications of radiation injury to genitourinary tissue is an essential aspect to the good practice of oncology. Use of modern radiation techniques and an understanding of genitourinary tissue tolerance furnish the practicing physician with clear guidelines for the safe use of radiation therapy.

Long-term renal toxicity related to total-body irradiation in bone marrow transplantation is associated with hypertension, anemia, decreased glomerular filtration rate, hematuria, and proteinuria. These findings are caused by subendothelial widening of the glomerular basement membrane, endothelial cell dropout, glomerular arteriolar intimal thickening, and tubular atrophy. These effects are dose dependent. In a review of bone marrow transplantation patients receiving total-body irradiation with 14 Gy, it was noted that the incidence of nephropathy decreased with increased shielding of the kidneys.[27] Of the patients without shielding of the kidneys, 30% developed nephropathy. When the kidneys were partially shielded, reducing the dosage by 15%, the fraction of patients developing nephropathy decreased to 15%. When the shielding was increased and the dosage was reduced by 30%, none of the patients developed nephropathy.[27] These patients are more susceptible to radiation-induced renal injury secondary to the use of higher doses of chemotherapy, aminoglycosides, and antifungal medications, as well as infections and the development of graft-versus-host disease.

Diagnosis, Treatment, and Prevention of Nephrotoxicity of Cancer Therapeutic Agents

With the advent of effective cytotoxic chemotherapy, attention has turned to the side effects of these widely used agents (Table 129-1). These side effects include tumor lysis syndrome, paraneoplastic glomerulonephritis, obstructive uropathy, and nephrotoxicity with renal failure and electrolyte disturbances. These are more common in the geriatric population secondary to polypharmacy or drug interactions and comorbid conditions. Also, nephrotoxicity with these agents is more common in bone marrow transplantation, secondary to high-dose chemotherapy, polypharmacy, and total-body irradiation. In the following sections, we describe commonly used agents that cause serious renal toxicity. Table 129-2 lists other agents that less commonly cause renal side effects. Table 129-3 lists the mechanism of renal injury for some of the drugs. Another important aspect related to prevention of nephrotoxicity involves the interaction among drugs. Drug interactions, by decreasing liver metabolism or renal clearance, can increase the serum concentration of antineoplastic agents. This increase can cause unexpected nephrotoxicity, even though the correct doses have been prescribed. A careful review of the patient's medications is essential in the prevention of renal toxicity. Table 129-4 describes some of these drug interactions. Also important is a baseline evaluation of the patient's renal function because several drugs may need a dose adjustment in the presence of renal insufficiency (Table 129-5).

Table 129-1 Therapeutic Agents Associated With Nephrotoxicity

Alkylating agent
AZQ (diaziquone)
Carboplatin
Cisplatin
Cyclophosphamide
Ifosfamide
Nitrosoreas (streptozocin, carmustine, lomustine)
Oxaliplatin
Antitumor antibiotic
Mitomycin C
Plicamycin
Antimetabolite
5-Azacytidine
Clofarabine
Gemcitabine
High-dose methotrexate
Folate antagonist
Pemetrexed
Monoclonal antibody
Bevacizumab
Cetuximab
Biologic agent
Aldesleukin (IL-2)
Interferon
Other
Asparaginase
Cyclosporine
Gallium nitrate
Gefitinib
Imatinib
Pentostatin
Tacrolimus

Cisplatin

The introduction of cisplatin to the clinic highlighted the hazards that come about with failure to understand the renal complications of cytotoxic agents.[28] Effectively overcoming the renal toxicity that is the principal toxicity of cisplatin has allowed significant benefits to patients with many types of cancer. Development of platinum analogues has, in part, been motivated by the renal toxicity associated with cisplatin. Cisplatin, however,

Table 129-2 Clinical and Pathologic Features of Chemotherapy-Associated Nephrotoxicity

Drug	Type of Injury	Clinical Features	Urine Analysis	Time of Toxicity	Treatment/Outcome	Prevention
5-Azacytidine	Acute tubular	Renal tubular acidosis	Bland, hypoosmolar on therapy	Polyuria and rising creatinine 7-10 d postdose	Replace HCO_3, PO_4, Mg; recovery is complete	Daily creatinine, BUN, and electrolytes
Bevacizumab	Glomerulopathy	Proteinuria	Proteinuria	Increasing with cumulative dose	Discontinue if nephrotic syndrome; hold therapy if urinary protein	Monitor regularly
Carboplatin	Tubular	Mg wasting	Bland	Rising creatinine 5-10 d after therapy	Cessation of drug; dialysis as necessary; recovery usually incomplete	Avoid other nephrotoxic drugs; Mg may increase in patients previously treated with cisplatin
Cisplatin	Acute tubular	Mg wasting	Bland	Rising creatinine with cumulative dose	Cessation of drug; dialysis as necessary; recovery usually incomplete	Vigorous hydration; Cl diuresis, mannitol diuresis, Na thiosulfate; avoid aminoglycosides
Cyclosporine	Tubular and afferent arteriole vasoconstriction	Increased K and decreased Mg; renal tubular acidosis; edema; hypertension	Proteinuria	Rising creatinine from days to months after initiation of therapy	Cessation of drug; dialysis as necessary; recovery usually complete	Periodic drug level; follow-up creatinine, BUN, and electrolytes
AZQ (diaziquone)	Tubular and glomerular	Anuria, proteinuria, and renal tubular acidosis	Proteinuria	Rising creatinine 5-10 d after therapy	Cessation of drug; dialysis as necessary; recovery usually complete	Avoid doses >245 mg/m^2
Gallium nitrate	Glomerulopathy	Proteinuria and occasional azotemia	Proteinuria	Proteinuria followed by rising creatinine during and shortly after therapy days	Cessation of drug; recovery usually complete	Daily urine flow >2 L; avoid doses >300 mg/m^2/d for 7 consecutive d
Ifosfamide	Acute tubular	Oliguria	Bland	Rising creatinine within 1-2 d after therapy	Supportive dialysis; recovery usually complete	Oliguria may be increased in patients with prior cisplatin therapy; mesna
Interleukin-2	Prerenal azotemia	Oliguria and hypotension	Proteinuria and hematuria	Rising creatinine during therapy	Stop drug when creatinine ≥4.5 mg/dL or >4 mg/dL with acidosis, fluid overload or increased K; creatinine >1.5 mg/dL with oliguria; recovery usually within 1-2 weeks	Dopamine at renal doses and fluids
Methotrexate	Acute tubular	Oliguria	Bland	Rising creatinine within 1-2 d of dose	High-dose leucovorin based on methotrexate level; high-volume urine output and alkalinization; recovery is complete	Vigorous hydration and urine alkalinization; dose reduction on renal dysfunction; avoid aminoglycosides and nonsteroidal antiinflammatory; leucovorin
Plicamycin	Acute tubular	Abrupt renal failure	Mild proteinuria	Rising creatinine during dosing	Cessation of drug; re-treat, if recovery complete	Alternate-day dosing; check creatinine and BUN daily
Mitomycin C	Renal vascular lesions	Hypertension, anemia	Hematuria, proteinuria	Rising creatinine after 2 or more doses (12-40 weeks from start)	Permanent cessation of drug; SPA immunoperfusion and dialysis; poor recovery	Stop drug at cumulative dose of 60 mg
Nitrosoureas	Interstitial fibrosis, glomerular sclerosis	Late complications	Bland	Rising creatinine months to years after therapy	Supportive dialysis; recovery is complete	Stop BCNU at cumulative dose of 1200 mg/m^2
Streptozocin	Tubular	Proteinuria, occasionally severe	Proteinuria, aminoaciduria	Proteinuria followed by rising creatinine during dosing	Cessation of drug; recovery usually complete	Stop drug at first evidence of proteinuria; hydration will not prevent injury

Abbreviations: BCNU, carmustine; BUN, blood urea nitrogen; SPA, staphylococcal protein A.

Table 129-3 **Types of Renal Injury Caused by Cancer Chemotherapeutic Agents**

Pathologic Finding	Causative Agent
Acute glomerulonephritis	None reported
Acute tubular necrosis	Plicamycin Cisplatin (?)
Interstitial nephritis	Nitrosoureas
Membranous glomerulonephritis (protein losing)	Gallium nitrate (?) AZQ (diaziquone) Bevacizumab
Obstructive uropathy	Methotrexate (?)
Renal tubular acidosis	5-Azacytidine
Renal vasculitis	Mitomycin C

continues to be widely used as a major cancer drug because of its differential antitumor activity when compared with the available analogues. The study of cisplatin, the modification of its delivery, and the anticipation of and screening for nephrotoxicity provide a paradigm for the study of nephrotoxic agents in general.

The principal excretion route of cisplatin is renal. Nevertheless, only a small portion of the total cisplatin dose can be recovered in the urine in the first few days after therapy.[29] Much of the drug is irreversibly bound to protein, but active metabolites, the aquated diamino derivative, as well as the parent, are found in the ultrafiltrable plasma fraction. This plasma clearance is triphasic, with nearly all of the drug gone in 4 h, but with a terminal half-life of over 24 h. The primary lesion of cisplatin toxicity is necrosis of the proximal convoluted tubules. The severity of the nephrotoxicity can be modified by hydration. The strong emetic effects of cisplatin can, however, produce dehydration. These dual side effects—severe nausea and vomiting and primary nephrotoxicity exaggerated by dehydration—have been largely overcome with hydration schedules and the aggressive use of new antiemetics.[30,31]

A reduction in the glomerular filtration rate (GFR) is the primary cisplatin-induced injury that is measured clinically. Other complications include hypomagnesemia and modest amounts of proteinuria. The proteinuria associated with cisplatin nephrotoxicity is attributed to a tubular defect.[32] Hemolytic-uremic syndrome (HUS) has also been described, especially when cisplatin is combined with bleomycin.[33] Sequential measurement of the GFR is essential for monitoring of cisplatin toxicity. An accurate urine collection for inulin clearance is superior to 24-h urine collection for creatinine clearance, but we have used the serum creatinine concentration and calculation of the creatinine clearance. Assay of electrolytes, including calcium, magnesium, and phosphorus, has also been routinely made. For patients treated at The University of Texas M. D. Anderson Cancer Center (UTMDACC) in the Department of Genitourinary Medical Oncology, electrolytes, BUN, and creatinine are monitored prior to each dose of therapy. There is a minimum interval of 7 days between cisplatin doses. This interval is important because maximal nephrotoxicity frequently does not manifest itself in less than 7 days. A significant decline in the creatinine clearance, as measured by the Cockcroft formula, should result in a delay of therapy (Table 129-6).

Prevention of toxicity is important in patient care. Empiric observations, in both the laboratory and the clinic, demonstrate that hydration with the use of mannitol or hypertonic saline has significantly reduced the cisplatin-induced decline in renal function.[30,31] Although hypertonic saline is not commonly used, normal saline is important to provide abundant chloride ions. This diminishes the formation of the aquated species by mass action, thereby lessening the impact on renal function. Minimum urine flow should be sustained at 100 mL/h before cisplatin administration. Multiple clinical trials have demonstrated the effectiveness of using mannitol in different schedules. Conflicting reports exist regarding the use of furosemide (Lasix) and its ability to affect cisplatin's nephrotoxicity. Its use has generally been avoided at the UTMDACC.[34,35] More recently, amifostine (phosphorylated aminothiol prodrug) has been used in the prevention of nephrotoxicity by cisplatin. Amifostine is metabolized to WR-1065 and WR-33278, which reduce formation of deoxyribonucleic acid (DNA)–DNA crosslinks,[36] reverse platinum-DNA adducts,[37] and bind to oxygen free radicals. Several studies show that amifostine decreases the number of patients with a greater than 40% reduction in creatinine clearance or with a decrease in glomerular filtration secondary to cisplatin nephrotoxicity, from 30% to 40% to approximately 10%.[38-40] It has been noted that amifostine does not affect the response to chemotherapy. Certain chemotherapeutic agents and other nephrotoxic drugs can impact significantly on nephrotoxicity. Cisplatin is used frequently in combination with other agents, such as ifosfamide and methotrexate (MTX). The side effects seem to be greatly diminished by adequate hydration. Paclitaxel in combination with cisplatin has been associated with elevation of serum creatinine in the treatment of gynecologic cancers.[41] Concurrent aminoglycoside antibiotics have been reported to result in a significantly greater reduction in renal function.[42] Meticulous attention to detail, adequate hydration, and avoidance of these interactions are important.

Table 129-4 **Drug Interactions That Can Increase Serum Levels of Antineoplastic Agents or Add Renal Toxicity**

Capecitabine	Leucovorin
Carboplatin	Cyclophosphamide, aminoglycosides, topotecan
Cisplatin	Any nephrotoxic agent,[a] melphalan, paclitaxel,[b] rituximab, topotecan[b]
Cladribine	Cyclophosphamide (high dose)
Cyclophosphamide	Allopurinol
Cyclosporine	Any nephrotoxic agent,[a] vancomycin, melphalan, cimetidine, potassium-sparing diuretics, naproxen, sulindac, diclofenac, allopurinol, cytochrome P-450 inhibitors,[c] methotrexate
Etoposide	Aprepitant, cyclosporine, valspodar
Gefitinib	Cytochrome P-450 3A4 inhibitors
Gemcitabine	5-Fluorouracil
Ifosfamide	Cytochrome P-450 inhibitors,[c] aprepitant
Interleukin-2	Any nephrotoxic agent[a]
Melphalan	Buthionine
Methotrexate	Organic acids, penicillins, cisplatin, NSAIDs, amiodarone, aspirin, ciprofloxacin, cotrimoxazole, cyclosporine, doxycycline, mercaptopurine, probenecid, procarbazine
Mercaptopurine	Allopurinol, methotrexate, TPMT inhibitors
Mitomycin	5-Fluorouracil–related hemolytic-uremic syndrome
Streptozocin	Any nephrotoxic agent[a]
Tacrolimus	Any nephrotoxic agent,[a] cyclosporine, cisplatin, drugs metabolized through cytochrome P-450 3A
Thioguanine	TPMT inhibitors
Topotecan	Cisplatin,[b] carboplatin[b]
Trimetrexate	Cimetidine, cytochrome P-450 inhibitors[c]

Abbreviations: NSAIDs, nonsteroidal antiinflammatory drugs; TPMT, thiopurine methyltransferase.
[a]For example, aminoglycosides, amphotericin B, intravenous contrast, NSAIDs.
[b]Related to sequence of administration.
[c]Azoles antifungals, macrolides, calcium channel blockers, corticosteroids, grapefruit juice.

Methotrexate

Methotrexate (MTX), an agent dependent on renal glomerular filtration as its principal excretory route, can also induce renal toxicity.[43,44] Renal toxicity can be particularly devastating because prolonged exposure to MTX at elevated levels substantially increases toxicity in the bone marrow and the oral cavity of the alimen-

Table 129-5 ■ **Adjustment of Antineoplastic Agents Based on Renal Insufficiency**

Azacytidine	Unexplained increase in creatinine or blood urea nitrogen; delay treatment until back to baseline, then reduce dose by 50%
Blemomycin	Creatinine clearance 10-50 mL/min: reduce dose by 25% Creatinine clearance <10 mL/min: reduce dose by 50%
Capecitabine	Creatinine clearance 30-50 mL/min: reduce dose by 25% Creatinine clearance <30 mL/min: not recommended
Carboplatin	Adjust according to Calvert formula: Total dose (mg) = (target AUC) × (GFR + 25)
Carmustine	Creatinine clearance <60 mL/min: omit dose
Cisplatin	Creatinine clearance 10-50 mL/min: decrease dose by 25% Creatinine clearance <10 mL/min: decrease dose by 50%
Clofarabine	Use with extreme caution
Cyclophosphamide	Creatinine clearance 10-50 mL/min: reduce dose by 25% Creatinine clearance <10 mL/min: reduce dose by 50%
Cytarabine	Creatinine clearance <60 mL/min, use caution; may decrease dose or change schedule
Daunorubicin	Creatinine >3 mg/dL: decrease dose by 50%
Etoposide	Creatinine clearance 15-50 mL/min: decrease dose by 25% Creatinine clearance <15 mL/min: consider 50% dose reduction
Fludarabine	Creatinine clearance 30-70 mL/min: decrease dose by 20-50% Creatinine clearance <30 mL/min: not recommended
Gefitinib	Use caution with severe renal impairment
Gemcitabine	Use caution with severe renal impairment
Hydroxyurea	Creatinine clearance <10 mL/min: reduce dose by 80%
Ifosfamide	Creatinine clearance 46-60 mL/min: reduce dose by 20% Creatinine clearance 31-45 mL/min: reduce dose by 25% Creatinine clearance ≤30 mL/min: reduce dose by 30%
Lomustine	Creatinine clearance <60 mL/min: omit dose
Melphalan	Dose reduction may be necessary; IV: BUN >30 mg/dL or creatinine >1.5 mg/dL: consider 50% dose reduction
Mercaptopurine	Decrease dose or increase interval
Methotrexate	Creatinine clearance 10-50 mL/min: reduce dose by 50% Creatinine clearance <10-30 mL/min: avoid use
Mitomycin C	Creatinine clearance <10-60 mL/min: reduce dose by 25% Creatinine clearance <10 mL/min: reduce dose by 50%
Oxaliplatin	Use with caution in mild to severe renal impairment
Pemetrexed	Hold therapy if creatinine clearance <45 mL/min: patient with grade 3/4; nonhematologic toxicity should decrease dose by 25%
Pentostatin	Creatinine clearance <30-6 0 mL/min: dose reduction may be necessary
Plicamycin	Creatinine clearance 10-50 mL/min: reduce by 25% Creatinine clearance <10 mL/min: reduce dose by 50-70%
Procarbazine	Creatinine clearance <30 mL/min: omit dose
Ralitrexed	Creatinine clearance <25-30 mL/min: reduce dose by 50% Creatinine clearance <25 mL/min: omit dose
Streptozocin	Use with caution
Teniposide	Dose reduction may be necessary
Thiotepa	Dose reduction may be necessary
Topotecan	Creatinine clearance 20-39 mL/min: decrease dose to 0.75 mg/m^2 Creatinine clearance <20 mL/min: insufficient evidence
Tretinoin	Maximum dose of 25 mg/m^2
Trimetrexate	Hold therapy if creatinine >2.5 mg dL; dose adjustment may be necessary

Abbreviations: AUC, area under the curve; BUN, blood urea nitrogen; GFR, glomerular filtration rate; IV, intravenous.

Table 129-6 ■ **Cockcroft Formula**

$$\frac{(14 - \text{Age})\ \text{Weight}\ (\text{kg})}{72 \times \text{Serum creatinine}}$$

tary canal. The renal toxicity of MTX is a dose-dependent phenomenon. Renal failure has often been implicated in deaths associated with the use of this agent.

The nephrotoxicity of MTX is manifested primarily in the renal tubule, where extensive necrosis of the convoluted tubules occurs. The lesion has been termed crystalline hydronephrosis and has been attributed to deposition of the agent. The precipitation of MTX and its less soluble principal metabolite, 7-hydroxy-MTX, in the renal tubule, results in changes in preglomerular vascular pressure and a direct decrease in glomerular filtration.

Avoidance of MTX nephrotoxicity can be accomplished by selecting patients with normal renal function, ensuring adequate hydration, and alkalinizing the urine to pH 7 or higher. Prior to administration of MTX at doses of 100 mg/m^2 or greater, adequate renal function should be ensured by normal serum creatinine and minimum urinary flow of 100 mL/h. Urine should have a pH of 7 or higher, and leucovorin can be administered after MTX. MTX is highly protein bound and is not readily removed by dialysis.[33] Specific attention to interaction with other agents is important when administering MTX. Weak organic acids, such as salicylates or sulfisoxazole, increase MTX levels by displacing the drug from binding sites on plasma proteins. In addition, renal tubular transport is diminished by probenecid and salicylates. Specific avoidance of these agents reduces the risk of inducing nephrotoxicity or increasing other side effects.

Nitrosoureas

Each of the nitrosoureas (lomustine [CCNU], methyl-CCNU, BCNU) was predicted to have significant nephrotoxicity.[45,46] Initial small phase 1 and phase 2 trials failed to reveal evidence of renal compromise, but with their use in large phase 3 trials, drug-induced nephrotoxicity was encountered.[47-49] Unlike the nephrotoxicity associated with MTX and cisplatin, nitrosoureas cause interstitial nephritis. The specific mechanism by which this occurs is unclear. At present, limiting the total cumulative dose of the agents is the only way of preventing this; hydration does not appear to alter it. Monitoring such patients with serial urinalysis and serum creatinine concentrations appears to be the most reliable way to screen for nephrotoxicity.

Mitomycin C

Mitomycin C is an antibiotic isolated from *Streptomyces caespitosus.* Although this agent has significant activity against a variety of tumors, it has received rather limited use because of prolonged thrombocytopenia and unpredictable side effects, which are dose-limiting.

The unique clinical nephrotoxicity of mitomycin C is a striking HUS. This is sometimes manifested by early elevation of serum creatinine or anemia, with a rise in serum lactate acid dehydrogenase, indicating hemolysis. Patients receiving mitomycin C should be carefully monitored for HUS. Total cumulative doses of less than 30 mg/m^2 of body surface area are rarely, if ever, associated with HUS. The most difficult problem in managing the HUS of patients treated with mitomycin C is that it is sometimes difficult to anticipate because the onset can be delayed after the time of delivery of the agent.

Mitomycin C–induced nephrotoxicity can be prevented by limiting the cumulative dose to less than 30 mg/m^2 of body surface area. The use of steroids, which is believed to reduce the pulmonary toxicity of this agent, has not clearly demonstrated a role in reducing nephrotoxicity. Plasmapheresis appears to provide therapeutic benefit in selected patients, although only limited studies have been performed.[50,51]

Immunologic Agents

Interleukin-2 causes renal insufficiency by a direct toxic effect on the kidneys and by prerenal azotemia from capillary leak syndrome. This renal toxicity is commonly reversible after discontinuation of the drug, intravenous saline, albumin, pressors, and renal dose dopamine.[33]

Cyclosporine produces renal vasoconstriction primarily at the afferent arteriole, causing arterial hypertension, fluid retention, and, ultimately, renal dysfunction.[52] Acute nephrotoxicity is reversible with dose modification. In contrast, chronic administration may cause a slowly irreversible renal failure secondary to renal tubular fibrosis and afferent arteriopathy with proteinaceous material.[53]

Tacrolimus causes renal injury in a fashion similar to that of cyclosporine. In contrast to cyclosporine, however, it is less likely to cause arterial hypertension. Tacrolimus stimulates transforming growth factor $\alpha 1$ expression and inhibits matrix protein degradation.[54]

Other Agents

On the basis of preclinical studies, the anthracyclines daunorubicin and doxorubicin were predicted to cause renal toxicity.[55-57] Anthracycline-induced nephrotoxicity has not, however, been convincingly reported in clinical trials. Ifosfamide can cause proximal tubular dysfunction, distal renal tubular acidosis, nephrogenic diabetes insipidus, and the syndrome of inappropriate antidiuretic hormone release. Multiple new agents are associated with kidney toxicity, but data are limited. Fludarabine has been reported to cause urologic complications related to urinary tract infections in 12-22% of patients.[10,58,59] Abnormal renal function is observed in less than 5% of patients treated with fludarabine[10,59-61] and is related to tumor lysis syndrome. Paclitaxel has been associated with elevation of serum creatinine in about 18% of human immunodeficiency virus (HIV) patients treated for Kaposi sarcoma.[10,62,63] Gemcitabine is linked to sporadic renal failure associated with thrombotic microangiopathy.[64] The increase in the number of new agents, including monoclonal antibodies and small molecule inhibitors of tyrosine kinase inhibitors, requires special considerations.

Several monoclonal antibodies have been approved for clinical trials. Bevacizumab is noteworthy for its nephrotoxic profile with proteinuria observed in a significant fraction of patients, although renal failure has been uncommon to date.

Monitoring for Drug-Induced Nephrotoxicity

The principle that should guide clinicians in the use of potentially nephrotoxic agents in the treatment of cancer is close monitoring for the development of renal toxicity, its early detection, and its management. The wide range of renal insults induced by cytotoxic drugs complicates the selection of the appropriate study to monitor potential nephrotoxicity.[65] Clinicians apply similar screening studies to detect a wide range of renal insults from cytotoxic agents. The use of specific studies that focus on the nature of the cytotoxic injury induced by the specific agent is more likely to detect early injury. For example, tubular defects resulting from cisplatin nephrotoxicity are not directly correlated with reduction in the GFR, whereas hypermagnesiuria and hypomagnesemia are characteristic. Monitoring patients for nephrotoxicity for agents that can cause interstitial nephritis (nitrosoureas) or glomerular injury (mitomycin C) requires routine and frequent urinalyses. The appearance of microhematuria should lead physicians to further exclude drug-induced renal injury.

The most common renal functional abnormality as a result of cytotoxic therapy is a decline in GFR. The most frequently used measure of GFR is creatinine clearance. Creatinine clearance is less accurate than other measures of GFR but, for practical reasons, has been widely applied clinically.[66] A serial decline in creatinine clearance is a reliable index of worsening renal function. Significant limitations are encountered in estimating a creatinine clearance from serum creatinine alone, using predictive formulas (Cockcroft; Table 129-6). Use of such formulae has, however, been widely applied in clinical oncology, in view of the difficulties in collecting reliable 24-h urine specimens. The 24-h collection for creatinine clearance has been supplanted by the use of the Cockcroft formula at UTMDACC in the Department of Genitourinary Medical Oncology. No increase in the frequency of renal compromise associated with cisplatin administration has been noted since this procedure was adopted. A practical approach has been to follow only the serum creatinine concentrations. In the absence of any change in the serum creatinine concentration or calculated clearance (Cockcroft), no further study is required. In patients whose serum creatine concentration increases more than 0.4 mg/dL, further investigation of renal function is undertaken. An adjustment in dose or a change in therapy may then be ordered as required. Particular attention should be paid to the correct calculation of the renal function by adjusting for weight. The creatinine clearance calculated by the Cockcroft formula is sufficient in patients of average body habitus but may result in erroneous predictions in patients who are emaciated or in those with a large muscle mass. The wide fluctuations in weight that occur in patients undergoing cancer therapy require that the patients be weighed before each dose of chemotherapy and that doses be adjusted for changes in weight.

Selected References

The complete reference list can be found at www.CANCERMEDICINE8.com

1. Logothetis CJ, Samuels ML, Ogden SL, et al. Cyclophosphamide and sequential cisplatin for advanced seminoma: long-term follow-up in 52 patients. *J Urol.* 1987;138:789–794.
2. Logothetis CJ, Samuels ML, Selig DE, et al. Cyclic chemotherapy with cyclophosphamide, doxorubicin, and cisplatin plus vinblastine and bleomycin in advanced germinal tumors: results with 100 patients. *Am J Med.* 1986;81:219–228.
4. Stables DP. Percutaneous nephrostomy: techniques, indications and results. *Urol Clin North Am.* 1982;9:15–29.
6. Gillenwater JY. The pathophysiology of urinary obstructions. In: Harrison JH, editor. *Campbell's Urology.* 4th ed. Philadelphia: WB Saunders; 1979:377.
7. Gutmann FD, Boxer RJ. Pathophysiology and management of urinary tract obstruction. In: Rieselbach RE, Garnick MB, editors. *Cancer and the Kidney.* Philadelphia: Lea & Febiger; 1982:594–624.
9. Brade WP, Herdrich K, Varani, M. Ifosfamide—pharmacology, safety and therapeutic potential. *Cancer Treat Rep.* 1985;12: 1–47.
11. Drake MJ, Nixon PM, Crew J. Drug-induced bladder and urinary disorders. Incidence, prevention and management. *Drug Saf.* 1998;19:45–55.
12. Brugieres L, Hartmann O, Travagli JP, et al. Hemorrhagic cystitis following high-dose chemotherapy and bone marrow transplantation in children with malignancies: incidence, clinical course and outcome. *J Clin Oncol.* 1989;7:194–199.
13. Klingemann JD, Sheperd DE, Reece MJ, et al. Regimen-related acute toxicities: pathophysiology, risk factors, clinical evaluation and preventive strategies. *Bone Marrow Transplant.* 1994;14(Suppl 4):514–518.
14. Ringden Q, Remberger M, Ruutu T, et al. Increased risk of chronic graft-versus-host disease, obstructive bronchiolitis and alopecia with busulfan versus total-body irradiation. *Blood.* 1999;93:2196–2201.
16. Bedi A, Miller CB, Hanson JL, et al. Association of BK virus with failure of prophylaxis against hemorrhagic cystitis following bone marrow transplantation. *J Clin Oncol.* 1995;13:1103–1109.
17. Burman C, Kutcher GJ, Goitein M. Fitting of normal tissue tolerance data to an analytic function. *Int J Radiat Oncol Biol Phys.* 1991;21:123–135.
20. Kohno A, Takeyama K, Narabajashi M,

et al. Hemorrhagic cystitis associated with allogeneic and autologous bone marrow transplantation for malignant neoplasm in adults. *Jpn J Clin Oncol*. 1993;23:46–52.

21. Miller LJ, Chandler SW, Ippolit CM. Treatment of cyclophosphamide-induced hemorrhagic cystitis with prostaglandins. *Ann Pharmacother*. 1994;28:590–594.
22. Srivastava A, Nair SC, Srivastava VM, et al. Evaluation of uroprotective efficacy of amifostine against cyclophosphamide induced hemorrhagic cystitis. *Bone Marrow Transplant*. 1999;23:463–467.
23. Yazawa H, Nakada T, Sasawaga I, et al. Hyperbaric oxygenation therapy for cyclophosphamide induced hemorrhagic cystitis. *Int Urol Nephrol*. 1995;27:381–385.
24. Liu YK, Harty JI, Steinbok GS, et al. Treatment of radiation or cyclophosphamide induced cystitis using conjugated estrogens. *J Urol*. 1990;144:41–43.
25. Assreuy AM, Martins GJ, Moreira ME. Prevention of cyclophosphamide-induced hemorrhagic cystitis by glucosemannose binding plant lectins. *J Urol*. 1999;161:1988–1993.
27. Lawton CA, Cohen EP, Murray KJ, et al. Long-term results of selective renal shielding in patients undergoing total-body irradiation in preparation for bone marrow transplantation. *Bone Marrow Transplant*. 1997;20:1069–1074.
28. Walker EM, Gale GR. Methods of reduction of cisplatin nephrotoxicity. *Ann Clin Lab Sci*. 1981;11:397–410.
29. Speer RJ, Ridgway H, Hall LM. Coordination complexes of platinum as antitumor agents. *Cancer Chemother Rep*. 1979;59:629–641.
30. Ozols RF, Cordon BJ, Jacobs J, et al. High-dose cisplatin in hypertonic saline. *Ann Intern Med*. 1984;100:19–24.
31. Gonzales-Vitale JC, Hayes DM, Cvitkovic E, Sternberg SS. The renal pathology in clinical trial of cisplatinum (II) diamminodichloride. *Cancer*. 1977;39:1362–1371.
32. Buamah PK, Howell A, Whitby H, et al. Assessment of renal function during high-dose cisplatin therapy in patients with ovarian carcinoma. *Cancer Chemother Pharmacol*. 1982;8:281–284.
34. Pera MF, Harder HC. Effects of furosemide (FM)- and mannitol (MN)- induced diuresis on the nephrotoxicity and physiologic disposition of *cis*-dichlorodiamminoplatinum (CDDP) in rats. *Proc Am Assoc Cancer Res*. 1978;19:100.
35. Pera MF, Zook BC, Harder HC. Effects of mannitol or furosemide diuresis on the nephrotoxicity and physiological disposition of *cis*-diammineplatinum (II) in rats. *Cancer Res*. 1979;29:1269–1278.
36. De Neve WJ, Everett CK, Suminski JE, et al. Influence of WR-2721 on DNA's cross-linking by nitrogen mustard in normal mouse bone marrow and leukemia cells in vivo. *Cancer Res*. 1988;48:6002–6005.
37. Treskes M, Nijtmans LG, Fichtinger-Schepman AM, et al. Effects of the modulating agent WR2721 and its main metabolites on the formation and stability of cisplatin-DNA adducts in vitro in comparison to the effects of thiosulphate and diethyldithiocarbamate. *Biochem Pharmacol*. 1992;43:1013–1019.
38. Kemp G, Rose P, Lurain J, et al. Amifostine pretreatment for protection against cyclophosphamide-induced and cisplatin-induced toxicities: results of a randomized control trial in patients with advanced ovarian cancer. *J Clin Oncol*. 1996;14:2101–2112.
39. Alberts DS, Green S, Hannigan EV, et al. Improved therapeutic index of carboplatin plus cyclophosphamide versus cisplatin plus cyclophosphamide: final report by the Southwest Oncology Group of a phase III randomized trial in stage IV ovarian cancer. *J Clin Oncol*. 1992;10:706–717.
40. Schiller JH, Berry W, Storer B, et al. Phase II trial of amifostine, cisplatin and vinblastine for metastatic non-small cell lung cancer. *Proc Am Soc Clin Oncol*. 1995;14:356.
41. Merouani A, Davidson SA, Schrier RW. Increased nephrotoxicity of combination Taxol and cisplatin chemotherapy in gynecologic cancers as compared to cisplatin alone. *Am J Nephrol*. 1997;17:53–58.
42. Gonzales-Vitale JC, Hayes DM, Cvitkovic E, Sternberg SS. Acute renal failure after cis-dichlorodiammineplatinum (II) and gentamicin-cephalothin therapies. *Cancer Treat Rep*. 1978;62:693–698.
43. Evans BD, Rajn KS, Calvert AH, et al. Phase II study of JM8, a new platinum analog, in advanced ovarian carcinoma. *Cancer Treat Rep*. 1983;67:997–1000.
45. Denine EP, Harrison SD, Pechkam JC. Qualitative and quantitative toxicity of sublethal doses of methyl-CCNU in BDF1 mice. *Cancer Treat Rep*. 1977;61:409–417.
46. Carter SK, Broder L, Friedman M. Streptozotocin and metastatic insulinoma. *Ann Intern Med*. 1971;74:445–446.
47. Harmon WE, Cohen HJ, Schneeberger EE, Grupe WE. Chronic renal failure in children treated with methyl CCNU. *N Engl J Med*. 1979;300:1200–1203.
49. Ellis ME, Weiss RB, Kupermine M. Nephrotoxicity of lomustine. *Cancer Chemother Pharmacol*. 1985;15:174–175.
50. Cantrell JE, Philips TM, Schein PS. Carcinoma-associated hemolytic-uremic syndrome: a complication of mitomycin C chemotherapy. *J Clin Oncol*. 1985;3:723–734.
52. Elzinga L, Kelley VE, Houghton DC, Bennett WM. Fish oil vehicle for cyclosporine lowers renal thromboxanes and reduces experimental nephrotoxicity. *Transplant Proc*. 1987;19:1403–1406.
53. Bennet WM, de Mattos A, Meyer MM, et al. Chronic cyclosporine nephropathy: the Achilles' heel of immunosuppressive therapy. *Kidney Int*. 1996;50:1089–1100.
54. Bennet WM. The nephrotoxicity of new and old immunosuppressive drugs. *Ren Fail*. 1998;20:687–690.
55. Sternberg SS. Cross-striated fibrils and other ultra-structural alterations in glomeruli of rats with daunomycin nephrosis. *Lab Invest*. 1970;23:39–51.
56. Buss H, Lamberts B. The kidney glomerulus of the rat during experimental daunomycin nephrosis. A comparative transmission-scanning electron microscopic study. *Beitr Pathol*. 1973;148:360–387.
57. Serpick AA, Henderson ES. Observations on toxicity and clinical trials with daunomycin. *Pathol Biol*. 1967;15:909–912.
58. Keating MJ, Kantarjian H, Talpaz M, et al. Fludarabine: a new agent with major activity against chronic lymphocytic leukemia. *Blood*. 1989;74:19–25.
59. Puccio CA, Mittleman A, Lichtman SM, et al. A loading dose/continuous infusion schedule of fludarabine phosphate in chronic lymphocytic leukemia. *J Clin Oncol*. 1991;9:1562–1569.
60. Chun HG, Leylan-Jones B, Cheson BD. Fludarabine phosphate: a synthetic purine metabolite with significant activity against lymphoid malignancies. *J Clin Oncol*. 1991;9:175–188.
61. List AF, Kummett TD, Adams JD, et al. Tumor lysis syndrome complicating chronic lymphocytic leukemia with fludarabine phosphate. *Am J Med*. 1990;89:383–390.
62. Welles L, Saville MW, Lietzau J, et al. Phase II trial with dose titration of paclitaxel for the therapy of human immunodeficiency virus-associated Kaposi's sarcoma. *J Clin Oncol*. 1998;16:1112–1121.
64. Flombaum CD, Mouradian JA, Casper ES, et al. Thrombotic microangiopathy as a complication of long-term therapy with gemcitabine. *Am J Kidney Dis*. 1999;33:552–562.
65. Daugaard G, Abildgaard U. Evaluation of nephrotoxicity secondary to cytostatic agents. *Clin Rev Oncol Hematol*. 1992;13:215–240.
66. Kassirer JP, Harrington JT. Laboratory evaluation of renal function. In: Schrier RW, Gottschalk CW, editors. *Diseases of the Kidney*. Vol 1. Boston: Little, Brown; 1988:393–441.

130 Cardiac Complications

Michael S. Ewer, MD, MPH, JD ▪ Steven M. Ewer, MD ▪ Thomas Suter, MD

Patients with malignant neoplastic diseases often have coexisting cardiovascular disorders or may face serious cardiovascular complications of their disease.[1] The disorders may result from underlying conditions such as atherosclerosis, hypertension, or valvular abnormalities, or they may result directly from cancer or its treatment (Table 130-1). In addition, cardiovascular disorders that are unusual in patients not afflicted with cancer may be more common in the cancer patient and are sometimes unsuspected. At the same time, cardiovascular diseases common in the general population must not be overlooked in patients with cancer; the presentation of such entities may be altered, and thus the diagnosis more complex. Increased clinical scrutiny is therefore necessary in this population. Several clinical problems may also coexist and defy a simple explanation because of the complex interactions between the malignancy and the cardiovascular system; what affects the first often alters the second. This chapter will look at some of the more common cardiovascular complications of cancer and its treatment, and will also address some of the clinical dilemmas encountered in patients with cancer.

Table 130-1 ▪ Important Cardiovascular Complications of Cancer

Primary cardiac neoplasia
Malignancy
Cardiac tumors
Pericardial tumors
Metastatic cancer
Pericardial metastasis
Pericardial effusion
Pericardial tamponade
Myocardial metastasis
Cardiomyopathy
Arrhythmias
Tachyarrhythmias
Conduction system disease
Complication of cancer treatment
Coronary vasospasm
Myocardial infarction
Arrhythmias
Supraventricular
Ventricular
QT prolongation
Cardiomyopathy
Type I dysfunction (irreversible)
Chronic heart failure
Sudden cardiac death
Type II dysfunction (reversible)
Disorders of diastolic filling
Hypertension
Effects of radiation
Miscellaneous entities
Cardiac amyloidosis
Carcinoid heart disease
Thromboembolic phenomena

Evaluation of the Cardiovascular System in the Cancer Patient

The evaluation of the cardiovascular system in patients with cancer begins with a detailed history and a complete physical examination. Signs or symptoms suggestive of heart failure, dysrhythmia, ischemia, or pericardial disease—all of which are common syndromes in the cancer patient—trigger a more rigorous cardiovascular assessment. The individual approach should be targeted to include the specific clinical entities that are enumerated in Table 130-1. Based on these considerations, the history should include information regarding any signs or symptoms suggestive of pericardial diseases, coronary artery syndromes, heart failure, or arrhythmias; the physical examination should include careful assessment of blood pressure, peripheral edema, neck vein distention, cardiac and pulmonary auscultation and an estimation of the perfusion status. If clinical assessment of the patient indicates possible cardiac disease, diagnostic assessment of the heart is essential; the electrocardiogram and the chest x-ray now have been joined by cardiac ultrasound and more focused imaging modalities as crucial adjuncts in the evaluation of these patients. While a minority of patients will require invasive evaluation with coronary angiography, electrophysiology studies, or other studies for specific indications, the cornerstone of cardiovascular assessment in cancer patients includes some form of noninvasive cardiac imaging.

The cardiac ultrasound or echocardiogram has enjoyed the widest usage in evaluating cancer patients. It plays an important role in evaluating cardiac contractile dysfunction and assessing the integrity of cardiac structures.[2] A complete echocardiographic evaluation involves several complementary techniques, each of which provides information about a cardiac abnormality from a different vantage point. Transthoracic 2-D echocardiography provides information regarding large regions of the heart, and in some views, all four cardiac chambers can be seen and wall-motion abnormalities reflecting regional or global dysfunction can be assessed. Localized or loculated pericardial effusions as well as primary and metastatic tumors can be appreciated using 2-D echocardiography although other imaging modalities may also supplement and reinforce information initially obtained from the cardiac ultrasound.[3] In situations where ultrasound imaging is suboptimal, echo contrast agents may be employed to augment the echocardiographic interface. Such agents are increasingly being used and are generally regarded as safe.[4]

Spectral and color flow Doppler studies, which are usually performed as part of an echocardiographic evaluation, show the direction and velocity of blood flow in the cardiac chambers and across the valves. This information is graphically depicted and is often superimposed on the 2-D echocardiogram. Valvular lesions, intracardiac shunts, turbulent blood movement, and abnormal direction of blood flow are best evaluated using the Doppler study. Doppler studies provide important information regarding diastolic cardiac function, an area of cardiac imaging that is becoming increasingly important.

Transesophageal echocardiography provides a higher resolution view of certain cardiac structures than does the conventional transthoracic study. Although the technique is semi-invasive (the transducer has dimensions similar to those of a gastrointestinal endoscope and is passed into the midesophagus in a similar manner), the increased diagnostic sensitivity of the transesophageal studies often offsets this disadvantage. Transesophageal studies are especially useful in identifying vegetations and other valvular lesions or myocardial involvement of cancer, which may be extremely difficult to assess on transthoracic studies (Fig. 130-1). The transesophageal study, in part because of the position of the probe, is an important adjunct for the evaluation of posterior accumulations of fluid, as may be seen postoperatively; they are also of great value in defining and monitoring intracardiac masses and thrombi (Fig. 130-2). Additionally, intraoperative transesophageal echocardiography is helpful in documenting the extent of an inferior vena caval tumor as well as the result of resection of such tumors. 3-D echocardiography allows the 2-D image

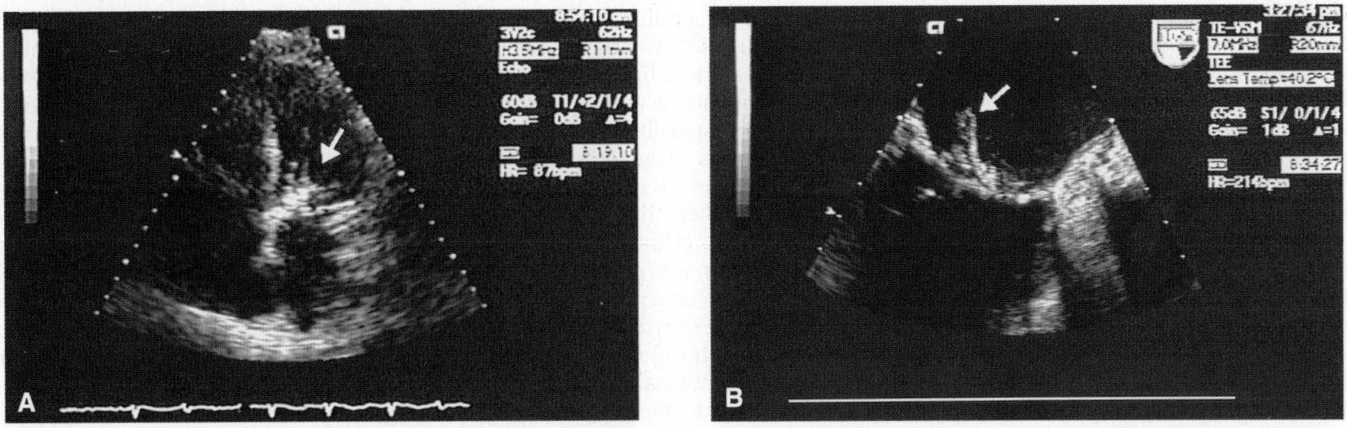

Figure 130-1 ■ Echocardiogram frames of a patient with infective endocarditis involving the mitral valve. (**A**) Nonspecific findings often seen on transthoracic studies, although suggestive of thickening of the leaflets, are not diagnostic for the valve infection. (**B**) Transesophageal image from the same patient recorded the same day, clearly showing the infected mitral valve leaflet.

to be rotated around a selected axis. The technique provides images of excellent resolution and aids with spatial orientation of cardiac structures. These techniques have now entered the mainstream of cardiac imaging and may provide vital information that was heretofore absent or suboptimal.[6]

Nuclear imaging techniques provide important information concerning both cardiac function and evaluation of the presence and degree of ischemic heart disease. The multigated (MUGA) cardiac blood-pool scan remains a common assessment tool for following left ventricular ejection fraction in patients being treated with agents known or suspected of being cardiotoxic. Nuclear imaging techniques may have a lower intra- and interobserver variability than do echocardiographic assessments. The technique, however, requires electrocardiographic gating that can be problematic in patients with dysrhythmia; additionally, MUGA scans acquire data over a period of several minutes, and therefore depend on patients being able to remain immobile during acquisition. Once the imaging data are acquired and stored in computer memory banks, these data can then be manipulated using one of several computer algorithms to provide an estimation of ejection fraction, information regarding wall-motion abnormalities, and parameters of cardiac relaxation (diastolic function). MUGA scans involve radiation exposure, and are more costly than are cardiac ultrasound examinations. While MUGA scans have previously been used to assess cardiac function in many large oncologic clinical trials, the improvement in cardiac ultrasound imaging, cost considerations, and the concerns regarding radiation exposure are providing an impetus toward the wider use of ultrasound in following patients enrolled in clinical trials using potentially cardiotoxic agents. Regardless of the method used, it must be emphasized that the results of any estimation of cardiac function are affected and modulated by many noncardiac factors, and that any alteration in cardiac function appreciated on such studies for a specific patient must be interpreted with some caution.[7] Furthermore, it should be noted that small changes in the left ventricular function (LVEF changes of 10 percentage points or less) frequently reflect conditions not associated with cancer or cancer treatment but rather physiological variation of the cardiac function or conditions unrelated to the cancer or its treatment (ie, metabolic state, degree of anemia, hormonal factors, viral infections and other conditions).

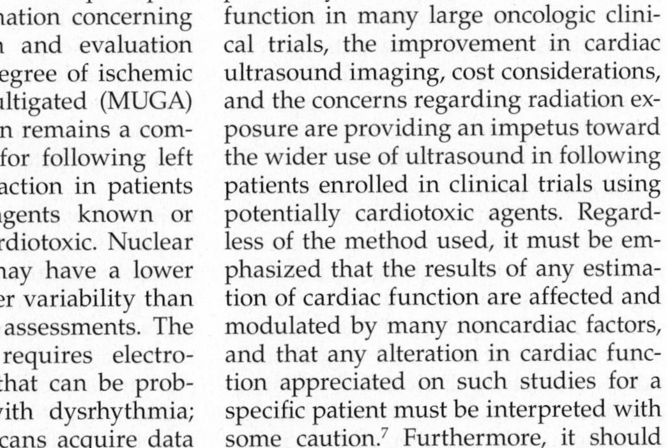

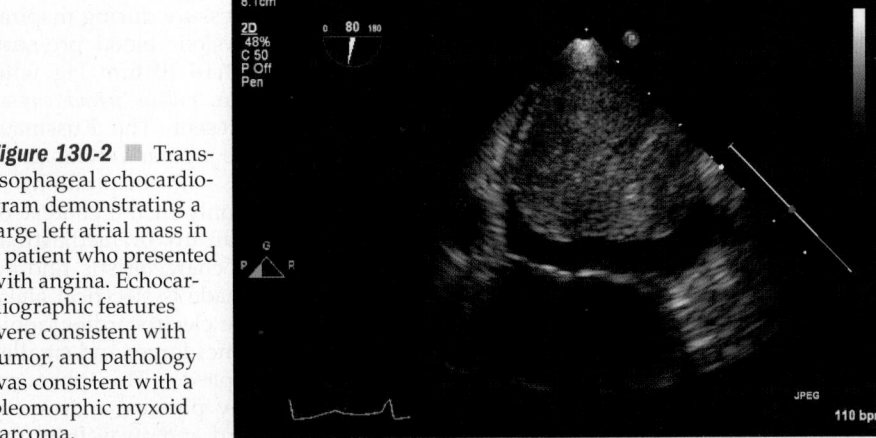

Figure 130-2 ■ Transesophageal echocardiogram demonstrating a large left atrial mass in a patient who presented with angina. Echocardiographic features were consistent with tumor, and pathology was consistent with a pleomorphic myxoid sarcoma.

Magnetic resonance imaging (MRI) can define pathologic lesions in and around the great vessels, and can delineate intracardiac and pericardial masses. The technique is also useful in identifying constrictive pericarditis.[8] The cost of MRI is decreasing but are still considerable, and problems related to long imaging times are gradually being resolved. Both rapid-acquisition MRI and MR angiography are making MRI techniques more suitable for routine use in cancer patients. Contrast-enhanced magnetic imaging of the heart is also expanding.[9] Such techniques have not yet replaced echocardiography and radionuclide imaging techniques.[10] Nevertheless, MR has become a much more readily available technique, and is now an established noninvasive imaging modality for the assessment of various cardiac disorders. To some extent it now can be considered the new gold standard for quantification of ventricular volumes, function and mass.[11] Cardiac computed tomography (CT) is increasingly being used as an imaging modality and, like MR, allows for excellent visualization of the pericardium and nearby extracardiac structures. Positron emission tomography (PET) has theoretical advantages over more traditional imaging techniques and also is gaining in acceptability and availability. It remains expensive and is not yet widely used to evaluate myocardial viability in the cancer patient.[12]

Metastatic Involvement of Cardiac Structures

Metastatic involvement of cardiac structures is common and is seen in approximately 8-10% of patients with cancer; the incidence is somewhat less in elderly patients.[13] Involvement may constitute an incidental finding at autopsy or may be the initial, catastrophic presentation of cancer. There are wide variations among primary disease sites and tumor types. Previously, except in cases of pericardial tamponade, it was unusual to diagnose cardiac involvement antemortem; newer imaging techniques have now made it possible to recognize cardiac involvement much earlier and to a far wider extent, often at a time when intervention can still be efficacious. Tumor spread to cardiac structures may be by direct invasion (ie, lung or esophagus), retrograde lymphatic spread (ie, lung, breast), or hematogenous seeding (ie, melanoma, leukemia, lymphoma). In view of the relatively high incidence of lung and breast cancers, these neoplasms are the most common etiologies of metastatic lesions in cardiac structures. Malignant melanoma, once metastatic, is particularly likely to involve cardiac structures.[14] It should be kept in mind that the biologic behavior of tumors is sufficiently unpredictable and that metastatic involvement is quite variable. While metastatic disease is much more common in the pericardium than in other cardiac structures, metastatic involvement has the potential to involve myocardial and endocardial sites. The heart therefore should be included in routine examinations that seek metastatic involvement. Among other malignancies, Hodgkin and non-Hodgkin lymphomas, leukemias, gastrointestinal and, gynecologic cancers (especially ovarian), multiple myeloma, and sarcoma all invade the pericardium.[15] In addition, renal cell cancer not infrequently spreads to the inferior vena cava and into the right atrium and right ventricle; these lesions often are amenable to surgical resection (Fig. 130-2).

Pericardial Involvement

Pericardial Effusion ■ Pericardial effusion in cancer patients may be malignant or nonmalignant in nature, and may be related to the tumor, its treatment, or to underlying cardiac or systemic disease. Malignant pericardial effusion is defined as an effusion associated with pathologic evidence for tumor invasion of the pericardium even though such cells may not be demonstrable by routine cytologic examination of the fluid. Pericardial effusion may also accumulate as a result of radiation, anticancer treatment, lymphatic obstruction, altered oncotic balance, or infection. Fluid may demonstrate considerable variability with regard to both the quantity of fluid that accumulates as well as the pressure exerted on the pericardium and the cardiac chambers. The rate of accumulation and the distensibility of the pericardial sac determine the hemodynamic effect and the symptoms of these effusions.[16] As little as 100 mL of fluid in the pericardial sac may cause symptoms in a patient with a scarred or infiltrated nondistensible parietal pericardium, whereas large effusions containing as much as 1 L may remain relatively indolent when the pericardial sac is elastic and the effusion accumulates gradually. Malignant pericardial effusion generally carries a poor prognosis.[17]

Normally, pericardial fluid is not static but is in equilibrium with other body fluids. Abnormal fluid build-up occurs when fluid enters the sac more rapidly than can be reabsorbed. This disequilibrium may occur when the efferent lymphatic vessels are obstructed, or when subcarinal lymph node metastases mechanically prevent effective drainage. Malignant effusions are usually serosanguinous or frankly bloody in content and often (but not always) contain cytologically identifiable cancer cells. When chylous effusions are malignant, the most likely cause is lymphoma; chylous effusions also have been reported following radiation for gynecologic malignancy.[18]

The onset of symptoms in patients with malignant pericardial effusion may be insidious. Indeed, many patients with large effusions are totally asymptomatic. Pericardial effusion may be suspected when the cardiac silhouette is enlarged on the chest radiograph. Decreased mean electrocardiographic QRS voltage also suggests a pericardial effusion, but other causes of decreased voltage are common in cancer patients, making such a finding less useful; a recent drop in voltage should raise suspicion of the presence of pericardial effusion and trigger additional evaluation. Pericardial effusions are often noted as incidental findings on radionuclide or other cardiac imaging studies, with the fluid appearing as a relatively inactive area separating the cardiac from the hepatic and pulmonary blood pools. Occasionally, a rocking motion of the heart suggesting hemodynamic compromise (cardiac tamponade) is noted on blood-pool scans. CT images of the chest also may demonstrate pericardial effusions but are not especially helpful for estimating the volume. CT of the chest is frequently used to evaluate pulmonary or mediastinal tumor involvement, and therefore may provide the first indication of an unsuspected pericardial effusion. Once suspected, the diagnosis of pericardial effusion is usually confirmed by echocardiography.[19-21] Once an effusion has been diagnosed, its progression or resolution may be followed with serial echocardiograms.

Differential Diagnosis ■ The etiology of a pericardial effusion in a cancer patient may not always be apparent.[22] The differential diagnosis is broad, and noninvasive evaluation is insufficient to establish the etiology. The patient's history is very helpful, and information regarding previous irradiation of the chest or previous nonspecific pericarditis with effusion or heart failure is especially pertinent.[22] High fever, leukocytosis, and prostration suggest septic pericarditis, whereas recent myocardial infarction could suggest an association with the ischemic event. When the cause of a pericardial effusion in the cancer patient remains unclear, diagnostic (cytologic, bacteriologic, chemical, and immunologic) analysis of a fluid specimen may be necessary. In some instances, the etiology of pericardial effusion remains elusive despite an aggressive attempt at evaluation; even pericardial biopsy does not always provide a definitive explanation. Interestingly, the serum cancer antigen 125 (CA 125) level may be elevated in patients with pericardial and pleural effusions, as well as in patients with heart failure, even in the absence of gynecologic malignancy[23,24]; conditions that irritate or inflame serosal surfaces appear to induce apparently normal mesothelial cells to express this antigen. Pericardioscopy has also been undertaken in selected patients to aid in the evaluation of patients with pericardial effusions by allowing direct visualization and targeted biopsy.[25]

Cardiac Tamponade ■ The accumulation of pericardial fluid may lead to an increase in global or localized intrapericardial pressure and compromise cardiac output, a condition known as cardiac tamponade.[26] Symptoms include dyspnea and exercise intolerance, and signs include hypotension, tachycardia, neck vein distension, hepatomegaly, and cardiogenic shock. Heart sounds are often, but not always, distant and difficult to auscultate, and pericardial friction rubs may or may not be present. Vague chest discomfort or fullness is frequently noted. Most patients with significantly increased intrapericardial pressure also demonstrate an exaggeration of the decrease in pulse pressure during inspiration; when the systolic blood pressure decreases more than 10 mm Hg with normal inspiration, *pulsus paradoxus* is deemed to be present. The Kussmaul sign (failure of the jugular venous pressure to decrease with inspiration) is seen more commonly in the context of constrictive pericarditis or mediastinal tumors. A highly characteristic finding of cardiac tamponade is electrical alternans, in which the electrocardiographic QRS voltage becomes larger and smaller on alternate complexes. This phenomenon is caused by physical movement of the heart toward and away from the electrode as the heart rocks back and forth within the fluid-containing pericardial sac. While electrical alternans is not always seen in cases of cardiac tamponade, when present it is a very helpful finding. Cardiac tamponade can almost always be diagnosed on the basis of the physical findings and noninvasive studies. Echocardiography usually confirms the diagnosis and estimates the extent of accumulated fluid, which may vary considerably in size. Systolic inward motion (collapse) of the right atrium is a sensitive but not specific finding; the finding is more specific when the collapse extends for more than one-third of the cardiac cycle. Diastolic collapse of the right ventricular wall becomes more pronounced as hemodynamic compromise progresses and is a much more specific finding. Doppler flow studies show exaggerated respiratory variation in tricuspid and mitral flow velocities. Cardiac catheterization is usually not required to confirm the diagnosis, but may show a graphic representation of pulsus paradoxus, and there may be elevation and ultimate equalization of the diastolic pressures in the cardiac chambers as tamponade progresses. When frank tamponade ensues, the pulse becomes weak or totally absent during inspiration, and patients develop symptoms of low-output cardiogenic shock. Death, sometimes preceded by profound bradycardia, may ensue if the tamponade is not resolved promptly.

Management of Malignant Pericardial Effusion and Pericardial Tamponade ■ The management of malignant pericardial effusion depends on a number of factors, including the likelihood of the tumor responding to local (surgical, radiotherapeutic, or intracavitary) or systemic anticancer therapy; the extent of and the symptoms attributable to the effusion; and the overall anticipated survival of the patient.[27,28] Patients with tumors highly likely to respond to the systemic therapy may proceed with their treatment; sometimes the malignant effusion resolves in responses to the systemic anticancer therapy alone. Pericardial effusion diagnosed in patients with tumors that are unlikely to respond to treatment, either because of the cell type or because the tumor has become refractory to chemotherapy, may require local intervention. In patients who have a more favorable oncologic prognosis and who are sufficiently strong to undergo general anesthesia and surgery, creation of a pleuropericardial window is both effective and generally considered the procedure of choice. Although the transthoracic and the subxyphoid approaches are equally efficacious, in-hospital mortality was significantly greater for patients treated with the subxyphoid approach.[29,30] Using either approach, the communication formed usually remains patent, and the larger surface area available in the pleural space permits more effective reabsorption of the excess fluid. Pericardial needle drainage may be required prior to surgery as a stabilizing measure in patients who have very large effusions or pretamponade that compromises cardiac output. Symptoms often resolve dramatically after removal of the fluid, allowing patients to again engage in activities that had become impossible.

Needle drainage is now almost always undertaken with either echocardiographic or radiologic confirmation of the position of the draining catheter.[31] Some patients experience transient left ventricular dysfunction after resolution of cardiac tamponade, and thus a period of careful monitoring is important.[32] The advantages of the pericardial window over percutaneous pericardiocentesis have not been fully evaluated, but some studies suggest little advantage to the more invasive pericardial window procedure. The advisability of routine drainage of large pericardial effusions in patients without tamponade has also been questioned; Merce et al. point out the low diagnostic yield and the lack of therapeutic benefit.[33] The clinical management of such patients should be determined by their overall performance status, oncologic prognosis, and by the expertise at the treatment center. Needle drainage, even when done with echocardiographic imaging is not innocuous, and instances of cardiac perforation with sudden death have been reported.

Sclerosis may be considered following needle drainage, but is now employed much less frequently than heretofore. A number of sclerosing agents have been studied, including hyperosmolar glucose, radioactive gold, bleomycin, sterile talc, doxycycline, and triethylenethiophosphoramide (thio-TEPA).[34,35] Doxycycline, used at a dose of 250-500 mg, has received considerable attention as an effective sclerosing agent.[36] In many instances daily draining of the fluid until the residual effusion is less than 50 mL without instilling a sclerosing agent is highly effective in preventing recurrent accumulations.[37] Balloon pericardiotomy has been largely replaced by surgical pericardiotomy, a surgical intervention that can often be accomplished with minimal invasion and which is often successful.[38]

Metastatic Involvement of the Myocardium

The spread of malignant tumors to the myocardium is rarely recognized in vivo since most patients with myocardial metastases remain asymptomatic. It is not uncommon, however, to find significant and even extensive myocardial involvement at autopsy. Many patients in whom metastatic disease to the myocardium is identified before death also have evidence of concomitant pericardial involvement.

The most dramatic manifestation of myocardial metastatic disease is sudden dysrhythmia.[39,40] Sudden cardiac death can occur in this setting but is unusual. Cardiac perforation and erosion of the coronary vessels with hemorrhage or infarction may also occur but are exceedingly rare. More commonly, patients with myocardial involvement demonstrate signs of loss of functioning muscle mass and present with progressive shortness of breath and exercise intolerance; a decreased ejection fraction is seen on echocardiograms or nuclear imaging studies. It needs to be remembered, however, that the pattern of ischemia or infarction seen on a standard electrocardiogram in patients with large metastatic lesions may be indistinguishable from the electrocardiographic changes encountered with myocardial infarction due to coronary occlusion (Fig. 130-3). ST-segment elevations, T-wave inversions, or Q waves may be seen in such cases, even when the coronary arteries are angiographically normal.[41]

The diagnosis of metastatic involvement of the myocardium is difficult to establish. A high degree of suspicion may prompt special imaging; MRI studies may be helpful in determining the presence and extent of metastatic myocardial disease. Although treatment of metastatic disease to the myocardium is usually supportive, large melanomas that had metastasized to the right ventricle have been successfully removed.[42,43]

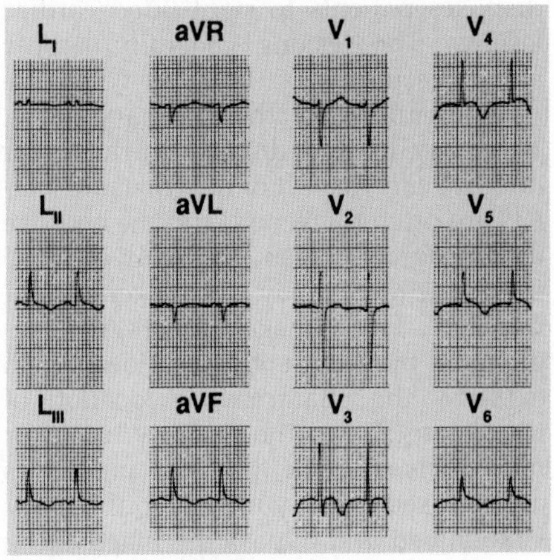

Figure 130-3 ■ Electrocardiogram suggesting ischemia in a 26-year-old man with documented (by MRI) myocardial metastatic disease and no history to suggest other causes of the electrocardiographic abnormality. Note T-wave inversions in the inferior leads (2, 3, and AVF) as well as in the precordial leads (V4-V6)

Cardiac Effects of Mediator Release, High-Output States, and Infiltrative Disorders in Cancer Patients

Metabolically active mediators are commonly associated with some forms of neoplastic diseases and frequently are the immediate cause of a patient's presenting signs and symptoms.[44] Such mediator-associated diseases, or paraneoplastic syndromes, may have a direct or indirect effect on the cardiovascular system.

Carcinoid Heart Disease

Carcinoid tumors arise from enterochromaffin cell-derived neuroendocrine tissue, most commonly in the gut or lungs; oncologic considerations regarding these tumors are considered elsewhere in this text. Carcinoid heart disease results from the long-term tumor release of biologically active mediators that stimulate the formation of a distinctive fibromuscular plaque that may destroy the integrity of the cardiac valves.[45-50] Carcinoid heart disease is seen most commonly in patients who have ileocecal carcinoid tumors that have metastasized to the liver. Rarely, it occurs in patients with bronchial or ovarian carcinoid tumors, and in those instances carcinoid heart disease may develop in the absence of hepatic metastases. The exact mechanism of plaque formation and cardiac injury remains elusive, but a number of possible mediators, including kinins, serotonin, 5-hydroxytryptophan, histamine, and prostaglandins, have been suggested; another as yet unidentified compound or combination of compounds may also contribute.[51]

Mediator release into the hepatic vein from metastatic liver disease predisposes patients to right-sided cardiac lesions. The lesions generally appear along the intima of the great veins, the right atrium, and the coronary sinus. The margins and distal (ventricular or downstream) aspect of the tricuspid leaflets are often thickened, and the chordae tendineae may also be involved. The pulmonic valve may be thickened and retracted. The damage appears to be aggravated by turbulent blood flow, which explains the characteristic location of the lesions. When the primary tumor or metastasis is in the lung, the mediators are released directly into the pulmonary venous bed and bypass the inactivating properties of lung tissue; left-sided valvular lesions are seen in such cases.[52] Left-sided lesions are less frequent than right-sided ones but are more likely to result in hemodynamic compromise. A review of surgically excised valves noted considerable variation in the histological appearance of the material; the excised valves predominantly (92%) came from the right side.[53]

The ultrastructure of the cardiac plaques has been studied extensively. The plaques are formed of smooth muscle cells embedded in a stroma of acid mucopolysaccharide and collagen and lack elastic fibers.[54] It has been postulated that the lesions, which resemble those seen after chronic endothelial irritation from long-term indwelling catheters, develop after repeated cycles of endothelial cell injury followed by healing.[55] Such lesions generally do not penetrate beyond the intima.

The most important consequence of carcinoid plaques is thickening and fibrosis of the valves with resultant distortion of the valvular apparatus and ring. Tricuspid regurgitation and pulmonic stenosis are typically seen, but in the case of progressive destruction, a rigid tricuspid valve with characteristic hemodynamic abnormalities reflecting both stenotic and regurgitant characteristics may be encountered. Significant pulmonic regurgitation is rare. Stiffening of the right atrium may be noted and contributes to the neck vein distention commonly seen in patients with the carcinoid syndrome. Finally, a high-output state, probably due to mediator release, has also been described.[56]

The clinical manifestations of carcinoid heart disease vary considerably. Some patients are able to tolerate the hemodynamic consequences of their valvular lesions well, whereas symptoms develop early in others, especially the aged or those with predisposing cardiac abnormalities.[57] Early symptoms include fatigue, dyspnea on exertion, and palpitations due to the high-output state, to dysrhythmias or to both. Later, symptoms of right-sided congestive heart failure, including edema, hepatomegaly, and sometimes ascites, predominate. Cardiac murmurs often predate symptoms, and the murmur of tricuspid regurgitation may be heard long before the hemodynamic effects become evident clinically. Most frequently, the murmur is appreciated as a loud, holosystolic, blowing sound heard along the left lower sternal border. The murmur may be augmented during inspiration. The murmur of pulmonic stenosis cannot always be distinguished from the often coexisting tricuspid regurgitation murmur; however, the pulmonic murmur is usually harsher and is appreciated most prominently in the second left intercostal space.

The chest radiograph may reveal prominence of the right ventricle. Unlike congenital pulmonic stenosis, which often includes poststenotic dilatation of the pulmonary trunk, this finding is usually not seen in carcinoid heart disease. Electrocardiographic findings include changes of right ventricular volume or pressure overload with or without right atrial abnormalities, right ventricular hypertrophy, right bundle-branch block, and/or right axis deviation; low voltage in the standard (limb) leads may also be seen.

Echocardiography is the most useful noninvasive tool for diagnosing carcinoid heart disease (Fig. 130-4). It not only identifies the valvular abnormality but, when coupled with Doppler ultrasonography studies, also can provide hemodynamic data for estimating the degree of valvular involvement.[58] Along with the thickening and loss of mobility of the tricuspid leaflets, increased flow velocity across the tricuspid valve during diastole is often evident. A regurgitant jet can be seen in the right atrium during systole. Furthermore, echocardiography can quantify the right atrial and right ventricular enlargement that is characteristic of this condition. Echocardiography has also been helpful in recognizing metastatic carcinoid tumors that involve the heart if those tumors are greater than 1 cm.[59]

The management of patients with carcinoid heart disease must be individualized and is often challenging. Although the carcinoid plaque is largely irreversible, controlling or eliminating the offending mediators can delay its progression. In this respect, treatment of the primary tumor or metastatic disease is crucial. Once the diagnosis is established, carcinoid heart disease is initially managed pharmacologically with diuretics, afterload reduction and salt restriction; the benefit of β-adrenergic blockade is unproven. Surgical intervention in the form of valvuloplasty or replacement is being considered more frequently than heretofore and with improved outcome.[48]

High-Output States and High-Output Cardiac Failure

Increased cardiac output occurs in many cancer patients and may be due to anemia, hyperthyroidism, primary or secondary aldosteronism, the syndrome of inappropriate antidiuretic hormone secretion, or the shunting of blood through tumors. High-output states also are relatively common in patients with multiple myeloma.[60] In addition, liver disease (nutritional cirrhosis or infectious hepatitis), fever, emotional excitement, and hypoxemia are also common causes of increased cardiac output and hyperdynamic states. High-output states are seen as well following treatment with a number of biologic response modifiers, including the interferons (possibly related to fever and the influenza-like reaction)

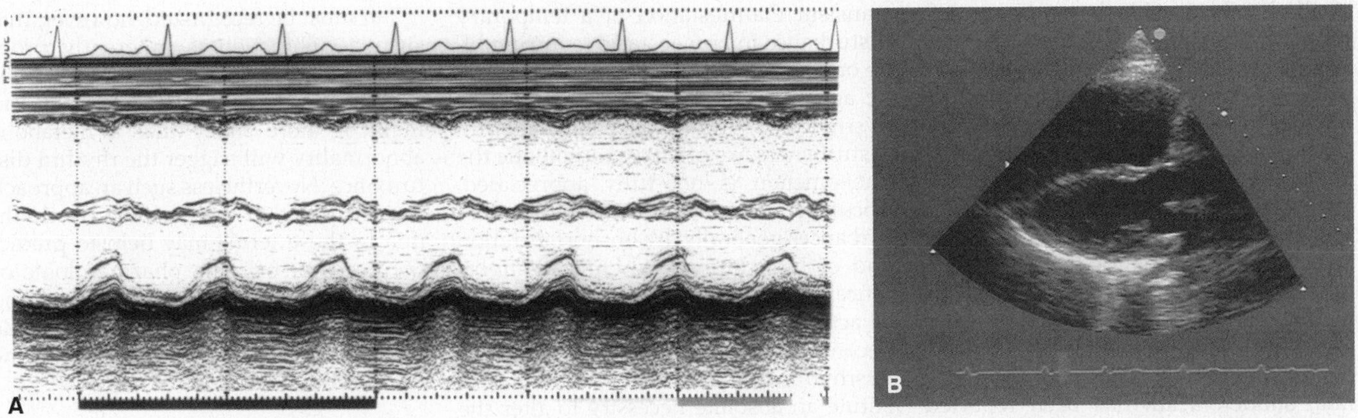

Figure 130-4 ■ Echocardiogram of a 47-year-old woman with long-standing carcinoid heart disease. (**A**) M-mode echocardiogram, showing right ventricle to be significantly enlarged and the septum showing paradoxical septal motion. These findings are characteristic of right ventricular volume and pressure overload. (**B**) The long-axis projection of the 2-D study from the same patient.

and interleukins; the phenomenon is usually self-limited and of short duration.

High-output states are associated with a moderately increased heart rate (usually 85-110 beats per minute, but sometimes higher) and with increased stroke volume. Physical examination typically reveals neck veins of normal appearance, since the preload is usually not increased. Peripheral pulses, however, are often bounding and have a rapid upstroke and fall; systolic blood pressure is elevated, and diastolic blood pressure often is reduced. Auscultation may reveal a systolic murmur and additionally may demonstrate a presystolic (S4) gallop. Pulmonary congestion is not uncommon in severe hyperdynamic states.

Echocardiography or radionuclide imaging is helpful in establishing the diagnosis. Two-dimensional studies show increased wall-motion in the long-axis, short-axis, and four-chamber views. In extreme cases, the images appear to suggest an almost total obliteration of the left ventricular cavity during systole; the ejection fraction is increased. MUGA cardiac blood-pool scans may also offer important data concerning the left ventricular ejection fraction and cardiac output. Right heart catheterization (most commonly undertaken with a flow-directed catheter) in conjunction with the measurement of cardiac output with thermodilution curves can confirm the diagnosis, but the procedure is rarely justified. It is important not to confuse this clinical picture with that of the more commonly encountered low-output congestive heart failure, with which it shares a number of characteristics. The treatment of high-output states should be directed toward the underlying cause; in the cancer patient metastatic disease with or without shunting, hyperthyroidism, hypoxia, anemia, and infection are the most common considerations. High-output states often respond to blood transfusion, diuretics, oxygen administration, or antipyretics. In selected cases, β-adrenergic blockers may be useful; digitalis preparations usually are not helpful, except as adjuncts in controlling the rate of ventricular response in patients with related or preexisting atrial fibrillation. Unless patients are symptomatic, the high-output state does not require specific therapy, and efforts should be directed at managing the underlying cause.

Cardiac Amyloidosis

Amyloidosis, or the deposition of amyloid proteins, may occur in a variety of organs including the heart, and may be caused by a number of pathologic processes.[61] Amyloid proteins are made up of fibrils consisting of antiparallel beta-pleated sheets that deposit in the interstitial spaces and are resistant to proteolysis. They are formed from a wide variety of precursor proteins.[61,62] Clinically significant cancer-related amyloidosis is encountered in patients with multiple myeloma and, less frequently, in patients with Hodgkin lymphoma. The amyloid protein associated with these diseases is known as AL amyloid, and is derived from light chain immunoglobulin (both Igλ and Igκ). AL amyloid accumulates in the atrial and ventricular myocardium and leads to either a restrictive or less commonly a dilated cardiomyopathy. Endocardial deposition resulting in valvular abnormalities has also been described.

Clinically, patients with cardiac amyloidosis experience fatigue and show signs of decreased cardiac output. Conduction abnormalities are seen and may be symptomatic; stress-precipitated syncope may be a precursor of sudden cardiac death.[63,64] Both systolic and diastolic function may be impaired. Restrictive cardiomyopathy can clinically be very difficult to distinguish from constrictive pericarditis; even findings at cardiac catheterization are not always conclusive in establishing the correct diagnosis. The chest radiograph shows a normal-sized or slightly enlarged cardiac shadow. When cardiac failure appears, pulmonary congestion or pleural effusion may be seen; the electrocardiogram characteristically shows decreased voltage, a pseudo-infarction pattern, and abnormalities of impulse formation or conduction. In one review, criteria for left ventricular hypertrophy were observed in 16% of the cases.[65] The echocardiogram is often helpful in suggesting the diagnosis of amyloidosis (Fig. 130-5). It may demonstrate a thickened septum and posterior wall with normal internal dimensions of the left ventricle; diastolic relaxation is often impaired. In addition, a spotted or stippled appearance is sometimes seen, and pericardial effusion is not uncommon. The paradox of left ventricular hypertrophy with decreased electrocardiographic voltage should suggest cardiac amyloidosis.[66] Antimyosin scintigraphy, showing left ventricular thickening and diffuse myocardial antimyosin uptake, has been reported to be highly suggestive of amyloid heart disease.[67]

Cardiac catheterization demonstrates elevated intracardiac pressures

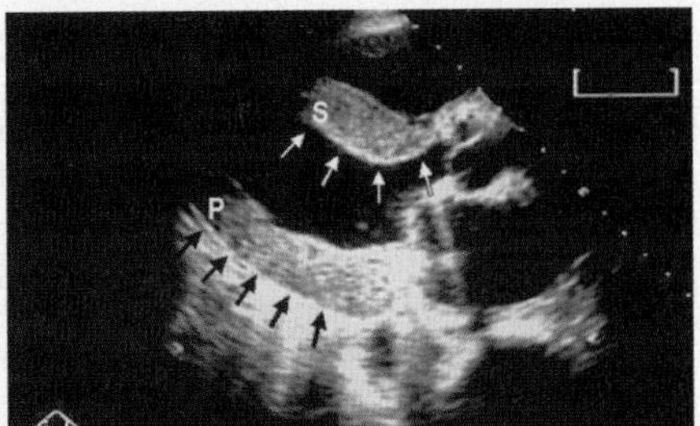

Figure 130-5 ■ Long-axis echocardiographic view from a patient with cardiac amyloid infiltration. Note thickened septum (S) and posterior wall (P) with stippled appearance (*arrows*).

in all chambers, with the minimum left ventricular pressure often increased to at least 10 mm Hg.[100]. The "dip and plateau" pattern seen on intraventricular pressure tracings in patients with constrictive pericarditis may be absent. Prominent papillary muscles are demonstrated with angiography. Endomyocardial biopsy with specimens stained with Congo red may be helpful in establishing the diagnosis.[68]

The therapeutic interventions for cardiac amyloidosis are limited. Cardiac glycosides may be especially dangerous in that they contribute to dysrhythmia; sudden death has been reported following their use.[69] Preload and afterload reduction using diuretics alone or in combination with angiotensin-converting enzyme (ACE) inhibitors, vasodilators, or long-acting nitroglycerin preparations also may be helpful. The use of β-adrenergic blockade has not been studied adequately. Clinical improvement may parallel control of the underlying process in patients with reactive forms of amyloidosis, and systemic treatment of myeloma may delay or alleviate the symptoms of myeloma-related cardiac amyloidosis. Intracardiac thrombosis is a significant risk in patients with amyloid infiltration. In one autopsy series thrombosis was encountered in 33% of patients coming to autopsy.[70] Anticoagulation in the presence of significant cardiac amyloidosis has been suggested. Therapy with a number of antineoplastic agents, including melphalan, cyclophosphamide, carmustine, and vincristine, have been attempted, as has hematopoietic stem cell transplantation.[62] Restrictive cardiomyopathy due to light chain deposition disease may, in rare cases, be reversible.[71] Cardiac transplantation has been undertaken in a patient with senile systemic amyloidosis and so the possibility exists for transplantation to treat amyloidosis of other etiologies.[72]

Cardiac Dysrhythmia in the Cancer Patient

Cardiac rhythm disturbances are common in cancer patients. These dysrhythmias may be caused by the tumor, but more often they are a consequence of anticancer treatment, the result of metabolic abnormalities, or from underlying heart disease. New onset atrial fibrillation, for example, may herald a pulmonary embolus in the hypercoagulable cancer patient. The rhythm disturbances seen in cancer patients are morphologically and functionally identical to those seen in patients without malignancy. In some settings, it is essential to suppress a cardiac dysrhythmia vigorously, whereas in others, rhythm disturbances may be a transient manifestation of a temporary disturbance in homeostasis requiring little or no intervention. Many antineoplastic agents are associated with transient dysrhythmia, and because such rhythm disturbances are often asymptomatic the phenomenon is not fully appreciated. These chemotherapy-related rhythm disturbances generally are of short duration and of little immediate clinical importance; while they may be an indication of actual myocardial damage that may become manifest only at a later time, the dysrhythmia itself usually does not constitute an absolute necessity to alter the chemotherapeutic regimen.

When faced with clinical decisions regarding which patients to treat, at what point in their management to initiate therapy, how long to continue treatment, and what form of therapy (pharmacologic or electrical) to use have been the focus of considerable debate. The wide assortment of antidysrhythmic drugs has not simplified these decisions. One useful approach is to distinguish dysrhythmias resulting from toxic substances or other metabolic abnormalities from those associated with structural abnormalities of the myocardium or other cardiac structures.[40]

Categories of Dysrhythmia: Primary (Structural) Versus Secondary (Metabolic)

The structural abnormalities within the heart that can result in cardiac abnormalities encompass a broad group of cardiac disorders. Ischemic heart disease, muscle hypertrophy, some forms of valvular disease, and infiltrative processes all fall within this group of disturbances. In the cancer patient, tumor infiltration, cell loss following chemotherapy, and fibrosis following radiation should also be included. When myocyte death is acute and involves a considerable portion of the myocardium, the rhythm may become unstable; severe dysrhythmias, both supraventricular and ventricular, may appear with little warning and progress catastrophically to hemodynamic instability and sudden cardiac death. While sudden arrhythmic death following cancer treatment is rare, it has been reported following cardiotoxic chemotherapy and radiation injury. Sudden death is more common in the presence of infiltrative processes such as amyloidosis.

Dysrhythmias in cancer patients also may be the result of nonstructural abnormalities that are seen often in cancer patients. Most commonly these include alterations in volume status, electrolyte disturbances, drug effects, and hormonal alterations, but other metabolic abnormalities that effect cardiac pacemaker and conduction tissue should also be considered.

It must be recognized, however, that such a distinction is inherently problematic in that structural abnormalities change the dysrhythmic threshold and make it more likely that a metabolic abnormality will trigger the rhythm disturbance. Nevertheless such an approach is useful in that categorizing dysrhythmia in these terms may help to predict the need for ongoing pharmacologic or electrical intervention and in selecting the specific agents most likely to provide satisfactory control or elimination of the dysrhythmia.

Treatment of Cardiac Rhythm Disturbances

Acute rhythm disturbances that result from metabolic abnormalities and that are not life threatening may be managed conservatively; in such cases, careful observation during treatment of the underlying metabolic abnormality may suffice. Active intervention is required when the dysrhythmia results in significant hemodynamic embarrassment, when the rhythm disturbance becomes life threatening, or when a protracted rhythm disturbance is of the type that results in an increased likelihood of a thromboembolic event. Such an approach may limit the likelihood of ongoing antidysrhythmic treatment for patients in whom the underlying cause of the dysrhythmia can be alleviated.

When structural abnormalities are involved, the control of a dysrhythmia is often more challenging. Hemodynamic instability, regardless of the underlying cause, constitutes a medical emergency requiring the use of advanced cardiac life-support protocols. Ventricular ectopy is seen commonly and ranges from isolated ventricular extrasystoles and benign accelerated idioventricular rhythm to malignant forms such as ventricular tachycardia and ventricular fibrillation. Coexisting conditions, such as fever or debilitation, which may augment tissue hypoxia, especially in anemic patients, predispose patients to ventricular ectopy. Unexpected death in cancer patients is usually attributed to dysrhythmia.

Once the decision has been made to treat a patient, the choice between pharmacologic intervention or the use of internal nonpharmacologic therapy such as implantable pacemakers or defibrillator, as well as the use of ablation therapy generally follows the usual guidelines for these therapies. In difficult cases, electrophysiologic studies or pharmacologic threshold analysis may be useful. Implantable devices increasingly are being used in cancer patients; malignant disease per se should not be considered a barrier to their use, but should be balanced with the patient's prognosis.

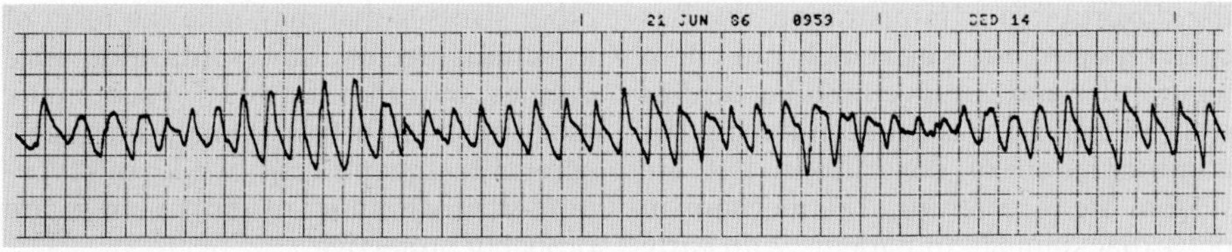

Figure 130-6 Rhythm strip of a patient with episodes of torsades de pointes. The previous rhythm strips showed prolongation of the QT interval.

An ever-increasing number of drugs are being implicated in causing a well-recognized variant form of ventricular tachycardia known as torsades de pointes. This polymorphic ventricular tachycardia (Fig. 130-6) is frequently preceded by a prolonged QT interval on the standard electrocardiogram. Antiarrhythmic drugs such as quinidine or procainamide, although used much less frequently than before, are still utilized for some patients and are associated with QT prolongation and torsades de pointes. This form of ventricular dysrhythmia is also associated with some antibiotics (erythromycin, clarithromycin, and pentamidine) psychotropic drugs (haloperidol), antiemetics, some forms of high-dose chemotherapy, and bone marrow transplantation.[73-75] Arsenic trioxide, which is most commonly used in the treatment of acute promyelocytic leukemia, also prolongs the QT interval, and patients should be observed carefully for QT prolongation during treatment with this agent.[76,77] Prompt recognition of this potentially malignant dysrhythmia and withdrawal of the offending agent may be the most appropriate therapy. Anecdotally, torsades de pointes may be more likely in African-Americans. QT prolongation has been reported to be more frequent in male patients as well as in those with hypokalemia. Serial monitoring of the QT interval is advised in high-risk individuals.[78] Table 130-2 lists the most important agents associated with QT prolongation.

The treatment of choice for torsades des pointes is intravenous magnesium sulfate; additional measures include isoproterenol infusion, and atropine. Maintenance of potassium and magnesium homeostasis may be helpful in preventing recurrences of this dysrhythmia; overdrive pacing, intravenous magnesium, or isoproterenol infusions may be used to revert the dysrhythmia back to a sinus mechanism.[79] Implantable defibrillators may be considered for patients in whom recurrent, hemodynamically significant tachydysrhythmias occur.[80]

Cardiac Complications of Chemotherapeutics

Nonsurgical therapies used to treat patients with cancer can damage the heart in a variety of ways. These therapies consist of chemical and biologic agents as well as physical agents such as ionizing radiation (Table 130-3). Individual modalities and combinations may act independently or synergistically; for example, the combination of cardiac irradiation and anthracyclines produces additive or synergistic toxicity. Damage resulting from cancer treatment may affect the pericardium, the myocardium, the vasculature, the conduction system, and the heart valves. Sometimes, the heart may incur subclinical damage, and a later insult or sequential stress may then trigger clinically relevant cardiac dysfunction.[81]

Table 130-2 Drugs That Prolong QT Interval and/or Induce Torsades de Pointes

Drugs with Established Risk	Drugs with Possible Risk
Amiodarone	Alfuzosin
Arsenic trioxide	Amantadine
Astemizole	Atazanavir
Bepridil	Azithromycin
Chloroquine	Chloral hydrate
Chlorpromazine	Clozapine
Cisapride	Dolasetron
Clarithromycin	Felbamate
Disopyramide	Flecainide
Dofetilide	Foscarnet
Domperidone	Fosphenytoin
Droperidol	Gatifloxacin
Erythromycin	Gemifloxacin
Halofantrine	Granisetron
Haloperidol	Indapamide
Ibutilide	Isradipine
Levomethadyl	Levofloxacin
Mesoridazine	Lithium
Methadone	Moexipril
Pentamidine	Moxifloxacin
Pimozide	Nicardipine
Probucol	Octreotide
Procainamide	Ofloxacin
Quinidine	Ondansetron
Sotalol	Paliperidone
Sparfloxacin	Perflutren lipid microspheres
Terfenadine	Quetiapine
Thioridazine	Ranolazine
	Risperidone
	Roxithromycin
	Sunitinib
	Tacrolimus
	Tamoxifen
	Telithromycin
	Tizanidine
	Vardenafil
	Venlafaxine
	Voriconazole

Source: Adapted from the Arizona Center for Education and Research on Therapeutics. www.torsades.org/medical-pros/drug-lists/drug-lists.cfm

Cardiotoxic anticancer agents may cause permanent or temporary contractile depression, ischemic disease, rhythm disturbances, and fluctuation in blood pressure. The discussion will review the subject of specific cardiotoxic anticancer agents according to this classification.

Agents With Myocardial Depressant Activity Several antineoplastic agents have been implicated as etiologic factors that cause

Table 130-3 Anticancer Agents Associated With Cardiotoxicity

- I. Type I chemotherapy-related cardiomyopathy
  - Anthracyclines
    - Doxorubicin
    - Pirarubicin
    - Idarubicin
    - Epirubicin
    - Daunorubicin
    - Liposomal formualtions
  - Anthraquinones
    - Mitoxantrone
  - Potential toxicity intensifiers
    - Cyclophosphamide
    - Ifosfamide
    - Mitomycin c
    - Etoposide
    - Melphalan
    - Vincristine
    - Bleomycin
    - Paclitaxel
- II. Type II chemotherapy-related cardiomyopathy
  - Trastuzumab
  - Lapatinib
  - Sunitinib
  - Sorafenib
  - Imatinib
- III. Antineoplastic agents associated with ischemia
  - 5-Fluorouracil (5-FU)
  - Capecitabine
  - Vinblastine
  - Vincristine
  - Bleomycin
  - Cisplatin
  - Biological response modifiers
- IV. Antineoplastic agents associated with hypotension
  - Interleukin-2
  - Homoharringtonine
- V. Antineoplastic agents associated with hypertension
  - Bevacizumab
  - Cisplatin
  - Sunitinib
  - Alemtuzumab
  - Gemtuzumab
  - Infliximab
  - Rituximab
  - Sorafenib
- VI. Miscellaneous
  - Paclitaxel (bradycardia)
  - α-Interferon
  - Arsenic trioxide (long QT/torsades des pointes)

myocyte dysfunction or death. The anthracyclines are the most widely studied, but other anthraquinones and agents affecting the myocyte through different mechanisms have also been implicated. From a functional standpoint, anticancer agents can be divided into two types, type I and type II, according to a number of characteristics.[82] Type I agents are associated with myocyte cellular damage that may progress to cell death; while some compensation and functional stabilization often takes place, the cellular damage, once it has progressed beyond a threshold, is permanent. Type I drugs involve damage that is cumulative dose-related, is associated with typical endomyocardial biopsy changes. Agents associated with type II treatment-related cardiac dysfunction cause myocyte dysfunction that resembles hibernation or stunning, and is more likely to be reversible. These agents do not demonstrate toxicity that is cumulative dose-related and they are not associated with the typical endomyocardial biopsy changes that are seen with anthracyclines. These differences are summarized in Table 130-4.

Type I Anticancer Treatment-Related Agents: Anthracyclines and Other Anthraquinolones The effects of anthracyclines on the heart have been the most extensively studied of all of the cardiotoxic agents; doxorubicin cardiotoxicity serves as a model for understanding anthracycline-associated and related type I cardiomyopathies.

Doxorubicin cardiotoxicity can be recognized early or late during a course of treatment, or it may surface months or even years after the completion of treatment. Early manifestations of toxicity include electrocardiographic abnormalities and myopericarditis. Significant early cardiac dysfunction is rare with current dosing regimens, but cases of heart failure occurring within weeks of the first administration of the drug have been reported.[83,84] Early toxicity is more likely to occur in elderly patients or in patients who have received large single doses, and has been reported more commonly in patients treated with daunorubicin than with doxorubicin. Sudden death following doxorubicin administration also has been reported but is extremely rare. Both ventricular and supraventricular cardiac dysrhythmias are often seen during the administration of doxorubicin but are seldom life threatening. The mechanism of cardiac damage in patients with early toxicity is uncertain, and treatment is supportive. Of considerable interest however, is the finding that markers of acute cardiac damage such as troponin T are increased following exposure to doxorubicin.[85] This suggests that early damage may be more important than had heretofore been appreciated; troponin release is an indicator of early cell death, and the beginning of an ongoing process that may go largely unrecognized in view of the vast ability of the heart to compensate for myocyte loss, and our inability to measure small changes in myocardial reserves with the usually utilized parameter of ejection fraction.[86] Early elevations in troponin I have been shown to correlate with cardiac abnormalities observed later, and may allow the stratification of patients who are at increased risk for subsequent cardiac damage with ongoing doxorubicin exposure. Such a differentiation would allow for more careful monitoring of such patients, but perhaps more importantly, might provide the opportunity to mitigate future damage by cardioprotection or by the consideration of alternate less cardiotoxic regimens.[87] Although these strategies have great potential, they have not yet been incorporated into standard patient protocols. Rather than categorizing doxorubicin cardiotoxicity as either early or late, it is now prudent to consider this as a single entity, whereby early damage and cell death is often initially well tolerated, but when such damage exceeds the cardiac mechanisms of compensation and remodeling may gradually evolve to a phase of decompensation with progressive heart failure, and may ultimately progress to cardiac death.

The concept of a continuum of the cardiac effects of doxorubicin, starting with the initial myocyte injury and evolving to a state of potential heart failure is supported by the shape of the dose-toxicity curve, the known risk factors, as well as other stresses that may take the form of infectious agents, other anticancer modalities or other factors.[88] Phenomena that stress or further damage the heart accelerate the process, while interventions that diminish oxidative stress are probably protective.

The cumulative dose relationship has been well established, and also fits this model. Clinical manifestations of cardiomyopathy are unusual when the cumulative dose is below 400 mg/m^2, but the risk becomes greater as the cumulative dose exceeds 450 mg/m^2 administered by the usual rapid-infusion schedule.[89] Cardiomyopathy may occur at lower doses when other cardiotoxic drugs are administered concomitantly (see later discussion); there is considerable inter-patient variability. It follows then that if cardiac decompensation occurs early, ie, less than 4 weeks from the last doxorubicin administration, it is much more likely to be serious or have a fatal outcome; patients who experience early toxicity probably have had more severe initial damage.

As noted above, doxorubicin cardiomyopathy may become manifest months, and even years, after an uncomplicated course of chemotherapy at or near the usual maximum recommended dose. Such late cardiomyopathy may involve additional insults or stresses such as viral infections.[81] The sequential stress, whatever its nature, might not have been of importance were it not for the fact that there had been considerable preexisting heart disease and a lack of reserve to compensate for the additional injury. Cardiac biopsy findings are rarely helpful as the tissue specimens most frequently show nonspecific changes; the doxorubicin damage is no longer recognizable, and the sequential stress may not demonstrate structural changes. Sequential stress or injury may explain some of the cases heretofore thought of as late cardiotoxicity. As the anthracyclines have been in use for more than 30 years, some of the patients cured of leukemias, lymphomas, sarcomas, and breast cancer may harbor subclinical cardiac damage that now makes them particularly prone to symptomatic heart failure in the event of additional cardiac insult. The effect of doxorubicin exposure on the genesis of coronary artery disease, myocardial infarction, and other cardiac injuries that occur with aging is unknown. In one review, 12 of 43 patients with doxorubicin-induced cardiomyopathy died due to progressive cardiac dysfunction.[90] Our understanding that cardiac damage, albeit subclinical, probably starts with the first exposure of an anthracycline, as well as the risk of subsequent or sequential stresses, makes the case for early and vigorous cardioprotection very compelling.[88,91]

Table 130-4 **Type I and Type II Treatment-Related Cardiac Dysfunction**

Type I (eg, Doxorubicin)	Type II (eg, Trastuzumab)
Celluar death	Celluar dysfunction
Damage starts with the first administration	
Biopsy changes (typical of anthracylines)	No typical anthracycline-like biopsy changes
Cumulative dose-related	Not cumulative dose related
Permanent damage	Predominantly reversible
Risk factors: combination CT, prior/concomitant RT, age, previous cardiac disease, hypertension	Risk factors: prior/concomitant anthracyclines or paclitaxel, age, previous cardiac disease, obesity (BMI > 25 kg/m^2)

Abbreviations: CT, chemotherapy; RT, radiation therapy; BMI, body mass index.

Mechanism of Anthracycline-Associated Cardiotoxicity ■ The mechanism of the cardiac damage caused by anthracycline exposure has not been fully elucidated, however free radical formation is believed to be an important factor. Free radicals can injure lipid structures in the myocardial cell, and the resultant peroxidation of these lipid structures impairs the function of the sarcoplasmic reticulum and mitochondria. Cardiac myocytes are more prone to these degenerative changes since they lack catalase and superoxide dismutase and thus are less able to metabolize free radicals than are other cells.[92] Cell necrosis is the end result of this damage. There is increasing evidence that the generation of the oxygen free radicals is mediated through an iron-doxorubicin complex.[93] Doxorubicinol, one of the principal metabolites of doxorubicin, has a greater effect on the calcium pump of the sarcoplasmic reticulum than does the parent doxorubicin, which suggests that the antitumor effect is distinct from the cardiotoxic effect.[94] It has been suggested that the level of atrial natriuretic peptide is increased in at least some patients with doxorubicin-associated cardiotoxicity, and this appears to correlate more with changes in diastolic than with changes in systolic function.[95]

Clinical Manifestations of Anthracycline-Associated Cardiotoxicity ■ The clinical manifestations of doxorubicin-related cardiomyopathy are indistinguishable from other forms of congestive heart failure. Patients may be asymptomatic in the early stages or may exhibit only minimal signs of cardiac dysfunction. In many patients, the first sign of a cardiac abnormality may be a failure to return to baseline cardiac rate in a timely manner following exertion. Resting tachycardia and loss of respiratory variation in heart rate may also be seen. As cardiac damage progresses, patients experience increasing dyspnea, with dyspnea at rest a poor prognostic sign.

The cardiac examination of a patient with fully developed cardiomyopathy often reveals an S_3 gallop, an enlarged area of cardiac dullness, an exaggerated increase in cardiac rate with minimal activity and, when pulmonary congestion ensues, diffuse rales. The chest radiograph shows nonspecific findings of an increased cardiac silhouette and engorged vasculature. Various degrees of pleural effusion may be noted. The electrocardiogram may show nonspecific repolarization changes. Blood chemistry values are being increasingly explored as markers of cardiac damage. The plasma level of B-type natriuretic peptide (BNP) is gaining importance as a parameter of cardiac dilation and strain, and is currently included in a number of oncologic trials that involve agents that are known to be or are possibly cardiotoxic.[96,97] The left ventricular ejection fraction remains the most frequently used noninvasive parameter with which to monitor the cardiac status in patients receiving doxorubicin or related agents.

The structural changes in myocardial tissue seen on examination of cardiac biopsy specimens can provide vital information concerning the toxicity of doxorubicin and related compounds.[91,98,99] Indeed, studying biopsy material is the best way to gauge cardiac damage at a time prior to the development of functional deterioration. In addition, in highly selected patients, it provides the essential information needed to decide whether to continue or terminate chemotherapy that includes cardiotoxic drugs. The procedure is generally regarded as safe, but nevertheless invasive; in one series of 1350 procedures, cardiac perforation with tamponade occurred in less than 0.6% of the patients, minor procedure-related problems were noted in 0.8% of the patients, and there were no reported deaths.[100] The cardiac biopsy specimens are graded according to ultrastructural changes seen by electron microscopy with both the degree and the extent of the abnormalities considered in determining the final grade. Cardiac biopsy grades not only measure the damage to the heart of an individual patient, it also serve to compare the cardiotoxic effects of other anthracyclines or different dosage schedules. With the presently used anthracycline regimens cardiac biopsy is now primarily a research tool.

Several groups of patients are known to be at greater risk of developing cardiac dysfunction at relatively lower cumulative doses of anthracyclines. Among these are elderly patients, pediatric patients, those with preexisting heart disease and hypertension. It is now postulated that any entity with diminished cardiac reserve, increased wall stress, or any condition in which patients are exposed to increased oxidative stress are probably at increased risk for cardiotoxicity of all anthracyclines. Included among these entities are aortic stenosis, hypertrophic and other cardiomyopathies. Ischemic heart disease may add some risk in that the increased metabolic needs produced by the chemotherapy may upset a precarious balance between oxygen supply and demand. Anecdotally, many patients with reduced baseline ejection fractions tolerate at least some doxorubicin, especially when used with adequate cardioprotection.[101] Despite some reports to the contrary, anthracyclines are generally not considered to be associated with coronary spasm or primary myocardial ischemia.[102] For patients in whom an increased risk is present, increased surveillance and consideration of cardiac-sparing regimens may be considered. Irradiation through portals that include the heart is a well-documented risk factor for cardiomyopathy developing at lower cumulative doses of doxorubicin than is usually seen, and patients who have undergone concomitant or sequential cardiac irradiation should be considered for cardioprotection or additional monitoring when high cumulative dosages are contemplated.[103,104]

A number of antineoplastic drugs have also been associated with increased anthracycline toxicity. Cyclophosphamide may augment the cardiotoxic effect of doxorubicin toxicity, a matter of particular clinical importance because the drugs are often used together. Although there is evidence both for and against the additive clinical cardiac toxicity of doxorubicin and cyclophosphamide in combination, cyclophosphamide at high doses is known to be independently cardiotoxic, and the combination is definitely more cardiotoxic in a monkey model. Dactinomycin, plicamycin, dacarbazine, and mitomycin C, all reportedly augment doxorubicin toxicity, but the evidence for the first three has not been persuasive.[105] On the other hand, mitomycin C appears to add substantially to the toxicity of doxorubicin, even when given after the completion of doxorubicin therapy.[106] Paclitaxel has also been reported to increase the cardiotoxic effect of doxorubicin. In one study, however, patients receiving the combination at cumulative doses of doxorubicin of below 340-380 mg/m^2 did not appear to demonstrate the additive effect.[107] The higher incidence of cardiac toxicity observed when the two drugs are administered within a short time may be due to the fact that the paclitaxel interferes with the pharmacokinetics of doxorubicin, leading to higher systemic levels of both doxorubicin and doxorubicinol, a metabolite.[108] Alternatively, the apparent increase in toxicity may simply be the result of increased surveillance using imperfect tests in patients undergoing frequent monitoring of cardiac function. Other anthracyclines and related agents, such as mitoxantrone (an anthraquinone), demonstrate intrinsic cardiac toxicity that is additive; as is noted below, changing from one anthracycline to another does not provide cardioprotection.[109,110]

Various strategies can lower the extent of doxorubicin cardiotoxicity. Limiting the cumulative dose is a strategy that grew out of the observation that clinically apparent cardiotoxicity is unusual at cumulative doses of less than 300 mg/m^2 and that the incidence is about 5% at a cumulative dose of 400 mg/m^2.[89]

Limiting the cumulative dosage to these levels in patients without risk factors helps to keep cardiotoxicity within an acceptable range. Dose-limitation also decreases the need for cardiac monitoring, as the likelihood of cardiotoxicity is lower; the risk of stopping effective therapy early because of false-positive testing results may exceed the benefits of such testing. Dose-limitation, however, does not take into consideration patients who are still responding after receiving the limiting dose. Most patients, including many who are at increased cardiac risk, tolerate 300 mg/m^2 of doxorubicin or the cardiotoxic equivalent of other anthracyclines.[101]

Encapsulating conventional anthracyclines in liposomes reduces the incidence and severity of cardiotoxicity.[111-113] Both pegylated and nonpegylated preparations have been studied, and the pegylated preparation is approved for the treatment of Kaposi sarcoma, multiple myeloma, and ovarian carcinoma in the United States; other indications are under consideration. The agent is effective in the treatment of breast cancer; comparisons of liposome-encapsulated and conventional doxorubicin in the treatment of that disease confirmed cardioprotection with comparable antitumor activity.[114,115] Pegylated liposomal doxorubicin appears to have a clinical efficacy similar to its parent compound in a subset of anthracycline-sensitive tumors.[116] Both pegylated and nonpegylated liposomal doxorubicin are clearly cardioprotective.[117,118] With the pegylated form, cardioprotection has been demonstrated both by cardiac biopsy as well as by noninvasive studies.[115] The degree of cardioprotection is difficult to quantify, but studies suggest that at least twice the number of cycles of pegylated liposomal doxorubicin can be given with the same degree of cardiotoxicity as is seen with the unprotected parent compound. The oncologic efficacy is not impaired, but the degree of stomatitis and hand-foot syndrome is higher.[119]

Modification of the dose schedule has been clearly shown to decrease anthracycline cardiotoxicity. Initially the effect was demonstrated for weekly administration; in comparison with the standard schedule (rapid-infusion, 21-28 day cycle), the weekly schedule allowed approximately 200 mg/m^2 more doxorubicin to be given than the usual amount tolerated. A series of trials of continuous-infusion doxorubicin were initiated using infusion times of 24-96 h, gauging the cardiotoxicity on the basis of endomyocardial biopsy findings.[120,121] Patients treated with continuous infusions showed a significantly lower incidence of high-grade endomyocardial pathology in their biopsy specimens despite receiving a significantly higher cumulative dose. Efficacy is not compromised, but infusions longer than 96 h are limited by increasingly troublesome mucositis and hand-foot syndrome.[122] Continuous infusion has also been evaluated in the pediatric population and has been shown to be cardioprotective.[123] The relative cardioprotection of various doxorubicin administration schedules is depicted in Table 130-5. The inconvenience of the portable infusion pumps and indwelling catheters that are required for continuous infusion and the trend to use lower cumulative dosages of doxorubicin has made many clinicians reluctant to use such schedules.

A number of compounds with possible cardioprotective properties have been investigated. The single approved cardiac protector to date is the iron chelator dexrazoxane. In a study of 92 patients randomly assigned to receive a doxorubicin-containing regimen (50 mg/m^2 doxorubicin with 500 mg/m^2 cyclophosphamide and 500 mg/m^2 fluorouracil given every 21 days) or the same regimen together with dexrazoxane, the investigators found a significant decrease in cardiotoxic effects demonstrated by ejection fraction measurements, biopsy grades, and clinical signs or symptoms of cardiac dysfunction.[124,125] Other toxicity and antitumor effects were unaffected. On the other hand, at least one subsequent study that confirmed the cardioprotective activity of dexrazoxane showed a possible decrease in antitumor effect as well.[126] There was no suggestion of diminished antineoplastic activity, however, in patients given dexrazoxane after they had received 300 mg/m^2 of doxorubicin.[127,128] Other studies have not found the efficacy of anthracyclines to be decreased by dexrazoxane. Additional studies are required before the relative risks and benefits of dexrazoxane can be placed in proper perspective. Dexrazox-

Table 130-5 **Relative Toxicities of Anthracycline: A Comparison of Relative Toxicities of Different Cardiotoxic Drugs and Dosage Schedules**

Drug	Schedule	Relative Myelosuppressive Potency of Single Dose Compared With Doxorubicin Administered by Standard Schedule	Approximate Relative Cardiotoxicity[a]	Cardiotoxicity Index Compared With Doxorubicin Administered by Standard Schedule[b]	Recommended Maximum Dose (mg/m^2)[c]
Doxorubicin	Rapid- infusion (20 min)	1	1	1	400
Doxorubicin	Weekly	1	0.73	0.73	550
Doxorubicin	24-h infusion	1	0.73	0.73	550
Doxorubicin	48-h infusion	1	0.62	0.62	650[d]
Doxorubicin	96-h infusion	1	0.5	0.5	800-1000[d]
Epirubicin	Rapid-infusion	0.67	0.66	0.44	900
Mitoxantrone	Rapid-infusion	5	0.5	2.5	160
Daunorubicin	Rapid-infusion	0.67	0.75[e]	0.5[e]	80[e]
Idarubicin	Rapid-infusion	5	0.53	2.67	150
Pirarubicin	Rapid-infusion	1	0.62	0.62	650[e]
Doxorubicin + dexrazoxane	Rapid-infusion	1[e]	0.5		800-1000[e]
Doxorubicin, 300 mg/m^2 + dexrazoxane	Rapid-infusion	1[e]	0.73[e]		550[e]

[a]Factor by which the cardiotoxic effects of the cumulative dose of rapid infusion doxorubicin can be compared with the cumulative dose of the agent, combination and schedule listed, when given at an equivalent myelosuppressive dose.

[b]Derived by dividing 400 mg/m^2, the recommended maximum dose of rapid-infusion doxorubicin, by the recommended maximum dose for the agent in question. The cardiotoxicity index represents a factor by which to multiply the cumulative dose of a drug administered to obtain an approximation of toxicity that might be expected had the resultant amount of doxorubicin been given by rapid infusion. For example, if a cumulative dose of 120 mg/m^2 mitoxantrone had been administered, the patient would be expected to demonstrate cardiac damage approximately equal to 300 mg/m^2 of doxorubicin given by rapid infusion (120 × 2.5 = 300). This value is useful when changing from one cardiotoxic regimen to another. When the sum of the products of the indexes and the cumulative doses administered exceeds 400, the risk of clinically significant cardiotoxicity exceeds 5%.

[c]Dose producing clinically significant congestive heart failure in 5% of patients.

[d]Less toxic by endomyocardial biopsy.

[e]Inadequate data.

ane has been studied in conjunction with epirubicin and mitoxantrone.[129,130] These studies suggest that dexrazoxane also reduces the cardiotoxicity of agents other than doxorubicin. Dexrazoxane is also used in children where there are special concerns regarding late toxicity.[131]

Cardiac Monitoring of Patients Receiving Doxorubicin ■ Most patients undergoing treatment for cancer, even aged patients and those with known cardiac disease, can tolerate at least some doxorubicin.[101] Patients with significant dilated cardiomyopathy and patients who have experienced cardiotoxicity from the prior use of an anthracycline or related drug are the major exceptions. Most patients with reduced ejection fractions as the result of prior myocardial infarctions tolerate doxorubicin when it is given with some form of cardioprotection, and when the cumulative dose remains below 300-400 mg/m^2; increased monitoring in those settings is prudent. Patients being considered for doxorubicin therapy generally undergo a cardiac evaluation usually consisting of a complete medical history and physical examination, chest roentgenogram, a determination of ejection fraction by using either a nuclear or an ultrasonographic technique, and a standard electrocardiogram. The routine testing of ejection fraction, however, is sometimes questioned, as basic studies and clinical assessment are usually sufficient in identifying patients at greatly increased risk; the preference of the authors is to obtain such measurements so that a basis for later comparison is available.[132-134] One analysis suggested that monitoring by nuclear scanning becomes cost effective in patients older than 40 years of age scheduled to receive cumulative doses of doxorubicin greater than 350 mg/m^2.[135] Echocardiographic studies are generally preferred in the pediatric population.

Patients without risk factors and who are without signs or symptoms suggesting cardiac compromise need not be reassessed before receiving a cumulative dose of 300-350 mg/m^2 by standard infusion or its equivalent in a less cardiotoxic schedule (Table 130-5). Thereafter, reassessment after each two additional cycles of treatment may be prudent, but the cost effectiveness of such a strategy has not been proven. When cumulative doses exceed those noted in Table 130-5, additional caution is suggested. Patients with risk factors for early toxicity may be monitored more closely. The most important precaution, however, is keeping track of the cumulative dose; at the upper ranges of the cumulative dosages suggested in Table 130-5, the risk of heart failure approaches 5% in the absence of other cardiac risk factors.

Patients who continue to have an ejection fraction above the lower limit of normal for the laboratory conducting the study, and who have not shown a decrease of more than 15% from the pretreatment value generally tolerate their next one or two cycles of doxorubicin well, up to a cumulative dosage of 400 mg/m^2. Patients whose ejection fractions fall below 45% are at increased risk. Patients with baseline ejection fractions between 45% and the lower limits of normal for the laboratory are considered at intermediate risk; in such patients, if the ejection fraction has not changed they may be treated up to 400 mg/m^2 with careful monitoring. For those whose ejection has either fallen by more than 15 percentage points or has fallen to a value below 45%, strong consideration should be made to stop doxorubicin and substitute alternative therapy using noncardiotoxic agents. The rare patients requiring further cardiotoxic therapy should be considered for cardiac biopsy to evaluate structural changes. A biopsy grade of 1.5 or higher constitutes a contraindication to continued treatment with an anthracycline.

Exercise testing to assess cardiac reserve in patients treated with anthracyclines was not found to correlate with cardiac biopsy results by some investigators, however, others consider it a useful modality. Although mean exercise ejection fractions do decrease with increasing cumulative dosages of anthracyclines, there is considerable overlap so as to preclude useful decision making on the basis of these tests.[136,137] Some investigators have also suggested that signal-averaged electrocardiography detect early cardiotoxicity damage in children.[138,139]

Other Anthracyclines and Related (Type I) Agents ■ Clinically, the cardiotoxic effects of daunorubicin, idarubicin, epirubicin, pirarubicin, and mitoxantrone are identical to those of doxorubicin. As is the case with oncologic efficacy of these agents, the cumulative dosages, expressed in mg/m^2 that causes cardiotoxicity, differs between the various agents. The cardiotoxicity of these agents has not been studied as extensively as has that of doxorubicin. Nevertheless, on the basis of ejection fractions and findings from cardiac biopsy specimen evaluation at equivalent oncologic doses, some data have emerged. Epirubicin is associated with a statistically significant decrease in the incidence of cardiac toxicity compared with that seen for doxorubicin given by rapid-infusion (Table 130-5).[140,141] The cardioprotection afforded by epirubicin, which is being used increasingly for the treatment of breast cancer, allows an additional margin of safety that may be especially important in populations at increased cardiac risk. Some investigations have suggested that the combination of paclitaxel and epirubicin causes less cardiotoxicity than the combination of doxorubicin and paclitaxel, and they attribute this to the fact that paclitaxel interferes less with the metabolism of epirubicin than with the parent compound.[142,143]

Mitoxantrone, an anthraquinone, is considered less cardiotoxic than doxorubicin in equi-myelosupressive dosages.[109,144] Although idarubicin is the least studied commercially available anthracycline, available data suggest that 150 mg/m^2 is a safe cumulative dose for patients who have not yet been exposed to an anthracycline.[145] Preliminary data for pirarubicin (THP doxorubicin), a doxorubicin analogue used extensively in Japan and France, suggest that the agent is significantly less cardiotoxic than doxorubicin given by standard-infusion schedules.[146]

Switching from one agent to another does not offer cardioprotection, and considerable care must be exercised when considering a new cardiotoxic treatment in a patient who has previously been treated with other type I cardiotoxic agents. The best approach when prescribing such agents in sequence is to calculate the fraction of the recommended maximum cumulative dose of the agent that has already been administered and use that fraction to estimate the remaining dosage that can be safely administered. If the sum of the individual fractions remains below unity, the likelihood of cardiotoxicity will remain acceptable. Converting the various cardiotoxic drug doses to the corresponding doses of rapidly administered doxorubicin allows comparisons (Table 130-5).

Type II Anticancer Treatment-Related Agents ■ Type II agents by definition do not demonstrate cumulative dose-related toxicity, and therefore the cardiotoxic expression is much less predictable. The best studied of these agents is trastuzumab, but other agents should also be considered in this grouping. Trastuzumab, a humanized monoclonal antibody directed against *HER2*, is effective for the treatment of breast cancers that overexpress this antigen (approximately 25-30% of breast cancers). Cardiomyopathy with a clinical expression initially thought to be similar to that seen for the cardiomyopathy produced by anthracyclines was observed in early clinical studies with trastuzumab and subsequently was noted in 28% of patients treated concurrently doxorubicin; 19% of these patients were deemed to have New York Heart Association class III or IV dysfunction. This finding led to a number of large multicenter trials that included more than 10,000 patients who received trastuzumab. A summary of the trials and their respective treatment

Table 130-6 **Summary of Cardiotoxicity in Adjuvant Trials Involving Trastuzumab**

Trial	No. of Patients	Entry Criteria	Arms	Reported Cardiac Events (%)	Reported Reversibility	Follow-up
NSABP B-31	2043	Node+	A) AC-T B) AC-TH	A) 0.8 B) 4.1	Yes	3 yr
BCIRG 006	3222	Node+ or high-risk node–Age<70	A) AC-T B) AC-TH C) TPH	A) 0.4 B) 1.9 C) 0.4	N/A	3 yr
NCCTG N9831	1944	Node+ or high-risk node–	A) AC-T B) AC-TH C) AC-TH	A) 0.3 B) 2.8 C) 3.3	Yes	3 yr
HERA	3386	Node+ or high-risk node–	A) Std B) Std-H	A) 3.6 B) 0.6	Yes	2 yr
FinHer	232	Node+ or high-risk node–Age <66	A) V/T-FAC B) V/T(H)-FAC	A) 3.4 B) 0	N/A	3 yr

Abbreviations: A, anthracycline; C cyclophosphamide; T, taxane; H, trastuzumab; P, carboplatin; Std, standard (neo)adjuvant regimen (94% contained anthracycline); V/T, vinorelbine or taxane; 5-FU, 5-fluorouracil; N/A, not applicable.

arms is shown in Table 130-6.[147,148] Several important conclusions have emerged from these trials, the most important from the perspective of cardiotoxicity are: (1) cardiac dysfunction in treatment arms that include an anthracycline followed by trastuzumab are higher than similar arms without trastuzumab; the difference, however, while less than 4% is nevertheless a topic of conern; (2) cardiac dysfunction for those that experience it following trastuzumab is largely but not invariably reversible; (3) cardiac deaths are extremely low; (4) regimens that include trastuzumab without pretreatment with an anthracycline have a much smaller incidence of cardiac dysfunction; and (5) the cardiotoxicity associated with trastuzumab while different from that of doxorubicin, is clinically indistinguishable using MUGA or echocardiographic parameters of decreased systolic function. An additional factor that emerges from these trials is that the interval between the anthracycline and trastuzumab may be a crucial factor.[134,149]

Although the precise mechanism of trastuzumab-induced cardiomyopathy is not well understood, its specific binding to HER2 and disruption of the ErbB-2 signaling pathway in the heart is thought to be the primary event. ErbB-2 (HER2/neu) belongs to the epidermal growth factor receptor (EGFR) family of receptor tyrosine kinases, of which there are four members: EGFR (ErbB-1), HER2/neu (ErbB-2), HER3 (ErbB-3), and HER4 (ErbB-4). These receptors are activated by the EGF family of ligands, including EGF itself and neuregulins, which are expressed in heart. Although ErbB-2 has no known ligand, binding of these EGF ligands to EGFR or ErbB-4 induces heterodimer formation with ErbB-2, triggers receptor autophosphorylation, and initiates downstream signaling. Among those pathways activated are Ras/Raf, PI3K/Akt, JNK, and MAPK, all important regulators of transcription in cardiac myocytes. An extensive body of work has implicated these pathways in cardiac development, maintenance of normal cardiac function, response to stress, hypertrophy, and regulation of apoptosis. Indeed, targeted deletion of ErbB-2 in murine models has demonstrated a specific role for this receptor in mediating the growth, repair and survival of cardiomyocytes after stress.[150] Temporary disruption of the ErbB-2 signaling pathway by trastuzumab thus results in an inadequate or even maladaptive response to cardiac stress that can lead to systolic dysfunction and congestive heart failure.[151]

The proposed mechanism could explain some of the clinical features observed regarding trastuzumab such as the increased toxicity when used concomitantly with anthracyclines, but minimal toxicity when used just prior to anthracycline administration. The additive effects on cardiac function when trastuzumab is given to patients previously exposed to an anthracyclines is conjectured to constitute a sequential stress whereby the underlying damage, even in the absence of clear abnormalities in ejection fraction sets the stage for the subsequent cardiac insult or the inability to fully repair potentially reversible anthracycline injury; when given in the absence of an anthracycline, the cardiac dysfunction related to trastuzumab appears to be largely reversible.[147,152,153] As it is an insult that involves an organ often previously damaged by exposure to an anthracycline, the dilemma of how great a portion of the observed dysfunction is likely to return arises. The question of temporarily holding trastuzumab, permanently stopping the drug, the risks of restarting after functional recovery, and effective short- and long-term monitoring of these patients is under consideration; at least one group has suggested guidelines.[134,154]

Other Type II Agents ■ In addition to trastuzumab, lapatinib, sunitinib, and imatinib all exhibit characteristics of cardiac dysfunction that are qualitatively similar to those described for trastuzumab; cardiotoxicity is reversible, biopsy changes are either absent or, in contrast to those of the anthracyclines, nonspecific, and there is no cumulative dose-related relationship. Lapatinib cardiac dysfunction was reported in 2.2% of patients previously treated with anthracyclines, and 1.5% of patients without prior exposure to cardiotoxic regimens; most patients (88%) experienced some degree of reversibility with regard to cardiac dysfunction.[155] Sunitinib has been associated with increased blood pressure that may be associated with the cardiac dysfunction observed with this agent. Further reviews of the cardiotoxicity of sunitinib are underway.[156]

Other Drugs That Demonstrate a Decrease in Cardiac Function ■ Significant decreases in myocardial function are occasionally noted for other agents that do not clearly fit within either type I or type II. Rarely α-interferon has been associated with a dramatic decrease in ejection fraction.[157] The mechanism is unknown; however, patients who survive the initial episode usually go on to recover cardiac function.[158] An unusual form of cardiac damage is associated with high-dose cyclophosphamide administration. When severe, the damage takes the form of a hemorrhagic myocarditis.[159] The process is often acute, is related to high individual doses (usually 4.5 g/m^2 or more) rather than to the cumulative dose, and is associated with decreased ejection fractions and mean QRS voltage. Although severe hemorrhagic myocarditis may be fatal, milder presentations may be asymptomatic and reversible.

Treatment Considerations of Patients With Treatment-Related Cardiac Failure or Dysfunction ■ The most important treatment consideration in patients who develop anthracycline-associated cardiac dysfunction is the avoidance of additional anthracyclines. Once established, anthracycline-associated cardiac dysfunction differs little from other forms of cardiomyopathy and it is usually treated in a similar way. The American College of Cardiology and the American Heart Association have issued guidelines for the diagnosis and management of chronic heart failure in adults.[160] Patients who have been treated with anthracyclines but show no symptoms of cardiac dysfunction should have other conditions that exacerbate cardiac dysfunction aggressively treated. Hypertension should be controlled and lifestyle changes encouraged. Pharmacologic intervention should also be considered for those who have ejection fractions below 40%. ACE inhibitors and β-adrenergic blockers may be appropriate for patients in stage A and stage B (Fig. 130-7). For patients in stage C, salt restriction and diuretics may be added. Digitalis preparations may offer symptomatic relief, but probably do not prolong life. When the cardiac damage becomes moderate or severe, is associated with left ventricular dilatation, or causes persistent cardiac dysrhythmias, anticoagulation (warfarin sodium titrated to maintain the prothrombin time at least 1.5 times control) or antiplatelet therapy (enteric-coated aspirin 81-324 mg) should be considered. There is no specific therapy for anthracycline-related cardiomyopathy. An underlying malignancy should not, however, be considered a contraindication to aggressive therapy and, in selected patients, mechanical assist devices and cardiac transplantation may be considered for those who have achieved oncologic stability or cure.[161] The cardiac failure associated with trastuzumab is different, in that there is evidence for recovery. Whether or not recovery is directly influenced by the specific therapy for congestive heart failure is uncertain; some patients have recovered without therapy. In any event, symptomatic patients should be treated aggressively.

Agents Associated With Myocardial Ischemia or Thromboembolic Events

A number of agents have the potential to cause myocardial ischemia, with or without frank myocardial infarction. The most extensively studied agent that causes this is 5-fluorouracil (5-FU), especially when the agent is administered in combination with cisplatin.[162] Capecitabine is currently used in the treatment of gastrointestinal and breast malignancy, and is an orally administered prodrug which is enzymatically converted to 5-FU. Myocardial infarction and dysrhythmia have been reported with both drugs.[163,164] The mechanism of the ischemia is uncertain, but coronary artery vasoactivity or spasm probably plays a role. Isolated cases of myocardial ischemia have also occurred after the administration of vinblastine, vincristine, bleomycin, cisplatin, and biologic response modifiers. The wide spectrum of ischemic responses suggests that ischemia accompanying anticancer treatment is more common than is generally appreciated. Nonspecific electrocardiographic changes may be seen in nearly half the patients treated with 5-FU, and as many as 16% show electrocardiographic evidence of ischemia including ST-segment depression or elevation and changes suggesting

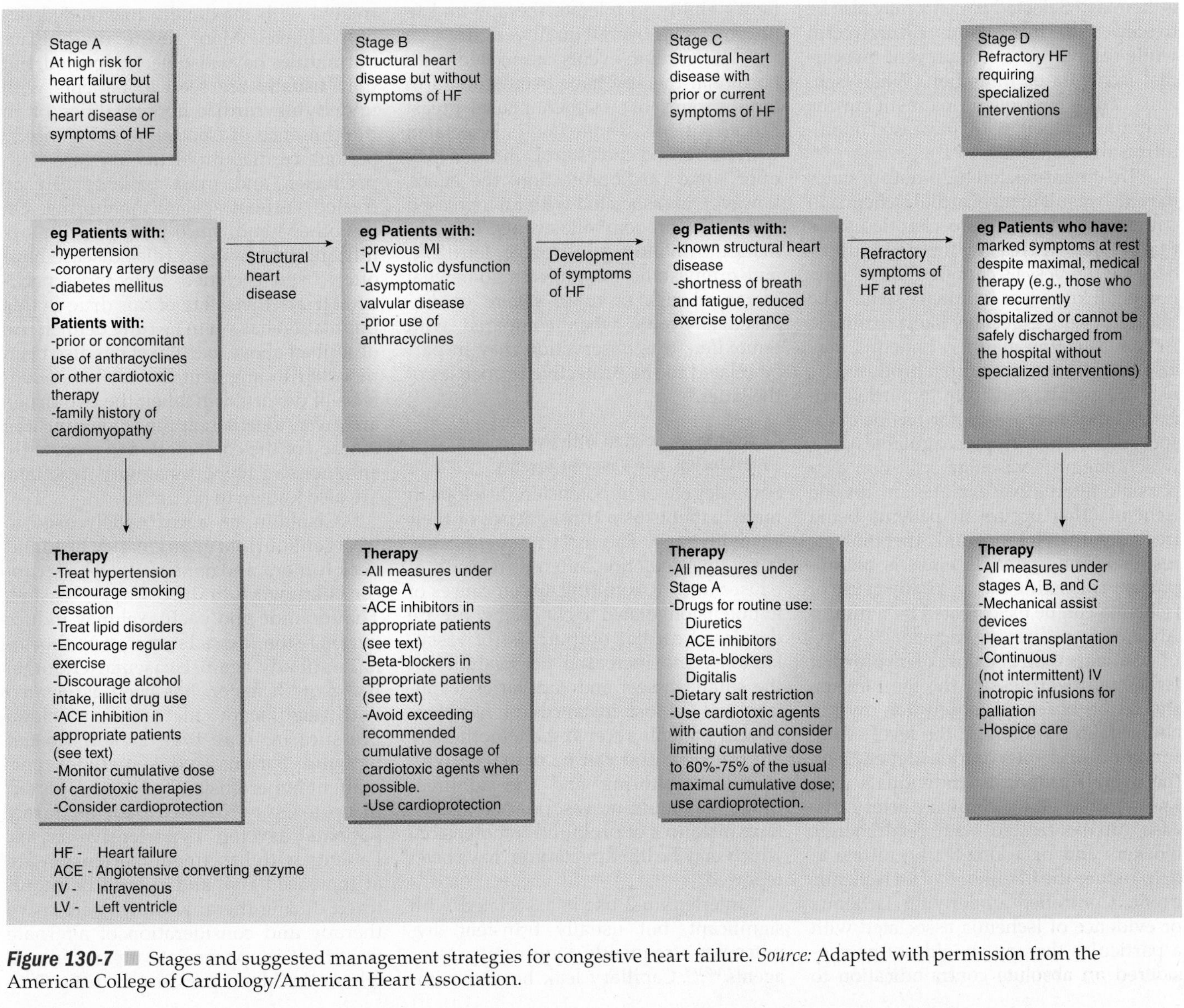

Figure 130-7 Stages and suggested management strategies for congestive heart failure. *Source:* Adapted with permission from the American College of Cardiology/American Heart Association.

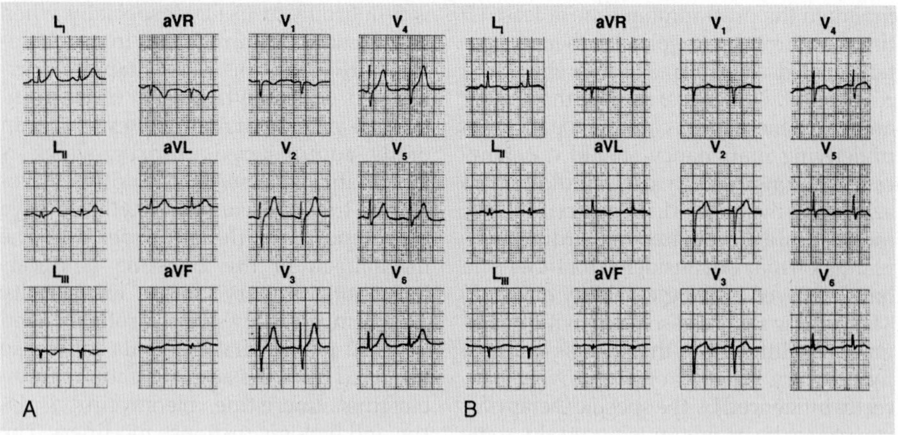

Figure 130-8 Electrocardiogram showing ischemic changes associated with 5-FU administration (**A**) Before treatment, and (**B**) Two days after treatment. Note the onset of lateral T-wave inversion after treatment.

myocardial infarction (Fig. 130-8). Many of the affected patients have underlying coronary artery disease, which suggests that preexisting coronary artery abnormalities augment the ischemic potential of 5-FU. The use of a calcium channel blocker has been reported to prevent the ischemia.[165] Selected patients may also be treated with intravenous nitroglycerin while receiving 5-FU to prevent myocardial ischemia or infarction. When ischemia can be controlled treatment may be continued, albeit with increased monitoring and caution.

Treatment-related high-output states may also result in myocardial ischemia in patients with fixed atherosclerotic lesions that preclude increasing the blood supply because the vessels cannot dilate, a phenomenon known as "coronary steal." The interferons are especially likely to initiate ischemia in this manner. Ischemia may also result from fever, often produced by biologic agents, and from hyperthyroidism. Tumor necrosis factor has been associated with a hypercoagulable state, which suggests vascular occlusion as a possible alternative explanation for the ischemia that occurs in patients being treated with cytokines and other biologic response modifiers. Anemia is an important coexisting factor, as any cause of ischemia can be exacerbated by a diminished oxygen-carrying capacity.

Patients with evidence of myocardial ischemia, regardless of the mechanism, should be observed closely for rhythm abnormalities, although the level of observation and intervention depends on the overall prognosis. Individuals with known preexisting coronary artery disease can be treated with β-adrenergic blockers and/or a long-acting nitrate to help reduce the likelihood of an ischemic event. Controlled underlying ischemia or evidence of ischemia associated with a particular therapy should not be considered an absolute contraindication to further treatment with the implicated agent or agents. Cancer patients with underlying coronary artery disease are often candidates for revascularization, and stress testing as well as coronary angiography with appropriate interventions may significantly improve the patient's ability to tolerate therapy and to improve their overall quality of life.

The cardiac events associated with hormonal therapy have been studied in large groups of postmenopausal breast cancer patients. Tamoxifen is associated with decreased cholesterol, and this may offer some cardioprotection; the agent, however, is associated with an increased risk of thromboembolic events. The aromatase inhibitors anastrozole, letrozole, and exemestane may have a somewhat increased risk of more severe cardiovascular events when compared with tamoxifen; this observation may in part be related to the protective properties of the latter.[166]

Agents Associated With Hypotension, Hypertension, and Vascular Toxicity

Some degree of hypotension develops in many patients as a consequence of their chemotherapy. The most frequent cause is volume depletion, often as a result of nausea and/or vomiting. Other causes of hypotension related to chemotherapy are decreased cardiac output, loss of vascular tone, and increased permeability of the small vessels and capillaries (capillary leak). Most instances of hypotension in patients receiving chemotherapy are transient and can be managed with careful monitoring and the administration of fluids or vasopressor agents. Rare instances of profound hypotension, which may be life threatening, have been reported.

Interleukin-2 use is associated with significant, but usually transient, hypotension, frequently requiring pressor agents.[167,168] Capillary leak has been implicated. Interleukin-2–related myocardial ischemia is possibly related to the hypotension, although a direct toxic effect has not been excluded. Interleukin-2 is also associated with an increased incidence of supraventricular dysrhythmias and myocarditis.[169] The vasodilation that occurs in response to interleukin-2 appears to be mediated by the release of nitric oxide. Evidence has suggested that NG-monomethyl-L-arginine, an inhibitor of nitric oxide synthase, reverses the hypotension caused by interleukin-2, lending support to the role of nitric oxide in the production of hypotension and indicating the therapeutic potential of NG-monomethyl-L-arginine as well.[170]

Homoharringtonine, an investigational agent used in the treatment of leukemias, is associated with dose-related, sometimes severe, hypotension arising immediately after its intravenous administration.[171] Intravenous epinephrine has been helpful in stabilizing patients in this setting.

Considerable interest has surrounded the possible cardiac effects of paclitaxel. In one study, asymptomatic bradycardia occurred in 29% of patients treated with maximally tolerated doses of paclitaxel. More severe rhythm abnormalities have also been reported, but they usually are seen in patients with underlying cardiac abnormalities or in the presence of electrolyte imbalance.[172] Serious cardiac problems are rare with paclitaxel, and most patients can be treated without special monitoring. On the other hand, since patients with significant underlying cardiac disease have often been excluded from most paclitaxel trials, the safety of this drug in this population has yet to be fully defined. As described above, paclitaxel has also been reported to augment the cardiotoxic effects of doxorubicin when the two drugs are given together; at the same time, the efficacy of the combination is reportedly enhanced.[173] Hypersensitivity reactions are also known to occur.[174]

Cisplatin, an agent widely used to treat genitourinary malignancy, head and neck tumors, and nonsmall cell lung cancer is known to induce a hypertension. Thalidomide and paclitaxel may induce hypotension. Bevacizumab, a monoclonal antibody against vascular endothelial growth factor, has been associated with significant increases in blood pressure in more than 25% of treated patients. Serious and sometimes permanent hypertension has been reported in up to 14% of treated patients; rarely patients develop hypertensive crises. Patients with baseline hypertension are at increased risk and should be monitored during therapy. Antihypertensive therapy and consideration of alternate treatment is appropriate for patients in whom the blood pressure is difficult to control. Sunitinib, alemtuzumab, gemtuzumab, infliximab, muromanoab-CD3, rituximab, and sorafenib are all associated with increased incidence of hypertension.

Cardiac Complications of Radiation Therapy

Links between radiation to the chest in the treatment for malignancy and subsequent heart disease have been clearly established. Inclusion of cardiac tissue in the radiation portals can lead to a broad spectrum of disease, which often presents decades after exposure. Recognition of these risks has led to dramatic improvements in radiation techniques over the years, but the degree to which the heart can be spared has not been fully determined, as long-term follow-up studies in patients treated with modern techniques are still underway.

The pathophysiology of ionizing radiation's cardiotoxic effects involves both DNA damage and generation of reactive oxygen species. Cells with higher turnover are more susceptible, particularly the vascular endothelium. Small vessel damage then leads to inflammation and ultimately fibrosis of cardiac tissue. All layers of the heart can be involved, leading to acute and chronic pericardial disease, accelerated coronary artery disease, cardiomyopathy, valvular disease and conduction system abnormalities. Secondary cardiac malignancies attributed to radiation therapy have even been reported.[175] The heart responds to the radiation insult over time with late-presentation and chronic progressive functional decline showing a direct correlation with the radiation fraction to the heart. Animal models have demonstrated a radiation dose-dependent chronic congestive myocardial failure that follows radiation damage to the myocardial microvasculature and that indirectly damages the coronary macrovasulature when coupled with cholesterol feeding; histologic examination shows a marked reduction in capillary density, myocardial degeneration and necrosis with interstitial fibrosis.[176,177] Cell kinetic studies show increased endothelial cell proliferation about 30-100 days postradiation. The morphologic changes in animal models parallel the drops in cardiac output and left ventricular ejection fraction. The slightly reduced cardiac function is maintained for many weeks due to a compensatory upregulation of cardiac β-adrenergic receptors; in the denervated heart the stroke volume and cardiac contractility show rapid and steady deterioration.

Human data on cardiac effects of radiation therapy have come mostly from patients with Hodgkin lymphoma and breast cancer, who historically received significant doses of cardiac radiation but also provided long-term follow-up. In contrast, survival in lung cancer is generally too poor to allow significant development of cardiac complications. Risk factors include total radiation dose (generally >35Gy), volume of the heart exposed, and specific techniques used, but other factors play a role, including age at the time of exposure (younger patients at higher risk), concurrent treatment with anthracycline-containing chemotherapy regimens, and traditional cardiac risk factors.

Radiation treatment for Hodgkin lymphoma carries the highest risk of cardiac complications due to proximity of mediastinal nodes to the heart, younger age at diagnosis, and good potential for long-term survival. The relative risk of fatal cardiac events has been reported as high as 7.2 after radiation-containing treatment.[178] As it may take years or even decades for radiation-related heart disease to clinically manifest, the discovery of major complications may not appear until late follow-up assessments are undertaken; in some instances this may be years or decades after the initial exposure. The most common complications are valvular lesions (predominantly regurgitant) and myocardial infarction, but also seen are restrictive cardiomyopathy, dysrhythmia and autonomic dysfunction. Pericardial disease has become less prevalent with better cardiac shielding and other technical improvements.[179]

Breast cancer cohorts provide us with the richest body of evidence regarding radiation effects on the heart, due both to overall disease prevalence and to the opportunity to compare right-sided versus left-sided disease. Several studies have utilized this natural control group to distinguish between systemic effects of chemotherapeutics and those of localized cardiac radiation. A strong correlation between radiation therapy and increased cardiovascular mortality was established by many early randomized trials.[180] Improved techniques, including better cardiac shielding, tangential fields, and respiratory gating have certainly reduced or delayed cardiac morbidity and mortality, but significant risk probably remains, especially for left-sided cancers. Inclusion of the right or left internal mammary lymph node chain in the radiation field increases cardiac exposure and has been shown to increase subsequent cardiovascular complications. Similar to the data for Hodgkin lymphoma, risk of cardiac events after radiation therapy increases with duration of follow-up, treatment with anthracyclines, and traditional cardiovascular risk factors.

Clinical manifestations of radiation cardiotoxicity are broad. Acute pericarditis can occur at the time of radiation treatment, and pericardial effusion is commonly seen in the acute and subacute setting, but can also be chronic. Distinction from malignant pericardial effusion can be difficult and occasionally necessitates fluid analysis by cytology. Cardiac tamponade is rare. Chronic inflammation can manifest as constrictive pericarditis, which can be challenging to diagnose and carries a grave prognosis unless the patient is well enough to undergo surgical pericardiectomy.

Coronary artery disease after radiation can present as angina, myocardial infarction or sudden death, and risk increases with time. At least two mechanisms appear to be involved in macrovascular disease. First, radiation induces thickening of the arterial wall secondary to intimal and adventitial proliferation; the luminal area is thereby reduced. Second, radiation greatly accelerates atherosclerosis and acts synergistically with that process to enhance cholesterol deposition and luminal ulceration.[181] Thus, as noted above, traditional cardiac risk factors such as smoking and dyslipidemia play a key cooperative role in the pathogenesis. By reason of its location, the left anterior descending artery is the most frequently affected.

The treatment of radiation-associated vascular injury is similar to the conventional treatment of ischemic cardiac disease; nitrates, β-adrenergic blockers, platelet inhibitors, and calcium channel blockers are the mainstays of pharmacological therapy. Invasive approaches for the management of ischemic heart disease are also often helpful; balloon angioplasty, however, often requires inflation pressures that are higher than those ordinarily used, and longer periods of balloon inflation may be required. Bypass surgery may prove more difficult than usual from a technical standpoint because of the smaller vascular lumens and because the surgeon must work in a previously irradiated field. Nevertheless, bypass surgery remains an important option for these patients.

The spectrum of radiation-induced cardiomyopathy includes diastolic dysfunction, restrictive cardiomyopathy, and systolic dysfunction. Small vessel ischemic disease and fibrosis are the predominant underlying pathology, with subsequent ventricular remodeling possible. Restrictive cardiomyopathy can be very difficult to distinguish from pericardial constriction—especially since both may be present in the same patient. Endomyocardial biopsy is sometimes employed prior to pericardiectomy to rule out coexisting myocardial disease, which carries a prohibitive operative mortality.

Valvular diseases, while common, are usually not severe. Nevertheless, they are progressive and can contribute to significant morbidity that accompanies the irradiated heart. The most common lesions found are tricuspid regurgitation, mitral regurgitation, and aortic regurgitation, but aortic stenosis is occasionally encountered.[182,183] Histologically, the valves show endocardial thickening resembling fibroelastosis.[184]

Radiation injury to the cardiac conduction system has also been noted and is usually suggested by abnormalities on the electrocardiogram. Nonspecific changes involving the P wave are frequently seen but may be due, in part, to concomitant radiation injury of the lung. Prolongation of the PR interval is often seen, as are supranodal and infranodal atrioventricular blocks. Complete heart block is occasionally encountered, and pacemaker implantation may prove lifesaving for such patients. Autonomic dysfunction can manifest with inappropriate sinus tachycardia, bradycardia, or inadequate heart rate response to exercise.

Selected References

The complete reference list can be found at www.CANCERMEDICINE8.com

1. Ewer MS, Benjamin RS, Yeh ET. Cardiac complications. In: Holland J, Frei E, editors. *Cancer Medicine.* 6 ed. Hamilton Ontario: BC Decker; 2003;2131–2149.
2. Feigenbaum H. *Echocardiography.* 5th ed. Philadelphia: Lea & Febiger; 1995.
6. Caiani EG, Corsi C, Sugeng L, et al. Improved quantification of left ventricular mass based on endo- and epicardial surface detection using real-time three-dimensional echocardiography. *Heart.* May 12, 2005.
7. Ewer M, Gibbs H, Swafford J, Benjamin R. Cardiotoxicity in patients receiving trastuzumab (Herceptin): primary toxicity, synergistic or sequential stress, or surveillance artifact? *Semin Oncol.* 1999;26(suppl 12):96–101.
8. Francone M, Dymarkowski S, Kalantzi M, J B. Magnetic rosonance imaging n the evaluation of the pericardium. A pictoral essay. *Radiol Med.* 2005;109(January–February):64–74.
9. Edelman R. Contrast-enhanced MR imaging of the heart: overview of the leterature. *Radiology.* 2004;232(September): 653–668.
10. Lawson M, Blackwell G, Pohost G. Cardiovascular magnetic resonance imaging: a review of principles and utilities. *Am Coll Cardial Curr J Rev.* 1994;4:7.
11. Kramer C. Current and future applications of cardiovascularmagneticresonanceimaging. *Cardiol Rev.* 2000;8(July–August):216–222.
20. Nugue O, Millaire A. Neoplastic versus nonmalignant pericardial effusion in patients with malignancies: etiology, diagnostic profile and clinical outcome. In: Seferociv P, Spodick D, Maisch B, editors. *Pericardiology.* Belgrade: Science Publichers; 2000:339–344.
21. Pozzoli M, Capomolla S, Pinna G, Cobelli F, Tavazzi L. Doppler echocardiography reliably predicts pulmonary artery wedge pressure in patients with chronic heart failure with and without mitral regurgitation. *J Am Coll Cardiol.* March 15, 1996;27(4):883–893.
22. Posner M, Cohen G, Skarin A. Pericardial disease in patients with cancer: the differentiation of malignant from idiopathic and radiation-induced pericarditis. *Am J Med.* 1981;71:407–413.
23. Eerdekens M, Nouwen E, Pollet D, Briers T, De Broe M. Placental alkaline phosphatase and cancer antigen-125 in sera of patients with benign and malignant diseases. *Clin Chem.* 1985;31:687–690.
24. Nagele H, Bahlo M, Klapdor R, Schaeperkoetter D, Rodiger W. CA 125 and its relation to cardiac function. *Am Heart J.* 1999;137:1039–1044.
25. Porte H, Janecki-Delebecq T, Finzi L, Metois D, Millaire A, Wurtz A. Pericardoscopy for primary management of pericardial effusion in cancer patients. *Eur J Cardiothorac Surg.* 1999(16):287–291.
26. Spodick D. Current concepts: acute cardiac tamponade. *N Engl J Med.* 2003;349:684–690.
27. Press O, Livingston R. Management of malignant pericardial effusion and tamponade. *JAMA.* 1987;257:1088–1092.
28. Vaitkus P, Herrmann H, LeWinter M. Treatment of malignant pericardial effusion. *JAMA.* 1994;272:59–64.
29. Liberman M, Labos C, Sampalis J, Sheiner N, Mulder D. Ten-year surgical experience with nontraumatic pericardial effusions: a comparison between the subxyphoid and transthoracic approaches to pericardial window. *Arch Surg.* 2005;140:191–195.
30. Tsang T, Seward J, Barnes M, et al. Outcomes of primary and secondary treatment of pericardial effusion in patients with malignancy. *Mayo Clin Proc.* 2000;75:248–253.
66. Carroll J, Gaasch W, McAdam K. Amyloid cardiomyopathy: Characterization by a distinctive voltage/mass relation. *Am J Cardiol.* 1982;49:9–13.
67. Lekakis J, Dimopoulos M, Nanas J. Antimyosin scintigraphy for detection of cardiac amyloidosis. *Am J Cardiol.* 1997;80:1491–1492.
68. Tzankov A, Polzl G, Mairinger T. Congo red-positive cardiac kappa-AL amyloidosis in plasmacytoma—case report and review of the literature. *Acta Med Austriaca.* 2003;30(1):29–32.
69. Rubinow A, Skinner M, Cohen AS. Digoxin sensitivity in amyloid cardiomyopathy. *Circulation.* June 1981;63(6):1285–1288.
70. Feng D, Edwards WD, Oh JK, et al. Intracardiac thrombosis and embolism in patients with cardiac amyloid. *Circulation.* 2007;116:2420–2426.
71. Nakamura H, Hashimot T, Taguchi T, et al. Chemoembolization. *Gan To Kagaku Ryoho.* 1987;14:1656–1663.
72. Fuchs U, Zittermann A, Suhr O, et al. Heart transplantation in a 68-year-old patient with senile systemic amyloidosis. *Am J Transplant.* May 2005;5:1159–1162.
83. Bristow M, Thompson P, Martin R, Mason J, Billingham M, Harrison D. Early anthracycline cardiotoxicity. *Am J Med.* 1978; 65:823–832.
84. Bristow M, Sageman W, Scott R, et al. Acute and chronic cardiovascular effects of doxorubicin in the dog: the cardiovascular pharmacology of drug-induced histamine release. *J Cardiovasc Pharmacol.* 1980;2:487–515.
85. Herman E, Lipshultz S, Rifai N, et al. Use of cardiac troponin T levels as an indicator of doxorubicin-induced cardiotoxicity. *Can Res.* 1998;38:195–197.
86. Ferretti G, Mandala M, Bria E, et al. Is cardiac troponin T serum level an accurate surrogate for acute doxorubicin-related myocardial injury? *Ann Oncol.* April 27, 2005;16:1403–1404.
87. Cardinale D, Sandri MT, Colombo A, et al. Prognostic value of troponin I in cardiac risk stratification of cancer patients undergoing high-dose chemotherapy. *Circulation.* June 8, 2004;109(22):2749–2754.
99. Mackay B, Ewer M, Carrasco C, Benjamin R. Assessment of anthracycline cardiomyopathy by endomyocardial biopsy. *Ultrastruct Pathol.* 1994;18:203–211.
100. Ewer M, Carrasco C, MacKay B, Ali M, Benjamin R. Cardiac biopsy procedures at a cancer center. Paper presented at: *Proc American Society of Clinical Oncology.* 1991;(abstract #1189) 10:336.
101. Ibrahim NK, Buzdar AU, Asmar L, Theriault RL, Hortobagyi GN. Doxorubicin-based adjuvant chemotherapy in elderly breast cancer patients: the M.D. Anderson experience, with long-term follow-up. *Ann Oncol.* December 2000;11:1597–1601.
102. Aydiner A, Bugra Z, Topuz E, Meric M. Acute myocardial infarction in man treated with epirubicin for non-Hodgkin lymphoma. *Am J Clin Oncol.* October 1995;18:444–448.
111. Rahman AM, Yusuf SW, Ewer MS. Anthracycline-induced cardiotoxicity and the cardiac-sparing effect of liposomal formulation. *Int J Nanomedicine.* 2007;2:567–583.
112. Ewer M, Martin F, Henderson I, Shapiro C, Benjamin R, Gabizon A. Cardiac safety of liposomal anthracyclines. *Semin Oncol.* 2004;31(Suppl 13):161–181.
113. Theodoulou M, Hudis C. Cardiac profiles of liposomal anthracyclines: greater cardiac safety versus conventional doxorubicin? *Cancer.* 2004;100:2052–2063.
114. Harris L, Batist G, Belt R, et al. The TLC D-99 Study Group. Liposome-encapsulated doxorubicin compared with conventional doxorubicin in a randomized multicenter trial as first-line therapy of metastatic breast carcinoma. *Cancer.* 2002;94:25–36.
115. Valero V, Buzdar A, Theriault R. Phase II trial of liposome-encapsulated doxorubicin, cyclophosphamide, and fluorouracil as first-line therapy in patients with metastatic breast cancer. *J Clin Oncol.* 1999;17:1425–1434.
116. Bafaloukos D, Papadimitriou C, Linardou H, et al. Combination of pegylated liposomal doxorubicin (PLD) and paclitaxel in patients with advanced soft tissue sarcoma: a phase II study of the Hellenic Cooperative Oncology Group. *Br J Cancer.* November 1, 2004;91:1639–1644.
130. Lopez M, Patrizia V. European trials with dexrazoxane in amelioration of doxorubicin and epirubicin-induced cardiotoxicity. *Semin Oncol.* 1998;25(suppl 10):55–60.
131. Lipschultz S, Colan S, Silverman L, et al. Dexrazoxane reduces incidence of doshurxorubicin-associated acute myocardiocyte injury in children with acute lymphoblastic leukemia (ALL.). *Proceedings of ASCO.* 2002.

131 Respiratory Complications

Vickie R. Shannon, MD ▪ George A. Eapen, MD ▪ Carlos A. Jimenez, MD ▪ Rodolfo C. Morice, MD ▪ Elizabeth L. Travis, PhD ▪ Lara Bashoura, MD ▪ Amar Safdar, MD, FACP ▪ Scott E. Evans, MD ▪ Roberto Adachi, MD ▪ Saadia A. Faiz, MD ▪ Diwakar D. Balachandran, MD ▪ Joseph L. Nates, MD, MBA, FCCM ▪ S. Egbert Pravinkumar, MD, FRCP ▪ Burton F. Dickey, MD

Introduction

The respiratory system is particularly susceptible to complications of cancer and cancer therapy. This vulnerability arises from the stringent architectural requirements for gas exchange, the continuous exposure of the respiratory tract to the external environment, and the severe symptoms that accompany respiratory compromise. Gas exchange requires patent airways, an effective musculoskeletal ventilatory pump, a thin alveolocapillary membrane, and adequate blood flow through the pulmonary circulation. In cancer patients, primary and metastatic tumors of the chest compromise major airways; malignant pleural effusions externally compress the lungs and impair diaphragmatic function; direct, hematogenous or lymphangitic spread of tumor replaces functioning lung parenchyma; resectional surgery reduces parenchymal volume and nonresectional surgery can transiently impair lung function; radiation therapy, chemotherapy, stem cell therapy and infection injure the vulnerable alveolocapillary membrane; tumors directly or indirectly compromise the musculoskeletal pump; venous thromboembolism and pulmonary vasculopathy obstruct blood flow through the lungs.

The respiratory system in normal persons contains considerable physiologic reserve, such that surgical loss of one lung is generally well tolerated. However in cancer patients, insults to multiple components of the respiratory system may result in progressive loss of physiologic reserve and the development of increasing dyspnea. Dyspnea is a very distressing symptom. Treatment should be directed at the underlying pathophysiologic process whenever possible, but when reversal of the underlying processes is not possible, palliation of dyspnea is mandatory. Other common symptoms leading to pulmonary consultation include cough, chest pain and hemoptysis.

In this chapter, we will discuss the pathophysiology, diagnosis and management of the major respiratory complications of cancer and its therapy. We begin with the direct effects of cancer on the lungs (airspace compromise and malignant pleural effusion), then consider the effects of cancer therapy on the lungs (postoperative respiratory failure, chemotherapy and radiation induced lung injury, pneumonia, and the complications of stem cell transplantation), review major indirect effects of cancer on the lungs (thromboembolism and respiratory pump compromise), and end with respiratory failure in the cancer patient.

Malignant Airway Obstruction

Malignant airspace disease may be central or peripheral, focal or diffuse, endoluminal, extraluminal or both. The dominant symptom complex associated with this process depends upon the location and extent of disease, which also dictates therapy.

Common Cancer Types and Clinical Presentation

The most common cause of malignant airway obstruction is direct extension from an adjacent tumor, particularly bronchogenic carcinoma. Esophageal and thyroid malignancies also frequently extend directly into the airways. Primary tumors of the major airways are relatively rare, with squamous cell carcinoma, adenoid cystic carcinoma and carcinoid tumors most often implicated.[1] Airway obstruction secondary to metastatic malignancies from renal, breast and thyroid sources has also been reported. Lymphomatous involvement of the central airways and extrinsic compression by malignant lymphadenopathy causing obstruction has also been described. Both endoluminal disease and extrinsic compression by tumor may severely compromise airway luminal diameter. Reduction in airway caliber and architectural distortion synergistically impair airflow obstruction and mucus clearance, leading to increased work of breathing and dyspnea.[2] Luminal narrowing of the trachea and mainstem bronchi in central airway obstruction leads to airflow limitation and an associated symptom complex that often includes dyspnea, cough, wheeze, stridor and atelectasis. Airway obstruction beyond the mainstem bronchi usually results in atelectasis, postobstructive pneumonitis, cough and dyspnea. Individual patient presentations range from asymptomatic discovery on staging workup to frank respiratory failure due to critical airway obstruction.[3] Exertional dyspnea typically occurs when tracheal diameter is reduced below 8 mm. Further reductions in tracheal diameter to <5 mm are usually associated with dyspnea at rest.[4] Chronic obstructive pulmonary disease (COPD) exacerbations or mucosal edema and increased secretions that accompany superimposed pneumonias may precipitate respiratory failure, even among patients with only moderate tumor-related airflow limitation. Symptoms may thus improve with measures directed at treating the infection or COPD exacerbation.

Differential Diagnosis

While critical airway obstruction is not usually a diagnostic challenge, the clinical presentation of subcritical obstruction can be. Stridor is usually pathognomonic of significant tracheal obstruction. Other findings, including dyspnea and wheezing, are prominent but nonspecific clinical symptoms that denote airflow limitation. Concurrent conditions, such as congestive heart failure, pleural effusions, and pulmonary emboli may produce similar symptoms, obscuring the diagnosis.

Diagnostic Evaluation

The diagnostic workup is aimed at establishing a definitive diagnosis, quantifying airflow limitation and delineating anatomic extent in an effort to optimize therapeutic strategies. The characteristic blunting noted in the flow-volume loop upon pulmonary function testing often provides the earliest indication of tracheal obstruction. However, this is a relatively insensitive test, with positive findings noted only with tracheal diameters below 10 mm.[5] Spirometry may precipitate frank respiratory failure in patients with severe airway obstruction, and therefore should be used with caution in this subgroup of patients. Rarely, deviation or compression of the trachea may be seen on plain chest radiographs. Plain chest films are otherwise useless in defining the anatomic extent of tumor or therapeutic options. Standard chest computed tomography as well as the latest iterations of low dose, multidetector scanners and advanced airway imaging techniques that allow multiplanar and three-dimensional reconstruction provide valuable additional information regarding the extent of the lesion and guidance in optimizing therapeutic strategies.[6] Bronchoscopy, either flexible or rigid, remains the gold standard in the workup of airway obstruction. Histologic confirmation of malignancy can be obtained at the time of the examination. Furthermore, bronchoscopy offers direct visualization of the lesion, which permits precise characterization of tumor vascularity and the extent of obstruction, as well as the degree of obstruction attributable to endoluminal versus extraluminal disease. Recent reports have also supported the use of endobronchial ultrasonography as an adjunctive tool in treatment planning.[7]

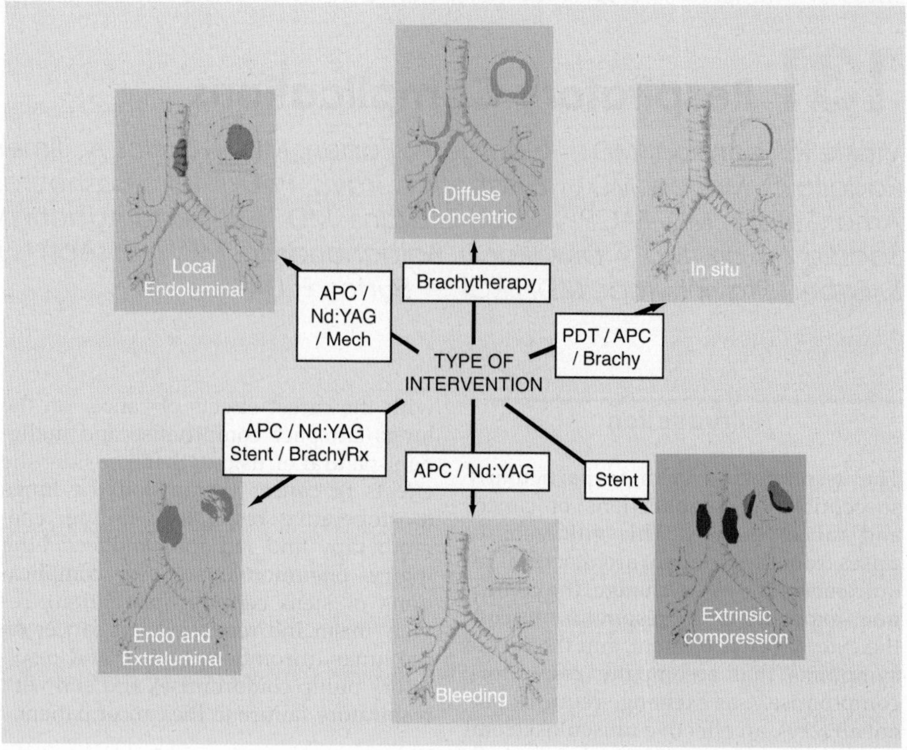

Figure 131-1 Approach to airway obstruction using interventional bronchoscopic therapy.

Management of Malignant Airway Obstruction

Tumor characteristics, including histologic type, stage and location, and patient attributes, such as urgency of presentation and performance status, dictate management. Therapeutic strategies vary based on the location and type of obstruction, as well as the local expertise and available institution-specific resources. Surgical resection provides the best prospect for long-term disease control and should be considered in all patients during the initial evaluation. Localized involvement of the small airways and lung parenchyma is best treated by surgical resection, if feasible. In many cases, however, external beam radiotherapy or systemic chemotherapy may be the only treatment options. Patients with central airway obstruction often present with either medically inoperable or surgically unresectable disease. While a comprehensive review of the various modalities is beyond the scope of this chapter, some basic principles are outlined (Fig. 131-1). In emergent cases, the barrel of the rigid bronchoscope may be used to mechanically core out the tumor and dilate the airways, providing palliation. Flexible bronchoscopy and balloon bronchoplasty may be used to dilate the airways in less urgent cases.[8] Electrocautery, argon plasma coagulation, laser therapy, cryotherapy, brachytherapy and photodynamic therapy, are reasonable approaches for predominantly endoluminal disease (Fig. 131-2). Extraluminal-predominant disease may be best treated with external beam radiotherapy and endobronchial stent placement (Fig. 131-3). Since most lesions are mixed with endo- and extraluminal components, multimodality therapy, using endobronchial laser therapy with mechanical debulking followed by stent placement and subsequent consolidation with external beam radiotherapy, for example, is quite common. Symptom palliation, resulting in reduction in levels of care, may be accomplished in most instances with the judicious application of endoscopic techniques.[9] Patients should be carefully evaluated with an early referral to an experienced bronchoscopist who can match the various therapeutic modalities available to the individual patient.

Malignant Pleural Effusions

The presence of malignant cells in pleural fluid is a common clinical problem in the cancer setting that signifies distant spread of tumor and, hence, advanced disease. Malignant pleural effusions thus have significant therapeutic and prognostic implications. Estimates of the incidence of malignant pleural effusions in the United States approach 150,000 cases annually.[10] Malignant pleural involvement without effusion occurs in up to 45% of patients with metastatic disease to the pleura.[11] In primary pleural malignancies, such as malignant mesothelioma, pleural effusions may also be absent. Almost any type of neoplasm can affect the pleura. Lung cancer accounts for up to half of all malignant effusions, followed in frequency by breast carcinoma and lymphoma. In 5-10% of patients, a primary tumor cannot be identified.[12,13] The incidence of mesothelioma, the most common primary pleural malignancy in the United States, varies widely with geographic location. Most pleural malignancies arise from tumor emboli to the visceral pleura. The parietal pleura may be secondarily involved presumably by seeding from the visceral pleura. Direct extensions of tumor from the lung, chest wall, mediastinal structures, or diaphragm, and hematogenous metastasis to the parietal pleura are other mechanisms that contribute to the genesis of malignant pleural fluid formation.[14] In addition to direct tumoral involvement of the pleura, malignant pleural effusions can result from lymphatic blockage anywhere between the parietal pleura and the mediastinal lymph nodes.[15] Elevations in the local production of vascular endothelial growth factor (VGEF), a potent mediator of increased vascular permeability, also plays a significant role in the formation of malignant pleural effusions.[16,17]

Seventeen percent of all pleural effusions in patients with cancer are "paramalignant," a term used for effusions that occur in the setting of cancer that are not caused by direct malignant in-

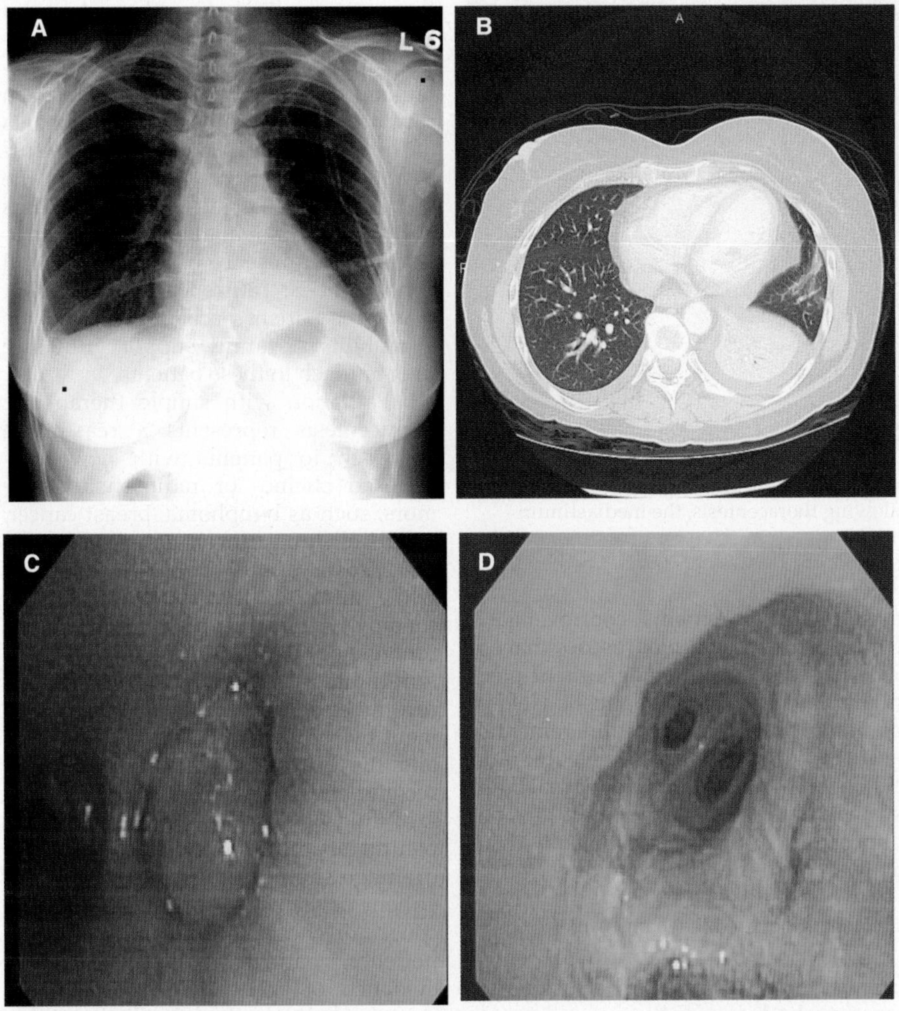

Figure 131-2 Left lower lobe collapse secondary to metastatic sarcoma **(A** and **B)**. Complete obstruction of the LLL basilar segments due to a large obstructing tumor was noted at bronchoscopy **(C)**, which was removed using snare forceps and argon plasma coagulation, revealing a patent distal airway **(D)**.

volvement of the pleural space.[14] These effusions develop as a result of local or systemic effects of the tumor, complications of cancer therapy, or concurrent nonmalignant disease.[18] Lymphatic obstruction is associated with both malignant and paramalignant effusions and is the most common cause of paramalignant effusions. Other common causes include bronchial obstruction, trapped lung, and pulmonary embolism.

Clinical Manifestations, Imaging Studies, and Diagnosis

Patients most commonly present with symptoms of progressive exertional dyspnea. Cough may also be a troubling symptom with large effusions. Constitutional symptoms are common signals of advanced disease and thus malaise, weight loss, and poor appetite are recurrent complaints, which may become more frequent as the performance status worsens. Hemoptysis and chest wall pain are less common symptoms that indicate endobronchial malignant disease and tumoral invasion of the chest wall.

Standard chest roentgenograms and bilateral decubitus films of the chest provide critical information in the initial evaluation of pleural effusions, including effusion size, position of the mediastinum and diaphragms, presence of loculations and air fluid levels within the pleural space, and characteristics of the underlying lung parenchyma. Lateral decubitus projections are useless in the evaluation of massive pleural effusions that obscure the entire hemithorax. Knowledge regarding the position of the mediastinum is imperative in therapeutic decision making. Large pleural effusions with contralateral mediastinal shift typically require prompt therapeutic thoracentesis, while those with a centered mediastinum or ipsilateral shift of the mediastinum should be approached cautiously (Figs. 131-4 and 131-5). In addition to pleural effusions, other disease processes that may cause an ipsilateral shift of the mediastinum or a centered mediastinum with hemithorax opacification include a frozen mediastinum associated with malignant mesothelioma or lymphoma, atelectasis related to occlusion of the ipsilateral central airway, or extensive tumoral infiltration of the ipsilateral lung simulating a large effusion.[18] Computed tomography (CT) is especially valuable in delineating alternate diagnoses and in identifying loculated effusions. In addition, CT offers better anatomical information of the chest wall, parietal and visceral pleura, mediastinal structures and lung parenchyma.[19] Ultrasonography is easy to learn and interpret and provides guidance in locating the optimal site for thoracentesis. This instrument is particularly helpful in the setting of loculated pleural effusions.[20] Positron emission tomography (PET) with 18-fluorodeoxyglucose is particularly helpful in highlighting extrapleural extension of disease associated with malignant mesothelioma. The utility of PET scanning in the evaluation

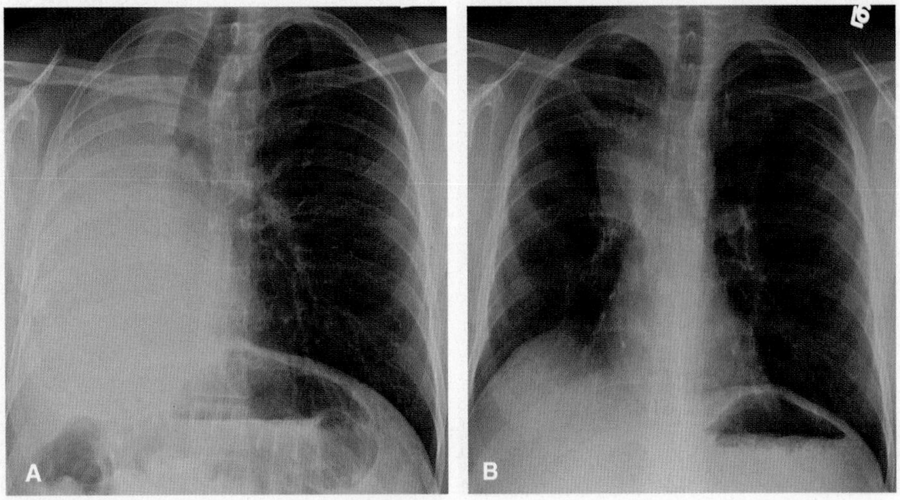

Figure 131-3 Complete opacification of the right thorax secondary to obstruction of the right mainstem bronchus by a large, predominantly extraluminal mass **(A)**. A wire stent was placed into the bronchus intermedius **(B)**, resulting in partial reexpansion of the right lung.

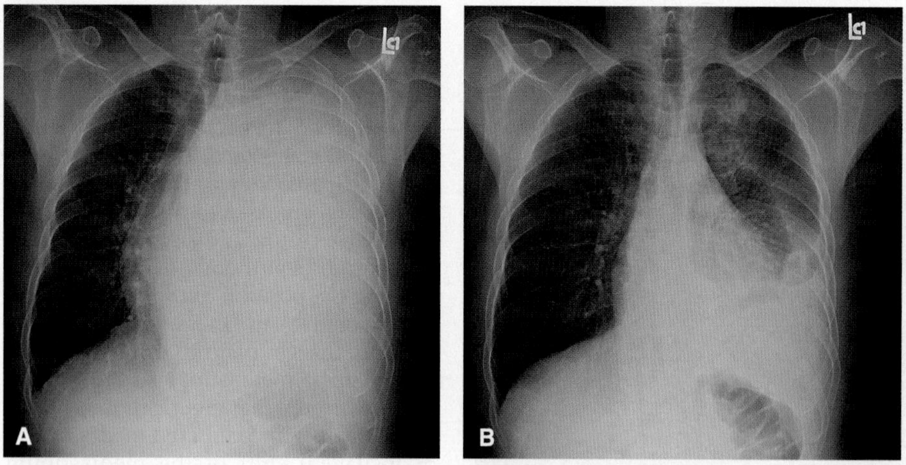

Figure 131-4 Large left-sided pleural effusion causing opacification of the left hemithorax and contralateral shift of the mediastinum **(A)**. Following thoracentesis, the mediastinum shifted back the midline **(B)**.

of other malignant pleural diseases has not been established. Magnetic resonance imaging (MRI) adds valuable information regarding extrapleural invasion of the chest wall, spine, nerves or mediastinal vascular structures, which is particularly useful when planning complex surgical procedures.[19] Chemical analysis reveals an exudative effusion in most cases, with only 5% of malignant pleural effusions being transudates.[18] The diagnostic cornerstone of malignant pleural effusion is the cytologic demonstration of malignant cells in the pleural fluid. Positive pleural fluid cytology is noted in 62% of cases.[21] Tumor marker measurements using flow cytometry improve the diagnostic yield of cytologically negative effusions by 33% and are particularly valuable when lymphoma, leukemia, or multiple myeloma are suspected.[22,23] Its role in the study of mesotheliomas remains controversial.[24] Pleural biopsies via pleuroscopy have a 95% sensitivity in the diagnosis of pleural malignancies. The diagnostic yield of pleuroscopy increases only incrementally (1%) when combined with pleural fluid cytology. By contrast, closed pleural biopsy has a diagnostic yield of only 44%, but improves to 77% when combined with an analysis of pleural fluid cytology.[21]

Management of Malignant Pleural Effusions

Because malignant pleural effusions often signal advanced disease and incurability, treatment efforts are frequently directed toward palliation. Hence, awareness of available therapeutic options tailored to individual patient needs is important. The patient's performance status and information regarding prior thoracenteses, including the volume of fluid evacuated, whether lung reexpansion and symptom palliation were obtained, and the time interval between repeated taps, are important components of the evaluation that help to guide further therapy. Performance status is the best predictor of survival in patients with recurrent malignant pleural effusions.[25] The presence of local chest wall abnormalities, future cancer treatment plans, the patient's preferences, and the availability of family support influence the approach to these patients.

Palliation with simple therapeutic thoracentesis represents a reasonable approach to patients with newly diagnosed chemo- or radiosensitive tumors, such as lymphoma, breast cancer, small-cell lung cancer, germ cell, ovarian, prostate, and thyroid neoplasms, while awaiting response to definitive therapy. After the initial clinical and roentgenographic evaluation, a symptom-limited therapeutic thoracentesis is recommended. A recent consensus statement by the American Thoracic Society and the European Respiratory Society recommends that not more than 1.0-1.5 L of fluid be slowly evacuated from the pleural space in one sitting and that drainage should be discontinued if the patient develops symptoms of dyspnea, cough, or chest discomfort.[10] In our experience, patients with radiographic evidence of contralateral mediastinal shift from large pleural effusions may safely tolerate the removal of 2-2.5 L of fluid in one sitting as long as there are no procedure-related symptoms of chest pain, cough, or dyspnea. However, large-volume pleural fluid drainage during a single procedure should be carried out

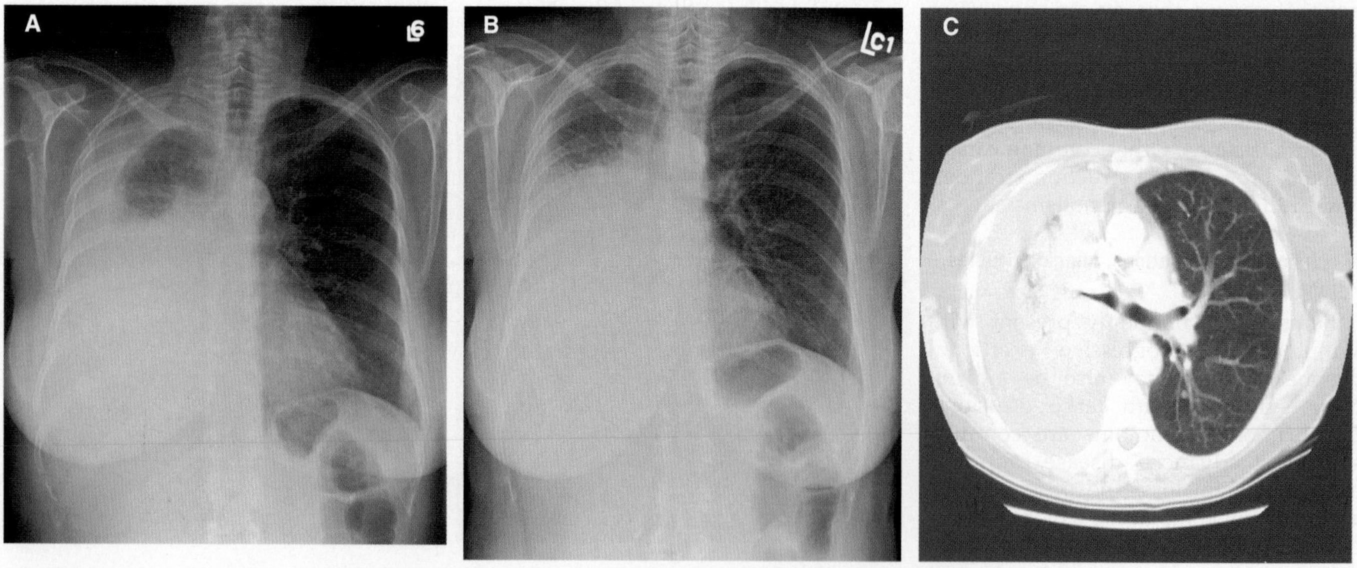

Figure 131-5 Large right-sided pleural effusion **(A)** with ipsilateral shift of the mediastinum following thoracentesis **(B)**, indicating volume loss secondary to atelectasis or mass. A CT scan of the chest **(C)** demonstrates a large mass compressing the right mainstem bronchus.

cautiously, especially when radiological studies reveal a centered or ipsilaterally shifted mediastinum. Measurement of pleural pressures during the evacuation of large amounts of fluid may reduce procedure-related complications.[26] Pleural pressure measurements may not be necessary in view of the safety of symptom-limited evacuation and its role requires further study. Lung reexpansion following thoracentesis may be assessed with posterior-anterior (PA) and lateral chest radiographs. Repeat thoracentesis spaced 1-2 days apart may be necessary to properly assess lung reexpansion associated with large effusions.[27] In 97% of patients, malignant pleural effusions will recur within 1 month, with most of these effusions reappearing within 1-3 days following fluid evacuation.[28] Patients with limited life expectances (<30 days), poor performance status, or those in which pleural fluid reaccumulation is slow are best treated with repeated therapeutic thoracentesis. Repeated thoracentesis is a reasonable approach for patients with malignancies that are expected to respond to chemotherapy and/or radiation therapy. However, frequent thoracentesis may trigger the production of local cytokines and fibrin, resulting in pleural fluid loculation, which not only complicates further thoracenteses, but also limits future modes of palliation.[29]

The use of indwelling pleural catheters has been increasingly accepted over the past few years as an alternative palliative option for patients with recurrent malignant effusions. Ideal candidates for this palliative modality include patients with life expectancies in excess of 30 days, and in whom prior thoracenteses effected symptomatic relief. Considerations for pleural catheter implantation are valid in this group of patients regardless of lung reexpansion following thoracentesis. Indwelling pleural catheters may be placed in an outpatient setting. Following documentation of proper catheter position, the patient, trained family members, or caregivers may drain the fluid intermittently at home. Daily pleural fluid drainage is recommended initially. During each session, which typically lasts less than 15 min, drainage should be continued until the patient develops cough, chest discomfort, or fluid flow stops spontaneously, presumably because the pleural space has been emptied. At our institution, 92% of patients treated with indwelling catheters reported significant relief of dyspnea, and 52% achieved effective pleurodesis. The mean time from catheter insertion to catheter removal was 32 days. Catheter-related complications were observed in only 4% of the patients, including one patient with empyema, and two patients with persistent pain at the insertion site. Only 6% of patients required additional drainage of fluid following removal of the catheter.[30] In a subgroup analysis, patients meeting criteria for a pleurodesis procedure achieved 70% effective pleurodesis after indwelling pleural catheter insertion.[31]

Traditionally, chemical pleurodesis has been the most widely used method to control recurrent malignant pleural effusions. Unfortunately, the lack of prospective studies precludes comparative analyses of efficacy, safety and cost of the existing chemical agents, and pleurodesis techniques. The results from available literature suggest that nonchemotherapeutic agents are more efficacious and the most cost-effective sclerosants.[10] Sterilized, asbestos-free talc is the preferred pleurodesing agent. Complications vary with the dose, size, and surface characteristics of the talc particles. Administration of more than 5 g of talc during one session or simultaneous bilateral pleurodesis is not recommended. The use of talc particles that are less than 5 mm in size has been associated with pulmonary injury, including acute pneumonitis and respiratory failure associated with Adult respiratory distress syndrome (ARDS), and should be avoided.[32] The safety of large-particle talc for pleurodesis was recently confirmed in a European multicenter trial in which no association with ARDS was identified.[33] The superiority of thoracoscopic talc insufflation over talc slurry as a method of administration of the sclerosant is a matter of debate. Success rates of >90% have been reported for both techniques, without significant differences in the rate of overall complications or disease recurrence.[10] The largest published prospective randomized trial comparing thoracoscopic talc insufflation and talc slurry included 501 patients with a performance status of 1 or 2. Results showed no difference in 30-day survival rates and pleurodesis success rates between chest tube talc slurry and thoracoscopic talc poudrage. Unexpected high morbidity and mortality rates were reported in both groups. A subset analysis suggested that thoracoscopic talc insufflation may be advantageous for patients with lung or breast cancer.[34] Based on the available information, our group considers all patients with a good performance status (ECOG 0, 1 or 2), and in whom symptomatic relief and lung reexpansion was achieved after initial drainage of the pleural fluid, for either indwelling pleural catheter placement or pleurodesis with pleuroscopic talc poudrage as the preferred palliative modalities.

Rarely, alternative modalities such as pleuroperitoneal shunts and parietal pleurectomy are used in the management of recurrent, symptomatic effusions following pleurodesis failures, or effusions associated with trapped lung. Chylous effusions associated with malignancy are controlled by treating the primary tumor. Prolonged loss of chyle, a protein-rich, fat-laden, and lymphocyte-predominant fluid, may result in lymphopenia, severe nutritional depletion, and water and electrolyte loss. Mortality due to chylothorax can be as high as 50%. Among those patients with recurrent symptomatic chylothorax and cancer relapse or progressive disease despite adequate treatment, parenteral alimentation and talc pleurodesis[35] or indwelling pleural catheter placement represent reasonable treatment alternatives.[36] Pleuroperitoneal shunt placement is an attractive option, since chyle is not lost but mobilized from the thorax to the peritoneum where it is reabsorbed, thus mitigating the risk of malnourishment and immune suppression. Unfortunately, the pleuroperitoneal shunt pump mechanism displaces only 1.5-2.5 mL at a time, making its use cumbersome. In addition, the incidence of obstruction of the pump is high. Peritoneal tumor seeding through the shunt is a theoretical concern, although this has not been clearly documented. Embolization of the thoracic duct represents an alternative strategy in the management of recurrent chylous effusions. This procedure appears to be well tolerated, but definitive evidence of its efficacy in the cancer population is not available. Parietal pleurectomy, decortication, or pleuropneumonectomy are associated with high mortality rates and do not provide better symptom control than other palliative options.[10] Utilization of compounds to block vascular endothelial growth factor (VEGF) either alone or in combination with other palliative modalities is promising. Theoretically, decreasing production of pleural fluid with VEGF blockade followed by drainage of the pleural effusion and instillation of a chemical agent to obtain pleural symphysis could accelerate pleurodesis and reduce hospital stay.[37]

In summary, in patients with limited life expectancies, modalities that offer the best chance for palliation of symptoms, the lowest procedure-related morbidity and mortality, and the shortest hospital stay represent a reasonable approach to the management of recurrent malignant effusions. A multidisciplinary approach (Fig. 131-6), involving oncology, pulmonary medicine, interventional radiology, and thoracic surgery, offers the best opportunities to achieve these goals.

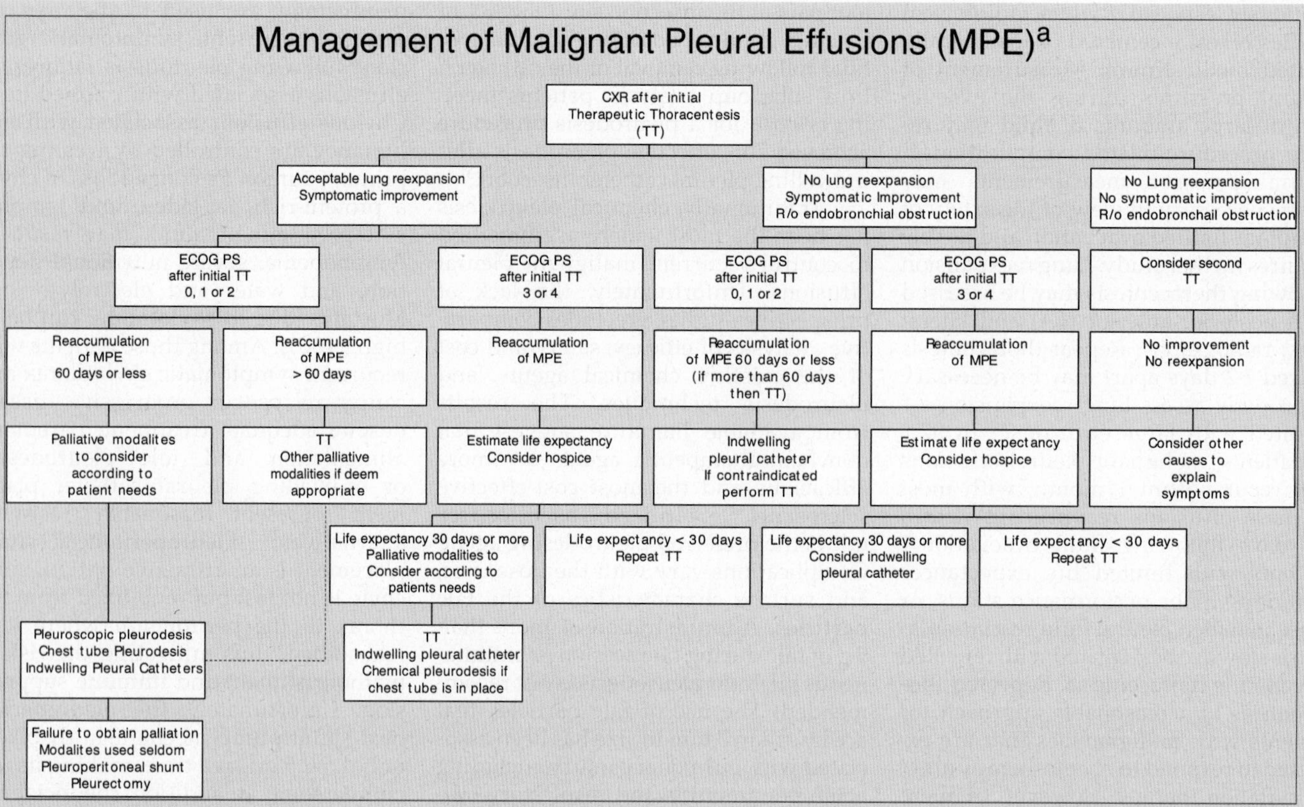

[a]Patients with chemo- or radiosensitivetumors on initial treatment (lymphome, breast cancer, small cell lung cancer, germ cell, ovarian, prostate and thyroid neoplams), may be candidates for therapeutic thomcentesis while awaiting systemic treatment results.

Figure 131-6 Management of malignant pleural effusions (MPE). *Abbreviation:* ECOG PS, Eastern Cooperative Oncology Group Performence Status

Postsurgical Respiratory Insufficiency

Diagnostic Evaluation

The initial approach to the patient with an anatomically resectable tumor includes strategies to determine the patient's functional operability and the predicted long-term pulmonary disability following the loss of the resected lung. This may be accomplished through pulmonary-specific testing as well as a general assessment aimed at identifying and optimizing control of any coexisting systemic diseases. The pulmonary evaluation consists of three sequential steps: (1) measurement of baseline pulmonary function; (2) quantitative radionuclide regional ventilation-perfusion pulmonary studies to calculate postoperative lung function; and (3) exercise testing for patients that do not meet acceptable results on the two previous steps.[38] Among the pulmonary function tests that have been used as predictors of postoperative outcome, reduced values of forced expiratory volume in 1 s (FEV_1) and diffusing capacity of the lung for carbon monoxide (DLCO) are the most reproducible and most frequently used for predicting complications of lung resection.[39] For decision making, values of FEV_1 reported as percent of predicted that take into account variations in patients' height, gender, and race are preferred over values reported in absolute units (L). In our laboratory, more than half of patients with an FEV_1 between 60% and 80% of predicted have an estimated postpneumonectomy FEV_1 by radionuclide studies that is below acceptable values for safe resection (<40% of predicted). Therefore, we recommend that only those patients with baseline FEV_1 and DLCO ≥80% of predicted and no clinical evidence of contralateral pulmonary disease, be considered for resection without further testing. All other patients should undergo a "split function" evaluation, which is a quantitative radionuclide assessment of regional lung ventilation and perfusion. In this study, the uptake of radioactive ions by various regions in each lung is measured by inhalation of ^{133}Xe and by intravenous administration of ^{133}Xe dissolved in saline or ^{99}Tc macroaggregates. The percentage of radioactivity contributed by each lung correlates with the contribution to the overall function by that lung. The predicted postoperative FEV_1 (FEV_1ppo) and predicted postoperative DLCO (DLCOppo) are calculated by subtracting the percent functional uptake of the region to be resected from the total uptake. Several investigators have documented the usefulness of split function studies for predicting both the risk of complications and the loss of pulmonary function after pulmonary resection.[40,41] In these studies, preoperative predicted values are closer to measured postoperative values for pneumonectomy and for resections involving more than three segments.[42] Pulmonary function remains relatively stable after pneumonectomy. Predictions for a smaller resection are less reliable, owing to a disproportionate early loss, followed by significant functional improvement with time.[43] Kearney et al also described a low FEV_1ppo as the only significant independent predictor of complications.[44] Other variables, including age ≥60, male sex, history of smoking, pneumonectomy, hypercarbia, (PCO_2 ≥45 mm Hg), desaturations on exercise oximetry ($SaO_2 \leq 90\%$), and a preoperative FEV1 ≤1 L were not predictive of complications. Markos et al[45] reported that a DLCOppo <40% of predicted was associated with higher morbidity and mortality and was the best predictor of postoperative respiratory failure.

In summary, an FEV_1 ppo and DLCOppo of ≥40% of predicted on split function studies represent criteria for lung resection, including pneumonectomy. Patients requiring lesser surgeries, such as a lobectomy, who do not meet these criteria, should undergo further evaluation with exercise testing before surgery can be undertaken.

The rationale for using exercise testing in these high-risk patients is based on two concepts: (1) lung function is not the only determinant of performance and (2) losses for lobectomies or lesser resections improve over time and tend to be overestimated by radiospirometric studies.[38] Exercise testing also offers the advantage of examining cardiopulmonary and musculoskeletal interactions during stress in a single study. The most validated form of exercise testing is cycle ergometry with incremental workloads to the symptom-limited maximum ($\dot{V}O_{2peak}$). Using this method, Smith et al found that only 1 of 10 patients with a $\dot{V}O_{2peak}$ >20 mL/kg/min developed complications postpoperatively, whereas all patients with a $\dot{V}O_{2peak}$ <15 mL/kg/min had complications.[46] We conducted two studies on patients that had been considered inoperable because of FEV_1 ≤40% of predicted postoperative FEV_1 ≤33% of predicted, and/or arterial PCO_2 ≥45 mm Hg. Patients that reached a $\dot{V}O_{2peak}$ ≥15 mL/kg/min underwent surgical treatment; others were referred to radiation and/or chemotherapy. All surgically treated patients were extubated within 24 h and the median time to discharge following surgery was 8 days. There were no in-hospital deaths, although reversible postoperative complications occurred in 40% of the patients. Moreover, a survival benefit among these high-risk patients treated surgically was noted.[47,48] More recently, we determined that values of $\dot{V}O_{2peak}$ expressed as percent of predicted more accurately estimated surgical risk and helped to maximize the number of patients that can safely undergo lung resection. We concluded that high-risk patients that achieve a VO_{2peak} ≥60% of predicted during exercise have an acceptable outcome after lung resection, even if VO_{2peak} <15 mL/Kg/min.[49] Our approach to preoperative assessment for lung resection is summarized in Figure 131-7. In addition to an estimation of surgical risk and postoperative function, the goals of preoperative assessment include the development of strategies to reduce the risk and maximize the number of patients that can benefit from surgical therapy. Finally, one must keep in mind that there is no test that will predict all complications and that the patient and the surgeon should make the final decision regarding the risk-benefit of surgical treatment.

Chemotherapy-Induced Lung Injury

Toxicities to the lung parenchyma, pleura, and pulmonary circulation are frequent sequelae of an ever-increasing number of drugs used in the treatment of cancer. In addition to the standard chemotherapeutic agents, interferons and novel molecular targeted therapies have emerged over the past decade as important anticancer agents, some of which may cause life-threatening lung injury. The response of the lungs to drug-induced injury is limited, resulting in stereotyped histopathologic lung injury patterns, of which interstitial lung diseases (ILDs) and alveolar processes are the most common. Pleural diseases (pleural effusions, fibrosis); drug-induced vascular disorders (thrombosis, pulmonary hypertension, pulmonary veno-occlusive disease-PVOD); mediastinal disease (lymphadenopathy, fibrosis) and airway disorders (bronchospasm, bronchiolitis obliterans with organizing pneumonia-BOOP) have also been described. A growing number of agents may cause type I hypersensitivity reactions with associated bronchospasm, which may manifest as an isolated adverse event or as a component of drug-induced anaphylaxis. Finally, individual chemotherapeutic agents may induce severe immune suppression. The often life-threatening pneumonias that emerge in this setting are discussed elsewhere in this section. Cancer agents within one therapeutic class may produce similar patterns of toxicity, although the frequency of lung injury caused by individual drugs within a particular therapeutic class may vary widely. Furthermore, lung injury caused by a single-agent may have more than one histopathologic feature.

Predisposing factors such as older age, cumulative dose, concomitant or sequential radiotherapy, oxygen administration, prior lung injury and the use of multidrug regimens vary with individual agents and may influence both the occurrence and latency period between drug exposure and clinical symptoms. Precise estimates of the incidence of lung injury caused by individual chemotherapeutic agents are incomplete, owing in part to the frequent use of complex multidrug and multimodality regimens. In addition, overlapping clinical and radiographic manifestations of lung injury caused by drug toxicity, infection and cancer relapse confound clinical distinctions between these entities.

Toxicity is typically assessed through clinical, radiographic, and histopathologic studies, although no single abnormality is pathognomonic. Symptom onset varies with the individual agents and may occur months to years following drug exposure, particularly following busulfan, bis-chloroethyl nitrosurea (BCNU), bleomycin, cyclophosphamide or gemcitabine administration.[50-53] High resolution CT (HRCT) scans may detect early abnormalities, however imaging findings are nonspecific. Interstitial and mixed alveolar-interstitial abnormalities typically localize to peripheral and lower lung zones, and are the most frequent radiographic findings on CT. Nodular lesions, reticular lines, septal thickening, mosaic patterns, and ground glass attenuation are also observed. With disease progression, radiographic manifestations of pulmonary fibrosis (traction bronchiectasis, honeycombing) predominates.

Bronchoalveolar lavage (BAL) with or without lung biopsies may be helpful in excluding competing diagnoses of infection or background disease. BAL findings of increased numbers of lym-

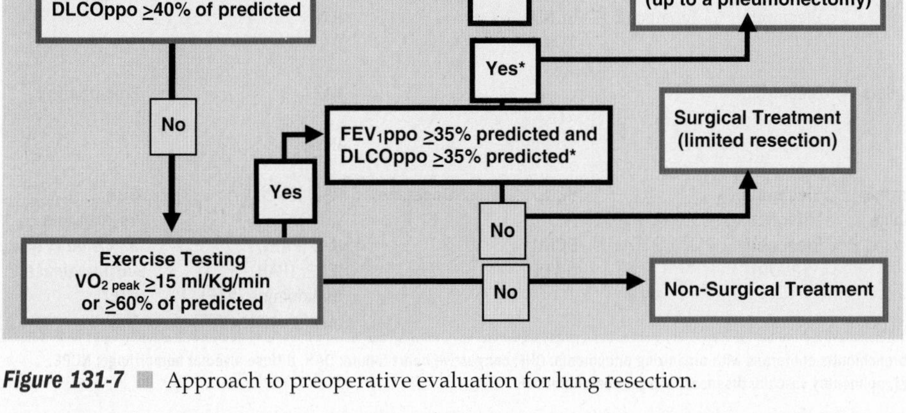

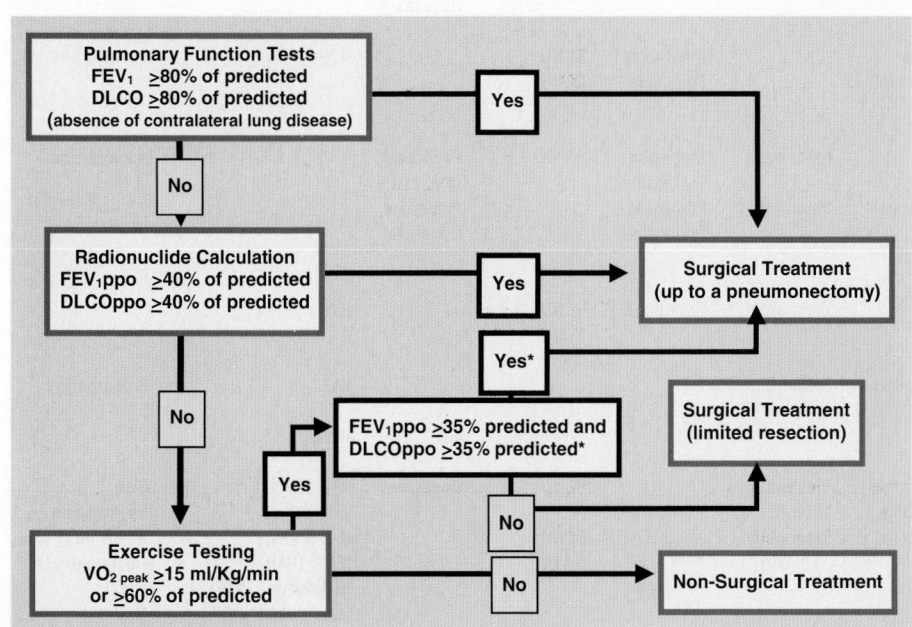

Figure 131-7 Approach to preoperative evaluation for lung resection.

phocytes, eosinophils, or dysplastic type II pneumocytes may aid in the diagnosis of chemotherapy-induced lung injury, although none of these findings are diagnostic. Decreased CD4/CD8 ratios on BAL fluid are also supportive findings, however ratios vary widely and cannot distinguish sufficiently between drug-induced versus other causes of ILD.[54] The diagnosis of DAH is supported by findings of progressively bloody BAL samples on sequential aliquots and/or cytologic evidence of increased numbers of hemosiderin-laden macrophages on BAL fluid. Serum elevations of the white blood cell (WBC) count, erythrocyte sedimentation rate, and C-reactive protein are also common but nonspecific findings.

Impairments in pulmonary function associated with toxicities involving the lung parenchyma are usually signaled by a reduction in the DLCO and the development of a restrictive ventilatory defect.[55-58] Although DLCO is generally accepted as the most sensitive parameter in assessing lung reactions to chemotherapy-related lung injury, its predictive potential for the detection of early change has been variable.[51,59] Near-complete normalization of pulmonary function within 2 years of drug exposure, on average, is common following some forms of chemotherapy-induced lung injury.[55,56,58]

With no available clinical, radiographic or histopathologic features that are reliably predictive of or diagnostic of drug-induced lung toxicity, the diagnosis is largely based on the temporal association between drug exposure and the development of pulmonary injury once competing diagnoses have been excluded. This section offers a brief overview of some of the clinically relevant pulmonary disease patterns induced by standard chemotherapeutic agents and the novel targeted molecular therapies (Tables 131-1 and 131-2).

Interstitial Lung Diseases

Interstitial Pneumonitis (IP) ■ An ever-enlarging list of chemotherapeutic agents has been associated with IP, of which bleomycin, busulfan, cyclophosphamide, carmusine, gemcitabine, methotrexate, rituximab, taxanes, interferons, and the tyrosine kinase inhibitors, gefitinib and erlotinib, have been most extensively studied.[60-70] Recent observations also document IP as a consequence of treatment with the rapamycin analogs, temsorilmus and everolimus.[71,72] IP progressing to fibrosis is a rare complication of platinum-based chemotherapy, in particular oxaliplatin.[73]

Nonspecific interstitial pneumonia (NSIP) represents the most frequent morphologic pattern of drug-induced IP. In most patients, a nonproductive cough and dyspnea develop insidiously, usually within weeks to months following drug exposure. Radiographic changes typically lag behind clinical symptoms by days to weeks but may occasionally occur as an early marker of lung injury. With the exception of methotrexate-associated hilar lymphadenopathy, the radiographic findings of IP are nonspecific for a particular chemotherapy agent.[74,75] Interstitial and mixed alveolar-interstitial abnormalities on chest imaging studies are the most frequent radiographic findings, which typically localize to the peripheral and lower lung zones. Nodular lesions, reticular lines, septal thickening, mosaic patterns, and ground glass attenuation are also observed. CT imaging is far superior to plain films in identifying interstitial lung disease. Other supportive findings include a reduction in DLCO and a restrictive defect on pulmonary function testing. Risk factors for IP vary with individual agents, but in general include advanced age, concurrent radiation or multiagent therapy, preexisting lung disease, and the need for high-inspired supplemental oxygen. Early pathologic changes associated with IP consist of damage to epithelial and endothelial cells, leading to edema of the alveolar interstitium. Alveolar edema and DAD are usual features of advanced IP, which may progress to end-stage fibrotic

Table 131-1 ■ **Major Clinical Syndromes and Histologic Patterns of Chemotherapy-Induced Lung Injury**

	Alkykating Agents	Antimetabolites/ Purine Analogs	Cytotoxic Antibiotics	Podophyllotoxins	Nitrosureas	Taxanes	Immunomodulators	Other
DAD/ARDS DAH	Busulfan, Cyclophosphamide	Methotrexate, Azathioprine, Ara-C, Fludarabine, Gemcitabine	Bleomycin mitomycin C		BCNU CCNU	Paclitaxel Docetaxel		ATRA
NCPE		Ara-C, Gemcitabine, Methotrexate, Pentostatin	Mitomycin C*			Paclitaxel Docetaxel	IL-2, TNF, IFN-γ	ATRA
NSIP	Busulfan, Cyclophosphamide, Oxaliplatin, Temozolamide	Methotrexate, Azathioprine, Fludarabine, Gemcitabine		Irinotecan Etoposide	BCNU CCNU		IFN-γ	Procarbazine
HP-like reaction	Cyclophosphamide	Methotrexate	Bleomycin	Etoposide Teniposide	BCNU	Paclitaxel Docetaxel		Procarbazine
Bronchospasm/ type 1 hypersensitivity reaction	Ifosphamide	Methotrexate, Gemcitabine	Mitomycin C*	Etoposide Teniposide		Paclitaxel Docetaxel		
BOOP	Busulfan, Cyclophosphamide, Oxaliplatin	Methotrexate	Bleomycin	Topotecan	BCNU CCNU		IFN-γ	
EP	Oxaliplatin	Methotrexate, Fludarabine	Bleomycin				IL-2	Procarbazine
Granulomatous reaction		Methotrexate					IFN-γ	
Pleural disease	Cyclophosphamide	Methotrexate, Azathioprine, Gemcitabine	Bleomycin Mitomycin C		BCNU	Docetaxel	IL-2, IFN-γ	ATRA Procarbazine
PVD		Zinostatin (PAH)	Bleomycin (PVOD)		BCNU (PVOD)		IL-2 (PAH), IFN-γ (PAH) thalidomide (VTE), lenalidomide (VTE)	Tamoxifen (VTE), L-asparaginase (VTE)

Abbreviations: ARDS, adult respiratory distress syndrome; BOOP, bronchiolitis obliterans with organizing pneumonia; CHF, congestive heart failure; DAH, diffuse alveolar hemorrhage; NCPE, noncardiogenic pulmonary edema; PF, pulmonary fibrosis; PVD/DVT, pulmonary vascular disease/deep venous thrombosis.

Table 131-2 **■ Major Clinical Syndromes and Histologic Patterns of Lung Injury Caused by Molecular Targeted Chemotherapeutic Agents**

Disorder	Monoclonal Antibody	Tyrosine Kinase Inhibitors	Rapamycin Inhibitors	Proteosome Inhibitors
NCPE with/without ARDS/PF	Rituximab Denileukin difitox	Gefitinib Erlotinib Imatinib	Everolimus	Bortezomib
Cardiogenic pulmonary edema	Bevacizumab	Sunitinib Sorafenib		
DAH	Bevacizumab	Sunitinib Sorafenib		
NSIP	Rituximab	Gefitinib Desatinib	Temsirolimus Everolimus	Bortezomib
Bronchospasm/airway disease (type 1 hypersensitivy reaction)?	Rituximab Transtuzumab Alemtuzumab Cetuximab Gemtuzumab			Bortezomib
BOOP	Rituximab Trastuzumab			
Infections		Gefitinib		
Pleural disease	Alemtuzumab	Desatinib		
PVD/DVT	Bevacizumab	Sunitinib Sorafenib		

lung despite corticosteroid therapy and drug withdrawal.

IP associated with bleomycin and several other chemotherapeutic agents has been carefully scrutinized and deserves specific attention. Up to 20% of bleomycin-treated patients develop clinically significant lung disease. The incidence of bleomycin-induced pneumonitis (BIP) appears to be dose-related, with higher rates associated with total cumulative doses above 450 U. An increased incidence and severity of BIP has been associated with age greater than 70 years, cumulative dose greater than 400 mg, bolus administration, multiagent therapy, multimodality therapy with concomitant or sequential radiation, high-inspired oxygen administration, and uremia.[76-83] BIP-related clinical symptoms of dry cough and exertional dyspnea typically evolve over months after bleomycin exposure and may be accompanied by early CT findings of bibasilar ground glass opacities that give way to linear and subpleural nodular lesions as the disease progresses (Fig. 131-8). Mortality rates are low (1-3%) but increase to 10% among patients with cumulative doses above 550 U. BCNU also causes dose-dependent lung toxicity with rates as high as 50% among patients whose cumulative dose exceeds 1500 mg/m^2.[82,84] The predilection for the middle and upper lobes distinguishes BCNU-induced IP. Intractable, upper lobe predominant fibrosis and pneumothorax may occur years after completion of therapy.[85] Late onset pneumonitis following busulfan and cyclophosphamide administration has also been reported. Radiographic evidence of IP is a frequent finding following temsirolimus therapy (up to 36% of treated patients), although nearly 50% of patients are clinically asymptomatic. IP following everolimus therapy occurs less frequently (3% of patients), however, the clinical presentation is often more severe, and may require mechanical ventilation. Adverse pulmonary reactions occur on average within the first 4 weeks of administration of either drug. IP has been described in 1-12% of single-agent paclitaxel recipients and up to 26% of patients after docetaxel monotherapy.[64,65] Although the pneumonitis is typically mild, severe reactions, progressing to pulmonary fibrosis and death have been reported with both drugs. The incidence of paclitaxel-related IP is much higher when given concurrently with radiation (47% of patients) or with other agents that potentiate lung toxicity, such as gemcitabine (33% of patients).[86-88]

Hypersensitivity Pneumonitis (HP) ■ Hypersensitivity-like reactions, including hypersensitivity pneumonitis have been described following treatment with methotrexate, bleomycin, etoposide, teniposide and the taxane agents.[61,84,89-93] Most patients present with fever, dyspnea, dry cough and BAL lymphocytosis following repeated exposure to the offending drug. Poorly formed noncaseating granulomas and mononuclear cell infiltration are typical histologic findings in subacute and chronic HP. Radiographic changes include homogeneous opacities with a predilection for the periphery and upper lobes, particularly in the chronic form of the disease. Methotrexate-induced HP has been extensively studied and supported by the presence of a helper T-lymphocyte alveolitis and granuloma formation on BAL fluid and biopsy specimens and by the presence of peripheral eosinophilia. Rechallenge with the drug, however, does not consistently result in disease recurrence, suggesting that a hypersensitivity response is not the sole mechanism of injury. Lung injury has been reported following oral, intravenous, intrathecal, and intramuscular routes of administration. Risk factors for methotrexate-induced lung injury are not well understood. Age, gender, total or cumulative dose of the drug, underlying lung disease, and radiation or oxygen therapy do not appear to confer an increased risk.[94,95] Clinical features of methotrexate-induced lung injury include dyspnea, dry cough, fatigue, fever, headache and interstitial pneumonitis that evolve over the first 3-4 weeks after drug exposure and may wax and wane without adjustments in therapy. Diffuse bilateral reticular infiltrates associated with unilateral or bilateral small to moderate effusions are common. Hilar adenopathy and pleural effusions occur in up to 10% of patients.

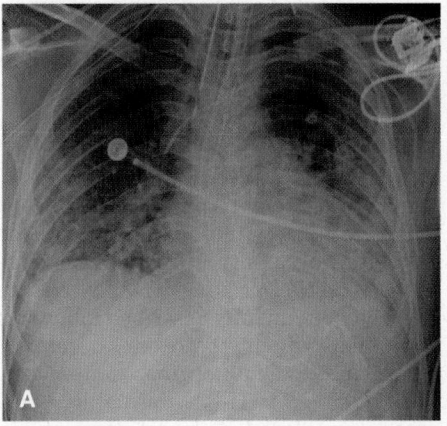

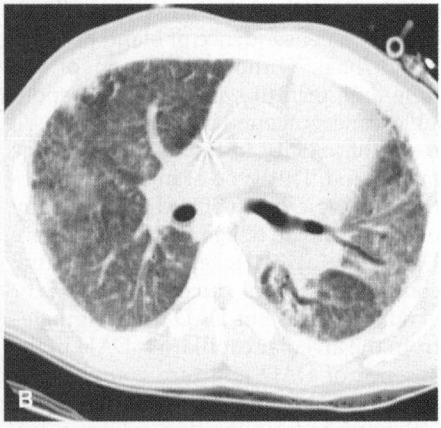

Figure 131-8 ■ A 32-year-old man treated with bleomycin-based chemotherapy for germ cell tumor developed respiratory distress following surgical resection of retroperitoneal lymph nodes. CXR **(A)** and CT scan **(B)** showed bilateral patchy reticulonodular and airspace disease. Work-up was consistent with ARDS associated with bleomycin toxicity, presumably triggered by hyperoxia during surgery.

Histologic evidence of ill-defined granulomas, together with a skin rash and radiographic findings of hilar adenopathy or pleural effusions may help to distinguish methotrexate-induced lung injury from other types of drug-induced HP. Overall, the prognosis for patients with chemotherapy-induced HP is very favorable. Complete resolution of clinical symptoms and radiographic findings is typical following steroid therapy in early-stage disease.

Alveolar Processes

Diffuse Alveolar Damage (DAD)/Adult Respiratory Distress Syndrome (ARDS) and Diffuse Alveolar Hemorrhage (DAH) ■ DAD, the histologic correlate of ARDS, frequently develops during severe lung injury. The most compelling causal associations of chemotherapy-induced DAD are with the alkylating agents (busulfan, cyclophosphamide), antibiotics (bleomycin, mitomycin C), antimetabolites (methotrexate, azathioprine, cytosine-arabinoside [Ara-C], fludarabine, gemcitabine) and nitrosureas (bis-chloroethyl nitrosurea [BCNU], chloroethyl-cyclohexyl nitrosurea [CCNU]). Bilateral heterogeneous ground glass opacities are early radiographic findings of ARDS, which may progress to diffuse opacification with irreversible lung damage, marked by architectural distortion, fibrosis and honeycomb lung. Multiagent protocols or the concurrent use of radiation or oxygen therapy potentiate both the risk and severity of lung injury, especially following therapy with bleomycin or bulsulfan.[75,96] Overall, the response to early drug withdrawal and initiation of corticosteriod therapy in the treatment of DAD has been variable. Progressive respiratory impairment, leading to respiratory failure and death has been reported with some agents (busulfan, cycophosphamide) despite drug withdrawal. Although drug-induced DAH may occur in association with capillaritis or as a consequence of bland alveolar hemorrhage without distortion of the lung architechture, most of the responsible cancer agents produce DAH as a result of toxicity to the alveolocapillary membrane. This type of injury produces the histologic lesion of DAD. Thus, many of the cytotoxic drugs that cause severe DAD may also trigger DAH. Bleeding commonly occurs during the early or exudative phase of DAD and originates from the alveolar capillaries. DAH in the absence of DAD is a rare complication of rituximab[97] and has been described following administration of vasculartargeting monoclonal antibodies (anti-VEGF), such as bevacizumab and the tyrosine kinase inhibitors, sorefinib and sunitenib.[98-100] Despite massive bleeds, hemoptysis is only seen in approximately 25% of patients.[98,101-103]

Noncardiogenic Pulmonary Edema (NCPE) ■ The antimetabolites (Ara-C, gemcitabine, methotrexate), all-trans retinoic acid (ATRA) and the biologic response modifiers (interleukin-2, tumor necrosis factor) are prominent causes of a bland pulmonary capillary leak syndrome. Pulmonary capillary leak with associated NCPE is also recognized during therapy with some of the monoclonal antibodies, notably denileukin difitox and imatinib mesylate administration. Drug-induced NCPE often occurs as an idiosyncratic reaction, unrelated to drug dosage or duration of therapy. Most reactions are mild and self-limited, although progression to ARDS with fatal outcomes occasionally occurs. The clinical and radiographic manifestations of NCPE are generally indistinguishable from other causes of pulmonary edema, although the presence of cardiomegaly, pulmonary vascular redistribution and kerley B lines on chest radiographs favors a cardiogenic etiology. Drug withdrawal, supplemental oxygen, and the judicious use of diuretics usually effect a rapid recovery. Rechallenge with the offending drug often results in recrudescence of symptoms.

Eosinophilic Pneumonia (EP) ■ Acute eosinophilic pneumonia has been documented following therapy with fludarabine, interleukin-2, methotrexate, bleomycin, procarbazine, and more recently, oxaloplatin.[95,104-106] BAL or peripheral blood eosinophilia are prominent features, which may promptly resolve following corticosteroid therapy. Radiographic changes occur abruptly and include homogeneous opacities with a predilection for the periphery and upper lobes. The "reverse pulmonary edema pattern" is seen only in a minority of patients.[107] Drug withdrawal and initiation of high-dose steroids are typically associated with favorable outcomes, although occasionally rapid progression to respiratory failure may occur despite therapy.

Pleural Disease

Pleural Effusions and Fibrosis ■ Drug-induced pleural disease is typically a component of a generalized pulmonary reaction that includes pulmonary infiltrates and effusions.[108] Pleuropulmonary reactions have been most frequently described following treatment with methotrexate, docetaxel, gemcitabine, azathioprine, mitomycin, interleukin-2, ATRA, dasatanib, and interferon-γ. Isolated pleural effusions are occasionally seen following methotrexate, docetaxel, and granulocyte-colony stimulating factor (GCSF) administration, and may resolve with discontinuation of therapy.[109,110] Pleural thickening may accompany pulmonary fibrosis as a late manifestation of cyclophosphamide, BCNU, or bleomycin toxicity.

Pulmonary Vascular Disorders (PVD)

Thromboembolic Disease, Pulmonary Hypertension, Pulmonary Veno-occlusive Disease ■ The adverse effects of chemotherapeutic agents on the pulmonary vasculature may result in thrombosis, pulmonary hypertension, or PVOD. The diagnosis of PVD is suggested by an isolated reduction in DLCO or a DLCO that is disproportionately decreased relative to other lung function parameters on pulmonary function testing. The prothrombotic effects of tamoxifen appear to be related to drug-related decrements in protein C and antithrombin III levels.[111] Combined therapy with tamoxifen and other chemotherapeutic agents, such as cyclophosphamide, methotrexate and 5-flurouracil confers a 3-fold increased risk of thromboembolic phenomenon.[112,113] Thromboembolic events, with rates ranging from 14% to 43% have been reported among recipients of thalidomide-based chemotherapy, given in combination with steroids, doxorubicin or BCNU.[114-116] The VEGF inhibitors, bevacizumab, sunitinib, and sorafenib, are also associated with thromboembolic events.[98-100] Zinostatin, an antitumor antibiotic, causes hypertrophy of the pulmonary vascular wall leading to pulmonary hypertension, possibly as a result of direct toxicity to the pulmonary endothelium.[107] More often, chemotherapy-related pulmonary hypertension emerges as a result of PVOD, a process characterized by fibrous obliteration of pulmonary venules and small pulmonary veins (see below). Although several drugs have been implicated in the development of PVOD, bleomycin and BCNU have been associated with the most incriminating data.[117,118]

Drug-Induced Airway Disease

Bronchospasm ■ Alterations in airway function are typically a component of drug-induced parenchymal reactions, but occasionally may be seen as isolated airway disease. Direct degranulation of mast cells causes bronchospasm following paclitaxel administration; for many of the other agents, the mechanism underlying bronchospasm is unclear. Paclitaxel is formulated in a highly allergenic polyoxyethylated castor oil solvent (Cremophor EL), which may educe mast cell activation and histamine release, triggering type 1-hypersensitivity reactions. Standard prophylaxis with histamine receptor antagonists and steroids has reduced the incidence of paclitaxel-induced bronchospasm from 30% to

2%.[119] Teniposide, a podophyllotoxin formulated in Cremaphor EL solvent, also causes prominent bronchospasm, presumably by the same mechanism.[120] Although vinorelbine and other vinca-alkyloids are rarely associated with lung toxicity, acute reactions characterized by cough, bronchospasm, flushing, dyspnea, abdominal pain, and hypotension have been described when these agents are given either concurrently or sequentially with mitomycin chemotherapy. Dyspnea associated with bronchospasm has also been reported as part of a type 1 infusion-related hypersensitivity reaction associated with monoclonal antibody therapy, particularly during retuximab, transtuzumab, alemtuzumab, cetuximab, and gemtuzumab administration. These hypersensitivity reactions may occasionally be sufficiently severe (eg, anaphylactoid reactions) to warrant aggressive therapy and discontinuation of the drug. Drug withdrawal coupled with supplemental oxygen, antihistamines, steroids and nebulized β-agonists generally result in favorable outcomes. Prophylaxis with steroids and antihistamines frequently permit successful rechallenge in selected cases.

Broncholitis Obliterans With Organizing Pneumonia (BOOP) ■ BOOP is common to a variety of pulmonary inflammatory disorders that develop following infection, connective tissue diseases, and lung or stem cell transplantation, but may also appear after exposure to certain drugs. Among the chemotherapeutic agents associated with this type of lung injury, bleomycin, cyclophosphamide, doxorubicin, methotrexate, busulfan, mitomycin C and the interferons have been most frequently reported.[75,121-123] Recent descriptions of drug-induced BOOP have also implicated rituximab and the oxaliplatin therapy.[124,125] Patients may present 4-8 weeks following therapy with a clinico-radiological syndrome of subacute pneumonia with patchy alveolar, and often migratory pulmonary opacities on imaging. Diffuse infiltrative opacities and focal pneumonia have also been described. A robust response to steroid therapy is expected; however, relapses may occur during steroid taper or withdrawal.

■ Other Clinicopathologic Syndromes

Granulomatous Disease ■ The development of noncaseating granulomas is a rare manifestation of drug-induced lung injury that has been described most often following methotrexate and interferon therapy.[126,127] Methotrexate-induced and interferon-induced granulomatous lymphadenopathy is indistinguishable from sarcoidosis. In addition to methotrexate and interferon, two other chemotherapeutic agents, procarbazine and sirolimus, may also incite a granulomatous pneumonitis with or without an associated bronchiolotis and interstitial inflammation that are seen in hypersensitivity pneumonitis. Drug withdrawal may result in disease regression.

Pulmonary Complications of Thoracic Radiation: Radiation Pneumonitis and Fibrosis

Radiation-induced lung injury (RILI) is the most common dose-limiting complication following thoracic radiation and chemoradiation regimens. Clinically significant lung toxicity has been reported in 5-20% of patients following thoracic radiation, although a precise estimate of radiation lung injury is unknown. Recent reports suggest that the incidence may be marginally lower among patients treated with radiation for breast cancer, in part owing to the different radiation methods used.[128] Radiation pneumonitis (RP) and radiation fibrosis (RF) represent acute and late phases of RILI, respectively, and are the most frequent forms of radiation toxicity. RP most commonly occurs in its classic form in which a predictable and dose-dependent lung injury is confined to the irradiated field. Early symptoms of classic RP include fever, dyspnea, and nonproductive cough, which typically develop insidiously over the initial 1-3 months and peak at 3-4 months after radiotherapy. Measurable changes in pulmonary function tests, including a reduction in lung volumes and diffusing capacity may be seen as early as 2-3 months after irradiation. A less predictable or sporadic form of RP has also been recognized.[129] Sporadic pneumonitis occurs in a minority (5%) of patients and is thought to represent a type of hypersensitivity pneumonitis characterized by a bilateral CD_4+ T-lymphocytic alveolitis that diffusely involves both lung fields. Hence, radiation changes on imaging studies may extend well beyond the irradiated field. Patients present at 1-3 months following thoracic irradiation with symptoms of dyspnea and dry cough that are disproportionate to the volume of lung irradiated. This form of pneumonitis and its associated symptoms typically abate in 6-8 weeks without any long-term sequelae.[129-131] Radiation recall pneumonitis describes a rare, but well recognized inflammatory reaction that occurs within a previously irradiated area of pulmonary tissue after application of certain pharmacological agents. Antineoplastic agents that have been most often implicated in this phenomenon include the antracyclines, taxanes tamoxifen and gemcitabine.[132-134] Lung injury in recall pneumonitis typically occurs shortly after administration of the inciting antineoplastic agent, which may be weeks to months following completion of radiotherapy. Standard treatment includes withdrawal of the precipitating agent. Systemic corticosteroid therapy has been tried with varied success.

RF develops in virtually all patients receiving radiotherapy, regardless of prior clinical manifestations of pneumonitis. This phase of radiation lung injury usually appears at 6 months and stabilizes over the ensuing year following thoracic irradiation injury. RF is characterized histopathologically by collagen deposition in the alveolar walls, collapse of air spaces, and an attendant loss of lung volume.

Early changes on conventional chest radiographs that suggest classical RP include diffuse haze and indistinct vascular margins within the irradiated filed. Patchy areas of consolidation with or without air-bronchograms coalesce over time to conform to the treatment portals, defying anatomic boundaries. Later, RF is signaled by the appearance of a well-demarcated area of volume loss, linear densities, bronchiectasis, retraction of the lung parenchyma, tenting and elevation of the hemidiaphragm, and ipsilateral pleural thickening. Pneumothorax and occasionally small pleural effusions may occur on the irradiated side. Radiation-related pleural effusions typically develop within 6 months of completion of radiotherapy. This observation, coupled with the absence of malignant cells on pleural fluid cytology, and clinical and radiographic evidence of pneumonitis, help to distinguish malignant from radiation-induced effusions. Pulmonary veno-occlusive disease has also been reported as a rare complication of radiation-induced lung toxicity. Recent reports of BOOP and eosinophilic pneumonia involving nonirradiated areas of the lung following breast radiation have also been documented.[135,136] Both entities may produce migratory pulmonary opacities on chest radiographs, which typically develop 1-3 months following radiotherapy. The presence of blood or tissue eosinophils, coupled with a prior history of asthma or atopy, favors the diagnosis of eosinophilic pneumonia.

Risk factors that influence the development of RILI include total dose, dose per fraction, irradiated lung volume, radiation portals and beam arrangements as well as physical characteristics of the irradiation. Pulmonary damage is almost always radiographically apparent with total doses of radiation that exceed 4000 cGy, whereas only subtle radiographic changes are seen at doses below 3000 cGy.[128] Multimodality regimens that combine radiation with chemotherapeutic agents such as mitomycin, cyclophosphamide, vincristine, adriamycin, bleomycin, gemcitabine, the taxanes and actinomycin D may not only potentiate an adverse radiation response in the lungs but shorten the latency period following radiation exposure.[137] Other factors affecting the development of lung injury and disease severity include preexisting lung disease, underlying pulmonary reserve, prior radiotherapy, and rapid steroid withdrawal.[138] Although data regarding optimal dose-fractionation and dose-volume relationships that mitigate lung injury are still evolving, it is generally agreed that a hyperfractionated course of radiation delivered to the smallest lung volume offers the lowest possibility of lung toxicity. Newer strategies, including conformal therapy and intensity-modulated radiation therapy (IMRT) have been developed to deliver adequate doses to the tumor while limiting exposure to normal lung. IMRT uses multiple radiation beams to generate dose distributions that tightly conform to irregularly shaped target volumes, ensuring that the entire tumor volume is adequately treated, while minimizing radiation to normal lung. Pneumonitis following IMRT does not appear as the traditional straight-edged infiltrate that is typically seen following conventional radiation and may, therefore, be more difficult to distinguish from competing disease entities such as infection or recurrence of the underlying malignancy.[139]

The pathophysiology of radiation-induced changes in the lung is poorly understood, due to the complexities of preexisting comorbidity, multimodality treatment regimens, lack of standardized scoring systems for RILI, and poor understanding of individual predisposing genetic factors. Whether pneumonitis and fibrosis represent a continuum or separate entities has been definitively resolved. Certain key regulatory genes and/or gene products, such as TGF-β, matrix metalloproteinases (MMPs), and tumor necrosis factor (TNF), are thought to be central in both pathological processes. TGF-β is a multifunctional cytokine regulator of cell growth and differentiation that stimulates the deposition of collagen and decreases its degradation, resulting in fibrosis. A clear relationship between plasma levels of TGF-β and radiation-induced pulmonary toxicity has been shown in preclinical and clinical studies.[140] In these studies, reductions in the expression of TGF-β_1 using various modifiers such as amifostine reduced the clinical and histologic manifestations of radiation pneumonitis and fibrosis.[141-143] More importantly, preselection of lung cancer patients for dose escalation using plasma TGF-β allowed identification of patients at low risk for complications to whom higher doses of radiation could be safely delivered.[140] One initiator of radiation lung damage that may be amenable to modulation is oxidative stress leading to the formation of reactive oxygen species.[141] Biological modifiers targeting oxidative damage, such as superoxide dismutase (SOD), a key enzyme in the defense against the superoxide radical, has been shown to protect the lung against radiation pneumonitis and fibrosis. A post irradiation hypoxic environment in the lung may be permissive and mediate sustained expression of inflammatory and fibrogenic cytokines, accounting for the appearance of lung fibrosis months to years after irradiation.[144] Genetic loci associated with susceptibility to RILI has been identified on specific chromosomes in mouse models, although none of the specific "susceptibility" genes has been identified.[145,146] Currently, there are no effective strategies for predicting the response of individual patients to treatment or susceptibility to injury. The identification of specific genes that confer an increased risk for RILI in individual patients would allow risk stratification for potential lung injury, and permit the use of more aggressive treatment protocols and higher tumor control in the less susceptible patients, while more susceptible patients could be treated with "targeted" therapies.

Other research efforts to improve the therapeutic index in radiotherapy have focused on the development of pharmacologic agents that selectively protect normal tissues from the damaging effects of radiation. Amifostine, a thiol-containing agent that exhibits remarkable cytoprotective properties, has been approved for clinical radiotherapy as a protector against radiation-induced xerostomia in patients with head and neck cancers.[147,148] In several recent clinical trials, amifostine-treated patients undergoing chemoradiation therapy for treatment of lung cancer experienced significantly fewer episodes of severe RP and esophagitis versus controls.[149,150] Notably, the cytoprotective effect of amifostine has been shown to occur without inducing tumor protection. With the exception of dysgeusia and transient hypotension that occurs in 7% of patients, the drug is generally well tolerated.

Fortunately, most cases of RP are subclinical or mild and require only expectant management and occasional antipyretics, antitussives and bronchodilators. Corticosteroids are indicated for moderate and severe cases and may result in dramatic improvements in symptoms. Although no large body of data detailing the efficacy of corticosteroids in the management of symptomatic RILI is currently available, a long clinical history of successful steroid use supports this practice. Guidelines for steroid administration in the treatment of RP have not been firmly established, although a regimen of prednisone given at 0.5-1 mg/kg of body weight is generally accepted. Steroids should be initiated once the diagnosis is reasonably certain and tapered according to clinical response over the ensuing weeks. In light of reports suggesting that rapid steroid taper may unmask latent radiation injury to the lung, a slow steroid taper is recommended. The late phase of pneumonitis may be refractory to even high-dose steroids. No benefit of steroids in the treatment of fibrotic lung disease has been shown and currently there are no effective strategies for intervening in this late sequela

Pulmonary Complications of Hematopoietic Stem Cell Transplantation

Hematopoietic stem cell transplantation (HSCT) is the only curative option for many patients with relapsed and high-risk hematologic malignancies. Despite advances in treatment regimens and supportive care, pulmonary complications occur in up to 60% of HSCT recipients, accounting for significant morbidity and mortality.[151,152] Like most aspects of transplantation care, pulmonary complications are conveniently divided into those that occur "early" (during the first 100 days after transplantation) and those that occur "late" (Table 131-3). These complications are primarily due to direct toxicities from conditioning regimens, delayed bone marrow recovery, prolonged immunosuppressive therapy, and graft-versus-host disease (GVHD). Infectious complications occur most commonly after allogeneic HSCT due to the high incidence of GVHD and prolonged use of immunosuppressive therapy. As successful prophylactic treatment strategies have effectively reduced the rates of infectious pulmonary complications, noninfectious pulmonary complications have emerged as a major cause of post-HSCT morbidity and mortality.

Pulmonary Infections in HSCT Patients

Pneumonia is a major cause of morbidity and mortality in HSCT, occurring in up to 80% of patients in some studies.[153,154] Compromised host defense following HSCT plays a principle role in the development of pneumonia. Early after transplantation (within the first 100 days), major alterations in host defense include neutropenia and the disruption of mucocutaneous barriers. Slow recovery of cellular immunity, hypogammaglobulinemia, and immunosuppressive treatment of GVHD are prominent late (>100 days following transplant) immune de-

Table 131-3 Pulmonary Complications After Hematopoietic Stem Cell Transplantation

	Early (<100 days)	Late (>100 days)
Infectious (pneumonia)	Bacterial, fungal , viral, protozoal pathogens	Bacterial, fungal, viral pathogens
Noninfectious	Pulmonary edema Idiopathic pneumonia syndrome Diffuse alveolar hemorrhage Engraftment syndrome Delayed pulmonary toxicity syndrome Rare disorders: secondary pulmonary alveolar proteinosis, pulmonary veno-occlusive disease	Restrictive lung disease Constrictive bronchiolitis Rare disorders: lymphocytic interstitial pneumonitis

fects. These underlying immunologic defects, both quantitative and qualitative, and the duration of the immunocompromised state may promote the emergence of pneumonias caused by opportunistic bacterial, fungal, and viral pathogens.

Bacterial Pneumonias Bacterial pneumonias are most common during the neutropenic preengraftment period, though they can occur at any time after HSCT with an overall incidence of 15%. Gram-negative enteric organisms, such as *Pseudomonas aeruginosa, Klebsiella pneumoniae, Enterobacter cloacae, Stenotrophomonas, Serratia, Proteus, Nocardia,* and *Citrobacter* species predominate during the first 100 days.[154,155] Gram-positive organisms, particularly *Staphylococcus aureus*, are also seen, but are usually associated with bacteremia from the universal use of central venous catheters. Encapsulated organisms, such as *Streptococcus pneumoniae* and *Haemophilus influenzae* play a larger role in the postengraftment period due to the prolonged impairment of humoral immunity. Hospital-acquired pneumonias are associated with higher mortality than community-acquired.[154] *Legionella pneumophila* has been reported as a cause of severe nosocomial pneumonia by several transplant centers.[156,157] The diagnosis of bacterial pneumonia is often difficult due to the nonspecific clinical presentation and the long differential diagnosis in HSCT patients. A chest radiograph is not a reliable method for primary detection of pneumonia due to its low sensitivity; a chest CT scan, in addition to being more sensitive for diagnosis, also helps direct the localization of invasive diagnostic procedures. Broad-spectrum antibiotics, including antipseudomonal coverage, should be initiated in all patients with suspected bacterial pneumonia, especially in the setting of neutropenia.

Viral Pneumonias Viral pneumonias are a major cause of morbidity and mortality after HSCT. The incidence of cytomegalovirus (CMV), the major viral pathogen causing pneumonia in the early post-transplant setting, has declined markedly due to effective prophylaxis and preemptive treatment.[158-160] CMV remains a problem, however, during the late phase of HSCT, with a current incidence of 2% in both allogeneic and autologous transplants. CMV-seropositive recipients are at highest risk, reflecting reactivation of latent virus.[160] Gancyclovir is currently the treatment of choice, and combination therapy with CMV immunoglobulin improved survival in nonrandomized prospective studies.[161,162] Despite treatment, mortality rates remain high, especially in patients with associated respiratory failure. Community-acquired viral respiratory infections are also important in HSCT recipients, with respiratory syncytial virus accounting for the majority.[163] Upper respiratory tract symptoms of fever, coryza and cough may progress to pneumonia in half of HSCT patients, which usually occurs as an early complication following transplantation. Mortality rates among those with respiratory syncytial virus (RSV) pneumonia approaches 80%, and initiation of treatment with aerosolized ribavirin and intravenous immunoglobulin initiated at the stage of upper respiratory infection is recommended to avoid progression.[164] Other viruses that less commonly affect the lungs include influenza, parainfluenza, herpes simplex, and adenovirus, often in association with seasonal outbreaks in the community. These can be diagnosed either by nasal washings or bronchoalveolar lavage.

Fungal Pneumonias Invasive aspergillosis remains an important problem among HSCT patients, with a rising incidence and high mortality. The major risk factors include allogeneic HSCT, immunosuppressive therapy, corticosteroid use, CMV disease, and GVHD.[165] A recent shift in the incidence of this disease from the preengraftment to the postengraftment period is attributed to the shorter duration of neutropenia, and delayed onsets of GVHD and CMV infection.[165] Other fungal infections occur less commonly, and are described below.

Miscellaneous Lung Infections The widespread use of prophylactic trimethoprim-sulfamethoxazole during the early transplant period has resulted in a significant decline in the incidence of *Pneumocystis* pneumonia, which is now primarily seen among sulfa-allergic patients receiving less effective prophylaxis.[166] Indolent infections with nontuberculous mycobacteria are relatively common at some transplant centers.[167]

Early Onset Noninfectious Complications of HSCT

Pulmonary Edema Diffuse pulmonary edema is one of the most common early complications after transplantation. Etiologies include increased hydrostatic capillary pressure associated with the administration of large volumes of fluid and cardiac dysfunction. Increased pulmonary capillary permeability leading to noncardiogenic pulmonary edema associated with the preconditioning regimen also occur.[152,168] Hydrostatic and permeability etiologies of post transplant pulmonary edema may be simultaneously present and overlap with other early-onset pulmonary complications. The abrupt onset of dyspnea, hypoxia and bilateral pulmonary infiltrates coupled with the absence of infection on diagnostic evaluation are supportive findings. Pleural effusions may accompany pulmonary edema. Bilateral pleural effusions associated with weight gain may be approached conservatively without the need for diagnostic thoracentesis.

Periengraftment Syndrome Fever, noncardiogenic pulmonary edema, erythematous skin rash, and hypoxemia, characterizes this syndrome which occurs during the neutrophil recovery phase following HSCT. Estimates of the reported incidence varies widely with disease definition and the population studied, but generally occurs in 5-10% of autologous HSCT recipients when stringent diagnostic criteria are used.[169,170,171] While the pathophysiology is not well understood, it appears to involve the release of proinflammatory cytokines during the engraftment period and endothelial damage from the conditioning regimen. Risk factors include the use of growth factors, number of infused mononuclear or CD34 positive cells, speed of neutrophil recovery, type of conditioning regimen, underlying disease, and peripheral blood as the source of stem cells. Some studies have shown improvement with corticosteroid therapy,[170] including a recent study in which corticosteroid prophylaxis decreased the risk of periengraftment syndrome without increasing the risk of infection.[172] Whereas the National Institutes of Health (NIH) sponsored Blood and Marrow Transplant Clinical Trials Network includes periengraftment syndrome within the definition of idiopathic pneumonia syndrome (see below), there may be value to considering it separately because of its responsiveness to corticosteroid therapy and lower mortality.[168]

Idiopathic Pneumonia Syndrome (IPS) ■ In 1993, a panel convened by the NIH proposed a broad working definition of IPS as widespread nonlobar radiographic infiltrates in the absence of congestive heart failure or evidence of lower respiratory tract infection.[173] IPS occurs in 10% of HSCT recipients, usually 14-90 days following transplantation. Mortality rates range from 50% to 70%.[174-176] Risk factors include transplantation for malignancy other than leukemia, older age, total body irradiation, type of pretransplant chemotherapy, high-grade GVHD, CMV-seropositive donor, HLA disparity, and lower performance status.[175] Possible etiologies of IPS include direct toxic effects of the chemoradiation conditioning regimen, occult infection, and the release of inflammatory cytokines. However, the association of IPS with the presence of acute GVHD after allogeneic transplantation suggests that alloreactive T-cell injury may also be an important contributor.[175,176] The clinical presentation is nonspecific, with symptoms of acute dyspnea, cough, and fever associated with diffuse infiltrates on chest radiograph. The diagnosis of IPS largely relies on the exclusion of infection in lower respiratory samples obtained from bronchoalveolar lavage. The nonspecific findings of diffuse alveolar damage and interstitial pneumonitis on histopathologic examination of tissue from lung biopsies are typically not helpful in directing therapy.[173,175] Although no randomized controlled trials of treatment for IPS are available, current standards include high-dose intravenous corticosteroids and supportive care, such as supplemental oxygen and broad-spectrum antibiotics. Recent preclinical and clinical data suggest a potential role for tumor necrosis factor-α (TNF-α) in the pathogenesis of IPS, and a randomized trial using etanercept, a TNF receptor fusion protein, is being conducted by the Blood and Marrow Transplant Clinical Trials Network.

Diffuse Alveolar Hemorrhage (DAH)

Posttransplant DAH, initially defined in autologous HSCT recipients, is characterized by widespread lung injury and diffuse radiographic infiltrates occurring in the absence of identifiable infection.[177] It is manifested bronchoscopically as progressively bloodier returns on bronchoalveolar lavage taken from three or more subsegmental bronchi. DAH is now known to occur in both allogeneic and autologous transplant recipients with equal frequency,[178-181] and the bronchoscopic criteria have expanded to include cytologic evidence of >20% hemosiderin-laden macrophages in the bronchoalveolar lavage fluid. These bronchoscopic criteria, however, may be seen in association with diffuse lung injury from a wide variety of causes in the posttransplant setting, and the diagnostic and therapeutic implications of DAH are unclear. In an autopsy study, bloody bronchoalveolar lavage fluid was neither sensitive nor specific for histologic evidence of DAH.[182] The bronchoscopic findings of DAH may simply represent an index of severity of alveolar injury and concomitant hemostatic defects rather than a separate syndrome, with prognosis and therapy more importantly determined by the underlying pathophysiologic process (engraftment syndrome, idiopathic pneumonia syndrome, sepsis, etc). The Blood and Marrow Transplant Clinical Trials Network has adopted this view and include DAH within the definition of idiopathic pneumonia syndrome.

Pulmonary Veno-occlusive Disease (PVOD)

PVOD is a very rare complication of HSCT in which progressive occlusion of pulmonary veins and venules caused by intimal proliferation and fibrosis leads to pulmonary hypertension.[183] High-dose chemotherapy and infections are implicated as causes of PVOD. The onset is typically insidious, with progressive dyspnea and fatigue occurring 6–8 weeks after transplant.[118,184] The diagnosis and treatment of PVOD are further described in the section entititled "Pulmonary Hypertension."

Late Onset Noninfectious Complications of HSCT

Posttransplantation Constrictive Bronchiolitis (PTCB) ■ Posttransplantation constrictive bronchiolitis is the most common pulmonary complication among long-term survivors of HSCT. It is a late manifestation of GVHD that leads to progressive respiratory insufficiency, and sometimes death. PTCB almost never occurs in the absence of GVHD, and thus only affects patients undergoing allogeneic transplant.[151,185,186] Due to the lack of uniform diagnostic criteria, its reported incidence varies from 10% to 26%. PTCB affects small airways, causing chronic inflammation, epithelial mucous metaplasia, submucosal scarring, smooth muscle hypertrophy, and concentric bronchiolar fibrosis. The most commonly identified risk factors are chronic GVHD, older age, viral infections during the first 100 days after transplant, the presence of airflow limitation before transplant, low serum IgG, and the use of methotrexate or busulfan in the conditioning regimen.[168,187] PTCB is generally accepted as a pulmonary manifestation of chronic GVHD. The recruitment of donor lymphocytes to the airways which then react against recipient alloantigens in host bronchiolar epithelial and mesenchymal cells is a putative mechanism in the pathogenesis of this disorder. A recent mouse model showed extensive perivascular and peribronchial inflammation with CD4 and CD8 T lymphocytes with histological features of airway obstruction consistent with bronchiolitis obliterans.[188] Approximately 80% of patients present with symptoms of progressive dyspnea, cough, and wheezing that typically develop insidiously within 6 months to 1 year following HSCT.[189] Earlier signs and symptoms occurring at 3 months post-HSCT have been described. Up to 20% of patients are asymptomatic. Chest radiographs are usually normal, but HRCT scans may show evidence of air trapping, thickened or dilated small airways, and mosaic attenuation. Bronchoscopy with BAL and transbronchial lung biopsy is generally not helpful in establishing the diagnosis. Pulmonary function tests (PFTs) are the primary tools used for diagnosis and follow-up. Evidence of airflow obstruction with reduction in forced expiratory volume in 1 s (FEV1) and FEV1/forced vital capacity (FVC) are supportive PFT findings, however, a consensus on the spirometric criteria for the diagnosis of PTCB following HSCT is lacking. The NIH consensus guidelines for diagnosing PTCB include: (1) FEV1/FVC <0.7 and FEV1 <75% of predicted; residual volume on PFTs >120% predicted; (2) evidence of air trapping, small airway thickening, or bronchiectasis on HRCT, or pathological confirmation of constrictive bronchiolitis; and (3) the absence of any infectious process on radiographic, laboratory or clinical testing.[190] These diagnostic criteria are typically associated with severe airflow obstruction and airway fibrosis which are late findings that are commonly refractory to therapeutic interventions.

Treatment options for PTCB have not been evaluated in any prospective trials. Augmentation of systemic immunosuppression with corticosteroids has traditionally been the mainstay of therapy.[176] However, two recent retrospective analyses, indicate that inhaled high-dose corticosteroid therapy is effective in stabilizing FEV_1 and significantly reducing symptoms.[191,192] A beneficial effect of azithromycin, possibly due to its antiinflammatory effects, has also been reported in a recent observational study[193] Lung transplantation is an option in selected patients. Chronic GVHD continues to be a major cause of mortality and morbidity in long-term survivors of HSCT, and PTCB is an important contributor. The clinical course and disease progression are variable, but persistent airflow obstruction is associated with a significantly increased risk of death.[185] Early detection of PTCB is crucial to improve survival. A recent 2-year international effort to improve the amount of properly conducted prospective trials in the management of chronic GVHD has been addressed in a series of guideline papers published by the NIH chronic GVHD Consensus Panel.

Cryptogenic Organizing Pneumonitis (COP)

Also known as idiopathic BOOP, COP occurs mostly in allogeneic HSCT recipients with GVHD or following CMV pneumonitis.[186,194] It is less common than PTCB, with an incidence of 1-2% in long-term survivors. Dry cough and dyspnea accompanied by patchy infiltrates on chest radiograph and CT scan are the predominant presenting signs and symptoms. The diagnosis is made with surgical lung biopsy. In the absence of HSCT, COP is usually responsive to corticosteroids; however, the response to steroids and prognosis of COP following HSCT is less favorable, with an overall case fatality of 20%.[168]

Delayed Pulmonary Toxicity Syndrome

This syndrome has been described in breast cancer patients following autologous HSCT. It is characterized by interstitial pneumonitis and fibrosis, and is thought to be due to the toxic effects of high-dose chemotherapy, including cyclophosphamide, cisplatin, and BCNU. Patients usually present around 10 weeks following transplantation with dry cough, dyspnea, and fever.[195] Pulmonary function testing reveals restrictive lung disease and a reduction in diffusing capacity. Steroid therapy is commonly beneficial and mortality rates are low.

Posttransplant Lymphoproliferative Disorder (PTLD)

Posttransplant lymphoproliferative disorder is an uncontrolled expansion of donor-derived EBV-infected B-lymphocytes that develops in response to inadequate cytotoxic T-cell function.[151,196] It occurs in approximately 1% of HSCT patients, usually within the first 4-12 months after transplanation. The lung is involved only 20% of the time, most commonly with ill-defined nodular infiltrates. PTLD has been successfully treated with donor leukocytes.

Pneumonia

Pulmonary infections frequently complicate cancer and its therapy, resulting in greater mortality than any other infectious complication of cancer.[197,198] Classic clinical indicators to suggest the presence of lower respiratory infections include the development of pulmonary parenchymal infiltrates, leukocytosis, fever, and expectoration of purulent secretions. However, as a consequence of impaired immune responses, these typical clinical observations may be absent in cancer patients with pneumonia. Therefore, a high index of suspicion is required to avoid overlooking the diagnosis. Further, early radiographic imaging, often including CT scanning, is indicated in cancer patients with unexplained clinical deterioration or new infiltrates on conventional imaging.

The diagnosis of pneumonia is confirmed by recovery of the likely pathogen from an otherwise sterile source (eg, blood, urine, pleural fluid) or isolation of a noncommensal organism in respiratory secretions. Although the utility of expectorated sputum in the diagnosis of pneumonia is debated, cytologically confirmed lower respiratory samples appear to be diagnostically useful. Fiberoptic bronchoscopy with BAL is considered the diagnostic tool of choice for obtaining lower respiratory samples. While this procedure is safe for most cancer patients, traditional culture methods yield the responsible pathogen in only 25-51% of cases.[199-202] The benefit of BAL may be enhanced by early bronchoscopic evaluation, particularly if obtained before the initiation of antimicrobial therapy. Microscopic examination of transbronchial biopsy specimens can identify angioinvasion of some commensal microbes (eg, *Aspergillus* spp.), but culture of biopsy material has not been proved diagnostically superior to BAL, and is precluded in many cancer patients by coagulopathy and/or thrombocytopenia. Culture results from BAL or biopsy can be difficult to interpret due to frequent colonization of the upper airway with nondisease associated microorganisms. Conversely, sterile respiratory tract cultures do not exclude an infectious etiology, particularly in the setting of recent administration of broad-spectrum antibiotics. Molecular techniques, including polymerase chain reaction (PCR) testing for pathogen genomic material or antigen detection methods (eg, serum galactomannan, urinary *Histoplasma* antigen), can also supplement the diagnostic evaluation.

Early and accurate diagnoses are critical to a successful outcome, although treatment should not be withheld while diagnostic interventions are undertaken. Antimicrobial selections are based on knowledge of the infecting pathogen, if available, pneumonia severity, underlying immune status and the presence of comorbid conditions[203,204] (see Chapter 137). Delays in appropriate antimicrobial therapy increase the risk of secondary complications and infection-associated deaths, especially in severely immunosuppressed individuals. Therefore, it is common practice to initiate empiric and/or preemptive antimicrobial therapy in patients in which the suspicion of infection is high. However, the clinician is cautioned to recall that cancer patients are prone to numerous causes of fever and pulmonary infiltrates other than infectious pneumonias, including toxicities of therapy, systemic inflammation associated with extrapulmonary infections, heart failure, parenchymal cancer involvement or intrapulmonary hemorrhage.

Venous Thromboembolism

Pulmonary embolism (PE) and deep venous thrombosis (DVT) are the two manifestations of venous thromboembolism (VTE), a common complication in cancer. Approximately 20% of VTE in the general population is associated with cancer, and cancer increases the risk for VTE about 5-fold. Therapy for cancer, including surgery, hospitalization, chemotherapy, hormonal therapy, growth factors, angiogenesis inhibitors, and central venous catheters (CVC), further heightens the risk of thrombosis.[205] For example, patients with cancer experience a 2-fold to 3-fold increase in the risk of VTE-associated with any surgical procedure; the incidence of VTE in postmenopausal women receiving chemotherapy and tamoxifen for breast cancer is 10%; and in renal cancer patients receiving thalidomide-based chemotherapy regimens the incidence of VTE is more than 40%. Although fatality rates directly attributable to VTE among cancer patients have not been firmly established, prospective analyses have demonstrated a 4- to 8-fold increase in VTE-associated mortality over patients without cancer.[206]

VTE has many clinical presentations, most of which are not specific. Algorithms and "score" systems developed to assist in the estimation of a pretest probability of VTE in the general population are useless in the cancer population, in which the mere presence of malignancy entails such a high risk. D-dimer assays are helpful screening tests with an excellent negative predictive value in both the noncancer and cancer setting. The likelihood of finding a normal D-dimer level among cancer patients, however, is less than 30%.[207] Venous ultrasound is the preferred method to diagnose DVT, although MRI and CT may be required in special circumstances, such as internal iliac vein or vena cava thrombosis. Ventilation/perfusion (V/Q) lung scans remain useful in the diagnosis of PE. The sensitivity and specificity of CT pulmonary angiography in the diagnosis of central thrombosis is equivalent if not superior to V/Q scans (Fig. 131-9). Furthermore, CT angiography offers the advantage of providing additional information regarding competing thoracic pathology that may confound the diagnosis of PE.[208]

VTE prophylaxis is of proven efficacy among at-risk patients and should be considered in almost every patient with cancer.[209] Thromboprophylaxis among cancer patients should follow current recommendations for medical and surgical patients in the general population, although some cancer-specific recommendations do exist. Low molecular weight heparins (LMWH) are the most studied agents in this population, and their use is encouraged. Cancer patients undergoing abdominal or pelvic surgery should receive LMWH[210,211] prophylaxis for at least 4 weeks.[212] Routine prophylaxis in cancer patients receiving chemotherapy is not recommended. Although there are no randomized clinical trials, a consensus statement based on expert opinion recommends active prophylaxis for patients with multiple myeloma receiving dexamethasone, doxorubicin or other chemotherapy, in combination with thalidomide or lenalidomide.[213] In the past, fixed, low dose warfarin and LMWH were regularly used for the prevention of CVC thrombosis. This practice was based on the results of older, open-label investigations. More recent, larger, and better-controlled studies contradict these findings.[214,215] and support the current opinion that no prophylaxis should be used for CVC thrombosis.

Initial therapy for established VTE follows general recommendations, as no cancer-specific treatment trials exist. Current recommendations include LMWH for most patients, unfractionated heparin (UFH) for patients with renal failure, thrombolysis in cases of massive PE, and IVC filters when there are clear contraindications for anticoagulation.[216]

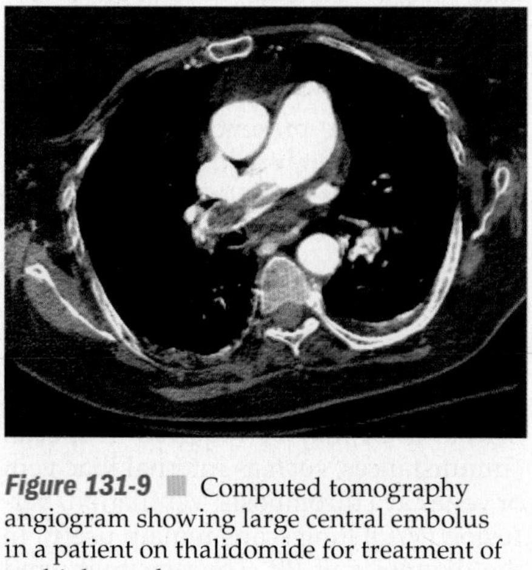

Figure 131-9 Computed tomography angiogram showing large central embolus in a patient on thalidomide for treatment of multiple myeloma.

Based on recent evidence, the long-term treatment or secondary prophylaxis of VTE in cancer patients should include at least 6 months of LMWH instead of warfarin.[217] Whether there is any added benefit in extending therapy beyond 6 months is currently the subject of ongoing studies.

Pulmonary Hypertension in the Cancer Patient

Pulmonary hypertension (PH), defined as a mean pulmonary artery pressure (mPAP) ≥25 mmHg at rest or ≥30 mm Hg during exercise, is an under-recognized problem in the cancer setting. Estimates of cancer-related pulmonary arterial hypertension (PAH) vary broadly with specific cancers, associated cancer therapies and the method of detection of PH. Transthoracic doppler echocardiography (TTE) provides an estimation of pulmonary artery systolic pressure (PASP) and serves as a noninvasive screening tool for PH. Confirmation requires right heart catherization (RHC), which can also be used to reliably assess associated hemodynamic impairments and to evaluate the vasoreactivity of the pulmonary circulation.[218,219] Nonspecific signs and symptoms of exertional dyspnea and fatigue early in the disease process render diagnostic evaluations notoriously difficult and result in substantial delays in treatment. Successful treatment of PAH requires high clinical suspicion, as advanced disease, signaled by syncope, angina, peripheral edema, abdominal distention, and hemodynamic instability is often refractory to therapy.

The WHO classification scheme from 2003 categorizes PH as PAH, pulmonary venous hypertension (PVH), hypoxic pulmonary hypertension, chronic thromboembolic pulmonary hypertension and pulmonary hypertension from miscellaneous causes. Cancer-related events impact each of these categories, giving rise to PH which both complicates and confounds cancer therapy. For example, prolonged hypoxia associated with ARDS, sepsis, pneumonia, or treatment-related lung injury are complications of cancer therapy that contributes to cancer-related microvascular arteriopathy and PAH. In addition, chronic obstructive lung disease and obstructive sleep apnea (OSA) frequently appear as comorbid illnesses in patients with lung and head and neck cancers and may be additional sources of refractory hypoxemia.[218-220] Hypothyroidism, an often a late sequela of head and neck irradiation, has also been linked to PAH.[221,222] Hypoventilation and hypoxemia associated with severe hypothyrodism may worsen existing PH.[223-225] Other cancer-related clinical disorders, notably, human immunodeficiency virus (HIV) infection, and chemotherapeutic agents, including carmustine, mitomycin, bleomycin and the immunomodulatory agents, interleukin-2 and interferon-γ, may incite substantial elevations in pulmonary artery pressures (PAPs) and PAH. An association between PH and portal hypertension, which occurs in up to 17% of patients with certain types of myeloproliferative disorders (MPD), such as polycythemia vera, myelofibrosis with myeloid metaplasia and essential thrombocythemia, is well described.[226] Increased rates of PAH are also observed among patients with MPD in the absence of portal hypertension, perhaps owing to the prothrombotic tendency and the propensity for vascular obstruction that characterizes this group of disorders.[226] Finally, leukemic patients with profound elevations in circulating myeloblasts or promyelocytes may develop PAH as a result of sludging of WBCs within the pulmonary microvasculature (the so-called "white clot" syndrome).[184,227-229]

PVH typically occurs as a result of decompensated left-sided valvular or myocardial disease that may be caused by a variety of cancer-related disorders. These include sepsis, arrhythmias, and myocardial toxicity secondary to chemoradiation therapy. In addition to primary cardiac disease, PVH may occur due to obstruction to postcapillary pulmonary veins caused by PVOD or external compression and/or entrapment of large pulmonary veins by adenopathy, neoplasms, or mediastinal fibrosis. Infection, chemotoxins, thoracic radiation and stem cell transplantation are postulated risk factors for PVOD, although no clear causal relationship has been established.[184,230,231] The prognosis for PVOD is poor. Although some patients may tolerate arterial vasodilators, fatal pulmonary edema precipitated by pulmonary vasodilator therapy has been observed. Hodgkin's lymphoma and germ cell tumors underlie most causes of PVH due to mediastinal compression. Fibrosing mediastinitis related to radiation and infection (*Aspergillous, Mycobacterium tuberculosis, Blastomycosis, Mucormycosis,* and *Cryptococcosis*) has also been reported.[232-234]

Arterial thrombosis due to massive pulmonary embolism may cause acute, catastrophic elevations in PAP associated with severe hypoxemia, cor pulmonale and sudden death. Submassive pulmonary embolism among patients with a preexisting cardiopulmonary disease may have an equally devastating outcome. Arterial thrombosis is typically caused by obstruction of the central pulmonary arteries by clot, although tumor, air, and fat may also become trapped in the pulmonary circulation, with equally catastrophic consequences. The cancer patient, for a variety of reasons, is at increased risk for the development of these unusual forms of pulmonary embolic disease, and the clinical and hemodynamic derangements may be indistinguishable from pulmonary thromboembolic disease.

The principal primary malignances involving the pulmonary vasculature are sarcomas. These rare and frequently fatal tumors typically arise from the main pulmonary arteries, although pulmonary venous sarcomas have also been described.[235] Patients with pulmonary arterial sarcomas often present with signs and symptoms that mimic chronic thromboembolic pulmonary hypertension (CTEPH) (dyspnea, chest pain, cough hemoptysis). However, associated findings of unexplained fever, weight loss, clubbing, anemia and elevated ESR should raise suspicion of malignancy. Secondary tumoral involvement of the pulmonary vascular bed may present as macrovascular central tumor emboli or smaller tumor cell aggregates that occlude small vessels. The latter may occur with or without lymphangiitic spread of disease. Choriocarcinomas and mucinous tumors originating in the breast, lung, gastrointestinal tract, and kidneys are associated with the highest rates of tumor embolization. Clinical symptoms of tumor emboli range from the abrupt onset of dyspnea, chest pain and cardiovascular collapse to subacute symptoms of cough, exertional dyspnea and exercise intolerance associated with unexplained pulmonary hypertension. Pulmonary tumor thrombotic microangiopathy (PTTM) is an unusual cause of malignancy-related pulmonary hypertension that is most often seen in patients with adenocarcinomas, particularly of the stomach. Patients present with severe, refractory pulmonary hypertension that rapidly progresses to sudden cardiovascular collapse and death. PTTM is characterized by severe obliterative fibrointimal hyperplasia that leads to massive reductions in the area of the pulmonary vascular bed. Histologic evidence of prominent intimal fibrosis of the arteries, focal fibrin emboli admixed with tumor cells and areas of recanalization helps to distinguish PTTM from tumor embolism. Findings on pulmonary microvascular cytology are diagnostically useful; however, the diagnosis of PTTM is most often made only at necropsy. No definitive treatment has thus far been identified.

Leukemic sequestration and leukocyte thrombus formation within the pulmonary microvasculature are rare complications of hyperleukocytosis (WBC >50,000/dL) and blast crisis associated with myeloid and lymphocytic leukemias. Patients typically present with dyspnea, nonproductive cough and hypoxemia associated with interstitial infiltrates and sighns of pulmonary hypertension and cor pulmonale. The clinical manifestations of macrovascular tumor emboli resemble acute pulmonary thromboembolic disease. Microvascular tumor embolization, however, typically presents with insidious symptoms of dyspnea, nonproductive cough, hypoxemia and severe pulmonary artery pressure elevations. Cor pulmonale and diffuse interstitial infiltrates, suggestive of lymphangitic spread of disease, are common findings that worsen the already poor prognosis (Fig. 131-10). Acute hypoxemic respiratory failure has also been reported following the initiation of chemotherapy for treatment of acute nonlymphocytic leukemia. This syndrome, known as leukemic cell lysis pneumopathy, typically occurs during the initial 48 h of treatment and is thought to be caused by chemotherapy-induced pulmonary leukostasis and perivascular hemorrhage. Measured PaO_2 may be artificially low in patients with hyperleukocytic leukemias in the absence of lung involvement, owing to leukocyte metabolism of oxygen within the arterial blood gas syringe. In this setting oxygen saturations obtained by pulse oximetry are normal. Rapid analysis of the arterial blood gas specimen kept on ice or the addition of cyanide to the blood gas syringe eliminates this problem.

Although in most major medical centers, CT angiography has replaced ventilation-perfusion scans in the evaluation of thromboembolic events, in the setting of suspected tumor emboli, ventilation-perfusion (V/Q) scans may be of greater diagnostic utility than the chest CT. Multiple subsegmental mismatched defects on V/Q scintigraphy are supportive findings. Pulmonary microvascular cytology of samples obtained from a wedged pulmonary artery catheter during RHC may offer additional support for tumor embolization.[236]

Evidenced-based algorithms are currently available in the management idiopathic PAH.[237,238] Caution in extrapolating these guidelines to other forms of PAH is warranted. No studies have addressed the utility of pulmonary vasodilator therapy in the management of cancer-related PH. Treatment of PH in this setting should address the underlying cause. Specific guidelines regarding the optimal use of vasopressor therapy in the critically ill cancer patient with PH and associated hemodynamic deterioration are also unavailable, but in the general population, the use of dobutamine, milrinone, inhaled nitric oxide, and intravenous prostacyclin have the greatest support in the literature.

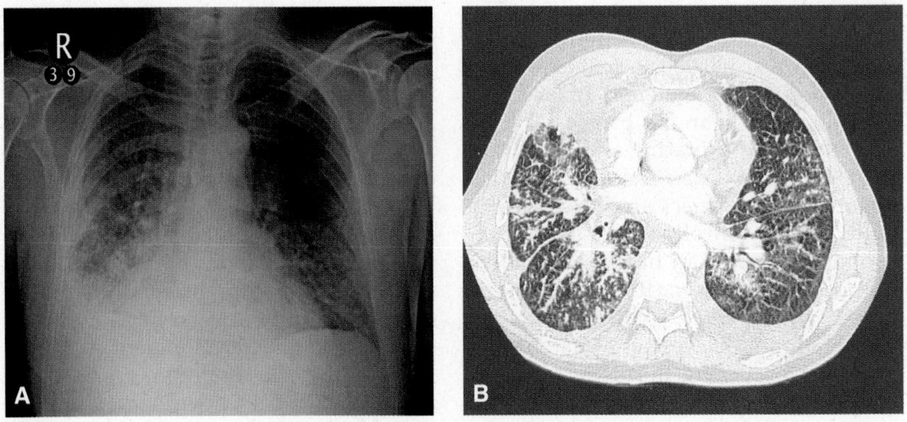

Figure 131-10 CXR **(A)** and chest CT **(B)** of a patient with primary bronchogenic carcinoma. The nodular perivascular and septal thickening in the absence of architectural distortion of the lung parenchymal is typical of lymphangitic spread of tumor.

Sleep Disorders, Chronobiology, and Cancer

Sleep-related complaints are common and but often unappreciated in cancer patients. A large cross-sectional series of 1012 patients with cancer documented the pervasiveness of sleep-related complaints, including fatigue (44%), leg restlessness (41%) insomnia (31%), and excessive sleepiness (28%).[239] Sleep disturbance and chronobiology have important implications throughout the continuum of care of the cancer patient, impacting cancer prevention, treatment and survivorship.

Cancer Prevention

Prolonged sleep duration and disturbed circadian rhythms of sleep are associated with increases in cancer risk. The Japanese Cohort Study, which collected data from over 100,000 patients, revealed excess cancer prevalence in patients who slept less than 5 h or greater than 9 h per night.[240] Rotating and nocturnal shift work may also increase the risk of cancer. The American Nurse Health Study, which enrolled over 70,000 respondents, found an increased relative risk of breast cancer (RR = 1.4) among nurses who worked rotating shifts for greater than 30 years. Melatonin, a naturally occurring hormone with oncostatic potential, is suppressed with nocturnal light exposure. The Lower urinary levels of melatonin metabolites found in these nurses were associated with an increased cancer risk.[241-243] There is increasing evidence to suggest that disturbed sleep has detrimental effects on the immune response. Cellular, hormonal and inflammatory mediators are also affected by sleep disruption.[244] Recent data suggest a reciprocal relationship between sleep and immunity. Oncogenesis may be promoted in the setting of impaired immune system-mediated tumor surveillance and the proinflammatory milieu consequent to sleep disruption and abnormal circadian rhythms.

Cancer Treatment

Disrupted sleep, a common symptom of cancer therapy, has important consequences on cancer treatment and symptoms, such as fatigue and pain. Excessive daytime sleepiness and fatigue are associated with increased plasma cytokines, such as IL-6. A good night's sleep can decrease the levels of this cytokine. Inflammatory mediators produced by specific cancer interventions or the cancer itself may exacerbate sleep disruption. For example, chemotherapy regimens used to treat breast cancer may induce elevations in vascular endothelial growth factor (VEGF) which is associated with disturbed sleep.[245] Sleep deprivation and, in particular, loss of rapid eye movement (REM) sleep, are known to be hyperalgesic. Thus, reduced sleep conditions, including REM sleep deprivation, which is common in many cancer patients, confer increased sensitivity to pain.[246] Studies in our center are underway to determine whether improved sleep quality will decrease the need for medications for cancer-related pain.

Primary sleep disorders, such as sleep-related movement disorders and sleep apnea also affect sleep quality in cancer patients. Restless leg syndrome and periodic leg movement disorders are often associated with insomnia and daytime hypersomnolence. These disorders are more common among certain cancer subgroups, perhaps due to anemia and peripheral neuropathy, with the latter being a common toxicity in platinum-based and taxane-based chemotherapies.[247,248]

The obstructive sleep apnea syndromes (OSAS) may also be more prevalent in certain cancers. Two small series reported a 76-91% incidence of OSAS in patients with tumors of the head and neck.[248] A growing body of literature suggests a link between head and neck cancers and the development of OSAS. Head and neck carcinomas presenting as OSAS have been documented in more than 30 case studies. In addition, OSAS occurring as a consequence of cancer therapy in this group of patients is also well described. Given the known link between opiod use and central sleep apnea, this form of sleep-disordered breathing may be a particular issue in patients with cancer, as many are on opiod medications for cancer-related pain.[249]

Chronobiology may play an important role in the treatment of cancer. Chronotherapy optimizes the effects of cancer therapy while minimizing toxicity by taking advantage of the differences in the circadian rhythm of the cell cycle of tumor cells versus host tissues. Human and animal studies have shown that not only are toxicities reduced and treatment outcomes improved, but dose intensity can be increased without enhanced side effect.[250,251]

Cancer Survivorship

Cancer survivors often complain of disturbed sleep, fatigue, and insomnia. A recent survey revealed that 51% of women treated for breast cancer reported nonspecific sleep difficulties and 19% met diagnostic criteria for insomnia.[252] Cognitive and behavioral therapy (CBT) is considered the treatment of choice for this disorder. CBT has been shown to improve symptoms of insomnia, decrease sedative-hypnotic medication use, and improve quality of life. CBT can also impact immune function by increasing levels of IL-1β and γ-interferon, which are thought to promote sleep.[253] The treatment of sleep disorders and circadian rhythm disturbance in patients with cancer, and the effect of this treatment on cancer-related symptoms, especially cancer-related fatigue, is an area of active research in our center and elsewhere. Studies are underway in our sleep laboratory to understand the effect of treating primary sleep disorders, such as limb movement disorder, sleep-disordered breathing and insomnia on cancer-related fatigue. Unraveling these critical, unanswered questions may facilitate our understanding of the complex and often-unrecognized relationships between sleep, chronobiology, and cancer.

Pulmonary Rehabilitation

Dyspnea and fatigue are pervasive symptoms that profoundly impact the quality of life of patients with cancer. Seventy percent of patients complain of fatigue during the course of cancer treatment, which may persist for years following the completion of therapy.[254,255] Rates of dyspnea approach 80% among patients with cancer and may be a marker of advanced disease.[256,257] The genesis of cancer-related dyspnea and fatigue emerges from overlapping and inherently multifactorial etiologies, including cancer and its therapy, hypoxia, anemia, inadequate nutrition, pychosocial factors, pain, altered energy and muscle metabolism and the release of endogenous inflammatory cytokines. Optimal management thus requires a multifaceted approach. Pulmonary rehabilitation (PR) represents a multidisciplinary strategy that incorporates exercise training, patient and family education, psychosocial and behavioral interventions and outcome assessment in the management of patients with chronic dyspnea and fatigue. This approach has been consistently shown to improve dyspnea and fatigue among patients with chronic obstructive lung disease and in the lung transplant setting, however, the benefits of PR in the cancer setting is largely unstudied. Several small reports have suggested that PR may counter chemotherapy-related fatigue, ameliorate performance status and reduce the length/frequency of hospitalizations among patients with cancer.[258-260] An increase in work rate and higher maximal oxygen consumption (VO_2max) claimed by two recent studies have also been suggested.[261,262] These findings, while intriguing, have not been investigated in any large, controlled trials to determine their impact, if any, on improving surgical resectability, or tolerance to aggressive chemoradiation therapy regimens. Several recent small studies have suggested that preoperative pulmonary rehabilitation may improve surgical outcomes and reduce hospital length of stay among patients with marginal lung function due to COPD who undergoing lung resection for lung cancer.[263-265] Our center has recently launched an investigation probing the utility of PR in facilitating eligibility for thoracic resection among lung cancer patients with anatomically resectable tumor, but whose poor performance status precludes surgery. Such studies may expand the role of PR in the management of patients with cancer.

Acute Respiratory Failure

The lung is a frequent target of life-threatening complications of cancer and its treatment. These complications often culminate in respiratory failure (ARF) which is the most common reason for ICU admission among adult patients with cancer. The predisposing conditions for both acute and chronic respiratory insufficiency in cancer patients can be divided into those that cause "lung" failure or "pump" failure. Lung failure is typically associated with ventilation/perfusion abnormalities, shunts, or alterations of alveolar-capillary diffusion and leads primarily to hypoxia, at least in its early stages. A classic example of lung failure is ARDS. Many of the diverse causes of ARDS in cancer, including surgery, infection, chemotherapy, radiotherapy, and complications related to stem cell transplantation have been discussed elsewhere in this chapter. Lung failure may also develop in the absence of ARDS as a consequence of ventilation/perfusion mismatch associated with pneumonia, atelectasis or pulmonary embolism, or as a result of shunt associated with pulmonary edema. Other common causes of lung failure are listed in Table 131-4. Pump failure, by contrast, results from primary failure of alveolar ventilation and leads to severe hypercapnea and acidosis with only mild hypoxemia. Conditions that compromise specific components of the ventilatory pump are prevalent causes of pump failure in patients with cancer. Multifactorial causes of ARF, such as severe COPD exacerbation with superimposed pneumonia may lead to both lung and pump failure. This mixed picture is a common source of respiratory failure in the cancer patient, which requires a systematic approach to each component of respiratory failure in an effort to logically devise treatment strategies. Both causes of respiratory failure in the cancer setting are discussed below.

Ventilatory Pump Insufficiency

The major components of the ventilatory pump include the respiratory controllers of the drive to breathe located in the central nervous system (CNS), the chest wall (including the respiratory muscles), and the pathways that connect the central controllers with the respiratory muscles (spinal and peripheral nerves). Primary failure of alveolar ventilation, also referred to as type II respiratory failure or ventilatory pump insufficiency, occurs when there is sufficient compromise of any of the components of the ventilatory pump. In the cancer setting, multiple contributors to neural and musculoskeletal dysfunction underlie the frequent development of pump failure. Pulmonary rehabilitation has been increasingly used in the management of patients with chronic respiratory insufficiency associated with pump failure.

Causes of Pump Failure

CNS Disorders: Impaired Drive ■ Isolated central depression of ventilatory drive is a rare cause of pump failure that may result from insults to the central nervous system, such as medullary tumors or infarction, or sedating or narcotic medications. Acquired central hypoventilation may occur following neurosurgical procedures for brainstem tumors, particularly those that are close to the floor of the fourth ventricle. Radiation to the base of the skull may have similar adverse effects. Occult hypothyroidism may also contribute to central hypoventilation and ventilatory failure, particularly in elderly women and following treatment for head and neck carcinoma. More often, respiratory failure owing to depressed central drive occurs as an additional insult, superimposed on chronic respiratory insufficiency. In this setting small doses of narcotic or sedating medications may have a profound effect on alveolar ventilation. Respiratory muscle fatigue may also contribute to central hypoventilation by sending inhibitory signals to the respiratory center in the CNS to reduce drive, thereby protecting muscles from injury and mitigating further muscle fatigue.

Peripheral Nervous System Disorders: Inadequate Neuromuscular Competence ■ Transmission of signals from the CNS to the respiratory muscles occurs via the spinal cord and peripheral nerves. Hence, conditions causing neuromuscular dysfunction, such as primary neurologic diseases, spinal cord lesions, neuromuscular blocking drugs and muscle weakness may precipitate ventilatory failure. Systemic anesthetics cause potent neuromuscular blockade and ventilatory depression. Other agents, including sedatives, anxiolytics, hypnotics, and aminoglycosides typically produce severe respiratory depression only in the setting of preexisting neuromuscular diseases such as myasthenia gravis and myasthenic paraneoplastic syndrome or after massive overdose. One exception to this principle is methadone, which may cause ventilatory insufficiency with chronic administration. Muscular weakness and fatigue are prominent complaints that may emerge from diverse etiologies among patients with cancer. Malnutrition and cachexia are well-known complications of advanced cancer, affecting approximately 40-80% of this population and contributing to 22% of cancer-related deaths.[266,267] One of the most relevant manifestations of cancer cachexia is muscle wasting, which contributes to markedly depressed strength and endurance of the skeletal muscles, including the diaphragm.[268] Overinflation of the thorax and flattened diaphragms associated with COPD, a common comorbidity of lung cancer, further contributes to compromised respiratory muscle performance and ventilatory failure. Electrolyte disturbances such as hypophosphatemia, hypokalemia, and hypomagnesemia frequently complicate chemotherapy and may cause profound muscle weakness in the cancer patient. In addition, many of the drugs used in the treatment of ventilatory failure, including beta-agonists, diuretics, and corticosteroids may exacerbate hypophosphatemia and aggravate muscle weakness. Chemotherapeutic agents and other drugs used in chancer treatment may also have deleterious effects on the neuromuscular system. Although corticosteroid-induced myopathy has been well described, the role of these drugs in potentiating respiratory muscle dysfunction has only recently been recognized.[269,270] Among the chemotherapeutic agents, vinca-alky-

Table 131-4 ■ **Lung versus Pump Failure in ARF: Characteristics and Underlying Causes**

	Lung Failure	Pump Failure
Characteristic feature(s)	Hypoxemia	Severe hypercapnea and acidosis: mild hypoxemia
Pathogenesis	Ventilation/perfusion mismatch Shunts Alterations in alveolar capillary membrane	Exhaustion of ventilatory pump (CNS, PNS or respiratory muscles)
Underlying Conditions	Acute lung injury/ARDS Pneumonia Atelectasis Pulmonary embolism/tumor emboli Lymphangitic spread of tumor Chemotherapy/radiation therapy Pulmonary leukostasis Transfusion-related lung injury Postoperative respiratory insufficiency	Coexisting COPD or OSA Intrinsic or extrinsic airway compression Head and neck malignancy causing OSA

Abbreviations: CNS, central nervous system; PNS, peripheral nervous system; OSA, obstructive sleep apnea.

loids, cisplatin, and the taxanes are most frequently associated with peripheral neurotoxicity. The clinical manifestations of these drugs on lung function may be subtle in the absence of predisposing factors, such as preexisting neuromuscular abnormalities. In addition to their CNS effects, the use of anesthetic agents, in particular, halothane, propofol, and nitrous oxide may induce respiratory depression by decreasing diaphragmatic contractility.[271,272] Injury to the phrenic nerve following surgery for head and neck cancer, or surgery to the anterior mediastinum, esophagus, or lungs may cause persistent diaphragmatic dysfunction and ventilatory failure. Loss of diaphragmatic function from direct phrenic nerve invasion by tumor may also be seen, particularly among patients with lymphoma or cancers of the lung, or head and neck. Diffuse neural dysfunction resulting from paraneoplastic syndromes is another cause of respiratory failure in the cancer setting. Lambert-Eaton myasthenic syndrome, which affects about 3% of patients with small-cell lung cancer, myasthenia gravis, which occurs in 10-15% of patients with thymoma, and demyelinating peripheral neuropathy, seen in 50% of patients with the osteosclerotic form of plasmacytoma are the most common types of paraneoplastic, disorders of the peripheral nervous system. These disorders typically have a subacute and debilitating course that may lead to ventilatory failure. Muscle fatigue, a pervasive problem with cancer, is central to the development of respiratory failure. An extensive list of factors may potentiate cancer-related muscle fatigue, including hypoperfusion states (cardiogenic, septic or hemorrhagic shock), excess lactate or hydrogen ion production, severe anemia and, thereby, respiratory failure.

Increased Work of Breathing: Increased Respiratory System Load and Chest Wall Abnormalities ■ A variety of cancer-related factors may result in acute or chronic escalations in the respiratory system load. Elevations in airway resistive workloads, characterized physiologically by abnormal airway resistance and increased elastance, are cardinal features of COPD, airway inflammation, airway edema or physical obstruction by mucous, blood or tumor. Upper airway obstruction caused by tracheal stenosis associated with prior intubation or radiation to the head and neck, and intubation with a small (<7.5 mm internal diameter) endotracheal tube also pose are also significant sources of increased airflow resistance, and precipitants of respiratory resistance. Increased minute ventilation, owing to factors that contribute to excess carbon dioxide production (fever, respiratory distress, infection) or increased dead space ventilation (pulmonary embolism preexisting lung disease, hypovolemia, PEEP) are also implicated. Abnormalities involving the chest wall and thoracic spine caused by tumor, radiation or surgery may cause increased chest wall elastic loads, increased work of breathing and respiratory failure.

Lung Failure (Pulmonary Edema, ARDS, ALI)

Pulmonary Edema/Acute Respiratory Distress Syndrome/Acute Lung Injury ■ The predilection for pulmonary edema in the setting of cancer arises from a broad array of insults to the lungs that may be sorted according to the underlying permeability characteristics of the microcirculation, and the presence or absence of diffuse alveolar damage histopathologically. In normal permeability pulmonary edema, increased hydrostatic pressure caused by an imbalance in Starling forces leads to fluid filtration into the lungs. Pulmonary edema of cardiogenic and neurogenic etiologies, as well as lung edema caused by lung reexpansion, lymphatic obstruction, and relief of upper airway obstruction are typically associated with normal microvascular permeability.

The histopathologic hallmark of increased microvascular permeability is the accumulation of proteinaceous fluid within the interstitum and alveoli resulting from a breach in the integrity of the alveolar and microvascular surfaces. Increased permeability pulmonary edema occurring in the absence of diffuse alveolar damage is referred to as capillary leak syndrome. In the cancer setting this type of pulmonary edema may occur following the administration of cytokines such as interferon, IL_2 which disrupt capillary endothelial integrity. These drugs may also cause direct toxicity to the myocardium, resulting in mixed or overlap edema associated with normal and increased permeability etiologies. Neurogenic and reexpansion pulmonary edema represent two other causes of mixed edema, which are frequently observed in the cancer setting. The frequent need for transfused blood products in the cancer setting predisposes the cancer patient to the syndrome of transfusion-related lung injury (TRALI), another form of noncardiogenic pulmonary edema. TRALI is characterized by the development of fever, hypotension, severe hypoxemia, and bilateral lung infiltrates which occur during or immediately following blood or blood product transfusion. Pulmonary hypertension with normal left ventricular end-diastolic pressures is also a cardinal feature of this syndrome. TRALI has been reported following transfusion of packed red blood cells, platelets, and granulocytes. The treatment is supportive. Resolution of clinical symptoms and radiographic changes typically occurs within 2-3 days of symptom onset without permanent pulmonary sequelae, although in 20% of patients symptoms and radiographic changes may persist for a week and may be associated with lung injury (ALI/ARDS—see below).[273,274]

Acute lung injury (ALI) and acute respiratory distress syndrome (ARDS) are terms used for varying severity of pulmonary edema accompanying the histopathologic finding of diffuse alveolar damage. ARDS is reserved for severe lung injury in which bilateral pulmonary infiltrates and severe hypoxemia (as defined by a ratio of the partial pressure of arterial oxygen to the fraction of inspired oxygen {PaO_2/FiO_2} <200) occur in the absence of clinical evidence of left atrial hypertension. ALI is reflective of a lesser injury, as indicated by a PaO_2/FiO_2 ration between 200 and 300. The list of cancer-related precipitating conditions associated with ARDS is extensive. An etiological dichotomy that sorts the causes of ARDS into conditions that provoke direct lung injury (pneumonia, gastric aspiration) and those that are associated with systemic diseases that promote indirect lung injury (sepsis, transfusion-related lung injury) provides a simplistic approach to ARDS, but is confounded by the fact that the inciting events are often multifactorial or unknown. Pathologically, ARDS is manifested by an early, exudative phase which is marked by diffuse alveolar damage (DAD), followed by fibroproliferative and recovery phases. Clinically, patients may present with acute respiratory failure and associated hypoxemia within 24–48 h of the predisposing event. Fever and leukocytosis, owing to the inflammatory response associated with lung injury may be prominent findings, even in the absence of infection. Although the radiographic changes in ARDS are not distinctive, the CXR is nonetheless important in ruling out competing diagnoses such as pneumothorax, infections, and congestive heart failure. Patchy areas of lung involvement may be seen as ground glass opacifications early on which may progress to diffuse areas of consolidation. Radiographic findings suggestive of cardiogenic pulmonary edema such as Kerley B lines, cardiomegaly, and apical vascular redistribution are typically absent.

Management of Respiratory Failure

Medical Therapy ■ The management of the critically ill cancer patient with respiratory failure involves aggressive supportive care as well as strategies that target the precipitating cause. Standard supportive measures include the provision of supplemental oxygen, inhaled bronchodilators, nutritional support, chest physiotherapy and pulmonary toilet, and the prudent use of diuretics, vasopressors, and antibiotics, where indicated. Although fluid loading augments oxygen consumption and tissue oxygen delivery, careful attention to fluid homeostasis is imperative, as a persistent positive fluid balance has been associated with a poor outcome.[278,279] More specific interventions, such as administration of helium-oxygen (heliox) mixtures may provide temporary relief of acute respiratory distress associated with proximal airway obstruction and serve as a bridge to more definitive therapy. Patients with DAH may benefit from the early use of high-dose steroids, DDAVP, and aggressive blood and blood product support.[280] Several studies have demonstrated significant reductions in bleeding episodes following administration of high-dose (90 μg/kg) recombinant Factor VII (rFactory VII) among patients with primary DAH or alveolar hemorrhage associated with pneumonia.[281] These findings have been questioned, however, in a recent prospective, randomized study, which failed to show a beneficial effect of rFactor VII relative to placebo in the management of post transplant bleeding complications.[282] Antifibrinolytics, such as aminocaproic acid, have been used to treat transplant-related DAH, although convincing evidence supporting this practice is not available.[283] The effect of activated protein C administration in reducing sepsis-related ARDS mortality has been exciting,[284,285] however, conflicting results in subgroup analysis and concerns regarding serious bleeding have limited the use of this drug.[286]

Advances in supportive care coupled with early identification and management of precipitating condition(s) and strategies that attenuate ventilator-associated lung injury have contributed to significant increases in ARDS-related survival rates over the past decade.[287] Several trials of high-dose corticosteroids for early-phase ARDS failed to demonstrate a survival benefit. A salutary effect of high-dose glucocorticoids given during the fibroproliferative phase of ARDS was suggested in several small studies,[288-290] though not borne out in a large, multicenter, NIH-sponsored (ARDS-Net), trial.[291] Moreover, in the ARDS-Net study, initiation of corticosteroid therapy more than 14 days after the onset of ARDS was associated with a significantly increased mortality at 60 and 180 days compared to placebo. The efficacy of other agents, such as anti-TNF-α, anti-interleukin-1, ketoconazole, prostaglandin E_1, prostacyclin, aerosolized surfactant, and inhaled nitric oxide in attenuating lung injury has been investigated in small clinical trials has not been proven.

Mechanical Ventilation

Noninvasive Ventilation (NIV) ■ Assisted ventilation is often required to manage ARF that is nonresponsive to conservative medical therapy. Newer modes of mechanical ventilation as well as the use of noninvasive ventilation (NIV) have shown promising results, and gained broad acceptance in the management of cancer patients with respiratory failure. The efficacy of NIV has been clearly demonstrated in several randomized, controlled studies in the management of pump failure[292,293] as well as selected cases of lung failure.[292] In a recent retrospective study of the outcome of cancer patients following ICU transfer for ARF, the use of NIV was associated with marked improvements in patient survival.[294] In addition, significant reductions in the need for conventional mechanical ventilation and declines in both ICU and post ICU hospital mortality have been linked to the use of intermittent NIV during the early stages of hypoxemic ARF (PaO_2/FiO_2 ratio <250).[295-297] Evidence favoring the early use of NPPV for ARF among immunocompromised patients is derived from several small studies which report reduced rates of endotracheal intubation, length of ICU stay, and ICU mortality.[295,298,299] Immunocompromised patients with respiratory failure who require mechanical ventilation have notoriously poor prognoses, with an estimated 1% increased risk for pneumonia per day of mechanical ventilation.[300] Thus, NPPV in this setting has quickly gained broad acceptance in the management of cancer patients with respiratory failure.

Invasive Mechanical Ventilation ■ Overdistension of the lungs at end-inspiration and repetitive collapse of the lungs at end exhalation that occurs with conventional mechanical ventilation at high tidal volumes may trigger further lung injury. This observation prompted the development of lung-protective ventilator strategies that mitigate alveolar overdistension and enhance recruitment of atelectatic alveoli, thereby reducing the incidence of ventilator-induced lung injury. Lung-protective ventilator strategies may be accomplished with conventional modes of ventilation such as assist-control and pressure-controlled ventilation with or without inverse ratio ventilation or alternative methods, such as biphasic positive airway pressure ventilation (BIPAP), airway pressure release ventilation (APRV), jet and high frequency oscillatory ventilation, and differential lung ventilation. None of these modes of ventilation have proven to be superior to conventional ventilatory strategies. Convincing evidence favoring the use of protective ventilator strategies is derived from the National Institute of Heath ARDS-Net trial where lower tidal volumes (6 mL/kg of predicted body weight) and limited static inspiratory pressures (<30 cm H_2O) resulted in a 22% improved survival compared to patients mechanically ventilated using higher tidal volumes and inflation pressures.[301,302] Other adjuncts to ventilator management of patients with ARF, including extracorporeal membrane oxygenation (ECMO) and partial liquid ventilation (PLV), prone positioning and surfactant instillation have been proposed, however the merits of these therapies over conventional treatment strategies have not been definitively proven. Early tracheostomy may be associated with improved outcomes in critically ill patients. Practice guidelines regarding the appropriate timing of tracheostomy in patients that require prolonged mechanical ventilation are based from a consensus statement, nearly 2 decades old, that suggested that tracheostomy be considered after 21 days of mechanical ventilation. Although these recommendations were only based on expert opinion, modern practice broadly continues to follow them. In a recent meta-analysis, an 8.5 day decrease in total mechanical ventilation days and a significant reduction in ICU length of stay were seen among patients that underwent early tracheostomy (within 7 days of initiation of invasive mechanical ventilation) compared to those in which tracheostomy was performed late, although mortality was not significantly altered.[303]

Respiratory Failure Outcomes

The mortality rate of critically ill cancer patients with respiratory failure is at least 3-fold higher than that of cancer patients without respiratory failure.[304-306] Conditions common to the critically ill cancer patient such as cardiac, renal or hepatic dysfunction, disseminated intravascular coagulation, hemodynamic instability, and the need for mechanical ventilation are independent predictive variables that portend a poor outcome.[304,305,307] Early reports documented mortality rates among mechanically ventilated cancer patients with ARF in excess of 90%, especially among patients with hematologic malignancies and recipients of hematopoietic transplants.[308-311] More recent investigations have offered a more favorable perspective, with mortality rates of 69-84%.[305,306,312,313] Survival gains may be attributable to better infection prophylaxis measures, improved transplantation techniques, standard use of preventive measures that mitigate aspiration, more aggressive use of hematopoietic growth factor support following transplantation and trends toward the use of peripheral stem cells rather than bone marrow as a source of donor stem cells. In addition, the newer ventilation strategies including NIV and lung-protective ventilator strategies may play a role in improved survival.[306] Finally, the implementation of programs for early identification and management of deteriorating patients on general hospital wards and improvements in ICU admission and triage criteria may not only contribute to overall improved ICU survival but also to the appropriate use of hospital resources.[314,315]

Selected References

The complete reference list can be found at www.CANCERMEDICINE8.com

8. Hautmann H, Gamarra F, Pfeifer KJ, et al. Fiberoptic bronchoscopic balloon dilatation in malignant tracheobronchial disease: indications and results. *Chest.* 2001;120:43–49.
18. Sahn S. Pleural diseases related to metastatic malignancies. *Eur Respir J.* 1997;10:1907–1913.
27. De Campos J, Vargas F, DeCampos E, et al. Thoracoscopy talc poudrage: a 15-year experience. *Chest.* 2001;119:801–806.
30. Alinsonorin CY, Jimenez CA, Ersoy YM, et al. Indwelling pleural catheters for management of recurrent malignant pleural effusions. *Am J Respir Crit Care Med.* 2003;167:A901.
36. Jimenez C, Mhatre A, Martinez C, et al. Use of an indwelling pleural catheter for the management of recurrent chylothorax in patients with cancer. *Chest.* 2007;132:1584–1590.
38. Bolliger CT, Wyser C, Roser H, et al. Lung scanning and exercise testing for the prediction of postoperative performance in lung resection candidates at increased risk for complications. *Chest.* 1995;108:341–348.
39. Datta D, Lahiri B. Preoperative evaluation of patients undergoing lung resection surgery. *Chest.* 2003;123:2096–2103.
42. Ali MK, Mountain CF, Ewer MS, et al. Predicting loss of pulmonary function after pulmonary resection for bronchogenic carcinoma. *Chest.* 1980;77:337–342.
47. Morice RC, Peters EJ, Ryan MB, et al. Exercise testing in the evaluation of patients at high risk for complications from lung resection. *Chest.* 1992;101:356–361.
53. Cooper J, White D, Matthay R. Drug-induced pulmonary disease. Part 1 Cytotoxic drugs. *Adv Intern Med.* 1986;42:231–268.
60. Steijfer S. Bleomycin-induced pneumonitis. *Chest.* 2001;120:617–624.
74. Camus P, Bonniaud P, Fanton A, et al. Drug-induced and iatrogenic infiltrative lung disease. *Clin Chest Med.* 2004;25:479–519, vi.
82. Sleijfer S. Bleomycin-induced pneumonitis. *Chest.* 2001;120:617–624.
96. Shannon V, Price K. Pulmonary complications of cancer therapy. *Anesthesiol Clin North America.* 1998;16:563–585.
103. Afessa B, Tefferi A, Litzow MR, et al. Diffuse alveolar hemorrhage in hematopoietic stem cell transplant recipients. *Am J Respir Crit Care Med.* 2002;166:641–645.
128. Marks LB, Yu X, Vujaskovic Z, et al. Radiation-induced lung injury. *Semin Radiat Oncol.* 2003;13:333–345.
152. Soubani A, Miller K, Hassoun P. Pulmonary complications of bone marrow transplantation. *Chest.* 1996;109(4):1066–1077.
153. Roychowdhury M, Pambuccian SE, Aslan DL, et al. Pulmonary complications after bone marrow transplantation: an autopsy study from a large transplantation center. *Arch Pathol Lab Med.* 2005;129:366–371.
168. Afessa B, Peters S. Major complications following hematopoietic stem cell transplantation. *Semin Respir Crit Care Med.* 2006;27:297–309.
171. Afessa B, Tefferi A, Litzow MR, et al. Outcome of diffuse alveolar hemorrhage in hematopoietic stem cell transplant recipients. *Am J Respir Crit Care Med.* 2002;166:1364–1368.
172. Mossad S, Kalaycio M, Sobecks R, et al. Steroids prevent engraftment syndrome after autologous hematopoietic stem cell transplantation without increasing the risk of infection. *Bone Marrow Transplant.* 2005;35:375–381.
175. Yanik G, Hellerstedt B, Custer J, et al. Etanercept (Enbrel) administration for idiopathic pneumonia syndrome after allogeneic hematopoietic stem cell transplantation. *Biol Blood Marrow Transplant.* 2002;8:395–400.
191. Bashoura L, Gupta S, Jain A, et al. Inhaled corticosteroids stabilize constrictive bronchiolitis after hematopoietic stem cell transplantation. *Bone Marrow Transplant.* 2008;41:63–67.
197. Safdar A, Armstrong D. Infectious morbidity in critically ill patients with cancer. *Crit Care Clin.* 2001;17:531–570, vii–viii.
202. Hohenthal U, Itala M, Salonen J, et al. Bronchoalveolar lavage in immunocompromised patients with haematological malignancy—value of new microbiological methods. *Eur J Haematol.* 2005;74:203–211.
203. Niederman MS, Mandell LA, Anzueto A, et al. Guidelines for the management of adults with community-acquired pneumonia. Diagnosis, assessment of severity, antimicrobial therapy, and prevention. *Am J Respir Crit Care Med.* 2001;163:1730–1754.
205. Bick RL. Cancer-associated thrombosis. *N Engl J Med.* 2003;349:109–111.
206. Lee AY, Levine MN. Venous thromboembolism and cancer: risks and outcomes. *Circulation.* 2003;107:I17–21.
207. ten Wolde M, Kraaijenhagen RA, Prins MH, et al. The clinical usefulness of D-dimer testing in cancer patients with suspected deep venous thrombosis. *Arch Intern Med.* 2002;162:1880–1884.
208. Moores LK, Jackson WL Jr, Shorr AF, et al. Meta-analysis: outcomes in patients with suspected pulmonary embolism managed with computed tomographic pulmonary angiography. *Ann Intern Med.* 2004;141:866–874.
212. Bergqvist D, Agnelli G, Cohen AT, et al. Duration of prophylaxis against venous thromboembolism with enoxaparin after surgery for cancer. *N Engl J Med.* 2002;346:975–980.
218. McGoon M, Gutterman D, Steen V, et al. American College of Chest Physicians. Screening, early detection, and diagnosis of pulmonary arterial hypertension: ACCP evidence-based clinical practice guidelines. *Chest.* 2004;126 (suppl 1):14S–34S.
220. Simonneau G, Galiè N, Rubin LJ, et al. Clinical classification of pulmonary hypertension. *J Am Coll Cardiol.* 2004;43:5S–12S.
248. Stepanski EJ, Burgess HJ. Sleep and cancer. *Sleep Med Clin.* 2007:2:67–75.
250. Ancoli-Israel S, Moore PJ, Jones V. The relationship between fatigue and sleep in cancer patients: a review. *Eur J Cancer Care.* 2001;10:245–255.
256. Edmonds P, Higginson I, Altmann D, et al. Is the presence of dyspnea a risk factor for morbidity in cancer patients? *J Pain Symptom Manage.* 2000;19:15–22.
260. Dimeo FC. Effects of exercise on cancer-related fatigue. *Cancer.* 2001;92:1689–1693.
265. Bobbio A, Chetta A, Ampollini L, et al. Preoperative pulmonary rehabilitation in patients undergoing lung resection for non-small cell lung cancer. *Eur J Cardiothorac Surg.* 2008;33:95–98.
275. Ware LB, Matthay MA. The acute respiratory distress syndrome. *N Engl J Med.* 2000;342:1334–1349.
280. Raptis A, Mavroudis D, Suffredini A. High-dose corticosteroid therapy for diffuse alveolar hemorrhage in allogenic bone marrow stem cell transplant recipients. *Bone Marrow Transplantation.* 1999;24:879–883.
284. Bernard GR, Vincent JL, Laterre PF, et al. Efficacy and safety of recombinant human activated protein C for severe sepsis. *N Engl J Med.* 2001;344:699–709.
285. Vincent J, Bernard G, Beale R, et al. Drotrecogin alfa (activated) treatment in severe sepsis from the global open-label trial ENHANCE: further evidence for survival and safety and implications for early treatment. *Crit Care Med.* 2005;33:2266–2277.
286. Abraham E, Laterre PF, Garg R et al. Drotrecogin alfa (activated) for adults with severe sepsis and a low risk of death. *N Engl J Med.* 2005;353:1332–1341.
291. Steinberg K, Hudson LD, Goodman RB, et al. Efficacy and safety of corticosteroids for persistent acute respiratory distress syndrome. *N Engl J Med.* 2006;354:1671–1684.
294. Azoulay E, Alberti C, Bornstain C, et al. Improved survival in cancer patients requiring mechanical ventilatory support: impact of noninvasive mechanical ventilatory support. *Crit Care Med.* 2001;29:519–525.
295. Hilbert G, Gruson D, Vargas F, et al. Noninvasive ventilation in immunosuppressed patients with pulmonary infiltrates, fever, and acute respiratory failure. *N Engl J Med.* 2001;344:481–487.
299. Caples S, Gay PC. Noninvasive positive pressure ventilation in the intensive care unit: a concise review. *Crit Care Med.* 2005;33:2651–2658.
301. Network TARDS. Ventilation with lower tidal volumes as compared with traditional tidal volumes for acute lung injury and the acute respiratory distress syndrome. *N Engl J Med.* 2000;42:1301–1308.
302. Brochard L, Roudot-Thoraval F, Roupie E, et al. Tidal volume reduction for prevention of ventilator-induced lung injury in acute respiratory distress syndrome. The Multicenter Trail Group on Tidal Volume reduction in ARDS. *Am J Respir Crit Care Med.* 1998;158:1831–1838.
306. Azoulay E, Thiery G, Chevret S, et al. The prognosis of acute respiratory failure in critically ill cancer patients. *Medicine.* (Baltimore) 2004;83:360–370.

132 Gastrointestinal and Hepatic Complications in Cancer Patients

Marta L. Davila, MD ■ Robert S. Bresalier, MD

Gastrointestinal (GI) complications are very common in patients undergoing cancer treatment. Some of these complications can be life threatening and require prompt and appropriate diagnosis and treatment. This chapter addresses the most significant GI issues in the cancer patient, and focuses on the evaluation and management of these problems.

Malignant Dysphagia

Patients with esophageal cancer will often present at an advanced, incurable stage. For those who are not candidates for chemoradiation or surgery and for those who develop recurrent dysphagia after treatment, a variety of endoscopic techniques have been developed to improve esophageal luminal patency (Table 132-1).

Esophageal Dilation

Esophageal dilation can be performed with through-the-scope balloons, mercury-filled rubber bougies, or wire-guided polyvinyl bougies (Savary-Gilliard dilators). Dilators can provide safe, temporary relief of dysphagia until definitive treatment is initiated.[1,2] Dilation, to be successful, must be repeated every few weeks.[1,2] The procedure carries a small risk of perforation, particularly with blind passage of Maloney dilators or in patients receiving concurrent radiation therapy.[3]

Laser Therapy

Laser energy produced by the neodymium:yttrium-aluminum-garnet (Nd:YAG) crystal, has been extensively used for the palliation of esophageal cancer.[4-7] The technique involves administration of laser energy by way of a quartz fiber guided through the biopsy channel of an endoscope. The laser beam is directed at the tumor with the goal of vaporizing the tissue and restoring luminal patency.[4] Treatment is usually accomplished in a retrograde fashion so that the distal end of the tumor is treated first. This approach may require prior esophageal dilation to allow passage of the endoscope. Early experiences revealed that if the most proximal end of the tumor was treated first, acute tissue edema occurred leading to the inability to advance the endoscope distally and possible premature cessation of treatment. Treatments can be performed every 2 days and are usually completed in 3-4 sessions.[4] Luminal patency can be achieved in up to 97% of patients with functional success (or the ability to ingest all necessary calories) in 70%.[4,6] Major complications include esophageal perforation (in fewer than 5% of patients), development of tracheoesophageal fistula, hemorrhage, and bacteremia.[8] Disadvantages of Nd:YAG laser therapy include difficulties in treating long, tortuous lesions or lesions located in the proximal esophagus, number of treatment sessions required and high cost.[7]

Table 132-1 ■ **Endoscopic Options in the Treatment of Malignant Dysphagia**

Esophageal dilation
Laser therapy with Nd:YAG
Photodynamic therapy
Self-expanding stents: Metal plastic

Photodynamic Therapy (PDT)

PDT uses a photosensitizing agent and low power laser to achieve tumor necrosis and luminal patency. Porfimer sodium (Photofrin) is the only photosensitizer approved by the Food and Drug Administration for the treatment of esophageal cancer. Photofrin is administered as an intravenous bolus at a dose of 2 mg/kg of body weight. After systemic injection, the photosensitizer is absorbed by all tissues, and selectively retained at a higher concentration by neoplastic tissue. Approximately 48 h after injection, patients are exposed to monochrome laser light at 630 nm via cylindrical diffuser attached to the tip of a quartz optical fiber placed through the accessory channel of an endoscope. The laser output is adjusted to deliver 300 J/cm at the diffuser tip.[9] The tip of the diffusing fibers is provided in several lengths to better match the length of the lesion being treated.

Laser light will initiate a photochemical reaction in the tissue leading to the formation of oxygen radicals, ischemia and tumor necrosis.[10] In a study comparing PDT with Nd:YAG, PDT was found to be superior in treating circumferential lesions in the upper third of the esophagus. For tumors longer than 8 cm, PDT was twice as effective as Nd:YAG in eradicating tumor, and lumens remained patent for a longer period of time, especially in patients with esophageal adenocarcinoma.[10] In a prospective, randomized, multicenter study involving 218 patients, treatment with both PDT and Nd:YAG had similar improvement in dysphagia and equivalent objective tumor response at week 1. The objective tumor response was significantly higher in the PDT treated group (32%) at one month compared to the Nd:YAG treated group (20%).[11] Trends for improved responses were seen with PDT for tumors located in the upper and lower third of the esophagus, in long tumors, and in patients who had prior therapy. PDT was associated with significantly fewer perforations compared to Nd:YAG laser (1% vs 7%), although there were more minor complications in the PDT treated group, with complications related to skin photosensitivity seen in 19% of patients.[11]

PDT can also be used effectively to treat tumor ingrowth or overgrowth in patients who had previous esophageal stenting.

Self-Expanding Stents

Peroral insertion of a plastic or a stainless steel reinforced endoprostheses served as a useful option in patients in need of palliation of dysphagia for over two decades.[12] Esophageal dilation is required to properly prepare the esophageal lumen for prosthesis deployment. Unfortunately, insertion of this type of endoprostheses was associated with a high complication rate including obstruction (14.5%), migration (3%), and perforation (2%), with a procedure related mortality of about 7%.[12]

Self-expanding metal stents (SEMS) were developed in the early 1990s in an attempt to decrease the complication rate and improve the ease of insertion.[13-15] SEMS are used increasingly as an effective nonsurgical option for the palliation of obstructive, advanced esophageal tumors. SEMS are made of a variety of metal alloys in different shapes and sizes to adjust to the length and position of the malignant stricture. Furthermore, approved devices are available in the uncovered, partially covered and fully covered designs. SEMS are placed under endoscopic guidance with or without

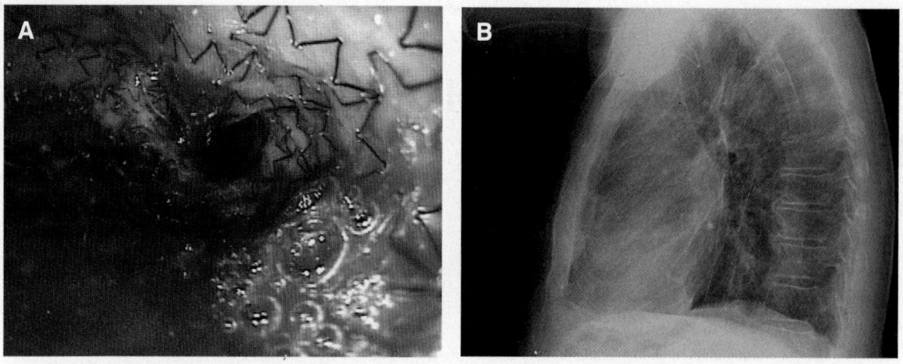

Figure 132-1 ■ Self-expanding esophageal stent. **(A)** Endoscopic view of a self-expanding stent deployed in the esophagus for treatment of an esophageal stricture. **(B)** Chest radiograph showing stent deployed in the esophagus.

fluoroscopy (Fig. 132-1). Once a metal stent is deployed, it cannot be removed.

In a study of 33 patients with inoperable esophageal cancer, all attempted insertions of expandable metal stents were successful, and the dysphagia scores were reduced from grades 3-4 to 0 or 1.[13] There were no perforations related to insertion, but dysphagia recurred in 6 patients (20%), due to stent migration, tumor overgrowth and food impaction. Similar results were seen in another study of 77 patients; with relief of dysphagia in over 90%, and a complication rate of 11%.[14] Advantages of SEMS include relative ease of insertion, larger stent diameters, and low risk of perforation with elimination of the need for excessive dilation. Disadvantages include high cost, tumor ingrowth and overgrowth, stent migration, maldeployment, inadequate expansion, airway obstruction, and hemorrhage.[15] The rate of tumor ingrowth has now been reduced with the introduction of stents covered by a polyurethane coating.[16] Covered stents are the device of choice in the management of patients with tracheoesophageal fistulas.[17] A recent additional option for palliation of esophageal cancer has resulted from the development of self-expanding plastic stents (SEPS). These stents require fluoroscopic guidance for placement. The advantage for the operator is that these stents can be repositioned or removed if necessary. SEPS have been reported to be as successful as metal stents in ease of deployment and palliation of dysphagia.[18] Another study, however, has reported a 25% deployment failure rate, and a 12.5% rate of early stent migration (within 72 h).[19] A prospective, randomized trial compared SEPS to SEMS in the treatment of malignant esophageal dysphagia.[20] No difference was seen in palliation of dysphagia between the two types of stents. Significantly more complications, especially late stent migration; however, were observed in the plastic stent group. No significant correlation between dilation or previous radiation therapy and the occurrence of complications was observed.[20]

In summary, there are several endoscopic approaches to the palliation of malignant dysphagia. Covered stents are the therapy of choice in patients with tracheoesophageal fistulas. In those without a fistula, endoscopic therapy should be individualized and based on location and features of the lesion, patient preference, and institutional expertise.

Esophagitis

Esophagitis can be caused by cytotoxic effects of chemotherapy, radiation, as well as by viral, fungal and bacterial organisms. Other causes of esophagitis include acid reflux disease, pill-induced injury, and graft-versus-host disease (GVHD) in hematopoietic cell transplant recipients (Table 132-2). When esophagitis is suspected, particularly in an immunocompromised patient, prompt evaluation with endoscopy with biopsies and/or brushings is indicated to allow for early diagnosis and therapy.[21]

Esophageal candidiasis is one of the most common infections in the immunocompromised host. Patients usually complain of odynophagia (pain on swallowing) and/or dysphagia (difficulties swallowing). The absence of oral thrush does not rule out the possibility of candida esophagitis. The diagnosis is usually made by endoscopic examination. On endoscopy, white plaque-like lesions with surrounding erythema can be seen covering the esophageal walls. Esophageal brushings confirm the presence of yeast or hyphal forms. The yeast may be seen invading mucosal cells on biopsy. Treatment requires systemic antifungal therapy.

Table 132-2 ■ **Causes of Esophagitis in the Cancer Patient**

Acid related
Infection
Fungal—*Candida*
Viral—CMV, HSV, VZV
Bacterial—polymicrobial from oral flora
Radiation
Pill-induced
GVHD

Abbreviations: CMV, cytomegalovirus; HSV, herpes simplex virus; VZV, varicella-zoster virus.

An empiric course in antifungal therapy is recommended in the immunosuppressed patients with symptoms of odynophagia and dysphagia. Endoscopy can be performed if symptoms do not improve after 72 h.[22] Fluconazole (100-200 mg daily for 14-21 days) is effective in eradicating the infection.[23] Itraconazole oral solution (200 mg daily) and voriconazole (200 mg twice daily) appear to be as effective as fluconazole in the treatment of esophageal candidiasis.[24,25] Furthermore, voriconazole may be used in the treatment of infections unresponsive or refractory to fluconazole therapy.[26] The new echinocandins (caspofungin, micafungin, and anidulafungin) are administered intravenously and are also effective for the treatment of Candida esophagitis.[27-29] Amphoterecin B (0.3-0.7 mg/kg daily) has fallen out of favor because of its toxicity when compared to the other antifungal drugs.

Viral infections of the esophagus are caused by herpes simplex virus (HSV), cytomegalovirus (CMV) and, rarely, varicella-zoster virus (VZV).[21] Patients usually present with odynophagia and dysphagia. Less frequent symptoms include nausea, vomiting, heartburn, epigastric pain, and fever. In the case of HSV esophagitis, some patients may have coexistent herpes labialis or oropharyngeal ulcers.[30] Diagnosis is made by endoscopy and biopsy (Fig. 132-2). In the early stage, HSV lesions may appear as small vesicles, although they are rarely seen. The vesicles eventually coalesce to form large ulcers which are usually less than 2 cm in size. The ulcers are well circumscribed with normal appearing intervening mucosa.[31] CMV will cause ulcers which are

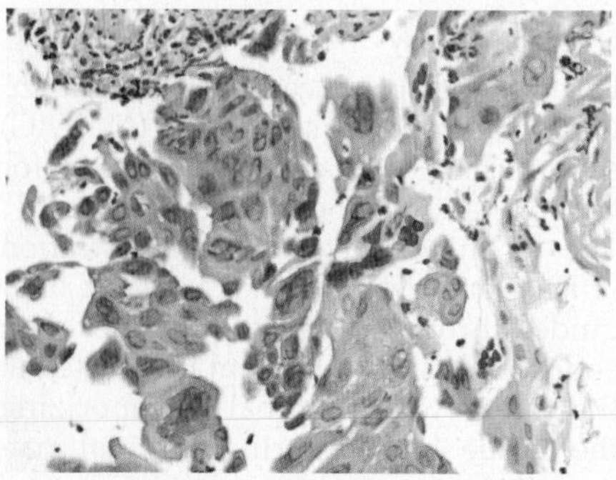

Figure 132-2 ■ Herpes simplex virus (HSV) esophagitis. High-power view of esophageal mucosa shows squamous cells with ground glass nuclear viral inclusions and multinucleated giant cells in a background of neutrophilic exudates. *Source*: Courtesy of Dr. T.T. Wu, MD Anderson Cancer Center.

linear or serpiginous and deeper than HSV-related ulcers. Exudates may also be present.[31] Biopsies taken from the edge of an HSV-related ulcer will show intranuclear inclusions and multinucleated giant cells. Inclusions can also be detected by immunohistochemistry, using monoclonal antibodies to HSV.[31] Viral cultures are helpful in identifying resistant strains in patients who do not respond to acyclovir. VZV can produce esophagitis in adults with herpes zoster, usually in the setting of disseminated infection.[21] Endoscopically, VZV ulcers are similar to those seen with HSV. On biopsy specimens, distinction from HSV will require immunohistochemistry or culture.

CMV infects endothelial cells and fibroblasts, but not epithelial cells as with HSV and VZV. Routine biopsies in a CMV-infected patient show intranuclear inclusions in fibroblasts and endothelial cells. Immunohistochemistry with anti-CMV antibodies is also helpful for diagnosis.

For patients with HSV esophagitis, acyclovir (orally or intravenously) is the therapy of choice. Foscarnet is reserved for those patients who are known to be resistant or do not respond to acyclovir.[32] VZV esophagitis is treated with intravenous acyclovir since these patients usually will have disseminated infection. After initial clinical improvement, patients can be switched to an oral agent such as valacyclovir. There is limited clinical experience with either valacyclovir or famciclovir in the immunocompromised host. Nonetheless, there are data that these drugs significantly accelerate the resolution of pain and reduce the duration of postherpetic neuralgia in immunocompetent adults when compared to acyclovir.[33,34] CMV esophagitis can be treated with intravenous ganciclovir (5 mg/kg BID) or foscarnet (90 mg/kg BID) for a total of 3-6 weeks.[35-37] There are anecdotal reports that oral valganciclovir is being used effectively to treat CMV esophagitis once odynophagia has improved with IV ganciclovir and patients can tolerate oral medication. Additional studies are needed in this area to make specific recommendations.

Bacterial esophagitis can occur in the immunocompromised patient and is usually polymicrobial and derived from oral flora. The diagnosis is made by endoscopic biopsies and treatment is broad-spectrum antibiotics.

Radiation esophagitis usually occurs during treatment of lung and esophageal cancers. The severity of esophagitis increases with radiation dose and with the use of certain chemotherapeutic agents such as doxorubicin, bleomycin, cyclophosphamide, and cisplatin.[38,39] Patients may complain of odynophagia, dysphagia, and chest pain. Endoscopy may reveal erythema, edema, and friability of the esophageal mucosa, as well as ulcerations with eventual stricture formation. Strictures can be managed with esophageal dilation. Medical therapy includes use of viscous lidocaine, H-2 blockers or proton pump inhibitors to prevent further acid-related injury.

Pill-induced esophagitis can occur in patients taking medication at bedtime with insufficient liquid or in the recumbent position. The most common medications associated with this disorder include potassium chloride, tetracyclines, aspirin, nonsteroidal antiinflammatory drugs, quinidine, iron, and alendronate. Injury is caused by prolonged contact of the caustic contents of the medication with the esophageal mucosa. Patients will often present with sudden onset of odynophagia which may be severe enough to make even the swallowing of saliva difficult and painful. Endoscopy is helpful in making a diagnosis; but more importantly, it serves to rule out other diagnoses such as infectious esophagitis and malignancy. On endoscopy, there is usually a discrete, single ulcer located in the proximal esophagus.[40] On occasion, the injury appears as a nodular, polypoid lesion suggestive of a neoplasm, or as a stricture[41,42] (Fig. 132-3). Esophageal biopsies are nonspecific and may show acute inflammatory changes only. There is no specific therapy for this disorder, since pill-induced ulcerations can heal spontaneously within a few days without any intervention. Strictures will require endoscopic dilation. The only recommendation is to avoid the inciting agent, if possible. If a patient needs to continue on medication, he or she should be instructed on drinking plenty of liquids with the medicine and avoiding a recumbent position after ingestion.

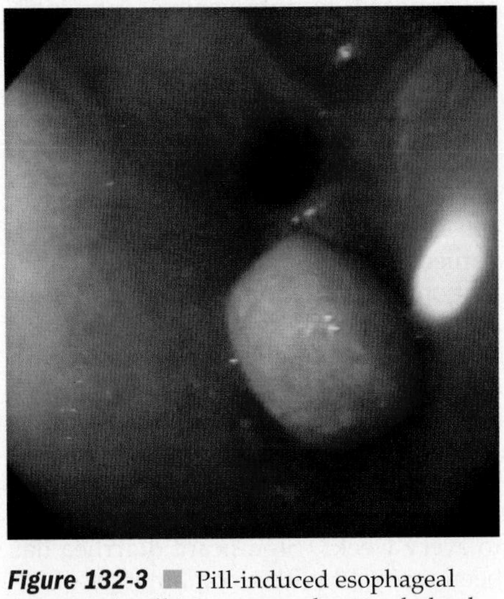

Figure 132-3 ■ Pill-induced esophageal damage. A pill is seen at endoscopy lodged above an esophageal stricture.

Neutropenic Enterocolitis or Typhlitis

Neutropenic enterocolitis or typhlitis (from the Greek word *typhlon*) is a clinical syndrome in neutropenic patients characterized by fever and right lower quadrant pain. This entity has received various names including necrotizing enterocolitis, neutropenic colitis, ileocecal syndrome, and cecitis.[43,44] Typhlitis was originally described in children following induction chemotherapy for acute leukemia.[45] It has subsequently been reported in adults with acute myeloid leukemia, acute lymphoblastic leukemia, multiple myeloma, aplastic anemia, myelodysplastic syndromes, granulocytopenias from other causes, acquired immunodeficiency syndrome, and following immunosuppressive therapy for solid malignancies and transplants.[46,47] The disease appears to be the result of a combination of factors including mucosal injury by cytotoxic drugs, neutropenia, and impaired host defense to intestinal organisms.[47] It has been postulated that the intact colonic mucosa cannot be maintained due to either leukemic infiltration or direct cytotoxic effect of chemotherapy. Bacterial invasion of the bowel wall ensues, facilitated by a decreased defense due to neutropenia. This is followed by production of bacterial endotoxins, with subsequent bacteremia, necrosis, and hemorrhage. The cecum is almost always affected but the disease can often extend into the terminal ileum and right and left colon.[46] The predilection for the cecum may be related to its distensibility and limited blood supply. Pathology may reveal edema of the mucosa or entire intestinal wall, mucosal ulcerations, focal hemorrhage and mucosal or transmural necrosis.[46] Rarely are leukemic or acute inflammatory infiltrates identified.[47] Various organisms, alone or in combination, have been identified in surgical specimens and peritoneal fluid, including gram-negative rods, gram-positive cocci, enterococci, *Clostridium septicum*, *Candida* and CMV.[45,46] *Clostridium difficile* toxin is occasionally detected in the stools.[45] Bacteremia and fungemia are frequently reported.[48]

Initial reports commented on the association of this entity with particular chemotherapeutic agents used in the treatment of leukemias and lymphomas, especially cytosine arabinoside (Ara-C), vincristine, doxorubicin, methotrexate, cyclophosphamide, etoposide (VP-16), daunomycin and prednisone.[45,46,48] More recently, other agents used in the treatment of ovarian, peritoneal, nonsmall-cell lung, squamous cell carcinoma of the lung, colorectal, and breast cancer have been implicated, including: vinorelbine, docetaxel, paclitaxel, carboplatin, cisplatin, gemcitabine, and 5-fluorouracil (5-FU).[49-56]

The true incidence of neutropenic enterocolitis is unknown. In a systematic review on the subject, involving 145 published articles, the authors report a 5.3% pooled incidence rate in adult patients hospitalized for the treatment of hematological malignancies, for high-dose chemotherapy in solid tumors or for aplastic anemia.[57]

Neutropenic enterocolitis should be suspected in any neutropenic patient presenting with fever and abdominal pain, particularly in the right lower quadrant, with or without rebound tenderness. Other presenting symptoms include abdominal distension, nausea, vomiting, and watery or bloody diarrhea. Peritoneal signs and shock can be present with bowel perforation. Symptoms often occur 10-14 days after initiation of cytotoxic chemotherapy.[58] Given that the clinical findings may be subtle and nonspecific, one must consider other entities in the differential diagnosis, including pseudomembranous colitis, colonic pseudoobstruction, acute appendicitis, ischemic colitis, inflammatory bowel disease and infectious colitis.

Imaging studies can be useful in supporting a diagnosis of typhlitis. CT is the preferred diagnostic modality over ultrasound and plain abdominal films.[45] Abnormal findings on CT imaging and ultrasonography include a fluid-filled, dilated cecum, a right lower quadrant inflammatory mass and pericecal fluid or inflammatory changes in the pericecal soft tissues.[45] Plain films of the abdomen may be nonspecific but, occasionally, a distended cecum with dilated adjacent small bowel loops, thumbprinting, or localized pneumatosis intestinalis is seen.[58] Barium enema or colonoscopy can be hazardous as they can precipitate perforation.

There have been no prospective randomized trials or high quality retrospective studies on the treatment of neutropenic enterocolitis. Therefore, a uniform management strategy cannot be recommended. The best strategy should be an individualized approach to each case given the wide spectrum of presentation. In those patients presenting without significant complications such as peritonitis, perforation or bleeding, nonsurgical management is a reasonable initial approach. Conservative management consists of bowel rest, nasogastric suction, total parenteral nutrition, and broad-spectrum antibiotic therapy.[45,57,59] Antibiotic coverage for *C. difficile* infection should be added if pseudomembranous colitis has not been excluded. Cytopenias and coagulopathy should be corrected. Recombinant granulocyte colony-stimulating factor (G-CSF) has been used to hasten recovery, since normalization of the leukocyte count may allow containment and healing of bowel lesions.[56-58]

Surgery has been recommended for patients with GI bleeding that persists despite correction of cytopenias and coagulopathy; for those with free intra-abdominal perforation or clinical deterioration during medical therapy, and to differentiate from other acute abdominal diseases for which surgery is indicated.[58,60]

Patients who develop neutropenic enterocolitis during chemotherapy are at risk for developing this complication during subsequent treatment. Patients should be allowed to heal completely and recover from enterocolitis before chemotherapy is again administered.

Diarrhea

Diarrhea is a common complication of cytotoxic therapy. It is most commonly described with fluoropyrimidines (particularly 5-FU), irinotecan, methotrexate and cisplatin. Diarrhea can be very debilitating and in severe cases it can lead to treatment delays, reduced quality of life, and diminished compliance. It is the dose-limiting factor and the major toxicity of regimens containing a fluoropyrimidine and/or irinotecan. The severity of chemotherapy-induced diarrhea is often described, particularly for study purposes, using the National Cancer Institute Common Toxicity Criteria (NCI CTC).[61] Grading is based on number of stools per day, presence of nocturnal stools, and the need for parenteral support or intensive care.

The severity of diarrhea with 5-FU is increased by the addition of leucovorin. Moreover, diarrhea can be worse when 5-FU is administered by bolus injection as opposed to intravenous infusion.[62] Other factors that appear to raise the risk of 5-FU induced diarrhea include female gender, the presence of unresected primary tumor, previous episode of chemotherapy-induced diarrhea, and treatment during the summer season.[63,64] Irinotecan can cause an early-onset diarrhea accompanied by abdominal cramping, lacrimation, salivation, and other symptoms that appear cholinergic-mediated. These symptoms can be effectively treated with atropine as well as loperamide.[65] The late diarrhea associated with irinotecan is unpredictable and can occur at all dose levels. It is seen less often when given in the every-three-week schedule compared to every week.[66] Significant diarrhea has been reported with a combination of irinotecan, 5-FU, and leucovorin compared to 5-FU and leucovorin alone.[67-69]

Radiation therapy can produce injury to the GI mucosa that peaks 1-2 weeks after irradiation. Worsening diarrhea can be seen when radiation is given in combination with chemotherapy, such as 5-FU in the treatment of rectal cancer.[70]

The treatment of chemotherapy or radiation-induced diarrhea involve aggressive oral rehydration and electrolyte replacement, and the use of pharmacologic agents to reduce fluid loss and decrease intestinal motility. Opioid agonists are the basics of therapy. Loperamide (Imodium) and diphenoxilate (Lomotil) are the most commonly used agents. For mild to moderate diarrhea, loperamide 4mg is given as the initial dose, followed by 2 mg every 4 h or after every stool. In severe cases or with irinotecan-induced diarrhea, a more aggressive regimen is needed with loperamide 4 mg initially followed by 2 mg every 2 h or 4 mg every 4 h until diarrhea-free for 12 h.[71,72] Careful observation of patients receiving these drugs is warranted because of their impairment of intestinal motility. If patients do not respond to opioids, octreotide, a synthetic long-acting somatostatin analog, has been used as second-line therapy. The recommended initial dose of octreotide is 100-150 μg subcutaneously three times a day or 25-50 μg/h intravenous infusion.[72,73] Octreotide can be titrated to higher doses (500-2500 μg three times daily) in nonresponders.[74,75] Other agents have been used as adjunctive therapy in the treatment of mild to moderate chemotherapy-induced diarrhea including absorbents such as kaolin and charcoal, deodorized tincture of opium (DTO), paregoric, and codeine.

Patients presenting with severe diarrhea, fever, or neutropenia should be admitted to the hospital for a diagnostic work-up and be treated aggressively with octreotide, intravenous fluids and antibiotics.[72]

For patients undergoing hematopoietic stem cell transplantation, diarrhea may be due to the conditioning regimen, GVHD or to an infection related to immunosuppressive therapy (Table 132-3). Diarrhea in the immediate posttransplantation period is generally the result of injury to the intestinal mucosa caused by the conditioning regimen. This regi-

***Table 132-3* ■ Differential Diagnosis of Diarrhea in the Cancer and Hematopoietic Cell Transplant Patient**

Chemotherapy related (fluoropyrimidine, irinotecan, methotrexate, cisplatin)
Radiation therapy
Conditioning regimen
GVHD
Infection
Bacterial (including *C. difficile*)
Viral (including CMV)

men includes total body irradiation and/or a combination of chemotherapy agents. Mucosal injury results in a secretory diarrhea that resolves with mucosal restitution, usually by the third week after treatment. After day 20, acute GVHD is the most common cause of diarrhea in this patients.[76] GVHD will be discussed separately in the next section.

If diarrhea is not directly the result of chemotherapy or radiation and particularly if it occurs in a hospital setting, *C. difficile* infection should be considered since this is the most common cause of infectious diarrhea in hospitalized patients.[77] Although commonly associated with use of antibiotic therapy, risk factors for *C difficile* diarrhea or colitis also include bowel surgery, immunocompromised state and any process that suppresses the normal flora including antifungal and chemotherapeutic agents. Cancer patients receiving chemotherapy appear predisposed to *C. difficile*-induced diarrhea even in the absence of antibiotics.[78,79] In a study of such patients, methotrexate, doxorubicin, and cyclophosphamide were the drugs most frequently associated with *C. difficile* infection.[79] Clinical presentation may vary from mild diarrhea without colitis, colitis with systemic manifestations, pseudomembranous colitis with or without protein-losing enteropathy, and fulminant colitis with development of toxic megacolon. The diagnosis is established by detecting the presence of *C. difficile* toxin in stool or by identifying pseudomembranous colitis on endoscopic evaluation (Fig. 132-4).

The stool-cytotoxin test is a tissue culture assay based on the induction of cell rounding by *C. difficile* toxin in stool filtrate. This assay is the "gold standard" because of its high sensitivity (94-100%) and specificity (99%).[80,81] The disadvantages of this assay are its high cost and the time needed to complete the assay, typically 2 or 3 days. More rapid and inexpensive assays with similar sensitivity (70-90%) and specificity (99%) are provided by a number of enzyme immunoassays (EIAs).[82] A stool culture for *C. difficile* is a less efficient method for establishing a laboratory diagnosis, since some strains of *C. difficile* are nontoxicogenic. In pseudomembranous colitis caused by *C. difficile* infection, sigmoidoscopy or colonoscopy reveals characteristic adherent yellow plaques that vary in diameter from 2 to 10 mm. The intervening mucosa typically appears normal or only mildly erythematous.[77]

The first step in the treatment is discontinuation of the inciting antibiotic. Standard therapy for *C. difficile*-associated diarrhea is oral metronidazole or oral vancomycin. Metronidazole 500 mg three times daily given orally or intravenously for 10-14 days is as effective as oral vancomycin 125 mg four times daily.[83,84] Metronidazole has advantages over vancomycin including lower cost and a reuction in the selection of vancomycin resistant enterococci. Metronidazole is therefore considered by many the initial therapy of choice in nonsevere cases. In patients with severe infection and signs of systemic toxicity, experts recommend initial therapy with vancomycin 125 mg orally four times daily and escalating the dose at 48-h intervals up to 500 mg four times daily if patients fail to improve. When patients do not respond to oral vancomycin, consideration should be given to adding intravenous metronidazole 500 mg ever 8 h or vancomycin retention enemas (0.5-1 g of vancomycin dissolved in 1-2 L of normal saline every 4-12 h).[85]

Relapse is common and may occur in up to 10-25% of cases. Relapses usually occur within 1-3 weeks after termination of initial therapy and are likely due to failure to eradicate the organism.[77,86] First relapses are treated with a second 10-14 day course of oral metronidazole or vancomycin.[77] If a patient relapses after a second course of antibiotics, different approaches have been suggested including tapering and pulsed antibiotic therapy and the use of anion-binding resins such as cholestyramine or cholestipol alone or in combination with vancomycin.[87,88]

In the posthematopoietic cell transplant patient, infectious diarrhea is relatively uncommon. In a prospective study of 296 patients following bone marrow transplantation, 126 (43%) developed acute diarrhea. Intestinal infection was found in 13%, with viruses being the most common organisms found (astrovirus, adenovirus, CMV, and rotavirus), followed by nosocomially-acquired bacteria (*C. difficile* and Aeromonas).[89] CMV deserves a special mention since it can cause diarrhea and bleeding because of mucosal ulceration.[90] The diagnosis of CMV is made by endoscopic biopsy (Fig. 132-5), which should be sent for immunohistochemistry and viral culture.[91] Infectious diarrhea related to *Salmonella*, *Shigella*, and *Campylobacter* species are very rare in hospitalized transplant patients. Diarrhea related to parasites (*Cryptosporidium*, *Giardia lamblia*, *Entamoeba histolytica*) is also a rare cause of diarrhea, and most of these patients are infected pretransplantation.[92-94]

Constipation

Constipation is a common problem in patients undergoing cancer treatment and is usually due to a combination of poor oral intake, decreased physical activity, and drugs such as opioid analgesics or antiemetic agents that slow intestinal transit time. Constipation has been reported with the vinka alkaloids, specially vincristine, and thalidomide.[95,96]

Impaction, bowel obstruction and colonic pseudoobstruction must be ruled out before starting therapy for constipation. Electrolyte abnormalities and other reversible causes should be corrected. Constipating drugs should be discontinued if possible. Laxatives, with or without stool softeners, can be used in

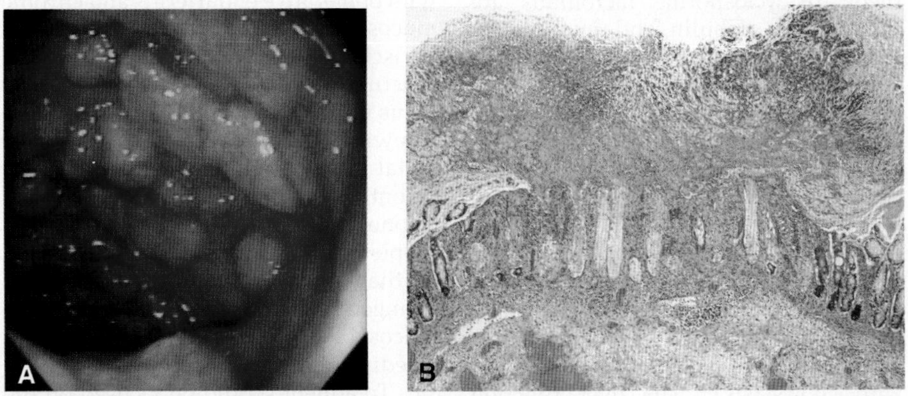

Figure 132-4 ■ Pseudomembranous colitis. **(A)** Pseudomembranes adherent to the colonic mucosa seen at colonoscopy. **(B)** Low power view of colonic mucosa shows a typical volcano (mushroom)-like appearance with luminal inflammatory exudates.

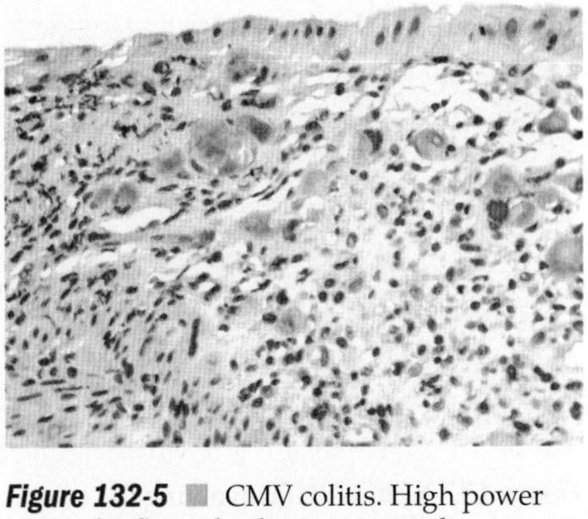

Figure 132-5 ■ CMV colitis. High power view of inflamed colonic mucosa demonstrates multiple viral inclusions in stroma cells. *Source*: Courtesy of Dr. T.T. Wu, MD Anderson Cancer Center.

the initial approach. Stimulant laxatives such as bisacodyl and senna work by altering electrolyte transport by the intestinal mucosa and increasing intestinal motor activity. If these agents are not effective, osmotic agents such as lactulose or sorbitol may be effective in improving stool frequency and consistency.[97] Polyethylene glycol solutions (without electrolytes) are available in powder form and have been found to be effective in improving chronic constipation.[97] The use of prokinetic agents, such as metoclopramide, to improve colonic transit has been disappointing.

GVHD

GVHD is divided into acute and chronic disease based upon the time of onset. Acute GVHD presents within the first 100 days of hematopoietic cell transplantation (HCT); whereas chronic is defined as the onset of disease after the first 100 days. The division at day 100 is artificial, and a continuum of clinical findings may be observed in patients with acute and chronic GVHD, as both commonly affect similar organs, principally the skin, liver and GI tract.

In acute GVHD, involvement of the GI tract is characterized by voluminous watery diarrhea and abdominal cramping. The diarrhea is secretory and can frequently become bloody.[98] Patients can also present with upper GI tract symptoms (dyspepsia, food intolerance, nausea, vomiting, and anorexia) in the absence of lower GI symptoms.[99] Biopsies are helpful in making the diagnosis. The most consistent histologic feature of GVHD is cell death (apoptosis)[100]; however, this finding is not specific and can be seen in other conditions. It is a topic of debate what area of the GI tract to target for endoscopic biopsies. Early literature suggested that rectal biopsies provide the highest diagnostic yield[101] (Fig. 132-6). Other studies have found that biopsies of the stomach[89] and small bowel[102,103] are most sensitive in the diagnosis of GVHD regardless of whether the patients present with upper or lower GI symptoms.

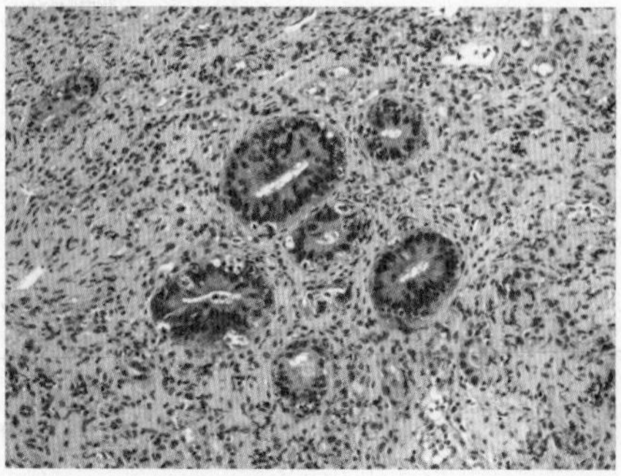

Figure 132-6 ■ GVHD involving the colon. The colonic mucosa shows prominent crypt apoptosis and focal crypt dropouts in a background of granulated tissue. *Source:* Courtesy of Dr. T.T. Wu, MD Anderson Cancer Center.

Until data from prospective studies are available, it may be best to routinely take biopsies from stomach, duodenum, and rectum when patients are referred for evaluation of potential GVHD.

In mild GVHD, the intestinal mucosa may appear grossly normal or have a mild granular appearance.[104] Moderate to severe GVHD is associated with granular, erythematous, and edematous mucosa; and in severe cases, mucosal ulceration or large areas of mucosal sloughing may be present.[105,106] Still, endoscopic findings are usually reported as having no correlation with histologic or clinical grading of GVHD severity.[102,107]

The liver is the second most commonly involved organ in acute GVHD. The earliest finding is commonly a rise in conjugated bilirubin and alkaline phosphatase. This reflects the underlying pathology in liver GVHD; that is, extensive bile duct damage with bile duct atypia and degeneration, epithelial cell dropout, and lymphocytic infiltration of small bile ducts leading to cholestasis.[108,109] Biopsy is the only method to diagnose GVHD of the liver, and to rule out other confounding diagnoses such veno-occlusive (VOD) disease, infection or drug toxicity. A liver biopsy may not be a feasible option, however, because of the risk of bleeding due to thrombocytopenia soon after hematopoietic cell transplant. A transjugular liver biopsy might be the preferred option, if a liver biopsy is deemed to be necessary for diagnosis. But this is rarely the case, since biopsies from skin of GI tract can be easily obtained, with less risk and a high diagnostic value.

For acute GVHD, the first and most effective treatment option is the use of corticosteroids.[110] Approximately 40% of patients will have a complete response.[111,112]

If high doses of steroids are not successful in controlling GVHD, second-line treatments are less successful. Among them are cyclosporine, tacrolimus, antithymocyte globulin and mycophenolate mofetil.[113,114] In those with acute GI GVHD, oral beclomethasone or oral budesonide may be more effective than systemic steroids alone.[115,116] For symptoms relief, octreotide is reported to control diarrhea in some patients with GVHD.[117]

In chronic GVHD, the skin, liver, GI tract and lungs are the principal organs affected. Liver histology will show lobular hepatitis, chronic hepatitis, and a reduction or absence of small bile ducts with cholestasis.[118] The liver function tests show elevations in bilirubin and alkaline phosphatase levels consistent with cholestasis. The oral mucosa is frequently involved and is commonly dry, resulting in ulceration and pain.[119] Involvement of the esophagus is the most common GI manifestation, with painful ulcerations, and formation of webs, rings, and strictures.[120,121] Involvement of small bowel and colon can occur, but it is significantly less frequent compared to the degree of involvement seen in acute GVHD. With intestinal involvement, patients can present with diarrhea, malabsorption, fibrosis of the submucosa, and sclerosis of the intestine.[121,122]

Ursodeoxycholic acid (UDCA) has been used in the treatment of refractory chronic GVHD of the liver. The rationale for its use is that GVHD of the liver shares many characteristics of primary biliary cirrhosis, a disease known to respond to this therapy. Treatment with UDCA results in a significant decrease in serum bilirubin, alkaline phosphatase and aspartate aminotransferase (AST) levels compared to baseline.[123,124] Discontinuation of the drug may result in prompt rise in the serum levels of all three markers.[123] The long-term efficacy of this treatment has not been studied.

Radiation Coloproctitis and Proctitis

Patients receiving radiation therapy to the abdomen and pelvis for the treatment of gynecologic, genitourinary, GI and other malignancies are at risk for developing acute and chronic intestinal injury. In the rectum and distal colon, acute radiation injury usually occurs within six weeks of therapy and is characterized by diarrhea, rectal urgency, tenesmus, and occasionally rectal bleeding. These symptoms usually resolve without therapy within 6 months.[125]

Chronic radiation proctitis or coloproctitis has a more delayed onset, occurring on average one year or later after exposure. Chronic injury is due to epithelial atrophy and fibrosis associated with obliterative endarteritis and chronic mucosal ischemia.[125] The end result is an ischemic segment of bowel prone to stricture formation and bleeding. Patients may complain of diarrhea, difficulties with defecation, bleeding, tenesmus, rectal urgency, and less commonly fecal incontinence. The diagnosis is made by colonoscopy or sigmoidoscopy. Endoscopic findings include mucosal edema, erythema, friability, and the presence of telangectasias. Severe cases may show mucosal ulcerations with or without bleeding and strictures.[125]

Treatment should be focused on the pattern of symptoms as patients may present with pain, diarrhea, tenesmus, obstruction, or bleeding. For patients with short, radiation-induced strictures, dilation by balloon, or Savary-Guillard dilators appears to be effective.[126] Sucralfate, administered orally or topically, has been reported to improve symptoms without causing significant adverse events.[127,128] Other treatments that have shown some benefit in small clinical trials include hyperbaric oxygen,[129] short-chain fatty acid enemas,[130] and rectal instillation of formaldehyde.[131] A variety of thermal endoscopic therapies have been used successfully to treat bleeding including Argon Plasma Coagulation (APC), argon and Nd:YAG lasers, bipolar electrocoagulation (BICAP) and heater probe. Among these modalities, APC has gained popularity because of ease of application, safe depth of penetration, low cost compared to lasers, and wide availability. APC uses energy transmitted to tissue by ionized argon gas. The benefits of APC treatment have been shown in several case series.[132-134] APC treated patients will have improvement in bleeding and anemia after a median of 2.9 endoscopic sessions.[135] Lasers such as argon and Nd:YAG are successful in controlling bleeding, but the equipment is expensive and not widely available. Bipolar electrocoagulation and heater probe are also effective but they may cause more tissue injury compared to APC or lasers. Surgery should be reserved for patients with uncontrollable symptoms such as obstruction due to strictures, pain or bleeding.

Acute Pancreatitis

Acute pancreatitis in cancer and post hematopoietic cell transplant patients can be caused by conditions found in the general population such as gallstones or alcohol. When managing these patients, it is important to take into consideration other etiologies including medications, chemotherapeutic agents, hypercalcemia and infections. Drug-induced pancreatitis has no distinguishing clinical features. A careful drug history and the exclusion of other etiologies are essential to make a diagnosis. Some of the most common drugs involved include metronidazole, sulfonamides, tetracycline, furosemide, thiazides, estrogen and tamoxifen.[136,137] These last two may act via the induction of hypertriglyceridemia.[138,139] During the course of chemotherapy, pancreatitis has been reported with azathioprine,[140] ifosfamide,[141] prednisone,[142] cytosine arabinoside,[143] and various regimens of combination chemotherapy including vinca alkaloids, methotrexate, mitomycin C, 5-FU, cyclophosphamide, cisplatin, and bleomycin. Causes of pancreatitis in immunocompromised patients include disseminated infections with CMV, VZV, adenovirus, and aspergillus.[144,145] Metastases to regional lymph nodes, producing ductal obstruction can cause pancreatitis, as can metastasis to the pancreas itself.[146,147]

In the evaluation of abdominal pain in patients with cancer, pancreatitis should be considered in the differential diagnosis. Evaluation should include a careful medication history, serum amylase and lipase levels, and imaging studies such as abdominal ultrasound to rule out gallstones or biliary obstruction, and CT scan to assess the severity of the inflammatory process and evaluate for associated complications.

Veno-Occlusive Disease (VOD) or Sinusoidal Obstruction Syndrome (SOS)

VOD or SOS is a clinical syndrome characterized by tender hepatomegaly, jaundice and weight gain. It is more often seen in patients following hematopoietic cell transplantation, but it can also occur following use of chemotherapeutic agents in the nontransplant setting, ingestion of alkaloid toxins, and after high-dose radiation therapy or liver transplantation.[148,149]

Recent advances in the study of the pathogenesis of this disease indicate that it is the sinusoidal, and not venous, endothelial cells that are the target of toxic injury.[150,151] Following injury, there is activation of the coagulation cascade and clot formation. Fibrin-related plugs, intracellular fluid entrapment and cellular debris progressively occlude sinusoids, (Fig. 132-7) causing intrahepatic post sinusoidal portal hypertension. In keeping with this concept, a new terminology has been coined for this entity: sinusoidal obstructive syndrome or SOS.[152]

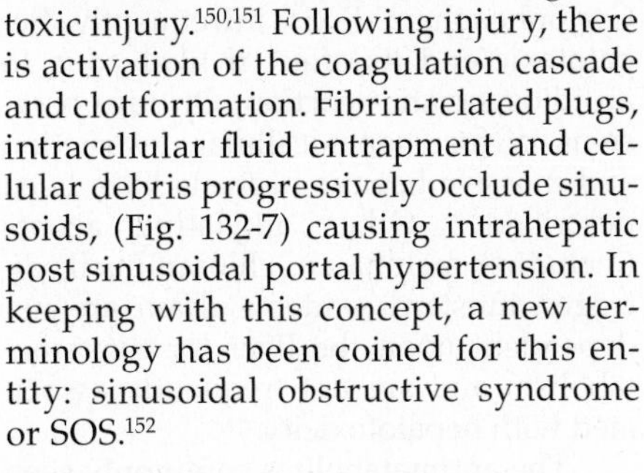

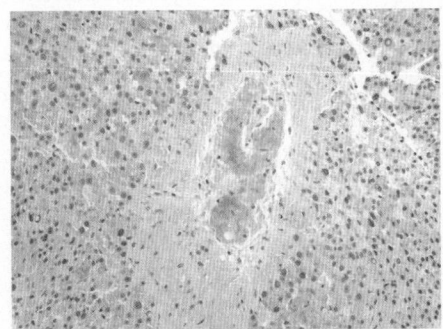

Figure 132-7 ■ VOD of the liver. The small hepatic vein demonstrates fibrous obliteration with fibrin deposits. The perivenular hepatocytes show prominent sinusoidal congestion. *Source*: Courtesy of Dr. T.T. Wu, MD Anderson Cancer Center.

Recognized pretransplant risk factors for the development of VOD/SOS include older transplant recipient age, poor performance status, female gender, donor-recipient HLA disparity, advanced malignancy, prior abdominal radiation, second myeloablative transplant, reduced pulmonary diffusion capacity (DLCO) and prior liver disease.[153-156]

The type and intensity of the transplant conditioning regimen is probably the greatest determining factor of risk for developing severe VOD/SOS. Risk increases with total body irradiation dose and use of certain drugs such as 6-mercaptopurine (6-MP), 6-thioguanine, actinomycin D, azathioprine, busulfan, cytosine arabinoside, cyclophosphamide, dacarbazine, gemtuzumab-ozogamicin, melphalan, oxaliplatin, and urethane.[152,153]

The classic presentation of VOD/SOS is characterized by weight gain caused by fluid retention, tender hepatomegaly and hyperbilirubinemia (Table 132-4) without any known cause.[157,158]

Diagnosis is usually based on signs and symptoms, having ruled out other conditions that can mimic the disease, particularly after stem cell transplantation; such as viral infection, GVHD, cholestasis secondary to sepsis, heart failure and tumor infiltration of the liver.[158]

In patients in whom the diagnosis is in question, and GVHD or infection needs to be excluded, a liver biopsy may be necessary. The transjugular access is probably the safest route to perform a liver biopsy and to measure hepatic venous pressure gradient (HVPG). Measurement of HVPG can help discriminate between GVHD and VOD/SOS since HPVG is greater in the latter.[159]

The clinical outcome of patients with VOD/SOS depends on the disease severity. Those with mild disease require no specific therapy despite evidence of liver biochemical abnormalities. Those with moderate disease will respond to sodium restriction, and diuretics. Severe VOD/SOS is associated with multiorgan failure and is usually fatal.[158]

Based on the histological presence of microthrombosis and fibrin deposition in the hepatic venules of patients with VOD/SOS, the principal specific therapy has been to promote fibrinolysis with or without anticoagulation.[160-162]

Table 132-4 ■ **Common Drugs Implicated in VOD/SOS**

• Dacarbazine	• Actinomycin D
• Azathioprine	• Cytosine arabinoside
• 6-MP	• Gemtuzumab-ozogamicin
• 6-thioguanine	• Melphalan
• Busulfan	• Oxaliplatin
• Cyclophosphamide	• Urethane

A number of treatment strategies have been used in severe VOD, including the use of alteplase (recombinant tissue-type plasminogen activator or tPA) alone or in combination with heparin, and defibrotide. Treatment with alteplase and heparin have resulted in a response rate of about 30% but has been associated with a significant risk of life-threatening hemorrhage, particularly in patients with multiorgan failure.[161] Defibrotide is a polydeoxyribonucleotide that has been found to have antithrombotic, antiischemic and thrombolytic properties without causing significant anticoagulation. Defibrotide given intravenously in doses ranging from 5 to 60 mg/kg per day for a minimum of 14 days, results in a response in about 42-55% of patients, without any significant treatment-related toxicity.[163,164] Predictors of survival with therapy included younger age, autologous stem cell transplantation and abnormal portal vein flow, while regimens based on busulfan and the present of encephalopathy predicted worse outcome.

Insertion of a transjugular intrahepatic portosystemic stent-shunt (TIPS) has been reported in small number of patients with severe VOD/SOS. TIPS was effective in improving portal pressure gradient; and in some patients, it was associated with clinical improvement of hepatic and renal symptoms. Nonetheless, these effects may be transient and may not improve overall survival.[165-167]

Orthotopic liver transplantation (OLT) has been reported anecdotally as a rescue therapy in patients with VOD/SOS after stem cell transplant, when there has been no response to medical therapy.[168,169] On the other hand, the majority of patients with severe VOD/SOS will not be capable of undergoing OLT, specially in the presence of malignancies and multiorgan failure. In summary, there are limited options in the treatment of severe VOD, and further studies are needed to demonstrate the optimum treatment strategy.

Drug Hepatotoxicity

Patients undergoing chemotherapy require careful assessment of liver function both prior to treatment and during therapy. If liver tests are abnormal, the etiology must be defined promptly and as clearly as possible. In addition to drug reactions, there are multiple potential causes of abnormal liver tests in the population undergoing chemotherapy including tumor progression, infection, or the presence of coexisting hepatic disease (Table 132-5).

Patients with preexisting liver disease may be more susceptible to drug-induced hepatotoxicity. Chemotherapy (including the use of monoclonal antibodies) can lead to reactivation of hepatitis B.[170-172] Risk factors for reactivation include hepatitis B surface antigen and hepatitis B e antigen seropositivity, detectable hepatitis B virus (HBV) DNA prior to chemotherapy, male sex, diagnosis of lymphoma or breast cancer, and use of steroids.[170,173,174] Prophylactic treatment with lamivudine appears to be beneficial in preventing viral reactivation, or reducing its severity, in patients undergoing cytotoxic chemotherapy.[175] The relationship between chemotherapy and hepetitis C virus (HCV) reactivation is less clear than for HBV infection. It appears the presence of HCV infection increases the risk of liver function tests abnormalities,[176] but severe flares of hepatitis are extremely rare.

Most hepatotoxic drug reactions are idiosyncratic and are due to either hypersensitivity mechanisms or host metabolic idiosyncrasy.[177] Features suggestive of drug toxicity include the lack of abnormalities prior to the introduction of the drug, clinical illness or biochemical abnormalities after drug administration, and resolution of those abnormalities after the drug is withdrawn.

Alkylating agents are uncommonly associated with hepatotoxicity. With the exception of cyclophosphamide and ifosfamide, patients receiving alkylating agents do not require a dose reduction. Cyclophosphamide is infrequently hepatotoxic and its effect if likely due to an idiosyncratic reaction. On rare occasions, diffuse hepatocellular destruction and massive hepatic necrosis have been described.[178] Other alkylating agents (including melphalan, chlorambucil, nitrogen mustard, and busulfan) are not dependent upon the liver for their metabolism and are not frequently associated with hepatotoxicity.

The antimetabolites commonly seen in clinical use include cytosine arabinoside Ara-C, 5-FU, 6-MP, azathioprine, 6-thioguanine, and methotrexate (MTX). Hepatic metabolism plays an important role in the processing of these drugs, and dose reductions are usually necessary in patients with liver dysfunction. Ara-C, used in the treatment of acute myelogenous leukemia (AML), has been on rare occasions associated with cholestasis, which appears reversible.[179] Only rare reports of hepatotoxicity have been noted with intravenous 5-FU, but hepatotoxicity has been reported more commonly when 5-FU is administered in combination with levamisole.[180] Intra-arterial administration of the 5-FU metabolite floxuridine (fluorodeoxyuridine [FudR]) has been associated with two types of toxicity: one suggestive of hepatocellular injury, and the second one consistent with sclerosing cholangitis, with stricturing of the intra and extrahepatic bile ducts, and elevations of alkaline phosphatase and bilirubin.[181-183]

Table 132-5 **Potential Causes of Hepatic Abnormalities in Cancer Patients**

Direct effects of the tumor
Hepatic metastases
Portal vein thrombosis
Indirect effects of the tumor
Paraneoplastic syndromes
Preexisting liver disease
Coexisting medical conditions
Chemotherapeutic drugs
GVHD
Infection

6-MP is often used for maintenance therapy in acute lymphoblastic leukemia (ALL). Two patterns of toxicity have been reported: hepatocellular injury and cholestasis.[184] Toxicity occurs more commonly when the daily dose of 2 mg/kg is exceeded. Azathioprine is a nitroimidazole derivative of 6-MP. Its toxicity is less frequent and less dose-dependent compared with 6-MP. Three different patterns of toxicity are described: a hypersensitivity reaction, a cholestatic reaction, and endothelial cell injury with development of elevated portal pressures, VOD/SOS, and peliosis hepatis.[185]

High-dose MTX therapy has been associated with reversible elevations in aminotransferases,[186] and patients taking chronic low dose methotrexate therapy for psoriasis or rheumatoid arthritis are at risk for developing hepatic fibrosis and cirrhosis. The risk is low in patients who receive less than 1.5 g of MTX as cumulative dose.[187] The antitumor antibiotics include doxorubicin and daunorubicin. Doxorubicin can cause hepatocellular injury and steatosis. Dose reduction has been recommended in patients with cholestasis to avoid greater toxicity.[188] Similar guidelines are followed for daunorubicin.

Combinations of 5-FU and oxaliplatin or irinotecan are used for neoadjuvant therapy in patients with colorectal cancer prior to the resection of liver metastases. These neoadjuvant regimens have been associated with steatosis, hepatic vascular injury, and nodular regenerative hyperplasia.[189-192]

In conclusion, chemotherapeutic agents alone or in combination with other drugs can cause a variety of toxic effects on the liver. Patients with underlying liver disease may be more susceptible to drug-induced hepatotoxicity. Careful monitoring of patients is critical in the prevention and treatment of hepatic complications of cancer chemotherapy.

Selected References

The complete reference list can be found at www.CANCERMEDICINE8.com

2. Moses FM, Peura DA, Wong RK, Johnson LF. Palliative dilation of esophageal carcinoma. *Gastrointest Endosc*. 1985;31:61–63.
4. Mellow MH, Pinkas H. Endoscopic laser therapy for malignancies affecting the esophagus and gastroesophageal junction. *Arch Intern Med*. 1985;145:1443–1446.
7. Fleischer D, Sivak MV Jr. Endoscopic Nd:YAG laser therapy as palliation for esophagogastric cancer. Parameters affecting initial outcome. *Gastroenterology*. 1985;89:827–831.
11. Lightdale CJ, Heler SK, Marcon NE, et al. Photodynamic therapy with porfimer sodium versus thermal ablation therapy with Nd:YAG laser for palliation of esophageal cancer: a multicenter randomized trial. *Gastrointest Endosc*. 1995;42:507–512.
14. Cowling MG, Hale H, Grundy A. Management of malignant oesophageal obstruction with self-expanding metallic stents. *Br J Surg*. 1998;85:264–266.
17. Raijman I, Siddique I, Ajani J, Lynch P. Palliation of malignant dysphagia and fistulae with coated expandable metal esophageal stents: experience with 101 patients. *Gastrointest Endosc*. 1998;48:172–179.
21. McDonald GB, Sharma P, Hackman RC, et al. Esophageal Infections in immunosuppressed patients after marrow transplantation. *Gastroenterology*. 1985;88:1111–1117.
22. Benson CA, Kaplan JE, Masur H, et al. Treating opportunistic infections among HIV-infected adults and adolescents: Recommendations from CDC, the National Institutes of Health, and the HIV Medicine Association/Infectious Disease Society of America. *MMWR Recomm Rep*. 2004;53(RR-15):1–112.
25. Ally R, Schurmann D, Kreisel W, et al. A randomized, double-blind, double-dummy, multicenter trial of voriconazole and fluconazole in the treatment of esophageal candidiasis in immunocompromised patients. *Clin Infect Dis*. 2001;33:1447–1454.
31. McBane RD, Gross JB Jr. Herpes esophagitis: clinical syndrome, endoscopic appearance, and diagnosis in 23 patients. *Gastrointest Endosc*. 1991;37:600–603.
36. Blanshard C, Benhamou Y, Dohin E, et al. Treatment of AIDS-associated gastrointestinal cytomegalovirus infection with foscarnet and ganciclovir: a randomized comparison. *J Infect Dis*. 1995;172:622–628.
37. Whitley RJ, Jacobson MA, Friedberg DN, et al. Guidelines for the treatment of cytomegalovirus diseases in patients with AIDS in the era of potent antiretroviral therapy: Recommendations of an international panel. *Arch Intern Med*. 1998;158:957–969.
40. Kikendall JW, Friedman AC, Oyewole MA, et al. Pill-induced esophageal injury: case reports and review of the medical literature. *Dig Dis Sci*. 1983;28:174–182.
43. Alt B, Glass NR, Sollinger H. Neutropenic enterocolitis in adults. Review of the literature and assessment of surgical intervention. *Am J Surg*. 1985;149:405–408.
45. Sloas MM, Flynn PM, Kaste SC, Patrick CC. Typhlitis in children with cancer: a 30-year experience. *Clin Infect Dis*. 1993;17:484–490.
46. Katz JA, Wagner ML, Gresik MV, et al. Typhlitis. An 18-year experience and postmortem review. *Cancer*. 1990;65:1041–1047.
57. Gorschlüter M, Mey U, Strehl J, et al. Neutropenic enterocolitis in adults: systematic analysis of evidence quality. *Eur J Haematol*. 2005;75:1–13.
60. Shamberger RC, Weinstein HJ, Delorey MJ, Levey RH. The medical and surgical management of typhlitis in children with acute nonlymphocytic (myelogenous) leukemia. *Cancer*. 1986;57:603–609.
67. Saltz LB, Cox JV, Blanke C, et al. Irinotecan plus fluorouracil and leucovorin for metastatic colorectal cancer. Irinotecan Study Group. *N Engl J Med*. 2000;343:905–914.
72. Benson AB, Ajani JA, Catalano RB, et al. Recommended guidelines for the treatment of cancer treatment-induced diarrhea. *J Clin Oncol*. 2004;22:2918–2926.
73. Harris AG, O'Dorisio TM, Woltering EA, et al. Consensus statement: octreotide dose titration in secretory diarrhea. Diarrhea Management Consensus Development Panel. *Dig Dis Sci*. 1995;40:1464–1473.
84. Bartlett JG. Antibiotic-associated diarrhea. *N Engl J Med*. 2002;346:334–349.
89. Cox GJ, Matsui SM, Lo RS, et al. Etiology and outcome of diarrhea after marrow transplantation: a prospective study. *Gastroenterology*. 1994;107:1398–1407.
97. Brandt LJ, Prather CM, Quigley EM, et al. Systematic review of the management of chronic constipation in North America. *Am J Gastroenterol*. 2005;100(S1):S5–S21.
98. Schwartz JM, Wolford JL, Thornquist MD, et al. Severe gastrointestinal bleeding after hematopoietic cell transplantation, 1987–1997: incidence, causes and outcome. *Am J Gastroenterol*. 2001;96:385–393.
106. Saito H, Oshimi K, Nagasako K, et al. Endoscopic appearance of the colon and small intestine of a patient with hemorrhagic enteric graft-vs.-host disease. *Dis Colon Rectum*. 1990;33:695–697.
110. Vogelsang GB, Lee L, Bensen-Kennedy DM. Pathogenesis and treatment of graft-versus-host disease after bone marrow transplant. *Annu Rev Med*. 2003;54:29–52.
114. Couriel D, Caldera H, Champlin R, Komanduri K. Acute graft-versus-host disease: pathophysiology, clinical manifestations, and management. *Cancer*. 2004;101:1936–1946.
121. Atkinson K. Chronic graft-versus-host disease. *Bone Marrow Transplant*. 1990;5:69–82.
123. Fried RH, Murakami CS, Fisher LD, et al. Ursodeoxycholic acid treatment of refractory chronic graft-versus-host disease of the liver. *Ann Intern Med*. 1992;116:624–629.
125. Babb RR. Radiation proctitis: a review. *Am J Gastroenterol*. 1996;91:1309–1311.
130. Al-Sabbagh R, Sinicrope FA, Sellin JH, et al. Evaluation of short-chain fatty acid enemas: treatment of radiation proctitis. *Am J Gastroenterol*. 1996;91:1814–1816.
136. Runzi M, Layer P. Drug-associated pancreatitis: facts and fiction. *Pancreas*. 1996;13:100–109.
144. Parenti DM, Steinberg W, Kang P. Infectious causes of acute pancreatitis. *Pancreas*. 1996;13:356–371.
148. Kumar S, DeLeve LD, Kamath PS, Tefferi A. Hepatic veno-occlusive disease (sinusoidal obstruction syndrome) after hematopoietic stem cell transplantation. *Mayo Clin Proc*. 2003;78:589–598.
151. DeLeve LD. Hepatic microvasculature in liver injury. *Semin Liver Dis*. 2007;27:390–400.
153. Carreras E, Bertz H, Arcese W, et al. Incidence and outcome of hepatic veno-occlusive disease after blood or marrow transplantation: a prospective cohort study of the European Group for Blood and Marrow Transplantation. European Group for Blood and Marrow Transplantation Chronic Leukemia Working Party. *Blood*. 1998;92:3599–3604.
158. McDonald GB, Hinds MS, Fisher LD, et al. Veno-occlusive disease of the liver and multiorgan failure after bone marrow transplantation: a cohort study of 355 patients. *Ann Intern Med*. 1993;118:255–267.
161. Bearman SI, Lee JL, Baron AE, McDonald GB. Treatment of hepatic venocclusive disease with recombinant human tissue plasminogen activator and heparin in 42 marrow transplant patients. *Blood*. 1997;89:1501–1506.
163. Richardson PG, Elias AD, Krishnan A, et al. Treatment of severe veno-occlusive disease with defibrotide: compassionate use results in response without significant toxicity in a high-risk population. *Blood*. 1998;92:737–744.
166. Fried MW, Connaghan DG, Sharma S, et al. Transjugular Intrahepatic portosystemic shunt for the management of severe venocclusive disease following bone marrow transplantation. *Hepatology*. 1996;24:588–591.
167. Azoulay D, Castaing D, Lemoine A, et al. Transjugular intrahepatic portosystemic shunt (TIPS) for severe veno-occlusive disease of the liver following bone marrow transplantation. *Bone Marrow Transplant*. 2000;25:987–992.
174. Yeo W, Zee B, Zhong S, et al. Comprehensive analysis of risk factors associating with Hepatitis B virus (HBV) reactivation in cancer patients undergoing cytotoxic chemotherapy. *Br J Cancer*. 2004;90:1306–1311.
175. Yeo W, Chan PK, Ho WM, et al. Lamivudine for the prevention of hepatitis B virus reactivation in hepatitis B s-Antigen seropositive cancer patients undergoing cytotoxic chemotherapy. *J Clin Oncol*. 2004;22:927–934.
177. Lee WM. Drug induced hepatotoxicity. *N Engl J Med*. 1995;333:1118–1127.
180. Moertel CG, Fleming TR, MacDonald JS, et al. Hepatic toxicity associated with fluorouracil plus levamisole adjuvant therapy. *J Clin Oncol*. 1993;11:2386–2390.
190. Rubbia-Brandt L, Audard V, Sartoretti P, et al. Severe hepatic sinusoidal obstruction associated with oxaliplatin-based chemotherapy in patients with metastatic colorectal cancer. *Ann Oncol*. 2004;15:460–466.
191. Vauthey JN, Pawlik TM, Ribero D, et al. Chemotherapy regimen predicts steatohepatitis and an increase in 90-day mortality after surgery for hepatic colorectal metastases. *J Clin Oncol*. 2006;24:2065–2072.

133 Oral Complications of Cancer and Their Treatment

Stephen T. Sonis, DMD, DMSc

The mouth is a frequent site of acute and chronic adverse side effects of cancer therapy. These may range broadly in their nature, incidence, severity, and course, but they uniformly and adversely affect patients' quality of life, ability to tolerate therapy, overall cost of treatment, and rehabilitation. Stomatotoxicity, which leads to the disruption of the integrity of the oral mucosa, also results in the mouth serving as a source for systemic or distant infection. Oral complications of cancer therapy are perceived as common in some cohorts such as patients with head and neck cancer (HNC), but relatively rare in others. This perception has been largely fueled by under-reporting, often by patients who understand that mentioning toxicity symptoms might result in subsequent compromise of their optimum anti-cancer treatment. While this phenomenon is not unique to oral complications, data surrounding the underestimates of oral toxicities are substantial. Additionally oral manifestations have been reported with many forms of developing therapies including cetuximab, bisphosphonates, and mTOR-inhibitors. It is also becoming increasingly clear that oral complications rarely occur in isolation. Rather, probably because of common biologic underpinnings, they often predictably occur with other regimen-related toxicities.

Overall, about 40% of patients being treated for cancers not of the head and neck develop some form of mouth-related problem, which range from xerostomia to mucositis.[1] The frequency escalates to more than 75% for patients being treated for HNC, those who develop graft-versus-host disease (GVHD), and patients receiving aggressive myeloablative chemotherapy regimens. The symptomatic and functional consequences of oral complications include increases in analgesics and antibiotics use, length of hospital stays, hospitalizations for pain and fluid management, nursing resource use, diagnostic treating, and need for parenteral feeding. The impact on charges and costs is dramatic. In a study population of patients receiving treatment for HNC and non-small cell lung cancer, the incremental cost of oral mucositis was found to be $17,244.[2] In the past, oral complications were largely considered to be inevitable, often were not recognized early, and were treated retrospectively rather than in a prospective or preventive manner. Significant progress has been made in the past decade to better define the biology and epidemiology of oral complications of treatment. As a result, interventions that target mechanisms have evolved, as has a better understanding of at risk populations.

Pretreatment Assessment

There is no question that the risk of many of the side effects that impact the mouth can be successfully mitigated by the elimination of existing sites of dental disease before anticancer treatment is initiated.[3-5] A pretreatment dental visit is strongly recommended as it serves a range of purposes. First, it provides an opportunity for the identification and elimination of sources of active and chronic dental or periodontal infections or chronic irritation when the patient is best able to tolerate treatment with the least risk of undesirable post-treatment sequelae, such as infection or osteonecrosis. Second, oral manifestations of the primary cancer may be detected. Third, it provides an opportunity for patient education and discussion regarding the impact of the cancer and its treatment on short- and long-term oral health. Fourth, for the patient about to undergo surgical intervention for tumors about the mouth, pretreatment evaluation is critical to optimize the fabrication of prostheses. The construction of protective appliances prior to the start of radiation therapy may reduce the impact of treatment on scatter-induced injury.

In a study of the effectiveness of dental screening, Woods and Sonis found that 72% of patients screened prior to bone marrow transplantation (BMT) demonstrated positive findings relative to latent dental infection, or mucosal irritation caused by faulty prostheses or dental restorations.[6] Results of another study in the same population suggested that one-third of the patients required oral care before transplantation.[7] Jham et al. reported that 57.9% of the 207 HNC patients they evaluated presented with pretreatment oral disease and that over 50% had dental pathology of such severity that tooth extraction was indicated.[6] Epstein and Stevenson-Moore noted similar findings in patients with nasopharyngeal cancer: 68% of dentate patients screened prior to treatment required extractions, primarily because of periodontal disease.[8] Studies by others further demonstrate that pre-chemotherapy intervention for abnormalities found on screening had a significant, favorable impact on morbidity relative to local infection and sepsis.[5] Importantly, effective dental screening with appropriate treatment, prior to the onset of cancer therapy results in significant cost savings by reducing the incidence of infection during periods of granulocytopenia.[9]

Timing of Assessment and Dental Treatment

If oral screening is performed close to the initiation of cancer therapy as to preclude dental intervention, the value of the process is nullified. The ideal interval between the completion of dental treatment, particularly extraction, and the initiation of radiation therapy has been the subject of much debate.[10] Nonetheless, given the rate by which wounds of the mouth heal, particularly extraction sites, it appears that a minimum of 2 weeks is acceptable and 3 weeks desirable. For patients about to undergo chemotherapy, sufficient time between the completion of dental treatment and the patient's anticipated granulocyte nadir (<500 cells/mL) is required. In general, non-emergent dental treatment should not be performed in a typical ambulatory setting if the patient is significantly thrombocytopenic (<100,000 platelets/mL).

Because of the acute onset of some hematologic malignancies and the need for immediate chemotherapy, pretreatment dental and oral screening in this high-risk population may not be possible. In these cases, oral assessment should be performed as close to the initiation of therapy as possible for two reasons: first, such an examination provides an important baseline for oral health; and second, the finding and elimination of active oral infection in this markedly myeloablated group is often critical to their overall clinical course. Eradication of identified sources of odontogenic infection should not be delayed, as there is significant data to support the conclusion that dental extractions may be performed safely in this group if they are managed well, preferably in a hospital setting.[11] The complication rate for extractions in patients with hematologic malignancies is reported to be 13%, with no effect on length of hospital stay or mortality. The most common complications include pain and bleeding. It is important to note that there is no evidence to suggest that an aggressive strategy of extraction of asymptomatic teeth has any benefit in the prevention of systemic infection.

Components of the pretreatment assessment include baseline data such as medical and dental histories; laboratory data—such as antibody status relative to herpes simplex type 1 virus—and a clinical assessment that should include an extra-oral examination of the head and neck, intra-oral soft tissue examination, periodontal disease screening, and dental evaluation. Radiographic evaluation should include those films that are necessary to definitively diagnose periodontal disease and caries, periapical pathology, and impacted teeth. It is also important to assess the patient's knowledge of, and motivation for dental maintenance. Teeth that demonstrate evidence of untreated periapical pathology, or advanced caries or periodontal disease should be eliminated.

Patients with removable prostheses should be encouraged to minimize their use or leave them out during their cancer therapy since even subtle mucosal trauma accelerates the risk and onset of mucositis. Similarly, the removal of orthodontic bands prior to the start of chemotherapy is an essential component in preventing trauma to atrophied mucosa.[1]

Oral Complications of Radiotherapy

Oral complications of radiation therapy are primarily the result of acute and chronic local tissue injury. In addition, radiation-induced xerostomia may result in secondary effects on the teeth and periodontium. The dose rate, total dose of radiation, and the size and structures within the radiation field are the major determinants of oral toxicity. As a result, patients being treated for tumors of the mouth, oropharynx, tongue, nasopharynx, and salivary glands are at highest risk. Patients with hypopharyngeal or laryngeal tumors are also often affected, although at a slightly lower rate. Brachytherapy tends to be more stomatotoxic than external beam irradiation. Although intensity-modulated radiation therapy (IMRT) (Chapter 77: Neoplasms of the Head and Neck) may spare some structures, its impact on oral mucosa is significant. Oral tissues that are directly affected by radiation include mucosa (epithelium and tissues in the lamina propria), salivary glands, bone, and muscle. In children, radiation that includes the jaws negatively affects craniofacial and dental development.[12-14]

Mucositis

Both radiation and chemotherapy can produce significant damage to the oral mucosa as a side effect of treatment. The term mucositis (ICD9 code 528.1) is preferred over stomatitis when describing mucosal injury caused by antineoplastic therapy as the latter is a generic term and can be associated with a range of infectious or traumatic etiologies unrelated to chemo- or radiotherapy. The severity and kinetics of radiation-induced oral mucositis are related to dose rate and total dose that target the oral mucosa. Local mucosal irritation, secondary infection, and xerostomia are factors that amplify the damaging effects of radiation to the tissue.

Three themes have characterized thinking relative to mucositis in the past 5 years: first, the pathobiology has been more fully defined; second, the commonality in mechanisms by which mucosal injury occurs has been applied to all parts of the alimentary canal, and third mucositis rarely occurs as an isolated toxicity.[15]

Historically, mucositis was viewed as the result of direct radiation or chemotherapy mediated injury to stem cells in the basal layer of the oral mucosa. It was proposed that these rapidly dividing cells were indiscriminately damaged resulting in atrophy and subsequent ulceration. Simultaneously, connective tissue injury was thought to lead to an increase in vascular permeability and tissue edema.[16] However, studies defining the mechanisms by which mucositis occurs reveal a process that is biologically more complex. Although epithelial stem cells are the ultimate mediators of mucosal injury, it is now clear that their demise occurs by indirect, as well as direct, mechanisms.[17] In fact, direct clonogenic cell death of these cells is insufficient to produce the extent of clinical injury that is typically observed. Rather, a sequence of events[18] triggered by the generation of reactive species in cells of the lamina propria produce a cascade of events in the endothelium, connective tissue, extra-cellular matrix, and the inflammatory infiltrate. This sequence begins almost immediately, following the initial exposure of the mucosa to radiation, and results in a range of molecular mediators and signals that permeate to the epithelium and cause injury, apoptosis, and necrosis.

Radiation-induced oral mucositis typically begins within the first 2 weeks of therapy, at cumulative doses of 10-20 Gy. Although clinical changes are observed at these doses, the cellular and tissue events producing these changes begin almost immediately following initial dosing (see below). Mucosal erythema, mild epithelial sloughing, and the formation of islands of hyperkeratosis characterize early changes of mucositis. These changes are accompanied by relatively mild symptoms characterized by a painful burning sensation that is analogous to a food burn such as that caused by hot cheese. Patients often have difficulty tolerating spicy foods. With the exception of the dorsal surface of the tongue, hard palate, and the gingiva, any mucosal surface of the mouth is susceptible. Most commonly affected areas are the buccal mucosa (cheeks), ventral and lateral surfaces of the tongue, and the floor of the mouth (Fig. 133-1). The soft palate and oropharynx are also frequently involved and are consistent drivers of symptoms associated with pain on swallowing. Consequently, patients may complain of a sore throat early in their treatment.

At cumulative doses of about 30 Gy, the integrity of the mucosa breaks down and ulceration occurs. Ulcers typically begin as isolated lesions, but then coalesce forming large, contiguous breaks in the mucosa, often covered by a collection of dead cells and bacteria in a pseudomembrane. In severe cases, the lesions may bleed (Fig. 133-2). Ulcerative mucositis is extremely painful. Not only do ulcers cover large mucosal surface areas, but they are also deep. Patients who have undergone radiation therapy and have developed mucositis describe this complication as the most significant of their treatment.[19] In many cases, mucositis results in breaks in radiation treatment, hospitalization for fluid support or pain management, and the need for parenteral feeding.[20] The incremental economic cost of oral mucositis in this population is significant.[2] It is important that patients about to begin treatment have some concept of the severity of mucosal in-

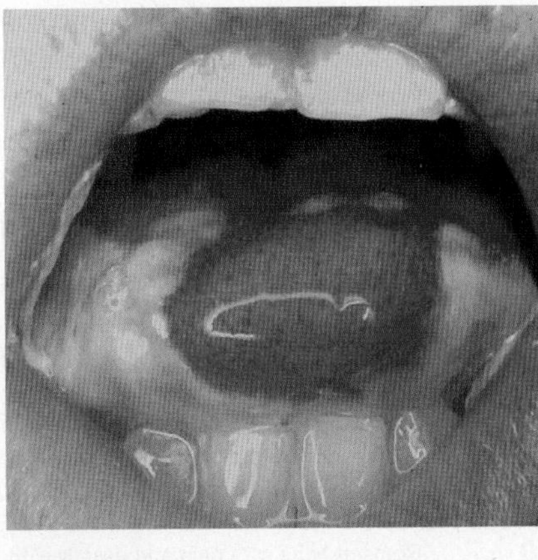

Figure 133-1 Severe oral mucositis with ulceration and pseudomembrane formation of the lateral and ventral surfaces of the tongue and buccal mucosa induced by myeloablative chemotherapy for conditioning prior to HSCT.

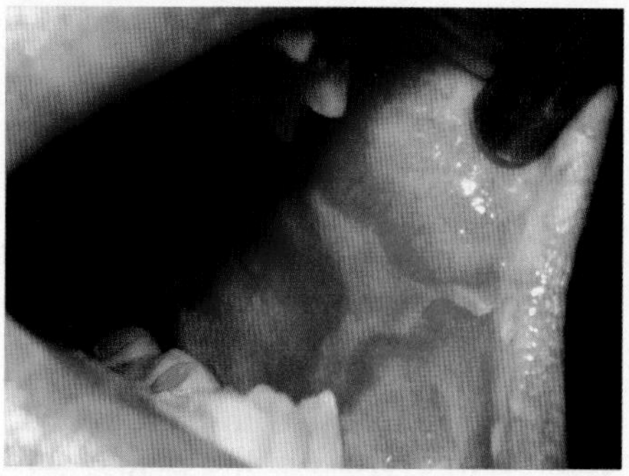

Figure 133-2 ■ Severe oral mucositis with ulceration, erythema, and pseudomembrane formation of the left buccal mucosa induced by radiation therapy for treatment of an oral carcinoma.

jury that they are likely to develop. The typical pretreatment characterization of mucositis as "mouth sores" seems to trivialize their significance to patients. It seems likely that a more realistic description and management plan would be advantageous. In most patients, ulcerative mucositis is self-limiting and resolves spontaneously 2-3 weeks following the completion of radiation.

Evaluation of Mucositis ■ Comparisons of the stomatotoxicity of treatment regimens and efficacy assessments of mucositis interventions have been hindered by the lack of a universally acceptable scoring system for the condition. A recent comprehensive review of mucositis by the Mucositis Study Section of the Multinational Association of Supportive Care in Cancer[15] lists 14 scales that are currently in use to grade mucositis. Measurement scales for mucositis fall into 3 major functional categories: those that are used to describe toxicity, those that are designed primarily for research, and those that are used as nursing management tools. Virtually all of the scales contain objective endpoints that focus on the extent of observed erythema and ulceration. Although some scales are limited to these objective findings, many add other elements that depend on symptomatic interpretation and patients' oral function, particularly associated with eating ability. Patient-reported scales have also been used to supplement clinician-based assessment.

Currently, the grading systems most commonly used to describe oral mucosal toxicity are the World Health Organization (WHO) and National Cancer Institute's common terminology criteria for adverse events (NCI-CTCAE) scales. The WHO scale combines objective findings of erythema and ulceration with the patients' ability to eat solids, liquids, or nothing by mouth (Table 133-1). The complexity of mucositis assessment is reflected by the fact that the NCI CTCAE version 3 has multiple scales that separately grade objective and functional findings for different clinical situations (radiation, chemotherapy, and hematopoietic stem cell transplantation (HSCT)). The lack of a universally accepted mucositis scale remains a barrier to easy comparisons of regimen-related toxicities and the effectiveness of new interventions.

Prevention and Treatment ■ There is currently no approved, active preventive or treatment intervention for radiation-induced mucositis in the United States. There is consensus that improved oral status may reduce the risk or severity of mucositis. Maintaining a high level of oral hygiene during treatment is thought to be beneficial.

Since mucosal injury is related to the extent of mucosa exposed to radiation, the use of midline radiation blocks[21] and three-dimensional radiation treatment[22] may reduce the extent of stomatotoxicity.

Benzydamine hydrochloride is a nonsteroidal rinse with anti-inflammatory, analgesic, and anesthetic properties that is approved for use in the prevention and treatment of radiation-induced mucositis in Canada, Australia, and Europe. Results of a number of studies suggest its efficacy in this application.[23-27] The MASCC panel recommended the use of benzydamine among patients receiving moderate dose radiotherapy.[28] There is no data to support its use in patients receiving concomitant chemotherapy.

A number of palliative barrier agents have been suggested to alleviate symptoms associated with oral mucositis. Gelclair, which has FDA approval as a device, purportedly forms a barrier on injured mucosa.[29] Sucralfate, an agent that has wide use in the treatment of gastric ulcers, forms a protein-drug complex on the site of ulcerated mucosa. Its use as a rinse in the treatment of mucositis has been reported in a number of studies, although its efficacy seems inconsistent.[29-33] It is specifically not recommended in the MASCC guidelines. A variety of topical agents exist for mucositis pain management. These include viscous lidocaine, benzocaine in Orabase, and suspensions of Benadryl in Kaopectate or milk of magnesia. Caphosol, a rinse originally developed as a tooth remineralizing solution for patients with xerostomia, is an electrolyte solution of sodium phosphate, calcium chloride, sodium chloride, and purified water, which purportedly lubricates the mucosa and thereby attenuates mucositis. The solution is approved as a device. There are no published randomized, blinded, placebo-controlled trials supporting its use in the HNC population. Oral aloe vera has been available for some time as a palliative agent. However it failed to demonstrate efficacy in a phase 2, double-blind, randomized, placebo controlled study.[34] Topical palliative rinses are typically effective only for mild forms of the condition. Systemic pain management following the WHO pain ladder is often necessary. Additionally, cold foods, such as ice cream or Popsicles, may be soothing. Patients should be instructed to remove dental prostheses.

The role of microbes on the severity and course of radiation-induced mucositis is unclear.[35] The strategy of mucosal decontamination as a mucositis intervention has produced conflicting results. Chlorhexidine gluconate rinses do not appear to have a role in mucositis prevention or treatment in radiation mucositis and, in fact, might exacerbate the condition.[28] Lozenges containing polymyxin E, tobramycin, and amphotericin have been studied and seem to of marginal value and are not recommended.[28]

The application of non-protein thiols as a mucositis intervention is currently under study.[36] Amifostine approved as cytoprotective agent for xerostomia (see below), may be effective in modulating mucositis. N-acetyl cysteine, used as a topical rinse, is currently undergoing evaluation in the prevention and attenuation of radiation-induced oral mucositis. If these agents prove to be efficacious, it seems likely that their success is due to a

Table 133-1 ■ **Staging and Management of Bisphosphonate-Associated Osteonecrosis of the Jaw**

Stage	Clinical Presentation	Management
At risk	No exposed bone	Patient education
1	Asymptomatic exposed bone with little soft tissue inflammation	Patient education; antibacterial rinses; careful follow-up
2	Exposed bone with pain, and usually with associated surrounding soft tissue inflammation or infection	Patient education; antibacterial rinses; antibiotics; superficial debridement of bone to dislodge loose fragments and smooth rough contours; careful follow-up
3	Exposed bone with pain and usually with associated soft tissue inflammation or infection; may see osteolysis extending to the inferior border of mandible or pathologic fracture; may see extraoral fistula	Patient education; bacterial rinses; antibiotics; palliative surgery; careful follow-up

Source: From Ruggiero SL and Woo SB. Bisphosphonate-related osteonecrosis of the jaws. Dent Clin N Am. 2008;52:111-128.

combination of antioxidant and cytoprotective activities.

A wide range of agents is currently in different stages of development as possible interventions for radiation-induced mucositis. The results of two phase 3 trials in which palifermin was tested for its efficacy in HNC populations suggest that it may have a role in this patient cohort. Additionally, vitamin E, growth factors (GM-CSF and members of the FGF super family), anti-inflammatory drugs, prostaglandins, cyclooxygenase inhibitors, glutamine, and a number of homeopathic medications are examples of the interventions under study.[37-39]

Xerostomia

Xerostomia is one of the most consistent and bothersome side effects of radiation therapy in which the salivary glands are included in the field of treatment.[16,40] Concomitant chemotherapy may exacerbate the effect. The effects of radiation on salivary flow are variable and symptoms of dry mouth may not correspond to observed salivary flow. Xerostomia is caused by the effects of radiation on acinar cells, especially of the serous glands (parotid).[41] Consequently, inflammation, degeneration, and fibrosis of the glandular parenchyma occur. The extent, duration, and degree of recovery are functions of the dose rate, total dose, and radiation port. Onset of xerostomia may be noted as early as 1 week following the start of radiation (cumulative dose of 10 Gy).[42] The saliva turns thick and ropey as serous function is diminished, but mucous production remains. Patients whose radiation to the ear and neck in cumulative doses of 60 Gy more often develop irreversible xerostomia, with an 80% loss in salivary gland function.[43] Spontaneous recovery is unlikely for patients with xerostomia persisting for 12 months or longer.[44] With lesser doses of radiation, however, inflammation and edema of glandular tissue often spontaneously disappear within a year of the completion of treatment.[45]

In addition to functional changes caused by xerostomia, such as dysphasia and alteration in taste, loss of saliva is also associated with a reduction in oral clearance, diminished salivary immunoglobulin A (IgA) levels, and salivary antibacterial enzymes. Consequently, patients with xerostomia are susceptible to increases in local oral infections including caries, periodontal disease, and candidiasis. Aggressive oral hygiene to reduce the tooth-borne bacterial load is critical to reducing the risk of dental disease.

Radiation-induced caries can be a common problem in patients with xerostomia.[46] Changes in salivary composition, decreases in buffering capacity, and loss of the cleansing action of saliva results in the accumulation of bacteria, increases in local cariogenic flora, and tooth decalcification with consequent caries development.[47-49] Typically, radiation caries presents with lesions at the cervical margins of teeth, which then rapidly progresses. Decalcification (white, chalky enamel) of the incisal edges of the teeth may also be noted. In addition to tooth loss, a major consequence of uncontrolled caries may be abscess formation in patients who are at risk for osteoradionecrosis (ORN).

Four goals should be considered for the prevention and treatment of xerostomia. Preservation of salivary function is critical. Whenever possible, tissue-sparing techniques aimed at minimizing the amount of salivary tissues exposed to direct radiation should be used. Whereas bilateral field radiation may result in an 80% reduction of salivary flow, mantle irradiation typically causes only a 30-40% decrease. Parotid sparing using three-dimensional treatment or intensity-modulated radiotherapy techniques offers the greatest change of glandular repair.[22] Stimulation of salivary flow should start simultaneously with XRT, as should an anticaries regimen to protect the dentition. Replacement of reduced secretions may be introduced as soon as needed.

Stimulation of salivary flow may be accomplished through local or systemic means. Sucrose-free lemon drops or sugarless chewing gum may be used. Cinnamon- or mint-flavored mints or gum should be avoided as they may irritate the mucosa.

Drug therapy may also help to stimulate parotid flow.[50] Of the cholinergic agents, pilocarpine has been best studied and found to stimulate parotid function, but not submandibular or sublingual gland function in patients with Sjögren syndrome and radiation-induced xerostomia.[51] Other agents such as bromhexine,[52] anetholtrithion,[53] bethanechol HCl, potassium iodide, neostigmine, and reserpine have been used for salivary stimulation,[50] but data substantiating their efficacy are scant. In contrast, substantial data exist to support the use of pilocarpine HCl tablets to stimulate salivary flow in patients with radiation-induced xerostomia.[54] In cases in which pilocarpine is used after patients have completed radiation treatment and are symptomatic, at least some residual salivary function must be present, and patients should be cautioned that clinically significant improvements in salivary flow may not be realized for up to 3 months following the initiation of treatment. Alternatively, pilocarpine may be prescribed to start simultaneously with radiation therapy. In either case, the typical dose of 5 mg given 3 times daily may be titrated depending on the patient's response and manifestation of side effects.

Amifostine, a non-protein, free-radical scavenger has been approved as a cytoprotective agent for salivary glands to prevent radiation-induced xerostomia.[55] The recommended dose for amifostine is 200 mg/m^2 administered once daily as a 3-minute infusion, starting 15-30 minutes prior to standard fraction radiation therapy.[56] The need for intravenous infusion, frequency of dosing, cost, and potential side effects have limited amifostine's adoption. A subcutaneous formulation is currently under study.[57]

Salivary replacement can be accomplished with the use of saliva substitutes or artificial saliva.[58] Most of these materials contain carboxymethylcellulose and may provide transient symptomatic relief of mucosal dryness. Saliva substitutes are available as over-the-counter rinses or sprays and are most effective if used before meals and at bedtime. A number of toothpastes and chewing gums have been developed specifically for use in patients with xerostomia.

Without question, the most effective protective agent for radiation-induced caries is the aggressive use of topical fluorides.[59] Topical fluoride supplements should be initiated at the start of radiation treatment. Continuation of fluoride following the completion of radiotherapy is critical, especially in patients who develop xerostomia. Fluorides for dental use come in 3 forms: rinses, gels applied by tooth brushing or in customized trays, and drops also used in trays molded to fit over patients' teeth. Patients in whom xerostomia is anticipated should have fluoride trays fabricated prior to the initiation of radiotherapy. Fluoride gel or drops are placed in the trays and applied by the patient each day. Use of tray-borne application can be supplemented with acidulated fluoride rinses; generally, the use of rinses in the morning and trays before sleep is most effective and easiest for patients. Acidulated fluorides tend to work best, although neutral fluoride rinses are available for patients with mucositis in whom acidulated material might be irritating, or for patients with porcelain prostheses in whom pitting of the restorations might occur. The supplemental use of a remineralizing toothpaste should also be considered.[60] Aggressive oral hygiene is to be encouraged, and patients should be seen by a dentist frequently. Regular dental visits are critical to insure early detection and intervention of caries and periodontal disease.

For patients who cannot tolerate trays because of gagging or mucositis, fluoride gels may be applied with a toothbrush, either as 1.1% sodium fluoride or as 0.4% stannous fluoride. The latter appears to be more efficacious. Patients should be instructed to avoid sucrose.

Loss of taste is a transient, but bothersome sequelae of head and neck radiation. The severity of taste loss increases rapidly up to doses of 30 Gy, but then usually plateaus.[61] Patients who receive doses of 30 Gy or more may lose their ability to distinguish salt or sweet tastes. Fortunately, hypogeusia is typically transient and taste begins to return within 1-2 months after the completion of treatment. Total recovery may take up to a year. If there does not seem to be progression to improvement following radiotherapy, candidiasis should be ruled out.

Osteoradionecrosis

Of all of the oral complications of head and neck radiation, perhaps the most significant is osteoradionecrosis.[62,63] First described in 1927, ORN results in the denudation of soft tissue and exposure and necrosis of bone.[64] Although not limited to the jaws, it frequently occurs at this site. ORN causes a painful, chronic, open, and foul-smelling wound that is typically of great distress to the patient. Most cases ultimately heal with conservative treatment, but the course is usually prolonged. Historically, ORN was attributed to a triad of trauma (often tooth extractions), radiation, and infection.[65] Subsequent studies suggest, however, that ORN represents a defect in wound healing rather than a true osteomyelitis.[66] The etiology appears to relate to diminished vascularization as a consequence of XRT.[67] Histologic changes of thickened arterial and arteriolar walls substantiate this hypothesis,[68] and the lack of culturable pathogenic microorganisms from active ORN lesions suggest the noninfectious nature of the process.[69]

No consensus exists concerning the overall frequency of ORN. Although reported ranges vary between 4% and 44%, approximately 15% appears to be the preponderant experience.[62,63,68] The mandible is involved more often than the maxilla, which probably reflects the difference in blood supply and vascularity of the two bones. Time until onset of ORN following XRT is controversial. Some authors have described ORN as early as 2 weeks after XRT,[68] whereas others report it as a late condition.[69] Most cases occur within the first 3 years after XRT (74%). Equally controversial is the rate at which ORN risk diminishes with time after the completion of XRT, although it seems clear that the risk never reaches zero.[70]

A number of risk factors for ORN have been positively identified. Men have been reported to have a risk for ORN that is 3-fold higher than women.[62] Patients who are edentulous are twice as likely as patients with teeth to develop ORN.[71,72] Furthermore, the frequency of ORN increases dramatically in individuals with active dental disease (eg, periodontal disease, caries, periapical disease, poorly fitting prostheses).[71] 50 percent of cases appear to be associated with tooth extraction following radiation. These findings strongly support pre-XRT dental evaluation and aggressive repair and removal of diseased teeth. The field size, dose rate, and total dose of XRT have a marked effect on the frequency of ORN. Patients who receive cumulative doses of 65 Gy or more to the mandible or maxilla are more likely to develop ORN than are patients receiving lesser doses.[63] For example, patients who receive 80 Gy or more are twice as likely to develop ORN compared to patients who are treated with 50-60 Gy. Use of three-dimensional radiation techniques has resulted in a slight reduction in ORN risk.[73] Patients with tumors that are adjacent or contiguous with bone are also at higher ORN risk.[74] It is likely that this finding is due to the inclusion of bone in the radiated field since the volume of bone exposed to XRT has a direct impact on ORN risk. Poor nutrition and immune status also appear to predispose to the condition. Diagnosis of ORN is usually based on clinical findings. In cases in which the diagnosis is questionable, magnetic resonance imaging may be of value.[75] In contrast, although scintigraphy with 99m technetium Tc-HDP may demonstrate positive findings, the overall specificity of this technique for ORN (57%) makes it less desirable.[75]

Treatment of ORN is based on the severity and chronicity of the condition. Fortunately, most lesions (up to 60%) eventually heal in approximately 6 months with conservative therapy consisting of local debridement, saliva irrigation, and oral antibiotics.[76] Although potassium phenoxymethyl penicillin (500 mg every 6 h) has demonstrated efficacy, the use of tetracycline (250 mg qid for 10 days followed by 250 mg bid for several months) has been suggested on the basis of tetracycline's predilection to be assimilated by bone.[77]

Lesions that show no improvement or demonstrate progression require more aggressive therapy. For these cases, surgical debridement and hyperbaric oxygen (HBO) may be indicated.[78,79] In extensive cases, radical resection of involved bone with immediate microvascular reconstruction has been used successfully in patients who have failed more conservative treatment, including HBO.[80,81]

Because most cases of intra-oral ORN are associated with dental disease and post-XRT extractions, eliminating potential sites of odontogenic pathology before the start of radiation is the basis for prevention. Teeth with periodontal disease, advanced caries with a risk of impingement on the dental pulp, fracture, or periapical disease should be removed before the initiation of XRT. Teeth adjacent to or involved in potential surgical sites (for tumor resection) also should be extracted. Because of the consequences of ORN, even suspiciously diseased teeth, especially in the XRT area, should be eliminated. The timing of dental extractions in patients being treated with XRT has been the subject of much analysis, discussion, and controversy; however, the consensus is that teeth should be extracted before XRT.[74] Ideally, a minimum 21-day healing period is desirable, although a shorter time may be dictated by circumstances. In either instance, extraction before XRT is much more desirable than extraction after the start of therapy, because a number of studies suggest that post-XRT extractions carry significant risk of ORN, no matter how long after XRT they are performed. In all cases, extraction should be performed as atraumatically as possible, with special care given to the soft tissue, primary closure if possible, and good local postoperative wound management. Perioperative use of antibiotics is also recommended.

Aggressive oral hygiene, use of fluorides, and dental care are important components in preventing the development of dental disease once XRT has started. If dental disease develops after XRT and a tooth is restorable, endodontic therapy is more desirable than extraction.[74,82] Inevitably, extractions are sometimes required of teeth in radiated fields. The risk of ORN in these cases has been reported to be reasonable (5.6%), even without the use of HBO. The efficacy of HBO in these cases is unresolved. One study found that, among patients having teeth removed within the first year following radiation, 98.5% of extraction sites treated pre- and postoperatively with HBO healed without complications. However, the efficacy of HBO reportedly decreased the farther out from where radiation extractions were performed. On the other hand, a recent randomized, placebo-controlled, double-blind trial in which patients were treated pre- and postoperatively with HBO failed to demonstrate any benefit.[83] Thus, the use of HBO, with its incurred cost and multiple visits, warrants additional study.

Oral Complications of Chemotherapy

Oral complications of cancer chemotherapy result from the effects of the drug acting on the oral mucosa (direct or primary stomatotoxicity), the patients' inability to contain local, minor oral disease during myelosuppression (indirect or secondary stomatotoxicity), or some combination of the two.

Risk Factors

Not all patients who undergo cancer chemotherapy are at equal risk to develop oral complications. This is especially true of oral mucositis. Although a number of variables have been identified that bear on the frequency and severity of oral problems, their predictive value, in general, has yet to be definitely defined. Risk factors can be divided into those that are associated with the patient and those that are related to the treatment regimen.[84]

Patient-related risk factors include tumor diagnosis, patient age, gender, body mass, genetics, the patient's oral condition before cancer therapy, the level of oral care during therapy, baseline xerostomia, and baseline neutrophil numbers. Patients with hematologic malignancies (ie, leukemia and lymphoma) are at greater risk of oral complications than are patients with non-head and neck solid tumors. For example, more than 66% of patients with leukemia and 33% of patients with non-Hodgkin lymphoma develop oral problems. It seems likely that tumor-related myelosuppression is at least partly the basis for this observation.[85] Almost all patients with tumors of the head and neck who receive local therapy develop problems after treatment.

The role of age as a risk factor for mucositis is unclear as there are few studies that compare the rate of mucositis among patients of varying ages with similar diagnoses. Among children, nadir of the neutrophil count, lower body weight, and higher peak creatinine levels have been observed to be associated with higher rates of mucositis.[86] Among adult patients with solid tumors being treated with 5-fluorouracil (5-FU), mucositis appears to be more severe and persistent among older persons.

Gender may affect risk. There are reports to suggest that women are more likely to have toxicities associated with 5-FU than are men.[87,88] This trend was also reported in patients receiving high-dose chemotherapy (BEAM) or high-dose melphalan followed by autologous HSCT.[89] A mechanism to explain this phenomenon has yet to be determined. Genetics may affect mucositis risk in at least two ways. Patients with genetic defects, which affect drug metabolism, are at increased risk for mucositis. For example, among a population of patients being treated with methotrexate for chronic myelogenous leukemia, increased toxicity (including mucositis) was observed in those individuals with lower methylenetetrahydrofolate reductase activity (TT genotype).[90] Similarly, deficiencies in dihydropyrimidine dehydrogenase (DPD)[88,91] predispose to toxicities mediated by 5- FU. Alternatively, genetics may affect and regulate the mechanisms, which provide the biological basis for chemotherapy-induced mucosal injury. For example, proinflammatory cytokine production varies among the population and is genetically controlled. These cytokines play a role and track closely with non-hematologic toxicities. Consequently, patients who are predisposed to be high producers of these proteins may also be at increased risk for mucositis and other toxicities. For example, among a cohort of allogeneic HSCT recipients, specific tumor necrosis factor polymorphisms conferred a relative risk (RR) of severe toxicities in excess of 17 fold.[92] The results of a recently reported study in a pediatric cohort being treated for a variety of malignancies suggest an association between ABO blood type. The RR of oropharyngeal mucositis was 2.86 among patients with type O compared to 0.47 for type A and 0.59 for type B.[93] Further study is needed to fully elucidate the impact of functional genes on mucosal injury, but it promises to be important in determining both risk and predicting responsiveness to mechanism-based interventions. It is generally agreed that patients whose pretreatment oral condition is poor are at greater risk for some, but not all, oral complications.[77,94] Chronic irritation for poorly fitting prostheses or faulty restorations predisposes patients to the development of ulcerative mucositis. Patients with advanced periodontal disease, pulpal disease, or low-grade soft-tissue infections such as those associated with partially erupted third molars (ie, wisdom teeth) are at increased risk for developing sepsis of oral origin once they become myelosuppressed. However, elevated risks of infection are not associated with asymptomatic radiographically demonstrable periapical lesions in endodontically treated teeth.[95]

The level of oral care during therapy has a marked influence on outcome relative to oral complications and infection.[96,97] The ability of the patients and their healthcare providers to reduce the load of oral bacterial flora favorably affects the risk of both local and systemic infection.[96] Aggressive techniques of oral hygiene, including mechanical debridement of the teeth and soft tissue, and antimicrobial rinses are effective.

Xerostomia prior to and during chemotherapy maybe associated with an increased risk of mucositis.[98] It has been suggested that alterations in the health of desiccated oral mucosa and an overall increase in the resident oral micro-flora may contribute to increasing the probability of mucositis. Studies evaluating treatment strategies aimed at replenishing saliva or mouth moisture have had very mixed results. The favorable effect of pilocarpine on chemotherapy-induced mucositis reported in 1 study was not replicated in a similar trial[99] or among recipients of autologous HSCT.[100] In contrast, the use of a mucosal lubricant was reported to be of value when used in conjunction with fluoride.[101] Clearly more investigation is needed before informed treatment decisions can be recommended.

The extent of mucositis correlates negatively with neutropenia. Baseline neutrophil counts of less than 4,000 are associated with higher rates of mucositis.[84] This finding may explain, in part, the observation of increased rates of mucositis among patients with hematologic malignancies.

Risk of complications also relates to the form, schedule, and dose of chemotherapy used.[15] Concomitant radiation, including TBI, also enhance the risk of oral problems. For example, the incidence of mucositis has been reported to be markedly lower in reduced intensity stem cell transplant recipients (30.9%) compared to patients who received conventional conditioning regimens (90.2%).[102] Significant differences exist in the degree of stomatotoxicity of drugs used for chemotherapy.[15] Drugs or regimens containing anthracyclines, taxanes, platinum, and 5-FU are consistently stomatotoxic. Conditioning regimens in which TBI is used also cause mucositis at high rates. There are 17 specific drugs or combinations in which oral mucositis rates (grade 3-4) affect a significant percentage of patients (>25%):

- Docetaxel/5-FU
- Docetaxel + XRT
- Paclitaxel + XRT
- Docetaxel + 5-FU
- Paclitaxel/5-FU + XRT
- Docetaxel/platinum + XRT
- Paclitaxel/platinum + XRT
- Docetaxel/platinum/5-FU
- Paclitaxel/platinum/5-FU
- Oxaliplatin + XRT
- Platinum/taxane + XRT
- Platinum/methotrexate/leucovorin
- 5-FU/platinum
- 5-FU/leucovorin/taxane
- Irinotecan/5-FU CI + XRT
- Ara-C/idarubicin/fludarabine
- Methotrexate
- Isofamide/etoposide
- Melphalan

In viewing the above list, it is important to remember that the incidence of oral complications, particularly mucositis, tends to be vastly underreported in terms of occurrence and severity. Virtually every chemotherapeutic agent in the current armamentarium has the potential to produce a stomatotoxic response in at least some portion of the treated population.

Repetitive, low-dose regimens tend to be less toxic than do bolus doses of the same agent. Toxicity that is secondary to radiation is dependent on cumulative dose; pulsed application of therapy does not significantly reduce stomatic changes.

Ulcerative mucositis usually occurs 5-8 days following the administration of chemotherapy and it lasts approximately 7-14 days. Lesions heal spontaneously and without scar formation. Chemotherapy-induced mucositis is confined to the movable oral mucosa: the mucosa of the cheeks, lateral and ventral tongue, inner aspects of the lips, floor of the mouth, and soft palate. Unlike radiation-induced mucositis, that produced by chemotherapy does not affect the hard palate or gingival. The dorsal surface of the tongue is also not affected. This observation is likely to be attributable to the differences in the character of the epithelium on each mucosal surface. Of the sites in the mouth, the buccal mucosa (cheeks), lateral and ventral surfaces of the tongue, and the floor of the mouth are the most commonly involved. In patients who receive multiple cycles of chemotherapy, lesions tend to reappear in the same sites. Numerous studies have confirmed that mucositis is not of infectious (particularly viral) origin. Although patients may also be at risk for herpes simplex infections, the lesions of viral stomatitis are quite distinct in appearance and behavior from those of mucositis.[103–105]

The biologic mechanisms, which underlie chemotherapy-induced mucositis, are currently the topic of intense investigation.[18,106] As noted above, mucositis was viewed as the result of nonspecific toxicity of chemotherapy directed against the rapidly dividing cells of the oral basal epithelium. Although data exist to support the hypothesis, the observation that agents could alter the course of mucositis with little or no epithelial activity suggests a more broadly based pathogenesis. It appears that mucositis represents a clinical outcome due to a complex interaction of local tissue toxicity (endothelium, connective tissue, and epithelium), the level of myelosuppression, and the local environment. Disruption of connective tissue and endothelial cells initiated by free radical formation likely leads to the activation of a range of transcription factors and increased expression of a number of genes that results in stimulation of proinflammatory cytokine production and tissue damage. Simultaneous activation of other signaling pathways and enzyme activation results in increases in ceramide, proteolytic enzymes, and other mediators of direct and indirect epithelial injury. Thus, in addition to clonogenic death of basal cells caused by direct DNA injury, secondary pathways produce a barrage of mechanisms that lead to apoptosis or necrosis. Therefore, the epithelium first becomes atrophic, as its renewal ceases, and then eventually completely breaks down to form an ulcer. It is noteworthy that in some patients, the extent of cumulative injury to the basal epithelium does not reach the threshold needed for ulceration to occur. In these patients, the thinned mucosa is mildly to moderately symptomatic (grade 1 mucositis). In cases when ulceration does occur, secondary colonization by oral bacteria (both gram positives and gram negatives) occurs. Cell wall products from these bacteria make their way into the underlying connective tissue where they effectively stimulate additional proinflammatory cytokine production by infiltrating macrophages.

The better understanding of the pathobiology of mucositis has served as the basis for the development of mechanistically based interventions.[107] The first of these agents to gain approval was palifermin (keratinocyte growth factor-1, Kepivance, Amgen) for the prevention and treatment of oral mucositis in patients receiving conditioning regimens in preparation for HSCT to treat hematologic malignancies. In a phase 3 trial in 212 HSCT recipients receiving a stomatotoxic conditioning regimen, palifermin, administered in multiple doses prior to and after transplantation was successful in significantly reducing the duration, incidence, and severity of oral mucositis, favorably affecting patient-reported quality of life outcomes, and in reducing days of opioid use and fever.[108] It seems likely that palifermin's effect was the consequence, not only of its ability to stimulate epithelial proliferation, but also because of its cytoprotective activates mediated through increased expression of mediating transcription factors. FGF20, another growth factor in the same superclass, demonstrated efficacy in the same study population in phase 2 trials.[109] Amifostine, a pleiotropic, free radical scavenger, has been reported to be efficacious in the HSCT population,[110] although other studies have not been positive. Of the 400,000 patients who develop mucositis each year in the United States, the HSCT population comprises only 5%. Consequently, extension of these and other agents to other tumor populations is a major objective.

Low-level (helium-neon) laser (λ = 632.8 nm) therapy (LLLT) has demonstrated some efficacy in reducing the severity and symptoms associated with oral mucositis.[28] While additional studies are needed to confirm its value, the cost and logistics of LLLT may limit its overall utility.

A number of cytoprotective strategies and agents have been suggested as mucositis interventions. Oral cryotherapy is inexpensive and without risk, its use for 30 minutes starting 5 minutes before the infusion of bolus 5-FU, edatrexate, or melphalan may be helpful in reducing the severity of mucositis.[28] Allopurinol does not significantly reduce oral toxicity in patients being treated with 5-FU. Recently a new formulation of L-glutamine (Saforis) demonstrated modest, but significant, efficacy in a phase 3 trial in a population of patients being treated for breast cancer.[111] Pentoxifylline has been evaluated in a number of studies with mixed results. The topical application of trefoil factor was reportedly beneficial in a recently reported phase 2 study performed in a colorectal cancer population.[112] Antioxidant therapy with vitamin E and beta-carotene has produced inconsistent results. While anticholinergics, such as pilocarpine and Pro-Banthine, may be of benefit, it is likely that they function as salivary stimulants.

Because the presence of oral microorganisms is thought to adversely affect the course of mucositis, antimicrobial therapy has been studied extensively as an approach to intervention.[35] In general, the weight of data suggest that reduction of the oral bacterial load through medication does not bear significantly on the incidence or severity of mucositis. The use of topical antimicrobials such as chlorhexidine gluconate has consistently failed to improve the frequency or course of mucositis in randomized, blinded trials.[28,35]

Palliation has been the most widely used approach for the management of mucositis. Saline 0.9% has been used for years and is more effective than hydrogen peroxide, and at least as good as "magic mouthwashes."[113] Barrier type palliatives such as sucralfate suspension and Gelclair are available, although their benefit has not been convincingly shown. Topical lidocaine or Benadryl in Kaopectate or milk of magnesia may offer some topical relief, but often do not eliminate the need for parenteral analgesia.

Ulceration Associated With mTOR-Inhibitor Use

Inhibitors of the mammalian target of rapamycin (mTOR) have demonstrated encouraging results in clinical trials as an intervention for advanced maligancies.[114] Oral ulceration is among the most significant dose-limiting toxicities associated with these agents[115] and has been reported as mucositis. However, the clinical course, behavior, appearance, and likely pathogenesis mTOR-inhibitor induced oral ulcers strongly suggests that they are profoundly different from mucositis induced by radiation or cytotoxic agents.

Unlike typical chemotherapy-induced mucositis, aphthous lesions present as discrete, ovoid, relatively shallow ulcers, and surrounded by a characteristic erythematous margin (Fig. 133-3). Lesions develop more quickly after drug administration and typically resolve spontaneously after an extremely painful course. Although randomized trials have not yet been performed, treatment approaches similar to those used for major aphthous stomatitis may be effective.

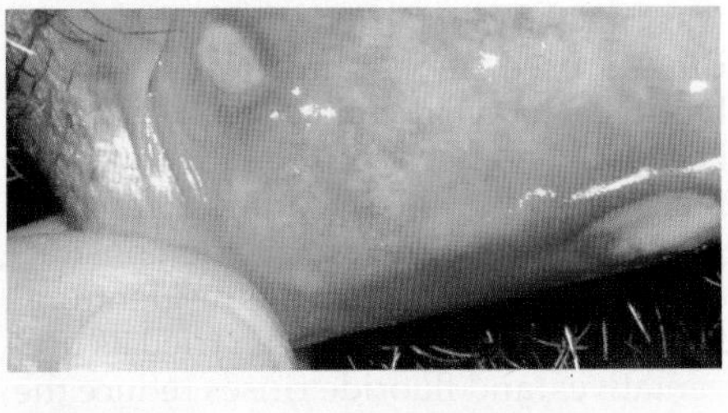

Figure 133-3 ■ Oral mucosal ulcers associated with the administration of an mTOR inhibitor. Note that the lesions are well-defined and oval with a central area of necrosis and an erythematous periphery reminiscent of aphthous stomatitis.

Osteonecrosis

Bisphosphonate administration concomitant with chemotherapy has been introduced as a strategy to reduce metastases to bone. Among patients being treated in this way, osteonecrosis of the jaws, particularly of the mandible (twice as common compared to maxilla) has been reported with increasing frequency.[116,117] The frequency of the condition has been reported to be between 4% and 7%. The presentation of osteonecrosis in this population varies in symptomatology. Although some patients experience pain, others do not. The majority of cases appear to be associated with dental manipulation, such as extraction, or soft tissue trauma. The mechanism underlying this pathology is yet to be defined, as is a full appreciation of the natural history of the condition. Conservative treatment seems to be most appropriate (Table 133-1). Presently, the most judicious strategy is to assure aggressive dental screening and treatment prior to the initiation of treatment so that the possible need for dental intervention is minimized.

Infections

Simultaneous with the breakdown of the oral epithelium, the patients' ability to deal with the abundant oral microbial flora is compromised by their myelosuppression. Thus, the mouth becomes an important source of bacteremia and sepsis in the granulocytopenic cancer patient, as well as locoregional secondary infection. These manifestations of indirect stomatotoxicity parallel the bone marrow status; hence, they are maximal at, or just proceeding toward the patient's granulocyte nadir. Systemic invasion of oral viridans streptococci are particularly common. Of these, Streptococcus mitus is associated with the most serious sequelae.

Fungal Infections ■ Local oral infections in myelosuppressed patients are attributable to fungal, viral, and bacterial organisms, in order of descending frequency. Candidiasis is the most frequent oral infection and may appear in its characteristic white, curdy form or as erythematous, macular lesions.[118] It most frequently occurs on the palate, tongue, and corners of the mouth. Poorly controlled oral candidiasis increases the risk of aspiration and the development of candidal esophagitis or fungemia. In addition, aspergillosis and mucormycosis are not uncommon in myelosuppressed patients; these lesions can appear as invasive oral ulcerations that are painful and may involve bone.

Since systemic candidiasis is associated with high rates of morbidity and mortality,[119] antifungal prophylaxis may be a reasonable consideration among patients in whom prolonged neutropenia is anticipated, ie, HSCT or stomatotoxic, myeloablative chemotherapy recipients. In general, topical agents are ineffective in this group. Treatment options include fluconazole, caspofungin, and micafungin.[120]

Topical antifungal prophylaxis directed against *Candida* may be beneficial for patients receiving head and neck radiation and promotes xerostomia and in patients who are immunosuppressed with steroids. The polyene antifungal agents (eg, nystatin) or the imidazole agents, clotrimazole (Mycelex) are equally efficacious. Nystatin is formulated as a thick, cherry-flavored suspension that is not a favorite of chemotherapy-nauseated individuals. Mycelex is dispensed as a troche. For pediatric patients, nystatin popsicles made by putting the drug plus water into an ice cube tray seems to work well. Two other imidazoles also are available: ketoconazole (Nizoral) and fluconazole (Diflucan); both have demonstrated efficacy for the prophylaxis and treatment of existing disease.[121,122] The requirement of an acidic environment for ketoconazole, however, may limit its usefulness in patients who have difficulty eating. Azole resistance may be of relevance in the treatment of fungal infections. Some of the candida species such as Candida glabriela and Candida krusei are inherently less sensitive to azole antifungal medications.[123]

The efficacy of chlorhexidine gluconate rinses as a topical antifungal agent is unclear.[115] Reports regarding its usefulness are inconsistent,[28] but in vivo data suggest that chlorhexidine reduces the activity of nystatin.[124,125] Hence, its simultaneous use with nystatin is not recommended.

While the use of surveillance cultures for predicting the presence or course of fungal infection has long been shown to be of little value,[126] PCR may have a role in the rapid diagnosis and speciation of oral candidal infections.[127]

Viral Infections ■ Herpes simplex virus type (HSV-1) is the most common oral viral infection in patients receiving chemotherapy or head and neck radiation and determination of antibody status is an important part of risk assessment. Oral HSV-1 infection can result from a primary infection with the virus or the reactivation of latent virus in a previously exposed host.[128] It is the latter that is most frequent in patients receiving cancer therapy. Individuals with prior HSV-1 exposure who are seropositive for the virus are at much greater risk than are patients who are negative. The most common manifestation of infection with HSV-1 is oral ulceration. While this may appear to be clinically similar to other forms of mucositis, it usually differs in its course and distribution.

The timing of HSV-1 infection in patients receiving chemotherapy or BMT is typically quite consistent.[129] Lesions generally are seen approximately 18 days following the start of therapy. This temporal relationship is important in differentiating lesions that likely result from HSV-1 from those that result from direct stomatotoxicity, which are noted 5-7 days after the start of treatment, and from secondary surface infection (usually bacterial) that are seen at the patient's maximum myelosuppression (ie, granulocyte nadir), which occurs around 12-14 days. Lesions can appear on any mucosal surface including the most heavily keratinized tissues of the hard palate and gingiva. Viral culture is the most definitive way to diagnose HSV-1 infection, and aggressive culturing is recommended, especially in patients who are seropositive. Systemic acyclovir remains the treatment of choice for prophylaxis and treatment of HSV infection.[120,130]

Herpes zoster also may present with oral lesions in patients who receive therapy for cancer.[105] These lesions tend to be crop-like. Although they begin as vesicular lesions, they quickly rupture and form painful, small, ulcerative lesions. Unlike those from HSV-1, these lesions usually are unilateral and linear, often following one of the branches of the fifth cranial nerve.

Bacterial Infections ■ The oral cavity may be a frequent source of local and systemic bacterial infection in the myelosuppressed patient with cancer, as evidenced by the increasing frequency of a-streptococcal infections among patients with granulocytopenic cancer.[131,132] Bacterial infections may be of soft tissue or gingival or odontogenic origin. Patients receiving cancer therapy often have increased numbers of oral organisms as a consequence of reduced hygiene and xerostomia. Additionally, the composition of the oral flora shifts from one in which gram-positive organisms predominate to one with an abundance of gram-negative pathogens.

Most often, odontogenic infections result from degeneration and infection of the dental pulp subsequent to bacterial invasion secondary to caries. Because of a patient's inability to mount an inflammatory response, conventional signs of dental infection (eg, abscess formation, swelling) are absent, and patients complain of localized tooth pain. Percussion or thermal sensitivity with clinical and/or radiographic evidence of caries progressing into the pulp is diagnostic. Neurotoxicity may cause dental pain that mimics odontogenic infection in patients receiving plant alkaloids. Odontogenic infections predominantly result from anaerobic species that are similar to those found in dental plaque. Treatment should consist of eliminating the source of infection, and in most cases, this involves tooth extraction. The safety of tooth extraction in the face of myelosuppression has been reported by a number of investigators.[133-135] These studies indicate that extraction may be performed with antibiotic coverage, platelet transfusion if needed, attention to tissue management, and good closure. Use of hemostatic agents such as Gelfoam in extraction sockets is discouraged, because they may act as foci of infection. Generally, platelet transfusion is not necessary for counts greater than 50,000 cells/mL. Systemic antibiotic coverage is indicated until the wound is epithelialized.

Gingival infections are relatively common in patients receiving myelosuppressive therapy. Some are localized, such as those that are associated with partially erupted third molars (ie, wisdom teeth), whereas others tend to be more diffuse. Acute gingival and periodontal infections are worse in patients with preexisting chronic gingival inflammation or periodontal disease. In addition, studies by Peterson[4] demonstrated that the periodontal health status of myelosuppressed patients influenced a shift from the normal oral flora to a composition rich in gram-negative bacteria.

The clinical appearance of acute gingival infections, which occur during periods of granulocytopenia, resembles that seen in acute necrotizing ulcerative gingivitis. Pain and loss of the gingival architecture, particularly necrosis of the interdental papillae, are characteristic. These lesions tend to be of a mixed bacterial nature, and include a variety of pathogens, such as Staphylococcus epidermidis, Pseudomonas aeruginosa, and bacteria typically associated with periodontal disease such as bacteroides and veillonella.

Treatment should include local debridement in addition to systemic antibiotics. Local culture of lesions may more useful than blood culture, because invasion of intact organisms may not occur. Empirical treatment is recommended regardless of culture results.

Mucosal infections in the myelosuppressed patient often are superimposed on ulcerated areas that have broken down as the result of direct stomatotoxicity. Ulcers may appear to be penetrating, with rounded borders and yellowish-white necrotic centers. Because of the lack of an inflammatory response, erythematous borders are usually absent. If the ulcerations are precipitated by trauma, secondary hematoma formation may occur in the patient with thrombocytopenia. Soft-tissue infections tend to be of gram-negative etiology, although HSV-1 must be ruled out. Treatment should include debridement, palliation, and antimicrobial therapy. Bacterial and viral cultures should be performed as well.

Preliminary data suggest that the mouth may seed indwelling lines with organisms, resulting in local-line infections and secondary sepsis. A correlation seems to exist between the presence of clinically significant mucositis α-hemolytic streptococcal positive blood cultures, and line infections and granulocytopenia.[136]

Strategies for the prevention of oral infection include eliminating sources of mucosal irritation and reducing the quantity of the local oral flora.[4] In addition, treatment of low-grade, asymptomatic infection before the start of therapy minimizes the risk of acute episodes once myelosuppression occurs. Reduction in the oral flora may be accomplished by mechanical and/or chemical means. Local debridement of the teeth can be accomplished with conventional toothbrushing; soft brushes should be used. Thrombocytopenia is not a contraindication to mechanical debridement if common sense is used. Brushing should be discontinued in the face of significant bleeding. Alternatively, cotton swabs or a towel-wrapped finger may be used to clean the teeth. Dental floss is an excellent adjuvant for cleaning but may be difficult for patients to use if they are unfamiliar with it. It also may be used until patients become profoundly thrombocytopenic. Essentially, anything that the patient or provider can use to physically wipe debris and microorganisms from the teeth will be beneficial. Cotton swabs, sponges, and rubber tips all may be of use.

Rinses are of varying degrees of help in maintaining oral hygiene. Any fluid that flushes the mouth, including water, will be of some help. Saline and diluted peroxide are frequently used. Generally, mouth rinses containing alcohol as their active agent cause burning of the atrophic mucosa and are not recommended. Mixed results have been reported with chlorhexidine gluconate rinses. No benefit of chlorhexidine over water was recently reported.[137] If chlorhexidine is used, its administration should be timed to avoid contact with nystatin, because the effects of the latter may be inactivated by chlorhexidine. Similarly, povidone iodine rinses have demonstrated efficacy in reducing the resident oral flora. Other drugs have been tried as preventatives, and fluoride rinses reduce the ability of oral bacteria to adhere to teeth. Consequently, they also may be helpful.

Patients with removable prostheses should be instructed to remove them during periods of myelosuppression. Oral bleeding during such periods most often is of gingival origin. Spontaneous gingival bleeding is a rare occurrence when platelet counts exceed 20,000 cells/mL. Slow oozing may be noted at lower platelet levels, especially in areas with preexisting periodontal disease. Local treatment of gingival bleeding includes initial debridement, nondisturbance of formed clots, and topical application of thrombin under pressure. Gingival bleeding usually is interpreted as evidence that the platelet count is low enough to allow other, more threatening hemorrhage.

Hematoma formation often occurs in areas of trauma, especially the buccal mucosa, alveolar mucosa, or edentulous areas. Areas of submucosal hemorrhage form bluish, blister-like areas, which then form a yellowish-white, tumor-like mass of fibrin. Epithelialization occurs beneath the mass. If bleeding occurs before healing is complete, topical therapy may include thrombin, microfibrillar collagen, or other hemostatic gel. Before healing is complete, the clot may serve as a focus for microbial growth. It should be checked daily and removed as soon as epithelialization is complete. Unchecked sublingual bleeding may cause respiratory embarrassment by elevating the tongue.

Oral Complications Associated With HSCT

Mucositis

The risk of mucositis in the HSCT population is largely dependent on the intensity of HSCT conditioning regimen. As many as three-quarters of patients who receive conventional conditioning regimens can be expected to develop the condition, while the frequency is markedly less among individuals receiving reduced intensity protocols. The inclusion of total-body irradiation increases the risk of developing mucositis.[138] As with other forms of chemotherapy-induced mucositis, lesions are localized to the movable oral mucosa and are most frequent in the floor of the mouth, lingual frenum, and labial and buccal mucosae (see Fig. 133-1). There appears to be no significant difference in either the onset of mucositis following transplantation or the duration of mucositis among recipients of autologous or allogeneic HSCT. Woo and colleagues reported a mean time of mucositis onset as 5 days following HSCT for autologous recipients, as compared to 6 days for allogeneic recipientsThe mean duration of mucositis for both groups was approximately 6 days, with resolution in 10-12 days. In another study in which autologous HSCT were performed in patients who received cyclophosphamide and TBI, the duration of WHO grade 3/4 mucositis was longer. Mucositis almost always resolves by 3 weeks after transplant, an important diagnostic observation when patients go on to develop GVHD. There is an association between absolute neutrophil count (ANC) and mucositis resolution. Unless patients have extremely severe lesions, mucositis usually spontaneously resolves with an ANC of greater than 500 cells/mL. However, it does not appear that the administration of either GCSF or GM-CSF prevent or minimize the mucositis development.

The mechanism of mucositis induction is discussed elsewhere in this chapter. It is important to note that the condition occurs independently of oral mucosal infections with either viral or fungal etiology. As noted above, palifermin has recently been approved for the prevention and treatment of oral mucositis in autologous HSCT recipients (see above).

Infection

Oral infection is a major cause of morbidity among HSCT recipients. Of special importance in this patient population is the oral cavity as a source of systemic or distant infection. The incidence of streptococcal infections in HSCT recipients has increased dramatically. One study demonstrated that bacteria of the Streptococcus viridans group were frequent isolates from infections associated with indwelling lines.[136] Consequently, pretreatment screening to identify and eliminate asymptomatic, dormant, or potential sources of dental infection or irritation should be mandated for BMT recipients.

In addition to bacterial infections, HSCT recipients are at risk for oral viral and fungal infections during the period of their granulocytopenia. As with other myelosuppressed patients, the clinical presentation of these infections in the BMT population often varies from the classic descriptions typically associated with these lesions. Consequently, early and aggressive culturing is mandated. Members of the herpes group account for most viral infections; herpes simplex, varicella, and herpes zoster are associated with oral infections in HSCT patients. The routine practice of acyclovir prophylaxis, however, generally has been discontinued. In addition, acyclovir resistant mucocutaneous herpes simplex infections have been reported in HSCT populations.[139] Candidiasis is the most common fungal infection, although both mucormycosis and aspergillosis have been reported. Lesions of the deep fungal infections generally present as nonhealing gingival ulcerations. Biopsy is the diagnostic method of choice.

Graft-versus-Host Disease

The mouth is a common site for manifestations of both acute and chronic GVHD.[140] Although there are relatively few reports on the oral manifestations of acute GVHD, 3 clinical patterns of oral lesions have been described by Barrett and Bilous[138] and are noted as early as 3 weeks following transplantation and almost 1 week after the onset of skin lesions (Fig. 133-4). Initially, multiple, small, white, papillated lesions present on the movable mucosa. These progress to the development of keratotic, white, lacey lesions that clinically resemble lichen planus and, in fact, have been described as lichenoid in appearance. Desquamative lesions may then develop. These also are similar to the lesions of erosive or bullous lichen planus, and unlike the other two forms, these tend to be symptomatic and require intervention.

The mouth is only second to the skin as a site for manifestations of chronic GVHD. The oral lesions of chronic GVHD appear approximately 3 months or later following transplantation. Approximately 70% of patients with GVHD develop oral lesions, which most typically are lichenoid in appearance. Symptomatic lesions usually present as erosive, vesiculobullous lesions of the oral mucosa, with peripheral areas of keratotic striations. Additionally, xerostomia is a frequent finding among patients with chronic GVHD. Both mucosal and salivary gland changes result from lymphocytic infiltration; the resulting tissue changes are analogous to those seen in other autoimmune changes in the mouth.

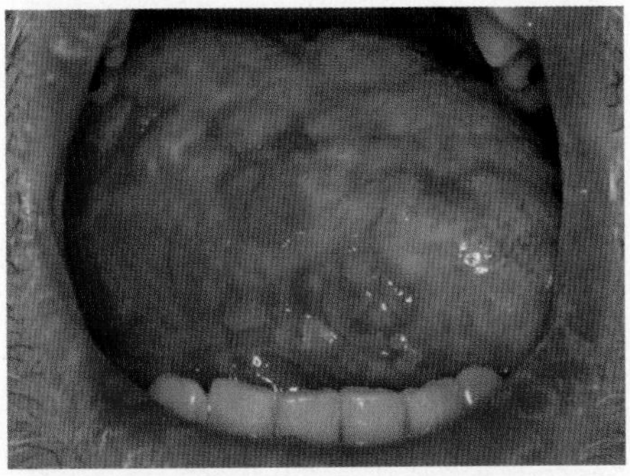

Figure 133-4 Oral manifestations of graft-vs-host disease characterized by mucosal blistering and lichenoid changes. *Source:* Courtesy of Dr. Nathaniel Treister.

Biopsy of the minor salivary glands of the lip appears to be an accurate and sensitive way to confirm the diagnosis of chronic GVHD, and it is more predictive than either biopsy of the buccal mucosa or the parotid gland.[141] Technically, minor salivary gland biopsy is easily performed in an office setting with local anesthesia and a minimum of tissue manipulation. Histologically, one notes acinar atrophy and/or destruction accompanied by a lymphocytic infiltrate that is rich in CD3+ T cells.

Lichenoid lesions generally respond to topical or systemic steroid therapy. Ultraviolet A light therapy reportedly has benefit in the treatment of severe, nonresponsive lesions.[142] Therapy for xerostomia was discussed earlier in this chapter. As with other patients having xerostomia, patients with GVHD are at increased risk for caries and should be managed accordingly.

Additional late effects of HSCT and GVHD also affect the mouth. Of sites for secondary malignancies in this population, the mouth is among the most common. Consequently, patients should receive routine and thorough oral examinations to screen for the development of squamous cell carcinoma. Pediatric HSCT has also been reported to be associated with significant long-term oral and craniofacial complications. Early referral and aggressive follow-up care by pediatric dental specialists is recommended.

Selected References

The complete reference list can be found at www.CANCERMEDICINE8.com

1. Sonis ST. Orthodontic management of selected medically compromised patients: cardiac disease, bleeding disorders, and asthma. *Semin Orthod*. 2004;10:277.
7. Jham BC, Reis PM, Miranda EL, et al. Oral health status of 207 head and neck cancer patients before, during and after radiotherapy. *Clin Oral Invest*. 2008;19–24.
8. Epstein JB, Stevenson-Moore P. Periodontal disease and periodontal management in patients with cancer. *Oral Oncol*. 2001; 613–619.
11. Haytac MC, Dogan MC, Antmen B. The results of a preventative dental program for pediatric patients with hematologic malignancies. *Oral Health Prev Dent*. 2004;2:59–65.
15. Sonis ST, Elting LS, Keefe D, et al. Perspectives on cancer therapy-induced mucosal injury: pathogenesis, measurement, epidemiology and consequences for patients. *Cancer*. 2004;100(9 Supp):1995.
18. Sonis ST. The pathobiology of mucositis. *Nat Rev Cancer*. 2004;4:277.

20. Trotti A, Bellm LA, Epstein JB, et al. Mucositis incidence, severity and associated outcomes in patients with head and neck cancer receiving radiotherapy with or without chemotherapy. *Radiother Oncol.* 2003;66:253.
22. Malouf JG, Aragon C, Henson BS, et al. Influence of parotid-sparing radiotherapy on xerostomia in head and neck cancer patients. *Cancer Detect Prev.* 2003;27:305.
27. Epstein JB, Silverman S, Passiarino DA, et al. Benzydamine HCL for prophylaxis of radiation-induced oral mucositis: results from a multicenter, randomized, double-blind, placebo-controlled clinical trial. *Cancer.* 2001;92;875–885.
29. Smith T. Gelclair: managing the symptoms of oral mucositis. *Hosp Med.* 2001;62:623–626.
33. Dodd MJ, Miaskowski C, Greenspan D, et al. Radiation-induced mucositis: a randomized clinical trial of micronized sucralfate versus salt and soda mouthwashes. *Cancer Invest.* 2003;21:21.
34. Su CK, Mehta V, Ravikumar L, et al. Phase II double-blind randomized study comparing oral aloe vera versus placebo to prevent radiation-related mucositis in patients with head and neck neoplasms. *Int J Radiat Oncol Biol Phys.* 2004;60:171–177.
35. Donnelly JP, Bellm LA, Epstein JB, et al. Antimicrobial therapy to prevent or treat oral mucositis. *Lancet Infect Dis.* 2003;3:405.
50. Vissink A, Burlage FR, Spijkervet FKL, et al. Prevention and treatment of the consequences of head and neck radiotherapy. *Crit Rev Oral Biol Med.* 2003;14:213.
51. Taylor SE. Efficacy and economic evaluation of pilocarpine in treating radiation-induced xerostomia. *Expert Opin Pharmacother.* 2003;4:1489.
56. Capizzi RL, Oster W. Chemoprotective and radioprotective effects of amifostine: an update of clinical trials. *Int J Hematol.* 2000;72:425–435.
57. Thorstad WL, Chao KS, Haughey B. Toxicity and compliance of subcutaneous amifostine in patients undergoing postoperative intensity-modulated radiation therapy for head and neck cancer. *Semin Oncol.* 2004;31:8.
60. Papas A, Russell D, Singh M, et al. Caries clinical trial of a remineralizing toothpaste in radiation patients. *Gerodontology.* 2008;25:76–88.
67. Aitasolo K. Bone tissue response to irradiation and treatment model of mandibular irradiation injury. *Acta Octolaryngol.* 1986;428(Suppl 1).
70. Epstein J, van der Meij E, McKenzie W, et al. Postradiation osteonecrosis of the mandible: a long-term follow-up study. *Oral Surg Oral Med Oral Pathol Oral Radiol Endod.* 1997;83:657.
73. Studer G, et al. Osteoradionecrosis of the mandible in patients treated with different fractionations. *Strahlenther Onkol.* 2004;180:233.
81. Curi MM, Dib LL, Kowalski LP. Management of refractory osteoradionecrosis of the jaws with surgery and adjunctive hyperbaric oxygen therapy. *Int J Oral Maxillofac Surg.* 2000;29:430–434.
82. Koga DH, Salvajol JV, Alves FA, et al. Dental extractions and radiotherapy in head and neck oncology: review of the literature. *Oral Dis.* 2008;14:40–44.
86. Cheng KK, Goggins B, Lee VW, et al. Risk factors for oral mucositis in children undergoing chemotherapy: a matched case-control study. *Oral Oncol.* 2009; In press.
88. Schwab M, Zanger UM, Marx C, et al. Role of genetic and nongenetic factors for fluourouracil treatment-related severe toxicity: a prospective clinical trial by the German 5-FU Toxixicity Study Group. *J Clin Oncol.* 2008;26:2131–2138.
89. Vokurka S, Bystricka E, Koza V, et al. Higher incidence of chemotherapy induced oral mucositis in females: a supplement of multivariate analysis to a randomized study. *Support Care Cancer.* 2006;14:974–976.
90. Ulrich CM, Yasui Y, Storb R, et al. Pharmacogenetics of methotrexate: toxicity among marrow transplantation patients varies with the methylenetetrahydrofolate reductase C677T polymorphism. *Blood.* 2001;98:231.
92. Bogunia-Kubik K, Polak M, Lange A. TNF polymorphisms are associated with toxic, but not GVHD allogeneic complications in the recipients of hematopoietic stem cell transplantation. *Bone Marrow Transplant.* 2003;32:617–622.
93. Otmani N, Alami R, Soulaymani A, et al. Sex, age and ABO blood groups in chemotherapy-induced oropharyngeal mucositis. *Minerva Stomatol.* 2008;57:505–509.
97. Cho SY, Cheng AC, Cheng MCK. Oral care for children with leukemia. *Hong Kong Med J.* 2000;6:203–208.
100. Lockhart PB, Brennan MT, Kent ML, et al. Randomized controlled trial of pilocarpine hydrochloride for the moderation of oral mucositis during autologous blood stem cell transplantation. *Bone Marrow Transplant.* 2005;35:713–720.
102. Ohbayashi Y, Imataki O, Ohnishi H, et al. Multivariate analysis of factors influencing oral mucositis in allogeneic hematopoietic stem cell transplantation. *Ann Hematol.* 2008;87:837–845.
106. Sonis ST. Pathobiology of oral mucositis: novel insights and opportunities. *J Support Oncol.* 2007;5:3–11.
107. Keefe DM, Sonis ST. Emerging drugs for chemotherapy-induced mucositis. *Expert Opin Emerg Drugs.* 2008;13:511–522.
114. Fasolo A, Sessa C. mTOR inhibitors in the treatment of cancer. *Exp Opin Invest Drugs.* 2008;17:1717–1734.
115. Vignot S, Faivre S, Aquirre D, et al. mTOR-targeted therapy of cancer with rapamycin derivatives. *Ann Oncol.* 2005;16:525–527.
117. Ruggiero SL, Methrota B. Bisphosphonate-related osteonecrosis of the jaw: diagnosis, prevention and treatment. *Ann Rev Med.* 2009, In press.
118. Worthington HV, Clarkson JE, Eden OB. Interventions for treatment of oral candidiasis for patients with cancer receiving treatment. *Cochrane Database Syst Rev.* 2007;18:CDOO1972.
119. Fisher BT, Zaouitis TE. Treatment of invasive candidiasis in immunocompromised pediatric patients. *Paediatr Drugs.* 2008;10:281–298.
120. Lerman MA, Laudenbach J, Marty FM, et al. Management of oral infections in cancer patients. *Dent Clin N Am.* 2008;52:129–153.
125. Epstein JB, Hancock PJ, Nantel S. Oral candidiasis in hematopoietic cell transplantation patients: an outcome-based analysis. *Oral Surg Oral Med Oral Pathol Oral Radiol Endo.* 2003;96:153.
127. Liquori G, Lucariello A, Colella G, et al. Rapid identification of Candida species in oral rinse solutions by PCR. *J Clin Pathol.* 2007;60:1035–1039.
128. Djuric M, Jankovic L, Jovanovic T, et al. Prevalence of oral herpes simplex virus reactivation in cancer patients: a comparison of different techniques of viral detection. *J Oral Pathol Med.* 2009;38:167–173.
130. Glenny AM, Fernandez MLM, Pavitt S, et al. Interventions for the prevention and treatment of herpes simplex virus in patients being treated for cancer. *Cochrane Database Syst Rev.* 2009:21:CD006706.
140. Imanguli MM, Alevizos I, Brown R, et al. Oral graft-versus-host disease. *Oral Dis.* 2008;14:396–412.

134 Gonadal Complications

Peter Kabos, MD ■ Catherine E. Klein, MD

The dramatic improvement in cancer therapy over the past 50 years is nowhere more evident than in the unprecedented survival now enjoyed by survivors of pediatric sarcomas and leukemias, and young adults with high-grade lymphomas, Hodgkin disease, and testicular tumors. Increasing numbers of premenopausal women with breast cancer are undergoing adjuvant chemotherapy, extending their survival sufficiently to justify concerns about their long-term reproductive health. Many of the new therapies allowing large numbers of long-term survivors to reach adulthood, have been associated with both temporary and permanent alterations in gonadal function, now recognized as among the most frequent significant side effects of modern cancer therapy. Women surviving cancer face symptoms of premature gonadal failure, including menopause, sterility, and presumably accelerated osteoporosis and possible early heart disease. Men experience subnormal fertility with oligo-azoospermia and subclinical Leydig cell dysfunction, which may correlate with the long-term effects of "andropause" including decreased bone density and lean muscle mass as well as decreased libido and increase in risk of coronary heart disease.

Recognition of these complications has resulted in better documentation of their frequency and severity, more effective patient counseling, and innovative approaches to attenuate or prevent the toxicity. Such interventions include hormonal manipulation, selection of alternative treatments, and pretreatment cryopreservation of germ cells, but they must be offered pre-therapy, and unfortunately many patients still report that they were uninformed of this potentially devastating outcome or of possible alternatives to the loss of fertility. As our cancer therapies continue to improve and the number of young cancer survivors increases, it will be vital for the practicing oncologist to address these issues in a timely and sensitive manner.

The Hypothalamic-Pituitary-Gonadal Axis

Regulation of the reproductive axis begins at the level of the hypothalamus, where neurosecretory cells synthesize, and release gonadotropin-releasing hormone (GnRH) in pulsatile fashion into the hypothalamic-hypophysial-portal circulation. In response, gonadotropes in the anterior pituitary synthesize and release the gonadotropins follicle stimulating hormone (FSH) and luteinizing hormone (LH), both of which ultimately control gonadal function. In women, ovarian follicles are stimulated by FSH to grow and mature; LH stimulates ovulation and corpus luteum formation. In men, FSH initiates, and in conjunction with high intratesticular testosterone, sustains spermatogenesis, whereas LH controls androgen synthesis by the testicular Leydig cells. In both men and women, gonadal failure results in increased LH, because of loss of the negative feedback of estrogen at the hypothalamus and pituitary in women and from decreases in both androgen and estrogen feedback in men. In response to decreased levels of sex steroids as well as the loss of inhibin, FSH levels are also elevated following gonadal damage. Serum gonadotropin and sex steroid values will differentiate between reproductive failure at the gonadal level or at the hypothalamic/pituitary level. Sex steroid levels will be low in both, but serum gonadotropin levels will be high in primary gonadal failure and low in those with hypothalamic or pituitary disease. Thus, the hallmark of primary gonadal failure from any cause is elevation of gonadotropin levels and this is the usual state in postpubertal patients receiving substantial doses of antineoplastic agents. Cranial radiation, on the other hand may result in significant hypothalamic-pituitary dysfunction and secondary gonadal failure with low serum levels of gonadotropins.

Historical Background

The effects of radiation and chemotherapy on gonadal function were recognized a century ago. Radiation sensitivity of the testes was reported in 1903, and a large literature on the topic accumulated over the next 50 years. Atomic Energy Commission studies of normal men, completed in the 1960s, confirmed the extraordinary sensitivity of spermatogonia to as little as 10 cGy of irradiation, a dose one-third that required in mice to produce equivalent damage.[1] Oocytes were more resistant but nevertheless displayed a reproducible, dose-dependent radiation sensitivity, which resulted in sterility and premature menopause at a frequency that increased with age. Data reported in 1939 demonstrated that a dose of 500 cGy delivered to human ovaries was associated with predictable amenorrhea that persisted for up to 18 months. All women over the age of 40 became permanently infertile.[2]

Initial reports documenting the detrimental effects of chemotherapy on human reproductive function were confirmed by a pathologic study of the testes obtained from 30 men who received nitrogen mustard in the 1940s. Twenty-seven of these men had significant testicular atrophy and absent spermatogenesis.[3]

The first convincing report of menstrual irregularities or amenorrhea in women in association with cancer therapy appeared in 1956.[4] Four young women treated with busulfan for chronic myelocytic leukemia developed menopausal symptoms within 3 months of starting therapy. Ovarian and endometrial histologic findings were consistent with primary ovarian failure. Soon after their introduction into medical use, nitrogen mustard, chlorambucil, and cyclophosphamide were recognized to do the same if administered in sufficient dose, and the list of chemotherapeutic agents with potential for testicular or ovarian toxicity continues to grow (Table 134-1).

Preclinical Studies

Although the effects of chemotherapy and radiation therapy on gonadal function have been well documented in humans, a number of preclinical models have permitted more detailed investigations into the mechanism of germ cell damage and possible methods to prevent it. Alkylating agents have been extensively studied in male rodents where they produce marked inhibition of DNA synthesis in differentiating spermatogonia, but spare the slowly dividing stem spermatogonia.[5] Similar findings have been reported in dogs and monkeys. The post-stem spermatogonial population displays a distinct species-specific and drug-specific variation in drug susceptibility. Few animal studies evaluating ovarian function have been published, as

Table 134-1 **Probability of Decreased Gonadal Function Associated With Commonly Used Antineoplastic Agents**

Frequency	Men	Women
Common	Cyclophosphamide	Cyclophosphamide
	Nitrogen mustard	Nitrogen mustard
	Procarbazine	Procarbazine
	Nitrosoureas	Nitrosoureas
		Busulfan
		Melphalan
		Thalidomide
Possible	Vinblastine	Vinblastine
	Etoposide	Etoposide
	Cisplatin	Cisplatin
	Carboplatin	Carboplatin
	Corticosteroids	Chlorambucil
	Ifosfamide	Hydroxyurea
	Interferon	Actinomycin D
	Cytosine arabinoside	Tamoxifen
	Thioguanine	Thioguanine
		Interferon
		Cytosine arabinoside
Rare	Vincristine	Methotrexate
	Doxorubicin	Doxorubicin
	Bleomycin	Bleomycin
	Methotrexate	Vincristine
	5-Fluorouracil	5-Fluorouracil
	Azathioprine	Dacarbazine
Inadequate information	Navelbine	Navelbine
	Taxanes	Taxanes
	Gemcitabine	Gemcitabine
	Interleukin	Imatinib
	Gefitinib	Ifosfamide
	Alemtuzumab	Imatinib
		Gefitinib
		Alemtuzumab

there are no well-accepted, reliable animal models for drug-induced female infertility. In female rats, alkylating agents appear to selectively target the medium and large follicles. Once the animal has become hypogonadal, the compensatory pituitary increases in gonadotropins may recruit the relatively resistant small follicles into the more sensitive pool, and if alkylating agent administration continues, thereby aggravate the damage.

In most animal systems, male infertility is reversible. In contrast to other alkylators, however, long-term administration of procarbazine to male rats results in permanent sterility. Although all alkylating agents are toxic to human gonads, the very high frequency of long-term infertility seen in survivors of Hodgkin disease treated with the mechlorethamine, vincristine (Oncovin), procarbazine, prednisone (MOPP) regimen suggests that procarbazine may be particularly toxic in humans as well (Table 134-2). Less is known about other classes of drugs; most have not been well studied in animals. In a cross-sectional study on the effects of doxorubicin, cytosine arabinoside, bleomycin, cyclophosphamide, hydroxyurea, vinblastine, and vincristine given as single injections to male mice, doxorubicin appeared to be the most toxic to stem cells. Presumably because of their relative specificity for the cell cycle S phase, antimetabolites have not been associated with long-term gonadal damage.

The direct in vivo effects of chemotherapy on the human ovary are not readily assessable. In order to make preclinical findings more relevant to humans, xenografting animal models are being developed. It is known that human primordial follicles undergo normal maturation in SCID mice, providing a good model. In one such model, subcutaneously grafted ovarian tissue into immunocompromised mice was validated with the use of cyclophosphamide.[6]

Effects of Chemotherapy on Gonadal Function

Effects in Boys

In contrast to the profound gonadal damage in adult men who receive nitrogen mustard therapy, early reports of therapy in prepubertal and pubertal boys suggested relative resistance of the less mature testicle to chemotherapy-induced effects. The reported frequency of significant testicular dysfunction, however, varies widely among studies. The vast majority of boys progress normally through puberty without the need for supplemental androgen.[7,8] Testicular volume may be reduced, however, and elevated LH levels attest to some degree of Leydig cell dysfunction.[9]

The prevalence of normal adult sperm counts in these patients (treated with single-agent cyclophosphamide), even years after therapy, has been reported in small case series of heterogeneous patient populations to range between 0% and 100%.[10,11] A review of cyclophosphamide administered orally in cumulative doses of 0.7-52 g revealed gonadal damage in 10 (16%) of 63 prepubertal boys, whereas 10 (67%) of 15 pubertal boys had evidence of gonadal dysfunction.[12] Boys are not, however, immune to the damage. Chlorambucil given alone or in combination with prednisone and azathioprine for the treatment of renal disease in patients aged 6-15 years produced azoospermia in 17 of 21 patients for up to 11 years after cessation of treatment.[13] MOPP chemotherapy given to boys with Hodgkin disease produces significant impairment in spermatogenesis at the time of puberty, a defect reported to last for years.[8,14]

In addition, although levels of LH, FSH, and serum testosterone following chemotherapy in prepubertal boys may be normal, testicular biopsies after combination chemotherapy for acute lymphoblastic leukemia or Hodgkin disease commonly show seminiferous tubular damage and interstitial fibrosis.[15]

Two major factors determine the degree of damage to testicular function among prepubertal boys receiving cytotoxic chemotherapy. The first is the cumulative dose of the drug administered, a relation especially clear for the alkylating agents. A meta-analysis was conducted of 30 studies comprising 456 patients who received cyclophosphamide alone or as part of combination chemotherapy for renal disease, Hodgkin disease, or leukemia, and who had no confounding exposure to either abdominal or gonadal irradiation. The analysis found that in addition to pubertal stage, the cumulative dose of cyclophosphamide profoundly affected the incidence of gonadal dysfunction assessed after reaching sexual maturity. Although fewer than 10% of prepubertal boys who received less than 400 mg/kg (total dose) of cyclophosphamide had gonadal dysfunction, the incidence rose to 30% in the group receiving 400-500 mg/kg and in the group receiving over 500 mg/kg.[16] The incidence of gonadal dysfunction ranged from 0% to 24% in prepubertal boys, but climbed to 68-95% in sexually mature men. Although a confounding effect of nutritional status may play some role, the critical factors in defining the extent of long-term damage to testicular spermatogenic epithelium in prepubertal boys undergoing chemotherapy with

Table 134-2 Gonadal Effects of Combination Chemotherapy

Disease	Regimen	n	Azospermia/ Amenorrhea (%)	References
Males				
Hodgkin disease	MOPP (adults)	150	73-95	16,17,21,29
	MOPP (pubertal)	18	78	16
	MOPP (boys)	27	14-80	16,156
	ABVD	13	0	16
	ChlVPP	13	87	18
	MVPP	210	84-100	23,24,27,33
	PACEBOM	12	0	69
	NOVP	21	5	151
	Stanford V	79	<85	30
Non-Hodgkin lymphoma	COPP	7	66-100	140
	VAPEC-B	14	14	31
	MACOP-B	15	0	69
Testis cancer	PVB	112	15-28	35,157
	PVB + Dox	36	17-39	36,37
	PEB	42	12	151
Acute leukemia	Standard dose	48	3-75	34
	High dose	104	14-32	34,79
Sarcomas	Dox/MTX (rt)	222	6-90	42,43,158
Females				
Ovarian cancer	P + others	66	0-8	68,72,159
Breast cancer	L-pam + FU	98	21-72	54,160
	CMF	549	54-96	153
	Mitomycin	15	26	52
Hodgkin disease	MOPP (adults)	95	55-71	153,160
	MOPP (pubertal)	15	7	16
	MVPP	72	36	8
	ABVD	24	0	28
	PACE BOM	15	0	66
	Stanford V	63	<60	30
Acute leukemia	Various	47	15	160
Non-Hodgkin lymphoma	Various	36	44	160
	High-dose	Case reports of pregnancies		145,154,155,160

Abbreviations: ABVD, Adriamycin (doxorubicin), bleomycin, vinblastine, dacarbazine; ChlVPP, chlorambucil, vinblastine, prednisone, procarbazine; CMF, cyclophosphamide, methotrexate, 5-fluorouracil; COPP, cyclophosphamide, vincristine, prednisone, procarbazine; 5-FU, 5-fluorouracil; MACOP-B, methotrexate, doxorubicin (Adriamycin), cyclophosphamide, vincristine (Oncovin), prednisone, bleomycin; MOPP, mechlorethamine, Oncovin (vincristine), prednisone, procarbazine; MVPP, mechlorethamine, vinblastine, prednisone, procarbazine; NOVP, mitoxantrone, vinblastine, vincristine, prednisone; PACE BOM, doxorubicin, cyclophosphamide, etoposide, bleomycin, vincristine, methotrexate, prednisolone; PEB, cisplatin (Platinol), etoposide, bleomycin; L-PAM, L-Phenylalanine mustard; PVB, Platinol (cisplatin), vinblastine, bleomycin; PVB + dox, cisplatin, vinblastine, bleomycin, doxorubicin; VAPEC-B, vincristine, doxorubicin, prednisone, etoposide, cyclophosphamide, bleomycin.

alkylating agents seems to be the drug dose and probably to a lesser extent the maturational stage of the testicle.

Unfortunately, there are many poorly understood exceptions to these general trends, and reliable predictions for any given patient are impossible. It cannot be assumed that even minimal doses of chemotherapy given to prepubertal children will not result in permanent sterility; the corollary is that infertility cannot be assured either, and men wanting to avoid conception need to bear this in mind.

Whether the function of Leydig cells is affected by chemotherapy in pubertal males is less clear. Gynecomastia associated with elevated FSH and LH levels was reported in 9 of 13 pubertal boys who received MOPP treatment.[17]

However, among four prepubertal boys similarly treated, all had normal basal and stimulated gonadotropin tests.[7] In addition, only two of 44 boys who recovered after therapy for acute lymphoblastic leukemia had abnormal testosterone responses to human chorionic gonadotropin (hCG) challenge, and gonadotropin secretion was normal in 29 of the 32 patients studied.[6] A more recent report on 40 men treated in childhood for Hodgkin disease found that 26 of 28 who received chemotherapy had elevated gonadotropin levels but normal serum testosterone levels and normal secondary sexual characteristics. Eleven of 13 tested were azoospermic. The study documented changes that persisted up to 17 years after therapy.[18] Follow-up of 17 adult survivors of childhood sarcoma documented azoospermia in 58%, oligospermia in another 30%, and normal testosterone in 94%. LH was elevated, however, in 40% of those with normal testosterone levels, and in 92% of their total cohort, suggesting some degree of Leydig cell insufficiency.[9] These data indicate that the seminiferous tubules are damaged by alkylating agents, generally in an age-dependent and dose-dependent manner, and that Leydig cell function may be subclinically affected in a large portion of men who appear to have normal testosterone levels after chemotherapy for childhood cancer.

Effects in Men

Administered as single agents, alkylating drugs produce permanent damage to the seminiferous epithelium. Cyclophosphamide administered in total doses of 9 g results in universal azoospermia. In total doses up to 18 g, the azoospermia is generally reversible.[19] As in animals, procarbazine appears to be the single most toxic chemotherapeutic agent to the adult male gonad. Although no studies of this drug as a single-agent are available, inferences can be drawn from multiple studies in Hodgkin disease in which patients received combination chemotherapy either with or without procarbazine. In one study all of 19 patients treated with the cyclophosphamide, vincristine (Oncovin), procarbazine, and prednisone (COPP) regimen remained oligospermic 11 years after therapy, whereas 7 of 10 treated with COPP minus the procarbazine had return of spermatogenesis within 3 years.[20,21]

Methotrexate causes minimal long-term reproductive toxicity. Little information is available with which to assess the potential harm from either vincristine or vinblastine, but that the former may be somewhat less toxic than the latter is inferred from the slightly lower incidence of infertility following MOPP therapy than that using mechlorethamine, vinblastine, procarbazine, and prednisone (MVPP). Although studies of single-agent daunorubicin are also not available, it appears to have minimal long-term effect when used in combination therapy not containing cyclophosphamide. When used with cyclophosphamide, however, daunorubicin appears to potentiate gonadal toxicity. Long-term administration of azathioprine to men with inflammatory bowel disease does not seem to affect semen quality. Hepatitis C patients treated long term with interferon have been reported to have normal gonadal hormone levels.

With the advent of curative combination chemotherapy, multiple reports have appeared indicating permanent infertility among survivors particularly of Hodgkin disease and the nonseminomatous testicular cancers. Complicating the interpretation of published studies is observation that even prior to therapy as many as 30% of young men presenting with Hodgkin disease and 50% with germ cell tumors are oligospermic,[22] and disorders of sperm motility and morphology are even more common.[23,24] Multivariate analysis in one study from Germany has found that elevated erythrocyte sedimentation rate and advanced stage are the best predictors of pre-therapy infertility among Hodgkin disease patients.[25]

Pretreatment FSH levels may provide a useful prognostic serum marker for subsequent spermatogenesis in young men with germ cell cancer.[26] MOPP or MOPP-like regimens to treat Hodgkin disease render all men infertile during therapy, and the recovery rate remains very poor (Table 134-2). In a prospective study of 37 men receiving the MVPP combination, 12 had low sperm counts before beginning treatment, but all of 14 studied after two cycles were azoospermic. All of 27 remained azoospermic in the first 12 months after treatment.[27] Follow-up of men off therapy for more than 2 years finds only 5-15% ever regain spermatogenesis.[11] Studies comparing MOPP chemotherapy to that using doxorubicin (Adriamycin), bleomycin, vinblastine, and dacarbazine (ABVD) in the treatment of Hodgkin disease provide convincing evidence that the latter combination produces less gonadal toxicity.[28,29] Because it is equally effective in the induction of durable remissions, ABVD should be the treatment of choice for men who are concerned about preserving reproductive potential.

Although there are many fewer data for treatment of non-Hodgkin lymphomas, there is some evidence that the cyclophosphamide, vinblastine, prednisone regimen may be less toxic than MOPP.[21] An update on the Stanford V regimen (vinblastine, doxorubicin, vincristine, bleomycin, mustard, etoposide and prednisone) recently reported 19 conceptions in 13 male survivors.[30] A recent analysis of 14 men treated with vincristine, doxorubicin, prednisone, etoposide, cyclophosphamide, and bleomycin suggests this may be an effective, relatively non-toxic regimen for non-Hodgkin lymphoma.[31]

Survivors of leukemia fare somewhat better, provided that abdominal or testicular irradiation is avoided.[32] Kreuser and colleagues found 100% recovery during the second year of maintenance therapy among 10 patients aged 14-38 years treated with combination chemotherapy for acute leukemia.[33] From limited data available, both allogeneic and autologous bone marrow transplantation for leukemia significantly increase the risk for long-term infertility.[34]

Among young men with testicular tumors, there is even greater evidence of spermatogenic dysfunction before therapy than there is among Hodgkin disease patients. In a series of 41 patients studied prospectively, Drasga and colleagues reported that 77% were oligoazoospermic and 17% were azoospermic, leaving only 6% with adequate sperm counts to consider cryopreservation.[35] Abnormalities of sperm motility are at least as prevalent. Pretreatment testicular histology demonstrates spermatogenic arrest, hyalinized tubules, or totally absent tubules with only Sertoli cells evident.

The etiology of this phenomenon is unknown, but a relation to elevated hCG levels with a subsequent increase in estrogen production or to the increased local heat from the tumor has been hypothesized. Sperm autoimmunity may also impair fertility in these men. It has been suggested that the altered blood-testis barrier associated with an invasive cancer may lead to circulating sperm antigen and antibody formation. In widespread cancer, generalized wasting may also contribute to impaired spermatogenesis. Nevertheless, recovery of spermatogenesis following chemotherapy for testis cancer is not uncommon. Following 2 months of therapy with cisplatin, vinblastine, and bleomycin, with or without doxorubicin, 94% of men in Drasga's study were azoospermic. However, in contrast to the MOPP-treated Hodgkin disease patients, most studies show a time-dependent recovery of spermatogenesis, with nearly 50% of patients recovering some sperm production after 2 years (Table 134-2).[36,37] In a follow-up survey of 59 patients treated with two cycles of cisplatin-based adjuvant chemotherapy for stage I nonseminomatous testis cancer, there appeared to be no adverse effects on fertility or sexual activity.[37] Recovery seems to be, at least in part, related to the cumulative dose of cisplatin. In men who receive more than 400 mg/m^2, permanent infertility should be anticipated. Limited data suggest that ifosfamide in this setting may cause less irreversible infertility than its similarity to cyclophosphamide might predict.[38,39]

Japanese studies with high-dose chemotherapy including carboplatin, etoposide, and ifosfamide found recovery of spermatogenies in half of their small series of 27 patients and could find no association with the cumulative dose of drug administered.[40] Both abdominal radiation therapy and retroperitoneal lymph node dissection decrease further the likelihood of fertility in survivors of testicular tumors.

As in boys, Leydig cell function is more resistant and is usually well compensated; despite frequently elevated gonadotropin levels, few if any of these men require androgen replacement therapy.[14,21] Occasionally men with various forms of cancer develop gynecomastia as a result of cancer therapy, presumably from an imbalance of testosterone and estrogen production. Subclinical Leydig cell dysfunction may have poorly recognized sequelae, which are just now being considered. One Dutch center evaluated the cardiovascular morbidity in long-term survivors of metastatic testicular cancer and found an incidence of coronary heart disease seven times higher than expected, a high incidence of hypercholesterolemia and obesity, in conjunction with lower testosterone and elevated LH and FSH. They hypothesize a metabolic consequence of long-term gonadal toxicity from prior chemotherapy in this group of long-term survivors.[41]

Less well studied are the male survivors of other tumor types. Shamberger and colleagues reported that three of five patients who received adjuvant doxorubicin-based therapy for sarcoma recovered normal sperm counts, although concomitant irradiation of the abdomen and pelvis or thigh, or even more distant sites, reduced the recovery rate substantially in 20 other patients studied.[42] A similar study by Meistrich and colleagues estimated that 28% of men recovered adequate sperm counts after doxorubicin-based adjuvant treatment for osteosarcoma.[43]

Interferon-α therapy in men treated for hairy cell leukemia was associated with no change in serum gonadotropin levels or sexual function in 11 patients followed for a median of 10 months.[44] Interleukin-2 (IL-2) may suppress the hypothalamic-pituitary-gonadal axis.

In summary, most of the available data for adult male gonadal toxicity comes from studies of testicular cancer and lymphoma patients. A substantial portion of patients with Hodgkin disease or a testicular tumor is sub-fertile before any therapy is given. The older MOPP-like regimens for Hodgkin disease uniformly produce azoospermia. Fewer than 15% regain adequate spermatogenesis.

Fortunately, several newer regimens appear less toxic and equally effective. Many patients treated for testicular cancer recover fertility within 1-2 years of completing chemotherapy, although the odds of full recovery decrease as the dose of cisplatin increases above 400 mg/m^2, and if surgery or radiation therapy is part of the treatment strategy.

Effect in Prepubertal Girls

The ovarian effects of chemotherapy in prepubertal girls are variable and depend on the drug, dose, and duration of therapy. Unfortunately, much of the information comes from studies on survivors of childhood leukemias and brain tumors for which cranial radiation is part of the therapy, making hypothalamic disorders more difficult to exclude. Single-agent cyclophosphamide, used to treat nonmalignant disorders, causes either a delay in puberty or permanent sterility very rarely.[45] Most girls treated with procarbazine and nitrosoureas for brain tumors show biochemical evidence of primary ovarian dysfunction, but essentially all enter and progress normally through puberty. Ovarian function appears to return to normal over a period of years, and elevated gonadotropin levels decrease to baseline in most women. Little is reported about the gonadal toxicity suffered by girls treated for lymphomas, but 80% of those surviving combination therapies for acute lymphoblastic leukemia also proceed normally through puberty. One study has suggested that despite evidence for primary gonadal damage, menarche may actually appear prematurely.[46] In a large follow-up study of childhood cancer survivors, the risk of developing premature nonsurgical menopause was 13-fold higher in cancer survivors when compared with siblings,[47] with a cumulative incidence of 8% by age 40. This increase was associated with increasing doses of alkylating agents, radiation to the ovaries as well as diagnosis of Hodgkin lymphoma.

Histologically, however, prepubertal ovaries are significantly damaged by cancer chemotherapy. Follicular maturation arrest, stromal fibrosis, and a partially depleted ova population have all been reported following single-agent cyclophosphamide as well as cytosine arabinoside (ara-C)-based antileukemic therapy.

Lasting effects on uterine function appear rare; successful pregnancy with no increased risk for miscarriage is the rule.

Effects in Women

Because the human ovary is relatively inaccessible to biopsy, the effects of antineoplastic agents on the female gonad have been inferred from the incidence of amenorrhea, changes in gonadotropin levels, and long-term fertility rates and outcomes as measures of ovarian function. The few autopsy or biopsy series reported in women treated with cyclophosphamide for non-neoplastic diseases or with multiagent therapy for cancer consistently describe complete absence of ova and follicles, with tunica albuginea thickening and stromal hyalinization. One autopsy series of patients treated for acute leukemia showed no difference in the number of primary follicles, but secondary follicles were markedly depleted.[48] Clinically, women receiving these agents develop signs and symptoms of primary ovarian failure; vaginal dryness with dyspareunia, endometrial hypoplasia, decreased libido, hot flashes, oligomenorrhea evolving into amenorrhea, and low serum estrogen levels with compensatory elevations of serum FSH and LH levels.[49,50]

The precise frequency of permanent amenorrhea and infertility depends on the drug given and its total dose, concomitant radiation exposure and the age of the patient at the time therapy is administered. Among the single agents studied, alkylating agents are the most consistently associated with premature ovarian failure, mutagenesis, and teratogenesis. Although mechlorethamine (nitrogen mustard) may be the most toxic, cyclophosphamide is the agent best studied in this regard. Most series report that 50-75% of women treated with cyclophosphamide develop amenorrhea within a month of starting therapy.[51] There is, however, a striking age-related susceptibility. In one study, the total dose of cyclophosphamide received before the onset of amenorrhea was 5.2 g for patients over 40 years of age, 9.3 g for patients aged 30-39, and 20.4 g for patients aged 20-29. Menses returned in 50% of those under 40 years of age.[52] For women under the age of 40, return of menstrual function seems closely correlated with the dose of cyclophosphamide administered after the cessation of menses. This same study has suggested a race-specific variation in sensitivity.

L-phenylalanine mustard as adjuvant chemotherapy for women with premenopausal breast cancer causes significant, age-related loss of ovarian function. The National Surgical Adjuvant Breast and Bowel Project reported that 73% of the women between the ages of 40 and 49, but only 22% of the women under the age of 39, developed amenorrhea during therapy; elevated LH and FSH levels appeared only in the older age group.[53] Single-agent treatment with busulfan or chlorambucil is associated with well documented ovarian toxicity that is also age and dose-related.[54,55] Amenorrhea among women undergoing adjuvant combination chemotherapy for breast cancer has been well described, but the absence of a uniform definition for menopause has complicated interpretation of these data. Bines and colleagues have reviewed the literature and found the average rate of amenorrhea among women treated with standard cyclophosphamide, methotrexate and fluorouracil (CMF) is about 68% but that the reported incidence ranges from 20% to 100%.[56] Most reports suggest that few women under the age of 30 treated with Adriamycin-containing regimens experienced amenorrhea; about one-third of women aged 30-40 years and nearly all those over 40 years of age experienced amenorrhea. Epirubicin-containing regimens are probably similar. One recent report of adjuvant Taxotere with Adriamycin and cyclophosphamide resulted in a 61% rate of amenorrhea in a patient population whose average as was 49 years.[57]

Small series of patients treated with high-dose methotrexate as adjuvant therapy for sarcomas report that associated amenorrhea even during therapy is uncommon and that serum gonadotropin levels remain normal during and after therapy.[42]

Given in low doses to women with gestational trophoblastic tumors, methotrexate appears to exert no significant toxicity. One large survey from the United Kingdom found that menopause occurred on average 3 years earlier in women who had received chemotherapy than in those who did not.[58] Fluorouracil, daunorubicin, and bleomycin as single agents are probably also well tolerated.

Few data are available for etoposide, but some ovarian dysfunction has been reported among women receiving the drug for gestational tumors.[59]

Vincristine and vinblastine likewise appear to be infrequent, reversible causes of amenorrhea. Reliable data on the taxanes are lacking.

The nonsteroidal antiestrogen tamoxifen, although not as well characterized, appears to exert a mild estrogenic effect associated with decreased gonadotropin levels in both premenopausal and postmenopausal women treated for breast cancer. Menstrual irregularities are common among the former, but the incidence of persistent amenorrhea is unclear. Data concerning the use of aromatase inhibitors in premenopausal cancer patients are scarce. Among children with precocious puberty, these drugs suppress estrogen levels in a safe and reversible manner, decreasing menses and bone maturation. Successful pregnancies are well documented following anastrazole treatment of endometriosis. Therapeutic doses of interferon-alpha are associated with attenuated menstrual cycling in monkeys, but there are little data available to assess its risk for humans. Successful pregnancies have been reported among women on chronic interferon therapy for a variety of malignant and nonmalignant diseases.[60] Anecdotal reports have been published of successful pregnancy in women previously treated with imatinib.[61] Reliable information about the ovarian effects of most small molecule, protein kinase inhibitors is unavailable.

Similarly, there is no available information on the reproductive toxicity associated with angiogenesis inhibitors, farnesyl transferase inhibitors, or arsenic trioxide.

Most information concerning chemotherapeutic effects on gonadal function relates to combination chemotherapy. Best studied are women who have undergone chemotherapy for Hodgkin disease. The incidence of amenorrhea in women treated with MOPP, MVPP, or COPP ranges from 15% to 80%, with a median of 50% (Table 134-2).[20,26,62-65] Two-thirds of those women develop amenorrhea during therapy, and in the rest, menses cease gradually over the next several years. A clear dose-response relationship remains to be fully established. In at least one study, there appeared to be no difference between women receiving three cycles of MOPP and those receiving six.[66] Age at the time of treatment, however, has been shown to be an important variable affecting the incidence and time of onset of permanent amenorrhea. In general, 60-100% of patients over the age of 25 develop permanent amenorrhea during therapy. Ovarian failure occurs with the initiation of therapy in 5-30% of women under the age of 25, and an additional percentage will cease menstruation over the next several months. Even younger women should anticipate a greater than 50% likelihood of premature menopause within 5-10 years of therapy.[67] Preliminary reports suggest that such alternative Hodgkin disease regimens as ABVD or doxorubicin, cyclophosphamide, etoposide, bleomycin, vincristine, methotrexate, and prednisolone may have lower rates of prolonged amenorrhea.[27,68] Horning and colleagues have reported 24 conceptions among 19 women treated with the Stanford V regimen V (mechlorethamine, doxorubicin, vinblastine, vincristine, prednisone, bleomycin.[30] Women receiving methotrexate, doxorubicin cyclophosphamide, vincristine, prednisone, and bleomycin for aggressive lymphomas appear, in small series, to maintain fertility.[69] In a small study of women treated with four cycles of Mega-CHOP for non-Hodgkin lymphoma 12 of 13 women had recovery of ovarian function.[70] Eight of these patients conceived spontaneously, five women after GnRH cotreatment.

In a second study of women younger than age 40 receiving CHOP therapy for non-Hodgkin lymphoma, only 2 of 36 women developed ovarian failure as defined by loss of menstrual cycle.[71] Fifty percent of these women became pregnant in the first remission of their disease, with no difference seen with the use of fertility-preserving measures.

Other forms of combination chemotherapy for ovarian germ cell tumors and some sarcomas have provided additional information on post-chemotherapy reproductive potential. Women receiving cisplatin-containing therapy for germ cell tumors typically become amenorrheic during treatment, but over 90% restart menstruation within a few months after completing treatment.[72-75] Among women with breast cancer, who may have age-related decreased reproductive potential to begin with, 80% receiving cyclophosphamide, methotrexate, and 5-fluorouracil (CMF) become menopausal within 10 months of beginning therapy.[76,77] Those given doxorubicin and cyclophosphamide usually become anovulatory within 3 months, or sooner if they are perimenopausal.

Fertility Following High-Dose Chemotherapy

As more young patients are undergoing high-dose, myeloablative chemotherapy, case reports and small series have documented the recovery of fertility in very few patients. A retrospective survey of over 37,000 patients who have undergone one autologous or allogeneic stem cell transplant showed that only 0.6% of patients subsequently conceived.[78] Follow-up of 187 young women previously treated with bone marrow transplantation for either aplastic anemia or leukemia found the anticipated age-dependent effect of cyclophosphamide on ovarian function.[79]

Patients with aplastic anemia overall retained fertility better than the leukemia patients, and those under 26 years of age had the best prognosis. One recent report evaluated 30 women who had survived at least 18 months following bone marrow transplantation for acute leukemia. Of the ten who had received one transplant, four developed ovarian failure, six resumed spontaneous menstrual cycling, and five of those six became pregnant. Of the three pregnancies allowed to go to term, all resulted in a normal infant.[80] One small series has documented the recovery of spermatogenesis in 4 of 25 men aged 21 to 41 following allogeneic transplantation.[81] Total-body irradiation in addition to chemotherapy is also a major risk factor for infertility, and has been associated with 2-fold to 3-fold decrease in the probability of recovering ovarian function.[79] Conditioning regimens without radiation should be considered when fertility is an issue and alternatives are available. The likelihood of recovery of ovarian function can be increased by the use of hormone replacement therapy.[82]

Effects of Radiation Therapy on Gonadal Function

Effects in Men

Information concerning the gonadal sequelae of therapeutic irradiation in boys comes from the population of long-term survivors of childhood leukemia, in whom the high incidence of testicular relapse once led to the common practice of gonadal irradiation. After it was demonstrated that doses below 1200 cGy were insufficient to control disease, most protocols delivered 2400 cGy to both testes. At these doses, permanent Leydig cell damage occurred, puberty was delayed, testosterone levels were frequently diminished, and gonadotropin levels were increased in most patients.[66,83]

These data are in contrast to those showing effective control of testicular leukemia by high-dose methotrexate and normal progression through puberty, suggesting relatively normal Leydig cell function in boys receiving chemotherapy in childhood.[84]

In adults, single 400-600 cGy doses of testicular radiation may produce azoospermia for 5 years or longer.[1] Scatter from fractionated radiation to the pelvis or lower extremities may result in substantial testicular doses as well. Berthelsen evaluated men undergoing prophylactic radiotherapy for seminoma and found that two-thirds became azoospermic from the scatter dose estimated to be between 20 and 130 cGy.[85] Shapiro and colleagues have documented oligospermia/azoospermia lasting up to 24 months after as little as 27 cGy.[86]

Recovery occurs in the majority; series report 37-66% success rates in men wishing to conceive a pregnancy.[87] Adult Leydig cell dysfunction, with elevated LH values occurs at radiation doses greater than 2000-3000 cGy.

Fractionated radiation appears to produce tubular damage similar to that seen with single doses. In adults, as in children, Leydig cell dysfunction after 2400-3000 cGy can be significant enough to require hormonal replacement. Total-body irradiation for bone marrow transplantation conditioning is routinely associated with permanent azoospermia. Secondary infertility has been reported in association with radiation administered to the hypothalamus or pituitary in conjunction with chemotherapy for intracranial neoplasms.[88]

Whether there are permanent effects on the surviving germ cells of male patients receiving radiation therapy remains controversial. Animal models suggest an increased risk for common tumors following parental exposure to radiation and chemicals. Most studies have been unable to document equivalent findings in humans.[89]

Effects in Women

The radiation sensitivity of the human ovary has not been defined as precisely as that of the male testis. Radiosensitivity is related to the oogonial developmental stage at the time of exposure. Small primordial oocytes are considerably more sensitive than large follicles. As in men, ovarian sensitivity to radiation is also dose-dependent and age-dependent. In children, the younger the age at exposure, the more primordial follicles present, and hence the longer time to loss of fertility. In adult women, single doses of 500 cGy produce menstrual irregularities in women of all ages. For women over the age of 40,600 cGy reliably induces menopause. Women aged 20-30 years can tolerate up to 3000 cGy if the dose is fractionated over 6 weeks.[90] Uterine radiation in childhood increases risk for nulliparity, spontaneous abortions, and intrauterine growth retardation, so fertility is not assured even if ovarian function is preserved.

Protective Measures

Protection for Men

Current information suggests that the toxic effects of chemotherapy are most pronounced for adult men, in whom spermatogenesis reflects a more brisk mitotic rate relative to the prepubertal testis or the adult female ovary, where the rate of germ cell mitosis is less. Such a differential susceptibility is consistent with the observation that the majority of chemotherapeutic agents affect the most rapidly dividing cells. This observation has led to speculation that halting spermatogenesis through hormonal manipulation might ameliorate testicular damage.

A number of animal studies have tested this hypothesis. Both GnRH analogues and sex steroids have been administered, and although the rate of spermatogenesis can be decreased, a protective effect has not been unequivocally documented, and remains controversial, as reflected in recent ASCO guidelines.[91]

Although some degree of success has been reported in procarbazine rat, dog, and primate models, other studies have failed to demonstrate protection and have occasionally shown increased damage from such manipulation.[92-94] In clinical trials of men receiving chemotherapy for Hodgkin disease, two attempts using GnRH analogues have been unsuccessful.[95,96] Preserving fertility by hormonal manipulation has not been demonstrated. For men who desire fertility following combination chemotherapy for advanced Hodgkin disease, the ABVD regimen is clearly preferable to MOPP.[26] Use of GnRH analogues does not shorten the recovery time to spermatogenesis.[97] Masala et al. documented some protection with the use of testosterone in patients treated with cyclophosphamide.[98]

For men anticipating cancer therapy, an alternative to in vivo protection is semen cryopreservation. Studies have shown that the process of sperm cryopreservation is no more detrimental to sperm quality in cancer patients that it is in non-cancer controls.[99] In general, these men should bank semen every 3 days, or as often as possible, before anticancer therapy is initiated. Because of the high prevalence of abnormal pre-therapy semen analyses, many patients have been considered inappropriate for this endeavor, but successful impregnation has been achieved following artificial insemination using semen with quite low sperm counts and poor sperm motility.[100] This requires careful, endocrinologically monitored timing with the woman's ovulation, and impeccable technique in freezing, storing, and thawing; if those conditions are met, fertilization may be effective in up to 45% of cases. In addition, in vitro fertilization and subsequent implantation has been successful in cases of even lower sperm counts and motility.[101] With the advent of intracytoplasmic sperm injection the chance of conception can be greatly enhanced despite exceedingly low sperm counts. Most studies document a rate of azoospermia in cancer patients pretreatment on the order of 10%. Fertilization has been reported using spermatozoa retrieved by testicular biopsy and with sperm extracted from the vas deferens at the time of orchiectomy in several azoospermic testis cancer survivors.[102] Many centers nonetheless, report that the overall success rate among men who elect to preserve semen may be somewhat limited, and perhaps is influenced by factors other than semen quality. One series from Memorial Sloan-Kettering Cancer Center reported locating 48 of 69 men who had banked sperm, but at a median of 27 months posttreatment only 11 had attempted to use their sperm for artificial insemination. Of these, only three achieved successful pregnancies.[100,103] Other centers have documented even lower rates of cryopreserved sperm use.

Penile vibratory stimulation and electroejaculation may provide an option for pubertal boys.[104] Very preliminary studies of testicular circulatory isolation suggest that this mechanical procedure is protective in a rat model and might be feasible in human clinical trials.[105] None have been reported.

Testis sperm extraction is reported to recover spermatozoa in 55-85% of men with nonobstructive azoospermia of various etiologies. Damani and colleagues have reported a series of azoospermic men with a history of chemotherapy.

Spermatozoa were found in 15 of 23 (65%). A total of 26 intracytoplasmic sperm injection cycles were performed in 12 couples. Fertilization rate was 65%. All babies born to date have had normal neonatal examinations.[106]

Testicular tissue biopsy and cryopreservation is experimental, as is isolation of germ cells from testicular tissue for storage.

Gonadal shielding remains the mainstay of protection from therapeutic radiation. No convincing studies to suggest benefit from scrotal cooling are currently available.

Protection for Women

Analogous to the hypothesis for men, it has also been proposed that suppression of ovarian function by oral contraceptives or GnRH analogue might offer gonadal protection to cycling women about to undergo potentially sterilizing radiation or chemotherapy. Some animal models have validated the hypothesis, both in protection from radiation and in chemotherapy-induced ovarian damage.[107] Results of such trials in humans have been conflicting, however, and the number of patients studied remains small. Most promising of these reports is that of Chapman and Sutcliffe, who administered oral contraceptives to women anticipating receiving MVPP therapy for Hodgkin disease. Five of six women had resumption of normal menses at a mean follow-up of 26 months.[108] One small study of patients with Hodgkin disease given the GnRH analogue buserelin for 1 week prior to initiation of MVPP failed to show any difference in amenorrhea or menopausal symptoms when compared to controls.[96] Pacheco and colleagues have administered leuprolide acetate to 12 patients aged 15-20 anticipating treatment for lymphoma.[109] Pretreatment suppression was instituted with both subcutaneous daily injections and the depot injection to overcome the delay in suppression of ovarian function. Suppression was continued monthly with depot administration until one month after cessation of chemotherapy. All 12 treated patients resumed normal menstrual cycling within 6 months, compared to none of the four women in this study who did not receive leuprolide suppression. Three pregnancies were reported. Although the short pretreatment interval may compromise the effect of ovarian suppression in some reported series, urgent cancer therapy often precludes a more lengthy delay. A possible protective effect of oral contraceptives was documented by Behringer et al. Protective benefit with administration of progesterone remains controversial.

The introduction of in vitro fertilization led to early optimism for the potential of ovarian tissue cryopreservation to preserve fertility, but oocyte cryopreservation has had very limited success and only an occasional successful pregnancy has been reported (Table 134-3). The chance of a live birth per retrieved oocyte remains low at 3-5%.[110] Despite the recent improvements in technology that have increased, oocyte survival rates and subsequent fertilization rates, at this time it is probably not a feasible option for women anticipating sterilizing therapy. Human ovarian cortical slices containing primordial ova have been obtained laparoscopically and cryopreserved successfully. Recent reports indicate that such tissue can be autografted subsequently and returned to patients, thus restoring fertility. Follicles can be retrieved from the orthotopic site.[111] To date only two live births have been reported with this technique.[112,113]

Table 134-3 Options for Preservation of Fertility in Patients With Cancer

	Males	Status	Females	Status
Children	Testicular tissue cryopreservation	Unproven	Ovarian tissue cryopreservation	Unproven
Adults	GnRH analogue	Unproven	GnRH analog suppression	? Effective
			OCP suppression	Unproven
	Sperm cryopreservation	Accepted	Oocyte cryopreservation	Experimental
	Testicular sperm extraction	Experimental	Ovarian tissue cryopreservation	Available
			Embryo cryopreservation	Available
			Ovarian tissue transposition	Experimental

Abbreviations: GnRH analogue, gonadotropin-releasing hormone analogue; OCP, oral contraceptives.

In women with stable relationships, embryo cryopreservation has been successful and this has been offered to cancer patients. In general, superovulation is required before fertilization, and neither the time required nor the hormone manipulation necessary may be acceptable. In vitro fertilization without stimulation is a possible but less effective option. One case report of a woman with breast cancer who underwent successful in vitro fertilization and embryo cryopreservation after a natural cycle suggests that this might become a potential fertility-preserving tool. The implantation rates range from 8% to 30%. A wide range of survival of thawed embryos has been reported in the literature. The cumulative pregnancy rate can be more than 60%.[114] However, a number of ethical concerns remain to be addressed before this technique will gain widespread acceptance, including the appropriate disposal of unused "orphan" embryos, the potential for transmission of cancer, the use of donor sperm, and various religious issues.[115] Oocyte donations have been used on occasion with subsequent in vitro fertilization and successful pregnancy. Sauer and colleagues have described a young woman, amenorrheic following therapy for Hodgkin disease, who was impregnated with a donor ovum recovered after insemination and uterine lavage.[116] Both oocyte and embryo cryopreservation require a significant delay in initiating cancer treatment while ovarian stimulation is undertaken, and in many situations this may be medically and ethically unsound. Oocyte preservation remains challenging as these cells are highly sensitive to cryoinjury. Oktay et al in a recent meta-analysis documented a significantly lower live birth rate with frozen oocytes when compared to IVF performed with fresh oocytes (15.4% vs 38.4% respectively).[117] Ultra-rapid freezing methods for oocyte preservation may further improve outcomes.

Ovarian tissue preservation may prove an option that avoids delay in cancer treatment. Ovarian cortical tissue also has the advantage of containing large numbers of follicles and thereby increasing the potential for successful future pregnancies. The ovarian tissue can ultimately be transplanted back in to the patient thus restoring ongoing fertility. Transplanted tissue has been reported to restore normal menstrual cycling.[118]

Oktey and colleagues reported the first human embryo development after heterotopic transplantation of cryopreserved ovarian tissue.[119] Donnez et al. reported recently a live birth following orthotopic transplantation of cryopreserved ovarian tissue.[113] This technique may ultimately offer an option for young girls as well as sexually mature young women. Risk of reseeding metastatic cancer needs to be defined carefully and this technique is not suitable for patients with ovarian malignancies. Obviously, the ethical issues regarding the necessary clinical trials add further controversy to the technique.[120]

For patients undergoing pelvic radiation therapy, oophoropexy can be undertaken. Generally, this is done at the time of exploratory or staging laparotomy to move the ovaries either medially behind the uterine fundus or laterally out of the radiation port. Radiation exposure is decreased 90%, and hormonal function is preserved in 55-95% of patients; however, fertility is still compromised, possibly owing to the abnormal tuboovarian anatomy or radiation scatter. In a study of 22 patients with Hodgkin disease who had undergone oophoropexy, 1 of 2 receiving para-aortic and 1 of 12 receiving inverted-Y radiation therapy subsequently became pregnant.[121] In a study of 134 women who had undergone ovarian transposition, 126 of whom received radiation therapy, a total ovarian dose of 5 cGy was statistically associated with ovarian failure.[122] A small trial of laparoscopic propriosacral ovariopexy offers the possibility of a less invasive approach to fertility preservation.[123] One option in this setting is the transposition of only one ovary and removal of the second for cryopreservation.[124] Reports have shown no increase in stillbirths, congenital malformations, abnormal karyotypes, or cancers in the offspring.[125,126] Oktay and colleagues have recently reported the successful transplantation of ovarian tissue removed at the time of ovariectomy in a woman with cervical cancer. Frozen sections revealed no evident metastatic cancer, and fresh tissue was transplanted into her antecubital fossa before the initiation of her pelvic radiation.

Follow-up determined that the tissue was cycling normally, oocytes were retrieved, but in vitro fertilization was not successful.[127] Specific ovarian shielding may be useful in some cases.

Protection for Children

No proven methods for protection of future fertility in children are available at this time. Some centers offer ovarian tissue or testicular tissue cryopreservation as an experimental approach, but research in this area is fraught with ethical problems. Many excellent reviews of the technical and ethical issues of fertility preservation are available.[120,128]

Outcomes of Pregnancy

Chemotherapy

Case reports document successful conception and delivery of normal infants to patients who have received even the most aggressive of chemotherapy regimens; neither male nor female permanent infertility can be presumed following chemotherapy for cancer. This point must be reiterated in counseling both those patients who wish and those who do not wish to have children. For the latter, appropriate contraception should be encouraged. For those who do wish to have children, a common concern is for the potential adverse fetal outcomes. Several retrospective series have evaluated the outcome of pregnancy in women treated with chemotherapeutic agents as children or young adults who completed therapy and then became pregnant. Fewer data are available for women who conceived during active cancer treatment.

One large study evaluating offspring of children treated for a variety of cancers found that in a total of 286 subsequent pregnancies there was no increase in congenital anomalies, and chromosomal analysis was normal in 23 of 24 children tested.[129] Pregnancies in women previously treated for trophoblastic tumors also appear to have no associated increased risk of congenital anomalies, spontaneous abortions, or neonatal mortality.[130]

Holmes and Holmes evaluated women treated for Hodgkin disease and compared the 93 pregnancies in their chemotherapy-treated patients to 288 sibling-control pregnancies. Overall, there was no difference between the groups, although when the subgroup that received both radiation therapy and chemotherapy was analyzed separately, it appeared that combined treatment produced more spontaneous abortions in wives of male patients, and those female patients were slightly more likely to produce abnormal offspring than control women.[113]

Offspring of fathers treated with prior chemotherapy likewise appear to be normal. When large series are combined, nearly 1400 live-born children have been reported to have a congenital defect incidence of about 4%, not significantly different from the general population. Most of these anomalies represent common, nongenetic abnormalities.[131]

Further follow-up suggests that offspring growth, development, and school performance are probably normal. A National Cancer Institute study to address the question of cancer in offspring of treated patients found a slight and statistically insignificant excess of cancers in these children when compared to offspring of sibling-matched controls (0.3% vs 0.23%), numbers not different from those expected in the general population. When analyzed by age and sex, however, it appeared that there was an excess of cancers diagnosed in male offspring under age 5. Five cancers were detected in this group, compared to the 1.7 expected.[132] Some of these cancers may have represented familial clustering of known hereditary cancers, such as retinoblastoma or Wilms tumor.

Risk to the fetus exposed in utero to chemotherapy agents depends on gestational age and the drug and dose administered. Aminopterin, a known folate antagonist has been consistently associated with teratogenic effects, as would be predicted from the critical importance of folate in neurologic development. It may be concentrated in the amniotic fluid and is associated with up to a 100% incidence of fetal malformations, often in the central nervous system, when exposure occurs during the first trimester. Folate antagonists should not be administered during the first trimester. Other antimetabolites have rarely been associated with congenital abnormalities. First trimester exposure to 5-fluorouracil, cyclophosphamide, busulfan, and chlorambucil has been associated with low birth-weight in infants and other abnormalities on rare occasion.[133] Fetal myocardial necrosis has been reported following maternal administration of anthracyclines.[134] Imatinib has demonstrated teratogenicity in animal models, but case reports have documented successful pregnancies in women who conceive during treatment.[135] Rituxan given unintentionally to a pregnant woman resulted in an uncomplicated pregnancy delivering an apparently healthy infant. Interferon-a has been given safely during pregnancy in a small number of women.[136]

Whether the risk to the fetus is further increased with drug combinations is uncertain. Case reports and small series indicate that exposure in the second and third trimesters is associated with minimal risk to the fetus and that long-term development of these offspring is normal.[137,138] One study of 16 children exposed to maternal antileukemic therapy could detect no difference in peripheral blood, bone marrow, cytogenetics, physical examination, neurologic assessment, school performance, or intelligence test results when compared to sibling controls.[139] Nonteratogenic effects including low birth-weight, intrauterine growth retardation, and more subtle developmental abnormalities remain to be defined. In utero exposure to diethylstilbestrol has been linked to the development of genital clear cell carcinomas in the female offspring of these women, but other clear documentation of carcinogenesis from in utero exposure to chemotherapy is lacking. No information is available on the reproductive potential of these children.

Radiation Therapy

Most of what is known about the genetic effects of radiation therapy is inferred from data on survivors of atomic bomb exposure. Although extensive data have been accumulated in their offspring, interpretation of the data is clouded by a variety of factors, particularly the calculation of the actual gonadal dose. Nevertheless, it is apparent that the increase in untoward outcomes of pregnancies (major congenital defects, stillbirth, and death during the first week of life) is small, estimated at 0.00182/gonadal rem (roentgen-equivalent–man)—the quantity of any ionizing radiation equivalent to the biologic effect of 1 rad (cGy). Small head size has been reported in these offspring,[140] but has not been a consistent finding among offspring of women irradiated therapeutically during gestation.

Among women treated with radiation therapy below the diaphragm, preterm delivery in up to 20% of pregnancies and an excess of low birth-weight infants have been reported. That these adverse outcomes are often clustered in the first posttreatment year suggests they may result from local uterine or hormonal factors and may not be because of genetic defects.[140,141] One large study of Wilms tumor survivors found an increase in perinatal death and low birth-weight infants, findings that contributed to an overall 30% adverse outcome in these patients. These abnormalities were limited to women who had received pelvic radiation therapy, and were not seen among those who had been treated with chemotherapy alone.

In utero exposure to irradiation produces the greatest risk of teratogenesis during the period of organogenesis from the second to the eighth week, with growth retardation, eye problems, and microcephaly appearing as the predominant abnormalities. A safe dose has not yet been defined, but generally, a therapeutic abortion is recommended for any uterine dose of 10 cGy during the first trimester. Supradiaphragmatic irradiation is associated with considerable scatter to the fetus, much of which can probably be prevented with abdominal shielding. Local irradiation of the neck and axilla may be safe during the first trimester.[133] Data on future fertility and the risks of malignancy in the offspring are unavailable.

Psychosocial Issues

The psychosocial issues of disfigurement, loss of fertility, anxiety about birth defects, sexual performance, and recurrence of tumor all have important impacts on the single patient facing dating and mate-selection issues, as well as on married patients in a stable relationship, for whom the separation rate may be fourfold of that of the general population.[142-144] Sildenafil for the treatment of erectile dysfunction appears to be useful for the treatment of men following radiation therapy for prostate cancer. Studies have shown that 70-80% of men treated with either external beam or brachytherapy respond favorably.[145,146] Loss of libido is particularly common in women; when associated with vaginal dryness and dyspareunia, vaginal lubricants, and estrogen creams may be helpful. Although many sexual side effects can be ameliorated (estrogen replacement, reconstructive surgery), many cannot.[147,148] Effective counseling is critical in alleviating major morbidity in these patients and in allowing patients to feel open and hopeful regarding their problems. Early follow-up should include assessment of the hypothalamic-pituitary-gonadal axis (especially in total-body irradiated patients), thyroid function tests, and a check of serum gonadotropin levels to document spontaneous return of fertility. Excellent reviews are available for the interested reader seeking further information.[142,148,149]

For physician assessment of sexual functioning, Andersen has proposed a model that helps the provider address many issues before they arise.[142] It is only through specific inquiry and careful documentation of current and prior sexual functioning, including frequency of activity, libido, arousal, orgasm, and sensation of resolution, that the health professional can determine cancer therapy-related dysfunction. As in other areas of cancer medicine, such a role is highly demanding, but it often provides the patient much comfort and the caregiver great satisfaction, considering the challenges raised by the gonadal effects of cancer therapy.

Selected References

The complete reference list can be found at www.CANCERMEDICINE8.com

1. Clifton DK, Bremner WJ. The effect of testicular x-irradiation on spermatogenesis in man: a comparison with the mouse. *J Androl*. 1983;4:387–392.
8. Whitehead E, Shalet SM, Jones PH, et al. Gonadal function after combination chemotherapy for Hodgkin's disease in childhood. *Arch Dis Child*. 1982;47:287–291.
14. Aubier F, Flamant F, Caillaud JM, et al. Male gonadal function after chemotherapy for solid tumors in childhood. *J Clin Oncol*. 1989;7:304–309.
16. Rivkees SA, Crawford JD. The relationship of gonadal activity and chemotherapy-induced gonadal damage. *JAMA*. 1988;259:2123–2125.
21. Roeser HP, Stocks AE, Smith AJ. Testicular damage due to cytotoxic drugs and recovery after cessation of therapy. *Aust N Z J Med*. 1978;8:250–254.
25. Rueffer U, Breuer K, Josting A, et al. Male gonadal dysfunction in patients with Hodgkin's disease prior to treatment. *Ann Oncol*. 2001;12:1307–1311.
27. Whitehead E, Shalet SM, Blackledge G, et al. The effects of Hodgkin's disease and combination chemotherapy on gonadal function in the adult male. *Cancer*. 1982;49:418–422.
29. Viviani S, Santoro A, Ragni G, et al. Gonadal toxicity after combination chemotherapy for Hodgkin's disease: comparative results of MOPP vs ABVD. *Eur J Cancer Clin Oncol*. 1985;21:601–605.
33. Kreuser ED, Hetzel WD, Wolfgang H, et al. Reproductive and endocrine gonadal functions in adults following multidrug chemotherapy for acute lymphoblastic or undifferentiated leukemia. *J Clin Oncol*. 1988;6:588–595.
38. Dominik B, Burkhard FC, Mills R, et al. Fertility and sexual function following orchiectomy and 2 cycles of chemotherapy for stage I high risk nonseminomatous germ cell cancer. *J Urol*. 2001;165:441–444.
40. Ishikawa T, Kamidono S, Fujisawa M. Fertility after highdose chemotherapy for testicular cancer. *Urology*. 2004; 63:137–140.
42. Shamberger RC, Rosenberg SA, Siepp CA, Sherins RJ. Effects of high-dose methotrexate and vincristine on ovarian and testicular functions in patients undergoing post-operative adjuvant treatment of osteosarcoma. *Cancer Treat Rep*. 1981;65:739–746.
44. Schilsky RL, Davidson HS, Magid D, et al. Gonadal and sexual function in male patients with hairy cell leukemia: lack of adverse effects of recombinant alpha 2-interferon treatment. *Cancer Treat Rep*. 1987;71:179–181.
46. Quigley C, Cowell C, Jimenez M, et al. Normal or early development of puberty despite gonadal damage in children treated for acute lymphocytic leukemia. *N Engl J Med*. 1989;321:143–151.
47. Sklar CA, Mertens AC, Mitby P, et al. Premature menopause in survivors of childhood cancer: a report from the childhood cancer survivor study. *J Natl Cancer Inst*. July 5, 2006;98(13):890–896.
49. Chapman RM, Rees LH, Sutcliffe SB, et al. Cyclical combination chemotherapy and gonadal function. Lancet 1979;1:285–289.
51. Schilsky RL, Lewis BJ, Sherins RJ. Gonadal dysfunction in patients receiving chemotherapy for cancer. *Ann Intern Med*. 1980;93:109–114.
53. Fisher B, Sherman B, Rockette H. L-phenylalanine mustard in the management of premenopausal patients with primary breast cancer. *Cancer*. 1979;44:847–857.
56. Bines J, Oleske DM, Cobleigh MA. Ovarian function in premenopausal women treated with adjuvant chemotherapy for breast cancer. *J Clin Oncol*. 1996;14:1718–1729.
59. Choo YC, Chan SWY, Wong LC, Ma HK. Ovarian dysfunction in patients with gestational trophoblastic neoplasm treated with short intensive courses of etoposide. *Cancer*. 1985;55:2348–2352.
61. Hensley ML, Ford JM. Imatinib treatment: specific issues related to safety, fertility, and pregnancy. *Semin Hematol*. 2003;40(suppl 2):21–25.
64. Schilsky RL, Sherins RJ, Hubbard SM, et al. Long-term follow-up of ovarian function in women treated with MOPP chemotherapy for Hodgkin's disease. *Am J Med*. 1981;71:552–556.
66. Sherins RJ, Winokur S, DeVita VT, Vaitukaitis J. Surprisingly high risk of functional castration in women receiving chemotherapy for lymphoma [abstract]. *Clin Res*. 1975;23:343.
67. Waxman JHX, Terry YA, Wrigley PFM, et al. Gonadal function in Hodgkin's disease: long-term follow-up of chemotherapy. *Br Med J*. 1982;285:1612–1613.
68. Simmonds PD, Mead GM, Sweetenham JW, et al. PACE BOM chemotherapy: a 12-week regimen for advanced Hodgkin's disease. *Ann Oncol*. 1997;8:259–266.
70. Dann EJ, Epelbaum R, Avivi I, et al. Fertility and ovarian function are preserved in women treated with an intensified regimen of cyclophosphamide, adriamycin, vincristine and prednisone (Mega-CHOP) for non-Hodgkin lymphoma. *Hum Reprod*. 2005;20:2247–2249.
72. Gershenson DM. Menstrual and reproductive function after treatment with combination chemotherapy for malignant ovarian germ cell tumors. *J Clin Oncol*. 1988;6:270–275.
75. Pfleiderer A. Therapy of ovarian malignant germ cell tumors and granulosa tumors. *Int J Gynecol Pathol*. 1993;12:162–165.
79. Sanders JE, Buckner CD, Amos D, et al. Ovarian function following marrow transplantation for aplastic anemia or leukemia. *J Clin Oncol*. 1988;6:813–818.
81. Jacob A, Barker H, Goodman A, Holmes J. Recovery of spermatogenesis following bone marrow transplantation. *Bone Marrow Transplant*. 1998;22:277–279.
82. Liu J, Malhotra R, Voltarelli J, et al. Ovarian recovery after stem cell transplantation. *Bone Marrow Transplant*. 2008;41:275–278.
85. Berthelsen JG. Sperm counts and serum follicle-stimulating hormone levels before and after radiotherapy and chemotherapy in men with testicular germ cell cancer. *Fertil Steril*. 1984;41:281–286.
87. Ohl DA, Sonksen J. What are the chances of fertility and should sperm be banked? *Semin Urol Oncol*. 1996;14:36–44.
89. Hawkins MM. Is there evidence of a therapy-related increase in germ-cell mutation among childhood cancer survivors? *J Natl Cancer Inst*. 1991;83:1643–1650.
92. Glode LM, Shannon JM, Nett T. Protection of rat spermatogenic epithelium from damage induced by procarbazine chemotherapy. *Br J Cancer*. 1990;62:61–64.
94. da Cunha MF, Meistrich ML, Nader S. Absence of testicular protection by a gonadotropin-releasing hormone analogue against cyclophosphamide-induced testicular cytotoxicity in the mouse. *Cancer Res*. 1987;47:1093–1097.
95. Johnson DH, Line R, Hainsworth JD, et al. Effects of luteinizing hormone releasing hormone agonist given during combination chemotherapy on post-therapy fertility in male patients with lymphoma: preliminary observations. *Blood*. 1985;65:832–836.
97. Brennemann W, Brensing KA, Leipner N,et al. Attempted protection of spermatogenesis from irradiation in patients with seminoma by D-Tryptophan-6 luteinizing hormone releasing hormone. *Clin Invest*. 1994;72:838–842.
98. Raptopolou A, Siridopoulos P, Boumpas DT. Ovarian failure and strategies for fertility preservation in patients with systemic lupus erythematosus. *Ann Intern Med*. 1997;126:292–295.
99. Hallak J, Kolettis PN, Sekhon VS. Thomas AJ, Agarwal A.Sperm ryopreservation in patients with testicular cancer. *Urology*. 1999;54:894–899.
101. Davis OK, Graf MJ, Bedford JM. Pregnancy achieved through in vitro fertilization with cryopreserved semen from a man with Hodgkin's lymphoma. *Fertil Steril*. 1990;53:377–378.
104. Schmiegelow ML, Sommer P, Carlson E, et al. Penile vibratory stimulation and electroejaculation before anti-cancer therapy in two pubertal boys. *J Pediat Hematol Oncol*. 1998;20:429–430.
106. Damani MN, Masters V, Meng MV, et al. Postchemotherapy ejaculatory azoospermia: fatherhood with sperm from testis tissue with intracytoplasmic sperm injection. *J Clin Oncol*. 2002;20:930–936.
107. Jarrell J, YoungLai EV, McMahon A, et al. Effects of ionizing radiation and pretreatment with [D-Leu6, des-GlylO] luteinizing hormone-releasing hormone ethylamide on developing rat ovarian follicles. *Cancer Res*. 1987;47:5005–5008.
108. Chapman R, Sutcliffe SB. Protection of ovarian function by oral contraceptives in women receiving chemotherapy for Hodgkin's disease. *Blood*. 1981;58:849–851.
110. Oktay K, Cil AP, Bang H. Efficiency of oocyte cryopreservation: a meta-analysis. *Fertil Steril*. 2006;86:70–80.
112. Demeestere I, Simon P, Emiliani S, et al. Fertility preservation: successful transplantation of cryopreserved ovarian tissue in a young patient previously treated for Hodgkin's disease. *Oncologist*. 2007;12:1437–1442.
114. Son WY, Yoon SH, Yoon HJ, et al. Pregnancy outcome following transfer of human blastocysts vitrified on electron microscopy grids after induced collapse of the blastocoele. *Hum Reprod*. 2003;18:137–139.
116. Sauer MV, Guidice L, Macaso TM. Pregnancy following nonsurgical donor ovum transfer to a functionally agonadal woman. *Fertil Steril*. 1987;48:324–325.
119. Oktay K, Buyuk E, Veeck L, et al. Embryo development after heterotopic transplantation of cryopreserved ovarian tissue. *Lancet*. 2004;363:837–840.
120. Dudzinski JM. Ethical issues in fertility preservation for adolescent cancer survivors: oocyte and ovarian tissue cryopreservation. *J Pediatr Adolesc Gynecol*. 2004;17:97–102.

135 Endocrine Complications and Paraneoplastic Syndromes

Sai-Ching Jim Yeung, MD, PhD ■ *Robert F. Gagel, MD*

This chapter is divided in two major sections. The first focuses on endocrine complications in cancer patients; the second on endocrine paraneoplastic syndromes. Cancer and its treatment can lead to endocrine dysfunction or clinical and laboratory abnormalities that obscure or mimic endocrine diseases. Paraneoplastic syndromes are a group of diverse clinical syndromes seen in cancer patients caused by circulating biologic/humoral factors that include hormones, immunoglobulins, cytokines, and other agents.

Endocrine Complications

Hypothalamic–Pituitary Dysfunction

Radiotherapy is a common cause of hypothalamic–pituitary dysfunction in cancer patients. There is no strong direct evidence to implicate chemotherapy as a cause of permanent dysfunction of the anterior pituitary. Metastasis to the hypothalamic region or the pituitary gland is uncommon,[1] and clinical manifestations of endocrine dysfunction because of metastatic disease in this region are rare. However, benign tumors such as pituitary tumors and craniopharyngiomas frequently affect this anatomic region and cause endocrine dysfunction.

Development of radiation-induced hypothalamic dysfunction is insidious; hormonal deficiency can manifest years after radiation. In general, the rapidity of onset and severity of dysfunction depend on the total dose of radiation and the rate of delivery. The sequence and frequency of dysfunction among the axes of hypothalamic–pituitary functions vary. The somatotropic axis is the most susceptible, while the thyrotropic axis is the least susceptible (Fig. 135-1).[2-5] The diagnosis of hypothalamic–pituitary dysfunction requires vigilance of the physician because most presenting symptoms (eg, fatigue and weakness) are nonspecific and attributable to other causes common among cancer patients. A diagnostic screen for hypothalamic/pituitary dysfunction may include serum growth hormone (GH) and insulin-like growth factor-1 (IGF-1) measurement and evaluation for gonadal failure. Signs of overt hypopituitarism include hypoglycemia, hypotension, and hypothermia.

In children and adolescents, evaluation of sexual development is a useful diagnostic tool. Staging sexual development according to Tanner's criteria, menstrual history in girls and penile/testicular size in boys should be evaluated. In children who have had cranial irradiation, height and weight should be measured every 6 months. In children treated with spinal and craniospinal irradiation, local rather than general growth abnormalities may be present and, if so, require specific evaluation. Foot size is a reliable indicator of growth that can be easily measured.[6] Deviation from normal growth curves should be evaluated for growth hormone deficiency, hypothyroidism, and adrenal insufficiency. If the initial evaluation of GH, IGF-1, thyrotropin (TSH), and free thyroxine (T4) levels, and radiographic bone age reveal abnormality, then detailed dynamic testing to evaluate the hypothalamic/pituitary axes should be performed (Table 135-1).

In adults who have received cranial or head and neck irradiation, detection of hypothalamic–pituitary abnormalities is more challenging. One strategy to detect hypothalamic–pituitary abnormalities in adults consists of routine screening for GH deficiency and gonadal failure. It is recommended that measurements of IGF-1 and testosterone levels in males and documentation of menstrual history in females be obtained annually for 5 years, and then at 5-year intervals for another 10 years. Any abnormalities noted on the screening tests should be pursued with further dynamic testing to evaluate all the axes of hypothalamic–pituitary functions.

Thyroid Disorders

Thyroid disorders and abnormalities in thyroid function are commonly associated with cancer and its therapy.

Serum Thyroid Hormone-Binding Protein Abnormalities ■ The levels of thyroid hormone-binding proteins [thyroxine-binding globulin (TBG), prealbumin, and albumin] can be modified by sex hormone levels and nutritional factors; abnormalities of both are encountered frequently in cancer patients. Several chemotherapy drugs affect thyroid function test results. L-Asparaginase appears to reversibly inhibit synthesis of albumin and TBG,

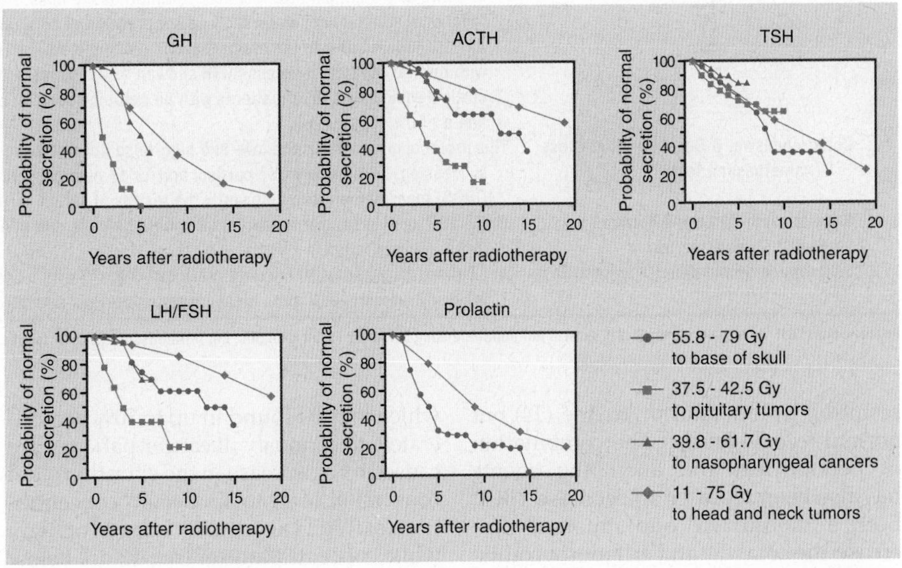

Figure 135-1 ■ Probability of normal pituitary hormone secretion over time after radiation exposure to the hypothalamic–pituitary areas. Data from four studies were replotted on this single figure. The first set of values (*closed circle*) are from Pai et al[3] where the patient received 55.8-79 Gy to the base of the skull. The second set of values (*solid square*) are from Shalet et al,[88] where patients with pituitary tumors were treated with 37.5-42.5 Gy. The third series (*open triangle*), from Lam et al,[2] shows the effect of radiation treatment for nasopharyngeal carcinoma with 39.8-61.7 Gy. The final series (*open diamond*) represents data from Samaan et al,[4] in which 11-75 Gy was administered to treat of head and neck tumors.

Table 135-1 **Dynamic Testing of the Hypothalamic/Pituitary Axes**

Test	Dose/Sampling	Contraindications
Growth hormone axis		
Insulin hypoglycemia	0.075-0.1 U regular insulin/kg IV to achieve glucose ≤40 mg/dL. Sample for glucose and GH at 0, 30, 45, 60, and 90 min	Coronary heart disease or seizures
Arginine	0.5 gm/kg (up to 30 gm) IV over 30 min. Sample for GH at 0, 30, 60, 90, and 120 min	Liver disease or renal disease
L-Dopa	500 mg by mouth. Sample for GH at 0, 30, 60, 90, and 120 min	Systolic blood pressure <100 mm Hg or age >60 years
Arginine and GHRH	Arginine dose as above. GHRH 1 µg/kg IV push. Sample for GH at 0, 30, 60, 90, and 120 min	Liver disease or renal disease
Clonidine Stimulation Protocol	Clonidine 0.15 mg/m² by mouth. Collect GH samples at baseline, 30, 60, 90, and 120 min	
Growth Hormone Releasing Hormone (GHRH) Stimulation Protocol	GHRH at 1.0 µg/kg body weight IV push. Collect GH samples at baseline, 15, 30, 45, 60, 90, and 120 min	
Growth Hormone Suppression Test	The test should be performed after an overnight fast with the patient maintained at bed rest. The patient should drink a solution of 100 g glucose. Collect GH samples at baseline, 60, and 120 min	
Adrenal axis		
ACTH Stimulation Test, 1 h	Cosyntropin 1 or 250 µg IM or IV. Draw blood for cortisol at 30 and 60 min after injection	
ACTH Stimulation Test, 48 h	Beginning at 9 a.m., obtain 24-h urine for 17-hydroxycorticosteroids (17-OHCS) and creatinine. Collect 24 h as on day 1. Beginning at 9 a.m., start IV and give 250 µg cosyntropin in 250 mL normal saline over 8 h every 8 h for 48 h. Alternatively, 40 IU of depot formulation of purified bovine ACTH in gelatin IM every 12 h for 48 h. Repeat 24-h urine as on days 1 and 2 Days 4 and 5: Collect 24-h urine as on previous days.	
Corticotropin-Releasing Hormone (CRH) Stimulation Test	Fast for at least 4 h prior to the test. Human CRH at 1.0 µg/kg IV bolus over 30 seconds. Blood samples should be collected at 15 minutes and 1 minute before CRH administration and at 15, 30, 45, 60, 90, and 120 minutes after for measurements of cortisol and ACTH	
Low-Dose Dexamethasone Test, overnight	Dexamethasone 1.0 mg (adult) or 20 µg/kg (children) PO between 11 p.m. and midnight. Serum cortisol is collected at 8-9 a.m. the next morning. A cortisol level <1.8 µg/dL essentially excludes Cushing syndrome	
Low-Dose Dexamethasone Test, 48-h	Serum cortisol is collected at 8-9 a.m. Dexamethasone 0.5 mg (adult) or 10 µg/kg (children) PO immediately after the cortisol is drawn and again every 6 h for 48 h. A second plasma cortisol is drawn at 9 a.m., 6 h after the last dexamethasone dose. Serum cortisol concentrations <1.8 µg/dL essentially exclude Cushing syndrome	
High-Dose Dexamethasone Test, 48-h	Serum cortisol is collected at 9 a.m. Dexamethasone is administered (2.0 mg; 50 µg/kg in children) every 6 h for 48 h. A second plasma cortisol is drawn at 9 a.m., 6 h after the last dexamethasone dose. Patients with functional adrenal adenomas show no suppression of cortisol levels in the 48-h sample relative to the initial (baseline) sample. About 78% of patients with pituitary source of excess ACTH showed >50% suppression of plasma cortisol while only 11% of patients with an ectopic source of excess ACTH had a >50% suppression	
Comprehensive, 6-Day, Low-/High-Dose Dexamethasone Test	This protocol incorporates the low- and high-dose dexamethasone tests in succession. 24-h urinary free cortisol and/or 17-hydroxycorticosteroid (17-OHCS) measurement can help verify the results of serum cortisol and ACTH	
Gonadotropin-Releasing Hormone (GnRH) Stimulation Test	GnRH 100 µg IV. A sample for serum LH should be collected at 40 min after GnRH administration	
Metyrapone Stimulation (Overnight) Test	At 11 p.m., metyrapone 30 mg/kg (maximum 3 g) PO with a snack. On the following morning, at 8 a.m., measure serum cortisol and 11-deoxycortisol	

Abbreviations: GH, growth hormone; GNRH, growth hormone-releasing hormone; IV, intravenous; IM, intramuscular; PO, by mouth.

resulting in low total thyroxine (T4) but normal free T4 levels.[7] The combination of podophyllin and alkylating agents has also been reported to decrease TBG.[8] Both 5-fluorouracil[9] and mitotane[10] increase the total T4 and triiodothyronine (T3) levels without suppressing TSH, suggesting that these drugs increase thyroid hormone binding capacity in the serum.

Euthyroid Sick Syndrome Alterations in thyroid hormone metabolism occur in patients with cancer and other serious systemic illnesses.[11] Low serum T3 levels, which may be found in up to 70% of moderately to seriously ill cancer patients, are caused by a decrease in the extrathyroidal conversion of T4 to T3. Serum concentrations of free T4 are usually normal or high, while concentrations of free T3 are below normal or low. The patients are clinically euthyroid, and serum TSH level and TRH stimulation test results are normal.

In most patients with euthyroid sick syndrome, T3, T4, and TSH levels are normal. Clinical manifestations of hypothyroidism are usually absent, but assessment may be confounded by obtundation, edema, and hypothermia that may accompany severe illness. Low free T4 levels in the context of euthyroid sick syndrome usually indicate a grave prognosis, with a mortality rate of more than 50%. Although it is generally accepted that thyroid hormone therapy has no benefit, in practice it is sometimes difficult to differentiate between the euthyroid sick syndrome and secondary hypothyroidism. Judicious replacement of thyroxine at physiologic levels in these uncommon patients may be appropriate if there are no contraindications (eg, active ischemic heart disease).

Hypothyroidism

Thyroidectomy ■ Thyroidectomy may be performed for a variety of oncologic reasons in the management of thyroid cancer, head and neck cancer, or thyroid metastasis. Thyroid replacement is needed in this group of patients. In thyroid cancer patients supraphysiologic doses of thyroid hormone are adjusted to suppress TSH without overt hyperthyroid symptoms. In others, the dose of thyroid hormone should be adjusted to keep TSH in the normal range.

Radiation ■ Irradiation is an important cause of hypothyroidism (primary, secondary, and tertiary). Radiation-induced primary hypothyroidism is caused by thyroid cell destruction, inhibition of cell division, vascular damage, and possibly an immune-mediated phenomenon. Factors that increase the risk of developing primary hypothyroidism includes a high-radiation dose to the vicinity of the thyroid gland, duration since therapy, lack of shielding of the thyroid during therapy, and combined irradiation and surgical treatments.[12]

The incidences of hypothyroidism after radiation therapy for various cancers and conditions are tabulated in Table 135-2.[4,12-22] A relationship between radiation dose and the prevalence of hypothyroidism is based on studies of patients with Hodgkin disease.[15,18] Long-term follow-up of patients treated with low-dose radiotherapy suggests that the threshold for causing clinically evident hypothyroidism is approximately 10 Gy. For Hodgkin disease patients who received >30 Gy, the actuarial risk of hypothyroidism was up to 45% 20 years after irradiation.[15] Patients with frank or subclinical hypothyroidism should receive thyroid hormone replacement therapy.

Chemotherapy ■ The diagnosis of hypothyroidism in 14% of BMT patients who received chemotherapy, but did not receive total-body irradiation,[23] suggests a causal relation between hypothyroidism and high-dose combination cytotoxic chemotherapy. This notion is also supported by studies that showed an increased incidence of primary hypothyroidism in patients treated with multiple combination drug regimens[24,25] with or without radiation.[24] L-Asparaginase, in addition to inhibition of TBG synthesis discussed earlier, may also inhibit TSH synthesis reversibly and lead to temporary hypothyroidism with decreased free T4 levels.[26]

Thyroid dysfunction is a recognized side effect of cytokine treatments. Treatment with interleukin-2 produces thyroid dysfunction in approximately 20-35% of patients.[27] These patients have hypothyroidism, hyperthyroidism, or hyperthyroidism followed by hypothyroidism.[28] Approximately 10% of interferon-treated patients develop primary hypothyroidism.[29] Pituitary enlargement secondary to interferon-induced hypothyroidism has also been reported.[30] Patients with antithyroid antibodies before therapy are at higher risk of cytokine-induced thyroid dysfunction.

Retinoid X receptor (RXR) ligands may be used in the treatment of certain malignancies such as cutaneous T-cell lymphoma. Bexarotene (an RXR-selective ligand) caused secondary hypothyroidism dose-dependently.[31] A single dose can rapidly suppress TSH in healthy subjects.[32] In addition to suppressing transcription of TSH by an RXR-mediated thyroid hormone-independent mechanism, bexarotene also increases metabolic clearance of thyroid hormones by a nondeiodinase-mediated pathway.[33]

Sunitinib is a multitarget small molecule inhibitor that inhibits platelet-derived growth factor receptors (PDGF-R) and vascular endothelial growth factor receptors (VEGF-R). Over 50% of sunitinib-treated patients have abnormal thyroid function tests. Most have symptomatic hypothyroidism.[34] Thyrotoxicosis can occur and is usually mild, self-limiting and rapidly progressed to hypothyroidism.[35] The mechanism of the antithyroid effect appears to be inhibition of peroxidase activity[36] as well as lymphocytic thyroiditis without circulating antithyroid antibodies.[37]

Sorafenib is another multitarget small molecule inhibitor that inhibits Raf kinase, PDGF-R, VEGF-R2 & 3, and c-Kit. About 20% of sorafenib-treated patients had thyroid dysfunction (predominantly hypothyroidism) and <10% needed thyroid hormone replacement.[38]

^{131}I-Containing Compounds ■ The use of ^{131}I for treatment of thyroid cancer requires a high serum TSH level. High-TSH level is achieved by either withholding thyroid hormone replacement or administration of recombinant human TSH. The use of ^{131}I-containing compounds in the treatment of other tumors may result in hypothyroidism. For instance, using high-dose (100-1,000 mCi) [^{131}I]-metaiodobenzylguanidine to treat unresectable pheochromocytoma may result in primary hypothyroidism.

Screening ■ Children who have received either head-and-neck or cranial irradiation should have a free T4 and a TSH measurement annually for 5 years and every 2 years thereafter. Early detection of abnormal T4 and TSH levels will permit medical intervention before hypothyroidism adversely affects physical and intellectual development and growth. In adults, neck irradiation for treatment of lymphoma and various head and neck tumors is associated with a high incidence of primary hypothyroidism. Patients who have received irradiation should have free T4 and TSH levels measured annually for 5 years, and then every other year for 10 years, and thereafter every 5 years for another 10 years. Once hypothyroidism is diagnosed, the patient should receive thyroid hormone replacement therapy.

Hyperthyroidism ■ Radiation-induced painless thyroiditis with hyperthyroxinemia is an uncommon side-effect of external beam radiotherapy to the head and neck area. Transient hyperthyroidism may occur as a result of inflammation and destruction of thyroid tissue with release of thyroglobulin (containing thyroxine or triiodothyronine) and is usually followed by hypothyroidism. Transient hyperthyroidism has been reported after mantle radiotherapy in Hodgkin disease patients, and occurs usually within 18 months of treatment.[39] A low uptake of radioiodine in most of these cases suggests a diagnosis of silent thyroiditis, but some have Graves disease. In one series of Hodgkin disease patient treated with radiation, the risk of Graves disease in these patients was estimated to be at least 7.2 times that in a healthy population.[15]

Ophthalmopathy, similar to that in Graves disease, has been reported within 18-84 months of high-dose radiotherapy to the neck for lymphoma, breast cancer, and nasopharyngeal or laryngeal cancer. Ophthalmopathy may occur without hyperthyroidism and in the absence of the human leukocyte antigen-B8.[40] This suggests that radiation-induced thyroid injury may induce an autoimmune process that is similar to Graves disease.

Thyroid Nodules and Cancers ■ Low-dose radiation increases the risk of thyroid nod-

Table 135-2 **Incidence of Hypothyroidism (Including Compensated Hypothyroidism) After Radiotherapy[a]**

Type of Malignancy or Conditions	Radiation Dose	% with Hypothyroidism
Hodgkin disease	30-60 Gy	30-50
Head and neck cancer	40-72 Gy	25-50
Lymphoma	20-40 Gy (median 36 Gy)	30-42
Breast carcinoma	?	15-21
Total-body irradiation in BMT	13.75-15 Gy	15-43

[a]Data based on Refs. 12 to 22.
Abbreviation: BMT, bone marrow transplantation.

ules and cancer. The association between thyroid cancer and low-dose irradiation has been extensively examined[41] and is discussed in Chapter 74. High-dose radiation therapy is also associated with an increased prevalence of thyroid nodules.[42] About 25% of patients who had received high-dose radiotherapy for childhood malignancies had palpable thyroid nodules 5-34 years after therapy.[43] Radiation-induced thyroid nodules are common sequelae of head and neck cancer treatments and are also found in breast cancer patients whose radiation field included the lower neck. High-dose radiation (>40 Gy) exposure to the thyroid increases the risk of thyroid cancer by approximately 3-fold in adults,[44] and approximately 13-fold in children.[45] The latent period from radiotherapy to the diagnosis of thyroid cancer can be up to 30 years. About 75-90% of radiation-induced thyroid cancers are papillary carcinomas. The frequency of palpable abnormalities increases with time after radiation, indicating a need for regular thyroid examination in such patients. Thyroid irregularities should be evaluated by ultrasonography and fine-needle aspiration biopsy. Figure 135-2 outlines the diagnostic approach to thyroid nodules in cancer patients.

Metastasis to the Thyroid ■ In autopsy series, the incidence of metastasis to the thyroid gland varies from 1.25% to 24%. The primary tumor site includes the kidney (33%), lung (16%), breast (16%), esophagus (9%), and uterus (7%).[46] Hypothyroidism secondary to metastatic infiltration and replacement of the thyroid by cancer is extremely rare. Thyrotoxicosis has been reported in patients with thyroid metastasis from lymphoma and pancreatic cancer. In these cases, the etiology of thyrotoxicosis is probably follicular destruction resulting in unregulated release of thyroid hormone and thyroglobulin. Intrathyroidal metastasis is most commonly treated by surgical removal of the lobe containing the metastatic cancer.

Energy Balance and Glucose Metabolism

Obesity and Metabolic Syndrome ■ Cancer treatments may lead to obesity and the metabolic syndrome.[47-49] The metabolic syndrome is a cluster of abnormalities consisting of central obesity, dyslipidemia, hyperglycemia, and hypertension that increases the risk of type 2 diabetes and cardiovascular disease. Obesity is a modifiable risk factor for carcinogenesis as well as cancer progression. The mechanisms by which obesity promotes cancer include: hyperinsulinemia due to insulin resistance, high IGF-1, adipokines, low adiponectin, increased production of estrogens by adipose tissue, and increased inflammation. Obesity in cancer survivors may place them at increased risk for poor disease outcomes.[47,50,51] Obesity increases the risk of colorectal and genitourinary second primary cancers.[52] Although low levels of physical activity in cancer survivors may have contributed to obesity, the pathophysiologic basis of the weight gain is unclear. Since obesity is an adverse prognostic factor for many cancers and it is a modifiable risk factor, this secondary obesity after cancer treatment needs to be addressed.

Diabetes Mellitus ■ Diabetes mellitus type 2 (DM2) is associated with an elevated risk of pancreatic, liver, colon, gastric, breast, and endometrial cancer.[53-58] Extensive epidemiologic data suggest important roles of diabetes in carcinogenesis[53-58] and cancer survival.[59] The strongest association is perhaps with pancreatic cancer.[60-64] Apart from the frequently coexisting obesity, the mechanisms by which diabetes promote cancer include: hyperinsulinemia, high IGF-1, and hyperglycemia. Hyperglycemia per se has a promoting effect on cancer proliferation. In male, cancer survivors with a fasting serum glucose concentration ≥126 mg/dL had a higher relative risk for hepatopancreatobiliary second primary cancer.[52] Evidence-based guidelines for the management of DM2 in cancer patients to optimize patient survival is lacking.

The administration of glucocorticoids (eg, in combination therapy regimens, for edema of brain metastasis, for prevention of transplant rejection, for graft-vs-host disease in BMT, and for nausea/vomiting) is probably the most common cause of diabetes mellitus in cancer patients. Therefore, patients who receive glucocorticoids must be periodically screened for diabetes with evaluation of fasting glucose levels during therapy. Treatment with streptozocin[65] or L-asparaginase[66] may result in insulin-deficient diabetes mellitus. Although there is no evidence of a delayed onset of diabetes mellitus following treatment with streptozocin, follow-up has been limited and short-term. For long-term survivors treated with streptozocin, periodic screening for delayed development of diabetes mellitus may be indicated. Diabetes mellitus may also develop as a consequence of serious pancreatitis secondary to treatment with L-asparaginase. Immunotherapy for cancer using cytokines such as interleukin-2 and interferons may cause toxicity to pancreatic β-cells and lead to insulin-dependent diabetes.[67] Tacrolimus, an immunosuppressive agent used to prevent graft-vs-host disease in BMT, also increases the incidence of diabetes, perhaps by damaging pancreatic β-cells.[68] Patients who received allogenic BMT are likely to be receiving both glucocorticoids, cyclosporine A and tacrolimus, and are particularly at risk for developing diabetes mellitus.[69] Management of the blood glucose levels would depend on the severity of the blood glucose level abnormality and on the underly-

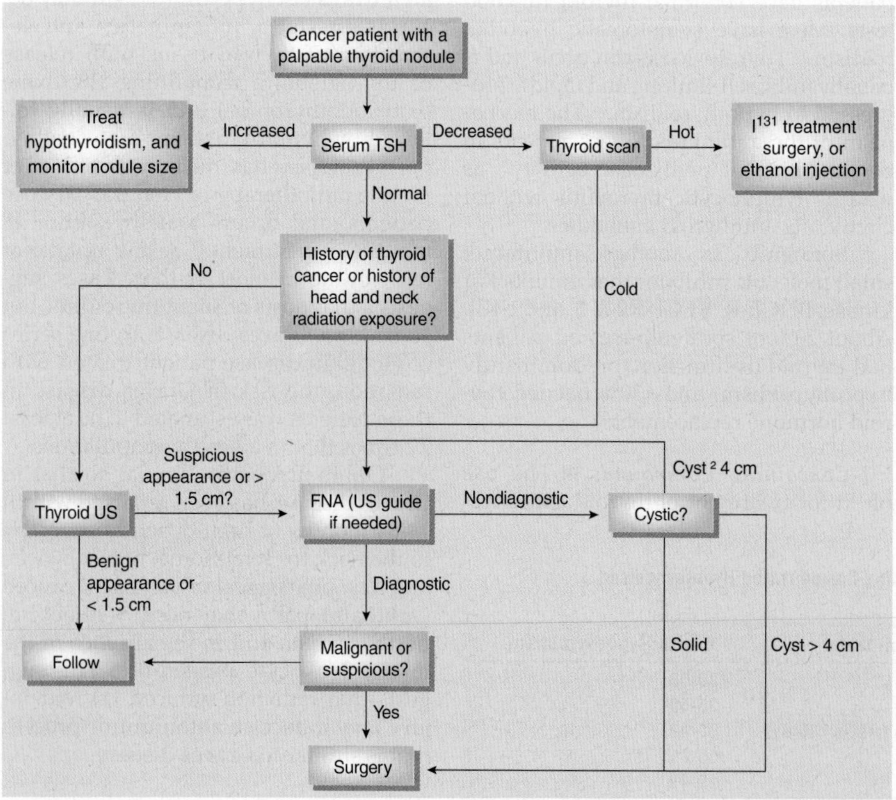

Figure 135-2 ■ Approach to a cancer patient with a thyroid nodule.

ing pathophysiologic mechanism of the increase in blood sugar. In general, insulin will be needed in patients who are insulin-deficient.

Metabolic Bone Diseases

Osteoporosis ■ Four groups of adult patients are at particular risk for accelerated bone loss and osteoporosis: (1) patients with lymphoma, myeloma, or leukemia, (2) women with breast cancer treated with cytotoxic chemotherapy frequently undergo an early menopause[70] and cannot receive estrogen-replacement therapy, (3) postmenopausal women with estrogen-receptor positive breast cancer, and (4) men with prostate cancer who are on antiandrogenic therapy and made hypogonadal. Normal bone remodeling involves a delicate balance between bone formation by osteoblasts and bone resorption by osteoclasts. Antineoplastic therapy is toxic to osteoblast function and decreases bone formation. Production by the tumor of hormonally active substances (eg, parathyroid hormone-related protein [PTHrP], lymphotoxin, interleukin-1, and interleukin-6) may contribute to the clinical picture of bone loss. In most cases, it is not clear whether bone loss is caused by antineoplastic therapy or by the underlying disease process and its effects (including cachexia, malnutrition, poor calcium, and vitamin D intake, or a combination of these). In patients with breast or prostate cancer, sex steroid hormone deficiency is the most important cause of bone loss. Bone loss is prominent in patients with several disorders (myeloma, leukemia, lymphoma) affecting hematopoietic cells, perhaps because of cytokine production and an intimate relationship of hematopoietic cells with bone-forming cells or the use of high dose or prolonged therapy with glucocorticords.

A number of drugs can induce osteoporosis.[71] In cancer patients, glucocorticoids, methotrexate, and cytotoxic drugs that cause renal loss of calcium, magnesium, or phosphorus (eg, platinum compounds, cyclophosphamide, ifosfamide) have significant impact on bone density. Osteoporosis (generalized or localized) is observed in children receiving methotrexate therapy for acute lymphoblastic leukemia (ALL).[72] The osteoporosis improves significantly after cessation of methotrexate therapy. Longitudinal study of ALL patients showed that the leukemic process, high-dose glucocorticoids, and hypomagnesemia (due to renal wastage following cyclical glucocorticoid and nephrotoxic chemotherapy or anti-infective agents) contributed to the impairment of calcium and vitamin D metabolism and decrease in bone mass at different stages of the treatment process.[73] Adjuvant chemotherapy for breast cancer (usually involving 5-fluorouracil, cyclophosphamide, and doxorubicin or methotrexate) is associated with low bone mass in premenopausal patients.[74] Bone loss during chemotherapy is substantial and may lead to increased risk of fracture. Post-treatment hypogonadism appears to be a major factor in these adult patients with osteoporosis. While tamoxifen has a slight protective effect on bone loss, the opposite is true for aromatase inhibitors. BMT usually involves treatment with high-dose cytotoxic drug, glucocorticoids, and immunosuppressive agents. In 24 patients who underwent BMT with high-dose chemotherapy, profound effects on bone biomarkers were observed.[75]

Prompt investigation of gonadal dysfunction in cancer survivors, and prompt replacement of gonadal steroids (in the absence of contraindications) in young hypogonadal men or women are recommended to decrease the risk of future bone fractures. The bone mass of long-term cancer survivors should be assessed when the patient is about 30 years old, the age at which most people have attained peak bone mass.[76] If bone mass is normal, no further evaluation is needed beyond the usual recommendations for prevention of osteoporosis. If it is abnormal (more than 2 standard deviations below), the patient should be referred for evaluation of the multiple reversible causes of osteoporosis.

A key point in the management of the osteoporosis syndrome in cancer patients is the use of bone mineral density measurement (eg, by dual-energy x-ray absorptiometry) to assess fracture risk and to monitor the effects of therapy. This measurement should be performed early in the course of management of the malignancy so that appropriate preventive measures can be implemented. The oncologist who is prescribing medications that are likely to decrease bone mass should consider active use of bisphosphonates (eg, alendronate, risedronate, or ibandronate), calcitonin, selective estrogen receptor modulators (SERMs), or teriparatide, in addition to a daily intake of 1200-1500 mg elemental calcium. Bisphosphonates are effective therapy for these patients. While osteoporosis in children with leukemia will frequently reverse because the children are in the formative years of bone development, in adults more active measures such as bisphosphonate or teriparatide therapy are necessary to prevent bone loss rather than waiting for the development of a fracture syndrome.

Another key point is correction of abnormal mineral and vitamin D metabolism by dietary supplements. Nutritional deficiency in teenagers and young adults result in lower bone mass. Treatment of hypocalcemia, hypomagnesemia, and vitamin D deficiency is integral to the successful therapy of osteoporosis in cancer patients. Recent studies document that clinically relevant vitamin D deficiency is present in 50% of the normal population; the percentage is almost certainly higher in patients undergoing cancer therapy.

Osteomalacia ■ Osteomalacia, a condition characterized by unmineralized bone matrix, is a rare complication of chemotherapy but should be considered in osteopenic patients and those with osteomalacic clinical syndrome (bone pain and proximal myopathy). The most common cause is a decrease in the serum calcium and/or phosphorus concentrations caused by nutritional deficiency and renal wasting of phosphorus and calcium. Patients who have received chemotherapeutic agents that cause hypophosphatemia, hypomagnesemia, or hypocalcemia are particularly at risk. Investigation of the levels of serum ionized calcium, phosphorus, magnesium, and vitamin D metabolites should be included in the initial evaluation. Appropriate replacement therapy of these vitamins and minerals should be instituted once deficiencies have been identified. Other contributing factors include systemic acidosis and drugs such as anticonvulsants and aluminum.[71] Tumor-induced osteomalacia will be addressed in the section that follows discussing paraneoplastic syndromes.

Ifosfamide causes tubular damage leading to renal phosphate wasting, hypophosphatemia, and rickets/osteomalacia.[77] The toxic effects of ifosfamide on renal tubular function include Fanconi syndrome in adults and children. Tubular damage is seen most commonly when ifosfamide is administered in doses of 50 g/m^2 or more, or when it is used in combination with cisplatin.[78] Rickets is reported most commonly in children. Estramustine, used in the treatment of prostate cancer, has been reported to increase bone resorption and at the same time cause hypocalcemia, hypophosphatemia, and secondary hyperparathyroidism.[79]

Adrenal Diseases

Adrenal Metastasis ■ Hematogenous metastasis to the adrenal glands is common, exceeded in frequency only by hematogenous metastasis to the lung, liver, and bone.[80] Autopsies have documented that 9-27% of patients who died from malignant illness had adrenal metastasis, with bilateral involvement in one-half to two-thirds of patients with adrenal metastasis.

The presence of adrenal metastasis may have important implications for diagnostic and therapeutic planning. When patients with cancer have an adrenal mass but no evidence of metastasis elsewhere, it is vital to determine whether this mass represents a metastatic deposit or a separate, unrelated adrenal lesion. Recent advances in imaging techniques have allowed the identification of adrenal lesions antemortem as part of the tumor-staging evaluation. The location of the adrenal glands in the perinephric fat allows the detection of almost all normal glands and contour-deforming masses as small as 5-10 mm. Computed tomography (CT) has a sensitivity and specificity in the detection of adrenal masses. Characteristics on CT examination that suggest adrenal metastasis rather than primary adrenal disease include heterogeneity, contrast enhancement, bilaterality, and size greater than 3 cm.[81]

Without other evidence of metastatic disease, whether the adrenal mass is actually a metastatic tumor is critical information in determining the appropriate therapy for the cancer. Evaluation of a patient who has a malignant adrenal mass should include a history and physical examination to elicit evidence of adrenal insufficiency, of Cushing syndrome, of mineralocorticoid excess, or of pheochromocytoma. Biochemical assessment should include a short ACTH stimulation test to rule out adrenal sufficiency. A 24-hours urine collection should be obtained to measure urinary free cortisol, aldosterone, catecholamines, and metanephrines. Pheochromocytoma must be excluded, especially if there is hypertension or an operative procedure of any type is contemplated. It has been reported that one-half of the patients who had a clinically unsuspected pheochromocytoma had clinical deterioration or even death immediately following a nonadrenal–related surgical procedure.[82]

If the biochemical assessment for pheochromocytoma is negative, CT-guided fine-needle aspiration should be considered. This procedure has a sensitivity of 85% in detecting cancer.[83] Magnetic resonance imaging (MRI) may be helpful in the diagnosis of pheochromocytoma. Functional scintigraphy using ^{131}I-6-iodomethyl-19-*nor*-cholesterol (NP-59) may be used in conjunction with CT and MRI to aid in the diagnosis of a unilateral adrenal mass greater than 2 cm.[84]

Adrenal Insufficiency ■ Despite the relatively high prevalence of adrenal infiltration by many common cancers, clinically evident adrenal hypofunction occurs infrequently, except when both adrenal glands are affected by metastatic disease.[85] It is estimated that more that 80% of adrenal tissue must be destroyed before corticosteroid production, under both basal and stress conditions, is impaired.[86] Because the clinical manifestations of adrenal insufficiency are nonspecific and overlap findings in cancer patients, a high index of suspicion is required to detect this treatable condition. The cachexia and weakness seen in patients with adrenal insufficiency can mimic the general wasting seen in patients with extensive metastatic disease. Electrolyte abnormalities can easily be explained by poor intake, malnutrition, side effects of chemotherapeutic agents, or paraneoplastic syndromes. Adrenal insufficiency may develop gradually and therefore be confused with cancer-associated cachexia.

Approximately 20-30% of the patients with bilateral adrenal metastasis will develop adrenal insufficiency.[85] These patients should all be evaluated by the ACTH stimulation test and should receive glucocorticoid- and mineralocorticoid-replacement therapy when adrenal insufficiency is suspected and until normal adrenal function is documented. Patients who are stable should receive 20 mg of hydrocortisone in the morning and 10 mg in early afternoon. In the event of circulatory instability, sepsis, emergency surgery, or other major complications, stress dosages of parenteral glucocorticoid should be given (eg, hydrocortisone succinate 100 mg intravenously every 8 hours).

Other causes of primary adrenal insufficiency in cancer patients include autoimmune adrenalitis, adrenal hemorrhage, and granulomatous diseases. Many cancer patients may be immunocompromised. For example, patients with leukemia or lymphoma or patients who have undergone BMT are immunocompromised. In these patients, infection of the adrenal glands by cytomegalovirus, mycobacteria, or fungi may lead to adrenal insufficiency.

Adrenal insufficiency may be drug induced. Etomidate,[85] a common intravenous anesthetic, and ketoconazole, an antifungal drug, both inhibit the production of cytochrome P450-dependent enzymes in the glucocorticoid synthetic pathway. Aminoglutethimide and metyrapone are drugs that inhibit enzymes in steroidogenesis, and may cause adrenal insufficiency when used in the treatment of prostate, breast, and adrenocortical cancers. Mitotane, structurally related to the insecticide dichlorodiphenyltrichloroethane (DDT), has selective toxicity for normal and neoplastic adrenocortical cells. Adrenal insufficiency is commonly observed when mitotane is administered in doses necessary to treat adrenocortical cancer; glucocorticoid replacement therapy is mandatory in such patients.[10] Increased protein binding may lead to an increased daily requirement of glucocorticoids during replacement therapy. Suramin, recently proposed as an anticancer agent based on its activity against the tumor growth factors, may also cause adrenal insufficiency.

Secondary adrenal insufficiency because of metastasis to the pituitary or hypothalamus may also occur. The most common cause of secondary adrenal hypofunction, however, is exogenous glucocorticoid therapy that suppresses the hypothalamic–pituitary-adrenal axis. A prolonged course of therapy may lead to hypothalamic–pituitary suppression lasting for many months. Short periods of steroid therapy (ie, 1, 2, or 4 weeks) in patients with leukemia and lymphoma suppress adrenal function for 2-4 days in most patients, and for longer in some patients. In patients who have received glucocorticoids for more than 2 weeks, a tapering period of 10-14 days should be considered. This is especially true for chemotherapy regimens that included high-dose glucocorticoids such as those used in the treatment of acute leukemia and lymphoma. In addition, patients who have been treated within the past year with prolonged glucocorticoid courses should receive stress dosages of glucocorticoid if acute medical or surgical complications occur (eg, neutropenic fever with hypotension, acute typhlitis). Irradiation of the hypothalamic–pituitary region causes ACTH deficiency and secondary adrenal insufficiency in 19-42% of treated patients (Fig. 135-1). Several diagnostic approaches have been used to evaluate secondary adrenal insufficiency, including basal 8 am serum cortisol measurements and dynamic tests with 1 μg of synthetic ACTH(1-24), insulin-induced hypoglycemia, or metyrapone.

Disorders of Growth Hormone Secretion and Growth

Childhood cancer or its treatment commonly impairs growth. Medulloblastoma and ALL, common childhood malignancies, are frequently treated with cranial or craniospinal irradiation and/or chemotherapy. Close to 40% of adult survivors of childhood brain cancer are below the 10th population percentile for height, and the risk factors for short stature are young age at diagnosis and radiation treatment affecting the hypothalamic–pituitary axis.[87] GH-deficiency and damage to the osseous growth plates are two common mechanisms of growth retardation.

Cranial irradiation may cause hypothalamic or pituitary dysfunction. The hypothalamus appears to be more radiosensitive than does the pituitary gland and may be damaged by lower radiation doses (<40 Gy). Higher doses (>40 Gy) are likely to damage both hypothalamic and pituitary function. Deficiency of one or more pituitary hormones following irradiation of the hypothalamic/pituitary area occurs in almost 100% of patients 5 years after irradiation (see Fig. 135-1).

GH deficiency is the most frequently noted deficiency and often the first deficiency to arise after cranial irradiation. Isolated GH deficiency following irradiation is common, and the effects are dose-related. At lower doses (20-24 Gy), the only effect may be an altered GH secretory pattern and subnormal response to insulin-induced hypoglycemia. With intermediate and higher doses, the GH response to arginine is impaired, and the frequency and amplitude of pulsatile GH secretion is decreased.[5] At doses up to 30 Gy, abnormal GH secretion and growth retardation are observed in more than 35% of patients, necessitating GH treatment.[88]

In addition to growth retardation caused by GH deficiency, craniospinal, or spinal irradiation for hematologic malignancy or central nervous system tumors and total-body irradiation prior to BMT may cause two other effects. First, irradiation affects the growth plates in vertebral bodies and in the pelvis and decreases vertebral growth. Second, irradiation causes resistance to GH or insulin-like growth factors.

Children treated with chemotherapy for malignancy frequently have a period of reduced growth velocity, followed by a "catch-up" growth phase. Systemic illness seems to be the most important component of growth retardation these children, although chemotherapy may play a significant role. Both growth velocity and height are lower in children who are treated with higher doses of chemotherapy and for a longer duration with combination chemotherapy than in those who receive regular therapy or less-intensive chemotherapy. If there is no catch-up growth after 1.5-2 years, it is important to exclude GH deficiency.

In adults, GH deficiency is thought to cause decreased bone and muscle mass, lower exercise capacity, increased adipose tissue, fatigue, a poor sense of well-being, impaired myocardial function, and increased cardiovascular risks. GH replacement may be indicated to improve the patients' quality of life and sense of well being,[89] but the concern over IGF-1-induced reactivation of malignant disease should be factored into the decision.

Disorders of Electrolyte/Mineral Metabolism

Hyponatremia ■ Risk factors for hyponatremia include treatment-induced nausea and vomiting, certain chemotherapy agents, hydration with hypotonic fluid, pain, opiates, and stress (both physical and psychological). In a prospective study of inpatient cancer patients, the incidence of hyponatraemia is 3.7% with sodium depletion and syndrome of inappropriate antidiuretic hormone (SIADH) each accounting for about one-third of all causes.[90] SIADH is characterized by low-serum osmolality and inappropriately high-urine osmolality in the absence of diuretics, heart failure, cirrhosis, adrenal insufficiency, and hypothyroidism. In cancer patients, SIADH may be caused by vasopressin secreted by tumors (eg, up to 15% of small-cell lung cancers), abnormal secretory stimuli (eg, intrathoracic infection, positive pressure ventilation), or cytotoxicity affecting paraventricular and supraoptic neurons. It is also possible that chemotherapy-induced lysis of vasopressin-containing cancer cells leads to or worsens SIADH. Drug-induced renal salt wasting or tumor-induced salt wasting (mediated by atrial natriuretic peptide)[91] can also cause hyponatremia, serum hypoosmolality, elevated urinary sodium, and urinary osmolality. These SIADH-like syndromes are difficult to distinguish from SIADH when signs and symptoms of fluid volume depletion are subtle or absent. Nonetheless, there are convincing reports that provide evidence of chemotherapy-induced hypothalamic or pituitary damage in the context of SIADH. There are at least seven reports associating vincristine with SIADH, and some of these reports document inappropriately high serum levels of vasopressin.[92] Vinblastine has also been reported to cause severe hyponatremia and SIADH.[92] The presumed mechanism of vinca alkaloid-induced SIADH is paraventricular or supraoptic cell microtubular damage.

Cyclophosphamide therapy has been associated with hyponatremia and SIADH. Autopsy findings in a case of fatal hyponatremia induced by cyclophosphamide (1800 mg/m^2) suggest that cyclophosphamide directly affects the hypothalamus.[93] Those findings included infundibular necrosis, decreased intra-axonal secretory granules, and depletion of posterior pituitary vasopressin. Patients treated with lower doses of cyclophosphamide also develop hyponatremia, hypotonicity, urinary hypertonicity, and increased plasma vasopressin levels. Damage to the renal tubules and resulting defects in salt and water transport may be the major cause of hyponatremia associated with low-dose cyclophosphamide therapy.[94]

There are many reports of cisplatin-induced hyponatremia caused by renal salt wasting.[95] Several reports claim that cisplatin induces SIADH. The mechanism of cisplatin-induced hyponatremia is unclear, but it has been suggested that renal toxic effects of cisplatin, ie, decreased papillary solute content, and maximal urinary osmolarity, are the major factors rather than a direct effect of cisplatin on vasopressin secretion. In a majority of the patients who have elevated vasopressin levels, the vasopressin levels became suppressed after correction of hypovolemia.[95] Therefore, the stimulus for vasopressin release in these patients was probably hypovolemia caused by renal salt wasting.

Figure 135-3 outlines the algorithm for evaluation and treatment of hyponatremia. For hypovolemia and sodium loss, fluid and sodium replacement are

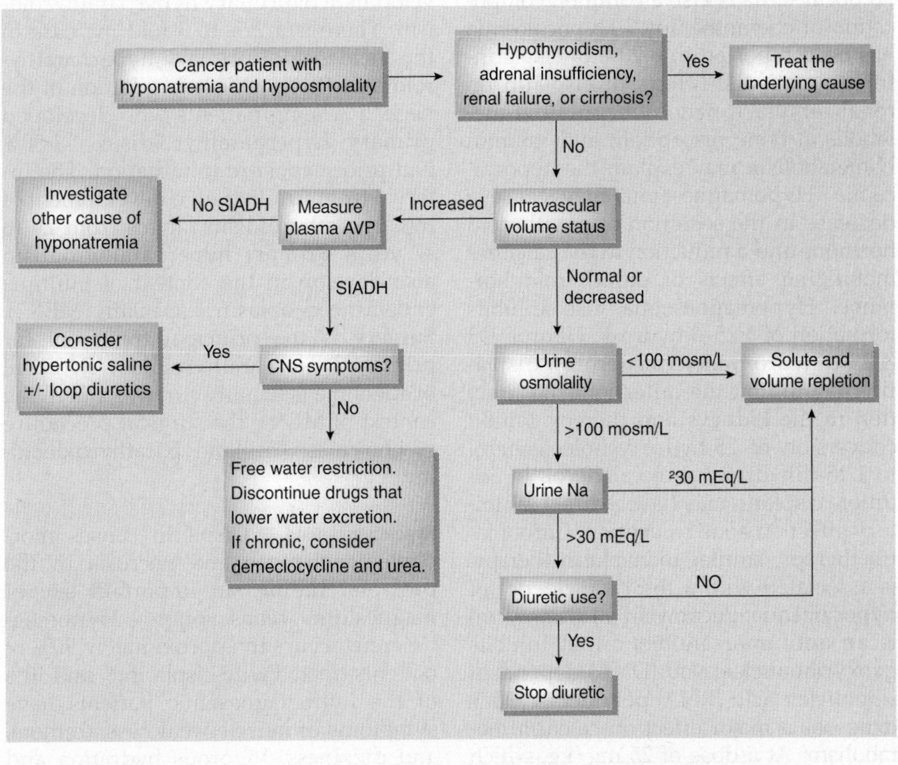

Figure 135-3 ■ Approach to evaluation of hyponatremia in a cancer patient.

the primary treatment. The AVP-receptor antagonists directly block the binding of AVP with its receptors. In clinical trials, conivaptan, lixivaptan, tolvaptan, and satavaptan effectively correct hyponatremia associated with SIADH, cirrhosis, or congestive heart failure, and this new class of drugs are likely to be useful for cancer-related hyponatremia.[96]

Hypernatremia ■ Hypernatremia secondary to central diabetes insipidus occurs frequently as a complication of neurosurgery or destruction by tumors of the anterior pituitary or the related hypothalamic nuclei. Nephrogenic diabetes insipidus can result from the effects of ifosfamide or streptozocin on tubular reabsorption of water. Ifosfamide has broad nephrotoxic effects, although tubular damage predominates. Distal tubular defects develop in about half of patients treated with ifosfamide. However, frank nephrogenic diabetes insipidus leading to hypernatremia is not common.[97] Streptozocin is another nephrotoxic drug; in addition to causing glomerular defects (proteinuria) and tubular defects (Fanconi syndrome), streptozocin therapy has been reported to cause nephrogenic diabetes insipidus.[98]

Hypocalcemia ■ Hypocalcemia may be one of the features of tumor lysis syndrome, which is discussed in Chapter 138. Hypocalcemia can also be caused by primary hypoparathyroidism after surgical procedures in the neck that sacrificed or damaged the parathyroid glands (eg, total laryngectomy, total thyroidectomy). Hypocalcemia is also a common complication of chemotherapy.[92] Hypocalcemia has been reported in 6-20% of cisplatin-treated patients. Effects of cisplatin on renal tubular function, magnesium metabolism, bone resorption, and vitamin D metabolism may explain the hypocalcemia. Hypomagnesemia may cause a decrease in the secretion of parathyroid hormone and a reduction in the calcium-mobilizing effects of parathyroid hormone. Hypomagnesemia also inhibits formation of 1,25-dihydroxy vitamin D3 (1,25-dihydroxycholecalciferol). Cisplatin may inhibit the mitochondrial function in the kidneys and thereby inhibit conversion of 25-hydroxycholecalciferol to 1,25-dihydroxy cholecalciferol. In addition, cisplatin may have a direct inhibitory effect on bone resorption. Carboplatin therapy, similar to cisplatin therapy, is associated with a 16-31% incidence of hypocalcemia. Plicamycin (mithramycin) is an antitumor antibiotic that inhibits deoxyribonucleic acid (DNA)-dependent ribonucleic acid (RNA) polymerase. This drug has a major effect on calcium metabolism. At a dose of 25 mg/kg, which is below the dose needed for antineoplastic effects, it inhibits bone resorption and lowers serum calcium concentration within 24-48 hours. Plicamycin inhibits basal- and thyroid hormone-stimulated osteoclast function by a mechanism that is unclear. The effect of plicamycin on osteoclast function has made plicamycin useful for treating Paget disease of the bone and osteoclast-mediated hypercalcemia associated with malignancy. The hypocalcemic effect of plicamycin, as well as its hepatic and renal toxicity, has limited its usefulness as an anticancer agent. Dactinomycin is another antitumor antibiotic that blocks DNA-directed RNA synthesis, causing hypocalcemia in animals. Dactinomycin also abolishes the calcium-mobilizing effect of thyroid hormone, presumably by interfering with osteoclast-mediated bone resorption. Asymptomatic hypomagnesemia, hypocalcemia, and hypoparathyroidism have also been reported in patients treated with a combination of doxorubicin and cytarabine.

Hypercalcemia ■ The incidence of hypercalcemia in cancer patients is approximately 1%.[99] Hypercalcemia in cancer patients is a poor prognostic sign associated with a short survival. The paraneoplastic syndrome of hypercalcemia of malignancy is discussed under "Endocrine Paraneoplastic Syndromes ('Ectopic' Hormone Production)." No chemotherapy has been identified as a cause of hypercalcemia. However, there is a clear association between low-dose (usually 2-7.5 Gy) external-beam irradiation of the head-and-neck area and subsequent development of primary hyperparathyroidism. There is a 2.5- to 3-fold increase in the incidence of primary hyperparathyroidism after low-dose irradiation of the neck.[100] Among patients who developed primary hyperparathyroidism, 14-30% had prior exposure to radiation. The interval from irradiation to development of hyperparathyroidism ranges from 29 to 47 years. Primary hyperparathyroidism also develop in the context of multiple endocrine neoplasm (especially MEN1). Surgery is the principal treatment for primary hyperparathyroidism. Removal of adenoma is usually curative, but in the context of MEN1, the surgical procedure of choice is 3.5-gland parathyroidectomy.[101]

Hypomagnesemia ■ Cisplatin causes morphologic changes and necrosis in the proximal tubule, an important site of magnesium reabsorption. Hypomagnesemia occurs in approximately 90% of patients treated with cisplatin,[102] and 10% of the hypomagnesemic patients have symptoms of muscle weakness, tremors, and dizziness. Vigorous hydration and the use of osmotic diuretics such as mannitol may prevent renal failure, but has little effect on renal magnesium wasting. Hypomagnesemia may persist long after cessation of cisplatin therapy. There are no large series in the literature addressing the incidence of hypomagnesemia, but the information from the manufacturer indicates that 60% of those taking cisplatin may be affected. Hypomagnesemia also occurs in patients who receive cyclophosphamide and carboplatin.

Disorders of Lipid Metabolism

Short-term lipid abnormalities caused by cancer therapy are generally of little clinical significance. However, major abnormalities can lead to acute complications. Interferons and vitamin A derivatives can cause significant increases in triglycerides that can lead to pancreatitis. Interferons cause hypertriglyceridemia by increasing hepatic and peripheral fatty acid production[103] and by suppressing hepatic triglyceride lipase.[104] Long-term treatment with interferon-α2 causes hypertriglyceridemia in approximately one-third of patients, most of whom had previous serum lipid abnormalities. Serum triglyceride levels of more than 1000 mg/dL are not unusual. In a case report, a therapeutic effect of diet and gemfibrozil was observed in the presence of continued interferon-α therapy.[105] All-*trans*-retinoic acid (tretinoin) and other derivatives, eg, 13-*cis*-retinoic acid (isotretinoin), have been used in the treatment of several malignancies, most notably head and neck cancers and acute promyelocytic leukemia. The effects on lipid metabolism are well characterized, although the mechanism of development of lipid abnormalities is less clear. These abnormalities include hypertriglyceridemia caused by elevated very-low-density lipoprotein levels, and hypercholesterolemia caused by increased low-density lipoprotein level. Retinoid-induced hypertriglyceridemia can cause stroke and pancreatitis. Hyperlipidemia associated with retinoid therapy has been treated with gemfibrozil or fish oil.

Sexual Dysfunction

Radiation treatment to the head may cause a broad spectrum of hypothalamic–pituitary abnormalities (Fig. 135-1). The resultant thyroid, GH, or adrenal deficiency may indirectly affect reproductive function. Sexual function is directly affected by hyperprolactinemia or gonadotropin deficiency, commonly observed in patients treated with >40 Gy of cranial irradiation.

Hyperprolactinemia occurs commonly (up to 50% incidence within 2 years) following head-and-neck irradiation with a median hypothalamic–pituitary radiation exposure of 50-57 Gy.[4]

Radiation damage to the hypothalamus leading to a loss of normal inhibition of prolactin secretion is the proposed mechanism of hyperprolactinemia. Hyperprolactinemia inhibits the secretion of gonadotropin by the pituitary and decreases the responsiveness of the pituitary to gonadotropin-releasing hormone, thereby causing secondary hypogonadism. Dopaminergic therapy can reverse this process, and it may be reasonable to proceed with a therapeutic trial if other anterior pituitary functions are normal.

Gonadotropin deficiency occurs commonly (up to 61%) in patients treated with irradiation for brain tumors.[106] In children, delayed puberty, absent menarche, and inadequate sexual development are significant problems related to gonadotropin deficiency. Early or even precocious puberty has been reported in patients treated with combined chemotherapy and cranial irradiation for ALL[107] or cranial irradiation for brain tumor.[108] This phenomenon occurs more frequently in female patients. Concomitant GH deficiency is frequently noted, although its role in the development of precocious puberty is unclear.

In adults, gonadotropin deficiency may cause sex-hormone deficiency and sexual dysfunction. Sex-hormone deficiency may alter libido and adversely affect bone and lipid metabolism. Sexual dysfunction and impotence need to be evaluated and appropriately treated. Figure 135-4 outlines a diagnostic algorithm for the evaluation of hypogonadism.

Gonadal complications were discussed in Chapter 134, and gonadal dysfunction caused by anticancer therapy has been reviewed.[92]

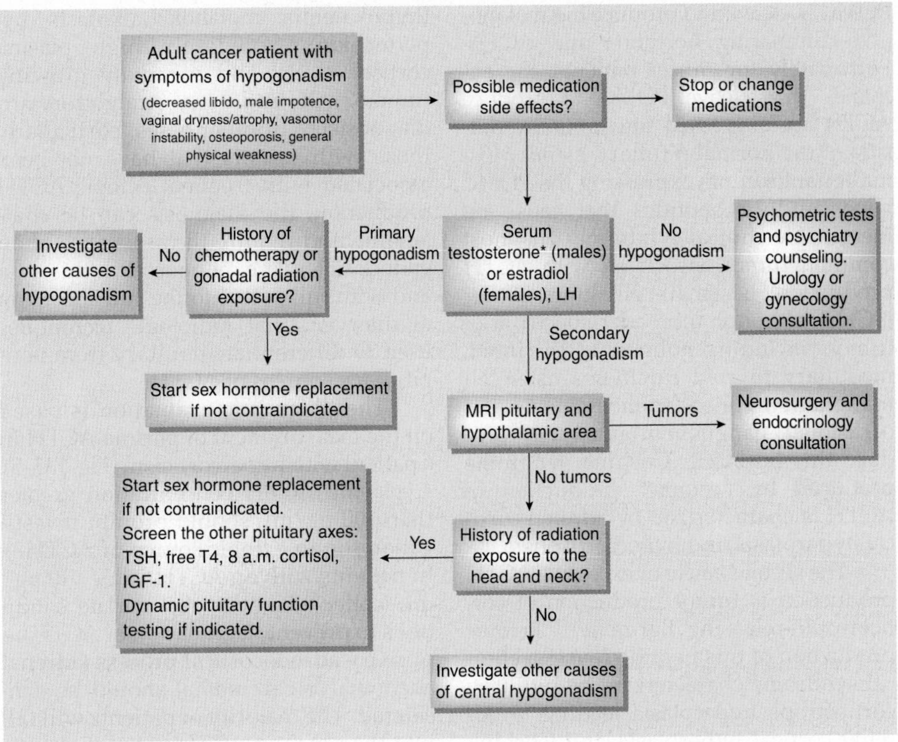

Figure 135-4 Approach to evaluation of hypogonadism in a cancer patient.

Endocrine Paraneoplastic Syndromes ("Ectopic" Hormone Production)

Among the more interesting and protean manifestations of cancer is the production of hormonal substances that produce unique clinical syndromes. These syndromes can be classified broadly into several different types. The first is the production of a hormonal substance by a cell type that normally produces the hormone. Examples include parathyroid hormone production by a parathyroid cancer, production of calcitonin by medullary thyroid carcinoma, and serotonin by carcinoid tumors. In each of these examples a malignancy of a differentiated cell type continues to produce its normal product, but does so in a manner that is largely independent of the normal regulatory processes. These clinical syndromes are discussed in the relevant chapters in this text that discuss these malignancies. The second type to be discussed in detail here is the "ectopic" production of a hormone by a cell type that does not normally produce the hormonal substance or produces it normally at very low levels. In some examples, the cell may have produced the hormonal product at an earlier stage in its development. An example of this is PTHrP production by a squamous cell carcinoma. PTHrP is normally expressed in differentiating squamous cells, but is not expressed or is expressed at low levels in differentiated squamous epithelium.[109] A second type of "ectopic" hormone production occurs in a hormone-producing cell whose machinery has been coopted to produce another hormone. An example of this is the production of ACTH by a wide spectrum of neuroendocrine tumor types, small-cell carcinoma of the lung being one example.

Production of peptides by neuroendocrine tumors comprises the most common of the "ectopic" hormone syndromes. Neuroendocrine cells are dispersed throughout nearly all organs. Prominent are lung, gastrointestinal tract, pancreas, thyroid gland, adrenal medulla, breast, prostate, and skin. These cells are most commonly derived from neural crest and produce biogenic amines and polypeptide hormones. The list of hormones produced by tumors derived from members of this group of neuroendocrine cells includes ACTH, calcitonin, vasoactive intestinal peptide (VIP), bombesin, growth hormone-releasing hormone (GHRH), pancreatic polypeptide, corticotropin-releasing hormone (CRH), neurotensin, somatostatin (SRIH), and other small peptides.

Defined Clinical Syndromes

There are clearly defined clinical ectopic hormone syndromes that occur with some frequency. Their recognition may help in the definition of the cancer type and lead to appropriate management approaches. In addition, these syndromes are a major cause of morbidity and mortality; treatment approaches are available for many of these syndromes and can improve both quality and duration of survival.

Ectopic ACTH Production Inappropriate secretion of ACTH, although uncommon, is an important cause of morbidity and mortality in certain types of malignancies. There are at least two different mechanisms: Ectopic ACTH production or ectopic production of CRH, the hypothalamic peptide that normally stimulates ACTH synthesis and release.

The most common cause of ectopic ACTH production is the expression of pro-opiomelanocortin (POMC) by a tumor. Post-translational processing of POMC normally proceeds down one of two mutually exclusive pathways.[110] The POMC precursor can be cleaved in two different ways to produce peptides with very different biologic activities. The pathway that leads to ACTH production and Cushing syndrome is one in which

POMC is cleaved to produce big melanocyte-stimulating hormone and ACTH. Fortunately for cancer patients, the enzymes that cleave POMC to produce ACTH are expressed uncommonly outside of the normal pituitary gland. Most malignant tumors expressing the *POMC* gene produce peptides that cause no identifiable clinical syndrome. The most common tumor associated with ACTH production is small-cell lung cancer (SCLC), although a broader spectrum of tumors including pulmonary carcinoid, medullary thyroid carcinoma, islet cell malignancy, pheochromocytoma, and occasional ganglioneuromas will produce this hormone. Cushing syndrome produced by "ectopic" production of ACTH is characterized by adrenal cortical hyperplasia and hypercortisolism.[111]

The second cause of excessive ACTH production is tumor production of corticotropin-releasing hormone.[112] Ectopic production of this peptide causes a clinical syndrome characterized by pituitary corticotrope hyperplasia leading to adrenal cortical hyperplasia and Cushing syndrome. Identification of excessive CRH production requires that the clinician consider this possibility and measure CRH in blood. Neoplasms that can produce CRH include medullary thyroid carcinoma, paragangliomas, prostate cancer, and islet cell neoplasms. There are examples of cancers that produce both ACTH and CRH.

Patients with ectopic ACTH syndrome may present with clinical features of Cushing syndrome—easy bruising, centripetal obesity, muscle wasting, hypertension, diabetes, and metabolic alkalosis predominate. Alternatively, patients with rapidly growing SCLC may present with a clinical syndrome characterized by wasting, muscle atrophy, profound hypokalemic metabolic alkalosis, and hypertension without the other clinical findings of Cushing syndrome.

The hallmark of ectopic ACTH syndrome is the finding of an elevated plasma ACTH concentration. However, in the differential diagnosis of hypercorticism with an elevated plasma ACTH concentration, the clinician should consider an ACTH producing pituitary tumor.[113] Differentiation between pituitary ACTH production (a primary pituitary tumor) and ectopic tumor production of ACTH or ectopic CRH production, mimicking a pituitary tumor, is among the most difficult diagnostic workups in the discipline of endocrinology. There are numerous examples where failure to correctly differentiate between ectopic ACTH production and a pituitary tumor producing ACTH has led to incorrect treatment.[114] In some cases, such as ectopic ACTH production by a SCLC, the clinical syndrome (hypokalemia, metabolic alkalosis, hypertension, exceedingly high plasma cortisol levels, and a rapidly growing tumor) will lead to a straightforward diagnosis).[115] In other cases, particularly those with tumors that have not been associated with frequent ectopic ACTH production, the diagnosis can be challenging and require the assistance of an endocrinologist experienced in this area and with full access to the full spectrum of interventional radiologic techniques used to differentiate pituitary from nonpituitary sources of ACTH.

The diagnostic evaluation is based on the measurement of plasma ACTH in a patient with hypercorticism (Fig. 135-5). A plasma ACTH concentration greater than 100 pg/mL should prompt investigation for an ectopic source of ACTH.[116] In patients with an ACTH value >10 pg/mL (collected under appropriate conditions to prevent degradation of ACTH), a primary adrenocortical process (adrenal adenoma or carcinoma) should be considered. The majority of patients will fall into the range of ACTH values between 10 and 100 pg/mL. The major differential diagnostic possibilities in these patients include a central (pituitary) or peripheral (ectopic) source of ACTH, with production of ectopic CRH by a tumor a rare possibility. Differentiation between central and peripheral sources of ACTH is accomplished by several approaches. The identification of a pituitary tumor by MRI provides a presumptive diagnosis of a pituitary source, although pituitary tumors that are nonfunctional or produce another hormonal product occur with some frequency. For this reason petrosal venous sinus sampling is often employed.[117] The diagnosis of ectopic CRH production can only be made by suspecting this diagnosis and measuring the plasma concentration of this peptide. It is also possible to use other approaches to diagnose ectopic ACTH syndrome. ACTH production from a tumor is not generally suppressed by a high-dose of dexamethasone. In patients with an ACTH > 10 pg/mL, administration of a single 8 mg oral dose of dexamethasone at 11:00 p.m. followed with measurement of serum cortisol level at 8:00 a.m. permits differentiation between central and peripheral sources.[111] In pituitary Cushing syndrome, dexamethasone will generally suppress ACTH by 50%; this strategy will not generally suppress ACTH production by a nonpituitary tumor. False-positive or false-negative results occur with each of these testing procedures.

Surgical removal or treatment of the tumor with chemotherapeutic agents is the primary therapy for an ACTH- or CRH-producing tumor. Patients with

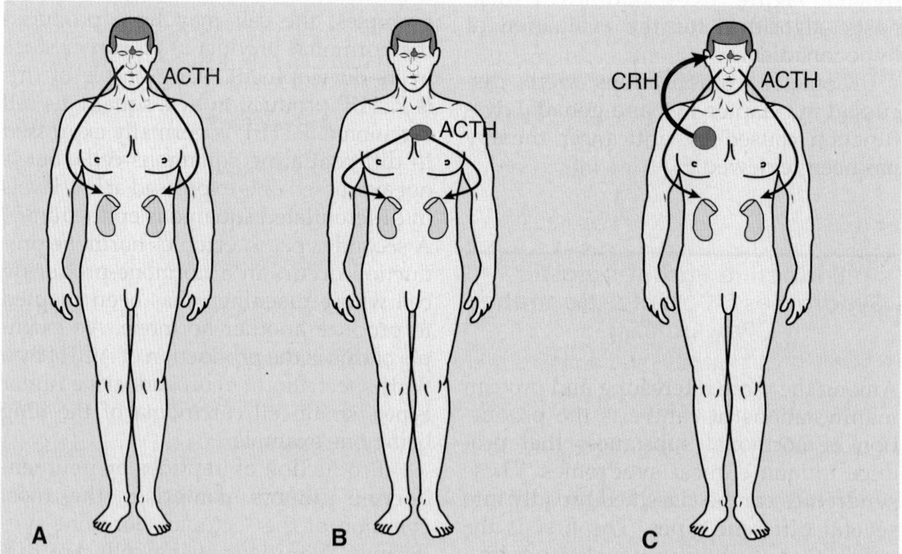

Figure 135-5 Differential diagnosis of adrenocorticotropin (ACTH)-dependent Cushing syndrome. It is difficult to differentiate between a pituitary (**A**) and ectopic (**B**) source of ACTH, the most common causes of ACTH-dependent Cushing syndrome. To differentiate with certainty, placement of catheters in veins draining the pituitary gland (inferior petrosal sinuses) combined with stimulation by exogenous corticotropin-releasing hormone permits differentiation with certainty (discussed in text). Ectopic corticotropin-releasing hormone (CRH) production by a tumor results in increased ACTH production by the pituitary gland (**C**). It is difficult to differentiate between ectopic CRH production and pituitary-dependent Cushing syndrome, necessitating the measurement of CRH in peripheral blood to make the diagnosis with certainty. Malignant tumors occasionally produce both CRH and ACTH, further complicating the diagnostic evaluation (not shown).

these tumors should have electrolyte abnormalities, diabetes mellitus, and hypertension corrected prior to a planned surgical procedure. Patients with long-standing Cushing syndrome and elevated plasma cortisol values have higher morbidity and mortality postoperatively. Preoperative treatment options include metyrapone (1-4 g/day orally; available only from the manufacturer), aminoglutethimide (250 mg orally four times per day with upward titration), or ketoconazole (200-400 mg twice a day orally).[118,119] Parenteral etomidate, used for sedation and induction of anesthesia, rapidly inhibits cortisol synthesis at subhypnotic-subhypnotic concentrations.[120] It is titrated from 0.3 to 4 mg/kg/hour to normalize serum cortisol measurements and has been used to rapidly reverse hypercorticism in a small number of patients. Replacement glucocorticoid therapy is needed when pharmacologic inhibitors of cortisol production are used to prevent adrenal insufficiency. If surgical removal of an ACTH- or CRH-producing tumor is not possible or inadvisable, chronic therapy with inhibitors of cortisol synthesis may be required. Alternatively, laparoscopic adrenalectomy with subsequent replacement of corticosteroids provides a rapid and generally safe approach to management of hypercorticism. This technique is probably underutilized as a therapeutic strategy for management of ectopic ACTH syndrome.

Patients with rapidly progressive SCLC and ectopic ACTH syndrome form a unique subset of patients because of the need to initiate chemotherapy on a timely basis. Unfortunately, these patients are also highly susceptible to opportunistic infections and initiation of therapy will often lead to death or serious morbidity related to infection.[121] The central dilemma in these patients is that a period of 1-2 weeks may be required for pharmacologic inhibitors of cortisol synthesis to normalize the serum cortisol (and a longer period may be required for normalization of immunity), a delay in the initiation of chemotherapy that is generally deemed unacceptable from an oncologic perspective. Laparoscopic adrenalectomy, a straightforward and well-tolerated technique following normalization of electrolyte abnormalities and hypertension, may provide a strategy for rapid normalization of excessive cortisol secretion. Prophylactic therapy for opportunistic infections caused by pneumocystis carinii or fungi should be considered if chemotherapy is initiated shortly after normalization of the serum cortisol.

Hypercalcemia Caused by Malignancy ■ Hypercalcemia is a common and serious cause of morbidity and mortality in cancer patients.

The most common causes of hypercalcemia in patients with cancer are PTHrP-mediated hypercalcemia, increased production of the active metabolite of vitamin D, calcitriol or 1,25 dihydroxy vitamin D3, and localized osteolytic hypercalcemia.[122,123] Ectopic production of PTH is a rare cause of cancer-associated hypercalcemia. Other causes of hypercalcemia, most notably primary hyperparathyroidism, should be considered in the cancer patient with hypercalcemia. Measurement of serum intact parathyroid hormone (iPTH) permits differentiation between hyperparathyroidism and a number of other causes of hypercalcemia. The combination of hypercalcemia and an elevated parathyroid hormone level combined with increased urinary calcium excretion provides reasonable evidence for primary hyperparathyroidism. Suppression of the iPTH below the normal range is found in PTHrP or calcitriol-mediated hypercalcemia. Other less common causes of hypercalcemia in cancer will be discussed below.

PTHrP ■ PTHrP is a small peptide in which 8 of the first 16 amino acids are identical to PTH. This small peptide causes hypercalcemia by binding to the PTH receptor and activating the expression of an osteoblast-specific cell surface protein, RANK ligand (RANKL). Interaction between RANKL and the RANK receptor on the osteoclast precursor causes increased osteoclast differentiation, bone resorption, and hypercalcemia. Other PTH-like actions of PTHrP include hypophosphatemia and increased urinary calcium excretion. PTHrP-mediated hypercalcemia is characterized by a suppressed iPTH level and a low or normal calcitriol level. This contrasts with the finding of elevated iPTH and calcitriol levels in primary hyperparathyroidism. PTHrP production is found commonly in squamous cell carcinomas; other tumors that produce it include: breast, neuroendocrine, renal, melanoma, and prostate tumors.

Calcitriol Production by Malignant Tumors ■ Lymphoma commonly produces calcitriol, leading to increased gastrointestinal absorption of calcium. Lymphomatous tissue, like granulomatous tissue seen in sarcoid, berylliosis, tuberculosis, and fungal infection, expresses 1α-hydroxylase, the enzyme that converts 25-hydroxy vitamin D3 to calcitriol. Clinical studies show that a high percentage of lymphoma patients have hypercalciuria at the time of diagnosis; a smaller percentage have frank hypercalcemia.[124] The characteristic clinical features of hypercalcemia in the context of lymphoma include a suppressed serum iPTH, a normal or slightly increased phosphorus level (caused by the suppression of PTH), hypercalciuria, absence of bone metastasis, and an elevated serum calcitriol level in approximately one-half of hypercalcemic patients.[124]

Localized Osteolytic Bone Resorption Causing Hypercalcemia ■ Certain malignancies metastasize to bone frequently and some cause hypercalcemia. Hypercalcemia associated with breast cancer and myeloma is common. In contrast, prostate cancer, despite its more frequent presence in bone, rarely produces hypercalcemia. Malignancies that cause hypercalcemia produce cytokines, PTHrP, or other factors that stimulate increased bone resorption.[122,123] Perhaps the best characterized is the production of PTHrP by breast carcinoma cells. There is compelling evidence in animal models that PTHrP production by breast cancer cells stimulates osteoclastic resorption and release of transforming growth factor (TGF)-β from normal bone. In this animal model TGF-β release from bone stimulates proliferation of breast carcinoma growth, setting up a loop in which PTHrP production not only stimulates increased osteoclastic resorption, but also accelerates growth of adjacent breast cancer.[125,126] Indeed, this thought process led to an examination of and subsequent approval of bisphosphonates, a class of drugs that inhibits osteoclast bone resorption, for prevention of breast cancer metastasis.[127,128]

In multiple myeloma several factors contribute to localized osteolysis. Increased expression of RANKL causing localized osteoclast proliferation appears to be the most important cause. Other factors that may contribute to osteoclast proliferation in myeloma are interleukin-6 and macrophage inflammatory protein 1α, although they appear to be less important than RANKL.[123]

Impact of Malignancy-Related Hypercalcemia ■ Severe hypercalcemia in the context of malignancy is associated with a shortened life span. The average survival for patients with severe and unresponsive hypercalcemia can be measured in weeks to months. The causes of death include complications of hypercalcemia (coma, renal failure) and progression of tumor. The development of hypercalcemia is often, although not always, an indicator of tumor progression in the face of adequate therapy. Since it is not always possible to predict which patients will respond to oncologic therapy, it is important to treat hypercalcemia in all newly diagnosed patients with cancer. Whether to continue to treat recurrent and/or refractory hypercalcemia is a decision that should be based on response of the causative tumor to oncologic therapy and the overall prognosis of the patient. Severe hypercalcemia frequently causes depression of cerebral function or coma, a clinical situation that may reduce suffering in a dying patient.

Therapy of Hypercalcemia ■ Dehydration is a common finding in hypercalcemic patients. Increased urine excretion of calcium causes a concentrating defect leading to increased fluid loss. Initial management should focus on the reversal of dehydration by infusion of a solution of normal saline at rates between 100 and 300 mL/hour. Hydration will commonly lower the serum calcium by 10-40% over a period of 6-12 hours. Patients with severe hypercalcemia, defined as a serum calcium concentration >13 mg/dL (3.25 mmol/L), an alteration of mental status, or evidence of renal dysfunction attributable to hypercalcemia should be treated with either intravenous pamidronate (60-90 mg over 4 hour) or zoledronate (4 mg over 30 minutes),[129] glucocorticoids (40-60 mg/day prednisone equivalent), or gallium nitrate (200 mg/m^2/day, infused daily for 7 days).[130,131] Salmon calcitonin may lower the serum calcium concentration by 1-2 mg/dL early in the treatment course, but is rarely effective long-term. These drugs are sometimes used in combination or sequentially in a patient who is poorly responsive. Glucocorticoids, which inhibit calcium absorption, are most commonly used as primary therapy for lymphoma, whereas bisphosphonate therapy is more likely to be effective in hypercalcemia associated with solid tumors. Zoledronate is generally more effective than pamidronate because of its increased potency.[132] Use of bisphosphonates for long-term treatment of bone metastasis has been associated with development of osteonecrosis of the jaw in 1-2.5% of treated patients. This has not been an issue in patients treated short-term for hypercalcemia associated with malignancy.

There are several new therapies for treatment of hypercalcemia in early stages of development that show considerable promise. A monoclonal antibody directed against RANKL prevents its interaction with the RANK receptor on osteoclast precursors, thereby reducing osteoclast-mediated bone resorption.[133] Preliminary studies with this antibody (denosumab) have shown it to be an effective inhibitor of bone resorption and clinical studies are currently underway to establish its efficacy in patients with hypercalcemia and bone metastasis.

Human Chorionic Gonadotropin ■ Human chorionic gonadotropin (HCG) is formed from two different protein subunits encoded by separate genes. The first is the α subunit that is shared by all members of the pituitary class of glycoprotein hormones including HCG, luteinizing hormone (LH), follicle-stimulating hormone (FSH), and thyroid-stimulating hormone (TSH). The second, the β subunit, is unique for each of these hormones. Production of HCG is found in trophoblastic tumors (choriocarcinomas, testicular embryonal carcinomas, and seminomas) and, uncommonly, in tumors of the lung and pancreas. In younger children, precocious puberty, caused by HCG stimulation of ovarian function, is seen. In adult males gynecomastia is a common occurrence. Hyperthyroidism may develop from an interaction of HCG with the thyroid-stimulating hormone receptor (TSHR) particularly when β-HCG is expressed at high levels.

Removal or effective therapy for the underlying tumor is the most effective therapy for clinical syndromes caused by excessive β-HCG production. Hyperthyroidism can be treated short-term with thionamide therapy if there is belief that chemotherapy or other strategies to treat the underlying malignancy are likely to be effective. In patients with less responsive tumors, thyroidectomy or radioactive iodine may be required.

Hypoglycemia ■ Tumor-induced hypoglycemia is an uncommon but challenging cause of morbidity for cancer patients. Three different clinical syndromes have been identified. First, insulin can be produced by islet cell malignancy. Islet cells tumors commonly produce low levels of insulin that are clinically insignificant until large tumor burdens, most commonly in the form of hepatic metastasis, develop. A second cause is insufficient gluconeogenesis, seen in patients with near complete replacement of hepatic parenchyma by tumor, interfering with or eliminating glucose production. The third form is caused by increased concentrations of insulin-like growth factor II (IGF-II), a peptide that activates the insulin receptor. This syndrome is most commonly seen in patients with fibrosarcomas, hemangiopericytomas, or hepatomas. In these patients, IGF-II levels are most commonly elevated, the result of a failure of IGF binding protein 3 (IGFBP3) and acid labile subunit to form a complex capable of binding IGF-II efficiently. The elevated circulating IGF-II activates the insulin receptor and causes hypoglycemia.[134-136]

The most common presentation for each of these clinical syndromes is fasting hypoglycemia and patients are most likely to develop symptoms during normal periods of fasting, particularly during nocturnal hours. Measurement of a plasma insulin, proinsulin, and C-peptide during a period of hypoglycemia is the most important diagnostic tool for separating the first clinical type (insulin production) from the second (replacement of liver by tumor) and third (IGF-II) types. The findings of elevated insulin, proinsulin, and C-peptide in the face of hypoglycemia (and the absence of any drugs that might stimulate insulin release from normal pancreas) make a compelling case for unregulated insulin production as a cause of the hypoglycemia. In contrast, insulin, proinsulin, and C-peptide levels will be low in tumor replacement of the liver or IGF-II–mediated hypoglycemia. Laboratory findings in IGF-II-mediated hypoglycemia include an elevated serum IGF-II, low or normal insulin, proinsulin, and C-peptide measurements, low IGF-I levels, and generally normal IGFBP3 or acid labile subunit measurements in the context of a large sarcoma or retroperitoneal tumor.

Surgical excision or antineoplastic therapy to reduce tumor mass is effective in insulin or IGF-II–mediated hypoglycemia; there is little effective therapy for hepatic replacement by tumor other than providing glucose. Hypoglycemia is treated with frequent meals. Patients may remain symptom-free by being awakened for caloric intake during nocturnal hours. A continuous infusion of 20% dextrose through a central venous line may be required to maintain normal blood glucose in patients, particularly those with hepatic replacement by tumors. Glucagon infusion (0.5-2 mg/hour) to stimulate hepatic gluconeogenesis is also an effective therapy for patients with insulin producing tumors or those with IGF-II–mediated hypoglycemia. It is important to document a response to glucagon (1 mg subcutaneously with measurement of plasma glucose at 30 and 60 minutes following injection) before trying this therapeutic approach. Glucagon can be administered in small volumes (1-5 mL over 24 hours), making it possible to use small infusion pumps.[137] Patients treated with glucagon may develop the characteristic rash associated with glucagonoma, necessitating discontinuance of this treatment modality. Other therapies that have been applied with periodic success include recombinant growth hormone (3-6 μg/kg subcutaneously daily) or glucocorticoids (20-40 mg prednisone equivalents per day). Octreotide or lanreotide have been used in patients with insulin-producing islet cell tumors, generally without success. The lack of success may relate to fact that somatostatin analogs currently available are more effective for inhibiting glucagon than insulin secretion. Diazoxide (3-8 mg/kg/day in 2-3 divided doses) has been used successfully to inhibit insulin secretion, but causes fluid retention, thereby limiting its usefulness at effective doses.

Hypoglycemia may also occur in patients with lactic acidosis in the context of end-stage leukemia or lymphoma. This clinical syndrome occurs in patients with end-stage or extensive disease and leukemic/lymphomatous involvement of the liver. It is hypothesized that lactic acid production by tumor cells exceeds the ability of the liver to clear it. The etiology of the hypoglycemia is unclear, but may result from impaired hepatic gluconeogenesis.[138]

SIADH ■ SIADH was discussed earlier (see "Disorders of Electrolyte/Mineral Metabolism: Hyponatremia") as a side effect of cancer therapy. In addition, approximately 15% of SCLC, 1% of other lung cancers, and 3% of squamous cell head-and-neck cancers produce vasopressin in an unregulated manner, leading to hyponatremia, hypoosmolality, increased urine sodium excretion, and an inappropriately high-urine osmolality relative to the plasma tonicity.[139] Other benign or malignant neoplasms that include primary brain tumors, hematologic neoplasms, skin tumors, and gastrointestinal, gynecologic, breast, and prostate cancers, and sarcomas, can also produce this clinical syndrome.

Most patients who develop this syndrome are asymptomatic. In cases where the serum sodium concentration falls <120 mEq/L, altered mental status and seizures may develop. In particular, women of reproductive age who develop hyponatremia may develop profound cerebral degeneration. Fluid restriction can be used effectively for short-term management, but treatment with demeclocycline (150-300 mg/day), an agent that inhibits the effects of vasopressin on the kidney, is preferable for long-term treatment. Vasopressin receptor antagonists, conivaptan, lixivaptan, tolvaptan, and satavaptan, have shown efficacy in clinical trials and at least one, conivaptan, is currently available in the United States in an intravenous form. Clinical trials of an orally administered form have shown evidence of efficacy.

Other Ectopic Hormone Syndromes

Tumor-Induced Osteomalacia ■ Severe hypophosphatemia caused by renal phosphate wasting is the hallmark of tumor-induced osteomalacia. This clinical syndrome is characterized by osteomalacia, caused by inadequate mineralization of osteoid, and moderate to severe proximal myopathy.[140] Tumors that produce this clinical syndrome include mesenchymal tumors (osteoblastomas, giant cell osteosarcomas, hemangiopericytomas, hemangiomas, nonossifying fibromas)[141] and, rarely, malignant tumors such as prostate or lung cancer. There is evidence that fibroblast growth factor-23, a member of the fibroblast growth factor family that is mutated in autosomal dominant osteomalacia,[142] is overexpressed by some neoplasms causing tumor-induced osteomalacia.[143] Oral or intravenous supplementation of phosphate combined with vitamin D therapy is generally effective for eradicating or improving clinical symptoms. Complete surgical removal of the tumor is generally curative.

Erythropoietin, Thrombopoietin, Leukopoietin, or Colony-Stimulating Factor Production ■ Polycythemia caused by ectopic erythropoietin production is a rare clinical syndrome. It is found in cerebellar hemangioblastoma, uterine fibroids, pheochromocytomas, and renal cell, ovarian, and hepatic cancers.[144,145] Treatment can include surgical or chemotherapy reduction of tumor mass or phlebotomy. Other less well-defined syndromes include production of thrombopoietin, leukopoietin, or colony-stimulating factor by some tumors. These conditions are treated by appropriate chemotherapy to reduce its size or by surgical removal.

Renin Production ■ Production of renin by renal (Wilms tumor, renal cell carcinoma, or hemangiopericytoma), lung (SCLC, adenocarcinoma), hepatic, pancreatic, or ovarian carcinomas can produce a clinical syndrome characterized by hypertension, hypokalemia, and evidence of increased aldosterone production.[146] Therapy with spironolactone, angiotensin-converting enzyme inhibitors, or angiotensin receptor antagonists may lower the blood pressure and normalize electrolyte abnormalities in patients in whom the tumor cannot be resected.

Growth Hormone and Prolactin ■ Acromegaly is a condition characterized by elevated growth hormone and IGF-1 values, most commonly caused by a pituitary tumor. There are uncommon examples of GH production by lung and gastric adenocarcinomas. Ectopic production of growth hormone releasing hormone, the hypothalamic peptide that normally regulates GH production by the pituitary,[147] has been demonstrated for islet cell tumors, bronchogenic carcinoids, and SCLC. Ectopic prolactin production is found rarely in gonadoblastoma,[148] lymphoma,[146] leukemia,[149] and colorectal cancer.[150] The clinical syndrome includes galactorrhea and amenorrhea in women and hypogonadism and gynecomastia in men. Dopamine agonists (bromocriptine, quinagolide, or cabergoline), effective for treatment of pituitary prolactinomas, are generally ineffective for treatment of ectopic prolactin production.

Selected References

The complete reference list can be found at www.CANCERMEDICINE8.com

1. Fassett DR, Couldwell WT. Metastases to the pituitary gland. *Neurosurg Focus.* 2004;16(4):E8.
2. Lam KS, Tse VK, Wang C, Yeung RT, Ho JH. Effects of cranial irradiation on hypothalamic-pituitary function—a 5-year longitudinal study in patients with nasopharyngeal carcinoma. *Q J Med.* 1991;78(286):165–176.
3. Pai HH, Thornton A, Katznelson L, et al. Hypothalamic/pituitary function following high-dose conformal radiotherapy to the base of skull: demonstration of a dose-effect relationship using dose-volume histogram analysis. *Int J Radiat Oncol Biol Phys.* 2001;49(4):1079–1092.
4. Samaan NA, Schultz PN, Yang KP, et al. Endocrine complications after radiotherapy for tumors of the head and neck. *J Lab Clin Med.* 1987;109(3):364–372.
5. Shalet SM. Disorders of the endocrine system due to radiation and cytotoxic chemotherapy. *Clin Endocrinol (Oxf).* 1983;19(5):637–659.
11. Chopra IJ. Clinical review 86: Euthyroid sick syndrome: is it a misnomer? *J Clin Endocrinol Metab.* 1997;82(2):329–334.
13. Grande C. Hypothyroidism following radiotherapy for head and neck cancer: multivariate analysis of risk factors. *Radiother Oncol.* 1992;25(1):31–36.
16. Constine LS, Donaldson SS, McDougall IR, Cox RS, Link MP, Kaplan HS. Thyroid dysfunction after radiotherapy in children with Hodgkin's disease. *Cancer.* 1984;53(4):878–883.
31. Sherman SI. Etiology, diagnosis, and treatment recommendations for central hypothyroidism associated with bexarotene therapy for cutaneous T-cell lymphoma. *Clin Lymphoma.* 2003;3(4):249–252.
32. Golden WM, Weber KB, Hernandez TL, Sherman SI, Woodmansee WW, Haugen BR. Single-dose rexinoid rapidly and specifically suppresses serum thyrotropin in normal subjects. *J Clin Endocrinol Metab.* 2007;92(1):124–130.
34. Rini BI, Tamaskar I, Shaheen P, et al. Hypothyroidism in patients with metastatic renal cell carcinoma treated with sunitinib. *J Natl Cancer Inst.* 2007;99(1):81–83.
38. Tamaskar I, Bukowski R, Elson P, et al. Thyroid function test abnormalities in patients with metastatic renal cell carcinoma treated with sorafenib. *Ann Oncol.* 2007.
42. Hancock SL, McDougall IR, Constine LS. Thyroid abnormalities after therapeutic external radiation. *Int J Radiat Oncol Biol Phys.* 1995;31(5):1165–1170.
49. Saquib N, Flatt SW, Natarajan L, et al. Weight gain and recovery of pre-cancer weight after breast cancer treatments: evidence from the women's healthy eating and living (WHEL) study. *Breast Cancer Res Treat.* 2007;105(2):177–186.
51. Kroenke CH, Chen WY, Rosner B, Holmes MD. Weight, weight gain, and survival after breast cancer diagnosis. *J Clin Oncol.* 2005;23(7):1370–1378.
53. Nilsen TI, Vatten LJ. Prospective study of colorectal cancer risk and physical activity, diabetes, blood glucose and BMI: explor-

ing the hyperinsulinaemia hypothesis. *Br J Cancer*. 2001;84(3):417–422.

54. Muti P, Quattrin T, Grant BJ, et al. Fasting glucose is a risk factor for breast cancer: a prospective study. *Cancer Epidemiol Biomarkers Prev*. 2002;11(11):1361–1368.
55. Verlato G, Zoppini G, Bonora E, Muggeo M. Mortality from site-specific malignancies in type 2 diabetic patients from Verona. *Diabetes Care*. 2003;26(4):1047–1051.
56. Richardson LC, Pollack LA. Therapy insight: influence of type 2 diabetes on the development, treatment and outcomes of cancer. *Nat Clin Pract Oncol*. 2005;2(1):48–53.
57. Coughlin SS, Calle EE, Teras LR, Petrelli J, Thun MJ. Diabetes mellitus as a predictor of cancer mortality in a large cohort of US adults. *Am J Epidemiol*. 2004;159(12):1160–1167.
62. Fisher WE. Diabetes: risk factor for the development of pancreatic cancer or manifestation of the disease? *World J Surg*. 2001;25(4):503–508.
63. Stolzenberg-Solomon RZ, Graubard BI, Chari S, et al. Insulin, glucose, insulin resistance, and pancreatic cancer in male smokers. *JAMA*. 2005;294(22):2872–2878.
69. Jindal RM, Sidner RA, Milgrom ML. Post-transplant diabetes mellitus. The role of immunosuppression. *Drug Saf*. 1997;16(4):242–257.
71. Jones G, Sambrook PN. Drug-induced disorders of bone metabolism. Incidence, management and avoidance. *Drug Saf*. 1994;10(6):480–489.
74. Bruning PF, Pit MJ, de Jong-Bakker M, van den Ende A, Hart A, van Enk A. Bone mineral density after adjuvant chemotherapy for premenopausal breast cancer. *Br J Cancer*. 1990;61(2):308–310.
76. Vassilopoulou-Sellin R, Brosnan P, Delpassand A, Zietz H, Klein MJ, Jaffe N. Osteopenia in young adult survivors of childhood cancer. *Med Pediatr Oncol*. 1999;32(4):272–278.
80. Abrams H, Spiro R, Goldstein N. Metastasis in carcinoma—one thousand autopsied cases. *Cancer*. 1950;3:74.
85. Redman BG, Pazdur R, Zingas AP, Loredo R. Prospective evaluation of adrenal insufficiency in patients with adrenal metastasis. *Cancer*. 1987;60(1):103–107.
87. Gurney JG, Ness KK, Stovall M, et al. Final height and body mass index among adult survivors of childhood brain cancer: childhood cancer survivor study. *J Clin Endocrinol Metab*. 2003;88(10):4731–4739.
88. Shalet SM, Clayton PE, Price DA. Growth and pituitary function in children treated for brain tumours or acute lymphoblastic leukaemia. *Horm Res*. 1988;30(2–3):53–61.
92. Yeung SC, Chiu AC, Vassilopoulou-Sellin R, Gagel RF. The endocrine effects of nonhormonal antineoplastic therapy. *Endocr Rev*. 1998;19(2):144–172.
96. Raftopoulos H. Diagnosis and management of hyponatremia in cancer patients. *Support Care Cancer*. 2007;15(12):1341–1347.
100. Cohen J, Gierlowski TC, Schneider AB. A prospective study of hyperparathyroidism in individuals exposed to radiation in childhood. *JAMA*. 1990;264(5):581–584.
102. Stewart AF, Keating T, Schwartz PE. Magnesium homeostasis following chemotherapy with cisplatin: a prospective study. *Am J Obstet Gynecol*. 1985;153(6):660–665.
109. Maioli E, Fortino V. The complexity of parathyroid hormone-related protein signalling. *Cell Mol Life Sci*. 2004;61(3):257–262.
111. Findling JW, Raff H. Diagnosis and differential diagnosis of Cushing's syndrome. *Endocrinol Metab Clin North Am*. 2001;30(3):729–747.
113. Newell-Price J. Cushing's syndrome. *Clin Med*. 2008;8(2):204–208.
119. Nieman LK, Ilias I. Evaluation and treatment of Cushing's syndrome. *Am J Med*. 2005;118(12):1340–1346.
122. Stewart AF. Clinical practice. Hypercalcemia associated with cancer. *N Engl J Med*. 2005;352(4):373–379.
123. Roodman GD. Mechanisms of bone metastasis. *N Engl J Med*. 2004;350(16):1655–1664.
125. Guise TA, Yin JJ, Thomas RJ, Dallas M, Cui Y, Gillespie MT. Parathyroid hormone-related protein (PTHrP)-(1-139) isoform is efficiently secreted in vitro and enhances breast cancer metastasis to bone in vivo. *Bone*. 2002;30(5):670–676.
129. Body JJ, Bartl R, Burckhardt P, et al. Current use of bisphosphonates in oncology. International Bone and Cancer Study Group. *J Clin Oncol*. 1998;16(12):3890–3899.
130. Chisholm MA, Mulloy AL, Taylor AT. Acute management of cancer-related hypercalcemia. *Ann Pharmacother*. 1996;30(5):507–513.
134. Baxter RC, Holman SR, Corbould A, Stranks S, Ho PJ, Braund W. Regulation of the insulin-like growth factors and their binding proteins by glucocorticoid and growth hormone in nonislet cell tumor hypoglycemia. *J Clin Endocrinol Metab*. 1995;80(9):2700–2708.
138. Sillos EM, Shenep JL, Burghen GA, Pui CH, Behm FG, Sandlund JT. Lactic acidosis: a metabolic complication of hematologic malignancies: case report and review of the literature. *Cancer*. 2001;92(9):2237–2246.
139. Flombaum CD. Metabolic emergencies in the cancer patient. *Semin Oncol*. 2000;27(3):322–334.
140. Kumar R. Tumor-induced osteomalacia and the regulation of phosphate homeostasis. *Bone*. 2000;27(3):333–338.
142. Shimada T, Mizutani S, Muto T, et al. Cloning and characterization of FGF23 as a causative factor of tumor-induced osteomalacia. *Proc Natl Acad Sci USA*. 2001;98(11):6500–6505.
145. Gold PJ, Fefer A, Thompson JA. Paraneoplastic manifestations of renal cell carcinoma. *Semin Urol Oncol*. 1996;14(4):216–222.
147. Doga M, Bonadonna S, Burattin A, Giustina A. Ectopic secretion of growth hormone-releasing hormone (GHRH) in neuroendocrine tumors: relevant clinical aspects. *Ann Oncol*. 2001;12(Suppl 2):S89–S94.

136 Treatment-Related Secondary Cancers

Susan R. Rheingold, MD ■ Alfred I. Neugut, MD, PhD ■ Thomas Uldrick, MD, MS ■
Anna T. Meadows, MD

Treatment-related secondary cancers have been an important concern in oncology since the late 1970's.[1] This chapter discusses the incidence and the etiologic factors responsible for treatment-related secondary malignant neoplasms (SMNs). Methods of long-term surveillance for individuals at high risk of developing SMNs are also suggested.

What was formerly a problem primarily in pediatric cancer survivors and for the survivors of the more curable adult cancers has become a more universal problem in the present-day practice of oncology. The 5-year survival rate for all cancers has increased steadily from 55% in 1973 to 66% today; reaching 79% in children. Second cancers now account for ~16% of incident cancers reported to the National Cancer Institute's Surveillance, Epidemiology, and End Results (SEER) Program.[2] When reviewing data on SMNs, consideration must be given to the definition. One can readily appreciate a "secondary cancer" that differs histologically, or molecularly, from the primary neoplasm. Reports and analyses of data have emphasized the importance of ruling out metastatic disease when a new tumor arises, but, traditionally, many registries consider tumors of the same histologic type in the second of paired organs to be "secondary cancers." Reports of multiple primaries should clearly state whether secondary cancers include or exclude nonmetastatic neoplasms in paired organs.

The frequency of SMNs may be expressed as an actuarial risk within a given cohort, as a relative risk when compared with a standard population, or as an attributable risk, with the latter reflecting the additional cases associated with a specific exposure or other etiology. Each of these methods has inherent limitations when attempting to ascribe causation, especially when several factors are implicated.

SMNs may result from the radiation therapy and chemotherapy used to treat a primary cancer. Studies of pediatric cancer survivors have provided much information concerning the relationship of therapy to SMNs because of the young age at diagnosis and the high cure rates following successful therapy.[3-5] As therapy becomes more intensive for adults and children, and as cure rates increase, we may expect a resultant increase in long-term toxicities, including SMNs.

Not all SMNs are exclusively treatment-related. Certain risk factors associated with the development of a first cancer, such as genetic predisposition, smoking or obesity, often play a role in the development of a second (Fig. 136-1). Patients with Li-Fraumeni syndrome, neurofibromatosis 1 (NF-1), and retinoblastoma are more likely to develop SMNs following chemotherapy and radiation therapy.[6,7] Gene polymorphisms for metabolizing enzymes and DNA repair pathways are a critical category of etiologic factors that are just being identified. For example, cytochrome P-450 and glutathione S-transferase or x-ray repair cross-complementing variants may be important determinants of whether exposure to a specific agent or radiation is associated with an increased likelihood of developing SMNs.[8-10] These and other factors will play a greater role in determining therapy in the future.

Incidence of Secondary Cancer

Overall, cancer is the second leading cause of death in the United States, exceeded only by heart disease. The National Cancer Institute SEER Program in its analysis from 1973 to 2000 found that cancer survivors had a 14% higher risk of developing a new malignancy than the general population and risk was found to be variable by age of primary cancer, race, and sex.[2] Childhood cancer survivors had 6 times the expected risk of developing a second cancer, which decreased consistently with age at primary diagnosis. Black patients had a higher risk of developing SMNs than their white counterparts. Not all of these additional neoplasms are treatment-related, but it should be recognized that a cancer survivor has approximately twice the probability of developing a new primary cancer than a cancer-free individual of the same age and sex.[1,11]

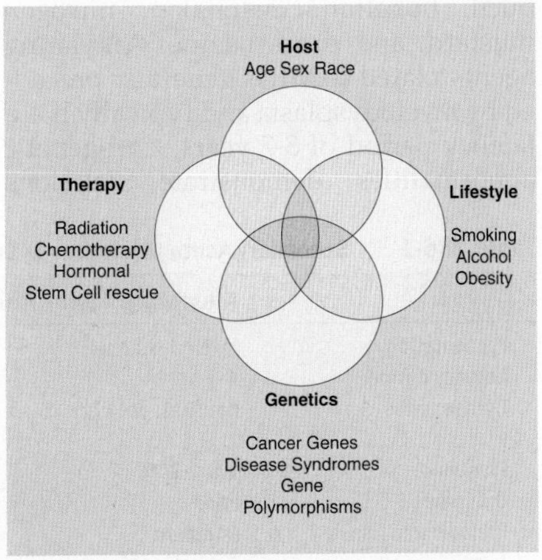

Figure 136-1 ■ Venn diagram depicting risk factors associated with the development of a second cancer

Clinical Characteristics

One question that often arises concerning SMNs is how they differ clinically from their de novo counterparts. Some SMNs are diagnosed earlier due to increased surveillance and better overall access to medical care, and thus have a better outcome. On the other hand some physicians focus on the primary neoplasm and neglect routine surveillance for secondary cancers.[12] Women who have survived cancer should at least have routine mammography screening, Papanicolaou (Pap) smears, and colorectal cancer screening, using the guidelines that would apply to any other woman in the general population. Men should undergo routine prostate and colorectal cancer screening. Counseling of survivors should include instructions for primary and secondary prevention of new malignancies and their risks.

Regardless of initial therapy some SMNs appear to be less amenable to treatment than primary tumors of the same histologic type. The best example of this is therapy-related acute myelogenous leukemia (tAML) for which the prognosis is worse than for de novo acute myelogenous leukemia (AML).[13] Molecular differences between de novo and tAML are the likely explanation for these findings.[14,15] On the other hand, treatment of some secondary tumors, such as osteosarcoma, is no different from that of a de novo primary tumor; the outcomes should also not differ.[16]

Ionizing Radiation

Radiation has long been associated with the development of primary cancers and, when used as treatment, imparts a risk for a secondary cancer. Typically, secondary tumors occur within or at the margin of the radiated field. Bone and soft tissue sarcomas are the most frequent SMNs following radiation therapy, but skin,[17] brain,[18] thyroid,[19] and breast cancers[20] also can occur.[4,5] Radiation doses less than 30 Gy, including total body irradiation (TBI), tend to be associated with skin, thyroid, and brain tumors, whereas doses greater than 30 Gy can evoke secondary sarcomas.[21-23] In the Late Effects Study Group, the median time to develop SMNs was 10 years following radiation, but some were seen as late as 30 years following exposure.[4] Similar results have been noted in other major cohort studies.[22,23] For many postradiation SMNs, the risk is higher if the radiation exposure occurs earlier in life or during periods of rapid growth of a tissue, such as bone sarcomas during adolescence. This is also seen with thyroid, breast, skin, brain, and stomach cancers.

Adolescent girls receiving mediastinal radiation therapy for Hodgkin disease (HD) develop breast cancer more often than do their adult counterparts.[24,25] Cells that have matured and are no longer proliferating appear to be less susceptible to the effects of radiation, although secondary lung, bladder, brain, and gastrointestinal tract cancer have been observed after irradiation.[26-29] Young women with (HD) who received doses as low as 4 Gy to the breast had a three-fold increase in developing breast cancer. The risk increased to eightfold if doses of radiation were > 40 Gy.[24] Breast cancer occurred following (HD) after a mean dose of 11.84 Gy to the breast, with a higher risk when the dose was delivered in fewer than 20 fractions compared with 20 fractions or more. In that study, the report by Travis and colleagues, and a report from the Childhood Cancer Survivor Study (CCSS), breast cancer risk was reduced following surgical castration or radiation to the pelvis.[20,24,25]

Dose-response relationships have also been found between radiation dose and sarcomas. A 40-fold increase in the risk of bone sarcomas was observed following 60 Gy or more.[30] Tenfold increases in the risk of soft tissue sarcoma were seen in retinoblastoma (RB) patients receiving 60 Gy or more, but even 5 Gy increased the risk twofold for this genetically predisposed group.[7] High-dose radiation appears not to increase the risk of leukemia or thyroid cancer.[19] This may be a result of cell killing or inactivation, with cells losing their ability to proliferate and thus their ability to sustain a malignant transformation. As has been observed with other sources of radiation exposure, radiation therapy and cigarette smoking may act in a synergistic fashion.[31] Radiotherapy doses > 15 Gy increase the risk of developing a secondary melanoma vs no or low-dose radiation.[17] A recent review of secondary central nevous system (CNS) tumors by the CCSS revealed a linear dose-response curve for radiation exposure and the risk of developing secondary glioma and meningioma.[18] For glioma, the risk was highest per Gy for children less than 5 years of age. The newer modalities of intensity-modulated radiation therapy and protons provide more focused radiation, but there exists some concern that overall scatter from the machines to the whole body may increase the risk of second cancers.[32]

Chemotherapy

Leukemia is the most common secondary cancer following treatment with chemotherapy. Although tAML and treatment-related myelodysplastic syndrome (tMDS) are the best established types of therapy-related SMNs, acute lymphoblastic leukemia (ALL) and chronic myelogenous leukemia have also been reported. Chemotherapy-induced myeloid leukemias are relatively resistant to subsequent therapy and have a cure rate of only 10-20%,[13] although molecular karyotype retains prognostic significance in tAML.[14]

Knowledge is accumulating concerning the mechanisms of leukemogenesis by topoisomerase II inhibitors and alkylating agents.[9,33-38] Table 136-1 summarizes the features of these chemotherapy-related leukemias. Alkylating agents include cyclophosphamide, ifosfamide, cisplatin, carboplatin, chlorambucil, busulfan, melphalan, nitrogen mustard, and procarbazine. Alkylating agent–related tAML is generally preceded by myelodysplasia and typically has a latency period of 3-7 years. Cytogenetic abnormalities demonstrate deletions on chromosome 5 or 7 and complex aberrant karyotypes.[9] Topoisomerase II inhibitors include the epipodophyllotoxins, etoposide, and teniposide, as well as the anthracyclines doxorubicin, daunorubicin, and mitoxantrone. Leukemia following epipodophyllotoxin therapy has a shorter latency period (usually 1-3 years) and is primarily associated with translocation of the *MLL* gene at chromosome band 11q23, and the AML1 gene at 21q22.[9] Chromosomal aberrations are usually balanced, and patients tend to have a more favorable response to treatment.[9,14]

Treatment for solid tumors, such as Hodgkin disease, Ewing sarcoma, and rhabdomyosarcoma, is associated with a dose-response relationship for alkylators and the risk of leukemia. Alkylating agents increase the risk of leukemia almost 5-fold, but that risk increases to almost 24-fold in patients receiving the highest doses.[34-36] Doxorubicin, together with high-dose alkylating agents, increases that risk further. In one study of childhood solid tumor survivors, exposure to ≥170 mg/m² of anthracycline had a three-fold increase in the risk of developing secondary leukemia relative to those who received <170 mg/m².[37]

A similar increase in risk of secondary leukemia has been reported with increasing doses of epipodophyllotoxins. Compared with those who received no epipodophyllotoxins, children treated for a variety of malignancies had an increased risk of developing a secondary leukemia by a factor of 3.7, 5.7, and 93 for cumulative doses of 2-3, 3-6, and >6 g/m², respectively.[37] The risk of tAML may also depend on the timing of epipodophyllotoxin administration. One study revealed an excess risk of leukemia in patients treated as children with weekly or twice-weekly epipodophyllotoxins compared with every other week, although more frequent dosing is associated with total higher dose.[38]

Two different studies have shown that alkylating agents may potentiate the risk of secondary bone cancers when used with radiation therapy.[22,30] The relative risk of secondary bone sarcomas

Table 136-1 Secondary Acute Myelogenous Leukemia

	Alkylating Agent Related	Epipodophyllotoxin Related
Presentation	Myelodysplasia	M4/M5 AML, some M1, M2
Latency period	4-7 yr	1-3 yr
Cytogenetics	del (5q), del (7q), -5, -7	Translocations, usually involving 11q23
Frequency	1 to >20%	2-12%
Outcome	Poor	Poor
Preleukemic phase	Common	Rare
Age	Typically older	Younger
Predisposition	Germline TP53 and NF1 mutations, *GSTT1 null genotype*	Unknown

Abbreviation: AML, acute myelogenous leukemia.

following radiation therapy was 2.7, but when alkylating agents were used as well, the relative risk rose to 4.7.[30] Relling and colleagues found an increased risk of tAML in children with ALL receiving granulocyte colony-stimulating factor (G-CSF) while receiving St. Jude's Total-X ALL therapy with etoposide, doxorubicin, and cyclophosphamide.[39]

High-Dose Therapy With Rescue

In this section, high-dose therapy followed by stem-cell rescue will be referred to as bone marrow transplantation (BMT). Although it is difficult to differentiate the role played by BMT compared with earlier therapy in the development of secondary cancers, several recent articles have attempted to shed light on the potentially important factors leading to cancer after allogeneic and autologous BMT for both malignant and nonmalignant disease. The cumulative incidence rates of secondary solid tumors increase sharply with time; 10 years following allogeneic BMT, the risk is 2-6%, and 15 years later, it increases to 7-15%,[40-42] whereas secondary leukemias/MDS tend to plateau by 10-15 years.[41] Malignant tumors of the head, neck, and skin; gastrointestinal tract carcinomas; brain tumors; soft tissue and bone sarcomas; and breast, uterine, and liver tumors have been seen. Risk factors for developing a secondary malignancy include age at the time of transplantation, development of graft versus host disease (GVHD), TBI, stem-cell source, and type of primary cancer. Multiple studies have shown that children <10 years of age with a variety of primary neoplasms have a 36-60 times higher risk of developing a secondary cancer when compared with older children undergoing BMT.[43] The risk of post-transplant malignancy in adults also appears to correlate inversely with age for many tumors, although there is an increased incidence of SMNs after autologous BMT for HD and non-Hodgkin lymphoma (NHL) patients older than 35 years.[44] Some studies have shown a decreased risk of developing a secondary cancer in patients who develop moderate to severe chronic GVHD whereas others noted an increased risk of developing squamous cell carcinomas of the skin and buccal cavity and thyroid carcinoma.[42,45] It is hypothesized that the chronic inflammation associated with GVHD predisposes patients to secondary tumors. Several articles have noted an increased risk of developing a secondary neoplasm post-BMT when the primary diagnosis is acute or chronic leukemia.[42] Recent studies found that the risk of developing a secondary breast, skin, or mucosal cancer after allogeneic BMT was higher (confidence intervals [CI] of 5-10% at 20 years) among patients who received TBI and those who underwent BMT at younger ages.[45,46] TBI has also been associated with thyroid and head and neck cancers. The contribution of prior treatment, conditioning regimen, immunosuppression, and means of stem-cell harvest, remain unclear.

Compared with allogeneic BMT, autologous BMT (auto-BMT) is associated with an increased risk of tMDS/AML.[43] Median time to developing tMDS/AML was 2 years post-BMT (range 0.6-9 years).[43,44] Actuarial risk estimates of developing tAML range from 3% to 20% in the first 5 years post-BMT for primary lymphomas and less for primary solid tumors. In different studies, the use of autologous stimulated peripheral blood stem-cells, prolonged duration of apheresis of stem-cells, prior radiation exposure and pretransplantation use of high-risk alkylating agents or greater than 4 chemotherapy regimens have been found to be independent risk factors for the development of tMDS/AML post–auto-BMT.[44,47]

Post-transplant lymphoproliferative disease (PTLD) accounts for almost half of the secondary malignancies diagnosed after allogeneic BMT. The majority of cases occur within 6-12 months of transplantation, but latency periods have been reported as long as 5 years post-BMT.[41,43,48] Risk factors for PTLD include acute and chronic GVHD, unrelated or human leukocyte antigen-disparate related donor, primary diagnosis of an immune deficiency, T cell-depleted graft, and antithymocyte globulin therapy.

Risk of Secondary Cancers After Treatment for Childhood Primary Neoplasms

Hodgkin Disease

Patients with HD treated with chemotherapy, radiation therapy, or a combination have an increased risk of developing SMNs.[49-53] Relative risks, based on comparison with cancer risk in age-matched individuals in the population, range from 2 to more than 50 and depend on the tissue of origin of the secondary cancer, as well as treatment.[26,49-52]

The overall cumulative incidence of SMNs, the majority of which are solid neoplasms, after treatment for childhood HD ranges between 2% and 27% by 30 years from diagnosis and depends primarily on the therapy received.

Thyroid cancer is the most common postradiation SMN in survivors of childhood and adolescent Hodgkin's disease.[5,21] As noted above, following radiation therapy, breast cancer is seen in females, with those over the age of 10 years at greatest risk.[20,24,42,50-52] There is also an increased risk of skin cancer within the radiation field. Recently, many pediatric centers have altered their therapy of Hodgkin disease to reflect differences in secondary cancer and gonadal toxicity in girls and boys, with girls receiving less chest irradiation and boys receiving less alkylating agent.[54]

Although radiation therapy for Hodgkin disease is associated with secondary solid tumors, chemotherapy is associated with the development of secondary leukemia. As many as 25% of secondary malignancies following treatment for Hodgkin disease are secondary leukemia or lymphoma.[35,51,52] Because mechlorethamine, Oncovin (vincristine), procarbazine, and prednisone (MOPP) regimens contain nitrogen mustard and procarbazine, they incur a greater risk of secondary leukemia than with either combination regimens containing cyclophosphamide or with doxorubicin, bleomycin, vinblastine, and dacarbazine (ABVD).[54] Higher doses and multiple alkylating agents also increase that risk; hence, the incidence of secondary leukemia is higher in patients who suffer a recurrence of Hodgkin disease and require re-treatment. Radiation therapy alone does not appear to increase the secondary leukemia risk.

Retinoblastoma

Retinoblastoma (RB) is the prototype of heritable cancers, with *RB1* on chromosome 13 being the first tumor suppressor gene cloned.[55] If both copies of *RB1* are lost or mutated, cancer develops.[56] Multiple tumors in both eyes and cancer in other organs, such as bone and soft tissue, have long been known in patients with the genetic form of this cancer. A recent study by Kleinerman et al of secondary cancers for patients with hereditary RB noted differences in the incidence of SMN at 50 years between RB survivors with the genetic form (36%) and those without evidence of the genetic form (6%).[7] Children who had received radiation therapy had a 40-year incidence of 30% for developing SMN both within and outside the radiation field compared to 9% in those who received no radiation.[7,57] Sarcomas are the most frequent second tumors; the majority of which are osteosarcomas. Leiomyosarcomas account for a third of the secondary soft tissue sarcomas followed by fibrosarcomas, histiocytomas, and rhabdomyosarcoma.[57] Patients with RB also appear to be at an increased risk of melanoma and brain tumors. Another recent report of hereditary RB survivors who did not receive radiotherapy revealed an increased risk of secondary epithelial neoplasms, such as lung and bladder cancer, and leiomyosarcoma years after the initial diagnosis.[58] All children with bilateral disease and approximately 10-15% of those with unilateral tumor are gene carriers and should be monitored for life for the development of sarcomas, adult carcinomas, and other neoplasms. Mutation analysis is now possible to determine which children with a negative family history and unilateral tumor are genetically predisposed so that they may also be followed more closely.

Pediatric Sarcomas

Recent studies show a consistent rate of secondary malignancies in patients treated with intensive chemotherapy for soft tissue and bone sarcomas. The cumulative risk of SMNs after therapy for Ewing sarcoma ranged from 3% at 10 years to more than 10% at 20 years.[59,60] Secondary sarcomas, related to radiation therapy in a dose-dependent manner, were noted 7-11 years after diagnosis and accounted for the majority of SMNs. Patients developed tAML and ALL 1 to 5 years after diagnosis. Rhabdomyosarcoma survivors, similar to the Ewing's sarcoma cohorts, developed SMNs with an identical latency period and a similar cumulative risk.[61] The rates were highest for patients who received both alkylating agents and radiation therapy. Survivors of osteosarcoma who develop secondary cancers may be at increased risk of having germline TP53 mutations, predisposing them to breast cancer and tMDS/AML.[62]

Acute Lymphoblastic Leukemia

Several reports have been published analyzing the risk of secondary malignancies following therapy for childhood ALL.[38,63,64] Children treated on Children's Cancer Group (CCG) protocols, Berlin-Frankfurt-Munster (BFM) protocols, and Dana-Farber Cancer Institute protocols have an estimated cumulative risk of SMNs at 15 years to be 2.5-3.3%. In a review of seven large series of SMNs after ALL therapy, the most common SMNs were CNS tumors (32%), tMDS/AML (17%), thyroid cancer (10%), lymphoma (8%), and skin cancer (8%).[65] Patients who received craniospinal radiation were at increased risk of CNS tumors, skin cancer, and thyroid cancer.[4,13,29] Underlying genetic factors, such as TP53 germline mutations, should be considered in children who develop SMNs following therapy for ALL.

Secondary brain tumors occurred after cranial radiation therapy for ALL in studies reported by the CCG and the St. Jude Children's Research Hospital.[4,29] In the latter report, the overall cumulative incidence was 1.4%. In multiple studies, a statistically significant increase in risk with increasing cranial radiation dose was noted.[4,29] Children treated on CCG protocols for ALL who received 18 Gy had a relative risk of developing a secondary brain tumor of 1.5, which increased to 3.9 in those who received 24 Gy.[4] Younger age increased the risk of secondary CNS tumors. Fortunately, in more recent pediatric ALL protocols, cranial radiation has been replaced by intensive intrathecal chemotherapy for children who have no evidence of CNS disease at diagnosis.

The risk of tMDS/AML in patients treated for ALL varies with the original protocol used and the dose and schedule of epipodophyllotoxins. Children receiving weekly or twice-weekly epipodophyllotoxins had a cumulative incidence of 12% of secondary AML.[38] In the BFM study, the development of tAML was not associated with the use of any specific cytotoxic agent and 12 of 16 children with tAML had not received epipodophyllotoxins.[63]

Wilms Tumor

The data from the National Wilms Tumor Study Group found an eightfold increase in SMNs in children treated for Wilms tumor between 1969 and 1991.[66] There was an excess of leukemia, as well as lymphomas and solid tumors. The secondary leukemias were primarily tAML and were diagnosed 1-6 years after original therapy. Similar latency periods were seen for lymphomas. Secondary solid tumors following treatment for Wilms tumor had a much longer latency period of 3-21 years. The solid tumors were primarily sarcomas and carcinomas (breast, thyroid, colon, hepatocellular, parotid), but there was also an increased incidence of brain tumors. Patients who had received abdominal radiation had twice the risk of secondary cancers compared with those who did not. The report also suggested that doxorubicin potentiates the radiation effect.

Neuroblastoma

As survival improves in childhood high-risk neuroblastoma (NBL), more SMNs are being detected. The median time from NBL diagnosis to development of an SMN is almost 20 years, with a range of 7-38 years and a cumulative incidence of about 2.0% at 20 years.[5,67] SMNs include thyroid and breast carcinoma, sarcomas, and ALL and AML. In a multivariate analysis, treatment with radiation was associated with a relative risk of 4.3 of developing an SMN, but no increased risk was associated with the administration of chemotherapy.[67] An independent association between NBL and later development of thyroid carcinoma may exist because a fivefold excess of radiation-induced thyroid cancer is seen after therapy for NBL. Survivors of NBL also have a significantly increased risk of developing renal cell carcinoma.[68]

Brain and CNS Tumors

Children and adolescents with primary brain tumors have a 15-year cumulative incidence of developing a secondary cancer of 5%.[69] Significantly elevated standardized incidence ratios (SIRs) have been noted for pathologically different brain tumors, t-MDS/AML, bone and soft tissue sarcomas, lymphomas, skin cancer, and salivary and thyroid gland carcinomas.[70] Development of secondary brain, bone, thyroid, and skin cancers is higher among patients whose up-front therapy included radiation.[70,71] Younger survivors of primary brain tumors are much more likely to develop secondary cancers than adults. The trend toward using more intensive chemotherapy including alkylators, in lieu of radiation therapy in very young children, can be expected to increase the number of secondary leukemias in this group, but decrease the risk of radiation-induced brain, thyroid, and skin tumors.[71] One-third of children who developed secondary tumors had an underlying genetic predisposition, such as Li-Fraumeni syndrome (leukemia, sarcomas), neurofibromatosis (leukemia, brain tumors), Gorlin syndrome (basal cell and brain tumors), and Gardner syndrome (desmoid tumors).[69] Children with neurofibromatosis type-1 who are predisposed to developing brain tumors, appear to have an increased risk of developing a pathologically different brain tumor when treated with radiation.[6] Using radiation is therefore cautioned in this population.

Risk of Secondary Cancers After Treatment for Adult Primary Neoplasms

Breast Cancer

Breast Cancer is the most common malignancy in women in the United States. Women with an initial breast cancer are at a significantly elevated risk of a second cancer in the contralateral breast[72] due to hormonal factors and genetic predisposition.[73] Estrogen is an established risk factor for breast cancer, and anti-estrogens and chemotherapy-induced menopause reduce the incidence of secondary breast cancer and improve survival.[74-76] Tamoxifen improves survival in women with early stage estrogen-receptor positive breast cancer,[77,78] but also carries a small absolute increase in the risk of endometrial cancer.[74,79,80]

In addition to tamoxifen associated endometrial cancer, an increase of radiation-induced solid tumors and chemo tMDS/AML have been observed in women treated for early stage breast cancer.

Postmastectomy radiation elevates the subsequent risk of ipsilateral lung cancer, particularly in women who smoke.[31,81-83] Similar increased risks have been observed for esophageal cancer following postmastectomy radiation.[84] Postirradiation sarcomas may also occur in the treatment field, with angiosarcoma being the most common histology.[85-88] Radiation therapy for an initial breast cancer does not appear to elevate the risk of contralateral breast cancer.[89] Women with a history of early stage breast cancer have a risk for second solid tumors that persists for decades[90] due to a combination of hormonal, genetic and treatment-related factors.

tMDS/AML may also occur after adjuvant chemotherapy for breast cancer. Alkylating agents increase the risk of tAML, although greater risk was seen in older regimens that included melphalan or experimental regimens that used high doses of cyclophosphamide.[91] Postmastectomy radiation potentiates the leukemogenic effects of alkylating agents.[92,93] Chemotherapy agents that inhibit topoisomerase II[94] are also associated with increased tAML risk when used as adjuvant therapy for breast cancer. This has been demonstrated with increased doses of doxorubicin, epirubicin[95] and mitoxantrone.[96]

G-CSF is increasingly used in the supportive care of women with breast cancer undergoing adjuvant chemotherapy,[97] and has been evaluated as a risk factor for tAML. In the National Surgical Adjuvant Breast and Bowel Project (NSABP) B-25 study, which compared doxorubicin plus varied doses of cyclophosphamide, there was an increased risk of tAML in those receiving higher cumulative doses of G-CSF (RR = 3.58, p = 0.02), even after adjusting for cyclophosphamide dose. However, these results were not statistically significant if women who developed metastatic breast cancer (and presumably received additional chemotherapy) before AML were censored in the analysis.[91] Two subsequent studies of the NCI SEER—Medicare linked database evaluated the risk of tAML in women older than 65 after receiving G-CSF in the management of localized breast cancer, and reported conflicting results regarding risk.[97,98] These latter studies were unable to establish G-CSF as a risk factor independent of the intensity of chemotherapy received.

Testicular Cancer

Testicular cancer is one of the most curable solid tumors, whether it occurs unilaterally or bilaterally. Etoposide and radiotherapy are commonly employed in the treatment of testicular cancer, and an increased risk of both solid tumors and tAML has been noted in studies of long-term survivors.[99] Increased risk of tAML has been associated with chemotherapy,[40,100,101] with the highest risk noted in patients receiving high doses of etoposide.[102] An increased risk of sarcomas and cancers occurring below the diaphragm have been noted[103] and are attributed to radiation therapy. Testicular cancer survivors who develop a second solid tumor have a comparable prognosis to men who develop the same primary cancer.

Second Cancers After Radiation Therapy for Prostate, Rectal, and Cervical Cancer

Treatment of localized prostate, rectal and cervical cancers may all include radiation therapy to the pelvis. Radiotherapy for prostate cancer slightly elevates the risk of SMN of other pelvic organs, with cancers developing many years after radiation therapy. Bladder cancer[27] and sarcoma[104,105] occur more frequently in men who are treated with radiotherapy than those treated with other modalities. An increased risk of rectal cancer is noted in some[104,105] but not all[27,106] epidemiologic studies. Radiation is commonly used in the management of rectal cancer, and the standardized incidence ratio of cervical and uterine cancer is increased in this population. Interestingly, the risk of prostate cancer is decreased after radiation therapy for rectal cancer.[107]

Women treated for cervical cancer are at increased risk of cancers associated with the human papillomavirus (HPV), such as ano-genital cancers, as well as tobacco related cancers, such as lung cancer and head and neck cancers. Furthermore, woman treated with pelvic irradiation are at increased risk of developing secondary rectal, bladder and ovarian cancers in the field, when compared to treatment with surgery alone.[108] While the absolute risk of radiation related SMNs is small, the risks of radiation therapy remain pertinent, especially when employed in younger patients.[109]

Other Solid Tumors

Evaluation of treatment-related SMNs after many other common solid tumors is limited by poor prognosis and limited survivorship, even when diagnosed early (ie, gastric, pancreatic, lung, esophageal and hepatocellular cancers). SMNs in other solid tumors are more likely due to other etiologic factors, such as smoking (ie, head and neck, lung and pancreatic cancer) or genetic syndromes (ie, hereditory nonpolyposis colorectal cancer [HNPCC], breast cancer) than to treatment. Lastly, some tumors, such as colon cancer and renal cell carcinoma, do not employ therapies known to be associated with second malignancies. Increased risk of SMNs after treatment for ovarian cancer was largely seen with alkylating agent based chemotherapy regimens that are no longer commonly used.[110]

Conclusion

Therapeutic options for secondary cancers are often compromised by the therapy for the first neoplasm, but early diagnosis can often lead to successful treatment of many secondary cancers. Identifying those who are at greater risk of multiple neoplasms can help health care providers institute more targeted monitoring for secondary neoplasms and counsel patients on the ways of reducing risks.

Many individuals at highest risk of therapy-related new cancers are already known, and several approaches to reducing their incidence are already under way. For instance, the knowledge that certain agents and regimens increase the risk of a secondary malignancy has prompted pediatric oncologists to modify therapy. Knowing that there are patients with genetic risk factors, such as those with the hereditary form of RB or neurofibromatosis who are at increased risk of developing second malignancies in the radiation field, has led to protocols substituting additional chemotherapeutic agents for radiation.

Wellness care for adult cancer survivors should also include surveillance for specific SMNs, as well as age appropriate cancer screening based on established guidelines. Research that focuses on the avoidance of known environmental carcinogens offers the hope that some neoplasms in multiple sites can be prevented. In this regard, survivors of childhood cancer are an excellent population in which to study the effectiveness of educational intervention techniques. Finally, study of the genetic changes in cancer in families with many affected members and of individuals with more than one primary tumor can increase our knowledge of the nature of the changes leading to transformation of a normal cell to malignancy. This may lead to the identification of more susceptible individuals and to the development of appropriate methods of surveillance and counseling.

Selected References

The complete reference list can be found at www.CANCERMEDICINE8.com

2. Curtis R, Freedman D, Ron E, et al. New malignancies among cancer survivors. SEER Cancer Registries, 197–2000. 2006;NIH Publ. #05-5302.
3. Meadows AT. **** second neoplasms in surviuos of childhood cancer: findings from the childhood cancer survivor study cohort J Clin Oncol 2009;272356–2362.
7. Kleinerman RA, Tucker MA, Tarone RE, et al. Risk of new cancers after radiotherapy in long-term survivors of retinoblastoma: an extended follow-up. *J Clin Oncol.* 2005;23:2272–2279.

9. Seedhouse C, Russell N. Advances in the understanding of susceptibility to treatment-related acute myeloid leukaemia. *Br J Haematol*. 2007;137:513–529.
12. Green RJ, Metlay JP, Propert K, et al. Surveillance for second primary colorectal cancer after adjuvant chemotherapy: an analysis of Intergroup 0089. *Ann Intern Med*. 2002;136:261–269.
13. Josting A, Wiedenmann S, Franklin J, et al. Secondary myeloid leukemia and myelodysplastic syndromes in patients treated for Hodgkin's disease: a report from the German Hodgkin's Lymphoma Study Group. *J Clin Oncol*. 2003;21:3440–3446.
14. Schoch C, Kern W, Schnittger S, Hiddemann W, Haferlach T. Karyotype is an independent prognostic parameter in therapy-related acute myeloid leukemia (t-AML): an analysis of 93 patients with t-AML in comparison to 1091 patients with de novo AML. *Leukemia*. 2004;18:120–125.
17. Guerin S, Dupuy A, Anderson H, et al. Radiation dose as a risk factor for malignant melanoma following childhood cancer. *Eur J Cancer*. 2003;39:2379–2386.
18. Neglia JP, Robison LL, Stovall M, et al. New primary neoplasms of the central nervous system in survivors of childhood cancer: a report from the Childhood Cancer Survivor Study. *J Natl Cancer Inst*. 2006;98:1528–1537.
19. Ronckers CM, Sigurdson AJ, Stovall M, et al. Thyroid cancer in childhood cancer survivors: a detailed evaluation of radiation dose response and its modifiers. *Radiat Res*. 2006;166:618–628.
20. Kenney LB, Yasui Y, Inskip PD, et al. Breast cancer after childhood cancer: a report from the Childhood Cancer Survivor Study. *Ann Intern Med*. 2004;141:590–597.
22. Menu-Branthomme A, Rubino C, Shamsaldin A, et al. Radiation dose, chemotherapy and risk of soft tissue sarcoma after solid tumours during childhood. *Int J Cancer*. 2004;110:87–93.
23. Henderson TO, Whitton J, Stovall M, et al. Secondary sarcomas in childhood cancer survivors: a report from the Childhood Cancer Survivor Study. *J Natl Cancer Inst*. 2007;99:300–308.
24. Travis LB, Hill DA, Dores GM, et al. Breast cancer following radiotherapy and chemotherapy among young women with Hodgkin disease. *JAMA*. 2003;290:465–475.
25. Bhatia S, Yasui Y, Robison LL, et al. High risk of subsequent neoplasms continues with extended follow-up of childhood Hodgkin's disease: report from the Late Effects Study Group. *J Clin Oncol*. 2003;21:4386–4394.
26. Swerdlow AJ, Schoemaker MJ, Allerton R, et al. Lung cancer after Hodgkin's disease: a nested case-control study of the relation to treatment. *J Clin Oncol*. 2001;19:1610–1618.
31. Neugut AI, Murray T, Santos J, et al. Increased risk of lung cancer after breast cancer radiation therapy in cigarette smokers. *Cancer*. 1994;73:1615–1620.
34. Bhatia S, Krailo MD, Chen Z, et al. Therapy-related myelodysplasia and acute myeloid leukemia after Ewing sarcoma and primitive neuroectodermal tumor of bone: a report from the Children's Oncology Group. *Blood*. 2007;109:46–51.
37. Le Deley MC, Leblanc T, Shamsaldin A, et al. Risk of secondary leukemia after a solid tumor in childhood according to the dose of epipodophyllotoxins and anthracyclines: a case-control study by the Societe Francaise d'Oncologie Pediatrique. *J Clin Oncol*. 2003;21:1074–1081.
38. Pui CH, Ribeiro RC, Hancock ML, et al. Acute myeloid leukemia in children treated with epipodophyllotoxins for acute lymphoblastic leukemia. *N Engl J Med*. 1991;325:1682–1687.
43. Baker KS, DeFor TE, Burns LJ, Ramsay NK, Neglia JP, Robison LL. New malignancies after blood or marrow stem-cell transplantation in children and adults: incidence and risk factors. *J Clin Oncol*. 2003;21:1352–1358.
44. Metayer C, Curtis RE, Vose J, et al. Myelodysplastic syndrome and acute myeloid leukemia after autotransplantation for lymphoma: a multicenter case-control study. *Blood*. 2003;101:2015–2023.
52. van Leeuwen FE, Klokman WJ, Veer MB, et al. Long-term risk of second malignancy in survivors of Hodgkin's disease treated during adolescence or young adulthood. *J Clin Oncol*. 2000;18:487–497.
57. Kleinerman RA, Tucker MA, Abramson DH, Seddon JM, Tarone RE, Fraumeni JF, Jr. Risk of soft tissue sarcomas by individual subtype in survivors of hereditary retinoblastoma. *J Natl Cancer Inst*. 2007;99:24–31.
60. Dunst J, Ahrens S, Paulussen M, et al. Second malignancies after treatment for Ewing's sarcoma: a report of the CESS-studies. *Int J Radiat Oncol Biol Phys*. 1998;42:379–384.
62. Malkin D, Li FP, Strong LC, et al. Germ line p53 mutations in a familial syndrome of breast cancer, sarcomas, and other neoplasms. *Science*. 1990;250:1233–1238.
63. Loning L, Zimmermann M, Reiter A, et al. Secondary neoplasms subsequent to Berlin-Frankfurt-Munster therapy of acute lymphoblastic leukemia in childhood: significantly lower risk without cranial radiotherapy. *Blood*. 2000;95:2770–2775.
65. Bhatia S, Sather HN, Pabustan OB, Trigg ME, Gaynon PS, Robison LL. Low incidence of second neoplasms among children diagnosed with acute lymphoblastic leukemia after 1983. *Blood*. 2002;99:4257–4264.
66. Breslow NE, Takashima JR, Whitton JA, Moksness J, D'Angio GJ, Green DM. Second malignant neoplasms following treatment for Wilm's tumor: a report from the National Wilms' Tumor Study Group. *J Clin Oncol*. 1995;13:1851–1859.
67. Rubino C, Adjadj E, Guerin S, et al. Long-term risk of second malignant neoplasms after neuroblastoma in childhood: role of treatment. *Int J Cancer*. 2003;107:791–796.
68. Bassal M, Mertens AC, Taylor L, et al. Risk of selected subsequent carcinomas in survivors of childhood cancer: a report from the Childhood Cancer Survivor Study. *J Clin Oncol*. 2006;24:476–483.
69. Broniscer A, Ke W, Fuller CE, Wu J, Gajjar A, Kun LE. Second neoplasms in pediatric patients with primary central nervous system tumors: the St. Jude Children's Research Hospital experience. *Cancer*. 2004;100:2246–2252.
70. Inskip PD. Multiple primary tumors involving cancer of the brain and central nervous system as the first or subsequent cancer. *Cancer*. 2003;98:562–570.
71. Peterson KM, Shao C, McCarter R, MacDonald TJ, Byrne J. An analysis of SEER data of increasing risk of secondary malignant neoplasms among long-term survivors of childhood brain tumors. *Pediatr Blood Cancer*. 2006;47:83–88.
76. Bertelsen L, Bernstein L, Olsen JH, et al. Effect of systemic adjuvant treatment on risk for contralateral breast cancer in the Women's Environment, Cancer and Radiation Epidemiology Study. *J Natl Cancer Inst*. 2008;100:32–40.
78. Fisher B, Jeong JH, Anderson S, Wolmark N. Treatment of axillary lymph node-negative, estrogen receptor-negative breast cancer: updated findings from National Surgical Adjuvant Breast and Bowel Project clinical trials. *J Natl Cancer Inst*. 2004;96:1823–1831.
82. Zablotska LB, Neugut AI. Lung carcinoma after radiation therapy in women treated with lumpectomy or mastectomy for primary breast carcinoma. *Cancer*. 2003;97:1404–1411.
83. Kaufman EL, Jacobson JS, Hershman DL, Desai M, Neugut AI. Effect of breast cancer radiotherapy and cigarette smoking on risk of second primary lung cancer. *J Clin Oncol*. 2008;26:392–398.
84. Zablotska LB, Chak A, Das A, Neugut AI. Increased risk of squamous cell esophageal cancer after adjuvant radiation therapy for primary breast cancer. *Am J Epidemiol*. 2005;161:330–337.
85. Yap J, Chuba PJ, Thomas R, et al. Sarcoma as a second malignancy after treatment for breast cancer. *Int J Radiat Oncol Biol Phys*. 2002;52:1231–1237.
87. Rubino C, Shamsaldin A, Le MG, et al. Radiation dose and risk of soft tissue and bone sarcoma after breast cancer treatment. *Breast Cancer Res Treat*. 2005;89:277–288.
90. Brown LM, Chen BE, Pfeiffer RM, et al. Risk of second non-hematological malignancies among 376,825 breast cancer survivors. *Breast Cancer Res Treat*. 2007;106:439–451.
91. Smith RE, Bryant J, DeCillis A, Anderson S. Acute myeloid leukemia and myelodysplastic syndrome after doxorubicin-cyclophosphamide adjuvant therapy for operable breast cancer: the National Surgical Adjuvant Breast and Bowel Project Experience. *J Clin Oncol*. 2003;21:1195–1204.
93. Yu GP, Schantz SP, Neugut AI, Zhang ZF. Incidences and trends of second cancers in female breast cancer patients: a fixed inception cohort-based analysis (United States). *Cancer Causes Control*. 2006;17:411–420.
97. Hershman D, Neugut AI, Jacobson JS, et al. Acute myeloid leukemia or myelodysplastic syndrome following use of granulocyte colony-stimulating factors during breast cancer adjuvant chemotherapy. *J Natl Cancer Inst*. 2007;99:196–205.
98. Patt DA, Duan Z, Fang S, Hortobagyi GN, Giordano SH. Acute myeloid leukemia after adjuvant breast cancer therapy in older women: understanding risk. *J Clin Oncol*. 2007;25:3871–3876.
99. Travis LB, Curtis RE, Storm H, et al. Risk of second malignant neoplasms among long-term survivors of testicular cancer. *J Natl Cancer Inst*. 1997;89:1429–1439.
100. Howard R, Gilbert E, Lynch CF, et al. Risk of leukemia among survivors of testicular cancer: a population-based study of 42,722 patients. *Ann Epidemiol*. 2008;18:416–421.
106. Kendal WS, Eapen L, Macrae R, Malone S, Nicholas G. Prostatic irradiation is not associated with any measurable increase in the risk of subsequent rectal cancer. *Int J Radiat Oncol Biol Phys*. 2006;65:661–668.
108. Chaturvedi AK, Engels EA, Gilbert ES, et al. Second cancers among 104,760 survivors of cervical cancer: evaluation of long-term risk. *J Natl Cancer Inst*. 2007;99:1634–1643.

137 Infections in Patients With Cancer

Kenneth V.I. Rolston, MD, FACP ■ Gerald P. Bodey, MD

Infection continues to be a common problem in patients with cancer.[1] The spectrum of infection continues to change.[2,3] Resistance among common bacterial and fungal pathogens is increasing and the pipeline for new drug development is relatively barren.[4] Fungal, viral, and some protozoal infections have increased in frequency, are often difficult to diagnose, are sometimes refractory to therapy, and are associated with substantial morbidity and mortality.[5,6] Consequently, infection prevention, reversal of the immunologic deficit(s) leading to infection, and antimicrobial stewardship are important aspects in the overall management of patients with cancer.

The frequency of infection is related to the type of underlying neoplastic disease. Nearly 80% of patients with acute leukemia, 75% of patients with lymphoma, and 50% of patients with multiple myeloma develop infection during the course of their disease. Serious infections also occur in patients with solid tumors.[7] Multiple episodes of infection in the same patient are not uncommon. It is often not possible to make a specific diagnosis, and empiric therapy is generally administered in high-risk patients who are suspected of having an infection. A thorough knowledge of the factors that predispose these patients toward the development of infections is essential.

Table 137-1 ■ **Defects in Host Defense Mechanisms and Common Infections Associated With Malignant Diseases**

Disease	Prominent Defect	Predominant Infections
Acute leukemia, aplastic anemia	Neutropenia	Gram-positive cocci, gram-negative bacilli, *Candida, Aspergillus, Fusarium, Tricho-sporon*
Hairy cell leukemia	Neutropenia, impaired lymphocyte function	Gram-negative bacilli, gram-positive cocci, mycobacteria (including nontuberculous)
Chronic lymphatic leukemia, multiple myeloma	Hypogammaglobulinemia	Encapsulated organisms, Streptococcus *pneumoniae; Haemophilus influenzae; Neisseria meningitides*
Hodgkin disease	Impaired T-lymphocyte response	*Pneumocystis, Cryptococcus, mycobacteria, Toxoplasma, Listeria, Cryptosporidium, Candida, cytomegalovirus*
Bone marrow, transplant recipients	Neutropenia, impaired cellular and humoral immunity	Gram-positive cocci, gram-negative bacilli, cytomegalovirus, *Candida, Aspergillus,* herpes viruses
Breast cancer	Tissue necrosis	Gram-positive cocci, gram-negative bacilli, anaerobes
Lung cancer	Local obstruction, tissue necrosis	Gram-positive cocci, gram-negative bacilli, anaerobes
Gynecologic malignancy	Local obstruction, tissue necrosis	Mixed aerobic and anaerobic enteric flora

Factors Responsible for Increased Susceptibility to Infections

Many factors increase the susceptibility of patients with cancer to infection. Each is associated with a unique set of infections, although there is some overlap between predisposing factors and certain infections. Multiple predisposing factors might exist in the same patient Table 137-1 lists the predominant defects in host defense mechanisms associated with various cancers and the infections associated with those defects.

Neutropenia

Neutropenia remains the most common predisposing factor.[8] Both the degree and the duration of neutropenia influence the development of infection. The currently accepted definition of neutropenia is an absolute neutrophil count of ≤500/mm³. Most serious infections, including bacteremias, develop during episodes of severe and prolonged neutropenia (Fig. 137-1). Patients with neutropenia often fail to develop the characteristic signs and symptoms of infection, because they are unable to mount an adequate inflammatory response. Common sites of infection in patients with neutropenia include the lung, oropharynx, blood, urinary tract, skin, and soft tissues, including the perirectal area. Infections are generally caused by organisms colonizing the patient, although some organisms are acquired after admission to the hospital.

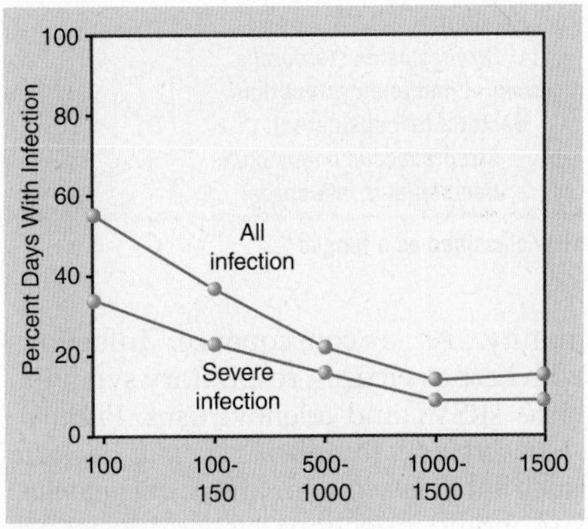

Figure 137-1 ■ Relationship between granulocyte count and infection in patients with acute leukemia. Percentage of days spent with infection is inversely related to the level of circulating granulocytes.

Hospital-acquired pathogens are more likely to be resistant to commonly used antimicrobial agents because of the pressure of heavy antibiotic usage.[9,10] Patients with adequate levels of circulating neutrophils may be susceptible to infection because of impaired neutrophil function. Defects include the inability to migrate to sites of inflammation, impaired phagocytosis, and reduced killing of ingested bacteria.

Not all patients with neutropenia have the same risk for developing infection or serious complications when they become febrile. High-, moderate-, and low-risk patients with neutropenia can be identified using clinical criteria/risk prediction rules during the initial phases of their febrile episode.[11,12] Many patients with solid tumors that are responding to antineoplastic therapy and in whom neutropenia is relatively short-lived (≤7 days) are considered low risk. These patients have a high response rate (>95%) to antibacterial therapy and a low complication rate (<2%). Strategies for their management, such as early discharge and outpatient antibiotic therapy, have been developed.[13-15]

Cellular Immune Dysfunction

Defects in the T-lymphocyte and/or mononuclear phagocytic system result in an increased susceptibility to infection. Cell-mediated immunity plays a primary role in protecting against intracellular pathogens. T4 lymphocytes, however, have an impact on practically all aspects of immunity as a consequence of their ability to induce specific immune responses in other cells.

T-lymphocyte function is impaired in a variety of disorders. Patients with Hodgkin disease also have evidence of impaired cell-mediated immunity, and, to a lesser degree, so do patients with chronic and acute lymphocytic leukemia. Immunosuppressive therapy with agents such as cyclosporine, tacrolimus, azathioprine, corticosteroids, certain cytotoxic agents (fludarabine and other purine analogues), and irradiation produces dysfunction in cellular immunity. These patients are especially susceptible to infection with intracellular organisms such as those listed in Table 137-2

Table 137-2 ■ Common Infectious Agents in Patients With Cancer

Neutropenia
Bacteria
Gram-positive organisms
Coagulase-negative staphylococci
Staphylococcus aureus (including MRSA)
Enterococcus spp. (including VRE)
Viridans group streptococci
β-Hemolytic streptococci
Corynebacterium jeikeium
Bacillus spp.
Stomatococcus mucilaginosus
Micrococcus spp.
Gram-negative organisms
Escherichia coli
Klebsiella pneumoniae
Pseudomonas aeruginosa
Enterobacter spp.
Citrobacter spp.
Serratia spp.
Pseudomonas (non-aeruginosa) spp.
Acinetobacter baumanni
Stenotrophomonas maltophilia
Fungi
Candida spp.
Aspergillus spp.
Zygomycetes
Fusarium spp.
Cellular Immune Dysfunction
Bacteria
Listeria monocytogenes
Rhodococcus equi
Salmonella spp.
Mycobacteria
Nocardia spp.
Legionella spp.
Fungi
Aspergillus spp.
Cryptococcus neoformans
Histoplasma capsulatum
Coccidioides immitis
Protozoa
Pneumocystis carinii P. jiroveci[a]
Toxoplasma gondii
Cryptosporidium spp.
Isospora belli
Viruses
Cytomegalovirus
Herpes simplex virus I and II
Varicella-zoster virus
Epstein-Barr virus
Human herpes virus-6
Community respiratory viruses
Helminth
Strongyloides stercoralis
Humoral immune dysfunction
Bacteria (encapsulated)
Streptococcus pneumoniae
Haemophilus influenzae

[a]Now classified as a fungus

Humoral Immune Dysfunction

The immune response that is mediated by antibodies, is referred to as humoral immunity. B lymphocytes are responsible for antibody production. In disorders such as multiple myeloma, Waldenstrom macroglobulinemia, and the various "heavy-chain diseases," overproduction of a specific subcomponent of an immunoglobulin occurs as a consequence of malignant proliferation of plasma cells or their precursors. As this pool of malignant plasma cells expands, it does so at the expense of normal cells, resulting in low levels of normal immunoglobulins. Hypogammaglobulinemia is also present in 30-40% of patients with chronic lymphocytic leukemia, and infection occurs in nearly 90% of these patients, as compared with only 15% in patients with normal gamma-globulin levels. Infection is the cause of death in approximately 60% of patients with multiple myeloma. Patients with multiple myeloma and chronic lymphocytic leukemia are especially susceptible to infections caused by encapsulated organisms such as *Streptococcus pneumoniae* and *Haemophilus influenzae* because specific opsonizing antibodies that play a major role in the defense against such pathogens are greatly reduced.

Marrow and Stem Cell Transplantation

Infection is one of the major complications of bone marrow and/or hematopoietic stem cell transplantation. During the initial period of neutropenia, patients are at risk of developing bacterial infections. Fungal infections caused by *Candida* spp. and *Aspergillus* spp. also occur during this period. The risk of these infections decreases after recovery of the neutrophil count, but neutrophil and macrophage function remain abnormal. Patients undergoing allogeneic transplantation also have suppressed cell-mediated immunity. As a consequence, infections with herpes viruses, respiratory syncytial virus sRSV), and adenoviruses, *Pneumocystis jiroveci, Toxoplasma gondii*, bacteria (such as *Legionella* spp., and *S. pneumoniae*) and mould infections (aspergillosis) are common. These infections generally occur after the initial period of neutropenia has elapsed, and patients remain at risk until the regenerating immune system matures and restores normal immunity. This depends a great deal on whether or not graft-versus-host disease (GVHD) can be prevented or controlled. Multiple (polymicrobial) infections are not uncommon in this setting.

Local Factors

Local factors, such as tumor metastases, that produce obstruction and operative procedures that result in disruption of normal anatomic barriers play an important role in infections occurring in patients with cancer. Pneumonia and pulmonary abscesses develop distal to tumors causing obstruction of major bronchi, and these infections respond poorly to antibiotic therapy, unless adequate drainage is established. Obstruction of the biliary tract can result in ascending cholangitis.[16] Urinary tract infections are common in patients with tumors, such as bladder or prostatic carcinoma, that obstruct a ureter or the bladder neck causing retention of urine. Hydronephrosis, pyonephrosis, chronic pyelonephritis, and cystitis are not uncommon complications in patients with cancer of the genitourinary tract (Table 137-3). In these situations, the infection is generally caused by one or more of the microorganisms colonizing the site of obstruction.

Damage to mucosal surfaces (particularly the gastrointestinal mucosa) occurs frequently as a result of antineoplastic chemotherapy and provides a portal of entry for infecting organisms such as viridans group streptococci, vancomycin-resistant enterococci (VRE), enteric gram-negative bacilli and *Candida* species. Radiation therapy results in depression of cell-mediated immunity, which can last for several months. Radiation also causes local tissue damage, which can predispose to secondary infection. Foreign bodies, such as urinary and venous catheters, also damage or circumvent normal anatomic barriers, thereby facilitating entry of microorganisms into tissues and the bloodstream.

Intravascular Devices

Central venous catheters are used extensively in patients who require frequent vascular access. These catheters (Hickman, Broviac, and long lines) can have multiple lumens, greatly facilitate a variety of functions, including the drawing of blood, and may remain in the same location for prolonged periods, ranging from several weeks to months. Three separate types of device-related infection have been described: infection of the entry site, tunnel infection, and catheter-related bacteremia or fungemia.[17] Gram-positive organisms predominate, but gram-negative bacilli are not infrequent. Fungemia is most often caused by

Table 137-3 Common Infections in Patients With Solid Tumors

Tumor Location	Infection Site or Type
Breast	Surgical wound infection; cellulitis or lymphangitis related to axillary node dissection; mastitis; breast abscess; bacteremia
Central nervous system (brain; meninges)	Surgical wound infection; epidural/subdural infection; brain abscess; meningitis/ventriculitis; proximal and distal end-shunt–related infections; aspiration pneumonia; urinary tract infection; bacteremia
Genitourinary and prostate	Cystitis; urethritis; acute/chronic pyelonephritis ± bacteremia; catheter-related complicated urinary tract infection (nephrostomy/stents); wound infection; acute/chronic prostatitis; epididymitis, orchitis; pelvic abscess
Hepatobiliary-pancreatic	Surgical wound infection; peritonitis; ascending cholangitis ± bacteremia; hepatic, pancreatic, or subdiaphragmatic abscess
Head and neck	Cellulitis; surgical wound infection; deep facial space infection; mastoiditis/osteomyelitis; sinusitis; aspiration/nosocomial pneumonia; bacteremia; suppurative intracranial phlebitis; meningitis; brain abscess; retropharyngeal and paravertebral abscesses
Musculoskeletal (muscles, bones, joints)	Surgical wound infections; skin and skin structure infection; pyomyositis; lymphangitis cartilage lymphadenitis; bursitis; synovitis; septic arthritis; osteomyelitis; wound infection; prosthesis related infections; bacteremia
Upper gastrointestinal	Esophagitis; tracheoesophageal fistula with pneumonitis/lung abscess; gastric perforation and abscess; feeding tube related infections; mediastinitis/osteomyelitis
Lower gastrointestinal	Surgical wound infection; intraabdominal or pelvic abscess; peritonitis (perforation); enterocolitis; urinary tract infection; perianal/perirectal infection; sacral/coccygeal osteomyelitis

Candida spp. Localized *Aspergillus* infection has also been described. Infections of shunts, stents, and prosthetic devices are also common.

Splenectomy

Splenectomy is associated with a lifelong risk of developing infections as a result of impaired antibody production and suboptimal removal of poorly opsonized pathogens. Most of these infections are caued by encapsulated pathogens such as *Streptococcus pneumoniae*, *Haemophilus influenzae*, and *Neisseria meningitides*, and by intraerythrocytic organisms such as *Babesia* spp. Lifelong penicillin prophylaxis after splenectomy has been recommended by some experts but the emergence of penicillin-resistant pneumococci has reduced the impact of this strategy.[18,19] Patients should be given the pneumococcal polyvalent capsular polysaccharide vaccine prior to splenectomy and every 3 years thereafter. Vaccination with *H. influenzae* type B conjugated polysaccharide vaccine and yearly influenza vaccination are also recommended. Quadrivalent meningococcal vaccination should only be administered during an epidemic of meningococcal infection.[19]

Chemotherapeutic Agents

Chemotherapeutic agents predispose to the development of infections by various mechanisms. Myelosuppressive agents produce neutropenia. Others interfere with cell-mediated and humoral immunity without producing profound myelosuppression. Agents such as fludarabine and other purine analogs, temozolomide, and monoclonal antibodies such as alemtuzumab and rituximab have profound effects on multiple components of host defenses, and are associated with unique infections.[20]

Bacterial Infections

Current data from the University of Texas, MD Anderson Cancer Center indicate that gram-positive organisms cause approximately 50-55% of documented infections in patients who have neutropenia (Table 137-4). Many other epidemiologic surveys focus only on bloodstream infections (SCOPE, EORTC).[3,21] These surveys give an incomplete and inaccurate picture of the overall spectrum because, (1) bloodstream infections account for only 15-25% of infections (other common sites are the respiratory tract, the urinary tract, the gastrointestinal tract and skin/skin structure), (2) bloodstream infections are predominantly gram-positive (65-75%), whereas (3) infections at other sites are predominantly gram-negative or have mixed flora.

In addition, 23% of bacterial infections in patients with hematologic malignancies, and 31% in patients with solid tumors are polymicrobial.[2,22] These infections including pneumonia, neutropenic enterocolitis, skin/skin structure infections (eg, perianal infections) are predominantly tissue based and are generally associated with greater morbidity and mortality than monomicrobial infections. When all sites (including monomicrobial and polymicrobial infections) are taken into account, a substantially different epidemiologic picture emerges, compared to that associated with bloodstream infections alone. The proportion of gram-positive infections decreases substantially (from 70-75% to 45-50%). This can influence the choice of agents used for prophylaxis and empiric therapy (eg, initial use of vancomycin, or monotherapy versus combination therapy). Consequently, clinicians should consider the entire spectrum of bacterial infections (not just bloodstream infections) when initiating empiric antibiotic therapy.[23]

Specific Bacterial Pathogens

Staphylococcus Spp.

Staphylococci are the most common organisms isolated from neutropenic and non-neutropenic cancer patients. Coagulase-negative staphylococci (particularly *Staphylococcus epidermidis*) are isolated more often than *S. homins*, and *S. haemolyticus*. Increased use of medical devices and other conditions that usurp natural barriers to infection (surgery, trauma, radiation) are primarily responsible for increased recovery of these organisms. Antimicrobial prophylaxis with fluoroquinolones (to which these organisms are generally resistant) might also account for this increase. The gastrointestinal tract also serves as an important source for coagulase-negative *staphylococcus* (CoNS) in febrile patients with neutropenia. *Staphylococcus aureus* is the second most common gram-positive species isolated from patients

Table 137-4 Distribution of Bacterial Infection in 3451 Febrile Episodes in Patients W ith Cancer Who Are Neutropenic

	1994-1995		1999-2000		2002-2003		2004-2005	
Infection Type	No.	%	No.	%	No.	%	No.	%
Microbiologically documented	189	28	207	30	262	26	301	27
Gram-positive	86	46	99	48	134	51	148	49
Gram-negative	54	28	51	25	51	20	61	20
Polymicrobial	49	26	51	25	71	27	30	30
Anaerobic	–	–	6	2	6	2	2	1
Clinically documented	107	16	93	13	210	21	287	26
Unexplained fever	373	56	390	57	521	53	511	47

with cancer. Of concern is the increasing rate of methicillin-resistance among *S. aureus* isolates which is now often >50% at many cancer treatment centers. The countrywide increase in community-acquired methicillin-resistant *Staphylococcus aureus* (CA-MRSA)ay require a change in guidelines and practice patterns for empiric therapy, and may result in an increased use of agents with activity against MRSA.[24] Data from quantitative cultures indicate that the majority of infections caused by CoNS are low-grade (≤10 colony forming units/mL) and might be associated with lower morbidity and mortality than *S. aureus*, for which high-grade infections (≥500 CFU/mL) are far more common.[25] Bacteremia (including catheter-related infection) is the most common manifestation of staphylococcal infection. Skin and soft-tissue infections, including surgical wound infections, are also relatively common. Serious complications including pneumonia, septic thrombophlebitis, endocarditis, lung and splenic abscesses, can occur, and occasionally can be fatal.

The treatment of staphylococcal infections should be guided by local susceptibility/resistance patterns. Most broad-spectrum agents used for empiric therapy in febrile patients with neutropenia are active against methicillin-susceptible isolates. Vancomycin remains the agent of choice for methicillin-resistant isolates although increasing numbers of vancomycin failures are being reported, even among vancomycin susceptible strains.[26] Older agents (tetracycline, minocycline, clindamycin, rifampin, trimethoprim/sulfamethoxazole) and some newer agents (quinupristin/dalfopristin, linezolid, daptomycin, dalbavancin, televancin) are also useful for the treatment of staphylococcal infections, although many have not been evaluated in patients with neutropenia.[27,28] Infected catheters should be removed, whenever feasible, although antibiotic therapy without catheter removal has also been shown to be successful. Recurrent infection will occur in 20-30% of patients in whom infected catheters are not removed.[29]

Streptococcus Spp.

Many streptococcal species are important pathogens in patients with cancer. *S. pneumoniae* causes infection primarily in patients who have undergone splenectomy, those with multiple myeloma, those with acute or chronic lymphocytic leukemia, and allogeneic stem cell transplant recipients.[30] The syndrome of overwhelming pneumococcal sepsis occurs in patients with splenectomy and often follows a fulminant course resulting in death. Disseminated intravascular coagulation may occur, and *S. pneumoniae* are often demonstrated in peripheral blood smears. Defects in antibody formation and clearing of the organisms from the bloodstream are probably responsible for this clinical syndrome. Prompt and effective antimicrobial therapy is critical. Penicillin G remains the drug of choice for the treatment of pneumococcal infections caused by susceptible strains. On the other hand, penicillin-resistant pneumococci are being reported with increasing frequency and need to be treated with alternative agents. Most penicillin-resistant strains are susceptible to the extended-spectrum cephalosporins (ceftriaxone, ceftazidime, cefepime). The carbapenems (imipenem, meropenem) are also active against penicillin-resistant strains. These strains are uniformly susceptible to vancomycin, which is often included in empiric regimens until the results of susceptibility testing become available. Newer generation quinolones (levofloxacin, moxifloxacin) have potent activity against penicillin-resistant pneumococci, and are being used with increasing frequency to treat these infections.[31]

Before the emergence of penicillin-resistance, high-risk patients were given a supply of antibiotics with antipneumococcal activity (eg, amoxicillin/clavulanic acid, Augmentin, which is also active against *H. influenzae*) so that they may initiate antibiotic therapy at the first sign of infection, prior to seeking medical attention. With current rates of penicillin-resistance running as high as 60%, the usefulness of this strategy has been severely limited. The newer generation quinolones have reliable activity against these organisms. Their use instead of amoxicillin/clavulanate might be prudent, but has not been fully evaluated.

α-Hemolytic (viridans) streptococci are important pathogens in patients with acute leukemia undergoing intensive chemotherapy and in allogeneic bone marrow transplant recipients.[32] α-Hemolytic streptococci colonize the oral cavity, and the most consistent predisposing factor for the development of infection appears to be high-dose chemotherapy with drugs, such as cytosine arabinoside, that induce severe mucosal damage, thereby facilitating entry of these organisms into the bloodstream. Other probable predisposing factors include antimicrobial prophylaxis, particularly with fluoroquinolones that might encourage the selection and overgrowth of these organisms, and the treatment of chemotherapy-induced gastritis with antacids or histamine type 2 (H2) antagonists.[33] *Streptococcus mitis*, *Streptococcus sanguis*, and *Streptococcus salivarius* are the predominant species. Bacteremia is the most common manifestation. In some patients, a rapidly progressive disseminated infection occurs involving the bloodstream,

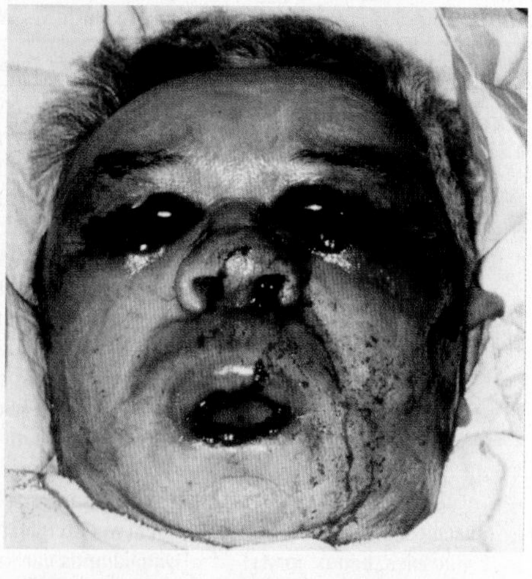

Figure 137-2 Invasive infection caused by α-hemolytic (viridans) streptococci. Note the hemorrhagic nature of the lesions in this patient with thrombocytopenia.

lungs, central nervous system, and skin (Fig. 137-2). Septic shock is often present, and the clinical picture resembles that of staphylococcal "toxic shock syndrome." This syndrome (which is also caused by *Streptococcus pyogenes*) has been termed the "toxicstrep syndrome" or the streptococcal toxic shock syndrome. Overwhelming infection produces substantial morbidity, and mortality in the range of 25-35% occurs despite prompt and aggressive antibiotic therapy. The use of clindamycin that blocks toxin production is recommended.

Of increasing concern are reports that 20-60% of α-hemolytic streptococci are now penicillin-resistant at some institutions. This has limited the utility of penicillin G and other penicillins for the prevention and treatment of such infections. All isolates are currently susceptible to vancomycin, although tolerance has been described, and the use of antibiotic combinations (vancomycin + rifampin ± gentamicin) is sometimes necessary. These organisms are also susceptible to the newer generation quinolones (gatifloxacin, moxifloxacin) daptomycin and linezolid, but clinical experience is limited.

β-Hemolytic streptococci belonging to Lance-field groups A, B, C, F, and G also cause infections in patients with cancer, but less often than *S. pneumoniae* and viridans streptococci. Like viridans streptococci, *S. pyogenes* has been associated with a rapidly progressive, toxic shock-like syndrome. The management of these infections is similar to that of other streptococcal infections. Penicillin G remains the drug of choice for susceptible isolates. Increasing resistance/tolerance to the penicillins is being described. Bactericidal combinations are recommended for the treatment of tolerant isolates.

Enterococcus Spp.

Enterococci are currently the third-most-common gram-positive organisms isolated from patients with neutropenia. This increased frequency is probably related to the increased use of extended-spectrum cephalosporins and other broad-spectrum agents to which these organisms are intrinsically resistant.[34] The most common infections caused by enterococci are those of the bloodstream, urinary tract, wounds, and intrasbdominal infections, although occasionally endocarditis, meningitis, pneumonia, and other infections may be seen. *Enterococcus faecalis* is the predominant species accounting for 60-70% of clinical isolates. Most isolates of *E. faecalis* are susceptible to clinically achievable concentrations of penicillin, ampicillin, and vancomycin although these agents may lack bactericidal activity. Consequently, synergistic combinations of these agents with aminoglycosides, such as gentamicin, are recommended for serious enterococcal infections.

Infections caused by *Enterococcus faecium* are rising, particularly in patients who are neutropenic and other patients who are immunosuppressed.[34] These isolates often express high-level resistance to the aminoglycosides, thereby eliminating the synergistic interaction with the penicillins, high-level resistance to ampicillin, and vancomycin. The most problematic infections occur when all these resistance patterns are seen within the same strains. Vancomycin resistance may now be seen in up to 35% of enterococcal isolates from high-risk populations. Risk factors for infection with VRE include gastrointestinal colonization with these strains, and the use of antimicrobial agents with significant activity against anaerobes (metronidazole, clindamycin, imipenem). The administration of vancomycin (both oral and parenteral) is also a frequently cited risk factor for subsequent colonization with VRE.[35] Infections caused by VRE are much more common in patients with severe neutropenia (acute leukemia; bone marrow transplantation prior to engraftment) and are seldom seen in patients with solid tumors.[36] VRE are associated more often with recurrent infections, higher rates of refractory infections, and serious morbidity and mortality.

Established therapeutic options for VRE include linezolid, daptomycin, and quinupristin/dalforpristin. Response rates are generally lower than those associated with susceptible enterococci.

Attempts at eradicating gastrointestinal colonization with VRE have been singularly unsuccessful. Thus, infection control measures to reduce the transmission of VRE are of over-riding importance. These measures are more aggressive than standard infection control practices and strict compliance by hospital personnel is a prerequisite for their success.[37]

Listeria monocytogenes

Listeria monocytogenes is a gram-positive bacillus that causes meningitis, encephalitis, septicemia, and endocarditis. The administration of fludarabine and prednisone is associated with an increased incidence of listeriosis in patients with chronic lymphocytic leukemia and may be the result of a depletion in CD4 cells.[38] Meningitis accounts for more than 60% of cases in patients with cancer, and septicemia without meningitis accounts for approximately 30%. Meningismus is present in only one-half of the cancer patients with meningitis, and, occasionally, the cerebrospinal fluid is normal. When pleocytosis is present, either neutrophils or mononuclear cells predominate. The organisms may be difficult to culture from the cerebrospinal fluid. Although these organisms are susceptible in vitro to various antibiotics, ampicillin or penicillin remains the drug of choice for therapy. These agents are frequently used in combination with an aminoglycoside, because experimental laboratory results have demonstrated synergism between penicillins and aminoglycosides against *L. monocytogenes*. If an aminoglycoside is administered for central nervous system infection, both systemic and intrathecal routes can be used. Although these organisms are susceptible, in vitro, to the extended-spectrum cephalosporins, these agents are not effective for the therapy of *L. monocytogenes* meningitis. Trimethoprim/sulfamethoxazole (TMP-SMX) is bactericidal against the majority of these isolates, and has been used successfully in patients with listeriosis who are allergic to penicillin, including those with *Listeria meningitis*. Newer quinolones (moxifloxacin) are active against L. monocytogenes, but clinical experience with these agents is lacking.

Enterobacteriaceae

The gastrointestinal tract serves as an important source of infection in patients who have neutropenia. Although the overall frequency of documented gram-negative infections has declined, the proportion of gram-negative infections caused by *Enterobacteriaceae* has remained remarkably constant.[39] Data from surveillance studies conducted at major cancer centers, both in the United States and Europe, indicate that *Enterobacteriaceae* cause approximately 65-80% of gram-negative infections in these patients, with *Escherichia coli* and *Klebsiella* spp. consistently being among the three most common species to be isolated. Thus, antimicrobial regimens used for prophylaxis and for empiric therapy in patients with neutropenia have stressed the need for potent activity against *Enterobacteriaceae* (and other gram-negative bacilli). The bloodstream is the most frequent site of infection, followed by the urinary tract and the lung. Central venous catheters and other vascular access devices can become secondarily seeded during episodes of bacteremia and can serve as a continuing source of infection. Fever is the only consistent manifestation of infection. Other manifestations depend on specific sites of infection (lung, urinary tract) and are often blunted in patients who are severely neutropenic and immunosuppressed. The majority of these infections respond to standard antimicrobial therapy. On the other hand, polymicrobial infections and infections that are complicated by deep tissue involvement (pneumonia, enterocolitis, perirectal infections), are associated with greater morbidity and mortality.[22,40] The emergence of resistance to β-lactam agents as a result of the production of type 1 and extended-spectrum β-lactamases is of great concern. The widespread use of fluoroquinolone prophylaxis has also resulted in the development of resistance among *E. coli* and other *Enterobacteriaceae.* Routine prophylaxis with the fluoroquinolones in patients with neutropenia is not recommended and should be considered only in patients whose risk of developing gram-negative infections is high.[41]

Pseudomonas aeruginosa

Pseudomonas aeruginosa has been a leading cause of infection in patients who have cancer with severe neutropenia. Pneumonia and bacteremia are the most common infections, but the urinary tract, skin and gastrointestinal tract are also sites of infection. It is also a cause of catheter-related infections.[42]

Skin lesions are present in approximately 20% of cases of bacteremia. *Ecthyma gangrenosum*, the characteristic skin lesion, may be located anywhere but is found most commonly in the axilla, groin, and perianal region. Single or multiple lesions at various stages might be present with extensive tissue damage (Fig. 137-3). *Ecthyma gangrenosum* may occur in the absence of detectable bacteremia. *P. aeruginosa* can be cultured from these lesions, and histologically, the lesions represent a bacterial vasculitis without thrombosis, with dense bacillary infiltration of the media and adventitia of blood vessels.

P. aeruginosa is widespread in the hospital environment. It thrives in moist areas, such as faucets, sink drains, shower stalls, hydrotherapy tanks, and water pitchers, and in respiratory equipment, such as respirators and nebulizers.

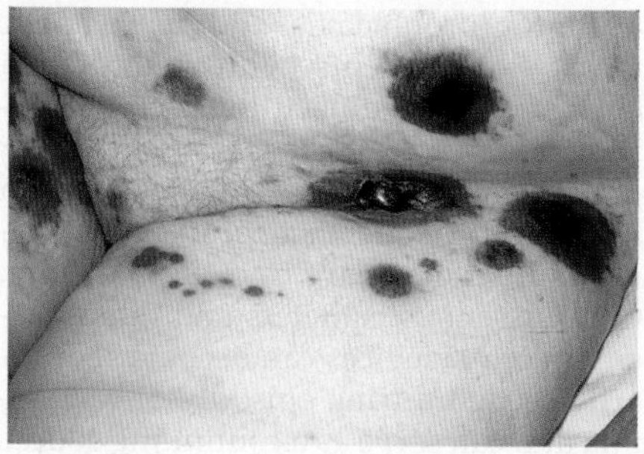

Figure 137-3 Multiple skin lesions (ecthyma gangrenosum) in a patient with *Pseudomonas aeruginosa* bacteremia.

It can also persist in soaps, shampoos, germicidal solutions, and ophthalmic solutions. Epidemics of *P. aeruginosa* infection have been observed in patients with cancer and approximately 25% of patients with acute leukemia are stool carriers of *P. aeruginosa*.

During the past 30 years, significant advances were made in the therapy of *P. aeruginosa* infections. Many potent antipseudomonal agents were developed including antipseudomonal penicillins (piperacillin ± tazobactam), extended spectrum cephalosporins (ceftazidime, cefepime), aminoglycosides (amikacin, tobramycin), monobactams (aztreonam), quinolones (ciprofloxacin), and carbapenems (imipenem, meropenem) The appropriate use of these agents resulted in response rates in the range of 80%.[43] Unfortunately, these advances are being eroded by the emergence of multidrug-resistant *P. aeruginosa* isolates with unique mechanisms of resistance.[9,10] Some of these isolates are susceptible only to agents such as colistin and polymyxin B which are not particularly useful in patients with neutropenia.[44]

Stenotrophomonas Spp.

Stenotrophomonas maltophilia are gram-negative bacilli that have emerged during the past decade as important nosocomial pathogens, particularly but not exclusively in patients with impaired host defense.[45] Moist hospital environments, such as sink drains and water faucets, are potential sources of infection. Broad-spectrum antimicrobial therapy and the presence of central venous catheters have been found to significantly increase the likelihood of infection.

Bacteremia (often related to central venous catheters) and pneumonia are the most common manifestations of infection. Urinary tract infection, skin and soft-tissue infection (including surgical wound infection), endocarditis, mastoiditis, and meningitis, have also been reported. Clinical manifestations of *S. maltophilia* infection are indistinguishable from those caused by other gram-negative rod infections. It is also often difficult to distinguish colonization from infection. Monotherapy using broad-spectrum agents, such as the carbapenems (imipenem, meropenem), to which *S. maltophilia* isolates are generally resistant, is a common form of therapy in patients with neutropenia. Empiric coverage against *S. maltophilia* should be considered in patients who fail to respond to such regimens. Approximately 70% of strains are susceptible to TMP-SMX, although increasing resistance to this agent is being reported. Alternative agents include ticarcillin/clavulanate, tigecycline, minocycline, rifampin, the newer fluoroquinolones, and some extended-spectrum cephalosporins. Most of these agents are less active than TMP-SMX, and susceptibility testing in each individual patient is recommended. Combination antibiotic therapy may be beneficial in patients from whom a relatively resistant strain has been isolated or who fail to respond to initial therapy with a single agent. High-dose therapy with TMP-SMX as used for the treatment of *Pneumocystis carinii* pneumonia, might be beneficial in some patients.[45]

Acinetobacter Spp.

Although infections caused by *Acinetobacter* spp. are relatively infrequent (approximately 4% of all gram-negative infections in patients who have cancer), infections of nearly all body sites (lungs, meninges, skin, heart valves, biliary tract, urinary tract, bones and joints, peritoneum, skin and soft tissue, and blood) have been reported. It may be difficult to distinguish infection from colonization.[46]

Outbreaks of infection caused by *Acinetobacter* spp. have been traced to intravascular access devices, contaminated respiratory therapy equipment, and contaminated bedding materials. Transmission via the hands of hospital personnel has been documented. In patients with cancer, up to 80% of bacteremic infections caused by *Acinetobacter* spp. are related to indwelling central venous catheters. Appropriate therapy includes the administration of antimicrobial agents to which the organisms are susceptible, and removal of the offending catheter in catheter-related infections. Multidrug resistance is common among these organisms and may complicate the treatment of serious infections.

Salmonella Spp.

Nearly 15% to 25% of serious *Salmonella* infections occur in patients with cancer. Patients with lymphoma, leukemia, or carcinoma of the gastrointestinal and genitourinary tract are most susceptible. *Salmonella typhimurium* and *Salmonella enteritidis* are the most frequently isolated species. Although gastroenteritis, which is usually self-limited, does occur in patients with cancer, about one-half of the infections involve other organ systems. Pneumonia, urinary tract infection, peritonitis, osteomyelitis, meningitis, and wound infection have been observed. Bacteremia and disseminated infections occur more frequently in patients with cancer than other patients with salmonellosis. A small percentage of patients continue to harbor *Salmonella* in stools or urine for periods >1 year following an acute infection, and are considered chronic carriers. Uncomplicated, nontyphoidal, *Salmonella* gastroenteritis generally requires no antibiotic therapy, but patients who are severely immunocompromised, who are at risk of developing bacteremia or disseminated infection might benefit from antibiotic therapy. The most reliable agents against *Salmonella* spp. are the fluoroquinolones, the extended-spectrum cephalosporins, and the carbapenems. Resistance to even these agents is being reported, and it may be prudent to administer more than one class of agent to seriously ill patients with salmonellosis until susceptibility determinations can be performed.

Clostridium difficile

Clostridium difficile is the leading infectious cause of diarrhea in cancer patients. Recently, a strain of *C. difficile* (NAP1) which produces increased levels of both toxins A and B has been identified.[47] This strain is associated with increased severity of illness, higher morbidity and mortality, and an increased risk of relapse and complications. Metronidazole and vancomycin remain the agents of choice for the treatment of *C. difficile*-associated disease (CDAD), although recent data suggest that vancomycin may be the preferred drug for patients with serious diseases.[48] Newer agents such as rifaximin and nitazoxamide have been used with some success to treat CDAD.[43] Investigational treatments include a toxin-binding polymer-tolevamer. Monoclonal antibodies, poorly absorbed antimicrobial agents such as ramoplanin, probiotics, and a *C. difficile* vaccine. Preventive measures include enforcements of strict infection control practices, appropriate antimicrobial usage, and improved environment cleaning methods.[49]

Mycobacterium Spp.

Protection against mycobacterial infection is mediated by cellular immunity. Mycobacterial infections, therefore, occur more frequently in patients with impairment of the cellular component of the host defense mechanisms (ie, Hodgkin disease). Infection is also frequent in patients with carcinoma of the head, neck, and lung. The diagnosis of tuberculosis is often difficult to establish with certainty because the usual manifestations of fever, weight loss, pulmonary infiltrates, and hepatosplenomegaly may be a result of neoplastic disease.

Anergy frequently occurs in patients with cellular immune defects, and positive tuberculin skin tests may be seen in only 10-30% of patients. The acid-fast stain is the only widely available test for a rapid presumptive diagnosis of tuberculosis. Traditional culture techniques, followed by biochemical testing, take up to 4-8 weeks to identify *M. tuberculosis*. This process is shortened considerably (1-3 weeks) by the use of radiometric culture methods followed by a deoxyribonucleic acid (DNA) probe for an *M. tuberculosis*-specific ribosomal ribonucleic acid (RNA) sequence. The DNA probe can be used in mycobacterial cultures but is not sensitive enough to detect organisms in clinical samples. Newer methods based on polymerase chain reaction (PCR) offer great promise and have the potential of providing a specific diagnosis within 24 h.

Standard therapy for drug-susceptible tuberculosis includes the administration of isoniazid, rifampin, and pyrazinamide daily for 2 months, followed by isoniazid and rifampin for 4 months, either daily or biweekly. Cure rates of greater than 95% are achieved by this regimen. Treatment with isoniazid, rifampin, ethambutol, and pyrazinamide three times a week for a period of 6 months is also effective. Because of the increasing frequency of drug resistance, the initial use of four-drug regimens is preferable until susceptibility determinations can be made. Cure rates of 90% can be achieved by using regimens containing isoniazid, rifampin, pyrazinamide, and ethambutol or streptomycin for 6-12 months in patients with an isoniazid-resistant isolate. Resistance to both isoniazid and rifampin markedly reduces the efficacy of therapeutic regimens, and failure rates of 40-70% have been reported. Quinolones, such as ofloxacin and ciprofloxacin, have been found to be useful in multidrugresistant (MDR) tuberculosis. Individualized drug regimens, based on results of susceptibility testing, should be employed, generally using at least three drugs to which the isolate is susceptible.[50] Directly observed therapy is recommended for all drug-resistant tuberculosis and for patients who are known to be noncompliant or unreliable.

Some patients with cancer are prone to developing infection with mycobacteria other than *M. tuberculosis*. Patients with hairy cell leukemia are particularly prone to developing disseminated infection caused by *Mycobacterium avium* intracellulare complex (MAC).[51] Recent data indicate that MAC infections are not uncommon in patients with solid tumors as well.[52] MAC infections are difficult to treat because the organisms are resistant to standard antituberculous agents. Commonly used agents include ethambutol, rifabutin, clarithromycin and azithromycin.[53] Refractory cases may respond to therapy with interferon-γ (IFN-γ) in combination with drug therapy. *Mycobacterium kansasii* also causes infection both in patients with hematologic malignancies and in patients with solid tumors.[54] Most patients have pulmonary disease, which is indistinguishable from that caused by *M. tuberculosis*. The organisms are generally susceptible to standard antituberculous agents, and most patients respond to therapy.

The pathogenic, rapidly growing mycobacteria (*Mycobacterium chelonae abscessus*, *M. chelonae* ssp. *chelonae* and *Mycobacterium fortuitum*) are environmental organisms commonly found in water and soil. The two most common infections caused by these organisms in patients with cancer include catheter-related bacteremia and pulmonary infection.[55,56] In the former, antibiotic therapy in addition to catheter removal is generally effective. In pulmonary or disseminated infection, prolonged therapy with combination regimens is necessary.[57] The organisms have variable susceptibility to agents such as the quinolones, the tetracyclines, the macrolides, amikacin, cephalosporins, and TMP-SMX.

Disease caused by mycobacteria can mimic cancer or present a diagnostic problem in patients with cancer who have been effectively treated and subsequently present with a pulmonary lesion. The assumption that this lesion is a metastatic or recurrent neoplasm should not be made, and patients should be carefully evaluated for tuberculosis or fungal infection before cancer chemotherapy is instituted.

Legionella pneumophila

Legionella pneumophila is an important cause of community-acquired and nosocomial pneumonia in healthy and immunosuppressed persons, including stem cell transplant recipients. Pleural effusion, empyema, and lung abscess formation, are recognized complications of *L. pneumophila* infection and occur more often in the immunosuppressed host.[58] Mortality rates as high as 80% have been documented in solid-organ transplant recipients and in others who are immunosuppressed.

A specific diagnosis of *L. pneumophila* infection might be difficult to establish. The organisms are fastidious and require selective culture media to promote growth (buffered charcoal yeast extract [BCYE] agar). Other diagnostic methods include serologic testing, direct fluorescent antibody staining, DNA probes, and the detection of urinary antigen.

Azithromycin and the fluoroquinolones are very active against *L. pneumophila* and are now the drugs of choice for the treatment of this infection.[59] Adding rifampin to azithromycin or a quinolone provides little benefit. The quinolones are the agents of choice for the treatment of legionellosis in patients receiving immunosuppressive therapy with cyclosporin or tacrolimus, because they do not alter the metabolism of cyclosporin or tacrolimus.

Fungal Infections

The setting in which fungal infection develops is complex, and multiple factors are responsible for the rapid increase in these infections. Frequently, this has been attributed to the widespread use of broad-spectrum antibiotics. Bacteria that inhibit the growth of *Candida* spp. are suppressed by antibiotic therapy permitting the overgrowth of *Candida* spp. Adrenal corticosteroids interfere with macrophage function, and the macrophage is one of the primary defenses against fungal invasion. Prolonged and severe neutropenia also predisposes to fungal infection. Neutrophils ingest and kill *Candida* spp. in vitro and serve as a major defense against systemic infection. The administration of adrenal corticosteroids interferes with macrophage function, allowing ingested spores to germinate. The administration of many cancer chemotherapeutic agents causes neutropenia, which facilitates establishment of infection by activated mycelia. The role of lymphocytes and lymphokines is complex and has not been fully elucidated. In the past, the majority of infections were caused by *Candida ablicans*, but in recent years *Candida tropicalis*, *Candida glabrata*, *Candida parapsilosis*, and other species have emerged as significant pathogens.[60]

Candida Spp.

Most superficial fungal infections of the oropharynx and gastrointestinal tract are caused by *C. albicans*. This infection is especially prevalent in patients receiving antitumor agents or radiotherapy that causes mucosal damage, patients receiving adrenal corticosteroids, and patients colonized with *Candida* spp. Patients with oropharyngeal candidiasis may have associated esophageal candidiasis that is asymptomatic.

The lesions appear as white or grayish white plaques surrounded by an erythematous halo (Fig. 137-4). The plaques are friable with a freely bleeding base. *Candida* plaques may occur in association with herpes simplex infection. Topical

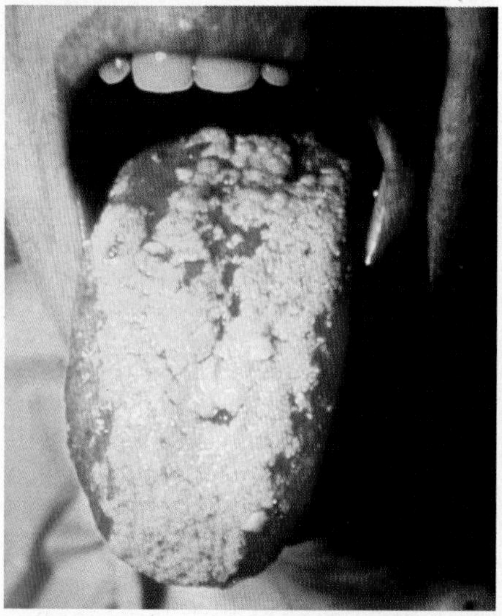

Figure 137-4 Severe oropharyngeal candidiasis in a patient with AIDS.

agents, such as nystatin, are of minimum benefit. Fluconazole and itraconazole solutions, are generally effective. *Candida esophagitis* produces dysphagia, often accompanied by retrosternal pain, nausea, and vomiting, and occasionally, gastrointestinal bleeding. It may be present with or without oral candidiasis. A characteristic cobblestone or moth-eaten appearance of the esophageal mucosa is present on barium-contrast radiographic studies (Fig. 137-5). These abnormalities, however, may be caused by other organisms, such as herpes simplex virus (HSV) and cytomegalovirus (CMV). Furthermore, in 25% of cases, the radiographic studies are negative. The diagnosis is established by esophagoscopy, which reveals characteristic ulcerations with pseudomembrane formation. Fluconazole is generally effective therapy. Newer triazoles (voriconazole, posaconazole) and the echinocandins (eg, caspofungin) are alternatives, but are seldom needed.

Systemic *Candida* infections may be localized to a single organ, but usually multiple organs are involved. Pulmonary infection is usually a manifestation of disseminated disease, but occasional primary infections of the lung do occur. It is difficult to establish the diagnosis of primary *Candida pneumonia* because there are no characteristic findings.[61] Isolation of *Candida* spp. from the sputum may represent contamination from the oropharynx. A substantial proportion of patients with urinary catheterization develop candiduria that often represents only colonization. Patients with surgery or abnormalities of the genitourinary tract, neutropenia or diabetes mellitus should always be treated with systemic therapy because they are at risk of serious *Candida* infection. *Candida* peritonitis may occur following intestinal perforation or in association with peritoneal catheters.

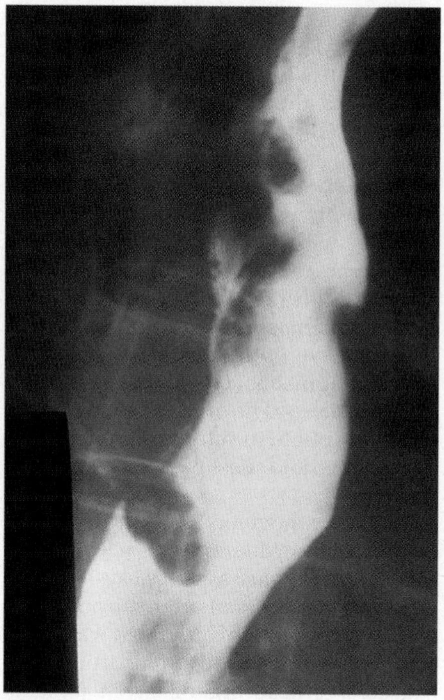

Figure 137-5 The characteristic "moth-eaten" appearance of the esophageal mucosa demonstrated on barium-swallow examination in a patient with esophageal candidiasis.

Disseminated candidiasis is found at autopsy examination in 20-30% of patients with acute leukemia, in 2% of patients with lymphoma, and in less than 1% of patients with metastatic cancer. Two patterns of organ involvement have been described. In one, occurring predominantly in patients with acute leukemia, the most frequent organs infected include the gastrointestinal tract, liver, spleen, and lungs. This pattern of involvement suggests the gastrointestinal tract as the primary site of origin. The second pattern of distribution predominantly involves the heart, kidneys, and lung, which is the pattern of distribution in animals following direct intravenous injection.

There are no characteristic physical signs and symptoms of disseminated candidiasis. Some patients present with the acute onset of tachycardia, tachypnea, and hypotension. Often, the only indications of this infection are a gradual worsening of the patient's clinical condition, associated with fever which is unresponsive to antibiotic therapy. Some patients have ocular infection causing blurred vision, pain, scotomata, or loss of visual acuity. Ocular lesions include white fluffy retinal exudates with vitreous haze or hemorrhage, hypopyon, or iritis, but these lesions are rarely found in patients with neutropenia. Nearly 10% of patients, especially those with severe neutropenia, develop characteristic erythematous macronodular skin lesions. In occasional patients, these skin lesions are associated with a myositis in which the patient has exquisitely tender muscles.

A chronic form of *Candida* infection known as hepatosplenic candidiasis—or, more appropriately, chronic disseminated candidiasis—has been described. This infection typically occurs in patients with acute leukemia undergoing chemotherapy while they are experiencing prolonged severe neutropenia. They develop fever that fails to respond to broad-spectrum antibiotics, as well as antifungal agents. After neutrophil recovery, they remain febrile and debilitated with substantial weight loss. Symptoms, including right upper quadrant or shoulder pain, may appear. Hepatosplenomegaly may be detected. Alkaline phosphatase concentration becomes highly elevated, and other liver function tests may also become abnormal. Ultrasonography, magnetic resonance imaging (MRI), or computed tomography (CT) of the liver and spleen reveals multiple lesions (Fig. 137-6). Other organs may also be infected and approximately 90% of the patients respond to fluconazole or lipid formulations of AMB.[62] Usually several weeks of therapy are required. This type of *Candida* infection has virtually disappeared from institutions where fluconazole is used prophylactically.

At many institutions *C. tropicalis* has surpassed *C. albicans* as the most common cause of disseminated infection.[63] It appears to be more virulent because only 3-15% of neutropenic patients colonized by *C. albicans* subsequently develop disseminated infection, as compared to 40-80% of those colonized by *C. tropicalis.* Skin lesions and myositis are associated more often with *C. tropicalis* infection. *C. parapsilosis* is less virulent than *C. albicans,* and infection is nearly always associated with intravascular catheters and parenteral nutrition. Colonization and infection caused by *C. krusei* and *C. glabrata* are associated with the use of fluconazole prophylaxis.[64] Unlike other *Candida* spp., *C. krusei* has been isolated from many foods and beverages, but

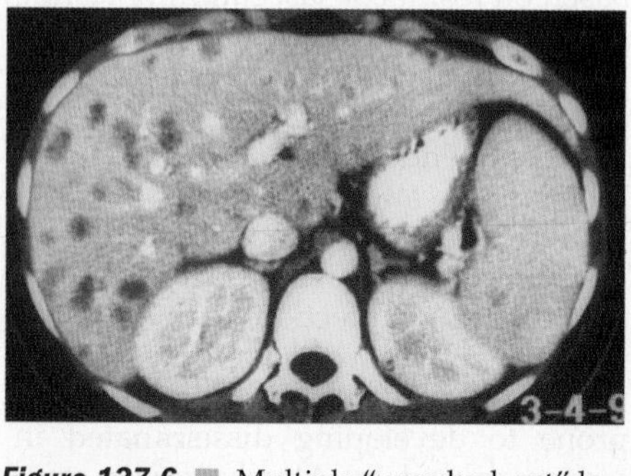

Figure 137-6 Multiple "punched-out" lesions in the liver, spleen, and kidneys in a patient with chronic disseminated candidiasis.

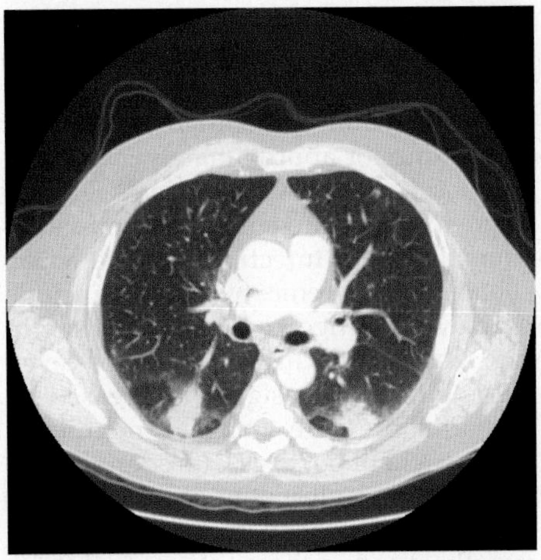

Figure 137-7 ■ Rounded pulmonary lesions with surrounding halo, compatible with invasive pulmonary aspergillosis.

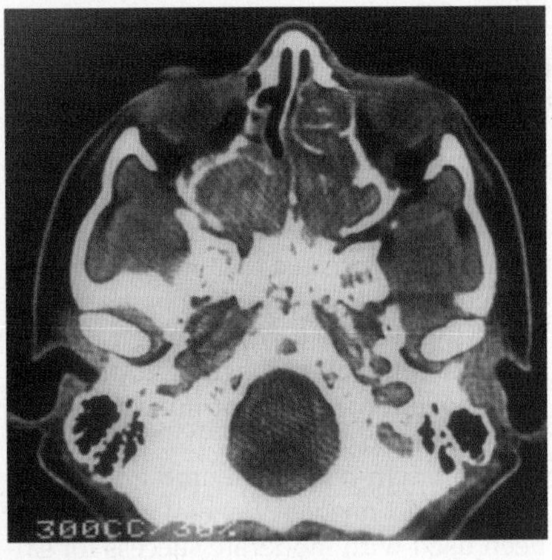

Figure 137-8 ■ Pansinusitis caused by *Aspergillus* spp. in an allogeneic bone marrow transplant recipient with persistent fever.

infrequently from healthy humans and is often a cause of candidemia among patients already receiving fluconazole or AMB as therapy or prophylaxis.[65] Patients who are azole naïve may also develop infections caused by nonalbicans *candida* species.[66]

The diagnosis of disseminated candidiasis is often not established before death. Only 50% of patients have abnormal chest radiographs at the onset of infection involving the lungs. *Candida* spp. are isolated from blood specimens of about 70% of patients with disseminated candidiasis. A variety of nonculture methods, including monoclonal antibodies to detect mannoproteins, enzyme-linked immunosorbent assay (ELISA) techniques to detect enolase, and PCR analyses have been developed, but none are reliable.[67] AMB has been effective for the treatment of disseminated candidiasis in patients with adequate neutrophil counts, due to acute toxicities including fever, chills, and headaches. It is seldome used anymore. The administration of AMB in lipid formulations (L-AMB) reduces the frequency of nephrotoxicity and allows for the administration of much higher daily doses. Fluconazole is as effective as AMB and is much less toxic.[68] *C. krusei* is inherently resistant to fluconazole and about 15% of isolates of *C. glabrata* are also resistant. Other agents available for therapy of *Candida* infections include itraconazole, voriconazole, posaconazole and the echinocandins.[69-72]

The therapy of disseminated candidiasis in patients with persistent neutropenia is often unsuccessful. The use of high-dose antifungal therapy (fluconazole, L-AMB or caspofungin) or combination therapy (eg, caspofungin and voriconazole) might offer some benefit in selected patients along with the use of hematopoietic growth factors (G-CSF, GM-CSF) and/or granulocyte transfusions.

■ *Aspergillus* Spp.

Aspergillosis is an increasing problem in patients with neutropenia and patients receiving chronic adrenal corticosteroid therapy. Recent studies report a frequency of 20-50% among patients with acute leukemia. This infection is also common in stem cell transplant recipients during the posttransplant period when they are neutropenic and later if they develop GVHD. The most common pathogen is *Aspergillus fumigatus*.[73] Other human pathogens include *Aspergillus terreus*, *Aspergillus flavus*, *Aspergillus niger*, *Aspergillus glaucus*, and *Aspergillus nidulans*. Infection is usually acquired by inhalation of spores, which are deposited in the paranasal sinuses or lungs. Outbreaks of aspergillosis have occurred on leukemic and bone marrow transplantation units, usually associated with construction within or adjacent to the hospital. Disturbance of dust above false ceilings represents a significant risk to susceptible patients, and they should be protected from such exposure.

More than 70% of infections involve the lungs, and approximately 35% of patients with pulmonary aspergillosis have hematogenous dissemination to other organs. Pulmonary infection may be manifested as necrotizing bronchopneumonia, hemorrhagic pulmonary infarction, solitary or miliary lung abscesses, lobar pneumonia, or bronchitis. A few patients will develop exsanguinating pulmonary hemorrhage early in the course of their infection. Often, the only evidence of infection is prolonged fever with pulmonary infiltrates that fail to respond to antibacterial therapy. High-resolution CT scanning of the lung is helpful in the early diagnosis of aspergillosis. Nodular lesions may be detected in the lungs of patients with normal chest radiographs. Characteristic findings in early stage disease are multiple nodules with a halo of surrounding ground-glass attenuation that represents hemorrhage surrounding a region of pulmonary infarction (Fig. 137-7). As healing occurs, the infarcted tissue becomes necrotic and retracts from the viable tissue leaving an air crescent.[74] Aspergillus sino-orbital infection is being diagnosed with increasing frequency in patients with acute leukemia and in marrow transplant recipients, accounting for at least 15% of cases of aspergillosis (Fig. 137-8). Signs and symptoms include fever, retro-orbital pain, headache, circumorbital erythema, nasal obstruction, and necrotic encrustation of the nasal septum, palate, or external nares. Infections may erode through the base of the skull and invade the brain or cause destruction of the paranasal and facial structures and the eye. About half the infections disseminate to other organs. The fungus can often be isolated from nasal cultures. It can be visualized histopathologically and often cultured from biopsy specimens.

Approximately 35% of infections are widely disseminated involving the lung, brain, gastrointestinal tract, liver, kidney, and thyroid. Aspergillus infection of the liver may cause multiple abscesses or vascular thrombosis and infarction, occasionally resulting in Budd–Chiari syndrome. The organism is seldom isolated from blood culture specimens of patients with disseminated disease.

Although central nervous system aspergillosis sometimes results from local extension of sinus infection, more often, it follows hematologic dissemination. Multiple lesions are usually present, with substantial vascular invasion leading to cerebral thrombosis, infarction, and abscess formation. These patients are lethargic and have focal neurologic signs indicative of the area of brain involvement. The cerebrospinal fluid is normal in most instances, although leukocytosis and increased protein concentrations may be found.

A localized form of aspergillosis has been described in association with intravascular catheters. *Aspergillus* spores may be deposited from the air at the time of insertion or may be impregnated in materials used for catheter dressings.[75] These infections are potentially serious because they can disseminate. Skin lesions, manifested as sharply defined black eschars, occur in about 5% of patients with disseminated infection. *Aspergillus stomatitis* occurs in patients with neutropenia.

Antemortem diagnosis of aspergillosis is difficult because the organism is cultured from clinical specimens of less than 30% of infected patients; hence, many infections are diagnosed only at autopsy examination. Although *Aspergillus* spp. can be cultured from normal, uninfected subjects and is a potential laboratory contaminant, if it is cultured from respiratory secretions of susceptible patients, there is a high probability of infection. Hyphal elements can be identified in infected sinus tissue biopsies, but the organism is cultured from only 75% of these cases. Galactomannan detection and PCR are promising methods for identifying infected patients.[76,77] Serial galactomannan assays may be useful for assessing response to therapy.

Voriconazole is considered the therapeutic agent of choice for invasive aspergillosis in most patients.[70,73,78] Liopsomal amphotericin B is considered an alternative to voriconazole.[73] Several agents have been used with moderate success for salvage therapy of invasive aspergillosis including the lipid formulation of amphotericin B, posaconazole, itraconazole, and the echinocandins caspofungin and micafungin.[73,79] Some refractory infections might respond to a change in the class of antifungal agent (eg, polyene to triazole or echinocandins), whereas othesr might respond to a combination of antifungal agents, but no controlled trials support these approaches.[73] Surgical resection might be warranted in some settings. Recovery from neutropenia and/or reversal of immunosuppression are critical, and responses are seldom seen in persistently neutropenic/immunosuppressed patients.

A major problem is the management of the patient who has recovered from pulmonary aspergillosis and who has a persistent cavity with or without a fungus ball. Acute pulmonary hemorrhage can occur, leading to death. Furthermore, the potential for reactivation of infection interferes with subsequent cancer chemotherapy. Surgical excision of the residual cavity should be given consideration, but that may not always be technically possible due to the presence of multiple cavities or the location of the lesion. Antifungal therapy should be administered during periods of neutropenia in patients with residual lesions to prevent reactivation. The appropriate duration of such therapy is unknown, but should be continued for a minimum of two courses.

Cryptococcus Spp.

Cryptococcosis is primarily a disease of patients with impaired cellular immunity; the organism is ubiquitous in animals and soil specimens. Infection begins in the lungs, where it may remain asymptomatic and resolve without therapy. Approximately 40% of infections in patients with cancer involve the lungs.[80] A variety of abnormalities may be found on chest radiographs, including miliary, nodular or cavitary lesions. Granulomas may be present in some cases. Primary cryptococcal pneumonia may follow a fulminant course, leading to the death of the patient within 1-2 weeks after onset of symptoms.

The most common form of cryptococcal infection is meningoencephalitis, accounting for approximately 50% of infections in patients with cancer. It is a consequence of hematogenous dissemination from the lung. Infection may be acute, subacute, or chronic. Symptoms include headache, vertigo, nausea, and vomiting; physical findings consist of fever, meningitis, stupor, signs of increased intracranial pressure, and focal neurologic defects. Leukocytosis (predominantly with lymphocytes), hypoglycorrhachia, and elevated protein concentrations are usually found in the cerebrospinal fluid. Yeast cells can be visualized in the cerebrospinal fluid of nearly 60% of patients. Crytpococcus neoformans usually is cultured easily from the cerebrospinal fluid of patients with meningitis. The serologic test for detection of cryptococcal antigen in cerebrospinal fluid and blood is useful for rapid diagnosis of this infection, especially in cases where the organism cannot be visualized.

Initial therapy of meningitis should consist of AMB plus 5-fluorocytosine for about 2 weeks. Subsequently, therapy can be continued with fluconazole for at least 10 weeks. Fluconazole can also be used as primary therapy for subacute and chronic infections of other sites. The echinocandins such as caspofungin are not active against *Cryptococcus* spp.

Other Opportunistic Fungi

A variety of fungi of low pathogenicity have been recognized as cause of significant infection in patients with cancer. These organisms include *Trichosporon* spp., the Zygomycetes, *Blastoschizomyces capitatus, Fusarium* spp., *Scedosporium* spp., *Geotrichum candidum*, and *Malassezia furfur.* Most of these infections occur sporadically, although there have been clusters of *Fusarium* infections at some institutions. The majority of patients who are infected have hematologic neoplasms, especially acute leukemia.

Zygomycosis is a rare infection with the most common pathogens being Mucor, Rhizopus, Absidia, and Rhizomucor species.[81] Pneumonia is the most common form of infection in patients with cancer, and occurs primarily in patients with hematologic malignancies. Some patients develop sinopulmonary, rhinocerebral, gastrointestinal, cutaneous, or disseminated infection. The clinical presentation of zygomycosis is often indistinguishable from aspergillosis. Zygomycosis should be considered in patients who are immunosuppressed and who develop sinusitis or invasive fungal infection after prolonged exposure to voriconazole, which is not active against these organisms.[82]

Like *Aspergillus* spp., Mucorales invade blood vessels, causing thrombosis and infarction. Aggressive surgical debridement is an important component of the therapy of sino-orbital infection and should be considered in patients with residual lesions after pulmonary infection. Patients with neutropenia uniformly fail to respond to therapy unless neutrophil recovery occurs. Posaconazole is a new agent with promising activity against the Zygomycetes.[71]

Trichosporon spp. cutaneum can cause disseminated infection, primarily in patients with hematologic neoplasms. The majority of patients have been severely neutropenic.[83] A few patients, especially those with adequate neutrophil counts, develop localized pneumonia without dissemination. There are no characteristic signs and symptoms suggestive of *Trichosporon* infection. A variety of skin lesions have been described, and skin lesions occur in approximately 30% of patients who are infected. Portals of entry include the gastrointestinal tract, respiratory tract, and intravenous catheter sites. *Trichosporon* infection is often associated with other concurrent opportunistic infections. Although these organisms may be susceptible to AMB, the azole compounds appear to be more effective therapeutic agents.

Fusarium spp. have emerged as significant pathogens in patients with neutropenia during the past decade.[84] Localized infections of the lung, sinuses, and skin occur, but most patients have disseminated infection. Cutaneous and subcutaneous skin lesions are frequent in disseminated infection. Like *Aspergillus* spp., these organisms invade blood vessels, causing thrombosis and infarction. Usually *Fusarium* spp. can be isolated readily from blood culture or tissue specimens. It may be difficult to distinguish *Fusarium* from some other fungi on histopathologic examination. Recovery from this infection depends on resolution of neutropenia, and currently available antifungal agents are at best only marginally effective. Encouraging results with posaconazole have been reported.

Empiric Therapy

The high frequency of fungal infections in patients with neutropenia and the inadequacy of diagnostic procedures have led to empiric administration of antifungal agents in patients who are suspected of having these infections. Empiric therapy should be considered in patients with neutrophil counts of less than 100/mm^3 for greater than 1 week who develop fever that fails to respond to 4-7 days of broad-spectrum antibacterial therapy. Other indications are indwelling catheters, chronic adrenal corticosteroid therapy, the presence of unexplained pulmonary infiltrates, and deteriorating renal or hepatic function. Lipid formulations of AMB, voriconazole or caspofungin may be used.[85,86] Patients who respond probably should remain on antifungal therapy for at least 1 or 2 weeks. Empiric antifungal therapy is not indicated for a majority of patients who have only transient or modest degrees of neutropenia.

Viral Infections

Viral infections are common following bone marrow transplant (BMT)/ human stem cell transplant (HSCT) and, to a lesser extent, among patients with leukemia and lymphoma. Herpes viruses are identified most frequently, especially HSV, varicella-zoster virus (VZV), and CMV. Community respiratory viruses, including RSV, influenza A and B, and parainfluenza viruses, are common among BMT recipients and patients with acute leukemia in whom upper respiratory tract infection can progress to pneumonitis, which is associated with a substantial mortality rate. Other viruses that can cause serious illness include Epstein-Barr virus (EBV), human herpes virus-6 (HHV-6), adenoviruses, hepatitis viruses, and polyoma viruses.[87]

HSV

Infections caused by HSV are the most common viral infections in patients with lymphoma and acute leukemia. These infections occur predominantly in patients with preexistent antibodies to HSV, most represent reactivation of endogenous latent infection. More than 80% of stem cell transplant recipients will have reactivation of latent HSV. Lesions caused by HSV are found most often on the lips and oral mucosa. Secondary infection with bacteria or fungi may occur. Localized bleeding may occur in patients with severe thrombocytopenia. Some patients develop chronic localized ulcers involving the nose, lips, or eyelids that begin as small papulovesicular lesions and gradually enlarge over several weeks. Herpetic lesions can extend from the oropharyngeal mucosa to involve the esophageal mucosa, producing symptoms that are indistinguishable from *Candida esophagitis*. Localized HSV lesions may also be seen in other areas of the body, such as the genital and perianal areas, and may become quite destructive. Dissemination of HSV infection is uncommon. The liver, spleen, adrenal glands, kidneys, pancreas, lungs, brain, and gastrointestinal tract may be involved in disseminated infection. Acyclovir, famciclovir, and valacyclovir are effective for the treatment of these infections. Because of the high frequency of mucocutaneous infections in acute leukemia patients undergoing induction chemotherapy and bone marrow transplant recipients who are seropositive, antiviral prophylaxis is indicated. Disseminated infection, encephalitis, and infection in immunocompromised patients generally require intravenous therapy with acyclovir (10 mg/kg q8h). Strains of HSV resistant to acyclovir may develop. In such cases, foscarnet is the treatment of choice. Cidofovir might also be useful in refractory infections.

VZV

Primary infection with VZV causes approximately 4 million cases of chicken pox in the United States each year. VZV remains latent in the sensory ganglia for the lifetime of the host, and reactivates in 15% of persons to cause herpes zoster.[88] Varicella has been recognized as a serious infection in children undergoing cancer chemotherapy. As it is highly contagious, it is especially hazardous, and epidemics have occurred in pediatric cancer facilities. Serious complications arise in approximately 5% of otherwise healthy children who develop varicella, but the fatality rate is less than 0.5%. Nearly 30% of children receiving cancer chemotherapy develop serious complications during varicella infection, with around 7% fatality rate. Characteristic manifestations of varicella include a generalized vesicular rash and fever. Lesions appear initially on the face and scalp and subsequently spread to the trunk and extremities. New lesions continue to appear as older lesions crust. Infection may be unduly prolonged in patients with cancer. The vesicles become hemorrhagic and necrotic in patients with thrombocytopenia. Around 10% of children develop a bacterial superinfection. Disseminated visceral infection may result in widespread pneumonia, and focal necrosis of the liver, pancreas, or adrenal glands. Fulminating encephalitis may develop. Dissemination generally develops within 1 week of the onset of skin lesions.

Herpes zoster occurs most often in patients with lymphoproliferative disorders. The infection is characterized by a unilateral vesicular rash in the distribution of one or two adjacent sensory dermatomes (Fig. 137-9). The thoracic, cervical, and lumbar dermatomes are most commonly involved. In approximately 20% of patients with cancer, herpes zoster lesions arise initially at sites where the tumor is in close proximity to a nerve trunk. In an additional 20% of the patients, eruption first appears at sites of recent radiation therapy. Initially, the lesions appear to be erythematous and maculopapular in nature but swiftly evolve into a vesicular rash. Vesicles may coalesce to form larger, bulbous lesions.

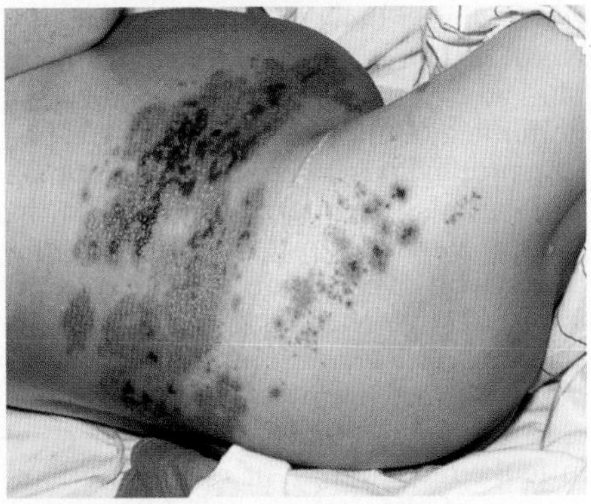

Figure 137-9 Typical vesicular rash caused by varicellazoster virus. Note the dermatomal distribution, and the hemorrhagic nature of lesions in this patient with thrombocytopenia.

Occasionally, patients develop a generalized varicelliform eruption, without localization. The rash is accompanied by pain (zoster-associated pain) that often precedes the eruption by 2-3 days, and can last for several weeks or even months. Postherpetic neuralgia is zoster-associated pain that persists beyond one month.

Cutaneous dissemination of herpes zoster occurs in approximately 35% of patients with cancer, as compared with only 4% of those without cancer. Therapy with adrenal corticosteroids, radiation, or antitumor agents facilitates dissemination. Visceral dissemination occurs infrequently but then commonly involves the gastrointestinal tract, liver, adrenals, pancreas, lungs, and brain, resulting in hepatitis, pneumonitis, and meningoencephalitis. Multiple episodes of herpes zoster are much more common in immunosuppressed individuals than in persons who are immunocompetent.

Laboratory confirmation of the diagnosis is not required for most cases of varicella. VZV can be recovered from the vesicular fluid for a few days after the onset of the eruption but is recovered infrequently from other sites. Cultures are positive 30-60% of the time. Detection of VZV antigens in skin scrapings using fluorescence microscopy, and detection of VZV DNA, in the cerebrospinal fluid or other tissues, using PCR, are more rapid and sensitive diagnostic techniques.

Therapy of VZV infection shortens viral shedding, accelerates healing of lesions and reduces the frequency of visceral disease.[89,90] Oral famciclovir and valacyclovir are more effective than acyclovir. Severe infections such as meningoencephalitis and pneumonitis require intravenous acyclovir therapy along with skilled supportive therapy. Significant mortality may occur despite these measures. Therapy with foscarnet or combination therapy with foscarnet and acyclovir should be considered for patients who fail to respond to acyclovir alone. The administration of varicella-zoster immune globulin is useful for postexposure prophylaxis in high-risk individuals and can also ameliorate established infection. Varicella-zoster immune globulin must be given within 96 h of exposure to be effective. Varicella vaccine is available for universal immunization and postexposure prophylaxis.[91,92] The vaccine is safe, immunogenic, and effective in leukemic children at risk for serious disease, if chemotherapy is interrupted for one week before and after administration; approximately 50% developed a mild rash. A 1-week course of antiviral therapy following exposure may be useful for patients who are at risk.

CMV

Although CMV infections occur sporadically among patients with cancer, especially among those with hematologic malignancies, they are a significant complication among HSCT recipients. Like other herpes viruses, CMV remains latent in tissues after recovery from initial infection. Up to 80% of patients who are seropositive and are undergoing HSCT reactivate latent infection and approximately 30% of seronegative recipients with seropositive donors acquire infection. The most common forms of infection in patients with cancer are pneumonia and gastroenteritis, but other infections include esophagitis, myocarditis, hepatitis, encephalitis, and retinitis.

Early detection of CMV infection is critical to optimal management. The isolation of virus from body fluids or tissues indicates infection but not always symptomatic disease. The CMV pp65 antigenemia assay using infected white blood cells or serum is a reliable, rapid, and sensitive test that is cost-effective. Real-time PCR for detection of CMV DNA in blood is an alternative that is also rapid and sensitive and is useful for diagnosing active disease and monitoring response to therapy.[93]

The usual therapy for established CMV infection has been ganciclovir.[94] In combination with intravenous immunoglobulin, it has been shown to improve survival in transplant recipients with CMV pneumonia or gastroenteritis. The dose-limiting toxicity of ganciclovir is the development of neutropenia, which can increase the risk of bacterial and fungal superinfections. Resistance to ganciclovir may occur during therapy because of viral mutations. Foscarnet is an acceptable alternative that does not cause neutropenia but is associated with nephrotoxicity. It has also been used in combination with ganciclovir. Cidofovir can also be used for treatment, but like foscarnet, causes nephrotoxicity. Unfortunately, the treatment of established infections such as CMV pneumonitis is not very satisfactory. Among patients with leukemia, the mortality rate among treated patients was approximately 60%.[95] Primary CMV infection can be prevented in CMV negative transplant recipients by using screened blood products from donors who are CMV negative. Because of the high risk of CMV infection in transplant recipients who are seropositive or whose donors are seropositive it is important to institute measures to prevent CMV disease. Two strategies are currently used to prevent CMV infection in patients who are seropositive and are at risk for reactivation. One is the prophylactic administration of ganciclovir. Although effective, prolonged ganciclovir administration often produces neutropenia. There is also evidence that prolonged ganciclovir prophylaxis inhibits the development of CMV-specific T-cell lymphocyte responses and promotes the occurrence of late CMV pneumonia.[96] The other approach involves preemptive therapy for subclinical CMV infection, on the basis of positive CMV antigenemia assays in blood or detection of CMV in bronchoalveolar lavage fluid.[97] This strategy has the advantage that it targets patients with subclinical CMV infection. Foscarnet can be used as an alternative for prophylaxis. Valganciclovir is an oral prodrug of ganciclovir that may prove to be useful for prophylaxis in some high-risk patients. Newer agents such as manibavir are being evaluated for CMV prophylaxis/preemptive therapy.[98]

HHV-6

HHV-6 is being recognized as an important pathogen in transplant recipients. Serologic reactivation accompanied by specific manifestations, including fever, rash, pneumonitis, hepatitis, myelosuppression, and neurologic dysfunction, have been described in recipients of bone marrow, kidney, and liver transplants. Ganciclovir and foscarnet inhibit viral replication, and therapy with these agents may be useful in patients with severe infections.[99]

EBV

Reactivation of EBV may occur after HSCT or following chemotherapy with purine analogues such as fludarabine. EBV infection may be responsible for Richter transformation or development of Hodgkin disease in patients with chronic lymphocytic leukemia. In recipients of bone marrow or solid-organ transplants, uncontrolled proliferation of EBV infected B cells may occur, producing posttransplant lymphoproliferative disorders (PTLD). In younger patients, a mononucleosis-like syndrome is a common presentation. Fever, sore throat, and lymphadenopathy are typical findings. Dissemination can occur from localized nodular lesions, and can be fulminant and rapidly fatal. Rituximab is recommended for the treatment of PTLD.

Community Respiratory Viral Infections

Community respiratory viruses can cause significant infection in patients with leukemia who are receiving chemotherapy and in HST recipients, accounting for approximately 30% of respiratory infections during the "flu" season. Although there are temporal and geographic variations, RSV accounts for approximately 35-50%, influenza 20-25%, and parainfluenza about 10-30% of infections. Rhinoviruses, picornaviruses, and adenoviruses have been detected less frequently.

RSV Infection

The presenting signs of RSV infection include fever, cough, rhinorrhea, and nasal congestion. As many as 40-60% of hospitalized patients progress to pneumonitis, which is associated with a mortality rate of about 60%.[100] Early therapy should be instituted for RSV pneumonia with inhaled ribavirin and probably intravenous immunoglobulin. The role of palivizumab, a monoclonal antibody, for therapy in these patients is uncertain.

Influenza

Most influenza infections are caused by influenza A. Approximately 60% of infections progress to pneumonia, and this is especially likely to occur among patients with severe lymphopenia.[101] A substantial proportion of these patients will have associated bacterial or fungal pneumonia. The mortality rate from influenza pneumonia is approximately 40% and is higher among elderly, patients with lymphopenia and those with concomitant infection. The impact of, oseltamivir and ribavirin therapy for influenza pneumonia in these patients is uncertain, but to be effective they must be administered early after onset. Annual immunization for patients, hospital staff and families is important. Nonetheless, antibody response to vaccination in patients receiving chemotherapy is often suboptimal.

Parainfluenza

Parainfluenza infections occur sporadically throughout the year. Infection progresses to pneumonia in 30-75% of patients who have leukemia and are and BMT recipients. As many as 30% of patients with pneumonia may not have upper respiratory symptoms. More than half of patients with pneumonia have concomitant pathogens. The mortality rate from pneumonia is 30-79%, and the efficacy of ribavirin is uncertain.

Hepatitis Viruses

Hepatitis B virus (HBV) infection is the most common cause of acute liver disease worldwide, and more than 300 million people have chronic infection with HBV. Chronic HBV infection leads to progressive liver disease, cirrhosis, and hepatocellular cancer. Hepatitis C virus (HCV) has been estimated to infect 100 million persons worldwide and 4 million in the United States. Eventually 10-15% of these individuals will develop cirrhosis (chronic HCV infection is the leading indication for liver transplantation), and some will develop hepatocellular carcinoma.[102] An association with HCV and non-Hodgkin lymphoma has been established.[103] Many patients with cancer develop elevation of transaminase levels indicating the presence of hepatitis, but it is often difficult to determine whether the disease is viral or drug induced. Although the current risk of transmission of HBV and HCV infection by the transfusion of screened blood is negligible, patients with acute leukemia and others who receive multiple transfusions may be at greater risk. The greatest threat to the safety of the blood supply is seronegative donors who donate blood during the infectious window period when they are undergoing seroconversion. Hepatitis can be a serious problem in patients with cancer for various reasons. Patients with impaired host defense mechanisms are more likely to develop fulminant infections. The presence of hepatitis may result in substantial delays in the administration of antineoplastic therapy. Several reports have focused on the phenomenon of reactivation of quiescent liver disease as a consequence of HBV following immunosuppressive or cytotoxic therapy.[104] The clinical picture is that of fulminant hepatic failure and some patients have required liver transplantation as a consequence. This syndrome has also been reported after withdrawal of low-dose methotrexate therapy, which has not been clearly established to be immunosuppressive.

Interferon-α (IFN-α) is currently the only approved treatment for HBV infection. The oral nucleoside analogue lamivudine produces substantial histologic improvement in many patients with chronic hepatitis.[105] The combination of pegylated IFN-α plus ribavirin produces sustained virologic responses in hepatitis C; approximately 50% in genotype 1 infections and 80% in other genotype infections.[106] Preexposure vaccination of persons at risk using recombinant hepatitis B vaccines affords protection against hepatitis B infection. Postexposure prophylaxis includes the administration of hepatitis B vaccine and hepatitis B immunoglobulin. Measures for preventing hepatitis C need to be developed.

Protozoal Infections

P. carinii and *T. gondii* are protozoal organisms (although *P. carinii* has been reclassified as a fungus) that are capable of causing serious infections in patients with cancer. Antitumor agents and adrenal corticosteroids facilitate the establishment of these infections.

P. carinii

Most cancer patients who develop this infection have evidence of immunosuppression, including a substantial number of children with acute leukemia who were in remission. PCP most often represents reactivation of latent infection but occasionally represents newly acquired infection. Recent reports indicate that cases of PCP in patients with solid tumors who have been treated with corticosteroids or temozolamide, appear to be increasing.[20,107-109]

PCP may be insidious in onset or may progress rapidly. The most frequent symptoms are unexplained fever, a nonproductive cough, and shortness of breath. The shortness of breath may occur initially only with exertion, but as the infection progresses, it is also present at rest, and the patient characteristically develops tachypnea, cyanosis, and tachycardia. Chest imaging often reveals more extensive pulmonary involvement than is suggested by the clinical findings. The most common finding is that of a diffuse interstitial infiltration involving most portions of the lung relatively evenly, although asymmetry may occur. Pleural effusions are very uncommon and may indicate the presence of another disease process.

Most patients with PCP have a dry cough and rarely produce sputum. Adequate amounts of sputum can be induced by having patients inhale a mist of hypertonic saline produced by an ultrasonic nebulizer for a period of 10-20 min. Staining of the sample can be done by a variety of stains that detect *P. carinii* (Gomori methenamine silver, toluidine blue O, Giemsa, polychrome methylene blue) (Fig. 137-10). Various invasive techniques for establishing the diagnosis of PCP are available. These include fiberoptic bronchoscopy with bronchoalveolar lavage and/or transbronchial lung biopsy. Needle lung biopsy and open lung biopsy are rarely necessary. The sensitivity and specificity of these procedures are greater than noninvasive techniques, but they are associated with complications, such as bleeding and pneumothorax. TMP-SMX represents the agent of choice for the treatment of PCP The daily intravenous dosage of TMP-SMX recommended for the treatment of PCP is trimethoprim, 15 mg/kg, and sulfamethoxazole, 75 mg/ kg. Pentamidine isethionate is administered by slow intravenous infusion at a dose of 4 mg/kg, as a single daily dose. For patients who are intolerant to, or who do not respond to, both TMP-SMX and pentamidine, the following alternatives exist. Oral dapsone-trimethoprim is useful in patients who have AIDS with mild to moderately severe PCP. A combination of clindamycin and primaquine has also been used to treat mild to moderately severe PCP in humans.[110] Another oral agent, atovaquone, has been approved for the treatment of mild to moderately severe PCP.[111] The use of corticosteroids as adjunctive therapy for patients with moderate to severe PCP reduces the occurrence of respiratory failure and of mortality.[112] TMP-SMX is highly successful in protecting children who are at high risk of acquiring PCP. Aerosolized pentamidine has found widespread use for the prevention of PCP particularly because it can be administered once a month. A small number of patients given aerosolized pentamidine will develop extrapulmonary (spleen, liver, bone marrow, eye) PCP. Other alternatives include intravenous pentamidine, dapsone, a combination of pyrimethamine and sulfadoxine (Fansidar), and atovaquone.

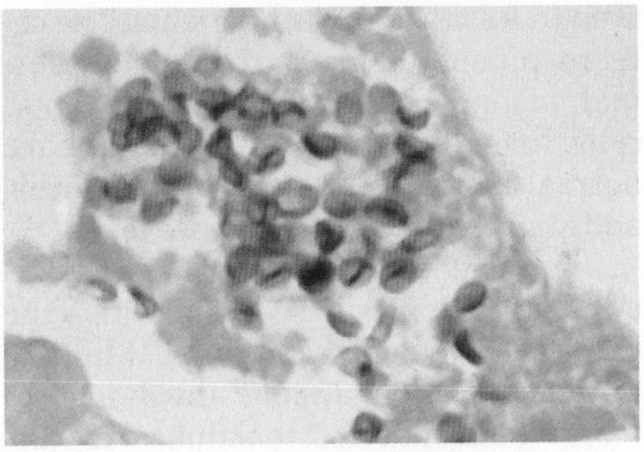

Figure 137-10 Gomori methenamine silver (GMS) stain from a bronchoalveolar lavage specimen demonstrating multiple organisms in an AIDS patient with *Pneumocystis carinii* pneumonia.

T. gondii

Toxoplasmosis is an infrequent infection even in patients who are immunosuppressed.[113] Nearly half of the patients with cancer who develop toxoplasmosis have underlying Hodgkin disease. Sixty percent of patients with lymphoma who develop toxoplasmosis have central nervous system disease; although other multiple organs may be infected.[114] Central nervous system disease may present as a nonspecific encephalopathy, diffuse meningoencephalitis, or a syndrome compatible with multiple space-occupying lesions. The usual signs and symptoms include drowsiness, disorientation, headache, vomiting, seizures, visual disturbances, and paresis. Fever and nuchal rigidity are seen in less than 50% of patients. The cerebrospinal fluid may be completely normal, or may contain a few white blood cells (usually lymphocytes), and have normal or slightly elevated protein levels and slightly decreased glucose levels.[115]

In patients who present with symptoms of toxoplasmic encephalitis, the CT scan is usually abnormal. Multiple intraparenchymal lesions involving cerebral hemispheres, thalamus, or cerebellum are seen. Contrast-enhancement may demonstrate a ring-like or nodular pattern.[116]

A large number of serologic tests for the detection of antibody to *T. gondii* are available. The most useful tests for the measurement of immunoglobulin (Ig) G antibody are the Sabin–Feldman dye test, the indirect fluorescent antibody (IFA) test, and the modified direct agglutination test. The methods available for detection of IgM antibodies include the IgM-IFA test and the double sandwich IgM-ELISA. IgG antibodies appear within 7-14 days of acquisition of infection, whereas IgM antibodies appear during the first week. IgG antibodies generally peak within 30-60 days and then begin to fall but persist for life. IgM antibodies rise rapidly, then fall to low levels, and disappear in a few months. The diagnosis of toxoplasmosis can also be established by demonstrating trophozoites in tissues, such as brain biopsy or endomyocardial biopsy specimens.

Toxoplasmosis can be treated successfully with a combination of pyrimethamine and sulfadiazine (or trisulfapyrimidines). The initial loading dose of pyrimethamine is 100-200 mg. This is followed by 25-50 mg daily for a period of 4-6 weeks. Sulfadiazine or trisulfapyrimidines are given at a dose of 6-8 g/d in four divided doses for 4-6 weeks. Folinic acid, 5 mg every other day, is generally administered in an attempt to reduce the myelosuppression associated with this regimen. Clindamycin has shown promise as an alternative to sulfadiazine in patients with toxoplasmosis and sulfonamide intolerance.[117] In combination with oral pyrimethamine, clindamycin seems comparable in efficacy to pyrimethamine and sulfadiazine. Atovaquone also appears promising for the treatment of cerebral toxoplasmosis, but relapse rates approach 50% when this agent is used alone. The new macrolides azithromycin, and clarithromycin have activity against *T. gondii*, but sufficient clinical data are lacking to recommend routine usage currently.

Other Parasitic Infections

Opportunistic infections, including the syndrome of hyperinfection with the nematode Strongyloides stercoralis, occur most often in patients with T-lymphocyte impairment. Usually, the parasite exists in the gut without causing severe disability. Patients with impaired host defenses or those receiving antitumor and/or immunosuppressive agents, however, may develop a serious infection. Large numbers of rhabditiform larvae may mature to filariform larvae and invade the gastrointestinal tract, causing ulceration. When hyperinfection occurs, pulmonary and gastrointestinal symptoms predominate.[118,119] Pulmonary manifestations include dyspnea, cough, hemoptysis, chest pain, and cyanosis. Migration of the larvae into the lungs produces a diffuse pulmonary infiltrate. Gastrointestinal manifestations include abdominal pain and/or distention, nausea, vomiting, diarrhea, hematochezia, and hematemesis. Fever, rash, headache, chills, and shock may also be present. Coexisting bacterial infections, which are generally caused by enteric gram-negative bacilli, are frequently present and may alert the astute clinician to the possibility of hyperinfection with *S. stercoralis*.

The crucial step in establishing the diagnosis of strongyloidiasis is the identification of larvae. They are usually demonstrated in stool samples and in pulmonary secretions. Duodenal aspiration might be necessary, if stool and pulmonary specimens fail to demonstrate larvae (Fig. 137-11). Eosinophilia is present in up to 50% of patients. Various immunologic tests are available including complement fixation tests, precipitin tests, indirect fluorescent antibody techniques, and direct passive hemagglutination tests. Thiabendazole (25 mg/kg twice daily for 2 days) is the agent of choice for the treatment of strongyloidiasis.[120] A longer duration of therapy (5-14 days) may be necessary in seriously ill patients and those with hyperinfection. Ivermectin alone or in combination with thiabendazole may have a therapeutic role in refractory infections.[121]

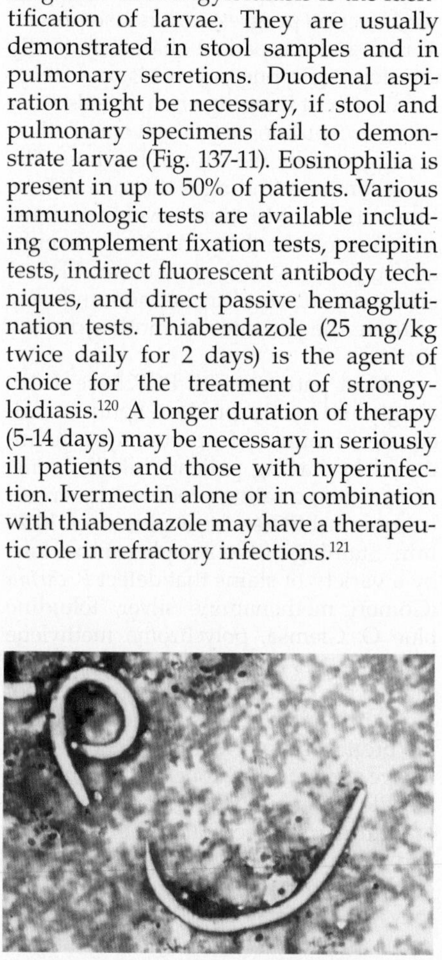

Figure 137-11 *Strongyloides stercoralis* larvae in a specimen obtained through duodenal aspiration. The patient had eosinophilia and chronic diarrhea.

Pulmonary Infections

The lung is a common site of infection in patients with cancer. The spectrum of pulmonary infection depends on the underlying immunologic deficit. In patients with neutropenia, bacterial infections predominate early. Most bacterial infections are mixed (polymicrobial) in nature with the following organisms being isolated frequently: *Staphylococcus aureus, Streptococcus pneumoniae*, the Enterobacteriaceae, *Pseudomonas aeruginosa*, and oral anaerobes. Secondary bacterial pathogens that emerge after prolonged antibacterial therapy include *Stenotrophomonas maltophilia, Acinetobacter* spp., other non-fermentative gram-negative bacilli, and multidrug-resistant *Pseudomonas aeruginosa*. Fungal infections tend to occur more often in patients with persistent neutropenia and include molds such as *Aspergillus* spp., *Fusarium* spp., and the Zygomycetes.[122] Community respiratory viruses also cause infections in patients with neutropenia particularly in the preengraftment phase following HSCT.

The spectrum of pulmonary infection in patients with impaired cellular immunity is quite different. *Legionella* spp. are the most common bacterial pathogens although other bacteria including *Rhodococcus equi, Nocardia* spp., and *Listeria monocytogenes* might occasionally be isolated. Mycobacterial infections (*M. tuberculosis* and nontuberculous mycobacteria) are also common particularly in patients with lymphoproliferative disorders, hairy cell leukemia, and those receiving cortisteroids or other immunosuppressive agents. *Aspergillus* spp. and the endemic fungi (*Cryptococcus neoformans, Histoplasma capsulatum, Coccoides immunities*) cause most of the fungal infections in this setting. Viral infections are predominantly caused by the herpes group of viruses with CMV being the most frequent. The community respiratory viruses are important causes of morbidity and mortality in high-risk subpopulations such as allogeneic HSCT recipients. *Pneumocystis jiroveci* also is a frequent cause of pneumonia in patients with impaired cellular immunity. In patients with impaired humoral immunity, infections caused by encapsulated organisms such as *S. pneumoniae* and *H. influenzae* are common. Of concern is the increase in resistant pneumococcal isolates. Recent surveys at the University of Texas MD Anderson Cancer Center have indicated that 36-47% of *S. pneumoniae* are not susceptible to penicillin.[123]

Patients with carcinoma of the lung or metastatic lung disease often develop focal pulmonary infections. This is generally due to partial obstruction of the airways leading to atelectasis and postobstructive pneumonia.[124] Occasionally, the infection may progress to empyema or lung abscess formation. These infections are predominantly polymicrobial (staphylococci, gram-negative bacilli, anaerobes) and are difficult to eradicate with antimicrobial therapy alone. Methods to overcome the obstruction (radiation, chemotherapy, stent placement, endobronchial brachytherapy) are usually necessary to ensure adequate drainage of the infected lung.

Patients with primary brain tumors or metastatic brain lesions often develop loss of the gag reflex that predisposes them to developing aspiration pneumonia. Damage to ciliary function, most often the result of radiation, also increases the likelihood of aspiration. These infections are also of mixed aerobic and anaerobic bacterial etiology and are caused by organisms colonizing the oropharynx and upper airways.

Certain infections can produce clinical and radiographic findings that are indistinguishable from those associated with neoplasms. Fungal and mycobacterial pathogens head the list of such organisms. These may cause diagnostic challenges in two specific settings: (1) patients with newly discovered pulmonary lesions in whom a neoplasm is suspected, and (2) patients with cancer who have received therapy, in whom a new pulmonary lesion (suspected to be metastatic) is seen.

For details of the various options and procedures commonly used to establish a diagnosis in patients with pulmonary infections, please refer to Chapter 131, Respiratory Complications.

Abdominal Infection

An acute abdomen is one of the most difficult problems for the physician caring for patients with cancer. Often, this occurs following the administration of chemotherapy when neutropenia and thrombocytopenia are complicating factors. Patients with neutropenia often cannot mount an adequate inflammatory response and, therefore, may have peritonitis without significant symptoms. Usually, they have abdominal pain, distention, and diminished to absent bowel sounds, but guarding and rebound may be absent. Adrenocorticosteroids can also mask the signs and symptoms of peritoneal inflammation. Some of the potential causes of acute abdomen in the immunocompromised host include appendicitis, cholecystitis, peritonitis, hepatic, splenic or ovarian abscesses, splenic infarcts, typhlitis, tumor lysis with perforation, and vinca alkaloid neuropathy.

Typhlitis or neutropenic enterocolitis is a disease that occurs in patients with neutropenia. The common presenting signs and symptoms include fever, abdominal pain, and diarrhea. More than 60% of patients have bloody diarrhea.[125] A substantial fraction of the patients have stomatitis, and 30% have vomiting. Physical examination reveals abdominal distention, tenderness often localized to the right lower quadrant, diminished to absent bowel sounds, and, infrequently, rebound tenderness. Septicemia is present in 70% of the patients, and the most common organisms are aerobic gram-negative bacteria. Some of the cases have been associated with infection caused by *Clostridium septicum*. Complications include perforation and peritonitis.[126]

The disease may be limited to the cecum, but it can involve the entire lower gastrointestinal tract. The cause is unknown, but neutropenia is clearly a prerequisite. Chemotherapeutic agents such as the taxanes also play a role because they also cause mucosal ulceration.[127]

Radiographic examination usually reveals evidence of a paralytic ileus with lack of bowel gas in the right lower quadrant, minimal distention of the terminal ileum, and thickening of the bowel wall. Ultrasonography or CT should be done to confirm the diagnosis and extent of disease. Initially, therapy should be supportive, consisting of nasogastric suction, intravenous fluids, and broad-spectrum antibiotics that include coverage for *P. aeruginosa* and anaerobes. Surgery is not indicated, unless it can be demonstrated that the process is localized and the patient is not responding to supportive therapy.[126] In a recent study, more than 70% of patients survived with medical therapy only.[125]

Perianal Infections

Perianal infections are estimated to occur in 6% of patients with hematologic neoplasms and are especially common in patients with acute monocytic and acute myelomonocytic leukemia, suggesting that leukemic infiltration of the tissues may play a role. A common predisposing factor is neutropenia, which is found in more than 90% of these patients. The major presenting symptom is pain that is aggravated by defecation. Most patients are febrile. The lesion is erythematous, indurated, and ulcerated. Abscess formation occurs infrequently, but there may be extensive necrosis and sloughing extending into the rectum. The infection often occurs at a site of a fissure or hemorrhoid.

Most of these infections are caused by aerobic gram-negative bacilli, especially *P. aeruginosa* and *Escherichia coli*. *Pseudomonas* infection can be especially devastating because the organism invades blood vessel walls causing a vasculitis that can lead to tissue necrosis. Anaerobic organisms play an important role in these infections, but are not often isolated.

Initial therapy should be symptomatic, consisting of sitz baths or warm compresses, stool softeners, analgesics, and broad-spectrum antibiotics. Gut-sterilizing oral antibiotic regimens may be of some value in reducing contamination of ulcers by fecal flora. If an abscess is present, it should be incised and drained.[128] Mortality from these infections has varied from 10% to 35%, with most deaths being a result of septic shock. In the patient with neutropenia, resolution of infection often depends on recovery of the neutrophil count. Some patients may respond to initial antibiotic therapy, only to develop superinfection with a resistant organism. Patients with hematologic diseases who recover from perianal infections caused by hemorrhoids or anal fissures should undergo surgical correction when they achieve a remission of their underlying disease; otherwise, they may experience recurrent infections at a later date.[129]

Skin Infections

Skin infections may occur secondary to necrotic tumor masses, postoperative wound infections, extravasation of vesicant drugs, infected intravascular catheters, folliculitis, infected decubitus ulcers, or as manifestations of systemic infection or embolic lesions secondary to endocarditis. Advanced squamous carcinomas of the skin, head and neck carcinomas, breast carcinomas, and sarcomas become necrotic and ulcerated and can serve as a focus of infection. Although initially these infections may be caused by gram-positive organisms, eventually superinfection with gram-negative bacilli occurs and is impossible to eradicate with antibiotic therapy alone. These infections can pose a serious threat to patients undergoing myelosuppressive chemotherapy because of the risk of septicemia when they become neutropenic.

Patients with neutropenia usually do not form abscesses at the site of skin infection but rather develop a spreading cellulitis, which often is associated with septicemia. A wide variety of aerobic gram-positive and gram-negative organisms can cause these infections, including CA-MRSA and skin contaminants such as *Bacillus* spp., *Corynebacterium jeikeium*, and *S. epidermidis*. Efforts should be made to aspirate material from these

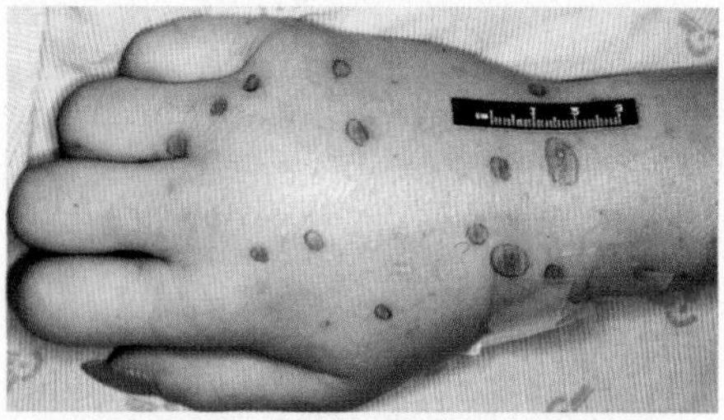

Figure 137-12 ■ Characteristic macronodular cutaneous lesions in a patient with acute leukemia and disseminated *Candida krusei* infection.

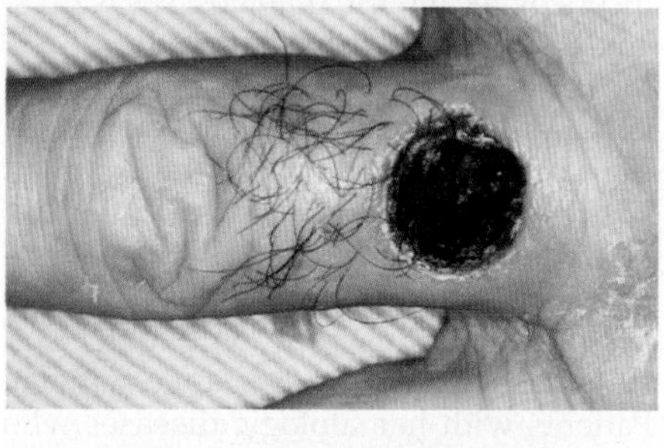

Figure 137-13 ■ Disseminated aspergillosis and mucormycosis are infrequently associated with sharply demarcated lesions covered by a black eschar.

infected sites, although cultures are frequently negative.

Systemic infections in patients with cancer may be associated with skin lesions. An important skin lesion is ecthyma gangrenosum, which characteristically is found in the perianal area, groin, or axilla. Nearly always, it is caused by *P. aeruginosa*, but other gram-negative bacilli including *Aeromonas* and *Serratia*, fungi including *Aspergillus* or *Mucorales*, or *S. aureus* may be the cause.

Several fungi cause skin lesions as a manifestation of systemic infection. Approximately 10% of patients with disseminated candidiasis develop characteristic macronodular skin lesions (Fig. 137-12). Disseminated aspergillosis and mucormycosis are infrequently associated with sharply demarcated lesions covered by a black eschar (Fig. 137-13). Skin lesions occur in cryptococcosis and histoplasmosis but are not characteristic. *Fusarium* causes a fungal infection that is frequently associated with a variety of skin lesions.

Catheter-Related Infections

Widespread use of intravascular catheters in patients with cancer has contributed to the changing spectrum of infection during the past decade. *S. epidermidis* has emerged as an important pathogen, and the frequency of *S. aureus* infection has increased substantially. Some of these infections are caused by *Bacillus* spp., *Corynebacterium jeikeium*, *Enterococcus*, *Enterobacter* spp., *Acinetobacter*, and fungi. Despite the widespread use of catheters, the infection rate seldom exceeds 15%, even in patients with neutropenia.

In the past, the recommended policy was to remove the catheter whenever a patient developed fever and especially when it was associated with septicemia. Recent experience indicates that many cases of septicemia can be successfully treated without the removal of the catheter.[130] Exceptions include fungi, *S. aureus*, *Acinetobacter*, *Pseudomonas* spp. *S. maltophilia*, the atypical mycobacteria, and whenever there is cellulitis at the catheter site. Nevertheless, if fever or bacteremia persists despite antibiotic therapy, catheters must always be removed. The most serious catheter-related infections are septic thrombophlebitis and endocarditis. Septic thrombophlebitis is characterized by microabscess formation within a cannulated vein, which may be associated with repeated septic embolization. The majority of these infections are caused by *S. aureus*, *Streptococcus*, *Bacteroides* spp., and enteric gram-negative bacilli. As many as 70% of infections occur without local signs. Septic emboli occur in as many as 50% of the patients. Surgical exploration of the vein is necessary if the patient fails to respond to appropriate antibiotic therapy shortly after removal of the infected catheter. Endocarditis in the patient with cancer presents no unique manifestations. The risk of endocarditis is greater in patients with valvular heart disease,and so catheters should not be routinely used in these patients for the administration of chemotherapy. Recently, antimicrobial impregnated catheters have become available that reduce the frequency of catheter-associated infections during short-term use.

Therapy of Infections in Patients With Neutropenia

General Principles

The practice of initiating empiric broad-spectrum antimicrobial therapy when a neutropenic patient becomes febrile immediately after procuring all relevant cultures is now a well-accepted standard.[41] Antibiotic therapy should be administered promptly, via the intravenous route, and at maximal therapeutic doses in order to achieve maximal efficacy. In general, an empiric regimen should provide a broad-pectrum of activity against gram-negative organisms including *P. aeruginosa*, and gram-positive pathogens. This is usually achieved by administering antibiotic combinations or broad-spectrum drugs used as single-agents (monotherapy). The increase in gram-positive infections has led to the inclusion of vancomycin or linezolid in some empiric regimens.[131]

In patients who are severely neutropenic, better results may be obtained if the pathogen is susceptible to both agents of a combination rather than to only one, regardless of the presence or absence of synergy.

Antibiotic selection is also influenced by the potential toxicity associated with various agents. The aminoglycosides have long been associated with significant nephrotoxicity and ototoxicity and require frequent monitoring of renal function and serum levels. Elderly patients or those with preexisting renal insufficiency are at greater risk for developing aminoglycoside-associated toxicity. The toxicity of the aminoglycosides can also be potentiated by other agents frequently used in patients with cancer. Although the β-lactam agents are associated with untoward reactions, such as hypersensitivity reactions and coagulation abnormalities, they are generally safer and better tolerated than aminoglycosides.

Local factors need to be considered when selecting antibiotics for initial empiric therapy. Certain pathogens may be endemic in a particular institution and must be included in the spectrum of the initial empiric regimen. Empiric therapy should include agents with antianaerobic activity in the case of intraabdominal and pelvic infections (Table 137-5). In addition, the susceptibility of various organisms may differ from one institution to another, and local susceptibility/

Table 137-5 ■ **Common Empiric Antibiotic Regimens for Febrile Neutropenic Patients**

Regimens for low-risk patients
→ Parenteral
Ceftriaxone or ertapenem + amikacin
Aztreonam + clindamycin
Quinolone + clindamycin
Ceftazidiem or cefepime
→ Oral
Quinolone + amoxicillin/clavulante
Quinolone + clindamycin or azithromycin
Moxifloxacin or levofloxacin
Regimens for moderate to high-risk patients
Aminoglycoside –containing regimens
Aminoglycoside + antipseudomonal pencicilllin/β-betamase inhibitors
Aminoglycoside + extended –spectrum cephalosporin
Aminoglycoside + carbapenem
Aminglyocoside + quinolone
Other regimens
Vancomycin + antipseudomonal penicillin/β-lactamase inhibitors
Vancomycin + extended-spectrum cephalosporin
Vancomycin + monobactam
Vancomycin + quinolone
Single-agent regimens (monotherapy)
Extended-spectrum cepahalsporin
Carbapenems
Antipseudomonal penicillin/β-lactamse inhibibor

resistance patterns must be kept in mind when designing empiric regimens.

Patient Evaluation

Antimicrobial therapy in febrile patients who are neutropenic needs to be administered promptly, and a delay of even a few hours can result in substantially increased mortality. Pretreatment evaluation of the patient should be performed as expeditiously as possible, yet it should be thorough. A careful interview for historic information and a physical examination must be performed. Particular attention should be paid to sites that are frequently infected, or serve as foci for the dissemination of infection. These include the oropharynx, lung, lower esophagus, perineum, paranasal sinuses, fingernails, and vascular catheter insertion sites. Prior to the initiation of empiric antibiotic therapy, at least two sets of blood cultures and cultures from other appropriate sites (ie, throat, urine, stool) should be obtained for bacterial and fungal pathogens. In patients with central venous catheters, cultures should be obtained from the catheters and from a peripheral site. Material exuding from infected catheter sites should also be sent for Gram staining and culture. In patients with neutropenia and pneumonia, radiographs may appear normal. CT scans of the chest or paranasal sinuses should be performed in patients in whom these sites are potential sources of infection. Other laboratory investigations include complete blood counts and determination of baseline values reflecting renal and hepatic function. These tests should be repeated at least twice a week while patients are receiving empiric antibiotic therapy. Imaging techniques, such as CT, MRI, ultrasonography, and radionuclide imaging, and invasive procedures, such as lung, liver, or skin biopsies, might be extremely useful at identifying sites of infection and isolating specific pathogens.

Initial Antibiotic Therapy

Table 137-5 lists antibiotic regimens that are frequently deployed in febrile patients with neutropenia. No single regimen is optimal, and the various factors discussed above need to be carefully considered before making a specific choice. The initial regimen may also need to be altered during the course of the febrile episode, depending on the susceptibility of microorganisms isolated from clinical specimens, the development of bacterial, fungal, or viral superinfections, or lack of apparent efficacy after administration of the regimen for 3 days. Combinations of aminoglycosides and antipseudomonal penicillins have been extensively evaluated and are generally associated with overall response rates in the range of 65-85%. Aminoglycosides are often used in combination with extended-spectrum cephalosporins (ceftazidime, cefepime) and other β-lactam agents (aztreonam, carbapenems, piperacillin + tazobactam).[41] Once-daily administration of aminoglycosides is associated with less toxicity than more frequent administration.[132] Care must be taken to ensure that the aminoglycoside is not the only active agent against any gram-negative bacilli that are isolated, because these agents are not effective by themselves in patients with neutropenia, even if the causative organisms are susceptible to them in vitro.

With the availability of broad-spectrum agents, such as carbapenems and extended-spectrum cephalosporins, it has become possible to initiate empiric therapy in febrile neutropenic patients using a single agent. Ceftazidime, imipenem/cilastatin, meropenem and piperacillin/tazobactam have been used alone as initial therapy and have produced response rates similar to those obtained with combination regimens (Table 137-6). Patients on single-agent therapy need to be carefully monitored and antibiotic changes made if the clinical situation or microbiologic data indicate the need.

With the increased incidence of gram-positive infections, many of which are caused by multidrug-resistant organisms, the inclusion of vancomycin, linezolid or daptomycin in the initial regimen might become necessary. Most gram-positive infections are associated with low mortality, and several studies show that vancomycin can be safely added to the initial regimen if no response is obtained after 48-72 h of therapy, or if a resistant organism is isolated, without adversely affecting the eventual outcome. Fulminant gram-positive infections caused by α-hemolytic streptococci, S. pyogenes, or other gram-positive organisms have been described. It might be prudent to include vancomycin in the initial empiric regimen in institutions or specific patient populations in whom these infections occur frequently.[41]

Recently, clinical vancomycin failures have been reported even in infections caused by organisms that are susceptible to it in vitro, presumably due to its diminishing bactericidal activity.[26,133] Newer agents with improved bactericidal activity (daptomycin, dalbavancin) are being developed, and need to be evaluated in patients who have cancer.

Low-Risk Patients

Antibiotic therapy for febrile patients who are neutropenic has traditionally been administered in the hospital because of the risk of infection-related and other complications. Recently, simple clinical criteria and statistically derived risk prediction rules have made it possible to identify low-risk subsets among such patients at the onset of a febrile episode.[11,12] This has enabled clinicians to evaluate not only the nature of antibiotic therapy (eg, combinations vs monotherapy) but also the setting (hospital, clinic, office, home) in which it is delivered.[134] Several alternative treatment strategies in low-risk febrile patients with neutropenia have been evaluated including (1) hospital based oral antibiotic therapy,[135,136] (2) initial hospitalization followed by early discharge on outpatient parenteral or oral antibiotics,[137] and (3) outpatient (parenteral or oral) antibiotic therapy for the entire febrile episode.[138]

This approach is associated with substantial cost saving, a lower incidence of nosocomial superinfections, and improved quality of life for patients and convenience for their families. Careful patient selection and daily follow-up are essential components of the success of this novel approach. The Infectious Dis-

Table 137-6 Antimicrobial Agents Commonly Used in Patients with Neutropenia

Aminoglycosides	
Amikacin	5 mg/kg q8h or 15-20 g/kg/d (single dose)
Antipseudomonal penicillins + β-lactamase inhibitor	
Piperacillin + tazobactam	3.375 g q6h, IV
Extended-spectrum cephalosporins	
Cefepime	1-2 g q8h, IV
Carbapenem	
Imipenem/cilastatin	500 mg q6h, IV
Meropenem	1 g q8h, IV
Monobactam	
Aztreonam	1.5-2.0 g q6-8h, IV
Quinolones	
Ciprofloxacin	200-400 mg q8h, IV
Levofloxacin	500 mg qd, IV
Moxifloxacin	400 mg qd, IV
Others	
Vancomycin	1 g q12h, IV
Trimethoprim-sulfamethoxazole	2.0-20.0 mg/kg/d (trimethoprim) IV q6h
Metronidazole	500 mg IV q6-8h
Linezolid	600 mg IV q12h
Daptomycin	4-6 mg/kg/d IV

Abbreviation: IV, intravenously.

eases Society of America and the National Comprehensive Cancer Network recently published guidelines for the treatment of febrile patients with neutropenia, which include suggestions for the outpatient management of low-risk patients.

Duration of Therapy

Some authorities recommend continuation of antibiotic therapy in patients with documented infections until recovery of the neutrophil count. This approach is expensive, as it actually represents prophylaxis after resolution of infection and may result in an increased number of superinfections requiring numerous modifications of antibacterial therapy and/or the addition of antifungal therapy. Another approach is to continue antibiotics until all sites of infection have resolved, the causative pathogen, if isolated, has been eradicated, the patient has been treated for a minimum of 7 days and has remained free of significant symptoms or signs of infection for at least 4 days. Antibiotic therapy may be discontinued safely at this point despite the persistence of neutropenia. This approach may be associated with a low relapse rate and fewer superinfections.

Unexplained Fever

The most perplexing group of patients are those with fever who display no clinical signs of infection and from whom no pathogen is isolated . Many of these patients respond to the initial antibacterial regimens, suggesting that they do have bacterial infections. The widespread use of prophylactic antibiotics to an extent, may be responsible for the failure to isolate the offending pathogens in such patients. Patients who remain febrile despite antibacterial therapy pose a difficult challenge. These patients may have bacterial infections that are resistant to therapy or infections by nonbacterial pathogens (fungi, viruses, parasites). Drug-related or tumor fever may also be present. Aggressive, often invasive, diagnostic maneuvers are sometimes necessary for the management of such patients. In patients unable to tolerate invasive diagnostic procedures, continuation of antibacterial therapy and the addition of empiric antifungal, antiviral, or antiparasitic therapy might be necessary.

Other Therapeutic Modalities

Nearly 15-25% of infections occurring in patients with neutropenia fail to respond to appropriate antimicrobial therapy. In most cases, profound neutropenia persists. There was considerable interest in the use of white blood cell transfusions in the 1960s and 1970s. Randomized trials in neutropenic patients with infections that failed to respond to appropriate therapy demonstrated that white blood cell transfusions increased the response rates. Interest waned because of the difficulties in obtaining sufficient donors, alloimmunization of recipients when random donors were used, and the possibility of transmitting CMV infection from transfused cells. The availability of the hematopoietic growth factors has rekindled interest because the administration of granulocyte colony-stimulating factor (G-CSF) to donors increases the number of neutrophils that can be collected. Preliminary clinical studies suggest that this approach to white blood cell collection has produced therapeutic benefit in about half the recipients.[139]

The administration of hematopoietic growth factors to patients receiving cancer chemotherapy reduces the severity and duration of neutropenia and, hence, the frequency of infectious complications. Guidelines for this use of these agents have been prepared by the American Society of Clinical Oncology.[140] The efficacy of these factors as adjuncts to antibiotic therapy for patients who are neutropenic after they have become infected has not been clearly established. It is reasonable to administer these agents to patients with neutrophil counts less than 500/mm^3 who develop pneumonia, septic shock, sepsis syndrome, or fungal infection, because these patients have a poor prognosis without recovery of their neutrophils. These agents should also be considered for patients with documented infections who are failing to respond to appropriate therapy after 24-48 h. IFN-γ may be beneficial for therapy with nonviral infections that are not responding to appropriate therapy.[141]

Infection Prevention

The two main strategies that are used for infection prevention are directed toward suppressing the endogenous microflora and preventing the acquisition of new organisms from environmental sources. Suppression of the endogenous microflora is usually achieved by using prophylactic antibiotic regimens during periods of severe myelosuppression. In patients who are at risk for fungal, viral, or protozoal infections or in centers where such infections are relatively common, prophylactic regimens generally also include agents active against these groups of organisms. The prevention of acquisition of new organisms is accomplished by various techniques, including strict hand-washing precautions, use of well-cooked foods, which reduces contamination with gram-negative bacteria, and various isolation techniques or protected environments.[142]

Antimicrobial Prophylaxis

Prophylactic antimicrobial regimens achieve a major reduction in the patients' microbial burden. Although most studies have shown a reduction in microbiologically documented infections and a reduction in the need for systemically administered antibiotics, the overall mortality has not been significantly altered. The quinolones (ciprofloxacin, levofloxacin) are the most commonly used agents for antibacterial chemoprophylaxis. The use of these agents has been associated with significant reductions in the frequency of gram-negative infections, but they have had little impact on or, or may actually increase the frequency of gram-positive infections (eg, *Staphylococcus* spp., viridans group streptococci).[143,144] Quinolone prophylaxis has also resulted in the emergence of quinolone resistance among enteric gram-negative bacilli including *E. coli*.[145] It is therefore not recommended for routine use in patients with neutropenia, but must be considered only in patients at high-risk for bacterial infection (ie, those with prolonged periods of neutropenia). TMP-SMX remains the agent of choice for PCP prophylaxis. Alternative (but less effective) agents include pentamidine, dapsone, and atovaquone.

Antifungal and Antiviral Prophylaxis

Increasing frequency of invasive fungal infections in high-risk patients has led to the use of antifungal prophylaxis. Fluconazole (and itraconazole) prophylaxis has been shown to decrease both superficial colonization and systemic *Candida* infections.[146,147] The selection of resistant species (*C. krusei*, *C. glabratta*) is a potential problem, although these organisms are also seen in "azole naïve" patients.[148,149] Prophylaxis against molds including *Aspergillus* spp. is less successful although newer agents such as micafungin, voriconazole and posaconazole, with more potent activity against molds than older agents have been evaluated.[150-152] Increased voriconazole administration has already been associated with the emergence of breakthrough zygomycotic infections, cautioning against the widespread adoption of this strategy.[82]

Prophylactic acyclovir has been shown to prevent reactivation of HSV infection in patients undergoing intensive chemotherapy (with or without radiation therapy) before HSCT or induction therapy for leukemia or lymphoma. Preemptive therapy (rather than prophylaxis) with ganciclovir or foscarnet is the current recommendation for high-risk patients with positive CMV antigenemia.[153]

Isolation

Reduction of the acquisition of new organisms has been attempted by putting patients at risk into reverse isolation. Patients are also given well-cooked foods and are asked to avoid fresh fruits and vegetables (eg, tomatoes, salads) that are naturally contaminated with gram-negative bacilli such as *P. aeruginosa*, *Klebsiella pneumoniae*, and *E. coli*. More elaborate regimens are expensive and time consuming and have not been shown to be more effective than strict adherence to hand-washing techniques.

Protected environments provide a combination of the two approaches, ie, the use of isolation units to protect the patient against nosocomial contamination plus antibiotic regimens to reduce the patient's endogenous flora. The protected environment generally consists of isolation units, which provide a barrier between the patient and the hospital environment, using aggressive decontamination techniques and filtered air. The patient's food is specially prepared or sterilized to minimize contamination. Disinfection of the patient is achieved by using intensive regimens, which include oral nonabsorbable antibiotics. Patients bathe with germicidal soaps and apply topical antibiotic ointments or sprays to areas of heavy microbial contamination.

Because attempts at suppressing the endogenous microflora and those at preventing the acquisition of organisms have not been overwhelmingly successful, other means for infection prevention need to be developed. The hematopoietic growth factors (granulocyte-macrophage [GM]-CSF and G-CSF) have been demonstrated to shorten the duration of neutropenia and to reduce the number of febrile days and of documented infections in selected subpopulations of patients with neutropenia. Current guidelines suggest that the primary use of these agents is not indicated in patients who were previously untreated and receiving most chemotherapy regimens.[140] The secondary administration of growth factors can decrease the probability of febrile neutropenia after a documented occurrence in an earlier cycle. It can also reduce the period of neutropenia and the frequency of infectious complications in patients undergoing high-dose cytotoxic therapy with autologous marrow transplantation.

Antimicrobial Stewardship

Antimicrobial resistance has been documented to result in increase morbidity, mortality, and cost of healthcare worldwide. Consequently, the appropriate use of antimicrobial agents for prophylaxis, empiric, preemptive, targeted, or maintenance therapy is an esstential part of the management of patients with cancer, particularly in an age where the development of novel antimicrobial agents is at a standstill.[4] The major goal of antimicrobial stewardship is to optimize antimicrobial usage while reducing unwanted consequences such as toxicity and the selection of resistant organisms. Strategies for effective antimicrobial stewardship are listed in Table 137-7. These strategies are best implemented by an independent, multidisciplinary, antimicrobial stewardship team (MAST).[154,155]

Table 137-7 Antimicrobial Stewardship Strategies

Continuing education for all healthcare providers
Guidelines/pathways for appropriate antimicrobial usage based on local microbiology and susceptibility/resistance
Formulary interventions restricting specific agents
Audits of antimicrobial usage with feedback to prescribers
Introduction of surveillance and decision support programs
Monitoring outcomes (morbidity, mortality, length of stay) and resistance patterns
Comprehensive infection control program

Perspectives

Despite substantial advances in supportive care, infection remains a serious complication for many patients with cancer. The spectrum of infection (bacterial, fungal, viral) continues to change, requiring continued vigilance, and new strategies for infection prevention and treatment. The emergence of multidrug-resistant bacterial pathogens (eg, MRSA, VRE, *Pseudomonas aeruginosa*, *S. maltophilia*, *Acinetobacter* spp.) has posed serious challenges, particularly in the area of new drug development as highlighted in the monograph published by the Infectious Diseases Society of America, entitled "Bad Bugs, No Drugs."[4] Disseminated fungal infections have become the leading cause of death in patients with hematologic malignancies, and in HSCT recipients. Although the armamentarium against fungi has expanded, resistant organisms (eg, *C. krusei*, *A. terreus*, *Zygomycetes*, *Scedosporium* spp., *Fusarium* spp.) have emerged. The early diagnosis and treatment of many invasive fungal infections, particularly in the setting of persistent neutropenia/immunosuppression remains unsatisfactory. Viral infections represent a growing threat particularly in patients with hematologic malignancies and HSCT recipients. Newly emerging global threats (such as SARS, avian influenza, West Nile virus, etc) can have a devastating impact on patients with cancer who are immunosuppressed. Reliable methods for the rapid diagnosis of these and other viral infections, and effective means for their prevention and treatment still need to be developed. Parasitic infections remain uncommon except in endemic areas. Although effective therapies are available, toxicity and the need for prolonged maintenance or suppressive therapy can be problematic.

The hematologic growth factors (G-CSF, GM-CSF) and other cytokines have had a significant impact in reducing the risk of infection in some patients with cancer. These agents may also be useful as therapeutic adjuncts in some infections that are refractory to antimicrobial therapy. Interest in granulocyte transfusions has been revived because it is now possible to transfer large numbers of granulocytes by stimulating their growth in normal donors using hematopoietic growth factors.

The development of risk assessment strategies has led to the recognition of a "low-risk" subset among patients with neutropenia. This has enabled clinicians to evaluate not only the nature of empiric therapy (eg, combination or monotherapy) but also the route of administration (IV or PO), and the setting in which such therapy is delivered (hospital, clinic, home). These strategies have resulted in substantial cost savings, reduction in healthcare associated (nosocomial) infections, and improved quality of life for patients and their families or caregivers. Protected environments, prophylactic programs, infection control strategies, and the CSFs have reduced the risk of infection in patients with cancer. The use of vaccines in high-risk patients affords protection against specific pathogens. Newer technologic advances should lead to further progress. Nonetheless, the recognition, prevention, diagnosis, and treatment of infections in patients with cancer will continue to challenge us in the foreseeable future, as we work toward the larger goal of eliminating cancer.

Selected References

The complete reference list can be found at www.CANCERMEDICINE8.com

3. Wisplinghoff H, Seifert H, Wenzel RP, Edmond MB. Current trends in the epidemiology of nosocomial bloodstream infections in patients with hematological malignancies and solid neoplasms in hospitals in the United States. *Clin Infect Dis.* 2003;36:1103–1110.
4. Bad Bugs, No Drugs. Infectious Diseases Society of America, July 2004. Available at:

http://www.idsociety.org/pa/ IDSA_Paper4_final_web.pdf

8. Bodey GP, Buckley M, Sathe YS, Freireich EJ. Quantitative relationships between circulating leukocytes and infection in patients with acute leukemia. *Ann Intern Med.* 1966;64:328–340.
12. Klastersky J, Paesmans M, Rubenstein E, et al. The MASCC Risk Index: a multinational scoring system to predict low-risk febrile neutropenic cancer patients. *J Clin Oncol.* 2000;18:3038–3051.
13. Rubenstein EB, Rolston K, Benjamin RS, et al. Outpatient treatment of febrile episodes in low-risk neutropenic patients with cancer. *Cancer.* 1993;71:3640–3646.
14. Kern WV. Risk Assessment and treatment of low-risk patients with febrile neutropenia. *Clin Infect Dis.* 2006;42:533–540.
19. Price VE, Dutta S, Blanchette VS, et al. The prevention and treatment of bacterial infections in children with asplenia or hyposplenia: practice considerations at the Hospital for Sick Children, Toronto. *Pediatr Blood Cancer.* 2006;46:597–603.
20. Su YB, Sohn S, Krown SE, et al. Selective CD4+ Lymphopenia in melanoma patients treated with temazolomide: a toxicity with therapeutic implications. *J Clin Oncol.* 2008;22:610–616.
22. Rolston KVI, Bodey GP, Safdar A. Polymicrobial infection in patients with cancer: an underappreciated and underreported entity. *Clin Infect Dis.* 2007;45:228–233.
23. Rolston KVI. Challenges in the treatment of infections caused by gram-positive and gram-negative bacteria in patients with cancer and neutropenia. *Clin Infect Dis.* 2005;40:S246–S252.
24. Stryjewski ME, Chambers HE. Skin and soft-tissue infections caused by community-acquired methicillin-resistant *Staphylococcus aureus. Clin Infect Dis.* 2008;46:S368–S377.
26. Skaoulas G, Moise-Broder PA, Schentag J, et al. Relationship of MIC and bactericidal activity to efficacy of vancomycin for treatment of methicillin-resistant *Staphylococcus aureus* bacteremia. *J Clin Microbiol.* 2004;42:2398–2402.
32. Han XY, Kamana M, Rolston KVI. Viridans streptococci isolated by culture from blood of cancer patients: clinical and microbiologic analysis of 50 cases. *J Clin Microbiol.* 2006;44:160–165.
34. Edmond MB, Ober JF, Weinbaum DL, et al. Vancomycin resistant Enterococcus faecium bacteremia: risk factors for infection. *Clin Infect Dis.* 1995;20:1126–1133.
36. Matar MJ, Tarrand J, Raad I, et al. Colonization and infection with vancomycin-resistant Enterococcus among patients with cancer. *Am J Infect Control.* 2006;34:534–536.
41. Hughes WT, Armstrong D, Bodey GP, et al. Guidelines for the use of antimicrobial agents in neutropenic patients with cancer. *Clin Infect Dis.* 2002;34:730–751.
44. Nguyen KA, Coyle EA, Tam VH, et al. Antibacterial activity of colistin (c) and Polymyxin B (PV) against multidrugresistant (MDR) Pseudomonas aeruginosa (PSA), Alcalignes Xylosoxidans (AX), and Stenotrophomonas maltophilia (SM) at a cancer Center [abstract]. In: Program and abstracts for the 44th Interscience Conference on Antimicrobial Agents and Chemotherapy; October 30–November 4, 2004; Washington, D.C.
46. Rolston KVI, Guan Z, Bodey GP, Elting L. Acinetobacter calcoaceticus septicemia in patients with cancer. *South Med J.* 1985;78:647–651.
50. Iseman MD. Treatment of multidrug-resistant tuberculosis. *N Engl J Med.* 1993;329:784–791.
53. Ward TT, Rimland D, Kauffman C. Randomized, open-label trial of azithromycin plus ethambutol vs clarithromycin plus ethambutol as therapy for Mycobacterium avium complex bacteremia in patients with human immunodeficiency virus infection. *Clin Infect Dis.* 1998;27:1278–1285.
60. Pfaller MA, Jones RN, Doern GV, et al. Bloodstream infections due to Candida species: SENTRY antimicrobial surveillance program in North America and Latin America, 1997–1998. *Antimicrob Agents Chemother.* 2000;44:747–751.
68. Rex JH, Bennet JE, Sugar AM, et al. A randomized trial comparing fluconazole with amphotericin B for the treatment of candidemia in patients without neutropenia. *N Engl J Med.* 1994;331:1325–1372.
69. Mora-Durate J, Betts R, Rotstein C, et al. Comparison of caspofungin and amphotericin B for invasive candidiasis. *N Engl J Med.* 2002;347:2020–2029.
73. Walsh TJ, Anaissie EJ, Denning DW, et al. Treatment of aspergillosis: Clinical Practice Guidelines of the Infectious Disease Society of America. *Clin Infect Dis.* 2008;46:327–360.
74. Caillot D, Couaillier JF, Bernard A, et al. Increasing volume and changing characteristics of invasive pulmonary aspergillosis on sequential thoracic computed tomography scans in patients with neutropenia. *J Clin Oncol.* 2001;19:253–259.
76. Herbrecht R, Letscher-Bru V, Oprea C, et al. Aspergillus galactomannan detection in the diagnosis of invasive aspergillosis in cancer patients. *J Clin Oncol.* 2002;20:1898–1906.
77. Francesconi A, Kasai M, Petraitiene, et al. Characterization and comparison of galactomannan enzyme immunoassay and quantitative real-time PCR assay for detection of Aspergillsu fumigatus in Cronchoalveolar lavage fluid from experimental invasive pulmonary aspergissosis. *J Clin Microbiol.* 2006;44:2475–2480.
78. . Herbrecht R, Denning DW, Patterson TF, et al. Voriconazole versus amphotericin B for primary therapy of invasive aspergillosis. *N Engl J Med.* 2002;347:408–415.
82. Kontoyiannis DP, Lionakis MS, Lewis RE, et al. Zygomycosis in a tertiary-care cancer center in the era of Aspergillusactive antifungal therapy: A case-control observational study of 27 recent cases. *J Infect Dis.* 2005;191:1350–1360.
84. . Raad I, Tarrand J, Hanna H, et al. Epidemiology, molecular mycology, and environmental sources of Fusarium infection in patients with cancer. *Infect Control Hosp Epidemoil.* 2002;23:532–537.
92. Oxman MN, Levin MJ, Johnson GR, et al. A vaccine to prevent herpes zoster and postherpetic neuralgia in older adults. *N Engl J Med.* 2005;352:2271–2284.
97. Zaia JA, Schmidt GM, Chao NJ, et al. Preemptive ganciclovir administration based solely on asymptomatic pulmonary cytomegalovirus infection in allogeneic bone marrow transplant recipients: long-term follow-up. *Biol Blood Marrow Transplant.* 1995;1:188–193.
98. Winston DJ, Young JAH, Pullarkat V, et al. Maribavir prophylaxis for prevention of cytomegalovirus infection in allogeneic stem cell transplant recipients: a multicenter, randomized, double-blind, placebo-controlled, dose-ranging study. *Blood.* 2008;111:5403–5410.
100. Whimbey E, Ghosh S. Respiratory syncytial virus infections in immunocompromised adults. In: Remington JS, Swartz MN, editors. *Current Clinical Topics in Infectious Diseases.* Boston: Blackwell Science; 2000:232–255.
112. Consensus statement on the use of corticosteroids as adjunctive therapy for Pneumocystis pneumonia in the acquired immunodeficiency syndrome. *N Engl J Med.* 1990;323:1500–1504.
123. Kumashi P, Girgawy E, Tarrand J, Rolston KV, Raad II, Safdar A. Streptococcus pneumoniae bacteremia in patients with cancer: disease characteristics and outcomes in the era of escalating drug resistance (1998–2002). *Medicine.* 2005;84:303–312.
124. Rolston KVI. Infections in patients with solid tumors. In: Rolston KVI, Rubenstein EB, editors. *Textbook of Febrile Neutropenia.* London: Martin Dunitz; 2001:91–109.
126. Badgwell BD, Cormier JN, Wray CJ. Challenges in surgical management of abdominal pain in the neutropenic cancer patient. *Ann Surg.* 2008;248:104–109.
130. O'Grady NP, Alexander M, Dellinger EP, et al. Guidelines for the prevention of intravascular catheter-related infections. *Am J Infect Control.* 2002;30:476–489.
135. Freifeld A, Marchigiani D, Walsh T, et al. A double-blind comparison of empirical oral and intravenous antibiotic therapy for low-risk febrile patients with neutropenia during cancer chemotherapy. *N Engl J Med.* 1999;341:305–311.
137. Klastersky J, Paesman M. Risk-adapted strategy for the management of febrile neutropenia in cancer patients. *Support Care Cancer.* 2007;15:477–482.
140. Smith TJ, Khatcheressian J, Lyman GH. Update of recommendations for the use of white blood cell growth factors: an evidence-based clinical practice guideline. *J Clin Oncol.* 2006;24:3187–3205.
143. Cruciani M, Rampazzo R, Malena M, et al. Prophylaxis with fluoroquinolones for bacterial infections in neutropenic patients. *Clin Infect Dis.* 1996;23:795–805.
151. Cornley OA, Maertens J, Winston DJ, et al. Posaconazole vs. fluconazole or itraconazole prophylaxis in patients with neutropenia. *N Engl J Med.* 2007;356:348–359.
154. Dellit TH, Owens RC, McGowan JE. Infectious Diseases Society of America and the Society for Healthcare Epidemiology of America Guidelines for Developing an Institutional Program to Enhance Antimicrobial Stewardship. *Clin Infect Dis.* 2007;44:159–177.

138 Oncologic Emergencies

Sai-Ching Jim Yeung, MD, PhD ▪ Carmen Escalante, MD

Introduction

An oncologic emergency may be defined as an acute condition that is caused by cancer or the treatment of cancer and that requires intervention as soon as possible to avoid mortality or severe permanent morbidity. Cancer patients are more likely than healthy individuals to require emergency health care. Cancer and its treatment can lead to emergency conditions. The debilitated physical status, altered hemostasis, and impaired immunity that can result from malignancy or treatment of malignancy make cancer patients more vulnerable than healthy people to accidents and mishaps in everyday life (trauma, burn, electrocution, environmental stresses). Because cancer patients have unique concerns different from those of the general population presenting to emergency care facilities, health care providers need to adapt to the special needs of cancer patients when caring for them.

The care of cancer patients with emergency conditions is evolving into a hybrid discipline—a cross between oncology and emergency medicine. There are many types of problems for which cancer patients present to an emergency care facility, and an in-depth discussion fills a volume by itself.[1-3] Because of page constraints and the fact that some relevant topics are covered in other chapters of this book, this chapter can cover only a short list of selected topics.

Approach to Acutely Ill Cancer Patients

Cancer patients often have complex medical problems in addition to their cancer diagnosis, such as coronary heart disease, diabetes mellitus, and chronic obstructive pulmonary disease. Some of these comorbid conditions may be attributable to the same risk factors for carcinogenesis (ie, old age, diet, cigarette smoking, or sedentary lifestyle). Regardless of the medical complexity, cancer patients presenting with acute emergencies should be approached in a manner similar to that used for patients without cancer. However, emergency care providers caring for cancer patients must also rapidly assess the extent of the malignancy, the response of the malignancy to current treatment, the overall prognosis, and the patient's and family's wishes so that an appropriate treatment plan can be formulated and carried out (Fig. 138-1).

First, the patient should be rapidly assessed. This assessment should include the chief complaint, a focused history, vital signs, and a quick overall physical assessment. If the patient is unable to relay the history of present illness, a family member/companion or caregiver may be able to relay pertinent information. Intervention for unstable vital signs should be initiated right away. In the case of cardiopulmonary arrest, appropriate guidelines should be followed (http://www.acls.net).[4] Once the patient is stabilized, a more thorough history and physical examination should be completed. For the majority of cancer patients with acute emergencies, a comprehensive evaluation is usually necessary. Depending on the clinical scenario, the acute event may be due to the cancer, cancer treatments, or comorbid conditions, all of which should be considered when developing a differential diagnosis of the acute problem.

Circulatory Oncologic Emergencies

Sudden Cardiopulmonary Arrest

Most deaths are preceded by cardiopulmonary arrest. Resuscitation is more likely to succeed when cardiopulmonary arrest results from an acute reversible insult (eg, pulmonary embolism, choking, aspiration, or cardiac arrhythmia) rather than from a steady decline from an irreversible condition (eg, hypoxia due to diffuse infiltration of lungs by cancer); this is true in cancer patients as well as in patients with other diseases. The success rate of resuscitation and the hospital discharge rate of resuscitated patients are similar for cancer patients and noncancer patients.[5] A meta-analysis of inpatient resuscitation (including cancer patients) estimated that the probability of successful resuscitation is one in three and the probability of being discharged alive is one in eight.[6] The mortality rate of cancer patients in intensive care is about 50%, which is similar to the mortality rate of severely ill noncancer patients.[7] If a cancer patient has good performance status and is not expected to die soon, reluctance to resuscitate the patient or ad-

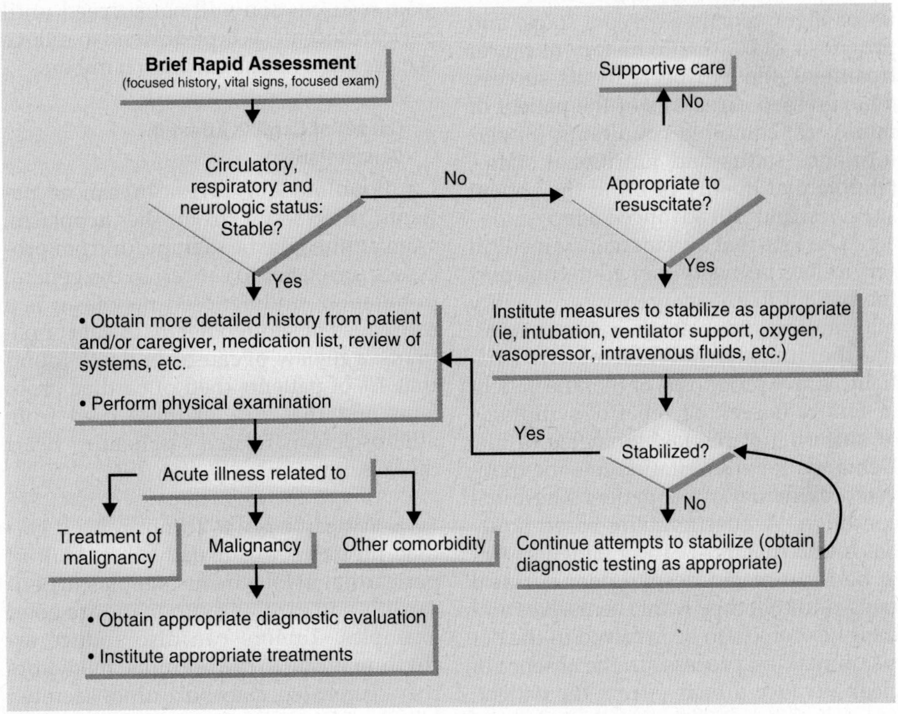

Figure 138-1 ▪ Approach to acutely ill cancer patients.

mit the patient to an intensive care unit is unjustified. A non–end stage cancer patient in cardiopulmonary arrest should be resuscitated with the same level of intense effort as any patient without cancer. However, when cardiopulmonary arrest occurs as the expected final event of a gradual decline and disintegration of bodily functions caused by cancer, resuscitation will generally not succeed.

Oncologists should ensure that advance directives (medical power of attorney, living will, and out-of-hospital do-not-resuscitate [DNR] orders) are discussed with patients and their families and that such orders or directives are carried out as the patient and family wish. Many informed patients readily sign living wills or appoint health care proxies. Timely recommendation of DNR status may avoid unnecessary trauma to patients, futile efforts and resources, and anguish for family members; timely recommendation of DNR status also provides time for open discussion to settle disagreements with patients or family.

When a cancer patient presents to a health care facility in cardiopulmonary arrest or impending arrest, the physician providing the emergency care may have never seen the patient before, and assessment of prognosis is difficult and quite often impossible. The decision to initiate or continue resuscitative efforts should be based on a rapid assessment of the patient's physical condition, a brief history of the events leading to or preceding the arrest, and any of the following factors that are known[8]: (1) duration of arrest, (2) initial cardiac rhythm, (3) rigor mortis or algor mortis, (4) type, stage, and prognosis of cancer, (5) history of cancer treatment and prospects for its success, (6) expressed directives of the patient or family, (7) comorbid conditions, (8) performance status and nutritional status, (9) potential quality of life if the patient survives, and (10) advanced age.

The fact that an emergency medical service has been summoned to transport the patient to an emergency care facility may indicate that death is unexpected, that the family has not yet accepted the patient's grave prognosis, or that the patient or family is seeking relief of symptoms or suffering at the last moments of life. Demands for resuscitation may be motivated by denial of the patient's terminal condition. A questionnaire-based study has found that most cancer patients want to be resuscitated despite poor survival rates, and that they want themselves and their next of kin to be involved in the decision-making process.[9] In the absence of clear advance directive from the patient, resuscitation may be needed to give the family "closure" by knowing that "everything possible has been done." However, resuscitation of patients with advanced refractory malignancies may be inappropriate when intubation and resuscitation will only prolong pain and suffering and waste health care resources without affecting outcome.

Special Consideration in Resuscitation of Cancer Patients

Most physicians and health care providers follow the resuscitation algorithms outlined in the advanced cardiac life support protocols (http://www.acls.net).[4] However, identification of specific causes of cardiopulmonary arrest may enable physicians to tailor resuscitative efforts to reverse or control the specific causes of arrest.

Carcinoid crisis (also referred to as acute carcinoid syndrome) is a good example of an uncommon but preventable and treatable cause of cardiopulmonary arrest in cancer patients. The crisis may be precipitated by anesthesia, biopsy, surgery, chemotherapy, or adrenergic drugs (eg, dopamine and epinephrine). Affected patients may develop refractory hypotension, arrhythmias, and bronchospasm due to massive release of serotonin and other vasoactive peptides from the tumor. Carcinoid crisis can be aborted or treated effectively with octreotide acetate (Sandostatin), a somatostatin analogue, 150-500 μg intravenously.[10] Cardiac tamponade is another case in which knowledge of the precipitating cause would help the physician to tailor the resuscitative effort. If a patient has pulseless electrical activity due to cardiac tamponade caused by malignant pericardial effusion, resuscitation will not succeed until pericardiocentesis is performed to relieve the pressure on the cardiac chambers.

Causes of Cardiac Arrest in Cancer Patients

Cardiopulmonary arrest in cancer patients may result from the neoplasm, from antineoplastic therapy, or from processes unrelated to cancer. In the general population, undiagnosed neoplasm is a rare cause of sudden death. In cancer patients, a review of causes of death found that 4% of patients died of cardiac problems and that 90% of these died from atherosclerosis-related ischemic heart disease.[11]

Tumor-Related Causes ■ Tumor-related cardiac problems are usually the result of pericardial involvement. Neoplastic pericarditis and cardiac tamponade are good examples. Tumors can also induce arrhythmias due to the hormone mediators they secrete (eg, catecholamines secreted by pheochromocytomas and serotonin secreted by carcinoid tumors) or due to direct mechanical irritation of the heart or pericardium. Arrhythmias associated with myocardial tumors,[12] coronary obstruction by tumor,[13] and massive tumor embolization[14] have all been reported as causes of sudden cardiopulmonary arrest. Cardiac amyloidosis can also lead to intractable congestive heart failure, arrhythmias, conduction disturbances, and sudden death.[15] Other tumor-related causes of cardiopulmonary arrest include malignancy-induced hemorrhage and malignancy-induced loss of ventilatory function (lymphangitic spread of tumor, airway obstruction, and loss of brain stem function).

Chemotherapy-Related Causes ■ Antineoplastic chemotherapeutic agents can cause complications leading to cardiopulmonary arrest. Angina, myocardial infarction, congestive heart failure, hypotension, arrhythmia, and sudden death have all been reported as complications of treatment with anticancer drugs.[16] Anthracyclines (doxorubicin, daunorubicin, and idarubicin), mitoxantrone, and mitomycin are known to injure cardiomyocytes, leading to cardiomyopathy. The long-term cardiotoxicity of anthracyclines is dependent on the cumulative dose. However, these drugs also cause acute side effects. Electrocardiographic and rhythm changes (mostly benign) have been noted in about 30% of patients treated with doxorubicin,[17] and sudden cardiopulmonary arrest has been reported in almost 1% of patients receiving doxorubicin.[18] Some of the molecular targets inhibited by new anticancer drugs (eg, imatinib, traztuzumab) are also important for cellular homeostasis of normal cardiomyocytes, particularly during exposure to other cytotoxic chemotherapy. Myocardial remodeling after cytotoxic myocardial damage can lead to progressive myocardial dysfunction over time and eventually manifest as cardiomyopathy and heart failure.[16] High-dose cyclophosphamide may cause acute problems of ventricular arrhythmia, cardiomyopathy, pericardial effusion, and cardiac arrest.[19] Fluorouracil has been associated with acute coronary vasospasm leading to angina and myocardial infarction.[20] Vasospasm or worsening angina in a patient receiving fluorouracil can be treated with calcium channel blockers. Hypotension, arrhythmia, and sudden death have also been reported with cytokines (interleukin-2 [IL-2], interferons) and monoclonal antibodies (discussed in the section "Systemic Reactions to Cytokines and Monoclonal Antibodies" later in this chapter).

Radiotherapy-Related Causes ■ Radiotherapy to the chest has adverse effects on the pericardium and heart.[21] Pericarditis may occur shortly or months to years after exposure of the chest to radiation. Radiotherapy can lead to pericardial effusion, tamponade, or pericardial fibrosis. The direct toxic effect of radiation on the heart can lead to electrocardiographic changes, including T-wave abnormalities and atrial arrhythmias. Exposure of the heart to radiation is also associated with accelerated atherosclerosis, coronary artery endarteritis, medial fibrosis, intimal proliferation, myocardial infarction, and sudden death.[22] Restrictive cardiomyopathy, arrhythmia, and valvular diseases are also significant problems after irradiation of the chest.

Arrhythmia

Arrhythmia is a common problem in cancer patients that leads to emergent evaluation. Arrhythmia may be related to malignancy or treatment of the malignancy, or it may be the result of other unrelated medical problems. Arrhythmia can lead to cardiopulmonary arrest and death; otherwise, the symptoms of arrhythmia can be subtle and intermittent. The symptoms are primarily due to the hemodynamic effects of the cardiac rhythm disturbance. Significant signs and symptoms include isolated or recurrent loss of consciousness (syncope), lightheadedness, dizziness, palpitation, chest pain, peripheral vascular embolization, dyspnea, and acute neurologic deficits (transient or persistent).

Sustained arrhythmia can be diagnosed electrographically with relative ease. However, arrhythmia is often transient, and transient or intermittent arrhythmia may present a diagnostic challenge. An electrocardiographic rhythm strip or a brief period of continuous monitoring does not exclude the possibility of a latent and potentially serious rhythm disturbance. When symptoms suggest arrhythmia (palpitation, syncope, etc), Holter monitoring for longer periods (24-48 hours) is indicated to try to capture the arrhythmic events and diagnose the problem. Analysis of cardiac rhythm may be more complicated in cancer patients than in noncancer patients because cancer patients often have exaggerated respiratory variations of the electrical axis and changes in mean QRS voltage that can be confused with heart rhythm irregularity. Such changes may be due to pleural or pericardial effusions, pulmonary surgery (pneumonectomy or lobectomy), or radiation-induced lung damage.

Primary Arrhythmia ■ Primary arrhythmia arises from cardiac and pericardial structures and may be caused by focal or diffuse abnormalities. Common causes of primary arrhythmia in all patients include ischemic disease; increased intracardiac pressure and wall stress; congestive, hypertrophic, and infiltrative cardiomyopathy; and fibrosis related to aging. In cancer patients, the major causes of primary arrhythmia are primary or metastatic intracardiac tumors, amyloid infiltration, myocarditis, pericarditis, pericardial constriction, and cardiomyopathy related to antitumor agents (especially anthracyclines and anti-HER2 therapy).[16,23]

Secondary Arrhythmia ■ Secondary arrhythmia arises from general toxic reactions to drugs; increased sympathetic states, such as those related to severe anxiety, hyperthyroidism, and mediator release (due to pheochromocytomas and carcinoid tumors); derangements of electrolyte metabolism; and radiation-induced heart damage. Some cancer drugs are arrhythmogenic; examples include anthracyclines, arsenic trioxide, 5-fluorouracil, irinotecan, gemcitabine, and interferon. A longer list of chemotherapeutic agents associated with arrhythmias is shown in Table 138-1. In addition to chemotherapeutic agents, antifungal agents, antiprotozoans, and antibiotics, which are commonly used to treat infectious complications of cancer patients, have also been associated with cardiac rhythm disturbances.

Table 138-1 ■ **Chemotherapeutic Drugs Associated With Arrhythmias**

Alkylating agents
Cisplatin
Ifosfamide
Cyclophosphamide
Busulfan
Carmustine
Anthracyclines
Daunorubicin
Doxorubicin
Idarubicin
Mitoxantrone
Antimetabolites
5-Fluorouracil
Gemcitabine
Topoisomerase I inhibitors
Irinotecan
Topoisomerase II inhibitors
Teniposide
Taxanes
Paclitaxel
Docetaxel
Vinca alkaloids
Vincristine
Vinblastine
Miscellaneous
Amsacrine
Arsenic trioxide
Asparaginase
Interferon
Tretinoin (retinoic acid)
Pentostatin

Treatment of Arrhythmia ■ Treatment of arrhythmia should be based on both urgency and etiology. For hemodynamically stable arrhythmias that are secondary in origin, immediate treatment should consist of correcting metabolic derangements (particularly achieving homeostasis of potassium, calcium, and magnesium) and discontinuing culprit drugs or substances. Specific treatment that is aimed at reversing the causative factor should be administered. When treatment aimed at controlling the cardiac rhythm is thought to be necessary, standard guidelines for management of arrhythmia may be followed.[4] Commonly used intravenous antiarrhythmic drugs are listed in Table 138-2.

Paroxysmal supraventricular tachycardia may be converted back into sinus rhythm in a considerable proportion of cases by vagal maneuvers. Adenosine administered as one or two doses of rapidly injected boluses under electrocardiographic monitoring is frequently effective in restoring sinus heart rhythm. The drug is also used to determine the mechanism of the arrhythmia when the diagnosis is unclear based on electrocardiographic strips; however, careful analysis of standard 12-lead electrocardiograms usually obviates the use of adenosine as a diagnostic tool.

Stable secondary arrhythmia is unlikely to deteriorate into a life-threatening or catastrophic problem. Frequently, secondary arrhythmia presents as either ventricular ectopy, sometimes in bigeminy or trigeminy or other coupled patterns, or supraventricular ectopy, most often as intermittent or sustained supraventricular tachycardia. Isolated premature ventricular complexes may not require any treatment. More complex forms of ventricular ectopy are often controlled by beta-adrenergic blockers, which do not have proarrhythmic properties. Amiodarone should be considered for patients with a low left ventricular ejection fraction, and should be used with caution for patients with hepatic insufficiency and patients with underlying thyroid diseases. Rarely, amiodarone can cause hypotension, bradycardia, and QT prolongation that may precipitate episodes of torsades de pointes. Except for beta-adrenergic blockers, many antiarrhythmic drugs, especially those in type 1A, 1C, and 3, are potentially proarrhythmic.[24] Cardiac monitoring during the initiation of antiarrhythmic therapy should be considered because cancer patients have an increased susceptibility to proarrhythmic side effects due to metabolic derangements and the concomitant use of or exposure to other proarrhythmic agents.

Supraventricular tachycardia is the most common arrhythmia in cancer patients. Sustained supraventricular arrhythmia in cancer patients is often difficult to terminate with drug therapy. While pharmacological agents are used to regulate or terminate the abnormal

Table 138-2 Commonly Used Intravenous Antiarrhythmic Drugs

Name	Class	Dose[a]	Indication[a]
Adenosine	Nucleoside	6 mg IV over <3 s followed by NS 20 mL bolus; second dose and third dose of 12 mg 2 min apart as needed	Narrow complex PSVT; PSVT due to AV node or sinus node reentry
Amiodarone	Class III antiarrhythmic	Cardiac arrest: 300 mg IVP; 150 mg IVP q 3-5 min up to 2.2 g/day	
		Stable wide-complex tachycardia: 150 mg IV over 10 min; repeat q 10 min as needed; maintenance infusion 0.5 mg/min; up to 2.2 g/day	Supraventricular or ventricular tachyarrhythmias; control of rapid atrial tachyarrhythmia in patients with low LVEF when digoxin is ineffective
Atropine	Anticholinergic	0.5-1 mg IVP q 3-5 min as needed , up to 0.04 mg/kg	Symptomatic sinus bradycardia; Mobitz type 1 AV block; asystole
Digoxin	Digitalis glycoside	Loading dose: 10-15 μg/kg lean body weight in divided doses	To slow ventricular response in A. fib. or A. flutter; PSVT
Diltiazem	Calcium channel blocker	0.25 mg/kg IV over 2 min; 2nd dose 0.35 mg/kg IV over 2 min in 15 min prn; maintenance: 5-15 mg/h by titration	To slow ventricular response in A. fib. or A. flutter; PSVT; to terminate AV nodal re-entrant tachycardia
Esmolol	β-blocker	0.5 mg/kg over 1 min; then infuse at 0.05 mg/kg/min; titrate up to maximum of 0.3 mg/kg/min	PSVT, A. fib. or A. flutter; Reduce incidence of VF in MI or USA
Ibutilide	Class III antiarrhythmic	1 mg IV over 10 min; repeat in 10 min prn	SVT including A. fib.A. flutter; effective for conversion of A. fib.flutter of relatively brief duration
Isoproterenol	β-agonist	Infuse 2-10 μg/min; titrate	Symptomatic bradycardia; torsades de pointes refractory to Mg; β-blocker overdose
Lidocaine	Local anesthetic	1-1.5 mg/kg IVP; repeat 0.5-0.75 mg/kg IVP q 5-10 min up to total of 3 mg/kg prn; maintenance: 30-50 μg/kg/min IV	VT or VF; wide-complex tachycardia; significant ventricular ectopy; torsades de pointes
Metoprolol	β-blocker	5 mg slow IVP q 5 min up to a total dose of 15 mg	PSVT, A. fib., or A. flutter; Reduce incidence of VF in MI or USA
Procainamide hydrochloride	Class IA antiarrhythmic	20-50 mg/min up to a total dose of 17 mg/kg	Recurrent VF or VT
Propranolol	β-blocker	0.1 mg/kg slow IVP in 3 divided doses 2-3 min apart	PSVT, A. fib., or A. flutter; Reduce incidence of VF in MI or USA
Quinidine gluconate	Class IA antiarrhythmic	Intermittent bolus doses of 80 mg every 5-10 min or 10 mg/min intravenous infusion up to 400 mg	Supraventricular and ventricular arrhythmias
Verapamil	Calcium channel blocker	2.5-5 mg IV over 2 min; repeat q 15-30 min prn up to a total dose of 20 mg	PSVT, A. fib., or A. flutter

Abbreviations: A. fib., atrial fibrillation; A. flutter, atrial flutter; AV, atrioventricular; IV, intravenously; IVP, intravenous push; LVEF, left ventricular ejection fraction; MI, myocardial infarction; NS, normal saline; prn, as needed; PSVT, paroxysmal supraventricular tachycardia; USA, unstable angina; VF, ventricular fibrillation; VT, ventricular tachycardia.
Source: From Ref. 4.

heart rhythm, elective, synchronized cardioversion under conscious sedation should be considered early and planned appropriately. The initial energy level for cardioversion recommended by the American Heart Association is 100 joules, but this level may not be high enough to convert atrial fibrillation. An initial shock with an energy level of 200 joules has been recommended by others for the conversion of atrial fibrillation.[25] Higher energy levels for cardioversion are appropriate when cancer patients have concomitant effusions or are significantly overweight. Lower initial energy levels (ie, 50-100 joules) should be used to convert atrial flutter. If sinus rhythm can be restored within 48 hours of the onset of supraventricular tachycardia, anticoagulation therapy may be avoided. However, the time of onset of the arrhythmia is not always clear, and the time of discovery of the arrhythmia cannot be presumed to be synchronous with the time of onset of arrhythmia. In the absence of clear evidence as to the time of arrhythmia onset, anticoagulation therapy should be administered prior to cardioversion. Transesophageal echocardiography may be used to exclude intracardiac thrombosis prior to elective synchronized cardioversion.

Arrhythmias that originate from structural cardiac abnormalities are much more difficult to control than arrhythmias of metabolic etiology, and this is especially true in cancer patients. Arrhythmias due to structural abnormalities are likely to persist over long periods and progress to higher-grade life-threatening arrhythmias. In the emergency setting, the therapeutic goals are stabilization of hemodynamic and respiratory status, discovery of correctable pathologic conditions, and control of symptoms. Depending on the etiology of the arrhythmia, emergent consultation with cardiologists and emergent diagnostic or interventional procedures may be required.

Patients with unstable arrhythmia should be treated with aggressive pharmacological or electrical interventions. The interventions should generally follow established algorithms or guidelines such as those recommended by the American Heart Association.[26] These interventions include administration of a vasopressor, such as vasopressin or epinephrine, to support blood pressure (if required); administration of antiarrhythmic drugs such as amiodarone, lidocaine, and procainamide; electrical cardioversion or defibrillation; airway management; ventilation with oxygen; administration of intravenous fluid; and chest compression (if required). Emergency treatment of torsades de pointes varies from the standard algorithms for other types of ventricular tachycardia; it entails expedient use of intravenous magnesium, electrical overdrive pacing or pharmacological overdrive with isoproterenol, and administration of phenytoin or lidocaine.

Tumor Lysis Syndrome

Tumor lysis syndrome (TLS) consists of severe hyperphosphatemia, hyperkalemia, hyperuricemia, azotemia, hypocalcemia, and metabolic acidosis (out of proportion to the degree of renal insufficiency) due to the massive release of cell contents and degradation products of dead tumor cells into the bloodstream. Acute TLS is caused by the death of a large number of neoplastic cells.[27] TLS usually occurs less than 72 hours after chemotherapy in patients with leukemia and lymphoma, but new therapeutic regimens and methods may alter the time of onset of TLS. TLS also has been reported in patients with nonhematologic malignancies, including small cell carcinomas, non–small cell lung cancer, breast cancer, and ovarian cancer.

We have chosen to discuss TLS immediately after the discussion of arrhythmia because the main acute cause of death in patients with TLS is arrhythmia secondary to the severe electrolyte abnormalities (especially hyperkalemia) and renal failure associated with this syndrome. Early recognition of metabolic abnormalities and prompt treatment can avoid fatal outcomes.

The symptoms of TLS are nonspecific. Common symptoms include nausea, vomiting, cloudy urine, weakness, fatigue, and arthralgia. Other signs and symptoms related to metabolic and electrolyte abnormalities include neuromuscular irritability, seizures, muscle weakness, and arrhythmias. Arrhythmia may cause sudden death in patients with TLS.[28] Hyperuricemia, hyperkalemia, and hypocalcemia may lead to cardiac arrhythmia, tetany, and sudden death. Precipitation of uric acid or calcium phosphate in the renal tubules may lead to acute renal failure. Hyponatremia and hypoalbuminemia at the time of diagnosis is associated with poor prognosis in patients, uric acid nephropathy resulting from TLS.[29]

TLS can occur spontaneously, but most commonly it occurs after chemotherapy (including glucocorticoid therapy alone in sensitive lymphomas), immunotherapy, and radiotherapy. Factors associated with increased risk of TLS include the type of malignancy (eg, Burkitt's lymphoma), good responsiveness of the malignancy to therapy, rapid cell turnover, and large tumor burden. Other risk factors are preexisting renal insufficiency, acute renal failure developing shortly after the treatment, and poor response to hydration. Pretreatment lactate dehydrogenase levels, which tend to correlate with tumor bulk in patients with stage C or D lymphoma, can predict the development of posttreatment azotemia, but pretreatment hyperuricemia is not predictive. A predictive scoring system for TLS has been proposed based on the data from acute myelocytic leukemia (AML) patients undergoing induction therapy.[30,31] The scoring system potentially can be used as part of a risk-based prophylaxis strategy against TLS. Preventive measures should be started early in patients at risk for TLS. Aggressive hydration with crystalloid fluid or normal saline up to 3 L/m^2/day may be required to maintain a urine output of at least 100 mL/hour with or without the help of loop or osmotic diuretics. The xanthine oxidase inhibitor allopurinol (100-300 mg orally per day) may prevent severe hyperuricemia. Other new xanthine oxidase inhibitors such as febuxostat and Y-700 may also be available soon. New biomarkers (cystatin-C, neutrophil gelatinase-associated lipocalin, kidney injury molecule 1) may identify patients with early significant renal damage before a significant increase in creatinine for aggressive intervention.

The diagnosis of TLS requires a high level of suspicion because there are few signs or symptoms in the early stage. Routine uric acid and electrolyte screening (including measurement of calcium and phosphorus levels) is indicated in patients with high tumor bulk or hematologic malignancies. Once diagnosed, patients with severe TLS should have continuous monitoring of hemodynamic and electrocardiographic parameters in an intensive care unit. The allopurinol dose may be increased up to 900 mg/day. Increased intravenous fluid hydration may be coupled with promotion of diuresis through administration of loop diuretics (eg, furosemide, 20-200 mg intravenously [IV] every 4-6 hours) and acetazolamide (250-500 mg IV daily). If aciduria is present, sodium bicarbonate or acetate infusion may be used to keep urine pH between 7.1 and 7.5. Recombinant urate oxidase (uricozyme or rasburicase, an enzyme that oxidizes uric acid to allantoin) (200 μg/kg IV over 30 minutes daily) may be used to prevent or treat urate nephropathy.[32] Frequent electrolyte measurements (every 4-6 hours) may be required. Hyperkalemia should be treated with insulin plus dextrose, calcium, and bicarbonate infusions along with oral potassium ion-exchange resins (sodium polystyrene sulfonate; Kayexalate). In hyperphosphatemic patients with hypocalcemia, the addition of an oral calcium-based compound (eg, calcium acetate [Phos-Lo] or calcium carbonate) will reduce phosphate absorption and enhance calcium absorption. Intravenous calcium infusion can potentially cause calcium phosphate precipitation in the presence of severe hyperphosphatemia and should be used cautiously. Dialysis may be required for patients with symptomatic hypocalcemia and a serum phosphorus level greater than 3.3 mmol/L (>10.2 mg/dL). Other indications for dialysis include persistent azotemia; persistent hyperkalemia, hyperuricemia, oliguria, or anuria despite diuretic use; refractory acidemia; and volume overload. Prompt dialysis should be instituted with continued careful monitoring until biochemical abnormalities resolve. Hemodialysis is the most common mode of dialysis; continuous arteriovenous hemodialysis with a high dialysate flow rate and continuous venovenous hemofiltration are also effective.

Pericardial Tamponade

Pericardial tamponade occurs when pericardial fluid accumulates to the point that hemodynamics are affected. Two mechanisms can lead to accumulation of excess fluid in the pericardial space in cancer patients: (1) obstruction of lymphatic drainage and (2) excess fluid secretion from tumor nodules on pericardial surfaces. A number of tumors can lead to pericardial tamponade. Mesothelioma is the most common malignancy that arises from the pericardium. Carcinoma of the lung and malignant thymoma may involve the pericardium by direct extension. More frequently, malignancies arrive at the pericardium by retrograde lymphangitic spread or hematogenous dissemination (eg, carcinomas of the lung and breast). Malignant melanoma is the malignancy most likely to metastasize to the heart. Lymphomas (both Hodgkin and non-Hodgkin), leukemias, and gastrointestinal neoplasms may also cause pericardial effusions.[33] Nonneoplastic causes of pericardial tamponade include pericardial abscess, Candida pericarditis, and complications of central venous catheterization.

Although malignant pericardial effusion is occasionally the first clinical manifestation of malignancy, it is usually a late finding in patients with known metastatic disease. Malignant pericardial effusion is associated with poor prognosis (median survival time: about 6 months; 1-year survival rate: 28%).[34] More than two-thirds of patients with malignant pericardial effusion are asymptomatic. In symptomatic patients, the most common complaints are shortness of breath, pleuritic chest pain, orthopnea, and general weakness. Findings on physical examination may vary from normal to hemodynamic collapse. Tachycardia, hypotension, jugular venous distention, organomegaly, and extremity edema may indicate compromised cardiac output. The classic findings of cardiac tamponade are determined by both the quantity of pericardial fluid and the rapidity of fluid accumulation. Pulsus paradoxus, an exaggeration of the usually normal decrease in systolic blood pressure with inspiration, is a classic but nonspecific finding of cardiac tamponade because it is seen also in patients with lung cancer, significant lung disease, or cor pulmonale.

Because the symptoms and physical findings of pericardial tamponade are often nonspecific, a definitive diagnosis usually requires additional testing. Electrical alternans in electrocardiographs, when present, is a very helpful finding. Plain chest radiographs may reveal widening of the mediastinum and cardiac silhouette (Fig. 138-2). Computed tomography (CT) or magnetic resonance (MR) imaging studies frequently detect pericardial effusions as an incidental finding. These studies provide information on the location (loculated or not) and size of pericardial effusions but do not ad-

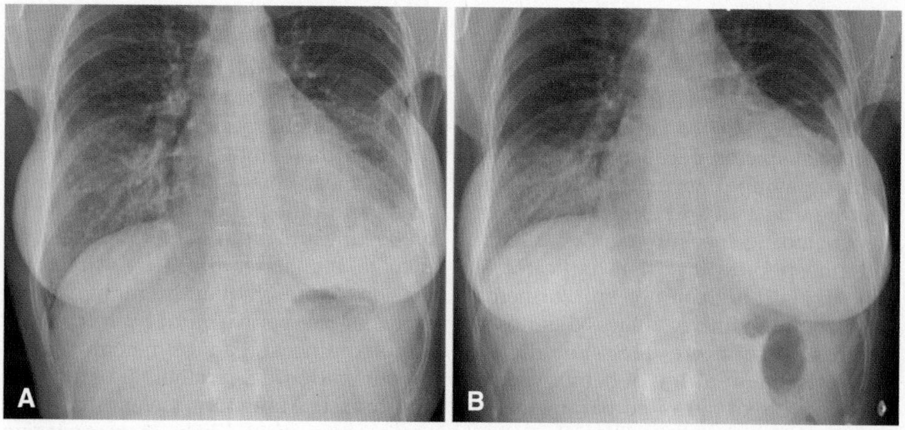

Figure 138-2 Chest radiographs of a breast cancer patient with pericardial tamponade. Widening of mediastinum and cardiac silhouette is evident **(B)** when compared with a prior chest radiograph **(A)**.

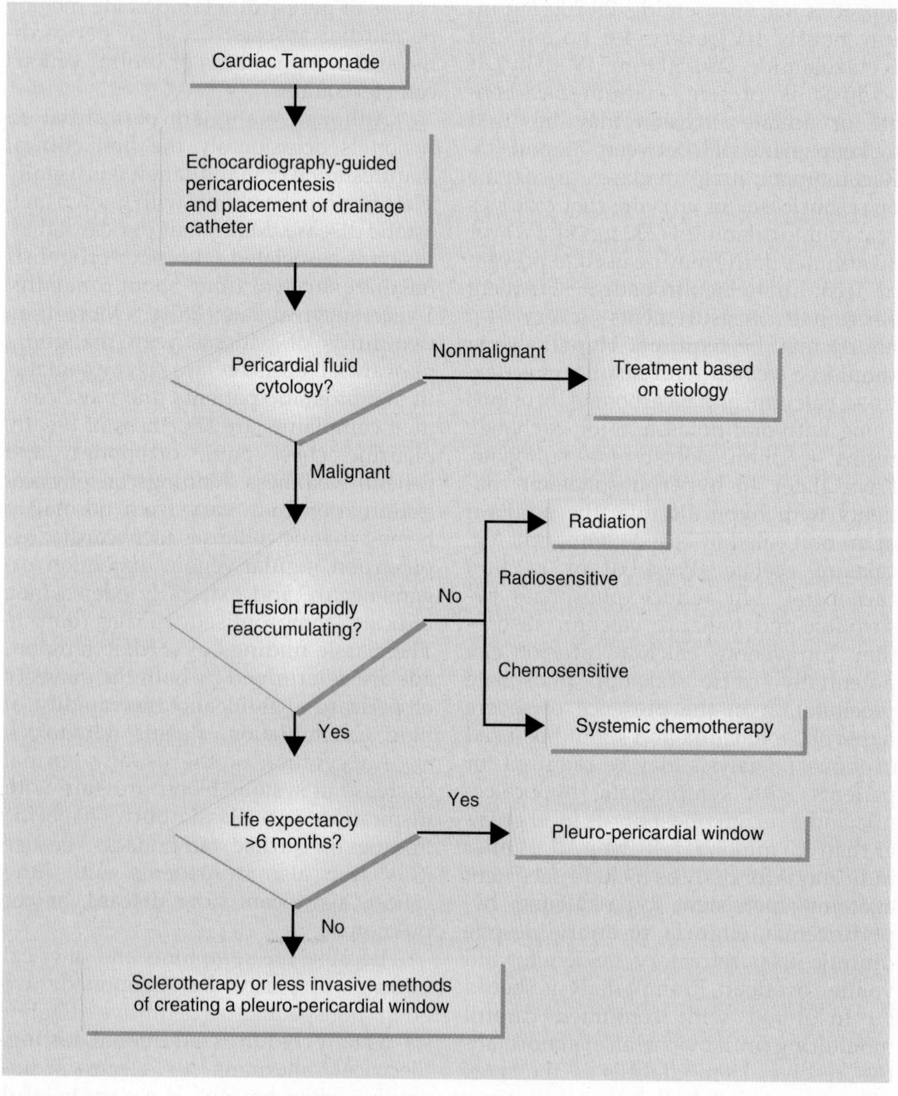

Figure 138-3 Algorithm for management of pericardial effusion.

equately assess the hemodynamic significance of the effusions. Two-dimensional echocardiography is the most useful test for diagnosing pericardial effusion and evaluating the hemodynamic significance of the effusion, ie, the presence of cardiac tamponade. Collapse or compression of the right atrium, diastolic collapse of the right ventricle, and cardiac "rocking" (a side-to-side or front-to-back movement of the heart) are often observed in cardiac tamponade. Alterations in the respiratory variation of flow patterns across the mitral valve as measured by Doppler shift are also helpful in evaluating the hemodynamic significance of pericardial effusions.

Initial management of a patient with malignant pericardial effusion depends on the patient's hemodynamic stability. Cytologic examination of pericardial fluid reveals metastatic disease in 70-80% of cancer patients with pericardial effusion. In patients with hemodynamic compromise, echocardiography-guided pericardiocentesis, with placement of a drainage catheter into the pericardial space, may be performed emergently in the emergency center or intensive care unit (Fig. 138-3). Complications are rare and may include massive pericardial bleeding (when a coronary artery is damaged) and pneumothorax (especially in patients with emphysema). Pericardial fluid can be drained from the catheter, and the catheter can remain in place until less than 50 mL of fluid is drained over 24 hours. Fibrinolytic agents may facilitate pericardial drainage and avoid repeat pericardiocentesis or replacement of the catheter when pericardial drainage subsides despite continued presence of pericardial fluid.[35]

However, pericardial fluid will usually reaccumulate after removal of the catheter.

Long-term management of malignant pericardial effusion focuses on preventing the reaccumulation of fluid, which occurs in more than 50% of patients. Because the long-term survival for most patients with malignant pericardial effusion is limited, an effective therapy that limits discomfort and is not associated with excessive risk to the patient should be employed. In patients with severe hemodynamic compromise and rapid fluid reaccumulation, the pleuro-pericardial window offers the most definitive therapy. Creation of a pleuro-pericardial window using one of a variety of approaches usually can avoid the need for repeated pericardiocentesis. The pleuro-pericardial window procedure is usually done in an operating room, but it can be performed in a hospital room or intensive care unit using local anesthesia. The use of a percutaneous intrapericardial balloon catheter to create a pleuro-pericardial window has had some success,[36] but results from large series of patients treated with this modality are not yet available. A laparoscopic transdiaphragmatic approach to create a pericardioperitoneal shunt has also been described.[37] In stable patients, systemic chemotherapy, pericardial radioactive colloid, or thoracic external-beam irradiation may be used for tumors that are still sensitive to these treatment modalities. Additional radiotherapy should be avoided in patients who have already had significant exposure of the heart to ionizing radiation. The use of local chemotherapeutic agents or agents given to sclerose the pericardium will prevent fluid reaccumulation in many patients,[38] but sclerotherapy can be very painful.

Acute Hemorrhage

In cancer patients, acute hemorrhage may result from the underlying malignancy or cancer treatment. Gastrointestinal bleeding and genitourinary bleeding are discussed in other chapters. Hemoptysis, which can rapidly compromise respiratory function, will be discussed later in this chapter. This section will cover some less frequent serious bleeding events: carotid arterial rupture, splenic rupture, and retroperitoneal hemorrhage.

The manifestations of acute hemorrhage depend on the rate and the site of bleeding. In most cases, the site of bleeding is obvious, but sometimes bleeding can be occult. Some patients may have only nonspecific clinical manifestations related to the bleeding organ, and some patients with substantial blood loss may have only signs and symptoms of hypovolemia and hypoperfusion (eg, tachycardia, hypotension, oliguria, and depressed mental status). It may be difficult to diagnose internal bleeding. Very often, diagnostic imaging studies or procedures, such as CT scans, ultrasonography, arteriography, or endoscopy, are necessary to make the correct diagnosis.

The primary objectives of management of acute hemorrhage are to rapidly identify the bleeding source and achieve hemostasis. In the acute setting, direct pressure to compress the bleeding vessel or site should be applied whenever feasible while the cardiopulmonary status is assessed expeditiously. Intravenous fluid resuscitation is vital in maintaining intravascular volume, cardiac output, and adequate vital organ perfusion. Isotonic crystalloid fluids (normal saline or lactated Ringer's solution, Plasmalyte, etc) should be used as first-line agents because colloids (eg, hetastarch) have not been proven to improve mortality rates.[39] Coagulopathy or thrombocytopenia should be corrected immediately by transfusion of blood products. The decision to transfuse red blood cells depends on the hemodynamic stability of the patient, persistence of hemorrhage, estimated blood loss, and presence of comorbid diseases (eg, coronary artery disease and cerebrovascular disease). Typed and cross-matched red blood cells are preferred, but non–cross-matched type-specific blood or type-O blood may have to be used in the case of massive life-threatening hemorrhage. Specific therapeutic procedures to control bleeding, such as embolization, balloon tamponade, or surgery, should be performed in a timely manner.

Carotid Artery Rupture ■ Most cases of carotid artery "blowout" or rupture occur in patients with head and neck cancers. Carotid artery rupture may be caused by direct tumor invasion or erosion into the carotid artery or by complications of cancer treatment, eg, postsurgical wound infection, postradiation necrosis, or orocutaneous fistula.

Carotid artery rupture usually occurs as a sudden and massive arterial spurting. Occasionally, ominous minor and transient bleeding episodes—so called sentinel bleeds—herald the massive blowout. In some cases, bleeding through a fistula into the esophagus or trachea may manifest as massive hematemesis or hemoptysis. Without prompt management, the patient's condition will rapidly deteriorate to hypotension, hypovolemic shock, loss of consciousness, and death.

Hemostasis is of utmost importance. Since neck vessels are accessible to direct manual compression, continuous firm compression should be applied at the site of the carotid artery rupture until the patient arrives at the operating room for surgical treatment. Crystalloid intravenous fluid resuscitation, prompt transfusion of blood products, and administration of vasopressors should be performed to maintain perfusion of vital organs. The bleeding very rarely stops spontaneously. Carotid artery rupture almost always requires surgical treatment. However, surgical ligation of the bleeding carotid artery is associated with high morbidity (25% of patients have neurologic sequelae) and high mortality (40%).[40] Intraluminal balloon occlusion with an intravascular catheter has been successful in controlling carotid bleeding in selected patients who are stable enough to undergo angiography.[41]

Splenic Rupture ■ The spleen is a fragile intraabdominal organ vulnerable to rupture. In most cases, splenic rupture results from trauma. Spontaneous splenic rupture is often associated with development of splenomegaly secondary to malaria and infectious mononucleosis in the general population. In cancer patients, spontaneous splenic rupture is relatively rare, and acute leukemia, non-Hodgkin's lymphoma, and chronic myelogenous leukemia are the most common malignancies associated with spontaneous splenic rupture. Other associated hematologic malignancies include hairy cell leukemia and Hodgkin's lymphoma. Metastases to the spleen in patients with solid tumors such as gastric, prostate, and lung cancer can also cause rupture. The mechanism of spontaneous splenic rupture is not clear. Minor trauma to the spleen may contribute in some cases. Other contributing factors include splenomegaly, infiltration of the splenic capsule by malignant cells, splenic infarction, thrombocytopenia, coagulopathy, anticoagulation therapy, and disseminated intravascular coagulation.

The typical clinical presentation of splenic rupture involves pain in the left shoulder or abdomen (left upper quadrant), tachycardia, and hypotension. The severity of the signs and symptoms may depend on the extent of bleeding. Diagnostic peritoneal lavage is rarely used in nontrauma cases; thus, the definitive diagnosis of splenic rupture relies on imaging studies. Contrast-enhanced CT is the diagnostic study of choice. It is accurate, noninvasive, and informative about the extent of splenic rupture and the severity of intraperitoneal or retroperitoneal hemorrhage. Using ultrasonography to diagnose splenic rupture[42] offers the advantages of availability and portability, and ultrasonography can be performed at bedside for hemodynamically unstable patients.

For patients with splenic rupture and hematologic malignancies, prompt splenectomy is necessary because the mortality rate for these patients is extremely high without surgery. In selected patients with contraindications to surgery, selective arterial embolization or external-beam irradiation of the ruptured site may provide control of bleeding.[43] Patients who are not surgical candidates should be treated with intravenous fluid administration, supplemental oxygen administration, pain control measures, blood transfusion, and correction of thrombocytopenia and coagulopathy.

Retroperitoneal Hemorrhage ■ Any damage to retroperitoneal organs or structures (ie, the kidneys, adrenal glands, duodenum, pancreas, major blood vessels, muscles, or bones) may cause retroperitoneal hemorrhage. Malignancies rarely cause spontaneous retroperitoneal hemorrhage; in the rare cases caused by malignancy, the culprit is usually renal cell carcinoma (primary or metastatic)[44] or an adrenal-gland tumor.[45] Anticoagulation therapy, thrombocytopenia, and coagulopathy are predisposing factors for spontaneous retroperitoneal hemorrhage. Retroperitoneal or intraperitoneal invasive procedures and placement of a central venous catheter through a femoral vessel can also cause severe retroperitoneal hemorrhage.

Retroperitoneal hemorrhage causes nonspecific signs and symptoms that may vary according to the rate of bleeding and the underlying disease. Patients may present with abdominal pain, a tender mass in the flank, tachycardia, and

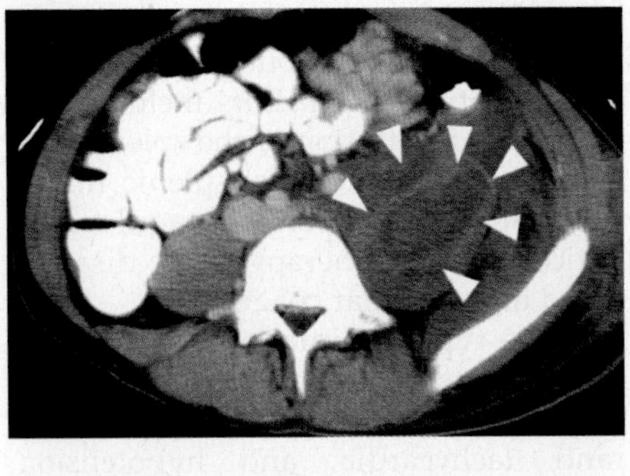

Figure 138-4 Retroperitoneal bleeding. The CT scan of the abdomen and pelvis of a thrombocytopenic leukemia patient showed a large inhomogeneous retroperitoneal collection (white arrowheads) consistent with a hematoma in the left psoas muscle displacing bowel loops to the right.

hypotension. Some may have hematuria or hematochezia if the blood somehow finds its way into the ureter or gastrointestinal tract. It is difficult to establish a diagnosis of retroperitoneal hemorrhage on the basis of clinical findings. Maintaining a high level of clinical suspicion and performing early imaging studies are keys to the successful treatment of retroperitoneal hemorrhage. CT of the abdomen and pelvis is the noninvasive study most commonly used to diagnose retroperitoneal bleeding (Fig. 138-4). Ultrasonography performed at the bedside may be useful to rapidly diagnose retroperitoneal bleeding.

The management of retroperitoneal hemorrhage depends on the severity of bleeding and the underlying cause. Stabilizing treatments for acute hemorrhage—such as intravenous fluid resuscitation, blood transfusion, and correction of coagulopathy and thrombocytopenia—should be started immediately. The patient should be monitored closely for hemodynamic stability and the presence of continued blood loss. In life-threatening situations, most patients require emergent laparotomy to remove the bleeding tumor or organ. Renal cell carcinomas are often hypervascular, and selective arterial embolization may control the bleeding of a renal lesion. External-beam radiation treatment of the bleeding tumor may be an option in hemodynamically stable patients with subacute bleeding and a relatively stable hematocrit.[46]

Superior Vena Cava Syndrome

Superior vena cava (SVC) syndrome refers to a constellation of signs and symptoms resulting from partial or complete obstruction of blood flow through the SVC to the right atrium. The obstruction may be caused by compression, invasion, thrombosis, or fibrosis of this vessel. Although SVC syndrome is traditionally considered a medical emergency and continues to be discussed as such, it is also well recognized that SVC syndrome rarely causes immediate, life-threatening complications.

Lung cancer is the leading cause of SVC syndrome; non-Hodgkin lymphoma is the second most common cause.[47] Although Hodgkin lymphoma commonly involves the mediastinum, it rarely causes SVC syndrome. Primary mediastinal malignancies like thymoma and germ cell tumors account for fewer than 2% of cases of SVC syndrome. Breast cancer is the most common metastatic disease that causes SVC syndrome.[48] Other metastatic cancers that may cause SVC syndrome include gastrointestinal adenocarcinomas, prostate adenocarcinomas, sarcomas, and melanomas. Nonmalignant causes of SVC syndrome include retrosternal goiter, pyogenic infections, sarcoidosis, teratoma, pleural calcification, silicosis, postradiation fibrosis, chemotherapy-induced fibrosis, constrictive pericarditis, and idiopathic mediastinal fibrosis.[47] An increasing cause of SVC syndrome in cancer patients is central venous catheter–induced thrombosis.

Obstruction of the SVC causes a rise in venous pressure in the SVC. Collateral venous circulation often flows through the azygos venous system. Obstruction below or at the entrance of the azygos veins forces blood to travel in the opposite direction down the azygos and chest wall veins to reach the inferior vena cava. Sudden obstruction of the SVC, which is rare, is a true emergency because the rapid elevation of pressure in the SVC causes increased intracranial pressure, resulting in cerebral edema, intracranial thrombosis or bleeding, and death. However, SVC syndrome most often develops insidiously over a few weeks.

Common symptoms of SVC syndrome are a sensation of fullness and pressure in the head, cough, dyspnea, chest pain, and dysphagia. More significant symptoms include visual disturbances, hoarseness, stupor, seizure, and syncope. Typical signs include venous distention of the neck and chest wall, nonpitting edema of the neck, facial edema, facial plethora, tongue edema, proptosis, retinal vessel dilatation, stridor, and upper-extremity edema. The signs and symptoms are exacerbated by lowering the upper body relative to the heart (ie, bending forward, stooping, or lying down).

CT, especially contrast-enhanced spiral CT, is the most useful radiographic study for diagnosing SVC obstruction. CT is able not only to reveal the site of obstruction and collateral flow but also to differentiate extrinsic compression of SVC by tumor from intravascular thrombus formation. More importantly, CT provides detailed information about the tumor mass and its relation to mediastinal structures, helping to guide a fine-needle aspiration biopsy or other diagnostic procedure if a histologic diagnosis has not previously been established. Other critical structures, such as the bronchi and the spinal cord, are also visualized on CT, and CT can exclude other emergent complications—such as proximal airway obstruction and pericardial effusion—that frequently coexist with SVC obstruction. Radionuclide venograms are useful for identifying the site of obstruction and visualizing the collateral circulation. MR imaging may be used instead of CT if intravenous iodine contrast is contraindicated. 3-D contrast-enhanced MR venography may be superior to CT, digital subtraction angiography, and Doppler ultrasonography in detecting and determining the extent of thrombo-occlusive disease in chest vessels.[49] Contrast angiography (with or without digital subtraction) for diagnosis of SVC syndrome is controversial and rarely indicated.

The method for establishing the histologic diagnosis of the malignancy may depend on the working diagnosis, location of the tumor, physical status of the patient, comorbid conditions, and available expertise of the health care facility. Percutaneous transthoracic biopsy with CT guidance is an effective and safe alternative to surgical biopsy by thoracotomy or mediastinoscopy. Percutaneous transthoracic biopsy provides a high diagnostic yield with low morbidity and mortality.[50] Bronchoscopy is another procedure commonly performed to diagnose the malignancy causing SVC syndrome. Bronchoscopy provides the diagnosis in up to 50% of patients with SVC syndrome and in most patients with SVC syndrome caused by small cell lung cancer. If accessible lymph nodes are present, excisional lymph node biopsy can help to establish the diagnosis with minimal morbidity in most cases. Excisional biopsy is preferred over fine-needle aspiration if lymphoma is suspected because the histologic classification of lymphoma is firmly based on lymph node architecture whereas needle aspiration can only reveal the cytologic features of the neoplastic cells.

More than 50% of patients with SVC syndrome become symptomatic before the primary diagnosis of malignancy is made. The emphasis in management of SVC syndrome has shifted from empirical radiotherapy to methodical diagnostic evaluation because emergent irradiation before biopsy may preclude proper interpretation of the biopsy specimen in 50% of cases (Fig. 138-5). The prognosis of patients with SVC syndrome primarily reflects the prognosis associated with the underlying disease. The common malig-

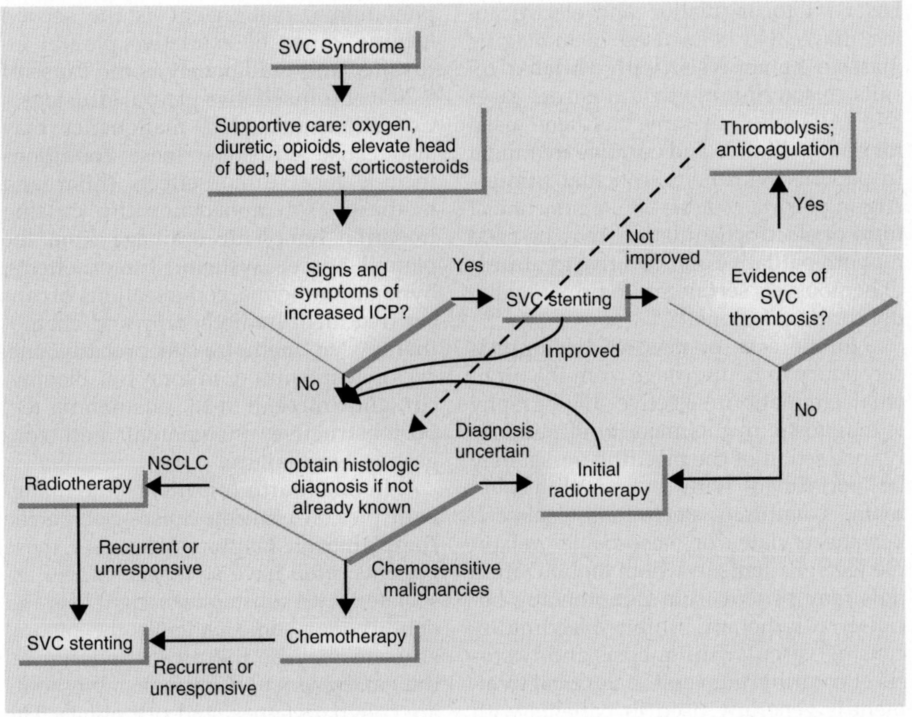

Figure 138-5 Algorithm for management of superior vena cava (SVC) syndrome.
Abbreviations: ICP, increased intracranial pressure; NSCLC, non–small cell lung cancer.

nant causes of SVC syndrome, such as small cell lung cancer and lymphoma, are chemosensitive and potentially curable even in the presence of SVC syndrome. The exception is that in rare emergent situations of impending airway obstruction or increased intracranial pressure, empiric radiotherapy or intravascular SVC stenting should be employed imm ediately. Supplemental oxygen, bed rest with upper body elevation, and sedation may help to lessen the symptoms by lowering venous pressure and cardiac output. The use of diuretics may transiently decrease edema, but the efficacy of diuretics has not been proven, and overdiuresis causes dehydration, which should be avoided in order to minimize the risk of thrombosis. Corticosteroids (eg, dexamethasone) may be useful in the presence of airway compromise or increased intracranial pressure.

Anticoagulation therapy in SVC syndrome is controversial despite the presence of superimposed thrombosis in up to 50% of patients with SVC syndrome. Anticoagulation and thrombolysis may be beneficial in certain situations, such as indwelling catheter–induced thrombosis or propagation of the thrombus into the brachiocephalic or subclavicular system. However, anticoagulation increases the risk of intracranial bleeding, especially when intracranial pressure is elevated, and anticoagulation may complicate or delay biopsy procedures for histologic diagnosis of the malignancy causing the SVC syndrome. Anticoagulation should be avoided until a clear indication for its use is identified.

Chemotherapy is the preferred initial treatment of SVC syndrome caused by tumors sensitive to chemotherapy, such as small cell lung cancer and lymphoma. Most small cell lung cancer patients experience partial or complete resolution of the signs and symptoms within a couple of weeks of initiation of chemotherapy. Although SVC obstruction occurs again in approximately 25% of cases, salvage chemotherapy or radiotherapy or the two modalities in combination can achieve prompt resolution of symptoms in most patients. Chemotherapy is also the treatment of choice for SVC syndrome secondary to non-Hodgkin's lymphoma because this treatment modality provides both local and systemic therapeutic activity. However, local consolidation with radiotherapy may be beneficial in patients with large cell lymphoma and large mediastinal masses.

Radiotherapy remains the principal treatment for many patients with SVC syndrome resulting from malignancy, especially those with SVC caused by recurrent disease after chemotherapy or tumors insensitive to chemotherapy, such as non–small cell lung cancer. Radiotherapy is also justified if a histologic diagnosis cannot be established in a timely manner. Emergent radiotherapy prior to completion of the histologic diagnostic evaluation may be indicated in rare life-threatening situations, such as airway obstruction, spinal cord compression, or increased intracranial pressure.[47] In general, external-beam radiotherapy for SVC syndrome is well tolerated, and most patients achieve relief of symptoms in about 1-3 weeks after the beginning of radiotherapy.

SVC stenting provides rapid symptomatic relief within a couple of days in the majority of patients and improves the quality of life. In cancer patients with SVC syndrome, these stents usually remain patent for the rest of the patient's life.[51] SVC stenting may provide relief of severe symptoms for patients while the histologic diagnosis of the malignancy causing SVC obstruction is being actively pursued. Stenting may also be indicated in patients in whom radiation or chemotherapy has not yet taken effect or in whom these modalities have failed. Some authors recommend stenting as first-line treatment to be performed early in the treatment of SVC syndrome.[52]

Respiratory Oncologic Emergencies

Massive Hemoptysis

Approximately 5% of hemoptysis episodes are considered massive. The definition of massive hemoptysis ranges from the expectoration of 100 mL of blood in a single episode to the expectoration of more than 600 mL of blood during 24 hours.[53,54] Airway bleeding leading to life-threatening airway obstruction, hypotension, aspiration, or anemia is also considered massive hemoptysis. Fatal hemorrhage occurs in about one third of patients with massive hemoptysis.[55] The higher the amount of blood expectorated, the higher the risk of death.[55] Other factors associated with increased risk of death include higher rate of hemoptysis, lower baseline pulmonary reserve, and higher amount of blood retained in the lungs. Death attributable to endobronchial and alveolar hemorrhage is usually due to asphyxiation rather than exsanguination.

The primary causes of massive hemoptysis in cancer patients are malignancy, infection, and hemostatic abnormalities. Massive hemoptysis may be caused by bronchogenic carcinoma and lung metastases from other malignancies. Bronchogenic carcinoma is the most common cause of massive hemoptysis in cancer patients over 40 years old. Fatal hemoptysis may be more common in necrotic squamous cell carcinoma of the lung than in other subtypes of lung cancer.[55,56] About 3% of lung cancer patients have fatal hemoptysis.[56] Hemoptysis secondary to lung metastases is most commonly associated with melanoma, breast, kidney, laryngeal, and colon cancers. Other tumors, such as esophageal tumors, may cause massive hemoptysis by direct extension to the tracheobronchial tree. In patients with hematologic malignancies and those who have undergone bone marrow transplantation, neutropenia or immunocompromise leads to increased risk of developing necrotizing, angioinvasive fungal infections (aspergillosis, mucormycosis) with massive pulmonary hemorrhage.[55] Hemostatic abnormalities such as severe thrombocytopenia and coagulopathy may result from malignancy or its treatments and contribute to the severity of pulmonary hemorrhage. Another factor that can contribute to massive pulmonary hemorrhage in cancer patients is lung injuries due to radiation or chemotherapeutic agents.

In addition to massive hemoptysis, the patient's symptoms may include hypotension, tachycardia, central cyanosis, clammy skin, dyspnea, or chest pain. The severity of the clinical presentation is dependent upon several factors—namely, the rate and duration of the bleeding, the degree of airway obstruction and pulmonary involvement, the patient's underlying performance status, and the status of chronic comorbid conditions. The airway should be protected, and intubation is recommended in patients with rapid bleeding, hemodynamic instability, ventilatory impairment, severe dyspnea, or hypoxia.[53] Patients with hemodynamic instability may require volume resuscitation, administration of supplemental oxygen, correction of underlying coagulopathies, and cough suppressants. For patients bleeding from one lung, lateral decubitus positioning with the affected lung in the dependent position may help to minimize aspiration to the unaffected side.

In the management of massive hemoptysis, the site of bleeding must be first identified. For unstable patients, unilateral intubation via the bronchoscope is performed. For massive right-sided pulmonary bleeding, the left mainstem bronchus is intubated over the bronchoscope. Unilateral intubation of the right lung in patients with massive left-sided bleeding is not recommended due to the risk of right upper lobe occlusion. In this scenario, an alternative is to use a double-lumen endotracheal tube to isolate the unaffected lung.

Bronchoscopic treatments for massive hemoptysis include administration of topical agents (thrombin, fibrinogen-thrombin), iced saline lavage, endobronchial tamponade, laser photocoagulation, and electrocautery. A balloon catheter may be used for endobronchial tamponade to alleviate bleeding. Rigid bronchoscopes offer improved airway control, offer greater ability to suction, and are more effective in removing large clots than fiberoptic scopes. The advantage of fiberoptic scopes is improved access and visualization of the distal airways. Laser photocoagulation and electrocautery have also been used in managing massive hemoptysis, with variable results. Neodymium-yttrium-garnet laser (Nd:YAG) phototherapy has been used for both palliative and curative treatment in patients with endobronchial tumors. Argon plasma coagulation, a noncontact form of electrocoagulation, may be used for both palliative and curative treatment of hemoptysis secondary to proximal endobronchial lesions.

In the case of massive hemoptysis secondary to hemorrhage from the bronchial circulation, selective angiography is diagnostic in the majority of patients. Embolization of the bleeding vessel may be performed with polyvinyl alcohol foam, Gianturco steel coils, isobutyl-2-cyanoacrylate, or absorbable gelatin pledgets. Patients in whom embolization fails may benefit from radiotherapy because radiotherapy inhibits bleeding by causing vascular thrombosis and necrosis of contributing vessels. Surgical treatment is generally used in patients with refractory hemoptysis in whom other treatment modalities and in patients with life-threatening cardiovascular compromise.[57]

Massive Pleural Effusion

Massive pleural effusions are described as those causing near-complete opacification of the hemithorax. Massive pleural effusions account for approximately 10% of effusions. About two-thirds of affected patients have underlying cancer.[58] The majority of patients with malignant pleural effusion have moderate- to large-volume effusions (500-2000 mL) (Fig. 138-6).

The majority (approximately 80% in total) of malignant pleural effusions are due to lung carcinoma (36%), breast carcinoma (25%), lymphoma (10%), and ovarian carcinoma (5%).[59] Adenocarcinoma accounts for 79% of cases of lung carcinoma that metastasize to the pleura.[60] In young adults, lymphoma is the most common cause of malignant pleural effusions.[60] Malignant effusions may appear serous, serosanguinous, or bloody. After

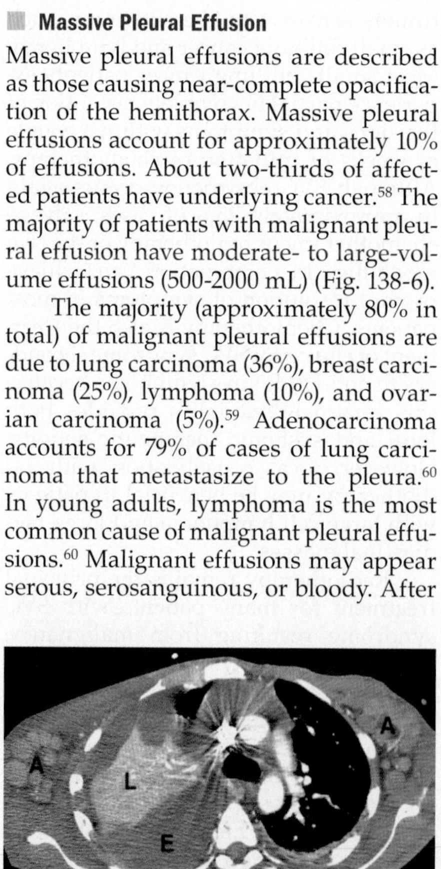

Figure 138-6 Massive pleural effusion. The CT scan of the chest of a patient with a massive pleural effusion is shown. L, collapsed lung; E, pleural effusion; A, extensive axillary lymphadenopathy.

pneumonia, malignancy is the second leading cause of exudative pleural effusions, and malignancy is the cause of 8-20% of transudative pleural effusions.[61] Conditions related to malignancy may also cause effusions; these conditions include local tumor effects (hilar and mediastinal lymphadenopathy causing impaired lymphatic drainage from the pleural space), systemic tumor effects, hypoalbuminemia, complications of cancer treatment [radiotherapy and chemotherapy (eg, methotrexate, procarbazine, cyclophosphamide, mitomycin, bleomycin, and interleukin-1)], pneumonia (eg, postobstructive pneumonia), and congestive heart failure.

In one fourth of patients, the malignant pleural effusion causes no specific complaints or symptoms. However, these patients often have advanced cancer associated with substantial weight loss and debility. For some patients, the pleural effusion may be the presenting sign of the malignancy. Common symptoms are cough, dyspnea, and orthopnea. The presence and severity of these symptoms depend on the volume and the rapidity of fluid accumulation. Fever is occasionally present and may be due to atelectasis or infection or pneumonia. Pleuritic chest pain and pleural friction rubs are not common; when present, they indicate extensive neoplastic involvement of the pleura, rib cage, and chest wall.

The presence of a pleural effusion is diagnosed by clinical examination and confirmed with radiography. On examination, patients with pleural effusion exhibit dullness to percussion, decreased breath sounds in the area of the effusion, and decreased diaphragmatic excursion and tactile and vocal fremitus on the affected side. Sometimes crackles may be auscultated immediately above the percussed dullness. Patients with large-volume effusions (>1500 mL) may have an inspiratory lag, contralateral tracheal deviation, and intercostal fullness. When the pleural effusion is caused by lung carcinoma, the effusion is generally on the same side as the primary lesion.[58]

The cause of a pleural effusion is generally diagnosed by thoracentesis. Thoracentesis is easily performed and is generally a safe procedure. For symptomatic patients, partial removal of the effusion may alleviate symptoms. Fluid analysis discriminates between exudative and transudative effusions and may be helpful in identifying the cause of the effusion.[62] Cytology is more sensitive than percutaneous pleural biopsy.[60,63] If these two less invasive procedures are nondiagnostic, other options for obtaining diagnostic material include bronchoscopy, pleuroscopy, video-assisted thoracoscopic surgery, and open pleural biopsy.

Treatment decisions are influenced by the severity of symptoms, the rate of fluid accumulation, the overall prognosis, the patient's performance status, and the responsiveness of the malignancy to treatment. Patients with massive pleural effusion and hemodynamic instability, significant dyspnea, hypoxemia, or mediastinal shift should be treated emergently by thoracentesis. Thoracostomy may be indicated depending on clinical and radiographic findings and the biochemical characteristics of the effusion.[64] Tube thoracostomy is recommended for patients with empyema or infected pleural fluid as confirmed by culture or microscopy (eg, Gram stain) and for patients with complicated parapneumonic effusions. Patients in whom thoracoscopic treatment fails and patients with chronic complicated parapneumonic effusions should be considered for open thoracotomy and decortication.

Pleurodesis may prevent effusions from recurring. In approximately 70% of patients with drainage of symptomatic malignant pleural effusion without pleurodesis, fluid reaccumulates within 30 days unless effective systemic chemotherapy is administered. The effective sclerosing agents, with success rates of 72-90%, are doxycycline, minocycline, bleomycin, and talc.[65,66] Pleurodesis should be considered in patients with symptomatic relief after thoracentesis. Life expectancy of more than several months should also be considered in deciding whether pleurodesis should be performed. Alternatives for patients with poor life expectancy may include repeated thoracentesis or placement of a chronic indwelling catheter (Denver catheter).[67]

Acute Airway Obstruction

Acute airway obstruction usually involves the upper airway. Upper airway obstruction may be due to malignant or nonmalignant causes. Tumors that can obstruct the upper airway by direct extension are primary tumors of the head and neck (base of tongue, larynx, hypopharynx, thyroid, or trachea) and mediastinum (lung cancer, thymoma). Tumors that can obstruct the upper airway by metastatic spread are tumors of the breast, esophagus, kidney, colon, melanoma, sarcoma, and mediastinal lymphoma. Airway obstruction may also be caused by tumor encroachment and by tumor-associated airway edema or hemorrhage. Nonmalignant causes of airway obstruction in cancer patients include food or foreign body aspiration (Fig. 138-7), airway edema, severe tracheomalacia, tracheal stenosis or stricture, and, rarely, infectious causes—fungal, viral, or bacterial. Severe acute upper airway obstruction can be caused by angioedema (drug-induced: eg, angiotensin

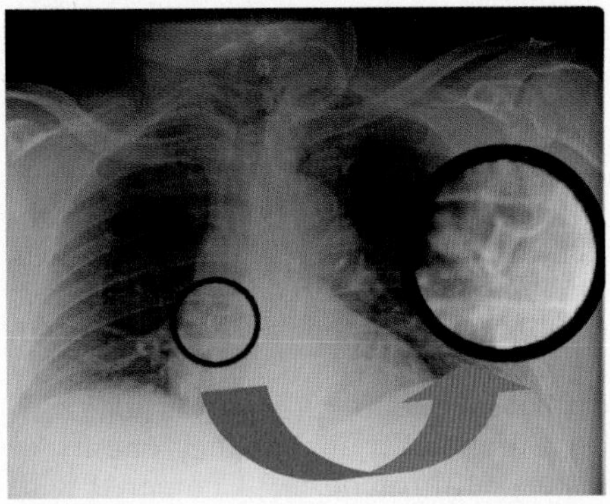

Figure 138-7 Foreign body in right mainstem bronchus. This patient underwent a laryngectomy for laryngeal cancer. He presented with a complaint of shortness of breath after his voice prosthesis fell inside his tracheal stoma. The prosthesis (*circled*) can be seen lodged in the right mainstem bronchus on this chest radiograph.

converting enzyme inhibitors, paclitaxel). The most common cause of lower airway obstruction is primary bronchogenic carcinoma. Other, rare causes of lower airway obstruction are metastases from cancers of the colon, breast, thyroid and kidney, melanoma, lymphoma, and sarcoma. Patients with primary carcinoid tumors of the gastrointestinal tract may experience severe airway obstruction (bronchospasm) due to release of hormone mediators.

Dyspnea may be the only early symptom of airway obstruction. When dyspnea occurs with exertion, the airway diameter is usually decreased to 8 mm, whereas when dyspnea occurs while the patient is at rest, the airway diameter is usually decreased to 5 mm, and this decrease often coincides with the development of stridor. As upper airway obstruction progresses, wheezing, orthopnea, tachycardia, diaphoresis, stridor, and intercostal muscle retraction may be noted. Stridor is an ominous finding that may be rapidly followed by bradycardia, cyanosis, obtundation, and death.

For patients with upper airway obstruction, the clinical examination is often accompanied by direct visualization via either laryngoscopy or bronchoscopy depending on the location of the lesion. Biopsy may be required. For patients with lower airway obstruction, chest radiographs identify the obstruction in 75% of cases. Bronchoscopy or fine-needle aspiration may be considered.

The oral cavity should be quickly visualized to exclude foreign body aspiration. In most cases of upper airway obstruction, the clinical examination provides the diagnosis. Laryngoscopy or bronchoscopy may be necessary to guide the endotracheal tube. Patients with obstructions involving the upper third of the trachea may require a low tracheotomy. Other supportive therapies are administration of corticosteroids, bronchodilators, and helium-oxygen mixtures. Other surgical interventions may be considered and are often dependent on the extent of the disease, the responsiveness of the malignancy to treatment, the patient's performance status, and comorbid conditions. For central airway obstruction, interventional pulmonary treatments may use rigid or flexible bronchoscopes and may include balloon bronchoplasty, placement of tracheobronchial stents, laser bronchoscopy, endobronchial argon plasma coagulation, cryosurgery, and brachytherapy.

Pneumothorax

Pneumothorax, air in the pleural space, occurs frequently in cancer patients. Most pneumothoraces in cancer patients are iatrogenic or occur spontaneously as a result of other medical conditions. The majority of pneumothoraces treated in hospitals are iatrogenic.[68] Procedures often associated with pneumothorax include percutaneous lung biopsy, transbronchial biopsy, insertion of central venous lines, and insertion of pulmonary artery catheters. Even nasogastric tube placement may occasionally cause pneumothorax. Secondary spontaneous pneumothorax is most commonly due to chronic obstructive pulmonary disease. Both primary and metastatic pulmonary neoplasms may result in pneumothorax. Chemotherapeutic agents associated with pneumothorax include bleomycin, carmustine, and lomustine. Infectious agents associated with pneumothorax include *Staphylococcus, Klebsiella,* and *Pseudomonas* species, *Pneumocystis carinii,* and *Mycobacterium* species. Rupture of mycetoma into the pleural space may result in pneumothorax and is associated with *Aspergillus fumigatus* infection, coccidioidomycosis, cryptococcosis, and mucormycosis.

The presence and severity of symptoms at presentation is related to the patient's underlying pulmonary status. Patients may present with respiratory distress, tachypnea, tachycardia, cyanosis, diaphoresis, and agitation. Patients with underlying lung disease are often unable to tolerate decreases in vital capacity or arterial PO2 and have a higher risk for developing respiratory failure secondary to pneumothorax.

Small pneumothoraces (<20%) are usually undetectable on physical examination. Dyspnea is often unrelated to the volume of pneumothorax; however, dyspnea and chest pain are present in almost all patients with a significant pneumothorax. Chest pain is frequently acute in onset and pleuritic, and located on the affected side. Cough, hemoptysis, orthopnea, and Horner's syndrome are less frequent symptoms. Examination usually demonstrates tachycardia, absent tactile fremitus, hyperresonance, and absent or decreased breath sounds on auscultation of the affected side. Patients with large or tension pneumothoraces may have contralateral deviation of the trachea, asymmetrical hyperexpansion, and decreased movement of the affected hemithorax. Patients with a tension pneumothorax may have elevated central venous, pulmonary artery, and right atrial pressures. Hypotension, severe hypoxemia and respiratory acidosis occur when increased central venous and intrapleural pressures impede venous return.

The diagnosis of pneumothorax is confirmed when an upright chest radiograph reveals a visceral pleural line with the absence of lung markings beyond the line. For patients with a small pneumothorax, the pleural line may be difficult to discern. Therefore, a good-quality radiograph and a bright light for viewing are needed to diagnose a small pneumothorax. Previous work has shown that one third of pneumothoraces are undetected on semi-erect and supine films.[69] In some cases, expiratory films may be helpful.

Patients with small pneumothoraces and minor symptoms may require close observation and supplemental oxygen. Serial chest radiographs should be obtained 3-6 hours after the initial radiograph. If there is no expansion of the pneumothorax, the patient may be discharged from observation with appropriate follow-up instructions and scheduled for repeat radiograph in 12-48 hours.[70]

For symptomatic pneumothoraces, rapidly expanding pneumothoraces, and pneumothoraces of more than 15% of the ipsilateral pleural space, catheter aspiration should be done. Most patients requiring chest tube placement for postbiopsy iatrogenic pneumothorax can be safely managed as an outpatient with small caliber chest tubes and Heimlich valves.[71] Patients with pneumothoraces that fail to reexpand or that recur following successful catheter aspirations require chest tube thoracostomy. Heimlich valves are often used. Tube thoracostomy is initially indicated in patients with a traumatic pneumothorax and hemothorax, patients with a pneumothorax occupying more than 15% of the ipsilateral pleural space with retained secretions, patients with lung infections on the affected side, and patients on mechanical ventilation. Patients with a persistent air leak due to bronchopleural fistula and patients with only partial lung expansion 5-7 days after a tube thoracostomy should be considered for thoracotomy with surgical repair. Pleurodesis with talc or other drugs may be indicated to prevent recurrence.[72]

Pulmonary Embolism

Pulmonary emboli can be difficult to diagnose in cancer patients because the signs and symptoms may be masked by the neoplastic process or complications of cancer treatments. In the general population, patients at high risk for development of deep venous thrombosis are patients with major trauma, patients undergoing orthopedic surgery, and patients undergoing abdominal surgery. The risk of pulmonary embolism is increased in patients with advanced age, recent myocardial infarction, cerebral vascular accident, immobility, malignancy, obesity, or history of thrombosis.[73] Compared with patients without malignancies, patients with cancer have greater rates of initial thrombosis, thrombosis recurrence, and fatal pulmonary embolism.[74] Patients with malignancy and no other underlying comorbid condition have a 15-20% risk of developing thromboembolic disease. Compared with patients without cancer undergoing similar procedures, cancer patients undergoing surgical procedures have two to three times the risk of developing postoperative venous thrombosis.[75]

In most cases, symptoms of pulmonary embolism are vague. The most common presenting symptom is dyspnea. Dyspnea, pleuritic chest pain, and tachypnea were present in 97% of patients with pulmonary embolism documented by angiography in the Prospective Investigation of Pulmonary Embolism Diagnosis study.[76,77] Patients with massive pulmonary embolism may have syncope. Angina may occur due to right ventricular ischemia. Hemoptysis may rarely occur and is associated with pulmonary infarction happening 12-36 hours after the thromboembolic event.

Most frequently, patients with pulmonary embolism have tachypnea and tachycardia. Sometimes, fever and a pleural rub may be detected. Deep venous thrombosis in the lower extremities occurs in fewer than half of all patients with pulmonary embolism. However, clinical examination of the lower extremities for evidence of thrombosis should be performed. Patients with suspected pulmonary embolism should have an oxygen saturation measurement done and may require measurement of arterial blood gases before supplemental oxygen is provided. A chest radiograph is most helpful in excluding other causes of pulmonary symptoms. An electrocardiogram commonly shows sinus tachycardia, inverted T waves, or nonspecific ST-T wave abnormalities. Right axis deviation, atrial arrhythmia, right bundle branch block, and P-pulmonale may occur, but the classical S1-Q3-T3 pattern is unusual. In cancer patients, d-dimer has a high negative predictive value and sensitivity for pulmonary embolism, and a normal d-dimer result can exclude pulmonary embolism.[78] In another study that included cancer patients, a d-dimer concentration >3000 ng/mL is associated with centrally located pulmonary emboli and death within 15 days.[79]

The radionuclide ventilation-perfusion (V/Q) scan was usually the initial test for diagnosing pulmonary embolism, but in the past decade high resolution CT pulmonary angiography or spiral CT has gained in popularity and replaced V/Q scan as the common diagnostic test for pulmonary embolism (Fig. 138-8). V/Q scan may be ordered if CT angiography is contraindicated because of renal dysfunction or iodine contrast dye hypersensitivity. Other diagnostic modalities for pulmonary embolism such as MR imaging, and pulmonary angiography are also available. Spiral CT and MR imaging have sensitivities and specificities of about 80% and 90%, respectively.[80,81] The negative predictive value of spiral CT angiography for pulmonary embolism is 98%.[82] However, thromboembolism in the distal pulmonary vasculature is not reliably detected with these modalities. Patients in whom pulmonary embolism is strongly suspected and who have negative findings on either spiral CT or MR imaging should be considered for pulmonary angiography, the gold standard for diagnosis.

Hemodynamically unstable patients should be stabilized. Interventions for stabilization may include administration of fluids and inotropic agents, usually guided by central venous monitoring in an intensive care setting. Oxygen administration by mask or endotracheal tube is necessary when massive pulmonary embolism occurs. In patients in whom pulmonary embolism is strongly suspected, heparin or low-molecular-weight heparin (LMWH) should be administered unless clinically contraindicated. When heparin is used, it is generally administered in a bolus injection of 5000-10,000 units, and then a continuous intravenous infusion of 1000-1500 units per hour is used with adjustments to maintain the activated partial thromboplastin time at

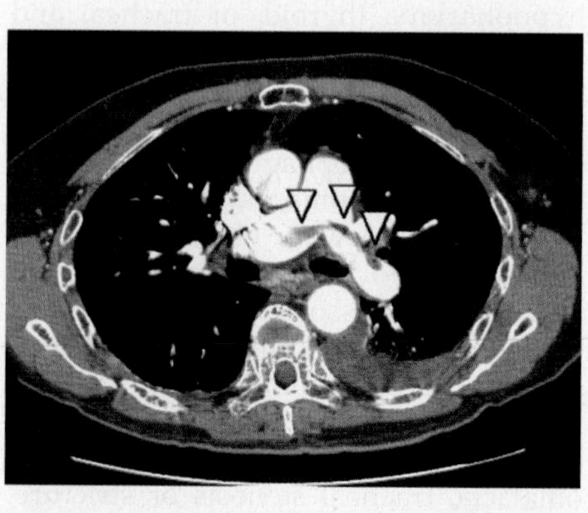

Figure 138-8 Saddle embolus. This CT scan shows a saddle embolus (below the three arrowheads) at the bifurcation into the pulmonary arteries.

1.5-2.0 times the baseline control value.[83] LMWH may be used and have the advantage of not requiring partial thromboplastin time monitoring and intravenous access. Moreover, the rate of bleeding complications with LMWH is the same as or less than that seen with unfractionated heparin.[84] The goal of anticoagulation therapy is to prevent thromboembolic recurrence. For cancer patients, it is recommended that anticoagulation therapy be continued until the malignancy is no longer active.[85] Compared with oral anticoagulant therapy, LMWH is less likely to interact with other drugs and chemotherapy, needs no monitoring, is associated with fewer recurrence of venous thromboembolism, and may prolong survival of cancer patients.[86] LMWH is the preferred anticoagulant for both initial and long-term treatment of VTE. Long-term treatment should be given for at least 6 months. Warfarin (maintaining international normalized ratio [INR] between 2 and 3) is acceptable when LMWH is unavailable.[131,132] Thrombolysis is generally considered in patients with massive pulmonary embolus and hemodynamic instability. Indications for use of thrombolytics are occlusion of more than 40% of the pulmonary vasculature by the thrombus,[87] right ventricular dysfunction according to echocardiography, and severe hypoxemia.[88] Compared to heparin alone, thrombolytic agents are associated with twice the rate of major complications and intracranial hemorrhage.[89] Thrombolytic therapy has been shown to result in acceleration of fibrinolysis and clot dissolution and improvement in both early and late cardiopulmonary function, but definite beneficial effect on mortality has not yet been shown by large-scale studies.[90] Surgical and catheter embolectomy is reserved for patients in whom usual approaches of clot removal fail.

Neurologic Oncologic Emergencies

Spinal Cord Compression

Spinal cord compression occurs in 1-5% of cancer patients and should be considered an emergency.[91] Treatment delays may result in irreversible consequences, including paralysis. In 95% of cases, spinal cord compression is caused by extradural metastases from tumors involving the vertebral column. Of these cases, 70% involve the thoracic spine, 20% involve the lumbosacral spine, and 10% involve the cervical spine. Metastasis to the thoracic vertebrae often causes lesser symptoms than does metastasis to the lumbar or cervical vertebrae. However, thoracic spine metastasis is frequently more important because of the vulnerable blood supply in this region and the fact that the spinal canal is narrowest here. Spinal cord compression occurs more frequently in patients with lung, breast, unknown primary, prostate, and renal cell cancer.

Back pain is the most common symptom in patients with spinal cord compression. Pain is often an early sign of spinal cord compression and may be present for months before the diagnosis. Patients may present with pain localized to the spine or radicular pain due to neural compression. The pain may worsen with movement, recumbence, coughing, sneezing, or straining. Pain that worsens with recumbence should increase the suspicion of epidural metastasis.

Muscle weakness follows pain and may be accompanied by sensory loss. Once symptoms of autonomic dysfunction, urinary retention, and constipation develop, spinal cord compression may result in rapid irreversible paralysis. Paralysis and urinary retention before treatment are the most significant factors associated with a poor outcome.

Tenderness and pain over the involved vertebral segments are elicited with palpation. Other clinical findings may include muscle weakness, abnormal muscle stretch reflexes and extensor plantar reflexes, and sensory loss in the distribution of the involved nerve roots. Leg ataxia may arise prior to muscle weakness and may occur without pain. Sensory loss occurs below the involved segment. Patients with autonomic dysfunction may have a palpable bladder, an increased postvoid urinary volume, or decreased rectal tone.

An accurate history and physical examination is essential in diagnosing spinal cord compression. The neurologic examination often identifies the suspicious areas of the spine, allowing for imaging efforts to be focused on these areas. Patients with spinal cord compression often have abnormalities on plain radiographs of the spine. The abnormalities encountered may include bony erosion and pedicle loss, partial or complete vertebral collapse, and paraspinous soft tissue masses. However, normal spine films do not exclude epidural metastasis.

MR tomography of the spine is the best method for evaluating epidural spinal cord compression (Fig. 138-9). Gadolinium enhancement may be used when there is suspicion of cord compression due to epidural abscess. Gadolinium enhances inflamed tissues and defines anatomic margins. Myelography requires an experienced physician. Myelography accompanied by CT may be performed with minimum patient discomfort. However, when metastatic disease completely blocks the spinal cord, myelography does not allow definition of the upper margin of tumor involvement.

Treatment of spinal cord compression aims to maintain normal neurologic function or, if symptoms are present, to improve neurologic function; to provide local tumor control, to stabilize the spine, and to provide appropriate pain control. Because bone is often affected and bony metastases cause significant pain, analgesics, especially narcotics, should be administered promptly and judiciously. Appropriate physical examination and diagnostic imaging often are delayed if pain control is inadequate.

For patients with suspected spinal cord compression, corticosteroid therapy should be administered. Dexamethasone is often used since it has good gastrointestinal absorption and has a 36-hour half-life. There is controversy as to whether a high-dose (100 mg) intravenous bolus followed by maintenance doses (usually 16 mg every 6 hours) is necessary. Other studies have suggested that lower doses are just as effective and cause fewer side effects.[92,93]

For most patients with spinal cord compression and a radiosensitive malignancy, radiotherapy alone is the standard initial treatment. The outcome of radiotherapy is directly related to the patient's neurologic status prior to treatment and the relative radiosensitivity of the malignancy.

Surgical decompression may also be an appropriate treatment option, especially in patients requiring spinal stability, in patients who have received radiotherapy in the area of the compression, when a tissue diagnosis is needed, and in patients with progression despite appropriate treatment with steroids and radiation. The

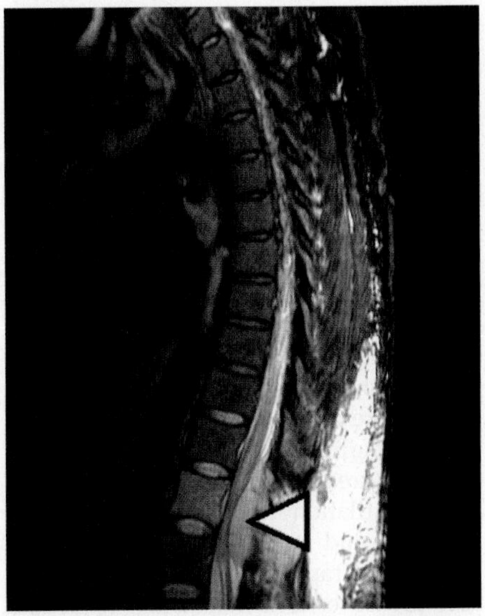

Figure 138-9 Spinal cord compression. This sagittal MRI of the spine demonstrates compression of the lower portion of the spinal cord by tumor (*arrowhead*). Metastatic disease in the vertebral body is also seen.

status of the patient's malignancy should also be taken into account when decisions are made regarding the appropriateness of surgical decompression. Surgical decompression may not be appropriate for patients with advanced malignancy and a limited life expectancy. However, for some of these patients, surgical compression may afford an improved quality of life. Anterior vertebral body resection with stabilization may offer the best choice but is a major surgical procedure and requires a skilled neurosurgical team, uninvolved adjacent vertebral bodies for spinal canal stabilization, and a patient with a good performance status and acceptable operative risks.

Chemotherapy may be effective in patients with a chemosensitive malignancy. It may also be used in combination with other treatment modalities. It is sometimes used as a treatment alternative when other treatment choices are not appropriate. For example, chemotherapy may be administered when a patient has increased operative risks or when radiotherapy has previously been administered in the affected area.

Brain Herniation

Patients with possible brain herniation should be rapidly assessed, and those with hemodynamic instability should be stabilized with appropriate therapies. Symptoms and physical findings suggestive of brain herniation include changes in the level of consciousness, papilledema, pupillary and eye movement irregularities, posturing, nausea, vomiting, and meningismus. Late clinical findings of brain herniation are hypertension, bradycardia, and the Cushing reflex. If there are findings suggestive of herniation or increased intracranial pressure, imaging studies should be performed. The first study generally done is noncontrast CT to exclude hemorrhage. MR imaging is a better imaging technique when herniation is present, but if a patient is unstable, CT may offer a safer venue until the patient is stabilized. In addition, CT can be performed quickly.

If clinical findings suggest increased intracranial pressure and the patient is unstable, treatment to decrease intracranial pressure should be instituted immediately, even before brain herniation is documented by imaging studies. Emergency treatments to treat or prevent herniation are hyperventilation and administration of mannitol and steroids. Hyperventilation is the most rapid in decreasing intracranial pressure. It is necessary to sedate and intubate the patient. Ventilation should achieve a PCO2 of 25-30 mm Hg. This maneuver causes vasoconstriction, decreasing cerebral blood volume, and subsequently decreased intracranial pressure. Decreased intracranial pressure secondary to hyperventilation is generally short-lived, and equilibration may occur within a few hours.

Mannitol, a hyperosmotic agent, becomes effective within minutes of administration and remains effective for several hours. Its usefulness may be due to formation of an osmotic gradient between the blood and brain, driving water from the brain across the blood-brain barrier into the blood. This proposed mechanism is controversial. Solutions of 20-25% mannitol are administered IV at a rate of 0.5-2.0 g/kg over 20-30 minutes. Additional doses may be necessary if the patient's clinical condition continues to deteriorate. Mannitol may induce a rebound increase in intracranial pressure, so it should be used cautiously.

Steroids should be administered and may be helpful especially when herniation is due to vasogenic edema. Dexamethasone is most commonly administered at an initial bolus dose of 40-100 mg IV, then 40-100 mg/day. Its onset of action occurs within hours, and its effect lasts several days. Dexamethasone may also be helpful in cancer patients when increased intracranial pressures are secondary to intracranial metastases or brain abscesses.[94] Neurosurgical intervention may be necessary if the patient has neurologic deterioration despite appropriate medical management. Treatment should be directed at the underlying cause once intracranial pressure is controlled.

Status Epilepticus

Status epilepticus is defined as more than 30 minutes of continuous seizure activity or two or more sequential seizures without full recovery between seizures. It can lead to devastating neurologic and systemic consequences, such as neuronal injury and cell death, neurogenic pulmonary edema, and rhabdomyolysis with renal failure.

The etiology of seizures in cancer patients may include structural, metabolic, infectious, and treatment-related causes. In a review of 50 cancer patients presenting to an emergency center with seizures, 16% had seizures due to a new structural lesion, and 52% had previously documented central nervous system lesions.[95] Seizures commonly occur in patients with intracranial tumors as a result of either metastatic disease or a primary brain tumor. The cancers that most commonly metastasize to the brain are lung cancer, breast cancer, melanoma, genitourinary malignancies, and gastrointestinal malignancies.

After a major seizure, neurologic function is suppressed, primarily owing to release of gamma-aminobutyric acid, an inhibitory endogenous neurotransmitter. Patients usually have a postictal phase that may last for 24 hours. Clinical findings after seizure activity may include bruising or tongue bites, signs of urinary or fecal incontinence, and increases in lactic acid and muscle enzyme levels. Patients may be confused or unresponsive following a major seizure. It is important to determine whether the patient has previously had seizures and, if so, the type of seizure and medications used for control. The status, extent, and treatment of the malignancy should also be reviewed.

If the event precipitating seizure activity cannot easily be determined, a diagnostic workup should be initiated. Evaluation may include measurement of electrolytes, serum glucose, calcium, and magnesium, and hepatic and renal function testing. A blood cell count, blood cultures, measurement of blood gases, electrocardiography, and drug screens may be appropriate. CT or MR imaging may be necessary. Lumbar puncture may also be indicated depending upon the suspected seizure precipitant, the patient's condition, and findings on imaging.[96]

Status epilepticus is a medical emergency, and when patients present with status epilepticus, airway, breathing, and circulation should be assessed immediately (Fig. 138-10). Anticonvulsant therapy with a short-acting intravenous benzodiazepine (lorazepam or diazepam) should be administered to halt seizure activity. Generally, lorazepam is used because of its more rapid onset of action and longer period of efficacy. Patients with status epilepticus require other anticonvulsants, usually phenytoin. Fosphenytoin and phenobarbital are generally considered second-line and third-line agents, respectively. The role of the new intravenous anticonvulsants such as levetiracetam has not been defined in the treatment of status epilepticus. For patients with continuing seizure activity despite anticonvulsant treatment, combination anticonvulsant therapy with complete sedation is required. These patients will require intubation, monitoring often in an intensive care setting, and electroencephalography.

Patients with seizures due to reversible medical causes should have correction of the reversible cause. These patients most likely will not require long-term anticonvulsant therapy. Patients with status epilepticus due to other causes will require prolonged treatment with an anticonvulsant. After a seizure, the unconscious patient should be placed on his or her side to help prevent aspiration and improve oxygenation. Airway suctioning and supplemental oxygen may be required.

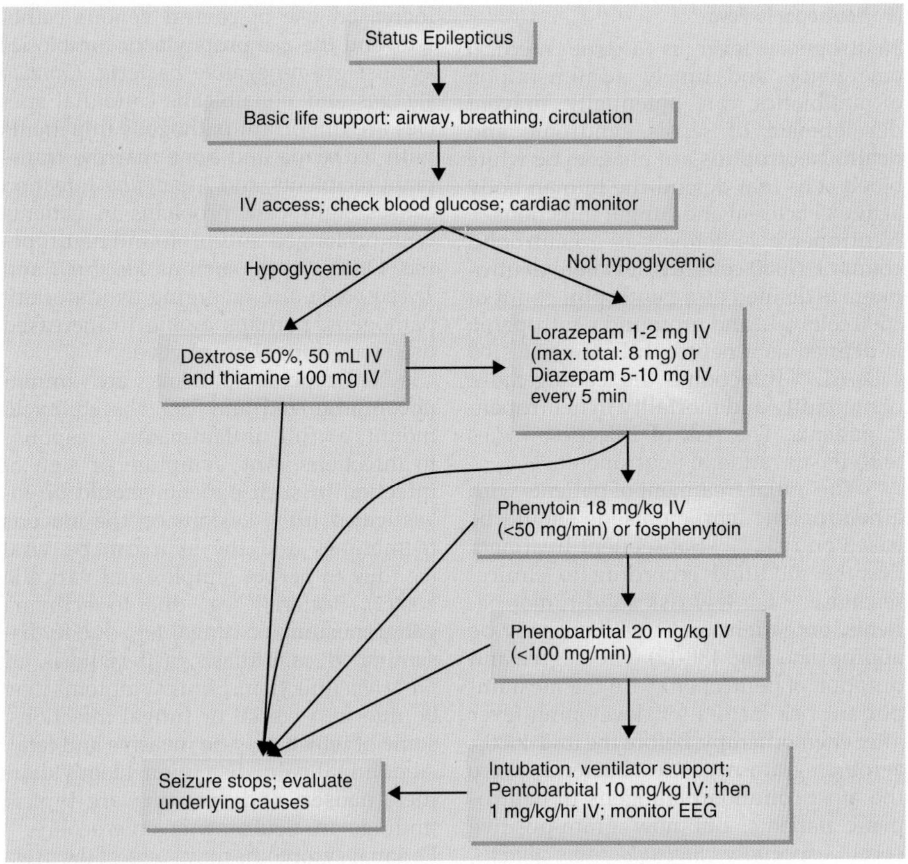

Figure 138-10 ■ Algorithm for management of status epilepticus.

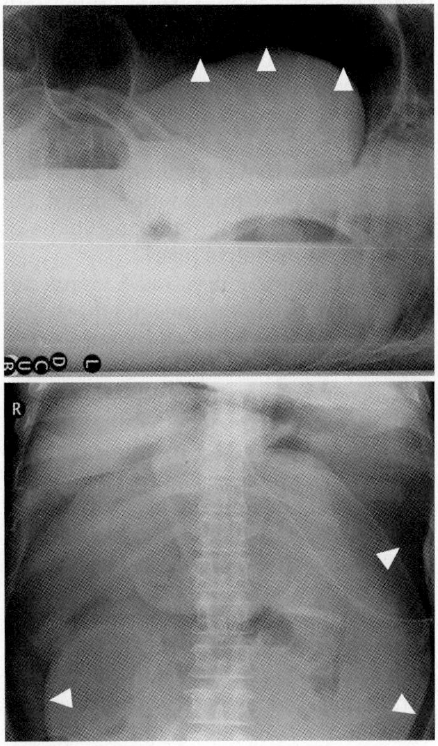

Figure 138-11 ■ Pneumoperitoneum. A 53-year-old man with multiple myeloma and amyloidosis involving the gastrointestinal tract, undergoing treatment with thalidomide and dexamethasone, presented with acute abdominal pain and abdominal distention. Abdominal radiographs showed intraperitoneal free air (*arrowheads*). Laparotomy revealed bowel perforation secondary to massive colonic distention.

Other Oncologic Emergencies

Perforated Bowel

Perforation along the gastrointestinal tract is a serious emergency. In cancer patients, the most common causes of perforation are spontaneous perforation secondary to tumor (primary[97,98] or metastatic[99]) and iatrogenic perforation secondary to endoscopy or cancer treatment.[100,101] If the wall of the gastrointestinal tract is significantly infiltrated or replaced by tumor, radiotherapy- or chemotherapy-induced tumor necrosis may lead to bowel perforation. Antiangiogenic therapies such as bevacizumab and small molecule inhibitors such as imatinib and sorafenib have been associated with bowel perforation.[102-104] Even when the wall of the gastrointestinal tract is not involved by tumor, severe gastroenteritis due to radiotherapy or chemotherapy may lead to severe bowel dilatation or distention and subsequent perforation. Bowel perforation can be caused by severe infections like typhlitis and neutropenic enterocolitis.[105] Perforation can also be caused by disease processes unrelated to cancer. For example, appendicitis, diverticulitis, peptic ulcer disease, ischemic bowel disease, and inflammatory bowel disease can lead to bowel perforation in cancer patients as well as noncancer patients.

Typically, perforation of the gastrointestinal tract causes acute or sudden onset of pain that prompts emergent evaluation. In cases of cervical esophageal perforation, symptoms at presentation may include neck pain, dysphagia, hoarseness, and subcutaneous emphysema. In thoracic esophageal perforation, upper abdominal rigidity, severe retrosternal chest pain, odynophagia, and hematemesis are common. In gastric perforation, acute onset of severe abdominal pain is usually the first symptom. The pain may be associated with nausea and vomiting, and in about 15% of patients, significant bleeding is present. Radiation of abdominal pain to the shoulders may occur because of irritation of the diaphragm. In cases of free perforation into the peritoneal cavity, abdominal distension and signs of peritonitis (severe rebound abdominal tenderness, guarding, and absent bowel sounds) may be present. In peritonitis, abdominal rigidity and rebound tenderness are present. In diffuse peritonitis, auscultation of the abdomen may yield few or no bowel sounds.

Fever and leukocytosis with left shift may be present in patients with peritonitis, mediastinitis, or abscess. However, the white blood cell count should be interpreted in the context of recent cytotoxic chemotherapy or use of neutrophil-stimulating cytokines. Amylase levels may be high in intestinal, esophageal, or gastric perforation, and lipase levels may be high in gastric perforation.

In cervical perforation, a plain radiograph of the neck in the lateral view may show air in the deep cervical tissues. Plain radiographs of the chest are also valuable in esophageal perforation as pneumomediastinum may be evident. Free air detected by plain radiographs (upright chest x-ray or abdominal series with upright or decubitus views) (Fig. 138-11) can provide evidence of bowel perforation in the acute abdomen. After a patient has been upright or in the left decubitus position for 10 minutes, a plain radiograph can detect as little as 1-2 mL of intraperitoneal free air. As for duodenal perforation, plain abdominal radiographs may show air in the retroperitoneal space or, if an oral contrast agent is used, retroperitoneal contrast collection. Other radiographic signs of perforation include outlining of both sides of the bowel wall by air and visualization of the hepatic ligament. If bowel perforation is highly suspected clinically and the initial studies do not show evidence of perforation, further study with oral contrast agents is indicated. A water-soluble contrast agent (eg, Gastrografin) is used initially as barium causes a severe inflammatory reaction when leaked into the peritoneal cavity. CT is very accurate in diagnosing bowel perforation and can provide detailed information about the location of perforation and the status of the surrounding structures.

Treatment of a perforated viscus can consist of expectant management, expectant management followed by surgery, or immediate surgery depending on the size and location of the perforating defect, the cause of perforation, whether the perforation is free or contained, the clinical course (development of sepsis), the patient's performance status and quality of life prior to the perforation, the prognosis based on the status of the malignant disease, and the presence of comorbid conditions that increase the risk of perioperative mortality. Nonsurgical treatment measures include nasogastric tube suction, administration of broad-spectrum intravenous antibiotics, intravenous hydration, parenteral nutrition, and close monitoring.[106] If the patient's condition deteriorates during expectant treatment, a decision to operate can be made. In general, perforations caused by peptic ulcer disease or by megacolon usually require emergent surgery. Factors associated with increased risk of perioperative mortality after peptic ulcer perforation include preoperative shock, long duration of perforation (>24 hours), and major medical illness.[107]

Neutropenic Fever

Neutropenic fever is a true medical emergency, and timely administration of antibiotics can potentially prevent development of sepsis syndrome and death. Neutrophils are phagocytic white blood cells that defend the human body against bacterial and fungal infections.[108] Neutropenia is defined as a neutrophil count of ≤1000 cells/μL, absolute neutropenia is defined as a neutrophil count of ≤500 cells/μL, and profound neutropenia is defined as a neutrophil count of ≤100 cells/μL.[108] Infection is the leading cause of morbidity and mortality in neutropenic patients. The risk of infection varies with the duration of neutropenia.[109]

The initial treatment of patients with a neutropenic febrile episode should be based on risk.[110,111] Subsequent treatment may be modified according to clinical response.[112] For low risk solid tumor patients, outpatient oral treatment may be appropriate (Fig. 138-12). The degree and duration of neutropenia are the most important risk factors for developing fever after chemotherapy. Before the mid-1980s, aerobic gram-negative bacteria were the most common pathogens in neutropenic patients, but now gram-positive cocci, especially *Staphylococcus aureus*, *Staphylococcus epidermidis*, and streptococcal species, have emerged as the most common pathogens in this population. Factors that contribute to the recent dominance of gram-positive bacterial infections are the increased use of chemotherapeutic agents that cause mucositis, increased use of central venous catheters, and the use prophylactic antibiotics against gram-negative bacteria. *Candida albicans* and nonalbicans candidial species are important pathogens in patients with leukemia and bone marrow transplant recipients, and *Aspergillus* infection causes significant problems in patients with prolonged and profound neutropenia. Other fungi, such as *Fusarium* and *Trichosporon*, are emerging as important pathogens, perhaps owing to increased use of antifungal prophylaxis.

Neutropenic patients are immunocompromized and lack the ability to mount a full inflammatory response to infections. Any symptom or sign of infection in such patients should be investigated fully. Lesions on the mucous membranes and the skin can be viral (eg, due to herpes simplex and varicella zoster), bacterial (eg, due to ecthyma gangrenosum), or fungal (eg, due to disseminated candidiasis, aspergillosis, or *Fusarium* infection). Sinus symptoms may be due to bacterial or fungal infections, some of which may be invasive and fatal. Abdominal pain, distention, bloody diarrhea, nausea, and vomiting are typical findings in neutropenic enterocolitis.[105] Perianal symptoms may suggest the presence of a perianal abscess. The spectrum of conditions that must be considered in the differential diagnosis of pulmonary disease in febrile neutropenic patients is broad: infection (viral, bacterial, fungal, and protozoan), radiation-induced pathologic conditions, chemotherapy-induced

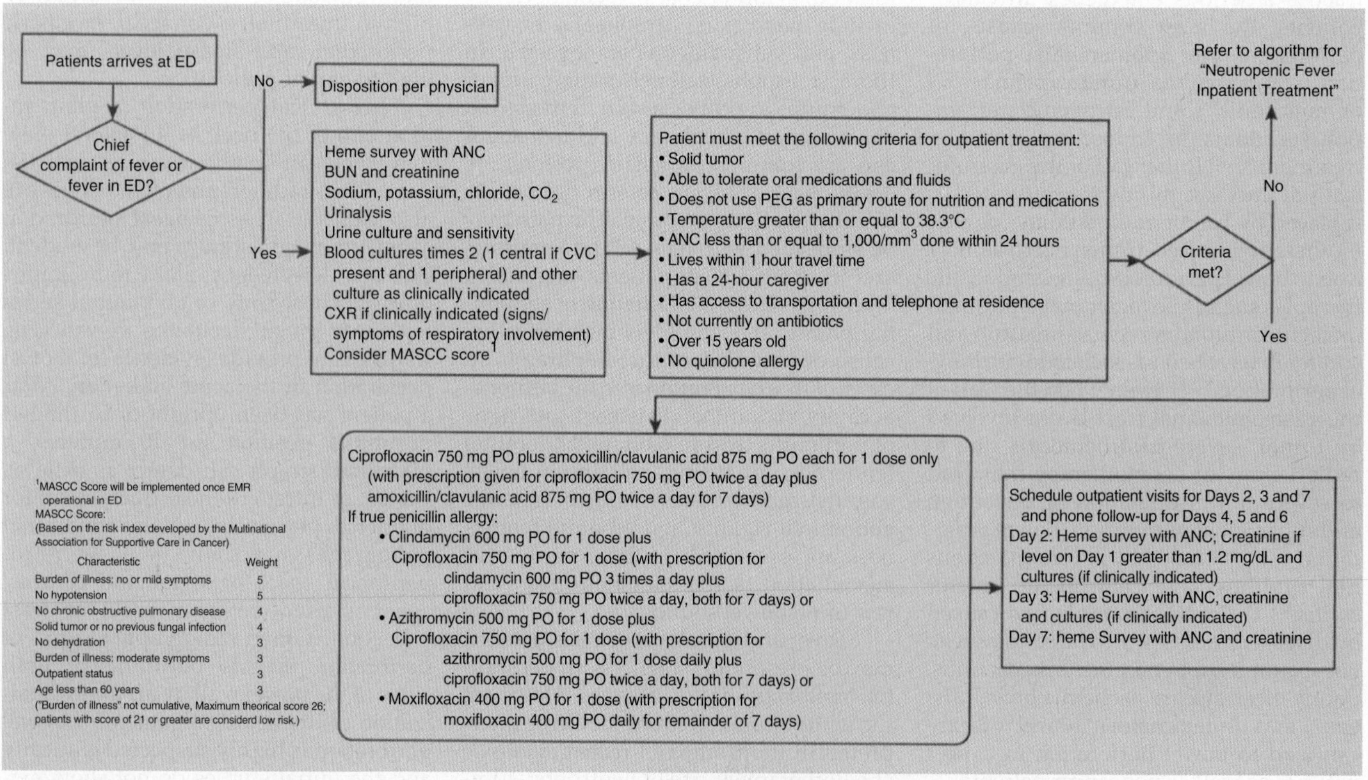

Figure 138-12 ■ Algorithm for outpatient management of solid tumor patients with neutropenic fever.

side effects, pulmonary hemorrhage, and pulmonary infarct. Physical findings in the chest are present in 30% of neutropenic patients with normal findings on chest radiography.[113] Correlation of pulmonary symptoms and findings on chest radiographs is a clinical challenge in neutropenic patients. In the majority of cases, neutropenic fever occurs in the absence of any clinically evident source of infection. Bacteremia in these patients may have resulted from translocation of organisms from the gastrointestinal tracts. Thus, the organism cultured is usually the major organism that has colonized the gastrointestinal tract of the patient.

Blood cultures may be helpful in neutropenic patients since they may provide a definitive diagnosis of the organism causing the infection and information about the sensitivity of the pathogen to antimicrobial agents. However, in persistently febrile patients receiving broad-spectrum antimicrobial drugs, less than 1% of blood cultures yield organisms. Sputum cultures should be obtained when a patient is expectorating. However, many neutropenic patients with documented pulmonary infection do not produce sputum. A positive sputum culture may provide the diagnosis of the agent causing the pulmonary infection. Any site with a localized sign of infection should be pursued with aspiration or biopsy for culture of pathogens since such culture may lead to a definite diagnosis and appropriate treatment. However, coexisting thrombocytopenia can be a contraindication to obtaining specimens or biopsy from some sites. Findings on chest radiography are abnormal in 17-25% of patients with neutropenic fever despite the absence of pulmonary signs or symptoms.[113] Classic methods such as direct examination of stained specimens, culture, and testing of antibiotic sensitivities are now complemented by molecular methods to detect microbial DNA (polymerase chain reaction in particular) and microbial antigen detection in body fluids or tissues. Polymerase chain reaction tests and antigen detection techniques for mycobacterial, *Aspergillus*, and some viral infections can help to diagnose a suspected infection early. These new detection methods offer rapid and sensitive diagnosiseven after antimicrobial therapy has been started. Serologic tests have also been helpful in identifying infections in neutropenic patients.

During the past few decades, the predominant organisms isolated from neutropenic patients with fever have changed gram-negative pathogens to gram-positive pathogens.[114] Because of the appearance of multi-drug-resistant organisms, antimicrobial therapy must be selected on the basis of the predominant pathogens and antimicrobial susceptibility patterns at each institution.[115]

Monotherapy with broad-spectrum beta-lactam antibiotics, including carbapenems or the fourth-generation cephalosporin cefepime, are established treatments. Empirical coverage for gram-negative bacilli is mandatory because gram-negative sepsis is associated with high mortality. Both double-agent therapy (aminoglycoside or fluoroquinolone plus beta-lactam) and monotherapy are acceptable.[116] All these regimens have an overall success rate of 60-80%. Empirical coverage for gram-positive organisms with vancomycin is acceptable if there is a suspected or documented infection with a gram-positive organism, like cellulitis or a central venous catheter–related infection, or if there is severe mucositis. If a febrile neutropenic patient does not respond to the initial broad-spectrum antibiotic therapy, vancomycin can be added because the presence of gram-positive bacterial infection is likely.[116] Teicoplanin and linezolid may be alternatives to vancomycin. If the fever persists after 4-7 days of broad-spectrum antibiotics, antifungal therapy is recommended. Fluconazole may be used as initial empirical therapy in patients who have not received prior antifungal prophylaxis. Amphotericin B is beneficial to three groups of patients: patients with persistent fever during broad-spectrum antibiotic treatment without antifungal prophylaxis, patients with persistent neutropenia for more than 15 days, and patients with a documented fungal infection. In some studies, hematopoietic growth factors shortened hospital stay and decreased the duration of neutropenia, but no reduction in the duration of fever or the rate of infection-related mortality was documented.[117,118]

Anaphylactic Reactions to Chemotherapy Drugs

Anaphylactic reactions to chemotherapy drugs are another important type of emergency in cancer patients. Urticaria and angioedema, the most common manifestations of anaphylaxis, occur in 90% of anaphylactic reactions. Other common manifestations are chest tightness, upper airway obstruction, abdominal pain, bronchospasm, and hypotension. Laryngeal edema causing upper airway obstruction is the most likely cause of death in anaphylaxis; hypotension is the second most likely cause.[119] Routes of drug administration, in order of decreasing severity of associated reactions, are intravenous, intra-arterial, intramuscular, subcutaneous, intradermal, oral, vaginal, rectal, and dermal.[119] In addition to the route of administration, factors known to affect the incidence or severity of hypersensitivity reactions include the class of the offending agent, the dose, the rate of infusion, the interval between doses, the cumulative dose, the number of previous exposures to the drug, and administration of prophylactic agents (the dose and timing of administration of the prophylactic agents and the thoroughness of the prevention plan). The three important elements in the treatment of anaphylaxis are early recognition, airway maintenance, and hemodynamic support. Recommendations for treatment of anaphylaxis are given in Table 138-3.[120-122]

Table 138-3 **Recommendations for Acute Management of Anaphylaxis in Adults**

1. Remove the antigen or delay the absorption of the antigen
2. Assess airway; intubate if there is evidence of laryngeal edema or impending severe airway obstruction
3. Administer epinephrine
   - In case of a less severe episode: 0.3 mg SQ, 1 mg/mL, repeated at 10- to 20-min intervals
   - In case of a more severe episode: 0.3-0.5 mg IM, 1 mg/mL, repeated at 5- to 10-min intervals
   - In case of shock or airway obstruction: 1 mg/100 mL IV, 0.01-0.02 mg/min, up to a total dose of 0.1 mg
   - In case of persistent shock: May repeat dose or start a drip. Add 1 mg to 500 mL normal saline and infuse at 2-10 μg/min
   - If patient is over 50 years old or has a history or cardiac problems and life-threatening symptoms exist: Test dose of 0.1-0.15 mg SQ or IM
4. Administer IV crystalloid fluid (normal saline or lactated Ringer's solution)
   In case of hypotension, administer 1 L over 15 min, then reassess; repeat as needed up to 3 L
5. Administer glucocorticoid:
   - Methylprednisolone 125 mg intravenous push; may repeat every 4 h if symptoms persist (alternative: hydrocortisone 500 mg, dexamethasone 20 mg, or other potent corticosteroids)
6. Administer antihistamine:
   Diphenhydramine 25-50 mg IV or IM; repeat every 2-4 h as needed
7. In case of resistant hypotension:
   - Military antishock trousers and Trendelenburg's position may be helpful
   - Infuse dopamine 5-20 μg/kg/min IV by titration
   - Administer naloxone 0.4-2.0 mg IV every 2 min (maximum 10 mg)
   - Administer cimetidine 300 mg IV or famotidine 20 mg IV
8. In case of beta-blocker-accentuated epinephrine-resistant anaphylaxis:
   - Administer glucagon 1-5 mg IV over 2-5 min
   - Administer terbutaline 0.25 mg SQ
   - Administer isoproterenol 2-10 μg/min IV by titration

Abbreviations: IM, intramuscularly; IV, intravenously; SQ, subcutaneously.
Source: Adapted from Refs. 120–122.

L-Asparaginase ■ L-asparaginase is an enzyme of bacterial origin. Multiple antigenic sites on this bacterial protein stimulate production of immunoglobulins. The risk of hypersensitivity reactions increases by 5-8% with each subsequent exposure and reaches about 33% with the fourth dose.[123] Both the *Escherichia coli* and *Erwinia chrysanthemi* forms of L-asparaginase can cause anaphylactic reactions. Fortunately, anaphylaxis occurs in fewer than 10% of treated patients, and death occurs in less than 1% of treated patients. Asparaginase covalently attached to polyethylene glycol, PEG-asparaginase, appears to decrease anaphylactic reactions

Risk factors for adverse reactions to L-asparaginase include high dosage (above 6000 IU/m^2/day),[124] previous exposure, intravenous administration,[125] a history of atopy or other drug allergy, and single-agent treatment with L-asparaginase.[126,127] Intradermal skin testing and test dosing are of no value in predicting adverse reactions to L-asparaginase.

Although reactions to L-asparaginase usually occur during and after the second week of treatment, preparations for immediate treatment of hypersensitivity reactions must be in place before every dose, including the first. Intramuscular administration is recommended because it is associated with a decreased incidence of anaphylactic reactions compared with intravenous administration.[125] Reactions to one form of L-asparaginase should prompt a change to another, less immunogenic preparation.

Taxanes ■ In early studies, the taxanes (paclitaxel and docetaxel) caused major hypersensitivity reactions in 10-30% of treated patients and minor reactions in approximately 40%.[128,129] The major hypersensitivity reactions are very similar to anaphylaxis (anaphylactoid reactions). Risk factors for hypersensitivity reactions with taxane infusion include short infusion schedules and fast infusion rates. Most major reactions occur within the first two doses. Reactions begin within 2-10 minutes of infusion and resolve within 15 minutes after the infusion is stopped. Manifestations of major hypersensitivity reactions are consistent with type 1 reactions and include urticaria, angioedema, dyspnea, bronchospasm, and hypotension.

Methods to prevent hypersensitivity reactions to taxanes include reducing the rate of infusion and administering prophylactic medications. One study showed that infusion of paclitaxel over 96 hours without prophylactic premedication caused no major reactions.[130] With shorter infusion times of 24 hours, 3 hours, or 1 hour, prophylaxis with appropriate premedications (steroids and histamine type 1 and 2 receptor antagonists) reduced the incidence of major reactions to about 3%.[129,131] The hypersensitivity reaction may be due to cremphor solvent, and taxane formulations without cremphor (eg, albumin-bound paclitaxel) may avoid this problem.

Teniposide and Etoposide ■ In adults, hypersensitivity reactions occur in about 7% of patients treated with teniposide[132] and about 3% of patients treated with etoposide.[133] In children, reactions to etoposide may occur more frequently than in adults.[134] Reactions can occur during the first exposure to these agents,[132] suggesting a nonimmunologic mechanism. On the other hand, the rate of reaction increases with increased cumulative doses of these agents, suggesting the development of an antibody-mediated reaction.[134] Reactions often occur during the first 10 minutes of infusion, sometimes after only a few milligrams have been infused, but they can also occur hours after administration. The hypersensitivity reactions seen are typical of a type 1 reaction, with angioedema, flushing, rashes, urticaria, bronchospasm, and hypotension. Teniposide can also cause a type 2 hemolytic reaction.

Procarbazine ■ Procarbazine causes type 1 hypersensitivity reactions in approximately 6-18% of treated patients,[135] and a case of type 3 reaction in the form of allergic alveolitis was reported.[136] Cutaneous manifestations are a maculopapular rash and urticaria typical of type 1 reactions. Patients who have a hypersensitivity reaction to procarbazine are unable to continue treatment because rechallenge causes recurrence of symptoms.

Platinum Compounds ■ Cisplatin produces type 1 hypersensitivity reactions and type 2 hypersensitivity reactions (hemolytic anemia).[137] The incidence of hypersensitivity reactions appears to be between 1% and 20%[138] with intravenous administration and between 10% and 25% with intravesicular administration.[139] Carboplatin also produces type 1 hypersensitivity reactions.[140] The type 1 reactions of both cisplatin and carboplatin appear to be mediated by immunoglobulin E and may be caused by the platinum atom in these compounds. Cross-reactivity among platinum analogues is possible. One review has suggested that six or more doses may be necessary to produce a hypersensitivity reaction.[141] Manifestations of hypersensitivity reactions caused by cisplatin and its analogues include rashes, urticaria, bronchospasm, and hypotension. Anaphylaxis may occur in 5% of treated patients.

Cyclophosphamide and Ifosfamide ■ Oral and intravenous cyclophosphamide and intravenous ifosfamide can produce type 1 reactions, which appear to be mediated by immunoglobulin E. Reactions to cyclophosphamide and ifosfamide may occur with the first or subsequent doses. Reported manifestations of cyclophosphamide- and ifosfamide-induced reactions include urticaria, rashes, angioedema, and anaphylaxis.[142-144]

Anthracyclines ■ Reported manifestations of hypersensitivity reactions induced by anthracyclines include rash, pruritus, urticaria, hypotension, and anaphylaxis. Intravenous daunorubicin and doxorubicin can cause type 1 reactions,[145] and type 1 reactions have been reported with intravesicular doxorubicin.[146] Oral or intravenous idarubicin has not been reported to produce type 1 reactions. It appears that cross-reactivity between anthracyclines is uncommon.

Systemic Reactions to Cytokines and Monoclonal Antibodies

Several cytokines (interferons, interleukins) and monoclonal antibodies have been approved for the treatment of specific malignancies. The toxic effects associated with cytokines may be serious. Monoclonal antibodies may induce massive release of cytokines, which may lead to fever, rigor, dyspnea, hypoxia, hypotension, or even death. Reactions to some of these biological agents have recently been reviewed.[147]

Interferons ■ Interferons (IFNs) are a family of proteins produced by cells in response to various stimuli. IFN-α is produced by macrophages and lymphocytes, IFN-β is produced by fibroblasts and epithelial cells, and IFN-γ is produced by natural killer cells, CD4- or CD8-positive lymphocytes, and lymphokine-activated killer cells. Recombinant forms of IFNs are used worldwide as therapy for viral infections, autoimmune diseases, and malignancies.

Acute adverse effects of IFN therapy occur during the first 2-8 hours after treatment, but these adverse effects rarely limit treatment. Flu-like symptoms, hypotension or hypertension, tachycardia, nausea, and vomiting are common side effects. With chronic administration, fatigue and anorexia can become severe, and significant weight loss (>10% body weight) can occur.[148] Anxiety, agitation, seizures, and coma have been reported with high-dose schedules and are reversible. These neurologic side effects and behavioral and cognitive changes may limit treatment. Mild granulocytopenia (about 50% reduction in cell counts) develops

Table 138-4 Antibody Therapies Approved by the U.S. Food and Drug Administration

Pharmaceutical Agent	Target Antigen	Type of Therapy	Cancer Type
Bevacizumab (Avastin)	VEGF	Monoclonal antibody, angiogenesis inhibitor	Colorectal cancer
Cetuximab (Erbitux)	EGFR	Monoclonal antibody, EGFR inhibitor	Colorectal cancer
Ibritumomab (Zevalin)		Radiolabeled monoclonal antibody	Non-Hodgkin lymphoma
Rituximab (Rituxan)	CD20	Monoclonal antibody	B-cell non-Hodgkin lymphoma
Tositumomab (Bexxar)		Radiolabeled monoclonal antibody	Follicular lymphoma
Trastuzumab (Herceptin)	HER2	Monoclonal antibody	Breast cancer
Gemtuzumab ozogamicin (Mylotarg)	CD33	Humanized antibody conjugated with calicheamicin	CD33-positive acute myeloid leukemia
Alemtuzuma (Campath-1H)	CD52	Humanized immunoglobulin G1 monoclonal antibody	B-cell chronic lymphocytic leukemia

gradually after the first week of treatment and is rapidly reversible upon drug discontinuation. Autoimmune and immune hemolytic anemia, myelosuppression, and thrombocytopenia may rarely be seen. Flu-like side effects may be managed with acetaminophen or nonsteroidal anti-inflammatory drugs. Other supportive care measures may be provided depending on the symptoms. In most patients, symptoms lessen with subsequent doses of IFN.

Interleukin-2 ■ Interleukin-2 (IL-2) is approved for the treatment of patients with metastatic renal cell carcinoma and melanoma. High-dose IL-2 therapy is associated with cardiovascular and hemodynamic adverse effects that resemble septic shock.[149] High-dose intravenous IL-2 therapy, which should be given in a hospital inpatient setting (sometimes with intensive care monitoring), can lead to hypotension, vascular leak syndrome, and respiratory insufficiency. Support of peripheral vascular resistance with vasopressors, endotracheal intubation, and fluid resuscitation may be necessary during therapy. Acute central nervous system side effects such as psychosis, disorientation, and behavioral changes may be seen with high-dose IL-2 therapy. Other neurologic side effects, such as seizures and coma, have been reported in patients with brain metastases. IL-2 treatment should be stopped as soon as neurologic side effects are observed. Guidelines for administration of high-dose IL-2 have been suggested.[150]

Lower-dose intravenous and subcutaneous IL-2 regimens can be administered in an ambulatory care setting with observation for several hours after administration. The severity of adverse effects of lower-dose therapy is dose dependent. Common symptoms include fever, chills, nausea, vomiting, anorexia, malaise, fatigue, myalgia, arthralgia, and pruritus. Prophylaxis includes acetaminophen 650-1000 mg 1 hour before therapy and 4 and 8 hours later and histamine type 1 and 2 receptor antagonists (eg, diphenhydramine 50 mg orally 1 hour before therapy and 25 mg 4, 8, and 12 hours later plus cimetidine 800 mg orally before therapy). Meperidine (25-50 mg intravenously) may be given as needed for rigor and chills during therapy. Various antiemetics may be used as needed. Recent works have identified angiopoietin-2 (Ang2) as a mediator of the vascular leak syndrome caused by high-dose IL-2 VLS, and the inhibition of Ang2 may be a therapeutic strategy to mitigate the vascular leak syndrome in patients receiving IL-2.[151]

Denileukin diftitox (Ontak) is an IL-2/diphtheria toxin fusion protein. The IL-2 portion of the molecule targets lymphoma cells by binding to the IL-2 receptor on the plasma membrane. Upon endocytosis, the diphtheria toxin is delivered to the lymphoma cells. Common side effects are nausea and vomiting, fever, and flu-like symptoms. Other significant side effects include the cytokine release syndrome and vascular leak syndrome.[152] Acute complaints reported on the first day of treatment include back pain, shortness of breath, flushing, rash, chest pain, difficulty swallowing, dizziness, and fainting. Only 2% of patients experience severe reactions. Slowing or terminating the infusion and administering antihistamines, corticosteroids, and epinephrine can relieve these reactions. Prophylactic treatment with systemic corticosteroids is recommended.[153]

Monoclonal Antibodies ■ The list of antibody pharmaceuticals has grown (Table 138-4). Although the incidence of reactions may vary among the agents, the general precautions and treatment of the antibody infusion syndrome are the same. Transient nausea, headache, fatigue, fever, chills, rash, wheezing, hypotension, arrhythmias, bronchospasm, and angioedema may reflect immune responses to immunoglobulin. Prophylactic treatment with acetaminophen and diphenhydramine may attenuate this antibody infusion syndrome. Reactions generally resolve with slowing or interruption of the infusion. The infusion of the antibody pharmaceutical may be interrupted and then restarted at 50% of the previous infusion rate when symptoms resolve.

Selected References

The complete reference list can be found at www.CANCERMEDICINE8.com

1. Yeung SC, Escalante CP, eds. *Oncologic Emergencies*. Hamilton, Canada: B. C. Decker; 2002.
2. Johnston PG, Spence RAJ, eds. *Oncologic Emergencies*. Oxford, UK: Oxford University Press; 2002.
3. Kosmidis PA, Schrijvers D, Andre F. *Handbook of Oncological Emergencies*. Philadelphia: Taylor & Francis Group; 2005.
4. *ACLS Provider Manual*. Dallas, TX: American Heart Association; 2001.
5. Hendrick JM, Pijls NH, van der Werf T, Crul JF. Cardiopulmonary resuscitation on the general ward: no category of patients should be excluded in advance. *Resuscitation*. 1990;20:163-171.
6. Ebell MH, Becker LA, Barry HC, Hagen M. Survival after in-hospital cardiopulmonary resuscitation. A meta-analysis. *J Gen Intern Med*. 1998;13:805-816.
9. Ackroyd R, Russon L, Newell R. Views of oncology patients, their relatives and oncologists on cardiopulmonary resuscitation (CPR): questionnaire-based study. *Palliat Med*. 2007;21:139-144.
10. Kvols LK. Therapy of the malignant carcinoid syndrome. *Endocrinol Metab Clin North Am*. 1989;18:557-568.
16. Zuppinger C, Timolati F, Suter TM. Pathophysiology and diagnosis of cancer drug induced cardiomyopathy. *Cardiovasc Toxicol*. 2007;7:61-66.
17. Bristow MR, Billingham ME, Mason JW, Daniels JR. Clinical spectrum of anthracycline antibiotic cardiotoxicity. *Cancer Treat Rep*. 1978;62:873-879.
21. Benoff LJ, Schweitzer P. Radiation therapy-induced cardiac injury [see comments]. *Am Heart J*. 1995;129:1193-1196.
23. Atallah E, Durand JB, Kantarjian H, Cortes J. Congestive heart failure is a rare event in patients receiving imatinib therapy. *Blood*. 2007;110:1233-1237.
26. Kern KB, Halperin HR, Field J. New guidelines for cardiopulmonary resuscitation and emergency cardiac care: changes in the management of cardiac arrest. *JAMA*. 2001;285:1267-1269.
27. Flombaum CD. Metabolic emergencies in the cancer patient. *Semin Oncol*. 2000;27:322-334.
29. Hsu HH, Chen YC, Tian YC, et al. Role of serum sodium in assessing hospital mortality in cancer patients with spontaneous tumour lysis syndrome inducing acute uric acid nephropathy. *Int J Clin Pract*. 2007.
30. Montesinos P, Lorenzo I, Martin G, et al. Tumor lysis syndrome in patients with acute myeloid leukemia: identification of risk factors and development of a predictive model. *Haematologica*. 2008;93:67-74.

31. Mato AR, Riccio BE, Qin L, et al. A predictive model for the detection of tumor lysis syndrome during AML induction therapy. *Leuk Lymphoma*. 2006;47:877-883.
34. Yonemori K, Kunitoh H, Tsuta K, et al. Prognostic factors for malignant pericardial effusion treated by pericardial drainage in solid-malignancy patients. *Med Oncol*. 2007;24:425-430.
35. Johnson KK, Soundarraj D, Patel P. Tenecteplase for malignant pericardial effusion. *Pharmacotherapy*. 2007;27:303-305.
41. Morrissey DD, Andersen PE, Nesbit GM, Barnwell SL, Everts EC, Cohen JI. Endovascular management of hemorrhage in patients with head and neck cancer. *Arch Otolaryngol Head Neck Surg*. 1997;123:15-19.
43. Athale UH, Kaste SC, Bodner SM, Ribeiro RC. Splenic rupture in children with hematologic malignancies. *Cancer*. 2000;88: 480-490.
48. Chen JC, Bongard F, Klein SR. A contemporary perspective on superior vena cava syndrome. *Am J Surg*. 1990;160:207-211.
52. Smayra T, Otal P, Chabbert V, et al. Long-term results of endovascular stent placement in the superior caval venous system. PG - 388-94. *Cardiovasc Intervent Radiol*. 2001;24:388-394.
53. Cahill BC, Ingbar DH. Massive hemoptysis. Assessment and management. *Clin Chest Med*. 1994;15:147-167.
57. Jougon J, Ballester M, Delcambre F, et al. Massive hemoptysis: what place for medical and surgical treatment. *Eur J Cardiothorac Surg*. 2002;22:345.
62. Light RW, Erozan YS, Ball WC, Jr. Cells in pleural fluid. Their value in differential diagnosis. *Arch Intern Med*. 1973;132: 854-860.
67. Putnam JB, Jr, Walsh GL, Swisher SG, et al. Outpatient management of malignant pleural effusion by a chronic indwelling pleural catheter. *Ann Thorac Surg*. 2000;69:369-375.
71. Gupta S, Hicks ME, Wallace MJ, Ahrar K, Madoff DC, Murthy R. Outpatient management of postbiopsy pneumothorax with small-caliber chest tubes: factors affecting the need for prolonged drainage and additional interventions. *Cardiovasc Intervent Radiol*. 2008;31:342-348.
73. Bick RL, Haas SK. International consensus recommendations. Summary statement and additional suggested guidelines. European Consensus Conference, November 1991. American College of Chest Physicians consensus statement of 1995. International Consensus Statement, 1997. *Med Clin North Am*. 1998;82:613-633.
74. Levitan N, Dowlati A, Remick SC, et al. Rates of initial and recurrent thromboembolic disease among patients with malignancy versus those without malignancy. Risk analysis using Medicare claims data. *Medicine (Baltimore)*. 1999;78:285-291.
78. King V, Vaze AA, Moskowitz CS, Smith LJ, Ginsberg MS. D-dimer assay to exclude pulmonary embolism in high-risk oncologic population: correlation with CT pulmonary angiography in an urgent care setting. *Radiology*. 2008;247:854-861.
79. Klok FA, Djurabi RK, Nijkeuter M, et al. High D-dimer level is associated with increased 15-d and 3 months mortality through a more central localization of pulmonary emboli and serious comorbidity. *Br J Haematol*. 2008;140:218-222.
80. Oudkerk M, van Beek EJ, Wielopolski P, et al. Comparison of contrast-enhanced magnetic resonance angiography and conventional pulmonary angiography for the diagnosis of pulmonary embolism: a prospective study. *Lancet*. 2002;359:1643-1647.
82. Tillie-Leblond I, Mastora I, Radenne F, et al. Risk of pulmonary embolism after a negative spiral CT angiogram in patients with pulmonary disease: 1-year clinical follow-up study. *Radiology*. 2002;223:461-467.
86. Ten Cate-Hoek AJ, Prins MH. Low molecular weight heparins in cancer Management and prevention of venous thromboembolism in patients with malignancies. *Thromb Res*. 2007.
87. Thrombolytic therapy in treatment: summary of an NIH Consensus Conference. *Br Med J*. 1980;280:1585-1587.
90. Goldhaber SZ. Thrombolysis in pulmonary embolism: a debatable indication. *Thromb Haemost*. 2001;86:444-451.
91. Byrne TN. Metastatic epidural cord compression. *Curr Neurol Neurosci Rep*. 2004;4:191-195.
102. Chiarugi M, Galatioto C, Lippolis PV, Seccia M. Multiple bowel perforations complicating imatinib treatment for advanced gastrointestinal stromal tumor. *J Am Coll Surg*. 2008;206:386-387.
104. Badgwell BD, Camp ER, Feig B, et al. Management of bevacizumab-associated bowel perforation: a case series and review of the literature. *Ann Oncol*. 2008;19: 577-582.
105. Bavaro MF. Neutropenic enterocolitis. *Curr Gastroenterol Rep*. 2002;4:297-301.
110. Kern WV. Risk assessment and risk-based therapeutic strategies in febrile neutropenia. *Curr Opin Infect Dis*. 2001;14:415-422.
111. Paesmans M. Risk factors assessment in febrile neutropenia. *Int J Antimicrob Agents*. 2000;16:107-111.
112. Kern WV. Modifications of therapy. *Int J Antimicrob Agents*. 2000;16:139-141.
115. Bodey GP, Rolston KV. Management of fever in neutropenic patients. *J Infect Chemother*. 2001;7:1-9.
116. Hughes WT, Armstrong D, Bodey GP, et al. 2002 guidelines for the use of antimicrobial agents in neutropenic patients with cancer. *Clin Infect Dis*. 2002;34:730-751.
117. Papadimitris C, Dimopoulos MA, Kostis E, et al. Outpatient treatment of neutropenic fever with oral antibiotics and granulocyte colony-stimulating factor. *Oncology*. 1999;57:127-130.
121. Gavalas M, Sadana A, Metcalf S. Guidelines for the management of anaphylaxis in the emergency department [see comments]. *J Accid Emerg Med*. 1998;15:96-98.
147. Albanell J, Baselga J. Systemic therapy emergencies. *Semin Oncol*. 2000;27:347-361.
150. Schwartzentruber DJ. Guidelines for the safe administration of high-dose interleukin-2. *J Immunother*. 2001;24:287-293.

139 Oncology Informatics

Edward P. Ambinder, MD

Health Care Policy, Quality Care, and Information Technology

As oncologists, we are experiencing unprecedented challenges to our research and therapeutic and practice management skills brought on by the necessity to manage the geometric increase in medical information, the striking changes in the clinical practice of oncology, and the urgent need to define and measure quality oncology care. The clinical oncologist must be a clinician, researcher, educator, businessperson, statistician, health care administrator, and informatician, who must interact with the whole patient, both as a specialist and as a primary-care physician. These skills must be assimilated into our daily clinical practice and research activities, while we continue to improve our evidence-based quality care and cost-effectiveness for a much more sophisticated consumer and payer.

Information management has become the most frustrating aspect of our professional life. Cancer patients receive intricate multimodality therapies for their complex diseases, requiring greater access to, and tracking of, detailed medical data. Disease management clinical guidelines and care plans for cancer patients require micromanagement and economic awareness of patient care.[1] Clinical trials, which demand intense documentation, must not only show progression free and overall survival benefits, but also display cost effectiveness and patient satisfaction.[2,3]

The digitalization of information, the ability to network or connect computers, and the rapid electronic interchange of information on a worldwide basis are recognized as the hallmark of a new order in society (Fig. 139-1). For oncologists to master these profound changes, it is necessary to embrace the medical tools of the Information Age. These tools include the computer, which acts as the information gateway and integrator, the Internet, which coordinates interactive information resources and personal socialization and communication, and the electronic health record (EHR), which is the translator and repository of our clinical information gathering. Information technology and personal computers have transformed every other profession and are now revolutionizing medicine as well.

Our chaotic health care system continues to confound our nation with inadequate funding for clinical care, research, and teaching; decreased reimbursements; a panoply of health care players with vested interests; and severe under use of information technology. Despite all the money invested in research, little is used for the more prosaic technology needed for gathering, analyzing, and making use of the collected data. Oncologists remain uncomfortable with the nexus of technology and medicine. We are taught by observation, textbooks, and by using our diagnostic skills with continued reliance on memory and experience.

Influential groups, including the Institute of Medicine,[4-6] the President's Information Technology Advisory Committee,[7] and the President's Cancer Council,[8] have released assessments of our health care system that highlight its many inadequacies and the need to apply advances in information technology to improve administrative and clinical processes. The reports criticize the variation of cancer treatments by locale, the lack of using guidelines and care plans based on best available evidence, the absence of tools to measure and monitor quality of care using core sets of quality measures or an EHR, and poor patient accrual to quality clinical trials. They also found major impediments for cancer patients to obtain compassionate psychosocial and palliative care. They stress the absence of any progress in restructuring health care to address both quality and cost concerns. Despite 10,000 clinical trials that are conducted annually that provide many medical advances, we do not efficiently translate this knowledge gained from research and development into routine clinical care, sometimes taking 15-20 years, and even then its adoption into routine clinical practice remains uneven.

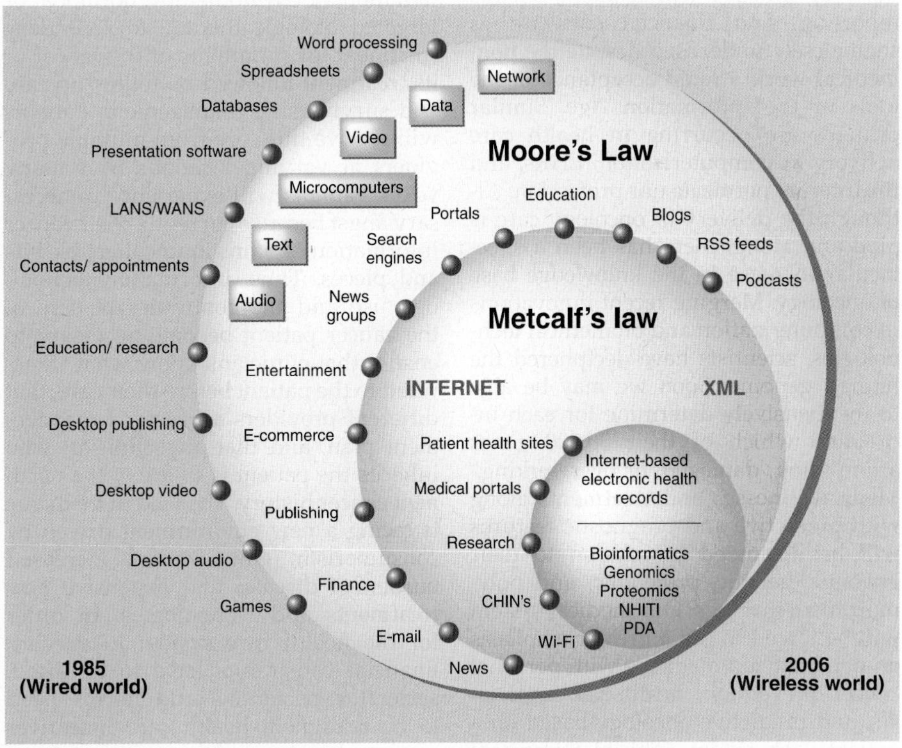

Figure 139-1 ■ The digitalization of medicine 1985-2009. This figure depicts the swift chronologic evolution of the oncologist's personal, professional, and oncologic uses of information technology from 1985 through 2009 using the unprecedented improvements in computer hardware as predicted by Moore's law and the rapid increases in networking communication efficiency as predicted by Metcalf's law. *Abbreviations:* CHIN, community health information networks; NANS, neighborhood area network system; NHITI, National Health-care Information Technology Initiative; RSS, Really Simple Syndication; XML, extensible markup language.

There is a convincing need for our health care system to methodically collect, analyze, and deliver medical evidence to physicians, payers, and patients.

Health care consumerism is an increasing fact of life that is fueled by the Internet and our economic prosperity. It is driven by individual autonomy; skepticism of our profession, government, managed care, and corporate dominance in health care; the women's health movement; alternative medicine; informed consent; increased malpractice litigation; Internet consumer information; consumer-directed drug advertisements; patient support groups; and patient-directed laboratory tests and procedures. Consumers usually do not understand health care quality and true cost; and they cannot easily navigate the complex health care system. Consumers are always better served when they navigate the health care system with physician assistance.

The delivery of patient care in the United States is disjointed, especially when considering the mobile society, patients who change practitioners and health plans every 3 years on average, the absence of any coordination of the patient's longitudinal medical record, and the lip service given to screening and prevention of disease. Health care delivery automation, with the exceptions of practice management, results reporting, and financial software, is shamelessly underused despite the nonmedical world's rapid acceptance of the tools of the Information Age. Similar changes are occurring in health care delivery as computerization, EHRs, and the Internet permeate our profession. Although the delivery of oncology care is plodding along, there has been a spectacular increase in the knowledge base of oncology. Merging recent innovations in computerization and biomedical technologies, scientists have deciphered the human genome. Soon we may be able to inexpensively determine for each individual which of their 30,000 genes are missing, damaged, or overworking.[9] Medical illnesses and treatments along with predictive and prognostic features will be discussed in relation to their genomic, genetic, proteomic, and polymorphism findings. Our medical system will be forced to put a greater emphasis on personalized medicine with personal cancer prevention, health-risk appraisals, and predictive oncology based on a patient's genetic data. This may translate into lower health care costs through earlier detection of cancer and more precision in choosing treatments.

If our health care system is to thrive in a rapidly changing medical universe, all the participants—providers, patients, administrators, researchers, educators, payers, industry, and the government—must understand the laws of the Information Age. By combining the huge cost-saving potential of computerization and Internet telecommunication, technology will provide a logical framework for health care.

With secured and confidential EHRs and the acceptance of Regional Health Information Organizations (RHIO) that electronically link, on a regional basis, all patients, practitioners, payers, hospitals, benefit managers, commercial laboratories, imaging centers, cancer registries, and drug stores, our health care system could become more cost-effective and efficient. Building on fundamental strengths and with a common spirit of compromise and sharing, we could look forward to a health care system that maintains its world leadership in the production of clinical and basic science oncologic research, and strives to achieve equivalent excellence in the delivery of oncologic health care and the oncologic education of health care providers and patients.

Cancer as a Chronic Disease

It is instructive to consider the care of cancer patients as a series of transitions from their primary treatment with surgery, radiation, or chemotherapy, hormonal or targeted biologic therapy to secondary treatment for symptoms of the cancer or its treatment followed by follow-up care and survivorship management. Patients will receive this care from multiple providers at varying locations over many years. Patients will experience unnecessary angst because currently their cancer information remains in uncollectible bits and pieces. Thus, information technology use and the continuity of care of the cancer patient become necessary to ensure that clinicians know what transpired to the patient before their care, that different providers agree on a management plan, and that any clinician who inherits the patient is aware of the pertinent cancer history. The field of medicine is facing a new environment driven by consumerism, globalization, increased burden of disease, and expensive new treatments and technologies. In order for the health care system to survive, financial constraints have to be lifted, societal expectations and norms need to be realigned, health care incentives need to be changed, a long-term view of health care must be accepted, and the ability to access and share critical information must be enabled. Today chronic care management remains costly, labor intensive, and plagued by wide variations in the effectiveness of care. Our care delivery and payment system must change from the episodic, acute type to the management and prevention of chronic disease using clinical standards and delivering quality care that can be easily measured and reported. All stakeholders must realign their involvement. Our patients must take more responsibility for their health. The payers must help our patients become healthier and obtain more efficient value from the health care system by incentivizing physician payments for prevention and chronic care coordination of chronically ill patients. Chronically ill patients will be empowered to take control of their diseases through disease management programs that improve outcomes and lower costs. Suppliers must work with all health care stakeholders to produce products that improve patient outcomes at lower costs. Our government needs to take a leadership role to encourage innovation and remove obstacles by providing adequate financing and national policy. Specialty disease and care management companies using sophisticated information systems need to share with providers and specialty nurses to work with the oncologist and the patient to identify subgroups of patients with high costs and disability. By implementing plans of care and home visits, addressing the psychosocial needs of our patients and having their nurses directly communicating with the oncologist, patient health will improve resulting in significant reductions in the cost of cancer care.

Recently the "medical home" concept, as defined by the Association of American Medical Colleges (AAMC) "as a model of care delivery that includes an ongoing relationship between a provider and patient, around the clock access to medical consultation, respect for the patient/family's cultural and religious beliefs, and a comprehensive approach to care and coordination of care through providers and community services" has been proposed as a working model for patients with chronic diseases (<http://www.aamc.org/newsroom/pressrel/2008/medicalhome.pdf>). In essence, the community oncologist presently functions as a medical home, coordinating care with other specialties, and serving as an intermediary for the cancer patient's rehabilitative, nutritional, psychosocial, durable medical, hospice, or home care needs. As the payers reimburse this component of care, oncologists will be rewarded for their efforts and the coordination of care of the cancer patient will significantly improve.

For the oncologist, profound improvements in our expectations for cancer patients based on expensive molecular-targeted drugs will continue to expand the number of cancer survivors (currently 10,400,000 in 2008) and their responsibility to provide cancer treatment and cancer summary reports to our patients who are becoming guardians of their medical records as the personal electronic health record (PHR) becomes part of the EHR. This will force changes in the reimbursement system that has emphasized payment for episodes of care and procedures to paying for prevention, continuity of care, quality documentation, using information technology effectively, and providing useful patient-specific reports as suggested by the Institute of Medicine in their report, Lost in Transition: From Cancer patient to Cancer Survivor (<http://www.iom.edu/?id=31512>). They defined four essential components of survivor care to include prevention, surveillance, intervention, and coordination.

Medical and Oncologic Informatics

Health care is an information-based science involving the gathering, synthesis, and implementation of information. Medical informatics is concerned with managing and using information in biomedicine and health care that is patient-specific (ie, EHRs) and knowledge-based (ie, information retrieval and decision support tools). Medical informatics uses information science and its technologies to deal with the "cognitive, information processing and communication tasks of medical practice, education, and research."[10] Medical oncology, with its strong emphasis on data collection and analysis, is positioned at the forefront of clinical trials requiring automated methods to record clinical signs, symptoms, toxicity, quality measures, and outcome. In its training programs, and carried over into clinical practice by its trainees, there is a heavy emphasis on research protocols requiring a time-oriented tabular flow sheet format that is ideal for computerization. Increasing documentation for cooperative groups, government bodies, insurance companies, pharmaceutical houses, and institutional review boards demands computerized records. Health care costs have escalated dramatically, particularly for cancer patients, who require complex diagnostic and therapeutic procedures, making them a prime target for cost-containment efforts by third-party payers and the federal government. Today, the computer is our most efficient tool for obtaining timely information. It has also become our most effective decision-making tool. The computer has become an integrated information device that has merged printers, scanners, facsimile machines (faxes), copiers, telephones, video and audio systems, and filing cabinets. Interested readers are referred to Shortliffe and Cimino for a comprehensive review of this field.[11]

As oncologists become more comfortable with computers and the electronic distribution of computer-based information, and as patients take more responsibility for their medical decisions, health care will use online computer-assisted communication among patients, medical databases, and physicians to replace a considerable part of the care now given in person.[12] Today's machines address the handling of data analysis by using intuitive interfaces. This digital information is then transmitted to output devices that can display the information. Table 139-1 lists these devices. In the future, computers will simulate the "whole-person paradigm," whereby data can be input by voice, pointing, writing, touching or gestures, and different languages can be freely translated. Table 139-2 summarizes the common types of software applications of interest to the oncologist.

Table 139-1 **Input and Output Devices for the Computer**

Device	Input Device	Output Device
35 mm slides projector	*	*
Barcode reader	*	
Cellular Phone	*	*
CD-ROM	*	*
Digital Pen	*	
DVD-ROM	*	*
Fax	*	*
Graphic pad	*	
Joystick	*	
Keyboard	*	
Microphone	*	
Keypad	*	
Music sound editing (MID1, MP3, iPOD, iPhone)	*	*
Monitor or video display terminal (VDT)		*
Mouse	*	
Medical imaging devices	*	*
Other computers	*	*
Overhead projection pads		*
Personal video recorder	*	*
PDA (personal digital assistant)	*	*
Printer (laser, dot matrix, or ink-jet)		*
Plotters		*
Radio	*	*
Scanner	*	
Storage device (disk or tape)	*	*
Tape recorder	*	*
Telephone	*	*
Television	*	*
Touch screen	*	
Trackball (stationary mouse)	*	
Track pad (stationary mouse)	*	
Video, still camera	*	*
Video recorder	*	*

Overview of Computerized Tools

Smartphones

Smartphones are hand-held devices that combine portability, computer processing power, pen-based or multi-touch interaction, and handwriting recognition. They also include personal organization programs, such as schedulers, calculators, reminder lists, address files, financial and travel tools, document and information retrieval capability, and wired and wireless communication by phone, modem, fax, or beeper. These devices can synchronize data with desktop computers and can use cellular modems for information updating and retrieval over the Internet to update all programs and databases. The oncologist uses these instruments to hold personal, financial, and patient medical data. Recently, these all-in-one devices have added instant messaging, Web access, beepers, mapping and location-based services and digital and video cameras, enhancing the oncologist's mobile communication tools. According to a recent American Society of Clinical Oncology survey, between 70% and 80% of members own and use Smartphones.[13] An updated list of Smartphone programs generated from the survey is provided in Table 139-3. Desktop programs can now seamlessly link to the Internet and Smartphones, providing selective information that is always available. As processing power and storage capabilities increase geometrically, any information available from computers or the Internet can be handled by these mobile devices. Recently, two inexpensive wireless protocols that facilitate wireless communications by defining protocols for security and authorization, and hardware and software designs, have become popular. The Bluetooth standard defines protocols for short-range communications between electronic devices; and the IEEE 802.11 or Wi-Fi (Wireless Fidelity) protocol defines a wireless local area network up to 1,500 feet per node, which permits access to the Internet at many public and corporate spaces at speeds up to 54 megabits per second in the 2.4 G Hz band. A new technology named "Wimax" has become available, positioned as a wide-area version of Wi-Fi having a maximum range of 30 miles. Apple's iPhone has revolutionized the Smartphone market not by just being an innovative phone, but by combining hardware, software, internet browser, multiple communication protocals and touch input to create the most versatile mobile device and a new software platform for developers. It has rapidly become the Smartphone of choice for physicians and with its App Store promises to be the mobile platform of choice for medical and well-

Table 139-2 ■ Medical Uses of the Computer

Uses	Examples	
Communications	Bulletin boards	Electronic mail
	Bibliographic databases Voice mail	Electronic forums
Database management system		
Medical records	Admission/discharges	Tumor registry
	Demographic information	Pain management tools
	Insurance eligibility	Protocol management
	Office records	Links to hospital databases
	Hospital records	Scheduling tests
	Bedside terminals	Cumulative drug dosing
	Patient monitoring	Orders
	Patient education/reminders	Blood products: history, matching, use
	Patient allergies	
	Body-surface-area calculation	Flow sheets
	Graphic data representation	Laboratory data
	Image analysis	Patient summaries
	Integrated patient care plans	Specialty encounters
	Clinical research protocols	Malpractice documentation
	Census reports	Legal documentation
Pharmacology management	Drug–drug interactions	Drug monitoring
	Patient drug list	Antibiotic screening
	Drug ordering	
Clinical decision support	Artificial intelligence	Computer-aided treatment
	Natural language processing	Medical decision making
	Computer-aided diagnosis	Consultation
Laboratory monitoring	Control and data analysis	
	Physiologic monitoring	
Management systems	Practice management	Resource management
	Quality assurance	Usage review
Office management	Electronic banking	Financial management
	Electronic billing	Inventory
	Accounts payable	Return visit reminders
	Accounts receivable	Patient schedules
	Financial analysis	Physician schedules
Graphics	Painting or bit-mapped	Drawing or vector-based or object-based
Image processing	Radiographic images	Pathologic images
	Radiation planning	
Presentation	Slides Handouts	Overhead projection pads
	Television projection systems	
Scanning	Documents Graphics	Optical character recognition
Statistics	Analysis of variance	Multivariate analysis
	Cluster analysis	Nonparametric tests
	Contingency tables	Path/latent variable analysis
	Correlation	
	Data handling	Regression
	Graphics	Reliability/test item analysis
	Linear programming	Survival analysis
Spreadsheets		
Word processing		
Publishing	Electronic textbooks	Electronic journals
Project management		
Programming		
Grant proposals		
Handicapped patients	Input and output devices	
Music		
Organizational charts		
Text retrieval or search	Medical literature	Medical databases
	Medical textbooks	
Education	Programmed instruction	Patient education
	Computer-aided instruction	Examinations
	Video simulation	Patient instructions
	Courseware	

ness software (<http://www.apple.com/iphone>). These networks allow one computer to talk to another computer, permitting electronic mail, exchanging files, sharing printers, telephony, videoconferencing, and accessing the Internet.

Internet

World Wide Web

No recent phenomenon has captured the world's and, in particular, the medical establishment's attention more swiftly than the Internet. It is the "Information Superhighway," the World Wide Web (WWW), with its linked matrix of information resources and its ability to network different computer systems and networks, all using the same wired or wireless interconnection technologies. Wilkins and Hovhanesian describe attributes of the Internet that have produced a societal paradigm shift.[14] Its most basic attribute is the capability to publish information that was formerly paper-based. Making this information interactive allows obtaining information that is now current, easily accessible, and at a single source. The information is stored in databases with self-servicing capabilities, whereby looking for information or filling out forms can take place without human assistance. Through two-way and real-time collaboration, the Internet becomes the virtual workplace where individual groups can share ideas synchronously in online meetings or asynchronously as in e-mail, bulletin boards, or news groups. With integration and knowledge management, information can finally be personalized, easily located, and is encyclopedic. This permits the neophyte to have access to the same information available to the experts, thus forever changing the relationship between patient and physician. This will translate into a joint community relationship of patients and physicians who will share in the collection and storage of medical data, as well as prevention and screening reminders for disease, heralding the Internet-based electronic patient health care record. This vision can be facilitated by incentives such as reduced insurance premiums for patients who participate in screening programs and reduced malpractice premiums for physicians who use electronic records.

The Internet, with 1,407,724,920 users worldwide in March 2008, representing a 21% penetration of the world's population[15] and growing at a rate of 3% per month, is a global, independent, but cooperative network of government, university, research laboratory, corporate, and private computers communicating by e-mail, bulletin boards, and discussion groups. It has the capability of permitting searches of database files and of retrieving information and software programs. It is fast becoming a post office, telephone system, and research library for its users. The reader is referred to the editorial "The Next Transformation in the Delivery of Health Care"[16] for an excellent overview of the Internet's indispensability for oncologists and physicians.

For collaborative Internet efforts, Usenet acts as a bulletin-board system that groups together Internet messages that pertain to a given topic, making discussion groups, newsletters, focused scientific groups, and subscription lists a reality. The information can be threaded

Table 139-3 ■ **PDA Applications of Interest to the Oncologist**

Type	Application	Location for Obtaining	Comment	Comment
Drug guides	Epocrates	http://www.epocrates.com	Combines drug information. Antibiotics, drug interactions, diagnostic information, clinical tables and clinical calculators	$
	Mobile PDR	http://www.pdr.net	Drug database & interactions	Free
	Mobile Micromedex	http://www.micromedex.com/mobilemicromedex	Drug database	$
	A to Z Drug facts	http://www.handheldmed.com (click on "products")	Drug database	$
	Lexi-Comp Onhand	http://www.store.lexi.com/lexistore	Drug database	$
	EDRUGSDATA HDB	http://www.pdacortex.com/eDrugsDataHDB_Pocket_PC_Download.htm	12,000 drugs. Requires HanDBase	$
Dosing, protocols and phemotherapy regimens	OncoMD	http://www.medicine.jbpub.com/oncomed	Cancer chemotherapy	$
	ChemoRxPlus	http://www.chemorxplus.com	Dosing calculator and protocol guide	Free
	Guide to Cancer Chemotherapeutic Regimens	http://healthcareprofessionals.orthobiotech.com/services/download.jsp	Protocol guide by cancer type	Free
	CAChemoRx	http://www.skyscape.com/EStore/ProductDetail.aspx?ProductID=1009	From Handbook of Cancer Chemotherapy	$
Chemotherapy regimens and cancer care	ChemoSrce	http://www.skyscape.com/EStore/ProductDetail.aspx?ProductID=1132&WT.mc_id=56789	Chemotherapy drugs, regimens and side effects	$
Clinical references	Journal Clinical Oncology	http://www.jco.org/misc/PDA.shtml	Tof C, Abstracts and Announcements	Subscription
	ASCO	http://www.asco.org/pda	PDA formatted site content	Members
	PIER PDA	http://www.acponline.org/pda/	The Physicians' Information and Education Resource from American College of Physicians. Has 355 diseases.	$
	JournaltoGo	http://www.journaltogo.com/	Find authoritative, evidence-based guidance to improve clinical care	Free
	5MCC/200	http://www.5mcc.com/handhelds.html or see Epocrates	Griffith's 5 Minute Clinical Consult 1000 medical conditions	$
	Washington Manual of Oncology	http://www.lww.com/pda		$
	NCI PDQ	http://www.cancer.gov	Download sections and place into PDA for a document reader (Silo at http://www.isilo.com)	Free
	Diagnosaurus	http://books.mcgraw-hill.com/medical/diagnosaurus/index.html	Differential diagnosis for medical and surgical conditions	Free
	Stedman's Medical Dictionary	http://www.Stedmans.com/product.cfm/320/210		$
	PocketMedicine	http://www.pocketmedicine.com	Clinical publications and treatment strategies	$
	Redi-reference Clinical Guidelines Handbook	http://www.redi-reference.com		$
	HaemOnc Rules	http://medeicine.com/my/palmsoft/	Collection of diagnostic and therapeutic algorithms and classifications	Free
	SurgOnco	http://www.pdamd.com/pdaorder/-/885030120699/item?oec-catalog-item-id=2492	MD Anderson Surgical Oncology Handbook	$
Staging	Cancer Staging and Treatment	http://www.palmgear.com search for "cancer staging"	Requires iSilo reader (http://www.isilo.com)	Free
	Cancer Staging Pocket Guide	http://healthcareprofessionals.orthobiotech.com/services/download.jsp		Free
	TNM Mobile Edition	http://www.wiley.com	Staging and staging Calculator	$
	AJCC TNM	http://www.skyscape.com	Staging (Springer-Verlag)	$
	EZTNM	http://www.skyscape.com	Staging Calculator (Springer-Verlag)	$
Prognosis and risk assessment	MSKCC: Prostate Cancer, RCC, Gastric Cancer & Sarcoma	http://www.mskcc.org/mskcc/html/5794.cfm	See also: http://www.nomograms.org	Free
	Cancer PRA	http://www.skyscape.com/EStore/ProductDetail.aspx?ProductID=1079	From The Handbook of Cancer Risk Assessment and Prevention	$
	MedRules	http://pbrain.hypermart.net/medrules.html		Free
	Adjuvant!	http://www.adjuvantonline.com	Breast and colon cancer	
	BreastCa	http://smi-web.stanford.edu/people/pcheng/breastca/index.html	Uses Gail and Claus models	Free
	BreastAssure	http://shop.store.yahoo.com/pilotgearsw/breastassure.html	Nottingham, Van Nuys Indices	$
	BRCA Guide	http://www.myriadtests.com/provider/brca.htm	Estimates probability of patient carrying BRCA1 or BRCA2 from Myriad genetic Laboratories	Free
	Lung Cancer Risk Assessment	http://www.mskcc.org/mskcc/html/12463.cfm	MSKCC	Free
	Partin Tables	http://urology.jhu.edu/Partin_tables	Prostate cancer	
Medical calculators	MedMath	http://smi-web.stanford.edu/people/pcheng/medmath/index.html	Contains 30 formulas	Free
	MedCalc	http://www.med-ia.ch/medcalc/		Free

(Continued)

Table 139-3 **PDA Applications of Interest to the Oncologist (*Continued*)**

Type	Application	Location for Obtaining	Comment	Comment
	ICU Math	http://www.freewarepalm.com/medical/icumath.shtml	50 calculators	Free
	Ca-Tools	http://www.cancer.org/docroot/COM/content/div_TX/COM_5_1x_The_ C-Tools_20.asp?SiteArea=	ACS & Texas Medical Assn Oncology items to prevent, diagnose and treat cancer	Free
	narcConvert	http://www.spazthecat.com	Converts one or more narcotics to equianalgesic doses of another drug	Free
Electronic medical records	Patientkeeper	http://www.patientkeeper.com		$
	ComChart	http://www.comchart.com		$
	ePatient	http://www.iatrosoft.com/		$
	eRecord System	http://www.erecordsystem.com/		$
Practice management	STAT E&M Coder	http://pda.surfnet.nl/palm/preview/34396.html	Assists evaluation and management coding for Medicare	$
	Pocket Med	http://www.pocketmed.org/	Medical billing software	$
Database	HanDBase	http://www.ddhsoftware,com/handbase	Create templates for any purpose	$
Anatomy	Netter's Anatomy	http://www.medicalwizards.com/client/productdesc.aspx?productid=62	Flash cards anatomy images	$
Other resources	pdaMD	http://www.pdamd.com		$
	AvantGo	http://avantgo.com		$
	Skyscape	http://www.skyscape.com		$
	Handheldmd.com	http://www.handheldmd.com		$
	Palmgear	http://www.palmgear.com		$
	Amazon	http://www.medicalamazon.com		$
	Collectivemed	http://www.collectivemed.com/pdasource.shtml		$
	Freewarepalm	http://www.freewarepalm.com		$
	MedicalPocketPC.com	http://www.medicalpocketpc.com		
	Health Palmpilot	http://www.healthypalmpilot.com		

on a related topic, distributed automatically to specific groups, deleted selectively by the system administrator, and can have expiration dates attached. The Web uses a client-server networking scheme that allows remote requests for data from any client personal computer to the host computer, which treats the requesting computer as if it were on its own local network. The Web displays its arrays of text, data, sounds, and video in an application called the browser. Microsoft's Explorer, the Mozilla Foundation's FireFox, and Apple's Safari are the most commonly used browsers. They use a graphical interface to search, retrieve, and display information from any Internet-linked source that is linked to the underlined words or images. They can also be used by anyone to publish information on the Web. It has provided a unified interface to the diverse protocols, data formats, and information archives used on the Internet. It attaches the Internet address of the computer that stores the documents desired, the document's location on that computer, and the language that computer understands to send the information back to the requester. Any information located anywhere in the world with an Internet connection can be interconnected, permitting users to travel through the information by clicking on the hyperlinked words. As of April 2008, the Internet had 165,719,150 sites containing information and administrative content, with 77% of sites having commercial information, and 9% having scientific and educational content.[17]

The Internet has become the principal method for communicating between oncologists. Most cancer cooperative groups use it for communication among their investigators. Some oncologists send their patients' computerized medical records with all reports and actual imaging studies to other physicians and hospitals over the Internet.

As the capability of sending 1-100 gigabytes per second of digital audio or video information on the Internet has become a reality, live transmission of scientific conferences on the Internet as virtual meetings with audio and video presentations and actual slides and posters are commonplace.

Oncologists who have a presence on the Web, and this now includes almost every practicing oncologist should periodically search Google for their listings and take control of the information that is readily available. Gorrindo and Groves recommend that physicians put forward information for their digital identity that is more likely to be seen in the first two pages of a Google search and push back unwanted material.[17] They also recommend having a Web page for your practice or professional activities. In addition, by using privacy settings on social network sites, being aggressive about slanderous material, talking to patients about how they are using the Internet and always being mindful of your Web presence, physicians should be able to better communicate with patients while balancing personal information.

Page Description Languages

Page description languages define the appearance and user interface of the browser screen. They are derived from Standard Generalized Markup Language (SGML). This is a metalanguage used by printers who originally scribbled notes on documents to instruct the typesetters and later codified these shortcuts for universal use. Hypertext Markup Language (HTML) was created as a computer-independent platform for the Internet, using tags to indicate the visual appearance and placement of text and pictures so all computer types see the same page. HTML uses angle-bracketed label tags that surround the text to which they apply and can be nested inside one another to multiple levels. For example, <BOLD>Name</BOLD> would produce **Name** on the screen. Although HTML is the most successful electronic publishing language to date, it can describe only the arrangement of text, images, and push buttons on a page. The deficiencies seen with HTML have all been rectified by the invention of Extensible Markup Language (XML), which combines more efficient processing and flexible linking.[18]

XML permits information to be self-describing, that is, what the information is, not just what it looks like. On the Internet, XML tags might tell the computer that a list of numbers represents the state of your bank account. Thus, the computer will know what the items are, how they are related, and how they should be dealt with. This opens up the possibility of facilitating the searching for and exchanging of scientific data, commercial products, and multilingual documents. It tells the computer how text, images, and video are placed on the screen, irrespective of whether the computer is a desktop PC or a SmartPhone. Thus, the oncologist could pull up a list of medications that the patient is taking and e-mail the list to a colleague, who could then paste the list into his or her hospital's own database record for this patient.

Like HTML, XML uses tags, like parentheses, that must precede and follow the item described; and like quotation marks, tag pairs can be nested inside one another to multiple levels, like a tree structure used to designate hierarchical relationships. These tags are labels that point to a definition in a combined thesaurus and dictionary. To indicate that a patient has a drug allergy to a given drug, the following XML notation would be used: <patient> <name> xxx </name> <drug-allergy>xxx </drug-allergy> </patient>. XML will offer four benefits: (1) A better way to search: Today, a keyword search can return thousands of possibilities. XML tags will filter data and return only the results desired. (2) A better way to distribute and track information: Today, it is difficult to republish content across many sites, and more difficult to track who is reading it. XML will make both feasible. (3) A better way to do business: Today, one can browse through catalogs online. XML tags will allow data to be customized. (4) A better way to do business on the road: Today, Internet graphics bog down and slow Internet connections. With XML, your computer will download only material tagged as text. XML permits specialized markup languages, such as terms for medical record fields in a database or a chemical markup language that graphically renders a molecular structure when a markup term is used. It also allows a choice of multiple linked sites and automatic updating of all links to a given site when that site changes location. Thus, XML will permit a more powerful and useful Internet that will have great value in simplifying medical information management. Thus, computers filled with different kinds of information, run by different companies, and connected to different Web sites could send messages behind the scenes to accomplish our tasks.

With XML as the alphabet and every item of information identified for its common meaning, every discipline, including medicine, will develop a specialized vocabulary for computers. By also having access to most of the information ever created, the Web will then become a semantic Web, as envisioned by its founder, Timothy Berners-Lee.[19] Thus the computer, already a master of mathematics, by using these Web agents, would understand not only the meaning of words and concepts, but also their logical relationships. This would also overcome our inability to easily translate jargon and significantly reduce foreign language barriers. As databases begin to use XML tags to give semantic meaning to their data fields, application-programming interfaces (API) that are short hooks of computer code that allow smaller programs to communicate with larger software operating systems like Windows will permit programmers to allow the operating system to automatically interact with the database on the Web site. As large medical database repositories use this technology, innovative linking of their data to other databases like our desktop EHRs will occur and the Internet will not just be used for human users to call up pre-formatted documents, but computers will be able to share data with other computers.

Messaging Standards

Messaging standards allow applications on the Internet to exchange information in a consistent and secure way. Computers have the capability to send the same information to individuals in e-mail, fax, pager, or voice-mail format. E-mail can exchange letters and documents from within a word-processing application. Directory services allow a common point of information storage for access by groups of users. Authentication insures that all communications are kept secure and private by using encryption techniques. Digital signatures attach a reliable approval signature to documents. Thus, documents can be securely handled, reviewed, and approved among work groups, facilitating scientific collaboration.

Electronic Publishing

Electronic publishing over the Internet is now common; abstracts, selected articles, or entire journals are made available on the date of publication. Aside from archiving issues, some journals permit subscribers to do full text searches, set up personal archives for saving articles and search results, and download articles in a printed format identical to the typeset pages. PubMed Central (<http://www.pubmedcentral.nih.gov>), BioMed Central (<http://www.biomedcentral.com>), and the Public Library of Science (PLOS) (http://www.plos.org) are digital archives of full-text medical journals that agree to make their contents freely available. They also include full-text from journals that are only published electronically. These examples are part of the open-access movement where universities and other institutions are granting itself a license to publish its own faculty's work, irrespective of publication anywhere else. Varmus has summarized the potential advantages of electronic publishing: open access, rapid and wide dissemination, reduced costs, and flexible publication formats,[20] creating healthy debate among the medical establishment.[21]

Search Engines

Computer technology today can increase accessibility to a collection of information. Tomorrow, it will make this information much more useful. Information refinement is an electronic, computer-based process that takes undifferentiated volumes of raw information and converts them into electronic form, extracts the content units, and recombines them into a new form that can be distributed in a variety of ways or recombined into new end products. Primitive refining today uses the literal terms of words, keywords, and synonym lists that rely on word indexes and the searching and indexing of keyword bases. It suffers from poor recall performance and poor precision. Future systems will be able to break all information into usable divisions, strip out the impurities, and turn the data into a basic form that can be reprocessed, refined, and transformed. Until these processes are refined, we rely on search engines (Table 139-4). The most popular search engine is Google (<http://www.google.com>), which can search the Internet for text, images, newsgroup information, news, product information and pricing, catalogs, directories, and scholarly books. Text can include words or phrases segregated by languages, file formats, dates, occurrences, current news specificity, page-specificity, or topic specificity. Images can be searched for related words or phrases, image size, image file types, color, or domains. Already Google has branched beyond Web searching to assist users to find information in product databases, e-mail archives, their own hard drives, and the printed book. Future search engines will search instant messages, music, video, and even conversations using voice-over Internet protocol (VOIP). Other search sites are competing with Google to become more accurate in searching or more effective in presenting search results. Amazon's A9 search engine (<http://www.a9.com>) presents the user with multiple panes, each of which contains a different type of search on a term. For example, it will divide a search for a term into text, pictures, references in books, references in reference books, or database of movies. Past searches can be bookmarked for future reference. My Yahoo's Search (<http://mysearch.yahoo.com>) searches preselected highly relevant sites that can be customized by the user or chosen by Yahoo. Sites can be sorted by categories. Searches can also be saved and new searches can include saved searches. Clusty (<http://www.clusty.com>) groups searches into fold-

Table 139-4 **Internet Portal Search Engines**

Site	Description	URL
Alta-Vista	Fast free-text searching Divides search results by categories; can save searches for review and re-execution	http://www.altavista.com
Amazon's A9		http://www.a9.com
Anonymizer		http://anonymizer.com
Answers.com	Provides direct answers to search queries	http://www.answers.com
AOL	Searches websites, phone numbers, business information	http://search.aol.com
Ask	Ask Jeevwa can; save searches for review and reexecute	http://www.ask.com
Bing	Searches internet, news, encyclopedia, dictionary, stock quotes, movies, and shopping	http://www.bing.com
Blinkx	Automatically searches the internet for words you are typing or reading	http://www.blinkx.com
BrightPlanet	Finds databases that cannot be crawled or indexed by surface web search engines	http://completeplanet.com
Clusty	Divides search results into folders by categories and permits preview of pages	http://www.clusty.com
Dogpile	Searches multiple search engines	http://www.dogpile.com
Euroseek	European source	http://www.euroseek.com
Excite	Concept searching	http://www.excite.com
Co.com	Basic search engine	http://go.com/
Google	Free-text, image searching; most popular site	http://www.google.com
Healia	Medical search engine	(http://www.healia.com
Hotbot	Searches multiple search engines simultaneously	http://hotbot.l.com
Kartoo	sites and gives results in visual form	http://kartoo.com
Lycos		http://www.lycos.com
Medical Health Line	Medical search engine	http://www.healthline.com
MedStory	Medical search engine	http://www.medstorv.com
Mooter	Categorizes search results in onscreen buttons and clusters	http://www.mooter.com
Northern Light	Free-text searches are categorized	http://www.northernlight.com
Shape	3D search engine that matches a drawn shape to images of similar forms	http://shape.cs.princeton.edu/search.html
Webcrawler	Metasearch engine	http://www.webcrawler.com
Yahoo	Subject guide and free-text searching	http://mysearch.yahoo.com

ers. Blinkx (<http:// www.blinkx.com>) creates a toolbar on your desktop that automatically scans the WWW and places in its own window Web links to words you type into your word processor or e-mail program or that are on a Web page. Microsoft's search engine (<http://www.bing.com>) searches the Internet, news, encyclopedia, dictionary, stock quotes, movies, and shopping.

Health-specific search engines such as Healia (http://www.healia.com), MedStory (<http://www.medstory.com>) and HealthLine (http://www.healthline.com) improve on existing search engines by searching not only the Internet, but health-specific sites such as PubMed and ClinicalTrials.gov using health-related taxonomies. These taxonomies may include Medlines' MEdical Subject Headings (MESH; http://www.nlm.nih.gov/mesh), Systematized Nomenclature of Medicine-Clinical Terms (SNOMED-CT; <http://www.ihtsdo.org/our-standards>) that is a clinical vocabulary, and the National Cancer Institute's (NCI) Thesaurus (http://ncit.nci.nih.gov). Other sites include health experts to refine the health terms and physicians (see Organized Wisdom at <http://www.organizedwisdom.com>).

Health Care Portals

Health care portals can be divided into three categories. First are the content-oriented sites, which divide nicely into four subgroups: patient-centric (<http://www.cancer.net>), provider-centric (<http://www.asco.org>), hybrids such as WebMD (<http://www.webmd.com>), and companies that have a product to sell, such as A.D.A. M. Software's Interactive Anatomy or Health Illustrated Encyclopedia (<http://www. adam.com>). These companies are comparable to publishers and information media. Second are the commerce sites, including Internet drugstores and global health care marketplaces that offer medical products and services. These companies compare with stores. Third are the transaction-based companies such as Emdeon that plan to reduce health care transaction costs by linking key health care constituencies, such as payers, providers, consumers, diagnostic agencies, and suppliers, providing patient enrollment, benefits administration, referral claims and tracking, third-party transactions, electronic prescriptions and reporting, and pharmacy benefit management. As a summary of the diverse cancer information available on the Internet, Table 139-5 lists topics available for each tumor type.

Table 139-5 **Professional and Patient Cancer Information on the Internet**

1. Overview for professional and patient cancers by body location/system
   Alphabetical list of cancers
2. Anatomy/physiology
3. Genetics, genetic testing, and causes
4. Risk factors
5. Self-risk assessment
6. Detection/screening information
   Specific tests
7. Prevention
8. Signs and symptoms
9. Diagnosis
   Procedures
   Imaging studies
   Laboratory studies
10. Cell classification
11. Staging
12. Guidelines
13. Clinical trials
    Open with eligibility and summary information
    Closed with abstracts/full-text citations
    Online access and data management
14. Types of therapy by stage/modality
15. Follow-up
16. Statistics
    Understanding
    Data sources
    By cancer type
17. Atlas incidence and mortality
18. Advocacy and support
19. Clinical research
20. Complementary and alternative medicine
21. Discussion groups
22. Disease classifications and coding
    ICD-9
    CPT
23. Educational programs/meetings
24. Headline and archived news
25. Pharmaceutical information
26. Public policy
27. Practice management, precertifications, seimbursements
28. Coping with cancer
    Advanced directives
    Supportive care and resources
    Side effects of cancer
    Complications caused by cancer
    Sexuality
    Survivorship
    Caregiver
    Financial
29. Toxicity criteria
30. Cancer literature
    PubMed
    Journal links
31. Research programs and funding
32. Patient tools
    Questions for your oncologist
    Medical record
    Personal diary
    Buddies
    Calendar
    Discussion groups
33. Resources
    Cancer centers and hospitals
    Foundations and Societies
    Government Agencies
    Medical dictionary
    Physician and facility finder

Because of the vastness, reliability, and ephemeral nature of Internet medical information, every oncologist needs to have an understanding of the basic issues related to information available on the Internet. It is important to know the expertise, conflicts of interests, and biases of the developers and sponsors of a site, as well as the site's purpose and intended audience. Is the original source of content identified, current, and valid? Is the user's confidentiality protected, and if not, who has access to information about the users?

Health 2.0/Web 2.0

The Internet has evolved beyond its interconnected web sites and static information generated by experts to a medium where relationships are established, information is aggregated and shared by experts and non-experts (user-generated content). Online communities have developed and patients are able to communicate their health care needs with caregivers and their offices and payers electronically as the Web becomes a desktop computer operating system like Windows or the Mac. Specific tools of the new Internet 2.0 are discussed below.

Blogs

Blogs—short for Web logs—and vlogs (video logs) are Web sites that are easy to set up. They provide information and opinion to audiences that are drawn by common interests. They have become personalized publishing sites of one's musings that can be constantly updated, utilize any form of electronic media, link to any Internet site, and can include online discussions without filters, oversight, or accountability. Blogs have become a genuine alternative to our mainstream information outlets. Suddenly everyone can become a publisher and a critic. Blogs have grown exponentially because of an innovation called the "permalink": a unique Web address for each posting, which remains accessible indefinitely, on every blog, not just the Web page, which can change frequently. Linking posts rapidly disseminates information, giving blogs almost a viral quality. With efficient blog search engines available, blogs have become a powerful "relationship generator" that can rapidly bring local, national, or worldwide attention to any subject. Blogs can host music, video, and photos. They are being used creatively as a substitute for e-mail, as project management software for collaborations in a company, as an up-to-date manual, and even by scientists as an experimental notebook since it is a written-down, date-stamped, and backed-up document. Blogs have become a major factor in medical communications. To locate blogs of interest, use <http://www.kinja.com>, <http://www. bloglines. com>, <http://www.feedster. com>, <http://www. technorati.com>, or <http://www.blogdex.net>. Blog sites that cater to the cancer patient include CaringBridge (<http://www.caringbridge. org/>) and TypePad (<http://www.typepad.com>. To create your own blog, go to Google's <http:// www.blogger.com> or Microsoft's <http://www.Spaces.MSN. com> and create a free account. Name your blog, study the templates, and choose a template for your blog. Write something interesting and then register at <http://www.Feedburner.com> to find out if anyone's reading your blog and which posts are liked best.

Really Simple Syndication

Using a software type known as RSS (Really Simple Syndication), custom-tailored bulletins that are continuously updated from thousands of sites can be linked to your blog or browser without having to manually visit each site. By clicking on one of these headlines on your site that is linked to the parent site, one can get the full story. Thus the user, not the Internet site, determines what information is seen and how often it is updated. RSS uses XML formats for the syndication of Internet content that can be read by a newsreader that is either a standalone program or part of a browser. Newsreaders can bring together the latest postings from your favorite blogs in a single place. RSS technology could be used to send a physician medical alerts and reminders, and since RSS readers can be embedded into database applications, users can automate database searching that gives constantly updated reports.

Shared Internet Resources

Sharing resources in large virtual communities is exemplified by sites such as Del.icio.us (http://del.icio.us), Flickr (http://www.flickr.com), and Digg (http://www.digg.com>) Del.icio.us and Digg let users choose, list, search for, tag with keywords, share with friends, and rate Internet sites. Flickr lets users post, organize, keyword tag, geotag and share pictures online. PeerClip (http://www. peerclip.com) is similar to Del.icio.us and Digg except that its participants are limited to health care personnel.

Social Networking

The two largest social networking sites for the general public are MySpace (http://myspace.com) and Facebook (http://www.facebook.com) and both have attracted many patients to create a presence on the Internet as well as to establish links to friends and business associates. Patient-oriented sites that include many of the features of MySpace and Facebook but include online journals, patient support group, some with physician guidance, and health-related information include MedHelp (http:// www.medhelp.com>), DailyStrength (http://www.dailvstrength.com), and PatientsLikeMe (http://www.patientslike me.com). Recently Twitter has become popular as a micro-blogging site sending and receiving short massages or "tweets" for repid communication between hugh numbers of people with similar interests (<http:www.twitter.com>).

Professional Networking

These sites can offer the ability to post questions to one's network or the larger community, join discussion forums, or review job postings. You can form connections with other members and be notified of any changes in their profiles. Linkedin (http://www.linkedin.com) is the largest site with over 20 million members. In health care, Sermo (http:// www.sermo.com) with 60,000 members is the largest and permits physicians, who must be verified, to post questions and answers on clinical topics. The site permits the pharmaceutical industry to monitor the topics without identification of physicians who are participating in the discussions. iMedExchange (http://www.imedexchange.com) allows members to discuss clinical topics but also has sections for business practice and personal interests. Within3 (http://www.within3.com) only networks and does not collect information discussed so it is used for both clinical and basic research discussions and for patient referrals.

Wiki

The new Internet can accumulate the collective wisdom of the entire online community using Wiki software. A Wiki is a Web site on which anyone with appropriate authority can post material, do searches, and make changes fast, without using arcane commands, and with the ability to track changes and revisions. Volunteers have posted 2,436,787 articles as of June 2008 in over 50 languages, creating the Wikipedia, the largest encyclopedia in the world. (<http://www.wikipedia.com>). This application can be used for creating textbooks, articles, manuals, catalogs, schedules, or structural database forms. Based on the principles of Wikipedia, a group of medical schools, governmental health institutes such as the NIH, CDC, FDA and others are creating Medpedia (<http://www.medpedia.com>), a free collaborative encyclopedia of health, medicine and the body.

Health Care Applications

Today, essential Internet health care applications include e-content with patients having almost equal access to medical information on par with the professionals. It includes e-connectivity linking all health care participants for clinical objectives, such as diagnostic and laboratory test reporting, EHRS, prescriptions, e-mail, and administrative purposes with appointments, billing inquiries, claims processing, eligibility, and referral authorizations; e-commerce with purchasing of drugs and medical advice; and e-care management with disease management and home monitoring of patients.

Personal Electronic Health Records (PHR)

One of the more persisting indictments of our health care system is the passive role taken by most patients. This has evolved because patients lack medical knowledge and judgment and find it difficult to compile their physician encounters, medical tests, medications and hospitalizations because few of their health care providers or institutions have functioning EHRs. Patients also have little need to concern themselves with the cost of their care and without access to appropriate comparative information are unable to consistently choose quality and cost-effective medical care.

Today, most patients have their health information managed by individual physicians and institutions and few have all this information available in any single location. However with secure accessibility of their medical information, the conversion of their paper medical records to electronic records available over the Internet, personal health information is starting to be managed by patients. Just as the Internet has simplified our ability to consolidate our financial information, media collections, and personal libraries, it will facilitate the development of the patient's PHR. Many of our patients have grown up with the Internet and are accustomed to communicating with others and storing personal data on the Internet. Having a PHR will become commonplace for them.[22,23] This PHR will enable patients to keep track of their medical history. This information can be stored online and accessed by any health care provider who is given permission by the patient to view the information. Content can range from simple demographic data to a complete medical history, physical findings, and tests assembled from many sources. The American Society of Clinical Oncology (ASCO), along with cancer advocacy and quality groups, is taking the first steps to encourage oncologists to provide parts of the PHR to all cancer patients with the creation of the Cancer Treatment Report and the Survivorship Care Plan.[24] As care and disease management activities become a larger component of the health care system, patients with chronic diseases like cancer will have more of their care given and monitored in their home with electronic resources and services requiring patients and their caregivers to maintain PHRs.

Today we have few standalone PHRs and even fewer PHRs that are integrated with EHRs. Integration over the Internet is key because it would then permit combining other patient services such as appointment scheduling, patient-physician emails, electronic prescriptions, and laboratory and imaging results. However, PHRs may become a major component of our health system sooner than we think. In December 2006, the Center for Disease Control and Prevention along with Wal-Mart, Intel and ten other large corporations—all fed up with the rising costs of health care and the lack of use of basic information technology tools in patient care, announced the development of a digital health record for all their employees that will be held in an electronic data repository linked to providers, hospitals, pharmacies, and patients so that "consumers coordinate their own health care among doctors, hospitals and pharmacies."[25] It would allow consumers and insurers to evaluate price and performance data reducing administration overhead, duplicative tests, and medical errors and permit physicians to measure, which treatments worked best. The coalition will use incentives and market pressures to induce health care participants who take care of these corporate employees to participate. The records will remain the property of the patient and using data that has eliminated all patient identities will be used for data mining. This plan needs to be watched closely since Wal-Mart is the largest corporation in the world, is the third largest pharmacy in the United States, is rapidly placing mini-clinics staffed by advanced practice nurses in their stores, is a master at effectively using information technology, and is making their employees the central figure in controlling their health information.

Recently Microsoft's HealthVault (http://www.healthvault.com) and Google's Google Health (http://www.google.com/health) have begun offering free sites for patients to store their medical data provided by cooperating physician offices, hospitals, commercial laboratories, pharmaceutical data hubs like Rxhub and Surescripts, payers, and medical device manufacturers to permit the patient to have a PHR populated with accurate medical data. Patients will be able to educate themselves about their medical conditions or medications taken using the search engines provided. Patients can be reminded when to take medication and if their medications have any potential serious drug interactions. Patients can also control this secured information to determine which health care provider or organization can have access to their data. The Centers for Medicare and Medicaid Services has instituted a PHR pilot in South Carolina that will provide patients with their Medicare claims data. When Walmart, Microsoft, Google, Medicare, and many national payers agree on something it is unusual and important and patient-centered health care is on the horizon. Many of our cancer patient advocacy groups are behind the concept. Thus, PHRs will be part of the EHR landscape whether just providing basic medical information, complete access to the EHR, medical reports or some other combination. ASCO's Chemotherapy Planning Reports and Cancer Treatment Summaries are the only reports for cancer patients to help them begin their PHR efforts.

Thus, with the increasing consumerism of the Internet, PHRs that are maintained by patients and EHRs that are maintained by physicians, cancer centers, and institutions have become available over the Internet to automatically synchronize updated patient information, and decision support reminders. This will permit the seamless electronic transfer of information from the patient to the physician for medical vetting and then on to all the other health care participants. Innovative desktop electronic records that permit easy customization for the physician's practice, Internet publishing, connectivity, and SmartPhone synchronization are appearing.

The Markle Foundation and most of the electronic PHR service providers in order to protect patient health information security and assuage patient fears, have recently signed the Connecting for Health guidelines that addresses authentication of consumers, audit trails, restrictions on identifying information, portability of patient data, security and system requirements, provisions for consumer consent, and policies for notifying patients when information is breached (http://www.connectingforhealth.org/).

Personally controlled online health data will transform the health care system and alter responsibilities and relationships between patients and physicians. Physicians will need to understand how to work with these new systems and decide how their office data will interact with the PHR. Large corporations involved in information technology will become new important players in the health care system. There will be many ramifications of this paradigm shift. To better understand this phenomenon, the reader is referred to articles by Steinbrook,[26]

Hartzband and Groopman,[27] and Mandl and Kohane.[28]

Electronic Patient-Physician Communication

As non-emergency communication between physicians and patients becomes commonplace, it is imperative that oncologists understand their new security and documentation responsibilities. The American Medical Informatics Association has published guidelines for electronic communication with patients that summarize turnaround time, privacy issues, sensitivity of subject matter, identification, protocol, and behavior (<http://www.amia. org/pubs/fpubl. html>).[29] Miller discusses the many issues that oncologists should consider when setting up programs to use the Internet for patient-physician communication.[30] Although many patients would like to use e-mail with their oncologists, many oncologists remain hesitant because of concerns about time commitment, reimbursement, confidentiality, and infrastructure. Our patients will prevail and all oncologists should encourage this technology and adopt practice-wide protocols for dealing with electronic messages from patients that ensure HIPAA compliance. This will lead to enhanced patient satisfaction and improve the quality of cancer care. Although it is not a complete Internet-based EHR, the Society of Gynecologic Oncologists' database (<http://www. sgodb.com/>) is a basic tumor registry that allows oncologists to track patients in their office using an application service provider (ASP) that specializes in information technology management, software, and database development from a remote, secure server.

Sites such as RelayHealth (<http:// www. relayhealth.com>) provide a secure and encrypted HIPAA-compliant site for e-mail with patients and other providers, e-prescriptions with drug-drug interactions, drug-disease interactions, and allergy checking, along with electronic billing of patients for these services and that are being reimbursed by some insurance carriers based on a RelayHealth pilot.[31] In contrast to free-form messages, it can use customized clinically structured, branched questions that generate concise, structured messages. Messages can be triaged automatically. Numerous academic health care networks have established Web sites that are providing Internet access for all transactions taking place between the patient, physician, hospital, clinic, commercial laboratory, imaging centers, and the payers, creating regional Regional Health Information Organizations.

Online patient self-reporting is a feasible long-term strategy for toxicity symptom monitoring during chemotherapy, even among patients with advanced cancer and high symptom burdens. However, as noted by Basch et al., without explicit reminders and clinician feedback, patients demonstrated limited voluntary interest in self-reporting between visits.[32]

Oncologists are beginning to evaluate their and their patients use of the Internet. Pereira and colleagues explored the use of the Internet by breast cancer patients.[33] They found that of the 107 surveys returned, 74% came from patients and 26% from family members. The majority of Internet users desired more information on their cancer (91%), checked into information given to them by their provider (66%), researched other treatment options (63%), and obtained information on alternative therapies (61%). Most were satisfied with their Internet experience and spoke to their physician about their findings. Chen and Siu discussed the impact of the media and the Internet on information gathering by Canadian patients and oncologists.[34] They concluded that cancer patients in Canada commonly search for information on the Internet. It did not seem to affect the oncologist-patient relationship. Helft and colleagues surveyed ASCO members on their Internet use with patients.[35] Responding oncologists indicated that 30% of their patients used the Internet to gain cancer information, adding 10 minutes to the clinical encounter. Forty-four percent noted that they had difficulty discussing Internet information and 9% felt threatened.

Strategic assistance is needed to provide guidance for patients to better understand their cancer and interpret this information on the Internet more effectively. Bichakjian and colleagues warn patients that too many sites found through using search engines have sparse, and at times inaccurate information about malignant melanoma.[36] They found that the majority of sites lacked complete basic melanoma information and 14% contained inaccuracies. It remains the duty of oncologists to be familiar with medical Internet sites and to educate their patients about linking only to sites that have reputable information. An issue of the British Medical Journal is devoted to the theme of evaluating the quality of health information on the Internet.[37] Thus oncologists must be prepared to guide their patients on the Internet. The National Library of Medicine (NLM) and the American College of Physicians (ACP) are using MedlinePlus (<http://www.medlineplus. gov>) as information, prepared therapy prescriptions to give patients appropriate Internet information for their medical conditions. Oncology.net (<http://www. oncology.net>), ASCO's site for cancer patients, is distributing cancer information prescription pads to oncologists to assist them with these endeavors.

Research Collaboration

The Internet is acting as a potent catalyst for scientific advances by permitting new ties among researchers at any worldwide site. Marshall and Haley discuss their experience with this Internet technology for setting up a research collaboration with 15 laboratories and clinics, collecting and maintaining an Internet database that was more efficient and secure than through conventional methods of paper, filing cabinets, and locked doors.[38] Colleagues can, with permission, be linked directly or by e-mail or fax to any computer on the Internet. Mountains of data, large electronic meetings, bulletin boards where questions can be answered almost instantaneously, and electronic journal publications are commonplace. Simon et al. discuss how electronic medical records (EMRs) can bridge patient care and research in oncology.[39]

File Sharing

As online file sharing has evolved, new methods are emerging to make it readily possible to exchange material online without using a central file server. Currently, the Internet requires a host computer to deal with any request for information from all computers (client computers). In the near future, any computer will be able to talk directly to any other computer without a host computer connection. This peer-to-peer sharing of information is based on the Simple Object Access Protocol (SOAP), which enables the network to become the computer. An operating system spanning the Internet permits any computer connected to the Internet to connect directly to any other computer, eliminating the need for host computers and opening up the possibility of computers sharing their unused processing power with other Internet users.[40]

With the appropriate adherence to HIPAA regulations, permission from the patient, the use of a controlled medical vocabulary like SNOMED (Systematized Nomenclature of Medicine), and universal identifiers for patients and physicians, it should be possible for a patient's latest medical data residing on multiple computers linked on the Internet to synchronize with a medical record in a given physician's office, giving the physician access to the latest patient medical data. Any doctor's office or hospital with a Web-connected computer will be able to share their stored records, via automated machine-to-machine processes, with any other doctor's office or hospital. An individual patient record would be maintained in a distributed fashion over the

Internet, obtainable and aggregated into a complete whole automatically and immediately on demand by any authorized Web-connected computer at any time and from anywhere. The evolving EMR will consist of many components linking patients, practices, clinics, imaging centers, hospitals, health plans, laboratories, and pharmacies over the Internet in a confidential, secure, and standardized format. We will use the Internet for practice management; scheduling, visits, procedures, and laboratory tests; documentation; referrals; prescriptions; patient eligibility for clinical trials; decision support; analyzing patterns of care; error checking; and e-mail communication.

Medical Information Management

Medical Education

Knowledge can be defined as the organization, analysis, and interpretation of data and observations that convey a higher degree of understanding. It is imperative that oncologists have direct access to knowledge for problem solving, and the ability to browse for curiosity's sake and to annotate and personalize knowledge. All major sources of oncologic information have become computerized. These include bibliographic information, such as CANCERLIT; factual information, such as Physician Data Query (PDQ); full text, such as this book; and knowledge bases, such as ONCOCIN.

Computerized Patient Records

In 1989, in order to improve the usefulness of the medical record, the computer-based patient record (CPR) was coined and defined by a committee of the Institute of Medicine of the National Academy of Sciences. Clinical oncology, with its emphasis on clinical trials and longitudinal data for its patients, would seem to be a natural target for automated records. Today, however, most oncologists still do not use EHRs because standards defining software tools, functions, or datasets are nonexistent; patient data remain insecure; physicians are expected to underwrite the costs of these technologies; software vendor viability is suspect; worries remain about how quickly programs can become obsolete; and one EMR program cannot easily exchange information with another.

Recently a snapshot of how physicians actually use and view EHRs was recently published.[41] It found that 4% of physicians were using a fully functional EHR and 13% used a basic system as defined in Table 139-6. These physicians who used EHRs believed that they improve the quality of care and are satisfying to use. However, both those who use these systems and those who do not feel that without significant financial incentives EHRs will not be widely adopted.

Recently, government and other concerned private parties have finally begun addressing these problems. With the maturing of computer, communication, and information technologies; acceptance by payers to reimburse for and the public to use electronic communication with their doctors; and the recognition of standards permitting cross-platform semantic understanding of data with information that is encrypted, secure, and authentic, oncologists must begin to participate in the defining of oncology tools, functions, and datasets as components of EMRs.

To help the oncologist, ASCO established an EHR Workgroup to direct ASCO's EHR initiatives and to help represent the needs of oncologists in health information technology. The Workgroup has begun to define components and functionalities of the oncology EHR. It has been able to get cooperation from many oncology EHR vendors to incorporate ASCO's Chemotherapy Treatment Plan and Treatment Summary reports into their products. These reports include (1) how oncologists plan to treat their patient's cancer; (2) a treatment summary given to the patient after completing treatment, which outlines their surgery, radiation, and chemotherapy treatments; and, (3) a plan for follow-up care, which describes how cancer survivors should monitor their health including guidance on screening tests, potential long-term side effects of therapies, and proposed follow-up visits.[42] The Workgroup has established a dedicated area for EHRs on the ASCO website at <http://www.asco.org/ehr>. An EHR Policy Roundtable was held for all oncology health care organizations early in 2007. Roundtable participants included cancer cooperative groups, cancer centers and academic institutions, government agencies, community and academic oncologists, cancer registry organizations, patient advocates, public and private insurance carriers, and vendors. In 2008, ASCO published The Oncology Electronic Health Record Field Guide: Selecting and Implementing an EHR that is a practical guide to help the oncologist purchase and implement an EHR (<http://www.asco.org/ehr>). The Field Guide is the only oncology-specific consumer manual developed to guide practitioners in a variety of settings—such as community-based, hospital outpatient, and academic—in the selection of current and future oncology-specific EHRs for clinical practice and management as well as quality-of-care measurement and improvement. The topics in this guide address core functionalities desired in an oncology-specific EHR and includes identifying an EHR project team; making a selection; building a budget; using the EHR to support quality of care and patient safety; and post-implementation management. At the end of each chapter, actionable tools and resources are made available to assist in the decision-making process. The Working Group began to define some important EHR functional elements that are unique in an oncology-specific EHR that are listed below:

- Tumor staging—Tumor-node-metastases (TNM) nomenclature and others
- Multidisciplinary and data-intensive workflow—pathology, lab, imaging
- Chemotherapy dosing and administration
- Toxicity assessment and management
- Clinical trial and protocol management
- Drug inventory management

Functionalities of the oncology EHR as defined by the Working Group are listed in Table 139-7. The Working Group has also summarized the financial, medication management and administrative incentives for purchasing an EHR in Table 139-8. The key oncology-specific documentation required in an oncology EHR is shown in Table 139-9. One of the major uses of the oncology EHR is to document and manage the chemotherapy administration process. The Workgroup has defined the workflow issues, guidelines for chemotherapy ordering, preparation and administration and appropriate alerts that should be functioning in an electronic chemotherapy administration module.[43,44]

Health care is being fundamentally changed by a coalition of forces, including employers reallocating benefit funding, health plan realignments, consumer action, and government mandates that will influence public policy to encourage the adoption of information and communication technologies. This will transform medicine by allowing gains in health care safety, efficiency, and cost savings.

Oncology practices have been hit hard by changes in Medicare and managed care. Oncologists are being forced to examine and control their costs, bet-

Table 139-6 **Core EHR Functionalities as Defined by the Institute of Medicine**

Core Functionalities	Other Functionalities
Health information and data	Electronic communication and connectivity
Results management	Patient support
Order entry and support	Administrative support
Decision support	Reporting and population health management

Source: Institute of Medicine. Key capabilities of an electronic health record system: letter report. Washington, DC: National Academies Press, 2003.

Table 139-7 EHR Functional Element Defined by ASCO's Electronic Health Record Workgroup

EHR Functional Element	How It Is Used in the Practice
View patient information	Review patient's symptoms or chief complaints, medication list, test results, and other clinical documentation
Gather data	Build electronic patient charts that are searchable. Build patient charts from customizable templates
Compile data	Pull together patient or practice population, histories, and graph it or map it for analysis. Report generation
Query patient or practice data to generate standard and/or custom reports	Assist in evaluating, diagnosing, and reviewing acute or chronic diseases and treatment regimens and provide appropriate clinical alerts and warnings based on established guidelines. Interoperability with other systems
Clinical decision support	Interact with internal practice management and other internal information systems (eg, laboratory information system – LIS); interface with external hospital, lab, imaging, pharmacies, and payers
Search capabilities	Query the database for reports on clinical issues and costs
Patient management	Manage the individual patient's acute and chronic diseases and conditions
Practice marketing	Provide information regarding types of services you perform most often. Provide analysis on your patients' clinical conditions, referral base, and patient population
Standardization	Standardize disease management goals and treatment regimens for patient groups within your practice
Billing and coding	Provide internal checks and balances with ICD and CPT codes to details of the patient encounter; integrate E&M coding and HCPCS codes. Order entry Order labs, imaging, referrals, and other non-medications
Chemotherapy ordering	Initiate chemotherapy orders, associated ancillary therapies, and dose modifications with proper authorization and confirmation
e-Prescribing	Authorize and manage prescription refills. Access formulary information. Route new prescriptions online to pharmacy
Communication	Communicate online with patients, colleagues, payers, hospitals, and pharmacies
Provide built-in compliance and regulatory guidance	Compliance
Clinical trials	Conduct research, registry, and clinical trial activities
Patient interaction	Incorporate information originating from the patient, including data from a personal health record (PHR) and medical and patient devices
Quality measurement	Use data to participate in quality measurement programs

ter track their inventories, and be more concerned with their billing and coding. They are also standardizing treatments and care plans, increasing documentation of the health care they provide, and measuring and collecting quality data for negotiations with payers—all processes requiring the right kind of computerized tools. As EHRs begin to address these requirements and seamlessly link with oncology-specific practice management software, all oncologists will have EMRs routinely deployed across all health care settings. The oncologist will be able to seamlessly create, maintain, edit, display, and manipulate all the data stored in the individual's record. Aggregates of data will be stored in a clinical data repository, which will serve as the storage facility database for EHRs, facilitating health research and clinical trials. Table 139-10 lists basic medical- and oncology-specific data elements for an EHR.

The Institute of Medicine study listed 12 key attributes of the CPR that have become the gold standard by which all EHRs are judged. These are listed in Table 139-11. In addition to these 12 attributes, more recent underpinnings have been identified as enablers of a robust EHR. These include the need for a minimum standardized clinical data dictionary to define the data elements required in the EHR and the need to support a controlled vocabulary that defines precisely how a term is used so that there is a uniform understanding of its meaning in clinical medicine. Further provisions will require that ambulatory medical records be created in oncology offices and that they be integrated seamlessly with hospital information systems, such that there is a virtual longitudinal record. Most likely, the set of technologies that make up the Internet will be used to provide the foundation for creating the EHR that will be shared by the patient, provider, and payer, with appropriate encryption, security, confidentiality, and audit trails. Fortunately, clinical message sending is being standardized around the Health Level Seven (HL-7) version 3 standard and XML. HL-7 permits the transfer of information that is vendor-, application-, and foreign language-neutral.

As oncologists become more focused on cancer screening and prevention, and as data management of clinical trials becomes automated, disease management will become an accepted part of our practice management, and the EHR will become indispensable. We will see collaborative online efforts to develop clinical pathways (multidisciplinary plans of care that standardize patient treatment) and bring decision support to the oncologist at the point of care. This will assist us in practicing more evidence-based medicine (bringing current scientific knowledge to the oncologist for point-of-care decision making). To reduce errors and enforce documentation of chemotherapy administration, Prescher-Hughes describes the setting up of practice protocol guidelines for the oncologist's office that are stored on the computer.[45] Table 139-12 lists elements of this protocol list.

Oncologists may be surprised that oncology and general medical practice have been criticized for not delivering state-of-the-art care. Specifically, these reports criticized the health care system for not using information technology effectively and not having a quality monitoring system capable of regular reporting on the quality of patient care. Government and payers, in their at-

Table 139-8 Financial, Medication Management, and Administrative Management Incentives for the Oncology EHR

Financial Incentives

- Measure and analyze office and clinician productivity. Cost reduction and savings can be realized over time.
- Identify hidden costs (how much you pay) for medical records staff and space against new revenues (how much that space would generate if you turned it into a lab or other revenue-generating space).
- Flag missing or insufficient documentation for payers.
- Receive alerts for billing errors and missing information.
- Use the correct billing code for diagnosis, procedure, treatment, and Evaluation and Management (E&M) support for billing decisions.
- Participate in quality monitoring and performance measurement.
- Reduce or eliminate transcription costs.
- Obtain malpractice insurance savings from many carriers.
- Simplify information gathering for correspondence, hospital admissions notes, pre-certifications, auditing, legal purposes, and patient chart requests.

Medication management incentives

- Embed clinical decision support, including chemotherapy dose ranges and maximum dose thresholds.
- Order lab tests, access results and have them auto-populate fields in the patient record (This is important! You want to minimize double entry.)
- Manage internal drug inventory.
- Standardize and automate the ordering process.
- Receive automatic alerts for allergies and adverse medication reactions, including drug-drug and drug-disease interactions.
- Calculate and modify doses based on evidence-based guidelines.
- Incorporate electronic prescribing (e-prescribing).

Administrative incentives

- Improve communication and workflow operations.
- Measure, track, and report on payer reimbursement.
- Manage patient schedules, no-shows, and reschedules.
- Eliminate lost charts.

Table 139-9 **Oncology-Specific Documentation Required in an Oncology EHR**

Provide menu-driven site/histology/pathology findings.
Manage patient response to treatment on flow sheets.
Document intent and goals of adjuvant/curative versus palliative therapy.
Document patient performance status per standardized guidelines.
Maintain list of co-morbid conditions and major toxicities expected to complicate chemotherapy.
Plan and manage chemotherapy/biotherapy regimens.
Manage and automate body surface area (BSA), starting doses, and dose adjustments.
Manage chemotherapy delivery – IV and oral, number of cycles, duration.
Document drug administration process.
Track duration of treatment and number of planned cycles.
Schedule and document radiation therapy and/or maintain results.
Assess pain and supportive care needs.
Manage patients on clinical trials.

tempts to make health care more efficient, are also looking at patterns of health care treatment and how to define and measure quality health care. To answer our critics, ASCO's National Initiative on Cancer Care Quality (NICCQ) was set up to develop a prototype for a national system that could monitor the quality of cancer care.[46] As part of its mission, the NICCQ has been able to define a dataset (data dictionary) for common cancers that, along with other oncology datasets, could be used as an oncology component of an EHR.

To help oncologists begin to measure quality in their offices, ASCO set up the Quality Oncology Practice Initiative (QOPI). The initiative assessed quality measures that included items derived from clinical guidelines, common sense items with high face validity and clinical relevance, and items related to physician-patient interactions. Its purpose was to become a tool for oncology offices to compare themselves with benchmarks reflecting quality cancer care and thereby become recognized by some type of certification. The QOPI presentation at ASCO's 2004 annual meeting used keypad technology to assess the interest of oncologists to measure quality care given in their offices by using computerized tools. Of the attendees, 50% already had a quality improvement effort, 13% used an EMR, 38% used some simple computer programs to gather patient data, 42% used seven or more standing orders for administering chemotherapy with 56% using guidelines in their standing order, 76% would participate in future QOPI initiatives, 84% wanted help in collecting aggregate practice data and physician-specific data, and 88% had Internet access in their offices.

Although 80% of cancer care in the United States is provided in the community setting, very little of the data collected is available. However, with appropriate financial incentives from the government and other payers to provide a seamless, cost-effective approach to managing medical information this data can be collected and benefit patients, providers, payers, government, and vendors. There is a consensus among those in informatics and in many governmental agencies (see below) that the time is right for the computer, communication, and information technologies to bring EHRs into our offices within 5 years. Oncologists must begin to educate themselves about using this technology so they have a role in its dissemination.

The ultimate goal of using these technologies is to have all of our medical information, practice management, and patient education needs in oncology accessible on our computer; to reduce unnecessary paperwork; to be reimbursed fairly for our work; and to contribute to the development of an efficient health care system based on evidence-based data that is responsive to the needs of all health care constituents. We must be able to incorporate patient-specific decision support and physician reminders into our point-of-care patient activities. Electronic links across care settings will not only facilitate collaborative and coordinated approaches among care givers, but also permit the real-time tracking and monitoring of the quality of our cancer care activities. The reader is referred to an excellent tutorial on the EMR at the American College of Physician's Website (<http://www.acponline.org/journals/news/apr04/emrs.htm#resources>) and the ASCO Website at <http//:www.asco.org/ehr for additional information on EHRs.

Currently ASCO notes that fewer than 5 % of clinical oncologists use EHRs in their practices because of the lack of IT products that support key oncology functions, interoperability standards and data definitions that an be used by vendors in development of oncology-specific EHRs. The NCI is engaged in development of the cancer Biomedical informatics Grid (caBIG), an information network dedicated to the discovery of new approaches for the detection, diagnosis , treatment, and prevention of cancer, ultimately improving patient outcomes. Recently, ASCO and the NCI, who both share common goals in promoting the development and use of EHRs by practicing oncologists, have agreed to through the "Clinical Oncology Requirements for the EHR" (CORE) project Jointly they will represent oncology in helping to define Medicare's EHR adoption incentive program and the planned development of certification requirements for an oncology-specific EHRs by the Certification Commission for Health information Technology (CCHIT).

Hospital Information Systems

Hospital information systems can be divided into six levels of organization. Level 1 encompasses billing and accounting applications. Level 2 includes departmental applications such as laboratory, radiology, pharmacy, materials management, and order management. Level 3 covers clinical orders applications such as point-of-care charting, clinical process and provider profiling, and communication with ancillary services such as home care and practice management. Level 4 has enterprise clinical care charting that includes master patient index, data warehouses, EMRs, and ambulatory charting. Level 5 encompasses a repository of member financial, clinical, and demographic data in an electronic data repository. Finally, level 6 has applications for analyzing health care outcomes and disease management.

Wirtschafter and colleagues implemented a computerized consultant extender for a breast cancer clinical protocol that used algorithms to produce a 95% compliance rate among 75 local physicians who used the system, as compared with a 64% rate for cancer center physicians who did not use the automated system.[47] ONCOCIN is an expert system, in use at Stanford University, for assisting oncologists to manage patients on chemotherapy protocols.[48,49] It is both a medical record and an advice system that records the course of the patient on a protocol, and it can assume an active role in adapting the protocol to the individual patient. It can determine drug doses based on time schedule, toxicity, and blood counts. When oncology patient care stipulated by the computer was compared with care given by oncology fellows, similar levels of competency were seen.

Numerous oncology medical records have been implemented at cancer centers to facilitate all aspects of patient care, to interact with hospital information systems and with data management offices, and to maintain patient and protocol charts. The CLIN system implemented at the Memorial Sloan-Kettering Cancer Center by Serber was one of the earliest systems that implemented an oncology protocol record with complete data management and statistical tools.[50] The OCIS (Oncology Clinical Information System) of the Johns Hopkins Hospital is a time-oriented tabular and graphic database with a meaningful grouping of related information that links patient data and procedural support.[51] It interconnects mainframe, minicomputers, and micro-

Table 139-10 ■ **Data Elements for Personal, Provider, and Oncology Medical Records**

Common Data Elements	Personal Health Data Elements	Provider Data Elements
Patient Identification elements	*	*
Emergency Contacts	*	*
Lifetime health history	*	*
Immunizations, allergies, family history, occupational history, environmental exposures, social history, medical history, treatments, procedures, medicines, outcomes		
Laboratory results	*	*
Emergency care information	*	*
Provider identification and contact information	*	*
Treatment plans and instructions	*	*
Health risk factor profile preventive services and results	*	*
Health insurance coverage information	*	*
Correspondence	*	*
Access and confidentiality information	*	*
Audit log	*	*
Self-care trackers: nutrition, activity, medication	*	*
Health care proxies, living wills, power of attorney	*	*
Sociodemographic identifiers gender, birthday, age, race/ethnicity, marital status, living arrangement, educational level, occupation		*
Legal consents or permission		*
Referral information		*
Reason for visit		*
External causes injury/illness		*
Symptoms		*
Physical exams		*
Assessment of patient signs and symptoms		*
Toxicity assessments		*
Diagnoses		*
Orders for lab, radiology and pharmacy		*
Laboratory results		*
Radiologic images and interpretations		*
Records of alerts, warnings and reminders		*
Operative reports		*
Vital signs		*
Treatment plans and instructions		*
Progress notes		*
Functional status		*
Discharge summaries		*
Outcome analyses		*
Provider notes		*
Protocols		*
Practice guidelines		*
Clinical decision-support programs		*
Referral history		*

<table>
<tr><th>Oncology Data</th><th>Elements</th></tr>
<tr><td>Historical</td><td>Surgery/procedure</td></tr>
<tr><td>Date diagnosis</td><td>Date</td></tr>
<tr><td>Cancer diagnosis</td><td>Procedure</td></tr>
<tr><td>Primary Site</td><td>Purpose</td></tr>
<tr><td>Subsite</td><td>Hospital</td></tr>
<tr><td>Laterality</td><td>Sentinal nodes</td></tr>
<tr><td>Prior Rx</td><td>Complications</td></tr>
<tr><td>Staging primary disease</td><td>Operative findings</td></tr>
<tr><td>Date staged</td><td>% Debulked</td></tr>
<tr><td>Geographic site</td><td>Surgeon</td></tr>
<tr><td>Primary location size</td><td>Time Procedure</td></tr>
<tr><td>Nodes</td><td>Estimated blood loss</td></tr>
<tr><td>Metastatic sites</td><td>Transfusion</td></tr>
<tr><td>T|N|M</td><td>Radiation therapy</td></tr>
<tr><td>Stage</td><td>Purpose</td></tr>
<tr><td>Tumor status</td><td>Location</td></tr>
<tr><td>Staging metastatic disease</td><td>Dose</td></tr>
<tr><td>Date</td><td>Start/End date</td></tr>
<tr><td>Site(s)</td><td>Response</td></tr>
<tr><td>Subsite</td><td>Progression date</td></tr>
<tr><td>Histology</td><td>Chemotherapy</td></tr>
<tr><td>Same as primary</td><td>Protocol name</td></tr>
<tr><td>in situ</td><td>Group</td></tr>
<tr><td>Residual</td><td>Protocol #</td></tr>
<tr><td>Lesion size</td><td>Patient #</td></tr>
<tr><td>Volume</td><td>Regimen (drugs)</td></tr>
<tr><td>Status</td><td>Purpose</td></tr>
<tr><td>Link with Primary (?)</td><td>Start/End date</td></tr>
<tr><td>Pathology</td><td>Ht Wt BSA</td></tr>
<tr><td>Date diagnosis</td><td>Response</td></tr>
<tr><td>Site</td><td>Cycles #</td></tr>
<tr><td>Gross</td><td>Cycle dates</td></tr>
<tr><td>Morphology</td><td>Progression date</td></tr>
<tr><td>Markers</td><td>Immunotherapy</td></tr>
<tr><td>Histology</td><td>Protocol name</td></tr>
<tr><td>Grade</td><td>Group</td></tr>
<tr><td>Maximum diameter</td><td>Protocol #</td></tr>
<tr><td>Volume</td><td>Patient #</td></tr>
<tr><td>Vascular involvement</td><td>Regimen (drugs)</td></tr>
<tr><td>Lymph involvement</td><td>Purpose</td></tr>
<tr><td>Margins</td><td>Start/end date</td></tr>
<tr><td>Character</td><td>Response</td></tr>
<tr><td>Size</td><td># Cycles</td></tr>
<tr><td>Synchrony</td><td>Cycle length</td></tr>
<tr><td>FISH</td><td>Progression date</td></tr>
<tr><td>DNA ploidy</td><td>Recurrence</td></tr>
<tr><td>Receptors</td><td>rT|rN|rM</td></tr>
<tr><td>Histochemistry</td><td>rStage</td></tr>
<tr><td>Genetics</td><td>Date</td></tr>
<tr><td>Currency</td><td>Site(s)</td></tr>
<tr><td>Current Rx modalities</td><td>Subsite</td></tr>
<tr><td>Status</td><td>Histology</td></tr>
<tr><td>Response</td><td>Same as primary</td></tr>
<tr><td>Rx intent</td><td>in situ</td></tr>
<tr><td>Rx toleration</td><td>Residual</td></tr>
<tr><td>Rx toxicity</td><td>Lesion size</td></tr>
<tr><td>Performance status</td><td>Volume</td></tr>
<tr><td>Pain level</td><td>Status</td></tr>
<tr><td>Fatigue level</td><td>Link with Primary (?)</td></tr>
<tr><td></td><td>Follow-up</td></tr>
<tr><td></td><td>Last date seen</td></tr>
<tr><td></td><td>DNR</td></tr>
<tr><td></td><td>Date of death</td></tr>
<tr><td></td><td>Autopsy findings</td></tr>
</table>

computers effectively to automate all aspects of cancer patient management.

Clinical Trials

To increase the number of patients accrued (now less than 3% of the national burden) and to simplify the data management requirements for cancer clinical trials, two recent innovations deserve comment. The NCI's Cancer Informatics Infrastructure permits oncologists and their patients to use their computers over the Internet to identify appropriate cancer clinical trials for their specific cancer diagnosis and to facilitate patient registration (<http://www.cancer.gov/clinicaltrials>). Another useful site is the American Cancer Society (<http://www.cancer.org/

Table 139-11 ■ Computer-Based Patient Record Attributes

1. Supports a problem list.
2. Has the ability to measure health status and functional levels.
3. Can document clinical reasoning and rationale.
4. Is a longitudinal computerized patient record (CPR) and has timely linkages with other patient records.
5. Guarantees confidentiality, privacy, and audit trails.
6. Offers continuous access for authorized users.
7. Supports simultaneously multiple user views into the CPR.
8. Supports timely access to local and remote information resources.
9. Facilitates clinical problem solving.
10. Supports direct data entry by physicians.
11. Supports practitioners in measuring costs and improving quality.
12. Has the flexibility to support existing or evolving needs of clinical specialties.

Table 139-12 ■ Physician Data Query (PDQ) Selections

1. Cancer information
    - Treatment by body system/site
    - Treatment by histologic tissue type
    - Treatment of childhood cancer
    - Prognosis
    - Staging
    - Supportive care
    - Rare tumor
    - Design of clinical tools
    - Cancer screening/detection (testing)
    - Prevention
    - Genetics
    - Complementary and alternative medicine
2. Late-breaking news in oncology
3. Physicians
4. Organizations
5. Protocols
    - Open
    - Study objectives
    - Patient eligibility
    - Treatment regimens
    - Dose and schedule modifications
    - Names of principal investigators and institutions
    - Closed
    - Abstracts
6. Investigational drug file
7. CANCERLIT searches

docroot/ETO/content/ETO_6_1X_Clinical_Trials_Matching_Service.asp>).

All phase 1, 2, and 3 cancer clinical trials approved by the NCI's Cancer Therapy Evaluation Program (CTEP) are now required to be reported to CTEP using the Clinical Data Update System (CDUS) that is based on coding standards approved by the International Conference on Harmonization Multidisciplinary Group 2 (<http://www.ich.org/cache/compo/276-254-1.html>). This group was established to recommend electronic standards for the transfer of regulatory information by evaluating and recommending open and nonproprietary standards that meet the requirements of regulatory authorities and pharmaceutical companies. The recommendations provide solutions for structured and personal messaging (free text), electronic data interchange, datasets, definitions that incorporate structured data formats, security to ensure confidentiality, data integrity, authentication, and non-repudiation. The datasets include protocol administrative information, patient demographics, treatment information, toxicity information, and response information. Further information about CTEP is available at <http://ctep.info.nih.gov> and for CDUS at <http://ctep.cancer.gov/reporting/cdus.html>.

Clinical Practice Guidelines

Clinical practice guidelines are systematically developed statements to assist the practitioner with clinical decisions about appropriate health care for specific clinical indications. With the upsurge in evidence-based medicine and systematic reviews, they have emerged as a health research tool to analyze and report patterns of care and clinical outcomes. In oncology, ASCO (<http://www. asco.org>) has developed clinical practice guidelines outlining appropriate methods of treatment and care that address specific clinical situations (disease-oriented) and the use of approved medical products, procedures, or tests (modality-oriented). In addition, ASCO has also published technology assessments that are used to determine if a procedure, device, or test is appropriate for broad-based conventional usage.

The National Comprehensive Cancer Network (NCCN) (<http://www.nccn.org>) has developed 90 specific guidelines for oncologic diseases, covering 93% of all tumor types and support modalities. The NCCN guidelines include screening, prevention, diagnosis, work-up, treatment, and follow-up components. In addition, the NCCN also provides the NCCN Drugs and Biologics Compendium™ that is recognized by Medicare for making reimbursement coverage decisions and the NCCN Chemotherapy Order Templates™ for standardizing the chemotherapy administration process. The NCCN and the American Cancer Society have collaborated on patient education versions of the NCCN guidelines for the common cancer types (<http://www.nccn.org/patients/patient_gls.asp>).

The goal of these techniques is to provide a means to measure an improvement in clinical outcome, in terms of survival, quality of life, treatment toxicity, patient satisfaction, and cost-effectiveness. Clinical practice guidelines will be incorporated into point-of-care oncologic practice by integrating them into oncologic electronic patient records, permitting analysis of patterns of care. In addition, computers will give creators of guidelines instant feedback from users when guidelines are not followed so that guidelines can be constantly assessed. Another useful site that is acting as a clearinghouse for all guidelines is the National Guidelines Clearinghouse (<http://www.guidelines.gov>).

Swanson and colleagues discuss using a practice-based computerized clinical information system to evaluate growth factor usage patterns and outcomes among oncologists in the community setting.[52] They found that ASCO's clinical guidelines were used mainly for reference purposes. They concluded that their system could accurately collect detailed information regarding practice patterns of oncologists and that ASCO's survey data significantly underreport the use of growth factors in the community and indicate that a substantial number of oncologists are not following these guidelines. However, despite these findings, guidelines will become a necessary part of our oncology practice tools and be incorporated as decision support tools in EHRs, as payers begin to require them for reimbursement certifications and documentation for using quality initiatives in our offices. Current guidelines do not take into account comparative effectiveness—which drug or procedure is better—or comparative cost-effectiveness. Oncologists will need these guidelines to be able to answer: What is the value of this treatment? Is it better than a less expensive treatment and who will pay? We must define effectiveness that today is usually defined by a regimen to prolong progression-free survival, since the overall survival benefit takes longer to assess and is compromised by patients receiving multiple regimens until they die. Oncologists must begin to discuss the cost of treatments with our patients because the payers are rapidly transferring the costs of our expensive treatments to the patient by dramatically increasing co-pays. Experts using cost-effectiveness analyses that incorporate patient-reported outcomes as well as quality of life evaluations must calculate cost components. Recently a GAO directive to CMS urged Medicare to set up a public-private commission to study and define these issues, and announcements from ASCO and NCCN indicated that they would begin to consider adding comparative effectiveness and cost-efficiencies to their guidelines.

Medical Informatics Standards

In order for computers to talk to other computers and exchange medical information, standards for transmitting electronic medical information are necessary. In its Consolidated Health Informatics (CHI) initiative, DHSS chose the five standards selected and mandated for sharing medical information among federal agencies: messaging standards from Health Level Seven Inc. (HL-7), retail pharmacy orders from the National Council for Prescription Drug Programs (NCDCP), the Institute of Electrical and Electronic Engineers (IEEE) 1073 series of standards for medical devices, Digital Imaging Communications in Medicine (DICOM) for images, and the Logical Observation Identifier Name codes (LOINC) for clinical laboratory results reporting. The American Society for Testing and Materials (<http://www.astm.org>) has developed the Continuity of Care Record that defines a core data set for defining data to be sent to providers to whom the patient is referred. The NLM licensed SNOMED-CT (Systematized Nomenclature of Medicine-Clinical Terms), which is a machine-readable, clinically rich lexicon using a controlled clinical vocabulary dataset maintained by the College of American Pathologists to standardize clinical communication. The NLM and Department of Health and Human Services (DHHS) have made SNOMED-CT available free to all physicians. The NCI has formulated a terminology and grading system for reporting adverse events covering medical, surgical, and radiation oncology events without regard to timing or cause of the event. This has become the standard dictionary for reporting adverse events and should become part of an oncology dataset for any oncologic EHR. In 2004, as the National Coordinator for Health Information Technology set a goal of having an electronic health care record in place for every American this decade and released "The Decade of Health Information Technology: Delivering Consumer-centric and Information-rich Health Care" (<http://www.hhs.gov/onchit/ framework>). Its key initiatives include working with the private sector for EHR product certification for minimal standards of functionality, security, and interoperability so physicians can make informed purchasing decisions; having CMS work on standards for electronic prescribing in Medicare; and having Health Resources and Services Administration providing seed money for implementation of community-based health information exchanges. The National Health Care Information Technology Infrastructure is summarized by Yasnoff and colleagues.[53]

Medical Literature Searching

The Unified Medical Language System (UMLS) project, undertaken by the National Library of Medicine, is designed to facilitate the retrieval and integration of information from many machine-readable information sources, including descriptions of the biomedical literature, clinical records, factual data banks, and medical knowledge bases. Further information is available at <http://www.nlm.nih.gov/research/umls/>. Like MESH, which is a controlled vocabulary of 21,000 terms culled from the medical literature and arranged in a series of tree structures, the UMLS is a highly structured language designed for a clinical database to define medical terminology more specifically. Thus, different software programs that describe signs and symptoms of a disease will use a common term and permit one program to communicate more easily with another. To the extent that an application conforms to the UMLS guidelines, it will be able to communicate with other UMLS systems.

Major Internet Resources of Interest to the Oncologist

The reader is referred to DIRLINE (Directory of Information Resources Online), produced by the NLM and available online at <http://www.nlm.nih.gov/pubs/factsheets/dirlinfs.html> for location and descriptive information about a wide variety of information resources, including organizations, research resources, projects, and databases concerned with health and biomedicine. More detailed summaries of the most popular medical and cancer-specific databases are given below.

Cancer Surveillance

It is essential to be able to measure cancer-related risk factors, health behaviors, health services, clinical outcomes, and cost from cancer incidence, morbidity, mortality, and survival statistics. The information and computer technologies combining statistical methodologies and national databases evaluating these parameters are readily available for analysis and are available on the Internet.

SEER

The NCI's Surveillance, Epidemiology, and End Results (SEER) tumor registry of cancer cases began in 1973 and collects cancer demographic information in the United States. The SEER program currently collects and publishes cancer incidence and survival data from 14 population-based cancer registries and 3 supplemental registries covering approximately 26% of the US population. Information on more than 3 million in situ and invasive cancer cases is included in the SEER database, and approximately 170,000 new cases are added each year. The SEER registries routinely collect data on patient demographics, primary tumor site, morphology, stage at diagnosis, first course of treatment, and follow-up for vital status. The SEER program is the only comprehensive source of population-based information in the United States that includes stage of cancer at the time of diagnosis and survival rates within each stage. The mortality data reported by SEER are provided by the National Center for Health Statistics. It is located at <http://seer.cancer.gov>.

Medical Claims

Medicare costs from claims data can be obtained from the Center for Medicare and Medicaid Services database on medical care and Medicare claims (<http://www.cms.gov/>).

National Cancer Database

The Commission on Cancer of the American College of Surgeons and the American Cancer Society produce the National Cancer Database. This database collects cancer registry data from hospitals and helps oncologists compare trends in the treatment of cancer and its outcomes by individual hospital or by state, regional, or national patterns of care (<http://www.facs.org/cancer/ncdb/index.html>).

Fraumeni and Rimer have inaugurated a series on the developing fields of cancer surveillance that uses these "geospatial databases," a term coined by them, to measure the progress of the National Cancer Program and to provide leads into the etiology and eventual control of cancer.[54] Researchers have combined the SEER database with the CMS Medicare claims files for the same patients.[55,56] This will help determine regional cancer treatment and staging procedure costs and the cost-effectiveness of screening and staging procedures, to compare hospital and outpatient costs of cancer care and to assist in outcome analyses and practice guidelines research.

Cancer.Gov

Cancer.gov (<http://www.cancer.gov/>) contains monthly updated information for professionals and patients on cancer, including PDQ, fact sheets, publications, and NCI news covering cancer treatment, detection, screening, prevention, rehabilitation, statistics, and quality of life issues, detailed information about ongoing clinical trials, and selected information from the Journal of the National Cancer Institute.

PubMed (MEDLINE)

Medical literature searching begins with the National Library of Medicine's PubMed site (http://www.ncbi.nlm.nih.gov/sites/entrez/). It uses the MEDLINE database, compiled since 1966, that contains more than 14,000,000 citations from the world's biomedical literature, with more than 60% containing abstracts since 1965 and 80% referring to English-language items. Approximately 4,500 of the world's 22,000 medical journals are currently indexed in MEDLINE. Each year

372,000 articles are added. Each article is referenced with carefully chosen key words and phrases from MESH terms so that one can call up a list of relevant titles and then obtain the most appropriate abstracts. To assist with searching for evidence-based medicine, a search filter for "systematic reviews" was added in 2002. The NLM links full text articles from about a quarter of the publishers represented on MEDLINE to PubMed. One of its most important features is the ability to search for "related articles" for more focused searching. The NLM Gateway site (<http://gateway.nlm.nih.gov/gw/Cmd>) allows users to search multiple NLM databases simultaneously, including MEDLINE, OLDMEDLINE, LOCATORplus, MEDLINEplus, DIRLINE, AIDS Meetings, and Health Services research meetings. A highly recommended tutorial for PubMed is located at <http://www.nlm.nih.gov/bsd/disted/pubmedtutorial/>.

Cancer Library

The CANCERLIT database (<http://www.cancer.gov/cancer_information/cancer_literature/>), compiled since 1976, contains more than 2,200,000 citations from the world's cancer literature beginning from 1963, with more than 60% containing abstracts. Approximately 4,000 medical resources are currently indexed in CANCERLIT, including journals, meeting proceedings, symposia, books, doctoral theses, and research project summaries. Each year an additional 96,000 records are added. Each article is referenced with appropriate MESH terms. CANCERLIT can be searched for cancer literature, clinical trials, and genetic services (<http://www.cancer.gov/search/cancer_literature>) or by topics (<http://www.cancer.gov/search/search_cancertopics.aspx>).

BIOSIS Produced by Biosis.org and Thomson Reuters, and available at <http://www.biosis.org>, this database contains 17 million citations from 1969 to the present, covering some 9,000 scientific journals and books, conferences, proceedings, and monographs.

EMBASE

This is EXCERPTA MEDICA's online database produced by Embase.com and Elsevier, which screens 5,000 journals published since 1974, making available more than 18 million citations. It is located at <http://www.embase.com/>.

HEALTHSTAR

This database includes patient outcomes and the effectiveness of procedures, programs, products, services, and processes, and nonclinical health care administration and planning aspects of health care delivery. It has 3.9 million records and adds 17,000 per month (<http://gateway.nlm.nih.gov/gw>).

ISI Journal Citation Reports

The ISI journal citation reports (JCR) uses the Science Citation Index to determine the frequency of literature citations for a given article and permits the tracking of all articles that cite common references in order to trace common work. Journals indexed are selected on the basis of several criteria, including citation analysis, resulting in coverage of the most significant publications in the scientific, technical, and biomedical literature. In addition to the more conventional retrieval methods, the JCR offers citation indexing, which permits searching by cited references. It is available at <http://www.isinet.com/isi/ products/citation/jcr/j crweb/index.html>.

Physician Data Query

Physician Data Query (PDQ) is the NCI's comprehensive database that contains information that has been evaluated by a panel of 70 experts and is updated on a quarterly basis. It contains the latest information about prognosis, staging, cellular classification, and state-of-the-art cancer treatments, clinical trials, screening, prevention, genetics, supportive care, and complementary and alternative medicines. It gives detailed summaries for the physician or layperson of the 90 major tumor types. Tumors may be searched by body system/site or histologic tissue/type. It lists more than 2,000 currently active protocols that use mostly standardized formats and 13,000 closed-treatment protocols, with detailed information on the study objectives, patient entry criteria, treatment regimens, and demographic information for cooperative groups and physicians involved with the protocols. In addition, PDQ makes available demographic information for approximately 17,000 cancer specialists and more than 1,500 organizations affiliated with societies that are related to cancer. It is readily available to physicians and their patients through telecommunication facilities or telephone (1-800-4-CANCER). The reader is referred to two excellent reviews for further information.[57,58] Table 139-12 lists the major categories of PDQ. It is used primarily by oncologists to ensure that the most current treatment methods are used to assist in making a clinical decision, and to find information about clinical trials. Less frequently, it is used to prepare for conferences or to confirm information from other sources. Other uses include referring a patient to an oncologic investigator in a specific location, finding an investigator who has access to a particular clinical trial, and seeking consultation from another physician (<http://cancer.gov/cancertopics/pdq>).

The Physicians' Information and Education Resource

The Physicians' Information and Education Resource (PIER) is a practical, evidence-based medical knowledge and guidance resource for their members (<http://pier.acponline.org/index>) It was developed by the ACP as a member benefit with 130 modules, covering both common and uncommon diseases including modules dealing with prevention and screening, diagnosis, consultation for diagnosis, hospitalization, drug and nondrug therapies, patient education, consultation management, follow-up, case scenarios, clinical alerts, glossaries, and references, along with legal and ethical issues, complementary/alternative medicine procedures, and what's new for that disease. It is presented electronically in a unique layered and telegraphic format designed for rapid access to clinical information. PIER is linked to other resources at the ACP's Web site and to many other Internet resources. Its uniqueness relates to its intention to mirror the way a physician thinks through a problem. In the disease modules, for example, there is a logical flow of information from diagnosis through management. Its structure and format allows its content to be readily integrated into other applications such as EMRs.

CCRIS

The Chemical Carcinogenesis Research Information System (CCRIS) contains carcinogenicity, tumor promotion, tumor inhibition, and mutagenicity test results derived from the scanning of primary journals, current awareness tools, NCI technical reports, review articles, and International Agency for Research on Cancer monographs published since 1976. It is located at <http://toxnet.nlm.nih.gov/>.

Clinical Research and Other Uses of Computers

Data Acquisition and Instrument Control

Data acquisition requires taking measured experimental data in wavelengths or analog form and converting the data to digital form by an analog-to-digital converter. With specialized computer software, it is possible to have the computer read this information, display it, analyze it, and make appropriate decisions automatically. The computer, by transforming itself into a voltmeter, frequency counter, oscilloscope, spectrum analyzer, or x-y recorder, can record sound, heat, light, pressure, and electrical signals. The most popular instrument control program is Lab View (<http://www.ni.com/labview/>).

Bioinformatics

In the last few decades, advances in molecular biology and the equipment available for research in this field have allowed the increasingly rapid sequencing of complete genomes of several species, including man. Popular sequence databases, such as the National Center for Biotechnology Information's GenBank (<http://www.ncbi.nlm.nih.gov>) and the European Bioinformatics Institute's EMBL Nucleotide Sequence Database <http://www.embl.org/> have been growing at exponential rates. This deluge of information has necessitated the careful storage, organization, and indexing of sequence information, whereby information science has been applied to biology to produce the field called Bioinformatics.

The simplest tasks used in bioinformatics concern the creation and maintenance of databases of biologic information. Nucleic acid sequences (and the protein sequences derived from them) comprise the majority of such databases. Although the storage and organization of millions of nucleotides is far from trivial, designing a database and developing an interface, whereby researchers can both access existing information and submit new entries is only the beginning. The most pressing tasks in bioinformatics involve the analysis of sequence information. Computational Biology is the name given to this process, and it involves finding the genes in the deoxyribonucleic acid (DNA) sequences of various organisms, developing methods to predict the structure and/or function of newly discovered proteins and structural ribonucleic acid (RNA) sequences, clustering protein sequences into families of related sequences and the development of protein models, and aligning similar proteins and generating phylogenetic trees to examine evolutionary relationships.

The process of evolution has produced DNA sequences that encode proteins with very specific functions. It is possible to predict the three-dimensional structure of a protein using algorithms that have been derived from our knowledge of physics, chemistry, and most importantly, from the analysis of other proteins with similar amino acid sequences. Using homology matrix analysis, the computer can compare sequences of numbers or letters. It, thus, can compare DNA sequences and perform DNA sequencing. Users can represent DNA sequences graphically or as text. Recombinant DNA molecules can be constructed on the screen. The program has a database of restriction enzymes that can cut DNA at specific base pairs. Thus, one can cut and splice DNA sequences and then analyze the results in the model. It is a means to bring the world of desktop publishing into the molecular biologist's world. Another useful tool is Oncomine that was created by Dr. Arul Chinnaiyan and is a proprietary compilation of microarray datasets from over 100 cancer studies allowing researchers to analyze data from disparate sources by normalizing data and making qualitative comparisons across datasets (<http://www.oncomine.org>).[59]

GenMAPP (Gene MicroArray Pathway Profiler) is a free computer program available at <http://www.genmapp.org> designed for viewing and analyzing gene expression data representing biological pathways and grouping of genes. It allows one to visualize gene expression data in a biological context with the graphical and more intuitive format of MAPPs that are computer-generated files that graphically show the biological relationship between genes or gene products. MAPPs can be represented in GenMAPP as metabolic pathways, signal transduction cascades, subcellular locations, gene families, or lists of genes associated with Gene Ontology categories. Each MAPP contains gene objects, which represent biological genes or gene products such as receptors, membranes and ribosomes, and the relationships among the objects. Each gene object on a MAPP is identified by a gene identifier from one of the GenMAPP-accepted gene ID systems.

The reader is referred to an article by Buetow for a description of the NCI's Center for Bioinformatics program.[60] For an excellent tutorial on how to use bioinformatics tools, the reader is referred to <http://www.ncbi.nlm.nih.gov/Coffeebreak>. For patients, an excellent resource that addresses the health implications of the Human Genome Project is the Genetics Home Reference (<http://ghr.nlm.nih.gov/ghr/page/Home>).[61]

caBIG

The National Cancer Institute Center for Bioinformatics (NCICB)-led enterprise, the cancer Biomedical Informatics Grid (caBIG™), supports the goal of optimally collecting and using cancer information for both research and quality initiatives as well as for best-practice patient care.[62] caBIG™ defines electronic oncologic content and uses pre-defined standards and interoperability as key elements in the optimal management of cancer information that distributes information easily with the ability to protect data and data integrity. caBIG™ supports the goals of cooperative groups and the overall conduct of clinical research by simplifying the analysis and sharing of information. In 2007, caBIG™ connected clinicians, researchers, and patients at more than 50 NCI-designated cancer centers and 30 other organizations in the public and private sectors. When fully mature, caBIG™ will be able to interface clinical research with clinical care, and the enabling of a "prototypic EHR" system through structured data collection to best serve the treatment needs of cancer patients.

Speakman and Reeves report that the NCI has begun to standardize treatment summaries for breast and colon cancer, electronic case report forms for demography, patient identification, patient enrollment, patient baseline assessment, adverse events, protocol deviations, and data elements for cancer care and research.[63] Deering and Dugan report on how caBIG™ is beginning to share its information technology for both cancer clinical and research data with vendors, cooperative groups, and institutions.[64]

Statistics

There is a plethora of statistical programs that combine the major procedures used in most analyses with the ability to display results instantly as charts or plots. Most programs permit the data to be read in from other programs and to be stored in tables, rectangular files, or matrices. After analysis, the results can be exported to other programs. Data can be sorted, selected, and rotated based on data values. Most programs include frequency distribution; data transformation; non-parametric statistics; cross-tabulation statistics; analysis of variance, correlation, and regression; and multivariate analysis.

All oncologists must become computer literate. A small investment in learning time and capital ($1,200 [US] to $3,000 [US]) will pay off handsomely. Oncologists will have easier access to patient data, less loss of records, greater medical knowledge, and more efficient updating of information. They would have immediate access to electronic textbooks and journals and easier communication from one's own office, using electronic mailboxes and modems, with other physicians' offices or the hospital. Thus, the computer has become the oncologist's "black bag."

Selected References

The complete reference list can be found at www.CANCERMEDICINE8.com

2. Gotay CC. Trial-related quality of life: using quality-of-life assessment to distinguish among cancer therapies. *Monogr Natl Cancer Inst*. 1996;20:1–6.

3. Weeks J. Taking quality of life into account in health economic analyses. *Monogr Natl Cancer Inst*. 1996;20:23–27.
4. Hewitt M, E J, editors. *Ensuring Quality Cancer Care. National Cancer Policy Board, Institute of Medicine and Commission on Life Sciences, National Research Council*. Washington, DC: National Academy Press; 1999.
6. Crossing the quality chasm: a new health system for the 21st century. Committee on Quality of Health Care in America. Institute of Medicine. Washington, DC: National Academy Press; 2001.
7. President's Information Technology Advisory Committee: Transforming health care through information technology. February 9, 2001. Available at: http://www.nitrd.gov/pubs/pitac/ pitac-hc-9feb01.pdf. Accessed May 23, 2008.
8. President's Cancer Panel: Voices of a broken system: real people, real problems. 2001. Available at: https://cissecure.nci.nih.gov/ncipubs/details.asp?pid=1060. Accessed June 23, 2005.
9. Stephenson J. Lab-on-a-chip shows promise in defining and diagnosing cancers. *JAMA*. 1999;282:1801–1802.
11. Shortliffe EH, Cimino JJ. Biomedical Informatics: Computer Applications in Health Care and Biomedicine (Health Informatics). New York: Springer; 2006.
13. Blumberg JW. PDA applications for physicians. ASCO Technology News. January 2004;4–6.
14. Wilkins A, Hovhanesian J. The virtual workplace. Healthc Inform. November 1999;66–70.
15. Internet World Stats. Available at http://www.internetworldstats.com/stats.htm. Accessed May 28, 2008.
17. Gorrindo T, Groves JE Web searching for information about physicians. JAMA. 2008;300:213–215.
19. Berners-Lee T, Hendler J, Lassila O. The semantic Web. Sci Am. 2001;284:35–43. Available at: http://www.sciam.com/article.cfm? articleID=00048144-10D2-1C70-84-A9809EC588EF21. Accessed June 23, 2008.
20. Varmus H. E-Biomed: a proposal for electronic publications in the biomedical sciences. Available at: http://www.nih.gov/about/ director/ebiomed/ebi.htm. Accessed June 23, 2005.
22. Kim MI, Johnson B. Personal health records: evaluation of functionality and utility. J Am Med Inform Assoc. 2002;9:171–180.
23. Halamka JD, Mandl KD, Tang PC. Early experiences with Personal Health Records. J Am Med Inform Assoc. 2008;15:1–13.
24. Ganz PA, Hahn EE. Implementing a survivorship care plan for patients with breast cancer. J Clin Oncol. 2008;26:759–767.
25. Wall Street Journal. 11/29/2006 page B1.
26. Steinbrook R. Personally controlled online health data-the next big thing in medical care. N Engl J Med. 2008;358:1653–1656.
27. Hartzband P, Groopman J. Off the record-avoiding the pitfalls of going electronic. N Engl J Med. 2008;358:1656–1658.
28. Mandl KD, Kohane IS. Teectonic shifts in the health information economy. N Engl J Med. 2008;358:1732–1737.
30. Miller RS. Effective use of the Internet for patient-physician communication. Education Book Amer Soc Clin Onc. 2006;376–379.
32. Basch E, Iasonos, A Barz A, et al. Long-term toxicity monitoring via electronic patient-reported outcomes in patients receiving chemotherapy. J Clin Oncol. 2007;25:5374–5380.
35. Helft PR, Hlubocky F, Daugherty CK. American oncologist's views of Internet use by cancer patients: a mail survey of American Society of Clinical Oncology members. J Clin Oncol. 2003;21:942–947.
37. Purcell GP, Wilson P. The quality of health information on the Internet. BMJ. 2002;324:557–558.
38. Marshall WW, Haley RW. Use of a secure Internet Web site for collaborative medical research. JAMA. 2000;284:1843–1849.
39. Simon GC, Agus DB, Hanna K. Using electronic medical records to bridge patient care and research in oncology. Am Soc Clin Oncol. Education Book. 2006;381–385.
41. DesRoches CM, Campbell EG, Rao SR, et al Electronic health records in ambulatory care – a national survey of physicians. N Engl J Med. 2008;359:50–60.
42. Earle CC, Schrag D, Woolf SH. The survivorship care plan: what, why, how and for whom. Am Soc Clin Oncol Education Book. 2006;525–531.
43. Shulman LN, Miller RS, Ambinder EP, Yu P, Cox J. Principles of safe practice using an oncology electronic EHR system for chemotherapy ordering, preparation and administration: Part 1 of a two part series. J Oncol Prac. 2008;4:203–206.
44. Shulman LN, Miller RS, Ambinder EP, Yu P, Cox J. Principles of safe practice using an oncology electronic EHR system for chemotherapy ordering, preparation and administration: Part 2 of a two part series. J Oncol Prac. 2008;4.
45. Prescher-Hughes DS. The nurse's forum: developing practice protocols. Oncologistics Fourth Quarter. 2003;11.
46. Schneider EC, Epstein AM, Malin JL, et al. Developing a system to assess the quality of cancer care: ASCO's National Initiative on Cancer Care Quality. JCO. 2004;22:2985–2991.
53. Yasnoff WA, Humphreys BL, Overhage JM, et al. A consensus action agenda for achieving the national health information infrastructure. J Am Med Inform Assoc. 2004;11:332–338.
55. Potosky AL, Riley GF, Lubitz JD, et al. Potential for cancer related health services research using a linked Medicare-tumor registry database. Med Care. 1993 ;31:732–748.
56. Earle CC, Neuman PJ, Gelber RD, et al. Impact of referral patterns on the use of chemotherapy for lung cancer. J Clin Oncol. 2002;20:1786–1792.
60. Buetow KH. The NCI Center for Bioinformatics (NCICB): building a foundation for in silico biomedical research. Cancer Invest. 2004;22:117–122.
61. Mitchell JA, Fun J, McCray AT. Design of genetics home reference: a new NLM consumer health resource. J Am Med Inform Assoc. 2004;11:439–447.
62. Whippen DW, Deering MJ, Ambinder EP. Advancing high-quality cancer care-cancer biomedical informatics grid supports personalized medicine and the electronic health record. J Oncol Prac. 2007;3:209–212.
63. Speakman J, Reeves D. Improving cancer care and research through the reuse of standardized electronic data. J Clin Oncol. 2008;26(May 20 suppl):abstr 17556.
64. Deering M, Duggan B. The National Cancer Institute's cancer Biomedical Informatics Grid (caBIG™): Linking research and care. J Clin Oncol. 2008;26(May 20 suppl):abstr 17539.v

Index

Note: Page numbers with f and t denote figures and tables, respectively.

8q24 region, 361–362
A rule, 264
AAH. *See* Atypical adenomatous hyperplasia (AAH)
AAV. *See* Adeno-associated virus (AAV)
ABC technique. *See* Avidin-biotin complex (ABC) technique
Abdomen
  aspiration cytology, 481
Abdominal infections, 1935
Abiraterone
  prostate cancer, 1248
abl, 78, 79, 81
Abortion
  breast cancer, 1396
Abraxane
  nanotechnology, 366, 368
Absolute risk, 381
ABVD, 32, 34, 1917
  Hodgkin lymphoma, 1623, 1631, 1637, 1638, 1639, 1640, 1642, 1643, 1710
  myelodysplastic syndrome, 1546
ACE. *See* Angiotensin-converting enzyme inhibitors
Acetabulum
  metastatic tumors to, 1790, 1790f
Acetaminophen
  for cancer pain, 868
  systemic reactions to, 1959
Acetazolamide, 1945
Acetylcholine, 1757
Acinetobacter, 1926
Acinic cell carcinoma, 985
Acquired hemophilia, 1815–1816
Acquired immune deficiency syndrome (AIDS), 1808–1809
  and cancer, 1696–1711, 1696t
    epidemiology, 1696–1697
Acquired von Willebrand syndrome (aVWS), 1815
Acral erythema (AE), 1783–1784, 1784f
  chemotherapeutic agents associated with, 1783t
Acral lentiginous melanoma (ALM), 1461–1462
Acromegaly, 1913
  treatment, 918f
ACS. *See* Anorexia/cachexia syndrome (ACS)
ACT. *See* Adoptive T-cell therapy (ACT)
ACTH *See* Adrenocorticotropic hormone (ACTH)
Actinic cheilitis, 1490
Actinic keratoses, 1487–1488, 1488f
  inflammation, 1783, 1783t
Actinomycin D
  Ewing sarcoma, 1509, 1732
  nephrotoxicity, 1826
  radiation-induced lung injury, 1860
  sinusoidal obstruction syndrome, 1877
  structure, 651f
  veno-occlusive disease, 1877
Active treatment
  adaptation to, 796–797
Acupuncture, 848–849, 850, 1761
Acute emesis, 1757
  prevention
    guidelines, 1761t
Acute generalized exanthematous pustulosis (AGEP), 1787
Acute lung injury (ALI), 1868
Acute lymphoblastic leukemia (ALL), 1591–1602, 1723, 1800, 1905, 1917, 1918. *See also* Acute lymphocytic leukemia
  8q24 rearrangements, 1594
  childhood, 1724–1725
  clinical signs and symptoms of, 1591–1592, 1592t
  cytochemistry, 1592
  cytogenetic and molecular abnormalities in, 1593–1594, 1593t
  del(9p21), abnormalities of, 1594
  diagnosis of, 1592–1595, 1593t
  E2A rearrangements (19q13), 1594
  epidemiology, 1591
  epigenetic microalterations in, 1595
  etiology, 1591
  fms-like tyrosine kinase 3, 1595
  gene expression microarrays, 1595
  gene rear arrangements, 1594
  immunophenotyping, 1592–1593
  mature B-cell, 1601–1602
  MLL rearrangements (11q23), 1594
  morphology, 1592
  NOTCH1, mutations of, 1594–1595
  numerical abnormalities in, 1593–1594
  Ph-positive, 1601
  prognostic factors, 1596, 1596t
  structural abnormalities in, 1594
  t(12;21) and del(12p), translocation of, 1594
  treatment, 1595–1601, 1595f
    pharmacogenetics, 1599–1600
Acute lymphocytic leukemia
  combination chemotherapy, 594
  hematopoietic cellular transplantation for, 785
  methotrexate, 614
  ophthalmic neoplasms, 908
  treatment, 559t
Acute myelofibrosis, 1690
Acute myelogenous leukemia, 218, 1800, 1915, 1916t, 1917, 1918, 1919
Acute myeloid leukemia (AML), 1559–1580
  chemotherapy regimens for, 1570, 1570t
  in children, 1725
  classification, 1559, 1560–1561
  complications, 1577–1578
  with cytogenetic abnormalities, 1561–1562, 1561f, 1562f
  diagnosis of, 1560–1561
  etiology, 1560
  hematopoietic cellular transplantation for, 784–785
  hematopoietic growth factors, 1576
  induction therapy of, 1569–1574
  karyotypic and molecular abnormalities in, 1563t
  with maturation, 1564
  without maturation, 1564
  with MDS-related changes, 1564
  methotrexate, 614
  minimal residual disease, 1564
  minimally differentiated, 1564
  with molecularly detected abnormalities, 1562–1563
  pathogenesis, 1560
  prognostic factors, 1568–1569
  relapsed and refractory AML, therapy of, 1574–1575, 1574t
Acute myeloid leukemia (AML) (*cont.*)
  signs and symptoms, 1567–1568, 1568t
  therapy-related, 1564
Acute myelosclerosis. *See* Acute myelofibrosis
Acute pancreatitis, 1877
Acute Panmyelosis with Myelofibrosis (APMF), 1567
Acute promyelocytic leukemia (APL), 1565, 1570, 1817, 1817f
  treatment of, 1575–1576, 1576t
Acute respiratory failure (ARF), 1867
  lung versus pump failure, 1867t
Acyclovir, 1939
  esophagitis, 1873
  viral infections, 1931
Adamantinoma, 1507–1511
Adaptation, 795–796, 795t
  to active treatment, 796–797
  on being a survivor, 797–798
  to increased genetic risk, 798–799
  to palliative care, 797
Adaptive allocation, 460
Adaptive dose-finding, 450
ADC. *See* Apparent diffusion coefficient (ADC)
Adeno-associated virus (AAV)
  gene delivery, 761
Adenocarcinoma, 1212
  anal neoplasms, 1202
  appendiceal, 1179
  of breast, 477f
  cervical, 1302–1303
    risk factors, 1301
  clear cell
    vagina, 1296–1297, 1296t
  endometrial papillary, 1327
  endometrial, 1327
  endometrioid, 1303
  of esophagus, 406
  of gallbladder, 1132
  of gastric cardia, 406
  lung, 1003
  mucinous
    cervix, 1302
  papillary serous
    ovaries, 481f
  of prostate, 1230f
  as single metastatic lesion, 1716
  small intestine, 1173–1174
  of unknown primary site, 1715–1717
    empiric chemotherapy for, 1717, 1717t
Adenoid cystic carcinoma, 913f, 985
Adenoma malignum
  of cervix, 1303
Adenomas
  sebaceous, 1494–1495
Adenomatous hyperplasia (AAH), 1230
Adenomatous polyposis coli, 92
  gastric cancer, 1090
Adenosine triphosphate (ATP)
  cachexia, 1751–1752
Adenosquamous carcinoma
  cervical, 1303
  endometrium, 1327
  lung, 1004
Adenovirus, 727
  gene delivery, 760
  oncolytic, 770–771

Adenovirus (*cont.*)
tumor-selective, 768
Adhesion molecules
multiple myeloma, 1670–1671, 1670f
Adhesion related kinase (Ark), 58
Adhesion, 143–144
Adjuvant chemotherapy
randomized studies, 561–562
Adjuvant therapy
melanoma, 1477–1499
A-Difluoromethylornithine, 1037
Adoptive cellular therapy (ACT), 179–180
current position of, 181
Adoptive T-cell therapy
distant metastatic melanoma, 1481, 1481f
Adrenal androgen synthesis inhibitors, 756
Adrenal cortex
steroid biosynthesis, 934f
Adrenal cortex neoplasms, 933–939
aldosterone producing, 934
benign vs. malignant, 936f
diagnosis, 934
differential diagnosis, 934–935
function inhibitors, 939
imaging, 935
MacFarlane classification, 936t
management, 936–938
algorithm, 938f
metastasis site, 936t
pathogenesis, 933–934
pathologic diagnosis, 936
staging, 935–936
Adrenal diseases, 1905–1906
Adrenal insufficiency, 1906
Adrenal metastasis, 1904–1906
Adrenicorticotropic hormone (ACTH), 1906
ectopic syndrome, 1909–1911, 1910f
Adrenocorticosteroids
abdominal infections, 1935
Adrenocorticotropic hormone (ACTH)
ectopic syndrome, 1007
secreting pituitary adenomas
ketoconazole, 919–921
Adriamycin
Ewing sarcoma, 1509
osteosarcoma, 1509
radiation-induced lung injury, 1860
thymomas, 1060
Adult respiratory distress syndrome (ARDS), 1853, 1858, 1867, 1868
Adult T-cell leukemia/lymphoma (ATLL), 1650
treatment, 1656
AE. *See* Acral erythema. (AE)
Aflatoxins, 229, 406
in liver, 1125
AFP. *See* Alpha-fetoprotein (AFP)
Age as a factor, 371–372
breast cancer, 238–239, 1394, 1407
colorectal cancer, 1180
incidence, 402f
incidence, 377f
invasive cancer, 375t
mortality, 375t, 377f
Age of onset
skin cancer, 262
xeroderma pigmentosum, 265f
Agency for Health Care and Policy Research (AHCPR), 866
outcome studies, 465–466
Agents
evaluation against targets, 579
preparation for clinical trials, 579
AGEP. *See* Acute generalized exanthematous pustulosis (AGEP)
Aggressive lymphomas, 1648–1649
allogeneic stem cell transplantation for, 1657
in first remission, 1656
autologous stem cell transplantation for, 1657
Aggressive lymphomas (*cont.*)
clinical prognostic factors in, 1652–1653
therapy
at advanced stage, 1655–1656
at early stage, 1655
salvage therapy, 1656–1657
Aging, 838–845
biology, 838–839
physiologic changes, 839
Agrin family, 59
AICAR. *See* Aminoimadazole-4-carboxamide ribonucleoside (AICAR)
AIDS. *See* Acquired immune deficiency syndrome (AIDS)
Air pollution
in head and neck neoplasms, 962
Airway obstruction
acute, 1951, 1951f
Akt, 49, 62
apoptosis substrates, 49f
breast cancer, 1449–1450
oncogenes, 84
Albumin
nanotechnology, 366
ALCL. *See* Anaplastic large-cell lymphoma (ALCL)
Alcohol, 402
breast cancer, 403, 1397
colorectal cancer, 403, 1180
head and neck neoplasms, 960–961
liver neoplasms, 1125
oral cancer, 406f
pancreatic neoplasms, 1146
Aldehyde dehydrogenase, 606
Alemtuzumab, 712, 1847
bronchospasm, 1859
chronic lymphocytic leukemia, 1614
minimal residual disease, 1616
mycosis fungoides/Sézary syndrome, 1666
Alendronate, 1905
bone metastasis, 1793
Aleukemic leukemia, 1561
Alexandria Cancer Registry, 311
ALI. *See* Acute lung injury
Alimentary tract dysfunction
cachexia, 1742
ALK, 79
Alkyl sulfonates, 635
Alkylating agents, 606, 633–644
cellular resistance to, 637–638
chemistry, 633
clinical pharmacology, 638–639
cytotoxicity, 636–637
in vivo resistance, 638
metabolism, 636–637
schedule effects, 563
toxicity, 639–641
ALL. *See* Acute lymphoblastic leukemia (ALL)
ALL1, 79
Allogeneic hematopoietic cellular transplantation
donor selection, 778
engraftment, 779
malignancies, 777
pretransplant therapy, 780–781
Allogeneic stem cell transplantation, 1708
hematopoietic, primary myelofibrosis, 1691
multiple myeloma, 1679–1680, 1679t, 1680t
Alloimmunization, 1803–1804, 1804t, 1805
Allopurinol, 629, 1945
oral complications, 1886
All-*trans* retinoic acid (ATRA), 1565, 1570, 1575, 1908
chemotherapy-induced lung injury, 1858
ALM. *See* Acral lentiginous melanoma (ALM)
Aloe vera
mucositis, 1882
Alopecia, 1779–1780
cause, 640–641
Alopecia (*cont.*)
chemotherapeutic agents associated with, 1779t
Alpha interferon, 1579, 1844. *See also* Interferon-a (IFN-a)
Alpha-1-antitrypsin deficiency
liver neoplasms, 1125
Alpha-beta tubulin dimer, 655f
Alpha-fetoprotein (AFP), 339
Alpha-hemolytic streptococci, 1924, 1924f
Alpha-particle radioimmunotherapy, 720
Alteplase
sinusoidal obstruction syndrome, 1878
veno-occlusive disease, 1878
Altretamine
hypersensitivity reactions, 1783
AMB. *See* Amphotericin B (AMB)
American Academy of Pain Medicine, 879
American Burkitt lymphoma
parasites, 316
American Cancer Society, 846, 851, 848
American Joint Commission on Cancer (AJCC), 1047, 1257
American Joint Committee on Cancer/Union Internationale Contre le Cancer, 1092, 1092t
American Pain Society, 879
American Society of Addiction Medicine, 879
American Society of Anesthesiologists
physical stages classification, 506t
American Society of Clinical Oncology (ASCO), 338
AMG 531, 691–692, 708
AMG 655, 692
Amifostine, 521
mucositis, 1882
nephrotoxicity, 1828
oral complications, 1886
radiation-induced lung injury, 1860
xerostomia, 1883
Amikacin
bacterial infections, 1926, 1927
Aminoglutethimide, 744, 1906, 1911
causing nail hyperpigmentation, 1780
Aminoglycoside
bacterial infections, 1925, 1926
neutropenia, 1837
Aminoimadazole-4-carboxamide ribonucleoside (AICAR), 607
5-Aminolevulinic acid
mycosis fungoides/Sézary syndrome, 1666
Aminopterin, 37, 618
Amiodarone, 1943, 1944
Amitriptyline
for cancer pain, 873
AML. *See* Acute myeloid leukemia (AML)
Amoxicillin
bacterial infections, 1924
for indolent NHL, 1653
Amphotericin B (AMB), 1931
candidiasis, 1929
cryptococcosis, 1930
esophagitis, 1872
zygomycosis, 1930
Amputation versus limb salvage
bone tumors, 1499–1501, 1500t
Amrubicin, 649
Amsacrine, 1574
Amsterdam criteria for cancer risk, 204t
Amyloidosis, 1683–1684, 1817
cardiac, 1837–1838, 1837f
Anabolic steroids
cachexia, 1749
Anagen effluvium
cutaneous reactions, 1779
Anal canal tumors
anal neoplasms, 1201
Anal intraepithelial neoplasia, 1194
Anal marginal cancer, 1200, 1201
Anal neoplasms, 1194–1202

Anal neoplasms (*cont.*)
anatomy, 1194
diagnosis, 1195
epidemiology, 1194
etiology, 1194
history, 1195, 1195t
inguinal node involvement, 1200–1201
metastatic disease treatment, 1201
pathology, 1195
prognostic factors, 1195–1198, 1197t
staging, 1195, 1196t
treatment, 1198–1200
Analytical test validation, 354
Anaphylaxis, 1957–1958, 1957t
Anaplastic astrocytoma, 890–891
Anaplastic large-cell lymphoma (ALCL), 1649
Anaplastic thyroid carcinoma, 931
therapy and prognosis, 931
Anastomosis
prostate cancer, 1238
Anastrazole, 33, 745
breast cancer, 1432
Androgen receptor (AR), 1231
Androgens
breast cancer, 1433
deprivation strategies, 751–752
inhibitors, 756
mechanism of action, 750
systemic levels, 750–751
Anemia, 1799, 1846
aplastic, 789
causes of, 1798t
Fanconi, 789
in chronic lymphocytic leukemia, 1618–1619
microangiopathic, 1799
sickle cell
Anesthesiologist, 826
Anetholtrithion
xerostomia, 1883
Aneuploid, 552
Aneurysmal bone cyst, 1505–1506, 1505f
Angiogenesis, 145, 475
gastric cancer, 1091
inhibition
interferons, 683t
markers
breast cancer, 1407–1408
multiple myeloma, 1671
and tumor, 277
Angiogenesis inhibitors
breast cancer, 1449
AngioimmunoblasticT-cell lymphoma, 1649
Angiomyolipoma, 1208–1209
Angiopoietin-1, 154
Angiopoietin-2, 154
systemic reactions to, 1959
Angiopoietins, 59, 154–155
Angiosarcoma
cardiac tumors, 1064
cutaneous, 1493
Angiostatin, 155–156, 156f
Angiotensin converting enzyme inhibitors
acute airway obstruction, 1951
Angiotensin receptor antagonists, 1913
Angiotensin-converting enzyme(ACE) inhibitors, 1838, 1845, 1913
Anidulafungin
esophagitis, 1872
Animal pharmacology, 579–580
Animal toxicology studies, 580
ANNA-1. *See* Antineuronal nuclear antibody
Anoikis, 43
Anorexia, 1740–1742. *See also* Cachexia
causes, 1740t
Anorexia/cachexia syndrome (ACS)
palliative care, 857–858
Antacids
bacterial infections, 1924
Anterosuperior mediastinal tumors
differential diagnosis of, 1058
Anthracenediones, 650–651
Anthracyclines, 1737, 1757, 1840–1843, 1942
cardiotoxicity, 649–650
causing anaphylaxis, 1958
encapsulated, 1536–1537
hyperthermia, 533
mechanism of resistance, 650
metabolic disease, 1535–1536
structure, 648f
targeting topoisomerase, 648–650
Anthraquinolones
cardiotoxicity, 1840
Antiadhesive agents
invasion, 146
Antiangiogenic therapy
invasion, 147
radiation therapy, 523
Antiarrhythmic drugs, 1944t
Anti-cachexia agents, 1754–1755
Anticholinergics, 1761
Anticipatory emesis, 1757
Anticoagulants
brain metastasis, 901
for coagulopathic complications, 1821–1822
Anticoagulation treatment
anticancer effects of, 1819
Anticonvulsants
brain metastasis, 901
for cancer pain, 873
Anti-CTLA4 antibodies, 715
Anti-CTLA4 therapy
distant metastatic melanoma, 1481, 1481t
Antidepressants, 805t
for cancer pain, 873
Antidotes, 1781
Antiemetics, 1757–1762
classes, 1758–1761
Antiestrogens, 741
breast cancer, 1433
side effects, 743–744
Antifungal prophylaxis, 1938–1939
Antigen-presenting cells, 178
Antigens
detection, 483
prostate-specific, 3, 376
tumor-associated, 725, 767–768
tumor-specific, 725
Antihistamines
for cancer pain, 874
hypersensitivity reactions, 1784
Anti-Hu, 1007
Anti-idiotypic antibodies, 710–711
Anti-inflammatory cytokines
cachexia, 1752
Anti-invasion therapy, 146f
Antimetabolites, 606–608
causing hyperpigmentation, 1782
Antimicrobial prophylaxis, 1938
Antimicrobial stewardship, 1939, 1939t
Antineoplastic agents
emetogenic potential, 1759t
Antineuronal nuclear antibody (ANNA-1), 1007
Antioxidants
cachexia, 1751
Antiretroviral therapy
for adult T-cell leukemia/lymphoma, 1656
Antisense, 764
Antithrombin III, 151
antiangiogenic confirmation of, 157
Antithymocyte globulin
GVHD, 1876
Anti-tumor activity mechanisms, 187–188
Antiviral prophylaxis, 1938–1939
Antracyclines
radiation-induced lung injury, 1859
Anxiety, causes in cancer patients, 802t, 802–803
treatment, 803t
APC, 92–93, 96f
genetic basis, 196–197
APC gene
colorectal cancer, 1181
Apixaban, 1821
APL. *See* Acute promyelocytic leukemia (APL)
Aplastic anemia, 789
APMF. *See* Acute panmyelosis with myelofibrosis
Apollon (Bruce), 45
Apomab, 692
Apoptosis, 40–50, 73
alternative forms, 48
-based therapies, 692
caspases, 40–43
cell proliferation, 33
gene therapy, 763
pathways, 44f
multidrug resistance, 602–603
protein domains, 42–48
radiation, 249, 522
resistance to, 128–129
signal transduction, 48–49
therapeutic opportunities, 49–50
Apparent diffusion coefficient (ADC), 323
Appendiceal neoplasms, 1177–1179
adenocarcinoma, 1179
carcinoids, 1177
mucoceles, 1178
pseudomyxoma peritonei, 1178–1179
Aprepitant, 1759, 1761, 1762
APRT, 265
Arabinoside, 30
Ara-C. *See* Cytosine arabinoside
ARF. *See* Acute respiratory failure
Arginase-1, 272
Aromatase inhibitors, 347, 744–749
adjuvant therapy, 746–747
breast cancer, 164, 1432–1433, 1438–1439
chemoprevention, 747–748
treatment, 745–745
first-generation, 744
neoadjuvant therapy, 747–748
resistance, 749
second-generation, 744
side effects, 748–749
third-generation, 744–745
Aromatic amines, 228
Arrhythmia, 1943
chemotherapeutic drugs associated with, 1943t
primary, 1943
secondary, 1943
treatment of, 1943
Artemin (ART), 59
Arterial blood gases
nonsmall-cell lung cancer, 1018
Arterial chemoembolization, 490–491, 491f
Arterial embolization, 490
Arterial infusion therapy, 490
Arterial thrombosis, 1820
Artificial sweeteners, 409
ASA. *See* Aspirin
Asbestos inhalation
malignant mesothelioma, 1044
Ascites, 2–3
ASCO. *See.* American Society of Clinical Oncology (ASCO)
ASCUS. *See* Atypical squamous cells of undetermined significance (ASCUS)
Aspartame, 409
Aspergillus, 1929–1930
Aspiration cytology, 481
Aspirin
for cancer pain, 867
essential thrombocytothemia, 1688
multiple myeloma, 1677
polycythemic vera, 1693, 1694
for venous thromboembolism, 1819

Astrocytoma
anaplastic, 890–891
AT/RT. *See* Atypical teratoid/rhabdoid tumor
Ataxia-telangiectasia
genetic basis, 210
Ataxia-telangiectasia mutation (ATM)
chronic lymphocytic leukemia, 1606
ATLL. *See* Adult T-cell leukemia/lymphoma (ATLL)
ATM, 29–30
ATM. *See* Ataxia telangiectasia mutation (ATM)
ATP. *See* Adenosine triphosphate (ATP)
ATRA syndrome, 1575
Atropine
diarrhea, 1874
Attributable risk, 382
Atypical adenomatous hyperplasia (AAH)
lung cancer, 1003
Atypical mole and melanoma syndrome, 1459
Atypical squamous cells of undetermined significance (ASCUS), 1304
Atypical teratoid/rhabdoid tumor (AT/RT), 1733
Augmentin
bacterial infections, 1924
Aurora kinases, 32–33
Autocrine mode, 51
Autocrine stimulation, 61
Autografting
multiple myeloma, 1678–1679
Autoimmune disorders
hematopoietic cellular transplantation for, 789
Autologous hematopoietic cellular transplantation
donor selection, 777–778
engraftment, 778–779
malignancies, 776–777
pretransplant therapy, 780
Autologous stem cell transplantation
for aggressive NHL, 1657
in first remission, 1656
for indolent NHL, 1655
multiple myeloma, 1678–1679, 1678f
Autonomic nerve blocks, 878
Autophagy, 48
Autopsy pathologist, role, 487
Auxiliary variables, 461–462
Avidin-biotin complex (ABC) technique, 482
Avipox virus, 727
aVWS. *See* Acquired von Willebrand syndrome (aVWS)
Axillary lymph node metastases
women with, 1716
Axitinib
breast cancer, 162
non-small cell lung cancer, 163
Axl, 58–59
Axl/SKY/MER family
ligands, 58–59
Azacitidine
epigenesis and human cancer, 173
myelodysplastic syndrome, 1553–1554, 1558
Azacytidine, 38, 626–627
structure, 626f
Azathioprine, 31, 1878
chemotherapy-induced lung injury, 1858
sinusoidal obstruction syndrome, 1877
veno-occlusive disease, 1877
Azithromycin, 1927
posttransplantation constrictive bronchiolitis, 1863
Aztreonam
bacterial infections, 1926
neutropenia, 1935

BAC. *See* Bronchioloalveolar carcinoma (BAC)
Back pain, 1764–1765
Bacteremia, 1924, 1926
Bacterial infections, 1887–1888, 1923
neutropenia, 1923t
Bacterial sepsis, 1808
Baculovirus IAP repeat (BIR), 42
Balanitis xerotica obliterans, 1255–1256
Balloon pericardiotomy, 1835
Bandolier, 852
Bandronate
for cancer pain, 874
Barium enema
colon cancer, 429
colorectal cancer, 1183
Bartholin gland carcinoma, 1294
Basal cell carcinoma (BCC), 267
morphea-like, 1491, 1492
pigmented, 1491f
of skin, 1491–1492, 1491f
vulva, 1294
Basal cell nevus syndrome (BCN), 262, 1491, 1492
Base excision repair, 232
Base pairing, 6, 6f
Basic fibroblast growth factor (bFGF), 35, 1091, 1700
Bayesian updating, 447–448
vs. frequentist interim analysis, 450–451
prior distributions, 448
BCC. *See* Basal cell carcinoma (BCC)
B-cell activating factor (BAFF)
multiple myeloma, 1671
B-cell chronic lymphocytic leukemia (B-CLL), 1604t
defective, 1606
Bcl-2, 73
cell life, 73f
family protein, 46–48, 47f, 603
homology, 42
multiple myeloma, 1673
Bcl-2
oncogenes, 84
Bcl-6, 1648
B-CLL. *See* B-cell Chronic lymphocytic leukemia (B-CLL)
Bcl-XL
multiple myeloma, 1673
BCN. *See* Basal cell nevus syndrome (BCN)
BCNU. *See* Bis-chloroethyl nitrosurea (BCNU)
Bcr/abl, 78, 81
BCR-ABL, 351
chronic myeloid leukemia, 1583, 1584–1585
BCRP. *See* Breast cancer resistance protein (BCRP)
BEACOPP
Hodgkin lymphoma, 1639, 1640, 1642, 1710
Becavizumab
breast cancer, 164
cerebrovascular ischemia, 165
colorectal cancer, 162
glioma, 165
-induced proteinuria, 166
non-small cell lung cancer, 162
pancreatic cancer, 165
renal cell cancer, 160
tumor angiogenesis, 168
Beckwith–Wiedemann syndrome, 304, 1728, 1735
Benadryl
oral complications, 1886
Bence Jones proteins (BJP), 1676
Bendamustine
chronic lymphocytic leukemia, 1614
clinical pharmacology, 639
Bendamustine-rituximab (BR)
chronic lymphocytic leukemia, 1616
Benign bone tumors, 1500
Benign breast disease, 1397–1398
Benign primary cardiac tumors, 1063–1064
Benign teratomas
of mediastinum, 1067
Benzamides, 1759
Benzocaine
for cancer pain, 874
mucositis, 1882
Benzodiazepine, 1761, 1762
neurologic complications, 1777
status epilepticus, 1954
Benzydamine hydrochloride
mucositis, 1882
Bereavement, 808
palliative care, 860–861
β-Adrenergic blockade, 1838
β-Adrenergic blockers, 1845, 1846, 1943
Beta carotene, 408
head and neck neoplasms, 962
Beta-cell lymphomas
interferons, 683
Betacellulin, 55
β-Endorphin, 864
β-Hemolytic streptococci, 1924
β-Hydroxy-β-methylbutyrate
cachexia, 1753
Betalactams, 1787
Bethanechol HCl
xerostomia, 1883
Bethesda guidelines for cancer risk, 204t
Bevacizumab, 714–715, 1846
adenocarcinoma of unknown primary site, 1717
for arterial thrombosis, 1820
chemotherapy-induced lung injury, 1858
colorectal cancer, 1192
Kaposi sarcoma, 1701
malignant mesothelioma, 1051
nephrotoxicity, 1830
prostate cancer, 1251
pulmonary vascular disorders, 1858
for venous thromboembolism, 1818
Bexarotene
mycosis fungoides/Sézary syndrome, 1663, 1666
Bexxar, 719
bFGF. *See* Basic fibroblast growth factor (bFGF)
Bicalutamide, 753–754
withdrawal, 755
Bile duct cancer, 1136–1142
causative factors, 1136–1137
clinical presentation, 1137–1138
diagnosis, 1138–1139
etiology, 1137
high-resolution helical computed tomography, 1138, 1139f
magnetic resonance imaging, 1139
pathology, 1138
ultrasonography, 1138–1139
Bilharzial bladder cancer, 311, 313f
progression of, 312–315
Billroth I gastroduodenostomy, 1097
Billroth II gastroduodenostomy, 1097
Bim protein, 46
Bio-bar code, 365
Biochemistry, 125–139
of cancer epigenetics, 133–134
of cell cycle, 137
of cell differentiation, 134–135
future directions, 137–139
of malignant transformation, 126–132
of signal transduction, 135–137
Biochemotherapy
distant metastatic melanoma, 1480–1481, 1480t
Bioenergetics, 129
Bioinformatics, 1979
Biologic therapies
for malignant mesothelioma, 1051
Biological barriers, to therapeutic action, 367
Biomarkers, 383–384, 461–462. *See also* *individual entries*
classification of, 348t

Biomarkers (*cont.*)
in drug development, 348–351
market and economic impact of, 354–357
Biopsy, 503–504
anal neoplasms, 1199–1200
of bone tumors, 1498–1499
core needle, 1499
excisional, 1499
fine needle, 1499
incisional open, 1499
cardiac, 1840, 1840t, 1841, 1842, 1843
cutting-core, 503
endomyocardial, 1838, 1840, 1842, 1847
excisional, 503
fine-needle aspiration, 1713
incisions, 503, 504, 504f
percutaneous, 496
soft tissue sarcomas, 1521–1522, 1522f
BIOSIS, 1968
Biphosphonates
bone tumors, 1501
for cancer pain, 875
multiple myeloma, 1675
BIR. *See* Baculovirus IAP repeat (BIR)
Bisacodyl
constipation, 1876
Bis-chloroethyl nitrosurea (BCNU)
for aggressive NHL, 1656
chemotherapy-induced lung injury, 1855, 1857, 1858
delayed pulmonary toxicity syndrome, 1863
pulmonary vascular disorders, 1858
Bismuth-Corlette classification
cholangiocarcinoma, 1141f
Bisodioxopiperazines, 646
Bisphosphonate, 1880
bone metastasis and, 1792, 1793, 1794, 1795
for cancer pain, 865, 874, 875
oral complications, 1880, 1882t, 1887
BJP. *See* Bence Jones proteins (BJP)
BL22, 721
Bladder cancer, 1219–1226, 1737
bilharzial, 312–315
clinical presentation, 1221
epidemiology, 1219
etiology, 1219
histologic distribution in Africa, 313t
investigation, 1221–1222
management
invasive, 1223–1225
non-muscle-invasive, 1222–1223
metastatic, 1225–1226
risk factors, 1223t
molecular determinants, 1219–1221
molecular imaging and, 331
noninvasive papillary tumors, 1219f
nutrition, 407
patho-biology, 1219–1221
prevention, 417
prognosis, 1222
schistosomiasis, 311–312
staging, 1221–1222, 1222f
uncommon histological variants, 1226
Bladder neck exposure and dissection
prostate cancer, 1237
Bladder outlet obstruction, 1824
Bleeding
management, 1106
Bleeding disorders, 1814–1817
Bleomycin, 30, 34, 589, 1835, 1845
acute pancreatitis, 1877
for aggressive NHL, 1656
causing hyperpigmentation, 1782f
causing nail hyperpigmentation, 1780
chemotherapy-induced lung injury, 1855, 1857, 1857f, 1858
for hemolytic uremic syndrome, 1820
Hodgkin lymphoma, 1631
for indolent NHL, 1654
Bleomycin (*cont.*)
Kaposi sarcoma, 1701
massive pleural effusion, 1950
for penile cancer, 1258
pregnancy and cancer, 834, 835
pulmonary fibrosis, 1737
radiation-induced lung injury, 33
thymomas, 1060
toxicity, 1284–1285
Blood
cellular elements of, 1798t
Blood bank, 1809–1810, 1810t
Blood component laboratory
future directions, 1809–1811
Bloom syndrome
genetic basis, 210
Blyeomycin
hyperthermia, 533
BM stromal cells (BMSCs)
multiple myeloma, 1670–1671, 1670f
BMSCs. *See* BM stromal cells (BMSCs)
BMT. *See* Bone marrow transplantation (BMT)
BNLI Trial, 1633
BNP. *See* B-type natriuretic peptide (BNP)
Body cavity
cytology, 480–481
Bone disease
multiple myeloma, 1674–1675
Bone lymphoma, 1512
Bone marrow
abnormal localization of immature precursors in, 1547
characteristic effects of drugs on, 1799t
cytokinetics, 560
stroma, in MDS, 1547
Bone marrow fibrosis
causes of, 1690t
Bone marrow transplantation (BMT), 1917
allogenic, 1917
autologous, 1917
dose effect, 561
in MDS patients', 1556–14
infection, 1922
Bone pain, adjuvants for
cancer pain, 874–875
Bone tumors, 1497–1515
biopsy, 1498–1488
evaluation, 1497–1498, 1498t
limb salvage versus amputation, 1499–1501, 1500t
in lower extremity, 1501
medical management, 1501–1515
radiotherapy, 1501
staging, 1498, 1498t, 1498f, 1499t
surgical margins, 1499
in upper extremity, 1501
BOOP. *See* Broncholitis obliterans with organizing pneumonia (BOOP)
Bortezomib, 1750
malignant mesothelioma, 1051
metabolic disease, 1537
multiple myeloma, 1677, 1681, 1682
neurologic complications, 1774
Bortezomimib, 1814
Bosutinib
chronic myeloid leukemia, 1587
Bourneville disease, 884
Bowen disease, 1489
Boys as cancer patients
gonadal complications in chemotherapy, 30–31
Brachial plexopathy, 1770–1771
Brachytherapy, 512–513
anal neoplasms, 1198, 1199
cervical cancer, 1314–1315
esophageal neoplasms, 1082
nonsmall-cell lung cancer, 1029
prostate cancer, 513f, 1236
retinoblastoma, 907
Bradford-Hill criteria, 234
BRAF
oncogenes, 84
BRAF mutations, 202
Bragg peak, 510
Brain
herniation, 1954
Brain metastasis, 899–903
clinical features, 900–901
pathophysiology, 899–900, 900f
stereotactic radiosurgery, 513f
treatment, 901–903, 901t
Brain stem gliomas (BSG), 1733
Brain toxicity
neurologic complications, 1774–1775
Brain tumors
radioimmunotherapy, 719
Branched-chain amino acids
cachexia, 1754
BRCA, 1918–1919
BRCA1, 98–100, 191–195, 318, 336, 337, 1345, 1394
pancreatic neoplasms, 1145
BRCA2, 98–100, 191–195, 212, 318, 336, 337, 362, 1345, 1394
pancreatic neoplasms, 1145
Brc-abl translocation, 339
Breakage-fusion-bridge (BFB) cycles, 359
Breast
adenocarcinoma, 477f
infiltrating ductal carcinoma, 1403f
medullary carcinoma, 1403f
mucinous carcinoma, 1404f
papillary carcinoma, 1402f
parasites, 314
tubular carcinoma, 1404f
Breast cancer resistance protein (BCRP), 598, 1577
Breast neoplasms, 15–16, 320f, 1393–1457
age-adjusted mortality
nutrition, 404f
aromatase inhibitors, 745–746, 748
aspiration cytology, 481
axillary dissection, 1419–1420
need, 1420–1421
biologic markers, 1414–1415
biopsy, 1412–1414, 1416–1419
bone marrow, 1408
breast conservation, 1416
contraindications, 1423
factors affecting outcome, 1424–1425
versus mastectomy, 1423
radiation, 1423–1424
breast self-examination, 1413–1414
chemoprevention, 1454–1456
chemotherapy, 1430–1432
classification, 1414–1415
cytotoxic chemotherapy, 1434–1435
combination chemotherapy, 1434
side effects, 1434–1435
diagnosis and screening, 1410–1414
differential diagnosis, 1414
ductal carcinoma in situ, 1421–1423
early stage
radiation, 1425–1426
elderly, 1452
endocrine therapy, 1432–1433, 1437–1438
epidemiology, 1393–1394
etiology, 237–247, 238t
growth regulation, 1399–1400, 1400f
hematopoietic cellular transplantation for, 788
hepatic arterial infusion chemotherapy, 1115t
hormonal action, 1433–1434
hormone therapy
side effects, 1434
hyperthermia, 537
inflammatory, 1451–1452
invasive
early stage, 1423
histologic types, 1402t

Breast neoplasms (cont.)
investigational markers, 1408–1409
isolated local-regional recurrence management, 1450
lifestyle changes, 1455–1456
lumpectomy, 1416, 1417
lymphatic invasion by, 1406f
male, 1451
mammography, 1411–1412
metastatic, 1442–1450
combination chemotherapy, 1448t
cytotoxic chemotherapy, 1446–1450
diagnostic evaluation, 1443
endocrine-sensitive, 1444–1445
HER2, 1445–1446
management, 1442–1450
symptomatic management, 1444
therapeutic guidelines, 1443
triple receptor-negative metastatic breast cancer, 1446
methotrexate, 615
molecular genetic alterations, 1408
clinical use, 1410
molecular imaging and, 318–321
molecular targets under investigation, 1450t
natural history, 1407–1410
neoadjuvant chemotherapy, 1430t
nonepithelial, 1404
nutrition, 403–405
osseous metastases, 1450–1451
outcome prediction and therapy responsiveness in, 337–338
palliative radiotherapy, 1429
pathology, 1401–1404
patient history, 1410
physical examinations, 1410–1411
pituitary function, 1433
postmastectomy radiation, 1427
after neoadjuvant chemotherapy, 1428–1429
indications, 1427–1428
modern, 1427
pregnancy and, 832–833, 1451
prevention, 414–415, 1452–1456
primary tumors, 1439–1442
progestin, 738–739
prognosis, 1407–1410
prognostic indices, 1409–1410
proliferative capacity, markers of, 1408
psychosocial aspects, 1416
radiation, 1429–1430
morbidity, 1430
risk assessment models, 1398–1399
risk factors, 1394–1399, 1394t
risk model, 1395t
risk of developing, 1393t
risk reduction options, 1453–1454
screening and early detection and molecular biomarkers, 336
screening in older patient, 844
screening, 422–425
evaluation, 424
options, 1453
physical examination, 424–425
randomized controlled trials, 423t
recommendations, 425
sentinel node dissection, 1420
staging, 1414–1415
surgery, 1416–1419
management, 1417f
systemic adjuvant therapy, 1435–1439
systemic therapy, 1430, 1432–1435
tamoxifen, 742, 742–743
technique and cosmetic considerations, 1416–1417, 1417f
tissue-specific biomarkers and, 342
TNM classification, 1415t
tumor characteristics, 1404–1407
tumor removal, 1418–1419
vaccine clinical trials, 729
Breast self-examination (BSE), 422, 424–425, 1413–1414
Breast–ovarian cancer syndrome
genetic basis, 191–195, 193f
Bromhexine
xerostomia, 1883
Bromocriptine, 917, 1913
growth hormone secreting pituitary adenomas, 919
Bromodeoxyuridine, 521
Bronchioloalveolar carcinoma (BAC)
lung, 1003–1004
Bronchogenic carcinoma, 1951
Bronchogenic cysts, 1064
Broncholitis obliterans with organizing pneumonia (BOOP), 1859
Bronchoscopic therapy
malignant airway obstruction, 1850, 1850f
Bronchoscopy
advances, 1010
electromagnetic navigation diagnostic, 1010
lung cancer, 1010
superior vena cava syndrome, 1948
Bronchospasm, 1858–1859
Bryostatin, 1787
BSE. *See* Breast self-examination (BSE)
BSG. *See* Brain stem gliomas (BSG)
B-type natriuretic peptide (BNP), 1841
Buccal mucosa, 969–970
Bupivacaine
for cancer pain, 874
Buprenorphine
for cancer pain, 871
Bupropion, 393
Burkitt leukemia, 1601–1602
Burkitt-like lymphoma, 1650
treatment, 1656
Burkitt lymphoma, 315–316, 1650
C-*myc* translocations, 78, 78f
Epstein-Barr virus, 293–294
parasites, 316
treatment, 1656
Burnout
in oncology staff, 808
Buschke–Loewenstein tumor, 1489, 1490
Buserelin
breast cancer, 1433
Business person, 829
Busulfan, 37, 635
causing hyperpigmentation, 1781
causing nail hyperpigmentation, 1780
chemotherapy-induced lung injury, 1855, 1858
clinical pharmacology, 639
for chronic myeloid leukemia, 1588
inducing hematuria, 1825
multiple myeloma, 1678
neurologic complications, 1774
pancytopenia, 1798
sinusoidal obstruction syndrome, 1877, 1878
structure, 635f
veno-occlusive disease, 1877, 1878
Butyrophenones, 1759

CA 125, 440
Cabergoline, 1913
growth hormone secreting pituitary adenomas, 919
caBIG™ (cancer Biomedical Informatics Grid), 1979
c-Abl, 516–517
11C-acetate
molecular imaging, 325, 328, 330
Cachexia, 1740, 1744t, 1755
biochemical and metabolic derangement, 1742–1748
enteral and parenteral nutrition, 1753–1754
etiology and mechanisms, 1740–1748
metabolic derangement, 1748
Cachexia (cont.)
palliative care, 857–858
pharmacologic management, 1748–1755
supportive care, 1748
treatment, 1748–1755
Cadherins, 143
CAK. *See* Cyclin-dependent kinase (CDK)-activating kinase (CAK)
Calcitonin, 1905, 1912
medullary thyroid carcinoma, 930
multiple myeloma, 1675
Calcitriol, 1911
bone metastasis, 1794
Calcium, 408
Calcium channel blockers, 1846, 1847
Calicheamicin, 717
CAM. *See* Complementary and alternative medicine (CAM)
Campath-1H, 712
Camptothecin, 652
small-cell lung cancer, 1038
structure, 652f
Cancer
bladder, 1737
cervical, 1919
as chronic disease, 1962
and chronic inflammation, 229
and coagulation system, relationship between, 1813–1814
functional screens for therapeutic target identification, 22–23
as local and systemic disease, 550–551
mouse models, 23–24
new cases, 374f
polygenetic etiology of, 550
prevention, 139, 234–236
prostate, 1919
rectal, 1919
secondary. *See* Secondary cancer
temporal progression, 141f
testicular, 1919
thyroid, 1917
thyroid nodules and, 1903–1904, 1904f
Cancer antigen 125 (CA125), 337, 339–340
Cancer antigen 15-3 (CA15-3), 340
Cancer antigen 19-9 (CA19-9), 340
Cancer antigen 27.29 (CA27.29), 340
Cancer-associated retinopathy (CAR), 912
Cancer biomarkers, 172–173, 335, 342
Cancer genome analysis, 113
Cancer.gov, 1977
Cancer pain, 863
addiction and drug abuse in patients, 879
anesthetic approaches, 876–877
assessment, 864–865
and treatment strategies, 866
cognitive-behavioral techniques for, 876t
common syndromes, 865–866
mechanisms, 864
neurophysiology, 864
neurosurgical approaches, 877–878, 877t
pharmacological approaches, 867–876
psychological and behavioral approaches, 876
syndromes, 866t
types, 865
Cancer pain management
barriers to, 863–864, 863t
guidelines for analgesic drug use in, 867t
WHO analgesic ladder for, 868f
Cancer risk modeling, 411
Cancer Statistics Review, 372
Cancer stem cell concept
vs. molecular classification, 550
Cancer study
enigmas, 550
Cancer therapy
cell differentiation, 38–39
Cancer vaccines
melanoma, 1478–1479

CANCERLIT database, 1978
Cancerophobia, 3
Candida, 1927–1929, 1928f
  esophagitis, 1872
Candidate tumor-suppressor genes, 99–100
Candidiasis, 1887
  chronic disseminated, 1928f
  disseminated, 1928
  esophageal, 1928f
  hepatosplenic, 1928
  oropharyngeal, 1928f
Cannabinoids, 1757, 1761
  cachexia, 1749
CAP chronic lymphocytic leukemia, 1614
Capacitabine
  colorectal cancer, 162
Capacitively coupled conduction current, 534
Capcetabine
  colorectal cancer, 1191
Capecitabine, 625, 1784, 1845
  breast cancer, 1447
  structure, 625f
Caphosol
  mucositis, 1882
Capillary hemangiomas
  pediatric ophthalmic neoplasms, 908–909
Capillary leak syndrome, 8
CAR. *See* Cancer-associated retinopathy (CAR)
Carbamazepine, 1761
  brain metastasis, 901
  for cancer pain, 873
Carbapenems
  bacterial infections, 1926
  neutropenia, 1935
Carboplatin, 32, 643, 889, 1574, 1757, 1908, 1916
  causing nail hyperpigmentation, 1780
  causing hyperpigmentation, 1782
  chemotherapy, 907
  distant metastatic melanoma, 1479
  malignant mesothelioma, 1050
  neuroblastoma, 1727
  non-small cell lung cancer, 163, 1030, 1031
  pharmacodynamics, 595
  poorly differentiated neuroendocrine carcinoma, 1720
  pregnancy and cancer, 835
  prostate cancer, 1249
  typhlitis, 1874
Carboplatinum
  prostate cancer, 1253
Carcino-embryonic antigen (CEA), 340
Carcinogen
  DNA dosimetry, 234
  metabolism, 228–229
Carcinogenesis
  chemical, 225–236
    examples, 225t
  multistage chemical, 226f
  radiation-induced
    experimental, 255–256
    genetic susceptibility, 256
    human epidemiologic studies, 256–259
    risk assessment, 259–260
Carcinoid heart disease, 1836, 1837f
Carcinoid tumors
  appendiceal, 1177
  lung, 1005
  ovaries, 1374
  small intestine, 1174–1175
Carcinoma
  basal cell, 1491–1492, 1491f
  bronchogenic, 1951
  choriocarcinoma, 1734
  embryonal, 1734
  hepatocellular, 1735
  medullary thyroid, 1495
  merkel cell, 1492–1493
  ovarian, 1842
  sebaceous, 1493–1494
  squamous cell, 1489–1491, 1489f
Carcinoma (*cont.*)
  verrucous, 1489, 1490
Carcinoma ex pleomorphic adenoma, 986
Carcinoma in situ, 1
  penis, 1256
CARD. *See* Caspase recruitment domains (CARD)
Cardiac arrest
  chemotherapy-related causes, 1942
  radiotherapy-related causes, 1942–1943
  tumor-related causes, 1942
Cardiac biopsy, 1840, 1840t, 1841, 1842, 1843
Cardiac blood-pool scan, 1833, 1837
Cardiac catheterization, 1836, 1837–1838
Cardiac complications, 1832–27, 1832t
  of cancer treatment, 1839–1847, 1839t
  of radiation therapy, 1847–1848
Cardiac dysrhythmia
  cardiac rhythm disturbances, treatment of, 1838–1839, 1839t
  categorids of, 1838
Cardiac failure
  in multiple myeloma, 1676
Cardiac fibromas, 1065
Cardiac rhythm disturbances
  treatment, 1838–1839, 1839t
Cardiac structures, metastatic involvement of, 1833f
Cardiac tamponade, 1834–1835
Cardiac tumors, 1063f
  benign primary, 1063–1064
  clinical features, 1062–1063
  diagnosis, 1063
  malignant primary, 1064
  metastatic, 1064
  pediatric, 1064–1065
Cardiomyopathy, 1840, 27
Cardiotoxic anticancer agents, 1839t
  with myocardial depressant activity, 1839–1840, 1840t
Cardiovascular system
  evaluation, 1832–1833, 1833f
Carinal resection, 1022
Carmustine, 635, 889, 1838
  causing hyperpigmentation, 1782
  multiple myeloma, 1676
  nephrotoxicity, 1826
  pancytopenia, 1798
Carney complex, 924, 1063, 1064t
Carotenoids, 408
Carotid artery rupture, 1947
Cartilage tumors, 1501–1503
Case control studies, 383, 422, 467
Casopitant, 1761
Caspase
  activation pathways, 41–42, 41f
  apoptosis, 40–43
  suppression
    IAP family protein, 46f
Caspase-8 antagonist, 50
Caspase recruitment domains (CARD), 42
  proteins, 44–45
Caspofungin, 1887, 1931
  aspergillosis, 1930
  candidiasis, 1928, 1929
  esophagitis, 1872
Castleman disease
  multicentric
    human herpesvirus, 296
Castration-resistant prostate cancer (CRPC), 755
Catenins, 1090
Cathepsin B
  cachexia, 1746
Catheter-related infections, 1936
CBE. *See* Clinical breast examination (CBE)
CC chemokines, 273
CCL2 (MCP-1), 273
CCNA. *See* Chloroethyl-cyclohexyl nitrosurea (CCNA)
CCRIS. *See* Chemical Carcinogenesis Research Information System (CCRIS)
CCSK. *See* Clear cell sarcoma of the kidney (CCSK)
CCT. *See* Combination chemotherapy (CCT)
CD28 molecules, 184
CD38 expression, 1611
CD4+ cells, 176, 177, 180
CD40 molecules, 181–182
2-CDA. *See* 2-Chlorodeoxyadenosine
CDC. *See* Centers for Disease Control and Prevention (CDC)
CDH1, 213–214, 214f
CDK. *See* Cyclin-dependent kinase (CDK)
CDKN2, 206
cDNA, 14–15
CEA. *See* Carcino-embryonic antigen (CEA)
CECs. *See* Circulating endothelial cells (CECs)
Cediranib
  non-small cell lung cancer, 163
Cefepime
  bacterial infections, 1924, 1926
  neutropenia, 1937
Ceftazidime
  bacterial infections, 1924, 1926
  neutropenia, 1936, 1937
Ceftriaxone
  bacterial infections, 1924
Celecoxib, 889, 1784
  cachexia, 1750
  molecular diagnostics, 337
  prostate neoplasms, 1242
Celiac axis block, 1105
Celiac sprue, 1173
Cell cycle
  checkpoints, 32
  control, 27–28
    gene therapy, 763
  cyclin-dependent kinase regulation, 27f
Cell death. *See also* Apoptosis
  pathway, 44f
  radiation, 249
Cell differentiation, 33–39, 134–135
  cancer therapy, 38–39
  cell proliferation, 33–34
  extracellular factors controlling, 35–36
  induction, 35t
Cell membrane
  changes, 130
Cell proliferation, 26–39
  apoptosis, 33
  cell differentiation, 33–34
  tumor growth, 26–27
Cell surface phenotype
  multiple myeloma, 1669
Cell survival, 129–130
  pathway, 44f
Cell-loss fraction. *See* Death fraction
Cellular immune dysfunction, 1921–1922
Cellular proliferation kinetics
  growth parameters assessment, 551–552
Cellular therapy products, generation of, 180
Cellulitis
  chemical, 1781
    chemotherapeutic agents associated with, 1781t
Centers for Disease Control and Prevention (CDC), and cancer epidemiology, 372
Central nervous system (CNS)
  prophylaxis, 1599, 1707
  tumors, 1732–1733
Central nervous system leukemia, 1578–1579
  metabolic abnormalities, 1579
  ophthalmic complications, 1579
Central nervous system neoplasms, 881–897
  chemotherapy, 888–889
  clinical presentation, 886
  computed tomography, 886
  diagnostic neuroimaging, 886–887
  epidemiology, 881

Central nervous system neoplasms (*cont.*)
experimental therapies, 889
familial syndromes, 883–885, 884t
magnetic resonance imaging, 886
molecular genetics, 882–883
neuroepithelial
histopathology, 885–886
radiation therapy, 888
risk factors, 881–882, 882t
supportive therapy, 889–890
surgery, 887–888
Cephalosporins, 1787
bacterial infections, 1926
neutropenia, 1936
CEPs. *See* Circulating endothelial progenitors (CEPs)
Cerebellar astrocytoma, 1733
Cerebrospinal fluid (CSF), 1578, 1768
cytology, 480–481
tumor markers, 1769t
Cerebrovascular complications
neurologic complications, 1776
Cervical condyloma, 298f
Cervical conization, 1311–1312
Cervical cytology
classification schemes, 434t
Cervical intraepithelial neoplasm
histopathology, 299f
Cervical neoplasms, 1919, 1299–1323
carcinoma in situ, 1316
concurrent chemoradiation, 1319–1320
epidemiology, 1299–1301
hyperthermia, 538–539
incidence, 375–376
invasive lesions, 1307–1313
diagnosis, 1308–1309
evaluation and staging, 1309–1310, 1309t
patterns of spread, 1307–1308
prognosis, 1310
surgery, 1311–1313
symptoms, 1308
metastatic, 1320–1321
molecular imaging and, 331
precancerous lesions, 1304–1307
during pregnancy, 833–834
prevention, 415–416
radiation therapy, 1313–1316
outcomes, 1315
recurrent, 1321–1323
relapse rates, 1309t
screening, 432–434
in older patients, 844
stage IA1, 1316
stage IA2, 1316
stage IB1 and IIA, 1316–1317
stage IB2, 1317–1319
stage IIB-IVA, 1319
Cervix
adenosquamous carcinoma, 1303
epithelial tumors
histologic classification, 1301–1303
lymphoepithelioma-like carcinoma, 1302, 1302f
nonsmall-cell neuroendocrine carcinoma, 1303, 1303f
papillary squamous cell carcinoma, 1302, 1302f
small-cell neuroendocrine carcinoma, 1303, 1303f
squamous cell carcinoma, 1301–1302, 1302f
verrucous carcinoma, 1302
Cetuximab, 712–713, 1787, 1880
bronchospasm, 1859
colorectal cancer, 162, 1192
immunotherapy, 187
personalized medicine, 351
CGH. *See* Comparative genomic hybridization (CGH)
Chagas disease, 1809
Charcoal for treatment of diarrhea, 1874
Checkpoints
CHEK2, 195
Chemical Carcinogenesis Research Information System (CCRIS), 1978
Chemical carcinogenesis, 225–236
examples, 225t
Chemical cellulites
chemotherapeutic agents associated with, 1781, 1781t
Chemical pleurodesis
malignant pleural effusion, 1853
Chemoimmunotherapy combinations
chronic lymphocytic leukemia, 1615
Chemokines, 273
Chemoprevention, 411–417
biology of, 411
incidence, 417
trials, 411–417
Chemoradiation
bleeding, 1106
Chemoreceptor trigger zone (CTZ), 1757
Chemotaxis, 53
Chemotherapeutic agents
activation, 588t
anaphylaxis, 1957–1958, 1957t
indications, 569t–576t
infection, 1923
nephrotoxicity, 1826–1830, 1826t, 1827t, 1828t, 1829t
Chemotherapy, 553
agents required for curve, 564t
anal neoplasms, 1198
antiangiogenic effects of, 158–159
for arterial thrombosis, 1820
for basal cell carcinoma, 1492
brain metastasis, 902–903
chronic low-dose, 147
chronic lymphocytic leukemia, 1612–1613
and combined therapy, for urethra, 1260
dermatologic complications, 1779–1787
distant metastatic melanoma, 1479–1480, 1480t
effects on gonadal function
in boys, 30–31
in men, 31–32
in prepubertal girls, 32–33
in women, 33–34
emetogenic, 1758, 1761, 1762
Ewing's sarcoma, 1532
Hodgkin lymphoma, 1623, 1634–1636, 1634t, 1635t, 1638t, 1640t, 1641t
hypothyroidism, 1903
intra-arterial, 907
for localized STS of extremities, 1529–1532
adjuvant, 1532
modification factors, 1531
preoperative, 1530–1531
with primary surgical resection, 1529–1530, 1529f, 1529t
low-risk, 1762
for malignant mesothelioma, 1050
metabolic disease, 1535, 1536
myelodysplastic syndrome, 1555–1556
neurologic complications, 1770
oral complications of, 1884–1888
bacterial infections, 1887–1888
fungal infections, 1887
risk factors, 1885–1886
viral infections, 1887
osteogenic sarcoma, 1532
osteosarcoma, 1731
penis, 1258
pharmacodynamic modeling of, 594–595
during pregnancy, 36–37
prostate cancer, 1243, 1248–1249
radiation therapy, 525t
renal tumors in children, 1729
retroperitoneal sarcomas, 1541
rhabdomyosarcoma, 1532
Chemotherapy (*cont.*)
for secondary cancer, 1916–1917
of solid tumors, and hematopoietic growth factors, 707
for squamous cell carcinoma, 1491
systemic, 907
thymomas, 1059–1060
thyroid carcinoma, 929
Chemotherapy-induced lung injury, 30t, 1855–1859, 1856t
Chemotherapy-induced nausea and vomiting (CINV), 1757, 1758f
prevention
recommendations, 1761
Chemotherapy-related pancytopenia, 1798
Chemotherapy response
kinetics of, 553–555
Chest radiograph
carcinoid heart disease, 1836
Chest wall, 1021
CHF. *See* Congestive heart failure (CHF)
Children as cancer patients
acute lymphoblastic in, 1724–1725
acute myeloid leukemia in, 1725
and adults
hematopoietic growth factors, 707
cancer and MMR, 203–204
exposed to cancer therapy in utero, 836
gonadal complications in
protection from, 36
Hodgkin disease in, 1725
non-Hodgkin lymphoma in, 1725
renal tumors in, 1728–1729
soft tissue sarcomas of, 1729–1730
Chimeric antigen receptors (CAR), 180
China, 314, 315
Chlamydia trachomatis, 1300
Chlorambucil, 30, 33, 37, 634–635, 1878, 1916
chronic lymphocytic leukemia, 1612, 1613, 1614
clinical pharmacology, 638–639
for indolent NHL, 1654
metabolism, 637
mycosis fungoides/Sézary syndrome, 1664
myelodysplastic syndrome, 1546
Waldenström macroglobulinemia, 1683
Chlorhexidine, 1888
Chlorhexidine gluconate, 1887
mucositis, 1882
2-Chlorodeoxyadenosine, 1574, 1786
chronic lymphocytic leukemia, 1613
Waldenström macroglobulinemia, 1683
Chloroethyl-cyclohexyl nitrosurea (CCNU)
chemotherapy-induced lung injury, 1858
Chloroquine
photosensitivity reactions, 1783
ChlVPP
Hodgkin lymphoma, 1631, 1639
Chocolate cysts, 909
Cholangiocarcinoma, 1129–1130, 1136–1137
Bismuth-Corlette classification, 1141f
distribution, 1137f
etiology, 1137
vs. hepatocellular carcinoma, 1137t
hilar, 1138–1142
intrahepatic
treatment, 1139–1140
liver neoplasms, 1130
epidemiology, 1129
natural history, 1130
risk factors, 1129
treatment, 1130
Cholangiography, 1139
Cholecystectomy, 1134–1136
Choline
molecular imaging, 324
Chondroblastic osteosarcoma, 1731, 1731f
Chondroblastoma, 1502
Chondromas, 1501–1502
Chondromyxoid fibroma, 1502–1503, 1503f

Chondrosarcoma, 1507–1508, 1507f, 1508t
clear cell, 1508
dedifferentiated, 1508
mesenchymal, 1508
CHOP, 1706, 1706t, 1707, 1709
acute lymphoblastic leukemia, 1601
for adult T-cell leukemia/lymphoma, 1656
for aggressive NHL, 1653, 1655–1656
bone lymphoma, 1512
for indolent NHL, 1654, 1655
for mantle cell lymphoma, 1656
mycosis fungoides/Sézary syndrome, 1665
Choriocarcinoma, 1266, 1734
methotrexate, 614–615
ovary, 1370
Choroidal melanoma, 910–912, 910f, 910t
Choroidal nevi, 909
Chromatin, 7
altered, 133, 172
formation, 170–171
Chromosomal abnormalities
radiation, 250
Chromosomal rearrangements, 76–78
molecularly characterized, 77t
Chromosomal translocations, 69, 79, 486t
Chromosome 11, 304
Chromosome 13, 88
Chromosome banding, 69
Chromosome microdissection FISH (micro-FISH), 108, 109f
Chronic disseminated candidiasis, 1928f
Chronic fibrosis, 1737
Chronic lymphocytic leukemia (CLL), 1604–1620
anemia in, 1618–1619
B-cell, 1604t
causation, 1605
clinical management, 1618–1619
clinical presentation, 1608
cytogenetics, 1606
defective B- and T-cell functions, 1606–1607
differential diagnosis, 1608
epidemiology, 1604–1605
familial, 1605
genetic basis, 218–219, 219f
hematopoietic cellular transplantation for, 786–787
hiatory of identification, 1604
immunobiology, 1605–1606
immunophenotype, 1605–1606
incidence, 1604–1605
infections in, 1618
at initial diagnosis
physical findings, 1608–1609
laboratory abnormalities, 1609
lymphocytes, 1607
minimum diagnostic requirements, 1608
molecular genetics, 1606–1607
monoclonal B-cell lymphocytosis, 1605
in monozygotic twins, 1605
morphology in peripheral blood smear, 1607, 1607t
natural history, 1609–1610
pathogenesis, 1605
prognosis, 1612, 1612t
psychosocial aspects, 1618
radiologic findings, 1609
salvage therapy, 1616–1617, 1616t
staging, 1610–1613, 1610t, 1611f
symptoms, 1608
thrombocytopenia in, 1619
treatment, 1612–1614, 1619–1620
variants, 1619
Chronic myeloid leukemia (CML), 81–82, 351, 1582, 1583f
and bcr-abl translocation, 339
clinical and hematologic characteristics, 1582–1583
cytogenetics, 1584
gleevec, 65
Chronic myeloid leukemia (CML) (*cont.*)
hematopoietic cellular transplantation for, 785–786
incidence and epidemiology, 1582
interferons, 683
molecular biology, 1584–1585
pathophysiology, 1583–1584
prognosis in, 1583
treatment, 1585–1589, 1589
Chronic myeloproliferative disorders
platelet-lowering agents, clinical properties of, 1686t
Cidofovir
viral infections, 1931
Cigarette smoking, 375
breast cancer, 1397
lung cancer, 1000
pancreatic neoplasms, 1146
Cilastatin
neutropenia, 1936
CIM. *See* Complementary and integrative medicine (CIM)
Cimetidine
systemic reactions to, 1959
Cingulotomy, 877
Cintredekin besudotox, 722
CINV. *See* Chemotherapy-induced nausea and vomiting (CINV)
CIPER, 45
Ciprofloxacin
acute lymphoblastic leukemia, 1597
bacterial infections, 1926
neutropenia, 1935
Circadian rhythm, 593
Circulating endothelial cells (CECs), 168
Circulating endothelial progenitors (CEPs), 168
Circulating tumor cells (CTCs), 343
Circulatory emergencies, 1941–1949
Cirrhosis
liver neoplasms, 1125
9-*Cis*-retinoic acid
Kaposi sarcoma, 1701
13-*Cis*-retinoic acid, 1728, 1908
Cisapride
anorexia, 1750
Cisplatin, 32, 34, 91, 163, 521, 889, 1757, 1823, 1845, 1846, 1907, 1908, 1916
acute pancreatitis, 1877
adenocarcinoma of unknown primary site, 1717
anal neoplasms, 1198, 1199, 1201
causing hyperpigmentation, 1782
causing nail hyperpigmentation, 1780
clinical trials, 641
delayed pulmonary toxicity syndrome, 1863
diarrhea, 1874
distant metastatic melanoma, 1479
epigenesis and human cancer
esophageal neoplasms, 1082t
gastric cancer, 1102, 1103, 1104
for hemolytic uremic syndrome, 1820
hypersensitivity reactions, 1783
hyperthermia, 533, 534
localized STS of extremities, 1532
malignant mesothelioma, 1050, 1051
myelodysplastic syndrome, 1546
nephrotoxicity, 1826, 1828
neuroblastoma, 1727
neurologic complications, 1773–1774
for nonbacterial thrombotic endocarditis, 1820
nonsmall-cell lung cancer, 1030, 1031, 1032
osteosarcoma, 1509, 1731
poorly differentiated carcinoma of unknown primary site, 1719
pregnancy and cancer, 833, 834, 835
prostate cancer, 1253
seminoma, 1069
small-cell lung cancer, 1039–1040
Cisplatin (*cont.*)
thymomas, 1059, 1060
toxicity, 606, 643
typhlitis, 1874
Cisplatinum
prostate cancer, 1253
CJD. *See* Creutzfeldt-Jakob disease (CJD)
c-kit ligand, 1804
Cladribine, 631, 1589
acute lymphoblastic leukemia, 1600
chronic lymphocytic leukemia, 1613
mycosis fungoides/Sézary syndrome, 1664
Clamshell incision for lung tumor resection, 1019
Clarithromycin, 1927
for indolent NHL, 1653
Clavulanate
bacterial infections, 1926
Clavulanic acid
bacterial infections, 1924
Clear cell carcinoma
endometrium, 1327–1328
Clear cell chondrosarcoma, 1508
Clear cell sarcoma of the kidney (CCSK), 1729
Clenbuterol
cachexia, 1751
CLIN system, 1974
Clindamycin, 1924
bacterial infections, 1925
PCNS lymphoma, 1708
Clinical breast examination (CBE), 422, 424–425
Clinical pathologist
role, 485–486
Clinical target volume
nonsmall-cell lung cancer, 1024
Clinical test validation, 354
Clinical trials
adaptive designs, 457–461
early, 580–581
phase I, 584
dose escalation, 582–584
patient selection, 584
schedule selection, 582
starting dose, 582
older patient, 842–843
phase 0, 580–581
Clinicopathologic staging schemes
for differentiated thyroid carcinoma, 925
CLL. *See* Chronic lymphocytic leukemia (CLL)
Clodronate
for cancer pain, 874
multiple myeloma, 1675
Clofarabine, 1574, 1784
acute lymphoblastic leukemia, 1600
Clonazepam
for cancer pain, 873
Clonidine, 393
for cancer pain, 873
Clonorchis sinensis, 315
Cloretazine, 1574
Clostridium difficile, 1873, 1874, 1926
and diarrhea, 1875
Clostridium septicum, 1873
Clotrimazole (Mycelex), 1887
Cluster of differntiation 44 (CD44), 1091
C-mer, 59
C-met, 57–58, 1091
11C-methionine
molecular imaging, 325
CMF, 33, 34
CML. *See* Chronic myeloid leukemia (CML)
CMV colitis, 1875, 1875f. *See also* Colitis
CMV. *See* Cytomegalovirus (CMV)
C-*myc* translocations
Burkitt lymphoma, 78, 78f
Coagulase-negative staphylococcus (CoNS), 1923, 1924
Coagulation factor deficiencies, 1816–1817

Coagulopathic complications, 1813–1822
  treatment, 1821–1822
Cochrane Review Organization, 851
Cockayne syndrome, 262, 266
Cockroft formula, 1828, 1829t, 1830
Codeine
  for cancer pain, 868–869
  diarrhea, 1874
Coding region, 5
Cohort studies, 382–383, 466–467
COL-3, 1703
Colitis
  CMV, 1875, 1875f
  pseudomembranous, 1875, 1875f
Collecting duct carcinoma, 1209
Colon cancer. *See also* Colorectal neoplasms
  chemoembolization, 1121t
  obstruction, 1188
  perforated, 1188
  screening and early detection and molecular biomarkers, 336
  screening in older patient, 844
  sigmoid, 1185–1186
  somatic *APC* mutations, 93–94
Colonoscopy
  colon cancer, 429–430
  colorectal cancer, 1183
Colony stimulating factor (CSF), 1798, 1913
Colony stimulating factor 1 (CSF-1), 53, 274
Colorectal metastases, 493
Colorectal neoplasms, 162
  adjuvant therapy, 1188–1190
  age
    incidence, 402f
  chemoembolization, 1121
  colonoscopy, 1183
  CT colonography, 1183
  development, 82f
  epidemiology, 1179–1180
  family history, 1180
  genetics, 195–206, 1180–1181
  guidelines, 431t
  laparoscopic colectomy, 1187–1188
  local recurrence, 1188
  lymphadenectomy, 1186–1187
  malignant polyp, 1184
    Haggitt classification, 1184t
  management, 1184–1188
  metastatic, 1191–1192
    treatment, 1115t
  mibiotic administration, 1184–1185
  molecular imaging and, 322–324
  nutrition, 402–3
  preoperative workup, 1183–1184
  prevention, 205
  prevention, 413–414, 425–431
  radioimmunotherapy, 719
  radiologic evaluation, 1183–1184
  resection margins, 1184, 1185f
  risk, 403f, 1180
  routine laboratory work, 1183
  screening
    recommendations, 431
    and surveillance, 1182–1183, 1183t
  signs and symptoms, 1182
  staging, 1184, 1184t
  surveillance following resection, 1188, 1188t
  synchronous distant metastases, 1188
  tissue-specific biomarkers and, 342
Combination chemotherapy (CCT), 564–565
  cytokinetics, 564
  drug resistance, 564
  experimental models, 565–566
  vs. holotherapy, 566t
  modulation, 565
  multiple myeloma, 1676
  vs myeloma therapies, 1677, 1677t
  synchronization, 564–565
Combinatorial immunotherapeutics, 187
Co-morbid medical conditions
  older patient, 840–841
Communication
  about bad news, 854–855
Community respiratory viral infections, 1932
Comparative genomic hybridization (CGH), 102, 108–109, 109f
  microarray based, 109–110, 110f, 359
Complementary and alternative medicine (CAM), 1761
  defined, 846
Complementary and integrative medicine (CIM), 846
  communication, importance of, 847–848
  and effective integration, 852
  rational stratetgy to approach, 849
  utilization, 846–847
Complete remission (CR), 1559, 1564, 1568, 1569, 1570, 1571
Comprehensive geriatric model, 842, 843f
Computed tomography (CT)
  colonography, 430–431
  Hodgkin lymphoma, 1629, 1629f
  malignant pleural effusion, 1851
Computer, medical uses of, 1964t
Computerized patient records (CPR), 1972–1974
Concomitant immunity, 176
Condyloma
  cervical, 298f
Confusions and hallucinations, 876
Congenital syndromes, 1512–1513
Congestive heart failure (CHF)
  management of, 1846f
  in multiple myeloma, 1676
Conivaptan, 1908, 1913
CoNS. *See* Coagulase-negative staphylococcus (CoNS)
Consortium of Academic Centers for Integrative Medicine, 846
Constipation, 875, 1875–1876
  palliative care, 855–856, 856t
Continuous reassessment method (CRM), 458–459
Contrast agents, nanoparticle, 366, 369
Conventional osteosarcoma, 1509–1510, 1509f
Coombs' test, 1547
COP. *See* Cryptogenic organizing pneumonitis (COP)
Coping, 796t
COPP, 31
Copy number abnormalities, 361f
  genome aberrations and, 361–362
Cordoba, 1508
Cordotomy, 877
Core needle biopsy, 1499. *See also* Biopsy
Coronary artery disease, 1847
Coronary heart disease, 743–744
Coronary steal, 1846
Corticosteroids, 1575, 1757, 1759, 1782, 1785
  for acquired hemophilia, 1816
  acute lymphoblastic leukemia, 1596
  brain metastasis, 901
  breast cancer, 1433–1434
  cachexia, 1748
  chemotherapy-induced lung injury, 1858
  chronic lymphocytic leukemia, 1612, 1613
  GVHD, 1876
  Hodgkin lymphoma, 1631
  hypersensitivity reactions, 1784
  multiple myeloma, 1675
  neurologic complications, 1774
  posttransplantation constrictive bronchiolitis, 1862
  primary myelofibrosis, 1691
  radiation-induced lung injury, 1860
  spinal cord compression, 1766
  thymomas, 1059
  Waldenström macroglobulinemia, 1683
Corticotropin releasing hormone (CRH), 1910
Cost-effectiveness analysis of modeling studies, 467
Costimulatory genes, 767
Costimulatory molecule genes
  direct injection of, 726
Coumadin
  multiple myeloma, 1677
Cowden disease, 924, 1494
Cowden syndrome
  genetic basis, 210–211
CPD. *See* Cyclobutane pyrimidine dimer (CPD)
CpG islands, 171, 172
CPR. *See* Computerized patient records (CPR)
Cranial and peripheral nerve metastases
  neurologic complications, 1770–1772
Cranial neuropathies, 1771t
C-reactive protein (CRP), 1687
Creutzfeldt-Jakob disease (CJD), 1809
CRH. *See* Corticotropin releasing hormone
Crises
  natural response to, 794t
Critical Path Initiative, 351, 353
CRM. *See* Continuous reassessment method (CRM)
Crohn's disease, 1173, 1180
CRP. *See* C-reactive protein (CRP)
CRPC. *See* Castration-resistant prostate cancer (CRPC)
CRS-207, 1051
Cryoablation
  liver neoplasms, 1128
Cryosurgery
  for squamous cell carcinoma, 1490
Cryotherapy
  retinoblastoma, 907
Cryptococcus, 1930
Cryptogenic organizing pneumonitis (COP), 1863
  chronic lymphocytic leukemia, 1613
CSF-1. *See* Colony stimulating factor 1 (CSF-1)
CTCs. *See* Circulating tumor cells (CTCs)
CTL. *See* Cytolytic T cells (CTL)
CTLA-4, 184
  anti-, 184, 187–188
CTZ. *See* Chemoreceptor trigger zone
Curcumin
  cachexia, 1750
Cushing syndrome, 934, 1910, 1910f, 1911
Cutaneous angiosarcoma, 1493
Cutaneous eruption of lymphocyte recovery (ELS), 1784–1785
Cutaneous mastocytosis (CM), 1579
Cutaneous reactions, 1779–1787
  causes, 1779t
  radiation-associated, 1782, 1782t
Cutting-core biopsy, 503
CVPP
  Hodgkin lymphoma, 1636, 1638
CXC chemokines, 273
Cyclin-dependent kinase (CDK), 27
  -activating kinase (CAK), 28
  activation, 31
  regulation, 27f
    cellcycle, 27f
Cyclin-dependent kinase inhibitor 2A (CDKN2A) locus, 92
Cyclobutane pyrimidine dimer (CPD), 263, 263f, 264f, 266t
Cyclooxygenase-2 (COX-2), 274
Cyclophosphamide, 30, 33, 32, 34, 37, 633–634, 1757, 1838, 1844, 1905, 1907, 1908, 1916, 1917, 1919, 1942
  for acquired hemophilia, 1816
  acute lymphoblastic leukemia, 1596
  acute pancreatitis, 1877
  for aggressive NHL, 1656
  antidiuresis, 640
  bladder toxicity, 640
  breast cancer, 164, 1448

Cyclophosphamide (*cont.*)
cardiotoxicity, 641, 1841, 1878
causing anaphylaxis, 1958
causing hyperpigmentation, 1782
causing nail hyperpigmentation, 1780
chemotherapy-induced lung injury, 1855, 1858
chronic lymphocytic leukemia, 1612, 1613, 1614, 23
clinical pharmacology, 638
delayed pulmonary toxicity syndrome, 1863
Ewing sarcoma, 1509, 1732
hyperthermia, 533
immunosuppression, 641
immunotherapy, 180
for indolent NHL, 1654
inducing hematuria, 1825
localized STS of extremities, 1531, 1532
massive pleural effusion, 1950
metabolism, 634f
multiple myeloma, 1676, 1678
mycosis fungoides/Sézary syndrome, 1664, 1665
neuroblastoma, 1727
photosensitivity reactions, 1783
pregnancy and cancer, 832, 833, 834, 835
prostate cancer, 1249, 1253
pulmonary vascular disorders, 1858
radiation-induced lung injury, 1859
renal tumors in children, 1729
rhabdomyosarcoma, 1730
sinusoidal obstruction syndrome, 1877
small cell lung cancer, 1035, 1037, 1039–1040
thymomas, 1060
typhlitis, 1873
veno-occlusive disease, 1877
Waldenström macroglobulinemia, 1683
Cyclosporin, 1927
neurologic complications, 1774
Cyclosporine, 782, 783, 1783
for acquired hemophilia, 1816
chemotherapy, 907
for hemolytic uremic syndrome, 1820
GVHD, 1876
multiple myeloma, 1678
nephrotoxicity, 1830
Cyclosporine A, 1577, 1904
Cylindromas, 985
Cymbalta
for cancer pain, 873
CYP 2B1. *See* Cytochrome P450 2B1 (CYP 2B1)
CYP. *See* Cytochrome P450 (CYP)
CYP3A4, 1735
Cyproheptadine
anorexia, 1754
Cyproterone acetate
breast cancer, 1434
Cystadenocarcinoma
mucinous, 1349f
serous, 1349f
Cysticercus fasciolaris, 316
Cystitis
hemorrhagic, 1825
etiology, 640
Cystosarcoma phyllodes, 1404f
Cytarabine, 889, 1569, 1784, 1908
acute lymphoblastic leukemia, 1596, 1597, 1599, 1600
for aggressive NHL, 1656
hypersensitivity reactions, 1783
for mantle cell lymphoma, 1656
myelodysplastic syndrome, 1556
neurologic complications, 1769, 1774
pregnancy and cancer, 835
schedule effects, 562
Cytochrome P450 (CYP), 227, 235, 389
Cytochrome P450 2B1 (CYP 2B1), 763
Cytogenetic abnormalities, in AML, 1561–1562, 1561f, 1562f
Cytogenetics
chronic lymphocytic leukemia, 1606
Cytokine genes, 766
direct injection of, 726
Cytokine therapy
miscellaneous reactions to, 26t
Cytokines, 181, 184, 186, 687t, 1942, 1955
anorexia, 1740–1741
cachexia, 1742
dermatologic complications, 1785–1786, 1786f
and hematopoietic growth factors, 686–709
immunostimlulants, 728
multiple myeloma, 1670–1671, 1670f
proinflammatory, 273
radiation, 521
systemic reactions to, 1958–1959
Cytokinetics, 550–557
Cytologic specimens
microscopic interpretation, 480
preparation, 479
Cytolytic T cells (CTL), 40
Cytomegalovirus (CMV), 1807–1808, 1808t, 1932
esophagitis, 1872, 1873
Cytopathologist, 479–481
Cytosine, 30
Cytosine arabinoside (Ara-C), 607, 625–626
acute pancreatitis, 1877
chemotherapy-induced lung injury, 1858
metabolism, 608f
myelodysplastic syndrome, 1555
neurologic complications, 1774
pregnancy and cancer, 832
sinusoidal obstruction syndrome, 1877, 1878
structure, 625f
typhlitis, 1873
veno-occlusive disease, 1877, 1878
Cytosine deaminase, 762–763
Cytotoxic therapy
reactions to, 1785t
Cytoxan
Ewing sarcoma, 1509

Dabigatran etexilate, 1821
Dacarbazine
cardiotoxicity, 1841
causing nail hyperpigmentation, 1780
immunotherapy, 187
localized STS of extremities, 1530, 1531
metabolic disease, 1536
sinusoidal obstruction syndrome, 1877
veno-occlusive disease, 1877
Dacryocystorhinostomy, 983
Dactinomycin, 1782, 1908
cardiotoxicity, 1841
causing nail hyperpigmentation, 1780
cutaneous reactions, 1779
hypersensitivity reactions, 1783
localized STS of extremities, 1532
renal tumors in children, 1729
rhabdomyosarcoma, 1730
DAD. *See* Diffuse alveolar damage (DAD)
DAH. *See* Diffuse alveolar hemorrhage (DAH)
Dalbavancin
bacterial infections, 1924
neutropenia, 1937
Dalforpristin, 1924, 1925
Danazol
myelodysplastic syndrome, 1555
DAP kinase, 43
Dapsone, 1785
Daptomycin
bacterial infections, 1924, 1925
neutropenia, 1937
Dasatanib, 1579
acute lymphoblastic leukemia, 1601
chemotherapy-induced lung injury, 1858
chronic myeloid leukemia, 1587
Dasatanib (*cont.*)
malignant mesothelioma, 1051
molecular diagnostics, 339
personalized medicine, 351
DAT (daunorubicin, ara-C, thioguanine), 1572
Data acquisition and instrument control, 1978–1979
Daunomycin, 648
activity, 649
dose, 648
typhlitis, 1873
Daunorubicin, 31, 33, 1570, 1916, 1942
acute lymphoblastic leukemia, 1596
cardiotoxicity, 1840, 1843
causing nail hyperpigmentation, 1780
nephrotoxicity, 1830
pregnancy and cancer, 835
DCC
gastric cancer, 1090
DCC gene
colorectal cancer, 1181
DCE-MRI. *See* Dynamic contrast-enhanced MRI
DCIS. *See* Ductal carcinoma in situ (DCIS)
DD. *See* Death domains (DD)
D-dimer, 1691
DDR. See Discoidin domain receptors (DDR)
DDTHF. *See* Dideazatetrahydrofolate (DDTHF)
de Guglielmo syndrome, 1566. *See also* Erythroleukemia
Death domains (DD)
proteins, 42–44
Death effector domains (DED), 41, 42, 44
Death-inducing signaling complex (DISC), 41
Decarbazine, 636
distant metastatic melanoma, 1479
Decision analysis, 456–457
Decitabine, 1571
epigenesis and human cancer, 173
myelodysplastic syndrome, 1555
DED. *See* Death effector domains (DED)
Dedifferentiated chondrosarcoma, 1508
Deep vein thrombosis (DVT), 1818, 1819
Defibrotide
sinusoidal obstruction syndrome, 1878
veno-occlusive disease, 1878
Dehydroepiandrosterone (DHEA), 1746
Dehydroepiandrosterone sulfate, 934
Dehydroxymethyl-epoxyquinomicin
cachexia, 1751
Delayed emesis guidelines, 1757, 1761t
prevention
Delayed pulmonary toxicity syndrome, 1863
Delirium, 806–807
behavioral symptoms, 806t
causes, 806t
medications for, 807t
palliative care, 859
Demeclocycline, 1913
Dendrimers, 368
Dendritic cells (DCs), 177
function, promoting, 181–182
Denileukin difitox, 721
chemotherapy-induced lung injury, 1858
systemic reactions to, 1959
Denys–Drash syndrome, 1728
Deodorized tincture of opium (DTO)
diarrhea, 1874
5′-Deoxy-5-Fluorouridine (5′-dFUrd)
cachexia, 1752
Deoxycoformycin, 629–630
Depression, 3, 803–805
evaluation, 804t
risk factors, 804t
Dermatofibrosarcoma protuberans (DFSP), 1493, 1493f, 1539
Dermatologic complications, 1779–1787
causes, 1779t
radiation-associated, 1782, 1782t

Dermoid cycts, 909
Descriptive studies, 422
Desipramine
for cancer pain, 873
Desmoid tumors, 197
Desmoplastic melanoma, 1469
and SLN biopsy, 1474–1475
Detectable preclinical phase, 419
Developmental stages, 796t
Dexamethasone, 1759, 1761, 1762
acute lymphoblastic leukemia, 1597
amyloidosis, 1955
brain herniation, 1954
cachexia, 1748
for cancer pain, 874, 875
multiple myeloma, 1677, 1680, 1681, 1955
neurologic complications, 1766, 1774
spinal cord compression, 1953
superior vena cava syndrome, 1949
venous thromboembolism, 1864
Dexrazoxane
cardiotoxicity, 1842–1843
Dextroamphetamine
for cancer pain, 874
DFSP. *See* Dermatofibrosarcoma protuberans (DFSP)
DHEA. *See* Dehydroepiandrosterone (DHEA)
DHFR. *See* Dihydrofolate reductase (DHFR)
Diabetes mellitus, 1904–1905
colorectal cancer, 1180
liver neoplasms, 1125
pancreatic neoplasms, 1144
type 2 (DM2), 1904
Diagnosis of cancer, 794–795
Diagnostic imaging
differentiated thyroid carcinoma, 927
Dianhydrogalacitol, 635
Diarrhea, 1874–1875
C. difficile-induced, 1875
chemotherapy-induced, 1874
differential diagnosis of, 1874t
GVHD and, 1874–1875, 1875t
radiation-induced, 1874
Diazepam
status epilepticus, 1954
Diaziquone, 1574, 1578
Diazoxide, 1913
Dibromodulcitol, 635
Dideazatetrahydrofolate (DDTHF), 618
Diet, 400–401
assessment, 400t
breast cancer, 239, 1396–1397
cervical cancer, 1301
colorectal cancer, 1180
head and neck neoplasms, 962
low fat, 401
Dietary fat
breast cancer, 239
pancreatic neoplasms, 1146
Dietary pattern
colorectal cancer, 403
Dietary supplements, 402
Diethylstilbestrol
prostate cancer, 1244
Differentiated thyroid cancer
clinicopathologic staging schemes, 925
management in special population, 929
pathogenesis, 923–924
postoperative adjuvant therapy, 926
radioiodine, 926
surgery, 925–926
Diffuse alveolar damage (DAD), 1858
Diffuse alveolar hemorrhage (DAH), 1858, 1862
Diffuse intravascular coagulation, 1801
Diffuse large B-cell lymphoma (DLBCL), 1647f, 1648–1649
Diffuse optical spectroscopic imaging (DOSI, 319
Diffusion-weighted imaging (DWI), 324
Digital clubbing, 1008
Digital rectal examination (DRE), 428, 435
Dihydrofolate reductase (DHFR), 611
Diltiazem, 1787
Dimethyl-benzanthracene (DMBA), 81
Dimethyl sulfoxide (DMSO), 1781
myelodysplastic syndrome, 1553
Diphenhydramine, 1760
systemic reactions to, 1959
Diphenoxilate
diarrhea, 1874
Diphenylhydramine, 1761
DISC. *See* Death-inducing signaling complex (DISC)
Discodermolide, 673
chemical structure, 674f
Discoidin domain receptors (DDR), 59–60
Discovery process
clinical observation, 568
evolution of, 568, 576–577
histocytotoxic effects, 568, 576
Disease occurrence, 371–372
Disseminated candidiasis, 1928
Disseminated intravascular coagulation, 1578, 1592, 1820–1821, 1821t, 1924
Distant metastatic melanoma, 1479–1484
chemotherapy, 1479–1480, 1480t
surgical excision of, 1482–1483
treatment, 1479
Distress
screening for, 799–802
standards of care for, 799t
DLBCL. *See* Diffuse large B-cell lymphoma (DLBC)
DLC. *See* Dynein light-chain (DLC)
DMBA. *See* Dimethyl-benzanthracene (DMBA)
DMSO. *See* Dimethyl sulfoxide (DMSO)
DNA
analysis, 9–10
damage, 229, 230, 231–232
radiation, 253–254
damage-induced checkpoints, 29–30
digestion, 8f
INDEX Flow cytometric analysis, 1726
ligases, 7
mediated transformation technique, 69
methylation, 37–38, 133–134
genes silenced, 38t
microarray analysis, 15, 17f
mismatches, 232
mismatch repair gene defects
HNPCC, 97–98
polymerase, 10f
low-fidelity, 264–265
polymorphisms, 12–13
radiation-induced damage, 515
recombinant, 7
repair, 134
radiotherapy, 517–518
repair genes, 230t
repair pathways, 231
sequencing, 10f
approaches, 111–112
sunlight-induced photoproducts, 263
topoisomerase damage, 646–647, 647f
DNA hypermethylation, 172, 172t
DNA methylation, 171f
altered, clinical implications of, 172–173
cancer biomarkers, 172–173
epigenetic therapy, 173
gene expression regulation mechanism and, 171
loss of, 172
Do not resuscitate (DNR), 1942
Dobutamine
pulmonary tumor thrombotic microangiopathy, 1865
Docetaxel, 664, 668, 889, 1761
administration, dose, schedule, 673
Docetaxel (*cont.*)
breast cancer, 162, 1446–1447, 1448
causing hyperpigmentation, 1782
causing nail hyperpigmentation, 1780
chemical structure, 664f
chemotherapy-induced lung injury, 1858
gastric cancer, 1104
hypersensitivity reactions, 1783
metabolic disease, 1536
neurologic complications, 1774
non-small cell lung cancer, 163
ovarian cancer, 1358
pregnancy and cancer, 833
prostate cancer, 1243, 1249, 1250, 1251, 1253
toxicity, 671–672
typhlitis, 1874
Dolasetron, 1759
Dopamine D2, 1757
Dopamine agonists
pituitary adenomas, 917
Dopamine receptor antagonists, 1759
Dorsal column stimulation, 878
Dorsal rhizotomy, 877
Dorsal root entry-zone lesion, 877
Dose effect
clinical trials, 560–561
sensitive tumors, 561
DOSI. *See* Diffuse optical spectroscopic imaging (DOSI)
Double effect principle, 878
Doxercalciferol
prostate neoplasms, 1242
Doxil, 1784
Doxorubicin, 30, 32, 34, 521, 648, 1493, 1782, 1784, 1878, 1905, 1908, 1916, 1917, 1918, 1919, 1942
activity, 649
acute lymphoblastic leukemia, 1601
adenocarcinoma of unknown primary site, 1717
anal neoplasms, 1201
breast cancer, 164, 1448
cardiac monitoring, 1843
cardiotoxicity, 1840, 1840t, 1841–1842, 1842t
causing hyperpigmentation, 1782
causing nail hyperpigmentation, 1780
cutaneous reactions, 1779
dose, 648
gastric cancer, 1102, 1103
hilar cholangiocarcinoma, 1141
hyperthermia, 534
Kaposi sarcoma, 1701
liver neoplasms, 1128, 1129
localized STS of extremities, 1530, 1531, 1532
malignant mesothelioma, 1051
metabolic disease, 1536, 1537
mycosis fungoides/Sézary syndrome, 1664, 1665
nanotechnology, 364, 369
nephrotoxicity, 1830
neuroblastoma, 1727
osteosarcoma, 1731
pegylated liposomal, 1842
pregnancy and cancer, 833, 834, 835
prostate cancer, 1253
pulmonary vascular disorders, 1858
renal tumors in children, 1729
small-cell lung cancer, 1037, 1039, 1040
thymomas, 1059, 1060
typhlitis, 1873
venous thromboembolism, 1864
Waldenström macroglobulinemia, 1683
Doxorubicinol
cardiotoxicity, 1841
Doxycycline, 1835
for indolent NHL, 1653
DRE. *See* Digital rectal examination (DRE)
Dronabinol
cachexia, 1749

Drug-conjugate export pumps
multidrug resistance, 601–602
Drug discovery
mechanism-based, 578
Drug-drug interactions, 593–594
Drug hepatotoxicity, 1878, 1878t
Drug-induced airway disease, 1858–1859
Drug-induced injury
repair, 590
Drug-monoclonal antibody conjugates, 717
Drug resistance, 559, 597–609
overcoming, 604–609
and pharmacogenomics, 603–604
tumor cell heterogeneity, 564
Drugs
action mechanisms, 587–590
administration, 562–563
continuous low-dose, 563
decreased accumulation, 597
intracellular activation, 588–589
membrane transport, 587–588
targets, 589–590
DTO. *See* Deodorized tincture of opium (DTO)
Ductal adenocarcinomas
prostate cancer, 1251–1252, 1252–1253
Ductal carcinoma in situ (DCIS), 1403f, 1421–1423
Duloxetine hydrochloride, 873
DVT. *See* Deep vein thrombosis (DVT)
DWI. *See* Diffusion-weighted imaging (DWI)
Dynamic contrast-enhanced MRI (DCE-MRI), 318, 321
Dynamic instability, 647
Dynamic markers, 348
Dynein light-chain (DLC), 47
Dysgerminomas
ovaries, 1365–1366
pregnancy, 1368
Dysphagia
gastric cancer, 1106–1107
malignant, 1871–1872
Dyspla nevus syndrome. *See* Atypical mole and melanoma syndrome
Dyspnea, 1849
acute airway obstruction, 1951
palliative care, 858–859
Dystrophin glycoprotein complex (DGC), 1747

E2F-1, 763
Early growth response (EGR-1) promoter, 769
Early response genes, 517
East Asian distomiasis, 315
Eastern Cooperative Oncology Group, 506t
Eaton-Lambert syndrome, 1007
EBRT. *See* External beam radiotherapy (EBRT)
Ebstein-Barr virus (EBV), 1932
EBV. *See* Ebstein-Barr virus (EBV)
E-cadherin, 1090
Eccrine squamous syringometaplasia (ESS), 1784
Echinocandins, 1929, 1930
Echocardiography, 1832, 1834, 1835
of carcinoid heart disease, 1836, 1837f
of cardiac amyloidosis, 1837–1838, 1837f
of infective endoicarditis, 1833f
of renal cell carcinoma, 1833f
ECP. *See* Extracorporeal photopheresis (ECP)
Ectopic ACTH production, 1909–1911, 1910f
Ectopic ACTH syndrome, 1007
Ectopic hormone production, 1909–1913
Edatrexate
oral complications, 1886
Edrocolomab, 713
EGF. *See* Epidermal growth factor (EGF)
EGFR. *See* Epidermal growth factor receptor
EGR-1. *See* Early growth response (EGR-1) promoter
EHE. *See* Epithelioid hemangioendothelioma (EHE)
EHR
administrative incentives, 1973t
financial incentives, 1973t
functionalities, 1972t, 1973T
medical management incentives, 1973t
oncology-specific documentation, 1974t
EIA protein
adenoviral, 770–771
Eicosapentaenoic acid (EPA)
cachexia, 1752–1753
eIF3-f, 1745
Elective lymph node dissection (ELND), 1469–1470, 1471f
Electrolyte disorders, 1907–1908
Electron microscopy
diagnosis of poorly differentiated neoplasms, 1714
role, 484–485
Electronic patient-physician communication, 1971
Eleutherobin, 673
chemical structure, 674f
ELISA. *See* Enzyme-linked immunosorbent assay (ELISA)
ELND. *See* Elective lymph node dissection (ELND)
ELS. *See* Cutaneous eruption of lymphocyte recovery
Eltrombopag, 1821
EMBASE, 1968
Embolization
bleeding, 1106
Embryonal carcinoma, 1265–1266, 1734
ovary, 1370
Emesis
types, 1757–1758
Emetogenic chemotherapy, 1758. *See also* Chemotherapy
EMH. *See* Extramedullary hematopoiesis (EMH)
Enchondroma, 1501–1502, 1502f
Enchondromatosis, 1512
Endocrine complications, 1901–1913
Endocrine glands, 915–922
Endocrine paraneoplastic syndromes, 1909–1913
Endogenous retroviruses, 279, 287–288
Endoluminal disease, 1850
Endometrial cancer
nutrition, 407
Endometrial hyperplasia, 1327
Endometrial neoplasms, 1325–1336
clinical and molecular features, 1331t
diagnosis, 1328
etiology, 241–243
nutrition, 407
oncogenes, 1330–1331
pathology, 1327–1328
prognosis, 1329–1331
radiation therapy, 1331–1333
risk factors, 1325–1327
screening, 440
staging, 1328–1329
treatment, 1331–1336
recurrent disease, 1333–1336
tumor-suppressor, 1330–1331
Endometrial papillary adenocarcinoma, 1327
Endometrial tumors, 744
Endometrioid adenocarcinoma
cervix, 1303
Endometrioid carcinoma, 1349f
Endometrium
adenocarcinoma, 1327
clear cell carcinoma, 1327–1328
mitotic activity, 241–242
Endomyocardial biopsy, 1838, 1840, 1842, 1847
Endoscopic cytology, 480
Endoscopic retrograde cholangiopancreatogram (ERCP), 1139, 1139f
Endoscopist, 824
Endoscopy
bleeding, 1106
Endostatin, 156–157
Energy
breast cancer, 403–404
colorectal cancer, 402, 403
Energy balance and glucose metabolism, 1904–1905
Engineered protein expression, 19
Enhanced permeation and retention (EPR), 366
Enostosis, 1504–1505, 1504f
Enterobacteriaceae, 1925
Enterococcus, 1925
Enucleation
retinoblastoma, 906
Envelope, 281–282
Environmental factors
breast cancer, 1397
Environmental tobacco smoke (ETS), 1000
head and neck neoplasms, 961
Enzyme
targets, 589
Enzyme-linked immunosorbent assay (ELISA), 19, 307, 1808
EORTC/Groupe d'Etude des Lymphomes de l'Adulte (GELA) H8F Trial, 1634
Eosinophilia
myelomonocytic leukemia with, 1565–1566
Eosinophilic pneumonia (EP), 1858
EP. *See* Eosinophilic pneumonia (EP)
Ependymoma, 894, 1733
Ephrin family, 59
Epidemiology, 371–384
nutritional, 380
proof, 384
Epidermal growth factor (EGF), 51, 55–56, 351
Epidermal growth factor receptor (EGFR), 1091
aberrations, 158, 338, 362
radiation, 521
Epidermal growth factor receptor inhibitors, 1787, 27f
Epigenesis and human cancer, 170
clinical implications of altered DNA methylation, 172–173
gene expression regulation mechanisms, 170–171
Epinephrine, 1846, 1944
Epipodophyllotoxins, 651–653, 1916, 1918
structure, 652f
Epiregulin, 55
Epirubicin, 648, 1919
activity, 649
for aggressive NHL, 1656
breast cancer, 1448
cardiotoxicity, 1843
dose, 648
gastric cancer, 1103
metabolic disease, 1536
pregnancy and cancer, 834
small-cell lung cancer, 1040
Epithelial and endothelial barriers, 367
Epithelial ovarian cancer, 1344–1364
etiology, 1344–1345
genetic risk, 1345–1346
prevention, 1345
Epithelioid hemangioendothelioma (EHE)
liver neoplasms, 1130–1131
Epithelioma cuniculatum, 1489
EPOCH, 1706t, 1707
Epothilone, 674
chemical structure, 674f
prostate cancer, 1249
Epoxide
structure, 635f

EPR. *See* Enhanced permeation and retention (EPR)
Epsilon aminocaproic acid
for disseminated intravascular coagulation, 1821
Epstein-Barr virus (EBV), 291–294
animal models, 293
Burkitt lymphoma, 293–294
cellular homologs, 291t
clinical aspects, 293
gene expression, 292
head and neck neoplasms, 961
Hodgkin disease, 294
Hodgkin lymphoma, 1623–1624, 1624f
leiomyosarcoma, 294
lymphoproliferative disease, 293
nasopharyngeal carcinoma, 294
T-cell lymphoma, 294
ER. *See* Estrogen receptor (ER)
ERB B1
oncogenes, 83
ERB B2, 362
oncogenes, 82–83
ERCC1. *See* Excision repair cross-complementation group 1 (ERCC1), 338
ERCP. *See* Endoscopic retrograde cholangiopancreatogram (ERCP)
ERK. *See* Extracellular signal-regulated kinase (ERK)
Erlotinib, 1787
adenocarcinoma of unknown primary site, 1717
liver neoplasms, 1129
molecular diagnostics, 341
non-small cell lung cancer, 163
Erysipelas, 178
Erythrocytosis
classification, 1693t
Erythroleukemia, 1562f, 1566. *See also* de Guglielmo syndrome
Erythromelalgia, 1688, 1688f
Erythromycin, 1761
Erythroplasia of Queyrat, 1256
Erythropoietin, 687–688, 687t, 708, 1557, 1687, 1750, 1913
ES. *See* Ewing sarcoma (ES)
ESHAP
mycosis fungoides/Sézary syndrome, 1665
Esophageal cancer
nutrition, 406
Esophageal candidiasis, 1928f
Esophageal dilation
malignant dysphagia, 1871
Esophageal neoplasms, 1074–1084, 1074t
biologic staging, 1078
bone scintigraphy, 1077
bronchoscopy, 1077
cervical@3 surgery, 1080–1081
chemoradiotherapy, 1083
randomized trials, 1079t
chemotherapy, 1082–1084
computed tomography, 1077
contrast radiography, 1077
diagnosis, 1076
distribution, 1074f
endoscopy, 1077
epidemiology, 1075–1076
etiology, 1075
long-term outcome, 1079f
lymph node staging map, 1078f
magnetic resonance imaging, 1077
minimally invasive surgical staging, 1077
neck ultrasonography, 1077
nutrition, 406
palliative therapy, 1084
photodynamic therapy, 1084,
positron emission tomography, 1077
presentation, 1077–1078
pretreatment assessment, 1076
prevention, 416–417
radiation therapy, 1081–1082
brachytherapy, 1082
staging, 1076
surgery, 1079–1084
therapy, 1078–1084
TNM staging, 1078
treatment, 1076
algorithm, 1076f
Esophagectomy, 1080
reconstruction after, 1081
Esophagitis, 1872–1873
graft-versus-host disease, 1872
causes of, 1872t
Candida, 1872
viral, 1872–1873
bacterial, 1873
radiation, 1873
infectious, 1873
pill-induced, 1873, 1873f
Candida, 1928f
Esophagus
adenocarcinoma of, 406
anatomy and histology, 1074
hyperthermia, 538
ESS. *See* Eccrine squamous syringometaplasia (ESS)
Essential thrombocythemia (ET), 1686–1689, 1687f, 1688f, 1688t
pregnancy in, 1689
and primary myelofibrosis, distinction between, 1687
and reactive thrombocytosis, distinction between, 1687
Esterase D, 88
Esthesioneuroblastoma, 983
Estramustine, 1905
prostate cancer, 1243, 1248, 1249, 1253
Estrogen, 739–741
acute pancreatitis, 1877
biosynthetic pathway, 739–740
breast cancer, 1395–1396, 1433
carcinogenic effects, 741
mechanism of action, 740–741
prostate cancer, 1248
sites of production, 740
Estrogen receptor (ER), 320
breast cancer, 1401
Estrogen therapy
endometrial cancer, 242–243
ET. *See* Essential thrombocythemia (ET)
Etanidazole
hyperthermia, 534
Ethambutol, 1927
Ethmoid sinuses
primary tumor staging characteristics, 981t
Ethnic groups, 376–378
breast cancer, 1394
mortality, 1393t
hepatitis C virus, 307
incidence, 379t
10-Ethyl-10-deazaaminopterin, 618
Etidronate
bone metastasis, 1793
Etomidate, 1906
Etoposide, 32, 651–652, 1574, 1577, 1761, 1916, 1917, 1919
acute lymphoblastic leukemia, 1596
for aggressive NHL, 1656
causing anaphylaxis, 1958
causing hyperpigmentation, 1782
chemotherapy, 907
gastric cancer, 1103
hyperthermia, 534
Kaposi sarcoma, 1701
mycosis fungoides/Sézary syndrome, 1665
myelodysplastic syndrome, 1546
neuroblastoma, 1727
nonsmall-cell lung cancer, 1030, 1031
Etoposide (*cont.*)
pharmacodynamics, 595
photosensitivity reactions, 1783
poorly differentiated neuroendocrine carcinoma, 1720
pregnancy and cancer, 834
prostate cancer, 1243, 1249, 1253
renal tumors in children, 1729
schedule effects, 563
small-cell lung cancer, 1037, 1039, 1040
thymomas, 1060
typhlitis, 1873
ETS. *See* Environmental tobacco smoke (ETS)
European Organization for the Research and Treatment of Cancer (EORTC) H7F Trial, 1633
Euthyroid sick syndrome, 1902
Ewing sarcoma (ES), 1508–1509, 1731–1732, 1918
adjuvant chemotherapy for, 1532
hematopoietic cellular transplantation for, 789
Excision margins, 478
Excision repair cross-complementation group 1 (ERCC1), 338
Excisional biopsy, 503, 1399. *See also* Biopsy
Excisional surgery
for basal cell carcinoma, 1492
for squamous cell carcinoma, 1490
Exemestane, 745
breast cancer, 1432
Exfoliative cytology, 480
External beam radiotherapy (EBRT), 510
anaplastic thyroid carcinoma, 931
cervical cancer, 13131314
differentiated thyroid carcinoma, 926–927
growth hormone secreting pituitary adenomas, 919
medullary thyroid carcinoma, 930
retinoblastoma, 906
thyroid carcinoma, 928–929
Extracellular matrix, 132
cell invasion, 143f
Extracellular signal-regulated kinase (ERK), 64
Extracolonial cancer, 202–203
Extracorporeal photopheresis (ECP)
mycosis fungoides/Sézary syndrome, 1666
Extrafascial hysterectomy, 1312
Extraim analyses, 461
Extraluminal-predominant disease, 1850
Extramammary Paget disease (EPD), 1494
Extramedullary hematopoiesis (EMH), 1689
Extranodal NK/T-cell lymphomas, 1649
Extraocular retinoblastoma, 907–908
Extrapleural pneumonectomy
for malignant mesothelioma, 1048–1049
Extravasation injury, 1780–1781, 1781t

18F-FACBC. *See* 18F, anti-1-amino-3-18F-fluorocyclobutane-1-carboxylic acid (18F-FACBC)
Face
squamous cell carcinoma, 477f
Factorial experiments, 454–456
Fadrozole, 744
Fallopian tube neoplasms, 1338–1342
clinical presentation, 1338
incidence and epidemiology, 1338
patterns of spread, 1339
preoperative diagnosis, 1338–1339
prognosis, 1339–1340, 1341–1342
sarcoma, 1386
staging and classification, 1339, 1339t
treatment, 1340–1341, 1340f
Famciclovir
viral infections, 1931
Familial adenomatous polyposis (FAP), 93, 336, 924, 1089, 1512–1513
colorectal cancer, 1181

Familial adenomatous polyposis (FAP) (*cont.*)
gastric cancer, 215
genetic basis, 195–197
prophylactic colectomy in, 196
Familial atypical multiple-mole melanoma (FAMMM) syndrome, 2061145
Familial chronic lymphocytic leukemia, 1605
Familial colorectal cancer
type X, 205–206
Familial gastric carcinoma
genetic basis, 213–215
Familial juvenile polyposis
genetic basis, 198
Familial medullary thyroid carcinoma (FMTC), 61
Familial neuroblastoma
genetic basis, 217–218
Familial nonmedullary carcinoma, 924
Familial non-syndromic colorectal cancer
genetic basis, 199
Familial pancreatic cancer
genetic basis, 212–213
Familial prostate cancer
genetic basis, 216–217
FAMMM. *See* Familial atypical multiple-mole melanoma syndrome (FAMMM)
Fanconi anemia
genetic basis, 211
hematopoietic cellular transplantation for, 789
Fanconi renal syndrome, 1737
18F, anti-1-amino-3-18F-fluorocyclobutane-1-carboxylic acid (18F-FACBC)
molecular imaging, 325
FAP. *See* Familial adenomatous polyposis (FAP)
Fas, 43
Fasaprepitant, 1761
Fat
breast cancer, 404
Fatigue
palliative care, 858
FDG. *See* Fluorodeoxy-D-glucose (FDG)
FDG-PET. *See* Fluorine-18-fluorodeoxyglucose positron emission tomographic scanning (FDF-PET)
118FDHT. *See* 16-[18F]fluoro-5-dihydrotestosterone (18FDHT)
18F-FDOPA. *See* L-3,4dihydroxy-6-(18)F-fluoro-phenylalanine (18F-FDOPA)
Febuxostat, 1945
Fecal occult blood testing (FOBT), 427–428
colorectal cancer, 1182
Femur
metastatic lesions to, 1790–1791
Fenretinide, 1345
Fentanyl
for cancer pain, 869–870
Fentora
for cancer pain, 870
Fertility
chemotherapy, 34, 1284
preservation of, 36t
Ferumoxtran-10, 1257
Ferumoxytol, 369
nanotechnology, 369
Fever of unexplained origin, 1938
Fever of unknown origin, 3
F-FDG. *See* 18F-labeled glucose analogue 2′-fluoro-2′-deoxyglucose (18F-FDG)
FGF. *See* Fibroblast growth factors (FGF)
FGF-1. *See* Fibroblast growth factor 1
FGF-2. *See* Fibroblast growth factor 2
FHIT, 82
Fiber
colorectal cancer, 403
Fiberoptic bronchoscopy, 1019
Fibroblast growth factor 1 (FGF-1), 153
Fibroblast growth factor 2 (FGF-2), 153
Fibroblast growth factors (FGF), 35, 56–57, 153
Fibroelastomas, 1064
Fibrosis, 1799, 1858
Fibrous dysplasia, 1503
Fibrous tumors, 1503–1504
FICTION, 106
Field cancer, 1002
File sharing, 1971–1972
Filgrastim, 1556–1557
Finasteride
prostate cancer, 1241, 1242
Fine needle aspiration (FNA), 503, 1499. *See also* Biopsy
biopsy, 1713
breast cancer, 1416
lung cancer, 1010
FISH. *See* Fluorescent in situ hybridization (FISH)
Fish oil, 408, 1908
FL. *See* Follicular lymphoma (FL)
18F-labeled glucose analogue 2′-fluoro-2′-deoxyglucose (18F-FDG)
molecular imaging, 318
Fleischner Society, 321
Flexible sigmoidoscopy
colon cancer, 428–429
colorectal cancer, 1183
Floor of mouth (FOM), 969f
squamous cell carcinoma, 969
Flow cytometry, 552
Floxuridine (FUDR), 1878
hepatic arterial infusion, 1117
18F-FLT. *See* 18F-3′-fluorothymidine (18F-FLT)
FLT-3 ligand, 705–706, 706t
Flt3 receptor, 53, 54
FLT3. *See* Fms-like tyrosine kinase 3 (FLT3)
Fluconazole, 1787, 1887, 1938
acute lymphoblastic leukemia, 1597
candidiasis, 1928, 1929
cryptococcosis, 1930
esophagitis, 1872
zygomycosis, 1930
Fludarabine, 630–631, 1574, 1577, 1786
acute lymphoblastic leukemia, 1600
chemotherapy-induced lung injury, 1858
chronic lymphocytic leukemia, 1615, 1619
for indolent NHL, 1654, 1655
mycosis fungoides/Sézary syndrome, 6
myelodysplastic syndrome, 1555, 1556
nephrotoxicity, 130
viral infections, 1932
Waldenström macroglobulinemia, 1683
Fludarabine-cyclophosphamide-rituximab (FCR)
chronic lymphocytic leukemia, 1615, 1620
Fludarabine monophosphate (Fludara)
chronic lymphocytic leukemia, 1613
Fludarabine-rituximab (FR)
chronic lymphocytic leukemia, 1615
Fluorescence in situ hybridization (FISH), 102, 105–106, 1577, 1715
chronic lymphocytic leukemia, 1606
multiple myeloma, 1672
myelodysplastic syndrome, 1546
Fluorescence spectroscopy, 1306–1307
18F-Fluoride
molecular imaging, 325
Fluorides
xerostomia, 1883
Fluorine-18-fluorodeoxyglucose positron emission tomographic (FDG-PET) scanning
Hodgkin lymphoma, 1630
16-[18F]fluoro-5-dihydrotestosterone (18FDHT)
molecular imaging, 325
5-Fluorocracil (5-FU), 33, 37, 621–625, 621f, 1198, 1488, 1492, 1165, 1782, 1784, 1845, 1878, 1902, 1905
actinic keratosis, 1783
acute pancreatitis, 1877
adenocarcinoma of unknown primary site, 1717
5-Fluorocracil (5-FU) (*cont.*)
anabolism, 622
anal neoplasms, 1199
catabolism, 623
causing hyperpigmentation, 1781
causing nail hyperpigmentation, 1780
colorectal cancer, 1188–1189
diarrhea, 1874
gastric cancer, 1102, 1103
hilar cholangiocarcinoma, 1141
mechanisms of action, 623–624
metabolism, 608f
neuroendocrine carcinoma of unknown primary site, 1719
neurologic complications, 1774
oral complications, 1885, 1886
pharmacokinetics, 622–623
pregnancy and cancer, 833
prostate cancer, 1243
pulmonary vascular disorders, 1858
resistance, 624
thymomas, 1060
typhlitis, 1874
5-Fluorocytosine, 1930
Fluorodeoxy-D-glucose (FDG), 489
Fluorodeoxyuridine (FudR), 1878
Fluoropyrimidines
schedule effects, 562–563
8F-3′-fluorothymidine (18F-FLT)
molecular imaging, 320, 323–324
Fluoroquinolone
bacterial infections, 1926
Fluorouracil, 1942
colorectal cancer, 162
Fluoxymesterone
primary myelofibrosis, 1691
Flutamide, 753
breast cancer, 1434
photosensitivity reactions, 1783
withdrawal, 755
18F-FMISO. *See* 18F-misonidazole
18F-misonidazole (18F-FMISO)
molecular imaging, 327
Fms-like tyrosine kinase 3 (FLT3), 1595
FMTC. *See* Familial medullary thyroid carcinoma (FMTC)
FNA. *See* Fine-needle aspiration (FNA)
FOBT. *See* Fecal occult blood testing (FOBT)
Folate, 403, 407–408
Folate antagonists, 611–619
historical overview, 611
pharmacogenomics, 613
FOLFIRI (folinic acid, 5-FU, irinotecan)
colorectal cancer, 1191–1192
FOLFOX (folinic acid, 5-FU, oxaliplatin)
colorectal cancer, 1191
Folinic acid
protozoal infections, 1934
Follicle-stimulating hormone (FSH), 1912
Follicular adenomas and carcinomas, 923
Follicular carcinomas, 924
Follicular large-cell lymphoma, 1656
Follicular lymphoma (FL), 1646, 1646f
International Prognostic Index (FLIPI), 1653t
FOM. *See* Floor of Mouth(FOM)
Food, 402
contamination, 408
environmental contaminants, 408–409
natural, 408
organic, 408
Forkhead box O (FOXO). *See* FOXO transcription factor, 1745
Formestane, 744
breast cancer, 1432
Fosaprepitant, 1761
Foscarnet
viral infections, 1932
Fosphenytoin
status epilepticus, 1954

Fotemustine
  causing hyperpigmentation, 1782
4-1BB, 182
  anti-, 182
  ligand (4-1BBL), 182
FOXO transcription factor, 1745
Free radical-mediated drug cytotoxicity, 606
Frequentist/Bayesian comparison, 449
Frequentist interim analysis
  vs. Bayesian updating, 450–451
Fresh frozen plasma, transfusion of, 1805
FSH. *See* Follicle-stimulating hormone (FSH)
FUDR. *See* Floxuridine (FUDR)
FudR. *See* Fluorodeoxyuridine (FudR)
Fulvestrant, 743
  breast cancer, 1433
Fungal infections, 1887, 1927–1931
Furosemide, 1787, 1945
  acute pancreatitis, 1877
  nephrotoxicity, 1828
Fusarium, 1930, 1936
Fusion genes, 76–77, 360

G0 checkpoint, 28–29
G1 phase checkpoint, 29f
GABA. *See* Gamma-amin-obutyric acid
Gabapentin
  for cancer pain, 873
Gadolinium
  spinal cord compression, 1953
Gag, 281
Gain-of-function approach, 22–23
Gallbladder neoplasms, 1132–1136
  chemotherapy, 1136
  clinical presentation, 1133
  diagnosis, 1133–1134
  etiology, 1132
  high-resolution helical computed tomography, 1134f
  lymphatic drainage, 1133f
  multidisciplinary approaches, 1136
  palliation, 1136
  pathology, 1132–1133
  radiation therapy, 1136
  resection, 1134–1136
  staging, 1134t
  surgical decision making, 1135f
  treatment, 1134–1136
Gallium nitrate, 1912
Gallstones, 1132
Gamma-amin-obutyric acid (GABA), 1757
Gamma radiation-related pancytopenia, 1798
Ganciclovir
  esophagitis, 1873
  PCNS lymphoma, 1708
  viral infections, 1932
Gardner syndrome, 93, 924, 1517
Gas chromatography/mass spectroscopy (GC/MS)
  tobacco smoke, 234
Gastrectomy, 1096
Gastric cancer
  familial, 213–215
  nutrition, 406
Gastric cardia
  adenocarcinoma of, 406
Gastric neoplasms, 1086–1108
  adjuvant therapy, 1098–1101, 1100t
  cellular adhesion, 1090–1091
  chemoradiation
    incompletely resected disease, 1099
    postoperative, 1099–1100
    preoperative, 1101
  chemotherapy
    combination, 1102–1104
    postoperative, 1098
    preoperative, 1101
  clinical manifestations, 1088
  electron micrograph, 485f
Gastric neoplasms (*cont.*)
  endoscopic mucosal resection, 1093
  epidemiology, 1086
  etiology, 1086–1087
  hereditary, 1089
  histology, 1087–1088
  hypermethylation, 1089–1090
  intraoperative radiotherapy, 1100
  intraperitoneal therapy, 1098–1099
  irradiation and supportive care, 1100–1101
  localization, 1088
  luminal resection, 1094
  microsatellites, 1090
  molecular biology, 1088–1092
  multivisceral resection, 1096
  node dissection, 1094–1096
  nutrition, 1107
  obstruction, 1106–1107
  pathologic and clinical staging, 1092–1093
  prevention, 416–417
  proximal, 1087
  reconstruction, 1097–1098
  SEER data, 1086f
  spread pattern, 1088
  surgical resection, 1093
  symptoms
    management, 1104–1107
  systemic therapy, 1102–1104
  therapy, 1093–1098
  transcription factors, 1091
  tumor-suppressor genes, 1090
Gastric outlet obstruction
  pancreatic neoplasms, 1164–1165
Gastro-esophageal cancer
  molecular imaging and, 328
Gastrografin, 1956
Gastrohepatic ligament, 1096
Gastrointestinal complications, 1871–1878
Gastrointestinal neoplasms
  methotrexate, 615
  vaccine clinical trials, 729
Gastrointestinal stromal tumors (GIST), 1538–1539, 1539f, 1540f
  genetic basis, 215
  outcome prediction and therapy responsiveness in, 339
  small intestine, 1175–1176
Gastrointestinal toxicity
  vinca alkaloids, 663
Gatekeeper genes, 225
Gatifloxacin
  bacterial infections, 1924
GBV. *See* Hepatitis GB virus
G-CSF. *See* Granulocyte colony-stimulating factor (G-CSF)
GC/MS. *See* Gas chromatography/mass spectroscopy (GC/MS)
Gefitinib
  personalized medicine, 351
Gelclair
  mucositis, 1882
  oral complications, 1886
GEM. *See* Genetically engineers mouse models (GEMM)
Gemcitabine, 588–589, 627
  adenocarcinoma of unknown primary site, 1717
  breast cancer, 1447
  chemotherapy-induced lung injury, 1855, 1858
  gallbladder cancer, 1136
  malignant mesothelioma, 1050, 1051
  metabolic disease, 1536
  mycosis fungoides/Sézary syndrome, 1664
  nephrotoxicity, 1830
  neurologic complications, 1774
  nonsmall-cell lung cancer, 163, 1029, 1030, 1031
  pancreatic neoplasms, 165, 1159–1160, 1166–1169
Gemcitabine (*cont.*)
  radiation-induced lung injury, 1859
  schedule effects, 562
  testis cancer, 1282
  typhlitis, 1874
Gemfibrozil, 1908
Gemtuzumab, 1847
  bronchospasm, 1859
Gemtuzumab-ozogamicin, 717, 1570, 1574, 1576
  sinusoidal obstruction syndrome, 1877
  veno-occlusive disease, 1877
Gender
  breast cancer, 1394
  invasive cancer, 375t
  mortality, 373, 375t
Gene(s)
  activation, 78
  amplification, 76
  cloning, 7–8
  delivery systems, 759–762
    nonviral, 761–762
  DNA methylation, 38t
  expression, 5, 6f, 14–17, 18–22
  functional components, 5
  fusion, 78–80, 78f
  immunomodulatory, 766
  probes, 8–9
  radiation, 253–254, 256
  structure, 5–7
  transfer, 69
Gene-environment interactions, 227–228, 235f
Gene expression profiling, 110–111
Gene therapy, 759–774
  radiation therapy, 522–523
  retroviral vectors, 288
Genetic Information Nondiscrimination Act (GINA), 221–222
Genetic predisposition, 190–224
  breast cancer, 245–246, 1394–1395
  family history, importance of, 190–191, 380
  head and neck neoplasms, 961
  skin cancer, 263–268
Genetic risk
  adaptation to, 798–799
Genetically engineers mouse models (GEMM), 23
Genital infections
  defined, 298
Genitourinary interventions, 494
Genitourinary neoplasms
  methotrexate, 615
Genodermatoses
  genetic basis, 209–212
Genome aberrations, 362f
  clinical outcomes and, 362
  contributing to cancer pathophysiology, 360–361
  copy number abnormalities and, 361–362
  formation mechanisms, 359
  technologies for anatomy assessment and, 359–360
Genomic and chromosomal aberrations, 102–123
  new methods, 105–113
  nomenclature, 103–105
Genomic Identification of Significant Targets in Cancer (GISTIC), 360–361
Genomic markers, 348
Genomic stability genes, 97, 100f
Genotype–phenotype heterogeneity, 203
Gentamicin
  bacterial infections, 1924, 1925
Geographic variation descuptive studies of, 379
Geriatric assessment, 840, 842
The German Hodgkin Study Group HD7 Trial, 1633
The German Hodgkin Study Group HD10 Trial, 1634

Germ cell tumors, 1734
benign, 1734
extragonadal, 1286–1287
of indeterminate behavior, 1734
mixed
ovaries, 1370–1371
ovaries, 1364–1365
of thymomas, 1057–1058
treatment, 1734–1735
Germ cell tumor syndrome
unrecognized, 1287
Germline biomarkers, novel, 341
Germonomas, 1734
Gestational trophoblastic neoplasia, 1376–1382
classification, 1376–1377
clinical presentation, 1378–1379
diagnosis, 1378–1379
epidemiology, 1376
etiology, 1376
hCG follow-up and relapse, 1382
management
algorithm, 1380f
high-risk, 1381
low-risk, 1380–1381
stages II and III, 1381
stages IV, 1381–1382
molecular pathogenesis, 1377–1378
quiescent, 1382
risk assessment, 1379
risk factors, 1376
staging, 1379
subsequent pregnancies, 1382
therapy, 1382
GGR. *See* Global genome repair (GGR)
GH. *See* Growth hormone (GH)
Ghana, 311
Ghrelin
anorexia, 1741
cachexia, 1754
Giant cell tumors, 1504
Giant congential nevi, 1459
GINA. *See* Genetic Information Nondiscrimination Act (GINA)
Ginger, 849, 1761
Gingival hypertrophy, 1562f
Gingival infections, 1888
Gingival mucosa, 969–970
GIST. *See* Gastrointestinal stromal tumor (GIST)
GISTIC. *See* Genomic Identification of Significant Targets in Cancer (GISTIC)
GITR, 183–184
anti-, 183
ligation (GITRL), 183
Glassy-cell carcinoma, 1303f
Gleevec, 65, 339, 635
Glial cell line-derived neurotrophic factor (GDNF), 59
Glioblastoma, 61, 890–891
Glioblastoma multiforme, 369
hyperthermia, 538
Glioma, 165
low-grade, 891–893
Global genome repair (GGR), 263
Glottic cancer, 976–977, 977f
Glucagon, 1912
Glucocorticoids, 756, 1904, 1905, 1906, 1912
myelodysplastic syndrome, 1555
prostate cancer, 1248
Glutamine
cachexia, 1754
Glutathione
alkylating agents, 637
Glutathione peroxidase (GSHPx), 606
Glutathione S-transferase (GST)-M1, 1735
Glutathione S-transferase (GST)-T1, 1735
Glycolipids, 130
Glycoproteins, 130
Glycosyl transferase, 130–132
GM-CSF. *See* Granulocyte–Machrophage colony-stimulating factor (GM–CSF)
GNEF. *See* Guanine nucleotide exchange factor (GNEF)
Goldenhar syndrome, 833
Gompertzian curve, 553
Gompertzian growth, 551, 554
etiology of, 556–557
Gonadoblastomas, 1734
Gonadotropin deficiency, 1909
Gorlin's syndrome. *See* Nevoid basal cell carcinoma (NBCCS)
Goserelin
breast cancer, 1433
Graft failure, 781–782
Graft rejection, 781
Graft-versus-host disease (GVHD), 776, 782–783, 1876, 1876f, 1889, 1917
clinical staging and grading, 782t(GVHD)
and diarrhea, 1874–1875, 1874t
esophagitis, 1872
transfusion-associated, 1806
Graft-versus-leukemia (GVL), 777
Graft-versus-malignancy (GVM), 776
Graft-vs-host disease (GVHD), 1572, 1573
Grains, 401
colorectal cancer, 403
Granisetron, 1759
for cancer pain, 875
Granulocyte colony-stimulating factor (G-CSF), 688–689, 689f, 708, 1576, 1597, 1800, 1801, 1919
chemotherapy-induced lung injury, 1858
typhlitis, 1874
Granulocyte–macrophage colony-stimulating factor (GM–CSF), 688, 688t, 1555, 1556, 1576, 1800, 1801
Granulocyte-monocyte colony-stimulating factor, 1687
Granulomatous disease, 1859
Granulosa cell tumor, 1372f
Granulosa-stromal cell tumors, 1371–1372
Granzyme B, 41
Grb2, 61
Great vessels, tumors of, 1065
Gross tumor volume
nonsmall-cell lung cancer, 1024
Growth factor(s)
abnormalities, 60
cachexia, 1749
classification, 52–60
hepatitis B virus, 304
inhibition of downstream signaling, 66
modes of action, 51f
multiple myeloma, 1670–1671
oncogenes, 71
radiation, 521
to alleviate secondary effects of cancer therapy, 66–67
Growth factor receptors
aberrations, 60–61
oncogenes, 71–73
tyrosine kinase, 51–52
Growth fraction, 552, 559–560
Growth hormone (GH), 1901, 1913
secretion disorders, 1906–1907
Growth hormone releasing peptide-2 (GHRP-2), 1749
Growth parameters assessment, 551–552
Growth patterns
cancer study enigma, 551
Growth stimulation plus two-step oncogenesis, 285f, 286
GSHPx. *See* Glutathione peroxidase (GSHPx)
Guanine nucleotide exchange factor (GNEF), 63
Guanosine triphosphate (GTP)-binding proteins, 73
Guided imagery, 1761
GVHD. *See* Graft-*versus*-host disease (GVHD)
GVL. *See* Graft-*versus*-leukemia (GVL)
GVM. *See* Graft-*versus*-malignancy (GVM)
Gynecologic oncologist, 827–828
Gynecologic sarcomas, 1384–1391
chemotherapy, 1389
clinical profile, 1384–1385
combination therapy, 1390–1391
hormone therapy, 1388
malignant mixed mullerian tumors (MMMT), 1388–1389
nonuterine, 1386
patterns of spread, 1385–1386
postsurgical therapy, 1388
prognosis, 1386
sarcoma-like variants, 1385
single-agent therapy, 1389
surgery, 1386–1388

H-2 blockers, 1873
HAART. *See* Highly active antiretroviral therapy
HAART. *See* Highly active antiretroviral therapy
Hairy cell leukemia,
interferons, 683
Haloperidol, 1757, 1759
for cancer pain, 874
neurologic complications, 1777
Halsted's theory, 550
HAMA. *See* Human anti–mouse antibodies
Hamartomas, 904
Hamartomatous polyposis syndromes, 199t
Hand-and-foot syndrome, 1784f
Haplotype map (HapMap), 348–349
HapMap. *See* Haplotype map, 348
HAT. *See* Histone acetyltransferases (HAT)
Hazards over time, 452–454
HB. *See* Hepatitis B
HBIg. *See* Hepatitis B immunoglobulin (HBIg)
HBsAG vaccines, 305
HBV. *See* Hepatitis B virus (HBV)
HBx protein, 304–305
HCC. *See* Hepatocellular carcinoma (HCC)
hCG. *See* Human chorionic gonadotropin (hCG)
HCV. *See* Hepatitis C virus (HCV)
HD. *See* Hodgkin disease (HD)
HDAC. *See* Histone deacetylase (HDAC)
HDGC. *See* Hereditary diffuse gastric cancer (HDGC)
Head and neck neoplasms, 959–997
accelerated and hyperfractionated radiotherapy, 991
anatomy, 963–964
clinical tumor staging characteristics, 966t
combined surgery and radiotherapy, 992
concomitant chemotherapy and radiation, 993–994, 993t
curative radiotherapy, 990–991
diagnosis and staging, 964–966
epidemiology, 959–962
hyperthermia, 537–538
incidence, 959
induction chemotherapy, 992–993, 993t
intensity-modulated radiotherapy, 989–990
intensity-modulated whole pelvic radiation therapy, 512f
metastasis, 988
methotrexate, 615
molecular imaging and, 327
mortality, 960
nodal levels, 964f
oral premalignancy, 411–412, 966–967
pathologic assessment, 962–963
prevalence, 959–960
radiation therapy, 988–992
recurrent and metastatic disease

Head and neck neoplasms (*cont.*)
recurrent and metastatic disease (*cont.*)
angiogenesis, 996
chemoprevention, 997
cytotoxic chemotherapy, 994–995
epidermal growth factor receptor, 995–996
gene therapy, 997
intracellular signaling, 996–997
novel therapeutics, 995
tissue hypoxia, 997
risk factors, 960–962
sarcoma, 988
systemic therapy, 992–997
treatment, 966
Head and neck squamous cell carcinomas (HNSCC), 327, 959–997
Health 2.0/Web 2.0, 1969–1972
Health care
applications, 1970
consumerism, 1962
portals, 1968–1969, 1968t
Health Insurance Portability and Accountability Act (HIPAA), 222, 466
HEALTHSTAR, 1978
heat shock proteins (HSPs), 529
Heath on the Net Foundation, 852
Heavy-chain diseases, 1683
Helicobacter pylori, 270, 406, 1145
head and neck neoplasms, 961
Hemangioendothelioma, 1511
Hemangioma
capillary, 908–909
of bone, 1504
Hematologic complications, 1797–1811
Hematologic malignancy
genetic basis, 218–221
radioimmunotherapy, 718
Hematologic neoplasia, 1069
Hematopathologist
role, 486
Hematopoeitic stem cell transplantation
for hemolytic uremic syndrome, 1820
Hematopoiesis, 1797–1798, 1797f
cell-mediated suppression of, 1799
clinical use of, 706–708
growth factors and, 686–687, 686f, 687t
IL-1 and, 692
normal, 1797
Hematopoietic cellular transplantation, 776–789
allogeneic, 777, 778, 779
autologous, 776–777, 777–778, 778–779
complications, 781
indications, 784–
methods, 776
selection, 779–780
Hematopoietic growth factors, 1576
drug resistance, circumvention of, 1577
immune modulation, 1576–1577
Hematopoietic stem cell transplantation (HSCT), 1810
mycosis fungoides/Sézary syndrome, 1665, 1665t
oral complications associated with, 1888–1889
pulmonary complications after, 1860–1863, 1861t
Hematuria
drug-induced, 1825
radiation-induced, 1825
Hemochromatosis
liver neoplasms, 1125
Hemolytic anemia, elevated liver enzymes and low platelet count (HELLP) syndrome, 832
Hemolytic streptococci, 1924, 1924f
Hemolytic uremic syndrome (HUS), 1820, 1820f, 1828, 1829
Hemoptysis
fatal, 1949
massive, 1949–1950
Hemorrhage, 1688
acute, 1947–1948
management, 1106
retroperitoneal, 1947–1948, 1948f
Hemorrhagic cystitis, 1825
etiology, 640
Hemostasis
physiology of, 1813, 1813f
Hemostatic abnormalities, 1814t
Heparin
for disseminated intravascular coagulation, 1821
for venous thromboembolism, 1818, 1819
Heparin. *See also* Low-molecular weight heparin
multiple myeloma, 1677
pulmonary embolism, 1953
sinusoidal obstruction syndrome, 1878
veno-occlusive disease, 1878
Heparin-induced thrombocytopenia (HIT), 1819–1820
Hepatic arterial infusion chemotherapy, 1115–1118
Hepatic arterial infusion floxuridine, 1117
Hepatic complications, 1871–1878
causes of, 1878t
Hepatic intra-arterial brachytherapy, 491
Hepatic metastasis, 493–494, 1190–1191
adjuvant therapy, 1191
conversion therapy, 1190–1191
neoadjuvant therapy, 1191
Hepatic toxicity
decrease, 1117
Hepatic vascular interventions, 490–492
Hepatitis B immunoglobulin (HBIg), 305
Hepatitis B virus (HBV), 302–307, 406, 1807, 1933
DNA, 303–304
hepatocellular carcinoma, 302–305
hepatocytic hyperplasia, 305
liver neoplasms, 1124–1125
treatment, 306–307
vaccines, 305
Hepatitis C virus (HCV), 307–309, 406, 1933
hepatocellular carcinoma, 307–308
liver neoplasms, 1124–1125
risk factors, 307
Hepatitis GB virus (GBV), 1807–1808, 1808t
Hepatitis viruses, 302–309, 303t, 1933
Hepatoblastoma, 1735
Hepatocellular carcinoma (HCC), 492–493, 1124–1129, 1735
chemoembolization, 1120t
hepatitis B virus, 302–305
liver neoplasms
clinical presentation, 1126
diagnosis, 1126–1127
early, 1126
epidemiology, 1124
hormonal factors, 1125
local-regional treatment modalities, 1128
natural history, 1126
orthotopic liver transplantation, 1127–1128
pathology, 1125–1126
progenitor cell, 1126
risk factors, 1124–1125
staging, 1127
surgical resection, 1127
systemic treatment, 1129
treatment, 1127–1129
vascular invasion, 1126
molecular imaging and, 328–329
screening, 306–307
Hepatocyte growth factor, 57–58
Hepatoma, 165
Hepatosplenic candidiasis, 1928
Hepatosplenic γ/δ T-cell lymphoma, 1649
Hepsulfam, 635
structure, 635f
HER2. *See* Human epidermal growth factor 2 (HER2)
Her2/neu, 1091
Herbicides, 408–409
HerbmedPro, 850
Herceptin, 338, 710
Hereditary cancer syndromes, available genetic testing for, 222t
Hereditary diffuse gastric cancer, 1089
familial gastric cancer, 213–214
Hereditary gastric carcinoma, 213
Hereditary non-polyposis colon cancer, 336
Hereditary nonpolyposis colorectal cancer (HNPCC), 1089, 1181
DNA mismatch repair gene defects, 97–98
genetic basis, 199–206
Hereditary papillary renal carcinoma (HPRC), 61
Herpes simplex virus (HSV), 1931
cervical cancer, 1299–1300
esophagitis, 1872, 1872f, 1873
gene delivery, 760–761
Herpes simplex virus (HSV-1), 1887
Herpes simplex viruses-thymidine kinase (HSV-tk), 762
Herpesviruses, 291–296
oncogenic features, 291
properties, 291
Herpes zoster, 1887, 1931
Heterocyclic amines, 229
Heterotypic cell-cell interactions, 143–144
Heterotypic cell-matrix interactions, 144
Hexamethylene bisacetamide (HMBA), 38
Hexamethylmelamine, 636
Hexokinase, 1742
HGML. *See* Hypertext Markup Language (HGML)
HGS-ETR2, 692
HHV-6. *See* Human herpes virus-6 (HHV-6)
HIDAC. *See* High-dose ara-C (HIDAC)
Hierarchical modeling, 451–452
in trial design, 452
HIF-1. *See* Hypoxia inducible factor-1 (HIF-1)
HIF-1 α. *See* Hypoxia inducible factor -1 α. (HIF-1 α)
High-dose ara-C (HIDAC), 1570, 1571, 1572, 1574, 1575, 1577, 1578, 1579
High-dose chemotherapy
mycosis fungoides/Sézary syndrome, 1665–1666, 1665t
High-dose therapy
stem cells, 562
High-fiber diet
breast cancer, 239
High-grade surface osteosarcoma, 1510
Highly active antiretroviral therapy (HAART), 1696–1697, 1699, 1702, 1705
Hodgkin lymphoma with HIV, 1642
Highly aggressive lymphomas, 1650
High-output cardiac failures, 1836–1837
High-output states, 1836–1837
Hilar cholangiocarcinoma, 1138
chemotherapy, 1141–1142
internal radiotherapy, 1142
interventional radiology, 1142
liver transplantation, 1141
palliation, 1141
prognosis, 1140
radiotherapy, 1141
resection, 1140
treatment, 1140–1141
HILP. *See* Hyperthermic isolated limb perfusion (HILP)
HIPAA. *See* Health Insurance Portability and Accountability Act (HIPAA)
Histamine, 1579, 1757, 1836
bronchospasm, 1858
systemic reactions to, 1959

Histamine H1 receptors, 1757
Histamine type 2 (H2) antagonist
  bacterial infections, 1924
Histologic transformation
  indolent NHL, 1655
Histone acetyltransferases (HAT), 36
Histone deacetylase (HDAC), 36
Histone deacetylase (HDAC) inhibitors, 37f, 50
  mycosis fungoides/Sézary syndrome, 1666
Histones, 170–171
  nucleosomes, 37f
HIT. *See* Heparin-induced thrombocytopenia (HIT)
HIV. *See* Human immune virus (HIV)
HL. *See* Hodgkin's lymphoma (HL)
HMBA. *See* Hexamethylene bisacetamide (HMBA)
HNPCC. *See* Hereditary nonpolyposis colorectal cancer (HNPCC)
HNSCC. *See* Head and neck squamous cell carcinoma (HNSCC)
Hodgkin disease (HD), 1917
  in children, 1725
  and non-Hodgkin's lymphoma, 220
Hodgkin lymphoma, 1622–1643)
  AIDS, 1709–1710
  chemotherapy, 1623, 1634–1636, 1634t, 1635t, 1638t, 1640t, 1641t
  computed tomography, 1629, 1629f
  CS I-II, 1631, 1632, 1635, 1636–1637, 1639
  cytogenetic abnormalities, 1627
  elderly patients with, 1642–44
  epidemiology, 1623–1624
  Epstein-Barr virus, 294
  etiology, 1623–1624
  hematopoietic cellular transplantation for, 787–788
  histopathology, 1627
  history, 1622–1623
  immunologic abnormalities, 1627–1630, 1629f, 1629t
  in HIV patients, 1642
  lymphocyte-depleted, 1625
  lymphocyte predominant, 1623, 1624, 1625, 1626, 1626f
  lymphocyte-rich classical, 1625–1626, 1625f, 1626f
  mantle irradiation alone, 1636–1637
  mixed cellularity, 1624–1625, 1624f
  molecylar biology, 1627
  mortality, 1630, 1630t
  nodular lymphocyte predominant, 1626–1627, 1637
  nodular sclerosis, 1623, 1625, 1625f, 1627, 1629f, 1636, 1637, 1641
  pathology, 1624–1626
  during pregnancy, 834
  radiation therapy, 1622–1623, 1636–1639, 1638t
  randomized clinical trials, 1629–1639
  Reed-Sternberg cells, 1624, 1625f
  relapse pattern, 1628
  staging, 1628–1630, 1629t
  treatment
    advanced, 1639–1642, 1640t, 1641t
    stage I-II, 1630–1636, 1630t, 1632t, 1633t, 1634t, 1635t
Holotherapy, 566
Homogeneous staining regions (HSRs), 104
Homoharringtonine, 1574, 1846
Homologous recombination, 254
Homotypic cell-cell interactions, 143
Hormonal aberration
  cachexia, 1747
Hormonal risk factors
  breast cancer, 238t
  endometrial cancer, 242t
  ovarian cancer, 243t
Hormone(s)
  breast cancer, 1395–1396
Hormone receptors and breast cancer, 337
Hormone therapy
  breast cancer, 240–241, 241f
  prostate cancer, 1242–1243, 1246–1247
  secondary, 1247–1248
Horner syndrome, 1028
Hospital information systems, 1974–1975
Host defense, 1921t
Host-tumor drug interactions, 603
HP. *See* Hypersensitivity pneumonitis (HP)
HPRC. *See* Hereditary papillary renal carcinoma (HPRC)
HPV. *See* Human papilloma virus (HPV)
HSCT. *See* Hematopoietic stem cell transplantation (HSCT)
HSPs. *See* heat shock proteins (HSPs)
HSRs. *See* Homogeneous staining regions (HSRs)
HSV. *See* Herpes simplex virus (HSV)
HSV-tk. *See* Herpes simplex viruses -thymidine kinase (HSV-tk)
HTLV-1. *See* Human T-cell lymphotrophic virus type I (HTLV-1)
HTLV-2. *See* Human T-cell lymphotrophic virus type II (HTLV-2)
HU. *See* Hydroxyurea (HU)
HuE10, 45
Human anti–mouse antibodies (HAMA), 8
Human chorionic gonadotropin (hCG), 339, 1912
Human epidermal growth factor receptor 2 (HER2), 338, 351
Human genome, 348–349
Human Genome Project, 344
Human herpes virus-6 (HHV-6), 1932
Human herpesvirus
  genes, 295t
  Kaposi sarcoma, 296
  multicentric Castleman disease, 296
  primary effusion lymphoma, 296
Human immune virus (HIV), 300
  cervical cancer, 1299
  patients
    Hodgkin lypmoma in, 1642
Human immune virus-2 (HIV-2), 1809
Human papilloma virus (HPV), 299–301, 299f, 299t
  anal neoplasms, 1194
  cervical cancer, 300, 1299–1300
  head and neck neoplasms, 961
  histopathology, 298f
  surrogate markers, 300–301
Human T-cell lymphotrophic virus type I (HTLV-1), 1809
Human T-cell lymphotrophic virus type II (HTLV-2), 1809
Human transcription and gene expression profiling, 349
Humoral immune dysfunction, 1922
Hürthle cell neoplasms, 925
HUS. *See* Hemolytic uremic syndrome (HUS)
Hyaluronidase
  causing nail hyperpigmentation, 1781
Hybrid capture II test, 300
Hybrid leukemias, 1567
Hybridization, 8–9
Hydrazine sulphate
  cachexia, 1750
Hydrazines, 636
Hydrocortisone, 1906
Hydromorphone
  for cancer pain, 869
5-Hydroxytryptamine 3 (5-HT3), 1757, 1758–1759, 1761, 1762
5-Hydroxytryptophan, 1836
Hydroxyurea (HU), 30, 521, 631–632, 635, 1578, 1782
  causing hyperpigmentation, 1782
  causing nail hyperpigmentation, 1780
  essential thrombocytothemia, 1689
Hydroxyurea (HU) (*cont.*)
  for chronic myeloid leukemia, 1588
  polycythemic vera, 1693
  primary myelofibrosis, 1691
Hydroxyzine
  for cancer pain, 874
Hyperadrenalism, 3
Hypercalcemia, 1674–1675, 1908
  calcitriol-mediated, 1911
  localized osteolytic bone resorption and, 1911
  of malignancy, 1007, 1796, 1911–1912
    impact, 1911–1912
  PTHrP-mediated, 1911
  therapy of, 1912
Hypercortisolism, 934
Hyperdiploidy, 1594
Hyperinsulinemia
  colorectal cancer, 1180
  pancreatic neoplasms, 1144–1145
Hyperleukocytosis, 1577–1578
Hypernatremia, 1908
Hyperosmolar glucose, 1835
Hyperparathyroidism, 3
Hyperpigmentation, 1781–1782, 1781t, 1782f
Hyperplastic polyps, 215
Hyperprolactinemia, 1908–1909
Hypersensitivity pneumonitis (HP), 1857–1858
Hypersensitivity reactions, 1783
Hyperthermia
  biology, 528–529
  cellular and tissue responses to, 529
  chemotherapy and, 533–534
  clinical, 536–540
    adult soft tissue sarcoma, 539
    thermal dose and outcome, relationship between, 536–537
    trial overview, 537–539
  cytotoxicity, 529
  definition, 528
  effects on tumor metabolism and oxygenation, 530–531
  gene therapy and, 534
  immunologic effects of, 531–533
    tumor cell sensitization, 532–533
  and metastases, 533
  normal tissue damage from, 531
  physics
    electromagnetic heating, 534–535
    noninvasive thermometry, 535–536
    ultrasound heating, 535
  physiological responses to, 529–531, 529f
  radiation and, 533
  temperature measurement during, 535
  thermal cytotoxicity enhancement, physiologic approaches to
    pH modification, 531
  whole body hyperthermia (WBH), 531f
Hyperthermic isolated limb perfusion (HILP), 1476–1477, 1533
  adjuvant setting, 1477
  morbidity, 1477
  toxicity, 1477
Hyperthermic perfusion
  for malignant mesothelioma, 1050
Hyperthyroidism, 1903
Hypertrophic pulmonary osteoarthropathy, 1008
Hyperviscosity, 1675
Hypnosis, 1761
Hypocalcemia, 1908
Hypogammaglobulinomia, 1056
Hypoglycemia, 1912
Hypogonadism, 876
Hypomagnesemia, 1908
Hyponatremia, 1907–1908, 1907f
Hypopharynx, 972–973, 972f
  primary tumor staging characteristics, 972t
Hypophysectomy, 877
Hypothalamic-pituitary-gonadal axis, 29
  dysfunction, 1901, 1901f, 1902t

Hypothyroidism, 1737, 1903–1904, 1903t
Hypoxia inducing factor-1 (HIF-1), 157, 520
Hypoxia inducible factor -1 α (HIF-1 α), 275
Hypoxia, 277
Hypoxia-induced apoptosis, 166–167
Hysterectomy
  extrafascial, 1312
  radical, 1312–1313

I1307K Ashkenazi mutation
  genetic basis, 197
IAP. *See* Inhibitors-of-apoptosis (IAP)
IARC. *See* International Agency for Research on Cancer (IARC)
Ibandronate, 1905
IBC. *See* Inflammatory breast cancer (IBC)
Ibritumomab
  for indolent NHL, 1654
Ibuprofen, 1747
  cachexia, 1750
131I-containing compounds, 1903
Idarubicin, 1570, 1574, 1942, 648
  cardiotoxicity, 1843
  causing nail hyperpigmentation, 1780
  dose, 648
  myelodysplastic syndrome, 1556
Idiopathic pneumonia syndrome (IPS), 1862
Idraparinux, 1822
IFN-α. *See* Interferon-α (IFN-α)
IFN-γ. *See* Interferon-γ (IFN-γ)
Ifosfamide, 32, 635, 1761, 1823, 1878, 1905, 1908, 1916
  acute pancreatitis, 1877
  bladder toxicity, 640
  causing anaphylaxis, 1958
  causing hyperpigmentation, 1782
  causing nail hyperpigmentation, 1780
  Ewing sarcoma, 1732
  inducing hematuria, 1825
  localized STS of extremities, 1530, 1531
  metabolic disease, 1535–1536
  nephrotoxicity, 1830
  neuroblastoma, 1727
  nonsmall-cell lung cancer, 1031
  osteosarcoma, 1509
  prostate cancer, 1253
  thymomas, 1059, 1060
IGF-1. *See* Insulin-growth factor-1 (IGF-1)
IGF-1/P13K/Akt/mTOR/P70S6K pathway, 1745
IGF-1/PI3K/Akt pathway, 1745
IGFBP. *See* Insulin-like growth factor-binding proteins (IGFBP)
IGFR. *See* Insulin-like growth factor and receptor (IGFR)
IgV gene mutation
  chronic lymphocytic leukemia, 1607
IgVH mutation
  chronic lymphocytic leukemia, 1611
IkB kinase (IKK), 62
IKK. *See* IkB kinase (IKK)
IL. *See* Interleukin (IL)
ILI. *See* Isolated limb infusion
Imatinab
  personalized medicine, 351
Imatinib, 33, 1585, 1787, 1493, 1761, 1942
  action, 83f
  acute lymphoblastic leukemia, 1601
  chemotherapy-induced lung injury, 1858
  for chronic myeloid leukemia, 1585–1587, 1586t
  gastrointestinal stromal tumors, 1538, 1539
  genetic predisposition, 215
  malignant mesothelioma, 1051
  molecular diagnostics, 339
  personalized medicine, 355
  pregnancy and cancer, 836
  prostate cancer, 1251
Imidazole, 1887
Imipenem
  bacterial infections, 1924, 1925, 1926
  neutropenia, 1937
Imipramine
  for cancer pain, 873
Imiquimod, 1488
  immunotherapy, 181
Immature teratomas
  ovaries, 1368–1370
Immune effector cells, 682
Immune precipitation, 19
Immune-related adverse events (irAEs), 188
Immune suppression
  tumor and, 276–277
Immune suppression mediators, 177
Immune system, transfusion of, 1805–1806
Immune tolerance, 176
Immunobiology
  chronic lymphocytic leukemia, 1605–1606
Immunoblotting, 18–19, 20f
Immunocytochemistry
  limitations, 483–484
Immunoediting, 175–176, 276
Immunoglobulin M monoclonal gammopathy, 1682
Immunohistochemistry, 478
  role, 482–484
Immunologic agents
  nephrotoxicity, 1830
Immunomodulatory genes, 766
Immunoperoxidase staining
  unknown primary site, 1713–1714, 1714t
Immunophenotype
  chronic lymphocytic leukemia, 1605–1606
Immunostimlulants, 728
Immunosuppression, 1805–1806
Immunosurveillance, 175
Immunotherapy, 183f
  anti-tumor activity mechanisms, 187–188
  chronic lymphocytic leukemia, 1617
  clinical effectiveness of, 178–186
  combinatorial immunotherapeutics, 187
  early failures and lessons, 176–177
  history of, 175–178
  renal cell carcinoma, 1207
Impaired drive, 1867
IMRT. *See* Intensity-modulated radiotherapy (IMRT)
In vitro fertilization (IVF), 35, 36
In vitro translation, 19, 20
Incidence of cancer
  age, 371f, 372, 377f
  chemoprevention, 417
  colorectal cancer
    age, 402f
  ethnic groups, 379t
  race, 378f, 379t
Incisional biopsy, 503
Incisional open biopsy, 1499. *See also* Biopsy
IND mechanisms, 353
Indium
  131I-tositumomab (Bexxar), 719
Indoleamine 2,3-dioxygenase, 177
Indolent lymphomas, 1646–1647, 1646f
  autologous stem cell transplantation for, 1655
  clinical prognostic factors in, 1653
  therapy
    at advanced stage, 1654
    at early stage, 1653–1654
Indomethacin, 1747
  cachexia, 1750
Indonesia, 315
Inducible promoters, 768–769
Induction chemotherapy
  and malignant mesothelioma, 1050
Induction therapy
  acute lymphoblastic leukemia, 1596–1597
  acute myeloid leukemia, 1569–1574
Induction
  cell differentiation, 134–135
Indwelling pleural catheters
  malignant pleural effusion, 1853
Infection, 1921–1940
  neutropenia, 1923t, 1936–1938
  prevention, 1938
  susceptibility, 1921–1923
Infectious agents, 1922t
  head and neck neoplasms, 961
Infectious diseases
  pancreatic neoplasms, 1145–1146
Infective endoicarditis
  echocardiography, 1833f
Infiltrating ductal carcinoma
  breast, 1403f
Inflammation
  chronic, 270, 272
  response, 270
  therapeutic applications for, 277
  tumorigenesis and, 275–277
Inflammatory bowel disease
  colorectal cancer, 1180
  genetic basis, 206
Inflammatory breast cancer (IBC)
  breast cancer, 1451–1452
Infliximab, 1847
Influenza infections, 1932
Inhaled nitric oxide
  pulmonary tumor thrombotic microangiopathy, 1865
Inherited cancer syndromes
  colorectal cancer, 1181
  pancreatic neoplasms, 1145
Inhibitors of apoptosis (IAP), 33, 45–46
Insertional mutagenesis, 71, 285f, 286
Insular carcinomas, 925
Insulin, 57
  cachexia, 1754
  synthesis, 57
Insulin-like growth factor (IGF)
  cachexia, 1749–1750
Insulin-growth factor-1 (IGF-1), 57, 1231, 1692
  breast cancer, 1396
  multiple myeloma, 1671
  prostate cancer, 383–384, 1901, 1904, 1907
Insulin-like growth factor and receptor (IGFR)
  breast cancer, 1449
Insulin-like growth factor-binding proteins (IGFBP), 57
Insulin receptor-related receptor (IRR), 57
Intact parathyroid hormone (iPTH), 1911
Integrative genome analysis, 112–113
Integrins, 144
Intensity modulated radiation therapy (IMRT), 512, 512f, 959–997, 1024–1025, 1766
  anal neoplasms, 1199
  respiratory complications, 1860
  thyroid carcinoma, 927
Intercalating drugs
  targeting topoisomerases, 648–651
Intercalation, 589
Interferon (IFN), 679–684
  angiogenesis inhibition, 683t
  antitumor action, 680–682
  for chronic myeloid leukemia, 1588–1589
  gene expression, 681t
  humans, 682–284
  induced genes, 680–682
  induction, 679
  pleiotropic biologic effects, 681t
  receptors, 679–680
  side effects, 684, 684t)
  signal transduction, 680, 680f
  systemic reactions to, 1958–1959
Interferon-a (IFN-a), 32, 155. *See also* Alpha interferon
  cutaneous reactions, 1779, 1785–1786
  hepatitis B virus, 306

Interferon-a (IFN-a) (*cont.*)
melanoma
adjuvant setting, 1477
clinical trials, 1477
mechanism of action, 1477–1478, 1478f
multiple myeloma, 1680
mycosis fungoides/Sézary syndrome, 1666
renal cell cancer, 160
soft tissue sarcomas, 1533
systemic reactions to, 1958)
Waldenström macroglobulinemia, 1683
Interferon-α2, 1908
Interferon-α2A (IFNα2A), 1689, 1694
Interferon-α-2b, 1493
Interferon-b
systemic reactions to, 1958
Interferon-γ (IFN-γ), 1743, 1927, 1938
Waldenström macroglobulinemia, 1683
Interleukin (IL), 686
Interleukin-1 (IL-1), 692–693, 693t, 1576, 1742, 1740, 1804
cytokines, 273
massive pleural effusion, 1950
multiple myeloma, 1674
Interleukin 1B (IL-1B), 1811
Interleukin-1β (IL-1 β), 273
multiple myeloma, 1671
Interleukin-2 (IL-2), 32, 178, 179, 180, 693–694, 694t, 1493, 1576–1577, 1700, 1703, 17041846, 1903, 1904
chemotherapy-induced lung injury, 1858
cutaneous reactions, 1779, 1785–1786, 1786f
diphtheria toxin fusion protein
distant metastatic melanoma, 1480
in-transit metastasis, 1476
mycosis fungoides/Sézary syndrome, 1666
nephrotoxicity, 1830)
PCNS lymphoma, 1708
renal cell cancer, 160
satellite metastasis, 1476
systemic reactions to, 1959
Interleukin-3 (IL-3), 694–695, 694t, 708, 1576, 1687, 1688, 1692, 1804
Interleukin-4 (IL-4), 695–696, 695t
Interleukin-5 (IL-5), 696, 696t
Interleukin-6 (IL-6), 696–697, 696t, 708, 1687, 1700, 1703, 1742–1743, 1804, 1811
multicentric Castleman disease, 1709
multiple myeloma, 1671, 1673, 1674, 1675, 1676
Interleukin-7 (IL-7), 697–698, 697t
Interleukin-8 (IL-8), 155, 698, 698t
Interleukin-9 (IL-9), 698–699, 698t
Interleukin-10 (IL-10), 699, 699t, 1700, 1703, 1704
multiple myeloma, 1671
Interleukin-11 (IL-11), 699–700, 700t, 708, 1804
Interleukin-12 (IL-12), 700–701, 700t
Interleukin-13 (IL-13), 695–696, 695t
Interleukin-15 (IL-15), 701, 701t
Interleukin-15 (IL-15)
multiple myeloma, 1671
Interleukin-16 (IL-16), 701, 701t
Interleukin-17 (IL-17), 701–702, 702t
cytokines, 277
Interleukin-18 (IL-18), 702, 702t
Interleukin-19 (IL-19), 702, 702t
Interleukin-20 (IL-20), 702, 703t
Interleukin-21 (IL-21), 702–703, 703t
Interleukin-21 (IL-21)
multiple myeloma, 1671
Interleukin-22 (IL-22), 703, 703t
Interleukin-23 (IL-23), 703, 703t
Interleukin-24 (IL-24), 703–704, 704t
Interleukin-25 (IL-25), 704, 704t
Interleukin-26 (IL-26), 704, 704t
Interleukin-27 (IL-27), 704–705, 705t
Interleukin-28 (IL-28), 705, 705t
Interleukin-29 (IL-29), 705, 705t
Interleukin-31 (IL-31), 705, 705t
Interleukin-32 (IL-32), 705, 706t
Interleukin-33 (IL-33), 705, 706t
Interleukin-35 (IL-35), 705, 706t
Intermittent dosing, 563
Internal target volume
nonsmall cell lung cancer, 1024
International Agency for Research on Cancer (IARC), 372
classification, 384
International Bone Marrow Treatment Registry (IBMTR) studies, 1587
International Mesothelioma Interest Group (IMIG), 1047
International Prognostic Index (IPI), 1652–1653, 1652t, 1705
Interstitial brachytherapy
cervical cancer, 1314–1315
Interstitial pneumonitis (IP), 1856–1859
Interventional radiology, 490–496
genitourinary, 494
hepatic vascular, 490–492
palliative therapy, 495
thoracic, 494–495
Intestinal T-cell lymphoma, 1649
Intracavitary radiation therapy
cervical cancer, 1314
Intracellular regulators, 36–37
Intracrine mode, 51
Intraepithelial neoplasia, 1
In-transit metastasis (ITM), 1466, 1476–1477, 1476f
Intraocular retinoblastoma, 906–907
Intrapleural photodynamic therapy
for malignant mesothelioma, 1050
Intrathecal pump implantation, 878
Intravascular devices
infection, 1922–1923
Intravenous immunoglobulin (IVIg)
for acquired hemophilia, 1816
Intravesical BCG
bladder cancer, 731
Introns, 6
Invasion of cancer, 141–148
proteolysis, 144
Invasive carcinoma
recognizing, 483
Invasive mechanical ventilation, 1869
Inversion, 105
Investigational New Drug application
preparation, 580, 580t
Iododeoxyuridine, 521
131I-6-iodomethyl-19-nor-cholesterol (NP-59), 1906
Iohexol, 1787
IOM. *See* Institute of Medicine (IOM), 847
Ionizing radiation, 248–260, 1847
molecular events following, 515
IP. *See* Interstitial pneumonitis (IP)
IPI. *See* International Prognostic Index (IPI)
Ipilimumab
immunotherapy, 187
IPS. *See* Idiopathic pneumonia syndrome (IPS)
iPTH. *See* Intact parathyroid hormone (iPTH)
Irinotecan, 653, 1761
adenocarcinoma of unknown primary site, 1717
colorectal cancer, 162, 1189
diarrhea, 1874
gastric cancer, 1104
small-cell lung cancer, 1039
thymomas, 1060
Iris nevi and melanomas, 910
IRR. *See* Insulin receptor-related receptor (IRR)
Irradiation, lethal
hematopoietic growth factors, 707
ISI journal citation reports, 1978
Isochromosome, 82
Isolated limb infusion (ILI), 1477
Isolation, 1939
Isoniazid, 1927
Isotretinoin, 1491, 1908
131I-tositumomab
for indolent NHL, 1654
131I-tositumomab (Bexxar), 719
ITM. *See* In-transit metastasis (ITM)
Itraconazole
acute lymphoblastic leukemia, 1597
aspergillosis, 1930
candidiasis, 1928, 1929
esophagitis, 1872
IVF. *See* In vitro fertilization (IVF)
Ivor Lewis procedure, 1094
Ixabepilone
administration, dose and schedule, 675–676
breast cancer, 1447–1449
clinical indications, 674
clinical pharmacology, 674–675
drug interactions, 675
mechanisms of resistance, 674
toxicity, 675

JAK. *See* Janus kinase (JAK)
Janus kinase (JAK), 273
Janus kinase 2 (JAK2) inhibitors, 1816
Japan, 314, 315
Jaundice, 2
Jejunal interposition, 1097
JM-216, 643
JNK. *See* Jun kinase (JNK)
John's wort, 849
JPA. *See* Juvenile pilocytic astrocytoma
Jun kinase (JNK), 1746
Jun N-terminal kinase (JNK)/stress-activated protein kinase (SAPK), 64
Juvenile pilocytic astrocytoma (JPA), 1733
Juvenile polyposis, familial
genetic basis, 198
Juxtamembrane sequence, 52

Kaolin
diarrhea, 1874
Kaposi sarcoma (KS), 1697–1703, 1698f, 1699t, 1701f
human herpesvirus, 296
interferons, 683
penis, 1255f, 1256, 1842
Kaposin, 295
Karnofsky rating, 506t
Karyotypic and molecular abnormalities, in AML, 1563t
Keratoacanthoma, 1488–1489, 1489f
Ketamine
for cancer pain, 875
Ketoconazole, 756, 1761, 1887, 1906, 1911
growth hormone secreting pituitary adenomas, 920
prostate cancer, 1248
Kidney
uncommon cancers of, 1208–1210
Kinases
oncogenes, 80
Kinetics, 550–557
of cellular proliferation
growth parameters assessment, 551
of chemotherapy response, 553–555
Kinins, 1836
KISS approach, 454
Kit ligand, 53
KIT
thymomas, 1060
KIT-pdgfra
oncogenes, 83
KLG, 60
Klinefelter's syndrome, 1068–1069
Korea, 315

K-*ras*, 82, 338
  colorectal cancer, 1181
Krukenberg tumor
  ovaries, 1374
KS. *See* Kaposi sarcoma (KS)
Kupffer cells, 271
Kussmaul sign, 1834
Kuwait, 312

L-3,4dihydroxy-6-(18)F-fluoro-phenylalanine
  (18F-FDOPA), 332
Lacrimal gland tumors, 913
Lactate dehydrogenase (LDH), 339
Lactic acid
  glucose metabolism, 1742
Lactotrophs, 917
Lactulose
  constipation, 1876
Lamivudine, 1878
  hepatitis B virus, 306
Lamotrigine
  for cancer pain, 873
Langerhans cell histiocytosis, 1506–1507, 1507f
Lanreotide, 1913
Laparoscopic cholecystectomies, 1135
Laparoscopic colectomy
  colorectal cancer, 1187–1188
Lapatinib
  cardiotoxicity, 1844
  pregnancy and cancer, 833
Large cell carcinoma
  lung, 1004
Large cell neuroendocrine carcinoma LCNEC)
  lung, 1004
Laryngeal cancer
  nutrition, 405–406
Laryngopharyngeal reflux
  head and neck neoplasms, 961–962
Larynx, 973–975, 974f
  anatomy, 963–964
  primary tumor staging characteristics, 973t
Larynx cancer
  nutrition, 405
Laser therapy
  malignant dysphagia, 1871
Lasix
  nephrotoxicity, 1828
L-asparaginase, 1577, 1817, 1903, 1904
  acute lymphoblastic leukemia, 1596, 1597,
    1600, 1601
  causing anaphylaxis, 1958
  hypersensitivity reactions, 1783
Lauren classification
  gastric cancer, 1088
Laxatives, 1875
Lazy S shaped incision, 1019
LCIS. *See* Lobular carcinoma in situ (LCIS)
LCNEC. *See* Large cell neuroendocrine
  carcinoma (LCNEC)
LDH. *See* Lactate dehydrogenase (LDH)
Leader sequence, 280–282
Legionella pneumophila, 1927
Leiomyosarcoma (LMS)
  Epstein-Barr virus, 294
  radiation therapy, 1388
Lenalidomide
  multiple myeloma, 1677, 1682
  multiple myeloma, 1680–1681
  myelodysplastic syndrome, 1555
  venous thromboembolism, 1818, 1864
Lentigo maligna melanoma (LMM), 1461
Leptin
  anorexia, 1741
Leptomeningeal metastasis, 1766–1770, 1767f,
    1767t
  diagnosis, 1768
  pathophysiology, 1766–1768
  symptoms and signs, 1768
  treatment, 1769
Letrozole, 745, 1846
  breast cancer, 1432
Leucovorin, 624–625
  colorectal cancer, 162
  diarrhea, 1874
  gastric cancer, 1103, 1104
  neurologic complications, 1769
Leukapheresis, 1578
  chronic lymphocytic leukemia, 1617
Leukemia
  acute, 1676, 1723
  acute lymphoblastic, 1723
  acute lymphocytic
    methotrexate, 614
  acute myeloid. *See* Acute myeloid leukemia
  acute promyelocytic, 1565
  categorization, 483
  central nervous system, 1578–1579
  chronic lymphocytic, 1604–1620
  erythroleukemia, 1562f
  hematopoietic growth factors, 707
  hybrid, 1567
  mast cell, 1579
  megakaryocytic, 1562f, 1567
  monoclonal antibodies, 710–712
  monocytic, 1562f, 1566
  myelomonocytic, 1562f, 1565–1566
  ovaries, 1374
  precursor B-lymphoblastic, 1650
  precursor T-lymphoblastic, 1650, 1650f
  during pregnancy, 835–836
  promyelocytic, 1562f
  radiation-induced, 257
  targeted toxins, 721–722
  vaccines, 731
Leukemia inhibitory factor (LIF), 1743, 1804
Leukemic cell lysis pneumopathy, 1865
Leukocyte
  collection/administration, 1801
  transfusion, 1800
    clinical studies, 1800–1801
Leukocyte tyrosine kinase (LTK), 60
Leukocytosis, 1800
Leukopenia, 1800
  causes of, 1798t
  clinical studies, 1800–1801
Leukoplakia, 1490
Leukopoietin, 1913
Leukopoor/single-donor blood components,
    1811
Leukoreduced red blood cells (LRBCs), 1800
Leuprolide
  breast cancer, 1433
Levofloxacin
  acute lymphoblastic leukemia, 1597
  bacterial infections, 1924
  neutropenia, 1938
Levorphanol
  for cancer pain, 870
Lewis lung carcinoma, 151, 155, 156f, 474f
Leydig cell tumor, 1267
L-glutamine (Saforis)
  oral complications, 1886
LH. *See* Luteinizing hormone
Lidocaine, 1944
  for cancer pain, 874
  mucositis, 1882
  oral complications, 1886
LIF. *See* Leukemia inhibitory factor (LIF)
Life expectancy, 838, 839t
Lifestyle
  colorectal cancer, 1180
Li-Fraumeni syndrome, 90, 206, 885, 1089, 1517,
    1731, 1737
Limb salvage versus amputation
  bone tumors, 1499–1501, 1500t
Linezolid
  bacterial infections, 1924, 1925
  neutropenia, 1936, 1937
Lipid metabolism disorders, 1908
Lipid kinases, 136
Lipid-mobilizing factor (LMF), 1743
Lipoid cell tumor
  ovaries, 1373
Lipolytic factors
  cachexia, 1743
Lipomatous septal hypertrophy, 1064
Liposomal amphotericin B, 1930
Liposomal modified drugs
  dermatologic complications, 1786
Liposomes, 367, 368
  and hyperthermia, 529–530
Lips
  squamous cell carcinoma, 967
Lisofylline
  cachexia, 1750
Listeria monocytogenes, 1925
Listeria vectors, 727
Liver
  laparoscopic biopsy, 501f
Liver metastasis, 1109–1122
  adjuvant chemotherapy, 1112–1114
  chemoembolization, 1120–1121
  computed tomography, 1110f
  cryoablation, 1118
  embolization, 1119–1120
  imaging, 1109
  magnetic resonance imaging, 1109
  neoadjuvant chemotherapy, 1114
  percutaneous ethanol injection, 1121–1122
  positron emission tomography, 1110
  primary site, 1109t
  radiation therapy, 1121
  radiofrequency ablation, 1118–1119
  resection, 1110–1112
  systemic chemotherapy, 1114–1115
  ultrasonography, 1109–1110
Liver neoplasms, 406, 1124–1131
  cholangiocarcinomas
    epidemiology, 1129
    natural history, 1130
    risk factors, 1129
    treatment, 1130
  cholangiocellular carcinoma, 1130
  epithelioid hemangioendothelioma,
      1130–1131
  hepatocellular carcinoma, 1124–1129
    clinical presentation, 1126
    diagnosis, 1126–1127
    early, 1126
    epidemiology, 1124
    hormonal factors, 1125
    local-regional treatment modalities, 1128
    natural history, 1126
    orthotopic liver transplantation, 1127–1128
    pathology, 1125–1126
    progenitor cell, 1126
    risk factors, 1124–1125
    staging, 1127
    surgical resection, 1127
    systemic treatment, 1129
    treatment, 1127–1129
    vascular invasion, 1126
  primary hepatic angiosarcoma, 1130
Liver transplantation
  hilar cholangiocarcinoma, 1141
Livin (ML-IAP), 45
Lixivaptan, 1908, 1913
LMB-2, 721–722
LMF. *See* Lipid-mobilizing factor (LMF)
LMM. *See* Lentigo maligna melanoma (LMM)
LMS. *See* Leiomyosarcoma (LMS)
LMWH. *See* Low-molecular weight heparin
    (LMWH)
Lobectomy, 1020–1021
Lobular carcinoma in situ (LCIS), 1403f
  breast cancer, 1454
Local anesthetics
  for cancer pain, 874
Local excision
  anal neoplasms, 1198

Local tissue ablation, 491–492
Localized STS of extremities, treatment for, 1523–1532
  amputation, 1524
  chemotherapy, 1529–1532
  limb-sparing treatment, 1524, 1524t
  radiotherapy, 1525–1529
  regional lymph nodes, management of, 1524–1525
  satisfactory surgical margins to omit radiotherapy, 1524
  surgery, 1523–1524
Locoregional disease
  radiation therapy, 1479
Lomustine, 635, 889
Long terminal repeat, 279–280
Loop electrical excision procedure
  for HPV, 301
Loop reconstruction, 1097
Loperamide
  diarrhea, 1874
Lorazepam
  for cancer pain, 875
  status epilepticus, 1954
Loss of genomic imprinting, 134
Low molecular weight heparin (LMWH)
  venous thromboembolism, 1864
Lower urinary tract obstruction, 1825
Low-grade glioma, 891–893
Low-grade intramedullary osteosarcoma, 1510, 1510f
Low-molecular weight heparin (LMWH). *See also* Heparin
  for venous thromboembolism, 1818, 1819
  pulmonary embolism, 1952
L-phenylalanine mustard, 33
LRBCs. *See* Leukoreduced red blood cells (LRBCs)
Lumbosacral plexopathy, 1771–1772
Lumpectomy
  breast cancer, 1416, 1417
Lung ablation, 494–495
Lung cancer
  genetic basis, 217
  nutrition, 405
  outcome prediction and therapy responsiveness in, 338
  tissue-specific biomarkers and, 342
  vaccine clinical trials, 731
Lung chemoembolization, 495
Lung neoplasms
  adenocarcinoma, 1003
  adenosquamous carcinoma, 1004
  aspiration cytology, 481
  atypical adenomatous hyperplasia, 1003
  carcinoid tumors, 1005
  clinical presentation, 1005
  computed tomography, 1009
  computed tomography, 438
  diagnosis and staging, 1008–1011
  distant metastases, 1006
  electron micrograph, 485f
  environmental causes, 1001
  epidemiology, 999
  etiology, 999
  familial predisposition, 1000–1001
  guidelines, 1015–1016
  historical note, 999
  incidence, 375
  initiation, 82
  intrathoracic spread, 1005–1006, 1006t
  invasive studies, 1010
  invasive tumors, 1003–1005
  large cell carcinoma, 1004
  large cell neuroendocrine carcinoma, 1004
  methotrexate, 615
  molecular pathogenesis, 1001
  noninvasive studies, 1009
Lung neoplasms (*cont.*)
  nutrition, 405
  operative staging, 1010–1011
  paraneoplastic manifestations, 1006–1008, 1007t
  pathology, 1002
  performance status, 1015
  precursor lesions, 1002–1003
  premalignancy
    molecular abnormalities, 1001–1002
  prevention, 437–439
  primary
    prevention, 412–413
  sarcomatoid carcinomas, 1004–1005
  screening, 437–439, 1011–1012
    recommendations, 439
  second primary cancer, 1002
  secondary
    prevention, 413
  signs and symptoms, 1006
  small cell lung carcinoma, 1005
  squamous cell carcinoma, 1004
  squamous dysplasia, 1003
  staging, 1012–1016
  undifferentiated, 477f
  in women, 1000
Lung premalignancy, 412–413
Luteinizing hormone (LH), 1912
Lycopene, 408
  prostate neoplasms, 1242
Lyme disease, 1809
Lymph node
  aspiration cytology, 481
  axillary
    breast cancer, 1404–1405
  map definition, 1014t
  regional
    clinical tumor staging characteristics, 966t
Lymph node management, regional
  penis, 1257–1258
Lymphadenectomy, 1490
  colorectal cancer, 1186–1187
  non-SLN involvement following, 1471–1472
Lymphangioma
  pediatric ophthalmic neoplasms, 909
Lymphatic mapping, 1470, 1471f
  complications of, 1475
  morbidity, 1475
  patient selection, 1473–1474
  technical considerations, 1475
Lymphocyte-depleted Hodgkin lymphoma, 1625
Lymphocyte-rich classical Hodgkin lymphoma, 1625–1626, 1625f, 1626f
Lymphocytosis, 1609
Lymphodepletion, 180–181
Lymphoepithelioma, 1057
Lymphoepithelioma-like carcinoma
  cervix, 1302, 1302f
Lymphokine-activated killer cells, 179–180
Lymphoma
  adult T-cell leukemia/lymphoma, 1650
  beta-cell
    interferons, 683
  Burkitt, 1650, 1656
  Burkitt-like, 1650, 1656
  cardiac tumors, 1064
  categorization, 483
  diffuse large B-cell, 1647f, 1648–1649
  follicular, 1646, 1646f
  human herpesvirus, 296
  indolent, 1646–1647, 1646f
  interferons, 683
  lymphoplasmacytic, 1647
  mantle cell, 787, 1605, 1648, 1656
  marginal zone, 1645, 1647–1648, 1654–1655
  methotrexate, 614
  molecular imaging and, 325–327
  monoclonal antibodies, 710–712
Lymphoma (*cont.*)
  non-Hodgkin, 1645–1657
  outcome prediction and therapy responsiveness in, 339
  ovaries, 1374
  parasites, 315
  PCNS, 1708–1709
  peripheral T-cell, 1649
  precursor B-lymphoblastic, 1650
  precursor T-lymphoblastic, 1650, 1650f
  radioimmunotherapy, 718–719
  small intestine, 1176–1177
  small lymphocytic, 1647, 1647f
  targeted toxins, 721–722
  T-cell
    Epstein-Barr virus, 294
  vaccines, 731
Lymphoplasmacytic lymphoma, 1647
Lyn, 516–517
Lynch syndrome
  cardinal features, 200t
  genetic basis, 199–206
  prostate cancer in, 216–217
  type II, 1346
Lytic enzymes, 132

MAC. *See* Mycobacterium avium intracellulare complex (MAC)
Machrophage colony-stimulating factor (M–CSF), 689–690, 689t
Macroadenomas, 915
Macrolides
  bacterial infections, 1926
Macrophages, 270–271, 276
MAFbx. *See* Muscle atrophy F-box (MAFbx), 1745
Maffucci syndrome, 1512
Magnetic induction heating, 534
Magnetic nanoparticles (MNPs), 369
Magnetic resonance imaging (MRI), 425, 1833, 1833f
  lung cancer, 1009
  malignant pleural effusion, 1852
Maintenance therapy
  multiple myeloma, 1680
Malaria
  parasites, 315–316
Malignant airway obstruction, 1849–1850
  clinical presentation, 1849
  diagnostic evaluation, 1849–1850
  differential diagnosis, 1849
  management, 1850, 1850f, 1850f
Malignant conversion, 227
Malignant dysphagia, 1871–1872
  treatment, 1871t
Malignant effusion, 2
Malignant germ cell tumor
  clinical features, 1068
  epidemiology, 1067–1068
  etiology, 1067
  histopathology, 1068
Malignant melanoma. *See* Melanoma
Malignant mesothelioma
  vs. carcinomas, 483
  diagnosis, 1045, 1046
  etiology, 1044–1045
  genetic predisposition to, 1045
  historical perspective, 1044
  incidence and epidemiology, 1044
  pathogenesis, 1045f
  pleural, 1044, 1047t
  prognostic factors, 1046
  staging, 1046–1047
  symptoms and signs, 1045
  treatment and surgical options, 1047–1051, 1048t
Malignant mixed müllerian tumors (MMMT)
  radiation therapy, 1388–1389

Malignant myelosclerosis, *See* Acute myelofibrosis
Malignant pericardial effusion, 1834–1835
  differential diagnosis, 1834
  management of, 1835
Malignant peripheral nerve sheath tumors (MPNST), 1517
Malignant pleural effusions (MPE), 1850–1853
  diagnosis, 1851–1852, 1852f
  imaging, 1851–1852
  management, 1852–1853, 1854t
Malignant primary tumors, 1064
Mammalian target of rapamycin (mTOR)
  breast cancer, 1449–1450
  gastric cancer, 1091–1092
  renal cell carcinoma, 1208
Mammalian target of rapamycin (mTOR) inhibitors, 1880, 1886
MammaPrint, 338
Mammography, 422–424
  parenchymal pattern
    breast cancer, 1398
m-Amsacrine
  acute lymphoblastic leukemia, 1596
Mannitol
  brain herniation, 1954
  nephrotoxicity, 1828
Mantle cell lymphoma (MCL), 787, 1605, 1648
  treatment, 1656
MAP. *See* MYH-associated polyposis (MAP)
MAPK. *See* Mitogen activated protein kinase (MAPK)
MAPs. *See* Microtubule-associated proteins (MAPs)
Marginal cost per year of life saved (MCYLS), 421
Marginal zone lymphomas (MZLs), 1645, 1647–1648, 1654–1655
Marijuana
  head and neck neoplasms, 962
Mass spectrometry, 19, 21f
Massage, 847, 1761
Mast cell growth factor, 53
Mast cell leukemia, 1579
Matrix metalloproteinase (MMP), 144, 273, 274
Matrix metalloproteinase-9 (MMP-9), 272
Maxillary sinuses
  malignant primary tumors
    AJCC staging, 981t
Maxillectomy, 982
Mazabraud's syndrome, 1503
m-BACOD, 1706, 1706t
MBL. *See* Monoclonal B-cell lymphocytosis
MCC. *See* Merkel cell carcinoma
McCune-Albright syndrome, 1503
MCD. *See* Multicentric Castleman disease (MCD)
MCHD. *See* Mixed cellularity Hodgkin lymphoma (MCHD)
MCL. *See* Mantle cell lymphoma (MCL)
Mcl-1
  multiple myeloma, 1673
MCP-1 (CCL2), 273
M-CSF. *See* Machrophage colony-stimulating factor (M-CSF)
MCV. *See* Merkel cell polyomavirus (MCV)
MCYLS. *See* Marginal cost per year of life saved (MCYLS)
MDS. *See* Myelodysplastic syndrome (MDS)
MDSCs. *See* Myeloid-derived suppressor cells (MDSCs)
Meat, as cause of colorectal cancer, 401–402
Mechanical impedence mismatch, 366
Mechlorethamine, 33, 34
  cutaneous reactions, 1779
  pregnancy and cancer, 834
Median sternotomy, 1019
Mediastinal germ cell tumor
  pretreatment evaluation and staging, 1069
Mediastinal radiation, 410
Mediastinoscopy
  lung cancer, 1010
Mediastinotomy
  lung cancer, 1010
Mediastinum
  benign, 1067
  diagnostic evaluation, 1072
  pathologic evaluation, 1072
  poorly differentiated carcinoma of, 1072
  treatment, 1072
Mediators
  cardiac effects of, 1836–1838
Medical informatics standards, 1976–1977
Medical information management, 1972–1977
  clinical practice guidelines, 1976
  clinical trials, 1975–1976
  computer-based patient record attributes, 1976t
  computerized patient records (CPR), 1972–1974
  data elements, 1975t
  hospital information systems, 1974–1975
  medical education, 1972
  medical literature searching, 1977
  standards of, 1976–1977
Medical literature searching, 1977
Medical oncologist, 826–827
Medical oncology, principles of, 541–548, 541t, 542t, 547t
Medicolegal issues
  genetic basis, 222–223
Medroxyprogesterone acetate
  cachexia, 1748
Medullary carcinoma
  breast, 1403f
Medullary thyroid carcinoma (MTC), 929–930, 1495
  calcitonin, 930
  external-beam radio therapy, 930
  prophylactic surgery, 930
  surgery, 930
Megakaryocyte growth and development factor (MGDF), 1576
Megakaryocytic leukemia, 1562f, 1567
Megastrol acetate, 1749
  cachexia, 1748
MEK. *See* Mitogen/extracellular-signal-regulated kinase kinase (MEK)
Melanocytomas, 909
Melanoma, 262, 1459–1485, 1735
  acral lentiginous, 1461–1462
  adjuvant therapy, 1477–1479
  anal neoplasms, 1201–1202
  biomarkers, 1484–1485
  biopsy, 1460–1461
  clinical presentation, 1460
  desmoplastic, 1469
  distant metastatic, 1479–1484
  end-stage primary cutaneous melanoma, treatment for
    wide local excision, 1467–1468, 1468f, 1468t
  environmental factors, 1459
  epidemiology, 1459
  etiology, 1459
  familial atypical multiple-mole, 1145
  future directions, 1485
  gentic factors, 1460
  host factors, 1459–1460
  hyperthermia, 538
  lentigo maligna, 1461
  to lymph nodes from unknown primary sites, 1467
  malignant, 117–123, 206–207, 477f, 1834
  metastatic
    interferons, 684
Melanoma (*cont.*)
  molecular imaging and, 327
  mucosal, 1468–1469
  nodular malignant, 1461
  pathology, 1461–1462, 1461f
    genetics and molecular, 1462–1467
  during pregnancy, 1469
  recurrent, 713f
  regional lymph nodes, management of, 1469–1474
  screening, 442–443
  SLN biopsy for. *See* Sentinal node biopsy, for melanoma
  staging of, 1462–1467, 1463–1467t, 1464f, 1465f, 1467f
  superficial spreading, 1461, 1461f
  uveal, 1484
  vaccine clinical trials, 728–729
  vagina, 1297
  vulva, 1294–1295
Melatonin
  cachexia, 1754
Melphalan, 635, 1838, 1878, 1916, 1919
  causing nail hyperpigmentation, 1780
  clinical pharmacology, 638
  for aggressive NHL, 1656
  hyperthermia, 533, 534
  multiple myeloma, 1676, 1677, 1678, 1680, 1682
  myelodysplastic syndrome, 1546
  oral complications, 1886
  sinusoidal obstruction syndrome, 1877
  soft tissue sarcomas, 1533
  veno-occlusive disease, 1877
  Waldenström macroglobulinemia, 1683
Membrane metalloproteinases, 1703
Memorial-Sloan Kettering Cancer Center, 852
MEMS. *See* Micro-electro-mechanical systems (MEMS)
MEN. See Multiple endocrine neoplasia (MEN)
Men as cancer patients
  gonadal complications in
    chemotherapy, 31–32
    protection from, 35
    radiation therapy, 34
  with skeletal metastases
    unknown primary site, 1716
MEN1. *See* Multiple endocrine neoplasia type 1 (MEN1)
MEN2. *See* Multiple endocrine neoplasia type 2 (MEN2)
Menarche
  breast cancer, 237–238
Meningioma, 895–897
Meningitis
  methotrexate, 615
Meningoencephalitis, 1930, 1931
Menogaril
  causing nail hyperpigmentation, 1780
Menopause
  breast cancer, 1395, 1407
Meperidine
  for cancer pain, 871
  systemic reactions to, 1959
Mercaptoethane sulfonate, 640
Mercaptopurine
  pregnancy and cancer, 835
6-Mercaptopurine (6-MP), 628–629, 1878
  sinusoidal obstruction syndrome, 1877
  veno-occlusive disease, 1877
Mercury, 1787
Merkel cell carcinoma (MCC), 1492–1493, 1711
Merkel cell polyomavirus (MCV), 1711
Meropenem
  neutropenia, 1937
Mesenchymal chondrosarcoma, 1508
Mesenchymal stem cells (MSC), 34–35
Mesna
  inducing hematuria, 1825

Mesothelin (SMRP)
  malignant mesothelioma, 1046
Mesothelioma, 1850
Messaging standards, 1967
Met, 61
Metabolic bone diseases, 1905
Metabolic disease, treatment for, 1533–1537
  chemotherapy for, 1535
    dose-response relationship, 1536
    individualizing, 1535
  clinical problem, 1533, 1533f
  resection of, 1533–1535, 1534f, 1534t, 1535f
Metabolic encephalopathy
  neurologic complications, 1776–1777, 1776t
Metabolic syndrome, 1904
  pancreatic neoplasms, 1144–1145
Metabolomics, 137–138
[131I]-Metaiodobenzylguanidine, 1903
Metallothionein, 643
Metastasis, 141–148
  adhesion, 143–144
  adrenal, 1905–1906
  bone, management of, 1792–1796
  bone pain, 866
  brain, 1484. *See* Brain metastasis
  breast carcinoma, 1793f, 1794f, 1795f
  breast neoplasms
    combination chemotherapy, 1448t
    cytotoxic chemotherapy, 1446–1450
    diagnostic evaluation, 1443
    endocrine-sensitive, 1444–1445
    HER2, 1445–1446
    management, 1442–1450
    symptomatic management, 1444
    therapeutic guidelines, 1443
    triple receptor-negative metastatic breast cancer, 1446
  cardiac tumors, 1064
  chemotherapy, 929
  colorectal, 493
  cranial and peripheral nerve, 1770–1772
  disease management, 931
  disease therapy
  external-beam radiation, 928
  gastrointestinal, 1483
  hepatic, 493–494
  integrins, 144
  leptomeningeal, 1766–1770
  liver, 1483
  lung carcinoma, 1791f, 1792f
  melanoma
    interferons, 684
  microdissection, 145f
  molecular events underlying, 141–142
  neuroendocrine, 493
  ophthalmic neoplasms, 912)
  placental, 836, 836t
  prostate carcinoma, 1789f
  pulmonary, 1483
  radioiodine, 927
  recurrent distant, 1483–1484
  renal cell carcinoma, 1791f, 1792f, 1792f
  site of origin, 482
  spinal, 1763–1766
  subcutaneous and lymph node, 1483
  surgery, 927
  therapeutic targets, 146t
  to thyroid, 1904
  thyroid carcinoma, 1788f, 1795f
  tumor-host interactions, 142–143, 142t
  tumor-stromal interactions, 142–143
Metastatic disease
  to bone, 1511–1511, 1511t, 1512t
  radiation therapy, 1484
  surgery for, 1482–1483
Metastatic involvement
  of cardiac structures, 1833f
  of myocardium, 1835, 1835f
Metastatic neoplasm
  small intestine, 1177
Metastatic tumors
  ovaries, 1374
Methadone
  for cancer pain, 870–871
  prostate cancer, 1251
Methotrexate (MTX), 31, 33, 34, 607, 782, 889, 1784, 1823, 1878, 1905
  acute lymphoblastic leukemia, 1597, 1599, 1600
  acute pancreatitis, 1877
  adverse effects, 615–617
  antifolate resistance, 617–618
  catabolism, 613f
  causing hyperpigmentation, 1782
  causing nail hyperpigmentation, 1780
  chemotherapy-induced lung injury, 1858
  clinical application, 614
  combination chemotherapy with, 614t
  diarrhea, 1874
  dosage scheduled, 614t
  drug interactions, 613
  -induced granulomatous lumphadenopathy, 1859
  localized STS of extremities, 1532
  for mantle cell lymphoma, 1656
  massive pleural effusion, 1950
  mechanism of action, 611–612
  metabolism, 607f
  mycosis fungoides/Sézary syndrome, 1664
  neoplastic disease treatment, 614–615
  nephrotoxicity, 1828–1829
  neurologic complications, 1769, 1773
  osteosarcoma, 1509
  PCNS lymphoma, 1708
  pharmacokinetics, 612–613
  photosensitivity reactions, 1783
  pregnancy and cancer, 835
  pulmonary vascular disorders, 1858
  schedule effects, 562
  sites of action, 611f
  small-cell lung cancer, 1039
  supportive care, 616t
  thymomas, 1060
  typhlitis, 1873
Methotrexate-associated hilar lymphadenopathy
  interstitial pneumonitis, 1856
Methotrexate-induced lung injury
  hypersensitivity pneumonitis, 1858
Methotrimeprazine
  for cancer pain, 873
Methyldropa, 1803
MethyLight analysis, 342
Methylmethacrylate
  bone metastasis, 1791
Methylphenidate
  for cancer pain, 874
Methylprednisolone
  for cancer pain, 874
Metochlopramide, 1757, 1762, 1759
  anorexia, 1750
  for cancer pain, 875
  constipation, 1876
Metronidazole
  acute pancreatitis, 1877
  bacterial infections, 1925, 1926
  C. difficile-induced diarrhea, 1875
  for indolent NHL, 1653
Metyrapone, 1911
M-FISH. *See* Multiplex fluorescence in situ hybridization (M-FISH)
MGDF. *See* Megakaryocyte growth and development factor (MGDF)
MGUS. *See* Monoclonal gammopathy of unclear significance (MGUS)
Micafungin, 1887
  esophagitis, 1872
Microarray analysis
  DNA, 15, 17f
Microarray Gene Expression Data (MGED) Society, 344
Microarrays, 365
Microarray technology, 223
Microdissection
  invasion, 145f
Micro-electro-mechanical systems (MEMS), 365
micro-FISH. *See* Chromosome microdissection FISH
Microfluidic systems, 365
Microgliomatosis. See Reticulum cell sarcoma
Micro RNA, 138–139
Microscopic sections
  preparation, 476–479
    frozen, 476
    permanent, 476
Microtubule-associated proteins (MAPs), 656
Microtubule-associated proteins kinase kinase (MKK), 64
Microtubule organizing center (MTOC), 655
Microtubule-targeted drugs, 608–609
Microtubule-targeting natural products, 655–677
  and tubulin depolymerization, 676–677
  and tubulin polymerization, 673–676
Midazolam, 1761
Mifepristone
  breast cancer, 1434
Migratory thrombophlebitis, 1817–1818
  lung cancer, 1008
Milrinone
  pulmonary tumor thrombotic microangiopathy, 1865
Mind-body practices, 849–850
  and connection, 847
Mineral metabolism disorders, 1907–1908
Mineralocorticoids, 1906
Minerals, 408
Minimal deviation, 126
Minimally differentiated AML, 1564
Minimal residual disease (MRD), 1564, 1577, 1600, 1612, 1616
  neuroblastoma, 1727–1728
Minocycline, 1924
  bacterial infections, 1926
Mismatch repair genes
  colorectal cancer, 1181
Mismatch repair mutations (MMR)
  Lynch syndrome, 200–206
Mismatch repair pathway, 97f
Mithramycin, 1908
  multiple myeloma, 1675
Mitimycin C
  nephrotoxicity, 1829–1830
Mitochondria
  apoptosis, 41–42
Mitogen activated protein kinase (MAPK), 1746
  signaling, 516
Mitogen/extracellular-signal-regulated kinase kinase (MEK), 64, 66
Mitogenic signaling, 53
Mitomycin, 1942
  causing nail hyperpigmentation, 1780
  massive pleural effusion, 950
Mitomycin C, 521, 635
  acute pancreatitis, 1877
  anal neoplasms, 1198
  cardiotoxicity, 1841
  chemotherapy-induced lung injury, 1858
  gastric cancer, 1090, 1102
  for hemolytic uremic syndrome, 1820
  hilar cholangiocarcinoma, 1141
  hyperthermia, 533
  radiation-induced lung injury, 1859
  structure, 635f
Mitosis. *See* Cellular proliferation
Mitotane, 1902, 1906
Mitotic index, 552

Mitotic kinesins
and tubular polymerization, 676–677
Mitoxantrone, 650, 1574, 1577, 1916, 1919, 1942
cardiotoxicity, 1843
causing nail hyperpigmentation, 1780
chronic lymphocytic leukemia, 1615
for indolent NHL, 1654
prostate cancer, 1248, 1249
structure, 650f
Mixed cellularity Hodgkin lymphoma (MCHD), 1624–1625, 1624f
Mixed germ cell tumors
ovaries, 1370–1371
MKK. *See* Microtubule-associated proteins kinase kinase kinase kinase (MKK)
MLH1
methylation and transcriptional silencing of, 202
ML-IAP. *See* Livin (ML-IAP)
MMMT. *See* Malignant mixed mullerian tumors (MMMT)
M-mode echocardiography, 1837f
MMP. *See* Matrix metalloproteinases (MMP)
MMTV. *See* Mouse mammary tumor virus (MMTV)
MNPs. *See* Magnetic nanoparticles (MNPs)
Modafinil Provigil, 874
Modeling studies, 467–468
Modified vaccina Ankara (MVA), 727
Mohs surgery
for basal cell carcinoma, 1492
for squamous cell carcinoma, 1490
Molar pregnancy
management, 1379–1380
Molecular biomarkers, 335
for monitoring cancer, 339–340
novel biomarkers, 340–341
for screening and early detection, 335–337
Molecular classification
vs. cancer stem cell concept, 550
Molecular cytogenetics and microarrays
genome aberrations and, 359
Molecular diagnostics. *See* Molecular biomarkers, 335
Molecular genetics
analysis, 1715–1717
chronic lymphocytic leukemia, 1606–1607
Molecularly detected abnormalities, in AML, 1562–1563
Molecular pathologist
role, 486–487
Molecular profiling, 348, 1715
Molecular targets
cancer treatment, 558t
MOMP, 1623
Monobactams
bacterial infections, 1926
Monoclonal antibodies, 710–715, 710t, 1713, 1878and growth factor signaling, 65
chronic lymphocytic leukemia, 1614
immunoperoxidase staining, 482f
systemic reactions to, 1959, 1959t
Monoclonal B-cell lymphocytosis (MBL)
of chronic lymphocytic leukemia, 1605
Monoclonal gammopathies
classification, 1669t
Monoclonal gammopathy of unclear significance (MGUS)
multiple myeloma, 1668
Monoclonal serotherapy, 710–723
barriers to, 715–716
Monocytic leukemia, 1562f, 1566
MOPP, 30, 32, 34, 1917
Hodgkin lymphoma, 1623, 1630, 1631, 1635, 1637, 1638, 1639, 1643
myelodysplastic syndrome, 1546
MORAb-009, 1051
Morphea-like basal cell carcinoma, 1491, 1492
Morphine
for cancer pain, 869
Mortality, 375
age, 371f, 372, 375t, 377f
gender, 373t, 374f, 375t
race, 378f, 381f
Mouse mammary tumor virus (MMTV), 56, 69
Moxifloxacin
bacterial infections, 1924, 1925, 1926
Mozambique, 311, 312, 314
MPE. *See* Malignant pleural effusions (MPE)
MPN. *See* Myeloproliferative neoplasms (MPN)
MPNST. *See* Malignant peripheral nerve sheath tumors (MPNST)
MRD. *See* Minimal residual disease (MRD)
MRI. *See* Magnetic resonance imaging (MRI)
MRNA transcript analysis, 14–17
MRP. *See* Multidrug resistance protein (MRP)
MSC. *See* Mesenchymal stem cells (MSC)
MSH2, 202, 222
MTC. *See* Medullary thyroid carcinoma (MTC)
MTOC. *See* Microtubule organizing center (MTOC)
mTOR. *See* Mammalian target of rapamycin (mTOR)
MTX. *See* Methotrexate
Mucinous adenocarcinoma
cervix, 1302
Mucinous carcinoma
breast, 1404f
Mucinous cystadenocarcinoma, 1349f
Mucins, 130, 131
Mucoceles
appendiceal tumors, 1178
Mucocutaneous bleeding, 1688, 1815
Mucoepidermoid carcinoma, 985
Mucosal infections, 1888–1889
Mucosal melanoma, 1468–1469
Mucositis, 1881–1882, 1882t
evaluation, 1882
in HSCT recipients, 1888–1889
prevention, 1882
treatment, 1882
ulcerative, 1885
MUGA color flow Doppler studies, 1832, 1837, 1844
Muir-Torre syndrome, 1494–1495
Multicentric Castleman disease (MCD), 1705
human herpesvirus, 296
Multidisciplinary management, 823–829
Multidrug resistance
apoptotic pathways, 602–603
drug-conjugate export pumps, 601–602
topoisomerase poisons, 600–601
Multidrug-resistance protein (MRP), 598, 599, 1566, 1577
Multifocal extraovarian serous carcinoma, 1716
Multifocal myoclonus, 875–876
Multimodality therapy
for malignant mesothelioma, 1049–1050
Multiparameter flow cytometry, 1577
Multiple endocrine neoplasia (MEN), 61
Multiple endocrine neoplasia type 1 (MEN1)
genetic basis, 207
Multiple endocrine neoplasia type 2 (MEN2)
genetic basis, 207
Multiple endocrine neoplasia type 2a (MEN 2a), 75
Multiple endocrine neoplasia type 2b (MEN 2b), 1495
Multiple mucosal neuromas, 1495
Multiple myeloma, 114–117, 1668–1684, 1789f, 1794f, 1795f
adhesion molecules, 1670–1671, 1670f
apoptotic signaling, 1673f, 1682
BM stromal cells, 1670–1671, 1670f
cell surface phenotype, 1669
cellular origin of, 1669
clinical features, 1668, 1669t
complications, 1674–1676
Multiple myeloma (*cont.*)
cytokines, 1670–1671, 1670f
diagnostic criteria, 1668, 1668t
Durie–Salmon staging system, 1673, 1673t
epidemiology, 1668
future directions, 1681–1682
gene expression models, 118f
genetic basis, 219–220, 220f
hematopoietic cellular transplantation for, 788
labeling index, 1668, 1674
laboratory features, 1668–1669, 20t
molecular pathogenesis of, 1671–1673
monoclonal gammopathy of unclear significance, 1668
prognostic factors, 1673–1674
recurrent infections, 1675
relapsed disease, 1680–1681
treatment, 1676–1680
tumor cell identification, 1672f
Multiple osteochondromatosis, 1513, 1513f
Multiple viral coinfections
hepatitis virus, 309
Multiplex fluorescence in situ hybridization (M-FISH), 107, 108f
Multistage chemical carcinogenesis, 226f
Mupirocin, 1782
MuRF1. *See* Muscle ring finger 1 (MuRF1), 1745
Muromanoab-CD3, 1847
Muscarinic, 1757
Muscle atropy F-box (MAFbx), 1745
Muscle ring finger 1 (MuRF1), 1745
Musculoskeletal ablation, 495
Music therapy, 1761
Mustard, 32
Mutagenesis
radiation, 249–250
Mutations
and genome aberrations, 359
toward resistance to destruction, 553
Mutator phenotype, 231, 232–234
MUTYH mutation and colorectal cancer, 197–198
MVA. *See* Modified vaccina ankara (MVA)
MVPP, 31, 32
Myasthenia gravis, 1056
Myc, 158
Mycobacterial infection, 1926–1927
Mycobacterium avium intracellulare complex (MAC), 1927
Mycobacterium kansasii, 1927
Mycobacterium tuberculosis, 1927
Mycophenolate mofetil
GVHD, 1876
Mycosis fungoides/Sézary syndrome, 1659–1667
diagnosis, 1660
epidemiology, 1659
etiology, 1659
natural history, 1659–1660
pathogenesis, 1659
pathology, 1659, 1659f
prognosis, 1660–1662
staging, 1660–1662, 1661t
therapy, 1662–1667, 1662f, 1664t, 1665t
Myelodysplastic syndrome (MDS), 1544–1558, 1571
classification, 1544–1545, 1545t
clinical and laboratory features, 1550–1552
clonal origin, 1546
bone marrow microenvironment, 1547
in vitro progenitor growth characteristics, 1546
signal transduction, 1547–1548
cytogenetics in, 1548–1550, 1548t, 1549t, 1550f
diagnosis of, 1552–1553
etiology, 1545–1546
hematopoietic cellular transplantation for, 785

Myelodysplastic syndrome (*cont.*)
history, 1544
morphologic and functional cellular abnormalities in, 1551t
pathobiology, 1546–9
treatment, 1553–1557, 1553t
clinical management, 1557, 1557f
future directions, 1557–1558
Myeloid-derived suppressor cells (MDSCs), 178, 275
Myeloid growth factors, 1801
Myeloid leukemia
in multiple myeloma, 1676
Myeloid sarcoma, 1564
Myeloma, 1512
interferons, 683
multiple. *See* Multiple myeloma
Myelomonocytic leukemia, 1562f, 1565
with eosinophilia, 1565–1566
Myeloproliferative disorders, 1816
Myeloproliferative neoplasms (MPN), 1686–1694
Myelosuppression, 776
vinca alkaloids, 663
MYH-associated polyposis (MAP)
colorectal cancer, 1181
Myocardium
metastatic involvement of, 1835, 1835f
Myostatin, 1747
Myostatin inhibitors
cachexia, 1751–1755
Myxoid liposarcoma, 79
Myxomas, 1063–1064
MZLs. *See* Marginal zone lymphomas (MZLs)

NAACCR. *See* North American Association of Central Cancer Registries (NAACCR)
N-acetyl cysteine
mucositis, 1882
NAD(P)H:quinone oxidoreductase (NQO1), 1735
Nails, 1780
hyperpigmentation, 1781–1782, 1781t
Naloxone
for cancer pain, 876
neurologic complications, 1777
NANBH. *See* Non-A Non-B hepatitis (NANBH)
Nanocells, 369
Nanoshell approach, 367
Nanoshuttle, 367
Nanotechnology, 138, 364. *See also* Nanovectors
historical perspective on, 364
laboratory applications in diagnostics and research, 364–365
nanoparticle contrast agents, 369
for therapeutic implants, 369–370
Nanovectors
first generation, 366
first generation therapeutic, 368
second generation, 366–367
second generation therapeutic, 368–369
third generation, 367–368
third generation therapeutic, 369
utilization, as carriers of therapeutic agents and imaging contrasts, 365–368
Nanowires, 365
Nasopharyngeal carcinoma
Epstein-Barr virus, 294
Nasopharynx, 978–980
primary tumor staging characteristics, 974t
National Association of Attorneys General (NAAG), 863
National Cancer Data Base (NCDB), 372, 1977
National Cancer Institute (NCI), 364, 372, 846, 851
National Cancer Institute Drug Discovery Program process, 576–577
National Center for Complementary and Alternative Medicine, 846
National Comprehensive Cancer Network (NCCN), 340, 865
The National Institute for Health and Clinical Excellence (NICE), 355
National Institutes of Health (NIH), 848
National Program of Cancer Registries (NPCR), 372
Natural killer (NK) cells, 40
Natural Medicines Comprehensive Database, 851
Nausea
anticipatory, 1762
breakthrough, 1762
pathophysiology, 1757, 1758f
prevention
guidelines, 1761t
radiation-induced, 1762
and vomiting, 875
Nausea and vomiting, 856–857
NB. *See* Nuclear bodies (NB)
NBI-3001, 722
NBL. *See* Neuroblastoma (NBL)
NBTE. *See* Nonbacterial thrombotic endocarditis (NBTE)
NCCN. *See* National Comprehensive Cancer Network (NCCN)
NCDB. *See* National Cancer Data Base (NCDB)
NCI. *See* National Cancer Institute (NCI)
NCPE. *See* Noncardiogenic pulmonary edema
Near-infrared (NIR) imaging, 319
Neck. *See also* Head and neck neoplasms
anatomy, 964
Needle drainage, 1835
Negative predictive value
screening test, 420
NEH. *See* Neutrophilic eccrine hidradenitis (NEH)
Nelarabine
acute lymphoblastic leukemia, 1600
Neoplasms. *See also individual entries*
in AIDS, 1696–1711
myeloproliferative, 1686–1694
poorly differentiated, 1713–1714
Neoplastic mast cell disease, 1578–1579
Neoplastic meningitis
methotrexate, 615
Neoplastic transformation, 299
in vitro, 250–251
Neopterin, 1746
Neostigmine
xerostomia, 1883
Neovascularization, 145
Nephrotoxicity
of cancer therapeutic agents, 1826–1830, 1826t, 1827t, 1828t, 1829t
monitoring, 1830
NER. *See* Nucleotide excision repair (NER)
Nerve growth factor (NGF), 51
Neuroblastoma (NBL)
in children, 1725–1727
DNA INDEX, 1726
minimal residual disease therapy, 1727–1728
MYCN, 1726
treatment, 1727
familial, 217–218
hematopoietic cellular transplantation for, 789, 1918
Neuroendocrine carcinomas, 983
poorly differentiated, 1720
of unknown primary site, 1719–1720
Neuroendocrine cells, 1228
Neuroendocrine metastases, 493
Neuroendocrine tumor
metastatic, 481f
molecular imaging and, 332
prostate cancer, 1252
Neurofibromas, 1065
Neurofibromatosis type 1 (NF1), 95–96, 883–884, 1733
genetic basis, 207–208
Neurofibromatosis type 2 (NF2), 96, 884
genetic basis, 208
Neurokinin-1 (NK-1), 1757, 1759–1761
Neuroleptics, atypical, 874
Neurologic complications, 1763–1777, 1763t, 1764t, 1772t, 1775t
cerebrovascular complications, 1776
cranial and peripheral nerve metastases, 1770–1772
metabolic encephalopathy, 1776–1777
nonmetastatic complications, 1772–1776
paraneoplastic neurologic syndromes, 1777
Neurologic emergencies, 1953–1954
Neuropathic pain, 865
Neuropathies
in multiple myeloma, 1676
Neuropeptidergic circuit dysregulation
anorexia, 1741–1742
Neuropeptide Y (NPY), 1741
Neurostimulant drugs
for cancer pain, 874
Neurostimulatory procedures, 877–878
Neurosurgeon, 828
Neurotoxicity
vinca alkaloids, 661–662
Neurotrophin family, 58
Neurovascular bundle dissection
prostate cancer, 1237
Neurturin (NTN), 59
Neutrons, 510
Neutropenia, 1921
antibiotics, 1936t
antimicrobial agents, 1937t
bacterial infection, 1923t
hematopoietic growth factors, 707–708
infection, 1936–1938
Neutropenic enterocolitis. *See* Typhlitis
Neutropenic fever, 1956–1957
management, 1956f
Neutrophilic eccrine hidradenitis (NEH), 1784
Neutrophils, 270
Nevoid basal cell carcinoma syndrome (NBCCS)
genetic basis, 208–209
New anticancer agents, 568, 569t–576t
New Drug Application (NDA)
investigational preparation, 580, 580t
NF-κB, 48–49, 272, 273, 274, 275, 277, 1627, 1681, 1744, 1746, 1750
apoptosis-suppressing, 49
NGF. *See* Nerve growth factor (NGF)
NG-monomethyl-l-arginine, 1846
NHEJ. *See* Nonhomologous end-joining (NHEJ)
NHL. *See* Non-Hodgkin lymphoma (NHL)
Nicotine, 389
addiction
pathophysiology, 391–392
susceptibility to, 392
NIH. *See* National Institutes of Health (NIH)
Nikolskyís sign, 1787
Nilatinib
acute lymphoblastic leukemia, 1601
chronic myeloid leukemia, 1587
molecular diagnostics, 339
Nimustine, 636
NIR imaging. *See* Near-infrared (NIR) imaging
Nitazoxamide
bacterial infections, 1926
Nitrates, 1847
9-Nitrocamptothecin (9NC)
metabolic disease, 1537
Nitrogen mustard, 33, 633–635, 1878, 1916, 1917
alkylation mechanism, 634f
hyperthermia, 533

Nitrogen mustard (cont.)
mycosis fungoides/Sézary syndrome, 1662–1663
Nitroglycerin, 1838
Nitrosoureas, 33, 635–636
clinical pharmacology, 639
hypersensitivity reactions, 1783
hyperthermia, 533, 534
myelodysplastic syndrome, 1546
nephrotoxicity, 1829
renal toxicity, 640
structure, 635f
NK-1. See Neurokinin-1 (NK-1)
NK cells. See Natural killer (NK) cells
NK-κB. See Nuclear factor kappa B (NK-κB)
NLPHD. See Nodular lymphocyte predominant Hodgkin lymphoma (NLPHD)
Nodular lymphocyte predominant Hodgkin lymphoma (NLPHD), 1626–1627, 1637
Nodular malignant melanoma, 1461
Nodular sclerosis (NS), 1623, 1625, 1625f, 1627, 1629f, 1636, 1637, 1641
Non-A Non-B hepatitis (NANBH), 1807
Nonbacterial thrombotic endocarditis (NBTE), 1820(NBTE)
lung cancer, 1008
Noncardiogenic pulmonary edema (NCPE)
chemotherapy-induced lung injury, 1858
Non cell-autonomous suppression, 177–178
Nonepithelial ovarian cancer, 1364–1374
Non-Hodgkin lymphoma (NHL), 165, 1645–1657
adult T-cell leukemia/lymphoma, 1650
AIDS, 1703–1709, 1705t, 1707t
Burkitt, 1650, 1656
Burkitt-like, 1650, 1656
cell surface phenotype, 1653
in children, 1725
classification, 1646t
detection of, 1651–1652
differential diagnosis, 1650–1651, 1651t
diffuse large B-cell, 1647f, 1648–1649
epidemiology, 1645–1646, 1645t
etiology, 1645
gene expression profiling, 1653
hematopoietic cellular transplantation for, 787–789
immunobiology, 1646–1650
indolent, 1646–1647, 1646f, 1654
leukemic phase, 1608
lymphoplasmacytic, 1647
mantle cell, 1648, 1656
marginal zone, 1645, 1647–1648, 1654–1655
natural history, 1646–1650
pathology, 1646–1650
peripheral T-cell, 1649
precursor B-lymphoblastic, 1650
precursor T-lymphoblastic, 1650, 1650f
during pregnancy, 834–835
prognosis, 1652–1653
sites of disease at presentation, 1650–1651, 1651t
small lymphocytic, 1647, 1647f
staging system for, 1651–1652, 1651t
Nonhomologous end-joining (NHEJ), 254
Nonintercalating topoisomerase-targeting drugs, 651–653
Noninvasive ventilation, 1869
Nonmedical professionals, 826–829
Non-myeloablative allogenic stem cell transplantation, 1708
for adult T-cell leukemia/lymphoma, 1656
Non-myeloid growth factors, 708
Nonopioid analgesics
cancer pain, 867–868, 868t
Nonosseous sarcomas
cytogenetic aberrations in, 1519t
Nonseminomatous germ cell tumors, 1265
Nonseminomatous tumors
management of, 1071f
syndromes with, 1068–1069
treatment of, 1070–1072, 1070t
Non-small cell neuroendocrine carcinoma
cervical, 1303, 1303f
Non-small cell lung cancer (NSCLC)
advanced
first-line chemotherapy, 1030–1031
second-line chemotherapy, 1031
anesthesia, 1019
antiangiogenic therapy for, 163
arterial blood gases, 1018
cardiac function, 1017
chemoradiotherapy, 1026–1027
chemotherapy, 1029–1034
adjuvant, 1032
combination, 1029–1030
combined modality, 1031–1032
in elderly, 1032–1033
neoadjuvant, 1031–1032
preoperative, 1026–1027
chest exploration, 1020
diffusing capacity, 1018–1019
incisions, 1019–1020
malignant pleural effusions, 1023
management, 1036f
molecular imaging and, 321–322
molecular predictive markers, 1035
molecular prognostic markers, 1034–1035
molecular targeted therapy, 1033–1034, 1035t
oxygen consumption, 1018
pulmonary function, 1018, 1018f
pulmonary hypertension, 1019
radiotherapy, 1023–1029
brachytherapy, 1029
medically inoperable lesions, 1025
postoperative, 1026
stage I and II, 1025–1026
unresectable stage III, 1027–1028
satellite lesions, 1023
staging, 1012–1013
standard surgical procedures, 1020–1021
surgery, 1017–1023
high-risk patients, 1023
metastatic disease, 1023
N2 diseases, 1023
positive margins, 1023
preoperative assessment, 1017–1019
synchronous and metachronous lung primaries, 1022–1023
therapy, 1016–1034
VEGFR TKIs with chemotherapy for, 162–163
xenon scanning, 1018
Nonspecific interstitial pneumonia (NSIP), 1856
Nonsteroidal anti-inflammatory drugs (NSAIDs), 867–868
essential thrombocytothemia, 1688
Osteoid osteoma, 1505
systemic reactions to, 1959
North American Association of Central Cancer Registries (NAACCR), 372
North American Trial, 1050
Northern blotting, 14
Nortriptyline, 393
Nose, 980–984
anatomy, 964
malignant tumor histology, 981t
NOTCH1, mutations of, 1594–1595
Novel molecular biomarkers, 343
NPCR. See National Program of Cancer Registries (NPCR)
NPM, 79
NPY. See Neuropeptide Y (NPY), 1741
NSAIDs. See Nonsteroidal anti-inflammatory drugs (NSAIDs)
NSCLC. See Non-small-cell lung cancer (NSCLC)
NSIP. See Nonspecific interstitial pneumonia (NSIP)
N-telopeptide (NTx)
bone metastasis, 1793
Nuclear bodies (NB), 42
Nuclear factor kappa B. See NF-κB
Nucleoside analogues
cutaneous reactions, 1786
Nucleosomes, 170–171, 170f
histones, 37f
Nucleotide excision repair (NER), 232, 263, 265
Nucleotide sequences, 5, 10–11
Numerical and structural aberrations
genomes and, 359
Nutrition, 398–410
gastric cancer, 1107
older patient, 841
Nutritionist, 828–829
Nystatin, 1787, 1887

Obesity, 1904
breast cancer, 403–404, 1397
liver neoplasms, 1125
pancreatic neoplasms, 1144–1145
Observational studies, 466–467
Obsessive compulsive disorder, 802–803
OCCAM. See Office of Cancer Complementary and Alternative Medicine (OCCAM)
Occupational exposure, 382
Occupations
head and neck neoplasms, 962
Occurrence, 375
OCIS (Oncology Clinical Information System), 1974–1975
OCT. See Optical coherence tomography (OCT)
Octreotide, 1912
diarrhea, 1874
growth hormone secreting pituitary adenomas, 919
GVHD, 1876
thymomas, 1059
Ocular disease
adult ophthalmic neoplasms, 909–912, 911t
pediatric ophthalmic neoplasms, 904–908
Ocular lymphoid tumors, 912
Odds ratio, 381
Odontogenic infections, 1888
Office of Cancer Complementary and Alternative Medicine (OCCAM), 846, 851
Olanzapine
for cancer pain, 874
Older patient
assessment, 840
chemotherapy, 844–845
clinical trials, 842–843
cognition, 841
co-morbid medical conditions, 840–841
evaluation, 840
frail, 839–840
functional status, 840
nutrition, 841
polypharmacy, 841–842
psychological state and social support, 841
radiation therapy, 844
screening, 844
treatment tolerance, 844–845
Olfactory neuroblastoma, 983
Oligodendrogliomas, 891–893
Oligosaccharide processing enzymes, 130–132
Olive oil, 408
Ollier disease, 1512
Omega-3 fatty acids, 408
Omental bursectomy, 1096
ONCOCIN system, 1974

Oncogenes, 68–84, 70t, 232–233, 255
activation, 74, 74f
amplification, 76t
capture, 284–286, 285f
discovery, 68–70
endometrial cancer, 1330–1331
hepatitis B virus, 304
mutation, 74–76
and protein overexpression and constitutive phosphorylation, 80
retroviral, 68
as target of new drugs, 82–84
Oncogenesis
mechanisms, 284–288
Oncolink, University of Pennsylvania, 851
Oncologist, 825–828, 826–827
internet resources to, 1977–1978
Cancer.gov, 1977
cancer library, 1978
cancer surveillance, 1977
CCRIS, 1978
EMBASE, 1978
HEALTHSTAR, 1978
ISI journal citation reports, 1978
medical claims, 1977
National Cancer Database, 1977
Physician Data Query, 1978
PIER, 1978
PubMed (MEDLINE), 1977–1978
SEER, 1977
Oncology, clinical
molecular imaging in, 318
treatment guideline in, 799f
Oncology informatics, 1961–1979, 1961f
Oncology staff, 828–829
stress and burnout in, 808
Oncolytic herpes simplex virus-1, 771–772
Oncolytic reovirus, 772–773
Oncotype Dx®, 337, 338
Ondansetron, 1759, 1759, 1761
for cancer pain, 875
Oophorectomy, 1345
Opana, 870
Operative fixation, 1500
OPG. *See* Osteoprotegrin (OPG)
Ophthalmic neoplasms, 904–913, 904t
acute lymphocytic leukemia, 908
adult oncology, 909–913
pediatric oncology, 904–909
retinoblastoma, 904–908
Ophthalmopathy, 1903
Opiate, 1757
Opioid analgesics
cancer pain, 868–871, 869t
Opioid rotations
for cancer pain, 871–872
Opisthorchis sinensis, 1137
Opisthorchis viverrini, 315, 1137
Optical coherence tomography (OCT), 319–320
Optimal experimental design, 454
Oral cancer
alcohol, 406f
nutrition, 405–406
screening, 443
smoking, 406f
Oral cavity
anatomy, 963
Oral cavity carcinoma, 967–970, 968f, 970f
nutrition, 405
primary tumor staging, 967t
Oral complications, 1880–1889
associated with HSCT, 1888–1889
of chemotherapy, 1884–1888
pretreatment assessment, 1880–1881
of radiotherapy, 1881–1884
Oral contraceptives
breast cancer, 239–240
cervical cancer, 1301
endometrial cancer, 243, 1325
ovarian cancer, 244
Oral leukoplakia, 411–412
Oral transmucosal fentanyl citrate (OTFC), 870
Orbital disease
adult ophthalmic neoplasms, 912–913
pediatric ophthalmic neoplasms, 908–909
ORN. *See* Osteoradionecrosis (ORN)
Oropharyngeal cancer
nutrition, 405–406
Oropharyngeal candidiasis, 1928f
Oropharynx, 970–972, 971f
primary tumor staging, 970t
Oropharynx cancer
nuitrition, 405
Orthotopic liver transplantation
hepatitis B virus, 306
liver neoplasms, 1127–1128
Osseous metastases
breast cancer, 1450–1451
Osteoblastoma, 1505
Osteochondroma, 1503
Osteoclastogenesis, 1674f
Osteofibrous dysplasia, 1503–1504
Osteogenic sarcoma
adjuvant chemotherapy for, 1532
methotrexate, 615
Osteogenic tumors, 1504–1505, 1504f
Osteoid osteoma, 1505
Osteomalacia, 1905
tumor-induced, 1913
Osteonecrosis, 1882t, 1887
Osteonectin
inflammation, 276
Osteopenia
corticosteroid-induced, 1796
Osteopontin
malignant mesothelioma, 1045–1046
Osteoporosis, 743, 1905
hematopoietic cellular transplantation for, 789
Osteoprotegrin (OPG)
hypercalcemia, 1675
Osteoradionecrosis (ORN), 1883, 1884
Osteosarcoma, 90–91, 1509, 1509t, 1730–1731
chondroblastic, 1731, 1731f
conventional, 1509–1510, 1509f
high-grade surface, 1510
low-grade intramedullary, 1510, 1510f
Pagetoid, 1510–1511
parosteal, 1510
periosteal, 1510
post-radiation, 1511
secondary, 1510–1511
small cell, 1510
Ototoxicity, 1773
Outcomes research, 464–472
history, 464–466
study designs, 466–468
Ovarian ablation
breast cancer, 1432, 1438
Ovarian cancer, 60, 165, 1344–1374, 1842
advanced
survival, 1364
cause, 243–244
classification, 1348–1350
clinical features, 1350
complementary markers, 1352
diagnosis, 1350–1351
early screening and detection, 337
epithelial, 1344–1361
hematopoietic cellular transplantation for, 788
hormonal therapy, 1364
immunotherapy, 1363
molecular imaging and, 329–330
nutrition, 407
palliative radiotherapy, 1364
patterns of spread, 1350
Ovarian cancer (*cont.*)
during pregnancy, 835
prognosis, 1346–1347
risk, 1351–1352
screening, 440–442, 1351
staging, 1353, 1353t
symptoms, 2
treatment, 1353–1359
Ovaries
carcinoid, 1374
choriocarcinoma, 1370
dysgerminomas, 1365–1366
embryonal carcinoma, 1370
germ cell tumors, 1364–1365
immature teratomas, 1368–1370
Krukenberg tumor, 1374
leukemia, 1374
lipoid cell tumor, 1373
lymphoma, 1374
metastatic tumors, 1374
mixed germ cell tumors, 1370–1371
papillary carcinoma, 1349f
papillary serous adenocarcinoma, 481f
sarcoma, 1373, 1386
Sertoli-Leydig cell tumors, 1373
small cell carcinoma, 1373
Overlap syndrome, 1552
Overwhelming pneumococcal sepsis syndrome, 1924
Ovulation, start of
breast cancer, 238
OX40, 183
ligand (OX40L), 183
Oxaliplatin, 643–644, 1773
broncholitis obliterans with organizing pneumonia, 1859
chemotherapy-induced lung injury, 1856
colorectal cancer, 162, 1189
neurologic complications
sinusoidal obstruction syndrome, 1877
testis cancer, 1282
veno-occlusive disease, 1877
Oxaloplatin
chemotherapy-induced lung injury, 1858
Oxycodone
for cancer pain, 869
Oxymorphone
for cancer pain, 870

P107, 90
P130, 90
P16INK4A, 92
P19ARF, 92, 94f
P21, 763
P38 MAP kinase, 64
p53 gene, 32, 90–92, 91f, 265
colorectal cancer, 1181
gastric cancer, 1090
p53, 157–158, 232t, 233, 763
Packed red blood cells (PRBCs), 1800
Paclitaxel, 667–668, 889, 1761, 1846
acute airway obstruction, 1951
administration, dose, schedule, 672–673
anaplastic thyroid carcinoma, 931
breast cancer, 162, 1446–1447, 1448
bronchospasm, 1858
cardiotoxicity, 1841, 1843
causing nail hyperpigmentation, 1781
chemical structure, 664f
gastric cancer, 1104
hypersensitivity reactions, 1783
Kaposi sarcoma, 1701
malignant mesothelioma, 1050
nanothechnology, 368, 369
nephrotoxicity, 1830
neurologic complications, 1774

Paclitaxel (*cont.*)
non-small cell lung cancer, 163, 1030, 1031
ovarian cancer, 1357–1358
personalized medicine, 351
photosensitivity reactions, 1783
poorly differentiated neuroendocrine carcinoma, 1720
pregnancy and cancer, 833, 835
prostate cancer, 1243, 1249
-related interstitial pneumonitis, 1857
small-cell lung cancer, 1040
testis cancer, 1282
toxicity, 669–671
typhlitis, 1874
Page description languages, 1966–1967
Paget's disease, 1255
vulva, 1290
Pagetoid osteosarcoma, 1510–1511
PAH. *See* Polycyclic aromatic hydrocarbons (PAH)
Pain
definition of, 863
management, 1105
Palate
soft, 972
Palivizumab
viral infections, 1932
Palliative care, 854
adaptation to, 797
barriers, 861
bereavement, 860–861
communication, 854–855
goals of care, 855
grief, 860–861
history of, 854
hospice, 861
internet resources, 861t
symptom management, 855–859
terminal phase, 859–860
whole patient assessment, 854
Palliative therapy, 495
Palonosetron, 1759–1759, 1762
Pamidronate, 1912
bone metastasis, 1793, 1794, 1795
multiple myeloma, 1675
Pancoast syndrome, 1006, 1028
Pancreas
parasites, 315
Pancreatic adenocarcinoma
molecular imaging and, 331–332
Pancreatic cancer, 165
familial, 212–213
nutrition, 406
Pancreatic neoplasms, 1144–1170
acinar cell, 1148
adjuvant therapy, 1156–1158
biliary drainage, 1151
chemotherapy, 1165, 1166
clinical manifestations, 1148–1149
clinical trials, 1169–1170
cytotoxic agents, 1169
diagnostic evaluation, 1149–1151
dietary factors, 1146
disease
chemoradiation, 1161–1163
radiotherapy technique, 1163–1164
stereotactic body radiotherapy, 1163
environmental factors, 1146
epidemiology, 1144
gastric outlet obstruction, 1164–1165
histopathology, 1146–1147
imaging, 1149–1150
laparoscopic staging, 1151
localized potentially resectable disease
treatment, 1151–1161
locally advanced
management algorithm, 1149f
metastases, 1170
treatment, 1165–1170
molecular agents, 1167–1168
Pancreatic neoplasms (*cont.*)
molecular pathology, 1147
neoadjuvant therapy, 1158–1159
novel molecular agents, 1169
nutrition, 406–407
occupational exposures, 1146
pathology, 1146–1148
prognosis, 1155–1156
pylorus preservation, 1154
reconstruction, 1154
staging, 1155, 1155t
stem cell model, 1148
syndromes, 3
tissue acquisition, 1150–1151
tobacco, 1146
treatment
locally advanced disease, 1161–1165
tumor biology, 1147–1148
tumor microenvironment, 1148
vascular resection, 1153–1154
Pancreaticoduodenectomy, 1152–1153, 1153f
Pancreatitis
pancreatic neoplasms, 1145
Pancytopenia
causes of, 1798–1799
Panitumumab, 713
colorectal cancer, 162
PANOREX (edrocolomab), 713
Pansinusitis, 1929f
Papillary carcinoma, 924
breast, 1402f
ovary, 1349f
Papillary serous adenocarcinoma
ovaries, 481f
Papillary squamous cell carcinoma
cervix, 1302, 1302f
Papillomaviruses, 298–301
Pap smear, 300
Papua New Guinea, 316
PAR2. *See* Protease-activated receptor 2 (PAR2)
Parainfluenza infections, 1932–1933
Paranasal sinuses, 980–984
anatomy, 964
malignant tumor distribution, 980t
malignant tumor histology, 981t
Paraneoplastic neurologic syndromes
neurologic complications, 1777, 1777t
Paraneoplastic syndromes, 3
Parasites, 311–317
cancer, 316–317
Parasitic diseases, 1809
Parasitic infections, 1934, 1934f
Parathyroid hormone-related protein (PTHrP), 1788, 1909, 1911
Paregoric diarrhea, 1874
Parenchyma, 473
Parosteal osteosarcoma, 1510
Parotid glands, 985
Paroxetine
for cancer pain, 873
Paroxysmal supraventricular tachycardia, 1943
Passive smoking, 1000
Patch testing, 1787
Patient-controlled analgesia, 1019
for cancer pain, 873
Patients
adaptation, 795–796. *See* Boys as cancer patients, Girls as cancer patients, men as cancer patients, Older patients, Women as cancer patients
PBPPI
administration, dose and schedule, 673
clinical pharmacology, 669
toxicity, 673
PBSC. *See* Peripheral blood stem cells (PBSC)
P. carinii, 1933
PCD. *See* Programmed cell death (PCD)
PCI. *See* Prophylactic cranial irradiation (PCI)
PCNSL. *See* Primary central nervous system lymphoma (PCNSL)
PD-1, 184–185, 185–186
PDGF. *See* Platelet-derived growth factor family (PDGF)
PD-L1, 185
PD-L2, 185
PDQ. *See* Physician Data Query
PDT. *See* Photodynamic therapy
PDTC. *See* Pyrrolidine dithiocarbamate (PDTC)
PE. *See* Pulmonary embolism (PE)
Pediatric bone tumors, 1730–1732
Pediatric cancer, 26t
distribution, 1723f
mortality, 1724f
Pediatric oncologist, 828
Pediatric oncology
epidemiology, 1724
ophthalmic neoplasms, 904–909
principles, 1723–1738
Pediatric sarcomas, 1918
Pediatric tumors, 1064–1065
Pedigree analysis
ovarian cancer, 1345–1346
Pegylated drugs
dermatologic complications, 1786
Pegylated liposomal doxorubicin, 1842. *See also* Doxorubicin
PEIT. *See* Percutaneous ethanol intra tumora ablation (PEIT)
Pelvic lymphadenectomy, 1258
Pemetrexed
malignant mesothelioma, 1050
Penicillin, 1803
Penicillin G
bacterial infections, 1924
Penis, 1255–1259, 1257t
prognosis, 1258
surgical treatment, 1257
Pentamidine
protozoal infections, 1933
Pentazocine
for cancer pain, 871
Pentostatin
chronic lymphocytic leukemia, 1613, 23
mycosis fungoides/Sézary syndrome, 1664
Pentostatin-cyclophosphamide-rituximab (PCR)
chronic lymphocytic leukemia, 1616, 1620
Pentoxifylline
cachexia, 1750
oral complications, 1886
Per genes, 33
Percentage of labeled mitoses (PLM) curve, 552
Percutaneous biliary drainage, 495
Percutaneous biliary stenting, 495
Percutaneous biopsy, 496
Percutaneous ethanol injection (PEI), 491–492
Percutaneous ethanol intra tumora ablation (PEIT)
liver neoplasms, 1128
Percutaneous nephrostomy, 1823
Perforated bowel, 1955–1956
Perianal infections, 1935
Pericardial cysts, 1064
Pericardial effusion
malignant, 1834–1835
Pericardial tamponade, 1834–1835, 1945–1947, 1946f
management of, 1835
Periengraftment syndrome, 1861–1862
Periosteal osteosarcoma, 1510
Peripheral blood, 1561
Peripheral blood stem cell (PBSC), 1572
autotransplantation, 1810–1811
dose effect, 561
infusion, in MDS patients', 1556
Peripheral conversion, 177
Peripheral nerve blocks, 877

Peripheral nerve stimulation, 878
Peripheral nervous system disorders, 1867–1868
Peripheral neuropathy, 866
Peripheral T-cell lymphomas (PTCLs), 1649
Peritoneal carcinomatosis
  women with, 1716
Peritoneal papillary serous carcinoma, 1716
Peroxisome proliferator-activated receptor gamma coactivator-1 (PGC-1), 1743, 1745–1746
Persephin (PSP), 59
Personal electronic health records (PHR), 1970–1971
Personalized medicine, 347
  biomarkers and drug development, 348–351
  market and economic impact of biomarkers, 354–357
  regulatory path, 354
  translational medicine and drug development, 351–354
Pertuzumab, 714
Pesticides, 408–409
PET. *See* Positron emission tomography (PET)
Peutz–Jeghers syndrome (PJS), 1145, 1173, 1181
  genetic basis, 198–199
PGC-1. *See* Peroxisome proliferator-activated receptor (PPAR) gamma coactivator-1 (PGC-1), 1743
PGE2, 272, 274
PGK1, 265
P-glycoprotein-dependent multidrug resistance, 598–599, 604–605
PG-TXL, 368
Phagocytosis, 271
Pharmacodynamic biomarkers, 352
Pharmacodynamic end points
  assays for, 579
Pharmacodynamics, 594–595
  defined, 594
Pharmacokinetics
  defined, 590–591
  interpatient variability, 592–593, 592t
  intrapatient variability, 593
  linear models, 591
  nonlinear models, 591–592
  principles, 590–594
Pharmacological audit trail, 352
Pharynx
  anatomy, 963
  wall, 972
Phase 0 studies. *See* IND mechanisms
Ph chromosome, 1584
Phenobarbital
  brain metastasis, 901
  status epilepticus, 1954
Phenothiazines, 1759
  for cancer pain, 873–874
Phenylketonuria, 262
Phenytoin, 1761, 1944
  brain metastasis, 901
Philadelphia chromosome, 69, 82
Phosphatases
  oncogenes, 80–81
Photodynamic therapy (PDT)
  esophageal neoplasms, 1084
  malignant dysphagia, 1871
Photofrin
  malignant dysphagia, 1871
Photolithography, 364, 365f
Photons, 510
Photoproducts
  recognition, 265
Photosensitivity reactions, 1782–1783, 1782t
Phototherapy
  mycosis fungoides/Sézary syndrome, 1663
PHR. *See* Personal electronic health records (PHR)
Phyllodes tumor, 1404f
Physical activity, 401
  breast cancer, 1396
  colorectal cancer, 402–403
Physical dependence, 879
Physician Data Query (PDQ), 1978
Physicians' Information and Education Resource (PIER), 1978
PI-3-kinase
  breast cancer, 1449–1450
  signaling, 63
  survival signaling, 62
PI3K Isoforms
  oncogenes, 81
PIER. *See* Physicians' Information and Education Resource (PIER)
PIF. *See* Proteolysis-inducing factor (PIF)
PIGF. *See* Placenta-derived growth factor (PIGF)
PIK3CA
  oncogenes, 84
Pilocarpine
  oral complications, 1885, 1886
Piperacillin
  bacterial infections, 1926
  neutropenia, 1936
Pirarubicin
  cardiotoxicity, 1843
Pituitary adenomas, 915
  ACTH secreting, 919–921
  gonadotropin secreting, 921
  growth hormone secreting, 918–919
  Hardy's classification, 916f
  prolactin-secreting, 916–918
  silent ACTH-secreting, 921
  TSH-secreting, 921–922
PIXY321, 708
PJS. *See* Peutz–Jeghers syndrome (PJS)
PKC. *See* Protein kinase C (PKC)
Place … *of wellness*, 852
Placenta-derived growth factor (PIGF), 55
Planning target volume
  nonsmall-cell lung cancer, 1024
Plasma cell dyscrasias, 1682–1684
Plasma cell tumors, 1668–1684
Plasmacytomas, 1682
Plasma protein profiling, 349, 350
Plasmid, 7
Plasminogen activator family, 144
Plasmodium berghei, 316
Plasmodium falciparum, 315, 316
Platelet(s)
  abnormalities of, 1801
  alloantigens, 1804
  function, abnormalities of, 1801–1802
  lypholized whole, 1804–1805
  multiple-donor, 1802
  radio-labeling, 1803
  recovery, factors affecting, 1803
  single-donor, 1802
  transfusion, 1802–1804
    clinical factors, 1803
    laboratory factors, 1803
    prophylactic, 1802
    support, 1802
    therapeutic, 1802
Platelet-derived growth factor family (PDGF), 52–54
  oncogenes, 71
Platelet inhibitors, 1847
Plateletpheresis, 1805
Platins
  nonmetastatic complications, 1773–1774
Platinum analogues, 643–644
Platinum antitumor agents, 641–644
  cellular resistance to, 642–643
  structure, 642f
Platinum compounds, 606, 1905
  causing anaphylaxis, 1958
  ovarian cancer, 1356–1357
PLC-gamma, 62
Pleural effusion, 1858
  massive, 1950–1951, 1950f
Pleurectomy
  for malignant mesothelioma, 1048, 1048f
Pleurodesis, 1951
Plicamycin, 1908
  cardiotoxicity, 1841
PLL. *See* Prolymphocytic leukemia (PLL)
PLM curve. *See* Percentage of labeled mitoses curve
PMF. *See* Primary myelofibrosis (PMF)
PML oncogenic domains (POD), 42
PML/RARA, 79
PMP. *See* Pseudomyxoma peritonei (PMP)
PMRT. *See* Progressive muscle relaxation therapy (PMRT)
Pneumonectomy, 1020–1021
Pneumonia, 1863
  bacterial, 1861
  fungal, 1861
  viral, 1861
Pneumonitis, 1737, 1932
Pneumothorax, 1951–1952
POD. *See* PML oncogenic domains (POD)
Podophyllotoxin
  structure, 652f
Point mutations, 74f
Pol, 281
Pol H, 264
Polychthemia, 1913
Polyclonal antibodies, 1714
Polycyclic aromatic hydrocarbons (PAH), 387
Polycystic ovary syndrome, 1325
Polycythemic vera (PV), 1691–1694, 1692t, 1693t, 1694t
Polygenetic etiology
  of cancer, 550
Polymerase chain reaction, 11–12, 11f, 15–16
  myelodysplastic syndrome, 1546
Polymorphisms
  colorectal cancer, 1181–1182
Polypharmacy
  older patient, 841–842
Polyps, 426
POMC. *See* Pro-opiomelamocortin (POMC)
Porphyria, 262
Portal vein embolization, 492, 492f
Posaconazole
  aspergillosis, 1930, 1938
  candidiasis, 1928, 1929
  zygomycosis, 1930
Positive predictive value (PPV), 347, 448
  screening test, 420
Positron emission tomography (PET), 489, 1139, 1833
  lung cancer, 1009
  malignant pleural effusion, 1851–1852
  PCNS lymphoma, 1708
Posterolateral thoracotomy, 1019
Postmastectomy pain, 866
Post-radiation osteosarcoma, 1511
Post-remission therapy
  acute lymphoblastic leukemia, 1597–1599, 1598t
  acute myeloid leukemia, 1571
Postsurgical respiratory insufficiency, 1854–1855, 1855f
Post-thoracotomy pain, 866
Posttranslational modifications, 18
Posttransplant lymphoproliferative disease (PTLD), 784, 1863, 1917
Posttransplantation constrictive bronchiolitis (PTCB), 1862–1863
Potassium iodide
  xerostomia, 1883
Potassium phenoxymethyl penicillin
  osteoradionecrosis, 1884
Poxvirus, 727
PPV. *See* Positive predictive value (PPV)

pRB protein, 90f, 904–905
PRBCs. *See* Packed red blood cells (PRBCs)
PRCA. *See* Pure red cell aplasia (PRCA)
Precocious puberty, 1909
Precursor B-lymphoblastic leukemia/lymphoma, 1650
Precursor T-lymphoblastic leukemia/lymphoma, 1650
Predictive biomarkers, 352, 353, 354, 355
Predictive probabilities, 449–451
Prednisolone
  acute lymphoblastic leukemia, 1597
  for indolent NHL, 1654
  pregnancy and cancer, 835
Prednisone, 32, 34, 756
  acute lymphoblastic leukemia, 1597
  acute pancreatitis, 1877
  for aggressive NHL, 1656
  for cancer pain, 874
  chronic lymphocytic leukemia, 1613
  for indolent NHL, 1654
  multiple myeloma, 1676, 1677
  mycosis fungoides/Sézary syndrome, 1665
  pregnancy and cancer, 834, 835
  primary myelofibrosis, 1691
  prostate cancer, 1243, 1248, 1249
  thymomas, 1060
  typhlitis, 1873
  Waldenström macroglobulinemia, 1683
Pregnancy
  breast cancer, 1451
  cancer diagnosis and staging, 830–831
  cancer treatment, 831
  chemotherapy during, 36–37
  drugs during, 832t
  dysgerminomas, 1368
  in essential thrombocytothemia, 1688
  melanoma and, 1469
  multidisciplinary approach for cancer patients, 836t
  radiation therapy during, 37
  tumor types, 831t
Preoperative preparation, 506
Prepubertal girls
  gonadal complications in chemotherapy, 32–33
Prevention, 410, 502–503
  public health guidelines, 399t–400t, 401–402
Primary bone sarcomas, 1500–1501, 1507–1511
Primary central nervous system lymphoma (PCNSL), 894–895
Primary germ cell tumors
  of thorax, 1067–1072
Primary myelofibrosis (PMF), 1688t, 1689–1691, 1690f, 1690t
  and essential thrombocytothemia, distinction between, 1687
Primary physician, 823–824
Primary prophylaxis, 707
Prior probabilities
  and Bayesian updating, 448
PRKAR1A, 1063
Pro-Banthine
  oral complications, 1886
Probenecid
  nephrotoxicity, 1829
Probiotics
  bacterial infections, 1926
Procainamide, 1944
Procarbazine, 33, 636, 889, 1916, 1917
  causing anaphylaxis, 1958
  chemotherapy-induced lung injury, 1858
  hypersensitivity reactions, 1783
  -induced granulomatous disease, 1859
  massive pleural effusion, 1950
  myelodysplastic syndrome, 1546
  neurologic complications, 1774
  pregnancy and cancer, 834
Prochlorperazine, 1757, 1759, 1762
  for cancer pain, 875
Proctitis, 1876–1877
Professional networking, 1969
Progesterone receptors
  breast cancer, 1401
Progestin, 737–739
  anti-progestins, 739
  breast cancer, 1433
  mechanism of action, 737
  metastatic breast cancers, 738–739
  physiologic actions, 737–738
  prostate cancer, 1248
  sites of production, 737
  synthesis, 737
  synthetic, 738
  uterine cancer, 739
Programmed cell death (PCD), 40
  oncogenes, 73–74
Progressive cancer, 410
Progressive muscle relaxation therapy (PMRT), 1761
Proinflammatory-cytokine inhibitors and antibodies
  cachexia, 1752
Prolactin, 1913
Proliferative inflammatory atrophy (PIA), 1230
Prolymphocytic leukemia (PLL), 1607f, 1608
Promethazine, 1761
Promotor region, 5
Promyelocytic leukemia, 1562f
Pro-opiomelamocortin (POMC), 1910–1911
Prophylactic cranial irradiation (PCI)
  small-cell lung cancer, 1038
Prophylactic surgery
  genetic basis, 193–194
  medullary thyroid carcinoma, 930
Prorton pump inhibitors, 1873
Prostacyclin
  pulmonary tumor thrombotic microangiopathy, 1865
Prostaglandin elevation
  cachexia, 1747–1748
Prostaglandins, 1836
Prostate cancer, 326f, 340, 376, 1250f, 1919
  5α-reductase inhibitors, 757
  algorithm for localized, 1234t, 1242
  androgen deprivation, 751–752
  antiandrogen withdrawal, 756
  biochemical recurrence of, 1245
  biology of
    cancer histologic features, 1230–1231
    molecular pathogenesis, 1231–1232
    normal anatomic and histologic features, 1228–1229, 1228f, 1229f
    premalignant lesions, 1229–1230
  cause, 244
  chemoprevention, 1241–1242
  clinical presentations, 1252–1253
  combined androgen blockade, 752
  early detection and disease identification, 1232–1233
  estrogen, 753
  familial, 216–217
  growth factors implicated in, 1231t
  histologic variants, 1251–1252, 1252t
  hormonal axis and therapeutic agents in, 1246f
  hormonal therapy, 752f
  immediate delayed androgen ablation, 754–755
  intermittent androgen suppression,, 754
  interstitial brachytherapy, 513f
  LHRH agonists, 751–752
  locally advanced, 1242–1244
    castrate-resistant, 1244
  mechanism of androgen action, 750
  metastatic, 1244–1251
    castrate-resistant disease, 1247
    diagnosis, 1245–1246
Prostate cancer (*cont.*)
    palliative care, 1251
    prognosis, 1247–1251
    therapies, 1246–1247
  molecular imaging and, 324–325
  nutrition, 405
  prevention, 415, 434–437
  screening, 435–437
    recommendations, 437
  screening and early detection and molecular biomarkers, 335–336
  screening in older patient, 844
  second-line hormone therapy, 755–757
  staging of, 1233–1238, 1233t, 1234t
    curative therapy, 1235–1236
    therapy options and applications, 1234–1235
  treatment outcomes for early disease, 1238–1241
    complications, 1239–1241
  vaccine
    clinical trials, 729–731
Prostate specific antigens (PSA), 3, 376, 435–436, 1713, 1714
  prostate cancer, 1228, 1232
  velocity (PSAV), 1232–1233
    as predictor after diagnosis, 1240–1241
Prostatic acid phosphatase (PAP), 1228
Prostatic intraepithelial neoplasia (PIN), 1229–1230
PROSTVAC, 767
Protease-activated receptor 2 (PAR2), 1813–1814
Proteases, 274
Protein
  analysis, 18–22
  identification and detection, 20f
Protein kinase, 136
Protein kinase C (PKC)
  signaling, 516
Protein phosphatase, 136–137
Protein sequencing, 19
Protein synthesis, 129, 129f
Proteoglycans, 130, 131–132
Proteolysis, 144
Proteolysis-inducing factor (PIF), 1743–1744
Proteomic profiling, human, 349–350
Protocols, in clinical trials, 446–447
Proton radiotherapy, 1024–1025
Protons, 510
Proto-oncogenes, 69, 71, 87
Protozoal infections, 1933–1934
PRX302, 722
PSA. *See* Prostate specific antigens (PSA)
Pseudoaddiction, 879
Pseudoephedrine, 1787
Pseudomembranous colitis, 1875, 1875f. *See also* Colitis
Pseudomonas aeruginosa, 1925–1926, 1926f
Pseudomyxoma peritonei (PMP)
  appendiceal tumors, 1178–1179
Psoralen
  mycosis fungoides/Sézary syndrome, 1663
Psychiatric disorders, 802–807
Psychological issues, 796–799, 879
Psycho-oncology, 793–808, 828
  historical perspective, 793–794, 794t
Psychosocial distress
  recognition of, 799–802
Psychosocial issues
  gonadal complications, 37–38
PTCB. *See* Posttransplantation constrictive bronchiolitis (PTCB)
PTCLs. *See* Peripheral T-cell lymphomas (PTCLs)
PTEN, 210–211
  breast cancer, 191
PTEN/MMAC tumor suppressor, 63

PTLD. *See* Posttransplant lymphoproliferative disease (PTLD)
PTTM. *See* Pulmonary tumor thrombotic microangiopathy (PTTM)
Puberty
  delayed, 1909
  precocious, 1909
Public health guidelines
  for prevention, 401
Pulmonary aspergillosis, 1929
Pulmonary edema, 1861, 1868
  noncardiogenic, 1858
Pulmonary embolism (PE), 1818, 1952–1953, 1953f
Pulmonary fibrosis, 1737
Pulmonary hypertension (PH), 1858
  in cancer patients, 1864–1865, 1865f
  nonsmall-cell lung cancer, 1019
Pulmonary infections, 1934–1935
Pulmonary rehabilitation (PR), 1866
Pulmonary tumor thrombotic microangiopathy (PTTM), 1865
Pulmonary vascular disorders (PVD), 1858
Pulmonary veno-occlusive disease (PVOD), 1858, 1862
Pulse oximetry, 1578
Pure red cell aplasia (PRCA), 1056
Purine analogs, 628–632
  -alkylating agent combinations
    chronic lymphocytic leukemia, 1614–23
  chronic lymphocytic leukemia, 1613–1614
Purine antimetabolites, 627f
Purine nucleoside catabolism inhibitors, 629f
Purine synthesis
  inhibitors, 618
PV. *See* Polycythemic vera (PV)
PVD. *See* Pulmonary vascular disorders (PVD)
PVOD. *See* Pulmonary veno-occlusive disease (PVOD)
Pyrazinamide, 1927
Pyridoxine, 1784
Pyrimethamine
  protozoal infections, 1933, 1934
Pyrimidine, 265
Pyrimidine analogs, 621–627
Pyrrolidine dithiocarbamate (PDTC)
  cachexia, 1751

QOL. *See* Quality-of-life (QOL)
Quackwatch, 851
Quality-adjusted life years (QALYs), 355, 467
Quality measurement, 470–471
Quality-of-care, 468
Quality-of-life (QOL), 468–469, 807–808
Quinagolide, 1913
Quinine, 1577
Quinolones
  bacterial infections, 1926, 1927
  protozoal infections, 1933
Quinupristin, 1924
  bacterial infections, 1925

Racial groups, 376–378, 381f
  incidence, 378f, 379t
  mortality, 378f
RAD51, 191
Radiation
  absorbed dose, 510
  adaptive responses, 253
  breast cancer, 1397
  bystander effects, 252–253, 253f
  cellular and tissue effects, 249–255
  cellular response to, 513–514
  dose response, 523–524
  growth, 515
  head and neck neoplasms, 962
  hypothyroidism, 1903
  induced carcinogenesis
Radiation (*cont.*)
    experimental, 255–256
    genetic susceptibility, 256
    human epidemiologic studies, 256–259
    risk assessment, 259–260
  -induced genomic instability, 251–252
  induced secondary tumors, 258
  injury, 248–249
  ionizing, 1847, 1916
  leukemia, 257
  low-dose exposures, 258–259
  molecular mechanisms, 253–255
  nephritis, 1826
  oncologist, 827
  oncology, 510–526
    clinical, 523–525
  physical basis, 510
  during pregnancy, 831
  response modifiers, 621
  stress-signaling pathways, 515
  survival analysis, 514
  survival curve analysis, 515
  types, 510
Radiation coloproctitis, 1876–1877
Radiation fibrosis (RF), 1859–1860
Radiation-induced lung injury (RILI), 1859–1860
Radiation-induced nausea and vomiting (RINV), 1762
Radiation pneumonitis (RP), 1859–1860
Radiation therapy, 1765, 1766
  adjuvant therapy, 524–525
  anal neoplasms, 1199
  antiangiogenic effects of, 159
  antiangiogenic therapy, 523
  for basal cell carcinoma, 1492
  biologic basis, 513–526
  bone tumors, 1501
  brain metastasis, 901
  cardiac complications of, 1847–1848
  chemotherapy, 525t
  chronic lymphocytic leukemia, 1617
  dermatologic complications, 1782, 1782t
  DNA repair, 517–518
  effects on gonadal function
    in men, 34
    in women, 34–35
  gene therapy, 522–523
  hematopoietic growth factors, 707
  Hodgkin lymphoma, 1622–1623, 1636–1639, 1638t
  and hypothalamic-pituitary dysfunction, 1901
  Kaposi sarcoma, 1701
  for localized STS of extremities, 1525–1529, 1531–1532
    delivery, 1527–1529
    dose fractionation, 1525
    dose-volume histograms, 1525
    external beam, 1525
    sequencing, 1527, 1528f, 1528t
    target volume, 1525–1527, 10f
    three-dimensional, 1525
  locoregional disease, 1479
  for malignant mesothelioma, 1049
  metastatic therapy, 1484
  multiple myeloma, 1677–1678
  mycosis fungoides/Sézary syndrome, 1663–1664
  neurologic complications, 1769, 1774–1776
  oral complications of, 1881–1884
  palliative, 525
  penis, 1258
  during pregnancy, 37
  prophylactic, 525
  prostate cancer
    chemotherapy, 1243–1244
    hormone therapy, 1242–1243
    palliative care, 1251
    postprostatectomy radiation, 1244
Radiation therapy (*cont.*)
  renal tumors in children, 1729
  retroperitoneal sarcomas, 1540–1541
  seminoma, 1069
  sequelae, 525–526
  for squamous cell carcinoma, 1490–1491
  thymomas, 1058–1059
  urethra, 1259–1260
Radiative phased array fields, 534–535
Radical hysterectomy, 1312–1313
Radical mastectomies, 550
Radical prostatectomy, 1243–1244
  prostate cancer, 1236, 1236f, 1238
Radioactive gold, 1835
Radiofrequency ablation (RFA)
  Osteoid osteoma, 1505
Radiofrequency thermoablation (RFA)
  liver neoplasms, 1128
Radioimmunotherapy, 717–720
  alpha-particle, 720
  improved, 719
  of lymphoma, 718–719
  pretargeting, 719–720
  of solid tumors, 719
Radioiodine
  for differentiated thyroid carcinoma, 926
  thyroid carcinoma, 927–928
Radioisotope
  alpha emitters, 718
  beta emitters, 717–718
  selection, 717
Radiologic techniques
  for cancer screening and early detection, 336–337
Radionuclide imaging
  high-output cardiac failure, 1837
Radiosurgery
  brain metastasis, 901–902
Raf, 64, 66
  signaling, 515–516
Raloxifene, 743
  for arterial thrombosis, 1820
  breast cancer, 1455
Ramoplantin
  bacterial infections, 1926
Randomized trials, 422, 446, 466
RANKL, 276
Ranpirnase
  malignant mesothelioma, 1051
Rapamycin
  chemotherapy-induced lung injury, 1856
  multiple myeloma, 1682
RAR. *See* Retinoic acid receptors (RAR)
RARA, 79
Ras, 63, 157
  MAP kinase cascade, 64
  oncogenes, 84
  signaling, 515–516
  signaling downstream, 64
Rate difference, 381
Rate ratio, 381
Razoxane
  localized STS of extremities, 1531
RB. *See* Retinoblastoma (RB)
RB1, 88, 88f
  cloning, 89
Rb growth control pathway deregulation, 32
Rbl gene, 905
Rb tumor-suppressor gene, 31–32
RCC. *See* Renal cell carcinoma (RCC)
Reactive mast cell hyperplasia, 1578
Reactive oxygen species (ROS), 1746
  and Reactive nitrogen species (RNS), 274–275
Reactive thrombocytosis (RT)
  and essential thrombocytothemia, distinction between, 1687
Receptor tyrosine kinase (RTK), 51–52
  intracellular effects, 61f
  invasion, 146
Recombinant DNA, 7

Recombinant factor VIIa (rFVIIa), 1821
Recombinant fusion protein therapy
  mycosis fungoides/Sézary syndrome, 1666
Recombinant growth hormone, 1912
Recombinant immunoblot test (RIBA)
  hepatitis C virus, 307
Recombinant proteins
  large-scale production, 20–21
Recombinant vaccinia virus, 767
Rectal neoplasms, 1919
  abdominal perineal resection, 1186
  adjuvant chemotherapy, 1190
  local excision, 1186
  low anterior resection, 1186
  neoadjuvant chemotherapy, 1190
  radiation therapy, 1190
  synchronous and metachronous lesions, 1186
Recurrence
  prevention, 410
Red cell(s)
  abnormalities of, 1799–1800
  growth factors, 1799
  transfusion, 1799–1800
Red meat, 402
5α-Reductase inhibitors, 757
Reese–Ellsworth classification, 906
Rehabilitation specialist, 828
Relapsed aggressive lymphoma
  in non-HIV infected individuals, 1707–1708
Relapsed disease, 1680–1681
Relative risk, 381
Renal ablation, 494
Renal arterial embolization, 494
Renal cell carcinoma, 160, 1204–1210, 1729
  clinical presentation, 1204
  echocardiography, 1833f
  epidemiology, 1204
  genetic basis, 215–216
  grade, 1205
  hematopoietic cellular transplantation for, 789
  metastatic disease, 1206
    surgery in patients with, 1206–1207
    systemic therapy for, 1207–1208
  molecular imaging and, 330–331, 330f
  pathology, 1204–1205
  prognostic features, 1205
  RF ablation, 494f
  staging, 1205, 1205t
  treatment, 1205–1206
Renal failure
  in multiple myeloma, 1675–1676
Renal medullary carcinoma, 1209–1210
Renal oncocytoma, 1209
Renal pelvis/ureter tumors, 1212–1218
  AJCC TNM classification, 1214t
  bladder cancer, associated with, 1213
  chemotherapy, 1216–1217
  clinical presentation, 1213
  cytology, 1213
  endoscopy, 1214
  epidemiology, 1212
  etiology, 1212
  pathobiology, 1212–1213
  prognosis, 1214–1215, 1215t
  radiological study, 1213–1214
  radiotherapy, 1216
  staging, 1214
  surgery, 1215–1216
Renal tumors
  in children, 1728–1729
Renin production, 1913
Replication-competent viruses
  combination chemotherapy/radiotherapy with, 774
  therapeutic gene delivery with, 773–774
Reproductive factors
  cervical cancer, 1300–1301
Research and development, in biomarkers
  economic value to, 354–355
Research collaboration, 1971
Reserpine
  xerostomia, 1883
Respiratory complications, 1849–1870
  invasive mechanical ventilation, 1869
  management, 1868–1869
  noninvasive ventilation, 1869
  outcomes, 1869–1870
Respiratory depression, 876
Response Evaluation in Solid Tumors (RECIST) criteria, 187
Restriction endonucleases, 7
Restriction fragment length polymorphism (RFLP maps), 348
Resuscitation, 1942
Resveratrol
  cachexia, 1750, 1751
RET
  oncogenes, 84
Reticulum cell sarcoma, 912
Retinoblastoma (RB), 87–90, 904–908, 904f, 905f, 907f, 1733–1734, 1917–1918
  diagnostic testing, 905–906
  extraocular, 907–908
  genetic basis, 208
  genetic testing, 905, 905t
  intraocular, 906–907, 906t
  molecular biology of, 904–905
  second malignancies, 908
  signs and symptoms, 905
Retinoblastoma protein, 89–90
Retinoblastoma syndrome, 1513
Retinoic acid, 889
Retinoic acid receptors (RAR), 36
  fusion proteins, 36f
Retinoids, 1307, 1728
Retinoid X receptor (RXR), 1903
Retromolar trigone, 970
Retroperitoneal hemorrhage, 1947–1948, 1948f
Retroperitoneal sarcomas (RPS), 1539–1541
Retroviral oncogenes, 68
Retroviral transduction, 69f
Retroviral vectors, 288
Retroviruses
  endogenous, 279, 287–288
  gene delivery, 759–760
  life cycle, 281f
  structure, 280f
Retuximab
  bronchospasm, 1859
Reverse phase protein lysate arrays (RPPA), 341, 341f
Reverse transcriptase polymerase chain reaction (RT-PCR), 1564, 1565, 1577, 1715
  hepatitis C virus, 307
Reverse transcription, 283f
Reversible posterior leukoencephalopathy syndrome (RPLS), 166
Revlimid
  multiple myeloma, 1677, 1682
RFA. *See* Radiofrequency thermoablation (RFA)
RFLP maps. *See* Restriction fragment length polymorphism (RFLP) maps
rFVIIa. *See* Recombinant factor VIIa (rFVIIa)
Rhabdoid tumor of the kidney (RTK), 1729
Rhabdomyomas, 1064, 1065
Rhabdomyosarcoma, 1729–1730, 1918
  adjuvant chemotherapy for, 1532
  pediatric ophthalmic neoplasms, 909
RIBA. *See* Recombinant immunoblot test (RIBA)
Ribavirin
  viral infections, 1932
Ribozymes, 17, 764–765
Richter syndrome, 1647f, 1609–1610, 1609f
Rifabutin, 1927
Rifampin, 1761, 1924, 1926, 1927
Rifaximin
  bacterial infections, 1926
RILI. *See* Radiation-induced lung injury (RILI)
RINV. *See* Radiation-induced nausea and vomiting (RINV)
Risedronate, 1905
Risk, 374
Risperidon
  for cancer pain, 874
Risperidone
  neurologic complications, 1777
Rituxan, 37
Rituximab, 711–712, 1847
  for acquired hemophilia, 1816
  acute lymphoblastic leukemia, 1600, 1602
  for aggressive NHL, 1653, 1655, 1657
  bone lymphoma, 1512
  broncholitis obliterans with organizing pneumonia, 1859
  chronic lymphocytic leukemia, 1614, 1619
  immunotherapy, 187
  for indolent NHL, 1653
  for mantle cell lymphoma, 1656
  molecular diagnostics, 339
  personalized medicine, 355
  pregnancy and cancer, 835
  viral infections, 1932
  Waldenström macroglobulinemia, 1683
Rivaroxaban, 1821
RNA
  5-fluorouracil, 623–624
RNAi, 765–766
RNA interference, 17
  and loss-of-function genetics, 22–23
Robustness principle, 448
Romiplostim, 1821
Ron/Stk, 58
Ropivacaine
  for cancer pain, 874
ROS. *See* Reactive oxygen species (ROS)
Rosenthal Center at Columbia University, 851
Rothmund-Thomson syndrome, 1513
Rous sarcoma virus (RSV), 68, 1932–1933
  oncogenic region, 87
Roux-en-Y reconstruction, 1097
RP. *See* Radiation pneumonitis (RP)
RPLS. *See* Reversible posterior leukoencephalopathy syndrome
RPPA. *See* Reverse phase protein lysate arrays (RPPA)
RPS. *See* Retroperitoneal sarcomas (RPS)
RSS. *See* Really simple syndication (RSS)
RSV. *See* Rous sarcoma virus (RSV)
RTK. *See* Receptor tyrosine kinase (RTK)
RT-PCR. *See* Reverse transcriptase polymerase chain reaction (RT-PCR)
RUNX3
  gastric cancer, 1090
RXR. *See* Retinoid X receptor
RYK, 60

Saccharin, 409
Saccharomyces cerevisiae, 727
SAGE. *See* Serial analysis of gene expression (SAGE)
Salicylate
  nephrotoxicity, 1829
Salivary glands, 985–988
  anatomy, 985
  chemotherapy, 987
  diagnosis, 985
  histopathology, 985–986
  malignant tumors, 985t
  neutron radiotherapy, 987
  primary tumors staging, 986t
  prognosis, 986–988
  staging, 986

Salmonella, 727, 1926
Salt, 402
Salvage chemotherapy
  high-dose chemotherapy as initial, 1280–1281
  testis cancer, 1279
Salvage therapy
  acute lymphoblastic leukemia, 1600–1601, 1601t
  for aggressive NHL, 1656–1657
  chronic lymphocytic leukemia, 1616–1617, 1616t
  Hodgkin lymphoma, 1642–1643
  Waldenström macroglobulinemia, 1683
Sample size
  selection, 456–457
SAPK. *See* Stress-activated protein kinase (SAPK)
Sarcoma(s), 79, 90–91
  anal neoplasms, 1202
  chondroblastic osteosarcoma, 1731, 1731f
  chondrosarcoma, 1507–1508, 1507f, 1508t
  Ewing's, 1508–1509, 1731–1732, 1918
  head and neck neoplasms, 988
  Kaposi's, 1842
  osteosarcoma, 1509–1511, 1509f, 1509t, 1510f, 1730–1731
  ovaries, 1373
  pediatric, 1918
  primary bone, 1500–1501, 1507–1511
  rhabdomyosarcoma, 1918
  vascular, 1511
  vulva, 1295
Sarcomatoid carcinomas
  lung, 1004–1005
  prostate cancer, 1252, 1253
Satavaptan, 1908, 1913
Satellite metastasis, 8
  local recurrence versus, 1476, 1476f
SBRT. *See* Stereotactic body radiation therapy (SBRT)
Scaffolding proteins, 62
Scapula
  metastatic lesions to, 1791
SCC. *See* Spinal cord compression (SCC)
SCF. *See* Stem cell factor (SCF)
ScFv(FRP5)-ETA, 722
Schistosoma haematobium, 311, 312, 313, 314, 315
Schistosoma japonicum, 314, 315
Schistosoma mansoni, 312, 313, 314, 315
SCLC. *See* Small cell lung carcinoma (SCLC)
Sclerosis, 1835
Scopolamine, 1761
  for cancer pain, 875
Screening, 419–444
  biases, 421–422
  cost effectiveness, 420–421
  criteria, 419
  hypothyroidism, 1903
  recommendations, 426t
Screening test, 419–421
  effectiveness, 420–421
SCT. *See* Stem cell transplantation (SCT)
Sebaceous adenoma, 1494–1495
Sebaceous carcinoma, 1493–1494
Secondary cancer, 1915–1919.
  chemotherapy, 1916–1917
  clinical characteristics, 1915
  high-dose therapy with rescue, 1917
  incidence of, 1915
  ionizing radiation, 1916
  risk after adult primary neoplasms treatment, 1918–1919
  risk after childhood primary neoplasms treatment, 1917–1918
Secondary malignant neoplasms (SMNs), 1915, 1916, 1917, 1918, 1919
Secondary osteosarcoma, 1510–1511
Secondary prophylaxis, 707
Secondary structure, 14
Sedation, 875
  in imminently dying, 878
Seed and soil hypothesis, 276
SEER. *See* Surveillance, Epidemiology, and End Results (SEER)
Seizures, 2
Selectins, 143–144
Selective ER modulators (SERMS), 741
  side effects, 743–744
Selective estrogen receptor modulators (SERMs), 1905
  breast cancer, 1433
Selective gene expression, 767
Selective serotonin reuptake inhibitor (SSRI), 593
Selenium, 408
  prostate cancer, 405
  prostate neoplasms, 1242
Self-expanding metal stents (SEMS), 1871–1872
Self-expanding plastic stents (SEPS), 1872
Self-expanding stents
  malignant dysphagia, 1871–1872, 1872t
Self seeding, growth by, 556
Seminal vesicles exposure and dissection
  prostate cancer, 1237
Seminoma, 1265
  chemotherapy, 1279
  malignant germ cell tumor, 1068
  treatment, 1069–1070, 1070t, 1269f, 1273–1274
SEMS. *See* Self-expanding metal stents (SEMS)
Semustine, 636
Sensitivity, 447
  screening test, 420
Sentinal node (SNL) biopsy, for melanoma, 1470, 1471f
  after previous wide local excision, 1474
  complications of, 1475
  desmoplastic melanoma and, 1474–1475
  goals and benefits of, 1470
  imaging considerations, 1474
  in regional disease control, 1472
  morbidity, 1475
  pathologic analysis of, 1472
  patient selection, 1474–1475
  in potential cure, 1473, 1473f
  predictors of, 1472, 1472t
  prognostic significance, 1471
  submicroscopic disease, clinical relevance of, 1472–1473
  technical considerations, 1475–1476
SEPS. *See* Self-expanding plastic stents (SEPS)
  sequencing and genome aberrations, 359–360
Serial analysis of gene expression (SAGE), 15, 16f
SERMs. *See* Selective estrogen receptor modulators (SERMS)
Serotonin, 1758–1759, 1836
  anorexia, 1740
Serous cystadenocarcinoma, 1349f
Sertoli cell tumor, 1267
Sertoli-Leydig cell tumors
  ovaries, 1373
Serum and urine biomarkers, 342–343
Serum response element (SRE), 64
Serum response factor (SRF), 64
Serum thyroglobulin monitoring
  differentiated thyroid carcinoma, 927
Serum thyroid hormone-binding protein abnormalities, 1901–1902
Severe combined immunodeficiency
  hematopoietic cellular transplantation for, 789
Sex and age based mortality, 377f
Sex cord-stromal tumors, 1267, 1371, 1372t
Sexual behavior
  cervical cancer, 1300
Sexual dysfunction, 1908–1909
Sézary cells, 1608
Sézary syndrome. *See* Mycosis fungoides/Sézary syndrome
SIADH. *See* Syndrome of inappropriate antidiuretic hormone (SIADH)
Sickle cell anemia
  hematopoietic cellular transplantation for, 789
Sideroblastic anemia
  in multiple myeloma, 1676
Sigmoidoscopy
  flexible
    colon cancer, 428–429
    colorectal cancer, 1183
Signal transduction, 135–137
  apoptosis, 48–49
  cancer therapy, 65–67
  in MDS patients', 1547–1548
  oncogenes, 73
Significance testing for aberrant copy number (STAC), 361
Simple bone cyst, 1506, 1506f
Simple object access protocol (SOAP), 1971
Sinerem®, 327
Single nucleotide polymorphisms (SNPs), 13, 348, 349
  genotyping arrays, 110
Single-photon emission computed tomography (SPECT)
  PCNS lymphoma, 1708
Single-walled carbon nanotubes (SWNTs), 368–369
Sinusoidal obstruction syndrome (SOS), 1877–1878
  treatment, 1877t
SIO. *See* Society for Integrative Oncology (SIO)
Sirolimus
  -induced granulomatous disease, 1859
SJS. *See* Stevens-Johnson syndrome (SJS)
Skeletal complications and metastases, 1788–1796
  hypercalcemia of malignancy, 1796
  medical management of bone metastases, 1792–1796
  pathogenesis, 1788–1789
  surgical management, 1789–1790
Skeletal metastases
  men with, 1716
Skin infections, 1935–1936, 1936f
Skin neoplasms, 262–263, 1487t
  age of onset, 262
  basal cell carcinoma, 1491–1492, 1491f
  genetic factors, 263–268
  metastases to, 1495
  prevention, 416
  screening, 442–443
  squamous cell carcinoma, 477f, 1489f
  sunlight, 262–263
  ultraviolet radiation genesis, 1487
  verrucous carcinoma, 1489, 1490
SKY. *See* Spectral karyotyping (SKY)
Sleep disorders, 1865–1866
Sleeve pneumonectomy, 1021, 1021f
SLF. *See* Steel factor (SLF)
Small cell carcinoma
  ovaries, 1373
  prostate cancer, 1230, 1252, 1253
Small cell lung carcinoma (SCLC)
  chemotherapy, 1038–1042
    alternating and sequential, 1040
    brain metastases, 1041
    combination, 1039
    dose escalation, 1039–1040
    dose response, 1039
    induction duration, 1040–1041
    management, 1041
    second-line, 1041–1042
    targeted therapy, 1042

Small cell lung carcinoma (*cont.*)
  hematopoietic cellular transplantation for, 789
  lung, 1005
  prognostic factors, 1015
  radiotherapy, 1037–1038
    with chemotherapy, 1037
    fractionation, 1037
    prophylactic cranial irradiation, 1038
    total tolerable dose, 1037–1038
  staging, 1013–1015
  subacute sensory neuropathy, 1008
  surgery, 1035–1037
  therapy, 1035–1042
Small cell osteosarcoma, 1510
Small cell neuroendocrine carcinoma
  cervical, 1303, 1303f
Small intestine neoplasms, 1172–1177
  clinical presentation, 1172
  computed tomography, 1172
  diagnostic imaging, 1172–1173
  endoscopic ultrasonography, 1172
  treatment, 1173
Small lymphocytic lymphoma, 1647, 1647f
SMNs. *See* Secondary malignant neoplasms (SMNs)
Smoking, 386–396
  cervical cancer, 1301
  lung cancer, 999–1000
  oral cancer, 406f
  passive, 1000
SN50, 1750
SNPs. *See* Single nucleotide polymorphisms (SNPs)
SOAP. *See* Simple Object Access Protocol (SOAP)
Social worker, 829
Society for Integrative Oncology (SIO), 846
Socioeconomic status, 376–378
  breast cancer, 1395
Sodium bicarbonate
  causing nail hyperpigmentation, 1781
Sodium dodecyl sulfate-polyacrylamide gel electrophoresis, 18
Sodium thiosulfate
  causing nail hyperpigmentation, 1781
Soft tissue sarcoma (STS), 1517–1542
  biopsy, 1521–1522, 1522f
  clinical presentation, 1518–1519
  etiology, 1517–1518
  functional outcome and morbidity, 1541–1542
  histologic grading, 1519–1520, 1520f
  histopathologic classification, 1519, 1519t
  imaging, 1520–1521, 1520f, 1521f
  localized STS of extremities, treatment for. *See* localized STS of extremities, treatment for
  locally advanced disease, treatment for, 1533
  local recurrence, management of, 1537, 1538f
  metabolic disease, treatment for. *See* metabolic disease, treatment for
  prognostic factors, 1522–1523, 1523f, 1523t
  screening, 1518
  sites of origin, 1518, 1518f
  staging, 1522, 1522t
Soft tissue sarcoma, adult
  hyperthermia, 539
Soft tissue sarcoma, of childhood, 1729–1730
Sojourn time, 419
Solar keratoses, 1487–1488, 1488f
Solid tumors, 1919
  infection, 1923t
  radioimmunotherapy, 719
  serotherapy of, 712–715
Solitary thyroid nodule
  diagnostic evaluation, 923
Somatic *APC* mutations
  sporadic colon tumors, 93–94
Somatic cell genetic studies
  tumorigenesis, 87
Somatic mutations, 87
Somatic pain, 865
Somatostatin, 1749
Somatostatin receptors (SSTRs), 332
Sonographer, 824
Sorafenib, 1847, 1903
  breast cancer, 164
  chemotherapy-induced lung injury, 1858
  distant metastatic melanoma, 1482
  hepatoma, 165
  liver neoplasms, 1129
  malignant mesothelioma, 1051
  non-small cell lung cancer, 162
  pulmonary vascular disorders, 1858
  renal cell cancer, 160
Sorbitol
  constipation, 1876
SOS. *See* Sinusoidal obstruction syndrome
Southern blotting, 9–10, 9f
Southwest Native American
  gallbladder cancer, 1132
Soy, 408
Soy isoflavones
  prostate neoplasms, 1242
Specificity, 447
  screening test, 420
Specimens
  handling, 476
  obtaining, 476, 479
SPECT. *See* Single-photon emission computed tomography
Spectral Doppler studies, 1832
Spectral karyotyping (SKY), 102, 107, 108f
Spermatocytic seminoma, 1264, 1266
Spinal cord
  metastatic lesions to, 1791–1792
Spinal cord compression (SCC), 1765t, 1766f, 1953–1954, 1953f
  clinical findings and diagnosis, 1764–1766
  pathophysiology, 1764
  radiation therapy, 1766
  surgery, 1766
  treatment, 1765–1766
Spinal cord toxicity
  neurologic complications, 1775–1776
Spinal cord tumors, 897
Spirocerca lupi, 316
Spironolactone, 1913
Splanchnic nerve block, 878
Spleen rupture, 1947
Splenectomy, 1691
  chronic lymphocytic leukemia, 1617
  infection, 1923
Splenomegaly
  in primary myelofibrosis, 1690, 1691f
Splicing, 14
Spontaneous bleeding, 1815
Spreading pigmented actinic keratosis, 1488
Sputum cytology
  lung cancer, 1009
Squamous cell carcinoma, 60, 267, 1212
  cervix, 1301–1302, 1302f
  head and neck
    recurrent and metastatic disease
      angiogenesis, 996
      chemoprevention, 997
      cytotoxic chemotherapy, 994–995
      epidermal growth factor receptor, 995–996
      gene therapy, 997
      intracellular signaling, 996–997
      novel therapeutics, 995
      tissue hypoxia, 997
  invasive, 1489f
  lung, 1004
  penis, 1256–1257, 1260f
  skin, 477f, 1489–1491, 1489f
Squamous cell carcinoma (*cont.*)
  of unknown primary site, 1717–1718
    cervical lymph nodes, 1718
    inguinal lymph nodes, 1718
    metastatic, 1718
  vagina
    staging, 1296t
  vulva, 1291
Squamous carcinoma-in-situ, 1255
Squamous cell meoplasia
  AIDS, 1710–1711
Squamous dysplasia
  lung cancer, 1003
SRE. *See* Serum response element (SRE)
SRF. *See* Serum response factor (SRF)
SRS. *See* Stereotactic radiosurgery (SRS)
SRT. *See* Stereotactic radiotherapy (SRT)
SS1P, 722
SSIP, 1051
SSM. *See* Superficial spreading melanoma (SSM)
SSRI. *See* Selective serotonin reuptake inhibitor (SSRI)
SST. *See* Superior sulcus tumors (SST)
SSTRs. *See* Somatostatin receptors (SSTRs)
St. John's wort, 849
Staging, 504–505
Standing posterioranterior chest radiograph
  Hodgkin lymphoma, 1629, 1629f
Staphylococcus, 1923–1924
Stathmokinetic technique, 552
Statins
  prostate neoplasms, 1242
Status epilepticus, 1954, 1955f
Steel factor (SLF), 53
Stem cell factor (SCF), 53, 690–691, 690t, 708
Stem cells, 34–35, 478
Stem cell transplantation (SCT)
  acute myeloid leukemia, 1572–1574
  allogenic, 1598–1599, 1598t, 1600, 1708
  chronic lymphocytic leukemia, 1617
  chronic myeloid leukemia, 1587–1588
  infection, 1922
  non-myeloablative allogenic, 1708
Stenotrophomonas maltophilia, 1926
Stents
  self-expanding, 1871–1872, 1872t
Step-down heating, 529
Stereotactic body radiation therapy (SBRT), 513
  nonsmall-cell lung cancer, 1026
  pancreatic neoplasms, 1163
Stereotactic radiosurgery (SRS), 513
Stereotactic radiotherapy (SRT), 513
Sterile talc, 1835
Steroid hormone receptors
  breast cancer, 1408
Steroids
  acute lymphoblastic leukemia, 1597, 1599, 1600
  brain herniation, 1954
  bronchospasm, 1858
  chemotherapy-induced lung injury, 1858
  nephrotoxicity, 1829
  PCNS lymphoma, 1708
  pulmonary vascular disorders, 1858
Stevens-Johnson syndrome (SJS), 1787
Stewart–Treves syndrome, 1493
Stimulatory antibodies, 182–184
Stomach cancer
  incidence, 375–376
  nutrition, 406
Stomatitis, 1780
Stool-cytotoxin test, 1875
Streptococcus, 1924, 1924f
Streptococcus pyogenes, 178
Streptomycin, 1927
Streptozocin, 1904, 1908

Stress
  in oncology staff, 808
Stress-activated protein kinase (SAPK), 64, 516–517
Stroma, 473
  generation, 474–475, 474f
Stromal cell derived growth factor (SDF-1)
  multiple myeloma, 1671
Strontium-89, 875
Subacute sensory neuropathy, 1008
Subcutaneous panniculitis-like T-cell lymphoma, 1649
Suberoylanilide hydroxamic acid, 1051
Subglottic cancer, 976–977
Sublingual glands, 985
Submandibular glands, 985
Submaxillary glands, 985
Sucralfate
  mucositis, 1882
  oral complications, 1886
Sudden cardiopulmonary arrest, 1941–1942
Sugar, 401, 409
Suicide, 805–806
  risk factors, 805t
Suicide genes, 763
Sulfadiazine
  PCNS lymphoma, 1708
  protozoal infections, 1933, 1934
Sulfamethoxazole, 1924
  protozoal infections, 1933
Sulfisoxazole
  nephrotoxicity, 1829
Sulfonamides
  acute pancreatitis, 1877
Sulindac
  prostate neoplasms, 1242
Sunburn cell
  apoptotic, 262
Sunitinib, 1847, 1903
  breast cancer, 164
  cardiotoxicity, 1844
  chemotherapy-induced lung injury, 1858
  molecular diagnostics, 339
  non-small cell lung cancer, 162
  pulmonary vascular disorders, 1858
  renal cell cancer, 160
  tumor angiogenesis, 168
Sunlight-induced photoproducts
  DNA, 263
Superficial spreading melanoma (SSM), 1461, 1461f
Superior sulcus tumors (SST)
  non-small cell lung cancer, 1028–1029
Superior vena cava (SVC) syndrome, 496, 1005–1006, 1067, 1068, 1948–1949
  management, 1949f
  non-small cell lung cancer, 1028
  small-cell lung cancer, 1041
Superlamycin
  personalized medicine, 356
SupF, 265
Supplements
  dietary, 402
Suppressing agent, 395
Supraglottic cancer, 975–976, 976f
Supraventricular tachycardia, 1943–1944
  paroxysmal, 1943
Suramin, 1752, 1906
  neurologic complications, 1774
  photosensitivity reactions, 1783
Surgery
  followed by radiation
    for malignant mesothelioma, 1049
  medullary thyroid carcinoma, 930
  during pregnancy, 831
  thyroid carcinoma, 927
Surgical oncology, 499–508, 825–826
  future of, 508
  history of, 499–501
  in the modern era, 501–502
  multidisciplinary management, 501–502
Surgical pathologist
  report, 479
  role, 475–476
Surveillance, 372–378
  data validity, 374–375
Surveillance, Epidemiology, and End Results (SEER), 372, 1977
Survival, 378
  adaptation to, 797–798
  diet, 409–410
Surviving family members
  grief in, 808
SVC. *See* Superior vena cava syndrome (SVC)
Sweeteners
  artificial, 409
SWNTs. *See* Single-walled carbon nanotubes (SWNTs)
SWOG/CALGB Study, 1633
Syndecan-1, 1670
Syndrome of ectopic ACTH, 1007
Syndrome of inappropriate antidiuretic hormone (SIADH), 1006–1007, 1907, 1913
Synovial sarcoma, 1542
Systemic chemotherapy
  mycosis fungoides/Sézary syndrome, 1664, 1664t
Systemic mast cell disease (SMCD), 1579
Systemic retinoids
  mycosis fungoides/Sézary syndrome, 1666
Systemic therapy
  during pregnancy, 831–832

TAA. *See* Tumor-associated antigens (TAA)
TACE. *See* Transarterial chemoembolization (TACE)
Tacrolimus, 782, 783, 1904
  bacterial infections, 1926
  GVHD, 1876
  nephrotoxicity, 1830
Taenia taeniaformis, 316
TA-GVHD. *See* Transfusion-associated GVHD (TA-GVHD)
Taipei, 315
Taiwan, 315
T-ALL. *See* T cell acute lymphoblastic leukemia (T-ALL)
tAML. *See* Therapy-related acute myelogenous leukemia (tAML)
Tamoxifen, 50, 133, 741–743, 593, 846, 889, 1918–1919
  acute pancreatitis, 1877
  adjuvant setting, 742
  for arterial thrombosis, 1820
  breast cancer, 164, 1437–1438, 1454–1455
  breast cancer, 742
    prevention, 742–743
  chemotherapy, 742
  clinical pharmacology, 741–742
  endometrial cancer, 1325–1326
  for hemolytic uremic syndrome, 1820
  mode of action, 741
  molecular diagnostics, 337
  personalized medicine, 347
  pregnancy and cancer, 833
  pulmonary vascular disorders, 1858
  radiation-induced lung injury, 1859
TAMs. *See* Tumor-associated machrophages (TAMs)
Tanzania, 311
Tapentadol
  for cancer pain, 868
Targeted therapy
  distant metastatic melanoma, 1481–1482
  for malignant mesothelioma, 1051
Targeted toxins, 720
  for leukemia, 721–722
  for lymphoma, 721–722
  pharmacology, 723
  for solid tumors, 722
  toxicities of, 722–723
Targeting and nanoparticles, 365–366
Taxane, 664–673, 1577
  abdominal infections, 1935
  adenocarcinoma of unknown primary site, 1717
  administration, dose, schedule, 672–673
  breast cancer, 1447
  causing anaphylaxis, 1958
  clinical indications, 663–664
  clinical pharmacology, 668
  comparative pharmacokinetics, 667t
  drug interactions, 668–669
  Kaposi sarcoma, 1701
  mechanisms of action, 664–666
  mechanisms of resistance, 666–667
  neurologic complications, 1774
  poorly differentiated carcinoma of unknown primary site, 1719
  pregnancy and cancer, 834
  radiation-induced lung injury, 1860
  toxicity, 669–672
Taxane chemotherapy
  prostate cancer, 1251
Taxane nanoparticles, 368
Taxol
  distant metastatic melanoma, 1479
  hyperthermia, 534
Taxotere
  personalized medicine, 351
Tazobactam
  bacterial infections, 1926
T cell acute lymphoblastic leukemia (T-ALL), 78
T-cell chronic lymphocytic leukemia (T-CLL), 1608
  adult, 1608
  defective, 1606
T-cell lymphoma
  Epstein-Barr virus, 294
T-cell prolymphocytic leukemia (T-PLL)
  alemtuzumab, 712
T cell receptors (TCRs), 177, 180, 1594
T cells, 179
  function, directly promoting, 182
Tcl-1, 78
T-CLL. *See* T-cell Chronic lymphocytic leukemia (T-CLL)
TCM. *See* Traditional Chinese medicine (TCM)
TCR. *See* Transcription-coupled repair (TCR)
Tea, 409
Tegafur
  causing hyperpigmentation, 1781
Televancin
  bacterial infections, 1924
Telomerase, 30
Temazolamide, 636, 889
  epigenesis and human cancer, 173
  mycosis fungoides/Sézary syndrome, 1664
Temsirolimus
  renal cell cancer, 160
Teniposide, 652, 1916
  acute lymphoblastic leukemia, 1596
  bronchospasm, 1859
  causing anaphylaxis, 1958
  chemotherapy, 907
  hypersensitivity reactions, 1783
TER. *See* Thermal enhancement ratio (TER)
Teratoma, 1266, 1823
  benign, 1067
  immature, 1734
    ovaries, 1368–1370
  mature, 1734
Terbinafine, 1787
Teriparatide, 1905
Testicular cancer, 1919
  molecular imaging and, 330

Testicular neoplasms, 439–440, 1263–1287
  AJCC staging, 1269t
  chemotherapy
    toxicity, 1282–1285
  clinical presentation, 1267–1268
  epidemiology, 1263–1264
  hematopoietic cellular transplantation for, 789
  pathology, 1264–1267
  post-chemotherapy surgery, 1277–1280
  radiation therapy
    toxicity, 1285–1286
  screening, 439–440
    recommendations, 440
  staging, 1268
  therapy, 1269–1274
    carcinoma in situ, 1269–1270
    disseminated disease, 1274–1277
    late relapse, 1282
    multiply recurrent germ cell cancer, 1281–1282
    nonseminoma, 1270–1271
    seminoma, 1273–1274
Tetracycline, 1924
  acute pancreatitis, 1877
  osteoradionecrosis, 1884
Tetraplatin, 643
TGF-alpha. *See* Transforming growth factor-alpha
TGF-beta. *See* Transforming growth factor-beta
T. gondii, 1933–1934
Thalamic stimulation, 878
Thalassemia
  hematopoietic cellular transplantation for, 789
Thalidomide, 889, 1846
  cachexia, 1751
  Kaposi sarcoma, 1701
  malignant mesothelioma, 1051
  multiple myeloma, 1677, 1679, 1680
  primary myelofibrosis, 1691
  venous thromboembolism, 1818, 1864
Thallium, 1787
Therapeutic cytapheresis, 1805
Therapeutic disruption, of tumor microenvironment, 147
Therapeutic genes, 762–769
Therapeutic leukopheresis, 1805
Therapeutic lymph node dissection (TLND), 1469
Therapy-related acute myelogenous leukemia (tAML), 1915, 1916, 1917, 1918, 1919
Therapy-related AML, 1564
Thermal enhancement ratio (TER), 533
Thermotolerance, 529
Thiabendazole
  protozoal infections, 1934
Thiamine
  neurologic complications, 1777
Thiazides
  acute pancreatitis, 1877
Thioguanine, 629
  pregnancy and cancer, 835
6-Thioguanine, 1878
  sinusoidal obstruction syndrome, 1877
  veno-occlusive disease, 1877
Thioinosine monophosphate, 628
Thiopurine methyltransferase (TPMT), 350
Thiopurines
  metabolic activation, 628f
Thiotepa, 635
  causing hyperpigmentation, 1782
  causing nail hyperpigmentation, 1780
  clinical pharmacology, 639
  neurologic complications, 1769
Thoracic interventions, 494–495
Thoracoscopy
  lung cancer, 1010
Thoracostomy, 1951
  anterior, 1019
  axillary, 1019
Thorax
  primary germ cell tumors, 1067–1072
Thrombin
  central prothrombotic roles of, 1814f
Thrombocythemia
  essential, 1686–1689
Thrombocytopathies, 1815–1816
Thrombocytopenia, 1801, 1814–1815, 1815t
  causes of, 1798t, 1801t
  in chronic lymphocytic leukemia, 1619
  differential diagnosis, 1815t
  heparin-induced, 1818, 1819–1820
Thrombocytosis, 1801
  interferons, 683
Thromboembolic disease, 1858
Thromboembolism, 744
Thrombophlebitis
  migratory
    lung cancer, 1008
Thrombopoiesis, 1799
Thrombopoietic agents, 708
Thrombopoietic agonists
  for coagulopathic complications, 1821
Thrombopoietin, 691–692, 691t 1913
Thrombotic complications, 1817–1819, 1818t
Thrombotic thrombocytopenic purpura (TTP), 783, 1820, 1820f
Thymic carcinoid and neuroendocrine tumors, 1057
Thymic carcinomas, 1053t, 1057
  chemotherapy of, 1060
Thymic lymphomas, 1057
Thymidine, 1577
Thymidine labeling index (TLI), 552
Thymidylate synthase, 624
Thymidylate synthetase
  inhibitors, 618
Thymomas, 1053–1060, 1054f, 1055f
  anatomic pathogenesis, 1053
  associated disorders, 1056t
  clinical features of, 1056
  combination chemotherapy and, 1060t
  etiology and epidemiology, 1053
  history, 1053
  paraneoplastic syndromes, 1056
  pathology of, 1053–1054
  single agents in, 1059t
  staging of, 1058, 1058t
  therapy, 1058–1060
  World Health Organization (WHO) classification of, 1054–1056, 1055t
Thyroid
  metastases to, 1904
Thyroid cancer, 1917
  131I-containing compounds for, 1903
  molecular imaging and, 328
Thyroid carcinoma
  anaplastic, 931
  chemotherapy, 929
  diagnostic imaging, 927
  differentiated. *See* Differentiated thyroid carcinoma
  external beam radiotherapy (EBRT), 926
  external-beam radiation, 928–927
  medullary thyroid carcinoma, 929–930
  metastatic disease therapy, 927
  pathogenesis, 924–925
  radioiodine, 927–928
  serum thyroglobulin monitoring, 927
  surgery, 927, 930
  thyroid hormone, 926
Thyroidectomy, 1903
Thyroid disorders, 1901–1902
Thyroid hormone
  differentiated thyroid carcinoma, 926
Thyroid neoplams, 61, 923
  fine needle aspiration, 481f
  during pregnancy, 833
  radiation-induced, 258
  solitary thyroid nodule, 923
Thyroid nodules, 1903–1904, 1904f
Thyroid stimulating hormone (TSH), 923, 1903, 1912
Ticarcillin
  bacterial infections, 1926
TIE. *See* Tyrosine kinase with immunoglobulin and epidermal growth factor (TIE)
Tigecycline
  bacterial infections, 1926
TIMP. *See* Tissue inhibitor of metalloproteinase (TIMP)
Tissue inhibitor of metalloproteinase (TIMP), 144
Tissue sections
  microscopic interpretation, 476–477
Tissue-specific biomarkers, 341–342
TLI. *See* Thymidine labeling index (TLI)
TLND. *See* Therapeutic lymph node dissection (TLND)
TLRs. *See* Toll-like receptors (TLRs)
TLS. *See* Tumor lysis syndrome (TLS)
T-lymphocyte function, 1921–1922
TMP-SMX. *See* Trimethoprim/sulfamethoxazole (TMP-SMX)
TMPT. *See* Thiopurine methyltransferase (TMPT)
TNBC. *See* Triple receptor-negative metastatic breast cancer (TNBC)
TNF receptors. *See* Tumor necrosis factor (TNF) receptors
TNF-α. *See* Tumor necrosis factor-α (TNF-α)
TNF-a. *See* Tumor necrosis factor-a (TNF-a)
TNFR. *See* Tumor necrosis factor receptor (TNFR)
TNF-related apoptosis-inducing ligand (TRAIL), 692
Tobacco
  carcinogens in, 387–388
    biomarkers, 391
    and DNA adducts, 390–391
    and tobacco-related cancers, 388
  colorectal cancer, 1180
  harm reduction, 394–395
  head and neck neoplasms, 960
  tumor induction, mechanism, 388–390
  use
    prevention and cessation, 392–393
    treatment of, 393–394
Tobacco-induced cancers
  overview, 386–396
  chemoprevention of, 395–396
Tobacco smoke, 90, 231
  environmental, 1000
  gas chromatography/mass spectroscopy, 234
  head and neck neoplasms, 961
Tobacco-specific nitrosamines, 387
Tobacco use
  Lynch syndrome, 205
Tobramycin
  bacterial infections, 1926
Tocopherols, 407
Tolerance, 878–879
Toll-like receptor (TLR), 181, 275
Tolvaptan, 1908, 1913
Tongue
  base, 971–972
  squamous cell carcinoma, 967–969
Tonsils, 970–971
Topical chemotherapy
  mycosis fungoides/Sézary syndrome, 1662–1663
Topical retinoids
  mycosis fungoides/Sézary syndrome, 1663

Topoisomerase, 589
biology, 645
catalysis, 646f
DNA strand cleavage, 645f
how drugs poison, 645–646
intercalating drugs targeting, 648–651
targeting resistance, 647
Topoisomerase I inhibitors
adenocarcinoma of unknown primary site, 1717
Topoisomerase II poisons, 605–606
Topoisomerase poisons
multidrug resistance, 600–601
Topotecan, 652–653, 1570, 1574
adenocarcinoma of unknown primary site, 1717
small-cell lung cancer, 1039
Toremifene, 743
breast cancer, 1433
prostate neoplasms, 1242
Toronto consensus, 848
Torsades de pointes, 1839, 1839t
Tositumomab (Bexxar), 719
Total-body irradiation, 34, 1798, 1825, 1826
Total gastrectomy, 1097–1098
Toxic shock syndrome, 1924
Toxicstrep syndrome, 1924
Toxohormone-L, 1743
TP53, 192. *See also* Tumor protein P53
polymorphism, 201
T-PLL. *See* T-cell prolymphocytic leukemia (T-PLL)
Tpo, 1687, 1688
Trabectidin
clinical pharmacology, 639
metabolic disease, 1537
Traditional Chinese medicine (TCM), 850
TRAIL. *See* Tumor necrosis factor-related apoptosis inducing ligand (TRAIL)
TRAIL receptors, 43f
Tramadol
for cancer pain, 868
Transactivation, 286–287
Transarterial chemoembolization (TACE)
liver neoplasms, 1128
Transcriptionally targeted oncolytic viruses, 773
Transcription-coupled repair (TCR), 263
Transcription factors
cell proliferation and differentiation, 34
oncogenes, 73
Transcription therapy, 36
Transcriptome, 5
Transcutaneous electrical nerve stimulation (TENS), 878
Transdermal fentanyl
for cancer pain, 869–870
Transesophageal echocardiography, 1832, 1833f
Transfection assay, 69, 71f
Transformation, 7, 298
Transformed cells
immortality, 127–128
Transforming growth factor-alpha (TGF-alpha), 60
Transforming growth factor-beta (TGF-beta), 35, 186, 272, 274
multiple myeloma, 1671
Transfusion-associated GVHD (TA-GVHD)
definition, 1806
prevention, 1806–1807
recommendations, 1807
Transitional cell carcinomas (TCC). *See* Urothelial carcinomas (UC)
Transjugular intrahepatic portosystemic shunts, 496
Transjugular intrahepatic portosystemic stent-shunt, 1878
Translational research and drug development, 351–352
Translocation, 105
Transmembrane domain, 52
TransMID, 722
Transplacental malignancy, 836
Transplantation
hematopoietic growth factors, 707
Transpupillary thermotherapy
retinoblastoma, 906
Transrectal ultrasonography (TRUS)
prostate cancer, 436–437
Trans-retinoic acid
myelodysplastic syndrome, 1558
Transsphenoidal surgery
growth hormone secreting pituitary adenomas, 919
Transthoracic echocardiography, 1832, 1833f
Transtuzumab
bronchospasm, 1859
Transvaginal sonography (TVS), 337
Trastuzumab, 713–714, 1845, 1942
cardiotoxicity, 1843–1844, 1844t
molecular diagnostics, 338
personalized medicine, 347, 351, 355
pregnancy and cancer, 833
Treg, 277
Treg suppressive capacity, targeting, 186
Tretinoin, 1908
Triazenes, 636
Triazole, 1930
Trichilemmoma, 1494
Trichosomoides crassicauda, 316
Trichosporon, 1930
Trichothiodystrophy (TTD), 262, 267
Triethylenethiophosphoramide (thio-TEPA), 1835
Trigger-point injections
for cancer pain, 877
Trilostane (Modrenal), 743
Trimethoprim, 1924
protozoal infections, 1933
Trimethoprim/sulfamethoxazole (TMP-SMX), 1708
acute lymphoblastic leukemia, 1597
bacterial infections, 1926, 1927
protozoal infections, 1933
Trimetrexate, 618
Triple receptor-negative metastatic breast cancer (TNBC), 1446
Triple-helix formation, 763–764
Trisomy 8, 82
Trisulfapyrimidines
protozoal infections, 1934
Trousseau syndrome, 1817–1818
Troxacitabine, 1574
Tryptophan
Anorexia, 1754
TSH. *See* Thyroid stimulating hormone (TSH)
TSP-1, 155
TTD. *See* Trichothiodystrophy (TTD)
TTP. *See* Thrombotic thrombocytopenic purpura (TTP)
Tubacin
multiple myeloma, 1682
Tuberous sclerosis, 884–885
Tubular carcinoma
breast, 1404f
Tubulin
personalized medicine, 351
Tubulin binders
schedule effects, 563
Tubulin dimer, 655f
TUCAN, 44
Tumor(s), 271
angiogenesis and, 277
benign bone, 1500
brain, 1918
burden of, 1466
cartilage, 1501–1503, 1502f
CNS, 1918, 1732–1733
fibrous, 1503–1504
Tumor(s) (*cont.*)
germ-cell, 1734
giant cell, 1504
grading, staging, prognosis, 478–479
growth and angiogenesis, 150–152, 150f, 152f
initiation and promotion, 275–276
of liver, 1735
mass, 149–150
non-angiogenic, 149
osteogenic, 1504–1505, 1504f
pediatric bone, 1730–1732
plasma cell, 1668–1684
progression, 276
recurrence of, 1825–1826
renal
in children, 1728–1729
solid, 1919
structure, 473–474
thickness, 1464
ulceration, 1464, 1464, 1466
Wilms', 1728, 1729, 1918
Tumor angiogenesis, 149–168
antiangiogenic therapy
clinical advances in, 158–160, 159t
clinical studies, 166–168, 167t
toxicities of, 165–166
anticancer therapy, 160–165
biology, 152
endogenous inhibitors of, 155
growth of tumor, 150–152, 150f, 152f
history, 150
inhibitors versus vascular targeting agents, 158
oncogenes as regulators of, 157–158
regulators of, 151t, 152–158
Tumor-associated antigens (TAA), 725
Tumor-associated macrophages (TAMs), 271–272, 276, 277
genes, 767–768
Tumor burden, 559
Tumor cell migration, 144–145
Tumor cells
checkpoint defects, 30–31
migration, 144–145
Tumor development
genetic basis, 86–87
Tumor grade
penis, 1258
Tumor growth
cell proliferation, 26–27
Tumor-host interactions, 142–143, 142t
Tumor hypoxia, 560
importance of, 519–520
Tumorigenesis
somatic cell genetic studies, 87
Tumor infiltrating lymphocytes (TILs), 180, 181
Tumor initiation, 225, 226
Tumor lysis syndrome (TLS), 1592, 1944–1945
Tumor necrosis factor, 179
chemotherapy-induced lung injury, 1858
Tumor necrosis factor-α (TNF-α), 273, 276, 1740, 1746
cachexia, 1742
multiple myeloma, 1671, 1674
soft tissue sarcomas, 1533
Tumor necrosis factor-a (TNF-a), 1811
Tumor necrosis factor receptor (TNFR), 41, 1627
Tumor necrosis factor-related apoptosis inducing ligand (TRAIL), 43, 1732
Tumor parasitism
cachexia, 1748
Tumor progression, 227, 233f
Tumor promotion, 226–227
Tumor protein P53 (TP53), 1606–1607
Tumor-reactive lymphocytes (TRLs), 180
Tumor-selective promoters/enhancers, 768
Tumor-selective retroviruses, 768
Tumor-specific antigens, 725

Tumor-specific chromosomal abnormalities, 1714–1715
Tumor-stromal interactions, 142–143
Tumor spread
  patterns, 505–506
Tumor suppressor
  endometrial cancer, 1330–1331
Tumor suppressor genes, 86–101, 100f, 232–233, 254–255
  gastric cancer, 1090
  hepatitis B virus, 304
Tumor vasculature
  rationale for targeting, 149–150
  therapeutic approaches to targeting, 158–159
Tumor viruses, 279–289
  classification, 279
  replication cycle, 282–284
  structure, 279–280
Tumstatin, 151, 155, 157
Turcot syndrome, 924
TVS. *See* Transvaginal sonography (TVS)
Two-dimensional echocardiography, 1832, 1833, 1837f
Type 1 antineuronal nuclear antibody (ANNA-1), 1007
Typhlitis, 1873–1874
Tyro3 (sky), 58
Tyrosine kinase, 54f, 1091
  growth factor receptors, 51–52
Tyrosine kinase inhibitors, 1703
  chemotherapy-induced lung injury, 1858
  cutaneous reactions, 1786
  and growth factor signaling, 65–66
Tyrosine kinase receptors
  signaling pathways, 61–62
Tyrosine kinase with immunoglobulin and epidermal growth factor (TIE), 59

Ubiquitin and protein substrate, 1744–1745
UDCA. *See* Ursodeoxycholic acid (UDCA)
UFH. *See* Unfractionated heparin (UFH)
Ufo, 58
Uganda, 311, 316
UGT1A1. *See* Uridine diphosphate-glucurono-syltransferase, 350
Ulceration, 7
  tumor, 1464, 1464, 1466
Ulcerative colitis, 1173
Ulcerative mucositis1885
Ultrasmall superparamagnetic iron oxide (USPIO), 320, 327
Ultrasonography
  malignant pleural effusion, 1851
Ultrasound Screening, 425
Ultraviolet (UV) photolithography, 364
Ultraviolet radiation (UVR)
  carcinogenesis, 262–268
    prevention, 268
  in pathogenesis of skin cancers, 1487
Ultraviolet recall reaction, 1782
Uncoupling of proteins, 1743
Undifferentiated malignant tumors, 482
Unfractionated heparin (UFH)
  venous thromboembolism, 1818, 1819, 1864
Unicameral bone cyst, 1506, 1506f
United Nations Scientific Committee on the Effects of Atomic Radiation (UNSCEAR 2000), 256
Unknown primary site, 1713–1721, 1720t
  future directions, 1720–1721
UNSCEAR 2000. *See* United Nations Scientific Committee on the Effects of Atomic Radiation
Unusual tumors, 204
Upper extremities
  metastatic lesions to, 1791
Uremia, 1816
Ureteral obstruction, 1823
Urethane
  sinusoidal obstruction syndrome, 1877
  veno-occlusive disease, 1877
Urethra, 1259–1261, 1259t
  female, 1259
  male, 1260
  prognosis, 1260
  prostate cancer, 1237–1238
  surgical management, 1259, 1260
Uridine diphosphate-glucuronosyltransferase (UGT1A1), 350
Urinary infection
  and schistosomiasis, 312
Urinary tract obstruction, 1823
  lower, 1825
  management algorithm, 1824–1825
Urologic complications, 1823–1830
Urothelial carcinomas (UC), 1212
Ursodeoxycholic acid (UDCA)
  GVHD, 1876
USPIO. *See* Ultrasmall superparamagnetic iron oxide (USPIO)
Uterine cervix
  epithelial cancer
    natural history, 1304
Uterine myometrial tumors, 1386
Uterine neoplasms
  incidence, 375–376
Uterine papillary serous carcinoma, 1327, 1327f
Uveal lymphoid infiltration, 912
Uveal melanoma, 1484
UV photoproducts
  excision, 263–264
  mutagenicity, 264–265
UVR. *See* Ultraviolet radiation (UVR)

Vaccines
  agonist peptides, 726
  allogeneic whole-tumor-cell, 726
  anti-idiotypes, 726
  autologous whole-tumor-cell, 726
  bacterial vectors, 727
  CEA, 729
  cervical neoplasia, 1307
  with chemotherapy, 732
  clinical trials, 728–732
  combination therapy, 732–733
  dendritic cell, 727–728
  design and delivery
    antigen cascade, 733733
    prime-and-boost immunization strategies, 734
    regulatory t cells, 733
    route of, 734
    T-cell activation, mechanism of, 733
  DNA vectors, 727
  dose scheduling of, 733
  with hormone therapy, 732
  issues in cancer, 734
  paradigm shifts, 734–735
  peptides, 726
  with radiation, 732
  replication-competent vectors, 727
  replication-defective, 727
  targets, 725
  types, 725–728
  vectors, 726–727
  whole tumor cell, 725–726
  yeast vectors, 727
Vaccinia virus, 727
  recombinant, 767
Vacular endothelial cell growth factor (VEGF), 277
Vagina
  clear cell adenocarcinoma, 1296–1297, 1296t
  lymphatic drainage, 1296f
  melanoma, 1297
  sarcoma, 1386
  squamous cell carcinoma
    staging, 1296t
Vaginal cancer, 1295
  treatment, 1276t
Valacyclovir
  esophagitis, 1873
  viral infections, 1931
Valerian, 849
Valproic acid, 873
Valvular diseases, 1847
Vancomycin, 1922
  bacterial infections, 1923, 1924, 1925, 1926
  C. difficile-induced diarrhea, 1875
  neutropenia, 1936, 1937
Vancomycin-resistant enterococci (VRE), 1925
Vandetanib
  non-small cell lung cancer, 163
  tumor angiogenesis, 168
Varenicline, 393
Varicella-zoster virus (VZV), 1931–1932, 1931f
  esophagitis, 1872, 1873
Vascular endothelial cell growth factor (VEGF), 54–55, 275, 1091, 1698, 1700, 1814, 1850, 1853
  biological function of, 154
  family, 153
  multiple myeloma, 1671
  pathway inhibitors, 158, 159t
    as anticancer therapy, 160–165, 166–168
    biomarkers for, 167–168, 167t
  radiation therapy, 523
  renal cell carcinoma, 1207–1208
  signal transduction, 153–154, 154f
  TKIs with chemotherapy, 163
Vascular endothelial growth factor-A (VEGF-A), 475
Vascular endothelial growth factor (VEGF)-related factor (VRF), 55
Vascular leak syndrome (VLS), 723
Vasodilators, 1838
Vasopressin, 1944
Vatalanib
  malignant mesothelioma, 1051
  non-small cell lung cancer, 162
VCAM-1, 272
Vegetables, 401
  breast cancer, 404
  colorectal cancer, 403
  head and neck neoplasms, 962
  pancreatic neoplasms, 1146
VEGF. *See* Vascular endothelial cell growth factor (VEGF)
Vena cava filters, 495–496
Venal caval syndrome, 496
Veno-occlusive disease (VOD), 1877–1878, 1877f
  treatment, 1877t
Venous stenosis, 496
Venous thromboembolism (VTE), 1818–1819, 1863–1864, 1864f
Ventilatory pump insufficiency, 1867
Verapamil, 1577
  hyperthermia, 534
Veridex, 343
  molecular diagnostics, 343
Verrucous carcinoma, 313f
  cervix, 1302
  penis, 1255f, 1256, 1256f
  skin, 1489, 1490
  vulva, 1294
VICOB-P
  mycosis fungoides/Sézary syndrome, 1665
Vicristine
  acute lymphoblastic leukemia, 1596
Vinblastine, 30, 32, 33, 34, 656, 660, 889, 1761, 1845
  cutaneous reactions, 1779
  distant metastatic melanoma, 1479
  Kaposi sarcoma, 1701
  thymomas, 1060